19th Edition

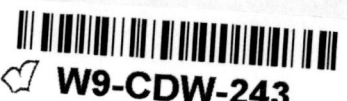

HARRISON'S™ PRINCIPLES OF INTERNAL MEDICINE

EDITORS OF PREVIOUS EDITIONS

T. R. Harrison
Editor-in-Chief, Editions 1, 2, 3, 4, 5

W. R. Resnick
Editor, Editions 1, 2, 3, 4, 5

M. M. Wintrobe
Editor, Editions 1, 2, 3, 4, 5
Editor-in-Chief, Editions 6, 7

G. W. Thorn
Editor, Editions 1, 2, 3, 4, 5, 6, 7
Editor-in-Chief, Edition 8

R. D. Adams
Editor, Editions 2, 3, 4, 5, 6, 7, 8, 9, 10

P. B. Beeson
Editor, Editions 1, 2

I. L. Bennett, Jr.
Editor, Editions 3, 4, 5, 6

E. Braunwald
Editor, Editions 6, 7, 8, 9, 10, 12, 13, 14, 16, 17
Editor-in-Chief, Editions 11, 15

K. J. Isselbacher
Editor, Editions 6, 7, 8, 10, 11, 12, 14
Editor-in-Chief, Editions 9, 13

R. G. Petersdorf
Editor, Editions 6, 7, 8, 9, 11, 12
Editor-in-Chief, Edition 10

J. D. Wilson
Editor, Editions 9, 10, 11, 13, 14
Editor-in-Chief, Edition 12

J. B. Martin
Editor, Editions 10, 11, 12, 13, 14

A. S. Fauci
Editor, Editions 11, 12, 13, 15, 16, 18
Editor-in-Chief, Editions 14, 17

R. Root
Editor, Edition 12

D. L. Kasper
Editor, Editions 13, 14, 15, 17, 18
Editor-in-Chief, Editions 16, 19

S. L. Hauser
Editor, Editions 14, 15, 16, 17, 18

D. L. Longo
Editor, Editions 14, 15, 16, 17
Editor-in-Chief, Edition 18

J. L. Jameson
Editor, Editions 15, 16, 17, 18

J. Loscalzo
Editor, Editions 17, 18

19th Edition

HARRISON'S™

PRINCIPLES OF INTERNAL MEDICINE

EDITORS

Dennis L. Kasper, MD
William Ellery Channing Professor of Medicine, Professor of Microbiology and Immunobiology, Department of Microbiology and Immunobiology, Harvard Medical School; Division of Infectious Diseases, Brigham and Women's Hospital
Boston, Massachusetts

Anthony S. Fauci, MD
Chief, Laboratory of Immunoregulation;
Director, National Institute of Allergy and Infectious Diseases,
National Institutes of Health
Bethesda, Maryland

Stephen L. Hauser, MD
Robert A. Fishman Distinguished Professor and Chairman, Department of Neurology, University of California, San Francisco
San Francisco, California

Dan L. Longo, MD
Professor of Medicine, Harvard Medical School; Senior Physician, Brigham and Women's Hospital; Deputy Editor, *New England Journal of Medicine,* Boston, Massachusetts

J. Larry Jameson, MD, PhD
Robert G. Dunlop Professor of Medicine; Dean, Perelman School of Medicine at the University of Pennsylvania; Executive Vice President, University of Pennsylvania for the Health System
Philadelphia, Pennsylvania

Joseph Loscalzo, MD, PhD
Hersey Professor of the Theory and Practice of Medicine, Harvard Medical School; Chairman, Department of Medicine, and Physician-in-Chief, Brigham and Women's Hospital
Boston, Massachusetts

VOLUME II

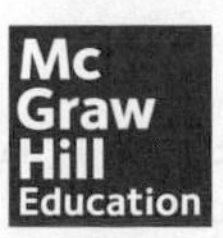

New York Chicago San Francisco Athens London Madrid Mexico City
Milan New Delhi Singapore Sydney Toronto

Note: Dr. Fauci's work as editor and author was performed outside the scope of his employment as a U.S. government employee. This work represents his personal and professional views and not necessarily those of the U.S. government.

Harrison's™
PRINCIPLES OF INTERNAL MEDICINE
Nineteenth Edition

1 2 3 4 5 6 7 8 9 10 DOW/DOW 19 18 17 16 15

Two Volume Set ISBN 978-0-07-180215-4; MHID 0-07-180215-0
Volume 1 ISBN 978-0-07-180213-0; MHID 0-07-180213-4
Volume 2 ISBN 978-0-07-180214-7; MHID 0-07-180214-2
DVD ISBN 978-0-07-184876-3; MHID 0-07-184876-2
eBook ISBN 978-0-07-1802161; MHID 0-07-180216-9

FOREIGN LANGUAGE EDITIONS

Arabic (13e): McGraw-Hill Libri Italia srl (1996)
Albanian (17e): Tabernakul Publishing, Skopje, Macedonia
Chinese Long Form (15e): McGraw-Hill International, Enterprises, Inc., Taiwan
Chinese Short Form (15e): McGraw-Hill Education (Asia), Singapore
Croatian (16e): Placebo, Split, Croatia
French (16e, 18e): Medecine-Sciences Flammarion, Paris, France
German (17e, 18e): ABW Wissenschaftsverlagsgesellschaft GmbH, Berlin, Germany
Greek (17e): Parissianos, S.A., Athens, Greece
Italian (17e, 18e): The McGraw-Hill Companies, Srl, Milan, Italy
Japanese (17e, 18e): MEDSI-Medical Sciences International Ltd, Tokyo, Japan
Korean (17e, 18e): McGraw-Hill Korea, Inc., Seoul, Korea
Macedonian (17e): Tabernakul Publishing, Skopje, Macedonia
Polish (17e): Czelej Publishing Company, Lubin, Poland
Portuguese (17e, 18e): McGraw-Hill Interamericana Editores, SA de C.V., Mexico City, Mexico
Romanian (17e): Editura All, Bucharest, Romania
Serbian (15e): Publishing House Romanov, Bosnia & Herzegovina, Republic of Serbska
Spanish (17e, 18e): McGraw-Hill Interamericana Editores, SA de C.V., Mexico City, Mexico
Turkish (17e): Nobel Tip Kitabevleri, Ltd., Istanbul, Turkey
Vietnamese (15e): McGraw-Hill Education (Asia), Singapore

This book was set in Minion Pro by Cenveo® Publisher Services. The editors were James F. Shanahan and Kim J. Davis. The production manager was Jeffrey Herzich. Project management was provided by Tania Andrabi, Cenveo Publisher Services. The index was prepared by Susan Hunter. The text designer was Alan Barnett of alan barnett design; the cover design was by Anthony Landi.

R.R. Donnelley and Sons, Inc., was printer and binder.

Li ary of Congress Cataloging-in-Publication Data

Harris 's principles of internal medicine. — 19th edition / editors, Dennis L. Kasper, Anthony S. Fauci, Stephen L. Hauser, an L. Longo, J. Larry Jameson, Joseph Loscalzo.
p. ; c
Principl f internal medicine
Includes i x.
ISBN 978-0 180213-0 (hardback : alk. paper)—ISBN 0-07-180213-4 (hardback : alk. paper)
I. Kasper, nis L., editor. II. Title: Principles of internal medicine.
[DNLM: 1. Int l Medicine. WB 115]
RC46
616—dc23

NOTICE

COVER ILLUSTRATION

Budding HIV particle, computer artwork *(Credit: Animate4.com Ltd. / Science Source)*

CONTENTS

PART 4 Regenerative Medicine

PART 5 Aging

PART 6 Nutrition and Weight Loss

PART 7 Oncology and Hematology

SECTION 1 NEOPLASTIC DISORDERS

SECTION 2 HEMATOPOIETIC DISORDERS

SECTION 3 DISORDERS OF HEMOSTASIS

PART 8 Infectious Diseases

SECTION 1 BASIC CONSIDERATIONS IN INFECTIOUS DISEASES

SECTION 2 CLINICAL SYNDROMES: COMMUNITY-ACQUIRED INFECTIONS

SECTION 3 CLINICAL SYNDROMES: HEALTH CARE–ASSOCIATED INFECTIONS

SECTION 4 APPROACH TO THERAPY FOR BACTERIAL DISEASES

SECTION 5 DISEASES CAUSED BY GRAM-POSITIVE BACTERIA

SECTION 6 DISEASES CAUSED BY GRAM-NEGATIVE BACTERIA

SECTION 7 MISCELLANEOUS BACTERIAL INFECTIONS

SECTION 8 MYCOBACTERIAL DISEASES

SECTION 9 SPIROCHETAL DISEASES

SECTION 10 DISEASES CAUSED BY RICKETTSIAE, MYCOPLASMAS, AND CHLAMYDIAE

SECTION 11 VIRAL DISEASES: GENERAL CONSIDERATIONS

SECTION 12 INFECTIONS DUE TO DNA VIRUSES

SECTION 13 INFECTIONS DUE TO DNA AND RNA RESPIRATORY VIRUSES

SECTION 14 INFECTIONS DUE TO HUMAN IMMUNODEFICIENCY VIRUS AND OTHER HUMAN RETROVIRUSES

CONTENTS

CONTENTS

SECTION 3 DISORDERS OF RHYTHM

SECTION 4 DISORDERS OF THE HEART

SECTION 5 CORONARY AND PERIPHERAL VASCULAR DISEASE

PART 11 Disorders of the Respiratory System

SECTION 1 DIAGNOSIS OF RESPIRATORY DISORDERS

SECTION 2 DISEASES OF THE RESPIRATORY SYSTEM

CONTENTS

PART 12 Critical Care Medicine

SECTION 1 RESPIRATORY CRITICAL CARE

SECTION 2 SHOCK AND CARDIAC ARREST

SECTION 3 NEUROLOGIC CRITICAL CARE

SECTION 4 ONCOLOGIC EMERGENCIES

PART 13 Disorders of the Kidney and Urinary Tract

PART 14 Disorders of the Gastrointestinal System

SECTION 1 DISORDERS OF THE ALIMENTARY TRACT

SECTION 2 LIVER AND BILIARY TRACT DISEASE

CONTENTS

SECTION 2 REPRODUCTIVE ENDOCRINOLOGY

SECTION 3 OBESITY, DIABETES MELLITUS, AND METABOLIC SYNDROME

SECTION 4 DISORDERS OF BONE AND MINERAL METABOLISM

SECTION 5 DISORDERS OF INTERMEDIARY METABOLISM

PART 17 Neurologic Disorders

SECTION 1 DIAGNOSIS OF NEUROLOGIC DISORDERS

SECTION 2 DISEASES OF THE CENTRAL NERVOUS SYSTEM

CONTENTS

SECTION 3 NERVE AND MUSCLE DISORDERS

SECTION 4 CHRONIC FATIGUE SYNDROME

SECTION 5 PSYCHIATRIC AND ADDICTION DISORDERS

PART 18 Poisoning, Drug Overdose, and Envenomation

PART 19 Disorders Associated with Environmental Exposures

James L. Abbruzzese, MD
Chief, Division of Medical Oncology, Department of Medicine; Associate Director, Clinical Research, Duke Cancer Institute, Durham, North Carolina [120e]

Manal F. Abdelmalek, MD, MPH
Associate Professor of Medicine, Division of Gastroenterology and Hepatology, Duke University, Durham, North Carolina [364]

Jamil Aboulhosn, MD
Assistant Professor of Medicine; Director Ahmanson/UCLA Adult Congenital Heart Disease Center, David Geffen School of Medicine, University of California, Los Angeles, Los Angeles, California [282]

John C. Achermann, MD, PhD, MB
Wellcome Trust Senior Research Fellow in Clinical Science, University College London; Professor of Paediatric Endocrinology, UCL Institute of Child Health, University College London, London, United Kingdom [410]

John W. Adamson, MD
Clinical Professor, Division of Hematology/Oncology, Department of Medicine, University of California at San Diego, San Diego, California [77, 126]

Rizwan Ahmed, MD
General Surgery Resident, Department of General Surgery, Johns Hopkins Hospital, Baltimore, Maryland [353, 354]

Praveen Akuthota, MD
Assistant Professor of Medicine, Harvard Medical School; Beth Israel Deaconess Medical Center, Boston, Massachusetts [310]

Anthony A. Amato, MD
Professor of Neurology, Harvard Medical School; Vice-Chairman, Department of Neurology, Brigham and Women's Hospital, Boston, Massachusetts [459-462e]

Michael J. Aminoff, MD, DSc, FRCP
Professor of Neurology, School of Medicine, University of California, San Francisco, San Francisco, California [30, 31, 442e]

Neil M. Ampel, MD
Professor of Medicine, University of Arizona; Staff Physician, Southern Arizona Veterans Affairs Health Care System, Tucson, Arizona [237]

Kenneth C. Anderson, MD
Kraft Family Professor of Medicine, Harvard Medical School; Chief, Jerome Lipper Multiple Myeloma Center, Dana-Farber Cancer Institute, Boston, Massachusetts [136, 138e]

Rosa M. Andrade, MD
Department of Medicine, Division of Infectious Diseases, University of California, San Diego, San Diego, California [247]

Elliott M. Antman, MD
Professor of Medicine, Cardiovascular Division, Department of Medicine, Brigham and Women's Hospital; Associate Dean for Clinical/Translational Research, Harvard Medical School, Boston, Massachusetts [293, 295]

Frederick R. Appelbaum, MD
Director, Division of Clinical Research, Fred Hutchinson Cancer Research Center, Seattle, Washington [139e]

Cesar A. Arias, MD, PhD, MSc
Associate Professor of Medicine, Microbiology and Molecular Genetics; Director, Laboratory for Antimicrobial Research, University of Texas Medical School at Houston, Houston, Texas; Director, Molecular Genetics and Antimicrobial Unit; Co-Director, International Center for Microbial Genomics, Universidad, El Bosque, Bogota, Colombia [174]

Wiebke Arlt, MD, DSc, FRCP, FMedSci
Professor of Medicine, Centre for Endocrinology, Diabetes and Metabolism, School of Clinical and Experimental Medicine, University of Birmingham; Consultant Endocrinologist, University Hospital Birmingham, Birmingham, United Kingdom [406]

Katrina Armstrong, MD, MS
Jackson Professor of Clinical Medicine, Physician in Chief, Massachusetts General Hospital, Boston Massachusetts [4]

Valder R. Arruda, MD, PhD
Associate Professor, Division of Hematology, Department of Pediatrics, Perelman School of Medicine, University of Pennsylvania, Philadelphia, Pennsylvania [141]

Andrew W. Artenstein, MD
Professor of Medicine, Tufts University School of Medicine, Boston, Massachusetts; Adjunct Professor of Medicine and Health Services, Policy and Practice, Alpert Medical School, Brown University, Providence, Rhode Island; Chair, Department of Medicine, Baystate Health, Springfield, Massachusetts [152e]

Anthony Atala, MD
Professor and Director, Wake Forest Institute for Regenerative Medicine, Wake Forest School of Medicine, Winston-Salem, North Carolina [92e]

John C. Atherton, MD, FRCP
Professor of Gastroenterology and Dean of the School of Medicine, University of Nottingham, Nottingham, United Kingdom [188]

Paul S. Auerbach, MD, MS, FACEP, FAWM
Redich Family Professor of Surgery, Division of Emergency Medicine, Stanford University School of Medicine, Stanford, California [474]

K. Frank Austen, MD
AstraZeneca Professor of Respiratory and Inflammatory Diseases, Director, Inflammation and Allergic Diseases Research Section, Harvard Medical School; Brigham and Women's Hospital, Boston, Massachusetts [376]

Eric H. Awtry, MD
Cardiology Division, Boston Medical Center, Boston, Massachusetts [289e, 290e]

Jamil Azzi, MD
Instructor in Medicine, Harvard Medical School; Associate Physician, Brigham and Women's Hospital, Boston, Massachusetts [337]

Bruce R. Bacon, MD
James F. King, MD Endowed Chair in Gastroenterology; Professor of Internal Medicine, Saint Louis University Liver Center, Saint Louis University School of Medicine, St. Louis, Missouri [365, 367e]

Lindsey R. Baden, MD
Associate Professor of Medicine, Harvard Medical School; Dana-Farber Cancer Institute, Brigham and Women's Hospital, Boston, Massachusetts [215e]

Natalie J. Badowski, MD
Division of Emergency Medicine, Stanford University School of Medicine, Stanford, California [474]

John R. Balmes, MD
Professor of Medicine, University of California, San Francisco; Professor, School of Public Health, University of California, Berkeley; Chief, Division of Occupational and Environmental Medicine, San Francisco General Hospital, San Francisco, California [311]

Manisha Balwani, MD, MS
Assistant Professor, Department of Genetics and Genomic Sciences, Mount Sinai School of Medicine of New York University, New York, New York [430]

Peter A. Banks, MD
Professor of Medicine, Harvard Medical School; Senior Physician, Division of Gastroenterology, Brigham and Women's Hospital, Boston, Massachusetts [370, 371]

Robert L. Barbieri, MD
Kate Macy Ladd Professor of Obstetrics, Gynecology and Reproductive Biology, Harvard Medical School; Chair, Department of Obstetrics and Gynecology, Brigham and Women's Hospital, Boston, Massachusetts [8]

Alan G. Barbour, MD
Professor of Medicine and Microbiology and Molecular Genetics, University of California Irvine, Irvine, California [209]

Joanne M. Bargman, MD, FRCPC
Professor of Medicine, University of Toronto; Staff Nephrologist, University Health Network, Toronto, Canada [335]

Tamar F. Barlam, MD, MSc
Associate Professor of Medicine, Infectious Disease Section, Boston University School of Medicine, Boston, Massachusetts [147, 183e]

Peter J. Barnes, DM, DSc, FMedSci, FRS
Head of Respiratory Medicine, Imperial College, London, United Kingdom [309]

Richard J. Barohn, MD
Chairman, Department of Neurology; Gertrude and Dewey Ziegler Professor of Neurology, University of Kansas Medical Center, Kansas City, Kansas [459]

Rebecca M. Baron, MD
Assistant Professor of Medicine, Harvard Medical School; Associate Physician, Brigham and Women's Hospital, Division of Pulmonary and Critical Care Medicine, Department of Medicine, Boston, Massachusetts [154, 312]

Miriam Baron Barshak, MD
Assistant Professor, Harvard Medical School; Associate Physician, Massachusetts General Hospital, Boston, Massachusetts [154, 159, 312]

Shehzad Basaria, MD
Men's Health: Aging and Metabolism, Brigham and Women's Hospital, Boston, Massachusetts [7e]

Robert C. Basner, MD
Professor of Clinical Medicine, Division of Pulmonary, Allergy, and Critical Care Medicine, Columbia University College of Physicians and Surgeons, New York, New York [Appendix]

Buddha Basnyat, MD, MSc, FACP, FRCP (Edinburgh)
Director, Oxford University Clinical Research Unit, Patan Academy of Health Sciences; Medical Director, Nepal International Clinic, Kathmandu, Nepal [476e]

Shari S. Bassuk, ScD
Epidemiologist, Division of Preventive Medicine, Brigham and Women's Hospital, Boston, Massachusetts [413]

John F. Bateman, PhD
Director, Cell Biology, Murdoch Children's Research Institute, Melbourne, Victoria, Australia; Murdoch Children's Research Institute, Parkville, Victoria, Australia [427]

David W. Bates, MD, MSc
Professor of Medicine, Harvard Medical School; Chief, General Internal Medicine and Primary Care Division, Brigham and Women's Hospital; Medical Director, Clinical and Quality Analysis, Partners HealthCare System, Inc., Boston, Massachusetts [12e]

Robert P. Baughman, MD
Department of Internal Medicine, University of Cincinnati Medical Center, Cincinnati, Ohio [390]

M. Flint Beal, MD
University Professor of Neurology and Neuroscience; Neurologist, New York Presbyterian Hospital; Weill Cornell Medical College, New York, New York [444e, 455]

Laurence H. Beck, MD, PhD
Assistant Professor of Medicine, Boston University School of Medicine, Boston, Massachusetts [340]

Christian D. Becker, MD, PhD, FCCP
Assistant Professor, Department of Internal Medicine, Division of Pulmonary, Critical Care and Sleep Medicine, Icahn School of Medicine at Mount Sinai New York, New York [485e]

Nicholas J. Beeching, MA, BM BCh, FRCP, FRACP, FFTM RCPS(Glasg), DCH, DTM&H
Senior Lecturer (Clinical) in Infectious Diseases, Liverpool School of Tropical Medicine; Clinical Director, Tropical and Infectious Disease Unit, Royal Liverpool University Hospital; NIHR Health Protection Research Unit in Emerging and Zoonotic Infections, Liverpool; Honorary Consultant, Public Health England and Honorary Civilian Consultant in Infectious Diseases, Army Medical Directorate, United Kingdom [194e]

Doron Behar, MD, PhD
Institute of Genetics, Rambam Health Care Campus, Haifa, Israel [85e]

Robert S. Benjamin, MD
P. H. and Faye E. Robinson Distinguished Professor of Medicine, Department of Sarcoma Medical Oncology, The University of Texas M.D. Anderson Cancer Center, Houston, Texas [119e]

Michael H. Bennett, MD, MBBS, MM (Clin Epi)
Conjoint Associate Professor in Anesthesia and Hyperbaric Medicine; Faculty of Medicine, University of New South Wales; Academic Head of Department, Wales Anaesthesia, Prince of Wales Hospital, Sydney, Australia [477e]

Edward J. Benz, Jr., MD
Richard and Susan Smith Professor of Medicine; Professor of Genetics, Harvard Medical School; President and CEO, Dana-Farber Cancer Institute; Director and Principal Investigator, Dana-Farber/Harvard Cancer Center; Boston, Massachusetts [127]

Jean Bergounioux, MD, PhD, PhC
Pediatric Intensive Care Unit, Hôpital Raymond-Poincaré, Université de Versailles-Saint Quentin, Garches, France [191]

John L. Berk, MD
Associate Professor of Medicine, Boston University School of Medicine; Clinical Director, Amyloidosis Center, Boston Medical Center, Boston, Massachusetts [137]

Aaron S. Bernstein, MD, MPH
Instructor, Harvard Medical School; Associate Director, Center for Health and the Global Environment, Harvard School of Public Health; Pediatric Hospitalist, Boston Children's Hospital, Boston, Massachusetts [151e]

Joseph R. Betancourt, MD, MPH
Associate Professor of Medicine, Harvard Medical School; Director, The Disparities Solutions Center, Massachusetts General Hospital, Boston, Massachusetts [16e]

Atul K. Bhan, MD, MBBS
Professor of Pathology, Harvard Medical School, Department of Pathology, Massachusetts General Hospital, Boston, Massachusetts [366e]

Shalender Bhasin, MBBS
Professor of Medicine, Harvard Medical School; Director, Research Program in Men's Health: Aging and Metabolism; Director, Boston Claude D. Pepper Older Americans Independence Center; Site Director, Harvard Catalyst Clinical Research Center at BWH, Brigham and Women's Hospital, Boston, Massachusetts [7e, 411]

Deepak L. Bhatt, MD, MPH
Professor of Medicine, Harvard Medical School; Chief of Cardiology, VA Boston Healthcare System; Senior Physician, Brigham and Women's Hospital; Senior Investigator, TIMI Study Group, Boston, Massachusetts [296e, 297e]

Roby P. Bhattacharyya, MD, PhD
Instructor in Medicine, Harvard Medical School; Assistant in Medicine, Division of Infectious Disease, Massachusetts General Hospital, Boston, Massachusetts [146]

David R. Bickers, MD
Carl Truman Nelson Professor and Chair, Department of Dermatology, Columbia University Medical Center, New York, New York [75]

Henry J. Binder, MD
Professor Emeritus of Medicine, Senior Research Scientist, Yale University, New Haven, Connecticut [349, 350e]

William R. Bishai, MD, PhD
Professor and Co-Director, Center for Tuberculosis Research, Department of Medicine, Division of Infectious Diseases, Johns Hopkins University School of Medicine, Baltimore, Maryland [175]

Bruce R. Bistrian, MD, PhD, MPH
Professor of Medicine, Harvard Medical School; Chief, Clinical Nutrition, Beth Israel Deaconess Medical Center, Boston, Massachusetts [98e]

Martin J. Blaser, MD
Muriel and George Singer Professor of Medicine; Professor of Microbiology; Director, Human Microbiome Program, New York University Langone Medical Center, New York, New York [188, 192]

Chantal P. Bleeker-Rovers, MD, PhD
Department of Internal Medicine, Radboud University Nijmegen Medical Center, Nijmegen, The Netherlands [26]

Gijs Bleijenberg, PhD
Professor Emeritus, Expert Centre for Chronic Fatigue, Radboud University Medical Centre, Nijmegen, The Netherlands [464e]

Clara D. Bloomfield, MD
Distinguished University Professor; William G. Pace, III Professor of Cancer Research; Cancer Scholar and Senior Advisor, The Ohio State University Comprehensive Cancer Center; Arthur G. James Cancer Hospital and Richard J. Solove Research Institute, Columbus, Ohio [132]

Richard S. Blumberg, MD
Chief, Division of Gastroenterology, Hepatology and Endoscopy, Brigham and Women's Hospital, Harvard Medical School, Boston, Massachusetts [351]

Jean L. Bolognia, MD
Professor, Department of Dermatology, Yale University School of Medicine, New Haven, Connecticut [72]

Joseph V. Bonventre, MD, PhD
Samuel A. Levine Professor of Medicine, Harvard Medical School; Chief, Renal Division; Chief, Division of Biomedical Engineering, Brigham and Women's Hospital, Boston, Massachusetts [333e, 334]

George J. Bosl, MD
Professor of Medicine, Weill Cornell Medical College; Chair, Department of Medicine; Patrick M. Byrne Chair in Clinical Oncology, Memorial Sloan-Kettering Cancer Center, New York, New York [116]

Joshua A. Boyce, MD
Professor of Medicine and Pediatrics; Albert L. Sheffer Professor of Medicine, Harvard Medical School; Director, Inflammation and Allergic Disease Research Section, Brigham and Women's Hospital, Boston, Massachusetts [376]

Eugene Braunwald, MD, MA (Hon), ScD (Hon), FRCP
Distinguished Hersey Professor of Medicine, Harvard Medical School; Founding Chairman, TIMI Study Group, Brigham and Women's Hospital, Boston, Massachusetts [50, 288, 294]

Irwin M. Braverman, MD
Professor Emeritus; Senior Research Scientist, Department of Dermatology, Yale University School of Medicine, New Haven, Connecticut [72]

Otis W. Brawley, MD, FACP
Professor of Hematology, Medical Oncology, Medicine and Epidemiology, Emory University; Chief Medical and Scientific Officer, American Cancer Society, Atlanta, Georgia [100]

Joel G. Breman, MD, DTPH
Senior Scientific Advisor, Fogarty International Center, National Institutes of Health, Bethesda, Maryland [248, 250e]

George J. Brewer, MD
Morton S. and Henrietta K. Sellner Emeritus, Professor of Human Genetics, Emeritus Professor of Internal Medicine, University of Michigan Medical School; Senior Vice President for Research and Development, Adeona Pharmaceuticals, Inc., Ann Arbor, Michigan [429]

Josephine P. Briggs, MD
Director, National Center for Complementary and Alternative Medicine (NCCAM) at the National Institutes of Health (NIH), Bethesda, Maryland [14e]

F. Richard Bringhurst, MD
Associate Professor of Medicine, Harvard Medical School; Physician, Massachusetts General Hospital, Boston, Massachusetts [423]

Steven M. Bromley, MD
Director, Outpatient Services, Virtua Neuroscience, Voorhees, New Jersey; Director, Bromley Neurology, PC, Audubon, New Jersey [42]

Darron R. Brown, MD
Professor of Medicine, Microbiology and Immunology, Division of Infectious Diseases, Simon Cancer Center, Indiana University School of Medicine, Indianapolis, Indiana [222]

Kevin E. Brown, MD, MRCp, FRCPath
Virus Reference Department, Public Health England, London, United Kingdom [221]

Robert H. Brown, Jr., MD, PhD
Chairman, Department of Neurology, University of Massachusetts Medical School, Worchester, Massachusetts [452, 462e]

Amy E. Bryant, PhD
Affiliate Assistant Professor, University of Washington School of Medicine, Seattle, Washington; Research Scientist, Veterans Affairs Medical Center, Boise, Idaho [179]

Christopher M. Burns, MD
Associate Professor, Department of Medicine, Section of Rheumatology, Geisel School of Medicine at Dartmouth, Dartmouth Hitchcock Medical Center, Lebanon, New Hampshire [431e]

David M. Burns, MD
Professor Emeritus, Department of Family and Preventive Medicine, University of California, San Diego School of Medicine, San Diego, California [470]

Stephen B. Calderwood, MD
Morton N. Swartz, MD Academy Professor of Medicine (Microbiology and Immunobiology), Harvard Medical School; Chief, Division of Infectious Diseases, Massachusetts General Hospital, Boston, Massachusetts [160]

Michael Camilleri, MD
Atherton and Winifred W. Bean Professor; Professor of Medicine, Pharmacology, and Physiology, Mayo Clinic College of Medicine, Rochester, Minnesota [55]

Christopher P. Cannon, MD
Professor of Medicine, Harvard Medical School; Senior Physician, Cardiovascular Division, Brigham and Women's Hospital, Boston, Massachusetts [294]

Jonathan R. Carapetis, MBBS, PhD, FRACP, FAFPHM
Director, Telethon Kids Institute, The University of Western Australia, Crawley, Western Australia [381]

Kathryn M. Carbone, MD
Deputy Scientific Director, Division of Intramural Research, National Institute of Dental and Craniofacial Research, Bethesda, Maryland [231e]

Brian I. Carr, MD, PhD, FRCP
IRCCS de Bellis National Center for GI Diseases, Castellana Grotte, BA, Italy [111]

John D. Carter, MD
Professor of Medicine, Division of Rheumatology; Director, University of South Florida Morsani College of Medicine, Tampa, Florida [384]

Arturo Casadevall, MD, PhD
Chair, Department of Microbiology and Immunology, Albert Einstein College of Medicine, Bronx, New York [239]

Agustin Castellanos, MD, FACC, FAHA
Professor of Medicine; Director, Clinical Electrophysiology, University of Miami Miller School of Medicine, Cardiovascular Division, Miami, Florida [327]

Bartolomo R. Celli, MD
Professor of Medicine, Harvard Medical School, Staff Physician, Division of Pulmonary and Critical Care Medicine, Brigham and Women's Hospital, Boston, Massachusetts [323]

Murali Chakinala, MD
Associate Professor of Medicine, Division of Pulmonary and Critical Care Medicine, Washington University School of Medicine, St. Louis, Missouri [279]

Anil Chandraker, MBChB, FRCP
Associate Professor of Medicine, Harvard Medical School; Medical Director of Kidney and Pancreas Transplantation; Interim Director, Schuster Family Transplantation Research Center, Brigham and Women's Hospital, Boston, Massachusetts [337]

Lan X. Chen, MD, PhD
Penn Presbyterian Medical Center, Philadelphia, Pennsylvania [395]

Yuan-Tsong Chen, MD, PhD
Duke University Medical Center, Division of Medical Genetics, Department of Pediatrics, Durham, North Carolina [433e]

Glenn M. Chertow, MD, MPH
Norman S. Coplon/Satellite Healthcare Professor of Medicine; Chief, Division of Nephrology, Stanford University School of Medicine, Palo Alto, California [336]

John S. Child, MD, FACC, FAHA, FASE
Streisand Professor of Medicine and Cardiology; Director, Ahmanson-UCLA Adult Congenital Heart Disease Center; Director, UCLA Adult Noninvasive Cardiodiagnostics Laboratory Ronald Reagan-UCLA Medical Center, Geffen School of Medicine, University of California, Los Angeles (UCLA), Los Angeles, California [282]

Augustine M. K. Choi, MD
Chairman, Department of Medicine, Weill Cornell Medical College, Physician-in-Chief, New York-Presbyterian Hospital-Weill Cornell Medical Center, New York, New York [305, 307, 322]

Raymond T. Chung, MD
Associate Professor of Medicine, Harvard Medical School; Director of Hepatology and Liver Center; Vice Chief, Gastroenterology, Massachusetts General Hospital, Boston, Massachusetts [368]

Jeffrey W. Clark, MD
Associate Professor of Medicine, Harvard Medical School; Medical Director, Clinical Trials Core, Dana-Farber Harvard Cancer Center; Massachusetts General Hospital, Boston, Massachusetts [102e]

Jeffrey I. Cohen, MD
Chief, Laboratory of Clinical Infectious Diseases, National Institute of Allergy and Infectious Diseases, National Institutes of Health, Bethesda, Maryland [218, 228]

Yehuda Z. Cohen, MD
Clinical Fellow, Department of Medicine, Division of Infectious Diseases and Center for Virology and Vaccine Research, Beth Israel Deaconess Medical Center; Harvard Medical School, Boston, Massachusetts [224]

Ronit Cohen-Poradosu, MD
Senior Physician, Infectious Diseases Unit, Tel Aviv Sourasky Medical Center, Tel Aviv, Israel [201]

Francis S. Collins, MD, PhD
Director, National Institutes of Health, Bethesda, Maryland [101e]

Wilson S. Colucci, MD, FAHA, FACC
Thomas J. Ryan Professor of Medicine, Boston University School of Medicine; Chief of Cardiovascular Medicine, Boston Medical Center, Boston, Massachusetts [289e, 290e]

Laura K. Conlin, PhD
Scientific Director, CytoGenomics Lab, The Children's Hospital of Philadelphia, Assistant Professor of Pathology and Laboratory Medicine, University of Pennsylvania, Philadelphia, Pennsylvania [83e]

Darwin L. Conwell, MD, MS
Professor of Medicine, The Ohio State University College of Medicine; Director, Division of Gastroenterology, Hepatology and Nutrition; The Ohio State University Wexner Medical Center, Columbus, Ohio [370, 371]

Michael J. Corbel, PhD, DSc, FRCPath
Retired (previously Head, Division of Bacteriology, National Institute for Biological Standards and Control, Hertfordshire, United Kingdom) [194e]

William E. Corcoran, V, MD
Staff Anesthesiologist, Allcare Clinical Associates; Medical Director of Analgesia and Sedation, Mission Health; Patient Safety Officer, Mission Health, Asheville, North Carolina [481e]

Kathleen E. Corey, MD, MPH
Clinical and Research Fellow, Harvard Medical School; Fellow, Gastrointestinal Unit, Massachusetts General Hospital, Boston, Massachusetts [59]

Lawrence Corey, MD
Professor, Medicine and Laboratory Medicine, University of Washington; President Emeritus, Fred Hutchinson Cancer Research Center; Member, Vaccine and Infectious Disease Division; Principal Investigator, HIV Vaccine Trials Network, Fred Hutchinson Cancer Research Center, Seattle, Washington [216]

Jorge Cortes, MD
D. B. Lane Cancer Research Distinguished Professor for Leukemia Research; Deputy Chairman; Section Chief of AML and CML, The University of Texas M.D. Anderson Cancer Center, Houston, Texas [133]

Felicia Cosman, MD
Professor of Medicine, Columbia University College of Physicians and Surgeons, New York, New York [425]

Mark A. Creager, MD
Professor of Medicine, Harvard Medical School; Simon C. Fireman Scholar in Cardiovascular Medicine; Director, Vascular Center, Brigham and Women's Hospital, Boston, Massachusetts [301-303]

Leslie J. Crofford, MD
Professor, Division of Rheumatology and Immunology, Vanderbilt University, Nashville, Tennessee; Chief, Division of Rheumatology, University of Kentucky, Lexington, Kentucky [396]

Jennifer M. Croswell, MD, MPH
Medical Officer, Center for Oncology Prevention Trials Research Group, Division of Cancer Prevention, National Cancer Institute, Bethesda, Maryland [100]

Philip E. Cryer, MD
Professor of Medicine Emeritus, Washington University in St. Louis; Physician, Barnes-Jewish Hospital, St. Louis, Missouri [420]

David Cunningham, MD, MB, ChB, FRCP
Professor, Head of Gastrointestinal/Lymphoma Unit; Director of Clinical Research, Royal Marsden NHS Trust, London, United Kingdom [112]

Gary C. Curhan, MD
Professor of Medicine, Harvard Medical School, Professor of Epidemiology, Harvard School of Public Health, Channing Division of Network Medicine/Renal Division, Brigham and Women's Hospital, Boston, Massachusetts [342]

Brendan D. Curti, MD
Director, Biotherapy Program, Robert W. Franz Cancer Research Center, Providence Portland Medical Center, Portland, Oregon [105]

John J. Cush, MD
Professor of Medicine and Rheumatology, Baylor University Medical Center; Director of Clinical Rheumatology, Baylor Research Institute, Dallas, Texas [393]

Charles A. Czeisler, MD, PhD
Frank Baldino, Jr., PhD Professor of Sleep Medicine, Professor of Medicine and Director, Division of Sleep Medicine, Harvard Medical School; Chief, Division of Sleep and Circadian Disorders, Departments of Medicine and Neurology, Brigham and Women's Hospital, Boston, Massachusetts [38]

Marinos C. Dalakas, MD
Professor of Neurology, University of Athens Medical School, Athens, Greece; Thomas Jefferson University, Philadelphia, Pennsylvania [388]

Josep Dalmau, MD, PhD
ICREA Professor, Institut d'Investigació Biomèdica August Pi i Sunyer, University of Barcelona, Barcelona, Spain; Adjunct Professor, University of Pennsylvania, Philadelphia, Pennsylvania [122]

Daniel F. Danzl, MD
University of Louisville, Department of Emergency Medicine, Louisville, Kentucky [478e, 479e]

Robert B. Daroff, MD
Professor and Chair Emeritus, Department of Neurology, Case Western Reserve University School of Medicine; University Hospitals–Case Medical Center, Cleveland, Ohio [28]

Charles E. Davis, MD
Professor of Pathology and Medicine, Emeritus, University of California, San Diego School of Medicine; Director Emeritus, Microbiology, University of California, San Diego Medical Center, San Diego, California [245e]

Stephen N. Davis, MBBS, FRCP
Theodore E. Woodward Professor and Chairman of the Department of Medicine, University of Maryland School of Medicine; Physician-in-Chief, University of Maryland Medical Center, Baltimore, Maryland [420]

Rafael de Cabo, PhD
Senior Investigator, Experimental Gerontology Section, TGB, National Institute on Aging, National Institutes of Health, Baltimore, Maryland [94e]

Lisa M. DeAngelis, MD
Professor of Neurology, Weill Cornell Medical College; Chair, Department of Neurology, Memorial Sloan Kettering Cancer Center, New York, New York [118]

John Del Valle, MD
Professor and Senior Associate Chair of Medicine, Department of Internal Medicine, University of Michigan School of Medicine, Ann Arbor, Michigan [348]

Marie B. Demay, MD
Professor of Medicine, Harvard Medical School; Physician, Massachusetts General Hospital, Boston, Massachusetts [423]

Bradley M. Denker, MD
Associate Professor of Medicine, Harvard Medical School; Renal Division, Beth Israel Deaconess Medical Center; Chief of Nephrology and Associate Chief of Medical Specialties, Harvard Vanguard Medical Associates, Boston, Massachusetts [61]

David W. Denning, MBBS, FRCP, FRCPath, FMedSci
Professor of Medicine and Medical Mycology; Director, National Aspergillosis Centre, The University of Manchester and Wythenshawe Hospital, Manchester, United Kingdom [241]

Robert J. Desnick, MD, PhD
Dean for Genetics and Genomics, Professor and Chairman Emeritus, Department of Human Genetics and Genomic Sciences, Icahn School of Medicine at Mount Sinai, New York, New York [430]

Richard A. Deyo, MD, MPH
Kaiser Permanente Professor of Evidence-Based Family Medicine, Department of Family Medicine, Department of Medicine, Department of Public Health and Preventive Medicine, Oregon Institute of Occupational Health Sciences; Oregon Health and Science University; Clinical Investigator, Kaiser Permanente Center for Health Research, Portland, Oregon [22]

Betty Diamond, MD
The Feinstein Institute for Medical Research, North Shore LIJ Health System; Center for Autoimmunity and Musculoskeletal Diseases, Manhasset, New York [377e]

Marcelo F. Di Carli, MD
Professor, Department of Radiology, Harvard Medical School; Chief, Division of Nuclear Medicine and Molecular Imaging; Executive Director, Noninvasive Cardiovascular Imaging Program, Brigham and Women's Hospital, Boston, Massachusetts [270e, 271e]

Anna Mae Diehl, MD
Florence McAlister Professor of Medicine; Chief, Division of Gastroenterology, Duke University, Durham, North Carolina [364]

Jules L. Dienstag, MD
Carl W. Walter Professor of Medicine and Dean for Medical Education, Harvard Medical School; Physician, Gastrointestinal Unit, Department of Medicine, Massachusetts General Hospital, Boston, Massachusetts [360-362, 366e, 368]

William P. Dillon, MD
Professor and Executive Vice-Chair; Chief, Section of Neuroradiology, Department of Radiology and Biomedical Imaging, University of California, San Francisco, San Francisco, California [440e, 441e]

Charles A. Dinarello, MD
Professor of Medicine and Immunology, University of Colorado Denver, Aurora, Colorado; Professor of Experimental Medicine, Radboud University Medical Center, Nijmegen, The Netherlands [23]

Raphael Dolin, MD
Maxwell Finland Professor of Medicine (Microbiology and Molecular Genetics), Harvard Medical School; Beth Israel Deaconess Medical Center; Brigham and Women's Hospital, Boston, Massachusetts [215e, 223, 224]

Susan M. Domchek, MD
Basser Professor of Oncology, Abramson Cancer Center, University of Pennsylvania, Philadelphia, Pennsylvania [84]

Richard L. Doty, PhD, MA
Director, Smell and Taste Center; Professor, Department of Otorhinolaryngology: Head and Neck Surgery, Perelman School of Medicine, University of Pennsylvania, Philadelphia, Pennsylvania [42]

Vanja C. Douglas, MD
Assistant Professor of Clinical Neurology and Sara and Evan Williams Foundation Endowed Neurohospitalist Chair, University of California, San Francisco, San Francisco, California [29]

Daniel B. Drachman, MD
Professor of Neurology and Neuroscience, W. W. Smith Charitable Trust Professor of Neuroimmunology, Department of Neurology, Johns Hopkins School of Medicine, Baltimore, Maryland [461]

David F. Driscoll, PhD
Associate Professor of Medicine, University of Massachusetts Medical School, Worchester, Massachusetts [98e]

Thomas D. DuBose, Jr., MD, MACP
Emeritus Professor of Internal Medicine and Nephrology, Wake Forest University School of Medicine, Winston-Salem, North Carolina [64e, 66]

J. Stephen Dumler, MD
Professor, Division of Medical Microbiology, Department of Pathology, Johns Hopkins University School of Medicine, Baltimore, Maryland [211]

Andrea Dunaif, MD
Charles F. Kettering Professor of Endocrinology and Metabolism and Vice-Chair for Research, Department of Medicine, Feinberg School of Medicine, Northwestern University, Chicago, Illinois [6e]

Samuel C. Durso, MD, MBA
Mason F. Lord Professor of Medicine; Director, Division of Geriatric Medicine and Gerontology, Johns Hopkins University School of Medicine, Baltimore, Maryland [45, 46e]

Janice P. Dutcher, MD
Associate Director, Cancer Research Foundation of New York, Chappaqua, New York; Former Professor, New York Medical College, Valhalla, New York [331]

Johanna Dwyer, DSc, RD
Jean Mayer USDA Human Nutrition Research Center on Aging; Professor, Tufts Medical Center and Director, Frances Stern Nutrition Center, Tufts Medical Center, Boston, Massachusetts [95e]

Jeffrey S. Dzieczkowski, MD
Physician, St. Alphonsus Regional Medical Center; Medical Director, Coagulation Clinic, Saint Alphonsus Medical Group, International Medicine and Travel Medicine, Boise, Idaho [138e]

Kim A. Eagle, MD
Albion Walter Hewlett Professor of Internal Medicine; Chief of Clinical Cardiology; Director, Frankel Cardiovascular Center, University of Michigan Health System, Ann Arbor, Michigan [9]

James A. Eastham, MD
Chief, Urology Service, Florence and Theodore Baumritter/Enid Ancell Chair of Urologic Oncology, Department of Surgery, Sidney Kimmel Center for Prostate and Urologic Cancers, Memorial Sloan Kettering Cancer Center, New York, New York [115]

Robert H. Eckel, MD
Professor of Medicine, Division of Endocrinology, Metabolism and Diabetes, Division of Cardiology; Professor of Physiology and Biophysics, Charles A. Boettcher, II Chair in Atherosclerosis, University of Colorado School of Medicine, Anschutz Medical Campus, Director Lipid Clinic, University of Colorado Hospital, Aurora, Colorado [422]

John E. Edwards, Jr., MD
Professor of Medicine, David Geffen School of Medicine, University of California, Los Angeles (UCLA), Los Angeles, California; Chief, Division of Infectious Diseases, Harbor/UCLA Medical Center, Torrance, California [235, 240]

David A. Ehrmann, MD
Professor, Department of Medicine, Section of Endocrinology, Diabetes, and Metabolism, The University of Chicago Pritzker School of Medicine, Chicago, Illinois [68]

Andrew J. Einstein, MD, PhD
Victoria and Esther Aboodi Assistant Professor of Medicine; Director, Cardiac CT Research; Co-Director, Cardiac CT and MRI, Department of Medicine, Cardiology Division, Department of Radiology, Columbia University College of Physicians and Surgeons, New York-Presbyterian Hospital, New York, New York [Appendix]

Ezekiel J. Emanuel, MD, PhD
Chair, Department of Medical Ethics and Health Policy, Levy University Professor, Perelman School of Medicine and Wharton School, University of Pennsylvania, Philadelphia, Pennsylvania [10]

John W. Engstrom, MD
Betty Anker Fife Distinguished Professor and Vice-Chairman; Neurology Residency Program Director, University of California, San Francisco, San Francisco, California [22, 454]

Moshe Ephros, MD
Clinical Associate Professor, Faculty of Medicine, Technion-Israel Institute of Technology; Pediatric Infectious Disease Unit, Carmel Medical Center; Haifa, Israel [197]

Jonathan A. Epstein, MD
William Wikoff Smith Professor; Chair, Department of Cell and Developmental Biology; Scientific Director, Penn Cardiovascular Institute, Perelman School of Medicine, University of Pennsylvania, Philadelphia, Pennsylvania [265e]

Aaron C. Ermel, MD
Assistant Research Professor; Assistant Professor of Clinical Medicine, Department of Internal Medicine, Division of Infectious Disease, Indiana University School of Medicine, Indianapolis, Indiana [222]

Tim Evans, MD, PhD
Senior Director, Health, Nutrition and Population, The World Bank Group, Washington, DC [13e]

Christopher H. Fanta, MD
Professor of Medicine, Harvard Medical School; Pulmonary and Critical Care Division, Brigham and Women's Hospital; Director, Partners Asthma Center, Boston, Massachusetts [48]

Paul Farmer, MD, PhD
Kolokotrones University Professor, Harvard University; Chair, Department of Global Health and Social Medicine, Harvard Medical School; Chief, Division of Global Health Equity, Brigham and Women's Hospital; Co-Founder, Partners In Health, Boston, Massachusetts [2]

Anthony S. Fauci, MD
Chief, Laboratory of Immunoregulation; Director, National Institute of Allergy and Infectious Diseases, National Institutes of Health, Bethesda, Maryland [1, 225e, 226, 261e, 372e, 385, 386e]

Murray J. Favus, MD
Professor of Medicine, Department of Medicine, Section of Endocrinology, Diabetes and Metabolism, Director Bone Program, University of Chicago Pritzker School of Medicine, Chicago, Illinois [426e]

David P. Faxon, MD
Vice Chair of Medicine for Strategic Planning, Department of Medicine, Brigham and Women's Hospital; Senior Lecturer, Harvard Medical School, Boston, Massachusetts [272, 296e, 297]

Darren R. Feldman, MD
Associate Professor in Medicine, Weill Cornell Medical Center; Assistant Attending, Genitourinary Oncology Service, Memorial Sloan-Kettering Cancer Center, New York, New York [116]

David T. Felson, MD, MPH
Professor of Medicine and Epidemiology; Chair, Clinical Epidemiology Unit, Boston University School of Medicine, Boston, Massachusetts [394]

Luigi Ferrucci, MD, PhD
Scientific Director, National Institute of Aging, National Institutes of Health, Baltimore, Maryland [11]

Howard L. Fields, MD, PhD
Professor, Department of Neurology, University of California, San Francisco, San Francisco, California [18]

Gregory A. Filice, MD
Professor of Medicine, Medical School, and Adjunct Professor of Epidemiology and Community Health, School of Public Health, University of Minnesota; Chief, Infectious Disease Section, Veterans Affairs Healthcare System, Minneapolis, Minnesota [199]

Robert W. Finberg, MD
Chair, Department of Medicine, University of Massachusetts Medical School, Worcester, Massachusetts [104, 169]

Joyce Fingeroth, MD
Professor of Medicine and MAPS, Division of Infectious Disease, University of Massachusetts Medical School, Worcester, Massachusetts [169]

Kurt Fink, MD
Palo Alto Medical Foundation, Palo Alto, California [481e]

Alain Fischer, MD, PhD
Director of INSERM U768; Director of Imagine Institute; Professor of Immunology and Pediatric Hematology; Université Paris Descartes, Paris, France [374, 375e]

Jeffrey S. Flier, MD
Caroline Shields Walker Professor of Medicine and Dean, Harvard Medical School, Boston, Massachusetts [415e]

Agnes B. Fogo, MD
John L. Shapiro Professor of Pathology; Professor of Medicine and Pediatrics, Vanderbilt University Medical Center, Nashville, Tennessee [62e]

Larry C. Ford, MD
Clinical Infectious Diseases, Intermountain Healthcare, Provo, Utah [44]

Jane E. Freedman, MD
Professor of Medicine, University of Massachusetts Medical School, Worcester, Massachusetts [142]

Roy Freeman, MD
Professor of Neurology, Harvard Medical School; Director, Center for Autonomic and Peripheral Nerve Disorders, Beth Israel Deaconess Medical Center, Boston, Massachusetts [27]

Gyorgy Frendl, MD, PhD, FCCM
Assistant Professor; Director of Surgical Critical Care Research Center, Department of Anesthesiology, Perioperative Critical Care and Pain Medicine, Harvard Medical School; Brigham and Women's Hospital, Boston, Massachusetts [481e]

Carl E. Freter, MD, PhD, FACP
Professor of Medicine; Director, Division of Hematology and Oncology; Associate Director, Cancer Center, Saint Louis University, St. Louis, Missouri [125]

Lawrence S. Friedman, MD
Professor of Medicine, Harvard Medical School; Professor of Medicine, Tufts University School of Medicine; Assistant Chief of Medicine, Massachusetts General Hospital, Boston, Massachusetts; Anton R. Fried, MD Chair, Department of Medicine, Newton-Wellesley Hospital, Newton, Massachusetts [59]

Sonia Friedman, MD
Associate Professor of Medicine, Harvard Medical School; Associate Physician, Brigham and Women's Hospital, Boston, Massachusetts [351]

Anne L. Fuhlbrigge, MD, MS
Assistant Professor of Medicine, Harvard Medical School, Pulmonary and Critical Care Division; Brigham and Women's Hospital, Boston, Massachusetts [307]

Andre D. Furtado, MD
Assistant Professor, Department of Radiology, School of Medicine, University of Pittsburgh, Pittsburgh, Pennsylvania [441e]

Nicholas B. Galifianakis, MD, MPH
Assistant Clinical Professor, Surgical Movement Disorders Center, Department of Neurology, University of California, San Francisco, San Francisco, California [33e]

John I. Gallin, MD
Director, Clinical Center, National Institutes of Health, Bethesda, Maryland [80]

Charlotte A. Gaydos, DrPh
Professor of Medicine, Johns Hopkins University, Division of Infectious Diseases, Baltimore, Maryland [213]

J. Michael Gaziano, MD, MPH
Professor of Medicine, Harvard Medical School; Chief, Division of Aging, Brigham and Women's Hospital; Director, Massachusetts Veterans Epidemiology Center, Boston VA Healthcare System, Boston, Massachusetts [266e]

Thomas A. Gaziano, MD, MSc
Assistant Professor of Medicine, Harvard Medical School; Assistant Professor, Health Policy and Management, Center for Health Decision Sciences, Harvard School of Public Health; Faculty Co-Leader, Chronic and Cardiovascular Diseases Working Group, Harvard Institute for Global Health, Harvard University; Associate Physician in Cardiovascular Medicine, Department of Cardiology, Brigham and Women's Hospital, Boston, Massachusetts [266e]

Susan L. Gearhart, MD
Associate Professor, Surgery, Johns Hopkins Medical Institutions, Baltimore, Maryland [353]

Robert H. Gelber, MD
Clinical Professor of Medicine and Dermatology, University of California, San Francisco, San Francisco, California [203]

Jeffrey M. Gelfand, MD, MAS
Assistant Professor of Clinical Neurology, Department of Neurology, University of California, San Francisco, San Francisco, California [29]

Alfred L. George, Jr., MD
Magerstadt Professor and Chair, Department of Pharmacology, Feinberg School of Medicine, Northwestern University, Chicago, Illinois [332e]

Dale N. Gerding, MD
Professor of Medicine, Department of Medicine, Loyola University Chicago Stritch School of Medicine, Maywood, Illinois; Research Physician, Edward Hines Jr. Veterans Affairs Hospital, Hines, Illinois [161]

Michael D. Geschwind, MD, PhD
Associate Professor of Neurology, Memory and Aging Center, University of California, San Francisco, San Francisco, California [33e]

Marc G. Ghany, MD, MHSc
Staff Physician, Liver Diseases Branch, National Institute of Diabetes and Digestive and Kidney Diseases, National Institutes of Health, Bethesda, Maryland [367]

Michael Giladi, MD, MSc
Associate Professor of Medicine, Sackler Faculty of Medicine, Tel Aviv University; The Infectious Disease Unit and the Bernard Pridan Laboratory for Molecular Biology of Infectious Diseases, Tel Aviv Medical Center, Tel Aviv, Israel [197]

Roger I. Glass, MD, PhD
Director, Fogarty International Center, Bethesda, Maryland [227]

Eli Glatstein, MD
Professor and Vice Chairman, Department of Radiation Oncology, Hospital of the University of Pennsylvania, Philadelphia, Pennsylvania [263e]

Peter J. Goadsby, MD, PhD, DSc, FRACp, FRCP
Professor, NIHR-Wellcome Trust Clinical Research Facility, King's College, London, United Kingdom; Professor, Department of Neurology, University of California, San Francisco, San Francisco, California [21, 447]

Morton F. Goldberg, MD, FACS, FAOS
Director Emeritus and Joseph Green Professor of Ophthalmology, Wilmer Eye Institute, Johns Hopkins University School of Medicine and Johns Hopkins Hospital, Baltimore, Maryland [40e]

Ary L. Goldberger, MD
Professor of Medicine, Harvard Medical School; Wyss Institute for Biologically Inspired Engineering, Harvard University; Beth Israel Deaconess Medical Center, Boston, Massachusetts [268, 269e, 278e]

David Goldblatt, MB, ChB, PhD
Professor of Vaccinology and Immunology; Consultant in Paediatric Immunology; Director of Clinical Research and Development; Director, NIHR Biomedical Research Centre, Institute of Child Health; University College London; Great Ormond Street Hospital for Children NHS Trust, London, United Kingdom [171]

Samuel Z. Goldhaber, MD
Professor of Medicine, Harvard Medical School; Director, Thrombosis Research Group, Brigham and Women's Hospital, Boston, Massachusetts [300]

Ralph Gonzales, MD, MSPH
Professor of Medicine, University of California, San Francisco, San Francisco, California [44]

Douglas S. Goodin, MD
Professor, Department of Neurology, School of Medicine, University of California, San Francisco, San Francisco, California [458]

Jeffrey I. Gordon, MD
Dr. Robert J. Glaser Distinguished University Professor and Director, Center for Genome Sciences and Systems Biology, Washington University School of Medicine, St. Louis, Missouri [86e]

Maria Luisa Gorno-Tempini, MD, PhD
Professor, Department of Neurology; Language Neurobiology Lab, Memory and Aging Center; Dyslexia Center, University of California, San Francisco, San Francisco, California [37e]

Peter A. Gottlieb, MD
Professor of Pediatrics and Medicine, Barbara Davis Center, University of Colorado School of Medicine, Aurora, Colorado [409]

Gregory A. Grabowski, MD
Adjunct Professor of Pediatrics and Molecular Genetics, Biochemistry, and Microbiology, University of Cincinnati College of Medicine; Division of Human Genetics Cincinnati Children's Hospital Medical Center, Cincinnati, Ohio; Chief Scientific Officer, Synageva BioPharma Corp., Lexington, Massachusetts [432e]

Yonatan H. Grad, MD, PhD
Assistant Professor of Immunology and Infectious Diseases, Harvard School of Public Health; Associate Physician, Division of Infectious Diseases, Brigham and Women's Hospital, Boston, Massachusetts [146]

Christine Grady, RN, PhD
Chief, Department of Bioethics, National Institutes of Health Clinical Center, Bethesda, Maryland [17e]

Alexander R. Green, MD, MPH
Assistant Professor of Medicine, Harvard Medical School; Associate Director, The Disparities Solutions Center, Massachusetts General Hospital, Boston, Massachusetts [16e]

Norton J. Greenberger, MD
Clinical Professor of Medicine, Harvard Medical School; Senior Physician, Division of Gastroenterology, Brigham and Women's Hospital, Boston, Massachusetts [369-371]

Michael F. Greene, MD
Professor of Obstetrics, Gynecology and Reproductive Biology, Harvard Medical School; Vincent Department of Obstetrics and Gynecology, Massachusetts General Hospital, Boston, Massachusetts [124e]

Daryl R. Gress, MD, FAAN, FCCM, FNCS
Associate Professor of Neurology, University of Virginia, Charlottesville, Virginia [330]

Rasim Gucalp, MD
Professor of Clinical Medicine, Albert Einstein College of Medicine; Associate Chairman for Educational Programs, Department of Oncology; Director, Hematology/Oncology Fellowship, Montefiore Medical Center, Bronx, New York [331]

Kalpana Gupta, MD, MPH
Associate Professor, Department of Medicine, Boston University School of Medicine; Chief, Section of Infectious Diseases, VA Boston Healthcare System, Boston, Massachusetts [162]

John G. Haaga, PhD
Deputy Associate Director, Behavioral and Social Research Program, National Institute on Aging, National Institutes of Health, Bethesda, Maryland [93e]

Chadi A. Hage, MD
Assistant Professor of Medicine, Thoracic Transplant Program, Indiana University Health, Indianapolis, Indiana [236]

Bevra Hannahs Hahn, MD
Professor Emerita Division of Rheumatology, University of California, Los Angeles, Los Angeles, California [378]

Colin N. Haile, MD, PhD
Assistant Professor, Menninger Department of Psychiatry and Behavioral Sciences, Baylor College of Medicine; Michael E. DeBakey VA Medical Center, Houston, Texas [468e]

Janet E. Hall, MD, MSc
Professor of Medicine, Harvard Medical School and Associate Chief, Reproductive Endocrine Unit, Massachusetts General Hospital, Boston, Massachusetts [69, 412, 414]

Jesse B. Hall, MD, FCCP
Professor of Medicine, Anesthesia and Critical Care; Chief, Section of Pulmonary and Critical Care Medicine, University of Chicago, Chicago, Illinois [321]

Scott A. Halperin, MD
Professor of Pediatrics and Microbiology and Immunology Head, Pediatric Infectious Diseases, Director, Canadian Center for Vaccinology, Dalhousie University, Halifax, Nova Scotia, Canada [185]

R. Doug Hardy, MD
Infectious Diseases Specialists, PA; Medical City Dallas Hospital and Medical City Children's Hospital, Dallas; Baylor Regional Medical Center, Plano, Texas [212]

Rudy A. Hartskeerl, PhD
Director WHO/FAO/OIE and National Leptospirosis Reference Centre, KIT Biomedical Research, KIT (Royal Tropical Institute), Amsterdam, The Netherlands [208]

William L. Hasler, MD
Professor, Division of Gastroenterology, University of Michigan Health System, Ann Arbor, Michigan [54, 344]

Stephen L. Hauser, MD
Robert A. Fishman Distinguished Professor and Chairman, Department of Neurology, University of California, San Francisco, San Francisco, California [1, 437, 443e, 444e, 455, 456, 458, 460]

Barton F. Haynes, MD
Frederic M. Hanes Professor of Medicine and Immunology, Departments of Medicine and Immunology; Director, Duke Human Vaccine Institute, Duke University School of Medicine, Durham, North Carolina [372e]

Douglas C. Heimburger, MD, MS
Professor of Medicine, Associate Director for Education and Training, Vanderbilt Institute for Global Health, Vanderbilt University School of Medicine, Nashville, Tennessee [97]

J. Claude Hemphill, III, MD, MAS
Professor of Neurology and Neurological Surgery, University of California, San Francisco; Chief of Neurology, San Francisco General Hospital, San Francisco, California [330, 446]

Patrick H. Henry, MD
Clinical Adjunct Professor of Medicine, University of Iowa, Iowa City, Iowa [79]

Katherine A. High, MD
William H. Bennett Professor of Pediatrics, Perelman School of Medicine, University of Pennsylvania; Investigator, Howard Hughes Medical Institute, The Children's Hospital of Philadelphia, Philadelphia, Pennsylvania [91e, 141]

Christine E. Hill-Kayser, MD
Assistant Professor of Radiation Oncology, Perelman School of Medicine, University of Pennsylvania, Philadelphia, Pennsylvania [263e]

Ikuo Hirano, MD
Professor of Medicine, Division of Gastroenterology, Northwestern University Feinberg School of Medicine, Chicago, Illinois [53, 347]

Martin S. Hirsch, MD
Professor of Medicine, Harvard Medical School; Professor of Immunology and Infectious Diseases, Harvard School of Public Health; Physician, Massachusetts General Hospital, Boston, Massachusetts [219]

Helen H. Hobbs, MD
Professor, Internal Medicine and Molecular Genetics, University of Texas Southwestern Medical Center; Investigator, Howard Hughes Medical Institute, Dallas, Texas [421]

Judith S. Hochman, MD
Harold Snyder Family Professor of Cardiology, Clinical Chief, Leon Charney Division of Cardiology, Co-Director, NYU-HHC Clinical and Translational Science Institute; Director, Cardiovascular Clinical Research Center, New York University School of Medicine, New York, New York [326]

A. Victor Hoffbrand, DM
Emeritus Professor of Haematology, University College, London; Honorary Consultant Haematologist, Royal Free Hospital, London, United Kingdom [128]

L. John Hoffer, MD, PhD
Professor, Faculty of Medicine, McGill University; Senior Physician, Divisions of Internal Medicine and Endocrinology, Lady Davis Institute for Medical Research, Jewish General Hospital, Montreal, Quebec, Canada [98e]

Charles W. Hoge, MD
Senior Scientist, Center for Psychiatry and Neuroscience, Walter Reed Army Institute of Research, Silver Spring, Maryland [471e]

Elizabeth L. Hohmann, MD
Associate Professor of Medicine and Infectious Diseases, Harvard Medical School; Massachusetts General Hospital, Boston, Massachusetts [176]

Steven M. Holland, MD
Chief, Laboratory of Clinical Infectious Diseases, National Institute of Allergy and Infectious Diseases, National Institutes of Health, Bethesda, Maryland [80, 204]

King K. Holmes, MD, PhD
Chair, Global Health; Professor of Medicine and Global Health; Adjunct Professor, Epidemiology; Director, Center for AIDS and STD; University of Washington School of Medicine; Head, Infectious Diseases Section, Harborview Medical Center, Seattle, Washington [163]

Jay H. Hoofnagle, MD
Director, Liver Diseases Research Branch, National Institute of Diabetes and Digestive and Kidney Diseases, National Institutes of Health, Bethesda, Maryland [357]

David C. Hooper, MD
Professor, Harvard Medical School; Chief, Infection Control Unit; Associate Chief, Division of Infectious Diseases, Massachusetts General Hospital, Boston, Massachusetts [170]

Robert J. Hopkin, MD
Associate Professor, Cincinnati Children's Hospital Medical Center, Cincinnati, Ohio [432e]

Leora Horn, MD, MSc
Assistant Professor, Division of Hematology and Medical Oncology, Vanderbilt University School of Medicine, Nashville, Tennessee [107]

Jonathan C. Horton, MD, PhD
William F. Hoyt Professor of Neuro-ophthalmology, Professor of Ophthalmology, Neurology and Physiology, University of California, San Francisco School of Medicine, San Francisco, California [39]

Howard Hu, MD, MPH, ScD
Dean; Professor of Environmental Health, Epidemiology and Global Health, Dalla Lana School of Public Health; Professor of Medicine, University of Toronto, Toronto, Ontario, Canada [472e]

Deborah T. Hung, MD, PhD
Associate Professor of Microbiology and Molecular Genetics, Assistant Professor of Medicine, Harvard Medical School; Brigham and Women's Hospital; Massachusetts General Hospital, Boston, Massachusetts; Co-director, Infectious Disease Initiative, Broad Institute of Harvard University and Massachusetts Institute of Technology, Cambridge, Massachusetts [146]

Sharon A. Hunt, MD, FACC
Professor of Medicine, Cardiovascular Medicine, Stanford University, Palo Alto, California [281]

Charles G. Hurst, MD
Chief, Chemical Casualty Care Division, United States Medical Research Institute of Chemical Defense, APG-Edgewood Area, Maryland [262e]

Ashraf S. Ibrahim, PhD
Professor, Department of Medicine, Geffen School of Medicine, University of California, Los Angeles (UCLA); Division of Infectious Diseases, Los Angeles Biomedical Research Institute at Harbor–UCLA Medical Center, Torrance, California [242]

David H. Ingbar, MD
Professor of Medicine, Pediatrics, and Physiology; Director, Pulmonary Allergy, Critical Care and Sleep Division, University of Minnesota School of Medicine, Minneapolis, Minnesota [326]

Alan C. Jackson, MD, FRCPC
Professor of Medicine (Neurology) and of Medical Microbiology, University of Manitoba; Section Head of Neurology, Winnipeg Regional Health Authority, Winnipeg, Manitoba, Canada [232]

Lisa A. Jackson, MD, MPH
Senior Investigator, Group Health Research Institute, Seattle, Washington [148]

Danny O. Jacobs, MD, MPH, FACS
Executive Vice President, Provost, and Dean of the School of Medicine; Thomas N. and Gleaves T. James Distinguished Chair, The University of Texas Medical Branch at Galveston, Galveston, Texas [20, 355, 356]

Richard F. Jacobs, MD
Robert H. Fiser, Jr., MD Endowed Chair in Pediatrics; Professor and Chairman, Department of Pediatrics, University of Arkansas for Medical Sciences; President, Arkansas Children's Hospital Research Institute, Little Rock, Arkansas [195]

J. Larry Jameson, MD, PhD
Robert G. Dunlop Professor of Medicine; Dean, Perelman School of Medicine at the University of Pennsylvania; Executive Vice President, University of Pennsylvania for the Health System, Philadelphia, Pennsylvania [1, 56, 82, 84, 121, 399-403, 405, 410, 411, 436e]

Robert T. Jensen, MD
Chief, Cell Biology Section, National Institutes of Diabetes, Digestive and Kidney Diseases, National Institutes of Health, Bethesda, Maryland [113]

Roy M. John, MBBS, PhD, FRCP
Assistant Professor of Medicine, Harvard Medical School; Department of Medicine, Brigham and Women's Hospital, Boston, Massachusetts [277]

Savio John, MD
Assistant Professor of Medicine, Division of Gastroenterology and Hepatology, State University of New York Upstate Medical University, Syracuse, New York [58]

David H. Johnson, MD
Donald W. Seldin Distinguished Chair in Internal Medicine; Professor and Chairman, Department of Internal Medicine, University of Texas Southwestern School of Medicine, Dallas, Texas [107]

James R. Johnson, MD
Professor of Medicine, University of Minnesota, Minneapolis, Minnesota [186]

Stuart Johnson, MD
Associate Professor of Medicine, Loyola University Chicago Stritch School of Medicine; Staff Physician, Edward Hines Jr. VA Hospital, Hines, Illinois [161]

S. Clairborne Johnston, MD, PhD
Dean, Dell Medical School; Frank Denius Distinguished Dean's Chair in Medical Leadership; Vice President for Medical Affairs, University of Texas, Austin, Austin, Texas [446]

S. Andrew Josephson, MD
Associate Professor; Vice Chairman, Department of Neurology, University of California, San Francisco, San Francisco, California [34, 329e, 463e]

Harald Jüppner, MD
Professor of Pediatrics, Endocrine Unit and Pediatric Nephrology Unit, Massachusetts General Hospital, Boston, Massachusetts [424]

Peter J. Kahrilas, MD
Gilbert H. Marquardt Professor of Medicine, Feinberg School of Medicine, Northwestern University, Chicago, Illinois [53, 347]

Gail Kang, MD
San Francisco, California [33e]

Hagop Kantarjian, MD
Chairman, Leukemia Department; Professor of Leukemia, The University of Texas M.D. Anderson Cancer Center, Houston, Texas [133]

Adolf W. Karchmer, MD
Professor of Medicine, Harvard Medical School, Division of Infectious Diseases, Beth Israel Deaconess Medical Center, Boston, Massachusetts [155]

Dennis L. Kasper, MD, MA
William Ellery Channing Professor of Medicine, Professor of Microbiology and Immunobiology, Department of Microbiology and Immunobiology, Harvard Medical School; Division of Infectious Diseases, Brigham and Women's Hospital, Boston, Massachusetts [1, 144, 147, 159, 183e, 201]

Lloyd H. Kasper, MD
Professor of Microbiology/Immunology and Medicine, Geisel School of Medicine, Dartmouth College, Hanover, New Hampshire [253]

Daniel L. Kastner, MD, PhD
Scientific Director, National Human Genome Research Institute, National Institutes of Health, Bethesda, Maryland [392]

Carol A. Kauffman, MD
Professor of Internal Medicine, University of Michigan Medical School; Chief, Infectious Diseases Section, Veterans Affairs Ann Arbor Healthcare System, Ann Arbor, Michigan [243]

Elaine T. Kaye, MD
Assistant Clinical Professor of Dermatology, Harvard Medical School; Boston Children's Hospital, Boston, Massachusetts [24, 25e]

Kenneth M. Kaye, MD
Associate Professor of Medicine, Harvard Medical School; Division of Infectious Diseases, Brigham and Women's Hospital, Boston, Massachusetts [24, 25e]

John A. Kessler, MD
Davee Professor of Stem Cell Biology, Department of Neurology, Feinberg School of Medicine, Northwestern University, Chicago, Illinois [90e]

Jay S. Keystone, MD, FRCPC, MSc(CTM)
Professor of Medicine, University of Toronto, Toronto, Ontario, Canada [149]

Sundeep Khosla, MD
Professor of Medicine and Physiology, College of Medicine, Mayo Clinic, Rochester, Minnesota [65]

Elliott Kieff, MD, PhD
Harriet Ryan Albee Professor of Medicine, Harvard Medical School; Brigham and Women's Hospital, Boston, Massachusetts [214e]

Anthony A. Killeen, MD, PhD
Professor, Department of Laboratory Medicine and Pathology, University of Minnesota, Minneapolis, Minnesota [480e]

Kami Kim, MD
Professor, Departments of Medicine, Pathology, and Microbiology and Immunology, Albert Einstein College of Medicine, Bronx, New York [253]

Charles H. King, MD, MS
Professor, Center for Global Health and Diseases, School of Medicine, Case Western Reserve University, Cleveland, Ohio [259]

Lindsay King, MD, MPH
Advanced Transplant/Hepatology Fellow, Department of Medicine, Gastrointestinal Unit, Massachusetts General Hospital, Boston, Massachusetts [483e]

Talmadge E. King, Jr., MD
Professor and Chair, Department of Medicine, University of California, San Francisco, San Francisco, California [315]

Louis V. Kirchhoff, MD, MPH
Professor, Departments of Internal Medicine (Infectious Diseases) and Epidemiology, University of Iowa; Staff Physician, Department of Veterans Affairs Medical Center, Iowa City, Iowa [252]

Priya S. Kishnani, MD
Professor of Pediatrics, Division Chief, Medical Genetics, Duke University Medical Center, Durham, North Carolina [433e]

Rob Knight, PhD
Professor, Howard Hughes Medical Institute; Departments of Chemistry and Biochemistry and Computer Science, Biofrontiers Institute, University of Colorado, Boulder, Colorado [86e]

Minoru S. H. Ko, MD, PhD
Mitsunada Sakaguchi Professor and Chair, Department of Systems Medicine, Keio University School of Medicine, Tokyo, Japan [88]

Barbara A. Konkle, MD
Professor of Medicine, Hematology, University of Washington; Director, Translational Research, Puget Sound Blood Center, Seattle, Washington [78, 140]

Peter Kopp, MD
Associate Professor, Division of Endocrinology, Metabolism and Molecular Science and Center for Genetic Medicine, Northwestern University Feinberg School of Medicine, Chicago, Illinois [82]

Walter J. Koroshetz, MD
National Institute of Neurological Disorders and Stroke, National Institutes of Health, Bethesda, Maryland [165]

Thomas R. Kosten, MD
J. H. Waggoner Professor of Psychiatry, Pharmacology, Immunology, Neuroscience, Baylor College of Medicine, Houston, Texas [468e]

Theodore A. Kotchen, MD
Professor Emeritus, Department of Medicine; Associate Dean for Clinical Research, Medical College of Wisconsin, Milwaukee, Wisconsin [298]

Camille Nelson Kotton, MD, FIDSA
Clinical Director, Transplant and Immunocompromised Host Infectious Diseases, Infectious Diseases Division, Massachusetts General Hospital; Harvard Medical School, Boston, Massachusetts [219]

Phyllis E. Kozarsky, MD
Professor of Medicine and Infectious Diseases, Emory University School of Medicine, Atlanta, Georgia [149]

Barnett S. Kramer, MD, MPH, FACP
Director, Division of Cancer Prevention, National Cancer Institute, Bethesda, Maryland [100]

Joel Kramer, PsyD
Professor of Neuropsychology in Neurology; Director of Neuropsychology, Memory and Aging Center, University of California, San Francisco, San Francisco, California [37e]

Stephen M. Krane, MD
Persis, Cyrus and Marlow B. Harrison Distinguished Professor of Medicine, Harvard Medical School; Massachusetts General Hospital, Boston, Massachusetts [423]

Alexander Kratz, MD, MPH, PhD
Associate Professor of Clinical Pathology and Cell Biology, Columbia University College of Physicians and Surgeons; Director, Core Laboratory, Columbia University Medical Center and the New York Presbyterian Hospital; Director, the Allen Hospital Laboratory, New York, New York [Appendix]

Peter J. Krause, MD
Senior Research Scientist, Yale School of Public Health; Yale School of Medicine, New Haven, Connecticut [249]

John P. Kress, MD
Professor of Medicine, Director, Medical Intensive Care Unit, University of Chicago, Chicago, Illinois [321]

Stephen Krieger, MD
Assistant Professor, Department of Neurology; Director, Neurology Residency Program, Icahn School of Medicine at Mount Sinai; Attending Physician, The Corinne Goldsmith Dickinson Center for MS, New York, New York [486e]

Patricia A. Kritek, MD, EdM
Associate Professor, Division of Pulmonary and Critical Care Medicine, University of Washington, Seattle, Washington [48, 305, 308e]

Henry M. Kronenberg, MD
Professor of Medicine, Harvard Medical School; Chief, Endocrine Unit, Massachusetts General Hospital, Boston, Massachusetts [423]

Jens H. Kuhn, MD, PhD, MS
Principal, Tunnell Government Services (TGS), Inc.; Lead Virologist, Integrated Research Facility at Fort Detrick (IRF-Frederick); TGS IRF-Frederick Team Leader, NIH/NIAID/DCR, Fort Detrick, Frederick, Maryland [233, 234]

Robert F. Kushner, MD, MS
Professor of Medicine, Northwestern University Feinberg School of Medicine, Chicago, Illinois [416]

Raymond Y. Kwong, MD, MPH
Associate Professor of Medicine, Harvard Medical School; Director of Cardiac Magnetic Resonance Imaging, Cardiovascular Division, Department of Medicine, Brigham and Women's Hospital, Boston, Massachusetts [270e, 271e]

Loren Laine, MD
Professor of Medicine, Yale University School of Medicine, New Haven, Connecticut; VA Connecticut Healthcare System, West Haven, Connecticut [57]

Neil K. Lakdawala, MD
Instructor in Medicine, Harvard Medical School; Associate Physician, Cardiovascular Medicine, Brigham and Women's Hospital; Boston VA Healthcare; Boston, Massachusetts [287]

Anil K. Lalwani, MD
Professor and Vice Chair for Research; Director, Division of Otology, Neurotology and Skull Base Surgery; Director, Columbia Cochlear Implant Center, Columbia University College of Physicians and Surgeons, New York, New York [43]

H. Clifford Lane, MD
Clinical Director, National Institute of Allergy and Infectious Diseases, National Institutes of Health, Bethesda, Maryland [226, 261e]

Carol A. Langford, MD, MHS
Harold C. Schott Endowed Chair; Director, Center for Vasculitis Care and Research, Department of Rheumatic and Immunologic Diseases, Cleveland Clinic, Cleveland, Ohio [385, 386e, 389, 397, 398]

Regina C. LaRocque, MD, MPH
Assistant Professor of Medicine, Harvard Medical School; Assistant Physician, Massachusetts General Hospital, Boston, Massachusetts [160]

Wei C. Lau, MD, FAHA
Emeritus Associate Professor, Department of Anesthesiology, Section Cardiovascular Anesthesiology, University of Michigan Health System Cardiovascular Center, Ann Arbor, Michigan [9]

Leslie P. Lawley, MD
Assistant Professor, Department of Dermatology, School of Medicine, Emory University, Atlanta, Georgia [71]

Thomas J. Lawley, MD
William P. Timmie Professor of Dermatology, Dean, Emory University School of Medicine, Atlanta, Georgia [70, 71, 73, 76e]

David G. Le Couteur, MD, PhD, FRACP
Professor of Geriatric Medicine, Director of the Centre for Education and Research on Ageing, University of Sydney and Sydney Research, Sydney, Australia [94e]

William M. Lee, MD
Professor of Internal Medicine; Meredith Mosle Chair in Liver Diseases, University of Texas Southwestern Medical Center at Dallas, Dallas, Texas [361]

Charles Lei, MD
Assistant Professor, Department of Emergency Medicine, Vanderbilt University Medical Center, Nashville, Tennessee [474]

Jane A. Leopold, MD
Associate Professor of Medicine, Harvard Medical School; Brigham and Women's Hospital, Boston, Massachusetts [272, 297e]

Nelson Leung, MD
Associate Professor of Medicine, Division of Nephrology and Hypertension, Division of Hematology, Mayo Clinic Rochester, Rochester, Minnesota [341]

Bruce D. Levy, MD
Associate Professor of Medicine, Harvard Medical School; Pulmonary and Critical Care Medicine, Brigham and Women's Hospital, Boston, Massachusetts [322]

Julia B. Lewis, MD
Professor, Department of Medicine, Division of Nephrology, Vanderbilt University Medical Center, Nashville, Tennessee [338]

Peter Libby, MD
Mallinckrodt Professor of Medicine, Harvard Medical School; Chief, Cardiovascular Medicine, Brigham and Women's Hospital, Boston, Massachusetts [265e, 291e, 292e]

Richard W. Light, MD
Professor of Medicine, Division of Allergy, Pulmonary, and Critical Care Medicine, Vanderbilt University, Nashville, Tennessee [316, 317]

Julie Lin, MD, MPH
Lecturer on Medicine, Harvard Medical School; Associate Physician, Renal Division, Brigham and Women's Hospital, Boston, Massachusetts, Boston, Massachusetts [61]

Yusen E. Lin, PhD, MBA
Professor and Director, Center for Environmental Laboratory Services; National Kaohsiung Normal University, Kaohsiung, Taiwan [184]

Robert Lindsay, MD, PhD
Chief, Internal Medicine; Professor of Clinical Medicine, Helen Hayes Hospital, West Haverstraw, New York [425]

Marc E. Lippman, MD, MACP, FRCP
Kathleen and Stanley Glaser Professor, Department of Medicine, Deputy Director, Sylvester Comprehensive Cancer Center, University of Miami Miller School of Medicine, Miami, Florida [108]

Peter E. Lipsky, MD
Charlottesville, Virginia [377e]

Kathleen D. Liu, MD, PhD, MAS
Associate Professor, Division of Nephrology, Department of Medicine, Division of Critical Care Medicine, Department of Anesthesiology, University of California, San Francisco, San Francisco, California [336]

Bernard Lo, MD
President, The Greenwall Foundation, New York; Professor of Medicine Emeritus and Director Emeritus of the Program in Medical Ethics, University of California, San Francisco, San Francisco, California [17e]

Dan L. Longo, MD
Professor of Medicine, Harvard Medical School; Senior Physician, Brigham and Women's Hospital; Deputy Editor, *New England Journal of Medicine*, Boston, Massachusetts [1, 77, 79, 81e, 89e, 99, 102e, 103e, 121, 123e, 124e, 125, 134, 135e, 136, 225e]

Nicola Longo, MD, PhD
Professor and Chief, Division of Medical Genetics, Departments of Pediatrics and Pathology; Medical Co-Director, Biochemical Genetics Laboratory, ARUP Laboratories, University of Utah, Salt Lake City, Utah [434e, 435e]

Joseph Loscalzo, MD, PhD
Hersey Professor of the Theory and Practice of Medicine, Harvard Medical School; Chairman, Department of Medicine; Physician-in-Chief, Brigham and Women's Hospital, Boston, Massachusetts [1, 49-52, 87e, 142, 264, 265e, 267, 283-287, 293, 295, 301-304]

Christine M. Lovly, MD, PhD
Academic, Vanderbilt Ingram Cancer Center, Vanderbilt University School of Medicine, Nashville, Tennessee [107]

Phillip A. Low, MD, FRACP, FRCP(Hon)
Robert D. and Patricia E. Kern Professor of Neurology, Mayo Clinic, College of Medicine, Rochester, Minnesota [454]

Daniel H. Lowenstein, MD
Dr. Robert B. and Mrs. Ellinor Aird Professor of Neurology; Director, Epilepsy Center, University of California, San Francisco, San Francisco, California [437, 438e, 445]

Elyse E. Lower, MD
Medical Oncology and Hematology, University of Cincinnati, Oncology Hematology Care, Inc., Cincinnati, Ohio [390]

Franklin D. Lowy, MD
Professor of Medicine and Pathology, Columbia University College of Physicians and Surgeons, New York, New York [172]

Sheila A. Lukehart, PhD
Professor, Departments of Medicine and Global Health, University of Washington, Seattle, Washington [206, 207e]

Lucio Luzzatto, MD, FRCP, FRCPath
Professor of Hematology, University of Genova, Genova; Scientific Director, Istituto Toscano Tumori, Florence, Italy [129]

Lawrence C. Madoff, MD
Professor of Medicine, University of Massachusetts Medical School, Worcester, Massachusetts; Director, Division of Epidemiology and Immunization, Massachusetts Department of Public Health, Jamaica Plain, Massachusetts [157, 166e, 167e]

Adel A. F. Mahmoud, MD, PhD
Professor in Molecular Biology and Public Policy, Princeton University, Princeton, New Jersey [259]

Ronald V. Maier, MD
Jane and Donald D. Trunkey Professor and Vice-Chair, Surgery, University of Washington; Surgeon-in-Chief, Harborview Medical Center, Seattle, Washington [324]

Mark E. Mailliard, MD
Frederick F. Paustian Professor; Chief, Division of Gastroenterology and Hepatology, Department of Internal Medicine, University of Nebraska College of Medicine, Omaha, Nebraska [363]

Mahmoud Malas, MD, MHS, FACS
Associate Professor of Surgery, Johns Hopkins University; Director of Endovascular Surgery; Director of The Vascular and Endovascular Clinical Research Center, Johns Hopkins Bayview Medical Center, Baltimore, Maryland [354]

Hari R. Mallidi, MD
Associate Professor of Surgery and Chief, Division of Transplant and Assist Devices; Lester and Sue Smith Endowed Chair in Surgery, Baylor College of Medicine, Houston, Texas [281]

Susan J. Mandel, MD, MPH
Professor of Medicine; Associate Chief, Division of Endocrinology, Diabetes and Metabolism, Perelman School of Medicine, University of Pennsylvania, Philadelphia, Pennsylvania [405]

Brian F. Mandell, MD, PhD
Professor and Chairman of Medicine, Cleveland Clinic Lerner College of Medicine, Department of Rheumatic and Immunologic Disease, Cleveland Clinic, Cleveland, Ohio [397]

Lionel A. Mandell, MD, FRCPC
Professor of Medicine, McMaster University, Hamilton, Ontario, Canada [153]

Douglas L. Mann, MD
Lewin Chair and Chief, Cardiovascular Division; Professor of Medicine, Cell Biology and Physiology, Washington University School of Medicine, Cardiologist-in-Chief, Barnes Jewish Hospital, St. Louis, Missouri [279]

JoAnn E. Manson, MD, DrPH
Professor of Medicine and the Elizabeth Fay Brigham Professor of Women's Health, Harvard Medical School; Chief, Division of Preventive Medicine, Brigham and Women's Hospital, Boston, Massachusetts [413]

Eleftheria Maratos-Flier, MD
Professor of Medicine, Harvard Medical School; Division of Endocrinology, Beth Israel Deaconess Medical Center, Boston, Massachusetts [415e]

Guido Marcucci, MD
Professor of Medicine; John B. and Jane T. McCoy Chair in Cancer Research; Associate Director of Translational Research, Comprehensive Cancer Center, The Ohio State University College of Medicine, Columbus, Ohio [132]

Daniel B. Mark, MD, MPH
Professor of Medicine, Duke University Medical Center; Director, Outcomes Research, Duke Clinical Research Institute, Durham, North Carolina [3]

Alexander G. Marneros, MD, PhD
Assistant Professor, Department of Dermatology, Harvard Medical School; Cutaneous Biology Research Center, Massachusetts General Hospital, Boston, Massachusetts [75]

Jeanne M. Marrazzo, MD, MPH
Professor of Medicine, Division of Allergy and Infectious Diseases, University of Washington, Seattle, Washington [163]

Thomas Marrie, MD
Dean, Faculty of Medicine; Professor, Department of Medicine, Dalhousie University, Halifax, Nova Scotia, Canada [211]

Gary J. Martin, MD
Raymond J. Langenbach, MD Professor of Medicine; Vice Chairman for Faculty Affairs, Department of Medicine, Northwestern University Feinberg School of Medicine, Chicago, Illinois [4]

Joseph B. Martin, MD, PhD
Edward R. and Anne G. Lefler Professor, Department of Neurobiology, Harvard Medical School, Boston, Massachusetts [437]

Susan Maslanka, PhD
Enteric Diseases Laboratory Branch, Centers for Disease Control and Prevention, Atlanta, Georgia [178]

Henry Masur, MD
Chief, Critical Care Medicine Department, Clinical Center, National Institutes of Health, Bethesda, Maryland [244]

Jeremy Matloff, MD
Fellow, Department of Gastroenterology, Icahn School of Medicine at Mount Sinai, New York, New York [485e, 486e]

Robert J. Mayer, MD
Faculty Vice President for Academic Affairs, Dana-Farber Cancer Institute; Stephen B. Kay Family Professor of Medicine, Harvard Medical School, Boston, Massachusetts [109, 110]

Alexander J. McAdam, MD, PhD
Associate Professor of Pathology, Harvard Medical School; Medical Director, Infectious Diseases Diagnostic Laboratory, Children's Hospital of Boston, Boston, Massachusetts [150e]

Calvin O. McCall, MD
Associate Professor, Department of Dermatology, Virginia Commonwealth University Medical Center, Richmond, Virginia; Chief, Dermatology Section, Hunter Holmes McGuire Veterans Affairs Medical Center, Richmond, Virginia [71, 76e]

John F. McConville, MD
Associate Professor of Medicine and Director, Internal Medicine Residency Program, University of Chicago, Chicago, Illinois [318]

Corey A. McGraw, MD
Assistant Professor, The Saul R. Korey Department of Neurology, Albert Einstein College of Medicine, Yeshiva University, New York, New York [486e]

Kevin T. McVary, MD, FACS
Professor and Chairman, Division of Urology, Southern Illinois University School of Medicine, Springfield, Illinois [67]

Mandeep R. Mehra, MD, FACC, FACP
Professor of Medicine, Harvard Medical School; Executive Director, Center for Advanced Heart Disease, Brigham and Women's Hospital; Co-Director, Brigham and Women's Hospital Heart and Vascular Center, Boston, Massachusetts [280]

Nancy K. Mello,† PhD
Professor of Psychology (Neuroscience), Harvard Medical School, Boston, Massachusetts; Director, Alcohol and Drug Abuse Research Center, McLean Hospital, Belmont, Massachusetts [469e]

Shlomo Melmed, MD
Senior Vice President and Dean of the Medical Faculty, Cedars-Sinai Medical Center, Los Angeles, California [401e-403]

Jack H. Mendelson,† MD
Professor of Psychiatry (Neuroscience), Harvard Medical School, Belmont, Massachusetts [469e]

Robert O. Messing, MD
Professor, Division of Pharmacology and Toxicology, College of Pharmacy; Associate Director, Waggoner Center for Alcohol and Addiction Research, University of Texas at Austin, Austin, Texas [465e]

M.-Marsel Mesulam, MD
Professor of Neurology, Psychiatry and Psychology, Cognitive Neurology and Alzheimer's Disease Center, Northwestern University Feinberg School of Medicine, Chicago, Illinois [36]

Gregory F. Michaud, MD
Assistant Professor of Medicine, Harvard Medical School; Brigham and Women's Hospital, Boston, Massachusetts [276]

Susan Miesfeldt, MD
Medical Oncology, Medical Director, Cancer Risk and Prevention Clinic, Maine Medical Center, Scarborough, Maine [84]

Edgar L. Milford, MD
Associate Professor of Medicine, Harvard Medical School; Director, Tissue Typing Laboratory, Brigham and Women's Hospital, Boston, Massachusetts [337]

Bruce L. Miller, MD
A. W. and Mary Margaret Clausen Distinguished Professor of Neurology, University of California, San Francisco School of Medicine, San Francisco, California [34, 35, 37e, 448, 453e]

Samuel I. Miller, MD
Professor, Departments of Microbiology, Medicine and Genome Sciences, University of Washington, Seattle, Washington [190]

Simon J. Mitchell, MB ChB, PhD, FUHM, FANZCA
Associate Professor, Department of Anaesthesiology, University of Auckland and Auckland City Hospital, Auckland, New Zealand [477e]

Babak Mokhlesi, MD, MSc
Professor of Medicine, Department of Medicine, Section of Pulmonary and Critical Care; Director, Sleep Disorders Center and Sleep Fellowship Program, University of Chicago, Chicago, Illinois [318]

Thomas A. Moore, MD, FACP, FIDSA
Chairman, Department of Infectious Diseases, Ochsner Health System, New Orleans, Louisiana [246e]

Pat J. Morin, PhD
Senior Director, Scientific Review and Grants Administration, American Association for Cancer Research, Philadelphia, Pennsylvania [101e]

Alison Morris, MD, MS
Associate Professor, Departments of Medicine and Immunology; Director, University of Pittsburgh HIV Lung Research Center, Division of Pulmonary, Allergy, and Critical Care Medicine, University of Pittsburgh School of Medicine, Pittsburgh, Pennsylvania [244]

Charles A. Morris, MD, MPH
Instructor in Medicine, Harvard Medical School; Staff Physician, Brigham and Women's Hospital, Boston, Massachusetts [482e, 484e]

David A. Morrow, MD, MPH
Associate Professor of Medicine, Harvard Medical School; Director, Levine Cardiac Intensive Care Unit; Senior Investigator, TIMI Study Group, Brigham and Women's Hospital, Boston, Massachusetts [19]

William J. Moss, MD, MPH
Professor, Departments of Epidemiology, International Health, and Molecular Microbiology and Immunology, Johns Hopkins Bloomberg School of Public Health, Baltimore, Maryland [229]

Robert J. Motzer, MD
Professor of Medicine, Joan and Sanford Weill College of Medicine of Cornell University D. Attending Physician, Genitourinary Oncology Service, Memorial Sloan-Kettering Cancer Center, New York, New York [114, 116]

David B. Mount, MD
Assistant Professor of Medicine, Harvard Medical School; Renal Division, Brigham and Women's Hospital, Renal Division, Boston VA Healthcare System, Boston, Massachusetts [63, 64e]

Haralampos M. Moutsopoulos, MD, FACP, FRCP(hc), Master ACR
Professor and Director, Department of Pathophysiology, Medical School, National University of Athens, Athens, Greece [379, 383, 387]

Robert S. Munford, MD
Senior Clinician, Laboratory of Clinical Infectious Diseases, National Institute of Allergy and Infectious Diseases, National Institutes of Health, Bethesda, Maryland [325]

Nikhil C. Munshi, MD
Professor of Medicine, Harvard Medical School; Boston VA Healthcare System; Director of Basic and Correlative Sciences; Associate Director, Jerome Lipper Myeloma Center, Dana-Farber Cancer Institute, Boston, Massachusetts [136]

John R. Murphy, PhD
Professor of Medicine and Microbiology; Director ad interim, National Emerging Infectious Diseases Laboratories Institute, Boston University School of Medicine, Boston, Massachusetts [175]

Timothy F. Murphy, MD
SUNY Distinguished Professor; Director, Clinical and Translational Research Center, University at Buffalo, the State University of New York, Buffalo, New York [182]

Barbara E. Murray, MD
J. Ralph Meadows Professor and Director, Division of Infectious Diseases, University of Texas Medical School, Houston, Texas [174]

Joseph A. Murray, MD
Professor of Medicine, Departments of Internal Medicine and Immunology, Mayo Clinic, Rochester, Minnesota [55]

Mark B. Mycyk, MD
Associate Professor, Department of Emergency Medicine, Northwestern University Feinberg School of Medicine; Associate Professor, Department of Emergency Medicine, Rush University School of Medicine; Research Director, Toxikon Consortium; Attending Physician, Department of Emergency Medicine, Cook County Hospital, Chicago, Illinois [473e]

Robert J. Myerburg, MD
Professor, Departments of Medicine and Physiology, Division of Cardiology; AHA Chair in Cardiovascular Research, University of Miami Miller School of Medicine, Miami, Florida [327]

Avindra Nath, MD
Chief, Section of Infections of the Nervous System; Clinical Director, National Institute of Neurological Disorders and Stroke (NINDS), National Institutes of Health, Bethesda, Maryland [165]

Edward T. Naureckas, MD
Professor of Medicine, and Director, Pulmonary Function Laboratory, and Adult Cystic Fibrosis Laboratory, Section of Pulmonary and Critical Care Medicine, University of Chicago, Chicago, Illinois [306e]

Eric G. Neilson, MD
Lewis Landsberg Dean, and Vice President, Medical Affairs, Feinberg School of Medicine, Northwestern University, Chicago, Illinois [62e, 332e, 338]

Emily Page Nelson, MD
Clinical Instructor, Department of Anesthesiology, Perioperative, and Pain Medicine, Brigham and Women's Hospital, Boston, Massachusetts [484e]

Gerald T. Nepom, MD, PhD
Professor (Affiliate), University of Washington School of Medicine; Director, Benaroya Research Institute at Virginia Mason; Director, Immune Tolerance Network, Seattle, Washington [373e]

†Deceased

Eric J. Nestler, MD, PhD
Nash Family Professor and Chair, Department of Neuroscience; Director, Friedman Brain Institute, Ichan School of Medicine at Mount Sinai, New York, New York [465e]

Hartmut P. H. Neumann, MD
Universitaet Freiburg, Medizinische Universitaetsklinik, Freiburg im Breisgau, Germany [407]

Joseph P. Newhouse, PhD
John D. MacArthur Professor of Health Policy and Management, Department of Health Care Policy, Harvard Medical School; Faculty, John F. Kennedy School of Government, Harvard School of Public Health, Faculty of Arts and Sciences, Harvard University, Boston, Massachusetts [15e]

Jonathan Newmark, MD
Colonel, Medical Corps, U.S. Army; Deputy Joint Program Executive Officer, Medical Systems, Joint Program Executive Office for Chemical/Biological Defense, U.S. Department of Defense, Falls Church, Virginia; Adjunct Professor of Neurology, F. Edward Hebert School of Medicine, Uniformed Services University of the Health Sciences, Bethesda, Maryland [262e]

Rathel L. Nolan, III, MD
Professor, Department of Medicine, Division of Infectious Diseases, University of Mississippi Medical Center, Jackson, Mississippi [238]

Robert L. Norris, MD
Professor, Department of Surgery; Chief, Division of Emergency Medicine, Stanford University School of Medicine, Stanford, California [474]

Scott A. Norton, MD, MPH, MSc
Chief of Dermatology, Children's National Health Systems, Washington, DC [475]

Thomas B. Nutman, MD
Head, Helminth Immunology Section, Head, Clinical Parasitology Unit, Laboratory of Parasitic Diseases, National Institute of Allergy and Infectious Diseases, National Institutes of Health, Bethesda, Maryland [257, 258]

Jose A. Obeso, MD
Professor of Neurology and Director, CIINAC, Hospital de Madrid; Medical School, CEU-San Pablo, Madrid, Spain [449]

Katherine L. O'Brien, MD, MPH
Professor, Department of International Health, Bloomberg School of Public Health, Johns Hopkins University, Baltimore, Maryland [171]

Max R. O'Donnell, MD, MPH
Assistant Professor of Medicine and Epidemiology, Division of Pulmonary, Allergy, and Critical Care Medicine, Columbia University Medical Center, New York, New York [205e]

Nigel O'Farrell, MD, MSc, FRCP
Ealing Hospital, London, United Kingdom [198e]

Jennifer Ogar, MS CCC-SLP
Speech-Language Pathologist, Memory and Aging Center, University of California, San Francisco, San Francisco, California [37e]

Patrick T. O'Gara, MD
Professor of Medicine, Harvard Medical School; Director, Clinical Cardiology, Brigham and Women's Hospital, Boston, Massachusetts [51e, 267, 283-286]

C. Warren Olanow, MD, FRCPC, FRCP(hon)
Henry P. and Georgette Goldschmidt Professor and Chairman Emeritus, Department of Neurology; Professor, Department of Neuroscience, Mount Sinai School of Medicine, New York, New York [449]

Andrew B. Onderdonk, PhD
Professor of Pathology, Harvard Medical School; Brigham and Women's Hospital, Boston, Massachusetts [150e]

Chung Owyang, MD
H. Marvin Pollard Professor of Internal Medicine; Chief, Division of Gastroenterology, University of Michigan Health System, Ann Arbor, Michigan [344, 352]

Umesh D. Parashar, MBBS, MPH
Lead, Viral Gastroenteritis Epidemiology Team, Division of Viral Diseases, National Center for Immunization and Respiratory Diseases, Centers for Disease Control and Prevention, Atlanta, Georgia [227]

Shreyaskumar R. Patel, MD
Robert R. Herring Distinguished Professor of Medicine; Center Medical Director, Sarcoma Center, The University of Texas M.D. Anderson Cancer Center, Houston, Texas [119e]

David L. Paterson, MD, PhD
Professor of Medicine, University of Queensland Centre for Clinical Research; Royal Brisbane and Women's Hospital, Brisbane, Australia [187]

Gustav Paumgartner, MD
Professor Emeritus of Medicine, University of Munich, Munich, Germany [369]

M. Luisa Pedro-Botet, MD, PhD
Professor of Medicine, Autonomous University of Barcelona; Infectious Diseases Section (Senior Consultant), Germans Trias i Pujol University Hospital, Badalona, Barcelona, Spain [184]

David A. Pegues, MD
Professor of Medicine, Division of Infectious Diseases, Perelman School of Medicine, University of Pennsylvania, Philadelphia, Pennsylvania [190]

Anton Y. Peleg, MBBS, PhD, MPH, FRACP
Associate Professor, Department of Infectious Diseases and Microbiology, The Alfred Hospital and Monash University, Melbourne, Victoria, Australia [187]

Florencia Pereyra, MD
Instructor in Medicine, Harvard Medical School; Associate Physician, Infectious Disease Division, Brigham and Women's Hospital, Boston, Massachusetts [166e, 167e]

Michael A. Pesce, PhD
Professor Emeritus of Pathology and Cell Biology, Columbia University College of Physicians and Surgeons; Director, Biochemical Genetics Laboratory, Columbia University Medical Center, New York Presbyterian Hospital, New York, New York [Appendix]

Clarence J. Peters, MD
John Sealy Distinguished University Chair in Tropical and Emerging Virology; Professor, Department of Microbiology and Immunology; Department of Pathology; Director for Biodefense, Center for Biodefense and Emerging Infectious Diseases, University of Texas Medical Branch, Galveston, Texas [233]

Gerald B. Pier, PhD
Professor of Medicine (Microbiology and Immunobiology), Harvard Medical School; Brigham and Women's Hospital, Division of Infectious Diseases, Boston, Massachusetts [145e]

Richard J. Pollack, PhD
Instructor, Department of Immunology and Infectious Disease, Harvard School of Public Health, Boston, Massachusetts; Senior Environmental Public Health Officer, Department of Environmental Health and Safety, Harvard University, Cambridge, Massachusetts; President and Chief Scientific Officer, IdentifyUS LLC, Newton, Massachusetts [475]

Martin R. Pollak, MD
Professor of Medicine, Harvard Medical School; Beth Israel Deaconess Medical Center, Boston, Massachusetts [339]

Andrew J. Pollard, PhD, FRCPCH
Professor of Paediatric Infection and Immunity, Department of Paediatrics, University of Oxford, Oxford, United Kingdom [180]

Reuven Porat, MD
Professor of Medicine, Department of Internal Medicine, Tel Aviv Souarsky Medical Center; Sackler Faculty of Medicine, Tel Aviv University, Tel Aviv, Israel [23]

Daniel A. Portnoy, PhD
Professor, Department of Molecular and Cell Biology and the School of Public Health, University of California, Berkeley, Berkeley, California [176]

John T. Potts, Jr., MD
Jackson Distinguished Professor of Clinical Medicine, Harvard Medical School; Physician-in-Chief and Director of Research Emeritus, Massachusetts General Hospital, Boston, Massachusetts [424]

Lawrie W. Powell, MD, PhD
Professor of Medicine, The University of Queensland; Director, Centre for the Advancement of Clinical Research, Royal Brisbane and Women's Hospital, Brisbane, Australia [428]

Alvin C. Powers, MD
Joe C. Davis Chair in Biomedical Science; Professor of Medicine, Molecular Physiology and Biophysics; Director, Vanderbilt Diabetes Center; Chief, Division of Diabetes, Endocrinology, and Metabolism, Vanderbilt University School of Medicine, Nashville, Tennessee [417-419]

Daniel S. Pratt, MD
Assistant Professor of Medicine, Harvard Medical Center; Massachusetts General Hospital, Boston, Massachusetts [58, 358]

Michael B. Prentice, MB ChB, PhD, MRCP(UK), FRCPath, FFPRCPI
Professor of Medical Microbiology, Departments of Microbiology and Pathology, University College Cork, Cork, Ireland [196]

Darwin J. Prockop, MD, PhD
Director and Professor, Institute for Regenerative Medicine, Texas A&M Health Science Center College of Medicine at Scott & White, Temple, Texas [427]

Stanley B. Prusiner, MD
Director, Institute for Neurodegenerative Diseases; Professor, Department of Neurology, University of California, San Francisco, San Francisco, California [444e, 453e]

Thomas C. Quinn, MD
Professor of Medicine, Johns Hopkins University, Baltimore, Maryland; Senior Investigator, National Institute of Allergy and Infectious Diseases, National Institutes of Health, Bethesda, Maryland [213]

Gil Rabinovici, MD
Associate Professor in Neurology, Memory and Aging Center, University of California, San Francisco, San Francisco, California [37e]

Daniel J. Rader, MD
Seymour Gray Professor of Molecular Medicine; Chair, Department of Genetics; Chief, Division of Translational Medicine and Human Genetics, Department of Medicine, Perelman School of Medicine at the University of Pennsylvania, Philadelphia, Pennsylvania [421]

Kaitlin Rainwater-Lovett, PhD, MPH
Research Fellow, Division of Infectious Diseases, Department of Pediatrics, Johns Hopkins University School of Medicine, Baltimore, Maryland [229]

Sanjay Ram, MBBS
Associate Professor of Medicine, Division of Infectious Diseases and Immunology, University of Massachusetts Medical School, Worcester, Massachusetts [181]

Reuben Ramphal, MD
Adjunct Professor of Medicine, Division of Infectious Diseases and Global Medicine, University of Florida College of Medicine, Gainesville, Florida [189]

Agam K. Rao, MD
Medical Officer, Division of Foodborne, Waterborne, and Environmental Diseases, Centers for Disease Control and Prevention, Atlanta, Georgia [178]

Beth Rapaport, MD
Attending Physician, Elmhurst Hospital Center, Mount Sinai Medical Affiliate, Elmhurst, New York [486e]

Kumanan Rasanathan, MBChB, MPH, FAFPHM
Technical Officer, Department of Ethics, Equity, Trade, and Human Rights, World Health Organization, Geneva, Switzerland [13e]

Neil H. Raskin, MD
Department of Neurology, University of California, San Francisco, San Francisco, California [21, 447]

Anis Rassi, Jr., MD, PhD, FACC, FACP, FAHA
Scientific Director, Anis Rassi Hospital, Goiânia, Brazil [252]

James P. Rathmell, MD
Henry Knowles Beecher Professor of Anesthesiology, Harvard Medical School; Executive Vice Chair and Chief, Division of Pain Medicine, Department of Anesthesia, Critical Care and Pain Medicine, Massachusetts General Hospital, Boston, Massachusetts [18]

Mario C. Raviglione, MD
Director, Global TB Programme, World Health Organization, Geneva, Switzerland [202]

Divya Reddy, MBBS, MPH
Faculty, Department of Medicine, Pulmonary Division, Albert Einstein College of Medicine; Montefiore Medical Center, Bronx, New York [205e]

Susan Redline, MD, MPH
Peter C. Farrell Professor of Sleep Medicine, Harvard Medical School; Brigham and Women's Hospital; Beth Israel Deaconess Medical Center, Boston, Massachusetts [319]

Sharon L. Reed, MD, MSCTM, D(ABMM)
Professor of Pathology and Medicine; Director, Microbiology Laboratory, University of California, San Diego School of Medicine, La Jolla, California [245e, 247]

Susan E. Reef, MD
Medical Epidemiologist, Centers for Disease Control and Prevention, Atlanta, Georgia [230e]

John J. Reilly, Jr., MD
Jack D. Myers Professor of Medicine and Chair, Department of Medicine; Vice Chair for Clinical Affairs, University of Pittsburgh, Pittsburgh, Pennsylvania [308e, 314]

John T. Repke, MD, FACOG
University Professor and Chairman, Department of Obstetrics and Gynecology, Pennsylvania State University College of Medicine; Obstetrician-Gynecologist In-Chief, The Milton S. Hershey Medical Center, Hershey, Pennsylvania [8]

Victor I. Reus, MD
Department of Psychiatry, University of California, San Francisco School of Medicine; Langley Porter Neuropsychiatric Institute, San Francisco, California [466]

Joseph J. Rhatigan, MD
Assistant Professor, Harvard Medical School, Harvard School of Public Health; Associate Chief, Division of Global Health Equity, Brigham and Women's Hospital, Boston, Massachusetts [2]

Peter A. Rice, MD
Professor of Medicine, Division of Infectious Diseases and Immunology, University of Massachusetts Medical School, Worcester, Massachusetts [181]

Elizabeth Robbins, MD
Clinical Professor of Pediatrics, University of California, San Francisco, San Francisco, California [443e]

Gary L. Robertson, MD
Emeritus Professor of Medicine, Northwestern University School of Medicine, Chicago, Illinois [404]

Russell G. Robertson, MD
Professor of Family Medicine, Chicago Medical School, Rosalind Franklin University of Medicine and Science, Chicago, Illinois [56]

Dan M. Roden, MD
William Stokes Professor of Experimental Therapeutics; Professor of Medicine and Pharmacology, Assistant Vice-Chancellor for Personalized Medicine, Director, Oates Institute for Experimental Therapeutics, Vanderbilt University School of Medicine, Nashville, Tennessee [5]

James A. Romano, Jr., PhD, DABT
Principal Senior Life Scientist Advisor, Tunnell Government Services, Inc., Rockville, Maryland [262e]

Karen L. Roos, MD
John and Nancy Nelson Professor of Neurology; Professor of Neurological Surgery, Indiana University School of Medicine, Indianapolis, Indiana [164]

Allan H. Ropper, MD, FRCP, FACP
Professor of Neurology, Harvard Medical School; Raymond D. Adams Master Clinician; Executive Vice Chair, Department of Neurology, Brigham and Women's Hospital, Boston, Massachusetts [328, 456, 457e]

Jonathan E. Rosenberg, MD
Associate Attending; Section Chief, Non-Prostate Program, Division of Solid Tumor Oncology, Department of Medicine, Memorial Sloan-Kettering Cancer Center, New York, New York [114]

Roger N. Rosenberg, MD
Zale Distinguished Chair and Professor of Neurology, Department of Neurology, University of Texas Southwestern Medical Center, Dallas, Texas [450, 451e]

Myrna R. Rosenfeld, MD, PhD
Department of Neurology, Hospital Clínic/IDIBAPS, Barcelona, Spain [122]

Michael A. Rubin, MD, PhD
Assistant Professor of Medicine, University of Utah School of Medicine, Salt Lake City, Utah [44]

Steven A. Rubin, PhD
Acting Principal Investigator, Center for Biologics Evaluation and Research, Food and Drug Administration, Bethesda, Maryland [231e]

Robert M. Russell, MD
Professor Emeritus of Medicine and Nutrition, Tufts University, Boston, Massachusetts; Office of Dietary Supplements, National Institutes of Health, Bethesda, Maryland [96e]

Thomas A. Russo, MD, CM
Staff Physician, Western New York VA Healthcare System; Professor of Medicine and Microbiology and Immunology; Vice Chair of Medicine; Head, Division of Infectious Disease, University at Buffalo, State University of New York, Buffalo, New York [186, 200]

Anna E. Rutherford, MD, MPH
Assistant Professor, Harvard Medical School; Associate Physician, Brigham and Women's Hospital, Boston, Massachusetts [483e]

Edward T. Ryan, MD, FACP, FIDSA, FASTMH
Professor of Medicine, Harvard Medical School; Professor of Immunology and Infectious Diseases, Harvard School of Public Health; Director, Global Infectious Diseases, Division of Infectious Diseases, Massachusetts General Hospital, Boston, Massachusetts [160, 193]

Sean Sadikot, MD
Department of Internal Medicine, Critical Care and Pulmonary Disease, Hackensack University Medical Center, Hackensack, New Jersey [485e, 486e]

David J. Salant, MD
Professor of Medicine, Boston University School of Medicine; Chief, Section of Nephrology, Boston Medical Center, Boston, Massachusetts [340]

Martin A. Samuels, MD
Professor of Neurology, Harvard Medical School; Chair, Department of Neurology, Brigham and Women's Hospital, Boston, Massachusetts [439e, 463e]

Philippe J. Sansonetti, MD
Professor, Collège de France; Institut Pasteur, Paris, France [191]

Clifford B. Saper, MD, PhD
James Jackson Putnam Professor of Neurology and Neuroscience, Harvard Medical School; Chairman, Department of Neurology, Beth Israel Deaconess Medical Center, Boston, Massachusetts [38]

Jussi J. Saukkonen, MD
Associate Professor of Medicine, Section of Pulmonary, Allergy, and Critical Care Medicine, Boston University School of Medicine, Boston, Massachusetts [205e]

Edward A. Sausville, MD, PhD
Professor of Medicine, University of Maryland School of Medicine; Associate Director for Clinical Research, Marlene and Stewart Greenbaum Cancer Center, Baltimore, Maryland [103e]

Mohamed H. Sayegh, MD
Raja N. Khuri Dean, Faculty of Medicine; Professor of Medicine and Immunology; Vice President of Medical Affairs, American University of Beirut, Beirut, Lebanon; Senior Lecturer, Harvard Medical School; Schuster Family Transplantation Center, Brigham and Women's Hospital, Boston, Massachusetts [337]

David T. Scadden, MD
Gerald and Darlene Professor of Medicine; Co-Chair, Harvard Stem Cell Institute; Co-chair, Department of Stem Cell and Regenerative Biology, Harvard Medical School; Director, Center for Regenerative Medicine; Chief, Hematologic Malignancies, Cancer Center, Massachusetts General Hospital, Boston, Massachusetts [89e]

Thomas E. Scammell, MD
Professor, Harvard Medical School; Beth Israel Deaconess Medical Center; Boston Children's Hospital, Boston, Massachusetts [38]

Anthony H. V. Schapira, MD, DSc, FRCP, FMedSci
Chair and Professor of Clinical Neurosciences, UCL Institute of Neurology, London, United Kingdom [449]

Howard I. Scher, MD
Professor of Medicine, Joan and Sanford Weill College of Medicine of Cornell University; D. Wayne Calloway Chair in Urologic Oncology; Attending Physician and Chief, Genitourinary Oncology Service, Department of Medicine, Memorial Sloan-Kettering Cancer Center, New York, New York [114, 115]

Anne Schuchat, MD
RADM, U.S. Public Health Service; Assistant Surgeon General, National Center for Immunization and Respiratory Diseases, Centers for Disease Control and Prevention, Atlanta, Georgia [148]

Marc A. Schuckit, MD
Distinguished Professor of Psychiatry, University of California, San Diego School of Medicine, La Jolla, California [467]

H. Ralph Schumacher, Jr., MD
Professor of Medicine, Division of Rheumatology, University of Pennsylvania, School of Medicine, Philadelphia, Pennsylvania [395]

Gordon E. Schutze, MD, FAAP
Professor of Pediatrics; Vice-Chairman for Educational Affairs; Martin I. Lorin, MD Chair in Medical Education, Department of Pediatrics, Section of Retrovirology, Vice President, Baylor International Pediatric AIDS Initiative at Texas Children's Hospital, Baylor College of Medicine, Texas Children's Hospital, Houston, Texas [195]

Richard M. Schwartzstein, MD
Ellen and Melvin Gordon Professor of Medicine and Medical Education, Harvard Medical School; Associate Division Chief, Division of Pulmonary, Critical Care, and Sleep Medicine, Beth Israel Deaconess Medical Center, Boston, Massachusetts [47e]

William W. Seeley, MD
Associate Professor of Neurology and Pathology, Memory and Aging Center, University of California, San Francisco, San Francisco, California [35, 448]

Michael V. Seiden, MD, PhD
Chief Medical Officer, McKesson Specialty Health, The Woodlands, Texas [117]

Julian L. Seifter, MD
Associate Professor of Medicine, Harvard Medical School; Brigham and Women's Hospital, Boston, Massachusetts [343]

David C. Seldin, MD, PhD
Professor, Departments of Medicine and Microbiology; Chief, Section of Hematology-Oncology; Director, Amyloidosis Center, Boston University School of Medicine; Boston Medical Center, Boston, Massachusetts [137]

Ankoor Shah, MD
Assistant Professor, Department of Medicine, Division of Rheumatology and Immunology, Duke University Medical Center, Durham, North Carolina [380]

Steven D. Shapiro, MD
Jack D. Myers Professor and Chair, Department of Medicine, University of Pittsburgh, Pittsburgh, Pennsylvania [314]

Erica S. Shenoy, MD, PhD
Instructor in Medicine, Harvard Medical School; Assistant Chief, Infection Control Unit, Massachusetts General Hospital, Boston, Massachusetts [170]

Kanade Shinkai, MD, PhD
Assistant Professor, Department of Dermatology, University of California, San Francisco, San Francisco, California [74]

William Silen, MD
Johnson and Johnson Professor Emeritus of Surgery, Harvard Medical School, Auburndale, Massachusetts [20]

Edwin K. Silverman, MD, PhD
Professor of Medicine, Harvard Medical School; Chief, Channing Division of Network Medicine, Department of Medicine, Brigham and Women's Hospital, Boston, Massachusetts [314]

Karl Skorecki, MD, FRCP(C), FASN
Annie Chutick Professor in Medicine (Nephrology); Director, Rappaport Research Institute, Technion-Israel Institute of Technology; Director of Medical and Research Development, Rambam Health Care Campus, Haifa, Israel [85e, 335]

Wade S. Smith, MD, PhD
Professor of Neurology, Daryl R. Gress Endowed Chair of Neurocritical Care and Stroke; Director, University of California, San Francisco Neurovascular Service, San Francisco, California [330, 446]

Elizabeth Smyth, MB BAO, MSc
Department of Gastrointestinal Oncology, Royal Marsden NHS Foundation Trust, London and Sutton, United Kingdom [112]

Kelly A. Soderberg, PhD, MPH
Associate Director, Duke Center for HIV/AIDS Vaccine Immunology-Immunogen Discovery, Duke Human Vaccine Institute, Duke University, Durham, North Carolina [372e]

Scott D. Solomon, MD
Professor, Harvard Medical School; Director, Noninvasive Cardiology, Brigham and Women's Hospital, Boston, Massachusetts [270e, 271e]

Julian Solway, MD
Walter L. Palmer Distinguished Service Professor of Medicine and Pediatrics; Associate Dean for Translational Medicine, Biological Sciences Division; Vice Chair for Research, Department of Medicine; Chair, Committee on Molecular Medicine, University of Chicago, Chicago, Illinois [306e, 318]

Michael F. Sorrell, MD
Robert L. Grissom Professor of Medicine, Department of Internal Medicine, University of Nebraska Medical Center, Omaha, Nebraska [363]

Eric J. Sorscher, MD
Professor, Departments of Medicine and Genetics, Gwaltney Chair for Medical Research; Director, Gregory Fleming James Cystic Fibrosis Research Center, University of Alabama at Birmingham, Birmingham, Alabama [313]

Frank E. Speizer, MD
E. H. Kass Distinguished Professor of Medicine, Harvard Medical School; Channing Division of Network Medicine, Department of Medicine, Brigham and Women's Hospital; Professor of Environmental Science, Department of Environmental Health, Harvard School of Public Health, Boston, Massachusetts [311]

Brad Spellberg, MD
Professor of Medicine; Associate Medical Director for Inpatient Services, Harbor–UCLA Medical Center and Los Angeles Biomedical Research Institute, Torrance, California [242]

Nancy B. Spinner, PhD, FACMG
Professor of Pathology and Laboratory Medicine, Perelman School of Medicine, University of Pennsylvania; Chief, Division of Genomic Diagnostics, Children's Hospital of Philadelphia, Philadelphia, Pennsylvania [83e]

Jerry L. Spivak, MD
Professor of Medicine and Oncology, Hematology Division, Johns Hopkins University School of Medicine, Baltimore, Maryland [131]

David D. Spragg, MD
Associate Professor, Department of Medicine, Johns Hopkins University; Director, Electrophysiology Laboratory, Johns Hopkins Bayview Medical Center, Baltimore, Maryland [273e-275]

E. William St. Clair, MD
Professor of Medicine and Immunology, Department of Medicine, Duke University Medical Center, Durham, North Carolina [380]

Allen C. Steere, MD
Professor of Medicine, Harvard Medical School; Massachusetts General Hospital, Boston, Massachusetts [210]

Robert S. Stern, MD
Carl J. Herzog Professor of Dermatology, Harvard Medical School; Chair, Department of Dermatology, Beth Israel Deaconess Medical Center, Boston, Massachusetts [74]

Dennis L. Stevens, MD, PhD
Professor of Medicine, University of Washington School of Medicine, Seattle, Washington [156, 179]

Lynne Warner Stevenson, MD
Professor of Medicine, Harvard Medical School; Director, Heart Failure Program, Brigham and Women's Hospital, Boston, Massachusetts [287]

William G. Stevenson, MD
Brigham and Women's Hospital; Cardiovascular Division, Department of Medicine, Harvard Medical School, Boston, Massachusetts [276, 277]

John H. Stone, MD, MPH
Professor of Medicine, Harvard Medical School; Director, Clinical Rheumatology, Massachusetts General Hospital, Boston, Massachusetts [391e]

Stephanie Studenski, MD, MPH
Director, Longitudinal Studies Section, Intramural Research Program, National Institute on Aging, National Institutes of Health, Baltimore, Maryland [11]

Lewis Sudarsky, MD
Associate Professor of Neurology, Harvard Medical School; Director of Movement Disorders, Brigham and Women's Hospital, Boston, Massachusetts [32]

Donna C. Sullivan, PhD
Professor, Department of Medicine, Division of Infectious Diseases, University of Mississippi Medical School, Jackson, Mississippi [238]

Shyam Sundar, MD, FRCP, FNA
Professor of Medicine, Institute of Medical Sciences, Banaras Hindu University, Varanasi, India [251]

Neeraj K. Surana, MD, PhD
Instructor in Pediatrics, Harvard Medical School; Assistant in Medicine, Boston Children's Hospital, Boston, Massachusetts [144]

Paolo M. Suter, MD, MS
Professor, Clinic and Policlinic of Internal Medicine, University Hospital, Zurich, Switzerland [96e]

Richard M. Suzman, PhD
Director, Behavioral and Social Research Program, National Institute on Aging, National Institutes of Health, Bethesda, Maryland [93e]

Robert A. Swerlick, MD
Alicia Leizman Stonecipher Professor and Chair of Dermatology, Emory University School of Medicine, Atlanta, Georgia [76e]

Homayoun Tabandeh, MD
Retina-Vitreous Associates Medical Group, Los Angeles, California [40e]

Geoffrey Tabin, MD
John and Marva Warnock Presidential Professor, University of Utah School of Medicine; Director, International Ophthalmology Division, John A. Moran Eye Center; Director, Himalayan Cataract Project, Salt Lake City, Utah [476e]

Maria Carmela Tartaglia, MD
Assistant Professor, Tanz Centre for Research in Neurodegenerative Diseases, University of Toronto, Toronto, Ontario, Canada [37e]

Joel D. Taurog, MD
Professor of Internal Medicine, Rheumatic Diseases Division, University of Texas Southwestern Medical Center at Dallas, Dallas, Texas [384]

Ayalew Tefferi, MD
Professor of Medicine and Hematology, Mayo Clinic, Rochester, Minnesota [135e]

Stephen C. Textor, MD
Professor of Medicine, Division of Nephrology and Hypertension, Mayo Clinic, Rochester, Minnesota [299, 341]

Rajesh V. Thakker, MD, FMedSci, FR
May Professor of Medicine, Academic Endocrine Unit, University of Oxford; O.C.D.E.M., Churchill Hospital, Headington, Oxford, United Kingdom [408]

C. Louise Thwaites, MD, MBBS
Oxford University Clinical Research Unit, Hospital for Tropical Diseases, Ho Chi Minh City, Vietnam [177]

Zelig A. Tochner, MD
Professor of Radiation Oncology, University of Pennsylvania School of Medicine; Medical Director, Proton Therapy Center, Philadelphia, Pennsylvania [263e]

Gordon F. Tomaselli, MD
Michel Mirowski, MD Professor of Cardiology; Professor of Medicine and Cellular and Molecular Medicine; Chief, Division of Cardiology, Johns Hopkins University, Baltimore, Maryland [273e-275]

Karina A. Top, MD, MS
Assistant Professor of Pediatrics, Dalhousie University, Halifax, Nova Scotia, Canada [185]

Mark Topazian, MD
Professor of Medicine, Mayo Clinic, Rochester, Minnesota [345, 346e]

Barbara W. Trautner, MD, PhD
Assistant Professor, Section of Infectious Diseases, Department of Medicine, Baylor College of Medicine; Houston VA Health Services Research and Development Center of Excellence, Houston, Texas [162]

Jeffrey M. Trent, PhD, FACMG
President and Research Director, Translational Genomics Research Institute, Phoenix, Arizona; Van Andel Research Institute, Grand Rapids, Michigan [101e]

Elbert P. Trulock, III, MD
Rosemary and I. Jerome Flance Professor in Pulmonary Medicine, Washington University School of Medicine, St. Louis, Missouri [320e]

Kenneth L. Tyler, MD
Reuler-Lewin Family Professor and Chair of Neurology; Professor of Medicine, Immunology, and Microbiology, University of Colorado School of Medicine, Aurora, Colorado; Neurologist, Denver Veterans Affairs Medical Center, Denver, Colorado [164]

Athanasios G. Tzioufas, MD
Professor, Department of Pathophysiology, School of Medicine, National University of Athens, Athens, Greece [383]

Walter J. Urba, MD, PhD
Director of Research, Earle A. Chiles Research Institute, Providence Cancer Center, Portland, Oregon [105]

Jos W. M. van der Meer, MD, PhD
Professor of Medicine; Head, Department of General Internal Medicine, Radboud University Nijmegen Medical Centre, Nijmegen, The Netherlands [26, 464e]

Edouard G. Vannier, PharmD, PhD
Assistant Professor, Division of Geographic Medicine and Infectious Diseases, Department of Medicine, Tufts Medical Center and Tufts University School of Medicine, Boston, Massachusetts [249]

Gauri R. Varadhachary, MD
Professor, Department of Gastrointestinal Medical Oncology, The University of Texas M.D. Anderson Cancer Center, Houston, Texas [120e]

John Varga, MD
John Hughes Professor of Medicine, Northwestern University Feinberg School of Medicine, Chicago, Illinois [382]

Christy A. Varughese, PharmD
Infectious Disease Specialist, Department of Pharmacy, Massachusetts General Hospital, Boston, Massachusetts [170]

Panayiotis G. Vlachoyiannopoulos, MD
Professor of Medicine-Immunology, Department of Pathophysiology, Medical School, National University of Athens, Athens, Greece [379]

Bert Vogelstein, MD
Investigator, Howard Hughes Medical Institute; Director, Ludwig Center at the Sidney Kimmel Comprehensive Cancer Center; Clayton Professor of Oncology and Pathology; Johns Hopkins Medical Institutions, Baltimore, Maryland [101e]

Everett E. Vokes, MD
John E. Ultmann Professor; Chairman, Department of Medicine; Physician-in-Chief, University of Chicago Medical Center, Chicago, Illinois [106]

Tamara J. Vokes, MD
Professor, Department of Medicine, Section of Endocrinology, University of Chicago, Chicago, Illinois [426e]

Jiři F. P. Wagenaar, MD, PhD
Senior Scientist, WHO/FAO/OIE and National Leptospirosis Reference Centre, KIT Biomedical Research, KIT (Royal Tropical Institute), Amsterdam, The Netherlands [208]

Sushrut S. Waikar, MD, MPH
Associate Professor, Harvard Medical School; Director, Renal Ambulatory Services, Brigham and Women's Hospital, Boston, Massachusetts [334]

Matthew K. Waldor, MD, PhD
Edward H. Kass Professor of Medicine, Channing Laboratory, Brigham and Women's Hospital; Harvard Medical School and Howard Hughes Medical Institute, Boston, Massachusetts [193]

David H. Walker, MD
The Carmage and Martha Walls Distinguished University Chair in Tropical Diseases; Professor and Chairman, Department of Pathology; Executive Director, Center for Biodefense and Emerging Infectious Diseases, University of Texas Medical Branch, Galveston, Texas [211]

Mark F. Walker, MD
Associate Professor, Neurology, Case Western Reserve University; Cleveland VA Medical Center, Cleveland, Ohio [28]

Fred Wang, MD
Professor of Medicine, Harvard Medical School and Brigham and Women's Hospital, Boston, Massachusetts [214e, 220e]

John W. Warren, MD
Professor of Medicine, University of Maryland School of Medicine, Baltimore, Maryland [60e]

Aaron B. Waxman, MD, PhD, FACP, FCCP
Associate Professor of Medicine, Harvard Medical School; Executive Director, Center for Pulmonary-Heart Diseases, Brigham and Women's Hospital Heart and Vascular Center, Boston, Massachusetts [304]

Michael E. Wechsler, MD, MMSc
Professor of Medicine; Director, Asthma Program, National Jewish Health, Denver, Colorado [310]

Anthony P. Weetman, MD, DSc
University of Sheffield, School of Medicine Sheffield, United Kingdom [405]

Robert A. Weinstein, MD
The C. Anderson Hedberg, MD Professor of Internal Medicine, Rush Medical College; Chief Academic Officer, Cook County Health and Hospitals System, Chicago, Illinois [168]

Jeffrey I. Weitz, MD, FRCP(C), FACP
Professor of Medicine and Biochemistry, McMaster University; Executive Director, Thrombosis and Atherosclerosis Research Institute, Hamilton, Ontario, Canada [143]

Peter F. Weller, MD
Chief, Infectious Disease Division; Chief, Allergy and Inflammation Division; Beth Israel Deaconess Medical Center, Boston, Massachusetts [254 258, 260]

Andrew Wellman, MD, PhD
Assistant Professor of Medicine, Division of Sleep Medicine, Harvard Medical School; Brigham and Women's Hospital, Boston, Massachusetts [319]

Patrick Y. Wen, MD
Professor of Neurology, Harvard Medical School; Director, Center for Neuro-Oncology, Dana-Farber Cancer Institute; Director, Division of Neuro-Oncology, Department of Neurology, Brigham and Women's Hospital; Dana-Farber Cancer Institute, Boston, Massachusetts [118]

Michael R. Wessels, MD
John F. Enders Professor of Pediatrics; Professor of Medicine, Harvard Medical School; Chief, Division of Infectious Diseases, Boston Children's Hospital, Boston, Massachusetts [173]

L. Joseph Wheat, MD
President and Medical Director, MiraVista Diagnostics, LLC, Indianapolis, Indiana [236]

A. Clinton White, Jr., MD
Paul R. Stalnaker Distinguished Professor; Director, Infectious Disease Division, Department of Internal Medicine, University of Texas Medical Branch, Galveston, Texas [260]

Nicholas J. White, DSc, MD, FRCP, F Med Sci, FRS
Professor of Tropical Medicine, Faculty of Tropical Medicine, Mahidol University, Mahidol-Oxford Research Unit, Bangkok, Thailand [248, 250e]

Richard J. Whitley, MD
Distinguished Professor of Pediatrics; Loeb Eminent Scholar Chair in Pediatrics; Professor of Microbiology, Medicine and Neurosurgery, The University of Alabama at Birmingham, Birmingham, Alabama [217]

Bruce U. Wintroub, MD
Professor and Chair, Department of Dermatology, University of California, San Francisco, San Francisco, California [74]

Andrea S. Wolf, MD, MPH
Assistant Professor, and Director, Women's Lung Cancer Program, Mt. Sinai Medical Center, New York, New York [482e]

Allan W. Wolkoff, MD
The Herman Lopata Chair in Liver Disease Research; Professor of Medicine and Anatomy and Structural Biology; Associate Chair of Medicine for Research; Chief, Division of Gastroenterology and Liver Diseases; Director, Marion Bessin Liver Research Center, Albert Einstein College of Medicine and Montefiore Medical Center, Bronx, New York [359]

John B. Wong, MD
Professor of Medicine, Tufts University School of Medicine; Chief, Division of Clinical Decision Making, Department of Medicine, Tufts Medical Center, Boston, Massachusetts [3]

Louis Michel Wong Kee Song, MD
Associate Professor, Division of Gastroenterology and Hepatology, Mayo Clinic College of Medicine, Rochester, Minnesota [345, 346e]

Robert L. Wortmann, MD, FACP, MACR
Professor Emeritus, Department of Medicine, Geisel School of Medicine at Dartmouth, Lebanon, New Hampshire [431e]

Shirley H. Wray, MD, PhD, FRCP
Professor of Neurology, Harvard Medical School; Master Clinician, Department of Neurology, Massachusetts General Hospital, Boston, Massachusetts [41e]

Richard G. Wunderink, MD
Professor, Pulmonary and Critical Care, Northwestern University Feinberg School of Medicine, Chicago, Illinois [153]

Kim B. Yancey, MD
Professor and Chair, Department of Dermatology, University of Texas Southwestern Medical Center in Dallas, Dallas, Texas [70, 73]

Janet A. Yellowitz, DMD, MPH
Associate Professor; Director, Geriatric Dentistry, University of Maryland Dental School, Baltimore, Maryland [46e]

Lam Minh Yen, MD
Director, Tetanus Intensive Care Unit, Hospital for Tropical Diseases, Ho Chi Minh City, Vietnam [177]

Maria A. Yialamas, MD
Assistant Professor of Medicine, Harvard Medical School; Associate Program Director, Internal Medicine Residency, Brigham and Women's Hospital, Boston, Massachusetts [481e, 483e]

Neal S. Young, MD
Chief, Hematology Branch, National Heart, Lung and Blood Institute; Director, NIH Center for Human Immunology, Autoimmunity and Inflammation, National Institutes of Health, Bethesda, Maryland [130]

Victor L. Yu, MD
Professor of Medicine, Department of Medicine, University of Pittsburgh Medical Center, Pittsburgh, Pennsylvania [184]

Jing Zhou, MD, PhD, FASN
Director, Laboratory of Molecular Genetics and Developmental Biology of Disease, Renal Division; Director, Center for Polycystic Kidney Disease Research, Brigham and Women's Hospital; Harvard Medical School, Boston, Massachusetts [339]

Werner Zimmerli, MD
Professor of Medicine, Basel University; Interdisciplinary Unit of Orthopaedic Infection, Kantonspital Basselland, Liestal, Switzerland [158]

Laura A. Zimmerman, MPH
Epidemiologist, Centers for Disease Control and Prevention, Atlanta, Georgia [230e]

PREFACE

The Editors are pleased to present the 19th edition of *Harrison's Principles of Internal Medicine.* Since the first edition was published 65 years ago, virtually every area of medicine and medical education has evolved remarkably, and many new fields have emerged.

While retaining the founding goals of *Harrison's*, this edition has been modified extensively in light of the varied needs of the book's readers and the diverse methods and formats by which information is now acquired and applied. The focus of medical education worldwide is shifting from the classic structure/function/disease approach to an integrated, often case-based approach in which basic and population sciences are specifically linked to the practical diagnosis and management of disease. Many of the updates and changes described here have been undertaken with the modern educational and clinical environments in mind.

This new edition offers a thoroughly updated presentation of the classic pathophysiologic basis of clinical medicine and details the cutting-edge methods and tools that are now available for the assessment of symptoms and the effective management of diseases in the modern patient-care environment. The text is supplemented by germane new photographs, radiographs, illustrations, atlases, patient-care algorithms, tables, and practical demonstrative videos.

In the interest of producing the most practical format possible for the 19th edition, a new system of referencing has been used. Detailed bibliographic listings, with summaries of articles' relevance to practice, appear in the online edition, replacing the general and limited collection of Suggested Readings that appeared in the prior print editions.

The 19th edition of *Harrison's* is designed for accessibility and flexibility. The print textbook is available in two volumes. Volume 1 focuses on the foundations of medicine and the understanding and assessment of cardinal disease manifestations; Volume 2 focuses on specific diseases, by system. This functional division will be helpful to students who are mastering the basis of clinical medicine and to clinicians who are more focused on gaining an advanced understanding of mechanisms and patient care in specific diseases. In terms of digital media, *Harrison's* is now available as an eBook on multiple platforms, as an enhanced "app" developed especially for tablet and smartphone devices that offer high-definition resolution of multimedia content and interactive features, and as an updated online edition. All of these options provide access to our numerous e-chapters as well as to videos and atlases. Additional resources include the *Harrison's Self-Assessment and Board Review*, a useful study guide based on information in the 19th edition, and the *Harrison's Manual of Medicine*, a pocket version of *Harrison's Principles of Internal Medicine.* A new *Harrison's* collection of case vignettes emphasizing differential diagnostic considerations in the assessment of cardinal manifestations will also be available.

Advances in medical science have been spectacular since *Harrison's* was first published in 1949. At that time, peptic ulcer disease was thought to be caused by stress, nearly every tumor that was not resected resulted in death, rheumatic heart disease was widely prevalent, and hepatitis B and HIV infection were unknown. In the intervening years, both the infectious cause of and the cure for peptic ulcer disease were identified; advances in diagnosis and treatment made it possible to cure two-thirds of cancers; rheumatic heart disease virtually disappeared; atherosclerotic coronary artery disease waxed and then—at least in part through management of modifiable risk factors—began to wane; hepatitis B and its consequences, cirrhosis and hepatocellular carcinoma, became preventable by a vaccine; and HIV, first viewed as a uniformly fatal worldwide scourge, became a treatable chronic disease. Notably, emerging and reemerging diseases have presented significant challenges to medical research and practice, while a new understanding of systems-wide concepts such as the microbiome offers exciting new possibilities for understanding and managing health and disease in ways never before possible.

Of particular note in this 19th edition are critical updates in the classic chapter on HIV/AIDS, which offers both a clinically pragmatic focus and a comprehensive and analytical approach to pathogenesis. The updates cover the latest treatment protocols and address the issue of combination prevention modalities, making the chapter the most up-to-date and comprehensive treatise on HIV disease available.

Several other chapters likewise reflect the rapid pace of advancement in the field of immune-related diseases and their treatment. In this regard, Chapter 372e, "Introduction to the Immune System," serves as a mini-textbook of immunology for use in immunology courses. In addition, a new chapter on IgG4-mediated disease summarizes an important and newly recognized constellation of entities.

Readers will find expanded coverage of the neurodegenerative diseases, highlighting advances in their classification and management and delineating the new understanding of mechanisms responsible for the deposition and spread of pathogenic protein aggregates in these disorders. The chapter on chronic hepatitis discusses in detail the dramatic new discoveries in the use of direct-acting antiviral agents for the treatment of hepatitis C virus disease; these agents are responsible for some of the most exciting therapeutic advances in medicine today.

The rapidly expanding application of genetic knowledge to medicine is covered in many chapters, including a new chapter on microbial genomics and infectious diseases and substantially updated chapters on the human microbiome and chromosomal genetic disorders. Other new chapters address timely topics such as the impact of climate change on disease, infections in U.S. veterans returning from foreign wars, and advances in contraception and the treatment of infertility. Another topic of increasing interest, the impact of aging on health and disease, is addressed by several chapters, including a newly authored chapter on the biology of aging. A new chapter on men's health complements the updated chapter on women's health. New chapters also address diverse topics including the emerging field of tissue engineering, the examination of the comatose patient, the management of heart failure, the major characteristics of helminths and helminthic infections, specific cardiac valvular disorders, venous and lymphatic diseases of the extremities, renovascular disease, late complications of diabetes, chronic myeloid leukemia, heat-related illnesses, fatigue, polyglandular failure syndromes, and nonalcoholic fatty liver disease and nonalcoholic steatohepatitis.

Supplementing new content and updates on diseases and patient care, new videos in this edition cover sleep disorders, tissue engineering, noninvasive cardiac imaging, examination of the comatose patient, and myasthenia gravis and other diseases of the neuromuscular junction. New atlases for this edition address noninvasive imaging, percutaneous revascularization, and gastrointestinal endoscopy.

We have many people to thank for their efforts in producing this book. First, the authors have done a superb job of producing authoritative chapters that synthesize vast amounts of scientific and clinical data to create state-of-the-art descriptions of medical disorders encompassed by internal medicine. In today's information-rich, rapidly evolving environment, they have ensured that this information is current. Helpful suggestions and critical input have been provided by a number of colleagues; particularly notable was the advice of Chung Owyang on the Gastroenterology Section. We are most grateful to our colleagues in each of our editorial offices who have kept track of the work in its various phases and facilitated communication with the authors, with the McGraw-Hill Education staff, and among the editors: Patricia Conrad, Patricia L. Duffey, Gregory K. Folkers, Julie B. McCoy, Elizabeth Robbins, Anita Rodriguez, and Stephanie Tribuna.

The staff at McGraw-Hill Education has been a constant source of support and expertise. James Shanahan, Associate Publisher for McGraw-Hill Education's Professional Publishing Division, has been a superb and insightful partner to the editors, guiding the development of the book and its related products in new formats. Kim Davis, as Associate Managing Editor, has adeptly ensured that the complex production of this multi-authored textbook proceeded smoothly and efficiently. Dominik Pucek oversaw the production of the new procedural videos. Jeffrey Herzich ably served as production manager for this new edition.

We are privileged to have compiled this 19th edition and are enthusiastic about all that it offers our readers. We learned much in the process of editing *Harrison's* and hope that you will find this edition a uniquely valuable educational resource.

THE EDITORS

SECTION 1 NEOPLASTIC DISORDERS

99 Approach to the Patient with Cancer

Dan L. Longo

The application of current treatment techniques (surgery, radiation therapy, chemotherapy, and biologic therapy) results in the cure of nearly two of three patients diagnosed with cancer. Nevertheless, patients experience the diagnosis of cancer as one of the most traumatic and revolutionary events that has ever happened to them. Independent of prognosis, the diagnosis brings with it a change in a person's self-image and in his or her role in the home and workplace. The prognosis of a person who has just been found to have pancreatic cancer is the same as the prognosis of the person with aortic stenosis who develops the first symptoms of congestive heart failure (median survival, ~8 months). However, the patient with heart disease may remain functional and maintain a self-image as a fully intact person with just a malfunctioning part, a diseased organ ("a bum ticker"). By contrast, the patient with pancreatic cancer has a completely altered self-image and is viewed differently by family and anyone who knows the diagnosis. He or she is being attacked and invaded by a disease that could be anywhere in the body. Every ache or pain takes on desperate significance. Cancer is an exception to the coordinated interaction among cells and organs. In general, the cells of a multicellular organism are programmed for collaboration. Many diseases occur because the specialized cells fail to perform their assigned task. Cancer takes this malfunction one step further. Not only is there a failure of the cancer cell to maintain its specialized function, but it also strikes out on its own; the cancer cell competes to survive using natural mutability and natural selection to seek advantage over normal cells in a recapitulation of evolution. One consequence of the traitorous behavior of cancer cells is that the patient feels betrayed by his or her body. The cancer patient feels that he or she, and not just a body part, is diseased.

THE MAGNITUDE OF THE PROBLEM

No nationwide cancer registry exists; therefore, the incidence of cancer is estimated on the basis of the National Cancer Institute's Surveillance, Epidemiology, and End Results (SEER) database, which tabulates cancer incidence and death figures from 13 sites, accounting for about 10% of the U.S. population, and from population data from the U.S. Census Bureau. In 2014, 1.665 million new cases of invasive cancer (855,220 men, 810,320 women) were diagnosed, and 585,720 persons (310,010 men, 275,710 women) died from cancer. The percent distribution of new cancer cases and cancer deaths by site for men and women is shown in Table 99-1. Cancer incidence has been declining by about 2% each year since 1992. Cancer is the cause of one in four deaths in the United States.

The most significant risk factor for cancer overall is age; two-thirds of all cases were in those older than age 65 years. Cancer incidence increases as the third, fourth, or fifth power of age in different sites. For the interval between birth and age 49 years, 1 in 29 men and 1 in 19 women will develop cancer; for the interval between ages 50 and 59 years, 1 in 15 men and 1 in 17 women will develop cancer; for the interval between ages 60 and 69 years, 1 in 6 men and 1 in 10 women will develop cancer; and for people age 70 and older, 1 in 3 men and 1 in 4 women will develop cancer. Overall, men have a 44% risk of developing cancer at some time during their lives; women have a 38% lifetime risk.

TABLE 99-1 DISTRIBUTION OF CANCER INCIDENCE AND DEATHS FOR 2014

Male			Female		
Sites	%	Number	Sites	%	Number
Cancer Incidence					
Prostate	27	233,000	Breast	29	232,670
Lung	14	116,000	Lung	13	108,210
Colorectal	8	71,830	Colorectal	8	65,000
Bladder	7	56,390	Endometrial	6	52,630
Melanoma	5	43,890	Thyroid	6	47,790
Kidney	4	39,140	Lymphoma	4	32,530
Lymphoma	4	38,270	Melanoma	4	32,210
Oral cavity	4	30,220	Kidney	3	24,780
Leukemia	4	30,100	Pancreas	3	22,890
Liver	3	24,600	Leukemia	3	22,280
All others	20	171,780	All others	21	169,330
All sites	100	855,220	All sites	100	810,320
Cancer Deaths					
Lung	28	86,930	Lung	26	72,330
Prostate	10	29,480	Breast	15	40,000
Colorectal	8	26,270	Colorectal	9	24,040
Pancreas	7	20,170	Pancreas	7	19,420
Liver	5	15,870	Ovary	5	14,270
Leukemia	5	14,040	Leukemia	4	10,050
Esophagus	4	12,450	Endometrial	3	8,590
Bladder	4	11,170	Lymphoma	3	8,520
Lymphoma	3	10,470	Liver	3	7,130
Kidney	3	8,900	CNS	2	6,230
All others	23	74,260	All others	23	65,130
All sites	100	310,010	All sites	100	275,710

Source: From R Siegel et al: Cancer statistics, 2014. CA Cancer J Clin 64:9, 2014.

Cancer is the second leading cause of death behind heart disease. Deaths from heart disease have declined 45% in the United States since 1950 and continue to decline. Cancer has overtaken heart disease as the number one cause of death in persons younger than age 85 years. Incidence trends over time are shown in Fig. 99-1. After a 70-year period of increase, cancer deaths began to decline in 1990–1991 (Fig. 99-2). Between 1990 and 2010, cancer deaths decreased by 21% among men and 12.3% among women. The magnitude of the decline is illustrated in Fig. 99-3. The five leading causes of cancer deaths are shown for various populations in Table 99-2. The 5-year survival for white patients was 39% in 1960–1963 and 69% in 2003–2009. Cancers are more often deadly in blacks; the 5-year survival was 61% for the 2003–2009 interval; however, the racial differences are narrowing over time. Incidence and mortality vary among racial and ethnic groups (Table 99-3). The basis for these differences is unclear.

CANCER AROUND THE WORLD

In 2008, 12.7 million new cancer cases and 7.6 million cancer deaths were estimated worldwide, according to estimates of GLOBOCAN 2008, developed by the International Agency for Research on Cancer (IARC). When broken down by region of the world, ~45% of cases were in Asia, 26% in Europe, 14.5% in North America, 7.1% in Central/South America, 6% in Africa, and 1% in Australia/New Zealand (Fig. 99-4). Lung cancer is the most common cancer and the most common cause of cancer death in the world. Its

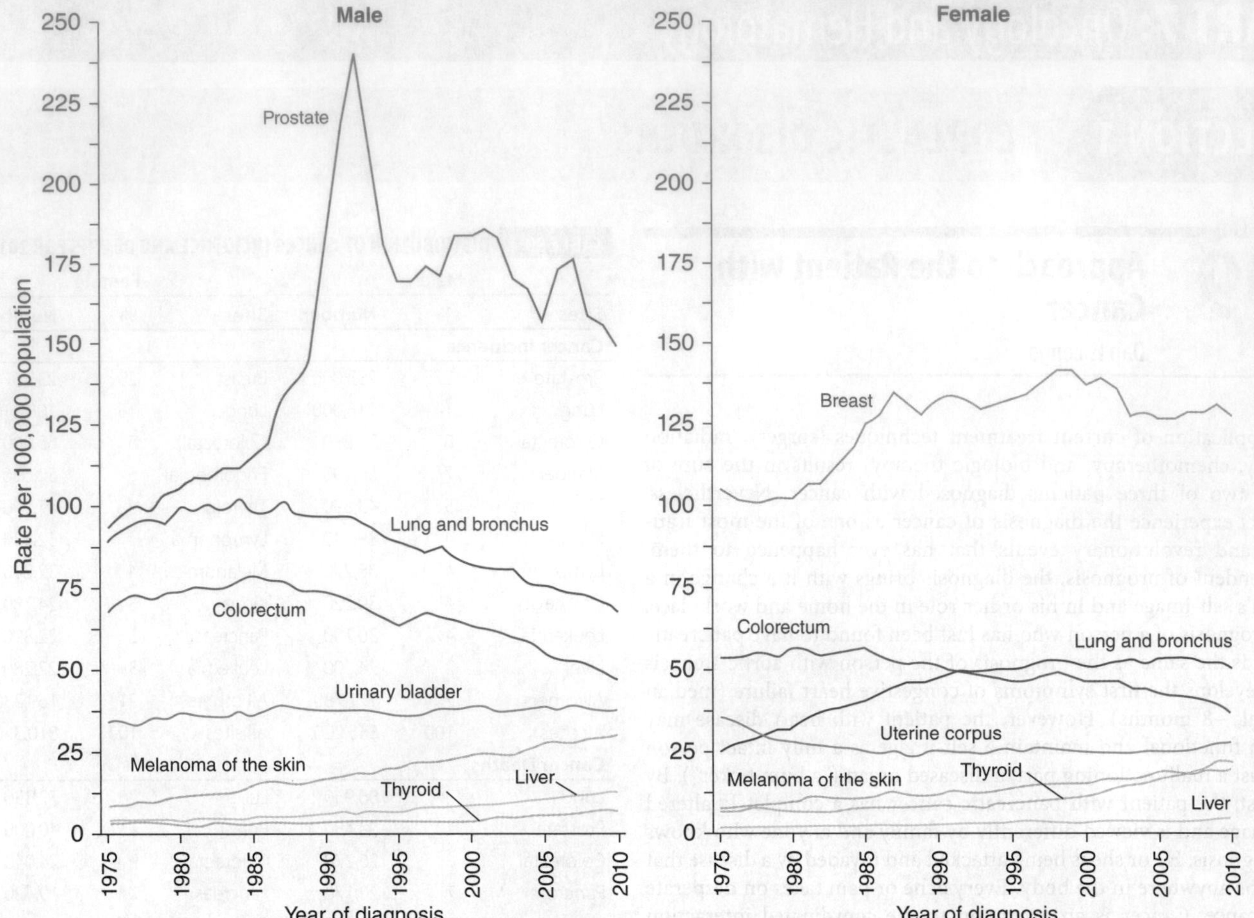

FIGURE 99-1 Incidence rates for particular types of cancer over the last 35 years in men (*A*) and women (*B*). *(From R Siegel et al: CA Cancer J Clin 64:9, 2014.)*

incidence is highly variable, affecting only 2 per 100,000 African women but as many as 61 per 100,000 North American men. Breast cancer is the second most common cancer worldwide; however, it ranks fifth as a cause of death behind lung, stomach, liver, and colorectal cancer. Among the eight most common forms of cancer, lung (2-fold), breast (3-fold), prostate (2.5-fold), and colorectal (3-fold) cancers are more common in more developed countries than in less developed countries. By contrast, liver (2-fold), cervical (2-fold), and esophageal (2- to 3-fold) cancers are more common in less developed countries. Stomach cancer incidence is similar in more and less developed countries but is much more common in Asia than North America or Africa. The most common cancers in Africa are cervical, breast, and liver cancers. It has been estimated that nine modifiable risk factors are responsible for more than one-third of cancers worldwide. These include smoking, alcohol consumption, obesity, physical inactivity, low fruit and vegetable consumption, unsafe sex, air pollution, indoor smoke from household fuels, and contaminated injections.

PATIENT MANAGEMENT

Important information is obtained from every portion of the routine history and physical examination. The duration of symptoms may reveal the chronicity of disease. The past medical history may alert the physician to the presence of underlying diseases that may affect the choice of therapy or the side effects of treatment. The social history may reveal occupational exposure to carcinogens or habits, such as smoking or alcohol consumption, that may influence the course of disease and its treatment. The family history may suggest an underlying familial cancer predisposition and point out the need to begin surveillance or other preventive therapy for unaffected siblings of the patient. The review of systems may suggest early symptoms of metastatic disease or a paraneoplastic syndrome.

DIAGNOSIS

The diagnosis of cancer relies most heavily on invasive tissue biopsy and should never be made without obtaining tissue; no noninvasive diagnostic test is sufficient to define a disease process as cancer. Although in rare clinical settings (e.g., thyroid nodules), fine-needle aspiration is an acceptable diagnostic procedure, the diagnosis generally depends on obtaining adequate tissue to permit careful evaluation of the histology of the tumor, its grade, and its invasiveness and to yield further molecular diagnostic information, such as the expression of cell-surface markers or intracellular proteins that typify a particular cancer, or the presence of a molecular marker, such as the t(8;14) translocation of Burkitt's lymphoma. Increasing evidence links the expression of certain genes with the prognosis and response to therapy **(Chaps. 101e and 102e)**.

Occasionally a patient will present with a metastatic disease process that is defined as cancer on biopsy but has no apparent primary site of disease. Efforts should be made to define the primary site based on age, sex, sites of involvement, histology and tumor markers, and personal and family history. Particular attention should be focused on ruling out the most treatable causes **(Chap. 120e)**.

Once the diagnosis of cancer is made, the management of the patient is best undertaken as a multidisciplinary collaboration among the primary care physician, medical oncologists, surgical oncologists, radiation oncologists, oncology nurse specialists, pharmacists, social workers, rehabilitation medicine specialists, and a number of other consulting professionals working closely with each other and with the patient and family.

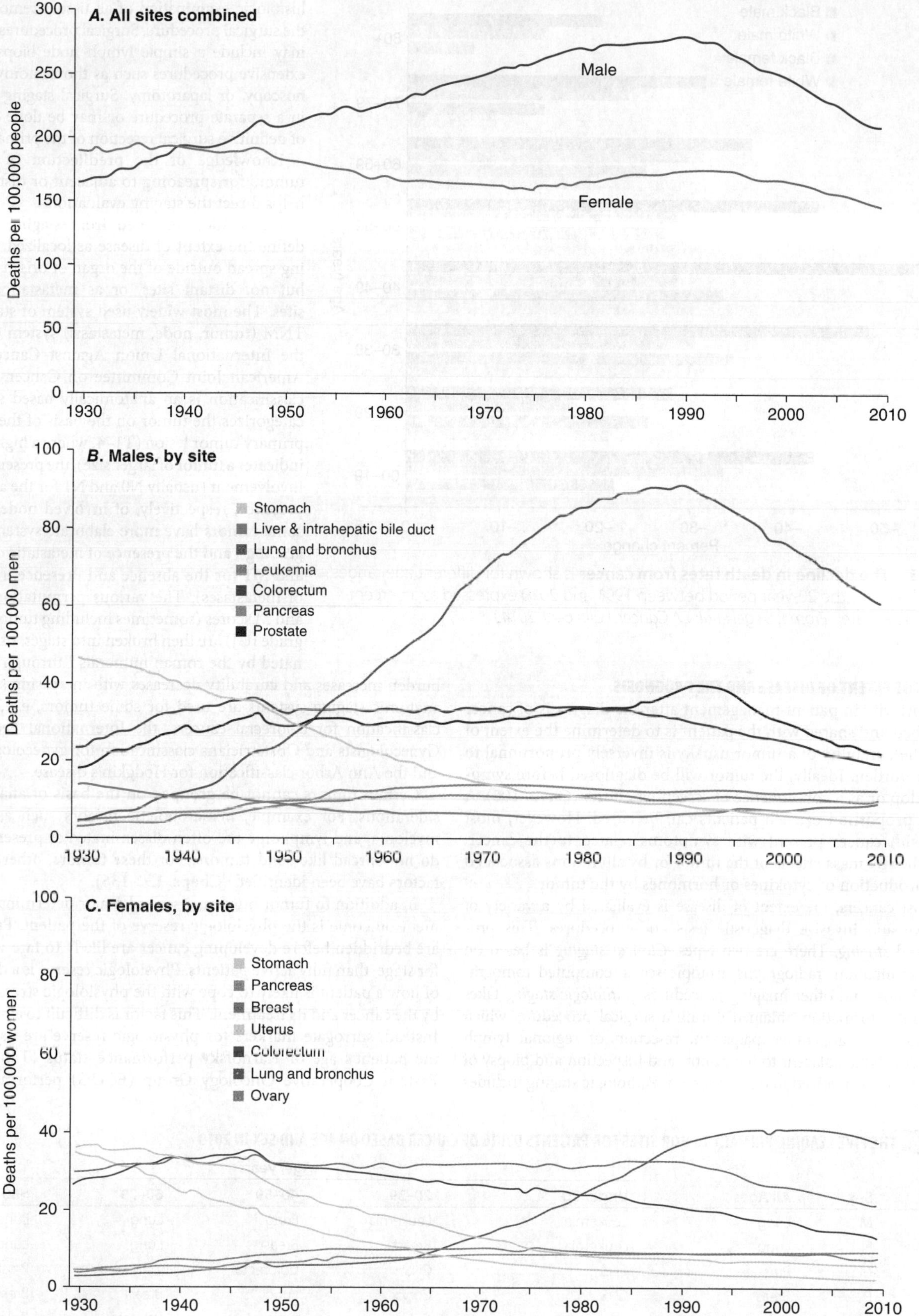

FIGURE 99-2 Eighty-year trend in cancer death rates for (*A*) women and (*B*) men by site in the United States, 1930–2010. Rates are per 100,000 age-adjusted to the 2000 U.S. standard population. All sites combined (*A*), individual sites in men (*B*) and individual sites in women (*C*) are shown. *(From R Siegel et al: CA Cancer J Clin 64:9, 2014.)*

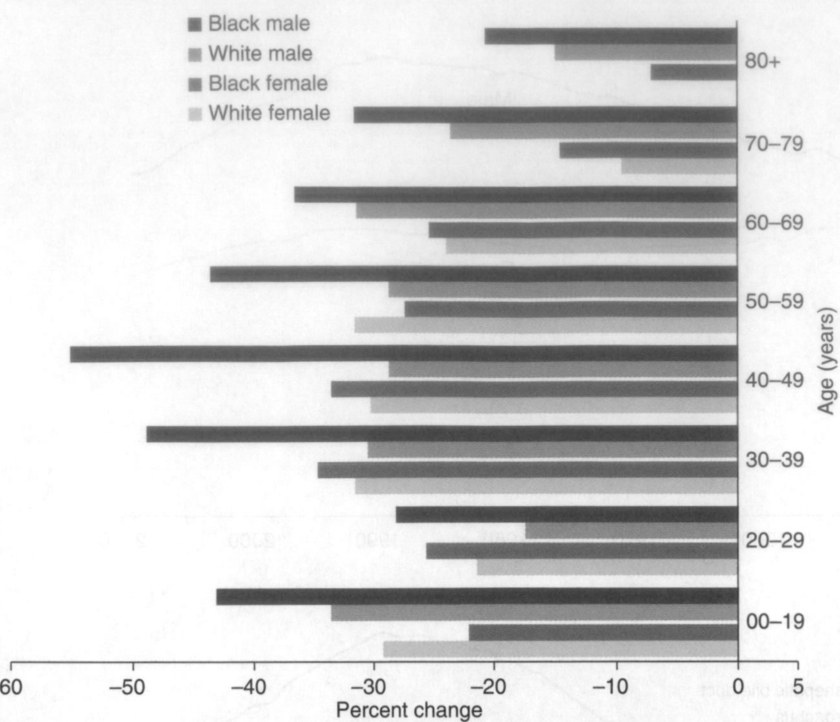

FIGURE 99-3 The decline in death rates from cancer is shown for different age ranges by sex and race for the 20-year period between 1991 and 2010 expressed as a percentage of the 1991 rate. *(From R Siegel et al: CA Cancer J Clin 64:9, 2014.)*

histologic examination of all tissues removed during the surgical procedure. Surgical procedures performed may include a simple lymph node biopsy or more extensive procedures such as thoracotomy, mediastinoscopy, or laparotomy. Surgical staging may occur in a separate procedure or may be done at the time of definitive surgical resection of the primary tumor.

Knowledge of the predilection of particular tumors for spreading to adjacent or distant organs helps direct the staging evaluation.

Information obtained from staging is used to define the extent of disease as localized, as exhibiting spread outside of the organ of origin to regional but not distant sites, or as metastatic to distant sites. The most widely used system of staging is the TNM (tumor, node, metastasis) system codified by the International Union Against Cancer and the American Joint Committee on Cancer. The TNM classification is an anatomically based system that categorizes the tumor on the basis of the size of the primary tumor lesion (T1–4, where a higher number indicates a tumor of larger size), the presence of nodal involvement (usually N0 and N1 for the absence and presence, respectively, of involved nodes, although some tumors have more elaborate systems of nodal grading), and the presence of metastatic disease (M0 and M1 for the absence and presence, respectively, of metastases). The various permutations of T, N, and M scores (sometimes including tumor histologic grade [G]) are then broken into stages, usually designated by the roman numerals I through IV. Tumor burden increases and curability decreases with increasing stage. Other anatomic staging systems are used for some tumors, e.g., the Dukes classification for colorectal cancers, the International Federation of Gynecologists and Obstetricians classification for gynecologic cancers, and the Ann Arbor classification for Hodgkin's disease.

Certain tumors cannot be grouped on the basis of anatomic considerations. For example, hematopoietic tumors such as leukemia, myeloma, and lymphoma are often disseminated at presentation and do not spread like solid tumors. For these tumors, other prognostic factors have been identified (Chaps. 132-136).

In addition to tumor burden, a second major determinant of treatment outcome is the physiologic reserve of the patient. Patients who are bedridden before developing cancer are likely to fare worse, stage for stage, than fully active patients. Physiologic reserve is a determinant of how a patient is likely to cope with the physiologic stresses imposed by the cancer and its treatment. This factor is difficult to assess directly. Instead, surrogate markers for physiologic reserve are used, such as the patient's age or Karnofsky performance status (Table 99-4) or Eastern Cooperative Oncology Group (ECOG) performance status

DEFINING THE EXTENT OF DISEASE AND THE PROGNOSIS

The first priority in patient management after the diagnosis of cancer is established and shared with the patient is to determine the extent of disease. The curability of a tumor usually is inversely proportional to the tumor burden. Ideally, the tumor will be diagnosed before symptoms develop or as a consequence of screening efforts (Chap. 100). A very high proportion of such patients can be cured. However, most patients with cancer present with symptoms related to the cancer, caused either by mass effects of the tumor or by alterations associated with the production of cytokines or hormones by the tumor.

For most cancers, the extent of disease is evaluated by a variety of noninvasive and invasive diagnostic tests and procedures. This process is called *staging*. There are two types. *Clinical staging* is based on physical examination, radiographs, isotopic scans, computed tomography (CT) scans, and other imaging procedures; *pathologic staging* takes into account information obtained during a surgical procedure, which might include intraoperative palpation, resection of regional lymph nodes and/or tissue adjacent to the tumor, and inspection and biopsy of organs commonly involved in disease spread. Pathologic staging includes

TABLE 99-2 THE FIVE LEADING PRIMARY TUMOR SITES FOR PATIENTS DYING OF CANCER BASED ON AGE AND SEX IN 2010

			Age, years				
Rank	Sex	All Ages	Under 20	20–39	40–59	60–79	>80
1	M	Lung	Leukemia	Leukemia	Lung	Lung	Lung
	F	Lung	Leukemia	Breast	Breast	Lung	Lung
2	M	Prostate	CNS	CNS	Colorectal	Colorectal	Prostate
	F	Breast	CNS	Cervix	Lung	Breast	Breast
3	M	Colorectal	Bone sarcoma	Colorectal	Liver	Prostate	Colorectal
	F	Colorectal	Bone sarcoma	Leukemia	Colorectal	Colorectal	Colorectal
4	M	Pancreas	Soft tissue sarcoma	Lymphoma	Pancreas	Pancreas	Bladder
	F	Pancreas	Soft tissue sarcoma	Colorectal	Ovary	Pancreas	Pancreas
5	M	Liver	Lymphoma	Lung	Esophagus	Liver	Pancreas
	F	Ovary	Liver	CNS	Pancreas	Ovary	Lymphoma

Abbreviations: CNS, central nervous system; F, female; M, male.

Source: From R Siegel et al: Cancer statistics, 2014. CA Cancer J Clin 64:9, 2014.

TABLE 99-3 CANCER INCIDENCE AND MORTALITY IN RACIAL AND ETHNIC GROUPS, UNITED STATES, 2006–2010

Site	Sex	White	Black	Asian/Pacific Islander	American Indian[a]	Hispanic
Incidence per 100,000 Population						
All	M	548.1	601.0	326.1	441.1	426.8
	F	436.2	395.9	282.6	372.0	330.8
Breast		127.3	118.4	84.7	90.3	91.1
Colorectal	M	50.9	62.5	40.8	51.7	47.3
	F	38.6	46.7	31.0	42.7	32.6
Kidney	M	21.6	23.0	10.6	30.6	20.5
	F	11.2	12.2	5.1	17.5	11.5
Liver	M	8.7	14.9	21.3	17.8	11.5
	F	2.9	4.4	8.0	8.0	6.9
Lung	M	82.9	94.7	48.8	70.2	45.9
	F	57.1	50.7	27.6	41.3	26.5
Prostate		138.6	220.0	75.0	104.1	124.2
Cervix		7.2	10.3	6.7	9.7	10.9
Deaths per 100,000 Population						
All	M	217.3	276.6	132.4	191.0	152.2
	F	153.6	171.2	92.1	139.0	101.3
Breast		22.7	30.8	11.5	15.5	14.8
Colorectal	M	19.2	28.7	13.1	18.7	16.1
	F	13.6	19.0	9.7	15.4	10.2
Kidney	M	5.9	5.7	3.0	9.5	5.1
	F	2.6	2.6	1.2	4.4	2.3
Liver	M	7.1	11.8	14.4	13.2	12.3
	F	2.9	4.1	6.0	6.1	5.4
Lung	M	65.7	78.5	35.5	49.6	31.3
	F	42.7	37.2	18.4	33.1	14.1
Prostate		21.3	50.9	10.1	20.7	19.2
Cervix		2.1	4.2	1.9	3.5	2.9

[a]Based on Indian Health Service delivery areas.

Abbreviations: F, female; M, male.

Source: From R Siegel R et al: Cancer statistics, 2014. CA Cancer J Clin 64:9, 2014.

(Table 99-5). Older patients and those with a Karnofsky performance status <70 or ECOG performance status ≥3 have a poor prognosis unless the poor performance is a reversible consequence of the tumor.

Increasingly, biologic features of the tumor are being related to prognosis. The expression of particular oncogenes, drug-resistance genes, apoptosis-related genes, and genes involved in metastasis is being found to influence response to therapy and prognosis. The presence of selected cytogenetic abnormalities may influence survival. Tumors with higher growth fractions, as assessed by expression of proliferation-related markers such as proliferating cell nuclear antigen, behave more aggressively than tumors with lower growth fractions. Information obtained from studying the tumor itself will increasingly be used to influence treatment decisions. Host genes involved in drug metabolism can influence the safety and efficacy of particular treatments.

Enormous heterogeneity has been noted by studying tumors; we have learned that morphology is not capable of discerning certain distinct subsets of patients whose tumors have different sets of abnormalities. Tumors that look the same by light microscopy can be very different. Similarly, tumors that look quite different from one another histologically can share genetic lesions that predict responses to treatments. Furthermore, tumor cells vary enormously within a single patient even though the cells share a common origin.

MAKING A TREATMENT PLAN

From information on the extent of disease and the prognosis and in conjunction with the patient's wishes, it is determined whether the treatment approach should be curative or palliative in intent. Cooperation among the various professionals involved in cancer treatment is of the utmost importance in treatment planning. For some cancers, chemotherapy or chemotherapy plus radiation therapy delivered before the use of definitive surgical treatment (so-called neoadjuvant therapy) may improve the outcome, as seems to be the case for locally advanced breast cancer and head and neck cancers. In certain settings in which combined-modality therapy is intended, coordination among the medical oncologist, radiation oncologist, and surgeon is crucial to achieving optimal results. Sometimes the chemotherapy and radiation therapy need to be delivered sequentially, and other times concurrently. Surgical procedures may precede or follow other treatment approaches. It is best for the treatment plan either to follow a standard protocol precisely or else to be part of an ongoing clinical research protocol evaluating new treatments. Ad hoc modifications of standard protocols are likely to compromise treatment results.

The choice of treatment approaches was formerly dominated by the local culture in both the university and the practice settings. However, it is now possible to gain access electronically to standard treatment protocols and to every approved clinical research study in North America through a personal computer interface with the Internet.[1]

[1]The National Cancer Institute maintains a database called PDQ (Physician Data Query) that is accessible on the Internet under the name CancerNet at *www.cancer.gov/cancertopics/pdq/cancerdatabase*. Information can be obtained through a facsimile machine using CancerFax by dialing 301-402-5874. Patient information is also provided by the National Cancer Institute in at least three formats: on the Internet via CancerNet at *www.cancer.gov*, through the CancerFax number listed above, or by calling 1-800-4-CANCER. The quality control for the information provided through these services is rigorous.

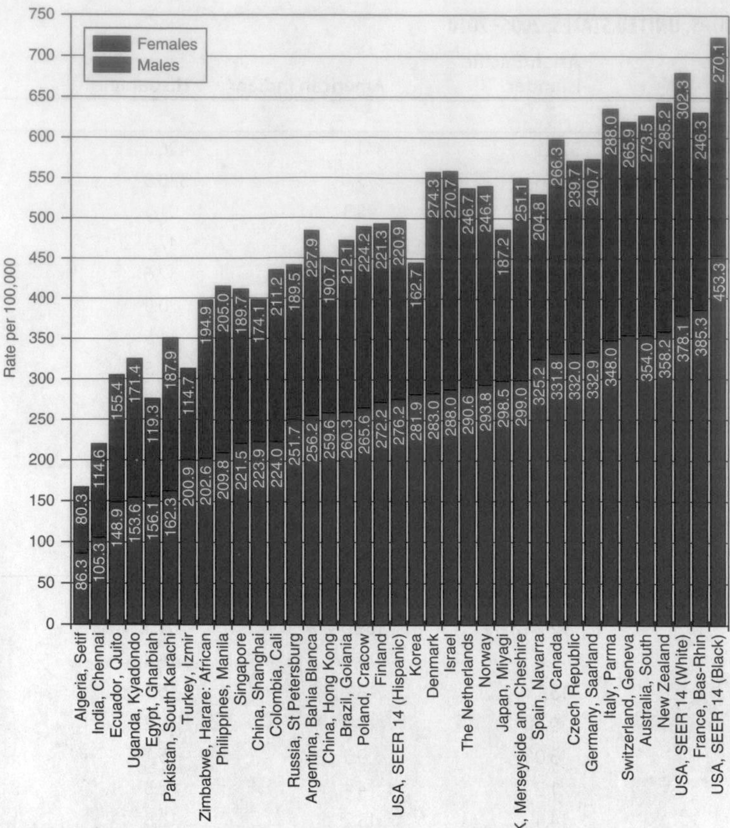

FIGURE 99-4 Worldwide overall annual cancer incidence, mortality, and 5-year prevalence for the period of 1993–2001. *(Adapted from A Jemal et al: Cancer Epidemiol Biomarkers Prev 19:1893, 2010.)*

The skilled physician also has much to offer the patient for whom curative therapy is no longer an option. Often a combination of guilt and frustration over the inability to cure the patient and the pressure of a busy schedule greatly limit the time a physician spends with a patient who is receiving only palliative care. Resist these forces. In addition to the medicines administered to alleviate symptoms (see below), it is important to remember the comfort that is provided by holding the patient's hand, continuing regular examinations, and taking time to talk.

TABLE 99-4 KARNOFSKY PERFORMANCE INDEX

Performance Status	Functional Capability of the Patient
100	Normal; no complaints; no evidence of disease
90	Able to carry on normal activity; minor signs or symptoms of disease
80	Normal activity with effort; some signs or symptoms of disease
70	Cares for self; unable to carry on normal activity or do active work
60	Requires occasional assistance but is able to care for most needs
50	Requires considerable assistance and frequent medical care
40	Disabled; requires special care and assistance
30	Severely disabled; hospitalization is indicated, although death is not imminent
20	Very sick; hospitalization is necessary; active supportive treatment is necessary
10	Moribund, fatal processes progressing rapidly
0	Dead

MANAGEMENT OF DISEASE AND TREATMENT COMPLICATIONS

Because cancer therapies are toxic (Chap. 103e), patient management involves addressing complications of both the disease and its treatment as well as the complex psychosocial problems associated with cancer. In the short term during a course of curative therapy, the patient's functional status may decline. Treatment-induced toxicity is less acceptable if the goal of therapy is palliation. The most common side effects of treatment are nausea and vomiting (see below), febrile neutropenia (Chap. 104), and myelosuppression (Chap. 103e). Tools are now available to minimize the acute toxicity of cancer treatment.

New symptoms developing in the course of cancer treatment should always be assumed to be reversible until proven otherwise. The fatalistic attribution of anorexia, weight loss, and jaundice to recurrent or progressive tumor could result in a patient dying from a reversible intercurrent cholecystitis. Intestinal obstruction may be due to reversible adhesions rather than progressive tumor. Systemic infections, sometimes with unusual pathogens, may be a consequence of the immunosuppression associated with cancer therapy. Some drugs used to treat cancer or its complications (e.g., nausea) may produce central nervous system symptoms that look like metastatic disease or may mimic paraneoplastic syndromes such as the syndrome of inappropriate antidiuretic hormone. A definitive diagnosis should be pursued and may even require a repeat biopsy.

A critical component of cancer management is assessing the response to treatment. In addition to a careful physical examination in which all sites of disease are physically measured and recorded in a flow chart by date, response assessment usually requires periodic repeating of imaging tests that were abnormal at the time of staging. If imaging tests have become normal, repeat biopsy of previously involved tissue is performed to document complete response by pathologic criteria. Biopsies are not usually required if there is macroscopic residual disease. A *complete response* is defined as disappearance of all evidence of disease, and a *partial response* as >50% reduction in the sum of the products of the perpendicular diameters of all measurable lesions. The determination of partial response may also be based on a 30% decrease in the sums of the longest diameters of lesions (Response Evaluation Criteria in Solid Tumors [RECIST]). *Progressive disease* is defined as the appearance of any new lesion or an increase of >25% in the sum of the products of the perpendicular diameters of all measurable lesions (or an increase of 20% in the sums of the longest diameters by RECIST). Tumor shrinkage or growth that does not meet any of these criteria is considered *stable disease*. Some sites of involvement (e.g., bone) or patterns of involvement (e.g., lymphangitic lung or diffuse pulmonary infiltrates) are considered unmeasurable. No response is complete without biopsy documentation of their resolution, but partial responses may exclude their assessment unless clear objective progression has occurred.

TABLE 99-5 THE EASTERN COOPERATIVE ONCOLOGY GROUP (ECOG) PERFORMANCE SCALE

ECOG Grade 0: Fully active, able to carry on all predisease performance without restriction
ECOG Grade 1: Restricted in physically strenuous activity but ambulatory and able to carry out work of a light or sedentary nature, e.g., light housework, office work
ECOG Grade 2: Ambulatory and capable of all self-care but unable to carry out any work activities. Up and about more than 50% of waking hours
ECOG Grade 3: Capable of only limited self-care, confined to bed or chair more than 50% of waking hours
ECOG Grade 4: Completely disabled. Cannot carry on any self-care. Totally confined to bed or chair
ECOG Grade 5: Dead

Source: From MM Oken et al: Am J Clin Oncol 5:649, 1982.

TABLE 99-6 TUMOR MARKERS

Tumor Markers	Cancer	Nonneoplastic Conditions
Hormones		
Human chorionic gonadotropin	Gestational trophoblastic disease, gonadal germ cell tumor	Pregnancy
Calcitonin	Medullary cancer of the thyroid	
Catecholamines	Pheochromocytoma	
Oncofetal Antigens		
α Fetoprotein	Hepatocellular carcinoma, gonadal germ cell tumor	Cirrhosis, hepatitis
Carcinoembryonic antigen	Adenocarcinomas of the colon, pancreas, lung, breast, ovary	Pancreatitis, hepatitis, inflammatory bowel disease, smoking
Enzymes		
Prostatic acid phosphatase	Prostate cancer	Prostatitis, prostatic hypertrophy
Neuron-specific enolase	Small-cell cancer of the lung, neuroblastoma	
Lactate dehydrogenase	Lymphoma, Ewing's sarcoma	Hepatitis, hemolytic anemia, many others
Tumor-Associated Proteins		
Prostate-specific antigen	Prostate cancer	Prostatitis, prostatic hypertrophy
Monoclonal immunoglobulin	Myeloma	Infection, MGUS
CA-125	Ovarian cancer, some lymphomas	Menstruation, peritonitis, pregnancy
CA 19-9	Colon, pancreatic, breast cancer	Pancreatitis, ulcerative colitis
CD30	Hodgkin's disease, anaplastic large-cell lymphoma	—
CD25	Hairy cell leukemia, adult T cell leukemia/lymphoma	—

Abbreviation: MGUS, monoclonal gammopathy of uncertain significance.

Tumor markers may be useful in patient management in certain tumors. Response to therapy may be difficult to gauge with certainty. However, some tumors produce or elicit the production of markers that can be measured in the serum or urine, and in a particular patient, rising and falling levels of the marker are usually associated with increasing or decreasing tumor burden, respectively. Some clinically useful tumor markers are shown in Table 99-6. Tumor markers are not in themselves specific enough to permit a diagnosis of malignancy to be made, but once a malignancy has been diagnosed and shown to be associated with elevated levels of a tumor marker, the marker can be used to assess response to treatment.

The recognition and treatment of depression are important components of management. The incidence of depression in cancer patients is ~25% overall and may be greater in patients with greater debility. This diagnosis is likely in a patient with a depressed mood (dysphoria) and/or a loss of interest in pleasure (anhedonia) for at least 2 weeks. In addition, three or more of the following symptoms are usually present: appetite change, sleep problems, psychomotor retardation or agitation, fatigue, feelings of guilt or worthlessness, inability to concentrate, and suicidal ideation. Patients with these symptoms should receive therapy. Medical therapy with a serotonin reuptake inhibitor such as fluoxetine (10–20 mg/d), sertraline (50–150 mg/d), or paroxetine (10–20 mg/d) or a tricyclic antidepressant such as amitriptyline (50–100 mg/d) or desipramine (75–150 mg/d) should be tried, allowing 4–6 weeks for response. Effective therapy should be continued at least 6 months after resolution of symptoms. If therapy is unsuccessful, other classes of antidepressants may be used. In addition to medication, psychosocial interventions such as support groups, psychotherapy, and guided imagery may be of benefit.

Many patients opt for unproven or unsound approaches to treatment when it appears that conventional medicine is unlikely to be curative. Those seeking such alternatives are often well educated and may be early in the course of their disease. Unsound approaches are usually hawked on the basis of unsubstantiated anecdotes and not only cannot help the patient but may be harmful. Physicians should strive to keep communications open and nonjudgmental, so that patients are more likely to discuss with the physician what they are actually doing. The appearance of unexpected toxicity may be an indication that a supplemental therapy is being taken.[2]

LONG-TERM FOLLOW-UP/LATE COMPLICATIONS

At the completion of treatment, sites originally involved with tumor are reassessed, usually by radiography or imaging techniques, and any persistent abnormality is biopsied. If disease persists, the multidisciplinary team discusses a new salvage treatment plan. If the patient has been rendered disease-free by the original treatment, the patient is followed regularly for disease recurrence. The optimal guidelines for follow-up care are not known. For many years, a routine practice has been to follow the patient monthly for 6–12 months, then every other month for a year, every 3 months for a year, every 4 months for a year, every 6 months for a year, and then annually. At each visit, a battery of laboratory and radiographic and imaging tests were obtained on the assumption that it is best to detect recurrent disease before it becomes symptomatic. However, where follow-up procedures have been examined, this assumption has been found to be untrue. Studies of breast cancer, melanoma, lung cancer, colon cancer, and lymphoma have all failed to support the notion that asymptomatic relapses are more readily cured by salvage therapy than symptomatic relapses. In view of the enormous cost of a full battery of diagnostic tests and their manifest lack of impact on survival, new guidelines are emerging for less frequent follow-up visits, during which the history and physical examination are the major investigations performed.

As time passes, the likelihood of recurrence of the primary cancer diminishes. For many types of cancer, survival for 5 years without recurrence is tantamount to cure. However, important medical problems can occur in patients treated for cancer and must be examined (Chap. 125). Some problems emerge as a consequence of the disease and some as a consequence of the treatment. An understanding of these disease- and treatment-related problems may help in their detection and management.

Despite these concerns, most patients who are cured of cancer return to normal lives.

SUPPORTIVE CARE

In many ways, the success of cancer therapy depends on the success of the supportive care. Failure to control the symptoms of cancer and its treatment may lead patients to abandon curative therapy. Of equal importance, supportive care is a major determinant of quality of life. Even when life cannot be prolonged, the physician must strive to preserve its quality. Quality-of-life measurements have become common endpoints of clinical research studies. Furthermore, palliative care has been shown to be cost-effective when approached in an organized fashion. A credo for oncology could be to cure sometimes, to extend life often, and to comfort always.

Pain Pain occurs with variable frequency in the cancer patient: 25–50% of patients present with pain at diagnosis, 33% have pain associated with treatment, and 75% have pain with progressive disease. The pain may have several causes. In ~70% of cases, pain is caused by the tumor itself—by invasion of bone, nerves, blood vessels, or mucous

[2]Information about unsound methods may be obtained from the National Council Against Health Fraud, Box 1276, Loma Linda, CA 92354, or from the Center for Medical Consumers and Health Care Information, 237 Thompson Street, New York, NY 10012.

membranes or obstruction of a hollow viscus or duct. In ~20% of cases, pain is related to a surgical or invasive medical procedure, to radiation injury (mucositis, enteritis, or plexus or spinal cord injury), or to chemotherapy injury (mucositis, peripheral neuropathy, phlebitis, steroid-induced aseptic necrosis of the femoral head). In 10% of cases, pain is unrelated to cancer or its treatment.

Assessment of pain requires the methodical investigation of the history of the pain, its location, character, temporal features, provocative and palliative factors, and intensity (Chap. 18); a review of the oncologic history and past medical history as well as personal and social history; and a thorough physical examination. The patient should be given a 10-division visual analogue scale on which to indicate the severity of the pain. The clinical condition is often dynamic, making it necessary to reassess the patient frequently. Pain therapy should not be withheld while the cause of pain is being sought.

A variety of tools are available with which to address cancer pain. About 85% of patients will have pain relief from pharmacologic intervention. However, other modalities, including antitumor therapy (such as surgical relief of obstruction, radiation therapy, and strontium-89 or samarium-153 treatment for bone pain), neurostimulatory techniques, regional analgesia, or neuroablative procedures, are effective in an additional 12% or so. Thus, very few patients will have inadequate pain relief if appropriate measures are taken. A specific approach to pain relief is detailed in Chap. 10.

Nausea Emesis in the cancer patient is usually caused by chemotherapy (Chap. 103e). Its severity can be predicted from the drugs used to treat the cancer. Three forms of emesis are recognized on the basis of their timing with regard to the noxious insult. *Acute emesis*, the most common variety, occurs within 24 h of treatment. *Delayed emesis* occurs 1–7 days after treatment; it is rare, but, when present, usually follows cisplatin administration. *Anticipatory emesis* occurs before administration of chemotherapy and represents a conditioned response to visual and olfactory stimuli previously associated with chemotherapy delivery.

Acute emesis is the best understood form. Stimuli that activate signals in the chemoreceptor trigger zone in the medulla, the cerebral cortex, and peripherally in the intestinal tract lead to stimulation of the vomiting center in the medulla, the motor center responsible for coordinating the secretory and muscle contraction activity that leads to emesis. Diverse receptor types participate in the process, including dopamine, serotonin, histamine, opioid, and acetylcholine receptors. The serotonin receptor antagonists ondansetron and granisetron are the most effective drugs against highly emetogenic agents, but they are expensive.

As with the analgesia ladder, emesis therapy should be tailored to the situation. For mildly and moderately emetogenic agents, prochlorperazine, 5–10 mg PO or 25 mg PR, is effective. Its efficacy may be enhanced by administering the drug before the chemotherapy is delivered. Dexamethasone, 10–20 mg IV, is also effective and may enhance the efficacy of prochlorperazine. For highly emetogenic agents such as cisplatin, mechlorethamine, dacarbazine, and streptozocin, combinations of agents work best and administration should begin 6–24 h before treatment. Ondansetron, 8 mg PO every 6 h the day before therapy and IV on the day of therapy, plus dexamethasone, 20 mg IV before treatment, is an effective regimen. Addition of oral aprepitant (a substance P/neurokinin 1 receptor antagonist) to this regimen (125 mg on day 1, 80 mg on days 2 and 3) further decreases the risk of both acute and delayed vomiting. Like pain, emesis is easier to prevent than to alleviate.

Delayed emesis may be related to bowel inflammation from the therapy and can be controlled with oral dexamethasone and oral metoclopramide, a dopamine receptor antagonist that also blocks serotonin receptors at high dosages. The best strategy for preventing anticipatory emesis is to control emesis in the early cycles of therapy to prevent the conditioning from taking place. If this is unsuccessful, prophylactic antiemetics the day before treatment may help. Experimental studies are evaluating behavior modification.

Effusions Fluid may accumulate abnormally in the pleural cavity, pericardium, or peritoneum. Asymptomatic malignant effusions may not require treatment. Symptomatic effusions occurring in tumors responsive to systemic therapy usually do not require local treatment but respond to the treatment for the underlying tumor. Symptomatic effusions occurring in tumors unresponsive to systemic therapy may require local treatment in patients with a life expectancy of at least 6 months.

Pleural effusions due to tumors may or may not contain malignant cells. Lung cancer, breast cancer, and lymphomas account for ~75% of malignant pleural effusions. Their exudative nature is usually gauged by an effusion/serum protein ratio of ≥0.5 or an effusion/serum lactate dehydrogenase ratio of ≥0.6. When the condition is symptomatic, thoracentesis is usually performed first. In most cases, symptomatic improvement occurs for <1 month. Chest tube drainage is required if symptoms recur within 2 weeks. Fluid is aspirated until the flow rate is <100 mL in 24 h. Then either 60 units of bleomycin or 1 g of doxycycline is infused into the chest tube in 50 mL of 5% dextrose in water; the tube is clamped; the patient is rotated on four sides, spending 15 min in each position; and, after 1–2 h, the tube is again attached to suction for another 24 h. The tube is then disconnected from suction and allowed to drain by gravity. If <100 mL drains over the next 24 h, the chest tube is pulled, and a radiograph is taken 24 h later. If the chest tube continues to drain fluid at an unacceptably high rate, sclerosis can be repeated. Bleomycin may be somewhat more effective than doxycycline but is very expensive. Doxycycline is usually the drug of first choice. If neither doxycycline nor bleomycin is effective, talc can be used.

Symptomatic pericardial effusions are usually treated by creating a pericardial window or by stripping the pericardium. If the patient's condition does not permit a surgical procedure, sclerosis can be attempted with doxycycline and/or bleomycin.

Malignant ascites is usually treated with repeated paracentesis of small volumes of fluid. If the underlying malignancy is unresponsive to systemic therapy, peritoneovenous shunts may be inserted. Despite the fear of disseminating tumor cells into the circulation, widespread metastases are an unusual complication. The major complications are occlusion, leakage, and fluid overload. Patients with severe liver disease may develop disseminated intravascular coagulation.

Nutrition Cancer and its treatment may lead to a decrease in nutrient intake of sufficient magnitude to cause weight loss and alteration of intermediary metabolism. The prevalence of this problem is difficult to estimate because of variations in the definition of cancer cachexia, but most patients with advanced cancer experience weight loss and decreased appetite. A variety of both tumor-derived factors (e.g., bombesin, adrenocorticotropic hormone) and host-derived factors (e.g., tumor necrosis factor, interleukins 1 and 6, growth hormone) contribute to the altered metabolism, and a vicious cycle is established in which protein catabolism, glucose intolerance, and lipolysis cannot be reversed by the provision of calories.

It remains controversial how to assess nutritional status and when and how to intervene. Efforts to make the assessment objective have included the use of a prognostic nutritional index based on albumin levels, triceps skinfold thickness, transferrin levels, and delayed-type hypersensitivity skin testing. However, a simpler approach has been to define the threshold for nutritional intervention as <10% unexplained body weight loss, serum transferrin level <1500 mg/L (150 mg/dL), and serum albumin <34 g/L (3.4 g/dL).

The decision is important, because it appears that cancer therapy is substantially more toxic and less effective in the face of malnutrition. Nevertheless, it remains unclear whether nutritional intervention can alter the natural history. Unless some pathology is affecting the absorptive function of the gastrointestinal tract, enteral nutrition provided orally or by tube feeding is preferred over parenteral supplementation. However, the risks associated with the tube may outweigh the benefits. Megestrol acetate, a progestational agent, has been advocated as a pharmacologic intervention to improve nutritional status. Research in this area may provide more tools in the future as cytokine-mediated mechanisms are further elucidated.

Psychosocial Support The psychosocial needs of patients vary with their situation. Patients undergoing treatment experience fear, anxiety, and depression. Self-image is often seriously compromised by deforming surgery and loss of hair. Women who receive cosmetic advice that enables them to look better also feel better. Loss of control over how one spends time can contribute to the sense of vulnerability. Juggling the demands of work and family with the demands of treatment may create enormous stresses. Sexual dysfunction is highly prevalent and needs to be discussed openly with the patient. An empathetic health care team is sensitive to the individual patient's needs and permits negotiation where such flexibility will not adversely affect the course of treatment.

Cancer survivors have other sets of difficulties. Patients may have fears associated with the termination of a treatment they associate with their continued survival. Adjustments are required to physical losses and handicaps, real and perceived. Patients may be preoccupied with minor physical problems. They perceive a decline in their job mobility and view themselves as less desirable workers. They may be victims of job and/or insurance discrimination. Patients may experience difficulty reentering their normal past life. They may feel guilty for having survived and may carry a sense of vulnerability to colds and other illnesses. Perhaps the most pervasive and threatening concern is the ever-present fear of relapse (the Damocles syndrome).

Patients in whom therapy has been unsuccessful have other problems related to the end of life.

Death and Dying The most common causes of death in patients with cancer are infection (leading to circulatory failure), respiratory failure, hepatic failure, and renal failure. Intestinal blockage may lead to inanition and starvation. Central nervous system disease may lead to seizures, coma, and central hypoventilation. About 70% of patients develop dyspnea preterminally. However, many months usually pass between the diagnosis of cancer and the occurrence of these complications, and during this period, the patient is severely affected by the possibility of death. The path of unsuccessful cancer treatment usually occurs in three phases. First, there is optimism at the hope of cure; when the tumor recurs, there is the acknowledgment of an incurable disease, and the goal of palliative therapy is embraced in the hope of being able to live with disease; finally, at the disclosure of imminent death, another adjustment in outlook takes place. The patient imagines the worst in preparation for the end of life and may go through stages of adjustment to the diagnosis. These stages include denial, isolation, anger, bargaining, depression, acceptance, and hope. Of course, patients do not all progress through all the stages or proceed through them in the same order or at the same rate. Nevertheless, developing an understanding of how the patient has been affected by the diagnosis and is coping with it is an important goal of patient management.

It is best to speak frankly with the patient and the family regarding the likely course of disease. These discussions can be difficult for the physician as well as for the patient and family. The critical features of the interaction are to reassure the patient and family that everything that can be done to provide comfort will be done. They will not be abandoned. Many patients prefer to be cared for in their homes or in a hospice setting rather than a hospital. The American College of Physicians has published a book called *Home Care Guide for Cancer: How to Care for Family and Friends at Home* that teaches an approach to successful problem-solving in home care. With appropriate planning, it should be possible to provide the patient with the necessary medical care as well as the psychological and spiritual support that will prevent the isolation and depersonalization that can attend in-hospital death.

The care of dying patients may take a toll on the physician. A "burnout" syndrome has been described that is characterized by fatigue, disengagement from patients and colleagues, and a loss of self-fulfillment. Efforts at stress reduction, maintenance of a balanced life, and setting realistic goals may combat this disorder.

End-of-Life Decisions Unfortunately, a smooth transition in treatment goals from curative to palliative may not be possible in all cases because of the occurrence of serious treatment-related complications or rapid disease progression. Vigorous and invasive medical support for a reversible disease or treatment complication is assumed to be justified. However, if the reversibility of the condition is in doubt, the patient's wishes determine the level of medical care. These wishes should be elicited before the terminal phase of illness and reviewed periodically. Information about advance directives can be obtained from the American Association of Retired Persons, 601 E Street, NW, Washington, DC 20049, 202-434-2277, or Choice in Dying, 250 West 57th Street, New York, NY 10107, 212-366-5540. Some states allow physicians to assist patients who choose to end their lives. This subject is challenging from an ethical and a medical point of view. Discussions of end-of-life decisions should be candid and involve clear informed consent, waiting periods, second opinions, and documentation. A full discussion of end-of-life management is in Chap. 10.

100 Prevention and Early Detection of Cancer

Jennifer M. Croswell, Otis W. Brawley, Barnett S. Kramer

Improved understanding of carcinogenesis has allowed cancer prevention and early detection (also known as cancer control) to expand beyond the identification and avoidance of carcinogens. Specific interventions to prevent cancer in those at risk, and effective screening for early detection of cancer, are the goals.

Carcinogenesis is not an event but a process, a continuum of discrete tissue and cellular changes over time resulting in aberrant physiologic processes. Prevention concerns the identification and manipulation of the biologic, environmental, social, and genetic factors in the causal pathway of cancer.

EDUCATION AND HEALTHFUL HABITS

Public education on the avoidance of identified risk factors for cancer and encouraging healthy habits contributes to cancer prevention and control. The clinician is a powerful messenger in this process. The patient-provider encounter provides an opportunity to teach patients about the hazards of smoking, the features of a healthy lifestyle, use of proven cancer screening methods, and avoidance of excessive sun exposure.

SMOKING CESSATION

Tobacco smoking is a strong, modifiable risk factor for cardiovascular disease, pulmonary disease, and cancer. Smokers have an approximately 1 in 3 lifetime risk of dying prematurely from a tobacco-related cancer, cardiovascular, or pulmonary disease. Tobacco use causes more deaths from cardiovascular disease than from cancer. Lung cancer and cancers of the larynx, oropharynx, esophagus, kidney, bladder, pancreas, and stomach are all tobacco-related.

The number of cigarettes smoked per day and the level of inhalation of cigarette smoke are correlated with risk of lung cancer mortality. Light- and low-tar cigarettes are not safer, because smokers tend to inhale them more frequently and deeply.

Those who stop smoking have a 30–50% lower 10-year lung cancer mortality rate compared to those who continue smoking, despite the fact that some carcinogen-induced gene mutations persist for years after smoking cessation. Smoking cessation and avoidance would save more lives than any other public health activity.

The risk of tobacco smoke is not limited to the smoker. Environmental tobacco smoke, known as secondhand or passive smoke, causes lung cancer and other cardiopulmonary diseases in nonsmokers.

Tobacco use prevention is a pediatric issue. More than 80% of adult American smokers began smoking before the age of 18 years. Approximately 20% of Americans in grades 9 through 12 have smoked a cigarette in the past month. Counseling of adolescents and young adults is critical to prevent smoking. A clinician's simple advice can be of benefit. Providers should query patients on tobacco use and offer smokers assistance in quitting.

Current approaches to smoking cessation recognize smoking as an addiction (Chap. 470). The smoker who is quitting goes through identifiable stages that include contemplation of quitting, an action phase in which the smoker quits, and a maintenance phase. Smokers who quit completely are more likely to be successful than those who gradually reduce the number of cigarettes smoked or change to lower-tar or lower-nicotine cigarettes. More than 90% of the Americans who have successfully quit smoking did so on their own, without participation in an organized cessation program, but cessation programs are helpful for some smokers. The Community Intervention Trial for Smoking Cessation (COMMIT) was a 4-year program showing that light smokers (<25 cigarettes per day) were more likely to benefit from simple cessation messages and cessation programs than those who did not receive an intervention. Quit rates were 30.6% in the intervention group and 27.5% in the control group. The COMMIT interventions were unsuccessful in heavy smokers (<25 cigarettes per day). Heavy smokers may need an intensive broad-based cessation program that includes counseling, behavioral strategies, and pharmacologic adjuncts, such as nicotine replacement (gum, patches, sprays, lozenges, and inhalers), bupropion, and/or varenicline.

The health risks of cigars are similar to those of cigarettes. Smoking one or two cigars daily doubles the risk for oral and esophageal cancers; smoking three or four cigars daily increases the risk of oral cancers more than eightfold and esophageal cancer fourfold. The risks of occasional use are unknown.

Smokeless tobacco also represents a substantial health risk. Chewing tobacco is a carcinogen linked to dental caries, gingivitis, oral leukoplakia, and oral cancer. The systemic effects of smokeless tobacco (including snuff) may increase risks for other cancers. Esophageal cancer is linked to carcinogens in tobacco dissolved in saliva and swallowed. The net effects of e-cigarettes on health are poorly studied. Whether they aid in smoking cessation or serve as a "gateway" for nonsmoking children to acquire a smoking habit is debated.

PHYSICAL ACTIVITY

Physical activity is associated with a decreased risk of colon and breast cancer. A variety of mechanisms have been proposed. However, such studies are prone to confounding factors such as recall bias, association of exercise with other health-related practices, and effects of preclinical cancers on exercise habits (reverse causality).

DIET MODIFICATION

International epidemiologic studies suggest that diets high in fat are associated with increased risk for cancers of the breast, colon, prostate, and endometrium. These cancers have their highest incidence and mortalities in Western cultures, where fat composes an average of one-third of the total calories consumed.

Despite correlations, dietary fat has not been proven to cause cancer. Case-control and cohort epidemiologic studies give conflicting results. In addition, diet is a highly complex exposure to many nutrients and chemicals. Low-fat diets are associated with many dietary changes beyond simple subtraction of fat. Other lifestyle changes are also associated with adherence to a low-fat diet.

In observational studies, dietary fiber is associated with a reduced risk of colonic polyps and invasive cancer of the colon. However, cancer-protective effects of increasing fiber and lowering dietary fat have not been proven in the context of a prospective clinical trial. The putative protective mechanisms are complex and speculative. Fiber binds oxidized bile acids and generates soluble fiber products, such as butyrate, that may have differentiating properties. Fiber does not increase bowel transit times. Two large prospective cohort studies of >100,000 health professionals showed no association between fruit and vegetable intake and risk of cancer.

The Polyp Prevention Trial randomly assigned 2000 elderly persons, who had polyps removed, to a low-fat, high-fiber diet versus routine diet for 4 years. No differences were noted in polyp formation.

The U.S. National Institutes of Health Women's Health Initiative, launched in 1994, was a long-term clinical trial enrolling >100,000 women age 45–69 years. It placed women in 22 intervention groups. Participants received calcium/vitamin D supplementation; hormone replacement therapy; and counseling to increase exercise, eat a low-fat diet with increased consumption of fruits, vegetables, and fiber, and cease smoking. The study showed that although dietary fat intake was lower in the diet intervention group, invasive breast cancers were not reduced over an 8-year follow-up period compared to the control group. No reduction was seen in the incidence of colorectal cancer in the dietary intervention arm. The difference in dietary fat averaged ~10% between the two groups. Evidence does not currently establish the anticarcinogenic value of vitamin, mineral, or nutritional supplements in amounts greater than those provided by a balanced diet.

ENERGY BALANCE

Risk of cancer appears to increase as body mass index increases beyond 25 kg/m^2. Obesity is associated with increased risk for cancers of the colon, breast (female postmenopausal), endometrium, kidney (renal cell), and esophagus, although causality has not been established.

In observational studies, relative risks of colon cancer are increased in obesity by 1.5–2 for men and 1.2–1.5 for women. Obese postmenopausal women have a 30–50% increased relative risk of breast cancer. An unproven hypothesis for the association is that adipose tissue serves as a depot for aromatase that facilitates estrogen production.

SUN AVOIDANCE

Nonmelanoma skin cancers (basal cell and squamous cell) are induced by cumulative exposure to ultraviolet (UV) radiation. Intermittent acute sun exposure and sun damage have been linked to melanoma, but the evidence is inconsistent. Sunburns, especially in childhood and adolescence, may be associated with an increased risk of melanoma in adulthood. Reduction of sun exposure through use of protective clothing and changing patterns of outdoor activities can reduce skin cancer risk. Sunscreens decrease the risk of actinic keratoses, the precursor to squamous cell skin cancer, but melanoma risk may not be reduced. Sunscreens prevent burning, but they may encourage more prolonged exposure to the sun and may not filter out wavelengths of energy that cause melanoma.

Educational interventions to help individuals assess their risk of developing skin cancer have some impact. In particular, appearance-focused behavioral interventions in young women can decrease indoor tanning use and other UV exposures. Self-examination for skin pigment characteristics associated with skin cancer, such as freckling, may be useful in identifying people at high risk. Those who recognize themselves as being at risk tend to be more compliant with sun-avoidance recommendations. Risk factors for melanoma include a propensity to sunburn, a large number of benign melanocytic nevi, and atypical nevi.

CANCER CHEMOPREVENTION

Chemoprevention involves the use of specific natural or synthetic chemical agents to reverse, suppress, or prevent carcinogenesis before the development of invasive malignancy.

Cancer develops through an accumulation of tissue abnormalities associated with genetic and epigenetic changes, and growth regulatory pathways that are potential points of intervention to prevent cancer. The initial changes are termed *initiation*. The alteration can be inherited or acquired through the action of physical, infectious, or chemical carcinogens. Like most human diseases, cancer arises from an interaction between genetics and environmental exposures (Table 100-1). Influences that cause the initiated cell and its surrounding tissue microenvironment to progress through the carcinogenic process and change phenotypically are termed *promoters*. Promoters include hormones such as androgens, linked to prostate cancer, and estrogen, linked to breast and endometrial cancer. The distinction between an initiator and promoter is indistinct; some components of cigarette smoke are "complete carcinogens," acting as both initiators and promoters. Cancer can be prevented or controlled through interference with the factors that cause cancer initiation, promotion, or progression. Compounds of interest in chemoprevention often have antimutagenic, hormone modulation, anti-inflammatory, antiproliferative, or proapoptotic activity (or a combination).

TABLE 100-1 SUSPECTED CARCINOGENS

Carcinogens[a]	Associated Cancer or Neoplasm
Alkylating agents	Acute myeloid leukemia, bladder cancer
Androgens	Prostate cancer
Aromatic amines (dyes)	Bladder cancer
Arsenic	Cancer of the lung, skin
Asbestos	Cancer of the lung, pleura, peritoneum
Benzene	Acute myelocytic leukemia
Chromium	Lung cancer
Diethylstilbestrol (prenatal)	Vaginal cancer (clear cell)
Epstein-Barr virus	Burkitt's lymphoma, nasal T cell lymphoma
Estrogens	Cancer of the endometrium, liver, breast
Ethyl alcohol	Cancer of the breast, liver, esophagus, head and neck
Helicobacter pylori	Gastric cancer, gastric MALT lymphoma
Hepatitis B or C virus	Liver cancer
Human immunodeficiency virus	Non-Hodgkin's lymphoma, Kaposi's sarcoma, squamous cell carcinomas (especially of the urogenital tract)
Human papilloma virus	Cancers of the cervix, anus, oropharynx
Human T cell lymphotropic virus type 1 (HTLV-1)	Adult T cell leukemia/lymphoma
Immunosuppressive agents (azathioprine, cyclosporine, glucocorticoids)	Non-Hodgkin's lymphoma
Ionizing radiation (therapeutic or diagnostic)	Breast, bladder, thyroid, soft tissue, bone, hematopoietic, and many more
Nitrogen mustard gas	Cancer of the lung, head and neck, nasal sinuses
Nickel dust	Cancer of the lung, nasal sinuses
Diesel exhaust	Lung cancer (miners)
Phenacetin	Cancer of the renal pelvis and bladder
Polycyclic hydrocarbons	Cancer of the lung, skin (especially squamous cell carcinoma of scrotal skin)
Radon gas	Lung cancer
Schistosomiasis	Bladder cancer (squamous cell)
Sunlight (ultraviolet)	Skin cancer (squamous cell and melanoma)
Tobacco (including smokeless)	Cancer of the upper aerodigestive tract, bladder
Vinyl chloride	Liver cancer (angiosarcoma)

[a]Agents that are thought to act as cancer initiators and/or promoters.

CHEMOPREVENTION OF CANCERS OF THE UPPER AERODIGESTIVE TRACT

Smoking causes diffuse epithelial injury in the oral cavity, neck, esophagus, and lung. Patients cured of squamous cell cancers of the lung, esophagus, oral cavity, and neck are at risk (as high as 5% per year) of developing second cancers of the upper aerodigestive tract. Cessation of cigarette smoking does not markedly decrease the cured cancer patient's risk of second malignancy, even though it does lower the cancer risk in those who have never developed a malignancy. Smoking cessation may halt the early stages of the carcinogenic process (such as metaplasia), but it may have no effect on late stages of carcinogenesis. This "field carcinogenesis" hypothesis for upper aerodigestive tract cancer has made "cured" patients an important population for chemoprevention of second malignancies.

Oral human papilloma virus (HPV) infection, particularly HPV-16, increases the risk for cancers of the oropharynx. This association exists even in the absence of other risk factors such as smoking or alcohol use (although the magnitude of increased risk appears greater than additive when HPV infection and smoking are both present). Oral HPV infection is believed to be largely sexually acquired. Although no direct evidence currently exists to confirm the hypothesis, the introduction of the HPV vaccine may eventually reduce oropharyngeal cancer rates.

Oral leukoplakia, a premalignant lesion commonly found in smokers, has been used as an intermediate marker of chemopreventive activity in smaller shorter-duration, randomized, placebo-controlled trials. Response was associated with upregulation of retinoic acid receptor-β (RAR-β). Therapy with high, relatively toxic doses of isotretinoin (13-*cis*-retinoic acid) causes regression of oral leukoplakia. However, the lesions recur when the therapy is withdrawn, suggesting the need for long-term administration. More tolerable doses of isotretinoin have not shown benefit in the prevention of head and neck cancer. Isotretinoin also failed to prevent second malignancies in patients cured of early-stage non-small cell lung cancer; mortality rates were actually increased in current smokers.

Several large-scale trials have assessed agents in the chemoprevention of lung cancer in patients at high risk. In the α-tocopherol/β-carotene (ATBC) Lung Cancer Prevention Trial, participants were male smokers, age 50–69 years at entry. Participants had smoked an average of one pack of cigarettes per day for 35.9 years. Participants received α-tocopherol, β-carotene, and/or placebo in a randomized, two-by-two factorial design. After median follow-up of 6.1 years, lung cancer incidence and mortality were statistically significantly increased in those receiving β-carotene. α-Tocopherol had no effect on lung cancer mortality, and no evidence suggested interaction between the two drugs. Patients receiving α-tocopherol had a higher incidence of hemorrhagic stroke.

The β-Carotene and Retinol Efficacy Trial (CARET) involved 17,000 American smokers and workers with asbestos exposure. Entrants were randomly assigned to one of four arms and received β-carotene, retinol, and/or placebo in a two-by-two factorial design. This trial also demonstrated harm from β-carotene: a lung cancer rate of 5 per 1000 subjects per year for those taking placebo and of 6 per 1000 subjects per year for those taking β-carotene.

The ATBC and CARET results demonstrate the importance of testing chemoprevention hypotheses thoroughly before their widespread implementation because the results contradict a number of observational studies. The Physicians' Health Trial showed no change in the risk of lung cancer for those taking β-carotene; however, fewer of its participants were smokers than those in the ATBC and CARET studies.

CHEMOPREVENTION OF COLON CANCER

Many colon cancer prevention trials are based on the premise that most colorectal cancers develop from adenomatous polyps. These trials use adenoma recurrence or disappearance as a surrogate endpoint (not yet validated) for colon cancer prevention. Early clinical trial results suggest that nonsteroidal anti-inflammatory drugs (NSAIDs), such as piroxicam, sulindac, and aspirin, may prevent adenoma formation or cause regression of adenomatous polyps. The mechanism of action of NSAIDs is unknown, but they are presumed to work through the cyclooxygenase pathway. Although two randomized controlled trials (the Physicians' Health Study and the Women's Health Study) did not show an effect of aspirin on colon cancer or adenoma incidence in persons with no previous history of colonic lesions after 10 years of therapy, these trials did show an approximately 18% relative risk reduction for colonic adenoma incidence in persons with a previous history of adenomas after 1 year. Pooled findings from observational cohort studies do demonstrate a 22% and 28% relative reduction in colorectal cancer and adenoma incidence, respectively, with regular aspirin use, and a well-conducted meta-analysis of four randomized controlled trials (albeit primarily designed to examine aspirin's effects on cardiovascular events) found that aspirin at doses of at least 75 mg resulted in a 24% relative reduction in colorectal cancer incidence after 20 years, with no clear increase in efficacy at higher doses. Cyclooxygenase-2 (COX-2) inhibitors have also been considered for colorectal cancer and polyp prevention. Trials with COX-2 inhibitors were initiated, but an increased risk of cardiovascular events in those taking the COX-2 inhibitors was noted, suggesting that these agents are not suitable for chemoprevention in the general population.

Epidemiologic studies suggest that diets high in calcium lower colon cancer risk. Calcium binds bile and fatty acids, which cause proliferation of colonic epithelium. It is hypothesized that calcium reduces intraluminal exposure to these compounds. The randomized controlled Calcium Polyp Prevention Study found that calcium supplementation decreased the absolute risk of adenomatous polyp recurrence by 7% at 4 years; extended observational follow-up demonstrated a 12% absolute risk reduction 5 years after cessation of treatment. However, in the Women's Health Initiative, combined use of calcium carbonate and vitamin D twice daily did not reduce the incidence of invasive colorectal cancer compared with placebo after 7 years.

The Women's Health Initiative demonstrated that postmenopausal women taking estrogen plus progestin have a 44% lower relative risk of colorectal cancer compared to women taking placebo. Of >16,600 women randomized and followed for a median of 5.6 years, 43 invasive colorectal cancers occurred in the hormone group and 72 in the placebo group. The positive effect on colon cancer is mitigated by the modest increase in cardiovascular and breast cancer risks associated with combined estrogen plus progestin therapy.

A case-control study suggested that statins decrease the incidence of colorectal cancer; however, several subsequent case-control and cohort studies have not demonstrated an association between regular statin use and a reduced risk of colorectal cancer. No randomized controlled trials have addressed this hypothesis. A meta-analysis of statin use showed no protective effect of statins on overall cancer incidence or death.

CHEMOPREVENTION OF BREAST CANCER

Tamoxifen is an antiestrogen with partial estrogen agonistic activity in some tissues, such as endometrium and bone. One of its actions is to upregulate transforming growth factor β, which decreases breast cell proliferation. In randomized placebo-controlled trials to assess tamoxifen as adjuvant therapy for breast cancer, tamoxifen reduced the number of new breast cancers in the opposite breast by more than a third. In a randomized placebo-controlled prevention trial involving >13,000 pre- and postmenopausal women at high risk, tamoxifen decreased the risk of developing breast cancer by 49% (from 43.4 to 22 per 1000 women) after a median follow-up of nearly 6 years. Tamoxifen also reduced bone fractures; a small increase in risk of endometrial cancer, stroke, pulmonary emboli, and deep vein thrombosis was noted. The International Breast Cancer Intervention Study (IBIS-I) and the Italian Randomized Tamoxifen Prevention Trial also demonstrated a reduction in breast cancer incidence with tamoxifen use. A trial comparing tamoxifen with another selective estrogen receptor modulator, raloxifene, in postmenopausal women showed that raloxifene is comparable to tamoxifen in cancer prevention. This trial only included postmenopausal women. Raloxifene was associated with more invasive breast cancers and a trend toward more noninvasive breast cancers, but fewer thromboembolic events than tamoxifen; the drugs are similar in risks of other cancers, fractures, ischemic heart disease, and stroke. Both tamoxifen and raloxifene (the latter for postmenopausal women only) have been approved by the U.S. Food and Drug Administration (FDA) for reduction of breast cancer in women at high risk for the disease (1.66% risk at 5 years based on the Gail risk model: *http://www.cancer.gov/bcrisktool/*).

Because the aromatase inhibitors are even more effective than tamoxifen in adjuvant breast cancer therapy, it has been hypothesized that they would be more effective in breast cancer prevention. A randomized, placebo-controlled trial of exemestane reported a 65% relative reduction (from 5.5 to 1.9 per 1000 women) in the incidence of invasive breast cancer in women at elevated risk after a median follow-up of about 3 years. Common adverse effects included arthralgias, hot flashes, fatigue, and insomnia. No trial has directly compared aromatase inhibitors with selective estrogen receptor modulators for breast cancer chemoprevention.

CHEMOPREVENTION OF PROSTATE CANCER

Finasteride and dutasteride are 5-α-reductase inhibitors. They inhibit conversion of testosterone to dihydrotestosterone (DHT), a potent stimulator of prostate cell proliferation. The Prostate Cancer Prevention Trial (PCPT) randomly assigned men age 55 years or older at average risk of prostate cancer to finasteride or placebo. All men in the trial were being regularly screened with prostate-specific antigen (PSA) levels and digital rectal examination. After 7 years of therapy, the incidence of prostate cancer was 18.4% in the finasteride arm, compared with 24.4% in the placebo arm, a statistically significant difference. However, the finasteride group had more patients with tumors of Gleason score 7 and higher compared with the placebo arm (6.4 vs 5.1%). Reassuringly, long-term (10–15 years) follow-up did not reveal any statistically significant differences in overall mortality between all men in the finasteride and placebo arms or in men diagnosed with prostate cancer; differences in prostate cancer in favor of finasteride persisted.

Dutasteride has also been evaluated as a preventive agent for prostate cancer. The Reduction by Dutasteride of Prostate Cancer Events (REDUCE) trial was a randomized double-blind trial in which approximately 8200 men with an elevated PSA (2.5–10 ng/mL for men age 50–60 years and 3–10 ng/mL for men age 60 years or older) and negative prostate biopsy on enrollment received daily 0.5 mg of dutasteride or placebo. The trial found a statistically significant 23% relative risk reduction in the incidence of biopsy-detected prostate cancer in the dutasteride arm at 4 years of treatment (659 cases vs 858 cases, respectively). Overall, across years 1 through 4, there was no difference between the arms in the number of tumors with a Gleason score of 7 to 10; however, during years 3 and 4, there was a statistically significant difference in tumors with Gleason score of 8 to 10 in the dutasteride arm (12 tumors vs 1 tumor, respectively).

The clinical importance of the apparent increased incidence of higher-grade tumors in the 5-α-reductase inhibitor arms of these trials is controversial. It may likely represent an increased sensitivity of PSA and digital rectal exam for high-grade tumors in men receiving these agents. The FDA has analyzed both trials, and it determined that the use of a 5-α-reductase inhibitor for prostate cancer chemoprevention would result in one additional high-grade (Gleason score 8 to 10) prostate cancer for every three to four lower-grade (Gleason score <6) tumors averted. Although it acknowledged that detection bias may have accounted for the finding, it stated that it could not conclusively dismiss a causative role for 5-α-reductase inhibitors. These agents are therefore not FDA-approved for prostate cancer prevention.

Because all men in both the PCPT and REDUCE trials were being screened and because screening approximately doubles the rate of prostate cancer, it is not known if finasteride or dutasteride decreases the risk of prostate cancer in men who are not being screened.

Several favorable laboratory and observational studies led to the formal evaluation of selenium and α-tocopherol (vitamin E) as potential prostate cancer preventives. The Selenium and Vitamin E Cancer Prevention Trial (SELECT) assigned 35,533 men to receive 200 μg/d selenium, 400 IU/d α-tocopherol, selenium plus vitamin E, or placebo. After a median follow-up of 7 years, a trend toward an increased risk of developing prostate cancer was observed for those men taking vitamin E alone as compared to the placebo arm (hazard ratio 1.17; 95% confidence interval, 1.004–1.36).

VACCINES AND CANCER PREVENTION

A number of infectious agents cause cancer. Hepatitis B and C are linked to liver cancer; some HPV strains are linked to cervical, anal, and head and neck cancer; and *Helicobacter pylori* is associated with gastric adenocarcinoma and gastric lymphoma. Vaccines to protect against these agents may reduce the risk of their associated cancers.

The hepatitis B vaccine is effective in preventing hepatitis and hepatomas due to chronic hepatitis B infection.

A quadrivalent HPV vaccine (covering HPV strains 6, 11, 16, and 18) and a bivalent vaccine (covering HPV strains 16 and 18) are available for use in the United States. HPV types 16 and 18 cause cervical and anal cancer; reduction in these HPV types could prevent >70% of cervical cancers worldwide. HPV types 6 and 11 cause genital papillomas. For individuals not previously infected with these HPV strains, the vaccines demonstrate high efficacy in preventing persistent strain-specific HPV infections; however, the trials and substudies that evaluated the vaccines' ability to prevent cervical and anal cancer relied on surrogate outcome measures (cervical or anal intraepithelial neoplasia [CIN/AIN] I, II, and III), and the degree of durability of the immune response beyond 5 years is not currently known. The vaccines do not appear to impact preexisting infections and the efficacy appears to be markedly lower for populations that had previously been exposed to vaccine-specific HPV strains. The vaccine is recommended in the United States for females and males age 9–26 years.

SURGICAL PREVENTION OF CANCER

Some organs in some individuals are at such high risk of developing cancer that surgical removal of the organ at risk may be considered. Women with severe cervical dysplasia are treated with laser or loop electrosurgical excision or conization and occasionally even hysterectomy. Colectomy is used to prevent colon cancer in patients with familial polyposis or ulcerative colitis.

Prophylactic bilateral mastectomy may be chosen for breast cancer prevention among women with genetic predisposition to breast cancer. In a prospective series of 139 women with *BRCA1* and *BRCA2* mutations, 76 chose to undergo prophylactic mastectomy and 63 chose close surveillance. At 3 years, no cases of breast cancer had been diagnosed in those opting for surgery, but eight patients in the surveillance group had developed breast cancer. A larger (n = 639) retrospective cohort study reported that three patients developed breast cancer after prophylactic mastectomy compared with an expected incidence of 30–53 cases: a 90–94% reduction in breast cancer risk. Postmastectomy breast cancer–related deaths were reduced by 81–94% for high-risk women compared with sister controls and by 100% for moderate-risk women when compared with expected rates.

Prophylactic oophorectomy may also be employed for the prevention of ovarian and breast cancers among high-risk women. A prospective cohort study evaluating the outcomes of *BRCA* mutation carriers demonstrated a statistically significant association between prophylactic oophorectomy and a reduced incidence of ovarian or primary peritoneal cancer (36% relative risk reduction, or a 4.5% absolute difference). Studies of prophylactic oophorectomy for prevention of breast cancer in women with genetic mutations have shown relative risk reductions of approximately 50%; the risk reduction may be greatest for women having the procedure at younger (i.e., <50 years) ages.

All of the evidence concerning the use of prophylactic mastectomy and oophorectomy for prevention of breast and ovarian cancer in high-risk women has been observational in nature; such studies are prone to a variety of biases, including case selection bias, family relationships between patients and controls, and inadequate information about hormone use. Thus, they may give an overestimate of the magnitude of benefit.

CANCER SCREENING

Screening is a means of detecting disease early in asymptomatic individuals, with the goal of decreasing morbidity and mortality. While screening can potentially reduce disease-specific deaths and has been shown to do so in cervical, colon, lung, and breast cancer, it is also subject to a number of biases that can suggest a benefit when actually there is none. Biases can even mask net harm. Early detection does not in itself confer benefit. Cause-specific mortality, rather than survival after diagnosis, is the preferred endpoint (see below).

Because screening is done on asymptomatic, healthy persons, it should offer substantial likelihood of benefit that outweighs harm. Screening tests and their appropriate use should be carefully evaluated before their use is widely encouraged in screening programs, as a matter of public policy.

A large and increasing number of genetic mutations and nucleotide polymorphisms have been associated with an increased risk of cancer. Testing for these genetic mutations could in theory define a high-risk population. However, most of the identified mutations have very low penetrance and individually provide minimal predictive accuracy. The ability to predict the development of a particular cancer may some day present therapeutic options as well as ethical dilemmas. It may eventually allow for early intervention to prevent a cancer or limit its severity. People at high risk may be ideal candidates for chemoprevention and screening; however, efficacy of these interventions in the high-risk population should be investigated. Currently, persons at high risk for a particular cancer can engage in intensive screening. While this course is clinically reasonable, it is not known if it reduces mortality in these populations.

TABLE 100-2 ASSESSMENT OF THE VALUE OF A DIAGNOSTIC TEST[a]

	Condition Present	Condition Absent
Positive test	*a*	*b*
Negative test	*c*	*d*
a = true positive		
b = false positive		
c = false negative		
d = true negative		
Sensitivity	The proportion of persons with the condition who test positive: $a/(a + c)$	
Specificity	The proportion of persons without the condition who test negative: $d/(b + d)$	
Positive predictive value (PPV)	The proportion of persons with a positive test who have the condition: $a/(a + b)$	
Negative predictive value	The proportion of persons with a negative test who do not have the condition: $d/(c + d)$	
Prevalence, sensitivity, and specificity determine PPV		

$$\text{PPV} = \frac{\text{prevalence} \times \text{sensitivity}}{(\text{prevalence} \times \text{sensitivity}) + (1 - \text{prevalence})(1 - \text{specificity})}$$

[a]For diseases of low prevalence, such as cancer, poor specificity has a dramatic adverse effect on PPV such that only a small fraction of positive tests are true positives.

The Accuracy of Screening A screening test's accuracy or ability to discriminate disease is described by four indices: sensitivity, specificity, positive predictive value, and negative predictive value (Table 100-2). *Sensitivity*, also called the true-positive rate, is the proportion of persons with the disease who test positive in the screen (i.e., the ability of the test to detect disease when it is present). *Specificity*, or 1 minus the false-positive rate, is the proportion of persons who do not have the disease that test negative in the screening test (i.e., the ability of a test to correctly identify that the disease is not present). The *positive predictive value* is the proportion of persons who test positive that actually have the disease. Similarly, *negative predictive value* is the proportion testing negative that do not have the disease. The sensitivity and specificity of a test are independent of the underlying prevalence (or risk) of the disease in the population screened, but the predictive values depend strongly on the prevalence of the disease.

Screening is most beneficial, efficient, and economical when the target disease is common in the population being screened. Specificity is at least as important to the ultimate feasibility and success of a screening test as sensitivity.

Potential Biases of Screening Tests Common biases of screening are lead time, length-biased sampling, and selection. These biases can make a screening test seem beneficial when actually it is not (or even causes net harm). Whether beneficial or not, screening can create the false impression of an epidemic by increasing the number of cancers diagnosed. It can also produce a shift in the proportion of patients diagnosed at an early stage and inflate survival statistics without reducing mortality (i.e., the number of deaths from a given cancer relative to the number of those at risk for the cancer). In such a case, the *apparent* duration of survival (measured from date of diagnosis) increases without lives being saved or life expectancy changed.

Lead-time bias occurs whether or not a test influences the natural history of the disease; the patient is merely diagnosed at an earlier date. Survival *appears* increased even if life is not really prolonged. The screening test only prolongs the time the subject is aware of the disease and spends as a patient.

Length-biased sampling occurs because screening tests generally can more easily detect slow-growing, less aggressive cancers than fast-growing cancers. Cancers diagnosed due to the onset of symptoms between scheduled screenings are on average more aggressive, and treatment outcomes are not as favorable. An extreme form of length bias sampling is termed *overdiagnosis*, the detection of "pseudo disease." The reservoir of some undetected slow-growing tumors is large. Many of these tumors fulfill the histologic criteria of cancer but will never become clinically significant or cause death. This problem is compounded by the fact that the most common cancers appear most frequently at ages when competing causes of death are more frequent.

Selection bias must be considered in assessing the results of any screening effort. The population most likely to seek screening may differ from the general population to which the screening test might be applied. In general, volunteers for studies are more health conscious and likely to have a better prognosis or lower mortality rate, irrespective of the screening result. This is termed the *healthy volunteer effect*.

Potential Drawbacks of Screening Risks associated with screening include harm caused by the screening intervention itself, harm due to the further investigation of persons with positive tests (both true and false positives), and harm from the treatment of persons with a true-positive result, whether or not life is extended by treatment (e.g., even if a screening test reduces relative cause-specific mortality by 20–30%, 70–80% of those diagnosed still go on to die of the target cancer). The diagnosis and treatment of cancers that would never have caused medical problems can lead to the harm of unnecessary treatment and give patients the anxiety of a cancer diagnosis. The psychosocial impact of cancer screening can also be substantial when applied to the entire population.

Assessment of Screening Tests Good clinical trial design can offset some biases of screening and demonstrate the relative risks and benefits of a screening test. A randomized controlled screening trial with cause-specific mortality as the endpoint provides the strongest support for a screening intervention. Overall mortality should also be reported to detect an adverse effect of screening and treatment on other disease outcomes (e.g., cardiovascular disease). In a randomized trial, two like populations are randomly established. One is given the usual standard of care (which may be no screening at all) and the other receives the screening intervention being assessed. The two populations are compared over time. Efficacy for the population studied is established when the group receiving the screening test has a better cause-specific mortality rate than the control group. Studies showing a reduction in the incidence of advanced-stage disease, improved survival, or a stage shift are weaker (and possibly misleading) evidence of benefit. These latter criteria are early indicators but not sufficient to establish the value of a screening test.

Although a randomized, controlled screening trial provides the strongest evidence to support a screening test, it is not perfect. Unless the trial is population-based, it does not remove the question of generalizability to the target population. Screening trials generally involve thousands of persons and last for years. Less definitive study designs are therefore often used to estimate the effectiveness of screening practices. However, every nonrandomized study design is subject to strong confounders. In descending order of strength, evidence may also be derived from the findings of internally controlled trials using intervention allocation methods other than randomization (e.g., allocation by birth date, date of clinic visit); the findings of analytic observational studies; or the results of multiple time series studies with or without the intervention.

Screening for Specific Cancers Screening for cervical, colon, and breast cancer is beneficial for certain age groups. Depending on age and smoking history, lung cancer screening can also be beneficial in specific settings. Special surveillance of those at high risk for a specific cancer because of a family history or a genetic risk factor may be prudent, but few studies have assessed the influence on mortality. A number of organizations have considered whether or not to endorse routine use of certain screening tests. Because these groups have not used the same criteria to judge whether a screening test should be endorsed, they have arrived at different recommendations. The American Cancer Society (ACS) and the U.S. Preventive Services Task Force (USPSTF) publish screening guidelines (Table 100-3); the American Academy of Family Practitioners (AAFP) generally follow/endorse the USPSTF recommendations; and the American College of Physicians (ACP) develops recommendations based on structured reviews of other organizations' guidelines.

BREAST CANCER Breast self-examination, clinical breast examination by a caregiver, mammography, and magnetic resonance imaging (MRI) have all been variably advocated as useful screening tools.

A number of trials have suggested that annual or biennial screening with mammography or mammography plus clinical breast examination in normal-risk women older than age 50 years decreases breast cancer mortality. Each trial has been criticized for design flaws. In most trials, breast cancer mortality rate is decreased by 15–30%. Experts disagree on whether average-risk women age 40–49 years should receive regular screening (Table 100-3). The U.K. Age Trial, the only randomized trial of breast cancer screening to specifically evaluate the impact of mammography in women age 40–49 years, found no statistically significant difference in breast cancer mortality for screened women versus controls after about 11 years of follow-up (relative risk 0.83; 95% confidence interval 0.66–1.04); however, <70% of women received screening in the intervention arm, potentially diluting the observed effect. A meta-analysis of eight large randomized trials showed a 15% relative reduction in mortality (relative risk 0.85; 95% confidence interval 0.75–0.96) from mammography screening for women age 39–49 years after 11–20 years of follow-up. This is equivalent to a number needed to invite to screening of 1904 over 10 years to prevent one breast cancer death. At the same time, nearly half of women age 40–49 years screened annually will have false-positive mammograms necessitating further evaluation, often including biopsy. Estimates of overdiagnosis range from 10 to 40% of diagnosed invasive cancers. In the United States, widespread screening over the last several decades has not been accompanied by a reduction in incidence of metastatic breast cancer despite a large increase in early-stage disease, suggesting a substantial amount of overdiagnosis at the population level.

No study of breast self-examination has shown it to decrease mortality. A randomized controlled trial of approximately 266,000 women in China demonstrated no difference in breast cancer mortality between a group that received intensive breast self-exam instruction and reinforcement/reminders and controls at 10 years of follow-up. However, more benign breast lesions were discovered and more breast biopsies were performed in the self-examination arm.

Genetic screening for *BRCA1* and *BRCA2* mutations and other markers of breast cancer risk has identified a group of women at high risk for breast cancer. Unfortunately, when to begin and the optimal frequency of screening have not been defined. Mammography is less sensitive at detecting breast cancers in women carrying *BRCA1* and *BRCA2* mutations, possibly because such cancers occur in younger women, in whom mammography is known to be less sensitive. MRI screening may be more sensitive than mammography in women at high risk due to genetic predisposition or in women with very dense breast tissue, but specificity may be lower. An increase in overdiagnosis may accompany the higher sensitivity. The impact of MRI on breast cancer mortality with or without concomitant use of mammography has not been evaluated in a randomized controlled trial.

CERVICAL CANCER Screening with Papanicolaou (Pap) smears decreases cervical cancer mortality. The cervical cancer mortality rate has fallen substantially since the widespread use of the Pap smear. With the onset of sexual activity comes the risk of sexual transmission of HPV, the fundamental etiologic factor for cervical cancer. Screening guidelines recommend regular Pap testing for all women who have reached the age of 21 (prior to this age, even in individuals that have begun sexual activity, screening may cause more harm than benefit). The recommended interval for Pap screening is 3 years. Screening more frequently adds little benefit but leads to important harms, including unnecessary procedures and overtreatment of transient lesions. Beginning at age 30, guidelines also offer the alternative of combined Pap smear and HPV testing for women. The screening interval for women who test normal using this approach may be lengthened to 5 years.

An upper age limit at which screening ceases to be effective is not known, but women age 65 years with no abnormal results in the previous 10 years may choose to stop screening. Screening should be

TABLE 100-3 SCREENING RECOMMENDATIONS FOR ASYMPTOMATIC SUBJECTS NOT KNOWN TO BE AT INCREASED RISK FOR THE TARGET CONDITION[a]

Cancer Type	Test or Procedure	USPSTF	ACS
Breast	Self-examination	"D"	Women ≥20 years: Breast self-exam is an option
	Clinical examination	Women ≥40 years: "I" (as a stand-alone without mammography)	Women 20–39 years: Perform every 3 years Women ≥40 years: Perform annually
	Mammography	Women 40–49 years: The decision should be an individual one, and take patient context/values into account ("C") Women 50–74 years: Every 2 years ("B") Women ≥75 years: "I"	Women ≥40 years: Screen annually for as long as the woman is in good health
	Magnetic resonance imaging (MRI)	"I"	Women with >20% lifetime risk of breast cancer: Screen with MRI plus mammography annually Women with 15–20% lifetime risk of breast cancer: Discuss option of MRI plus mammography annually Women with <15% lifetime risk of breast cancer: Do not screen annually with MRI
Cervical	Pap test (cytology)	Women 21–65 years: Screen every 3 years ("A") Women <21 years: "D" Women >65 years, with adequate, normal prior Pap screenings: "D" Women after total hysterectomy for noncancerous causes: "D"	Women 21–29 years: Screen every 3 years Women 30–65 years: Acceptable approach to screen with cytology every 3 years (see HPV test below) Women <21 years: No screening Women >65 years: No screening following adequate negative prior screening Women after total hysterectomy for noncancerous causes: Do not screen
	HPV test	Women 30–65 years: Screen in combination with cytology every 5 years if woman desires to lengthen the screening interval (see Pap test, above) ("A") Women <30 years: "D" Women >65 years, with adequate, normal prior Pap screenings: "D" Women after total hysterectomy for noncancerous causes: "D"	Women 30–65 years: Preferred approach to screen with HPV and cytology co-testing every 5 years (see Pap test above) Women <30 years: Do not use HPV testing Women >65 years: No screening following adequate negative prior screening Women after total hysterectomy for noncancerous causes: Do not screen
Colorectal	Sigmoidoscopy	Adults 50–75 years: every 5 years in combination with high-sensitivity FOBT every 3 years ("A")[b] Adults 76–85 years: "C" Adults ≥85 years: "D"	Adults ≥50 years: Screen every 5 years
	Fecal occult blood testing (FOBT)	Adults 50–75 years. Annually, for high-sensitivity FOBT ("A") Adults 76–85 years: "C" Adults ≥85 years: "D"	Adults ≥50 years: Screen every year
	Colonoscopy	Adults 50–75 years: every 10 years ("A") Adults 76–85 years: "C" Adults ≥85 years: "D"	Adults ≥50 years: Screen every 10 years
	Fecal DNA testing	"I"	Adults ≥50 years: Screen, but interval uncertain
	Fecal immuno-chemical testing (FIT)	"I"	Adults ≥50 years: Screen every year
	CT colonography	"I"	Adults ≥50 years: Screen every 5 years
Lung	Low-dose computed tomography (CT) scan	Adults 55–80 years, with a ≥30 pack-year smoking history, still smoking or have quit within past 15 years. Discontinue once a person has not smoked for 15 years or develops a health problem that substantially limits life expectancy or the ability to have curative lung surgery: "B"	Men and women, 55–74 years, with ≥30 pack-year smoking history, still smoking or have quit within past 15 years: Discuss benefits, limitations, and potential harms of screening; only perform screening in facilities with the right type of CT scanner and with high expertise/specialists
Ovarian	CA-125	"D"	There is no sufficiently accurate test proven effective in the early detection of ovarian cancer. For women at high risk of ovarian cancer and/or who have unexplained, persistent symptoms, the combination of CA-125 and transvaginal ultrasound with pelvic exam may be offered.
	Transvaginal ultrasound	"D"	

(Continued)

TABLE 100-3 SCREENING RECOMMENDATIONS FOR ASYMPTOMATIC SUBJECTS NOT KNOWN TO BE AT INCREASED RISK FOR THE TARGET CONDITION[a] (CONTINUED)

Cancer Type	Test or Procedure	USPSTF	ACS
Prostate	Prostate-specific antigen (PSA)	Men, all ages: "D"	Starting at age 50, men should talk to a doctor about the pros and cons of testing so they can decide if testing is the right choice for them. If African American or have a father or brother who had prostate cancer before age 65, men should have this talk starting at age 45. How often they are tested will depend on their PSA level.
	Digital rectal examination (DRE)	No individual recommendation	As for PSA; if men decide to be tested, they should have the PSA blood test with or without a rectal exam
Skin	Complete skin examination by clinician or patient	"I"	Self-examination monthly; clinical exam as part of routine cancer-related checkup

[a]Summary of the screening procedures recommended for the general population by the USPSTF and the ACS. These recommendations refer to asymptomatic persons who are not known to have risk factors, other than age or gender, for the targeted condition. [b]USPSTF lettered recommendations are defined as follows: "A": The USPSTF recommends the service, because there is high certainty that the net benefit is substantial; "B": The USPSTF recommends the service, because there is high certainty that the net benefit is moderate or moderate certainty that the net benefit is moderate to substantial; "C": The USPSTF recommends selectively offering or providing this service to individual patients based on professional judgment and patient preferences; there is at least moderate certainty that the net benefit is small; "D": The USPSTF recommends against the service because there is moderate or high certainty that the service has no net benefit or that the harms outweigh the benefits; "I": The USPSTF concludes that the current evidence is insufficient to assess the balance of benefits and harms of the service.

Abbreviations: ACS, American Cancer Society; USPSTF, U.S. Preventive Services Task Force.

discontinued in women who have undergone a hysterectomy for noncancerous reasons.

Although the efficacy of the Pap smear in reducing cervical cancer mortality has never been directly confirmed in a randomized, controlled setting, a clustered randomized trial in India evaluated the impact of one-time cervical visual inspection and immediate colposcopy, biopsy, and/or cryotherapy (where indicated) versus counseling on cervical cancer deaths in women age 30–59 years. After 7 years of follow-up, the age-standardized rate of death due to cervical cancer was 39.6 per 100,000 person-years in the intervention group versus 56.7 per 100,000 person-years in controls.

COLORECTAL CANCER Fecal occult blood testing (FOBT), digital rectal examination (DRE), rigid and flexible sigmoidoscopy, colonoscopy, and computed tomography (CT) colonography have been considered for colorectal cancer screening. A meta-analysis of four randomized controlled trials demonstrated a 15% relative reduction in colorectal cancer mortality with FOBT. The sensitivity for FOBT is increased if specimens are rehydrated before testing, but at the cost of lower specificity. The false-positive rate for rehydrated FOBT is high; 1–5% of persons tested have a positive test. Only 2–10% of those with occult blood in the stool have cancer. The high false-positive rate of FOBT dramatically increases the number of colonoscopies performed.

Fecal immunochemical tests appear to have higher sensitivity for colorectal cancer than nonrehydrated FOBT tests. Fecal DNA testing is an emerging testing modality; it may have increased sensitivity and comparable specificity to FOBT and could potentially reduce harms associated with follow-up of false-positive tests. The body of evidence on the operating characteristics and effectiveness of fecal DNA tests in reducing colorectal cancer mortality is limited.

Two meta-analyses of five randomized controlled trials of sigmoidoscopy (i.e., the NORCCAP, SCORE, PLCO, Telemark, and U.K. trials) found an 18% relative reduction in colorectal cancer incidence and a 28% relative reduction in colorectal cancer mortality. Participant ages ranged from 50 to 74 years, with follow-up ranging from 6 to 13 years. Diagnosis of adenomatous polyps by sigmoidoscopy should lead to evaluation of the entire colon with colonoscopy. The most efficient interval for screening sigmoidoscopy is unknown, but an interval of 5 years is often recommended. Case-control studies suggest that intervals of up to 15 years may confer benefit; the U.K. trial demonstrated benefit with one-time screening.

One-time colonoscopy detects ~25% more advanced lesions (polyps >10 mm, villous adenomas, adenomatous polyps with high-grade dysplasia, invasive cancer) than one-time FOBT with sigmoidoscopy; comparative *programmatic* performance of the two modalities over time is not known. Perforation rates are about 3/1000 for colonoscopy and 1/1000 for sigmoidoscopy. Debate continues on whether colonoscopy is too expensive and invasive and whether sufficient provider capacity exists to be recommended as the preferred screening tool in standard-risk populations. Some observational studies suggest that efficacy of colonoscopy to decrease colorectal cancer mortality is primarily limited to the left side of the colon.

CT colonography, if done at expert centers, appears to have a sensitivity for polyps ≥6 mm comparable to colonoscopy. However, the rate of extracolonic findings of abnormalities of uncertain significance that must nevertheless be worked up is high (~15–30%); the long-term cumulative radiation risk of repeated colonography screenings is also a concern.

LUNG CANCER Chest x-ray and sputum cytology have been evaluated in several randomized lung cancer screening trials. The most recent and largest (n = 154,901) of these, one substudy of the Prostate, Lung, Colorectal, and Ovarian (PLCO) cancer screening trial, found that, compared with usual care, annual chest x-ray did not reduce the risk of dying from lung cancer (relative risk 0.99; 95% confidence interval 0.87–1.22) after 13 years. Low-dose CT has also been evaluated in several randomized trials. The largest and longest of these, the National Lung Screening Trial (NLST), was a randomized controlled trial of screening for lung cancer in approximately 53,000 persons age 55–74 years with a 30+ pack-year smoking history. It demonstrated a statistically significant relative reduction of about 15–20% in lung cancer mortality in the CT arm compared to the chest x-ray arm (or about 3 fewer deaths per 1000 people screened with CT). However, the harms include the potential radiation risks associated with multiple scans, the discovery of incidental findings of unclear significance, and a high rate of false-positive test results. Both incidental findings and false-positive tests can lead to invasive diagnostic procedures associated with anxiety, expense, and complications (e.g., pneumo- or hemothorax after lung biopsy). The NLST was performed at experienced screening centers, and the balance of benefits and harms may differ in the community setting at less experienced centers.

OVARIAN CANCER Adnexal palpation, transvaginal ultrasound (TVUS), and serum CA-125 assay have been considered for ovarian cancer screening. A large randomized controlled trial has shown that an annual screening program of TVUS and CA-125 in average-risk women does not reduce deaths from ovarian cancer (relative risk 1.21; 95% confidence interval 0.99–1.48). Adnexal palpation was dropped early in the study because it did not detect any ovarian cancers that were not detected by either TVUS or CA-125. The risks and costs associated with the high number of false-positive results are impediments to routine use of these modalities for screening. In the PLCO trial, 10% of participants had a false-positive result from TVUS or CA-125, and one-third of these women underwent a major surgical procedure; the ratio of surgeries to screen-detected ovarian cancer was approximately 20:1.

PROSTATE CANCER The most common prostate cancer screening modalities are DRE and serum PSA assay. An emphasis on PSA screening has caused prostate cancer to become the most common nonskin cancer diagnosed in American males. This disease is prone to lead-time bias, length bias, and overdiagnosis, and substantial debate continues among experts as to whether screening should be offered unless the patient specifically asks to be screened. Virtually all organizations stress the importance of informing men about the uncertainty regarding screening efficacy and the harms associated with screening. Prostate cancer screening clearly detects many asymptomatic cancers, but the ability to distinguish tumors that are lethal but still curable from those that pose little or no threat to health is limited, and randomized trials indicate that the effect of PSA screening on prostate cancer mortality across a population is, at best, small. Men older than age 50 years have a high prevalence of indolent, clinically insignificant prostate cancers (about 30–50% of men, increasing further as men age).

Two major randomized controlled trials of the impact of PSA screening on prostate cancer mortality have been published. The PLCO Cancer Screening Trial was a multicenter U.S. trial that randomized almost 77,000 men age 55–74 years to receive either annual PSA testing for 6 years or usual care. At 13 years of follow-up, no statistically significant difference in the number of prostate cancer deaths were noted between the arms (rate ratio 1.09; 95% confidence interval 0.87–1.36). Approximately 50% of men in the control arm received at least one PSA test during the trial, which may have potentially diluted a small effect.

The European Randomized Study of Screening for Prostate Cancer (ERSPC) was a multinational study that randomized approximately 182,000 men between age 50 and 74 years (with a predefined "core" screening group of men age 55–69 years) to receive PSA testing or no screening. Recruitment and randomization procedures, as well as actual frequency of PSA testing, varied by country. After a median follow-up of 11 years, a 20% relative reduction in the risk of prostate cancer death in the screened arm was noted in the "core" screening group. The trial found that 1055 men would need to be invited to screening, and 37 cases of prostate cancer detected, to avert 1 death from prostate cancer. Of the seven countries included in the mortality analysis, two demonstrated statistically significant reductions in prostate cancer deaths, whereas five did not. There was also an imbalance in treatment between the two study arms, with a higher proportion of men with clinically localized cancer receiving radical prostatectomy in the screening arm and receiving it at experienced referral centers.

Treatments for low-stage prostate cancer, such as surgery and radiation therapy, can cause significant morbidity, including impotence and urinary incontinence. In a trial conducted in the United States after the initiation of widespread PSA testing, random assignment to radical prostatectomy compared with "watchful waiting" did not result in a statistically significant decrease in prostate cancer deaths (absolute risk reduction 2.7%; 95% confidence interval–1.3 to 6.2%).

SKIN CANCER Visual examination of all skin surfaces by the patient or by a health care provider is used in screening for basal and squamous cell cancers and melanoma. No prospective randomized study has been performed to look for a mortality decrease. Unfortunately, screening is associated with a substantial rate of overdiagnosis.

101e Cancer Genetics

Pat J. Morin, Jeffrey M. Trent, Francis S. Collins, Bert Vogelstein

This is a digital-only chapter. It is available on the DVD that accompanies this book, as well as on Access Medicine/Harrison's Online, and the eBook and "app" editions of HPIM 19e.

CANCER IS A GENETIC DISEASE

Cancer arises through a series of somatic alterations in DNA that result in unrestrained cellular proliferation. Most of these alterations involve actual sequence changes in DNA (i.e., mutations). They may originate as a consequence of random replication errors, exposure to carcinogens (e.g., radiation), or faulty DNA repair processes. While most cancers arise sporadically, familial clustering of cancers occurs in certain families that carry a germline mutation in a cancer gene.

102e Cancer Cell Biology

Jeffrey W. Clark, Dan L. Longo

This is a digital-only chapter. It is available on the DVD that accompanies this book, as well as on Access Medicine/Harrison's Online, and the eBook and "app" editions of HPIM 19e.

Cancers are characterized by unregulated cell division, avoidance of cell death, tissue invasion, and the ability to metastasize. A neoplasm is *benign* when it grows in an unregulated fashion without tissue invasion. The presence of unregulated growth and tissue invasion is characteristic of *malignant* neoplasms. Cancers are named based on their origin: those derived from epithelial tissue are called *carcinomas*, those derived from mesenchymal tissues are *sarcomas*, and those derived from hematopoietic tissue are *leukemias, lymphomas*, and *plasma cell dyscrasias* (including *multiple myeloma*).

Cancers nearly always arise as a consequence of genetic alterations, the vast majority of which begin in a single cell and therefore are monoclonal in origin. However, because a wide variety of genetic and epigenetic changes can occur in different cells within malignant tumors over time, most cancers are characterized by marked heterogeneity in the populations of cells. This heterogeneity significantly complicates the treatment of most cancers because it is likely that there are subsets of cells that will be resistant to therapy and will therefore survive and proliferate even if the majority of cells are killed.

103e Principles of Cancer Treatment

Edward A. Sausville, Dan L. Longo

This is a digital-only chapter. It is available on the DVD that accompanies this book, as well as on Access Medicine/Harrison's Online, and the eBook and "app" editions of HPIM 19e.

CANCER PRESENTATION

Cancer in a localized or systemic state is a frequent item in the differential diagnosis of a variety of common complaints. Although not all forms of cancer are curable at diagnosis, affording patients the greatest opportunity for cure or meaningful prolongation of life is greatly aided by diagnosing cancer at the earliest point possible in its natural history and defining treatments that prevent or retard its systemic spread. Indeed, certain forms of cancer, notably breast, colon, and possibly lung cancers in certain patients, can be prevented by screening appropriately selected asymptomatic patients; screening is arguably the earliest point in the spectrum of possible cancer-related interventions where cure is possible.

104 Infections in Patients with Cancer

Robert W. Finberg

Infections are a common cause of death and an even more common cause of morbidity in patients with a wide variety of neoplasms. Autopsy studies show that most deaths from acute leukemia and half of deaths from lymphoma are caused directly by infection. With more intensive chemotherapy, patients with solid tumors have also become more likely to die of infection. Fortunately, an evolving approach to prevention and treatment of infectious complications of cancer has decreased infection-associated mortality rates and will probably continue to do so. This accomplishment has resulted from three major steps:

1. The practice of using "early empirical" antibiotics reduced mortality rates among patients with leukemia and bacteremia from 84% in 1965 to 44% in 1972. Recent studies suggest that the mortality rate due to infection in febrile neutropenic patients dropped to <10% by 2013. This dramatic improvement is attributed to early intervention with appropriate antimicrobial therapy.
2. "Empirical" antifungal therapy has also lowered the incidence of disseminated fungal infection, with dramatic decreases in mortality rates. An antifungal agent is administered—on the basis of likely fungal infection—to neutropenic patients who, after 4–7 days of antibiotic therapy, remain febrile but have no positive cultures.
3. Use of antibiotics for afebrile neutropenic patients as broad-spectrum prophylaxis against infections has decreased both mortality and morbidity even further. The current approach to treatment of severely neutropenic patients (e.g., those receiving high-dose chemotherapy for leukemia or high-grade lymphoma) is based on initial prophylactic therapy at the onset of neutropenia, subsequent "empirical" antibacterial therapy targeting the organisms whose involvement is likely in light of physical findings (most often fever alone), and finally "empirical" antifungal therapy based on the known likelihood that fungal infection will become a serious issue after 4–7 days of broad-spectrum antibacterial therapy.

A physical predisposition to infection in patients with cancer (Table 104-1) can be a result of the neoplasm's production of a break in the skin. For example, a squamous cell carcinoma may cause local invasion of the epidermis, which allows bacteria to gain access to subcutaneous tissue and permits the development of cellulitis. The artificial closing of a normally patent orifice can also predispose to infection; for example, obstruction of a ureter by a tumor can cause urinary tract infection, and obstruction of the bile duct can cause cholangitis. Part of the host's normal defense against infection depends on the continuous emptying of a viscus; without emptying, a few bacteria that are present as a result of bacteremia or local transit can multiply and cause disease.

A similar problem can affect patients whose lymph node integrity has been disrupted by radical surgery, particularly patients who have had radical node dissections. A common clinical problem following radical mastectomy is the development of cellulitis (usually caused by streptococci or staphylococci) because of lymphedema and/or inadequate lymph drainage. In most cases, this problem can be addressed by local measures designed to prevent fluid accumulation and breaks in the skin, but antibiotic prophylaxis has been necessary in refractory cases.

A life-threatening problem common to many cancer patients is the loss of the reticuloendothelial capacity to clear microorganisms after splenectomy, which may be performed as part of the management of hairy cell leukemia, chronic lymphocytic leukemia (CLL), and chronic myelogenous leukemia (CML) and in Hodgkin's disease. Even after curative therapy for the underlying disease, the lack of a spleen predisposes such patients to rapidly fatal infections. The loss of the spleen through trauma similarly predisposes the normal host to overwhelming infection throughout life. The splenectomized patient should be counseled about the risks of infection with certain organisms, such as the protozoan *Babesia* (Chap. 249) and *Capnocytophaga canimorsus*, a bacterium carried in the mouths of animals (Chaps. 167e and 183e). Because encapsulated bacteria (*Streptococcus pneumoniae*, *Haemophilus influenzae*, and *Neisseria meningitidis*) are the organisms most commonly associated with postsplenectomy sepsis, splenectomized persons should be vaccinated (and revaccinated; Table 104-2 and Chap. 148) against the capsular polysaccharides of these organisms. Many clinicians recommend giving splenectomized patients a small supply of antibiotics effective against *S. pneumoniae*, *N. meningitidis*, and *H. influenzae* to avert rapid, overwhelming sepsis in the event that they cannot present for medical attention immediately after the onset of fever or other signs or symptoms of bacterial infection. A few tablets of amoxicillin/clavulanic acid (or levofloxacin if resistant strains of *S. pneumoniae* are prevalent locally) are a reasonable choice for this purpose.

TABLE 104-1 DISRUPTION OF NORMAL BARRIERS THAT MAY PREDISPOSE TO INFECTIONS IN PATIENTS WITH CANCER

Type of Defense	Specific Lesion	Cells Involved	Organism	Cancer Association	Disease
Physical barrier	Breaks in skin	Skin epithelial cells	Staphylococci, streptococci	Head and neck, squamous cell carcinoma	Cellulitis, extensive skin infection
Emptying of fluid collections	Occlusion of orifices: ureters, bile duct, colon	Luminal epithelial cells	Gram-negative bacilli	Renal, ovarian, biliary tree, metastatic diseases of many cancers	Rapid, overwhelming bacteremia; urinary tract infection
Lymphatic function	Node dissection	Lymph nodes	Staphylococci, streptococci	Breast cancer surgery	Cellulitis
Splenic clearance of microorganisms	Splenectomy	Splenic reticuloendothelial cells	*Streptococcus pneumoniae, Haemophilus influenzae, Neisseria meningitidis, Babesia, Capnocytophaga canimorsus*	Hodgkin's disease, leukemia	Rapid, overwhelming sepsis
Phagocytosis	Lack of granulocytes	Granulocytes (neutrophils)	Staphylococci, streptococci, enteric organisms, fungi	Acute myeloid and acute lymphocytic leukemias, hairy cell leukemia	Bacteremia
Humoral immunity	Lack of antibody	B cells	*S. pneumoniae, H. influenzae, N. meningitidis*	Chronic lymphocytic leukemia, multiple myeloma	Infections with encapsulated organisms, sinusitis, pneumonia
Cellular immunity	Lack of T cells	T cells and macrophages	*Mycobacterium tuberculosis, Listeria*, herpesviruses, fungi, intracellular parasites	Hodgkin's disease, leukemia, T cell lymphoma	Infections with intracellular bacteria, fungi, parasites; virus reactivation

TABLE 104-2 VACCINATION OF CANCER PATIENTS RECEIVING CHEMOTHERAPY[a]

	Use in Indicated Patients		
Vaccine	**Intensive Chemotherapy**	**Hodgkin's Disease**	**Hematopoietic Stem Cell Transplantation**
Diphtheria-tetanus[b]	Primary series and boosters as necessary	No special recommendation	3 doses given 6–12 months after transplantation
Poliomyelitis[c]	Complete primary series and boosters	No special recommendation	3 doses given 6–12 months after transplantation
Haemophilus influenzae type b conjugate	Primary series and booster for children	Single dose for adults	3 doses given 6–12 months after transplantation (separated by 1 month)
Human papillomavirus (HPV)	Quadrivalent HPV vaccine is approved for males and females 9–26 years of age. Check Centers for Disease Control and Prevention (CDC) website *(www.cdc.gov/vaccines)* for updated recommendations.	Quadrivalent HPV vaccine is approved for males and females 9–26 years of age. Check CDC website *(www.cdc.gov/vaccines)* for updated recommendations.	Quadrivalent HPV vaccine is approved for males and females 9–26 years of age. Check CDC website *(www.cdc.gov/vaccines)* for updated recommendations.
Hepatitis A	As indicated for normal hosts on the basis of occupation and lifestyle	As indicated for normal hosts on the basis of occupation and lifestyle	As indicated for normal hosts on the basis of occupation and lifestyle
Hepatitis B	Same as for normal hosts	As indicated for normal hosts on the basis of occupation and lifestyle	3 doses given 6–12 months after transplantation
Pneumococcal conjugate vaccine (PCV13) Pneumococcal polysaccharide vaccine (PPSV23)[d]	Finish series prior to chemotherapy if possible	Patients with splenectomy should receive PPSV23.	Three doses of PCV13, beginning 3–6 months after transplantation, are followed by a dose of PPSV23 at least 8 weeks later. A second PPSV23 dose can be given 5 years later.
Quadrivalent meningococcal vaccine[e]	Should be administered to splenectomized patients and to patients living in endemic areas, including college students in dormitories	Should be administered to splenectomized patients and to patients living in endemic areas, including college students in dormitories. An additional dose can be given after 5 years.	Should be administered to splenectomized patients and to patients living in endemic areas, including college students in dormitories. An additional dose can be given after 5 years.
Influenza	Seasonal immunization	Seasonal immunization	Seasonal Immunization (A seasonal dose is recommended and can be given as early as 4 months after transplantation; if given <6 months after transplantation, an additional dose is recommended.)
Measles/mumps/rubella	Contraindicated	Contraindicated during chemotherapy	After 24 months in patients without graft-versus-host disease
Varicella-zoster virus[f]	Contraindicated[g]	Contraindicated	Contraindicated (CDC recommends use on a case-by-case basis following reevaluation.)

[a]The latest recommendations by the Advisory Committee on Immunization Practices and the CDC guidelines can be found at *http://www.cdc.gov/vaccines*. [b]A single dose of TDaP (tetanus–diphtheria–acellular pertussis), followed by a booster dose of Td (tetanus-diphtheria) every 10 years, is recommended for adults. [c]Live-virus vaccine is contraindicated; inactivated vaccine should be used. [d]Two types of vaccine are used to prevent pneumococcal disease. A conjugate vaccine active against 13 serotypes (13-valent pneumococcal conjugate vaccine, or PCV13) is currently administered in three separate doses to all children. A polysaccharide vaccine active against 23 serotypes (23-valent pneumococcal polysaccharide vaccine, or PPSV23) elicits titers of antibody lower than those achieved with the conjugate vaccine, and immunity may wane more rapidly. Because the ablative chemotherapy given to recipients of hematopoietic stem cell transplants (HSCTs) eradicates immunologic memory, revaccination is recommended for all such patients. Vaccination is much more effective once immunologic reconstitution has occurred; however, because of the need to prevent serious disease, pneumococcal vaccine should be administered 6–12 months after transplantation in most cases. Because PPSV23 includes serotypes not present in PCV13, HSCT recipients should receive a dose of PPSV23 at least 8 weeks after the last dose of PCV13. Although antibody titers from PPSV23 clearly decay, experience with multiple doses of PPSV23 is limited, as are data on the safety, toxicity, or efficacy of such a regimen. For this reason, the CDC currently recommends the administration of one additional dose of PPSV23 at least 5 years after the last dose to immunocompromised patients, including transplant recipients, as well as patients with Hodgkin's disease, multiple myeloma, lymphoma, or generalized malignancies. Beyond this single additional dose, further doses are not recommended at this time.
[e]Meningococcal conjugate vaccine MenACWY is recommended for adults ≤55 years old, and meningococcal polysaccharide vaccine (MPSV4) is recommended for those ≥56 years old.
[f]Includes both varicella vaccine for children and zoster vaccine for adults. [g]Contact the manufacturer for more information on use in children with acute lymphocytic leukemia.

The level of suspicion of infections with certain organisms should depend on the type of cancer diagnosed (Table 104-3). Diagnosis of multiple myeloma or CLL should alert the clinician to the possibility of hypogammaglobulinemia. While immunoglobulin replacement therapy can be effective, in most cases prophylactic antibiotics are a cheaper, more convenient method of eliminating bacterial infections in CLL patients with hypogammaglobulinemia. Patients with acute lymphocytic leukemia (ALL), patients with non-Hodgkin's lymphoma, and all cancer patients treated with high-dose glucocorticoids (or glucocorticoid-containing chemotherapy regimens) should receive antibiotic prophylaxis for *Pneumocystis* infection (Table 104-3) for the duration of their chemotherapy. In addition to exhibiting susceptibility to certain infectious organisms, patients with cancer are likely to manifest their infections in characteristic ways. For example, fever—generally a sign of infection in normal hosts—continues to be a reliable indicator in neutropenic patients. In contrast, patients receiving glucocorticoids and agents that impair T cell function and cytokine secretion may have serious infections in the absence of fever. Similarly, neutropenic patients commonly present with cellulitis without purulence and with pneumonia without sputum or even x-ray findings (see below).

The use of monoclonal antibodies that target B and T cells as well as drugs that interfere with lymphocyte signal transduction events is associated with reactivation of latent infections. The use of rituximab, the antibody to CD20 (a B cell surface protein), is associated with the development of reactivation tuberculosis as well as other latent viral infections, including hepatitis B and cytomegalovirus (CMV) infection. Like organ transplant recipients (Chap. 169), patients with latent bacterial disease (like tuberculosis) and latent viral disease (like herpes simplex or zoster) should be carefully monitored for reactivation disease.

SYSTEM-SPECIFIC SYNDROMES

SKIN-SPECIFIC SYNDROMES

Skin lesions are common in cancer patients, and the appearance of these lesions may permit the diagnosis of systemic bacterial or fungal infection. While cellulitis caused by skin organisms such as

TABLE 104-3 INFECTIONS ASSOCIATED WITH SPECIFIC TYPES OF CANCER

Cancer	Underlying Immune Abnormality	Organisms Causing Infection
Multiple myeloma	Hypogammaglobulinemia	*Streptococcus pneumoniae, Haemophilus influenzae, Neisseria meningitidis*
Chronic lymphocytic leukemia	Hypogammaglobulinemia	*S. pneumoniae, H. influenzae, N. meningitidis*
Acute myeloid or lymphocytic leukemia	Granulocytopenia, skin and mucous membrane lesions	Extracellular gram-positive and gram-negative bacteria, fungi
Hodgkin's disease	Abnormal T cell function	Intracellular pathogens (*Mycobacterium tuberculosis, Listeria, Salmonella, Cryptococcus, Mycobacterium avium*); herpesviruses
Non-Hodgkin's lymphoma and acute lymphocytic leukemia	Glucocorticoid chemotherapy, T and B cell dysfunction	*Pneumocystis*
Colon and rectal tumors	Local abnormalities[a]	*Streptococcus bovis* biotype 1 (bacteremia)
Hairy cell leukemia	Abnormal T cell function	Intracellular pathogens (*M. tuberculosis, Listeria, Cryptococcus, M. avium*)

[a]The reason for this association is not well defined.

TABLE 104-4 ORGANISMS LIKELY TO CAUSE INFECTIONS IN GRANULOCYTOPENIC PATIENTS

Gram-Positive Cocci	
Staphylococcus epidermidis	*Staphylococcus aureus*
Viridans *Streptococcus*	*Enterococcus faecalis*
Streptococcus pneumoniae	
Gram-Negative Bacilli	
Escherichia coli	*Serratia* spp.
Klebsiella spp.	*Acinetobacter* spp.[a]
Pseudomonas aeruginosa	*Stenotrophomonas* spp.
Enterobacter spp.	*Citrobacter* spp.
Non-*aeruginosa Pseudomonas* spp.[a]	
Gram-Positive Bacilli	
Diphtheroids	JK bacillus[a]
Fungi	
Candida spp.	*Mucor/Rhizopus*
Aspergillus spp.	

[a]Often associated with intravenous catheters.

Streptococcus or *Staphylococcus* is common, neutropenic patients—i.e., those with <500 functional polymorphonuclear leukocytes (PMNs)/μL—and patients with impaired blood or lymphatic drainage may develop infections with unusual organisms. Innocent-looking macules or papules may be the first sign of bacterial or fungal sepsis in immunocompromised patients (Fig. 104-1). In the neutropenic host, a macule progresses rapidly to ecthyma gangrenosum (see Fig. 25e-35), a usually painless, round, necrotic lesion consisting of a central black or gray-black eschar with surrounding erythema. Ecthyma gangrenosum, which is located in nonpressure areas (as distinguished from necrotic lesions associated with lack of circulation), is often associated with *Pseudomonas aeruginosa* bacteremia (Chap. 189) but may be caused by other bacteria.

Candidemia (Chap. 240) is also associated with a variety of skin conditions (see Fig. 25e-38) and commonly presents as a maculopapular rash. Punch biopsy of the skin may be the best method for diagnosis.

Cellulitis, an acute spreading inflammation of the skin, is most often caused by infection with group A *Streptococcus* or *Staphylococcus aureus*, virulent organisms normally found on the skin (Chap. 156). Although cellulitis tends to be circumscribed in normal hosts, it may spread rapidly in neutropenic patients. A tiny break in the skin may lead to spreading cellulitis, which is characterized by pain and erythema; in the affected patients, signs of infection (e.g., purulence) are often lacking. What might be a furuncle in a normal host may require amputation because of uncontrolled infection in a patient presenting with leukemia. A dramatic response to an infection that might be trivial in a normal host can mark the first sign of leukemia. Fortunately, granulocytopenic patients are likely to be infected with certain types of organisms (Table 104-4); thus the selection of an antibiotic regimen is somewhat easier than it might otherwise be (see "Antibacterial Therapy," below). It is essential to recognize cellulitis early and to treat it aggressively. Patients who are neutropenic or who have previously received antibiotics for other reasons may develop cellulitis with unusual organisms (e.g., *Escherichia coli*, *Pseudomonas*, or fungi). Early treatment, even of innocent-looking lesions, is essential to prevent necrosis and loss of tissue. Debridement to prevent spread may sometimes be necessary early in the course of disease, but it can often be performed after chemotherapy, when the PMN count increases.

A

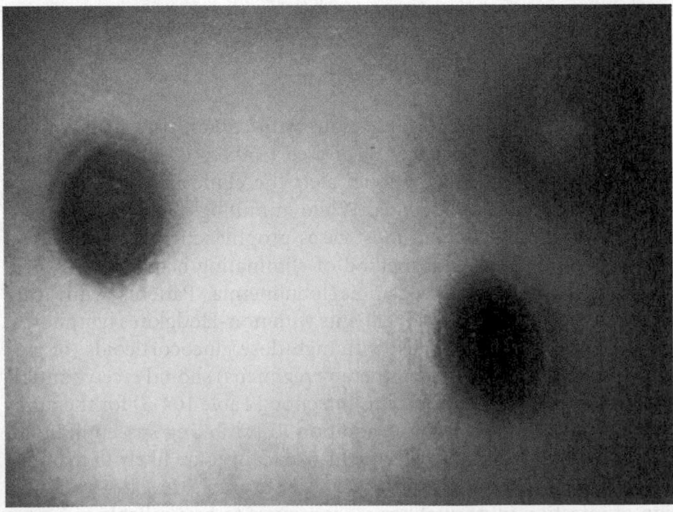

B

FIGURE 104-1 ***A.*** Papules related to *Escherichia coli* bacteremia in a patient with acute lymphocytic leukemia. ***B.*** The same lesions on the following day.

Sweet syndrome, or *febrile neutrophilic dermatosis,* was originally described in women with elevated white blood cell (WBC) counts. The disease is characterized by the presence of leukocytes in the lower dermis, with edema of the papillary body. Ironically, this disease now is usually seen in neutropenic patients with cancer, most often in association with acute myeloid leukemia (AML) but also in association with a variety of other malignancies. Sweet syndrome usually presents as red or bluish-red papules or nodules that may coalesce and form sharply bordered plaques (see Fig. 25e-41). The edema may suggest vesicles, but on palpation the lesions are solid, and vesicles probably never arise in this disease. The lesions are most common on the face, neck, and arms. On the legs, they may be confused with erythema nodosum (see Fig. 25e-40). The development of lesions is often accompanied by high fevers and an elevated erythrocyte sedimentation rate. Both the lesions and the temperature elevation respond dramatically to glucocorticoid administration. Treatment begins with high doses of glucocorticoids (prednisone, 60 mg/d) followed by tapered doses over the next 2–3 weeks.

Data indicate that *erythema multiforme* (see Fig. 25e-25) with mucous membrane involvement is often associated with herpes simplex virus (HSV) infection and is distinct from Stevens-Johnson syndrome, which is associated with drugs and tends to have a more widespread distribution. Because cancer patients are both immunosuppressed (and therefore susceptible to herpes infections) and heavily treated with drugs (and therefore subject to Stevens-Johnson syndrome [see Fig. 46e-4]), both of these conditions are common in this population.

Cytokines, which are used as adjuvants or primary treatments for cancer, can themselves cause characteristic rashes, further complicating the differential diagnosis. This phenomenon is a particular problem in bone marrow transplant recipients (Chap. 169), who, in addition to having the usual chemotherapy-, antibiotic-, and cytokine-induced rashes, are plagued by graft-versus-host disease.

CATHETER-RELATED INFECTIONS

Because IV catheters are commonly used in cancer chemotherapy and are prone to cause infection (Chap. 168), they pose a major problem in the care of patients with cancer. Some catheter-associated infections can be treated with antibiotics, whereas in others the catheter must be removed (Table 104-5). If the patient has a "tunneled" catheter (which consists of an entrance site, a subcutaneous tunnel, and an exit site), a red streak over the subcutaneous part of the line (the tunnel) is grounds for immediate device removal. Failure to remove catheters under these circumstances may result in extensive cellulitis and tissue necrosis.

More common than tunnel infections are exit-site infections, often with erythema around the area where the line penetrates the skin. Most authorities (Chap. 172) recommend treatment (usually with vancomycin) for an exit-site infection caused by coagulase-negative *Staphylococcus.* Treatment of coagulase-positive staphylococcal infection is associated with a poorer outcome, and it is advisable to remove the catheter if possible. Similarly, most clinicians remove catheters associated with infections due to *P. aeruginosa* and *Candida* species, because such infections are difficult to treat and bloodstream infections with these organisms are likely to be deadly. Catheter infections caused by *Burkholderia cepacia, Stenotrophomonas* species, *Agrobacterium* species, *Acinetobacter baumannii, Pseudomonas* species other than *aeruginosa,* and carbapenem-resistant Enterobacteriaceae are likely to be very difficult to eradicate with antibiotics alone. Similarly, isolation of *Bacillus, Corynebacterium,* and *Mycobacterium* species should prompt removal of the catheter.

GASTROINTESTINAL TRACT–SPECIFIC SYNDROMES

Upper Gastrointestinal Tract Disease

INFECTIONS OF THE MOUTH The oral cavity is rich in aerobic and anaerobic bacteria (Chap. 201) that normally live in a commensal relationship with the host. The antimetabolic effects of chemotherapy cause a breakdown of mucosal host defenses, leading to ulceration of the mouth and the potential for invasion by resident bacteria. Mouth ulcerations afflict most patients receiving cytotoxic chemotherapy and have been associated with viridans streptococcal bacteremia. *Candida* infections of the mouth are very common. Fluconazole is clearly effective in the treatment of both local infections (thrush) and systemic infections (esophagitis) due to *Candida albicans.* Other azoles (e.g., voriconazole) as well as echinocandins offer similar efficacy as well as activity against the fluconazole-resistant organisms that are associated with chronic fluconazole treatment (Chap. 240).

Noma (*cancrum oris*), commonly seen in malnourished children, is a penetrating disease of the soft and hard tissues of the mouth and adjacent sites, with resulting necrosis and gangrene. It has a counterpart in immunocompromised patients and is thought to be due to invasion of the tissues by *Bacteroides, Fusobacterium,* and other normal inhabitants of the mouth. Noma is associated with debility, poor oral hygiene, and immunosuppression.

TABLE 104-5 APPROACH TO CATHETER INFECTIONS IN IMMUNOCOMPROMISED PATIENTS

Clinical Presentation or Isolated Pathogen	Catheter Removal	Antibiotics	Comments
Evidence of Infection, Negative Blood Cultures			
Exit-site erythema	Not necessary if infection responds to treatment	Usually, begin treatment for gram-positive cocci.	Coagulase-negative staphylococci are most common.
Tunnel-site erythema	Required	Treat for gram-positive cocci pending culture results.	Failure to remove the catheter may lead to necrosis of the involved area requiring skin grafts in the future.
Blood Culture–Positive Infections			
Coagulase-negative staphylococci	Line removal optimal but may be unnecessary if patient is clinically stable and responds to antibiotics	Usually, start with vancomycin. Linezolid, quinupristin/dalfopristin, and daptomycin are alternative agents.	If there are no contraindications to line removal, this course of action is optimal. If the line is removed, antibiotics may not be necessary.
Other gram-positive cocci (e.g., *Staphylococcus aureus, Enterococcus*); gram-positive rods (*Bacillus, Corynebacterium* spp.)	Recommended	Treat with antibiotics to which the organism is sensitive, with duration based on the clinical setting.	The incidence of metastatic infections following *S. aureus* infection and the difficulty of treating enterococcal infection make line removal the recommended course of action. In addition, gram-positive rods do not respond readily to antibiotics alone.
Gram-negative bacteria	Recommended	Use an agent to which the organism is shown to be sensitive.	Organisms like *Stenotrophomonas, Pseudomonas,* and *Burkholderia* are notoriously hard to treat, as are carbapenem-resistant organisms.
Fungi	Recommended	—	Fungal infections of catheters are extremely difficult to treat.

Viruses, particularly HSV, are a prominent cause of morbidity in immunocompromised patients, in whom they are associated with severe mucositis. The use of acyclovir, either prophylactically or therapeutically, is of value.

ESOPHAGEAL INFECTIONS The differential diagnosis of esophagitis (usually presenting as substernal chest pain upon swallowing) includes herpes simplex and candidiasis, both of which are readily treatable.

Lower Gastrointestinal Tract Disease Hepatic candidiasis (Chap. 240) results from seeding of the liver (usually from a gastrointestinal source) in neutropenic patients. It is most common among patients being treated for AML and usually presents symptomatically around the time the neutropenia resolves. The characteristic picture is that of persistent fever unresponsive to antibiotics, abdominal pain and tenderness or nausea, and elevated serum levels of alkaline phosphatase in a patient with hematologic malignancy who has recently recovered from neutropenia. The diagnosis of this disease (which may present in an indolent manner and persist for several months) is based on the finding of yeasts or pseudohyphae in granulomatous lesions. Hepatic ultrasound or CT may reveal bull's-eye lesions. MRI scans reveal small lesions not visible by other imaging modalities. The pathology (a granulomatous response) and the timing (with resolution of neutropenia and an elevation in granulocyte count) suggest that the host response to *Candida* is an important component of the manifestations of disease. In many cases, although organisms are visible, cultures of biopsied material may be negative. The designation *hepatosplenic candidiasis* or *hepatic candidiasis* is a misnomer because the disease often involves the kidneys and other tissues; the term *chronic disseminated candidiasis* may be more appropriate. Because of the risk of bleeding with liver biopsy, diagnosis is often based on imaging studies (MRI, CT). Treatment should be directed to the causative agent (usually *C. albicans* but sometimes *Candida tropicalis* or other less common *Candida* species).

Typhlitis *Typhlitis* (also referred to as necrotizing colitis, neutropenic colitis, necrotizing enteropathy, ileocecal syndrome, and cecitis) is a clinical syndrome of fever and right-lower-quadrant (or generalized abdominal) tenderness in an immunosuppressed host. This syndrome is classically seen in neutropenic patients after chemotherapy with cytotoxic drugs. It may be more common among children than among adults and appears to be much more common among patients with AML or ALL than among those with other types of cancer. Physical examination reveals right-lower-quadrant tenderness, with or without rebound tenderness. Associated diarrhea (often bloody) is common, and the diagnosis can be confirmed by the finding of a thickened cecal wall on CT, MRI, or ultrasonography. Plain films may reveal a right-lower-quadrant mass, but CT with contrast or MRI is a much more sensitive means of diagnosis. Although surgery is sometimes attempted to avoid perforation from ischemia, most cases resolve with medical therapy alone. The disease is sometimes associated with positive blood cultures (which usually yield aerobic gram-negative bacilli), and therapy is recommended for a broad spectrum of bacteria (particularly gram-negative bacilli, which are likely to be found in the bowel flora). Surgery is indicated in the case of perforation.

***Clostridium difficile*–Induced Diarrhea** Patients with cancer are predisposed to the development of *C. difficile* diarrhea (Chap. 161) as a consequence of chemotherapy alone. Thus, they may test positive for *C. difficile* even without receiving antibiotics. Obviously, such patients are also subject to *C. difficile*–induced diarrhea as a result of antibiotic pressure. *C. difficile* should always be considered as a possible cause of diarrhea in cancer patients who have received either chemotherapy or antibiotics.

CENTRAL NERVOUS SYSTEM–SPECIFIC SYNDROMES

Meningitis The presentation of meningitis in patients with lymphoma or CLL and in patients receiving chemotherapy (particularly with glucocorticoids) for solid tumors suggests a diagnosis of cryptococcal or listerial infection. As noted previously, splenectomized patients are susceptible to rapid, overwhelming infection with encapsulated bacteria (including *S. pneumoniae*, *H. influenzae*, and *N. meningitidis*). Similarly, patients who are antibody-deficient (e.g., those with CLL, those who have received intensive chemotherapy, or those who have undergone bone marrow transplantation) are likely to have infections caused by these bacteria. Other cancer patients, however, because of their defective cellular immunity, are likely to be infected with other pathogens (Table 104-3). Central nervous system (CNS) tuberculosis should be considered, especially in patients from countries where tuberculosis is highly prevalent in the population.

Encephalitis The spectrum of disease resulting from viral encephalitis is expanded in immunocompromised patients. A predisposition to infections with intracellular organisms similar to those encountered in patients with AIDS (Chap. 226) is seen in cancer patients receiving (1) high-dose cytotoxic chemotherapy, (2) chemotherapy affecting T cell function (e.g., fludarabine), or (3) antibodies that eliminate T cells (e.g., anti-CD3, alemtuzumab, anti-CD52) or cytokine activity (anti–tumor necrosis factor agents or interleukin 1 receptor antagonists). Infection with varicella-zoster virus (VZV) has been associated with encephalitis that may be caused by VZV-related vasculitis. Chronic viral infections may also be associated with dementia and encephalitic presentations. A diagnosis of progressive multifocal leukoencephalopathy (Chap. 164) should be considered when a patient who has received chemotherapy (rituximab in particular) presents with dementia (Table 104-6). Other abnormalities of the CNS that may be confused with infection include normal-pressure hydrocephalus and vasculitis resulting from CNS irradiation. It may be possible to differentiate these conditions by MRI.

Brain Masses Mass lesions of the brain most often present as headache with or without fever or neurologic abnormalities. Infections associated with mass lesions may be caused by bacteria (particularly *Nocardia*), fungi (particularly *Cryptococcus* or *Aspergillus*), or parasites (*Toxoplasma*). Epstein-Barr virus (EBV)–associated lymphoma may also present as single—or sometimes multiple—mass lesions of the brain. A biopsy may be required for a definitive diagnosis.

PULMONARY INFECTIONS

Pneumonia (Chap. 153) in immunocompromised patients may be difficult to diagnose because conventional methods of diagnosis depend on the presence of neutrophils. Bacterial pneumonia in neutropenic patients may present without purulent sputum—or, in fact, without any sputum at all—and may not produce physical findings suggestive of chest consolidation (rales or egophony).

In granulocytopenic patients with persistent or recurrent fever, the chest x-ray pattern may help to localize an infection and thus to determine which investigative tests and procedures should be undertaken and which therapeutic options should be considered (Table 104-7). In this setting, a simple chest x-ray is a screening tool; because the impaired host response results in less evidence of consolidation or infiltration, high-resolution CT is recommended for the diagnosis of pulmonary infections. The difficulties encountered in the management of pulmonary infiltrates relate in part to the difficulties of performing diagnostic procedures on the patients involved. When platelet counts can be increased to adequate levels by transfusion,

TABLE 104-6 DIFFERENTIAL DIAGNOSIS OF CENTRAL NERVOUS SYSTEM INFECTIONS IN PATIENTS WITH CANCER

	Underlying Predisposition	
Findings on CT or MRI	**Prolonged Neutropenia**	**Defects in Cellular Immunity**[a]
Mass lesions	*Aspergillus, Nocardia,* or *Cryptococcus* brain abscess	Toxoplasmosis, Epstein-Barr virus lymphoma (rare)
Diffuse encephalitis	Progressive multifocal leukoencephalopathy (JC virus)	Infection with varicella-zoster virus, cytomegalovirus, herpes simplex virus, human herpesvirus type 6, JC virus, *Listeria*

[a]High-dose glucocorticoid therapy, cytotoxic chemotherapy.

TABLE 104-7 DIFFERENTIAL DIAGNOSIS OF CHEST INFILTRATES IN IMMUNOCOMPROMISED PATIENTS

	Cause of Pneumonia	
Infiltrate	**Infectious**	**Noninfectious**
Localized	Bacteria (including *Legionella*, mycobacteria)	Local hemorrhage or embolism, tumor
Nodular	Fungi (e.g., *Aspergillus* or *Mucor*), *Nocardia*	Recurrent tumor
Diffuse	Viruses (especially cytomegalovirus), *Chlamydia*, *Pneumocystis*, *Toxoplasma gondii*, mycobacteria	Congestive heart failure, radiation pneumonitis, drug-induced lung injury, lymphangitic spread of cancer

microscopic and microbiologic evaluation of the fluid obtained by endoscopic bronchial lavage is often diagnostic. Lavage fluid should be cultured for *Mycoplasma*, *Chlamydia*, *Legionella*, *Nocardia*, more common bacterial pathogens, fungi, and viruses. In addition, the possibility of *Pneumocystis* pneumonia should be considered, especially in patients with ALL or lymphoma who have not received prophylactic trimethoprim-sulfamethoxazole (TMP-SMX). The characteristics of the infiltrate may be helpful in decisions about further diagnostic and therapeutic maneuvers. Nodular infiltrates suggest fungal pneumonia (e.g., that caused by *Aspergillus* or *Mucor*). Such lesions may best be approached by visualized biopsy procedures. It is worth noting that while bacterial pneumonias classically present as lobar infiltrates in normal hosts, bacterial pneumonias in granulocytopenic hosts present with a paucity of signs, symptoms, or radiographic abnormalities; thus, the diagnosis is difficult.

Aspergillus species (Chap. 241) can colonize the skin and respiratory tract or cause fatal systemic illness. Although this fungus may cause aspergillomas in a previously existing cavity or may produce allergic bronchopulmonary disease in some patients, the major problem posed by this genus in neutropenic patients is invasive disease, primarily due to *Aspergillus fumigatus* or *Aspergillus flavus*. The organisms enter the host following colonization of the respiratory tract, with subsequent invasion of blood vessels. The disease is likely to present as a thrombotic or embolic event because of this ability of the fungi to invade blood vessels. The risk of infection with *Aspergillus* correlates directly with the duration of neutropenia. In prolonged neutropenia, positive surveillance cultures for nasopharyngeal colonization with *Aspergillus* may predict the development of disease.

Patients with *Aspergillus* infection often present with pleuritic chest pain and fever, which are sometimes accompanied by cough. Hemoptysis may be an ominous sign. Chest x-rays may reveal new focal infiltrates or nodules. Chest CT may reveal a characteristic halo consisting of a mass-like infiltrate surrounded by an area of low attenuation. The presence of a "crescent sign" on chest x-ray or chest CT, in which the mass progresses to central cavitation, is characteristic of invasive *Aspergillus* infection but may develop as the lesions are resolving.

In addition to causing pulmonary disease, *Aspergillus* may invade through the nose or palate, with deep sinus penetration. The appearance of a discolored area in the nasal passages or on the hard palate should prompt a search for invasive *Aspergillus*. This situation is likely to require surgical debridement. Catheter infections with *Aspergillus* usually require both removal of the catheter and antifungal therapy.

Diffuse interstitial infiltrates suggest viral, parasitic, or *Pneumocystis* pneumonia. If the patient has a diffuse interstitial pattern on chest x ray, it may be reasonable, while considering invasive diagnostic procedures, to institute empirical treatment for *Pneumocystis* with TMP-SMX and for *Chlamydia*, *Mycoplasma*, and *Legionella* with a quinolone or azithromycin. Noninvasive procedures, such as staining of induced sputum smears for *Pneumocystis*, serum cryptococcal antigen tests, and urine testing for *Legionella* antigen, may be helpful. Serum galactomannan and β-D-glucan tests may be of value in diagnosing *Aspergillus* infection, but their utility is limited by their lack of sensitivity and specificity. The presence of an elevated level of β-D-glucan in the serum of a patient being treated for cancer who is not receiving prophylaxis against *Pneumocystis* suggests the diagnosis of *Pneumocystis* pneumonia. Infections with viruses that cause only upper respiratory symptoms in immunocompetent hosts, such as respiratory syncytial virus (RSV), influenza viruses, and parainfluenza viruses, may be associated with fatal pneumonitis in immunocompromised hosts. CMV reactivation occurs in cancer patients receiving chemotherapy, but CMV pneumonia is most common among HSCT recipients (Chap. 169). Polymerase chain reaction testing now allows rapid diagnosis of viral pneumonia, which can lead to treatment in some cases (e.g., influenza). Multiplex studies that can detect a wide array of viruses in the lung and upper respiratory tract are now available and will lead to specific diagnoses of viral pneumonias.

Bleomycin is the most common cause of chemotherapy-induced lung disease. Other causes include alkylating agents (such as cyclophosphamide, chlorambucil, and melphalan), nitrosoureas (carmustine [BCNU], lomustine [CCNU], and methyl-CCNU), busulfan, procarbazine, methotrexate, and hydroxyurea. Both infectious and noninfectious (drug- and/or radiation-induced) pneumonitis can cause fever and abnormalities on chest x-ray; thus, the differential diagnosis of an infiltrate in a patient receiving chemotherapy encompasses a broad range of conditions (Table 104-7). The treatment of radiation pneumonitis (which may respond dramatically to glucocorticoids) or drug-induced pneumonitis is different from that of infectious pneumonia, and a biopsy may be important in the diagnosis. Unfortunately, no definitive diagnosis can be made in ~30% of cases, even after bronchoscopy.

Open-lung biopsy is the gold standard of diagnostic techniques. Biopsy via a visualized thoracostomy can replace an open procedure in many cases. When a biopsy cannot be performed, empirical treatment can be undertaken; a quinolone or an erythromycin derivative (azithromycin) and TMP-SMX are used in the case of diffuse infiltrates, and an antifungal agent is administered in the case of nodular infiltrates. The risks should be weighed carefully in these cases. If inappropriate drugs are administered, empirical treatment may prove toxic or ineffective; either of these outcomes may be riskier than biopsy.

CARDIOVASCULAR INFECTIONS

Patients with Hodgkin's disease are prone to persistent infections by *Salmonella*, sometimes (and particularly often in elderly patients) affecting a vascular site. The use of IV catheters deliberately lodged in the right atrium is associated with a high incidence of bacterial endocarditis, presumably related to valve damage followed by bacteremia. Nonbacterial thrombotic endocarditis (marantic endocarditis) has been described in association with a variety of malignancies (most often solid tumors) and may follow bone marrow transplantation as well. The presentation of an embolic event with a new cardiac murmur suggests this diagnosis. Blood cultures are negative in this disease of unknown pathogenesis.

ENDOCRINE SYNDROMES

Infections of the endocrine system have been described in immunocompromised patients. *Candida* infection of the thyroid may be difficult to diagnose during the neutropenic period. It can be defined by indium-labeled WBC scans or gallium scans after neutrophil counts increase. CMV infection can cause adrenalitis with or without resulting adrenal insufficiency. The presentation of a sudden endocrine anomaly in an immunocompromised patient can be a sign of infection in the involved end organ.

MUSCULOSKELETAL INFECTIONS

Infection that is a consequence of vascular compromise, resulting in gangrene, can occur when a tumor restricts the blood supply to muscles, bones, or joints. The process of diagnosis and treatment of such infection is similar to that in normal hosts, with the following caveats:

1. *In terms of diagnosis*, a lack of physical findings resulting from a lack of granulocytes in the granulocytopenic patient should make the clinician more aggressive in obtaining tissue rather than more willing to rely on physical signs.
2. *In terms of therapy*, aggressive debridement of infected tissues may be required. However, it is usually difficult to operate on patients

who have recently received chemotherapy, both because of a lack of platelets (which results in bleeding complications) and because of a lack of WBCs (which may lead to secondary infection). A blood culture positive for *Clostridium perfringens*—an organism commonly associated with gas gangrene—can have a number of meanings (Chap. 179). *Clostridium septicum* bacteremia is associated with the presence of an underlying malignancy. Bloodstream infections with intestinal organisms such as *Streptococcus bovis* biotype 1 and *C. perfringens* may arise spontaneously from lower gastrointestinal lesions (tumor or polyps); alternatively, these lesions may be harbingers of invasive disease. The clinical setting must be considered in order to define the appropriate treatment for each case.

RENAL AND URETERAL INFECTIONS

Infections of the urinary tract are common among patients whose ureteral excretion is compromised (Table 104-1). *Candida*, which has a predilection for the kidney, can invade either from the bloodstream or in a retrograde manner (via the ureters or bladder) in immunocompromised patients. The presence of "fungus balls" or persistent candiduria suggests invasive disease. Persistent funguria (with *Aspergillus* as well as *Candida*) should prompt a search for a nidus of infection in the kidney.

Certain viruses are typically seen only in immunosuppressed patients. BK virus (polyomavirus hominis 1) has been documented in the urine of bone marrow transplant recipients and, like adenovirus, may be associated with hemorrhagic cystitis.

ABNORMALITIES THAT PREDISPOSE TO INFECTION

(Table 104-1)

THE LYMPHOID SYSTEM

It is beyond the scope of this chapter to detail how all the immunologic abnormalities that result from cancer or from chemotherapy for cancer lead to infections. Disorders of the immune system are discussed in other sections of this book. As has been noted, patients with antibody deficiency are predisposed to overwhelming infection with encapsulated bacteria (including *S. pneumoniae*, *H. influenzae*, and *N. meningitidis*). Infections that result from the lack of a functional cellular immune system are described in Chap. 226. It is worth mentioning, however, that patients undergoing intensive chemotherapy for any form of cancer will have not only defects due to granulocytopenia but also lymphocyte dysfunction, which may be profound. Thus, these patients—especially those receiving glucocorticoid-containing regimens or drugs that inhibit either T cell activation (calcineurin inhibitors or drugs like fludarabine, which affect lymphocyte function) or cytokine induction—should be given prophylaxis for *Pneumocystis* pneumonia.

Patients receiving treatment that eliminates B cells (e.g., with anti-CD20 antibodies or rituximab) are especially vulnerable to intercurrent viral infections. The incidence of progressive multifocal leukoencephalopathy (caused by JC virus) is elevated in these patients.

THE HEMATOPOIETIC SYSTEM

Initial studies in the 1960s revealed a dramatic increase in the incidence of infections (fatal and nonfatal) among cancer patients with a granulocyte count of <500/μL. The use of prophylactic antibacterial agents has reduced the number of bacterial infections, but 35–78% of febrile neutropenic patients being treated for hematologic malignancies develop infections at some time during chemotherapy. Aerobic pathogens (both gram-positive and gram-negative) predominate in all series, but the exact organisms isolated vary from center to center. Infections with anaerobic organisms are uncommon. Geographic patterns affect the types of fungi isolated. Tuberculosis and malaria are common causes of fever in the developing world and may present in this setting as well.

Neutropenic patients are unusually susceptible to infection with a wide variety of bacteria; thus, antibiotic therapy should be initiated promptly to cover likely pathogens if infection is suspected. Indeed, early initiation of antibacterial agents is mandatory to prevent deaths. Like most immunocompromised patients, neutropenic patients are threatened by their own microbial flora, including gram-positive and gram-negative organisms found commonly on the skin and mucous membranes and in the bowel (Table 104-4). Because treatment with narrow-spectrum agents leads to infection with organisms not covered by the antibiotics used, the initial regimen should target all pathogens likely to be the initial causes of bacterial infection in neutropenic hosts. As noted in the algorithm shown in Fig. 104-2, administration of antimicrobial agents is routinely continued until neutropenia resolves—i.e., the granulocyte count is sustained above 500 μL for at least 2 days. In some cases, patients remain febrile after resolution of neutropenia. In these instances, the risk of sudden death from overwhelming bacteremia is greatly reduced, and the following diagnoses should be seriously considered: (1) fungal infection, (2) bacterial abscesses or undrained foci of infection, and (3) drug fever (including reactions to antimicrobial agents as well as to chemotherapy or cytokines). In the proper setting, viral infection or graft-versus-host disease should be considered. In clinical practice, antibacterial therapy is usually discontinued when the patient is no longer neutropenic and all evidence of bacterial disease has been eliminated. Antifungal agents are then discontinued if there is no evidence of fungal disease. If the patient remains febrile, a search for viral diseases or unusual pathogens is conducted while unnecessary cytokines and other drugs are systematically eliminated from the regimen.

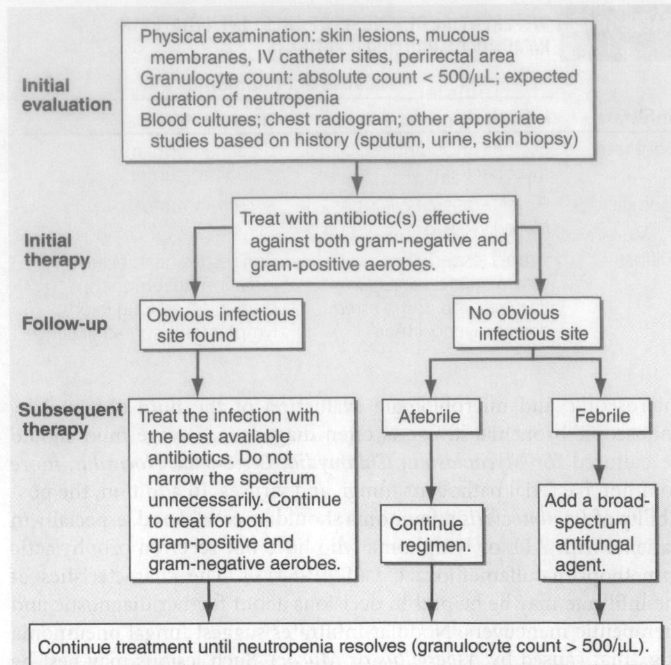

FIGURE 104-2 Algorithm for the diagnosis and treatment of fever and neutropenia.

TREATMENT INFECTIONS IN CANCER PATIENTS

ANTIBACTERIAL THERAPY

Hundreds of antibacterial regimens have been tested for use in patients with cancer. The major risk of infection is related to the degree of neutropenia seen as a consequence of either the disease or the therapy. Many of the relevant studies have involved small populations in which the outcomes have generally been good, and most have lacked the statistical power to detect differences among the regimens studied. Each febrile neutropenic patient should be approached as a unique problem, with particular attention given to previous infections and recent antibiotic exposures. Several general guidelines are useful in the initial treatment of neutropenic patients with fever (Fig. 104-2):

1. In the initial regimen, it is necessary to use antibiotics active against both gram-negative and gram-positive bacteria (Table 104-4).
2. Monotherapy with an aminoglycoside or an antibiotic lacking good activity against gram-positive organisms (e.g., ciprofloxacin or aztreonam) is not adequate in this setting.
3. The agents used should reflect both the epidemiology and the antibiotic resistance pattern of the hospital.
4. If the pattern of resistance justifies its use, a single third-generation cephalosporin constitutes an appropriate initial regimen in many hospitals.
5. Most standard regimens are designed for patients who have not previously received prophylactic antibiotics. The development of fever in a patient who has received antibiotics affects the choice of subsequent therapy, which should target resistant organisms and organisms known to cause infections in patients being treated with the antibiotics already administered.
6. Randomized trials have indicated the safety of oral antibiotic regimens in the treatment of "low-risk" patients with fever and neutropenia. Outpatients who are expected to remain neutropenic for <10 days and who have no concurrent medical problems (such as hypotension, pulmonary compromise, or abdominal pain) can be classified as low risk and treated with a broad-spectrum oral regimen.
7. Several large-scale studies indicate that prophylaxis with a fluoroquinolone (ciprofloxacin or levofloxacin) decreases morbidity and mortality rates among afebrile patients who are anticipated to have neutropenia of long duration.

Commonly used antibiotic regimens for the treatment of febrile patients in whom prolonged neutropenia (>7 days) is anticipated include (1) ceftazidime or cefepime, (2) piperacillin/tazobactam, or (3) imipenem/cilastatin or meropenem. All three regimens have shown equal efficacy in large trials. All three are active against *P. aeruginosa* and a broad spectrum of aerobic gram-positive and gram-negative organisms. Imipenem/cilastatin has been associated with an elevated rate of *C. difficile* diarrhea, and many centers reserve carbapenem antibiotics for treatment of gram-negative bacteria that produce extended-spectrum β-lactamases; these limitations make carbapenems less attractive as an initial regimen. Despite the frequent involvement of coagulase-negative staphylococci, the initial use of vancomycin or its automatic addition to the initial regimen has not resulted in improved outcomes, and the antibiotic does exert toxic effects. For these reasons, only judicious use of vancomycin is recommended—for example, when there is good reason to suspect the involvement of coagulase-negative staphylococci (e.g., the appearance of erythema at the exit site of a catheter or a positive culture for methicillin-resistant *S. aureus* or coagulase-negative staphylococci). Because the sensitivities of bacteria vary from hospital to hospital, clinicians are advised to check their local sensitivities and to be aware that resistance patterns can change quickly, necessitating a change in approach to patients with fever and neutropenia. Similarly, infection control services should monitor for basic antibiotic resistance and for fungal infections. The appearance of a large number of *Aspergillus* infections, in particular, suggests the possibility of an environmental source that requires further investigation and remediation.

The initial antibacterial regimen should be refined on the basis of culture results (Fig. 104-2). Blood cultures are the most relevant basis for selection of therapy; surface cultures of skin and mucous membranes may be misleading. In the case of gram-positive bacteremia or another gram-positive infection, it is important that the antibiotic be optimal for the organism isolated. Once treatment with broad-spectrum antibiotics has begun, it is not desirable to discontinue all antibiotics because of the risk of failing to treat a potentially fatal bacterial infection; the addition of more and more antibacterial agents to the regimen is not appropriate unless there is a clinical or microbiologic reason to do so. Planned progressive therapy (the serial, empirical addition of one drug after another without culture data) is not efficacious in most settings and may have unfortunate consequences. Simply adding another antibiotic for fear that a gram-negative infection is present is a dubious practice. The synergy exhibited by β-lactams and aminoglycosides against certain gram-negative organisms (especially *P. aeruginosa*) provides the rationale for using two antibiotics in this setting, but recent analyses suggest that efficacy is not enhanced by the addition of aminoglycosides, while toxicity may be increased. Mere "double coverage," with the addition of a quinolone or another antibiotic that is not likely to exhibit synergy, has not been shown to be of benefit and may cause additional toxicities and side effects. Cephalosporins can cause bone marrow suppression, and vancomycin is associated with neutropenia in some healthy individuals. Furthermore, the addition of multiple cephalosporins may induce β-lactamase production by some organisms; cephalosporins and double β-lactam combinations should probably be avoided altogether in *Enterobacter* infections.

ANTIFUNGAL THERAPY

Fungal infections in cancer patients are most often associated with neutropenia. Neutropenic patients are predisposed to the development of invasive fungal infections, most commonly those due to *Candida* and *Aspergillus* species and occasionally those caused by *Mucor, Rhizopus, Fusarium, Trichosporon, Bipolaris*, and others. Cryptococcal infection, which is common among patients taking immunosuppressive agents, is uncommon among neutropenic patients receiving chemotherapy for AML. Invasive candidal disease is usually caused by *C. albicans* or *C. tropicalis* but can be caused by *C. krusei, C. parapsilosis*, and *C. glabrata*.

For decades, it has been common clinical practice to add amphotericin B to antibacterial regimens if a neutropenic patient remains febrile despite 4–7 days of treatment with antibacterial agents. The rationale for this empirical addition is that it is difficult to culture fungi before they cause disseminated disease and that mortality rates from disseminated fungal infections in granulocytopenic patients are high. Before the introduction of newer azoles into clinical practice, amphotericin B was the mainstay of antifungal therapy. The insolubility of amphotericin B has resulted in the marketing of several lipid formulations that are less toxic than the amphotericin B deoxycholate complex. Echinocandins (e.g., caspofungin) are useful in the treatment of infections caused by azole-resistant *Candida* strains as well as in therapy for aspergillosis and have been shown to be equivalent to liposomal amphotericin B for the empirical treatment of patients with prolonged fever and neutropenia. Newer azoles have also been demonstrated to be effective in this setting. Although fluconazole is efficacious in the treatment of infections due to many *Candida* species, its use against serious fungal infections in immunocompromised patients is limited by its narrow spectrum: it has no activity against *Aspergillus* or against several non-*albicans Candida* species. The broad-spectrum azoles (e.g., voriconazole and posaconazole) provide another option for the treatment of *Aspergillus* infections (Chap. 241), including CNS infection. Clinicians should be aware that the spectrum of each azole is somewhat different and that no drug can be assumed to be efficacious against all fungi. *Aspergillus terreus* is resistant to amphotericin B. Although voriconazole is active against *Pseudallescheria boydii*, amphotericin B is not; however, voriconazole has no activity against *Mucor*. Posaconazole, which is administered orally, is useful as a prophylactic agent in patients with prolonged neutropenia. Studies in progress are assessing the use of these agents in combinations. **For a full discussion of antifungal therapy, see Chap. 235.**

ANTIVIRAL THERAPY

The availability of a variety of agents active against herpes-group viruses, including some new agents with a broader spectrum of activity, has heightened focus on the treatment of viral infections, which pose a major problem in cancer patients. Viral diseases caused by the herpes group are prominent. Serious (and sometimes fatal) infections due to HSV and VZV are well documented in patients receiving chemotherapy. CMV may also cause serious disease, but fatalities from CMV infection are more common in HSCT recipients. The roles of human herpesvirus (HHV)-6, HHV-7, and HHV-8 (Kaposi's sarcoma–associated herpesvirus) in cancer patients are still being defined (Chap. 219). EBV lymphoproliferative disease (LPD) can occur in patients receiving chemotherapy but is much more common among transplant recipients (Chap. 169). While clinical experience is most extensive with acyclovir, which can be used therapeutically or prophylactically, a number of derivative drugs offer advantages over this agent (Chap. 215e).

In addition to the herpes group, several respiratory viruses (especially RSV) may cause serious disease in cancer patients. Although influenza vaccination is recommended (see below), it may be ineffective in this patient population. The availability of antiviral drugs with activity against influenza viruses gives the clinician additional options for the prophylaxis and treatment of these patients (Chaps. 215e and 224).

OTHER THERAPEUTIC MODALITIES

Another way to address the problems posed by the febrile neutropenic patient is to replenish the neutrophil population. Although granulocyte transfusions may be effective in the treatment of refractory gram-negative bacteremia, they do not have a documented role in prophylaxis. Because of the expense, the risk of leukoagglutinin reactions (which has probably been decreased by improved cell-separation procedures), and the risk of transmission of CMV from unscreened donors (which has been reduced by the use of filters), granulocyte transfusion is reserved for patients whose condition is unresponsive to antibiotics. This modality is efficacious for documented gram-negative bacteremia refractory to antibiotics, particularly in situations where granulocyte numbers will be depressed for only a short period. The demonstrated usefulness of granulocyte colony-stimulating factor in mobilizing neutrophils and advances in preservation techniques may make this option more useful than in the past.

A variety of cytokines, including granulocyte colony-stimulating factor and granulocyte-macrophage colony-stimulating factor, enhance granulocyte recovery after chemotherapy and consequently shorten the period of maximal vulnerability to fatal infections. The role of these cytokines in routine practice is still a matter of some debate. Most authorities recommend their use only when neutropenia is both severe and prolonged. The cytokines themselves may have adverse effects, including fever, hypoxemia, and pleural effusions or serositis in other areas (Chap. 372e).

Once neutropenia has resolved, the risk of infection decreases dramatically. However, depending on what drugs they receive, patients who continue on chemotherapeutic protocols remain at high risk for certain diseases. Any patient receiving more than a maintenance dose of glucocorticoids (e.g., in many treatment regimens for diffuse lymphoma) should also receive prophylactic TMP-SMX because of the risk of *Pneumocystis* infection; those with ALL should receive such prophylaxis for the duration of chemotherapy.

PREVENTION OF INFECTION IN CANCER PATIENTS

EFFECT OF THE ENVIRONMENT

Outbreaks of fatal *Aspergillus* infection have been associated with construction projects and materials in several hospitals. The association between spore counts and risk of infection suggests the need for a high-efficiency air-handling system in hospitals that care for large numbers of neutropenic patients. The use of laminar-flow rooms and prophylactic antibiotics has decreased the number of infectious episodes in severely neutropenic patients. However, because of the expense of such a program and the failure to show that it dramatically affects mortality rates, most centers do not routinely use laminar flow to care for neutropenic patients. Some centers use "reverse isolation," in which health care providers and visitors to a patient who is neutropenic wear gowns and gloves. Since most of the infections these patients develop are due to organisms that colonize the patients' own skin and bowel, the validity of such schemes is dubious, and limited clinical data do not support their use. Hand washing by all staff caring for neutropenic patients should be required to prevent the spread of resistant organisms.

The presence of large numbers of bacteria (particularly *P. aeruginosa*) in certain foods, especially fresh vegetables, has led some authorities to recommend a special "low-bacteria" diet. A diet consisting of cooked and canned food is satisfactory to most neutropenic patients and does not involve elaborate disinfection or sterilization protocols. However, there are no studies to support even this type of dietary restriction. Counseling of patients to avoid leftovers, deli foods, undercooked meat, and unpasteurized dairy products is recommended.

PHYSICAL MEASURES

Although few studies address this issue, patients with cancer are predisposed to infections resulting from anatomic compromise (e.g., lymphedema resulting from node dissections after radical mastectomy). Surgeons who specialize in cancer surgery can provide specific guidelines for the care of such patients, and patients benefit from common-sense advice about how to prevent infections in vulnerable areas.

IMMUNOGLOBULIN REPLACEMENT

Many patients with multiple myeloma or CLL have immunoglobulin deficiencies as a result of their disease, and all allogeneic bone marrow transplant recipients are hypogammaglobulinemic for a period after transplantation. However, current recommendations reserve intravenous immunoglobulin replacement therapy for those patients with severe (<400 mg of total IgG/dL), prolonged hypogammaglobulinemia and a history of repeated infections. Antibiotic prophylaxis has been shown to be cheaper and is efficacious in preventing infections in most CLL patients with hypogammaglobulinemia. Routine use of immunoglobulin replacement is not recommended.

SEXUAL PRACTICES

The use of condoms is recommended for severely immunocompromised patients. Any sexual practice that results in oral exposure to feces is not recommended. Neutropenic patients should be advised to avoid any practice that results in trauma, as even microscopic cuts may result in bacterial invasion and fatal sepsis.

ANTIBIOTIC PROPHYLAXIS

Several studies indicate that the use of oral fluoroquinolones prevents infection and decreases mortality rates among severely neutropenic patients. Prophylaxis for *Pneumocystis* is mandatory for patients with ALL and for all cancer patients receiving glucocorticoid-containing chemotherapy regimens.

VACCINATION OF CANCER PATIENTS

In general, patients undergoing chemotherapy respond less well to vaccines than do normal hosts. Their greater need for vaccines thus leads to a dilemma in their management. Purified proteins and inactivated vaccines are almost never contraindicated and should be given to patients even during chemotherapy. For example, all adults should receive diphtheria–tetanus toxoid boosters at the indicated times as well as seasonal influenza vaccine. However, if possible, vaccination should not be undertaken concurrent with cytotoxic chemotherapy. If patients are expected to be receiving chemotherapy for several months and vaccination is indicated (e.g., influenza vaccination in the fall), the vaccine should be given midcycle—as far apart in time as possible from the antimetabolic agents that will prevent an immune response. The meningococcal and pneumococcal polysaccharide vaccines should be given to patients before splenectomy, if possible. The *H. influenzae* type b conjugate vaccine should be administered to all splenectomized patients.

In general, live virus (or live bacterial) vaccines should not be given to patients during intensive chemotherapy because of the risk of disseminated infection. Recommendations on vaccination are summarized in Table 104-2 (see *www.cdc.gov/vaccine* for updated recommendations).

105 Cancer of the Skin

Walter J. Urba, Brendan D. Curti

MELANOMA

Pigmented lesions are among the most common findings on skin examination. The challenge is to distinguish cutaneous melanomas, which account for the overwhelming majority of deaths resulting from skin cancer, from the remainder, which are usually benign. Cutaneous melanoma can occur in adults of all ages, even young individuals, and people of all colors; its location on the skin and its distinct clinical features make it detectable at a time when complete surgical excision is possible. Examples of malignant and benign pigmented lesions are shown in Fig. 105-1.

EPIDEMIOLOGY

Melanoma is an aggressive malignancy of melanocytes, pigment-producing cells that originate from the neural crest and migrate to the skin, meninges, mucous membranes, upper esophagus, and eyes. Melanocytes in each of these locations have the potential for malignant transformation. Cutaneous melanoma is predominantly a malignancy of white-skinned people (98% of cases), and the incidence correlates with latitude of residence, providing strong evidence for the role of sun exposure. Men are affected slightly more than women (1.3:1), and the median age at diagnosis is the late fifties. Dark-skinned populations (such as those of India and Puerto Rico), blacks, and East Asians also develop melanoma, albeit at rates 10–20 times lower than those in whites. Cutaneous melanomas in these populations are diagnosed more often at a higher stage, and patients tend to have worse outcomes. Furthermore, in nonwhite populations, there is a much higher frequency of acral (subungual, plantar, palmar) and mucosal melanomas. In 2014, more than 76,000 individuals in the United States were expected to develop melanoma, and approximately 9700 were expected to die. There will be nearly 50,000 annual deaths worldwide as a result of melanoma. Data from the Connecticut Tumor Registry support an unremitting increase in the incidence and mortality of melanoma. In the past 60 years, there have been 17-fold and 9-fold increases in incidence for men and women, respectively. In the same six decades, there has been a tripling of mortality rates for men and doubling for women. Mortality rates begin to rise at age 55, with the greatest increase in men age >65 years. Of particular concern is the increase in rates among women <40 years of age. Much of this increase is believed to be associated with a greater emphasis on tanned skin as a marker of beauty, the increased availability and use of indoor tanning beds, and exposure to intense ultraviolet (UV) light in childhood. These statistics highlight the need to promote prevention and early detection.

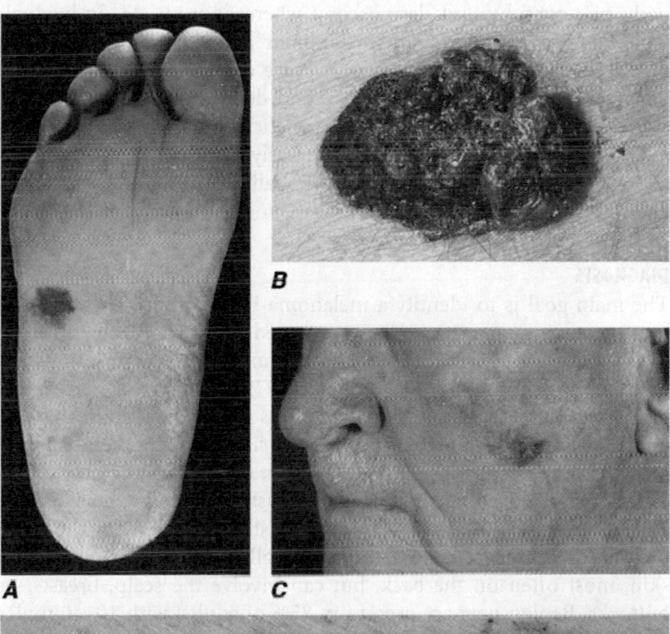

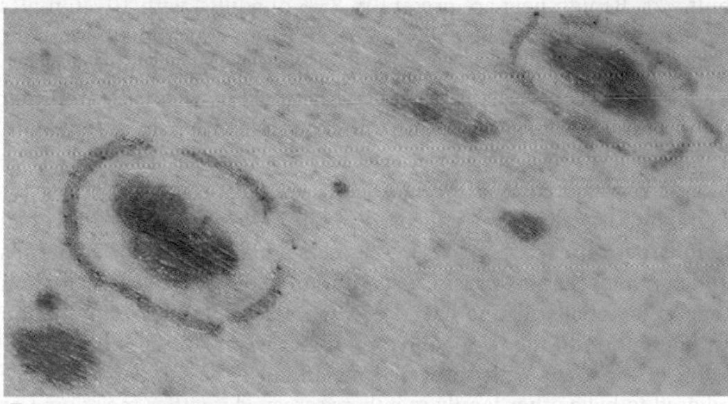

FIGURE 105-1 Atypical and malignant pigmented lesions. The most common melanoma is superficial spreading melanoma (not pictured). ***A.*** Acral lentiginous melanoma is the most common melanoma in blacks, Asians, and Hispanics and occurs as an enlarging hyperpigmented macule or plaque on the palms and soles. Lateral pigment diffusion is present. ***B.*** Nodular melanoma most commonly manifests as a rapidly growing, often ulcerated or crusted black nodule. ***C.*** Lentigo maligna melanoma occurs on sun-exposed skin as a large, hyperpigmented macule or plaque with irregular borders and variable pigmentation. ***D.*** Dysplastic nevi are irregularly pigmented and shaped nevomelanocytic lesions that may be associated with familial melanoma.

RISK FACTORS

Presence of Nevi The risk of developing melanoma is related to genetic, environmental, and host factors (Table 105-1). The strongest risk factors for melanoma are the presence of multiple benign or atypical nevi and a family or personal history of melanoma. The presence of melanocytic nevi, common or dysplastic, is a marker for increased risk of melanoma. Nevi have been referred to as precursor lesions because they can transform into melanomas; however, the actual risk for any specific nevus is exceedingly low. About one-quarter of melanomas are histologically associated with nevi, but the majority arise de novo. The number of clinically atypical moles may vary from one to several hundred, and they usually differ from one another in appearance. The borders are often hazy and indistinct, and the pigment pattern is more highly varied than that in benign acquired nevi. Individuals with clinically atypical moles and a strong family history of melanoma have been reported to have a >50% lifetime risk for developing melanoma and warrant close follow-up with a dermatologist. Of the 90% of patients whose disease is sporadic (i.e., who lack a family history of melanoma), ~40% have clinically atypical moles, compared with an estimated 5–10% of the population at large.

Congenital melanocytic nevi, which are classified as small (≤1.5 cm), medium (1.5–20 cm), and giant (>20 cm), can be precursors for melanoma. The risk is highest for the giant melanocytic nevus, also called the bathing trunk nevus, a rare malformation that affects 1 in 30,000–100,000 individuals. Since the lifetime risk of melanoma development is estimated to be as high as 6%, prophylactic excision early in life is prudent. This usually requires staged removal with coverage

TABLE 105-1 FACTORS ASSOCIATED WITH INCREASED RISK OF MELANOMA
Total body nevi (higher number = higher risk)
Dysplastic nevi (10-fold increased risk)
Family or personal history
Ultraviolet exposure/sunburns/tanning booths
Light skin/hair/eye color
Poor tanning ability
Freckling
CDKN2A, CDK4, MITF mutations
MC1R variants

by split-thickness skin grafts. Surgery cannot remove all at-risk nevus cells, as some may penetrate into the muscles or central nervous system (CNS) below the nevus. Small- to medium-size congenital melanocytic nevi affect approximately 1% of persons; the risk of melanoma developing in these lesions is not known but appears to be relatively low. The management of small- to medium-size congenital melanocytic nevi remains controversial.

Personal and Family History Once diagnosed, patients with melanoma require a lifetime of surveillance because their risk of developing another melanoma is 10 times that of the general population. First-degree relatives have a higher risk of developing melanoma than do individuals without a family history, but only 5–10% of all melanomas are truly familial. In familial melanoma, patients tend to be younger at first diagnosis, lesions are thinner, survival is improved, and multiple primary melanomas are common.

Genetic Susceptibility Approximately 20–40% of cases of hereditary melanoma (0.2–2% of all melanomas) are due to germline mutations in the cell cycle regulatory gene cyclin-dependent kinase inhibitor 2A (*CDKN2A*). In fact, 70% of all cutaneous melanomas have mutations or deletions affecting the *CDKN2A* locus on chromosome 9p21. This locus encodes two distinct tumor-suppressor proteins from alternate reading frames: p16 and ARF ($p14^{ARF}$). The p16 protein inhibits CDK4/6-mediated phosphorylation and inactivation of the retinoblastoma (RB) protein, whereas ARF inhibits MDM2 ubiquitin-mediated degradation of p53. The end result of the loss of *CDKN2A* is inactivation of two critical tumor-suppressor pathways, RB and p53, which control entry of cells into the cell cycle. Several studies have shown an increased risk of pancreatic cancer among melanoma-prone families with *CDKN2A* mutations. A second high-risk locus for melanoma susceptibility, *CDK4*, is located on chromosome 12q13 and encodes the kinase inhibited by p16. *CDK4* mutations, which also inactivate the RB pathway, are much rarer than *CDKN2A* mutations. Germline mutations in the melanoma lineage-specific oncogene microphthalmia-associated transcription factor (*MITF*) predispose to both familial and sporadic melanomas.

The melanocortin-1 receptor (*MC1R*) gene is a moderate-risk inherited melanoma susceptibility factor. Solar radiation stimulates the production of melanocortin (α-melanocyte-stimulating hormone [α-MSH]), the ligand for *MC1R*, which is a G-protein-coupled receptor that signals via cyclic AMP and regulates the amount and type of pigment produced. *MC1R* is highly polymorphic, and among its 80 variants are those that result in partial loss of signaling and lead to the production of red/yellow pheomelanins, which are not sun-protective and produce red hair, rather than brown/black eumelanins that are photoprotective. This red hair color (RHC) phenotype is associated with fair skin, red hair, freckles, increased sun sensitivity, and increased risk of melanoma. In addition to its weak UV shielding capacity relative to eumelanin, increased pheomelanin production in patients with inactivating polymorphisms of *MC1R* also provides a UV-independent carcinogenic contribution to melanomagenesis via oxidative damage.

A number of other more common, low-penetrance polymorphisms that have small effects on melanoma susceptibility include other genes related to pigmentation, nevus count, immune responses, DNA repair, metabolism, and the vitamin D receptor.

PREVENTION AND EARLY DETECTION

Primary prevention of melanoma and nonmelanoma skin cancer (NMSC) is based on protection from the sun. Public health initiatives, such as the SunSmart program that started in Australia and now is operative in Europe and the United States, have demonstrated that behavioral change can decrease the incidence of NMSC and melanoma. Preventive measures should start early in life because damage from UV light begins early despite the fact that cancers develop years later. Biological factors are increasingly being understood, such as tanning addiction, which is postulated to involve stimulation of reward centers in the brain involving dopamine pathways, and cutaneous secretion of β-endorphins after UV exposure, and may represent another area for preventive intervention. Regular use of broad-spectrum sunscreens that block UVA and UVB with a sun protection factor (SPF) of at least 30 and protective clothing should be encouraged. Avoidance of tanning beds and midday (10:00 A.M. to 2:00 P.M.) sun exposure is recommended.

Secondary prevention comprises education, screening, and early detection. Patients should be educated in the clinical features of melanoma (ABCDEs; see following "Diagnosis" section) and advised to report any growth or other change in a pigmented lesion. Brochures are available from the American Cancer Society, the American Academy of Dermatology, the National Cancer Institute, and the Skin Cancer Foundation. Self-examination at 6- to 8-week intervals may enhance the likelihood of detecting change. Although the U.S. Preventive Services Task Force states that evidence is insufficient to recommend for or against skin cancer screening, a full-body skin exam seems to be a simple, practical way to approach reducing the mortality rate for skin cancer. Depending on the presence or absence of risk factors, strategies for early detection can be individualized. This is particularly true for patients with clinically atypical moles (dysplastic nevi) and those with a personal history of melanoma. For these individuals, surveillance should be performed by the dermatologist and include total-body photography and dermoscopy where appropriate. Individuals with three or more primary melanomas and families with at least one invasive melanoma and two or more cases of melanoma and/or pancreatic cancer among first- or second-degree relatives on the same side of the family may benefit from genetic testing. Precancerous and in situ lesions should be treated early. Early detection of small tumors allows the use of simpler treatment modalities with higher cure rates and lower morbidity.

DIAGNOSIS

The main goal is to identify a melanoma before tumor invasion and life-threatening metastases have occurred. Early detection may be facilitated by applying the ABCDEs: *a*symmetry (benign lesions are usually symmetric); *b*order irregularity (most nevi have clear-cut borders); *c*olor variegation (benign lesions usually have uniform light or dark pigment); *d*iameter >6 mm (the size of a pencil eraser); and *e*volving (any change in size, shape, color, or elevation or new symptoms such as bleeding, itching, and crusting). Benign nevi usually appear on sun-exposed skin above the waist, rarely involving the scalp, breasts, or buttocks; atypical moles usually appear on sun-exposed skin, most often on the back, but can involve the scalp, breasts, or buttocks. Benign nevi are present in 85% of adults, with 10–40 moles scattered over the body; atypical nevi can be present in the hundreds.

The entire skin surface, including the scalp and mucous membranes, as well as the nails should be examined in each patient. Bright room illumination is important, and a hand lens is helpful for evaluating variation in pigment pattern. Any suspicious lesions should be biopsied, evaluated by a specialist, or recorded by chart and/or photography for follow-up. A focused method for examining individual lesions, dermoscopy, employs low-level magnification of the epidermis and may allow a more precise visualization of patterns of pigmentation than is possible with the naked eye. Complete physical examination with attention to the regional lymph nodes is part of the initial evaluation in a patient with suspected melanoma. The patient should be advised to have other family members screened if either melanoma or clinically atypical moles (dysplastic nevi) are present. Patients who fit into high-risk groups should be instructed to perform monthly self-examinations.

Biopsy Any pigmented cutaneous lesion that has changed in size or shape or has other features suggestive of malignant melanoma is a candidate for biopsy. An excisional biopsy with 1- to 3-mm margins is suggested. This facilitates pathologic assessment of the lesion, permits accurate measurement of thickness if the lesion is melanoma, and constitutes definitive treatment if the lesion is benign. For lesions that are large or on anatomic sites where excisional biopsy may not be feasible (such as the face, hands, and feet), an incisional biopsy through the most nodular or darkest area of the lesion is acceptable; this should include the vertical growth phase of the primary tumor, if present. Incisional biopsy does not appear to facilitate the spread of melanoma. For suspicious lesions, every attempt should be made to preserve the ability to assess the deep and peripheral margins and to perform immunohistochemistry. Shave biopsies are an acceptable alternative, particularly if the suspicion of malignancy is low, but they should be deep and include underlying fat; cauterization should be avoided. The biopsy should be read by a pathologist experienced in pigmented lesions, and the report should include Breslow thickness, mitoses per square millimeter for lesions ≤1 mm, presence or absence of ulceration, and peripheral and deep margin status. Breslow thickness is the greatest thickness of a primary cutaneous melanoma measured on the slide from the top of the epidermal granular layer, or from the ulcer base, to the bottom of the tumor. To distinguish melanomas from benign nevi in cases with challenging histology, fluorescence in situ hybridization (FISH) with multiple probes and comparative genome hybridization (CGH) can be helpful.

CLINICAL CLASSIFICATION

Four major types of cutaneous melanoma have been recognized (Table 105-2). In three of these types—*superficial spreading melanoma, lentigo maligna melanoma*, and *acral lentiginous melanoma*—the lesion has a period of superficial (so-called radial) growth during which it increases in size but does not penetrate deeply. It is during this period that the melanoma is most capable of being cured by surgical excision. The fourth type—*nodular melanoma* —does not have a recognizable radial growth phase and usually presents as a deeply invasive lesion that is capable of early metastasis. When tumors begin to penetrate deeply into the skin, they are in the so-called vertical growth phase. Melanomas with a radial growth phase are characterized by irregular and sometimes notched borders, variation in pigment pattern, and variation in color. An increase in size or change in color is noted by the patient in 70% of early lesions. Bleeding, ulceration, and pain are late signs and are of little help in early recognition. Superficial spreading melanoma is the most common variant observed in the white population. The back is the most common site for melanoma in men. In women, the back and the lower leg (from knee to ankle) are common sites. Nodular melanomas are dark brown-black to blue-black nodules. Lentigo maligna melanoma usually is confined to chronically sun-damaged sites in older individuals. Acral lentiginous melanoma occurs on the palms, soles, nail beds, and mucous membranes. Although this type occurs in whites, it occurs most frequently (along with nodular melanoma) in blacks and East Asians. A fifth type of melanoma, *desmoplastic melanoma*, is associated with a fibrotic response, neural invasion, and a greater tendency for local recurrence. Occasionally, melanomas appear clinically to be amelanotic, in which case the diagnosis is established microscopically after biopsy of a new or a changing skin nodule. Melanomas can also arise in the mucosa of the head and neck (nasal cavity, paranasal sinuses and oral cavity), the gastrointestinal tract, the CNS, the female genital tract (vulva, vagina), and the uveal tract of the eye.

Although cutaneous melanoma subtypes are clinically and histopathologically distinct, this classification does not have independent prognostic value. Histologic subtype is not part of American Joint Committee on Cancer (AJCC) staging, although the College of American Pathologists (CAP) recommends inclusion in the pathology report. Newer classifications will increasingly emphasize molecular features of each melanoma (see below). The molecular analysis of individual melanomas will provide a basis for distinguishing benign nevi from melanomas, and determination of the mutational status of the tumor will help elucidate the molecular mechanisms of tumorigenesis and be used to identify targets that will guide therapy.

PATHOGENESIS AND MOLECULAR CLASSIFICATION

Considerable evidence from epidemiologic and molecular studies suggests that cutaneous melanomas arise via multiple causal pathways. There are both environmental and genetic components. UV solar radiation causes genetic changes in the skin, impairs cutaneous immune function, increases the production of growth factors, and induces the formation of DNA-damaging reactive oxygen species that affect keratinocytes and melanocytes. A comprehensive catalog of somatic mutations from a human melanoma revealed more than 33,000 base mutations with damage to almost 300 protein-coding segments compared with normal cells from the same patient. The dominant mutational signature reflected DNA damage due to UV light exposure. The melanoma also contained previously described driver mutations (i.e., mutations that confer selective clonal growth advantage and are implicated in oncogenesis). These driver mutations affect pathways that promote cell proliferation and inhibit normal pathways of apoptosis in response to DNA repair (see below). The altered melanocytes accumulate DNA damage, and selection occurs for all the attributes that constitute the malignant phenotype: invasion, metastasis, and angiogenesis.

An understanding of the molecular changes that occur during the transformation of normal melanocytes into malignant melanoma would not only help classify patients but also would contribute to the understanding of etiology and aid the development of new therapeutic options. A genome-wide assessment of melanomas classified into four groups based on their location and degree of exposure to the sun has confirmed that there are distinct genetic pathways in the development of melanoma. The four groups were cutaneous melanomas on skin without chronic sun-induced damage, cutaneous melanomas with chronic sun-induced damage, mucosal melanomas, and acral melanomas. Distinct patterns of DNA alterations were noted that varied with the site of origin and were independent of the histologic subtype of the tumor. Thus, although the genetic changes are diverse, the overall pattern of mutation, amplification, and loss of cancer genes indicates they have convergent effects on key biochemical pathways involved in proliferation, senescence, and apoptosis. The *p16* mutation that affects cell cycle arrest and the *ARF* mutation that results in defective apoptotic responses to genotoxic damage were described earlier. The proliferative pathways affected were the mitogen-activated protein (MAP) kinase and phosphatidylinositol 3' kinase/AKT pathways (Fig. 105-2).

TABLE 105-2 HISTOLOGIC SUBTYPES OF MALIGNANT MELANOMA

Type	Site	Average Age at Diagnosis, Years	Duration of Known Existence, Years	Color
Lentigo maligna melanoma	Sun-exposed surfaces, particularly malar region of cheek and temple	70	5–20 or longer[a]	In flat portions, shades of brown and tan predominate, but whitish gray occasionally present; in nodules, shades of reddish brown, bluish gray, bluish black
Superficial spreading melanoma	Any site (more common on upper back and, in women, lower legs)	40–50	1–7	Shades of brown mixed with bluish red (violaceous), bluish black, reddish brown, and often whitish pink, and the border of lesion is at least in part visibly and/or palpably elevated
Nodular melanoma	Any	40–50	Months–<5 years	Reddish blue (purple) or bluish black; either uniform in color or mixed with brown or black
Acral lentiginous melanoma	Palm, sole, nail bed, mucous membrane	60	1–10	In flat portions, dark brown predominantly; in raised lesions (plaques), brown-black or blue-black predominantly

[a]During much of this time, the precursor stage, lentigo maligna, is confined to the epidermis.

Source: Adapted from AJ Sober, in NA Soter, HP Baden (eds): *Pathophysiology of Dermatologic Diseases*. New York, McGraw-Hill, 1984.

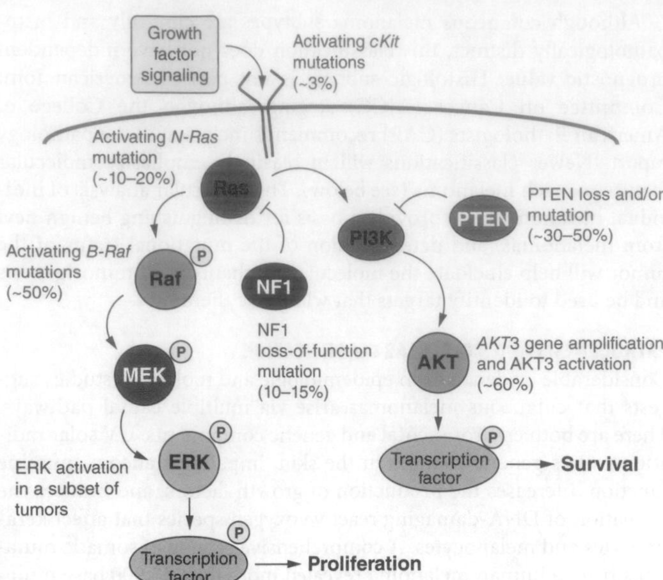

FIGURE 105-2 Major pathways involved in melanoma. The MAP kinase and PI3K/AKT pathways, which promote proliferation and inhibit apoptosis, respectively, are subject to mutations in melanoma. ERK, extracellular signal-regulated kinase; MEK, mitogen-activated protein kinase kinase; NF-1; neurofibromatosis type 1 gene; PTEN, phosphatase and tensin homolog.

RAS and *BRAF*, members of the MAP kinase pathway, which classically mediates the transcription of genes involved in cell proliferation and survival, undergo somatic mutation in melanoma and thereby generate potential therapeutic targets. *N-RAS* is mutated in approximately 20% of melanomas, and somatic activating *BRAF* mutations are found in most benign nevi and 40–60% of melanomas. Neither mutation by itself appears to be sufficient to cause melanoma; thus, they often are accompanied by other mutations. The *BRAF* mutation is most commonly a point mutation (T→A nucleotide change) that results in a valine-to-glutamate amino acid substitution (V600E). V600E *BRAF* mutations do not have the standard UV signature mutation (pyrimidine dimer); they are more common in younger patients and are present in most melanomas that arise on sites with intermittent sun exposure and are less common in melanomas from chronically sun-damaged skin.

Melanomas also harbor mutations in *AKT* (primarily in *AKT3*) and *PTEN* (phosphatase and tensin homolog). *AKT* can be amplified, and *PTEN* may be deleted or undergo epigenetic silencing that leads to constitutive activation of the PI3K/AKT pathway and enhanced cell survival by antagonizing the intrinsic pathway of apoptosis. Loss of *PTEN*, which dysregulates AKT activity, and mutation of *AKT3* both prolong cell survival through inactivation of BAD, Bc12-antagonist of cell death, and activation of the forkhead transcription factor FOXO1, which leads to synthesis of prosurvival genes. A loss-of-function mutation in *NF1*, which can affect both MAP kinase and PI3K/AKT pathways, has been described in 10–15% of melanomas. In melanoma, these two signaling pathways (MAP kinase and PI3K/AKT) enhance tumorigenesis, chemoresistance, migration, and cell cycle dysregulation. Targeted agents that inhibit these pathways have been developed, and some are available for clinical use (see below). Optimal treatment of patients with melanoma may require simultaneous inhibition of both MAPK and PI3K pathways as well as promotion of immune eradication of malignancy.

PROGNOSTIC FACTORS

The prognostic factors of greatest importance to a newly diagnosed patient are included in the staging classification (Table 105-3). The best predictor of metastatic risk is the lesion's Breslow thickness. The Clark level, which defines melanomas on the basis of the layer of skin to which a melanoma has invaded, does not add significant prognostic information and has minimal influence on treatment decisions. The anatomic site of the primary is also prognostic; favorable sites are the forearm and leg (excluding the feet), and unfavorable sites include the scalp, hands, feet, and mucous membranes. In general, women with stage I or II disease have better survival than men, perhaps in part because of earlier diagnosis; women frequently have melanomas on the lower leg, where self-recognition is more likely and the prognosis is better. The effect of age is not straightforward. Older individuals, especially men over 60, have worse prognoses, a finding that has been explained in part by a tendency toward later diagnosis (and thus thicker tumors) and in part by a higher proportion of acral melanomas in men. However, there is a greater risk of lymph node metastasis in young patients. Other important adverse factors recognized via the staging classification include high mitotic rate, presence of ulceration, microsatellite lesions and/or in-transit metastases, evidence of nodal involvement, elevated serum lactate dehydrogenase (LDH), and presence and site of distant metastases.

STAGING

Once the diagnosis of melanoma has been made, the tumor must be staged to determine the prognosis and treatment. Staging helps determine prognosis and aids in treatment selection. The current melanoma staging criteria and estimated 15-year survival by stage are depicted in Table 105-3. The clinical stage of the patient is determined after the pathologic evaluation of the melanoma skin lesion and clinical/radiologic assessment for metastatic disease. Pathologic staging also includes the microscopic evaluation of the regional lymph nodes obtained at sentinel lymph node biopsy or completion lymphadenectomy as indicated. All patients should have a complete history, with attention to symptoms that may represent metastatic disease such as malaise, weight loss, headaches, visual changes, and pain, and physical examination directed to the site of the primary melanoma, looking for persistent disease or for dermal or subcutaneous nodules that could represent satellite or in-transit metastases, and to the regional draining lymph nodes, CNS, liver, and lungs. A complete blood count (CBC), complete metabolic panel, and LDH should be performed. Although these are low-yield tests for uncovering occult metastatic disease, a microcytic anemia would raise the possibility of bowel metastases, particularly in the small bowel, and an unexplained elevated LDH should prompt a more extensive evaluation, including computed tomography (CT) scan or possibly a positron emission tomography (PET) (or CT/PET combined) scan. If signs or symptoms of metastatic disease are present, appropriate diagnostic imaging should be performed. At initial presentation, more than 80% of patients will have disease confined to the skin and a negative history and physical exam, in which case imaging is not indicated.

TREATMENT MELANOMA

MANAGEMENT OF CLINICALLY LOCALIZED MELANOMA (STAGE I, II)

For a newly diagnosed cutaneous melanoma, wide surgical excision of the lesion with a margin of normal skin is necessary to remove all malignant cells and minimize possible local recurrence. The following margins are recommended for a primary melanoma: in situ, 0.5–1.0 cm; invasive up to 1 mm thick, 1 cm; >1.01–2 mm, 1–2 cm; and >2 mm, 2 cm. For lesions on the face, hands, and feet, strict adherence to these margins must give way to individual considerations about the constraints of surgery and minimization of morbidity. In all instances, however, inclusion of subcutaneous fat in the surgical specimen facilitates adequate thickness measurement and assessment of surgical margins by the pathologist. Topical imiquimod also has been used, particularly for lentigo maligna, in cosmetically sensitive locations.

Sentinel lymph node biopsy (SLNB) is a valuable staging tool that has replaced elective regional nodal dissection for the evaluation of regional nodal status. SLNB provides prognostic information and

TABLE 105-3 STAGING CRITERIA FOR MELANOMA

Pathologic and TNM Stage	Thickness, mm	Ulceration	No. of Involved Lymph Nodes	Nodal Involvement	15-Year Survival Estimate (%)
0					98
Tis	In situ	No	0	None	
IA					92
T1a	<1	No, mitosis <1/mm	0	None	
IB					80
T1b	<1	Yes or mitosis >1/mm	0	None	
T2a	1.01–2	No	0	None	
IIA					62
T2b	1.01–2	Yes	0	None	
T3a	2.01–4	No	0	None	
IIB					51
T3b	2.01–4	Yes	0	None	
T4a	>4	No	0	None	
IIC					37
T4b	>4	Yes	0	None	
IIIA					68
N1a	T1-4a	No	1	Microscopic	
N2a	T1-4a	No	2 or 3	Microscopic	
IIIB					38
N1a	Any	Yes	1	Microscopic	
N2a	Any	Yes	2 or 3	Microscopic	
N1b	Any	Yes or no	1	Macroscopic	
N2b	Any	Yes or no	2 or 3	Macroscopic	
N2c	Any	Yes or no	In-transit metastases/satellites, no nodal involvement		
IIIC					22
N1b	Any	Yes or no	1	Macroscopic	
N2b	Any	Yes or no	2 or 3	Macroscopic	
N2c	Any	Yes or no	In-transit metastases/satellites, no nodal Involvement		
N3	Any	Yes or no	4+ metastatic nodes, matted nodes or in-transit metastases/satellites, with metastatic nodes		
IV		Distant metastasis			<10
M1a		Skin, subcutaneous			
M1b		Lung			
M1c		Other visceral site			
		Elevated lactate dehydrogenase			

helps identify patients at high risk for relapse who may be candidates for adjuvant therapy. The initial (sentinel) draining node(s) from the primary site is (are) identified by injecting a blue dye and a radioisotope around the primary site. The sentinel node(s) then is (are) identified by inspection of the nodal basin for the blue-stained node and/or the node with high uptake of the radioisotope. The identified nodes are removed and subjected to careful histopathologic analysis with serial section using hematoxylin and eosin stains as well as immunohistochemical stains (e.g., S100, HMB45, and MelanA) to identify melanocytes.

Not every patient requires a SLNB. Patients whose melanomas are ≤0.75 mm thick have <5% risk of sentinel lymph node (SLN) disease and do not require a SLNB. Patients with tumors >1 mm thick generally undergo SLNB. For melanomas 0.76–1.0 mm thick, SLNB may be considered for lesions with high-risk features such as ulceration, high mitotic index, or lymphovascular invasion, but wide excision alone is the usual definitive therapy. Most other patients with clinically negative lymph nodes should undergo a SLNB. Patients whose SLNB is negative are spared a complete node dissection and its attendant morbidities, and can simply be followed or, based on the features of the primary melanoma, be considered for adjuvant therapy or a clinical trial. The current standard of care for all patients with a positive SLN is to perform a complete lymphadenectomy; however, ongoing clinical studies will determine whether patients with small-volume SLN metastases can be managed safely without additional surgery. Patients with microscopically positive lymph nodes should be considered for adjuvant therapy with interferon or enrollment in a clinical trial.

MANAGEMENT OF REGIONALLY METASTATIC MELANOMA (STAGE III)

Melanomas may recur at the edge of the scar or graft, as satellite metastases, which are separate from but within 2 cm of the scar; as in-transit metastases, which are recurrences >2 cm from the primary lesion but not beyond the regional nodal basin; or, most commonly, as metastasis to a draining lymph node basin. Each of these presentations is managed surgically, following which there is the possibility of long-term disease-free survival. Isolated limb perfusion or infusion with melphalan and hyperthermia are options for patients with extensive cutaneous regional recurrences in an extremity. High complete response rates have been reported and significant palliation of symptoms can be achieved, but there is no change in overall survival.

Patients rendered free of disease after surgery may be at high risk for a local or distant recurrence and should be considered for adjuvant therapy. Radiotherapy can reduce the risk of local recurrence after lymphadenectomy, but does not affect overall survival. Patients with large nodes (>3–4 cm), four or more involved lymph nodes, or extranodal spread on microscopic examination should be considered for radiation. Systemic adjuvant therapy is indicated primarily for patients with stage III disease, but high-risk, node-negative patients (>4 mm thick or ulcerated lesions) and patients with completely resected stage IV disease also may benefit. Either interferon α2b (IFN-α2b), which is given at 20 million units/m^2 IV 5 days a week for 4 weeks followed by 10 million units/m^2 SC three times a week for 11 months (1 year total), or subcutaneous peginterferon α2b (6 μg/kg per week for 8 weeks followed by 3 μg/kg per week for a total of 5 years) is acceptable adjuvant therapy. Treatment is accompanied by significant toxicity, including a flu-like illness, decline in performance status, and the development of depression. Side effects can be managed in most patients by appropriate treatment of symptoms, dose reduction, and treatment interruption. Sometimes IFN must be permanently discontinued before all of the planned doses are administered because of unacceptable toxicity. The high-dose regimen is significantly more toxic than peginterferon, but the latter requires 4 additional years of therapy. Adjuvant treatment with IFN improves disease-free survival, but its impact on overall survival remains controversial. Enrollment in a clinical trial is appropriate for these patients, many of whom will otherwise be observed without treatment either because they are poor candidates for IFN or because the patient (or their oncologist) does not believe the beneficial effects of IFN outweigh the toxicity. The recently approved immunotherapy and targeted agents are being evaluated in the adjuvant setting.

TREATMENT METASTATIC DISEASE

At diagnosis, most patients with melanoma will have early-stage disease; however, some will present with metastases, and others will develop metastases after initial therapy. Patients with a history of melanoma who develop signs or symptoms suggesting recurrent disease should undergo restaging that includes physical examination, CBC, complete metabolic panel, LDH, and appropriate diagnostic imaging that may include a magnetic resonance image (MRI) of the brain and total-body PET/CT or CT scans of the chest, abdomen, and pelvis. Distant metastases (stage IV), which may involve any organ, commonly involve the skin and lymph nodes as well as viscera, bone, or the brain. Historically, metastatic melanoma was considered incurable; median survival ranges from 6 to 15 months, depending on the organs involved. The prognosis is better for patients with skin and subcutaneous metastases (M1a) than for lung (M1b) and worst for those with metastases to liver, bone, and brain (M1c). An elevated serum LDH is a poor prognostic factor and places the patient in stage M1c regardless of the site of the metastases (Table 105-3). Although historical data suggest that the 15-year survival of patients with M1a, M1b, and M1c disease is less than 10%, there is optimism that newer therapies will increase the number of melanoma patients with long-term survival, especially patients with M1a and M1b disease.

The treatment for patients with stage IV melanoma has changed dramatically in the past 2 years. Two new classes of therapeutic agents for melanoma have been approved by the U.S. Food and Drug Administration (FDA). The immune T cell checkpoint inhibitor, ipilimumab, and three new oral agents that target the MAP kinase pathway: the BRAF inhibitors, vemurafenib and dabrafenib, and the MEK inhibitor, trametinib, are now available, so patients with stage IV disease now have multiple therapeutic options (Table 105-4).

TABLE 105-4 TREATMENT OPTIONS FOR METASTATIC MELANOMA

Surgery: Metastasectomy for small number of lesions

Immunotherapy:

- Interleukin 2
- Immune checkpoint blockade
  - FDA approved
    - Anti-CTLA-4: ipilimumab
  - Experimental
    - Anti-PD-1: nivolumab, lambrolizumab
    - Anti-PD-L1

Molecular targeted therapy:

- BRAF inhibitor: vemurafenib, dabrafenib
- MEK inhibitor: trametinib

Chemotherapy: dacarbazine, temozolomide, paclitaxel, albumin-bound paclitaxel (Abraxane), carboplatin

Patients with oligometastatic disease should be referred to a surgical oncologist for consideration of metastasectomy, because they may experience long-term disease-free survival after surgery. Patients with solitary metastases are the best candidates, but surgery increasingly is being used even for patients with metastases at more than one site. Patients rendered free of disease can be considered for IFN therapy or a clinical trial because their risk of developing additional metastases is very high. Surgery can also be used as an adjunct to immunotherapy when only a few of many metastatic lesions prove resistant to systemic therapy.

IMMUNOTHERAPY

The cytokine interleukin 2 (IL-2 or aldesleukin) has been approved to treat patients with melanoma since 1995. IL-2 is used to treat stage IV patients who have a good performance status and is administered at centers with experience managing IL-2-related toxicity. Patients require hospitalization in an intensive care unit–like setting to receive high-dose IL-2 600,000 or 720,000 IU every 8 h for up to 14 doses (one cycle). Patients continue treatment until they achieve maximal benefit, usually 4–6 cycles. Treatment is associated with long-term disease-free survival (probable cures) in 5% of treated patients. The mechanism by which IL-2 causes tumor regression has not been identified, but it is presumed that IL-2 induces melanoma-specific T cells that eliminate tumor cells by recognizing specific antigens. Rosenberg and his colleagues at the National Cancer Institute (NCI) have combined adoptive transfer of in vitro–expanded tumor-infiltrating lymphocytes with high-dose IL-2 in patients who were preconditioned with nonmyeloablative chemotherapy (sometimes combined with total-body irradiation). Tumor regression was observed in more than 50% of patients with IL-2-refractory metastatic melanoma.

Immune checkpoint blockade with monoclonal antibodies to the inhibitory immune receptors CTLA-4 and PD-1 has shown promising clinical efficacy. An array of inhibitory receptors are upregulated during an immune response. An absolute requirement to ensure proper regulation of a normal immune response, the continued expression of inhibitory receptors during chronic infection (hepatitis, HIV) and in cancer patients denotes exhausted T cells with limited potential for proliferation, cytokine production, or cytotoxicity (Fig. 105-3). Checkpoint blockade with a monoclonal antibody results in improved T cell function with eradication of tumor cells in preclinical animal models. Ipilimumab, a fully human IgG antibody that binds CTLA-4 and blocks inhibitory signals, was the first treatment of any kind to improve survival in patients with metastatic melanoma. A full course of therapy is four IV outpatient infusions of ipilimumab 3 mg/kg every 3 weeks. Although response rates were low (~10%) in randomized clinical trials, survival of both previously treated and untreated patients was improved, and ipilimumab was approved by the FDA in March 2011.

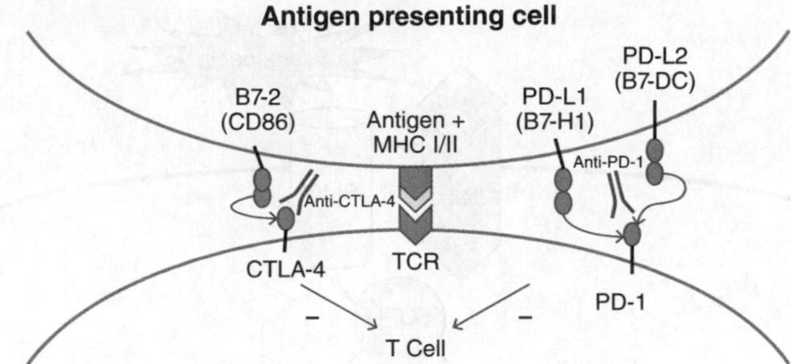

FIGURE 105-3 Inhibitory regulatory pathways that influence T cell function, memory, and lifespan after engagement of the T cell receptor by antigen presented by antigen-presenting cells in the context of MHC I/II. CTLA-4 and PD-1 are part of the CD28 family and have inhibitory effects that can be mitigated by antagonistic antibodies to the receptors or ligand, resulting in enhanced T cell function and antitumor effects. CTLA-4, cytotoxic T lymphocyte antigen-4; MHC, major histocompatibility complex; PD-1, programmed death-1; PD-L1, programmed death ligand-1; PD-L2, programmed death ligand-2; TCR, T cell receptor.

In addition to its antitumor effects, ipilimumab's interference with normal regulatory mechanisms produced a novel spectrum of side effects that resembled autoimmunity. The most common immune-related adverse events were skin rash and diarrhea (sometimes severe, life-threatening colitis), but toxicity could involve most any organ (e.g., hypophysitis, hepatitis, nephritis, pneumonitis, myocarditis, neuritis). Vigilance and early treatment with steroids that do not appear to interfere with the antitumor effects are required to manage these patients safely. Widespread use of ipilimumab has not been completely embraced by the oncology community because of the low objective response rate, significant toxicity (including death), and high cost (drug cost alone for a course of therapy is approximately $120,000 in 2013). Despite these reservations, ipilimumab's overall survival benefit (17% of patients alive at 7 years) indicates that treatment should be strongly considered for all eligible patients.

Chronic T cell activation also leads to induction of PD-1 on the surface of T cells. Expression of one of its ligands, PD-L1, on tumor cells can protect them from immune destruction (Fig. 105-3). Early trials attempting to block the PD-1.PD-L1 axis by IV administration of anti-PD-1 or anti-PD-L1 have shown substantial clinical activity in patients with advanced melanoma (and lung cancer) with significantly less toxicity than ipilimumab. Anti-PD-1 therapy looks promising, but is not currently available except by participation in clinical trials. Intriguingly, preliminary results from a clinical trial indicate that blocking both inhibitory pathways with ipilimumab and anti-PD-1 leads to superior antitumor activity than treatment with either agent alone. The main benefit to patients from immune-based therapy (IL-2, ipilimumab, and anti-PD-1) is the durability of the responses achieved. Although the percentage of patients whose tumors regress following immunotherapy is lower than the response rate after targeted therapy (see below), the durability of immunotherapy-induced responses (>10 years in some cases) appears to be superior to responses after targeted therapy and suggests that many of these patients have been cured.

TARGETED THERAPY

RAF and MEK inhibitors of the MAP kinase pathway are a new and exciting approach for patients whose melanomas harbor a *BRAF* mutation. The high frequency of oncogenic mutations in the RAS-RAF-MEK-ERK pathway, which delivers proliferation and survival signals from the cell surface to the cytoplasm and nucleus, has led to the development of inhibitors to BRAF and MEK. Two BRAF inhibitors, vemurafenib and dabrafenib, have been approved for the treatment of stage IV patients whose melanomas harbor a mutation at position 600 in the gene for *BRAF*. The oral BRAF inhibitors cause tumor regression in approximately 50% of patients, and overall survival is improved compared to treatment with chemotherapy. Treatment is accompanied by manageable side effects that differ from those following immunotherapy or chemotherapy. A class-specific complication of BRAF inhibition is the development of numerous skin lesions, some of which are well-differentiated squamous cell skin cancers (seen in up to a quarter of patients). Patients should be co-managed with a dermatologist as these skin cancers will need excision. Metastases have not been reported, and treatment can be continued safely following simple excision. Long term results following treatment with BRAF inhibitors are not yet available, but the current concern is that over time the vast majority of patients will relapse and eventually die from drug-resistant disease. There are a number of mechanisms by which resistance develops, usually via maintenance of MAP kinase signaling; however, mutations in the *BRAF* gene that affect binding of the inhibitor are not among them. The MEK inhibitor trametinib has activity as a single agent, but appears to be less effective than either of the BRAF inhibitors. Combined therapy with the BRAF inhibitor and MEK inhibitor showed improved progression-free survival compared to BRAF inhibitor therapy alone; and, interestingly, the neoplastic skin lesions that were so troubling with BRAF inhibition alone did not occur. Although the durability of responses following combined therapy remains to be determined, its use in metastatic melanoma is FDA approved. Activating mutations in the c-kit receptor tyrosine kinase are found in a minority of cutaneous melanomas with chronic sun damage, but more commonly in mucosal and acral lentiginous subtypes. Overall, the number of patients with *c-kit* mutations is exceedingly small, but when present, they are largely identical to mutations found in gastrointestinal stromal tumors (GISTs); melanomas with activating *c-kit* mutations can have clinically meaningful responses to imatinib.

CHEMOTHERAPY

No chemotherapy regimen has ever been shown to improve survival in metastatic melanoma, and the advances in immunotherapy and targeted therapy have relegated chemotherapy to the palliation of symptoms. Drugs with antitumor activity include dacarbazine (DTIC) or its orally administered analog temozolomide (TMZ), cisplatin and carboplatin, the taxanes (paclitaxel alone or albumin-bound and docetaxel), and carmustine (BCNU), which have reported response rates of 12–20%.

INITIAL APPROACH TO PATIENT WITH METASTATIC DISEASE

Upon diagnosis of stage IV disease, whether by biopsy or diagnostic imaging, a sample of the patient's tumor needs to undergo molecular testing to determine whether a druggable mutation (e.g., *BRAF*) is present. Analysis of a metastatic lesion is preferred, but any biopsy will suffice because there is little discordance between primary and metastatic lesions. Treatment algorithms start with the tumor's *BRAF* status. For *BRAF* "wild-type" tumors, immunotherapy is recommended. For patients whose tumors harbor a *BRAF* mutation, initial therapy with either a BRAF inhibitor or immunotherapy is acceptable. Molecular testing may also include *N-RAS* and *c-kit* in appropriate tumors.

The majority of patients still die from their melanoma, despite improvements in therapy. Therefore, enrollment in a clinical trial is always an important consideration, even for previously untreated patients. Most patients with stage IV disease will eventually progress despite advances in therapy, and many, because of disease burden, poor performance status, or concomitant illness, will be unsuitable for therapy. Therefore, a major focus of care should be the timely integration of palliative care and hospice.

FOLLOW-UP

Skin examination and surveillance at least once a year are recommended for all patients with melanoma. The National Comprehensive Cancer Network (NCCN) guidelines for patients with stage IA–IIA melanoma recommend a comprehensive history and physical examination every 6–12 months for 5 years, and then annually as clinically indicated. Particular attention should be paid to the draining lymph nodes in stage I–III patients as resection of lymph node recurrences may still be curative. A CBC, LDH, and chest x-ray are recommended at the physician's discretion, but are ineffective tools for the detection of occult metastases. Routine imaging for metastatic disease is not recommended at this time. For patients with higher stage disease (IIB–IV), imaging (chest x-ray, CT, and/or PET/CT scans) every 4–12 months can be considered. Because no discernible survival benefit has been demonstrated for routine surveillance, it is reasonable to perform scans only if clinically indicated.

NONMELANOMA SKIN CANCER

Nonmelanoma skin cancer (NMSC) is the most common cancer in the United States. Although tumor registries do not routinely gather data on the incidence of basal cell and squamous cell skin cancers, it is estimated that the annual incidence is 1.5–2 million cases in the United States. Basal cell carcinomas (BCCs) account for 70–80% of NMSCs. Squamous cell carcinomas (SCCs), which comprise ~20% of NMSCs, are more significant because of their ability to metastasize and account for 2400 NMSC deaths annually. There has also been an increase in the incidence of nonepithelial skin cancer, especially Merkel cell carcinoma, with nearly 5000 new diagnoses and 3000 deaths annually.

PATHOPHYSIOLOGY AND ETIOLOGY

The most significant cause of BCC and SCC is UV exposure, whether through direct exposure to sunlight or by artificial UV light sources (tanning beds). Both UVA and UVB can induce DNA damage through free radical formation (UVA) or induction of pyrimidine dimers (UVB). The sun emits energy across the UV spectrum, whereas tanning bed equipment typically emits 97% UVA and 3% UVB. DNA damage induced by UV irradiation can result in cell death or repair of damaged DNA by nucleotide excision repair (NER). Inherited disorders of NER, such as xeroderma pigmentosum, are associated with a greatly increased incidence of skin cancer and help to establish the link between UV-induced DNA damage, inadequate DNA repair, and skin cancer. The genes damaged most commonly by UV in BCC involve the Hedgehog pathway (Hh). In SCC, *p53* and *N-RAS* are commonly affected. There is a dose-response relationship between tanning bed use and the incidence of skin cancer. As few as four tanning bed visits per year confers a 15% increase in BCC and an 11% increase in SCC and melanoma. Tanning bed use as a teenager or young adult confers greater risk than comparable exposure in older individuals. Other associations include blond or red hair, blue or green eyes, a tendency to sunburn easily, and an outdoor occupation. The incidence of NMSC increases with decreasing latitude. Most tumors develop on sun-exposed areas of the head and neck. The risk of lip or oral SCC is increased with cigarette smoking. Human papillomaviruses and UV radiation may act as cocarcinogens.

Solid organ transplant recipients on chronic immunosuppression have a 65-fold increase in SCC and a 10-fold increase in BCC. The frequency of skin cancer is proportional to the level and duration of immunosuppression and the extent of sun exposure before and after transplantation. SCCs in this population also demonstrate higher rates of local recurrence, metastasis, and mortality. There is increasing use of tumor necrosis factor (TNF) antagonists to treat inflammatory bowel disease and autoimmune disorders such as rheumatoid and psoriatic arthritis. TNF antagonists may also confer an increased risk of NMSC. BRAF-targeted therapy can induce SCCs including keratoacanthoma-type SCCs in keratinocytes, with preexisting *H-RAS* overexpression present in approximately 60% of patients.

Other risk factors include HIV infection, ionizing radiation, thermal burn scars, and chronic ulcerations. Albinism, xeroderma pigmentosum, Muir-Torre syndrome, Rombo's syndrome, Bazex-Dupré-Christol syndrome, dyskeratosis congenita, and basal cell nevus syndrome (Gorlin syndrome) also increase the incidence of NMSC. Mutations in Hh genes encoding the tumor-suppressor patched homolog 1 (*PTCH1*) and smoothened homolog (*SMO*) occur in BCC. Aberrant *PTCH1* signaling is propagated by the nuclear transcription factors Gli1 and Gli2, which are salient in the development of BCC and have led to the FDA approval of an oral SMO inhibitor, vismodegib, to treat advanced inoperable or metastatic BCC (Fig. 105-4). Vismodegib also reduces the incidence of BCC in patients with basal cell nevus syndrome who have *PTCH1* mutations, affirming the importance of Hh in the onset of BCC.

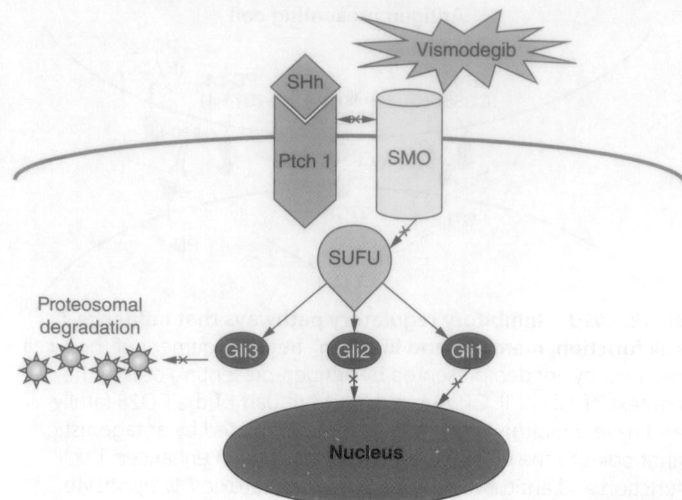

FIGURE 105-4 Influence of vismodegib on the hedgehog (Hh) pathway. Normally, one of three Hh ligands (sonic [SHh], Indian, or desert) binds to patched homolog 1 (PTCH1), causing its degradation and release of smoothened homolog (SMO). The downstream events of SMO release are the activation of Gli1, Gli2, and Gli3 through the transcriptional regulator known as SUFU. Gli1 and Gli2 translocate to the nucleus and promote gene transcription. Vismodegib is an SMO antagonist that decreases the interaction between SMO and PTCH1, resulting in decreased Hh pathway signaling, gene transcription, and cell division. The downstream Hh pathway events inhibited by vismodegib are indicated in red.

CLINICAL PRESENTATION

Basal Cell Carcinoma BCC arises from epidermal basal cells. The least invasive of BCC subtypes, superficial BCC, consists of often subtle, erythematous scaling plaques that slowly enlarge and are most commonly seen on the trunk and proximal extremities (Fig. 105-5). This BCC subtype may be confused with benign inflammatory dermatoses, especially nummular eczema and psoriasis. BCC also can present as a small, slowly growing pearly nodule, often with tortuous telangiectatic vessels on its surface, rolled borders, and a central crust (nodular BCC). The occasional presence of melanin in this variant of nodular BCC (pigmented BCC) may lead to confusion with melanoma. Morpheaform (fibrosing), infiltrative, and micronodular BCC, the most invasive and potentially aggressive subtypes, manifest as solitary, flat or slightly depressed, indurated whitish, yellowish, or pink scar-like plaques. Borders are typically indistinct, and lesions can be subtle; thus, delay in treatment is common, and tumors can be more extensive than expected clinically.

Squamous Cell Carcinoma Primary *cutaneous SCC* is a malignant neoplasm of keratinizing epidermal cells. SCC has a variable clinical course, ranging from indolent to rapid growth kinetics, with the potential for metastasis to regional and distant sites. Commonly, SCC appears as an ulcerated erythematous nodule or superficial erosion on sun-exposed skin of the head, neck, trunk, and extremities (Fig. 105-5). It may also appear as a banal, firm, dome-shaped papule or rough-textured plaque. It is commonly mistaken for a wart or callous when the inflammatory response to the lesion is minimal. Clinically visible overlying telangiectasias are uncommon, although dotted or coiled vessels are a hallmark of SCC when viewed through a dermatoscope.

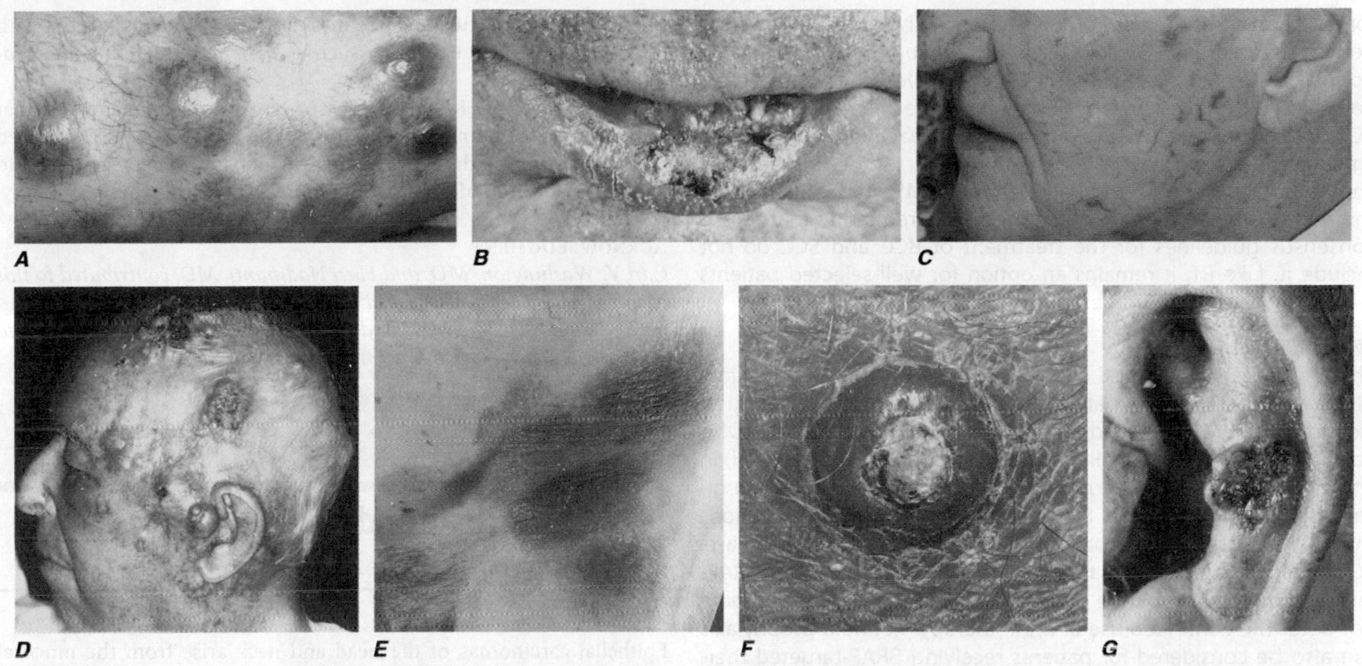

FIGURE 105-5 Cutaneous neoplasms. ***A.*** Non-Hodgkin's lymphoma involves the skin with typical violaceous, "plum-colored" nodules. ***B.*** Squamous cell carcinoma is seen here as a hyperkeratotic crusted and somewhat eroded plaque on the lower lip. Sun-exposed skin in areas such as the head, neck, hands, and arms represent other typical sites of involvement. ***C.*** Actinic keratoses consist of hyperkeratotic erythematous papules and patches on sun-exposed skin. They arise in middle-aged to older adults and have some potential for malignant transformation. ***D.*** Metastatic carcinoma to the skin is characterized by inflammatory, often ulcerated dermal nodules. ***E.*** Mycosis fungoides is a cutaneous T cell lymphoma, and plaque-stage lesions are seen in this patient. ***F.*** Keratoacanthoma is a low-grade squamous cell carcinoma that presents as an exophytic nodule with central keratinous debris. ***G.*** This basal cell carcinoma shows central ulceration and a pearly, rolled telangiectatic tumor border.

The margins of this tumor may be ill defined, and fixation to underlying structures may occur ("tethering").

A very rapidly growing but low-grade form of SCC, called keratoacanthoma (KA), typically appears as a large dome-shaped papule with a central keratotic crater. Some KAs regress spontaneously without therapy, but because progression to metastatic SCC has been documented, KAs should be treated in the same manner as other types of cutaneous SCC. KAs are also associated with medications that target *BRAF* mutations and occur in 15–25% of patients receiving these medications.

Actinic keratoses and *cheilitis* (actinic keratoses occurring on the lip), both premalignant forms of SCC, present as hyperkeratotic papules on sun-exposed areas. The potential for malignant degeneration in untreated lesions ranges from 0.25 to 20%. SCC in situ, also called *Bowen's disease*, is the intraepidermal form of SCC and usually presents as a scaling, erythematous plaque. As with invasive SCC, SCC in situ most commonly arises on sun-damaged skin, but can occur anywhere on the body. Bowen's disease forming secondary to infection with human papillomavirus (HPV) can arise on skin with minimal or no prior sun exposure, such as the buttock or posterior thigh. Treatment of premalignant and in situ lesions reduces the subsequent risk of invasive disease.

NATURAL HISTORY

Basal Cell Carcinoma The natural history of BCC is that of a slowly enlarging, locally invasive neoplasm. The degree of local destruction and risk of recurrence vary with the size, duration, location, and histologic subtype of the tumor. Location on the central face, ears, or scalp may portend a higher risk. Small nodular, pigmented, cystic, or superficial BCCs respond well to most treatments. Large lesions and micronodular, infiltrative, and morpheaform subtypes may be more aggressive. The metastatic potential of BCC is low (0.0028–0.1% in immunocompetent patients), but the risk of recurrence or a new primary NMSC is about 40% over 5 years.

Squamous Cell Carcinoma The natural history of SCC depends on tumor and host characteristics. Tumors arising on sun-damaged skin have a lower metastatic potential than do those on non-sun-exposed areas. Cutaneous SCC metastasizes in 0.3–5.2% of individuals, most frequently to regional lymph nodes. Tumors occurring on the lower lip and ear develop regional metastases in 13 and 11% of patients, respectively, whereas the metastatic potential of SCC arising in scars, chronic ulcerations, and genital or mucosal surfaces is higher. Recurrent SCC has a much higher potential for metastatic disease, approaching 30%. Large, poorly differentiated, deep tumors with perineural or lymphatic invasion, multifocal tumors, and those arising in immunosuppressed patients often behave aggressively.

TREATMENT BASAL CELL CARCINOMA

Treatments used for BCC include electrodesiccation and curettage (ED&C), excision, cryosurgery, radiation therapy (RT), laser therapy, Mohs micrographic surgery (MMS), topical 5-fluorouracil, photodynamic therapy (PDT), and topical immunomodulators such as imiquimod. The therapy chosen depends on tumor characteristics including depth and location, patient age, medical status, and patient preference. ED&C remains the most commonly employed method for superficial, minimally invasive nodular BCCs and low-risk tumors (e.g., a small tumor of a less aggressive subtype in a favorable location). Wide local excision with standard margins is usually selected for invasive, ill-defined, and more aggressive subtypes of tumors, or for cosmetic reasons. MMS, a specialized type of surgical excision that provides the best method for tumor removal while preserving uninvolved tissue, is associated with cure rates >98%. It is the preferred modality for lesions that are recurrent, in high-risk or cosmetically sensitive locations (including recurrent tumors in these locations), and in which maximal tissue conservation is critical (e.g., the eyelids, lips, ears, nose, and digits). RT can cure patients not considered surgical candidates and can be used as a surgical adjunct in high-risk tumors. Younger patients may not be good candidates for RT because of the risks of long-term carcinogenesis and radiodermatitis. Imiquimod can be used to treat superficial and smaller nodular BCCs, although it is not FDA-approved for nodular BCC. Topical 5-fluorouracil therapy should be limited to superficial BCC. PDT, which uses selective activation of a photoactive drug by visible light, has been used in patients with numerous tumors. Intralesional chemotherapy (5-fluorouracil and IFN) for NMSC has existed since the mid-twentieth century, but is used so infrequently that recent consensus guidelines for the treatment of BCC and SCC do not include it. Like RT, it remains an option for well-selected patients who cannot or will not undergo surgery.

SQUAMOUS CELL CARCINOMA

Therapy for cutaneous SCC should be based on the size, location, histologic differentiation, patient age, and functional status. Surgical excision and MMS are standard treatments. Cryosurgery and ED&C have been used for premalignant lesions and small, superficial, in situ primary tumors. Lymph node metastases are treated with surgical resection, RT, or both. Systemic chemotherapy combinations that include cisplatin can palliate patients with advanced disease. SCC and keratoacanthomas that develop in patients receiving BRAF-targeted therapy should be excised, but their development should not deter the continued use of BRAF therapy. Retinoid prophylaxis can also be considered for patients receiving BRAF-targeted therapy, although no prospective studies have been completed thus far.

PREVENTION

The general principles for prevention are those described for melanoma earlier. Unique strategies for NMSC include active surveillance for patients on immunosuppressive medications or BRAF-targeted therapy. Chemoprophylaxis using synthetic retinoids and immunosuppression reduction when possible may be useful in controlling new lesions and managing patients with multiple tumors.

OTHER NONMELANOMA CUTANEOUS MALIGNANCIES

Neoplasms of cutaneous adnexae and sarcomas of fibrous, mesenchymal, fatty, and vascular tissues make up the remaining 1–2% of NMSCs.

Merkel cell carcinoma (MCC) is a neural crest–derived highly aggressive malignancy with mortality rates approaching 33% at 3 years. An oncogenic Merkel cell polyomavirus is present in 80% of tumors. Many patients have detectable cellular or humoral immune responses to polyoma viral proteins, although this immune response is insufficient to eradicate the malignancy. Survival depends on extent of disease: 90% survive with local disease, 52% with nodal involvement, and only 10% with distant disease at 3 years. MCC incidence tripled over the last 20 years with an estimated 1600 cases per year in the United States. Immunosuppression can increase incidence and diminish prognosis. MCC lesions typically present as an asymptomatic rapidly expanding bluish-red/violaceous tumor on sun-exposed skin of older white patients. Treatment is surgical excision with sentinel lymph node biopsy for accurate staging in patients with localized disease, often followed by adjuvant RT. Patients with extensive disease can be offered systemic chemotherapy; however, there is no convincing survival benefit. Whenever possible a clinical trial should be considered for this rare but aggressive NMSC, especially in light of the potential for new treatments directed at the oncogenic virus that causes this malignancy.

Extramammary Paget's disease is an uncommon apocrine malignancy arising from stem cells of the epidermis that are characterized histologically by the presence of Paget cells. These tumors present as moist erythematous patches on anogenital or axillary skin of the elderly. Outcomes are generally good with site-directed surgery, and 5-year disease specific survival is approximately 95% with localized disease. Advanced age and extensive disease at presentation are factors that confer diminished prognosis. RT or topical imiquimod can be considered for more extensive disease. Local management may be challenging because these tumors often extend far beyond clinical margins; surgical excision with MMS has the highest cure rates. Similarly, MMS is the treatment of choice in other rare cutaneous tumors with extensive subclinical extension such as *dermatofibromasarcoma protuberans*.

Kaposi's sarcoma (KS) is a soft tissue sarcoma of vascular origin that is induced by the human herpesvirus 8. The incidence of KS increased dramatically during the AIDS epidemic, but has now decreased tenfold with the institution of highly active antiretroviral therapy.

ACKNOWLEDGMENT

Carl V. Washington, MD, and Hari Nadiminti, MD, contributed to this chapter in the 18th edition, and material from that chapter is included here. Claudia Taylor, MD, and Steven Kolker, MD, provided valued feedback and suggested many improvements to this chapter.

106 Head and Neck Cancer

Everett E. Vokes

Epithelial carcinomas of the head and neck arise from the mucosal surfaces in the head and neck and typically are squamous cell in origin. This category includes tumors of the paranasal sinuses, the oral cavity, and the nasopharynx, oropharynx, hypopharynx, and larynx. Tumors of the salivary glands differ from the more common carcinomas of the head and neck in etiology, histopathology, clinical presentation, and therapy. They are rare and histologically highly heterogeneous. **Thyroid malignancies are described in Chap. 405.**

INCIDENCE AND EPIDEMIOLOGY

The number of new cases of head and neck cancers (oral cavity, pharynx, and larynx) in the United States was 53,640 in 2013, accounting for about 3% of adult malignancies; 11,520 people died from the disease. The worldwide incidence exceeds half a million cases annually. In North America and Europe, the tumors usually arise from the oral cavity, oropharynx, or larynx. The incidence of oropharyngeal cancers is increasing in recent years. Nasopharyngeal cancer is more commonly seen in the Mediterranean countries and in the Far East, where it is endemic in some areas.

ETIOLOGY AND GENETICS

Alcohol and tobacco use are the most significant risk factors for head and neck cancer, and when used together, they act synergistically. Smokeless tobacco is an etiologic agent for oral cancers. Other potential carcinogens include marijuana and occupational exposures such as nickel refining, exposure to textile fibers, and woodworking.

Some head and neck cancers have a viral etiology. Epstein-Barr virus (EBV) infection is frequently associated with nasopharyngeal cancer, especially in endemic areas of the Mediterranean and Far East. EBV antibody titers can be measured to screen high-risk populations. Nasopharyngeal cancer has also been associated with consumption of salted fish and in-door pollution.

In Western countries, the human papilloma virus (HPV) is associated with a rising incidence of tumors arising from the oropharynx, i.e., the tonsillar bed and base of tongue. Over 50% of oropharyngeal tumors are caused by HPV in the United States. HPV 16 is the dominant viral subtype, although HPV 18 and other oncogenic subtypes are seen as well. Alcohol- and tobacco-related cancers, on the other hand, have decreased in incidence. HPV-related oropharyngeal cancer occurs in a younger patient population and is associated with increased numbers of sexual partners and oral sexual practices. It is associated with a better prognosis, especially for nonsmokers.

Dietary factors may contribute. The incidence of head and neck cancer is higher in people with the lowest consumption of fruits and vegetables. Certain vitamins, including carotenoids, may be protective if included in a balanced diet. Supplements of retinoids, such as *cis*-retinoic acid, have not been shown to prevent head and neck cancers (or lung cancer) and may increase the risk in active smokers. No specific risk factors or environmental carcinogens have been identified for salivary gland tumors.

HISTOPATHOLOGY, CARCINOGENESIS, AND MOLECULAR BIOLOGY

Squamous cell head and neck cancers are divided into well-differentiated, moderately well-differentiated, and poorly differentiated categories. Poorly differentiated tumors have a worse prognosis than well-differentiated tumors. For nasopharyngeal cancers, the less common differentiated squamous cell carcinoma is distinguished from nonkeratinizing and undifferentiated carcinoma (lymphoepithelioma) that contains infiltrating lymphocytes and is commonly associated with EBV.

Salivary gland tumors can arise from the major (parotid, submandibular, sublingual) or minor salivary glands (located in the submucosa of the upper aerodigestive tract). Most parotid tumors are benign, but half of submandibular and sublingual gland tumors and most minor salivary gland tumors are malignant. Malignant tumors include mucoepidermoid and adenoid cystic carcinomas and adenocarcinomas.

The mucosal surface of the entire pharynx is exposed to alcohol- and tobacco-related carcinogens and is at risk for the development of a premalignant or malignant lesion. Erythroplakia (a red patch) or leukoplakia (a white patch) can be histopathologically classified as hyperplasia, dysplasia, carcinoma in situ, or carcinoma. However, most head and neck cancer patients do not present with a history of premalignant lesions. Multiple synchronous or metachronous cancers can also be observed. In fact, over time, patients with early-stage head and neck cancer are at greater risk of dying from a second malignancy than from a recurrence of the primary disease.

Second head and neck malignancies are usually not therapy-induced; they reflect the exposure of the upper aerodigestive mucosa to the same carcinogens that caused the first cancer. These second primaries develop in the head and neck area, the lung, or the esophagus. Thus, computed tomography (CT) screening for lung cancer in heavy smokers who have already developed a head and neck cancer should be considered. Rarely, patients can develop a radiation therapy–induced sarcoma after having undergone prior radiotherapy for a head and neck cancer.

Much progress has been made in describing the molecular features of head and neck cancer. These features have allowed investigators to describe the genetic and epigenetic alterations and the mutational spectrum of these tumors. Early reports demonstrated frequent overexpression of the epidermal growth factor receptor (EGFR). Overexpression was shown to correlate with poor prognosis. However, it has not proved to be a good predictor of tumor response to EGFR inhibitors, which are successful in only about 10–15% of patients. *p53* mutations are also found frequently with other major affected oncogenic driver pathways including the mitotic signaling and Notch pathways and cell cycle regulation. The PI3K pathway is frequently altered, especially in HPV-positive tumors, where it is the only mutated cancer gene identified to date. Overall, these alterations affect mitogenic signaling, genetic stability, cellular proliferation, and differentiation. HPV is known to act through inhibition of the *p53* and *RB* tumor-suppressor genes, thereby initiating the carcinogenic process, and has a mutational spectrum distinct from alcohol- and tobacco-related tumors.

CLINICAL PRESENTATION AND DIFFERENTIAL DIAGNOSIS

Most tobacco-related head and neck cancers occur in patients older than age 60 years. HPV-related malignancies are frequently diagnosed in younger patients, usually in their forties or fifties, whereas EBV-related nasopharyngeal cancer can occur in all ages, including teenagers. The manifestations vary according to the stage and primary site of the tumor. Patients with nonspecific signs and symptoms in the head and neck area should be evaluated with a thorough otolaryngologic exam, particularly if symptoms persist longer than 2–4 weeks. Males are more frequently affected than women by head and neck cancers, including HPV-positive tumors.

Cancer of the nasopharynx typically does not cause early symptoms. However, it may cause unilateral serous otitis media due to obstruction of the eustachian tube, unilateral or bilateral nasal obstruction, or epistaxis. Advanced nasopharyngeal carcinoma causes neuropathies of the cranial nerves due to skull base involvement.

Carcinomas of the oral cavity present as nonhealing ulcers, changes in the fit of dentures, or painful lesions. Tumors of the tongue base or oropharynx can cause decreased tongue mobility and alterations in speech. Cancers of the oropharynx or hypopharynx rarely cause early symptoms, but they may cause sore throat and/or otalgia. HPV-related tumors frequently present with neck lymphadenopathy as the first sign.

Hoarseness may be an early symptom of laryngeal cancer, and persistent hoarseness requires referral to a specialist for indirect laryngoscopy and/or radiographic studies. If a head and neck lesion treated initially with antibiotics does not resolve in a short period, further workup is indicated; to simply continue the antibiotic treatment may be to lose the chance of early diagnosis of a malignancy.

Advanced head and neck cancers in any location can cause severe pain, otalgia, airway obstruction, cranial neuropathies, trismus, odynophagia, dysphagia, decreased tongue mobility, fistulas, skin involvement, and massive cervical lymphadenopathy, which may be unilateral or bilateral. Some patients have enlarged lymph nodes even though no primary lesion can be detected by endoscopy or biopsy; these patients are considered to have carcinoma of unknown primary (Fig. 106-1). If the enlarged nodes are located in the upper neck and the tumor cells are of squamous cell histology, the malignancy probably arose from a mucosal surface in the head or neck. Tumor cells in supraclavicular lymph nodes may also arise from a primary site in the chest or abdomen.

The physical examination should include inspection of all visible mucosal surfaces and palpation of the floor of the mouth and of the tongue and neck. In addition to tumors themselves, leukoplakia (a white mucosal patch) or erythroplakia (a red mucosal patch) may be observed; these "premalignant" lesions can represent hyperplasia, dysplasia, or carcinoma in situ and require biopsy. Further examination should be performed by a specialist. Additional staging procedures include CT of the head and neck to identify the extent of the disease. Patients with lymph node involvement should have CT scan of the chest and upper abdomen to screen for distant metastases. In heavy smokers, the CT scan of the chest can also serve as a screening tool to rule out a second lung primary tumor. A positron emission tomography (PET) scan may also be administered and can help to identify or exclude distant metastases. The definitive staging procedure is an

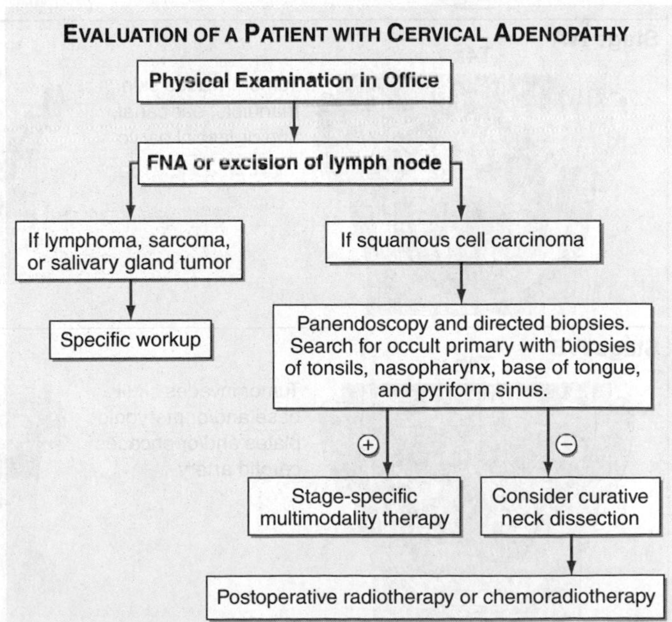

FIGURE 106-1 Evaluation of a patient with cervical adenopathy without a primary mucosal lesion; a diagnostic workup. FNA, fine-needle aspiration.

endoscopic examination under anesthesia, which may include laryngoscopy, esophagoscopy, and bronchoscopy; during this procedure, multiple biopsy samples are obtained to establish a primary diagnosis, define the extent of primary disease, and identify any additional premalignant lesions or second primaries.

Head and neck tumors are classified according to the tumor-node-metastasis (TNM) system of the American Joint Committee on Cancer (Fig. 106-2). This classification varies according to the specific anatomic subsite. In general, primary tumors are classified as T1 to T3 by increasing size, whereas T4 usually represents invasion of another structure such as bone, muscle, or root of tongue. Lymph nodes are staged by size, number, and location (ipsilateral vs contralateral to the primary). Distant metastases are found in <10% of patients at initial diagnosis and are more common in patients with advanced lymph node stage; microscopic involvement of the lungs, bones, or liver is more common, particularly in patients with advanced neck lymph node disease. Modern imaging techniques may increase the number of patients with clinically detectable distant metastases in the future.

In patients with lymph node involvement and no visible primary, the diagnosis should be made by lymph node excision (Fig. 106-1). If

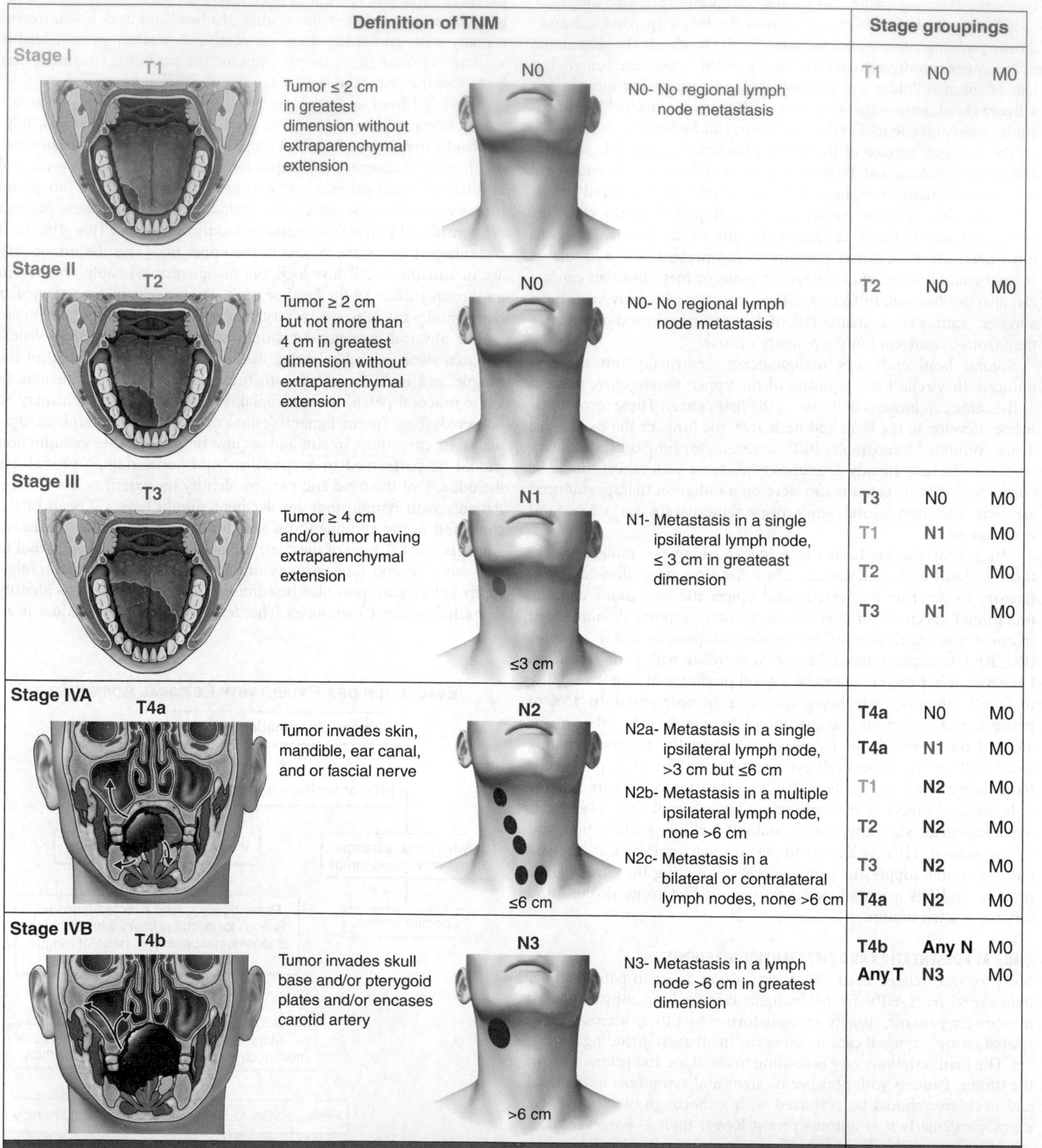

Stage	Definition of TNM: T		Definition of TNM: N		Stage groupings		
Stage I	T1	Tumor ≤ 2 cm in greatest dimension without extraparenchymal extension	N0	N0- No regional lymph node metastasis	T1	N0	M0
Stage II	T2	Tumor ≥ 2 cm but not more than 4 cm in greatest dimension without extraparenchymal extension	N0	N0- No regional lymph node metastasis	T2	N0	M0
Stage III	T3	Tumor ≥ 4 cm and/or tumor having extraparenchymal extension	N1 (≤3 cm)	N1- Metastasis in a single ipsilateral lymph node, ≤ 3 cm in greateast dimension	T3	N0	M0
					T1	N1	M0
					T2	N1	M0
					T3	N1	M0
Stage IVA	T4a	Tumor invades skin, mandible, ear canal, and or fascial nerve	N2 (≤6 cm)	N2a- Metastasis in a single ipsilateral lymph node, >3 cm but ≤6 cm; N2b- Metastasis in a multiple ipsilateral lymph node, none >6 cm; N2c- Metastasis in a bilateral or contralateral lymph nodes, none >6 cm	T4a	N0	M0
					T4a	N1	M0
					T1	N2	M0
					T2	N2	M0
					T3	N2	M0
					T4a	N2	M0
Stage IVB	T4b	Tumor invades skull base and/or pterygoid plates and/or encases carotid artery	N3 (>6 cm)	N3- Metastasis in a lymph node >6 cm in greatest dimension	T4b	Any N	M0
					Any T	N3	M0
Stage IVC			M1		Any T	Any N	M1

FIGURE 106-2 Tumor-node-metastasis (TNM) staging system.

the results indicate squamous cell carcinoma, a panendoscopy should be performed, with biopsy of all suspicious-appearing areas and directed biopsies of common primary sites, such as the nasopharynx, tonsil, tongue base, and pyriform sinus. HPV-positive tumors especially can have small primary tumors that spread early to locoregional lymph nodes.

TREATMENT HEAD AND NECK CANCER

Patients with head and neck cancer can be grossly categorized into three clinical groups: those with localized disease, those with locally or regionally advanced disease (lymph node positive), and those with recurrent and/or metastatic disease. Comorbidities associated with tobacco and alcohol abuse can affect treatment outcome and define long-term risks for patients who are cured of their disease.

LOCALIZED DISEASE

Nearly one-third of patients have localized disease, that is, T1 or T2 (stage I or stage II) lesions without detectable lymph node involvement or distant metastases. These patients are treated with curative intent by either surgery or radiation therapy. The choice of modality differs according to anatomic location and institutional expertise. Radiation therapy is often preferred for laryngeal cancer to preserve voice function, and surgery is preferred for small lesions in the oral cavity to avoid the long-term complications of radiation, such as xerostomia and dental decay. Overall 5-year survival is 60–90%. Most recurrences occur within the first 2 years following diagnosis and are usually local.

LOCALLY OR REGIONALLY ADVANCED DISEASE

Locally or regionally advanced disease—disease with a large primary tumor and/or lymph node metastases—is the stage of presentation for >50% of patients. Such patients can also be treated with curative intent, but not with surgery or radiation therapy alone. Combined-modality therapy including surgery, radiation therapy, and chemotherapy is most successful. It can be administered as induction chemotherapy (chemotherapy before surgery and/or radiotherapy) or as concomitant (simultaneous) chemotherapy and radiation therapy. The latter is currently most commonly used and supported by the best evidence. Five-year survival rates exceed 50% in many trials, but part of this increased survival may be due to an increasing fraction of study populations with HPV-related tumors who carry a better prognosis. HPV testing of newly diagnosed tumors is now performed for most patients at the time of diagnosis, and clinical trials for HPV-related tumors are focused on exploring reductions in treatment intensity, especially radiation dose, in order to ameliorate long-term toxicities (fibrosis, swallowing dysfunction).

In patients with intermediate-stage tumors (stage III and early stage IV), concomitant chemoradiotherapy can be administered either as a primary treatment for patients with unresectable disease, to pursue an organ-preserving approach, or in the postoperative setting for intermediate-stage resectable tumors.

Induction Chemotherapy In this strategy, patients receive chemotherapy (current standard is a three-drug regimen of docetaxel, cisplatin, and fluorouracil [5-FU]) before surgery and radiation therapy. Most patients who receive three cycles show tumor reduction, and the response is clinically "complete" in up to half of patients. This "sequential" multimodality therapy allows for organ preservation (omission of surgery) in patients with laryngeal and hypopharyngeal cancer, and it has been shown to result in higher cure rates compared with radiotherapy alone.

Concomitant Chemoradiotherapy With the concomitant strategy, chemotherapy and radiation therapy are given simultaneously rather than in sequence. Tumor recurrences from head and neck cancer develop most commonly locoregionally (in the head and neck area of the primary and draining lymph nodes). The concomitant approach is aimed at enhancing tumor cell killing by radiation therapy in the presence of chemotherapy (radiation enhancement) and is a conceptually attractive approach for bulky tumors. Toxicity (especially mucositis, grade 3 or 4 in 70–80%) is increased with concomitant chemoradiotherapy. However, meta-analyses of randomized trials document an improvement in 5-year survival of 8% with concomitant chemotherapy and radiation therapy. Results seem more favorable in recent trials as more active drugs or more intensive radiotherapy schedules are used. In addition, concomitant chemoradiotherapy produces better laryngectomy-free survival (organ preservation) than radiation therapy alone in patients with advanced larynx cancer. The use of radiation therapy together with cisplatin has also produced improved survival in patients with advanced nasopharyngeal cancer. The outcome of HPV-related cancers seems to be especially favorable following cisplatin-based chemoradiotherapy.

The success of concomitant chemoradiotherapy in patients with unresectable disease has led to the testing of a similar approach in patients with resected intermediate-stage disease as a postoperative therapy. Concomitant chemoradiotherapy produces a significant improvement over postoperative radiation therapy alone for patients whose tumors demonstrate higher risk features, such as extracapsular spread beyond involved lymph nodes, involvement of multiple lymph nodes, or positive margins at the primary site following surgery.

A monoclonal antibody to EGFR (cetuximab) increases survival rates when administered during radiotherapy. EGFR blockade results in radiation sensitization and has milder systemic side effects than traditional chemotherapy agents, although an acneiform skin rash is commonly observed. Nevertheless, the integration of cetuximab into current standard chemoradiotherapy regimens has failed to show additional improvement in survival and is not recommended.

RECURRENT AND/OR METASTATIC DISEASE

Five to ten percent of patients present with metastatic disease, and 30–50% of patients with locoregionally advanced disease experience recurrence, frequently outside the head and neck region. Patients with recurrent and/or metastatic disease are, with few exceptions, treated with palliative intent. Some patients may require local or regional radiation therapy for pain control, but most are given chemotherapy. Response rates to chemotherapy average only 30–50%; the durations of response are short, and the median survival time is 8–10 months. Therefore, chemotherapy provides transient symptomatic benefit. Drugs with single-agent activity in this setting include methotrexate, 5-FU, cisplatin, paclitaxel, and docetaxel. Combinations of cisplatin with 5-FU, carboplatin with 5-FU, and cisplatin or carboplatin with paclitaxel or docetaxel are frequently used.

EGFR-directed therapies, including monoclonal antibodies (e.g., cetuximab) and tyrosine kinase inhibitors (TKIs) of the EGFR signaling pathway (e.g., erlotinib or gefitinib), have single-agent activity of approximately 10%. Side effects are usually limited to an acneiform rash and diarrhea (for the TKIs). The addition of cetuximab to standard combination chemotherapy with cisplatin or carboplatin and 5-FU was shown to result in a significant increase in median survival. Drugs targeting specific mutations are under investigation, but no such strategy has yet been shown to be feasible in head and neck cancer.

COMPLICATIONS

Complications from treatment of head and neck cancer are usually correlated to the extent of surgery and exposure of normal tissue structures to radiation. Currently, the extent of surgery has been limited or completely replaced by chemotherapy and radiation therapy as the primary approach. Acute complications of radiation include mucositis and dysphagia. Long-term complications include xerostomia, loss of taste, decreased tongue mobility, second malignancies, dysphagia, and neck fibrosis. The complications of chemotherapy vary with the regimen used but usually include myelosuppression, mucositis, nausea and vomiting, and nephrotoxicity (with cisplatin).

The mucosal side effects of therapy can lead to malnutrition and dehydration. Many centers address issues of dentition before starting treatment, and some place feeding tubes to ensure control of hydration and nutrition intake. About 50% of patients develop hypothyroidism from the treatment; thus, thyroid function should be monitored.

SALIVARY GLAND TUMORS

Most benign salivary gland tumors are treated with surgical excision, and patients with invasive salivary gland tumors are treated with surgery and radiation therapy. These tumors may recur regionally; adenoid cystic carcinoma has a tendency to recur along the nerve tracks. Distant metastases may occur as late as 10–20 years after the initial diagnosis. For metastatic disease, therapy is given with palliative intent, usually chemotherapy with doxorubicin and/or cisplatin. Identification of novel agents with activity in these tumors is a high priority.

107 Neoplasms of the Lung

Leora Horn, Christine M. Lovly, David H. Johnson

Lung cancer, which was rare prior to 1900 with fewer than 400 cases described in the medical literature, is considered a disease of modern man. By the mid-twentieth century, lung cancer had become epidemic and firmly established as the leading cause of cancer-related death in North America and Europe, killing over three times as many men as prostate cancer and nearly twice as many women as breast cancer. This fact is particularly troubling because lung cancer is one of the most preventable of all of the major malignancies. Tobacco consumption is the primary cause of lung cancer, a reality firmly established in the mid-twentieth century and codified with the release of the U.S. Surgeon General's 1964 report on the health effects of tobacco smoking. Following the report, cigarette use started to decline in North America and parts of Europe, and with it, so did the incidence of lung cancer. To date, the decline in lung cancer is seen most clearly in men; only recently has the decline become apparent among women in the United States. Unfortunately, in many parts of the world, especially in countries with developing economies, cigarette use continues to increase, and along with it, the incidence of lung cancers is also rising. Although tobacco smoking remains the primary cause of lung cancer worldwide, approximately 60% of new lung cancers in the United States occur in former smokers (smoked ≥100 cigarettes per lifetime, quit ≥1 year), many of whom quit decades ago, or never smokers (smoked <100 cigarettes per lifetime). Moreover, one in five women and one in 12 men diagnosed with lung cancer have never smoked. Given the magnitude of the problem, it is incumbent that every internist has a general knowledge of lung cancer and its management.

EPIDEMIOLOGY

Lung cancer is the most common cause of cancer death among American men and women. More than 225,000 individuals will be diagnosed with lung cancer in the United States in 2013, and over 150,000 individuals will die from the disease. The incidence of lung cancer peaked among men in the late 1980s and has plateaued in women. Lung cancer is rare below age 40, with rates increasing until age 80, after which the rate tapers off. The projected lifetime probability of developing lung cancer is estimated to be approximately 8% among males and approximately 6% among females. The incidence of lung cancer varies by racial and ethnic group, with the highest age-adjusted incidence rates among African Americans. The excess in age-adjusted rates among African Americans occurs only among men, but examinations of age-specific rates show that below age 50, mortality from lung cancer is more than 25% higher among African American than Caucasian women. Incidence and mortality rates among Hispanics and Native and Asian Americans are approximately 40–50% those of whites.

RISK FACTORS

Cigarette smokers have a 10-fold or greater increased risk of developing lung cancer compared to those who have never smoked. A deep sequencing study suggested that one genetic mutation is induced for every 15 cigarettes smoked. The risk of lung cancer is lower among persons who quit smoking than among those who continue smoking; former smokers have a ninefold increased risk of developing lung cancer compared to men who have never smoked versus the 20-fold excess in those who continue to smoke. The size of the risk reduction increases with the length of time the person has quit smoking, although generally even long-term former smokers have higher risks of lung cancer than those who never smoked. Cigarette smoking has been shown to increase the risk of all the major lung cancer cell types. Environmental tobacco smoke (ETS) or second-hand smoke is also an established cause of lung cancer. The risk from ETS is less than from active smoking, with about a 20–30% increase in lung cancer observed among never smokers married for many years to smokers, in comparison to the 2000% increase among continuing active smokers.

Although cigarette smoking is the cause of the majority of lung cancers, several other risk factors have been identified, including occupational exposures to asbestos, arsenic, bischloromethyl ether, hexavalent chromium, mustard gas, nickel (as in certain nickel-refining processes), and polycyclic aromatic hydrocarbons. Occupational observations also have provided insight into possible mechanisms of lung cancer induction. For example, the risk of lung cancer among asbestos-exposed workers is increased primarily among those with underlying asbestosis, raising the possibility that the scarring and inflammation produced by this fibrotic nonmalignant lung disease may in many cases (although likely not in all) be the trigger for asbestos-induced lung cancer. Several other occupational exposures have been associated with increased rates of lung cancer, but the causal nature of the association is not as clear.

The risk of lung cancer appears to be higher among individuals with low fruit and vegetable intake during adulthood. This observation led to hypotheses that specific nutrients, in particular retinoids and carotenoids, might have chemopreventative effects for lung cancer. However, randomized trials failed to validate this hypothesis. In fact, studies found the incidence of lung cancer was increased among smokers with supplementation. Ionizing radiation is also an established lung carcinogen, most convincingly demonstrated from studies showing increased rates of lung cancer among survivors of the atom bombs dropped on Hiroshima and Nagasaki and large excesses among workers exposed to alpha irradiation from radon in underground uranium mining. Prolonged exposure to low-level radon in homes might impart a risk of lung cancer equal or greater than that of ETS. Prior lung diseases such as chronic bronchitis, emphysema, and tuberculosis have been linked to increased risks of lung cancer as well.

Smoking Cessation Given the undeniable link between cigarette smoking and lung cancer (not even addressing other tobacco-related illnesses), physicians must promote tobacco abstinence. Physicians also must help their patients who smoke to stop smoking. Smoking cessation, even well into middle age, can minimize an individual's subsequent risk of lung cancer. Stopping tobacco use before middle age avoids more than 90% of the lung cancer risk attributable to tobacco. However, there is little health benefit derived from just "cutting back." Importantly, smoking cessation can even be beneficial in individuals with an established diagnosis of lung cancer, as it is associated with improved survival, fewer side effects from therapy, and an overall improvement in quality of life. Moreover, smoking can alter the metabolism of many chemotherapy drugs, potentially adversely altering the toxicities and therapeutic benefits of the agents. Consequently, it is important to promote smoking cessation even *after* the diagnosis of lung cancer is established.

Physicians need to understand the essential elements of smoking cessation therapy. The individual must want to stop smoking and must be willing to work hard to achieve the goal of smoking abstinence. Self-help strategies alone only marginally affect quit rates, whereas individual and combined pharmacotherapies in combination with counseling can significantly increase rates of cessation. Therapy with an antidepressant (e.g., bupropion) and nicotine replacement therapy (varenicline, a $\alpha_4\beta_2$ nicotinic acetylcholine receptor partial agonist) are approved by the U.S. Food and Drug Administration (FDA) as first-line treatments for nicotine dependence. However, both drugs have been reported to increase suicidal ideation and must be used with caution. In a randomized trial, varenicline was shown to be more efficacious than bupropion or placebo. Prolonged use of varenicline beyond the initial induction phase proved useful in maintaining smoking abstinence. Clonidine and nortriptyline are recommended as second-line treatments. Of note, reducing cigarettes smoked before quit day and quitting abruptly, with no prior reduction, yield comparable quit rates. Therefore, patients can be given the choice to quit in either of these ways (Chap. 470).

Inherited Predisposition to Lung Cancer Exposure to environmental carcinogens, such as those found in tobacco smoke, induce or facilitate the transformation from bronchoepithelial cells to the malignant phenotype. The contribution of carcinogens on transformation is modulated by polymorphic variations in genes that affect aspects of carcinogen metabolism. Certain genetic polymorphisms of the P450 enzyme system, specifically CYP1A1, and chromosome fragility are associated with the development of lung cancer. These genetic variations occur at relatively high frequency in the population, but their contribution to an individual's lung cancer risk is generally low. However, because of their population frequency, the overall impact on lung cancer risk could be high. In addition, environmental factors, as modified by inherited modulators, likely affect specific genes by deregulating important pathways to enable the cancer phenotype.

First-degree relatives of lung cancer probands have a two- to threefold excess risk of lung cancer and other cancers, many of which are not smoking-related. These data suggest that specific genes and/or genetic variants may contribute to susceptibility to lung cancer. However, very few such genes have yet been identified. Individuals with inherited mutations in *RB* (patients with retinoblastoma living to adulthood) and *p53* (Li-Fraumeni syndrome) genes may develop lung cancer. Common gene variants involved in lung cancer have been recently identified through large, collaborative, genome-wide association studies. These studies identified three separate loci that are associated with lung cancer (5p15, 6p21, and 15q25) and include genes that regulate acetylcholine nicotinic receptors and telomerase production. A rare germline mutation (T790M) involving the epidermal growth factor receptor (EGFR) maybe be linked to lung cancer susceptibility in never smokers. Likewise, a susceptibility locus on chromosome 6q greatly increases risk lung cancer risk among light and never smokers. Although progress has been made, there is a significant amount of work that remains to be done in identifying heritable risk factors for lung cancer. Currently no molecular criteria are suitable to select patients for more intense screening programs or for specific chemopreventative strategies.

PATHOLOGY

The World Health Organization (WHO) defines lung cancer as tumors arising from the respiratory epithelium (bronchi, bronchioles, and alveoli). The WHO classification system divides epithelial lung cancers into four major cell types: small-cell lung cancer (SCLC), adenocarcinoma, squamous cell carcinoma, and large-cell carcinoma; the latter three types are collectively known as non-small-cell carcinomas (NSCLCs) (Fig. 107-1). Small-cell carcinomas consist of small cells with scant cytoplasm, ill-defined cell borders, finely granular nuclear chromatin, absent or inconspicuous nucleoli, and a high mitotic count. SCLC may be distinguished from NSCLC by the presence of neuroendocrine markers including CD56, neural cell adhesion molecule (NCAM), synaptophysin, and chromogranin. In North America, adenocarcinoma is the most common histologic type of lung cancer. Adenocarcinomas possess glandular differentiation or mucin production and may show acinar, papillary, lepidic, or solid features or a mixture of these patterns. Squamous cell carcinomas of the lung are morphologically identical to extrapulmonary squamous cell carcinomas and cannot be distinguished by immunohistochemistry alone. Squamous cell tumors show keratinization and/or intercellular bridges that arise from bronchial epithelium. The tumor tends to consists of sheets of cells rather than the three-dimensional groups of cells characteristic of adenocarcinomas. Large-cell carcinomas comprise less than 10% of lung carcinomas. These tumors lack the cytologic and architectural features of small-cell carcinoma and glandular or squamous differentiation. Together these four histologic types account for approximately 90% of all epithelial lung cancers.

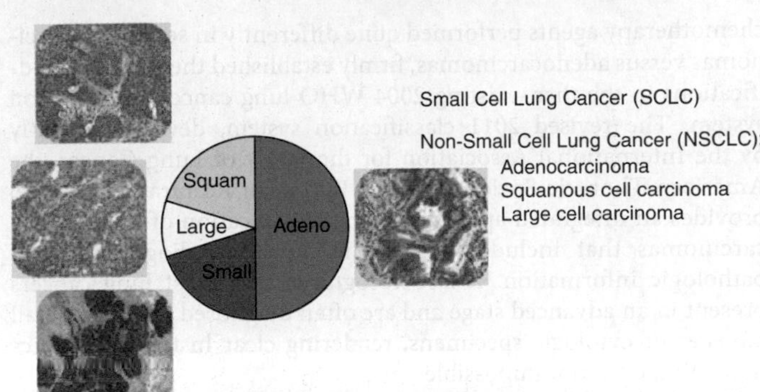

FIGURE 107-1 Traditional histologic view of lung cancer.

All histologic types of lung cancer can develop in current and former smokers, although squamous and small-cell carcinomas are most commonly associated with heavy tobacco use. Through the first half of the twentieth century, squamous carcinoma was the most common subtype of NSCLC diagnosed in the United States. However, with the decline in cigarette consumption over the past four decades, adenocarcinoma has become the most frequent histologic subtype of lung cancer in the United States as both squamous carcinoma and small-cell carcinoma are on the decline. In lifetime never smokers or former light smokers (<10 pack-year history), women, and younger adults (<60 years), adenocarcinoma tends to be the most common form of lung cancer.

Historically, the major pathologic distinction was simply between SCLC and NSCLC, because these tumors have quite different natural histories and therapeutic approaches (see below). Likewise, until fairly recently, there was no apparent need to distinguish among the various subtypes of NSCLC because there were no clear differences in therapeutic outcome based on histology alone. However, this perspective radically changed in 2004 with the recognition that a small percentage of lung adenocarcinomas harbored mutation in *EGFR* that rendered those tumors exquisitely sensitive to inhibitors of the EGFR tyrosine kinases (e.g., gefitinib and erlotinib). This observation, coupled with the subsequent identification of other "actionable" molecular alterations (Table 107-1) and the recognition that some active

TABLE 107-1 DRIVER MUTATIONS IN NON-SMALL-CELL LUNG CANCER (NSCLC)

Gene	Alteration	Frequency in NSCLC	Typical Histology
AKT1	Mutation	1%	Adenocarcinoma, squamous
ALK	Rearrangement	3–7%	Adenocarcinoma
BRAF	Mutation	1–3%	Adenocarcinoma
DDR2	Mutation	~4%	Squamous
EGFR	Mutation	10–35%	Adenocarcinoma
FGFR1	Amplification	~20%	Squamous
HER2	Mutation	2–4%	Adenocarcinoma
KRAS	Mutation	15–25%	Adenocarcinoma
MEK1	Mutation	1%	Adenocarcinoma
MET	Amplification	2–4%	Adenocarcinoma
NRAS	Mutation	1%	Adenocarcinoma
PIK3CA	Mutation	1–3%	Squamous
PTEN	Mutation	4–8%	Squamous

chemotherapy agents performed quite differently in squamous carcinomas versus adenocarcinomas, firmly established the need for modifications in the then-existing 2004 WHO lung cancer classification system. The revised 2011 classification system, developed jointly by the International Association for the Study of Lung Cancer, the American Thoracic Society, and the European Respiratory Society, provides an integrated approach to the classification of lung adenocarcinomas that includes clinical, molecular, radiographic, and pathologic information. It also recognizes that most lung cancers present in an advanced stage and are often diagnosed based on small biopsies or cytologic specimens, rendering clear histologic distinctions difficult if not impossible.

Previously, in the 2004 classification system, tumors *failing* to show definite glandular or squamous morphology in a small biopsy or cytologic specimen were simply classified as *non-small-cell carcinoma, not otherwise specified.* However, because the distinction between adenocarcinoma and squamous carcinoma is now viewed as critical to optimal therapeutic decision making, the modified classification approach recommends these lesions be further characterized using a limited special stain workup. This distinction can be achieved using a single marker for adenocarcinoma (thyroid transcription factor-1 or napsin-A) plus a squamous marker (p40 or p63) and/or mucin stains. The modified classification system also recommends preservation of sufficient specimen material for appropriate molecular testing necessary to help guide therapeutic decision making (see below).

Another significant modification to the WHO classification system is the discontinuation of the terms *bronchioloalveolar carcinoma* and *mixed-subtype adenocarcinoma.* The term *bronchioloalveolar carcinoma* was dropped due to its inconsistent use and because it caused confusion in routine clinical care and research. As formerly used, the term encompassed at least five different entities with diverse clinical and molecular properties. The terms *adenocarcinoma in situ* and *minimally invasive adenocarcinoma* are now recommended for small solitary adenocarcinomas (≤3 cm) with either pure lepidic growth (term used to describe single-layered growth of atypical cuboidal cells coating the alveolar walls) or predominant lepidic growth with ≤5 mm invasion. Individuals with these entities experience 100% or near 100% 5-year disease-free survival with complete tumor resection. *Invasive adenocarcinomas,* representing more than 70–90% of surgically resected lung adenocarcinomas, are now classified by their predominant pattern: lepidic, acinar, papillary, and solid patterns. Lepidic-predominant subtype has a favorable prognosis, acinar and papillary have an intermediate prognosis, and solid-predominant has a poor prognosis. The terms *signet ring* and *clear cell adenocarcinoma* have been eliminated from the variants of invasive lung adenocarcinoma, whereas the term *micropapillary,* a subtype with a particularly poor prognosis, has been added. Although *EGFR* mutations are encountered most frequently in nonmucinous adenocarcinomas with a lepidic- or papillary-predominant pattern, most adenocarcinoma subtypes can harbor *EGFR* or *KRAS* mutations. The same is true of *ALK, RET,* and *ROS1* rearrangements. What was previously termed *mucinous bronchioloalveolar carcinoma* is now called *invasive mucinous adenocarcinoma.* These tumors generally lack *EGFR* mutations and show a strong correlation with *KRAS* mutations. Overall, the revised WHO reclassification of lung cancer addresses important advances in diagnosis and treatment, most importantly, the critical advances in understanding the specific genes and molecular pathways that initiate and sustain lung tumorigenesis resulting in new "targeted" therapies with improved specificity and better antitumor efficacy.

IMMUNOHISTOCHEMISTRY

The diagnosis of lung cancer most often rests on the morphologic or cytologic features correlated with clinical and radiographic findings. Immunohistochemistry may be used to verify neuroendocrine differentiation within a tumor, with markers such as neuron-specific enolase (NSE), CD56 or NCAM, synaptophysin, chromogranin, and Leu7. Immunohistochemistry is also helpful in differentiating primary from metastatic adenocarcinomas; thyroid transcription factor-1 (TTF-1), identified in tumors of thyroid and pulmonary origin, is positive in over 70% of pulmonary adenocarcinomas and is a reliable indicator of primary lung cancer, provided a thyroid primary has been excluded. A negative TTF-1, however, does not exclude the possibility of a lung primary. TTF-1 is also positive in neuroendocrine tumors of pulmonary and extrapulmonary origin. Napsin-A (Nap-A) is an aspartic protease that plays an important role in maturation of surfactant B7 and is expressed in cytoplasm of type II pneumocytes. In several studies, Nap-A has been reported in >90% of primary lung adenocarcinomas. Notably, a combination of Nap-A and TTF-1 is useful in distinguishing primary lung adenocarcinoma (Nap-A positive, TTF-1 positive) from primary lung squamous cell carcinoma (Nap-A negative, TTF-1 negative) and primary SCLC (Nap-A negative, TTF-1 positive). Cytokeratins 7 and 20 used in combination can help narrow the differential diagnosis; nonsquamous NSCLC, SCLC, and mesothelioma may stain positive for CK7 and negative for CK20, whereas squamous cell lung cancer often will be both CK7 and CK20 negative. p63 is a useful marker for the detection of NSCLCs with squamous differentiation when used in cytologic pulmonary samples. Mesothelioma can be easily identified ultrastructurally, but it has historically been difficult to differentiate from adenocarcinoma through morphology and immunohistochemical staining. Several markers in the last few years have proven to be more helpful including CK5/6, calretinin, and Wilms tumor gene-1 (*WT-1*), all of which show positivity in mesothelioma.

MOLECULAR PATHOGENESIS

Cancer is a disease involving dynamic changes in the genome. As proposed by Hanahan and Weinberg, virtually all cancer cells acquire six hallmark capabilities: self-sufficiency in growth signals, insensitivity to antigrowth signals, evading apoptosis, limitless replicative potential, sustained angiogenesis, and tissue invasion and metastasis. The order in which these hallmark capabilities are acquired appears quite variable and can differ from tumor to tumor. Events leading to acquisition of these hallmarks can vary widely, although broadly, cancers arise as a result from accumulations of gain-of-function mutations in oncogenes and loss-of-function mutations in tumor-suppressor genes. Further complicating the study of lung cancer, the sequence of events that lead to disease is clearly different for the various histopathologic entities.

The exact cell of origin for lung cancers is not clearly defined. Whether one cell of origin leads to all histologic forms of lung cancer is unclear. However, for lung adenocarcinoma, evidence suggests that type II epithelial cells (or alveolar epithelial cells) have the capacity to give rise to tumors. For SCLC, cells of neuroendocrine origin have been implicated as precursors.

For cancers in general, one theory holds that a small subset of the cells within a tumor (i.e., "stem cells") are responsible for the full malignant behavior of the tumor. As part of this concept, the large bulk of the cells in a cancer are "offspring" of these cancer stem cells. While clonally related to the cancer stem cell subpopulation, most cells by themselves cannot regenerate the full malignant phenotype. The stem cell concept may explain the failure of standard medical therapies to eradicate lung cancers, even when there is a clinical complete response. Disease recurs because therapies do not eliminate the stem cell component, which may be more resistant to chemotherapy. Precise human lung cancer stem cells have yet to be identified.

Lung cancer cells harbor multiple chromosomal abnormalities, including mutations, amplifications, insertions, deletions, and translocations. One of the earliest sets of oncogenes found to be aberrant was the MYC family of transcription factors (*MYC, MYCN,* and *MYCL*). *MYC* is most frequently activated via gene amplification or transcriptional dysregulation in both SCLC and NSCLC. Currently, there are no MYC-specific drugs.

Among lung cancer histologies, adenocarcinomas have been the most extensively catalogued for recurrent genomic gains and losses as well as for somatic mutations (Fig. 107-2). While multiple different kinds of aberrations have been found, a major class involves "driver mutations," which are mutations that occur in genes encoding signaling proteins that when aberrant, drive initiation and maintenance of tumor cells. Importantly, driver mutations can serve as potential Achilles' heels for tumors, if their gene products can be targeted

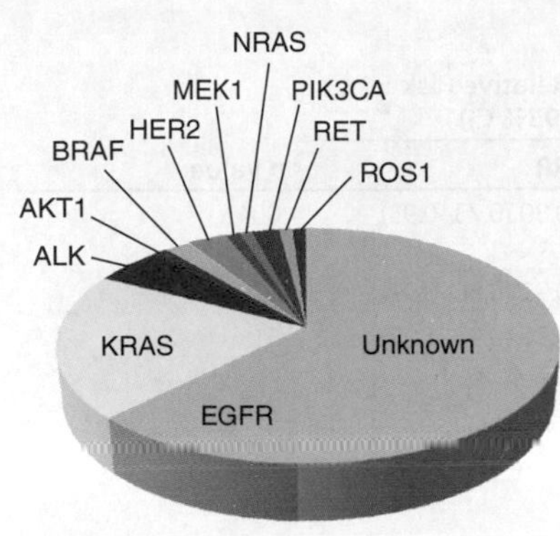

Frequency of driver mutations in NSCLC	
AKT1	1%
ALK	3–7%
BRAF	1–3%
EGFR	10–35%
HER2	2–4%
KRAS	15–25%
MEK1	1%
NRAS	1%
PIK3CA	[illegible]
RET	1–2%
ROS1	1–2%

FIGURE 107-2 Driver mutations in adenocarcinomas.

appropriately. For example, one set of mutations involves EGFR, which belongs to the ERBB (HER) family of protooncogenes, including *EGFR* (ERBB1), *HER2/neu* (ERBB2), *HER3* (ERBB3), and *HER4* (ERBB4). These genes encode cell-surface receptors consisting of an extracellular ligand-binding domain, a transmembrane structure, and an intracellular tyrosine kinase (TK) domain. The binding of ligand to receptor activates receptor dimerization and TK autophosphorylation, initiating a cascade of intracellular events, and leading to increased cell proliferation, angiogenesis, metastasis, and a decrease in apoptosis. Lung adenocarcinomas can arise when tumors express mutant *EGFR*. These same tumors display high sensitivity to small-molecule EGFR TK inhibitors (TKIs). Additional examples of driver mutations in lung adenocarcinoma include the GTPase *KRAS*, the serine-threonine kinase *BRAF*, and the lipid kinase *PIK3CA*. More recently, more subsets of lung adenocarcinoma have been identifed as defined by the presence of specific chromsomal rearrangements resulting in the abberant activation of the TKs ALK, ROS1, and RET. Notably, most driver mutations in lung cancer appear to be mutually exclusive, suggesting that acquisition of one of these mutations is sufficient to drive tumorigenesis. Although driver mutations have mostly been found in adenocarinomas, three potential molecular targets recently have been identified in squamous cell lung carcinomas: *FGFR1* amplification, *DDR2* mutations, and *PIK3CA* mutations/*PTEN* loss (Table 107-1). Together, these potentially "actionable" defects occur in up to 50% of squamous carcinomas.

A large number of tumor-suppressor genes have also been identified that are inactivated during the pathogenesis of lung cancer. These include *TP53, RB1, RASSF1A, CDKN2A/B, LKB1* (*STK11*), and *FHIT*. Nearly 90% of SCLCs harbor mutations in *TP53* and *RB1*. Several tumor-suppressor genes on chromosome 3p appear to be involved in nearly all lung cancers. Allelic loss for this region occurs very early in lung cancer pathogenesis, including in histologically normal smoking-damaged lung epithelium.

EARLY DETECTION AND SCREENING

In lung cancer, clinical outcome is related to the stage at diagnosis, and hence, it is generally assumed that early detection of occult tumors will lead to improved survival. Early detection is a process that involves screening tests, surveillance, diagnosis, and early treatment. Screening refers to the use of simple tests across a healthy population in order to identify individuals who harbor asymptomatic disease. For a screening program to be successful, there must be a high burden of disease within the target population; the test must be sensitive, specific, accessible, and cost effective; and there must be effective treatment that can reduce mortality. With any screening procedure, it is important to consider the possible influence of *lead-time bias* (detecting the cancer earlier without an effect on survival), *length-time bias* (indolent cancers are detected on screening and may not affect survival, whereas aggressive cancers are likely to cause symptoms earlier in patients and are less likely to be detected), and *overdiagnosis* (diagnosing cancers so slow growing that they are unlikely to cause the death of the patient) (Chap. 100).

Because a majority of lung cancer patients present with advanced disease beyond the scope of surgical resection, there is understandable skepticism about the value of screening in this condition. Indeed, randomized controlled trials conducted in the 1960s to 1980s using screening chest x-rays (CXR), with or without sputum cytology, reported no impact on lung cancer–specific mortality in patients characterized as high risk (males age ≥45 years with a smoking history). These studies have been criticized for their design, statistical analyses, and outdated imaging modalities. The results of the more recently conducted Prostate, Lung, Colorectal and Ovarian Cancer Screening Trial (PLCO) are consistent with these earlier reports. Initiated in 1993, participants in the PLCO lung cancer screening trial received annual CXR screening for 4 years, whereas participants in the usual care group received no interventions other than their customary medical care. The diagnostic follow-up of positive screening results was determined by participants and their physicians. The PLCO trial differed from previous lung cancer screening studies in that women and never smokers were eligible. The study was designed to detect a 10% reduction in lung cancer mortality in the interventional group. A total of 154,901 individuals between 55 and 74 years of age were enrolled (77,445 assigned to annual CXR screenings; 77,456 assigned to usual care). Participant demographics and tumor characteristics were well balanced between the two groups. Through 13 years of follow-up, cumulative lung cancer incidence rates (20.1 vs 19.2 per 10,000 person-years; rate ratio [RR], 1.05; 95% confidence interval [CI], 0.98–1.12) and lung cancer mortality (n = 1213 vs n = 1230) were identical between the two groups. The stage and histology of detected cancers in the two groups also were similar. These data corroborate previous recommendations *against* CXR screening for lung cancer.

In contrast to CXR, low-dose, noncontrast, thin-slice spiral chest computed tomography (LDCT) has emerged as an effective tool to screen for lung cancer. In nonrandomized studies conducted in the 1990s, LDCT scans were shown to detect more lung nodules and cancers than standard CXR in selected high-risk populations (e.g., age ≥60 years and a smoking history of ≥10 pack-years). Notably, up to 85% of the lung cancers discovered in these trials were classified as stage I disease and therefore considered potentially curable with surgical resection.

These data prompted the National Cancer Institute (NCI) to initiate the National Lung Screening Trial (NLST), a randomized study designed to determine if LDCT screening could reduce mortality from lung cancer in high-risk populations as compared with standard posterior anterior CXR. High-risk patients were defined as individuals between 55 and 74 years of age, with a ≥30 pack-year history of cigarette smoking; former smokers must have quit within the previous 15 years. Excluded from the trial were individuals with a previous lung cancer diagnosis, a history of hemoptysis, an unexplained weight loss of >15 lb in the preceding year, or a chest CT within 18 months of enrollment. A total of 53,454 persons were enrolled and randomized to annual screening yearly for three years (LDCT screening, n = 26,722; CXR screening, n = 26,732). Any noncalcified nodule measuring ≥4 mm in any diameter found on LDCT and CXR images with any noncalcified nodule or mass were classified as "positive." Participating radiologists had the option of not calling a final screen positive if a noncalcified nodule had been stable on the three screening exams. Overall, 39.1% of participants in the LDCT group and 16% in the CXR group had at least one positive screening result. Of those who screened positive, the false-positive rate was 96.4% in the LDCT group and 94.5% in the CXR group. This was consistent across all three rounds. In the LDCT group, 1060 cancers were identified compared with 941 cancers in the CXR group (645 vs 572 per 100,000 person-years; RR, 1.13; 95% CI, 1.03 to 1.23). Nearly twice as many early-stage IA cancers were detected in the LDCT group compared with the CXR group (40% vs 21%). The overall rates of lung cancer death were 247 and 309 deaths per 100,000 participants in the LDCT and CXR groups, respectively, representing a 20% reduction in lung cancer mortality in the LDCT-screened population (95% CI, 6.8–26.7%; $p = .004$). Compared with the CXR group, the rate of death in the LDCT group from *any* cause was reduced by 6.7% (95% CI, 1.2–13.6; $p = .02$) (Table 107-2). The

TABLE 107-2 RESULTS OF NATIONAL LUNG SCREENING TRIAL

	Event Number		Rates of Events per 100,000 Person-Years		Relative Risk (95% CI)	
	LDCT (n = 26,772)	CXR (n = 26,732)	LDCT	CXR	RR	*p* Value
Lung cancer mortality	356	443	247	309	0.80 (0.73–0.93)	.004
All-cause mortality	1877	2000	1303	1395	0.93 (0.86–0.99)	.02
Mortality not due to lung cancer	1521	1557	1056	1086	0.99 (0.95–1.02)	.51

Abbreviations: CI, confidence interval; CXR, chest x-ray; LDCT, low-dose computed tomography; RR, rate ratio.

Source: Modified from PB Bach et al: JAMA 307:2418, 2012.

number needed to screen (NNTS) to prevent one lung cancer death was calculated to be 320.

LDCT screening for lung cancer comes with known risks including a high rate of false-positive results, false-negative results, potential for unnecessary follow-up testing, radiation exposure, overdiagnosis, changes in anxiety and quality of life, and substantial financial costs. By far the biggest challenge confronting the use of CT screening is the high false-positive rate. False positives can have a substantial impact on patients through the expense and risk of unneeded further evaluation and emotional stress. The management of these patients usually consists of serial CT scans over time to see if the nodules grow, attempted fine-needle aspirates, or surgical resection. At $300 per scan (NCI estimated cost), the outlay for initial LDCT alone could run into the billions of dollars annually, an expense that only further escalates when factoring in various downstream expenditures an individual might incur in the assessment of positive findings. A formal cost-effectiveness analysis of the NLST is expected soon that should help resolve this crucial concern.

Despite the aforementioned caveats, screening of individuals who meet the NLST criteria for lung cancer risk (or in some cases, modified versions of these criteria) seems warranted, provided comprehensive multidisciplinary coordinated care and follow-up similar to those provided to NLST participants are available. Algorithms to improve candidate selection are under development. When discussing the option of LDCT screening, use of absolute risks rather than relative risks is helpful because studies indicate the public can process absolute terminology more effectively than relative risk projections. A useful guide has been developed by the NCI to help patients and physicians assess the benefits and harms of LDCT screening for lung cancer (Table 107-3). Finally, even a small negative effect of screening on smoking behavior (either lower quit rates or higher recidivism) could easily offset the potential gains in a population. Fortunately no such impact has been reported to date. Nonetheless, smoking cessation must be included as an indispensable component of any screening program.

TABLE 107-3 THE BENEFITS AND HARMS OF LDCT SCREENING FOR LUNG CANCER BASED ON NLST DATA

	LDCT	CXR
Benefits: How Did CT Scans Help Compared To CXR?		
4 in 1000 fewer died from lung cancer	13 in 1000	17 in 1000
5 in 1000 fewer died from all causes	70 in 1000	75 in 1000
Harms: What Problems Did CT Scans Cause Compared to CXR?		
223 in 1000 had at least 1 false alarm	365 in 1000	142 in 1000
18 in 1000 had a false alarm leading to an invasive procedure	25 in 1000	7 in 1000
2 in 1000 had a major complication from an invasive procedure	3 in 1000	1 in 1000

Abbreviations: CXR, chest x-ray; LDCT, low-dose computed tomography; NLST, National Lung Screening Trial.

Source: Modified from S Woloshin et al: N Engl J Med 367:1677, 2012.

CLINICAL MANIFESTATIONS

Over half of all patients diagnosed with lung cancer present with locally advanced or metastatic disease at the time of diagnosis. The majority of patients present with signs, symptoms, or laboratory abnormalities that can be attributed to the primary lesion, local tumor growth, invasion or obstruction of adjacent structures, growth at distant metastatic sites, or a paraneoplastic syndrome (Tables 107-4 and 107-5). The prototypical lung cancer patient is a current or former smoker of either sex, usually in the seventh decade of life. A history of chronic cough with or without hemoptysis in a current or former smoker with chronic obstructive pulmonary disease (COPD) age 40 years or older should prompt a thorough investigation for lung cancer even in the face of a normal CXR. A persistent pneumonia without constitutional symptoms and unresponsive to repeated courses of antibiotics also should prompt an evaluation for the underlying cause. Lung cancer arising in a lifetime never smoker is more common in women and East Asians. Such patients also tend to be younger than their smoking counterparts at the time of diagnosis. The clinical presentation of lung cancer in never smokers tends to mirror that of current and former smokers.

Patients with central or endobronchial growth of the primary tumor may present with cough, hemoptysis, wheeze, stridor, dyspnea, or postobstructive pneumonitis. Peripheral growth of the primary tumor may cause pain from pleural or chest wall involvement, dyspnea on a restrictive basis, and symptoms of a lung abscess resulting from tumor cavitation. Regional spread of tumor in the thorax (by contiguous growth or by metastasis to regional lymph nodes) may cause tracheal obstruction, esophageal compression with dysphagia, recurrent laryngeal paralysis with hoarseness, phrenic nerve palsy with elevation of the hemidiaphragm and dyspnea, and sympathetic nerve paralysis with Horner's syndrome (enophthalmos, ptosis, miosis, and anhydrosis). Malignant pleural effusions can cause pain, dyspnea, or cough. Pancoast (or superior sulcus tumor) syndromes result from local extension of a tumor growing in the apex of the lung with involvement of the eighth cervical and first and second thoracic nerves, and present with shoulder pain that characteristically radiates in the ulnar

TABLE 107-4 PRESENTING SIGNS AND SYMPTOMS OF LUNG CANCER

Symptom and Signs	Range of Frequency
Cough	8–75%
Weight loss	0–68%
Dyspnea	3–60%
Chest pain	20–49%
Hemoptysis	6–35%
Bone pain	6–25%
Clubbing	0–20%
Fever	0–20%
Weakness	0–10%
Superior vena cava obstruction	0–4%
Dysphagia	0–2%
Wheezing and stridor	0–2%

Source: Reproduced with permission from MA Beckles: Chest 123:97-104, 2003.

TABLE 107-5 CLINICAL FINDINGS SUGGESTIVE OF METASTATIC DISEASE

Symptoms elicited in history	• Constitutional: weight loss >10 lb • Musculoskeletal: focal skeletal pain • Neurologic: headaches, syncope, seizures, extremity weakness, recent change in mental status
Signs found on physical examination	• Lymphadenopathy (>1 cm) • Hoarseness, superior vena cava syndrome • Bone tenderness • Hepatomegaly (>13 cm span) • Focal neurologic signs, papilledema • Soft-tissue mass
Routine laboratory tests	• Hematocrit, <40% in men; <35% in women • Elevated alkaline phosphatase, GGT, SGOT, and calcium levels

Abbreviations: GGT, gamma-glutamyltransferase; SGOT, serum glutamic-oxaloacetic transaminase.

Source: Reproduced with permission from GA Silvestri et al: Chest 123(1 Suppl):147S, 2003.

distribution of the arm, often with radiologic destruction of the first and second ribs. Often Horner's syndrome and Pancoast syndrome coexist. Other problems of regional spread include superior vena cava syndrome from vascular obstruction; pericardial and cardiac extension with resultant tamponade, arrhythmia, or cardiac failure; lymphatic obstruction with resultant pleural effusion; and lymphangitic spread through the lungs with hypoxemia and dyspnea. In addition, lung cancer can spread transbronchially, producing tumor growth along multiple alveolar surfaces with impairment of gas exchange, respiratory insufficiency, dyspnea, hypoxemia, and sputum production. Constitutional symptoms may include anorexia, weight loss, weakness, fever, and night sweats. Apart from the brevity of symptom duration, these parameters fail to clearly distinguish SCLC from NSCLC or even from neoplasms metastatic to lungs.

Extrathoracic metastatic disease is found at autopsy in more than 50% of patients with squamous carcinoma, 80% of patients with adenocarcinoma and large-cell carcinoma, and greater than 95% of patients with SCLC. Approximately one-third of patients present with symptoms as a result of distant metastases. Lung cancer metastases may occur in virtually every organ system, and the site of metastatic involvement largely determines other symptoms. Patients with brain metastases may present with headache, nausea and vomiting, seizures, or neurologic deficits. Patients with bone metastases may present with pain, pathologic fractures, or cord compression. The latter may also occur with epidural metastases. Individuals with bone marrow invasion may present with cytopenias or leukoerythroblastosis. Those with liver metastases may present with hepatomegaly, right upper quadrant pain, fever, anorexia, and weight loss. Liver dysfunction and biliary obstructions are rare. Adrenal metastases are common but rarely cause pain or adrenal insufficiency unless they are large.

Paraneoplastic syndromes are common in patients with lung cancer, especially those with SCLC, and may be the presenting finding or the first sign of recurrence. In addition, paraneoplastic syndromes may mimic metastatic disease and, unless detected, lead to inappropriate palliative rather than curative treatment. Often the paraneoplastic syndrome may be relieved with successful treatment of the tumor. In some cases, the pathophysiology of the paraneoplastic syndrome is known, particularly when a hormone with biological activity is secreted by a tumor. However, in many cases, the pathophysiology is unknown. Systemic symptoms of anorexia, cachexia, weight loss (seen in 30% of patients), fever, and suppressed immunity are paraneoplastic syndromes of unknown etiology or at least not well defined. Weight loss greater than 10% of total body weight is considered a bad prognostic sign. Endocrine syndromes are seen in 12% of patients; hypercalcemia resulting from ectopic production of parathyroid hormone (PTH), or more commonly, PTH-related peptide, is the most common life-threatening metabolic complication of malignancy, primarily occurring with squamous cell carcinomas of the lung. Clinical symptoms include nausea, vomiting, abdominal pain, constipation, polyuria, thirst, and altered mental status.

Hyponatremia may be caused by the syndrome of inappropriate secretion of antidiuretic hormone (SIADH) or possibly atrial natriuretic peptide (ANP). SIADH resolves within 1-4 weeks of initiating chemotherapy in the vast majority of cases. During this period, serum sodium can usually be managed and maintained above 128 mEq/L via fluid restriction. Demeclocycline can be a useful adjunctive measure when fluid restriction alone is insufficient. Vasopressin receptor antagonists like tolvaptan also have been used in the management of SIADH. However, there are significant limitations to the use of tolvaptan including liver injury and overly rapid correction of the hyponatremia, which can lead to irreversible neurologic injury. Likewise, the cost of tolvaptan may be prohibitive (as high as $300 per tablet in some areas). Of note, patients with ectopic ANP may have worsening hyponatremia if sodium intake is not concomitantly increased. Accordingly, if hyponatremia fails to improve or worsens after 3–4 days of adequate fluid restriction, plasma levels of ANP should be measured to determine the causative syndrome.

Ectopic secretion of ACTH by SCLC and pulmonary carcinoids usually results in additional electrolyte disturbances, especially hypokalemia, rather than the changes in body habitus that occur in Cushing's syndrome from a pituitary adenoma. Treatment with standard medications, such as metyrapone and ketoconazole, is largely ineffective due to extremely high cortisol levels. The most effective strategy for management of the Cushing's syndrome is effective treatment of the underlying SCLC. Bilateral adrenalectomy may be considered in extreme cases.

Skeletal–connective tissue syndromes include clubbing in 30% of cases (usually NSCLCs) and hypertrophic primary osteoarthropathy in 1–10% of cases (usually adenocarcinomas). Patients may develop periostitis, causing pain, tenderness, and swelling over the affected bones and a positive bone scan. Neurologic-myopathic syndromes are seen in only 1% of patients but are dramatic and include the myasthenic Eaton-Lambert syndrome and retinal blindness with SCLC, whereas peripheral neuropathies, subacute cerebellar degeneration, cortical degeneration, and polymyositis are seen with all lung cancer types. Many of these are caused by autoimmune responses such as the development of anti-voltage-gated calcium channel antibodies in Eaton-Lambert syndrome. Patients with this disorder present with proximal muscle weakness, usually in the lower extremities, occasional autonomic dysfunction, and rarely, cranial nerve symptoms or involvement of the bulbar or respiratory muscles. Depressed deep tendon reflexes are frequently present. In contrast to patients with myasthenia gravis, strength improves with serial effort. Some patients who respond to chemotherapy will have resolution of the neurologic abnormalities. Thus, chemotherapy is the initial treatment of choice. Paraneoplastic encephalomyelitis and sensory neuropathies, cerebellar degeneration, limbic encephalitis, and brainstem encephalitis occur in SCLC in association with a variety of antineuronal antibodies such as anti-Hu, anti-CRMP5, and ANNA-3. Paraneoplastic cerebellar degeneration may be associated with anti-Hu, anti-Yo, or P/Q calcium channel autoantibodies. Coagulation or thrombotic or other hematologic manifestations occur in 1–8% of patients and include migratory venous thrombophlebitis (Trousseau's syndrome), nonbacterial thrombotic (marantic) endocarditis with arterial emboli, and disseminated intravascular coagulation with hemorrhage, anemia, granulocytosis, and leukoerythroblastosis. Thrombotic disease complicating cancer is usually a poor prognostic sign. Cutaneous manifestations such as dermatomyositis and acanthosis nigricans are uncommon (1%), as are the renal manifestations of nephrotic syndrome and glomerulonephritis (≤1%).

DIAGNOSING LUNG CANCER

Tissue sampling is required to confirm a diagnosis in all patients with suspected lung cancer. In patients with suspected metastatic disease, a biopsy of the most distant site of disease is preferred for tissue confirmation. Given the greater emphasis placed on molecular testing for NSCLC patients, a core biopsy is preferred to ensure adequate tissue for analysis. Tumor tissue may be obtained via minimally invasive techniques such as bronchial or transbronchial biopsy during fiberoptic bronchoscopy, by fine-needle aspiration or percutaneous biopsy using image guidance, or via endobronchial ultrasound (EBUS) guided biopsy. Depending on the location, lymph node sampling may occur via transesophageal endoscopic ultrasound-guided biopsy (EUS), EBUS, or blind biopsy. In patients with clinically palpable disease such as a lymph node or skin metastasis, a biopsy may be obtained. In patients with suspected metastatic disease, a diagnosis may be confirmed by percutaneous biopsy of a soft tissue mass, lytic bone lesion, bone marrow, pleural or liver lesion, or an adequate cell block obtained from a malignant pleural effusion. In patients with a suspected malignant pleural effusion, if the initial thoracentesis is negative, a repeat thoracentesis is warranted. Although the majority of pleural effusions are due to malignant disease, particularly if they are exudative or bloody, some may be parapneumonic. In the absence of distant disease, such patients should be considered for possible curative treatment.

The diagnostic yield of any biopsy depends on several factors including location (accessibility) of the tumor, tumor size, tumor type, and technical aspects of the diagnostic procedure including the experience level of the bronchoscopist and pathologist. In general, central lesions such as squamous cell carcinomas, small-cell carcinomas, or endobronchial lesions such as carcinoid tumors are more readily diagnosed by bronchoscopic examination, whereas peripheral lesions such as adenocarcinomas and large-cell carcinomas are more amenable to transthoracic biopsy. Diagnostic accuracy for SCLC versus NSCLC for most specimens is excellent, with lesser accuracy for subtypes of NSCLC.

Bronchoscopic specimens include bronchial brush, bronchial wash, bronchioloalveolar lavage, transbronchial fine-needle aspiration (FNA), and core biopsy. For more accurate histologic classification, mutation analysis, or investigational purposes, reasonable efforts (e.g., a core needle biopsy) should be made to obtain more tissue than what is contained in a routine cytology specimen obtained by FNA. Overall sensitivity for combined use of bronchoscopic methods is approximately 80%, and together with tissue biopsy, the yield increases to 85–90%. Like transbronchial core biopsy specimens, transthoracic core biopsy specimens are also preferred. Sensitivity is highest for larger lesions and peripheral tumors. In general, core biopsy specimens, whether transbronchial, transthoracic, or EUS-guided, are superior to other specimen types. This is primarily due to the higher percentage of tumor cells with fewer confounding factors such as obscuring inflammation and reactive nonneoplastic cells.

Sputum cytology is inexpensive and noninvasive but has a lower yield than other specimen types due to poor preservation of the cells and more variability in acquiring a good-quality specimen. The yield for sputum cytology is highest for larger and centrally located tumors such as squamous cell carcinoma and small-cell carcinoma histology. The specificity for sputum cytology averages close to 100%, although sensitivity is generally <70%. The accuracy of sputum cytology improves with increased numbers of specimens analyzed. Consequently, analysis of at least three sputum specimens is recommended.

STAGING LUNG CANCER

Lung cancer staging consists of two parts: first, a determination of the location of the tumor and possible metastatic sites (anatomic staging), and second, an assessment of a patient's ability to withstand various antitumor treatments (physiologic staging). All patients with lung cancer should have a complete history and physical examination, with evaluation of all other medical problems, determination of performance status, and history of weight loss. The most significant dividing line is between those patients who are candidates for surgical resection and those who are inoperable but will benefit from chemotherapy, radiation therapy, or both. Staging with regard to a patient's potential for surgical resection is principally applicable to NSCLC.

ANATOMIC STAGING OF PATIENTS WITH LUNG CANCER

The accurate staging of patients with NSCLC is essential for determining the appropriate treatment in patients with resectable disease and avoiding unnecessary surgical procedures in patients with advanced disease (Fig. 107-3). All patients with NSCLC should undergo initial

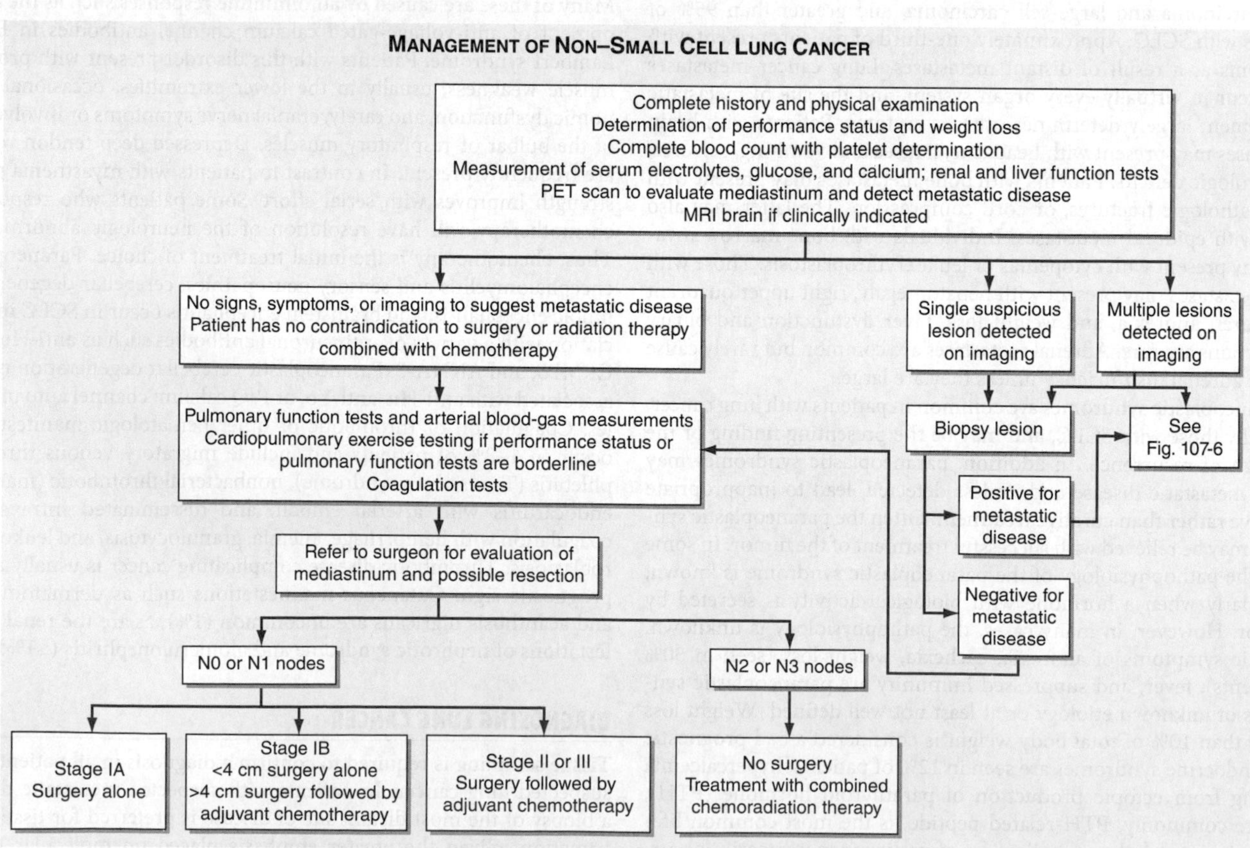

FIGURE 107-3 Algorithm for management of non-small-cell lung cancer. MRI, magnetic resonance imaging; PET, positron emission tomography.

radiographic imaging with CT scan, positron emission tomography (PET), or preferably CT-PET. PET scanning attempts to identify sites of malignancy based on glucose metabolism by measuring the uptake of ^{18}F-fluorodeoxyglucose (FDG). Rapidly dividing cells, presumably in the lung tumors, will preferentially take up ^{18}F-FDG and appear as a "hot spot." To date, PET has been mostly used for staging and detection of metastases in lung cancer and in the detection of nodules >15 mm in diameter. Combined ^{18}F-FDG PET-CT imaging has been shown to improve the accuracy of staging in NSCLC compared to visual correlation of PET and CT or either study alone. CT-PET has been found to be superior in identifying pathologically enlarged mediastinal lymph nodes and extrathoracic metastases. A standardized uptake value (SUV) of >2.5 on PET is highly suspicious for malignancy. False negatives can be seen in diabetes, in lesions <8 mm, and in slow growing tumors (e.g., carcinoid tumors or well-differentiated adenocarcinoma). False positives can be seen in certain infections and granulomatous disease (e.g., tuberculosis). Thus, PET should never be used alone to diagnose lung cancer, mediastinal involvement, or metastases. Confirmation with tissue biopsy is required. For brain metastases, magnetic resonance imaging (MRI) is the most effective method. MRI can also be useful in selected circumstances, such as superior sulcus tumors to rule out brachial plexus involvement, but in general, MRI does not play a major role in NSCLC staging.

In patients with NSCLC, the following are contraindications to potential curative resection: extrathoracic metastases, superior vena cava syndrome, vocal cord and, in most cases, phrenic nerve paralysis, malignant pleural effusion, cardiac tamponade, tumor within 2 cm of the carina (potentially curable with combined chemoradiotherapy), metastasis to the contralateral lung, metastases to supraclavicular lymph nodes, contralateral mediastinal node metastases (potentially curable with combined chemoradiotherapy), and involvement of the main pulmonary artery. In situations where it will make a difference in treatment, abnormal scan findings require tissue confirmation of malignancy so that patients are not precluded from having potentially curative therapy.

The best predictor of metastatic disease remains a careful history and physical examination. If signs, symptoms, or findings from the physical examination suggest the presence of malignancy, then sequential imaging starting with the most appropriate study should be performed. If the findings from the clinical evaluation are negative, then imaging studies beyond CT-PET are unnecessary and the search for metastatic disease is complete. More controversial is how one should assess patients with known stage III disease. Because these patients are more likely to have asymptomatic occult metastatic disease, current guidelines recommend a more extensive imaging evaluation including imaging of the brain with either CT scan or MRI. In patients in whom distant metastatic disease has been ruled out, lymph node status needs to be assessed via a combination of radiographic imaging and/or minimally invasive techniques such as those mentioned above and/or invasive techniques such as mediastinoscopy, mediastinotomy, thoracoscopy, or thoracotomy. Approximately one-quarter to one-half of patients diagnosed with NSCLC will have mediastinal lymph node metastases at the time of diagnosis. Lymph node sampling is recommended in all patients with enlarged nodes detected by CT or PET scan and in patients with large tumors or tumors occupying the inner third of the lung. The extent of mediastinal lymph node involvement is important in determining the appropriate treatment strategy: surgical resection followed by adjuvant chemotherapy versus combined chemoradiation alone (see below). A standard nomenclature for referring to the location of lymph nodes involved with lung cancer has evolved (Fig. 107-4).

In SCLC patients, current staging recommendations include a CT scan of the chest and abdomen (because of the high frequency of hepatic and adrenal involvement), MRI of the brain (positive in 10% of asymptomatic patients), and radionuclide bone scan if symptoms or signs suggest disease involvement in these areas (Fig. 107-5). Although there are less data on the use of CT-PET in SCLC, the most recent American College of Chest Physicians Evidence-Based Clinical Practice Guidelines recommend PET scans in patients with clinical stage I SCLC who are being considered for curative intent surgical resection. In addition, invasive mediastinal staging and extrathoracic imaging (head MRI/CT and PET or abdominal CT plus bone scan) is also recommended for patients with clinical stage I SCLC if curative intent surgical resection is contemplated. Some practice guidelines also recommend the use of PET scanning in the staging of SCLC patients who are potential candidates for the addition of thoracic radiotherapy to chemotherapy. Bone marrow biopsies and aspirations are rarely performed now given the low incidence of isolated bone marrow metastases. Confirmation of metastatic disease, ipsilateral or contralateral lung nodules, or metastases beyond the mediastinum may be achieved by the same modalities recommended earlier for patients with NSCLC.

If a patient has signs or symptoms of spinal cord compression (pain, weakness, paralysis, urinary retention), a spinal CT or MRI scan and examination of the cerebrospinal fluid cytology should be performed. If metastases are evident on imaging, a neurosurgeon should be consulted for possible palliative surgical resection and/or a radiation oncologist should be consulted for palliative radiotherapy to the site of compression. If signs or symptoms of leptomeningitis develop at any time in a patient with lung cancer, an MRI of the brain and spinal cord should be performed, as well as a spinal tap, for detection of malignant cells. If the spinal tap is negative, a repeat spinal tap should be considered. There is currently no approved therapy for the treatment of leptomeningeal disease.

STAGING SYSTEM FOR NON-SMALL-CELL LUNG CANCER

The tumor-node-metastasis (TNM) international staging system provides useful prognostic information and is used to stage all patients with NSCLC. The various T (tumor size), N (regional node involvement), and M (presence or absence of distant metastasis) are combined to form different stage groups (Tables 107-6 and 107-7). The previous edition of the TNM staging system for lung cancer was developed based on a relatively small database of patients from a single institution. The latest seventh edition of the TNM staging system went into effect in 2010 and developed using a much more robust database of more than 100,000 patients with lung cancer who were treated in multiple countries between 1990 and 2000. Data from 67,725 patients with NSCLC were then used to reevaluate the prognostic value of the TNM descriptors (Table 107-8). The major distinction between the sixth and seventh editions of the international staging systems is within the T classification; T1 tumors are divided into tumors ≤2 cm in size, as these patients were found to have a better prognosis compared to patients with tumors >2 cm but ≤3 cm. T2 tumors are divided into those that are >3 cm but ≤5 cm and those that are >5 cm but ≤7 cm. Tumors that are >7 cm are considered T3 tumors. T3 tumors also include tumors with invasion into local structures such as chest wall and diaphragm and additional nodules in the same lobe. T4 tumors include tumors of any size with invasion into mediastinum, heart, great vessels, trachea, or esophagus or multiple nodules in the ipsilateral lung. No changes have been made to the current classification of lymph node involvement (N). Patients with metastasis may be classified as M1a (malignant pleural or pericardial effusion, pleural nodules, or nodules in the contralateral lung) or M1b (distant metastasis; e.g., bone, liver, adrenal, or brain metastasis). Based on these data, approximately one-third of patients have localized disease that can be treated with curative attempt (surgery or radiotherapy), one-third have local or regional disease that may or may not be amenable to a curative attempt, and one-third have metastatic disease at the time of diagnosis.

STAGING SYSTEM FOR SMALL-CELL LUNG CANCER

In patients with SCLC, it is now recommended that both the Veterans Administration system and the American Joint Committee on Cancer/International Union Against Cancer seventh edition system (TNM) be used to classify the tumor stage. The Veterans Administration system is a distinct two-stage system dividing patients into those with limited- or extensive-stage disease. Patients with limited-stage disease (LD) have cancer that is confined to the ipsilateral hemithorax and can be encompassed within a tolerable radiation port. Thus, contralateral

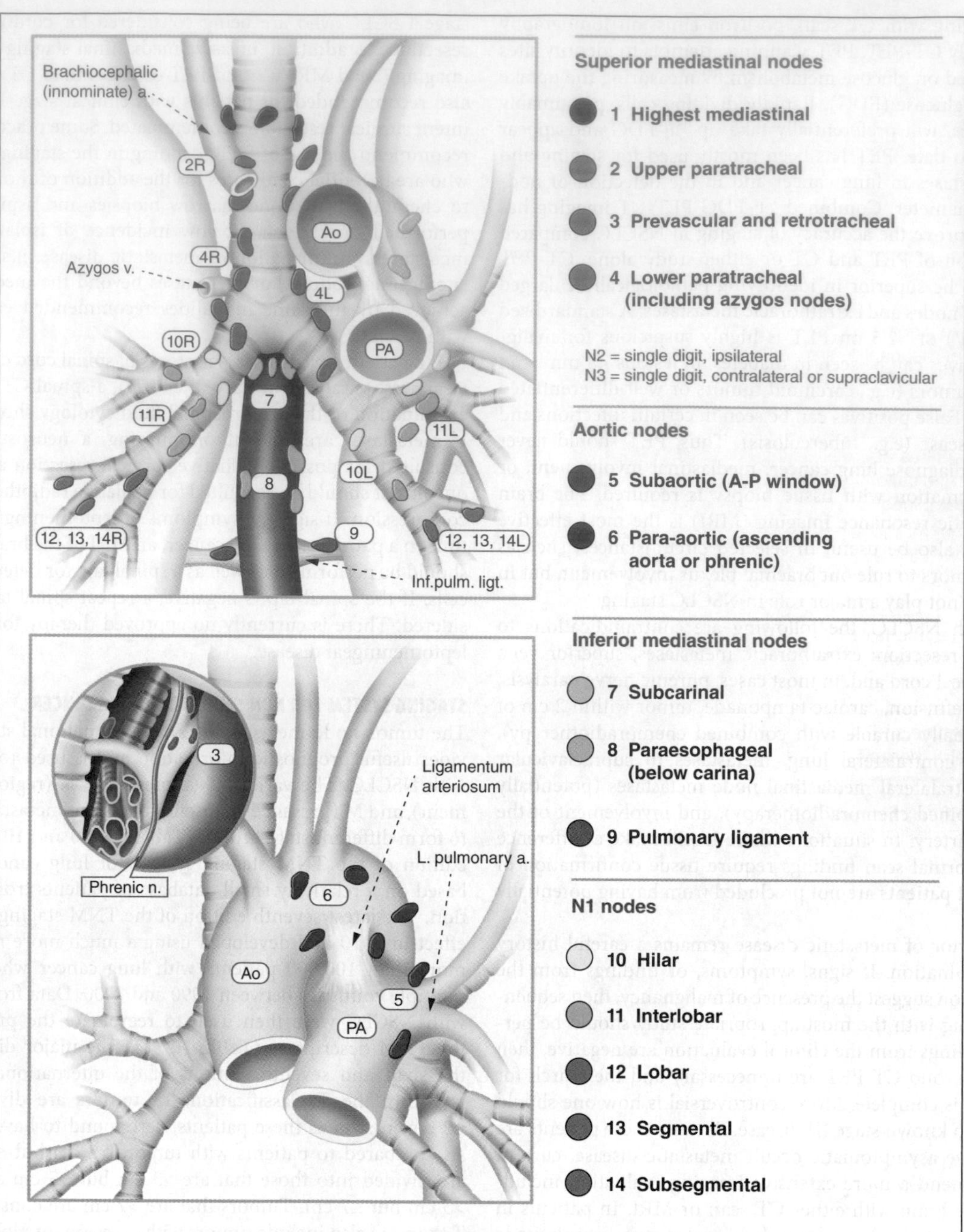

FIGURE 107-4 Lymph node stations in staging non-small-cell lung cancer. The International Association for the Study of Lung Cancer (IASLC) lymph node map, including the proposed grouping of lymph node stations into "zones" for the purposes of prognostic analyses. a., artery; Ao, aorta; Inf. pulm. ligt., inferior pulmonary ligament; n., nerve; PA, pulmonary artery; v., vein.

supraclavicular nodes, recurrent laryngeal nerve involvement, and superior vena caval obstruction can all be part of LD. Patients with extensive-stage disease (ED) have overt metastatic disease by imaging or physical examination. Cardiac tamponade, malignant pleural effusion, and bilateral pulmonary parenchymal involvement generally qualify disease as ED, because the involved organs cannot be encompassed safely or effectively within a single radiation therapy port. Sixty to 70% of patients are diagnosed with ED at presentation. The TNM staging system is preferred in the rare SCLC patient presenting with what appears to be clinical stage I disease (see above).

PHYSIOLOGIC STAGING

Patients with lung cancer often have other comorbid conditions related to smoking including cardiovascular disease and COPD. To improve their preoperative condition, correctable problems (e.g., anemia, electrolyte and fluid disorders, infections, cardiac disease, and arrhythmias) should be addressed, appropriate chest physical therapy should be instituted, and patients should be encouraged to stop smoking. Because it is not always possible to predict whether a lobectomy or pneumonectomy will be required until the time of operation, a conservative approach is to restrict surgical resection to patients who could potentially tolerate a pneumonectomy. Patients with a forced expiratory volume in 1 s (FEV_1) of greater than 2 L or greater than 80% of predicted can tolerate a pneumonectomy, and those with an FEV_1 greater than 1.5 L have adequate reserve for a lobectomy. In patients with borderline lung function but a resectable tumor, cardiopulmonary exercise testing could be performed as part of the physiologic evaluation. This test allows an estimate of the maximal oxygen consumption (Vo_{2max}). A Vo_{2max} <15 mL/(kg·min) predicts for a higher risk of postoperative complications. Patients deemed unable to tolerate lobectomy or pneumonectomy from a pulmonary functional standpoint may be candidates for more limited resections, such as wedge or anatomic segmental resection, although such procedures are associated with significantly higher rates of local

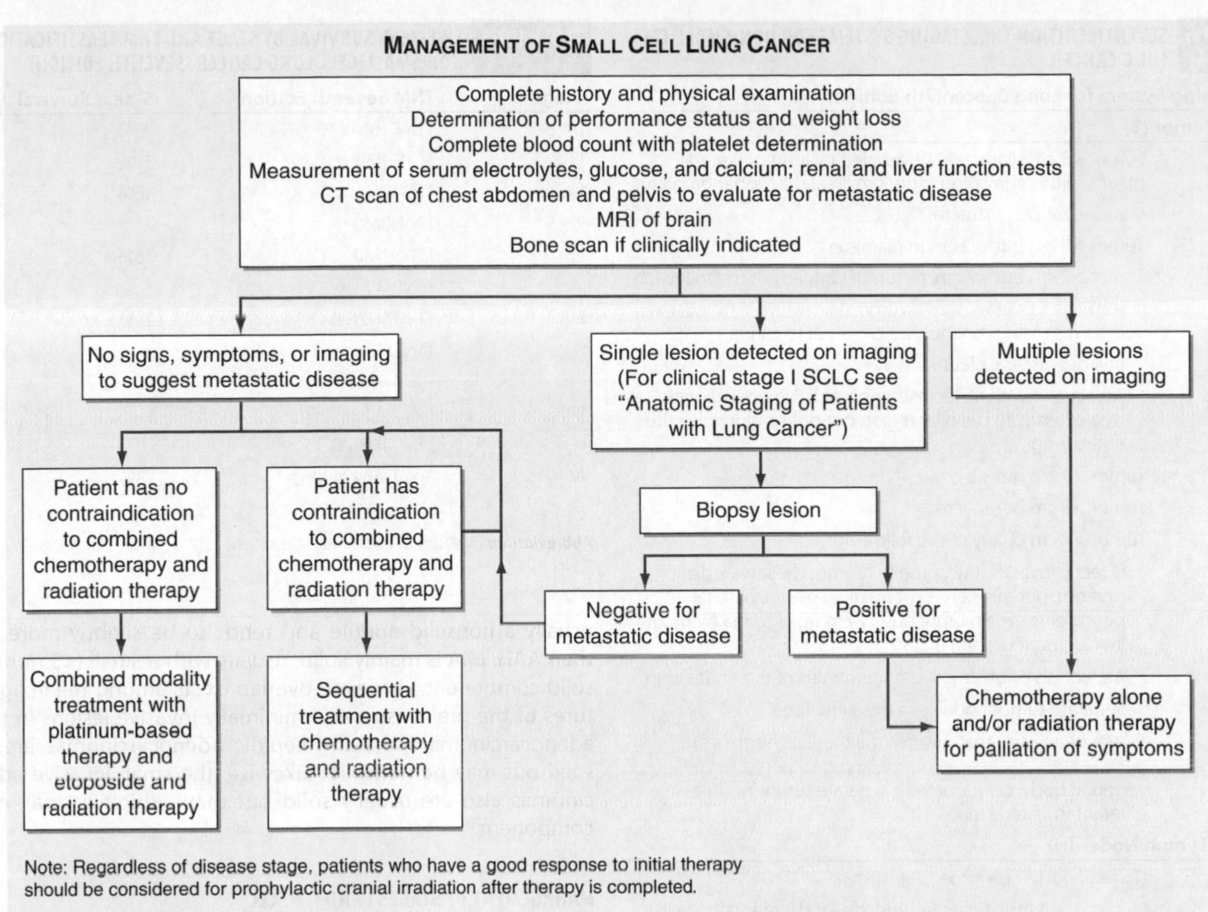

FIGURE 107-5 Algorithm for management of small-cell lung cancer. CT, computed tomography; MRI, magnetic resonance imaging.

recurrence and a trend toward decreased overall survival. All patients should be assessed for cardiovascular risk using American College of Cardiology and American Heart Association guidelines. A myocardial infarction within the past 3 months is a contraindication to thoracic surgery because 20% of patients will die of reinfarction. An infarction in the past 6 months is a relative contraindication. Other major contraindications include uncontrolled arrhythmias, an FEV_1 of less than 1 L, CO_2 retention (resting Pco_2 >45 mmHg), DL_{co} <40%, and severe pulmonary hypertension.

TREATMENT NON-SMALL-CELL LUNG CANCER

The overall treatment approach to patients with NSCLC is shown in Fig. 107-3.

OCCULT AND STAGE 0 CARCINOMAS

Patients with severe atypia on sputum cytology have an increased risk of developing lung cancer compared to those without atypia. In the uncommon circumstance where malignant cells are identified in a sputum or bronchial washing specimen but the chest imaging appears normal (TX tumor stage), the lesion must be localized. More than 90% of tumors can be localized by meticulous examination of the bronchial tree with a fiberoptic bronchoscope under general anesthesia and collection of a series of differential brushings and biopsies. Surgical resection following bronchoscopic localization has been shown to improve survival compared to no treatment. Close follow-up of these patients is indicated because of the high incidence of second primary lung cancers (5% per patient per year).

SOLITARY PULMONARY NODULE AND "GROUND-GLASS" OPACITIES

A solitary pulmonary nodule is defined as an x-ray density completely surrounded by normal aerated lung with circumscribed margins, of any shape, usually 1–6 cm in greatest diameter. The approach to a patient with a solitary pulmonary nodule is based on an estimate of the probability of cancer, determined according to the patient's smoking history, age, and characteristics on imaging (Table 107-9). Prior CXRs and CT scans should be obtained if available for comparison. A PET scan may be useful if the lesion is greater than 7–8 mm in diameter. If no diagnosis is apparent, Mayo investigators reported that clinical characteristics (age, cigarette smoking status, and prior cancer diagnosis) and three radiologic characteristics (nodule diameter, spiculation, and upper lobe location) were independent predictors of malignancy. At present, only two radiographic criteria are thought to predict the benign nature of a solitary pulmonary nodule: lack of growth over a period >2 years and certain characteristic patterns of calcification. Calcification alone, however, does not exclude malignancy; a dense central nidus, multiple punctuate foci, and "bulls eye" (granuloma) and "popcorn ball" (hamartoma) calcifications are highly suggestive of a benign lesion. In contrast, a relatively large lesion, lack of or asymmetric calcification, chest symptoms, associated atelectasis, pneumonitis, or growth of the lesion revealed by comparison with an old x-ray or CT scan or a positive PET scan may be suggestive of a malignant process and warrant further attempts to establish a histologic diagnosis. An algorithm for assessing these lesions is shown in Fig. 107-6.

Since the advent of screening CTs, small "ground-glass" opacities (GGOs) have often been observed, particularly as the increased sensitivity of CTs enables detection of smaller lesions. Many of these GGOs, when biopsied, are found to be atypical adenomatous hyperplasia (AAH), adenocarcinoma in situ (AIS), or minimally invasive adenocarcinoma (MIA). AAH is usually a nodule of <5 mm and is minimally hazy, also called nonsolid or ground glass (i.e., hazy slightly increased attenuation, no solid component, and preservation of bronchial and vascular margins). On thin-section CT, AIS is

TABLE 107-6 SEVENTH EDITION TNM STAGING SYSTEMS FOR NON-SMALL-CELL LUNG CANCER

TNM Staging System for Lung Cancer (7th Edition)	
Primary Tumor (T)	
T1	Tumor ≤3 cm diameter, surrounded by lung or visceral pleura, without invasion more proximal than lobar bronchus
T1a	Tumor ≤2 cm in diameter
T1b	Tumor >2 cm but ≤ 3 cm in diameter
T2	Tumor >3 cm but ≤7 cm, or tumor with any of the following features:
	Involves main bronchus, ≥2 cm distal to carina
	Invades visceral pleura
	Associated with atelectasis or obstructive pneumonitis that extends to the hilar region but does not involve the entire lung
T2a	Tumor >3 cm but ≤5 cm
T2b	Tumor >5 cm but ≤7 cm
T3	Tumor >7 cm or any of the following:
	Directly invades any of the following: chest wall, diaphragm, phrenic nerve, mediastinal pleura, parietal pericardium, main bronchus <2 cm from carina (without involvement of carina)
	Atelectasis or obstructive pneumonitis of the entire lung
	Separate tumor nodules in the same lobe
T4	Tumor of any size that invades the mediastinum, heart, great vessels, trachea, recurrent laryngeal nerve, esophagus, vertebral body, carina, or with separate tumor nodules in a different ipsilateral lobe
Regional Lymph Nodes (N)	
N0	No regional lymph node metastases
N1	Metastasis in ipsilateral peribronchial and/or ipsilateral hilar lymph nodes and intrapulmonary nodes, including involvement by direct extension
N2	Metastasis in ipsilateral mediastinal and/or subcarinal lymph node(s)
N3	Metastasis in contralateral mediastinal, contralateral hilar, ipsilateral or contralateral scalene, or supraclavicular lymph node(s)
Distant Metastasis (M)	
M0	No distant metastasis
M1	Distant metastasis
M1a	Separate tumor nodule(s) in a contralateral lobe; tumor with pleural nodules or malignant pleural or pericardial effusion
M1b	Distant metastasis (in extrathoracic organs)

Abbreviation: TNM, tumor-node-metastasis.

Source: Reproduced with permission from P Goldstraw et al: J Thorac Oncol 2:706, 2007.

TABLE 107-7 SEVENTH EDITION TNM STAGING SYSTEMS FOR NON-SMALL-CELL LUNG CANCER

Stage groupings			
Stage IA	T1a-T1b	N0	M0
Stage IB	T2a	N0	M0
Stage IIA	T1a,T1b,T2a	N1	M0
	T2b	N0	M0
Stage IIB	T2b	N1	M0
	T3	N0	M0
Stage IIIA	T1a,T1b,T2a,T2b	N2	M0
	T3	N1,N2	M0
	T4	N0,N1	M0
Stage IIIB	T4	N2	M0
	Any T	N3	M0
Stage IV	Any T	Any N	M1a or M1b

Abbreviation: TNM, tumor-node-metastasis.

Source: Reproduced with permission from P Goldstraw P et al: J Thorac Oncol 2:706, 2007.

TABLE 107-8 FIVE-YEAR SURVIVAL BY STAGE AND TNM CLASSIFICATION OF NON-SMALL-CELL LUNG CANCER (SEVENTH EDITION)

Stage	TNM Seventh Edition	5-Year Survival (%)
IA	T1a-T1bN0M0	73%
IB	T2aN0M0	58%
IIA	T1a-T2aN1M0	46%
	T2bN0M0	
IIB	T2bN1M0	36%
	T3N0M0	
IIIA	T1a-T3N2M0	24%
	T3N1M0	
	T4N0-1M0	
IIIB	T4N2M0	9%
	T1a-T4N3M0	
IV	Any T Any N plus	13%
	M1a or M1b	

Abbreviation: TNM, tumor-node-metastasis.

usually a nonsolid nodule and tends to be slightly more opaque than AAH. MIA is mainly solid, usually with a small (<5 mm) central solid component. However, overlap exists among the imaging features of the preinvasive and minimally invasive lesions in the lung adenocarcinoma spectrum. Lepidic adenocarcinomas are usually solid but may be nonsolid. Likewise, the small invasive adenocarcinomas also are usually solid but may exhibit a small nonsolid component.

MANAGEMENT OF STAGES I AND II NSCLC

Surgical Resection of Stage I and II NSCLC Surgical resection, ideally by an experienced thoracic surgeon, is the treatment of choice for patients with clinical stage I and II NSCLC who are able to tolerate the procedure. Operative mortality rates for patients resected by thoracic or cardiothoracic surgeons are lower compared to general surgeons. Moreover, survival rates are higher in patients who undergo resection in facilities with a high surgical volume compared to those performing fewer than 70 procedures per year, even though the higher-volume facilities often serve older and less socioeconomic advantaged populations. The improvement in survival is most evident in the immediate postoperative period. The extent of resection is a matter of surgical judgment based on findings at exploration. In patients with stage IA NSCLC, lobectomy is superior to wedge resection with respect to rates of local recurrence. There is also a trend toward improvement in overall survival. In patients with comorbidities, compromised pulmonary reserve, and small peripheral lesions, a limited resection, wedge resection, and segmentectomy (potentially by video-assisted thoracoscopic surgery) may be reasonable surgical option. Pneumonectomy is reserved for patients with central tumors and should be performed only in

TABLE 107-9 ASSESSMENT OF RISK OF CANCER IN PATIENTS WITH SOLITARY PULMONARY NODULES

	Risk		
Variable	**Low**	**Intermediate**	**High**
Diameter (cm)	<1.5	1.5–2.2	≥2.3
Age (years)	<45	45–60	>60
Smoking status	Never smoker	Current smoker (<20 cigarettes/d)	Current smoker (>20 cigarettes/d)
Smoking cessation status	Quit ≥7 years ago or quit	Quit <7 years ago	Never quit
Characteristics of nodule margins	Smooth	Scalloped	Corona radiata or spiculated

Source: Reproduced with permission from D Ost et al: N Engl J Med 348:2535, 2003.

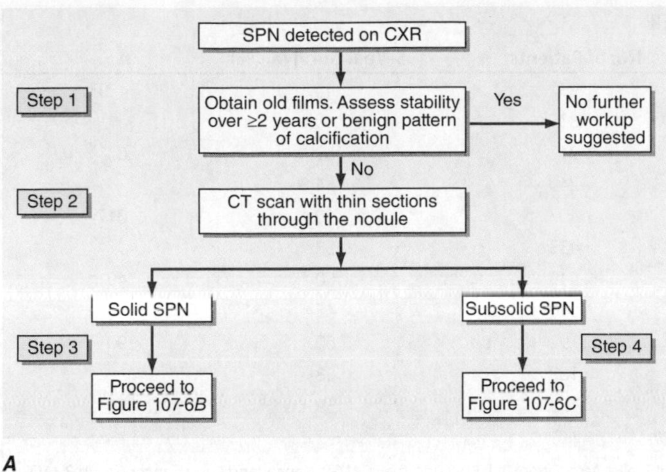

A

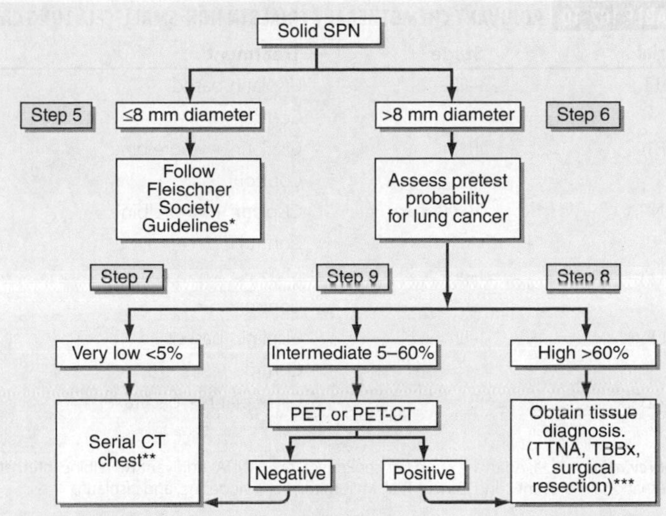

*Fleischner society guidelines; modified from: H. MacMahon, et al: *Radiology* 2005; 237;395–400

Nodule size (a):	Low-risk patient (b):	High-risk patient (c):
≤4 mm	No follow-up needed (d)	Follow-up at 12 months; if unchanged, no further follow-up
>4–6 mm	Follow-up CT at 12 months; if unchanged, no further follow-up	Follow-up CT at 6–12 months; then 18–24 months if no change
>6–8 mm	Follow-up CT at 6–12 months, then 18–24 months if no change	Follow-up CT at 3–6 months, then 9–12 and 24 months if no change
>8 mm	Follow-up CT at 3, 9, and 24 months; dynamic contrast-enhanced CT, PET, and/or biopsy	Same as low-risk patient

(a) Average of largest and smallest axial diameters of the nodule
(b) No smoking history and absence of other risk factors
(c) Previous or current smoking history or other risk factors
(d) Risk of malignancy (<0.1%) is substantially lower than for an asymptomatic smoker

**ACCP guidelines (see MK Gould et al: *Chest* 2007;132(suppl 3):108s-130S.
***Consider patient preference, severity of medical comorbidities, center specific expertise prior to tissue diagnosis.

B

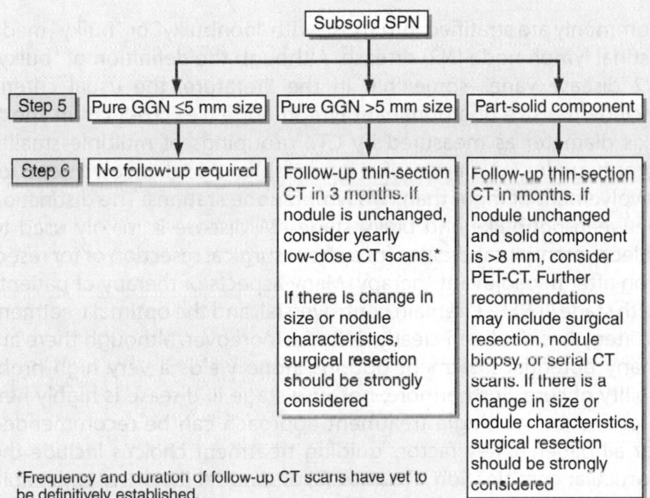

C

FIGURE 107-6 *A.* Algorithm for evaluation of solitary pulmonary nodule (SPN). *B.* Algorithm for evaluation of solid SPN. *C.* Algorithm for evaluation of semisolid SPN. CT, computed tomography; CXR, chest radiograph; GGN, ground-glass nodule; PET, positron emission tomography; TTBx, transbronchial biopsy; TTNA, transthoracic needle biopsy. *(Adapted from VK Patel et al: Chest 143:840, 2013.)*

patients with excellent pulmonary reserve. The 5-year survival rates are 60–80% for patients with stage I NSCLC and 40–50% for patients with stage II NSCLC.

Accurate pathologic staging requires adequate segmental, hilar, and mediastinal lymph node sampling. Ideally this includes a mediastinal lymph node dissection. On the right side, mediastinal stations 2R, 4R, 7, 8R, and 9R should be dissected; on the left side, stations 5, 6, 7, 8L, and 9L should be dissected. Hilar lymph nodes are typically resected and sent for pathologic review, although it is helpful to specifically dissect and label level 10 lymph nodes when possible. On the left side, level 2 and sometimes level 4 lymph nodes are generally obscured by the aorta. Although the therapeutic benefit of nodal dissection versus nodal sampling is controversial, a pooled analysis of three trials involving patients with stages I to IIIA NSCLC demonstrated a superior 4-year survival in patients undergoing resection and a complete mediastinal lymph node dissection compared with lymph node sampling. Moreover, complete mediastinal lymphadenectomy added little morbidity to a pulmonary resection for lung cancer when carried out by an experienced thoracic surgeon.

Radiation Therapy in Stages I and II NSCLC There is currently no role for postoperative radiation therapy in patients following resection of stage I or II NSCLC. However, patients with stage I and II disease who either refuse or are not suitable candidates for surgery should be considered for radiation therapy with *curative* intent. Stereotactic body radiation therapy (SBRT) is a relatively new technique used to treat patients with isolated pulmonary nodules (≤5 cm) who are not candidates for or refuse surgical resection. Treatment is typically administered in three to five fractions delivered over 1–2 weeks. In uncontrolled studies, disease control rates are >90%, and 5-year survival rates of up to 60% have been reported with SBRT. By comparison, survival rates typically range from 13 to 39% in patients with stage I or II NSCLC treated with standard external-beam radiotherapy. Cryoablation is another technique occasionally used to treat small, isolated tumors (i.e., ≤3 cm). However, very little data exist on long-term outcomes with this technique.

Chemotherapy in Stages I and II NSCLC Although a landmark meta-analysis of cisplatin-based adjuvant chemotherapy trials in patients with resected stages I to IIIA NSCLC (the Lung Adjuvant Cisplatin Evaluation [LACE] Study) demonstrated a 5.4% improvement in 5-year survival for adjuvant chemotherapy compared to surgery alone, the survival benefit was seemingly confined to patients with stage II or III disease **(Table 107-10)**. By contrast, survival was actually worsened in stage IA patients with the application of adjuvant therapy. In stage IB, there was a modest improvement in survival of questionable clinical significance. Adjuvant chemotherapy was

TABLE 107-10 ADJUVANT CHEMOTHERAPY TRIALS IN NON-SMALL-CELL LUNG CANCER

Trial	Stage	Treatment	No. of Patients	5-Year Survival (%)	p
IALT	I–III	Cisplatin-based	932	44.5	< .03
		Control	835	40.4	
BR10	IB–II	Cisplatin + vinorelbine	242	69	.03
		Control	240	54	
ANITA	IB–IIIA	Cisplatin + vinorelbine	407	60	.017
		Control	433	58	
ALPI	I–III	MVP	548	50	.49
		Control	540	45	
BLT	I–III	Cisplatin-based	192	60	.90
		Control	189	58	
CALGB	IB	Carboplatin + paclitaxel	173	59	.10
			171	57	

Abbreviations: ALPI, Adjuvant Lung Cancer Project Italy; ANITA, Adjuvant Navelbine International Trialist Association; BLT, Big Lung Trial; CALGB, Cancer and Lung Cancer Group B; IALT, International Adjuvant Lung Cancer Trial; MVP, mitomycin, vindesine, and cisplatin.

also detrimental in patients with poor performance status (Eastern Cooperative Oncology Group [ECOG] performance status = 2). These data suggest that adjuvant chemotherapy is best applied in patients with resected stage II or III NSCLC. There is no apparent role for adjuvant chemotherapy in patients with resected stage IA or IB NSCLC. A possible exception to the prohibition of adjuvant therapy in this setting is the stage IB patient with a resected lesion ≥4 cm.

As with any treatment recommendation, the risks and benefits of adjuvant chemotherapy should be considered on an individual patient basis. If a decision is made to proceed with adjuvant chemotherapy, in general, treatment should be initiated 6–12 weeks after surgery, assuming the patient has fully recovered, and should be administered for no more than four cycles. Although a cisplatin-based chemotherapy is the preferred treatment regimen, carboplatin can be substituted for cisplatin in patients who are unlikely to tolerate cisplatin for reasons such as reduced renal function, presence of neuropathy, or hearing impairment. No specific chemotherapy regimen is considered optimal in this setting, although platinum plus vinorelbine is most commonly used.

Neoadjuvant chemotherapy, which is the application of chemotherapy administered *before* an attempted surgical resection, has been advocated by some experts on the assumption that such an approach will more effectively extinguish occult micrometastases compared to postoperative chemotherapy. In addition, it is thought that preoperative chemotherapy might render an inoperable lesion resectable. With the exception of superior sulcus tumors, however, the role of neoadjuvant chemotherapy in stage I to III disease is not well defined. However, a meta-analysis of 15 randomized controlled trials involving more than 2300 patients with stage I to III NSCLC suggested there may be a modest 5-year survival benefit (i.e., ~5%) that is virtually identical to the survival benefit achieved with postoperative chemotherapy. Accordingly, neoadjuvant therapy may prove useful in selected cases (see below). A decision to use neoadjuvant chemotherapy should always be made in consultation with an experienced surgeon.

In should be noted that all patients with resected NSCLC are at high risk of recurrence, most of which occurs within 18–24 months of surgery, or developing a second primary lung cancer. Thus, it is reasonable to follow these patients with periodic imaging studies. Given the results of the NLST, periodic CT scans appear to be the most appropriate screening modality. Based on the timing of most recurrences, some guidelines recommend a contrasted chest CT scan every 6 months for the first 3 years after surgery, followed by yearly CT scans of the chest without contrast thereafter.

MANAGEMENT OF STAGE III NSCLC

Management of patients with stage III NSCLC usually requires a combined-modality approach. Patients with stage IIIA disease commonly are stratified into those with "nonbulky" or "bulky" mediastinal lymph node (N2) disease. Although the definition of "bulky" N2 disease varies somewhat in the literature, the usual criteria include the size of a dominant lymph node (i.e., >2–3 cm in short-axis diameter as measured by CT), groupings of multiple smaller lymph nodes, evidence of extracapsular nodal involvement, or involvement of more than two lymph node stations. The distinction between nonbulky and bulky stage IIIA disease is mainly used to select potential candidates for *upfront* surgical resection or for resection after neoadjuvant therapy. Many aspects of therapy of patients with stage III NSCLC remain controversial, and the optimal treatment strategy has not been clearly defined. Moreover, although there are many potential treatment options, none yields a very high probability of cure. Furthermore, because stage III disease is highly heterogeneous, no single treatment approach can be recommended for all patients. Key factors guiding treatment choices include the particular combination of tumor (T) and nodal (N) disease, the ability to achieve a complete surgical resection if indicated, and the patient's overall physical condition and preferences. For example, in carefully selected patients with limited stage IIIA disease where involved mediastinal lymph nodes can be completed resected, initial surgery followed by postoperative chemotherapy (with or without radiation therapy) may be indicated. By contrast, for patients with clinically evident bulky mediastinal lymph node involvement, the standard approach to treatment is concurrent chemoradiotherapy. Nevertheless, in some cases, the latter group of patients may be candidates for surgery following chemoradiotherapy.

Absent and Nonbulky Mediastinal (N2, N3) Lymph Node Disease For the subset of stage IIIA patients initially thought to have clinical stage I or II disease (i.e., pathologic involvement of mediastinal [N2] lymph nodes is *not* detected preoperatively), surgical resection is often the treatment of choice. This is followed by adjuvant chemotherapy in patients with microscopic lymph node involvement in a resection specimen. Postoperative radiation therapy (PORT) may also have a role for those with close or positive surgical margins. Patients with tumors involving the chest wall or proximal airways within 2 cm of the carina with hilar lymph node involvement (but not N2 disease) are classified as having T3N1 stage IIIA disease. They too are best managed with surgical resection, if technically feasible, followed by adjuvant chemotherapy if completely resected. Patients with tumors exceeding 7 cm in size also are now classified as T3 and are consider stage IIIA if tumor has spread to N1 nodes. The appropriate initial management of these patients involves surgical resection when feasible, provided the mediastinal staging is negative, followed by adjuvant chemotherapy for those who achieve complete tumor resection. Patients with T3N0 or T3N1 disease due to the presence of satellite nodules within the same lobe as the primary tumor also are candidates for surgery, as are patients with ipsilateral nodules in another lobe and negative mediastinal nodes (IIIA, T4N0 or T4N1). Although data regarding adjuvant chemotherapy in the latter subsets of patients are limited, it is often recommended.

Patients with T4N0-1 were reclassified as having stage IIIA tumors in the seventh edition of the TNM system. These patients may have involvement of the carina, superior vena cava, or a vertebral body and yet still be candidates for surgical resection in selected circumstances. The decision to proceed with an attempted resection must be made in consultation with an experienced thoracic surgeon often in association with a vascular or cardiac surgeon and an orthopedic surgeon depending on tumor location. However, if an incomplete resection is inevitable or if there is evidence of N2 involvement (stage IIIB), surgery for T4 disease is contraindicated. Most T4 lesions are best treated with chemoradiotherapy.

The role of PORT in patients with completely resected stage III NSCLC is controversial. To a large extent, the use of PORT is dictated by the presence or absence of N2 involvement and, to a lesser degree, by the biases of the treating physician. Using the Surveillance, Epidemiology, and End Results (SEER) database, a recent meta-analysis of PORT identified a significant increase in survival in patients with N2 disease but not in patients with N0 or N1 disease. An earlier analysis by the PORT Meta-analysis Trialist Group using an older database produced similar results.

Known Mediastinal (N2, N3) Lymph Node Disease When pathologic involvement of mediastinal lymph nodes is documented preoperatively, a combined-modality approach is recommended assuming the patient is a candidate for treatment with curative intent. These patients are at high risk for both local and distant recurrence if managed with resection alone. For patients with stage III disease who are not candidates for initial surgical resection, *concurrent* chemoradiotherapy is most commonly used as the initial treatment. Concurrent chemoradiotherapy has been shown to produce superior survival compared to *sequential* chemoradiotherapy; however, it also is associated with greater host toxicities (including fatigue, esophagitis, and neutropenia). Therefore, for patients with a good performance status, concurrent chemoradiotherapy is the preferred treatment approach, whereas sequential chemoradiotherapy may be more appropriate for patients with a performance status that is not as good. For patients who are *not* candidates for a combined-modality treatment approach, typically due to a poor performance status or a comorbidity that makes chemotherapy untenable, radiotherapy alone may provide a modest survival benefit in addition to symptom palliation.

For patients with potentially resectable N2 disease, it remains uncertain whether surgery after neoadjuvant chemoradiotherapy improves survival. In an NCI-sponsored Intergroup randomized trial comparing concurrent chemoradiotherapy alone to concurrent chemoradiotherapy followed by attempted surgical resection, no survival benefit was observed in the trimodality arm compared to the bimodality therapy. In fact, patients subjected to a pneumonectomy had a worse survival outcome. By contrast, those treated with a lobectomy appeared to have a survival advantage based on a retrospective subset analysis. Thus, in carefully selected, otherwise healthy patients with nonbulky mediastinal lymph node involvement, surgery may be a reasonable option if the primary tumor can be fully resected with a lobectomy. This is not the case if a pneumonectomy is required to achieve complete resection.

Superior Sulcus Tumors (Pancoast Tumors) Superior sulcus tumors represent a distinctive subset of stage III disease. These tumors arise in the apex of the lung and may invade the second and third ribs, the brachial plexus, the subclavian vessels, the stellate ganglion, and adjacent vertebral bodies. They also may be associated with Pancoast syndrome, characterized by pain that may arise in the shoulder or chest wall or radiate to the neck. Pain characteristically radiates to the ulnar surface of the hand. Horner's syndrome (enophthalmos, ptosis, miosis, and anhydrosis) due to invasion of the paravertebral sympathetic chain may be present as well. Patients with these tumors should undergo the same staging procedures as all patients with stage II and III NSCLC. Neoadjuvant chemotherapy or combined chemoradiotherapy followed by surgery is reserved for those without N2 involvement. This approach yields excellent survival outcomes (>50% 5-year survival in patients with an R0 resection). Patients with N2 disease are less likely to benefit from surgery and can be managed with chemoradiotherapy alone. Patients presenting with metastatic disease can be treated with radiation therapy (with or without chemotherapy) for symptom palliation.

MANAGEMENT OF METASTATIC NSCLC

Approximately 40% of NSCLC patients present with advanced, stage IV disease at the time of diagnosis. These patients have a poor median survival (4–6 months) and a 1-year survival of 10% when managed with best supportive care alone. In addition, a significant number of patients who first presented with early-stage NSCLC will eventually relapse with distant disease. Patients who have recurrent disease have a better prognosis than those presenting with metastatic disease at the time of diagnosis. Standard medical management, the judicious use of pain medications, and the appropriate use of radiotherapy and chemotherapy form the cornerstone of management. Chemotherapy palliates symptoms, improves the quality of life, and improves survival in patients with stage IV NSCLC, particularly in patients with good performance status. In addition, economic analysis has found chemotherapy to be cost-effective palliation for stage IV NSCLC. However, the use of chemotherapy for NSCLC requires clinical experience and careful judgment to balance potential benefits and toxicities. Of note, the early application of palliative care in conjunction with chemotherapy is associated with improved survival and a better quality of life.

First-Line Chemotherapy for Metastatic or Recurrent NSCLC A landmark meta-analysis published in 1995 provided the earliest meaningful indication that chemotherapy could provide a survival benefit in metastatic NSCLC as opposed to supportive care alone. However, the survival benefit was seemingly confined to cisplatin-based chemotherapy regimens (hazard ratio 0.73; 27% reduction in the risk of death; 10% improvement in survival at 1 year). These data launched two decades of clinical research aimed at detecting the optimal chemotherapy regimen for advanced NSCLC. For the most part, however, these efforts proved unsuccessful because the overwhelming majority of randomized trials showed no major survival improvement with any one regimen versus another (Table 107-11). On the other hand, differences in progression-free survival, cost, side effects, and schedule were frequently observed. These first-line studies were later extended to elderly patients, where doublet chemotherapy was found to improve overall survival compared to single agents in the "fit" elderly (e.g., elderly patients with no major comorbidities) and in patients with an ECOG performance status of 2. An ongoing debate in the treatment of patients with advanced NSCLC is the appropriate duration of platinum-based chemotherapy. Several large phase III randomized trials have failed to show a meaningful benefit for increasing the duration of platinum-based doublet chemotherapy beyond four to six cycles. In fact, longer duration of chemotherapy has been associated with increased toxicities and impaired quality of life. Therefore, prolonged front-line therapy (beyond four to six cycles) with platinum-based regimens is not recommended. Maintenance therapy following initial platinum-based therapy is discussed below.

Although specific tumor histology was once considered irrelevant to treatment choice in NSCLC, with the recent recognition that selected chemotherapy agents perform quite differently in squamous versus adenocarcinomas, accurate determination of histology has become essential. Specifically, in a landmark randomized phase III trial, patients with nonsquamous NSCLC were found to have an improved survival when treated with cisplatin and pemetrexed compared to cisplatin and gemcitabine. By contrast, patients with squamous carcinoma had an improved survival when treated with cisplatin and gemcitabine. This survival difference is thought to be related to the differential expression of thymidylate synthase (TS),

TABLE 107-11 FIRST-LINE CHEMOTHERAPY TRIALS FOR METASTATIC NON-SMALL-CELL LUNG CANCER

Trial	Regimen	No. of Patients	RR (%)	Median Survival (months)
ECOG1594	Cisplatin + paclitaxel	288	21	7.8
	Cisplatin + gemcitabine	288	22	8.1
	Cisplatin + docetaxel	289	17	7.4
	Carboplatin + paclitaxel	290	17	8.1
TAX-326	Cisplatin + docetaxel	406	32	11.3
	Cisplatin + vinorelbine	394	25	10.1
	Carboplatin + docetaxel	404	24	9.4
EORTC	Cisplatin + paclitaxel	159	32	8.1
	Cisplatin + gemcitabine	160	37	8.9
	Paclitaxel + gemcitabine	161	28	6.7
ILCP	Cisplatin + gemcitabine	205	30	9.8
	Carboplatin + paclitaxel	204	32	9.9
	Cisplatin + vinorelbine	203	30	9.5
SWOG	Cisplatin + vinorelbine	202	28	8.0
	Carboplatin + paclitaxel	206	25	8.0
FACS	Cisplatin + irinotecan	145	31	13.9
	Carboplatin + paclitaxel	145	32	12.3
	Cisplatin + gemcitabine	146	30	14.0
	Cisplatin + vinorelbine	145	33	11.4
Scagliotti	Cisplatin + gemcitabine	863	28	10.3
	Cisplatin + pemetrexed	862	31	10.3
iPASS[a]	Carboplatin + paclitaxel	608	32	17.3
	Gefitinib	609	43%	18.6

[a]Enrolled selected patients: 18 years of age or older, had histologic or cytologically confirmed stage IIIB or IV non-small-cell lung cancer with histologic features of adenocarcinoma (including bronchioloalveolar carcinoma), were nonsmokers (defined as patients who had smoked <100 cigarettes in their lifetime) or former light smokers (those who had stopped smoking at least 15 years previously and had a total of ≤10 pack-years of smoking), and had had no previous chemotherapy or biologic or immunologic therapy.

Abbreviations: ECOG, Eastern Cooperative Oncology Group; EORTC, European Organization for Research and Treatment of Cancer; ILCP, Italian Lung Cancer Project; SWOG, Southwest Oncology Group; FACS, Follow-up After Colorectal Surgery; iPASS, Iressa Pan-Asian Study.

one of the targets of pemetrexed, between tumor types. Squamous cancers have a much higher expression of TS compared to adenocarcinomas, accounting for their lower responsiveness to pemetrexed. By contrast, the activity of gemcitabine is not impacted by the levels of TS. Bevacizumab, a monoclonal antibody against VEGF, has been shown to improve response rate, progression-free survival, and overall survival in patients with advanced disease when combined with chemotherapy (see below). However, bevacizumab cannot be given to patients with squamous cell histology NSCLC because of their tendency to experience serious hemorrhagic effects.

Agents That Inhibit Angiogenesis Bevacizumab, a monoclonal antibody directed against VEGF, was the first antiangiogenic agent approved for the treatment of patients with advanced NSCLC in the United States. This drug primarily acts by blocking the growth of new blood vessels, which are required for tumor viability. Two randomized phase III trials of chemotherapy with or without bevacizumab had conflicting results. The first trial, conducted in North America, compared carboplatin plus paclitaxel with or without bevacizumab in patients with recurrent or advanced nonsquamous NSCLC and reported a significant improvement in response rate, progression-free survival, and overall survival in patients treated with chemotherapy plus bevacizumab versus chemotherapy alone. Bevacizumab-treated patients had a significantly higher incidence of toxicities. The second trial, conducted in Europe, compared cisplatin/gemcitabine with or without bevacizumab in patients with recurrent or advanced nonsquamous NSCLC and reported a significant improvement in progression-free survival but no improvement in overall survival for bevacizumab-treated patients. A randomized phase III trial compared carboplatin/pemetrexed and bevacizumab to carboplatin/paclitaxel and bevacizumab as first-line therapy in patients with recurrent or advanced nonsquamous NSCLC and reported no significant difference in progression-free survival or overall survival between treatment groups. Therefore, currently carboplatin/paclitaxel and bevacizumab or carboplatin/pemetrexed and bevacizumab are appropriate regimens for first-line treatment for stage IV nonsquamous NSCLC patients. Of note, there are many small-molecule inhibitors of VEGFR; however, these VEGFR TKIs have not proven to be effective in the treatment of NSCLC.

Maintenance Therapy for Metastatic NSCLC Maintenance chemotherapy in nonprogressing patients (patients with a complete response, partial response, or stable disease) is a controversial topic in the treatment of NSCLC. Conceptually, there are two types of maintenance strategies: (1) switch maintenance therapy, where patients receive four to six cycles of platinum-based chemotherapy and are switched to an entirely different regimen; and (2) continuation maintenance therapy, where patients receive four to six cycles of platinum-based chemotherapy and then the platinum agent is discontinued but the agent it is paired with is continued (Table 107-12). Two studies investigated switch maintenance single-agent chemotherapy with docetaxel or pemetrexed in nonprogressing patients following treatment with first-line platinum-based chemotherapy. Both trials randomized patients to immediate single-agent therapy versus observation and reported improvements in progression-free and overall survival. In both trials, a significant portion of patients in the observation arm did not receive therapy with the agent under investigation upon disease progression; 37% of study patients never received docetaxel in the docetaxel study and 81% of patients never received pemetrexed in the pemetrexed study. In the trial of maintenance docetaxel versus observation, survival was identical to the treatment group in the subset of patients who received docetaxel on progression, indicating this is an active agent in NSCLC. These data are not available for the pemetrexed study. Two additional trials evaluated switch maintenance therapy with erlotinib after platinum-based chemotherapy in patients with advanced

TABLE 107-12 MAINTENANCE THERAPY TRIALS

Group	CT	No. of Patients	Survival OS (months)	PFS (months)
Switch Maintenance				
Fidias	Immediate docetaxel	153	12.3	5.7
	Delayed docetaxel	156	9.7	2.7
Ciuleanu	Pemetrexed	444	13.4	4.3
	BSC	222	10.6	2.6
Paramount	Pemetrexed	472	13.9	4.1
	BSC	297	11.0	2.8
ATLAS	Bev + erlotinib	384	15.9	4.8
	Bev + placebo	384	13.9	3.8
SATURN	Erlotinib	437	12.3	2.9
	Placebo	447	11.1	2.6
Continuation Maintenance				
ECOG4599	Bev 15 mg/kg	444	12.3	6.2
	BSC	434	10.3	4.5
AVAiL	Bev 15 mg/kg	351	13.4	6.5
	Bev 7.5 mg/kg	345	13.6	6.7
	Placebo	347	13.1	6.1
POINTBREAK	Pemetrexed + Bev 15 mg/kg			8.6
	Bev 15 mg/kg			6.9

Abbreviations: Bev, bevacizumab; BSC, best supportive care; CT, chemotherapy; OS, overall survival; PFS, progression-free survival.

NSCLC and reported an improvement in progression-free survival and overall survival in the erlotinib treatment group. Currently, maintenance pemetrexed or erlotinib following platinum-based chemotherapy in patients with advanced NSCLC are approved by the U.S. FDA. However, maintenance therapy is not without toxicity and, at this time, should be considered on an individual patient basis.

Targeted Therapies for Select Molecular Cohorts of NSCLC As the efficacy of traditional cytotoxic chemotherapeutic agents plateaued in NSCLC, there was a critical need to define novel therapeutic treatment strategies. These novel strategies have largely been based on the identification of somatic driver mutations within the tumor. These driver mutations occur in genes encoding signaling proteins that, when aberrant, drive initiation and maintenance of tumor cells. Importantly, driver mutations can serve as Achilles' heels for tumors, if their gene products can be targeted therapeutically with small-molecule inhibitors. For example, *EGFR* mutations have been detected in 10–15% of North American patients diagnosed with NSCLC. *EGFR* mutations are associated with younger age, light (<10 pack-year) and nonsmokers, and adenocarcinoma histology. Approximately 90% of these mutations are exon 19 deletions or exon 21 L858R point mutations within the EGFR TK domain, resulting in hyperactivation of both EGFR kinase activity and downstream signaling. Lung tumors that harbor activating mutations within the EGFR kinase domain display high sensitivity to small-molecule EGFR TKIs. Erlotinib and afatinib are FDA-approved oral small-molecule TKIs that inhibit EGFR. Outside the United States, gefitinib also is available. Several large, international, phase III studies have demonstrated improved response rates, progression-free survival, and overall survival in patients with *EGFR* mutation–positive NSCLC patients treated with an EGFR TKI as compared with standard first-line chemotherapy regimens (Table 107-13).

Although response rates with EGFR TKI therapy are clearly superior in patients with lung tumors harboring activating EGFR kinase domain mutations, the EGFR TKI erlotinib is also FDA approved for second- and third-line therapy in patients with advanced NSCLC *irrespective* of tumor genotype. The reason for this apparent discrepancy is that erlotinib was initially evaluated in lung cancer *before* the discovery of *EGFR* activating mutations. In fact, *EGFR* mutations were initially identified in lung cancer by studying the tumors of patients who had dramatic responses to this agent. With the rapid pace of scientific discovery, additional driver mutations in lung cancer have been identified and targeted therapeutically with impressive clinical results. For example, chromosomal rearrangements involving the anaplastic lymphoma kinase (*ALK*) gene on chromosome 2 have been found in ~3–7% of NSCLC. The result of these *ALK* rearrangements is hyperactivation of the ALK TK domain. Similar to EGFR, *ALK* rearrangements are typically (but not exclusively) associated with younger age, light (<10 pack-year) and nonsmokers, and adenocarcinoma histology. Remarkably, *ALK* rearrangements were initially described in lung cancer in 2007, and by 2011, the first ALK inhibitor, crizotinib, received FDA approval for patients with lung tumors harboring *ALK* rearrangements.

TABLE 107-13 RESULTS OF PHASE III TRIALS COMPARING CHEMOTHERAPY AND FIRST-LINE EGFR TKI IN *EGFR* MUTATION–POSITIVE PATIENTS

Study	Therapy	No. of Patients	ORR (%)	PFS (months)
IPASS	CbP	129	47	6.3
	Gefitinib	132	71	9.3
EURTAC	CG	87	15	5.2
	Erlotinib	86	58	9.7
OPTIMAL	CG	72	36	4.6
	Erlotinib	82	83	13.1
NEJOO2	CG	114	31	5.4
	Gefitinib	114	74	10.8
WJTOG3405	CD	89	31	6.3
	Gefitinib	88	62	9.2
LUX LUNG 3	CP	115	23	6.9
	Afatinib	230	56	11.1

Abbreviations: CbP, carboplatin and paclitaxel; CD, cisplatin and docetaxel; CG, cisplatin and gemcitabine; CP, cisplatin and paclitaxel; ORR, overall response rate; PFS, progression-free survival.

In addition to *EGFR* and *ALK*, other driver mutations have been discovered with varying frequencies in NSCLC, including *KRAS, BRAF, PIK3CA, NRAS, AKT1, MET, MEK1* (*MAP2K1*), *ROS1*, and *RET*. Mutations within the *KRAS* GTPase are found in approximately 20% of lung adenocarcinomas. To date, however, no small-molecule inhibitors are available to specifically target mutant *KRAS*. Each of the other driver mutations occurs in less than 1–3% of lung adenocarcinomas. The great majority of the driver mutations are mutually exclusive, and there are ongoing clinical studies for their specific inhibitors. For example, the BRAF inhibitor vemurafenib and the RET inhibitor cabozantinib have already demonstrated efficacy in patients with lung cancer harboring *BRAF* mutations or *RET* gene fusions, respectively. Most of these mutations are present in adenocarcinoma; however, mutations that may be linked to future targeted therapies in squamous cell carcinomas are emerging. In addition, there are active research efforts aimed at defining novel targetable mutations in lung cancer as well as defining mechanisms of acquired resistance to small molecule inhibitors used in the treatment of patients with NSCLC.

Second-Line Chemotherapy and Beyond Second-line therapy for advanced NSCLC was almost never recommended until a seminal study in 2000 showed that docetaxel improved survival compared to supportive care alone. As first-line chemotherapy regimens improve, a substantial number of patients will maintain a good performance status and a desire for further therapy when they develop recurrent disease. Currently, several agents are FDA approved for second-line use in NSCLC including docetaxel, pemetrexed, erlotinib (approved for second-line therapy regardless of tumor genotype), and crizotinib (for patients with *ALK*-mutant lung cancer only). Most of the survival benefit for any of these agents is realized in patients who maintain a good performance status.

Immunotherapy For more than 30 years, the investigation of vaccines and immunotherapies in lung cancer has yielded little in the way of meaningful benefit. Recently, however, this perception has changed based on preliminary results of studies using monoclonal antibodies that activate antitumor immunity through blockade of immune checkpoints. For example, ipilimumab, a monoclonal antibody directed at cytotoxic T lymphocyte antigen-4 (CTLA-4), was studied in combination with paclitaxel plus carboplatin in patients with both SCLC and NSCLC. There appeared to be a small but not statistically significant advantage to the combination when ipilimumab was instituted after several cycles of chemotherapy. A randomized phase III trial in SCLC is under way to validate these data. Antibodies to the T cell programmed cell death receptor 1 (PD-1), nivolumab and pembrolizumab, have been shown to produce responses in lung cancer, renal cell cancer, and melanoma. Many of these responses have had very long duration (i.e., >1 year). Monoclonal antibodies to the PD-1 ligand (anti-PDL-1), which may be expressed on the tumor cell, have also been shown to produce responses in patients with melanoma and lung cancer. Preliminary studies in melanoma suggest that the combination of ipilimumab and nivolumab could produce higher response rates compared to either agent alone. A similar strategy is being investigated in SCLC patients. Further evaluation of these agents in both NSCLC and SCLC is ongoing in combination with already approved chemotherapy and targeted agents.

Supportive Care No discussion of the treatment strategies for patients with advanced lung cancer would be complete without a mention of supportive care. Coincident with advances in chemotherapy and targeted therapy was a pivotal study that demonstrated that the early integration of palliative care with standard treatment strategies improved both quality of life and mood for patients with advanced lung cancer. Aggressive pain and symptom control is an important component for optimal treatment of these patients.

SURGERY FOR LIMITED-DISEASE SMALL-CELL LUNG CANCER

SCLC is a highly aggressive disease characterized by its rapid doubling time, high growth fraction, early development of disseminated disease, and dramatic response to first-line chemotherapy and radiation. In general, surgical resection is *not* routinely recommended for patients because even patients with LD-SCLC still have occult micrometastases. However, the most recent American College of Chest Physicians Evidence-Based Clinical Practice Guidelines recommend surgical resection over nonsurgical treatment in SCLC patients with clinical stage I disease after a thorough evaluation for distant metastases and invasive mediastinal stage evaluation (grade 2C). After resection, these patients should receive platinum-based adjuvant chemotherapy (grade 1C). If the histologic diagnosis of SCLC is made in patients on review of a resected surgical specimen, such patients should receive standard SCLC chemotherapy as well.

CHEMOTHERAPY

Chemotherapy significantly prolongs survival in patients with SCLC. Four to six cycles of platinum-based chemotherapy with either cisplatin or carboplatin plus either etoposide or irinotecan has been the mainstay of treatment for nearly three decades and is recommended over other chemotherapy regimens irrespective of initial stage. Cyclophosphamide, doxorubicin (Adriamycin), and vincristine (CAV) may be an alternative for patients who are unable to tolerate a platinum-based regimen. Despite response rates to first-line therapy as high as 80%, the median survival ranges from 12 to 20 months for patients with LD and from 7 to 11 months for patients with ED. Regardless of disease extent, the majority of patients relapse and develop chemotherapy-resistant disease. Only 6–12% of patients with LD-SCLC and 2% of patients with ED-SCLC live beyond 5 years. The prognosis is especially poor for patients who relapse within the first 3 months of therapy; these patients are said to have *chemotherapy-resistant disease*. Patients are said to have *sensitive disease* if they relapse more than 3 months after their initial therapy and are thought to have a somewhat better overall survival. These patients also are thought to have the greatest potential benefit from second-line chemotherapy (Fig. 107-7). Topotecan is the only FDA-approved agent for second-line therapy in patients with SCLC. Topotecan has only modest activity and can be given either intravenously or orally. In one randomized trial, 141 patients who were not considered candidates for further IV chemotherapy were randomized to receive either oral topotecan or best supportive care. Although the response rate to oral topotecan was only 7%, overall survival was significantly better in patients receiving chemotherapy (median survival time, 26 weeks vs 14 weeks; $p = .01$). Moreover, patients given topotecan had a slower decline in quality of life than did those not receiving chemotherapy. Other agents with similar low levels of activity in the second-line setting include irinotecan, paclitaxel, docetaxel, vinorelbine, oral etoposide, and gemcitabine. Clearly novel treatments for this all too common disease are desperately needed.

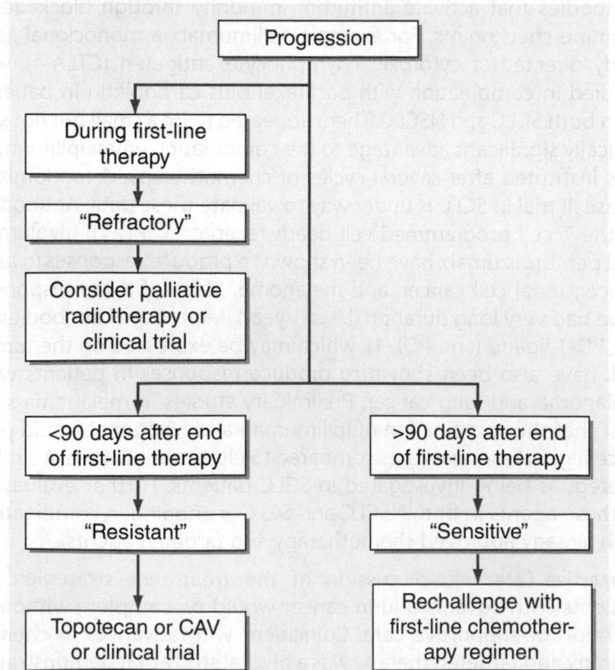

FIGURE 107-7 Management of recurrent small-cell lung cancer (SCLC). CAV, cyclophosphamide, doxorubicin, and vincristine. *(Adapted with permission from JP van Meerbeeck et al: Lancet 378:1741, 2011.)*

THORACIC RADIATION THERAPY

Thoracic radiation therapy (TRT) is a standard component of induction therapy for good performance status and limited-stage SCLC patients. Meta-analyses indicate that chemotherapy combined with chest irradiation improves 3-year survival by approximately 5% as compared with chemotherapy alone. The 5-year survival rate, however, remains disappointingly low at ~10–15%. Most commonly, TRT is combined with cisplatin and etoposide chemotherapy due to a superior toxicity profile as compared to anthracycline-containing chemotherapy regimens. As observed in locally advanced NSCLC, *concurrent* chemoradiotherapy is more effective than *sequential* chemoradiation but is associated with significantly more esophagitis and hematologic toxicity. Ideally TRT should be administered with the first two cycles of chemotherapy because later application appears slightly less effective. If for reasons of fitness or availability, this regimen cannot be offered, TRT should follow induction chemotherapy. With respect to fractionation of TRT, twice-daily 1.5-Gy fractioned radiation therapy has been shown to improve survival in LD-SCLC patients but is associated with higher rates of grade 3 esophagitis and pulmonary toxicity. Although it is feasible to deliver once-daily radiation therapy doses up to 70 Gy concurrently with cisplatin-based chemotherapy, there are no data to support equivalency of this approach compared with the 45-Gy twice-daily radiotherapy dose. Therefore, the current standard regimen of a 45-Gy dose administered in 1.5-Gy fractions twice daily for 30 days is being compared with higher-dose regimens in two phase III trials, one in the United States and one in Europe. Patients should be carefully selected for concurrent chemoradiation therapy based on good performance status and adequate pulmonary reserve. The role of radiotherapy in ED-SCLC is largely restricted to palliation of tumor-related symptoms such as bone pain and bronchial obstruction.

PROPHYLACTIC CRANIAL IRRADIATION

Prophylactic cranial irradiation (PCI) should be considered in all patients with either LD-SCLC or ED-SCLC who have responded well to initial therapy. A meta-analysis including seven trials and 987 patients with LD-SCLC who had achieved a complete remission after upfront chemotherapy yielded a 5.4% improvement in overall survival for patients treated with PCI. In patients with ED-SCLC who have responded to first-line chemotherapy, a prospective randomized phase III trial showed that PCI reduced the occurrence of symptomatic brain metastases and prolonged disease-free and overall survival compared to no radiation therapy. Long-term toxicities, including deficits in cognition, have been reported after PCI but are difficult to sort out from the effects of chemotherapy or normal aging.

SUMMARY

The management of NSCLC has undergone major change in the past decade. To a lesser extent, the same is true for SCLC. For patients with early-stage disease, advances in radiotherapy and surgical procedures as well as new systemic therapies have greatly improved prognosis in both diseases. For patients with advanced disease, major progress in understanding tumor genetics has led to the development of

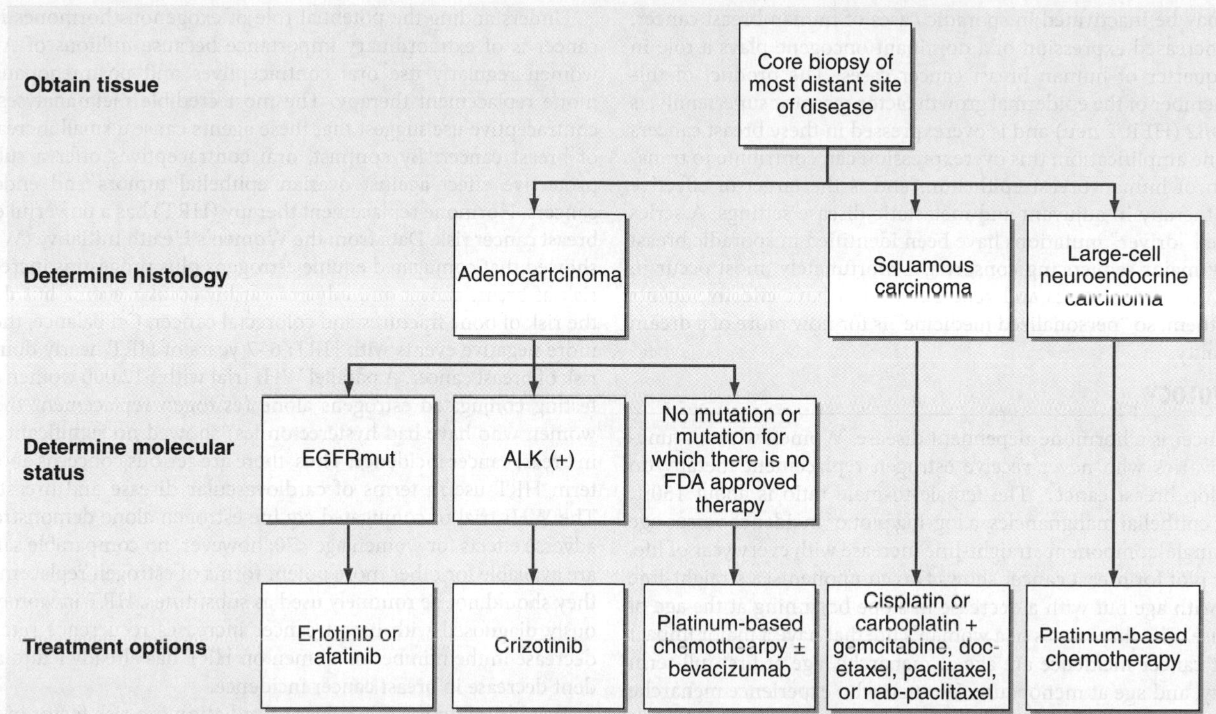

FIGURE 107-8 Approach to first-line therapy in a patient with stage IV non-small-cell lung cancer (NSCLC). EGFRmut, *EGFR* mutation; FDA, Food and Drug Administration.

targeted inhibitors based specifically on the tumor's molecular profile. Furthermore, increased understanding of how to activate the immune system to drive antitumor immunity is proving to be a promising therapeutic strategy for some patients with advanced lung cancer. In Fig. 107-8, we propose an algorithm of the treatment approach for patient with stage IV NSCLC. However, the reality is that the majority of patients treated with targeted therapies or chemotherapy eventually develop resistance, which provides strong motivation for further research and enrollment of patients onto clinical trials in this rapidly evolving area.

108 Breast Cancer

Marc E. Lippman

Breast cancer is a malignant proliferation of epithelial cells lining the ducts or lobules of the breast. In the year 2014, about 180,000 cases of invasive breast cancer and 40,000 deaths will occur in the United States. In addition, about 2000 men will be diagnosed with breast cancer. Epithelial malignancies of the breast are the most common cause of cancer in women (excluding skin cancer), accounting for about one-third of all cancer in women. As a result of improved treatment and earlier detection, the mortality rate from breast cancer has begun to decrease very substantially in the United States. This Chapter will not consider rare malignancies presenting in the breast, such as sarcomas and lymphomas, but will focus on the epithelial cancers.

GENETIC CONSIDERATIONS

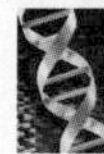

Human breast cancer is a clonal disease; a single transformed cell—the product of a series of somatic (acquired) or germline mutations—is eventually able to express full malignant potential. Thus, breast cancer may exist for a long period as either a noninvasive disease or an invasive but nonmetastatic disease. These facts have significant clinical ramifications.

Not more than 10% of human breast cancers can be linked directly to germline mutations. Several genes have been implicated in familial cases. The Li-Fraumeni syndrome is characterized by inherited mutations in the *p53* tumor-suppressor gene, which lead to an increased incidence of breast cancer, osteogenic sarcomas, and other malignancies. Inherited mutations in *PTEN* have also been reported in breast cancer.

Another tumor-suppressor gene, *BRCA1*, has been identified at the chromosomal locus 17q21; this gene encodes a zinc finger protein, and the protein product functions as a transcription factor and is involved in gene repair. Women who inherit a mutated allele of this gene from either parent have at least a 60–80% lifetime chance of developing breast cancer and about a 33% chance of developing ovarian cancer. The risk is higher among women born after 1940, presumably due to promotional effects of hormonal factors. Men who carry a mutant allele of the gene have an increased incidence of prostate cancer and breast cancer. A fourth gene, termed *BRCA2*, which has been localized to chromosome 13q12, is also associated with an increased incidence of breast cancer in men and women.

Germline mutations in *BRCA1* and *BRCA2* can be readily detected; patients with these mutations should be counseled appropriately. All women with strong family histories for breast cancer should be referred to genetic screening programs, particularly women of Ashkenazi Jewish descent who have a high likelihood of a specific founder *BRCA1* mutation (substitution of adenine for guanine at position 185).

Even more important than the role these genes play in inherited forms of breast cancer may be their role in sporadic breast cancer. A *p53* mutation is present in nearly 40% of human breast cancers as an acquired defect. Acquired mutations in *PTEN* occur in about 10% of the cases. *BRCA1* mutation in sporadic primary breast cancer has not been reported. However, decreased expression of *BRCA1* mRNA (possibly via gene methylation) and abnormal cellular location of the BRCA1 protein have been found in some breast cancers. Loss of heterozygosity of *BRCA1* and *BRCA2* suggests that tumor-suppressor activity may be inactivated in sporadic cases of human breast cancer. Finally, increased expression of a dominant oncogene plays a role in about a quarter of human breast cancer cases. The product of this gene, a member of the epidermal growth factor receptor superfamily, is called *erbB2* (HER/2 neu) and is overexpressed in these breast cancers due to gene amplification; this overexpression can contribute to transformation of human breast epithelium and is the target of effective systemic therapy in adjuvant and metastatic disease settings. A series of acquired "driver" mutations have been identified in sporadic breast cancer by major sequencing consortia. Unfortunately, most occur in no more than 5% of cases and generally do not have effective agents to target them, so "personalized medicine" is for now more of a dream than a reality.

EPIDEMIOLOGY

Breast cancer is a hormone-dependent disease. Women without functioning ovaries who never receive estrogen replacement therapy do not develop breast cancer. The female-to-male ratio is about 150:1. For most epithelial malignancies, a log-log plot of incidence versus age shows a single-component straight-line increase with every year of life. A similar plot for breast cancer shows two components: a straight-line increase with age but with a decrease in slope beginning at the age of menopause. The three dates in a woman's life that have a major impact on breast cancer incidence are age at menarche, age at first full-term pregnancy, and age at menopause. Women who experience menarche at age 16 years have only 50–60% of the breast cancer risk of a woman having menarche at age 12 years; the lower risk persists throughout life. Similarly, menopause occurring 10 years before the median age of menopause (52 years), whether natural or surgically induced, reduces lifetime breast cancer risk by about 35%. Women who have a first full-term pregnancy by age 18 years have a 30–40% lower risk of breast cancer compared with nulliparous women. Thus, length of menstrual life—particularly the fraction occurring before first full-term pregnancy—is a substantial component of the total risk of breast cancer. These three factors (menarche, age of first full-term pregnancy, and menopause) can account for 70–80% of the variation in breast cancer frequency in different countries. Also, duration of maternal nursing correlates with substantial risk reduction independent of either parity or age at first full-term pregnancy.

International variation in incidence has provided some of the most important clues on hormonal carcinogenesis. A woman living to age 80 years in North America has one chance in nine of developing invasive breast cancer. Asian women have one-fifth to one-tenth the risk of breast cancer of women in North America or Western Europe. Asian women have substantially lower concentrations of estrogens and progesterone. These differences cannot be explained on a genetic basis because Asian women living in a Western environment have sex steroid hormone concentrations and risks identical to those of their Western counterparts. These migrant women, and more notably their daughters, also differ markedly in height and weight from Asian women in Asia; height and weight are critical regulators of age of menarche and have substantial effects on plasma concentrations of estrogens.

The role of diet in breast cancer etiology is controversial. While there are associative links between total caloric and fat intake and breast cancer risk, the exact role of fat in the diet is unproven. Increased caloric intake contributes to breast cancer risk in multiple ways: earlier menarche, later age at menopause, and increased postmenopausal estrogen concentrations reflecting enhanced aromatase activities in fatty tissues. On the other hand, central obesity is both a risk factor for occurrence and recurrence of breast cancer. Moderate alcohol intake also increases the risk by an unknown mechanism. Folic acid supplementation appears to modify risk in women who use alcohol but is not additionally protective in abstainers. Recommendations favoring abstinence from alcohol must be weighed against other social pressures and the possible cardioprotective effect of moderate alcohol intake. Chronic low-dose aspirin use is associated with a decreased incidence of breast cancer. Depression is also associated with both occurrence and recurrence of breast cancer.

Understanding the potential role of exogenous hormones in breast cancer is of extraordinary importance because millions of American women regularly use oral contraceptives and postmenopausal hormone replacement therapy. The most credible meta-analyses of oral contraceptive use suggest that these agents cause a small increased risk of breast cancer. By contrast, oral contraceptives offer a substantial protective effect against ovarian epithelial tumors and endometrial cancers. Hormone replacement therapy (HRT) has a powerful effect on breast cancer risk. Data from the Women's Health Initiative (WHI) trial showed that conjugated equine estrogens plus progestins increased the risk of breast cancer and adverse cardiovascular events but decreased the risk of bone fractures and colorectal cancer. On balance, there were more negative events with HRT; 6–7 years of HRT nearly doubled the risk of breast cancer. A parallel WHI trial with >12,000 women enrolled testing conjugated estrogens alone (estrogen replacement therapy in women who have had hysterectomies) showed no significant increase in breast cancer incidence. Thus, there are serious concerns about long-term HRT use in terms of cardiovascular disease and breast cancer. The WHI trial of conjugated equine estrogen alone demonstrated few adverse effects for women age <70; however, no comparable safety data are available for other more potent forms of estrogen replacement, and they should not be routinely used as substitutes. HRT in women previously diagnosed with breast cancer increases recurrence rates. Rapid decrease in the number of women on HRT has already led to a coincident decrease in breast cancer incidence.

In addition to the other factors, radiation is a risk factor in younger women. Women who have been exposed before age 30 years to radiation in the form of multiple fluoroscopies (200–300 cGy) or treatment for Hodgkin's disease (>3600 cGy) have a substantial increase in risk of breast cancer, whereas radiation exposure after age 30 years appears to have a minimal carcinogenic effect on the breast.

EVALUATION OF BREAST MASSES IN MEN AND WOMEN

Because the breasts are a common site of potentially fatal malignancy in women, examination of the breast is an essential part of the physical examination. Unfortunately, internists frequently do not examine breasts in men, and in women, they are apt to defer this evaluation to gynecologists. Because of the plausible association between early detection and improved outcome, it is the duty of every physician to identify breast abnormalities at the earliest possible stage and to institute a diagnostic workup. Women should be trained in breast self-examination (BSE). Although breast cancer in men is unusual, unilateral lesions should be evaluated in the same manner as in women, with the recognition that gynecomastia in men can sometimes begin unilaterally and is often asymmetric.

Virtually all breast cancer is diagnosed by biopsy of a nodule detected either on a mammogram or by palpation. Algorithms have been developed to enhance the likelihood of diagnosing breast cancer and reduce the frequency of unnecessary biopsy (Fig. 108-1).

THE PALPABLE BREAST MASS

Women should be strongly encouraged to examine their breasts monthly. A potentially flawed study from China has suggested that BSE does not alter survival, but given its safety, the procedure should still be encouraged. At worst, this practice increases the likelihood of detecting a mass at a smaller size when it can be treated with more limited surgery. Breast examination by the physician should be performed in good light so as to see retractions and other skin changes. The nipple and areolae should be inspected, and an attempt should be made to elicit nipple discharge. All regional lymph node groups should be examined, and any lesions should be measured. Physical examination alone cannot exclude malignancy. Lesions with certain features are more likely to be cancerous (hard, irregular, tethered or fixed, or painless lesions). A negative mammogram in the presence of a persistent lump in the breast does not exclude malignancy. Palpable lesions require additional diagnostic procedures, including biopsy.

In premenopausal women, lesions that are either equivocal or nonsuspicious on physical examination should be reexamined in 2–4

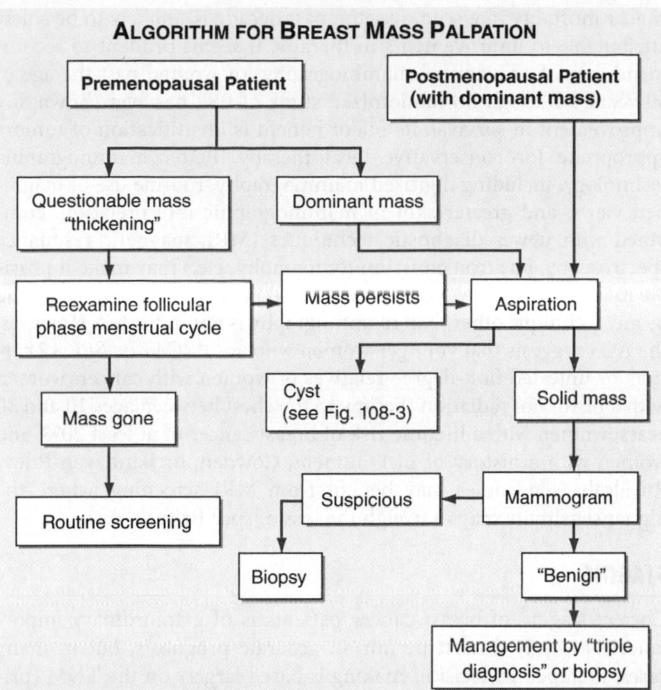

FIGURE 108-1 Approach to a palpable breast mass.

weeks, during the follicular phase of the menstrual cycle. Days 5–7 of the cycle are the best time for breast examination. A dominant mass in a postmenopausal woman or a dominant mass that persists through a menstrual cycle in a premenopausal woman should be aspirated by fine-needle biopsy or referred to a surgeon. If nonbloody fluid is aspirated, the diagnosis (cyst) and therapy have been accomplished together. Solid lesions that are persistent, recurrent, complex, or bloody cysts require mammography and biopsy, although in selected patients the so-called triple diagnostic technique (palpation, mammography, aspiration) can be used to avoid biopsy (Figs. 108-1, 108-2, and 108-3). Ultrasound can be used in place of fine-needle aspiration to distinguish cysts from solid lesions. Not all solid masses are detected by ultrasound; thus, a palpable mass that is not visualized on ultrasound must be presumed to be solid.

Several points are essential in pursuing these management decision trees. First, risk-factor analysis is not part of the decision structure. No constellation of risk factors, by their presence or absence, can be used to exclude biopsy. Second, fine-needle aspiration should be used only in centers that have proven skill in obtaining such specimens and analyzing them. The likelihood of cancer is low in the setting of a "triple negative" (benign-feeling lump, negative mammogram, and negative fine-needle aspiration), but it is not zero. The patient and physician

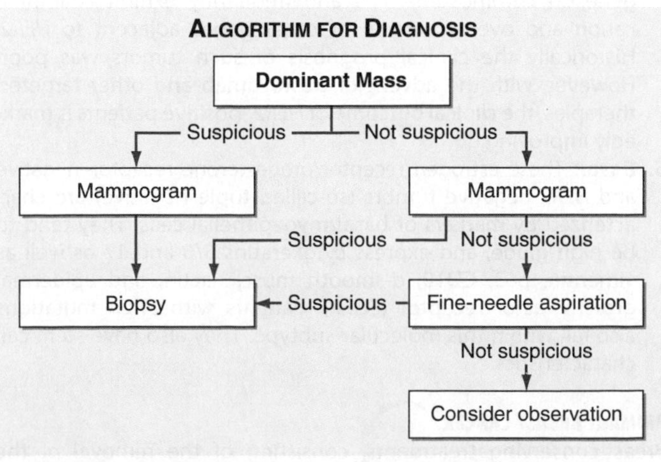

FIGURE 108-2 The "triple diagnosis" technique.

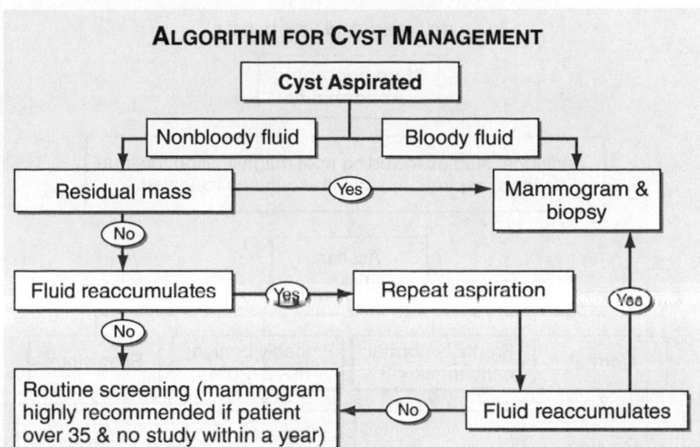

FIGURE 108-3 Management of a breast cyst.

must be aware of a 1% risk of false negatives. Third, additional technologies such as magnetic resonance imaging (MRI), ultrasound, and sestamibi imaging cannot be used to exclude the need for biopsy, although in unusual circumstances, they may provoke a biopsy.

THE ABNORMAL MAMMOGRAM

Diagnostic mammography should not be confused with *screening mammography*, which is performed after a palpable abnormality has been detected. Diagnostic mammography is aimed at evaluating the rest of the breast before biopsy is performed or occasionally is part of the triple-test strategy to exclude immediate biopsy.

Subtle abnormalities that are first detected by screening mammography should be evaluated carefully by compression or magnified views. These abnormalities include clustered microcalcifications, densities (especially if spiculated), and new or enlarging architectural distortion. For some nonpalpable lesions, ultrasound may be helpful either to identify cysts or to guide biopsy. If there is no palpable lesion and detailed mammographic studies are unequivocally benign, the patient should have routine follow-up appropriate to the patient's age. It cannot be stressed too strongly that in the presence of a breast lump a negative mammogram does not rule out cancer.

If a nonpalpable mammographic lesion has a low index of suspicion, mammographic follow-up in 3–6 months is reasonable. Workup of indeterminate and suspicious lesions has been rendered more complex by the advent of stereotactic biopsies. Morrow and colleagues have suggested that these procedures are indicated for lesions that require biopsy but are likely to be benign—that is, for cases in which the procedure probably will eliminate additional surgery. When a lesion is more probably malignant, open biopsy should be performed with a needle localization technique. Others have proposed more widespread use of stereotactic core biopsies for nonpalpable lesions on economic grounds and because diagnosis leads to earlier treatment planning. However, stereotactic diagnosis of a malignant lesion does not eliminate the need for definitive surgical procedures, particularly if breast conservation is attempted. For example, after a breast biopsy with needle localization (i.e., local excision) of a stereotactically diagnosed malignancy, reexcision may still be necessary to achieve negative margins. To some extent, these issues are decided on the basis of referral pattern and the availability of the resources for stereotactic core biopsies. A reasonable approach is shown in Fig. 108-4.

BREAST MASSES IN THE PREGNANT OR LACTATING WOMAN

During pregnancy, the breast grows under the influence of estrogen, progesterone, prolactin, and human placental lactogen. Lactation is suppressed by progesterone, which blocks the effects of prolactin. After delivery, lactation is promoted by the fall in progesterone levels, which leaves the effects of prolactin unopposed. The development of a dominant mass during pregnancy or lactation should never be attributed to hormonal changes. A dominant mass must be treated with the same concern in a pregnant woman as any other. Breast

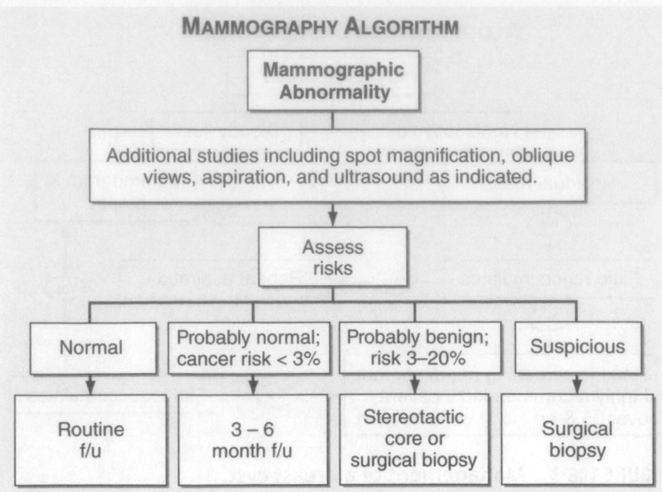

FIGURE 108-4 Approaches to abnormalities detected by mammogram.

cancer develops in 1 in every 3000–4000 pregnancies. Stage for stage, breast cancer in pregnant patients is no different from premenopausal breast cancer in nonpregnant patients. However, pregnant women often have more advanced disease because the significance of a breast mass was not fully considered and/or because of endogenous hormone stimulation. Persistent lumps in the breast of pregnant or lactating women *cannot* be attributed to benign changes based on physical findings; such patients should be promptly referred for diagnostic evaluation.

BENIGN BREAST MASSES

Only about 1 in every 5–10 breast biopsies leads to a diagnosis of cancer, although the rate of positive biopsies varies in different countries and clinical settings. (These differences may be related to interpretation, medico-legal considerations, and availability of mammograms.) The vast majority of benign breast masses are due to "fibrocystic" disease, a descriptive term for small fluid-filled cysts and modest epithelial cell and fibrous tissue hyperplasia. However, fibrocystic disease is a histologic, not a clinical, diagnosis, and women who have had a biopsy with benign findings are at greater risk of developing breast cancer than those who have not had a biopsy. The subset of women with ductal or lobular cell proliferation (about 30% of patients), particularly the small fraction (3%) with atypical hyperplasia, have a fourfold greater risk of developing breast cancer than those women who have not had a biopsy, and the increase in the risk is about ninefold for women in this category who also have an affected first-degree relative. Thus, careful follow-up of these patients is required. By contrast, patients with a benign biopsy without atypical hyperplasia are at little risk and may be followed routinely.

SCREENING

Breast cancer is virtually unique among the epithelial tumors in adults in that screening (in the form of annual mammography) improves survival. Meta-analysis examining outcomes from every randomized trial of mammography conclusively shows a 25–30% reduction in the chance of dying from breast cancer with annual screening after age 50 years; the data for women between ages 40 and 50 years are almost as positive; however, since the incidence is much lower in younger women, there are more false positives. While controversy continues to surround the assessment of screening mammography, the preponderance of data strongly supports the benefits of screening mammography. New analyses of older randomized studies have occasionally suggested that screening may not work. While the design defects in some older studies cannot be retrospectively corrected, most experts, including panels of the American Society of Clinical Oncology and the American Cancer Society (ACS), continue to believe that screening conveys substantial benefit. Furthermore, the profound drop in breast cancer mortality rate seen over the past decade is unlikely to be solely attributable to improvements in therapy. It seems prudent to recommend annual or biannual mammography for women past the age of 40 years. Although no randomized study of BSE has ever shown any improvement in survival, its major benefit is identification of tumors appropriate for conservative local therapy. Better mammographic technology, including digitized mammography, routine use of magnified views, and greater skill in mammographic interpretation, combined with newer diagnostic techniques (MRI, magnetic resonance spectroscopy, positron emission tomography, etc.) may make it possible to identify breast cancers even more reliably and earlier. Screening by any technique other than mammography is not indicated. However, the ACS suggests that younger women who are *BRCA1* or *BRCA2* carriers or untested first-degree relatives of women with cancer; women with a history of radiation therapy to the chest between ages 10 and 30 years; women with a lifetime risk of breast cancer of at least 20%; and women with a history of Li-Fraumeni, Cowden, or Bannayan-Riley-Ruvalcaba syndromes may benefit from MRI screening, where the higher sensitivity may outweigh the loss of specificity.

STAGING

Correct staging of breast cancer patients is of extraordinary importance. Not only does it permit an accurate prognosis, but in many cases, therapeutic decision-making is based largely on the TNM (primary tumor, regional nodes, metastasis) classification (Table 108-1). Comparison with historic series should be undertaken with caution, as the staging has changed several times in the past 20 years. The current staging is complex and results in significant changes in outcome by stage as compared with prior staging systems.

TREATMENT BREAST CANCER

One of the most exciting aspects of breast cancer biology has been its subdivision into at least five subtypes based on gene expression profiling.

1. **Luminal A:** The luminal tumors express cytokeratins 8 and 18, have the highest levels of estrogen receptor expression, tend to be low grade, are most likely to respond to endocrine therapy, and have a favorable prognosis. They tend to be less responsive to chemotherapy.
2. **Luminal B:** Tumor cells are also of luminal epithelial origin, but with a gene expression pattern distinct from luminal A. Prognosis is somewhat worse that luminal A.
3. **Normal breast–like:** These tumors have a gene expression profile reminiscent of nonmalignant "normal" breast epithelium. Prognosis is similar to the luminal B group. This subtype is somewhat controversial and may represent contamination of the sample by normal mammary epithelium.
4. ***HER2* amplified:** These tumors have amplification of the *HER2* gene on chromosome 17q and frequently exhibit coamplification and overexpression of other genes adjacent to *HER2*. Historically the clinical prognosis of such tumors was poor. However, with the advent of trastuzumab and other targeted therapies, the clinical outcome of *HER2* -positive patients is markedly improving.
5. **Basal:** These estrogen receptor/progesterone receptor–negative and *HER2*-negative tumors (so-called triple negative) are characterized by markers of basal/myoepithelial cells. They tend to be high grade, and express cytokeratins 5/6 and 17 as well as vimentin, p63, CD10, α-smooth muscle actin, and epidermal growth factor receptor (EGFR). Patients with *BRCA* mutations also fall within this molecular subtype. They also have stem cell characteristics.

PRIMARY BREAST CANCER

Breast-conserving treatments, consisting of the removal of the primary tumor by some form of lumpectomy with or without irra-

TABLE 108-1 STAGING OF BREAST CANCER

Primary Tumor (T)			
T0	No evidence of primary tumor		
TIS	Carcinoma in situ		
T1	Tumor ≤2 cm		
T1a	Tumor >0.1 cm but ≤0.5 cm		
T1b	Tumor >0.5 but ≤1 cm		
T1c	Tumor >1 cm but ≤2 cm		
T2	Tumor >2 cm but ≤5 cm		
T3	Tumor >5 cm		
T4	Extension to chest wall, inflammation, satellite lesions, ulcerations		
Regional Lymph Nodes (N)			
PN0(i−)	No regional lymph node metastasis histologically, negative IHC		
PN0(i+)	No regional lymph node metastasis histologically, positive IHC, no IHC cluster greater than 0.2 mm		
PN0(mol−)	No regional lymph node metastasis histologically, negative molecular findings (RT-PCR)		
PN0(mol+)	No regional lymph node metastasis histologically, positive molecular findings (RT-PCR)		
PN1	Metastasis in one to three axillary lymph nodes, or in internal mammary nodes with microscopic disease detected by sentinel lymph node dissection but not clinically apparent		
PN1mi	Micrometastasis (>0.2 mm, none >2 mm)		
PN1a	Metastasis in one to three axillary lymph nodes		
PN1b	Metastasis in internal mammary nodes with microscopic disease detected by sentinel lymph node dissection but not *clinically apparent*[a]		
PN1c	Metastasis in one to three axillary lymph nodes and in internal mammary lymph nodes with microscopic disease detected by sentinel lymph node dissection but not clinically apparent.[a] (If associated with greater than three positive axillary lymph nodes, the internal mammary nodes are classified as pN3b to reflect increased tumor burden.)		
pN2	Metastasis in four to nine axillary lymph nodes, or in clinically apparent internal mammary lymph nodes in the *absence* of axillary lymph node metastasis		
pN3	Metastasis in 10 or more axillary lymph nodes, or in infraclavicular lymph nodes, or in clinically apparent[a] ipsilateral internal mammary lymph nodes in the *presence* of 1 or more positive axillary lymph nodes; or in more than 3 axillary lymph nodes with clinically negative microscopic metastasis in internal mammary lymph nodes; or in ipsilateral subcarinal lymph nodes		
Distant Metastasis (M)			
M0	No distant metastasis		
M1	Distant metastasis (includes spread to ipsilateral supraclavicular nodes)		
Stage Grouping			
Stage 0	TIS	N0	M0
Stage I	T1	N0	M0
Stage IIA	T0	N1	M0
	T1	N1	M0
	T2	N0	M0
Stage IIB	T2	N1	M0
	T3	N0	M0
Stage IIIA	T0	N2	M0
	T1	N2	M0
	T2	N2	M0
	T3	N1, N2	M0
Stage IIIB	T4	N0, N1, N2	M0
Stage IIIC	Any T	N3	M0
Stage IV	Any T	Any N	M1

[a]Clinically apparent is defined as detected by imaging studies (excluding lymphoscintigraphy) or by clinical examination.

Abbreviations: IHC, immunohistochemistry; RT-PCR, reverse transcriptase polymerase chain reaction.

Source: Used with permission of the American Joint Committee on Cancer (AJCC), Chicago, Illinois. The original source for this material is the *AJCC Cancer Staging Manual,* 7th ed. New York, Springer, 2010; *www.springeronline.com*.

diating the breast, result in a survival that is as good as (or slightly superior to) that after extensive surgical procedures, such as mastectomy or modified radical mastectomy, with or without further irradiation. Postlumpectomy breast irradiation greatly reduces the risk of recurrence in the breast. While breast conservation is associated with a possibility of recurrence in the breast, 10-year survival is at least as good as that after more extensive surgery. Postoperative radiation to regional nodes following mastectomy is also associated with an improvement in survival. Because radiation therapy can also reduce the rate of local or regional recurrence, it should be strongly considered following mastectomy for women with high-risk primary tumors (i.e., T2 in size, positive margins, positive nodes). At present, nearly one-third of women in the United States are managed by lumpectomy. Breast-conserving surgery is not suitable for all patients: it is not generally suitable for tumors >5 cm (or for smaller tumors if the breast is small), for tumors involving the nipple-areola complex, for tumors with extensive intraductal disease involving multiple quadrants of the breast, for women with a history of collagen-vascular disease, and for women who either do not have the motivation for breast conservation or do not have convenient access to radiation therapy. However, these groups probably do not account for more than one-third of patients who are treated with mastectomy. Thus, a great many women still undergo mastectomy who could safely avoid this procedure and probably would if appropriately counseled.

Sentinel lymph node biopsy (SLNB) is generally the standard of care for women with localized breast cancer and clinically negative axilla. If SLNB is negative, more extensive axillary surgery is not required, avoiding much of the risk of lymphedema following more extensive axillary dissections. In the presence of minimal involvement of a sentinel lymph node, further axillary surgery is not required.

An extensive intraductal component is a predictor of recurrence in the breast, and so are several clinical variables. Both axillary lymph node involvement and involvement of vascular or lymphatic channels by metastatic tumor in the breast are associated with a higher risk of relapse in the breast but are not contraindications to breast-conserving treatment. When these patients are excluded, and when lumpectomy with negative tumor margins is achieved, breast conservation is associated with a recurrence rate in the breast of 5% or less. The survival of patients who have recurrence in the breast is somewhat worse than that of women who do not. Thus, recurrence in the breast is a negative prognostic variable for long-term survival. However, recurrence in the breast is not the *cause* of distant metastasis. If recurrence in the breast caused metastatic disease, then women treated with lumpectomy, who have a higher rate of recurrence in the breast, should have poorer survival than women treated with mastectomy, and they do not. Most patients should consult with a radiation oncologist before making a final decision concerning local therapy. However, a multimodality clinic in which the surgeon, radiation oncologist, medical oncologist, and other caregivers cooperate to evaluate the patient and develop a treatment plan is usually considered a major advantage by patients.

Adjuvant Therapy The use of systemic therapy after local management of breast cancer substantially improves survival. More than half of the women who would otherwise die of metastatic breast cancer remain disease-free when treated with the appropriate systemic regimen. These data have grown more and more impressive with longer follow-up and more effective regimens.

PROGNOSTIC VARIABLES The most important prognostic variables are provided by *tumor staging*. The size of the tumor and the status of the axillary lymph nodes provide reasonably accurate information on the likelihood of tumor relapse. The relation of pathologic stage to 5-year survival is shown in Table 108-2. For most women, the need for adjuvant therapy can be readily defined on this basis alone. In the absence of lymph node involvement, involvement of microvessels (either capillaries or lymphatic channels) in tumors is nearly equivalent to lymph node involvement. The greatest controversy concerns women with intermediate prognoses. *There is rarely justification for adjuvant chemotherapy in most women with tumors <1 cm in size whose axillary lymph nodes are negative. HER2-positive tumors are a potential exception.* Detection of breast cancer cells either in the circulation or bone marrow is associated with an increased relapse rate. The most exciting development in this area is the use of gene expression arrays to analyze patterns of tumor gene expression. Several groups have independently defined gene sets that reliably predict disease-free and overall survival far more accurately than any single prognostic variable including the Oncotype DX® analysis of 21 genes. Also, the use of such standardized risk assessment tools such as Adjuvant! Online (*www.adjuvantonline.com*) is very helpful. These tools are highly recommended in otherwise ambiguous circumstances.

Estrogen receptor status and progesterone receptor status are of prognostic significance. Tumors that lack either or both of these receptors are more likely to recur than tumors that have them.

Several *measures of tumor growth rate* correlate with early relapse. S-phase analysis using flow cytometry is the most accurate measure. Indirect S-phase assessments using antigens associated with the cell cycle, such as PCNA (Ki67), are also valuable. Tumors with a high proportion (more than the median) of cells in S-phase pose a greater risk of relapse; chemotherapy offers the greatest survival benefit for these tumors. Assessment of DNA content in the form of ploidy is of modest value, with nondiploid tumors having a somewhat worse prognosis.

Histologic classification of the tumor has also been used as a prognostic factor. Tumors with a poor nuclear grade have a higher risk of recurrence than tumors with a good nuclear grade. Semiquantitative measures such as the Elston score improve the reproducibility of this measurement.

Molecular changes in the tumor are also useful. Tumors that overexpress *erbB2* (HER2/neu) or have a mutated *p53* gene have a worse prognosis. Particular interest has centered on *erbB2* overexpression as measured by immunohistochemistry or fluorescence in situ hybridization. Tumors that overexpress *erbB2* are more likely to respond to doxorubicin-containing regimens; *erbB2* overexpression also predicts those tumors that will respond to HER2/neu antibodies (trastuzumab) (Herceptin) and HER2/neu kinase inhibitors.

Other variables that have also been used to evaluate prognosis include proteins associated with invasiveness, such as type IV collagenase, cathepsin D, plasminogen activator, plasminogen activator receptor, and the metastasis-suppressor gene *nm23*. None of these has been widely accepted as a prognostic variable for therapeutic decision-making. One problem in interpreting these prognostic variables is that most of them have not been examined in a study using a large cohort of patients.

ADJUVANT REGIMENS Adjuvant therapy is the use of systemic therapies in patients whose known disease has received local therapy but who are at risk of relapse. Selection of appropriate adjuvant chemotherapy or hormone therapy is highly controversial in some situations. Meta-analyses have helped to define broad limits for therapy but do not help in choosing optimal regimens or in choosing a regimen for certain subgroups of patients. A summary of recommendations is shown in Table 108-3. In general, premenopausal women for whom any form of adjuvant systemic therapy is indicated should receive multidrug chemotherapy. Antihormone therapy improves survival in premenopausal patients who are estrogen receptor positive and should be added following completion of chemotherapy. Prophylactic surgical or medically induced castration may also be associated with a substantial survival benefit (primarily in estrogen receptor–positive patients) but is not widely used in this country.

Data on postmenopausal women are also controversial. The impact of adjuvant chemotherapy is quantitatively less clear-cut than in premenopausal patients, particularly in estrogen receptor–positive cases, although survival advantages have been shown. The first decision is whether chemotherapy or endocrine therapy should be used. While adjuvant endocrine therapy (aromatase inhibitors and tamoxifen) improves survival regardless of axillary lymph node status, the improvement in survival is modest for patients in whom multiple lymph nodes are involved. For this reason, it has been usual to give chemotherapy to postmenopausal patients who have no medical contraindications and who have more than one positive lymph node; hormone therapy is commonly given subsequently. For postmenopausal women for whom systemic therapy is warranted but who have a more favorable prognosis (based more commonly on analysis such as the Oncotype DX methodology), hormone therapy may be used alone. Large clinical trials have

TABLE 108-2 5-YEAR SURVIVAL RATE FOR BREAST CANCER BY STAGE

Stage	5-Year Survival, %
0	99
I	92
IIA	82
IIB	65
IIIA	47
IIIB	44
IV	14

Source: Modified from data of the National Cancer Institute: Surveillance, Epidemiology, and End Results (SEER).

TABLE 108-3 SUGGESTED APPROACHES TO ADJUVANT THERAPY

Age Group	Lymph Node Status[a]	Estrogen Receptor (ER) Status	Tumor	Recommendation
Premenopausal	Positive	Any	Any	Multidrug chemotherapy + tamoxifen if ER-positive + trastuzumab in HER2/neu-positive tumors
Premenopausal	Negative	Any	>2 cm, or 1–2 cm with other poor prognostic variables	Multidrug chemotherapy + tamoxifen if ER-positive + trastuzumab in HER2/neu-positive tumors. Consider Oncotype or similar testing.
Postmenopausal	Positive	Negative	Any	Multidrug chemotherapy + trastuzumab in HER2/neu-positive tumors
Postmenopausal	Positive	Positive	Any	Aromatase inhibitors and tamoxifen with or without chemotherapy + trastuzumab in HER2/neu-positive tumors
Postmenopausal	Negative	Positive	>2 cm, or 1–2 cm with other poor prognostic variables	Aromatase inhibitors and tamoxifen + trastuzumab in HER2/neu-positive tumors
Postmenopausal	Negative	Negative	>2 cm, or 1–2 cm with other poor prognostic variables	Consider multidrug chemotherapy + trastuzumab in HER2/neu-positive tumors

[a]As determined by pathologic examination.

shown superiority for aromatase inhibitors over tamoxifen alone in the adjuvant setting, although tamoxifen appears essentially equivalent in women who are obese and therefore presumably have higher endogenous concentrations of estrogen. Unfortunately the optimal plan is unclear. Tamoxifen for 5 years followed by an aromatase inhibitor, the reverse strategy, or even switching to an aromatase inhibitor after 2–3 years of tamoxifen has been shown to be better than tamoxifen alone. Continuation of tamoxifen for 10 years yields further benefit and is a reasonable decision for women with less favorable prognoses. Unfortunately, multiple studies have revealed very suboptimal adherence to long-term adjuvant endocrine regimens, and every effort should be made to encourage their continuous use. No valid information currently permits selection among the three clinically approved aromatase inhibitors. Concomitant use of bisphosphonates is almost always warranted; however, it is not finally settled as to whether their prophylactic use increases survival in addition to just decreasing recurrences in bone.

Most comparisons of adjuvant chemotherapy regimens show little difference among them, although small advantages for doxorubicin-containing regimens and "dose-dense" regimens are usually seen.

One approach—so-called neoadjuvant chemotherapy—involves the administration of adjuvant therapy before definitive surgery and radiation therapy. Because the objective response rates of patients with breast cancer to systemic therapy in this setting exceed 75%, many patients will be "downstaged" and may become candidates for breast-conserving therapy. However, overall survival has not been improved using this approach as compared with the same drugs given postoperatively. Patients who achieve a pathologic complete remission after neoadjuvant chemotherapy not unexpectedly have a substantially improved survival. The neoadjuvant setting also provides a wonderful opportunity for the evaluation of new agents. For example, a second HER2 targeting antibody, pertuzumab, has been shown to provide additional benefit when combined with trastuzumab in the neoadjuvant setting.

Other adjuvant treatments under investigation include the use of taxanes, such as paclitaxel and docetaxel, and therapy based on alternative kinetic and biologic models. In such approaches, high doses of single agents are used separately in relatively dose-intensive cycling regimens. Node-positive patients treated with doxorubicin-cyclophosphamide for four cycles followed by four cycles of a taxane have a substantial improvement in survival compared with women receiving doxorubicin-cyclophosphamide alone, particularly in women with estrogen receptor–negative tumors. In addition, administration of the same drug combinations at the same dose but at more frequent intervals (every 2 weeks with cytokine support as compared with the standard every 3 weeks) is even more effective. Among the 25% of women whose tumors overexpress HER2/neu, addition of trastuzumab given concurrently with a taxane and then for a year after chemotherapy produces significant improvement in survival. Although longer follow-up will be important, this is now the standard care for most women with HER2/neu-positive breast cancers. Cardiotoxicity, immediate and long-term, remains a concern, and further efforts to exploit non-anthracycline-containing regimens are being pursued. Very-high-dose therapy with stem cell transplantation in the adjuvant setting has not proved superior to standard-dose therapy and should not be routinely used.

A variety of exciting approaches are close to adoption, and the literature needs to be followed attentively. Tyrosine kinase inhibitors such as lapatinib and additional HER2 targeting antibodies such as pertuzumab are very promising. Finally, as described in the next section, a novel class of agents targeting DNA repair—the so-called poly-ADP ribose polymerase (PARP) inhibitors—is likely to have a major effect on breast cancers either caused by *BRCA1* or *BRCA2* mutations or sharing similar defects in DNA repair in their etiology.

SYSTEMIC THERAPY OF METASTATIC DISEASE

About one-third of patients treated for apparently localized breast cancer develop metastatic disease. Although a small number of these patients enjoy long remissions when treated with combinations of systemic and local therapy, most eventually succumb to metastatic disease. The median survival for all patients diagnosed with metastatic breast cancer is less than 3 years. Soft tissue, bony, and visceral (lung and liver) metastases each account for approximately one-third of sites of initial relapses. However, by the time of death, most patients will have bony involvement. Recurrences can appear at any time after primary therapy. A very cruel fact about breast cancer recurrences is that at least half of all breast cancer recurrences occur >5 years after initial therapy. It is now clear that a variety of host factors can influence recurrence rates, including depression and central obesity, and these diseases should be managed as aggressively as possible.

Because the diagnosis of metastatic disease alters the outlook for the patient so drastically, it should rarely be made without a confirmatory biopsy. Every oncologist has seen patients with tuberculosis, gallstones, sarcoidosis, or other nonmalignant diseases misdiagnosed and treated as though they had metastatic breast cancer or even second malignancies such as multiple myeloma thought to be recurrent breast cancer. This is a catastrophic mistake and justifies biopsy for virtually every patient at the time of initial suspicion of metastatic disease. Furthermore, there are well-documented changes in hormone receptor status that can occur and substantially alter treatment decisions.

The choice of therapy requires consideration of local therapy needs, the overall medical condition of the patient, and the hormone receptor status of the tumor, as well as clinical judgment. Because therapy of systemic disease is palliative, the potential toxicities of therapies should be balanced against the response rates. Several variables influence the response to systemic therapy. For example, the presence of estrogen and progesterone receptors is a strong indication for endocrine therapy. On the other hand, patients with short disease-free intervals, rapidly progressive visceral disease, lymphangitic pulmonary disease, or intracranial disease are unlikely to respond to endocrine therapy.

In many cases, systemic therapy can be withheld while the patient is managed with appropriate local therapy. Radiation therapy and occasionally surgery are effective at relieving the symptoms of metastatic disease, particularly when bony sites are involved. Many patients with bone-only or bone-dominant disease have a relatively indolent course. Under such circumstances, systemic chemotherapy has a modest effect, whereas radiation therapy may be effective for long periods. Other systemic treatments, such as strontium-89 and/or bisphosphonates, may provide a palliative benefit without inducing objective responses. Most patients with metastatic disease, and certainly all who have bone involvement, should receive concurrent bisphosphonates. Because the goal of therapy is to maintain well-being for as long as possible, emphasis should be placed on avoiding the most hazardous complications of metastatic disease, including pathologic fracture of the axial skeleton and spinal cord compression. New back pain in patients with cancer should be explored aggressively on an emergent basis; to wait for neurologic symptoms is a potentially catastrophic error. Metastatic involvement of endocrine organs can cause profound dysfunction, including adrenal insufficiency and hypopituitarism. Similarly, obstruction of the biliary tree or other impaired organ function may be better managed with a local therapy than with a systemic approach.

Many patients are inappropriately treated with toxic regimens into their last days of life. Often oncologists are unwilling to have the difficult conversations that are required with patients nearing the end of life, and not uncommonly, patients and families can pressure physicians into treatments with very little survival value. Palliative care consultation and realistic assessment of treatment expectations need to be reviewed with patients and families. We urge consideration of palliative care consultations for patients who have received at least two lines of therapy for metastatic disease.

Endocrine Therapy Normal breast tissue is estrogen dependent. Both primary and metastatic breast cancer may retain this phenotype. The best means of ascertaining whether a breast cancer is hormone dependent is through analysis of estrogen and progesterone receptor levels on the tumor. Tumors that are positive for the estrogen receptor and negative for the progesterone receptor have a response rate of ~30%. Tumors that are positive for both receptors have a response rate approaching 70%. If neither receptor is present, the objective response rates are <5%. Receptor analyses provide information as to the correct ordering of endocrine therapies as opposed to chemotherapy. Because of their lack of toxicity and because some patients whose receptor analyses are reported as negative respond to endocrine therapy, an endocrine treatment should be attempted in virtually every patient with metastatic breast cancer. Potential endocrine therapies are summarized in Table 108-4. The choice of endocrine therapy is usually determined by toxicity profile and availability. In most postmenopausal patients, the initial endocrine therapy should be an aromatase inhibitor rather than tamoxifen. For the subset of postmenopausal women who are estrogen receptor–positive but also HER2/neu-positive, response rates to aromatase inhibitors are substantially higher than to tamoxifen. Aromatase inhibitors are not used in premenopausal women because their hypothalamus can respond to estrogen deprivation by producing gonadotropins that promote estrogen synthesis. Newer "pure" antiestrogens that are free of agonistic effects are also effective. Cases in which tumors shrink in response to tamoxifen withdrawal (as well as withdrawal of pharmacologic doses of estrogens) have been reported. A series of studies with aromatase inhibitors, tamoxifen, and fulvestrant have all shown that the addition of everolimus to the hormonal treatment can lead to significant benefit after progression on the endocrine agent alone. Everolimus (an mTOR inhibitor) in coordination with endocrine agents is now being explored as front-line therapy and in the adjuvant setting. Endogenous estrogen formation may be blocked by analogues of

TABLE 108-4 ENDOCRINE THERAPIES FOR BREAST CANCER

Therapy	Comments
Castration	For premenopausal women
Surgical	
LHRH agonists	
Antiestrogens	
Tamoxifen	Useful in pre- and postmenopausal women[a]
"Pure" antiestrogens	Responses in tamoxifen-resistant and aromatase inhibitor–resistant patients[a]
Surgical adrenalectomy	Rarely used second-line choice
Aromatase inhibitors	Low toxicity; now first choice for metastatic disease[a]
High-dose progestogens	Common fourth-line choice after aromatase inhibitors, tamoxifen, and fulvestrant
Hypophysectomy	Rarely used
Additive androgens or estrogens	Plausible fourth-line therapies; potentially toxic

[a]Consider retreatment with Everolimus in combination for disease progression

Abbreviation: LHRH, luteinizing hormone–releasing hormone.

luteinizing hormone–releasing hormone in premenopausal women. Additive endocrine therapies, including treatment with progestogens, estrogens, and androgens, may also be tried in patients who respond to initial endocrine therapy; the mechanism of action of these latter therapies is unknown. Patients who respond to one endocrine therapy have at least a 50% chance of responding to a second endocrine therapy. It is not uncommon for patients to respond to two or three sequential endocrine therapies; however, combination endocrine therapies do not appear to be superior to individual agents, and combinations of chemotherapy with endocrine therapy are not useful. The median survival of patients with metastatic disease is approximately 2 years, although many patients, particularly older persons and those with hormone-dependent disease, may respond to endocrine therapy for 3–5 years or longer.

Chemotherapy Unlike many other epithelial malignancies, breast cancer responds to multiple chemotherapeutic agents, including anthracyclines, alkylating agents, taxanes, and antimetabolites. Multiple combinations of these agents have been found to improve response rates somewhat, but they have had little effect on duration of response or survival. The choice among multidrug combinations frequently depends on whether adjuvant chemotherapy was administered and, if so, what type. Although patients treated with adjuvant regimens such as cyclophosphamide, methotrexate, and fluorouracil (CMF regimens) may subsequently respond to the same combination in the metastatic disease setting, most oncologists use drugs to which the patients have not been previously exposed. Once patients have progressed after combination drug therapy, it is most common to treat them with single agents. Given the significant toxicity of most drugs, the use of a single effective agent will minimize toxicity by sparing the patient exposure to drugs that would be of little value. No method to select the drugs most efficacious for a given patient has been demonstrated to be useful.

Most oncologists use either an anthracycline or paclitaxel following failure with the initial regimen. However, the choice has to be balanced with individual needs. One randomized study has suggested that docetaxel may be superior to paclitaxel. A nanoparticle formulation of paclitaxel (Abraxane) is also effective.

The use of a humanized antibody to *erbB2* (trastuzumab [Herceptin]) combined with paclitaxel can improve response rate and survival for women whose metastatic tumors overexpress *erbB2*. A novel antibody conjugate (ADC) that links trastuzumab to a cytotoxic agent has been approved for management of HER2-positive breast cancer. The magnitude of the survival extension is modest in patients with metastatic disease. Similarly, the use of bevacizumab

(Avastin) has improved the response rate and response duration to paclitaxel. Objective responses in previously treated patients may also be seen with gemcitabine, vinca alkaloids, capecitabine, vinorelbine, and oral etoposide, as well as a new class of agents, epothilones. There are few comparative trials of one agent versus another in metastatic disease. It is a sad fact that choices are often influenced by aggressive marketing of new very expensive agents that have not been shown to be superior to other generic agents. Platinum-based agents have become far more widely used in both the adjuvant and advanced disease settings for some breast cancers, particularly those of the "triple-negative" subtype.

HIGH DOSE CHEMOTHERAPY INCLUDING AUTOLOGOUS BONE MARROW TRANSPLANTATION Autologous bone marrow transplantation combined with high doses of single agents can produce objective responses even in heavily pretreated patients. However, such responses are rarely durable and do not alter the clinical course for most patients with advanced metastatic disease.

STAGE III BREAST CANCER

Between 10 and 25% of patients present with so-called locally advanced, or stage III, breast cancer at diagnosis. Many of these cancers are technically operable, whereas others, particularly cancers with chest wall involvement, inflammatory breast cancers, or cancers with large matted axillary lymph nodes, cannot be managed with surgery initially. Although no randomized trials have shown any survival benefit for neoadjuvant regimens as compared to adjuvant therapy, this approach has gained widespread use. More than 90% of patients with locally advanced breast cancer show a partial or better response to multidrug chemotherapy regimens that include an anthracycline. Early administration of this treatment reduces the bulk of the disease and frequently makes the patient a suitable candidate for salvage surgery and/or radiation therapy. These patients should be managed in multimodality clinics to coordinate surgery, radiation therapy, and systemic chemotherapy. Such approaches produce long-term disease-free survival in about 30–50% of patients. The neoadjuvant setting is also an ideal time to evaluate the efficacy of novel treatments because the effect on the tumor can be directly assessed.

BREAST CANCER PREVENTION

Women who have one breast cancer are at risk of developing a contralateral breast cancer at a rate of approximately 0.5% per year. When adjuvant tamoxifen or an aromatase inhibitor is administered to these patients, the rate of development of contralateral breast cancers is reduced. In other tissues of the body, tamoxifen has estrogen-like effects that are beneficial, including preservation of bone mineral density and long-term lowering of cholesterol. However, tamoxifen has estrogen-like effects on the uterus, leading to an increased risk of uterine cancer (0.75% incidence after 5 years on tamoxifen). Tamoxifen also increases the risk of cataract formation. The Breast Cancer Prevention Trial (BCPT) revealed a >49% reduction in breast cancer among women with a risk of at least 1.66% taking the drug for 5 years. Raloxifene has shown similar breast cancer prevention potency but may have different effects on bone and heart. The two agents have been compared in a prospective randomized prevention trial (the Study of Tamoxifen and Raloxifene [STAR] trial). The agents are approximately equivalent in preventing breast cancer with fewer thromboembolic events and endometrial cancers with raloxifene; however, raloxifene did not reduce noninvasive cancers as effectively as tamoxifen, so no clear winner has emerged. A newer selective estrogen receptor modulator (SERM), lasofoxifene, has been shown to reduce cardiovascular events in addition to breast cancer and fractures, and further studies of this agent should be watched with interest. It should be recalled that prevention of contralateral breast cancers in women diagnosed with *one* cancer is a reasonable surrogate for breast cancer prevention because these are second primaries not recurrences. In this regard, the aromatase inhibitors are all considerably more effective than tamoxifen; however, they are not approved for primary breast cancer prevention. It remains puzzling that agents with the safety profile of raloxifene, which can reduce breast cancer risk by 50% with additional benefits in preventing osteoporotic fracture, are still so infrequently prescribed. They should be far more commonly offered to women than they are.

NONINVASIVE BREAST CANCER

Breast cancer develops as a series of molecular changes in the epithelial cells that lead to ever more malignant behavior. Increased use of mammography has led to more frequent diagnoses of noninvasive breast cancer. These lesions fall into two groups: ductal carcinoma in situ (DCIS) and lobular carcinoma in situ (lobular neoplasia). The management of both entities is controversial.

Ductal Carcinoma In Situ Proliferation of cytologically malignant breast epithelial cells within the ducts is termed *DCIS*. Atypical hyperplasia may be difficult to differentiate from DCIS. At least one-third of patients with untreated DCIS develop invasive breast cancer within 5 years. However, many low-grade DCIS lesions do not appear to progress over many years; therefore, many patients are overtreated. Unfortunately there is no reliable means of distinguishing patients who require treatment from those who may be safely observed. For many years, the standard treatment for this disease was mastectomy. However, treatment of this condition by lumpectomy and radiation therapy gives survival that is as good as the survival for invasive breast cancer treated by mastectomy. In one randomized trial, the combination of wide excision plus irradiation for DCIS caused a substantial reduction in the local recurrence rate as compared with wide excision alone with negative margins, although survival was identical in the two arms. No studies have compared either of these regimens to mastectomy. Addition of tamoxifen to any DCIS surgical/radiation therapy regimen further improves local control. Data for aromatase inhibitors in this setting are not available.

Several prognostic features may help to identify patients at high risk for local recurrence after either lumpectomy alone or lumpectomy with radiation therapy. These include extensive disease; age <40; and cytologic features such as necrosis, poor nuclear grade, and comedo subtype with overexpression of *erbB2*. Some data suggest that adequate excision with careful determination of pathologically clear margins is associated with a low recurrence rate. When surgery is combined with radiation therapy, recurrence (which is usually in the same quadrant) occurs with a frequency of ≤10%. Given the fact that half of these recurrences will be invasive, about 5% of the initial cohort will eventually develop invasive breast cancer. A reasonable expectation of mortality for these patients is about 1%, a figure that approximates the mortality rate for DCIS managed by mastectomy. Although this train of reasoning has not formally been proved valid, it is reasonable to recommend that patients who desire breast preservation, and in whom DCIS appears to be reasonably localized, be managed by adequate surgery with meticulous pathologic evaluation, followed by breast irradiation and tamoxifen. For patients with localized DCIS, axillary lymph node dissection is unnecessary. More controversial is the question of what management is optimal when there is any degree of invasion. Because of a significant likelihood (10–15%) of axillary lymph node involvement even when the primary lesion shows only microscopic invasion, it is prudent to do at least a sentinel lymph node sampling for all patients with any degree of invasion. Further management is dictated by the presence of nodal spread.

Lobular Neoplasia Proliferation of cytologically malignant cells within the lobules is termed *lobular neoplasia*. Nearly 30% of patients who have had adequate local excision of the lesion develop breast cancer (usually infiltrating ductal carcinoma) over the next 15–20 years. Ipsilateral and contralateral cancers are equally common. Therefore, lobular neoplasia may be a premalignant lesion that suggests an elevated risk of subsequent breast cancer, rather than a form of malignancy itself, and aggressive local management seems unreasonable. Most patients should be treated with an SERM or an aromatase inhibitor (for postmenopausal women) for 5 years and followed with careful annual mammography and semiannual physical examinations. Additional molecular analysis of these lesions may make it possible to discriminate between patients who are at risk of further progression and require additional therapy and those in whom simple follow-up is adequate.

MALE BREAST CANCER

Breast cancer is about 1/150th as frequent in men as in women; 1720 men developed breast cancer in 2006. It usually presents as a unilateral lump in the breast and is frequently not diagnosed promptly. Given the small amount of soft tissue and the unexpected nature of the problem, locally advanced presentations are somewhat more common. When male breast cancer is matched to female breast cancer by age and stage, its overall prognosis is identical. Although gynecomastia may initially be unilateral or asymmetric, any unilateral mass in a man older than age 40 years should receive a careful workup including biopsy. On the other hand, bilateral symmetric breast development rarely represents breast cancer and is almost invariably due to endocrine disease or a drug effect. It should be kept in mind, nevertheless, that the risk of cancer is much greater in men with gynecomastia; in such men, gross asymmetry of the breasts should arouse suspicion of cancer. Male breast cancer is best managed by mastectomy and axillary lymph node dissection or SLNB. Patients with locally advanced disease or positive nodes should also be treated with irradiation. Approximately 90% of male breast cancers contain estrogen receptors, and approximately 60% of cases with metastatic disease respond to endocrine therapy. No randomized studies have evaluated adjuvant therapy for male breast cancer. Two historic experiences suggest that the disease responds well to adjuvant systemic therapy, and, if not medically contraindicated, the same criteria for the use of adjuvant therapy in women should be applied to men.

The sites of relapse and spectrum of response to chemotherapeutic drugs are virtually identical for breast cancers in either sex.

FOLLOW-UP OF BREAST CANCER PATIENTS

Despite the availability of sophisticated and expensive imaging techniques and a wide range of serum tumor marker tests, survival is not influenced by early diagnosis of relapse. Surveillance guidelines are given in Table 108-5. Despite pressure from patients and their families, routine computed tomography scans (or other imaging) are not recommended.

TABLE 108-5 BREAST CANCER SURVEILLANCE GUIDELINES

Test	Frequency
Recommended	
History; eliciting symptoms; physical examination	q3–6 months × 3 years; q6–12 months × 2 years; then annually
Breast self-examination	Monthly
Mammography	Annually
Pelvic examination	Annually (particularly for patients on SERMs)
Patient education about symptoms of recurrence	Ongoing
Coordination of care	Ongoing
Not Recommended	
Complete blood count	
Serum chemistry studies	
Chest radiographs	
Bone scans	
Ultrasound examination of the liver	
Computed tomography of chest, abdomen, or pelvis	
Tumor markers CA 15-3, CA 27-29, CEA	

Abbreviations: CEA, carcinoembryonic antigen; SERM, selective estrogen receptor modulator.

Source: Recommended Breast Cancer Surveillance Guidelines, ASCO Education Book, Fall, 1997.

109 Upper Gastrointestinal Tract Cancers

Robert J. Mayer

Upper gastrointestinal cancers include malignancies arising in the esophagus, stomach, and small intestine.

ESOPHAGEAL CANCER

INCIDENCE AND ETIOLOGY

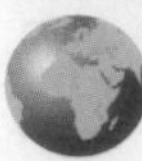

Cancer of the esophagus is an increasingly common and extremely lethal malignancy. The diagnosis was made in 18,170 Americans in 2014 and led to 15,450 deaths. Almost all esophageal cancers are either squamous cell carcinomas or adenocarcinomas; the two histologic subtypes have a similar clinical presentation but different causative factors.

Worldwide, squamous cell carcinoma is the more common cell type, having an incidence that rises strikingly in association with geographic location. It occurs frequently within a region extending from the southern shore of the Caspian Sea on the west to northern China on the east, encompassing parts of Iran, central Asia, Afghanistan, Siberia, and Mongolia. Familial increased risk has been observed in regions with high incidence, although gene associations are not yet defined. High-incidence "pockets" of the disease are also present in such disparate locations as Finland, Iceland, Curaçao, southeastern Africa, and northwestern France. In North America and western Europe, the disease is more common in blacks than whites and in males than females; it appears most often after age 50 and seems to be associated with a lower socioeconomic status. Such cancers generally arise in the cervical and thoracic portions of the esophagus.

A variety of causative factors have been implicated in the development of squamous cell cancers of the esophagus (Table 109-1). In the United States, the etiology of such cancers is primarily related to excess alcohol consumption and/or cigarette smoking. The relative risk increases with the amount of tobacco smoked or alcohol consumed, with these factors acting synergistically. The consumption of whiskey is linked to a higher incidence than the consumption of wine or beer. Squamous cell esophageal carcinoma has also been associated with the ingestion of nitrates, smoked opiates, and fungal toxins in pickled vegetables, as well as mucosal damage caused by such physical insults as long-term exposure to extremely hot tea, the ingestion of lye, radiation-induced strictures, and chronic achalasia. The presence of an esophageal web in association with glossitis and iron deficiency (i.e., Plummer-Vinson or Paterson-Kelly syndrome) and congenital

TABLE 109-1 SOME ETIOLOGIC FACTORS ASSOCIATED WITH SQUAMOUS CELL CANCER OF THE ESOPHAGUS

- Excess alcohol consumption
- Cigarette smoking
- Other ingested carcinogens
  - Nitrates (converted to nitrites)
  - Smoked opiates
  - Fungal toxins in pickled vegetables
- Mucosal damage from physical agents
  - Hot tea
  - Lye ingestion
  - Radiation-induced strictures
  - Chronic achalasia
- Host susceptibility
- Esophageal web with glossitis and iron deficiency (i.e., Plummer-Vinson or Paterson-Kelly syndrome)
- Congenital hyperkeratosis and pitting of the palms and soles (i.e., tylosis palmaris et plantaris)
- ? Dietary deficiencies of selenium, molybdenum, zinc, and vitamin A

TABLE 109-2 SOME ETIOLOGIC FACTORS ASSOCIATED WITH ADENOCARCINOMA OF THE ESOPHAGUS

Chronic gastroesophageal reflux
Obesity
Barrett's esophagus
Male sex
Cigarette smoking

hyperkeratosis and pitting of the palms and soles (i.e., tylosis palmaris et plantaris) have each been linked with squamous cell esophageal cancer, as have dietary deficiencies of molybdenum, zinc, selenium, and vitamin A. Patients with head and neck cancer are at increased risk of squamous cell cancer of the esophagus.

For unclear reasons, the incidence of squamous cell esophageal cancer has decreased somewhat in both the black and white populations in the United States over the past 40 years, whereas the rate of adenocarcinoma has risen sevenfold, particularly in white males (male-to-female ratio of 6:1). Whereas squamous cell cancers comprised the vast majority of esophageal cancers in the United States as recently as 40–50 years ago, more than 75% of esophageal tumors are now adenocarcinomas, with the incidence of this histologic subtype continuing to increase rapidly. Understanding the cause for this increase is the focus of current investigation.

Several strong etiologic associations have been observed to account for the development of adenocarcinoma of the esophagus (Table 109-2). Such tumors arise in the distal esophagus in association with chronic gastric reflux, often in the presence of Barrett's esophagus (replacement of the normal squamous epithelium of the distal esophagus by columnar mucosa), which occurs more commonly in obese individuals. Adenocarcinomas arise within dysplastic columnar epithelium in the distal esophagus. Even before frank neoplasia is detectable, aneuploidy and *p53* mutations are found in the dysplastic epithelium. These adenocarcinomas behave clinically like gastric adenocarcinomas, although they are not associated with *Helicobacter pylori* infections. Approximately 15% of esophageal adenocarcinomas overexpress the *HER2/neu* gene.

CLINICAL FEATURES

About 5% of esophageal cancers occur in the upper third of the esophagus (cervical esophagus), 20% in the middle third, and 75% in the lower third. Squamous cell carcinomas and adenocarcinomas cannot be distinguished radiographically or endoscopically.

Progressive dysphagia and weight loss of short duration are the initial symptoms in the vast majority of patients. Dysphagia initially occurs with solid foods and gradually progresses to include semisolids and liquids. By the time these symptoms develop, the disease is already very advanced, because difficulty in swallowing does not occur until >60% of the esophageal circumference is infiltrated with cancer. Dysphagia may be associated with pain on swallowing (odynophagia), pain radiating to the chest and/or back, regurgitation or vomiting, and aspiration pneumonia. The disease most commonly spreads to adjacent and supraclavicular lymph nodes, liver, lungs, pleura, and bone. Tracheoesophageal fistulas may develop, primarily in patients with upper and mid-esophageal tumors. As with other squamous cell carcinomas, hypercalcemia may occur in the absence of osseous metastases, probably from parathormone-related peptide secreted by tumor cells (Chap. 121).

DIAGNOSIS

Attempts at endoscopic and cytologic screening for carcinoma in patients with Barrett's esophagus, while effective as a means of detecting high-grade dysplasia, have not yet been shown to reduce the likelihood of death from esophageal adenocarcinoma. Esophagoscopy should be performed in all patients suspected of having an esophageal abnormality, to both visualize and identify a tumor and also to obtain histopathologic confirmation of the diagnosis. Because the population of persons at risk for squamous cell carcinoma of the esophagus (i.e., smokers and drinkers) also has a high rate of cancers of the lung and the head and neck region, endoscopic inspection of the larynx, trachea, and bronchi should also be carried out. A thorough examination of the fundus of the stomach (by retroflexing the endoscope) is imperative as well. The extent of tumor spread to the mediastinum and para-aortic lymph nodes should be assessed by computed tomography (CT) scans of the chest and abdomen and by endoscopic ultrasound. Positron emission tomography scanning provides a useful assessment of the presence of distant metastatic disease, offering accurate information regarding spread to mediastinal lymph nodes, which can be helpful in defining radiation therapy fields. Such scans, when performed sequentially, appear to provide a means of making an early assessment of responsiveness to preoperative chemotherapy.

TREATMENT ESOPHAGEAL CANCER

The prognosis for patients with esophageal carcinoma is poor. Approximately 10% of patients survive 5 years after the diagnosis; thus, management focuses on symptom control. Surgical resection of all gross tumor (i.e., total resection) is feasible in only 45% of cases, with residual tumor cells frequently present at the resection margins. Such esophagectomies have been associated with a postoperative mortality rate of approximately 5% due to anastomotic fistulas, subphrenic abscesses, and cardiopulmonary complications. Although debate regarding the comparative benefits of transthoracic versus transhiatal resections has continued, experienced thoracic surgeons are now favoring minimally invasive transthoracic esophagectomies. Endoscopic resections of superficial squamous cell cancers or adenocarcinomas are being examined but have not yet been shown to result in a similar likelihood of survival as observed with conventional surgical procedures. Similarly, the value of endoscopic ablation of dysplastic lesions in an area of Barrett's esophagus on reducing subsequent mortality from esophageal carcinoma is uncertain. Some experts have advocated fundoplication surgery (i.e., the removal of the gastroesophageal junction) as a means of cancer prevention in patients with Barrett's esophagus; again, objective data are not yet available to fully assess the risks versus benefits of this invasive procedure. About 20% of patients who survive a total surgical resection live for 5 years. The evaluation of chemotherapeutic agents in patients with esophageal carcinoma has been hampered by ambiguity in the definition of "response" and the debilitated physical condition of many treated individuals, particularly those with squamous cell cancers. Nonetheless, significant reductions in the size of measurable tumor masses have been reported in 15–25% of patients given single-agent treatment and in 30–60% of patients treated with drug combinations that include cisplatin. In the small subset of patients whose tumors overexpress the *HER2/neu* gene, the addition of the monoclonal antibody trastuzumab (Herceptin) appears to further enhance the likelihood of benefit, particularly in patients with gastroesophageal lesions. The use of the antiangiogenic agent bevacizumab (Avastin) seems to be of limited value in the setting of esophageal cancer. Combination chemotherapy and radiation therapy as the initial therapeutic approach, either alone or followed by an attempt at operative resection, seems to be beneficial. When administered along with radiation therapy, chemotherapy produces a better survival outcome than radiation therapy alone. The use of preoperative chemotherapy and radiation therapy followed by esophageal resection appears to prolong survival compared with surgery alone according to several randomized trials and a meta-analysis; some reports suggest that no additional benefit accrues when surgery is added if significant shrinkage of tumor has been achieved by the chemoradiation combination.

For the incurable, surgically unresectable patient with esophageal cancer, dysphagia, malnutrition, and the management of tracheoesophageal fistulas are major issues. Approaches to palliation include repeated endoscopic dilatation, the surgical placement of a gastrostomy or jejunostomy for hydration and feeding, endoscopic placement of an expansive metal stent to bypass the tumor, and radiation therapy.

GASTRIC ADENOCARCINOMA

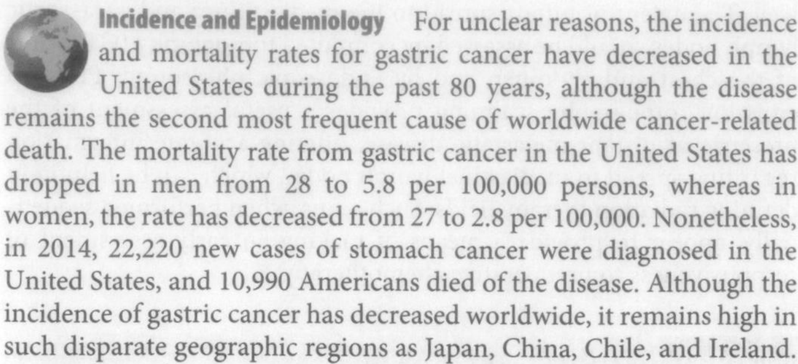

Incidence and Epidemiology For unclear reasons, the incidence and mortality rates for gastric cancer have decreased in the United States during the past 80 years, although the disease remains the second most frequent cause of worldwide cancer-related death. The mortality rate from gastric cancer in the United States has dropped in men from 28 to 5.8 per 100,000 persons, whereas in women, the rate has decreased from 27 to 2.8 per 100,000. Nonetheless, in 2014, 22,220 new cases of stomach cancer were diagnosed in the United States, and 10,990 Americans died of the disease. Although the incidence of gastric cancer has decreased worldwide, it remains high in such disparate geographic regions as Japan, China, Chile, and Ireland.

The risk of gastric cancer is greater among lower socioeconomic classes. Migrants from high- to low-incidence nations maintain their susceptibility to gastric cancer, whereas the risk for their offspring approximates that of the new homeland. These findings suggest that an environmental exposure, probably beginning early in life, is related to the development of gastric cancer, with dietary carcinogens considered the most likely factor(s).

Pathology About 85% of stomach cancers are adenocarcinomas, with 15% due to lymphomas, gastrointestinal stromal tumors (GISTs), and leiomyosarcomas. Gastric adenocarcinomas may be subdivided into two categories: a *diffuse type*, in which cell cohesion is absent, so that individual cells infiltrate and thicken the stomach wall without forming a discrete mass; and an *intestinal type*, characterized by cohesive neoplastic cells that form glandlike tubular structures. The diffuse carcinomas occur more often in younger patients, develop throughout the stomach (including the cardia), result in a loss of distensibility of the gastric wall (so-called *linitis plastica*, or "leather bottle" appearance), and carry a poorer prognosis. Diffuse cancers have defective intercellular adhesion, mainly as a consequence of loss of expression of E-cadherin. Intestinal-type lesions are frequently ulcerative, more commonly appear in the antrum and lesser curvature of the stomach, and are often preceded by a prolonged precancerous process, often initiated by *H. pylori* infection. Although the incidence of diffuse carcinomas is similar in most populations, the intestinal type tends to predominate in the high-risk geographic regions and is less likely to be found in areas where the frequency of gastric cancer is declining. Thus, different etiologic factor(s) are likely involved in these two subtypes. In the United States, ~30% of gastric cancers originate in the distal stomach, ~20% arise in the midportion of the stomach, and ~40% originate in the proximal third of the stomach. The remaining 10% involve the entire stomach.

Etiology The long-term ingestion of high concentrations of nitrates found in dried, smoked, and salted foods appears to be associated with a higher risk. The nitrates are thought to be converted to carcinogenic nitrites by bacteria (Table 109-3). Such bacteria may be introduced exogenously through the ingestion of partially decayed foods, which are consumed in abundance worldwide by the lower socioeconomic classes. Bacteria such as *H. pylori* may also contribute to this effect by causing chronic inflammatory atrophic gastritis, loss of gastric acidity, and bacterial growth in the stomach. Although the risk for developing gastric cancer is thought to be sixfold higher in people infected with *H. pylori*, it remains uncertain whether eradicating the bacteria after infection has already occurred actually reduces this risk. Loss of acidity may occur when acid-producing cells of the gastric antrum have been removed surgically to control benign peptic ulcer disease or when achlorhydria, atrophic gastritis, and even pernicious anemia develop in the elderly. Serial endoscopic examinations of the stomach in patients with atrophic gastritis have documented replacement of the usual gastric mucosa by intestinal-type cells. This process of intestinal metaplasia may lead to cellular atypia and eventual neoplasia. Because the declining incidence of gastric cancer in the United States primarily reflects a decline in distal, ulcerating, intestinal-type lesions, it is conceivable that better food preservation and the availability of refrigeration for all socioeconomic classes have decreased the dietary ingestion of exogenous bacteria. *H. pylori* has not been associated with the diffuse, more proximal form of gastric carcinoma or with cancers arising at the gastroesophageal junction or in the distal esophagus. Approximately 10–15% of adenocarcinomas appearing in the proximal stomach, the gastroesophageal junction, and the distal esophagus overexpress the *HER2/neu* gene; individuals whose tumors demonstrate this overexpression benefit from treatment directed against this target (i.e., trastuzumab [Herceptin]).

TABLE 109-3 NITRATE-CONVERTING BACTERIA AS A FACTOR IN THE CAUSATION OF GASTRIC CARCINOMA[a]

Exogenous sources of nitrate-converting bacteria:
Bacterially contaminated food (common in lower socioeconomic classes, who have a higher incidence of the disease; diminished by improved food preservation and refrigeration)
Helicobacter pylori infection
Endogenous factors favoring growth of nitrate-converting bacteria in the stomach:
Decreased gastric acidity
Prior gastric surgery (antrectomy) (15- to 20-year latency period)
Atrophic gastritis and/or pernicious anemia
? Prolonged exposure to histamine H_2-receptor antagonists

[a]Hypothesis: Dietary nitrates are converted to carcinogenic nitrites by bacteria.

Several additional etiologic factors have been associated with gastric carcinoma. Gastric ulcers and adenomatous polyps have occasionally been linked, but data on a cause-and-effect relationship are unconvincing. The inadequate clinical distinction between benign gastric ulcers and small ulcerating carcinomas may, in part, account for this presumed association. The presence of extreme hypertrophy of gastric rugal folds (i.e., Ménétrier's disease), giving the impression of polypoid lesions, has been associated with a striking frequency of malignant transformation; such hypertrophy, however, does not represent the presence of true adenomatous polyps. Individuals with blood group A have a higher incidence of gastric cancer than persons with blood group O; this observation may be related to differences in the mucous secretion, leading to altered mucosal protection from carcinogens. A germline mutation in the E-cadherin gene (*CDH1*), inherited in an autosomal dominant pattern and coding for a cell adhesion protein, has been linked to a high incidence of occult diffuse-type gastric cancers in young asymptomatic carriers. Duodenal ulcers are not associated with gastric cancer.

Clinical Features Gastric cancers, when superficial and surgically curable, usually produce no symptoms. As the tumor becomes more extensive, patients may complain of an insidious upper abdominal discomfort varying in intensity from a vague, postprandial fullness to a severe, steady pain. Anorexia, often with slight nausea, is very common but is not the usual presenting complaint. Weight loss may eventually be observed, and nausea and vomiting are particularly prominent in patients whose tumors involve the pylorus; dysphagia and early satiety may be the major symptoms caused by diffuse lesions originating in the cardia. There may be no early physical signs. A palpable abdominal mass indicates long-standing growth and predicts regional extension.

Gastric carcinomas spread by direct extension through the gastric wall to the perigastric tissues, occasionally adhering to adjacent organs such as the pancreas, colon, or liver. The disease also spreads via lymphatics or by seeding of peritoneal surfaces. Metastases to intraabdominal and supraclavicular lymph nodes occur frequently, as do metastatic nodules to the ovary (Krukenberg's tumor), periumbilical region ("Sister Mary Joseph node"), or peritoneal cul-de-sac (Blumer's shelf palpable on rectal or vaginal examination); malignant ascites may also develop. The liver is the most common site for hematogenous spread of tumor.

The presence of iron-deficiency anemia in men and of occult blood in the stool in both sexes mandates a search for an occult gastrointestinal tract lesion. A careful assessment is of particular importance in patients with atrophic gastritis or pernicious anemia. Unusual clinical features associated with gastric adenocarcinomas include migratory thrombophlebitis, microangiopathic hemolytic anemia, diffuse seborrheic keratoses (so-called Leser-Trélat sign), and acanthosis nigricans.

Diagnosis The use of double-contrast radiographic examinations has been supplanted by esophagogastroscopy and CT scanning for the evaluation of patients with epigastric complaints.

Gastric ulcers identified at the time of such endoscopic procedure may appear benign but merit biopsy in order to exclude a malignancy. Malignant gastric ulcers must be recognized before they penetrate into surrounding tissues, because the rate of cure of early lesions limited to the mucosa or submucosa is >80%. Because gastric carcinomas are difficult to distinguish clinically or endoscopically from gastric lymphomas, endoscopic biopsies should be made as deeply as possible, due to the submucosal location of lymphoid tumors.

The staging system for gastric carcinoma is shown in Table 109-4.

TABLE 109-4 STAGING SYSTEM FOR GASTRIC CARCINOMA

			Data from ACS in the United States	
Stage	**TNM**	**Features**	**No. of Cases, %**	**5-Year Survival, %**
0	T_{is}N0M0	Node negative; limited to mucosa	1	90
IA	T1N0M0	Node negative; invasion of lamina propria or submucosa	7	59
IB	T2N0M0 T1N1M0	Node negative; invasion of muscularis propria	10	44
II	T1N2M0 T2N1M0	Node positive; invasion beyond mucosa but within wall	17	29
		or		
	T3N0M0	Node negative; extension through wall		
IIIA	T2N2M0 T3N1-2M0	Node positive; invasion of muscularis propria or through wall	21	15
IIIB	T4N0-1M0	Node negative; adherence to surrounding tissue	14	9
IIIC	T4N2-3M0	>3 nodes positive; invasion of serosa or adjacent structures		
	T3N3M0	7 or more positive nodes; penetrates wall without invading serosa or adjacent structures		
IV	T4N2M0	Node positive; adherence to surrounding tissue	30	3
		or		
	T1-4N0-2-M1	Distant metastases		

Abbreviations: ACS, American Cancer Society; TNM, tumor, node, metastasis.

TREATMENT GASTRIC ADENOCARCINOMA

Complete surgical removal of the tumor with resection of adjacent lymph nodes offers the only chance for cure. However, this is possible in less than a third of patients. A subtotal gastrectomy is the treatment of choice for patients with distal carcinomas, whereas total or near-total gastrectomies are required for more proximal tumors. The inclusion of extended lymph node dissection in these procedures appears to confer an added risk for complications without providing a meaningful enhancement in survival. The prognosis following complete surgical resection depends on the degree of tumor penetration into the stomach wall and is adversely influenced by regional lymph node involvement and vascular invasion, characteristics found in the vast majority of American patients. As a result, the probability of survival after 5 years for the 25–30% of patients able to undergo complete resection is ~20% for distal tumors and <10% for proximal tumors, with recurrences continuing for at least 8 years after surgery. In the absence of ascites or extensive hepatic or peritoneal metastases, even patients whose disease is believed to be incurable by surgery should be offered resection of the primary lesion. Reduction of tumor bulk is the best form of palliation and may enhance the probability of benefit from subsequent therapy. In high-incidence regions such as Japan and Korea, where the use of endoscopic screening programs has identified patients with superficial tumors, the use of laparoscopic gastrectomy has gained popularity. In the United States and western Europe, the use of this less invasive surgical approach remains investigational.

Gastric adenocarcinoma is a relatively radioresistant tumor, and the adequate control of the primary tumor requires doses of external-beam irradiation that exceed the tolerance of surrounding structures, such as bowel mucosa and spinal cord. As a result, the major role of radiation therapy in patients has been palliation of pain. Radiation therapy alone after a complete resection does not prolong survival. In the setting of surgically unresectable disease limited to the epigastrium, patients treated with 3500–4000 cGy did not live longer than similar patients not receiving radiotherapy; however, survival was prolonged slightly when 5-fluorouracil (5-FU) plus leucovorin was given in combination with radiation therapy (3-year survival 50% vs 41% for radiation therapy alone). In this clinical setting, the 5-FU likely functions as a radiosensitizer.

The administration of combinations of cytotoxic drugs to patients with advanced gastric carcinoma has been associated with partial responses in 30–50% of cases; responders appear to benefit from treatment. Such drug combinations have generally included cisplatin combined with epirubicin or docetaxel and infusional 5-FU or capecitabine, or with irinotecan. Despite the encouraging response rates, complete remissions are uncommon, the partial responses are transient, and the overall impact of multidrug therapy on survival has been limited; the median survival time for patients treated in this manner remains less than 12 months. As with adenocarcinomas arising in the esophagus, the addition of bevacizumab (Avastin) to chemotherapy regimens in treating gastric cancer appears to provide limited benefit. However, preliminary results utilizing another antiangiogenic compound—ramucirumab (Cyranza)—in the treatment of gastric cancer are encouraging. The use of adjuvant chemotherapy alone following the complete resection of a gastric cancer has only minimally improved survival. However, combination chemotherapy administered before and after surgery (*perioperative treatment*) as well as postoperative chemotherapy combined with radiation therapy reduces the recurrence rate and prolongs survival.

PRIMARY GASTRIC LYMPHOMA

Primary lymphoma of the stomach is relatively uncommon, accounting for <15% of gastric malignancies and ~2% of all lymphomas. The stomach is, however, the most frequent extranodal site for lymphoma, and gastric lymphoma has increased in frequency during the past

35 years. The disease is difficult to distinguish clinically from gastric adenocarcinoma; both tumors are most often detected during the sixth decade of life; present with epigastric pain, early satiety, and generalized fatigue; and are usually characterized by ulcerations with a ragged, thickened mucosal pattern demonstrated by contrast radiographs or endoscopic appearance. The diagnosis of lymphoma of the stomach may occasionally be made through cytologic brushings of the gastric mucosa but usually requires a biopsy at gastroscopy or laparotomy. Failure of gastroscopic biopsies to detect lymphoma in a given case should not be interpreted as being conclusive, because superficial biopsies may miss the deeper lymphoid infiltrate. The macroscopic pathology of gastric lymphoma may also mimic adenocarcinoma, consisting of either a bulky ulcerated lesion localized in the corpus or antrum or a diffuse process spreading throughout the entire gastric submucosa and even extending into the duodenum. Microscopically, the vast majority of gastric lymphoid tumors are lymphomas of B-cell origin. Histologically, these tumors may range from well-differentiated, superficial processes (mucosa-associated lymphoid tissue [MALT]) to high-grade, large-cell lymphomas. Like gastric adenocarcinoma, infection with *H. pylori* increases the risk for gastric lymphoma in general and MALT lymphomas in particular. Large-cell lymphomas of the stomach spread initially to regional lymph nodes (often to Waldeyer's ring) and may then disseminate.

TREATMENT PRIMARY GASTRIC LYMPHOMA

Primary gastric lymphoma is a far more treatable disease than adenocarcinoma of the stomach, a fact that underscores the need for making the correct diagnosis. Antibiotic treatment to eradicate *H. pylori* infection has led to regression of about 75% of gastric MALT lymphomas and should be considered before surgery, radiation therapy, or chemotherapy is undertaken in patients having such tumors. A lack of response to such antimicrobial treatment has been linked to a specific chromosomal abnormality, i.e., t(11;18). Responding patients should undergo periodic endoscopic surveillance because it remains unclear whether the neoplastic clone is eliminated or merely suppressed, although the response to antimicrobial treatment is quite durable. Subtotal gastrectomy, usually followed by combination chemotherapy, has led to 5-year survival rates of 40–60% in patients with localized high-grade lymphomas. The need for a major surgical procedure has been questioned, particularly in patients with preoperative radiographic evidence of nodal involvement, for whom chemotherapy (CHOP [cyclophosphamide, doxorubicin, vincristine, and prednisone]) plus rituximab is highly effective therapy. A role for radiation therapy is not defined because most recurrences develop at distant sites.

GASTRIC (NONLYMPHOID) SARCOMA

Leiomyosarcomas and GISTs make up 1–3% of gastric neoplasms. They most frequently involve the anterior and posterior walls of the gastric fundus and often ulcerate and bleed. Even those lesions that appear benign on histologic examination may behave in a malignant fashion. These tumors rarely invade adjacent viscera and characteristically do not metastasize to lymph nodes, but they may spread to the liver and lungs. The treatment of choice is surgical resection. Combination chemotherapy should be reserved for patients with metastatic disease. All such tumors should be analyzed for a mutation in the c-*kit* receptor. GISTs are unresponsive to conventional chemotherapy; yet ~50% of patients experience objective response and prolonged survival when treated with imatinib mesylate (Gleevec) (400–800 mg PO daily), a selective inhibitor of the c-*kit* tyrosine kinase. Many patients with GIST whose tumors have become refractory to imatinib subsequently benefit from sunitinib (Sutent) or regorafenib (Stivarga), other inhibitors of the c-*kit* tyrosine kinase.

TUMORS OF THE SMALL INTESTINE

Small-bowel tumors comprise <3% of gastrointestinal neoplasms. Because of their rarity and inaccessibility, a correct diagnosis is often delayed. Abdominal symptoms are usually vague and poorly defined, and conventional radiographic studies of the upper and lower intestinal tract often appear normal. Small-bowel tumors should be considered in the differential diagnosis in the following situations: (1) recurrent, unexplained episodes of crampy abdominal pain; (2) intermittent bouts of intestinal obstruction, especially in the absence of inflammatory bowel disease (IBD) or prior abdominal surgery; (3) intussusception in the adult; and (4) evidence of chronic intestinal bleeding in the presence of negative conventional and endoscopic examination. A careful small-bowel barium study should be considered in such a circumstance; the diagnostic accuracy may be improved by infusing barium through a nasogastric tube placed into the duodenum (enteroclysis). Alternatively, capsule endoscopic procedures have been used.

BENIGN TUMORS

The histology of benign small-bowel tumors is difficult to predict on clinical and radiologic grounds alone. The symptomatology of benign tumors is not distinctive, with pain, obstruction, and hemorrhage being the most frequent symptoms. These tumors are usually discovered during the fifth and sixth decades of life, more often in the distal rather than the proximal small intestine. The most common benign tumors are adenomas, leiomyomas, lipomas, and angiomas.

Adenomas These tumors include those of the islet cells and Brunner's glands as well as polypoid adenomas. *Islet cell adenomas* are occasionally located outside the pancreas; the associated syndromes are discussed in Chap. 113. *Brunner's gland adenomas* are not truly neoplastic but represent a hypertrophy or hyperplasia of submucosal duodenal glands. These appear as small nodules in the duodenal mucosa that secrete a highly viscous alkaline mucus. Most often, this is an incidental radiographic finding not associated with any specific clinical disorder.

Polypoid Adenomas About 25% of benign small-bowel tumors are polypoid adenomas (see Table 110-2). They may present as single polypoid lesions or, less commonly, as papillary villous adenomas. As in the colon, the sessile or papillary form of the tumor is sometimes associated with a coexisting carcinoma. Occasionally, patients with Gardner's syndrome develop premalignant adenomas in the small bowel; such lesions are generally in the duodenum. Multiple polypoid tumors may occur throughout the small bowel (and occasionally the stomach and colorectum) in the Peutz-Jeghers syndrome. The polyps are usually hamartomas (juvenile polyps) having a low potential for malignant degeneration. Mucocutaneous melanin deposits as well as tumors of the ovary, breast, pancreas, and endometrium are also associated with this autosomal dominant condition.

Leiomyomas These neoplasms arise from smooth-muscle components of the intestine and are usually intramural, affecting the overlying mucosa. Ulceration of the mucosa may cause gastrointestinal hemorrhage of varying severity. Cramping or intermittent abdominal pain is frequently encountered.

Lipomas These tumors occur with greatest frequency in the distal ileum and at the ileocecal valve. They have a characteristic radiolucent appearance and are usually intramural and asymptomatic, but on occasion cause bleeding.

Angiomas While not true neoplasms, these lesions are important because they frequently cause intestinal bleeding. They may take the form of telangiectasia or hemangiomas. Multiple intestinal telangiectasias occur in a nonhereditary form confined to the gastrointestinal tract or as part of the hereditary Osler-Rendu-Weber syndrome. Vascular tumors may also take the form of isolated hemangiomas, most commonly in the jejunum. Angiography, especially during bleeding, is the best procedure for evaluating these lesions.

MALIGNANT TUMORS

While rare, small-bowel malignancies occur in patients with long-standing regional enteritis and celiac sprue as well as in individuals with AIDS. Malignant tumors of the small bowel are frequently associated with fever, weight loss, anorexia, bleeding, and a palpable abdominal mass. After ampullary carcinomas (many of which arise from biliary or pancreatic ducts), the most frequently occurring small-bowel malignancies are adenocarcinomas, lymphomas, carcinoid tumors, and leiomyosarcomas.

ADENOCARCINOMAS

The most common primary cancers of the small bowel are adenocarcinomas, accounting for ~50% of malignant tumors. These cancers occur most often in the distal duodenum and proximal jejunum, where they tend to ulcerate and cause hemorrhage or obstruction. Radiologically, they may be confused with chronic duodenal ulcer disease or with Crohn's disease if the patient has long-standing regional enteritis. The diagnosis is best made by endoscopy and biopsy under direct vision. Surgical resection is the treatment of choice with suggested postoperative adjuvant chemotherapy options generally following treatment patterns used in the management of colon cancer.

LYMPHOMAS

Lymphoma in the small bowel may be primary or secondary. A diagnosis of a primary intestinal lymphoma requires histologic confirmation in a clinical setting in which palpable adenopathy and hepatosplenomegaly are absent and no evidence of lymphoma is seen on chest radiograph, CT scan, or peripheral blood smear or on bone marrow aspiration and biopsy. Symptoms referable to the small bowel are present, usually accompanied by an anatomically discernible lesion. Secondary lymphoma of the small bowel consists of involvement of the intestine by a lymphoid malignancy extending from involved retroperitoneal or mesenteric lymph nodes (Chap. 134).

Primary intestinal lymphoma accounts for ~20% of malignancies of the small bowel. These neoplasms are non-Hodgkin's lymphomas; they usually have a diffuse, large-cell histology and are of T cell origin. Intestinal lymphoma involves the ileum, jejunum, and duodenum, in decreasing frequency—a pattern that mirrors the relative amount of normal lymphoid cells in these anatomic areas. The risk of small-bowel lymphoma is increased in patients with a prior history of malabsorptive conditions (e.g., celiac sprue), regional enteritis, and depressed immune function due to congenital immunodeficiency syndromes, prior organ transplantation, autoimmune disorders, or AIDS.

The development of localized or nodular masses that narrow the lumen results in periumbilical pain (made worse by eating) as well as weight loss, vomiting, and occasional intestinal obstruction. The diagnosis of small-bowel lymphoma may be suspected from the appearance on contrast radiographs of patterns such as infiltration and thickening of mucosal folds, mucosal nodules, areas of irregular ulceration, or stasis of contrast material. The diagnosis can be confirmed by surgical exploration and resection of involved segments. Intestinal lymphoma can occasionally be diagnosed by peroral intestinal mucosal biopsy, but because the disease mainly involves the lamina propria, full-thickness surgical biopsies are usually required.

Resection of the tumor constitutes the initial treatment modality. While postoperative radiation therapy has been given to some patients following a total resection, most authorities favor short-term (three cycles) systemic treatment with combination chemotherapy. The frequent presence of widespread intraabdominal disease at the time of diagnosis and the occasional multicentricity of the tumor often make a total resection impossible. The probability of sustained remission or cure is ~75% in patients with localized disease but is ~25% in individuals with unresectable lymphoma. In patients whose tumors are not resected, chemotherapy may lead to bowel perforation.

A unique form of small-bowel lymphoma, diffusely involving the entire intestine, was first described in oriental Jews and Arabs and is referred to as *immunoproliferative small intestinal disease* (IPSID), *Mediterranean lymphoma*, or *α heavy chain disease*. This is a B cell tumor. The typical presentation includes chronic diarrhea and steatorrhea associated with vomiting and abdominal cramps; clubbing of the digits may be observed. A curious feature in many patients with IPSID is the presence in the blood and intestinal secretions of an abnormal IgA that contains a shortened α heavy chain and is devoid of light chains. It is suspected that the abnormal α chains are produced by plasma cells infiltrating the small bowel. The clinical course of patients with IPSID is generally one of exacerbations and remissions, with death frequently resulting from either progressive malnutrition and wasting or the development of an aggressive lymphoma. The use of oral antibiotics such as tetracycline appears to be beneficial in the early phases of the disorder, suggesting a possible infectious etiology. Combination chemotherapy has been administered during later stages of the disease, with variable results. Results are better when antibiotics and chemotherapy are combined.

CARCINOID TUMORS

Carcinoid tumors arise from argentaffin cells of the crypts of Lieberkühn and are found from the distal duodenum to the ascending colon, areas embryologically derived from the midgut. More than 50% of intestinal carcinoids are found in the distal ileum, with most congregating close to the ileocecal valve. Most intestinal carcinoids are asymptomatic and of low malignant potential, but invasion and metastases may occur, leading to the carcinoid syndrome (Chap. 113).

LEIOMYOSARCOMAS

Leiomyosarcomas often are >5 cm in diameter and may be palpable on abdominal examination. Bleeding, obstruction, and perforation are common. Such tumors should be analyzed for the expression of mutant c *kit* receptor (defining GIST), and in the presence of metastatic disease, justifying treatment with imatinib mesylate (Gleevec) or, in imatinib-refractory patients, sunitinib (Sutent) or regorafenib (Stivarga).

110 Lower Gastrointestinal Cancers

Robert J. Mayer

Lower gastrointestinal cancers include malignant tumors of the colon, rectum, and anus.

COLORECTAL CANCER

INCIDENCE

Cancer of the large bowel is second only to lung cancer as a cause of cancer death in the United States: 136,830 new cases occurred in 2014, and 50,310 deaths were due to colorectal cancer. The incidence rate has decreased significantly during the past 25 years, likely due to enhanced and more compliantly followed screening practices. Similarly, mortality rates in the United States have decreased by approximately 25%, resulting largely from earlier detection and improved treatment.

POLYPS AND MOLECULAR PATHOGENESIS

Most colorectal cancers, regardless of etiology, arise from adenomatous polyps. A polyp is a grossly visible protrusion from the mucosal surface and may be classified pathologically as a nonneoplastic hamartoma (e.g., *juvenile polyp*), a hyperplastic mucosal proliferation (*hyperplastic polyp*), or an adenomatous polyp. Only adenomas are clearly premalignant, and only a minority of adenomatous polyps evolve into cancer. Adenomatous polyps may be found in the colons of ~30% of middle-aged and ~50% of elderly people; however, <1% of polyps ever become malignant. Most polyps produce no symptoms and remain clinically undetected. Occult blood in the stool is found in <5% of patients with polyps.

A number of molecular changes are noted in adenomatous polyps and colorectal cancers that are thought to reflect a multistep process in the evolution of normal colonic mucosa to life-threatening invasive carcinoma. These developmental steps toward carcinogenesis include, but are not restricted to, point mutations in the K-*ras* protooncogene; hypomethylation of DNA, leading to gene activation; loss of DNA (*allelic loss*) at the site of a tumor-suppressor gene (the adenomatous polyposis coli [*APC*] gene) on the long arm of chromosome 5 (5q21); allelic loss at the site of a tumor-suppressor gene located on chromosome 18q (the deleted in colorectal cancer [*DCC*] gene); and allelic loss at chromosome 17p, associated with mutations in the *p53* tumor-suppressor gene (see Fig. 101e-2). Thus, the altered proliferative pattern of the colonic mucosa, which results in progression to a polyp and then to carcinoma, may involve the mutational activation of an oncogene followed by and coupled with the loss of genes that normally suppress tumorigenesis. It remains uncertain whether the genetic aberrations always occur in a defined order. Based on this model, however, cancer is believed to develop only in those polyps in which most (if not all) of these mutational events take place.

Clinically, the probability of an adenomatous polyp becoming a cancer depends on the gross appearance of the lesion, its histologic features, and its size. Adenomatous polyps may be pedunculated (stalked) or sessile (flat-based). Invasive cancers develop more frequently in sessile polyps. Histologically, adenomatous polyps may be tubular, villous (i.e., papillary), or tubulovillous. Villous adenomas, most of which are sessile, become malignant more than three times as often as tubular adenomas. The likelihood that any polypoid lesion in the large bowel contains invasive cancer is related to the size of the polyp, being negligible (<2%) in lesions <1.5 cm, intermediate (2–10%) in lesions 1.5–2.5 cm, and substantial (10%) in lesions >2.5 cm in size.

Following the detection of an adenomatous polyp, the entire large bowel should be visualized endoscopically because synchronous lesions are noted in about one-third of cases. Colonoscopy should then be repeated periodically, even in the absence of a previously documented malignancy, because such patients have a 30–50% probability of developing another adenoma and are at a higher-than-average risk for developing a colorectal carcinoma. Adenomatous polyps are thought to require >5 years of growth before becoming clinically significant; colonoscopy need not be carried out more frequently than every 3 years for the vast majority of patients.

ETIOLOGY AND RISK FACTORS

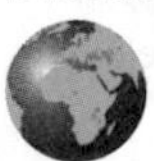

Risk factors for the development of colorectal cancer are listed in Table 110-1.

Diet The etiology for most cases of large-bowel cancer appears to be related to environmental factors. The disease occurs more often in upper socioeconomic populations who live in urban areas. Mortality from colorectal cancer is directly correlated with per capita consumption of calories, meat protein, and dietary fat and oil as well as elevations in the serum cholesterol concentration and mortality from coronary artery disease. Geographic variations in incidence largely are unrelated to genetic differences, since migrant groups tend to assume the large-bowel cancer incidence rates of their adopted countries. Furthermore, population groups such as Mormons and Seventh Day Adventists, whose lifestyle and dietary habits differ somewhat from those of their neighbors, have significantly lower-than-expected incidence and mortality rates for colorectal cancer. The incidence of colorectal cancer has increased in Japan since that nation has adopted a more "Western" diet. At least three hypotheses have been proposed to explain the relationship to diet, none of which is fully satisfactory.

TABLE 110-1 RISK FACTORS FOR THE DEVELOPMENT OF COLORECTAL CANCER

Diet: Animal fat
Hereditary syndromes
- Polyposis coli
- MYH-associated polyposis
- Nonpolyposis syndrome (Lynch's syndrome)

Inflammatory bowel disease
Streptococcus bovis bacteremia
? Tobacco use

ANIMAL FATS One hypothesis is that the ingestion of animal fats found in red meats and processed meat leads to an increased proportion of anaerobes in the gut microflora, resulting in the conversion of normal bile acids into carcinogens. This provocative hypothesis is supported by several reports of increased amounts of fecal anaerobes in the stools of patients with colorectal cancer. Diets high in animal (but not vegetable) fats are also associated with high serum cholesterol, which is also associated with enhanced risk for the development of colorectal adenomas and carcinomas.

INSULIN RESISTANCE The large number of calories in Western diets coupled with physical inactivity has been associated with a higher prevalence of obesity. Obese persons develop insulin resistance with increased circulating levels of insulin, leading to higher circulating concentrations of insulin-like growth factor type I (IGF-I). This growth factor appears to stimulate proliferation of the intestinal mucosa.

FIBER Contrary to prior beliefs, the results of randomized trials and case-controlled studies have *failed* to show any value for dietary fiber or diets high in fruits and vegetables in preventing the recurrence of colorectal adenomas or the development of colorectal cancer.

The weight of epidemiologic evidence, however, implicates diet as being the major etiologic factor for colorectal cancer, particularly diets high in animal fat and in calories.

HEREDITARY FACTORS AND SYNDROMES

Up to 25% of patients with colorectal cancer have a family history of the disease, suggesting a hereditary predisposition. Inherited large-bowel cancers can be divided into two main groups: the well-studied but uncommon polyposis syndromes and the more common nonpolyposis syndromes (Table 110-2).

Polyposis Coli Polyposis coli (familial polyposis of the colon) is a rare condition characterized by the appearance of thousands of adenomatous polyps throughout the large bowel. It is transmitted as an autosomal

TABLE 110-2 HEREDITABLE (AUTOSOMAL DOMINANT) GASTROINTESTINAL POLYPOSIS SYNDROMES

Syndrome	Distribution of Polyps	Histologic Type	Malignant Potential	Associated Lesions
Familial adenomatous polyposis	Large intestine	Adenoma	Common	None
Gardner's syndrome	Large and small intestines	Adenoma	Common	Osteomas, fibromas, lipomas, epidermoid cysts, ampullary cancers, congenital hypertrophy of retinal pigment epithelium
Turcot's syndrome	Large intestine	Adenoma	Common	Brain tumors
MYH-associated polyposis	Large intestine	Adenoma	Common	None
Nonpolyposis syndrome (Lynch's syndrome)	Large intestine (often proximal)	Adenoma	Common	Endometrial and ovarian tumors (most frequently) gastric, genitourinary, pancreatic, biliary cancers (less frequently)
Peutz-Jeghers syndrome	Small and large intestines, stomach	Hamartoma	Rare	Mucocutaneous pigmentation; tumors of the ovary, breast, pancreas, endometrium
Juvenile polyposis	Large and small intestines, stomach	Hamartoma, rarely progressing to adenoma	Rare	Various congenital abnormalities

dominant trait; the occasional patient with no family history probably developed the condition due to a spontaneous mutation. Polyposis coli is associated with a deletion in the long arm of chromosome 5 (including the *APC* gene) in both neoplastic (somatic mutation) and normal (germline mutation) cells. The loss of this genetic material (i.e., allelic loss) results in the absence of tumor-suppressor genes whose protein products would normally inhibit neoplastic growth. The presence of soft tissue and bony tumors, congenital hypertrophy of the retinal pigment epithelium, mesenteric desmoid tumors, and ampullary cancers in addition to the colonic polyps characterizes a subset of polyposis coli known as *Gardner's syndrome*. The appearance of malignant tumors of the central nervous system accompanying polyposis coli defines *Turcot's syndrome*. The colonic polyps in all these conditions are rarely present before puberty but are generally evident in affected individuals by age 25. If the polyposis is not treated surgically, colorectal cancer will develop in almost all patients before age 40. Polyposis coli results from a defect in the colonic mucosa, leading to an abnormal proliferative pattern and impaired DNA repair mechanisms. Once the multiple polyps are detected, patients should undergo a total colectomy. Medical therapy with nonsteroidal anti-inflammatory drugs (NSAIDs) such as sulindac and selective cyclooxygenase-2 inhibitors such as celecoxib can decrease the number and size of polyps in patients with polyposis coli; however, this effect on polyps is only temporary, and the use of NSAIDs has not been shown to reduce the risk of cancer. Colectomy remains the primary therapy/prevention. The offspring of patients with polyposis coli, who often are prepubertal when the diagnosis is made in the parent, have a 50% risk for developing this premalignant disorder and should be carefully screened by annual flexible sigmoidoscopy until age 35. Proctosigmoidoscopy is a sufficient screening procedure because polyps tend to be evenly distributed from cecum to anus, making more invasive and expensive techniques such as colonoscopy or barium enema unnecessary. Testing for occult blood in the stool is an inadequate screening maneuver. If a causative germline *AP C* mutation has been identified in an affected family member, an alternative method for identifying carriers is testing DNA from peripheral blood mononuclear cells for the presence of the specific *APC* mutation. The detection of such a germline mutation can lead to a definitive diagnosis before the development of polyps.

MYH-Associated Polyposis MYH-associated polyposis (MAP) is a rare autosomal recessive syndrome caused by a biallelic mutation in the *MUT4H* gene. This hereditary condition may have a variable clinical presentation, resembling polyposis coli or colorectal cancer occurring in younger individuals without polyposis. Screening and colectomy guidelines for this syndrome are less clear than for polyposis coli, but annual to biennial colonoscopic surveillance is generally recommended starting at age 25–30.

Hereditary Nonpolyposis Colon Cancer Hereditary nonpolyposis colon cancer (HNPCC), also known as *Lynch's syndrome*, is another autosomal dominant trait. It is characterized by the presence of three or more relatives with histologically documented colorectal cancer, one of whom is a first-degree relative of the other two; one or more cases of colorectal cancer diagnosed before age 50 in the family; and colorectal cancer involving at least two generations. In contrast to polyposis coli, HNPCC is associated with an unusually high frequency of cancer arising in the proximal large bowel. The median age for the appearance of an adenocarcinoma is <50 years, 10–15 years younger than the median age for the general population. Despite having a poorly differentiated, mucinous histologic appearance, the proximal colon tumors that characterize HNPCC have a better prognosis than sporadic tumors from patients of similar age. Families with HNPCC often include individuals with multiple primary cancers; the association of colorectal cancer with either ovarian or endometrial carcinomas is especially strong in women, and an increased appearance of gastric, small-bowel, genitourinary, pancreaticobiliary, and sebaceous skin tumors has been reported as well. It has been recommended that members of such families undergo annual or biennial colonoscopy beginning at age 25 years, with intermittent pelvic ultrasonography and endometrial biopsy for afflicted women; such a screening strategy has not yet been validated. HNPCC is associated with germline mutations of several genes, particularly *hMSH2* on chromosome 2 and *hMLH1* on chromosome 3. These mutations lead to errors in DNA replication and are thought to result in DNA instability because of defective repair of DNA mismatches resulting in abnormal cell growth and tumor development. Testing tumor cells through molecular analysis of DNA or immunohistochemical staining of paraffin-fixed tissue for "microsatellite instability" (sequence changes reflecting defective mismatch repair) in patients with colorectal cancer and a positive family history for colorectal or endometrial cancer may identify probands with HNPCC.

INFLAMMATORY BOWEL DISEASE

(Chap. 351) Large-bowel cancer is increased in incidence in patients with long-standing inflammatory bowel disease (IBD). Cancers develop more commonly in patients with ulcerative colitis than in those with granulomatous (i.e., Crohn's) colitis, but this impression may result in part from the occasional difficulty of differentiating these two conditions. The risk of colorectal cancer in a patient with IBD is relatively small during the initial 10 years of the disease, but then appears to increase at a rate of ~0.5–1% per year. Cancer may develop in 8–30% of patients after 25 years. The risk is higher in younger patients with pancolitis.

Cancer surveillance strategies in patients with IBD are unsatisfactory. Symptoms such as bloody diarrhea, abdominal cramping, and obstruction, which may signal the appearance of a tumor, are similar to the complaints caused by a flare-up of the underlying disease. In patients with a history of IBD lasting ≥15 years who continue to experience exacerbations, the surgical removal of the colon can significantly reduce the risk for cancer and also eliminate the target organ for the underlying chronic gastrointestinal disorder. The value of such surveillance techniques as colonoscopy with mucosal biopsies and brushings for less symptomatic individuals with chronic IBD is uncertain. The lack of uniformity regarding the pathologic criteria that characterize dysplasia and the absence of data that such surveillance reduces the development of lethal cancers have made this costly practice an area of controversy.

OTHER HIGH-RISK CONDITIONS

***Streptococcus bovis* Bacteremia** For unknown reasons, individuals who develop endocarditis or septicemia from this fecal bacterium have a high incidence of occult colorectal tumors and, possibly, upper gastrointestinal cancers as well. Endoscopic or radiographic screening appears advisable.

Tobacco Use Cigarette smoking is linked to the development of colorectal adenomas, particularly after >35 years of tobacco use. No biologic explanation for this association has yet been proposed.

PRIMARY PREVENTION

Several orally administered compounds have been assessed as possible inhibitors of colon cancer. The most effective class of chemopreventive agents is aspirin and other NSAIDs, which are thought to suppress cell proliferation by inhibiting prostaglandin synthesis. Regular aspirin use reduces the risk of colon adenomas and carcinomas as well as death from large-bowel cancer; such use also appears to diminish the likelihood for developing additional premalignant adenomas following successful treatment for a prior colon carcinoma. This effect of aspirin on colon carcinogenesis increases with the duration and dosage of drug use. Oral folic acid supplements and oral calcium supplements appear to reduce the risk of adenomatous polyps and colorectal cancers in case-controlled studies. The value of vitamin D as a form of chemoprevention is under study. Antioxidant vitamins such as ascorbic acid, tocopherols, and β-carotene are ineffective at reducing the incidence of subsequent adenomas in patients who have undergone the removal of a colon adenoma. Estrogen replacement therapy has been associated with a reduction in the risk of colorectal cancer in women, conceivably by an effect on bile acid synthesis and composition or by decreasing synthesis of IGF-I.

The rationale for colorectal cancer screening programs is that the removal of adenomatous polyps will prevent colorectal cancer, and that earlier detection of localized, superficial cancers in asymptomatic individuals will increase the surgical cure rate. Such screening programs are particularly important for individuals with a family history of the disease in first-degree relatives. The relative risk for developing colorectal cancer increases to 1.75 in such individuals and may be even higher if the relative was afflicted before age 60. The prior use of proctosigmoidoscopy as a screening tool was based on the observation that 60% of early lesions are located in the rectosigmoid. For unexplained reasons, however, the proportion of large-bowel cancers arising in the rectum has been decreasing during the past several decades, with a corresponding increase in the proportion of cancers in the more proximal descending colon. As such, the potential for proctosigmoidoscopy to detect a sufficient number of occult neoplasms to make the procedure cost-effective has been questioned.

Screening strategies for colorectal cancer that have been examined during the past several decades are listed in Table 110-3.

Many programs directed at the early detection of colorectal cancers have focused on digital rectal examinations and fecal occult blood (i.e., stool guaiac) testing. The digital examination should be part of any routine physical evaluation in adults older than age 40 years, serving as a screening test for prostate cancer in men, a component of the pelvic examination in women, and an inexpensive maneuver for the detection of masses in the rectum. However, because of the proximal migration of colorectal tumors, its value as an overall screening modality for colorectal cancer has become limited. The development of the fecal occult blood test has greatly facilitated the detection of occult fecal blood. Unfortunately, even when performed optimally, the fecal occult blood test has major limitations as a screening technique. About 50% of patients with documented colorectal cancers have a negative fecal occult blood test, consistent with the intermittent bleeding pattern of these tumors. When random cohorts of asymptomatic persons have been tested, 2–4% have fecal occult blood-positive stools. Colorectal cancers have been found in <10% of these "test-positive" cases, with benign polyps being detected in an additional 20–30%. Thus, a colorectal neoplasm will not be found in most asymptomatic individuals with occult blood in their stool. Nonetheless, persons found to have fecal occult blood-positive stool routinely undergo further medical evaluation, including sigmoidoscopy and/or colonoscopy—procedures that are not only uncomfortable and expensive but also associated with a small risk for significant complications. The added cost of these studies would appear justifiable if the small number of patients found to have occult neoplasms because of fecal occult blood screening could be shown to have an improved prognosis and prolonged survival. Prospectively controlled trials have shown a statistically significant reduction in mortality rate from colorectal cancer for individuals undergoing annual stool guaiac screening. However, this benefit only emerged after >13 years of follow-up and was extremely expensive to achieve, because all positive tests (most of which were falsely positive) were followed by colonoscopy. Moreover, these colonoscopic examinations quite likely provided the opportunity for cancer prevention through the removal of potentially premalignant adenomatous polyps because the eventual development of cancer was reduced by 20% in the cohort undergoing annual screening.

With the appreciation that the carcinogenic process leading to the progression of the normal bowel mucosa to an adenomatous polyp and then to a cancer is the result of a series of molecular changes, investigators have examined fecal DNA for evidence of mutations associated with such molecular changes as evidence of the occult presence of precancerous lesions or actual malignancies. Such a strategy has been tested in more than 4000 asymptomatic individuals whose stool was assessed for occult blood and for 21 possible mutations in fecal DNA; these study subjects also underwent colonoscopy. Although the fecal DNA strategy suggested the presence of more advanced adenomas and cancers than did the fecal occult blood testing approach, the overall sensitivity, using colonoscopic findings as the standard, was less than 50%, diminishing enthusiasm for further pursuit of the fecal DNA screening strategy.

The use of imaging studies to screen for colorectal cancers has also been explored. Air contrast barium enemas had been used to identify sources of occult blood in the stool prior to the advent of fiberoptic endoscopy; the cumbersome nature of the procedure and inconvenience to patients limited its widespread adoption. The introduction of computed tomography (CT) scanning led to the development of virtual (i.e., CT) colonography as an alternative to the growing use of endoscopic screening techniques. Virtual colonography was proposed as being equivalent in sensitivity to colonoscopy and being available in a more widespread manner because it did not require the same degree of operator expertise as fiberoptic endoscopy. However, virtual colonography requires the same cathartic preparation that has limited widespread acceptance of endoscopic colonoscopy, is diagnostic but not therapeutic (i.e., patients with suspicious findings must undergo a subsequent endoscopic procedure for polypectomy or biopsy), and, in the setting of general radiology practices, appears to be less sensitive as a screening technique when compared with endoscopic procedures.

With the appreciation of the inadequacy of fecal occult blood testing alone, concerns about the practicality of imaging approaches, and the wider adoption of endoscopic examinations by the primary care community, screening strategies in asymptomatic persons have changed. At present, both the American Cancer Society and the National Comprehensive Cancer Network suggest either fecal occult blood testing annually coupled with flexible sigmoidoscopy every 5 years or colonoscopy every 10 years beginning at age 50 in asymptomatic individuals with no personal or family history of polyps or colorectal cancer. The recommendation for the inclusion of flexible sigmoidoscopy is strongly supported by the recently published results of three randomized trials performed in the United States, the United Kingdom, and Italy, involving more than 350,000 individuals, which consistently showed that periodic (even single) sigmoidoscopic examinations, after more than a decade of median follow-up, lead to an approximate 21% reduction in the development of colorectal cancer and a more than 25% reduction in mortality from the malignant disease. Less than 20% of participants in these studies underwent a subsequent colonoscopy. In contrast to the cathartic preparation required before colonoscopic procedures, which is only performed by highly trained specialists, flexible sigmoidoscopy requires only an enema as preparation and can be accurately performed by nonspecialty physicians or physician-extenders. The randomized screening studies using flexible sigmoidoscopy led to the estimate that approximately 650 individuals needed to be screened to prevent one colorectal cancer death; this contrasts with the data for mammography where the number of women needing to be screened to prevent one breast cancer death is 2500, reinforcing the efficacy of endoscopic surveillance for colorectal cancer screening. Presumably the benefit from the sigmoidoscopic screening is the result of the identification and removal of adenomatous polyps; it is intriguing that this benefit has been achieved using a technique that leaves the proximal half of the large bowel unvisualized.

It remains to be seen whether surveillance colonoscopy, which has gained increasing popularity in the United States for colorectal cancer screening, will prove to be more effective than flexible sigmoidoscopy. Ongoing randomized trials being conducted in Europe are addressing

TABLE 110-3 SCREENING STRATEGIES FOR COLORECTAL CANCER

Digital rectal examination
Stool testing
• Occult blood
• Fecal DNA
Imaging
• Contrast barium enema
• Virtual (i.e., computed tomography colonography)
Endoscopy
• Flexible sigmoidoscopy
• Colonoscopy

this issue. Although flexible sigmoidoscopy only visualizes the distal half of the large bowel, leading to the assumption that colonoscopy represents a more informative approach, colonoscopy has been reported as being less accurate for screening the proximal rather than the distal colon, perhaps due to technical considerations but also possibly because of a greater frequency of serrated (i.e., "flat") polyps in the right colon, which are more difficult to identify. At present, colonoscopy performed every 10 years has been offered as an alternative to annual fecal occult blood testing with periodic (every 5 years) flexible sigmoidoscopy. Colonoscopy has been shown to be superior to double-contract barium enema and also to have a higher sensitivity for detecting villous or dysplastic adenomas or cancers than the strategy using occult fecal blood testing and flexible sigmoidoscopy. Whether colonoscopy performed every 10 years beginning at age 50 is medically superior and economically equivalent to flexible sigmoidoscopy remains to be determined.

CLINICAL FEATURES

Presenting Symptoms Symptoms vary with the anatomic location of the tumor. Because stool is relatively liquid as it passes through the ileocecal valve into the right colon, cancers arising in the cecum and ascending colon may become quite large without resulting in any obstructive symptoms or noticeable alterations in bowel habits. Lesions of the right colon commonly ulcerate, leading to chronic, insidious blood loss without a change in the appearance of the stool. Consequently, patients with tumors of the ascending colon often present with symptoms such as fatigue, palpitations, and even angina pectoris and are found to have a hypochromic, microcytic anemia indicative of iron deficiency. Because the cancers may bleed intermittently, a random fecal occult blood test may be negative. As a result, the unexplained presence of iron-deficiency anemia in any adult (with the possible exception of a premenopausal, multiparous woman) mandates a thorough endoscopic and/or radiographic visualization of the entire large bowel (Fig. 110-1).

Because stool becomes more formed as it passes into the transverse and descending colon, tumors arising there tend to impede the passage of stool, resulting in the development of abdominal cramping, occasional obstruction, and even perforation. Radiographs of the abdomen often reveal characteristic annular, constricting lesions ("apple-core" or "napkin-ring") (Fig. 110-2).

Cancers arising in the rectosigmoid are often associated with hematochezia, tenesmus, and narrowing of the caliber of stool; anemia is an infrequent finding. While these symptoms may lead patients and their physicians to suspect the presence of hemorrhoids, the development of rectal bleeding and/or altered bowel habits demands a prompt digital rectal examination and proctosigmoidoscopy.

Staging, Prognostic Factors, and Patterns of Spread The prognosis for individuals having colorectal cancer is related to the depth of tumor penetration into the bowel wall and the presence of both regional lymph node involvement and distant metastases. These variables are incorporated into the staging system introduced by Dukes and subsequently applied to a TNM classification method, in which T represents the depth of tumor penetration, N the presence of lymph node involvement, and M the presence or absence of distant metastases (Fig. 110-3). Superficial lesions that do not involve regional lymph nodes and do not penetrate through the submucosa (T1) or the muscularis (T2) are designated as *stage I* (T1–2N0M0) disease; tumors that penetrate through the muscularis but have not spread to lymph nodes are *stage II* disease (T3-4N0M0); regional lymph node involvement defines *stage III* (TXN1-2M0) disease; and metastatic spread to sites such as liver, lung, or bone indicates *stage IV* (TXNXM1) disease. Unless gross evidence of metastatic disease is present, disease stage cannot be determined accurately before surgical resection and pathologic analysis of the operative specimens. It is not clear whether the detection of nodal metastases by special immunohistochemical molecular techniques has the same prognostic implications as disease detected by routine light microscopy.

Most recurrences after a surgical resection of a large-bowel cancer occur within the first 4 years, making 5-year survival a fairly reliable indicator of cure. The likelihood for 5-year survival in patients with colorectal cancer is stage-related (Fig. 110-3). That likelihood has improved during the past several decades when similar surgical stages have been compared. The most plausible explanation for this improvement is more thorough intraoperative and pathologic staging. In particular, more exacting attention to pathologic detail has revealed that the prognosis following the resection of a colorectal cancer is not related merely to the presence or absence of regional lymph node involvement; rather, prognosis may be more precisely gauged by the number of involved lymph nodes (one to three lymph nodes ["N1"] vs four or more lymph nodes ["N2"]) and the number of nodes examined. A minimum of 12 sampled lymph nodes is thought necessary to

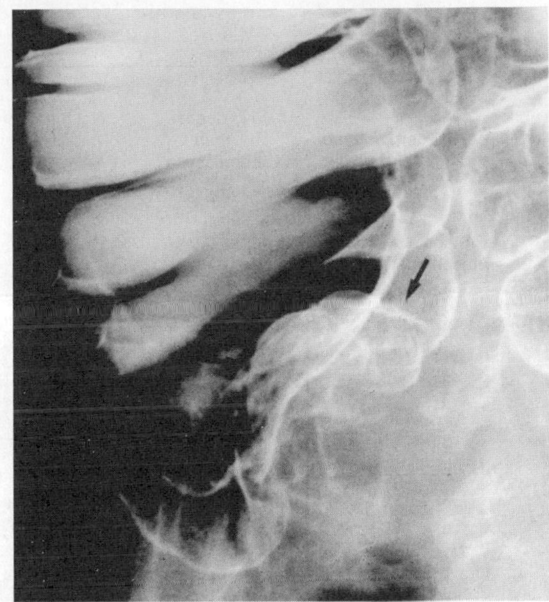

FIGURE 110-1 Double-contrast air-barium enema revealing a sessile tumor of the cecum in a patient with iron-deficiency anemia and guaiac-positive stool. The lesion at surgery was a stage II adenocarcinoma.

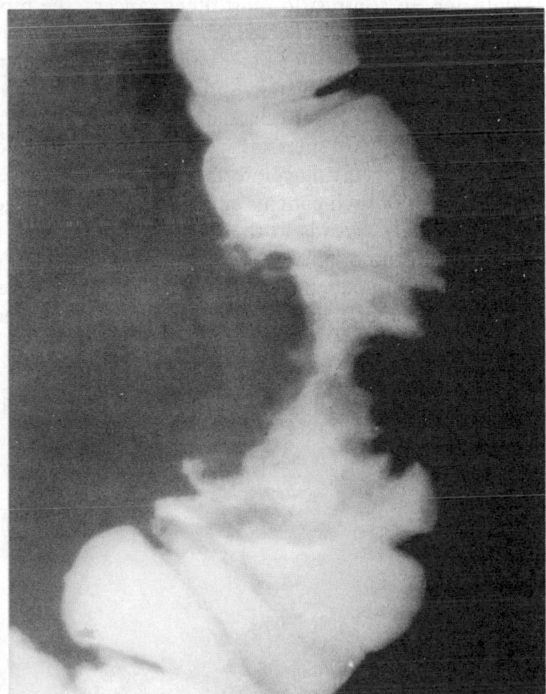

FIGURE 110-2 Annular, constricting adenocarcinoma of the descending colon. This radiographic appearance is referred to as an "apple-core" lesion and is always highly suggestive of malignancy.

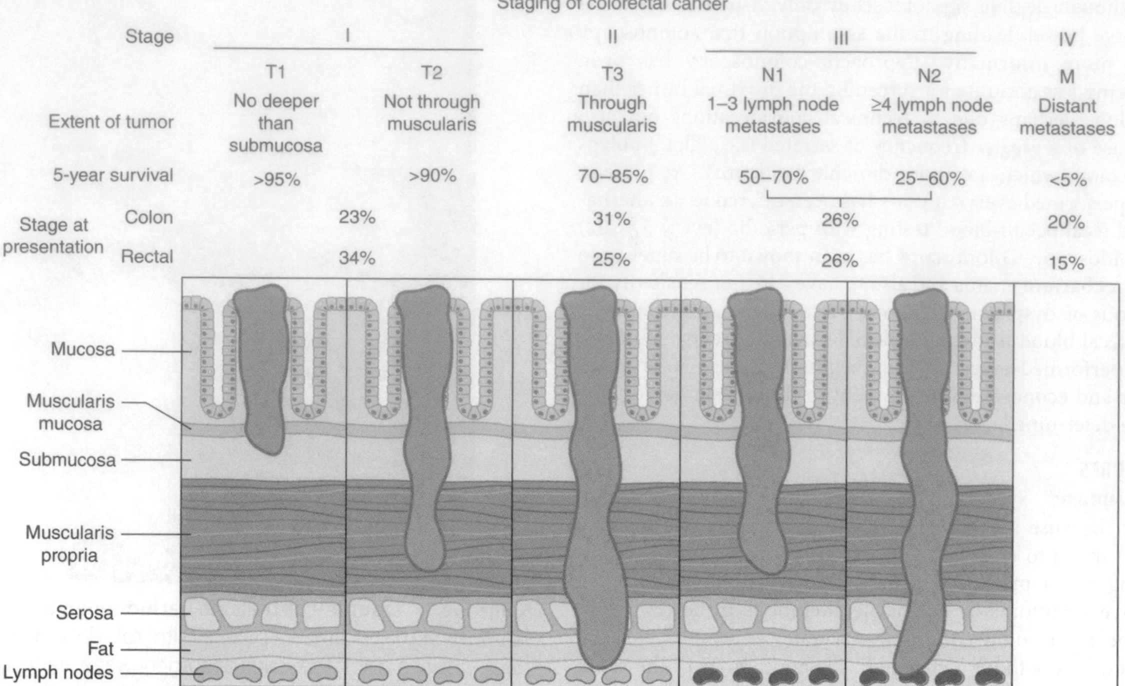

FIGURE 110-3 Staging and prognosis for patients with colorectal cancer.

accurately define tumor stage, and the more nodes examined, the better. Other predictors of a poor prognosis after a total surgical resection include tumor penetration through the bowel wall into pericolic fat, poorly differentiated histology, perforation and/or tumor adherence to adjacent organs (increasing the risk for an anatomically adjacent recurrence), and venous invasion by tumor (Table 110-4). Regardless of the clinicopathologic stage, a preoperative elevation of the plasma carcinoembryonic antigen (CEA) level predicts eventual tumor recurrence. The presence of aneuploidy and specific chromosomal deletions, such as a mutation in the *b-raf* gene in tumor cells, appears to predict for a higher risk for metastatic spread. Conversely, the detection of microsatellite instability in tumor tissue indicates a more favorable outcome. In contrast to most other cancers, the prognosis in colorectal cancer is not influenced by the size of the primary lesion when adjusted for nodal involvement and histologic differentiation.

Cancers of the large bowel generally spread to regional lymph nodes or to the liver via the portal venous circulation. The liver represents the most frequent visceral site of metastasis; it is the initial site of distant spread in one-third of recurring colorectal cancers and is involved in more than two-thirds of such patients at the time of death. In general, colorectal cancer rarely spreads to the lungs, supraclavicular lymph nodes, bone, or brain without prior spread to the liver. A major exception to this rule occurs in patients having primary tumors in the distal rectum, from which tumor cells may spread through the paravertebral venous plexus, escaping the portal venous system and thereby reaching the lungs or supraclavicular lymph nodes without hepatic involvement. The median survival after the detection of distant metastases has ranged in the past from 6–9 months (hepatomegaly, abnormal liver chemistries) to 24–30 months (small liver nodule initially identified by elevated CEA level and subsequent CT scan), but effective systemic therapy is significantly improving this prognosis.

Efforts to use gene expression profiles to identify patients at risk of recurrence or those particularly likely to benefit from adjuvant therapy have not yet yielded practice-changing results. Despite a burgeoning literature examining a host of prognostic factors, pathologic stage at diagnosis remains the best predictor of long-term prognosis. Patients with lymphovascular invasion and high preoperative CEA levels are likely to have a more aggressive clinical course.

TABLE 110-4 PREDICTORS OF POOR OUTCOME FOLLOWING TOTAL SURGICAL RESECTION OF COLORECTAL CANCER

Tumor spread to regional lymph nodes
Number of regional lymph nodes involved
Tumor penetration through the bowel wall
Poorly differentiated histology
Perforation
Tumor adherence to adjacent organs
Venous invasion
Preoperative elevation of CEA titer (>5 ng/mL)
Aneuploidy
Specific chromosomal deletion (e.g., mutation in the *b-raf* gene)

Abbreviation: CEA, carcinoembryonic antigen.

TREATMENT COLORECTAL CANCER

Total resection of tumor is the optimal treatment when a malignant lesion is detected in the large bowel. An evaluation for the presence of metastatic disease, including a thorough physical examination, biochemical assessment of liver function, measurement of the plasma CEA level, and a CT scan of the chest, abdomen, and pelvis, should be performed before surgery. When possible, a colonoscopy of the entire large bowel should be performed to identify synchronous neoplasms and/or polyps. The detection of metastases should not preclude surgery in patients with tumor-related symptoms such as gastrointestinal bleeding or obstruction, but it often prompts the use of a less radical operative procedure. The necessity for a primary tumor resection in asymptomatic individuals with metastatic disease is an area of controversy. At the time of laparotomy, the entire peritoneal cavity should be examined, with thorough inspection of the liver, pelvis, and hemidiaphragm and careful palpation of the full length of the large bowel. Following recovery from a complete resection, patients should be observed carefully for 5 years by semiannual physical examinations and blood chemistry measurements. If a complete colonoscopy was not performed preoperatively, it should be carried out within the first several postoperative months. Some authorities favor measuring plasma CEA levels at 3-month intervals because of the sensitivity of this test as a marker for otherwise undetectable tumor recurrence. Subsequent endoscopic surveillance of the large bowel, probably at triennial intervals, is indicated, because patients who have been cured of one colorectal cancer have a 3–5% probability of developing an additional bowel cancer during their lifetime and a >15% risk for the development of adenomatous polyps. Anastomotic ("suture-line") recurrences are infrequent in colorectal cancer patients, provided the surgical resection margins are adequate and free of tumor. The value of periodic CT scans of the abdomen, assessing for an early, asymptomatic indication of tumor recurrence, is an area of uncertainty, with some experts recommending the test be performed annually for the first 3 postoperative years.

Radiation therapy to the pelvis is recommended for patients with rectal cancer because it reduces the 20–25% probability of regional recurrences following complete surgical resection of stage II or III tumors, especially if they have penetrated through the serosa. This alarmingly high rate of local disease recurrence is believed to be due to the fact that the contained anatomic space within the pelvis limits the extent of the resection and because the rich lymphatic network of the pelvic side wall immediately adjacent to the rectum facilitates the early spread of malignant cells into surgically inaccessible tissue. The use of sharp rather than blunt dissection of rectal cancers (*total mesorectal excision*) appears to reduce the likelihood of local disease recurrence to ~10%. Radiation therapy, either pre- or postoperatively, further reduces the likelihood of pelvic recurrences but does not appear to prolong survival. Combining radiation therapy with 5-fluorouracil (5-FU)-based chemotherapy, preferably prior to surgical resection, lowers local recurrence rates and improves overall survival. Preoperative radiotherapy is indicated for patients with large, potentially unresectable rectal cancers; such lesions may shrink enough to permit subsequent surgical removal. Radiation therapy is not effective as the primary treatment of colon cancer.

Systemic therapy for patients with colorectal cancer has become more effective. 5-FU remains the backbone of treatment for this disease. Partial responses are obtained in 15–20% of patients. The probability of tumor response appears to be somewhat greater for patients with liver metastases when chemotherapy is infused directly into the hepatic artery, but intraarterial treatment is costly and toxic and does not appear to appreciably prolong survival. The concomitant administration of folinic acid (leucovorin) improves the efficacy of 5-FU in patients with advanced colorectal cancer, presumably by enhancing the binding of 5-FU to its target enzyme, thymidylate synthase. A threefold improvement in the partial response rate is noted when folinic acid is combined with 5-FU; however, the effect on survival is marginal, and the optimal dose schedule remains to be defined. 5-FU is generally administered intravenously but may also be given orally in the form of capecitabine (Xeloda) with seemingly similar efficacy.

Irinotecan (CPT-11), a topoisomerase 1 inhibitor, prolongs survival when compared to supportive care in patients whose disease has progressed on 5-FU. Furthermore, the addition of irinotecan to 5-FU and leucovorin (LV) (e.g., FOLFIRI) improves response rates and survival of patients with metastatic disease. The *FOLFIRI regimen* is as follows: irinotecan, 180 mg/m^2 as a 90-min infusion on day 1; LV, 400 mg/m^2 as a 2-h infusion during irinotecan administration; immediately followed by 5-FU bolus, 400 mg/m^2, and 46-h continuous infusion of 2.4–3 g/m^2 every 2 weeks. Diarrhea is the major side effect from irinotecan. Oxaliplatin, a platinum analogue, also improves the response rate when added to 5-FU and LV (FOLFOX) as initial treatment of patients with metastatic disease. The *FOLFOX regimen* is as follows: 2-h infusion of LV (400 mg/m^2 per day) followed by a 5-FU bolus (400 mg/m^2 per day) and 22-h infusion (1200 mg/m^2) every 2 weeks, together with oxaliplatin, 85 mg/m^2 as a 2-h infusion on day 1. Oxaliplatin frequently causes a dose-dependent sensory neuropathy that often but not always resolves following the cessation of therapy. FOLFIRI and FOLFOX are equal in efficacy. In metastatic disease, these regimens may produce median survivals of 2 years.

Monoclonal antibodies are also effective in patients with advanced colorectal cancer. Cetuximab (Erbitux) and panitumumab (Vectibix) are directed against the epidermal growth factor receptor (EGFR), a transmembrane glycoprotein involved in signaling pathways affecting growth and proliferation of tumor cells. Both cetuximab and panitumumab, when given alone, have been shown to benefit a small proportion of previously treated patients, and cetuximab appears to have therapeutic synergy with such chemotherapeutic agents as irinotecan, even in patients previously resistant to this drug; this suggests that cetuximab can reverse cellular resistance to cytotoxic chemotherapy. The antibodies are not effective in the approximate 40% subset of colon tumors that contain mutated K-*ras*. The use of both cetuximab and panitumumab can lead to an acne-like rash, with the development and severity of the rash being correlated with the likelihood of antitumor efficacy. Inhibitors of the EGFR tyrosine kinase such as erlotinib (Tarceva) or sunitinib (Sutent) do not appear to be effective in colorectal cancer.

Bevacizumab (Avastin) is a monoclonal antibody directed against the vascular endothelial growth factor (VEGF) and is thought to act as an antiangiogenesis agent. The addition of bevacizumab to irinotecan-containing combinations and to FOLFOX initially appeared to significantly improve the outcome observed with chemotherapy alone, but subsequent studies have suggested a lesser degree of benefit. The use of bevacizumab can lead to hypertension, proteinuria, and an increased likelihood of thromboembolic events.

Patients with solitary hepatic metastases without clinical or radiographic evidence of additional tumor involvement should be considered for partial liver resection, because such procedures are associated with 5-year survival rates of 25–30% when performed on selected individuals by experienced surgeons.

The administration of 5-FU and LV for 6 months after resection of tumor in patients with stage III disease leads to a 40% decrease in recurrence rates and 30% improvement in survival. The likelihood of recurrence has been further reduced when oxaliplatin has been combined with 5-FU and LV (e.g., FOLFOX); unexpectedly, the addition of irinotecan to 5-FU and LV as well as the addition of either bevacizumab or cetuximab to FOLFOX did not significantly enhance outcome. Patients with stage II tumors do not appear to benefit appreciably from adjuvant therapy, with the use of such treatment generally restricted to those patients having biologic characteristics (e.g., perforated tumors, T4 lesions, lymphovascular invasion) that place them at higher likelihood for recurrence. The addition of oxaliplatin to adjuvant treatment for patients older than age 70 and those with stage II disease does not appear to provide any therapeutic benefit.

In rectal cancer, the delivery of preoperative or postoperative combined-modality therapy (5-FU plus radiation therapy) reduces the risk of recurrence and increases the chance of cure for patients with stage II and III tumors, with the preoperative approach being better tolerated. The 5-FU acts as a radiosensitizer when delivered together with radiation therapy. Life-extending adjuvant therapy is used in only about half of patients older than age 65 years. This age bias is unfortunate because the benefits and likely the tolerance of adjuvant therapy in patients age ≥65 years appear similar to those seen in younger individuals.

CANCERS OF THE ANUS

Cancers of the anus account for 1–2% of the malignant tumors of the large bowel. Most such lesions arise in the anal canal, the anatomic area extending from the anorectal ring to a zone approximately halfway between the pectinate (or dentate) line and the anal verge. Carcinomas arising proximal to the pectinate line (i.e., in the transitional zone between the glandular mucosa of the rectum and the squamous epithelium of the distal anus) are known as *basaloid*, *cuboidal*, or *cloacogenic* tumors; about one-third of anal cancers have this histologic pattern. Malignancies arising distal to the pectinate line have squamous histology, ulcerate more frequently, and constitute ~55% of anal cancers. The prognosis for patients with basaloid and squamous cell cancers of the anus is identical when corrected for tumor size and the presence or absence of nodal spread.

The development of anal cancer is associated with infection by human papillomavirus, the same organism etiologically linked to cervical cancer. The virus is sexually transmitted. The infection may lead to anal warts (condyloma acuminata), which may progress to anal intraepithelial neoplasia and on to squamous cell carcinoma. The risk for anal cancer is increased among homosexual males, presumably related to anal intercourse. Anal cancer risk is increased in both men and women with AIDS, possibly because their immunosuppressed state permits more severe papillomavirus infection. Vaccination against human papilloma viruses may reduce the eventual risk for anal cancer. Anal cancers occur most commonly in middle-aged persons and are more frequent in women than men. At diagnosis, patients may experience bleeding, pain, sensation of a perianal mass, and pruritus.

Radical surgery (abdominal-perineal resection with lymph node sampling and a permanent colostomy) was once the treatment of choice for this tumor type. The 5-year survival rate after such a procedure was 55–70% in the absence of spread to regional lymph nodes and <20% if nodal involvement was present. An alternative therapeutic approach combining external beam radiation therapy with concomitant chemotherapy (5-FU and mitomycin C) has resulted in biopsy-proven disappearance of all tumor in >80% of patients whose initial lesion was <3 cm in size. Tumor recurrences develop in <10% of these patients, meaning that ~70% of patients with anal cancers can be cured with nonoperative treatment and without the need for a colostomy. Surgery should be reserved for the minority of individuals who are found to have residual tumor after being managed initially with radiation therapy combined with chemotherapy.

111 Tumors of the Liver and Biliary Tree

Brian I. Carr

HEPATOCELLULAR CARCINOMA

INCIDENCE

Hepatocellular carcinoma (HCC) is one of the most common malignancies worldwide. The annual global incidence is approximately 1 million cases, with a male-to-female ratio of approximately 4:1 (1:1 without cirrhosis to 9:1 in many high-incidence countries). The incidence rate equals the death rate. In the United States, approximately 22,000 new cases are diagnosed annually, with 18,000 deaths. The death rates in males in low-incidence countries such as the United States are 1.9 per 100,000 per year; in intermediate areas such as Austria and South Africa, they range from 5.1–20; and in high-incidence areas such as in the Orient (China and Korea), they are as high as 23.1–150 per 100,000 per year (Table 111-1). The incidence of HCC in the United States is approximately 3 per 100,000 persons, with significant gender, ethnic, and geographic variations. These numbers are rapidly increasing and may be an underestimate. Approximately 4 million chronic hepatitis C virus (HCV) carriers are in the United States alone. Approximately 10% of them, or 400,000, are likely to develop cirrhosis. Approximately 5%, or 20,000, of these patients may develop HCC annually. Add to this the two other common predisposing factors—hepatitis B virus (HBV) and chronic alcohol consumption—and 60,000 new HCC cases annually seem possible. Future advances in HCC survival will likely depend in part on immunization strategies for HBV (and HCV) and earlier diagnosis by screening of patients at risk of HCC development.

Current Directions With the U.S. HCV epidemic, HCC is increasing in most states, and obesity-associated liver disease (nonalcoholic steatohepatitis [NASH]) is increasingly recognized as a cause.

TABLE 111-1 AGE-ADJUSTED INCIDENCE RATES FOR HEPATOCELLULAR CARCINOMA

	Persons per 100,000 per Year	
Country	**Male**	**Female**
Argentina	6.0	2.5
Brazil, Recife	9.2	8.3
Brazil, Sao Paulo	3.8	2.6
Mozambique	112.9	30.8
South Africa, Cape: Black	26.3	8.4
South Africa, Cape: White	1.2	0.6
Senegal	25.6	9.0
Nigeria	15.4	3.2
Gambia	33.1	12.6
Burma	25.5	8.8
Japan	7.2	2.2
Korea	13.8	3.2
China, Shanghai	34.4	11.6
India, Bombay	4.9	2.5
India, Madras	2.1	0.7
Great Britain	1.6	0.8
France	6.9	1.2
Italy, Varese	7.1	2.7
Norway	1.8	1.1
Spain, Navarra	7.9	4.7

EPIDEMIOLOGY

There are two general types of epidemiologic studies of HCC—those of country-based incidence rates (Table 111-1) and those of migrants. Endemic hot spots occur in areas of China and sub-Saharan Africa, which are associated both with high endemic hepatitis B carrier rates as well as mycotoxin contamination of foodstuffs (aflatoxin B_1), stored grains, drinking water, and soil. Environmental factors are important, for example, Japanese in Japan have a higher incidence than Japanese living in Hawaii, who in turn have a higher incidence than those living in California.

ETIOLOGIC FACTORS

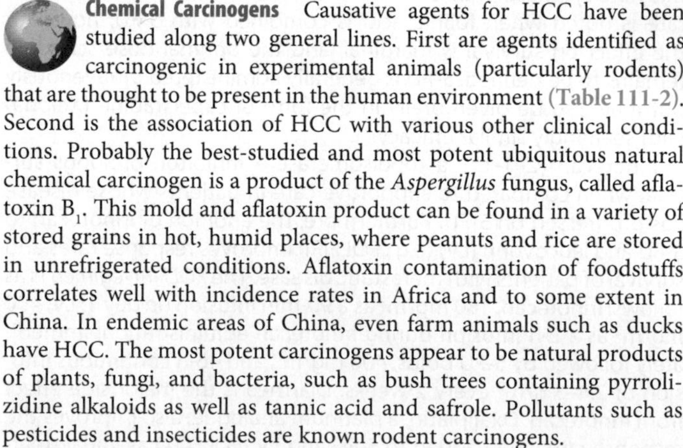

Chemical Carcinogens Causative agents for HCC have been studied along two general lines. First are agents identified as carcinogenic in experimental animals (particularly rodents) that are thought to be present in the human environment (Table 111-2). Second is the association of HCC with various other clinical conditions. Probably the best-studied and most potent ubiquitous natural chemical carcinogen is a product of the *Aspergillus* fungus, called aflatoxin B_1. This mold and aflatoxin product can be found in a variety of stored grains in hot, humid places, where peanuts and rice are stored in unrefrigerated conditions. Aflatoxin contamination of foodstuffs correlates well with incidence rates in Africa and to some extent in China. In endemic areas of China, even farm animals such as ducks have HCC. The most potent carcinogens appear to be natural products of plants, fungi, and bacteria, such as bush trees containing pyrrolizidine alkaloids as well as tannic acid and safrole. Pollutants such as pesticides and insecticides are known rodent carcinogens.

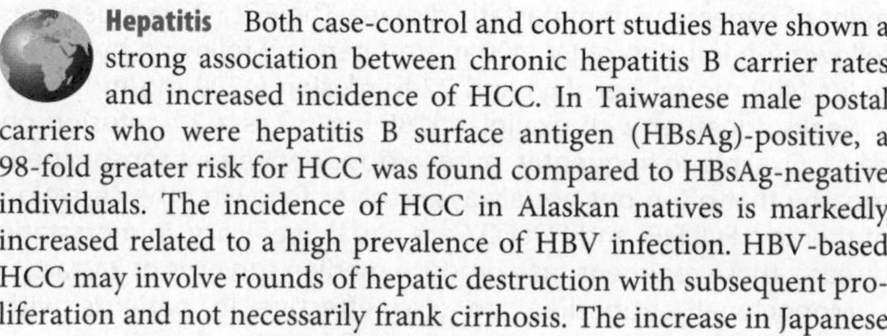

Hepatitis Both case-control and cohort studies have shown a strong association between chronic hepatitis B carrier rates and increased incidence of HCC. In Taiwanese male postal carriers who were hepatitis B surface antigen (HBsAg)-positive, a 98-fold greater risk for HCC was found compared to HBsAg-negative individuals. The incidence of HCC in Alaskan natives is markedly increased related to a high prevalence of HBV infection. HBV-based HCC may involve rounds of hepatic destruction with subsequent proliferation and not necessarily frank cirrhosis. The increase in Japanese

TABLE 111-2 FACTORS ASSOCIATED WITH AN INCREASED RISK OF DEVELOPING HEPATOCELLULAR CARCINOMA

Common	Unusual
Cirrhosis from any cause	Primary biliary cirrhosis
Hepatitis B or C chronic infection	Hemochromatosis
Ethanol chronic consumption	α_1 Antitrypsin deficiency
NASH/NAFL	Glycogen storage diseases
Aflatoxin B_1 or other mycotoxins	Citrullinemia
	Porphyria cutanea tarda
	Hereditary tyrosinemia
	Wilson's disease

Abbreviations: NAFL, nonalcoholic fatty liver; NASH, nonalcoholic steatohepatitis.

TABLE 111-3 HEPATOCELLULAR CARCINOMA CLINICAL PRESENTATION (N = 547)

Symptom	No. of Patients (%)
No symptom	129 (24)
Abdominal pain	219 (40)
Other (workup of anemia and various diseases)	64 (12)
Routine physical exam finding, elevated LFTs	129 (24)
Weight loss	112 (20)
Appetite loss	59 (11)
Weakness/malaise	83 (15)
Jaundice	30 (5)
Routine CT scan screening of known cirrhosis	92 (17)
Cirrhosis symptoms (ankle swelling, abdominal bloating, increased girth, pruritus, GI bleed)	98 (18)
Diarrhea	7 (1)
Tumor rupture	1
Patient Characteristics	
Mean age (yr)	56 ± 13
Male:Female	3:1
Ethnicity	
White	72%
Middle Eastern	10%
Asian	13%
African American	5%
Cirrhosis	81%
No cirrhosis	19%
Tumor Characteristics	
Hepatic tumor numbers	
1	20%
2	25%
3 or more	65%
Portal vein invasion	75%
Unilobar	25%
Bilobar	75%

Abbreviations: CT, computed tomography; GI, gastrointestinal; LFT, liver function test.

HCC incidence rates in the last three decades is thought to be from hepatitis C. A large-scale World Health Organization (WHO)-sponsored intervention study is currently under way in Asia involving HBV vaccination of the newborn. HCC in African blacks is not associated with severe cirrhosis but is poorly differentiated and very aggressive. Despite uniform HBV carrier rates among the South African Bantu, there is a ninefold difference in HCC incidence between Mozambicans living along the coast and inland. These differences are attributed to the additional exposure to dietary aflatoxin B_1 and other carcinogenic mycotoxins. A typical interval between HCV-associated transfusion and subsequent HCC is approximately 30 years. HCV-associated HCC patients tend to have more frequent and advanced cirrhosis, but in HBV-associated HCC, only half the patients have cirrhosis, with the remainder having chronic active hepatitis (Chap. 362).

Other Etiologic Conditions The 75–85% association of HCC with underlying cirrhosis has long been recognized, more typically with macronodular cirrhosis in Southeast Asia, but also with micronodular cirrhosis (alcohol) in Europe and the United States (Chap. 365). It is still not clear whether cirrhosis itself is a predisposing factor to the development of HCC or whether the underlying causes of the cirrhosis are actually the carcinogenic factors. However, ~20% of U.S. patients with HCC do not have underlying cirrhosis. Several underlying conditions are associated with an increased risk for cirrhosis-associated HCC (Table 111-2), including hepatitis, alcohol, autoimmune chronic active hepatitis, cryptogenic cirrhosis, and NASH. A less common association is with primary biliary cirrhosis and several metabolic diseases including hemochromatosis, Wilson's disease, α_1 antitrypsin deficiency, tyrosinemia, porphyria cutanea tarda, glycogenesis types 1 and 3, citrullinemia, and orotic aciduria. The etiology of HCC in those 20% of patients who have no cirrhosis is currently unclear, and their HCC natural history is not well-defined.

Current Directions Many patients have multiple etiologies, and the interactions of HBV, HCV, alcohol, smoking, and aflatoxins are just beginning to be explored.

CLINICAL FEATURES

Symptoms These include abdominal pain, weight loss, weakness, abdominal fullness and swelling, jaundice, and nausea (Table 111-3). Presenting signs and symptoms differ somewhat between high- and low-incidence areas. In high-risk areas, especially in South African blacks, the most common symptom is abdominal pain; by contrast, only 40–50% of Chinese and Japanese patients present with abdominal pain. Abdominal swelling may occur as a consequence of ascites due to the underlying chronic liver disease or may be due to a rapidly expanding tumor. Occasionally, central necrosis or acute hemorrhage into the peritoneal cavity leads to death. In countries with an active surveillance program, HCC tends to be identified at an earlier stage, when symptoms may be due only to the underlying disease. Jaundice is usually due to obstruction of the intrahepatic ducts from underlying liver disease. Hematemesis may occur due to esophageal varices from the underlying portal hypertension. Bone pain is seen in 3–12% of patients, but necropsies show pathologic bone metastases in ~20% of patients. However, 25% of patients may be asymptomatic.

Physical Signs Hepatomegaly is the most common physical sign, occurring in 50–90% of the patients. Abdominal bruits are noted in 6–25%, and ascites occurs in 30–60% of patients. Ascites should be examined by cytology. Splenomegaly is mainly due to portal hypertension. Weight loss and muscle wasting are common, particularly with rapidly growing or large tumors. Fever is found in 10–50% of patients, from unclear cause. The signs of chronic liver disease may often be present, including jaundice, dilated abdominal veins, palmar erythema, gynecomastia, testicular atrophy, and peripheral edema. Budd-Chiari syndrome can occur due to HCC invasion of the hepatic veins, with tense ascites and a large tender liver (Chap. 365).

Paraneoplastic Syndromes Most paraneoplastic syndromes in HCC are biochemical abnormalities without associated clinical consequences. They include hypoglycemia (also caused by end-stage liver failure), erythrocytosis, hypercalcemia, hypercholesterolemia, dysfibrinogenemia, carcinoid syndrome, increased thyroxin-binding globulin, changes in secondary sex characteristics (gynecomastia, testicular atrophy, and precocious puberty), and porphyria cutanea tarda. Mild hypoglycemia occurs in rapidly growing HCC as part of terminal illness, and profound hypoglycemia may occur, although the cause is unclear. Erythrocytosis occurs in 3–12% of patients and hypercholesterolemia in 10–40%. A high percentage of patients have thrombocytopenia associated with their fibrosis or leukopenia, resulting from portal hypertension, and not from cancer infiltration of bone marrow, as in other tumor types. Furthermore, large HCCs have normal or high platelet levels (thrombocytosis), as in ovarian and other gastrointestinal cancers, probably related to elevated interleukin 6 (IL-6) levels.

STAGING

Multiple clinical staging systems for HCC have been described. A widely used one has been the American Joint Committee on Cancer (AJCC) tumor-node-metastasis (TNM) classification. However, the Cancer of the Liver Italian Program (CLIP) system is now popular because it takes cirrhosis into account, based on the original Okuda system (Table 111-4). Patients with Okuda stage III disease have a dire prognosis because they usually cannot be curatively resected, and the condition of their liver typically precludes chemotherapy. Other staging systems have been proposed, and a consensus is needed. They are all based on combining the prognostic features of liver damage with those of tumor aggressiveness and include the Barcelona Clinic Liver Cancer (BCLC) system from Spain (Fig. 111-1), which is externally validated and incorporates baseline survival estimates; the Chinese University Prognostic Index (CUPI); the important and simple Japan Integrated Staging Score (JIS); and SLiDe, which stands for *s* tage, *li* ver damage, and *de* s-γ-carboxy prothrombin. CLIP and BCLC appear most popular in the West, whereas JIS is favored in Japan. Each system has its champions. The best prognosis is for stage I, solitary tumors less than 2 cm in diameter without vascular invasion. Adverse prognostic features include ascites, jaundice, vascular invasion, and elevated α fetoprotein (AFP). Vascular invasion in particular has profound effects

TABLE 111-4 CLIP AND OKUDA STAGING SYSTEMS FOR HEPATOCELLULAR CARCINOMA

CLIP Classification

	Points		
Variables	**0**	**1**	**2**
i. Tumor number	Single	Multiple	–
Hepatic replacement by tumor (%)	<50	<50	>50
ii. Child-Pugh score	A	B	C
iii. α Fetoprotein level (ng/mL)	<400	≥400	–
iv. Portal vein thrombosis (CT)	No	Yes	–

CLIP stages (score = sum of points): CLIP 0, 0 points; CLIP 1, 1 point; CLIP 2, 2 points; CLIP 3, 3 points.

Okuda Classification

Tumor Extent[a]		Ascites		Albumin (g/L)		Bilirubin (mg/dL)	
≥50%	<50	+	–	≤3	>3	≥ 3	<3
(+)	(–)	(+)	(–)	(+)	(–)	(+)	(–)

Okuda stages: stage 1, all (–); stage 2, 1 or 2 (+); stage 3, 3 or 4 (+).

[a]Extent of liver occupied by tumor.

Abbreviation: CLIP, Cancer of the Liver Italian Program.

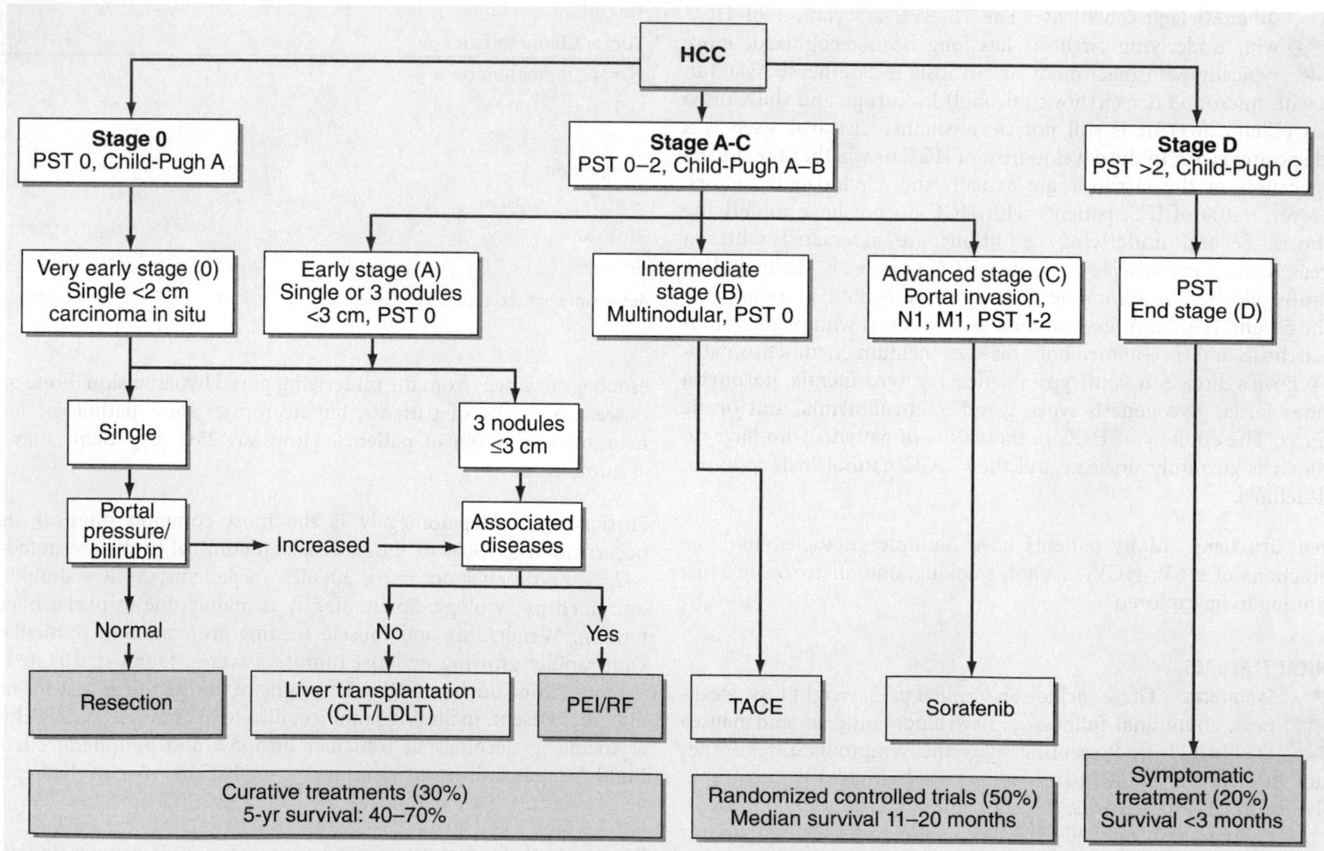

FIGURE 111-1 Barcelona Clinic Liver Cancer (BCLC) staging classification and treatment schedule. Patients with very early hepatocellular carcinoma (HCC) (stage 0) are optimal candidates for resection. Patients with early HCC (stage A) are candidates for radical therapy (resection, liver transplantation [LT], or local ablation via percutaneous ethanol injection [PEI] or radiofrequency [RF] ablation). Patients with intermediate HCC (stage B) benefit from transcatheter arterial chemoembolization (TACE). Patients with advanced HCC, defined as presence of macroscopic vascular invasion, extrahepatic spread, or cancer-related symptoms (Eastern Cooperative Oncology Group performance status 1 or 2) (stage C), benefit from sorafenib. Patients with end-stage disease (stage D) will receive symptomatic treatment. Treatment strategy will transition from one stage to another on treatment failure or contraindications for the procedures. CLT, cadaveric liver transplantation; LDLT, living donor liver transplantation; PST, Performance Status Test. *(Modified from JM Llovet et al: JNCI 100:698, 2008.)*

on prognosis and may be microscopic or macroscopic (visible on computed tomography [CT] scans). Most large tumors have microscopic vascular invasion, so full staging can usually be made only after surgical resection. Stage III disease contains a mixture of lymph node–positive and–negative tumors. Stage III patients with positive lymph node disease have a poor prognosis, and few patients survive 1 year. The prognosis of stage IV is poor after either resection or transplantation, and 1-year survival is rare.

New Directions Consensus is needed on staging. These systems will soon be refined or upended by proteomics.

APPROACH TO THE PATIENT: Hepatocellular Carcinoma

HISTORY AND PHYSICAL

The history is important in evaluating putative predisposing factors, including a history of hepatitis or jaundice, blood transfusion, or use of intravenous drugs. A family history of HCC or hepatitis should be sought and a detailed social history taken to include job descriptions for industrial exposure to possible carcinogenic drugs as well as contraceptive hormones. Physical examination should include assessing stigmata of underlying liver disease such as jaundice, ascites, peripheral edema, spider nevi, palmar erythema, and weight loss. Evaluation of the abdomen for hepatic size, masses or ascites, hepatic nodularity and tenderness, and splenomegaly is needed, as is assessment of overall performance status and psychosocial evaluation.

SEROLOGIC ASSAYS

AFP is a serum tumor marker for HCC; however, it is only increased in approximately one-half of U.S. patients. The lens culinaris agglutinin-reactive fraction of AFP (AFP-L3) assay is thought to be more specific. The other widely used assay is that for des γ-carboxy prothrombin (DCP), a protein induced by vitamin K absence (PIVKA-2). This protein is increased in as many as 80% of HCC patients but may also be elevated in patients with vitamin K deficiency; it is always elevated after warfarin use. It may also predict for portal vein invasion. Both AFP-L3 and DCP are U.S. Food and Drug Administration (FDA) approved. Many other assays have been developed, such as glypican-3, but none have greater aggregate sensitivity and specificity. In a patient presenting with either a new hepatic mass or other indications of recent hepatic decompensation, carcinoembryonic antigen (CEA), vitamin B_{12}, AFP, ferritin, PIVKA-2, and antimitochondrial antibody should be measured, and standard liver function tests should be performed, including prothrombin time (PT), partial thromboplastin time (PTT), albumin, transaminases, γ-glutamyl transpeptidase, and alkaline phosphatase. γ-Glutamyl transpeptidase and alkaline phosphatase may be particularly important in the 50% of HCC patients who have low AFP levels. Decreases in platelet count and white blood cell count may reflect portal hypertension and associated hypersplenism. Hepatitis A, B, and C serology should be measured. If HBV or HCV serology is positive, quantitative measurements of HBV DNA or HCV RNA are needed.

New Directions Newer biomarkers are being evaluated, especially tissue- and serum-based genomics profiling. Newer plasma biomarkers include glypican-3, osteopontin, insulin-like growth factor I, and vascular endothelial growth factor. However, they are still in process of validation. Furthermore, the commercial availability of kits for isolating circulating tumor cells is permitting the molecular profiling of HCCs without the need for further tissue biopsy.

RADIOLOGY

An ultrasound examination of the liver is an excellent screening tool. The two characteristic vascular abnormalities are hypervascularity of the tumor mass (neovascularization or abnormal tumor-feeding arterial vessels) and thrombosis by tumor invasion of otherwise normal portal veins. To determine tumor size and extent and the presence of portal vein invasion accurately, a helical/triphasic CT scan of the abdomen and pelvis, with fast-contrast bolus technique, should be performed to detect the vascular lesions typical of HCC. Portal vein invasion is normally detected as an obstruction and expansion of the vessel. A chest CT is used to exclude metastases. Magnetic resonance imaging (MRI) can also provide detailed information, especially with the newer contrast agents. Ethiodol (Lipiodol) is an ethiodized oil emulsion retained by liver tumors that can be delivered by hepatic artery injection (5–15 mL) for CT imaging 1 week later. For small tumors, Ethiodol injection is very helpful before biopsy because the histologic presence of the dye constitutes proof that the needle biopsied the mass under suspicion. A prospective comparison of triphasic CT, gadolinium-enhanced MRI, ultrasound, and fluorodeoxyglucose positron emission tomography (FDG-PET) showed similar results for CT, MRI, and ultrasound; PET imaging appears to be positive in only a subset of HCC patients. Abdominal CT versus MRI/CT uses a faster single breath-hold, is less complex, and is less dependent on patient cooperation. MRI requires a longer examination, and ascites can cause artifacts, but MRI is better able to distinguish dysplastic or regenerative nodules from HCC. Imaging criteria have been developed for HCC that do not require biopsy proof, as they have >90% specificity. The criteria include nodules >1 cm with arterial enhancement and portal venous washout and, for small tumors, specified growth rates on two scans performed less than 6 months apart (Organ Procurement and Transplant Network). Nevertheless, explant pathology after liver transplant for HCC has shown that ~20% of patients diagnosed without biopsy did not actually have a tumor.

New Directions The altered tumor vascularity that is a consequence of molecularly targeted therapies is the basis for newer imaging techniques including contrast-enhanced ultrasound (CEUS) and dynamic MRI.

PATHOLOGIC DIAGNOSIS

Histologic proof of the presence of HCC is obtained through a core liver biopsy of the liver mass under ultrasound guidance, as well as random biopsy of the underlying liver. Bleeding risk is increased compared to other cancers because (1) the tumors are hypervascular and (2) patients often have thrombocytopenia and decreased liver-dependent clotting factors. Bleeding risk is further increased in the presence of ascites. Tracking of tumor has an uncommon problem. Fine-needle aspirates can provide sufficient material for diagnosis of cancer, but core biopsies are preferred. Tissue architecture allows the distinction between HCC and adenocarcinoma. Laparoscopic approaches can also be used. For patients suspected of having portal vein involvement, a core biopsy of the portal vein may be performed safely. If positive, this is regarded as an exclusion criterion for transplantation for HCC.

New Directions Immunohistochemistry has become mainstream. Prognostic subgroupings are being defined based on growth signaling pathway proteins and genotyping strategies, including a prognostically significant five-gene profile score. Furthermore, molecular profiling of the underlying liver has provided evidence for a "field-effect" of cirrhosis in generating recurrent or new HCCs after primary resection. In addition, characteristics of HCC stem cells have been identified and include EpCAM, CD44, and CD90 expression, which may form the basis of stem cell therapeutic targeting strategies.

SCREENING HIGH-RISK POPULATIONS

There are two goals of screening, both in patients at increased risk for developing HCC, such as those with cirrhosis. The first goal is to detect smaller tumors that are potentially curable by ablation. The second goal is to enhance survival, compared with patients who were not diagnosed by surveillance. Evidence from Taiwan has shown a survival advantage to population screening in HBV-positive patients, and other evidence has shown its efficacy in diagnosis for HCV. Prospective studies in high-risk populations showed that ultrasound was more sensitive than AFP elevations alone, although most practitioners request both tests at 6-month intervals for HBV and HCV carriers, especially in the presence of cirrhosis or worsening of liver function tests. However, an Italian study in patients with cirrhosis identified a yearly HCC incidence of 3% but showed no increase in the rate of detection of potentially curable tumors with aggressive screening. Prevention strategies including universal vaccination against hepatitis are more likely to be effective than screening efforts. Despite absence of formal guidelines, most practitioners obtain 6-month AFP and ultrasound (cheap and ubiquitous, even in poor countries) or CT (more sensitive, especially in overweight patients, but more costly) studies when following high-risk patients (HBV carriers, HCV cirrhosis, family history of HCC).

Current Directions Cost-benefit analysis is not yet convincing, even though screening is intuitively sound. However, studies from areas with high HBV carrier rates have shown a survival benefit for screening as a result of earlier stage at diagnosis. A definitive clinical trial on screening is unlikely, due to difficulties in obtaining informed consent for patients who are not to be screened. γ-Glutamyl transpeptidase appears useful for detecting small tumors.

PREVENTION

Prevention strategies can only be planned when the causes of a cancer are known or strongly suspected. This is true of few human cancers, with significant exceptions being smoking and lung cancer, papilloma virus and cancer of the cervix uteri, and cirrhosis of any cause or dietary contamination by aflatoxin B_1 for HCC. Aflatoxin B_1 is one of the most potent known chemical carcinogens and is a product of the *Aspergillus* mold that grows on peanuts and rice when stored in hot and humid climates. The obvious strategy is to refrigerate these foodstuffs when stored and to conduct surveillance programs for elevated aflatoxin B_1 levels, as happens in the United States, but not usually in Asia. HBV is commonly transmitted from mother to fetus in Asia (except Japan), and neonatal HBV vaccination programs have resulted in a big decrease in adolescent HBV and, thus, in predicted HCC rates. There are millions of HBV and HCV carriers (4 million with HCV in the United States) who are already infected. Nucleoside analogue–based chemoprevention (entecavir) of HBV-mediated HCC in Japan resulted in a fivefold decrease in HCC incidence over 5 years in cirrhotic but not in noncirrhotic HBV patients. More powerful and effective HCV therapies promise the possibility of prevention of HCV-based HCC in the future.

TREATMENT HEPATOCELLULAR CARCINOMA

Most HCC patients have two liver diseases, cirrhosis and HCC, each of which is an independent cause of death. The presence of cirrhosis usually places constraints on resection surgery, ablative therapies, and chemotherapy. Thus patient assessment and treatment planning have to take the severity of the nonmalignant liver disease into account. The clinical management choices for HCC can be complex (**Fig. 111-2, Tables 111-5 and 111-6**). The natural history of HCC is highly variable. Patients presenting with advanced tumors (vascular invasion, symptoms, extrahepatic spread) have a median survival of ~4 months, with or without treatment. Treatment results from the literature are difficult to interpret. Survival is not always a measure of the efficacy of therapy because of the adverse effects on survival of the underlying liver disease. A multidisciplinary team, including a hepatologist, interventional radiologist, surgical oncologist, resection surgeon, transplant surgeon, and medical oncologist, is important for the comprehensive management of HCC patients.

TNM STAGES I AND II HCC

Early-stage tumors are successfully treated using various techniques, including surgical resection, local ablation (thermal, radiofrequency [RFA], or microwave ablation (MWA]), and local injection therapies (Table 111-6). Because the majority of patients with HCC suffer from a field defect in the cirrhotic liver, they are at risk for subsequent multiple primary liver tumors. Many will also have significant underlying liver disease and may not tolerate major surgical loss of hepatic parenchyma, and they may be eligible for orthotopic liver transplant (OLTX). Living related donor transplants have increased in popularity, resulting in absence of waiting for a transplant. An important principle in treating early-stage HCC in the nontransplant

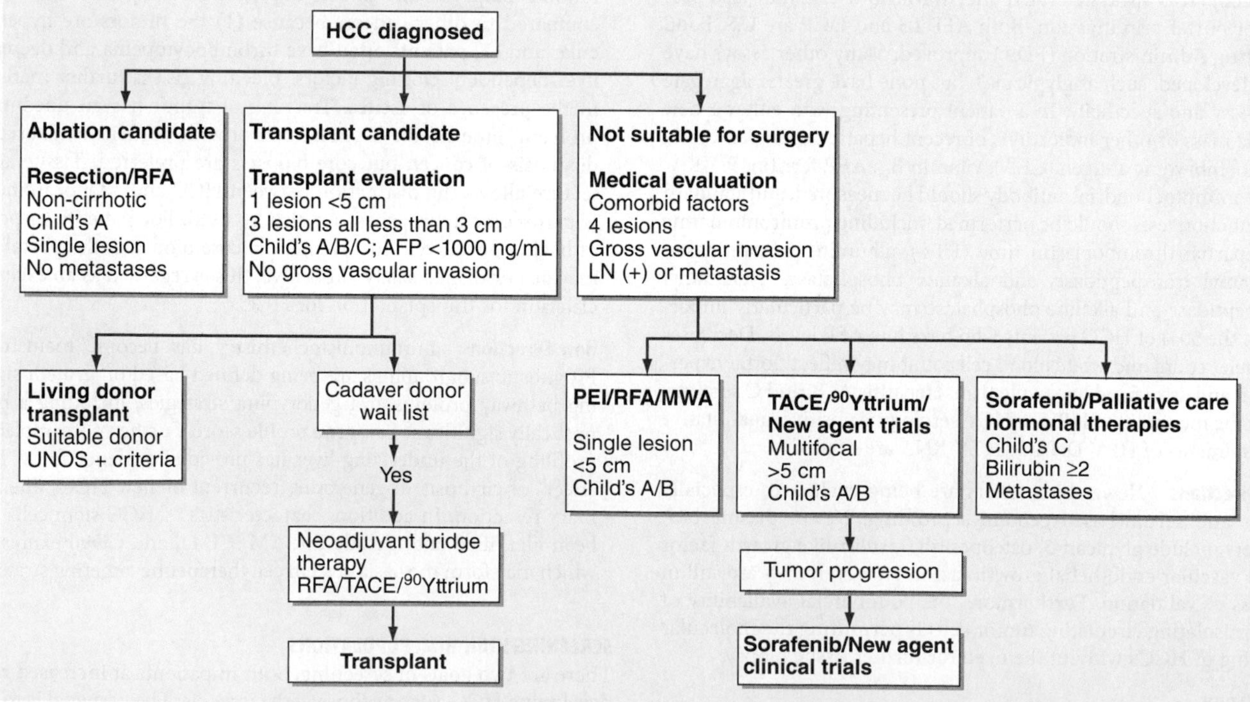

FIGURE 111-2 Hepatocellular carcinoma (HCC) treatment algorithm. The initial clinical evaluation is aimed at assessing the extent of the tumor and the underlying functional compromise of the liver by cirrhosis. Patients are classified as having resectable disease or unresectable disease or as being candidates for transplantation. AFP, α fetoprotein; LN, lymph node; MWA, microwave ablation; OLTX, orthotopic liver transplantation; PEI, percutaneous ethanol injection; RFA, radiofrequency ablation; TACE, transcatheter arterial chemoembolization; UNOS, United Network for Organ Sharing. Child's A/B/C refers to the Child-Pugh classification of liver failure.

TABLE 111-5 TREATMENT OPTIONS FOR HEPATOCELLULAR CARCINOMA

Surgery
Resection
Liver transplantation
Local Ablative Therapies
Radiofrequency ablation (RFA)
Microwave ablation (MWA)
Cryosurgery
Percutaneous ethanol injection (PEI)
Regional Therapies: Hepatic Artery Transcatheter Treatments
Transarterial chemotherapy
Transarterial embolization
Transarterial chemoembolization
Transarterial drug-eluting beads
Transarterial radiotherapies:
^{90}Yttrium microspheres
^{131}Iodine– Ethiodol
Proton beam radiation
Conformal External-Beam Radiation and Intensity-Modulated Radiation Therapy
Systemic therapies
Molecularly targeted therapies (sorafenib, etc.)
Chemotherapy
Immunotherapy
Hormonal therapy + growth control
Supportive Therapies

setting is to use liver-sparing treatments and to focus on treatment of both the tumor and the cirrhosis.

Surgical Excision The risk of major hepatectomy is high (5–10% mortality rate) due to the underlying liver disease and the potential for liver failure, but acceptable in selected cases and highly dependent on surgical experience. The risk is lower in high-volume centers. Preoperative portal vein occlusion can sometimes be performed to cause atrophy of the HCC-involved lobe and compensatory hypertrophy of the noninvolved liver, permitting safer resection. Intraoperative ultrasound is useful for planning the surgical approach. The ultrasound can image the proximity of major vascular structures that may be encountered during the dissection. In cirrhotic patients, any major liver surgery can result in liver failure. The Child-Pugh classification of liver failure is still a reliable prognosticator for tolerance of hepatic surgery, and only Child A patients should be considered for surgical resection. Child B and C patients with stages I and II HCC should be referred for OLTX if appropriate, as well as patients with ascites or a recent history of variceal bleeding. Although open surgical excision is the most reliable, the patient may be better served with a laparoscopic approach to resection, using RFA, MWA, or percutaneous ethanol injection (PEI). No adequate comparisons of these different techniques have been undertaken, and the choice of treatment is usually based on physician skill. However, RFA has been shown to be superior to PEI in necrosis induction for tumors <3 cm in diameter and is thought to be equivalent to open resection and, thus, is the treatment of first choice for these small tumors. As tumors get larger than 3 cm, especially ≥5 cm, the effectiveness of RFA-induced necrosis diminishes. The combination of transcatheter arterial chemoembolization (TACE) with RFA has shown superior results to TACE alone in a prospective, randomized trial. Although vascular invasion is a preeminent negative prognostic factor, microvascular invasion in small tumors appears not to be a negative factor.

Local Ablation Strategies RFA uses heat to ablate tumors. The maximum size of the probe arrays allows for a 7-cm zone of necrosis, which would be adequate for a 3- to 4-cm tumor. The heat reliably kills cells within the zone of necrosis. Treatment of tumors close to the main portal pedicles can lead to bile duct injury and obstruction. This limits the location of tumors that are anatomically suited for this technique. RFA can be performed percutaneously with CT or ultrasound guidance, or at the time of laparoscopy with ultrasound guidance.

Local Injection Therapy Numerous agents have been used for local injection into tumors, most commonly ethanol (PEI). The relatively soft HCC within the hard background cirrhotic liver allows for injection of large volumes of ethanol into the tumor without diffusion into the hepatic parenchyma or leakage out of the liver. PEI causes direct destruction of cancer cells, but it is not selective for cancer and will destroy normal cells in the vicinity. However, it usually requires multiple injections (average three), in contrast to one for RFA. The maximum size of tumor reliably treated is 3 cm, even with multiple injections.

CURRENT DIRECTIONS Resection and RFA each obtain similar results. However, a distinction has been made between the causes and prevention strategies needed to prevent early versus late tumor recurrences after resection. Early recurrence has been linked to tumor invasion factors, especially microvascular tumor invasion with elevated transaminases, whereas late recurrence has been associated with cirrhosis and virus hepatitis factors and, thus, the development of new tumors. See the section on virus-directed adjuvant therapy below.

Liver Transplantation (OLTX) A viable option for stages I and II tumors in the setting of cirrhosis is OLTX, with survival approaching that for noncancer cases. OLTX for patients with a single lesion ≤5 cm or three or fewer nodules, each ≤3 cm (Milan criteria), resulted in excellent tumor-free survival (≥70% at 5 years). For advanced HCC, OLTX has been abandoned due to high tumor recurrence rates. Priority scoring for OLTX previously led to HCC patients waiting too long for their OLTX, resulting in some tumors becoming too advanced during the patient's wait for a donated liver. A variety of therapies were used as a "bridge" to OLTX, including RFA, TACE, and hepatic arterial ^{90}Y-radioembolization. These pretransplant treatments allow patients to remain on the waiting list longer, giving them greater opportunities to be transplanted, because they can stabilize the tumor and prevent it from

TABLE 111-6 SOME RANDOMIZED CLINICAL TRIALS INVOLVING TRANSHEPATIC ARTERY CHEMOEMBOLIZATION (TACE) FOR HEPATOCELLULAR CARCINOMA

Author	Year	Agents 1	Agents 2	Survival Effect
Kawaii	1992	Doxorubicin + Embo	Embo	No
Chang	1994	Cisplatin + Embo	Embo	No
Hatanaka	1995	Cisplatin, doxorubicin, + Embo	Same + Lipiodol	No
Uchino	1993	Cisplatin, doxorubicin, + oral FU	Same + Tamoxifen	No
Lin	1988	Embo	Embo + IV FU	No
Yoshikawa	1994	Epirubicin + Ethiodol	Epirubicin	No
Pelletier	1990	Doxorubicin + Gelfoam	None	No
Trinchet	1995	Cisplatin + Gelfoam	None	No
Bruix	1998	Coils + Gelfoam	None	No
Pelletier	1998	Cisplatin + Ethiodol	None	No
Trinchet	1995	Cisplatin + Gelfoam	None	No
Lo	2002	Cisplatin + Ethiodol	None	Yes
Llovet	2002	Doxorubicin + Ethiodol	None	Yes

Abbreviations: Embo, embolization; FU, 5-fluorouracil.

growing in the months until a donor liver becomes available. What remains unclear, however, is whether this translates into prolonged survival after transplant. Further, it is not known whether patients who have had their tumor(s) treated preoperatively follow the recurrence pattern predicted by their tumor status at the time of transplant (i.e., post–local ablative therapy), or if they follow the course set by their tumor parameters present before such treatment. The United Network for Organ Sharing (UNOS) point system for priority scoring of OLTX recipients now includes additional points for patients with HCC. The success of living related donor liver transplantation programs has also led to patients receiving transplantation earlier for HCC and often with greater than minimal tumors.

CURRENT DIRECTIONS Expanded criteria for larger HCCs beyond the Milan criteria (one lesion <5 cm or three lesions, each <3 cm), such as the University of California, San Francisco (UCSF) criteria (single lesion ≤6.5 cm or two lesions ≤4.5 cm with a total diameter ≤8 cm; 1- and 5-year survival rates of 90 and 75%, respectively), are being increasingly accepted by various UNOS areas for OLTX with satisfactory longer-term survival comparable to Milan criteria results. Furthermore, downstaging of HCCs that are too large for the Milan criteria by medical therapy (TACE) is increasingly recognized as acceptable treatment before OLTX with equivalent outcomes to patients who originally were within Milan criteria. Within-criteria patients with AFP levels >1000 ng/mL have exceptionally high post-OLTX recurrence rates. Also, the use of "salvage" OLTX after recurrent HCC after resection has produced conflicting outcomes. Shortages of organs combined with advances in resection safety have led to increasing use of resection for patients with good liver function.

Adjuvant Therapy The role of adjuvant chemotherapy for patients after resection or OLTX remains unclear. Both adjuvant and neoadjuvant approaches have been studied, but no clear advantage in disease-free or overall survival has been found. However, a meta-analysis of several trials revealed a significant improvement in disease-free and overall survival. Although analysis of postoperative adjuvant systemic chemotherapy trials demonstrated no disease-free or overall survival advantage, single studies of TACE and neoadjuvant ^{131}I-Ethiodol showed enhanced survival after resection.

Antiviral therapy, instead of anticancer therapy, has been successful in decreasing postresection tumor recurrences in the postresection adjuvant setting. Nucleoside analogues in HBV-based HCC and peg-interferon plus ribavirin for HCV-based HCC have both been effective in reducing recurrence rates.

CURRENT DIRECTIONS A large adjuvant trial examining resection and transplantation, with or without sorafenib (see below) is in progress. The success of viral therapies in decreasing HCC recurrence after resection is part of a broader focus on the tumor microenvironment (stroma, blood vessels, inflammatory cells, and cytokines) as mediators of HCC progression and as targets for new therapies.

TNM STAGES III AND IV HCC

Fewer surgical options exist for stage III tumors involving major vascular structures. In patients without cirrhosis, a major hepatectomy is feasible, although prognosis is poor. Patients with Child A cirrhosis may be resected, but a lobectomy is associated with significant morbidity and mortality rates, and long-term prognosis is poor. Nevertheless, a small percentage of patients will achieve long-term survival, justifying an attempt at resection when feasible. Because of the advanced nature of these tumors, even successful resection can be followed by rapid recurrence. These patients are not considered candidates for transplantation because of the high tumor recurrence rates, unless their tumors can first be downstaged with neoadjuvant therapy. Decreasing the size of the primary tumor allows for less surgery, and the delay in surgery allows for extrahepatic disease to manifest on imaging studies and avoid unhelpful OLTX. The prognosis is poor for stage IV tumors, and no surgical treatment is recommended.

Systemic Chemotherapy A large number of controlled and uncontrolled clinical studies have been performed with most of the major classes of cancer chemotherapy. No single agent or combination of agents given systemically reproducibly leads to even a 25% response rate or has any effect on survival.

Regional Chemotherapy In contrast to the dismal results of systemic chemotherapy, a variety of agents given via the hepatic artery have activity for HCC confined to the liver (Table 111-6). Two randomized controlled trials have shown a survival advantage for TACE in a selected subset of patients. One used doxorubicin, and the other used cisplatin. Despite the fact that increased hepatic extraction of chemotherapy has been shown for very few drugs, some drugs such as cisplatin, doxorubicin, mitomycin C, and possibly neocarzinostatin, produce substantial objective responses when administered regionally. Few data are available on continuous hepatic arterial infusion for HCC, although pilot studies with cisplatin have shown encouraging responses. Because the reports have not usually stratified responses or survival based on TNM staging, it is difficult to know long-term prognosis in relation to tumor extent. Most of the studies on regional hepatic arterial chemotherapy also use an embolizing agent such as Ethiodol, gelatin sponge particles (Gelfoam), starch (Spherex), or microspheres. Two products are composed of microspheres of defined size ranges—Embospheres (Biospheres) and Contour SE—using particles of 40–120, 100–300, 300–500, and 500–1000 μm in size. The optimal diameter of the particles for TACE has yet to be defined. Consistently higher objective response rates are reported for arterial administration of drugs together with some form of hepatic artery occlusion compared with any form of systemic chemotherapy to date. The widespread use of some form of embolization in addition to chemotherapy has added to its toxicities. These include a frequent but transient fever, abdominal pain, and anorexia (all in >60% of patients). In addition, >20% of patients have increased ascites or transient elevation of transaminases. Cystic artery spasm and cholecystitis are also not uncommon. However, higher responses have also been obtained. The hepatic toxicities associated with embolization may be ameliorated by the use of degradable starch microspheres, with 50–60% response rates. Two randomized studies of TACE versus placebo showed a survival advantage for treatment (Table 111-6). In addition, it is not clear that formal oncologic CT response criteria are adequate for HCC. A loss of vascularity on CT without size change may be an index of loss of viability and thus of response to TACE. A major problem that TACE trials have had in showing a survival advantage is that many HCC patients die of their underlying cirrhosis, not the tumor. Nevertheless, two randomized controlled trials, one using doxorubicin and the other using cisplatin, showed a survival advantage for TACE versus placebo (Table 111-6). However, improving quality of life is a legitimate goal of regional therapy. Drug-eluting beads using doxorubicin (DEB-TACE) have been claimed to produce equivalent survival with less toxicity, but this strategy has not been tested in a randomized trial.

Kinase Inhibitors A survival advantage has been observed for the oral multikinase inhibitor, sorafenib (Nexavar), versus placebo in two randomized trials. It targets both the Raf mitogenic pathway and the vascular endothelial growth factor receptor (VEGFR) endothelial vasculogenesis pathway. However, tumor responses were negligible, and the survival in the treatment arm in Asians was less than the placebo arm in the Western trial (Table 111-7). Sorafenib has considerable toxicity, with 30–40% of patients requiring "drug holidays," dose reductions, or cessation of therapy. The most common toxicities include fatigue, hypertension, diarrhea, mucositis, and skin changes, such as the painful hand-foot syndrome, hair loss, and itching, each in 20–40% of patients. Several "look-alike" new agents that also target angiogenesis have either proved to be inferior or more toxic. These include sunitinib, brivanib, linifanib, everolimus, and bevacizumab (Table 111-8). The idea of angiogenesis alone as a major HCC therapeutic target may need revision.

New Therapies Although prolonged survival has been reported in phase II trials using newer agents, such as bevacizumab plus

TABLE 111-7 TARGETED THERAPIES IN HEPATOCELLULAR CARCINOMA: TRIALS

Phase III	Target	Survival (mo)
Sorafenib vs placebo	Raf, VEGFR, PDGFR	10.7 vs 7.9
Sorafenib vs placebo (Asians)	Raf, VEGFR, PDGFR	6.5 vs 4.2

Abbreviations: PDGFR, platelet-derived growth factor receptor; Raf, rapidly accelerated fibrosarcoma; VEGFR vascular endothelial growth factor receptor.

erlotinib, the data from a phase III trial were disappointing. Several forms of *radiation therapy* have been used in the treatment of HCC, including external-beam radiation and conformal radiation therapy. Radiation hepatitis remains a dose-limiting problem. The pure beta emitter ^{90}Yttrium attached to either glass (TheraSphere) or resin (SIR-Spheres) microspheres injected into a major branch hepatic artery has been assessed in phase II trials of HCC and has encouraging tumor control and survival effects with minimal toxicities. Randomized phase III trials comparing it to TACE have yet to be completed. The main attractiveness of ^{90}Yttrium therapy is its safety in the presence of major branch portal vein thrombosis, where TACE is dangerous or contraindicated. Furthermore, external-beam radiation has been reported to be safe and useful in the control of major branch portal or hepatic vein invasion (thrombosis) by tumors. The studies have all been small. Vitamin K has been assessed in clinical trials at high dosage for its HCC-inhibitory actions. This idea is based on the characteristic biochemical defect in HCC of elevated plasma levels of immature prothrombin (DCP or PIVKA-2), due to a defect in the activity of prothrombin carboxylase, a vitamin K–dependent enzyme. Two vitamin K randomized controlled trials from Japan show decreased tumor occurrence, but a major phase III trial aimed at limiting postresection recurrence was not successful.

CURRENT DIRECTIONS A number of new kinase inhibitors are being evaluated for HCC (**Tables 111-9 and 111-10**). These include the biologicals, such as Raf kinase and vascular endothelial growth factor (VEGF) inhibitors, and agents that target various steps of the cell growth pathway. Current hopes focus particularly on the Met pathway inhibitors such as tivantinib and several IGF receptor antagonists. ^{90}Yttrium looks promising and without chemotherapy toxicities. It is particularly attractive because, unlike TACE, it seems safe in the presence of portal vein thrombosis, a pathognomonic feature of HCC aggressiveness. The bottleneck of liver donors for OLTX is at last widening with increasing use of living donors, and criteria for OLTX for larger HCCs are slowly expanding. Patient participation in clinical trials assessing new therapies is encouraged (*www.clinicaltrials.gov*).

The main effort now is the evaluation of combinations of the compounds listed in Tables 111-7 to 111-9 that target different pathways, as well as the combination of any of these targeted therapies, but especially sorafenib, with TACE or ^{90}Yttrium radioembolization. Combining TACE with sorafenib appears to be safe in phase II studies with promising survival data, but randomized studies are still in progress. The same is true for intra-arterial ^{90}Yttrium plus sorafenib as therapy for HCC and as bridge to transplant therapy.

TABLE 111-8 PROMISING TARGETED THERAPIES THAT FAILED THEIR CLINICAL TRIAL GOALS

Sunitinib
Brivanib
Linifanib
Everolimus
Erlotinib
ThermaDox
Oncolytic virus JX-594
Bevacizumab
Bevacizumab plus erlotinib vs sorafenib
Sorafenib plus erlotinib vs sorafenib

TABLE 111-9 NEW TARGETED AGENTS AND THEIR TARGETS IN CURRENT CLINICAL TRIALS

Targets	Inhibitors
EGF receptor	Erlotinib
	Gefitinib
	Cetuximab
	Panitumumab
cMET	Tivantinib (ARQ197)
	EMD1204831
	Cabozantinib
VEGF receptor	Bevacizumab
	Regorafenib
	Brivanib
	Cediranib
	Sunitinib
FGF1 receptor	AEW54
	R1507 (MAb)
	Linsitinib (OSI-906)
	Brivanib
TRAIL-R1 (proapoptosis)	Mapatumumab
PDGF receptor	Sorafenib
	Dovitinib
	Linifanib
IGF-I receptor	IMC-A12
	B11B022
	Cixutumumab
Ubiquitin-proteasome	Bortezomib

Abbreviations: EGF, epidermal growth factor; FGF1, fibroblast growth factor 1; IGF-I, insulin-like growth factor I; PDGF, platelet-derived growth factor; VEGF, vascular endothelial growth factor.

SIGNIFICANCE AND EVALUATION OF RESPONSES TO NONSURGICAL THERAPIES Tumor growth or spread is considered a poor prognostic sign and evidence of treatment failure. By contrast, patients receiving chemotherapy are judged to have a response if there is shrinkage of tumor size. Lack of response/size decrease has been thought of as treatment failure. Three considerations in HCC management have completely changed the views concerning nonshrinkage after therapy. First, the correlation between response to chemotherapy and survival is poor in various tumors; in some tumors, such as ovarian cancer and small-cell lung cancer, substantial tumor shrinkage on chemotherapy is followed by rapid

TABLE 111-10 SOME NOVEL MEDICAL TREATMENTS FOR HEPATOCELLULAR CARCINOMA

EGF receptor antagonists: erlotinib, gefitinib, lapatinib, cetuximab, brivanib
Multikinase antagonists: sorafenib, sunitinib
VEGF antagonist: bevacizumab
VEGFR antagonist: ABT-869 (linifanib)
mTOR antagonists: sirolimus, temsirolimus, everolimus
Proteasome inhibitors: bortezomib
Vitamin K
^{131}I–Ethiodol (lipiodol)
^{131}I–Ferritin
^{90}Yttrium microspheres (TheraSphere, SIR-Spheres)
^{166}Holmium, ^{188}Rhenium
Three-dimensional conformal radiation
Proton beam high-dose radiotherapy
Gamma knife, CyberKnife
New targets: inhibitors of cyclin dependent kinases (Cdk), TRAIL induction caspases, and stem cells

Abbreviations: EGF, epidermal growth factor; mTOR, mammalian target of rapamycin; VEGF, vascular endothelial growth factor; VEGFR, vascular endothelial growth factor receptor.

tumor regrowth. Second, the Sorafenib HCC Assessment Randomized Protocol (SHARP) phase III trial of sorafenib versus placebo for unresectable HCC showed that survival could be significantly enhanced in the treatment arm with only 2% of the patients having tumor response but 70% of patients having disease stabilization. This observation has led to a reconsideration of the usefulness of response and the significance of disease stability. Third, HCC is a typically highly vascular tumor, and the vascularity is considered to be a measure of tumor viability. As a result, the Response Evaluation Criteria in Solid Tumors (RECIST) have been modified to mRECIST, which requires measurement of vascular/viable tumor on the CT or MRI scan. A partial response is defined as a 30% decrease in the sum of diameters of viable (arterially enhancing) target tumors. The need for semiquantitation of tumor vascularity on scans has led to the introduction of diffusion-weighted MRI imaging. Tissue-specific imaging agents such as gadoxetic acid (Primovist or Eovist) and the move to functional and genetic imaging mark a shift in approaches. Furthermore, plasma AFP response may be a biologic marker of radiologic response.

TREATMENT SUMMARY

Long-term survival is associated with resection or ablation or transplantation, all of which can yield >70% 5-year survival. Liver transplant is the only therapy that can treat the tumor and the underlying liver disease simultaneously and may be the most important advance in HCC therapy in 50 years. Unfortunately, it benefits only patients with limited size tumors without macrovascular portal vein invasion. Untreated patients with multinodular asymptomatic tumors without vascular invasion or extrahepatic spread have a median survival of approximately 16 months. Chemoembolization (TACE) improves their median survival to 19–20 months and is considered standard therapy for these patients, who represent the majority of HCC patients, although ^{90}Yttrium therapy may provide similar results with less toxicity. Patients with advanced-stage disease, vascular invasion, or metastases have a median survival of around 6 months. Among this group, outcomes may vary according to their underlying liver disease. It is this group at which kinase inhibitors are directed.

SUMMARY (TABLE 111-5)

The Most Common Modes of Patient Presentation

1. A patient with known history of hepatitis, jaundice, or cirrhosis, with an abnormality on ultrasound or CT scan, or rising AFP or DCP (PIVKA-2)
2. A patient with an abnormal liver function test as part of a routine examination
3. Radiologic workup for liver transplant for cirrhosis
4. Symptoms of HCC including cachexia, abdominal pain, or fever

History and Physical Examination

1. Clinical jaundice, asthenia, itching (scratches), tremors, or disorientation
2. Hepatomegaly, splenomegaly, ascites, peripheral edema, skin signs of liver failure

Clinical Evaluation

1. Blood tests: full blood count (splenomegaly), liver function tests, ammonia levels, electrolytes, AFP and DCP (PIVKA-2), Ca^{2+} and Mg^{2+}; hepatitis B, C, and D serology (and quantitative HBV DNA or HCV RNA, if either is positive); neurotensin (specific for fibrolamellar HCC)
2. Triphasic dynamic helical (spiral) CT scan of liver (if inadequate, then follow with an MRI); chest CT scan; upper and lower gastrointestinal endoscopy (for varices, bleeding, ulcers); and brain scan (only if symptoms suggest)
3. Core biopsy: of the tumor and separate biopsy of the underlying liver

Therapy (Tables 111-5 and 111-6)

1. HCC <2 cm: RFA, PEI, or resection
2. HCC >2 cm, no vascular invasion: liver resection, RFA, or OLTX
3. Multiple unilobar tumors or tumor with vascular invasion: TACE or sorafenib
4. Bilobar tumors, no vascular invasion: TACE with OLTX for patients with tumor response
5. Extrahepatic HCC or elevated bilirubin: sorafenib or bevacizumab plus erlotinib (combination agent trials are in progress)

OTHER PRIMARY LIVER TUMORS

FIBROLAMELLAR HCC (FL-HCC)

This rarer variant of HCC has a quite different biology than adult-type HCC. None of the known HCC causative factors seem important here. It is typically a disease of younger adults, often teenagers and predominantly females. It is AFP-negative, but patients typically have elevated blood neurotensin levels, normal liver function tests, and no cirrhosis. Radiology is similar for HCC, except that characteristic adult-type portal vein invasion is less common. Although it is often multifocal in the liver, and therefore not resectable, metastases are common, especially to lungs and locoregional lymph nodes, but survival is often much better than with adult-type HCC. Resectable tumors are associated with 5-year survival ≥50%. Patients often present with a huge liver or unexplained weight loss, fever, or elevated liver function tests on routine evaluations. These huge masses suggest quite slow growth for many tumors. Surgical resection is the best management option, even for metastases, as these tumors respond much less well to chemotherapy than adult-type HCC. Although several series of OLTX for FL-HCC have been reported, the patients seem to die from tumor recurrences, with a 2- to 5-year lag compared with OLTX for adult-type HCC. Anecdotal responses to gemcitabine plus cisplatin-TACE are reported.

Epithelioid Hemangioendothelioma (EHE) This rare vascular tumor of adults is also usually multifocal and can also be associated with prolonged survival, even in the presence of metastases, which are commonly in the lung. There is usually no underlying cirrhosis. Histologically, these tumors are usually of borderline malignancy and express factor VIII, confirming their endothelial origin. OLTX may produce prolonged survival.

Cholangiocarcinoma (CCC) CCC typically refers to mucin-producing adenocarcinomas (different from HCC) that arise from the biliary tract and have features of cholangiocyte differentiation. They are grouped by their anatomic site of origin, as intrahepatic (IHC), perihilar (central, ~65% of CCCs), and peripheral (or distal, ~30% of CCCs). IHC is the second most common primary liver tumor. Depending on the site of origin, they have different features and require different treatments. They arise on the basis of cirrhosis less frequently than HCC, but may complicate primary biliary cirrhosis. However, cirrhosis and both primary biliary cirrhosis and HCV predispose to IHC. Nodular tumors arising at the bifurcation of the common bile duct are called *Klatskin* tumors and are often associated with a collapsed gallbladder, a finding that mandates visualization of the entire biliary tree. The approach to management of central and peripheral CCC is quite different. Incidence is increasing. Although most CCCs have no obvious cause (etiology unknown), a number of predisposing factors have been identified. Predisposing diseases include primary sclerosing cholangitis (10–20% of primary sclerosing cholangitis [PSC] patients), an autoimmune disease, and liver fluke in Asians, especially *Opisthorchis viverrini* and *Clonorchis sinensis*. CCC seems also to be associated with any cause of chronic biliary inflammation and injury, with alcoholic liver disease, choledocholithiasis, choledochal cysts (10%), and Caroli's disease (a rare inherited form of bile duct ectasia). CCC most typically presents as painless jaundice, often with pruritus or weight loss. Diagnosis is made by biopsy, percutaneously for peripheral liver lesions, or more commonly via endoscopic retrograde cholangiopancreatography (ERCP) under direct vision for central lesions. The tumors often stain positively for cytokeratins 7, 8, and 19 and negatively for cytokeratin 20. However, histology alone cannot usually distinguish CCC from metastases from colon or pancreas primary tumors. Serologic tumor markers appear to be nonspecific, but CEA, CA 19-9, and CA-125 are often elevated in CCC patients and are useful for following response to therapy. Radiologic evaluation typically starts with ultrasound, which is very useful in visualizing dilated bile ducts, and then proceeds with either MRI or magnetic resonance cholangiopancreatography (MRCP) or helical CT scans. Invasive cholangiopancreatography (ERCP) is then needed to define the biliary tree and obtain a biopsy or is needed therapeutically to decompress an obstructed biliary tree with internal stent placement. If that fails, then percutaneous biliary drainage will be needed, with the biliary drainage flowing into an external bag. Central tumors often invade the porta hepatis, and locoregional lymph node involvement by tumor is frequent. Incidence has been increasing in recent decades; few patients survive 5 years. The usual treatment is surgical, but combination systemic chemotherapy may be effective. After complete surgical resection for IHC, 5-year survival is 25–30%. Combination radiation therapy with liver transplant has produced a 5-year recurrence-free survival rate of 65%.

TREATMENT CHOLANGIOCARCINOMA

Hilar CCC is resectable in ~30% of patients and usually involves bile duct resection and lymphadenectomy for prognostication. Typical survival is approximately 24 months, with recurrences being mainly in the operative bed but with ~30% in the lungs and liver. Distal CCC, which involves the main ducts, is normally treated by resection of the extrahepatic bile ducts, often with pancreaticoduodenectomy. Survival is similar. Due to the high rates of locoregional recurrences or positive surgical margins, many patients receive postoperative adjuvant radiotherapy. Its effect on survival has not been assessed. Intraluminal brachyradiotherapy has also shown some promise. However, photodynamic therapy enhanced survival in one study. In this technique, sodium porfimer is injected intravenously and then subjected to intraluminal red light laser photoactivation. OLTX has been assessed for treatment of unresectable CCC. Five-year survival was ~20%, so enthusiasm waned. However, neoadjuvant radiotherapy with sensitizing chemotherapy has shown better survival rates for CCC treated by OLTX and is currently used by UNOS for perihilar CCC <3 cm with neither intrahepatic or extrahepatic metastases. A 12-center data collection study of 287 patients with perihilar CCC confirmed the benefit of this approach in a subset of patients, with a 53% 5-year survival rate but with 10% patient dropout before transplantation. The patients had neoadjuvant external radiation with radiosensitizing therapy. Patients with tumors >3 cm had significantly shorter survival. Multiple chemotherapeutic agents have been assessed for activity and survival in unresectable CCC. Most have been inactive. However, both systemic and hepatic arterial gemcitabine have shown promising results. The combination of cisplatin plus gemcitabine has produced a survival advantage compared with gemcitabine alone in a 410-patient randomized controlled phase III trial for patients with locally advanced or metastatic CCC and is now considered standard therapy for unresectable CCC. Median overall survival in the combination arm was 11.7 months versus 8.1 months for gemcitabine alone. Significant responses were seen mainly in patients with IHC and gallbladder cancer. However, neither surgery for lymph node–positive disease nor regional chemotherapy in nonsurgical patients has shown any survival advantage thus far. Several case series have shown safety and some responses for hepatic arterial chemotherapy with gemcitabine, drug-eluting beads, and ^{90}Yttrium microspheres, but no convincing clinical trials are available. Clinical trials are under way with targeted therapies. Bevacizumab plus erlotinib gave a 10% partial response rate with median overall survival of 9.9 months. A sorafenib trial yielded an overall survival of 4.4 months, but 50% of the patients had received previous chemotherapy. Patients with unresectable tumors should be treated in clinical trials.

GALLBLADDER CANCER

Gallbladder (GB) cancer has an even worse prognosis than CCC, with a typical survival of ~6 months or less. Women are affected much more commonly than men (4:1), unlike HCC or CCC, and GB cancer occurs more frequently than CCC. Most patients have a history of antecedent gallstones, but very few patients with gallstones develop GB cancer (~0.2%). GB cancer presents similarly to CCC and is often diagnosed unexpectedly during gallstone or cholecystitis surgery. Presentation is typically that of chronic cholecystitis, chronic right upper quadrant pain, and weight loss. Useful but nonspecific serum markers include CEA and CA 19-9. CT scans or MRCP typically reveal a GB mass. The mainstay of treatment is surgical, either simple or radical cholecystectomy for stage I or II disease, respectively. Survival rates are near 100% at 5 years for stage I, and range from 60–90% at 5 years for stage II. More advanced GB cancer has worse survival, and many patients are unresectable. Adjuvant radiotherapy, used in the presence of local lymph node disease, has not been shown to enhance survival. Chemotherapy is not useful in advanced or metastatic GB cancer.

CARCINOMA OF THE AMPULLA OF VATER

This tumor arises within 2 cm of the distal end of the common bile duct and is mainly (90%) an adenocarcinoma. Locoregional lymph nodes are commonly involved (50%), and the liver is the most frequent site for metastases. The most common clinical presentation is jaundice, and many patients also have pruritus, weight loss, and epigastric pain. Initial evaluation is performed with an abdominal ultrasound to assess vascular involvement, biliary dilation, and liver lesions. This is followed by a CT scan or MRI and especially MRCP. The most effective therapy is resection by pylorus-sparing pancreaticoduodenectomy, an aggressive procedure resulting in better survival rates than with local resection. Survival rates are ~25% at 5 years in operable patients with involved lymph nodes and 50% in patients without involved nodes. Unlike CCC, approximately 80% of patients are thought to be resectable at diagnosis. Adjuvant chemotherapy or radiotherapy has not been shown to enhance survival. For metastatic tumors, chemotherapy is currently experimental.

TUMORS METASTATIC TO THE LIVER

These are predominantly from colon, pancreas, and breast primary tumors but can originate from any organ primary. Ocular melanomas are prone to liver metastasis. Tumor spread to the liver normally carries a poor prognosis for that tumor type. Colorectal and breast hepatic metastases were previously treated with continuous hepatic arterial infusion chemotherapy. However, more effective systemic drugs for each of these two cancers, especially the addition of oxaliplatin to colorectal cancer regimens, have reduced the use of hepatic artery infusion therapy. In a large randomized study of systemic versus infusional plus systemic chemotherapy for resected colorectal metastases to the liver, the patients receiving infusional therapy had no survival advantage, mainly due to extrahepatic tumor spread. ^{90}Yttrium resin beads are approved in the United States for treatment of colorectal hepatic metastases. The role of this modality, either alone or in combination with chemotherapy, is being evaluated in many centers. Palliation may be obtained from chemoembolization, PEI, or RFA.

BENIGN LIVER TUMORS

Three common benign tumors occur and all are found predominantly in women. They are *hemangiomas, adenomas,* and *focal nodular hyperplasia* (FNH). FNH is typically benign, and usually no treatment is needed. Hemangiomas are the most common and are entirely benign. Treatment is unnecessary unless their expansion causes symptoms. Adenomas are associated with contraceptive hormone use. They can cause pain and can bleed or rupture, causing acute problems. Their main interest for the physician is a low potential for malignant change and a 30% risk of bleeding. For this reason, considerable effort has gone into differentiating these three entities radiologically. On discovery of a liver mass, patients are usually advised to stop taking sex steroids, because adenoma regression may then occasionally occur. Adenomas can often be large masses ranging from 8–15 cm. Due to their size and definite, but low, malignant potential and potential for bleeding, adenomas are typically resected. The most useful diagnostic differentiating tool is a triphasic CT scan performed with HCC fast bolus protocol for arterial-phase imaging, together with subsequent delayed venous-phase imaging. Adenomas usually do not appear on the basis of cirrhosis, although both adenomas and HCCs are intensely vascular on the CT arterial phase and both can exhibit hemorrhage (40% of adenomas). However, adenomas have smooth, well-defined edges, and enhance homogeneously, especially in the portal venous phase on delayed images, when HCCs no longer enhance. FNHs exhibit a characteristic central scar that is hypovascular on the arterial-phase and hypervascular on the delayed-phase CT images. MRI is even more sensitive in depicting the characteristic central scar of FNH.

112 Pancreatic Cancer

Elizabeth Smyth, David Cunningham

Pancreatic cancer is the fourth leading cause of cancer death in the United States and is associated with a poor prognosis. Endocrine tumors affecting the pancreas are discussed in Chap. 113. Infiltrating ductal adenocarcinomas, the subject of this Chapter, account for the vast majority of cases and arise most frequently in the head of pancreas. At the time of diagnosis, 85–90% of patients have inoperable or metastatic disease, which is reflected in the 5-year survival rate of only 6% for all stages combined. An improved 5-year survival of up to 24% may be achieved when the tumor is detected at an early stage and when complete surgical resection is accomplished.

EPIDEMIOLOGY

Pancreatic cancer represents 3% of all newly diagnosed malignancies in the United States. The most common age group at diagnosis is 65–84 years for both sexes. Pancreatic cancer was estimated to have been diagnosed in approximately 45,220 patients and accounted for approximately 38,460 deaths in 2013. Although survival rates have almost doubled over the past 35 years for this disease, overall survival remains low.

GLOBAL CONSIDERATIONS

An estimated 278,684 cases of pancreatic cancer occur annually worldwide (the thirteenth most common cancer globally), with up to 60% of these cases diagnosed in more developed countries. It remains the eighth most common cause of cancer death in men and the ninth most common in women. The incidence is highest in the United States and western Europe and lowest in parts of Africa and South Central Asia. However, increasing rates of obesity, diabetes, and tobacco use in addition to access to diagnostic radiology in the developing world are likely to increase incidence rates in these countries. In this situation, consideration of the cost implications of adoption of current treatment paradigms in resource-constrained environments will be necessary. Primary prevention such as limiting tobacco use and avoiding obesity may be more cost effective than improvements in treatment of preexisting disease.

RISK FACTORS

Cigarette smoking may be the cause of up to 20–25% of all pancreatic cancers and is the most common environmental risk factor for this disease. A longstanding history of type 1 or type 2 diabetes also appears to be a risk factor; however, diabetes may also occur in association with pancreatic cancer, possibly confounding this interpretation. Other risk factors may include obesity, chronic pancreatitis, and ABO blood group status. Alcohol does not appear to be a risk factor unless excess consumption gives rise to chronic pancreatitis.

GENETIC AND MOLECULAR CONSIDERATIONS

Pancreatic cancer is associated with a number of well-defined molecular hallmarks. The four genes most commonly mutated or inactivated in pancreatic cancer are *KRAS* (predominantly codon 12, in 60–75% of pancreatic cancers), the tumor-suppressor genes *p16* (deleted in 95% of tumors), *p53* (inactivated or mutated in 50–70% of tumors), and *SMAD4* (deleted in 55% of tumors). The pancreatic cancer precursor lesion pancreatic intraepithelial neoplasia (PanIN) acquires these genetic abnormalities in a progressive manner associated with increasing dysplasia; initial *KRAS* mutations are followed by *p16* loss and finally *p53* and *SMAD4* alterations. *SMAD4* gene inactivation is associated with a pattern of widespread metastatic disease in advanced-stage patients and poorer survival in patients with surgically resected pancreatic adenocarcinoma.

Up to 16% of pancreatic cancers may be inherited. Germline mutations in the following genes are associated with a significantly increased risk of pancreatic cancer and other cancers: (1) *STK11* gene (Peutz-Jeghers syndrome), which carries a 132-fold increased lifetime risk of pancreatic cancer above the general population; (2) *BRCA2* (increased risk of breast, ovarian, and pancreatic cancer); (3) *p16/CDKN2A* (familial atypical multiple mole melanoma), which carries an increased risk of melanoma and pancreatic cancer; (4) *PALB2*, which confers an increased risk of breast and pancreatic cancer; (5) *hMLH1* and *MSH2* (Lynch syndrome), which carries an increased risk of colon and pancreatic cancer; and (6) *ATM* (ataxia-telangiectasia), which carries an increased risk of breast cancer, lymphoma, and pancreatic cancer. Familial pancreatitis and an increased risk of pancreatic cancer are associated with mutations of the *PRSS1* (serine protease 1) gene. However, for most familial pancreatic syndromes, the underlying genetic cause remains unexplained. The absolute number of affected first-degree relatives is also correlated with increased cancer risk, and patients with at least two first-degree relatives with pancreatic cancer should be considered to have familial pancreatic cancer until proven otherwise.

The desmoplastic stroma surrounding pancreatic adenocarcinoma functions as a mechanical barrier to chemotherapy and secretes compounds essential for tumor progression and metastasis. Key mediators of these functions include the activated pancreatic stellate cell and the glycoprotein SPARC (secreted protein acidic and rich in cysteine), which is expressed in 80% of pancreatic ductal adenocarcinomas. Targeting this extracellular environment has become increasingly important in the treatment of advanced disease.

SCREENING AND PRECURSOR LESIONS

Screening is not routinely recommended because the incidence of pancreatic cancer in the general population is low (lifetime risk 1.3%), putative tumor markers such as carbohydrate antigen 19-9 (CA19-9) and carcinoembryonic antigen (CEA) have insufficient sensitivity, and computed tomography (CT) has inadequate resolution to detect pancreatic dysplasia. Endoscopic ultrasound (EUS) is a more promising screening tool, and preclinical efforts are focused on identifying biomarkers that may detect pancreatic cancer at an early stage. Consensus practice recommendations based largely on expert opinion have chosen a threshold of greater than fivefold increased risk for developing pancreatic cancer to select individuals who may benefit from screening. This includes people with two or more first-degree relatives with pancreatic cancer, patients with Peutz-Jeghers syndrome, and *BRCA* 2, *p16*, and hereditary nonpolyposis colorectal cancer (HNPCC) mutation carriers with one or more affected first-degree relatives.

PanIN represents a spectrum of small (<5 mm) neoplastic but noninvasive precursor lesions of the pancreatic ductal epithelium demonstrating mild, moderate, or severe dysplasia (PanIN 1–3, respectively); however, not all PanIN lesions will progress to frank invasive malignancy. Cystic pancreatic tumors such as intraductal mucinous papillary neoplasms (IPMNs) and mucinous cystic neoplasms (MCNs) are increasingly detected radiologically and are frequently asymptomatic. Main duct IPMNs are more likely to occur in older persons and have higher malignant potential than branched duct IPMNs (invasive cancer in 45% vs 18% of resected lesions, respectively). In contrast, MCNs are solitary lesions of the distal pancreas that do not communicate with the duct system. MCNs have an almost exclusive female distribution (95%). The rate of invasive cancer in resected MCNs is lower (<18%) with increased rates associated with larger tumors or the presence of nodules.

CLINICAL FEATURES

Clinical Presentation Obstructive jaundice occurs frequently when the cancer is located in the head of the pancreas. This may be accompanied by symptoms of abdominal discomfort, pruritus, lethargy, and weight loss. Less common presenting features include epigastric pain, backache, new-onset diabetes mellitus, and acute pancreatitis caused by pressure effects on the pancreatic duct. Nausea and vomiting, resulting from gastroduodenal obstruction, may also be a symptom of this disease.

Physical Signs Patients can present with jaundice and cachexia, and scratch marks may be present. Of patients with operable tumors, 25% have a palpable gallbladder (Courvoisier's sign). Physical signs related to the development of distant metastases include hepatomegaly, ascites, left supraclavicular lymphadenopathy (Virchow's node), and periumbilical nodules (Sister Mary Joseph's nodes).

DIAGNOSIS

Diagnostic Imaging Patients who present with clinical features suggestive of pancreatic cancer undergo imaging to confirm the presence of a tumor and to establish whether the mass is likely to be inflammatory or malignant in nature. Other imaging objectives include the local and distant staging of the tumor, which will determine resectability and provide prognostic information. Dual-phase, contrast-enhanced spiral CT is the imaging modality of choice (Fig. 112-1). It provides accurate visualization of surrounding viscera, vessels, and lymph nodes, thus determining tumor resectability. Intestinal infiltration and liver and lung metastases are also reliably depicted on CT. There is no advantage of magnetic resonance imaging (MRI) over CT in predicting tumor resectability, but selected cases may benefit from MRI to characterize the nature of small indeterminate liver lesions and to evaluate the cause of biliary dilatation when no obvious mass is seen on CT. Endoscopic retrograde cholangiopancreatography (ERCP) is useful for revealing small pancreatic lesions, identifying stricture or obstruction in pancreatic or common bile ducts, and facilitating stent placement; however, it is associated with a risk of pancreatitis (Fig. 112-2). Magnetic resonance cholangiopancreatography (MRCP) is a noninvasive method for accurately depicting the level and degree of bile and pancreatic duct dilatation. EUS is highly sensitive in detecting lesions less than 3 cm in size (more sensitive than CT for lesions <2 cm) and is useful as a local staging tool for assessing vascular invasion and lymph node involvement. Fluorodeoxyglucose positron emission tomography (FDG-PET) should be considered before surgery or radical chemoradiotherapy (CRT), because it is superior to conventional imaging in detecting distant metastases.

Tissue Diagnosis and Cytology Preoperative confirmation of malignancy is not always necessary in patients with radiologic appearances consistent with operable pancreatic cancer. However, EUS-guided fine-needle aspiration is the technique of choice when there is any doubt, and also for use in patients who require neoadjuvant treatment. It has an accuracy of approximately 90% and has a smaller risk of intraperitoneal dissemination compared with the percutaneous route.

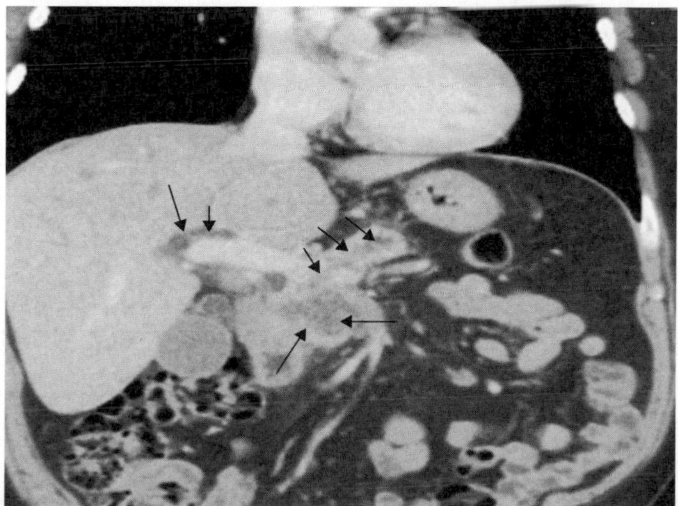

FIGURE 112-1 Coronal computed tomography showing pancreatic cancer and dilated intrahepatic and pancreatic ducts (*arrows*).

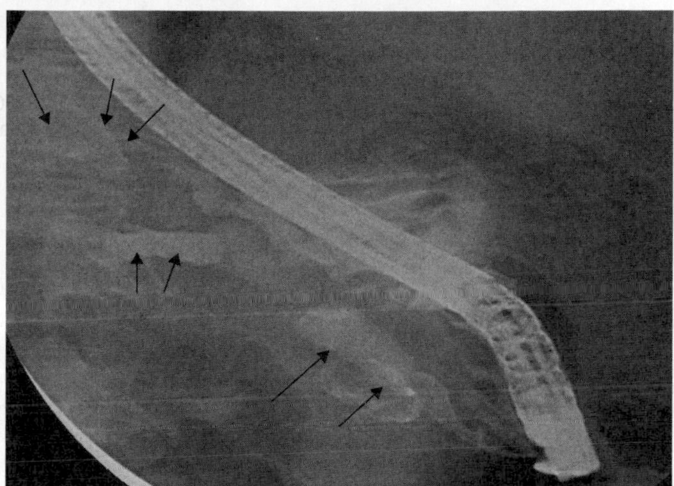

FIGURE 112-2 Endoscopic retrograde cholangiopancreatography showing contrast in dilated pancreatic duct (*arrows*).

Percutaneous biopsy of the pancreatic primary or liver metastases is only acceptable in patients with inoperable or metastatic disease. ERCP is a useful method for obtaining ductal brushings, but the sensitivity of ERCP for diagnosis ranges from 35 to 70%.

Serum Markers Tumor-associated CA19-9 is elevated in approximately 70–80% of patients with pancreatic carcinoma but is not recommended as a routine diagnostic or screening test because its sensitivity and specificity are inadequate for accurate diagnosis. Preoperative CA19-9 levels correlate with tumor stage, and postresection CA19-9 level has prognostic value. It is an indicator of asymptomatic recurrence in patients with completely resected tumors and is used as a biomarker of response in patients with advanced disease undergoing chemotherapy. A number of studies have established a high pretreatment CA19-9 level as an independent prognostic factor.

STAGING

The American Joint Committee on Cancer (AJCC) tumor-node-metastasis (TNM) staging of pancreatic cancer takes into account the location and size of the tumor, the involvement of lymph nodes, and distant metastasis. This information is then combined to assign a stage (Fig. 112-3). From a practical standpoint, patients are grouped according to whether the cancer is resectable, locally advanced (unresectable, but without distant spread), or metastatic.

TREATMENT PANCREATIC CANCER

RESECTABLE DISEASE

Approximately 10% of patients present with localized nonmetastatic disease that is potentially suitable for surgical resection. Approximately 30% of patients have R1 resection (microscopic residual disease) following surgery. Those who undergo R0 resection (no microscopic or macroscopic residual tumor) and who receive adjuvant treatment have the best chance of cure, with an estimated median survival of 20–23 months and a 5-year survival of approximately 20%. Outcomes are more favorable in patients with small (<3 cm), well-differentiated tumors and lymph node–negative disease.

Patients should have surgery in dedicated pancreatic centers that have lower postoperative morbidity and mortality rates. The standard surgical procedure for patients with tumors of the pancreatic head or uncinate process is a pylorus-preserving pancreaticoduodenectomy (modified Whipple's procedure). The procedure of choice for tumors of the pancreatic body and tail is a distal pancreatectomy, which routinely includes splenectomy.

Postoperative treatment improves long-term outcomes in this group of patients. Adjuvant chemotherapy comprising six cycles of gemcitabine is common practice worldwide based on data from three randomized controlled trials (Table 112-1). The Charité

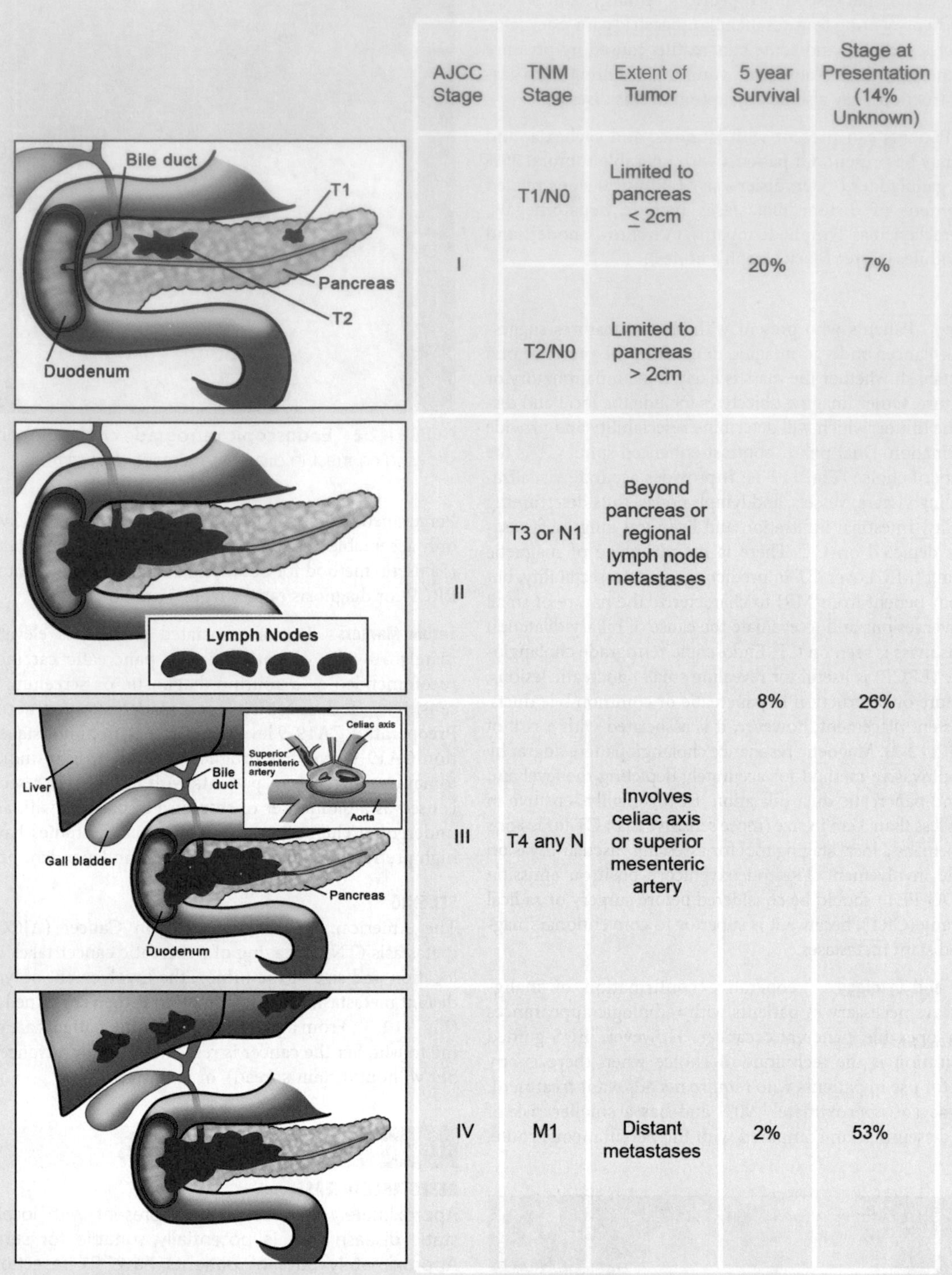

FIGURE 112-3 Staging of pancreatic cancer, and survival according to stage. AJCC, American Joint Committee on Cancer. *(Illustration by Stephen Millward.)*

TABLE 112-1 PHASE III STUDIES OF ADJUVANT CHEMOTHERAPY IN RESECTED PANCREATIC CANCER

			Survival	
Study	**Comparator Arm**	**No. of Patients**	**PFS/DFS (months)**	**Median Survival (months)**
ESPAC-1, Neoptolemos et al: N Engl J Med 350:1200, 2004	Chemotherapy (folinic acid + bolus 5-FU) vs no chemotherapy	289	PFS 15.3 vs 9.4. (p = .02)	20.1 vs 15.5 (HR 0.71; 95% CI 0.55–0.92; p = .009)
CONKO 001, Oettle et al: JAMA 297:267, 2007	Gemcitabine vs observation	368	Median DFS 13.4 vs 6.9 (p <.001)	22.1 vs 20.2 (p = .06)
ESPAC-3, Neoptolemos et al: JAMA 304:1073, 2010	5-FU/LV vs gemcitabine	1088		23 vs 23.6 (HR 0.94; 95% CI 0.81–1.08, p = .39)

Abbreviations: CI, confidence interval; CONKO, Charité Onkologie; DFS, disease-free survival; ESPAC, European Study Group for Pancreatic Cancer; 5-FU, 5-fluorouracil; HR, hazard ratio; LV, leucovorin; PFS, progression-free survival.

TABLE 112-2 SELECTED PHASE III STUDIES EVALUATING CHEMOTHERAPY TREATMENT IN ADVANCED PANCREATIC CANCER

Study	Comparator Arm	No. of Patients	Survival	
			PFS (months)	Median Survival (months)
Moore et al: J Clin Oncol 26:1960, 2007	Gemcitabine vs gemcitabine + erlotinib	569	3.55 vs 3.75 (HR 0.77; 95% CI 0.64–0.92; $p = .004$)	5.91 vs 6.24 (HR 0.82; 95% CI 0.69–0.99; $p = .038$)
Cunningham et al: J Clin Oncol 27:5513, 2009	Gemcitabine vs gemcitabine + capecitabine (GEM-CAP)	533	3.8 vs 5.3 (HR 0.78; 95% CI 0.66–0.93; $p = .004$)	6.2 vs 7.1 (HR 0.86; 95% CI 0.72–1.02; $p = .08$)
Von Hoff et al: N Engl J Med 369:1691, 2013	Gemcitabine vs gemcitabine + nab-paclitaxel	861	3.7 vs 5.5 (HR 0.69; 95% CI 0.58–0.82; $p < .001$)	6.7 vs 8.5 (HR 0.72; 95% CI 0.62–0.83; $p < .001$)
Conroy et al: N Engl J Med 364:1817, 2011	Gemcitabine vs FOLFIRINOX	342	3.3 vs 6.4 (HR 0.47; 95% CI 0.37–0.59; $p < .001$)	6.8 vs 11.1 (HR 0.57; 95% CI 0.45–0.73; $p < .001$)

Onkologie trial (CONKO 001) found that the use of gemcitabine after complete resection significantly delayed the development of recurrent disease compared with surgery alone. The European Study Group for Pancreatic Cancer 3 (ESPAC-3) trial, which investigated the benefit of adjuvant 5-fluorouracil/folinic acid (5-FU/FA) versus gemcitabine, revealed no survival difference between the two drugs. However, the toxicity profile of adjuvant gemcitabine was superior to 5-FU/FA by virtue of its lower incidence of stomatitis and diarrhea. Adjuvant radiotherapy is not commonly used in Europe based on the negative results of the ESPAC-1 study. Adjuvant 5-FU-based CRT with gemcitabine before and after radiotherapy as used in the Radiation Therapy Oncology Group (RTOG) 97-04 trial is preferred in the United States. This approach may be most beneficial in patients with bulky tumors involving the pancreatic head.

INOPERABLE LOCALLY ADVANCED DISEASE

Approximately 30% of patients present with locally advanced, unresectable, but nonmetastatic pancreatic carcinoma. The median survival with gemcitabine is 9 months. Patients who respond to chemotherapy or who achieve stable disease after 3–6 months of gemcitabine have frequently been offered consolidation radiotherapy. However, a large, phase III, randomized controlled trial, LAP-07, did not demonstrate any improvement in survival for patients treated with CRT after 4 months of disease control on either gemcitabine or a gemcitabine/erlotinib combination.

METASTATIC DISEASE

Approximately 60% of patients with pancreatic cancer present with metastatic disease. Patients with poor performance status do not usually benefit from chemotherapy. Gemcitabine was the standard treatment with a median survival of 6 months and a 1-year survival rate of only 20%. The addition of nab-paclitaxel (an albumin bound nanoparticle formulation of paclitaxel) to gemcitabine results in significantly improved 1-year survival compared to gemcitabine alone (35% vs 22%, $p < .001$). Capecitabine, an oral fluoropyrimidine, has also been combined with gemcitabine (GEM-CAP) in a phase III trial that showed an improvement in response rate and progression-free survival over single-agent gemcitabine, but no overall survival benefit. However, pooling of two other randomized controlled trials with this trial in a meta-analysis resulted in a survival advantage with GEM-CAP. Addition of erlotinib, a small-molecule epidermal growth factor receptor inhibitor, produced a statistically significant but clinically marginal benefit when added to gemcitabine in the advanced disease setting. A phase III trial limited to good performance status patients with metastatic pancreatic cancer showed improved survival with the combination of 5-FU/FA, irinotecan, and oxaliplatin (FOLFIRINOX) compared with gemcitabine, but with increased toxicity (Table 112-2).

FUTURE DIRECTIONS

The early detection and future treatment of pancreatic cancer relies on an improved understanding of molecular pathways involved in the development of this disease. This will ultimately lead to the discovery of novel agents and the identification of patient groups who are likely to benefit most from targeted therapy.

ACKNOWLEDGMENT

Dr. Irene Chong is acknowledged for her work on this chapter in the 18th edition.

113 Endocrine Tumors of the Gastrointestinal Tract and Pancreas

Robert T. Jensen

GENERAL FEATURES OF GASTROINTESTINAL NEUROENDOCRINE TUMORS

Gastrointestinal (GI) neuroendocrine tumors (NETs) are tumors derived from the diffuse neuroendocrine system of the GI tract; that system is composed of amine- and acid-producing cells with different hormonal profiles, depending on the site of origin. The tumors historically are divided into GI-NETs (in the GI tract) (also frequently called *carcinoid tumors*) and pancreatic neuroendocrine tumors (pNETs), although newer pathologic classifications have proposed that they all be classified as GI-NETs. The term *GI-NET* has been proposed to replace the term *carcinoid*; however, the term *carcinoid* is widely used, and many are not familiar with this change. Accordingly, this chapter will use the term *GI NETs* (carcinoids). These tumors originally were classified as APUDomas (for *a*mine *p*recursor *u*ptake and *d*ecarboxylation), as were pheochromocytomas, melanomas, and medullary thyroid carcinomas, because they share certain cytochemical features as well as various pathologic, biologic, and molecular features (Table 113-1). It was originally proposed that APUDomas had a similar embryonic origin from neural crest cells, but it is now known the peptide-secreting cells are not of neuroectodermal origin. Nevertheless, the concept of APUDomas is useful because these tumors have important similarities as well as some differences (Table 113-1). In this section, the areas of similarity between pNETs and GI-NETs (carcinoids) will be discussed together, and areas in which there are important differences will be discussed separately.

CLASSIFICATION/PATHOLOGY/TUMOR BIOLOGY OF NETs

NETs generally are composed of monotonous sheets of small round cells with uniform nuclei, and mitoses are uncommon. They can be identified tentatively on routine histology; however, these tumors are now recognized principally by their histologic staining patterns due to shared cellular proteins. Historically, silver staining was used, and

TABLE 113-1 GENERAL CHARACTERISTICS OF GASTROINTESTINAL NEUROENDOCRINE TUMORS (GI-NETs [CARCINOIDS], PANCREATIC NEUROENDOCRINE TUMORS [pNETs])

A. Share general neuroendocrine cell markers (identification used for diagnosis)
   1. Chromogranins (A, B, C) are acidic monomeric soluble proteins found in the large secretory granules. Chromogranin A is the most widely used.
   2. Neuron-specific enolase (NSE) is the γ-γ dimer of the enzyme enolase and is a cytosolic marker of neuroendocrine differentiation.
   3. Synaptophysin is an integral membrane glycoprotein of 38,000 molecular weight found in small vesicles of neurons and neuroendocrine tumors.

B. Pathologic similarities
   1. All are APUDomas showing *a*mine *p*recursor *u*ptake and *d*ecarboxylation.
   2. Ultrastructurally, they have dense-core secretory granules (>80 nm).
   3. Histologically, they generally appear similar with few mitoses and uniform nuclei.
   4. Frequently synthesize multiple peptides/amines, which can be detected immunocytochemically but may not be secreted.
   5. Presence or absence of clinical syndrome or type cannot be predicted by immunocytochemical studies.
   6. Histologic classifications (grading, TNM classification) have prognostic significance. Only invasion or metastases establish malignancy.

C. Similarities of biologic behavior
   1. Generally slow growing, but some are aggressive.
   2. Most are well-differentiated tumors having low proliferative indices.
   3. Secrete biologically active peptides/amines, which can cause clinical symptoms.
   4. Generally have high densities of somatostatin receptors, which are used for both localization and treatment.
   5. Most (>70%) secrete chromogranin A, which is frequently used as a tumor marker.

D. Similarities/differences in molecular abnormalities
   1. Similarities
      a. Uncommon—mutations in common oncogenes (*ras, jun, fos,* etc).
      b. Uncommon—mutations in common tumor-suppressor genes (*p53*, retinoblastoma).
      c. Alterations at MEN 1 locus (11q13) (frequently foregut, less commonly mid/hindgut NETs) and p16^{INK4a} (9p21) occur in a proportion (10–45%).
      d. Methylation of various genes occurs in 40–87% (*ras*-associated domain family I, p14, p16, O^6-methylguanine methyltransferases, retinoic acid receptor β).
   2. Differences
      a. pNETs—loss of 1p (21%), 3p (8–47%), 3q (8–41%), 11q (21–62%), 6q (18–68%), Y (45%). Gains at 17q (10–55%), 7q (16–68%), 4q (33%), 18 (up to 45%).
      b. GI-NETs (carcinoids)—loss of 18q (38–88%), >18p (33–43%), >9p, 16q21 (21–23%). Gains at 17q, 19p (57%), 4q (33%), 14q (20%), 5 (up to 36%).
      c. pNETs: *ATRX/DAXX* mutations in 43%, MEN 1 mutations in 44%, mTor mutations (14%); uncommon in midgut GI-NETs (0–2%).

Abbreviations: *ATRX*, alpha-thalassemia X-lined mental retardation protein; *DAXX*, death domain associated protein; *MEN 1*, multiple endocrine neoplasia type 1; TNM, tumor, node, metastasis.

tumors were classified as showing an argentaffin reaction if they took up and reduced silver or as being argyrophilic if they did not reduce it. Currently, immunocytochemical localization of chromogranins (A, B, C), neuron-specific enolase, and synaptophysin, which are all neuroendocrine cell markers, is used (Table 113-1). Chromogranin A is the most widely used.

Ultrastructurally, these tumors possess electron-dense neurosecretory granules and frequently contain small clear vesicles that correspond to synaptic vesicles of neurons. NETs synthesize numerous peptides, growth factors, and bioactive amines that may be ectopically secreted, giving rise to a specific clinical syndrome (Table 113-2). The diagnosis of the specific syndrome requires the clinical features of the disease (Table 113-2) and cannot be made from the immunocytochemistry results alone. The presence or absence of a specific clinical syndrome also cannot be predicted from the immunocytochemistry alone (Table 113-1). Furthermore, pathologists cannot distinguish between benign and malignant NETs unless metastasis or invasion is present.

GI-NETs (carcinoids) frequently are classified according to their anatomic area of origin (i.e., foregut, midgut, hindgut) because tumors with similar areas of origin share functional manifestations, histochemistry, and secretory products (Table 113-3). Foregut tumors generally have a low serotonin (5-HT) content; are argentaffin-negative but argyrophilic; occasionally secrete adrenocorticotropic hormone (ACTH) or 5-hydroxytryptophan (5-HTP), causing an atypical carcinoid syndrome (Fig. 113-1); are often multihormonal; and may metastasize to bone. They uncommonly produce a clinical syndrome due to the secreted products. Midgut carcinoids are argentaffin-positive, have a high serotonin content, most frequently cause the typical carcinoid syndrome when they metastasize (Table 113-3, Fig. 113-1), release serotonin and tachykinins (substance P, neuropeptide K, substance K), rarely secrete 5-HTP or ACTH, and less commonly metastasize to bone. Hindgut carcinoids (rectum, transverse and descending colon) are argentaffin-negative, are often argyrophilic, rarely contain serotonin or cause the carcinoid syndrome (Fig. 113-1, Table 113-3), rarely secrete 5-HTP or ACTH, contain numerous peptides, and may metastasize to bone.

pNETs can be classified into nine well-established specific functional syndromes (Table 113-2), six additional very rare specific functional syndromes (less than five cases described), five possible specific functional syndromes (pNETs secreting calcitonin, neurotensin, pancreatic polypeptide, ghrelin) (Table 113-2), and nonfunctional pNETs. Other functional hormonal syndromes due to nonpancreatic tumors (usually intraabdominal in location) have been described only rarely and are not included in (Table 113-2). These include secretion by intestinal and ovarian tumors of peptide tyrosine tyrosine (PYY), which results in altered motility and constipation, and ovarian tumors secreting renin or aldosterone causing alterations in blood pressure or somatostatin causing diabetes or reactive hypoglycemia. Each of the functional syndromes listed in Table 113-2 is associated with symptoms due to the specific hormone released. In contrast, nonfunctional pNETs release no products that cause a specific clinical syndrome. "Nonfunctional" is a misnomer in the strict sense because those tumors frequently ectopically secrete a number of peptides (pancreatic polypeptide [PP], chromogranin A, ghrelin, neurotensin, α subunits of human chorionic gonadotropin, and neuron-specific enolase); however, they cause no specific clinical syndrome. The symptoms caused by nonfunctional pNETs are entirely due to the tumor per se. pNETs frequently ectopically secrete PP (60–85%), neurotensin (30–67%), calcitonin (30–42%), and to a lesser degree, ghrelin (5–65%). Whereas a few studies have proposed their secretion can cause a specific functional syndrome, most studies support the conclusion that their ectopic secretion is not associated with a specific clinical syndrome, and thus they are listed in Table 113-2 as possible clinical syndromes.

TABLE 113-2 GASTROINTESTINAL NEUROENDOCRINE TUMOR SYNDROMES

Name	Biologically Active Peptide(s) Secreted	Incidence (New Cases/10^6 Population/Year)	Tumor Location	Malignant, %	Associated with MEN 1, %	Main Symptoms/Signs
I. Established Specific Functional Syndromes						
A. Carcinoid syndrome due to GI-NET						
Carcinoid syndrome	Serotonin, possibly tachykinins, motilin, prostaglandins	0.5–2	Midgut (75–87%) Foregut (2–33%) Hindgut (1–8%) Unknown (2–15%)	95–100	Rare	Diarrhea (32–84%) Flushing (63–75%) Pain (10–34%) Asthma (4–18%) Heart disease (11–41%)
B. Well-established functional pNET syndromes						
Zollinger-Ellison syndrome	Gastrin	0.5–1.5	Duodenum (70%) Pancreas (25%) Other sites (5%)	60–90	20–25	Pain (79–100%) Diarrhea (30–75%) Esophageal symptoms (31–56%)
Insulinoma	Insulin	1–2	Pancreas (>99%)	<10	4–5	Hypoglycemic symptoms (100%)
VIPoma (Verner-Morrison syndrome, pancreatic cholera, WDHA)	Vasoactive intestinal peptide	0.05–0.2	Pancreas (90%, adult) Other (10%, neural, adrenal, periganglionic)	40–70	6	Diarrhea (90–100%) Hypokalemia (80–100%) Dehydration (83%)
Glucagonoma	Glucagon	0.01–0.1	Pancreas (100%)	50–80	1–20	Rash (67–90%) Glucose intolerance (38–87%) Weight loss (66–96%)
Somatostatinoma	Somatostatin	Rare	Pancreas (55%) Duodenum/jejunum (44%)	>70	45	Diabetes mellitus (63–90%) Cholelithiasis (65–90%) Diarrhea (35–90%)
GRFoma	Growth hormone–releasing hormone	Unknown	Pancreas (30%) Lung (54%) Jejunum (7%) Other (13%)	>60	16	Acromegaly (100%)
ACTHoma	ACTH	Rare	Pancreas (4–16% all ectopic Cushing's)	>95	Rare	Cushing's syndrome (100%)
pNET causing carcinoid syndrome	Serotonin, ?tachykinins	Rare (43 cases)	Pancreas (<1% all carcinoids)	60–88	Rare	Same as carcinoid syndrome above
pNET causing hypercalcemia	PTHrP Others unknown	Rare	Pancreas (rare cause of hypercalcemia)	84	Rare	Abdominal pain due to hepatic metastases
II. Rare Specific Functional Syndromes						
pNET secreting renin	Renin	Rare	Pancreas	Unknown	No	Hypertension
pNET secreting luteinizing hormone	Luteinizing hormone	Rare	Pancreas	Unknown	No	Anovulation, virilization (female); reduced libido (male)
pNET secreting erythropoietin	Erythropoietin	Rare	Pancreas	100	No	Polycythemia
pNET secreting IGF-II	Insulin-like growth factor II	Rare	Pancreas	Unknown	No	Hypoglycemia
pNET secreting GLP-1	Glucagon-like peptide-1	Rare	Pancreas	Unknown	No	Hypoglycemia, diabetes
pNET secreting enteroglucagon	Enteroglucagon	Rare	Pancreas, small intestine	Unknown	Rare	Small intestinal hypertrophy, intestinal stasis, malabsorption
III. Possible Specific Functional pNET Syndromes						
pNET secreting calcitonin	Calcitonin	Rare	Pancreas (rare cause of hypercalcitonemia)	>80	16	Diarrhea (50%)
pNET secreting neurotensin	Neurotensin	Rare	Pancreas (100%)	Unknown	No	Motility disturbances, vascular symptoms
pNET secreting pancreatic polypeptide (PPoma)	Pancreatic polypeptide	1–2	Pancreas	>60	18–44	Watery diarrhea
pNET secreting ghrelin	Ghrelin	Rare	Pancreas	Unknown	No	Effects on appetite, body weight
IV. Nonfunctional Syndrome pNET						
PPoma/nonfunctional[a]	None	1–2	Pancreas (100%)	>60	18–44	Weight loss (30–90%) Abdominal mass (10–30%) Pain (30–95%)

Abbreviations: ACTH, adrenocorticotropic hormone; GRFoma, growth hormone–releasing factor secreting pancreatic endocrine tumor; IGF-II, insulin-like growth factor II; MEN, multiple endocrine neoplasia; pNET, pancreatic neuroendocrine tumor; PPoma, tumor secreting pancreatic polypeptide; PTHrP, parathyroid hormone–related peptide; VIPoma, tumor secreting vasoactive intestinal peptide; WDHA, *w*atery *d*iarrhea, *h*ypokalemia, and *a*chlorhydria syndrome.

[a]Pancreatic polypeptide–secreting tumors (PPomas) are listed in two places because most authorities classify these as not associated with a specific hormonal syndrome (nonfunctional); however, rare cases of watery diarrhea proposed to be due to PPomas have been reported.

TABLE 113-3 GI-NET (CARCINOID) LOCATION, FREQUENCY OF METASTASES, AND ASSOCIATION WITH THE CARCINOID SYNDROME

	Location (% of Total)	Incidence of Metastases	Incidence of Carcinoid Syndrome
Foregut			
Esophagus	<0.1	—	—
Stomach	4.6	10	9.5
Duodenum	2.0	—	3.4
Pancreas	0.7	71.9	20
Gallbladder	0.3	17.8	5
Bronchus, lung, trachea	27.9	5.7	13
Midgut			
Jejunum	1.8	{58.4	9
Ileum	14.9		9
Meckel's diverticulum	0.5	—	13
Appendix	4.8	38.8	<1
Colon	8.6	51	5
Liver	0.4	32.	—
Ovary	1.0	2 32	50
Testis	<0.1	—	50
Hindgut			
Rectum	13.6	3.9	—

Abbreviation: GI-NET, gastrointestinal neuroendocrine tumor.

Source: Location is from the PAN-SEER data (1973–1999), and incidence of metastases is from the SEER data (1992–1999), reported by IM Modlin et al: Cancer 97:934, 2003. Incidence of carcinoid syndrome is from 4349 cases studied from 1950–1971, reported by JD Godwin: Cancer 36:560, 1975.

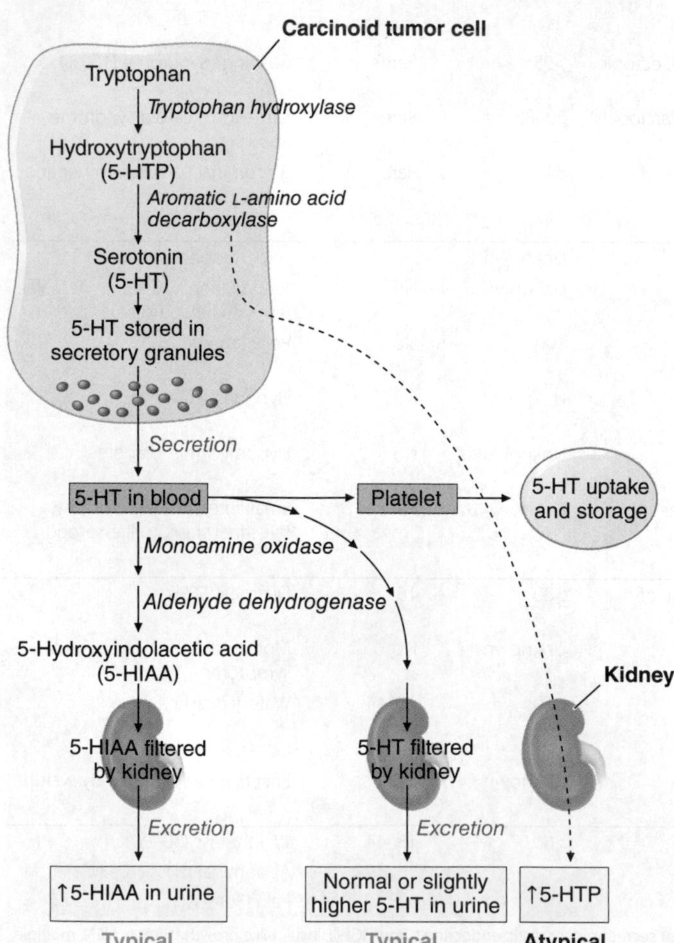

FIGURE 113-1 Synthesis, secretion, and metabolism of serotonin (5-HT) in patients with typical and atypical carcinoid syndromes. 5-HIAA, 5-hydroxyindolacetic acid.

Because a large proportion of nonfunctional pNETs (60–90%) secrete PP, these tumors are often referred to as PPomas (Table 113-2).

GI-NETs (carcinoids) can occur in almost any GI tissue (Table 113-3); however, at present, most (70%) have their origin in one of three sites: bronchus, jejunoileum, or colon/rectum. In the past, GI-NET (carcinoids) most frequently were reported in the appendix (i.e., 40%); however, the bronchus/lung, rectum, and small intestine are now the most common sites. Overall, the GI tract is the most common site for these tumors, accounting for 64%, with the respiratory tract a distant second at 28%. Both race and sex can affect the frequency as well as the distribution of GI-NETs (carcinoids). African Americans have a higher incidence of carcinoids. Race is particularly important for rectal carcinoids, which are found in 41% of Asians/Pacific Islanders with NETs compared to 32% of American Indians/Alaskan natives, 26% of African Americans, and 12% of white Americans. Females have a lower incidence of small intestinal and pancreatic carcinoids.

The term *pancreatic neuroendocrine* or *endocrine tumor*, although widely used and therefore retained here, is also a misnomer, strictly speaking, because these tumors can occur either almost entirely in the pancreas (insulinomas, glucagonomas, nonfunctional pNETs, pNETs causing hypercalcemia) or at both pancreatic and extrapancreatic sites (gastrinomas, VIPomas [vasoactive intestinal peptide], somatostatinomas, GRFomas [growth hormone–releasing factor]). pNETs are also called islet cell tumors; however, the use of this term is discouraged because it is not established that they originate from the islets, and many can occur at extrapancreatic sites.

Whereas the classification of GI neuroendocrine tumors into foregut, midgut, or hindgut is widely used and generally useful because the NETs within these areas have many similarities, they also have marked differences, particularly in biologic behavior, and it has not proved useful for prognostic purposes. More general classifications have been developed that allow NETs with similar features in different locations to be compared, have proven prognostic value, and are widely used. New classification systems have been developed for both GI-NETs (carcinoids) and pNETs by the World Health Organization (WHO), European Neuroendocrine Tumor Society (ENETS), and the American Joint Committee on Cancer/International Union Against Cancer (AJCC/UICC). Although there are some differences between these different classification systems, each uses similar information, and it is now recommended that the basic data underlying the classification be included in all standard pathology reports. These classification systems divide NETs from all sites into those that are well differentiated (low grade [G1] or intermediate grade [G2]) and those that are poorly differentiated (high grade [G3] divided into either small-cell carcinoma or large-cell neuroendocrine carcinoma). In these classification systems, both pNETs and GI-NETs (carcinoids) are classified as neuroendocrine tumors, and the old term of carcinoid is equivalent to well-differentiated neuroendocrine tumors of the GI tract. These classification systems are based on not only the differentiation of the NET, but also a grading system assessing proliferative indices (Ki-67 and the mitotic count). NETs are considered low grade (ENETS G1) if the Ki-67 is <3% and the mitotic count is <2 mitoses/high-power field (HPF), intermediate grade (ENETS G2) if the Ki-67 is 3–20% and the mitotic count is 2–20 mitoses/HPF, and high grade (ENETS G3) if the Ki-67 is >20% and the mitotic count is >20 mitoses/HPF. In addition to the grading system, a TNM classification has been proposed that is based on the level of tumor invasion, tumor size, and tumor extent (see Table 113-4 for an example with pNETs and appendiceal GI-NETs [carcinoids]). Because of the proven prognostic value of these classification and grading systems, as well as the fact that NETs with different classifications/grades respond differently to treatments, the systems are now essential for the management of all NETs.

In addition to these classification/grading systems, a number of other factors have been identified that provide important prognostic information that can guide treatment (Table 113-5).

The exact incidence of GI-NETs (carcinoids) or pNETs varies according to whether only symptomatic tumors or all tumors are considered. The incidence of clinically significant carcinoids is 7–13 cases/million population per year, whereas any malignant carcinoids

TABLE 113-4 COMPARISON OF THE CRITERIA FOR THE TUMOR CATEGORY IN THE ENETS AND SEVENTH EDITION AJCC TNM CLASSIFICATIONS OF PANCREATIC AND APPENDICEAL NETs

	ENETS TNM	AJCC/UICC TNM
pNETs		
T1	Confined to pancreas, <2 cm	Confined to pancreas, <2 cm
T2	Confined to pancreas, 2–4 cm	Confined to pancreas, >2 cm
T3	Confined to pancreas, >4 cm, or invasion of duodenum or bile duct	Peripancreatic spread, but without major vascular invasion (truncus coeliacus, superior mesenteric artery)
T4	Invasion of adjacent organs or major vessels	Major vascular invasion
Appendiceal NETs		
T1	≤1 cm; invasion of muscularis propria	T1a, ≤1 cm; T1b, >1–2 cm
T2	≤2 cm and <3 mm invasion of subserosa/mesoappendix	>2–4 cm or invasion of cecum
T3	>2 cm or >3 mm invasion of subserosa/mesoappendix	>4 cm or invasion of ileum
T4	Invasion of peritoneum/other organs	Invasion of peritoneum/other organs

Abbreviations: AJCC, American Joint Committee on Cancer; ENETS, European Neuroendocrine Tumor Society; NET, neuroendocrine tumor; pNET, pancreatic neuroendocrine tumor; TNM, tumor, node, metastasis; UICC, International Union Against Cancer.

Source: Modified from DS Klimstra: Semin Oncol 40:23, 2013 and G Kloppel et al: Virchow Arch 456:595, 2010.

at autopsy are reported in 21–84 cases/million population per year. The incidence of GI-NETs (carcinoids) is approximately 25–50 cases per million in the United States, which makes them less common than adenocarcinomas of the GI tract. However, their incidence has increased sixfold in the last 30 years. In an analysis of 35,825 GI-NETs (carcinoids) (2004) from the U.S. Surveillance, Epidemiology, and End Results (SEER) database, their incidence was 5.25/100,000 per year, and the 29-year prevalence was 35/100,000. Clinically significant pNETs have a prevalence of 10 cases/million population, with insulinomas, gastrinomas, and nonfunctional pNETs having an incidence of 0.5–2 cases/million population per year (Table 113-2). pNETs account for 1–10% of all tumors arising in the pancreas and 1.3% of tumors in the SEER database, which consists primarily of malignant tumors. VIPomas are 2–8 times less common, glucagonomas are 17–30 times less common, and somatostatinomas are the least common. In autopsy studies, 0.5–1.5% of all cases have a pNET; however, in less than 1 in 1000 cases was a functional tumor thought to occur.

Both GI-NETs (carcinoids) and pNETs commonly show malignant behavior (Tables 113-2 and 113-3). With pNETs, except for insulinomas in which <10% are malignant, 50–100% in different series are malignant. With GI-NETs (carcinoids), the percentage showing malignant behavior varies in different locations (Table 113-3). For the three most common sites of occurrence, the incidence of metastases varies greatly from the jejunoileum (58%), lung/bronchus (6%), and rectum (4%) (Table 113-3). With both GI-NETs (carcinoids) and pNETs, a number of factors (Table 113-5) are important prognostic factors in determining survival and the aggressiveness of the tumor. Patients with pNETs (excluding insulinomas) generally have a poorer prognosis than do patients with GI-NETs (carcinoids). The presence of liver metastases is the single most important prognostic factor in single and multivariate analyses for both GI-NETs (carcinoids) and pNETs. Particularly important in the development of liver metastases is the size of the primary tumor. For example, with small intestinal carcinoids, which are the most common cause of the carcinoid syndrome due to metastatic disease in the liver (Table 113-2), metastases occur in 15–25% if the tumor is <1 cm in diameter, 58–80% if it is 1–2 cm in diameter, and >75% if it is >2 cm in diameter. Similar data exist for gastrinomas and other pNETs; the size of the primary tumor is an independent predictor of the development of liver metastases.

TABLE 113-5 PROGNOSTIC FACTORS IN NEUROENDOCRINE TUMORS

I. Both GI-NETs (carcinoids) and pNETs
Symptomatic presentation ($p < .05$)
Presence of liver metastases ($p < .001$)
Extent of liver metastases ($p < .001$)
Presence of lymph node metastases ($p < .001$)
Development of bone or extrahepatic metastases ($p < .01$)
Depth of invasion ($p < .001$)
Rapid rate of tumor growth
Elevated serum alkaline phosphatase levels ($p = .003$)
Primary tumor site ($p < .001$)
Primary tumor size ($p < .005$)
High serum chromogranin A level ($p < .01$)
Presence of one or more circulating tumor cells ($p < .001$)
Various histologic features
Tumor differentiation ($p < .001$)
High growth indices (high Ki-67 index, PCNA expression)
High mitotic counts ($p < .001$)
Necrosis present
Presence of cytokeratin 19 ($p < .02$)
Vascular or perineural invasion
Vessel density (low microvessel density, increased lymphatic density)
High CD10 metalloproteinase expression (in series with all grades of NETs)
Flow cytometric features (i.e., aneuploidy)
High VEGF expression (in low-grade or well-differentiated NETs only)
WHO, ENETS, AJCC/UICC, and grading classification
Presence of a pNET rather than GI-NET associated with poorer prognosis ($p = .0001$)
Older age ($p < .01$)
II. GI-NETs (Carcinoids)
Location of primary: appendix < lung, rectum < small intestine < pancreas
Presence of carcinoid syndrome
Laboratory results (urinary 5-HIAA levels [$p < .01$], plasma neuropeptide K [$p < .05$], serum chromogranin A [$p < .01$])
Presence of a second malignancy
Male sex ($p < .001$)
Molecular findings (TGF-α expression [$p < .05$], chr 16q LOH or gain chr 4p [$p < .05$])
WHO, ENETS, AJCC/UICC, and grading classification
Molecular findings (gain in chr 14, loss of 3p13 [ileal carcinoid], upregulation of Hoxc6)
III. pNETs
Location of primary: duodenal (gastrinoma) better than pancreatic
Ha-*ras* oncogene or p53 overexpression
Female gender
MEN 1 syndrome absent
Presence of nonfunctional tumor (some studies, not all)
WHO, ENETS, AJCC/UICC, and grading classification
Various histologic features: IHC positivity for c-KIT, low cyclin B1 expression ($p < .01$), loss of PTEN or of tuberous sclerosis-2 IHC, expression of fibroblast growth factor-13
Laboratory findings (increased chromogranin A in some studies; gastrinomas—increased gastrin level)
Molecular findings (increased HER2/*neu* expression [$p = .032$], chr 1q, 3p, 3q, or 6q LOH [$p = .0004$], EGF receptor overexpression [$p = .034$], gains in chr 7q, 17q, 17p, 20q; alterations in the VHL gene [deletion, methylation]; presence of FGFR4-G388R single-nucleotide polymorphism)

Abbreviations: 5-HIAA, 5-hydroxyindoleacetic acid; AJCC, American Joint Committee on Cancer; chr, chromosome; EGF, epidermal growth factor; FGFR, fibroblast growth factor receptor; GI-NET, gastrointestinal neuroendocrine tumor; IHC, immunohistochemistry; Ki-67, proliferation-associated nuclear antigen recognized by Ki-67 monoclonal antibody; LOH, loss of heterozygosity; MEN, multiple endocrine neoplasia; NET, neuroendocrine tumor; PCNA, proliferating cell nuclear antigen; pNET, pancreatic neuroendocrine tumor; PTEN, phosphatase and tensin homologue deleted from chromosome 10; TGF-α, transforming growth factor α; TNM, tumor, node, metastasis; UICC, International Union Against Cancer; VEGF, vascular endothelial growth factor; WHO, World Health Organization.

The presence of lymph node metastases or extrahepatic metastases; the depth of invasion; the rapid rate of growth; various histologic features (differentiation, mitotic rates, growth indices, vessel density, vascular endothelial growth factor [VEGF], and CD10 metalloproteinase expression); necrosis; presence of cytokeratin; elevated serum alkaline phosphatase levels; older age; presence of circulating tumor cells; and flow cytometric results, such as the presence of aneuploidy, are all important prognostic factors for the development of metastatic disease (Table 113-5). For patients with GI-NETs (carcinoids), additional associations with a worse prognosis include the development of the carcinoid syndrome (especially the development of carcinoid heart disease), male sex, the presence of a symptomatic tumor or greater increases in a number of tumor markers (5-hydroxyindolacetic acid [5-HIAA], neuropeptide K, chromogranin A), and the presence of various molecular features. With pNETs or gastrinomas, a worse prognosis is associated with female sex, overexpression of the Ha-*ras* oncogene or p53, the absence of multiple endocrine neoplasia type 1 (MEN 1), higher levels of various tumor markers (i.e., chromogranin A, gastrin), and presence of various histologic features (immunohistochemistry for c-KIT, low cyclin B1, loss of PTEN/TSC-2, expression of fibroblast growth factor-13) and various molecular features (Table 113-5). The TNM classification systems and the grading systems (G1–G3) have important prognostic value.

A number of diseases due to various genetic disorders are associated with an increased incidence of NETs (Table 113-6). Each one is caused by a loss of a possible tumor-suppressor gene. The most important is MEN 1, which is an autosomal dominant disorder due to a defect in a 10-exon gene on 11q13, which encodes for a 610-amino-acid nuclear protein, menin (Chap. 408). Patients with MEN 1 develop hyperparathyroidism due to parathyroid hyperplasia in 95–100% of cases, pNETs in 80–100%, pituitary adenomas in 54–80%, adrenal adenomas in 27–36%, bronchial carcinoids in 8%, thymic carcinoids in 8%, gastric carcinoids in 13–30% of patients with Zollinger-Ellison syndrome, skin tumors (angiofibromas [88%], collagenomas [72%]), central nervous system (CNS) tumors (meningiomas [<8%]), and smooth-muscle tumors (leiomyomas, leiomyosarcomas [1–7%]). Among patients with MEN 1, 80–100% develop nonfunctional pNETs (most are microscopic with 0–13% large/symptomatic), and functional pNETs occur in 20–80% in different series, with a mean of 54% developing Zollinger-Ellison syndrome, 18% insulinomas, 3% glucagonomas, 3% VIPomas, and <1% GRFomas or somatostatinomas. MEN 1 is present in 20–25% of all patients with Zollinger-Ellison syndrome, 4% of patients with insulinomas, and a low percentage (<5%) of patients with other pNETs.

TABLE 113-6 GENETIC SYNDROMES ASSOCIATED WITH AN INCREASED INCIDENCE OF NEUROENDOCRINE TUMORS (NETS) (GI-NETS [CARCINOIDS] OR PNETS)

Syndrome	Location of Gene Mutation and Gene Product	NETs Seen/Frequency
Multiple endocrine neoplasia type 1 (MEN 1)	11q13 (encodes 610-amino-acid protein, menin)	80–100% develop pNETS (microscopic), 20–80% (clinical): (nonfunctional > gastrinoma > insulinoma)
		GI-NETs (Carcinoids): gastric (13–30%), bronchial/thymic (8%)
von Hippel–Lindau disease	3q25 (encodes 213-amino-acid protein)	12–17% develop pNETS (almost always nonfunctional)
von Recklinghausen's disease (neurofibromatosis 1 [NF-1])	17q11.2 (encodes 2485-amino-acid protein, neurofibromin)	0–10% develop pNETs, primarily duodenal somatostatinomas (usually nonfunctional)
		Rarely insulinoma, gastrinoma
Tuberous sclerosis	9q34 (TSCI) (encodes 1164-amino-acid protein, hamartin), 16p13 (TSC2) (encodes 1807-amino-acid protein, tuberin)	Uncommonly develop pNETS (nonfunctional and functional [insulinoma, gastrinoma])

Abbreviations: GI, gastrointestinal; PNETs, pancreatic neuroendocrine tumors.

Three phacomatoses associated with NETs are von Hippel–Lindau disease (VHL), von Recklinghausen's disease (neurofibromatosis type 1 [NF-1]), and tuberous sclerosis (Bourneville's disease) (Table 113-6). VHL is an autosomal dominant disorder due to defects on chromosome 3p25, which encodes for a 213-amino-acid protein that interacts with the elongin family of proteins as a transcriptional regulator (Chaps. 118, 339, 407, and 408). In addition to cerebellar hemangioblastomas, renal cancer, and pheochromocytomas, 10–17% develop a pNET. Most are nonfunctional, although insulinomas and VIPomas have been reported. Patients with NF-1 (von Recklinghausen's disease) have defects in a gene on chromosome 17q11.2 that encodes for a 2845-amino-acid protein, neurofibromin, which functions in normal cells as a suppressor of the *ras* signaling cascade (Chap. 118). Up to 10% of these patients develop an upper GI-NET (carcinoid), characteristically in the periampullary region (54%). Many are classified as somatostatinomas because they contain somatostatin immunocytochemically; however, they uncommonly secrete somatostatin and rarely produce a clinical somatostatinoma syndrome. NF-1 has rarely been associated with insulinomas and Zollinger-Ellison syndrome. NF-1 accounts for 48% of all duodenal somatostastinomas and 23% of all ampullary GI-NETs (carcinoids). Tuberous sclerosis is caused by mutations that alter either the 1164-amino-acid protein hamartin (TSC1) or the 1807-amino-acid protein tuberin (TSC2) (Chap. 118). Both hamartin and tuberin interact in a pathway related to phosphatidylinositol 3-kinases and mammalian target of rapamycin (mTOR) signaling cascades. A few cases including nonfunctional and functional pNETs (insulinomas and gastrinomas) have been reported in these patients (Table 113-6). Mahvash disease is associated with the development of α-cell hyperplasia, hyperglucagonemia, and the development of NF pNETs and is due to a homozygous P86S mutation of the human glucagon receptor.

Mutations in common oncogenes (*ras, myc, fos, src, jun*) or common tumor-suppressor genes (*p53*, retinoblastoma susceptibility gene) are not commonly found in either pNETs or GI-NETs (carcinoids) (Table 113-1). However, frequent (70%) gene amplifications in *MDM2, MDM4,* and *WIPI* inactivating the p53 pathway are noted in well-differentiated pNETs, and the retinoblastoma pathway is altered in the majority of pNETs. In addition to these genes, additional alterations that may be important in their pathogenesis include changes in the *MEN1* gene, *p16/MTS1* tumor-suppressor gene, and *DPC4/Smad4* gene; amplification of the HER-2/*neu* protooncogene; alterations in transcription factors (Hoxc6 [GI carcinoids]), growth factors, and their receptors; methylation of a number of genes that probably results in their inactivation; and deletions of unknown tumor-suppressor genes as well as gains in other unknown genes (Table 113-1). The clinical antitumor activity of everolimus, an mTOR inhibitor, and sunitinib, a tyrosine kinase inhibitor (PDGFR, VEGFR1, VEGFR2, c-KIT, FLT-3), support the importance of the mTOR-AKT pathway and tyrosine kinase receptors in mediating growth of malignant NETs (especially pNETs). The importance of the mTOR pathway in pNET growth is further supported by the finding that a single-nucleotide polymorphism (FGFR4-G388R, in fibroblast growth factor receptor 4) affects selectivity to the mTOR inhibitor and can result in significantly higher risk of advanced pNET stage and liver metastases (Table 113-5). Comparative genomic hybridization, genome-wide allelotyping studies, and genome-wide single-nucleotide polymorphism analyses have shown that chromosomal losses and gains are common in pNETs and GI-NETs (carcinoids), but they differ between these two NETs, and some have prognostic significance (Table 113-5). Mutations in the *MEN1* gene are probably particularly important. Loss of heterozygosity at the MEN 1 locus on chromosome 11q13 is noted in 93% of sporadic pNETs (i.e., in patients without MEN 1) and in 26–75% of sporadic GI-NETs (carcinoids). Mutations in the *MEN1* gene are reported in 31–34% of sporadic gastrinomas. Exomic sequencing of sporadic pNETs found that the most frequently altered gene was

MEN1, occurring in 44% of patients, followed by mutations in 43% of patients in genes encoding for two subunits of a transcription/chromatin remodeling complex consisting of DAXX (death-domain-associated protein) and ATRX (α-thalassemia/mental retardation syndrome X-linked) and in 15% of patients in the mTOR pathway. The presence of a number of these molecular alterations in pNETs or GI-NETs (carcinoids) correlates with tumor growth, tumor size, and disease extent or invasiveness and may have prognostic significance (Table 113-5).

GI-NETs (CARCINOIDS) AND CARCINOID SYNDROME

CHARACTERISTICS OF THE MOST COMMON GI-NETs (CARCINOIDS)

Appendiceal NETs (Carcinoids) Appendiceal NETs (carcinoids) occur in 1 in every 200–300 appendectomies, usually in the appendiceal tip, have an incidence of 0.15/100,000 per year, comprise 2–5% of all GI-NETs (carcinoids), and comprise 32–80% of all appendiceal tumors. Most (i.e., >90%) are <1 cm in diameter without metastases in older studies, but more recently, 2–35% have had metastases (Table 113-3). In the SEER data of 1570 appendiceal carcinoids, 62% were localized, 27% had regional metastases, and 8% had distant metastases. The risk of metastases increases with size, with those <1 cm having a 0 to <10% risk of metastases and those >2 cm having a 25–44% risk. Besides tumor size, other important prognostic factors for metastases include basal location, invasion of mesoappendix, poor differentiation, advanced stage or WHO/ENETS classification, older age, and positive resection margins. The 5-year survival is 88–100% for patients with localized disease, 78–100% for patients with regional involvement, and 12–28% for patients with distal metastases. In patients with tumors <1 cm in diameter, the 5-year survival is 95–100%, whereas it is 29% if tumors are >2 cm in diameter. Most tumors are well-differentiated G1 tumors (87%) (Table 113-4), with the remainder primarily well-differentiated G2 tumors (13%); poorly differentiated G3 tumors are uncommon (<1%). Their percentage of the total number of carcinoids decreased from 43.9% (1950–1969) to 2.4% (1992–1999). Appendiceal goblet cell (GC) NETs (carcinoids)/carcinomas are a rare subtype (<5%) that are mixed adeno-neuroendocrine carcinomas. They are malignant and are thought to comprise a distinct entity; they frequently present with advanced disease and are recommended to be treated as adenocarcinomas, not carcinoid tumors.

SMALL INTESTINAL NETs (CARCINOIDS)

Small intestinal (SI) NETs (carcinoids) have a reported incidence of 0.67/100,000 in the United States, 0.32/100,000 in England, and 1.12/100,000 in Sweden and comprise >50% of all SI tumors. There is a male predominance (1.5:1), and race affects frequency, with a lower frequency in Asians and greater frequency in African Americans. The mean age of presentation is 52–63 years, with a wide range (1–93 years). Familial SI carcinoid families exist but are very uncommon. These are frequently multiple, 9–18% occur in the jeunum, 70–80% are present in the ileum, and 70% occur within 6 cm (2.4 in.) of the ileocecal valve. Forty percent are <1 cm in diameter, 32% are 1–2 cm, and 29% are >2 cm. They are characteristically well differentiated; however, they are generally invasive, with 1.2% being intramucosal in location, 27% penetrating the submucosa, and 20% invading the muscularis propria. Metastases occur in a mean of 47–58% (range 20–100%). Liver metastases occur in 38%, to lymph nodes in 37% and more distant in 20–25%. They characteristically cause a marked fibrotic reaction, which can lead to intestinal obstruction. Tumor size is an important variable in the frequency of metastases. However, even small NETs (carcinoids) of the small intestine (<1 cm) have metastases in 15–25% of cases, whereas the proportion increases to 58–100% for tumors 1–2 cm in diameter. Carcinoids also occur in the duodenum, with 31% having metastases. Duodenal tumors <1 cm virtually never metastasize, whereas 33% of those >2 cm had metastases. SI NETs (carcinoids) are the most common cause (60–87%) of the carcinoid syndrome and are discussed in a later section (Table 113-7). Important prognostic factors are listed in (Table 113-5), and particularly important are the tumor extent, proliferative index by grading, and stage (Table 113-4). The overall survival at 5 years is 55–75%; however, it varies markedly with disease extent, being 65–90% with localized disease, 66–72% with regional involvement, and 36–43% with distant disease.

TABLE 113-7 CLINICAL CHARACTERISTICS IN PATIENTS WITH CARCINOID SYNDROME

	Percentage (Range)	
	At Presentation	**During Course of Disease**
Symptoms/signs		
Diarrhea	32–93%	68–100%
Flushing	23–100%	45–96%
Pain	10%	34%
Asthma/wheezing	4–14%	3–18%
Pellagra	0–7%	0–5%
None	12%	22%
Carcinoid heart disease present	11–40%	14–41%
Demographics		
Male	46–59%	46–61%
Age		
Mean	57 yrs	59.2 yrs
Range	25–79 yrs	18–91 yrs
Tumor location		
Foregut	5–14%	0–33%
Midgut	57–87%	60–100%
Hindgut	1–7%	0–8%
Unknown	2–21%	0–26%

Rectal NETs (Carcinoids) Rectal NETs (carcinoids) comprise 27% of all GI-NETs (carcinoids) and 16% of all NETs and are increasing in frequency. In the U.S. SEER data, they currently have an incidence of 0.86/100,000 per year (up from 0.2/100,000 per year in 1973) and represent 1–2% of all rectal tumors. They are found in approximately 1 in every 1500/2500 proctoscopies/colonoscopies or 0.05–0.07% of individuals undergoing these procedures. Nearly all occur between 4 and 13 cm above the dentate line. Most are small, with 66–80% being <1 cm in diameter, and rarely metastasize (5%). Tumors between 1 and 2 cm can metastasize in 5–30%, and those >2 cm, which are uncommon, in >70%. Most invade only to the submucosa (75%), with 2.1% confined to the mucosa, 10% to the muscular layer, and 5% to adjacent structures. Histologically, most are well differentiated (98%) with 72% ENETS/WHO grade G1 and 28% grade G2 (Table 113-4). Overall survival is 88%; however, it is very much dependent of the stage, with 5-year survival of 91% for localized disease, 36–49% for regional disease, and 20–32% for distant disease. Risk factors are listed in Table 113-5 and particularly include tumor size, depth of invasion, presence of metastases, differentiation, and recent TNM classification and grade.

Bronchial NETs (Carcinoids) Bronchial NETs (carcinoids) comprise 25–33% of all well-differentiated NETs and 90% of all the poorly differentiated NETs found, likely due to a strong association with smoking. Their incidence ranges from 0.2 to 2/100,000 per year in the United States and European countries and is increasing at a rate of 6% per year. They are slightly more frequent in females and in whites compared with those of Hispanic/Asian/African descent, and are most commonly seen in the sixth decade of life, with a younger age of presentation for typical carcinoids (45 years) compared to atypical carcinoids (55 years).

A number of different classifications of bronchial GI-NETs (carcinoids) have been proposed. In some studies, they are classified into four categories: typical carcinoid (also called bronchial carcinoid tumor, Kulchitsky cell carcinoma I [KCC-I]), atypical carcinoid (also called well-differentiated neuroendocrine carcinoma [KC-II]), intermediate small-cell neuroendocrine carcinoma, and small-cell neuroendocarcinoma

(KC-III). Another proposed classification includes three categories of lung NETs: benign or low-grade malignant (typical carcinoid), low-grade malignant (atypical carcinoid), and high-grade malignant (poorly differentiated carcinoma of the large-cell or small-cell type). The WHO classification includes four general categories: typical carcinoid, atypical carcinoid, large-cell neuroendocrine carcinoma, and small-cell carcinoma. The ratio of typical to atypical carcinoids is 8–10:1, with the typical carcinoids comprising 1–2% of lung tumors, atypical 0.1–0.2%, large-cell neuroendocrine tumors 0.3%, and small-cell lung cancer 9.8% of all lung tumors. These different categories of lung NETs have different prognoses, varying from excellent for typical carcinoid to poor for small-cell neuroendocrine carcinomas. The occurrence of large-cell and small-cell lung carcinoids, but not typical or atypical lung carcinoids, is related to tobacco use. The 5-year survival is very much influenced by the classification of the tumor, with survival of 92–100% for patients with a typical carcinoid, 61–88% with an atypical carcinoid, 13–57% with a large-cell neuroendocrine tumor, and 5% with a small-cell lung cancer.

Gastric NET (Carcinoids) Gastric NETs (carcinoids) account for 3 of every 1000 gastric neoplasms and 1.3–2% of all carcinoids, and their relative frequency has increased three- to fourfold over the last five decades (2.2% in 1950 to 9.6% in 2000–2007, SEER data). At present, it is unclear whether this increase is due to better detection with the increased use of upper GI endoscopy or to a true increase in incidence. Gastric NETs (carcinoids) are classified into three different categories, and this has important implications for pathogenesis, prognosis, and treatment. Each originates from gastric enterochromaffin-like (ECL) cells, one of the six types of gastric neuroendocrine cells, in the gastric mucosa. Two subtypes are associated with hypergastrinemic states, either chronic atrophic gastritis (type I) (80% of all gastric NETs [carcinoids]) or Zollinger-Ellison syndrome, which is almost always a part of the MEN 1 syndrome (type II) (6% of all cases). These tumors generally pursue a benign course, with type I uncommonly (<10%) associated with metastases, whereas type II tumors are slightly more aggressive, with 10–30% associated with metastases. They are usually multiple, small, and infiltrate only to the submucosa. The third subtype of gastric NETs (carcinoids) (type III) (sporadic) occurs without hypergastrinemia (14–25% of all gastric carcinoids) and has an aggressive course, with 54–66% developing metastases. Sporadic carcinoids are usually single, large tumors; 50% have atypical histology, and they can be a cause of the carcinoid syndrome. Five-year survival is 99–100% in patients with type I, 60–90% in patients with type II, and 50% in patients with type III gastric NETs (carcinoids).

CLINICAL PRESENTATION OF NETs (CARCINOIDS)

GI/Lung NET (Carcinoid) Without the Carcinoid Syndrome The age of patients at diagnosis ranges from 10 to 93 years, with a mean age of 63 years for the small intestine and 66 years for the rectum. The presentation is diverse and is related to the site of origin and the extent of malignant spread. In the appendix, NETs (carcinoids) usually are found incidentally during surgery for suspected appendicitis. SI NETs (carcinoids) in the jejunoileum present with periodic abdominal pain (51%), intestinal obstruction with ileus/invagination (31%), an abdominal tumor (17%), or GI bleeding (11%). Because of the vagueness of the symptoms, the diagnosis usually is delayed approximately 2 years from onset of the symptoms, with a range up to 20 years. Duodenal, gastric, and rectal NETs (carcinoids) are most frequently found by chance at endoscopy. The most common symptoms of rectal carcinoids are melena/bleeding (39%), constipation (17%), and diarrhea (12%). Bronchial NETs (carcinoids) frequently are discovered as a lesion on a chest radiograph, and 31% of the patients are asymptomatic. Thymic NETs (carcinoids) present as anterior mediastinal masses, usually on chest radiograph or computed tomography (CT) scan. Ovarian and testicular NETs (carcinoids) usually present as masses discovered on physical examination or ultrasound. Metastatic NETs (carcinoids) in the liver frequently presents as hepatomegaly in a patient who may have minimal symptoms and nearly normal liver function test results.

GI-NETs (CARCINOIDS) WITH SYSTEMIC SYMPTOMS DUE TO SECRETED PRODUCTS

GI/lung NETs (carcinoids) immunocytochemically can contain numerous GI peptides: gastrin, insulin, somatostatin, motilin, neurotensin, tachykinins (substance K, substance P, neuropeptide K), glucagon, gastrin-releasing peptide, vasoactive intestinal peptide (VIP), PP, ghrelin, other biologically active peptides (ACTH, calcitonin, growth hormone), prostaglandins, and bioactive amines (serotonin). These substances may or may not be released in sufficient amounts to cause symptoms. In various studies of patients with GI-NETs (carcinoids), elevated serum levels of PP were found in 43%, motilin in 14%, gastrin in 15%, and VIP in 6%. Foregut NETs (carcinoids) are more likely to produce various GI peptides than are midgut NETs (carcinoids). Ectopic ACTH production causing Cushing's syndrome is seen increasingly with foregut carcinoids (respiratory tract primarily) and, in some series, has been the most common cause of the ectopic ACTH syndrome, accounting for 64% of all cases. Acromegaly due to growth hormone–releasing factor release occurs with foregut NETs (carcinoids), as does the somatostatinoma syndrome, but rarely occurs with duodenal NETs (carcinoids). The most common systemic syndrome with GI-NETs (carcinoids) is the carcinoid syndrome, which is discussed in detail in the next section.

CARCINOID SYNDROME

Clinical Features The cardinal features from a number of series at presentation as well as during the disease course are shown in Table 113-7. Flushing and diarrhea are the two most common symptoms, occurring in a mean of 69–70% of patients initially and in up to 78% of patients during the course of the disease. The characteristic flush is of sudden onset; it is a deep red or violaceous erythema of the upper body, especially the neck and face, often associated with a feeling of warmth and occasionally associated with pruritus, lacrimation, diarrhea, or facial edema. Flushes may be precipitated by stress; alcohol; exercise; certain foods, such as cheese; or certain agents, such as catecholamines, pentagastrin, and serotonin reuptake inhibitors. Flushing episodes may be brief, lasting 2–5 min, especially initially, or may last hours, especially later in the disease course. Flushing usually is associated with metastatic midgut NETs (carcinoids) but can also occur with foregut NETs (carcinoids). With bronchial NETs (carcinoids), the flushes frequently are prolonged for hours to days, reddish in color, and associated with salivation, lacrimation, diaphoresis, diarrhea, and hypotension. The flush associated with gastric NETs (carcinoids) can also be reddish in color, but with a patchy distribution over the face and neck, although the classic flush seen with midgut NETs (carcinoids) can also be seen with gastric NETs (carcinoids). It may be provoked by food and have accompanying pruritus.

Diarrhea usually occurs with flushing (85% of cases). The diarrhea usually is described as watery, with 60% of patients having <1 L/d of diarrhea. Steatorrhea is present in 67%, and in 46%, it is >15 g/d (normal <7 g). Abdominal pain may be present with the diarrhea or independently in 10–34% of cases.

Cardiac manifestations occur initially in 11–40% (mean 26%) of patients with carcinoid syndrome and in 14–41% (mean 30%) at some time in the disease course. The cardiac disease is due to the formation of fibrotic plaques (composed of smooth-muscle cells, myofibroblasts, and elastic tissue) involving the endocardium, primarily on the right side, although lesions on the left side also occur occasionally, especially if a patent foramen ovale exists. The dense fibrous deposits are most commonly on the ventricular aspect of the tricuspid valve and less commonly on the pulmonary valve cusps. They can result in constriction of the valves, and pulmonic stenosis is usually predominant, whereas the tricuspid valve is often fixed open, resulting in regurgitation predominating. Overall, in patients with carcinoid heart disease, 90–100% have tricuspid insufficiency, 43–59% have tricuspid stenosis, 50–81% have pulmonary insufficiency, 25–59% have pulmonary stenosis, and 11% (0–25%) left-side lesions. Up to 80% of patients with cardiac lesions develop heart failure. Lesions on the left side are much less extensive, occur in 30% at autopsy, and most frequently affect the mitral valve. Up to 80% of patients with cardiac lesions have evidence of heart failure. At diagnosis in various series, 27–43% of patients are in New York Heart Association class I, 30–40% are in class II, 13–31% are in class III, and 3–12% are in class IV. At present, carcinoid heart disease is reported to be decreasing in frequency and severity, with mean occurrence in 20% of patients and occurrence in as few as 3–4% in some reports. Whether this decrease is due to the widespread use of somatostatin analogues, which control the release of bioactive agents thought involved in mediating the heart disease, is unclear.

Other clinical manifestations include wheezing or asthma-like symptoms (8–18%), pellagra-like skin lesions (2–25%), and impaired cognitive function. A variety of noncardiac problems due to increased fibrous tissue have been reported, including retroperitoneal fibrosis causing urethral obstruction, Peyronie's disease of the penis, intraabdominal fibrosis, and occlusion of the mesenteric arteries or veins.

Pathobiology Carcinoid syndrome occurred in 8% of 8876 patients with GI-NETs (carcinoids), with a rate of 1.7–18.4% in different studies. It occurs only when sufficient concentrations of products secreted by the tumor reach the systemic circulation. In 91–100% of cases, this occurs after distant metastases to the liver. Rarely, primary GI-NETs (carcinoids) with nodal metastases with extensive retroperitoneal invasion, pNETs (carcinoids) with retroperitoneal lymph nodes, or NETs (carcinoids) of the lung or ovary with direct access to the systemic circulation can cause the carcinoid syndrome without hepatic metastases. All GI-NETs (carcinoids) do not have the same propensity to metastasize and cause the carcinoid syndrome (Table 113-3). Midgut NETs (carcinoids) account for 57–67% of cases of carcinoid syndrome, foregut NETs (carcinoids) for 0–33%, hindgut for 0–8%, and an unknown primary location for 2–26% (Tables 113-3 and 113-7).

One of the main secretory products of GI-NETs (carcinoids) involved in the carcinoid syndrome is serotonin (5-HT) (Fig. 113-1), which is synthesized from tryptophan. Up to 50% of dietary tryptophan can be used in this synthetic pathway by tumor cells, and this can result in inadequate supplies for conversion to niacin; hence, some patients (2.5%) develop pellagra-like lesions. Serotonin has numerous biologic effects, including stimulating intestinal secretion with inhibition of absorption, stimulating increases in intestinal motility, and stimulating fibrogenesis. In various studies, 56–88% of all GI-NETs (carcinoids) were associated with serotonin overproduction; however, 12–26% of the patients did not have the carcinoid syndrome. In one study, platelet serotonin was elevated in 96% of patients with midgut NETs (carcinoids), 43% with foregut tumors, and 0% with hindgut tumors. In 90–100% of patients with the carcinoid syndrome, there is evidence of serotonin overproduction. Serotonin is thought to be predominantly responsible for the diarrhea. Patients with the carcinoid syndrome have increased colonic motility with a shortened transit time and possibly a secretory/absorptive alteration that is compatible with the known actions of serotonin in the gut mediated primarily through 5-HT_3 and, to a lesser degree, 5-HT_4 receptors. Serotonin receptor antagonists (especially 5-HT_3 antagonists) relieve the diarrhea in many, but not all, patients. A tryptophan 5-hydroxylase inhibitor, LX-1031, which inhibits serotonin synthesis in peripheral tissues, is reported to cause a 44% decrease in bowel movement frequency and a 20% improvement in stool form in patients with the carcinoid syndrome. Additional studies suggest that tachykinins may be important mediators of diarrhea in some patients. In one study, plasma tachykinin levels correlated with symptoms of diarrhea. Serotonin does not appear to be involved in the flushing because serotonin receptor antagonists do not relieve flushing. In patients with gastric carcinoids, the characteristic red, patchy pruritic flush is thought due to histamine release because H_1 and H_2 receptor antagonists can prevent it. Numerous studies have shown that tachykinins (substance P, neuropeptide K) are stored in GI-NETs (carcinoids) and released during flushing. However, some studies have demonstrated that octreotide can relieve the flushing induced by pentagastrin in these patients without altering the stimulated increase in plasma substance P, suggesting that other mediators must be involved in the flushing. A correlation between plasma tachykinin levels (but not substance P levels) and flushing has been reported. Prostaglandin release could be involved in mediating either the diarrhea or flush, but conflicting data exist. Both histamine and serotonin may be responsible for the wheezing as well as the fibrotic reactions involving the heart, causing Peyronie's disease and intraabdominal fibrosis.

The exact mechanism of the heart disease remains unclear, although increasing evidence supports a central role for serotonin. Patients with heart disease have higher plasma levels of neurokinin A, substance P, plasma atrial natriuretic peptide (ANP), pro-brain natriuretic peptide, chromogranin A, and activin A as well as higher urinary 5-HIAA excretion.

The valvular heart disease caused by the appetite-suppressant drug dexfenfluramine is histologically indistinguishable from that observed in carcinoid disease. Furthermore, ergot containing dopamine receptor agonists used for Parkinson's disease (pergolide, cabergoline) cause valvular heart disease that closely resembles that seen in the carcinoid syndrome. Furthermore, in animal studies, the formation of valvular plaques/fibrosis occurs after prolonged treatment with serotonin as well as in animals with a deficiency of the 5-HIAA transporter gene, which results in an inability to inactivate serotonin. Metabolites of fenfluramine, as well as the dopamine receptor agonists, have high affinity for serotonin receptor subtype 5-HT_{2B} receptors, whose activation is known to cause fibroblast mitogenesis. Serotonin receptor subtypes $5\text{-HT}_{1B,1D,2A,2B}$ normally are expressed in human heart valve interstitial cells. High levels of 5-HT_{2B} receptors are known to occur in heart valves and occur in cardiac fibroblasts and cardiomyocytes. Studies of cultured interstitial cells from human cardiac valves have demonstrated that these valvulopathic drugs induce mitogenesis by activating 5-HT_{2B} receptors and stimulating upregulation of transforming growth factor β and collagen biosynthesis. These observations support the conclusion that serotonin overproduction by GI-NETs (carcinoids) is important in mediating the valvular changes, possibly by activating 5-HT_{2B} receptors in the endocardium. Both the magnitude of serotonin overproduction and prior chemotherapy are important predictors of progression of the heart disease, whereas patients with high plasma levels of ANP have a worse prognosis. Plasma connective tissue growth factor levels are elevated in many fibrotic conditions; elevated levels occur in patients with carcinoid heart disease and correlate with the presence of right ventricular dysfunction and the extent of valvular regurgitation in patients with GI-NETs (carcinoids).

Patients may develop either a typical or, rarely, an atypical carcinoid syndrome (Fig. 113-1). In patients with the typical form, which characteristically is caused by midgut NETs (carcinoids), the conversion of tryptophan to 5-HTP is the rate-limiting step (Fig. 113-1). Once 5-HTP is formed, it is rapidly converted to 5-HT and stored in secretory granules of the tumor or in platelets. A small amount remains in plasma and is converted to 5-HIAA, which appears in large amounts in the urine. These patients have an expanded serotonin pool size, increased blood and platelet serotonin, and increased urinary 5-HIAA. Some GI-NETs (carcinoids) cause an atypical carcinoid syndrome that is thought to be due to a deficiency in the enzyme dopa decarboxylase; thus, 5-HTP cannot be converted to 5-HT (serotonin), and 5-HTP is secreted into the bloodstream (Fig. 113-1). In these patients, plasma serotonin levels are normal but urinary levels may be increased because some 5-HTP is converted to 5-HT in the kidney. Characteristically, urinary 5-HTP and 5-HT are increased, but urinary 5-HIAA levels are only slightly elevated. Foregut carcinoids are the most likely to cause an atypical carcinoid syndrome; however, they also can cause a typical carcinoid syndrome.

One of the most immediate life-threatening complications of the carcinoid syndrome is the development of a carcinoid crisis. This is more common in patients who have intense symptoms or have greatly increased urinary 5-HIAA levels (i.e., >200 mg/d). The crisis may occur spontaneously; however, it is usually provoked by procedures such as anesthesia, chemotherapy, surgery, biopsy, endoscopy, or radiologic examinations such as during biopsies, hepatic artery embolization, and vessel catheterization. It can be provoked by stress or procedures as mild as repeated palpation of the tumor during physical examination. Patients develop intense flushing, diarrhea, abdominal pain, cardiac abnormalities including tachycardia, hypertension, or hypotension, and confusion or stupor. If not adequately treated, this can be a terminal event.

DIAGNOSIS OF THE CARCINOID SYNDROME AND GI-NETs (CARCINOIDS)

The diagnosis of carcinoid syndrome relies on measurement of urinary or plasma serotonin or its metabolites in the urine. The measurement of 5-HIAA is used most frequently. False-positive elevations may occur if the patient is eating serotonin-rich foods such as bananas, pineapples, walnuts, pecans, avocados, or hickory nuts or is taking certain medications (cough syrup containing guaifenesin, acetaminophen, salicylates, serotonin reuptake inhibitors, or L-dopa). The normal range for daily urinary 5-HIAA excretion is 2–8 mg/d. Serotonin overproduction was noted in 92% of patients with carcinoid syndrome in one study, and in another study, 5-HIAA had 73% sensitivity and 100% specificity for carcinoid syndrome. Serotonin overproduction is *not* synonymous with the presence of clinical carcinoid syndrome because 12–26% of patients with serotonin overproduction do not have clinical evidence of the carcinoid syndrome.

Most physicians use only the urinary 5-HIAA excretion rate; however, plasma and platelet serotonin levels, if available, may provide additional information. Platelet serotonin levels are more sensitive than urinary 5-HIAA but are not generally available. A single plasma 5-HIAA determination was found to correlate with the 24-h urinary values, raising the possibility that this could replace the standard urinary collection because of its greater convenience and avoidance of incomplete or improper collections. Because patients with foregut NETs (carcinoids) may produce an atypical carcinoid syndrome, if this syndrome is suspected and the urinary 5-HIAA is minimally elevated or normal, other urinary metabolites of tryptophan, such as 5-HTP and 5-HT, should be measured (Fig. 113-1).

Flushing occurs in a number of other diseases, including systemic mastocytosis, chronic myeloid leukemia with increased histamine release, menopause, reactions to alcohol or glutamate, and side effects of chlorpropamide, calcium channel blockers, and nicotinic acid. None of these conditions cause increased urinary 5-HIAA.

The diagnosis of carcinoid tumor can be suggested by the carcinoid syndrome, recurrent abdominal symptoms in a healthy-appearing individual, or the discovery of hepatomegaly or hepatic metastases associated with minimal symptoms. Ileal NETs (carcinoids), which make up 25% of all clinically detected carcinoids, should be suspected in patients with bowel obstruction, abdominal pain, flushing, or diarrhea.

Serum chromogranin A levels are elevated in 56–100% of patients with GI-NETs (carcinoids), and the level correlates with tumor bulk. Serum chromogranin A levels are not specific for GI-NETs (carcinoids) because they are also elevated in patients with pNETs and other NETs. Furthermore, a major problem is caused by potent acid antisecretory drugs such as proton pump inhibitors (omeprazole and related drugs) because they almost invariably cause elevation of plasma chromogranin A levels; the elevation occurs rapidly (3–5 days) with continued use, and the elevated levels overlap with the levels seen in many patients with NETs. Plasma neuron-specific enolase levels are also used as a marker of GI-NETs (carcinoids) but are less sensitive than chromogranin A, being increased in only 17–47% of patients. Newer markers have been proposed including pancreastatin (a chromogranin A breakdown product) and activin A. The former is not affected by proton pump inhibitors; however, its sensitivity and specificity are not established. Plasma activin elevations are reported to correlate with the presence of cardiac disease with a sensitivity of 87% and specificity of 57%.

TREATMENT CARCINOID SYNDROME AND NONMETASTATIC GASTROINTESTINAL NEUROENDOCRINE TUMORS (CARCINOIDS)

CARCINOID SYNDROME

Treatment includes avoiding conditions that precipitate flushing, dietary supplementation with nicotinamide, treatment of heart failure with diuretics, treatment of wheezing with oral bronchodilators, and control of the diarrhea with antidiarrheal agents such as loperamide and diphenoxylate. If patients still have symptoms, serotonin receptor antagonists or somatostatin analogues (Fig. 113-2) are the drugs of choice.

There are 14 subclasses of serotonin receptors, and antagonists for many are not available. The 5-HT_1 and 5-HT_2 receptor antagonists methysergide, cyproheptadine, and ketanserin have all been used to control the diarrhea but usually do not decrease flushing. The use of methysergide is limited because it can cause or enhance retroperitoneal fibrosis. Ketanserin diminishes diarrhea in 30–100% of patients. 5-HT_3 receptor antagonists (ondansetron, tropisetron, alosetron) can control diarrhea and nausea in up to 100% of patients and occasionally ameliorate the flushing. A combination of histamine H_1 and H_2 receptor antagonists (i.e., diphenhydramine and cimetidine or ranitidine) may control flushing in patients with foregut carcinoids. The tryptophan 5-hydoxylase inhibitor telotristat etiprate decreased bowel frequency in 44% and improved stool consistency in 20%.

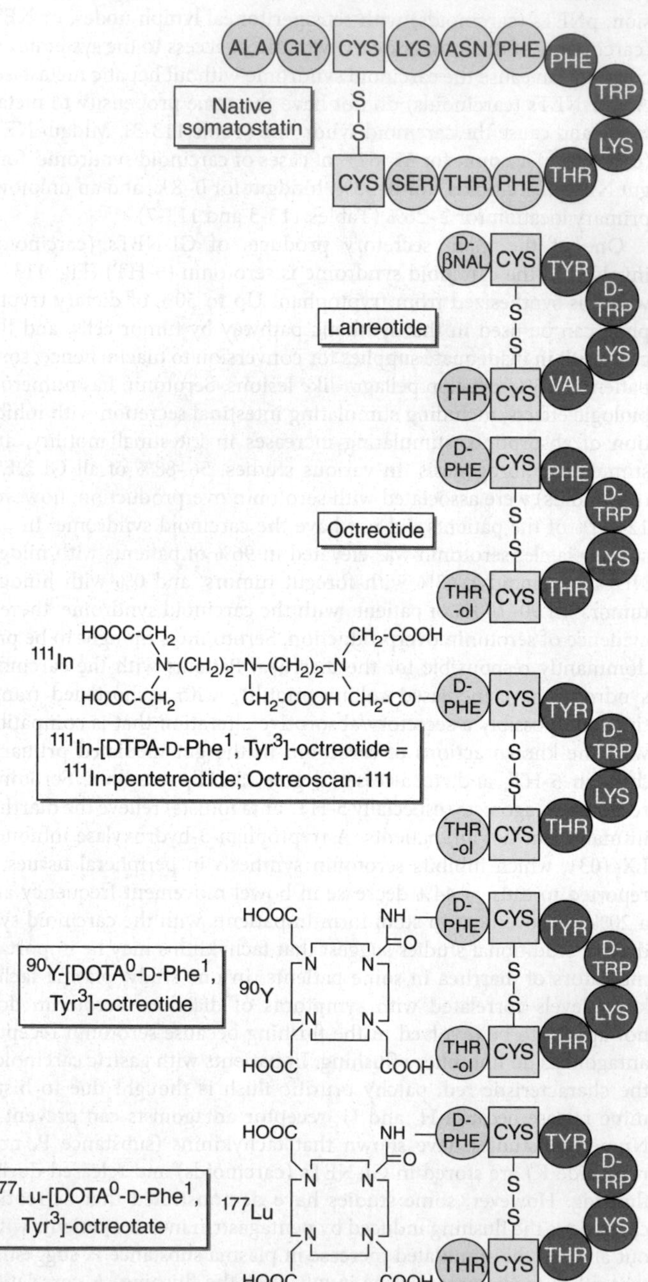

FIGURE 113-2 Structure of somatostatin and synthetic analogues used for diagnostic or therapeutic indications.

Synthetic analogues of somatostatin (octreotide, lanreotide) are now the most widely used agents to control the symptoms of patients with carcinoid syndrome (Fig. 113-2). These drugs are effective at relieving symptoms and decreasing urinary 5-HIAA levels in patients with this syndrome. Octreotide-LAR and lanreotide-SR/autogel (Somatuline) (sustained-release formulations allowing monthly injections) control symptoms in 74% and 68% of patients, respectively, with carcinoid syndrome and show a biochemical response in 51% and 64%, respectively. Patients with mild to moderate symptoms usually are treated initially with octreotide 100 μg SC every 8 h and then begun on the long-acting monthly depot forms (octreotide LAR or lanreotide-autogel). Forty percent of patients escape control after a median time of 4 months, and the depot dosage may have to be increased as well as supplemented with the shorter-acting formulation, SC octreotide. Pasireotide (SOM230) is a somatostatin analogue with broader selectivity (high-affinity somatostatin receptors [sst_1, sst_2, sst_3, sst_5]) than octreotide/lanreotide (sst_2, sst_5). In a phase II study of patients with refractory carcinoid syndrome, pasireotide controlled symptoms in 27%.

Carcinoid heart disease is associated with a decreased mean survival (3.8 years), and therefore, it should be sought for and carefully assessed in all patients with carcinoid syndrome. Transthoracic echocardiography remains a key element in establishing the diagnosis of carcinoid heart disease and determining the extent and type of cardiac abnormalities. Treatment with diuretics and somatostatin analogues can reduce the negative hemodynamic effects and secondary heart failure. It remains unclear whether long-term treatment with these drugs will decrease the progression of carcinoid heart disease. Balloon valvuloplasty for stenotic valves or cardiac valve surgery may be required.

In patients with carcinoid crises, somatostatin analogues are effective at both treating the condition and preventing their development during known precipitating events such as surgery, anesthesia, chemotherapy, and stress. It is recommended that octreotide 150–250 μg SC every 6 to 8 h be used 24–48 h before anesthesia and then continued throughout the procedure.

Currently, sustained-release preparations of both octreotide (octreotide-LAR [long-acting release], 10, 20, 30 mg) and lanreotide (lanreotide-PR [prolonged release, lanreotide-autogel], 60, 90, 120 mg) are available and widely used because their use greatly facilitates long-term treatment. Octreotide-LAR (30 mg/month) gives a plasma level ≥1 ng/mL for 25 days, whereas this requires three to six injections a day of the non-sustained-release form. Lanreotide-autogel (Somatuline) is given every 4–6 weeks.

Short-term side effects occur in up to one-half of patients. Pain at the injection site and side effects related to the GI tract (59% discomfort, 15% nausea, diarrhea) are the most common. They are usually short-lived and do not interrupt treatment. Important long term side effects include gallstone formation, steatorrhea, and deterioration in glucose tolerance. The overall incidence of gallstones/biliary sludge in one study was 52%, with 7% having symptomatic disease that required surgical treatment.

Interferon α is reported to be effective in controlling symptoms of the carcinoid syndrome either alone or combined with hepatic artery embolization. With interferon α alone, the clinical response rate is 30–70%, and with interferon α with hepatic artery embolization, diarrhea was controlled for 1 year in 43% and flushing was controlled in 86%. Side effects develop in almost all patients, with the most frequent being a flu-like syndrome (80–100%), followed by anorexia and fatigue, even though these frequently improve with continued treatment. Other more severe side effects include bone marrow toxicity, hepatotoxicity, autoimmune disorders, and rarely CNS side effects (depression, mental disorders, visual problems).

Hepatic artery embolization alone or with chemotherapy (chemoembolization) has been used to control the symptoms of carcinoid syndrome. Embolization alone is reported to control symptoms in up to 76% of patients, and chemoembolization (5-fluorouracil, doxorubicin, cisplatin, mitomycin) controls symptoms in 60–75% of patients. Hepatic artery embolization can have major side effects, including nausea, vomiting, pain, and fever. In two studies, 5–7% of patients died from complications of hepatic artery occlusion.

Other drugs have been used successfully in small numbers of patients to control the symptoms of carcinoid syndrome. Parachlorophenylanine can inhibit tryptophan hydroxylase and therefore the conversion of tryptophan to 5-HTP. However, its severe side effects, including psychiatric disturbances, make it intolerable for long-term use. α-Methyldopa inhibits the conversion of 5-HTP to 5-HT, but its effects are only partial.

Peptide radioreceptor therapy (using radiotherapy with radiolabeled somatostatin analogues), the use of radiolabeled microspheres, and other methods for treatment of advanced metastatic disease may facilitate control of the carcinoid syndrome and are discussed in a later section dealing with treatment of advanced disease.

GI-NETs (CARCINOIDS) (NONMETASTATIC)

Surgery is the only potentially curative therapy. Because with most GI-NETs (carcinoids), the probability of metastatic disease increases with increasing size, the extent of surgical resection is determined accordingly. With appendiceal NETs (carcinoids) <1 cm, simple appendectomy was curative in 103 patients followed for up to 35 years. With rectal NETs (carcinoids) <1 cm, local resection is curative. With SI NETs (carcinoids) <1 cm, there is not complete agreement. Because 15–69% of SI NETs (carcinoids) this size have metastases in different studies, some recommend a wide resection with en bloc resection of the adjacent lymph-bearing mesentery. If the tumor is >2 cm for rectal, appendiceal, or SI NETs (carcinoids), a full cancer operation should be done. This includes a right hemicolectomy for appendiceal NETs (carcinoids), an abdominoperineal resection or low anterior resection for rectal NETs (carcinoids), and an en bloc resection of adjacent lymph nodes for SI NETs (carcinoids). For appendiceal NETs (carcinoids) 1–2 cm in diameter, a simple appendectomy is proposed by some, whereas others favor a formal right hemicolectomy. For 1–2 cm rectal NETs (carcinoids), it is recommended that a wide, local, full-thickness excision be performed.

With type I or II gastric NETs (carcinoids), which are usually <1 cm, endoscopic removal is recommended. In type I or II gastric carcinoids, if the tumor is >2 cm or if there is local invasion, some recommend total gastrectomy, whereas others recommend antrectomy in type I to reduce the hypergastrinemia, which has led to regression of the carcinoids in a number of studies. For types I and II gastric NETs (carcinoids) of 1–2 cm, there is no agreement, with some recommending endoscopic treatment followed by chronic somatostatin treatment and careful follow-up and others recommending surgical treatment. With type III gastric NETs (carcinoids) >2 cm, excision and regional lymph node clearance are recommended. Most tumors <1 cm are treated endoscopically.

Resection of isolated or limited hepatic metastases may be beneficial and will be discussed in a later section on treatment of advanced disease.

PANCREATIC NEUROENDOCRINE TUMORS

Functional pNETs usually present clinically with symptoms due to the hormone-excess state (Table 113-2). Only late in the course of the disease does the tumor per se cause prominent symptoms such as abdominal pain. In contrast, all the symptoms due to nonfunctional pNETs are due to the tumor per se. The overall result of this is that some functional pNETs may present with severe symptoms with a small or undetectable primary tumor, whereas nonfunctional tumors usually present late in the disease course with large tumors, which are frequently metastatic. The mean delay between onset of continuous symptoms and diagnosis of a functional pNET syndrome is 4–7 years. Therefore, the diagnoses frequently are missed for extended periods.

TREATMENT PANCREATIC NEUROENDOCRINE TUMOR (GENERAL POINTS)

Treatment of pNETs requires two different strategies. First, treatment must be directed at the hormone-excess state such as the gastric acid hypersecretion in gastrinomas or the hypoglycemia in insulinomas. Ectopic hormone secretion usually causes the presenting symptoms and can cause life-threatening complications. Second, with all the tumors except insulinomas, >50% are malignant (Table 113-2); therefore, treatment must also be directed against the tumor per se. Because in many patients these tumors are not surgically curable due to the presence of advanced disease at diagnosis, surgical resection for cure, which addresses both treatment aspects, is often not possible.

GASTRINOMA (ZOLLINGER-ELLISON SYNDROME)

A gastrinoma is an NET that secretes gastrin; the resultant hypergastrinemia causes gastric acid hypersecretion (Zollinger-Ellison syndrome [ZES]). The chronic hypergastrinemia results in marked gastric acid hypersecretion and growth of the gastric mucosa with increased numbers of parietal cells and proliferation of gastric ECL cells. The gastric acid hypersecretion characteristically causes peptic ulcer disease (PUD), often refractory and severe, as well as diarrhea. The most common presenting symptoms are abdominal pain (70–100%), diarrhea (37–73%), and gastroesophageal reflux disease (GERD) (30–35%); 10–20% of patients have diarrhea only. Although peptic ulcers may occur in unusual locations, most patients have a typical duodenal ulcer. Important observations that should suggest this diagnosis include PUD with diarrhea; PUD in an unusual location or with multiple ulcers; PUD refractory to treatment or persistent; PUD associated with prominent gastric folds; PUD associated with findings suggestive of MEN 1 (endocrinopathy, family history of ulcer or endocrinopathy, nephrolithiases); and PUD without *Helicobacter pylori* present. *H. pylori* is present in >90% of idiopathic peptic ulcers but is present in <50% of patients with gastrinomas. Chronic unexplained diarrhea also should suggest ZES.

Approximately 20–25% of patients with ZES have MEN 1 (MEN1/ZES), and in most cases, hyperparathyroidism is present before the ZES develops. These patients are treated differently from those without MEN 1 (sporadic ZES); therefore, MEN 1 should be sought in all patients with ZES by family history and by measuring plasma ionized calcium and prolactin levels and plasma hormone levels (parathormone, growth hormone).

Most gastrinomas (50–90%) in sporadic ZES are present in the duodenum, followed by the pancreas (10–40%) and other intraabdominal sites (mesentery, lymph nodes, biliary tract, liver, stomach, ovary). Rarely, the tumor may involve extraabdominal sites (heart, lung cancer). In MEN 1/ZES the gastrinomas are also usually in the duodenum (70–90%), followed by the pancreas (10–30%), and are almost always multiple. About 60–90% of gastrinomas are malignant (Table 113-2) with metastatic spread to lymph nodes and liver. Distant metastases to bone occur in 12–30% of patients with liver metastases.

Diagnosis The diagnosis of ZES requires the demonstration of inappropriate fasting hypergastrinemia, usually by demonstrating hypergastrinemia occurring with an increased basal gastric acid output (BAO) (hyperchlorhydria). More than 98% of patients with ZES have fasting hypergastrinemia, although in 40–60% the level may be elevated less than tenfold. Therefore, when the diagnosis is suspected, a fasting gastrin is usually the initial test performed. It is important to remember that potent gastric acid suppressant drugs such as proton pump inhibitors (PPIs) (omeprazole, esomeprazole, pantoprazole, lansoprazole, rabeprazole) can suppress acid secretion sufficiently to cause hypergastrinemia; because of their prolonged duration of action, these drugs have to be tapered or frequently discontinued for a week before the gastrin determination. Withdrawal of PPIs should be performed carefully because PUD complications can rapidly develop in some patients and is best done in consultation with GI units with experience in this area. The widespread use of PPIs can confound the diagnosis of ZES by raising a false-positive diagnosis by causing hypergastrinemia in a patient being treated with idiopathic PUD (without ZES) and lead to a false-negative diagnosis because at routine doses used to treat patients with idiopathic PUD, PPIs control symptoms in most ZES patients and thus mask the diagnosis. If ZES is suspected and the gastrin level is elevated, it is important to show that it is increased when gastric pH is ≤2.0 because physiologically hypergastrinemia secondary to achlorhydria (atrophic gastritis, pernicious anemia) is one of the most common causes of hypergastrinemia. Nearly all ZES patients have a fasting pH ≤2 when off antisecretory drugs. If the fasting gastrin is >1000 pg/mL (increased tenfold) and the pH is ≤2.0, which occurs in 40–60% of patients with ZES, the diagnosis of ZES is established after the possibility of retained antrum syndrome has been ruled out by history. In patients with hypergastrinemia with fasting gastrins <1000 pg/mL (<10-fold increased) and gastric pH ≤2.0, other conditions, such as *H. pylori* infections, antral G-cell hyperplasia/hyperfunction, gastric outlet obstruction, and, rarely, renal failure, can masquerade as ZES. To establish the diagnosis in this group, a determination of BAO and a secretin provocative test should be done. In patients with ZES without previous gastric acid–reducing surgery, the BAO is usually (>90%) elevated (i.e., >15 mEq/h). The secretin provocative test is usually positive, with the criterion of a >120-pg/mL increase over the basal level having the highest sensitivity (94%) and specificity (100%). Unfortunately the diagnosis of ZES is becoming increasing more difficult. This is due not only to the widespread use of PPIs (leading to false-positive results as well as masking ZES presentation), but also recent studies demonstrate than many of the commercial gastrin kits that are used by most laboratories to measure fasting serum gastrin levels are not reliable. In one study, 7 of the 12 tested commercial gastrin kits inaccurately assessed the true serum concentration of gastrin primarily because the antibodies used had inappropriate specificity for the different circulating forms of gastrin and were not adequately validated. Both underestimation and overestimation of fasting serum gastrin levels occurred using these commercial kits. To circumvent this problem, it is either necessary to use one of the five reliable kits identified or, alternatively, to refer the patient to a center with expertise in making the diagnosis in your area, or if this is not possible, to contact such a center and use the gastrin assay they recommend. An accurate gastrin assay is essential for accurate measurement of fasting serum gastrin level as well as for assessing gastrin levels during the secretin provocative test, and thus, the diagnosis of ZES cannot reliably be made without one.

TREATMENT ZOLLINGER-ELLISON SYNDROME

Gastric acid hypersecretion in patients with ZES can be controlled in almost every case by oral gastric antisecretory drugs. Because of their long duration of action and potency, which allows dosing once or twice a day, the PPIs (H^+, K^+-ATPase inhibitors) are the drugs of choice. Histamine H_2-receptor antagonists are also effective, although more frequent dosing (q 4–8 h) and high doses are required. In patients with MEN 1/ZES with hyperparathyroidism, correction of the hyperparathyroidism increases the sensitivity to gastric antisecretory drugs and decreases the basal acid output. Long-term treatment with PPIs (>15 years) has proved to be safe and effective, without development of tachyphylaxis. Although patients with ZES, especially those with MEN 1/ZES, more frequently develop gastric NETs (carcinoids), no data suggest that the long-term use of PPIs increases this risk in these patients. With long-term PPI use in ZES patients, vitamin B_{12} deficiency can develop; thus, vitamin B_{12} levels should be assessed during follow-up. Epidemiologic studies suggest that long-term PPI use may be associated with an increased incidence of bone fractures; however, at present, there is no such report in ZES patients.

With the increased ability to control acid hypersecretion, more than 50% of patients who are not cured (>60% of patients) will die from tumor-related causes. At presentation, careful imaging studies are essential to localize the extent of the tumor to determine the appropriate treatment. A third of patients present with hepatic metastases, and in <15% of those patients, the disease is limited, so that surgical resection may be possible. Surgical short-term cure is possible in 60% of all patients without MEN 1/ZES or liver metastases (40% of all patients) and in 30% of patients long term. In patients with MEN 1/ZES, long-term surgical cure is rare because the tumors are multiple, frequently with lymph node metastases. Surgical studies demonstrate that successful resection of the gastrinoma not only decreases the chances of developing liver metastases but also increases the disease-related survival rate. Therefore, all patients with gastrinomas without MEN 1/ZES or a medical condition that limits life expectancy should undergo surgery by a surgeon experienced in the treatment of these disorders.

INSULINOMAS

An insulinoma is an NET of the pancreas that is thought to be derived from beta cells that ectopically secrete insulin, which results in hypoglycemia. The average age of occurrence is 40–50 years old. The most common clinical symptoms are due to the effect of the hypoglycemia on the CNS (neuroglycemic symptoms) and include confusion, headache, disorientation, visual difficulties, irrational behavior, and even coma. Also, most patients have symptoms due to excess catecholamine release secondary to the hypoglycemia, including sweating, tremor, and palpitations. Characteristically, these attacks are associated with fasting.

Insulinomas are generally small (>90% are <2 cm) and usually not multiple (90%); only 5–15% are malignant, and they almost invariably occur only in the pancreas, distributed equally in the pancreatic head, body, and tail.

Insulinomas should be suspected in all patients with hypoglycemia, especially when there is a history suggesting that attacks are provoked by fasting, or with a family history of MEN 1. Insulin is synthesized as proinsulin, which consists of a 21-amino-acid α chain and a 30-amino-acid β chain connected by a 33-amino-acid connecting peptide (C peptide). In insulinomas, in addition to elevated plasma insulin levels, elevated plasma proinsulin levels are found, and C-peptide levels are elevated.

Diagnosis The diagnosis of insulinoma requires the demonstration of an elevated plasma insulin level at the time of hypoglycemia. A number of other conditions may cause fasting hypoglycemia, such as the inadvertent or surreptitious use of insulin or oral hypoglycemic agents, severe liver disease, alcoholism, poor nutrition, and other extrapancreatic tumors. Furthermore, postprandial hypoglycemia can be caused by a number of conditions that confuse the diagnosis of insulinoma. Particularly important here is the increased occurrence of hypoglycemia after gastric bypass surgery for obesity, which is now widely performed. A new entity, insulinomatosis, was described that can cause hypoglycemia and mimic insulinomas. It occurs in 10% of patients with persistent hyperinsulinemic hypoglycemia and is characterized by the occurrence of multiple macro-/microadenomas expressing insulin, and it is not clear how to distinguish this entity from insulinoma preoperatively. The most reliable test to diagnose insulinoma is a fast up to 72 h with serum glucose, C-peptide, proinsulin, and insulin measurements every 4–8 h. If at any point the patient becomes symptomatic or glucose levels are persistently below <2.2 mmol/L (40 mg/dL), the test should be terminated, and repeat samples for the above studies should be obtained before glucose is given. Some 70–80% of patients will develop hypoglycemia during the first 24 h, and 98% by 48 h. In nonobese normal subjects, serum insulin levels should decrease to <43 pmol/L (<6 μU/mL) when blood glucose decreases to <2.2 mmol/L (<40 mg/dL) and the ratio of insulin to glucose is <0.3 (in mg/dL). In addition to having an insulin level >6 μU/mL when blood glucose is <40 mg/dL, some investigators also require an elevated C-peptide and serum proinsulin level, an insulin/glucose ratio >0.3, and a decreased plasma β-hydroxybutyrate level for the diagnosis of insulinomas. Surreptitious use of insulin or hypoglycemic agents may be difficult to distinguish from insulinomas. The combination of proinsulin levels (normal in exogenous insulin/hypoglycemic agent users), C-peptide levels (low in exogenous insulin users), antibodies to insulin (positive in exogenous insulin users), and measurement of sulfonylurea levels in serum or plasma will allow the correct diagnosis to be made. The diagnosis of insulinoma has been complicated by the introduction of specific insulin assays that do not also interact with proinsulin, as do many of the older radioimmunoassays (RIAs), and therefore give lower plasma insulin levels. The increased use of these specific insulin assays has resulted in increased numbers of patients with insulinomas having lower plasma insulin values (<6 μU/mL) than levels proposed to be characteristic of insulinomas by RIA. In these patients, the assessment of proinsulin and C-peptide levels at the time of hypoglycemia is particularly helpful for establishing the correct diagnosis. An elevated proinsulin level when the fasting glucose level is <45 mg/dL is sensitive and specific.

TREATMENT INSULINOMAS

Only 5–15% of insulinomas are malignant; therefore, after appropriate imaging (see below), surgery should be performed. In different studies, 75–100% of patients are cured by surgery. Before surgery, the hypoglycemia can be controlled by frequent small meals and the use of diazoxide (150–800 mg/d). Diazoxide is a benzothiadiazide whose hyperglycemic effect is attributed to inhibition of insulin release. Its side effects are sodium retention and GI symptoms such as nausea. Approximately 50–60% of patients respond to diazoxide. Other agents effective in some patients to control the hypoglycemia include verapamil and diphenylhydantoin. Long-acting somatostatin analogues such as octreotide and lanreotide are acutely effective in 40% of patients. However, octreotide must be used with care because it inhibits growth hormone secretion and can alter plasma glucagon levels; therefore, in some patients, it can worsen the hypoglycemia.

For the 5–15% of patients with malignant insulinomas, these drugs or somatostatin analogues are used initially. In a small number of patients with insulinomas, some with malignant tumors, mammalian target of rapamycin (mTOR) inhibitors (everolimus, rapamycin) are reported to control the hypoglycemia. If they are not effective, various antitumor treatments such as hepatic arterial embolization, chemoembolization, chemotherapy, and peptide receptor radiotherapy have been used (see below).

Insulinomas, which are usually benign (>90%) and intrapancreatic in location, are increasingly resected using a laparoscopic approach, which has lower morbidity rates. This approach requires that the insulinoma be localized on preoperative imaging studies.

GLUCAGONOMAS

A glucagonoma is NET of the pancreas that secretes excessive amounts of glucagon, which causes a distinct syndrome characterized by dermatitis, glucose intolerance or diabetes, and weight loss. Glucagonomas principally occur between 45 and 70 years of age. The tumor is clinically heralded by a characteristic dermatitis (migratory necrolytic erythema) (67–90%), accompanied by glucose intolerance (40–90%), weight loss (66–96%), anemia (33–85%), diarrhea (15–29%), and thromboembolism (11–24%). The characteristic rash usually starts as an annular erythema at intertriginous and periorificial sites, especially in the groin or buttock. It subsequently becomes raised, and bullae form; when the bullae rupture, eroded areas form. The lesions can wax and wane. The development of a similar rash in patients receiving glucagon therapy suggests that the rash is a direct effect of the hyperglucagonemia. A characteristic laboratory finding is hypoaminoacidemia, which occurs in 26–100% of patients.

Glucagonomas are generally large tumors at diagnosis (5–10 cm). Some 50–80% occur in the pancreatic tail. From 50 to 82% have evidence of metastatic spread at presentation, usually to the liver. Glucagonomas are rarely extrapancreatic and usually occur singly.

Two new entities have been described that can also cause hyperglucagonemia and may mimic glucagonomas. Mahvah disease is due to a homozygous P86S mutation of the human glucagon receptor. It is associated with the development of α-cell hyperplasia, hyperglucagonemia, and the development of nonfunctioning pNETs. A second disease called *glucagon cell adenomatosis* can mimic glucagonoma syndrome clinically and is characterized by the presence of hyperplastic islets staining positive for glucagon instead of a single glucagonoma.

Diagnosis The diagnosis is confirmed by demonstrating an increased plasma glucagon level. Characteristically, plasma glucagon levels exceed 1000 pg/mL (normal is <150 pg/mL) in 90%; 7% are between 500 and 1000 pg/mL, and 3% are <500 pg/mL. A trend toward lower levels at diagnosis has been noted in the last decade. A plasma glucagon level >1000 pg/mL is considered diagnostic of glucagonoma. Other diseases causing increased plasma glucagon levels include cirrhosis, diabetic ketoacidosis, celiac disease, renal insufficiency, acute pancreatitis, hypercorticism, hepatic insufficiency, severe stress, and prolonged fasting or familial hyperglucagonemia, as well as danazol treatment. With the exception of cirrhosis, these disorders do not increase plasma glucagon >500 pg/mL.

Necrolytic migratory erythema is not pathognomonic for glucagonoma and occurs in myeloproliferative disorders, hepatitis B infection, malnutrition, short-bowel syndrome, inflammatory bowel disease, zinc deficiency, and malabsorption disorders.

TREATMENT GLUCAGONOMAS

In 50–80% of patients, hepatic metastases are present, and so curative surgical resection is not possible. Surgical debulking in patients with advanced disease or other antitumor treatments may be beneficial (see below). Long-acting somatostatin analogues such as octreotide and lanreotide improve the skin rash in 75% of patients and may improve the weight loss, pain, and diarrhea, but usually do not improve the glucose intolerance.

SOMATOSTATINOMA SYNDROME

The somatostatinoma syndrome is due to an NET that secretes excessive amounts of somatostatin, which causes a distinct syndrome characterized by diabetes mellitus, gallbladder disease, diarrhea, and steatorrhea. There is no general distinction in the literature between a tumor that contains somatostatin-like immunoreactivity (somatostatinoma) and does (11–45%) or does not (55–90%) produce a clinical syndrome (somatostatinoma syndrome) by secreting somatostatin. In a review of 173 cases of somatostatinomas, only 11% were associated with the somatostatinoma syndrome. The mean age is 51 years. Somatostatinomas occur primarily in the pancreas and small intestine, and the frequency of the symptoms and occurrence of the somatostatinoma syndrome differ in each. Each of the usual symptoms is more common in pancreatic than in intestinal somatostatinomas: diabetes mellitus (95% vs 21%), gallbladder disease (94% vs 43%), diarrhea (92% vs 38%), steatorrhea (83% vs 12%), hypochlorhydria (86% vs 12%), and weight loss (90% vs 69%). The somatostatinoma syndrome occurs in 30–90% of pancreatic and 0–5% of SI somatostatinomas. In various series, 43% of all duodenal NETs contain somatostatin; however, the somatostatinoma syndrome is rarely present (<2%). Somatostatinomas occur in the pancreas in 56–74% of cases, with the primary location being the pancreatic head. The tumors are usually solitary (90%) and large (mean size 4.5 cm). Liver metastases are common, being present in 69–84% of patients. Somatostatinomas are rare in patients with MEN 1, occurring in only 0.65%.

Somatostatin is a tetradecapeptide that is widely distributed in the CNS and GI tract, where it functions as a neurotransmitter or has paracrine and autocrine actions. It is a potent inhibitor of many processes, including release of almost all hormones, acid secretion, intestinal and pancreatic secretion, and intestinal absorption. Most of the clinical manifestations are directly related to these inhibitory actions.

Diagnosis In most cases, somatostatinomas have been found by accident either at the time of cholecystectomy or during endoscopy. The presence of psammoma bodies in a duodenal tumor should particularly raise suspicion. Duodenal somatostatin-containing tumors are increasingly associated with von Recklinghausen's disease (NF-1) (Table 113-6). Most of these tumors (>98%) do not cause the somatostatinoma syndrome. The diagnosis of the somatostatinoma syndrome requires the demonstration of elevated plasma somatostatin levels.

TREATMENT SOMATOSTATINOMAS

Pancreatic tumors are frequently (70–92%) metastatic at presentation, whereas 30–69% of SI somatostatinomas have metastases. Surgery is the treatment of choice for those without widespread hepatic metastases. Symptoms in patients with the somatostatinoma syndrome are also improved by octreotide treatment.

VIPOMAS

VIPomas are NETs that secrete excessive amounts of vasoactive intestinal peptide (VIP), which causes a distinct syndrome characterized by large-volume diarrhea, hypokalemia, and dehydration. This syndrome also is called Verner-Morrison syndrome, pancreatic cholera, and WDHA syndrome for *w*atery *d*iarrhea, *h*ypokalemia, and *a*chlorhydria, which some patients develop. The mean age of patients with this syndrome is 49 years; however, it can occur in children, and when it does, it is usually caused by a ganglioneuroma or ganglioneuroblastoma.

The principal symptoms are large-volume diarrhea (100%) severe enough to cause hypokalemia (80–100%), dehydration (83%), hypochlorhydria (54–76%), and flushing (20%). The diarrhea is secretory in nature, persisting during fasting, and is almost always >1 L/d and in 70% is >3 L/d. In a number of studies, the diarrhea was intermittent initially in up to half the patients. Most patients do not have accompanying steatorrhea (16%), and the increased stool volume is due to increased excretion of sodium and potassium, which, with the anions, accounts for the osmolality of the stool. Patients frequently have hyperglycemia (25–50%) and hypercalcemia (25–50%).

VIP is a 28-amino-acid peptide that is an important neurotransmitter, ubiquitously present in the CNS and GI tract. Its known actions include stimulation of SI chloride secretion as well as effects on smooth-muscle contractility, inhibition of acid secretion, and vasodilatory effects, which explain most features of the clinical syndrome.

In adults, 80–90% of VIPomas are pancreatic in location, with the rest due to VIP-secreting pheochromocytomas, intestinal carcinoids, and rarely ganglioneuromas. These tumors are usually solitary, 50–75% are in the pancreatic tail, and 37–68% have hepatic metastases at diagnosis. In children <10 years old, the syndrome is usually due to ganglioneuromas or ganglioblastomas and is less often malignant (10%).

Diagnosis The diagnosis requires the demonstration of an elevated plasma VIP level and the presence of large-volume diarrhea. A stool volume <700 mL/d is proposed to exclude the diagnosis of VIPoma. When the patient fasts, a number of diseases can be excluded that can cause marked diarrhea because the high volume of diarrhea is not sustained during the fast. Other diseases that can produce a secretory large-volume diarrhea include gastrinomas, chronic laxative abuse, carcinoid syndrome, systemic mastocytosis, rarely medullary thyroid cancer, diabetic diarrhea, sprue, and AIDS. Among these conditions, only VIPomas caused a marked increase in plasma VIP. Chronic surreptitious use of laxatives/diuretics can be particularly difficult to detect clinically. Hence, in a patient with unexplained chronic diarrhea, screens for laxatives should be performed; they will detect many, but not all, laxative abusers. Elevated plasma levels of VIP should not be the only basis of the diagnosis of VIPomas because they can occur with some diarrheal states including inflammatory bowel disease, post small bowel resection, and radiation enteritis. Furthermore, nesidioblastosis can mimic VIPomas by causing elevated plasma VIP levels, diarrhea, and even false-positive location in the pancreatic region on somatostatin receptor scintigraphy.

TREATMENT VIPOMAS

The most important initial treatment in these patients is to correct their dehydration, hypokalemia, and electrolyte losses with fluid and electrolyte replacement. These patients may require 5 L/d of fluid and >350 mEq/d of potassium. Because 37–68% of adults with VIPomas have metastatic disease in the liver at presentation, a significant number of patients cannot be cured surgically. In these patients, long-acting somatostatin analogues such as octreotide and lanreotide are the drugs of choice.

Octreotide/lanreotide will control the diarrhea short- and long-term in 75–100% of patients. In nonresponsive patients, the combination of glucocorticoids and octreotide/lanreotide has proved helpful in a small number of patients. Other drugs reported to be helpful in small numbers of patients include prednisone (60–100 mg/d), clonidine, indomethacin, phenothiazines, loperamide, lidamidine, lithium, propranolol, and metoclopramide. Treatment of advanced disease with cytoreductive surgery, embolization, chemoembolization, chemotherapy, radiotherapy, radiofrequency ablation, and peptide receptor radiotherapy may be helpful (see below).

NONFUNCTIONAL PANCREATIC NEUROENDOCRINE TUMORS (NF-pNETs)

NF-pNETs are NETs that originate in the pancreas and either secrete no products or their products do not cause a specific clinical syndrome. Their symptoms are due entirely to the tumor per se. NF-pNETs secrete chromogranin A (90–100%), chromogranin B (90–100%), α-HCG (human chorionic gonadotropin) (40%), neuron-specific enolase (31%), and β-HCG (20%), and because 40–90% secrete PP, they are also often called PPomas. Because the symptoms are due to the tumor mass, patients with NF-pNETs usually present late in the disease course with invasive tumors and hepatic metastases (64–92%), and the tumors are usually large (72% >5 cm). NF-pNETs are usually solitary except in patients with MEN 1, in which case they are multiple. They occur primarily in the pancreatic head. Even though these tumors do not cause a functional syndrome, immunocytochemical studies show that they synthesize numerous peptides and cannot be distinguished from functional pNETs by immunocytochemistry. In MEN 1, 80–100% of patients have microscopic NF-pNETs, but they become large or symptomatic in a minority (0–13%) of cases. In VHL, 12–17% develop NF-pNETs, and in 4%, they are ≥3 cm in diameter.

The most common symptoms are abdominal pain (30–80%), jaundice (20–35%), and weight loss, fatigue, or bleeding; 10–35% are found incidentally. The average time from the beginning of symptoms to diagnosis is 5 years.

Diagnosis The diagnosis is established by histologic confirmation in a patient without either the clinical symptoms or the elevated plasma hormone levels of one of the established syndromes. The principal difficulty in diagnosis is to distinguish an NF-pNET from a nonendocrine pancreatic tumor, which is more common, as well as from a functional pNET. Even though chromogranin A levels are elevated in almost every patient, this is not specific for this disease as it can be found in functional pNETs, GI-NETs (carcinoids), and other neuroendocrine disorders. Plasma PP elevations should strongly suggest the diagnosis in a patient with a pancreatic mass because it is usually normal in patients with pancreatic adenocarcinomas. Elevated plasma PP is not diagnostic of this tumor because it is elevated in a number of other conditions, such as chronic renal failure, old age, inflammatory conditions, alcohol abuse, pancreatitis, hypoglycemia, postprandially, and diabetes. A positive somatostatin receptor scan in a patient with a pancreatic mass should suggest the presence of pNET/NF-pNET rather than a nonendocrine tumor.

TREATMENT NONFUNCTIONAL PANCREATIC NEUROENDOCRINE TUMORS (NF-pNETs)

Overall survival in patients with sporadic NF-pNET is 30–63% at 5 years, with a median survival of 6 years. Unfortunately, surgical curative resection can be considered only in a minority of these patients because 64–92% present with diffuse metastatic disease. Treatment needs to be directed against the tumor per se using the various modalities discussed below for advanced disease. The treatment of NF-pNETs in either MEN 1 patients or patients with VHL is controversial. Most recommend surgical resection for any tumor >2–3 cm in diameter; however, there is no consensus on smaller NF-pNETs in these inherited disorders, with most recommending careful surveillance of these patients. The treatment of small sporadic, asymptomatic NF-pNETs (≤2 cm) is also controversial. Most of these are low- or intermediate-grade lesions, and <7% are malignant. Some advocate a nonoperative approach with careful, regular follow-up, whereas other recommend an operative approach with specially consideration for a laparoscopic surgical approach.

GRFOMAS

GRFomas are NETs that secrete excessive amounts of growth hormone–releasing factor (GRF) that cause acromegaly. GRF is a 44-amino-acid peptide, and 25–44% of pNETs have GRF immunoreactivity, although it is uncommonly secreted. GRFomas are lung tumors in 47–54% of cases, pNETs in 29–30%, and SI carcinoids in 8–10%; up to 12% occur at other sites. Patients have a mean age of 38 years, and the symptoms usually are due to either acromegaly or the tumor per se. The acromegaly caused by GRFomas is indistinguishable from classic acromegaly. The pancreatic tumors are usually large (>6 cm), and liver metastases are present in 39%. They should be suspected in any patient with acromegaly and an abdominal tumor, a patient with MEN 1 with acromegaly, or a patient without a pituitary adenoma with acromegaly or associated with hyperprolactinemia, which occurs in 70% of GRFomas. GRFomas are an uncommon cause of acromegaly. GRFomas occur in <1% of MEN 1 patients. The diagnosis is established by performing plasma assays for GRF and growth hormone. Most GRFomas have a plasma GRF level >300 pg/mL (normal <5 pg/mL men, <10 pg/mL women). Patients with GRFomas also have increased plasma levels of insulin-like growth factor type I (IGF-I) similar to those in classic acromegaly. Surgery is the treatment of choice if diffuse metastases are not present. Long-acting somatostatin analogues such as octreotide and lanreotide are the agents of choice, with 75–100% of patients responding.

OTHER RARE PANCREATIC NEUROENDOCRINE TUMOR SYNDROMES

Cushing's syndrome (ACTHoma) due to a pNET occurs in 4–16% of all ectopic Cushing's syndrome cases. It occurs in 5% of cases of sporadic gastrinomas, almost invariably in patients with hepatic metastases, and is an independent poor prognostic factor. Paraneoplastic hypercalcemia due to pNETs releasing parathyroid hormone–related peptide (PTHrP), a PTH-like material, or unknown factor, is rarely reported. The tumors are usually large, and liver metastases are usually present. Most (88%) appear to be due to release of PTHrP. pNETs occasionally can cause the carcinoid syndrome. A number of very rare pNET syndromes involving a few cases (less than five) have been described; these include a renin-producing pNET in a patient presenting with hypertension; pNETs secreting luteinizing hormone, resulting in masculinization or decreased libido; a pNET secreting erythropoietin, resulting in polycythemia; pNETs secreting IGF-II, causing hypoglycemia; and pNETs secreting enteroglucagon, causing small intestinal hypertrophy, colonic/SI stasis, and malabsorption (Table 113-2). A number of other possible functional pNETs have been proposed, but most authorities classify these as unclear or as a nonfunctional pNET because in each case numerous patients have been described with similar plasma hormone elevations that do not cause any symptoms. These include pNETs secreting calcitonin, neurotensin (neurotensinoma), PP (PPoma), and ghrelin (Table 113-2).

TUMOR LOCALIZATION

Localization of the primary tumor and knowledge of the extent of the disease are essential to the proper management of all GI-NETs (carcinoids) and pNETs. Without proper localization studies, it is not possible to determine whether the patient is a candidate for surgical resection (curative or cytoreductive) or requires antitumor treatment, to determine whether the patient is responding to antitumor therapies, or to appropriately classify/stage the patient's disease to assess prognosis.

Numerous tumor localization methods are used in both types of NETs, including cross-sectional imaging studies (CT, magnetic resonance imaging [MRI], transabdominal ultrasound), selective angiography, somatostatin receptor scintigraphy (SRS), and positron emission tomography. In pNETs, endoscopic ultrasound (EUS) and functional localization by measuring venous hormonal gradients are also reported to be useful. Bronchial carcinoids are usually detected by standard chest radiography and assessed by CT. Rectal, duodenal, colonic, and gastric carcinoids are usually detected by GI endoscopy. Because of their wide availability, CT and MRI are generally initially used to determine the location of the primary NETs and the extent of disease. NETs are hypervascular tumors, and with both MRI and CT, contrast enhancement is essential for maximal sensitivity, and it is recommended that generally triple-phase scanning be used. The ability of cross-sectional imaging and, to a lesser extent, SRS to detect NETs is a function of NET size. With CT and MRI, <10% of tumors <1 cm in diameter are detected, 30–40% of tumors 1–3 cm are detected, and >50% of tumors >3 cm are detected. Many primary GI-NETs (carcinoids) are small, as are insulinomas and duodenal gastrinomas, and are frequently not detected by cross-sectional imaging, whereas most other pNETs present late in the course of their disease and are large (>4 cm). Selective angiography is more sensitive, localizing 60–90% of all NETs; however, it is now used infrequently. For detecting liver metastases, CT and MRI are more sensitive than ultrasound, and with recent improvements, 5–25% of patients with liver metastases will be missed by CT and/or MRI.

pNETs, as well as GI-NETs (carcinoids), frequently (>80%) overexpress high-affinity somatostatin receptors in both the primary tumors and the metastases. Of the five types of somatostatin receptors (sst_{1-5}), radiolabeled octreotide binds with high affinity to sst_2 and sst_5, has a lower affinity for sst_3, and has a very low affinity for sst_1 and sst_4. Between 80 and 100% of GI-NETs (carcinoids) and pNETs possess sst_2, and many also have the other four sst subtypes. Interaction with these receptors can be used to treat these tumors as well as to localize NETs by using radiolabeled somatostatin analogues (SRS). In the United States, [^{111}In-DTPA-D-Phe^1]octreotide (octreoscan) is generally used with gamma camera detection using single-photon emission computed tomography (SPECT) imaging. Numerous studies, primarily in Europe, using gallium-68-labeled somatostatin analogues and positron emission tomography (PET) detection, demonstrate even greater sensitivity than with SRS with ^{111}In-labeled somatostatin analogues. Although not yet approved in the United States, there are a number of centers starting to use this approach. Because of its sensitivity and ability to localize tumor throughout the body, SRS is the initial imaging modality of choice for localizing both the primary tumor and metastatic NETs. SRS localizes tumor in 73–95% of patients with GI-NETs (carcinoids) and in 56–100% of patients with pNETs, except insulinomas. Insulinomas are usually small and have low densities of sst receptors, resulting in SRS being positive in only 12–50% of patients with insulinomas. SRS identifies >90–95% of patients with liver metastases due to NETs. Figure 113-3 shows an example of the increased sensitivity of SRS in a patient with a GI-NET (carcinoid) tumor. The CT scan showed a single liver metastasis, whereas the SRS demonstrated three metastases in the liver in multiple locations. Occasional false-positive responses with SRS can occur (12% in one study) because numerous other normal tissues as well as diseases can have high densities of sst receptors, including granulomas (sarcoid, tuberculosis, etc.), thyroid diseases (goiter, thyroiditis), and activated lymphocytes (lymphomas, wound infections). If liver metastases are identified by SRS, to plan the proper treatment, either a CT or an MRI (with contrast enhancement) is recommended to assess the size and exact location of the metastases because SRS does not provide information on tumor size. For pNETs in the pancreas, EUS is highly sensitive, localizing 77–100% of insulinomas, which occur almost exclusively within the pancreas. Endoscopic ultrasound is less sensitive for extrapancreatic tumors. It is increasingly used in patients with MEN 1, and to a lesser extent VHL, to detect small pNETs not seen with other modalities or for serial pNET assessments to determine size changes or rapid growth in patients in whom surgery is deferred. EUS with cytologic evaluation also is used frequently to distinguish an NF-pNET from a pancreatic adenocarcinoma or another nonendocrine pancreatic tumor. Not infrequently patients present with liver metastases due to an NET and the primary site is unclear. Occult small intestinal NETs (carcinoids) are increasingly detected by double-balloon enteroscopy or capsule endoscopy.

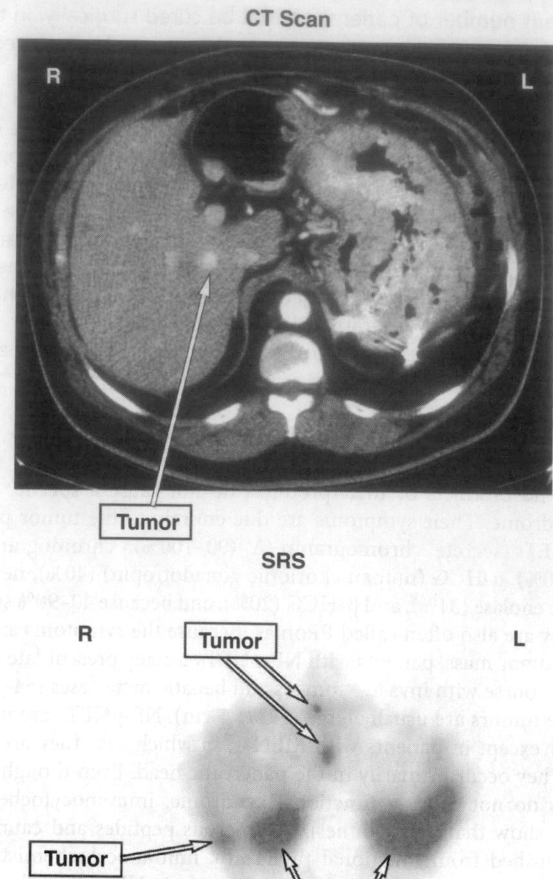

FIGURE 113-3 Ability of computed tomography (CT) scanning (*top*) or somatostatin receptor scintigraphy (SRS) (*bottom*) to localize metastatic carcinoid in the liver.

Insulinomas frequently overexpress receptors for glucagon-like peptide-1 (GLP-1), and radiolabeled GLP-1 analogues have been developed that can detect occult insulinomas not localized by other imaging modalities. Functional localization by measuring hormonal gradients is now uncommonly used with gastrinomas (after intra-arterial secretin injections) but is still frequently used in insulinoma patients in whom other imaging studies are negative (assessing hepatic vein insulin concentrations post-intra-arterial calcium injections). Functional localization measuring hormone gradients in insulinomas or gastrin gradients in gastrinoma is a sensitive method, being positive in 80–100% of patients. The intra-arterial calcium test may also allow differentiation of the cause of the hypoglycemia and indicate whether it is due to an insulinoma or a nesidioblastosis. The latter entity is becoming increasingly important because hypoglycemia after gastric bypass surgery for obesity is increasing in frequency, and it is primarily due to nesidioblastosis, although it can occasionally be due to an insulinoma.

PET and use of hybrid scanners such as CT and SRS may have increased sensitivity. PET scanning with ^{18}F-fluoro-DOPA in patients with carcinoids or with ^{11}C-5-HTP in patients with pNETs or GI-NETs (carcinoids) has greater sensitivity than cross-sectional imaging studies and may be used increasingly in the future. PET scanning for GI-NETs is not currently approved in the United States.

TREATMENT ADVANCED DISEASE (DIFFUSE METASTATIC DISEASE)

The single most important prognostic factor for survival is the presence of liver metastases (Fig. 113-4). For patients with foregut carcinoids without hepatic metastases, the 5-year survival in one

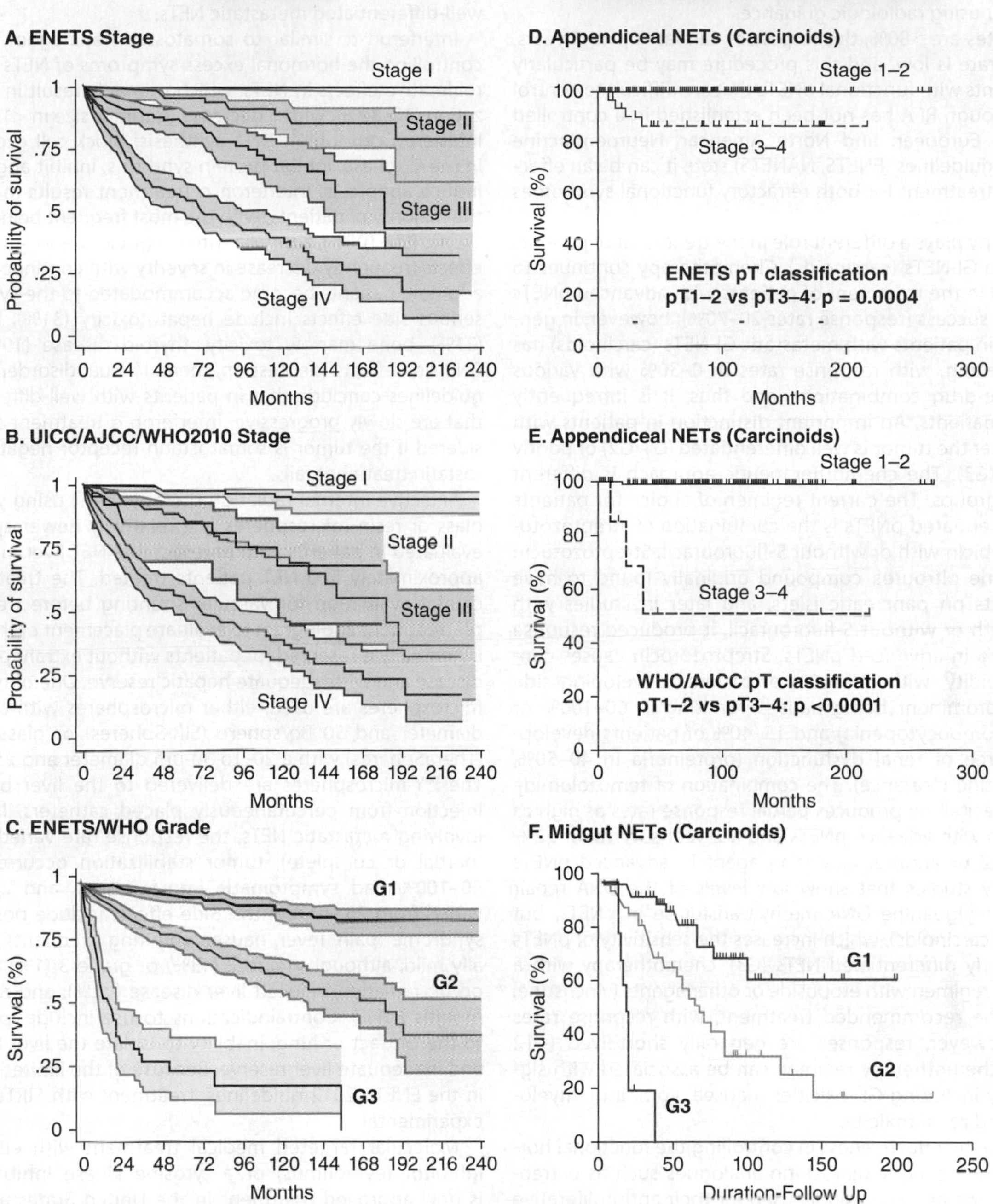

FIGURE 113-4 Survival (Kaplan-Meier plots) of patients with pancreatic neuroendocrine tumors (pNETs; n = 1072) (*A–C*) or gastrointestinal neuroendocrine tumors (GI-NETs; carcinoids) (appendix, n = 138; midgut, n = 238) (*D–F*) stratified according to recent proposed classification and grading systems. *(Panels A–C are drawn from data in G Rindi et al: J Natl Cancer Inst 104:764, 2012; panels D and E are drawn from data in M Volante et al: Am J Surg Pathol 37:606, 2013; and panel F is drawn from data in MS Khan: Br J Cancer 108:1838, 2013.)*

study was 95%, and with distant metastases, it was 20% (Fig. 113-4). With gastrinomas, the 5-year survival without liver metastases is 98%; with limited metastases in one hepatic lobe, it is 78%; and with diffuse metastases, 16% (Fig. 113-4). In a large study of 156 patients (67 pNETs, rest carcinoids), the overall 5-year survival rate was 77%; it was 96% without liver metastases, 73% with liver metastases, and 50% with distant disease. Another very important prognostic factor is whether the NET is well-differentiated (G1/G2) or poorly differentiated (<1% of all NETs) (G3). Well-differentiated NETs have a 5-year survival of 50–80%, whereas poorly differentiated NETs have a 5-year survival of only 0–15%.

Therefore, treatment for advanced metastatic disease is an important challenge. A number of different modalities are reported to be effective, including cytoreductive surgery (surgically or by radiofrequency ablation [RFA]), treatment with chemotherapy, somatostatin analogues, interferon α, hepatic embolization alone or with chemotherapy (chemoembolization), molecular targeted therapy, radiotherapy with radiolabeled beads/microspheres, peptide radioreceptor therapy (PRRT), and liver transplantation.

SPECIFIC ANTITUMOR TREATMENTS

Cytoreductive surgery is considered if either all of the visible metastatic disease or at last 90% is thought resectable; however, unfortunately, this is possible in only the 9–22% of patients who present with limited hepatic metastases. Although no randomized studies have proven that it extends life, results from a number of studies suggest that it may increase survival; therefore, it is recommended, if possible. RFA can be applied to NET liver metastases if they are limited in number (usually less than five) and size (usually <3.5 cm in diameter). It can be used at the time of surgery (either general or laparoscopic) or using radiologic guidance.

Response rates are >80%, the responses can last up to 3 years, the morbidity rate is low, and this procedure may be particularly helpful in patients with functional pNETs that are difficult to control medically. Although RFA has not been established in a controlled trial, both the European and North American Neuroendocrine Tumor Society guidelines (ENETS, NANETS) state it can be an effective antitumor treatment for both refractory functional syndromes and for palliative treatment.

Chemotherapy plays a different role in the treatment of patients with pNETs and GI-NETs (carcinoids). Chemotherapy continues to be widely used in the treatment of patients with advanced pNETs with moderate success (response rates 20–70%); however, in general, its results in patients with metastatic GI-NETs (carcinoids) has been disappointing, with response rates of 0–30% with various two- and three-drug combinations, and thus, it is infrequently used in these patients. An important distinction in patients with pNETs is whether the tumor is well differentiated (G1/G2) or poorly differentiated (G3). The chemotherapeutic approach is different for these two groups. The current regimen of choice for patients with well-differentiated pNETs is the combination of streptozotocin and doxorubicin with or without 5-fluorouracil. Streptozotocin is a glucosamine nitrourea compound originally found to have cytotoxic effects on pancreatic islets, and later in studies with doxorubicin with or without 5-fluorouracil, it produced response rates of 20–45% in advanced pNETs. Streptozotocin causes considerable morbidity, with 70–100% of patients developing side effects (most prominent being nausea/vomiting in 60–100% or leukopenia/thrombocytopenia) and 15–40% of patients developing some degree of renal dysfunction (proteinuria in 40–50%, decreased creatine clearance). The combination of temozolomide (TMZ) with capecitabine produces partial response rates as high as 70% in patients with advance pNETs and a 2-year survival of 92%. The use of TMZ or another alkylating agent in advanced pNETs is supported by studies that show low levels of the DNA repair enzyme O^6-methylguanine DNA methyltransferase in pNETs, but not in GI-NETs (carcinoids), which increases the sensitivity of pNETs to TMZ. In poorly differentiated NETs (G3), chemotherapy with a cisplatin-based regimen with etoposide or other agents (vincristine, paclitaxel) is the recommended treatment, with response rates of 40–70%; however, responses are generally short-lived (<12 months). This chemotherapy regimen can be associated with significant toxicity including GI toxicities (nausea, vomiting), myelosuppression, and renal toxicity.

In addition to the effectiveness in controlling the functional hormonal state, long-acting somatostatin analogues such as octreotide and lanreotide are increasingly used for their antiproliferative effects. Whereas somatostatin analogues rarely decrease tumor size (i.e., 0–17%), these drugs have tumoristatic effects, stopping additional growth in 26–95% of patients with NETs. In a randomized, double-blind study in patients with metastatic midgut carcinoids (PROMID study) octreotide-LAR demonstrated a marked lengthening of time to progression (14.3 vs 6 months, $p = .000072$). This improvement was seen in patients with limited liver involvement. This study did not assess whether such treatment will extend survival. A double-blind, randomized, placebo-controlled, phase III study in patients with well-differentiated, metastatic, inoperable pNETs (45%) or GI-NETs (carcinoids) (55%) (CLARINET study) showed that monthly treatment with lanreotide-autogel reduced tumor progression or death by 53%. Somatostatin analogues can induce apoptosis in GI-NETs (carcinoids), which probably contributes to their tumoristatic effects. Treatment with somatostatin analogues is generally well-tolerated, with most side effects being mild and uncommonly leading to stopping the drug. Potential long-term side effects include diabetes/glucose intolerance, steatorrhea, and the development of gallbladder sludge/gallstones (10–80%), although only 1% of patients develop symptomatic gallbladder disease. Because of these phase III studies, somatostatin analogues are generally recommended as first-line treatment for patients with well-differentiated metastatic NETs.

Interferon α, similar to somatostatin analogues, is effective at controlling the hormonal excess symptoms of NETs and has antiproliferative effects in NETs, which primarily result in disease stabilization (30–80%), with a decrease in tumor size in <15% of patients. Interferon can inhibit DNA synthesis, block cell cycle progression in the G_1 phase, inhibit protein synthesis, inhibit angiogenesis, and induce apoptosis. Interferon α treatment results in side effects in the majority of patients, with the most frequent being a flu-like syndrome (80–100%), anorexia with weight loss, and fatigue. These side effects frequently decrease in severity with continued treatment. In addition, patients become accommodated to the symptoms. More serious side effects include hepatotoxicity (31%), hyperlipidemia (31%), bone marrow toxicity, thyroid disease (19%), and rarely CNS side effects (depression, mental/visual disorders). ENETS 2012 guidelines conclude that in patients with well-differentiated NETs that are slowly progressive, interferon α treatment should be considered if the tumor is somatostatin receptor negative or if somatostatin treatment fails.

Selective internal radiation therapy (SIRT) using yttrium-90 (^{90}Y) glass or resin microspheres is a relatively newer approach being evaluated in patients with unresectable NET liver metastases, with approximately 500 NET patients treated. The treatment requires careful evaluation for vascular shunting before treatment and a pretreatment angiogram to evaluate placement of the catheter and is generally is reserved for patients without extrahepatic metastatic disease and with adequate hepatic reserve. One of two types of ^{90}Y microspheres are used: either microspheres with a 20- to 60-μm diameter and 50 Bq/sphere (SIR-Spheres) or glass microspheres (TheraSpheres) with a 20- to 30-μm diameter and 2500 Bq/sphere. The ^{90}Y-microspheres are delivered to the liver by intra-arterial injection from percutaneously placed catheters. In four studies involving metastatic NETs, the response rate varied from 50–61% (partial or complete), tumor stabilization occurred in 22–41%, 60–100% had symptomatic improvement, and overall survival varied from 25–70 months. Side effects include postembolization syndrome (pain, fever, nausea/vomiting [frequent]), which is usually mild, although grade 2 (43%) or grade 3 (1%) symptoms can occur; radiation-induced liver disease (<1%); and radiation pneumonitis (<1%). Contraindications to use include excess shunting to the GI tract or lung, inability to isolate the liver arterial supply, and inadequate liver reserve. Because of the limited data available in the ENETS 2012 guidelines, treatment with SIRTs is considered experimental.

Molecular targeted medical treatment with either an mTOR inhibitor (everolimus) or a tyrosine kinase inhibitor (sunitinib) is now approved treatment in the United States and Europe for patients with metastatic unresectable pNET, each supported by a phase III, double-blind, prospective, placebo-controlled trial. mTOR is a serine-threonine kinase that plays an important role in proliferation, cell growth, and apoptosis in both normal and neoplastic cells. Activation of the mTOR cascade is important in mediating NET cell growth, especially in pNETs. A number of mTOR inhibitors have shown promising antitumor activity in NETs including everolimus and temsirolimus, with the former undergoing a phase III trial (RADIANT-3) involving 410 patients with advance progressive pNETs. Everolimus caused significant improvement in progression-free survival (11 vs 4.6 months, $p < .001$) and increased by a factor of 3.7 the proportion of patients progression-free at 18 months (37% vs 9%). Everolimus treatment was associated with frequent side effects, causing a twofold increase in adverse events, with the most frequent being grade 1 or 2. Grade 3 or 4 side effects included hematologic, GI (diarrhea), stomatitis, or hypoglycemia occurring in 3–7% of patients. Most grade 3 or 4 side effects were controlled by dose reduction or drug interruption. The ENETS 2012 guidelines conclude that everolimus, similar to sunitinib (below), should be considered as a first-line treatment in selected cases of well-differentiated pNETs that are unresectable. NETs, like other normal and neoplastic cells, frequently possess multiple types of the 20 different tyrosine kinase (TK) receptors that are known and mediate the action of different growth factors. Numerous studies demonstrate that TK receptors in normal and neoplastic tissues as well as NETs are especially important in mediating cell growth, angiogenesis, differentiation, and apoptosis. Whereas a number of TK inhibitors show antiproliferative activity in NETs only sunitinib has undergone a phase III controlled trial. Sunitinib is an orally active small-molecule inhibitor of TK receptors (PDGFRs, VEGFR-1, VEGFR-2, c-KIT, FLT-3). In a phase III study in which 171 patients with progressive, metastatic, nonresectable pNETs were treated with sunitinib (37.5 mg/d) or placebo, sunitinib treatment caused a doubling of progression-free survival (11.4 vs 4.5 months, $p < .001$), an increase in objective tumor response rate (9% vs 0%, $p = .007$), and an increase in overall survival. Sunitinib treatment was associated with an overall threefold increase in side effects, although most were grade 1 or 2. The most frequent grade 3 or 4 side effects were neutropenia (12%) and hypertension (9.6%), which were controlled by dose reduction or temporary interruption. There is no consensus regarding the order of sunitinib or everolimus use in patients with advanced, well-differentiated, progressive pNETs.

PRRT for NETs involves treatment with radiolabeled somatostatin analogues. The success of this approach is based on the finding that somatostatin receptors (sst) are overexpressed or ectopically expressed by 60–100% of all NETs, which allows the targeting of cytotoxic, radiolabeled somatostatin receptor ligands.

Three different radionuclides are being used. High doses of [^{111}In-DTPA-D-Phe^{1}]octreotide, which emits γ-rays, internal conversion, and Auger electrons; ^{90}yttrium, which emits high-energy β-particles coupled by a DOTA chelating group to octreotide or octreotate; and ^{177}lutetium-coupled analogues, which emit both, are all in clinical studies. At present, the ^{177}lutetium-coupled analogues are the most widely used. ^{111}Indium-, ^{90}yttrium-, and ^{177}lutetium-labeled compounds caused tumor stabilization in 41–81%, 44–88%, and 23–40%, respectively, and a decrease in tumor size in 8–30%, 6–37%, and 38%, respectively, of patients with advanced metastatic NETs. In one large study involving 504 patients with malignant NETs, ^{177}lutetium-labeled analogues produced a reduction of tumor size of >50% in 30% of patients (2% complete) and tumor stabilization in 51% of patients. An effect on survival has not been established. At present, PRRT is not approved for use in either the United States or Europe, but because of the above promising results, a large phase III study is now being conducted in both the United States and Europe. The ENETS 2012, NANETS 2010, Nordic 2010, and European Society for Medical Oncology (ESMO) guidelines list PRRT as an experimental or investigational treatment at present.

The use of liver transplantation has been abandoned for treatment of most metastatic tumors to the liver. However, for metastatic NETs, it is still a consideration. Among 213 European patients with NETs (50% functional NETs) who had liver transplantation from 1982 to 2009, the overall 5-year survival was 52% and disease free-survival was 30%. In various studies, the postoperative mortality rate is 10–14%. These results are similar to the United Network for Organ Sharing data in the United States in which 150 NET patients had liver transplants and the 5-year survival was 49%. In various studies, important prognostic factors for a poor outcome include a major resection performed in addition at the time of the liver transplant; poor tumor differentiation; hepatomegaly; age >45 years; a primary NET in the duodenum or pancreas; the presence of extrahepatic metastatic disease or extensive liver involvement (>50%); Ki-67 proliferative index >10%; and abnormal E-cadherin staining. The ENETS 2012 guidelines conclude that liver transplantation should be viewed as providing palliative care, with cure an exception, and recommend it be reserved for patients with life-threatening hormonal disturbances refractory to other treatments or for selected patients with a nonfunctional tumor with diffuse liver metastatic disease refractory to all other treatments.

114 Bladder and Renal Cell Carcinomas

Howard I. Scher, Jonathan E. Rosenberg, Robert J. Motzer

BLADDER CANCER

Transitional cell epithelium lines the urinary tract from the renal pelvis to the ureter, urinary bladder, and the proximal two-thirds of the urethra. Cancers can occur at any point: 90% of malignancies develop in the bladder, 8% in the renal pelvis, and 2% in the ureter or urethra. Bladder cancer is the fourth most common cancer in men and the thirteenth in women, with an estimated 72,570 new cases and 15,210 deaths in the United States predicted for the year 2013. The almost 5:1 ratio of incidence to mortality reflects the higher frequency of the less lethal superficial variants compared to the more lethal invasive and metastatic variants. The incidence is roughly four times higher in men than in women and twofold higher in white men than in black men, with a median age of 65 years.

Once diagnosed, urothelial tumors exhibit polychronotropism, which is the tendency to recur over time in new locations in the urothelial tract. As long as urothelium is present, continuous monitoring is required.

EPIDEMIOLOGY

Cigarette smoking is believed to contribute to up to 50% of urothelial cancers in men and nearly 40% in women. The risk of developing a urothelial cancer in male smokers is increased two- to fourfold relative to nonsmokers and continues for 10 years or longer after cessation. Other implicated agents include aniline dyes, the drugs phenacetin and chlornaphazine, and external beam radiation. Chronic cyclophosphamide exposure also increases risk, whereas vitamin A supplements appear to be protective. Exposure to *Schistosoma haematobium*, a parasite found in many developing countries, is associated with an increase in both squamous and transitional cell carcinomas of the bladder.

PATHOLOGY

Clinical subtypes are grouped into three categories: 75% are superficial, 20% invade muscle, and 5% are metastatic at presentation. Staging of the tumor within the bladder is based on the pattern of growth and depth of invasion. The revised tumor, node, metastasis (TNM) staging system is illustrated in Fig. 114-1. About half of invasive tumors presented originally as superficial lesions that later progressed. Tumors are also rated by grade. Low-grade (highly differentiated) tumors rarely progress to a higher stage, whereas high-grade tumors do.

More than 95% of urothelial tumors in the United States are transitional cell in origin. Pure squamous cancers with keratinization constitute 3%, adenocarcinomas 2%, and small cell tumors (often with paraneoplastic syndromes) <1%. Adenocarcinomas develop primarily in the urachal remnant in the dome of the bladder or in the periurethral tissues. Paragangliomas, lymphomas, and melanomas are rare. Of the transitional cell tumors, low-grade papillary lesions that grow on a central stalk are most common. These tumors are very friable, have a tendency to bleed, and have a high risk for recurrence, yet they rarely progress to the more lethal invasive variety. In contrast, carcinoma in situ (CIS) is a high-grade tumor that is considered a precursor of the more lethal muscle-invasive disease.

PATHOGENESIS

The multicentric nature of the disease and high recurrence suggests a field effect in the urothelium that results in a predisposition to develop cancer. Molecular genetic analyses suggest that the superficial and invasive lesions develop along distinct molecular pathways. Low-grade noninvasive papillary tumors harbor constitutive activation of the receptor tyrosine kinase-Ras signal transduction pathway and high frequencies of fibroblast growth factor receptor 3 and phosphoinositide-3 kinase α subunit mutations. In contrast, CIS and invasive tumors have a higher frequency of *TP53* and *RB* gene alterations. Within all clinical stages, including Tis, T1, and T2 or greater lesions, tumors with alterations in *p53*, *p21*, and/or *RB* have a higher probability of recurrence, metastasis, and death from disease.

CLINICAL PRESENTATION, DIAGNOSIS, AND STAGING

Hematuria occurs in 80–90% of patients and often reflects exophytic tumors. The bladder is the most common source of gross hematuria (40%), but benign cystitis (22%) is a more common cause than bladder cancer (15%) (Chap. 61). Microscopic hematuria is more commonly of prostate origin (25%); only 2% of bladder cancers produce microscopic hematuria. Once hematuria is documented, a urinary cytology, visualization of the urothelial tract by computed tomography (CT) or magnetic resonance urogram or intravenous pyelogram, and cystoscopy are recommended if no other etiology is found. Screening asymptomatic individuals for hematuria increases the diagnosis of tumors at an early stage but has not been shown to prolong life. After hematuria, irritative symptoms are the next most common presentation. Ureteral obstruction may cause flank pain. Symptoms of metastatic disease are rarely the first presenting sign.

The endoscopic evaluation includes an examination under anesthesia to determine whether a palpable mass is present. A flexible endoscope is inserted into the bladder, and bladder barbotage for cytology is performed. Visual inspection includes mapping the location, size, and number of lesions, as well as a description of the growth pattern (solid vs papillary). All visible tumors should be resected, and a sample of the muscle underlying the tumor should be obtained to assess the depth of invasion. Normal-appearing areas are biopsied at random to ensure no CIS is present. A notation is made as to whether a tumor was completely or incompletely resected. Selective catheterization and visualization of the upper tracts should be performed if the cytology is positive and no disease is visible in the bladder. Ultrasonography, CT, and/or magnetic resonance imaging (MRI) are used to determine whether a tumor extends to perivesical fat (T3) and to document nodal spread. Distant metastases are assessed by CT of the chest and abdomen, MRI, or radionuclide imaging of the skeleton.

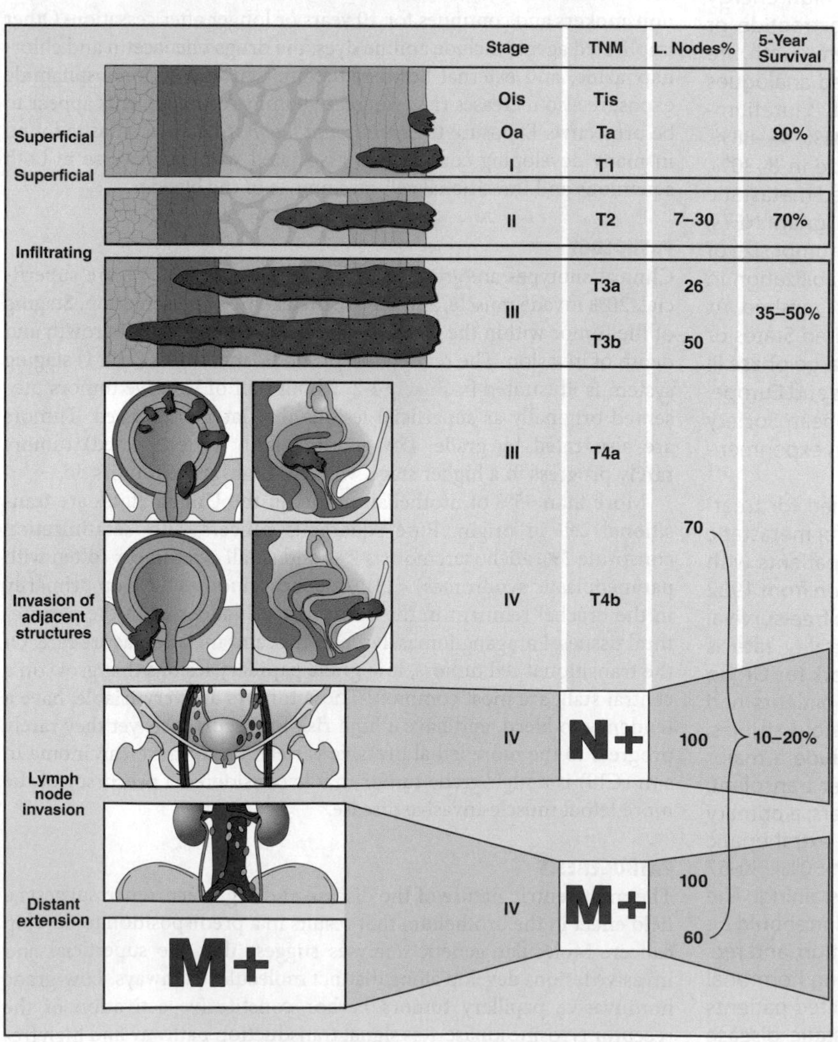

	Stage	TNM	L. Nodes%	5-Year Survival
Superficial	Ois	Tis		
	Oa	Ta		90%
Superficial	I	T1		
	II	T2	7–30	70%
Infiltrating	III	T3a	26	35–50%
		T3b	50	
	III	T4a		
Invasion of adjacent structures	IV	T4b	70	
Lymph node invasion	IV	N+	100	10–20%
Distant extension	IV	M+	100	
M+			60	

FIGURE 114-1 Bladder staging. TNM, tumor, node, metastasis.

TREATMENT BLADDER CANCER

Management depends on whether the tumor invades muscle and whether it has spread to the regional lymph nodes and beyond. The probability of spread increases with increasing T stage.

NON–MUSCLE-INVASIVE DISEASE

At a minimum, the management is complete endoscopic resection with or without intravesical therapy. The decision to recommend intravesical therapy depends on the histologic subtype, number of lesions, depth of invasion, presence or absence of CIS, and antecedent history. Recurrences develop in upward of 50% of cases, of which 5–20% progress to a more advanced stage. In general, solitary papillary lesions are managed by transurethral surgery alone. CIS and recurrent disease are treated by transurethral surgery followed by intravesical therapy.

Intravesical therapies are used in two general contexts: as an adjuvant to a complete endoscopic resection to prevent recurrence or to eliminate disease that cannot be controlled by endoscopic resection alone. Intravesical treatments are advised for patients with diffuse CIS, recurrent disease, >40% involvement of the bladder surface by tumor, or T1 disease. The standard therapy, based on randomized comparisons, is Bacillus Calmette-Guérin (BCG) in six weekly instillations, often followed by maintenance administrations for ≥1 year. Other agents with activity include mitomycin C, interferon, and gemcitabine. The side effects of intravesical therapies include dysuria, urinary frequency, and, depending on the drug, myelosuppression or contact dermatitis. Rarely, intravesical BCG may produce a systemic illness associated with granulomatous infections in multiple sites requiring antituberculin therapy.

Following the endoscopic resection, patients are monitored for recurrence at 3-month intervals during the first year. Recurrence may develop anywhere along the urothelial tract, including the renal pelvis, ureter, or urethra. Persistent disease in the bladder and new tumors are treated with a second course of BCG or intravesical chemotherapy with valrubicin or gemcitabine. In some cases, cystectomy is recommended. Tumors in the ureter or renal pelvis are typically managed by resection during retrograde examination or, in some cases, by instillation through the renal pelvis. Prostatic urethral tumors may require cystoprostatectomy if the tumor cannot be resected completely.

MUSCLE-INVASIVE DISEASE

The treatment of a tumor that has invaded muscle can be separated into control of the primary tumor and systemic chemotherapy to treat micrometastatic disease. Radical cystectomy is the standard treatment in the United States, although in selected cases, a bladder-sparing approach is used. This approach includes complete endoscopic resection; partial cystectomy; or a combination of resection, systemic chemotherapy, and external beam radiation therapy. In some countries, external beam radiation therapy is considered standard. In the United States, it is generally limited to those patients deemed unfit for cystectomy, those with unresectable local disease, or as part of an experimental bladder-sparing approach.

Indications for cystectomy include muscle-invading tumors not suitable for segmental resection; non–muscle-invasive tumors unsuitable for conservative management (e.g., due to multicentric and frequent recurrences resistant to intravesical instillations); high-grade T1 tumors especially if associated with CIS; and bladder symptoms (e.g., frequency or hemorrhage) that impair quality of life.

Radical cystectomy is major surgery that requires appropriate preoperative evaluation and management. It involves removal of the bladder and pelvic lymph nodes and creation of a conduit or reservoir for urinary flow. Grossly abnormal lymph nodes are evaluated by frozen section. If metastases are confirmed, the procedure is often aborted. In males, radical cystectomy includes the removal of the prostate, seminal vesicles, and proximal urethra. Impotence is universal unless the nerves responsible for erectile function are preserved. In females, the procedure includes removal of the bladder, urethra, uterus, fallopian tubes, ovaries, anterior vaginal wall, and surrounding fascia.

Several options are frequently used for urinary diversion. Ileal conduits bring urine directly from the ureter to the abdominal wall. Some patients receive either a continent cutaneous reservoir constructed from detubularized bowel or an orthotopic neobladder. Approximately 25% of men receive a neobladder, leading to 85–90% continence during the day. Cutaneous reservoirs are drained by intermittent catheterization. Contraindications to a neobladder include renal insufficiency, an inability to self-catheterize, or CIS or an exophytic tumor in the urethra. Diffuse CIS in the bladder is a relative contraindication based on the risk of a urethral recurrence. Concurrent ulcerative colitis or Crohn's disease may hinder the use of bowel.

A partial cystectomy may be considered when the disease is limited to the dome of the bladder, a ≥2 cm margin can be achieved, there is no associated CIS, and the bladder capacity is adequate after resection. This occurs in 5–10% of cases. Carcinomas in the ureter or in the renal pelvis are treated with nephroureterectomy with a bladder cuff to remove the tumor.

The probability of recurrence following surgery is based on pathologic stage, presence or absence of lymphatic or vascular invasion, and nodal spread. Among those whose cancers recur, the recurrence develops in a median of 1 year. Long-term outcomes vary by pathologic stage and histology (Table 114-1). The number of lymph nodes removed is also prognostic, whether or not the nodes contained tumor.

Chemotherapy (described below) has been shown to prolong the survival of patients with muscle-invasive disease when combined with definitive treatment of the bladder by radical cystectomy or radiation therapy. Presurgical (or neoadjuvant) chemotherapy has been the most thoroughly explored, and increases the cure rate by 5–15%, whereas postsurgical (adjuvant) chemotherapy has not been proven definitively beneficial. For the majority of patients, chemotherapy alone is inadequate to eradicate the disease. Use of neoadjuvant chemotherapy is increasing, although it still remains underused. Experimental studies are evaluating bladder preservation strategies by combining chemotherapy and radiation therapy in patients whose tumors were endoscopically removed.

METASTATIC DISEASE

The primary goal of metastatic disease treatment is to achieve complete remission with chemotherapy alone or with a combined-modality approach of chemotherapy followed by surgical resection of residual disease. One can define a goal in terms of cure or palliation on the basis of the probability of achieving a complete response to chemotherapy using prognostic factors, such as Karnofsky performance status (KPS) (<80%) and whether the pattern of spread is nodal or visceral (liver, lung, or bone). For those with zero, one, or two risk factors, the probability of complete remission is 38, 25, and 5%, respectively, and median survival is 33, 13.4, and 9.3 months, respectively. Patients who have low KPS or who have visceral disease or bone metastases rarely achieve long-term survival. The toxicities also vary as a function of risk, and treatment-related mortality rates are as high as 3–4% using some combinations in these poor-risk patient groups. For most patients, treatment is palliative, aimed at delaying or relieving cancer-related symptoms, because few patients experience durable complete remissions.

CHEMOTHERAPY

A number of chemotherapeutic drugs have activity as single agents; cisplatin, paclitaxel, and gemcitabine are considered most active. Standard therapy consists of two-, three-, or four-drug combinations. Overall response rates of >50% have been reported using combinations such as methotrexate, vinblastine, doxorubicin, and cisplatin (MVAC); gemcitabine and cisplatin (GC); or gemcitabine, paclitaxel, and cisplatin (GPC). MVAC was considered standard, but the toxicities of neutropenia and fever, mucositis, diminished renal and auditory function, and peripheral neuropathy led to the development of alternative regimens. At present, GC is used more commonly than MVAC based on the results of a comparative trial of MVAC versus GC that showed less neutropenia and fever and less mucositis for the GC regimen with similar response rates and median overall survival. Anemia and thrombocytopenia were more common with GC. GPC is not more effective than GC.

Chemotherapy has also been tested in the neoadjuvant and adjuvant settings. In a randomized trial, patients receiving three cycles of neoadjuvant MVAC followed by cystectomy had a significantly better median (6.2 years) and 5-year survival (57%) compared to cystectomy alone (median survival 3.8 years; 5-year survival 42%). Similar results were obtained in an international study of three cycles of cisplatin, methotrexate, and vinblastine (CMV) followed by either radical cystectomy or radiation therapy. The decision to administer adjuvant therapy is based on recurrence risk after cystectomy. Studies of adjuvant chemotherapy have been underpowered, and most closed for lack of accrual. One underpowered study using the GPC regimen suggested that adjuvant treatment improved survival, although many patients never received chemotherapy for metastases. Another underpowered study did not show a benefit for GC chemotherapy. Therefore, preoperative chemotherapy is preferred when medically appropriate. Indications for adjuvant chemotherapy in patients who did not receive neoadjuvant treatment include nodal disease, extravesical tumor extension, or vascular invasion in the resected specimen.

The management of bladder cancer is summarized in Table 114-2.

CARCINOMA OF THE RENAL PELVIS AND URETER

About 5000 cases of renal pelvis and ureter cancer occur each year; nearly all are transitional cell carcinomas similar to bladder cancer in biology and appearance. This tumor is associated with chronic phenacetin abuse and aristolochic acid consumption in Chinese herbal preparations; aristolochic acid also seems to be associated with Balkan nephropathy, a chronic interstitial nephritis endemic in Bulgaria, Greece, Bosnia-Herzegovina,

TABLE 114-1 SURVIVAL FOLLOWING SURGERY FOR BLADDER CANCER

Pathologic Stage	5-Year Survival, %	10-Year Survival, %
T2,N0	89	87
T3a,N0	78	76
T3b,N0	62	61
T4,N0	50	45
Any T,N1	35	34

TABLE 114-2 MANAGEMENT OF BLADDER CANCER

Nature of Lesion	Management Approach
Non–muscle-invasive disease	Endoscopic removal, usually with intravesical therapy
Muscle-invasive disease	Cystectomy ± systemic chemotherapy (before or after surgery)
Metastatic disease	Curative or palliative chemotherapy (based on prognostic factors) ± surgery

and Romania. In addition, upper tract urothelial carcinoma is linked to hereditary nonpolyposis colorectal cancer.

The most common symptom is painless gross hematuria, and the disease is usually detected on imaging during the workup for hematuria. Patterns of spread are like bladder cancer. For low-grade disease localized to the renal pelvis and ureter, nephroureterectomy (including excision of the distal ureter with a portion of the bladder) is associated with 5-year survival of 80–90%. More invasive or poorly differentiated tumors are more likely to recur locally and to metastasize. Metastatic disease is treated with the chemotherapy used in bladder cancer, and the outcome is similar to that of metastatic bladder cancer.

RENAL CELL CARCINOMA

Renal cell carcinomas account for 90–95% of malignant neoplasms arising from the kidney. Notable features include resistance to cytotoxic agents, infrequent responses to biologic response modifiers such as interleukin (IL) 2, robust activity to antiangiogenesis targeted agents, and a variable clinical course for patients with metastatic disease, including anecdotal reports of spontaneous regression.

EPIDEMIOLOGY

The incidence of renal cell carcinoma continues to rise and is now nearly 65,000 cases annually in the United States, resulting in 13,700 deaths. The male-to-female ratio is 2:1. Incidence peaks between the ages of 50 and 70 years, although this malignancy may be diagnosed at any age. Many environmental factors have been investigated as possible contributing causes; the strongest association is with cigarette smoking. Risk is also increased for patients who have acquired cystic disease of the kidney associated with end-stage renal disease and for those with tuberous sclerosis. Most cases are sporadic, although familial forms have been reported. One is associated with von Hippel-Lindau (VHL) syndrome. VHL syndrome is an autosomal dominant disorder. Genetic studies identified the *VHL* gene on the short arm of chromosome 3. Approximately 35% of individuals with VHL disease develop clear cell renal cell carcinoma. Other associated neoplasms include retinal hemangioma, hemangioblastoma of the spinal cord and cerebellum, pheochromocytoma, neuroendocrine tumors and cysts, and cysts in the epididymis of the testis in men and the broad ligament in women.

PATHOLOGY AND GENETICS

Renal cell neoplasia represents a heterogeneous group of tumors with distinct histopathologic, genetic, and clinical features ranging from benign to high-grade malignant (Table 114-3). They are classified on the basis of morphology and histology. Categories include clear cell carcinoma (60% of cases), papillary tumors (5–15%), chromophobe tumors (5–10%), oncocytomas (5–10%), and collecting or Bellini duct tumors (<1%). Papillary tumors tend to be bilateral and multifocal. Chromophobe tumors have a more indolent clinical course, and oncocytomas are considered benign neoplasms. In contrast, Bellini duct carcinomas, which are thought to arise from the collecting ducts within the renal medulla, are rare but often very aggressive. Clear cell tumors, the predominant histology, are found in >80% of patients who develop metastases. Clear cell tumors arise from the epithelial cells of the proximal tubules and usually show chromosome 3p deletions. Deletions of 3p21–26 (where the *VHL* gene maps) are identified in patients with familial as well as sporadic tumors. *VHL* encodes a tumor suppressor protein that is involved in regulating the transcription of vascular endothelial growth factor (VEGF), platelet-derived growth factor (PDGF), and a number of other hypoxia-inducible proteins. Inactivation of *VHL* leads to overexpression of these agonists of the VEGF and PDGF receptors, which promote tumor angiogenesis and tumor growth. Agents that inhibit proangiogenic growth factor activity show antitumor effects. Enormous genetic variability has been documented in tumors from individual patients. Although the tumors have a clear clonal origin and often contain *VHL* mutations in common, different portions of the primary tumor and different metastatic sites may have wide variation in genetic lesions they contain. This tumor heterogeneity may underlie the emergence of treatment resistance.

TABLE 114-3 CLASSIFICATION OF EPITHELIAL NEOPLASMS ARISING FROM THE KIDNEY

Carcinoma Type	Growth Pattern	Cell of Origin	Cytogenetics
Clear cell	Acinar or sarcomatoid	Proximal tubule	3p-, 5q+, 14q-
Papillary	Papillary or sarcomatoid	Proximal tubule	+7, +17, -Y
Chromophobe	Solid, tubular, or sarcomatoid	Distal tubules/cortical collecting duct	Whole arm losses (1, 2, 6, 10, 13, 17, and 21)
Oncocytic	Tumor nests	Cortical collecting duct	Undetermined
Collecting duct	Papillary or sarcomatoid	Medullary collecting duct	Undetermined

CLINICAL PRESENTATION

The presenting signs and symptoms include hematuria, abdominal pain, and a flank or abdominal mass. Other symptoms are fever, weight loss, anemia, and a varicocele. The tumor is most commonly detected as an incidental finding on a radiograph. Widespread use of radiologic cross-sectional imaging procedures (CT, ultrasound, MRI) contributes to earlier detection, including incidental renal masses detected during evaluation for other medical conditions. The increasing number of incidentally discovered low-stage tumors has contributed to an improved 5-year survival for patients with renal cell carcinoma and increased use of nephron-sparing surgery (partial nephrectomy). A spectrum of paraneoplastic syndromes has been associated with these malignancies, including erythrocytosis, hypercalcemia, nonmetastatic hepatic dysfunction (Stauffer's syndrome), and acquired dysfibrinogenemia. Erythrocytosis is noted at presentation in only about 3% of patients. Anemia, a sign of advanced disease, is more common.

The standard evaluation of patients with suspected renal cell tumors includes a CT scan of the abdomen and pelvis, chest radiograph, urine analysis, and urine cytology. If metastatic disease is suspected from the chest radiograph, a CT of the chest is warranted. MRI is useful in evaluating the inferior vena cava in cases of suspected tumor involvement or invasion by thrombus. In clinical practice, any solid renal masses should be considered malignant until proven otherwise; a definitive diagnosis is required. If no metastases are demonstrated, surgery is indicated, even if the renal vein is invaded. The differential diagnosis of a renal mass includes cysts, benign neoplasms (adenoma, angiomyolipoma, oncocytoma), inflammatory lesions (pyelonephritis or abscesses), and other primary or metastatic cancers. Other malignancies that may involve the kidney include transitional cell carcinoma of the renal pelvis, sarcoma, lymphoma, and Wilms' tumor. All of these are less common causes of renal masses than is renal cell cancer.

STAGING AND PROGNOSIS

Staging is based on the American Joint Committee on Cancer (AJCC) staging system (Fig. 114-2). Stage I tumors are <7 cm in greatest diameter and confined to the kidney, stage II tumors are ≥7 cm and confined to the kidney, stage III tumors extend through the renal capsule but are confined to Gerota's fascia (IIIa) or involve a single hilar lymph node (N1), and stage IV disease includes tumors that have invaded adjacent organs (excluding the adrenal gland) or involve multiple lymph nodes or distant metastases. The 5-year survival rate varies by stage: >90% for stage I, 85% for stage II, 60% for stage III, and 10% for stage IV.

TREATMENT RENAL CELL CARCINOMA

LOCALIZED TUMOR

The standard management for stage I or II tumors and selected cases of stage III disease is radical or partial nephrectomy. A radical nephrectomy involves en bloc removal of Gerota's fascia and

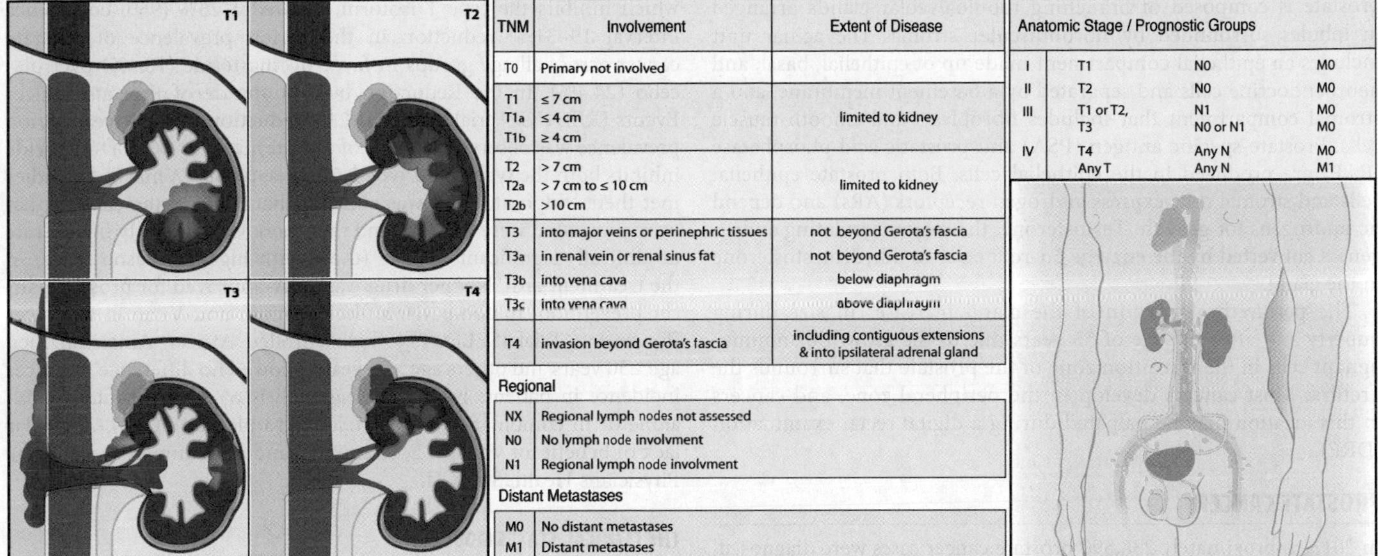

TNM	Involvement	Extent of Disease
T0	Primary not involved	
T1	≤ 7 cm	limited to kidney
T1a	≤ 4 cm	
T1b	≥ 4 cm	
T2	> 7 cm	limited to kidney
T2a	> 7 cm to ≤ 10 cm	
T2b	>10 cm	
T3	into major veins or perinephric tissues	not beyond Gerota's fascia
T3a	in renal vein or renal sinus fat	not beyond Gerota's fascia
T3b	into vena cava	below diaphragm
T3c	into vena cava	above diaphragm
T4	invasion beyond Gerota's fascia	including contiguous extensions & into ipsilateral adrenal gland
Regional		
NX	Regional lymph nodes not assessed	
N0	No lymph node involvment	
N1	Regional lymph node involvment	
Distant Metastases		
M0	No distant metastases	
M1	Distant metastases	

Anatomic Stage / Prognostic Groups			
I	T1	N0	M0
II	T2	N0	M0
III	T1 or T2,	N1	M0
	T3	N0 or N1	M0
IV	T4	Any N	M0
	Any T	Any N	M1

FIGURE 114-2 Renal cell carcinoma staging. TNM, tumor, node, metastasis.

its contents, including the kidney, the ipsilateral adrenal gland in some cases, and adjacent hilar lymph nodes. The role of a regional lymphadenectomy is controversial. Extension into the renal vein or inferior vena cava (stage III disease) does not preclude resection even if cardiopulmonary bypass is required. If the tumor is resected, half of these patients have prolonged survival.

Nephron-sparing approaches via open or laparoscopic surgery may be appropriate for patients who have only one kidney, depending on the size and location of the lesion. A nephron-sparing approach can also be used for patients with bilateral tumors. Partial nephrectomy techniques are applied electively to resect small masses for patients with a normal contralateral kidney. Adjuvant therapy following this surgery does not improve outcome, even in cases with a poor prognosis.

ADVANCED DISEASE

Surgery has a limited role for patients with metastatic disease. Long-term survival may occur in patients who relapse after nephrectomy in a solitary site that is removed. One indication for nephrectomy with metastases at initial presentation is to alleviate pain or hemorrhage of a primary tumor. Also, a cytoreductive nephrectomy before systemic treatment improves survival for carefully selected patients with stage IV tumors.

Metastatic renal cell carcinoma is refractory to chemotherapy. Cytokine therapy with IL-2 or interferon α (IFN-α) produces regression in 10–20% of patients. IL-2 produces durable complete remission in a small proportion of cases. In general, cytokine therapy is considered unsatisfactory for most patients.

The situation changed dramatically when two large-scale randomized trials established a role for antiangiogenic therapy, as predicted by the genetic studies. These trials separately evaluated two orally administered antiangiogenic agents, sorafenib and sunitinib, that inhibited receptor tyrosine kinase signaling through the VEGF and PDGF receptors. Both showed efficacy as second-line treatment following progression during cytokine treatment, resulting in approval by regulatory authorities for the treatment of advanced renal cell carcinoma. A randomized phase III trial comparing sunitinib to IFN-α showed superior efficacy for sunitinib with an acceptable safety profile. The trial resulted in a change in the standard first-line treatment from IFN to sunitinib. Sunitinib is usually given orally at a dose of 50 mg/d for 4 out of 6 weeks. Pazopanib and axitinib are newer agents of the same class. Pazopanib was compared to sunitinib in a randomized first-line phase III trial. Efficacy was similar, and there was less fatigue and skin toxicity, resulting in better quality of life scores for pazopanib compared with sunitinib. Temsirolimus and everolimus, inhibitors of the mammalian target of rapamycin (mTOR), show activity in patients with untreated poor-prognosis tumors and in sunitinib/sorafenib-refractory tumors. Patients benefit from the sequential use of axitinib and everolimus following progression to sunitinib or pazopanib first-line therapy.

The prognosis of metastatic renal cell carcinoma is variable. In one analysis, no prior nephrectomy, a KPS <80, low hemoglobin, high corrected calcium, and abnormal lactate dehydrogenase were poor prognostic factors. Patients with zero, one or two, and three or more factors had a median survival of 24, 12, and 5 months, respectively. These tumors may follow an unpredictable and protracted clinical course. It may be best to document progression before considering systemic treatment.

115 Benign and Malignant Diseases of the Prostate

Howard I. Scher, James A. Eastham

Benign and malignant changes in the prostate increase with age. Autopsies of men in the eighth decade of life show hyperplastic changes in >90% and malignant changes in >70% of individuals. The high prevalence of these diseases among the elderly, who often have competing causes of morbidity and mortality, mandates a risk-adapted approach to diagnosis and treatment. This can be achieved by considering these diseases as a series of states. Each state represents a distinct clinical milestone for which therapy(ies) may be recommended based on current symptoms, the risk of developing symptoms, or death from disease in relation to death from other causes within a given time frame. For benign proliferative disorders, symptoms of urinary frequency, infection, and potential for obstruction are weighed against the side effects and complications of medical or surgical intervention. For prostate malignancies, the risks of developing the disease, symptoms, or death from cancer are balanced against the morbidities of the recommended treatments and preexisting comorbidities.

ANATOMY

The prostate is located in the pelvis and is surrounded by the rectum, the bladder, the periprostatic and dorsal vein complexes and neurovascular bundles that are responsible for erectile function, and the urinary sphincter that is responsible for passive urinary control. The prostate is composed of branching tubuloalveolar glands arranged in lobules surrounded by fibromuscular stroma. The acinar unit includes an epithelial compartment made up of epithelial, basal, and neuroendocrine cells and separated by a basement membrane, and a stromal compartment that includes fibroblasts and smooth-muscle cells. Prostate-specific antigen (PSA) and prostatic acid phosphatase (PAP) are produced in the epithelial cells. Both prostate epithelial cells and stromal cells express androgen receptors (ARs) and depend on androgens for growth. Testosterone, the major circulating androgen, is converted by the enzyme 5α-reductase to dihydrotestosterone in the gland.

The periurethral portion of the gland increases in size during puberty and after the age of 55 years due to the growth of nonmalignant cells in the transition zone of the prostate that surrounds the urethra. Most cancers develop in the peripheral zone, and cancers in this location may be palpated during a digital rectal examination (DRE).

PROSTATE CANCER

In 2013, approximately 238,590 prostate cancer cases were diagnosed, and 29,720 men died from prostate cancer in the United States. The absolute number of prostate cancer deaths has decreased in the past 5 years, which has been attributed by some to the widespread use of PSA-based detection strategies. However, the benefit of screening on survival is unclear. The paradox of management is that although 1 in 6 men will eventually be diagnosed with the disease, and the disease remains the second leading cause of cancer deaths in men, only 1 man in 30 with prostate cancer will die of his disease.

EPIDEMIOLOGY

Epidemiologic studies show that the risk of being diagnosed with prostate cancer increases by a factor of two if one first-degree relative is affected and by four if two or more are affected. Current estimates are that 40% of early-onset and 5–10% of all prostate cancers are hereditary. Prostate cancer affects ethnic groups differently. Matched for age, African-American males have both a higher incidence of prostate cancer and larger tumors and more worrisome histologic features than white males. Polymorphic variants of the AR, the cytochrome P450 C17, and the steroid 5α-reductase type II (SRD5A2) genes have been implicated in the variations in incidence.

The prevalence of autopsy-detected cancers is similar around the world, while the incidence of clinical disease varies. Thus, environmental and dietary factors may play a role in prostate cancer growth and progression. High consumption of dietary fats, such as α-linoleic acid or the polycyclic aromatic hydrocarbons that form when red meats are cooked, is believed to increase risk. Similar to breast cancer in Asian women, the risk of prostate cancer in Asian men increases when they move to Western environments. Protective factors include consumption of the isoflavonoid genistein (which inhibits 5α-reductase) found in many legumes, cruciferous vegetables that contain the isothiocyanate sulforaphane, retinoids such as lycopene found in tomatoes, and inhibitors of cholesterol biosynthesis (e.g., statin drugs). The development of prostate cancer is a multistep process. One early change is hypermethylation of the *GSTP1* gene promoter, which leads to loss of function of a gene that detoxifies carcinogens. The finding that many prostate cancers develop adjacent to a lesion termed proliferative inflammatory atrophy (PIA) suggests a role for inflammation.

PREVENTION

Currently no drugs or dietary supplements are approved by the U.S. Food and Drug Administration (FDA) for prevention of prostate cancer, nor are any recommended by the major clinical guidelines. Although statins may have some protective effect, the potential risks outweigh the benefits given the small number of men who die of prostate cancer. The results from several large, double-blind, randomized chemoprevention trials established 5α-reductase inhibitors (5ARI) as the most likely therapy to reduce the future risk of a prostate cancer diagnosis. The Prostate Cancer Prevention Trial (PCPT), in which men older than age 55 years received placebo or the 5ARI finasteride, which inhibits the type 1 isoform, showed a 25% (95% confidence interval 19–31%) reduction in the period prevalence of prostate cancer across all age groups in favor of finasteride (18.4%) over placebo (24.4%). In the Reduction by Dutasteride of Prostate Cancer Events (REDUCE) trial, a similar 23% reduction in the 4-year period prevalence was observed in favor of dutasteride ($p = .001$). Dutasteride inhibits both the type 1 and type 2 5ARI isoforms. While both studies met their endpoint, there was concern that most of the cancers that were prevented were low risk and that there was a slightly higher rate of clinically significant cancers (those with higher Gleason score) in the treatment arm. Neither drug was FDA-approved for prostate cancer prevention. In comparison, the Selenium and Vitamin E Cancer Prevention Trial (SELECT), which enrolled African-American men age ≥50 years and others age ≥55 years, showed no difference in cancer incidence in patients receiving vitamin E (4.6%) or selenium (4.9%) alone or in combination (4.6%) relative to placebo (4.4%). A similar lack of benefit for vitamin E, vitamin C, and selenium was seen in the Physicians Health Study II.

THE CLINICAL STATES MODEL

The prostate cancer continuum—from the appearance of a preneoplastic and invasive lesion localized to the prostate, to a metastatic lesion that results in symptoms and, ultimately, mortality—can span decades. To facilitate disease management, competing risks are considered in the context of a series of clinical states (Fig. 115-1). The states are defined operationally on the basis of whether or not a cancer diagnosis has been established and, for those with a diagnosis, whether or not metastases are detectable on imaging studies and the measured level of testosterone in the blood. With this approach, an individual resides in only one state and remains in that state until he has progressed. At each assessment, the decision to offer treatment and the specific form of treatment are based on the risk posed by the cancer relative to competing causes of mortality that may be present in that individual. It follows that the more advanced the disease, the greater is the need for treatment.

For those without a cancer diagnosis, the decision to undergo testing to detect a cancer is based on the individual's estimated life expectancy and, separately, the probability that a clinically significant cancer may be present. For those with a prostate cancer diagnosis, the clinical states model considers the probability of developing symptoms or dying from prostate cancer. Thus, a patient with localized prostate cancer who has had all cancer removed surgically remains in the state of localized disease as long as the PSA remains undetectable. The time within a state becomes a measure of the efficacy of an intervention, although the effect may not be assessable for years. Because many men with active cancer are not at risk for metastases, symptoms, or death, the clinical states model allows a distinction between *cure*—the elimination of all cancer cells, the primary therapeutic objective when treating most cancers—and *cancer control*, in which the tempo of the illness is altered and symptoms are controlled until the patient dies of other causes. These can be equivalent therapeutically from a patient standpoint if the patient has not experienced symptoms of the disease or the treatment needed to control it. Even when a recurrence is documented, immediate therapy is not always necessary. Rather, as at the time of diagnosis, the need for intervention is based on the tempo of the illness as it unfolds in the individual, relative to the risk-to-benefit ratio of the therapy being considered.

SCREENING AND DIAGNOSIS

Physical Examination The need to pursue a diagnosis of prostate cancer is based on symptoms, an abnormal DRE, or, more typically, a change in or an elevated serum PSA. The urologic history should focus on symptoms of outlet obstruction, continence, potency, or change in ejaculatory pattern.

The DRE focuses on prostate size and consistency and abnormalities within or beyond the gland. Many cancers occur in the peripheral zone and may be palpated on DRE. Carcinomas are characteristically hard, nodular, and irregular, while induration may also be due to benign prostatic hypertrophy (BPH) or calculi. Overall, 20–25% of men with an abnormal DRE have cancer.

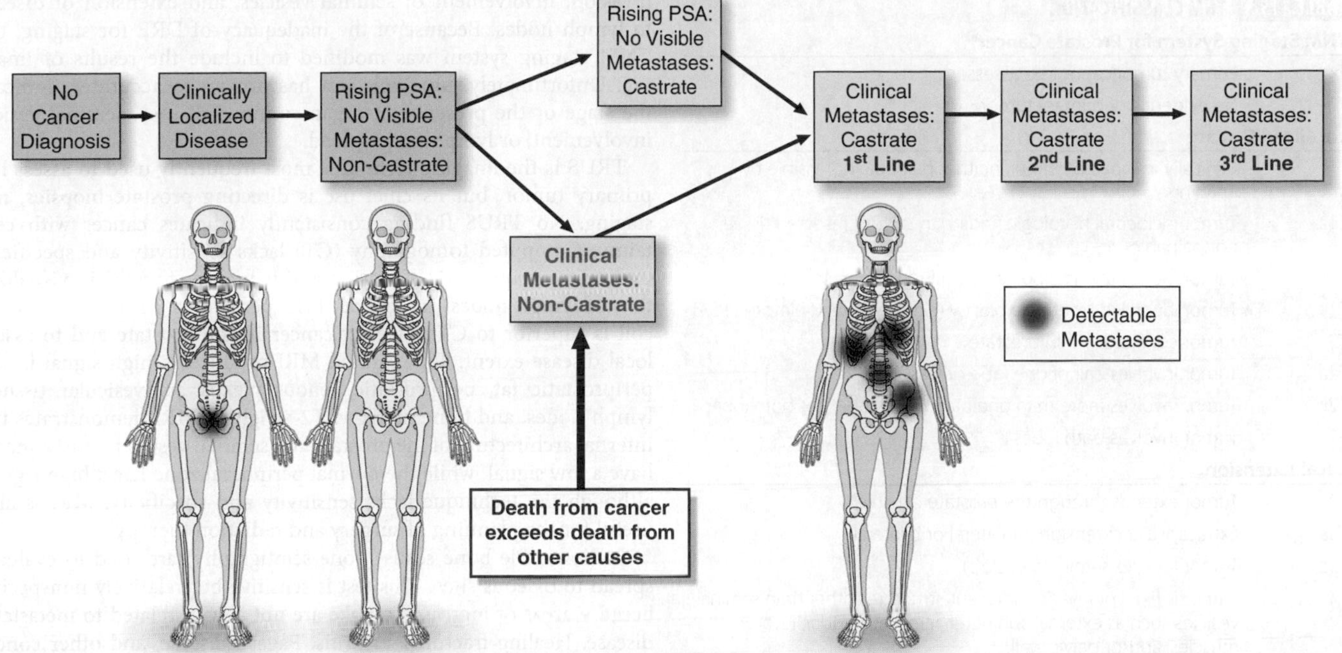

FIGURE 115-1 Clinical states of prostate cancer. PSA, prostate-specific antigen.

Prostate-Specific Antigen PSA (kallikrein-related peptidase 3; *KLK3*) is a kallikrein-related serine protease that causes liquefaction of seminal coagulum. It is produced by both nonmalignant and malignant epithelial cells and, as such, is prostate-specific, not prostate cancer–specific. Serum levels may also increase from prostatitis and BPH. Serum levels are not significantly affected by DRE, but the performance of a prostate biopsy can increase PSA levels up to tenfold for 8–10 weeks. PSA circulating in the blood is inactive and mainly occurs as a complex with the protease inhibitor α_1-antichymotrypsin and as free (unbound) PSA forms. The formation of complexes between PSA, α_2-macroglobulin, or other protease inhibitors is less significant. Free PSA is rapidly eliminated from the blood by glomerular filtration with an estimated half-life of 12–18 h. Elimination of PSA bound to α_1-antichymotrypsin is slow (estimated half-life of 1–2 weeks) because it too is largely cleared by the kidneys. Levels should be undetectable after about 6 weeks if the prostate has been removed. Immunohistochemical staining for PSA can be used to establish a prostate cancer diagnosis.

PSA-BASED SCREENING AND EARLY DETECTION PSA testing was approved by the U.S. FDA in 1994 for early detection of prostate cancer, and the widespread use of the test has played a significant role in the proportion of men diagnosed with early-stage cancers: more than 70–80% of newly diagnosed cancers are clinically organ-confined. The level of PSA in blood is strongly associated with the risk and outcome of prostate cancer. A single PSA measured at age 60 is associated (area under the curve [AUC] of 0.90) with lifetime risk of death from prostate cancer. Most prostate cancer deaths (90%) occur among men with PSA levels in the top quartile (>2 ng/mL), although only a minority of men with PSA >2 ng/mL will develop lethal prostate cancer. Despite this and mortality rate reductions reported from large randomized prostate cancer screening trials, routine use of the test remains controversial.

The U.S. Preventive Services Task Force (USPSTF) reviewed the evidence for screening for prostate cancer and made a clear recommendation against screening. By giving a grade of "D" in the recommendation statement that was based on this review, the USPSTF concluded that "there is moderate or high certainty that this service has no net benefit or that the harms outweigh the benefits." Whether the harms of screening, overdiagnosis, and overtreatment are justified by the benefits in terms of reduced prostate cancer mortality is open to reasonable doubt. In response to the USPSTF, the American Urological Association (AUA) updated their consensus statement regarding prostate cancer screening. They concluded that the quality of evidence for the benefits of screening was moderate, and evidence for harm was high for men age 55–69 years. For men outside this age range, evidence was lacking for benefit, but the harms of screening, including overdiagnosis and overtreatment, remained. The AUA recommends shared decision making considering PSA-based screening for men age 55–69, a target age group for whom benefits may outweigh harms. Outside this age range, PSA-based screening as a routine test was not recommended based on the available evidence. The entire guideline is available at *www.AUAnet.org/education/guidelines/prostate-cancer-detection.cfm*.

The PSA criteria used to recommend a diagnostic prostate biopsy have evolved over time. However, based on the commonly used cut point for prostate biopsy (a total PSA ≥4 ng/mL), most men with a PSA elevation do not have histologic evidence of prostate cancer at biopsy. In addition, many men with PSA levels below this cut point harbor cancer cells in their prostate. Information from the PCPT demonstrates that there is no PSA below which the risk of prostate cancer is zero. Thus, the PSA level establishes the likelihood that a man will harbor cancer if he undergoes a prostate biopsy. The goal is to increase the sensitivity of the test for younger men more likely to die of the disease and to reduce the frequency of detecting cancers of low malignant potential in elderly men more likely to die of other causes. Patients with symptomatic prostatitis should have a course of antibiotics before biopsy. However, the routine use of antibiotics in an asymptomatic man with an elevated PSA level is strongly discouraged.

Prostate Biopsy A diagnosis of cancer is established by an image-guided needle biopsy. Direct visualization by transrectal ultrasound (TRUS) or magnetic resonance imaging (MRI) assures that all areas of the gland are sampled. Contemporary schemas advise an extended-pattern 12-core biopsy that includes sampling from the peripheral zone as well as a lesion-directed palpable nodule or suspicious image-guided sampling. Men with an abnormal PSA and negative biopsy are advised to undergo a repeat biopsy.

BIOPSY PATHOLOGY Each core of the biopsy is examined for the presence of cancer, and the amount of cancer is quantified based on the length of the cancer within the core and the percentage of the core involved. Of the cancers identified, >95% are adenocarcinomas; the rest are squamous or transitional cell tumors or, rarely, carcinosarcomas. Metastases to the prostate are rare, but in some cases colon cancers or transitional cell tumors of the bladder invade the gland by direct extension.

TABLE 115-1 TNM CLASSIFICATION

TNM Staging System for Prostate Cancer[a]	
Tx	Primary tumor cannot be assessed
T0	No evidence of primary tumor
Localized Disease	
T1	Clinically inapparent tumor, neither palpable nor visible by imaging
T1a	Tumor incidental histologic finding in ≤5% of resected tissue; not palpable
T1b	Tumor incidental histologic finding in >5% of resected tissue
T1c	Tumor identified by needle biopsy (e.g., because of elevated PSA)
T2	Tumor confined within prostate[b]
T2a	Tumor involves half of one lobe or less
T2b	Tumor involves more than one half of one lobe, not both lobes
T2c	Tumor involves both lobes
Local Extension	
T3	Tumor extends through the prostate capsule[c]
T3a	Extracapsular extension (unilateral or bilateral)
T3b	Tumor invades seminal vesicle(s)
T4	Tumor is fixed or invades adjacent structures other than seminal vesicles such as external sphincter, rectum, bladder, levator muscles, and/or pelvic wall.
Metastatic Disease	
N1	Positive regional lymph nodes
M1	Distant metastases

[a]Revised from SB Edge et al (eds): *AJCC Cancer Staging Manual*, 7th ed. New York, Springer, 2010. [b]Tumor found in one or both lobes by needle biopsy, but not palpable or reliably visible by imaging, is classified as T1c. [c]Invasion into the prostatic apex or into (but not beyond) the prostatic capsule is classified not as T3 but as T2.

Abbreviations: PSA, prostate-specific antigen; TNM, tumor, node, metastasis.

When prostate cancer is diagnosed, a measure of histologic aggressiveness is assigned using the *Gleason grading system*, in which the dominant and secondary glandular histologic patterns are scored from 1 (well-differentiated) to 5 (undifferentiated) and summed to give a total score of 2–10 for each tumor. The most poorly differentiated area of tumor (i.e., the area with the highest histologic grade) often determines biologic behavior. The presence or absence of perineural invasion and extracapsular spread is also recorded.

Prostate Cancer Staging The tumor, node, metastasis (TNM) staging system includes categories for cancers identified solely on the basis of an abnormal PSA (T1c), those that are palpable but clinically confined to the gland (T2), and those that have extended outside the gland (T3 and T4) (**Table 115-1, Fig. 115-2**). DRE alone is inaccurate in determining the extent of disease within the gland, the presence or absence of capsular invasion, involvement of seminal vesicles, and extension of disease to lymph nodes. Because of the inadequacy of DRE for staging, the TNM staging system was modified to include the results of imaging. Unfortunately, no single test has proven to accurately indicate the stage or the presence of organ-confined disease, seminal vesicle involvement, or lymph node spread.

TRUS is the imaging technique most frequently used to assess the primary tumor, but its chief use is directing prostate biopsies, not staging. No TRUS finding consistently indicates cancer with certainty. Computed tomography (CT) lacks sensitivity and specificity to detect extraprostatic extension and is inferior to MRI in visualization of lymph nodes. In general, MRI performed with an endorectal coil is superior to CT to detect cancer in the prostate and to assess local disease extent. T1-weighted MRI produces a high signal in the periprostatic fat, periprostatic venous plexus, perivesicular tissues, lymph nodes, and bone marrow. T2-weighted MRI demonstrates the internal architecture of the prostate and seminal vesicles. Most cancers have a low signal, while the normal peripheral zone has a high signal, although the technique lacks sensitivity and specificity. MRI is also useful for the planning of surgery and radiation therapy.

Radionuclide bone scans (bone scintigraphy) are used to evaluate spread to osseous sites. This test is sensitive but relatively nonspecific because areas of increased uptake are not always related to metastatic disease. Healing fractures, arthritis, Paget's disease, and other conditions will also cause abnormal uptake. True-positive bone scans are uncommon when the PSA is <10 ng/mL unless the tumor is high grade.

TREATMENT — TREATMENT OF PROSTATE CANCER BY CLINICAL STATE

CLINICALLY LOCALIZED PROSTATE CANCER

Clinically localized prostate cancers are those that appear to be nonmetastatic after staging studies are performed. Patients with clinically localized disease are managed by radical prostatectomy, radiation therapy, or active surveillance. Choice of therapy requires the consideration of several factors: the presence of symptoms, the probability that the untreated tumor will adversely affect the quality or duration of survival and thus require treatment, and the probability that the tumor can be cured by single-modality therapy directed at the prostate or that it will require both local and systemic therapy to achieve cure.

Data from the literature do not provide clear evidence for the superiority of any one treatment relative to another. Comparison of outcomes of various forms of therapy is limited by the lack of prospective trials, referral bias, the experience of the treating teams, and differences in endpoints and cancer control definitions. Often, PSA relapse-free survival is used because an effect on metastatic progression

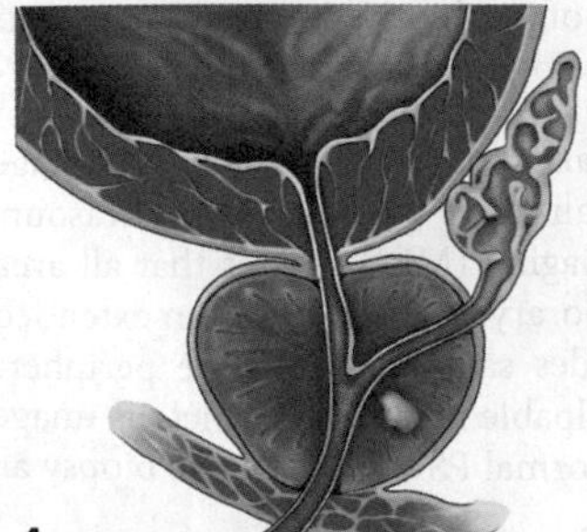

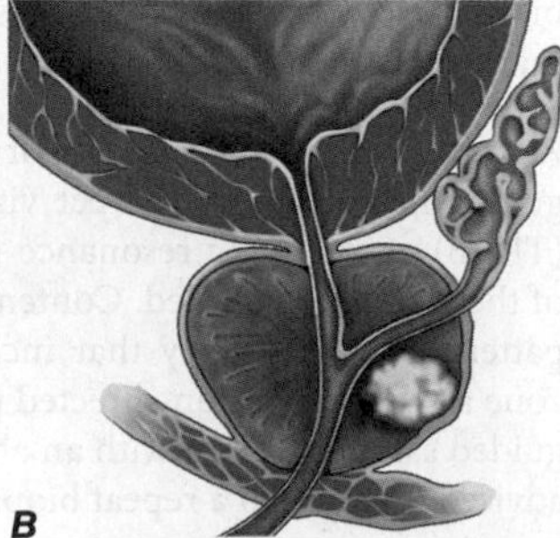

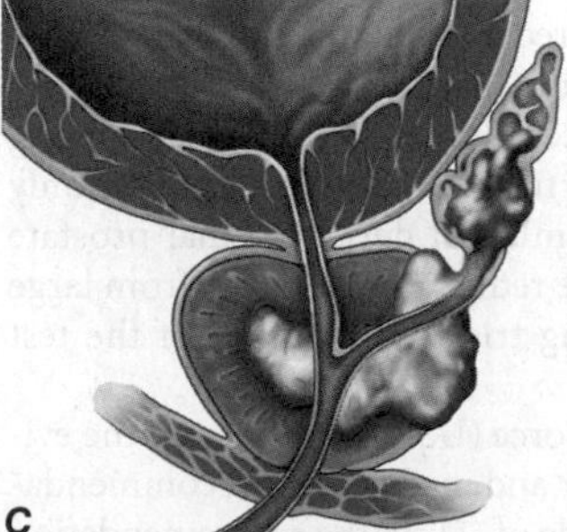

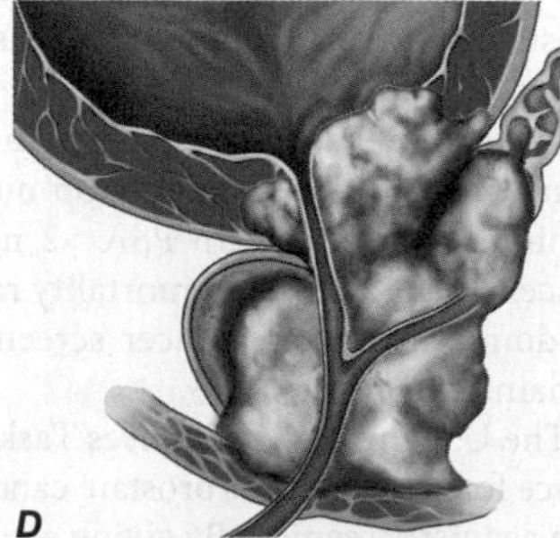

FIGURE 115-2 T stages of prostate cancer. *(A)* T1—Clinically inapparent tumor, neither palpable nor visible by imaging; *(B)* T2—Tumor confined within prostate; *(C)* T3—Tumor extends through prostate capsule and may invade the seminal vesicles; *(D)* T4—Tumor is fixed or invades adjacent structures. Eighty-one percent of patients present with local disease (T1 and T2), which is associated with a 5-year survival rate of 100%. An additional 12% of patients present with regional disease (T3 and T4 without metastases), which is also associated with a 100% survival rate after 5 years. Four percent of patients present with distant disease (T4 with metastases), which is associated with a 28% 5-year survival rate. (Three percent of patients are ungraded, and this group is associated with a 73% 5-year survival rate.) *(Data from AJCC, http://seer.cancer.gov/statfacts/html/prost.html. Figure © 2014 Memorial Sloan-Kettering Cancer Center; used with permission.)*

or survival may not be apparent for years. After radical surgery to remove all prostate tissue, PSA should become undetectable in the blood within 6 weeks. If PSA remains or becomes detectable after radical prostatectomy, the patient is considered to have persistent disease. After radiation therapy, in contrast, PSA does not become undetectable because the remaining nonmalignant elements of the gland continue to produce PSA even if all cancer cells have been eliminated. Similarly, cancer control is not well defined for a patient managed by active surveillance because PSA levels will continue to rise in the absence of therapy. Other outcomes are time to objective progression (local or systemic), cancer-specific survival, and overall survival; however, these outcomes may take years to assess.

The more advanced the disease, the lower the probability of local control and the higher the probability of systemic relapse. More important is that within the categories of T1, T2, and T3 disease are cancers with a range of prognoses. Some T3 tumors are curable with therapy directed solely at the prostate, and some T1 lesions have a high probability of systemic relapse that requires the integration of local and systemic therapy to achieve cure. For T1c cancers in particular, stage alone is inadequate to predict outcome and select treatment; other factors must be considered.

Nomograms To better assess risk and guide treatment selection, many groups have developed prognostic models or nomograms that use a combination of the initial clinical T stage, biopsy Gleason score, and baseline PSA. Some use discrete cut points (PSA <10 or ≥10 ng/mL; Gleason score of ≤6, 7, or ≥8); others employ nomograms that use PSA and Gleason score as continuous variables. More than 100 nomograms have been reported to predict the probability that a clinically significant prostate cancer is present, disease extent (organ-confined vs non–organ-confined, node-negative or -positive), or the probability of success of treatment for specific local therapies using pretreatment variables. Considerable controversy exists over what constitutes "high risk" based on a predicted probability of success or failure. In these situations, nomograms and predictive models can only go so far. Exactly what probability of success or failure would lead a physician to recommend and a patient to seek alternative approaches is controversial. As an example, it may be appropriate to recommend radical surgery for a younger patient with a low probability of cure. Nomograms are being refined continually to incorporate additional clinical parameters, biologic determinants, and year of treatment, which can also affect outcomes, making treatment decisions a dynamic process.

Treatment-Related Adverse Events The frequency of adverse events varies by treatment modality and the experience of the treating team. For example, following radical prostatectomy, incontinence rates range from 2–47% and impotence rates range from 25–89%. Part of the variability relates to how the complication is defined and whether the patient or physician is reporting the event. The time of the assessment is also important. After surgery, impotence is immediate but may reverse over time, while with radiation therapy impotence is not immediate but may develop over time. Of greatest concern to patients are the effects on continence, sexual potency, and bowel function.

Radical Prostatectomy The goal of radical prostatectomy is to excise the cancer completely with a clear margin, to maintain continence by preserving the external sphincter, and to preserve potency by sparing the autonomic nerves in the neurovascular bundle. The procedure is advised for patients with a life expectancy of 10 years or more and is performed via a retropubic or perineal approach or via a minimally invasive robotic-assisted or hand-held laparoscopic approach. Outcomes can be predicted using postoperative nomograms that consider pretreatment factors and the pathologic findings at surgery. PSA failure is usually defined as a value greater than 0.1 or 0.2 ng/mL. Specific criteria to guide the choice of one approach over another are lacking. Minimally invasive approaches offer the advantage of a shorter hospital stay and reduced blood loss. Rates of cancer control, recovery of continence, and recovery of erectile function are comparable between open and minimally invasive approaches. The individual surgeon rather than the surgical approach used is most important in determining outcomes after surgery.

Neoadjuvant hormonal therapy has also been explored in an attempt to improve the outcomes of surgery for high-risk patients, using a variety of definitions. The results of several large trials testing 3 or 8 months of androgen depletion before surgery showed that serum PSA levels decreased by 96%, prostate volumes decreased by 34%, and margin positivity rates decreased from 41% to 17%. Unfortunately, hormones did not produce an improvement in PSA relapse–free survival. Thus, neoadjuvant hormonal therapy is not recommended.

Factors associated with incontinence following radical prostatectomy include older age and urethral length, which impacts the ability to preserve the urethra beyond the apex and the distal sphincter. The skill and experience of the surgeon are also factors. Recovery of erectile function is associated with younger age, quality of erections before surgery, and the absence of damage to the neurovascular bundles. In general, erectile function begins to return about 6 months after surgery if both neurovascular bundles are preserved. Potency is reduced by half if at least one neurovascular bundle is sacrificed. Overall, with the availability of drugs such as phosphodiesterase-5 (PDE5) inhibitors, intraurethral inserts of alprostadil, and intracavernosal injections of vasodilators, many patients recover satisfactory sexual function.

Radiation Therapy Radiation therapy is given by external beam, by radioactive sources implanted into the gland, or by a combination of the two techniques.

EXTERNAL-BEAM RADIATION THERAPY Contemporary external-beam radiation therapy requires three-dimensional conformal treatment plans to maximize the dose to the prostate and to minimize the exposure of the surrounding normal tissue. Intensity-modulated radiation therapy (IMRT) permits shaping of the dose and allows the delivery of higher doses to the prostate and a further reduction in normal tissue exposure than three-dimensional conformal treatment alone. These advances have enabled the safe administration of doses >80 Gy and resulted in higher local control rates and fewer side effects.

Cancer control after radiation therapy has been defined by various criteria, including a decline in PSA to <0.5 or 1 ng/mL, "nonrising" PSA values, and a negative biopsy of the prostate 2 years after completion of treatment. The current standard definition of biochemical failure (the Phoenix definition) is a rise in PSA by ≥2 ng/mL higher than the lowest PSA achieved. The date of failure is "at call" and not backdated.

Radiation dose is critical to the eradication of prostate cancer. In a representative study, a PSA nadir of <1.0 ng/mL was achieved in 90% of patients receiving 75.6 or 81.0 Gy versus 76% and 56% of those receiving 70.2 and 64.8 Gy, respectively. Positive biopsy rates at 2.5 years were 4% for those treated with 81 Gy versus 27% and 36% for those receiving 75.6 and 70.2 Gy, respectively.

Overall, radiation therapy is associated with a higher frequency of bowel complications (mainly diarrhea and proctitis) than surgery. The frequency relates directly to the volume of the anterior rectal wall receiving full-dose treatment. In one series, grade 3 rectal or urinary toxicities were seen in 2.1% of patients who received a median dose of 75.6 Gy, whereas grade 3 urethral strictures requiring dilatation developed in 1% of cases, all of whom had undergone a transurethral resection of the prostate (TURP). Pooled data show that the frequency of grade 3 and 4 toxicities is 6.9% and 3.5%, respectively, for patients who received >70 Gy. The frequency of erectile dysfunction is related to the age of the patient, the quality of erections pretreatment, the dose administered, and the time of assessment. Postradiation erectile dysfunction is related to a disruption of the vascular supply and not the nerve fibers.

Neoadjuvant hormone therapy before radiation therapy has the aim of decreasing the size of the prostate and, consequently, reducing the exposure of normal tissues to full-dose radiation, increasing local control rates, and decreasing the rate of systemic failure.

Short-term hormone therapy can reduce toxicities and improve local control rates, but long-term treatment (2–3 years) is needed to prolong the time to PSA failure and lower the risk of metastatic disease in men with high-risk cancers. The impact on survival has been less clear.

BRACHYTHERAPY Brachytherapy is the direct implantation of radioactive sources (seeds) into the prostate. It is based on the principle that the deposition of radiation energy in tissues decreases as a function of the square of the distance from the source (Chap. 103e). The goal is to deliver intensive irradiation to the prostate, minimizing the exposure of the surrounding tissues. The current standard technique achieves a more homogeneous dose distribution by placing seeds according to a customized template based on imaging assessment of the cancer and computer-optimized dosimetry. The implantation is performed transperineally as an outpatient procedure with real-time imaging.

Improvements in brachytherapy techniques have resulted in fewer complications and a marked reduction in local failure rates. In a series of 197 patients followed for a median of 3 years, 5-year actuarial PSA relapse–free survival for patients with pretherapy PSA levels of 0–4, 4–10, and >10 ng/mL were 98%, 90%, and 89%, respectively. In a separate report of 201 patients who underwent posttreatment biopsies, 80% were negative, 17% were indeterminate, and 3% were positive. The results did not change with longer follow-up. Nevertheless, many physicians feel that implantation is best reserved for patients with good or intermediate prognostic features.

Brachytherapy is well tolerated, although most patients experience urinary frequency and urgency that can persist for several months. Incontinence has been seen in 2–4% of cases. Higher complication rates are observed in patients who have undergone a prior TURP, whereas those with obstructive symptoms at baseline are at a higher risk for retention and persistent voiding symptoms. Proctitis has been reported in <2% of patients.

Active Surveillance Although prostate cancer is the most common form of cancer affecting men in the United States, patients are being diagnosed earlier and more frequently present with early-stage disease. Active surveillance, described previously as *watchful waiting* or *deferred therapy*, is the policy of monitoring the illness at fixed intervals with DREs, PSA measurements, and repeat prostate biopsies as indicated until histopathologic or serologic changes correlative of progression warrant treatment with curative intent. It evolved from studies that evaluated predominantly elderly men with well-differentiated tumors who demonstrated no clinically significant progression for protracted periods, recognition of the contrast between incidence and disease-specific mortality, the high prevalence of autopsy cancers, and an effort to reduce overtreatment. A recent screening study estimated that between 50–100 men with low-risk disease would need to be treated to prevent one prostate cancer–specific death.

Arguing against active surveillance are the results of a Swedish randomized trial of radical prostatectomy versus active surveillance. With a median follow-up of 6.2 years, men treated by radical surgery had a lower risk of prostate cancer death relative to active surveillance patients (4.6% vs 8.9%) and a lower risk of metastatic progression (hazard ratio 0.63). Case selection is critical, and determining clinical parameters predictive of cancer aggressiveness that can be used to reliably select men most likely to benefit from active surveillance is an area of intense study. In one prostatectomy series, it was estimated that 10–15% of those treated had "insignificant" disease. One set of criteria includes men with clinical T1c tumors that are biopsy Gleason grade 6 or less involving three or fewer cores, each of them having less than 50% involvement by tumor and a PSA density of less than 0.15.

Concerns about active surveillance include the limited ability to predict pathologic findings by needle biopsy even when multiple cores are obtained, the recognized multifocality of the disease, and the possibility of a missed opportunity to cure the disease. Nomograms to help predict which patients can safely be managed by active surveillance continue to be refined, and as their predictive accuracy improves, it can be anticipated that more patients will be candidates.

RISING PSA AFTER DEFINITIVE LOCAL THERAPY

This term is applied to a group of patients in whom the sole manifestation of disease is a rising PSA after surgery and/or radiation therapy. By definition, there is no evidence of disease on an imaging study. For these patients, the central issue is whether the rise in PSA results from persistent disease in the primary site, systemic disease, or both. In theory, disease in the primary site may still be curable by additional local treatment.

The decision to recommend radiation therapy after prostatectomy is guided by the pathologic findings at surgery, because imaging studies such as CT and bone scan are typically uninformative. Some recommend a choline-11 positron emission tomography (PET) scan, but availability in the United States is limited. Others recommend that a biopsy of the urethrovesical anastomosis be obtained before considering radiation, whereas others treat empirically based on risk. Factors that predict for response to salvage radiation therapy are a positive surgical margin, lower Gleason score in the radical prostatectomy specimen, long interval from surgery to PSA failure, slow PSA doubling time, absence of disease in the lymph nodes, and a low (<0.5–1 ng/mL) PSA value at the time of radiation treatment. Radiation therapy is generally not recommended if the PSA was persistently elevated after surgery, which usually indicates that the disease has spread outside of the area of the prostate bed and is unlikely to be controlled with radiation therapy. As is the case for other disease states, nomograms to predict the likelihood of success are available.

For patients with a rising PSA after radiation therapy, salvage local therapy can be considered if the disease was "curable" at the time of diagnosis, if persistent disease has been documented by a biopsy of the prostate, and if no metastatic disease is seen on imaging studies. Unfortunately, case selection is poorly defined in most series, and morbidities are significant. Options include salvage radical prostatectomy, salvage cryotherapy, salvage radiation therapy, and salvage irreversible electroporation.

The rise in PSA after surgery or radiation therapy may indicate subclinical or micrometastatic disease with or without local recurrence. In these cases, the need for treatment depends, in part, on the estimated probability that the patient will develop clinically detectable metastatic disease on a scan and in what time frame. That immediate therapy is not always required was shown in a series where patients who developed a biochemical recurrence after radical prostatectomy received no systemic therapy until metastatic disease was documented. Overall, the median time to metastatic progression by imaging was 8 years, and 63% of the patients with rising PSA values remained free of metastases at 5 years. Factors associated with progression included the Gleason score of the radical prostatectomy specimen, time to recurrence, and PSA doubling time. For those with Gleason grade ≥8, the probability of metastatic progression was 37%, 51%, and 71% at 3, 5, and 7 years, respectively. If the time to recurrence was <2 years and PSA doubling time was long (>10 months), the proportions with metastatic disease at the same time intervals were 23%, 32%, and 53%, versus 47%, 69%, and 79% if the doubling time was short (<10 months). PSA doubling times are also prognostic for survival. In one series, all patients who succumbed to disease had PSA doubling times of 3 months or less.

Most physicians advise treatment if the PSA doubling time is 12 months or less. A difficulty with predicting the risk of metastatic spread, symptoms, or death from disease in the rising PSA state is that most patients receive some form of therapy before the development of metastases. Nevertheless, predictive models continue to be refined.

METASTATIC DISEASE: NONCASTRATE

The state of *noncastrate metastatic prostate cancer* includes men with metastases visible on an imaging study and noncastrate levels of testosterone (>150 ng/dL). The patient may be newly diagnosed or have a recurrence after treatment for localized disease. Symptoms of metastatic disease include pain from osseous spread, although many patients are asymptomatic despite extensive spread. Less common are symptoms related to marrow compromise (myelophthisis), spinal cord compression, or a coagulopathy.

Standard treatment is to deplete/lower androgens by medical or surgical means and/or to block androgen binding to the AR with antiandrogens. More than 90% of male hormones originate in the testes; <10% are synthesized in the adrenal gland. Surgical orchiectomy is the "gold standard" but is rarely used due to the availability of effective medical therapies and the more widespread use of hormones on an intermittent basis by which patients are treated for defined periods of time, following which the treatments are intentionally discontinued (discussed further below) **(Fig. 115-3)**.

Testosterone-Lowering Agents Medical therapies that lower testosterone levels include the gonadotropin-releasing hormone (GnRH) agonists/antagonists, 17,20-lyase inhibitors, CYP17 inhibitors, estrogens, and progestational agents. Of these, GnRH analogues such as leuprolide acetate and goserelin acetate initially produce a rise in luteinizing hormone and follicle-stimulating hormone, followed by a downregulation of receptors in the pituitary gland, which effects a chemical castration. They were approved on the basis of randomized comparisons showing an improved safety profile (specifically, reduced cardiovascular toxicities) relative to diethylstilbestrol (DES), with equivalent potency. The initial rise in testosterone may result in a clinical flare of the disease. As such, these agents are relatively contraindicated in men with significant obstructive symptoms, cancer-related pain, or spinal cord compromise. GnRH antagonists such as degarelix achieve castrate levels of testosterone within 48 h without the initial rise in serum testosterone and do not cause a flare in the disease. Estrogens such as DES are rarely used due to the risk of vascular complications such as fluid retention, phlebitis, embolic events, and stroke. Progestational agents alone are less efficacious.

Agents that lower testosterone are associated with an androgen-depletion syndrome that includes hot flushes, weakness, fatigue, loss of libido, impotence, sarcopenia, anemia, change in personality, and depression. Changes in lipids, obesity, and insulin resistance, along with an increased risk of diabetes and cardiovascular disease, can also occur, mimicking the metabolic syndrome. A decrease in bone density may also result that worsens over time and results in an increased risk of clinical fractures. This is a particular concern, often underappreciated, for men with preexisting osteopenia secondary to hypogonadism or glucocorticoid or alcohol use. Baseline fracture risk can be assessed using the Fracture Risk Assessment Scale (FRAX), and to minimize fracture risk, patients are advised to take calcium and vitamin D supplementation, along with a bisphosphonate or the RANK ligand inhibitor, denosumab.

Antiandrogens First generation nonsteroidal antiandrogens such as flutamide, bicalutamide, and nilutamide block ligand binding to the AR and were initially approved to block the disease flare that may occur with the rise in serum testosterone associated with GnRH agonist therapy. When antiandrogens are given alone, testosterone levels typically increase above baseline, but relative to testosterone-lowering therapies, they cause fewer hot flushes, less of an effect on libido, less muscle wasting, fewer personality changes, and less bone loss. Gynecomastia remains a significant problem but can be alleviated in part by tamoxifen.

Most reported randomized trials suggest that the cancer-specific outcomes are inferior when antiandrogens are used alone. Bicalutamide, even at 150 mg (three times the recommended dose), was associated with a shorter time to progression and inferior survival compared to surgical castration for patients with established metastatic disease. Nevertheless, some men may accept the trade-off of a potentially inferior cancer outcome for an improved quality of life.

Combined androgen blockade, the administration of an antiandrogen plus a GnRH analogue or surgical orchiectomy, and triple androgen blockade, which includes the addition of a 5ARI, have not

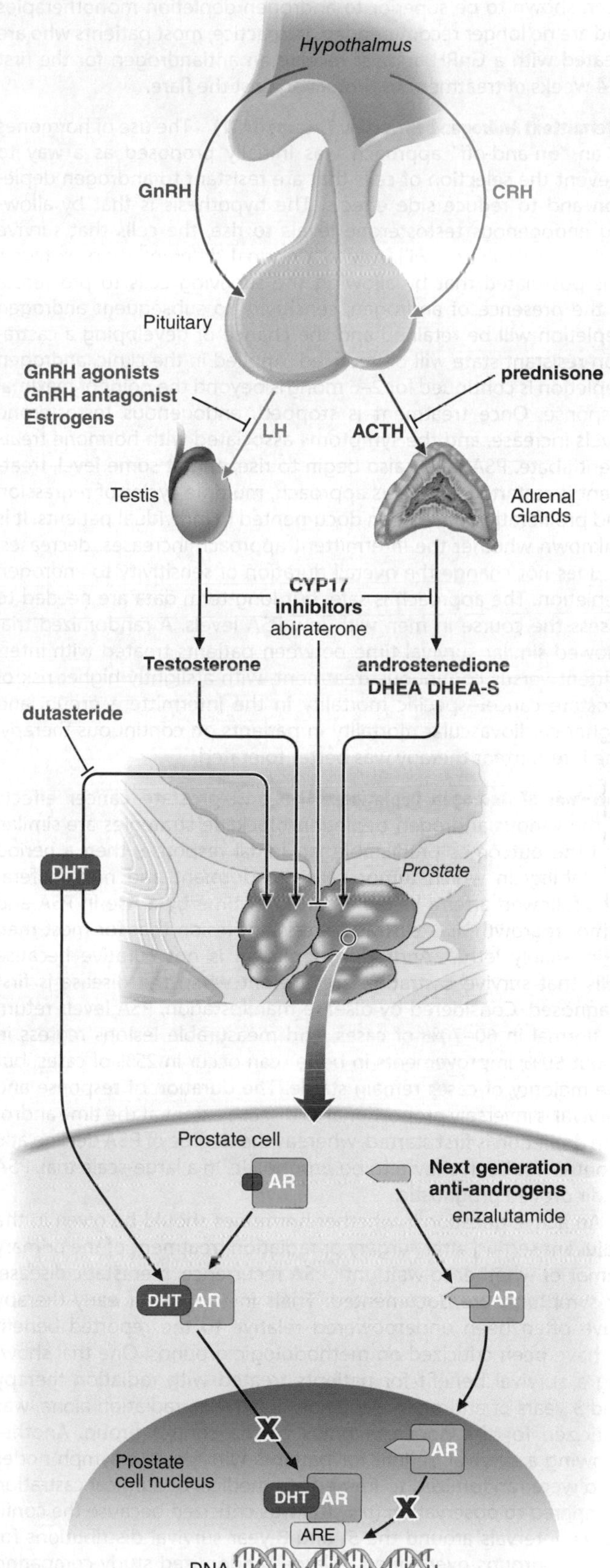

FIGURE 115-3 Sites of action of different hormone therapies. ACTH, adrenocorticotropic hormone; AR, androgen receptor; ARE, androgen-response element; CRH, corticotropin-releasing hormone; DHEA, dehydroepiandrosterone; DHEA-S, dehydroepiandrosterone sulphate; DHT, dihydrotestosterone; GnRH, gonadotropin-releasing hormone; LH, luteinizing hormone.

been shown to be superior to androgen depletion monotherapies and are no longer recommended. In practice, most patients who are treated with a GnRH agonist receive an antiandrogen for the first 2–4 weeks of treatment to protect against the flare.

Intermittent Androgen Deprivation Therapy (IADT) The use of hormones in an "on-and-off" approach was initially proposed as a way to prevent the selection of cells that are resistant to androgen depletion and to reduce side effects. The hypothesis is that by allowing endogenous testosterone levels to rise, the cells that survive androgen depletion will induce a normal differentiation pathway. It is postulated that by allowing the surviving cells to proliferate in the presence of androgen, sensitivity to subsequent androgen depletion will be retained and the chance of developing a castration-resistant state will be reduced. Applied in the clinic, androgen depletion is continued for 2–6 months beyond the point of maximal response. Once treatment is stopped, endogenous testosterone levels increase, and the symptoms associated with hormone treatment abate. PSA levels also begin to rise, and at some level, treatment is restarted. With this approach, multiple cycles of regression and proliferation have been documented in individual patients. It is unknown whether the intermittent approach increases, decreases, or does not change the overall duration of sensitivity to androgen depletion. The approach is safe, but long-term data are needed to assess the course in men with low PSA levels. A randomized trial showed similar survival time between patients treated with intermittent versus continuous treatment, with a slightly higher risk of prostate cancer–specific mortality in the intermittent group, and higher cardiovascular mortality in patients on continuous therapy. The intermittent therapy was better tolerated.

Outcomes of Androgen Depletion The anti–prostate cancer effects of the various androgen depletion/blockade strategies are similar, and the outcomes predictable: an initial response, then a period of stability in which tumor cells are dormant and nonproliferative, followed after a variable period of time by a rise in PSA and tumor regrowth as a castration-resistant lesion that for most men is invariably lethal. Androgen depletion is not curative because cells that survive castration are present when the disease is first diagnosed. Considered by disease manifestation, PSA levels return to normal in 60–70% of cases, and measurable lesions regress in about 50%; improvements in bone scan occur in 25% of cases, but the majority of cases remain stable. The duration of response and survival is inversely proportional to disease extent at the time androgen depletion is first started, whereas the degree of PSA decline at 6 months has been shown to be prognostic. In a large-scale trial, PSA nadir proved prognostic.

An active question is whether hormones should be given in the adjuvant setting after surgery or radiation treatment of the primary tumor or whether to wait until PSA recurrence, metastatic disease, or symptoms are documented. Trials in support of early therapy have often been underpowered relative to the reported benefit or have been criticized on methodologic grounds. One trial showing a survival benefit for patients treated with radiation therapy and 3 years of androgen depletion, relative to radiation alone, was criticized for the poor outcomes of the control group. Another showing a survival benefit for patients with positive lymph nodes who were randomized to immediate medical or surgical castration compared to observation ($p = .02$) was criticized because the confidence intervals around the 5- and 8-year survival distributions for the two groups overlapped. A large randomized study comparing early to late hormone treatment (orchiectomy or GnRH analogue) in patients with locally advanced or asymptomatic metastatic disease showed that patients treated early were less likely to progress from M0 to M1 disease, to develop pain, and to die of prostate cancer. This trial was criticized because therapy was delayed "too long" in the late-treatment group. Noteworthy is that the American Society of Clinical Oncology Guidelines recommend deferring treatment until the disease has recurred and the prognosis has been reassessed. These guidelines do not support immediate therapy.

METASTATIC DISEASE: CASTRATE

Castration-resistant prostate cancer (CRPC) is defined as disease that progresses despite androgen suppression by medical or surgical therapies where the measured levels of testosterone are 50 ng/mL or lower. The rise in PSA indicates continued signaling through the AR signaling axis, the result of a series of oncogenic changes that include overexpression of androgen biosynthetic enzymes that can lead to increased intratumoral androgens, and overexpression of the receptor itself that enables signaling to occur even in the setting of low levels of androgen. The majority of CRPC cases are not "hormone-refractory," and considering them as such can deny patients safe and effective treatment. CRPC can manifest in many ways. For some, it is a rise in PSA with no change in radiographs and no new symptoms. In others, it is a rising PSA and progression in bone with or without symptoms of disease. Still others will show soft tissue disease with or without osseous metastases, and others have visceral spread.

For the individual patient, it is first essential to ensure that a castrate status be documented. Patients receiving an antiandrogen alone, whose serum testosterone levels are elevated, should be treated first with a GnRH analogue or orchiectomy and observed for response. Patients on an antiandrogen in combination with a GnRH analogue should have the antiandrogen discontinued, because approximately 20% will respond to the selective discontinuation of the antiandrogen.

Chemotherapy and New Agents Through 2009, docetaxel was the only systemic therapy proven to prolong life. As a single agent, the drug produced PSA declines in 50% of patients, measurable disease regression in 25%, and improvement in both preexisting pain and prevention of future cancer-related pain. Since then, six agents with diverse mechanisms of action that target the tumor itself or other aspects of the metastatic process have been proven to prolong life and were FDA approved. The first was sipuleucel-T, the first biologic approach shown to prolong life in which antigen-presenting cells are activated ex vivo, pulsed with antigen, and reinfused. The second, cabazitaxel, a non–cross-resistant taxane, was shown to be superior to mitoxantrone in the post-docetaxel setting. This was followed by the CYP17 inhibitor abiraterone acetate, which lowers androgen levels in the tumor, adrenal glands, and testis, and the next-generation antiandrogen enzalutamide, which not only has a higher binding affinity to the AR relative to first-generation compounds, but uniquely inhibits nuclear location and DNA binding of the receptor complex. Both abiraterone acetate and enzalutamide were first approved for postchemotherapy treated patients on the basis of placebo-controlled phase III trials—a further indication that these tumors are not uniformly hormone-refractory. The indication for abiraterone acetate was later expanded to the prechemotherapy setting, based on a second trial using a co-primary endpoint of radiographic progression–free survival and overall survival. Similar results were seen with enzalutamide, for which an expanded indication is also anticipated. Alpharadin (radium-223 chloride), an alpha-emitting bone-seeking radioisotope, has been shown to prolong life in patients with symptoms related to osseous disease. The alpharadin result validated the bone microenvironment as a therapeutic target independent of direct effects on the tumor itself, as no declines in PSA were observed in the trial. Notable is that in addition to a survival benefit, the drug also reduced the development of significant skeletal events.

Other bone-targeted agents, such as the bisphosphonates and the RANK ligand inhibitor denosumab, protect against bone loss associated with androgen depletion and also reduce skeletal-related events by targeting bone osteoclasts. In one trial, denosumab was shown to be superior to zoledronic acid with respect to skeletal-related events, but had a slightly higher frequency of osteonecrosis of the jaw.

In clinical practice, most men seek to avoid chemotherapy and are first treated with a biologic agent and/or newer hormonal agent approved for this indication. It is crucial to the management of the individual patient to define therapeutic objectives before initiating treatment, as there are defined standards of care for different disease manifestations. For example, sipuleucel-T is not indicated for patients with symptoms or visceral disease because the effects on the disease occur late. Similarly, alpharadin is not indicated for patients with disease that is predominantly in soft tissue or who have osseous disease that is not causing symptoms.

Pain Management Management of pain secondary to osseous metastatic disease is a critical part of therapy. Optimal palliation requires assessing whether the symptoms are from metastases that threaten or that are already affecting the spinal cord, the cauda equina, or the base of the skull, which are best treated with external-beam radiation, as are single sites of pain. Neurologic symptoms require emergency evaluation because loss of function may be permanent if not addressed quickly. Because the disease is often diffuse, palliation at one site is often followed by the emergence of symptoms in a separate site that had not received radiation. In these cases, bone-seeking radioisotopes such as alpharadin or the beta emitter ^{153}Sm-EDTMP (Quadramet) can be considered in addition to abiraterone acetate, docetaxel, and mitoxantrone, each of which is formally approved for the palliation of pain due to prostate cancer metastases.

BENIGN DISEASE

BENIGN PROSTATIC HYPERTROPHY

BPH is a pathologic process that contributes to the development of lower urinary tract symptoms in men. Such symptoms, arising from lower urinary tract dysfunction, are further subdivided into obstructive symptoms (urinary hesitancy, straining, weak stream, terminal dribbling, prolonged voiding, incomplete emptying) and irritative symptoms (urinary frequency, urgency, nocturia, urge incontinence, small voided volumes). Lower urinary tract symptoms and other sequelae of BPH are not just due to a mass effect, but are also likely due to a combination of the prostatic enlargement and age related detrusor dysfunction.

TREATMENT BENIGN PROSTATIC HYPERTROPHY

The symptoms are generally measured using a validated, reproducible index that is designed to determine disease severity and response to therapy—the AUA's Symptom Index (AUASI), also adopted as the International Prostate Symptom Score (IPSS) (**Table 115-2**). Serial AUASI is particularly useful in following patients as they are treated with various forms of therapy. Asymptomatic patients do not require treatment regardless of the size of the gland, whereas patients with an inability to urinate, gross hematuria, recurrent infection, or bladder stones may require surgery. In patients with symptoms, uroflowmetry can identify those with normal flow rates who are unlikely to benefit from treatment, and bladder ultrasound can identify those with high postvoid residuals who may need intervention. Pressure-flow (urodynamic) studies detect primary bladder dysfunction. Cystoscopy is recommended if hematuria is documented and to assess the urinary outflow tract before surgery. Imaging of the upper tracts is advised for patients with hematuria, a history of calculi, or prior urinary tract problems.

Symptomatic relief is the most common reason men seek treatment for BPH, and therefore the goal of therapy for BPH is usually relief of these symptoms. Alpha-adrenergic receptor antagonists are thought to treat the dynamic aspect of BPH by reducing sympathetic tone of the bladder outlet, thereby decreasing resistance and improving urinary flow. 5ARIs are thought to treat the static aspect of BPH by reducing prostate volume and having a similar, albeit delayed effect. They have also proven to be beneficial in the prevention of BPH progression, as measured by prostate volume, the risk of developing acute urinary retention, and the risk of having BPH-related surgery. The use of an alpha-adrenergic receptor antagonist and a 5ARI as combination therapy seeks to provide symptomatic relief while preventing progression of BPH.

Another class of medications that has shown improvement in lower urinary tract symptoms secondary to BPH is PDE5 inhibitors, used currently in the treatment of erectile dysfunction. All three of the PDE5 inhibitors available in the United States, sildenafil, vardenafil, and tadalafil, appear to be effective in the treatment of symptoms secondary to BPH. The use of PDE5 inhibitors is not without controversy, however, given the fact that short-acting phosphodiesterase inhibitors such as sildenafil need to be dosed separately from alpha blockers such as tamsulosin because of potential hypotensive effects. Newer classes of pharmacologic agents have been used to treat symptoms secondary to BPH. Symptoms due to BPH often coexist with symptoms due to overactive bladder, and the most common pharmacologic agents for the treatment of overactive bladder symptoms are anticholinergics. This has led to multiple studies evaluating the efficacy of anticholinergics for the treatment of lower urinary tract symptoms secondary to BPH. Surgical therapy is now considered second-line therapy and is usually reserved for patients after a trial of medical therapy. The goal of surgical therapy is to reduce the size of the prostate, effectively reducing resistance to urine flow.

Surgical approaches include TURP, transurethral incision, or removal of the gland via a retropubic, suprapubic, or perineal approach. Also used are transurethral ultrasound-guided laser-induced prostatectomy (TULIP), stents, and hyperthermia.

TABLE 115-2 AUA SYMPTOM INDEX

	AUA Symptom Score (Circle 1 Number on Each Line)					
Questions to Be Answered	Not at All	Less Than 1 Time in 5	Less Than Half the Time	About Half the Time	More Than Half the Time	Almost Always
Over the past month, how often have you had a sensation of not emptying your bladder completely after you finished urinating?	0	1	2	3	4	5
Over the past month, how often have you had to urinate again less than 2 h after you finished urinating?	0	1	2	3	4	5
Over the past month, how often have you found you stopped and started again several times when you urinated?	0	1	2	3	4	5
Over the past month, how often have you found it difficult to postpone urination?	0	1	2	3	4	5
Over the past month, how often have you had a weak urinary stream?	0	1	2	3	4	5
Over the past month, how often have you had to push or strain to begin urination?	0	1	2	3	4	5
Over the past month, how many times did you most typically get up to urinate from the time you went to bed at night until the time you got up in the morning?	(None)	(1 time)	(2 times)	(3 times)	(4 times)	(5 times)
Sum of 7 circled numbers (AUA Symptom Score): ____						

Abbreviation: AUA, American Urological Association.

Source: MJ Barry et al: J Urol 148:1549, 1992. Used with permission.

116 Testicular Cancer

Robert J. Motzer, Darren R. Feldman, George J. Bosl

Primary germ cell tumors (GCTs) of the testis arising by the malignant transformation of primordial germ cells constitute 95% of all testicular neoplasms. Infrequently, GCTs arise from an extragonadal site, including the mediastinum, retroperitoneum, and, very rarely, the pineal gland. This disease is notable for the young age of the afflicted patients, the totipotent capacity for differentiation of the tumor cells, and its curability; approximately 95% of newly diagnosed patients are cured. Experience in the management of GCTs leads to improved outcome.

INCIDENCE AND EPIDEMIOLOGY

The incidence of testicular GCT is now approximately 8000 cases annually in the United States, resulting in nearly 400 deaths. The tumor occurs most frequently in men between the ages of 20 and 40 years. A testicular mass in a male ≥50 years should be regarded as a lymphoma until proved otherwise. GCT is at least four to five times more common in white than in African-American males, and a higher incidence has been observed in Scandinavia and New Zealand than in the United States.

ETIOLOGY AND GENETICS

Cryptorchidism is associated with a several-fold higher risk of GCT. Abdominal cryptorchid testes are at a higher risk than inguinal cryptorchid testes. Orchiopexy should be performed before puberty, if possible. Early orchiopexy reduces the risk of GCT and improves the ability to save the testis. An abdominal cryptorchid testis that cannot be brought into the scrotum should be removed. Approximately 2% of men with GCTs of one testis will develop a primary tumor in the other testis. Testicular feminization syndromes and family history increase the risk of testicular GCT, and Klinefelter's syndrome is associated with mediastinal GCT.

An isochromosome of the short arm of chromosome 12 [i(12p)] is pathognomonic for GCT. Excess 12p copy number, either in the form of i(12p) or as increased 12p on aberrantly banded marker chromosomes, occurs in nearly all GCTs, but the gene(s) on 12p involved in the pathogenesis are not yet defined.

CLINICAL PRESENTATION

A painless testicular mass is pathognomonic for a testicular malignancy. More commonly, patients present with testicular discomfort or swelling suggestive of epididymitis and/or orchitis. In this circumstance, a trial of antibiotics is reasonable. However, if symptoms persist or a residual abnormality remains, then testicular ultrasound examination is indicated.

Ultrasound of the testis is indicated whenever a testicular malignancy is considered and for persistent or painful testicular swelling. If a testicular mass is detected, a radical inguinal orchiectomy should be performed. Because the testis develops from the gonadal ridge, its blood supply and lymphatic drainage originate in the abdomen and descend with the testis into the scrotum. An inguinal approach is taken to avoid breaching anatomic barriers and permitting additional pathways of spread.

Back pain from retroperitoneal metastases is common and must be distinguished from musculoskeletal pain. Dyspnea from pulmonary metastases occurs infrequently. Patients with increased serum levels of human chorionic gonadotropin (hCG) may present with gynecomastia. A delay in diagnosis is associated with a more advanced stage and possibly worse survival.

The staging evaluation for GCT includes a determination of serum levels of α fetoprotein (AFP), hCG, and lactate dehydrogenase (LDH). After orchiectomy, a computed tomography (CT) scan of the chest, abdomen, and pelvis is generally performed. Stage I disease is limited to the testis, epididymis, or spermatic cord. Stage II disease is limited to retroperitoneal (regional) lymph nodes. Stage III disease is disease outside the retroperitoneum, involving supradiaphragmatic nodal sites or viscera. The staging may be "clinical"—defined solely by physical examination, blood marker evaluation, and radiographs—or "pathologic"—defined by an operative procedure.

The regional draining lymph nodes for the testis are in the retroperitoneum, and the vascular supply originates from the great vessels (for the right testis) or the renal vessels (for the left testis). As a result, the lymph nodes that are involved first by a right testicular tumor are the interaortocaval lymph nodes just below the renal vessels. For a left testicular tumor, the first involved lymph nodes are lateral to the aorta (para-aortic) and below the left renal vessels. In both cases, further retroperitoneal nodal spread is inferior, contralateral, and, less commonly, above the renal hilum. Lymphatic involvement can extend cephalad to the retrocrural, posterior mediastinal, and supraclavicular lymph nodes. Treatment is determined by tumor histology (seminoma versus nonseminoma) and clinical stage (Fig. 116-1).

PATHOLOGY

GCTs are divided into nonseminoma and seminoma subtypes. Nonseminomatous GCTs are most frequent in the third decade of life and can display the full spectrum of embryonic and adult cellular differentiation. This entity comprises four histologies: embryonal carcinoma, teratoma, choriocarcinoma, and endodermal sinus (yolk sac) tumor. Choriocarcinoma, consisting of both cytotrophoblasts and syncytiotrophoblasts, represents malignant trophoblastic differentiation and is invariably associated with secretion of hCG. Endodermal sinus tumor is the malignant counterpart of the fetal yolk sac and is associated with secretion of AFP. Pure embryonal carcinoma may secrete AFP or hCG, or both; this pattern is biochemical evidence of differentiation. Teratoma is composed of somatic cell types derived from two or more germ layers (ectoderm, mesoderm, or endoderm). Each of these histologies may be present alone or in combination with others. Nonseminomatous GCTs tend to metastasize early to sites such as the retroperitoneal lymph nodes and lung parenchyma. Sixty percent of patients present with disease limited to the testis (stage I), 20% with retroperitoneal metastases (stage II), and 20% with more extensive supradiaphragmatic nodal or visceral metastases (stage III).

Seminoma represents approximately 50% of all GCTs, has a median age in the fourth decade, and generally follows a more indolent clinical course. Eighty percent of patients present with stage I disease, approximately 10% with stage II disease, and 10% with stage III disease; lung or other visceral metastases are rare. When a tumor contains both seminoma and nonseminoma components, patient management is directed by the more aggressive nonseminoma component.

TUMOR MARKERS

Careful monitoring of the serum tumor markers AFP and hCG is essential in the management of patients with GCT, because these markers are important for diagnosis, as prognostic indicators, in monitoring treatment response, and in the early detection of relapse. Approximately 70% of patients presenting with disseminated nonseminomatous GCT have increased serum concentrations of AFP and/or hCG. Although hCG concentrations may be increased in patients with either nonseminoma or seminoma histology, the AFP concentration is increased only in patients with nonseminoma. The presence of an increased AFP level in a patient whose tumor shows only seminoma indicates that an occult nonseminomatous component exists, and the patient should be treated for nonseminomatous GCT. LDH levels are less specific than AFP or hCG but are increased in 50–60% patients with metastatic nonseminoma and in up to 80% of patients with advanced seminoma.

AFP, hCG, and LDH levels should be determined before and after orchiectomy. Increased serum AFP and hCG concentrations decay according to first-order kinetics; the half-life is 24–36 h for hCG and 5–7 days for AFP. AFP and hCG should be assayed serially during and after treatment. The reappearance of hCG and/or AFP or the failure of these markers to decline according to the predicted half-life is an indicator of persistent or recurrent tumor.

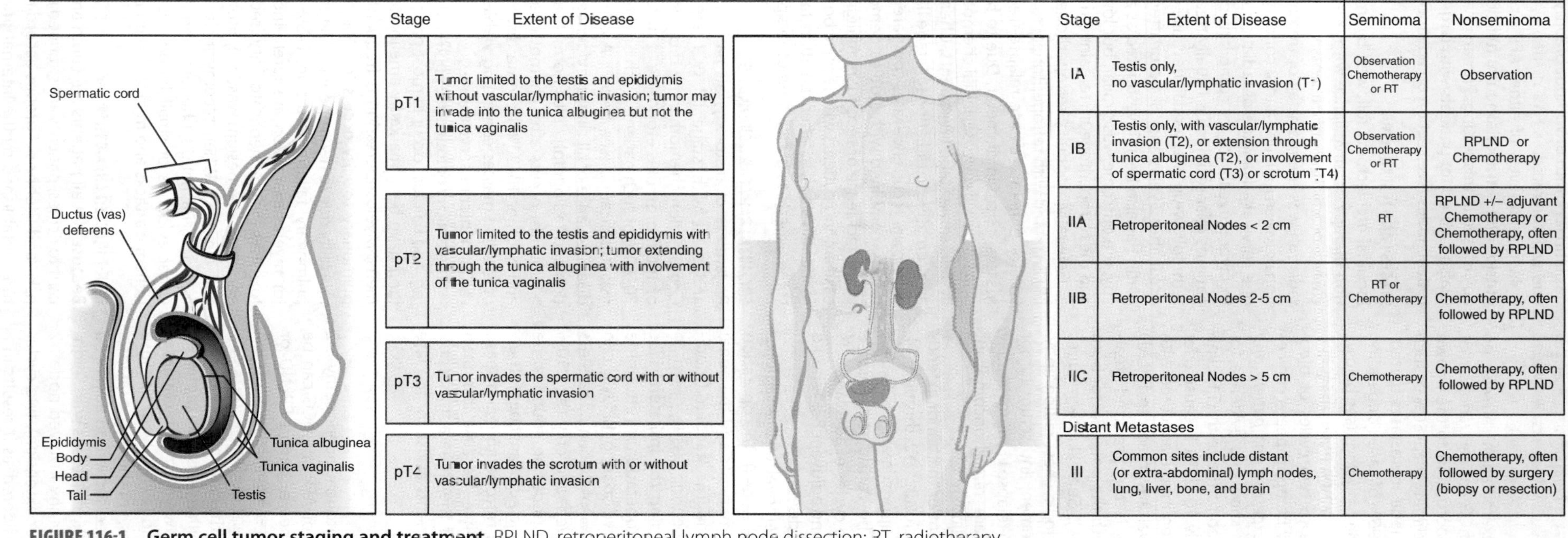

Stage	Extent of Disease
pT1	Tumor limited to the testis and epididymis without vascular/lymphatic invasion; tumor may invade into the tunica albuginea but not the tunica vaginalis
pT2	Tumor limited to the testis and epididymis with vascular/lymphatic invasion; tumor extending through the tunica albuginea with involvement of the tunica vaginalis
pT3	Tumor invades the spermatic cord with or without vascular/lymphatic invasion
pT4	Tumor invades the scrotum with or without vascular/lymphatic invasion

Stage	Extent of Disease	Treatment Option: Seminoma	Treatment Option: Nonseminoma
IA	Testis only, no vascular/lymphatic invasion (T1)	Observation Chemotherapy or RT	Observation
IB	Testis only, with vascular/lymphatic invasion (T2), or extension through tunica albuginea (T2), or involvement of spermatic cord (T3) or scrotum (T4)	Observation Chemotherapy or RT	RPLND or Chemotherapy
IIA	Retroperitoneal Nodes < 2 cm	RT	RPLND +/– adjuvant Chemotherapy or Chemotherapy, often followed by RPLND
IIB	Retroperitoneal Nodes 2-5 cm	RT or Chemotherapy	Chemotherapy, often followed by RPLND
IIC	Retroperitoneal Nodes > 5 cm	Chemotherapy	Chemotherapy, often followed by RPLND
Distant Metastases			
III	Common sites include distant (or extra-abdominal) lymph nodes, lung, liver, bone, and brain	Chemotherapy	Chemotherapy, often followed by surgery (biopsy or resection)

FIGURE 116-1 Germ cell tumor staging and treatment. RPLND, retroperitoneal lymph node dissection; RT, radiotherapy.

TREATMENT TESTICULAR CANCER

STAGE I NONSEMINOMA

Patients with radiographs and physical examination showing no evidence of disease and serum AFP and hCG concentrations that are either normal or declining to normal according to the known half-life have clinical stage I disease. Approximately 20–50% of such patients will have retroperitoneal lymph node metastases (pathologic stage II) but will still be cured in over 95% of cases. Depending on risk of relapse, which is determined by the pathology (see below), surveillance, a nerve-sparing retroperitoneal lymph node dissection (RPLND), or adjuvant chemotherapy (one to two cycles of bleomycin, etoposide, and cisplatin [BEP]) may be appropriate choices depending on *the availability of surgical expertise and patient and physician preference.* If the primary tumor shows no evidence for lymphatic or vascular invasion and is limited to the testis (T1, clinical stage IA), then the risk of relapse is only 10–20%. Because over 80% of patients with clinical stage IA nonseminoma are cured with orchiectomy alone and there is no survival advantage to RPLND (or adjuvant chemotherapy), surveillance is the preferred treatment option. This avoids overtreatment with the potential for both acute and long-term toxicities (see below). Surveillance requires patients to be carefully followed with periodic chest radiography, physical examination, CT scan of the abdomen, and serum tumor marker determinations. The median time to relapse is approximately 7 months, and late relapses (>2 years) are rare. Noncompliant patients can be considered for RPLND or adjuvant BEP.

If lymphatic or vascular invasion is present or the tumor extends *through* the tunica, spermatic cord, or scrotum (T2 through T4, clinical stage IB), then the risk of relapse is approximately 50%, and RPLND and adjuvant chemotherapy can be considered. Relapse rates are reduced to 3–5% after one to two cycles of adjuvant BEP. All three approaches (surveillance, RPLND, and adjuvant BEP) should cure >95% of patients with clinical stage IB disease.

RPLND is the standard operation for removal of the regional lymph nodes of the testis (retroperitoneal nodes). The operation removes the lymph nodes draining the primary site and the nodal groups adjacent to the primary landing zone. The standard (modified bilateral) RPLND removes all node-bearing tissue down to the bifurcation of the great vessels, including the ipsilateral iliac nodes. The major long-term effect of this operation is retrograde ejaculation with resultant infertility. Nerve-sparing RPLND can preserve anterograde ejaculation in ~90% of patients. Patients with pathologic stage I disease are observed, and only the <10% who relapse require additional therapy. If nodes are found to be involved at RPLND, then a decision regarding adjuvant chemotherapy is made on the basis of the extent of retroperitoneal disease (see "Stage II Nonseminoma" below). Hence, because less than 20% of patients require chemotherapy, of the three approaches, RPLND results in the lowest number of patients at risk for the late toxicities of chemotherapy.

STAGE II NONSEMINOMA

Patients with limited, ipsilateral retroperitoneal adenopathy ≤2 cm in largest diameter and normal levels of AFP and hCG can be treated with either a modified bilateral nerve-sparing RPLND or chemotherapy. The local recurrence rate after a properly performed RPLND is very low. Depending on the extent of disease, the postoperative management options include either surveillance or two cycles of adjuvant chemotherapy. Surveillance is the preferred approach for patients with resected "low-volume" metastases (tumor nodes ≤2 cm in diameter *and* <6 nodes involved) because the probability of relapse is one-third or less. For those who relapse, risk-directed chemotherapy is indicated (see section on advanced GCT below). Because relapse occurs in ≥50% of patients with "high-volume" metastases (>6 nodes involved, *or* any involved node >2 cm in largest diameter, *or* extranodal tumor extension), two cycles of adjuvant chemotherapy should be considered, as it results in a cure in ≥98% of patients. Regimens consisting of etoposide plus cisplatin (EP) with or without bleomycin every 3 weeks are effective and well tolerated.

Increased levels of either AFP or hCG imply metastatic disease outside the retroperitoneum; full-dose (not adjuvant) chemotherapy is used in this setting. Primary management with chemotherapy is also favored for patients with larger (>2 cm) or bilateral retroperitoneal nodes (see section on advanced GCT below).

STAGES I AND II SEMINOMA

Inguinal orchiectomy followed by immediate retroperitoneal radiation therapy or surveillance with treatment at relapse both result in cure in nearly 100% of patients with stage I seminoma. Historically, radiation was the mainstay of treatment, but the reported association between radiation and secondary malignancies and the absence of a survival advantage of radiation over surveillance has led many to favor surveillance for compliant patients. Approximately 15% of patients relapse, which is usually treated with chemotherapy. Long-term follow-up is essential, because approximately 30% of relapses occur after 2 years and 5% occur after 5 years. A single dose of carboplatin has also been investigated as an alternative to radiation therapy; the outcome was similar, but long-term safety data are lacking, and the retroperitoneum remained the most frequent site of relapse.

Generally, nonbulky retroperitoneal disease (stage IIA and small IIB) is treated with retroperitoneal radiation therapy. Approximately 90% of patients achieve relapse-free survival with retroperitoneal masses <3 cm in diameter. Due to higher relapse rates after radiation for bulkier disease, initial chemotherapy is preferred for all stage IIC and some stage IIB patients. Chemotherapy has been studied as an alternative to radiation for stage IIA and small stage IIB seminoma with lower recurrence rates compared with historical controls. These results, combined with studies demonstrating a threefold increase in the incidence of secondary malignancies and cardiovascular disease among patients who receive both radiation and chemotherapy (patients relapsing after radiation fall into this category), have led some experts to prefer chemotherapy for all stage II seminomas.

CHEMOTHERAPY FOR ADVANCED GCT

Regardless of histology, all patients with stage IIC and stage III and most with stage IIB GCT are treated with chemotherapy. Combination chemotherapy programs based on cisplatin at doses of 100 mg/m^2 plus etoposide at doses of 500 mg/m^2 per cycle cure 70–80% of such patients, with or without bleomycin, depending on risk stratification (see below). A complete response (the complete disappearance of all clinical evidence of tumor on physical examination and radiography plus normal serum levels of AFP and hCG for ≥1 month) occurs after chemotherapy alone in ~60% of patients, and another 10–20% become disease free with surgical resection of residual masses containing viable GCT. Lower doses of cisplatin result in inferior survival rates.

The toxicity of four cycles of the BEP is substantial. Nausea, vomiting, and hair loss occur in most patients, although nausea and vomiting have been markedly ameliorated by modern antiemetic regimens. Myelosuppression is frequent, and symptomatic bleomycin pulmonary toxicity occurs in ~5% of patients. Treatment-induced mortality due to neutropenia with septicemia or bleomycin-induced pulmonary failure occurs in 1–3% of patients. Dose reductions for myelosuppression are rarely indicated. Long-term permanent toxicities include nephrotoxicity (reduced glomerular filtration and persistent magnesium wasting), ototoxicity, peripheral neuropathy, and infertility. When bleomycin is administered by weekly bolus injection, Raynaud's phenomenon appears in 5–10% of patients. Other evidence of small blood vessel damage, such as transient ischemic attacks and myocardial infarction, is seen less often.

RISK-DIRECTED CHEMOTHERAPY

Because not all patients are cured and treatment may cause significant toxicities, patients are stratified into "good-risk," "intermediate-risk," and "poor-risk" groups according to pretreatment clinical features established by the International Germ Cell Cancer Consensus Group (Table 116-1). For good-risk patients, the goal is to achieve

TABLE 116-1 INTERNATIONAL GERM CELL CANCER CONSENSUS GROUP RISK CLASSIFICATION FOR ADVANCED GERM CELL TUMORS

Risk	Nonseminoma	Seminoma
Good	Gonadal or retroperitoneal primary site Absent nonpulmonary visceral metastases AFP <1000 ng/mL β-hCG <5000 mIU/mL LDH <1.5 × upper limit or normal (ULN)	Any primary site Absent nonpulmonary visceral metastases Any LDH, hCG
Intermediate	Gonadal or retroperitoneal primary site Absent nonpulmonary visceral metastases AFP 1000–10,000 ng/mL β-hCG 5000–50,000 mIU/mL LDH 1.5–10 × ULN	Any primary site Presence of nonpulmonary visceral metastases Any LDH, hCG
Poor	Mediastinal primary site Presence of nonpulmonary visceral metastases AFP >10,000 ng/mL β-hCG >50,000 mIU/mL LDH >10 × ULN	No patients classified as poor prognosis

Abbreviations: AFP, α fetoprotein; hCG, human chorionic gonadotropin; LDH, lactate dehydrogenase.

Source: From International Germ Cell Cancer Consensus Group.

maximum efficacy with minimal toxicity. For intermediate- and poor-risk patients, the goal is to identify more effective therapy with tolerable toxicity.

The marker cut offs are included in the TNM (primary tumor, regional nodes, metastasis) staging of GCT. Hence, TNM stage groupings are based on both anatomy (site and extent of disease) and biology (marker status and histology). Seminoma is either good- or intermediate-risk, based on the absence or presence of nonpulmonary visceral metastases. No poor-risk category exists for seminoma. Marker levels and primary site play no role in defining risk for seminoma. Nonseminomas have good-, intermediate-, and poor-risk categories based on the primary site of the tumor, the presence or absence of nonpulmonary visceral metastases, and marker levels.

For ~90% of patients with good-risk GCTs, four cycles of EP or three cycles of BEP produce durable complete responses, with minimal acute and chronic toxicity, and a low relapse rate. Pulmonary toxicity is absent when bleomycin is not used and is rare when therapy is limited to 9 weeks; myelosuppression with neutropenic fever is less frequent; and the treatment mortality rate is negligible. Approximately 75% of intermediate-risk patients and 50% of poor-risk patients achieve durable complete remission with four cycles of BEP, and no regimen has proved superior.

POSTCHEMOTHERAPY SURGERY Resection of residual metastases after the completion of chemotherapy is an integral part of therapy. If the initial histology is nonseminoma and the marker values have normalized, all sites of residual disease should be resected. In general, residual retroperitoneal disease requires a modified bilateral RPLND. Thoracotomy (unilateral or bilateral) and neck dissection are less frequently required to remove residual mediastinal, pulmonary parenchymal, or cervical nodal disease. Viable tumor (seminoma, embryonal carcinoma, yolk sac tumor, or choriocarcinoma) will be present in 15%, mature teratoma in 40%, and necrotic debris and fibrosis in 45% of resected specimens. The frequency of teratoma or viable disease is highest in residual mediastinal tumors. If necrotic debris or mature teratoma is present, no further chemotherapy is necessary. If viable tumor is present but is completely excised, two additional cycles of chemotherapy are given.

If the initial histology is pure seminoma, mature teratoma is rarely present, and the most frequent finding is necrotic debris. For residual retroperitoneal disease, a complete RPLND is technically difficult due to extensive postchemotherapy fibrosis. Observation is recommended when no radiographic abnormality exists on CT scan. Positive findings on a positron emission tomography (PET) scan correlate with viable seminoma in residua and mandate surgical excision or biopsy.

SALVAGE CHEMOTHERAPY

Of patients with advanced GCT, 20–30% fail to achieve a durable complete response to first-line chemotherapy. A combination of vinblastine, ifosfamide, and cisplatin (VeIP) will cure approximately 25% of patients as a second-line therapy. Patients are more likely to achieve a durable complete response if they had a testicular primary tumor and relapsed from a prior complete remission to first-line cisplatin-containing chemotherapy. Substitution of paclitaxel for vinblastine (TIP) in this setting was associated with durable remission in nearly two-thirds of patients. In contrast, for patients with a primary mediastinal nonseminoma or who did not achieve a complete response with first-line chemotherapy, then VeIP standard-dose salvage therapy is rarely beneficial. Such patients are usually managed with high-dose chemotherapy and/or surgical resection.

Chemotherapy consisting of dose-intensive, high-dose carboplatin plus high-dose etoposide, with peripheral blood stem cell support, induces a complete response in 25–40% of patients who have progressed after ifosfamide-containing salvage chemotherapy. Approximately one-half of the complete responses will be durable. High-dose therapy is standard of care for this patient population and has been suggested as the treatment of choice for all patients with relapsed or refractory disease. Paclitaxel is active when incorporated into high-dose combination programs. Cure is still possible in some relapsed patients.

EXTRAGONADAL GCT

The prognosis and management of patients with extragonadal GCT depends on the tumor histology and site of origin. All patients with a diagnosis of extragonadal GCT should have a testicular ultrasound examination. Nearly all patients with retroperitoneal or mediastinal seminoma achieve a durable complete response to BEP or EP. The clinical features of patients with primary retroperitoneal nonseminoma GCT are similar to those of patients with a primary tumor of testis origin, and careful evaluation will find evidence of a primary testicular GCT in about two-thirds of cases. In contrast, a primary mediastinal nonseminomatous GCT is associated with a poor prognosis; one-third of patients are cured with standard therapy (four cycles of BEP). Patients with newly diagnosed mediastinal nonseminoma are considered to have poor-risk disease and should be considered for clinical trials testing regimens of possibly greater efficacy. In addition, mediastinal nonseminoma is associated with hematologic disorders, including acute myelogenous leukemia, myelodysplastic syndrome, and essential thrombocytosis unrelated to previous chemotherapy. These hematologic disorders are very refractory to treatment. Nonseminoma of any primary site may change into other malignant histologies such as embryonal rhabdomyosarcoma or adenocarcinoma. This is called *malignant transformation.* i(12p) has been identified in the transformed cell type, indicating GCT clonal origin.

A group of patients with poorly differentiated tumors of unknown histogenesis, midline in distribution, and not associated with secretion of AFP or hCG has been described; a few (10–20%) are cured by standard cisplatin-containing chemotherapy. An i(12p) is present in ~25% of such tumors (the fraction that are cisplatin-responsive), confirming their origin from primitive germ cells. This finding is also predictive of the response to cisplatin-based chemotherapy and resulting long-term survival. These tumors are heterogeneous; neuroepithelial tumors and lymphoma may also present in this fashion.

Infertility is an important consequence of the treatment of GCTs. Preexisting infertility or impaired fertility is often present. Azoospermia and/or oligospermia are present at diagnosis in at least 50% of patients with testicular GCTs. Ejaculatory dysfunction is associated with RPLND, and germ cell damage may result from cisplatin-containing chemotherapy. Nerve-sparing techniques to preserve the retroperitoneal sympathetic nerves have made retrograde ejaculation less likely in the subgroups of patients who are candidates for this operation. Spermatogenesis does recur in some patients after chemotherapy. However, because of the significant risk of impaired reproductive capacity, semen analysis and cryopreservation of sperm in a sperm bank should be recommended to all patients before treatment.

117 Gynecologic Malignancies

Michael V. Seiden

OVARIAN CANCER

INCIDENCE AND PATHOLOGY

Cancer arising in or near the ovary is actually a collection of diverse malignancies. This collection of malignancies, often referred to as "ovary cancer," is the most lethal gynecologic malignancy in the United States and other countries that routinely screen women for cervical neoplasia. In 2014, it was estimated that there were 21,980 cases of ovarian cancer with 14,270 deaths in the United States. The ovary is a complex and dynamic organ and, between the ages of approximately 11 and 50 years, is responsible for follicle maturation associated with egg maturation, ovulation, and cyclical sex steroid hormone production. These complex and linked biologic functions are coordinated through a variety of cells within the ovary, each of which possesses neoplastic potential. By far the most common and most lethal of the ovarian neoplasms arise from the ovarian epithelium or, alternatively, the neighboring specialized epithelium of the fallopian tube, uterine corpus, or cervix. Epithelial tumors may be benign (50%), malignant (33%), or of borderline malignancy (16%). Age influences risk of malignancy; tumors in younger women are more likely benign. The most common of the ovarian epithelial malignancies are serous tumors (50%); tumors of mucinous (25%), endometrioid (15%), clear cell (5%), and transitional cell histology or Brenner tumor (1%) represent smaller proportions of epithelial ovarian tumors. In contrast, stromal tumors arise from the steroid hormone–producing cells and likewise have different phenotypes and clinical presentations largely dependent on the type and quantity of hormone production. Tumors arising in the germ cell are most similar in biology and behavior to testicular tumors in males (Chap. 116).

Tumors may also metastasize to the ovary from breast, colon, appendiceal, gastric, and pancreatic primaries. Bilateral ovarian masses from metastatic mucin-secreting gastrointestinal cancers are termed *Krukenberg tumors.*

OVARIAN CANCER OF EPITHELIAL ORIGIN

Epidemiology and Pathogenesis A female has approximately a 1 in 72 lifetime risk (1.6%) of developing ovarian cancer, with the majority of affected women developing epithelial tumors. Each of the histologic variants of epithelial tumors is distinct with unique molecular features. As a group of malignancies, epithelial tumors of the ovary have a peak incidence in women in their sixties, although age at presentation can range across the extremes of adult life, with cases being reported in women in their twenties to nineties. Each histologic subtype of ovarian cancer likely has its own associated risk factors. Serous cancer, the most common type of epithelial ovarian cancer, is seen with increased frequency in women who are nulliparous or have a history of use of talc agents applied to the perineum; other risk factors include obesity and probably hormone replacement therapy. Protective factors include the use of oral contraceptives, multiparity, and breast-feeding. These protective factors are thought to work through suppression of ovulation and perhaps the associated reduction of ovulation associated inflammation of the ovarian epithelium or, alternatively, the serous epithelium located within the fimbriae of the fallopian tube. Other protective factors, such as fallopian tube ligation, are thought to protect the ovarian epithelium (or perhaps the distal fallopian tube fimbriae) from carcinogens that migrate from the vagina to the tubes and ovarian surface epithelium. Mucinous tumors are more frequent in women with a history of cigarette smoking, whereas endometrioid and clear cell tumors are more frequent in women with a history of endometriosis.

Considerable evidence now suggests that the precursor cell to serous carcinoma of the ovary might actually arise in the fimbria of the fallopian tube with extension or metastasis to the ovarian surface or capture of preneoplastic or neoplastic exfoliating tubal cells into an involuting ovarian follicle around the time of ovulation. Careful histologic and molecular analysis of tubal epithelium demonstrates molecular and histologic abnormalities, termed serous tubular intraepithelial carcinoma (STIC) lesions, in a high proportion of women undergoing risk-reducing salpingo-oophorectomies in the context of high-risk germline mutations in *BRCA1* and *BRCA2*, as well as a modest proportion of women with ovarian cancer in the absence of such mutations.

Genetic Risk Factors A variety of genetic syndromes substantially increase a woman's risk of developing ovarian cancer. Approximately 10% of women with ovarian cancer have a germline mutation in one of two DNA repair genes: *BRCA1* (chromosome 17q12-21) or *BRCA2* (chromosome 13q12-13). Individuals inheriting a single copy of a mutant allele have a very high incidence of breast and ovarian cancer. Most of these women have a family history that is notable for multiple cases of breast and/or ovarian cancer, although inheritance through male members of the family can camouflage this genotype through several generations. The most common malignancy in these women is breast carcinoma, although women harboring germline *BRCA1* mutations have a marked increased risk of developing ovarian malignancies in their forties and fifties with a 30–50% lifetime risk of developing ovarian cancer. Women harboring a mutation in *BRCA2* have a lower penetrance of ovarian cancer with perhaps a 20–40% chance of developing this malignancy, with onset typically in their fifties or sixties. Women with a *BRCA2* mutation also are at slightly increased risk of pancreatic cancer. Likewise women with mutations in the DNA mismatch repair genes associated with Lynch syndrome, type 2 (*MSH2, MLH1, MLH6, PMS1, PMS2*) may have a risk of ovarian cancer as high as 1% per year in their forties and fifties. Finally, a small group of women with familial ovarian cancer may have mutations in other *BRCA*-associated genes such as *RAD51, CHK2*, and others. Screening studies in this select population suggest that current screening techniques, including serial evaluation of the CA-125 tumor marker and ultrasound, are insufficient at detecting early-stage and curable disease, so women with these germline mutations are advised to undergo prophylactic removal of ovaries and fallopian tubes typically after completing childbearing and ideally before age 35–40 years. Early prophylactic oophorectomy also protects these women from subsequent breast cancer with a reduction of breast cancer risk of approximately 50%.

Presentation Neoplasms of the ovary tend to be painless unless they undergo torsion. Symptoms are therefore typically related to compression of local organs or due to symptoms from metastatic disease. Women with tumors localized to the ovary do have an increased incidence of symptoms including pelvic discomfort, bloating, and perhaps changes in a woman's typical urinary or bowel pattern. Unfortunately, these symptoms are frequently dismissed by either the woman or her health care team. It is believed that high-grade tumors metastasize early in the neoplastic process. Unlike other epithelial malignancies,

TABLE 117-1 STAGING AND SURVIVAL IN GYNECOLOGIC MALIGNANCIES

Stage	Ovarian	5-Year Survival, %	Endometrial	5-Year Survival, %	Cervix	5-Year Survival, %
0	—		—		Carcinoma in situ	100
I	Confined to ovary	90–95	Confined to corpus	89	Confined to uterus	85
II	Confined to pelvis	70–80	Involves corpus and cervix	73	Invades beyond uterus but not to pelvic wall	65
III	Intraabdominal spread	20–50	Extends outside the uterus but not outside the true pelvis or to lymph nodes	52	Extends to pelvic wall and/or lower third of vagina, or hydronephrosis	35
IV	Spread outside abdomen	1–5	Extends outside the true pelvis or involves the bladder or rectum	17	Invades mucosa of bladder or rectum or extends beyond the true pelvis	7

these tumors tend to exfoliate throughout the peritoneal cavity and thus present with symptoms associated with disseminated intraperitoneal tumors. The most common symptoms at presentation include a multimonth period of progressive complaints that typically include some combination of heartburn, nausea, early satiety, indigestion, constipation, and abdominal pain. Signs include the rapid increase in abdominal girth due to the accumulation of ascites that typically alerts the patient and her physician that the concurrent gastrointestinal symptoms are likely associated with serious pathology. Radiologic evaluation typically demonstrates a complex adnexal mass and ascites. Laboratory evaluation usually demonstrates a markedly elevated CA-125, a shed mucin (Muc 16) associated with, but not specific for, ovarian cancer. Hematogenous and lymphatic spread are seen but are not the typical presentation. Ovarian cancers are divided into four stages, with stage I tumors confined to the ovary, stage II malignancies confined to the pelvis, and stage III tumors confined to the peritoneal cavity (Table 117-1). These three stages are subdivided, with the most common presentation, stage IIIC, defined as tumors with bulky intraperitoneal disease. About 60% of women present with stage IIIC disease. Stage IV disease includes women with parenchymal metastases (liver, lung, spleen) or, alternatively, abdominal wall or pleural disease. The 40% not presenting with stage IIIC disease are roughly evenly distributed among the other stages, although mucinous and clear cell tumors are overrepresented in stage I tumors.

Screening Ovarian cancer is the fifth most lethal malignancy in women in the United States. It is curable in early stages, but seldom curable in advanced stages; hence, the development of effective screening strategies is of considerable interest. Furthermore, the ovary is well visualized with a variety of imaging techniques, most notably transvaginal ultrasound. Early-stage tumors often produce proteins that can be measured in the blood such as CA-125 and HE-4. Nevertheless, the incidence of ovarian cancer in the middle-aged female population is low, with only approximately 1 in 2000 women between the ages of 50 and 60 carrying an asymptomatic and undetected tumor. Thus effective screening techniques must be sensitive but, more importantly, highly specific to minimize the number of false-positive results. Even a screening test with 98% specificity and 50% sensitivity would have a positive predictive value of only about 1%. A large randomized study of active screening versus usual standard care demonstrated that a screening program consisting of six annual CA-125 measurements and four annual transvaginal ultrasounds in a population of women age 55–74 was not effective at reducing death from ovarian cancer and was associated with significant morbidity in the screened arm due to complications associated with diagnostic testing in the screened group. Although ongoing studies are evaluating the utility of alternative screening strategies, currently screening of normal-risk women is not recommended outside of a clinical trial.

TREATMENT OVARIAN CANCER

In women presenting with a localized ovarian mass, the principal diagnostic and therapeutic maneuver is to determine if the tumor is benign or malignant and, in the event that the tumor is malignant, whether the tumor arises in the ovary or is a site of metastatic disease. Metastatic disease to the ovary can be seen from primary tumors of the colon, appendix, stomach (Krukenberg tumors), and breast. Typically women undergo a unilateral salpingo-oophorectomy, and if pathology reveals a primary ovarian malignancy, then the procedure is followed by a hysterectomy, removal of the remaining tube and ovary, omentectomy, and pelvic node sampling along with some random biopsies of the peritoneal cavity. This extensive surgical procedure is performed because approximately 30% of tumors that by visual inspection appear to be confined to the ovary have already disseminated to the peritoneal cavity and/or surrounding lymph nodes.

If there is evidence of bulky intraabdominal disease, a comprehensive attempt at maximal tumor cytoreduction is attempted even if it involves partial bowel resection, splenectomy, and in certain cases more extensive upper abdominal surgery. The ability to debulk metastatic ovarian cancer to minimal visible disease is associated with an improved prognosis compared with women left with visible disease. Patients without gross residual disease after resection have a median survival of 39 months, compared with 17 months for those left with macroscopic tumor. Once tumors have been surgically debulked, women receive therapy with a platinum agent, typically a taxane. Debate continues as to whether this therapy should be delivered intravenously or, alternatively, whether some of the therapy should be delivered directly into the peritoneal cavity via a catheter. Three randomized studies have demonstrated improved survival with intraperitoneal therapy, but this approach is still not widely accepted due to technical challenges associated with this delivery route and increased toxicity. In women who present with bulky intraabdominal disease, an alternative approach is to treat with platinum plus a taxane for several cycles before attempting a surgical debulking procedure (neoadjuvant therapy). Subsequent surgical procedures are more effective at leaving the patient without gross residual tumor and appear to be less morbid. Two studies have demonstrated that the neoadjuvant approach is associated with an overall survival that is comparable to the traditional approach of primary surgery followed by chemotherapy.

With optimal debulking surgery and platinum-based chemotherapy (usually carboplatin dosed to an area under the curve [AUC] of 6 plus paclitaxel 175 mg/m^2 by 3-h infusion in 21-day cycles), 70% of women who present with advanced-stage tumors respond, and 40–50% experience a complete remission with normalization of their CA-125, computed tomography (CT) scans, and physical examination. Unfortunately, a small proportion of women who obtain a complete response to therapy will remain in remission. Disease recurs within 1–4 years from the completion of their primary therapy in 75% of the complete responders. CA-125 levels often increase as a first sign of relapse; however, data are not clear that early intervention in relapsing patients influences survival. Recurrent disease is effectively managed, but not cured, with a variety of chemotherapeutic agents. Eventually all women with recurrent disease develop chemotherapy-refractory disease at which point refractory ascites, poor bowel motility, and obstruction or pseudoobstruction due to a tumor-infiltrated aperistaltic bowel are common. Limited surgery to relieve intestinal obstruction, localized radiation therapy to relieve pressure or pain from masses, or palliative chemotherapy may be helpful. Agents with >15% response rates include gemcitabine, topotecan, liposomal doxorubicin, pemetrexed, and bevacizumab. Approximately 10% of ovarian cancers are HER2/neu positive, and trastuzumab may induce responses in this subset.

Five-year survival correlates with the stage of disease: stage I, 85–90%; stage II, 70–80%; stage III, 20–50%; and stage IV, 1–5% (Table 117-1). Low-grade serous tumors are molecularly distinct from high-grade serous tumors and are, in general, poorly responsive to chemotherapy. Targeted therapies focused on inhibiting kinases downstream of *RAS* and *BRAF* are being tested. Patients with tumors of low malignant potential are managed by surgery; chemotherapy and radiation therapy do not improve survival.

OVARIAN SEX CORD AND STROMAL TUMORS

Epidemiology, Presentation, and Predisposing Syndromes Approximately 7% of ovarian neoplasms are stromal or sex cord tumors, with approximately 1800 cases expected each year in the United States. Ovarian stromal tumors or sex cord tumors are most common in women in their fifties or sixties, but tumors can present in the extremes of age, including the pediatric population. These tumors arise from the mesenchymal components of the ovary, including steroid-producing cells as well as fibroblasts. Essentially all of these tumors are of low malignant potential and present as unilateral solid masses. Three clinical presentations are common: the detection of an abdominal mass; abdominal pain due to ovarian torsion, intratumoral hemorrhage, or rupture; or signs and symptoms due to hormonal production by these tumors.

The most common hormone-producing tumors include thecomas, granulosa cell tumor, or juvenile granulosa tumors in children. These estrogen-producing tumors often present with breast tenderness as well as isosexual precocious pseudopuberty in children, menometrorrhagia, oligomenorrhea, or amenorrhea in premenopausal women, or alternatively as postmenopausal bleeding in older women. In some women, estrogen-associated secondary malignancies, such as endometrial or breast cancer, may present as synchronous malignancies. Alternatively, endometrial cancer may serve as the presenting malignancy with evaluation subsequently identifying a unilateral solid ovarian neoplasm that proves to be an occult granulosa cell tumor. Sertoli-Leydig tumors often present with hirsutism, virilization, and occasionally Cushing's syndrome due to increased production of testosterone, androstenedione, or other 17-ketosteroids. Hormonally inert tumors include fibroma that presents as a solitary mass often in association with ascites and occasionally hydrothorax also known as Meigs' syndrome. A subset of these tumors present in individuals with a variety of inherited disorders that predispose them to mesenchymal neoplasia. Associations include juvenile granulosa cell tumors and perhaps Sertoli-Leydig tumors with Ollier's disease (multiple enchondromatosis) or Maffucci's syndrome, ovarian sex cord tumors with annular tubules with Peutz-Jeghers syndrome, and fibromas with Gorlin's disease. Essentially all granulosa tumors and a minority of juvenile granulosa cell tumors and thecomas have a defined somatic point mutation in the *FOXL2* gene at C134W generated by replacement of cysteine with a guanine at position 402. About 30% of Sertoli-Leydig tumors harbor a mutation in the RNA-processing gene *DICER* in the RNAIIIb domain.

TREATMENT SEX CORD TUMORS

The mainstay of treatment for sex cord tumors is surgical resection. Most women present with tumors confined to the ovary. For the small subset of women who present with metastatic disease or develop evidence of tumor recurrence after primary resection, survival is still typically long, often in excess of a decade. Because these tumors are slow growing and relatively refractory to chemotherapy, women with metastatic disease are often debulked because disease is usually peritoneal-based (as with epithelial ovarian cancer). Definitive data that surgical debulking of metastatic or recurrent disease prolongs survival are lacking, but ample data document women who have survived years or, in some cases, decades after resection of recurrent disease. In addition, large peritoneal-based metastases also have a proclivity for hemorrhage, sometimes with catastrophic complications. Chemotherapy is occasionally effective, and women tend to receive regimens designed to treat epithelial or germ cell tumors. Bevacizumab has some activity in clinical trials but is not approved for this specific indication. These tumors often produce high levels of müllerian inhibiting substance (MIS), inhibin, and, in the case of Sertoli-Leydig tumors, α fetoprotein (AFP). These proteins are detectable in serum and can be used as tumor markers to monitor women for recurrent disease because the increase or decrease of these proteins in the serum tends to reflect the changing bulk of systemic tumor.

GERM CELL TUMORS OF THE OVARY

Germ cell tumors, like their counterparts in the testis, are cancers of germ cells. These totipotent cells contain the programming for differentiation to essentially all tissue types, and hence the germ cell tumors include a histologic menagerie of bizarre tumors, including benign teratomas and a variety of malignant tumors, such as immature teratomas, dysgerminomas, yolk sac malignancies, and choriocarcinomas. Benign teratoma (or dermoid cyst) is the most common germ cell neoplasm of the ovary and often presents in young woman. These tumors include a complex mixture of differentiated tissue including tissues from all three germ layers. In older women, these differentiated tumors can develop malignant transformation, most commonly squamous cell carcinomas. Malignant germ cell tumors include dysgerminomas, yolk sac tumors, immature teratomas, and embryonal carcinoma and choriocarcinomas. There are no known genetic abnormalities that unify these tumors. A subset of dysgerminomas harbor mutations in *c-Kit* oncogenes (as seen in gastrointestinal stromal tumors [GIST]), whereas a subset of germ cell tumors have isochromosome 12 abnormalities, as seen in testicular malignancies. In addition, a subset of dysgerminomas is associated with dysgenetic ovaries. Identification of a dysgerminoma arising in genotypic XY gonads is important in that it highlights the need to identify and remove the contralateral gonad due to risk of gonadoblastoma.

Presentation Germ cell tumors can present at all ages, but the peak age of presentation tends to be in females in their late teens or early twenties. Typically these tumors will become large ovarian masses, which eventually present as palpable low abdominal or pelvic masses. Like sex cord tumors, torsion or hemorrhage may present urgently or emergently as acute abdominal pain. Some of these tumors produce elevated levels of human chorionic gonadotropin (hCG), which can lead to isosexual precocious puberty when tumors present in younger girls. Unlike epithelial ovarian cancer, these tumors have a higher proclivity for nodal or hematogenous metastases. As with testicular tumors, some of these tumors tend to produce AFP (yolk sac tumors) or hCG (embryonal carcinoma, choriocarcinomas, and some dysgerminomas) that are reliable tumor markers.

TREATMENT GERM CELL TUMORS

Germ cell tumors typically present in women who are still of child-bearing age, and because bilateral tumors are uncommon (except in dysgerminoma, 10–15%), the typical treatment is unilateral oophorectomy or salpingo-oophorectomy. Because nodal metastases to pelvic and para-aortic nodes are common and may affect treatment choices, these nodes should be carefully inspected and, if enlarged, should be resected if possible. Women with malignant germ cell tumors typically receive bleomycin, etoposide, and cisplatin (BEP) chemotherapy. In the majority of women, even those with advanced-stage disease, cure is expected. Close follow-up without adjuvant therapy of women with stage I tumors is reasonable if there is high confidence that the patient and health care team are committed to compulsive and careful follow-up, as chemotherapy at the time of tumor recurrence is likely to be curative.

Dysgerminoma is the ovarian counterpart of testicular seminoma. The 5-year disease-free survival is 100% in early-stage patients and 61% in stage III disease. Although the tumor is highly radiation-sensitive, radiation produces infertility in many patients. BEP chemotherapy is as effective or more so without causing infertility. The use of BEP following incomplete resection is associated with a 2-year disease-free survival rate of 95%. This chemotherapy is now the treatment of choice for dysgerminoma.

FALLOPIAN TUBE CANCER

Transport of the egg to the uterus occurs via transit through the fallopian tube, with the distal ends of these tubes composed of fimbriae that drape about the ovarian surface and capture the egg as it erupts from the ovarian cortex. Fallopian tube malignancies are typically serous tumors. Previous teaching was that these malignancies were rare, but more careful histologic examination suggests that many "ovarian malignancies" might actually arise in the distal fimbria of the fallopian tube (see above). These women often present with adnexal masses, and like ovarian cancer, these tumors spread relatively early throughout the peritoneal cavity and respond to platinum and taxane therapy and have a natural history that is essentially identical to ovarian cancer (Table 117-1).

CERVICAL CANCER

GLOBAL CONSIDERATIONS

Cervical cancer is the second most common and most lethal malignancy in women worldwide likely due to the widespread infection with high-risk strains of human papillomavirus (HPV) and limited utilization of or access to Pap smear screening in many nations throughout the world. Nearly 500,000 cases of cervical cancer are expected worldwide, with approximately 240,000 deaths annually. Cancer incidence is particularly high in women residing in Central and South America, the Caribbean, and southern and eastern Africa. Mortality rate is disproportionately high in Africa. In the United States, 12,360 women were diagnosed with cervical cancer and 4020 women died in 2014. Developed countries have looked at high-technology screening techniques for HPV involving automated polymerase chain reaction in thin preps that identify dysplastic cytology as well as high-risk HPV genetic material. Visual inspection of the cervix coated with acetic acid has demonstrated the ability to reduce mortality from cervical cancer with potential broad applicability in low-resource environments. The development of effective vaccines for high-risk HPV types makes it imperative to determine economical, socially acceptable, and logistically feasible strategies to deliver and distribute this vaccine to girls and boys before their engagement in sexual activity.

HPV INFECTION AND PREVENTIVE VACCINATION

HPV is the primary neoplastic-initiating event in the vast majority of women with invasive cervical cancer. This double-strand DNA virus infects epithelium near the transformation zone of the cervix. More than 60 types of HPV are known, with approximately 20 types having the ability to generate high-grade dysplasia and malignancy. HPV-16 and -18 are the types most frequently associated with high-grade dysplasia and targeted by both U.S. Food and Drug Administration–approved vaccines. The large majority of sexually active adults are exposed to HPV, and most women clear the infection without specific intervention. The 8-kilobase HPV genome encodes seven early genes, most notably *E6* and *E7*, which can bind to *RB* and *p53*, respectively. High-risk types of HPV encode *E6* and *E7* molecules that are particularly effective at inhibiting the normal cell cycle checkpoint functions of these regulatory proteins, leading to immortalization but not full transformation of cervical epithelium. A minority of woman will fail to clear the infection with subsequent HPV integration into the host genome. Over the course of as short as months but more typically years, some of these women develop high-grade dysplasia. The time from dysplasia to carcinoma is likely years to more than a decade and almost certainly requires the acquisition of other poorly defined genetic mutations within the infected and immortalized epithelium.

Risk factors for HPV infection and, in particular, dysplasia include a high number of sexual partners, early age of first intercourse, and history of venereal disease. Smoking is a cofactor; heavy smokers have a higher risk of dysplasia with HPV infection. HIV infection, especially when associated with low CD4+ T cell counts, is associated with a higher rate of high-grade dysplasia and likely a shorter latency period between infection and invasive disease. The administration of highly active antiretroviral therapy reduces the risk of high-grade dysplasia associated with HPV infection.

Currently approved vaccines include the recombinant proteins to the late proteins, L1 and L2, of HPV-16 and -18. Vaccination of women before the initiation of sexual activity dramatically reduces the rate of HPV-16 and -18 infection and subsequent dysplasia. There is also partial protection against other HPV types, although vaccinated women are still at risk for HPV infection and still require standard Pap smear screening. Although no randomized trial data demonstrate the utility of Pap smears, the dramatic drop in cervical cancer incidence and death in developed countries employing wide-scale screening provides strong evidence for its effectiveness. In addition, even visual inspection of the cervix with preapplication of acetic acid using a "see and treat" strategy has demonstrated a 30% reduction in cervical cancer death. The incorporation of HPV testing by polymerase chain reaction or other molecular techniques increases the sensitivity of detecting cervical pathology but at the cost of identifying many women with transient infections who require no specific medical intervention.

CLINICAL PRESENTATIONS

The majority of cervical malignancies are squamous cell carcinomas associated with HPV. Adenocarcinomas are also HPV-related and arise deep in the endocervical canal; they are typically not seen by visual inspection of the cervix and thus are often missed by Pap smear screening. A variety of rarer malignancies including atypical epithelial tumors, carcinoids, small cell carcinomas, sarcomas, and lymphomas have also been reported.

The principal role of Pap smear testing is the detection of asymptomatic preinvasive cervical dysplasia of squamous epithelial lining. Invasive carcinomas often have symptoms or signs including postcoital spotting or intermenstrual cycle bleeding or menometrorrhagia. Foul-smelling or persistent yellow discharge may also be seen. Presentations that include pelvic or sacral pain suggest lateral extension of the tumor into pelvic nerve plexus by either the primary tumor or a pelvic node and are signs of advanced-stage disease. Likewise, flank pain from hydronephrosis from ureteral compression or deep venous thrombosis from iliac vessel compression suggests either extensive nodal disease or direct extension of the primary tumor to the pelvic sidewall. The most common finding of physical exam is a visible tumor on the cervix.

TREATMENT CERVICAL CANCER

Scans are not part of the formal clinical staging of cervical cancer yet are very useful in planning appropriate therapy. CT can detect hydronephrosis indicative of pelvic sidewall disease but is not accurate at evaluating other pelvic structures. Magnetic resonance imaging (MRI) is more accurate at estimating uterine extension and paracervical extension of disease into soft tissues typically bordered by broad and cardinal ligaments that support the uterus in the central pelvis. Positron emission tomography (PET) scan is the most accurate technique for evaluating the pelvis and more importantly nodal (pelvic, para-aortic, and scalene) sites for disease.

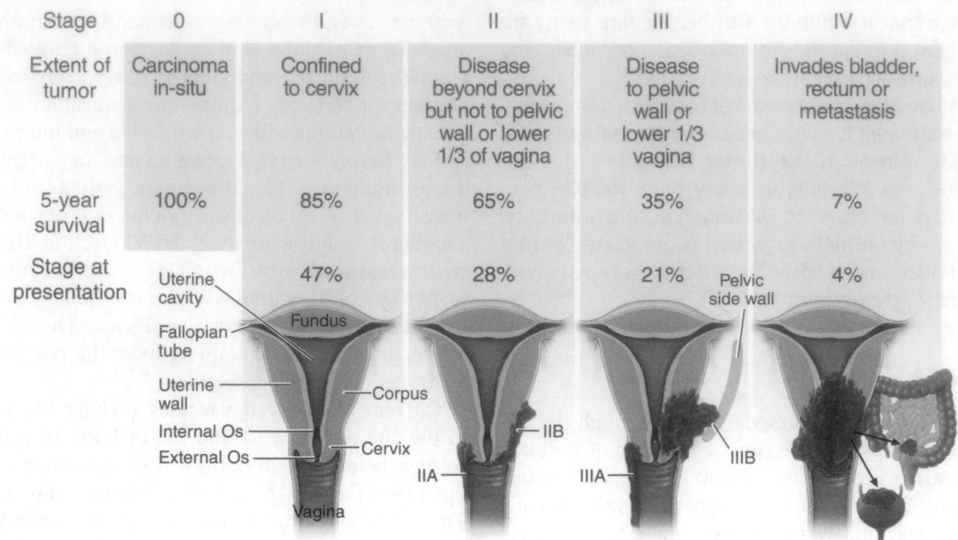

FIGURE 117-1 **Anatomic display of the stages of cervix cancer** defined by location, extent of tumor, frequency of presentation, and 5-year survival.

This technique seems more prognostic and accurate than CT, MRI, or lymphangiogram, especially in the para-aortic region.

Stage I cervical tumors are confined to the cervix, whereas stage II tumors extend into the upper vagina or paracervical soft tissue (Fig. 117-1). Stage III tumors extend to the lower vagina or the pelvic sidewalls, whereas stage IV tumors invade the bladder or rectum or have spread to distant sites. Very small stage I cervical tumors can be treated with a variety of surgical procedures. In young women desiring to maintain fertility, radical trachelectomy removes the cervix with subsequent anastomosis of the upper vagina to the uterine corpus. Larger cervical tumors confined to the cervix can be treated with either surgical resection or radiation therapy in combination with cisplatin-based chemotherapy with a high chance of cure. Larger tumors that extend regionally down the vagina or into the paracervical soft tissues or the pelvic sidewalls are treated with combination chemotherapy and radiation therapy. The treatment of recurrent or metastatic disease is unsatisfactory due to the relative resistance of these tumors to chemotherapy and currently available biological agents, although bevacizumab, a monoclonal antibody that is said to inhibit tumor-associated angiogenesis, has demonstrated clinically meaningful activity in the management of metastatic disease.

UTERINE CANCER

EPIDEMIOLOGY

Several different tumor types arise in uterine corpus. Most tumors arise in the glandular lining and are endometrial adenocarcinomas. Tumors can also arise in the smooth muscle; most are benign (uterine leiomyoma), with a small minority of tumors being sarcomas. The endometrioid histologic subtype of endometrial cancer is the most common gynecologic malignancy in the United States. In 2014, an estimated 52,630 women were diagnosed with cancer of the uterine corpus, with 8590 deaths from the disease. Development of these tumors is a multistep process, with estrogen playing an important early role in driving endometrial gland proliferation. Relative overexposure to this class of hormones is a risk factor for the subsequent development of endometrioid tumors. In contrast, progestins drive glandular maturation and are protective. Hence, women with high endogenous or pharmacologic exposure to estrogens, especially if unopposed by progesterone, are at high risk for endometrial cancer. Obese women, women treated with unopposed estrogens, or women with estrogen-producing tumors (such as granulosa cell tumors of the ovary) are at higher risk for endometrial cancer. In addition, treatment with tamoxifen, which has antiestrogenic effects in breast tissue but estrogenic effects in uterine epithelium, is associated with an increased risk of endometrial cancer. Events such as the loss of the *PTEN* tumor suppressor gene with activation and often additional mutations in the PIK-3CA/AKT pathways likely serve as secondary events in carcinogenesis. The Cancer Genome Atlas Research Network has demonstrated that endometrioid tumors can be divided into four subgroups: ultramutated, microsatellite instability hypermutated, copy number low, and copy number high subgroups. These groups have different natural histories; therapy for these subgroups may eventually be individualized. Serous tumors of the uterine corpus represent approximately 5–10% of epithelial tumors of the uterine corpus and possess distinct molecular characteristics that are most similar to those seen in serous tumors arising in the ovary or fallopian tube.

Women with a mutation in one of a series of DNA mismatch repair genes associated with the Lynch syndrome, also known as hereditary nonpolyposis colon cancer (HNPCC), are at increased risk for endometrioid endometrial carcinoma. These individuals have germline mutations in *MSH2*, *MLH1*, and in rare cases *PMS1* and *PMS2*, with resulting microsatellite instability and hypermutation. Individuals who carry these mutations typically have a family history of cancer and are at markedly increased risk for colon cancer and modestly increased risk for ovarian cancer and a variety of other tumors. Middle-aged women with HNPCC carry a 4% annual risk of endometrial cancer and a relative overall risk of approximately 200-fold as compared to age-matched women without HNPCC.

PRESENTATIONS

The majority of women with tumors of the uterine corpus present with postmenopausal vaginal bleeding due to shedding of the malignant endometrial lining. Premenopausal women often will present with atypical bleeding between typical menstrual cycles. These signs typically bring a woman to the attention of a health care professional, and hence the majority of women present with early-stage disease with the tumor confined to the uterine corpus. Diagnosis is typically established by endometrial biopsy. Epithelial tumors may spread to pelvic or para-aortic lymph nodes. Pulmonary metastases can appear later in the natural history of this disease but are very uncommon at initial presentation. Serous tumors tend to have patterns of spread much more reminiscent of ovarian cancer with many patients presenting with disseminated peritoneal disease and sometimes ascites. Some women presenting with uterine sarcomas will present with pelvic pain. Nodal metastases are uncommon with sarcomas, which are more likely to present with either intraabdominal disease or pulmonary metastases.

TREATMENT UTERINE CANCER

Most women with endometrial cancer have disease that is localized to the uterus (75% are stage I, Table 117-1), and definitive treatment typically involves a hysterectomy with removal of the ovaries and fallopian tubes. The resection of lymph nodes does not improve outcome but does provide prognostic information. Node involvement defines stage III disease, which is present in 13% of patients. Tumor grade and depth of invasion are the two key prognostic variables in early-stage tumors, and women with low-grade and/or minimally invasive tumors are typically observed after definitive surgical therapy. Patients with high-grade tumors or tumors that are deeply invasive (stage IB, 13%) are at higher risk for pelvic recurrence or recurrence at the vaginal cuff, which is typically prevented by vaginal vault brachytherapy.

Women with regional metastases or metastatic disease (3% of patients) with low-grade tumors can be treated with progesterone. Poorly differentiated tumors are typically resistant to hormonal manipulation and thus are treated with chemotherapy. The role of chemotherapy in the adjuvant setting is currently under investigation. Chemotherapy for metastatic disease is delivered with palliative intent. Drugs that effectively target and inhibit signaling of the AKT-mTOR pathway are currently under investigation.

Five-year survival is 89% for stage I, 73% for stage II, 52% for stage III, and 17% for stage IV disease (Table 117-1).

GESTATIONAL TROPHOBLASTIC TUMORS

GLOBAL CONSIDERATIONS

Gestational trophoblastic diseases represent a spectrum of neoplasia from benign hydatidiform mole to choriocarcinoma due to persistent trophoblastic disease associated most commonly with molar pregnancy but occasionally seen after normal gestation. The most common presentations of trophoblastic tumors are partial and complete molar pregnancies. These represent approximately 1 in 1500 conceptions in developed Western countries. The incidence widely varies globally, with areas in Southeast Asia having a much higher incidence of molar pregnancy. Regions with high molar pregnancy rates are often associated with diets low in carotene and animal fats.

RISK FACTORS

Trophoblastic tumors result from the outgrowth or persistence of placental tissue. They arise most commonly in the uterus but can also arise in other sites such as the fallopian tubes due to ectopic pregnancy. Risk factors include poorly defined dietary and environmental factors as well as conceptions at the extremes of reproductive age, with the incidence particularly high in females conceiving younger than age 16 or older than age 50. In older women, the incidence of molar pregnancy might be as high as one in three, likely due to increased risk of abnormal fertilization of the aged ova. Most trophoblastic neoplasms are associated with complete moles, diploid tumors with all genetic material from the paternal donor (known as parental disomy). This is thought to occur when a single sperm fertilizes an enucleate egg that subsequently duplicates the paternal DNA. Trophoblastic proliferation occurs with exuberant villous stroma. If pseudopregnancy extends out past the 12th week, fluid progressively accumulates within the stroma, leading to "hydropic changes." There is no fetal development in complete moles.

Partial moles arise from the fertilization of an egg with two sperm; hence two-thirds of genetic material is paternal in these triploid tumors. Hydropic changes are less dramatic, and fetal development can often occur through late first trimester or early second trimester at which point spontaneous abortion is common. Laboratory findings will include excessively high hCG and high AFP. The risk of persistent gestational trophoblastic disease after partial mole is approximately 5%. Complete and partial moles can be noninvasive or invasive. Myometrial invasion occurs in no more than one in six complete moles and a lower portion of partial moles.

PRESENTATION OF INVASIVE TROPHOBLASTIC DISEASE

The clinical presentation of molar pregnancy is changing in developed countries due to the early detection of pregnancy with home pregnancy kits and the very early use of Doppler and ultrasound to evaluate the early fetus and uterine cavity for evidence of a viable fetus. Thus, in these countries, the majority of women presenting with trophoblastic disease have their moles detected early and have typical symptoms of early pregnancy including nausea, amenorrhea, and breast tenderness. With uterine evacuation of early complete and partial moles, most women experience spontaneous remission of their disease as monitored by serial hCG levels. These women require no chemotherapy. Patients with persistent elevation of hCG or rising hCG after evacuation have persistent or actively growing gestational trophoblastic disease and require therapy. Most series suggest that between 15 and 25% of women will have evidence of persistent gestational trophoblastic disease after molar evacuation.

In women who lack access to prenatal care, presenting symptoms can be life threatening including the development of preeclampsia or even eclampsia. Hyperthyroidism can also be seen. Evacuation of large moles can be associated with life-threatening complications including uterine perforation, volume loss, high-output cardiac failure, and adult respiratory distress syndrome (ARDS).

For women with evidence of rising hCG or radiologic confirmation of metastatic or persistent regional disease, prognosis can be estimated through a variety of scoring algorithms that identify those women at low, intermediate, and high risk for requiring multiagent chemotherapy. In general, women with widely metastatic nonpulmonary disease, very elevated hCG, and prior normal antecedent term pregnancy are considered at high risk and typically require multiagent chemotherapy for cure.

TREATMENT INVASIVE TROPHOBLASTIC DISEASE

The management for a persistent and rising hCG after evacuation of a molar conception is typically chemotherapy, although surgery can play an important role for disease that is persistently isolated in the uterus (especially if childbearing is complete) or to control hemorrhage. For women wishing to maintain fertility or with metastatic disease, the preferred treatment is chemotherapy. Chemotherapy is guided by the hCG level, which typically drops to undetectable levels with effective therapy. Single-agent treatment with methotrexate or dactinomycin cures 90% of women with low-risk disease. Patients with high-risk disease (high hCG levels, presentation 4 or more months after pregnancy, brain or liver metastases, failure of methotrexate therapy) are typically treated with multiagent chemotherapy (e.g., etoposide, methotrexate, and dactinomycin alternating with cyclophosphamide and vincristine [EMA-CO]), which is typically curative even in women with extensive metastatic disease. Cisplatin, bleomycin, and either etoposide or vinblastine are also active combinations. Survival in high-risk disease exceeds 80%. Cured women may get pregnant again without evidence of increased fetal or maternal complications.

118 Primary and Metastatic Tumors of the Nervous System

Lisa M. DeAngelis, Patrick Y. Wen

Primary brain tumors are diagnosed in approximately 52,000 people each year in the United States. At least one-half of these tumors are malignant and associated with a high mortality. Glial tumors account for about 30% of all primary brain tumors, and 80% of those are malignant. Meningiomas account for 35%, vestibular schwannomas 10%, and central nervous system (CNS) lymphomas about 2%. Brain metastases are three times more common than all primary brain tumors combined and are diagnosed in approximately 150,000 people each year. Metastases to the leptomeninges and epidural space of the spinal cord each occur in approximately 3–5% of patients with systemic cancer and are also a major cause of neurologic disability.

APPROACH TO THE PATIENT: Primary and Metastatic Tumors of the Nervous System

CLINICAL FEATURES

Brain tumors of any type can present with a variety of symptoms and signs that fall into two categories: general and focal; patients often have a combination of the two (Table 118-1). General or nonspecific symptoms include headache, with or without nausea or vomiting, cognitive difficulties, personality change, and gait disorder. Generalized symptoms arise when the enlarging tumor and its surrounding edema cause an increase in intracranial pressure or direct compression of cerebrospinal fluid (CSF) circulation leading to hydrocephalus. The classic headache associated with a brain tumor is most evident in the morning and improves during the day, but this particular pattern is actually seen in a minority of patients. Headaches are often holocephalic but can be ipsilateral to the side of a tumor. Occasionally, headaches have features of a typical migraine with unilateral throbbing pain associated with visual scotoma. Personality changes may include apathy and withdrawal from social circumstances, mimicking depression. Focal or lateralizing findings include hemiparesis, aphasia, or visual field defect. Lateralizing symptoms are typically subacute and progressive. A visual field defect is often unnoticed by the patient; its presence may only be revealed after it leads to an injury such as an automobile accident occurring in the blind visual field. Language difficulties may be mistaken for confusion. Seizures are a common presentation of brain tumors, occurring in about 25% of patients with brain metastases or malignant gliomas but can be the presenting symptom in up to 90% of patients with a low-grade glioma. All seizures that arise from a brain tumor will have a focal onset whether or not it is apparent clinically.

TABLE 118-1 SYMPTOMS AND SIGNS AT PRESENTATION OF BRAIN TUMORS

	High-Grade Glioma (%)	Low-Grade Glioma (%)	Meningioma (%)	Metastases (%)
Generalized				
Impaired cognitive function	50	10	30	60
Hemiparesis	40	10	36	60
Headache	50	40	37	50
Lateralizing				
Seizures	20	70+	17	18
Aphasia	20	<5	—	18
Visual field deficit	—	—	—	7

NEUROIMAGING

Cranial MRI is the preferred diagnostic test for any patient suspected of having a brain tumor and should be performed with gadolinium contrast administration. Computed tomography (CT) scan should be reserved for those patients unable to undergo magnetic resonance imaging (MRI; e.g., pacemaker). Malignant brain tumors—whether primary or metastatic—typically enhance with gadolinium and may have central areas of necrosis; they are characteristically surrounded by edema of the neighboring white matter. Low-grade gliomas usually do not enhance with gadolinium and are best appreciated on fluid-attenuated inversion recovery (FLAIR) MRIs. Meningiomas have a characteristic appearance on MRI because they are dural-based with a dural tail and compress but do not invade the brain. Dural metastases or a dural lymphoma can have a similar appearance. Imaging is characteristic for many primary and metastatic tumors and sometimes will suffice to establish a diagnosis when the location precludes surgical intervention (e.g., brainstem glioma). Functional MRI is useful in presurgical planning to define eloquent sensory, motor, or language cortex. Positron emission tomography (PET) is useful in determining the metabolic activity of the lesions seen on MRI; MR perfusion and spectroscopy can provide information on blood flow or tissue composition. These techniques may help distinguish tumor progression from necrotic tissue as a consequence of treatment with radiation and chemotherapy or identify foci of high-grade tumor in an otherwise low-grade-appearing glioma.

Neuroimaging is the only test necessary to diagnose a brain tumor. Laboratory tests are rarely useful, although patients with metastatic disease may have elevation of a tumor marker in their serum that reflects the presence of brain metastases (e.g., β human chorionic gonadotropin [β-hCG] from testicular cancer). Additional testing such as cerebral angiogram, electroencephalogram (EEG), or lumbar puncture is rarely indicated or helpful.

TREATMENT BRAIN TUMORS

Therapy of any intracranial malignancy requires both symptomatic and definitive treatments. Definitive treatment is based on the specific tumor type and includes surgery, radiotherapy, and chemotherapy. However, symptomatic treatments apply to brain tumors of any type. Most high-grade malignancies are accompanied by substantial surrounding edema, which contributes to neurologic disability and raised intracranial pressure. Glucocorticoids are highly effective at reducing perilesional edema and improving neurologic function, often within hours of administration. Dexamethasone has been the glucocorticoid of choice because of its relatively low mineralocorticoid activity. Initial doses are typically 12–16 mg/d in divided doses given orally or IV (both are equivalent). Although glucocorticoids rapidly ameliorate symptoms and signs, their long-term use causes substantial toxicity including insomnia, weight gain, diabetes mellitus, steroid myopathy, and personality changes. Consequently, a taper is indicated as definitive treatment is administered and the patient improves.

Patients with brain tumors who present with seizures require antiepileptic drug therapy. There is no role for prophylactic antiepileptic drugs in patients who have not had a seizure. The agents of choice are those drugs that do not induce the hepatic microsomal enzyme system. These include levetiracetam, topiramate, lamotrigine, valproic acid, and lacosamide (Chap. 445). Other drugs, such as phenytoin and carbamazepine, are used less frequently because they are potent enzyme inducers that can interfere with both glucocorticoid metabolism and the metabolism of chemotherapeutic agents needed to treat the underlying systemic malignancy or the primary brain tumor. Venous thromboembolic disease occurs in 20–30% of patients with high-grade gliomas and brain metastases. Therefore, prophylactic anticoagulants should be used during hospitalization and in nonambulatory patients. Those who have had either a deep vein thrombosis or pulmonary embolus can receive therapeutic doses of anticoagulation safely and without increasing the risk for hemorrhage into the tumor. Inferior vena cava filters are reserved for patients with absolute contraindications to anticoagulation such as recent craniotomy.

PRIMARY BRAIN TUMORS

PATHOGENESIS

No underlying cause has been identified for the majority of primary brain tumors. The only established risk factors are exposure to ionizing radiation (meningiomas, gliomas, and schwannomas) and immunosuppression (primary CNS lymphoma). Evidence for an association with exposure to electromagnetic fields including cellular telephones, head injury, foods containing *N*-nitroso compounds, or occupational risk factors are unproven. A small minority of patients have a family history of brain tumors. Some of these familial cases are associated with genetic syndromes (Table 118-2).

As with other neoplasms, brain tumors arise as a result of a multistep process driven by the sequential acquisition of genetic alterations. These include loss of tumor-suppressor genes (e.g., *p53* and phosphatase and tensin homolog on chromosome 10 [*PTEN*]) and amplification and overexpression of protooncogenes such as the epidermal growth factor receptor (*EGFR*) and the platelet-derived growth factor receptors (*PDGFR*). The accumulation of these genetic abnormalities results in uncontrolled cell growth and tumor formation.

Important progress has been made in understanding the molecular pathogenesis of several types of brain tumors, including glioblastoma and medulloblastoma. Morphologically indistinguishable glioblastomas can be separated into four subtypes defined by molecular profiling: (1) classical, characterized by overactivation of the EGFR pathway; (2) proneural, characterized by overexpression of PDGFRA, mutations of the isocitrate dehydrogenase (*IDH*) 1 and 2 genes, and expression of neural markers; (3) mesenchymal, defined by expression of mesenchymal markers and loss of *NF1*; and (4) neural, characterized by overactivity of EGFR and expression of neural markers. The clinical implications of these subtypes are under study. Medulloblastoma is the other primary brain tumor that has been highly analyzed, and four molecular subtypes have also been identified: (1) the Wnt subtype is defined by a mutation in β-catenin and has an excellent prognosis; (2) the SHH subtype has mutations in *PTCH1*, *SMO*, *GLI2*, or *SUFU* and has an intermediate prognosis; (3) group 3 has elevated MYC expression and has the worst prognosis; and (4) group 4 is characterized by isochromosome 17q. Targeted therapeutics are under development for some of the medulloblastoma subtypes, especially the SHH group.

INTRINSIC "MALIGNANT" TUMORS

ASTROCYTOMAS

These are infiltrative tumors with a presumptive glial cell of origin. The World Health Organization (WHO) classifies astrocytomas into four prognostic grades based on histologic features: grade I (pilocytic astrocytoma, subependymal giant cell astrocytoma); grade II (diffuse astrocytoma); grade III (anaplastic astrocytoma); and grade IV (glioblastoma). Grades I and II are considered low-grade astrocytomas, and grades III and IV are considered high-grade astrocytomas.

Low-Grade Astrocytoma These tumors occur predominantly in children and young adults.

GRADE I ASTROCYTOMAS Pilocytic astrocytomas (WHO grade I) are the most common tumor of childhood. They occur typically in the cerebellum but may also be found elsewhere in the neuraxis, including the optic nerves and brainstem. Frequently they appear as cystic lesions

TABLE 118-2 GENETIC SYNDROMES ASSOCIATED WITH PRIMARY BRAIN TUMORS

Syndrome	Inheritance	Gene/Protein	Associated Tumors
Cowden's syndrome	AD	Mutations of *PTEN* (ch10p23)	Dysplastic cerebellar gangliocytoma (Lhermitte-Duclos disease), meningioma, astrocytoma Breast, endometrial, thyroid cancer, trichilemmomas
Familial schwannomatosis	Sporadic Hereditary	Mutations in *INI1/SNF5* (ch22q11)	Schwannomas, gliomas
Gardner's syndrome	AD	Mutations in *APC* (ch5q21)	Medulloblastoma, glioblastoma, craniopharyngioma Familial polyposis, multiple osteomas, skin and soft tissue tumors
Gorlin syndrome (basal cell nevus syndrome)	AD	Mutations in *Patched 1* gene (ch9q22.3)	Medulloblastomas Basal cell carcinoma
Li-Fraumeni syndrome	AD	Mutations in *p53* (ch17p13.1)	Gliomas, medulloblastomas Sarcomas, breast cancer, leukemias, others
Multiple endocrine neoplasia 1 (Werner's syndrome)	AD	Mutations in *Menin* (ch11q13)	Pituitary adenoma, malignant schwannomas Parathyroid and pancreatic islet cell tumors
Neurofibromatosis type 1 (NF1)	AD	Mutations in *NF1*/neurofibromin (ch17q12-22)	Schwannomas, astrocytomas, optic nerve gliomas, meningiomas Neurofibromas, neurofibrosarcomas, others
Neurofibromatosis type 2 (NF2)	AD	Mutations in *NF2*/merlin (ch22q12)	Bilateral vestibular schwannomas, astrocytomas, multiple meningiomas, ependymomas
Tuberous sclerosis (TSC) (Bourneville disease)	AD	Mutations in *TSC1/TSC2* (ch9q34/16)	Subependymal giant-cell astrocytoma, ependymomas, glioma, ganglioneuroma, hamartoma
Turcot syndrome	AD AR	Mutations in *APC*[a] (ch5) hMLH1 (ch3p21)	Gliomas, medulloblastomas Adenomatous colon polyps, adenocarcinoma
von Hippel–Lindau (VHL)	AD	Mutations in *VHL* gene (ch3p25)	Hemangioblastomas Retinal angiomas, renal cell carcinoma, pheochromocytoma, pancreatic tumors and cysts, endolymphatic sac tumors of the middle ear

[a]Various DNA mismatch repair gene mutations may cause a similar clinical phenotype, also referred to as Turcot syndrome, in which there is a predisposition to nonpolyposis colon cancer and brain tumors.

Abbreviations: AD, autosomal dominant; APC, adenomatous polyposis coli; AR, autosomal recessive; ch, chromosome; PTEN, phosphatase and tensin homologue; TSC, tuberous sclerosis complex.

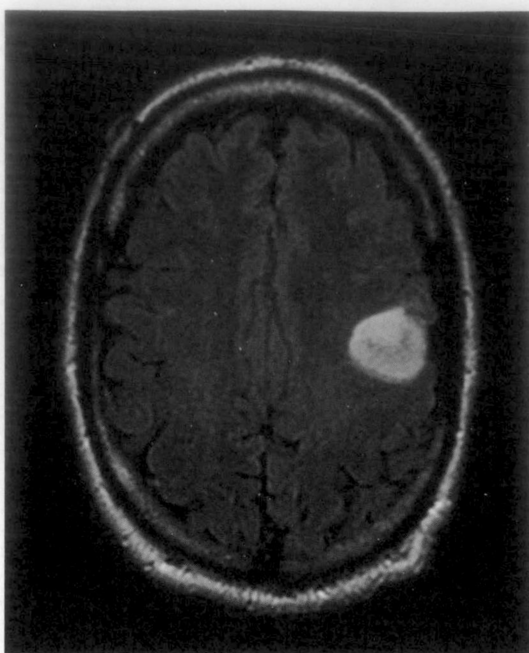

FIGURE 118-1 Fluid-attenuated inversion recovery (FLAIR) MRI of a left frontal low-grade astrocytoma. This lesion did not enhance.

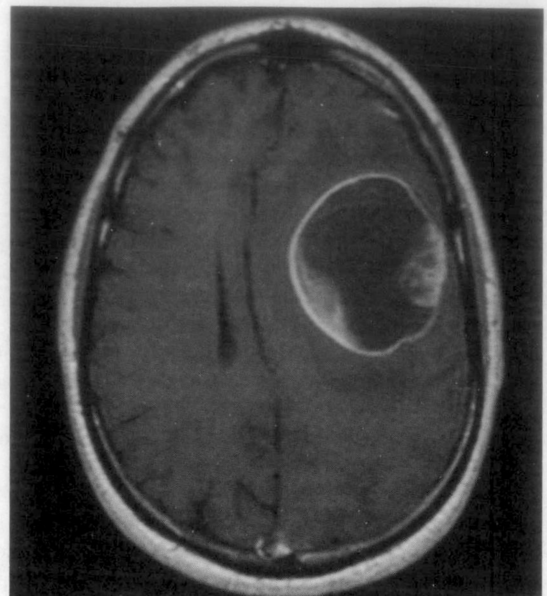

FIGURE 118-2 Postgadolinium T1 MRI of a large cystic left frontal glioblastoma.

with an enhancing mural nodule. These are well-demarcated lesions that are potentially curable if they can be resected completely. Giant-cell subependymal astrocytomas are usually found in the ventricular wall of patients with tuberous sclerosis. They often do not require intervention but can be treated surgically or with inhibitors of the mammalian target of rapamycin (mTOR).

GRADE II ASTROCYTOMAS These are infiltrative tumors that usually present with seizures in young adults. They appear as nonenhancing tumors with increased T2/FLAIR signal (Fig. 118-1). If feasible, patients should undergo maximal surgical resection, although complete resection is rarely possible because of the invasive nature of the tumor. Radiation therapy (RT) is helpful, but there is no difference in overall survival between RT administered postoperatively or delayed until the time of tumor progression. There is increasing evidence that chemotherapeutic agents such as temozolomide, an oral alkylating agent, can be helpful in some patients. The tumor transforms to a malignant astrocytoma in the majority of patients, leading to variable survival with a median of about 5 years.

High-Grade Astrocytoma

GRADE III (ANAPLASTIC) ASTROCYTOMA These account for approximately 15–20% of high-grade astrocytomas. They generally present in the fourth and fifth decades of life as variably enhancing tumors. Treatment is the same as for glioblastoma, consisting of maximal safe surgical resection followed by RT with concurrent and adjuvant temozolomide or by RT and adjuvant temozolomide alone.

GRADE IV ASTROCYTOMA (GLIOBLASTOMA) Glioblastoma accounts for the majority of high-grade astrocytomas. They are the most common malignant primary brain tumor, with over 10,000 cases diagnosed each year in the United States. Patients usually present in the sixth and seventh decades of life with headache, seizures, or focal neurologic deficits. The tumors appear as ring-enhancing masses with central necrosis and surrounding edema (Fig. 118-2). These are highly infiltrative tumors, and the areas of increased T2/FLAIR signal surrounding the main tumor mass contain invading tumor cells. Treatment involves maximal surgical resection followed by partial-field external-beam RT (6000 cGy in thirty 200-cGy fractions) with concomitant temozolomide, followed by 6–12 months of adjuvant temozolomide. With this regimen, median survival is increased to 14.6 months compared to only 12 months with RT alone, and 2-year survival is increased to 27%, compared to 10% with RT alone. Patients whose tumor contains the DNA repair enzyme O^6-methylguanine-DNA methyltransferase (MGMT) are relatively resistant to temozolomide and have a worse prognosis compared to those whose tumors contain low levels of MGMT as a result of silencing of the MGMT gene by promoter hypermethylation. Implantation of biodegradable polymers containing the chemotherapeutic agent carmustine into the tumor bed after resection of the tumor also produces a modest improvement in survival.

Despite optimal therapy, glioblastomas invariably recur. Treatment options for recurrent disease may include reoperation, carmustine wafers, and alternate chemotherapeutic regimens. Reirradiation is rarely helpful. Bevacizumab, a humanized vascular endothelial growth factor (VEGF) monoclonal antibody, has activity in recurrent glioblastoma, increasing progression-free survival and reducing peritumoral edema and glucocorticoid use (Fig. 118-3). Treatment decisions for patients with recurrent glioblastoma must be made on an individual basis, taking into consideration such factors as previous therapy, time to relapse, performance status, and quality of life. Whenever feasible, patients with recurrent disease should be enrolled in clinical trials. Novel therapies undergoing evaluation in patients with glioblastoma include targeted molecular agents directed at receptor tyrosine kinases and signal transduction pathways; antiangiogenic agents, especially those directed at the VEGF receptors; chemotherapeutic agents that cross the blood-brain barrier more effectively than currently available drugs; gene therapy; immunotherapy; and infusion of radiolabeled drugs and targeted toxins into the tumor and surrounding brain by means of convection-enhanced delivery.

The most important adverse prognostic factors in patients with high-grade astrocytomas are older age, histologic features of glioblastoma, poor Karnofsky performance status, and unresectable tumor. Patients whose tumor contains an unmethylated MGMT promoter resulting in the presence of the repair enzyme in tumor cells and resistance to temozolomide also have a worse prognosis.

Gliomatosis Cerebri Rarely, patients may present with a highly infiltrating, nonenhancing tumor of variable histologic grade involving more than two lobes of the brain. These tumors may be indolent initially, but will eventually behave aggressively and have a poor outcome. Treatment involves RT and temozolomide chemotherapy.

OLIGODENDROGLIOMA

Oligodendrogliomas account for approximately 15–20% of gliomas. They are classified by the WHO into well-differentiated oligodendrogliomas (grade II) or anaplastic oligodendrogliomas (AOs) (grade III). Tumors with oligodendroglial components have distinctive pathologic

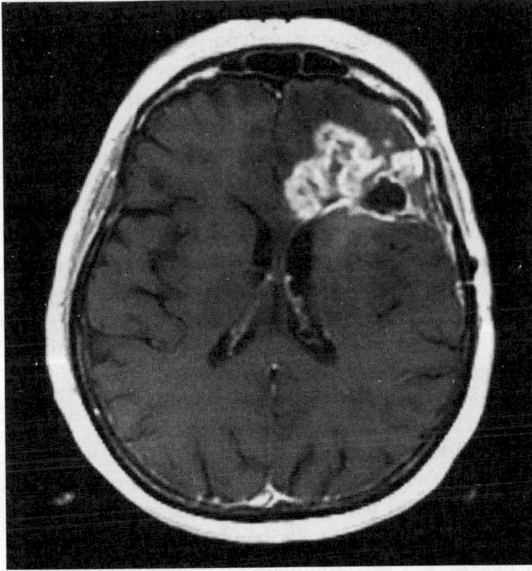

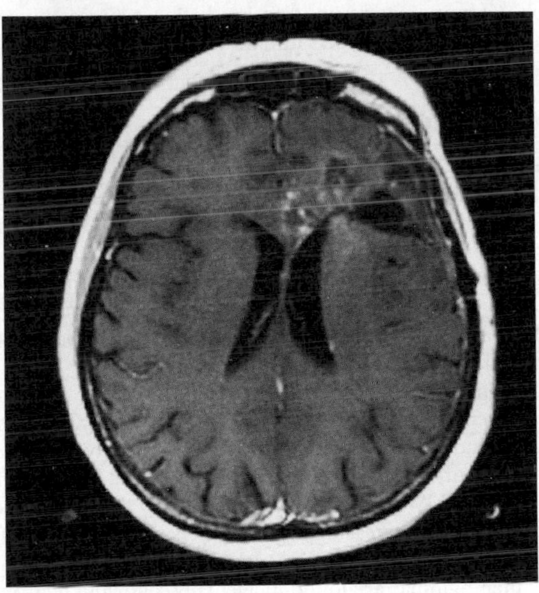

FIGURE 118-3 Postgadolinium T1 MRI of a recurrent glioblastoma before (*A*) and after (*B*) administration of bevacizumab. Note the decreased enhancement and mass effect.

features such as perinuclear clearing—giving rise to a "fried-egg" appearance—and a reticular pattern of blood vessel growth. Some tumors have both an oligodendroglial as well as an astrocytic component. These mixed tumors, or oligoastrocytomas (OAs), are also classified into well-differentiated OA (grade II) or anaplastic oligoastrocytomas (AOAs) (grade III).

Grade II oligodendrogliomas and OAs are generally more responsive to therapy and have a better prognosis than pure astrocytic tumors. These tumors present similarly to grade II astrocytomas in young adults. The tumors are nonenhancing and often partially calcified. They should be treated with surgery and, if necessary, RT and chemotherapy. Patients with oligodendrogliomas have a median survival in excess of 10 years.

AOs and AOAs present in the fourth and fifth decades as variably enhancing tumors. They are more responsive to therapy than grade III astrocytomas. Co-deletion of chromosomes 1p and 19q, mediated by an unbalanced translocation of 19p to 1q, occurs in 61–89% of patients with AO and 14–20% of patients with AOA. Tumors with the 1p and 19q co-deletion are particularly sensitive to chemotherapy with procarbazine, lomustine (cyclohexylchloroethylnitrosourea [CCNU]), and vincristine (PCV) or temozolomide, as well as to RT. Median survival of patients with AO or AOA is approximately 3–6 years, but those with co-deleted tumors can have a median survival of 10–14 years if treated with RT and chemotherapy.

EPENDYMOMAS

Ependymomas are tumors derived from ependymal cells that line the ventricular surface. They account for approximately 5% of childhood tumors and frequently arise from the wall of the fourth ventricle in the posterior fossa. Although adults can have intracranial ependymomas, they occur more commonly in the spine, especially in the filum terminale of the spinal cord where they have a myxopapillary histology. Ependymomas that can be completely resected are potentially curable. Partially resected ependymomas will recur and require irradiation. The less common anaplastic ependymoma is more aggressive and is treated with resection and RT; chemotherapy has limited efficacy. Subependymomas are slow-growing benign lesions arising in the wall of ventricles that often do not require treatment.

OTHER LESS COMMON GLIOMAS

Gangliogliomas and pleomorphic xanthoastrocytomas occur in young adults. They behave as more indolent forms of grade II gliomas and are treated in the same way. Brainstem gliomas usually occur in children or young adults. Despite treatment with RT and chemotherapy, the prognosis is poor, with a median survival of only 1 year. Gliosarcomas contain both an astrocytic as well as a sarcomatous component and are treated in the same way as glioblastomas.

PRIMARY CENTRAL NERVOUS SYSTEM LYMPHOMA

Primary central nervous system lymphoma (PCNSL) is a rare non-Hodgkin lymphoma accounting for less than 3% of primary brain tumors. For unclear reasons, its incidence is increasing, particularly in immunocompetent individuals.

PCNSL in immunocompetent patients usually consists of a diffuse large B cell lymphoma. PCNSL may also occur in immunocompromised patients, usually those infected with the human immunodeficiency virus (HIV) or organ transplant recipients on immunosuppressive therapy. PCNSL in immunocompromised patients is typically large cell with immunoblastic and more aggressive features. These patients are usually severely immunocompromised, with CD4 counts of less than 50/mL. The Epstein-Barr virus (EBV) frequently plays an important role in the pathogenesis of HIV-related PCNSL.

Immunocompetent patients with PCNSL are older (median 60 years) compared to patients with HIV-related PCNSL (median 31 years). PCNSL usually presents as a mass lesion, with neuropsychiatric symptoms, symptoms of increased intracranial pressure, lateralizing signs, or seizures.

On contrast-enhanced MRI, PCNSL usually appears as a densely enhancing tumor (Fig. 118-4). Immunocompetent patients have solitary lesions more often than immunosuppressed patients. Frequently there is involvement of the basal ganglia, corpus callosum, or periventricular region. Although the imaging features are often characteristic, PCNSL can sometimes be difficult to differentiate from high-grade gliomas, infections, or demyelination. Stereotactic biopsy is necessary to obtain a histologic diagnosis. Whenever possible, glucocorticoids should be withheld until after the biopsy has been obtained because they have a cytolytic effect on lymphoma cells and may lead to nondiagnostic tissue. In addition, patients should be tested for HIV and the extent of disease should be assessed by performing PET or CT of the body, MRI of the spine, CSF analysis, and slit-lamp examination of the eye. Bone marrow biopsy and testicular ultrasound are occasionally performed.

TREATMENT PRIMARY CENTRAL NERVOUS SYSTEM LYMPHOMA

PCNSL is more sensitive to glucocorticoids, chemotherapy, and RT than other primary brain tumors. Durable complete responses and long-term survival are possible with these treatments. High-dose methotrexate, a folate antagonist that interrupts DNA synthesis, produces response rates ranging from 35–80% and median

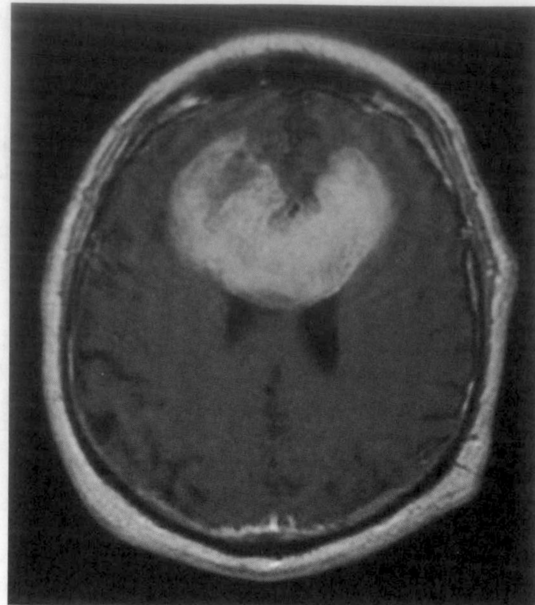

FIGURE 118-4 Postgadolinium T1 MRI demonstrating a large bifrontal primary central nervous system lymphoma (PCNSL). The periventricular location and diffuse enhancement pattern are characteristic of lymphoma.

survival of up to 50 months. The combination of methotrexate with other chemotherapeutic agents such as cytarabine increases the response rate to 70–100%. The addition of whole-brain RT to methotrexate-based chemotherapy prolongs progression-free survival but not overall survival. Furthermore, RT is associated with delayed neurotoxicity, especially in patients over the age of 60 years. As a result, full-dose RT is frequently omitted, but there may be a role for reduced-dose RT. The anti-CD20 monoclonal antibody rituximab has activity in PCNSL and is often incorporated into the chemotherapy regimen. For some patients, high-dose chemotherapy with autologous stem cell rescue may offer the best chance of preventing relapse. At least 50% of patients will eventually develop recurrent disease. Treatment options include RT for patients who have not had prior irradiation, re-treatment with methotrexate, as well as other agents such as temozolomide, rituximab, procarbazine, topotecan, and pemetrexed. High-dose chemotherapy with autologous stem cell rescue may have a role in selected patients with relapsed disease.

PCNSL IN IMMUNOCOMPROMISED PATIENTS

PCNSL in immunocompromised patients often produces multiple ring-enhancing lesions that can be difficult to differentiate from metastases and infections such as toxoplasmosis. The diagnosis is usually established by examination of the CSF for cytology and EBV DNA, toxoplasmosis serologic testing, brain PET imaging for hypermetabolism of the lesions consistent with tumor instead of infection, and, if necessary, brain biopsy. Since the advent of highly active antiretroviral drugs, the incidence of HIV-related PCNSL has declined. These patients may be treated with whole-brain RT, high-dose methotrexate, and initiation of highly active antiretroviral therapy. In organ transplant recipients, reduction of immunosuppression may improve outcome.

MEDULLOBLASTOMAS

Medulloblastomas are the most common malignant brain tumor of childhood, accounting for approximately 20% of all primary CNS tumors among children. They arise from granule cell progenitors or from multipotent progenitors from the ventricular zone. Approximately 5% of children have inherited disorders with germline mutations of genes that predispose to the development of medulloblastoma. Gorlin syndrome, the most common of these inherited disorders, is due to mutations in the patched-1 (*PTCH-1*) gene, a key component in the sonic hedgehog pathway. Turcot syndrome, caused by mutations in the adenomatous polyposis coli (*APC*) gene and familial adenomatous polyposis, has also been associated with an increased incidence of medulloblastoma. Histologically, medulloblastomas are highly cellular tumors with abundant dark staining, round nuclei, and rosette formation (Homer-Wright rosettes). They present with headache, ataxia, and signs of brainstem involvement. On MRI they appear as densely enhancing tumors in the posterior fossa, sometimes associated with hydrocephalus. Seeding of the CSF is common. Treatment involves maximal surgical resection, craniospinal irradiation, and chemotherapy with agents such as cisplatin, lomustine, cyclophosphamide, and vincristine. Approximately 70% of patients have long-term survival but usually at the cost of significant neurocognitive impairment. A major goal of current research is to improve survival while minimizing long-term complications.

PINEAL REGION TUMORS

A large number of tumors can arise in the region of the pineal gland. These typically present with headache, visual symptoms, and hydrocephalus. Patients may have Parinaud syndrome characterized by impaired upgaze and accommodation. Some pineal tumors such as pineocytomas and benign teratomas can be treated simply by surgical resection. Germinomas respond to irradiation, whereas pineoblastomas and malignant germ cell tumors require craniospinal radiation and chemotherapy.

EXTRINSIC "BENIGN" TUMORS

MENINGIOMAS

Meningiomas are diagnosed with increasing frequency as more people undergo neuroimaging for various indications. They are now the most common primary brain tumor, accounting for approximately 35% of the total. Their incidence increases with age. They tend to be more common in women and in patients with neurofibromatosis type 2. They also occur more commonly in patients with a past history of cranial irradiation.

Meningiomas arise from the dura mater and are composed of neoplastic meningothelial (arachnoidal cap) cells. They are most commonly located over the cerebral convexities, especially adjacent to the sagittal sinus, but can also occur in the skull base and along the dorsum of the spinal cord. Meningiomas are classified by the WHO into three histologic grades of increasing aggressiveness: grade I (benign), grade II (atypical), and grade III (malignant).

Many meningiomas are found incidentally following neuroimaging for unrelated reasons. They can also present with headaches, seizures, or focal neurologic deficits. On imaging studies they have a characteristic appearance usually consisting of a partially calcified, densely enhancing extraaxial tumor arising from the dura (Fig. 118-5). Occasionally they may have a dural tail, consisting of thickened, enhanced dura extending like a tail from the mass. The main differential diagnosis of meningioma is a dural metastasis.

If the meningioma is small and asymptomatic, no intervention is necessary and the lesion can be observed with serial MRI studies. Larger, symptomatic lesions should be resected. If complete resection is achieved, the patient is cured. Incompletely resected tumors tend to recur, although the rate of recurrence can be very slow with grade I tumors. Tumors that cannot be resected, or can only be partially removed, may benefit from treatment with external-beam RT or stereotactic radiosurgery (SRS). These treatments may also be helpful in patients whose tumor has recurred after surgery. Hormonal therapy and chemotherapy are currently unproven.

Rarer tumors that resemble meningiomas include hemangiopericytomas and solitary fibrous tumors. These are treated with surgery and RT but have a higher propensity to recur locally or metastasize systemically.

SCHWANNOMAS

These are generally benign tumors arising from the Schwann cells of cranial and spinal nerve roots. The most common schwannomas, termed *vestibular schwannomas* or *acoustic neuromas*, arise from the

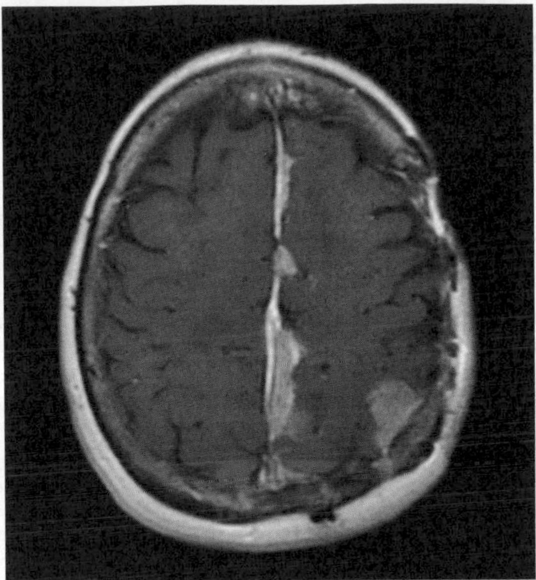

FIGURE 118-5 Postgadolinium T1 MRI demonstrating multiple meningiomas along the falx and left parietal cortex.

vestibular portion of the eighth cranial nerve and account for approximately 9% of primary brain tumors. Patients with neurofibromatosis type 2 have a high incidence of vestibular schwannomas that are frequently bilateral. Schwannomas arising from other cranial nerves, such as the trigeminal nerve (cranial nerve V), occur with much lower frequency. Neurofibromatosis type 1 is associated with an increased incidence of schwannomas of the spinal nerve roots.

Vestibular schwannomas may be found incidentally on neuroimaging or present with progressive unilateral hearing loss, dizziness, tinnitus, or less commonly, symptoms resulting from compression of the brainstem and cerebellum. On MRI they appear as densely enhancing lesions, enlarging the internal auditory canal and often extending into the cerebellopontine angle (Fig. 118-6). The differential diagnosis includes meningioma. Very small, asymptomatic lesions can be observed with serial MRIs. Larger lesions should be treated with surgery or SRS. The optimal treatment will depend on the size of the tumor, symptoms, and the patient's preference. In patients with small vestibular schwannomas and relatively intact hearing, early surgical intervention increases the chance of preserving hearing.

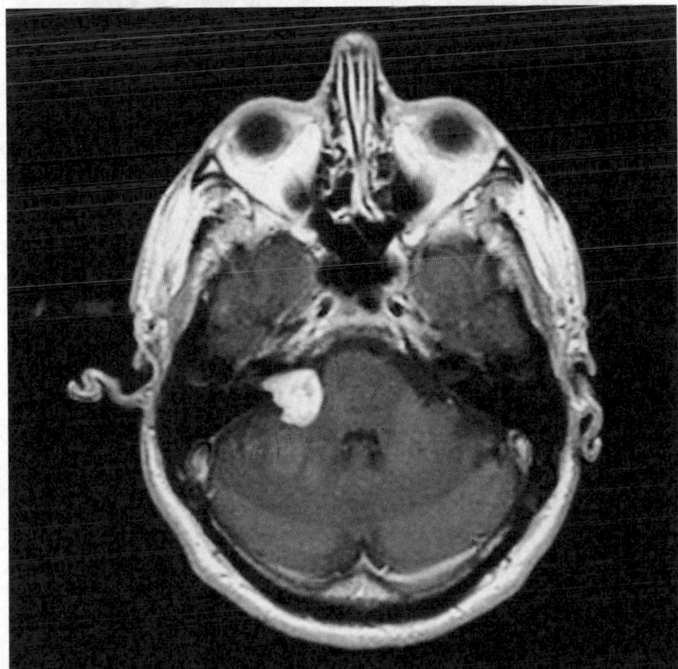

FIGURE 118-6 Postgadolinium MRI of a right vestibular schwannoma. The tumor can be seen to involve the internal auditory canal.

PITUITARY TUMORS (CHAP. 401e)

These account for approximately 9% of primary brain tumors. They can be divided into functioning and nonfunctioning tumors. Functioning tumors are usually microadenomas (<1 cm in diameter) that secrete hormones and produce specific endocrine syndromes (e.g., acromegaly for growth hormone–secreting tumors, Cushing syndrome for adrenocorticotropic hormone [ACTH]-secreting tumors, and galactorrhea, amenorrhea, and infertility for prolactin-secreting tumors). Nonfunctioning pituitary tumors tend to be macroadenomas (>1 cm) that produce symptoms by mass effect, giving rise to headaches, visual impairment (such as bitemporal hemianopia), and hypopituitarism. Prolactin-secreting tumors respond well to dopamine agonists such as bromocriptine and cabergoline. Other pituitary tumors usually require treatment with surgery and sometimes RT or radiosurgery and hormonal therapy.

CRANIOPHARYNGIOMAS

Craniopharyngiomas are rare, usually suprasellar, partially calcified, solid, or mixed solid-cystic benign tumors that arise from remnants of Rathke's pouch. They have a bimodal distribution, occurring predominantly in children but also between the ages of 55 and 65 years. They present with headaches, visual impairment, and impaired growth in children and hypopituitarism in adults. Treatment involves surgery, RT, or a combination of the two.

OTHER BENIGN TUMORS

Dysembryoplastic Neuroepithelial Tumors (DNTs) These are benign, supratentorial tumors, usually in the temporal lobe. They typically occur in children and young adults with a long-standing history of seizures. Surgical resection is curative.

Epidermoid Cysts These consist of squamous epithelium surrounding a keratin-filled cyst. They are usually found in the cerebellopontine angle and the intrasellar and suprasellar regions. They may present with headaches, cranial nerve abnormalities, seizures, or hydrocephalus. Imaging studies demonstrate extraaxial lesions with characteristics that are similar to CSF but have restricted diffusion. Treatment involves surgical resection.

Dermoid Cysts Like epidermoid cysts, dermoid cysts arise from epithelial cells that are retained during closure of the neural tube. They contain both epidermal and dermal structures such as hair follicles, sweat glands, and sebaceous glands. Unlike epidermoid cysts, these tumors usually have a midline location. They occur most frequently in the posterior fossa, especially the vermis, fourth ventricle, and suprasellar cistern. Radiographically, dermoid cysts resemble lipomas, demonstrating T1 hyperintensity and variable signal on T2. Symptomatic dermoid cysts can be treated with surgery.

Colloid Cysts These usually arise in the anterior third ventricle and may present with headaches, hydrocephalus, and, very rarely, sudden death. Surgical resection is curative, or a third ventriculostomy may relieve the obstructive hydrocephalus and be sufficient therapy.

NEUROCUTANEOUS SYNDROMES (PHAKOMATOSES)

A number of genetic disorders are characterized by cutaneous lesions and an increased risk of brain tumors. Most of these disorders have an autosomal dominant inheritance with variable penetrance.

NEUROFIBROMATOSIS TYPE 1 (NF1) (von RECKLINGHAUSEN'S DISEASE)

NF1 is an autosomal dominant disorder with an incidence of approximately 1 in 2600–3000. Approximately one-half the cases are familial; the remainder are caused by new mutations arising in patients with unaffected parents. The *NF1* gene on chromosome 17q11.2 encodes a protein, neurofibromin, a guanosine triphosphatase (GTPase)-activating protein (GAP) that modulates signaling through the ras pathway. Mutations of *NF1* result in a large number of nervous system tumors including neurofibromas, plexiform neurofibromas, optic nerve gliomas, astrocytomas, and meningiomas. In addition to neurofibromas, which appear as multiple, soft, rubbery cutaneous tumors, other cutaneous manifestations of NF1 include café-au-lait spots and axillary freckling. NF1 is also associated with hamartomas of the iris termed Lisch nodules, pheochromocytomas, pseudoarthrosis of the tibia, scoliosis, epilepsy, and mental retardation.

NEUROFIBROMATOSIS TYPE 2 (NF2)

NF2 is less common than NF1, with an incidence of 1 in 25,000–40,000. It is an autosomal dominant disorder with full penetrance. As with NF1, approximately one-half the cases arise from new mutations. The *NF2* gene on 22q encodes a cytoskeletal protein, merlin (moesin, ezrin, radixin-like protein) that functions as a tumor suppressor. NF2 is characterized by bilateral vestibular schwannomas in over 90% of patients, multiple meningiomas, and spinal ependymomas and astrocytomas. Treatment of bilateral vestibular schwannomas can be challenging because the goal is to preserve hearing for as long as possible. These patients may also have diffuse schwannomatosis that may affect the cranial, spinal, or peripheral nerves; posterior subcapsular lens opacities; and retinal hamartomas.

TUBEROUS SCLEROSIS (BOURNEVILLE DISEASE)

This is an autosomal dominant disorder with an incidence of approximately 1 in 5000–10,000 live births. It is caused by mutations in either the *TSC1* gene, which maps to chromosome 9q34 and encodes a protein termed hamartin, or the *TSC2* gene, which maps to chromosome 16p13.3 and encodes the protein tuberin. Hamartin forms a complex with tuberin, which inhibits cellular signaling through the mTOR, and acts as a negative regulator of the cell cycle. Patients with tuberous sclerosis may have seizures, mental retardation, adenoma sebaceum (facial angiofibromas), shagreen patch, hypomelanotic macules, periungual fibromas, renal angiomyolipomas, and cardiac rhabdomyomas. These patients have an increased incidence of subependymal nodules, cortical tubers, and subependymal giant-cell astrocytomas (SEGA). Patients frequently require anticonvulsants for seizures. SEGAs do not always require therapeutic intervention, but the most effective therapy is with the mTOR inhibitors sirolimus or everolimus, which often decrease seizures as well as SEGA size.

TUMORS METASTATIC TO THE BRAIN

Brain metastases arise from hematogenous spread and frequently either arise from a lung primary or are associated with pulmonary metastases. Most metastases develop at the gray matter–white matter junction in the watershed distribution of the brain where intravascular tumor cells lodge in terminal arterioles. The distribution of metastases in the brain approximates the proportion of blood flow such that about 85% of all metastases are supratentorial and 15% occur in the posterior fossa. The most common sources of brain metastases are lung and breast carcinomas; melanoma has the greatest propensity to metastasize to the brain, being found in 80% of patients at autopsy Table 118-3). Other tumor types such as ovarian and esophageal carcinoma rarely metastasize to the brain. Prostate and breast cancer also have a propensity to metastasize to the dura and can mimic meningioma. Leptomeningeal metastases are common from hematologic malignancies and also breast and lung cancers. Spinal cord compression primarily arises in patients with prostate and breast cancer, tumors with a strong propensity to metastasize to the axial skeleton.

TABLE 118-3 FREQUENCY OF NERVOUS SYSTEM METASTASES BY COMMON PRIMARY TUMORS

	Brain %	LM %	ESCC %
Lung	41	17	15
Breast	19	57	22
Melanoma	10	12	4
Prostate	1	1	10
GIT	7	—	5
Renal	3	2	7
Lymphoma	<1	10	10
Sarcoma	7	1	9
Other	11	—	18

Abbreviations: ESCC, epidural spinal cord compression; GIT, gastrointestinal tract; LM, leptomeningeal metastases.

DIAGNOSIS OF METASTASES

Brain metastases are best visualized on MRI, where they usually appear as well-circumscribed lesions (Fig. 118-7). The amount of perilesional edema can be highly variable, with large lesions causing minimal edema and sometimes very small lesions causing extensive edema. Enhancement may be in a ring pattern or diffuse. Occasionally,

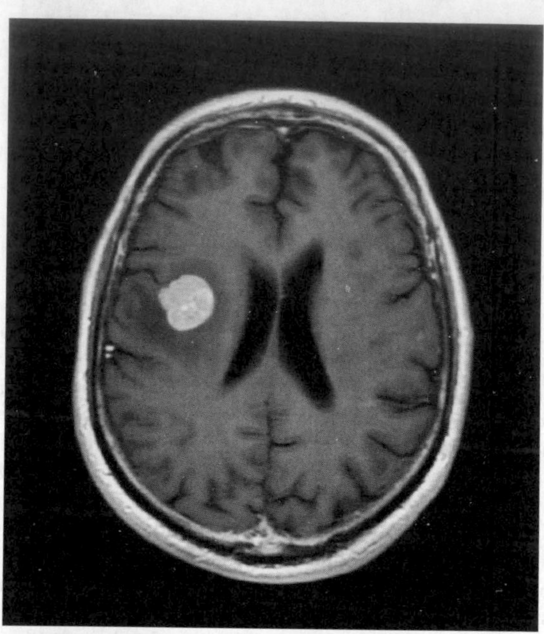

A

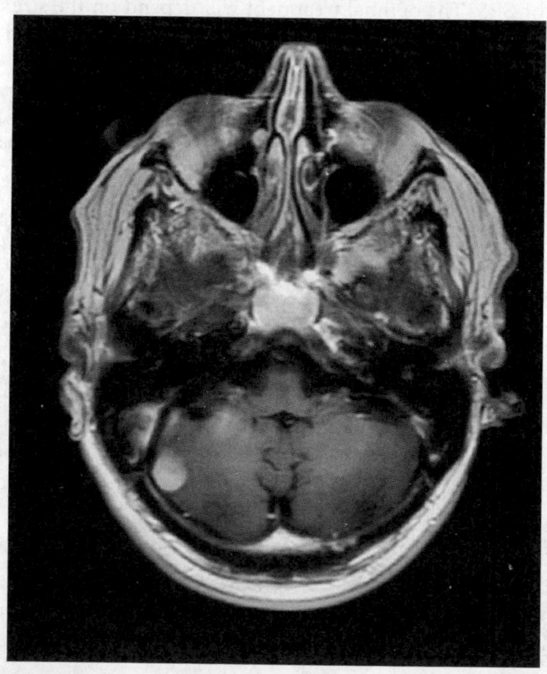

B

FIGURE 118-7 Postgadolinium T1 MRI of multiple brain metastases from non-small-cell lung cancer involving the right frontal (***A***) and right cerebellar (***B***) hemispheres. Note the diffuse enhancement pattern and absence of central necrosis.

intracranial metastases will hemorrhage; although melanoma, thyroid, and kidney cancer have the greatest propensity to hemorrhage, the most common cause of a hemorrhagic metastasis is lung cancer because it accounts for the majority of brain metastases. The radiographic appearance of brain metastasis is nonspecific, and similar-appearing lesions can occur with infection including brain abscesses and also with demyelinating lesions, sarcoidosis, radiation necrosis in a previously treated patient, or a primary brain tumor that may be a second malignancy in a patient with systemic cancer. However, biopsy is rarely necessary for diagnosis in most patients because imaging alone in the appropriate clinical situation usually suffices. This is straightforward for the majority of patients with brain metastases because they have a known systemic cancer. However, in approximately 10% of patients, a systemic cancer may present with a brain metastasis, and if there is not an easily accessible systemic site to biopsy, then a brain lesion must be removed for diagnostic purposes.

TREATMENT TUMORS METASTATIC TO THE BRAIN

DEFINITIVE TREATMENT

The number and location of brain metastases often determine the therapeutic options. The patient's overall condition and the current or potential control of the systemic disease are also major determinants. Brain metastases are single in approximately one-half of patients and multiple in the other half.

RADIATION THERAPY

The standard treatment for brain metastases has been whole-brain radiotherapy (WBRT) usually administered to a total dose of 3000 cGy in 10 fractions. This affords rapid palliation, and approximately 80% of patients improve with glucocorticoids and RT. However, it is not curative. Median survival is only 4–6 months. More recently, SRS delivered through a variety of techniques including the gamma knife, linear accelerator, proton beam, and CyberKnife all can deliver highly focused doses of RT, usually in a single fraction. SRS can effectively sterilize the visible lesions and afford local disease control in 80–90% of patients. In addition, there are some patients who have clearly been cured of their brain metastases using SRS, whereas this is distinctly rare with WBRT. However, SRS can be used only for lesions 3 cm or less in diameter and should be confined to patients with only one to three metastases. The addition of WBRT to SRS improves disease control in the nervous system but does not prolong survival.

SURGERY

Randomized controlled trials have demonstrated that surgical extirpation of a single brain metastasis followed by WBRT is superior to WBRT alone. Removal of two lesions or a single symptomatic mass, particularly if compressing the ventricular system, can also be useful. This is particularly useful in patients who have highly radioresistant lesions such as renal carcinoma. Surgical resection can afford rapid symptomatic improvement and prolonged survival. WBRT administered after complete resection of a brain metastasis improves disease control but does not prolong survival.

CHEMOTHERAPY

Chemotherapy is rarely useful for brain metastases. Metastases from certain tumor types that are highly chemosensitive, such as germ cell tumors or small-cell lung cancer, may respond to chemotherapeutic regimens chosen according to the underlying malignancy. Increasingly, there are data demonstrating responsiveness of brain metastases to chemotherapy including small molecule–targeted therapy when the lesion possesses the target. This has been best illustrated in patients with lung cancer harboring EGFR mutations that sensitize them to EGFR inhibitors. Antiangiogenic agents such as bevacizumab may also prove efficacious in the treatment of CNS metastases.

LEPTOMENINGEAL METASTASES

Leptomeningeal metastases are also identified as carcinomatous meningitis, meningeal carcinomatosis, or in the case of specific tumors, leukemic or lymphomatous meningitis. Among the hematologic malignancies, acute leukemia is the most common to metastasize to the subarachnoid space, and in lymphomas the aggressive diffuse lymphomas can metastasize to the subarachnoid space frequently as well. Among solid tumors, breast and lung carcinomas and melanoma most frequently spread in this fashion. Tumor cells reach the subarachnoid space via the arterial circulation or occasionally through retrograde flow in venous systems that drain metastases along the bony spine or cranium. In addition, leptomeningeal metastases may develop as a direct consequence of prior brain metastases and can develop in almost 40% of patients who have a metastasis resected from the cerebellum.

CLINICAL FEATURES

Leptomeningeal metastases are characterized clinically by multilevel symptoms and signs along the neuraxis. Combinations of lumbar and cervical radiculopathies, cranial neuropathies, seizures, confusion, and encephalopathy from hydrocephalus or raised intracranial pressure can be present. Focal deficits such as hemiparesis or aphasia are rarely due to leptomeningeal metastases unless there is direct brain infiltration, and they are more often associated with coexisting brain lesions. New-onset limb pain in patients with breast cancer, lung cancer, or melanoma should prompt consideration of leptomeningeal spread.

LABORATORY AND IMAGING DIAGNOSIS

Leptomeningeal metastases are particularly challenging to diagnose because identification of tumor cells in the subarachnoid compartment may be elusive. MRI can be definitive in patients when there are clear tumor nodules adherent to the cauda equina or spinal cord, enhancing cranial nerves, or subarachnoid enhancement on brain imaging (Fig. 118-8). Imaging is diagnostic in approximately 75% of patients and is more often positive in patients with solid tumors. Demonstration of tumor cells in the CSF is definitive and often considered the gold standard. However, CSF cytologic examination is positive in only 50% of patients on the first lumbar puncture and still misses 10% after three CSF samples. CSF cytologic examination is most useful in hematologic malignancies. Accompanying CSF abnormalities include an elevated protein concentration and an elevated white count. Hypoglycorrhachia is noted in less than 25% of patients but is useful when present. Identification of tumor markers or molecular confirmation of clonal proliferation with techniques such as flow cytometry within the CSF can also be definitive when present. Tumor markers are usually specific to solid tumors, and chromosomal or molecular markers are most useful in patients with hematologic malignancies. New technologies, such as rare cell capture, may enhance identification of tumor cells in the CSF.

TREATMENT LEPTOMENINGEAL METASTASES

The treatment of leptomeningeal metastasis is palliative because there is no curative therapy. RT to the symptomatically involved areas, such as skull base for cranial neuropathy, can relieve pain and sometimes improve function. Whole-neuraxis RT has extensive toxicity with myelosuppression and gastrointestinal irritation as well as limited effectiveness. Systemic chemotherapy with agents that can penetrate the blood-CSF barrier may be helpful. Alternatively, intrathecal chemotherapy can be effective, particularly in hematologic malignancies. This is optimally delivered through an intraventricular cannula (Ommaya reservoir) rather than by lumbar puncture. Few drugs can be delivered safely into the subarachnoid space, and they have a limited spectrum of antitumor activity, perhaps accounting for the relatively poor response to this approach. In addition, impaired CSF flow dynamics can compromise intrathecal drug delivery. Surgery has a limited role in the treatment of leptomeningeal metastasis, but placement of a ventriculoperitoneal shunt can relieve raised intracranial pressure. However, it compromises delivery of chemotherapy into the CSF.

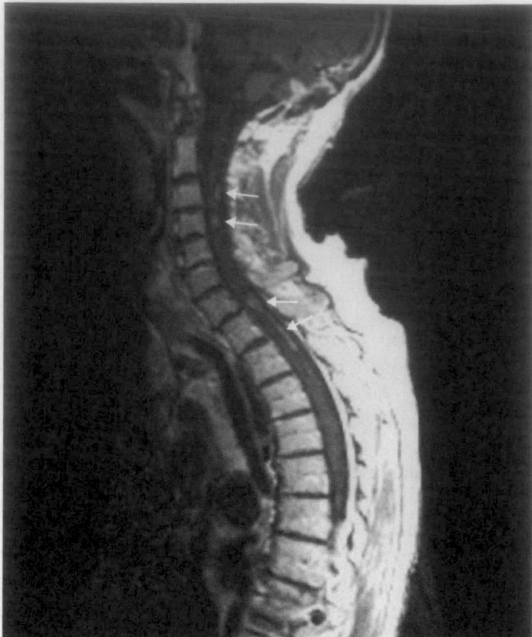
A

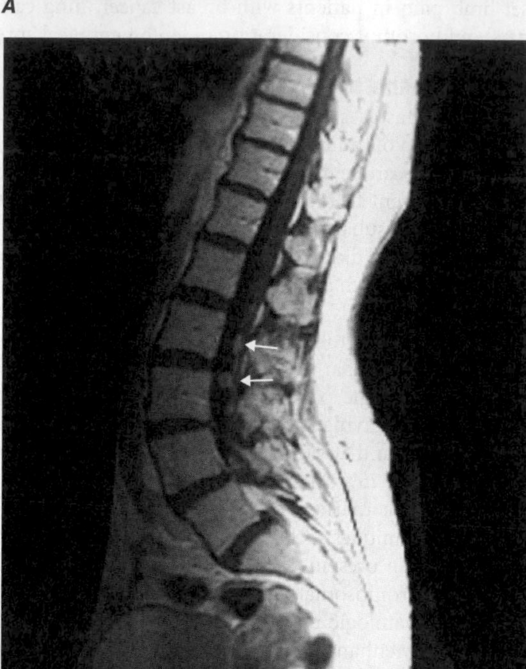
B

FIGURE 118-8 Postgadolinium MRI images of extensive leptomeningeal metastases from breast cancer. Nodules along the dorsal surface of the spinal cord (***A***) and cauda equina (***B***) are seen.

EPIDURAL METASTASIS

Epidural metastasis occurs in 3–5% of patients with a systemic malignancy and causes neurologic compromise by compressing the spinal cord or cauda equina. The most common cancers that metastasize to the epidural space are those malignancies that spread to bone, such as breast and prostate. Lymphoma can cause bone involvement and compression, but it can also invade the intervertebral foramens and cause spinal cord compression without bone destruction. The thoracic spine is affected most commonly, followed by the lumbar and then cervical spine.

CLINICAL FEATURES

Back pain is the presenting symptom of epidural metastasis in virtually all patients; the pain may precede neurologic findings by weeks or months. The pain is usually exacerbated by lying down; by contrast, arthritic pain is often relieved by recumbency. Leg weakness is seen in about 50% of patients, as is sensory dysfunction. Sphincter problems are present in about 25% of patients at diagnosis.

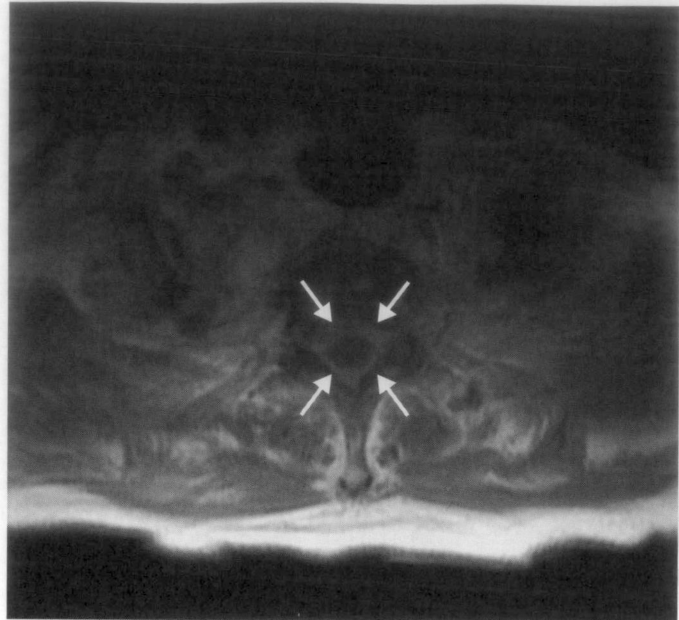

FIGURE 118-9 Postgadolinium T1 MRI showing circumferential epidural tumor around the thoracic spinal cord from esophageal cancer.

DIAGNOSIS

Diagnosis is established by imaging, with MRI of the complete spine being the best test (Fig. 118-9). Contrast is not needed to identify spinal or epidural lesions. Any patient with cancer who has severe back pain should undergo an MRI. Plain films, bone scans, or even CT scans may show bone metastases, but only MRI can reliably delineate epidural tumor. For patients unable to have an MRI, CT myelography should be performed to outline the epidural space. The differential diagnosis of epidural tumor includes epidural abscess, acute or chronic hematomas, and rarely, extramedullary hematopoiesis.

TREATMENT EPIDURAL METASTASIS

Epidural metastasis requires immediate treatment. A randomized controlled trial demonstrated the superiority of surgical resection followed by RT compared to RT alone. However, patients must be able to tolerate surgery, and the surgical procedure of choice is a complete removal of the mass, which is typically anterior to the spinal canal, necessitating an extensive approach and resection. Otherwise, RT is the mainstay of treatment and can be used for patients with radiosensitive tumors, such as lymphoma, or for those unable to undergo surgery. Chemotherapy is rarely used for epidural metastasis unless the patient has minimal to no neurologic deficit and a highly chemosensitive tumor such as lymphoma or germinoma. Patients generally fare well if treated before there is severe neurologic deficit. Recovery after paraparesis is better after surgery than with RT alone, but survival is often short due to widespread metastatic tumor.

NEUROLOGIC TOXICITY OF THERAPY

TOXICITY FROM RADIOTHERAPY

RT can cause a variety of toxicities in the CNS. These are usually described based on their relationship in time to the administration of RT: acute (occurring within days of RT), early delayed (months), or late delayed (years). In general, the acute and early delayed syndromes resolve and do not result in persistent deficits, whereas the late delayed toxicities are usually permanent and sometimes progressive.

Acute Toxicity Acute cerebral toxicity usually occurs during RT to the brain. RT can cause a transient disruption of the blood-brain barrier, resulting in increased edema and elevated intracranial pressure. This is usually manifest as headache, lethargy, nausea, and vomiting and can be both prevented and treated with the administration of glucocorticoids. There is no acute RT toxicity that affects the spinal cord.

Early Delayed Toxicity Early delayed toxicity is usually apparent weeks to months after completion of cranial irradiation and is likely due to focal demyelination. Clinically it may be asymptomatic or take the form of worsening or reappearance of a preexisting neurologic deficit. At times a contrast-enhancing lesion can be seen on MRI/CT that can mimic the tumor for which the patient received the RT. For patients with a malignant glioma, this has been described as "pseudoprogression" because it mimics tumor recurrence on MRI but actually represents inflammation and necrotic debris engendered by effective therapy. This is seen with increased frequency when chemotherapy, particularly temozolomide, is given concurrently with RT. Pseudoprogression can resolve on its own or, if very symptomatic, may require resection. A rare form of early delayed toxicity is the somnolence syndrome that occurs primarily in children and is characterized by marked sleepiness.

In the spinal cord, early delayed RT toxicity is manifest as a Lhermitte symptom with paresthesias of the limbs or along the spine when the patient flexes the neck. Although frightening, it is benign, resolves on its own, and does not portend more serious problems.

Late Delayed Toxicity Late delayed toxicities are the most serious because they are often irreversible and cause severe neurologic deficits. In the brain, late toxicities can take several forms, the most common of which include radiation necrosis and leukoencephalopathy. Radiation necrosis is a focal mass of necrotic tissue that is contrast enhancing on CT/MRI and may be associated with significant edema. This may appear identical to pseudoprogression but is seen months to years after RT and is always symptomatic. Clinical symptoms and signs include seizure and lateralizing findings referable to the location of the necrotic mass. The necrosis is caused by the effect of RT on cerebral vasculature with resultant fibrinoid necrosis and occlusion of the blood vessels. It can mimic tumor radiographically, but unlike tumor, it is typically hypometabolic on a PET scan and has reduced perfusion on perfusion MR sequences. It may require resection for diagnosis and treatment unless it can be managed with glucocorticoids. There are rare reports of improvement with hyperbaric oxygen or anticoagulation, but the usefulness of these approaches is questionable.

Leukoencephalopathy is seen most commonly after WBRT as opposed to focal RT. On T2 or FLAIR MR sequences, there is diffuse increased signal seen throughout the hemispheric white matter, often bilaterally and symmetrically. There tends to be a periventricular predominance that may be associated with atrophy and ventricular enlargement. Clinically, patients develop cognitive impairment, gait disorder, and later urinary incontinence, all of which can progress over time. These symptoms mimic those of normal pressure hydrocephalus, and placement of a ventriculoperitoneal shunt can improve function in some patients but does not reverse the deficits completely. Increased age is a risk factor for leukoencephalopathy but not for radiation necrosis. Necrosis appears to depend on an as yet unidentified predisposition.

Other late neurologic toxicities include endocrine dysfunction if the pituitary or hypothalamus was included in the RT port. An RT-induced neoplasm can occur many years after therapeutic RT for either a prior CNS tumor or a head and neck cancer; accurate diagnosis requires surgical resection or biopsy. In addition, RT causes accelerated atherosclerosis, which can cause stroke either from intracranial vascular disease or carotid plaque from neck irradiation.

The peripheral nervous system is relatively resistant to RT toxicities. Peripheral nerves are rarely affected by RT, but the plexus is more vulnerable. Plexopathy develops more commonly in the brachial distribution than in the lumbosacral distribution. It must be differentiated from tumor progression in the plexus, which is usually accomplished with CT/MR imaging of the area or PET scan demonstrating tumor infiltrating the region. Clinically, tumor progression is usually painful, whereas RT-induced plexopathy is painless. Radiation plexopathy is also more commonly associated with lymphedema of the affected limb. Sensory loss and weakness are seen in both.

TABLE 118-4 NEUROLOGIC SIGNS CAUSED BY AGENTS COMMONLY USED IN PATIENTS WITH CANCER

Acute encephalopathy (delirium)	Seizures
Methotrexate (high-dose IV, IT)	Methotrexate
Cisplatin	Etoposide (high-dose)
Vincristine	Cisplatin
Asparaginase	Vincristine
Procarbazine	Asparaginase
5-Fluorouracil (± levamisole)	Nitrogen mustard
Cytarabine (high-dose)	Carmustine
Nitrosoureas (high-dose or arterial)	Dacarbazine (intraarterial or high-dose)
Ifosfamide	Busulfan (high-dose)
Etoposide (high-dose)	Myelopathy (intrathecal drugs)
Bevacizumab (PRES)	Methotrexate
Chronic encephalopathy (dementia)	Cytarabine
Methotrexate	Thiotepa
Carmustine	Peripheral neuropathy
Cytarabine	Vinca alkaloids
Fludarabine	Cisplatin
Visual loss	Procarbazine
Tamoxifen	Etoposide
Gallium nitrate	Teniposide
Cisplatin	Cytarabine
Fludarabine	Taxanes
Cerebellar dysfunction/ataxia	Suramin
5-Fluorouracil (± levamisole)	Bortezomib
Cytarabine	
Procarbazine	

Abbreviations: IT, intrathecal; IV, intravenous; PRES, posterior reversible encephalopathy syndrome.

TOXICITY FROM CHEMOTHERAPY

Neurotoxicity is second to myelosuppression as the dose-limiting toxicity of chemotherapeutic agents (Table 118-4). Chemotherapy causes peripheral neuropathy from a number of commonly used agents, and the type of neuropathy can differ, depending on the drug. Vincristine causes paresthesias but little sensory loss and is associated with motor dysfunction, autonomic impairment (frequently ileus), and rarely cranial nerve compromise. Cisplatin causes large fiber sensory loss resulting in sensory ataxia but little cutaneous sensory loss and no weakness. The taxanes also cause a predominately sensory neuropathy. Agents such as bortezomib and thalidomide also cause neuropathy.

Encephalopathy and seizures are common toxicities from chemotherapeutic drugs. Ifosfamide can cause a severe encephalopathy, which is reversible with discontinuation of the drug and the use of methylene blue for severely affected patients. Fludarabine also causes a severe global encephalopathy that may be permanent. Bevacizumab and other anti-VEGF agents can cause posterior reversible encephalopathy syndrome. Cisplatin can cause hearing loss and less frequently vestibular dysfunction. Immunotherapy with anti-CTLA-4 monoclonal antibodies, such as ipilimumab, can cause an autoimmune hypophysitis.

119e Soft Tissue and Bone Sarcomas and Bone Metastases

Shreyaskumar R. Patel, Robert S. Benjamin

This is a digital-only chapter. It is available on the DVD that accompanies this book, as well as on Access Medicine/Harrison's Online, and the eBook and "app" editions of HPIM 19e.

Sarcomas are rare (<1% of all malignancies) mesenchymal neoplasms that arise in bone and soft tissues. These tumors are usually of mesodermal origin, although a few are derived from neuroectoderm, and they are biologically distinct from the more common epithelial malignancies. Sarcomas affect all age groups; 15% are found in children <15 years of age, and 40% occur after age 55 years. Sarcomas are one of the most common solid tumors of childhood and are the fifth most common cause of cancer deaths in children. Sarcomas may be divided into two groups, those derived from bone and those derived from soft tissues.

120e Carcinoma of Unknown Primary

Gauri R. Varadhachary, James L. Abbruzzese

This is a digital-only chapter. It is available on the DVD that accompanies this book, as well as on Access Medicine/Harrison's Online, and the eBook and "app" editions of HPIM 19e.

Carcinoma of unknown primary (CUP) is a biopsy-proven malignancy for which the anatomic site of origin remains unidentified after an intensive search. CUP is one of the 10 most frequently diagnosed cancers worldwide, accounting for 3–5% of all cancers. Most investigators limit CUP to epithelial cancers and do not include lymphomas, metastatic melanomas, and metastatic sarcomas because these cancers have specific histology- and stage-based treatments that guide management.

The emergence of sophisticated imaging, robust immunohistochemistry (IHC), and genomic and proteomic tools has challenged the "unknown" designation. Additionally, effective targeted therapies in several cancers have moved the paradigm from empiricism to considering a personalized approach to CUP management. The reasons cancers present as CUP remain unclear. One hypothesis is that the primary tumor either regresses after seeding the metastasis or remains so small that it is not detected. It is possible that CUP falls on the continuum of cancer presentation where the primary has been contained or eliminated by the natural body defenses. Alternatively, CUP may represent a specific malignant event that results in an increase in metastatic spread or survival relative to the primary. Whether the CUP metastases truly define a clone that is genetically and phenotypically unique to this diagnosis remains to be determined.

121 Paraneoplastic Syndromes: Endocrinologic/Hematologic

J. Larry Jameson, Dan L. Longo

Neoplastic cells can produce a variety of products that can stimulate hormonal, hematologic, dermatologic, and neurologic responses. *Paraneoplastic syndromes* is the term used to refer to the disorders that accompany benign or malignant tumors but are not directly related to mass effects or invasion. Tumors of neuroendocrine origin, such as small-cell lung carcinoma (SCLC) and carcinoids, produce a wide array of peptide hormones and are common causes of paraneoplastic syndromes. However, almost every type of tumor has the potential to produce hormones or to induce cytokine and immunologic responses. Careful studies of the prevalence of paraneoplastic syndromes indicate that they are more common than is generally appreciated. The signs, symptoms, and metabolic alterations associated with paraneoplastic disorders may be overlooked in the context of a malignancy and its treatment. Consequently, atypical clinical manifestations in a patient with cancer should prompt consideration of a paraneoplastic syndrome. The most common endocrinologic and hematologic syndromes associated with underlying neoplasia will be discussed here.

ENDOCRINE PARANEOPLASTIC SYNDROMES

Etiology Hormones can be produced from eutopic or ectopic sources. *Eutopic* refers to the expression of a hormone from its normal tissue of origin, whereas *ectopic* refers to hormone production from an atypical tissue source. For example, adrenocorticotropic hormone (ACTH) is expressed eutopically by the corticotrope cells of the anterior pituitary, but it can be expressed ectopically in SCLC. Many hormones are produced at low levels from a wide array of tissues in addition to the classic endocrine source. Thus, ectopic expression is often a quantitative change rather than an absolute change in tissue expression. Nevertheless, the term *ectopic expression* is firmly entrenched and conveys the abnormal physiology associated with hormone production by neoplastic cells. In addition to high levels of hormones, ectopic expression typically is characterized by abnormal regulation of hormone production (e.g., defective feedback control) and peptide processing (resulting in large, unprocessed precursors).

A diverse array of molecular mechanisms has been suggested to cause ectopic hormone production. In rare instances, genetic rearrangements explain aberrant hormone expression. For example, translocation of the parathyroid hormone (*PTH*) gene can result in high levels of PTH expression in tissues other than the parathyroid gland because the genetic rearrangement brings the *PTH* gene under the control of atypical regulatory elements. A related phenomenon is well documented in many forms of leukemia and lymphoma, in which somatic genetic rearrangements confer a growth advantage and alter cellular differentiation and function (Chap. 134). Although genetic rearrangements cause selected cases of ectopic hormone production, this mechanism is rare, as many tumors are associated with excessive production of numerous peptides. Cellular dedifferentiation probably underlies most cases of ectopic hormone production. Many cancers are poorly differentiated, and certain tumor products, such as human chorionic gonadotropin (hCG), parathyroid hormone–related protein (PTHrP), and α fetoprotein, are characteristic of gene expression at earlier developmental stages. In contrast, the propensity of certain cancers to produce particular hormones (e.g., squamous cell carcinomas produce PTHrP) suggests that dedifferentiation is partial or that selective pathways are derepressed. These expression profiles probably reflect epigenetic modifications that alter transcriptional repression, microRNA expression, and other pathways that govern cell differentiation.

In SCLC, the pathway of differentiation has been relatively well defined. The neuroendocrine phenotype is dictated in part by the basic-helix-loop-helix (bHLH) transcription factor human achaete-scute homologue 1 (hASH-1), which is expressed at abnormally high

TABLE 121-1 PARANEOPLASTIC SYNDROMES CAUSED BY ECTOPIC HORMONE PRODUCTION

Paraneoplastic Syndrome	Ectopic Hormone	Typical Tumor Types[a]
Common		
Hypercalcemia of malignancy	Parathyroid hormone–related protein (PTHrP)	Squamous cell (head and neck, lung, skin), breast, genitourinary, gastrointestinal
	1,25-dihydroxyvitamin D	Lymphomas
	Parathyroid hormone (PTH) (rare)	Lung, ovary
	Prostaglandin E_2 (PGE_2) (rare)	Renal, lung
Syndrome of inappropriate antidiuretic hormone secretion (SIADH)	Vasopressin	Lung (squamous, small cell), gastrointestinal, genitourinary, ovary
Cushing's syndrome	Adrenocorticotropic hormone (ACTH)	Lung (small cell, bronchial carcinoid, adenocarcinoma, squamous), thymus, pancreatic islet, medullary thyroid carcinoma
	Corticotropin-releasing hormone (CRH) (rare)	Pancreatic islet, carcinoid, lung, prostate
	Ectopic expression of gastric inhibitory peptide (GIP), luteinizing hormone (LH)/human chorionic gonadotropin (hCG), other G protein–coupled receptors (rare)	Macronodular adrenal hyperplasia
Less Common		
Non–islet cell hypoglycemia	Insulin-like growth factor type II (IGF-II)	Mesenchymal tumors, sarcomas, adrenal, hepatic, gastrointestinal, kidney, prostate
	Insulin (rare)	Cervix (small-cell carcinoma)
Male feminization	hCG[b]	Testis (embryonal, seminomas), germinomas, choriocarcinoma, lung, hepatic, pancreatic islet
Diarrhea or intestinal hypermotility	Calcitonin[c]	Lung, colon, breast, medullary thyroid carcinoma
	Vasoactive intestinal peptide (VIP)	Pancreas, pheochromocytoma, esophagus
Rare		
Oncogenic osteomalacia	Phosphatonin (fibroblast growth factor 23 [FGF23])	Hemangiopericytomas, osteoblastomas, fibromas, sarcomas, giant cell tumors, prostate, lung
Acromegaly	Growth hormone–releasing hormone (GHRH)	Pancreatic islet, bronchial, and other carcinoids
	Growth hormone (GH)	Lung, pancreatic islet
Hyperthyroidism	Thyroid-stimulating hormone (TSH)	Hydatidiform mole, embryonal tumors, struma ovarii
Hypertension	Renin	Juxtaglomerular tumors, kidney, lung, pancreas, ovary

[a]Only the most common tumor types are listed. For most ectopic hormone syndromes, an extensive list of tumors has been reported to produce one or more hormones. [b]hCG is produced eutopically by trophoblastic tumors. Certain tumors produce disproportionate amounts of the hCG α or hCG β subunit. High levels of hCG rarely cause hyperthyroidism because of weak binding to the TSH receptor. [c]Calcitonin is produced eutopically by medullary thyroid carcinoma and is used as a tumor marker.

levels in SCLC associated with ectopic ACTH. The activity of hASH-1 is inhibited by hairy enhancer of split 1 (HES-1) and by Notch proteins, which also are capable of inducing growth arrest. Thus, abnormal expression of these developmental transcription factors appears to provide a link between cell proliferation and differentiation.

Ectopic hormone production would be merely an epiphenomenon associated with cancer if it did not result in clinical manifestations. Excessive and unregulated production of hormones such as ACTH, PTHrP, and vasopressin can lead to substantial morbidity and complicate the cancer treatment plan. Moreover, the paraneoplastic endocrinopathies may be a presenting clinical feature of underlying malignancy and prompt the search for an unrecognized tumor.

A large number of paraneoplastic endocrine syndromes have been described, linking overproduction of particular hormones with specific types of tumors. However, certain recurring syndromes emerge from this group (Table 121-1). The most common paraneoplastic endocrine syndromes include hypercalcemia from overproduction of PTHrP and other factors, hyponatremia from excess vasopressin, and Cushing's syndrome from ectopic ACTH.

HYPERCALCEMIA CAUSED BY ECTOPIC PRODUCTION OF PTHRP

(See also Chap. 424)

Etiology Humoral hypercalcemia of malignancy (HHM) occurs in up to 20% of patients with cancer. HHM is most common in cancers of the lung, head and neck, skin, esophagus, breast, and genitourinary tract and in multiple myeloma and lymphomas. There are several distinct humoral causes of HHM, but it is caused most commonly by overproduction of PTHrP. In addition to acting as a circulating humoral factor, bone metastases (e.g., breast, multiple myeloma) may produce PTHrP, leading to local osteolysis and hypercalcemia. PTHrP may also affect the initiation and progression of tumors by acting through pro-survival and chemokine pathways.

PTHrP is structurally related to PTH and binds to the PTH receptor, explaining the similar biochemical features of HHM and hyperparathyroidism. PTHrP plays a key role in skeletal development and regulates cellular proliferation and differentiation in other tissues, including skin, bone marrow, breast, and hair follicles. The mechanism of PTHrP induction in malignancy is incompletely understood; however, tumor-bearing tissues commonly associated with HHM normally produce PTHrP during development or cell renewal. PTHrP expression is stimulated by hedgehog pathways and Gli transcription factors that are active in many malignancies. Transforming growth factor β (TGF-β), which is produced by many tumors, also stimulates PTHrP, in part by activating the Gli pathway. Mutations in certain oncogenes, such as *Ras*, also can activate PTHrP expression. In adult T cell lymphoma, the transactivating Tax protein produced by human T cell lymphotropic virus 1 (HTLV-1) stimulates PTHrP promoter activity. Metastatic lesions to bone are more likely to produce PTHrP than are metastases in other tissues, suggesting that bone produces factors (e.g., TGF-β) that enhance PTHrP production or that PTHrP-producing metastases have a selective growth advantage in bone. PTHrP activates the pro-survival AKT pathway and the chemokine receptor CXCR4. Thus, PTHrP production can be stimulated by mutations in oncogenes, altered expression of viral or cellular transcription factors, and local growth factors. In addition to its role in HHM, the PTHrP pathway may also provide a potential target for therapeutic intervention to impede cancer growth.

Another relatively common cause of HHM is excess production of 1,25-dihydroxyvitamin D. Like granulomatous disorders associated with hypercalcemia, lymphomas can produce an enzyme that converts 25-hydroxyvitamin D to the more active 1,25-dihydroxyvitamin D, leading to enhanced gastrointestinal calcium absorption. Other causes of HHM include tumor-mediated production of osteolytic cytokines and inflammatory mediators.

Clinical Manifestations The typical presentation of HHM is a patient with a known malignancy who is found to be hypercalcemic on routine laboratory tests. Less often, hypercalcemia is the initial presenting feature of malignancy. Particularly when calcium levels are markedly increased (>3.5 mmol/L [>14 mg/dL]), patients may experience fatigue, mental status changes, dehydration, or symptoms of nephrolithiasis.

Diagnosis Features that favor HHM, as opposed to primary hyperparathyroidism, include known malignancy, recent onset of hypercalcemia, and very high serum calcium levels. Like hyperparathyroidism, hypercalcemia caused by PTHrP is accompanied by hypercalciuria and hypophosphatemia. Patients with HHM typically have metabolic alkalosis rather than hyperchloremic acidosis, as is seen in hyperparathyroidism. Measurement of PTH is useful to exclude primary hyperparathyroidism; the PTH level should be suppressed in HHM. An elevated PTHrP level confirms the diagnosis, and it is increased in ~80% of hypercalcemic patients with cancer. 1,25-Dihydroxyvitamin D levels may be increased in patients with lymphoma.

TREATMENT HUMORAL HYPERCALCEMIA OF MALIGNANCY

The management of HHM begins with removal of excess calcium in the diet, medications, or IV solutions. Saline rehydration (typically 200–500 mL/h) is used to dilute serum calcium and promote calciuresis; exercise caution in patients with cardiac, hepatic, or renal insufficiency. Forced diuresis with furosemide (20–80 mg IV in escalating doses) or other loop diuretics can enhance calcium excretion but provides relatively little value except in life-threatening hypercalcemia. When used, loop diuretics should be administered only after complete rehydration and with careful monitoring of fluid balance. Oral phosphorus (e.g., 250 mg Neutra-Phos 3–4 times daily) should be given until serum phosphorus is >1 mmol/L (>3 mg/dL). Bisphosphonates such as pamidronate (60–90 mg IV), zoledronate (4–8 mg IV), and etidronate (7.5 mg/kg per day PO for 3–7 consecutive days) can reduce serum calcium within 1–2 days and suppress calcium release for several weeks. Bisphosphonate infusions can be repeated, or oral bisphosphonates can be used for chronic treatment. Dialysis should be considered in severe hypercalcemia when saline hydration and bisphosphonate treatments are not possible or are too slow in onset. Previously used agents such as calcitonin and mithramycin have little utility now that bisphosphonates are available. Calcitonin (2–8 U/kg SC every 6–12 h) should be considered when rapid correction of severe hypercalcemia is needed. Hypercalcemia associated with lymphomas, multiple myeloma, or leukemia may respond to glucocorticoid treatment (e.g., prednisone 40–100 mg PO in four divided doses).

ECTOPIC VASOPRESSIN: TUMOR-ASSOCIATED SIADH

(See also Chap. 63)

Etiology Vasopressin is an antidiuretic hormone normally produced by the posterior pituitary gland. Ectopic vasopressin production by tumors is a common cause of the syndrome of inappropriate antidiuretic hormone (SIADH), occurring in at least half of patients with SCLC. SIADH also can be caused by a number of nonneoplastic conditions, including central nervous system (CNS) trauma, infections, and medications (Chap. 404). Compensatory responses to SIADH, such as decreased thirst, may mitigate the development of hyponatremia. However, with prolonged production of excessive vasopressin, the osmostat controlling thirst and hypothalamic vasopressin secretion may become reset. In addition, intake of free water, orally or intravenously, can quickly worsen hyponatremia because of reduced renal diuresis.

Tumors with neuroendocrine features, such as SCLC and carcinoids, are the most common sources of ectopic vasopressin production, but it also occurs in other forms of lung cancer and with CNS lesions, head and neck cancer, and genitourinary, gastrointestinal, and ovarian cancers. The mechanism of activation of the vasopressin gene in these tumors is unknown but often involves concomitant expression of the adjacent oxytocin gene, suggesting derepression of this locus.

Clinical Manifestations Most patients with ectopic vasopressin secretion are asymptomatic and are identified because of the presence of hyponatremia on routine chemistry testing. Symptoms may include weakness, lethargy, nausea, confusion, depressed mental status, and seizures. The severity of symptoms reflects the rapidity of onset as well as the severity of hyponatremia. Hyponatremia usually develops slowly but may be exacerbated by the administration of IV fluids or the institution of new medications.

Diagnosis The diagnostic features of ectopic vasopressin production are the same as those of other causes of SIADH (Chaps. 63 and 404). Hyponatremia and reduced serum osmolality occur in the setting of an inappropriately normal or increased urine osmolality. Urine sodium excretion is normal or increased unless volume depletion is present. Other causes of hyponatremia should be excluded, including renal, adrenal, or thyroid insufficiency. Physiologic sources of vasopressin stimulation (CNS lesions, pulmonary disease, nausea), adaptive circulatory mechanisms (hypotension, heart failure, hepatic cirrhosis), and medications, including many chemotherapeutic agents, also should be considered as possible causes of hyponatremia. Vasopressin measurements are not usually necessary to make the diagnosis.

TREATMENT ECTOPIC VASOPRESSIN: TUMOR-ASSOCIATED SIADH

Most patients with ectopic vasopressin production develop hyponatremia over several weeks or months. The disorder should be corrected gradually unless mental status is altered or there is risk of seizures. Treatment of the underlying malignancy may reduce ectopic vasopressin production, but this response is slow if it occurs at all. Fluid restriction to less than urine output, plus insensible losses, is often sufficient to correct hyponatremia partially. However, strict monitoring of the amount and types of liquids consumed or administered intravenously is required for fluid restriction to be effective. Salt tablets and saline are not helpful unless volume depletion is also present. Demeclocycline (150–300 mg orally three to four times daily) can be used to inhibit vasopressin action on the renal distal tubule, but its onset of action is relatively slow (1–2 weeks). Conivaptan, a nonpeptide V_2-receptor antagonist, can be administered either PO (20–120 mg bid) or IV (10–40 mg) and is particularly effective when used in combination with fluid restriction in euvolemic hyponatremia. Tolvaptan (15 mg PO daily) is another vasopressin antagonist. The dose can be increased to 30–60 mg/d based on response. Severe hyponatremia (Na <115 meq/L) or mental status changes may require treatment with hypertonic (3%) or normal saline infusion together with furosemide to enhance free water clearance. The rate of sodium correction should be slow (0.5–1 meq/L per hour) to prevent rapid fluid shifts and the possible development of central pontine myelinolysis.

CUSHING'S SYNDROME CAUSED BY ECTOPIC ACTH PRODUCTION

(See also Chap. 406)

Etiology Ectopic ACTH production accounts for 10–20% of cases of Cushing's syndrome. The syndrome is particularly common in neuroendocrine tumors. SCLC is the most common cause of ectopic ACTH, followed by bronchial and thymic carcinoids, islet cell tumors, other carcinoids, and pheochromocytomas. Ectopic ACTH production is caused by increased expression of the proopiomelanocortin (*POMC*) gene, which encodes ACTH, along with melanocyte-stimulating hormone (MSH), β lipotropin, and several other peptides. In many tumors, there is abundant but aberrant expression of the *POMC* gene from an internal promoter, proximal to the third exon, which encodes ACTH. However, because this product lacks the signal sequence necessary for protein processing, it is not secreted. Increased production of ACTH arises instead from less abundant, but unregulated, *POMC* expression from the same promoter site used in the pituitary. However, because the tumors lack many of the enzymes needed to process the POMC polypeptide, it is typically released as multiple large, biologically inactive fragments along with relatively small amounts of fully processed, active ACTH.

Rarely, corticotropin-releasing hormone (CRH) is produced by pancreatic islet cell tumors, SCLC, medullary thyroid cancer, carcinoids, or prostate cancer. When levels are high enough, CRH can cause pituitary corticotrope hyperplasia and Cushing's syndrome. Tumors that produce CRH sometimes also produce ACTH, raising the possibility of a paracrine mechanism for ACTH production.

A distinct mechanism for ACTH-independent Cushing's syndrome involves ectopic expression of various G protein–coupled receptors in the adrenal nodules. Ectopic expression of the gastric inhibitory peptide (GIP) receptor is the best-characterized example of this mechanism. In this case, meals induce GIP secretion, which inappropriately stimulates adrenal growth and glucocorticoid production.

Clinical Manifestations The clinical features of hypercortisolemia are detected in only a small fraction of patients with documented ectopic ACTH production. Patients with ectopic ACTH syndrome generally exhibit less marked weight gain and centripetal fat redistribution, probably because the exposure to excess glucocorticoids is relatively brief and because cachexia reduces the propensity for weight gain and fat deposition. The ectopic ACTH syndrome is associated with several clinical features that distinguish it from other causes of Cushing's syndrome (e.g., pituitary adenomas, adrenal adenomas, iatrogenic glucocorticoid excess). The metabolic manifestations of ectopic ACTH syndrome are dominated by fluid retention and hypertension, hypokalemia, metabolic alkalosis, glucose intolerance, and occasionally steroid psychosis. The very high ACTH levels often cause increased pigmentation, and melanotrope-stimulating hormone (MSH) activity derived from the POMC precursor peptide is also increased. The extraordinarily high glucocorticoid levels in patients with ectopic sources of ACTH can lead to marked skin fragility and easy bruising. In addition, the high cortisol levels often overwhelm the renal 11β-hydroxysteroid dehydrogenase type II enzyme, which normally inactivates cortisol and prevents it from binding to renal mineralocorticoid receptors. Consequently, in addition to the excess mineralocorticoids produced by ACTH stimulation of the adrenal gland, high levels of cortisol exert activity through the mineralocorticoid receptor, leading to severe hypokalemia.

Diagnosis The diagnosis of ectopic ACTH syndrome is usually not difficult in the setting of a known malignancy. Urine free cortisol levels fluctuate but are typically greater than two to four times normal, and the plasma ACTH level is usually >22 pmol/L (>100 pg/mL). A suppressed ACTH level excludes this diagnosis and indicates an ACTH-independent cause of Cushing's syndrome (e.g., adrenal or exogenous glucocorticoid). In contrast to pituitary sources of ACTH, most ectopic sources of ACTH do not respond to glucocorticoid suppression. Therefore, high-dose dexamethasone (8 mg PO) suppresses 8:00 A.M. serum cortisol (50% decrease from baseline) in ~80% of pituitary ACTH-producing adenomas but fails to suppress ectopic ACTH in ~90% of cases. Bronchial and other carcinoids are well-documented exceptions to these general guidelines, as these ectopic sources of ACTH may exhibit feedback regulation indistinguishable from pituitary adenomas, including suppression by high-dose dexamethasone, and ACTH responsiveness to adrenal blockade with metyrapone. If necessary, petrosal sinus catheterization can be used to evaluate a patient with ACTH-dependent Cushing's syndrome when the source of ACTH is unclear. After CRH stimulation, a 3:1 petrosal sinus:peripheral ACTH ratio strongly suggests a pituitary ACTH source. Imaging studies (computed tomography or magnetic resonance imaging) are also useful in the evaluation of suspected carcinoid lesions, allowing biopsy and characterization of hormone production using special stains. If available, positron emission tomography or octreotide scanning may identify some sources of ACTH production.

TREATMENT CUSHING'S SYNDROME CAUSED BY ECTOPIC ACTH PRODUCTION

The morbidity associated with the ectopic ACTH syndrome can be substantial. Patients may experience depression or personality changes because of extreme cortisol excess. Metabolic derangements, including diabetes mellitus and hypokalemia, can worsen fatigue. Poor wound healing and predisposition to infections can complicate the surgical management of tumors, and opportunistic infections caused by organisms such as *Pneumocystis carinii* and mycoses are often the cause of death in patients with ectopic ACTH production. These patients likely have increased risk of venous thromboembolism reflecting the combination of malignancy and altered coagulation factor profiles. Depending on prognosis and treatment plans for the underlying malignancy, measures to reduce cortisol levels are often indicated. Treatment of the underlying malignancy may reduce ACTH levels but is rarely sufficient to reduce cortisol levels to normal. Adrenalectomy is not practical for most of these patients but should be considered during surgery for the malignancy or if the underlying tumor is not resectable and the prognosis is otherwise favorable (e.g., carcinoid). Medical therapy with ketoconazole (300–600 mg PO bid), metyrapone (250–500 mg PO every 6 h), mitotane (3–6 g PO in four divided doses, tapered to maintain low cortisol production), or other agents that block steroid synthesis or action is often the most practical strategy for managing the hypercortisolism associated with ectopic ACTH production. Glucocorticoid replacement should be provided to prevent adrenal insufficiency (Chap. 406). Unfortunately, many patients eventually progress despite medical blockade.

TUMOR-INDUCED HYPOGLYCEMIA CAUSED BY EXCESS PRODUCTION OF IGF-II

(See also Chap. 120) Mesenchymal tumors, hemangiopericytomas, hepatocellular tumors, adrenal carcinomas, and a variety of other large tumors have been reported to produce excessive amounts of insulin-like growth factor type II (IGF-II) precursor, which binds weakly to insulin receptors and more strongly to IGF-I receptors, leading to insulin-like actions. The gene encoding IGF-II resides on a chromosome 11p15 locus that is normally imprinted (that is, expression is exclusively from a single parental allele). Biallelic expression of the IGF-II gene occurs in a subset of tumors, suggesting loss of methylation and loss of imprinting as a mechanism for gene induction. In addition to increased IGF-II production, IGF II bioavailability is increased due to complex alterations in circulating binding proteins. Increased IGF-II suppresses growth hormone (GH) and insulin, resulting in reduced IGF binding protein 3 (IGFBP-3), IGF-I, and acid-labile subunit (ALS). The reduction in ALS and IGFBP-3, which normally sequester IGF-II, causes it to be displaced to a small circulating complex that has greater access to insulin target tissues. For this reason, circulating IGF-II levels may not be markedly increased despite causing hypoglycemia. In addition to IGF-II–mediated hypoglycemia, tumors may occupy enough of the liver to impair gluconeogenesis.

In most cases, a tumor causing hypoglycemia is clinically apparent (usually >10 cm in size) and hypoglycemia develops in association with fasting. The diagnosis is made by documenting low serum glucose and suppressed insulin levels in association with symptoms of hypoglycemia. Serum IGF-II levels may not be increased (IGF-II assays may not detect IGF-II precursors). Increased IGF-II mRNA expression is found in most of these tumors. Any medications associated with hypoglycemia should be eliminated. Treatment of the underlying malignancy, if possible, may reduce the predisposition to hypoglycemia. Frequent meals and IV glucose, especially during sleep or fasting, are often necessary to prevent hypoglycemia. Glucagon and glucocorticoids have also been used to enhance glucose production.

HUMAN CHORIONIC GONADOTROPIN

hCG is composed of α and β subunits and can be produced as intact hormone, which is biologically active, or as uncombined biologically inert subunits. Ectopic production of intact hCG occurs most often in association with testicular embryonal tumors, germ cell tumors, extragonadal germinomas, lung cancer, hepatoma, and pancreatic islet tumors. Eutopic production of hCG occurs with trophoblastic malignancies. hCG α subunit production is particularly common in lung cancer and pancreatic islet cancer. In men, high hCG levels stimulate steroidogenesis and aromatase activity in testicular Leydig cells, resulting in increased estrogen production and the development of gynecomastia. Precocious puberty in boys or gynecomastia in men should prompt measurement of hCG and consideration of a testicular tumor or another source of ectopic hCG production. Most women are asymptomatic. hCG is easily measured. Treatment should be directed at the underlying malignancy.

ONCOGENIC OSTEOMALACIA

Hypophosphatemic oncogenic osteomalacia, also called tumor-induced osteomalacia (TIO), is characterized by markedly reduced serum phosphorus and renal phosphate wasting, leading to muscle weakness, bone pain, and osteomalacia. Serum calcium and PTH levels are normal, and 1,25-dihydroxyvitamin D is low. Oncogenic osteomalacia is usually caused by benign mesenchymal tumors, such as hemangiopericytomas, fibromas, and giant cell tumors, often of the skeletal extremities or head. It has also been described in sarcomas and in patients with prostate and lung cancer. Resection of the tumor reverses the disorder, confirming its humoral basis. The circulating phosphaturic factor is called *phosphatonin*—a factor that inhibits renal tubular reabsorption of phosphate and renal conversion of 25-hydroxyvitamin D to 1,25-dihydroxyvitamin D. Phosphatonin has been identified as fibroblast growth factor 23 (FGF23). FGF23 levels are increased in some, but not all, patients with osteogenic osteomalacia. FGF23 forms a ternary complex with the klotho protein and renal FGF receptors to reduce renal phosphate reabsorption. Treatment involves removal of the tumor, if possible, and supplementation with phosphate and vitamin D. Octreotide treatment reduces phosphate wasting in some patients with tumors that express somatostatin receptor subtype 2. Octreotide scans may also be useful in detecting these tumors.

HEMATOLOGIC SYNDROMES

The elevation of granulocyte, platelet, and eosinophil counts in most patients with myeloproliferative disorders is caused by the proliferation of the myeloid elements due to the underlying disease rather than to a paraneoplastic syndrome. The paraneoplastic hematologic syndromes in patients with solid tumors are less well characterized than are the endocrine syndromes because the ectopic hormone(s) or cytokines responsible have not been identified in most of these tumors (Table 121-2). The extent of the paraneoplastic syndromes parallels the course of the cancer.

ERYTHROCYTOSIS

Ectopic production of erythropoietin by cancer cells causes most paraneoplastic erythrocytosis. The ectopically produced erythropoietin stimulates the production of red blood cells (RBCs) in the bone marrow and raises the hematocrit. Other lymphokines and hormones produced by cancer cells may stimulate erythropoietin release but have not been proved to cause erythrocytosis.

Most patients with erythrocytosis have an elevated hematocrit (>52% in men, >48% in women) that is detected on a routine blood count. Approximately 3% of patients with renal cell cancer, 10% of patients with hepatoma, and 15% of patients with cerebellar hemangioblastomas have erythrocytosis. In most cases, the erythrocytosis is asymptomatic.

Patients with erythrocytosis due to a renal cell cancer, hepatoma, or CNS cancer should have measurement of red cell mass. If the red cell mass is elevated, the serum erythropoietin level should be measured. Patients with an appropriate cancer, elevated erythropoietin levels, and no other explanation for erythrocytosis (e.g., hemoglobinopathy that causes increased O_2 affinity; Chap. 77) have the paraneoplastic syndrome.

TABLE 121-2 PARANEOPLASTIC HEMATOLOGIC SYNDROMES

Syndrome	Proteins	Cancers Typically Associated with Syndrome
Erythrocytosis	Erythropoietin	Renal cancers, hepatocarcinoma, cerebellar hemangioblastomas
Granulocytosis	G-CSF, GM-CSF, IL-6	Lung cancer, gastrointestinal cancer, ovarian cancer, genitourinary cancer, Hodgkin's disease
Thrombocytosis	IL-6	Lung cancer, gastrointestinal cancer, breast cancer, ovarian cancer, lymphoma
Eosinophilia	IL-5	Lymphoma, leukemia, lung cancer
Thrombophlebitis	Unknown	Lung cancer, pancreatic cancer, gastrointestinal cancer, breast cancer, genitourinary cancer, ovarian cancer, prostate cancer, lymphoma

Abbreviations: G-CSF, granulocyte colony-stimulating factor; GM-CSF, granulocyte-macrophage colony-stimulating factor; IL, interleukin.

TREATMENT ERYTHROCYTOSIS

Successful resection of the cancer usually resolves the erythrocytosis. If the tumor cannot be resected or treated effectively with radiation therapy or chemotherapy, phlebotomy may control any symptoms related to erythrocytosis.

GRANULOCYTOSIS

Approximately 30% of patients with solid tumors have granulocytosis (granulocyte count >8000/μL). In about half of patients with granulocytosis and cancer, the granulocytosis has an identifiable nonparaneoplastic etiology (infection, tumor necrosis, glucocorticoid administration, etc.). The other patients have proteins in urine and serum that stimulate the growth of bone marrow cells. Tumors and tumor cell lines from patients with lung, ovarian, and bladder cancers have been documented to produce granulocyte colony-stimulating factor (G-CSF), granulocyte-macrophage colony-stimulating factor (GM-CSF), and/or interleukin 6 (IL-6). However, the etiology of granulocytosis has not been characterized in most patients.

Patients with granulocytosis are nearly all asymptomatic, and the differential white blood cell count does not have a shift to immature forms of neutrophils. Granulocytosis occurs in 40% of patients with lung and gastrointestinal cancers, 20% of patients with breast cancer, 30% of patients with brain tumors and ovarian cancers, 20% of patients with Hodgkin's disease, and 10% of patients with renal cell carcinoma. Patients with advanced-stage disease are more likely to have granulocytosis than are those with early-stage disease.

Paraneoplastic granulocytosis does not require treatment. The granulocytosis resolves when the underlying cancer is treated.

THROMBOCYTOSIS

Some 35% of patients with thrombocytosis (platelet count >400,000/μL) have an underlying diagnosis of cancer. IL-6, a candidate molecule for the etiology of paraneoplastic thrombocytosis, stimulates the production of platelets in vitro and in vivo. Some patients with cancer and thrombocytosis have elevated levels of IL-6 in plasma. Another candidate molecule is thrombopoietin, a peptide hormone that stimulates megakaryocyte proliferation and platelet production. The etiology of thrombocytosis has not been established in most cases.

Patients with thrombocytosis are nearly all asymptomatic. Thrombocytosis is not clearly linked to thrombosis in patients with cancer. Thrombocytosis is present in 40% of patients with lung and gastrointestinal cancers; 20% of patients with breast, endometrial, and ovarian cancers; and 10% of patients with lymphoma. Patients with thrombocytosis are more likely to have advanced-stage disease and have a poorer prognosis than do patients without thrombocytosis. In ovarian cancer, IL-6 has been shown to directly promote tumor growth. Paraneoplastic thrombocytosis does not require treatment other than treatment of the underlying tumor.

EOSINOPHILIA

Eosinophilia is present in ~1% of patients with cancer. Tumors and tumor cell lines from patients with lymphomas or leukemia may produce IL-5, which stimulates eosinophil growth. Activation of IL-5 transcription in lymphomas and leukemias may involve translocation of the long arm of chromosome 5, to which the genes for IL-5 and other cytokines map.

Patients with eosinophilia are typically asymptomatic. Eosinophilia is present in 10% of patients with lymphoma, 3% of patients with lung cancer, and occasional patients with cervical, gastrointestinal, renal, and breast cancer. Patients with markedly elevated eosinophil counts (>5000/μL) can develop shortness of breath and wheezing. A chest radiograph may reveal diffuse pulmonary infiltrates from eosinophil infiltration and activation in the lungs.

TREATMENT EOSINOPHILIA

Definitive treatment is directed at the underlying malignancy: Tumors should be resected or treated with radiation or chemotherapy. In most patients who develop shortness of breath related to eosinophilia, symptoms resolve with the use of oral or inhaled glucocorticoids. IL-5 antagonists exist but have not been evaluated in this clinical setting.

THROMBOPHLEBITIS

Deep venous thrombosis and pulmonary embolism are the most common thrombotic conditions in patients with cancer. Migratory or recurrent thrombophlebitis may be the initial manifestation of cancer. Nearly 15% of patients who develop deep venous thrombosis or pulmonary embolism have a diagnosis of cancer (Chap. 142). The coexistence of peripheral venous thrombosis with visceral carcinoma, particularly pancreatic cancer, is called *Trousseau's syndrome*.

Pathogenesis Patients with cancer are predisposed to thromboembolism because they are often at bed rest or immobilized, and tumors may obstruct or slow blood flow. Postoperative deep venous thrombosis is twice as common in cancer patients who undergo surgery. Chronic IV catheters also predispose to clotting. In addition, clotting may be promoted by release of procoagulants or cytokines from tumor cells or associated inflammatory cells or by platelet adhesion or aggregation. The specific molecules that promote thromboembolism have not been identified.

Chemotherapeutic agents, particularly those associated with endothelial damage, can induce venous thrombosis. The annual risk of venous thrombosis in patients with cancer receiving chemotherapy is about 11%, sixfold higher than the risk in the general population. Bleomycin, L-asparaginase, thalidomide analogues, cisplatin-based regimens, and high doses of busulfan and carmustine are all associated with an increased risk.

In addition to cancer and its treatment causing secondary thrombosis, primary thrombophilic diseases may be associated with cancer. For example, the antiphospholipid antibody syndrome is associated with a wide range of pathologic manifestations (Chap. 379). About 20% of patients with this syndrome have cancers. Among patients with cancer and antiphospholipid antibodies, 35–45% develop thrombosis.

Clinical Manifestations Patients with cancer who develop deep venous thrombosis usually develop swelling or pain in the leg, and physical examination reveals tenderness, warmth, and redness. Patients who present with pulmonary embolism develop dyspnea, chest pain, and syncope, and physical examination shows tachycardia, cyanosis, and hypotension. Some 5% of patients with no history of cancer who have a diagnosis of deep venous thrombosis or pulmonary embolism will have a diagnosis of cancer within 1 year. The most common cancers associated with thromboembolic episodes include lung, pancreatic, gastrointestinal, breast, ovarian, and genitourinary cancers; lymphomas; and brain tumors. Patients with cancer who undergo surgical procedures requiring general anesthesia have a 20–30% risk of deep venous thrombosis.

Diagnosis The diagnosis of deep venous thrombosis in patients with cancer is made by impedance plethysmography or bilateral compression ultrasonography of the leg veins. Patients with a noncompressible venous segment have deep venous thrombosis. If compression ultrasonography is normal and there is a high clinical suspicion for deep venous thrombosis, venography should be done to look for a luminal filling defect. Elevation of D-dimer is not as predictive of deep venous thrombosis in patients with cancer as it is in patients without cancer; elevations are seen in people over age 65 years without concomitant evidence of thrombosis, probably as a consequence of increased thrombin deposition and turnover in aging.

Patients with symptoms and signs suggesting a pulmonary embolism should be evaluated with a chest radiograph, electrocardiogram, arterial blood gas analysis, and ventilation-perfusion scan. Patients with mismatched segmental perfusion defects have a pulmonary embolus. Patients with equivocal ventilation-perfusion findings should be evaluated as described above for deep venous thrombosis in their legs. If deep venous thrombosis is detected, they should be anticoagulated. If deep venous thrombosis is not detected, they should be considered for a pulmonary angiogram.

Patients without a diagnosis of cancer who present with an initial episode of thrombophlebitis or pulmonary embolus need no additional tests for cancer other than a careful history and physical examination. In light of the many possible primary sites, diagnostic testing in asymptomatic patients is wasteful. However, if the clot is refractory to standard treatment or is in an unusual site or if the thrombophlebitis is migratory or recurrent, efforts to find an underlying cancer are indicated.

TREATMENT THROMBOPHLEBITIS

Patients with cancer and a diagnosis of deep venous thrombosis or pulmonary embolism should be treated initially with IV unfractionated heparin or low-molecular-weight heparin for at least 5 days, and warfarin should be started within 1 or 2 days. The warfarin dose should be adjusted so that the international normalized ratio (INR) is 2–3. Patients with proximal deep venous thrombosis and a relative contraindication to heparin anticoagulation (hemorrhagic brain metastases or pericardial effusion) should be considered for placement of a filter in the inferior vena cava (Greenfield filter) to prevent pulmonary embolism. Warfarin should be administered for 3–6 months. An alternative approach is to use low-molecular-weight heparin for 6 months. Patients with cancer who undergo a major surgical procedure should be considered for heparin prophylaxis or pneumatic boots. Breast cancer patients undergoing chemotherapy and patients with implanted catheters should be considered for prophylaxis. Guidelines recommend that hospitalized patients with cancer and patients receiving a thalidomide analogue receive prophylaxis with low-molecular-weight heparin or low-dose aspirin. Use of prophylaxis routinely during chemotherapy is controversial and not recommended by the American Society of Clinical Oncology.

Cutaneous paraneoplastic syndromes are discussed in Chap. 72. Neurologic paraneoplastic syndromes are discussed in Chap. 122.

Acknowledgment

The authors acknowledge the contributions of Bruce E. Johnson to prior versions of this chapter.

122 Paraneoplastic Neurologic Syndromes and Autoimmune Encephalitis

Josep Dalmau, Myrna R. Rosenfeld

Paraneoplastic neurologic disorders (PNDs) are cancer-related syndromes that can affect any part of the nervous system (Table 122-1). They are caused by mechanisms other than metastasis or by any of the complications of cancer such as coagulopathy, stroke, metabolic and nutritional conditions, infections, and side effects of cancer therapy. In 60% of patients, the neurologic symptoms precede the cancer diagnosis. Clinically disabling PNDs occur in 0.5–1% of all cancer patients, but they affect 2–3% of patients with neuroblastoma or small-cell lung cancer (SCLC) and 30–50% of patients with thymoma or sclerotic myeloma.

PATHOGENESIS

Most PNDs are mediated by immune responses triggered by neuronal proteins (onconeuronal antigens) expressed by tumors. In PNDs of the central nervous system (CNS), many antibody-associated immune responses have been identified (Table 122-2). These antibodies react with the patient's tumor, and their detection in serum or cerebrospinal fluid (CSF) usually predicts the presence of cancer. When the antigens are intracellular, most syndromes are associated with extensive infiltrates of CD4+ and CD8+ T cells, microglial activation, gliosis, and variable neuronal loss. The infiltrating T cells are often in close contact with neurons undergoing degeneration, suggesting a primary pathogenic role. T cell–mediated cytotoxicity may contribute directly to cell death in these PNDs. Thus both humoral and cellular immune mechanisms participate in the pathogenesis of many PNDs. This complex immunopathogenesis may underlie the resistance of many of these conditions to therapy.

In contrast to the disorders associated with immune responses against intracellular antigens, those associated with antibodies to antigens expressed on the neuronal cell surface of the CNS or at the neuromuscular junction are more responsive to immunotherapy (Table 122-3, Fig. 122-1). These disorders occur with and without a cancer association and may affect children and young adults, and there is increasing evidence that they are mediated by the antibodies.

Other PNDs are likely immune-mediated, although their antigens are unknown. These include several syndromes of inflammatory neuropathies and myopathies. In addition, many patients with typical PND syndromes are antibody-negative.

TABLE 122-1 PARANEOPLASTIC SYNDROMES OF THE NERVOUS SYSTEM

Classic Syndromes: Usually Occur with Cancer Association	Nonclassic Syndromes: May Occur with and Without Cancer Association
Encephalomyelitis	Brainstem encephalitis
Limbic encephalitis	Stiff-person syndrome
Cerebellar degeneration (adults)	Necrotizing myelopathy
Opsoclonus-myoclonus	Motor neuron disease
Subacute sensory neuronopathy	Guillain-Barré syndrome
Gastrointestinal paresis or pseudo-obstruction	Subacute and chronic mixed sensory-motor neuropathies
Dermatomyositis (adults)	Neuropathy associated with plasma cell dyscrasias and lymphoma
Lambert-Eaton myasthenic syndrome	Vasculitis of nerve
Cancer- or melanoma-associated retinopathy	Pure autonomic neuropathy
	Acute necrotizing myopathy
	Polymyositis
	Vasculitis of muscle
	Optic neuropathy
	BDUMP

Abbreviation: BDUMP, bilateral diffuse uveal melanocytic proliferation.

TABLE 122-2 ANTIBODIES TO INTRACELLULAR ANTIGENS, SYNDROMES, AND ASSOCIATED CANCERS

Antibody	Associated Neurologic Syndrome(s)	Tumors
Anti-Hu (ANNA1)	Encephalomyelitis, subacute sensory neuronopathy	SCLC
Anti-Yo (PCA1)	Cerebellar degeneration	Ovary, breast
Anti-Ri (ANNA2)	Cerebellar degeneration, opsoclonus, brainstem encephalitis	Breast, gynecologic, SCLC
Anti-Tr	Cerebellar degeneration	Hodgkin's lymphoma
Anti-CRMP5 (CV2)	Encephalomyelitis, chorea, optic neuritis, uveitis, peripheral neuropathy	SCLC, thymoma, other
Anti-Ma proteins	Limbic, hypothalamic, brainstem encephalitis	Testicular (Ma2), other (Ma)
Anti-amphiphysin	Stiff-person syndrome, encephalomyelitis	Breast, SCLC
Recoverin, bipolar cell antibodies, others[a]	Cancer-associated retinopathy (CAR) Melanoma-associated retinopathy (MAR)	SCLC (CAR), melanoma (MAR)
Anti-GAD	Stiff-person, cerebellar syndromes, limbic encephalitis	Infrequent tumor association (thymoma)

[a]A variety of target antigens have been identified.

Abbreviations: CRMP, collapsing response-mediator protein; SCLC, small-cell lung cancer.

TABLE 122-3 ANTIBODIES TO CELL SURFACE OR SYNAPTIC ANTIGENS, SYNDROMES, AND ASSOCIATED TUMORS

Antibody	Neurologic Syndrome	Tumor Type When Associated
Anti-AChR (muscle)[a]	Myasthenia gravis	Thymoma
Anti-AChR (neuronal)[a]	Autonomic ganglionopathy	SCLC
Anti-VGCC[b]	LEMS, cerebellar degeneration	SCLC
Anti-NMDAR[a]	Anti-NMDAR encephalitis	Teratoma in young women (children and men rarely have tumors)
Anti-LGI1[c]	Limbic encephalitis, hyponatremia, faciobrachial tonic or dystonic seizures	Rarely thymoma
Anti-Caspr2[c]	Morvan's syndrome, neuromyotonia	Thymoma, prostate cancer
Anti-$GABA_BR$[d]	Limbic encephalitis, seizures	SCLC, neuroendocrine
Anti-$GABA_AR$[d]	Encephalitis with prominent seizures and status epilepticus; less often opsoclonus and stiff-person syndrome	Rarely thymoma
Anti-AMPAR[d]	Limbic encephalitis with relapses	SCLC, thymoma, breast
Glycine receptor[d]	Encephalomyelitis with rigidity, stiff-person syndrome	Rarely, thymoma, lung cancer
Anti-DPPX[d]	Agitation, myoclonus, tremor, seizures, hyperekplexia, encephalomyelitis with rigidity	No cancer, but frequent diarrhea or cachexia suggesting paraneoplasia

[a]A direct pathogenic role of these antibodies has been demonstrated. [b]Anti-VGCC antibodies are pathogenic for LEMS. [c]Previously named voltage-gated potassium channel antibodies (VGKC); currently included under the term VGKC-complex proteins. Of note, the significance of antibodies to VGKC-complex proteins other than LGI1 and Caspr2 is uncertain (the antigens are unknown, and the response to immunotherapy is variable) [d]These antibodies are strongly suspected to be pathogenic.

Abbreviations: AChR, acetylcholine receptor; AMPAR, α-amino-3-hydroxy-5-methylisoxazole-4-propionic acid receptor; Caspr2, contactin-associated protein-like 2; DPPX, dipeptidyl-peptidase-like protein-6; $GABA_BR$, γ-aminobutyric acid B receptor; GAD, glutamic acid decarboxylase; LEMS, Lambert-Eaton myasthenic syndrome; LGI1, leucine-rich glioma-inactivated 1; NMDAR, *N*-methyl-D-aspartate receptor; SCLC, small-cell lung cancer; VGCC, voltage-gated calcium channel.

PART 7 Oncology and Hematology

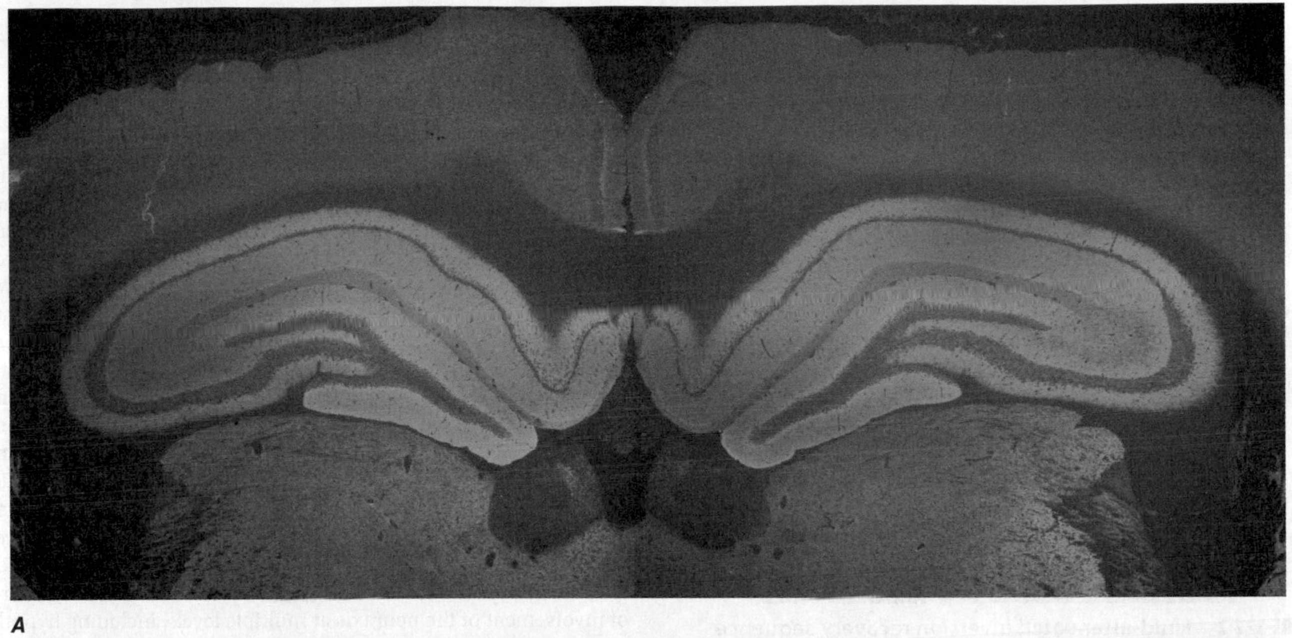

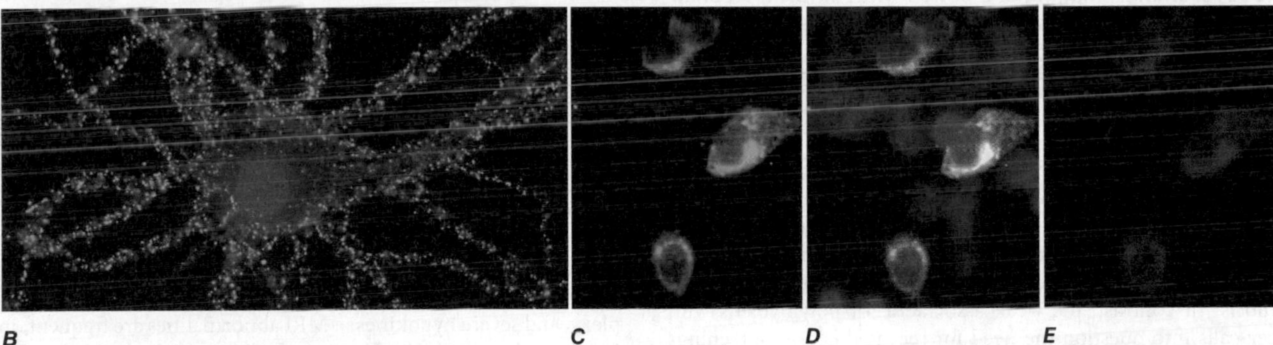

FIGURE 122-1 Antibodies to the GluN1 subunit of the *N*-methyl-D-aspartate (NMDA) receptor in a patient with anti NMDA receptor encephalitis and ovarian teratoma. (***A***) Coronal section of rat brain immunolabeled (green fluorescence) with the patient's antibodies. The reactivity predominates in the hippocampus, which is highly enriched in NMDA receptors. (***B***) This image shows the antibody reactivity with cultures of rat hippocampal neurons; the intense green immunolabeling is due to the antibodies against the GluN1 subunit of NMDA receptors. (***C–E***) Images of HEK cells (a human kidney cell line) transfected to express NMDA receptors, showing reactivity with patient's antibodies (***C***) and with a commercial monoclonal antibody against NMDA receptors (***E***); the patient's antibody reactivity co-labels only the cells that express NMDA receptors (***D***). *(From J Dalmau et al: Lancet Neurol 7:1091, 2008; with permission.)*

For still other PNDs, the cause remains quite obscure. These include, among others, several neuropathies that occur in the terminal stages of cancer and a number of neuropathies associated with plasma cell dyscrasias or lymphoma without evidence of inflammatory infiltrates or deposits of immunoglobulin, cryoglobulin, or amyloid.

APPROACH TO THE PATIENT: **Paraneoplastic Neurologic Disorders**

Three key concepts are important for the diagnosis and management of PNDs. First, it is common for symptoms to appear before the presence of a tumor is known; second, the neurologic syndrome usually develops rapidly, producing severe deficits in a short period of time; and third, there is evidence that prompt tumor control improves the neurologic outcome. Therefore, the major concern of the physician is to recognize a disorder promptly as paraneoplastic and to identify and treat the tumor.

PND OF THE CENTRAL NERVOUS SYSTEM AND DORSAL ROOT GANGLIA

When symptoms involve brain, spinal cord, or dorsal root ganglia, the suspicion of PND is usually based on a combination of clinical, radiologic, and CSF findings. Presence of antineuronal antibodies (Tables 122-2 and 122-3) may help in the diagnosis, but only 60–70% of PNDs of the CNS and less than 20% of those involving the peripheral nervous system have neuronal or neuromuscular junction antibodies that can be used as diagnostic tests.

Magnetic resonance imaging (MRI) and CSF studies are important to rule out neurologic complications due to the direct spread of cancer, particularly metastatic and leptomeningeal disease. In most PNDs, the MRI findings are nonspecific. Paraneoplastic limbic encephalitis is usually associated with characteristic MRI abnormalities in the mesial temporal lobes (see below), but similar findings can occur with other disorders (e.g., nonparaneoplastic autoimmune limbic encephalitis and human herpesvirus type 6 [HHV-6] encephalitis) (Fig. 122-2). The CSF profile of patients with PND of the CNS or dorsal root ganglia typically consists of mild to moderate pleocytosis (<200 mononuclear cells, predominantly lymphocytes), an increase in the protein concentration, and a variable presence of oligoclonal bands. There are no specific electrophysiologic tests that are diagnostic of PND. Moreover, a biopsy of the affected tissue is often difficult to obtain, and although useful to rule out other disorders (e.g., metastasis) the pathologic findings are not specific for PND.

PND OF NERVE AND MUSCLE

If symptoms involve peripheral nerve, neuromuscular junction, or muscle, the diagnosis of a specific PND is usually established on clinical, electrophysiologic, and pathologic grounds. The clinical

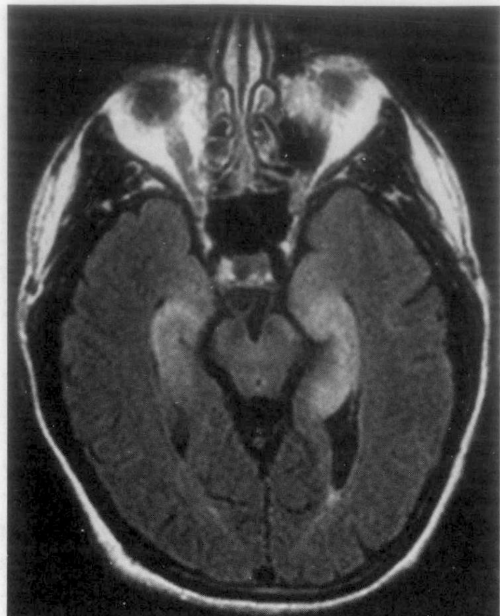

FIGURE 122-2 Fluid-attenuated inversion recovery sequence magnetic resonance imaging of a patient with limbic encephalitis and LGI1 antibodies. Note the abnormal hyperintensity involving the medial aspect of the temporal lobes.

history, accompanying symptoms (e.g., anorexia, weight loss), and type of syndrome dictate the studies and degree of effort needed to demonstrate a neoplasm. For example, the frequent association of Lambert-Eaton myasthenic syndrome (LEMS) with SCLC should lead to a chest and abdomen computed tomography (CT) or body positron emission tomography (PET) scan and, if negative, periodic tumor screening for at least 3 years after the neurologic diagnosis. In contrast, the weak association of polymyositis with cancer calls into question the need for repeated cancer screenings in this situation. Serum and urine immunofixation studies should be considered in patients with peripheral neuropathy of unknown cause; detection of a monoclonal gammopathy suggests the need for additional studies to uncover a B cell or plasma cell malignancy. In paraneoplastic neuropathies, diagnostically useful antineuronal antibodies are limited to anti-CV_2/CRMP5 and anti-Hu.

For any type of PND, if antineuronal antibodies are negative, the diagnosis relies on the demonstration of cancer and the exclusion of other cancer-related or independent neurologic disorders. Combined CT and PET scans often uncover tumors undetected by other tests. For germ cell tumors of the testis and teratomas of the ovary, ultrasound and CT or MRI of the abdomen and pelvis may reveal tumors undetectable by PET.

SPECIFIC PARANEOPLASTIC NEUROLOGIC SYNDROMES

PARANEOPLASTIC ENCEPHALOMYELITIS AND FOCAL ENCEPHALITIS

The term *encephalomyelitis* describes an inflammatory process with multifocal involvement of the nervous system, including brain, brainstem, cerebellum, and spinal cord. It is often associated with dorsal root ganglia and autonomic dysfunction. For any given patient, the clinical manifestations are determined by the areas predominantly involved, but pathologic studies almost always reveal abnormalities beyond the symptomatic regions. Several clinicopathologic syndromes may occur alone or in combination: (1) *cortical encephalitis*, which may present as "epilepsia partialis continua"; (2) *limbic encephalitis*, characterized by confusion, depression, agitation, anxiety, severe short-term memory deficits, partial complex seizures, and sometimes dementia (the MRI usually shows unilateral or bilateral medial temporal lobe abnormalities, best seen with T2 and fluid-attenuated inversion recovery sequences); (3) *brainstem encephalitis*, resulting in eye movement disorders (nystagmus, opsoclonus, supranuclear or nuclear paresis), cranial nerve paresis, dysarthria, dysphagia, and central autonomic dysfunction; (4) *cerebellar gait and limb ataxia*; (5) *myelitis*, which may cause lower or upper motor neuron symptoms, myoclonus, muscle rigidity, and spasms; and (6) *autonomic dysfunction* as a result of involvement of the neuraxis at multiple levels, including hypothalamus, brainstem, and autonomic nerves (see Paraneoplastic Peripheral Neuropathies, below). Cardiac arrhythmias, postural hypotension, and central hypoventilation are frequent causes of death in patients with encephalomyelitis.

Paraneoplastic encephalomyelitis and focal encephalitis are usually associated with SCLC, but many other cancers have been implicated. Patients with SCLC and these syndromes usually have anti-Hu antibodies in serum and CSF. Anti-CRMP5 antibodies occur less frequently; some of these patients may develop chorea, uveitis, or optic neuritis. Antibodies to Ma proteins are associated with limbic, hypothalamic, and brainstem encephalitis and occasionally with cerebellar symptoms (Fig. 122-3); some patients develop hypersomnia, cataplexy, and severe hypokinesia. MRI abnormalities are frequent, including those described with limbic encephalitis and variable involvement of the hypothalamus, basal ganglia, or upper brainstem. The oncologic associations of these antibodies are shown in Table 122-2.

TREATMENT ENCEPHALOMYELITIS AND FOCAL ENCEPHALITIS

Most types of paraneoplastic encephalitis and encephalomyelitis respond poorly to treatment. Stabilization of symptoms or partial neurologic improvement may occasionally occur, particularly if there is a satisfactory response of the tumor to treatment. Controlled trials of therapy are lacking, but many experts recommend treatment initially with glucocorticoids. If there is

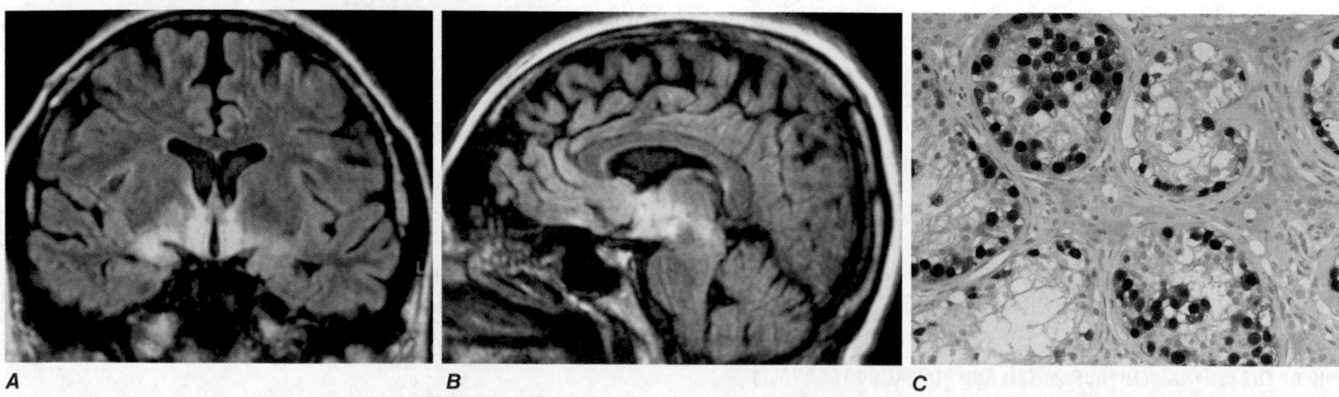

FIGURE 122-3 Magnetic resonance imaging (MRI) and tumor of a patient with anti-Ma2-associated encephalitis. (***A* and *B***) Fluid-attenuated inversion recovery MRI sequences showing abnormal hyperintensities in the medial temporal lobes, hypothalamus, and upper brainstem. (***C***) This image corresponds to a section of the patient's orchiectomy incubated with a specific marker (Oct4) of germ cell tumors. The positive (*brown*) cells correspond to an intratubular germ cell neoplasm.

no response within several days, one can advance to intravenous immunoglobulin (IVIg) or plasma exchange, and then to immunosuppression with either rituximab or cyclophosphamide. Approximately 30% of patients with anti-Ma2-associated encephalitis respond to treatment of the tumor (usually a germ cell neoplasm of the testis) and immunotherapy.

ENCEPHALITIDES WITH ANTIBODIES TO CELL-SURFACE OR SYNAPTIC PROTEINS (TABLE 122-3)

These disorders are important for three reasons: (1) they can occur with and without tumor association, (2) some syndromes predominate in young individuals and children, and (3) despite the severity of the symptoms patients usually respond to treatment of the tumor, if found, and immunotherapy (e.g., glucocorticoids, IVIg, plasma exchange, rituximab, or cyclophosphamide).

Encephalitis with N-methyl-D-aspartate (NMDA) receptor antibodies (Fig. 122-1) usually occurs in young women and children, but men and older patients of both sexes can be affected. The disorder has a characteristic pattern of symptom progression that includes a prodrome resembling a viral process, followed in a few days by the onset of severe psychiatric symptoms, memory loss, seizures, decreased level of consciousness, abnormal movements (orofacial, limb, and trunk dyskinesias, dystonic postures), autonomic instability, and frequent hypoventilation. Monosymptomatic episodes, such as pure psychosis, occur in 4% of the patients. Clinical relapses occur in 12–24% of patients (12% during the first 2 years after initial presentation). Most patients have intrathecal synthesis of antibodies, likely by infiltrating plasma cells in brain and meninges (Fig. 122-4*A*). The syndrome is often misdiagnosed as a viral or idiopathic encephalitis, neuroleptic malignant syndrome, or encephalitis lethargica, and many patients are initially evaluated by psychiatrists with the suspicion of acute psychosis. The detection of an associated teratoma is dependent on age and gender: 46% of female patients 12 years or older have uni- or bilateral ovarian teratomas, whereas less than 7% of girls younger than 12 have a teratoma (Fig. 122-4*B*). In male patients, the detection of a tumor is rare. Patients older than 45 years are more frequently male; about 20% of these patients have tumors (e.g., cancer of the breast, ovary, or lung).

Encephalitis with leucine-rich glioma-inactivated 1 (LGI1) antibodies predominates in patients older than 50 years (65% male) and frequently presents with memory loss and seizures (limbic encephalopathy), along with hyponatremia and sleep dysfunction. In a small number of patients, the encephalitis is preceded by or occurs with myoclonic-like movements called faciobrachial dystonic or tonic seizures. Less than 10% of patients have thymoma.

Encephalitis with contactin-associated protein-like 2 (Caspr2) antibodies predominates in patients older than 50 years and is associated with Morvan's syndrome (encephalitis, insomnia, confusion, hallucinations, autonomic dysfunction, and neuromyotonia) and, less frequently, with limbic encephalitis, neuromyotonia, and neuropathic pain. About 30–40% of patients have thymoma.

Encephalitis with γ-aminobutyric acid type B ($GABA_B$) receptor antibodies is usually associated with limbic encephalitis and seizures. In rare instances, patients develop cerebellar symptoms and opsoclonus. Fifty percent of patients have SCLC or a neuroendocrine tumor of the lung. Patients may have additional antibodies to glutamic acid decarboxylase (GAD), which are of unclear significance. Other antibodies to nonneuronal proteins are often found in these patients as well as in patients with α-amino-3-hydroxy-5-methylisoxazole-4-propionic acid (AMPA) receptor antibodies, indicating a general tendency to autoimmunity.

Encephalitis with GABAA receptor antibodies may affect children and adults. When antibodies are present at high titer in serum and CSF, the disorder associates with prominent seizures and status epilepticus, often requiring pharmacologically induced coma. Low titer antibodies in serum are often associated with other autoimmune conditions, and the spectrum of symptoms is wider, including encephalitis, seizures, opsoclonus, or stiff-person syndrome. Most patients do not have an underlying tumor, but some may have thymoma.

Encephalitis with AMPA receptor antibodies affects middle-aged women, who develop acute limbic dysfunction or, less frequently, prominent psychiatric symptoms; 70% of the patients have an underlying tumor in the lung, breast, or thymus. Neurologic relapses may occur; these also respond to immunotherapy and are not necessarily associated with tumor recurrence.

Encephalitis with glycine receptor (GlyR) antibodies has been described in adults with progressive encephalomyelitis with rigidity and myoclonus (PERM) and stiff-person spectrum of symptoms (with or without GAD antibodies). The disorder usually occurs without tumor association, although some patients have lung cancer, thymoma, or Hodgkin's lymphoma.

Encephalitis with dipeptidyl-peptidase-like protein-6 (or DPPX) antibodies results in symptoms of CNS hyperexcitability including agitation, hallucinations, paranoid delusions, tremor, myoclonus, nystagmus, seizures, and sometimes hyperekplexia. Some patients develop progressive encephalomyelitis with rigidity and myoclonus. Diarrhea, other gastrointestinal symptoms, and substantial loss of weight often suggest the presence of an underlying tumor, but no tumor association has been identified. The disorder responds to immunotherapy.

PARANEOPLASTIC CEREBELLAR DEGENERATION

This disorder is often preceded by a prodrome that may include dizziness, oscillopsia, blurry or double vision, nausea, and vomiting. A few

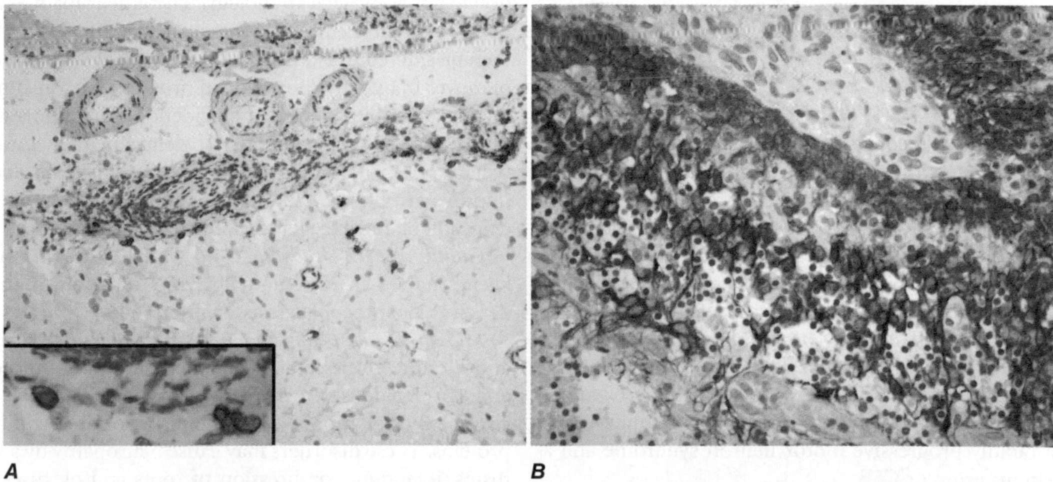

FIGURE 122-4 Pathologic findings in anti–*N*-methyl-D-aspartate (NMDA) receptor encephalitis. Infiltrates of plasma cells (brown cells; stained for CD138) in the meninges and brain of a patient (***A***); the inset is a magnification of some plasma cells. (***B***) Neurons and neuronal processes in the teratoma of a patient (brown cells; stained with MAP2); these neurons express NMDA receptors (not shown). *(From E Martinez-Hernandez et al: Neurology 77:589, 2011, with permission.)*

days or weeks later, patients develop dysarthria, gait and limb ataxia, and variable dysphagia. The examination usually shows downbeating nystagmus and, rarely, opsoclonus. Brainstem dysfunction, upgoing toes, or a mild neuropathy may occur. Early in the course, MRI studies are usually normal; later, the MRI reveals cerebellar atrophy. The disorder results from extensive degeneration of Purkinje cells, with variable involvement of other cerebellar cortical neurons, deep cerebellar nuclei, and spinocerebellar tracts. The tumors more frequently involved are SCLC, cancer of the breast and ovary, and Hodgkin's lymphoma.

Anti-Yo antibodies in patients with breast and gynecologic cancers and anti-Tr antibodies in patients with Hodgkin's lymphoma are the two immune responses typically associated with prominent or pure cerebellar degeneration. Antibodies to P/Q-type voltage-gated calcium channels (VGCC) occur in some patients with SCLC and cerebellar dysfunction; only some of these patients develop LEMS. A variable degree of cerebellar dysfunction can be associated with virtually any of the antibodies and PND of the CNS shown in Table 122-2.

A number of single case reports have described neurologic improvement after tumor removal, plasma exchange, IVIg, cyclophosphamide, rituximab, or glucocorticoids. However, most patients with paraneoplastic cerebellar degeneration do not improve with treatment.

PARANEOPLASTIC OPSOCLONUS-MYOCLONUS SYNDROME

Opsoclonus is a disorder of eye movement characterized by involuntary, chaotic saccades that occur in all directions of gaze; it is frequently associated with myoclonus and ataxia. Opsoclonus-myoclonus may be cancer-related or idiopathic. When the cause is paraneoplastic, the tumors involved are usually cancer of the lung and breast in adults, neuroblastoma in children, and ovarian teratoma in adolescents and young women. The pathologic substrate of opsoclonus-myoclonus is unclear, but studies suggest that disinhibition of the fastigial nucleus of the cerebellum is involved. Most patients do not have antineuronal antibodies. A small subset of patients with ataxia, opsoclonus, and other eye-movement disorders develop anti-Ri antibodies; in rare instances, muscle rigidity, laryngeal spasms, autonomic dysfunction, and dementia also occur. The tumors most frequently involved in anti-Ri-associated syndromes are breast and ovarian cancer. If the tumor is not successfully treated, the syndrome in adults often progresses to encephalopathy, coma, and death. In addition to treating the tumor, symptoms may respond to immunotherapy (glucocorticoids, plasma exchange, and/or IVIg).

At least 50% of children with opsoclonus-myoclonus have an underlying neuroblastoma. Hypotonia, ataxia, behavioral changes, and irritability are frequent accompanying symptoms. Neurologic symptoms often improve with treatment of the tumor and glucocorticoids, adrenocorticotropic hormone (ACTH), plasma exchange, IVIg, and rituximab. Many patients are left with psychomotor retardation and behavioral and sleep problems.

PARANEOPLASTIC SYNDROMES OF THE SPINAL CORD

The number of reports of paraneoplastic spinal cord syndromes, such as *subacute motor neuronopathy* and *acute necrotizing myelopathy*, has decreased in recent years. This may represent a true decrease in incidence, due to improved and prompt oncologic interventions, or the identification of nonparaneoplastic etiologies. Some patients with cancer develop *upper* or *lower motor neuron dysfunction* or both, resembling amyotrophic lateral sclerosis. It is unclear whether these disorders have a paraneoplastic etiology or simply coincide with the presence of cancer. There are isolated case reports of cancer patients with motor neuron dysfunction who had neurologic improvement after tumor treatment. A search for lymphoma should be undertaken in patients with a rapidly progressive motor neuron syndrome and a monoclonal protein in serum or CSF.

Paraneoplastic myelitis may present with upper or lower motor neuron symptoms, segmental myoclonus, and rigidity, and can be the first manifestation of encephalomyelitis. *Neuromyelitis optica (NMO) with aquaporin 4 antibodies* may occur in rare instances as a paraneoplastic manifestation of a cancer.

PARANEOPLASTIC STIFF-PERSON SYNDROME

This disorder is characterized by progressive muscle rigidity, stiffness, and painful spasms triggered by auditory, sensory, or emotional stimuli. Rigidity mainly involves the lower trunk and legs, but it can affect the upper extremities and neck. Sometimes, only one extremity is affected (*stiff-limb syndrome*). Symptoms improve with sleep and general anesthetics. Electrophysiologic studies demonstrate continuous motor unit activity. The associated antibodies target proteins (GAD, amphiphysin) involved in the function of inhibitory synapses using γ-aminobutyric acid (GABA) or glycine as neurotransmitters. The presence of amphiphysin antibodies usually indicates a paraneoplastic etiology related to SCLC and breast cancer. By contrast, GAD antibodies may occur in some cancer patients but are much more frequently present in the nonparaneoplastic disorder. GlyR antibodies may occur in some patients with stiff-person syndrome; these antibodies are also detectable in patients with PERM.

Optimal treatment of stiff-person syndrome requires therapy of the underlying tumor, glucocorticoids, and symptomatic use of drugs that enhance GABA-ergic transmission (diazepam, baclofen, sodium valproate, tiagabine, vigabatrin). IVIg and plasma exchange are transiently effective in some patients.

PARANEOPLASTIC SENSORY NEURONOPATHY OR DORSAL ROOT GANGLIONOPATHY

This syndrome is characterized by sensory deficits that may be symmetric or asymmetric, painful dysesthesias, radicular pain, and decreased or absent reflexes. All modalities of sensation and any part of the body including face and trunk can be involved. Specialized sensations such as taste and hearing can also be affected. Electrophysiologic studies show decreased or absent sensory nerve potentials with normal or near-normal motor conduction velocities. Symptoms result from an inflammatory, likely immune-mediated, process that targets the dorsal root ganglia, causing neuronal loss and secondary degeneration of the posterior columns of the spinal cord. The dorsal and, less frequently, the anterior nerve roots and peripheral nerves may also be involved. This disorder often precedes or is associated with encephalomyelitis and autonomic dysfunction and has the same immunologic and oncologic associations (Hu antibodies, SCLC).

As with anti-Hu-associated encephalomyelitis, the therapeutic approach focuses on prompt treatment of the tumor. Glucocorticoids occasionally produce clinical stabilization or improvement. The benefit of IVIg and plasma exchange is not proven.

PARANEOPLASTIC PERIPHERAL NEUROPATHIES

These disorders may develop any time during the course of the neoplastic disease. Neuropathies occurring at late stages of cancer or lymphoma usually cause mild to moderate sensorimotor deficits due to axonal degeneration of unclear etiology. These neuropathies are often masked by concurrent neurotoxicity from chemotherapy and other cancer therapies. In contrast, the neuropathies that develop in the early stages of cancer frequently show a rapid progression, sometimes with a relapsing and remitting course, and evidence of inflammatory infiltrates and axonal loss or demyelination. If demyelinating features predominate (Chaps. 459 and 460), IVIg, plasma exchange, or glucocorticoids may improve symptoms. Occasionally anti-CRMP5 antibodies are present; detection of anti-Hu suggests concurrent dorsal root ganglionitis.

Guillain-Barré syndrome and *brachial plexitis* have occasionally been reported in patients with lymphoma, but there is no clear evidence of a paraneoplastic association (Chap. 460).

Malignant monoclonal gammopathies include: (1) multiple myeloma and sclerotic myeloma associated with IgG or IgA monoclonal proteins; and (2) Waldenström's macroglobulinemia, B cell lymphoma, and chronic B cell lymphocytic leukemia associated with IgM monoclonal proteins. These disorders may cause neuropathy by a variety of mechanisms, including compression of roots and plexuses by metastasis to vertebral bodies and pelvis, deposits of amyloid in peripheral nerves, and paraneoplastic mechanisms. The paraneoplastic variety has several distinctive features. Approximately half of patients with sclerotic myeloma develop a sensorimotor neuropathy with predominantly motor deficits, resembling a chronic inflammatory demyelinating neuropathy (Chap. 460); some patients develop elements of the POEMS syndrome (*p*olyneuropathy, *o*rganomegaly, *e*ndocrinopathy, *M* protein, *s*kin changes). Treatment of the plasmacytoma or sclerotic lesions usually improves the neuropathy. In contrast, the sensorimotor or sensory neuropathy associated with multiple myeloma is more refractory to treatment. Between 5 and 10% of patients with Waldenström's macroglobulinemia develop a distal symmetric sensorimotor neuropathy with predominant involvement of large sensory fibers. These patients may have IgM antibodies in their serum against myelin-associated glycoprotein and various gangliosides (Chap. 460). In addition to treating the Waldenström's macroglobulinemia, other therapies may improve the neuropathy, including plasma exchange, IVIg, chlorambucil, cyclophosphamide, fludarabine, or rituximab.

Vasculitis of the nerve and muscle causes a painful symmetric or asymmetric distal axonal sensorimotor neuropathy with variable proximal weakness. It predominantly affects elderly men and is associated with an elevated erythrocyte sedimentation rate and increased CSF protein concentration. SCLC and lymphoma are the primary tumors involved. Glucocorticoids and cyclophosphamide often result in neurologic improvement.

Peripheral nerve hyperexcitability (*neuromyotonia*, or *Isaacs' syndrome*) is characterized by spontaneous and continuous muscle fiber activity of peripheral nerve origin. Clinical features include cramps, muscle twitching (fasciculations or myokymia), stiffness, delayed muscle relaxation (pseudomyotonia), and spontaneous or evoked carpal or pedal spasms. The involved muscles may be hypertrophic, and some patients develop paresthesias and hyperhidrosis. CNS dysfunction, including mood changes, sleep disorder, hallucinations, and autonomic symptoms may occur. The electromyogram (EMG) shows fibrillations; fasciculations; and doublet, triplet, or multiplet single-unit (myokymic) discharges that have a high intraburst frequency. Some patients have Caspr2 antibodies in the context of Morvan's syndrome, but most cases of isolated neuromyotonia are antibody negative. The disorder often occurs without cancer; if paraneoplastic, benign and malignant thymomas and SCLC are the usual tumors. Phenytoin, carbamazepine, and plasma exchange improve symptoms.

Paraneoplastic autonomic neuropathy usually develops as a component of other disorders, such as LEMS and encephalomyelitis. It may rarely occur as a pure or predominantly autonomic neuropathy with cholinergic or adrenergic dysfunction at the pre- or postganglionic levels. Patients can develop several life-threatening complications, such as gastrointestinal paresis with pseudo-obstruction, cardiac dysrhythmias, and postural hypotension. Other clinical features include abnormal pupillary responses, dry mouth, anhidrosis, erectile dysfunction, and problems in sphincter control. The disorder occurs in association with several tumors, including SCLC, cancer of the pancreas or testis, carcinoid tumors, and lymphoma. Because autonomic symptoms can be the presenting feature of encephalomyelitis, serum anti-Hu and anti-CRMP5 antibodies should be sought. Antibodies to ganglionic (alpha3-type) neuronal acetylcholine receptors are the cause of autoimmune autonomic ganglionopathy, a disorder that frequently occurs without cancer association (Chap. 454).

LAMBERT-EATON MYASTHENIC SYNDROME

LEMS is discussed in Chap. 461.

MYASTHENIA GRAVIS

Myasthenia gravis is discussed in Chap. 461.

POLYMYOSITIS-DERMATOMYOSITIS

Polymyositis and dermatomyositis are discussed in detail in Chap. 388.

ACUTE NECROTIZING MYOPATHY

Patients with this syndrome develop myalgias and rapid progression of weakness involving the extremities and the pharyngeal and respiratory muscles, often resulting in death. Serum muscle enzymes are elevated, and muscle biopsy shows extensive necrosis with minimal or absent inflammation and sometimes deposits of complement. The disorder occurs as a paraneoplastic manifestation of a variety of cancers including SCLC and cancer of the gastrointestinal tract, breast, kidney, and prostate, among others. Glucocorticoids and treatment of the underlying tumor rarely control the disorder.

PARANEOPLASTIC VISUAL SYNDROMES

This group of disorders involves the retina and, less frequently, the uvea and optic nerves. The term *cancer-associated retinopathy* is used to describe paraneoplastic cone and rod dysfunction characterized by photosensitivity, progressive loss of vision and color perception, central or ring scotomas, night blindness, and attenuation of photopic and scotopic responses in the electroretinogram (ERG). The most commonly associated tumor is SCLC. Melanoma-associated retinopathy affects patients with metastatic cutaneous melanoma. Patients develop acute onset of night blindness and shimmering, flickering, or pulsating photopsias that often progress to visual loss. The ERG shows reduced b waves with normal dark adapted a waves. Paraneoplastic optic neuritis and uveitis are very uncommon and can develop in association with encephalomyelitis. Some patients with paraneoplastic uveitis and optic neuritis have anti-CRMP5 antibodies.

Some paraneoplastic retinopathies are associated with serum antibodies that specifically react with the subset of retinal cells undergoing degeneration, supporting an immune-mediated pathogenesis (Table 122 2). Paraneoplastic retinopathies usually fail to improve with treatment, although rare responses to glucocorticoids, plasma exchange, and IVIg have been reported.

123e Thymoma

Dan L. Longo

This is a digital-only chapter. It is available on the DVD that accompanies this book, as well as on Access Medicine/Harrison's Online, and the eBook and "app" editions of HPIM 19e.

The thymus is derived from the third and fourth pharyngeal pouches and is located in the anterior mediastinum. It is composed of epithelial and stromal cells derived from the pharyngeal pouch and lymphoid precursors derived from mesodermal cells. It is the site to which bone marrow precursors that are committed to differentiate into T cells migrate to complete their differentiation. Like many organs, it is organized into functional regions, in this case the cortex and the medulla. The cortex of the thymus contains ~85% of the lymphoid cells, and the medulla contains ~15%. It appears that the primitive bone marrow progenitors enter the thymus at the corticomedullary junction and migrate first through the cortex toward the periphery of the gland and then toward the medulla as they mature. Medullary thymocytes have a phenotype that cannot be distinguished readily from that of mature peripheral blood and lymph node T cells.

Several things can go wrong with the thymus, but thymic abnormalities are very rare. If the thymus does not develop properly, serious deficiencies in T-cell development ensue and severe immunodeficiency is seen (e.g., DiGeorge syndrome, Chap. 374). If a lymphoid cell within the thymus becomes neoplastic, the disease that develops is a lymphoma. The majority of lymphoid tumors that develop in the thymus are derived from the precursor T cells, and the tumor is a precursor T-cell lymphoblastic lymphoma (Chap. 134). Rare B cells exist in the thymus, and when they become neoplastic, the tumor is a mediastinal (thymic) B cell lymphoma (Chap. 134). Hodgkin's disease, particularly the nodular sclerosing subtype, often involves the anterior mediastinum. Extranodal marginal zone (mucosa-associated lymphoid tissue [MALT]) lymphomas have been reported to involve the thymus in the setting of Sjögren's syndrome or other autoimmune disorders, and the lymphoma cells often express IgA instead of IgM on their surface. Castleman's disease can involve the thymus. Germ cell tumors and carcinoid tumors occasionally may arise in the thymus. If the epithelial cells of the thymus become neoplastic, the tumor that develops is a *thymoma*.

124e Neoplasia During Pregnancy

Michael F. Greene, Dan L. Longo

This is a digital-only chapter. It is available on the DVD that accompanies this book, as well as on Access Medicine/Harrison's Online, and the eBook and "app" editions of HPIM 19e.

Cancer complicates ~1 in every 1000 pregnancies. Of all the cancers that occur in women, less than 1% complicate pregnancies. The four cancers that most commonly complicate pregnancies are cervical cancer, breast cancer, melanoma, and lymphomas (particularly Hodgkin's lymphoma); however, virtually every form of cancer has been reported in pregnant women. In addition to cancers developing in other organs of the mother, gestational trophoblastic tumors can arise from the placenta. The problem of cancer in a pregnant woman is complex. One must take into account (1) the possible influence of the pregnancy on the natural history of the cancer, (2) effects on the mother and fetus of complications from the malignancy (e.g., anorexia, nausea, vomiting, malnutrition), (3) potential effects of diagnostic and staging procedures, and (4) potential effects of cancer treatments on both the mother and the developing fetus. Generally, the management that optimizes maternal physiology is also best for the fetus. However, the dilemma occasionally arises that what is best for the mother may be harmful to the fetus, and what is best for the fetus may compromise the ultimate prognosis for the mother. The best way to approach management of a pregnant woman with cancer is to ask, "What would we do for this woman in this clinical situation if she was not pregnant? Now, which, if any, of those plans need to be modified because she is pregnant?"

125 Late Consequences of Cancer and Its Treatment

Carl E. Freter, Dan L. Longo

There are over 10 million American cancer survivors. The vast majority of these will bear some mark of their cancer and its treatment, and a large proportion will experience long-term consequences including medical problems, psychosocial dysfunction, economic hardship, sexual dysfunction, and discrimination regarding employment and insurance. Many of these problems are directly related to cancer treatment. As patients survive longer from more types of malignancies, we are increasingly recognizing the biologic toll our very imperfect therapies take in terms of morbidity and mortality. The human face of these consequences of therapy confronts the cancer specialist who treats them every day. Although long-term survivors of childhood leukemias, Hodgkin's lymphoma, and testicular cancer, as examples, have taught us much about the consequences of cancer treatment, we keep learning more as patients survive longer with newer therapies. Newer "targeted" chemotherapy drugs have their own, often unique, long-term toxicities about which we remain in a learning process. Cancer "survivorship" clinics are increasing to expressly follow patients for long-term toxicities of cancer treatment.

The pace of developing therapies that mitigate treatment-related consequences has been slow, partly due to an understandable aversion to alter regimens that work and partly due to a lack of new, effective, less toxic therapeutic agents with less "collateral damage" to replace known agents with known toxicities. The types of damage from cancer treatment vary. Often, a final common pathway is irreparable damage to DNA. Surgery can create dysfunction, including blind gut loops with absorption problems and loss of function of removed body parts. Radiation may damage end-organ function, for example, loss of potency in prostate cancer patients, pulmonary fibrosis, and neurocognitive impairment, and may act as a direct carcinogen. Cancer chemotherapy can be a direct carcinogen and has a kaleidoscope of other toxicities discussed in this chapter. Table 125-1 lists the late effects of cancer treatment.

TABLE 125-1 LATE EFFECTS OF CANCER THERAPY

Surgical Procedure		**Effect**
Amputation		Functional loss
Lymph node dissection		Risk of lymphedema
Ostomy		Psychosocial impact
Splenectomy		Risk of sepsis
Adhesions		Risk of obstruction
Bowel anastomoses		Malabsorption syndromes
Radiation Therapy		**Effect**
Organ		
Bone		Premature termination of growth, osteonecrosis
Soft tissues		Atrophy, fibrosis
Brain		Neuropsychiatric deficits, cognitive dysfunction
Thyroid		Hypothyroidism, Graves' disease, cancer
Salivary glands		Dry mouth, caries, dysgeusia
Eyes		Cataracts
Heart		Pericarditis, myocarditis, coronary artery disease
Lung		Pulmonary fibrosis
Kidney		Decreased function, hypertension
Liver		Decreased function
Intestine		Malabsorption, stricture
Gonads		Infertility, premature menopause
Any		Secondary neoplasia
Chemotherapy		**Effect**
Organ	**Drug**	
Bone	Glucocorticoids	Osteoporosis, avascular necrosis
Brain	Methotrexate, cytarabine, others	Neuropsychiatric deficits, cognitive decline?
Peripheral nerves	Vincristine, platinum, taxanes	Neuropathy, hearing loss
Eyes	Glucocorticoids	Cataracts
Heart	Anthracyclines, trastuzumab	Cardiomyopathy
Lung	Bleomycin	Pulmonary fibrosis
	Methotrexate	Pulmonary hypersensitivity
Kidney	Platinum, others	Decreased function, hypomagnesemia
Liver	Various	Altered function
Gonads	Alkylating agents, others	Infertility, premature menopause
Bone marrow	Various	Aplasia, myelodysplasia, secondary leukemia

The first goal of therapy is to eradicate or control the malignancy. Late treatment consequences are, indeed, testimony to the increasing success of such treatment. Their occurrence sharply underlines the necessity to develop more effective therapies with less long-term morbidity and mortality. At the same time, a sense of perspective and relative risk is necessary; fear of long-term complications should not prevent the application of effective, particularly curative, cancer treatment.

CARDIOVASCULAR DYSFUNCTION

CHEMOTHERAPEUTIC AGENTS

Cardiovascular toxicity of cancer chemotherapeutic agents includes dysrhythmias, cardiac ischemia, cardiomyopathic congestive heart failure (CHF), pericardial disease, and peripheral vascular disease. Because these cardiac toxicities are difficult to distinguish from disease that is not associated with cancer treatment, clear etiologic implication of cancer chemotherapeutic agents may be difficult. Cardiovascular complications occurring in an unexpected clinical setting in patients who have undergone cancer therapy are often important in raising suspicion. Dose-dependent myocardial toxicity of anthracyclines with characteristic myofibrillar dropout is pathologically pathognomonic on endomyocardial biopsy. Anthracycline cardiotoxicity occurs through a root mechanism of chemical free radical damage. Fe^{3+}-doxorubicin complexes damage DNA, nuclear and cytoplasmic membranes, and mitochondria. About 5% of patients receiving >450–550 mg/m^2 of doxorubicin will develop CHF. Cardiotoxicity in relation to the dose of anthracycline is clearly not a step function, but rather a continuous function, and occasional patients are seen with CHF at substantially lower doses. Advanced age, other concomitant cardiac disease, hypertension, diabetes, and thoracic radiation therapy are all important cofactors in promoting anthracycline-associated CHF. The risk of cardiac failure appears to be substantially lower when doxorubicin is administered by continuous infusion. Anthracycline-related CHF is difficult to reverse and has a mortality rate as high as 50%, making prevention crucial. Some anthracyclines such as mitoxantrone are associated with less cardiotoxicity, and continuous-infusion regimens and liposomally encapsulated doxorubicin are associated with less cardiotoxicity. Dexrazoxane, an intracellular iron chelator, may limit anthracycline toxicity, but the concern of limiting chemotherapeutic efficacy has somewhat limited its use. Monitoring patients for cardiac toxicity typically involves periodic gated nuclear cardiac blood pool ejection fraction testing (multigated acquisition scan [MUGA]) or cardiac ultrasonography. More recently, cardiac magnetic resonance imaging (MRI) has been used, but MRI is not standard or widespread. Testing is performed more frequently at higher cumulative doses, with additional risk factors, and certainly for any newly developing CHF or other symptoms of cardiac dysfunction.

After anthracyclines, trastuzumab is the next most frequent cardiotoxic drug currently in use. Trastuzumab is frequently used as adjuvant breast cancer therapy, sometimes in conjunction with anthracyclines, which is believed to result in additive or possibly synergistic toxicity. In contrast to anthracyclines, cardiotoxicity is not dose-related, is usually reversible, is not associated with pathologic changes of anthracyclines on cardiac myofibrils, and has a different biochemical mechanism inhibiting intrinsic cardiac repair mechanisms. Toxicity is typically routinely monitored every three to four doses using functional cardiac testing as mentioned earlier for anthracyclines.

Other cardiotoxic drugs include lapatinib, phosphoramide mustards (cyclophosphamide), ifosfamide, interleukin 2, ponatinib, imatinib, and sunitinib.

RADIATION THERAPY

Radiation therapy that includes the heart can cause interstitial myocardial fibrosis, acute and chronic pericarditis, valvular disease, and accelerated premature atherosclerotic coronary artery disease. Repeated or high (>6000 cGy) radiation doses are associated with greater risk, as is concomitant or distant cardiotoxic cancer chemotherapy exposure. Symptoms of acute pericarditis, which peaks about 9 months after treatment, include dyspnea, chest pain, and fever. Chronic constrictive pericarditis may develop 5–10 years following radiation therapy. Cardiac valvular disease includes aortic insufficiency from fibrosis or papillary muscle dysfunction resulting in mitral regurgitation. A threefold increased risk of fatal myocardial infarction is associated with mantle field radiation with accelerated coronary artery disease. Carotid radiation similarly increases the risk of embolic stroke.

TREATMENT CHEMOTHERAPEUTIC/RADIATION-INDUCED CARDIOVASCULAR DISEASE

Therapy for chemotherapeutic/radiation-induced cardiovascular disease is essentially the same as therapy for disease not associated with cancer treatment. Discontinuation of the offending agent is the first step. Diuretics, fluid and sodium restriction, and antiarrhythmic agents are often useful for acute symptoms. Afterload reduction with angiotensin-converting enzyme (ACE) inhibitors or, in some cases, β-adrenergic blockers (carvedilol) often is of significant benefit, and digitalis may be helpful as well.

A hybrid discipline of "cardio-oncology" has been developing in clinics to expressly follow chemotherapy-treated patients for cardiotoxicity. The goals are early intervention using more sensitive techniques, management of cardiotoxicity before it becomes symptomatic, and using clinical trials to identify cardioprotective strategies.

PULMONARY DYSFUNCTION

CHEMOTHERAPEUTIC AGENTS

Bleomycin generates activated free radical oxygen species and causes pneumonitis associated with a radiographic or interstitial ground-glass appearance diffusely throughout both lungs, often worse in the lower lobes. A nonproductive cough with or without fever may be an early sign. This toxicity is dose-related and dose-limiting. The diffusion capacity of the lungs for carbon dioxide (DL_{CO}) is a sensitive measure of toxicity and recovery, and a baseline value is generally obtained for future comparison prior to bleomycin therapy. Additive or synergistic risk factors include age, prior lung disease, and concomitant use of other chemotherapy, lung irradiation, and high concentrations of inspired oxygen. Other chemotherapeutic agents notable for pulmonary toxicity include mitomycin, nitrosoureas, doxorubicin with radiation, gemcitabine combined with weekly docetaxel, methotrexate, and fludarabine. High-dose alkylating agents, cyclophosphamide, ifosfamide, and melphalan are frequently used in the hematopoietic stem cell transplant setting, often with whole-body radiation. This therapy may result in severe pulmonary fibrosis and/or pulmonary venoocclusive disease.

RADIATION THERAPY

Risk factors for radiation pneumonitis include advanced age, poor performance status, preexisting compromised pulmonary function, and radiation volume and dose. The dose "threshold" is thought to be in the range of 5 to 20 Gy. Hypoxemia and dyspnea on exertion are characteristic. Fine, high-pitched "Velcro rales" may be an accompanying physical finding, and fever, cough, and pleuritic chest pain are common symptoms. The DL_{CO} is the most sensitive measure of pulmonary functional impairment, and ground-glass infiltrates often correspond with relatively sharp edges to the irradiated volume, although the pneumonitis may progress beyond the field and even occasionally involve the contralateral unirradiated lung.

TREATMENT PULMONARY DYSFUNCTION

Chemotherapy- and radiation-induced pneumonitis is generally very corticosteroid responsive, except in the case of nitrosoureas. Prednisone 1 mg/kg is often used to control acute symptoms and pulmonary dysfunction with a generally slow taper. Prolonged glucocorticoid therapy requires gastrointestinal protection with proton pump inhibitors, management of hyperglycemia, heightened infection management, and treatment of steroid-induced osteoporosis. Antibiotics, bronchodilators, oxygen in only necessary doses, and diuretics may all play an important role in management of pneumonitis, and consultation with a pulmonologist should be routinely undertaken. Amifostine has been studied as a pulmonary radioprotectant, with inconclusive results, and is associated with skin rash, fatigue, and nausea; hence, it is not considered standard therapy at this time. Transforming growth factor β (TGF-β) is believed to be a major inducer of radiation fibrosis and represents a therapeutic target for development of anti-TGF-β therapies.

NEUROLOGIC DYSFUNCTION

CHEMOTHERAPEUTIC AGENTS

Chemotherapy- and radiation-induced neurologic dysfunction is unfortunately increasing in both incidence and severity as a result of improved supportive care leading to more aggressive regimens and longer cancer survivorship allowing the development of late toxicity. Direct effects on myelin, glial cells, and neurons have all been implicated, with alterations in cellular cytoskeleton, axonal transport, and cellular metabolism as mechanisms.

Vinca alkaloids produce a characteristic "stocking-glove" neuropathy with numbness and tingling advancing to loss of motor function, which is highly dose related. Distal sensorimotor polyneuropathy prominently involves loss of deep tendon reflexes with initially loss of pain and temperature sensation, followed by proprioceptive and vibratory loss. This requires careful patient history and physical examination by experienced oncologists to decide when the drug must be stopped due to toxicity. Milder toxicity often slowly completely resolves. Vinca alkaloids may sometimes be associated with jaw claudication, autonomic neuropathy, ileus, cranial nerve palsies, and, in severe cases, encephalopathy, seizures, and coma.

Cisplatin is associated with sensorimotor neuropathy and hearing loss, especially at doses >400 mg/m^2, requiring audiometry in patients with preexisting hearing compromise. Carboplatin is often substituted in such cases given its lesser effect on hearing.

Many of the agents that target kinase enzymes in tumor cells and 5-fluorouracil congeners produce dysesthesias and painful hands and feet known as hand-foot syndrome or palmar-plantar erythrodysesthesia. Symptoms usually abate when the agent is stopped.

Neurocognitive dysfunction has been well described in childhood survivors of acute lymphoblastic leukemia (ALL) treatment, including intrathecal methotrexate or cytosine arabinoside in conjunction with prophylactic cranial irradiation. Methotrexate alone may cause acute leukoencephalopathy characterized by somnolence and confusion that is often reversible. Acute toxicity is dose related, especially at doses >3 g/m^2, with younger patients being at greater risk. Subacute methotrexate toxicity occurs weeks after therapy and is often ameliorated with glucocorticoid therapy. Chronic methotrexate toxicity (leukoencephalopathy) develops months or years after treatment and is characterized clinically as progressive loss of cognitive function and focal neurologic signs, which are irreversible, promoted by synchronous or metachronous radiation therapy, and more pronounced at a younger age.

Neurocognitive decline following chemotherapy alone occurs notably in breast cancer patients receiving adjuvant chemotherapy; this has been referred to as "chemo brain." It is clinically associated with impaired memory, learning, attention, and speed of information processing. There is no clear mechanistic explanation for its cause and no clearly effective therapy. This entity is justifiably attracting more attention and clearly needs to be studied to develop effective therapy or prophylaxis.

Many cancer patients experience intrusive or debilitating concerns about cancer recurrence following successful therapy. In addition, these patients may experience job, insurance, stress, relationship, financial, and sexual difficulties. Oncologists need to ask about and address these issues explicitly with patients and provide appropriate counseling or support systems. Suicidal ideation and suicide have an increased incidence in cancer patients and survivors.

RADIATION THERAPY

Acute radiation central nervous system (CNS) toxicity occurs within weeks; is characterized by nausea, drowsiness, hypersomnia, and ataxia; and is most often associated with recovery. Early delayed toxicity occurring weeks to 3 months following therapy is associated with similar symptoms as acute toxicity and is pathologically associated with reversible demyelination. Chronic, late radiation injury occurs 9 months to up to 10 years following therapy. Focal necrosis is a common pathologic finding, and glucocorticoid therapy may be helpful. Diffuse radiation injury is associated with global CNS neurologic dysfunction and diffuse white matter changes on computed tomography (CT) or MRI. Pathologically, small vessel changes are prominent. Glucocorticoids may be symptomatically useful but do not alter the course. Necrotizing encephalopathy is the most severe form of radiation injury and almost always is associated with chemotherapy, notably methotrexate.

Cranial radiation may also be associated with an array of endocrine abnormalities with disruption of normal pituitary/hypothalamic axis function, and a high index of suspicion needs to be maintained to identify and treat this toxicity.

Radiation-associated spinal cord injury (myelopathy) is highly dose-dependent and rarely occurs with modern radiation therapy. An early, self-limited form involving electric sensations down the spine on neck flexion (Lhermitte's sign) is seen 6–12 weeks after treatment and generally resolves over weeks. Peripheral nerve toxicity is quite rare owing to relative radiation resistance.

HEPATIC DYSFUNCTION

CHEMOTHERAPEUTIC AGENTS

Long-term hepatic damage from standard chemotherapy regimens is rare. Long-term methotrexate or high-dose chemotherapy alone or with radiation therapy, for example, in preparative regimens for bone marrow transplantation, may result in venoocclusive disease of the liver. This potentially lethal complication classically presents with anicteric ascites, elevated alkaline phosphatase, and hepatosplenomegaly. Pathologically, there is venous congestion, epithelial cell proliferation, and hepatocyte atrophy progressing to frank fibrosis. Frequent monitoring of liver function tests during any chemotherapy is necessary to avoid both idiosyncratic and expected toxicities.

Certain nucleoside drugs have been associated with hepatic dysfunction; however, this complication is rare in oncology.

RADIATION THERAPY

Hepatic radiation damage depends on dose, volume, fractionation, preexisting liver disease, and synchronous or metachronous chemotherapy. In general, radiation doses to the liver >1500 cGy can produce hepatic dysfunction with a steep dose-injury curve. Radiation-induced liver disease closely mimics hepatic venoocclusive disease.

RENAL/BLADDER DYSFUNCTION

Cisplatin produces reversible decrements in renal function, but may also produce severe irreversible toxicity in the presence of renal disease and may predispose to accentuated damage with subsequent renal insults. Cyclophosphamide and ifosfamide, as prodrugs primarily activated in the liver, have cleavage products (acrolein) that can produce hemorrhagic cystitis. This can be prevented with the free radical scavenger MESNA (mercaptoethane sulfonate), which is required for ifosfamide administration. Hemorrhagic cystitis caused by these agents may predispose to bladder cancer.

REPRODUCTIVE AND ENDOCRINE DYSFUNCTION

CHEMOTHERAPEUTIC AGENTS

Alkylating agents are associated with the highest rates of male and female infertility, which is directly dependent on age, dose, and duration of treatment. The age at treatment is an important determinant of fertility outcome, with prepubertal patients having the highest tolerance. Ovarian failure is age related, and females who resume menses after treatment are still at increased risk for premature menopause. Males generally have reversible azoospermia during lower intensity alkylator chemotherapy, and long-term infertility is associated with doses of cyclophosphamide >9 g/m^2 and with high-intensity therapy, such as that used in hematopoietic stem cell transplantation. Males undergoing potentially sterilizing chemotherapy should be offered sperm banking. Gonadotropin-releasing hormone (GnRH) analogs remain experimental to preserve ovarian function. Assisted reproductive technologies can be helpful to couples with chemotherapy-induced infertility.

RADIATION THERAPY

Testicles and ovaries in prepubertal patients are less sensitive to radiation damage; spermatogenesis is affected by low doses of radiation, and complete azoospermia occurs at 600–700 cGy. Leydig cell dysfunction, in contrast, occurs at <2000 cGy, and hence, endocrine function is lost at much higher radiation doses than spermatogenesis. Erectile dysfunction occurs in up to 80% of men treated with external-beam radiation therapy for prostate cancer. Sildenafil may be useful in reversing erectile dysfunction. Ovarian function damage with radiation is age related and occurs at doses of 150–500 cGy. Premature induction of menopause can have serious medical and psychological sequelae. Hormone replacement therapy is often contraindicated (as in estrogen receptor–positive breast cancer). Attention must be paid to maintenance of bone mass with calcium and vitamin D supplements and oral bisphosphonates, and bone mass should be monitored using bone density determinations. Paroxetine, clonidine, pregabalin, and other drugs may be useful in symptomatically controlling hot flashes.

Long-term survivors of childhood cancer (e.g., ALL) who have received cranial radiation may have altered leptin biology and growth hormone deficiency, leading to obesity and reduced strength, exercise tolerance, and bone density.

Radiation therapy to the neck (e.g., in Hodgkin's lymphoma) may lead to hypothyroidism, Graves' disease, thyroiditis, and thyroid malignancies. Thyroid-stimulating hormone (TSH) is followed routinely in such patients to prevent hypothyroidism, and to suppress persistently elevated levels of TSH which may cause or drive thyroid cancer.

OCULAR COMPLICATIONS

Cataracts may be caused by glucocorticoids, depending on duration and dose; radiation therapy; and uncommonly tamoxifen. Orbital radiation therapy may cause blindness.

ORAL COMPLICATIONS

Radiation therapy can produce xerostomia (dry mouth), with an attendant increase in caries and poor dentition. Taste and appetite may be suppressed. Bisphosphonate use may result in osteonecrosis of the jaw.

RAYNAUD'S PHENOMENON

Up to 40% of patients treated with bleomycin may develop Raynaud's phenomenon as a result of an unknown mechanism.

SECOND MALIGNANCIES

Second malignancies in patients cured of cancer are a major cause of death, and treated cancer patients must be monitored for their occurrence. The induction of second malignancies is governed by the complex interplay of a number of factors including age, gender, environmental exposures, genetic susceptibility, and cancer treatment itself. In a number of settings, the events leading to the primary cancer themselves increase the risk of second malignancies. Patients with lung cancer are at increased risk of esophageal and head and neck cancers, and vice versa, due to shared risk factors including alcohol and tobacco abuse. Indeed, the risk of developing a second primary head and neck, esophageal, or lung cancer is also increased in these patients. Patients with breast cancer are at increased risk of breast cancer in the opposite breast. Patients with Hodgkin's lymphoma are at risk for non-Hodgkin's lymphomas. Genetic cancer syndromes (e.g., multiple endocrine neoplasia or Li-Fraumeni, Lynch's, Cowden's, and Gardner's syndromes) are examples of genetically based second malignancies of specific types. Cancer treatment itself does not appear to be responsible for the risk of these secondary malignancies. Deficient DNA repair can greatly increase the risk of cancers from DNA-damaging agents, as in ataxia-telangiectasia. Importantly, the risk of treatment-related second malignancies is at least additive and often synergistic with combined chemotherapy and radiation therapy, and hence for such combined-therapy treatment approaches, it is important to establish the necessity of each in the treatment program. All of these patients require special surveillance or, in some cases, prophylactic surgery as part of appropriate treatment and follow-up.

CHEMOTHERAPEUTIC AGENTS

Chemotherapy is significantly associated with two fatal second malignancies, acute leukemia and myelodysplastic syndromes. Two types of leukemia have been described; in patients treated with alkylating agents, acute myeloid leukemia is associated with deletions in chromosome 5 or 7. The lifetime risk is about 1–5%, is increased by radiation therapy, and increases with age. The incidence of these leukemias peaks at 4–6 years, with risk returning close to baseline at 10 years. The other type of acute myeloid leukemia is related to therapy with topoisomerase inhibitors, is associated with chromosome 10q23 translocations, has an incidence of <1%, and generally occurs 1.5–3 years after treatment. Both of these acute myeloid leukemias are refractory to treatment and have a high mortality. The development of myelodysplastic syndromes is increased following chemotherapy, and these are often associated with leukemic progression and a dismal prognosis.

RADIATION THERAPY

Patients receiving radiation have an increasing and lifelong risk of second malignancies that is 1–2% in the second decade following treatment but increases to >25% after 25 years. These malignancies include cancers of the thyroid and breast, sarcomas, and CNS cancers, which often tend to be aggressive and have a poor prognosis. An example of organ-, age-, and sex-dependent radiation-induced secondary malignancy is breast cancer, in which the risk is small with radiation in women under age 30 but increases about 20-fold over baseline in women over 30. A 25-year-old woman treated with mantle radiation for Hodgkin's lymphoma has a 29% actuarial risk of developing breast cancer by age 55.

HORMONAL THERAPY

Treatment of breast cancer with tamoxifen for 5 years or longer is associated with a 1–2% risk of endometrial cancer. Surveillance is generally effective at finding these cancers at an early stage. The risk of mortality from tamoxifen-induced endometrial cancer is low compared to the benefit of tamoxifen as adjuvant therapy for breast cancer.

IMMUNOSUPPRESSIVE THERAPY

Immunosuppressive therapy, as used in allogeneic bone marrow transplantation, particularly with T cell depletion using antithymocyte globulin or other means, increases the risk of Epstein Barr virus–associated

TABLE 125-2 LONG-TERM TREATMENT EFFECTS BY CANCER TYPE

Cancer Type	Late Effects
Pediatric cancers	Majority have at least one late effect
	30% with moderate/severe problems
	Cardiovascular: radiation, anthracyclines
	Lungs: radiation
	Skeletal abnormalities: radiation
	Psychological, cognitive, and sexual problems
	Second neoplasms significant cause of death
Hodgkin's lymphoma	Thyroid dysfunction: radiation
	Premature coronary artery disease: radiation
	Gonadal dysfunction: chemotherapy
	Postsplenectomy sepsis
	Myelodysplasia
	Acute myeloid leukemia
	Non-Hodgkin's lymphomas
	Breast cancer, lung cancer, and melanoma
	Fatigue, psychological and sexual problems
	Peripheral neuropathy
Non-Hodgkin's lymphoma	Myelodysplasia
	Acute leukemia
	Bladder cancer
	Peripheral neuropathy
Acute leukemia	Second malignancies: hematologic, solid tumors
	Neuropsychiatric dysfunction
	Subnormal growth
	Thyroid abnormalities
	Infertility
Bone marrow stem cell transplantation	Infertility
	Graft-versus-host disease (allogeneic transplant)
	Psychosexual dysfunction.
Head and neck cancer	Poor dentition, dry mouth, poor nutrition: radiation
Breast cancer	Tamoxifen: endometrial cancer, blood clots
	Aromatase inhibitors: osteoporosis, arthritis
	Cardiomyopathy: anthracycline ± radiation, trastuzumab
	Acute leukemia
	Hormone deficiency symptoms: hot flashes, vaginal dryness, dyspareunia
	Psychosocial dysfunction
	"Chemo brain"
Testicular cancer	Raynaud's phenomenon
	Renal dysfunction
	Pulmonary dysfunction
	Retrograde ejaculation: surgery
	15% sexual dysfunction
Colon cancer	Major risk is second colon cance.
	Quality of life high in survivors
Prostate cancer	Impotence
	Urinary incontinence (0–15%)
	Chronic proctitis, prostatitis/cystitis: radiation

B cell lymphoproliferative disorder. The incidence at 10 years after T cell depletion is 9–12%. Discontinuing immunosuppressive therapy, if possible, is often associated with complete disease regression.

RECOMMENDATIONS FOR FOLLOW-UP

All former cancer patients should be followed indefinitely. This is most often done by oncologists, but demographic changes suggest that more primary care physicians will need to be trained in the follow-up of treated cancer patients in remission. Cancer patients need to be educated about signs and symptoms of recurrence and potentially adverse effects related to therapy. Localized pain or palpable abnormality in a previously radiated field should prompt radiographic evaluation. Screening tests, when available and validated, should be used on a routine and regular basis (e.g., mammography and Pap smear), particularly in patients receiving radiation to specific organs. Annual mammography should start no later than 10 years after breast radiation. Patients receiving radiation fields encompassing thyroid tissue should have regular thyroid exams and TSH testing. Patients treated with alkylating agents or topoisomerase inhibitors should have a complete blood count every 6–12 months, and cytopenias, abnormal cells on peripheral smear, or macrocytosis should be evaluated with bone marrow biopsy and aspirate, to include cytogenetics, flow cytometry, or fluorescence in situ hybridization (FISH) studies as appropriate.

As the population of cancer survivors lives longer and grows, cancer survivorship has become an increasingly recognized subject, and the Institute of Medicine and National Research Council have published a monograph entitled *From Cancer Patient to Cancer Survivor: Lost in Transition.* The monograph proposes a plan that would inform clinicians caring for cancer survivors in complete detail of their previous treatments, complications thereof, signs and symptoms of late effects, and recommended screening and follow-up procedures. Table 125-2 lists long-term treatment effects by cancer type.

OUTLOOK

Clearly, the challenge for the future is to combine chemotherapy, targeted agents, biologic therapies, radiation, and surgery to produce better outcomes with less toxicity, including late effects of therapy. This is easily said but less easily accomplished. As treatment becomes more effective in new patient populations (ovarian, bladder, anal, and laryngeal cancers, for example), we will expect to discover new populations at risk for late effects. These populations will need to be followed carefully, so that such effects are recognized and treated. Cancer survivors represent an underused resource for prevention studies. Childhood cancer survivors, especially, suffer multiple chronic health impairments. The incidence of these late treatment consequences appears to have no plateau with age, throwing in stark relief the necessity of close monitoring and therapies with fewer late consequences of treatment.

126 Iron Deficiency and Other Hypoproliferative Anemias

John W. Adamson

Anemias associated with normocytic and normochromic red cells and an inappropriately low reticulocyte response (reticulocyte index <2–2.5) are *hypoproliferative anemias*. This category includes early iron deficiency (before hypochromic microcytic red cells develop), acute and chronic inflammation (including many malignancies), renal disease, hypometabolic states such as protein malnutrition and endocrine deficiencies, and anemias from marrow damage. Marrow damage states are discussed in Chap. 130.

Hypoproliferative anemias are the most common anemias, and in the clinic, iron deficiency anemia is the most common of these followed by the anemia of inflammation. The anemia of inflammation, similar to iron deficiency, is related in part to abnormal iron metabolism. The anemias associated with renal disease, inflammation, cancer, and hypometabolic states are characterized by a suboptimal erythropoietin response to the anemia.

IRON METABOLISM

Iron is a critical element in the function of all cells, although the amount of iron required by individual tissues varies during development. At the same time, the body must protect itself from free iron, which is highly toxic in that it participates in chemical reactions that generate free radicals such as singlet O_2 or OH^-. Consequently, elaborate mechanisms have evolved that allow iron to be made available for physiologic functions while at the same time conserving this element and handling it in such a way that toxicity is avoided.

The major role of iron in mammals is to carry O_2 as part of hemoglobin. O_2 is also bound by myoglobin in muscle. Iron is a critical element in iron-containing enzymes, including the cytochrome system in mitochondria. Iron distribution in the body is shown in Table 126-1. Without iron, cells lose their capacity for electron transport and energy metabolism. In erythroid cells, hemoglobin synthesis is impaired, resulting in anemia and reduced O_2 delivery to tissue.

THE IRON CYCLE IN HUMANS

Figure 126-1 outlines the major pathways of internal iron exchange in humans. Iron absorbed from the diet or released from stores circulates in the plasma bound to *transferrin*, the iron transport protein. Transferrin is a bilobed glycoprotein with two iron binding sites. Transferrin that carries iron exists in two forms—*monoferric* (one iron atom) or *diferric* (two iron atoms). The turnover (half-clearance time) of transferrin-bound iron is very rapid—typically 60–90 min. Because almost all of the iron transported by transferrin is delivered to the erythroid marrow, the clearance time of transferrin-bound iron from the circulation is affected most by the plasma iron level and the erythroid marrow activity. When erythropoiesis is markedly stimulated, the pool of erythroid cells requiring iron increases and the clearance time of iron from the circulation decreases. The half-clearance time of iron in

TABLE 126-1 BODY IRON DISTRIBUTION

	Iron Content, mg	
	Adult Male, 80 kg	Adult Female, 60 kg
Hemoglobin	2500	1700
Myoglobin/enzymes	500	300
Transferrin iron	3	3
Iron stores	600–1000	0–300

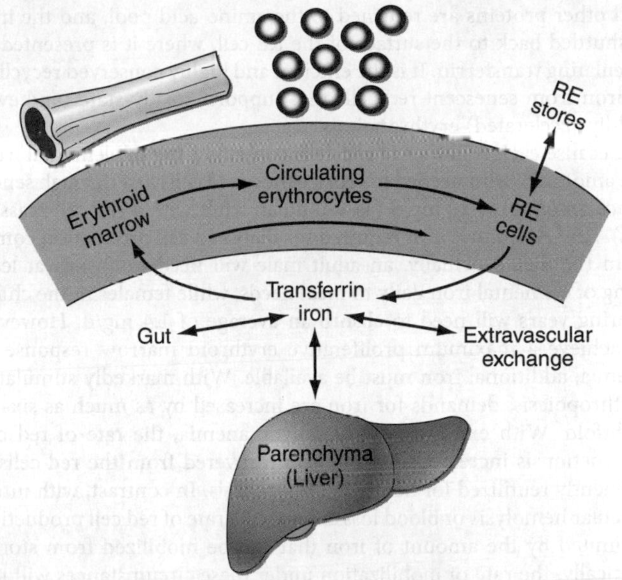

FIGURE 126-1 Internal iron exchange. Normally 80% of iron passing through the plasma transferrin pool is recycled from senescent red cells. Absorption of approximately 1 mg/d is required from the diet in men, and 1.4 mg/d in women to maintain homeostasis. As long as transferrin saturation is maintained between 20 and 60% and erythropoiesis is not increased, use of iron stores is not required. However, in the event of blood loss, dietary iron deficiency, or inadequate iron absorption, up to 40 mg/d of iron can be mobilized from stores. RE, reticuloendothelial.

the presence of iron deficiency is as short as 10–15 min. With suppression of erythropoiesis, the plasma iron level typically increases and the half-clearance time may be prolonged to several hours. Normally, the iron bound to transferrin turns over 6–8 times per day. Assuming a normal plasma iron level of 80–100 μg/dL, the amount of iron passing through the transferrin pool is 20–24 mg/d.

The iron-transferrin complex circulates in the plasma until it interacts with specific *transferrin receptors* on the surface of marrow erythroid cells. Diferric transferrin has the highest affinity for transferrin receptors; apotransferrin (not carrying iron) has very little affinity. Although transferrin receptors are found on cells in many tissues within the body—and all cells at some time during development will display transferrin receptors—the cell having the greatest number of receptors (300,000–400,000/cell) is the developing erythroblast.

Once the iron-bearing transferrin interacts with its receptor, the complex is internalized via clathrin-coated pits and transported to an acidic endosome, where the iron is released at the low pH. The iron is then made available for heme synthesis while the transferrin-receptor complex is recycled to the surface of the cell, where the bulk of the transferrin is released back into circulation and the transferrin receptor reanchors into the cell membrane. At this point a certain amount of the transferrin receptor protein may be released into circulation and can be measured as soluble transferrin receptor protein. Within the erythroid cell, iron in excess of the amount needed for hemoglobin synthesis binds to a storage protein, *apoferritin*, forming *ferritin*. This mechanism of iron exchange also takes place in other cells of the body expressing transferrin receptors, especially liver parenchymal cells where the iron can be incorporated into heme-containing enzymes or stored. The iron incorporated into hemoglobin subsequently enters the circulation as new red cells are released from the bone marrow. The iron is then part of the red cell mass and will not become available for reutilization until the red cell dies.

In a normal individual, the average red cell life span is 120 days. Thus, 0.8–1% of red cells are replaced each day. At the end of its life span, the red cell is recognized as senescent by the cells of the *reticuloendothelial (RE) system*, and the red cell undergoes phagocytosis. Once within the RE cell, the ingested hemoglobin is broken down, the globin and other proteins are returned to the amino acid pool, and the iron is shuttled back to the surface of the RE cell, where it is presented to circulating transferrin. It is the efficient and highly conserved recycling of iron from senescent red cells that supports steady-state (and even mildly accelerated) erythropoiesis.

Because each milliliter of red cells contains 1 mg of elemental iron, the amount of iron needed to replace those red cells lost through senescence amounts to 20 mg/d (assuming an adult with a red cell mass of 2 L). Any additional iron required for daily red cell production comes from the diet. Normally, an adult male will need to absorb at least 1 mg of elemental iron daily to meet needs, while females in the childbearing years will need to absorb an average of 1.4 mg/d. However, to achieve a maximum proliferative erythroid marrow response to anemia, additional iron must be available. With markedly stimulated erythropoiesis, demands for iron are increased by as much as six- to eightfold. With extravascular hemolytic anemia, the rate of red cell destruction is increased, but the iron recovered from the red cells is efficiently reutilized for hemoglobin synthesis. In contrast, with intravascular hemolysis or blood loss anemia, the rate of red cell production is limited by the amount of iron that can be mobilized from stores. Typically, the rate of mobilization under these circumstances will not support red cell production more than 2.5 times normal. If the delivery of iron to the stimulated marrow is suboptimal, the marrow's proliferative response is blunted, and hemoglobin synthesis is impaired. The result is a hypoproliferative marrow accompanied by microcytic, hypochromic anemia.

Whereas blood loss or hemolysis places a demand on the iron supply, inflammatory conditions interfere with iron release from stores and can result in a rapid decrease in the serum iron (see below).

NUTRITIONAL IRON BALANCE

The balance of iron in humans is tightly controlled and designed to conserve iron for reutilization. There is no regulated excretory pathway for iron, and the only mechanisms by which iron is lost are blood loss (via gastrointestinal bleeding, menses, or other forms of bleeding) and the loss of epithelial cells from the skin, gut, and genitourinary tract. Normally, the only route by which iron comes into the body is via absorption from food or from medicinal iron taken orally. Iron may also enter the body through red cell transfusions or injection of iron complexes. The margin between the amount of iron available for absorption and the requirement for iron in growing infants and the adult female is narrow; this accounts for the great prevalence of iron deficiency worldwide—currently estimated at one-half billion people.

The amount of iron required from the diet to replace losses averages approximately 10% of body iron content a year in men and 15% in women of childbearing age. Dietary iron content is closely related to total caloric intake (approximately 6 mg of elemental iron per 1000 calories). Iron bioavailability is affected by the nature of the foodstuff, with heme iron (e.g., red meat) being most readily absorbed. In the United States, the average iron intake in an adult male is 15 mg/d with 6% absorption; for the average female, the daily intake is 11 mg/d with 12% absorption. An individual with iron deficiency can increase iron absorption to approximately 20% of the iron present in a meat-containing diet but only 5–10% of the iron in a vegetarian diet. As a result, one-third of the female population in the United States has virtually no iron stores. Vegetarians are at an additional disadvantage because certain foodstuffs that include phytates and phosphates reduce iron absorption by approximately 50%. When ionizable iron salts are given together with food, the amount of iron absorbed is reduced. When the percentage of iron absorbed from individual food items is compared with the percentage for an equivalent amount of ferrous salt, iron in vegetables is only about one-twentieth as available, egg iron one-eighth, liver iron one-half, and heme iron one-half to two-thirds.

Infants, children, and adolescents may be unable to maintain normal iron balance because of the demands of body growth and lower dietary intake of iron. During the last two trimesters of pregnancy, daily iron requirements increase to 5–6 mg, and iron supplements are strongly recommended for pregnant women in developed countries.

Iron absorption takes place largely in the proximal small intestine and is a carefully regulated process. For absorption, iron must be taken up by the luminal cell. That process is facilitated by the acidic contents of the stomach, which maintains the iron in solution. At the brush border of the absorptive cell, the ferric iron is converted to the ferrous form by a ferrireductase. Transport across the membrane is accomplished by divalent metal transporter type 1 (DMT-1, also known as natural resistance macrophage-associated protein type 2 [Nramp 2] or DCT-1). DMT-1 is a general cation transporter. Once inside the gut cell, iron may be stored as ferritin or transported through the cell to be released at the basolateral surface to plasma transferrin through the membrane-embedded iron exporter, ferroportin. The function of ferroportin is negatively regulated by hepcidin, the principal iron regulatory hormone. In the process of release, iron interacts with another ferroxidase, hephaestin, which oxidizes the iron to the ferric form for transferrin binding. Hephaestin is similar to ceruloplasmin, the copper-carrying protein.

Iron absorption is influenced by a number of physiologic states. Erythroid hyperplasia stimulates iron absorption even in the face of normal or increased iron stores, and hepcidin levels are inappropriately low. Thus, patients with anemias associated with high levels of ineffective erythropoiesis absorb excess amounts of dietary iron. The molecular mechanism underlying this relationship is not known. Over time, this may lead to iron overload and tissue damage. In iron deficiency, hepcidin levels are also low and iron is much more efficiently absorbed; the contrary is true in states of secondary iron overload. The normal individual can reduce iron absorption in situations of excessive intake or medicinal iron intake; however, while the percentage of iron absorbed goes down, the absolute amount goes up. This accounts for the acute iron toxicity occasionally seen when children ingest large numbers of iron tablets. Under these circumstances, the amount of iron absorbed exceeds the transferrin binding capacity of the plasma, resulting in free iron that affects critical organs such as cardiac muscle cells.

IRON-DEFICIENCY ANEMIA

Iron deficiency is one of the most prevalent forms of malnutrition. Globally, 50% of anemia is attributable to iron deficiency and accounts for approximately 841,000 deaths annually worldwide. Africa and parts of Asia bear 71% of the global mortality burden; North America represents only 1.4% of the total morbidity and mortality associated with iron deficiency.

STAGES OF IRON DEFICIENCY

The progression to iron deficiency can be divided into three stages (Fig. 126-2). The first stage is *negative iron balance*, in which the demands for (or losses of) iron exceed the body's ability to absorb iron from the diet. This stage results from a number of physiologic mechanisms, including blood loss, pregnancy (in which the demands for red cell production by the fetus outstrip the mother's ability to provide iron), rapid growth spurts in the adolescent, or inadequate dietary iron intake. Blood loss in excess of 10–20 mL of red cells per day is greater than the amount of iron that the gut can absorb from a normal diet. Under these circumstances, the iron deficit must be made up by mobilization of iron from RE storage sites. During this period, iron stores—reflected by the serum ferritin level or the appearance of stainable iron on bone marrow aspirations—decrease. As long as iron stores are present and can be mobilized, the serum iron, total iron-binding capacity (TIBC), and red cell protoporphyrin levels remain within normal limits. At this stage, red cell morphology and indices are normal.

When iron stores become depleted, the serum iron begins to fall. Gradually, the TIBC increases, as do red cell protoporphyrin levels. By definition, marrow iron stores are absent when the serum ferritin level is <15 μg/L. As long as the serum iron remains within the normal

	Normal	Negative iron balance	Iron-deficient erythropoiesis	Iron-deficiency anemia
Iron stores / Erythron iron				
Marrow iron stores	1-3+	0-1+	0	0
Serum ferritin (μg/L)	50-200	<20	<15	<15
TIBC (μg/dL)	300-360	>360	>380	>400
SI (μg/dL)	50-150	NL	<50	<30
Saturation (%)	30-50	NL	<20	<10
Marrow sideroblasts (%)	40-60	NL	<10	<10
RBC protoporphyrin (μg/dL)	30-50	NL	>100	>200
RBC morphology	NL	NL	NL	Microcytic/hypochromic

FIGURE 126-2 Laboratory studies in the evolution of iron deficiency. Measurements of marrow iron stores, serum ferritin, and total iron-binding capacity (TIBC) are sensitive to early iron-store depletion. Iron-deficient erythropoiesis is recognized from additional abnormalities in the serum iron (SI), percent transferrin saturation, the pattern of marrow sideroblasts, and the red blood cell (RBC) protoporphyrin level. Patients with iron-deficiency anemia demonstrate all the same abnormalities plus hypochromic microcytic anemia. *(From RS Hillman, CA Finch: The Red Cell Manual, 7th ed. Philadelphia, F.A.Davis and Co., 1996, with permission.)*

range, hemoglobin synthesis is unaffected despite the dwindling iron stores. Once the transferrin saturation falls to 15–20%, hemoglobin synthesis becomes impaired. This is a period of *iron-deficient erythropoiesis*. Careful evaluation of the peripheral blood smear reveals the first appearance of microcytic cells, and if the laboratory technology is available, one finds hypochromic reticulocytes in circulation. Gradually, the hemoglobin and hematocrit begin to fall, reflecting *iron-deficiency anemia*. The transferrin saturation at this point is 10–15%.

When moderate anemia is present (hemoglobin 10–13 g/dL), the bone marrow remains hypoproliferative. With more severe anemia (hemoglobin 7–8 g/dL), hypochromia and microcytosis become more prominent, target cells and misshapen red cells (poikilocytes) appear on the blood smear as cigar- or pencil-shaped forms, and the erythroid marrow becomes increasingly ineffective. Consequently, with severe prolonged iron deficiency anemia, erythroid hyperplasia of the marrow develops, rather than hypoproliferation.

CAUSES OF IRON DEFICIENCY

Conditions that increase demand for iron, increase iron loss, or decrease iron intake or absorption can produce iron deficiency (Table 126-2).

CLINICAL PRESENTATION OF IRON DEFICIENCY

Certain clinical conditions carry an increased likelihood of iron deficiency. Pregnancy, adolescence, periods of rapid growth, and an intermittent history of blood loss of any kind should alert the clinician to possible iron deficiency. A cardinal rule is that the appearance of iron deficiency in an adult male means gastrointestinal blood loss until proven otherwise. Signs related to iron deficiency depend on the severity and chronicity of the anemia in addition to the usual signs of anemia—fatigue, pallor, and reduced exercise capacity. *Cheilosis* (fissures at the corners of the mouth) and *koilonychia* (spooning of the fingernails) are signs of advanced tissue iron deficiency. The diagnosis of iron deficiency is typically based on laboratory results.

TABLE 126-2 CAUSES OF IRON DEFICIENCY

Increased Demand for Iron
Rapid growth in infancy or adolescence
Pregnancy
Erythropoietin therapy
Increased Iron Loss
Chronic blood loss
Menses
Acute blood loss
Blood donation
Phlebotomy as treatment for polycythemia vera
Decreased Iron Intake or Absorption
Inadequate diet
Malabsorption from disease (sprue, Crohn's disease)
Malabsorption from surgery (gastrectomy and some forms of bariatric surgery)
Acute or chronic inflammation

LABORATORY IRON STUDIES

Serum Iron and Total Iron-Binding Capacity The serum iron level represents the amount of circulating iron bound to transferrin. The TIBC is an indirect measure of the circulating transferrin. The normal range for the serum iron is 50–150 μg/dL; the normal range for TIBC is 300–360 μg/dL. Transferrin saturation, which is normally 25–50%, is obtained by the following formula: serum iron × 100 ÷ TIBC. Iron-deficiency states are associated with saturation levels below 20%. There is a diurnal variation in the serum iron. A transferrin saturation % >50% indicates that a disproportionate amount of the iron bound to transferrin is being delivered to nonerythroid tissues. If this persists for an extended time, tissue iron overload may occur.

Serum Ferritin Free iron is toxic to cells, and the body has established an elaborate set of protective mechanisms to bind iron in various tissue compartments. Within cells, iron is stored complexed to protein as ferritin or hemosiderin. Apoferritin binds to free ferrous iron and stores it in the ferric state. As ferritin accumulates within cells of the RE system, protein aggregates are formed as hemosiderin. Iron in ferritin or hemosiderin can be extracted for release by the RE cells, although hemosiderin is less readily available. Under steady-state conditions, the serum ferritin level correlates with total body iron stores; thus, the serum ferritin level is the most convenient laboratory test to estimate iron stores. The normal value for ferritin varies according to the age and gender of the individual (Fig. 126-3). Adult males have serum

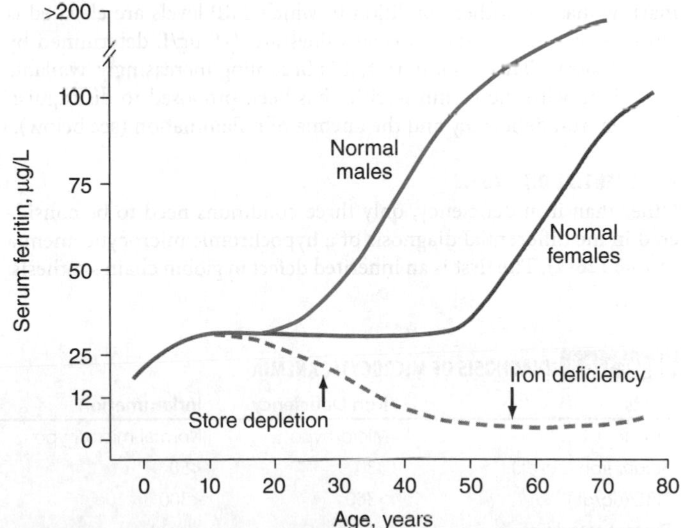

FIGURE 126-3 Serum ferritin levels as a function of sex and age. Iron store depletion and iron deficiency are accompanied by a decrease in serum ferritin level below 20 μg/L. *(From RS Hillman et al: Hematology in Clinical Practice, 5th ed. New York, McGraw-Hill, 2011, with permission.)*

TABLE 126-3 IRON STORE MEASUREMENTS

Iron Stores	Marrow Iron Stain, 0–4+	Serum Ferritin, μg/L
0	0	<15
1–300 mg	Trace to 1+	15–30
300–800 mg	2+	30–60
800–1000 mg	3+	60–150
1–2 g	4+	>150
Iron overload	—	>500–1000

ferritin values averaging 100 μg/L, while adult females have levels averaging 30 μg/L. As iron stores are depleted, the serum ferritin falls to <15 μg/L. Such levels are diagnostic of absent body iron stores.

Evaluation of Bone Marrow Iron Stores Although RE iron stores can be estimated from the iron stain of a bone marrow aspirate or biopsy, the measurement of serum ferritin has largely supplanted these procedures for determination of storage iron (Table 126-3). The serum ferritin level is a better indicator of iron overload than the marrow iron stain. However, in addition to storage iron, the marrow iron stain provides information about the effective delivery of iron to developing erythroblasts. Normally, when the marrow smear is stained for iron, 20–40% of developing erythroblasts—called *sideroblasts*—will have visible ferritin granules in their cytoplasm. This represents iron in excess of that needed for hemoglobin synthesis. In states in which release of iron from storage sites is blocked, RE iron will be detectable, and there will be few or no sideroblasts. In the myelodysplastic syndromes, mitochondrial dysfunction can occur, and accumulation of iron in mitochondria appears in a necklace fashion around the nucleus of the erythroblast. Such cells are referred to as *ringed sideroblasts*.

Red Cell Protoporphyrin Levels Protoporphyrin is an intermediate in the pathway to heme synthesis. Under conditions in which heme synthesis is impaired, protoporphyrin accumulates within the red cell. This reflects an inadequate iron supply to erythroid precursors to support hemoglobin synthesis. Normal values are <30 μg/dL of red cells. In iron deficiency, values in excess of 100 μg/dL are seen. The most common causes of increased red cell protoporphyrin levels are absolute or relative iron deficiency and lead poisoning.

Serum Levels of Transferrin Receptor Protein Because erythroid cells have the highest numbers of transferrin receptors of any cell in the body, and because transferrin receptor protein (TRP) is released by cells into the circulation, serum levels of TRP reflect the total erythroid marrow mass. Another condition in which TRP levels are elevated is absolute iron deficiency. Normal values are 4–9 μg/L determined by immunoassay. This laboratory test is becoming increasingly available and, along with the serum ferritin, has been proposed to distinguish between iron deficiency and the anemia of inflammation (see below).

DIFFERENTIAL DIAGNOSIS

Other than iron deficiency, only three conditions need to be considered in the differential diagnosis of a hypochromic microcytic anemia (Table 126-4). The first is an inherited defect in globin chain synthesis: the thalassemias. These are differentiated from iron deficiency most readily by serum iron values; normal or increased serum iron levels and transferrin saturation are characteristic of the thalassemias. In addition, the red blood cell distribution width (RDW) index is generally normal in thalassemia and elevated in iron deficiency.

The second condition is the anemia of inflammation (AI; also referred to as the anemia of chronic disease) with inadequate iron supply to the erythroid marrow. The distinction between true iron-deficiency anemia and AI is among the most common diagnostic problems encountered by clinicians (see below). Usually, AI is normocytic and normochromic. The iron values usually make the differential diagnosis clear, as the ferritin level is normal or increased and the percent transferrin saturation and TIBC are typically below normal.

Finally, the myelodysplastic syndromes represent the third and least common condition. Occasionally, patients with myelodysplasia have impaired hemoglobin synthesis with mitochondrial dysfunction, resulting in impaired iron incorporation into heme. The iron values again reveal normal stores and more than an adequate supply to the marrow, despite the microcytosis and hypochromia.

TREATMENT IRON-DEFICIENCY ANEMIA

The severity and cause of iron-deficiency anemia will determine the appropriate approach to treatment. As an example, symptomatic elderly patients with severe iron-deficiency anemia and cardiovascular instability may require red cell transfusions. Younger individuals who have compensated for their anemia can be treated more conservatively with iron replacement. The foremost issue for the latter patient is the precise identification of the cause of the iron deficiency.

For the majority of cases of iron deficiency (pregnant women, growing children and adolescents, patients with infrequent episodes of bleeding, and those with inadequate dietary intake of iron), oral iron therapy will suffice. For patients with unusual blood loss or malabsorption, specific diagnostic tests and appropriate therapy take priority. Once the diagnosis of iron-deficiency anemia and its cause is made, there are three major therapeutic approaches.

RED CELL TRANSFUSION

Transfusion therapy is reserved for individuals who have symptoms of anemia, cardiovascular instability, and continued and excessive blood loss from whatever source and who require immediate intervention. The management of these patients is less related to the iron deficiency than it is to the consequences of the severe anemia. Not only do transfusions correct the anemia acutely, but the transfused red cells provide a source of iron for reutilization, assuming they are not lost through continued bleeding. Transfusion therapy will stabilize the patient while other options are reviewed.

ORAL IRON THERAPY

In the asymptomatic patient with established iron-deficiency anemia, treatment with oral iron is usually adequate. Multiple preparations are available, ranging from simple iron salts to complex iron compounds designed for sustained release throughout the small intestine (Table 126-5). Although the various preparations

TABLE 126-4 DIAGNOSIS OF MICROCYTIC ANEMIA

Tests	Iron Deficiency	Inflammation	Thalassemia	Sideroblastic Anemia
Smear	Micro/hypo	Normal micro/hypo	Micro/hypo with targeting	Variable
Serum iron (μg/dL)	<30	<50	Normal to high	Normal to high
TIBC (μg/dL)	>360	<300	Normal	Normal
Percent saturation	<10	10–20	30–80	30–80
Ferritin (μg/L)	<15	30–200	50–300	50–300
Hemoglobin pattern on electrophoresis	Normal	Normal	Abnormal with β thalassemia; can be normal with α thalassemia	Normal

Abbreviation: TIBC, total iron-binding capacity.

TABLE 126-5 ORAL IRON PREPARATIONS

Generic Name	Tablet (Iron Content), mg	Elixir (Iron Content), mg in 5 mL
Ferrous sulfate	325 (65)	300 (60)
	195 (39)	90 (18)
Extended release	525 (105)	
Ferrous fumarate	325 (107)	
	195 (64)	100 (33)
Ferrous gluconate	325 (39)	300 (35)
Polysaccharide iron	150 (150)	100 (100)
	50 (50)	

contain different amounts of iron, they are generally all absorbed well and are effective in treatment. Some come with other compounds designed to enhance iron absorption, such as ascorbic acid. It is not clear whether the benefits of such compounds justify their costs. Typically, for iron replacement therapy, up to 200 mg of elemental iron per day is given, usually as three or four iron tablets (each containing 50–65 mg elemental iron) given over the course of the day. Ideally, oral iron preparations should be taken on an empty stomach, since food may inhibit iron absorption. Some patients with gastric disease or prior gastric surgery require special treatment with iron solutions, because the retention capacity of the stomach may be reduced. The retention capacity is necessary for dissolving the shell of the iron tablet before the release of iron. A dose of 200 mg of elemental iron per day should result in the absorption of iron up to 50 mg/d. This supports a red cell production level of two to three times normal in an individual with a normally functioning marrow and appropriate erythropoietin stimulus. However, as the hemoglobin level rises, erythropoietin stimulation decreases, and the amount of iron absorbed is reduced. The goal of therapy in individuals with iron-deficiency anemia is not only to repair the anemia, but also to provide stores of at least 0.5–1 g of iron. Sustained treatment for a period of 6–12 months after correction of the anemia will be necessary to achieve this.

Of the complications of oral iron therapy, gastrointestinal distress is the most prominent and is seen in 15–20% of patients. Abdominal pain, nausea, vomiting, or constipation may lead to noncompliance. Although small doses of iron or iron preparations with delayed release may help somewhat, the gastrointestinal side effects are a major impediment to the effective treatment of a number of patients.

The response to iron therapy varies, depending on the erythropoietin stimulus and the rate of absorption. Typically, the reticulocyte count should begin to increase within 4–7 days after initiation of therapy and peak at 1–1½ weeks. The absence of a response may be due to poor absorption, noncompliance (which is common), or a confounding diagnosis. A useful test in the clinic to determine the patient's ability to absorb iron is the *iron tolerance test*. Two iron tablets are given to the patient on an empty stomach, and the serum iron is measured serially over the subsequent 2 h. Normal absorption will result in an increase in the serum iron of at least 100 μg/dL. If iron deficiency persists despite adequate treatment, it may be necessary to switch to parenteral iron therapy.

PARENTERAL IRON THERAPY

Intravenous iron can be given to patients who are unable to tolerate oral iron; whose needs are relatively acute; or who need iron on an ongoing basis, usually due to persistent gastrointestinal blood loss. Parenteral iron use has been increasing rapidly in the last several years with the recognition that recombinant erythropoietin (EPO) therapy induces a large demand for iron—a demand that frequently cannot be met through the physiologic release of iron from RE sources or oral iron absorption. The safety of parenteral iron—particularly iron dextran—has been a concern. The serious adverse reaction rate to intravenous high-molecular-weight iron dextran is 0.7%. Fortunately, newer iron complexes are available in the United States, such as ferumoxytol (Feraheme), sodium ferric gluconate (Ferrlecit), iron sucrose (Venofer), and ferric carboxymaltose (Injectafer), that have much lower rates of adverse effects. Ferumoxytol delivers 510 mg of iron per injection; ferric gluconate 125 mg per injection, ferric carboxymaltose 750 mg per injection, and iron sucrose 200 mg per injection.

Parenteral iron is used in two ways: one is to administer the total dose of iron required to correct the hemoglobin deficit and provide the patient with at least 500 mg of iron stores; the second is to give repeated small doses of parenteral iron over a protracted period. The latter approach is common in dialysis centers, where it is not unusual for 100 mg of elemental iron to be given weekly for 10 weeks to augment the response to recombinant EPO therapy. The amount of iron needed by an individual patient is calculated by the following formula:

$$\text{Body weight (kg)} \times 2.3 \times (15 - \text{patient's hemoglobin, g/dL}) + 500 \text{ or } 1000 \text{ mg (for stores)}.$$

In administering intravenous iron dextran, anaphylaxis is a concern. Anaphylaxis is much rarer with the newer preparations. The factors that have correlated with an anaphylactic-like reaction include a history of multiple allergies or a prior allergic reaction to dextran (in the case of iron dextran). Generalized symptoms appearing several days after the infusion of a large dose of iron can include arthralgias, skin rash, and low-grade fever. These may be dose-related, but they do not preclude the further use of parenteral iron in the patient. To date, patients with sensitivity to iron dextran have been safely treated with other parenteral iron preparations. If a large dose of iron dextran is to be given (>100 mg), the iron preparation should be diluted in 5% dextrose in water or 0.9% NaCl solution. The iron solution can then be infused over a 60- to 90-min period (for larger doses) or at a rate convenient for the attending nurse or physician. Although a test dose (25 mg) of parenteral iron dextran is recommended, in reality a slow infusion of a larger dose of parenteral iron solution will afford the same kind of early warning as a separately injected test dose. Early in the infusion of iron, if chest pain, wheezing, a fall in blood pressure, or other systemic symptoms occur, the infusion of iron should be stopped immediately.

OTHER HYPOPROLIFERATIVE ANEMIAS

In addition to mild to moderate iron-deficiency anemia, the hypoproliferative anemias can be divided into four categories: (1) chronic inflammation, (2) renal disease, (3) endocrine and nutritional deficiencies (hypometabolic states), and (4) marrow damage (Chap. 130). With chronic inflammation, renal disease, or hypometabolism, endogenous EPO production is inadequate for the degree of anemia observed. For the anemia of chronic inflammation, the erythroid marrow also responds inadequately to stimulation, due in part to defective *iron reutilization*. As a result of the lack of adequate EPO stimulation, an examination of the peripheral blood smear will disclose only an occasional polychromatophilic ("shift") reticulocyte. In cases of iron deficiency or marrow damage, appropriate elevations in endogenous EPO levels are typically found, and shift reticulocytes will be present on the blood smear.

ANEMIA OF ACUTE AND CHRONIC INFLAMMATION/INFECTION (AI)

AI—which encompasses inflammation, infection, tissue injury, and conditions (such as cancer) associated with the release of proinflammatory cytokines—is one of the most common forms of anemia seen clinically. It is the most important anemia in the differential diagnosis of iron deficiency, because many of the features of the anemia are brought about by inadequate iron delivery to the marrow, despite the presence of normal or increased iron stores. This is reflected by a low serum iron, increased red cell protoporphyrin, a hypoproliferative marrow, transferrin saturation in the range of 15–20%, and a normal or increased serum ferritin. The serum ferritin values are often the most distinguishing features between true iron-deficiency anemia and the iron-restricted erythropoiesis associated with inflammation. Typically, serum ferritin values increase threefold over basal levels

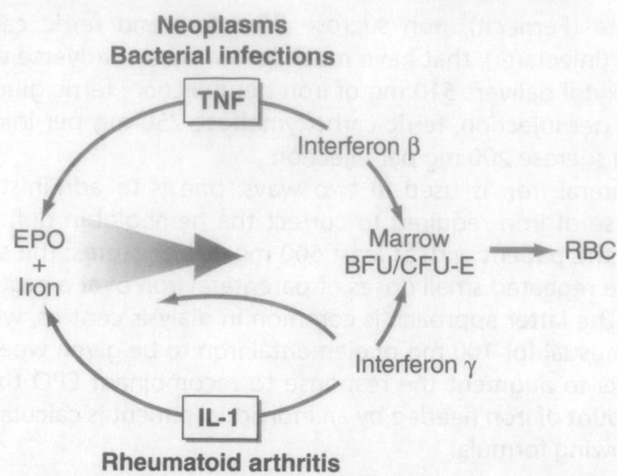

FIGURE 126-4 Suppression of erythropoiesis by inflammatory cytokines. Through the release of tumor necrosis factor (TNF) and interferon γ (IFN-γ), neoplasms and bacterial infections suppress erythropoietin (EPO) production and the proliferation of erythroid progenitors (erythroid burst-forming units and erythroid colony-forming units [BFU/CFU-E]). The mediators in patients with vasculitis and rheumatoid arthritis include interleukin 1 (IL-1) and IFN-γ. The *red arrows* indicate sites of inflammatory cytokine inhibitory effects. RBC, red blood cell.

in the face of inflammation. These changes are due to the effects of inflammatory cytokines and hepcidin, the key iron regulatory hormone, acting at several levels of erythropoiesis (Fig. 126-4).

Interleukin 1 (IL-1) directly decreases EPO production in response to anemia. IL-1, acting through accessory cell release of interferon γ (IFN-γ), suppresses the response of the erythroid marrow to EPO—an effect that can be overcome by EPO administration in vitro and in vivo. In addition, tumor necrosis factor (TNF), acting through the release of IFN-γ by marrow stromal cells, also suppresses the response to EPO. Hepcidin, made by the liver, is increased in inflammation via an IL-6 mediated pathway, and acts to suppress iron absorption and iron release from storage sites. The overall result is a chronic hypoproliferative anemia with classic changes in iron metabolism. The anemia is further compounded by a mild to moderate shortening in red cell survival.

With chronic inflammation, the primary disease will determine the severity and characteristics of the anemia. For example, many patients with cancer also have anemia that is typically normocytic and normochromic. In contrast, patients with long-standing active rheumatoid arthritis or chronic infections such as tuberculosis will have a microcytic, hypochromic anemia. In both cases, the bone marrow is hypoproliferative, but the differences in red cell indices reflect differences in the availability of iron for hemoglobin synthesis. Occasionally, conditions associated with chronic inflammation are also associated with chronic blood loss. Under these circumstances, a bone marrow aspirate stained for iron may be necessary to rule out absolute iron deficiency. However, the administration of iron in this case will correct the iron deficiency component of the anemia and leave the inflammatory component unaffected.

The anemia associated with acute infection or inflammation is typically mild but becomes more pronounced over time. Acute infection can produce a decrease in hemoglobin levels of 2–3 g/dL within 1 or 2 days; this is largely related to the hemolysis of red cells near the end of their natural life span. The fever and cytokines released exert a selective pressure against cells with more limited capacity to maintain the red cell membrane. In most individuals, the mild anemia is reasonably well tolerated, and symptoms, if present, are associated with the underlying disease. Occasionally, in patients with preexisting cardiac disease, moderate anemia (hemoglobin 10–11 g/dL) may be associated with angina, exercise intolerance, and shortness of breath. The erythropoietic profile that distinguishes the anemia of inflammation from the other causes of hypoproliferative anemias is shown in Table 126-6.

TABLE 126-6 DIAGNOSIS OF HYPOPROLIFERATIVE ANEMIAS

Tests	Iron Deficiency	Inflammation	Renal Disease	Hypometabolic States
Anemia	Mild to severe	Mild	Mild to severe	Mild
MCV (fL)	60–90	80–90	90	90
Morphology	Normo-microcytic	Normocytic	Normocytic	Normocytic
SI (μg/dL)	<30	<50	Normal	Normal
TIBC (μg/dL)	>360	<300	Normal	Normal
Saturation (%)	<10	10–20	Normal	Normal
Serum ferritin (μg/L)	<15	30–200	115–150	Normal
Iron stores	0	2–4+	1–4+	Normal

Abbreviations: MCV, mean corpuscular volume; SI, serum iron; TIBC, total iron-binding capacity.

ANEMIA OF CHRONIC KIDNEY DISEASE (CKD)

Progressive CKD is usually associated with a moderate to severe hypoproliferative anemia; the level of the anemia correlates with the stage of CKD. Red cells are typically normocytic and normochromic, and reticulocytes are decreased. The anemia is primarily due to a failure of EPO production by the diseased kidney and a reduction in red cell survival. In certain forms of acute renal failure, the correlation between the anemia and renal function is weaker. Patients with the hemolytic-uremic syndrome increase erythropoiesis in response to the hemolysis, despite renal failure requiring dialysis. Polycystic kidney disease also shows a smaller degree of EPO deficiency for a given level of renal failure. By contrast, patients with diabetes or myeloma have more severe EPO deficiency for a given level of renal failure.

Assessment of iron status provides information to distinguish the anemia of CKD from the other forms of hypoproliferative anemia (Table 126-6) and to guide management. Patients with the anemia of CKD usually present with normal serum iron, TIBC, and ferritin levels. However, those maintained on chronic hemodialysis may develop iron deficiency from blood loss through the dialysis procedure. Iron must be replenished in these patients to ensure an adequate response to EPO therapy (see below).

ANEMIA IN HYPOMETABOLIC STATES

Patients who are starving, particularly for protein, and those with a variety of endocrine disorders that produce lower metabolic rates, may develop a mild to moderate hypoproliferative anemia. The release of EPO from the kidney is sensitive to the need for O_2, not just O_2 levels. Thus, EPO production is triggered at lower levels of blood O_2 content in disease states (such as hypothyroidism and starvation) where metabolic activity, and thus O_2 demand, is decreased.

Endocrine Deficiency States The difference in the levels of hemoglobin between men and women is related to the effects of androgen and estrogen on erythropoiesis. Testosterone and anabolic steroids augment erythropoiesis; castration and estrogen administration to males decrease erythropoiesis. Patients who are hypothyroid or have deficits in pituitary hormones also may develop a mild anemia. Pathogenesis may be complicated by other nutritional deficiencies because iron and folic acid absorption can be affected by these disorders. Usually, correction of the hormone deficiency reverses the anemia.

Anemia may be more severe in Addison's disease, depending on the level of thyroid and androgen hormone dysfunction; however, anemia may be masked by decreases in plasma volume. Once such patients are given cortisol and volume replacement, the hemoglobin level may fall rapidly. Mild anemia complicating hyperparathyroidism may be due to decreased EPO production as a consequence of the renal effects of hypercalcemia or to impaired proliferation of erythroid progenitors.

Protein Starvation Decreased dietary intake of protein may lead to mild to moderate hypoproliferative anemia; this form of anemia may be prevalent in the elderly. The anemia can be more severe in patients with a greater degree of starvation. In marasmus, where patients are both protein and calorie deficient, the release of EPO is impaired in proportion to the reduction in metabolic rate; however, the degree of anemia may be masked by volume depletion and becomes apparent after refeeding. Deficiencies in other nutrients (iron, folate) may also complicate the clinical picture but may not be apparent at diagnosis. Changes in the erythrocyte indices on refeeding should prompt evaluation of iron, folate, and B_{12} status.

Anemia in Liver Disease A mild hypoproliferative anemia may develop in patients with chronic liver disease from nearly any cause. The peripheral blood smear may show spur cells and stomatocytes from the accumulation of excess cholesterol in the membrane from a deficiency of lecithin-cholesterol acyltransferase. Red cell survival is shortened, and the production of EPO is inadequate to compensate. In alcoholic liver disease, nutritional deficiencies are common and complicate the management. Folate deficiency from inadequate intake, as well as iron deficiency from blood loss and inadequate intake, can alter the red cell indices.

TREATMENT HYPOPROLIFERATIVE ANEMIAS

Many patients with hypoproliferative anemias experience recovery of normal hemoglobin levels when the underlying disease is appropriately treated. For those in whom such reversals are not possible—such as patients with end-stage kidney disease, cancer, and chronic inflammatory diseases—symptomatic anemia requires treatment. The two major forms of treatment are transfusions and EPO.

TRANSFUSIONS

Thresholds for transfusion should be determined based on the patient's symptoms. In general, patients without serious underlying cardiovascular or pulmonary disease can tolerate hemoglobin levels above 7–8 g/dL and do not require intervention until the hemoglobin falls below that level. Patients with more physiologic compromise may need to have their hemoglobin levels kept above 11 g/dL. Usually, a unit of packed red cells increases the hemoglobin level by 1 g/dL. Transfusions are associated with certain infectious risks (Chap. 138e), and chronic transfusions can produce iron overload. Importantly, the liberal use of blood has been associated with increased morbidity and mortality, particularly in the intensive care setting. Therefore, in the absence of documented tissue hypoxia, a conservative approach to the use of red cell transfusions is preferable.

ERYTHROPOIETIN (EPO)

EPO is particularly useful in anemias in which endogenous EPO levels are inappropriately low, such as CKD or AI. Iron status must be evaluated and iron replaced to obtain optimal effects from EPO. In patients with CKD, the usual dose of EPO is 50–150 U/kg three times a week intravenously. Hemoglobin levels of 10–12 g/dL are usually reached within 4–6 weeks if iron levels are adequate; 90% of these patients respond. Once a target hemoglobin level is achieved, the EPO dose can be decreased. A decrease in hemoglobin level occurring in the face of EPO therapy usually signifies the development of an infection or iron depletion. Aluminum toxicity and hyperparathyroidism can also compromise the response to EPO. When an infection intervenes, it is best to interrupt the EPO therapy and rely on transfusions to correct the anemia until the infection is adequately treated. The dose of EPO needed to correct chemotherapy-induced anemia in patients with cancer is higher, up to 300 U/kg three times a week, and only approximately 60% of patients respond. Because of evidence that there is an increased risk of thromboembolic complications and tumor progression with EPO administration, the risks and benefits of using EPO in such patients must be weighed carefully, and the target hemoglobin should be that necessary to avoid transfusions.

Longer-acting preparations of EPO can reduce the frequency of injections. Darbepoetin alfa, a molecularly modified EPO with additional carbohydrate, has a half-life in the circulation that is three to four times longer than recombinant human EPO, permitting weekly or every other week dosing.

127 Disorders of Hemoglobin

Edward J. Benz, Jr.

Hemoglobin is critical for normal oxygen delivery to tissues; it is also present in erythrocytes in such high concentrations that it can alter red cell shape, deformability, and viscosity. Hemoglobinopathies are disorders affecting the structure, function, or production of hemoglobin. These conditions are usually inherited and range in severity from asymptomatic laboratory abnormalities to death in utero. Different forms may present as hemolytic anemia, erythrocytosis, cyanosis, or vasoocclusive stigmata.

PROPERTIES OF THE HUMAN HEMOGLOBINS

HEMOGLOBIN STRUCTURE

Different hemoglobins are produced during embryonic, fetal, and adult life (Fig. 127-1). Each consists of a tetramer of globin polypeptide chains: a pair of α-like chains 141 amino acids long and a pair of β-like chains 146 amino acids long. The major adult hemoglobin, HbA, has the structure $\alpha_2\beta_2$. HbF ($\alpha_2\gamma_2$) predominates during most of gestation, and HbA$_2$ ($\alpha_2\delta_2$) is minor adult hemoglobin. Embryonic hemoglobins need not be considered here.

Each globin chain enfolds a single heme moiety, consisting of a protoporphyrin IX ring complexed with a single iron atom in the ferrous state (Fe^{2+}). Each heme moiety can bind a single oxygen molecule; a molecule of hemoglobin can transport up to four oxygen molecules.

The amino acid sequences of the various globins are highly homologous to one another. Each has a highly helical *secondary structure.* Their globular *tertiary structures* cause the exterior surfaces to be rich in polar (hydrophilic) amino acids that enhance solubility, and the interior to be lined with nonpolar groups, forming a hydrophobic pocket into which heme is inserted. The tetrameric *quaternary structure* of HbA contains two αβ dimers. Numerous tight interactions (i.e., $\alpha_1\beta_1$ contacts) hold the α and β chains together. The complete tetramer is held together by interfaces (i.e., $\alpha_1\beta_2$ contacts) between the α-like chain of one dimer and the non-α chain of the other dimer.

The hemoglobin tetramer is highly soluble, but individual globin chains are insoluble. Unpaired globin precipitates, forming inclusions that damage the cell and can trigger apoptosis. Normal globin chain synthesis is balanced so that each newly synthesized α or non-α globin chain will have an available partner with which to pair.

Solubility and reversible oxygen binding are the key properties deranged in hemoglobinopathies. Both depend most on the hydrophilic surface amino acids, the hydrophobic amino acids lining the heme pocket, a key histidine in the F helix, and the amino acids forming the $\alpha_1\beta_1$ and $\alpha_1\beta_2$ contact points. Mutations in these strategic regions tend to be the ones that alter oxygen affinity or solubility.

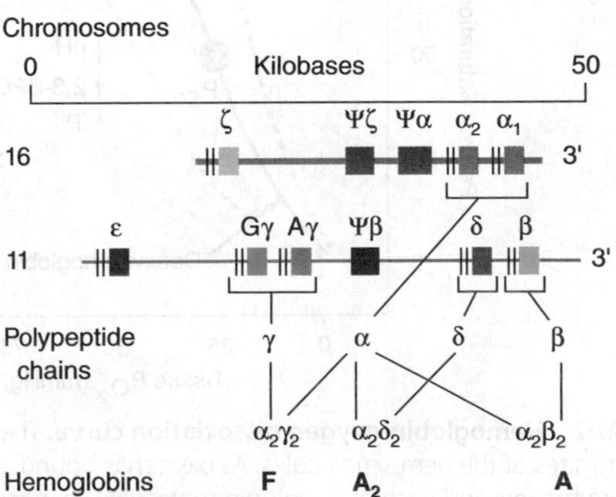

FIGURE 127-1 The globin genes. The α-like genes (α, ζ) are encoded on chromosome 16; the β-like genes (β, γ, δ, ε) are encoded on chromosome 11. The ζ and ε genes encode embryonic globins.

To support oxygen transport, hemoglobin must bind O_2 efficiently at the partial pressure of oxygen (Po_2) of the alveolus, retain it in the circulation, and release it to tissues at the Po_2 of tissue capillary beds. Oxygen acquisition and delivery over a relatively narrow range of oxygen tensions depend on a property inherent in the tetrameric arrangement of heme and globin subunits within the hemoglobin molecule called *cooperativity* or *heme-heme interaction.*

At low oxygen tensions, the hemoglobin tetramer is fully deoxygenated (Fig. 127-2). Oxygen binding begins slowly as O_2 tension rises. However, as soon as some oxygen has been bound by the tetramer, an abrupt increase occurs in the slope of the curve. Thus, hemoglobin molecules that have bound some oxygen develop a higher oxygen affinity, greatly accelerating their ability to combine with more oxygen. This S-shaped oxygen equilibrium curve (Fig. 127-2), along which substantial amounts of oxygen loading *and unloading* can occur over a narrow range of oxygen tensions, is physiologically more useful than the high-affinity hyperbolic curve of individual monomers.

Oxygen affinity is modulated by several factors. The Bohr effect is the ability of hemoglobin to deliver more oxygen to tissues at low pH. It arises from the stabilizing action of protons on deoxyhemoglobin, which binds protons more readily than oxyhemoglobin because the latter is a weaker acid (Fig. 127-2). Thus, hemoglobin has a lower oxygen affinity at low pH. The major small molecule that alters oxygen affinity in humans is 2,3-bisphosphoglycerate (2,3-BPG; formerly 2,3-DPG), which lowers oxygen affinity when bound to hemoglobin. HbA has a reasonably high affinity for 2,3-BPG. HbF does not bind 2,3-BPG, so it tends to have a higher oxygen affinity in vivo. Hemoglobin also binds nitric oxide reversibly; this interaction influences vascular tone, but its clinical relevance remains incompletely understood.

Proper oxygen transport depends on the tetrameric structure of the proteins, the proper arrangement of hydrophilic and hydrophobic amino acids, and interaction with protons or 2,3-BPG.

DEVELOPMENTAL BIOLOGY OF HUMAN HEMOGLOBINS

Red cells first appearing at about 6 weeks after conception contain the embryonic hemoglobins Hb Portland ($\zeta_2\gamma_2$), Hb Gower I ($\zeta_2\varepsilon_2$), and Hb Gower II ($\alpha_2\varepsilon_2$). At 10–11 weeks, fetal hemoglobin (HbF; $\alpha_2\gamma_2$) becomes predominant. The switch to nearly exclusive synthesis of adult hemoglobin (HbA; $\alpha_2\beta_2$) occurs at about 38 weeks (Fig. 127-1). Fetuses and newborns therefore require α-globin but not β-globin for normal gestation. A major advance in understanding the HbF to HbA transition has been the demonstration that the transcription factor Bcl11a plays a pivotal role in its regulation. Small amounts of HbF are produced during postnatal life. A few red cell clones called *F cells* are progeny of a small pool of immature committed erythroid precursors (BFU-e) that retain the ability to produce HbF. Profound erythroid stresses, such as severe hemolytic anemias, bone marrow transplantation, or cancer chemotherapy, cause more of the F-potent BFU-e to be recruited. HbF levels thus tend to rise in some patients with sickle cell anemia or thalassemia. This phenomenon probably explains the ability of hydroxyurea to increase levels of HbF in adults. Agents such as butyrate and histone deacetylase inhibitors can also activate fetal globin genes partially after birth.

GENETICS AND BIOSYNTHESIS OF HUMAN HEMOGLOBIN

The human hemoglobins are encoded in two tightly linked gene clusters; the α-like globin genes are clustered on chromosome 16 and the β-like genes on chromosome 11 (Fig. 127-1). The α-like cluster consists of two α-globin genes and a single copy of the ζ gene. The non-α gene cluster consists of a single ε gene, the Gγ and Aγ fetal globin genes, and the adult δ and β genes.

Important regulatory sequences flank each gene. Immediately upstream are typical promoter elements needed for the assembly of the transcription initiation complex. Sequences in the 5′ flanking region of the γ and the β genes appear to be crucial for the correct developmental regulation of these genes, whereas elements that function like classic enhancers and silencers are in the 3′ flanking regions. The locus control region (LCR) elements located far upstream appear to control the overall level of expression of each cluster. These elements achieve their regulatory effects by interacting with *trans*-acting transcription factors. Some of these factors are ubiquitous (e.g., Sp1 and YY1), while others are more or less limited to erythroid cells or hematopoietic cells (e.g., GATA-1, NFE-2, and EKLF). The LCR controlling the α-globin gene cluster is modulated by a SWI/SNF-like protein called *ATRX*; this protein appears to influence chromatin remodeling and DNA methylation. The association of α thalassemia with mental retardation and myelodysplasia in some families appears to be related to mutations in the ATRX pathway. This pathway also modulates genes specifically expressed during erythropoiesis, such

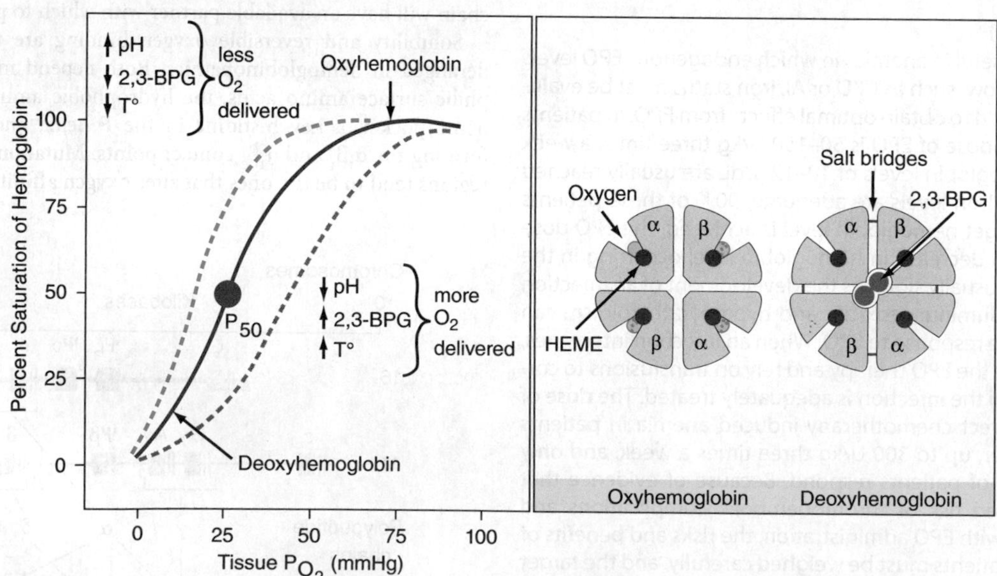

FIGURE 127-2 Hemoglobin-oxygen dissociation curve. The hemoglobin tetramer can bind up to four molecules of oxygen in the iron-containing sites of the heme molecules. As oxygen is bound, 2,3-bisphosphoglycerate (2,3-BPG) and carbon dioxide (CO_2) are expelled. Salt bridges are broken, and each of the globin molecules changes its conformation to facilitate oxygen binding. Oxygen release to the tissues is the reverse process, with salt bridges being formed and 2,3-BPG and CO_2 bound. Deoxyhemoglobin does not bind oxygen efficiently until the cell returns to conditions of higher pH, the most important modulator of O_2 affinity (Bohr effect). When acid is produced in the tissues, the dissociation curve shifts to the right, facilitating oxygen release and CO_2 binding. Alkalosis has the opposite effect, reducing oxygen delivery.

as those that encode the enzymes for heme biosynthesis. Normal red blood cell (RBC) differentiation requires the coordinated expression of the globin genes with the genes responsible for heme and iron metabolism. RBC precursors contain a protein, α-hemoglobin-stabilizing protein (AHSP), that enhances the folding and solubility of α globin, which is otherwise easily denatured, leading to insoluble precipitates. These precipitates play an important role in the thalassemia syndromes and certain unstable hemoglobin disorders. Polymorphic variation in the amounts and/or functional capacity of AHSP might explain some of the clinical variability seen in patients inheriting identical thalassemia mutations.

CLASSIFICATION OF HEMOGLOBINOPATHIES

There are five major classes of hemoglobinopathies (Table 127-1). *Structural hemoglobinopathies* occur when mutations alter the amino acid sequence of a globin chain, altering the physiologic properties of the variant hemoglobins and producing the characteristic clinical abnormalities. The most clinically relevant variant hemoglobins polymerize abnormally, as in sickle cell anemia, or exhibit altered solubility or oxygen-binding affinity. *Thalassemia syndromes* arise from mutations that impair production or translation of globin mRNA, leading to deficient globin chain biosynthesis. Clinical abnormalities are attributable to the inadequate supply of hemoglobin and the imbalances in the production of individual globin chains, leading to premature destruction of erythroblasts and RBC. *Thalassemic hemoglobin variants* combine features of thalassemia (e.g., abnormal globin biosynthesis) and of structural hemoglobinopathies (e.g., an abnormal amino acid sequence). *Hereditary persistence of fetal hemoglobin* (HPFH) is characterized by synthesis of high levels of fetal hemoglobin in adult life. *Acquired hemoglobinopathies* include modifications of the hemoglobin molecule by toxins (e.g., acquired methemoglobinemia) and clonal abnormalities of hemoglobin synthesis (e.g., high levels of HbF production in preleukemia and α thalassemia in myeloproliferative disorders).

TABLE 127-1 CLASSIFICATION OF HEMOGLOBINOPATHIES

I. Structural hemoglobinopathies—hemoglobins with altered amino acid sequences that result in deranged function or altered physical or chemical properties
   - A. Abnormal hemoglobin polymerization—HbS, hemoglobin sickling
   - B. Altered O_2 affinity
     - 1. High affinity—polycythemia
     - 2. Low affinity—cyanosis, pseudoanemia
   - C. Hemoglobins that oxidize readily
     - 1. Unstable hemoglobins—hemolytic anemia, jaundice
     - 2. M hemoglobins—methemoglobinemia, cyanosis

II. Thalassemias—defective biosynthesis of globin chains
   - A. α Thalassemias
   - B. β Thalassemias
   - C. δβ, γδβ, αβ Thalassemias

III. Thalassemic hemoglobin variants—structurally abnormal Hb associated with coinherited thalassemic phenotype
   - A. HbE
   - B. Hb Constant Spring
   - C. Hb Lepore

IV. Hereditary persistence of fetal hemoglobin—persistence of high levels of HbF into adult life

V. Acquired hemoglobinopathies
   - A. Methemoglobin due to toxic exposures
   - B. Sulfhemoglobin due to toxic exposures
   - C. Carboxyhemoglobin
   - D. HbH in erythroleukemia
   - E. Elevated HbF in states of erythroid stress and bone marrow dysplasia

EPIDEMIOLOGY

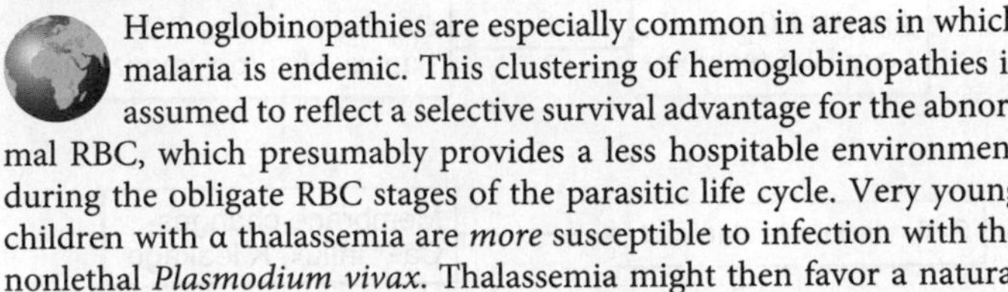

Hemoglobinopathies are especially common in areas in which malaria is endemic. This clustering of hemoglobinopathies is assumed to reflect a selective survival advantage for the abnormal RBC, which presumably provides a less hospitable environment during the obligate RBC stages of the parasitic life cycle. Very young children with α thalassemia are *more* susceptible to infection with the nonlethal *Plasmodium vivax*. Thalassemia might then favor a natural protection against infection with the more lethal *Plasmodium falciparum*.

Thalassemias are the most common genetic disorders in the world, affecting nearly 200 million people worldwide. About 15% of African Americans are silent carriers for α thalassemia; α thalassemia trait (minor) occurs in 3% of African American and in 1–15% of persons of Mediterranean origin. β Thalassemia has a 10–15% incidence in individuals from the Mediterranean and Southeast Asia and 0.8% in African Americans. The number of severe cases of thalassemia in the United States is about 1000. Sickle cell disease is the most common structural hemoglobinopathy, occurring in heterozygous form in ~8% of African Americans and in homozygous form in 1 in 400. Between 2 and 3% of African Americans carry a hemoglobin C allele.

INHERITANCE AND ONTOGENY

Hemoglobinopathies are autosomal codominant traits—thus, compound heterozygotes who inherit a different abnormal mutant allele from each parent exhibit composite features of each. For example, patients inheriting sickle β thalassemia exhibit features of β thalassemia and sickle cell anemia. The α chain is present in HbA, HbA_2, and HbF; α-chain mutations thus cause abnormalities in all three. The α-globin hemoglobinopathies are symptomatic in utero and after birth because normal function of the α-globin gene is required throughout gestation and adult life. In contrast, infants with β-globin hemoglobinopathies tend to be asymptomatic until 3–9 months of age, when HbA has largely replaced HbF. Prevention or partial reversion of the switch should thus be an effective therapeutic strategy for β-chain hemoglobinopathies.

DETECTION AND CHARACTERIZATION OF HEMOGLOBINOPATHIES—GENERAL METHODS

Electrophoretic techniques are still widely used for hemoglobin analysis. Electrophoresis at pH 8.6 on cellulose acetate membranes is especially simple, inexpensive, and reliable for initial screening. Agar gel electrophoresis at pH 6.1 in citrate buffer is often used as a complementary method because each method detects different variants. Some important variants are electrophoretically silent. These mutant hemoglobins can usually be characterized by more specialized techniques such as mass spectroscopy, which is rapidly replacing electrophoresis for initial analysis.

Quantitation of the hemoglobin profile is often desirable. HbA_2 is frequently elevated in β thalassemia trait and depressed in iron deficiency. HbF is elevated in HPFH, some β thalassemia syndromes, and occasional periods of erythroid stress or marrow dysplasia. For characterization of sickle cell trait, sickle thalassemia syndromes, or HbSC disease, and for monitoring the progress of exchange transfusion therapy to lower the percentage of circulating HbS, quantitation of individual hemoglobins is also required. In most laboratories, quantitation is performed only if the test is specifically ordered. Complete characterization, including amino acid sequencing or gene cloning and sequencing, is readily available from several reference laboratories.

Because some variants can comigrate with HbA or HbS (sickle hemoglobin), electrophoretic assessment should always be regarded as incomplete unless functional assays for hemoglobin sickling, solubility, or oxygen affinity are also performed, as dictated by the clinical presentation. The best sickling assays involve measurement of the degree to which the hemoglobin sample becomes insoluble, or gelated, as it is deoxygenated (i.e., sickle solubility test). Unstable hemoglobins are detected by their precipitation in isopropanol or after heating to 50°C. High-O_2 affinity and low-O_2 affinity variants are detected

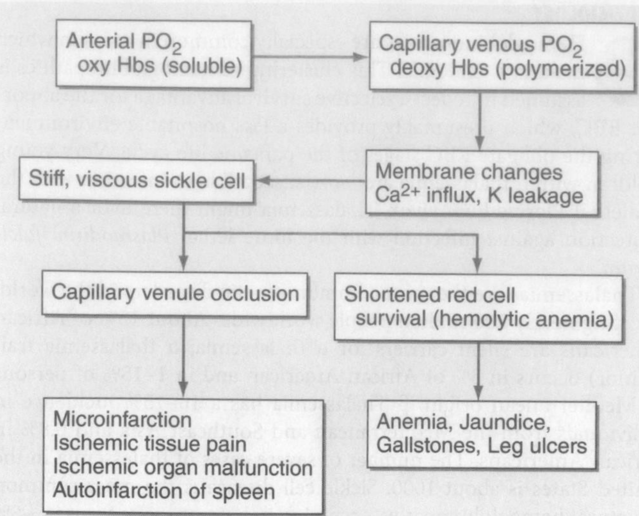

FIGURE 127-3 Pathophysiology of sickle cell crisis.

by quantitating the P_{50}, the partial pressure of oxygen at which the hemoglobin sample becomes 50% saturated with oxygen. Direct tests for the percent carboxyhemoglobin and methemoglobin, using spectrophotometric techniques, can readily be obtained from most clinical laboratories on an urgent basis.

Laboratory evaluation remains an adjunct, rather than the sole diagnostic aid. Diagnosis is best established by recognition of a characteristic history, physical findings, peripheral blood smear morphology, and abnormalities of the complete blood cell count (e.g., profound microcytosis with minimal anemia in thalassemia trait).

STRUCTURALLY ABNORMAL HEMOGLOBINS

SICKLE CELL SYNDROMES

The sickle cell syndromes are caused by a mutation in the β-globin gene that changes the sixth amino acid from glutamic acid to valine. HbS ($\alpha_2\beta_2^{6\ Glu\to Val}$) polymerizes reversibly when deoxygenated to form a gelatinous network of fibrous polymers that stiffen the RBC membrane, increase viscosity, and cause dehydration due to potassium leakage and calcium influx (Fig. 127-3). These changes also produce the sickle shape. Sickled cells lose the pliability needed to traverse small capillaries. They possess altered "sticky" membranes that are abnormally adherent to the endothelium of small venules. These abnormalities provoke unpredictable episodes of microvascular vasoocclusion and premature RBC destruction (hemolytic anemia). Hemolysis occurs because the spleen destroys the abnormal RBC. The rigid adherent cells clog small capillaries and venules, causing tissue ischemia, acute pain, and gradual end-organ damage. This venooc-clusive component usually dominates the clinical course. Prominent manifestations include episodes of ischemic pain (i.e., painful crises) and ischemic malfunction or frank infarction in the spleen, central nervous system, bones, joints, liver, kidneys, and lungs (Fig. 127-3).

Several sickle syndromes occur as the result of inheritance of HbS from one parent and another hemoglobinopathy, such as β thalassemia or HbC ($\alpha_2\beta_2^{6\ Glu\to Lys}$), from the other parent. The prototype disease, sickle cell anemia, is the homozygous state for HbS (Table 127-2).

Clinical Manifestations of Sickle Cell Anemia Most patients with sickling syndromes suffer from hemolytic anemia, with hematocrits from 15 to 30%, and significant reticulocytosis. Anemia was once thought to exert protective effects against vasoocclusion by reducing blood viscosity. However, natural history and drug therapy trials suggest that an *increase* in the hematocrit and feedback inhibition of reticulocytosis might be beneficial, even at the expense of increased blood viscosity. The role of adhesive reticulocytes in vasoocclusion might account for these paradoxical effects.

Granulocytosis is common. The white count can fluctuate substantially and unpredictably during and between painful crises, infectious episodes, and other intercurrent illnesses.

Vasoocclusion causes protean manifestations. Intermittent episodes of vasoocclusion in connective and musculoskeletal structures produce ischemia manifested by acute pain and tenderness, fever, tachycardia, and anxiety. These recurrent episodes, called *painful crises*, are the most common clinical manifestation. Their frequency and severity vary greatly. Pain can develop almost anywhere in the body and may last from a few hours to 2 weeks. Repeated crises requiring hospitalization (>3 episodes per year) correlate with reduced survival in adult life, suggesting that these episodes are associated with accumulation of chronic end-organ damage. Provocative factors include infection, fever, excessive exercise, anxiety, abrupt changes in temperature, hypoxia, or hypertonic dyes.

Repeated microinfarction can destroy tissues having microvascular beds prone to sickling. Thus, splenic function is frequently lost within the first 18–36 months of life, causing susceptibility to infection, particularly by pneumococci. Acute venous obstruction of the spleen (*splenic sequestration crisis*), a rare occurrence in early childhood, may require emergency transfusion and/or splenectomy to prevent trapping of the entire arterial output in the obstructed spleen. Occlusion of retinal vessels can produce hemorrhage, neovascularization, and eventual detachments. Renal papillary necrosis invariably produces isosthenuria. More widespread renal necrosis leads to renal failure in adults, a common late cause of death. Bone and joint ischemia can lead to aseptic necrosis, especially of the femoral or humeral heads; chronic arthropathy; and unusual susceptibility to osteomyelitis, which may be caused by organisms, such as *Salmonella*, rarely encountered in other settings. The *hand-foot syndrome* is caused by painful infarcts of the digits and dactylitis. Stroke is especially common in children; a small subset tends to suffer repeated episodes. Stroke is less common in adults and is often hemorrhagic. A particularly painful complication in males is priapism, due to infarction of the penile venous outflow tracts; permanent impotence is a frequent consequence. Chronic lower leg ulcers probably arise from ischemia and superinfection in the distal circulation.

Acute chest syndrome is a distinctive manifestation characterized by chest pain, tachypnea, fever, cough, and arterial oxygen desaturation. It can mimic pneumonia, pulmonary emboli, bone marrow infarction and embolism, myocardial ischemia, or in situ lung infarction. Acute chest syndrome is thought to reflect in situ sickling within the lung, producing pain and temporary pulmonary dysfunction. Often it is difficult or impossible to distinguish among other possibilities. Pulmonary infarction and pneumonia are the most frequent underlying or concomitant conditions in patients with this syndrome. Repeated episodes of acute chest pain correlate with reduced survival. Acutely, reduction in arterial oxygen saturation is especially ominous because it promotes sickling on a massive

TABLE 127-2 CLINICAL FEATURES OF SICKLE HEMOGLOBINOPATHIES

Condition	Clinical Abnormalities	Hemoglobin Level, g/L (g/dL)	MCV, fL	Hemoglobin Electrophoresis
Sickle cell trait	None; rare painless hematuria	Normal	Normal	HbS/A: 40/60
Sickle cell anemia	Vasoocclusive crises with infarction of spleen, brain, marrow, kidney, lung; aseptic necrosis of bone; gallstones; priapism; ankle ulcers	70–100 (7–10)	80–100	HbS/A: 100/0 HbF: 2–25%
S/β° thalassemia	Vasoocclusive crises; aseptic necrosis of bone	70–100 (7–10)	60–80	HbS/A: 100/0 HbF: 1–10%
S/β+ thalassemia	Rare crises and aseptic necrosis	100–140 (10–14)	70–80	HbS/A: 60/40
Hemoglobin SC	Rare crises and aseptic necrosis; painless hematuria	100–140 (10–14)	80–100	HbS/A: 50/0 HbC: 50%

scale. Chronic acute or subacute pulmonary crises lead to pulmonary hypertension and cor pulmonale, an increasingly common cause of death as patients survive longer. Considerable controversy exists about the possible role played by free plasma HbS in scavenging nitrogen dioxide (NO_2), thus raising pulmonary vascular tone. Trials of sildenafil to restore NO_2 levels were terminated because of adverse effects.

Chronic subacute central nervous system damage in the absence of an overt stroke is a distressingly common phenomenon beginning in early childhood. Modern functional imaging techniques have pinpointed circulatory dysfunction due to a likely CNS sickle vasculopathy; these changes correlate with an array of cognitive and behavioral abnormalities in children and young adults. It is important to be aware of these often subtle changes because they can complicate clinical management or be misinterpreted as "difficult patient" behaviors.

Sickle cell syndromes are remarkable for their clinical heterogeneity. Some patients remain virtually asymptomatic into or even through adult life, while others suffer repeated crises requiring hospitalization from early childhood. Patients with sickle thalassemia and sickle-HbE tend to have similar, slightly milder symptoms, perhaps because of the ameliorating effects of production of other hemoglobins within the RBC. Hemoglobin SC disease, one of the more common variants of sickle cell anemia, is frequently marked by lesser degrees of hemolytic anemia and a greater propensity for the development of retinopathy and aseptic necrosis of bones. In most respects, however, the clinical manifestations resemble sickle cell anemia. Some rare hemoglobin variants actually aggravate the sickling phenomenon.

The clinical variability in different patients inheriting the same disease-causing mutation (sickle hemoglobin) has made sickle cell disease the focus of efforts to identify modifying genetic polymorphisms in other genes that might account for the heterogeneity. The complexity of the data obtained thus far has dampened the expectation that genome-wide analysis will yield individualized profiles that predict a patient's clinical course. Nevertheless, a number of interesting patterns have emerged from these modifying gene analyses. For example, genes affecting the inflammatory response or cytokine expression appear to be modifying candidates. Genes that affect transcriptional regulation of lymphocytes may also be involved.

Clinical Manifestations of Sickle Cell Trait Sickle cell trait is often asymptomatic. Anemia and painful crises are rare. An uncommon but highly distinctive symptom is painless hematuria often occurring in adolescent males, probably due to papillary necrosis. Isosthenuria is a more common manifestation of the same process. Sloughing of papillae with urethral obstruction has been reported, as have isolated cases of massive sickling or sudden death due to exposure to high altitudes or extremes of exercise and dehydration. Avoidance of dehydration or extreme physical stress should be advised.

Diagnosis Sickle cell syndromes are suspected on the basis of hemolytic anemia, RBC morphology (Fig. 127-4), and intermittent episodes of ischemic pain. Diagnosis is confirmed by hemoglobin electrophoresis, mass spectroscopy, and the sickling tests already discussed. Thorough characterization of the exact hemoglobin profile of the patient is important, because sickle thalassemia and hemoglobin SC disease have distinct prognoses or clinical features. Diagnosis is usually established in childhood, but occasional patients, often with compound heterozygous states, do not develop symptoms until the onset of puberty, pregnancy, or early adult life. Genotyping of family members and potential parental partners is critical for genetic counseling. Details of the childhood history establish prognosis and need for aggressive or experimental therapies. Factors associated with increased morbidity and reduced survival include more than three crises requiring hospitalization per year, chronic neutrophilia, a history of splenic sequestration or hand-foot syndrome, and second episodes of acute chest syndrome. Patients with a history of cerebrovascular accidents are at higher risk for repeated episodes and require partial exchange transfusion and especially close monitoring using Doppler carotid flow measurements. Patients with severe or repeated episodes of acute chest syndrome may need lifelong transfusion support, using partial exchange transfusion, if possible.

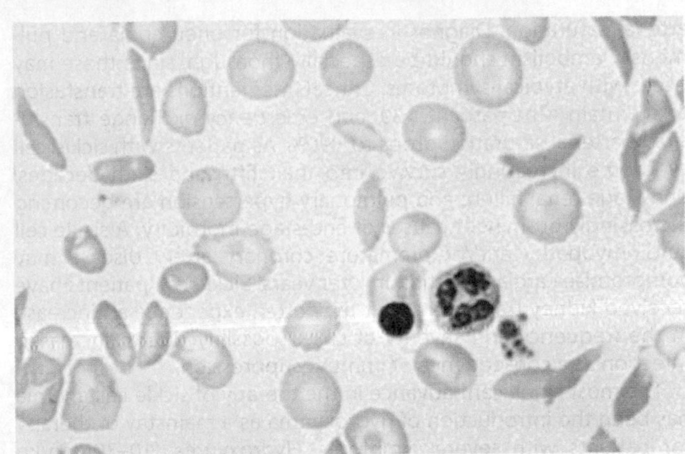

FIGURE 127-4 Sickle cell anemia. The elongated and crescent-shaped red blood cells seen on this smear represent circulating irreversibly sickled cells. Target cells and a nucleated red blood cell are also seen.

TREATMENT SICKLE CELL SYNDROMES

Patients with sickle cell syndromes require ongoing continuity of care. Familiarity with the pattern of symptoms provides the best safeguard against excessive use of the emergency room, hospitalization, and habituation to addictive narcotics. Additional preventive measures include regular slit-lamp examinations to monitor development of retinopathy; antibiotic prophylaxis appropriate for splenectomized patients during dental or other invasive procedures; and vigorous oral hydration during or in anticipation of periods of extreme exercise, exposure to heat or cold, emotional stress, or infection. Pneumococcal and *Haemophilus influenzae* vaccines are less effective in splenectomized individuals. Thus, patients with sickle cell anemia should be vaccinated early in life.

The management of an acute painful crisis includes vigorous hydration, thorough evaluation for underlying causes (such as infection), and aggressive analgesia administered by a standing order and/or patient-controlled analgesia (PCA) pump. Morphine (0.1–0.15 mg/kg every 3–4 h) should be used to control severe pain. Bone pain may respond as well to ketorolac (30–60 mg initial dose, then 15–30 mg every 6–8 h). Inhalation of nitrous oxide can provide short-term pain relief, but great care must be exercised to avoid hypoxia and respiratory depression. Nitrous oxide also elevates O_2 affinity, reducing O_2 delivery to tissues. Its use should be restricted to experts. Many crises can be managed at home with oral hydration and oral analgesia. Use of the emergency room should be reserved for especially severe symptoms or circumstances in which other processes, e.g., infection, are strongly suspected. Nasal oxygen should be used as appropriate to protect arterial saturation. Most crises resolve in 1–7 days. Use of blood transfusion should be reserved for extreme cases: transfusions do not shorten the duration of the crisis.

No tests are definitive to diagnose acute painful crisis. Critical to good management is an approach that recognizes that most patients reporting crisis symptoms do indeed have crisis or another significant medical problem. Diligent diagnostic evaluation for underlying causes is imperative, even though these are found infrequently. In adults, the possibility of aseptic necrosis or sickle arthropathy must be considered, especially if pain and immobility become repeated or chronic at a single site. Nonsteroidal anti-inflammatory agents are often effective for sickle cell arthropathy.

Acute chest syndrome is a medical emergency that may require management in an intensive care unit. Hydration should be monitored carefully to avoid the development of pulmonary edema, and oxygen therapy should be especially vigorous for protection of arterial saturation. Diagnostic evaluation for pneumonia and pulmonary embolism should be especially thorough, since these may occur with atypical symptoms. Critical interventions are transfusion to maintain a hematocrit >30, and emergency exchange transfusion if arterial saturation drops to <90%. As patients with sickle cell syndrome increasingly survive into their fifth and sixth decades, end-stage renal failure and pulmonary hypertension are becoming increasingly prominent causes of end-stage morbidity. A sickle cell cardiomyopathy and/or premature coronary artery disease may compromise cardiac function in later years. Sickle cell patients have received kidney transplants, but they often experience an increase in the frequency and severity of crises, possibly due to increased infection as a consequence of immunosuppression.

The most significant advance in the therapy of sickle cell anemia has been the introduction of hydroxyurea as a mainstay of therapy for patients with severe symptoms. Hydroxyurea (10–30 mg/kg per day) increases fetal hemoglobin and may also exert beneficial effects on RBC hydration, vascular wall adherence, and suppression of the granulocyte and reticulocyte counts; dosage is titrated to maintain a white cell count between 5000 and 8000/μL. White cells and reticulocytes may play a major role in the pathogenesis of sickle cell crisis, and their suppression may be an important side benefit of hydroxyurea therapy.

Hydroxyurea should be considered in patients experiencing repeated episodes of acute chest syndrome or with more than three crises per year requiring hospitalization. The utility of this agent for reducing the incidence of other complications (priapism, retinopathy) is under evaluation, as are the long-term side effects. To date, however, minimal risk of bone marrow dyscrasias or other neoplasms has been documented. Hydroxyurea offers broad benefits to most patients whose disease is severe enough to impair their functional status, and it may improve survival. HbF levels increase in most patients within a few months.

The antitumor drug 5-azacytidine was the first agent found to elevate HbF. It never achieved widespread use because of concerns about acute toxicity and carcinogenesis. However, low doses of the related agent 5-deoxyazacytidine (decitabine) can elevate HbF with more acceptable toxicity.

Bone marrow transplantation can provide definitive cures but is known to be effective and safe only in children. Clinical trials studying partially myeloablative conditioning regimens ("mini" transplants) are likely to support more widespread use of this modality in older patients. Prognostic features justifying bone marrow transplant are the presence of repeated crises early in life, a high neutrophil count, or the development of hand-foot syndrome. Children at risk for stroke can now be identified through the use of Doppler ultrasound techniques. Prophylactic exchange transfusion appears to substantially reduce the risk of stroke in this population. Children who do suffer a cerebrovascular accident should be maintained for at least 3–5 years on a program of vigorous exchange transfusion, as the risk of second strokes is extremely high.

Gene therapy for sickle cell anemia is being intensively pursued, but no safe measures are currently available. The development of newer methods of direct gene correction in situ (e.g., zinc finger nucleases, or "CRISPR" [clustered regularly interspaced short palindromic repeats] technology) could well find clinical use in these patients. Experimental methods of derepressing HbF by interfering with Bcl11a are also being explored.

UNSTABLE HEMOGLOBINS

Amino acid substitutions that reduce solubility or increase susceptibility to oxidation result in unstable hemoglobins that precipitate, forming inclusion bodies injurious to the RBC membrane. Representative mutations are those that interfere with contact points between the α and β subunits (e.g., Hb Philly [$\beta^{35Tyr\to Phe}$]), alter the helical segments (e.g., Hb Genova [$\beta^{28Leu\to Pro}$]), or disrupt interactions of the hydrophobic pockets of the globin subunits with heme (e.g., Hb Köln [$\beta^{98Val\to Met}$]) (Table 127-3). The inclusions, called *Heinz bodies*, are clinically detectable by staining with supravital dyes such as crystal violet. Removal of these inclusions by the spleen generates pitted, rigid cells that have shortened life spans, producing hemolytic anemia of variable severity, sometimes requiring chronic transfusion support. Splenectomy may be needed to correct the anemia. Leg ulcers and premature gallbladder disease due to bilirubin loading are frequent stigmata.

TABLE 127-3 REPRESENTATIVE ABNORMAL HEMOGLOBINS WITH ALTERED SYNTHESIS OR FUNCTION

Designation	Mutation	Population	Main Clinical Effects[a]
Sickle or S	$\beta^{6Glu\to Val}$	African	Anemia, ischemic infarcts
C	$\beta^{6Glu\to Lys}$	African	Mild anemia; interacts with HbS
E	$\beta^{26Glu\to Lys}$	Southeast Asian	Microcytic anemia, splenomegaly, thalassemic phenotype
Köln	$\beta^{98Val\to Met}$	Sporadic	Hemolytic anemia, Heinz bodies when splenectomized
Yakima	$\beta^{99Asp\to His}$	Sporadic	Polycythemia
Kansas	$\beta^{102Asn\to Lys}$	Sporadic	Mild anemia
M Iwata	$\beta^{87His\to Tyr}$	Sporadic	Methemoglobinemia

[a]See text for details.

Unstable hemoglobins occur sporadically, often by spontaneous new mutations. Heterozygotes are often symptomatic because a significant Heinz body burden can develop even when the unstable variant accounts for only a portion of the total hemoglobin. Symptomatic unstable hemoglobins tend to be β-globin variants, because sporadic mutations affecting only one of the four α globins alleles would generate only 20–30% abnormal hemoglobin.

HEMOGLOBINS WITH ALTERED OXYGEN AFFINITY

High-affinity hemoglobins (e.g., Hb Yakima [$\beta^{99Asp\to His}$]) bind oxygen more readily but deliver less O_2 to tissues at normal capillary Po_2 levels (Fig. 127-2). Mild tissue hypoxia ensues, stimulating RBC production and erythrocytosis (Table 127-3). In extreme cases, the hematocrits can rise to 60–65%, increasing blood viscosity and producing typical symptoms (headache, somnolence, or dizziness). Phlebotomy may be required. Typical mutations alter interactions within the heme pocket or disrupt the Bohr effect or salt-bond site. Mutations that impair the interaction of HbA with 2,3-BPG can increase O_2 affinity because 2,3-BPG binding lowers O_2 affinity.

Low-affinity hemoglobins (e.g., Hb Kansas [$\beta^{102Asn\to Lys}$]) bind sufficient oxygen in the lungs, despite their lower oxygen affinity, to achieve nearly full saturation. At capillary oxygen tensions, they lose sufficient amounts of oxygen to maintain homeostasis at a low hematocrit (Fig. 127-2) (*pseudoanemia*). Capillary hemoglobin desaturation can also be sufficient to produce clinically apparent cyanosis. Despite these findings, patients usually require no specific treatment.

METHEMOGLOBINEMIAS

Methemoglobin is generated by oxidation of the heme iron moieties to the ferric state, causing a characteristic bluish-brown muddy color resembling cyanosis. Methemoglobin has such high oxygen affinity that virtually no oxygen is delivered. Levels >50–60% are often fatal.

Congenital methemoglobinemia arises from globin mutations that stabilize iron in the ferric state (e.g., HbM Iwata [$\alpha^{87His\to Tyr}$], Table 127-3) or from mutations that impair the enzymes that reduce methemoglobin to hemoglobin (e.g., methemoglobin reductase, NADP diaphorase). Acquired methemoglobinemia is caused by toxins that oxidize heme iron, notably nitrate and nitrite-containing compounds, including drugs commonly used in cardiology and anesthesiology.

DIAGNOSIS AND MANAGEMENT OF PATIENTS WITH UNSTABLE HEMOGLOBINS, HIGH-AFFINITY HEMOGLOBINS, AND METHEMOGLOBINEMIA

Unstable hemoglobin variants should be suspected in patients with nonimmune hemolytic anemia, jaundice, splenomegaly, or premature biliary tract disease. Severe hemolysis usually presents during infancy as neonatal jaundice or anemia. Milder cases may present in adult life with anemia or only as unexplained reticulocytosis, hepatosplenomegaly, premature biliary tract disease, or leg ulcers. Because spontaneous mutation is common, family history of anemia may be absent. The peripheral blood smear often shows anisocytosis, abundant cells with punctate inclusions, and irregular shapes (i.e., poikilocytosis).

The two best tests for diagnosing unstable hemoglobins are the Heinz body preparation and the isopropanol or heat stability test. Many unstable Hb variants are electrophoretically silent. A normal electrophoresis does not rule out the diagnosis. Mass spectroscopy or direct gene analysis will provide a definitive diagnosis.

Severely affected patients may require transfusion support for the first 3 years of life, because splenectomy before age 3 is associated with a significantly higher immune deficit. Splenectomy is usually effective thereafter, but occasional patients may require lifelong transfusion support. After splenectomy, patients can develop cholelithiasis and leg ulcers, hypercoagulable states, and susceptibility to overwhelming sepsis. Splenectomy should thus be avoided or delayed unless it is the only alternative. Precipitation of unstable hemoglobins is aggravated by oxidative stress, e.g., infection and antimalarial drugs, which should be avoided where possible.

High-O_2 affinity hemoglobin variants should be suspected in patients with erythrocytosis. The best test for confirmation is measurement of the P_{50}. A high-O_2 affinity hemoglobin causes a significant left shift (i.e., lower numeric value of the P_{50}); confounding conditions, e.g., tobacco smoking or carbon monoxide exposure, can also lower the P_{50}.

High-affinity hemoglobins are often asymptomatic; rubor or plethora may be telltale signs. When the hematocrit approaches 60%, symptoms of high blood viscosity and sluggish flow (headache, lethargy, dizziness, etc.) may be present. These persons may benefit from judicious phlebotomy. Erythrocytosis represents an appropriate attempt to compensate for the impaired oxygen delivery by the abnormal variant. Overzealous phlebotomy may stimulate increased erythropoiesis or aggravate symptoms by thwarting this compensatory mechanism. The guiding principle of phlebotomy should be to improve oxygen delivery by reducing blood viscosity and increasing blood flow rather than restoration of a normal hematocrit. Phlebotomy-induced modest iron deficiency may aid in control.

Low-affinity hemoglobins should be considered in patients with cyanosis or a low hematocrit with no other reason apparent after thorough evaluation. The P_{50} test confirms the diagnosis. Counseling and reassurance are the interventions of choice.

Methemoglobin should be suspected in patients with hypoxic symptoms who appear cyanotic but have a Pao_2 sufficiently high that hemoglobin should be fully saturated with oxygen. A history of nitrite or other oxidant ingestions may not always be available; some exposures may be inapparent to the patient, and others may result from suicide attempts. The characteristic muddy appearance of freshly drawn blood can be a critical clue. The best diagnostic test is methemoglobin assay, which is usually available on an emergency basis.

Methemoglobinemia often causes symptoms of cerebral ischemia at levels >15%; levels >60% are usually lethal. Intravenous injection of 1 mg/kg of methylene blue is effective emergency therapy. Milder cases and follow-up of severe cases can be treated orally with methylene blue (60 mg three to four times each day) or ascorbic acid (300–600 mg/d).

THALASSEMIA SYNDROMES

The thalassemia syndromes are inherited disorders of α- or β-globin biosynthesis. The reduced supply of globin diminishes production of hemoglobin tetramers, causing hypochromia and microcytosis. Unbalanced accumulation of α and β subunits occurs because the synthesis of the unaffected globins proceeds at a normal rate. Unbalanced chain accumulation dominates the clinical phenotype. Clinical severity varies widely, depending on the degree to which the synthesis of the affected globin is impaired, altered synthesis of other globin chains, and coinheritance of other abnormal globin alleles.

CLINICAL MANIFESTATIONS OF β THALASSEMIA SYNDROMES

Mutations causing thalassemia can affect any step in the pathway of globin gene expression: transcription, processing of the mRNA precursor, translation, and posttranslational metabolism of the β-globin polypeptide chain. The most common forms arise from mutations that derange splicing of the mRNA precursor or prematurely terminate translation of the mRNA.

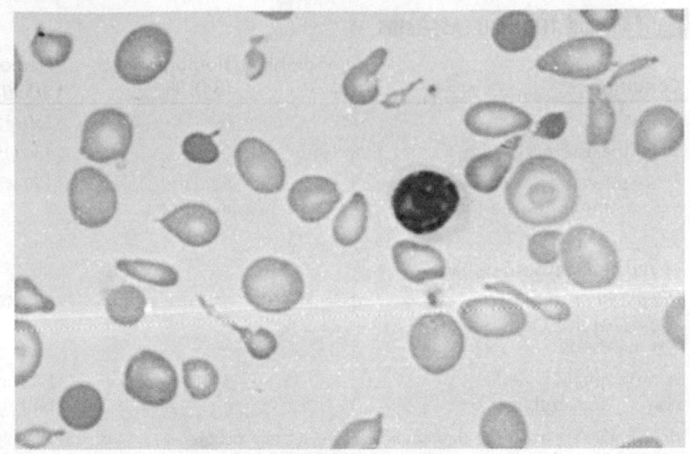

FIGURE 127-5 β Thalassemia intermedia. Microcytic and hypochromic red blood cells are seen that resemble the red blood cells of severe iron-deficiency anemia. Many elliptical and teardrop-shaped red blood cells are noted.

Hypochromia and microcytosis characterize all forms of β thalassemia because of the reduced amounts of hemoglobin tetramers (Fig. 127-5). In heterozygotes (β thalassemia trait), this is the only abnormality seen. Anemia is minimal. In more severe homozygous states, unbalanced α- and β-globin accumulation causes accumulation of highly insoluble unpaired α chains. They form toxic inclusion bodies that kill developing erythroblasts in the marrow. Few of the proerythroblasts beginning erythroid maturation survive. The surviving RBCs bear a burden of inclusion bodies that are detected in the spleen, shortening the RBC life span and producing severe hemolytic anemia. The resulting profound anemia stimulates erythropoietin release and compensatory erythroid hyperplasia, but the marrow response is sabotaged by the ineffective erythropoiesis. Anemia persists. Erythroid hyperplasia can become exuberant and produce masses of extramedullary erythropoietic tissue in the liver and spleen.

Massive bone marrow expansion deranges growth and development. Children develop characteristic "chipmunk" facies due to maxillary marrow hyperplasia and frontal bossing. Thinning and pathologic fracture of long bones and vertebrae may occur due to cortical invasion by erythroid elements and profound growth retardation. Hemolytic anemia causes hepatosplenomegaly, leg ulcers, gallstones, and high-output congestive heart failure. The conscription of caloric resources to support erythropoiesis leads to inanition, susceptibility to infection, endocrine dysfunction, and in the most severe cases, death during the first decade of life. Chronic transfusions with RBCs improve oxygen delivery, suppress the excessive ineffective erythropoiesis, and prolong life, but the inevitable side effects, notably iron overload, often prove fatal by age 30 years.

Severity is highly variable. Known modulating factors are those that ameliorate the burden of unpaired α-globin inclusions. Alleles associated with milder synthetic defects and coinheritance of α thalassemia trait reduce clinical severity by reducing accumulation of excess α globin. HbF persists to various degrees in β thalassemias. γ-Globin gene chains can substitute for β chains, generating more hemoglobin and reducing the burden of α-globin inclusions. The terms *β thalassemia major* and *β thalassemia intermedia* are used to reflect the clinical heterogeneity. Patients with β thalassemia major require intensive transfusion support to survive. Patients with β thalassemia intermedia have a somewhat milder phenotype and can survive without transfusion. The terms *β thalassemia minor* and *β thalassemia trait* describe asymptomatic heterozygotes for β thalassemia.

THALASSEMIA SYNDROMES

The four classic α thalassemias, most common in Asians, are α thalassemia-2 trait, in which one of the four α-globin loci is deleted;

TABLE 127-4 THE α THALASSEMIAS

Condition	Hemoglobin A, %	Hemoglobin H (β4), %	Hemoglobin Level, g/L (g/dL)	MCV, fL
Normal	97	0	150 (15)	90
Silent thalassemia: –α/αα	98–100	0	150 (15)	90
Thalassemia trait: –α/–α homozygous α-thal-2[a] or ––/αα heterozygous α-thal-1[a]	85–95	Rare red blood cell inclusions	120–130 (12–13)	70–80
Hemoglobin H disease: ––/–α heterozygous α-thal-1/α-thal-2	70–95	5–30	60–100 (6–10)	60–70
Hydrops fetalis: ––/–– homozygous α-thal-1	0	5–10[b]	Fatal in utero or at birth	

[a]When both α alleles on one chromosome are deleted, the locus is called α-thal-1; when only a single α allele on one chromosome is deleted, the locus is called α-thal-2. [b]90–95% of the hemoglobin is hemoglobin Barts (tetramers of γ chains).

α thalassemia-1 trait, with two deleted loci; HbH disease, with three loci deleted; and hydrops fetalis with Hb Barts, with all four loci deleted (Table 127-4). Nondeletion forms of α thalassemia also exist.

α Thalassemia-2 trait is an asymptomatic, silent carrier state. *α Thalassemia-1 trait* resembles β thalassemia minor. Offspring doubly heterozygous for α thalassemia-2 and α thalassemia-1 exhibit a more severe phenotype called *HbH disease*. Heterozygosity for a deletion that removes both genes from the same chromosome (*cis* deletion) is common in Asians and in those from the Mediterranean region, as is homozygosity for α thalassemia-2 (*trans* deletion). Both produce asymptomatic hypochromia and microcytosis.

In *HbH disease*, HbA production is only 25–30% normal. Fetuses accumulate some unpaired γ chains (Hb Barts; γ-chain tetramers). In adults, unpaired β chains accumulate and are soluble enough to form β_4 tetramers called HbH. HbH forms few inclusions in erythroblasts and precipitates in circulating RBC. Patients with HbH disease have thalassemia intermedia characterized by moderately severe hemolytic anemia but milder ineffective erythropoiesis. Survival into midadult life without transfusions is common.

The homozygous state for the α thalassemia-1 *cis* deletion (hydrops fetalis) causes total absence of α-globin synthesis. No physiologically useful hemoglobin is produced beyond the embryonic stage. Excess γ globin forms tetramers called *Hb Barts* (γ_4), which has a very high oxygen affinity. It delivers almost no O_2 to fetal tissues, causing tissue asphyxia, edema (hydrops fetalis), congestive heart failure, and death in utero. α Thalassemia-2 trait is common (15–20%) among people of African descent. The *cis* α thalassemia-1 deletion is almost never seen, however. Thus, α thalassemia-2 and the *trans* form of α thalassemia-1 are very common, but HbH disease and hydrops fetalis are rare.

It has been known for some time that some patients with myelodysplasia or erythroleukemia produce RBC clones containing HbH. This phenomenon is due to mutations in the ATRX pathway that affect the LCR of the α-globin gene cluster.

DIAGNOSIS AND MANAGEMENT OF THALASSEMIAS

The diagnosis of β-thalassemia major is readily made during childhood on the basis of severe anemia accompanied by the characteristic signs of massive ineffective erythropoiesis: hepatosplenomegaly, profound microcytosis, a characteristic blood smear (Fig. 127-5), and elevated levels of HbF, HbA_2, or both. Many patients require chronic hypertransfusion therapy designed to maintain a hematocrit of at least 27–30% so that erythropoiesis is suppressed. Splenectomy is required if the annual transfusion requirement (volume of RBCs per kilogram of body weight per year) increases by >50%. Folic acid supplements may be useful. Vaccination with Pneumovax in anticipation of eventual splenectomy is advised, as is close monitoring for infection, leg ulcers, and biliary tract disease. Many patients develop endocrine deficiencies as a result of iron overload. Early endocrine evaluation is required for glucose intolerance, thyroid dysfunction, and delayed onset of puberty or secondary sexual characteristics.

Patients with β thalassemia intermedia exhibit similar stigmata but can survive without chronic hypertransfusion. Management is particularly challenging because a number of factors can aggravate the anemia, including infection, onset of puberty, and development of splenomegaly and hypersplenism. Some patients may eventually benefit from splenectomy. The expanded erythron can cause absorption of excessive dietary iron and hemosiderosis, even without transfusion. Some patients eventually become transfusion dependent.

β Thalassemia minor (i.e., thalassemia trait) usually presents as profound microcytosis and hypochromia with target cells, but only minimal or mild anemia. The mean corpuscular volume is rarely >75 fL; the hematocrit is rarely <30–33%. Hemoglobin analysis classically reveals an elevated HbA_2 (3.5–7.5%), but some forms are associated with normal HbA_2 and/or elevated HbF. Genetic counseling and patient education are essential. Patients with β thalassemia trait should be warned that their blood picture resembles iron deficiency and can be misdiagnosed. They should eschew empirical use of iron, yet iron deficiency requiring replacement therapy can develop during pregnancy or from chronic bleeding.

Persons with α thalassemia trait may exhibit mild hypochromia and microcytosis usually without anemia. HbA_2 and HbF levels are normal. Affected individuals usually require only genetic counseling. HbH disease resembles β thalassemia intermedia, with the added complication that the HbH molecule behaves like moderately unstable hemoglobin. Patients with HbH disease should undergo splenectomy if excessive anemia or a transfusion requirement develops. Oxidative drugs should be avoided. Iron overload leading to death can occur in more severely affected patients.

PREVENTION

Antenatal diagnosis of thalassemia syndromes is now widely available. DNA diagnosis is based on polymerase chain reaction (PCR) amplification of fetal DNA, obtained by amniocentesis or chorionic villus biopsy followed by hybridization to allele-specific oligonucleotide probes or direct DNA sequencing.

THALASSEMIC STRUCTURAL VARIANTS

Thalassemic structural variants are characterized by both defective synthesis and abnormal structure.

HEMOGLOBIN LEPORE

Hb Lepore $[\alpha_2(\delta\beta)_2]$ arises by an unequal crossover and recombination event that fuses the proximal end of the δ-gene with the distal end of the closely linked β-gene. It is common in the Mediterranean basin. The resulting chromosome contains only the fused δβ gene. The Lepore (δβ) globin is synthesized poorly because the fused gene is under the control of the weak δ-globin promoter. Hb Lepore alleles have a phenotype like β thalassemia, except for the added presence of 2–20% Hb Lepore. Compound heterozygotes for Hb Lepore and a classic β thalassemia allele may also have severe thalassemia.

HEMOGLOBIN E

HbE (i.e., $\alpha_2\beta_2^{26Glu\rightarrow Lys}$) is extremely common in Cambodia, Thailand, and Vietnam. The gene has become far more prevalent in the United States as a result of immigration of Asian persons, especially in California, where HbE is the most common variant detected. HbE is mildly unstable but not enough to affect RBC life span significantly. Heterozygotes resemble individuals with a mild β-thalassemia trait. Homozygotes have somewhat more marked abnormalities but are asymptomatic. Compound heterozygotes for

HbE and a β thalassemia gene can have β thalassemia intermedia or β thalassemia major, depending on the severity of the coinherited thalassemic gene.

The β^E allele contains a single base change in codon 26 that causes the amino acid substitution. This mutation also activates a cryptic RNA splice site, generating a structurally abnormal globin mRNA that cannot be translated, from about 50% of the initial pre-mRNA molecules. The remaining 40–50% are normally spliced and generate functional mRNA that is translated into β^E-globin because the mature mRNA carries the base change that alters codon 26.

Genetic counseling of the persons at risk for HbE should focus especially on the interaction of HbE with β thalassemia, because HbE homozygosity is a condition associated with mildly asymptomatic microcytosis, hypochromia, and hemoglobin levels rarely <100 g/L (<10 g/dL).

HEREDITARY PERSISTENCE OF FETAL HEMOGLOBIN

HPFH is characterized by continued synthesis of high levels of HbF in adult life. No deleterious effects are apparent, even when all of the hemoglobin produced is HbF. These rare patients demonstrate convincingly that prevention or reversal of the fetal to adult hemoglobin switch would provide effective therapy for sickle cell anemia and β thalassemia.

ACQUIRED HEMOGLOBINOPATHIES

The two most important acquired hemoglobinopathies are carbon monoxide poisoning and methemoglobinemia (see above). Carbon monoxide has a higher affinity for hemoglobin than does oxygen; it can replace oxygen and diminish O_2 delivery. Chronic elevation of carboxyhemoglobin levels to 10 or 15%, as occurs in smokers, can lead to secondary polycythemia. Carboxyhemoglobin is cherry red in color and masks the development of cyanosis usually associated with poor O_2 delivery to tissues.

Abnormalities of hemoglobin biosynthesis have also been described in blood dyscrasias. In some patients with myelodysplasia, erythroleukemia, or myeloproliferative disorders, elevated HbF or a mild form of HbH disease may also be seen. The abnormalities are not severe enough to alter the course of the underlying disease.

TREATMENT TRANSFUSIONAL HEMOSIDEROSIS

Chronic blood transfusion can lead to bloodborne infection, alloimmunization, febrile reactions, and lethal iron overload (Chap. 138e). A unit of packed RBCs contains 250–300 mg iron (1 mg/mL). The iron assimilated by a single transfusion of 2 units of packed RBCs is thus equal to a 1- to 2-year oral intake of iron. Iron accumulates in chronically transfused patients because no mechanisms exist for increasing iron excretion: an expanded erythron causes especially rapid development of iron overload because accelerated erythropoiesis promotes excessive absorption of dietary iron. Vitamin C should not be supplemented because it generates free radicals in iron excess states.

Patients who receive >100 units of packed RBCs usually develop hemosiderosis. The ferritin level rises, followed by early endocrine dysfunction (glucose intolerance and delayed puberty), cirrhosis, and cardiomyopathy. Liver biopsy shows both parenchymal and reticuloendothelial iron. The superconducting quantum-interference device (SQUID) is accurate at measuring hepatic iron but not widely available. Cardiac toxicity is often insidious. Early development of pericarditis is followed by dysrhythmia and pump failure. The onset of heart failure is ominous, often presaging death within a year (Chap. 428).

The decision to start long-term transfusion support should also prompt one to institute therapy with iron-chelating agents. Deferoxamine (Desferal) is for parenteral use. Its iron-binding kinetics require chronic slow infusion via a metering pump. The constant presence of the drug improves the efficiency of chelation and protects tissues from occasional releases of the most toxic fraction of iron—low-molecular-weight iron—which may not be sequestered by protective proteins.

Deferoxamine is relatively nontoxic. Occasional cataracts, deafness, and local skin reactions, including urticaria, occur. Skin reactions can usually be managed with antihistamines. Negative iron balance can be achieved, even in the face of a high transfusion requirement, but this alone does not prevent long-term morbidity and mortality in chronically transfused patients. Irreversible end-organ deterioration develops at relatively modest levels of iron overload, even if symptoms do not appear for many years thereafter. To enjoy a significant survival advantage, chelation must begin before 5–8 years of age in β thalassemia major.

Deferasirox is an oral iron-chelating agent. Single daily doses of 20–30 mg/kg deferasirox produced reductions in liver iron concentration comparable to deferoxamine in long-term transfused adult and pediatric patients. Deferasirox produces some elevations in liver enzymes and slight but persistent increases in serum creatinine, without apparent clinical consequence. Other toxicities are similar to those of deferoxamine. Its toxicity profile is acceptable, although long-term effects are still being evaluated.

EXPERIMENTAL THERAPIES

BONE MARROW TRANSPLANTATION, GENE THERAPY, AND MANIPULATION OF HbF

Bone marrow transplantation provides stem cells able to express normal hemoglobin; it has been used in a large number of patients with β thalassemia and a smaller number of patients with sickle cell anemia. Early in the course of disease, before end-organ damage occurs, transplantation is curative in 80–90% of patients. In highly experienced centers, the treatment-related mortality is <10%. Because survival into adult life is possible with conventional therapy, the decision to transplant is best made in consultation with specialized centers.

Gene therapy of thalassemia and sickle cell disease has proved to be an elusive goal, but experimental advances are raising expectations.

Reestablishing high levels of fetal hemoglobin synthesis should ameliorate the symptoms of β-chain hemoglobinopathies. Cytotoxic agents such as hydroxyurea and cytarabine promote high levels of HbF synthesis, probably by stimulating proliferation of the primitive HbF-producing progenitor cell population (i.e., F cell progenitors). Unfortunately, this regimen has not yet been effective in β thalassemia. Butyrates stimulate HbF production, but only transiently. Pulsed or intermittent administration has been found to sustain HbF induction in the majority of patients with sickle cell disease. It is unclear whether butyrates will have similar activity in patients with β thalassemia.

APLASTIC AND HYPOPLASTIC CRISIS IN PATIENTS WITH HEMOGLOBINOPATHIES

Patients with hemolytic anemias sometimes exhibit an alarming decline in hematocrit during and immediately after acute illnesses. Bone marrow suppression occurs in almost everyone during acute and chronic inflammatory illnesses. In patients with short RBC life spans, suppression can affect RBC counts more dramatically. These hypoplastic crises are usually transient and self-correcting before intervention is required.

Aplastic crisis refers to a profound cessation of erythroid activity in patients with chronic hemolytic anemias. It is associated with a rapidly falling hematocrit. Episodes are usually self-limited. Aplastic crises are caused by infection with a particular strain of parvovirus, B19A. Children infected with this virus usually develop permanent immunity. Aplastic crises do not often recur and are rarely seen in adults. Management requires close monitoring of the hematocrit and reticulocyte count. If anemia becomes symptomatic, transfusion support is indicated. Most crises resolve spontaneously within 1–2 weeks.

128 Megaloblastic Anemias

A. Victor Hoffbrand

The megaloblastic anemias are a group of disorders characterized by the presence of distinctive morphologic appearances of the developing red cells in the bone marrow. The marrow is usually hypercellular and the anemia is based on ineffective erythropoiesis. The cause is usually a deficiency of either cobalamin (vitamin B_{12}) or folate, but megaloblastic anemia may occur because of genetic or acquired abnormalities that affect the metabolism of these vitamins or because of defects in DNA synthesis not related to cobalamin or folate (Table 128-1). Cobalamin and folate absorption and metabolism are described next, followed by the biochemical basis, clinical and laboratory features, causes, and treatment of megaloblastic anemia.

COBALAMIN

Cobalamin (vitamin B_{12}) exists in a number of different chemical forms. All have a cobalt atom at the center of a corrin ring. In nature, the vitamin is mainly in the 2-deoxyadenosyl (ado) form, which is located in mitochondria. It is the cofactor for the enzyme methylmalonyl coenzyme A (CoA) mutase. The other major natural cobalamin is methylcobalamin, the form in human plasma and in cell cytoplasm. It is the cofactor for methionine synthase. There are also minor amounts of hydroxocobalamin to which methyl- and adocobalamin are converted rapidly by exposure to light.

DIETARY SOURCES AND REQUIREMENTS

Cobalamin is synthesized solely by microorganisms. Ruminants obtain cobalamin from the foregut, but the only source for humans is food of animal origin, e.g., meat, fish, and dairy products. Vegetables, fruits, and other foods of nonanimal origin are free from cobalamin unless they are contaminated by bacteria. A normal Western diet contains 5–30 μg of cobalamin daily. Adult daily losses (mainly in the urine and feces) are 1–3 μg (~0.1% of body stores), and because the body does not have the ability to degrade cobalamin, daily requirements are also about 1–3 μg. Body stores are of the order of 2–3 mg, sufficient for 3–4 years if supplies are completely cut off.

ABSORPTION

Two mechanisms exist for cobalamin absorption. One is passive, occurring equally through buccal, duodenal, and ileal mucosa; it is rapid but extremely inefficient, with <1% of an oral dose being absorbed by this process. The normal physiologic mechanism is active; it occurs through the ileum and is efficient for small (a few micrograms) oral doses of cobalamin, and it is mediated by gastric intrinsic factor (IF). Dietary cobalamin is released from protein complexes by enzymes in the stomach, duodenum, and jejunum; it combines rapidly with a salivary glycoprotein that belongs to the family of cobalamin-binding proteins known as haptocorrins (HCs). In the intestine, the haptocorrin is digested by pancreatic trypsin and the cobalamin is transferred to IF.

TABLE 128-1 CAUSES OF MEGALOBLASTIC ANEMIA

Cobalamin deficiency or abnormalities of cobalamin metabolism (see Tables 128-3, 128-4)
Folate deficiency or abnormalities of folate metabolism (see Table 128-5)
Therapy with antifolate drugs (e.g., methotrexate)
Independent of either cobalamin or folate deficiency and refractory to cobalamin and folate therapy:
Some cases of acute myeloid leukemia, myelodysplasia
Therapy with drugs interfering with synthesis of DNA (e.g., cytosine arabinoside, hydroxyurea, 6-mercaptopurine, azidothymidine [AZT])
Orotic aciduria (responds to uridine)
Thiamine-responsive

IF (gene at chromosome 11q13) is produced in the gastric parietal cells of the fundus and body of the stomach, and its secretion parallels that of hydrochloric acid. Normally, there is a vast excess of IF. The IF-cobalamin complex passes to the ileum, where IF attaches to a specific receptor (cubilin) on the microvillus membrane of the enterocytes. Cubilin also is present in yolk sac and renal proximal tubular epithelium. Cubilin appears to traffic by means of amnionless (AMN), an endocytic receptor protein that directs sublocalization and endocytosis of cubilin with its ligand IF-cobalamin complex. The cobalamin-IF complex enters the ileal cell, where IF is destroyed. After a delay of about 6 h, the cobalamin appears in portal blood attached to transcobalamin (TC) II.

Between 0.5 and 5 μg of cobalamin enter the bile each day. This binds to IF, and a major portion of biliary cobalamin normally is reabsorbed together with cobalamin derived from sloughed intestinal cells. Because of the appreciable amount of cobalamin undergoing enterohepatic circulation, cobalamin deficiency develops more rapidly in individuals who malabsorb cobalamin than it does in vegans, in whom reabsorption of biliary cobalamin is intact.

TRANSPORT

Two main cobalamin transport proteins exist in human plasma; they both bind cobalamin—one molecule for one molecule. One HC, also known as TC I, is closely related to other cobalamin-binding HCs in milk, gastric juice, bile, saliva, and other fluids. The gene *TCNL* is at chromosome 11q11-q12.3. These HCs differ from each other only in the carbohydrate moiety of the molecule. TC I is derived primarily from the specific granules in neutrophils. Normally, it is about two-thirds saturated with cobalamin, which it binds tightly. TC I does not enhance cobalamin entry into tissues. Glycoprotein receptors on liver cells are involved in the removal of TC I from plasma, and TC I may play a role in the transport of cobalamin analogues (which it binds more effectively than IF) to the liver for excretion in bile.

The other major cobalamin transport protein in plasma is transcobalamin, also known as TC II. The gene is on chromosome 22q11-q13.1. As for IF and HC, there are nine exons. The three proteins are likely to have a common ancestral origin. TC II is synthesized by liver and by other tissues, including macrophages, ileum, and vascular endothelium. It normally carries only 20–60 ng of cobalamin per liter of plasma and readily gives up cobalamin to marrow, placenta, and other tissues, which it enters by receptor-mediated endocytosis involving the TC II receptor and megalin (encoded by the *LRP-2* gene). The TC II cobalamin is internalized by endocytosis via clathrin-coated pits; the complex is degraded, but the receptor probably is recycled to the cell membrane as is the case for transferrin. Export of "free" cobalamin is via the ATP-binding cassette drug transporter alias multidrug resistance protein 1.

FOLATE

DIETARY FOLATE

Folic (pteroylglutamic) acid is a yellow, crystalline, water-soluble substance. It is the parent compound of a large family of natural folate compounds, which differ from it in three respects: (1) they are partly or completely reduced to di- or tetrahydrofolate (THF) derivatives, (2) they usually contain a single carbon unit (Table 128-2), and (3) 70–90% of natural folates are folate-polyglutamates.

Most foods contain some folate. The highest concentrations are found in liver, yeast, spinach, other greens, and nuts (>100 μg/100 g). The total folate content of an average Western diet is ~250 μg daily, but the amount varies widely according to the type of food eaten and the method of cooking. Folate is easily destroyed by heating, particularly in large volumes of water. Total body folate in the adult is ~10 mg, with the liver containing the largest store. Daily adult requirements are ~100 μg, and so stores are sufficient for only 3–4 months in normal adults and severe folate deficiency may develop rapidly.

ABSORPTION

Folates are absorbed rapidly from the upper small intestine. The absorption of folate polyglutamates is less efficient than that of monoglutamates; on average, ~50% of food folate is absorbed. Polyglutamate

TABLE 128-2 BIOCHEMICAL REACTIONS OF FOLATE COENZYMES

Reaction	Coenzyme Form of Folate Involved	Single Carbon Unit Transferred	Importance
Formate activation	THF	–CHO	Generation of 10-formyl-THF
Purine synthesis			
Formation of glycinamide ribonucleotide	5,10-Methylene-THF	–CHO	Formation of purines needed for DNA, RNA synthesis, but reactions probably not rate-limiting
Formylation of aminoimidazole carboxamide ribonucleotide (AICAR)	10-Formyl (CHO)THF		
Pyrimidine synthesis			
Methylation of deoxyuridine monophosphate (dUMP) to thymidine monophosphate (dTMP)	5,10-Methylene-THF	$-CH_3$	Rate limiting in DNA synthesis Oxidizes THF to DHF Some breakdown of folate at the C-9–N-10 bond
Amino acid interconversion			
Serine–glycine interconversion	THF	$=CH_2$	Entry of single carbon units into active pool
Homocysteine to methionine	5-Methyl(M)THF	$-CH_3$	Demethylation of 5-MTHF to THF; also requires cobalamin, flavine adenine dinucleotide, ATP, and adenosylmethionine
Forminoglutamic acid to glutamic acid in histidine catabolism	THF	HN–CH=	

Abbreviations: DHF, dihydrofolate; THF, tetrahydrofolate.

forms are hydrolyzed to the monoglutamate derivatives either in the lumen of the intestine or within the mucosa. All dietary folates are converted to 5-methylTHF (5-MTHF) within the small intestinal mucosa before entering portal plasma. The monoglutamates are actively transported across the enterocyte by a proton-coupled folate transporter (PCFT, SCL46A1). This is situated at the apical brush border and is most active at pH 5.5, which is about the pH of the duodenal and jejunal surface. Genetic mutations of this protein underlie hereditary malabsorption of folate (see below). Pteroylglutamic acid at doses >400 μg is absorbed largely unchanged and converted to natural folates in the liver. Lower doses are converted to 5-MTHF during absorption through the intestine.

About 60–90 μg of folate enters the bile each day and is excreted into the small intestine. Loss of this folate, together with the folate of sloughed intestinal cells, accelerates the speed with which folate deficiency develops in malabsorption conditions.

TRANSPORT

Folate is transported in plasma; about one-third is loosely bound to albumin, and two-thirds is unbound. In all body fluids (plasma, cerebrospinal fluid, milk, bile), folate is largely, if not entirely, 5-MTHF in the monoglutamate form. Three types of folate-binding protein are involved. A reduced folate transporter (RFC, SLC19A1) is the major route of delivery of plasma folate (5-MTHF) to cells. Two folate receptors, FR2 and FR3 embedded in the cell membrane by a glycosyl phosphatidylinositol anchor, transport folate into the cell via receptor-mediated endocytosis. The third protein, PCFT, transports folate at low pH from the vesicle to the cell cytoplasm. The reduced folate transporter also mediates uptake of methotrexate by cells.

BIOCHEMICAL FUNCTIONS

Folates (as the intracellular polyglutamate derivatives) act as coenzymes in the transfer of single-carbon units (Fig. 128-1 and Table 128-2). Two of these reactions are involved in purine synthesis and one in pyrimidine synthesis necessary for DNA and RNA replication. Folate is also a coenzyme for methionine synthesis, in which methylcobalamin is also involved and in which THF is regenerated. THF is the acceptor of single carbon units newly entering the active pool via conversion of serine to glycine. Methionine, the other product of the methionine synthase reaction, is the precursor for *S*-adenosylmethionine (SAM), the universal methyl donor involved in >100 methyltransferase reactions (Fig. 128-1).

During thymidylate synthesis, 5,10-methylene-THF is oxidized to DHF (dihydrofolate). The enzyme DHF reductase converts this to THF. The drugs methotrexate, pyrimethamine, and (mainly in bacteria) trimethoprim inhibit DHF reductase and so prevent formation of active THF coenzymes from DHF. A small fraction of the folate coenzyme is not recycled during thymidylate synthesis but is degraded at the C9-N10 bond.

BIOCHEMICAL BASIS OF MEGALOBLASTIC ANEMIA

The common feature of all megaloblastic anemias is a defect in DNA synthesis that affects rapidly dividing cells in the bone marrow. All conditions that give rise to megaloblastic changes have in common a disparity in the rate of synthesis or availability of the four immediate precursors of DNA: the deoxyribonucleoside triphosphates (dNTPs)—dA(adenine)TP and dG(guanine)TP (purines), dT(thymine)TP and dC(cytosine) TP (pyrimidines). In deficiencies of either folate or cobalamin, there is failure to convert deoxyuridine monophosphate (dUMP) to deoxythymidine monophosphate (dTMP), the precursor of dTTP (Fig 128-1). This is the case because folate is needed as the coenzyme 5,10-methylene-THF polyglutamate for conversion of dUMP to dTMP; the availability of 5,10-methylene-THF is reduced in either cobalamin or folate deficiency. An alternative theory for megaloblastic anemia in cobalamin or folate deficiency is misincorporation of uracil into DNA because of a buildup of deoxyuridine triphosphate (dUTP) at the DNA replication fork as a consequence of the block in conversion of dUMP to dTMP.

COBALAMIN-FOLATE RELATIONS

Folate is required for many reactions in mammalian tissues. Only two reactions in the body are known to require cobalamin. Methylmalonyl CoA isomerization requires adocobalamin, and the methylation of homocysteine to methionine requires both methylcobalamin and 5-MTHF (Fig. 128-1). This reaction is the first step in the pathway by which 5-MTHF, which enters bone marrow and other cells from plasma, is converted into all the intracellular folate coenzymes. The coenzymes are all polyglutamated (the larger size aiding retention in the cell), but the enzyme folate polyglutamate synthase can use only THF, not MTHF, as substrate. In cobalamin deficiency, MTHF accumulates in plasma, and intracellular folate concentrations fall due to failure of formation of THF, the substrate on which folate polyglutamates are built. This has been termed *THF starvation*, or the *methylfolate trap*.

This theory explains the abnormalities of folate metabolism that occur in cobalamin deficiency (high serum folate, low cell folate, positive purine precursor aminoimidazole carboxamide ribonucleotide [AICAR] excretion; Table 128-2) and also why the anemia of cobalamin deficiency responds to folic acid in large doses.

CLINICAL FEATURES

Many symptomless patients are detected through the finding of a raised mean corpuscular volume (MCV) on a routine blood count. The main clinical features in more severe cases are those of anemia. Anorexia is

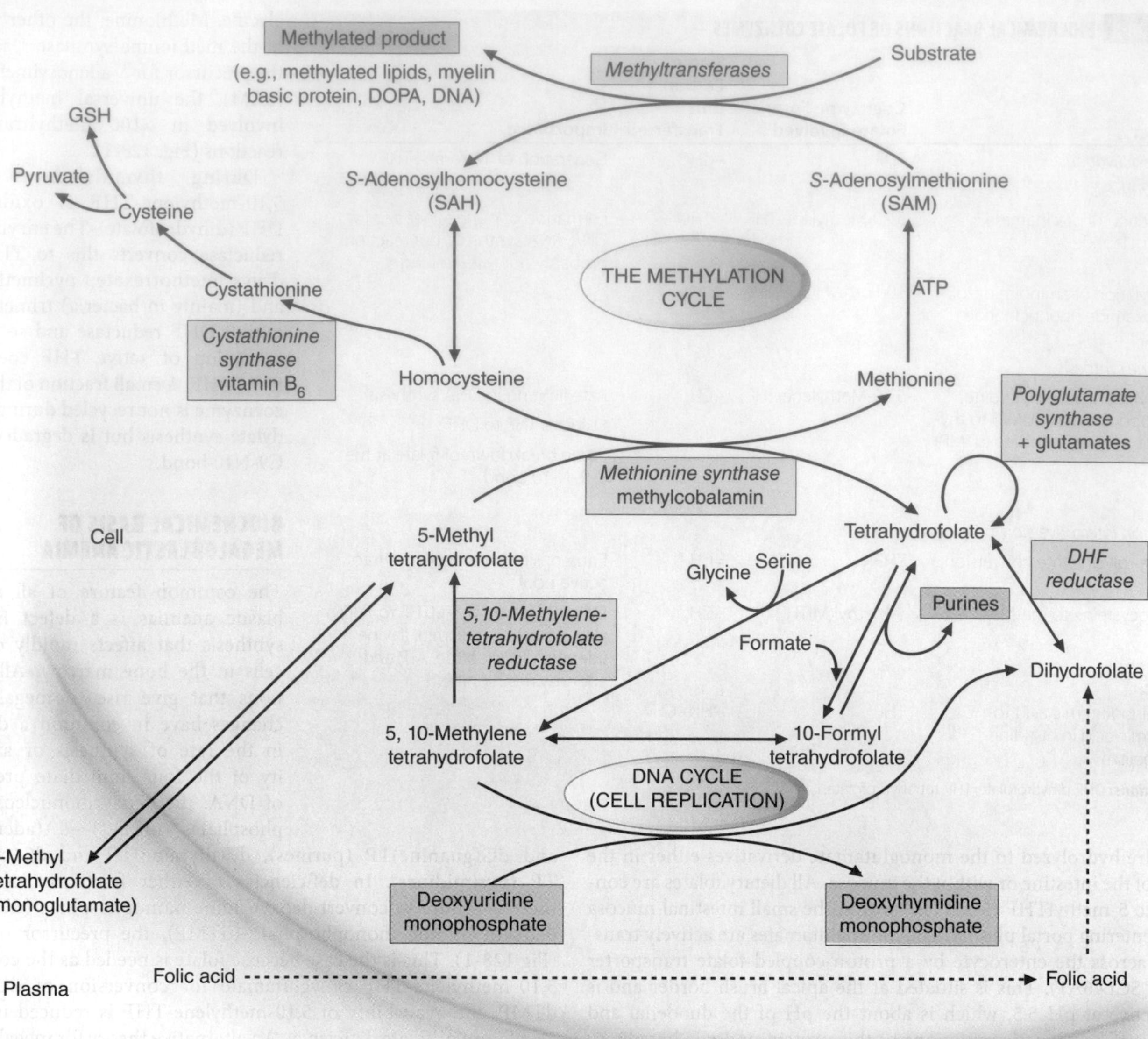

FIGURE 128-1 The role of folates in DNA synthesis and in formation of *S*-adenosylmethionine (SAM), which is involved in numerous methylation reactions. DHF, dihydrofolate; GSH, glutathione. *(Reprinted from AV Hoffbrand et al [eds]:* Postgraduate Haematology, *5th ed. Oxford, UK, Blackwell Publishing, 2005; with permission.)*

usually marked, and there may be weight loss, diarrhea, or constipation. Glossitis, angular cheilosis, a mild fever in more severely anemic patients, jaundice (unconjugated), and reversible melanin skin hyperpigmentation also may occur with a deficiency of either folate or cobalamin. Thrombocytopenia sometimes leads to bruising, and this may be aggravated by vitamin C deficiency or alcohol in malnourished patients. The anemia and low leukocyte count may predispose to infections, particularly of the respiratory and urinary tracts. Cobalamin deficiency has also been associated with impaired bactericidal function of phagocytes.

GENERAL TISSUE EFFECTS OF COBALAMIN AND FOLATE DEFICIENCIES

Epithelial Surfaces After the marrow, the next most frequently affected tissues are the epithelial cell surfaces of the mouth, stomach, and small intestine and the respiratory, urinary, and female genital tracts. The cells show macrocytosis, with increased numbers of multinucleate and dying cells. The deficiencies may cause cervical smear abnormalities.

Complications of Pregnancy The gonads are also affected, and infertility is common in both men and women with either deficiency. Maternal folate deficiency has been implicated as a cause of prematurity, and both folate deficiency and cobalamin deficiency have been implicated in recurrent fetal loss and neural tube defects, as discussed below.

Neural Tube Defects Folic acid supplements at the time of conception and in the first 12 weeks of pregnancy reduce by ~70% the incidence of neural tube defects (NTDs) (anencephaly, meningomyelocele, encephalocele, and spina bifida) in the fetus. Most of this protective effect can be achieved by taking folic acid, 0.4 mg daily, at the time of conception.

The incidence of cleft palate and harelip also can be reduced by prophylactic folic acid. There is no clear simple relationship between maternal folate status and these fetal abnormalities, although overall the lower the maternal folate, the greater the risk to the fetus. NTDs also can be caused by antifolate and antiepileptic drugs.

An underlying maternal folate metabolic abnormality has also been postulated. One abnormality has been identified: reduced activity of the enzyme 5,10-methylene-THF reductase (MTHFR) (Fig. 128-1) caused by a common C677T polymorphism in the *MTHFR* gene. In one study, the prevalence of this polymorphism was found to be higher than in controls in the parents of NTD fetuses and in the fetuses themselves: homozygosity for the TT mutation was found in 13% of cases compared with 5% of control subjects. The polymorphism codes for a thermolabile form of MTHFR. The homozygous state results in a lower mean serum and red cell folate level compared with control subjects, as well as significantly higher serum homocysteine levels. Tests for mutations in other enzymes possibly associated with NTDs, e.g., methionine synthase and serine–glycine hydroxymethylase, have been negative. Serum vitamin B_{12} levels are also lower in the sera of mothers of NTD infants than in controls. In addition, maternal TC II receptor polymorphisms are associated with increased risk of NTD births. There are, however, no studies showing dietary fortification with vitamin B_{12} reduces the incidence of NTDs.

Cardiovascular Disease Children with severe homocystinuria (blood levels ≥100 μmol/L) due to deficiency of one of three enzymes, methionine synthase, MTHFR, or cystathionine synthase (Fig. 128-1), have vascular disease, e.g., ischemic heart disease, cerebrovascular disease, or pulmonary embolus, as teenagers or in young adulthood. Lesser degrees of raised serum homocysteine and low levels of serum folate and homozygous inherited mutations of MTHFR have been found to be associated with cerebrovascular, peripheral vascular, and coronary heart disease and with deep vein thrombosis. Prospective randomized trials of lowering homocysteine levels with supplements of folic acid, vitamin B_{12}, and vitamin B_6 against placebo over a 5-year period in patients with vascular disease or diabetes have not, however, shown a reduction of first event fatal or nonfatal myocardial infarction, nor have these supplements reduced the risk of recurrent cardiovascular disease after an acute myocardial infarct. Meta-analysis showed an 18% reduction in strokes but no significant prevention of death from any cause. Venous thrombosis has been reported to be more frequent in vitamin B_{12}–deficient subjects than in controls. This was ascribed to raised plasma homocysteine levels in vitamin B_{12} deficiency.

Malignancy Prophylactic folic acid in pregnancy has been found in some but not all studies to reduce the subsequent incidence of acute lymphoblastic leukemia (ALL) in childhood. A significant negative association has also been found with the *MTHFR* C677T polymorphism and leukemias with mixed lineage leukemia (MLL) translocations, but a positive association with hyperdiploidy in infants with ALL or acute myeloid leukemia or with childhood ALL. A second polymorphism in the *MTHFR* gene, A1298C, is also strongly associated with hyperdiploid leukemia. There are various positive and negative associations between polymorphisms in folate-dependent enzymes and the incidence of adult ALL. The C677T polymorphism is thought to lead to increased thymidine pools and "better quality" of DNA synthesis by shunting one-carbon groups toward thymidine and purine synthesis. This may explain its reported association with a lower risk for colorectal cancer. Most but not all studies suggest that prophylactic folic acid also protects against colon adenomas. Other tumors that have been associated with folate polymorphisms or status include follicular lymphoma, breast cancer, and gastric cancer. A meta-analysis of 50,000 individuals given folic acid or placebo in cardiovascular or colon adenoma prevention trials found that folic acid supplementation did not substantially increase or decrease the incidence of site-specific cancer during the first 5 years of treatment. Because folic acid may "feed" tumors, it probably should be avoided in those with established tumors unless there is severe megaloblastic anemia due to folate deficiency.

Neurologic Manifestations Cobalamin deficiency may cause a bilateral peripheral neuropathy or degeneration (demyelination) of the posterior and pyramidal tracts of the spinal cord and, less frequently, optic atrophy or cerebral symptoms.

The patient, more frequently male, presents with paresthesias, muscle weakness, or difficulty in walking and sometimes dementia, psychotic disturbances, or visual impairment. Long-term nutritional cobalamin deficiency in infancy leads to poor brain development and impaired intellectual development. Folate deficiency has been suggested to cause organic nervous disease, but this is uncertain, although methotrexate injected into the cerebrospinal fluid may cause brain or spinal cord damage.

An important clinical problem is the nonanemic patient with neurologic or psychiatric abnormalities and a low or borderline serum cobalamin level. In such patients, it is necessary to try to establish whether there is significant cobalamin deficiency, e.g., by careful examination of the blood film, tests for serum gastrin level and for antibodies to IF or parietal cells, along with serum methylmalonic acid (MMA) measurement if available. A trial of cobalamin therapy for at least 3 months will usually also be needed to determine whether the symptoms improve.

The biochemical basis for cobalamin neuropathy remains obscure. Its occurrence in the absence of methylmalonic aciduria in TC II deficiency suggests that the neuropathy is related to the defect in homocysteine-methionine conversion. Accumulation of S-adenosylhomocysteine in the brain, resulting in inhibition of transmethylation reactions, has been suggested.

Psychiatric disturbance is common in both folate and cobalamin deficiencies. This, like the neuropathy, has been attributed to a failure of the synthesis of SAM, which is needed in methylation of biogenic amines (e.g., dopamine) as well as that of proteins, phospholipids, and neurotransmitters in the brain (Fig. 128-1). Associations between lower serum folate or cobalamin levels and higher homocysteine levels and the development of decreased cognitive function and dementia in Alzheimer's disease have been reported. A meta-analysis of randomized, placebo-controlled trials of homocysteine-lowering B-vitamin supplementation of individuals with and without cognitive impairment, however, showed that supplementation with vitamin B_{12}, vitamin B_6, and folic acid alone or in combination did not improve cognitive function. It is unknown whether prolonged treatment with these B vitamins can reduce the risk of dementia in later life.

HEMATOLOGIC FINDINGS

PERIPHERAL BLOOD

Oval macrocytes, usually with considerable anisocytosis and poikilocytosis, are the main feature (Fig. 128-2*A*). The MCV is usually >100 fL unless a cause of microcytosis (e.g., iron deficiency or thalassemia trait) is present. Some of the neutrophils are hypersegmented (more than five nuclear lobes). There may be leukopenia due to a reduction in granulocytes and lymphocytes, but this is usually $>1.5 \times 10^9$/L; the platelet count may be moderately reduced, rarely to $<40 \times 10^9$/L. The severity of all these changes parallels the degree of anemia. In a nonanemic patient, the presence of a few macrocytes and hypersegmented neutrophils in the peripheral blood may be the only indication of the underlying disorder.

BONE MARROW

In a severely anemic patient, the marrow is hypercellular with an accumulation of primitive cells due to selective death by apoptosis of more mature forms. The erythroblast nucleus maintains a primitive appearance despite maturation and hemoglobinization of the cytoplasm. The cells are larger than normoblasts, and an increased number of cells with eccentric lobulated nuclei or nuclear fragments may be present (Fig. 128-2*B*). Giant and abnormally shaped metamyelocytes and enlarged hyperpolyploid megakaryocytes are characteristic. In severe cases, the accumulation of primitive cells may mimic acute myeloid leukemia, whereas in less anemic patients, the changes in the marrow may be difficult to recognize. The terms *intermediate*, *mild*, and *early* have been used. The term *megaloblastoid* does not mean mildly megaloblastic. It is used to describe cells with both immature-appearing nuclei and defective hemoglobinization and is usually seen in myelodysplasia.

CHROMOSOMES

Bone marrow cells, transformed lymphocytes, and other proliferating cells in the body show a variety of changes, including random breaks, reduced contraction, spreading of the centromere, and exaggeration of secondary chromosomal constrictions and overprominent satellites. Similar abnormalities may be produced by antimetabolite drugs (e.g., cytosine arabinoside, hydroxyurea, and methotrexate) that interfere with either DNA replication or folate metabolism and that also cause megaloblastic appearances.

INEFFECTIVE HEMATOPOIESIS

There is an accumulation of unconjugated bilirubin in plasma due to the death of nucleated red cells in the marrow (ineffective erythropoiesis). Other evidence for this includes raised urine urobilinogen, reduced haptoglobins and positive urine hemosiderin, and a raised

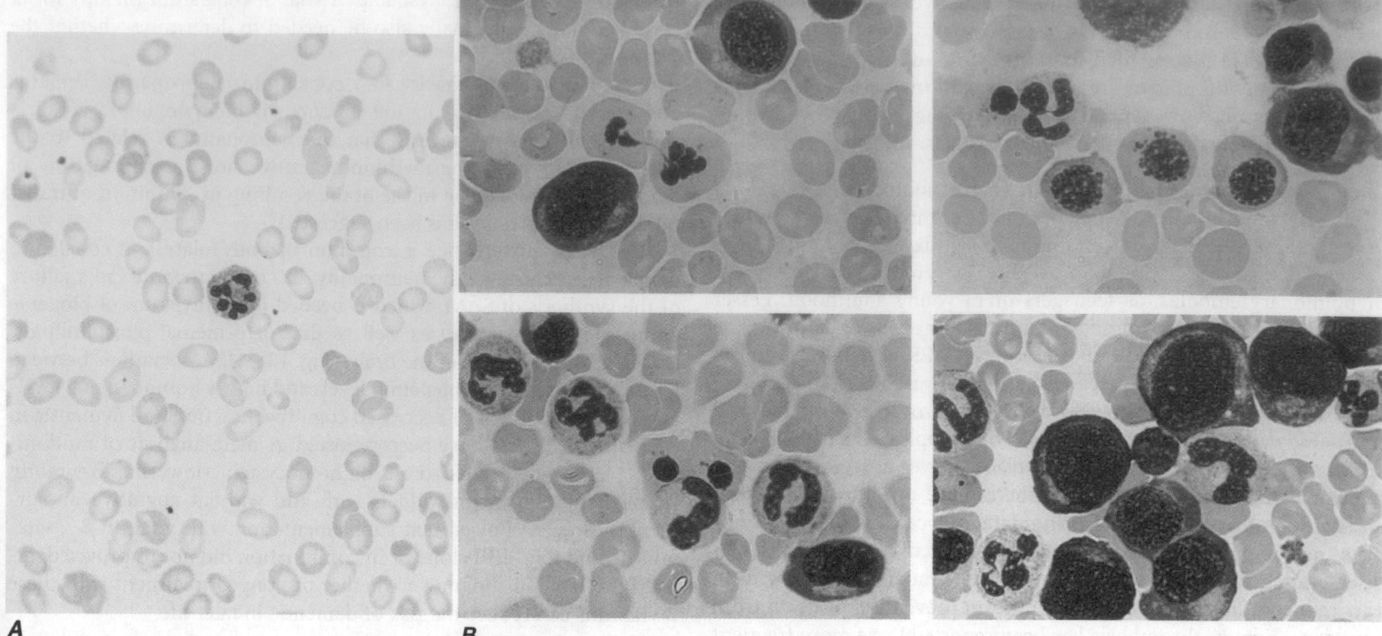

FIGURE 128-2 ***A.*** The peripheral blood in severe megaloblastic anemia. ***B.*** The bone marrow in severe megaloblastic anemia. *(Reprinted from AV Hoffbrand et al [eds]: Postgraduate Haematology, 5th ed. Oxford, UK, Blackwell Publishing, 2005; with permission.)*

serum lactate dehydrogenase. A weakly positive direct antiglobulin test due to complement can lead to a false diagnosis of autoimmune hemolytic anemia.

CAUSES OF COBALAMIN DEFICIENCY

Cobalamin deficiency is usually due to malabsorption. The only other cause is inadequate dietary intake.

INADEQUATE DIETARY INTAKE

Adults Dietary cobalamin deficiency arises in vegans who omit meat, fish, eggs, cheese, and other animal products from their diet. The largest group in the world consists of Hindus, and it is likely that many millions of Indians are at risk of deficiency of cobalamin on a nutritional basis. Subnormal serum cobalamin levels are found in up to 50% of randomly selected, young, adult Indian vegans, but the deficiency usually does not progress to megaloblastic anemia since the diet of most vegans is not totally lacking in cobalamin and the enterohepatic circulation of cobalamin is intact. Dietary cobalamin deficiency may also arise rarely in nonvegetarian individuals who exist on grossly inadequate diets because of poverty or psychiatric disturbance.

Infants Cobalamin deficiency has been described in infants born to severely cobalamin-deficient mothers. These infants develop megaloblastic anemia at about 3–6 months of age, presumably because they are born with low stores of cobalamin and because they are fed breast milk with low cobalamin content. The babies have also shown growth retardation, impaired psychomotor development, and other neurologic sequelae.

GASTRIC CAUSES OF COBALAMIN MALABSORPTION

See Tables 128-3 and 128-4.

Pernicious Anemia Pernicious anemia (PA) may be defined as a severe lack of IF due to gastric atrophy. It is a common disease in north Europeans but occurs in all countries and ethnic groups. The overall incidence is about 120 per 100,000 population in the United Kingdom (UK). The ratio of incidence in men and women among whites is ~1:1.6, and the peak age of onset is 60 years, with only 10% of patients being <40 years of age. However, in some ethnic groups, notably black individuals and Latin Americans, the age at onset of PA is generally lower. The disease occurs more commonly than by chance

TABLE 128-3 CAUSES OF COBALAMIN DEFICIENCY SUFFICIENTLY SEVERE TO CAUSE MEGALOBLASTIC ANEMIA

Nutritional	Vegans
Malabsorption	Pernicious anemia
Gastric causes	Congenital absence of intrinsic factor or functional abnormality
	Total or partial gastrectomy
Intestinal causes	Intestinal stagnant loop syndrome: jejunal diverticulosis, ileocolic fistula, anatomic blind loop, intestinal stricture, etc.
	Ileal resection and Crohn's disease
	Selective malabsorption with proteinuria
	Tropical sprue
	Transcobalamin II deficiency
	Fish tapeworm

TABLE 128-4 MALABSORPTION OF COBALAMIN MAY OCCUR IN THE FOLLOWING CONDITIONS BUT IS NOT USUALLY SUFFICIENTLY SEVERE AND PROLONGED TO CAUSE MEGALOBLASTIC ANEMIA

Gastric causes
- Simple atrophic gastritis (food cobalamin malabsorption)
- Zollinger-Ellison syndrome
- Gastric bypass surgery
- Use of proton pump inhibitors

Intestinal causes
- Gluten-induced enteropathy
- Severe pancreatitis
- HIV infection
- Radiotherapy
- Graft-versus-host disease

Deficiencies of cobalamin, folate, protein, ?riboflavin, ?nicotinic acid

Therapy with colchicine, para-aminosalicylate, neomycin, slow-release potassium chloride, anticonvulsant drugs, metformin, phenformin, cytotoxic drugs

Alcohol

in close relatives and in persons with other organ-specific autoimmune diseases, e.g., thyroid diseases, vitiligo, hypoparathyroidism, and Addison's disease. It is also associated with hypogammaglobulinemia, with premature graying or blue eyes, and persons of blood group A. An association with human leukocyte antigen (HLA) 3 has been reported in some but not all series and, in those with endocrine disease, with HLA-B8, -B12, and -BW15. Life expectancy is normal in women once regular treatment has begun. Men have a slightly subnormal life expectancy as a result of a higher incidence of carcinoma of the stomach than in control subjects. Gastric output of hydrochloric acid, pepsin, and IF is severely reduced. The serum gastrin level is raised, and serum pepsinogen I levels are low.

Gastric Biopsy A single endoscopic examination is recommended if PA is diagnosed. Gastric biopsy usually shows atrophy of all layers of the body and fundus, with loss of glandular elements, an absence of parietal and chief cells and replacement by mucous cells, a mixed inflammatory cell infiltrate, and perhaps intestinal metaplasia. The infiltrate of plasma cells and lymphocytes contains an excess of CD4 cells. These are directed against gastric H/K-ATPase. The antral mucosa is usually well preserved. *Helicobacter pylori* infection occurs infrequently in PA, but it has been suggested that *H. pylori* gastritis occurs at an early phase of atrophic gastritis and presents in younger patients as iron-deficiency anemia but in older patients as PA. *H. pylori* is suggested to stimulate an autoimmune process directed against parietal cells, with the *H. pylori* infection then being gradually replaced, in some individuals, by an autoimmune process.

Serum Antibodies Two types of IF immunoglobulin G antibody may be found in the sera of patients with PA. One, the "blocking," or type I, antibody, prevents the combination of IF and cobalamin, whereas the "binding," or type II, antibody prevents attachment of IF to ileal mucosa. Type I occurs in the sera of ~55% of patients, and type II in 35%. IF antibodies cross the placenta and may cause temporary IF deficiency in a newborn infant. Patients with PA also show cell-mediated immunity to IF. Type I antibody has been detected rarely in the sera of patients without PA but with thyrotoxicosis, myxedema, Hashimoto's disease, or diabetes mellitus and in relatives of PA patients. IF antibodies also have been detected in gastric juice in ~80% of PA patients. These gastric antibodies may reduce absorption of dietary cobalamin by combining with small amounts of remaining IF.

Parietal cell antibody is present in the sera of almost 90% of adult patients with PA but is frequently present in other subjects. Thus, it occurs in as many as 16% of randomly selected female subjects age >60 years. The parietal cell antibody is directed against the α and β subunits of the gastric proton pump (H^+,K^+-ATPase).

JUVENILE PERNICIOUS ANEMIA

This usually occurs in older children and resembles PA of adults. Gastric atrophy, achlorhydria, and serum IF antibodies are all present, although parietal cell antibodies are usually absent. About one-half of these patients show an associated endocrinopathy such as autoimmune thyroiditis, Addison's disease, or hypoparathyroidism; in some, mucocutaneous candidiasis occurs.

CONGENITAL INTRINSIC FACTOR DEFICIENCY OR FUNCTIONAL ABNORMALITY

An affected child usually presents with megaloblastic anemia in the first to third year of life; a few have presented as late as the second decade. The child usually has no demonstrable IF but has a normal gastric mucosa and normal secretion of acid. The inheritance is autosomal recessive. Parietal cell and IF antibodies are absent. Variants have been described in which the child is born with IF that can be detected immunologically but is unstable or functionally inactive, unable to bind cobalamin or to facilitate its uptake by ileal receptors.

GASTRECTOMY

After total gastrectomy, cobalamin deficiency is inevitable, and prophylactic cobalamin therapy should be commenced immediately after the operation. After partial gastrectomy, 10–15% of patients also develop this deficiency. The exact incidence and time of onset are most influenced by the size of the resection and the preexisting size of cobalamin body stores.

FOOD COBALAMIN MALABSORPTION

Failure of release of cobalamin from binding proteins in food is believed to be responsible for this condition, which is more common in the elderly. It is associated with low serum cobalamin levels, with or without raised serum levels of MMA and homocysteine. Typically, these patients have normal cobalamin absorption, as measured with crystalline cobalamin, but show malabsorption when a modified test using food-bound cobalamin is used. The frequency of progression to severe cobalamin deficiency and the reasons for this progression are not clear.

INTESTINAL CAUSES OF COBALAMIN MALABSORPTION

Intestinal Stagnant Loop Syndrome Malabsorption of cobalamin occurs in a variety of intestinal lesions in which there is colonization of the upper small intestine by fecal organisms. This may occur in patients with jejunal diverticulosis, enteroanastomosis, or an intestinal stricture or fistula or with an anatomic blind loop due to Crohn's disease, tuberculosis, or an operative procedure.

Ileal Resection Removal of ≥1.2 m of terminal ileum causes malabsorption of cobalamin. In some patients after ileal resection, particularly if the ileocecal valve is incompetent, colonic bacteria may contribute further to the onset of cobalamin deficiency.

Selective Malabsorption of Cobalamin with Proteinuria (Imerslund's Syndrome; Imerslund-Gräsbeck Syndrome; Congenital Cobalamin Malabsorption; Autosomal Recessive Megaloblastic Anemia; MGA1) This autosomally recessive disease is the most common cause of megaloblastic anemia due to cobalamin deficiency in infancy in Western countries. More than 200 cases have been reported, with familial clusters in Finland, Norway, the Middle East, and North Africa. The patients secrete normal amounts of IF and gastric acid but are unable to absorb cobalamin. In Finland, impaired synthesis, processing, or ligand binding of cubilin due to inherited mutations is found. In Norway, mutation of the gene for *AMN* has been reported. Other tests of intestinal absorption are normal. Over 90% of these patients show nonspecific proteinuria, but renal function is otherwise normal and renal biopsy has not shown any consistent renal defect. A few have shown aminoaciduria and congenital renal abnormalities, such as duplication of the renal pelvis.

Tropical Sprue Nearly all patients with acute and subacute tropical sprue show malabsorption of cobalamin; this may persist as the principal abnormality in the chronic form of the disease, when the patient may present with megaloblastic anemia or neuropathy due to cobalamin deficiency. Absorption of cobalamin usually improves after antibiotic therapy and, in the early stages, folic acid therapy.

Fish Tapeworm Infestation The fish tapeworm (*Diphyllobothrium latum*) lives in the small intestine of humans and accumulates cobalamin from food, rendering the cobalamin unavailable for absorption. Individuals acquire the worm by eating raw or partly cooked fish. Infestation is common around the lakes of Scandinavia, Germany, Japan, North America, and Russia. Megaloblastic anemia or cobalamin neuropathy occurs only in those with a heavy infestation.

Gluten-Induced Enteropathy Malabsorption of cobalamin occurs in ~30% of untreated patients (presumably those in whom the disease extends to the ileum). Cobalamin deficiency is not severe in these patients and is corrected with a gluten-free diet.

Severe Chronic Pancreatitis In this condition, lack of trypsin is thought to cause dietary cobalamin attached to gastric non-IF (R) binder to be unavailable for absorption. It also has been proposed that in pancreatitis, the concentration of calcium ions in the ileum falls below the level needed to maintain normal cobalamin absorption.

HIV Infection Serum cobalamin levels tend to fall in patients with HIV infection and are subnormal in 10–35% of those with AIDS.

Malabsorption of cobalamin not corrected by IF has been shown in some, but not all, patients with subnormal serum cobalamin levels. Cobalamin deficiency sufficiently severe to cause megaloblastic anemia or neuropathy is rare.

Zollinger-Ellison Syndrome Malabsorption of cobalamin has been reported in the Zollinger-Ellison syndrome. It is thought that there is a failure to release cobalamin from R-binding protein due to inactivation of pancreatic trypsin by high acidity, as well as interference with IF binding of cobalamin.

Radiotherapy Both total-body irradiation and local radiotherapy to the ileum (e.g., as a complication of radiotherapy for carcinoma of the cervix) may cause malabsorption of cobalamin.

Graft-versus-Host Disease This commonly affects the small intestine. Malabsorption of cobalamin due to abnormal gut flora, as well as damage to ileal mucosa, is common.

Drugs The drugs that have been reported to cause malabsorption of cobalamin are listed in Table 105-4. However, megaloblastic anemia due to these drugs is rare.

ABNORMALITIES OF COBALAMIN METABOLISM

Congenital Transcobalamin II Deficiency or Abnormality Infants with TC II deficiency usually present with megaloblastic anemia within a few weeks of birth. Serum cobalamin and folate levels are normal, but the anemia responds to massive (e.g., 1 mg three times weekly) injections of cobalamin. Some cases show neurologic complications. The protein may be present but functionally inert. Genetic abnormalities found include mutations of an intra-exonic cryptic splice site, extensive deletion, single nucleotide deletion, nonsense mutation, and an RNA editing defect. Malabsorption of cobalamin occurs in all cases, and serum immunoglobulins are usually reduced. Failure to institute adequate cobalamin therapy or treatment with folic acid may lead to neurologic damage.

Congenital Methylmalonic Acidemia and Aciduria Infants with this abnormality are ill from birth with vomiting, failure to thrive, severe metabolic acidosis, ketosis, and mental retardation. Anemia, if present, is normocytic and normoblastic. The condition may be due to a functional defect in either mitochondrial methylmalonyl CoA mutase or its cofactor adocobalamin. Mutations in the methylmalonyl CoA mutase are not responsive, or only poorly responsive, to treatment with cobalamin. A proportion of infants with failure of adocobalamin synthesis respond to cobalamin in large doses. Some children have combined methylmalonic aciduria and homocystinuria due to defective formation of both cobalamin coenzymes. This usually presents in the first year of life with feeding difficulties, developmental delay, microcephaly, seizures, hypotonia, and megaloblastic anemia.

Acquired Abnormality of Cobalamin Metabolism: Nitrous Oxide Inhalation Nitrous oxide (N_2O) irreversibly oxidizes methylcobalamin to an inactive precursor; this inactivates methionine synthase. Megaloblastic anemia has occurred in patients undergoing prolonged N_2O anesthesia (e.g., in intensive care units). A neuropathy resembling cobalamin neuropathy has been described in dentists and anesthetists who are exposed repeatedly to N_2O. Methylmalonic aciduria does not occur as adocobalamin is not inactivated by N_2O.

CAUSES OF FOLATE DEFICIENCY

(Table 128-5)

NUTRITIONAL

Dietary folate deficiency is common. Indeed, in most patients with folate deficiency a nutritional element is present. Certain individuals are particularly prone to have diets containing inadequate amounts of folate (Table 128-5). In the United States and other countries where fortification of the diet with folic acid has been adopted, the prevalence of folate deficiency has dropped dramatically and is now almost restricted to high-risk groups with increased folate needs. Nutritional folate deficiency occurs in kwashiorkor and scurvy and in infants with repeated infections or those who are fed solely on goats' milk, which has a low folate content.

TABLE 128-5 CAUSES OF FOLATE DEFICIENCY

Dietary[a]
Particularly in: old age, infancy, poverty, alcoholism, chronic invalids, and the psychiatrically disturbed; may be associated with scurvy or kwashiorkor
Malabsorption
Major causes of deficiency
Tropical sprue, gluten-induced enteropathy in children and adults, and in association with dermatitis herpetiformis, specific malabsorption of folate, intestinal megaloblastosis caused by severe cobalamin or folate deficiency
Minor causes of deficiency
Extensive jejunal resection, Crohn's disease, partial gastrectomy, congestive heart failure, Whipple's disease, scleroderma, amyloid, diabetic enteropathy, systemic bacterial infection, lymphoma, sulfasalazine (Salazopyrin)
Excess utilization or loss
Physiologic
Pregnancy and lactation, prematurity
Pathologic
Hematologic diseases: chronic hemolytic anemias, sickle cell anemia, thalassemia major, myelofibrosis
Malignant diseases: carcinoma, lymphoma, leukemia, myeloma
Inflammatory diseases: tuberculosis, Crohn's disease, psoriasis, exfoliative dermatitis, malaria
Metabolic disease: homocystinuria
Excess urinary loss: congestive heart failure, active liver disease
Hemodialysis, peritoneal dialysis
Antifolate drugs[b]
Anticonvulsant drugs (phenytoin, primidone, barbiturates), sulfasalazine
Nitrofurantoin, tetracycline, antituberculosis (less well documented)
Mixed causes
Liver diseases, alcoholism, intensive care units

[a]In severely folate-deficient patients with causes other than those listed under Dietary, poor dietary intake is often present. [b]Drugs inhibiting dihydrofolate reductase are discussed in the text.

MALABSORPTION

Malabsorption of dietary folate occurs in tropical sprue and in gluten-induced enteropathy. In the rare congenital recessive syndrome of selective malabsorption of folate due to mutation of the proton-coupled folate transporter (PCFT), there is an associated defect of folate transport into the cerebrospinal fluid, and these patients show megaloblastic anemia, which responds to physiologic doses of folic acid given parenterally but not orally. They also show mental retardation, convulsions, and other central nervous system abnormalities. Minor degrees of malabsorption may also occur after jejunal resection or partial gastrectomy, in Crohn's disease, and in systemic infections, but in these conditions, if severe deficiency occurs, it is usually largely due to poor nutrition. Malabsorption of folate has been described in patients receiving sulfasalazine (Salazopyrin), cholestyramine, and triamterene.

EXCESS UTILIZATION OR LOSS

Pregnancy Folate requirements are increased by 200–300 μg to ~400 μg daily in a normal pregnancy, partly because of transfer of the vitamin to the fetus but mainly because of increased folate catabolism due to cleavage of folate coenzymes in rapidly proliferating tissues. Megaloblastic anemia due to this deficiency is prevented by prophylactic folic acid therapy. It occurred in 0.5% of pregnancies in the UK and other Western countries before prophylaxis with folic acid, but the incidence is much higher in countries where the general nutritional status is poor.

Prematurity A newborn infant, whether full term or premature, has higher serum and red cell folate concentrations than does an adult. However, a newborn infant's demand for folate has been estimated to be up to 10 times that of adults on a weight basis, and the neonatal folate level falls rapidly to the lowest values at about 6 weeks of age. The falls are steepest and are liable to reach subnormal levels in premature babies, a number of whom develop megaloblastic anemia responsive to folic acid at about 4–6 weeks of age. This occurs particularly in the smallest babies (<1500 g birth weight) and those who have feeding difficulties or infections or have undergone multiple exchange transfusions. In these babies, prophylactic folic acid should be given.

Hematologic Disorders Folate deficiency frequently occurs in chronic hemolytic anemia, particularly in sickle cell disease, autoimmune hemolytic anemia, and congenital spherocytosis. In these and other conditions of increased cell turnover (e.g., myelofibrosis, malignancies), folate deficiency arises because it is not completely reutilized after performing coenzyme functions.

Inflammatory Conditions Chronic inflammatory diseases such as tuberculosis, rheumatoid arthritis, Crohn's disease, psoriasis, exfoliative dermatitis, bacterial endocarditis, and chronic bacterial infections cause deficiency by reducing the appetite and increasing the demand for folate. Systemic infections also may cause malabsorption of folate. Severe deficiency is virtually confined to the patients with the most active disease and the poorest diet.

Homocystinuria This is a rare metabolic defect in the conversion of homocysteine to cystathionine. Folate deficiency occurring in most of these patients may be due to excessive utilization because of compensatory increased conversion of homocysteine to methionine.

Long-Term Dialysis Because folate is only loosely bound to plasma proteins, it is easily removed from plasma by dialysis. In patients with anorexia, vomiting, infections, and hemolysis, folate stores are particularly likely to become depleted. Routine folate prophylaxis is now given.

Congestive Heart Failure, Liver Disease Excess urinary folate losses of >100 μg per day may occur in some of these patients. The explanation appears to be release of folate from damaged liver cells.

ANTIFOLATE DRUGS

A large number of epileptics who are receiving long-term therapy with phenytoin or primidone, with or without barbiturates, develop low serum and red cell folate levels. The exact mechanism is unclear. Alcohol may also be a folate antagonist, as patients who are drinking spirits may develop megaloblastic anemia that will respond to normal quantities of dietary folate or to physiologic doses of folic acid only if alcohol is withdrawn. Macrocytosis of red cells is associated with chronic alcohol intake even when folate levels are normal. Inadequate folate intake is the major factor in the development of deficiency in spirit-drinking alcoholics. Beer is relatively folate-rich in some countries, depending on the technique used for brewing.

The drugs that inhibit DHF reductase include methotrexate, pyrimethamine, and trimethoprim. Methotrexate has the most powerful action against the human enzyme, whereas trimethoprim is most active against the bacterial enzyme and is likely to cause megaloblastic anemia only when used in conjunction with sulfamethoxazole in patients with preexisting folate or cobalamin deficiency. The activity of pyrimethamine is intermediate. The antidote to these drugs is folinic acid (5-formyl-THF).

CONGENITAL ABNORMALITIES OF FOLATE METABOLISM

Some infants with congenital defects of folate enzymes (e.g., cyclohydrolase or methionine synthase) have had megaloblastic anemia.

DIAGNOSIS OF COBALAMIN AND FOLATE DEFICIENCIES

The diagnosis of cobalamin or folate deficiency has traditionally depended on the recognition of the relevant abnormalities in the peripheral blood and analysis of the blood levels of the vitamins.

COBALAMIN DEFICIENCY

Serum Cobalamin This is measured by an automated enzyme-linked immunosorbent assay (ELISA) or competitive-binding luminescence assay (CBLA). Normal serum levels range from 118–148 pmol/L (160–200 ng/L) to ~738 pmol/L (1000 ng/L). In patients with megaloblastic anemia due to cobalamin deficiency, the level is usually <74 pmol/L (100 ng/L). In general, the more severe the deficiency, the lower is the serum cobalamin level. In patients with spinal cord damage due to the deficiency, levels are very low even in the absence of anemia. Values between 74 and 148 pmol/L (100 and 200 ng/L) are regarded as borderline. They may occur, for instance, in pregnancy, in patients with megaloblastic anemia due to folate deficiency. They may also be due to heterozygous, homozygous, or compound heterozygous mutations of the gene *TCN1* that codes for haptocorrin (transcobalamin I). There is no clinical or hematologic abnormality. The serum cobalamin level is sufficiently robust, cost-effective, and most convenient to rule out cobalamin deficiency in the vast majority of patients suspected of having this problem. However, problems have arisen with commercial CBLA assays involving intrinsic factor in PA patients with intrinsic antibodies in serum. These antibodies may cause false normal serum vitamin B_{12} levels in up to 50% of cases tested. Where clinical indications of PA are strong, a normal serum vitamin B_{12} does not rule out the diagnosis. Serum MMA levels will be elevated in PA (see below).

Serum Methylmalonate and Homocysteine In patients with cobalamin deficiency sufficient to cause anemia or neuropathy, the serum MMA level is raised. Sensitive methods for measuring MMA and homocysteine in serum have been introduced and recommended for the early diagnosis of cobalamin deficiency, even in the absence of hematologic abnormalities or subnormal levels of serum cobalamin. Serum MMA levels fluctuate, however, in patients with renal failure. Mildly elevated serum MMA and/or homocysteine levels occur in up to 30% of apparently healthy volunteers, with serum cobalamin levels up to 258 pmol/L (350 ng/L) and normal serum folate levels; 15% of elderly subjects, even with cobalamin levels >258 pmol/L (>350 ng/L), have this pattern of raised metabolite levels. These findings bring into question the exact cutoff points for normal MMA and homocysteine levels. It is also unclear at present whether these mildly raised metabolite levels have clinical consequences.

Serum homocysteine is raised in both early cobalamin and folate deficiency but may be raised in other conditions, e.g., chronic renal disease, alcoholism, smoking, pyridoxine deficiency, hypothyroidism, and therapy with steroids, cyclosporine, and other drugs. Levels are also higher in serum than in plasma, in men than in premenopausal women, in women taking hormone replacement therapy or in oral contraceptive users, and in elderly persons and patients with several inborn errors of metabolism affecting enzymes in trans sulfuration pathways of homocysteine metabolism. Thus, homocysteine levels must be carefully interpreted for diagnosis of cobalamin or folate deficiency.

Tests for the Cause of Cobalamin Deficiency Only vegans, strict vegetarians, or people living on a totally inadequate diet will become vitamin B_{12} deficient because of inadequate intake. Studies of cobalamin absorption once were widely used, but difficulty in obtaining radioactive cobalamin and ensuring that IF preparations are free of viruses has made these tests obsolete. Tests to diagnose PA include serum gastrin, which is raised; serum pepsinogen I, which is low in PA (90–92%) but also in other conditions; and gastric endoscopy. Tests for IF and parietal cell antibodies are also used, as well as tests for individual intestinal diseases.

FOLATE DEFICIENCY

Serum Folate This is also measured by an ELISA technique. In most laboratories, the normal range is from 11 nmol/L (2 μg/L) to ~82 nmol/L (15 μg/L). The serum folate level is low in all folate-deficient patients. It also reflects recent diet. Because of this, serum folate may be low before there is hematologic or biochemical evidence of deficiency. Serum folate rises in severe cobalamin deficiency because of the block in conversion of MTHF to THF inside cells; raised levels have also been reported in the intestinal stagnant loop syndrome due to absorption of bacterially synthesized folate.

Red Cell Folate The red cell folate assay is a valuable test of body folate stores. It is less affected than the serum assay by recent diet and traces of hemolysis. In normal adults, concentrations range from 880–3520 μmol/L (160–640 μg/L) of packed red cells. Subnormal levels occur in patients with megaloblastic anemia due to folate deficiency but also in nearly two-thirds of patients with severe cobalamin deficiency. False-normal results may occur if a folate-deficient patient has received a recent blood transfusion or if a patient has a raised reticulocyte count. Serum homocysteine assay is discussed earlier.

Tests for the Cause of Folate Deficiency The diet history is important. Tests for transglutaminase antibodies are performed to confirm or exclude celiac disease. If positive, duodenal biopsy is needed. An underlying disease causing increased folate breakdown should also be excluded.

TREATMENT COBALAMIN AND FOLATE DEFICIENCY

It is usually possible to establish which of the two deficiencies, folate or cobalamin, is the cause of the anemia and to treat only with the appropriate vitamin. In patients who enter the hospital severely ill, however, it may be necessary to treat with both vitamins in large doses once blood samples have been taken for cobalamin and folate assays and a bone marrow biopsy has been performed (if deemed necessary). Transfusion is usually unnecessary and inadvisable. If it is essential, packed red cells should be given slowly, one or two units only, with the usual treatment for heart failure if present. Potassium supplements have been recommended to obviate the danger of the hypokalemia but are not necessary. Occasionally, an excessive rise in platelets occurs after 1–2 weeks of therapy. Antiplatelet therapy, e.g., aspirin, should be considered if the platelet count rises to >800 × 10^9/L.

COBALAMIN DEFICIENCY

It is usually necessary to treat patients who have developed cobalamin deficiency with lifelong regular cobalamin injections. In the UK, the form used is hydroxocobalamin; in the United States, cyanocobalamin. In a few instances, the underlying cause of cobalamin deficiency can be permanently corrected, e.g., fish tapeworm, tropical sprue, or an intestinal stagnant loop that is amenable to surgery. The indications for starting cobalamin therapy are a well-documented megaloblastic anemia or other hematologic abnormalities and neuropathy due to the deficiency. Patients with borderline serum cobalamin levels but no hematologic or other abnormality may be followed to make sure that the cobalamin deficiency does not progress (see below). If malabsorption of cobalamin or rises in serum MMA levels have been demonstrated, however, these patients also should be given regular maintenance cobalamin therapy. Cobalamin should be given routinely to all patients who have had a total gastrectomy or ileal resection. Patients who have undergone gastric reduction for control of obesity or who are receiving long-term treatment with proton pump inhibitors should be screened and, if necessary, given cobalamin replacement.

Replenishment of body stores should be complete with six 1000-μg IM injections of hydroxocobalamin given at 3- to 7-day intervals. More frequent doses are usually used in patients with cobalamin neuropathy, but there is no evidence that they produce a better response. Allergic reactions are rare and may require desensitization or antihistamine or glucocorticoid cover. For maintenance therapy, 1000 μg hydroxocobalamin IM once every 3 months is satisfactory. Because of the poorer retention of cyanocobalamin, protocols generally use higher and more frequent doses, e.g., 1000 μg IM, monthly, for maintenance treatment.

Because a small fraction of cobalamin can be absorbed passively through mucous membranes even when there is complete failure of physiologic IF-dependent absorption, large daily oral doses (1000–2000 μg) of cyanocobalamin have been used in PA for replacement and maintenance of normal cobalamin status in, e.g., food malabsorption of cobalamin. Sublingual therapy has also been proposed for those in whom injections are difficult because of a bleeding tendency and who may not tolerate oral therapy. If oral therapy is used, it is important to monitor compliance, particularly with elderly, forgetful patients. This author prefers parenteral therapy for initial treatment, particularly in severe anemia or if a neuropathy is present, and for maintenance.

For treatment of patients with subnormal serum vitamin B_{12} (B_{12}) levels with a normal MCV and no hypersegmentation of neutrophils, a negative IF antibody test in the absence of tests of B_{12} absorption is problematic. Some (perhaps 15%) cases may be due to TC I (HC) deficiency. Homocysteine and/or MMA measurements may help, but in the absence of these tests and with otherwise normal gastrointestinal function, repeat serum B_{12} assay after 6–12 months may help one decide whether to start cobalamin therapy.

Vitamin B_{12} injections are used in a wide variety of diseases, often neurologic, despite normal serum B_{12} and folate levels and a normal blood count and in the absence of randomized, double-blind, controlled trials. These conditions include multiple sclerosis and chronic fatigue syndrome/myalgic encephalomyelitis (ME). It seems probable that any benefit is due to the placebo effect of a usually painless, pink injection. In ME, oral B_{12} therapy, despite providing equally large amounts of B_{12}, has not been beneficial, supporting the view of the effect of the injections being placebo only.

FOLATE DEFICIENCY

Oral doses of 5–15 mg folic acid daily are satisfactory, as sufficient folate is absorbed from these extremely large doses even in patients with severe malabsorption. The length of time therapy must be continued depends on the underlying disease. It is customary to continue therapy for about 4 months, when all folate-deficient red cells will have been eliminated and replaced by new folate-replete populations.

Before large doses of folic acid are given, cobalamin deficiency must be excluded and, if present, corrected; otherwise cobalamin neuropathy may develop despite a response of the anemia of cobalamin deficiency to folate therapy. Studies in the United States, however, suggest that there is no increase in the proportion of individuals with low serum cobalamin levels and no anemia since food fortification with folic acid, but it is unknown if there has been a change in incidence of cobalamin neuropathy.

Long-term folic acid therapy is required when the underlying cause of the deficiency cannot be corrected and the deficiency is likely to recur, e.g., in chronic dialysis or hemolytic anemias. It may also be necessary in gluten-induced enteropathy that does not respond to a gluten-free diet. Where mild but chronic folate deficiency occurs, it is preferable to encourage improvement in the diet after correcting the deficiency with a short course of folic acid. In any patient receiving long-term folic acid therapy, it is important to measure the serum cobalamin level at regular (e.g., once-yearly) intervals to exclude the coincidental development of cobalamin deficiency.

Folinic Acid (5-Formyl-THF) This is a stable form of fully reduced folate. It is given orally or parenterally to overcome the toxic effects of methotrexate or other DHF reductase inhibitors, e.g., trimethoprim or cotrimoxazole.

PROPHYLACTIC FOLIC ACID

Prophylactic folic acid is used in chronic dialysis patients and in parenteral feeds. Prophylactic folic acid has been used to reduce homocysteine levels to prevent cardiovascular disease and for cognitive function in the elderly, but there are no firm data to show any benefit.

Pregnancy In over 70 countries (but none in Europe), food is fortified with folic acid (in grain or flour) to reduce the risk of NTDs. Nevertheless, folic acid, 400 μg daily, should be given as a supplement before and throughout pregnancy to prevent megaloblastic anemia and reduce the incidence of NTDs, even in countries with fortification of the diet. The levels of fortification provide up to 400 μg daily on average in Chile, but in most countries, it is nearer to 200 μg, so periconceptual folic acid is still needed. Studies in early pregnancy show significant lack of compliance with the folic acid supplements, emphasizing the benefit of food fortification. Supplemental folic acid reduces the incidence of birth defects in babies born to diabetic mothers. In women who have had a previous fetus with an NTD, 5 mg daily is recommended when pregnancy is contemplated and throughout the subsequent pregnancy.

Infancy and Childhood The incidence of folate deficiency is so high in the smallest premature babies during the first 6 weeks of life that folic acid (e.g., 1 mg daily) should be given routinely to those weighing <1500 g at birth and to larger premature babies who require exchange transfusions or develop feeding difficulties, infections, or vomiting and diarrhea.

The World Health Organization currently recommends routine supplementation with iron and folic acid in children in countries where iron deficiency is common and child mortality, largely due to infectious diseases, is high. However, some studies suggest that in areas where malaria rates are high, this approach may increase the incidence of severe illness and death. Even where malaria is rare, there appears to be no survival benefit.

MEGALOBLASTIC ANEMIA NOT DUE TO COBALAMIN OR FOLATE DEFICIENCY OR ALTERED METABOLISM

This may occur with many antimetabolic drugs (e.g., hydroxyurea, cytosine arabinoside, 6-mercaptopurine) that inhibit DNA replication. Antiviral nucleoside analogues used in treatment of HIV infection may also cause macrocytosis and megaloblastic marrow changes. In the rare disease orotic aciduria, two consecutive enzymes in purine synthesis are defective. The condition responds to therapy with uridine, which bypasses the block. In thiamine-responsive megaloblastic anemia, there is a genetic defect in the high-affinity thiamine transport (*SLC19A2*) gene. This causes defective RNA ribose synthesis through impaired activity of transketolase, a thiamine-dependent enzyme in the pentose cycle. This leads to reduced nucleic acid production. It may be associated with diabetes mellitus and deafness and the presence of many ringed sideroblasts in the marrow. The explanation is unclear for megaloblastic changes in the marrow in some patients with acute myeloid leukemia and myelodysplasia.

129 Hemolytic Anemias and Anemia Due to Acute Blood Loss

Lucio Luzzatto

DEFINITIONS

A finite life span is a distinct characteristic of red cells. Hence, a logical, time-honored classification of anemias is in three groups: (1) decreased production of red cells, (2) increased destruction of red cells, and (3) acute blood loss. Decreased production is covered in Chaps. 126, 128, and 130; increased destruction and acute blood loss are covered in this chapter.

All patients who are anemic as a result of either increased destruction of red cells or acute blood loss have one important element in common: the anemia results from overconsumption of red cells from the peripheral blood, whereas the supply of cells from the bone marrow is normal (indeed, it is usually increased). On the other hand, these two groups differ in that physical loss of red cells from the bloodstream or *from* the body itself, as in acute hemorrhage, is fundamentally different from destruction of red cells *within* the body, as in hemolytic anemias.

TABLE 129-1 CLASSIFICATION OF HEMOLYTIC ANEMIAS[a]

	Intracorpuscular Defects	Extracorpuscular Factors
Hereditary	Hemoglobinopathies Enzymopathies Membrane-cytoskeletal defects	Familial (atypical) hemolytic-uremic syndrome
Acquired	Paroxysmal nocturnal hemoglobinuria (PNH)	Mechanical destruction (microangiopathic) Toxic agents Drugs Infectious Autoimmune

[a]Hereditary causes correlate with intracorpuscular defects, because these defects are due to inherited mutations; the one exception is PNH, because the defect is due to an acquired somatic mutation. Similarly, acquired causes correlate with extracorpuscular factors, because mostly these factors are exogenous; the one exception is familial hemolytic-uremic syndrome (HUS; often referred to as atypical HUS), because here an inherited abnormality allows complement activation to be excessive, with bouts of production of membrane attack complex capable of destroying normal red cells.

Therefore, the clinical aspects and pathophysiology of anemia in these two groups of patients are quite different, and they will be considered separately.

HEMOLYTIC ANEMIAS

With respect to primary etiology, anemias due to increased destruction of red cells, which we know as hemolytic anemias (HAs), may be *inherited* or *acquired*; from a clinical point of view, they may be more *acute* or more *chronic*, and they may vary from mild to very severe; the site of hemolysis may be predominantly *intravascular* or *extravascular*. With respect to mechanisms, HAs may be due to *intracorpuscular* causes or to *extracorpuscular* causes (Table 129-1). But before reviewing the individual types of HA, it is appropriate to consider what they have in common.

GENERAL CLINICAL AND LABORATORY FEATURES

The clinical presentation of a patient with anemia is greatly influenced in the first place by whether the onset is abrupt or gradual, and HAs are no exception. A patient with autoimmune HA or with favism may be a medical emergency, whereas a patient with mild hereditary spherocytosis or with cold agglutinin disease may be diagnosed after years. This is due in large measure to the remarkable ability of the body to adapt to anemia when it is slowly progressing (Chap. 77).

What differentiates HAs from other anemias is that the patient has signs and symptoms arising directly from hemolysis (Table 129-2). At the clinical level, the main sign is *jaundice*; in addition, the patient may report discoloration of the urine. In many cases of HA, the spleen is enlarged, because it is a preferential site of hemolysis; and in some cases, the liver may be enlarged as well. In all severe congenital forms of HA, there may also be skeletal changes due to overactivity of the bone marrow (although they are never as severe as they are in thalassemia).

TABLE 129-2 FEATURES COMMON TO MOST PATIENTS WITH A HEMOLYTIC DISORDER

General examination	Jaundice, pallor
Other physical findings	Spleen may be enlarged; bossing of skull in severe congenital cases
Hemoglobin level	From normal to severely reduced
MCV, MCH	Usually increased
Reticulocytes	Increased
Bilirubin	Increased (mostly unconjugated)
LDH	Increased (up to 10 time normal with intravascular hemolysis)
Haptoglobin	Reduced to absent (if hemolysis in part intravascular)

Abbreviations: LDH, lactate dehydrogenase; MCH, mean corpuscular hemoglobin; MCV, mean corpuscular volume.

The laboratory features of HA are related to hemolysis per se and the erythropoietic response of the bone marrow. Hemolysis regularly produces an increase in unconjugated bilirubin and aspartate aminotransferase (AST) in the serum; urobilinogen will be increased in both urine and stool. If hemolysis is mainly intravascular, the telltale sign is hemoglobinuria (often associated with hemosiderinuria); in the serum, there is hemoglobin, lactate dehydrogenase (LDH) is increased, and haptoglobin is reduced. In contrast, the bilirubin level may be normal or only mildly elevated. The main sign of the erythropoietic response by the bone marrow is an increase in reticulocytes (a test all too often neglected in the initial workup of a patient with anemia). Usually the increase will be reflected in both the percentage of reticulocytes (the more commonly quoted figure) and the absolute reticulocyte count (the more definitive parameter). The increased number of reticulocytes is associated with an increased mean corpuscular volume (MCV) in the blood count. On the blood smear, this is reflected in the presence of macrocytes; there is also polychromasia, and sometimes one sees nucleated red cells. In most cases, a bone marrow aspirate is not necessary in the diagnostic workup; if it is done, it will show erythroid hyperplasia. In practice, once an HA is suspected, specific tests will usually be required for a definitive diagnosis of a specific type of HA.

GENERAL PATHOPHYSIOLOGY

The mature red cell is the product of a developmental pathway that brings the phenomenon of differentiation to an extreme. An orderly sequence of events produces synchronous changes, whereby the gradual accumulation of a huge amount of hemoglobin in the cytoplasm (to a final level of 340 g/L, i.e., about 5 m*M*) goes hand in hand with the gradual loss of cellular organelles and of biosynthetic abilities. In the end, the erythroid cell undergoes a process that has features of apoptosis, including nuclear pyknosis and actual loss of the nucleus. However, the final result is more altruistic than suicidal; the cytoplasmic body, instead of disintegrating, is now able to provide oxygen to all cells in the human organism for some remaining 120 days of the red cell life span.

As a result of this unique process of differentiation and maturation, intermediary metabolism is drastically curtailed in mature red cells (Fig. 129-1); for instance, cytochrome-mediated oxidative phosphorylation has been lost with the loss of mitochondria (through a process of physiologic autophagy); therefore, there is no backup to anaerobic glycolysis, which in the red cell is the only provider of adenosine triphosphate (ATP). Also the capacity of making protein has been lost with the loss of ribosomes. This places the cell's limited metabolic apparatus at risk, because if any protein component deteriorates, it cannot be replaced, as it would be in most other cells; and in fact the activity of most enzymes gradually decreases as red cells age. At the same time, during their long time in circulation, various red cell components inevitably accumulate damage; in senescent red cells, the membrane protein band 3 molecules (see below and Fig. 129-1), having bound hemichromes on their intracellular domains, tend to cluster. Now they bind anti–band 3 IgG antibodies (present in most people) and C3 complement fragments; thus they become opsonized and are eventually removed by phagocytosis in the reticuloendothelial system.

Another consequence of the relative simplicity of red cells is that they have a very limited range of ways to manifest distress under hardship; in essence, any sort of metabolic failure will eventually lead either to structural damage to the membrane or to failure of the cation pump. In either case, the life span of the red cell is reduced, which is the definition of a *hemolytic disorder*. If the rate of red cell destruction exceeds the capacity of the bone marrow to produce more red cells, the hemolytic disorder will manifest as HA.

Thus, the essential pathophysiologic process common to all HAs is an increased red cell turnover; and in many HAs, this is due at least in part to an acceleration of the senescence process described above. The gold standard for proving that the life span of red cells is reduced (compared to the normal value of about 120 days) is a *red cell survival* study, which can be carried out by labeling the red cells with ^{51}Cr and measuring residual radioactivity over several days or weeks: however, this classic test is now available in very few centers, and it is rarely necessary.

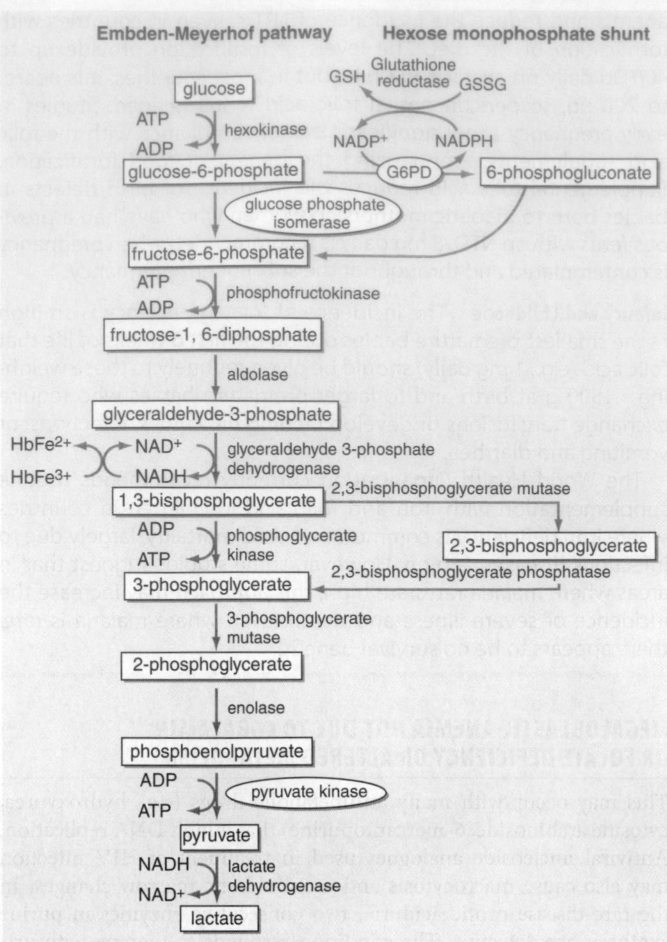

FIGURE 129-1 Red blood cell (RBC) metabolism. The Embden-Meyerhof pathway (glycolysis) generates ATP for energy and membrane maintenance. The generation of NADPH maintains hemoglobin in a reduced state. The hexose monophosphate shunt generates NADPH that is used to reduce glutathione, which protects the red cell against oxidant stress. Regulation of 2,3-bisphosphoglycerate levels is a critical determinant of oxygen affinity of hemoglobin. Enzyme deficiency states in order of prevalence: glucose 6-phosphate dehydrogenase (G6PD) > pyruvate kinase > glucose-6-phosphate isomerase > rare deficiencies of other enzymes in the pathway. The more common enzyme deficiencies are encircled.

If the hemolytic event is transient, it does not usually cause any long-term consequences, except for an increased requirement for erythropoietic factors, particularly folic acid. However, if hemolysis is recurrent or persistent, the increased bilirubin production favors the formation of gallstones. If a considerable proportion of hemolysis takes place in the spleen, as is often the case, splenomegaly may become increasingly a feature, and hypersplenism may develop, with consequent neutropenia and/or thrombocytopenia.

The increased red cell turnover also has metabolic consequences. In normal subjects, the iron from effete red cells is very efficiently recycled by the body; however, with chronic intravascular hemolysis, the persistent hemoglobinuria will cause considerable iron loss, needing replacement. With chronic extravascular hemolysis, the opposite problem, iron overload, is more common, especially if the patient needs frequent blood transfusions. Chronic iron overload will cause secondary hemochromatosis; this will cause damage particularly to the liver, eventually leading to cirrhosis, and to the heart muscle, eventually causing heart failure.

Compensated Hemolysis Versus Hemolytic Anemia Red cell destruction is a potent stimulus for erythropoiesis, which is mediated by erythropoietin (EPO) produced by the kidney. This mechanism is so effective that in many cases the increased output of red cells from the bone marrow can fully balance an increased destruction of red cells. In such cases, we say that hemolysis is *compensated*. The pathophysiology of compensated hemolysis is similar to what we have just described, except there is no anemia. This notion is important from the diagnostic point of view, because a patient with a hemolytic condition, even an inherited one, may present without anemia; and it is also important from the point of view of management, because compensated hemolysis may become "decompensated," i.e., anemia may suddenly appear, in certain circumstances, for instance in pregnancy, folate deficiency, or renal failure interfering with adequate EPO production. Another general feature of chronic HAs is seen when any intercurrent condition, such as an acute infection, depresses erythropoiesis. When this happens, in view of the increased rate of red cell turnover, the effect will be predictably much more marked than in a person who does not have hemolysis. The most dramatic example is infection by parvovirus B19, which may cause a rather precipitous fall in hemoglobin—an occurrence sometimes referred to as *aplastic crisis*.

INHERITED HEMOLYTIC ANEMIAS

There are three essential components in the red cell: (1) hemoglobin, (2) the membrane-cytoskeleton complex, and (3) the metabolic machinery necessary to keep hemoglobin and the membrane-cytoskeleton complex in working order. Diseases caused by abnormalities of hemoglobin, or hemoglobinopathies, are covered in Chap. 127. Here we will deal with diseases of the other two components.

Hemolytic Anemias due to Abnormalities of the Membrane-Cytoskeleton Complex The detailed architecture of the red cell membrane is complex, but its basic design is relatively simple (Fig. 129-2). The lipid bilayer incorporates phospholipids and cholesterol, and it is spanned by a number of proteins that have their hydrophobic transmembrane domain(s) embedded in the membrane; most of these proteins also extend to both the outside (extracellular domains) and the inside of the cell (cytoplasmic domains). Other proteins are tethered to the membrane through a glycosylphosphatidylinositol (GPI) anchor; these have only an extracellular domain, and they include ion channels, receptors for complement components, and receptors for other ligands. The most abundant red cell membrane proteins are glycophorins and the so-called *band 3*, an anion transporter. The extracellular domains of many of these proteins are heavily glycosylated, and they carry antigenic determinants that correspond to blood groups. Underneath the membrane, and tangential to it, is a network of other proteins that make up the cytoskeleton. The main cytoskeletal protein is spectrin, the basic unit of which is a dimer of α-spectrin and β-spectrin. The membrane is physically linked to the cytoskeleton by a third set of proteins (including ankyrin and the so-called *band 4.1* and *band 4.2*), which thus make these two structures intimately connected to each other.

The membrane-cytoskeleton complex is so integrated that, not surprisingly, an abnormality of almost any of its components will be disturbing or disruptive, causing structural failure, which results ultimately in hemolysis. These abnormalities are almost invariably inherited mutations; thus, diseases of the membrane-cytoskeleton complex belong to the category of inherited HAs. Before the red cells lyse, they often exhibit more or less specific morphologic changes that alter the normal biconcave disk shape. Thus, the majority of the diseases in this group have been known for over a century as *hereditary spherocytosis* and *hereditary elliptocytosis*. Over the past 20 years, their molecular basis has been elucidated; it has emerged that both conditions can arise from mutations in several genes with considerable overlap (Fig. 129-3).

HEREDITARY SPHEROCYTOSIS (HS) This is a relatively common type of genetically determined HA, with an estimated frequency of at least 1 in 5000. Its identification is credited to Minkowksy and Chauffard, who, at the end of the nineteenth century, reported families who had the presence of numerous spherocytes in the peripheral blood (Fig 129-4A). In vitro studies revealed that the red cells were abnormally susceptible to lysis in hypotonic media; indeed, the presence of *osmotic fragility* became the main diagnostic test for HS. Today we know that HS, thus defined, is genetically heterogeneous; i.e., it can arise from a variety of mutations in one of several genes (Table 129-3). It has been also recognized that the inheritance of HS is not always autosomal dominant (with the patient being heterozygous); indeed, some of the most severe forms are instead autosomal recessive (with the patient being homozygous).

Clinical presentation and diagnosis The spectrum of clinical severity of HS is broad. Severe cases may present in infancy with severe anemia, whereas mild cases may present in young adults or even later in life. The main clinical findings are jaundice, an enlarged spleen, and often gallstones; indeed, it may be the finding of gallstones in a young person that triggers diagnostic investigations.

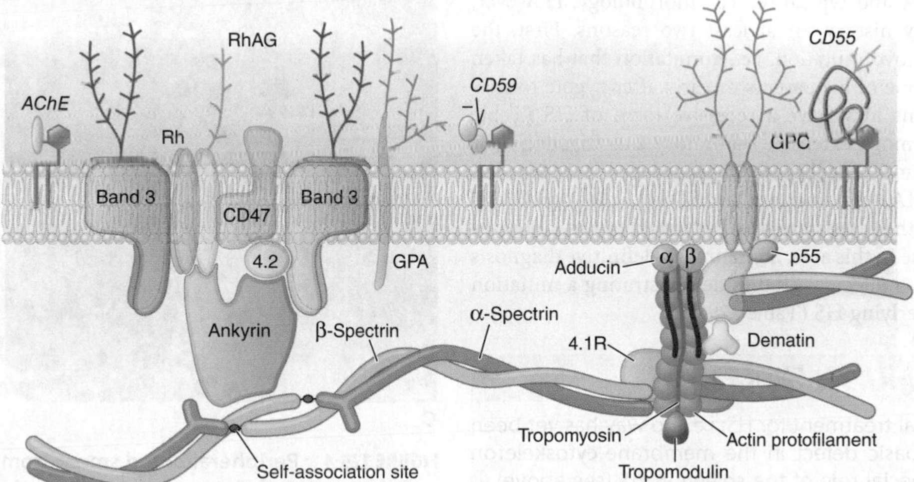

FIGURE 129-2 The red cell membrane. In this figure, one sees, within the lipid bilayer, several membrane proteins, of which band 3 (anion exchanger 1 [AE1]) is the most abundant; the α-β spectrin dimers that associate to form most of the cytoskeleton; and several proteins (e.g., ankyrin) that connect the membrane to the cytoskeleton. In addition, as examples of glycosylphosphatidylinositol (GPI)-linked proteins, one sees acetylcholinesterase (AChE) and the two complement-regulatory proteins CD59 and CD55. The (nonrealistic) shapes of the protein moieties of the GPI-linked proteins are meant to indicate that they can be very different from each other and that, unlike with the other membrane proteins shown, the entire polypeptide chain is extracellular. Branched lines symbolize carbohydrate moiety of proteins. The molecules are obviously not drawn to the same scale. Additional explanations can be found in the text. *(From N Young et al: Clinical Hematology. Copyright Elsevier, 2006; with permission.)*

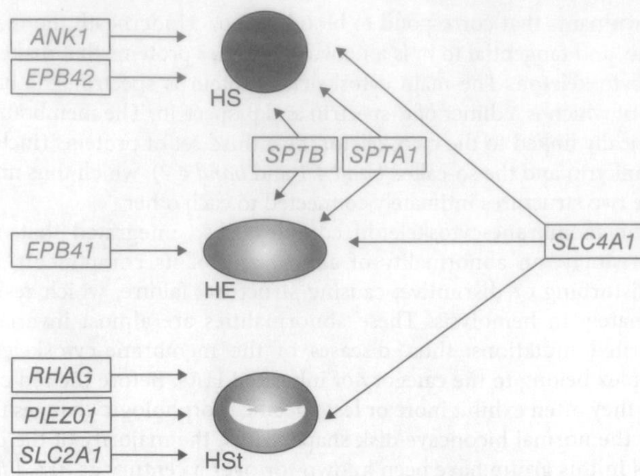

FIGURE 129-3 Hereditary spherocytosis (HS), hereditary elliptocytosis (HE), and hereditary stomatocytosis (HSt) are three morphologically distinct forms of congenital hemolytic anemia. It has emerged that each one can arise from mutation of one of several genes and that different mutations of the same gene can give one or another form. (See also Table 129-3.)

The variability in clinical manifestations that is observed among patients with HS is largely due to the different underlying molecular lesions (Table 129-3). Not only are mutations of several genes involved, but also individual mutations of the same gene can also give very different clinical manifestations. In milder cases, hemolysis is often compensated (see above), and this may cause variation in time even in the same patient, due to the fact that intercurrent conditions (e.g., pregnancy, infection) may cause decompensation. The anemia is usually normocytic, with the characteristic morphology that gives the disease its name. An increased mean corpuscular hemoglobin concentration (MCHC) on an ordinary blood count report should raise the suspicion of HS, because HS is almost the only condition in which this abnormality occurs. It has been apparent for a long time that the spleen plays a special role in HS through a dual mechanism. On one hand, like in many other HAs, the spleen itself is a major site of destruction; on the other hand, transit through the splenic circulation makes the defective red cells more spherocytic and, therefore, accelerates their demise, even though that may take place elsewhere.

When there is a family history, it is usually easy to make a diagnosis based on features of HA and typical red cell morphology. However, there may be no family history for at least two reasons. First, the patient may have a de novo mutation, i.e., a mutation that has taken place in a germ cell of one of his parents or early after zygote formation. Second, the patient may have a recessive form of HS (Table 129-3). In such cases, more extensive laboratory investigations are required, including osmotic fragility, the acid glycerol lysis test, the eosin-5′-maleimide (EMA)–binding test, and SDS-gel electrophoresis of membrane proteins; these tests are usually carried out in laboratories with special expertise in this area. Sometimes a definitive diagnosis can be obtained only by molecular studies demonstrating a mutation in one of the genes underlying HS (Table 129-3).

TREATMENT HEREDITARY SPHEROCYTOSIS

We do not have a causal treatment for HS; i.e., no way has yet been found to correct the basic defect in the membrane-cytoskeleton structure. Given the special role of the spleen in HS (see above), it has long been thought that an almost obligatory therapeutic measure was splenectomy. Because this operation may have more than trivial consequences, today we have more articulate recommendations, based on disease severity (having found out, whenever possible, about the outcome of splenectomy in the patient's relatives with HS), as follows. In mild cases, avoid splenectomy. Delay splenectomy until puberty in moderate cases or until 4–6 years of age in severe cases. Antipneumococcal vaccination before splenectomy is imperative, whereas penicillin prophylaxis after splenectomy is controversial. Along with splenectomy, cholecystectomy should not be regarded as automatic; it should be carried out, usually by the laparoscopic approach, when clinically indicated.

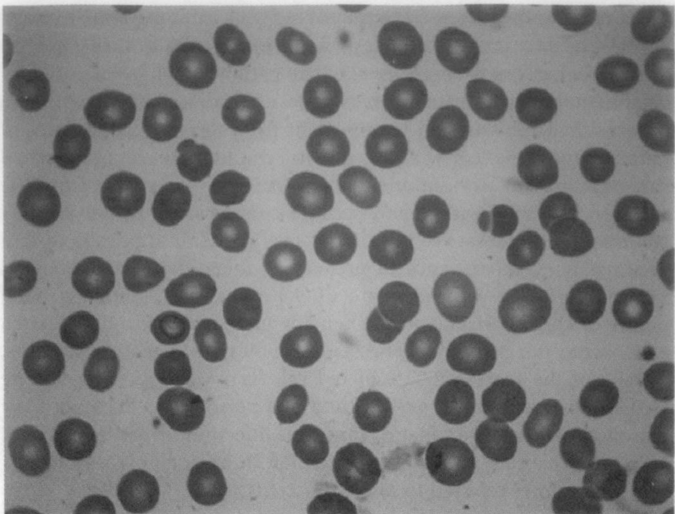
A

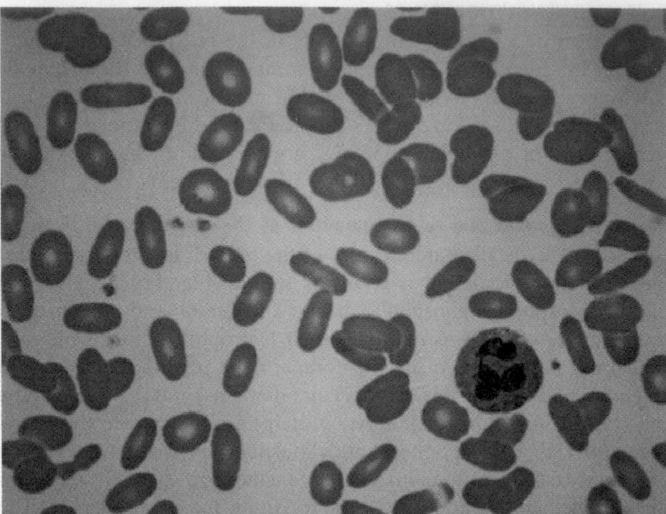
B

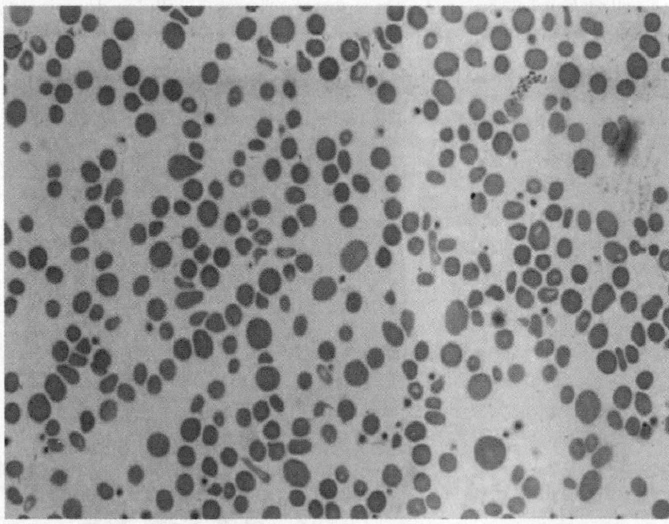
C

FIGURE 129-4 Peripheral blood smear from patients with membrane-cytoskeleton abnormalities. ***A.*** Hereditary spherocytosis. ***B.*** Hereditary elliptocytosis, heterozygote. ***C.*** Elliptocytosis, with both alleles of the α-spectrin gene mutated.

TABLE 129-3 INHERITED DISEASES OF THE RED CELL MEMBRANE-CYTOSKELETON COMPLEX

Gene	Chromosomal Location	Protein Produced	Disease(s) with Certain Mutations (Inheritance)	Comments
SPTA1	1q22-q23	α-Spectrin	HS (recessive)	Rare
			HE (dominant)	Mutations of this gene account for about 65% of HE. More severe forms may be due to coexistence of an otherwise silent mutant allele.
SPTB	14q23-q24.1	β-Spectrin	HS (dominant)	Rare
			HE (dominant)	Mutations of this gene account for about 30% of HE, including some severe forms.
ANK1	8p11.2	Ankyrin	HS (dominant)	May account for majority of HS.
SLC4A1	17q21	Band 3; also known as AE (anion exchanger) or AE1	HS (dominant)	Mutations of this gene may account for about 25% of HS.
			Southeast Asia ovalocytosis (dominant)	Polymorphic mutation (deletion of 9 amino acids); clinically asymptomatic; protective against *Plasmodium falciparum*.
			Stomatocytosis	Certain specific missense mutations shift protein function from anion exchanger to cation conductance.
EPB41	1p33-p34.2	Band 4.1	HE (dominant)	Mutations of this gene account for about 5% of HE, mostly with prominent morphology but no hemolysis in heterozygotes; severe hemolysis in homozygotes.
EPB42	15q15-q21	Band 4.2	HS (recessive)	Mutations of this gene account for about 3% of HS.
RHAG	6p21.1-p11	Rhesus antigen	Chronic nonspherocytic hemolytic anemia (recessive)	Very rare; associated with total loss of all Rh antigens. A specific mutation causes overhydrated stomatocytosis.
PIEZO1	16q23-q24	PIEZO1	Dehydrated hereditary stomatocytosis (dominant)	Also known as xerocytosis with pseudohyperkalemia. Patients may present with perinatal edema. PIEZO1 is a mechanosensitive cation channel.

Abbreviations: HE, hereditary elliptocytosis; HS, hereditary spherocytosis.

HEREDITARY ELLIPTOCYTOSIS (HE) HE is at least as heterogeneous as HS, both from the genetic point of view (Table 129-3, Fig. 129-3) and from the clinical point of view. Again, it is the shape of the red cells (Fig. 129-4B) that gives the name to the condition, but there is no direct correlation between the elliptocytic morphology and clinical severity. In fact, some mild or even asymptomatic cases may have nearly 100% elliptocytes, whereas in severe cases, all kinds of bizarre poikilocytes can predominate. Clinical features and recommended management are similar to those outlined above for HS. Although the spleen may not have the specific role it has in HS, in severe cases, splenectomy may be beneficial. The prevalence of HE causing clinical disease is similar to that of HS. However, an in-frame deletion of nine amino acids in the *SLC4A1* gene encoding band 3, causing the so-called *Southeast Asia ovalocytosis*, has a frequency of up to 7% in certain populations, presumably as a result of malaria selection; it is asymptomatic in heterozygotes and probably lethal in homozygotes.

Disorders of Cation Transport These rare conditions with autosomal dominant inheritance are characterized by increased intracellular sodium in red cells, with concomitant loss of potassium; indeed, they are sometimes discovered through the incidental finding, in a blood test, of a high serum K^+ (*pseudohyperkalemia*). In patients from some families, the cation transport disturbance is associated with gain of water; as a result, the red cells are overhydrated (low MCHC), and on a blood smear, the normally round-shaped central pallor is replaced by a linear-shaped central pallor, which has earned this disorder the name *stomatocytosis* (Fig. 129-3). In patients from other families, instead, the red cells are dehydrated (high MCHC), and their consequent rigidity has earned this disorder the name *xerocytosis*. One would surmise that in these disorders the primary defect may be in a cation transporter; indeed, xerocytosis results from mutations in *PIEZO1*. In other patients with stomatocytosis, mutations are found in other genes also related to solute transport (Table 129-3), including *SLC4A1* (encoding band 3), the Rhesus gene *RHAG*, and the glucose transporter gene *SLC2A1* responsible for a special form called cryohydrocytosis. Hemolysis can vary from relatively mild to quite severe. From the practical point of view, it is important to know that in stomatocytosis, splenectomy is strongly contraindicated because it has been followed in a significant proportion of cases by severe thromboembolic complications.

Enzyme Abnormalities When there is an important defect in the membrane or in the cytoskeleton, hemolysis is a direct consequence of the fact that the very structure of the red cell is abnormal. Instead, when one of the enzymes is defective, the consequences will depend on the precise role of that enzyme in the metabolic machinery of the red cell, which, in first approximation, has two important functions: (1) to provide energy in the form of ATP and (2) to prevent oxidative damage to hemoglobin and to other proteins by providing sufficient reductive potential; the key molecule for this is NADPH.

ABNORMALITIES OF THE GLYCOLYTIC PATHWAY Because red cells, in the course of their differentiation, have sacrificed not only their nucleus and their ribosomes, but also their mitochondria, they rely exclusively on the anaerobic portion of the glycolytic pathway for producing energy in the form of ATP. Most of the ATP is required by the red cell for cation transport against a concentration gradient across the membrane. If this fails, due to a defect of any of the enzymes of the glycolytic pathway (Table 129-4), the result will be hemolytic disease.

Pyruvate kinase deficiency Abnormalities of the glycolytic pathway are all inherited and all rare. Among them, deficiency of pyruvate kinase (PK) is the least rare, with an estimated prevalence in most populations of the order of 1:10,000. However, very recently, a polymorphic PK mutation (E277K) was found in some African populations, with heterozygote frequencies of 1–7%, suggesting that this may be another malaria-related polymorphism. The clinical picture of homozygous (or compound biallelic) PK deficiency is that of an HA that often presents in the newborn with neonatal jaundice; the jaundice persists, and it is usually associated with a very high reticulocytosis. The anemia is of variable severity; sometimes it is so severe as to require regular blood transfusion treatment, whereas sometimes it is mild, bordering on a nearly compensated hemolytic disorder. As a result, the diagnosis may be delayed, and in some cases, it is made, for instance, in a young woman during her first pregnancy, when the anemia may get worse. The delay in diagnosis may be also helped by the fact that the anemia is remarkably well tolerated, because the metabolic block at the last step in glycolysis causes an increase in bisphosphoglycerate (or DPG; Fig. 129-1), a major effector of the hemoglobin-oxygen dissociation curve; thus, the oxygen delivery to the tissues is enhanced, a remarkable compensatory feat.

TABLE 129-4 RED CELL ENZYME ABNORMALITIES CAUSING HEMOLYSIS

	Enzyme (Acronym)	Chromosomal Location	Prevalence of Enzyme Deficiency (Rank)	Clinical Manifestations Extra-Red Cell	Comments
Glycolytic Pathway					
	Hexokinase (HK)	10q22	Very rare		Other isoenzymes known
	Glucose 6-phosphate isomerase (G6PI)	19q31.1	Rare (4)[a]	NM, CNS	
	Phosphofructokinase (PFK)	12q13	Very rare	Myopathy	
	Aldolase	16q22-24	Very rare		
	Triose phosphate isomerase (TPI)	12p13	Very rare	CNS (severe), NM	
	Glyceraldehyde 3-phosphate dehydrogenase (GAPD)	12p13.31-p13.1	Very rare	Myopathy	
	Diphosphoglycerate mutase (DPGM)	7q31-q34	Very rare		Erythrocytosis rather than hemolysis
	Phosphoglycerate kinase (PGK)	Xq13	Very rare	CNS, NM	May benefit from splenectomy
	Pyruvate kinase (PK)	1q21	Rare (2)[a]		May benefit from splenectomy
Redox					
	Glucose 6-phosphate dehydrogenase (G6PD)	Xq28	Common (1)[a]	Very rarely granulocytes	In almost all cases, only AHA from exogenous trigger
	Glutathione synthase	20q11.2	Very rare	CNS	
	γ-Glutamylcysteine synthase	6p12	Very rare	CNS	
	Cytochrome b5 reductase	22q13.31-qter	Rare	CNS	Methemoglobinemia rather than hemolysis
Nucleotide Metabolism					
	Adenylate kinase (AK)	9q34.1	Very rare	CNS	
	Pyrimidine 5′-nucleotidase (P5N)	3q11-q12	Rare (3)[a]		May benefit from splenectomy

[a]The numbers from (1) to (4) indicate the ranking order of these enzymopathies in terms of frequency.

Abbreviations: AHA, acquired hemolytic anemia; CNS, central nervous system; NM, neuromuscular.

TREATMENT PYRUVATE KINASE DEFICIENCY

The management of PK deficiency is mainly supportive. In view of the marked increase in red cell turnover, oral folic acid supplements should be given constantly. Blood transfusion should be used as necessary, and iron chelation may have to be added if the blood transfusion requirement is high enough to cause iron overload. In these patients, who have more severe disease, splenectomy may be beneficial. There is a single case report of curative treatment of PK deficiency by bone marrow transplantation from an HLA-identical PK-normal sibling. This seems a viable option for severe cases when a sibling donor is available. Rescue of inherited PK deficiency through lentiviral-mediated human PK gene transfer has been successful in mice. Prenatal diagnosis has been carried out in a mother who had already had an affected child.

Other glycolytic enzyme abnormalities All of these defects are rare to very rare (Table 129-4), and all cause hemolytic anemia with varying degrees of severity. It is not unusual for the presentation to be in the guise of severe neonatal jaundice, which may require exchange transfusion; if the anemia is less severe, it may present later in life, or it may even remain asymptomatic and be detected incidentally when a blood count is done for unrelated reasons. The spleen is often enlarged. When other systemic manifestations occur, they can involve the central nervous system (sometimes entailing severe mental retardation, particularly in the case of triose phosphate isomerase deficiency), the neuromuscular system, or both. This is not altogether surprising, if we consider that these are housekeeping genes. The *diagnosis* of hemolytic anemia is usually not difficult, thanks to the triad of normomacrocytic anemia, reticulocytosis, and hyperbilirubinemia. Enzymopathies should be considered in the differential diagnosis of any chronic Coombs-negative hemolytic anemia. Unlike with membrane disorders where the red cells show characteristic morphologic abnormalities, in most cases of glycolytic enzymopathies, these are conspicuous by their absence. A definitive diagnosis can be made only by demonstrating the deficiency of an individual enzyme by quantitative assays; these are carried out in only a few specialized laboratories. If a particular molecular abnormality is already known in the family, then one could test directly for that defect at the DNA level, thus bypassing the need for enzyme assays. Of course the time may be getting nearer when a patient will present with her or his exome already sequenced, and we will need to concentrate on which genes to look up within the file. The principles for the management of these conditions are similar as for PK deficiency. In one case of phosphoglycerate kinase deficiency, allogeneic bone marrow transplantation (BMT) effectively controlled the hematologic manifestations but did not reverse neurologic damage.

ABNORMALITIES OF REDOX METABOLISM

Glucose 6-phosphate dehydrogenase (G6PD) deficiency G6PD is a housekeeping enzyme critical in the redox metabolism of all aerobic cells (Fig. 129-1). In red cells, its role is even more critical, because it is the only source of NADPH, which directly and via glutathione (GSH) defends these cells against oxidative stress (Fig. 129-5). G6PD deficiency is a prime example of an HA due to interaction between

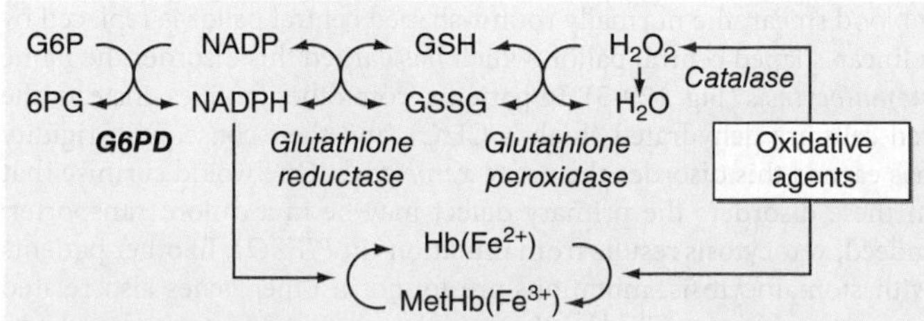

FIGURE 129-5 Diagram of redox metabolism in the red cell. 6PG, 6-phosphogluconate; G6P, glucose 6-phosphate; G6PD, glucose 6-phosphate dehydrogenase; GSH, reduced glutathione; GSSG, oxidized glutathione; Hb, hemoglobin; MetHb, methemoglobin; NADP, nicotinamide adenine dinucleotide phosphate; NADPH, reduced nicotinamide adenine dinucleotide phosphate.

an intracorpuscular cause and an extracorpuscular cause, because in the majority of cases hemolysis is triggered by an exogenous agent. Although a decrease in G6PD activity is present in most tissues of G6PD-deficient subjects, in other cells, the decrease is much less marked than in red cells, and it does not seem to impact on clinical expression.

GENETIC CONSIDERATIONS

The *G6PD* gene is X-linked, and this has important implications. First, because males have only one *G6PD* gene (i.e., they are hemizygous for this gene), they must be either normal or G6PD deficient. By contrast, females, who have two *G6PD* genes, can be either normal or deficient (homozygous) or intermediate (heterozygous). As a result of the phenomenon of X chromosome inactivation, heterozygous females are genetic mosaics, with a highly variable ratio of G6PD-normal to G6PD-deficient cells and an equally variable degree of clinical expression; some heterozygotes can be just as affected as hemizygous males. The enzymatically active form of G6PD is either a dimer or a tetramer of a single protein subunit of 514 amino acids. G6PD-deficient subjects have been found invariably to have mutations in the coding region of the *G6PD* gene (Fig. 129-5). Almost all of the approximately 180 different mutations known are single missense point mutations, entailing single amino acid replacements in the G6PD protein. In most cases, these mutations cause G6PD deficiency by decreasing the in vivo stability of the protein; thus, the physiologic decrease in G6PD activity that takes place with red cell aging is greatly accelerated. In some cases, an amino acid replacement can also affect the catalytic function of the enzyme.

Among these mutations, those underlying chronic nonspherocytic hemolytic anemia (CNSHA; see below) are a discrete subset. This much more severe clinical phenotype can be ascribed in some cases to adverse qualitative changes (for instance, a decreased affinity for the substrate, glucose 6-phosphate) or simply to the fact that the enzyme deficit is more extreme, because of a more severe instability of the enzyme. For instance, a cluster of mutations map at or near the dimer interface, and clearly they compromise severely the formation of the dimer.

Epidemiology G6PD deficiency is widely distributed in tropical and subtropical parts of the world (Africa, Southern Europe, the Middle East, Southeast Asia, and Oceania) (Fig. 129-6) and wherever people from those areas have migrated. A conservative estimate is that at least 400 million people have a *G6PD* deficiency gene. In several of these areas, the frequency of a *G6PD* deficiency gene may be as high as 20% or more. It would be quite extraordinary for a trait that causes significant pathology to spread widely and reach high frequencies in many populations without conferring some biologic advantage. Indeed, G6PD is one of the best-characterized examples of genetic polymorphisms in the human species. Clinical field studies and in vitro experiments strongly support the view that G6PD deficiency has been selected by *Plasmodium falciparum* malaria, by virtue of the fact that it confers a relative resistance against this highly lethal infection. Different G6PD variants underlie G6PD deficiency in different parts of the world. Some of the more widespread variants are G6PD Mediterranean on the shores of that sea, in the Middle East, and in India; G6PD A– in Africa and in Southern Europe; G6PD Vianchan and G6PD Mahidol in Southeast Asia; G6PD Canton in China; and G6PD Union worldwide. The heterogeneity of polymorphic G6PD variants is proof of their independent origin, and it supports the notion that they have been selected by a common environmental agent, in keeping with the concept of convergent evolution (Fig. 129-6).

Clinical manifestations The vast majority of people with G6PD deficiency remain clinically asymptomatic throughout their lifetime; however, all of them have an increased risk of developing neonatal jaundice (NNJ) and a risk of developing acute HA (AHA) when challenged by a number of oxidative agents. NNJ related to G6PD deficiency is very rarely present at birth; the peak incidence of clinical onset is between day 2 and day 3, and in most cases, the anemia is not severe. However, NNJ can be very severe in some G6PD-deficient babies, especially in association with prematurity, infection, and/or environmental factors (such as naphthalene-camphor balls, which are used in babies' bedding and clothing), and the risk of severe NNJ is also increased by the coexistence of a monoallelic or biallelic mutation in the uridyl transferase gene (*UGT1A1*; the same mutations are associated with Gilbert's syndrome). If inadequately managed, NNJ associated with G6PD deficiency can produce kernicterus and permanent neurologic damage.

AHA can develop as a result of three types of triggers: (1) fava beans, (2) infections, and (3) drugs (Table 129-5). Typically, a hemolytic attack starts with malaise, weakness, and abdominal or lumbar pain. After an interval of several hours to 2–3 days, the patient develops jaundice and often dark urine. The onset can be extremely abrupt, especially with favism in children. The anemia is moderate to extremely severe, usually normocytic and normochromic, and due partly to intravascular hemolysis; hence, it is associated with hemoglobinemia, hemoglobinuria, high LDH, and low or absent plasma haptoglobin. The blood film shows anisocytosis, polychromasia, and spherocytes typical of hemolytic anemias. The most typical feature of G6PD deficiency is the presence of bizarre poikilocytes, with red cells that appear to have unevenly distributed hemoglobin ("hemighosts") and red cells that appear to have had parts of them bitten away ("bite cells" or "blister cells") (Fig. 129-7). A classical test, now rarely carried out, is supravital staining with methyl violet, which, if done promptly, reveals the presence of Heinz bodies (consisting of precipitates of denatured hemoglobin and hemichromes), which are regarded as a signature of oxidative damage to red cells (they are also seen with unstable hemoglobins). LDH is high, and so is the unconjugated

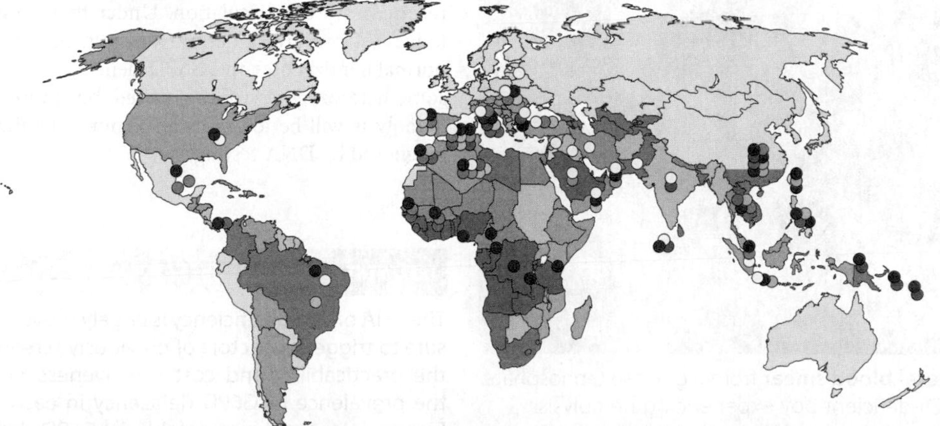

FIGURE 129-6 Epidemiology of glucose 6-phosphate dehydrogenase (G6PD) deficiency throughout the world. The different shadings indicate increasingly high levels of prevalence, up to about 20%; the different colored symbols indicate individual genetic variants of G6PD, each one having a different mutation. *(From L Luzzato et al, in C Scriver et al [eds]: The Metabolic & Molecular Bases of Inherited Disease, 8th ed. New York, McGraw-Hill, 2001.)*

TABLE 129-5 DRUGS THAT CARRY RISK OF CLINICAL HEMOLYSIS IN PERSONS WITH GLUCOSE 6-PHOSPHATE DEHYDROGENASE DEFICIENCY

	Definite Risk	Possible Risk	Doubtful Risk
Antimalarials	Primaquine Dapsone/chlorproguanil[a]	Chloroquine	Quinine
Sulphonamides/sulphones	Sulfamethoxazole Others Dapsone	Sulfasalazine Sulfadimidine	Sulfisoxazole Sulfadiazine
Antibacterial/antibiotics	Cotrimoxazole Nalidixic acid Nitrofurantoin Niridazole	Ciprofloxacin Norfloxacin	Chloramphenicol *p*-Aminosalicylic acid
Antipyretic/analgesics	Acetanilide Phenazopyridine	Acetylsalicylic acid high dose (>3 g/d)	Acetylsalicylic acid (<3 g/d) Acetaminophen Phenacetin
Other	Naphthalene Methylene blue Rasburicase	Vitamin K analogues Ascorbic acid (>1 g)	Doxorubicin Probenecid

[a]Marketed as Lapdap from 2003 to 2008.

bilirubin, indicating that there is also extravascular hemolysis. The most serious threat from AHA in adults is the development of acute renal failure (this is exceedingly rare in children). Once the threat of acute anemia is over and in the absence of comorbidity, full recovery from AHA associated with G6PD deficiency is the rule.

Although it was primaquine (PQ) that led to the discovery of G6PD deficiency, this drug has not been very prominent subsequently, because it is not necessary for the treatment of life-threatening *P. falciparum* malaria. Today there is a revival of interest in PQ because it is the only effective agent for eliminating the gametocytes of *P. falciparum* (thus preventing further transmission) and eliminating the hypnozoites of *Plasmodium vivax* (thus preventing endogenous relapse). In countries aiming to eliminate malaria, there may be a call for mass administration of PQ; this ought to be associated with G6PD testing. At the other end of the historic spectrum, the latest addition to the list of potentially hemolytic drugs (Table 129-5) is rasburicase; again G6PD testing ought to be made mandatory before giving this drug because fatal cases have been reported in newborns with kidney injury and in adults with tumor lysis syndrome.

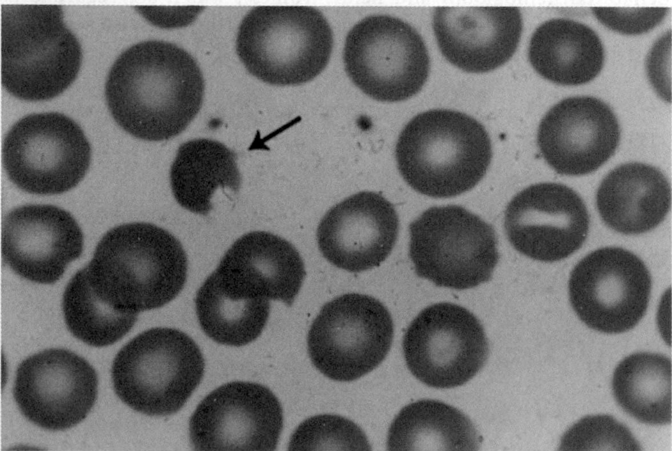

FIGURE 129-7 Peripheral blood smear from a glucose 6-phosphate dehydrogenase (G6PD)-deficient boy experiencing hemolysis. Note the red cells that are misshapen and called "bite" cells. *(From MA Lichtman et al: Lichtman's Atlas of Hematology: http://www.accessmedicine.com. Copyright © The McGraw-Hill Companies, Inc. All rights reserved.)*

A very small minority of subjects with G6PD deficiency have *chronic nonspherocytic hemolytic anemia* (CNSHA) of variable severity. The patient is nearly always a male, usually with a history of NNJ, who may present with anemia, unexplained jaundice, or gallstones later in life. The spleen may be enlarged. The severity of anemia ranges in different patients from borderline to transfusion dependent. The anemia is usually normomacrocytic, with reticulocytosis. Bilirubin and LDH are increased. Although hemolysis is, by definition, chronic in these patients, they are also vulnerable to acute oxidative damage, and therefore the same agents that can cause AHA in people with the ordinary type of G6PD deficiency will cause severe exacerbations in people with CNSHA associated with G6PD deficiency. In some cases of CNSHA, the deficiency of G6PD is so severe in granulocytes that it becomes rate-limiting for their oxidative burst, with consequent increased susceptibility to some bacterial infections.

Laboratory diagnosis The suspicion of G6PD deficiency can be confirmed by semiquantitative methods often referred to as screening tests, which are suitable for population studies and can correctly classify male subjects, in the steady state, as G6PD normal or G6PD deficient. However, in clinical practice, a diagnostic test is usually needed when the patient has had a hemolytic attack; this implies that the oldest, most G6PD-deficient red cells have been selectively destroyed, and young red cells, having higher G6PD activity, are being released into the circulation. Under these conditions, only a quantitative test can give a definitive result. In males, this test will identify normal hemizygotes and G6PD-deficient hemizygotes; among females, some heterozygotes will be missed, but those who are at most risk of hemolysis will be identified. Of course, G6PD deficiency also can be diagnosed by DNA testing.

TREATMENT G6PD DEFICIENCY

The AHA of G6PD deficiency is largely preventable by avoiding exposure to triggering factors of previously screened subjects. Of course, the practicability and cost-effectiveness of screening depend on the prevalence of G6PD deficiency in each individual community. Favism is entirely preventable in G6PD-deficient subjects by not eating fava beans. Drug-induced hemolysis can be prevented by testing for G6PD deficiency before prescribing; in most cases, one can use alternative drugs. When AHA develops and once its cause is recognized, in most cases, no specific treatment is needed. However, if the anemia is severe, it may be a medical emergency, especially in children, requiring immediate action, including blood transfusion. This has been the case with an antimalarial drug combination containing dapsone (called Lapdap, introduced in 2003) that has caused severe acute hemolytic episodes in children with malaria in several African countries; after a few years, the drug was taken off the market. If there is acute renal failure, hemodialysis may be necessary, but if there is no previous kidney disease, recovery is the rule. The management of NNJ associated with G6PD deficiency is no different from that of NNJ due to other causes.

In cases with CNSHA, if the anemia is not severe, regular folic acid supplements and regular hematologic surveillance will suffice. It will be important to avoid exposure to potentially hemolytic drugs, and blood transfusion may be indicated when exacerbations occur, mostly in concomitance with intercurrent infection. In rare patients, regular blood transfusions may be required, in which case appropriate iron chelation should be instituted. Unlike in HS, there is no evidence of selective red cell destruction in the spleen; however, in practice, splenectomy has proven beneficial in severe cases.

Other abnormalities of the redox system As mentioned above, GSH is a key player in the defense against oxidative stress. Inherited defects of GSH metabolism are exceedingly rare, but each one can give rise to chronic HA (Table 129-4). A rare, peculiar, usually self-limited severe HA of the first month of life, called *infantile poikilocytosis*, may be associated with deficiency of glutathione peroxidase (GSHPX) due not to an inherited abnormality, but to transient nutritional deficiency of selenium, an element essential for the activity of GSHPX.

PYRIMIDINE 5′-NUCLEOTIDASE (P5N) DEFICIENCY P5N is a key enzyme in the catabolism of nucleotides arising from the degradation of nucleic acids that takes place in the final stages of erythroid cell maturation. How exactly its deficiency causes HA is not well understood, but a highly distinctive feature of this condition is a morphologic abnormality of the red cells known as *basophilic stippling*. The condition is rare, but it probably ranks third in frequency among red cell enzyme defects (after G6PD deficiency and PK deficiency). The anemia is lifelong, of variable severity, and may benefit from splenectomy.

Familial (Atypical) Hemolytic-Uremic Syndrome The term *familial (atypical) hemolytic-uremic syndrome* is used to designate a group of rare disorders, mostly affecting children, characterized by microangiopathic HA with presence of fragmented erythrocytes in the peripheral blood smear, thrombocytopenia (usually mild), and acute renal failure. (The word *atypical* is part of the phrase for historical reasons; it was hemolytic-uremic syndrome [HUS] caused by infection with *Escherichia coli* producing the Shiga toxin that was regarded as *typical*). The genetic basis of atypical HUS (aHUS) has been elucidated. Studies of >100 families have revealed that those family members who developed HUS had mutations in any one of several genes encoding complement regulatory proteins: complement factor H (*CFH*), CD46 or membrane cofactor protein (*MCP*), complement factor I (*CFI*), complement component C3, complement factor B (*CFB*), and thrombomodulin. Thus, whereas all other inherited HAs are due to intrinsic red cell abnormalities, this group is unique in that hemolysis results from an inherited defect external to red cells (Table 129-1). Because the regulation of the complement cascade has considerable redundancy, in the steady state, any of the above abnormalities can be tolerated. However, when an intercurrent infection or some other trigger activates complement through the alternative pathway, the deficiency of one of the complement regulators becomes critical. Endothelial cells get damaged, especially in the kidney; at the same time, and partly as a result of this, there will be brisk hemolysis (thus, the more common Shiga toxin–related HUS [Chap. 149] can be regarded as a phenocopy of aHUS). aHUS is a severe disease, with up to 15% mortality in the acute phase and up to 50% of cases progressing to end-stage renal disease. Not infrequently, aHUS undergoes spontaneous remission; but because its basis is an inherited abnormality, it is not surprising that, given renewed exposure to a trigger, the syndrome will tend to recur; when it does, the prognosis is always serious. The standard treatment has been plasma exchange, which will supply the deficient complement regulator. The anti-C5 complement inhibitor eculizumab (see below) was found to greatly ameliorate the microangiopathic picture, with improvement in platelet counts and in renal function, thus abrogating the need for plasma exchange. It remains to be seen for how long eculizumab treatment will have to be continued in individual patients and whether it will influence the controversial issue of kidney (and liver) transplantation.

ACQUIRED HEMOLYTIC ANEMIA

Mechanical Destruction of Red Cells Although red cells are characterized by the remarkable deformability that enables them to squeeze through capillaries narrower than themselves for thousands of times in their lifetime, there are at least two situations in which they succumb to shear, if not to wear and tear; the result is intravascular hemolysis, resulting in hemoglobinuria (Table 129-6). One situation is acute and self-inflicted, *march hemoglobinuria*. Why sometimes a marathon runner may develop this complication, whereas on another occasion, this does not happen, we do not know (perhaps her or his footwear needs attention). A similar syndrome may develop after prolonged barefoot ritual dancing or intense playing of bongo drums. The other situation is chronic and iatrogenic (it has been called *microangiopathic hemolytic anemia*). It takes place in patients with prosthetic heart valves, especially when paraprosthetic regurgitation is present. If the hemolysis consequent on mechanical trauma to the red cells is mild, and if the supply of iron is adequate, the loss may be largely compensated; if more

TABLE 129-6 DISEASES AND CLINICAL SITUATIONS WITH PREDOMINANTLY INTRAVASCULAR HEMOLYSIS

	Onset/Time Course	Main Mechanism	Appropriate Diagnostic Procedure	Comments
Mismatched blood transfusion	Abrupt	Nearly always ABO incompatibility	Repeat cross-match	
Paroxysmal nocturnal hemoglobinuria (PNH)	Chronic with acute exacerbations	Complement (C)-mediated destruction of CD59(−) red cells	Flow cytometry to display a CD59(−) red cell population	Exacerbations due to C activation through any pathway
Paroxysmal cold hemoglobinuria (PCH)	Acute	Immune lysis of normal red cells	Test for Donath-Landsteiner antibody	Often triggered by viral infection
Septicemia	Very acute	Exotoxins produced by *Clostridium perfringens*	Blood cultures	Other organisms may be responsible
Microangiopathic	Acute or chronic	Red cell fragmentation	Red cell morphology on blood smear	Different causes ranging from endothelial damage to hemangioma to leaky prosthetic heart valve
March hemoglobinuria	Abrupt	Mechanical destruction	Targeted history taking	
Favism	Acute	Destruction of older fraction of G6PD-deficient red cells	G6PD assay	Triggered by ingestion of large dish of fava beans, but trigger can be infection or drug instead

Abbreviation: G6PD, glucose 6-phosphate dehydrogenase.

than mild anemia develops, reintervention to correct regurgitation may be required.

Infection By far the most frequent infectious cause of HA, in endemic areas, is malaria (Chap. 248). In other parts of the world, the most frequent direct cause is probably Shiga toxin–producing *E. coli* O157:H7, now recognized as the main etiologic agent of HUS, which is more common in children than in adults (Chap. 149). Life-threatening intravascular hemolysis, due to a toxin with lecithinase activity, occurs with *Clostridium perfringens* sepsis, particularly following open wounds, septic abortion, or as a disastrous accident due to a contaminated blood unit. Rarely, and if at all in children, HA is seen with sepsis or endocarditis from a variety of organisms. In addition, bacterial and viral infections can cause HA by indirect mechanisms (see above section on G6PD deficiency and Table 129-6).

Immune Hemolytic Anemias These can arise through at least two distinct mechanisms. (1) There is a true autoantibody directed against a red cell antigen, i.e., a molecule present on the surface of red cells. (2) When an antibody directed against a certain molecule (e.g., a drug) reacts with that molecule, red cells may get caught in the reaction, whereby they are damaged or destroyed. Because the antibodies involved differ in optimum reactivity temperatures, they are classified in the time-honored categories of "cold" and "warm" (Table 129-7). Autoantibody-mediated HAs may be seen in isolation (when they are called *idiopathic*) or as part of a systemic autoimmune disorder such as systemic lupus erythematosus. Here we discuss the most distinctive clinical pictures.

AUTOIMMUNE HEMOLYTIC ANEMIA (AIHA) Once a red cell is coated by an autoantibody (see [1] above), it will be destroyed by one or more mechanisms. In most cases, the Fc portion of the antibody will be recognized by the Fc receptor of macrophages, and this will trigger erythrophagocytosis. Thus, destruction of red cells will take place wherever macrophages are abundant, i.e., in the spleen, liver, or bone marrow; this is called *extravascular hemolysis* (Fig. 129-8). Because of the special anatomy of the spleen, this organ is particularly efficient in trapping antibody-coated red cells, and often this is the predominant site of red cell destruction. In some cases, the nature of the antibody is such (usually an IgM antibody) that the antigen-antibody complex on the surface of red cells is able to activate complement (C); as a result, a large amount of membrane attack complex will form, and the red cells may be destroyed directly; this is known as *intravascular hemolysis*.

Clinical features AIHA is a serious condition; without appropriate treatment, it may have a mortality of approximately 10%. The onset is often abrupt and can be dramatic. The hemoglobin level can drop, within days, to as low as 4 g/dL; the massive red cell removal will produce jaundice; and sometimes the spleen is enlarged. When this triad is present, the suspicion of AIHA must be high. When hemolysis is (in part) intravascular, the telltale sign will be hemoglobinuria, which the patient may report or about which we must enquire or test for. The diagnostic test for AIHA is the direct antiglobulin test developed in 1945 by R. R. A. Coombs and known since by this name. The beauty of this test is that it detects directly the pathogenetic mediator of the disease, i.e., the presence of antibody on the red cells themselves. When the test is positive, it clinches the diagnosis; when it is negative, the diagnosis is unlikely. However, the sensitivity of the Coombs test varies depending on the technique that is used, and in doubtful cases, a repeat in a specialized lab is advisable; the term *Coombs-negative AIHA* is a last resort. In some cases, the autoantibody has a defined identity; it may be specific for an antigen belonging to the Rhesus system (it is often anti-e). In many cases, it is regarded as "nonspecific" because it reacts with virtually all types of red cells.

When AIHA develops in a person who is already known to have, for instance, systemic lupus or chronic lymphocytic leukemia (Table 129-7), we call it a complication; conversely, when AIHA presents on its own, it may be a pointer to an underlying condition that we ought to seek out. In both cases, what brings about AIHA remains, as in other autoimmune disorders, obscure. In some cases, AIHA can be associated, on first presentation or subsequently, with autoimmune thrombocytopenia (Evans' syndrome).

TABLE 129-7 CLASSIFICATION OF ACQUIRED IMMUNE HEMOLYTIC ANEMIAS

	Type of Antibody	
Clinical Setting	**Cold, Mostly IgM, Optimal Temperature 4–30°C**	**Warm, Mostly IgG, Optimal Temperature 37°C; or Mixed**
Primary	CAD	AIHA (idiopathic)
Secondary to viral infection	EBV	HIV
	CMV	Viral vaccines
	Other	
Secondary to other infection	Mycoplasma infection: paroxysmal cold hemoglobinuria	
Secondary to/associated with other disease	CAD in:	AIHA in:
	Waldenström's disease	SLE
	Lymphoma	CLL
		Other malignancy
		Chronic inflammatory disorders (e.g., IBD)
		After allogeneic HSCT
Secondary to drugs: drug-induced immune hemolytic anemia	Small minority (e.g., with lenalidomide)	Majority: currently most common culprit drugs are cefotetan, ceftriaxone, piperacillin
	Drug-dependent: antibody destroys red cells only when drug present (e.g., rarely penicillin)	
	Drug-independent: antibody can destroy red cells even when drug no longer present (e.g., methyldopa)	

Abbreviations: AIHA, autoimmune hemolytic anemia; CAD, cold agglutinin disease; CLL, chronic lymphocytic leukemia; CMV, cytomegalovirus; EBV, Epstein-Barr virus; HIV, human immunodeficiency virus; HSCT, hematopoietic stem cell transplantation; IBD, inflammatory bowel disease; SLE, systemic lupus erythematosus.

TREATMENT AUTOIMMUNE HEMOLYTIC ANEMIA

Severe acute AIHA can be a medical emergency. The immediate treatment almost invariably includes transfusion of red cells. This may pose a special problem because, if the antibody involved is nonspecific, all of the blood units cross-matched will be incompatible. In these cases, it is often correct, paradoxically, to transfuse incompatible blood, with the rationale being that the transfused red cells will be destroyed no less but no more than the patient's own red cells, but in the meantime, the patient stays alive. A situation like this requires close liaison and understanding between the clinical unit treating the patient and the blood transfusion/serology lab. Whenever the anemia is not immediately life-threatening, blood transfusion should be withheld (because compatibility problems may increase with each unit of blood transfused), and medical treatment started immediately with prednisone (1 mg/kg per day), which will produce a remission promptly in at least one-half of patients. Rituximab (anti-CD20) was regarded as second-line treatment, but it is increasingly likely that a relatively low dose (100 mg/wk × 4) of rituximab together with prednisone will become a first-line standard. It is especially encouraging that this approach seems to reduce the rate of relapse, a common occurrence in AIHA. For patients who do relapse or are refractory to medical treatment, one may have to consider splenectomy, which, although it does not cure the disease, can produce significant benefit by removing a major site of hemolysis, thus improving the anemia and/or reducing the need for other therapies (e.g., the dose of prednisone). Since the introduction of rituximab, azathioprine, cyclophosphamide, cyclosporine, and intravenous immunoglobulin have become second- or third-line agents. In very rare severe refractory cases, either autologous or allogeneic hematopoietic stem cell transplantation may have to be considered.

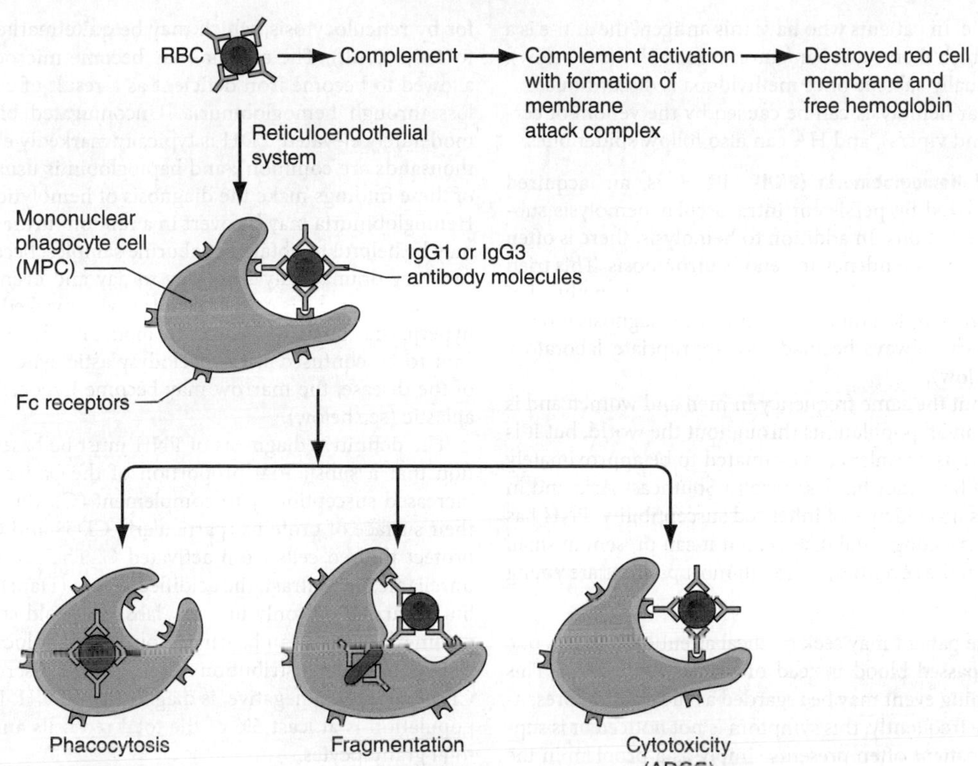

FIGURE 129-8 Mechanism of antibody-mediated immune destruction of red blood cells (RBCs). ADCC, antibody-dependent cell-mediated cytotoxicity. *(From N Young et al: Clinical Hematology. Philadelphia, Elsevier, 2006; with permission.)*

PAROXYSMAL COLD HEMOGLOBINURIA (PCH) PCH is a rather rare form of AIHA occurring mostly in children, usually triggered by a viral infection, usually self-limited, and characterized by the involvement of the so-called Donath-Landsteiner antibody. In vitro, this antibody has unique serologic features; it has anti-P specificity and binds to red cells only at a low temperature (optimally at 4°C), but when the temperature is shifted to 37°C, lysis of red cells takes place in the presence of complement. Consequently, in vivo there is intravascular hemolysis, resulting in hemoglobinuria. Clinically the differential diagnosis must include other causes of hemoglobinuria (Table 129-6), but the presence of the Donath-Landsteiner antibody will prove PCH. Active supportive treatment, including blood transfusion, is needed to control the anemia; subsequently, recovery is the rule.

COLD AGGLUTININ DISEASE (CAD) This designation is used for a form of chronic AIHA that usually affects the elderly and has special clinical and pathologic features. First, the term *cold* refers to the fact that the autoantibody involved reacts with red cells poorly or not at all at 37°C, whereas it reacts strongly at lower temperatures. As a result, hemolysis is more prominent the more the body is exposed to the cold. The antibody is usually IgM; usually it has an anti-I specificity (the I antigen is present on the red cells of almost everybody), and it may have a very high titer (1:100,000 or more has been observed). Second, the antibody is produced by an expanded clone of B lymphocytes, and sometimes its concentration in the plasma is high enough to show up as a spike in plasma protein electrophoresis, i.e., as a monoclonal gammopathy. Third, because the antibody is IgM, CAD is related to Waldenström's macroglobulinemia (WM) (Chap. 136), although in most cases, the other clinical features of this disease are not present. Thus, CAD must be regarded as a form of WM (i.e., as a low-grade mature B cell lymphoma) that manifests at an earlier stage precisely because the unique biologic properties of the IgM that it produces give the clinical picture of chronic HA.

In mild forms of CAD, avoidance of exposure to cold may be all that is needed to enable the patient to have a reasonably comfortable quality of life; but in more severe forms, the management of CAD is not easy. Blood transfusion is not very effective because donor red cells are I positive and will be rapidly removed. Immunosuppressive/cytotoxic treatment with azathioprine or cyclophosphamide can reduce the antibody titer, but clinical efficacy is limited, and in view of the chronic nature of the disease, the side effects may prove unacceptable. Unlike in AIHA, prednisone and splenectomy are ineffective. Plasma exchange will remove antibody and is, therefore, in theory, a rational approach, but it is laborious and must be carried out at frequent intervals if it is to be beneficial. The management of CAD has changed significantly with the advent of rituximab; although its impact on CAD is not as great as on AIHA, up to 60% of patients respond, and remissions may be more durable with a rituximab-fludarabine combination. Given the long clinical course of CAD, it remains to be seen with what schedule or periodicity these agents will need to be administered.

Toxic Agents and Drugs A number of chemicals with oxidative potential, whether medicinal or not, can cause hemolysis even in people who are not G6PD deficient (see above). Examples are hyperbaric oxygen (or 100% oxygen), nitrates, chlorates, methylene blue, dapsone, cisplatin, and numerous aromatic (cyclic) compounds. Other chemicals may be hemolytic through nonoxidative, largely unknown mechanisms; examples include arsine, stibine, copper, and lead. The HA caused by lead poisoning is characterized by basophilic stippling; it is in fact a phenocopy of that seen in P5N deficiency (see above), suggesting it is mediated at least in part by lead inhibiting this enzyme.

In these cases, hemolysis appears to be mediated by a direct chemical action on red cells. But drugs can cause hemolysis through at least two other mechanisms. (1) A drug can behave as a hapten and induce antibody production; in rare subjects, this happens, for instance, with penicillin. Upon a subsequent exposure, red cells are caught, as innocent bystanders, in the reaction between penicillin and antipenicillin antibodies. Hemolysis will subside as soon as penicillin administration is stopped. (2) A drug can trigger, perhaps through mimicry, the production of an antibody against a red cell antigen. The best known example is methyldopa, an antihypertensive agent no longer in use, which in a small fraction of patients stimulated the production of the

Rhesus antibody anti-e. In patients who have this antigen, the anti-e is a true autoantibody, which then causes an autoimmune HA (see below). Usually this will gradually subside once methyldopa is discontinued.

Severe intravascular hemolysis can be caused by the venom of certain snakes (cobras and vipers), and HA can also follow spider bites.

Paroxysmal Nocturnal Hemoglobinuria (PNH) PNH is an acquired chronic HA characterized by persistent intravascular hemolysis subject to recurrent exacerbations. In addition to hemolysis, there is often pancytopenia and a distinct tendency to venous thrombosis. This triad makes PNH a truly unique clinical condition; however, when not all of these three features are manifest on presentation, the diagnosis is often delayed, although it can always be made by appropriate laboratory investigations (see below).

PNH has about the same frequency in men and women and is encountered in all populations throughout the world, but it is a rare disease; its prevalence is estimated to be approximately 5 per million (it may be somewhat less rare in Southeast Asia and in the Far East). There is no evidence of inherited susceptibility. PNH has never been reported as a congenital disease, but it can present in small children or as late as in the seventies, although most patients are young adults.

CLINICAL FEATURES The patient may seek medical attention because, one morning, she or he passed blood instead of urine (Fig. 129-9). This distressing or frightening event may be regarded as the classical presentation; however, more frequently, this symptom is not noticed or is suppressed. Indeed, the patient often presents simply as a problem in the differential diagnosis of *anemia*, whether symptomatic or discovered incidentally. Sometimes, the anemia is associated from the outset with neutropenia, thrombocytopenia, or both, thus signaling an element of bone marrow failure (see below). Some patients may present with recurrent attacks of severe abdominal pain defying a specific diagnosis and eventually found to be related to thrombosis. When thrombosis affects the hepatic veins, it may produce acute hepatomegaly and ascites, i.e., a full-fledged Budd-Chiari syndrome, which, in the absence of liver disease, ought to raise the suspicion of PNH.

The *natural history* of PNH can extend over decades. Without treatment, the median survival is estimated to be about 8–10 years; in the past, the most common cause of death has been venous thrombosis, followed by infection secondary to severe neutropenia and hemorrhage secondary to severe thrombocytopenia. Rarely (estimated 1–2% of all cases), PNH may terminate in acute myeloid leukemia. On the other hand, full spontaneous recovery from PNH has been documented, albeit rarely.

LABORATORY INVESTIGATIONS AND DIAGNOSIS The most consistent blood finding is anemia, which may range from mild to moderate to very severe. The anemia is usually normomacrocytic, with unremarkable red cell morphology. If the MCV is high, it is usually largely accounted for by reticulocytosis, which may be quite marked (up to 20%, or up to 400,000/μL). The anemia may become microcytic if the patient is allowed to become iron deficient as a result of chronic urinary blood loss through hemoglobinuria. Unconjugated bilirubin is mildly or moderately elevated; LDH is typically markedly elevated (values in the thousands are common); and haptoglobin is usually undetectable. All of these findings make the diagnosis of hemolytic anemia compelling. Hemoglobinuria may be overt in a random urine sample; if it is not, it may be helpful to obtain serial urine samples, because hemoglobinuria can vary dramatically from day to day and even from hour to hour. The bone marrow is usually cellular, with marked to massive erythroid hyperplasia, often with mild to moderate dyserythropoietic features (not to be confused with myelodysplastic syndrome). At some stage of the disease, the marrow may become hypocellular or even frankly aplastic (see below).

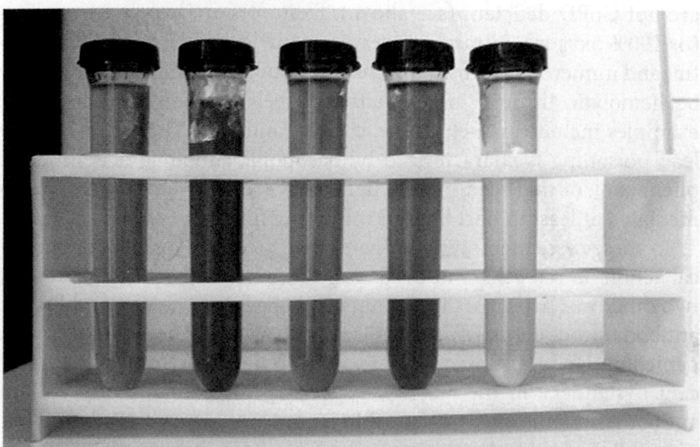

FIGURE 129-9 Consecutive urine samples from a patient with paroxysmal nocturnal hemoglobinuria (PNH). The variation in the severity of hemoglobinuria within hours is probably unique to this condition.

The definitive diagnosis of PNH must be based on the demonstration that a substantial proportion of the patient's red cells have an increased susceptibility to complement (C), due to the deficiency on their surface of proteins (particularly CD59 and CD55) that normally protect the red cells from activated C. The sucrose hemolysis test is unreliable; in contrast, the acidified serum (Ham) test is highly reliable but is carried out only in a few labs. The gold standard today is flow cytometry, which can be carried out on granulocytes as well as on red cells. A bimodal distribution of cells, with a discrete population that is CD59 and CD55 negative, is diagnostic of PNH. In PNH patients, this population is at least 5% of the total red cells and at least 20% of the total granulocytes.

PATHOPHYSIOLOGY Hemolysis in PNH is mainly intravascular and is due to an intrinsic abnormality of the red cell, which makes it exquisitely sensitive to activated C, whether it is activated through the alternative pathway or through an antigen-antibody reaction. The former mechanism is mainly responsible for chronic hemolysis in PNH; the latter explains why the hemolysis can be dramatically exacerbated in the course of a viral or bacterial infection. Hypersusceptibility to C is due to deficiency of several protective membrane proteins (Fig. 129-10), of which CD59 is the most important, because it hinders the insertion into the membrane of C9 polymers. The molecular basis for the deficiency of these proteins has been pinpointed not to a defect in any of the respective genes, but rather to the shortage of a unique glycolipid molecule, GPI (Fig. 129-2), which, through a peptide bond, anchors these proteins to the surface membrane of cells. The shortage of GPI is due in turn to a mutation in an X-linked gene, called *PIG-A*, required for an early step in GPI biosynthesis. In virtually each patient, the *PIG-A* mutation is different. This is not surprising, because these mutations are not inherited; rather, each one takes place de novo in a hemopoietic stem cell (i.e., they are somatic mutations). As a result, the patient's marrow is a mosaic of mutant and nonmutant cells, and the peripheral blood always contains both PNH cells and normal (non-PNH) cells. Thrombosis is one of the most immediately life-threatening complications of PNH and yet one of the least understood in its pathogenesis. It could be that deficiency of CD59 on the PNH platelet causes inappropriate platelet activation; however, other mechanisms are possible.

BONE MARROW FAILURE (BMF) AND RELATIONSHIP BETWEEN PNH AND APLASTIC ANEMIA (AA) It is not unusual that patients with firmly established PNH have a previous history of well-documented AA; indeed, BMF preceding overt PNH is probably the rule rather than the exception. On the other hand, sometimes a patient with PNH becomes less hemolytic and more pancytopenic and ultimately has the clinical picture of AA. Because AA is probably an organ-specific autoimmune disease, in which T cells cause damage to hematopoietic stem cells, the same may be true of PNH, with the specific proviso that the damage spares PNH stem cells. *PIG-A* mutations can be demonstrated in normal people, and there is evidence from mouse models that PNH stem cells do not expand when the rest of the bone marrow is normal. Thus, we can visualize PNH as always having two components: failure of normal hematopoiesis and massive expansion of a PNH clone. Findings supporting this notion include skewing of the T cell repertoire and the demonstration of GPI-reactive T cells in patients with PNH.

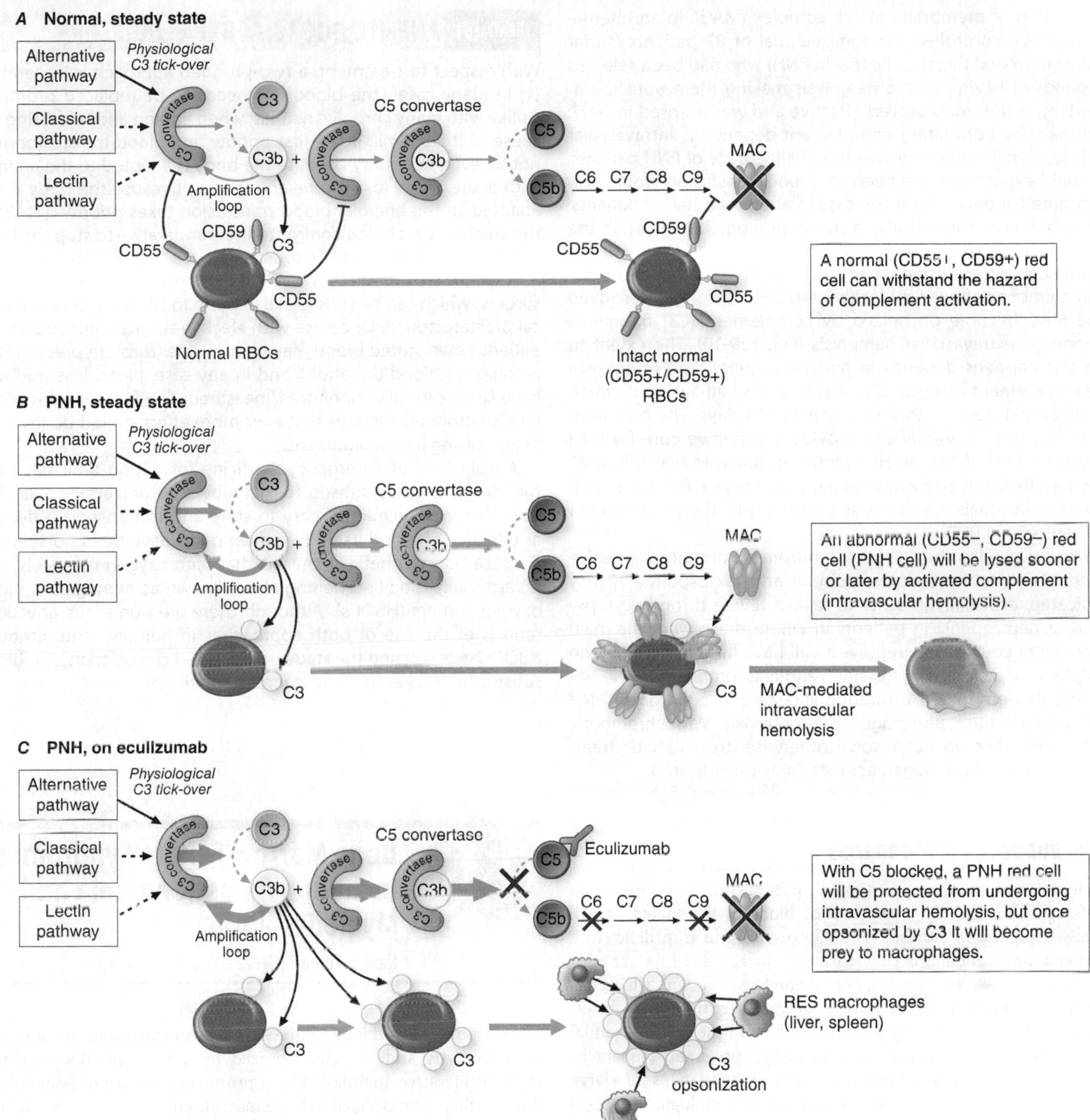

FIGURE 129-10 The complement cascade and the fate of red cells. ***A.*** Normal red cells are protected from complement activation and subsequent hemolysis by CD55 and CD59. These two proteins, being GPI-linked, are missing from the surface of PNH red cells as a result of a somatic mutation of the X-linked *PIG-A* gene that encodes a protein required for an early step of the GPI molecule biosynthesis. ***B.*** In the steady state, PNH erythrocytes suffer from spontaneous (tick-over) complement activation, with consequent intravascular hemolysis through formation of the membrane attack complex (MAC); when extra complement is activated through the classical pathway, an exacerbation of hemolysis will result. ***C.*** On eculizumab, PNH erythrocytes are protected from hemolysis from the inhibition of C5 cleavage; however, upstream complement activation may lead to C3 opsonization and possible extravascular hemolysis. GPI, glycosylphosphatidylinositol; PNH, paroxysmal nocturnal hemoglobinuria. *(From L Luzzatto et al: Haematologica 95:523, 2010.)*

TREATMENT PAROXYSMAL NOCTURNAL HEMOGLOBINURIA

Unlike other acquired hemolytic anemias, PNH may be a lifelong condition, and most patients receive supportive treatment only, including transfusion of filtered red cells[1] whenever necessary, which, for some patients, means quite frequently. Folic acid supplements (at least 3 mg/d) are mandatory; the serum iron should be checked periodically, and iron supplements should be administered as appropriate. Long-term glucocorticoids are not indicated because there is no evidence that they have any effect on chronic hemolysis; in fact, they are contraindicated because their side effects are considerable and potentially dangerous. A major advance in the management of PNH has been the development of a humanized monoclonal antibody, eculizumab, which binds to the complement component C5 near the site that, when cleaved, will trigger the distal part of the complement cascade leading to

[1]Now that filters with excellent retention of white cells are routinely used, the traditional washing of red cells, aiming to avoid white cell reactions triggering hemolysis, is no longer necessary and is wasteful.

the formation of membrane attack complex (MAC). In an international, placebo-controlled, randomized trial of 87 patients (so far the only controlled therapeutic trial in PNH) who had been selected on grounds of having severe hemolysis making them transfusion-dependent, eculizumab proved effective and was licensed in 2007. Eculizumab, by abrogating complement-dependent intravascular hemolysis, significantly improves the quality of life of PNH patients. One would expect that the need for blood transfusion would also be abrogated; indeed, this is the case in about one-half of patients, in many of whom there is also a rise in hemoglobin levels. In the remaining patients, however, the anemia remains sufficiently severe to require blood transfusion. One reason for this is that, once the distal complement pathway is blocked, red cells no longer destroyed by the MAC become opsonized by complement (C3) fragments and undergo extravascular hemolysis (Fig. 129-10). The extent to which this happens depends in part on a genetic polymorphism of the complement receptor CR1. Based on its half-life, eculizumab must be administered intravenously every 14 days. The only form of treatment that currently can provide a definitive cure for PNH is allogeneic BMT. When an HLA-identical sibling is available, BMT should be offered to any young patient with severe PNH; the availability of eculizumab has decreased significantly the proportion of patients receiving BMT.

For patients with the PNH-AA syndrome, immunosuppressive treatment with antithymocyte globulin and cyclosporine A may be indicated, especially in order to relieve severe thrombocytopenia and/or neutropenia in patients in whom these were the main problem(s); of course, this treatment will have little or no effect on hemolysis. Any patient who has had venous thrombosis or who has a genetically determined thrombophilic state in addition to PNH should be on regular anticoagulant prophylaxis. With thrombotic complications that do not resolve otherwise, thrombolytic treatment with tissue plasminogen activator may be indicated.

ANEMIA DUE TO ACUTE BLOOD LOSS

Blood loss causes anemia by two main mechanisms: (1) by the direct loss of red cells; and (2) if the loss of blood is protracted, it will gradually deplete iron stores, eventually resulting in iron deficiency. The latter type of anemia is covered in Chap. 126; here we are concerned with the former type, i.e., *posthemorrhagic anemia*, which follows *acute* blood loss. This can be *external* (e.g., after trauma or obstetric hemorrhage) or *internal* (e.g., from bleeding in the gastrointestinal tract, rupture of the spleen, rupture of an ectopic pregnancy, subarachnoid hemorrhage). In any of these cases, after the sudden loss of a large amount of blood, there are three clinical/pathophysiologic stages. (1) At first, the dominant feature is hypovolemia, which poses a threat particularly to organs that normally have a high blood supply, like the brain and the kidneys; therefore, loss of consciousness and acute renal failure are major threats. It is important to note that at this stage an ordinary blood count will not show anemia, because the hemoglobin concentration is not affected. (2) Next, as an emergency response, baroreceptors and stretch receptors will cause release of vasopressin and other peptides, and the body will shift fluid from the extravascular to the intravascular compartment, producing hemodilution; thus, the hypovolemia gradually converts to anemia. The degree of anemia will reflect the amount of blood lost. If after 3 days the hemoglobin is, for example, 7 g/dL, it means that about half of the entire blood has been lost. (3) Provided bleeding does not continue, the bone marrow response will gradually ameliorate the anemia.

The diagnosis of acute posthemorrhagic anemia (APHA) is usually straightforward, although sometimes internal bleeding episodes (e.g., after a traumatic injury), even when large, may not be immediately obvious. Whenever an abrupt fall in hemoglobin has taken place, whatever history is given by the patient, APHA should be suspected. Supplementary history may have to be obtained by asking the appropriate questions, and appropriate investigations (e.g., a sonogram or an endoscopy) may have to be carried out.

TREATMENT ANEMIA DUE TO ACUTE BLOOD LOSS

With respect to treatment, a two-pronged approach is imperative. (1) In many cases, the blood lost needs to be replaced promptly. Unlike with many chronic anemias, when finding and correcting the cause of the anemia is the first priority and blood transfusion may not be even necessary because the body is adapted to the anemia, with acute blood loss the reverse is true; because the body is not adapted to the anemia, blood transfusion takes priority. (1) While the emergency is being confronted, it is imperative to stop the hemorrhage and to eliminate its source.

A special type of APHA is blood loss during and immediately after surgery, which can be substantial (e.g., up to 2 L in the case of a radical prostatectomy). Of course with elective surgical procedures, the patient's own stored blood may be available (through preoperative autologous blood donation), and in any case, blood loss ought to have been carefully monitored/measured. The fact that this blood loss is iatrogenic dictates that ever more effort should be invested in optimizing its management.

A Holy Grail of emergency medicine for a long time has been the idea of a blood substitute that would be universally available, suitable for all recipients, easy to store and to transport, safe, and as effective as blood itself. Two main paths have been pursued: (1) fluorocarbon synthetic chemicals that bind oxygen reversibly, and (2) artificially modified hemoglobins, known as hemoglobin-based oxygen carriers (HBOCs). Although there are numerous anecdotal reports of the use of both approaches in humans, and although HBOCs have reached the stage of phase 2–3 clinical trials, no "blood substitute" has yet become standard treatment.

130 Bone Marrow Failure Syndromes Including Aplastic Anemia and Myelodysplasia

Neal S. Young

The hypoproliferative anemias are normochromic, normocytic, or macrocytic and are characterized by a low reticulocyte count. Hypoproliferative anemia is also a prominent feature of hematologic diseases that are described as bone marrow failure states; these include aplastic anemia, myelodysplastic syndrome (MDS), pure red cell aplasia (PRCA), and myelophthisis. Anemia in these disorders is often not a solitary or even the major hematologic finding. More frequent in bone marrow failure is *pancytopenia*: anemia, leukopenia, and thrombocytopenia. Low blood counts in the marrow failure diseases result from deficient hematopoiesis, as distinguished from blood count depression due to peripheral destruction of red cells (hemolytic anemias), platelets (idiopathic thrombocytopenic purpura [ITP] or due to splenomegaly), and granulocytes (as in the immune leukopenias). Marrow damage and dysfunction also may be secondary to infection, inflammation, or cancer.

Hematopoietic failure syndromes are classified by dominant morphologic features of the bone marrow (Table 130-1). Although practical distinction among these syndromes usually is clear, some processes are so closely related that the diagnosis may be complex. Patients may seem to suffer from two or three related diseases simultaneously, or one diagnosis may appear to evolve into another. Many of these syndromes share an immune-mediated mechanism of marrow destruction and some element of genomic instability resulting in a higher rate of malignant transformation.

It is important that the internist and general practitioner recognize the marrow failure syndromes, as their prognosis may be poor if the

TABLE 130-1 DIFFERENTIAL DIAGNOSIS OF PANCYTOPENIA

Pancytopenia with Hypocellular Bone Marrow	
Acquired aplastic anemia	
Constitutional aplastic anemia (Fanconi anemia, dyskeratosis congenita)	
Some myelodysplasia	
Rare aleukemic leukemia	
Some acute lymphoid leukemia	
Some lymphomas of bone marrow	
Pancytopenia with Cellular Bone Marrow	
Primary bone marrow diseases	Secondary to systemic diseases
Myelodysplasia	Systemic lupus erythematosus
Paroxysmal nocturnal hemoglobinuria	Hypersplenism
	B_{12}, folate deficiency
Myelofibrosis	Overwhelming infection
Some aleukemic leukemia	Alcohol
Myelophthisis	Brucellosis
Bone marrow lymphoma	Sarcoidosis
Hairy cell leukemia	Tuberculosis
	Leishmaniasis
Hypocellular Bone Marrow ± Cytopenia	
Q fever	
Legionnaires' disease	
Anorexia nervosa, starvation	
Mycobacterium	

patient is untreated; effective therapies are often available but sufficiently complicated in their choice and delivery so as to warrant the care of a hematologist or oncologist.

APLASTIC ANEMIA

DEFINITION

Aplastic anemia is pancytopenia with bone marrow hypocellularity. Acquired aplastic anemia is distinguished from iatrogenic aplasia, marrow hypocellularity after intensive cytotoxic chemotherapy for cancer. Aplastic anemia can also be constitutional: the genetic diseases Fanconi anemia and dyskeratosis congenita, although frequently associated with typical physical anomalies and the development of pancytopenia early in life, can also present as marrow failure in normal-appearing adults. Acquired aplastic anemia is often stereotypical in its manifestations, with the abrupt onset of low blood counts in a previously well young adult; seronegative hepatitis or a course of an incriminated medical drug may precede the onset. The diagnosis in these instances is uncomplicated. Sometimes blood count depression is moderate or incomplete, resulting in anemia, leukopenia, and thrombocytopenia in some combination. Aplastic anemia is related to both paroxysmal nocturnal hemoglobinuria (PNH; Chap. 129) and to MDS, and in some cases, a clear distinction among these disorders may not be possible.

EPIDEMIOLOGY

The incidence of acquired aplastic anemia in Europe and Israel is two cases per million persons annually. In Thailand and China, rates of five to seven per million have been established. In general, men and women are affected with equal frequency, but the age distribution is biphasic, with the major peak in the teens and twenties and a second rise in older adults.

ETIOLOGY

The origins of aplastic anemia have been inferred from several recurring clinical associations (Table 130-2); unfortunately, these relationships are not reliable in an individual patient and may not be etiologic. In addition, although most cases of aplastic anemia are idiopathic, little other than history separates these cases from those with a presumed etiology such as a drug exposure.

TABLE 130-2 CLASSIFICATION OF APLASTIC ANEMIA AND SINGLE CYTOPENIAS

Acquired	Inherited
Aplastic Anemia	
Secondary	Fanconi anemia
Radiation	Dyskeratosis congenita
Drugs and chemicals	Shwachman-Diamond syndrome
Regular effects	Reticular dysgenesis
Idiosyncratic reactions	Amegakaryocytic thrombocytopenia
Viruses	Familial aplastic anemias
Epstein Barr virus (infectious mononucleosis)	Preleukemia (monosomy 7, etc.)
Hepatitis (non-A, non-B, non-C hepatitis)	Nonhematologic syndrome (Down, Dubowitz, Seckel)
Parvovirus B19 (transient aplastic crisis, PRCA)	
HIV-1 (AIDS)	
Immune diseases	
Eosinophilic fasciitis	
Hyperimmunoglobulinemia	
Large granular lymphocytosis (LGL)	
Thymoma/thymic carcinoma	
Graft-versus-host disease in immunodeficiency	
Paroxysmal nocturnal hemoglobinuria (PNH)	
Pregnancy	
Idiopathic	
Cytopenias	
PRCA (see Table 130-4)	Congenital PRCA (Diamond-Blackfan anemia)
Neutropenia/agranulocytosis	
Idiopathic	Kostmann syndrome
Drugs, toxins	Shwachman-Diamond syndrome
LGL	Reticular dysgenesis
Pure white cell aplasia (+/− thymoma)	
Thrombocytopenia	
Drugs, toxins	Amegakaryocytic thrombocytopenia
Idiopathic amegakaryocytic	Thrombocytopenia with absent radii

Abbreviation: PRCA, pure red cell aplasia.

Radiation Marrow aplasia is a major acute sequela of radiation. Radiation damages DNA; tissues dependent on active mitosis are particularly susceptible. Nuclear accidents involve not only power plant workers but also employees of hospitals, laboratories, and industry (food sterilization, metal radiography, etc.), as well as innocents exposed to stolen, misplaced, or misused sources. Whereas the radiation dose can be approximated from the rate and degree of decline in blood counts, dosimetry by reconstruction of the exposure can help to estimate the patient's prognosis and also to protect medical personnel from contact with radioactive tissue and excreta. MDS and leukemia, but probably not aplastic anemia, are late effects of radiation.

Chemicals Benzene is a notorious cause of bone marrow failure: epidemiologic, clinical, and laboratory data link benzene to aplastic anemia, acute leukemia, and blood and marrow abnormalities. For leukemia, incidence is correlated with cumulative exposure, but susceptibility must also be important, because only a minority of even heavily exposed workers develop myelotoxicity. The employment history is important, especially in industries where benzene is used for a secondary purpose, usually as a solvent. Benzene-related blood diseases have declined with regulation of industrial exposure. Although benzene is no longer generally available as a household solvent, exposure to its metabolites occurs in the normal diet and in the environment. The association between marrow failure and other chemicals is much less well substantiated.

TABLE 130-3 SOME DRUGS AND CHEMICALS ASSOCIATED WITH APLASTIC ANEMIA

Agents that regularly produce marrow depression as major toxicity in commonly used doses or normal exposures:

- Cytotoxic drugs used in cancer chemotherapy: *alkylating agents, antimetabolites, antimitotics,* some antibiotics

Agents that frequently but not inevitably produce marrow aplasia:

- *Benzene*

Agents associated with aplastic anemia but with a relatively low probability:

- *Chloramphenicol*
- Insecticides
- Antiprotozoals: *quinacrine* and chloroquine, mepacrine
- Nonsteroidal anti-inflammatory drugs (including *phenylbutazone,* indomethacin, ibuprofen, sulindac, aspirin)
- Anticonvulsants (*hydantoins, carbamazepine,* phenacemide, felbamate)
- Heavy metals (*gold,* arsenic, bismuth, mercury)
- Sulfonamides: some antibiotics, antithyroid drugs (methimazole, methylthiouracil, propylthiouracil), antidiabetes drugs (tolbutamide, chlorpropamide), carbonic anhydrase inhibitors (acetazolamide and methazolamide)
- Antihistamines (*cimetidine,* chlorpheniramine)
- D-Penicillamine
- Estrogens (in pregnancy and in high doses in animals)

Agents whose association with aplastic anemia is more tenuous:

- Other antibiotics (streptomycin, tetracycline, methicillin, mebendazole, trimethoprim/sulfamethoxazole, flucytosine)
- Sedatives and tranquilizers (chlorpromazine, prochlorperazine, piperacetazine, chlordiazepoxide, meprobamate, methyprylon)
- Allopurinol
- Methyldopa
- Quinidine
- Lithium
- Guanidine
- Potassium perchlorate
- Thiocyanate
- Carbimazole

Note: Terms set in italics show the most consistent association with aplastic anemia.

Drugs (Table 130-3) Many chemotherapeutic drugs have marrow suppression as a major toxicity; effects are dose dependent and will occur in all recipients. In contrast, idiosyncratic reactions to a large and diverse group of drugs may lead to aplastic anemia without a clear dose-response relationship. These associations rest largely on accumulated case reports until a large international study in Europe in the 1980s quantitated drug relationships, especially for nonsteroidal analgesics, sulfonamides, thyrostatic drugs, some psychotropics, penicillamine, allopurinol, and gold. Association does not equal causation: a drug may have been used to treat the first symptoms of bone marrow failure (antibiotics for fever or the preceding viral illness) or provoked the first symptom of a preexisting disease (petechiae by nonsteroidal anti-inflammatory agents administered to the thrombocytopenic patient). In the context of total drug use, idiosyncratic reactions, although individually devastating, are rare events. Risk estimates are usually lower when determined in population-based studies. Furthermore, the low absolute risk is also made more obvious: even a 10- or 20-fold increase in risk translates, in a rare disease, to just a handful of drug-induced aplastic anemia cases among hundreds of thousands of exposed persons.

Infections Hepatitis is the most common preceding infection, and posthepatitis marrow failure accounts for approximately 5% of etiologies in most series. Patients are usually young men who have recovered from a bout of liver inflammation 1 to 2 months earlier; the subsequent pancytopenia is very severe. The hepatitis is seronegative (non-A, non-B, non-C) and possibly due to an as yet undiscovered infectious agent. Fulminant liver failure in childhood also follows seronegative hepatitis, and marrow failure occurs at a high rate in these patients. Aplastic anemia can rarely follow infectious mononucleosis. Parvovirus B19, the cause of transient aplastic crisis in hemolytic anemias and of some PRCAs (see below), does not usually cause generalized bone marrow failure. Mild blood count depression is frequent in the course of many viral and bacterial infections but resolves with the infection.

Immunologic Diseases Aplasia is a major consequence and the inevitable cause of death in *transfusion-associated graft-versus-host disease* (GVHD) that can occur after infusion of nonirradiated blood products to an immunodeficient recipient. Aplastic anemia is strongly associated with the rare collagen vascular syndrome *eosinophilic fasciitis* that is characterized by painful induration of subcutaneous tissues (Chap. 382). Thymoma and hypoimmunoglobulinemia are occasional associations with aplastic anemia. Pancytopenia with marrow hypoplasia can also occur in systemic lupus erythematosus (SLE).

Pregnancy Aplastic anemia very rarely may occur and recur during pregnancy and resolve with delivery or with spontaneous or induced abortion.

Paroxysmal Nocturnal Hemoglobinuria An acquired mutation in the *PIG-A* gene in a hematopoietic stem cell is required for the development of PNH, but *PIG-A* mutations probably occur commonly in normal individuals. If the PIG-A mutant stem cell proliferates, the result is a clone of progeny deficient in glycosylphosphatidylinositol-linked cell surface membrane proteins (Chap. 129). Small clones of deficient cells can be detected by sensitive flow cytometry tests in one-half or more of patients with aplastic anemia at the time of presentation. Functional studies of bone marrow from PNH patients, even those with mainly hemolytic manifestations, show evidence of defective hematopoiesis. Patients with an initial clinical diagnosis of PNH, especially younger individuals, may later develop frank marrow aplasia and pancytopenia; patients with an initial diagnosis of aplastic anemia may suffer from hemolytic PNH years after recovery of blood counts.

Constitutional Disorders Fanconi anemia, an autosomal recessive disorder, manifests as congenital developmental anomalies, progressive pancytopenia, and an increased risk of malignancy. Chromosomes in Fanconi anemia are peculiarly susceptible to DNA cross-linking agents, the basis for a diagnostic assay. Patients with Fanconi anemia typically have short stature, café au lait spots, and anomalies involving the thumb, radius, and genitourinary tract. At least 16 different genetic defects (all but one with an identified gene) have been defined; the most common, type A Fanconi anemia, is due to a mutation in *FANCA*. Most of the Fanconi anemia gene products form a protein complex that activates FANCD2 by monoubiquitination to play a role in the cellular response to DNA damage and especially interstrand cross-linking.

Dyskeratosis congenita is characterized by the triad of mucous membrane leukoplasia, dystrophic nails, reticular hyperpigmentation, and with the development of aplastic anemia in childhood. Dyskeratosis is due to mutations in genes of the telomere repair complex, which acts to maintain telomere length in replicating cells: the X-linked variety is due to mutations in the *DKC1* (*dyskerin*) gene; the more unusual autosomal dominant type is due to mutation in *TERC*, which encodes an RNA template, and *TERT*, which encodes the catalytic reverse transcriptase, telomerase. Mutations in *TNF2*, a component of the shelterin complex, proteins that bind the telomere DNA, also occur.

In Shwachman-Diamond syndrome, presentation is early in life with neutropenia with pancreatic insufficiency and malabsorption; most patients have compound heterozygous mutations in *SBDS* that may affect both ribosomal biogenesis (as in Diamond-Blackfan anemia; see below) and marrow stroma function.

While these constitutional syndromes can on occasion present in adults, genetic mutations are also risk factors for bone marrow failure. In the recently recognized telomeropathies, mutations in *TERT* and *TERC* have subtle effects on hematopoietic function. Typical presentations include not only severe but also moderate aplastic anemia, which can be chronic and not progressive, and isolated macrocytic anemia or thrombocytopenia. Physical anomalies are usually not found in the patient, although early hair graying is a clue to the diagnosis. A careful family history may disclose pulmonary fibrosis and hepatic cirrhosis. Specific involvement of the bone marrow, liver, and lung is highly variable, as is penetrance of clinical phenotype, both within families and among kindreds. Variable penetrance means that *TERT* and *TERC* mutations represent risk factors for marrow failure, as family members with the same mutations may have normal or only slight hematologic abnormalities but more subtle evidence of (compensated) hematopoietic insufficiency.

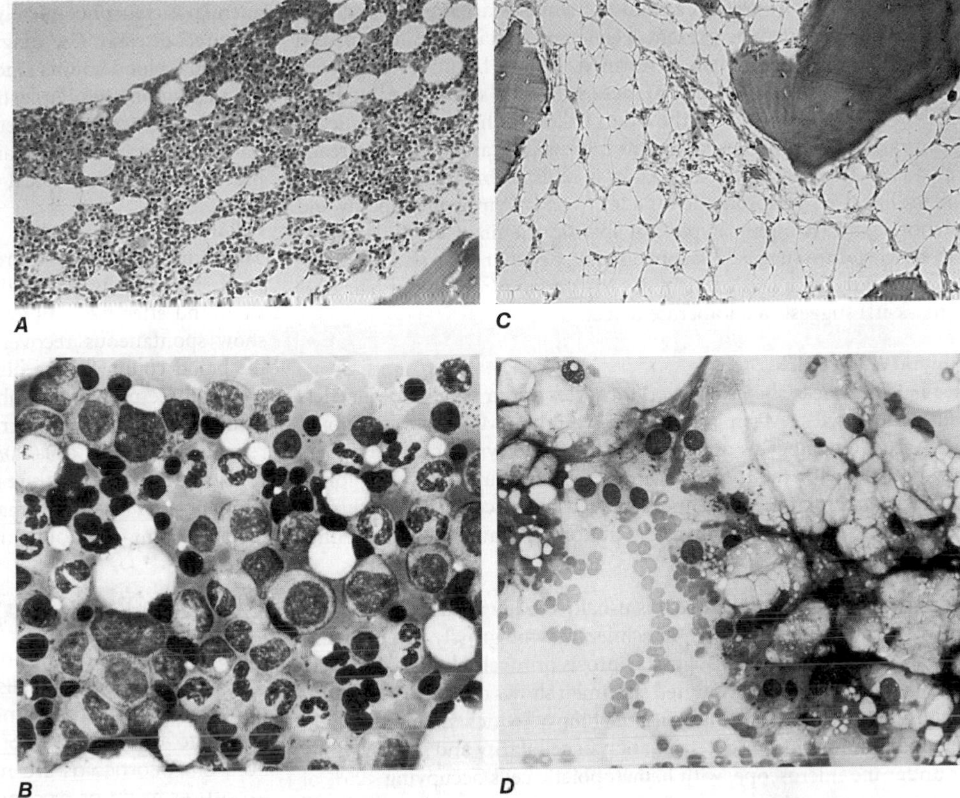

FIGURE 130-1 Normal and aplastic bone marrow. ***A.*** Normal bone marrow biopsy. ***B.*** Normal bone marrow aspirate smear. The marrow is normally 30–70% cellular, and there is a heterogeneous mix of myeloid, erythroid, and lymphoid cells. ***C.*** Aplastic anemia biopsy. ***D.*** Marrow smear in aplastic anemia. The marrow shows replacement of hematopoietic tissue by fat and only residual stromal and lymphoid cells.

PATHOPHYSIOLOGY

Bone marrow failure results from severe damage to the hematopoietic cell compartment. In aplastic anemia, replacement of the bone marrow by fat is apparent in the morphology of the biopsy specimen (Fig. 130-1) and magnetic resonance imaging (MRI) of the spine. Cells bearing the CD34 antigen, a marker of early hematopoietic cells, are greatly diminished, and in functional studies, committed and primitive progenitor cells are virtually absent; in vitro assays have suggested that the stem cell pool is reduced to ≤1% of normal in severe disease at the time of presentation.

An intrinsic stem cell defect exists for the constitutional aplastic anemias: cells from patients with Fanconi anemia exhibit chromosome damage and death on exposure to certain chemical agents. Telomeres are short in some patients with aplastic anemia, due to heterozygous mutations in genes of the telomere repair complex. Telomeres may also shorten physiologically in acquired marrow failure due to replicative demands on a limited stem cell pool.

Drug Injury Extrinsic damage to the marrow follows massive physical or chemical insults such as high doses of radiation and toxic chemicals. For the more common idiosyncratic reaction to modest doses of medical drugs, altered drug metabolism has been invoked as a likely mechanism. The metabolic pathways of many drugs and chemicals, especially if they are polar and have limited water solubility, involve enzymatic degradation to highly reactive electrophilic compounds; these intermediates are toxic because of their propensity to bind to cellular macromolecules. For example, derivative hydroquinones and quinolones are responsible for benzene-induced tissue injury. Excessive generation of toxic intermediates or failure to detoxify the intermediates may be genetically determined and apparent only on specific drug challenge; the complexity and specificity of the pathways imply multiple susceptibility loci and would provide an explanation for the rarity of idiosyncratic drug reactions.

Immune-Mediated Injury The recovery of marrow function in some patients prepared for bone marrow transplantation with antilymphocyte globulin first suggested that aplastic anemia might be immune mediated. Consistent with this hypothesis was the frequent failure of simple bone marrow transplantation from a syngeneic twin, without conditioning cytotoxic chemotherapy, which also argued both *against* simple stem cell absence as the cause and *for* the presence of a host factor producing marrow failure. Laboratory data support an important role for the immune system in aplastic anemia. Blood and bone marrow cells of patients can suppress normal hematopoietic progenitor cell growth, and removal of T cells from aplastic anemia bone marrow improves colony formation in vitro. Increased numbers of activated cytotoxic T cell clones are observed in aplastic anemia patients and usually decline with successful immunosuppressive therapy; type 1 cytokines are implicated; and interferon γ (IFN-γ) induces Fas expression on CD34 cells, leading to apoptotic cell death. The early immune system events in aplastic anemia are not well understood, but an oligoclonal, T cell response implies antigenic stimulus. The rarity of aplastic anemia despite common exposures (medicines, seronegative hepatitis) suggests that genetically determined features of the immune response can convert a normal physiologic response into a sustained abnormal autoimmune process, including polymorphisms in histocompatibility antigens, cytokine genes, and genes that regulate T cell polarization and effector function.

CLINICAL FEATURES

History Aplastic anemia can appear abruptly or insidiously. Bleeding is the most common early symptom; a complaint of days to weeks of easy bruising, oozing from the gums, nose bleeds, heavy menstrual flow, and sometimes petechiae will have been noticed. With thrombocytopenia, massive hemorrhage is unusual, but small amounts of bleeding in the central nervous system can result in catastrophic intracranial or retinal hemorrhage. Symptoms of anemia are also frequent, including lassitude, weakness, shortness of breath, and a pounding sensation in the ears. Infection is an unusual first symptom in aplastic anemia (unlike in agranulocytosis, where pharyngitis, anorectal infection, or frank sepsis occurs early). A striking feature of aplastic anemia is the restriction of symptoms to the hematologic system, and patients often feel and look remarkably well despite drastically reduced blood counts. Systemic complaints and weight loss should point to other etiologies of pancytopenia. Prior drug use, chemical exposure, and preceding viral illnesses must often be elicited with repeated questioning. A family history of hematologic diseases or blood abnormalities, of pulmonary or liver fibrosis, or of early hair graying points to a telomeropathy.

Physical Examination Petechiae and ecchymoses are typical, and retinal hemorrhages may be present. Pelvic and rectal examinations can often be deferred but, when performed, should be undertaken with great gentleness to avoid trauma; these will often show bleeding from the cervical os and blood in the stool. Pallor of the skin and mucous membranes is common except in the most acute cases or those already transfused. Infection on presentation is unusual but may occur if the patient has been symptomatic for a few weeks. Lymphadenopathy and splenomegaly are highly atypical of aplastic anemia. Café au lait spots and short stature suggest Fanconi anemia; peculiar nails and leukoplakia suggest dyskeratosis congenita; early graying (and use of hair dyes to mask it!) suggests a telomerase defect.

LABORATORY STUDIES

Blood The smear shows large erythrocytes and a paucity of platelets and granulocytes. Mean corpuscular volume (MCV) is commonly increased. Reticulocytes are absent or few, and lymphocyte numbers may be normal or reduced. The presence of immature myeloid forms suggests leukemia or MDS; nucleated red blood cells (RBCs) suggest marrow fibrosis or tumor invasion; abnormal platelets suggest either peripheral destruction or MDS.

Bone Marrow The bone marrow is usually readily aspirated but dilute on smear, and the fatty biopsy specimen may be grossly pale on withdrawal; a "dry tap" instead suggests fibrosis or myelophthisis. In severe aplasia, the smear of the aspirated specimen shows only red cells, residual lymphocytes, and stromal cells; the biopsy (which should be >1 cm in length) is superior for determination of cellularity and shows mainly fat under the microscope, with hematopoietic cells occupying <25% of the marrow space; in the most serious cases, the biopsy is virtually all fat. The correlation between marrow cellularity and disease severity is imperfect, in part because marrow cellularity declines physiologically with aging. Additionally, some patients with moderate disease by blood counts will have empty iliac crest biopsies, whereas "hot spots" of hematopoiesis may be seen in severe cases. If an iliac crest specimen is inadequate, cells may also be obtained by aspiration from the sternum. Residual hematopoietic cells should have normal morphology, except for mildly megaloblastic erythropoiesis; megakaryocytes are invariably greatly reduced and usually absent. Granulomas may indicate an infectious etiology of the marrow failure.

Ancillary Studies Chromosome breakage studies of peripheral blood using diepoxybutane or mitomycin C should be performed on children and younger adults to exclude Fanconi anemia. Very short telomere length (available commercially) strongly suggests the presence of a telomerase or shelterin mutation, which can be pursued by family studies and nucleotide sequencing. Chromosome studies of bone marrow cells are often revealing in MDS and should be negative in typical aplastic anemia. Flow cytometry offers a sensitive diagnostic test for PNH. Serologic studies may show evidence of viral infection, such as Epstein-Barr virus and HIV. Posthepatitis aplastic anemia is seronegative. The spleen size should be determined by computed tomography (CT) scanning or ultrasound if the physical examination of the abdomen is unsatisfactory. Occasionally MRI may be helpful to assess the fat content of vertebrae in order to distinguish aplasia from MDS.

DIAGNOSIS

The diagnosis of aplastic anemia is usually straightforward, based on the combination of pancytopenia with a fatty bone marrow. Aplastic anemia is a disease of the young and should be a leading diagnosis in the pancytopenic adolescent or young adult. When pancytopenia is secondary, the primary diagnosis is usually obvious from either history or physical examination: the massive spleen of alcoholic cirrhosis, the history of metastatic cancer or SLE, or miliary tuberculosis on chest radiograph (Table 130-1).

Diagnostic problems can occur with atypical presentations and among related hematologic diseases. Although pancytopenia is most common, some patients with bone marrow hypocellularity have depression of only one or two of three blood lines, with later progression to pancytopenia. The bone marrow in constitutional aplastic anemia is morphologically indistinguishable from the aspirate in acquired disease. The diagnosis can be suggested by family history, abnormal blood counts since childhood, or the presence of associated physical anomalies. Aplastic anemia may be difficult to distinguish from the hypocellular variety of MDS: MDS is favored by finding morphologic abnormalities, particularly of megakaryocytes and myeloid precursor cells, and typical cytogenetic abnormalities (see below).

PROGNOSIS

The natural history of severe aplastic anemia is rapid deterioration and death. Historically, provision first of RBC and later of platelet transfusions and effective antibiotics were of some benefit, but few patients show spontaneous recovery. The major prognostic determinant is the blood count. Severe disease has been defined by the presence of two of three parameters: absolute neutrophil count <500/μL, platelet count <20,000/μL, and corrected reticulocyte count <1% (or absolute reticulocyte count <60,000/μL). In the era of effective immunosuppressive therapies, absolute numbers of reticulocytes (>25,000/μL) and lymphocytes (>1000/μL) may be better predictors of response to treatment and long-term outcome.

TREATMENT APLASTIC ANEMIA

Severe acquired aplastic anemia can be cured by replacement of the absent hematopoietic cells (and the immune system) by stem cell transplant, or it can be ameliorated by suppression of the immune system to allow recovery of the patient's residual bone marrow function. Glucocorticoids are not of value as primary therapy. Suspect exposures to drugs or chemicals should be discontinued; however, spontaneous recovery of severe blood count depression is rare, and a waiting period before beginning treatment may not be advisable unless the blood counts are only modestly depressed.

HEMATOPOIETIC STEM CELL TRANSPLANTATION

This is the best therapy for the younger patient with a fully histocompatible sibling donor (Chap. 139e). Human leukocyte antigen (HLA) typing should be ordered as soon as the diagnosis of aplastic anemia is established in a child or younger adult. In transplant candidates, transfusion of blood from family members should be avoided so as to prevent sensitization to histocompatibility antigens, but limited numbers of blood products probably do not greatly affect outcome. For allogeneic transplant from fully matched siblings, long-term survival rates for children are approximately 90%. Transplant morbidity and mortality are increased among adults, due to the higher risk of chronic GVHD and serious infections.

Most patients do not have a suitable sibling donor. Occasionally, a full phenotypic match can be found within the family and serve as well. Far more available are other alternative donors, either unrelated but histocompatible volunteers or closely but not perfectly matched family members. High-resolution matching at HLA and more effective conditioning regimens and GVHD prophylaxis have led to improved survival rates in patients who proceed to alternative donor transplant, in some series approximating results with conventional sibling donors. Patients will be at risk for late complications, especially a higher rate of cancer, if radiation is used as a component of conditioning.

IMMUNOSUPPRESSION

The standard regimen of antithymocyte globulin (ATG) in combination with cyclosporine induces hematologic recovery (independence from transfusion and a leukocyte count adequate to prevent infection) in 60–70% of patients. Children do especially well, whereas older adult patients often suffer complications due to the presence of comorbidities. An early robust hematologic response correlates with long-term survival. Improvement in granulocyte number is generally apparent within 2 months of treatment. Most recovered patients continue to have some degree of blood count depression, the MCV remains elevated, and bone marrow cellularity returns toward normal very slowly if at all. Relapse (recurrent pancytopenia) is frequent, often occurring as cyclosporine is discontinued; most, but not all, patients respond to reinstitution of immunosuppression, but some responders become dependent on continued cyclosporine administration. Development of MDS, with typical marrow morphologic or cytogenetic abnormalities, occurs in approximately 15% of treated patients, usually but not invariably associated with a return of pancytopenia, and some patients develop leukemia. A laboratory diagnosis of PNH can generally be made at the time of presentation of aplastic anemia by flow cytometry; recovered patients may have frank hemolysis if the PNH clone expands. Bone marrow examinations should be performed if there is an unfavorable change in blood counts.

Horse ATG is administered as intravenous infusions over 4 days. ATG binds to peripheral blood cells; therefore, platelet and granulocyte numbers may decrease further during active treatment. Serum sickness, a flulike illness with a characteristic cutaneous eruption and arthralgia, often develops approximately 10 days after initiating treatment. Methylprednisolone is administered with ATG to ameliorate the immune consequences of heterologous protein infusion. Excessive or extended glucocorticoid therapy is associated with avascular joint necrosis. Cyclosporine is administered orally at an initial high dose, with subsequent adjustment according to blood levels obtained every 2 weeks; rough levels should be between 150 and 200 ng/mL. The most important side effects are nephrotoxicity, hypertension, seizures, and opportunistic infections, especially *Pneumocystis jiroveci* (prophylactic treatment with monthly inhaled pentamidine is recommended).

Most patients with aplastic anemia lack a suitable marrow donor, and immunosuppression is the treatment of choice. Overall survival is equivalent with transplantation and immunosuppression. However, successful transplant cures marrow failure, whereas patients who recover adequate blood counts after immunosuppression remain at risk of relapse and malignant evolution. Because of excellent results in children and younger adults, allogeneic transplant should be performed if a suitable sibling donor is available. Increasing age and the severity of neutropenia are the most important factors weighing in the decision between transplant and immunosuppression in adults who have a matched family donor: older patients do better with ATG and cyclosporine, whereas transplant is preferred if granulocytopenia is profound.

Outcomes following both transplant and immunosuppression have improved with time. High doses of cyclophosphamide, without stem cell rescue, have been reported to produce durable hematologic recovery, without relapse or evolution to MDS, but this treatment can produce sustained severe fatal neutropenia, and response is often delayed.

OTHER THERAPIES

The effectiveness of androgens has not been verified in controlled trials, but occasional patients will respond or even demonstrate blood count dependence on continued therapy. Sex hormones upregulate telomerase gene activity in vitro, which is possibly also their mechanism of action in improving marrow function. For patients with moderate disease, especially if a telomere defect is present, or those with severe pancytopenia in whom immunosuppression has failed, a 3- to 4-month trial is appropriate.

Hematopoietic growth factors (HGFs) such as erythropoietin and granulocyte colony-stimulating factor (G-CSF) are not definitive therapy for severe aplastic anemia, and even their roles as adjuncts to immunosuppression are not clear. In research protocols, thrombopoietin mimetics have shown surprising activity in patients with refractory aplastic anemia, with patterns of blood count recovery suggesting that they act as stem cell stimulants.

SUPPORTIVE CARE

Meticulous medical attention is required so that the patient may survive to benefit from definitive therapy or, having failed treatment, to maintain a reasonable existence in the face of pancytopenia. First and most important, infection in the presence of severe neutropenia must be aggressively treated by prompt institution of parenteral, broad-spectrum antibiotics, usually ceftazidime or a combination of an aminoglycoside, cephalosporin, and semisynthetic penicillin. Therapy is empirical and must not await results of culture, although specific foci of infection such as oropharyngeal or anorectal abscesses, pneumonia, sinusitis, and typhlitis (necrotizing colitis) should be sought on physical examination and with radiographic studies. When indwelling plastic catheters become contaminated, vancomycin should be added. Persistent or recrudescent fever implies fungal disease: *Candida* and *Aspergillus* are common, especially after several courses of antibacterial antibiotics. A major reason for the improved prognosis in aplastic anemia has been the development of better antifungal drugs and the timely institution of such therapy when infection is suspected. Granulocyte transfusions using G-CSF–mobilized peripheral blood may be effective in the treatment of overwhelming or refractory infections. Hand washing, the single best method of preventing the spread of infection, remains a neglected practice. Nonabsorbed antibiotics for gut decontamination are poorly tolerated and not of proven value. Total reverse isolation does not reduce mortality from infections.

Both platelet and erythrocyte numbers can be maintained by transfusion. Alloimmunization historically limited the usefulness of platelet transfusions and is now minimized by several strategies, including use of single donors to reduce exposure and physical or chemical methods to diminish leukocytes in the product; HLA-matched platelets are often effective in patients refractory to random donor products. Inhibitors of fibrinolysis such as aminocaproic acid have not been shown to relieve mucosal oozing; the use of low-dose glucocorticoids to induce "vascular stability" is unproven and not recommended. Whether platelet transfusions are better used prophylactically or only as needed remains unclear. Any rational regimen of prophylaxis requires transfusions once or twice weekly to maintain the platelet count >10,000/μL (oozing from the gut increases precipitously at counts <5000/μL). Menstruation should be suppressed either by oral estrogens or nasal follicle-stimulating hormone/luteinizing hormone (FSH/LH) antagonists. Aspirin and other nonsteroidal anti-inflammatory agents inhibit platelet function and must be avoided.

RBCs should be transfused to maintain a normal level of activity, usually at a hemoglobin value of 70 g/L (90 g/L if there is underlying cardiac or pulmonary disease); a regimen of 2 units every 2 weeks will replace normal losses in a patient without a functioning bone marrow. In chronic anemia, the iron chelators, deferoxamine and deferasirox, should be added at approximately the fiftieth transfusion to avoid secondary hemochromatosis.

PURE RED CELL APLASIA

Other, more restricted forms of marrow failure occur, in which only a single circulating cell type is affected and the marrow shows corresponding absence or decreased numbers of specific precursor cells: aregenerative anemia as in PRCA (see below), thrombocytopenia with amegakaryocytosis (Chap. 140), and neutropenia without marrow myeloid cells in agranulocytosis (Chap. 80). In general, and in contrast to aplastic anemia and MDS, the unaffected lineages appear quantitatively and qualitatively normal. Agranulocytosis, the most frequent of these syndromes, is usually a complication of medical drug use (with agents similar to those related to aplastic anemia), either by a mechanism of direct chemical toxicity or by immune destruction. Agranulocytosis has an incidence similar to aplastic anemia but is especially frequent among older adults and in women. The syndrome should resolve with discontinuation of exposure, but significant mortality is attached to neutropenia in the older and often previously unwell patient. Both pure white cell aplasia (agranulocytosis without incriminating drug exposure) and amegakaryocytic thrombocytopenia are exceedingly rare and, like PRCA, appear to be due to destructive antibodies or lymphocytes and can respond to immunosuppressive therapies. In all of the single-lineage failure syndromes, progression to pancytopenia or leukemia is unusual.

TABLE 130-4 CLASSIFICATION OF PURE RED CELL APLASIA

Self-limited
Transient erythroblastopenia of childhood
Transient aplastic crisis of hemolysis (acute B19 parvovirus infection)
Fetal red blood cell aplasia
Nonimmune hydrops fetalis (in utero B19 parvovirus infection)
Hereditary pure red cell aplasia
Congenital pure red cell aplasia (Diamond-Blackfan anemia)
Acquired pure red cell aplasia
Cancer
Thymoma
Lymphoid malignancies (and more rarely other hematologic diseases)
Paraneoplastic to solid tumors
Connective tissue disorders with immunologic abnormalities
Systemic lupus erythematosus, juvenile rheumatoid arthritis, rheumatoid arthritis
Multiple endocrine gland insufficiency
Viruses
Persistent B19 parvovirus, hepatitis, adult T cell leukemia virus, Epstein-Barr virus
Pregnancy
Drugs
Especially phenytoin, azathioprine, chloramphenicol, procainamide, isoniazid
Antibodies to erythropoietin
Idiopathic

DEFINITION AND DIFFERENTIAL DIAGNOSIS

PRCA is characterized by anemia, reticulocytopenia, and absent or rare erythroid precursor cells in the bone marrow. The classification of PRCA is shown in Table 130-4. In adults, PRCA is acquired. An identical syndrome can occur constitutionally: Diamond-Blackfan anemia, or congenital PRCA, is diagnosed at birth or in early childhood and often responds to glucocorticoid treatment; mutations in ribosome protein genes are etiologic. Temporary red cell failure occurs in transient aplastic crisis of hemolytic anemias due to acute parvovirus infection (Chap. 221) and in transient erythroblastopenia of childhood, which occurs in normal children.

CLINICAL ASSOCIATIONS AND ETIOLOGY

PRCA has important associations with immune system diseases. A small minority of cases occur with a thymoma. More frequently, red cell aplasia can be the major manifestation of large granular lymphocytosis or complicate chronic lymphocytic leukemia. Some patients may be hypogammaglobulinemic. Infrequently (compared to agranulocytosis), PRCA can be due to an idiosyncratic drug reaction. Subcutaneous administration of erythropoietin (EPO) has provoked PRCA mediated by neutralizing antibodies.

Like aplastic anemia, PRCA results from diverse mechanisms. Antibodies to RBC precursors are frequently present in the blood, but T cell inhibition is probably the more common immune mechanism. Cytotoxic lymphocyte activity restricted by histocompatibility locus or specific for human T cell leukemia/lymphoma virus I–infected cells and natural killer cell activity inhibitory of erythropoiesis have been demonstrated in particularly well-studied individual cases.

PERSISTENT PARVOVIRUS B19 INFECTION

Chronic parvovirus infection is an important, treatable cause of PRCA. This common virus causes a benign exanthem of childhood (fifth disease) and a polyarthralgia/arthritis syndrome in adults. In patients with underlying hemolysis (or any condition that increases demand for RBC production), parvovirus infection can cause a transient aplastic crisis and an abrupt but temporary worsening of the anemia due to failed erythropoiesis. In normal individuals, acute infection is resolved by production of neutralizing antibodies to the virus, but in the setting of congenital, acquired, or iatrogenic immunodeficiency, persistent viral infection may occur. The bone marrow shows red cell aplasia and the presence of giant pronormoblasts (Fig. 130-2), which is the cytopathic sign of B19 parvovirus infection. Viral tropism for human erythroid progenitor cells is due to its use of erythrocyte P antigen as a cellular receptor for entry. Direct cytotoxicity of virus causes anemia if demands on erythrocyte production are high; in normal individuals, the temporary cessation of red cell production is not clinically apparent, and skin and joint symptoms are mediated by immune complex deposition.

TREATMENT PURE RED CELL APLASIA

History, physical examination, and routine laboratory studies may disclose an underlying disease or a drug exposure. Thymoma should be sought by radiographic procedures. Tumor excision

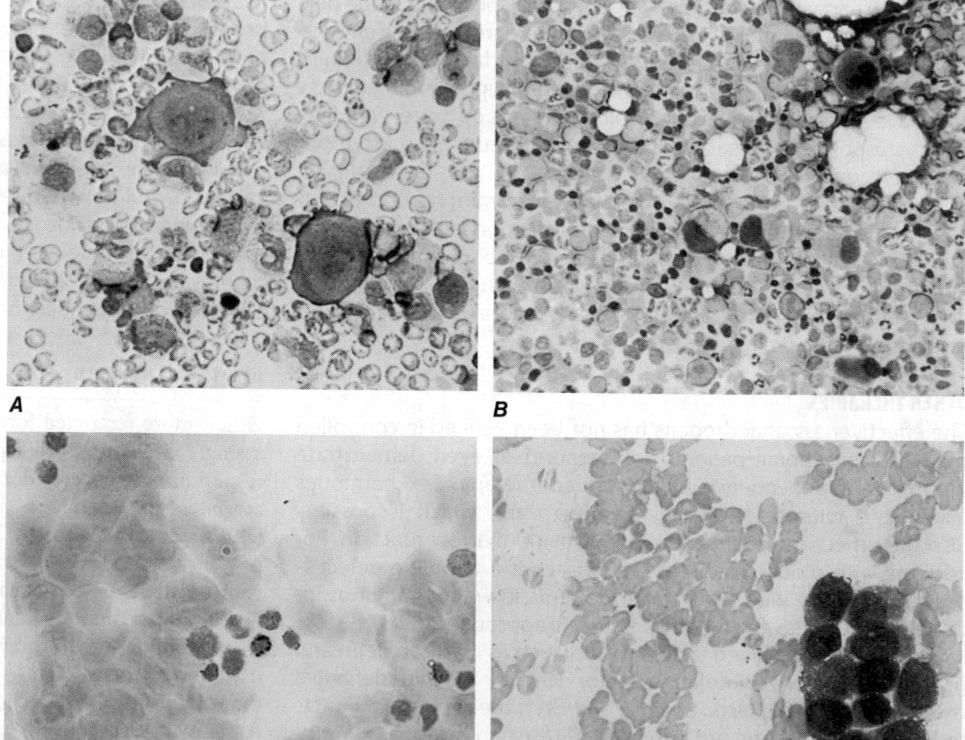

FIGURE 130-2 Pathognomonic cells in marrow failure syndromes. ***A.*** Giant pronormoblast, the cytopathic effect of B19 parvovirus infection of the erythroid progenitor cell. ***B.*** Uninuclear megakaryocyte and microblastic erythroid precursors typical of the 5q–myelodysplasia syndrome. ***C.*** Ringed sideroblast showing perinuclear iron granules. ***D.*** Tumor cells present on a touch preparation made from the marrow biopsy of a patient with metastatic carcinoma.

is indicated, but anemia does not necessarily improve with surgery. The diagnosis of parvovirus infection requires detection of viral DNA sequences in the blood (IgG and IgM antibodies are commonly absent). The presence of erythroid colonies has been considered predictive of response to immunosuppressive therapy in idiopathic PRCA.

Red cell aplasia is compatible with long-term survival with supportive care alone: a combination of erythrocyte transfusions and iron chelation. For persistent B19 parvovirus infection, almost all patients respond to intravenous immunoglobulin therapy (e.g., 0.4 g/kg daily for 5 days), although relapse and retreatment may be expected, especially in patients with AIDS. The majority of patients with idiopathic PRCA respond favorably to immunosuppression. Most first receive a course of glucocorticoids. Also effective are cyclosporine, ATG, azathioprine, and cyclophosphamide.

MYELODYSPLASIA

DEFINITION

The myelodysplastic syndromes (MDS) are a heterogeneous group of hematologic disorders broadly characterized by both (1) cytopenias due to bone marrow failure and (2) a high risk of development of acute myeloid leukemia (AML). Anemia, often with thrombocytopenia and neutropenia, occurs with dysmorphic (abnormal appearing) and usually cellular bone marrow, which is evidence of ineffective blood cell production. In patients with "low-risk" MDS, marrow failure dominates the clinical course. In other patients, myeloblasts are present at diagnosis, chromosomes are abnormal, and the "high risk" is due to leukemic progression. MDS may be fatal due to the complications of pancytopenia or the incurability of leukemia, but a large proportion of patients will die of concurrent disease, the comorbidities typical in an elderly population. A clinically useful nosology of these often confusing entities was first developed by the French-American-British Cooperative Group in 1983. Five entities were defined: refractory anemia (RA), refractory anemia with ringed sideroblasts (RARS), refractory anemia with excess blasts (RAEB), refractory anemia with excess blasts in transformation (RAEB-t), and chronic myelomonocytic leukemia (CMML). The World Health Organization (WHO) classification (2002) recognized that the distinction between RAEB-t and AML is arbitrary and grouped them together as acute leukemia and that CMML behaves as a myeloproliferative disease; the WHO classification also separated refractory anemias with dysmorphic change restricted to erythroid lineage from those with multilineage changes. In a 2008 revision, specific categories for unilineage dysplasias were added (**Table 130-5**).

TABLE 130-5 WORLD HEALTH ORGANIZATION (WHO) CLASSIFICATION OF MYELODYSPLASTIC SYNDROMES/NEOPLASMS

Name	WHO Estimated Proportion of Patients with MDS	Peripheral Blood: Key Features	Bone Marrow: Key Features
Refractory cytopenias with unilineage dysplasia (RCUD):			
Refractory anemia (RA)	10–20%	Anemia <1% of blasts	Unilineage erythroid dysplasia (in ≥10% of cells) <5% blasts
Refractory neutropenia (RN)	<1%	Neutropenia <1% blasts	Unilineage granulocytic dysplasia <5% blasts
Refractory thrombocytopenia (RT)	<1%	Thrombocytopenia <1% blasts	Unilineage megakaryocytic dysplasia <5% blasts
Refractory anemia with ringed sideroblasts (RARS)	3–11%	Anemia No blasts	Unilineage erythroid dysplasia ≥15% of erythroid precursors are ringed sideroblasts <5% blasts
Refractory cytopenias with multilineage dysplasia (RCMD)	30%	Cytopenia(s) <1% blasts No Auer rods	Multilineage dysplasia ± ringed sideroblasts <5% blasts No Auer rods
Refractory anemia with excess blasts, type 1 (RAEB-1)	40%	Cytopenia(s) <5% blasts No Auer rods	Unilineage or multilineage dysplasia
Refractory anemia with excess blasts, type 2 (RAEB-2)		Cytopenia(s) 5–19% blasts ± Auer rods	Unilineage or multilineage dysplasia 10–19% blasts ± Auer rods
MDS associated with isolated del(5q) [del(5q)]	Uncommon	Anemia Normal or high platelet count <1% blasts	Isolated 5q31 chromosome deletion Anemia; hypolobated megakaryocytes <5% blasts
Childhood MDS, including refractory cytopenia of childhood (*provisional*) (RCC)	<1%	Pancytopenia	<5% marrow blasts for RCC Marrow usually hypocellular
MDS, unclassifiable (MDS-U)	?	Cytopenia ≤1% blasts	Does not fit other categories Dysplasia <5% blasts If no dysplasia, MDS-associated karyotype

Note: If peripheral blood blasts are 2–4%, the diagnosis is RAEB-1 even if marrow blasts are <5%. If Auer rods are present, the WHO considers the diagnosis RAEB-2 if the blast proportion is <20% (even if <10%), or acute myeloid leukemia (AML) if at least 20% blasts. For all subtypes, peripheral blood monocytes are <1 × 10^9/L. Bicytopenia may be observed in RCUD subtypes, but pancytopenia with unilineage marrow dysplasia should be classified as MDS-U. Therapy-related MDS (t-MDS), whether due to alkylating agents or topoisomerase II inhibitors (t-MDS/t-AML) is now included in the WHO classification of myeloid neoplasms. The listing in this table excludes MDS/myeloproliferative neoplasm overlap categories, such as chronic myelomonocytic leukemia, juvenile myelomonocytic leukemia, and the provisional entity RARS with thrombocytosis.

Abbreviation: MDS, myelodysplastic syndrome.

The diagnosis of MDS may be a challenge, because sometimes subtle clinical and pathologic features must be distinguished and precise diagnostic categorization requires a hematopathologist knowledgeable in the latest classification scheme. Nonetheless, it is important that the internist and primary care physician be sufficiently familiar with MDS to expedite referral to a hematologist, both because many new therapies are now available to improve hematopoietic function and the judicious use of supportive care can improve the patient's quality of life.

EPIDEMIOLOGY

Idiopathic MDS is a disease of the elderly; the mean age at onset is older than 70 years. There is a slight male preponderance. MDS is a relatively common form of bone marrow failure, with reported incidence rates of 35 to >100 per million persons in the general population and 120 to >500 per million in the older adult. MDS is rare in children, but monocytic leukemia can be seen. Secondary or therapy-related MDS is not age related. Rates of MDS have increased over time, due to better recognition of the syndrome by physicians and an aging population.

ETIOLOGY AND PATHOPHYSIOLOGY

MDS is associated with environmental exposures such as radiation and benzene; other risk factors have been reported inconsistently. Secondary MDS occurs as a late toxicity of cancer treatment, usually a combination of radiation and the radiomimetic alkylating agents such as busulfan, nitrosourea, or procarbazine (with a latent period of 5–7 years) or the DNA topoisomerase inhibitors (2-year latency). Acquired aplastic anemia, Fanconi anemia, and other constitutional marrow failure diseases can evolve into MDS. However, the typical MDS patient does not have a suggestive environmental exposure history or a preceding hematologic disease. MDS is a disease of aging, suggesting random cumulative intrinsic and environmental damage to marrow cells.

MDS is a clonal hematopoietic stem cell disorder characterized by disordered cell proliferation and impaired differentiation, resulting in cytopenias and risk of progression to leukemia. Both chromosomal and genetic instability have been implicated, and both are likely aging-related. Cytogenetic abnormalities are found in approximately one-half of patients, and some of the same specific lesions are also seen in frank leukemia; aneuploidy (chromosome loss or gain) is more frequent than translocations. More sensitive assays, such as comparative genomic hybridization and single nucleotide polymorphism arrays, reveal chromosomal abnormalities in a large proportion of patients with normal conventional cytogenetics. Accelerated telomere attrition may destabilize the genome in marrow failure and predispose to acquisition of chromosomal lesions. Cytogenetic abnormalities are not random (loss of all or part of 5, 7, and 20, trisomy of 8) and may be related to etiology (11q23 following topoisomerase II inhibitors). The type and number of cytogenetic abnormalities strongly correlate with the probability of leukemic transformation and survival.

Genomics has illuminated the role of point mutations in the pathophysiology of MDS. Recurrent somatic mutations, acquired in the abnormal marrow cells and absent in the germline, have been identified in almost 100 genes. Many of the same genes are also mutated in AML without MDS, whereas others are distinctive in subtypes of MDS. A prominent example of the latter is the discovery of mutations in genes of the RNA splicing machinery, especially *SF3B1*, which strongly associate with sideroblastic anemia. Some mutations correlate with prognosis: spliceosome defects with favorable outcome, and mutations in *EZH2, TP53, RUNX1*, and *ASXL1* with poor outcome. Mutations and cytogenetic abnormalities are not independent: *TP53* mutations associate with complex cytogenetic abnormalities and *TET2* mutations with normal cytogenetics. Correlation and exclusion in the pattern of mutations indicate a functional genomic architecture. Analysis of deep sequencing results in patients whose MDS evolved to AML has shown evidence of clonal succession, with founder clones acquiring further mutations that allow clonal dominance. Furthermore, the prevalence of abnormal cells by morphology underestimates bone marrow involvement by MDS clones, as cells normal in appearance are apparently derived from the abnormal clones. Both presenting and evolving hematologic manifestations result from the accumulation of multiple genetic lesions: loss of tumor-suppressor genes, activating oncogene mutations, epigenetic pathways that affect mRNA processing and methylation status, or other harmful alterations. Pathophysiology has been linked to mutations and chromosome abnormalities in some specific MDS syndromes. The 5q– deletion leads to heterozygous loss of a ribosomal protein gene that is also mutant in Diamond-Blackfan anemia, and both are characterized by deficient erythropoiesis. An immune pathophysiology may underlie trisomy 8 MDS, in which patients often experience improved blood counts after immunosuppressive therapy; there is T cell activity directed to hematopoietic progenitors, which the cytogenetically aberrant clone resists. However, in general for MDS, the role of the immune system and its cells and cytokines; the role of the hematopoietic stem cell niche, the microenvironment, and cell-cell interactions; the fate of normal cells in the Darwinian competitive environment of the dysplastic marrow; and how mutant cells produce marrow failure in MDS are not well understood.

CLINICAL FEATURES

Anemia dominates the early course. Most symptomatic patients complain of the gradual onset of fatigue and weakness, dyspnea, and pallor, but at least one-half the patients are asymptomatic, and their MDS is discovered only incidentally on routine blood counts. Previous chemotherapy or radiation exposure is an important historic fact. Fever and weight loss should point to a myeloproliferative rather than myelodysplastic process. MDS in childhood is rare and, when diagnosed, increases the likelihood of an underlying genetic disease. Children with Down syndrome are susceptible to MDS, and a family history may indicate a hereditary form of sideroblastic anemia, Fanconi anemia, or a telomeropathy. Inherited *GATA2* mutations, as in the MonoMAC syndrome (with increased susceptibility to viral, mycobacteria, and fungal infections, as well as deficient numbers of monocytes, natural killer cells, and B lymphocytes), also cause MDS in young patients.

The physical examination is remarkable for signs of anemia; approximately 20% of patients have splenomegaly. Some unusual skin lesions, including Sweet syndrome (febrile neutrophilic dermatosis), occur with MDS. Accompanying autoimmune syndromes are not infrequent. In the younger patient, stereotypical anomalies point to a constitutional syndrome (short stature, abnormal thumbs in Fanconi anemia; early graying in the telomeropathies; cutaneous warts in *GATA2* deficiency).

LABORATORY STUDIES

Blood Anemia is present in most cases, either alone or as part of bi- or pancytopenia; isolated neutropenia or thrombocytopenia is more unusual. Macrocytosis is common, and the smear may be dimorphic with a distinctive population of large red blood cells. Platelets are also large and lack granules. In functional studies, they may show marked abnormalities, and patients may have bleeding symptoms despite seemingly adequate numbers. Neutrophils are hypogranulated; have hyposegmented, ringed, or abnormally segmented nuclei; contain Döhle bodies; and may be functionally deficient. Circulating myeloblasts usually correlate with marrow blast numbers, and their quantity is important for classification and prognosis. The total white blood cell count (WBC) is usually normal or low, except in chronic myelomonocytic leukemia. As in aplastic anemia, MDS can be associated with a clonal population of PNH cells. Genetic testing is commercially available for constitutional syndromes.

Bone Marrow The bone marrow is usually normal or hypercellular, but in about 20% of cases, it is sufficiently hypocellular to be confused with aplasia. No single characteristic feature of marrow morphology distinguishes MDS, but the following are commonly observed: dyserythropoietic changes (especially nuclear abnormalities) and ringed sideroblasts in the erythroid lineage; hypogranulation and hyposegmentation in granulocytic precursors, with an increase in myeloblasts; and megakaryocytes showing reduced numbers of or disorganized

TABLE 130-6 INTERNATIONAL PROGNOSTIC SCORING SYSTEM (IPSS)

	Score Value				
Prognostic Variable	**0**	**0.5**	**1**	**1.5**	**2**
Bone marrow blasts (%)	<5%	5–10%		11–20%	21–30%
Karyotype[a]	Good	Intermediate	Poor		
Cytopenia[b] (lineages affected)	0 or 1	2 or 3			
Risk Group Scores	**Score**				
Low	0				
Intermediate-1	0.5–1				
Intermediate-2	1.5–2				
High	≥2.5				

[a]Good, normal, –Y, del(5q), del (20q); poor, complex (≥3 abnormalities) or chromosome 7 abnormalities; intermediate, all other abnormalities. [b]Cytopenias defined as hemoglobin <100 g/L, platelet count <100,000/μL, and absolute neutrophil count <1500/μL.

nuclei. Megaloblastic nuclei associated with defective hemoglobinization in the erythroid lineage are common. Prognosis strongly correlates with the proportion of marrow blasts. Cytogenetic analysis and fluorescent in situ hybridization can identify chromosomal abnormalities.

DIFFERENTIAL DIAGNOSIS

Deficiencies of vitamin B_{12} or folate should be excluded by appropriate blood tests; vitamin B_6 deficiency can be assessed by a therapeutic trial of pyridoxine if the bone marrow shows ringed sideroblasts. Marrow dysplasia can be observed in acute viral infections, drug reactions, or chemical toxicity but should be transient. More difficult are the distinctions between hypocellular MDS and aplasia or between refractory anemia with excess blasts and early acute leukemia. The WHO considers the presence of 20% blasts in the marrow as the criterion that separates AML from MDS. In young patients, underlying, predisposing genetic diseases should be considered (see above).

PROGNOSIS

The median survival varies greatly from years for patients with 5q– or sideroblastic anemia to a few months in refractory anemia with excess blasts or severe pancytopenia associated with monosomy 7; an International Prognostic Scoring System (IPSS; Table 130-6) assists in making predictions. Even "low-risk" MDS has significant morbidity and mortality. Most patients die as a result of complications of pancytopenia and not due to leukemic transformation; perhaps one-third will succumb to other diseases unrelated to their MDS. Precipitous worsening of pancytopenia, acquisition of new chromosomal abnormalities on serial cytogenetic determination, increase in the number of blasts, and marrow fibrosis are all poor prognostic indicators. The outlook in therapy-related MDS, regardless of type, is extremely poor, and most patients will progress within a few months to refractory AML.

TREATMENT MYELODYSPLASIA

Historically, the therapy of MDS has been unsatisfactory, but new drugs recently have been approved for this disease. Several regimens appear to not only improve blood counts but to delay onset of leukemia and to improve survival. The choice of therapy for an individual patient, administration of treatment, and management of toxicities are complicated and require hematologic expertise.

Only hematopoietic stem cell transplantation offers cure of MDS. The current survival rate in selected patient cohorts is ~50% at 3 years and is improving. Results using unrelated matched donors are now similar to those obtained using siblings, and patients in their 50s and 60s have been successfully transplanted. Nevertheless, treatment-related mortality and morbidity increase with recipient age. Complicating the decision to undertake transplant is that the high-risk patient, for whom the procedure is most obviously indicated, has a high probability of a poor outcome from transplant-related mortality or disease relapse, whereas the low-risk patient, who is more likely to tolerate transplant, also may do well for years with less aggressive therapies.

MDS has been regarded as particularly refractory to cytotoxic chemotherapy regimens, and as in AML in the older adult, drug toxicity is frequent and often fatal, and remissions if achieved are brief. Low doses of cytotoxic drugs have been administered for their "differentiation" potential, and from this experience, drug therapies have emerged based on pyrimidine analogues. These new drugs are classified as epigenetic modulators, believed to act through a demethylating mechanism to alter gene regulation and allow differentiation to mature blood cells from the abnormal MDS stem cell (although global methylation status has not correlated with clinical efficacy). Azacitidine and decitabine are two epigenetic modifiers frequently used in bone marrow failure clinics. Azacitidine improves blood counts and survival in MDS, compared to best supportive care. Azacitidine is usually administered subcutaneously, daily for 7 days, at 4-week intervals, for at least four cycles before assessing for response. Overall, generally improved blood counts with a decrease in transfusion requirements occurred in ~50% of patients in published trials. Response is dependent on continued drug administration, and most patients eventually will no longer respond and experience recurrent cytopenias or progression to AML. Decitabine is closely related to azacitidine and more potent; 30–50% of patients show responses in blood counts, with a duration of response of almost a year. Decitabine is usually administered by continuous intravenous infusion in regimens of varying doses and durations of 3 to 10 days in repeating cycles. The major toxicity of azacitidine and decitabine is myelosuppression, leading to worsened blood counts. Other symptoms associated with cancer chemotherapy frequently occur. Demethylating agents are frequently used in the high-risk patient who is not a candidate for stem cell transplant. In the lower risk patient, they are also effective, but alternative therapies should be considered.

Lenalidomide, a thalidomide derivative with a more favorable toxicity profile, is particularly effective in reversing anemia in MDS patients with 5q– syndrome; not only do a high proportion of these patients become transfusion independent with normal or near-normal hemoglobin levels, but their cytogenetics also become normal. The drug has many biologic activities, and it is unclear which is critical for clinical efficacy. Lenalidomide is administered orally. Most patients will improve within 3 months of initiating therapy. Toxicities include myelosuppression (worsening thrombocytopenia and neutropenia, necessitating blood count monitoring) and an increased risk of deep vein thrombosis and pulmonary embolism.

Immunosuppression, as used in aplastic anemia, also may produce sustained independence from transfusion and improve survival. ATG, cyclosporine, and the anti-CD52 monoclonal antibody alemtuzumab are especially effective in younger MDS patients (<60 years old) with more favorable IPSS scores and who bear the histocompatibility antigen HLA-DR15.

HGFs can improve blood counts but, as in most other marrow failure states, have been most beneficial to patients with the least severe pancytopenia. EPO alone or in combination with G-CSF can improve hemoglobin levels, but mainly in those with low serum EPO levels who have no or only a modest need for transfusions. Survival does not appear to be improved by G-CSF treatment alone but may be enhanced by erythropoietin and amelioration of anemia. G-CSF treatment alone failed to improve survival in a controlled trial.

The same principles of supportive care described for aplastic anemia apply to MDS. Despite improvements in drug therapy, many patients will be anemic for years. RBC transfusion support should be accompanied by iron chelation to prevent secondary hemochromatosis.

MYELOPHTHISIC ANEMIAS

Fibrosis of the bone marrow (see Fig. 129-2), usually accompanied by a characteristic blood smear picture called *leukoerythroblastosis*, can occur as a primary hematologic disease, called *myelofibrosis* or *myeloid metaplasia* (Chap. 131), and as a secondary process, called *myelophthisis.* Myelophthisis, or secondary myelofibrosis, is reactive. Fibrosis can be a response to invading tumor cells, usually an epithelial cancer of breast, lung, or prostate origin or neuroblastoma. Marrow fibrosis may occur with infection of mycobacteria (both *Mycobacterium tuberculosis* and *Mycobacterium avium*), fungi, or HIV and in sarcoidosis. Intracellular lipid deposition in Gaucher's disease and obliteration of the marrow space related to absence of osteoclast remodeling in congenital osteopetrosis also can produce fibrosis. Secondary myelofibrosis is a late consequence of radiation therapy or treatment with radiomimetic drugs. Usually the infectious or malignant underlying processes are obvious. Marrow fibrosis can also be a feature of a variety of hematologic syndromes, especially chronic myeloid leukemia, multiple myeloma, lymphomas, myeloma, and hairy cell leukemia.

The pathophysiology has three distinct features: proliferation of fibroblasts in the marrow space (myelofibrosis); the extension of hematopoiesis into the long bones and into extramedullary sites, usually the spleen, liver, and lymph nodes (myeloid metaplasia); and ineffective erythropoiesis. The etiology of the fibrosis is unknown but most likely involves dysregulated production of growth factors: platelet-derived growth factor and transforming growth factor β have been implicated. Abnormal regulation of other hematopoietins would lead to localization of blood-producing cells in nonhematopoietic tissues and uncoupling of the usually balanced processes of stem cell proliferation and differentiation. Myelofibrosis is remarkable for pancytopenia despite very large numbers of circulating hematopoietic progenitor cells.

Anemia is dominant in secondary myelofibrosis, usually normocytic and normochromic. The diagnosis is suggested by the characteristic leukoerythroblastic smear (see Fig. 129-1). Erythrocyte morphology is highly abnormal, with circulating nucleated RBCs, teardrops, and shape distortions. WBC numbers are often elevated, sometimes mimicking a leukemoid reaction, with circulating myelocytes, promyelocytes, and myeloblasts. Platelets may be abundant and are often of giant size. Inability to aspirate the bone marrow, the characteristic "dry tap," can allow a presumptive diagnosis in the appropriate setting before the biopsy is decalcified.

The course of secondary myelofibrosis is determined by its etiology, usually a metastatic tumor or an advanced hematologic malignancy. Treatable causes must be excluded, especially tuberculosis and fungus. Transfusion support can relieve symptoms.

131 Polycythemia Vera and Other Myeloproliferative Neoplasms

Jerry L. Spivak

The World Health Organization (WHO) classification of the chronic myeloproliferative neoplasms (MPNs) includes eight disorders, some of which are rare or poorly characterized (Table 131-1) but all of which share an origin in a multipotent hematopoietic progenitor cell; overproduction of one or more of the formed elements of the blood without significant dysplasia; and a predilection to extramedullary hematopoiesis, myelofibrosis, and transformation at varying rates to acute leukemia. Within this broad classification, however, significant phenotypic heterogeneity exists. Some diseases such as chronic myelogenous leukemia (CML), chronic neutrophilic leukemia (CNL), and chronic eosinophilic leukemia (CEL) express primarily a myeloid phenotype, whereas in other diseases, such as polycythemia vera (PV), primary myelofibrosis (PMF), and essential thrombocytosis (ET), erythroid or megakaryocytic hyperplasia predominates. The latter three disorders, in contrast to the former three, also appear capable of transforming into each other.

TABLE 131-1 WORLD HEALTH ORGANIZATION CLASSIFICATION OF CHRONIC MYELOPROLIFERATIVE NEOPLASMS

Chronic myeloid leukemia, bcr-abl–positive
Chronic neutrophilic leukemia
Chronic eosinophilic leukemia, not otherwise specified
Polycythemia vera
Primary myelofibrosis
Essential thrombocytosis
Mastocytosis
Myeloproliferative neoplasms, unclassifiable

Such phenotypic heterogeneity has a genetic basis; CML is the consequence of the balanced translocation between chromosomes 9 and 22 [t(9;22)(q34;11)]; CNL has been associated with a t(15;19) translocation; and CEL occurs with a deletion or balanced translocations involving the *PDGFRα* gene. By contrast, to a greater or lesser extent, PV, PMF, and ET are characterized by a mutation, V617F, that causes constitutive activation of JAK2, a tyrosine kinase essential for the function of the erythropoietin and thrombopoietin receptors but not the granulocyte colony-stimulating factor receptor. This important distinction is also reflected in the natural histories of CML, CNL, and CEL, which are usually measured in years, and their high rate of leukemic transformation. By contrast, the natural history of PV, PMF, and ET is usually measured in decades, and transformation to acute leukemia is uncommon in PV and ET in the absence of exposure to mutagenic drugs. This chapter, therefore, will focus only on PV, PMF, and ET, because their clinical and genetic overlap is substantial even though their clinical courses are distinctly different.

The other chronic myeloproliferative neoplasms will be discussed in Chaps. 133 and 135e.

POLYCYTHEMIA VERA

PV is a clonal disorder involving a multipotent hematopoietic progenitor cell in which phenotypically normal red cells, granulocytes, and platelets accumulate in the absence of a recognizable physiologic stimulus. The most common of the chronic MPNs, PV occurs in 2.5 per 100,000 persons, sparing no adult age group and increasing with age to rates over 10/100,000. Familial transmission is infrequent, and women predominate among sporadic cases.

ETIOLOGY

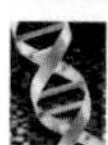

The etiology of PV is unknown. Although nonrandom chromosome abnormalities such as deletion 20q and trisomy 8 and 9 have been documented in up to 30% of untreated PV patients, unlike CML, no consistent cytogenetic abnormality has been associated with the disorder. However, a mutation in the autoinhibitory pseudokinase domain of the tyrosine kinase JAK2—that replaces valine with phenylalanine (V617F), causing constitutive kinase activation—appears to have a central role in the pathogenesis of PV.

JAK2 is a member of an evolutionarily well-conserved, nonreceptor tyrosine kinase family and serves as the cognate tyrosine kinase for the erythropoietin and thrombopoietin receptors. It also functions as an obligate chaperone for these receptors in the Golgi apparatus and is responsible for their cell-surface expression. The conformational change induced in the erythropoietin and thrombopoietin receptors following binding to their respective cognate ligands, erythropoietin or thrombopoietin, leads to JAK2 autophosphorylation, receptor phosphorylation, and phosphorylation of proteins involved in cell proliferation, differentiation, and resistance to apoptosis. Transgenic animals lacking *JAK2* die as embryos from severe anemia. Constitutive activation of JAK2, on the other hand, explains the erythropoietin hypersensitivity, erythropoietin-independent erythroid colony formation, rapid terminal differentiation, increase in Bcl-X_L expression, and apoptosis resistance in the absence of erythropoietin that characterize the in vitro behavior of PV erythroid progenitor cells.

Importantly, the *JAK2* gene is located on the short arm of chromosome 9, and loss of heterozygosity on chromosome 9p due to mitotic recombination is the most common cytogenetic abnormality in PV. The segment of 9p involved contains the *JAK2* locus, and loss of heterozygosity in this region leads to homozygosity for *JAK2* V617F. More than 95% of PV patients express this mutation, as do approximately 50% of PMF and ET patients. Homozygosity for the mutation occurs in approximately 30% of PV patients and 60% of PMF patients but is rare in ET. Over time, a portion of PV *JAK2* V617F heterozygotes become homozygotes due to mitotic recombination, but usually not after 10 years of the disease. Most PV patients who do not express *JAK2* V617F express a mutation in exon 12 of the kinase and are not clinically different from those who do, nor do *JAK2* V617F heterozygotes differ clinically from homozygotes. Interestingly, the predisposition to acquire mutations in *JAK2* appears to be associated with a specific *JAK2* gene haplotype, GGCC. *JAK2* V617F is the basis for many of the phenotypic and biochemical characteristics of PV such as elevation of the leukocyte alkaline phosphatase (LAP) score; however, it cannot solely account for the entire PV phenotype and is probably not the initiating lesion in the three MPNs. First, PV patients with the same phenotype and documented clonal disease lack any mutation of *JAK2*. Second, ET and PMF patients have the same mutation but different clinical phenotypes. Third, familial PV can occur without the mutation, even when other members of the same family express it. Fourth, not all the cells of the malignant clone express *JAK2* V617F. Fifth, *JAK2* V617F has been observed in patients with long-standing idiopathic erythrocytosis. Sixth, in some patients, *JAK2* V617F appears to be acquired after another mutation. Finally, in some *JAK2* V617F–positive PV or ET patients, acute leukemia can occur in a *JAK2* V617F–negative progenitor cell. However, although *JAK2* V617F alone may not be sufficient to cause PV, it appears essential for the transformation of ET to PV, although not for its transformation to PMF.

CLINICAL FEATURES

Although isolated thrombocytosis, leukocytosis, or splenomegaly may be the initial presenting manifestation of PV, most often the disorder is first recognized by the incidental discovery of a high hemoglobin or hematocrit. With the exception of aquagenic pruritus, no symptoms distinguish PV from other causes of erythrocytosis.

Uncontrolled erythrocytosis causes hyperviscosity, leading to neurologic symptoms such as vertigo, tinnitus, headache, visual disturbances, and transient ischemic attacks (TIAs). Systolic hypertension is also a feature of the red cell mass elevation. In some patients, venous or arterial thrombosis may be the presenting manifestation of PV. Any vessel can be affected; but cerebral, cardiac, or mesenteric vessels are most commonly involved. Intraabdominal venous thrombosis is particularly common in young women and may be catastrophic if a sudden and complete obstruction of the hepatic vein occurs. Indeed, PV should be suspected in any patient who develops hepatic vein thrombosis. Digital ischemia, easy bruising, epistaxis, acid-peptic disease, or gastrointestinal hemorrhage may occur due to vascular stasis or thrombocytosis. Erythema, burning, and pain in the extremities, a symptom complex known as erythromelalgia, are other complications of the thrombocytosis of PV due to increased platelet stickiness. Given the large turnover of hematopoietic cells, hyperuricemia with secondary gout, uric acid stones, and symptoms due to hypermetabolism can also complicate the disorder.

DIAGNOSIS

When PV presents with erythrocytosis in combination with leukocytosis, thrombocytosis, or splenomegaly or a combination of these, the diagnosis is apparent. However, when patients present with an elevated hemoglobin or hematocrit alone, the diagnostic evaluation is more complex because of the many diagnostic possibilities (Table 131-2). Furthermore, unless the hemoglobin level is ≥20 g/dL (hematocrit ≥60%), it is not possible to distinguish true erythrocytosis from disorders causing plasma volume contraction. This is because uniquely in PV, in contrast to other causes of true erythrocytosis, there is expansion of the plasma volume, which can mask the elevated red cell mass; thus, red cell mass and plasma volume determinations are necessary to establish the presence of an absolute erythrocytosis and to distinguish this from relative erythrocytosis due to a reduction in plasma volume alone (also known as *stress* or *spurious erythrocytosis* or *Gaisböck's syndrome*). Figure 77-18 illustrates a diagnostic algorithm for the evaluation of suspected erythrocytosis. Assay for *JAK2* mutations in the presence of a normal arterial oxygen saturation provides an alternative diagnostic approach to erythrocytosis when red cell mass and plasma volume determinations are not available; a normal serum erythropoietin level does not exclude the presence of PV, but an elevated erythropoietin level is more consistent with a secondary cause for the erythrocytosis.

TABLE 131-2 CAUSES OF ERYTHROCYTOSIS

Relative Erythrocytosis	
Hemoconcentration secondary to dehydration, diuretics, ethanol abuse, androgens, or tobacco abuse	
Absolute Erythrocytosis	
Hypoxia	**Tumors**
Carbon monoxide intoxication	Hypernephroma
High-oxygen-affinity hemoglobin	Hepatoma
High altitude	Cerebellar hemangioblastoma
Pulmonary disease	Uterine myoma
Right to left cardiac or vascular shunts	Adrenal tumors
Sleep apnea syndrome	Meningioma
Hepatopulmonary syndrome	Pheochromocytoma
Renal Disease	**Drugs**
Renal artery stenosis	Androgens
Focal sclerosing or membranous glomerulonephritis	Recombinant erythropoietin
Postrenal transplantation	**Familial (with normal hemoglobin function)**
Renal cysts	Erythropoietin receptor mutation
Bartter's syndrome	*VHL* mutations (Chuvash polycythemia)
	2,3-BPG mutation
	Polycythemia vera

Abbreviations: 2,3-BPG, 2,3-bisphosphoglycerate; VHL, von Hippel-Lindau.

Other laboratory studies that may aid in diagnosis include the red cell count, mean corpuscular volume, and red cell distribution width (RDW), particularly when the hematocrit or hemoglobin levels are less than 60% or 20 g/dL, respectively. Only three situations cause microcytic erythrocytosis: β thalassemia trait, hypoxic erythrocytosis, and PV. With β thalassemia trait, the RDW is normal, whereas with hypoxic erythrocytosis and PV, the RDW may be elevated due to associated iron deficiency. Today, however, the assay for *JAK2* V617F has superseded other tests for establishing the diagnosis of PV. Of course, in patients with associated acid-peptic disease, occult gastrointestinal bleeding may lead to a presentation with hypochromic, microcytic anemia, masking the presence of PV.

A bone marrow aspirate and biopsy provide no specific diagnostic information because these may be normal or indistinguishable from ET or PMF. Similarly, no specific cytogenetic abnormality is associated with the disease, and the absence of a cytogenetic marker does not exclude the diagnosis.

COMPLICATIONS

Many of the clinical complications of PV relate directly to the increase in blood viscosity associated with red cell mass elevation and indirectly to the increased turnover of red cells, leukocytes, and platelets with the attendant increase in uric acid and cytokine production. The latter appears to be responsible for constitutional symptoms. Peptic ulcer disease can also be due to *Helicobacter pylori* infection, the incidence of which is increased in PV, while the pruritus associated with this disorder may be a consequence of mast cell activation by *JAK2* V617F. A sudden increase in spleen size can be associated with painful splenic infarction. Myelofibrosis appears to be part of the natural history of the disease but is a reactive, reversible process that does not itself impede hematopoiesis and by itself has no prognostic significance. In approximately 15% of patients, however, myelofibrosis is accompanied by significant extramedullary hematopoiesis, hepatosplenomegaly, and transfusion-dependent anemia, which are manifestations of stem cell failure. The organomegaly can cause significant mechanical discomfort, portal hypertension, and progressive cachexia. Although the incidence of acute nonlymphocytic leukemia is increased in PV, the incidence of acute leukemia in patients not exposed to chemotherapy or radiation therapy is low. Interestingly, chemotherapy, including hydroxyurea, has been associated with acute leukemia in *JAK2* V617F–negative stem cells in some PV patients. *Erythromelalgia* is a curious syndrome of unknown etiology associated with thrombocytosis, primarily involving the lower extremities and usually manifested by erythema, warmth, and pain of the affected appendage and occasionally digital infarction. It occurs with a variable frequency and is usually responsive to salicylates. Some of the central nervous system symptoms observed in patients with PV, such as ocular migraine, appear to represent a variant of erythromelalgia.

Left uncontrolled, erythrocytosis can lead to thrombosis involving vital organs such as the liver, heart, brain, or lungs. Patients with massive splenomegaly are particularly prone to thrombotic events because the associated increase in plasma volume masks the true extent of the red cell mass elevation measured by the hematocrit or hemoglobin level. A "normal" hematocrit or hemoglobin level in a PV patient with massive splenomegaly should be considered indicative of an elevated red cell mass until proven otherwise.

TREATMENT POLYCYTHEMIA VERA

PV is generally an indolent disorder, the clinical course of which is measured in decades, and its management should reflect its tempo. Thrombosis due to erythrocytosis is the most significant complication and often the presenting manifestation, and maintenance of the hemoglobin level at ≤140 g/L (14 g/dL; hematocrit <45%) in men and ≤120 g/L (12 g/dL; hematocrit <42%) in women is mandatory to avoid thrombotic complications. Phlebotomy serves initially to reduce hyperviscosity by bringing the red cell mass into the normal range while further expanding the plasma volume. Periodic phlebotomies thereafter serve to maintain the red cell mass within the normal range and to induce a state of iron deficiency that prevents an accelerated reexpansion of the red cell mass. In most PV patients, once an iron-deficient state is achieved, phlebotomy is usually only required at 3-month intervals. Neither phlebotomy nor iron deficiency increases the platelet count relative to the effect of the disease itself, and thrombocytosis is not correlated with thrombosis in PV, in contrast to the strong correlation between erythrocytosis and thrombosis in this disease. The use of salicylates as a tonic against thrombosis in PV patients is not only potentially harmful if the red cell mass is not controlled by phlebotomy, but is also an unproven remedy. Anticoagulants are only indicated when a thrombosis has occurred and can be difficult to monitor if the red cell mass is substantially elevated owing to the artifactual imbalance between the test tube anticoagulant and plasma that occurs when blood from these patients is assayed for prothrombin or partial thromboplastin activity. Asymptomatic hyperuricemia (<10 mg/dL) requires no therapy, but allopurinol should be administered to avoid further elevation of the uric acid when chemotherapy is used to reduce splenomegaly or leukocytosis or to treat pruritus. Generalized pruritus intractable to antihistamines or antidepressants such as doxepin can be a major problem in PV; interferon α (IFN-α), psoralens with ultraviolet light in the A range (PUVA) therapy, and hydroxyurea are other methods of palliation. Asymptomatic thrombocytosis requires no therapy unless the platelet count is sufficiently high to cause bleeding due an acquired form of von Willebrand's disease in which there is adsorption and proteolysis of high-molecular-weight von Willebrand factor (VWF) multimers by the expanded platelet mass. Symptomatic splenomegaly can be treated with pegylated IFN-α. Pegylated IFN-α can also produce complete hematologic and molecular remissions in PV, and its role in this disorder is currently under investigation. Anagrelide, a phosphodiesterase inhibitor, can reduce the platelet count and, if tolerated, is preferable to hydroxyurea because it lacks marrow toxicity and is protective against venous thrombosis. A reduction in platelet number may be necessary for the treatment of erythromelalgia or ocular migraine if salicylates are not effective or if the platelet count is sufficiently high to increase the risk of hemorrhage but only to the degree that symptoms are alleviated. Alkylating agents and radioactive sodium phosphate (^{32}P) are leukemogenic in PV, and their use should be avoided. If a cytotoxic agent must be used, hydroxyurea is preferred, but this drug does not prevent either thrombosis or myelofibrosis in PV, is itself leukemogenic, and should be used for as short a time as possible. Previously, PV patients with massive splenomegaly unresponsive to reduction by chemotherapy or interferon required splenectomy. However, with the introduction of the nonspecific JAK2 inhibitor ruxolitinib, it has been possible in the majority of patients with PV complicated by myelofibrosis and myeloid metaplasia to reduce spleen size while at the same time alleviating constitutional symptoms to due to cytokine release. This drug is currently undergoing clinical trials in PV patients intolerant of hydroxyurea. In some patients with end-stage disease, pulmonary hypertension may develop due to fibrosis or extramedullary hematopoiesis. A role for allogeneic bone marrow transplantation in PV has not been defined.

Most patients with PV can live long lives without functional impairment when their red cell mass is effectively managed with phlebotomy alone. Chemotherapy is never indicated to control the red cell mass unless venous access is inadequate.

PRIMARY MYELOFIBROSIS

Chronic PMF (other designations include *idiopathic myelofibrosis, agnogenic myeloid metaplasia*, or *myelofibrosis with myeloid metaplasia*) is a clonal disorder of a multipotent hematopoietic progenitor cell of unknown etiology characterized by marrow fibrosis, extramedullary hematopoiesis, and splenomegaly. PMF is the least common chronic MPN, and establishing this diagnosis in the absence of a specific clonal marker is difficult because myelofibrosis and splenomegaly are also features of both PV and CML. Furthermore, myelofibrosis and splenomegaly also occur in a variety of benign and malignant disorders (Table 131-3), many of which are amenable to specific therapies not effective in PMF. In contrast to the other chronic MPNs and so-called acute or malignant myelofibrosis, which can occur at any age, PMF primarily afflicts men in their sixth decade or later.

ETIOLOGY

The etiology of PMF is unknown. Nonrandom chromosome abnormalities such as 9p, 20q−, 13q−, trisomy 8 or 9, or partial trisomy 1q are common, but no cytogenetic abnormality specific to the disease has been identified. *JAK2* V617F is present in approximately 50% of PMF patients, and mutations in the thrombopoietin receptor *Mpl* occur in about 5%. Most of the rest have mutations in the

TABLE 131-3 DISORDERS CAUSING MYELOFIBROSIS

Malignant	Nonmalignant
Acute leukemia (lymphocytic, myelogenous, megakaryocytic)	HIV infection
Chronic myeloid leukemia	Hyperparathyroidism
Hairy cell leukemia	Renal osteodystrophy
Hodgkin's disease	Systemic lupus erythematosus
Primary myelofibrosis	Tuberculosis
Lymphoma	Vitamin D deficiency
Multiple myeloma	Thorium dioxide exposure
Myelodysplasia	Gray platelet syndrome
Metastatic carcinoma	
Polycythemia vera	
Systemic mastocytosis	

calreticulin gene (*CALR*) that alter the carboxy-terminal portion of the gene product. The degree of myelofibrosis and the extent of extramedullary hematopoiesis are also not related. Fibrosis in this disorder is associated with overproduction of transforming growth factor β and tissue inhibitors of metalloproteinases, whereas osteosclerosis is associated with overproduction of osteoprotegerin, an osteoclast inhibitor. Marrow angiogenesis occurs due to increased production of vascular endothelial growth factor. Importantly, fibroblasts in PMF are polyclonal and not part of the neoplastic clone.

CLINICAL FEATURES

No signs or symptoms are specific for PMF. Many patients are asymptomatic at presentation, and the disease is usually detected by the discovery of splenic enlargement and/or abnormal blood counts during a routine examination. However, in contrast to its companion MPN, night sweats, fatigue, and weight loss are common presenting complaints. A blood smear will show the characteristic features of extramedullary hematopoiesis: teardrop-shaped red cells, nucleated red cells, myelocytes, and promyelocytes; myeloblasts may also be present (Fig. 131-1). Anemia, usually mild initially, is the rule, whereas the leukocyte and platelet counts are either normal or increased, but either can be depressed. Mild hepatomegaly may accompany the splenomegaly but is unusual in the absence of splenic enlargement; isolated lymphadenopathy should suggest another diagnosis. Both serum lactate dehydrogenase and alkaline phosphatase levels can be elevated. The LAP score can be low, normal, or high. Marrow is usually inaspirable due to the myelofibrosis (Fig. 131-2), and bone x-rays may reveal osteosclerosis. Exuberant extramedullary hematopoiesis can cause ascites; portal, pulmonary, or intracranial hypertension; intestinal or ureteral obstruction; pericardial tamponade; spinal cord compression; or skin nodules. Splenic enlargement can be sufficiently rapid to cause splenic infarction with fever and pleuritic chest pain. Hyperuricemia and secondary gout may ensue.

DIAGNOSIS

While the clinical picture described above is characteristic of PMF, all of the clinical features described can also be observed in PV or CML. Massive splenomegaly commonly masks erythrocytosis in PV, and reports of intraabdominal thrombosis in PMF most likely represent instances of unrecognized PV. In some patients with PMF, erythrocytosis has developed during the course of the disease. Furthermore, because many other disorders have features that overlap with PMF but respond to distinctly different therapies, the diagnosis of PMF is one of exclusion, which requires that the disorders listed in Table 131-3 be ruled out.

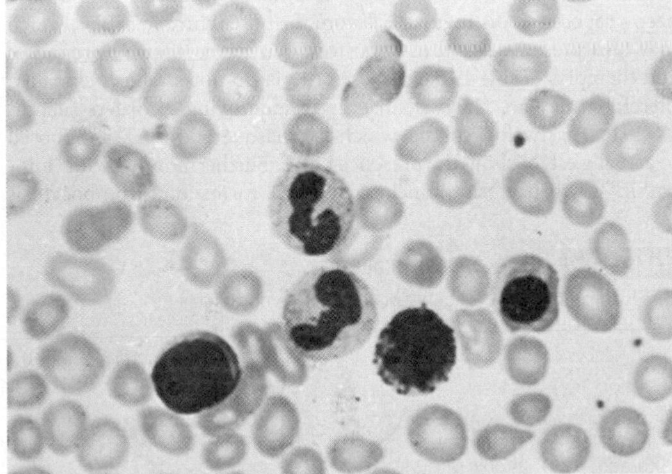

FIGURE 131-1 Teardrop-shaped red blood cells indicative of membrane damage from passage through the spleen, a nucleated red blood cell, and immature myeloid cells indicative of extramedullary hematopoiesis are noted. This peripheral blood smear is related to any cause of extramedullary hematopoiesis.

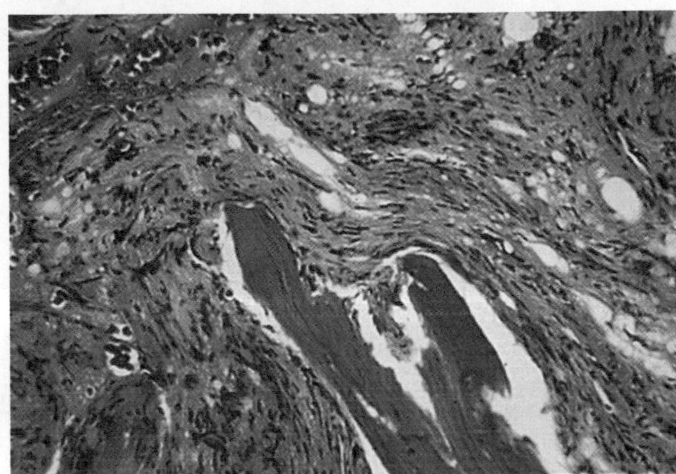

FIGURE 131-2 This marrow section shows the marrow cavity replaced by fibrous tissue composed of reticulin fibers and collagen. When this fibrosis is due to a primary hematologic process, it is called *myelofibrosis*. When the fibrosis is secondary to a tumor or a granulomatous process, it is called *myelophthisis*.

The presence of teardrop-shaped red cells, nucleated red cells, myelocytes, and promyelocytes establishes the presence of extramedullary hematopoiesis, while the presence of leukocytosis, thrombocytosis with large and bizarre platelets, and circulating myelocytes suggests the presence of an MPN as opposed to a secondary form of myelofibrosis (Table 131-3). Marrow is usually inaspirable due to increased marrow reticulin, but marrow biopsy will reveal a hypercellular marrow with trilineage hyperplasia and, in particular, increased numbers of megakaryocytes in clusters and with large, dysplastic nuclei. However, there are no characteristic bone marrow morphologic abnormalities that distinguish PMF from the other chronic MPNs. Splenomegaly due to extramedullary hematopoiesis may be sufficiently massive to cause portal hypertension and variceal formation. In some patients, exuberant extramedullary hematopoiesis can dominate the clinical picture. An intriguing feature of PMF is the occurrence of autoimmune abnormalities such as immune complexes, antinuclear antibodies, rheumatoid factor, or a positive Coombs' test. Whether these represent a host reaction to the disorder or are involved in its pathogenesis is unknown. Cytogenetic analysis of blood is useful both to exclude CML and for prognostic purposes, because complex karyotype abnormalities portend a poor prognosis in PMF. For unknown reasons, the number of circulating CD34+ cells is markedly increased in PMF (>15,000/μL) compared to the other chronic MPNs, unless they too develop myeloid metaplasia.

Importantly, approximately 50% of PMF patients, like patients with its companion myeloproliferative disorders PV and ET, express the *JAK2* V617F mutation, often as homozygotes. Such patients are usually older and have higher hematocrits than the patients who are *JAK2* V617F–negative, whereas PMF patients expressing an *MPL* mutation tend to be more anemic and have lower leukocyte counts. Somatic mutations in exon 9 of the calreticulin gene (*CALR*) have been found in a majority of patients with PMF and ET who lack mutations in either *JAK2* or *MPL*, and their clinical course appears to be more indolent than patients expressing either a *JAK2* or an *MPL* mutation.

COMPLICATIONS

Survival in PMF varies according to specific risk factors at diagnosis (Tables 131-4 and 131-5) but is shorter in most patients than in PV or ET patients. The natural history of PMF is one of increasing marrow failure with transfusion-dependent anemia and increasing organomegaly due to extramedullary hematopoiesis. As with CML, PMF can evolve from a chronic phase to an accelerated phase with constitutional symptoms and increasing marrow failure. About 10% of patients spontaneously transform to an aggressive form of acute leukemia for which therapy is usually ineffective. Additional important prognostic

TABLE 131-4 THREE CURRENT SCORING SYSTEMS FOR ESTIMATING PROGNOSIS IN PMF PATIENTS

Risk Factor	IPSS (2009)[a]	DIPSS (2010)[b]	DIPSS Plus (2011)[c]
Anemia (<10 g/dL)	X	X	X
Leukocytosis (>25,000/μL)	X	X	X
Peripheral blood blasts (≥1%)	X	X	X
Constitutional symptoms	X	X	X
Age (>65 years)	X	X	X
Unfavorable karyotype			X
Platelet count (<100,000/μL)			X
Transfusion dependence			X

[a]Blood 113:2895, 2009. [b]Blood 115:1703, 2010. [c]J Clin Oncol 29:392, 2011.

Note: The Dynamic International Prognostic Scoring System (DIPSS) was developed to determine if the International Prognostic Scoring System (IPSS) risk factors identified as important for survival at the time of primary myelofibrosis (PMF) diagnosis could also be used for risk stratification following their acquisition during the course of the disease. One point is assigned to each risk factor for IPSS scoring. For DIPSS, the same is true, but age >65 years, anemia, blood blasts, and constitutional symptoms are assigned 2 points each. The DIPSS Plus scoring system represents recognition that the addition of unfavorable karyotype, thrombocytopenia, and transfusion dependence improved the DIPSS risk stratification system for which additional points are assigned (Table 131-5). More recent studies suggest that mutational analysis of the *ASXL1*, *EZH2*, *SRSF2*, and *IDH1/2* genes further improves risk stratification for survival and leukemic transformation (Leukemia 27:1861, 2013).

factors for disease acceleration during the course of PMF include the presence of complex cytogenetic abnormalities, thrombocytopenia, and transfusion-dependent anemia. Most recently, mutations in the *ASXL1*, *EZH2*, *SRSF2*, and *IDH1/2* genes have been identified as risk factors for early death or transformation to acute leukemia and may prove to be more useful for PMF risk assessment than any clinical scoring system.

TREATMENT PRIMARY MYELOFIBROSIS

No specific therapy exists for PMF. The causes for anemia are multifarious and include ineffective erythropoiesis uncompensated by splenic extramedullary hematopoiesis, hemodilution due to splenomegaly, splenic sequestration, blood loss secondary to thrombocytopenia or portal hypertension, folic acid deficiency, systemic inflammation, and autoimmune hemolysis. Neither recombinant erythropoietin nor androgens such as danazol have proven to be consistently effective as therapy for anemia. Erythropoietin may worsen splenomegaly and will be ineffective if the serum erythropoietin level is >125 mU/L. Given the inflammatory milieu that characterizes PMF, corticosteroids can ameliorate anemia as well as constitutional symptoms such as fever, chills, night sweats, anorexia, and weight loss, and low-dose thalidomide together with prednisone has proved effective as well. Thrombocytopenia can be due to impaired marrow function, splenic sequestration, or autoimmune destruction and may also respond to low-dose thalidomide together with prednisone. Splenomegaly is by far the most distressing and intractable problem for PMF patients, causing abdominal pain, portal hypertension, easy satiety, and cachexia, whereas surgical removal of a massive spleen is associated with significant postoperative complications including mesenteric venous thrombosis, hemorrhage, rebound leukocytosis and thrombocytosis, and hepatic extramedullary hematopoiesis with no amelioration of either anemia or thrombocytopenia when present. For unexplained reasons, splenectomy also increases the risk of blastic transformation. Splenic irradiation is, at best, temporarily palliative and associated with a significant risk of neutropenia, infection, and subsequent operative hemorrhage if splenectomy is attempted. Allopurinol can control significant hyperuricemia, and bone pain can be alleviated by local irradiation. The role of IFN-α is still undefined; its side effects are more pronounced in the older individuals, and it may exacerbate the bone marrow failure. The JAK2 inhibitor, ruxolitinib, has proved effective in reducing splenomegaly and alleviating constitutional symptoms in a majority of advanced PMF patients while also prolonging survival, although it does not significantly influence the *JAK2* V617F allele burden. Although anemia and thrombocytopenia are its major side effects, these are dose-dependent, and with time, anemia stabilizes and thrombocytopenia may improve. Allogeneic bone marrow transplantation is the only curative treatment for PMF and should be considered in younger patients; nonmyeloablative conditioning regimens may permit hematopoietic cell transplantation to be extended to older individuals, but this approach is currently under investigation.

TABLE 131-5 IPSS AND DIPSS RISK STRATIFICATION SYSTEMS

	Number of Risk Factors		
Risk Categories[a]	IPSS	DIPSS	DIPSS PLUS
Low	0	0	0
Intermediate-1	1	1–2	1
Intermediate-2	2	3–4	2–3
High	≥3	>4	4–6

[a]The corresponding survival curves for each risk category can be found in the references cited in the footnotes of Table 131-4.

Abbreviations: DIPSS, Dynamic International Prognostic Scoring System; IPSS, International Prognostic Scoring System.

ESSENTIAL THROMBOCYTOSIS

Essential thrombocytosis (other designations include *essential thrombocythemia*, *idiopathic thrombocytosis*, *primary thrombocytosis*, and *hemorrhagic thrombocythemia*) is a clonal disorder of unknown etiology involving a multipotent hematopoietic progenitor cell manifested clinically by overproduction of platelets without a definable cause. ET is an uncommon disorder, with an incidence of 1–2/100,000 and a distinct female predominance. No clonal marker is available to consistently distinguish ET from the more common nonclonal, reactive forms of thrombocytosis (Table 131-6), making its diagnosis difficult. Once considered a disease of the elderly and responsible for significant morbidity due to hemorrhage or thrombosis, with the widespread use of electronic cell counters, it is now clear that ET can occur at any age in adults and often without symptoms or disturbances of hemostasis. There is an unexplained female predominance in contrast to PMF or the reactive forms of thrombocytosis where no sex difference exists. Because no specific clonal marker is available, clinical criteria have been proposed to distinguish ET from the other chronic MPNs, which may also present with thrombocytosis but have differing prognoses and therapies (Table 131-6). These criteria do not establish clonality; therefore, they are truly useful only in identifying disorders such as CML, PV, or myelodysplasia, which can masquerade as ET, as opposed to actually establishing the presence of ET. Furthermore, as with "idiopathic" erythrocytosis, nonclonal benign forms of thrombocytosis

TABLE 131-6 CAUSES OF THROMBOCYTOSIS

Tissue inflammation: collagen vascular disease, inflammatory bowel disease	Hemorrhage
Malignancy	Iron-deficiency anemia
Infection	Surgery
Myeloproliferative disorders: polycythemia vera, primary myelofibrosis, essential thrombocytosis, chronic myelogenous leukemia	Rebound: Correction of vitamin B_{12} or folate deficiency, post-ethanol abuse
Myelodysplastic disorders: 5q–syndrome, idiopathic refractory sideroblastic anemia	Hemolysis
Postsplenectomy or hyposplenism	Familial: Thrombopoietin overproduction, *MPL* mutations

exist (such as hereditary overproduction of thrombopoietin) that are not widely recognized because we currently lack adequate diagnostic tools. Approximately 50% of ET patients carry the *JAK2* V617F mutation, but its absence does not exclude the disorder.

ETIOLOGY

Megakaryocytopoiesis and platelet production depend on thrombopoietin and its receptor *Mpl*. As in the case of early erythroid and myeloid progenitor cells, early megakaryocytic progenitors require the presence of interleukin 3 (IL-3) and stem cell factor for optimal proliferation in addition to thrombopoietin. Their subsequent development is also enhanced by the chemokine stromal cell-derived factor 1 (SDF-1). However, megakaryocyte maturation requires thrombopoietin.

Megakaryocytes are unique among hematopoietic progenitor cells because reduplication of their genome is endomitotic rather than mitotic. In the absence of thrombopoietin, endomitotic megakaryocytic reduplication and, by extension, the cytoplasmic development necessary for platelet production are impaired. Like erythropoietin, thrombopoietin is produced in both the liver and the kidneys, and an inverse correlation exists between the platelet count and plasma thrombopoietic activity. Unlike erythropoietin, thrombopoietin is only constitutively produced, and the plasma thrombopoietin level is controlled by the size of its progenitor cell pool. Also, in contrast to erythropoietin, but like its myeloid counterparts, granulocyte and granulocyte-macrophage colony-stimulating factors, thrombopoietin not only enhances the proliferation of its target cells but also enhances the reactivity of their end stage product, the platelet. In addition to its role in thrombopoiesis, thrombopoietin also enhances the survival of multipotent hematopoietic stem cells and their bone marrow residence.

The clonal nature of ET was established by analysis of glucose-6-phosphate dehydrogenase isoenzyme expression in patients hemizygous for this gene, by analysis of X-linked DNA polymorphisms in informative female patients, and by the expression in patients of nonrandom, though variable, cytogenetic abnormalities. Although thrombocytosis is its principal manifestation, like the other chronic MPNs, a multipotent hematopoietic progenitor cell is involved in ET. Furthermore, a number of families have been described in which ET was inherited, in one instance as an autosomal dominant trait. In addition to ET, PMF and PV have also been observed in some kindreds. Like PMF, most patients who do not have *JAK2* mutations have *CALR* mutations.

CLINICAL FEATURES

Clinically, ET is most often identified incidentally when a platelet count is obtained during the course of a routine medical evaluation. Occasionally, review of previous blood counts will reveal that an elevated platelet count was present but overlooked for many years. No symptoms or signs are specific for ET, but these patients can have hemorrhagic and thrombotic tendencies expressed as easy bruising for the former and microvascular occlusive events for the latter such as erythromelalgia, ocular migraine, or a TIA. Physical examination is generally unremarkable except occasionally for mild splenomegaly. Splenomegaly is indicative of another MPN, in particular PV, PMF, or CML.

Anemia is unusual, but a mild neutrophilic leukocytosis is not. The blood smear is most remarkable for the number of platelets present, some of which may be very large. The large mass of circulating platelets may prevent the accurate measurement of serum potassium due to release of platelet potassium upon blood clotting. This type of hyperkalemia is a laboratory artifact and not associated with electrocardiographic abnormalities. Similarly, arterial oxygen measurements can be inaccurate unless thrombocythemic blood is collected on ice. The prothrombin and partial thromboplastin times are normal, whereas abnormalities of platelet function such as a prolonged bleeding time and impaired platelet aggregation can be present. However, despite much study, no platelet function abnormality is characteristic of ET, and no platelet function test predicts the risk of clinically significant bleeding or thrombosis.

The elevated platelet count may hinder marrow aspiration, but marrow biopsy usually reveals megakaryocyte hypertrophy and hyperplasia, as well as an overall increase in marrow cellularity. If marrow reticulin is increased, another diagnosis should be considered. The absence of stainable iron demands an explanation because iron deficiency alone can cause thrombocytosis, and absent marrow iron in the presence of marrow hypercellularity is a feature of PV.

Nonrandom cytogenetic abnormalities occur in ET but are uncommon, and no specific or consistent abnormality is notable, even those involving chromosomes 3 and 1, where the genes for thrombopoietin and its receptor *Mpl*, respectively, are located.

DIAGNOSIS

Thrombocytosis is encountered in a broad variety of clinical disorders (Table 131-6), in many of which production of cytokines is increased. The absolute level of the platelet count is not a useful diagnostic aid for distinguishing between benign and clonal causes of thrombocytosis. About 50% of ET patients express the *JAK2* V617F mutation. When *JAK2* V617F is absent, cytogenetic evaluation is mandatory to determine if the thrombocytosis is due to CML or a myelodysplastic disorder such as the 5q– syndrome. Because the bcr-abl translocation can be present in the absence of the Ph chromosome, and because bcr-abl reverse transcriptase polymerase chain reaction is associated with false positive results, fluorescence in situ hybridization (FISH) analysis for bcr-abl is the preferred assay in patients with thrombocytosis in whom a cytogenetic study for the Ph chromosome is negative. *CALR* mutations are present in most patients who do not have *JAK2* mutations, but diagnostic tools to detect these mutations are not yet widespread. Anemia and ringed sideroblasts are not features of ET, but they are features of idiopathic refractory sideroblastic anemia, and in some of these patients, the thrombocytosis occurs in association with *JAK2* V617F expression. Splenomegaly should suggest the presence of another MPN, and in this setting, a red cell mass determination should be performed because splenomegaly can mask the presence of erythrocytosis. Importantly, what appears to be ET can evolve into PV or PMF after a period of many years, revealing the true nature of the underlying MPN. There is sufficient overlap of the *JAK2* V617F neutrophil allele burden between ET and PV that this cannot be used as a distinguishing diagnostic feature; only a red cell mass and plasma volume determination can distinguish PV from ET, and importantly in this regard, 64% of *JAK2* V617F–positive ET patients actually were found to have PV when red cell mass and plasma volume determinations were performed.

COMPLICATIONS

Perhaps no other condition in clinical medicine has caused otherwise astute physicians to intervene inappropriately more often than thrombocytosis, particularly if the platelet count is $>1 \times 10^6/\mu L$. It is commonly believed that a high platelet count causes intravascular stasis and thrombosis; however, no controlled clinical study has ever established this association, and in patients younger than age 60 years, the incidence of thrombosis was not greater in patients with thrombocytosis than in age-matched controls, and tobacco use appears to be the most important risk factor for thrombosis in ET patients.

To the contrary, very high platelet counts are associated primarily with hemorrhage due to acquired von Willebrand's disease. This is not meant to imply that an elevated platelet count cannot cause symptoms in an ET patient, but rather that the focus should be on the patient, not the platelet count. For example, some of the most dramatic neurologic problems in ET are migraine-related and respond only to lowering of the platelet count, whereas other symptoms such as erythromelalgia respond simply to platelet cyclooxygenase-1 inhibitors such as aspirin or ibuprofen, without a reduction in platelet number. Still others may represent an interaction between an atherosclerotic vascular system and a high platelet count, and others may have no relationship to the platelet count whatsoever. Recognition that PV can present with thrombocytosis alone as well as the discovery of previously unrecognized causes of hypercoagulability (Chap. 142) make the older literature on the complications of thrombocytosis unreliable.

ET can also evolve into PMF, but whether this is a feature of ET or represents PMF presenting initially with isolated thrombocytosis is unknown.

TREATMENT ESSENTIAL THROMBOCYTOSIS

Survival of patients with ET is not different than for the general population. An elevated platelet count in an asymptomatic patient without cardiovascular risk factors requires no therapy. Indeed, before any therapy is initiated in a patient with thrombocytosis, the cause of symptoms must be clearly identified as due to the elevated platelet count. When the platelet count rises above $1 \times 10^6/\mu L$, a substantial quantity of high-molecular-weight von Willebrand multimers are removed from the circulation and destroyed by the enlarged platelet mass, resulting in an acquired form of von Willebrand's disease. This can be identified by a reduction in ristocetin cofactor activity. In this situation, aspirin could promote hemorrhage. Bleeding in this situation usually responds to ε-aminocaproic acid, which can be given prophylactically before and after elective surgery. Plateletpheresis is at best a temporary and inefficient remedy that is rarely required. Importantly, ET patients treated with ^{32}P or alkylating agents are at risk of developing acute leukemia without any proof of benefit; combining either therapy with hydroxyurea increases this risk. If platelet reduction is deemed necessary on the basis of symptoms refractory to salicylates alone, pegylated IFN-α, the quinazoline derivative, anagrelide, or hydroxyurea can be used to reduce the platelet count, but none of these is uniformly effective or without significant side effects. Hydroxyurea and aspirin are more effective than anagrelide and aspirin for prevention of TIAs but not more effective for the prevention of other types of arterial thrombosis and are actually less effective for venous thrombosis. The effectiveness of hydroxyurea in preventing TIAs is because it is an NO donor. Normalizing the platelet count also does not prevent either arterial or venous thrombosis. The risk of gastrointestinal bleeding is also higher when aspirin is combined with anagrelide.

As more clinical experience is acquired, ET appears more benign than previously thought. Evolution to acute leukemia is more likely to be a consequence of therapy than of the disease itself. In managing patients with thrombocytosis, the physician's first obligation is to do no harm.

132 Acute Myeloid Leukemia

Guido Marcucci, Clara D. Bloomfield

INCIDENCE

Acute myeloid leukemia (AML) is a neoplastic disease characterized by infiltration of the blood, bone marrow, and other tissues by proliferative, clonal undifferentiated cells of the hematopoietic system. These leukemias comprise a spectrum of malignancies that, untreated, range from rapidly fatal to slowly growing. In 2013, the estimated number of new AML cases in the United States was 14,590. The incidence of AML is ~3.5 per 100,000 people per year, and the age-adjusted incidence is higher in men than in women (4.5 vs 3.1). AML incidence increases with age; it is 1.7 in individuals age <65 years and 15.9 in those age >65 years. The median age at diagnosis is 67 years.

ETIOLOGY

Heredity, radiation, chemical and other occupational exposures, and drugs have been implicated in the development of AML. No direct evidence suggests a viral etiology.

Heredity Certain syndromes with somatic cell chromosome aneuploidy, such as trisomy 21 noted in Down syndrome, are associated with an increased incidence of AML. Inherited diseases with defective DNA repair, e.g., Fanconi anemia, Bloom syndrome, and ataxia-telangiectasia, are also associated with AML. Congenital neutropenia (Kostmann syndrome) is a disease with mutations in the genes encoding the granulocyte colony-stimulating factor (G-CSF) receptor and, often, neutrophil elastase that may evolve into AML. Germline mutations of CCAAT/enhancer-binding protein α (*CEBPA*), runt-related transcription factor 1 (*RUNX1*), and tumor protein p53 (*TP53*) have also been associated with a higher predisposition to AML in some series.

Radiation High-dose radiation, like that experienced by survivors of the atomic bombs in Japan or nuclear reactor accidents, increases the risk of myeloid leukemias that peaks 5–7 years after exposure. Therapeutic radiation alone seems to add little risk of AML but can increase the risk in people also exposed to alkylating agents.

Chemical and Other Exposures Exposure to benzene, a solvent used in the chemical, plastic, rubber, and pharmaceutical industries, is associated with an increased incidence of AML. Smoking and exposure to petroleum products, paint, embalming fluids, ethylene oxide, herbicides, and pesticides have also been associated with an increased risk of AML.

Drugs Anticancer drugs are the leading cause of therapy-associated AML. Alkylating agent–associated leukemias occur on average 4–6 years after exposure, and affected individuals have aberrations in chromosomes 5 and 7. Topoisomerase II inhibitor–associated leukemias occur 1–3 years after exposure, and affected individuals often have aberrations involving chromosome 11q23. Newer agents for treatment of other hematopoietic malignancies and solid tumors are also under scrutiny for increased risk of AML. Chloramphenicol, phenylbutazone, and, less commonly, chloroquine and methoxypsoralen can result in bone marrow failure that may evolve into AML.

CLASSIFICATION

The current categorization of AML uses the World Health Organization (WHO) classification (Table 132-1), which includes different biologically distinct groups based on clinical features and cytogenetic and molecular abnormalities in addition to morphology. In contrast to the previously used French-American-British (FAB) schema, the WHO classification places limited reliance on cytochemistry. A major difference between the WHO and the FAB systems is the blast cutoff for a diagnosis of AML as opposed to myelodysplastic syndrome (MDS); it is 20% in the WHO classification and 30% in the FAB. However, within the WHO classification, specific chromosomal rearrangements, i.e., t(8;21)(q22;q22), inv(16)(p13.1q22), t(16;16)(p13.1;q22), and t(15;17)(q22;q12), define AML even with <20% blasts.

Immunophenotype and Relevance to the WHO Classification The immunophenotype of human leukemia cells can be studied by multiparameter flow cytometry after the cells are labeled with monoclonal antibodies to cell-surface antigens. This can be important for separating AML from acute lymphoblastic leukemia (ALL) and identifying some subtypes of AML. For example, AML with minimal differentiation that is characterized by immature morphology and no lineage-specific cytochemical reactions may be diagnosed by flow-cytometric demonstration of the myeloid-specific antigens cluster designation (CD) 13 and/or 117. Similarly, acute megakaryoblastic leukemia can often be diagnosed only by expression of the platelet-specific antigens CD41 and/or CD61. Although flow cytometry is useful, widely used, and in some cases essential for the diagnosis of AML, it is supportive only in establishing the different subtypes of AML through the WHO classification.

Clinical Features and Relevance to the WHO Classification The WHO classification also considers clinical features in subdividing AML. For example, it identifies therapy-related AML as a separate entity that develops following prior therapy (e.g., alkylating agents, topoisomerase II inhibitors, ionizing radiation). It also identifies AML with

TABLE 132-1 WORLD HEALTH ORGANIZATION CLASSIFICATION OF ACUTE MYELOID LEUKEMIA (AML) AND RELATED NEOPLASMS[a]
AML with recurrent genetic abnormalities
AML with t(8;21)(q22;q22); *RUNX1-RUNX1T1*[b]
AML with inv(16)(pl3.1q22) or t(16;16)(p13.1;q22); *CBFB-MYH11*[b]
Acute promyelocytic leukemia with t(15;17)(q22;q12); *PML-RARA*[b]
AML with t(9;11)(p22;q23); *MLLT3-MLL*
AML with t(6;9)(p23;q34); *DEK-NUP214*
AML with inv(3)(q21q26.2) or t(3;3)(q21;q26.2); *RPN1-EVI1*
AML (megakaryoblastic) with t(1;22)(p13;q13); *RBM15-MKL1*
Provisional entity: AML with mutated NPM1
Provisional entity: AML with mutated CEBPA
AML with myelodysplasia-related changes
Therapy-related myeloid neoplasms
AML, not otherwise specified
AML with minimal differentiation
AML without maturation
AML with maturation
Acute myelomonocytic leukemia
Acute monoblastic and monocytic leukemia
Acute erythroid leukemia
Acute megakaryoblastic leukemia
Acute basophilic leukemia
Acute panmyelosis with myelofibrosis
Myeloid sarcoma
Myeloid proliferations related to Down syndrome
Transient abnormal myelopoiesis
Myeloid leukemia associated with Down syndrome
Blastic plasmacytoid dendritic cell neoplasm

[a]From SH Swerdlow et al (eds): *World Health Organization Classification of Tumours of Haematopoietic and Lymphoid Tissues*. Lyon, IARC Press, 2008. [b]Diagnosis is AML regardless of blast count.

myelodysplasia-related changes based in part on medical history of an antecedent MDS or myelodysplastic/myeloproliferative neoplasm. The clinical features likely contribute to the prognosis of AML and have therefore been included in the classification.

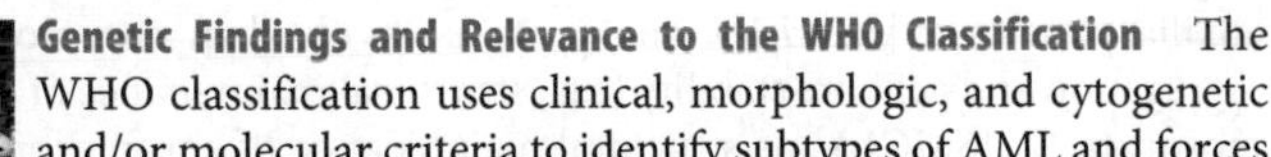

Genetic Findings and Relevance to the WHO Classification The WHO classification uses clinical, morphologic, and cytogenetic and/or molecular criteria to identify subtypes of AML and forces the clinician to take the appropriate steps to correctly identify the entity and thus tailor treatment(s) accordingly. The WHO classification is indeed the first AML classification that incorporates genetic (chromosomal and molecular) information. In this classification, subtypes of AML are recognized based on the presence or absence of specific recurrent genetic abnormalities. For example, the diagnosis of *acute promyelocytic leukemia* (APL) is based on the presence of either the t(15;17)(q22;q12) cytogenetic rearrangement or the *PML-RARA* fusion product of the translocation. A similar approach is taken with regard to core binding factor (CBF) AML that is now designated based on the presence of t(8;21)(q22;q22), inv(16)(p13.1q22), or t(16;16)(p13.1;q22) or the respective fusion products *RUNX1-RUNX1T1* and *CBFB-MYH11*.

The WHO classification incorporates cytogenetics in the AML classification by recognizing a category of AML with recurrent genetic abnormalities and a category of AML with myelodysplasia-related changes (Table 132-1). The latter category is diagnosed not only by morphologic changes, but also in part by selected myelodysplasia-related cytogenetic abnormalities (e.g., complex karyotypes and unbalanced and balanced changes involving, among others, chromosomes 5, 7, and 11). Only one cytogenetic abnormality has been invariably associated with specific morphologic features: t(15;17)(q22;q12) with APL. Other chromosomal abnormalities have been associated primarily with one morphologic/immunophenotypic group, including inv(16)(p13.1q22) with AML with abnormal bone marrow eosinophils; t(8;21)(q22;q22) with slender Auer rods, expression of CD19, and increased normal eosinophils; and t(9;11)(p22;q23), and other translocations involving 11q23, with monocytic features. Recurring chromosomal abnormalities in AML may also be associated with specific clinical characteristics. More commonly associated with younger age are t(8;21) and t(15;17), and with older age, del(5q) and del(7q). Myeloid sarcomas (see below) are associated with t(8;21), and disseminated intravascular coagulation (DIC) is associated with t(15;17).

The WHO classification also incorporates molecular abnormalities by recognizing fusion genes that are products of recurrent cytogenetic aberrations or have been found mutated and may be involved in leukemogenesis. For instance, t(15;17) results in the fusion gene *PML-RARA* that encodes a chimeric protein, promyelocytic leukemia (Pml)–retinoic acid receptor α (Rarα), which is formed by the fusion of the retinoic acid receptor α (*RARA*) gene from chromosome 17 and the promyelocytic leukemia (*PML*) gene from chromosome 15. The *RARA* gene encodes a member of the nuclear hormone receptor family of transcription factors. After binding retinoic acid, *RARA* can promote expression of a variety of genes. The 15;17 translocation juxtaposes *PML* with *RARA* in a head-to-tail configuration that is under the transcriptional control of *PML*. Three different breakpoints in the *PML* gene lead to various fusion protein isoforms. The Pml-Rarα fusion protein tends to suppress gene transcription and blocks differentiation of the cells. Pharmacologic doses of the Rarα ligand, all-*trans*-retinoic acid (tretinoin), relieve the block and promote hematopoietic cell differentiation (see below). Similar examples of molecular subtypes of the disease included in the category of AML with recurrent genetic abnormalities are those characterized by the leukemogenic fusion genes *RUNX1-RUNX1T1*, *CBFB-MYH11*, *MLLT3-MLL*, and *DEK-NUP214*, resulting, respectively, from t(8;21), inv(16) or t(16;16), t(9;11), and t(6;9)(p23;q34).

Two new provisional entities defined by the presence of gene mutations, rather than microscopic chromosomal abnormalities, have been added to the category of AML with recurrent genetic abnormalities: *AML with mutated nucleophosmin (nucleolar phosphoprotein B23, numatrin)* (*NPM1*) and *AML with mutated CEBPA*. AML with fms-related tyrosine kinase 3 (*FLT3*) mutations is not considered a distinct entity, although determining the presence of such mutations is recommended by WHO in patients with cytogenetically normal AML (CN-AML) because the relatively frequent *FLT3*-internal tandem duplication (ITD) carries a negative prognostic significance and therefore is clinically relevant. *FLT3* encodes a tyrosine kinase receptor important in the development of myeloid and lymphoid lineages. Activating mutations of *FLT3* are present in ~30% of adult AML patients due to ITDs in the juxtamembrane domain or point mutations of the activating loop of the kinase (called tyrosine kinase domain mutations). Aberrant activation of the *FLT3*-encoded protein provides increased proliferation and antiapoptotic signals to the myeloid progenitor cell. *FLT3*-ITD, the more common of the *FLT3* mutations, occurs preferentially in patients with CN-AML. The importance of identifying *FLT3*-ITD at diagnosis relates to the fact that not only is it a useful prognosticator but it also may predict response to specific treatment such as the tyrosine kinase inhibitors that are in clinical investigation.

PROGNOSTIC FACTORS

Several factors have been demonstrated to predict outcome of AML patients treated with chemotherapy, and they can be used for risk stratification and treatment guidance.

Chromosome findings at diagnosis are currently the most important independent prognostic factors. Several studies have categorized patients as having favorable, intermediate, or poor cytogenetic risk based on the presence of structural and/or numerical aberrations. Patients with t(15;17) have a very good prognosis (~85% cured), and those with t(8;21) and inv(16) have a good prognosis (~55% cured), whereas those with no cytogenetic abnormality have an intermediate outcome risk (~40% cured). Patients with a complex karyotype, t(6;9), inv(3), or −7 have a very poor prognosis. Another cytogenetic subgroup, the monosomal karyotype, has been suggested to adversely impact the outcome of AML patients other than those with t(15;17), t(8;21), or inv(16) or t(16;16). The monosomal karyotype subgroup is defined by the presence of at least two autosomal monosomies (loss of chromosomes other than Y or X) or a single autosomal monosomy with additional structural abnormalities.

For patients lacking prognostic cytogenetic abnormalities, such as those with CN-AML, outcome prediction uses mutated or aberrantly expressed genes. *NPM1* mutations without concurrent presence of *FLT3*-ITD, and *CEBPA* mutations, especially if concurrently present in two different alleles, have been shown to predict favorable outcome, whereas *FLT3*-ITD predicts poor outcome. Given the proven prognostic importance of *NPM1* and *CEBPA* mutations and *FLT3*-ITD, molecular assessment of these genes at diagnosis has been incorporated in AML management guidelines by the National Comprehensive Cancer Network (NCCN) and the European LeukemiaNet (ELN). The same markers have also been incorporated in the definitions of the genetic groups of the ELN standardized reporting system, which are based on both cytogenetic and molecular abnormalities and used for comparing clinical features and treatment response among subsets of patients reported in different studies (Table 132-2). More recently, the prognostic impact of the genetic groups recognized by the ELN reporting system has been demonstrated. Thus, these genetic groups may also be used for risk stratification and treatment guidance.

In addition to *NPM1* and *CEBPA* mutations and *FLT3*-ITD, other molecular aberrations (Table 132-3) may in the future be routinely used for prognostication in AML and incorporated in the WHO classification and the ELN reporting system. Among these prognostic mutated genes are those encoding receptor tyrosine kinases (e.g., v-kit Hardy-Zuckerman 4 feline sarcoma viral oncogene homolog [*KIT*]), transcription factors (i.e., *RUNX1* and Wilms tumor 1 [*WT1*]), and epigenetic modifiers (i.e., additional sex combs like transcriptional regulator 1 [*ASXL1*], DNA (cytosine-5-)-methyltransferase 3 alpha [*DNMT3A*], isocitrate dehydrogenase 1 (NADP+), soluble [*IDH1*] and isocitrate dehydrogenase 2 (NADP+), mitochondrial [*IDH2*], lysine (K)-specific methyltransferase 2A [*KMT2A*, also known as *MLL*], and tet methylcytosine dioxygenase 2 [*TET2*]). Although *KIT* mutations are almost exclusively present in CBF AML and impact adversely the outcome, the remaining markers have been reported primarily in CN-AML. These gene mutations have been shown to be associated with outcome in multivariable analyses independently from other prognostic factors. However, for some of them, the prognostic impact (e.g., *TET2* mutations) or the type (adverse vs favorable) of prognostic impact (e.g., *IDH1*, *IDH2*) has been found in the majority, but not in all, of the reported studies.

An independent prognostic impact remains to be determined for mutated genes that are either associated primarily with unfavorable

TABLE 132-2 EUROPEAN LEUKEMIANET RECOMMENDED STANDARDIZED REPORTING FOR CORRELATION OF CYTOGENETIC AND MOLECULAR GENETIC DATA IN AML WITH CLINICAL DATA[a]

Genetic Group	Subsets
Favorable	t(8;21)(q22;q22); *RUNX1-RUNX1T1*
	inv(16)(p13.1q22) or t(16;16)(p13.1;q22); *CBFB-MYH11*
	Mutated *NPM1* without *FLT3*-ITD (normal karyotype)
	Mutated *CEBPA* (normal karyotype)
Intermediate-I	Mutated *NPM1* and *FLT3*-ITD (normal karyotype)
	Wild-type *NPM1* and *FLT3*-ITD (normal karyotype)
	Wild-type *NPM1* without *FLT3*-ITD (normal karyotype)
Intermediate-II	t(9;11)(p22;q23); *MLLT3-MLL*
	Cytogenetic abnormalities not classified as favorable or adverse
Adverse	inv(3)(q21q26.2) or t(3;3)(q21;q26.2); *RPN1-EVI1*
	t(6;9)(p23;q34); *DEK-NUP214*
	t(v;11)(v;q23); *MLL* rearranged
	−5 or del(5q); −7; abn(17p); complex karyotype (≥3 abnormalities)

[a]H Döhner et al: Blood 115:453, 2010.

Abbreviation: ITD, internal tandem duplication.

TABLE 132-3 MOLECULAR PROGNOSTIC MARKERS IN AML

Gene Symbol	Gene Location	Prognostic Impact
Genes Included in the WHO Classification and ELN Reporting System		
NPM1 mutations	5q35.1	Favorable
CEBPA mutations	19q13.1	Favorable
FLT3-ITD	13q12	Adverse
Genes Encoding Receptor Tyrosine Kinases		
KIT mutation	4q12	Adverse
FLT3-TKD	13q12	Adverse
Genes Encoding Transcription Factors		
RUNX1 mutations	21q22.12	Adverse
WT1 mutations	11p13	Adverse
Genes Encoding Epigenetic Modifiers		
ASXL1 mutations	20q11.21	Adverse
DNMT3A mutations	2p23.3	Adverse
IDH mutations (*IDH1* and *IDH2*)	2q34 & 15q26.1	Adverse
MLL-PTD	11q23	Adverse
TET2 mutations	4q24	Adverse
Deregulated Genes		
BAALC overexpression	8q22.3	Adverse
ERG overexpression	21q22.3	Adverse
MN1 overexpression	22q12.1	Adverse
EVI1 overexpression	3q26.2	Adverse
Deregulated MicroRNAs		
miR-155 overexpression	21q21.3	Adverse
miR-3151 overexpression	8q22.3	Adverse
miR-181a overexpression	1q32.1 and 9q33.3	Favorable

Abbreviations: AML, acute myeloid leukemia; ELN, European LeukemiaNet; ITD, internal tandem duplication; PTD, partial tandem duplication; TKD, tyrosine kinase domain; WHO, World Health Organization.

cytogenetic aberrations (e.g., *TP53*) or are found with a relatively lower frequency in AML patients like those encoding epigenetic modifiers (e.g., enhancer of zeste 2 polycomb repressive complex 2 subunit [*EZH2*]), phosphatases (e.g., protein tyrosine phosphatase, non-receptor type 11 (*PTPN11*]), putative transcription factors (e.g., PHD finger protein 6 [*PHF6*]), splicing factors (e.g., U2 small nuclear RNA auxiliary factor 1 [*U2AF1*]), and proteins involved in chromosome segregation and genome stability (e.g., structural maintenance of chromosomes 1A [*SMC1A*] or structural maintenance of chromosomes 3 [*SMC3*]). Finally, other mutated genes are recognized as predictors of treatment response to distinct therapies rather than prognosticators; for example, neuroblastoma RAS viral (v-ras) oncogene homolog (*NRAS*) and Kirsten rat sarcoma viral oncogene homolog (*KRAS*) predict a better response to high-dose cytarabine in CBF AML.

In addition to gene mutations, deregulation of the expression levels of coding genes and of short noncoding RNAs (microRNAs) have been reported to provide prognostic information (Table 132-3). Overexpression of genes such as brain and acute leukemia, cytoplasmic (*BAALC*), v-ets avian erythroblastosis virus E26 oncogene homologue (avian) (*ERG*), meningioma (disrupted in balanced translocation) 1 (*MN1*), and MDS1 and EVI1 complex locus (*MECOM*, also known as *EVI1*) have been found to be predictive for poor outcome, especially in CN-AML. Similarly, deregulated expression levels of microRNAs, naturally occurring noncoding RNAs that have been shown to regulate the expression of proteins involved in hematopoietic differentiation and survival pathways by degradation or translation inhibition of target coding RNAs, have been associated with prognosis in AML. Overexpression of *miR-155* and *miR-3151* has been found to affect outcome adversely in CN-AML, whereas overexpression of *miR-181a* predicts a favorable outcome both in CN-AML and cytogenetically abnormal AML.

Because prognostic molecular markers in AML are not mutually exclusive and often occur concurrently (>80% patients have at least two or more prognostic gene mutations), the likelihood that distinct marker combinations may be more informative than single markers is being recognized.

Epigenetic changes (e.g., DNA methylation) and microRNAs are often involved in deregulation of genes involved in hematopoiesis, contribute to leukemogenesis, and are often associated with the previously discussed prognostic gene mutations. These changes not only have been shown to provide biologic insights into leukemogenic mechanisms, but also independent prognostic information. Indeed, it is anticipated that with the enormous progress made in DNA and RNA sequencing technology, additional genetic and epigenetic aberrations will soon be discovered and will contribute to classification and reporting systems and outcome risk determination in AML patients.

In addition to cytogenetics and/or molecular aberrations, several other factors are associated with outcome in AML. Age at diagnosis is one of the most important risk factors. Advancing age is associated with a poorer prognosis not only because of its influence on the ability to survive induction therapy due to coexisting comorbidities, but also because with each successive decade of age, a greater proportion of patients have an intrinsically more resistant disease. A prolonged symptomatic interval with cytopenias preceding diagnosis or a history of antecedent hematologic disorders including myeloproliferative neoplasms is often found in older patients and is a clinical feature associated with a lower complete remission (CR) rate and shorter survival time. The CR rate is lower in patients who have had anemia, leukopenia, and/or thrombocytopenia for >3 months before the diagnosis of AML when compared to those without such a history. Responsiveness to chemotherapy declines as the duration of the antecedent disorder(s) increases. AML developing after treatment with cytotoxic agents for other malignancies is usually difficult to treat successfully. Finally, it is likely that AML in older patients is also associated with poor outcome because of the presence of distinct biologic features that may increase the aggressiveness of the disease and reduce the likelihood of treatment response. The leukemic cells in older patients more commonly express the multidrug resistance 1 (MDR1) efflux pump that conveys resistance to natural product–derived agents such as the anthracyclines that are frequently incorporated into the initial treatment. In addition, older patients less frequently harbor favorable cytogenetic abnormalities [i.e., t(8;21), inv(16), and t(16;16)] and more frequently harbor adverse cytogenetic (e.g., complex and monosomal karyotypes) and/or molecular (e.g., *ASXL1*, *IDH2*, *RUNX1*, *TET2*) abnormalities.

Other factors independently associated with worse outcome are a low performance status that influences ability to survive induction therapy and thus respond to treatment and a high presenting leukocyte count that in some series is an adverse prognostic factor for attaining a CR. Among patients with hyperleukocytosis (>100,000/μL), early central nervous system bleeding and pulmonary leukostasis contribute to poor outcome with initial therapy.

Achievement of CR is associated with better outcome and longer survival. CR is defined after examination of both blood and bone marrow. The blood neutrophil count must be ≥1000/μL and the platelet count ≥100,000/μL. Hemoglobin concentration is not considered in determining CR. Circulating blasts should be absent. Although rare blasts may be detected in the blood during marrow regeneration, they should disappear on successive studies. The bone marrow should contain <5% blasts, and Auer rods should be absent. Extramedullary leukemia should not be present. Patients who achieve CR after one induction cycle have longer CR durations than those requiring multiple cycles.

CLINICAL PRESENTATION

Symptoms Patients with AML most often present with nonspecific symptoms that begin gradually or abruptly and are the consequence of anemia, leukocytosis, leukopenia or leukocyte dysfunction, or thrombocytopenia. Nearly half have had symptoms for ≤3 months before the leukemia was diagnosed.

Half of patients mention fatigue as the first symptom, but most complain of fatigue or weakness at the time of diagnosis. Anorexia and weight loss are common. Fever with or without an identifiable infection is the initial symptom in approximately 10% of patients. Signs of abnormal hemostasis (bleeding, easy bruising) are noted first in 5% of patients. On occasion, bone pain, lymphadenopathy, nonspecific cough, headache, or diaphoresis is the presenting symptom.

Rarely patients may present with symptoms from a myeloid sarcoma that is a tumor mass consisting of myeloid blasts occurring at anatomic sites other than bone marrow. Sites involved are most commonly the skin, lymph node, gastrointestinal tract, soft tissue, and testis. This rare presentation, often characterized by chromosome aberrations [e.g., monosomy 7, trisomy 8, *MLL* rearrangement, inv(16), trisomy 4, t(8;21)], may precede or coincide with AML.

Physical Findings Fever, splenomegaly, hepatomegaly, lymphadenopathy, sternal tenderness, and evidence of infection and hemorrhage are often found at diagnosis. Significant gastrointestinal bleeding, intrapulmonary hemorrhage, or intracranial hemorrhage occurs most often in APL. Bleeding associated with coagulopathy may also occur in monocytic AML and with extreme degrees of leukocytosis or thrombocytopenia in other morphologic subtypes. Retinal hemorrhages are detected in 15% of patients. Infiltration of the gingivae, skin, soft tissues, or meninges with leukemic blasts at diagnosis is characteristic of the monocytic subtypes and those with 11q23 chromosomal abnormalities.

Hematologic Findings Anemia is usually present at diagnosis and can be severe. The degree varies considerably, irrespective of other hematologic findings, splenomegaly, or duration of symptoms. The anemia is usually normocytic normochromic. Decreased erythropoiesis often results in a reduced reticulocyte count, and red blood cell (RBC) survival is decreased by accelerated destruction. Active blood loss also contributes to the anemia.

The median presenting leukocyte count is about 15,000/μL. Between 25 and 40% of patients have counts <5000/μL, and 20% have counts >100,000/μL. Fewer than 5% have no detectable leukemic cells in the blood. The morphology of the malignant cell varies in different subsets. In AML, the cytoplasm often contains primary (nonspecific) granules, and the nucleus shows fine, lacy chromatin with one or more nucleoli characteristic of immature cells. Abnormal rod-shaped granules called Auer rods are not uniformly present, but when they are, myeloid lineage is virtually certain (Fig. 132-1). Poor neutrophil function may be noted functionally by impaired phagocytosis and migration and morphologically by abnormal lobulation and deficient granulation.

Platelet counts <100,000/μL are found at diagnosis in ~75% of patients, and about 25% have counts <25,000/μL. Both morphologic and functional platelet abnormalities can be observed, including large and bizarre shapes with abnormal granulation and inability of platelets to aggregate or adhere normally to one another.

Pretreatment Evaluation Once the diagnosis of AML is suspected, a rapid evaluation and initiation of appropriate therapy should follow. In addition to clarifying the subtype of leukemia, initial studies should evaluate the overall functional integrity of the major organ systems, including the cardiovascular, pulmonary, hepatic, and renal systems (Table 132-4). Factors that have prognostic significance, either for achieving CR or for predicting the duration of CR, should also be assessed before initiating treatment, including cytogenetics and molecular markers (see above). Leukemic cells should be obtained from all patients and cryopreserved for future use as new tests and therapeutics become available. All patients should be evaluated for infection.

Most patients are anemic and thrombocytopenic at presentation. Replacement of the appropriate blood components, if necessary, should begin promptly. Because qualitative platelet dysfunction or the presence of an infection may increase the likelihood of bleeding, evidence of hemorrhage justifies the immediate use of platelet transfusion, even if the platelet count is only moderately decreased.

About 50% of patients have a mild to moderate elevation of serum uric acid at presentation. Only 10% have marked elevations, but renal precipitation of uric acid and the nephropathy that may result is a serious but uncommon complication. The initiation of chemotherapy may aggravate hyperuricemia, and patients are usually started immediately on allopurinol and hydration at diagnosis. Rasburicase (recombinant

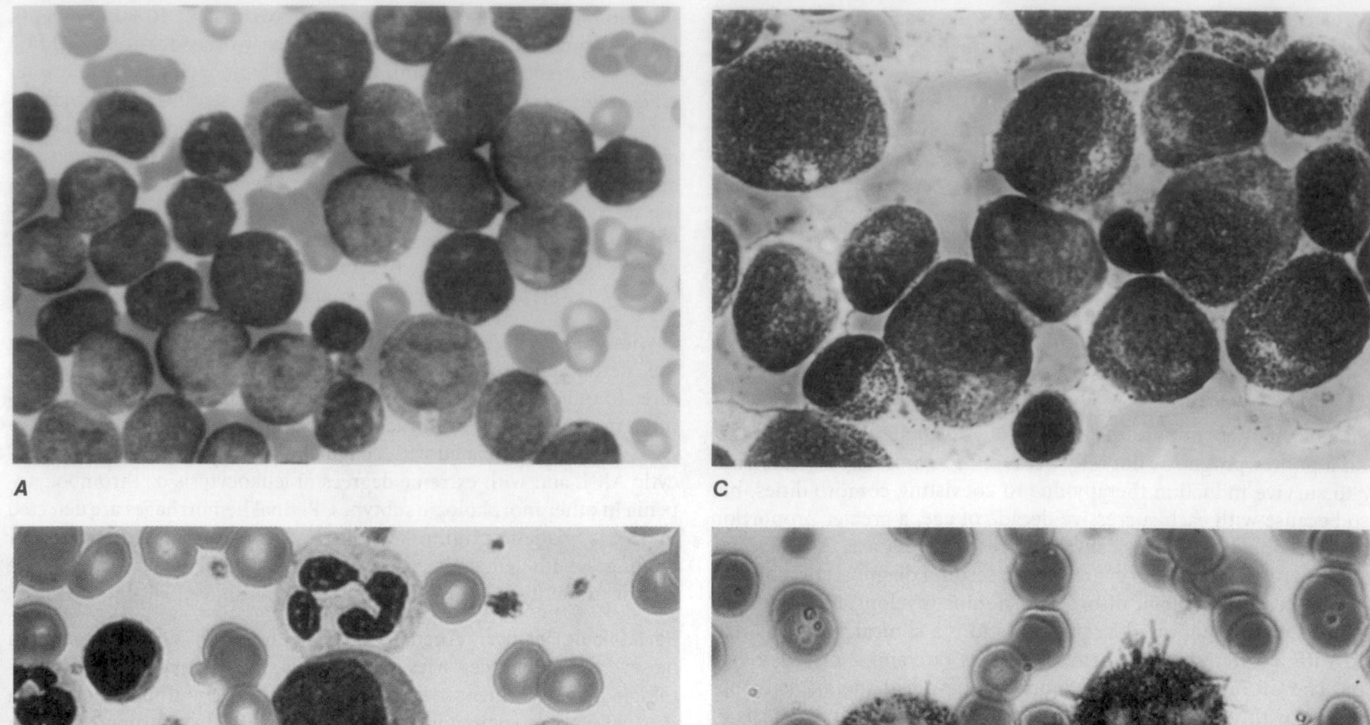

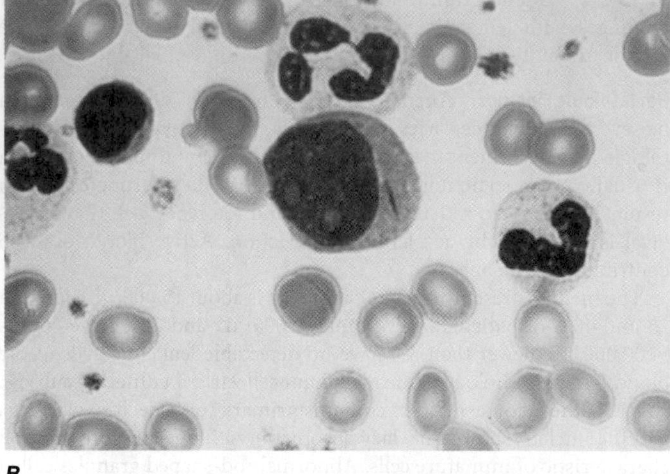

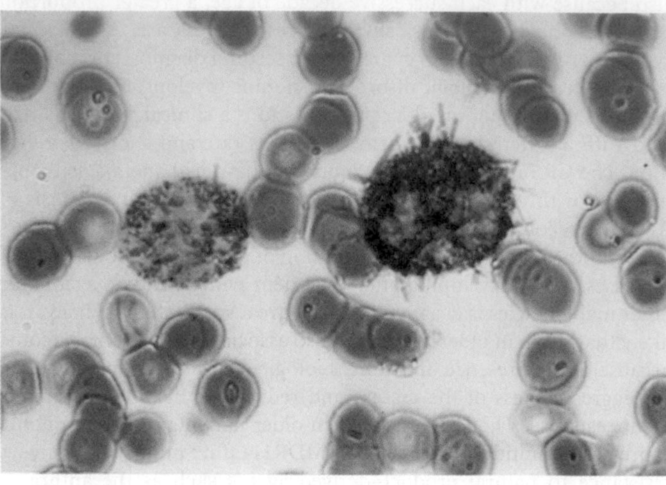

FIGURE 132-1 Morphology of acute myeloid leukemia (AML) cells. *A.* Uniform population of primitive myeloblasts with immature chromatin, nucleoli in some cells, and primary cytoplasmic granules. ***B.*** Leukemic myeloblast containing an Auer rod. ***C.*** Promyelocytic leukemia cells with prominent cytoplasmic primary granules. ***D.*** Peroxidase stain shows dark blue color characteristic of peroxidase in granules in AML.

uric oxidase) is also useful for treating uric acid nephropathy and often can normalize the serum uric acid level within hours with a single dose of treatment. The presence of high concentrations of lysozyme, a marker for monocytic differentiation, may be etiologic in renal tubular dysfunction, which could worsen other renal problems that arise during the initial phases of therapy.

TREATMENT ACUTE MYELOID LEUKEMIA

Treatment of the newly diagnosed patient with AML is usually divided into two phases, induction and postremission management (Fig. 132-2). The initial goal is to induce CR. Once CR is obtained, further therapy must be used to prolong survival and achieve cure. The initial induction treatment and subsequent postremission therapy are often chosen based on the patient's age. Intensifying therapy with traditional chemotherapy agents such as cytarabine and anthracyclines in younger patients (<60 years) appears to increase the cure rate of AML. In older patients, the benefit of intensive therapy is controversial; novel approaches for selecting patients predicted to be responsive to treatment and new therapies are being pursued.

INDUCTION CHEMOTHERAPY

The most commonly used CR induction regimens (for patients other than those with APL) consist of combination chemotherapy with cytarabine and an anthracycline (e.g., daunorubicin, idarubicin, mitoxantrone). Cytarabine is a cell cycle S-phase–specific antimetabolite that becomes phosphorylated intracellularly to an active triphosphate form that interferes with DNA synthesis. Anthracyclines are DNA intercalators. Their primary mode of action is thought to be inhibition of topoisomerase II, leading to DNA breaks.

In younger adults (age <60 years), cytarabine is used either at standard dose (100–200 mg/m^2) administered as a continuous intravenous infusion for 7 days or higher dose (2 g/m^2) administered intravenously every 12 h for 6 days. With standard-dose cytarabine, anthracycline therapy generally consists of daunorubicin (60–90 mg/m^2) or idarubicin (12 mg/m^2) intravenously on days 1, 2, and 3 (the 7 and 3 regimen). Other agents can be added (i.e., cladribine) when 60 mg/m^2 of daunorubicin is used.

High-dose cytarabine-based regimens have also been shown to induce high CR rates. When given in high doses, higher intracellular levels of cytarabine may be achieved, thereby saturating the cytarabine-inactivating enzymes and increasing the intracellular levels of 1-β-D-arabinofuranylcytosine-triphosphate, the active metabolite incorporated into DNA. Thus, higher doses of cytarabine may increase the inhibition of DNA synthesis and thereby overcome resistance to standard-dose cytarabine. With high-dose cytarabine, daunorubicin 60 mg/m^2 or idarubicin 12 mg/m^2 is generally used.

The hematologic toxicity of high-dose cytarabine-based induction regimens has typically been greater than that associated with 7 and 3 regimens. Toxicity with high-dose cytarabine also includes pulmonary toxicity and significant and occasionally irreversible

TABLE 132-4 INITIAL DIAGNOSTIC EVALUATION AND MANAGEMENT OF ADULT PATIENTS WITH AML

History
Increasing fatigue or decreased exercise tolerance (anemia)
Excess bleeding or bleeding from unusual sites (DIC, thrombocytopenia)
Fevers or recurrent infections (neutropenia)
Headache, vision changes, nonfocal neurologic abnormalities (CNS leukemia or bleed)
Early satiety (splenomegaly)
Family history of AML (Fanconi, Bloom, or Kostmann syndromes or ataxia-telangiectasia)
History of cancer (exposure to alkylating agents, radiation, topoisomerase II inhibitors)
Occupational exposures (radiation, benzene, petroleum products, paint, smoking, pesticides)
Physical Examination
Performance status (prognostic factor)
Ecchymosis and oozing from IV sites (DIC, possible acute promyelocytic leukemia)
Fever and tachycardia (signs of infection)
Papilledema, retinal infiltrates, cranial nerve abnormalities (CNS leukemia)
Poor dentition, dental abscesses
Gum hypertrophy (leukemic infiltration, most common in monocytic leukemia)
Skin infiltration or nodules (leukemia infiltration, most common in monocytic leukemia)
Lymphadenopathy, splenomegaly, hepatomegaly
Back pain, lower extremity weakness [spinal granulocytic sarcoma, most likely in t(8;21) patients]
Laboratory and Radiologic Studies
CBC with manual differential cell count
Chemistry tests (electrolytes, creatinine, BUN, calcium, phosphorus, uric acid, hepatic enzymes, bilirubin, LDH, amylase, lipase)
Clotting studies (prothrombin time, partial thromboplastin time, fibrinogen, D-dimer)
Viral serologies (CMV, HSV-1, varicella-zoster)
RBC type and screen
HLA typing for potential allogeneic HSCT
Bone marrow aspirate and biopsy (morphology, cytogenetics, flow cytometry, molecular studies for *NPM1* and *CEBPA* mutations and *FLT3*-ITD)
Cryopreservation of viable leukemia cells
Myocardial function (echocardiogram or MUGA scan)
PA and lateral chest radiograph
Placement of central venous access device
Interventions for Specific Patients
Dental evaluation (for those with poor dentition)
Lumbar puncture (for those with symptoms of CNS involvement)
Screening spine MRI (for patients with back pain, lower extremity weakness, paresthesias)
Social work referral for patient and family psychosocial support
Counseling for All Patients
Provide patients with information regarding their disease, financial counseling, and support group contacts

Abbreviations: AML, acute myeloid leukemia; BUN, blood urea nitrogen; CBC, complete blood count; CMV, cytomegalovirus; CNS, central nervous system; DIC, disseminated intravascular coagulation; HLA, human leukocyte antigen; HSCT, hematopoietic stem cell transplantation; HSV, herpes simplex virus; IV, intravenous; LDH, lactate dehydrogenase; MRI, magnetic resonance imaging; MUGA, multigated acquisition; PA, posteroanterior; RBC, red blood (cell) count.

cerebellar toxicity. All patients treated with high-dose cytarabine must be closely monitored for cerebellar toxicity. Full cerebellar testing should be performed before each dose, and further high-dose cytarabine should be withheld if evidence of cerebellar toxicity develops. This toxicity occurs more commonly in patients with renal impairment and in those older than age 60 years. The increased toxicity observed with high-dose cytarabine has limited the use of this therapy in older AML patients.

Incorporation of novel and molecular targeting agents into these regimens is currently under investigation. For patients with *FLT3*-ITD AML, trials with tyrosine kinase inhibitors are ongoing. Patients with CBF AML may benefit from the combination of gemtuzumab ozogamicin, a monoclonal CD33 antibody linked to the cytotoxic agent calicheamicin, with induction and consolidation chemotherapies. This agent, initially approved for older patients with relapsed disease, has been withdrawn from the U.S. market at the request of the U.S. Food and Drug Administration due to concerns about the product's toxicity, including myelosuppression, infusion toxicity, and venoocclusive disease and the clinical benefit of the initially recommended higher doses. However, the aforementioned recent results are encouraging and support the reintroduction of this agent into the therapeutic armamentarium for AML.

In older patients (age ≥60 years), the outcome is generally poor likely due to a higher induction treatment–related mortality rate and frequency of resistant disease, especially in patients with prior hematologic disorders (MDS or myeloproliferative syndromes) or who have received chemotherapy treatment for another malignancy or harbor cytogenetic and genetic abnormalities that adversely impact on clinical outcome. These patients should be considered for clinical trials. Alternatively, older patients can be also treated with the 7 and 3 regimen with standard-dose cytarabine and idarubicin (12 mg/m^2), daunorubicin (45–90 mg/m^2), or mitoxantrone (12 mg/m^2). For patients older than 65 years, higher dose daunorubicin (90 mg/m^2) has not shown benefit due to the increased toxicity and is not recommended. The combination of gemtuzumab ozogamicin with chemotherapy reduces the risk of relapse for patients age 50–70 years with previously untreated AML. Finally, older patients may be considered for single-agent therapies with clofarabine or hypomethylating agents (i.e., 5-azacitidine or decitabine). The latter are often used for patients unfit for more intensive therapies.

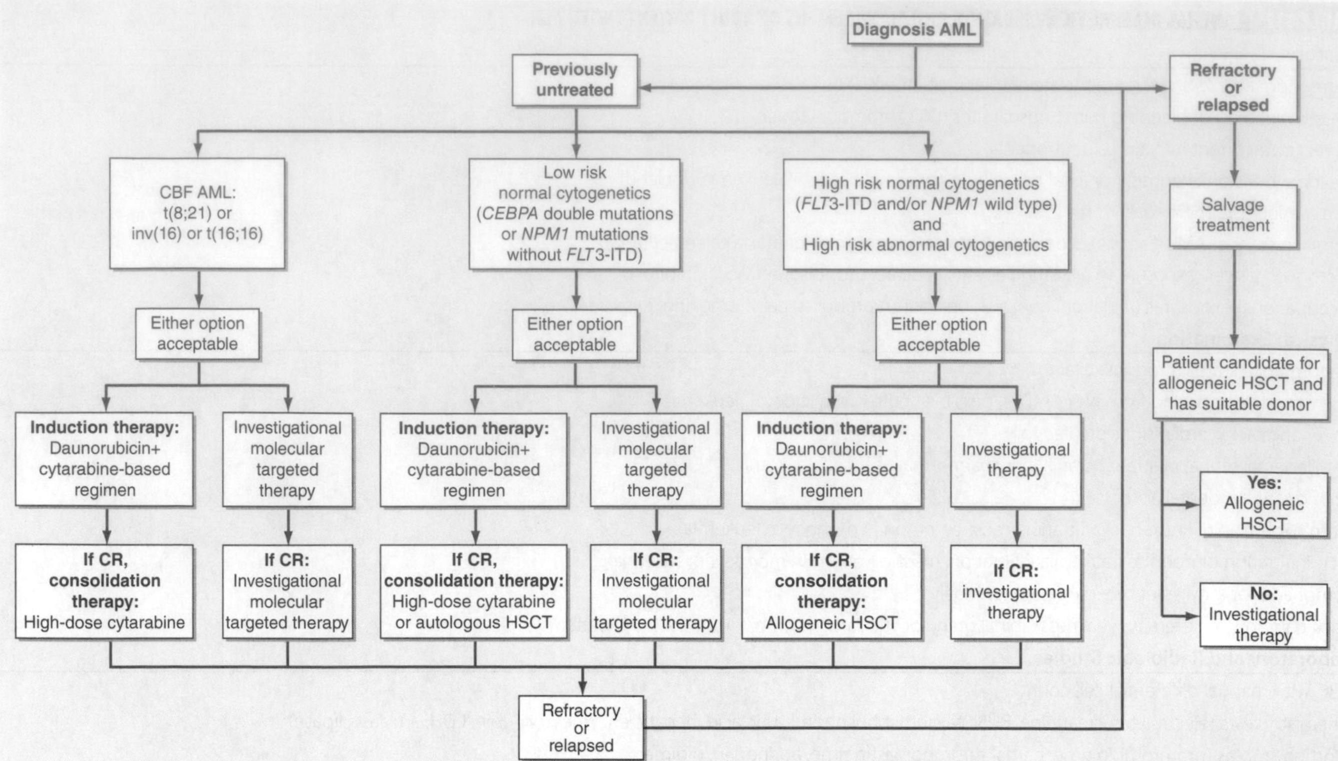

FIGURE 132-2 Flow chart for the therapy of newly diagnosed acute myeloid leukemia (AML). For all forms of AML except acute promyelocytic leukemia (APL), standard therapy includes a regimen based on a 7-day continuous infusion of cytarabine (100–200 mg/m^2 per day) and a 3-day course of daunorubicin (60–90 mg/m^2 per day) with or without additional drugs. Idarubicin (12–13 mg/m^2 per day) could be used in place of daunorubicin (not shown). Patients who achieve complete remission (CR) undergo postremission consolidation therapy, including sequential courses of high-dose cytarabine, autologous hematopoietic stem cell transplantation (HSCT), allogeneic HSCT, or novel therapies, based on their predicted risk of relapse (i.e., risk-stratified therapy). Patients with APL (see text for treatment) usually receive tretinoin and arsenic trioxide–based regimens with or without anthracycline-based chemotherapy and possibly maintenance with tretinoin. CBF, core binding factor; ITD, internal tandem duplication.

After one cycle of the 7 and 3 chemotherapy induction regimen, if persistence of leukemia is documented, the patient is usually retreated with the same agents (cytarabine and the anthracycline) for 5 and 2 days, respectively. Our recommendation, however, is to consider changing therapy in this setting.

POSTREMISSION THERAPY

Induction of a durable first CR is critical to long-term disease-free survival in AML. However, without further therapy, virtually all patients experience relapse. Thus, postremission therapy is designed to eradicate residual leukemic cells to prevent relapse and prolong survival. The type of postremission therapy in AML is often based on age and cytogenetic and molecular risk.

For younger patients, most studies include intensive chemotherapy and allogeneic or autologous hematopoietic stem cell transplantation (HSCT). In the postremission setting, high-dose cytarabine for three to four cycles is more effective than standard-dose cytarabine. The Cancer and Leukemia Group B (CALGB), for example, compared the duration of CR in patients randomly assigned after remission to four cycles of high (3 g/m^2, every 12 h on days 1, 3, and 5), intermediate (400 mg/m^2 for 5 days by continuous infusion), or standard (100 mg/m^2 per day for 5 days by continuous infusion) doses of cytarabine. A dose-response effect for cytarabine in patients with AML who were age ≤60 years was demonstrated. High-dose cytarabine significantly prolonged CR and increased the fraction cured in patients with favorable [t(8;21) and inv(16)] and normal cytogenetics, but it had no significant effect on patients with other abnormal karyotypes. As discussed, high-dose cytarabine has increased toxicity in older patients. Therefore, in this age group, for patients without CBF AML, exploration of attenuated chemotherapy regimens has been pursued. However, because the outcome of older patients is poor, allogeneic HSCT, when feasible, should be strongly considered. Postremission therapy is also a setting for introduction of new agents **(Table 132-5)**.

Autologous HSCT preceded by one to two cycles of high-dose cytarabine is also an option for intensive consolidation therapy. Autologous HSCT has been generally applied to AML patients in the context of a clinical trial or when the risk of repetitive intensive chemotherapy represents a higher risk than the autologous HSCT (e.g., in patients with severe platelet alloimmunization) or when other factors including patient age, comorbid conditions, and fertility are considered.

Allogeneic HSCT is used in patients age <70–75 years with a human leukocyte antigen (HLA)-compatible donor who have high-risk cytogenetics. Selected high-risk patients are also considered for alternative donor transplants (e.g., mismatched unrelated, haploidentical related, and unrelated umbilical cord donors). In patients with CN-AML and high-risk molecular features such as *FLT3*-ITD, allogeneic HSCT is best applied in the context of clinical trials because the impact of aggressive therapy on outcome is unknown. For older patients, exploration of reduced-intensity allogeneic HSCT has been pursued.

Trials comparing intensive chemotherapy and autologous and allogeneic HSCT have shown improved duration of remission with allogeneic HSCT compared to autologous HSCT or chemotherapy alone. However, overall survival is generally not different; the improved disease control with allogeneic HSCT is erased by the increase in fatal toxicity. In fact, relapse following allogeneic HSCT occurs in only a small fraction of patients, but treatment-related toxicity is relatively high; complications include venoocclusive disease, graft-versus-host disease (GVHD), and infections. Autologous HSCT can be administered in young and older patients and uses the same preparative regimens. Patients subsequently receive their own stem cells collected while in remission. The toxicity is relatively low with

TABLE 132-5 SELECTED AGENTS UNDER STUDY FOR THE TREATMENT OF ACUTE MYELOID LEUKEMIA

Class of Drugs	Examples of Agents in Class
Inhibitors of Mutant proteins	
Tyrosine kinase inhibitors	Dasatinib, midostaurin, quizartinib, sorafenib
IDH2 mutation inhibitor	AG-221
Epigenetic Targeting Compounds	
Demethylating agents	S110 (decitabine dinucleotide), oral azacitidine
Histone deacetylase inhibitors	Suberoylanilide hydroxamic acid (SAHA), MS275, LBH589
Inhibitors of Cell Proliferation	
Cell cycle inhibitors	Flavopiridol, CYC202 (R-roscovitine), SNS-032
Farnesyl transferase inhibitors	R115777, SCH66336
Aurora inhibitors	AZD1152, MLN-8237, AT9283
Inhibitors of Protein Synthesis and Degradation	
Aminopeptide inhibitors	Tosedostat
HSP-90 antagonists	17-Allylaminogeldanamycin (17-AAG), DMAG, or derivatives
Nedd8 activating enzyme (NAE) inhibitors	MLN4924
Cytotoxic Compounds	
Nucleoside analogues	Clofarabine, troxacitabine, elacytarabine, sapacitabine
Compounds with Immuno-Mediated Mechanisms	
Antibodies	CSL362 (anti-CD123), anti-CD33 (SGN33), anti-KIR
Immunomodulatory	Lenalidomide, interleukin 2, histamine dihydrochloride

autologous HSCT (5% mortality rate), but the relapse rate is higher than with allogeneic HSCT, due to the absence of the graft-versus-leukemia (GVL) effect seen with allogeneic HSCT and possible contamination of the autologous stem cells with residual tumor cells.

Prognostic factors may ultimately help to select the appropriate postremission therapy in patients in first CR. Our approach includes allogeneic HSCT in first CR for patients without favorable cytogenetics or genotype (e.g., patients who do not have *CEBPA* biallelic mutations or *NPM1* mutations without *FLT3*-ITD) and/or with other poor risk factors (e.g., an antecedent hematologic disorder or failure to attain remission with a single induction course). If a suitable HLA donor does not exist, investigational therapeutic approaches are considered. Indeed, postremission therapy is also a setting for introduction of new agents (Table 132-5). Because *FLT3*-ITD can be targeted with emerging novel inhibitors, patients with this molecular abnormality should be considered for clinical trials with these agents whenever possible.

Patients with the favorable CBF AML [i.e., t(8;21), inv(16), or t(16;16)] are treated with repetitive doses of high-dose cytarabine, which offers a high frequency of cure without the morbidity of transplant. Among AML patients with t(8;21) and inv(16), those with *KIT* mutations, who have a worse prognosis, may be considered for novel investigational studies, including tyrosine kinase inhibitors. The inclusion of gemtuzumab ozogamicin in induction and consolidation chemotherapy-based treatment has been reported to be beneficial in this subset of patients.

For patients in morphologic CR, immunophenotyping to detect minute populations of blasts or sensitive molecular assays (e.g., reverse transcriptase polymerase chain reaction [RT-PCR]) to detect AML-associated molecular abnormalities (e.g., *NPM1* mutation, the CBF AML *RUNX1/RUNX1T1* and *CBFB/MYH11* transcripts, the APL *PML/RARA* transcript), and the less sensitive metaphase cytogenetics or interphase cytogenetics by fluorescence in situ hybridization (FISH) to detect AML-associated cytogenetic aberrations, can be performed to assess whether clinically meaningful minimal residual disease (MRD) is present at sequential time points during or after treatment. Detection of MRD may be a reliable discriminator between patients who will continue in CR and those who are destined to experience disease recurrence and therefore require early therapeutic intervention before clinical relapse occurs. Although assessment of MRD in bone marrow and/or blood during CR is routinely used in the clinic to anticipate clinical relapse and initiate timely salvage treatment for APL patients, for other cytogenetic and molecular subtypes of AML, this is an area of current investigation.

SUPPORTIVE CARE

Measures geared to supporting patients through several weeks of neutropenia and thrombocytopenia are critical to the success of AML therapy. Patients with AML should be treated in centers expert in providing supportive measures. Multilumen right atrial catheters should be inserted as soon as patients with newly diagnosed AML have been stabilized. They should be used thereafter for administration of intravenous medications and transfusions, as well as for blood drawing.

Adequate and prompt blood bank support is critical to therapy of AML. Platelet transfusions should be given as needed to maintain a platelet count ≥10,000/μL. The platelet count should be kept at higher levels in febrile patients and during episodes of active bleeding or DIC. Patients with poor posttransfusion platelet count increments may benefit from administration of platelets from HLA-matched donors. RBC transfusions should be administered to keep the hemoglobin level >80 g/L (8 g/dL) in the absence of active bleeding, DIC, or congestive heart failure, which require higher hemoglobin levels. Blood products leukodepleted by filtration should be used to avert or delay alloimmunization as well as febrile reactions. Blood products should also be irradiated to prevent transfusion-associated GVHD. Cytomegalovirus (CMV)-negative blood products should be used for CMV-seronegative patients who are potential candidates for allogeneic HSCT. Leukodepleted products are also effective for these patients if CMV-negative products are not available.

Neutropenia (neutrophils <500/μL or <1000/μL and predicted to decline to <500/μL over the next 48 h) can be part of the initial presentation and/or a side effect of the chemotherapy treatment in AML patients. Thus, infectious complications remain the major cause of morbidity and death during induction and postremission chemotherapy for AML. Antibacterial (i.e., quinolones) and antifungal (i.e., posaconazole) prophylaxis in the absence of fever is likely to be beneficial. For patients who are herpes simplex virus or varicella-zoster seropositive, antiviral prophylaxis should be initiated (e.g., acyclovir, valacyclovir).

Fever develops in most patients with AML, but infections are documented in only half of febrile patients. Early initiation of empirical broad-spectrum antibacterial and antifungal antibiotics has significantly reduced the number of patients dying of infectious complications (Chap. 104). An antibiotic regimen adequate to treat gram-negative organisms should be instituted at the onset of fever in a neutropenic patient after clinical evaluation, including a detailed physical examination with inspection of the indwelling catheter exit site and a perirectal examination, as well as procurement of cultures and radiographs aimed at documenting the source of fever. Specific antibiotic regimens should be based on antibiotic sensitivity data obtained from the institution at which the patient is being treated. Acceptable regimens for empiric antibiotic therapy include monotherapy with imipenem-cilastatin, meropenem, piperacillin/tazobactam, or an extended-spectrum antipseudomonal cephalosporin (cefepime or ceftazidime). The combination of an aminoglycoside with an antipseudomonal penicillin (e.g., piperacillin) or an aminoglycoside in combination with an extended-spectrum antipseudomonal cephalosporin should be considered in complicated or resistant cases. Aminoglycosides should be avoided if possible in patients with renal insufficiency. Empirical vancomycin should be added in neutropenic patients with catheter-related infections, blood cultures positive for gram-positive bacteria before final identification and susceptibility testing, hypotension or shock, or known colonization with penicillin/cephalosporin-resistant pneumococci or methicillin-resistant *Staphylococcus aureus*. In special situations where decreased susceptibility to vancomycin, vancomycin-resistant organisms, or vancomycin toxicity is documented, other options including linezolid, daptomycin, and quinupristin/dalfopristin need to be considered.

Caspofungin (or a similar echinocandin), voriconazole, or liposomal amphotericin B should be considered for antifungal treatment if fever persists for 4–7 days following initiation of empiric antibiotic therapy. Amphotericin B has long been used for antifungal therapy. Although liposomal formulations have improved the toxicity profile of this agent, its use has been limited to situations with high risk of or documented mold infections. Caspofungin has been approved for empiric antifungal treatment. Voriconazole has also been shown to be equivalent in efficacy and less toxic than amphotericin B. Antibacterial and antifungal antibiotics should be continued until patients are no longer neutropenic, regardless of whether a specific source has been found for the fever.

Recombinant hematopoietic growth factors have been incorporated into clinical trials in AML. These trials have been designed to lower the infection rate after chemotherapy. Both G-CSF and granulocyte-macrophage colony-stimulating factor (GM-CSF) have reduced the median time to neutrophil recovery. This accelerated rate of neutrophil recovery, however, has not generally translated into significant reductions in infection rates or shortened hospitalizations. In most randomized studies, both G-CSF and GM-CSF have failed to improve the CR rate, disease-free survival, or overall survival. Although receptors for both G-CSF and GM-CSF are present on AML blasts, therapeutic efficacy is neither enhanced nor inhibited by these agents. The use of growth factors as supportive care for AML patients is controversial. We favor their use in elderly patients with complicated courses, those receiving intensive postremission regimens, patients with uncontrolled infections, or those participating in clinical trials.

TREATMENT FOR REFRACTORY OR RELAPSED AML

With the 7 and 3 regimen, 65–75% of younger and 50–60% of older patients with primary AML achieve CR. Two-thirds achieve CR after a single course of therapy, and one-third require two courses. Of patients who do not achieve CR, approximately 50% have a drug-resistant leukemia, and 50% do not achieve CR because of fatal complications of bone marrow aplasia or impaired recovery of normal stem cells. Patients with refractory disease after induction should be considered for salvage treatments, preferentially on clinical trials, before receiving allogeneic HSCT usually administered in patients who achieve a disease-free status. Because these patients are usually not cured even if they achieve second CR with salvage chemotherapy, allogeneic HSCT is a necessary therapeutic step.

In patients who relapse after achieving CR, the length of first CR is predictive of response to salvage chemotherapy treatment; patients with longer first CR (>12 months) generally relapse with drug-sensitive disease and have a higher chance of attaining a CR, even with the same chemotherapeutic agents used for first remission induction. Whether initial CR was achieved with one or two courses of chemotherapy and the type of postremission therapy may also predict achievement of second CR. Similar to patients with refractory disease, patients with relapsed disease are rarely cured by the salvage chemotherapy treatments. Therefore, patients who eventually achieve a second CR and are eligible for allogeneic HSCT should be transplanted.

Because achievement of a second CR with routine salvage therapies is relatively uncommon, especially in patients who relapse rapidly after achievement of first CR (<12 months), these patients and those lacking HLA-compatible donors or who are not candidates for allogeneic HSCT should be considered for innovative approaches on clinical trials (Table 132-5). The discovery of novel gene mutations and mechanisms of leukemogenesis that might represent actionable therapeutic targets has prompted the development of new targeting agents. In addition to kinase inhibitors for *FLT3*- and *KIT*-mutated AML, other compounds targeting the aberrant activity of mutant proteins (e.g., IDH2 inhibitors) or biologic mechanisms deregulating epigenetics (e.g., histone deacetylase and DNA methyltransferase inhibitors), cell proliferation (e.g., farnesyl transferase inhibitors), protein synthesis (e.g., aminopeptide inhibitors) and folding (e.g., heat shock protein inhibitors), and ubiquitination, or with novel cytotoxic mechanisms (e.g., clofarabine, sapacitabine), are being tested in clinical trials. Furthermore, approaches with antibodies targeting commonly expressed leukemia blasts (e.g., CD33) or leukemia initiating cells (e.g., CD123) and immunomodulatory agents (e.g., lenalidomide) are also under investigation. Once these compounds have demonstrated safety and activity as single agents, investigation of combinations with other molecular targeting compounds and/or chemotherapy should be pursued.

TREATMENT OF ACUTE PROMYELOCYTIC LEUKEMIA

APL is a highly curable subtype of AML, and approximately 85% of these patients achieve long-term survival with current approaches. APL has long been shown to be responsive to cytarabine and daunorubicin, but previously patients treated with these drugs alone frequently died from DIC induced by the release of granule components by the chemotherapy-treated leukemia cells. However, the prognosis of APL patients has changed dramatically from adverse to favorable with the introduction of tretinoin, an oral drug that induces the differentiation of leukemic cells bearing the t(15;17), where disruption of the *RARA* gene encoding a retinoid acid receptor occurs. Tretinoin decreases the frequency of DIC but produces another complication called the APL differentiation syndrome. Occurring within the first 3 weeks of treatment, it is characterized by fever, fluid retention, dyspnea, chest pain, pulmonary infiltrates, pleural and pericardial effusions, and hypoxemia. The syndrome is related to adhesion of differentiated neoplastic cells to the pulmonary vasculature endothelium. Glucocorticoids, chemotherapy, and/or supportive measures can be effective for management of the APL differentiation syndrome. Temporary discontinuation of tretinoin is necessary in cases of severe APL differentiation syndrome (i.e., patients developing renal failure or requiring admission to the intensive care unit due to respiratory distress). The mortality rate of this syndrome is about 10%.

Tretinoin (45 mg/m^2 per day orally until remission is documented) plus concurrent anthracycline-based (i.e., idarubicin or daunorubicin) chemotherapy appears to be among the most effective treatment for APL, leading to CR rates of 90–95%. The role of cytarabine in APL induction and consolidation is controversial. The addition of cytarabine, although not demonstrated to increase the CR rate, seemingly decreases the risk for relapse. Following achievement of CR, patients should receive at least two cycles of anthracycline-based chemotherapy.

Arsenic trioxide has significant antileukemic activity and is being explored as part of initial treatment in clinical trials of APL. In a randomized trial, arsenic trioxide improved outcome if used after achievement of CR and before consolidation therapy with anthracycline-based chemotherapy. Patients receiving arsenic trioxide are at risk of APL differentiation syndrome, especially when it is administered during induction or salvage treatment after disease relapse. In addition, arsenic trioxide may prolong the QT interval, increasing the risk of cardiac arrhythmias.

Given the progress made in APL resulting in high cure rates, in recent years the goal has been to identify patients with low risk of relapse (i.e., those presenting with a leukocyte count ≤10,000/μL) where attempts are being made to decrease the amount of therapy administered and to identify patients at greatest risk of relapse (i.e., those presenting with a leukocyte count ≥10,000/μL) where new approaches can be developed to increase cure. A study compared the gold standard (tretinoin plus chemotherapy) in newly diagnosed non-high-risk APL with a chemotherapy-free combination of tretinoin and arsenic trioxide. An equivalent outcome was demonstrated between the two arms, and the chemotherapy-free regimen will likely become a new standard for non-high-risk APL patients.

Combinations of tretinoin, arsenic trioxide, and/or chemotherapy and/or gemtuzumab ozogamicin have shown favorable responses in high-risk APL patients at diagnosis.

Assessment of residual disease by RT-PCR amplification of the t(15;17) chimeric gene product *PML-RARA* following the final cycle of chemotherapy is an important step in the management of APL patients. Disappearance of the signal is associated with long-term disease-free survival; its persistence documented by two consecutive tests performed 2 weeks apart invariably predicts relapse. Sequential monitoring of RT-PCR for *PML-RARA* is now considered standard for postremission monitoring of APL, especially in high-risk patients.

The benefit from maintenance therapy with tretinoin has been documented in some studies and not in others. Thus, the use of tretinoin depends on which regimen has been used for induction and consolidation treatment and the risk category of the patients, with those with high-risk disease seemingly benefiting the most from maintenance therapy.

Patients in molecular, cytogenetic, or clinical relapse should be salvaged with arsenic trioxide with or without tretinoin; it produces meaningful responses in up to 85% of patients and can be followed by autologous or, less frequently, especially if RT-PCR positive for *PML-RARA*, allogeneic HSCT.

133 Chronic Myeloid Leukemia

Hagop Kantarjian, Jorge Cortes

Chronic myeloid leukemia (CML) is a clonal hematopoietic stem cell disorder. The disease is driven by the *BCR-ABL1* chimeric gene product, a constitutively active tyrosine kinase, resulting from a reciprocal balanced translocation between the long arms of chromosomes 9 and 22, t(9;22) (q34;q11.2), cytogenetically detected as the Philadelphia chromosome (Ph) (Fig. 133-1). Untreated, the course of CML may be biphasic or triphasic, with an early indolent or chronic phase, followed often by an accelerated phase and a terminal blastic phase. Before the era of selective BCR-ABL1 tyrosine kinase inhibitors (TKIs), the median survival in CML was 3–7 years, and the 10-year survival rate was 30% or less. Introduced into CML therapy in 2000, TKIs have revolutionized the treatment, natural history, and prognosis of CML. Today, the estimated 10-year survival rate with imatinib mesylate, the first BCR-ABL1 TKI approved, is 85%. Allogeneic stem cell transplantation (SCT), a curative but risky treatment approach, is now offered as second- or third-line therapy after failure of TKIs.

INCIDENCE AND EPIDEMIOLOGY

CML accounts for 15% of all cases of leukemia. There is a slight male preponderance (male:female ratio 1.6:1). The median age at diagnosis is 55–65 years. It is uncommon in children; only 3% of patients with CML are younger than 20 years. CML incidence increases slowly with age, with a steeper increase after the age of 40–50 years. The annual incidence of CML is 1.5 cases per 100,000 individuals. In the United States, this translates into 4500–5000 new cases per year. The incidence of CML has not changed over several decades. By extrapolation, the worldwide annual incidence of CML is about 100,000 cases. With a median survival of 6 years before 2000, the disease prevalence in the United States was 20,000–30,000 cases. With TKI therapy, the annual mortality has been reduced from 10–20% to about 2%. Therefore, the prevalence of CML in the United States is expected to continue to increase (about 80,000 in 2013) and reach a plateau of approximately 180,000 cases around 2030. The worldwide prevalence will depend on the treatment penetration of TKIs and their effect on reduction of worldwide annual mortality. Ideally, with full TKI treatment penetration, the worldwide prevalence should plateau at 35 times the incidence, or around 3 million patients.

ETIOLOGY

There are no familial associations in CML. The risk of developing CML is not increased in monozygotic twins or in relatives of patients. No etiologic agents are incriminated, and no associations exist with exposures to benzene or other toxins, fertilizers, insecticides, or viruses. CML is not a frequent secondary leukemia following therapy of other cancers with alkylating agents and/or radiation. Exposure to ionizing radiation (e.g., nuclear accidents, radiation treatment for ankylosing spondylitis or cervical cancer) has increased the risk of CML, which peaks at 5–10 years after exposure and is dose-related. The median time to development of CML among atomic bomb survivors was 6.3 years. Following the Chernobyl accident, the incidence of CML did not increase, suggesting that only large doses of radiation can cause CML. Because of adequate protection, the risk of CML is not increased in individuals working in the nuclear industry or among radiologists in recent times.

PATHOPHYSIOLOGY

The t(9;22) (q34;q11.2) is present in more than 90% of classical CML cases. It results from a balanced reciprocal translocation between the long arms of chromosomes 9 and 22. It is present in hematopoietic cells (myeloid, erythroid, megakaryocytes, and monocytes; less often mature B lymphocytes; rarely mature T lymphocytes, but not stromal cells), but not in other cells in the human body. As a result of the translocation, DNA sequences from the cellular oncogene *ABL1* are translocated next to the major breakpoint cluster region (*BCR*) gene on chromosome 22, generating a hybrid oncogene, *BCR-ABL1*. This fusion gene codes for a novel oncoprotein of molecular weight 210 kDa, referred to as $p210^{BCR-ABL1}$ (Fig. 133-1*B*). This BCR-ABL1 oncoprotein exhibits constitutive kinase activity that leads to excessive proliferation and reduced apoptosis of CML cells, endowing them with a growth advantage over their normal counterparts. Over time, normal hematopoiesis is suppressed, but normal stem cells can persist and may reemerge following effective therapy, for example with TKIs. In Ph-positive acute lymphocytic leukemia (ALL) and in rare cases of CML, the breakpoint in *BCR* is more centromeric, in a region called the minor *BCR* region (*mBCR*). As a result, a shorter sequence of *BCR* is fused to *ABL1*, with a consequent smaller BCR-ABL1 oncoprotein, $p190^{BCR-ABL1}$. When occurring in Ph-positive CML, this translocation may predict for a worse outcome. A third rare breakpoint in *BCR* occurs telomeric to the major *BCR* region and is called *micro-BCR* (μ-BCR). It juxtaposes a larger fragment of the *BCR* gene to ABL1 and produces a larger $p230^{BCR-ABL1}$ oncoprotein, which is associated with a more indolent CML course.

The constitutive activation of *BCR-ABL1* results in autophosphorylation and activation of multiple downstream pathways that modify gene transcription, apoptosis, skeletal organization, and degradation of inhibitory proteins. These transduction pathways may involve RAS, mitogen-activated protein (MAP) kinases, signal transducers and activators of transcription (STAT), phosphatidylinositol-3-kinase (PI3k), MYC, and others. These interactions are mostly mediated through tyrosine phosphorylation and require binding of BCR-ABL1 to adapter proteins such as GRB-2, CRK, CRK-like (CRK-L) protein, and Src homology containing proteins (SHC). BCR-ABL1 TKIs bind to the *BCR-ABL1* kinase domain (KD), preventing the activation of transformation pathways and inhibiting downstream signaling. As a result, proliferation of CML cells is inhibited and apoptosis induced, leading to the reemergence of normal hematopoiesis. A plethora of signaling pathways have been implicated in BCR-ABL1-mediated cellular transformation. The emerging picture is a complex and redundant transformation network. An additional layer of complexity is related to differences in signal transduction between CML differentiated cells and early progenitors. Beta-catenin, Wnt1, Foxo3a, transforming growth factor β, interleukin-6, PP2A, SIRT1, and others have been implicated in CML stem cell survival.

Experimental models have established the causal relationship between the Ph-related *BCR-ABL1* molecular events and the development of CML. In animal models, expression of *BCR-ABL1* in normal hematopoietic cells produced CML-like disorders or lymphoid leukemia, demonstrating the leukemogenic potential of *BCR-ABL1* as a single oncogenic abnormality.

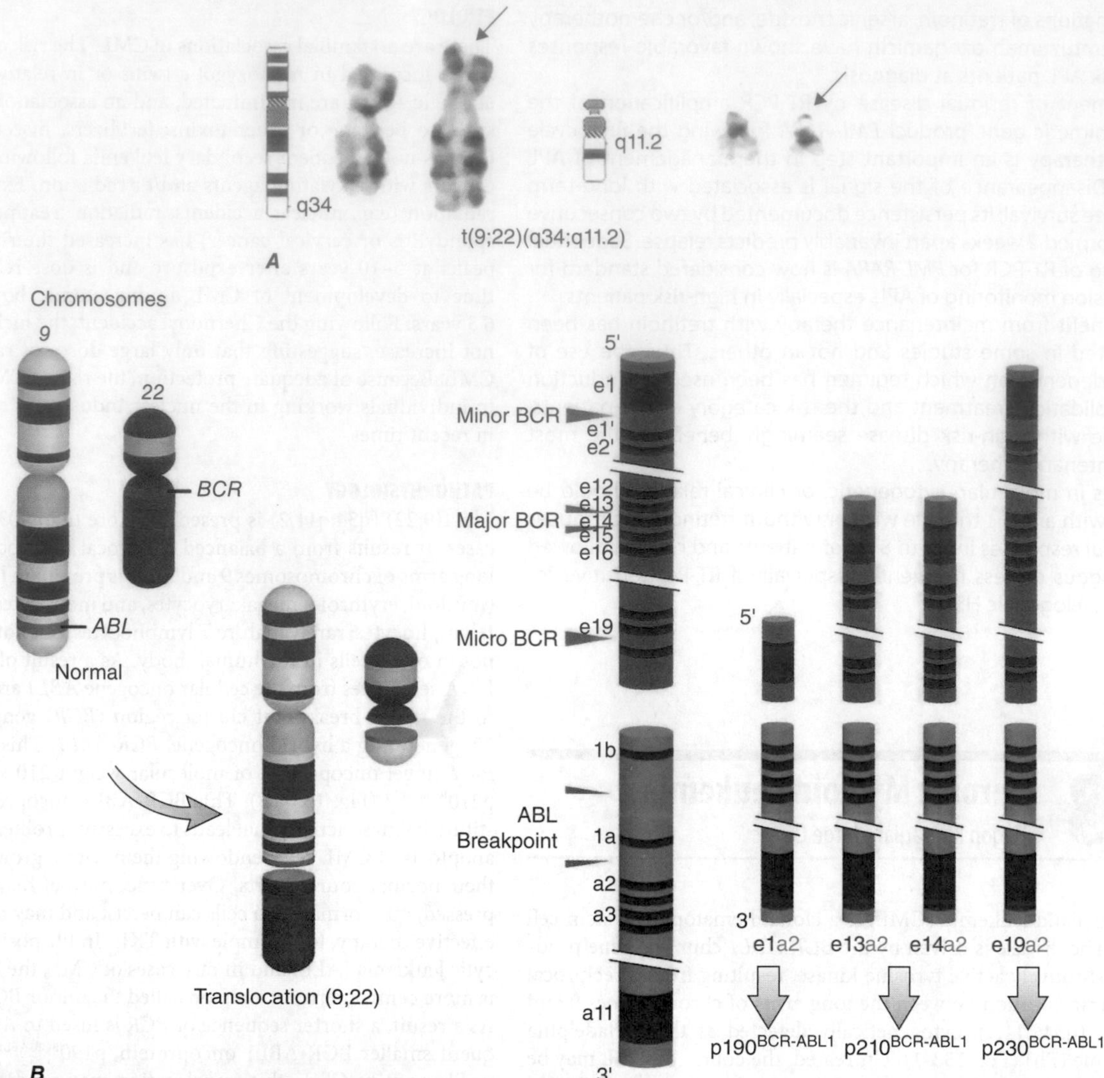

FIGURE 133-1 *A.* The Philadelphia (Ph) chromosome cytogenetic abnormality. *B.* Breakpoints in the long arms of chromosome 9 (*ABL* locus) and chromosome 22 (*BCR* regions) result in three different BCR-ABL oncoprotein messages, p210$^{BCR-ABL1}$ (most common message in chronic myeloid leukemia [CML]), p190$^{BCR-ABL1}$ (present in two-thirds of patients with Ph-positive acute lymphocytic leukemia; rare in CML), and p230$^{BCR-ABL1}$ (rare in CML and associated with an indolent course). *(© 2013 The University of Texas MD Anderson Cancer Center.)*

The cause of the *BCR-ABL1* molecular rearrangement is unknown. Molecular techniques that detect *BCR-ABL1* at a level of 1 in 10^8 identify this molecular abnormality in the blood of up to 25% of normal adults and 5% of infants, but 0% of cord blood samples. This suggests that *BCR-ABL1* is not sufficient to cause overt CML in the overwhelming majority of individuals in whom it occurs. Because CML develops in only 1.5 of 100,000 individuals annually, it is evident that additional molecular events or poor immune recognition of the rearranged cells are needed to cause overt CML.

CML is defined by the presence of *BCR-ABL1* abnormality in a patient with a myeloproliferative neoplasm. In some patients with a typical morphologic picture of CML, the Ph abnormality is not detectable by standard cytogenetic analysis, but fluorescence in situ hybridization (FISH) and molecular studies (polymerase chain reaction [PCR]) detect *BCR-ABL1*. These patients have a course similar to Ph-positive CML and respond to TKI therapy. Many of the remaining patients have atypical morphologic or clinical features and belong to other diagnostic groups, such as atypical CML or chronic myelomonocytic leukemia. These individuals do not respond to TKI therapy and have a poor prognosis with a median survival of about 2–3 years. Detection of mutations in the granulocyte colony-stimulating factor receptor (*CSF3R*) in chronic neutrophilic leukemia and in some cases of atypical CML and of mutations in *SETBP1* in atypical CML confirmed that they are distinct entities.

The mechanisms associated with the transition of CML from a chronic to accelerated-blastic phase are poorly understood. They are often associated with characteristic chromosomal abnormalities such as a double Ph, trisomy 8, isochromosome 17 or deletion of 17p (loss of *TP53*), 20q−, and others. Molecular events associated with transformation include mutations in *TP53*, retinoblastoma 1 (*RB1*), myeloid transcriptions factors like Runx1, and cell cycle regulators like p16. A plethora of other mutations or functional abnormalities have been implicated in blastic transformation, but no unifying theme has emerged other than that *BCR-ABL1* itself induces genetic instability that leads to the acquisition of additional mutations and eventually to blastic transformation. In this frame of thinking, one critical effect of TKIs is their ability to stabilize the CML genome, leading to a much reduced transformation rate. In particular, the previously observed sudden blastic transformations (i.e., abrupt transformation to blastic phase in a patient who had been in cytogenetic response) have become uncommon, occurring rarely in younger patients in the first 1–2 years of TKI therapy (usually sudden lymphoid blastic transformations). Sudden transformations beyond the third year of TKI therapy are rare in patients who continue on TKI therapy. Moreover, initial experience suggests that the course of CML has become significantly more indolent, even without cytogenetic responses, in patients on TKI-based therapy compared to previous experience with hydroxyurea/busulfan.

Among patients developing resistance to TKIs, several resistance mechanisms have been observed. The most clinically relevant one is the development of different *ABL1* kinase domain mutations that prevent the binding of TKIs to the catalytic site (ATP binding site) of the kinase. More than 100 *BCR-ABL1* mutations have now been described, many of which confer relative or absolute resistance to imatinib. This has resulted in the development of second-generation TKIs (i.e., dasatinib, nilotinib, bosutinib) and of a third-generation TKI (ponatinib) with selective efficacy against T315I, a mutation of the gatekeeper residue of the kinase that causes resistance to all other TKIs.

CLINICAL PRESENTATION

The presenting signs and symptoms in CML depend on the availability of and access to health care procedures, including physical exams and screening tests. In the United States, because of the easy access to health care screening and physical exams, 50–60% of patients are diagnosed on routine blood tests and have minimal symptoms at presentation, such as fatigue. In geographic locations where access to health care is more limited, patients often present with high CML burden including splenomegaly, anemia, and related symptoms (abdominal pain, weight loss, fatigue), as well as a higher frequency of high-risk CML. Presenting findings in patients diagnosed in the United States are shown in Table 133-1.

Symptoms Most patients with CML (90%) present in the indolent or chronic phase. Depending on the timing of diagnosis, patients are often asymptomatic (if the diagnosis is discovered during health care screening tests). Common symptoms, when present, are manifestations of anemia and splenomegaly. These may include fatigue, malaise, weight loss (if high leukemia burden), or early satiety and left upper quadrant pain or masses (from splenomegaly). Less common presenting findings include thrombotic or vasoocclusive events (from severe leukocytosis or thrombocytosis). These include priapism, cardiovascular complications, myocardial infarction, venous thrombosis, visual disturbances, dyspnea and pulmonary insufficiency, drowsiness, loss of coordination, confusion, or cerebrovascular accidents. Bleeding diatheses findings include retinal hemorrhages, gastrointestinal bleeding, and others. Patients who present with, or progress to, the accelerated or blastic phases have additional symptoms including unexplained fever, significant weight loss, severe fatigue, bone and joint aches, bleeding and thrombotic events, and infections.

TABLE 133-1 PRESENTING SIGNS AND SYMPTOMS OF NEWLY DIAGNOSED PHILADELPHIA CHROMOSOME–POSITIVE CHRONIC MYELOID LEUKEMIA IN CHRONIC PHASE

Parameter	Percentage
Age ≥60 years (median)	18 (46)
Female gender	35–45
Splenomegaly	30
Hepatomegaly	5
Lymphadenopathy	5
Other extramedullary disease	2
Hemoglobin <10 g/dL	10–15
Platelets	
>450 × 10^9 cells/L	30–35
<100 × 10^9 cells/L	3–5
White blood cells ≥50 × 10^9 cells/L	35–40
Marrow	
≥5% blasts	5
≥5% basophils	10–15
Peripheral blood	
≥3% blasts	8–10
≥7% basophils	10
Cytogenetic clonal evolution other than the Philadelphia chromosome	4–5
Sokal risk	
Low	60–65
Intermediate	25–30
High	10

Physical Findings Splenomegaly is the most common physical finding, occurring in 20–70% of patients depending on health care screening frequency. Other less common findings include hepatomegaly (10–20%), lymphadenopathy (5–10%), and extramedullary disease (skin or subcutaneous lesions). The latter indicates CML transformation if a biopsy confirms the presence of sheets of blasts. Other physical findings are manifestations of complications of high tumor burden described earlier (e.g., cardiovascular, cerebrovascular, bleeding). High basophil counts may be associated with histamine overproduction causing pruritus, diarrhea, flushing, and even gastrointestinal ulcers.

Hematologic and Marrow Findings In untreated CML, leukocytosis ranging from 10–500 × 10^9/L is common. The peripheral blood differential shows left-shifted hematopoiesis with predominance of neutrophils and the presence of bands, myelocytes, metamyelocytes, promyelocytes, and blasts (usually ≤5%). Basophils and/or eosinophils are frequently increased. Thrombocytosis is common, but thrombocytopenia is rare and, when present, suggests a worse prognosis, disease acceleration, or an unrelated etiology. Anemia is present in one-third of patients. Cyclic oscillations of counts are noted in 25% of patients without treatment. Biochemical abnormalities include a low leukocyte alkaline phosphatase score and high levels of vitamin B_{12}, uric acid, lactic dehydrogenase, and lysozyme. The presence of unexplained and sustained leukocytosis, with or without splenomegaly, should lead to a marrow examination and cytogenetic analysis.

The bone marrow is hypercellular with marked myeloid hyperplasia and a high myeloid-to-erythroid ratio of 15–20:1. Marrow blasts are 5% or less; when higher, they carry a worse prognosis or represent acceleration (if they are ≥15%). Increased reticulin fibrosis (by Snook's silver stain) is common, with 30–40% of patients demonstrating grade 3–4 reticulin fibrosis. This was considered adverse in the pre-TKI era. With TKI therapy, reticulin fibrosis resolves in most patients and is not an indicator of poor prognosis. Collagen fibrosis (Wright-Giemsa stain) is rare at diagnosis. Disease progression with a "spent phase" of myelofibrosis (myelophthisis, or burnt-out marrow) was common with busulfan therapy (20–30%) but is rare with TKI therapy.

Cytogenetic and Molecular Findings The diagnosis of CML is straightforward and depends on documenting t(9;22)(q34;q11.2), which is found in 90% of cases. This is known as the Philadelphia-chromosome abnormality (discovered in Philadelphia) and was initially identified as a shortened chromosome, later identified to be chromosome 22 (22q–) (Fig. 133-1). Some patients may have complex translocations (variant Ph) involving three or more translocations that include chromosomes 9 and 22 and one or more other chromosomes. Others may have a "masked Ph," involving translocations between chromosome 9 and a chromosome other than 22. The prognosis of these patients and their response to TKI therapy are similar to those in patients with Ph. About 5–10% of patients may have additional chromosomal abnormalities in the Ph-positive cells. These usually involve trisomy 8, a double Ph, isochromosome 17 or 17p deletion, 20q–, or others. This is referred to as clonal evolution and was historically a sign of adverse prognosis, particularly when trisomy 8, double Ph, or chromosome 17 abnormalities were noted.

Techniques such as FISH and PCR are now used to aid in the diagnosis of CML. They are more sensitive approaches to estimate the CML burden in patients on TKI therapy. They can be done on peripheral samples, and thus are less painful and more convenient. Patients with CML at diagnosis should have a FISH analysis to quantify the percentage of Ph-positive cells, if FISH is used to replace marrow cytogenetic analysis in monitoring response to therapy. FISH may not detect additional chromosomal abnormalities (clonal evolution); thus, a cytogenetic analysis is usually recommended at the time of diagnosis. The *BCR-ABL1* RNA message is usually one of two variants: e13a2 (formerly b2a2) and e14a2 (formerly b3a2). About 2–5% of patients may have other RNA fusion types (e.g., e1a2, e13a3, or e14a3). In these patients, the routine PCR primers may not amplify the *BCR-ABL1* transcripts, thus leading to false-negative results. Therefore, molecular studies at diagnosis are important to document the type and presence of *BCR-ABL1* transcripts to avoid erroneously "undetectable" *BCR-ABL1* transcripts on follow-up studies, with the misconception of a complete molecular response.

Both FISH and PCR studies can be falsely positive at low levels or falsely negative because of technical issues. Therefore, a diagnosis of CML must always rely on a marrow analysis with routine cytogenetics. The diagnostic bone marrow confirms the presence of the Ph chromosome, detects clonal evolution, i.e., chromosomal abnormalities in the Ph-positive cells (which may be prognostic), and also quantifies the percentage of marrow blasts and basophils. In 10% of patients, the percentage of marrow blasts and basophils can be significantly higher than in the peripheral blood, suggesting poorer prognosis or even disease transformation.

Monitoring patients on TKI therapy by cytogenetics, FISH, and molecular studies has become an important standard practice to assess response to therapy, emphasize compliance, evaluate possible treatment resistance, change TKI therapy, and order mutational analysis studies. It is thus important to recognize the comparability of these measures in monitoring response. A partial cytogenetic response is defined as the presence of 35% less Ph-positive metaphases by routine cytogenetic analysis. This is roughly equivalent to *BCR-ABL1* transcripts by the International Scale (IS) of 10% or less. A complete cytogenetic response refers to the absence of Ph-positive metaphases (0% Ph positivity). This is approximately equivalent to *BCR-ABL1* transcripts (IS) of 1% or less. A major molecular response refers to *BCR-ABL1* transcripts (IS) ≤0.1%, or roughly a 3-log or greater reduction of CML burden from baseline. A complete molecular response usually refers to *BCR-ABL1* transcripts (IS) <0.0032% (undetectable by current techniques), roughly equivalent to a more than 4.5-log reduction of CML burden from baseline.

Findings in CML Transformation Progression of CML is usually associated with leukocytosis resistant to therapy, increasing anemia, fever and constitutional symptoms, and increased blasts and basophils in the peripheral blood or marrow. Criteria of accelerated-phase CML, historically associated with median survival of less than 1.5 years, include the presence of 15% or more peripheral blasts, 30% or more peripheral blasts plus promyelocytes, 20% or more peripheral basophils, cytogenetic clonal evolution (presence of chromosomal abnormalities in addition to Ph), and thrombocytopenia $<100 \times 10^9/L$ (unrelated to therapy). About 5–10% of patients present with de novo accelerated phase or blastic phase. The prognosis of de novo accelerated phase with TKI therapy has improved significantly, with an estimated 8-year survival rate of 75%. The median survival of accelerated phase evolving from chronic phase has also improved from a historical median survival of 18 months to an estimated 4-year survival rate of 70% on TKI therapy. Therefore, the criteria for accelerated-phase CML should be revisited because most have lost much of their prognostic significance. Blastic-phase CML is defined by the presence of 30% or more peripheral or marrow blasts or the presence of sheets of blasts in extramedullary disease (usually skin, soft tissues, or lytic bone lesions). Blastic-phase CML is commonly myeloid (60%) but can present uncommonly as erythroid, promyelocytic, monocytic, or megakaryocytic. Lymphoid blastic phase occurs in about 25% of patients. Lymphoblasts are terminal deoxynucleotide transferase positive and peroxidase negative (although occasionally with low positivity up to 3–5%) and express lymphoid markers (CD10, CD19, CD20, CD22). However, they also often express myeloid markers (50–80%), resulting in diagnostic confusion. This is important because, unlike other morphologic blastic phases, lymphoid blastic-phase CML is quite responsive to anti-ALL-type chemotherapy (e.g., hyper-CVAD [cyclophosphamide, vincristine, doxorubicin, and dexamethasone]) in combination with TKIs.

PROGNOSIS AND CML COURSE

Before the imatinib era, the annual mortality in CML was 10% in the first 2 years and 15–20% thereafter. The median survival time in CML was 3–7 years (with hydroxyurea-busulfan and interferon α). Without a curative option of allogeneic SCT, the course of CML was inexorable toward transformation to, and death from, accelerated or blastic phases. The disease stability was unpredictable, with some patients demonstrating sudden transformation to a blastic phase. With imatinib therapy, the annual mortality in CML has decreased to 2% in the first 12 years of observation. Half of the deaths are from factors other than CML, such as old age, accidents, suicides, other cancers, and other medical conditions (e.g., infections, surgical procedures). The estimated 8- to 10-year survival rate is now 85%, or 93% if only CML-related deaths are considered (Fig. 133-2). The course of CML has also become quite predictable. In the first 2 years of TKI therapy, rare sudden transformations are still noted (1–2%), usually lymphoid blastic transformations that respond to combinations of chemotherapy and TKIs followed by allogeneic SCT. These may be explained by the intrinsic mechanisms of sudden transformation already existing in the CML clones before the start of therapy that were not amenable to TKI inhibition, in particular imatinib. Second-generation TKIs (nilotinib,

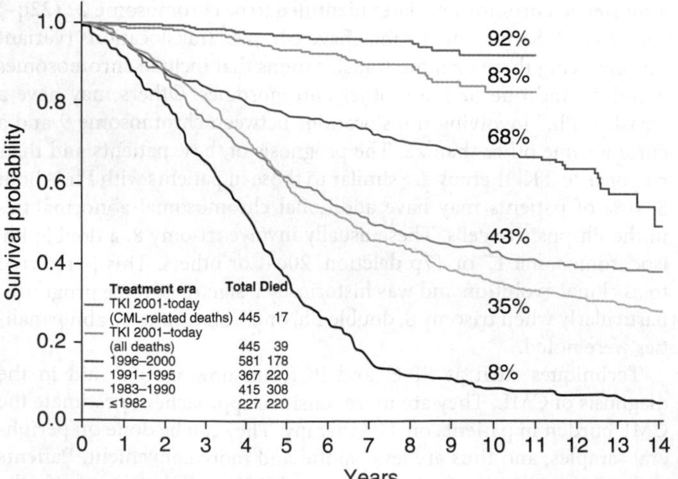

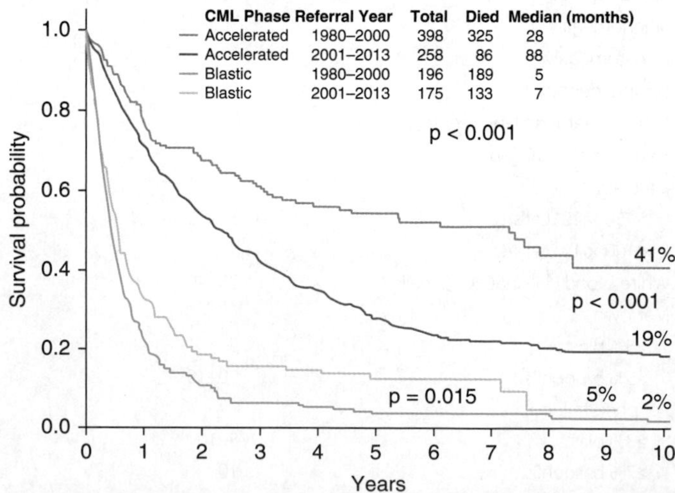

FIGURE 133-2 ***A.*** Survival in newly diagnosed chronic-phase chronic myeloid leukemia (CML) by era of therapy (M.D. Anderson Cancer Center experience from 1965 to present). Causes of non-CML deaths in 22 patients were other cancers (n = 7), postsurgical complications (n = 3), car accident (n = 2), suicide (n = 1), neurologic events (n = 3), cardiac (n = 3), pneumonia (n = 1), and unknown (n = 2). ***B.*** Survival in patients with accelerated- and blastic-phase CML referred to M.D. Anderson Cancer Center by era of therapy, demonstrating the significant survival benefit in the tyrosine kinase inhibitor (TKI) era in accelerated-phase CML but the modest benefit in blastic-phase CML. Referred cases included de novo and post-chronic-phase transformations.

dasatinib) used as frontline therapy have reduced the incidence of transformation in the first 2–3 years from 6–8% with imatinib to 2–4% with nilotinib or dasatinib. Disease transformation to accelerated or blastic phase is rare on continued TKI therapy, estimated at <1% annually in years 4–8 of follow-up on the original imatinib trials. Patients usually develop resistance in the form of cytogenetic relapse, followed by hematologic relapse and subsequent transformation, rather than the previously feared sudden transformations without the warning signals of cytogenetic-hematologic relapse.

Before the imatinib era, several pretreatment prognostic factors predicted for worse outcome in CML and have been incorporated into prognostic models and staging systems. These have included older age, significant splenomegaly, anemia, thrombocytopenia or thrombocytosis, high percentages of blasts and basophils (and/or eosinophils), marrow fibrosis, deletions in the long arm of chromosome 9, clonal evolution, and others. Different risk models and staging systems, derived from multivariate analyses, were proposed to define different risk groups. As with the introduction of cisplatin into testicular cancer therapy, the introduction of TKIs into CML therapy has nullified or lessened the prognostic impact of most of these prognostic factors and the significance of the CML models (e.g., Sokal, Hasford, European Treatment and Outcome Study [EUTOS]). Treatment related prognostic factors have emerged as the most important prognostic factors in the era of imatinib therapy. Achievement of complete cytogenetic response has become the major therapeutic endpoint and is the only endpoint associated with improvement in survival. Achievement of a major molecular response is associated with decreased risk of events (relapse) and CML progression, may predict for differences in event-free survival (depending on the definition of an event) and for small differences in transformation rates, but has not been associated with survival prolongation. Among patients in complete cytogenetic response, survival is similar independent of whether they achieve a major molecular response or not. This may be due to the efficacy of salvage TKI therapies, which are and should be implemented at the first evidence of cytogenetic relapse. Achievement of complete molecular response (undetectable *BCR-ABL1* transcripts), particularly when durable (>2 years), may offer the possibility of durable molecular response (molecular cure rather than functional cure) in the context of investigational trials and may allow temporary therapy interruption in women eager to have babies. The lack of achievement of major or complete molecular responses should not be considered as "failure" of a particular TKI therapy and/or an indication to change the TKI or to consider allogeneic SCT.

Pretreatment prognostic factors and prognostic models have lost much of their clinical relevance to define prognosis and to select different therapies. However TKI-associated therapeutic responses have gained major clinical relevance and dictate appropriate and careful monitoring of patients to optimize their treatment.

TREATMENT CHRONIC MYELOID LEUKEMIA

The introduction of TKI therapy, first in the form of imatinib mesylate in 2001, has revolutionized the treatment and prognosis in CML. Before 2000, allogeneic SCT was frontline therapy, when available, because of its potentially curative capacity. Otherwise, patients were offered interferon α therapy (approved for the treatment of CML in 1986), which had modest benefits (improving survival from a median of 3–4 years with hydroxyurea-busulfan to a median of 6–7 years), but also significant side effects. Other alternatives included hydroxyurea, busulfan, and other nonspecific chemotherapies. With TKI therapy, the estimated 10-year survival in CML is 85%. Since 2001, six agents have been approved by the U.S. Food and Drug Administration (FDA) for the treatment of CML. These include five oral BCR-ABL1-selective TKIs: imatinib (Gleevec), nilotinib (Tasigna), dasatinib (Sprycel), bosutinib (Bosulif), and ponatinib (Iclusig). Imatinib 400 mg orally daily, nilotinib 300 mg orally twice a day (on an empty stomach), and dasatinib 100 mg orally daily are approved for frontline therapy of CML. All three are also approved for salvage therapy (nilotinib 400 mg twice daily), in addition to bosutinib (500 mg daily) and ponatinib (45 mg daily). Imatinib, dasatinib (140 mg daily), bosutinib, and ponatinib are also approved for the treatment of CML transformation (accelerated and blastic phase), whereas nilotinib is only approved for chronic and accelerated phase. Dasatinib, nilotinib, and bosutinib are referred to as second-generation TKIs; ponatinib is referred to as a third-generation TKI. The sixth approved agent is omacetaxine (Synribo), a protein synthesis inhibitor with presumed more selective inhibition of the synthesis of the BCR-ABL1 oncoprotein. It is approved for the treatment of chronic- and accelerated-phase CML after failure of two or more TKIs, at 1.25 mg/m^2 subcutaneously twice a day for 14 days for induction and for 7 days for consolidation-maintenance. Nilotinib is similar in structure to imatinib but 30 times more potent. Dasatinib and bosutinib are dual SRC-ABL1 TKIs (dasatinib is reported to be 300 times more potent and bosutinib 30–50 times more potent than imatinib). Ponatinib is effective against wild-type and mutant *BCR-ABL1* clones. It is unique in being the only currently available BCR-ABL1 TKI that is active against T315I, a gatekeeper mutant resistant to the other four TKIs (Table 133-2).

Imatinib, nilotinib, and dasatinib are all acceptable frontline therapies in CML. The long-term results of imatinib are very favorable. The 8-year follow-up results show a cumulative complete cytogenetic response rate (occurring at least once) of 83%, with 60–65% of patients being in complete cytogenetic response at 5-year follow-up. The estimated 8-year event-free survival rate is 81%, and the overall survival rate is 85%. Among patients continuing on imatinib, the annual rate of transformation to accelerated-blastic phase in years 4–8 is <1%. In two randomized studies, one comparing nilotinib 300 mg twice daily or 400 mg twice daily with imatinib (ENEST-nd) and the other comparing dasatinib 100 mg daily with imatinib (DASISION), the second-generation TKIs were associated with better outcomes in early surrogate endpoints, including higher rates of complete cytogenetic responses (85–87% vs 77–82%), major molecular responses (65–76% vs 46–63%), and undetectable *BCR-ABL1* transcripts (IS) (32–37% vs 15–30%), and lower rates of transformation to accelerated-blastic phase (2–4% vs 6%). However, neither study showed a survival benefit with second-generation TKIs (median follow-up times of 4–5 years). This may be because salvage

TABLE 133-2 MEDICAL THERAPEUTIC OPTIONS IN CHRONIC MYELOID LEUKEMIA

Agent (Brand Name)	Approved Indications	Dose Schedule	Notable Toxicities
Imatinib mesylate (Gleevec)	All phases	400 mg daily	See text
Dasatinib (Sprycel)	All phases	First-line: 100 mg daily Salvage: 140 mg daily	Myelosuppression; pleural and pericardial effusions; pulmonary hypertension
Nilotinib (Tasigna)	All phases except blastic phase	First-line: 300 mg twice daily Salvage: 400 mg twice daily	Diabetes; vasoocclusive disease; pancreatitis
Bosutinib (Bosulif)	All phases except frontline	500 mg daily	Diarrhea
Ponatinib (Iclusig)	All phases except frontline	45 mg daily (may consider lower starting doses in the future, e.g., 30 mg daily)	Skin rashes, pancreatitis; vasoocclusive disease (10–20%)
Omacetaxine mepesuccinate (Synribo)	Failure ≥2 tyrosine kinase inhibitors	1.25 mg/m^2 subcutaneously twice daily for 14 days for induction; 7 days of maintenance every month	Myelosuppression

therapy with other TKIs (following close observation and treatment change at progression) provides highly effective salvage therapy that rebalances the negative effect of the relapse.

Salvage therapy in chronic phase with dasatinib, nilotinib, bosutinib, or ponatinib is associated with complete cytogenetic response rates of 30–60% of patients, depending on the salvage status (cytogenetic vs hematologic relapse), prior response to other TKIs, and the mutations at the time of relapse. Complete cytogenetic responses are generally durable, particularly in the absence of clonal evolution and mutations. Ponatinib is the only TKI active in the setting of T315I mutation, with complete cytogenetic response rates of 50–70%. The estimated 3- to 5-year survival rates with new TKIs as salvage are 70–80% (compared with <50% before their availability). For example, with dasatinib salvage after imatinib failure in chronic-phase CML, the major molecular response rates were 40–43%, the estimated 6-year survival rates were 74–83%, and progression-free survival rates were 40–51%. Thus, TKIs in the salvage setting have already reduced the annual mortality from the historical rate of 10–15% to ≤5%.

The goal of CML therapy is viewed differently in the context of research versus standard practice. In current practice, functional cure, defined as survival with CML similar to survival among normal individuals, is the current goal of therapy. CML is now considered an indolent disease, which, with appropriate TKI therapy, treatment compliance, careful monitoring, and early change to other TKIs as indicated, can be associated with close to normal survival. Therefore, in standard practice, achievement and maintenance of a complete cytogenetic response are the aims of therapy, because complete cytogenetic response is the only treatment-related factor associated with survival prolongation. Lack of achievement of a major molecular response (protects against events; associated with longer event-free survival) or of negative *BCR-ABL1* transcripts (offers the potential of TKI interruption on investigational studies) should not be considered indications to change TKI therapy or to consider allogeneic SCT. A general practice rule is to continue the particular TKI chosen at the most tolerable dose schedule not associated with grade 3–4 side effects or with bothersome chronic side effects, for as long as possible, until either cytogenetic relapse or the persistence of unacceptable side effects. These two factors (i.e., cytogenetic relapse and intolerable side effects as judged by the patient and treating physician) are the indicators of "failure" of a particular TKI therapy. Because of the increasing prevalence of CML (cost of TKI therapy) and the emerging long-term low rates of significant organ toxicities, the ultimate goal of CML therapy in the research setting is to achieve eradication of the disease (molecular cure) that is prolonged and durable, with recovery of nonneoplastic, nonclonal hematopoiesis off TKI therapy. The first step toward this aim is to obtain the highest rates of undetectable *BCR-ABL1* transcripts lasting for at least 2 or more years.

Recommendations provided by the National Comprehensive Cancer Network (NCCN) and by the European LeukemiaNet (ELN) discuss optimal/expected, suboptimal/warning, and failure response scenarios at different time points of TKI treatment duration. Unfortunately, they may have been misinterpreted in current practice, because oncologists often report that their aim of treatment is the achievement of major molecular response and disease eradication. Significantly, a substantial proportion of oncologists consider a change of TKI therapy in a patient in complete cytogenetic response if they note "loss of major molecular response" (increase of *BCR-ABL1* transcripts ([IS] from <0.1% to >0.1%). This perception may be the result of confusion regarding the NCCN and ELN guidelines, which have been updated often as a result of maturing data and have multiple treatment endpoint considerations. Although such endpoints have been suggested by these recommendations as possible criteria for failure, it is important to emphasize that no randomized study has yet shown that a change of TKI treatment in patients with complete cytogenetic response because of a loss of major molecular response, versus changing at the time of cytogenetic relapse, has been shown to improve survival. This is likely because of the high efficacy of salvage TKI therapy at the time of cytogenetic relapse.

Side effects of TKIs are generally mild to moderate, although with long-term TKI therapy, they could affect the patient's quality of life. Serious side effects occur in less than 5–10% of patients. With imatinib therapy, common mild to moderate side effects include fluid retention, weight gain, nausea, diarrhea, skin rashes, periorbital edema, bone or muscle aches, fatigue, and others (rates of 10–20%). In general, second-generation TKIs are associated with lower rates of these bothersome adverse events. However, dasatinib is associated with higher rates of myelosuppression (20–30%), particularly thrombocytopenia, and with pleural (10–25%) or pericardial effusions (≤5%). Nilotinib is associated with higher rates of hyperglycemia (10–20%), pruritus and skin rashes, and headaches. Nilotinib is also associated with rare events of pancreatitis (<5%). Bosutinib is associated with higher rates of early and self-limited gastrointestinal complications like diarrhea (50–70%). Ponatinib is associated with higher rates of skin rashes (10–15%), pancreatitis (5%), elevations of amylase/lipase (10%), and vasospastic/vasoocclusive events (10–20%). Nilotinib and dasatinib may cause prolongation of the QTc interval; therefore, they should be evaluated cautiously in patients with prolonged QTc interval on electrocardiogram (>470–480 ms), and drugs given for other medical conditions should have relatively smaller or no effects on QTc. These side effects can often be dose-dependent and are generally reversible with treatment interruptions and dose reductions. Dose reductions can be individualized. However, the lowest estimated effective doses of TKIs (from different studies and treatment practices) are imatinib 300 mg daily; nilotinib 200 mg twice daily; dasatinib 20 mg daily; bosutinib 300 mg daily; and ponatinib 15 mg daily.

With long-term follow-up, rare but clinically relevant serious toxicities are emerging. Renal dysfunction and renal failure (creatinine elevations >2–3 mg/dL) are observed in 2–3% of patients and reverse with TKI discontinuation and empirical use of other TKIs. Pulmonary hypertension has been reported with dasatinib (<1–2%) and should be considered in a patient with shortness of breath and a normal chest x-ray (echocardiogram with emphasis on measurement of pulmonary artery pressure). This may be reversible with dasatinib discontinuation and occasionally the use of sildenafil citrate. Systemic hypertension has been observed more often with ponatinib therapy, as well as other TKIs. Hyperglycemia and diabetes have been noted more frequently with nilotinib. Finally, mid- and small-vessel vasoocclusive and vasospastic events have been reported at low but significant rates with nilotinib and ponatinib and should be considered possibly TKI-related and represent indications to interrupt or reduce the dose of the TKI. These events include angina, coronary artery disease, myocardial infarction, peripheral arterial occlusive disease, transient ischemic attacks, cerebral vascular accidents, Raynaud's phenomenon, and accelerated atherosclerosis. Although these events are uncommon (<5%), they are clinically significant for the patient's long-term prognosis and occur at significantly higher rates than in the general population (5–20 times more often).

ALLOGENEIC STEM CELL TRANSPLANT

Allogeneic SCT, a curative modality in CML, is associated with long-term survival rates of 40–60% when implemented in the chronic phase. It is associated with early (1-year) mortality rates of 5–30%. Although the 5- to 10-year survival rates were reported to be around 50–60% (and considered as cure rates), about 10–15% of patients die in the subsequent 1–2 decades from subtle long-term complications of the transplant (rather than from CML relapse). These are related to chronic graft-versus-host disease (GVHD), organ dysfunction, development of second cancers, and hazard ratios for mortality higher than in the normal population. Other significant morbidities include infertility, chronic immune-mediated complications, cataracts, hip necrosis, and other morbidities affecting quality of life. The cure and early mortality rates in chronic-phase CML are also associated with several factors: patient age, duration of chronic phase, whether the donor is related or unrelated, degree of matching, preparative regimen, and others. In accelerated-phase

CML, the cure rates with allogeneic SCT are 20–40%, depending on the definition of acceleration. Patients with clonal evolution as the only criterion have cure rates of up to 40–50%. Patients undergoing allogeneic SCT in second chronic phase have cure rates of 40–50%. The cure rates with allogeneic SCT in blastic phase CML are ≤15%. Post–allogeneic SCT strategies are now implemented in the setting of molecular or cytogenetic relapse or in hematologic relapse/transformation. These include the use of TKIs for prevention or treatment of relapse, donor lymphocyte infusions, and second allogeneic SCTs, among others. TKIs appear to be highly successful at reinducing cytogenetic/molecular remissions in the setting of cytogenetic or molecular relapse after allogeneic SCT.

Choice and Timing of Allogeneic SCT Allogeneic SCT was considered first-line CML therapy before 2000. The maturing positive experience with TKIs has now relegated its use to after first-line TKI failures. An important question is the optimal timing and sequence of TKIs and allogeneic SCT (whether allogeneic SCT should be used as second- or third-line therapy). Among patients who present with or evolve to blastic phase, combinations of chemotherapy and TKIs should be used to induce remission, followed by allogeneic SCT as soon as possible. The same applies to patients who evolve from chronic to accelerated phase. Patients with de novo accelerated-phase CML may do well with long-term TKI therapy (estimated 8-year survival rate 75%); the timing of allogeneic SCT depends on their optimal response to TKI (achievement of complete cytogenetic response). Among patients who relapse in chronic phase, the treatment sequence depends on several factors: (1) patient age and availability of appropriate donors; (2) risk of allogeneic SCT; (3) presence or absence of clonal evolution and mutations; (4) patient's prior history and comorbidities; and (5) patient and physician preferences (Table 133-3). Patients with T315I mutations at relapse should be offered ponatinib and considered for allogeneic SCT (because of the short follow-up with ponatinib). Patients with mutations involving Y253H, E255K/V, and F359V/C/I respond better to dasatinib or bosutinib. Patients with mutations involving V299L, T315A, and F317L/F/I/C respond better to nilotinib. Comorbidities such as diabetes, hypertension, pulmonary hypertension, chronic lung disease, cardiac conditions, and pancreatitis may influence the choice for or against a particular TKI. Patients with clonal evolution, unfavorable mutations, or lack of major/complete cytogenetic

TABLE 133-3 GENERAL SUGGESTIONS REGARDING THE USE OF TYROSINE KINASE INHIBITORS (TKIS) AND ALLOGENEIC STEM CELL TRANSPLANTATION (SCT) IN CHRONIC MYELOID LEUKEMIA (CML)

CML Phase	Use of TKI	Consideration of Allogeneic SCT
Accelerated or blastic	Interim therapy to achieve minimal CML burden	As soon as possible (exception: de novo accelerated phase)
Imatinib failure in chronic phase; T315I mutation	Ponatinib to achieve minimal CML burden	Depends on longer term follow-up results of ponatinib efficacy
Imatinib failure in chronic phase; no clonal evolution, no mutations, good initial response	Second-line kinase inhibitors long-term	Third-line after second-line TKI failures
Imatinib failure in chronic phase; clonal evolution or mutations, or no cytogenetic response to second-line TKI	Interim therapy to achieve minimal CML burden	Second-line
Older patients (≥65–70 years) after imatinib failure in chronic phase	Salvage TKIs as longer-term therapy	May forgo allogeneic SCT in favor of good quality of life and survival in chronic phase

Note: Mutations involving Y253H, E255K/V, or F359V/C/I: prefer dasatinib or bosutinib. Mutations involving V299L, T315A, or F317L/F/I/C: prefer nilotinib.

response within 1 year of salvage TKI therapy have short remission durations and should consider allogeneic SCT as more urgent in the setting of salvage. Patients without clonal evolution or mutations at relapse and who achieve a complete cytogenetic response with TKI salvage, have long-lasting complete remissions and may delay the option of allogeneic SCT to third-line therapy. Finally, older patients (age 65–70 years or older) and those with high risk of mortality with allogeneic SCT may forgo this curative option for several years of disease control in chronic phase with or without cytogenetic response (Table 133-3). Historically, before the availability of TKIs, patients without cytogenetic response on interferon α or hydroxyurea had expected short median survival times (2–3 years) with expected rapid disease transformation. The maturing experience with TKIs suggests a different course, whereby patients may remain in chronic phase on TKI-based therapies (combinations including hydroxyurea, cytarabine, decitabine, and others), with or without cytogenetic response, for many years. Table 133-3 summarizes a general guidance to the choice of TKIs versus allogeneic SCT.

MONITORING THERAPY IN CML

Achievement of complete cytogenetic response by 12 months of imatinib therapy and its persistence later, the only consistent prognostic factor associated with survival, is now the main therapeutic endpoint in CML. Failure to achieve a complete cytogenetic response by 12 months or occurrence of later cytogenetic or hematologic relapse is considered as treatment failure and an indication to change therapy. Because salvage therapy with other TKIs reestablishes good outcome, it is important to ensure patient compliance to continued TKI therapy and change therapy at the first sign of cytogenetic relapse. Patients on frontline imatinib therapy should be closely monitored until documentation of complete cytogenetic response, at which time they can be monitored every 6 months with peripheral blood FISH and PCR studies (to check for concordance of results), or more frequently if there are concerns about changes in *BCR-ABL1* transcripts (e.g., every 3 months). Monitoring by molecular studies only is reasonable in patients who are in major molecular response. Cytogenetic relapse on imatinib is an indication of treatment failure and need to change TKI therapy. Mutational analysis in this instance helps in the selection of the next TKI and identifies mutations in 30–50% of patients. Mutational studies in patients in complete cytogenetic response (in whom there may be concerns of increasing *BCR-ABL1* transcripts) identify mutations in ≤5% and are therefore not indicated. Earlier response has been identified as a prognostic factor for long-term outcome, including achievement of partial cytogenetic response (*BCR-ABL1* transcripts ≤10%) by 3–6 months of therapy. Failure to achieve such a response on imatinib therapy has been associated with significantly worse survival in some studies (particularly when second-generation TKIs were not readily available as salvage therapy), but not in others (when they were).

The use of second-generation TKIs (nilotinib, dasatinib) as frontline therapy changed the monitoring approach slightly. Patients are expected to achieve complete cytogenetic response by 3–6 months of therapy. Failure to do so is associated with worse event-free survival, transformation rates, and survival. However, the 3- to 5-year estimated survival among such patients is still high, around 80–90%, which is better than what would be anticipated if such patients were offered allogeneic SCT at that time. Thus, this adverse response to therapy is considered a warning signal, but it is not known whether changing therapy to other TKIs at that time would improve longer term outcome.

TREATMENT OF ACCELERATED AND BLASTIC PHASES

Patients in accelerated or blastic phase may receive therapy with TKIs, preferably second- or third-generation TKIs (dasatinib, nilotinib, bosutinib, ponatinib), alone or in combination with chemotherapy, to reduce the CML burden, before undergoing allogeneic SCT. Response rates with single-agent TKIs range from 30 to 50% in accelerated phase and from 20 to 30% in blastic phase. Cytogenetic responses, particularly complete cytogenetic responses, are uncommon (10–30%) and transient in blastic phase. Studies of TKIs in combination with chemotherapy are ongoing; the general experience suggests that combined TKI-chemotherapy strategies increase the response rates and their durability and improve survival. In CML lymphoid blastic phase, the combination of anti-ALL chemotherapy with TKIs results in complete response rates of 60–70% and median survival times of 2–3 years (compared with historical response rates of 40–50% and median survival times of 12–18 months). This allows many patients to undergo allogeneic SCT in a state of minimal CML burden or secondary chronic phase, which are associated with higher cure rates. In CML nonlymphoid blastic phase, anti-AML chemotherapy combined with TKIs results in CR rates of 30–50% and median survival times of 9–12 months (compared with historical response rates of 20–30% and median survival times of 3–5 months). In accelerated phase, response to single TKIs is significant in conditions where "softer" accelerated phase criteria are considered (e.g., clonal evolution alone, thrombocytosis alone, significant splenomegaly or resistance to hydroxyurea, but without evidence of high blast and basophil percentages). In accelerated phase, combinations usually include TKIs with low-intensity chemotherapy such as low-dose cytarabine, low-dose idarubicin, decitabine, interferon α, hydroxyurea, or others.

OTHER TREATMENTS AND SPECIAL THERAPEUTIC CONSIDERATIONS

Interferon α Interferon α was a standard of care before 2000. Today, it is considered in combination with TKIs (an investigational approach), sometimes after CML failure on TKIs, occasionally in patients during pregnancy, or as part of investigational strategies with TKIs to eradicate residual molecular disease.

Chemotherapeutic Agents Hydroxyurea and busulfan were commonly used chemotherapeutic agents in the past. Hydroxyurea remains a safe and effective agent (at daily doses of 0.5–10 g) to reduce initial CML burden, as a temporary measure in between definitive therapies, or in combination with TKIs to sustain complete hematologic or cytogenetic responses. Busulfan is often used in allogeneic SCT preparative regimens. Because of its side effects (delayed myelosuppression, Addison-like disease, pulmonary and cardiac fibrosis, myelofibrosis), it is now only rarely used in the chronic management of CML. Low-dose cytarabine, decitabine, anthracyclines, 6-mercaptopurine, 6-thioguanine, thiotepa, anagrelide, and other agents are useful in different CML settings to control the disease burden.

Others Splenectomy is occasionally considered to alleviate symptoms of massive splenomegaly and/or hypersplenism. Splenic irradiation is rarely used, if at all, because of the postirradiation adhesions and complications. Leukapheresis is rarely used in patients presenting with extreme leukocytosis and leukostatic complications. Single doses of high-dose cytarabine or high doses of hydroxyurea, with tumor lysis management, may be as effective and less cumbersome.

Special Considerations Women with CML who become pregnant should discontinue TKI therapy immediately. Among 125 babies delivered to women with CML who discontinued TKI therapy as soon as the pregnancy was known, three babies were born with ocular, skeletal, and renal malformations, suggesting the uncommon teratogenicity of imatinib. There are no or little data with other TKIs. Control of CML during pregnancy can be managed with leukapheresis for severe symptomatic leukocytosis in the first trimester and with hydroxyurea subsequently until delivery. There are case reports of successful pregnancies and deliveries of normal babies with interferon α therapy and registry studies in essential thrombocytosis of its safety, but interferon α can be antiangiogenic and may increase the risk of spontaneous abortions.

Patients on TKI therapy may develop chromosomal abnormalities in the Ph-negative cells. These may involve loss of chromosome Y, trisomy 8, 20q–, chromosome 5 or 7 abnormalities, and others. Most chromosomal abnormalities disappear spontaneously on follow-up and may be indicative of the genetic instability of the hematopoietic stem cells that predispose the patient to develop CML in the first place. Rarely, abnormalities involving chromosomes 5 or 7 may be truly clonal and evolve into myelodysplastic syndrome or acute myeloid leukemia. This is thought to be part of the natural course of patients in whom CML was suppressed and who live long enough to develop other hematologic malignancies.

GLOBAL ASPECTS OF CHRONIC MYELOID LEUKEMIA

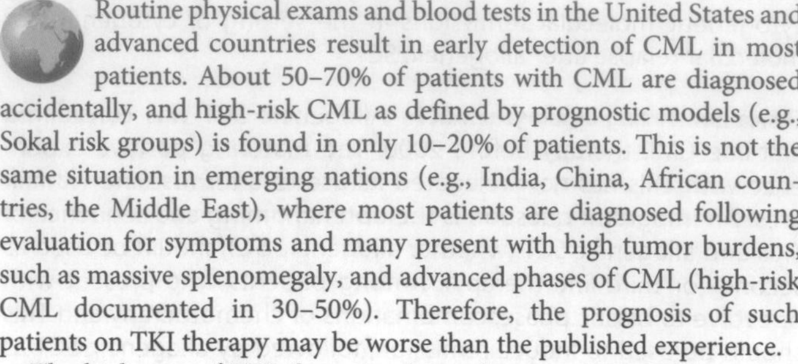

Routine physical exams and blood tests in the United States and advanced countries result in early detection of CML in most patients. About 50–70% of patients with CML are diagnosed accidentally, and high-risk CML as defined by prognostic models (e.g., Sokal risk groups) is found in only 10–20% of patients. This is not the same situation in emerging nations (e.g., India, China, African countries, the Middle East), where most patients are diagnosed following evaluation for symptoms and many present with high tumor burdens, such as massive splenomegaly, and advanced phases of CML (high-risk CML documented in 30–50%). Therefore, the prognosis of such patients on TKI therapy may be worse than the published experience.

The high cost of TKI therapies (annual costs of $90,000–$140,000 in the United States; lower but variable in the rest of the world) makes the general affordability of such treatments difficult. Although TKI treatment penetration is high in nations where cost of therapy is not an issue (e.g., Sweden, European Union), it may be less so in other nations, even in advanced ones like the United States, where out-of-pocket expenses may be prohibitive to a subset of patients (perhaps 10–20%). Based on the sales of imatinib worldwide and charity free drug supplies, it is estimated that less than 30% of patients are treated with imatinib (or other TKIs) consistently. Although the estimated 10-year survival in CML is 85% in single-institution studies (e.g., M.D. Anderson Cancer Center), in national studies in countries with TKI affordability (Sweden) (Figs. 133-2 and 133-3) or in company-sponsored studies (where all patients have access to TKIs throughout their care), the estimated 10-year survival worldwide, even 12 years after the introduction of TKI therapies, is likely to be less than 50%. The Surveillance, Epidemiology, and End Results (SEER) data from

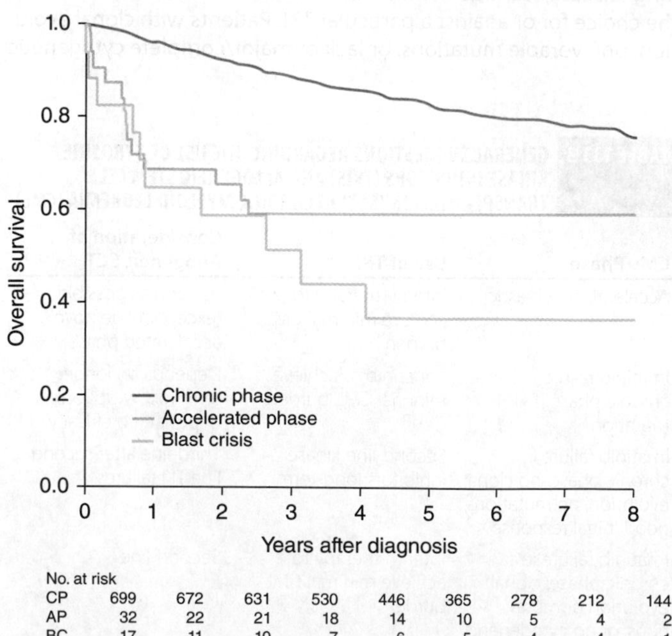

FIGURE 133-3 Survival in chronic (CP), accelerated (AP), and blastic crisis (BC) phases of chronic myeloid leukemia (CML) in the population-based Swedish national registry study. The accelerated- and blastic-phase cases are de novo presentations. The favorable outcome with de novo blastic phase may be due to use of 20% blasts or more to define blastic phase. *(With permission from Dr. Martin Hoglund, Swedish CML Registry, 2013.)*

the United States report an estimated 5-year survival rate of 60% in the era of TKIs.

The current high cost of TKI therapies poses two additional considerations. The first are the treatment pathways and guidelines in nations where TKIs may not be affordable by patients or the health care system. In these conditions, there are trends of pathways advocating frontline allogeneic SCT (a one-time cost of $30,000–$50,000) despite the associated mortality and morbidities. The second is the choice of frontline TKI therapy once imatinib becomes available in generic forms (hopefully at much lower annual prices, e.g., $2,000–$10,000). This will depend on the maturing data in randomized studies of second-generation TKIs versus imatinib in relation to important long-term outcome endpoints, particularly survival, but also event-free survival and transformation-free survival.

134 Malignancies of Lymphoid Cells

Dan L. Longo

Malignancies of lymphoid cells range from the most indolent to the most aggressive human malignancies. These cancers arise from cells of the immune system at different stages of differentiation, resulting in a wide range of morphologic, immunologic, and clinical findings. Insights on the normal immune system have allowed a better understanding of these sometimes confusing disorders.

Some malignancies of lymphoid cells almost always present as leukemia (i.e., primary involvement of bone marrow and blood), while others almost always present as lymphomas (i.e., solid tumors of the immune system). However, other malignancies of lymphoid cells can present as either leukemia or lymphoma. In addition, the clinical pattern can change over the course of the illness. This change is more often seen in a patient who seems to have a lymphoma and then develops the manifestations of leukemia over the course of the illness.

BIOLOGY OF LYMPHOID MALIGNANCIES: CONCEPTS OF THE WORLD HEALTH ORGANIZATION CLASSIFICATION OF LYMPHOID MALIGNANCIES

The classification of lymphoid cancers evolved steadily throughout the twentieth century. The distinction between leukemia and lymphoma was made early, and separate classification systems were developed for each. Leukemias were first divided into acute and chronic subtypes based on average survival. Chronic leukemias were easily subdivided into those of lymphoid or myeloid origin based on morphologic characteristics. However, a spectrum of diseases that were formerly all called *chronic lymphoid leukemia* has become apparent (Table 134-1). The acute leukemias were usually malignancies of blast cells with few identifying characteristics. When cytochemical stains became available, it was possible to divide these objectively into myeloid malignancies and acute leukemias of lymphoid cells. Acute leukemias of lymphoid cells have been subdivided based on morphologic characteristics by the French-American-British (FAB) group (Table 134-2). Using this system, lymphoid malignancies of small uniform blasts (e.g., typical childhood acute lymphoblastic leukemia) were called L1, lymphoid malignancies with larger and more variable size cells were called L2, and lymphoid malignancies of uniform cells with basophilic and sometimes vacuolated cytoplasm were called L3 (e.g., typical Burkitt's lymphoma cells). Acute leukemias of lymphoid cells have also been subdivided based on immunologic (i.e., T cell vs B cell) and cytogenetic abnormalities (Table 134-2). Major cytogenetic subgroups include the t(9;22) (e.g., Philadelphia chromosome–positive acute lymphoblastic leukemia) and the t(8;14) found in the L3 or Burkitt's leukemia.

TABLE 134-1 LYMPHOID DISORDERS THAT CAN PRESENT AS "CHRONIC LEUKEMIA" AND BE CONFUSED WITH TYPICAL B-CELL CHRONIC LYMPHOID LEUKEMIA

Follicular lymphoma	Prolymphocytic leukemia (B cell or T cell)
Splenic marginal zone lymphoma	Lymphoplasmacytic lymphoma
Nodal marginal zone lymphoma	Sézary's syndrome
Mantle cell lymphoma	Smoldering adult T-cell leukemia/lymphoma
Hairy cell leukemia	

TABLE 134-2 CLASSIFICATION OF ACUTE LYMPHOID LEUKEMIA (ALL)

Immunologic Subtype	% of Cases	FAB Subtype	Cytogenetic Abnormalities
Pre-B ALL	75	L1, L2	t(9;22), t(4;11), t(1;19)
T-cell ALL	20	L1, L2	14q11 or 7q34
B-cell ALL	5	L3	t(8;14), t(8;22), t(2;8)

Abbreviation: FAB, French-American-British classification.

Non-Hodgkin's lymphomas were separated from Hodgkin's lymphoma by recognition of the Sternberg-Reed cells early in the twentieth century. The histologic classification for non-Hodgkin's lymphomas has been one of the most contentious issues in oncology. Imperfect morphologic systems were supplanted by imperfect immunologic systems, and poor reproducibility of diagnosis has hampered progress. In 1999, the World Health Organization (WHO) classification of lymphoid malignancies was devised through a process of consensus development among international leaders in hematopathology and clinical oncology. The WHO classification takes into account morphologic, clinical, immunologic, and genetic information and attempts to divide non-Hodgkin's lymphomas and other lymphoid malignancies into clinical/pathologic entities that have clinical and therapeutic relevance. This system is presented in Table 134-3. This system is clinically relevant and has a higher degree of diagnostic accuracy than those used previously. The possibilities for subdividing lymphoid malignancies are extensive. However, Table 134-3 presents in bold those malignancies that occur in at least 1% of patients. Specific lymphoma subtypes will be dealt with in more detail below.

Lymphomas occurring in fewer than 1% of patients with lymphoproliferative diseases are discussed in Chap. 135e, and lymphomas associated with HIV infection are discussed in Chap. 226.

GENERAL ASPECTS OF LYMPHOID MALIGNANCIES

ETIOLOGY AND EPIDEMIOLOGY

The relative frequency of the various lymphoid malignancies is shown in Fig. 134-1. Chronic lymphoid leukemia (CLL) is the most prevalent form of leukemia in Western countries. It occurs most frequently in older adults and is exceedingly rare in children. In 2014, 15,720 new cases were diagnosed in the United States, but because of the prolonged survival associated with this disorder, the total prevalence is many times higher. CLL is more common in men than in women and more common in whites than in blacks. This is an uncommon malignancy in Asia. The etiologic factors for typical CLL are unknown.

In contrast to CLL, acute lymphoid leukemias (ALLs) are predominantly cancers of children and young adults. The L3 or Burkitt's leukemia occurring in children in developing countries seems to be associated with infection by the Epstein-Barr virus (EBV) in infancy. However, the explanation for the etiology of more common subtypes of ALL is much less certain. Childhood ALL occurs more often in higher socioeconomic subgroups. Children with trisomy 21 (Down's syndrome) have an increased risk for childhood ALL as well as acute myeloid leukemia (AML). Exposure to high-energy radiation in early childhood increases the risk of developing T-cell ALL.

The etiology of ALL in adults is also uncertain. ALL is unusual in middle-aged adults but increases in incidence in the elderly. However, AML is still much more common in older patients. Environmental exposures, including certain industrial exposures, exposure to agricultural chemicals, and smoking, might increase the risk of developing

TABLE 134-3 WHO CLASSIFICATION OF LYMPHOID MALIGNANCIES

B Cell	T Cell	Hodgkin's Lymphoma
Precursor B-cell neoplasm	Precursor T-cell neoplasm	Nodular lymphocyte-predominant Hodgkin's lymphoma
Precursor B lymphoblastic leukemia/lymphoma (precursor B-cell acute lymphoblastic leukemia) includes subtypes with recurrent genetic abnormalities	**Precursor T lymphoblastic lymphoma/leukemia (precursor T cell acute lymphoblastic leukemia)**	
Mature (peripheral) B-cell neoplasms	Mature (peripheral) T-cell neoplasms	Classical Hodgkin's lymphoma
B-cell chronic lymphocytic leukemia/small lymphocytic lymphoma	T-cell prolymphocytic leukemia	Nodular sclerosis classical Hodgkin's lymphoma
B-cell prolymphocytic leukemia	T-cell granular lymphocytic leukemia	Lymphocyte-rich classical Hodgkin's lymphoma
Lymphoplasmacytic lymphoma (Waldenström's macroglobulinemia)	Aggressive NK cell leukemia	Mixed-cellularity classical Hodgkin's lymphoma
Splenic marginal zone B-cell lymphoma (± villous lymphocytes)	Adult T-cell lymphoma/leukemia (HTLV-1+)	Lymphocyte-depletion classical Hodgkin's lymphoma
Hairy cell leukemia	Extranodal NK/T-cell lymphoma, nasal type	
Plasma cell myeloma/plasmacytoma	Enteropathy-type T-cell lymphoma	
Extranodal marginal zone B-cell lymphoma of MALT type	Hepatosplenic γδ T-cell lymphoma	
Mantle cell lymphoma	Subcutaneous panniculitis-like T-cell lymphoma	
Follicular lymphoma	Mycosis fungoides/Sézary's syndrome	
Nodal marginal zone B-cell lymphoma (± monocytoid B cells)	Anaplastic large cell lymphoma, primary cutaneous type	
Diffuse large B-cell lymphoma (including subtypes)	**Peripheral T-cell lymphoma, not otherwise specified (NOS)**	
Burkitt's lymphoma/Burkitt's cell leukemia	Angioimmunoblastic T-cell lymphoma	
Primary mediastinal large B-cell lymphoma	**Anaplastic large cell lymphoma, ALK+**	
Plasmablastic lymphoma	Primary cutaneous γδ T-cell lymphoma	
Primary effusion lymphoma		
Large B-cell lymphoma arising in HHV-8+ multicentric Castleman's disease		
Intravascular large B-cell lymphoma		
ALK+ large B-cell lymphoma		

Note: Malignancies in bold occur in at least 1% of patients.

Abbreviations: HHV, human herpesvirus; HTLV, human T-cell lymphotropic virus; MALT, mucosa-associated lymphoid tissue; NK, natural killer; WHO, World Health Organization.

Source: Adapted from SH Swerdlow et al: *WHO Classification of Tumours of Haematopoietic and Lymphoid Tissues*, 4th ed. World Health Organization, 2008.

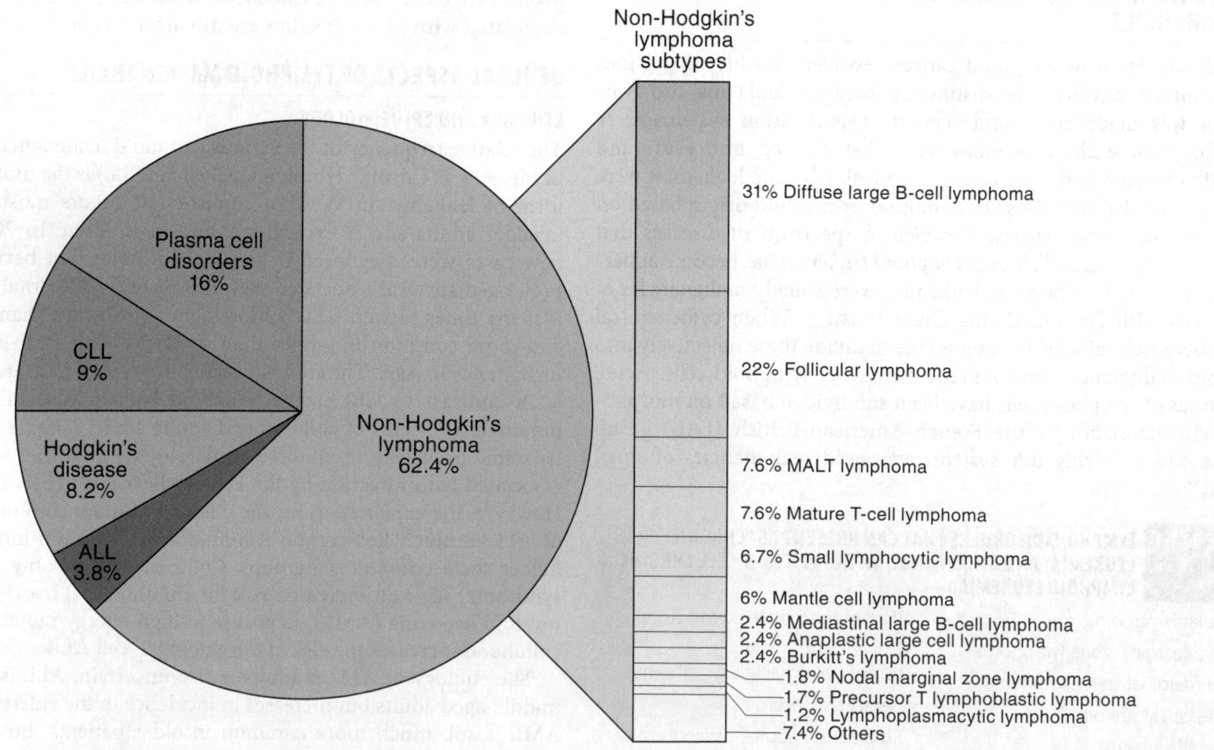

FIGURE 134-1 Relative frequency of lymphoid malignancies. ALL, acute lymphoid leukemia; CLL, chronic lymphoid leukemia; MALT, mucosa-associated lymphoid tissue.

ALL as an adult. ALL was diagnosed in 6020 persons and AML in 18,860 persons in the United States in 2014.

The preponderance of evidence suggests that Hodgkin's lymphoma is of B-cell origin. The incidence of Hodgkin's lymphoma appears fairly stable, with 9190 new cases diagnosed in 2014 in the United States. Hodgkin's lymphoma is more common in whites than in blacks and more common in males than in females. A bimodal distribution of age at diagnosis has been observed, with one peak incidence occurring in patients in their twenties and the other in those in their eighties. Some of the late age peak may be attributed to confusion among entities with similar appearance such as anaplastic large cell lymphoma and T-cell–rich B-cell lymphoma. Patients in the younger age groups diagnosed in the United States largely have the nodular sclerosing subtype of Hodgkin's lymphoma. Elderly patients, patients infected with HIV, and patients in Third World countries more commonly have mixed-cellularity Hodgkin's lymphoma or lymphocyte-depleted Hodgkin's lymphoma. Infection by HIV is a risk factor for developing Hodgkin's lymphoma. In addition, an association between infection by EBV and Hodgkin's lymphoma has been suggested. A monoclonal or oligoclonal proliferation of EBV-infected cells in 20–40% of the patients with Hodgkin's lymphoma has led to proposals for this virus having an etiologic role in Hodgkin's lymphoma. However, the matter is not settled definitively.

For unknown reasons, non-Hodgkin's lymphomas increased in frequency in the United States at the rate of 4% per year and increased 2–8% per year globally between 1950 and the late 1990s. The rate of increase in the past few years seems to be decreasing. About 70,800 new cases of non-Hodgkin's lymphoma were diagnosed in the United States in 2014 and nearly 360,000 cases worldwide. Non-Hodgkin's lymphomas are more frequent in the elderly and more frequent in men. Patients with both primary and secondary immunodeficiency states are predisposed to developing non-Hodgkin's lymphomas. These include patients with HIV infection; patients who have undergone organ transplantation; and patients with inherited immune deficiencies, the sicca syndrome, and rheumatoid arthritis.

The incidence of non-Hodgkin's lymphomas and the patterns of expression of the various subtypes differ geographically. T-cell lymphomas are more common in Asia than in Western countries, while certain subtypes of B-cell lymphomas such as follicular lymphoma are more common in Western countries. A specific subtype of non-Hodgkin's lymphoma known as the angiocentric nasal T/natural killer (NK) cell lymphoma has a striking geographic occurrence, being most frequent in Southern Asia and parts of Latin America. Another subtype of non-Hodgkin's lymphoma associated with infection by human T-cell lymphotropic virus (HTLV) 1 is seen particularly in southern Japan and the Caribbean (Chap. 225e).

A number of environmental factors have been implicated in the occurrence of non-Hodgkin's lymphoma, including infectious agents, chemical exposures, and medical treatments. Several studies have demonstrated an association between exposure to agricultural chemicals and an increased incidence of non-Hodgkin's lymphoma. Patients treated for Hodgkin's lymphoma can develop non-Hodgkin's lymphoma; it is unclear whether this is a consequence of the Hodgkin's lymphoma or its treatment. However, a number of non-Hodgkin's lymphomas are associated with infectious agents (Table 134-4). HTLV-1 infects T cells and leads directly to the development of adult T-cell lymphoma in a small percentage of infected patients. The cumulative lifetime risk of developing lymphoma in an infected patient is 2.5%. The virus is transmitted by infected lymphocytes ingested by nursing babies of infected mothers, bloodborne transmission, or sexually. The median age of patients with adult T-cell lymphoma is ~56 years, emphasizing the long latency. HTLV-1 is also the cause of tropical spastic paraparesis—a neurologic disorder that occurs somewhat more frequently than lymphoma and with shorter latency and usually from transfusion-transmitted virus (Chap. 225e).

EBV is associated with the development of Burkitt's lymphoma in Central Africa and the occurrence of aggressive non-Hodgkin's lymphomas in immunosuppressed patients in Western countries. The majority of primary central nervous system (CNS) lymphomas are associated with EBV. EBV infection is strongly associated with the occurrence of extranodal nasal T/NK cell lymphomas in Asia and South America. Infection with HIV predisposes to the development of aggressive, B-cell non-Hodgkin's lymphoma. This may be through overexpression of interleukin 6 by infected macrophages. Infection of the stomach by the bacterium *Helicobacter pylori* induces the development of gastric MALT (mucosa-associated lymphoid tissue) lymphomas. This association is supported by evidence that patients treated with antibiotics to eradicate *H. pylori* have regression of their MALT lymphoma. The bacterium does not transform lymphocytes to produce the lymphoma; instead, a vigorous immune response is made to the bacterium, and the chronic antigenic stimulation leads to the neoplasia. MALT lymphomas of the skin may be related to *Borrelia* sp. infections, those of the eyes to *Chlamydophila psittaci*, and those of the small intestine to *Campylobacter jejuni*.

TABLE 134-4 INFECTIOUS AGENTS ASSOCIATED WITH THE DEVELOPMENT OF LYMPHOID MALIGNANCIES

Infectious Agent	Lymphoid Malignancy
Epstein-Barr virus	Burkitt's lymphoma
	Post–organ transplant lymphoma
	Primary CNS diffuse large B-cell lymphoma
	Hodgkin's lymphoma
	Extranodal NK/T-cell lymphoma, nasal type
HTLV-1	Adult T-cell leukemia/lymphoma
HIV	Diffuse large B-cell lymphoma
	Burkitt's lymphoma
Hepatitis C virus	Lymphoplasmacytic lymphoma
Helicobacter pylori	Gastric MALT lymphoma
Human herpesvirus 8	Primary effusion lymphoma
	Multicentric Castleman's disease

Abbreviations: CNS, central nervous system; HIV, human immunodeficiency virus; HTLV, human T-cell lymphotropic virus; MALT, mucosa-associated lymphoid tissue; NK, natural killer.

Chronic hepatitis C virus infection has been associated with the development of lymphoplasmacytic lymphoma. Human herpesvirus 8 is associated with primary effusion lymphoma in HIV-infected persons and multicentric Castleman's disease, a diffuse lymphadenopathy associated with systemic symptoms of fever, malaise, and weight loss.

In addition to infectious agents, a number of other diseases or exposures may predispose to developing lymphoma (Table 134-5).

IMMUNOLOGY

All lymphoid cells are derived from a common hematopoietic progenitor that gives rise to lymphoid, myeloid, erythroid, monocyte, and megakaryocyte lineages. Through the ordered and sequential activation of a series of transcription factors, the cell first becomes committed to the lymphoid lineage and then gives rise to B and T cells. About 75% of all lymphoid leukemias and 90% of all lymphomas are of B-cell origin. A cell becomes committed to B-cell development when it begins to rearrange its immunoglobulin genes. The sequence of cellular changes,

TABLE 134-5 DISEASES OR EXPOSURES ASSOCIATED WITH INCREASED RISK OF DEVELOPMENT OF MALIGNANT LYMPHOMA

Inherited immunodeficiency disease	Autoimmune disease
Klinefelter's syndrome	Sjögren's syndrome
Chédiak-Higashi syndrome	Celiac sprue
Ataxia-telangiectasia syndrome	Rheumatoid arthritis and systemic lupus erythematosus
Wiskott-Aldrich syndrome	
Common variable immunodeficiency disease	Chemical or drug exposures
	Phenytoin
Acquired immunodeficiency diseases	Dioxin, phenoxy herbicides
Iatrogenic immunosuppression	Radiation
HIV-1 infection	Prior chemotherapy and radiation therapy
Acquired hypogammaglobulinemia	

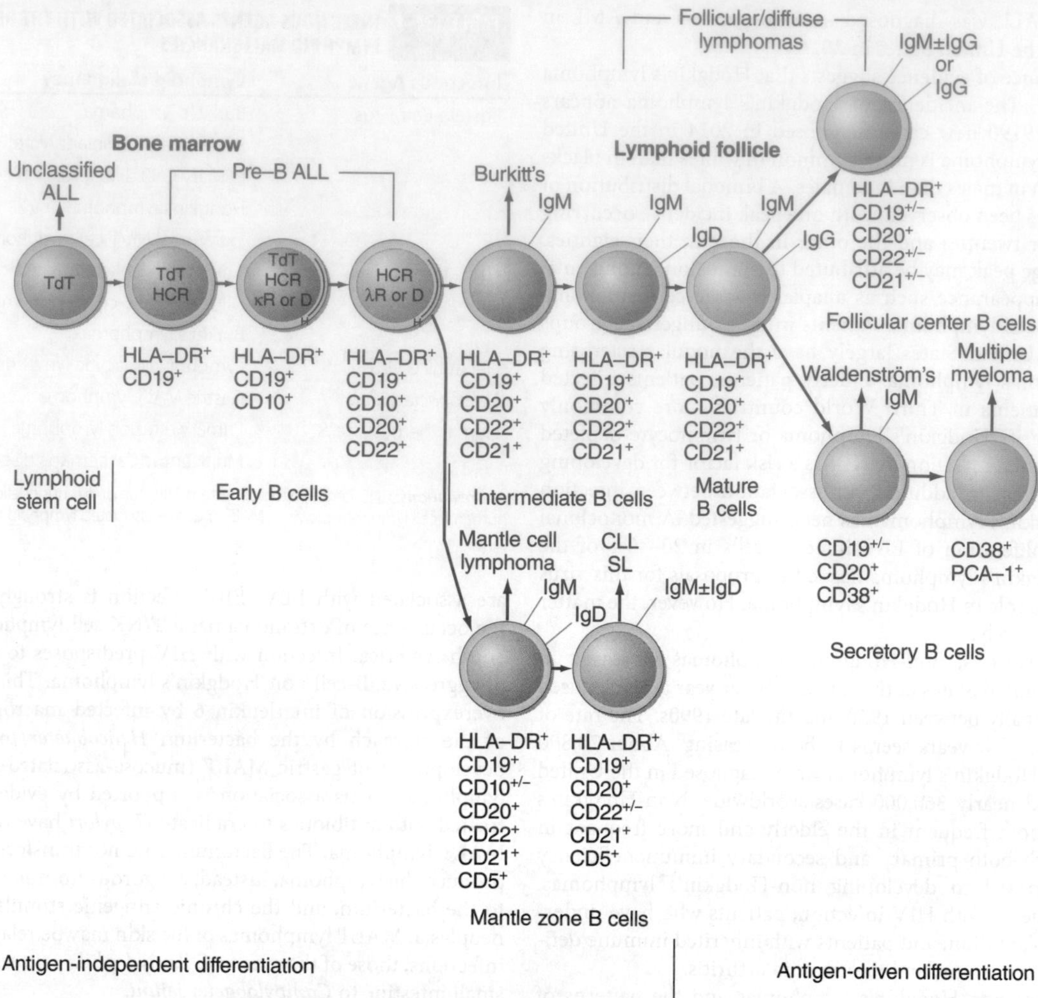

FIGURE 134-2 Pathway of normal B-cell differentiation and relationship to B-cell lymphomas. HLA-DR, CD10, CD19, CD20, CD21, CD22, CD5, and CD38 are cell markers used to distinguish stages of development. Terminal transferase (TdT) is a cellular enzyme. Immunoglobulin heavy chain gene rearrangement (HCR) and light chain gene rearrangement or deletion (κR or D, λR or D) occur early in B-cell development. The approximate normal stage of differentiation associated with particular lymphomas is shown. ALL, acute lymphoid leukemia; CLL, chronic lymphoid leukemia; SL, small lymphocytic lymphoma.

including changes in cell-surface phenotype, that characterizes normal B-cell development is shown in Fig. 134-2. A cell becomes committed to T-cell differentiation upon migration to the thymus and rearrangement of T-cell antigen receptor genes. The sequence of the events that characterize T-cell development is depicted in Fig. 134-3.

Although lymphoid malignancies often retain the cell-surface phenotype of lymphoid cells at particular stages of differentiation, this information is of little consequence. The so-called stage of differentiation of a malignant lymphoma does not predict its natural history. For example, the clinically most aggressive lymphoid leukemia is Burkitt's leukemia, which has the phenotype of a mature follicle center IgM-bearing B cell. Leukemias bearing the immunologic cell-surface phenotype of more primitive cells (e.g., pre-B ALL, CD10+) are less aggressive and more amenable to curative therapy than the "more mature" appearing Burkitt's leukemia cells. Furthermore, the apparent stage of differentiation of the malignant cell does not reflect the stage at which the genetic lesions that gave rise to the malignancy developed. For example, follicular lymphoma has the cell-surface phenotype of a follicle center cell, but its characteristic chromosomal translocation, the t(14;18), which involves juxtaposition of the antiapoptotic *bcl-2* gene next to the immunoglobulin heavy chain gene (see below), had to develop early in ontogeny as an error in the process of immunoglobulin gene rearrangement. Why the subsequent steps that led to transformation became manifest in a cell of follicle center differentiation is not clear.

The major value of cell-surface phenotyping is to aid in the differential diagnosis of lymphoid tumors that appear similar by light microscopy. For example, benign follicular hyperplasia may resemble follicular lymphoma; however, the demonstration that all the cells bear the same immunoglobulin light chain isotype strongly suggests the mass is a clonal proliferation rather than a polyclonal response to an exogenous stimulus.

Malignancies of lymphoid cells are associated with recurring genetic abnormalities. While specific genetic abnormalities have not been identified for all subtypes of lymphoid malignancies, it is presumed that they exist. Genetic abnormalities can be identified at a variety of levels including gross chromosomal changes (i.e., translocations, additions, or deletions); rearrangement of specific genes that may or may not be apparent from cytogenetic studies; and overexpression, underexpression, or mutation of specific oncogenes. Altered expression or mutation of specific proteins is particularly important. Many lymphomas contain balanced chromosomal translocations involving the antigen receptor genes; immunoglobulin genes on chromosomes 2, 14, and 22 in B cells; and T-cell antigen receptor genes on chromosomes 7 and 14 in T cells. The rearrangement of chromosome segments to generate mature antigen receptors must create a site of vulnerability to aberrant recombination. B cells are even more susceptible to acquiring mutations during their maturation in germinal centers; the generation of antibody of higher affinity requires the introduction of mutations into the variable region genes in the germinal centers. Other nonimmunoglobulin genes, e.g., *bcl-6*, may acquire mutations as well.

In the case of diffuse large B-cell lymphoma, the translocation t(14;18) occurs in ~30% of patients and leads to overexpression of the

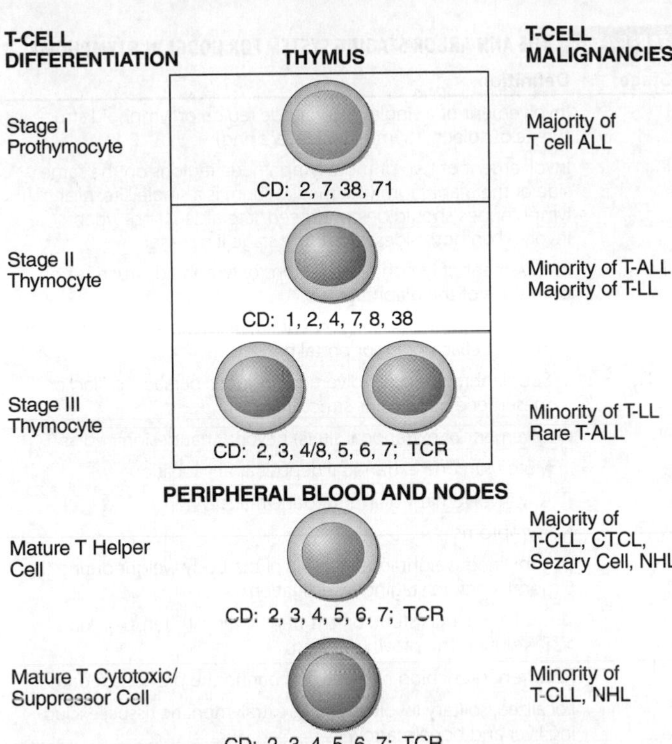

FIGURE 134-3 Pathway of normal T-cell differentiation and relationship to T-cell lymphomas. CD1, CD2, CD3, CD4, CD5, CD6, CD7, CD8, CD38, and CD71 are cell markers used to distinguish stages of development. T-cell antigen receptors (TCR) rearrange in the thymus, and mature T cells emigrate to nodes and peripheral blood. ALL, acute lymphoid leukemia; T-ALL, T-cell ALL; T-LL, T-cell lymphoblastic lymphoma; T-CLL, T-cell chronic lymphoid leukemia; CTCL, cutaneous T-cell lymphoma; NHL, non-Hodgkin's lymphoma.

bcl-2 gene found on chromosome 18. Some other patients without the translocation also overexpress the BCL-2 protein. This protein is involved in suppressing apoptosis—i.e., the mechanism of cell death most often induced by cytotoxic chemotherapeutic agents. A higher relapse rate has been observed in patients whose tumors overexpress the BCL-2 protein, but not in those patients whose lymphoma cells show only the translocation. Thus, particular genetic mechanisms have clinical ramifications.

Table 134-6 presents the most common translocations and associated oncogenes for various subtypes of lymphoid malignancies. In some cases, such as the association of the t(14;18) in follicular lymphoma, the t(2;5) in anaplastic large T/null cell lymphoma, the t(8;14) in Burkitt's lymphoma, and the t(11;14) in mantle cell lymphoma, the great majority of tumors in patients with these diagnoses display these abnormalities. In other types of lymphoma where a minority of the patients have tumors expressing specific genetic abnormalities, the defects may have prognostic significance. No specific genetic abnormalities have been identified in Hodgkin's lymphoma other than aneuploidy.

In typical B-cell CLL, trisomy 12 conveys a poorer prognosis. In ALL in both adults and children, genetic abnormalities have important prognostic significance. Patients whose tumor cells display the t(9;22) and translocations involving the *MLL* gene on chromosome 11q23 have a much poorer outlook than patients who do not have these translocations. Other genetic abnormalities that occur frequently in adults with ALL include the t(4;11) and the t(8;14). The t(4;11) is associated with younger age, female predominance, high white cell counts, and L1 morphology. The t(8;14) is associated with older age, male predominance, frequent CNS involvement, and L3 morphology. Both are associated with a poor prognosis. In childhood ALL, hyperdiploidy has been shown to have a favorable prognosis.

Gene profiling using array technology allows the simultaneous assessment of the expression of thousands of genes. This technology provides the possibility to identify new genes with pathologic importance in lymphomas, the identification of patterns of gene expression with diagnostic and/or prognostic significance, and the identification of new therapeutic targets. Recognition of patterns of gene expression is complicated and requires sophisticated mathematical techniques. Early successes using this technology in lymphoma include the identification of previously unrecognized subtypes of diffuse large B-cell lymphoma whose gene expression patterns resemble either those of follicular center B cells or activated peripheral blood B cells. Patients whose lymphomas have a germinal center B-cell pattern of gene expression have a considerably better prognosis than those whose lymphomas have a pattern resembling activated peripheral blood B cells. This improved prognosis is independent of other known prognostic factors. Similar information is being generated in follicular lymphoma and mantle cell lymphoma. The challenge remains to provide information from such techniques in a clinically useful time frame.

TABLE 134-6 CYTOGENETIC TRANSLOCATION AND ASSOCIATED ONCOGENES OFTEN SEEN IN LYMPHOID MALIGNANCIES

Disease	Cytogenetic Abnormality	Oncogene
CLL/small lymphocytic lymphoma	t(14;15)(q32;q13)	—
MALT lymphoma	t(11;18)(q21;q21)	*API2/MALT, BCL-10*
Precursor B-cell acute lymphoid leukemia	t(9;22)(q34;q11) or variant	*BCR/ABL*
	t(4;11)(q21;q23)	*AF4, MLLI*
	t(12;21)	*TEL, AML1*
Precursor acute lymphoid leukemia	t(9;22)	*BCR, ABL*
	t(1;19)	*E2A, PBX*
	t(17;19)	*HLF, E2A*
	t(5;14)	*HOX11L2, CTIP2*
Mantle cell lymphoma	t(11;14)(q13;q32)	*BCL-1, IgH*
Follicular lymphoma	t(14;18)(q32;q21)	*BCL-2, IgH*
Diffuse large cell lymphoma	t(3;-)(q27;-)[a]	*BCL-6*
	t(17;-)(p13;-)	*p53*
Burkitt's lymphoma, Burkitt's leukemia	t(8;-)(q24;-)[a]	*C-MYC*
CD30+ anaplastic large cell lymphoma	t(2;5)(p23;q35)	*ALK, NPM*
Lymphoplasmacytoid lymphoma	t(9;14)(p13;q32)	*PAX5, IgH*

[a]Numerous sites of translocation may be involved with these genes.

Abbreviations: CLL, chronic lymphoid leukemia; IgH, immunoglobulin heavy chain, MALT, mucosa-associated lymphoid tissue.

APPROACH TO THE PATIENT: Lymphoid Cell Malignancies

Regardless of the type of lymphoid malignancy, the initial evaluation of the patient should include performance of a careful history and physical examination. These will help confirm the diagnosis, identify those manifestations of the disease that might require prompt attention, and aid in the selection of further studies to optimally characterize the patient's status to allow the best choice of therapy. It is difficult to overemphasize the importance of a carefully done history and physical examination. They might provide observations that lead to reconsidering the diagnosis, provide hints at etiology, clarify the stage, and allow the physician to establish rapport with the patient that will make it possible to develop and carry out a therapeutic plan.

For patients with ALL, evaluation is usually completed after a complete blood count, chemistry studies reflecting major organ function, a bone marrow biopsy with genetic and immunologic studies, and a lumbar puncture. The latter is necessary to rule out occult CNS involvement. At this point, most patients would be ready to begin therapy. In ALL, prognosis is dependent on the genetic characteristics of the tumor, the patient's age, the white cell count, and the patient's overall clinical status and major organ function.

In CLL, the patient evaluation should include a complete blood count, chemistry tests to measure major organ function, serum protein electrophoresis, and a bone marrow biopsy. However, some physicians believe that the diagnosis would not always require a bone marrow biopsy. Patients often have imaging studies of the chest and abdomen looking for pathologic lymphadenopathy. Patients with typical B-cell CLL can be subdivided into three major prognostic groups. Those patients with only blood and bone marrow involvement by leukemia but no lymphadenopathy, organomegaly, or signs of bone marrow failure have the best prognosis. Those with lymphadenopathy and organomegaly have an intermediate prognosis, and patients with bone marrow failure, defined as hemoglobin <100 g/L (10 g/dL) or platelet count <100,000/μL, have the worst prognosis. The pathogenesis of the anemia or thrombocytopenia is important to discern. The prognosis is adversely affected when either or both of these abnormalities are due to progressive marrow infiltration and loss of productive marrow. However, either or both may be due to autoimmune phenomena or to hypersplenism that can develop during the course of the disease. These destructive mechanisms are usually completely reversible (glucocorticoids for autoimmune disease; splenectomy for hypersplenism) and do not influence disease prognosis.

Two popular staging systems have been developed to reflect these prognostic groupings (Table 134-7). Patients with typical B-cell CLL can have their course complicated by immunologic abnormalities, including autoimmune hemolytic anemia, autoimmune thrombocytopenia, and hypogammaglobulinemia. Patients with hypogammaglobulinemia benefit from regular (monthly) γ globulin administration. Because of expense, γ globulin is often withheld until the patient experiences a significant infection. These abnormalities do not have a clear prognostic significance and should not be used to assign a higher stage.

Two other features may be used to assess prognosis in B-cell CLL, but neither has yet been incorporated into a staging classification. At least two subsets of CLL have been identified based on the cytoplasmic expression of ZAP-70; expression of this protein, which is usually expressed in T cells, identifies a subgroup with poorer prognosis. A less powerful subsetting tool is CD38 expression. CD38+ tumors tend to have a poorer prognosis than CD38– tumors. A less easily measured feature, the presence of immunoglobulin variable region gene mutations, is also able to separate prognostic groups; patients with mutated immunoglobulin variable region genes respond better to treatment and have better survival than those with unmutated immunoglobulin variable region genes.

TABLE 134-7 STAGING OF TYPICAL B-CELL LYMPHOID LEUKEMIA

Stage	Clinical Features	Median Survival, Years
Rai System		
0: Low risk	Lymphocytosis only in blood and marrow	>10
I: Intermediate risk	Lymphocytosis + lymphadenopathy	7
II: Intermediate risk	Lymphocytosis + lymphadenopathy + splenomegaly ± hepatomegaly	
III: High risk	Lymphocytosis + anemia	1.5
IV: High risk	Lymphocytosis + thrombocytopenia	
Binet System		
A	Fewer than three areas of clinical lymphadenopathy; no anemia or thrombocytopenia	>10
B	Three or more involved node areas; no anemia or thrombocytopenia	7
C	Hemoglobin ≤10 g/dL and/or platelets <100,000/μL	2

TABLE 134-8 THE ANN ARBOR STAGING SYSTEM FOR HODGKIN'S LYMPHOMA

Stage	Definition
I	Involvement of a single lymph node region or lymphoid structure (e.g., spleen, thymus, Waldeyer's ring)
II	Involvement of two or more lymph node regions on the same side of the diaphragm (the mediastinum is a single site; hilar lymph nodes should be considered "lateralized" and, when involved on both sides, constitute stage II disease)
III	Involvement of lymph node regions or lymphoid structures on both sides of the diaphragm
III_1	Subdiaphragmatic involvement limited to spleen, splenic hilar nodes, celiac nodes, or portal nodes
III_2	Subdiaphragmatic involvement includes paraaortic, iliac, or mesenteric nodes plus structures in III_1
IV	Involvement of extranodal site(s) beyond that designated as "E"
	More than one extranodal deposit at any location
	Any involvement of liver or bone marrow
A	No symptoms
B	Unexplained weight loss of >10% of the body weight during the 6 months before staging investigation
	Unexplained, persistent, or recurrent fever with temperatures >38°C during the previous month
	Recurrent drenching night sweats during the previous month
E	Localized, solitary involvement of extralymphatic tissue, excluding liver and bone marrow

The initial evaluation of a patient with Hodgkin's lymphoma or non-Hodgkin's lymphoma is similar. In both situations, the determination of an accurate anatomic stage is an important part of the evaluation. Staging is done using the Ann Arbor staging system originally developed for Hodgkin's lymphoma (Table 134-8).

Evaluation of patients with Hodgkin's lymphoma will typically include a complete blood count; erythrocyte sedimentation rate; chemistry studies reflecting major organ function; computed tomography (CT) scans of the chest, abdomen, and pelvis; and a bone marrow biopsy. Neither a positron emission tomography (PET) scan nor a gallium scan is absolutely necessary for primary staging, but one performed at the completion of therapy allows evaluation of persisting radiographic abnormalities, particularly the mediastinum. Knowing that the PET scan or gallium scan is abnormal before treatment can help in this assessment. In most cases, these studies will allow assignment of anatomic stage and the development of a therapeutic plan.

In patients with non-Hodgkin's lymphoma, the same evaluation described for patients with Hodgkin's lymphoma is usually carried out. In addition, serum levels of lactate dehydrogenase (LDH) and β_2-microglobulin and serum protein electrophoresis are often included in the evaluation. Anatomic stage is assigned in the same manner as used for Hodgkin's lymphoma. However, the prognosis of patients with non-Hodgkin's lymphoma is best assigned using the International Prognostic Index (IPI) (Table 134-9). This is a powerful predictor of outcome in all subtypes of non-Hodgkin's lymphoma. Patients are assigned an IPI score based on the presence or absence of five adverse prognostic factors and may have none or all five of these adverse prognostic factors. Figure 134-4 shows the prognostic significance of this score in 1300 patients with all types of non-Hodgkin's lymphoma. With the addition of rituximab to CHOP (cyclophosphamide, doxorubicin, vincristine, and prednisone), treatment outcomes have improved and the original IPI has lost some of its discrimination power. A revised IPI has been proposed that better predicts outcome of rituximab plus chemotherapy-based programs (Table 134-9). CT scans are routinely used in the evaluation of patients with all subtypes of non-Hodgkin's lymphoma, but PET and

TABLE 134-9 INTERNATIONAL PROGNOSTIC INDEX FOR NON-HODGKIN'S LYMPHOMA

Five clinical risk factors:	
Age ≥60 years	
Serum lactate dehydrogenase levels elevated	
Performance status ≥2 (ECOG) or ≤70 (Karnofsky)	
Ann Arbor stage III or IV	
>1 site of extranodal involvement	
Patients are assigned a number for each risk factor they have	
Patients are grouped differently based on the type of lymphoma	
For diffuse large B-cell lymphoma:	
0, 1 factor = low risk:	35% of cases; 5-year survival, 73%
2 factors = low-intermediate risk:	27% of cases; 5-year survival, 51%
3 factors = high-intermediate risk:	22% of cases; 5-year survival, 43%
4, 5 factors = high risk:	16% of cases; 5-year survival, 26%
For diffuse large B-cell lymphoma treated with R-CHOP:	
0 factor = very good:	10% of cases; 5-year survival, 94%
1, 2 factors = good:	45% of cases; 5-year survival, 79%
3, 4, 5 factors = poor:	45% of cases; 5-year survival, 55%

Abbreviations: ECOG, Eastern Cooperative Oncology Group; R-CHOP, rituximab, cyclophosphamide, doxorubicin, vincristine, prednisone.

gallium scans are much more useful in aggressive subtypes such as diffuse large B-cell lymphoma than in more indolent subtypes such as follicular lymphoma or small lymphocytic lymphoma. Although the IPI does divide patients with follicular lymphoma into subsets with distinct prognoses, the distribution of such patients is skewed toward lower-risk categories. A follicular lymphoma–specific IPI (FLIPI) has been proposed that replaces performance status with hemoglobin level (<120 g/L [<12 g/dL]) and number of extranodal sites with number of nodal sites (more than four). Low risk (zero or one factor) was assigned to 36% of patients, intermediate risk (two factors) to 37%, and poor risk (more than two factors) to 27% of patients.

CLINICAL FEATURES, TREATMENT, AND PROGNOSIS OF SPECIFIC LYMPHOID MALIGNANCIES

PRECURSOR CELL B-CELL NEOPLASMS

Precursor B-Cell Lymphoblastic Leukemia/Lymphoma The most common cancer in childhood is B-cell ALL. Although this disorder can also present as a lymphoma in either adults or children, presentation as lymphoma is rare.

The malignant cells in patients with precursor B-cell lymphoblastic leukemia are most commonly of pre–B cell origin. Patients typically present with signs of bone marrow failure such as pallor, fatigue, bleeding, fever, and infection related to peripheral blood cytopenias. Peripheral blood counts regularly show anemia and thrombocytopenia but might show leukopenia, a normal leukocyte count, or leukocytosis based largely on the number of circulating malignant cells (Fig. 134-5). Extramedullary sites of disease are frequently involved in patients who present with leukemia, including lymphadenopathy, hepato- or splenomegaly, CNS disease, testicular enlargement, and/or cutaneous infiltration.

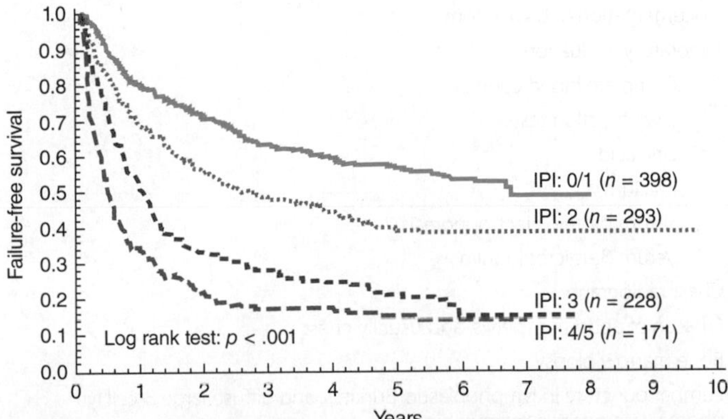

FIGURE 134-4 Relationship of International Prognostic Index (IPI) to survival. Kaplan-Meier survival curves for 1300 patients with various kinds of lymphoma stratified according to the IPI.

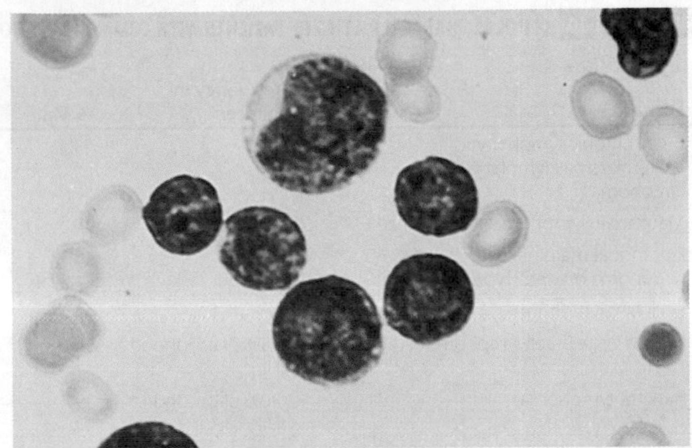

FIGURE 134-5 Acute lymphoblastic leukemia. The cells are heterogeneous in size and have round or convoluted nuclei, high nuclear/cytoplasmic ratio, and absence of cytoplasmic granules.

The diagnosis is usually made by bone marrow biopsy, which shows infiltration by malignant lymphoblasts. Demonstration of a pre–B cell immunophenotype (Fig. 134-2) and, often, characteristic cytogenetic abnormalities (Table 134-6) confirm the diagnosis. An adverse prognosis in patients with precursor B-cell ALL is predicted by a very high white cell count, the presence of symptomatic CNS disease, and unfavorable cytogenetic abnormalities. For example, t(9;22), frequently found in adults with B-cell ALL, has been associated with a very poor outlook. The bcr/abl kinase inhibitors have improved the prognosis.

TREATMENT PRECURSOR B-CELL LYMPHOBLASTIC LEUKEMIA

The treatment of patients with precursor B-cell ALL involves remission induction with combination chemotherapy, a consolidation phase that includes administration of high-dose systemic therapy and treatment to eliminate disease in the CNS, and a period of continuing therapy to prevent relapse and effect cure. The overall cure rate in children is 90%, whereas ~50% of adults are long-term disease-free survivors. This reflects the high proportion of adverse cytogenetic abnormalities seen in adults with precursor B-cell ALL.

Precursor B-cell lymphoblastic lymphoma is a rare presentation of precursor B-cell lymphoblastic malignancy. These patients often have a rapid transformation to leukemia and should be treated as though they had presented with leukemia. The few patients who present with the disease confined to lymph nodes have a high cure rate.

MATURE (PERIPHERAL) B-CELL NEOPLASMS

B-Cell Chronic Lymphoid Leukemia/Small Lymphocytic Lymphoma B-cell CLL/small lymphocytic lymphoma represents the most common lymphoid leukemia, and when presenting as a lymphoma, it accounts for ~7% of non-Hodgkin's lymphomas. Presentation can be as either leukemia or lymphoma. The major clinical characteristics of B-cell CLL/small lymphocytic lymphoma are presented in Table 134-10.

The diagnosis of typical B-cell CLL is made when an increased number of circulating lymphocytes (i.e., $>4 \times 10^9$/L and usually

TABLE 134-10 CLINICAL CHARACTERISTICS OF PATIENTS WITH COMMON TYPES OF NON-HODGKIN'S LYMPHOMA (NHL)

Disease	Median Age, Years	Frequency in Children	% Male	Stage I/II vs III/IV, %	B Symptoms, %	Bone Marrow Involvement, %	Gastrointestinal Tract Involvement, %	% Surviving 5 Years
B-cell chronic lymphocytic leukemia/small lymphocytic lymphoma	65	Rare	53	9 vs 91	33	72	3	51
Mantle cell lymphoma	63	Rare	74	20 vs 80	28	64	9	27
Extranodal marginal zone B-cell lymphoma of MALT type	60	Rare	48	67 vs 33	19	14	50	74
Follicular lymphoma	59	Rare	42	33 vs 67	28	42	4	72
Diffuse large B-cell lymphoma	64	~25% of childhood NHL	55	54 vs 46	33	16	18	46
Burkitt's lymphoma	31	~30% of childhood NHL	89	62 vs 38	22	33	11	45
Precursor T-cell lymphoblastic lymphoma	28	~40% of childhood NHL	64	11 vs 89	21	50	4	26
Anaplastic large T/null-cell lymphoma	34	Common	69	51 vs 49	53	13	9	77
Peripheral T-cell NHL	61	~5% of childhood NHL	55	20 vs 80	50	36	15	25

Abbreviation: MALT, mucosa-associated lymphoid tissue.

>10×10^9/L) is found (Fig. 134-6) that are monoclonal B cells expressing the CD5 antigen. Finding bone marrow infiltration by the same cells confirms the diagnosis. The peripheral blood smear in such patients typically shows many "smudge" or "basket" cells, nuclear remnants of cells damaged by the physical shear stress of making the blood smear. If cytogenetic studies are performed, trisomy 12 is found in 25–30% of patients. Abnormalities in chromosome 13 are also seen.

If the primary presentation is lymphadenopathy and a lymph node biopsy is performed, pathologists usually have little difficulty in making the diagnosis of small lymphocytic lymphoma based on morphologic findings and immunophenotype. However, even in these patients, 70–75% will be found to have bone marrow involvement and circulating monoclonal B lymphocytes are often present.

The differential diagnosis of typical B-cell CLL is extensive (Table 134-1). Immunophenotyping will eliminate the T-cell disorders and can often help sort out other B-cell malignancies. For example, only mantle cell lymphoma and typical B-cell CLL are usually CD5 positive. Typical B-cell small lymphocytic lymphoma can be confused with other B-cell disorders, including lymphoplasmacytic lymphoma (i.e., the tissue manifestation of Waldenström's macroglobulinemia), nodal marginal zone B-cell lymphoma, and mantle cell lymphoma. In addition, some small lymphocytic lymphomas have areas of large

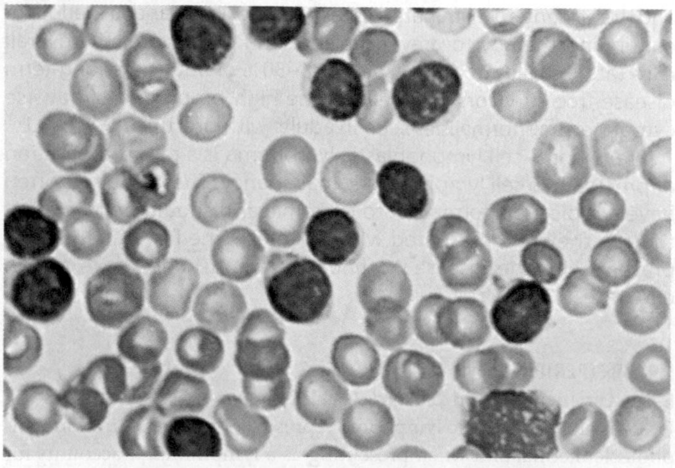

FIGURE 134-6 Chronic lymphocytic leukemia. The peripheral white blood cell count is high due to increased numbers of small, well-differentiated, normal-appearing lymphocytes. The leukemia lymphocytes are fragile, and substantial numbers of broken, smudged cells are usually also present on the blood smear.

cells that can lead to confusion with diffuse large B-cell lymphoma. An expert hematopathologist is vital for making this distinction.

Typical B-cell CLL is often found incidentally when a complete blood count is done for another reason. However, complaints that might lead to the diagnosis include fatigue, frequent infections, and new lymphadenopathy. The diagnosis of typical B-cell CLL should be considered in a patient presenting with an autoimmune hemolytic anemia or autoimmune thrombocytopenia. B-cell CLL has also been associated with red cell aplasia. When this disorder presents as lymphoma, the most common abnormality is asymptomatic lymphadenopathy, with or without splenomegaly. The staging systems predict prognosis in patients with typical B-cell CLL (Table 134-7). The evaluation of a new patient with typical B-cell CLL/small lymphocytic lymphoma will include many of the studies (Table 134-11) that are used in patients with other non-Hodgkin's lymphomas. In addition, particular attention needs to be given to detecting immune abnormalities such as autoimmune hemolytic anemia, autoimmune thrombocytopenia, hypogammaglobulinemia, and red cell aplasia. Molecular analysis of immunoglobulin gene sequences in CLL has demonstrated that about half the patients have tumors expressing mutated immunoglobulin genes and half have tumors expressing unmutated or germline immunoglobulin sequences. Patients with unmutated immunoglobulins tend to have a more aggressive clinical course and are less responsive to therapy. Unfortunately, immunoglobulin gene sequencing is not routinely available. CD38

TABLE 134-11 STAGING EVALUATION FOR NON-HODGKIN'S LYMPHOMA

- Physical examination
- Documentation of B symptoms
- Laboratory evaluation
  - Complete blood counts
  - Liver function tests
  - Uric acid
  - Calcium
  - Serum protein electrophoresis
  - Serum β_2-microglobulin
- Chest radiograph
- CT scan of abdomen, pelvis, and usually chest
- Bone marrow biopsy
- Lumbar puncture in lymphoblastic, Burkitt's, and diffuse large B-cell lymphoma with positive marrow biopsy
- Gallium scan (SPECT) or PET scan in large cell lymphoma

Abbreviations: CT, computed tomography; PET, positron emission tomography; SPECT, single-photon emission computed tomography.

expression is said to be low in the better-prognosis patients expressing mutated immunoglobulin and high in poorer-prognosis patients expressing unmutated immunoglobulin, but this test has not been confirmed as a reliable means of distinguishing the two groups. ZAP-70 expression correlates with the presence of unmutated immunoglobulin genes, but the assay is not yet standardized and widely available.

TREATMENT B-CELL CHRONIC LYMPHOID LEUKEMIA/ SMALL LYMPHOCYTIC LYMPHOMA

Patients whose presentation is typical B-cell CLL with no manifestations of the disease other than bone marrow involvement and lymphocytosis (i.e., Rai stage 0 and Binet stage A; Table 134-7) can be followed without specific therapy for their malignancy. These patients have a median survival >10 years, and some will never require therapy for this disorder. If the patient has an adequate number of circulating normal blood cells and is asymptomatic, many physicians would not initiate therapy for patients in the intermediate stage of the disease manifested by lymphadenopathy and/or hepatosplenomegaly. However, the median survival for these patients is ~7 years, and most will require treatment in the first few years of follow-up. Patients who present with bone marrow failure (i.e., Rai stage III or IV or Binet stage C) will require initial therapy in almost all cases. These patients have a serious disorder with a median survival of only 1.5 years. It must be remembered that immune manifestations of typical B-cell CLL should be managed independently of specific antileukemia therapy. For example, glucocorticoid therapy for autoimmune cytopenias and γ globulin replacement for patients with hypogammaglobulinemia should be used whether or not antileukemia therapy is given.

Patients who present primarily with lymphoma and have a low IPI score have a 5-year survival of ~75%, but those with a high IPI score have a 5-year survival of <40% and are more likely to require early therapy.

The most common treatments for patients with typical B-cell CLL/small lymphocytic lymphoma have been chlorambucil or fludarabine, alone or in combination. Chlorambucil can be administered orally with few immediate side effects, while fludarabine is administered IV and is associated with significant immune suppression. However, fludarabine is by far the more active agent and is the only drug associated with a significant incidence of complete remission. The combination of rituximab (375–500 mg/m^2 day 1), fludarabine (25 mg/m^2 days 2–4 on cycle 1 and days 1–3 in subsequent cycles), and cyclophosphamide (250 mg/m^2 with fludarabine) achieves complete responses in 69% of patients, and those responses are associated with molecular remissions in half of the cases. Half the patients experience grade III or IV neutropenia. For young patients presenting with leukemia requiring therapy, regimens containing fludarabine are the treatment of choice. Because fludarabine is an effective second-line agent in patients with tumors unresponsive to chlorambucil, the latter agent is often chosen in elderly patients who require therapy. Bendamustine, an alkylating agent structurally related to nitrogen mustard, is highly effective and is vying with fludarabine as the primary treatment of choice. Patients who present with lymphoma (rather than leukemia) are also highly responsive to bendamustine, and some patients will receive a combination chemotherapy regimen used in other lymphomas such as CVP (cyclophosphamide, vincristine, and prednisone) or CHOP plus rituximab. Alemtuzumab (anti-CD52) is an antibody with activity in the disease, but it kills both B and T cells and is associated with more immune compromise than rituximab. Young patients with this disease can be candidates for bone marrow transplantation. Allogeneic bone marrow transplantation can be curative but is associated with a significant treatment-related mortality rate. Mini-transplants using immunosuppressive rather than myeloablative doses of preparative drugs are being studied (Chap. 139e). The use of autologous transplantation in patients with this disorder has been discouraging.

At least two newer anti-CD20 monoclonal antibodies have become available, ofatumumab and obinutuzumab. Both have activity in previously treated patients. Agents targeting signaling pathways, such as ibrutinib, an irreversible inhibitor of Bruton's tyrosine kinase, and idelalisib, an inhibitor of phosphoinositide-3-kinase delta, also have antitumor effects. The ideal combination and sequence of these therapies have not been defined.

Extranodal Marginal Zone B-Cell Lymphoma of MALT Type Extranodal marginal zone B-cell lymphoma of MALT type (MALT lymphoma) makes up ~8% of non-Hodgkin's lymphomas. This small cell lymphoma presents in extranodal sites. It was previously considered a small lymphocytic lymphoma or sometimes a pseudolymphoma. The recognition that the gastric presentation of this lymphoma was associated with *H. pylori* infection was an important step in recognizing it as a separate entity. The clinical characteristics of MALT lymphoma are presented in Table 134-10.

The diagnosis of MALT lymphoma can be made accurately by an expert hematopathologist based on a characteristic pattern of infiltration of small lymphocytes that are monoclonal B cells and CD5 negative. In some cases, transformation to diffuse large B-cell lymphoma occurs, and both diagnoses may be made in the same biopsy. The differential diagnosis includes benign lymphocytic infiltration of extranodal organs and other small cell B-cell lymphomas.

MALT lymphoma may occur in the stomach, orbit, intestine, lung, thyroid, salivary gland, skin, soft tissues, bladder, kidney, and CNS. It may present as a new mass, be found on routine imaging studies, or be associated with local symptoms such as upper abdominal discomfort in gastric lymphoma. Most MALT lymphomas are gastric in origin. At least two genetic forms of gastric MALT exist: one (accounting for ~50% of cases) characterized by t(11;18)(q21;q21) that juxtaposes the amino terminal of the *API2* gene with the carboxy terminal of the *MALT1* gene creating an API2/MALT1 fusion product, and the other characterized by multiple sites of genetic instability including trisomies of chromosomes 3, 7, 12, and 18. About 95% of gastric MALT lymphomas are associated with *H. pylori* infection, and those that are do not usually express t(11;18). The t(11;18) usually results in activation of nuclear factor-κB (NF-κB), which acts as a survival factor for the cells. Lymphomas with t(11;18) translocations are genetically stable and do not evolve to diffuse large B-cell lymphoma. By contrast, t(11;18)-negative MALT lymphomas often acquire *BCL6* mutations and progress to aggressive histology lymphoma. MALT lymphomas are localized to the organ of origin in ~40% of cases and to the organ and regional lymph nodes in ~30% of patients. However, distant metastasis can occur—particularly with transformation to diffuse large B-cell lymphoma. Many patients who develop this lymphoma will have an autoimmune or inflammatory process such as Sjögren's syndrome (salivary gland MALT), Hashimoto's thyroiditis (thyroid MALT), *Helicobacter* gastritis (gastric MALT), *C. psittaci* conjunctivitis (ocular MALT), or *Borrelia* skin infections (cutaneous MALT).

Evaluation of patients with MALT lymphoma follows the pattern (Table 134-11) for staging a patient with non-Hodgkin's lymphoma. In particular, patients with gastric lymphoma need to have studies performed to document the presence or absence of *H. pylori* infection. Endoscopic studies including ultrasound can help define the extent of gastric involvement. Most patients with MALT lymphoma have a good prognosis, with a 5-year survival of ~75%. In patients with a low IPI score, the 5-year survival is ~90%, whereas it drops to ~40% in patients with a high IPI score.

TREATMENT MUCOSA-ASSOCIATED LYMPHOID TISSUE LYMPHOMA

MALT lymphoma is often localized. Patients with gastric MALT lymphomas who are infected with *H. pylori* can achieve remission in the 80% of cases with eradication of the infection. These remissions can be durable, but molecular evidence of persisting neoplasia is not infrequent. After *H. pylori* eradication, symptoms generally improve quickly, but molecular evidence of persistent disease may be present for 12–18 months. Additional therapy is not indicated unless progressive disease is documented. Patients with more extensive disease or progressive disease are most often treated with single-agent chemotherapy such as chlorambucil. Combination regimens that include rituximab are also highly effective. Coexistent diffuse large B-cell lymphoma must be treated with combination chemotherapy (see below). The additional acquired mutations that mediate the histologic progression also convey *Helicobacter* independence to the growth.

Mantle Cell Lymphoma Mantle cell lymphoma makes up ~6% of all non-Hodgkin's lymphomas. This lymphoma was previously placed in a number of other subtypes. Its existence was confirmed by the recognition that these lymphomas have a characteristic chromosomal translocation, t(11;14), between the immunoglobulin heavy chain gene on chromosome 14 and the *bcl-1* gene on chromosome 11, and regularly overexpress the BCL-1 protein, also known as cyclin D1. Table 134-10 shows the clinical characteristics of mantle cell lymphoma.

The diagnosis of mantle cell lymphoma can be made accurately by an expert hematopathologist. As with all subtypes of lymphoma, an adequate biopsy is important. The differential diagnosis of mantle cell lymphoma includes other small cell B-cell lymphomas. In particular, mantle cell lymphoma and small lymphocytic lymphoma share a characteristic expression of CD5. Mantle cell lymphoma usually has a slightly indented nucleus.

The most common presentation of mantle cell lymphoma is with palpable lymphadenopathy, frequently accompanied by systemic symptoms. The median age is 63 years, and men are affected four times as commonly as women. Approximately 70% of patients will be stage IV at the time of diagnosis, with frequent bone marrow and peripheral blood involvement. Of the extranodal organs that can be involved, gastrointestinal involvement is particularly important to recognize. Patients who present with lymphomatosis polyposis in the large intestine usually have mantle cell lymphoma. Table 134-11 outlines the evaluation of patients with mantle cell lymphoma. Patients who present with gastrointestinal tract involvement often have Waldeyer's ring involvement, and vice versa. The 5-year survival for all patients with mantle cell lymphoma is ~25%, with only occasional patients who present with a high IPI score surviving 5 years and ~50% of patients with a low IPI score surviving 5 years.

TREATMENT MANTLE CELL LYMPHOMA

Current therapies for mantle cell lymphoma are evolving. Patients with localized disease might be treated with combination chemotherapy followed by radiotherapy; however, these patients are exceedingly rare. For the usual presentation with disseminated disease, standard lymphoma treatments have been unsatisfactory, with the minority of patients achieving complete remission. Aggressive combination chemotherapy regimens followed by autologous or allogeneic bone marrow transplantation are frequently offered to younger patients. For the occasional elderly, asymptomatic patient, observation followed by single-agent chemotherapy might be the most practical approach. An intensive combination chemotherapy regimen originally used in the treatment of acute leukemia, HyperC-VAD (cyclophosphamide, vincristine, doxorubicin, dexamethasone, cytarabine, and methotrexate), in combination with rituximab, seems to be associated with better response rates, particularly in younger patients. Alternating two regimens, HyperC-VAD with rituximab added (R-HyperC-VAD) and rituximab plus high-dose methotrexate and cytarabine, can achieve complete responses in >80% of patients and an 8-year survival of 56%, comparable to regimens using high-dose therapy and autologous hematopoietic stem cell transplantation. Bendamustine plus rituximab has been found to induce complete responses in about 31% of patients, but the responses are generally not long lasting. Bortezomib and temsirolimus are single agents that induce transient partial responses in a minority of patients and are being added to primary combinations.

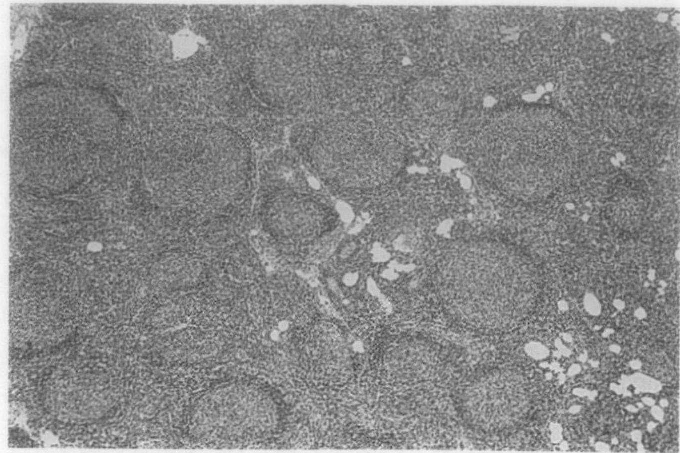

FIGURE 134-7 Follicular lymphoma. The normal nodal architecture is effaced by nodular expansions of tumor cells. Nodules vary in size and contain predominantly small lymphocytes with cleaved nuclei along with variable numbers of larger cells with vesicular chromatin and prominent nucleoli.

Follicular Lymphoma Follicular lymphomas make up 22% of non-Hodgkin's lymphomas worldwide and at least 30% of non-Hodgkin's lymphomas diagnosed in the United States. This type of lymphoma can be diagnosed accurately on morphologic findings alone and has been the diagnosis in the majority of patients in therapeutic trials for "low-grade" lymphoma in the past. The clinical characteristics of follicular lymphoma are presented in Table 134-10.

Evaluation of an adequate biopsy by an expert hematopathologist is sufficient to make a diagnosis of follicular lymphoma. The tumor is composed of small cleaved and large cells in varying proportions organized in a follicular pattern of growth (Fig. 134-7). Confirmation of B-cell immunophenotype and the existence of the t(14;18) and abnormal expression of BCL-2 protein are confirmatory. The major differential diagnosis is between lymphoma and reactive follicular hyperplasia. The coexistence of diffuse large B-cell lymphoma must be considered. Patients with follicular lymphoma are often subclassified into those with predominantly small cells, those with a mixture of small and large cells, and those with predominantly large cells. Although this distinction cannot be made simply or very accurately, these subdivisions do have prognostic significance. Patients with follicular lymphoma with predominantly large cells have a higher proliferative fraction, progress more rapidly, and have a shorter overall survival with simple chemotherapy regimens.

The most common presentation for follicular lymphoma is with new, painless lymphadenopathy. Multiple sites of lymphoid involvement are typical, and unusual sites such as epitrochlear nodes are sometimes seen. However, essentially any organ can be involved, and extranodal presentations do occur. Most patients do not have fevers, sweats, or weight loss, and an IPI score of 0 or 1 is found in ~50% of patients. Fewer than 10% of patients have a high (i.e., 4 or 5) IPI score. The staging evaluation for patients with follicular lymphoma should include the studies shown in Table 134-11.

TREATMENT FOLLICULAR LYMPHOMA

Follicular lymphoma is one of the malignancies most responsive to chemotherapy and radiotherapy. In addition, tumors in as many as 25% of the patients undergo spontaneous regression—usually transient—without therapy. In an asymptomatic patient, no initial treatment and watchful waiting can be an appropriate management strategy and is particularly likely to be adopted for older patients with advanced-stage disease. For patients who do require treatment, single-agent chlorambucil or cyclophosphamide or combination chemotherapy with CVP or CHOP is most frequently used. With adequate treatment, 50–75% of patients will achieve a complete remission. Although most patients relapse (median response duration is ~2 years), at least 20% of complete responders will remain in remission for >10 years. For the rare patients (15%) with localized follicular lymphoma, involved-field radiotherapy produces long-term disease-free survival in the majority.

A number of therapies have been shown to be active in the treatment of patients with follicular lymphoma. These include cytotoxic agents such as fludarabine, biologic agents such as interferon α, monoclonal antibodies with or without radionuclides, and lymphoma vaccines. In patients treated with a doxorubicin-containing combination chemotherapy regimen, interferon α given to patients in complete remission seems to prolong survival, but interferon toxicities can affect quality of life. The monoclonal antibody rituximab can cause objective responses in 35–50% of patients with relapsed follicular lymphoma, and radiolabeled antibodies appear to have response rates well in excess of 50%. The addition of rituximab to CHOP and other effective combination chemotherapy programs achieves prolonged overall survival and a decreased risk of histologic progression. Complete remissions can be noted in 85% or more of patients treated with R-CHOP, and median remission durations can exceed 6 or 7 years. Maintenance intermittent rituximab therapy can prolong remissions even further, although it is not completely clear that overall survival is prolonged. Some trials with tumor vaccines have been encouraging. Both autologous and allogeneic hematopoietic stem cell transplantations yield high complete response rates in patients with relapsed follicular lymphoma, and long-term remissions can occur in 40% or more of patients.

Patients with follicular lymphoma with a predominance of large cells have a shorter survival when treated with single-agent chemotherapy but seem to benefit from receiving an anthracycline-containing combination chemotherapy regimen plus rituximab. When their disease is treated aggressively, the overall survival for such patients is no lower than for patients with other follicular lymphomas, and the failure-free survival is superior.

Patients with follicular lymphoma have a high rate of histologic transformation to diffuse large B-cell lymphoma (5–7% per year). This is recognized ~40% of the time during the course of the illness by repeat biopsy and is present in almost all patients at autopsy. This transformation is usually heralded by rapid growth of lymph nodes—often localized—and the development of systemic symptoms such as fevers, sweats, and weight loss. Although these patients have a poor prognosis, aggressive combination chemotherapy regimens can sometimes cause a complete remission in the diffuse large B-cell lymphoma, at times leaving the patient with persisting follicular lymphoma. With more frequent use of R-CHOP to treat follicular lymphoma at diagnosis, it appears that the rate of histologic progression is decreasing. R-CHOP or bendamustine plus rituximab with intermittent rituximab maintenance for 2 years are the most commonly used treatment approaches.

Diffuse Large B-Cell Lymphoma Diffuse large B-cell lymphoma is the most common type of non-Hodgkin's lymphoma, representing approximately one-third of all cases. This lymphoma makes up the majority of cases in previous clinical trials of "aggressive" or "intermediate-grade" lymphoma. Table 134-10 shows the clinical characteristics of diffuse large B-cell lymphoma.

The diagnosis of diffuse large B-cell lymphoma can be made accurately by an expert hematopathologist (Fig. 134-8). Cytogenetic and molecular genetic studies are not necessary for diagnosis, but some evidence has accumulated that patients whose tumors overexpress the BCL-2 protein might be more likely to relapse than others. A subset of patients have tumors with mutations in *BCL6* and translocations involving *MYC*; these are called "double-hit" lymphomas and typically have more aggressive growth and are more poorly responsive to treatment than other diffuse large B-cell lymphomas. Patients with prominent mediastinal involvement are sometimes diagnosed as a separate subgroup having primary mediastinal diffuse large B-cell lymphoma. This latter group of patients has a younger median age (i.e., 37 years) and a female predominance (66%). Subtypes of diffuse large B-cell lymphoma, including those with an immunoblastic subtype and tumors with extensive fibrosis, are recognized by pathologists but do not appear to have important independent prognostic significance.

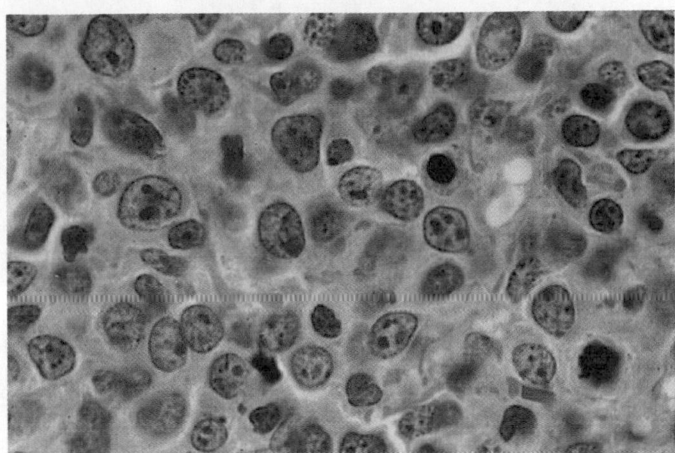

FIGURE 134-8 Diffuse large B-cell lymphoma. The neoplastic cells are heterogeneous but predominantly large cells with vesicular chromatin and prominent nucleoli.

Diffuse large B-cell lymphoma can present as either primary lymph node disease or at extranodal sites. More than 50% of patients will have some site of extranodal involvement at diagnosis, with the most common sites being the gastrointestinal tract and bone marrow, each being involved in 15–20% of patients. Essentially any organ can be involved, making a diagnostic biopsy imperative. For example, diffuse large B-cell lymphoma of the pancreas has a much better prognosis than pancreatic carcinoma but would be missed without biopsy. Primary diffuse large B-cell lymphoma of the brain is being diagnosed with increasing frequency. Other unusual subtypes of diffuse large B-cell lymphoma such as pleural effusion lymphoma and intravascular lymphoma have been difficult to diagnose and associated with a very poor prognosis.

Table 134-11 shows the initial evaluation of patients with diffuse large B-cell lymphoma. After a careful staging evaluation, ~50% of patients will be found to have stage I or II disease, and ~50% will have widely disseminated lymphoma. Bone marrow biopsy shows involvement by lymphoma in ~15% of cases, with marrow involvement by small cells more frequent than by large cells.

TREATMENT DIFFUSE LARGE B-CELL LYMPHOMA

The initial treatment of all patients with diffuse large B-cell lymphoma should be with a combination chemotherapy regimen. The most popular regimen in the United States is CHOP plus rituximab, although a variety of other anthracycline-containing combination chemotherapy regimens appear to be equally efficacious. Patients with stage I or nonbulky stage II disease can be effectively treated with three to four cycles of combination chemotherapy with or without subsequent involved-field radiotherapy. The need for radiation therapy is unclear. Cure rates of 70–80% in stage II disease and 85–90% in stage I disease can be expected.

For patients with bulky stage II, stage III, or stage IV disease, six to eight cycles of CHOP plus rituximab are usually administered. A large randomized trial showed the superiority of CHOP combined with rituximab over CHOP alone in elderly patients. A frequent approach would be to administer four cycles of therapy and then reevaluate. If the patient has achieved a complete remission after four cycles, two more cycles of treatment might be given and then therapy discontinued. Using this approach, 70–80% of patients can be expected to achieve a complete remission, and 50–70% of complete responders will be cured. The chances for a favorable response to treatment are predicted by the IPI. In fact, the IPI was developed based on the outcome of patients with diffuse large B-cell lymphoma treated with CHOP-like regimens. For the 35% of patients with a low IPI score of 0–1, the 5-year survival is >70%, whereas for the 20% of patients with a high IPI score of 4–5, the 5-year survival is ~20%. The addition of rituximab to CHOP has improved each of those numbers by ~15%. A number of other factors, including molecular features of the tumor, levels of circulating cytokines and soluble receptors, and other surrogate markers, have been shown to influence prognosis. However, they have not been validated as rigorously as the IPI and have not been uniformly applied clinically.

Because a number of patients with diffuse large B-cell lymphoma are either initially refractory to therapy or relapse after apparently effective chemotherapy, 30–40% of patients will be candidates for salvage treatment at some point. Alternative combination chemotherapy regimens can induce complete remission in as many as 50% of these patients, but long-term disease-free survival is seen in ≤10%. Autologous bone marrow transplantation is superior to salvage chemotherapy at usual doses and leads to long-term disease-free survival in ~40% of patients whose lymphomas remain chemotherapy-sensitive after relapse.

Burkitt's Lymphoma/Leukemia Burkitt's lymphoma/leukemia is a rare disease in adults in the United States, making up <1% of non-Hodgkin's lymphomas, but it makes up ~30% of childhood non-Hodgkin's lymphoma. Burkitt's leukemia, or L3 ALL, makes up a small proportion of childhood and adult acute leukemias. Table 134-10 shows the clinical features of Burkitt's lymphoma.

Burkitt's lymphoma can be diagnosed morphologically by an expert hematopathologist with a high degree of accuracy. The cells are homogeneous in size and shape (Fig. 134-9). Demonstration of a very high proliferative fraction and the presence of the t(8;14) or one of its variants, t(2;8) (*c-myc* and the λ light chain gene) or t(8;22) (*c-myc* and the κ light chain gene), can be confirmatory. Burkitt's cell leukemia is recognized by the typical monotonous mass of medium-sized cells with round nuclei, multiple nucleoli, and basophilic cytoplasm with cytoplasmic vacuoles. Demonstration of surface expression of immunoglobulin and one of the above-noted cytogenetic abnormalities is confirmatory.

Three distinct clinical forms of Burkitt's lymphoma are recognized: endemic, sporadic, and immunodeficiency-associated. Endemic and sporadic Burkitt's lymphomas occur frequently in children in Africa, and the sporadic form occurs in Western countries. Immunodeficiency-associated Burkitt's lymphoma is seen in patients with HIV infection.

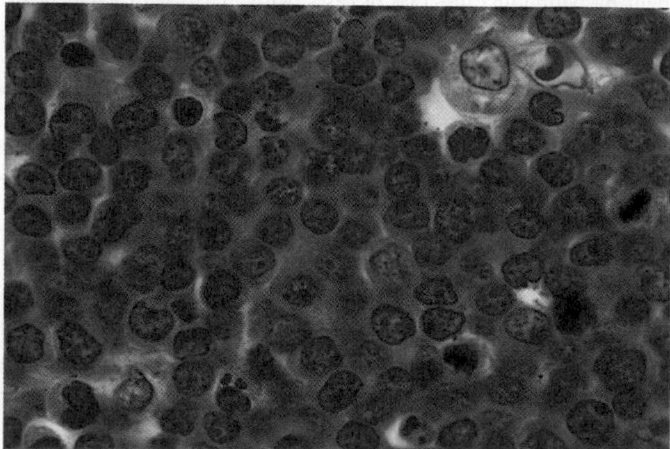

FIGURE 134-9 Burkitt's lymphoma. The neoplastic cells are homogeneous, medium-sized B cells with frequent mitotic figures, a morphologic correlate of high growth fraction. Reactive macrophages are scattered through the tumor, and their pale cytoplasm in a background of blue-staining tumor cells gives the tumor a so-called starry sky appearance.

Pathologists sometimes have difficulty distinguishing between Burkitt's lymphoma and diffuse large B-cell lymphoma. In the past, a separate subgroup of non-Hodgkin's lymphoma intermediate between the two was recognized. When tested, this subgroup could not be diagnosed accurately. Distinction between the two major types of B-cell aggressive non-Hodgkin's lymphoma can sometimes be made based on the extremely high proliferative fraction seen in patients with Burkitt's lymphoma (i.e., essentially 100% of tumor cells are in cycle) caused by *c-myc* deregulation.

Most patients in the United States with Burkitt's lymphoma present with peripheral lymphadenopathy or an intraabdominal mass. The disease is rapidly progressive and has a propensity to metastasize to the CNS. Initial evaluation should always include an examination of cerebrospinal fluid to rule out metastasis in addition to the other staging evaluations noted in Table 134-11. Once the diagnosis of Burkitt's lymphoma is suspected, a diagnosis must be made promptly, and staging evaluation must be accomplished expeditiously. This is the most rapidly progressive human tumor, and any delay in initiating therapy can adversely affect the patient's prognosis.

TREATMENT BURKITT'S LYMPHOMA

Treatment of Burkitt's lymphoma in both children and adults should begin within 48 h of diagnosis and involves the use of intensive combination chemotherapy regimens incorporating high doses of cyclophosphamide. Prophylactic therapy to the CNS is mandatory. Burkitt's lymphoma was one of the first cancers shown to be curable by chemotherapy. Today, cure can be expected in 70–80% of both children and young adults when effective therapy is administered precisely. Salvage therapy has been generally ineffective in patients in whom the initial treatment fails, emphasizing the importance of the initial treatment approach.

Other B-Cell Lymphoid Malignancies *B-cell prolymphocytic leukemia* involves blood and marrow infiltration by large lymphocytes with prominent nucleoli. Patients typically have a high white cell count, splenomegaly, and minimal lymphadenopathy. The chances for a complete response to therapy are poor.

Hairy cell leukemia is a rare disease that presents predominantly in older males. Typical presentation involves pancytopenia, although occasional patients will have a leukemic presentation. Splenomegaly is usual. The malignant cells appear to have "hairy" projections on light and electron microscopy and show a characteristic staining pattern with tartrate-resistant acid phosphatase. Bone marrow is typically not able to be aspirated, and biopsy shows a pattern of fibrosis with diffuse infiltration by the malignant cells. Patients with this disorder have monocytopenia and are prone to unusual infections, including infection by *Mycobacterium avium intracellulare*, and to vasculitic syndromes. Hairy cell leukemia is responsive to chemotherapy with interferon α, pentostatin, or cladribine, with the latter being the usually preferred treatment. Clinical complete remissions with cladribine occur in the majority of patients, and long-term disease-free survival is frequent. Many of these tumors have the V600E *BRAF* mutation and accordingly are responsive to BRAF inhibitors like vemurafenib.

Splenic marginal zone lymphoma involves infiltration of the splenic white pulp by small, monoclonal B cells. This is a rare disorder that can present as leukemia as well as lymphoma. Definitive diagnosis is often made at splenectomy, which is also an effective therapy. This is an extremely indolent disorder, but when chemotherapy is required, the most usual treatment has been chlorambucil.

Lymphoplasmacytic lymphoma is the tissue manifestation of Waldenström's macroglobulinemia (Chap. 136). Many of these tumors harbor a specific mutation, L265P, in *MYD88*, a change that leads to NF-κB activation. This type of lymphoma has been associated with chronic hepatitis C virus infection, and an etiologic association has been proposed. Patients typically present with lymphadenopathy, splenomegaly, bone marrow involvement, and occasionally peripheral blood involvement. The tumor cells do not express CD5. Patients often have a monoclonal IgM protein, high levels of which can dominate the clinical picture with the symptoms of hyperviscosity. Treatment of lymphoplasmacytic lymphoma can be aimed primarily at reducing the abnormal protein, if present, but will usually also involve chemotherapy. Chlorambucil, fludarabine, and cladribine have been used. The median 5-year survival for patients with this disorder is ~60%.

Nodal marginal zone lymphoma, also known as *monocytoid cell lymphoma*, represents ~1% of non-Hodgkin's lymphomas. This lymphoma has a slight female predominance and presents with disseminated disease (i.e., stage III or IV) in 75% of patients. Approximately one-third of patients have bone marrow involvement, and a leukemic presentation occasionally occurs. The staging evaluation and therapy should use the same approach as used for patients with follicular lymphoma. Approximately 60% of the patients with nodal marginal zone lymphoma will survive 5 years after diagnosis.

Other more uncommon B-cell malignancies are discussed in Chap. 135e.

PRECURSOR T-CELL MALIGNANCIES

Precursor T-Cell Lymphoblastic Leukemia/Lymphoma Precursor T-cell malignancies can present either as ALL or as an aggressive lymphoma. These malignancies are more common in children and young adults, with males more frequently affected than females.

Precursor T-cell ALL can present with bone marrow failure, although the severity of anemia, neutropenia, and thrombocytopenia is often less than in precursor B cell ALL. These patients sometimes have very high white cell counts, a mediastinal mass, lymphadenopathy, and hepatosplenomegaly. Precursor T-cell lymphoblastic lymphoma is most often found in young men presenting with a large mediastinal mass and pleural effusions. Both presentations have a propensity to metastasize to the CNS, and CNS involvement is often present at diagnosis.

TREATMENT PRECURSOR T-CELL LYMPHOBLASTIC LEUKEMIA/LYMPHOMA

Children with precursor T-cell ALL seem to benefit from very intensive remission induction and consolidation regimens. The majority of patients treated in this manner can be cured. Older children and young adults with precursor T-cell lymphoblastic lymphoma are also often treated with "leukemia-like" regimens. Patients who present with localized disease have an excellent prognosis. However, advanced age is an adverse prognostic factor. Adults with precursor T-cell lymphoblastic lymphoma who present with high LDH levels or bone marrow or CNS Involvement are often offered bone marrow transplantation as part of their primary therapy.

MATURE (PERIPHERAL) T-CELL DISORDERS

Mycosis Fungoides Mycosis fungoides is also known as *cutaneous T-cell lymphoma*. This lymphoma is more often seen by dermatologists than internists. The median age of onset is in the mid-fifties, and the disease is more common in males and in blacks.

Mycosis fungoides is an indolent lymphoma with patients often having several years of eczematous or dermatitic skin lesions before the diagnosis is finally established. The skin lesions progress from patch stage to plaque stage to cutaneous tumors. Early in the disease, biopsies are often difficult to interpret, and the diagnosis may only become apparent by observing the patient over time. In advanced stages, the lymphoma can spread to lymph nodes and visceral organs. Patients with this lymphoma may develop generalized erythroderma and circulating tumor cells, called *Sézary's syndrome*.

Rare patients with localized early-stage mycosis fungoides can be cured with radiotherapy, often total-skin electron beam irradiation. More advanced disease has been treated with topical glucocorticoids, topical nitrogen mustard, phototherapy, psoralen with ultraviolet A (PUVA), extracorporeal photopheresis, retinoids (bexarotene), electron beam radiation, interferon, antibodies, fusion toxins, histone deacetylase inhibitors, and systemic cytotoxic therapy. Unfortunately, these treatments are palliative.

Adult T-Cell Lymphoma/Leukemia Adult T-cell lymphoma/leukemia is one manifestation of infection by the HTLV-1 retrovirus. Patients can be infected through transplacental transmission, mother's milk, blood transfusion, and by sexual transmission of the virus. Patients who acquire the virus from their mother through breast milk are most likely to develop lymphoma, but the risk is still only 2.5% and the latency averages 55 years. Nationwide testing for HTLV-1 antibodies and the aggressive implementation of public health measures could theoretically lead to the disappearance of adult T-cell lymphoma/leukemia. Tropical spastic paraparesis, another manifestation of HTLV-1 infection (Chap. 225e), occurs after a shorter latency (1–3 years) and is most common in individuals who acquire the virus during adulthood from transfusion or sex.

The diagnosis of adult T-cell lymphoma/leukemia is made when an expert hematopathologist recognizes the typical morphologic picture, a T-cell immunophenotype (i.e., CD4 positive), and the presence in serum of antibodies to HTLV-1. Examination of the peripheral blood will usually reveal characteristic, pleomorphic abnormal CD4-positive cells with indented nuclei, which have been called "flower" cells (Fig. 134-10).

A subset of patients have a smoldering clinical course and long survival, but most patients present with an aggressive disease manifested by lymphadenopathy, hepatosplenomegaly, skin infiltration, pulmonary infiltrates, hypercalcemia, lytic bone lesions, and elevated LDH levels. The skin lesions can be papules, plaques, tumors, and ulcerations. Lung lesions can be either tumor or opportunistic infection in light of the underlying immunodeficiency in the disease. Bone marrow involvement is not usually extensive, and anemia and thrombocytopenia are not usually prominent. Although treatment with combination chemotherapy regimens can result in objective responses, true complete remissions are unusual, and the median survival of patients is ~7 months. A small phase II study reported a high response rate with interferon plus zidovudine and arsenic trioxide.

Anaplastic Large T/Null-Cell Lymphoma Anaplastic large T/null-cell lymphoma was previously usually diagnosed as undifferentiated carcinoma or malignant histiocytosis. Discovery of the CD30 (Ki-1) antigen and the recognition that some patients with previously unclassified malignancies displayed this antigen led to the identification of a new type of lymphoma. Subsequently, discovery of the t(2;5) and the resultant frequent overexpression of the anaplastic lymphoma kinase (ALK) protein confirmed the existence of this entity. This lymphoma accounts for ~2% of all non-Hodgkin's lymphomas. Table 134-10 shows the clinical characteristics of patients with anaplastic large T/null cell lymphoma.

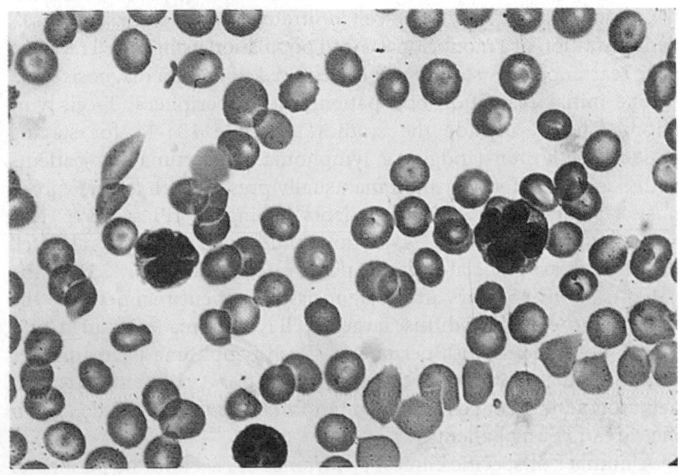

FIGURE 134-10 Adult T-cell leukemia/lymphoma. Peripheral blood smear showing leukemia cells with typical "flower-shaped" nucleus.

The diagnosis of anaplastic large T/null-cell lymphoma is made when an expert hematopathologist recognizes the typical morphologic picture and a T-cell or null-cell immunophenotype with CD30 positivity. Documentation of the t(2;5) and/or overexpression of ALK protein confirm the diagnosis. Some diffuse large B-cell lymphomas can also have an anaplastic appearance but have the same clinical course or response to therapy as other diffuse large B-cell lymphomas. A small percentage of anaplastic lymphomas are ALK negative.

Patients with anaplastic large T/null-cell lymphoma are typically young (median age, 33 years) and male (~70%). Some 50% of patients present in stage I/II, and the remainder present with more extensive disease. Systemic symptoms and elevated LDH levels are seen in about one-half of patients. Bone marrow and the gastrointestinal tract are rarely involved, but skin involvement is frequent. Some patients with disease confined to the skin have a different and more indolent disorder that has been termed *cutaneous anaplastic large T/null-cell lymphoma* and might be related to lymphomatoid papulosis.

TREATMENT ANAPLASTIC LARGE T/NULL-CELL LYMPHOMA

Treatment regimens appropriate for other aggressive lymphomas, such as diffuse large B-cell lymphoma, should be used in patients with anaplastic large T/null-cell lymphoma, with the exception that the B-cell–specific antibody, rituximab, is omitted. Surprisingly, given the anaplastic appearance, this disorder has the best survival rate of any aggressive lymphoma. The 5-year survival is >75%. While traditional prognostic factors such as the IPI predict treatment outcome, overexpression of the ALK protein is an important prognostic factor, with patients overexpressing this protein having a superior treatment outcome. The ALK inhibitor crizotinib appears highly active as well. In addition, the CD30 immunotoxin, brentuximab vedotin, is active in the disease.

Peripheral T-Cell Lymphoma The peripheral T-cell lymphomas make up a heterogeneous morphologic group of aggressive neoplasms that share a mature T-cell immunophenotype. They represent ~7% of all cases of non-Hodgkin's lymphoma. A number of distinct clinical syndromes are included in this group of disorders. Table 134-10 shows the clinical characteristics of patients with peripheral T-cell lymphoma.

The diagnosis of peripheral T-cell lymphoma, or any of its specific subtypes, requires an expert hematopathologist, an adequate biopsy, and immunophenotyping. Most peripheral T-cell lymphomas are CD4+, but a few will be CD8+, both CD4+ and CD8+, or have an NK cell immunophenotype. No characteristic genetic abnormalities have yet been identified, but translocations involving the T-cell antigen receptor genes on chromosomes 7 or 14 may be detected. The differential diagnosis of patients suspected of having peripheral T-cell lymphoma includes reactive T-cell infiltrative processes. In some cases, demonstration of a monoclonal T-cell population using T-cell receptor gene rearrangement studies will be required to make a diagnosis.

The initial evaluation of a patient with a peripheral T-cell lymphoma should include the studies in Table 134-11 for staging patients with non-Hodgkin's lymphoma. Unfortunately, patients with peripheral T-cell lymphoma usually present with adverse prognostic factors, with >80% of patients having an IPI score ≥2 and >30% having an IPI score ≥4. As this would predict, peripheral T-cell lymphomas are associated with a poor outcome, and only 25% of the patients survive 5 years after diagnosis. Treatment regimens are the same as those used for diffuse large B-cell lymphoma (omitting rituximab), but patients with peripheral T-cell lymphoma have a poorer response to treatment. Because of this poor treatment outcome, hematopoietic stem cell transplantation is often considered early in the care of young patients.

A number of specific clinical syndromes are seen in the peripheral T-cell lymphomas. *Angioimmunoblastic T-cell lymphoma* is one of the more common subtypes, making up ~20% of T-cell lymphomas. These patients typically present with generalized lymphadenopathy, fever, weight loss, skin rash, and polyclonal hypergammaglobulinemia. In some cases, it is difficult to separate patients with a reactive disorder from those with true lymphoma.

Extranodal T/NK-cell lymphoma of nasal type has also been called *angiocentric lymphoma* and was previously termed *lethal midline granuloma*. This disorder is more frequent in Asia and South America than in the United States and Europe. EBV is thought to play an etiologic role. Although most frequent in the upper airway, it can involve other organs. The course is aggressive, and patients frequently have the hemophagocytic syndrome. When marrow and blood involvement occur, distinction between this disease and leukemia might be difficult. Some patients will respond to aggressive combination chemotherapy regimens, but the overall outlook is poor.

Enteropathy-type intestinal T-cell lymphoma is a rare disorder that occurs in patients with untreated gluten-sensitive enteropathy. Patients are frequently wasted and sometimes present with intestinal perforation. The prognosis is poor. *Hepatosplenic γδ T-cell lymphoma* is a systemic illness that presents with sinusoidal infiltration of the liver, spleen, and bone marrow by malignant T cells. Tumor masses generally do not occur. The disease is associated with systemic symptoms and is often difficult to diagnose. Treatment outcome is poor. *Subcutaneous panniculitis-like T-cell lymphoma* is a rare disorder that is often confused with panniculitis. Patients present with multiple subcutaneous nodules, which progress and can ulcerate. Hemophagocytic syndrome is common. Response to therapy is poor. The development of the hemophagocytic syndrome (profound anemia, ingestion of erythrocytes by monocytes and macrophages, elevated ferritin levels) in the course of any peripheral T-cell lymphoma is generally associated with a fatal outcome.

HODGKIN'S LYMPHOMA

Classical Hodgkin's Lymphoma Hodgkin's lymphoma occurs in 9000 patients in the United States each year, and the disease does not appear to be increasing in frequency. Most patients present with palpable lymphadenopathy that is nontender; in most patients, these lymph nodes are in the neck, supraclavicular area, and axilla. More than half the patients will have mediastinal adenopathy at diagnosis, and this is sometimes the initial manifestation. Subdiaphragmatic presentation of Hodgkin's lymphoma is unusual and more common in older males. One-third of patients present with fevers, night sweats, and/or weight loss—B symptoms in the Ann Arbor staging classification (Table 134-8). Occasionally, Hodgkin's lymphoma can present as a fever of unknown origin. This is more common in older patients who are found to have mixed-cellularity Hodgkin's lymphoma in an abdominal site. Rarely, the fevers persist for days to weeks, followed by afebrile intervals and then recurrence of the fever. This pattern is known as *Pel-Ebstein fever*. Hodgkin's lymphoma can occasionally present with unusual manifestations. These include severe and unexplained itching, cutaneous disorders such as erythema nodosum and ichthyosiform atrophy, paraneoplastic cerebellar degeneration and other distant effects on the CNS, nephrotic syndrome, immune hemolytic anemia and thrombocytopenia, hypercalcemia, and pain in lymph nodes on alcohol ingestion.

The diagnosis of Hodgkin's lymphoma is established by review of an adequate biopsy specimen by an expert hematopathologist. In the United States, most patients have nodular sclerosing Hodgkin's lymphoma, with a minority of patients having mixed-cellularity Hodgkin's lymphoma. Lymphocyte-predominant and lymphocyte-depleted Hodgkin's lymphoma are rare. Mixed-cellularity Hodgkin's lymphoma or lymphocyte-depletion Hodgkin's lymphoma are seen more frequently in patients infected by HIV (Fig. 134-11). Hodgkin's lymphoma is a tumor characterized by rare neoplastic cells of B-cell origin (immunoglobulin genes are rearranged but not expressed) in a tumor mass that is largely polyclonal inflammatory infiltrate, probably a reaction to cytokines produced by the tumor cells. The differential diagnosis of a lymph node biopsy suspicious for Hodgkin's lymphoma includes inflammatory processes, mononucleosis, non-Hodgkin's lymphoma, phenytoin-induced adenopathy, and nonlymphomatous malignancies.

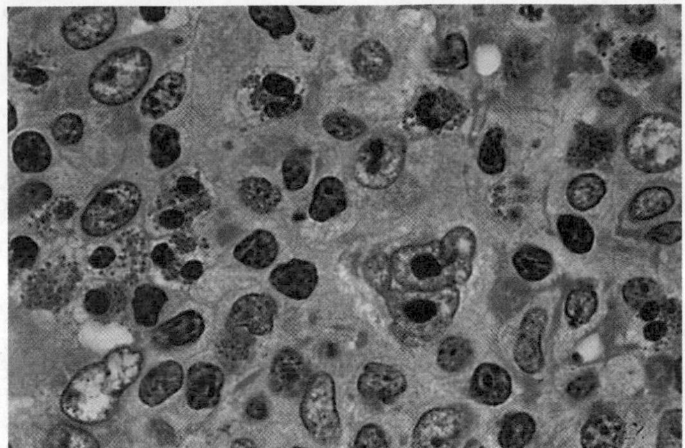

FIGURE 134-11 Mixed-cellularity Hodgkin's lymphoma. A Reed-Sternberg cell is present near the center of the field; a large cell with a bilobed nucleus and prominent nucleoli giving an "owl's eyes" appearance. The majority of the cells are normal lymphocytes, neutrophils, and eosinophils that form a pleomorphic cellular infiltrate.

The staging evaluation for a patient with Hodgkin's lymphoma would typically include a careful history and physical examination; complete blood count; erythrocyte sedimentation rate; serum chemistry studies including LDH; chest radiograph; CT scan of the chest, abdomen, and pelvis; and bone marrow biopsy. Many patients would also have a PET scan or a gallium scan. Although rarely used, a bipedal lymphangiogram can be helpful. PET and gallium scans are most useful to document remission. Staging laparotomies were once popular for most patients with Hodgkin's lymphoma but are now done rarely because of an increased reliance on systemic rather than local therapy.

TREATMENT CLASSICAL HODGKIN'S LYMPHOMA

Patients with localized Hodgkin's lymphoma are cured >90% of the time. In patients with good prognostic factors, extended-field radiotherapy has a high cure rate. Increasingly, patients with all stages of Hodgkin's lymphoma are treated initially with chemotherapy. Patients with localized or good-prognosis disease receive a brief course of chemotherapy followed by radiotherapy to sites of node involvement. Patients with more extensive disease or those with B symptoms receive a complete course of chemotherapy. The most popular chemotherapy regimen used in Hodgkin's lymphoma is a combination of doxorubicin, bleomycin, vinblastine, and dacarbazine (ABVD). Today, most patients in the United States receive ABVD, but a weekly chemotherapy regimen administered for 12 weeks called *Stanford V* is becoming increasingly popular, but it includes radiation therapy, which has been associated with life-threatening late toxicities such as premature coronary artery disease and second solid tumors. In Europe, a high-dose regimen called *BEACOPP* incorporating alkylating agents has become popular and might have a better response rate in very-high-risk patients. Long-term disease-free survival in patients with advanced disease can be achieved in >75% of patients who lack systemic symptoms and in 60–70% of patients with systemic symptoms.

Patients who relapse after primary therapy of Hodgkin's lymphoma can frequently still be cured. Patients who relapse after initial treatment with only radiotherapy have an excellent outcome when treated with chemotherapy. Patients who relapse after an effective chemotherapy regimen are usually not curable with subsequent chemotherapy administered at standard doses. However, patients with a long initial remission can be an exception to this rule. Autologous bone marrow transplantation can cure half of patients in whom effective chemotherapy regimens fail to induce durable remissions. The immunotoxin, brentuximab vedotin, a CD30-directed chemotherapy that selectively targets cells expressing CD30, is active in the salvage setting and is being integrated into ABVD for initial treatment.

Because of the very high cure rate in patients with Hodgkin's lymphoma, long-term complications have become a major focus for clinical research. In fact, in some series of patients with early-stage disease, more patients died from late complications of therapy than from Hodgkin's lymphoma itself. This is particularly true in patients with localized disease. The most serious late side effects include second malignancies and cardiac injury. Patients are at risk for the development of acute leukemia in the first 10 years after treatment with combination chemotherapy regimens that contain alkylating agents plus radiation therapy. The risk for development of acute leukemia appears to be greater after MOPP-like (mechlorethamine, vincristine, procarbazine, prednisone) regimens than with ABVD. The risk of development of acute leukemia after treatment for Hodgkin's lymphoma is also related to the number of exposures to potentially leukemogenic agents (i.e., multiple treatments after relapse) and the age of the patient being treated, with those age >60 years at particularly high risk. The development of carcinomas as a complication of treatment for Hodgkin's lymphoma has become a major problem. These tumors usually occur ≥10 years after treatment and are associated with use of radiotherapy. For this reason, young women treated with thoracic radiotherapy for Hodgkin's lymphoma should institute screening mammograms 5–10 years after treatment, and all patients who receive thoracic radiotherapy for Hodgkin's lymphoma should be discouraged from smoking. Thoracic radiation also accelerates coronary artery disease, and patients should be encouraged to minimize risk factors for coronary artery disease such as smoking and elevated cholesterol levels. Cervical radiation therapy increases the risk of carotid atherosclerosis and stroke.

A number of other late side effects from the treatment of Hodgkin's lymphoma are well known. Patients who receive thoracic radiotherapy are at very high risk for the eventual development of hypothyroidism and should be observed for this complication; intermittent measurement of thyrotropin should be made to identify the condition before it becomes symptomatic. Lhermitte's syndrome occurs in ~15% of patients who receive thoracic radiotherapy. This syndrome is manifested by an "electric shock" sensation into the lower extremities on flexion of the neck. Infertility is a concern for all patients undergoing treatment for Hodgkin's lymphoma. In both women and men, the risk of permanent infertility is age-related, with younger patients more likely to recover fertility. In addition, treatment with ABVD increases the chances to retain fertility.

Nodular Lymphocyte-Predominant Hodgkin's Lymphoma Nodular lymphocyte-predominant Hodgkin's lymphoma is now recognized as an entity distinct from classical Hodgkin's lymphoma. Previous classification systems recognized that biopsies from a subset of patients diagnosed as having Hodgkin's lymphoma contained a predominance of small lymphocytes and rare Reed-Sternberg cells (Fig. 134-11). A subset of these patients have tumors with nodular growth pattern and a clinical course that varied from that of patients with classical Hodgkin's lymphoma. This is an unusual clinical entity and represents <5% of cases of Hodgkin's lymphoma.

Nodular lymphocyte-predominant Hodgkin's lymphoma has a number of characteristics that suggest its relationship to non-Hodgkin's lymphoma. These include a clonal proliferation of B cells and a distinctive immunophenotype; tumor cells express J chain and display CD45 and epithelial membrane antigen (EMA) and do not express two markers normally found on Reed-Sternberg cells, CD30 and CD15. This lymphoma tends to have a chronic, relapsing course and sometimes transforms to diffuse large B-cell lymphoma.

The treatment of patients with nodular lymphocyte-predominant Hodgkin's lymphoma is controversial. Some clinicians favor no treatment and merely close follow-up. In the United States, most physicians will treat localized disease with radiotherapy and disseminated disease with regimens used for patients with classical Hodgkin's lymphoma. Regardless of the therapy used, most series report a long-term survival of >80%.

The most common condition that pathologists and clinicians might confuse with lymphoma is reactive, atypical lymphoid hyperplasia. Patients might have localized or disseminated lymphadenopathy and might have the systemic symptoms characteristic of lymphoma. Underlying causes include a drug reaction to phenytoin or carbamazepine. Immune disorders such as rheumatoid arthritis and lupus erythematosus, viral infections such as cytomegalovirus and EBV, and bacterial infections such as cat-scratch disease may cause adenopathy (Chap. 79). In the absence of a definitive diagnosis after initial biopsy, continued follow-up, further testing, and repeated biopsies, if necessary, constitute the appropriate approach, rather than instituting therapy.

Specific conditions that can be confused with lymphoma include *Castleman's disease*, which can present with localized or disseminated lymphadenopathy; some patients have systemic symptoms. The disseminated form is often accompanied by anemia and polyclonal hypergammaglobulinemia, and the condition has been associated with overproduction of interleukin 6 (IL-6), in some cases produced by human herpesvirus 8 infection. Patients with localized disease can be treated effectively with local therapy, whereas the initial treatment for patients with disseminated disease is usually with systemic glucocorticoids. IL-6-directed therapy (tocilizumab) has produced short-term responses. Rituximab appears to produce longer remissions than tocilizumab.

Sinus histiocytosis with massive lymphadenopathy (*Rosai-Dorfman disease*) usually presents with bulky lymphadenopathy in children or young adults. The disease is usually nonprogressive and self-limited, but patients can manifest autoimmune hemolytic anemia.

Lymphomatoid papulosis is a cutaneous lymphoproliferative disorder that is often confused with anaplastic large cell lymphoma involving the skin. The cells of lymphomatoid papulosis are similar to those seen in lymphoma and stain for CD30, and T-cell receptor gene rearrangements are sometimes seen. However, the condition is characterized by waxing and waning skin lesions that usually heal, leaving small scars. In the absence of effective communication between the clinician and the pathologist regarding the clinical course in the patient, this disease will be misdiagnosed. Since the clinical picture is usually benign, misdiagnosis is a serious mistake.

ACKNOWLEDGMENT

James Armitage was a coauthor of this chapter in prior editions, and substantial material from those editions has been included here.

135e Less Common Hematologic Malignancies

Ayalew Tefferi, Dan L. Longo

The most common lymphoid malignancies are discussed in Chap. 134, myeloid leukemias in Chaps. 132 and 133, myelodysplastic syndromes in Chap. 130, and myeloproliferative syndromes in Chap. 131. This chapter will focus on the more unusual forms of hematologic malignancy. Each of these entities accounts for less than 1% of hematologic neoplasms.

LYMPHOID MALIGNANCIES

Precursor B-cell and precursor T-cell neoplasms are discussed in Chap. 134. All the lymphoid tumors discussed here are mature B cell or T cell, natural killer (NK) cell neoplasms.

136 Plasma Cell Disorders

Nikhil C. Munshi, Dan L. Longo, Kenneth C. Anderson

The *plasma cell disorders* are monoclonal neoplasms related to each other by virtue of their development from common progenitors in the B-lymphocyte lineage. Multiple myeloma, Waldenström's macroglobulinemia, primary amyloidosis (Chap. 137), and the heavy chain diseases comprise this group and may be designated by a variety of synonyms such as *monoclonal gammopathies*, *paraproteinemias*, *plasma cell dyscrasias*, and *dysproteinemias*. Mature B lymphocytes destined to produce IgG bear surface immunoglobulin molecules of both M and G heavy chain isotypes with both isotypes having identical idiotypes (variable regions). Under normal circumstances, maturation to antibody-secreting plasma cells and their proliferation is stimulated by exposure to the antigen for which the surface immunoglobulin is specific; however, in the plasma cell disorders, the control over this process is lost. The clinical manifestations of all the plasma cell disorders relate to the expansion of the neoplastic cells, to the secretion of cell products (immunoglobulin molecules or subunits, lymphokines), and to some extent to the host's response to the tumor. **Normal development of B lymphocytes is discussed in Chap. 372e and depicted in Fig. 134-2.**

There are three categories of structural variation among immunoglobulin molecules that form antigenic determinants, and these are used to classify immunoglobulins. *Isotypes* are those determinants that distinguish among the main classes of antibodies of a given species and are the same in all normal individuals of that species. Therefore, isotypic determinants are, by definition, recognized by antibodies from a distinct species (heterologous sera) but not by antibodies from the same species (homologous sera). There are five heavy chain isotypes (M, G, A, D, E) and two light chain isotypes (κ, λ). *Allotypes* are distinct determinants that reflect regular small differences between individuals of the same species in the amino acid sequences of otherwise similar immunoglobulins. These differences are determined by allelic genes; by definition, they are detected by antibodies made in the same species. *Idiotypes* are the third category of antigenic determinants. They are unique to the molecules produced by a given clone of antibody-producing cells. Idiotypes are formed by the unique structure of the antigen-binding portion of the molecule.

Antibody molecules (Fig. 136-1) are composed of two heavy chains (~50,000 mol wt) and two light chains (~25,000 mol wt). Each chain has a constant portion (limited amino acid sequence variability) and a variable region (extensive sequence variability). The light and heavy chains are linked by disulfide bonds and are aligned so that their variable regions are adjacent to one another. This variable region forms the antigen recognition site of the antibody molecule; its unique structural features form idiotypes that are reliable markers for a particular clone of cells because each antibody is formed and secreted by a single clone. Because of the mechanics of the gene rearrangements necessary to specify the immunoglobulin variable regions (VDJ joining for the heavy chain, VJ joining for the light chain), a particular clone rearranges only one of the two chromosomes to produce an immunoglobulin molecule of only one light chain isotype and only one allotype (allelic exclusion) (Fig. 136-1). After exposure to antigen, the variable region may become associated with a new heavy chain isotype (class switch). Each clone of cells performs these sequential gene arrangements in a unique way. This results in each clone producing a unique immunoglobulin molecule. In most plasma cells, light chains are synthesized in slight excess, secreted as free light chains, and cleared by the kidney, but <10 mg of such light chains is excreted per day.

Electrophoretic analysis permits separation of components of the serum proteins (Fig. 136-2). The immunoglobulins move heterogeneously in an electric field and form a broad peak in the gamma region, which is usually increased in the sera of patients with plasma cell tumors. There is a sharp spike in this region called an *M component* (M for monoclonal). Less commonly, the M component may appear in the

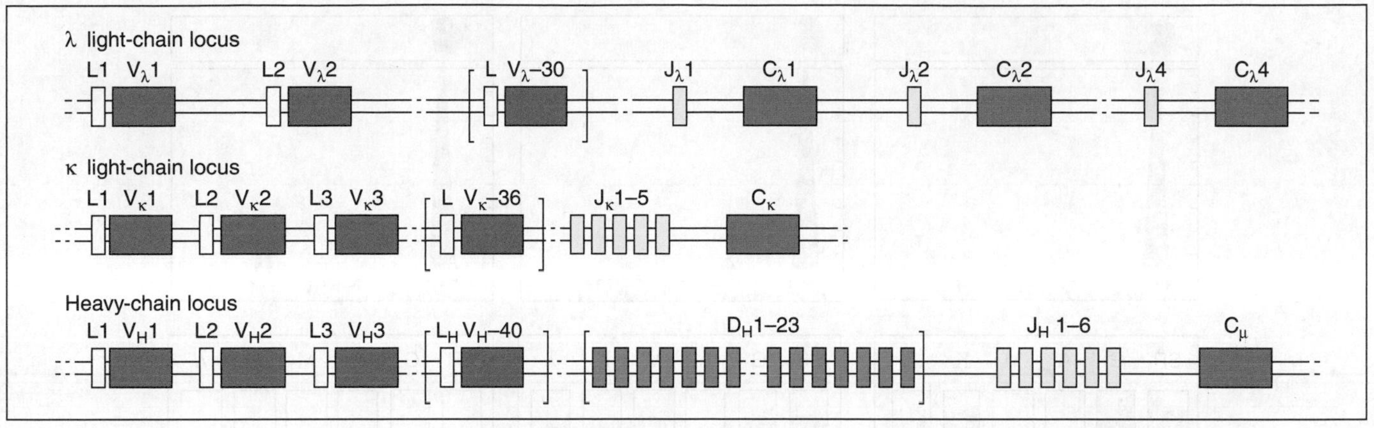

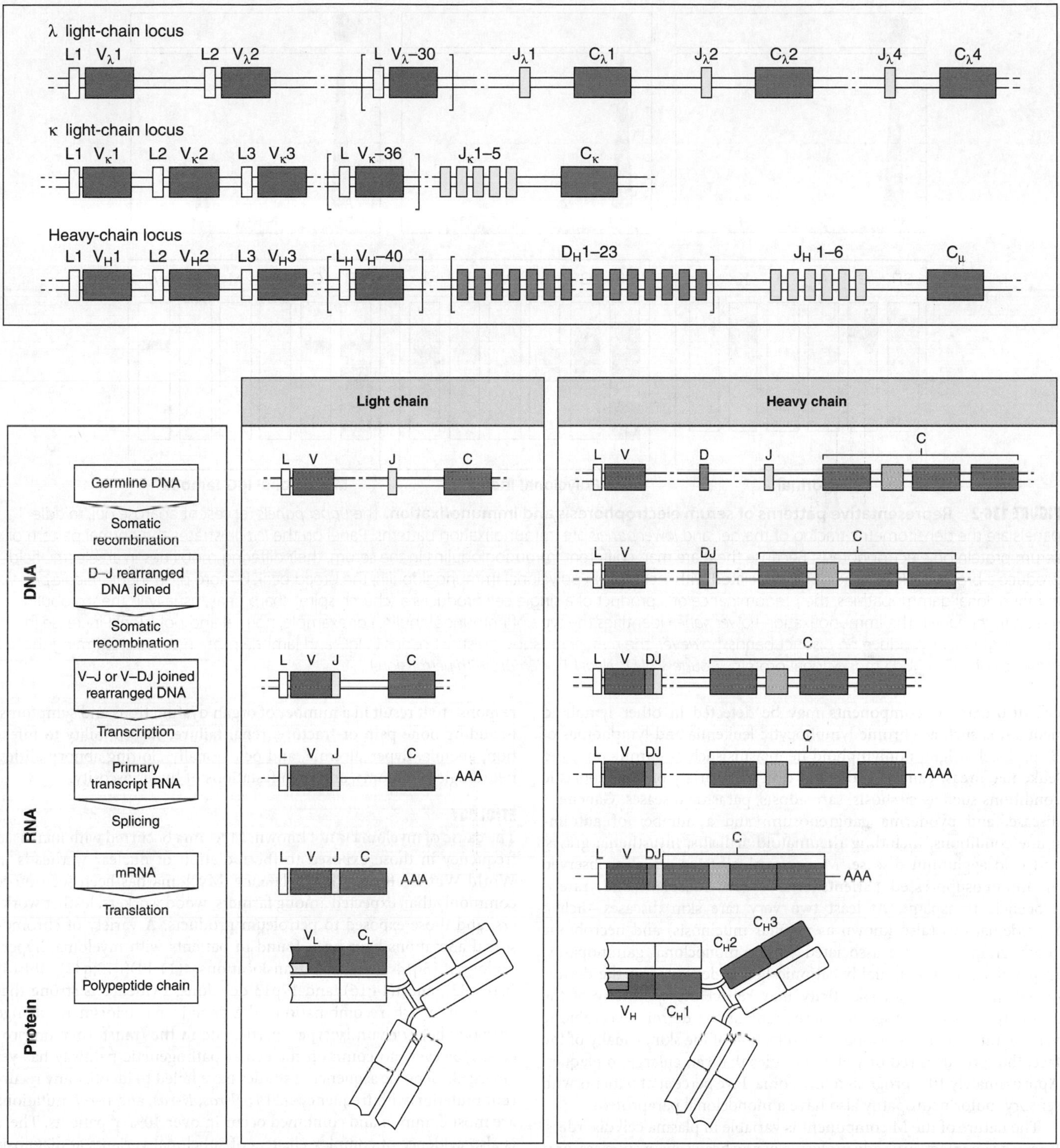

Light chain
Heavy chain

DNA
Germline DNA
Somatic recombination
D–J rearranged DNA joined
Somatic recombination
V–J or V–DJ joined rearranged DNA
Transcription

RNA
Primary transcript RNA
Splicing
mRNA
Translation

Protein
Polypeptide chain

L V J C
L V D J C
L V DJ C
L V J C
L V DJ C
L V J C AAA
L V DJ C AAA
L V J C AAA
L V DJ C AAA
V_L C_L
V_H C_H1 C_H2 C_H3

FIGURE 136-1 Immunoglobulin genetics and the relationship of gene segments to the antibody protein. The *top* portion of the figure is a schematic of the organization of the immunoglobulin genes, λ on chromosome 22, κ on chromosome 2, and the heavy chain locus on chromosome 14. The heavy chain locus is longer than 2 megabases, and some of the D region gene segments are only a few bases long, so the figure depicts the schematic relationship among the segments, not their actual size. The *bottom* portion of the figure outlines the steps in going from the noncontiguous germline gene segments to an intact antibody molecule. Two recombination events juxtapose the V-D-J (or V-J for light chains) segments. The rearranged gene is transcribed, and RNA splicing cuts out intervening sequences to produce an mRNA, which is then translated into an antibody light or heavy chain. The sites on the antibody that bind to antigen (the so called CDR3 regions) are encoded by D and J segments for heavy chains and the J segments for light chains. *(From K Murphy: Janeway's Immunobiology, 8th ed. Garland Science, 2011.)*

β_2 or α_2 globulin region. The monoclonal antibody must be present at a concentration of at least 5 g/L (0.5 g/dL) to be accurately quantitated by this method. This corresponds to ~10^9 cells producing the antibody. Confirmation of the type of immunoglobulin and that it is truly monoclonal is determined by immunoelectrophoresis that reveals a single heavy and/or light chain type. Hence immunoelectrophoresis and electrophoresis provide qualitative and quantitative assessment of the M component, respectively. Once the presence of an M component has been confirmed, the amount of M component in the serum is a reliable measure of the tumor burden, making M component an excellent tumor marker to manage therapy, yet it is not specific enough to be used to screen asymptomatic patients. In addition to the plasma

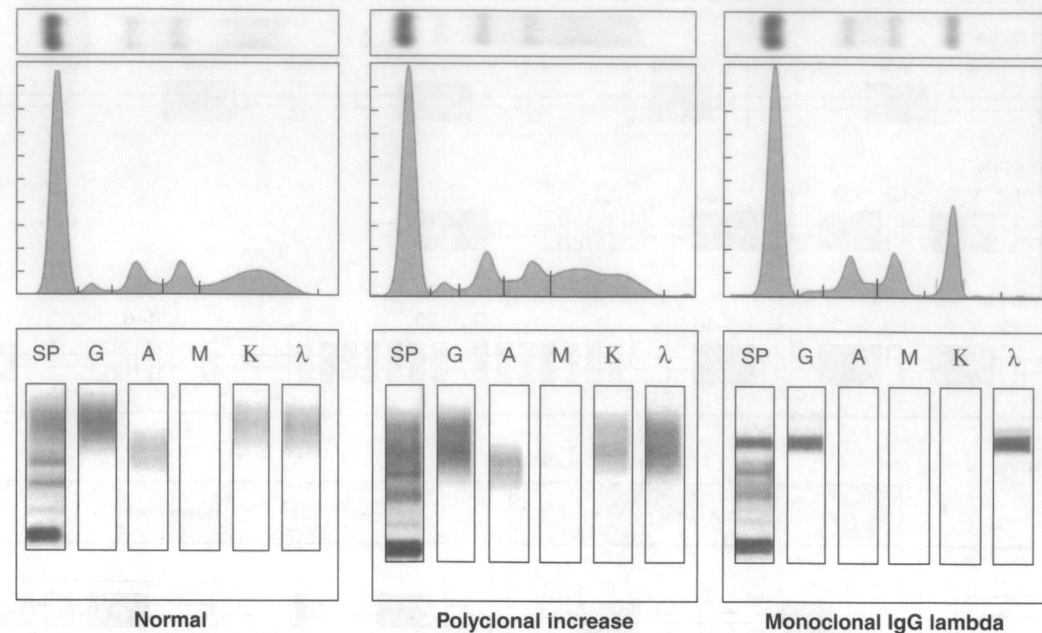

FIGURE 136-2 Representative patterns of serum electrophoresis and immunofixation. The *upper panels* represent agarose gel, middle panels are the densitometric tracing of the gel, and *lower panels* are immunofixation patterns. Panel on the *left* illustrates the normal pattern of serum protein on electrophoresis. Because there are many different immunoglobulins in the serum, their differing mobilities in an electric field produce a broad peak. In conditions associated with increases in polyclonal immunoglobulin, the broad peak is more prominent (*middle panel*). In monoclonal gammopathies, the predominance of a product of a single cell produces a "church spire" sharp peak, usually in the γ globulin region (*right panel*). The immunofixation (*lower panel*) identifies the type of immunoglobulin. For example, normal and polyclonal increase in immunoglobulins produce no distinct bands; however, the *right panel* shows distinct bands in IgG and lambda protein lanes, confirming the presence of IgG lambda monoclonal protein. *(Courtesy of Dr. Neal I. Lindeman; with permission.)*

cell disorders, M components may be detected in other lymphoid neoplasms such as chronic lymphocytic leukemia and lymphomas of B- or T-cell origin; nonlymphoid neoplasms such as chronic myeloid leukemia, breast cancer, and colon cancer; a variety of nonneoplastic conditions such as cirrhosis, sarcoidosis, parasitic diseases, Gaucher's disease, and pyoderma gangrenosum; and a number of autoimmune conditions, including rheumatoid arthritis, myasthenia gravis, and cold agglutinin disease. Monoclonal proteins are also observed in immunosuppressed patients after organ transplant and, rarely, allogeneic transplant. At least two very rare skin diseases—lichen myxedematosus (also known as papular mucinosis) and necrobiotic xanthogranuloma—are associated with a monoclonal gammopathy. In papular mucinosis, highly cationic IgG is deposited in the dermis of patients. This organ specificity may reflect the specificity of the antibody for some antigenic component of the dermis. Necrobiotic xanthogranuloma is a histiocytic infiltration of the skin, usually of the face, that produces red or yellow nodules that can enlarge to plaques. Approximately 10% progress to myeloma. Five percent of patients with sensory motor neuropathy also have a monoclonal paraprotein.

The nature of the M component is variable in plasma cell disorders. It may be an intact antibody molecule of any heavy chain subclass, or it may be an altered antibody or fragment. Isolated light or heavy chains may be produced. In some plasma cell tumors such as extramedullary or solitary bone plasmacytomas, less than one-third of patients will have an M component. In ~20% of myelomas, only light chains are produced and, in most cases, are secreted in the urine as Bence Jones proteins. The frequency of myelomas of a particular heavy chain class is roughly proportional to the serum concentration, and therefore, IgG myelomas are more common than IgA and IgD myelomas. In approximately 1% of patients with myeloma, biclonal or triclonal gammopathy is observed.

MULTIPLE MYELOMA

DEFINITION

Multiple myeloma represents a malignant proliferation of plasma cells derived from a single clone. The tumor, its products, and the host response to it result in a number of organ dysfunctions and symptoms, including bone pain or fracture, renal failure, susceptibility to infection, anemia, hypercalcemia, and occasionally clotting abnormalities, neurologic symptoms, and manifestations of hyperviscosity.

ETIOLOGY

The cause of myeloma is not known. Myeloma occurred with increased frequency in those exposed to the radiation of nuclear warheads in World War II after a 20-year latency. Myeloma has been seen more commonly than expected among farmers, wood workers, leather workers, and those exposed to petroleum products. A variety of chromosomal alterations have been found in patients with myeloma: hyperdiploidy, 13q14 deletions, translocations t(11;14)(q13;q32), t(4;14)(p16;q32), and t(14;16), and 17p13 deletions. Evidence is strong that errors in switch recombination—the genetic mechanism to change antibody heavy chain isotype—participate in the transformation process. However, no common molecular pathogenetic pathway has yet emerged. Genome sequencing studies have failed to identify any recurrent mutation with frequency >20%; *N-ras*, *K-ras*, and *B-raf* mutations are most common and combined occur in over 40% of patients. There is also evidence of complex clusters of subclonal variants at diagnosis that acquire additional mutations over time, indicative of genomic evolution that may drive disease progression. The neoplastic event in myeloma may involve cells earlier in B-cell differentiation than the plasma cell. Interleukin (IL) 6 may play a role in driving myeloma cell proliferation. It remains difficult to distinguish benign from malignant plasma cells based on morphologic criteria in all but a few cases (**Fig. 136-3**).

INCIDENCE AND PREVALENCE

An estimated 24,050 new cases of myeloma were diagnosed in 2014, and 11,090 people died from the disease in the United States. Myeloma increases in incidence with age. The median age at diagnosis is 70 years; it is uncommon under age 40. Males are more commonly affected than females, and blacks have nearly twice the incidence of whites. Myeloma accounts for 1.3% of all malignancies in whites and 2% in blacks, and 13% of all hematologic cancers in whites and 33% in blacks.

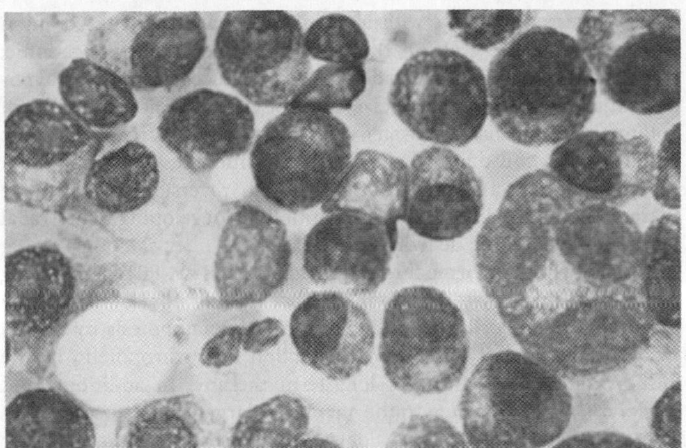

FIGURE 136-3 Multiple myeloma (marrow). The cells bear characteristic morphologic features of plasma cells, round or oval cells with an eccentric nucleus composed of coarsely clumped chromatin, a densely basophilic cytoplasm, and a perinuclear clear zone containing the Golgi apparatus. Binucleate and multinucleate malignant plasma cells can be seen.

GLOBAL CONSIDERATIONS

The incidence of myeloma is highest in African Americans and Pacific Islanders; intermediate in Europeans and North American whites; and lowest in people from developing countries including Asia. The higher incidence in more developed countries may result from the combination of a longer life expectancy and more frequent medical surveillance. Incidence of multiple myeloma in other ethnic groups including native Hawaiians, female Hispanics, American Indians from New Mexico, and Alaskan natives is higher relative to U.S. whites in the same geographic area. Chinese and Japanese populations have a lower incidence than whites. Immunoproliferative small-intestinal disease with alpha heavy chain disease is most prevalent in the Mediterranean area. Despite these differences in prevalence, the characteristics, response to therapy, and prognosis of myeloma are similar worldwide.

PATHOGENESIS AND CLINICAL MANIFESTATIONS

Multiple myeloma (MM) cells bind via cell-surface adhesion molecules to bone marrow stromal cells (BMSCs) and extracellular matrix (ECM), which triggers MM cell growth, survival, drug resistance, and migration in the bone marrow milieu (Fig. 136-4). These effects are due both to direct MM cell–BMSC binding and to induction of various cytokines, including IL-6, insulin-like growth factor type I (IGF-I), vascular endothelial growth factor (VEGF), and stromal cell–derived growth factor (SDF)-1α. Growth, drug resistance, and migration are mediated via Ras/Raf/mitogen-activated protein kinase, PI3K/Akt, and protein kinase C signaling cascades, respectively.

Bone pain is the most common symptom in myeloma, affecting nearly 70% of patients. Unlike the pain of metastatic carcinoma, which often is worse at night, the pain of myeloma is precipitated by movement. Persistent localized pain in a patient with myeloma usually signifies a pathologic fracture. The bone lesions of myeloma are caused by the proliferation of tumor cells, activation of osteoclasts that destroy bone, and suppression of osteoblasts that form new bone. The increased osteoclast activity is mediated by osteoclast activating factors (OAFs) made by the myeloma cells (OAF activity can be mediated by several cytokines, including IL-1, lymphotoxin, VEGF, receptor activator of NF-κB [RANK] ligand, macrophage inhibitory factor [MIP]-1α, and tumor necrosis factor [TNF]). The bone lesions are lytic in nature and are rarely associated with osteoblastic new bone formation due to their suppression by dickhoff-1 (DKK-1) produced by myeloma cells. Therefore, radioisotopic bone scanning is less useful in diagnosis than is plain radiography. The bony lysis results in substantial mobilization of calcium from bone, and serious acute and chronic complications of hypercalcemia may dominate the clinical picture (see below). Localized bone lesions may expand to the point that mass lesions may be palpated, especially on the skull (Fig. 136-5), clavicles, and sternum; and the collapse of vertebrae may lead to spinal cord compression. The next most common clinical problem in patients with myeloma is susceptibility to bacterial infections. The most common infections are pneumonias and pyelonephritis, and the most frequent pathogens are *Streptococcus pneumoniae*, *Staphylococcus aureus*, and *Klebsiella pneumoniae* in the lungs and *Escherichia coli* and other gram-negative organisms in the urinary tract. In ~25% of patients, recurrent infections are the presenting features, and >75%

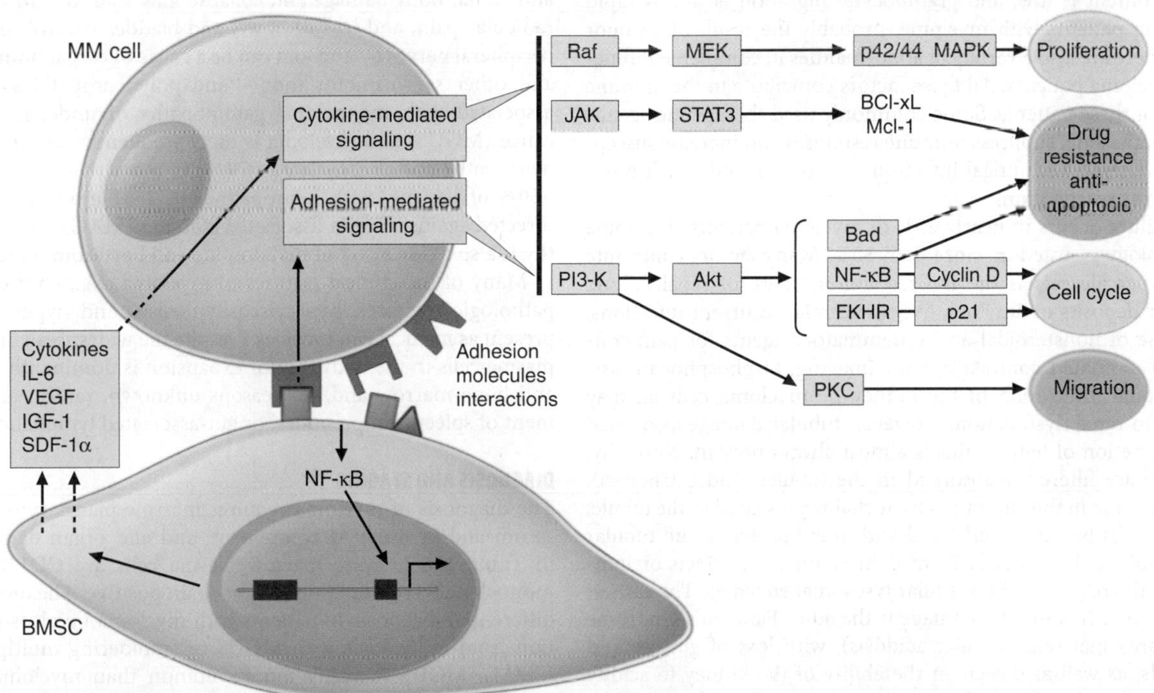

FIGURE 136-4 Pathogenesis of multiple myeloma. Multiple myeloma (MM) cells interact with bone marrow stromal cells (BMSCs) and extracellular matrix proteins via adhesion molecules, triggering adhesion-mediated signaling as well as cytokine production. This triggers cytokine-mediated signaling that provides growth, survival, and antiapoptotic effects as well as development of drug resistance.

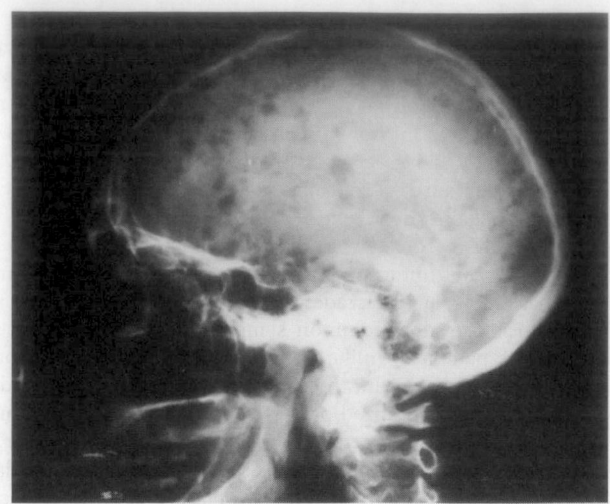

FIGURE 136-5 Bony lesions in multiple myeloma. The skull demonstrates the typical "punched out" lesions characteristic of multiple myeloma. The lesion represents a purely osteolytic lesion with little or no osteoblastic activity. *(Courtesy of Dr. Geraldine Schechter; with permission.)*

of patients will have a serious infection at some time in their course. The susceptibility to infection has several contributing causes. First, patients with myeloma have diffuse hypogammaglobulinemia if the M component is excluded. The hypogammaglobulinemia is related to both decreased production and increased destruction of normal antibodies. Moreover, some patients generate a population of circulating regulatory cells in response to their myeloma that can suppress normal antibody synthesis. In the case of IgG myeloma, normal IgG antibodies are broken down more rapidly than normal because the catabolic rate for IgG antibodies varies directly with the serum concentration. The large M component results in fractional catabolic rates of 8–16% instead of the normal 2%. These patients have very poor antibody responses, especially to polysaccharide antigens such as those on bacterial cell walls. Most measures of T-cell function in myeloma are normal, but a subset of CD4+ cells may be decreased. Granulocyte lysozyme content is low, and granulocyte migration is not as rapid as normal in patients with myeloma, probably the result of a tumor product. There are also a variety of abnormalities in complement functions in myeloma patients. All these factors contribute to the immune deficiency of these patients. Some commonly used therapeutic agents, e.g., dexamethasone, suppress immune responses and increase susceptibility to bacterial and fungal infection, and bortezomib predisposes to herpesvirus reactivation.

Renal failure occurs in nearly 25% of myeloma patients, and some renal pathology is noted in more than 50%. Many factors contribute to this. Hypercalcemia is the most common cause of renal failure. Glomerular deposits of amyloid, hyperuricemia, recurrent infections, frequent use of nonsteroidal anti-inflammatory agents for pain control, use of iodinated contrast dye for imaging, bisphosphonate use, and occasional infiltration of the kidney by myeloma cells all may contribute to renal dysfunction. However, tubular damage associated with the excretion of light chains is almost always present. Normally, light chains are filtered, reabsorbed in the tubules, and catabolized. With the increase in the amount of light chains presented to the tubule, the tubular cells become overloaded with these proteins, and tubular damage results either directly from light chain toxic effects or indirectly from the release of intracellular lysosomal enzymes. The earliest manifestation of this tubular damage is the adult Fanconi's syndrome (a type 2 proximal renal tubular acidosis), with loss of glucose and amino acids, as well as defects in the ability of the kidney to acidify and concentrate the urine. The proteinuria is not accompanied by hypertension, and the protein is nearly all light chains. Generally, very little albumin is in the urine because glomerular function is usually normal. When the glomeruli are involved, nonselective proteinuria is also observed. Patients with myeloma also have a decreased anion gap [i.e., $Na^+ - (Cl^- + HCO_3^-)$] because the M component is cationic, resulting in retention of chloride. This is often accompanied by hyponatremia that is felt to be artificial (pseudohyponatremia) because each volume of serum has less water as a result of the increased protein. Renal dysfunction due to light chain deposition disease, light chain cast nephropathy, and amyloidosis is partially reversible with effective therapy. Myeloma patients are susceptible to developing acute renal failure if they become dehydrated.

Normocytic and normochromic anemia occurs in ~80% of myeloma patients. It is usually related to the replacement of normal marrow by expanding tumor cells, to the inhibition of hematopoiesis by factors made by the tumor, to reduced production of erythropoietin by the kidney, and to the effects of long-term therapy. In addition, mild hemolysis may contribute to the anemia. A larger than expected fraction of patients may have megaloblastic anemia due to either folate or vitamin B_{12} deficiency. Granulocytopenia and thrombocytopenia are rare except when therapy-induced. Clotting abnormalities may be seen due to the failure of antibody-coated platelets to function properly; the interaction of the M component with clotting factors I, II, V, VII, or VIII; antibody to clotting factors; or amyloid damage of endothelium. Deep venous thrombosis is also observed with use of thalidomide, lenalidomide, or pomalidomide in combination with dexamethasone. Raynaud's phenomenon and impaired circulation may result if the M component forms cryoglobulins, and hyperviscosity syndromes may develop depending on the physical properties of the M component (most common with IgM, IgG3, and IgA paraproteins). Hyperviscosity is defined based on the relative viscosity of serum as compared with water. Normal relative serum viscosity is 1.8 (i.e., serum is normally almost twice as viscous as water). Symptoms of hyperviscosity occur at a level greater than 4 centipoise (cP), which is usually reached at paraprotein concentrations of ~40 g/L (4 g/dL) for IgM, 50 g/L (5 g/dL) for IgG3, and 70 g/L (7 g/dL) for IgA; however, depending on chemical and physical properties of the paraprotein molecule, it can occasionally be observed at lower levels.

Although neurologic symptoms occur in a minority of patients, they may have many causes. Hypercalcemia may produce lethargy, weakness, depression, and confusion. Hyperviscosity may lead to headache, fatigue, shortness of breath, exacerbation or precipitation of heart failure, visual disturbances, ataxia, vertigo, retinopathy, somnolence, and coma. Bony damage and collapse may lead to cord compression, radicular pain, and loss of bowel and bladder control. Infiltration of peripheral nerves by amyloid can be a cause of carpal tunnel syndrome and other sensorimotor mono- and polyneuropathies. Neuropathy associated with monoclonal gammopathy of undetermined significance (MGUS) and myeloma is more frequently sensory than motor neuropathy and is associated with IgM more than other isotypes. In >50% of patients with neuropathy, the IgM monoclonal protein is directed against myelin-associated globulin (MAG). Sensory neuropathy is also a side effect of thalidomide and bortezomib therapy.

Many of the clinical features of myeloma, e.g., cord compression, pathologic fractures, hyperviscosity, sepsis, and hypercalcemia, can present as medical emergencies. Despite the widespread distribution of plasma cells in the body, tumor expansion is dominantly within bone and bone marrow and, for reasons unknown, rarely causes enlargement of spleen, lymph nodes, or gut-associated lymphatic tissue.

DIAGNOSIS AND STAGING

The diagnosis of myeloma requires marrow plasmacytosis (>10%), a serum and/or urine M component, and end organ damage detailed in Table 136-1. Bone marrow plasma cells are CD138 and either monoclonal kappa or lambda light chain positive. The most important differential diagnosis in patients with myeloma involves their separation from individuals with MGUS or smoldering multiple myeloma (SMM). MGUS is vastly more common than myeloma, occurring in 1% of the population older than age 50 years and in up to 10% of individuals older than age 75 years. The diagnostic criteria for MGUS, SMM, and myeloma are described in Table 136-1. Although ~1% of patients per year with MGUS go on to develop myeloma, all

TABLE 136-1 DIAGNOSTIC CRITERIA FOR MULTIPLE MYELOMA, MYELOMA VARIANTS, AND MONOCLONAL GAMMOPATHY OF UNDETERMINED SIGNIFICANCE

Monoclonal Gammopathy of Undetermined Significance (MGUS)
M protein in serum <30 g/L
Bone marrow clonal plasma cells <10%
No evidence of other B cell proliferative disorders
No myeloma-related organ or tissue impairment (no end organ damage, including bone lesions)[a]
Smoldering Multiple Myeloma (Asymptomatic Myeloma)
M protein in serum ≥30 g/L *and/or*
Bone marrow clonal plasma cells ≥10%
No myeloma-related organ or tissue impairment (no end organ damage, including bone lesions)[a] or symptoms
Symptomatic Multiple Myeloma
M protein in serum and/or urine
Bone marrow (clonal) plasma cells[b] or plasmacytoma
Myeloma-related organ or tissue impairment (end organ damage, including bone lesions)
Nonsecretory Myeloma
No M protein in serum and/or urine with immunofixation
Bone marrow clonal plasmacytosis >10% or plasmacytoma
Myeloma-related organ or tissue impairment (end organ damage, including bone lesions)[a]
Solitary Plasmacytoma of Bone
No M protein in serum and/or urine[c]
Single area of bone destruction due to clonal plasma cells
Bone marrow not consistent with multiple myeloma
Normal skeletal survey (and magnetic resonance imaging of spine and pelvis if done)
No related organ or tissue impairment (no end organ damage other than solitary bone lesion)[a]
POEMS Syndrome
All of the following four criteria must be met:
1. Polyneuropathy
2. Monoclonal plasma cell proliferative disorder
3. Any one of the following: (a) sclerotic bone lesions; (b) Castleman's disease; (c) elevated levels of vascular endothelial growth factor (VEGF)
4. Any one of the following: (a) organomegaly (splenomegaly, hepatomegaly, or lymphadenopathy); (b) extravascular volume overload (edema, pleural effusion, or ascites); (c) endocrinopathy (adrenal, thyroid, pituitary, gonadal, parathyroid, and pancreatic); (d) skin changes (hyperpigmentation, hypertrichosis, glomeruloid hemangiomata, plethora, acrocyanosis, flushing, and white nails); (e) papilledema; (f) thrombocytosis/polycythemia[d]

[a]Myeloma-related organ or tissue impairment (end organ damage): calcium levels increased: serum calcium >0.25 mmol/L above the upper limit of normal or >2.75 mmol/L; renal insufficiency: creatinine >173 mmol/L; anemia: hemoglobin 2 g/dL below the lower limit of normal or hemoglobin <10 g/dL; bone lesions: lytic lesions or osteoporosis with compression fractures (magnetic resonance imaging or computed tomography may clarify); other: symptomatic hyperviscosity, amyloidosis, recurrent bacterial infections (>2 episodes in 12 months). [b]If flow cytometry is performed, most plasma cells (>90%) will show a "neoplastic" phenotype. [c]A small M component may sometimes be present. [d]These features should have no attributable other causes and have temporal relation with each other.

Abbreviation: POEMS, polyneuropathy, organomegaly, endocrinopathy, M-protein, and skin changes.

myeloma is preceded by MGUS. Non-IgG subtype, abnormal kappa/lambda free light chain ratio, and serum M protein >15 g/L (1.5 g/dL) are associated with higher incidence of progression of MGUS to myeloma. Absence of all three features predicts a 5% chance of progression, whereas higher risk MGUS with the presence of all three features predicts a 60% chance of progression over 20 years. The features responsible for higher risk of progression from SMM to MM are bone marrow plasmacytosis >10%, abnormal kappa/lambda free light chain ratio, and serum M protein >30 g/L (3 g/dL). Patients with only one of these three features have a 25% chance of progression to MM in 5 years, whereas patients with high-risk SMM with all three features have a 76% chance of progression. There are two important variants of myeloma—solitary bone plasmacytoma and solitary extramedullary plasmacytoma. These lesions are associated with an M component in <30% of the cases, they may affect younger individuals, and both are associated with median survivals of ≥10 years. Solitary bone plasmacytoma is a single lytic bone lesion without marrow plasmacytosis. Extramedullary plasmacytomas usually involve the submucosal lymphoid tissue of the nasopharynx or paranasal sinuses without marrow plasmacytosis. Both tumors are highly responsive to local radiation therapy. If an M component is present, it should disappear after treatment. Solitary bone plasmacytomas may recur in other bony sites or evolve into myeloma. Extramedullary plasmacytomas rarely recur or progress.

The clinical evaluation of patients with myeloma includes a careful physical examination searching for tender bones and masses. Chest and bone radiographs may reveal lytic lesions or diffuse osteopenia. Magnetic resonance imaging (MRI) offers a sensitive means to document extent of bone marrow infiltration and cord or root compression in patients with pain syndromes. A complete blood count with differential may reveal anemia. Erythrocyte sedimentation rate is elevated. Rare patients (~1%) may have plasma cell leukemia with >2000 plasma cells/μL. This may be seen in disproportionate frequency in IgD (12%) and IgE (25%) myelomas. Serum calcium, urea nitrogen, creatinine, and uric acid levels may be elevated. Protein electrophoresis and measurement of serum immunoglobulins and free light chains are useful for detecting and characterizing M spikes, supplemented by immunoelectrophoresis, which is especially sensitive for identifying low concentrations of M components not detectable by protein electrophoresis. A 24-h urine specimen is necessary to quantitate Bence Jones protein excretion. Serum alkaline phosphatase is usually normal even with extensive bone involvement because of the absence of osteoblastic activity. It is also important to quantitate serum β_2-microglobulin and albumin (see below).

The serum M component will be IgG in 53% of patients, IgA in 25%, and IgD in 1%; 20% of patients will have only light chains in serum and urine. Dipsticks for detecting proteinuria are not reliable at identifying light chains, and the heat test for detecting Bence Jones protein is falsely negative in ~50% of patients with light chain myeloma. Fewer than 1% of patients have no identifiable M component; these patients usually have light chain myeloma in which renal catabolism has made the light chains undetectable in the urine. In most of these patients, light chains can now be detected by serum free light chain assay. IgD myeloma may also present with light chain disease. About two-thirds of patients with serum M components also have urinary light chains. The light chain isotype may have an impact on survival. Patients secreting lambda light chains have a significantly shorter overall survival than those secreting kappa light chains. Whether this is due to some genetically important determinant of cell proliferation or because lambda light chains are more likely to cause renal damage and form amyloid than are kappa light chains is unclear. The heavy chain isotype may have an impact on patient management as well. About half of patients with IgM paraproteins develop hyperviscosity compared with only 2–4% of patients with IgA and IgG M components. Among IgG myelomas, it is the IgG3 subclass that has the highest tendency to form both concentration- and temperature-dependent aggregates, leading to hyperviscosity and cold agglutination at lower serum concentrations.

PROGNOSIS

Serum β_2-microglobulin is the single most powerful predictor of survival and can substitute for staging. β_2-Microglobulin is a protein of 11,000 mol wt with homologies to the constant region of immunoglobulins that is the light chain of the class I major histocompatibility antigens (HLA-A, -B, -C) on the surface of every cell. Patients with β_2-microglobulin levels <0.004 g/L have a median survival of 43 months, and those with levels >0.004 g/L have a survival of only 12 months. Combination of serum β_2-microglobulin and albumin levels forms the basis for a three-stage International Staging System (ISS) (Table 136-2) that predicts survival. With the use of high-dose therapy and the newer agents, the

TABLE 136-2 RISK STRATIFICATION IN MYELOMA

Chromosomal Abnormalities		
Method	**Standard Risk (80%) (expected survival 6–7+ years)**	**High Risk (20%) (expected survival 2–3 years)**
Karyotype	No chromosomal aberration	Any abnormality on conventional karyotype
FISH	t(11;14)	Del(17p)
	t(6:14)	t(4:14)
	Del(13)	t(14:16)
		t(14;20)
International Staging System		
	Stage	**Median Survival, Months**
β_2M <3.5, alb ≥3.5	I (28%)[a]	62
β_2M <3.5, alb <3.5 *or* β_2M = 3.5–5.5	II (39%)	44
β_2M >5.5	III (33%)	29

Other features suggesting high-risk disease:

- De novo plasma cell leukemia
- Extramedullary disease
- Elevated lactate dehydrogenate (LDH)
- High-risk gene expression profile

[a]Percentage of patients presenting at each stage.

Abbreviations: β_2M, serum β_2-microglobulin in mg/L; alb, serum albumin in g/dL; FISH, fluorescent in situ hybridization.

Durie-Salmon staging system is unable to predict outcome and thus is no longer used. High labeling index, circulating plasma cells, performance status, and high levels of lactate dehydrogenase are also associated with poor prognosis.

Other factors that may influence prognosis are the presence of cytogenetic abnormalities and hypodiploidy by karyotype, fluorescent in situ hybridization (FISH)–identified chromosome 17p deletion, and translocations t(4;14), (14;16), and t(14;20). Chromosome 13q deletion, previously thought to predict poor outcome, is not a predictor following the use of newer agents. Microarray profiling and comparative genomic hybridization have formed the basis for RNA- and DNA-based prognostic staging systems, respectively. The ISS system, along with cytogenetic changes, is the most widely used method for assessing prognosis (Table 136-2).

TREATMENT MULTIPLE MYELOMA

No specific intervention is indicated for patients with MGUS. Follow-up once a year or less frequently is adequate except in higher risk MGUS, where serum protein electrophoresis, complete blood count, creatinine, and calcium should be repeated every 6 months. A patient with MGUS and severe polyneuropathy is considered for therapeutic intervention if a causal relationship can be assumed, especially in absence of any other potential causes for neuropathy. Therapy can include plasmapheresis and occasionally rituximab in patients with IgM MGUS or myeloma-like therapy in those with IgG or IgA disease. About 10% of patients with myeloma are asymptomatic (SMM) and will have an indolent course demonstrating only very slow progression of disease over many years. For these patients, no specific therapeutic intervention is indicated, although early intervention with lenalidomide and dexamethasone may prevent progression from high-risk SMM to active MM. At present, patients with SMM only require antitumor therapy when the disease becomes symptomatic with development of anemia, hypercalcemia, progressive lytic bone lesions, renal dysfunction, or recurrent infections. Patients with solitary bone plasmacytomas and extramedullary plasmacytomas may be expected to enjoy prolonged disease-free survival after local radiation therapy at a dose of around 40 Gy. There is a low incidence of occult marrow involvement in patients with solitary bone plasmacytoma. Such patients are usually identified because their serum M component falls slowly or disappears initially, only to return after a few months. These patients respond well to systemic therapy.

Patients with symptomatic and/or progressive myeloma require therapeutic intervention. In general, such therapy is of two sorts: (1) systemic therapy to control the progression of myeloma and (2) symptomatic supportive care to prevent serious morbidity from the complications of the disease. Therapy can significantly prolong survival and improve the quality of life for myeloma patients.

The therapy of myeloma includes an initial induction regimen followed by consolidation and/or maintenance therapy and, on subsequent progression, management of relapsed disease. The therapy is partly dictated by the patient's age and comorbidities, which may affect a patient's ability to undergo high-dose therapy and transplantation.

Thalidomide (200 mg daily), when combined with dexamethasone, achieved responses in two-thirds of newly diagnosed MM patients. Subsequently, lenalidomide (25 mg/d on days 1–21 every 4 weeks), an immunomodulatory derivative of thalidomide, and bortezomib (1.3 mg/m^2 on days 1, 4, 8, and 11 every 3 weeks), a proteasome inhibitor, have each been combined with dexamethasone (40 mg once every week) and obtained high response rates (>80%) in newly diagnosed patients with MM. Importantly, their superior toxicity profile with improved efficacy has made them the preferred agents for induction therapy. Efforts to improve the fraction of patients responding and the degree of response have involved adding agents to the treatment regimen. The combination of lenalidomide, bortezomib, and dexamethasone achieves close to a 100% response rate and 30% complete response rate, making it one of the preferred induction regimens in transplant-eligible patients. Other similar three-drug combinations (bortezomib, thalidomide, and dexamethasone or bortezomib, cyclophosphamide, and dexamethasone) also achieve >90% response rate. Herpes zoster prophylaxis is indicated if bortezomib is used, and neuropathy attendant to bortezomib can be decreased both by its subcutaneous administration and administration on a weekly schedule. Lenalidomide use requires prophylaxis for deep vein thrombosis (DVT) with either aspirin or warfarin or low-molecular-weight heparin if patients are at a greater risk of DVT. In patients receiving lenalidomide, stem cells should be collected within 6 months, because the continued use of lenalidomide may compromise the ability to collect adequate numbers of stem cells. Initial therapy is continued until maximal cytoreduction. In patients who are transplant candidates, alkylating agents such as melphalan should be avoided because they damage stem cells, leading to decreased ability to collect stem cells for autologous transplant.

In patients who are not transplant candidates due to physiologic age >70 years, significant cardiopulmonary problems, or other comorbid illnesses, the same two- or three-drug combinations described above are considered standard of care as induction therapy. Previously, therapy consisting of intermittent pulses of melphalan, an alkylating agent, with prednisone (MP; melphalan, 0.25 mg/kg per day, and prednisone, 1 mg/kg per day for 4 days) every 4–6 weeks was used. However, a number of studies have combined novel agents with MP and reported superior response and survival outcomes. In patients >65 years old, combining thalidomide with MP (MPT) obtains higher response rates and overall survival compared with MP alone. Similarly, significantly improved response (71 vs 35%) and overall survival (3-year survival 72 vs 59%) were observed with the combination of bortezomib and MP compared with MP alone. Lenalidomide added to MP followed by lenalidomide maintenance also prolonged progression-free survival compared with MP alone. These combinations of novel agents with MP also achieve high complete response rates (MPT, ~15%; MP plus bortezomib, ~30%; MP plus lenalidomide, ~20%; and MP, ~2–4%). Although combinations of MP with newer agents are an alternative in these patients, most studies favor continuous therapy with non-MP-containing regimens (e.g., lenalidomide plus dexamethasone) due to longer term safety profile and efficacy.

Improvement in the serum M component may lag behind the symptomatic improvement. The fall in M component depends on the rate of tumor kill and the fractional catabolic rate of immunoglobulin, which in turn depends on the serum concentration (for IgG). Light chain excretion, with a functional half-life of ~6 h, may fall within the first week of treatment. Because urine light chain levels may relate to renal tubular function, they are not a reliable measure of tumor cell kill, especially in patients with renal dysfunction; however, improvements in serum free light chain measurement are often seen sooner. Although patients may not achieve complete remission, clinical responses may last for long periods of time.

High-dose therapy and consolidation/maintenance are standard practice in the majority of eligible patients. Randomized studies comparing standard-dose therapy to high-dose melphalan therapy (HDT) with hematopoietic stem cell support have shown that HDT can achieve high overall response rates, with up to 25–40% additional complete responses and prolonged progression-free and overall survival; however, few, if any, patients are cured. Although two successive HDTs (tandem transplantations) are more effective than single HDT, the benefit is only observed in the subset of patients who do not achieve a complete or very good partial response to the first transplantation, which is rare. Moreover, a randomized study failed to show any significant difference in overall survival between early transplantation after induction therapy versus delayed transplantation at relapse. These data allow an option to delay transplantation, especially with the availability of more agents and combinations. Allogeneic transplantations may also produce high response rates, but treatment-related mortality may be as high as 40%. Nonmyeloablative allogeneic transplantation can reduce toxicity but is recommended only under the auspices of a clinical trial to exploit an immune graft-versus-myeloma effect while avoiding attendant toxicity.

Maintenance therapy prolongs remissions following standard-dose regimens as well as HDT. Two phase 3 studies have demonstrated improved progression-free survival, and one study showed prolonged overall survival in patients receiving lenalidomide compared to placebo as maintenance therapy after HDT. In non-transplant candidates, another phase 3 study showed prolonged progression-free survival with lenalidomide maintenance after MP plus lenalidomide induction therapy. Although there is concern regarding an increased incidence of second primary malignancies in patients receiving lenalidomide maintenance, its benefits far outweigh the risk of progressive disease and death from myeloma. In patients with high-risk cytogenetics, lenalidomide and bortezomib have been combined and show promise as maintenance therapy after transplantation.

Relapsed myeloma can be treated with a number of agents including lenalidomide and/or bortezomib. These agents in combination with dexamethasone can achieve a partial response rate of up to 60% and a 10–15% complete response rate in patients with relapsed disease. The combination of bortezomib and liposomal doxorubicin is active in relapsed myeloma. Thalidomide, if not used as initial therapy, can achieve responses in refractory cases. The second-generation proteasome inhibitor carfilzomib and immunomodulatory agent pomalidomide have shown efficacy in relapsed and refractory MM, even MM refractory to lenalidomide and bortezomib. High-dose melphalan and stem cell transplantation, if not used earlier, also have activity as salvage therapy in patients with refractory disease.

The median overall survival of patients with myeloma is 7–8+ years, with subsets of younger patients surviving more than 10 years. The major causes of death are progressive myeloma, renal failure, sepsis, or therapy-related myelodysplasia. Nearly a quarter of patients die of myocardial infarction, chronic lung disease, diabetes, or stroke—all intercurrent illnesses related more to the age of the patient group than to the tumor.

Supportive care directed at the anticipated complications of the disease may be as important as primary antitumor therapy. Hypercalcemia generally responds well to bisphosphonates, glucocorticoid therapy, hydration, and natriuresis, and rarely requires calcitonin as well. Bisphosphonates (e.g., pamidronate 90 mg or zoledronate 4 mg once a month) reduce osteoclastic bone resorption and preserve performance status and quality of life, decrease bone-related complications, and may also have antitumor effects. Osteonecrosis of the jaw and renal dysfunction can occur in a minority of patients receiving aminobisphosphonate therapy. Treatments aimed at strengthening the skeleton such as fluorides, calcium, and vitamin D, with or without androgens, have been suggested, but are not of proven efficacy. Kyphoplasty or vertebroplasty should be considered in patients with painful collapsed vertebra. Iatrogenic worsening of renal function may be prevented by maintaining a high fluid intake to prevent dehydration and enhance excretion of light chains and calcium. In the event of acute renal failure, plasmapheresis is ~10 times more effective at clearing light chains than peritoneal dialysis; however, its role in reversing renal failure remains controversial. Importantly, reducing the protein load by effective antitumor therapy with agents such as bortezomib may result in improvement in renal function in over half of the patients. Use of lenalidomide in renal failure is possible but requires dose modification, because it is renally excreted. Urinary tract infections should be watched for and treated early. Plasmapheresis may be the treatment of choice for hyperviscosity syndromes. Although the pneumococcus is a dreaded pathogen in myeloma patients, pneumococcal polysaccharide vaccines may not elicit an antibody response. Prophylactic administration of intravenous γ globulin preparations is used in the setting of recurrent serious infections. Chronic oral antibiotic prophylaxis is not warranted. Patients developing neurologic symptoms in the lower extremities, severe localized back pain, or problems with bowel and bladder control may need emergency MRI and local radiation therapy and glucocorticoids if cord compression is identified. In patients in whom neurologic deficit is increasing or substantial, emergent surgical decompression may be necessary. Most bone lesions respond to analgesics and systemic therapy, but certain painful lesions may respond most promptly to localized radiation. The anemia associated with myeloma may respond to erythropoietin along with hematinics (iron, folate, cobalamin). The pathogenesis of the anemia should be established and specific therapy instituted, whenever possible.

WALDENSTRÖM'S MACROGLOBULINEMIA

In 1948, Waldenström described a malignancy of lymphoplasmacytoid cells that secreted IgM. In contrast to myeloma, the disease was associated with lymphadenopathy and hepatosplenomegaly, but the major clinical manifestation was hyperviscosity syndrome. The disease resembles the related diseases chronic lymphocytic leukemia, myeloma, and lymphocytic lymphoma. It originates from a post-germinal center B cell that has undergone somatic mutations and antigenic selection in the lymphoid follicle and has the characteristics of an IgM-bearing memory B cell. Waldenström's macroglobulinemia (WM) and IgM myeloma follow a similar clinical course, but therapeutic options are different. The diagnosis of IgM myeloma is usually reserved for patients with lytic bone lesions and predominant infiltration with CD138+ plasma cells in the bone marrow. Such patients are at greater risk of pathologic fractures than patients with WM.

A familial occurrence is common in WM, but its molecular bases are yet unclear. A distinct MYD88 L265P somatic mutation has been reported in over 90% of patients with WM and the majority of IgM MGUS. Presence of this mutation is now used as a diagnostic test to discriminate WM from marginal zone lymphomas (MZLs), IgM-secreting myeloma, and chronic lymphocytic leukemia (CLL) with plasmacytic differentiation. This mutation also explains the molecular pathogenesis of the disease, with involvement of Toll-like receptor (TLR) and interleukin 1 receptor (IL-1R) signaling leading to activation of IL-1R–associated kinase (IRAK) 4 and IRAK1 followed by nuclear factor-κB (NF-κB) activation. The disease is similar to myeloma in being slightly more common in men and occurring with increased incidence with increasing age (median 64 years). There have been reports that the IgM in some patients with macroglobulinemia may have specificity for myelin-associated glycoprotein (MAG), a protein that has been associated with demyelinating disease of the peripheral nervous system and may be lost earlier and to a greater extent than the better known myelin basic protein in patients with multiple sclerosis. Sometimes patients with macroglobulinemia develop a peripheral neuropathy, and half of these patients are positive for anti-MAG antibody. The neuropathy may precede the appearance of the neoplasm. There is speculation that the whole process begins with a viral infection that may elicit an antibody response that cross-reacts with a normal tissue component.

Like myeloma, the disease involves the bone marrow, but unlike myeloma, it does not cause bone lesions or hypercalcemia. Bone marrow shows >10% infiltration with lymphoplasmacytic cells (surface IgM+, CD19+, CD20+, and CD22+, rarely CD5+, but CD10– and CD23–) with an increase in number of mast cells. Like myeloma, an M component is present in the serum in excess of 30 g/L (3 g/dL), but unlike myeloma, the size of the IgM paraprotein results in little renal excretion, and only ~20% of patients excrete light chains. Therefore, renal disease is not common. The light chain isotype is kappa in 80% of the cases. Patients present with weakness, fatigue, and recurrent infections similar to myeloma patients, but epistaxis, visual disturbances, and neurologic symptoms such as peripheral neuropathy, dizziness, headache, and transient paresis are much more common in macroglobulinemia. Physical examination reveals adenopathy and hepatosplenomegaly, and ophthalmoscopic examination may reveal vascular segmentation and dilation of the retinal veins characteristic of hyperviscosity states. Patients may have a normocytic, normochromic anemia, but rouleaux formation and a positive Coombs' test are much more common than in myeloma. Malignant lymphocytes are usually present in the peripheral blood. About 10% of macroglobulins are cryoglobulins. These are pure M components and are not the mixed cryoglobulins seen in rheumatoid arthritis and other autoimmune diseases. Mixed cryoglobulins are composed of IgM or IgA complexed with IgG, for which they are specific. In both cases, Raynaud's phenomenon and serious vascular symptoms precipitated by the cold may occur, but mixed cryoglobulins are not commonly associated with malignancy. Patients suspected of having a cryoglobulin based on history and physical examination should have their blood drawn into a warm syringe and delivered to the laboratory in a container of warm water to avoid errors in quantitating the cryoglobulin.

TREATMENT WALDENSTRÖM'S MACROGLOBULINEMIA

Control of serious hyperviscosity symptoms such as an altered state of consciousness or paresis can be achieved acutely by plasmapheresis because 80% of the IgM paraprotein is intravascular. The median survival of affected individuals is ~50 months, similar to that of MM. However, many patients with WM have indolent disease that does not require therapy. Pretreatment parameters including older age, male sex, general symptoms, and cytopenias define a high-risk population. Treatment is usually not initiated unless the disease is symptomatic or increasing anemia, hyperviscosity, lymphadenopathy, or hepatosplenomegaly is present. Bortezomib and bendamustine are two agents with significant efficacy in WM. Rituximab (anti-CD20) can produce responses, alone or combined with either of these two agents. Rituximab can produce IgM flare, so its use is initially withheld in patients with high IgM levels. Fludarabine (25 mg/m^2 per day for 5 days every 4 weeks) and cladribine (0.1 mg/kg per day for 7 days every 4 weeks) are also highly effective single agents. With identification of the MYD88 mutation, BTK and IRAK1/4 inhibitors are being evaluated and show significant responses. Although high-dose therapy plus autologous transplantation is an option, its use has declined due to the availability of other effective agents.

POEMS SYNDROME

The features of this syndrome are *p*olyneuropathy, *o*rganomegaly, *e*ndocrinopathy, *M*-protein, and *s*kin changes (POEMS). Diagnostic criteria are described in Table 136-1. Patients usually have a severe, progressive sensorimotor polyneuropathy associated with sclerotic bone lesions from myeloma. Polyneuropathy occurs in ~1.4% of myelomas, but the POEMS syndrome is only a rare subset of that group. Unlike typical myeloma, hepatomegaly and lymphadenopathy occur in about two-thirds of patients, and splenomegaly is seen in one-third. The lymphadenopathy frequently resembles Castleman's disease histologically, a condition that has been linked to IL-6 overproduction. The endocrine manifestations include amenorrhea in women and impotence and gynecomastia in men. Hyperprolactinemia due to loss of normal inhibitory control by the hypothalamus may be associated with other central nervous system manifestations such as papilledema and elevated cerebrospinal fluid pressure and protein. Type 2 diabetes mellitus occurs in about one-third of patients. Hypothyroidism and adrenal insufficiency are occasionally noted. Skin changes are diverse: hyperpigmentation, hypertrichosis, skin thickening, and digital clubbing. Other manifestations include peripheral edema, ascites, pleural effusions, fever, and thrombocytosis. Not all the components of POEMS syndrome may be present initially.

The pathogenesis of the disease is unclear, but high circulating levels of the proinflammatory cytokines IL-1, IL-6, VEGF, and TNF have been documented, and levels of the inhibitory cytokine transforming growth factor β are lower than expected. Treatment of the myeloma may result in an improvement in the other disease manifestations.

Patients are often treated similarly to those with myeloma. Plasmapheresis does not appear to be of benefit in POEMS syndrome. Patients presenting with isolated sclerotic lesions may have resolution of neuropathic symptoms after local therapy for plasmacytoma with radiotherapy. Similar to multiple myeloma, novel agents and high-dose therapy with autologous stem cell transplantation have been pursued in selected patients and have been associated with prolonged progression-free survival.

HEAVY CHAIN DISEASES

The heavy chain diseases are rare lymphoplasmacytic malignancies. Their clinical manifestations vary with the heavy chain isotype. Patients have absence of light chain and secrete a defective heavy chain that usually has an intact Fc fragment and a deletion in the Fd region. Gamma, alpha, and mu heavy chain diseases have been described, but no reports of delta or epsilon heavy chain diseases have appeared. Molecular biologic analysis of these tumors has revealed structural genetic defects that may account for the aberrant chain secreted.

GAMMA HEAVY CHAIN DISEASE (FRANKLIN'S DISEASE)

This disease affects individuals of widely different age groups and countries of origin. It is characterized by lymphadenopathy, fever, anemia, malaise, hepatosplenomegaly, and weakness. It is frequently associated with autoimmune diseases, especially rheumatoid arthritis. Its most distinctive symptom is palatal edema, resulting from involvement of nodes in Waldeyer's ring, and this may progress to produce respiratory compromise. The diagnosis depends on the demonstration of an anomalous serum M component (often <20 g/L [<2 g/dL]) that reacts with anti-IgG but not anti–light chain reagents. The M component is typically present in both serum and urine. Most of the paraproteins have been of the γ_1 subclass, but other subclasses have been seen. The patients may have thrombocytopenia, eosinophilia, and nondiagnostic bone marrow that may show increased numbers of lymphocytes or plasma cells that do not stain for light chain. Patients usually have a rapid downhill course and die of infection; however, some patients have survived 5 years with chemotherapy. Therapy is indicated when symptomatic and involves chemotherapeutic combinations used in low-grade lymphoma. Rituximab has also been reported to show efficacy.

ALPHA HEAVY CHAIN DISEASE (SELIGMANN'S DISEASE)

This is the most common of the heavy chain diseases. It is closely related to a malignancy known as Mediterranean lymphoma, a disease that affects young persons in parts of the world where intestinal parasites are common, such as the Mediterranean, Asia, and South America. The disease is characterized by an infiltration of the lamina propria of the small intestine with lymphoplasmacytoid cells that secrete truncated alpha chains. Demonstrating alpha heavy chains is difficult because the alpha chains tend to polymerize and appear as a smear instead of a sharp peak on electrophoretic profiles. Despite the polymerization, hyperviscosity is not a common problem in alpha heavy chain disease. Without J chain–facilitated dimerization, viscosity does not increase dramatically. Light chains are absent from serum and urine. The patients present with chronic diarrhea, weight loss, and malabsorption and have extensive mesenteric and paraaortic adenopathy. Respiratory tract involvement occurs rarely. Patients may vary widely in their clinical course. Some may develop diffuse aggressive histologies of malignant lymphoma. Chemotherapy may produce long-term remissions. Rare patients appear to have responded to antibiotic therapy, raising the question of the etiologic role of antigenic stimulation, perhaps by some chronic intestinal infection. Chemotherapy plus antibiotics may be more effective than chemotherapy alone. Immunoproliferative small-intestinal disease (IPSID) is recognized as an infectious pathogen–associated human lymphoma that has association with *Campylobacter jejuni*. It involves mainly the proximal small intestine resulting in malabsorption, diarrhea, and abdominal pain. IPSID is associated with excessive plasma cell differentiation and produces truncated alpha heavy chain proteins lacking the light chains as well as the first constant domain. Early-stage IPSID responds to antibiotics (30–70% complete remission). Most untreated IPSID patients progress to lymphoplasmacytic and immunoblastic lymphoma. Patients not responding to antibiotic therapy are considered for treatment with combination chemotherapy used to treat low-grade lymphoma.

MU HEAVY CHAIN DISEASE

The secretion of isolated mu heavy chains into the serum appears to occur in a very rare subset of patients with CLL. The only features that may distinguish patients with mu heavy chain disease are the presence of vacuoles in the malignant lymphocytes and the excretion of kappa light chains in the urine. The diagnosis requires ultracentrifugation or gel filtration to confirm the nonreactivity of the paraprotein with the light chain reagents, because some intact macroglobulins fail to interact with these serums. The tumor cells seem to have a defect in the assembly of light and heavy chains, because they appear to contain both in their cytoplasm. There is no evidence that such patients should be treated differently from other patients with CLL (Chap. 134).

137 Amyloidosis

David C. Seldin, John L. Berk

GENERAL PRINCIPLES

Amyloidosis is the term for a group of protein folding disorders characterized by the extracellular deposition of insoluble polymeric protein fibrils in tissues and organs. A robust cellular machinery exists to chaperone proteins during the process of synthesis and secretion, to ensure that they achieve correct tertiary conformation and function, and to eliminate proteins that misfold. However, genetic mutation, incorrect processing, and other factors may favor misfolding, with consequent loss of normal protein function and intracellular or extracellular aggregation. Many diseases, ranging from cystic fibrosis to Alzheimer's disease, are now known to involve protein misfolding. In the amyloidoses, the aggregates are typically extracellular, and the misfolded protein subunits assume a common antiparallel, β-pleated sheet–rich structural conformation that leads to the formation of higher-order oligomers and then of fibrils with unique staining properties. The term *amyloid* was coined around 1854 by the pathologist Rudolf Virchow, who thought that these deposits resembled starch (Latin *amylum*) under the microscope.

Amyloid diseases, defined by the biochemical nature of the protein composing the fibril deposits, are classified according to whether they are systemic or localized, whether they are acquired or inherited, and their clinical patterns (Table 137-1). The standard nomenclature is *AX*, where *A* indicates amyloidosis and *X* represents the protein present in the fibril. This chapter focuses primarily on the systemic forms. *AL* refers to amyloid composed of immunoglobulin light chains (LCs); this disorder, formerly termed *primary systemic amyloidosis*, arises from a clonal B cell or plasma cell disorder and can be associated with myeloma or lymphoma. *AF* refers to the *familial amyloidoses*, which are most commonly due to mutations in transthyretin (TTR), the transport protein for thyroid hormone and retinol-binding protein. *AA* amyloid is composed of the acute-phase reactant protein serum amyloid A (SAA) and occurs in the setting of chronic inflammatory or infectious diseases; for this reason, this type was formerly known as *secondary amyloidosis*. *Aβ$_2$M* amyloid results from misfolded β$_2$-microglobulin, occurring in individuals with long-standing renal disease who have undergone dialysis, typically for years. *Aβ*, the most common form of localized amyloidosis, is found in the brain of patients with Alzheimer's disease after abnormal proteolytic processing and aggregation of polypeptides derived from the amyloid precursor protein.

Diagnosis and treatment of the amyloidoses rest upon the histopathologic identification of amyloid deposits and immunohistochemical, biochemical, or genetic determination of amyloid type (Fig. 137-1). In the systemic amyloidoses, the clinically involved organs can be biopsied, but amyloid deposits may be found in any tissue of the body. Historically, blood vessels of the gingiva or rectal mucosa were often examined, but the most easily accessible tissue—positive in more than 80% of patients with systemic amyloidosis—is fat. After local anesthesia, fat is aspirated from the abdominal pannus with a 16-gauge needle. Fat globules expelled onto a glass slide can be stained, thus avoiding a surgical procedure. If this material is negative, more invasive biopsies of the kidney, heart, liver, or gastrointestinal tract can be considered in patients in whom amyloidosis is suspected. The regular β-sheet structure of amyloid deposits exhibits a unique "apple green" birefringence by polarized light microscopy when stained with Congo red dye; other regular protein structures (e.g., collagen) appear white under these conditions. The 10-nm-diameter fibrils can also be visualized by electron microscopy of paraformaldehyde-fixed tissue. Once amyloid is found, the protein type must be determined by immunohistochemistry, immunoelectron microscopy, or extraction and biochemical analysis employing mass spectrometry; gene sequencing is used to identify mutants causing AF amyloid. The patient's history, physical findings, and clinical presentation, including age and ethnic origin, organ system involvement, underlying diseases, and family history, may provide helpful clues as to the type of amyloid. However, there can be considerable overlap in clinical presentations, and accurate typing is essential to guide appropriate therapy.

The mechanisms of fibril formation and tissue toxicity remain controversial. The "amyloid hypothesis," as it is currently understood, proposes that precursor proteins undergo a process of reversible unfolding or misfolding; misfolded proteins form oligomeric aggregates, higher-order polymers, and then fibrils that deposit in tissues. Accumulating evidence suggests that the oligomeric intermediates may constitute the most toxic species. Oligomers are more capable than large fibrils of interacting with cells and inducing formation of reactive oxygen species and stress signaling. Ultimately, the fibrillar tissue deposits are likely to interfere with normal organ function. A more sophisticated understanding of the mechanisms leading to amyloid formation and cell and tissue dysfunction will continue to provide new targets for therapies.

The clinical syndromes of the amyloidoses are associated with relatively nonspecific alterations in routine laboratory tests. Blood counts are usually normal, although the erythrocyte sedimentation rate is frequently elevated. Patients with glomerular kidney involvement generally have proteinuria, often in the nephrotic range, leading to

TABLE 137-1 AMYLOID PRECURSOR PROTEINS AND THEIR CLINICAL SYNDROMES

Designation	Precursor	Clinical Syndrome	Clinical Involvement
Systemic Amyloidoses			
AL	Immunoglobulin light chain	Primary or myeloma-associated[a]	Any
AH	Immunoglobulin heavy chain	Rare variant of primary or myeloma-associated	Any
AA	Serum amyloid A protein	Secondary; reactive[b]	Renal, other
Aβ_2M	β_2-Microglobulin	Hemodialysis-associated	Synovial tissue, bone
ATTR	Transthyretin	Familial (mutant) Age-related (wild type)	Cardiac, peripheral and autonomic nerves
AApoAI	Apolipoprotein AI	Familial	Hepatic, renal
AApoAII	Apolipoprotein AII	Familial	Renal
AGel	Gelsolin	Familial	Cornea, cranial nerves, skin, renal
AFib	Fibrinogen Aα	Familial	Renal
ALys	Lysozyme	Familial	Renal, hepatic
ALECT2	Leukocyte chemotactic factor 2	Undefined	Renal
Localized Amyloidoses			
Aβ	Amyloid β protein	Alzheimer's disease; Down syndrome	Central nervous system
ACys	Cystatin C	Cerebral amyloid angiopathy	Central nervous system, vascular
APrP	Prion protein	Spongiform encephalopathies	Central nervous system
AIAPP	Islet amyloid polypeptide (amylin)	Diabetes-associated	Pancreas
ACal	Calcitonin	Medullary carcinoma of the thyroid	Thyroid
AANF	Atrial natriuretic factor	Atrial fibrillation	Cardiac atria
APro	Prolactin	Endocrinopathy	Pituitary
ASgI	Semenogelin I	Age-related; incidental autopsy or biopsy finding	Seminal vesicles

[a]Localized AL deposits can occur in skin, conjunctiva, urinary bladder, and the tracheobronchial tree. [b]Secondary to chronic inflammation or infection or to a hereditary periodic fever syndrome such as familial Mediterranean fever.

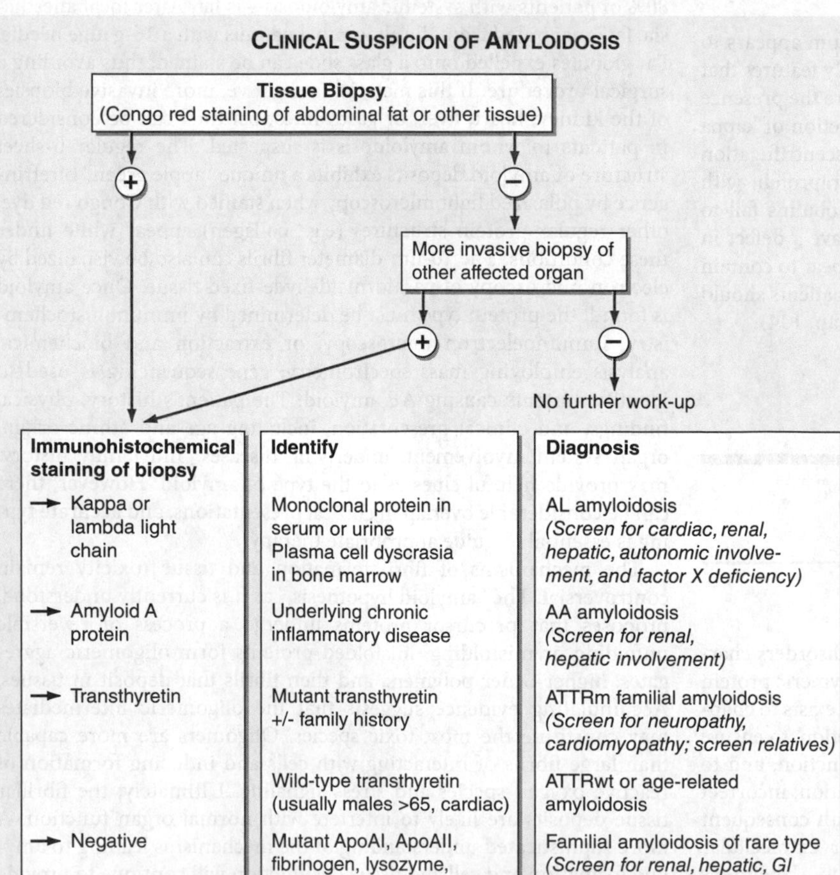

FIGURE 137-1 Algorithm for the diagnosis of amyloidosis and determination of type. Clinical suspicion: unexplained nephropathy, cardiomyopathy, neuropathy, enteropathy, arthropathy, and macroglossia. ApoAI, apolipoprotein AI; ApoAII, apolipoprotein AII; GI, gastrointestinal.

hypoalbuminemia that may be severe; patients with serum albumin levels below 2 g/dL generally have pedal edema or anasarca. Amyloid cardiomyopathy is characterized by concentric ventricular hypertrophy and diastolic dysfunction associated with elevation of brain natriuretic peptide or N-terminal pro–brain natriuretic peptide as well as troponin. These cardiac biomarkers can be used for disease staging, prognostication, and disease activity monitoring in patients with AL amyloidosis. Notably, renal insufficiency can falsely elevate levels of these biomarkers. Recently, biomarkers of cardiac remodeling—i.e., matrix metalloproteinases and tissue inhibitors of metalloproteinases—have been found to be altered in the serum of patients with amyloid cardiomyopathy. Electrocardiographic and echocardiographic features of amyloid cardiomyopathy are described below. Patients with liver involvement, even when advanced, usually develop cholestasis with an elevated alkaline phosphatase concentration but minimal alteration of the aminotransferases and preservation of synthetic function. In AL amyloidosis, endocrine organs may be infiltrated with fibrils, and hypothyroidism, hypoadrenalism, or even hypopituitarism can occur. Although none of these findings is specific for amyloidosis, the presence of abnormalities in multiple organ systems should raise suspicion regarding this diagnosis.

AL AMYLOIDOSIS

Etiology and Incidence AL amyloidosis is most frequently caused by a clonal expansion of bone-marrow plasma cells that secrete a monoclonal immunoglobulin LC depositing as amyloid fibrils in tissues. Whether the clonal plasma cells produce an LC that misfolds and leads to AL amyloidosis or an LC that folds properly, allowing the cells to inexorably expand over time and develop into multiple myeloma (Chap. 136), may depend upon primary sequence or other genetic or epigenetic factors. AL amyloidosis can occur with multiple myeloma or other B lymphoproliferative diseases, including non-Hodgkin's lymphoma (Chap. 134) and Waldenström's macroglobulinemia (Chap. 136). AL amyloidosis is the most common type of systemic amyloidosis diagnosed in North America. Its incidence has been estimated at 4.5 cases/100,000 population; however, ascertainment continues to be inadequate, and the true incidence may be much higher. AL amyloidosis, like other plasma cell diseases, usually occurs after age 40 and is often rapidly progressive and fatal if untreated.

Pathology and Clinical Features Amyloid deposits are usually widespread in AL amyloidosis and can be present in the interstitium of any organ outside the central nervous system. The amyloid fibril deposits are composed of full-length 23-kDa monoclonal immunoglobulin LCs as well as fragments. Accessory molecules co-deposited with LC fibrils (as well as with other amyloid fibrils) include serum amyloid P component, other proteins, glycosaminoglycans, and metal ions. Although all kappa and lambda LC subtypes have been identified in AL amyloid fibrils, lambda subtypes predominate. The lambda 6 subtype appears to have unique structural properties that predispose it to fibril formation, often in the kidney.

AL amyloidosis is often a rapidly progressive disease that presents as a pleiotropic set of clinical syndromes, recognition of which is key for initiation of the appropriate workup. Nonspecific symptoms of fatigue and weight loss are common; however, the diagnosis is rarely considered until symptoms referable to a specific organ develop. The kidneys are the most frequently involved organ and are affected in 70–80% of patients. Renal amyloidosis usually manifests as proteinuria, often in the nephrotic range and associated with hypoalbuminemia, secondary hypercholesterolemia and hypertriglyceridemia, and edema or anasarca. In some patients, interstitial rather than glomerular amyloid deposition can produce azotemia without proteinuria. The heart is the second most commonly affected organ (50–60% of patients), and cardiac involvement is the leading cause of death from AL amyloidosis. Early on, the electrocardiogram may show low voltage in the limb leads with a pseudo-infarct pattern. Echocardiographic features of disease include concentrically thickened ventricles and diastolic dysfunction with an abnormal strain pattern a "sparkly" appearance has been described but is often not seen with modern high-resolution echocardiographic techniques. Poor atrial contractility occurs even in sinus rhythm, and patients with cardiac amyloidosis are at risk for development of atrial thrombi and stroke. Cardiac MRI can show increased wall thickness, and characteristic enhancement of the subendocardium has been described following injection of gadolinium contrast. Nervous system symptoms include peripheral sensorimotor neuropathy and/or autonomic dysfunction manifesting as gastrointestinal motility disturbances (early satiety, diarrhea, constipation), impotence, orthostatic hypotension, and/or neurogenic bladder. Macroglossia (Fig. 137-2*A*), a pathognomonic sign of AL amyloidosis, is seen in only ~10% of patients. Liver involvement causes cholestasis and hepatomegaly. The spleen is frequently involved, and there may be functional hyposplenism in the absence of significant splenomegaly. Many patients experience "easy bruising" due to amyloid deposits in capillaries or deficiency of clotting factor X, which can bind to amyloid fibrils; cutaneous ecchymoses appear, particularly around the eyes, producing the "raccoon-eye" sign Fig. 137-2*B*), another uncommon but pathognomonic finding. Other findings include nail dystrophy (Fig. 137-2*C*), alopecia, and amyloid arthropathy with thickening of synovial membranes in the wrists and shoulders. The presence of a multisystemic illness or general fatigue along with any of these clinical syndromes should prompt a workup for amyloidosis.

Diagnosis Identification of an underlying clonal plasma cell or B lymphoproliferative process and a clonal LC are key to the diagnosis of AL amyloidosis. Serum protein electrophoresis and urine protein electrophoresis, although of value in multiple myeloma, are *not* useful screening tests if AL amyloidosis is suspected because the clonal LC or whole immunoglobulin often is not present in sufficient amounts to produce a monoclonal "M-spike" in the serum or LC (Bence Jones) protein in the urine. However, more than 90% of patients with AL amyloidosis have serum or urine monoclonal LC or whole immunoglobulin detectable by immunofixation electrophoresis of serum (SIFE) or urine (UIFE) (Fig. 137-3*A*) or by nephelometric measurement of "free" LCs (i.e., LCs circulating in monomeric form rather than in an immunoglobulin tetramer with heavy chain). Examining the ratio as well as the absolute amount of free LCs is essential, as renal insufficiency reduces LC clearance, elevating both isotypes. In addition, an increased percentage of plasma cells in the bone marrow—typically 5–30% of nucleated cells—is found in ~90% of patients. Kappa or lambda clonality should be demonstrated by flow cytometry, immunohistochemistry, or in situ hybridization for LC mRNA (Fig. 137-3*B*).

A monoclonal serum protein by itself is not diagnostic of amyloidosis, since monoclonal gammopathy of uncertain significance is common in older patients (Chap. 136). However, when monoclonal gammopathy of uncertain significance is found in patients with biopsy-proven amyloidosis, the AL type should be strongly suspected. Similarly, patients thought to have "smoldering myeloma" because of a modest elevation of bone-marrow plasma cells should be screened for AL amyloidosis if they have signs or symptoms of renal, cardiac, or neurologic disease. Accurate tissue amyloid typing is essential for appropriate treatment. Immunohistochemical staining of the amyloid deposits is useful if they bind one LC antibody in preference to the other; some AL deposits bind antibodies nonspecifically. Immunoelectron microscopy is more reliable, and mass spectrometry–based microsequencing of small amounts of protein extracted from fibril deposits can also be undertaken. In ambiguous cases, other forms of amyloidosis should be thoroughly excluded with appropriate genetic and other testing.

TREATMENT AL AMYLOIDOSIS

Extensive multisystemic involvement typifies AL amyloidosis, and the median survival period without treatment is usually only ~1–2 years from the time of diagnosis. Current therapies target the

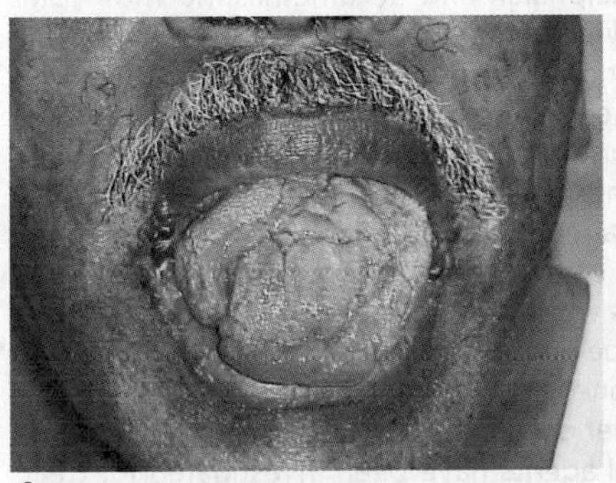

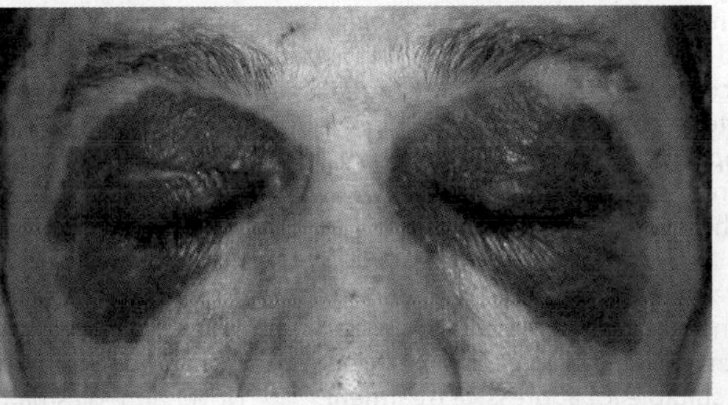

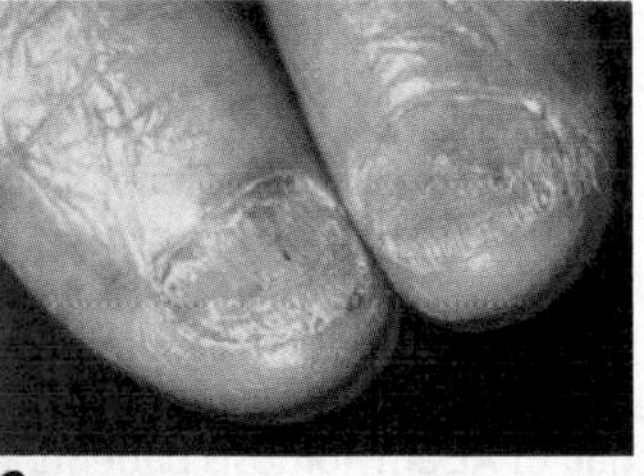

FIGURE 137-2 **Clinical signs of AL amyloidosis.** ***A.*** Macroglossia. ***B.*** Periorbital ecchymoses. ***C.*** Fingernail dystrophy.

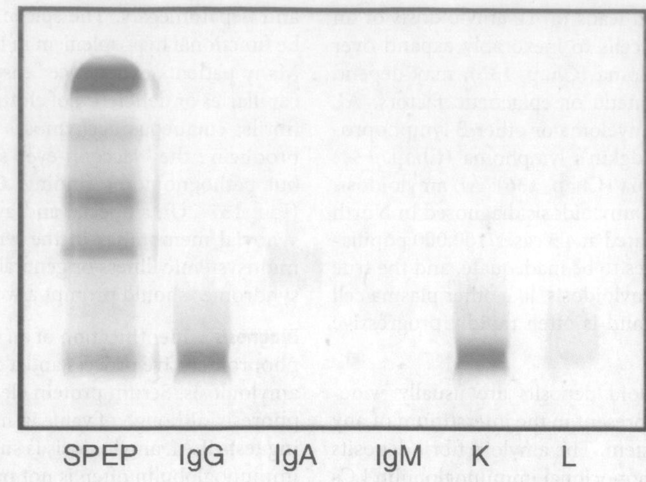

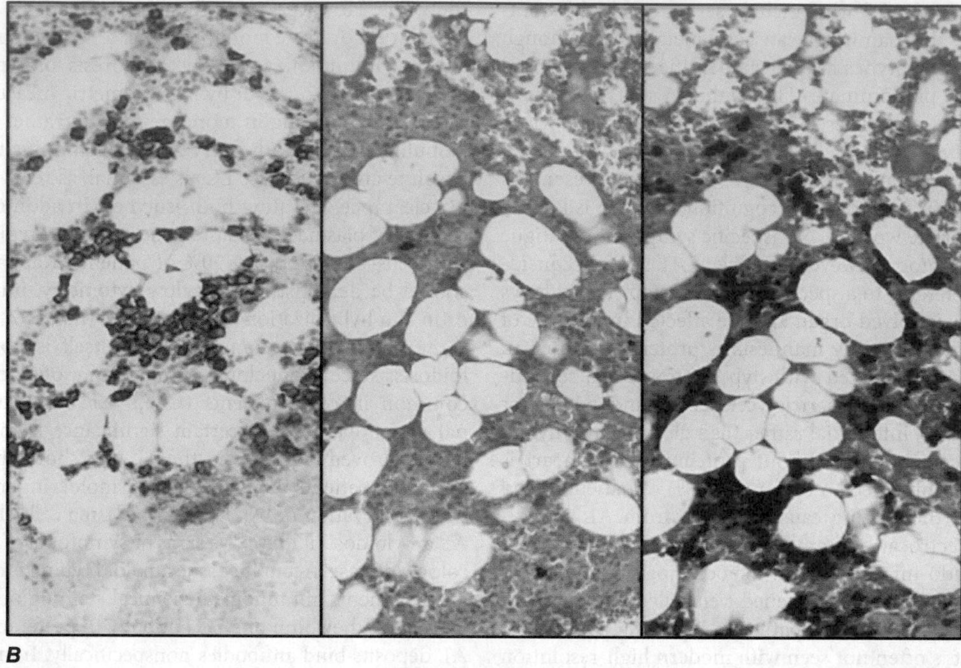

FIGURE 137-3 Laboratory features of AL amyloidosis. *A.* Serum immunofixation electrophoresis reveals an IgGκ monoclonal protein in this example; serum protein electrophoresis is often normal. ***B.*** Bone-marrow biopsy sections stained by immunohistochemistry with antibody to CD138 (syndecan, highly expressed on plasma cells) (*left*) or by in situ hybridization with fluorescein-tagged probes (Ventana Medical Systems) binding to κ mRNA (*center*) and λ mRNA (*right*) in plasma cells. *(Photomicrograph courtesy of C. O'Hara; with permission.)*

clonal bone-marrow plasma cells, using approaches employed for multiple myeloma. Treatment with oral melphalan and prednisone can decrease the plasma cell burden but rarely leads to complete hematologic remission, meaningful organ responses, or improved survival and is no longer widely used. The substitution of dexamethasone for prednisone produces a higher response rate and more durable remissions, although dexamethasone is not always well tolerated by patients with significant edema or cardiac disease. High-dose IV melphalan followed by autologous stem cell transplantation (HDM/SCT) produces complete hematologic responses in ~40% of treated patients, as determined by loss of clonal plasma cells in the bone marrow and disappearance of the monoclonal LC, as determined by SIFE/UIFE and free LC quantitation. Hematologic responses can be followed in the subsequent 6–12 months as improvements in organ function and quality of life. Hematologic responses appear to be more durable after HDM/SCT than in multiple myeloma, with remissions continuing in some patients beyond 15 years without additional treatment. Unfortunately, only about half of AL amyloidosis patients are suitable for aggressive treatment, and, even at specialized treatment centers, transplantation-related mortality rates are higher than those for other hematologic diseases because of impaired organ function. Amyloid cardiomyopathy, poor nutritional and performance status, and multiorgan disease contribute to excess morbidity and mortality. A bleeding diathesis resulting from adsorption of clotting factor X to amyloid fibrils also increases mortality rates; however, this syndrome occurs in only 5–10% of patients. A randomized multicenter trial conducted in France compared oral melphalan and dexamethasone with HDM/SCT and failed to show a benefit of dose-intensive treatment, although the transplantation-related mortality rate in this study was very high. It has become clear that careful selection of patients and expert peritransplantation management are essential in reducing transplantation-related mortality.

For patients with impaired cardiac function or arrhythmias due to amyloid involvement of the myocardium, the median survival period is only ~6 months without treatment. In these patients, cardiac transplantation can be performed and followed by HDM/SCT to eliminate the noxious clone and prevent amyloid deposition in the transplanted heart or other organs.

Novel anti–plasma cell agents have been investigated for treatment of plasma cell diseases. The immunomodulators thalidomide, lenalidomide, and pomalidomide display activity; dosing may need to be adjusted compared to their usage for myeloma. The proteasome inhibitor bortezomib has also been found to be effective in single-center and multicenter trials. Anti-fibril small molecules and humanized monoclonal antibodies are also being tested. Clinical trials are essential in improving therapy for this rare disease.

Supportive care is important for patients with any type of amyloidosis. For nephrotic syndrome, diuretics and supportive stockings can ameliorate edema; angiotensin-converting enzyme inhibitors should be used with caution and have not been shown to slow renal disease progression. Effective diuresis can be facilitated with albumin infusions to raise intravascular oncotic pressure. Congestive heart failure due to amyloid cardiomyopathy is best treated with diuretics; it is important to note that digitalis, calcium channel blockers, and beta blockers are relatively contraindicated as they can interact with amyloid fibrils and produce heart block and worsening heart failure. Amiodarone has been used for atrial and ventricular arrhythmias. Automatic implantable defibrillators have reduced effectiveness due to the thickened myocardium, but they may benefit some patients. Atrial ablation is an effective approach for atrial fibrillation. For conduction abnormalities, ventricular pacing may be indicated. Atrial contractile dysfunction is common in amyloid cardiomyopathy and is an indication for anticoagulation even in the absence of atrial fibrillation. Autonomic neuropathy can be treated with α agonists such as midodrine to support the blood pressure; gastrointestinal dysfunction may respond to motility or bulk agents. Nutritional supplementation, either oral or parenteral, is also important.

In localized AL disease, amyloid deposits can be produced by clonal plasma cells infiltrating local sites in the airways, bladder, skin, or lymph nodes (Table 137-1). These deposits may respond to surgical intervention or low-dose radiation therapy (typically only 20 Gy); systemic treatment generally is not appropriate. Patients should be referred to a center familiar with management of these rare manifestations of amyloidosis.

AA AMYLOIDOSIS

Etiology and Incidence AA amyloidosis can occur in association with almost any chronic inflammatory state (e.g., rheumatoid arthritis, inflammatory bowel disease, familial Mediterranean fever [Chap. 392], or other periodic fever syndromes) or chronic infections such as tuberculosis or subacute bacterial endocarditis. In the United States and Europe, AA amyloidosis has become less common, occurring in fewer than 2% of patients with these diseases, presumably because of advances in anti-inflammatory and antimicrobial therapies. It has also been described in association with Castleman's disease, and patients with AA amyloidosis should undergo CT scanning to look for such tumors as well as serologic and microbiologic studies. AA amyloidosis can also be seen without any identifiable underlying disease. AA is the only type of systemic amyloidosis that occurs in children.

Pathology and Clinical Features Organ involvement in AA amyloidosis usually begins in the kidneys. Hepatomegaly, splenomegaly, and autonomic neuropathy can also occur as the disease progresses; cardiomyopathy occurs, albeit rarely. The symptoms and signs of AA disease cannot be reliably distinguished from those of AL amyloidosis. AA amyloid fibrils are usually composed of an 8-kDa, 76-amino-acid *N*-terminal portion of the 12-kDa precursor protein SAA. This acute-phase apoprotein is synthesized in the liver and transported by high-density lipoprotein (HDL3) in the plasma. Several years of an underlying inflammatory disease causing chronic elevation of SAA levels usually precede fibril formation, although infections can lead to AA deposition more rapidly.

TREATMENT AA AMYLOIDOSIS

Primary therapy for AA amyloidosis consists of treatment of the underlying inflammatory or infectious disease. Treatment that suppresses or eliminates the inflammation or infection also decreases the SAA concentration. For familial Mediterranean fever, colchicine at a dose of 1.2–1.8 mg/d is the standard treatment. However, colchicine has not been helpful for AA amyloidosis of other causes or for other amyloidoses. Tumor necrosis factor and interleukin 1 antagonists can be effective in syndromes related to cytokine elevation. For this disease, there is also a fibril-specific agent: eprodisate was designed to interfere with the interaction of AA amyloid protein with glycosaminoglycans and to prevent or disrupt fibril formation. The drug is well tolerated and delays progression of AA renal disease. Randomized phase III clinical trials with eprodisate are ongoing; the drug is not otherwise available.

ATTR AND AF AMYLOIDOSIS

The familial amyloidoses are autosomal dominant diseases in which, beginning in midlife, a variant (FINE) plasma protein forms amyloid deposits. These diseases are rare, with an estimated incidence of <1 case/100,000 population in the United States, although founder effects in isolated areas of Portugal, Sweden, and Japan have led to a much higher incidence. The most common form of AF amyloidosis is ATTRm in the updated nomenclature, caused by mutation of the abundant plasma protein transthyretin (TTR, also known as *prealbumin*). More than 100 TTR mutations are known, and most are associated with ATTR amyloidosis. One variant, V122I, has a carrier frequency that may be as high as 4% in the African-American population and is associated with late-onset cardiac amyloidosis. The actual incidence and penetrance of disease in the African-American population is the subject of ongoing research, but ATTR amyloidosis warrants consideration in the differential diagnosis of African-American patients who present with concentric cardiac hypertrophy and evidence of diastolic dysfunction, particularly in the absence of a history of hypertension. Other familial amyloidoses, caused by variant apolipoproteins AI or AII, gelsolin, fibrinogen Aα, or lysozyme, are reported in only a few families worldwide. New amyloidogenic serum proteins continue to be identified periodically, including recently the leukocyte chemotactic factor LECT2, a cause of renal amyloidosis in Hispanic and Pakistani populations. To date, no mutation in the coding sequence for the LECT2 gene has been identified, so the heritability of ALECT2 is uncertain.

TTR deposits composed of unmutated fibrils occur with aging, and ATTRwt is being diagnosed with increasing frequency in Caucasian men >65 years of age with amyloid cardiomyopathy. Formerly termed senile systemic amyloidosis, ATTRwt has been found at autopsy in 25% of hearts from patients older than age 80 years. Why a wild type protein becomes amyloidogenic, and why patients bearing mutant TTR genes do not express disease until adulthood, remains a mystery.

Clinical Features and Diagnosis AF amyloidosis has a presentation that is variable but is usually consistent within kindreds affected by the same mutant protein. A family history makes AF disease more likely, but many patients present sporadically with new mutations. ATTR amyloidosis typically presents as a syndrome of familial amyloidotic polyneuropathy or familial amyloidotic cardiomyopathy. Peripheral neuropathy begins as a small-fiber lower-extremity sensory and motor neuropathy and progresses to the upper extremities. Autonomic neuropathy manifests as diarrhea with weight loss and orthostatic hypotension. Patients with TTR V30M, the most common mutation, have normal electrocardiograms but may develop conduction defects late in the disease. Patients with TTR T60A and several other mutations have myocardial thickening similar to that caused by AL amyloidosis, although heart failure is less common and long-term survival rates are usually better. Vitreous opacities caused by amyloid deposits are pathognomonic for ATTR amyloidosis.

Typical syndromes associated with other forms of AF disease include renal amyloidosis with mutant fibrinogen, lysozyme, or apolipoproteins; hepatic amyloidosis with apolipoprotein AI; and amyloidosis of cranial nerves and cornea with gelsolin. Patients with AF amyloidosis can present with clinical syndromes that mimic those of patients with AL disease. Rarely, AF carriers can develop AL disease or AF patients may have monoclonal gammopathy without AL.

Thus, it is important to screen both for plasma cell disorders and for mutations in patients with amyloidosis. Variant TTRs can usually be detected by isoelectric focusing, but DNA sequencing is now standard for diagnosis of ATTR and other AF mutations.

TREATMENT ATTR AMYLOIDOSIS

Without intervention, the survival period after onset of ATTR disease is 5–15 years. Orthotopic liver transplantation replaces the major source of variant TTR production with a source of normal TTR. While liver transplantation can slow disease progression and improve chances of survival, it does not reverse sensorimotor neuropathy. Liver transplants are most successful in young patients with early peripheral neuropathy; older patients with familial amyloidotic cardiomyopathy or advanced polyneuropathy often experience end-organ disease progression despite successful liver transplantation. Progressive disease has been attributed to accumulation of wild-type TTR in fibrillar deposits initiated by the mutant.

The rate-limiting step in ATTR amyloidosis is dissociation of the TTR tetramer into monomer followed by misfolding and aggregation. TTR tetramers can be stabilized by thyroxine binding or by small molecules such as the non-steroidal anti-inflammatory drug diflunisal or the rationally designed small-molecule therapeutic tafamidis. A placebo-controlled randomized trial of diflunisal demonstrated a reduction in the progression of polyneuropathy and maintenance of quality of life in patients with a wide variety of ATTR mutations who received the "repurposed" diflunisal. Tafamidis tested in a similar fashion in patients with the V30M ATTR mutation failed to meet its primary endpoints, but tafamidis was approved by the European Medicines Agency since most secondary endpoints favored the drug. These agents are now being investigated for effects on cardiomyopathy, and in ATTRwt. *In vitro* data and serendipitous observations in patients suggest that ATTRm disease can be ameliorated by "trans-suppression," in which a T119M TTR variant stabilizes tetramers that also contain amyloidogenic subunits. Interestingly, in a large population study in Denmark, 0.5% of participants were heterozygous for the T119M allele, and this small group had higher levels of TTR in their blood, a reduced incidence of cerebrovascular disease, and a 5- to 10-year survival advantage compared with participants lacking this allele.

Aβ_2M AMYLOIDOSIS

Aβ_2M amyloid is composed of β_2-microglobulin, the invariant chain of class I human leukocyte antigens, and produces rheumatologic manifestations in patients undergoing long-term hemodialysis. β_2-Microglobulin is excreted by the kidney, and levels become elevated in end-stage renal disease. The molecular mass of β_2M is 11.8 kDa—above the cutoff of some dialysis membranes. The incidence of this disease appears to be declining with the use of newer membranes in high-flow dialysis techniques. Aβ_2M amyloidosis usually presents as carpal tunnel syndrome, persistent joint effusions, spondyloarthropathy, or cystic bone lesions. Carpal tunnel syndrome is often the first symptom. In the past, persistent joint effusions accompanied by mild discomfort were found in up to 50% of patients who had undergone dialysis for >12 years. Involvement is bilateral, and large joints (shoulders, knees, wrists, and hips) are most frequently affected. The synovial fluid is noninflammatory, and β_2M amyloid can be found if the sediment is stained with Congo red. Although less common, visceral β_2M amyloid deposits do occasionally occur in the gastrointestinal tract, heart, tendons, and subcutaneous tissues of the buttocks. There is no specific therapy for Aβ_2M amyloidosis, but cessation of dialysis after renal allografting may lead to symptomatic improvement.

SUMMARY

A diagnosis of amyloidosis should be considered in patients with unexplained nephropathy, cardiomyopathy (particularly with diastolic dysfunction), neuropathy (either peripheral or autonomic), enteropathy, or the pathognomonic soft tissue findings of macroglossia or periorbital ecchymoses. Pathologic identification of amyloid fibrils can be made with Congo red staining of aspirated abdominal fat or of an involved-organ biopsy specimen. Accurate typing by a combination of immunologic, biochemical, and genetic testing is essential in selecting appropriate therapy (Fig. 137-1). Systemic amyloidosis should not be considered an untreatable condition, as anti–plasma cell chemotherapy is highly effective in AL disease and targeted therapies are being developed for AA and ATTR disease. Tertiary referral centers can provide specialized diagnostic techniques and access to clinical trials for patients with these rare diseases.

ACKNOWLEDGMENT

This chapter represents a revised version of a chapter that was co-authored by Dr. Martha Skinner and Dr. David Seldin in previous editions of Harrison's Principles of Internal Medicine.

138e Transfusion Biology and Therapy

Jeffery S. Dzieczkowski, Kenneth C. Anderson

This is a digital-only chapter. It is available on the DVD that accompanies this book, as well as on Access Medicine/Harrison's Online, and the eBook and "app" editions of HPIM 19e.

BLOOD GROUP ANTIGENS AND ANTIBODIES

The study of red blood cell (RBC) antigens and antibodies forms the foundation of transfusion medicine. Serologic studies initially characterized these antigens, but now the molecular composition and structure of many are known. Antigens, either carbohydrate or protein, are assigned to a blood group system based on the structure and similarity of the determinant epitopes. Other cellular blood elements and plasma proteins are also antigenic and can result in *alloimmunization*, the production of antibodies directed against the blood group antigens of another individual. These antibodies are called *alloantibodies*.

Antibodies directed against RBC antigens may result from "natural" exposure, particularly to carbohydrates that mimic some blood group antigens. Those antibodies that occur via natural stimuli are usually produced by a T cell–independent response (thus, generating no memory) and are IgM isotype. *Autoantibodies* (antibodies against autologous blood group antigens) arise spontaneously or as the result of infectious sequelae (e.g., from *Mycoplasma pneumoniae*) and are also often IgM. These antibodies are often clinically insignificant due to their low affinity for antigen at body temperature. However, IgM antibodies can activate the complement cascade and result in hemolysis. Antibodies that result from allogeneic exposure, such as transfusion or pregnancy, are usually IgG. IgG antibodies commonly bind to antigen at warmer temperatures and may hemolyze RBCs. Unlike IgM antibodies, IgG antibodies can cross the placenta and bind fetal erythrocytes bearing the corresponding antigen, resulting in hemolytic disease of the newborn, or *hydrops fetalis*.

Alloimmunization to leukocytes, platelets, and plasma proteins may also result in transfusion complications such as fevers and urticaria but generally does not cause hemolysis. Assay for these other alloantibodies is not routinely performed; however, they may be detected using special assays.

139e Hematopoietic Cell Transplantation

Frederick R. Appelbaum

This is a digital-only chapter. It is available on the DVD that accompanies this book, as well as on Access Medicine/Harrison's Online, and the eBook and "app" editions of HPIM 19e.

Bone marrow transplantation was the original term used to describe the collection and transplantation of hematopoietic stem cells, but with the demonstration that peripheral blood and umbilical cord blood are also useful sources of stem cells, *hematopoietic cell transplantation* has become the preferred generic term for this process. The procedure is usually carried out for one of two purposes: (1) to replace an abnormal but nonmalignant lymphohematopoietic system with one from a normal donor or (2) to treat malignancy by allowing the administration of higher doses of myelosuppressive therapy than would otherwise be possible. The use of hematopoietic cell transplantation has been increasing, both because of its efficacy in selected diseases and because of increasing availability of donors. The Center for International Blood and Marrow Transplant Research (*http://www.cibmtr.org*) estimates that about 65,000 transplants are performed each year.

SECTION 3 DISORDERS OF HEMOSTASIS

140 Disorders of Platelets and Vessel Wall

Barbara A. Konkle

Hemostasis is a dynamic process in which the platelet and the blood vessel wall play key roles. Platelets become activated upon adhesion to von Willebrand factor (VWF) and collagen in the exposed subendothelium after injury. Platelet activation is also mediated through shear forces imposed by blood flow itself, particularly in areas where the vessel wall is diseased, and is also affected by the inflammatory state of the endothelium. The activated platelet surface provides the major physiologic site for coagulation factor activation, which results in further platelet activation and fibrin formation. Genetic and acquired influences on the platelet and vessel wall, as well as on the coagulation and fibrinolytic systems, determine whether normal hemostasis or bleeding or clotting symptoms will result.

THE PLATELET

Platelets are released from the megakaryocyte, likely under the influence of flow in the capillary sinuses. The normal blood platelet count is 150,000–450,000/μL. The major regulator of platelet production is the hormone thrombopoietin (TPO), which is synthesized in the liver. Synthesis is increased with inflammation and specifically by interleukin 6. TPO binds to its receptor on platelets and megakaryocytes, by which it is removed from the circulation. Thus a reduction in platelet and megakaryocyte mass increases the level of TPO, which then stimulates platelet production. Platelets circulate with an average life span of 7–10 days. Approximately one-third of the platelets reside in the spleen, and this number increases in proportion to splenic size, although the platelet count rarely decreases to <40,000/μL as the spleen enlarges. Platelets are physiologically very active, but are anucleate, and thus have limited capacity to synthesize new proteins.

Normal vascular endothelium contributes to preventing thrombosis by inhibiting platelet function (Chap. 78). When vascular endothelium is injured, these inhibitory effects are overcome, and platelets adhere to the exposed intimal surface primarily through VWF, a large multimeric protein present in both plasma and in the extracellular matrix of the subendothelial vessel wall. Platelet adhesion results in the generation of intracellular signals that lead to activation of the platelet glycoprotein (Gp) IIb/IIIa ($\alpha_{IIb}\beta_3$) receptor and resultant platelet aggregation.

Activated platelets undergo release of their granule contents, which include nucleotides, adhesive proteins, growth factors, and procoagulants that serve to promote platelet aggregation and blood clot formation and influence the environment of the forming clot. During platelet aggregation, additional platelets are recruited to the site of injury, leading to the formation of an occlusive platelet thrombus. The platelet plug is stabilized by the fibrin mesh that develops simultaneously as the product of the coagulation cascade.

THE VESSEL WALL

Endothelial cells line the surface of the entire circulatory tree, totaling 1–6 × 10^{13} cells, enough to cover a surface area equivalent to about six tennis courts. The endothelium is physiologically active, controlling vascular permeability, flow of biologically active molecules and nutrients, blood cell interactions with the vessel wall, the inflammatory response, and angiogenesis.

The endothelium normally presents an antithrombotic surface (Chap. 78) but rapidly becomes prothrombotic when stimulated, which promotes coagulation, inhibits fibrinolysis, and activates platelets. In many cases, endothelium-derived vasodilators are also platelet inhibitors (e.g., nitric oxide) and, conversely, endothelium-derived vasoconstrictors (e.g., endothelin) can also be platelet activators. The net effect of vasodilation and inhibition of platelet function is to promote blood fluidity, whereas the net effect of vasoconstriction and platelet activation is to promote thrombosis. Thus, blood fluidity and hemostasis are regulated by the balance of antithrombotic/prothrombotic and vasodilatory/vasoconstrictor properties of endothelial cells.

DISORDERS OF PLATELETS

THROMBOCYTOPENIA

Thrombocytopenia results from one or more of three processes: (1) decreased bone marrow production; (2) sequestration, usually in an enlarged spleen; and/or (3) increased platelet destruction. Disorders of production may be either inherited or acquired. In evaluating a patient with thrombocytopenia, a key step is to review the peripheral blood smear and to first rule out "pseudothrombocytopenia," particularly in a patient without an apparent cause for the thrombocytopenia. Pseudothrombocytopenia (Fig. 140-1*B*) is an in vitro artifact resulting from platelet agglutination via antibodies (usually IgG, but also IgM and IgA) when the calcium content is decreased by blood collection in ethylenediamine tetraacetic (EDTA) (the anticoagulant present in tubes [purple top] used to collect blood for complete blood counts [CBCs]). If a low platelet count is obtained in EDTA-anticoagulated blood, a blood smear should be evaluated and a platelet count determined in blood collected into sodium citrate (blue top tube) or heparin (green top tube), or a smear of freshly obtained unanticoagulated blood, such as from a finger stick, can be examined.

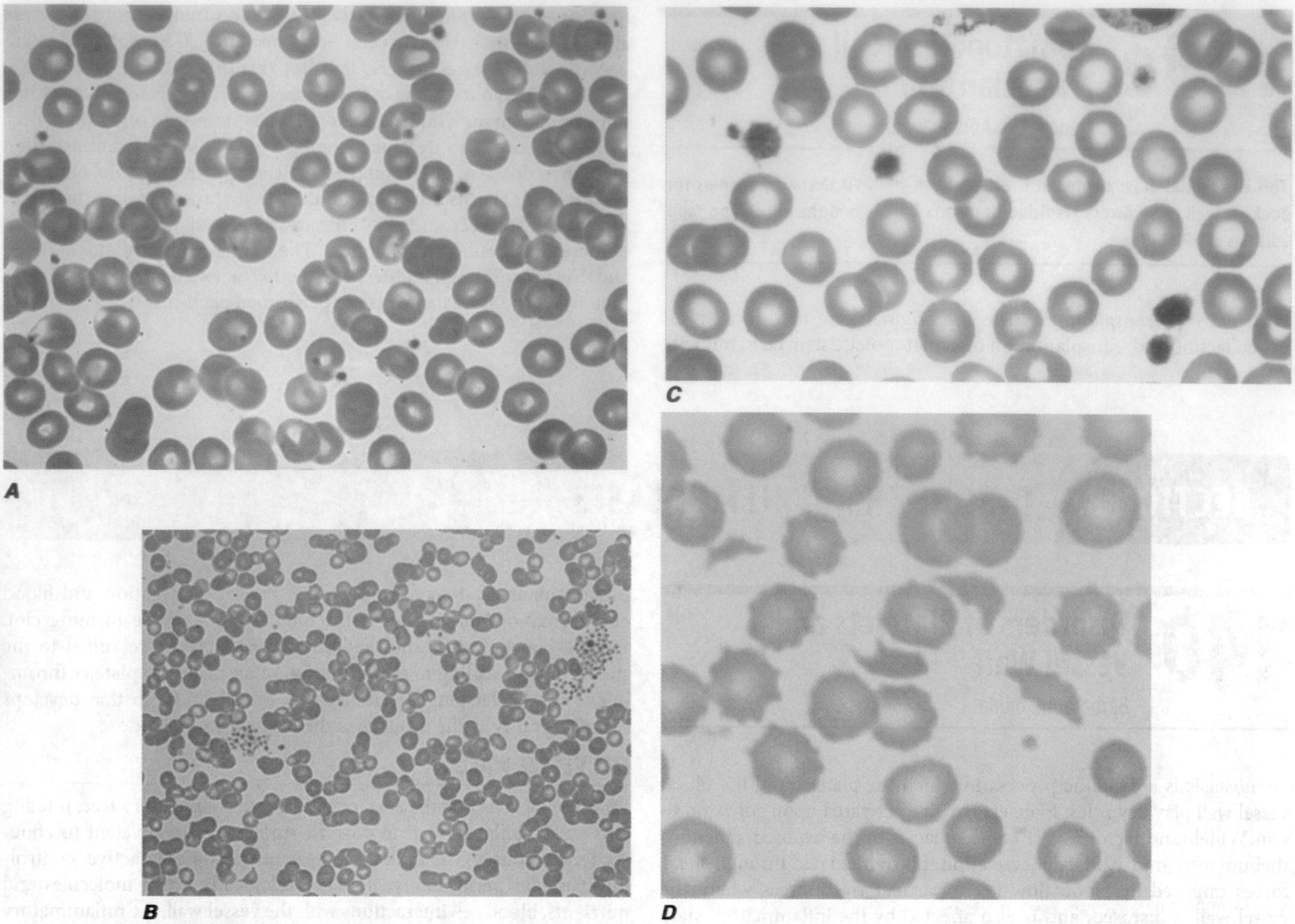

A B C D

FIGURE 140-1 Photomicrographs of peripheral blood smears. *A.* Normal peripheral blood. ***B.*** Platelet clumping in pseudothrombocytopenia. ***C.*** Abnormal large platelet in autosomal dominant macrothrombocytopenia. ***D.*** Schistocytes and decreased platelets in microangiopathic hemolytic anemia.

APPROACH TO THE PATIENT: Thrombocytopenia

The history and physical examination, results of the CBC, and review of the peripheral blood smear are all critical components in the initial evaluation of thrombocytopenic patients (Fig. 140-2). The overall health of the patient and whether he or she is receiving drug treatment will influence the differential diagnosis. A healthy young adult with thrombocytopenia will have a much more limited differential diagnosis than an ill hospitalized patient who is receiving multiple medications. Except in unusual inherited disorders, decreased platelet production usually results from bone marrow disorders that also affect red blood cell (RBC) and/or white blood cell (WBC) production. Because myelodysplasia can present with isolated thrombocytopenia, the bone marrow should be examined in patients presenting with isolated thrombocytopenia who are older than 60 years of age. While inherited thrombocytopenia is rare, any prior platelet counts should be retrieved and a family history regarding thrombocytopenia obtained. A careful history of drug ingestion should be obtained, including nonprescription and herbal remedies, because drugs are the most common cause of thrombocytopenia.

The physical examination can document an enlarged spleen, evidence of chronic liver disease, and other underlying disorders. Mild to moderate splenomegaly may be difficult to appreciate in many individuals due to body habitus and/or obesity but can be easily assessed by abdominal ultrasound. A platelet count of approximately 5000–10,000 is required to maintain vascular integrity in the microcirculation. When the count is markedly decreased, petechiae

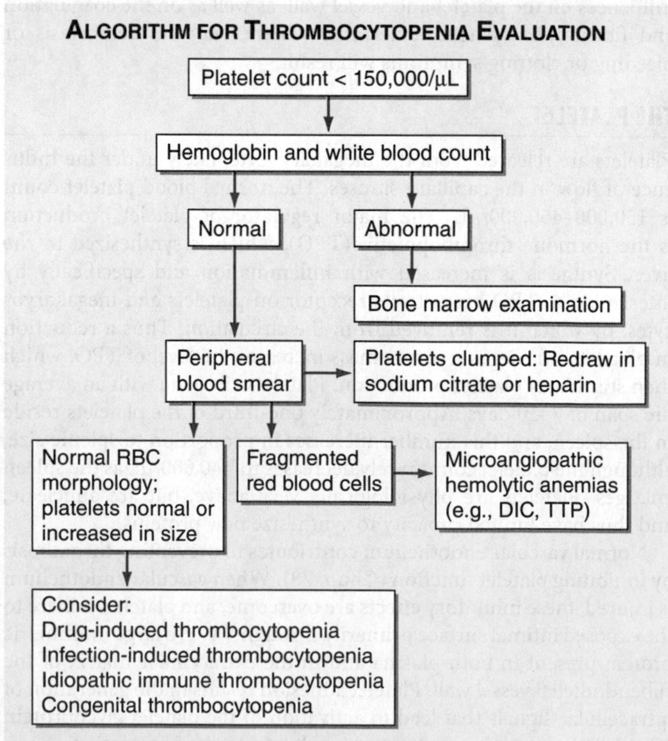

FIGURE 140-2 Algorithm for evaluating the thrombocytopenic patient. DIC, disseminated intravascular coagulation; RBC, red blood cell; TTP, thrombotic thrombocytopenic purpura.

first appear in areas of increased venous pressure, the ankles and feet in an ambulatory patient. Petechiae are pinpoint, nonblanching hemorrhages and are usually a sign of a decreased platelet number and not platelet dysfunction. Wet purpura, blood blisters that form on the oral mucosa, are thought to denote an increased risk of life-threatening hemorrhage in the thrombocytopenic patient. Excessive bruising is seen in disorders of both platelet number and function.

Infection-Induced Thrombocytopenia Many viral and bacterial infections result in thrombocytopenia and are the most common noniatrogenic cause of thrombocytopenia. This may or may not be associated with laboratory evidence of disseminated intravascular coagulation (DIC), which is most commonly seen in patients with systemic infections with gram-negative bacteria. Infections can affect both platelet production and platelet survival. In addition, immune mechanisms can be at work, as in infectious mononucleosis and early HIV infection. Late in HIV infection, pancytopenia and decreased and dysplastic platelet production are more common. Immune-mediated thrombocytopenia in children usually follows a viral infection and almost always resolves spontaneously. This association of infection with immune thrombocytopenic purpura is less clear in adults.

Bone marrow examination is often requested for evaluation of occult infections. A study evaluating the role of bone marrow examination in fever of unknown origin in HIV-infected patients found that for 86% of patients, the same diagnosis was established by less invasive techniques, notably blood culture. In some instances, however, the diagnosis can be made earlier; thus, a bone marrow examination and culture are recommended when the diagnosis is needed urgently or when other, less invasive methods have been unsuccessful.

Drug-Induced Thrombocytopenia Many drugs have been associated with thrombocytopenia. A predictable decrease in platelet count occurs after treatment with many chemotherapeutic drugs due to bone marrow suppression (Chap. 103e). Drugs that cause isolated thrombocytopenia and have been confirmed with positive laboratory testing are listed in Table 140-1, but all drugs should be suspect in a patient with thrombocytopenia without an apparent cause and should be stopped, or substituted, if possible. A helpful website, Platelets on the Internet (*http://www.ouhsc.edu/platelets/ditp.html*), lists drugs and supplements reported to have caused thrombocytopenia and the level of evidence supporting the association. Although not as well studied, herbal and over-the-counter preparations may also result in thrombocytopenia and should be discontinued in patients who are thrombocytopenic.

TABLE 140-1 DRUGS REPORTED AS DEFINITELY OR PROBABLY CAUSING ISOLATED THROMBOCYTOPENIA[a]

Abciximab	Mirtazapine
Acetaminophen	Naproxen
Amiodarone	Oxaliplatin
Amlodipine	Penicillin
Ampicillin	Phenytoin
Carbamazepine	Piperacillin
Ceftriaxone	Quinine
Cephamandole	Quinidine
Ciprofloxacin	Ranitidine
Diazepam	Rosiglitazone
Eptifibatide	Roxifiban
Furosemide	Sulfisoxazole
Gold	Suramin
Haloperidol	Tirofiban
Heparin	Tranilast
Ibuprofen	Trimethoprim/sulfamethoxazole
Lorazepam	Vancomycin

[a]Based on scoring requiring a compatible clinical picture and positive laboratory testing.

Source: Adapted from DM Arnold et al: J Thromb Hemost 11:169, 2013.

Classic drug-dependent antibodies are antibodies that react with specific platelet surface antigens and result in thrombocytopenia only when the drug is present. Many drugs are capable of inducing these antibodies, but for some reason, they are more common with quinine and sulfonamides. Drug-dependent antibody binding can be demonstrated by laboratory assays, showing antibody binding in the presence of, but not without, the drug present in the assay. The thrombocytopenia typically occurs after a period of initial exposure (median length 21 days), or upon reexposure, and usually resolves in 7–10 days after drug withdrawal. The thrombocytopenia caused by the platelet Gp IIb/IIIa inhibitory drugs, such as abciximab, differs in that it may occur within 24 h of initial exposure. This appears to be due to the presence of naturally occurring antibodies that cross-react with the drug bound to the platelet.

Heparin-Induced Thrombocytopenia Drug-induced thrombocytopenia due to heparin differs from that seen with other drugs in two major ways. (1) The thrombocytopenia is not usually severe, with nadir counts rarely <20,000/μL. (2) Heparin-induced thrombocytopenia (HIT) is not associated with bleeding and, in fact, markedly increases the risk of thrombosis. HIT results from antibody formation to a complex of the platelet-specific protein platelet factor 4 (PF4) and heparin. The anti-heparin/PF4 antibody can activate platelets through the FcγRIIa receptor and also activate monocytes and endothelial cells. Many patients exposed to heparin develop antibodies to heparin/PF4, but do not appear to have adverse consequences. A fraction of those who develop antibodies will develop HIT, and a portion of those (up to 50%) will develop thrombosis (HITT).

HIT can occur after exposure to low-molecular-weight heparin (LMWH) as well as unfractionated heparin (UFH), although it is more common with the latter. Most patients develop HIT after exposure to heparin for 5–14 days (Fig. 140-3). It occurs before 5 days in those who were exposed to heparin in the prior few weeks or months (<~100 days) and have circulating anti-heparin/PF4 antibodies. Rarely, thrombocytopenia and thrombosis begin several days after all heparin has been stopped (termed *delayed-onset HIT*). The "4T's" have been recommended to be used in a diagnostic algorithm for HIT: *t*hrombocytopenia, *t*iming of platelet count drop, *thrombosis* and other sequelae such as localized skin reactions, and o*t*her causes of thrombocytopenia not evident. Application of the 4T scoring system is very useful in excluding a diagnosis of HIT but will result in overdiagnosis of HIT in situations where thrombocytopenia and thrombosis due to other etiologies are common, such as in the intensive care unit. A scoring model based on broad expert opinion (the HIT Expert Probability [HEP] Score) has improved operating characteristics and may provide better utility as a scoring system.

LABORATORY TESTING FOR HIT HIT (anti-heparin/PF4) antibodies can be detected using two types of assays. The most widely available is an enzyme-linked immunoassay (ELISA) with PF4/polyanion complex as the antigen. Because many patients develop antibodies but do not develop clinical HIT, the test has a low specificity for the diagnosis

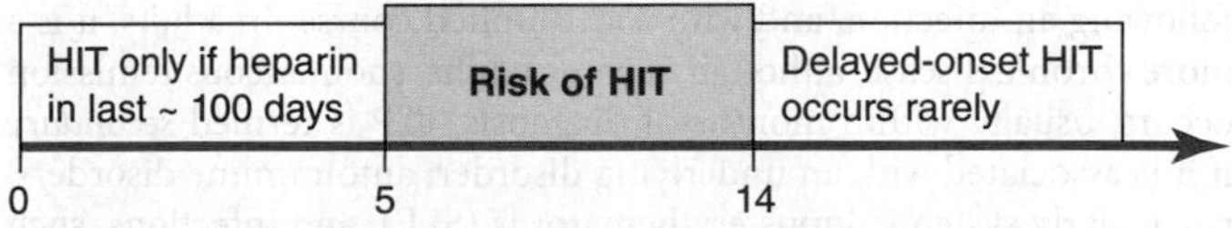

FIGURE 140-3 Time course of heparin-induced thrombocytopenia (HIT) development after heparin exposure. The timing of development after heparin exposure is a critical factor in determining the likelihood of HIT in a patient. HIT occurs early after heparin exposure in the presence of preexisting heparin/platelet factor 4 (PF4) antibodies, which disappear from circulation by ~100 days following a prior exposure. Rarely, HIT may occur later after heparin exposure (termed delayed-onset HIT). In this setting, heparin/PF4 antibody testing is usually markedly positive. HIT can occur after exposure to either unfractionated (UFH) or low-molecular-weight heparin (LMWH).

of HIT. This is especially true in patients who have undergone cardiopulmonary bypass surgery, where approximately 50% of patients develop these antibodies postoperatively. IgG-specific ELISAs increase specificity but may decrease sensitivity. The other assay is a platelet activation assay, most commonly the serotonin release assay, which measures the ability of the patient's serum to activate platelets in the presence of heparin in a concentration-dependent manner. This test has lower sensitivity but higher specificity than the ELISA. However, HIT remains a clinical diagnosis.

TREATMENT HEPARIN-INDUCED THROMBOCYTOPENIA

Early recognition is key in treatment of HIT, with prompt discontinuation of heparin and use of alternative anticoagulants if bleeding risk does not outweigh thrombotic risk. Thrombosis is a common complication of HIT, even after heparin discontinuation, and can occur in both the venous and arterial systems. Patients with higher anti-heparin/PF4 antibody titers may have a higher risk of thrombosis. In patients diagnosed with HIT, imaging studies to evaluate the patient for thrombosis (at least lower extremity duplex Doppler imaging) are recommended. Patients requiring anticoagulation should be switched from heparin to an alternative anticoagulant. The direct thrombin inhibitors (DTIs) argatroban and lepirudin are effective in HITT. The DTI bivalirudin and the antithrombin-binding pentasaccharide fondaparinux are also effective but not yet approved by the U.S. Food and Drug Administration (FDA) for this indication. Danaparoid, a mixture of glycosaminoglycans with anti-Xa activity, has been used extensively for the treatment of HITT; it is no longer available in the United States but is in other countries. HIT antibodies cross-react with LMWH, and these preparations should not be used in the treatment of HIT.

Because of the high rate of thrombosis in patients with HIT, anticoagulation should be considered, even in the absence of thrombosis. In patients with thrombosis, patients can be transitioned to warfarin, with treatment usually for 3–6 months. In patients without thrombosis, the duration of anticoagulation needed is undefined. An increased risk of thrombosis is present for at least 1 month after diagnosis; however, most thromboses occur early, and whether thrombosis occurs later if the patient is initially anticoagulated is unknown. Options include continuing anticoagulation until a few days after platelet recovery or for 1 month. Introduction of warfarin alone in the setting of HIT or HITT may precipitate thrombosis, particularly venous gangrene, presumably due to clotting activation and severely reduced levels of proteins C and S. Warfarin therapy, if started, should be overlapped with a DTI or fondaparinux and started after resolution of the thrombocytopenia and lessening of the prothrombotic state.

Immune Thrombocytopenic Purpura Immune thrombocytopenic purpura (ITP; also termed *idiopathic thrombocytopenic purpura*) is an acquired disorder in which there is immune-mediated destruction of platelets and possibly inhibition of platelet release from the megakaryocyte. In children, it is usually an acute disease, most commonly following an infection, and with a self-limited course. In adults, it is a more chronic disease, although in some adults, spontaneous remission occurs, usually within months of diagnosis. ITP is termed *secondary* if it is associated with an underlying disorder; autoimmune disorders, particularly systemic lupus erythematosus (SLE), and infections, such as HIV and hepatitis C, are common causes. The association of ITP with *Helicobacter pylori* infection is unclear.

ITP is characterized by mucocutaneous bleeding and a low, often very low, platelet count, with an otherwise normal peripheral blood cells and smear. Patients usually present either with ecchymoses and petechiae, or with thrombocytopenia incidentally found on a routine CBC. Mucocutaneous bleeding, such as oral mucosa, gastrointestinal, or heavy menstrual bleeding, may be present. Rarely, life-threatening, including central nervous system, bleeding can occur. Wet purpura (blood blisters in the mouth) and retinal hemorrhages may herald life-threatening bleeding.

LABORATORY TESTING IN ITP Laboratory testing for antibodies (serologic testing) is usually not helpful due to the low sensitivity and specificity of the current tests. Bone marrow examination can be reserved for those who have other signs or laboratory abnormalities not explained by ITP or in patients who do not respond to initial therapy. The peripheral blood smear may show large platelets, with otherwise normal morphology. Depending on the bleeding history, iron-deficiency anemia may be present.

Laboratory testing is performed to evaluate for secondary causes of ITP and should include testing for HIV infection and hepatitis C (and other infections if indicated). Serologic testing for SLE, serum protein electrophoresis, immunoglobulin levels to potentially detect hypogammaglobulinemia, selective testing for IgA deficiency or monoclonal gammopathies, and testing for *H. pylori* infection should be considered, depending on the clinical circumstance. If anemia is present, direct antiglobulin testing (Coombs' test) should be performed to rule out combined autoimmune hemolytic anemia with ITP (Evans' syndrome).

TREATMENT IMMUNE THROMBOCYTOPENIC PURPURA

The treatment of ITP uses drugs that decrease reticuloendothelial uptake of the antibody-bound platelet, decrease antibody production, and/or increase platelet production. The diagnosis of ITP does not necessarily mean that treatment must be instituted. Patients with platelet counts >30,000/μL appear not to have increased mortality related to the thrombocytopenia.

Initial treatment in patients without significant bleeding symptoms, severe thrombocytopenia (<5000/μL), or signs of impending bleeding (such as retinal hemorrhage or large oral mucosal hemorrhages) can be instituted as an outpatient using single agents. Traditionally, this has been prednisone at 1 mg/kg, although Rh_0(D) immune globulin therapy (WinRho SDF), at 50–75 μg/kg, is also being used in this setting. Rh_0(D) immune globulin must be used only in Rh-positive patients because the mechanism of action is production of limited hemolysis, with antibody-coated cells "saturating" the Fc receptors, inhibiting Fc receptor function. Monitoring patients for 8 h after infusion is now advised by the FDA because of the rare complication of severe intravascular hemolysis. Intravenous gamma globulin (IVIgG), which is pooled, primarily IgG antibodies, also blocks the Fc receptor system, but appears to work primarily through different mechanism(s). IVIgG has more efficacy than anti-Rh_0(D) in postsplenectomized patients. IVIgG is dosed at 1–2 g/kg total, given over 1–5 days. Side effects are usually related to the volume of infusion and infrequently include aseptic meningitis and renal failure. All immunoglobulin preparations are derived from human plasma and undergo treatment for viral inactivation.

For patients with severe ITP and/or symptoms of bleeding, hospital admission and combined-modality therapy is given using high-dose glucocorticoids with IVIgG or anti-Rh_0(D) therapy and, as needed, additional immunosuppressive agents. Rituximab, an anti-CD20 (B cell) antibody, has shown efficacy in the treatment of refractory ITP, although long-lasting remission only occurs in approximately 30% of patients.

Splenectomy has been used for treatment of patients who relapse after glucocorticoids are tapered. Splenectomy remains an important treatment option; however, more patients than previously thought will go into a remission over time. Observation, if the platelet count is high enough, or intermittent treatment with anti-Rh_0(D) or IVIgG, or initiation of treatment with a TPO receptor agonist (see below) may be a reasonable approach to see if the ITP will resolve. Vaccination against encapsulated organisms (especially pneumococcus, but also meningococcus and *Haemophilus influenzae*, depending on patient age and potential exposure) is recommended before splenectomy. Accessory spleen(s) are a very rare cause of relapse.

TPO receptor agonists are now available for the treatment of ITP. This approach stems from the finding that many patients with ITP do not have increased TPO levels, as was previously hypothesized. TPO levels reflect megakaryocyte mass, which is usually normal in ITP. TPO levels are not increased in the setting of platelet destruction. Two agents, one administered subcutaneously (romiplostim) and another orally (eltrombopag), are effective in raising platelet counts in patients with ITP and are recommended for adults at risk of bleeding who relapse after splenectomy or who have been unresponsive to at least one other therapy, particularly in those who have a contraindication to splenectomy. However, with the recognition that ITP will resolve spontaneously in some adult patients, short-term treatment with a TPO agonist can be considered before splenectomy in patients who need therapy.

Inherited Thrombocytopenia Thrombocytopenia is rarely inherited, either as an isolated finding or as part of a syndrome, and may be inherited in an autosomal dominant, autosomal recessive, or X-linked pattern. Many forms of autosomal dominant thrombocytopenia are now known to be associated with mutations in the nonmuscle myosin heavy chain *MYH9* gene. Interestingly, these include the May-Hegglin anomaly, and Sebastian, Epstein's, and Fechtner syndromes, all of which have distinct distinguishing features. A common feature of these disorders is large platelets (Fig. 140-1*C*). Autosomal recessive disorders include congenital amegakaryocytic thrombocytopenia, thrombocytopenia with absent radii, and Bernard-Soulier syndrome. The latter is primarily a functional platelet disorder due to absence of Gp Ib-IX-V, the VWF adhesion receptor. X-linked disorders include Wiskott-Aldrich syndrome and a dyshematopoietic syndrome resulting from a mutation in *GATA-1*, an important transcriptional regulator of hematopoiesis.

THROMBOTIC THROMBOCYTOPENIC PURPURA AND HEMOLYTIC-UREMIC SYNDROME

Thrombotic thrombocytopenic microangiopathies are a group of disorders characterized by thrombocytopenia, a microangiopathic hemolytic anemia evident by fragmented RBCs (Fig. 140-1*D*) and laboratory evidence of hemolysis, and microvascular thrombosis. They include thrombotic thrombocytopenic purpura (TTP) and hemolytic-uremic syndrome (HUS), as well as syndromes complicating bone marrow transplantation, certain medications and infections, pregnancy, and vasculitis. In DIC, although thrombocytopenia and microangiopathy are seen, a coagulopathy predominates, with consumption of clotting factors and fibrinogen resulting in an elevated prothrombin time (PT) and often activated partial thromboplastin time (aPTT). The PT and aPTT are characteristically normal in TTP or HUS.

Thrombotic Thrombocytopenic Purpura TTP and HUS were previously considered overlap syndromes. However, in the past few years, the pathophysiology of inherited and idiopathic TTP has become better understood and clearly differs from HUS. TTP was first described in 1924 by Eli Moschcowitz and characterized by a pentad of findings that include microangiopathic hemolytic anemia, thrombocytopenia, renal failure, neurologic findings, and fever. The full-blown syndrome is less commonly seen now, probably due to earlier diagnosis. The introduction of treatment with plasma exchange markedly improved the prognosis in patients, with a decrease in mortality from 85–100% to 10–30%.

The pathogenesis of inherited (Upshaw-Schulman syndrome) and idiopathic TTP is related to a deficiency of, or antibodies to, the metalloprotease ADAMTS13, which cleaves VWF. VWF is normally secreted as ultra-large multimers, which are then cleaved by ADAMTS13. The persistence of ultra-large VWF molecules is thought to contribute to pathogenic platelet adhesion and aggregation (Fig. 140-4). This defect alone, however, is not sufficient to result in TTP because individuals with a congenital absence of ADAMTS13 develop TTP only episodically. Additional provocative factors have not been defined. The level of ADAMTS13 activity, as well as antibodies, can now be detected by laboratory assays. Although assays with sufficient sensitivity and specificity to direct clinical management have yet to be clearly defined, ADAMTS13 activity levels of <10% are more clearly associated with idiopathic TTP.

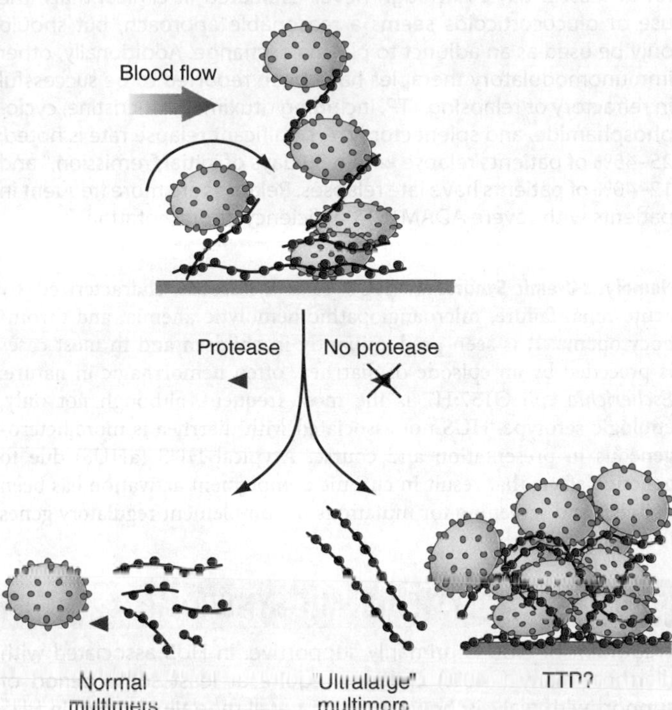

FIGURE 140-4 Pathogenesis of thrombotic thrombocytopenic purpura (TTP). Normally the ultra-high-molecular-weight multimers of von Willebrand factor (VWF) produced by the endothelial cells are processed into smaller multimers by a plasma metalloproteinase called ADAMTS13. In TTP, the activity of the protease is inhibited, and the ultra-high-molecular-weight multimers of VWF initiate platelet aggregation and thrombosis.

Idiopathic TTP appears to be more common in women than in men. No geographic or racial distribution has been defined. TTP is more common in patients with HIV infection and in pregnant women. TTP in pregnancy is not clearly related to ADAMTS13. Medication-related microangiopathic hemolytic anemia may be secondary to antibody formation (ticlopidine and possibly clopidogrel) or direct endothelial toxicity (cyclosporine, mitomycin C, tacrolimus, quinine), although this is not always so clear, and fear of withholding treatment, as well as lack of other treatment alternatives, results in broad application of plasma exchange. However, withdrawal, or reduction in dose, of endothelial toxic agents usually decreases the microangiopathy.

TREATMENT THROMBOTIC THROMBOCYTOPENIC PURPURA

TTP is a devastating disease if not diagnosed and treated promptly. In patients presenting with new thrombocytopenia, with or without evidence of renal insufficiency and other elements of classic TTP, laboratory data should be obtained to rule out DIC and to evaluate for evidence of microangiopathic hemolytic anemia. Findings to support the TTP diagnosis include an increased lactate dehydrogenase and indirect bilirubin, decreased haptoglobin, and increased reticulocyte count, with a negative direct antiglobulin test. The peripheral smear should be examined for evidence of schistocytes (Fig. 140-1*D*). Polychromasia is usually also present due to the increased number of young red blood cells, and nucleated RBCs are often present, which is thought to be due to infarction in the microcirculatory system of the bone marrow.

Plasma exchange remains the mainstay of treatment of TTP. ADAMTS13 antibody-mediated TTP (idiopathic TTP) appears to respond best to plasma exchange. Plasma exchange is continued until the platelet count is normal and signs of hemolysis are resolved for at least 2 days. Although never evaluated in clinical trials, the use of glucocorticoids seems a reasonable approach, but should only be used as an adjunct to plasma exchange. Additionally, other immunomodulatory therapies have been reported to be successful in refractory or relapsing TTP, including rituximab, vincristine, cyclophosphamide, and splenectomy. A significant relapse rate is noted; 25–45% of patients relapse within 30 days of initial "remission," and 12–40% of patients have late relapses. Relapses are more frequent in patients with severe ADAMTS13 deficiency at presentation.

Hemolytic-Uremic Syndrome HUS is a syndrome characterized by acute renal failure, microangiopathic hemolytic anemia, and thrombocytopenia. It is seen predominantly in children and in most cases is preceded by an episode of diarrhea, often hemorrhagic in nature. *Escherichia coli* O157:H7 is the most frequent, although not only, etiologic serotype. HUS not associated with diarrhea is more heterogeneous in presentation and course. Atypical HUS (aHUS) due to genetic defects that result in chronic complement activation has been defined, and screening for mutations in complement regulatory genes is available.

TREATMENT HEMOLYTIC-UREMIC SYNDROME

Treatment of HUS is primarily supportive. In HUS associated with diarrhea, many (~40%) children require at least some period of support with dialysis; however, the overall mortality is <5%. In HUS not associated with diarrhea, the mortality is higher, approximately 26%. Plasma infusion or plasma exchange has not been shown to alter the overall course. ADAMTS13 levels are generally reported to be normal in HUS, although occasionally they have been reported to be decreased. In patients with atypical HUS, eculizumab therapy increases the platelet count and preserves renal function.

THROMBOCYTOSIS

Thrombocytosis is almost always due to (1) iron deficiency; (2) inflammation, cancer, or infection (reactive thrombocytosis); or (3) an underlying myeloproliferative process (essential thrombocythemia or polycythemia vera) (Chap. 131) or, rarely, the 5q– myelodysplastic process (Chap. 130). Patients presenting with an elevated platelet count should be evaluated for underlying inflammation or malignancy, and iron deficiency should be ruled out. Thrombocytosis in response to acute or chronic inflammation has not been clearly associated with an increased thrombotic risk. In fact, patients with markedly elevated platelet counts (>1.5 million), usually seen in the setting of a myeloproliferative disorder, have an increased risk of bleeding. This appears to be due, at least in part, to acquired von Willebrand disease (VWD) due to platelet-VWF binding and removal from the circulation.

QUALITATIVE DISORDERS OF PLATELET FUNCTION

Inherited Disorders of Platelet Function Inherited platelet function disorders are thought to be relatively rare, although the prevalence of mild disorders of platelet function is unclear, in part because our testing for such disorders is suboptimal. Rare qualitative disorders include the autosomal recessive disorders Glanzmann's thrombasthenia (absence of the platelet Gp IIb/IIIa receptor) and Bernard-Soulier syndrome (absence of the platelet Gp Ib-IX-V receptor). Both are inherited in an autosomal recessive fashion and present with bleeding symptoms in childhood.

Platelet storage pool disorder (SPD) is the classic autosomal dominant qualitative platelet disorder. This results from abnormalities of platelet granule formation. It is also seen as a part of inherited disorders of granule formation, such as Hermansky-Pudlak syndrome. Bleeding symptoms in SPD are variable, but often are mild. The most common inherited disorders of platelet function prevent normal secretion of granule content and are termed *secretion defects*. Few of these abnormalities have been dissected at the molecular level but they likely result from various mutations..

TREATMENT INHERITED DISORDERS OF PLATELET DYSFUNCTION

Bleeding symptoms or prevention of bleeding in patients with severe platelet dysfunction frequently requires platelet transfusion. Care is taken to limit the risk of alloimmunization by limiting exposure, using HLA-matched leuko-depleted platelet concentrates for transfusion. Platelet disorders associated with milder bleeding symptoms frequently respond to desmopressin (1-deamino-8-D-arginine vasopressin [DDAVP]). DDAVP increases plasma VWF and factor VIII levels; it may also have a direct effect on platelet function. Particularly for mucosal bleeding symptoms, antifibrinolytic therapy (ε-aminocaproic acid or tranexamic acid) is used alone or in conjunction with DDAVP or platelet therapy.

Acquired Disorders of Platelet Function Acquired platelet dysfunction is common, usually due to medications, either intentionally as with antiplatelet therapy or unintentionally as with high-dose penicillins. Acquired platelet dysfunction occurs in uremia. This is likely multifactorial, but the resultant effect is defective adhesion and activation. The platelet defect is improved most by dialysis but may also be improved by increasing the hematocrit to 27–32%, giving DDAVP (0.3 μg/kg), or use of conjugated estrogens. Platelet dysfunction also occurs with cardiopulmonary bypass due to the effect of the artificial circuit on platelets, and bleeding symptoms respond to platelet transfusion. Platelet dysfunction seen with underlying hematologic disorders can result from nonspecific interference by circulating paraproteins or intrinsic platelet defects in myeloproliferative and myelodysplastic syndromes.

VON WILLEBRAND DISEASE

VWD is the most common inherited bleeding disorder. Estimates from laboratory data suggest a prevalence of approximately 1%, but data based on symptomatic individuals suggest that it is closer to 0.1% of the population. VWF serves two roles: (1) as the major adhesion molecule that tethers the platelet to the exposed subendothelium; and (2) as the binding protein for factor VIII (FVIII), resulting in significant prolongation of the FVIII half-life in circulation. The platelet-adhesive function of VWF is critically dependent on the presence of large VWF multimers, whereas FVIII binding is not. Most of the symptoms of VWD are "platelet-like" except in more severe VWD when the FVIII is low enough to produce symptoms similar to those found in FVIII deficiency (hemophilia A).

VWD has been classified into three major types, with four subtypes of type 2 (Table 140-2; Fig. 140-5). By far the most common type of VWD is type 1 disease, with a parallel decrease in VWF protein, VWF function, and FVIII levels, accounting for at least 80% of cases. Patients have predominantly mucosal bleeding symptoms, although postoperative bleeding can also be seen. Bleeding symptoms are very uncommon in infancy and usually manifest later in childhood with excessive bruising and epistaxis. Because these symptoms occur commonly in childhood, the clinician should particularly note bruising at sites unlikely to be traumatized and/or prolonged epistaxis requiring medical attention. Menorrhagia is a common manifestation of VWD. Menstrual bleeding resulting in anemia should warrant an evaluation for VWD and, if negative, functional platelet disorders. Frequently, mild type 1 VWD first manifests with dental extractions, particularly wisdom tooth extraction, or tonsillectomy.

Not all patients with low VWF levels have bleeding symptoms. Whether patients bleed or not will depend on the overall hemostatic balance they have inherited, along with environmental influences and the type of hemostatic challenges they experience. Although the inheritance of VWD is autosomal, many factors modulate both VWF levels and bleeding symptoms. These have not all been defined, but include blood type, thyroid hormone status, race, stress, exercise, and hormonal (both endogenous and exogenous) influences. Patients with type O blood have VWF protein levels of approximately one-half that of patients with AB blood type; and, in fact, the normal range for

TABLE 140-2 LABORATORY DIAGNOSIS OF VON WILLEBRAND DISEASE (VWD)

Type	aPTT	VWF Antigen	VWF Activity	FVIII Activity	Multimer
1	Nl or ↑	↓	↓	↓	Normal distribution, decreased in quantity
2A	Nl or ↑	↓	↓↓	↓	Loss of high- and intermediate-MW multimers
2B[a]	Nl or ↑	↓	↓↓	↓	Loss of high-MW multimers
2M	Nl or ↑	↓	↓↓	↓	Normal distribution, decreased in quantity
2N	↑↑	Nl or ↓[b]	Nl or ↓[b]	↓↓	Normal distribution
3	↑↑	↓↓	↓↓	↓↓	Absent

[a]Usually also decreased platelet count. [b]For type 2N, in the homozygous state, FVIII is very low; in the heterozygous state, it is only seen in conjunction with type 1 VWD.

Abbreviations: aPTT, activated partial thromboplastin time; F, factor; MW, molecular weight; Nl, normal; VWF, von Willebrand factor.

patients with type O blood overlaps that which has been considered diagnostic for VWD. A mildly decreased VWF level should be viewed more as a risk factor for bleeding than as an actual disease.

Patients with type 2 VWD have functional defects; thus, the VWF antigen measurement is significantly higher than the test of function. For types 2A, 2B, and 2M VWD, platelet-binding and/or collagen binding VWF activity is decreased. In type 2A VWD, the impaired function is due either to increased susceptibility to cleavage by ADAMTS13, resulting in loss of intermediate- and high-molecular-weight multimers, or to decreased secretion of these multimers by the cell. Type 2B VWD results from gain-of-function mutations that result in increased spontaneous binding of VWF to platelets in circulation, with subsequent clearance of this complex by the reticuloendothelial system. The resulting VWF in the patients' plasma lacks the highest molecular-weight multimers, and the platelet count is usually modestly reduced. Type 2M occurs as a consequence of a group of mutations that cause dysfunction but do not affect multimer structure.

Type 2N VWD is due to mutations in VWF that affect binding of FVIII. As FVIII is stabilized by binding to VWF, the FVIII in patients with type 2N VWD has a very short half-life, and the FVIII level is markedly decreased. This is sometimes termed *autosomal hemophilia*. Type 3 VWD, or severe VWD, describes patients with virtually no VWF protein and FVIII levels <10%. Patients experience mucosal and joint bleeding, surgery-related bleeding, and other bleeding symptoms. Some patients with type 3 VWD, particularly those with large VWF gene deletions, are at risk of developing antibodies to infused VWF.

Acquired VWD is a rare disorder, most commonly seen in patients with underlying lymphoproliferative disorders, including monoclonal gammopathies of underdetermined significance (MGUS), multiple myeloma, and Waldenström's macroglobulinemia. It is seen most commonly in the setting of MGUS and should be suspected in patients, particularly elderly patients, with a new onset of severe mucosal bleeding symptoms. Laboratory evidence of acquired VWD is found in some patients with aortic valvular disease. Heyde's syndrome (aortic stenosis with gastrointestinal bleeding) is attributed to the presence of angiodysplasia of the gastrointestinal tract in patients with aortic stenosis. The shear stress on blood passing through the stenotic aortic valve appears to produce a change in VWF, making it susceptible to serum proteases. Consequently, large multimer forms are lost, leading to an acquired type 2 VWD, but return when the stenotic valve is replaced.

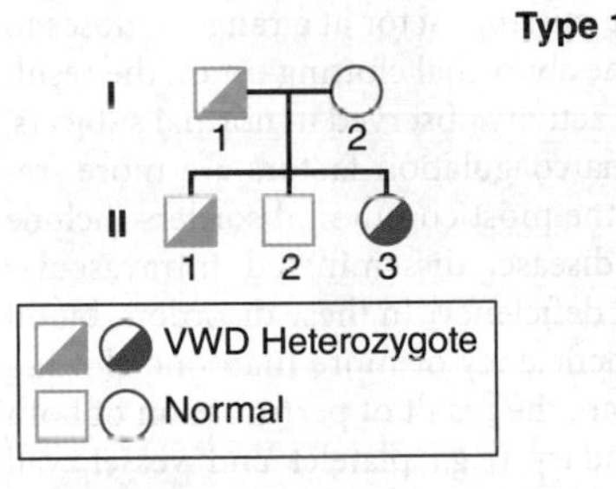

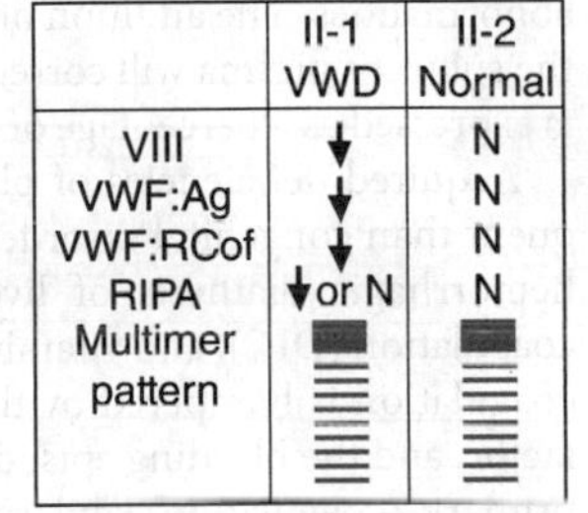

Type 1

	II-1 VWD	II-2 Normal
VIII	↓	N
VWF:Ag	↓	N
VWF:RCof	↓	N
RIPA	↓ or N	N
Multimer pattern		

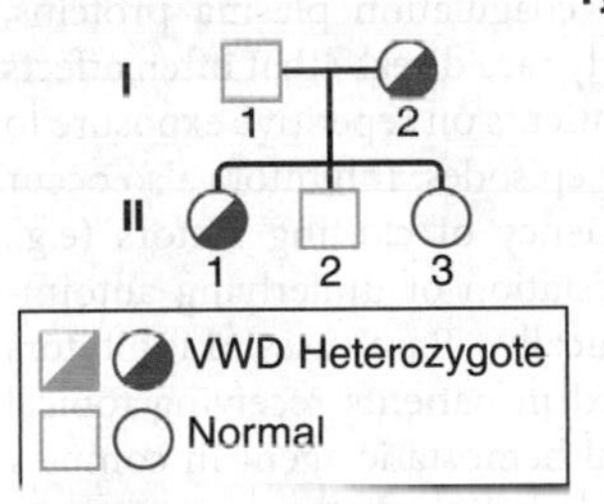

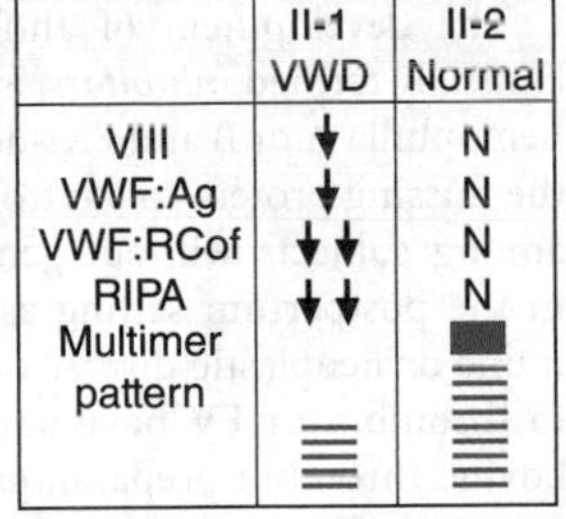

Type 2A

	II-1 VWD	II-2 Normal
VIII	↓	N
VWF:Ag	↓	N
VWF:RCof	↓↓	N
RIPA	↓↓	N
Multimer pattern		

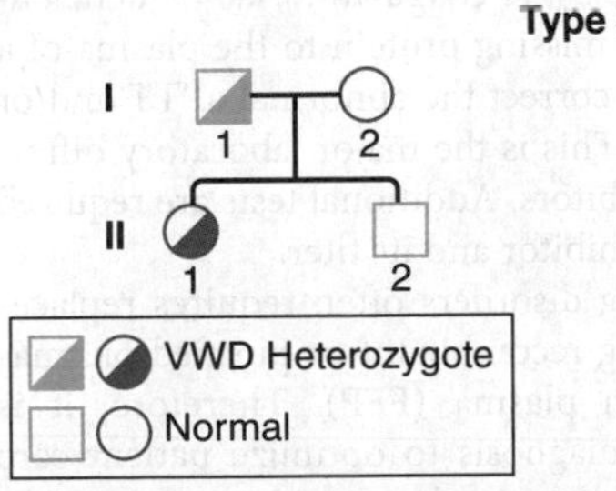

Type 2B

	II-1 VWD	II-2 Normal
VIII	↓	N
VWF:Ag	↓	N
VWF:RCof	↓↓	N
RIPA	↑	N
Multimer pattern		

FIGURE 140-5 Pattern of inheritance and laboratory findings in von Willebrand disease (VWD). The assays of platelet function include a coagulation assay of factor VIII bound and carried by von Willebrand factor (VWF), abbreviated as VIII; immunoassay of total VWF protein (VWF:Ag); bioassay of the ability of patient plasma to support ristocetin-induced agglutination of normal platelets (VWF:RCoF); and ristocetin-induced aggregation of patient platelets, abbreviated RIPA. The multimer pattern illustrates the protein bands present when plasma is electrophoresed in a polyacrylamide gel. The II-1 and II-2 columns refer to the phenotypes of the second-generation offspring.

TREATMENT VON WILLEBRAND DISEASE

The mainstay of treatment for type 1 VWD is DDAVP (desmopressin), which results in release of VWF and FVIII from endothelial stores. DDAVP can be given intravenously or by a high-concentration intranasal spray (1.5 mg/mL). The peak activity when given intravenously is approximately 30 min, whereas it is 2 h when given intranasally. The usual dose is 0.3 μg/kg intravenously or two squirts (one in each nostril) for patients >50 kg (one squirt for those <50 kg). It is recommended that patients with VWD be tested with DDAVP to assess their response before using it. In patients who respond well (increase in laboratory values of two- to fourfold), it can be used for procedures with minor to moderate risk of bleeding. Depending on the procedure, additional doses may be needed; it is usually given every 12–24 h. Less frequent dosing may result in less tachyphylaxis, which occurs when synthesis cannot compensate for the released stores. The major side effect of DDAVP is hyponatremia due to decreased free water clearance. This occurs most commonly in the very young and the very old, but fluid restriction should be advised for all patients for the 24 h following each dose.

Some patients with types 2A and 2M VWD respond to DDAVP such that it can be used for minor procedures. For the other subtypes, for type 3 disease, and for major procedures requiring longer periods of normal hemostasis, VWF replacement can be given. Virally inactivated VWF-containing factor concentrates are safer than cryoprecipitate as the replacement product.

Antifibrinolytic therapy using either ε-aminocaproic acid or tranexamic acid is an important therapy, either alone or in an adjunctive capacity, particularly for the prevention or treatment of mucosal bleeding. These agents are particularly useful in prophylaxis for dental procedures, with DDAVP for dental extractions and tonsillectomy, menorrhagia, and prostate procedures. It is contraindicated in the setting of upper urinary tract bleeding, due to the risk of ureteral obstruction.

DISORDERS OF THE VESSEL WALL

The vessel wall is an integral part of hemostasis, and separation of a fluid phase is artificial, particularly in disorders such as TTP or HIT that clearly involve the endothelium as well. Inflammation localized to the vessel wall, such as vasculitis, and inherited connective tissue disorders are abnormalities inherent to the vessel wall.

METABOLIC AND INFLAMMATORY DISORDERS Acute febrile illnesses may result in vascular damage. This can result from immune complexes containing viral antigens or the viruses themselves. Certain pathogens, such as the rickettsiae causing Rocky Mountain spotted fever, replicate in endothelial cells and damage them. Vascular purpura may occur in patients with polyclonal gammopathies but more commonly in those with monoclonal gammopathies, including Waldenström's macroglobulinemia, multiple myeloma, and cryoglobulinemia. Patients with mixed cryoglobulinemia develop a more extensive maculopapular rash due to immune complex–mediated damage to the vessel wall.

Patients with scurvy (vitamin C deficiency) develop painful episodes of perifollicular skin bleeding as well as more systemic bleeding symptoms. Vitamin C is needed to synthesize hydroxyproline, an essential constituent of collagen. Patients with Cushing's syndrome or on chronic glucocorticoid therapy develop skin bleeding and easy bruising due to atrophy of supporting connective tissue. A similar phenomenon is seen with aging, where following minor trauma, blood spreads superficially under the epidermis. This has been termed *senile purpura*. It is most common on skin that has been previously damaged by sun exposure.

Henoch-Schönlein, or anaphylactoid, purpura is a distinct, self-limited type of vasculitis that occurs in children and young adults. Patients have an acute inflammatory reaction with IgA and complement components in capillaries, mesangial tissues, and small arterioles leading to increased vascular permeability and localized hemorrhage. The syndrome is often preceded by an upper respiratory infection, commonly with streptococcal pharyngitis, or is triggered by drug or food allergies. Patients develop a purpuric rash on the extensor surfaces of the arms and legs, usually accompanied by polyarthralgias or arthritis, abdominal pain, and hematuria from focal glomerulonephritis. All coagulation tests are normal, but renal impairment may occur. Glucocorticoids can provide symptomatic relief but do not alter the course of the illness.

INHERITED DISORDERS OF THE VESSEL WALL Patients with inherited disorders of the connective tissue matrix, such as Marfan's syndrome, Ehlers-Danlos syndrome, and pseudoxanthoma elasticum, frequently report easy bruising. Inherited vascular abnormalities can result in increased bleeding. This is notably seen in hereditary hemorrhagic telangiectasia (HHT, or Osler-Weber-Rendu disease), a disorder where abnormal telangiectatic capillaries result in frequent bleeding episodes, primarily from the nose and gastrointestinal tract. Arteriovenous malformation (AVM) in the lung, brain, and liver may also occur in HHT. The telangiectasia can often be visualized on the oral and nasal mucosa. Signs and symptoms develop over time. Epistaxis begins, on average, at the age of 12 and occurs in >95% of affected individuals by middle age. Two genes involved in the pathogenesis are *eng* (endoglin) on chromosome 9q33-34 (so-called HHT type 1), associated with pulmonary AVM in 40% of cases, and *alk1* (activin-receptor-like kinase 1) on chromosome 12q13, associated with a much lower risk of pulmonary AVM.

ACKNOWLEDGMENT

Robert Handin, MD, contributed this chapter in the 16th edition and some materials from his chapter are included here.

141 Coagulation Disorders

Valder R. Arruda, Katherine A. High

Deficiencies of coagulation factors have been recognized for centuries. Patients with genetic deficiencies of plasma coagulation factors exhibit life-long recurrent bleeding episodes into joints, muscles, and closed spaces, either spontaneously or following an injury. The most common inherited factor deficiencies are the hemophilias, X-linked diseases caused by deficiency of factor (F) VIII (hemophilia A) or FIX (hemophilia B). Rare congenital bleeding disorders due to deficiencies of other factors, including FII (prothrombin), FV, FVII, FX, FXI, and FXIII, and fibrinogen are commonly inherited in an autosomal recessive manner (Table 141-1). Advances in characterization of the molecular bases of clotting factor deficiencies have contributed to better understanding of the disease phenotypes and may eventually allow more targeted therapeutic approaches through the development of small molecules, recombinant proteins, or cell and gene-based therapies.

Commonly used tests of hemostasis provide the initial screening for clotting factor activity (Fig. 141-1), and disease phenotype often correlates with the level of clotting activity. An isolated abnormal prothrombin time (PT) suggests FVII deficiency, whereas a prolonged activated partial thromboplastin time (aPTT) indicates most commonly hemophilia or FXI deficiency (Fig. 141-1). The prolongation of both PT and aPTT suggests deficiency of FV, FX, FII, or fibrinogen abnormalities. The addition of the missing factor at a range of doses to the subject's plasma will correct the abnormal clotting times; the result is expressed as a percentage of the activity observed in normal subjects.

Acquired deficiencies of plasma coagulation factors are more frequent than congenital disorders; the most common disorders include hemorrhagic diathesis of liver disease, disseminated intravascular coagulation (DIC), and vitamin K deficiency. In these disorders, blood coagulation is hampered by the deficiency of more than one clotting factor, and the bleeding episodes are the result of perturbation of both primary (coagulation) and secondary (e.g., platelet and vessel wall interactions) hemostasis.

The development of antibodies to coagulation plasma proteins, clinically termed *inhibitors*, is a relatively rare disease that often affects hemophilia A or B and FXI-deficient patients on repetitive exposure to the missing protein to control bleeding episodes. Inhibitors also occur among subjects without genetic deficiency of clotting factors (e.g., in the postpartum setting as a manifestation of underlying autoimmune or neoplastic disease or idiopathically). Rare cases of inhibitors to thrombin or FV have been reported in patients receiving topical bovine thrombin preparation as a local hemostatic agent in complex surgeries. The diagnosis of inhibitors is based on the same tests as those used to diagnose inherited plasma coagulation factor deficiencies. However, the addition of the missing protein to the plasma of a subject with an inhibitor does not correct the abnormal aPTT and/or PT tests (known as mixing tests). This is the major laboratory difference between deficiencies and inhibitors. Additional tests are required to measure the specificity of the inhibitor and its titer.

The treatment of these bleeding disorders often requires replacement of the deficient protein using recombinant or purified plasma-derived products or fresh-frozen plasma (FFP). Therefore, it is imperative to arrive at a proper diagnosis to optimize patient care without unnecessary exposure to suboptimal treatment and the risks of bloodborne disease.

HEMOPHILIA

PATHOGENESIS AND CLINICAL MANIFESTATIONS

Hemophilia is an X-linked recessive hemorrhagic disease due to mutations in the *F8* gene (hemophilia A or classic hemophilia) or *F9* gene (hemophilia B). The disease affects 1 in 10,000 males worldwide, in all ethnic groups; hemophilia A represents 80% of all cases. Male subjects

TABLE 141-1 GENETIC AND LABORATORY CHARACTERISTICS OF INHERITED COAGULATION DISORDERS

Clotting Factor Deficiency	Inheritance	Prevalence in General Population	Laboratory Abnormality[a] aPTT	PT	TT	Minimum Hemostatic Levels	Treatment	Plasma Half-Life
Fibrinogen	AR	1 in 1,000,000	+	+	+	100 mg/dL	Cryoprecipitate	2–4 d
Prothrombin	AR	1 in 2,000,000	+	+	–	20–30%	FFP/PCC	3–4 d
Factor V	AR	1 in 1,000,000	+/–	+/–	–	15–20%	FFP	36 h
Factor VII	AR	1 in 500,000	–	+	–	15–20%	FFP/PCC	4–6 h
Factor VIII	X-linked	1 in 5,000	+	–	–	30%	FVIII concentrates	8–12 h
Factor IX	X-linked	1 in 30,000	+	–	–	30%	FIX concentrates	18–24 h
Factor X	AR	1 in 1,000,000	+/–	+/–	–	15–20%	FFP/PCC	40–60 h
Factor XI	AR	1 in 1,000,000	+	–	–	15–20%	FFP	40–70 h
Factor XII	AR	ND	+	–	–	[b]	[b]	60 h
HK	AR	ND	+	–	–	[b]	[b]	150 h
Prekallikrein	AR	ND	+	–	–	[b]	[b]	35 h
Factor XIII	AR	1 in 2,000,000	–	–	+/–	2–5%	Cryoprecipitate/FXIII concentrates	11–14 d

[a]Values within normal range (–) or prolonged (+). [b]No risk for bleeding; treatment is not indicated.

Abbreviations: aPTT, activated partial thromboplastin time; AR, autosomal recessive; FFP, fresh-frozen plasma; HK, high-molecular-weight kininogen; ND, not determined; PCC, prothrombin complex concentrates; PT, prothrombin time; TT, thrombin time.

are clinically affected; women, who carry a single mutated gene, are generally asymptomatic. Family history of the disease is absent in ~30% of cases, and in these cases, 80% of the mothers are carriers of the de novo mutated allele. More than 500 different mutations have been identified in the *F8* or *F9* genes of patients with hemophilia A or B, respectively. One of the most common hemophilia A mutations results from an inversion of the intron 22 sequence, and it is present in 40% of cases of severe hemophilia A. Advances in molecular diagnosis now permit precise identification of mutations, allowing accurate diagnosis of women carriers of the hemophilia gene in affected families.

Clinically, hemophilia A and hemophilia B are indistinguishable. The disease phenotype correlates with the residual activity of FVIII or FIX and can be classified as severe (<1%), moderate (1–5%), or mild (6–30%). In the severe and moderate forms, the disease is characterized by bleeding into the joints (hemarthrosis), soft tissues, and muscles after minor trauma or even spontaneously. Patients with mild disease experience infrequent bleeding that is usually secondary to trauma. Among those with residual FVIII or FIX activity >25% of normal, the disease is discovered only by bleeding after major trauma or during routine presurgery laboratory tests. Typically, the global tests of coagulation show only an isolated prolongation of the aPTT assay. Patients with hemophilia have normal bleeding times and platelet counts. The diagnosis is made after specific determination of FVIII or FIX clotting activity.

Early in life, bleeding may present after circumcision or rarely as intracranial hemorrhages. The disease is more evident when children begin to walk or crawl. In the severe form, the most common bleeding manifestations are the recurrent hemarthroses, which can affect every joint but mainly affect knees, elbows, ankles, shoulders, and hips. Acute hemarthroses are painful, and clinical signs are local swelling and erythema. To avoid pain, the patient may adopt a fixed position, which leads eventually to muscle contractures. Very young children unable to communicate verbally show irritability and a lack of movement of the affected joint. Chronic hemarthroses are debilitating, with synovial thickening and synovitis in response to the intraarticular blood. After a joint has been damaged, recurrent bleeding episodes result in the clinically recognized "target joint," which then establishes a vicious cycle of bleeding, resulting in progressive joint deformity that in critical cases requires surgery as the only therapeutic option. Hematomas into the muscle of distal parts of the limbs may lead to external compression of arteries, veins, or nerves that can evolve to a compartment syndrome.

Bleeding into the oropharyngeal spaces, central nervous system (CNS), or retroperitoneum is life threatening and requires immediate therapy. Retroperitoneal hemorrhages can accumulate large quantities of blood with formation of masses with calcification and inflammatory tissue reaction (pseudotumor syndrome) and also result in damage to the femoral nerve. Pseudotumors can also form in bones, especially long bones of the lower limbs. Hematuria is frequent among hemophilia patients, even in the absence of genitourinary pathology. It is often self-limited and may not require specific therapy.

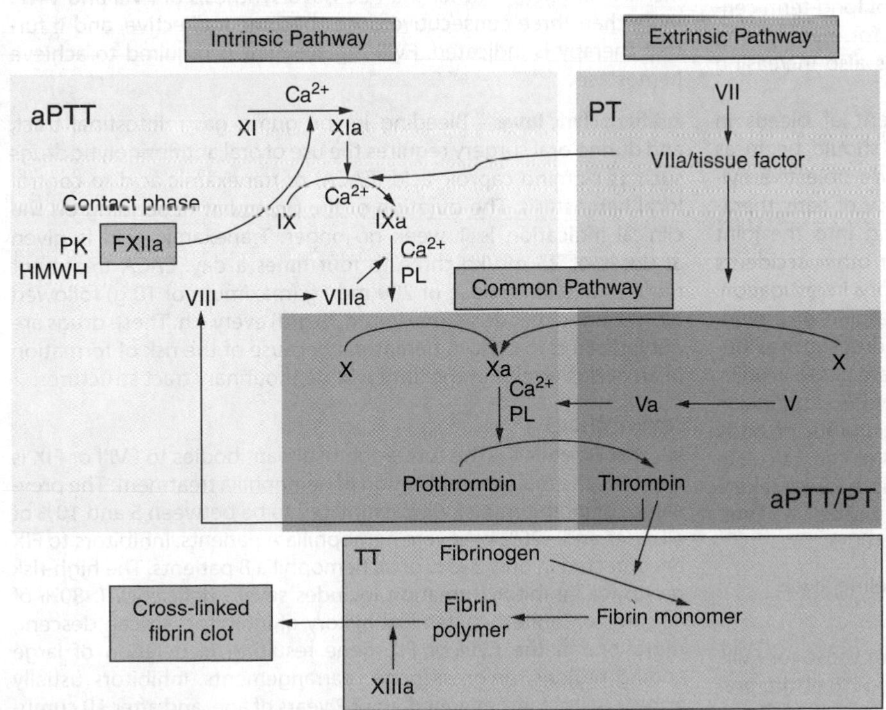

FIGURE 141-1 Coagulation cascade and laboratory assessment of clotting factor deficiency by activated partial prothrombin time (aPTT), prothrombin time (PT), thrombin time (TT), and phospholipid (PL).

TREATMENT HEMOPHILIA

Without treatment, severe hemophilia has a limited life expectancy. Advances in the blood fractionation industry during World War II resulted in the realization that plasma could be used to treat hemophilia, but the volumes required to achieve even modest elevation of circulating factor levels limit the utility of plasma infusion as an approach to disease management. The discovery in the 1960s that the cryoprecipitate fraction of plasma was enriched for FVIII, and the eventual purification of FVIII and FIX from plasma, led to the introduction of home infusion therapy with factor concentrates in the 1970s. The availability of factor concentrates resulted in a dramatic improvement in life expectancy and in quality of life for people with severe hemophilia. However, the contamination of the blood supply with hepatitis viruses and, subsequently, HIV resulted in widespread transmission of these bloodborne infections within the hemophilia population; complications of HIV and of hepatitis C are now the leading causes of death among U.S. adults with severe hemophilia. The introduction of viral inactivation steps in the preparation of plasma-derived products in the mid-1980s greatly reduced the risk of HIV and hepatitis, and the risks were further reduced by the successful production of recombinant FVIII and FIX proteins, both licensed in the 1990s. It is uncommon for hemophilic patients born after 1985 to have contracted either hepatitis or HIV, and for these individuals, life expectancy is approximately 65 years. In fact, since 1998, no evidence of new infections with viral hepatitis or HIV has been reported in patients using blood products.

Factor replacement therapy for hemophilia can be provided either in response to a bleeding episode or as a prophylactic treatment. Primary prophylaxis is defined as a strategy for maintaining the missing clotting factor at levels ~1% or higher on a regular basis in order to prevent bleeds, especially the onset of hemarthroses. Hemophilic boys receiving regular infusions of FVIII (3 days/week) or FIX (2 days/week) can reach puberty without detectable joint abnormalities. Prophylaxis has become gradually more common in young patients. The Centers for Disease Control and Prevention reported that 51% of children with severe hemophilia who are younger than age 6 years receive prophylaxis, increasing considerably from 33% in 1995. Although highly recommended, the high cost and difficulties in accessing peripheral veins in young patients and the potential infectious and thrombotic risks of long-term central vein catheters are important limiting factors for many young patients. Emerging data show that prophylaxis is also increasing among adults with severe hemophilia.

General considerations regarding the treatment of bleeds in hemophilia include the following: (1) Treatment should begin as soon as possible because symptoms often precede objective evidence of bleeding; because of the superior efficacy of early therapeutic intervention, classic symptoms of bleeding into the joint in a reliable patient, headaches, or automobile or other accidents require prompt replacement and further laboratory investigation. (2) Drugs that hamper platelet function, such as aspirin or aspirin-containing drugs, should be avoided; to control pain, drugs such as ibuprofen or propoxyphene are preferred. FVIII and FIX are dosed in units. One unit is defined as amount of FVIII (100 ng/mL) or FIX (5 μg/mL) in 1 mL of normal plasma. One unit of FVIII per kilogram of body weight increases the plasma FVIII level by 2%. One can calculate the dose needed to increase FVIII levels to 100% in a 70-kg severe hemophilia patient (<1%) using the simple formula below. Thus, 3500 units of FVIII will raise the circulating level to 100%.

$$\text{FVIII dose (IU)} = \text{Target FVIII levels} - \text{FVIII baseline levels} \\ \times \text{body weight (kg)} \times 0.5 \text{ unit/kg}$$

The doses for FIX replacement are different from those for FVIII, because FIX recovery after infusion is usually only 50% of the predicted value. Therefore, the formula for FIX replacement is as follows:

$$\text{FIX dose (IU)} = \text{Target FIX levels} - \text{FIX baseline levels} \\ \times \text{body weight (kg)} \times 1 \text{ unit/kg}$$

The FVIII half-life of 8–12 h requires injections twice a day to maintain therapeutic levels, whereas the FIX half-life is longer, ~24 h, so that once-a-day injection is sufficient. In specific situations such as after surgery, continuous infusion of factor may be desirable because of its safety in achieving sustained factor levels at a lower total cost.

Cryoprecipitate is enriched with FVIII protein (each bag contains ~80 IU of FVIII) and was commonly used for the treatment of hemophilia A decades ago; it is still in use in some developing countries, but because of the risk of bloodborne diseases, this product should be avoided in hemophilia patients when factor concentrates are available.

Mild bleeds such as uncomplicated hemarthroses or superficial hematomas require initial therapy with factor levels of 30–50%. Additional doses to maintain levels of 15–25% for 2 or 3 days are indicated for severe hemarthroses, especially when these episodes affect the "target joint." Large hematomas, or bleeds into deep muscles, require factor levels of 50% or even higher if the clinical symptoms do not improve, and factor replacement may be required for a period of 1 week or longer. The control of serious bleeds including those that affect the oropharyngeal spaces, CNS, and the retroperitoneum require sustained protein levels of 50–100% for 7–10 days. Prophylactic replacement for surgery is aimed at achieving normal factor levels (100%) for a period of 7–10 days; replacement can then be tapered depending on the extent of the surgical wounds. Oral surgery is associated with extensive tissue damage that usually requires factor replacement for 1–3 days coupled with oral antifibrinolytic drugs.

NONTRANSFUSION THERAPY IN HEMOPHILIA

DDAVP (1-Amino-8-D-Arginine Vasopressin) DDAVP is a synthetic vasopressin analog that causes a transient rise in FVIII and von Willebrand factor (VWF), but not FIX, through a mechanism involving release from endothelial cells. Patients with moderate or mild hemophilia A should be tested to determine if they respond to DDAVP before a therapeutic application. DDAVP at doses of 0.3 μg/kg body weight, over a 20-min period, is expected to raise FVIII levels by two- to threefold over baseline, peaking between 30 and 60 min after infusion. DDAVP does not improve FVIII levels in severe hemophilia A patients, because there are no stores to release. Repeated dosing of DDAVP results in tachyphylaxis because the mechanism is an increase in release rather than de novo synthesis of FVIII and VWF. More than three consecutive doses become ineffective, and if further therapy is indicated, FVIII replacement is required to achieve hemostasis.

Antifibrinolytic Drugs Bleeding in the gums, gastrointestinal tract, and during oral surgery requires the use of oral antifibrinolytic drugs such as ε-amino caproic acid (EACA) or tranexamic acid to control local hemostasis. The duration of the treatment depending on the clinical indication is 1 week or longer. Tranexamic acid is given at doses of 25 mg/kg three to four times a day. EACA treatment requires a loading dose of 200 mg/kg (maximum of 10 g) followed by 100 mg/kg per dose (maximum 30 g/d) every 6 h. These drugs are not indicated to control hematuria because of the risk of formation of an occlusive clot in the lumen of genitourinary tract structures.

COMPLICATIONS

Inhibitor Formation The formation of alloantibodies to FVIII or FIX is currently the major complication of hemophilia treatment. The prevalence of inhibitors to FVIII is estimated to be between 5 and 10% of all cases and ~20% of severe hemophilia A patients. Inhibitors to FIX are detected in only 3–5% of all hemophilia B patients. The high-risk group for inhibitor formation includes severe deficiency (>80% of all cases of inhibitors), familial history of inhibitor, African descent, mutations in the FVIII or FIX gene resulting in deletion of large coding regions, or gross gene rearrangements. Inhibitors usually appear early in life, at a median of 2 years of age, and after 10 cumulative days of exposure. However, intensive replacement therapy such as for major surgery, intracranial bleeding, or trauma increases the risk of inhibitor formation for patients of all ages and degree of clinical severity, which requires close laboratory monitoring in the following weeks.

The clinical diagnosis of an inhibitor is suspected when patients do not respond to factor replacement at therapeutic doses. Inhibitors increase both morbidity and mortality in hemophilia. Because early detection of an inhibitor is critical to a successful correction of the bleeding or to eradication of the antibody, most hemophilia centers perform annual screening for inhibitors. The laboratory test required to confirm the presence of an inhibitor is an aPTT with a mix (with normal plasma). In most hemophilia patients, a 1:1 mix with normal plasma completely corrects the aPTT. In inhibitor patients, the aPTT on a 1:1 mix is abnormally prolonged, because the inhibitor neutralizes the FVIII clotting activity of the normal plasma. The Bethesda assay uses a similar principle and defines the specificity of the inhibitor and its titer. The results are expressed in Bethesda units (BU), in which 1 BU is the amount of antibody that neutralizes 50% of the FVIII or FIX present in normal plasma after 2 h of incubation at 37°C. Clinically, inhibitor patients are classified as low responders or high responders, which provides guidelines for optimal therapy. Therapy for inhibitor patients has two goals: the control of acute bleeding episodes and the eradication of the inhibitor. For the control of bleeding episodes, low responders, those with titer <5 BU, respond well to high doses of human or porcine FVIII (50–100 U/kg), with minimal or no increase in the inhibitor titers. However, high-responder patients, those with initial inhibitor titer >10 BU or an anamnestic response in the antibody titer to >10 BU even if low titer initially, do not respond to FVIII or FIX concentrates. The control of bleeding episodes in high-responder patients can be achieved by using concentrates enriched for prothrombin, FVII, FIX, FX (prothrombin complex concentrates [PCCs] or activated PCCs [aPCCs]), and more recently recombinant activated factor VII (FVIIa) known as "bypass agents" (Fig. 141-1). The rates of therapeutic success have been higher for FVIIa than for PCC or aPCC. For eradication of the inhibitory antibody, immunosuppression alone is not effective. The most effective strategy is the immune tolerance induction (ITI) based on daily infusion of missing protein until the inhibitor disappears, typically requiring periods longer than 1 year, with success rates of approximately 60%. The management of patients with severe hemophilia and inhibitors resistant to ITI is challenging. The use of anti-CD20 monoclonal antibody (rituximab) combined with ITI was thought to be effective. Although this therapy may reduce the inhibitor titers in some cases, sustained eradication is uncommon and may require two to three infusions weekly of clotting factor concentrates.

Novel Therapeutic Approaches in Development for Hemophilia Clinical studies using long-acting clotting factors with prolonged half-lives are in the late phase of clinical testing, and these new generation products (for FVIII and FIX) may facilitate prophylaxis by requiring fewer injections to maintain circulating levels above 1%.

The use of recombinant interleukin 11 in patients with moderate or mild hemophilia A unresponsive to DDAVP has been tested in early-phase clinical trials and may be an alternate therapeutic strategy for clinical situations that require transient increases in FVIII levels.

Gene therapy trials for hemophilia B using adeno-associated viral vectors are ongoing, and initial data are promising (Chap. 91e).

INFECTIOUS DISEASES

Hepatitis C virus (HCV) infection is the major cause of morbidity and the second leading cause of death in hemophilia patients exposed to older clotting factor concentrates. The vast majority of young patients treated with plasma-derived products from 1970 to 1985 became infected with HCV. It has been estimated that >80% of patients older than 20 years of age are HCV antibody positive as of 2006. The comorbidity of the underlying liver disease in hemophilia patients is clear when these individuals require invasive procedures; correction of both genetic and acquired (secondary to liver disease) deficiencies may be needed. Infection with HIV also swept the population of patients using plasma-derived concentrates two decades ago. Co-infection of HCV and HIV, present in almost 50% of hemophilia patients, is an aggravating factor for the evolution of liver disease. The response to HCV antiviral therapy in hemophilia is restricted to <30% of patients and even poorer among those with both HCV and HIV infection. End-stage liver disease requiring organ transplantation may be curative for both the liver disease and for hemophilia.

EMERGING CLINICAL PROBLEMS IN AGING HEMOPHILIA PATIENTS

There has been continuous improvement of the management of hemophilia since the increase in the population of adults living beyond middle age in the developing world. The life expectancy of a patient with severe hemophilia is only ~10 years shorter than the general male population. In patients with mild or moderate hemophilia, life expectancy is approaching that of the male population without coagulopathy. Elderly hemophilia patients have different problems compared to the younger generation; they have more severe arthropathy and chronic pain, due to suboptimal treatment, and high rates of HCV and/or HIV infections.

Early data indicate that mortality from coronary artery disease is lower in hemophilia patients than the general male population. The underlying hypocoagulability probably provides a protective effect against thrombus formation, but it does not prevent atherogenesis. Similar to the general population, these patients are exposed to cardiovascular risk factors such as age, obesity, and smoking. Moreover, physical inactivity, hypertension, and chronic renal disease are commonly observed in hemophilia patients. In HIV patients on combined antiretroviral therapy, there may be a further increase in the risk of cardiovascular disease. Therefore, these patients should be carefully considered for preventive and therapeutic approaches to minimize the risk of cardiovascular disease.

Excessive replacement therapy should be avoided, and it is prudent to slowly infuse factor concentrates. Continuous infusion of clotting factor is preferable to bolus dosing in patients with cardiovascular risk factors undergoing invasive procedures. The management of an acute ischemic event and coronary revascularization should include the collaboration of hematologists and internists. The early assumption that hemophilia would protect against occlusive vascular disease may change in this aging population. Cancer is a common cause of mortality in aging hemophilia patients because they are at risk for HIV- and HCV-related malignancies. Hepatocellular carcinoma (HCC) is the most prevalent primary liver cancer and a common cause of death in HIV-negative patients. The recommendations for cancer screening for the general population should be the same for age-matched hemophilia patients. Among those with high-risk HCV, a semiannual or annual ultrasound and α fetoprotein are recommended for HCC. Screening for urogenital neoplasm in the presence of hematuria or hematochezia may be delayed due to the underlying bleeding disease, thus preventing early intervention. Multidisciplinary interaction should facilitate the attempts to ensure optimal cancer prevention and treatment recommendations for those with hemophilia.

MANAGEMENT OF CARRIERS OF HEMOPHILIA

Usually hemophilia carriers, with factor levels of ~50% of normal, have not been considered to be at risk for bleeding. However, a wide range of values (22–116%) have been reported due to random inactivation of the X chromosomes (*lyonization*). Therefore, it is important to measure the factor level of carriers to recognize those at risk of bleeding and to optimize preoperative and postoperative management. During pregnancy, both FVIII and FIX levels increase gradually until delivery. FVIII levels increase approximately two- to threefold compared to nonpregnant women, whereas an FIX increase is less pronounced. After delivery, there is a rapid fall in the pregnancy-induced rise of maternal clotting factor levels. This represents an imminent risk of bleeding that can be prevented by infusion of factor concentrate to levels of 50–70% for 3 days in the setting of vaginal delivery and up to 5 days for cesarean section. In mild cases, the use of DDAVP and/or antifibrinolytic drugs is recommended.

Factor XI is a zymogen of an active serine protease (FIXa) in the intrinsic pathway of blood coagulation that activates FIX (Fig. 141-1). There are two pathways for the formation of FXIa. In an aPTT-based assay, the protease is the result of activation by FXIIa in conjunction with high-molecular-weight kininogen and kallikrein. In vivo data suggest that thrombin is the physiologic activator of FXI. The generation of thrombin by the tissue factor/factor VIIa pathway activates FXI on the platelet surface that contributes to additional thrombin generation after the clot has formed and thus augments resistance to fibrinolysis through a thrombin-activated fibrinolytic inhibitor (TAFI).

Factor XI deficiency is a rare bleeding disorder that occurs in the general population at a frequency of one in a million. However, the disease is highly prevalent among Ashkenazi and Iraqi Jewish populations, reaching a frequency of 6% as heterozygotes and 0.1–0.3% as homozygotes. More than 65 mutations in the FXI gene have been reported, whereas fewer mutations (two to three) are found among affected Jewish populations.

Normal FXI clotting activity levels range from 70 to 150 U/dL. In heterozygous patients with moderate deficiency, FXI ranges from 20 to 70 U/dL, whereas in homozygous or double heterozygote patients, FXI levels are <1–20 U/dL. Patients with FXI levels <10% of normal have a high risk of bleeding, but the disease phenotype does not always correlate with residual FXI clotting activity. A family history is indicative of the risk of bleeding in the propositus. Clinically, the presence of mucocutaneous hemorrhages such as bruises, gum bleeding, epistaxis, hematuria, and menorrhagia are common, especially following trauma. This hemorrhagic phenotype suggests that tissues rich in fibrinolytic activity are more susceptible to FXI deficiency. Postoperative bleeding is common but not always present, even among patients with very low FXI levels.

FXI replacement is indicated in patients with severe disease required to undergo a surgical procedure. A negative history of bleeding complications following invasive procedures does not exclude the possibility of an increased risk for hemorrhage.

TREATMENT FACTOR XI DEFICIENCY

The treatment of FXI deficiency is based on the infusion of FFP at doses of 15–20 mL/kg to maintain trough levels ranging from 10 to 20%. Because FXI has a half-life of 40–70 h, the replacement therapy can be given on alternate days. The use of antifibrinolytic drugs is beneficial to control bleeds, with the exception of hematuria or bleeds in the bladder. The development of an FXI inhibitor was observed in 10% of severely FXI-deficient patients who received replacement therapy. Patients with severe FXI deficiency who develop inhibitors usually do not bleed spontaneously. However, bleeding following a surgical procedure or trauma can be severe. In these patients, FFP and FXI concentrates should be avoided. The use of PCC/aPCC or recombinant activated FVII has been effective.

RARE BLEEDING DISORDERS

Collectively, the inherited disorders resulting from deficiencies of clotting factors other than FVIII, FIX, and FXI (Table 141-1) represent a group of rare bleeding diseases. The bleeding symptoms in these patients vary from asymptomatic (dysfibrinogenemia or FVII deficiency) to life-threatening (FX or FXIII deficiency). There is no pathognomonic clinical manifestation that suggests one specific disease, but overall, in contrast to hemophilia, hemarthrosis is a rare event and bleeding in the mucosal tract or after umbilical cord clamping is common. Individuals heterozygous for plasma coagulation deficiencies are often asymptomatic. The laboratory assessment for the specific deficient factor following screening with general coagulation tests (Table 141-1) will define the diagnosis.

Replacement therapy using FFP or prothrombin complex concentrates (containing prothrombin, FVII, FIX, and FX) provides adequate hemostasis in response to bleeds or as prophylactic treatment. The use of PCC should be carefully monitored and avoided in patients with underlying liver disease, or those at high risk for thrombosis because of the risk of DIC.

FAMILIAL MULTIPLE COAGULATION DEFICIENCIES

There are several bleeding disorders characterized by the inherited deficiency of more than one plasma coagulation factor. To date, the genetic defects in two of these diseases have been characterized, and they provide new insights into the regulation of hemostasis by gene-encoding proteins outside blood coagulation.

Combined Deficiency of FV and FVIII Patients with combined FV and FVIII deficiency exhibit ~5% of residual clotting activity of each factor. Interestingly, the disease phenotype is a mild bleeding tendency, often following trauma. An underlying mutation has been identified in the endoplasmic reticulum/Golgi intermediate compartment (*ERGIC-53*) gene, a mannose-binding protein localized in the Golgi apparatus that functions as a chaperone for both FV and FVIII. In other families, mutations in the multiple coagulation factor deficiency 2 (*MCFD2*) gene have been defined; this gene encodes a protein that forms a Ca^{2+} -dependent complex with *ERGIC-53* and provides cofactor activity in the intracellular mobilization of both FV and FVIII.

Multiple Deficiencies of Vitamin K–Dependent Coagulation Factors Two enzymes involved in vitamin K metabolism have been associated with combined deficiency of all vitamin K–dependent proteins, including the procoagulant proteins prothrombin, VII, IX, and X and the anticoagulant proteins C and S. Vitamin K is a fat-soluble vitamin that is a cofactor for carboxylation of the gamma carbon of the glutamic acid residues in the vitamin K–dependent factors, a critical step for calcium and phospholipid binding of these proteins (Fig. 141-2). The enzymes γ-glutamylcarboxylase and epoxide reductase are critical for the metabolism and regeneration of vitamin K. Mutations in the genes encoding the γ-carboxylase (GGCX) or vitamin K epoxide reductase complex 1 (VKORC1) result in defective enzymes and thus in vitamin K–dependent factors with reduced activity, varying from 1 to 30% of normal. The disease phenotype is characterized by mild to severe bleeding episodes present from birth. Some patients respond to high doses of vitamin K. For severe bleeding, replacement therapy with FFP or PCC may be necessary to achieve full hemostatic control.

DISSEMINATED INTRAVASCULAR COAGULATION

DIC is a clinicopathologic syndrome characterized by widespread intravascular fibrin formation in response to excessive blood protease

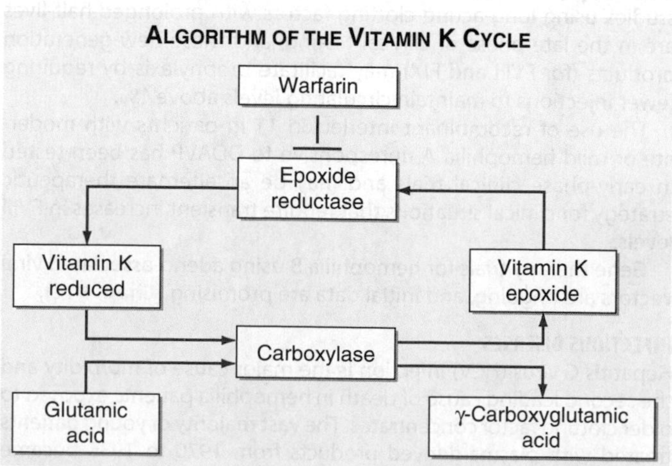

FIGURE 141-2 The vitamin K cycle. Vitamin K is a cofactor for the formation of γ-carboxyglutamic acid residues on coagulation proteins. Vitamin K–dependent γ-glutamylcarboxylase, the enzyme that catalyzes the vitamin K epoxide reductase, regenerates reduced vitamin K. Warfarin blocks the action of the reductase and competitively inhibits the effects of vitamin K.

TABLE 141-2 COMMON CLINICAL CAUSES OF DISSEMINATED INTRAVASCULAR COAGULATION

Sepsis	Immunologic Disorders
• Bacterial: Staphylococci, streptococci, pneumococci, meningococci, gram-negative bacilli	• Acute hemolytic transfusion reaction
• Viral	• Organ or tissue transplant rejection
• Mycotic	• Immunotherapy
• Parasitic	• Graft-versus-host disease
• Rickettsial	
Trauma and Tissue Injury	**Drugs**
• Brain injury (gunshot)	• Fibrinolytic agents
• Extensive burns	• Aprotinin
• Fat embolism	• Warfarin (especially in neonates with protein C deficiency)
• Rhabdomyolysis	• Prothrombin complex concentrates
	• Recreational drugs (amphetamines)
Vascular Disorders	**Envenomation**
• Giant hemangiomas (Kasabach-Merritt syndrome)	• Snake
• Large vessel aneurysms (e.g., aorta)	• Insects
Obstetrical Complications	**Liver Disease**
• Abruptio placentae	• Fulminant hepatic failure
• Amniotic fluid embolism	• Cirrhosis
• Dead fetus syndrome	• Fatty liver of pregnancy
• Septic abortion	
Cancer	**Miscellaneous**
• Adenocarcinoma (prostate, pancreas, etc.)	• Shock
• Hematologic malignancies (acute promyelocytic leukemia)	• Respiratory distress syndrome
	• Massive transfusion

activity that overcomes the natural anticoagulant mechanisms. There are several underlying pathologies associated with DIC (Table 141-2). The most common causes are bacterial sepsis, malignant disorders such as solid tumors or acute promyelocytic leukemia, and obstetric causes. DIC is diagnosed in almost one-half of pregnant women with abruptio placentae or with amniotic fluid embolism. Trauma, particularly to the brain, can also result in DIC. The exposure of blood to phospholipids from damaged tissue, hemolysis, and endothelial damage are all contributing factors to the development of DIC in this setting. Purpura fulminans is a severe form of DIC resulting from thrombosis of extensive areas of the skin; it affects predominantly young children following viral or bacterial infection, particularly those with inherited or acquired hypercoagulability due to deficiencies of the components of the protein C pathway. Neonates homozygous for protein C deficiency also present high risk for purpura fulminans with or without thrombosis of large vessels.

The central mechanism of DIC is the uncontrolled generation of thrombin by exposure of the blood to pathologic levels of tissue factor (Fig. 141-3). Simultaneous suppression of physiologic anticoagulant mechanisms and abnormal fibrinolysis further accelerate the process. Together, these abnormalities contribute to systemic fibrin deposition in small and midsize vessels. The duration and intensity of the fibrin deposition can compromise the blood supply of many organs, especially the lung, kidney, liver, and brain, with consequent organ failure. The sustained activation of coagulation results in consumption of clotting factors and platelets, which in turn leads to systemic bleeding. This is further aggravated by secondary hyperfibrinolysis. Studies in animals demonstrate that the fibrinolytic system is indeed suppressed at the time of maximal activation of coagulation. Interestingly, in patients with acute promyelocytic leukemia, a severe hyperfibrinolytic state often occurs in addition to the coagulation activation. The release of several proinflammatory cytokines such as interleukin 6 and tumor necrosis factor α plays a central role in mediating the coagulation defects in DIC and symptoms associated with systemic inflammatory response syndrome (SIRS).

Clinical manifestations of DIC are related to the magnitude of the imbalance of hemostasis, to the underlying disease, or to both. The most common findings are bleeding ranging from oozing from venipuncture sites, petechiae, and ecchymoses to severe hemorrhage from the gastrointestinal tract, lung, or into the CNS. In chronic DIC, the bleeding symptoms are discrete and restricted to skin or mucosal surfaces. The hypercoagulability of DIC manifests as the occlusion of vessels in the microcirculation and resulting organ failure. Thrombosis of large vessels and cerebral embolism can also occur. Hemodynamic complications and shock are common among patients with acute DIC. The mortality ranges from 30 to >80% depending on the underlying disease, the severity of the DIC, and the age of the patient.

The diagnosis of clinically significant DIC is based on the presence of clinical and/or laboratory abnormalities of coagulation or thrombocytopenia. The laboratory diagnosis of DIC should prompt a search for the underlying disease if it is not already apparent. There is no single test that establishes the diagnosis of DIC. The laboratory investigation should include coagulation tests (aPTT, PT, thrombin time [TT]) and markers of fibrin degradation products (FDPs), in addition to platelet and red cell count and analysis of the blood smear. These tests should be repeated over a period of 6–8 h because an initially mild abnormality can change dramatically in patients with severe DIC.

Common findings include the prolongation of PT and/or aPTT; platelet counts µ100,000/µL, or a rapid decline in platelet numbers; the presence of schistocytes (fragmented red cells) in the blood smear; and elevated levels of FDP. The most sensitive test for DIC is the FDP level. DIC is an unlikely diagnosis in the presence of normal levels of FDP. The D-dimer test is more specific for detection of fibrin—but not fibrinogen—degradation products and indicates that the cross-linked fibrin has been digested by plasmin. Because fibrinogen has a prolonged half-life, plasma levels diminish acutely only in severe cases of DIC. High-grade DIC is also associated with levels of antithrombin III or plasminogen activity <60% of normal.

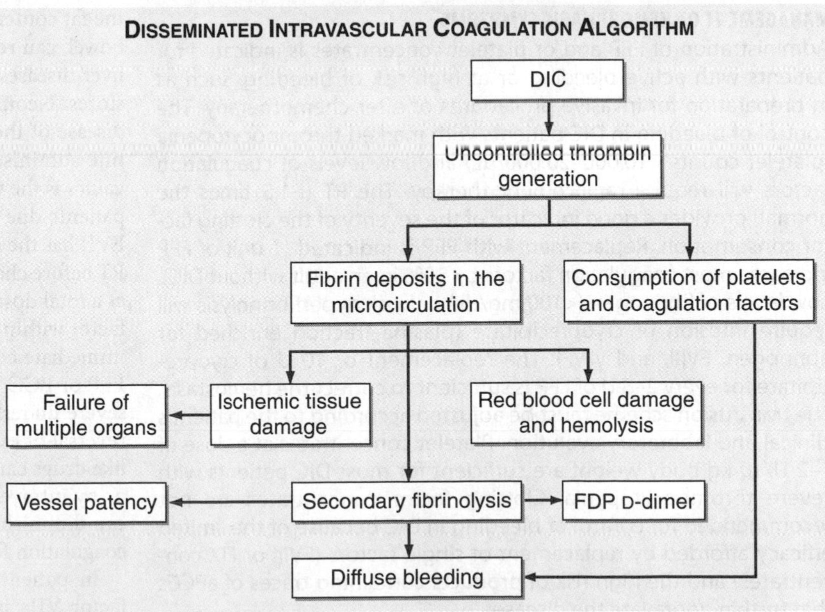

FIGURE 141-3 The pathophysiology of disseminated intravascular coagulation (DIC). Interactions between coagulation and fibrinolytic pathways result in bleeding and thrombosis in the microcirculation in patients with DIC. FDP, fibrin degradation product.

Chronic DIC Low-grade, compensated DIC can occur in clinical situations including giant hemangioma, metastatic carcinoma, or the dead fetus syndrome. Plasma levels of FDP or D-dimers are elevated. aPTT, PT, and fibrinogen values are within the normal range or high. Mild thrombocytopenia or normal platelet counts are also common findings. Red cell fragmentation is often detected but at a lower degree than in acute DIC.

Differential Diagnosis The differential diagnosis between DIC and severe liver disease is challenging and requires serial measurements of the laboratory parameters of DIC. Patients with severe liver disease are at risk for bleeding and manifest laboratory features including thrombocytopenia (due to platelet sequestration, portal hypertension, or hypersplenism), decreased synthesis of coagulation factors and natural anticoagulants, and elevated levels of FDP due to reduced hepatic clearance. However, in contrast to DIC, these laboratory parameters in liver disease do not change rapidly. Other important differential findings include the presence of portal hypertension or other clinical or laboratory evidence of an underlying liver disease.

Microangiopathic disorders such as thrombotic thrombocytopenic purpura present an acute clinical onset of illness accompanied by thrombocytopenia, red cell fragmentation, and multiorgan failure. However, there is no consumption of clotting factors or hyperfibrinolysis.

Over the last few years, several clinical trials on immune therapies for neoplasias using monoclonal antibodies or gene-modified T cells targeting tumor-specific antigens showed unwanted inflammatory responses with increased cytokine release. These complications are sometimes associated with increased D-dimers and decreased fibrinogen levels, cytopenias, and liver dysfunction; thus, careful screening tests for DIC are indicated.

TREATMENT DISSEMINATED INTRAVASCULAR COAGULATION

The morbidity and mortality associated with DIC are primarily related to the underlying disease rather than the complications of the DIC. The control or elimination of the underlying cause should therefore be the primary concern. Patients with severe DIC require control of hemodynamic parameters, respiratory support, and sometimes invasive surgical procedures. Attempts to treat DIC without accompanying treatment of the causative disease are likely to fail.

MANAGEMENT OF HEMORRHAGIC SYMPTOMS

Administration of FFP and/or platelet concentrates is indicated for patients with active bleeding or at high risk of bleeding, such as in preparation for invasive procedures or after chemotherapy. The control of bleeding in DIC patients with marked thrombocytopenia (platelet counts <10,000–20,000/μL) and low levels of coagulation factors will require replacement therapy. The PT (>1.5 times the normal) provides a good indicator of the severity of the clotting factor consumption. Replacement with FFP is indicated (1 unit of FFP increases most coagulation factors by 30% in an adult without DIC). Low levels of fibrinogen (<100 mg/dL) or brisk hyperfibrinolysis will require infusion of cryoprecipitate (plasma fraction enriched for fibrinogen, FVIII, and VWF). The replacement of 10 U of cryoprecipitate for every 2–3 U of FFP is sufficient to correct the hemostasis. The transfusion scheme must be adjusted according to the patient's clinical and laboratory evolution. Platelet concentrates at a dose of 1–2 U/10 kg body weight are sufficient for most DIC patients with severe thrombocytopenia. Clotting factor concentrates are not recommended for control of bleeding in DIC because of the limited efficacy afforded by replacement of single factors (FVIII or FIX concentrates) and the high risk of products containing traces of aPCCs that further aggravate the disease.

REPLACEMENT OF COAGULATION OR FIBRINOLYSIS INHIBITORS

Drugs to control coagulation such as heparin, antithrombin III (ATIII) concentrates, or antifibrinolytic drugs have all been tried in the treatment of DIC. Low doses of continuous-infusion heparin (5–10 U/kg per h) may be effective in patients with low-grade DIC associated with solid tumor, acute promyelocytic leukemia, or in a setting with recognized thrombosis. Heparin is also indicated for the treatment of purpura fulminans during the surgical resection of giant hemangiomas and during removal of a dead fetus. In acute DIC, the use of heparin is likely to aggravate bleeding. To date, the use of heparin in patients with severe DIC has no proven survival benefit. The use of antifibrinolytic drugs, EACA, or tranexamic acid to prevent fibrin degradation by plasmin may reduce bleeding episodes in patients with DIC and confirmed hyperfibrinolysis. However, these drugs can increase the risk of thrombosis, and concomitant use of heparin is indicated. Patients with acute promyelocytic leukemia or those with chronic DIC associated with giant hemangiomas are among the few patients who may benefit from this therapy. The use of protein C concentrates to treat purpura fulminans associated with acquired protein C deficiency or meningococcemia has been proven efficacious. The results from the replacement of ATIII in early-phase studies are promising but require further study.

Guidance for diagnosis and treatment of DIC had been proposed by the International Society of Thrombosis and Haemostasis. This initiative will permit more detailed clinical data on diagnosis and treatment of DIC. The clinical utility of these scoring systems and therapeutic recommendations contained in these guidelines is not yet known.

VITAMIN K DEFICIENCY Vitamin K–dependent proteins are a heterogenous group, including clotting factor proteins and also proteins found in bone, lung, kidney, and placenta. Vitamin K mediates posttranslational modification of glutamate residues to γ-carboxylglutamate, a critical step for the activity of vitamin K–dependent proteins for calcium binding and proper assembly to phospholipid membranes (Fig. 141-2). Inherited deficiency of the functional activity of the enzymes involved in vitamin K metabolism, notably the GGCX or VKORC1 (see above), results in bleeding disorders. The amount of vitamin K in the diet is often limiting for the carboxylation reaction; thus recycling of the vitamin K is essential to maintain normal levels of vitamin K–dependent proteins. In adults, low dietary intake alone is seldom reason for severe vitamin K deficiency but may become common in association with the use of broad-spectrum antibiotics. Disease or surgical interventions that affect the ability of the intestinal tract to absorb vitamin K, either through anatomic alterations or by changing the fat content of bile salts and pancreatic juices in the proximal small bowel, can result in significant reduction of vitamin K levels. Chronic liver diseases such as primary biliary cirrhosis also deplete vitamin K stores. Neonatal vitamin K deficiency and the resulting hemorrhagic disease of the newborn have been almost entirely eliminated by routine administration of vitamin K to all neonates. Prolongation of PT values is the most common and earliest finding in vitamin K–deficient patients due to reduction in prothrombin, FVII, FIX, and FX levels. FVII has the shortest half-life among these factors that can prolong the PT before changes in the aPTT. Parenteral administration of vitamin K at a total dose of 10 mg is sufficient to restore normal levels of clotting factor within 8–10 h. In the presence of ongoing bleeding or a need for immediate correction before an invasive procedure, replacement with FFP or PCC is required. The latter should be avoided in patients with severe underlying liver disorders due to high risk of thrombosis. The reversal of excessive anticoagulant therapy with warfarin or warfarin-like drugs can be achieved by minimal doses of vitamin K (1 mg orally or by intravenous injection) for asymptomatic patients. This strategy can diminish the risk of bleeding while maintaining therapeutic anticoagulation for an underlying prothrombotic state.

In patients with life-threatening bleeds, the use of recombinant factor VIIa in nonhemophilia patients on anticoagulant therapy has been shown to be effective at restoring hemostasis rapidly, allowing emergency surgical intervention. However, patients with underlying vascular disease, vascular trauma and other comorbidities are at risk for thromboembolic complications that affect both arterial and venous

TABLE 141-3 COAGULATION DISORDERS AND HEMOSTASIS IN LIVER DISEASE

Bleeding
Portal hypertension
Esophageal varices
Thrombocytopenia
Splenomegaly
Chronic or acute DIC
Decreased synthesis of clotting factors
Hepatocyte failure
Vitamin K deficiency
Systemic fibrinolysis
DIC
Dysfibrinogenemia
Thrombosis
Decreased synthesis of coagulation inhibitors: protein C, protein S, antithrombin
Hepatocyte failure
Vitamin K deficiency (protein C, protein S)
Failure to clear activated coagulation proteins (DIC)
Dysfibrinogenemia
Iatrogenic: Transfusion of prothrombin complex concentrates
Antifibrinolytic agents: EACA, tranexamic acid

Abbreviations: DIC, disseminated intravascular coagulation; EACA, ε-aminocaproic acid.

systems. Thus, the use of factor VIIa in this setting is limited to administration of low doses given for only a limited number of injections. Close monitoring for vascular complications is highly indicated.

COAGULATION DISORDERS ASSOCIATED WITH LIVER FAILURE The liver is central to hemostasis because it is the site of synthesis and clearance of most procoagulant and natural anticoagulant proteins and of essential components of the fibrinolytic system. Liver failure is associated with a high risk of bleeding due to deficient synthesis of procoagulant factors and enhanced fibrinolysis. Thrombocytopenia is common in patients with liver disease, and may be due to congestive splenomegaly (hypersplenism) or immune-mediated shortened platelet lifespan (primary biliary cirrhosis). In addition, several anatomic abnormalities secondary to underlying liver disease further promote the occurrence of hemorrhage (Table 141-3). Dysfibrinogenemia is a relatively common finding in patients with liver disease due to impaired fibrin polymerization. The development of DIC concomitant to chronic liver disease is not uncommon and may enhance the risk for bleeding. Laboratory evaluation is mandatory for an optimal therapeutic strategy, either to control ongoing bleeding or to prepare patients with liver disease for invasive procedures. Typically, these patients present with prolonged PT, aPTT, and TT depending on the degree of liver damage, thrombocytopenia, and normal or slight increase of FDP. Fibrinogen levels are diminished only in fulminant hepatitis, decompensated cirrhosis, or advanced liver disease, or in the presence of DIC. The presence of prolonged TT and normal fibrinogen and FDP levels suggest dysfibrinogenemia. FVIII levels are often normal or elevated in patients with liver failure, and decreased levels suggest superimposing DIC. Because FV is only synthesized in the hepatocyte and is not a vitamin K–dependent protein, reduced levels of FV may be an indicator of hepatocyte failure. Normal levels of FV and low levels of FVII suggest vitamin K deficiency. Vitamin K levels may be reduced in patients with liver failure due to compromised storage in hepatocellular disease, changes in bile acids, or cholestasis that can diminish the absorption of vitamin K. Replacement of vitamin K may be desirable (10 mg given by slow intravenous injection) to improve hemostasis.

Treatment with FFP is the most effective to correct hemostasis in patients with liver failure. Infusion of FFP (5–10 mL/kg; each bag contains ~200 mL) is sufficient to ensure 10–20% of normal levels of clotting factors but not correction of PT or aPTT. Even high doses of FFP (20 mL/kg) do not correct the clotting times in all patients. Monitoring for clinical symptoms and clotting times will determine if repeated doses are required 8–12 h after the first infusion. Platelet concentrates are indicated when platelet counts are <10,000–20,000/μL to control an ongoing bleed or immediately before an invasive procedure if counts are <50,000/μL. Cryoprecipitate is indicated only when fibrinogen levels are less than 100 mg/mL; dosing is six bags for a 70-kg patient daily. Prothrombin complex concentrate infusion in patients with liver failure should be avoided due to the high risk of thrombotic complications. The safety of the use of antifibrinolytic drugs to control bleeding in patients with liver failure is not yet well defined and should be avoided.

LIVER DISEASE AND THROMBOEMBOLISM The clinical bleeding phenotype of hemostasis in patients with stable liver disease is often mild or even asymptomatic. However, as the disease progresses, the hemostatic balance is less stable and more easily disturbed than in healthy individuals. Furthermore, the hemostatic balance is compromised by comorbid complications such as infections and renal failure (Fig. 141-4). Based on the clinical bleeding complications in patients with cirrhosis and laboratory evidence of hypocoagulation such as a prolonged PT/aPTT, it has long been assumed that these patients are protected against thrombotic disease. Cumulative clinical experience, however, has demonstrated that these patients are at risk for thrombosis, especially those with advanced liver disease. Although hypercoagulability could explain the occurrence of venous thrombosis, according to Virchow's

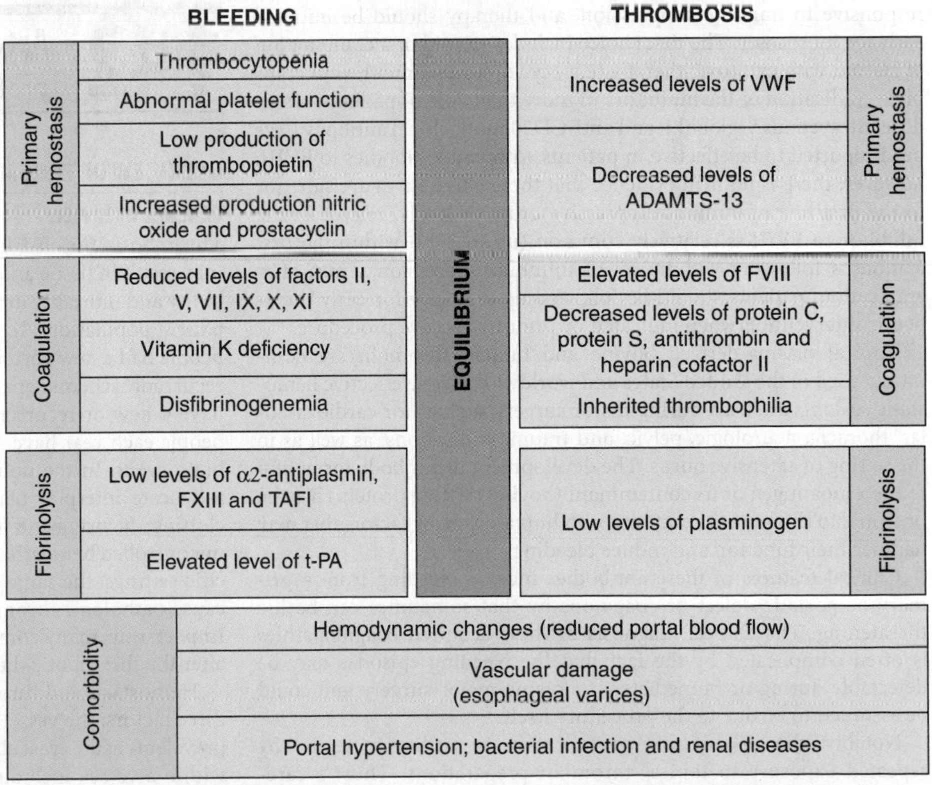

FIGURE 141-4 Balance of hemostasis in liver disease. TAFI, thrombin-activated fibrinolytic inhibitor; t-PA, tissue plasminogen activator; VWF, von Willebrand factor.

triad, hemodynamic changes and damaged vasculature may also be a contributing factor, and both processes may potentially also occur in patients with liver disease. Liver-related thrombosis, in particular, thrombosis of the portal and mesenteric veins, is common in patients with advanced cirrhosis. Hemodynamic changes, such as decreased portal flow, and evidence that inherited thrombophilia may enhance the risk for portal vein thrombosis in patients with cirrhosis suggest that hypercoagulability may play a role as well. Patients with liver disease develop deep vein thrombosis and pulmonary embolism at appreciable rates (ranging from 0.5 to 1.9%). The implication of these findings is relevant to the erroneous exclusion of thrombosis in patients with advanced liver disease, even in the presence of prolongation of routine clotting times, and caution should be advised on overcorrection of these laboratory abnormalities.

ACQUIRED INHIBITORS OF COAGULATION FACTORS An acquired inhibitor is an immune-mediated disease characterized by the presence of an autoantibody against a specific clotting factor. FVIII is the most common target of antibody formation, and is sometimes referred to as acquired hemophilia A, but inhibitors to prothrombin, FV, FIX, FX, and FXI are also reported. Acquired inhibitor to FVIII occurs predominantly in older adults (median age of 60 years), but occasionally in pregnant or postpartum women with no previous history of bleeding. In 50% of patients with inhibitors, no underlying disease is identified at the time of diagnosis. In the remaining patients, the causes are autoimmune diseases, malignancies (lymphomas, prostate cancer), dermatologic diseases, and pregnancy. Bleeding episodes occur commonly in soft tissues, the gastrointestinal or urinary tracts, and skin. In contrast to hemophilia, hemarthrosis is rare in these patients. Retroperitoneal hemorrhages and other life-threatening bleeding may appear suddenly. The overall mortality in untreated patients ranges from 8 to 22%, and most deaths occur within the first few weeks after presentation. The diagnosis is based on the prolonged aPTT with normal PT and TT. The aPTT remains prolonged after mixture of the test plasma with equal amounts of pooled normal plasma for 2 h at 37°C. The Bethesda assay using FVIII-deficient plasma as performed for inhibitor detection in hemophilia will confirm the diagnosis. Major bleeding is treated with bypass products such as PCC/aPCC or recombinant FVIIa. In contrast to hemophilia, inhibitors in nonhemophilic patients are typically responsive to immune suppression, and therapy should be initiated early for most cases. The first choice includes steroid or a combination of steroid with cytotoxic therapy (e.g., cyclophosphamide), with complete eradication of the inhibitors in more than 70% of patients. High-dose intravenous γ-globulin and anti-CD20 monoclonal antibody have been reported to be effective in patients with autoantibodies to FVIII; however, there is no firm evidence that these alternatives are superior to the first line of immunosuppressive drugs. Notably, relapse of the inhibitor to FVIII is relatively common (up to 20%) within the first 6 months following withdrawal of immunosuppression. Thus, after eradication, patients should be followed up regularly for early therapeutic intervention when indicated or prior to invasive procedure.

Topical plasma-derived bovine and human thrombin are commonly used in the United States and worldwide. These effective hemostatic sealants are used during major surgery such as for cardiovascular, thoracic, neurologic, pelvic, and trauma indications, as well as in the setting of extensive burns. The development of antibody formation to the xenoantigen or its contaminant (bovine clotting protein) has the potential to show cross-reactivity with human clotting factors that may hamper their function and induce bleeding.

Clinical features of these antibodies include bleeding from a primary hemostatic defect or coagulopathy that sometimes can be life threatening. The clinical diagnosis of these acquired coagulopathies is often complicated by the fact that the bleeding episodes may be detectable during or immediately following major surgery and could be assumed to be due to the procedure itself.

Notably, the risk of this complication is further increased by repeated exposure to topical thrombin preparations. Thus, a careful medical history of previous surgical interventions that may have occurred even decades earlier is critical to assessing risk.

The laboratory abnormalities are reflected by combined prolongation of the aPTT and PT that often fails to improve by transfusion of FFP and vitamin K. The abnormal laboratory tests cannot be corrected by mixing a test with equal parts of normal plasma that denotes the presence of inhibitory antibodies. The diagnosis of a specific antibody is obtained by the determination of the residual activity of human FV or other suspected human clotting factor. There are no commercially available assays specific for bovine thrombin coagulopathy.

There are no established treatment guidelines. Platelet transfusions have been used as a source of FV replacement for patients with FV inhibitors. Frequent injections of FFP and vitamin K supplementation may function as co-adjuvant rather than an effective treatment of the coagulopathy itself. Experience with recombinant FVIIa as a bypass agent is limited, and outcomes have been generally poor. Specific treatments to eradicate the antibodies based on immunosuppression with steroids, intravenous immunoglobulin, or serial plasmapheresis have been sporadically reported. Patients should be advised to avoid any topical thrombin sealant in the future.

Novel plasma-derived and recombinant human thrombin preparations for topical hemostasis have been approved by the U.S. Food and Drug Administration. These preparations have demonstrated hemostatic efficacy with reduced immunogenicity compared to the first generation of bovine thrombin products.

The presence of lupus anticoagulant can be associated with venous or arterial thrombotic disease. However, bleeding has also been reported in lupus anticoagulant; it is due to the presence of antibodies to prothrombin, which results in hypoprothrombinemia. Both disorders show a prolonged PTT that does not correct on mixing. To distinguish acquired inhibitors from lupus anticoagulant, note that the dilute Russell's viper venom test and the hexagonal-phase phospholipids test will be negative in patients with an acquired inhibitor and positive in patients with lupus anticoagulants. Moreover, lupus anticoagulant interferes with the clotting activity of many factors (FVIII, FIX, FXII, FXI), whereas acquired inhibitors are specific to a single factor.

142 Arterial and Venous Thrombosis

Jane E. Freedman, Joseph Loscalzo

OVERVIEW OF THROMBOSIS

GENERAL OVERVIEW

Thrombosis, the obstruction of blood flow due to the formation of clot, may result in tissue anoxia and damage, and it is a major cause of morbidity and mortality in a wide range of arterial and venous diseases and patient populations. In 2009 in the United States, an estimated 785,000 people had a new coronary thrombotic event, and about 470,000 had a recurrent ischemic episode. Each year, approximately 795,000 people have a new or recurrent stroke. It is estimated that 300,000–600,000 people each year have a pulmonary embolism or deep venous thrombotic event. In the nondiseased state, physiologic hemostasis reflects a delicate interplay between factors that promote and inhibit blood clotting, favoring the former. This response is crucial as it prevents uncontrolled hemorrhage and exsanguination following injury. In specific settings, the same processes that regulate normal hemostasis can cause pathologic thrombosis, leading to arterial or venous occlusion. Importantly, many commonly used therapeutic interventions may also alter the thrombotic–hemostatic balance adversely.

Hemostasis and thrombosis primarily involve the interplay among three factors: the vessel wall, coagulation proteins, and platelets. Many prevalent acute vascular diseases are due to thrombus formation within a vessel, including myocardial infarction, thrombotic cerebrovascular events, and venous thrombosis. Although the end result is vessel occlusion and tissue ischemia, the pathophysiologic processes governing these pathologies have similarities as well as distinct differences. While many of the pathways regulating thrombus formation are similar to those that regulate hemostasis, the processes triggering thrombosis and, often, perpetuating the thrombus may be distinct and can vary in different clinical and genetic settings. In venous thrombosis, primary hypercoagulable states reflecting defects in the proteins governing coagulation and/or fibrinolysis or secondary hypercoagulable states involving abnormalities of blood vessels and blood flow or stasis lead to thrombosis. By contrast, arterial thrombosis is highly dependent on the state of the vessel wall, the platelet, and factors related to blood flow.

ARTERIAL THROMBOSIS

OVERVIEW OF ARTERIAL THROMBOSIS

In arterial thrombosis, the platelets and abnormalities of the vessel wall typically play a key role in vessel occlusion. Arterial thrombus forms via a series of sequential steps in which platelets adhere to the vessel wall, additional platelets are recruited, and thrombin is activated (Fig. 142-1). The regulation of platelet adhesion, activation, aggregation, and recruitment will be described in detail below. In addition, while the primary function of platelets is regulation of hemostasis, our understanding of their role in other processes, such as immunity, wound healing, and inflammation, continues to grow.

ARTERIAL THROMBOSIS AND VASCULAR DISEASE

Arterial thrombosis is a major cause of morbidity and mortality both in the United States and, increasingly, worldwide. Although the rates have declined in the United States, the overall burden remains high and accounts for approximately 33% of deaths. Overall, coronary heart disease is estimated to cause about 1 of every 5 deaths in the United States. In addition to the 785,000 Americans who will have a new coronary event, an additional 195,000 silent first myocardial infarctions are projected to occur annually. Although the rate of strokes has fallen by a third, each year, about 795,000 people experience a new or recurrent stroke, although not all are caused by thrombotic occlusion of the vessel. Approximately 610,000 strokes are first events and 185,000 are recurrent events; it is estimated that 1 of every 18 deaths in the United States is due to stroke.

THE PLATELET

Many processes in platelets have parallels with other cell types, such as the presence of specific receptors and signaling pathways; however, unlike most cells, platelets lack a nucleus and are unable to adapt to changing biologic settings by altered gene transcription. Platelets sustain limited protein synthetic capacity from megakaryocyte-derived and intracellularly transported microRNA (miRNA) and messenger RNA (mRNA). Most of the molecules needed to respond to various stimuli, however, are maintained in storage granules and membrane compartments.

Platelets are disc-shaped, very small, anucleate cells (1–5 μm in diameter) that circulate in the blood at concentrations of 200–400,000/μL, with an average lifespan of 7–10 days. Platelets are derived from megakaryocytes, polyploidal hematopoietic cells found in the bone marrow. The primary regulator of platelet formation is thrombopoietin (TPO). The precise mechanism by which megakaryocytes produce and release fully formed platelets is unclear, but the process likely involves formation of proplatelets, pseudopod-like structures generated by the evagination of the cytoplasm from which platelets bud. Platelet granules are synthesized in megakaryocytes before thrombopoiesis and contain an array of prothrombotic, proinflammatory, and antimicrobial mediators. The two major types of platelet granules, alpha and dense, are distinguished by their size, abundance, and content. Alpha-granules contain soluble coagulation proteins, adhesion molecules, growth factors, integrins, cytokines, and inflammatory modulators. Platelet dense-granules are smaller than alpha-granules and less abundant. Whereas alpha-granules contain proteins that may be more important in the inflammatory response, dense-granules contain high concentrations of small molecules, including adenosine diphosphate (ADP) and serotonin, that influence platelet aggregation.

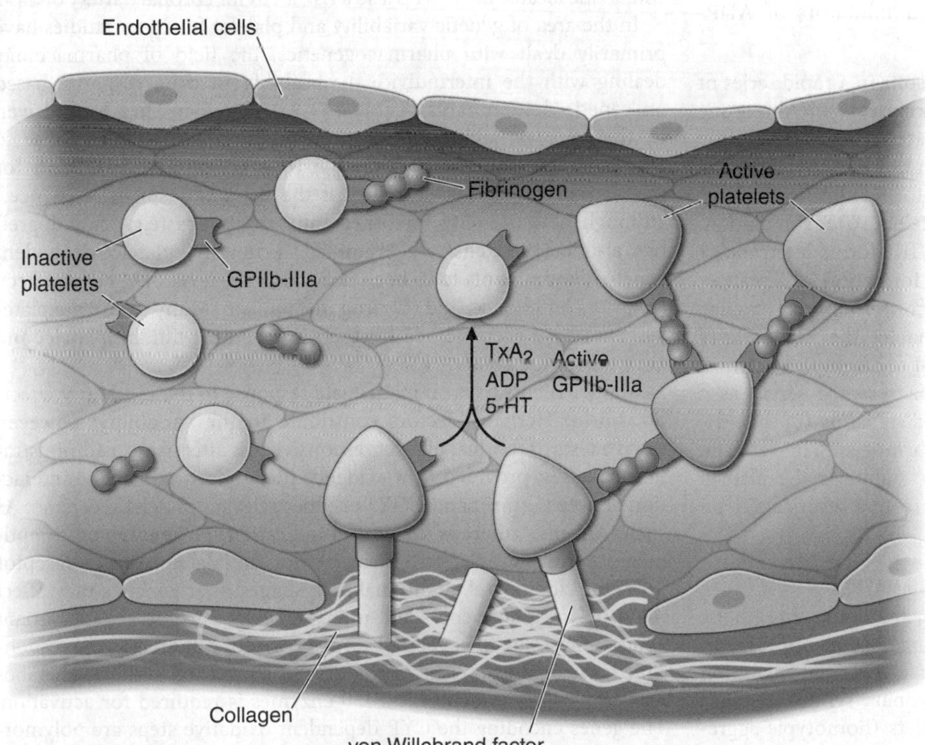

FIGURE 142-1 Platelet activation and thrombosis. Platelets circulate in an inactive form in the vasculature. Damage to the endothelium and/or external stimuli activates platelets that adhere to the exposed subendothelial von Willebrand factor and collagen. This adhesion leads to activation of the platelet, shape change, and the synthesis and release of thromboxane (TxA_2), serotonin (5-HT), and adenosine diphosphate (ADP). Platelet stimuli cause conformational change in the platelet integrin glycoprotein (GP) IIb/IIIa receptor, leading to the high-affinity binding of fibrinogen and the formation of a stable platelet thrombus.

Platelet Adhesion (See Fig. 142-1) The formation of a thrombus is initiated by the adherence of platelets to the damaged vessel wall. Damage exposes subendothelial components responsible for triggering platelet reactivity, including collagen, von Willebrand factor, fibronectin, and other adhesive proteins, such as vitronectin and thrombospondin. The hemostatic response may vary, depending on the extent of damage, the specific proteins exposed, and flow conditions. Certain proteins are expressed on the platelet surface that subsequently regulate collagen-induced platelet adhesion, particularly under flow conditions, and include glycoprotein (GP) IV, GPVI, and the integrin $\alpha_2\beta_1$. The platelet GPIb-IX-V complex adhesive receptor is central both to platelet adhesion and to the initiation of platelet activation. Damage to the blood vessel wall exposes subendothelial von Willebrand factor and collagen to the circulating blood. The GPIb-IX-V complex binds to the exposed von Willebrand factor, causing platelets to adhere (Fig. 142-1). In addition, the engagement of the GPIb-IX-V complex with ligand induces signaling pathways that lead to platelet activation. von Willebrand factor–bound GPIb-IX-V promotes a calcium-dependent conformational change in the GPIIb/IIIa receptor, transforming it from an inactive low-affinity state to an active high-affinity receptor for fibrinogen.

Platelet Activation The activation of platelets is controlled by a variety of surface receptors that regulate various functions in the activation process. Platelet receptors control many distinct processes and are stimulated by a wide variety of agonists and adhesive proteins that result in variable degrees of activation. In general terms, the stimulation of platelet receptors triggers two specific processes: (1) activation of internal signaling pathways that lead to further platelet activation and granule release and (2) the capacity of the platelet to bind to other adhesive proteins/platelets. Both of these processes contribute to the formation of a thrombus. Stimulation of nonthrombotic receptors results in platelet adhesion or interaction with other vascular cells including endothelial cells, neutrophils, and mononuclear cells.

Many families and subfamilies of receptors are found on platelets that regulate a variety of platelet functions. These include the seven transmembrane receptor family, which is the main agonist-stimulated receptor family. Several seven transmembrane receptors are found on platelets, including the ADP receptors, prostaglandin receptors, lipid receptors, and chemokine receptors. Receptors for thrombin comprise the major seven transmembrane receptors found on platelets. Among this last group, the first identified was the protease activation receptor 1 (PAR1). The PAR class of receptors has a distinct mechanism of activation that involves specific cleavage of the N-terminus of thrombin, which, in turn, acts as a ligand for the receptor. Other PAR receptors are present on platelets, including PAR2 (not activated by thrombin) and PAR4. Adenosine receptors are responsible for transduction of ADP-induced signaling events, which are initiated by the binding of ADP to purinergic receptors on the platelet surface. There are several distinct ADP receptors, classified as $P2X_1$, $P2Y_1$, and $P2Y_{12}$. The activation of both the $P2Y_{12}$ and $P2Y_1$ receptors is essential for ADP-induced platelet aggregation. The thienopyridine derivatives, clopidogrel and prasugrel, are clinically used inhibitors of ADP-induced platelet aggregation.

Platelet Aggregation Activation of platelets results in a rapid series of signal transduction events, including tyrosine kinase, serine/threonine kinase, and lipid kinase activation. In unstimulated platelets, the major platelet integrin GPIIb/IIIa is maintained in an inactive conformation and functions as a low-affinity adhesion receptor for fibrinogen. This integrin is unique as it is only expressed on platelets. After stimulation, the interaction between fibrinogen and GPIIb/IIIa forms intercellular connections between platelets, leading to the formation of a platelet aggregate (Fig. 142-1). A calcium-sensitive conformational change in the extracellular domain of GPIIb/IIIa enables the high-affinity binding of soluble plasma fibrinogen as a result of a complex network of inside-out signaling events. The GPIIb/IIIa receptor serves as a bidirectional conduit with GPIIb/IIIa-mediated signaling (outside-in) occurring immediately after the binding of fibrinogen. This leads to additional intracellular signaling that further stabilizes the platelet aggregate and transforms platelet aggregation from a reversible to an irreversible process (inside-out).

THE ROLE OF PLATELETS AND THROMBOSIS IN INFLAMMATION

Inflammation plays an important role during the acute thrombotic phase of acute coronary syndromes. In the setting of acute upper respiratory infections, people are at higher risk of myocardial infarction and thrombotic stroke. Patients with acute coronary syndromes have not only increased interactions between platelets (homotypic aggregates), but also increased interactions between platelets and leukocytes (heterotypic aggregates) detectable in circulating blood. These latter aggregates form when platelets are activated and adhere to circulating leukocytes. Platelets bind via P-selectin (CD62P) expressed on the surface of activated platelets to the leukocyte receptor, P-selectin glycoprotein ligand 1 (PSGL-1). This association leads to increased expression of CD11b/CD18 (Mac-1) on leukocytes, which itself supports interactions with platelets partially via bivalent fibrinogen linking this integrin with its platelet surface counterpart, GPIIb/IIIa. Platelet surface P-selectin also induces the expression of tissue factor on monocytes, which promotes fibrin formation.

In addition to platelet–monocyte aggregates, the immunomodulator, soluble CD40 ligand (CD40L or CD154), also reflects a link between thrombosis and inflammation. The CD40 ligand is a trimeric transmembrane protein of the tumor necrosis factor family and, with its receptor CD40, is an important contributor to the inflammatory process leading both to thrombosis and atherosclerosis. While many immunologic and vascular cells have been found to express CD40 and/or CD40 ligand, in platelets, CD40 ligand is rapidly translocated to the surface after stimulation and is upregulated in the newly formed thrombus. The surface-expressed CD40 ligand is cleaved from the platelet to generate a soluble fragment (soluble CD40 ligand).

Links have also been established among platelets, infection, immunity, and inflammation. Bacterial and viral infections are associated with a transient increase in the risk of acute thrombotic events, such as acute myocardial infarction and stroke. In addition, platelets contribute significantly to the pathophysiology and high mortality rates of sepsis. The expression, functionality, and signaling pathways of toll-like receptors (TLRs) have been established in platelets. Stimulation of platelet TLR2, TLR3, and TLR4 directly and indirectly activates the platelet's thrombotic and inflammatory responses, and live bacteria induce a proinflammatory response in platelets in a TLR2-dependent manner, suggesting a mechanism by which specific bacteria and bacterial components can directly activate platelet-dependent thrombosis.

GENETICS OF ARTERIAL THROMBOSIS

Some studies have associated arterial thrombosis with genetic variants (Table 142-1 *A*); however, the associations have been weak and not confirmed in larger series. Platelet count and mean platelet volume have been studied by genome-wide association studies (GWAS), and this approach identified signals located to noncoding regions. Of 15 quantitative trait loci associated with mean platelet volume and platelet count, one located at 12q24 is also a risk locus for coronary artery disease.

In the area of genetic variability and platelet function, studies have primarily dealt with pharmacogenetics, the field of pharmacology dealing with the interindividual variability in drug response based on genetic determinants (Table 142-2). This focus has been driven by the wide variability among individuals in terms of response to antithrombotic drugs and the lack of a common explanation for this variance. The best described is the issue of "aspirin resistance," although heterogeneity for other antithrombotics (e.g., clopidogrel) has also been extensively examined. Primarily, platelet-dependent genetic determinants have been defined at the level of (1) drug effect, (2) drug compliance, and (3) drug metabolism. Many candidate platelet genes have been studied for their interaction with antiplatelet and antithrombotic agents.

Many patients have an inadequate response to the inhibitory effects of aspirin. Heritable factors contribute to the variability; however, ex vivo tests of residual platelet responsiveness after aspirin administration have not provided firm evidence for a pharmacogenetic interaction between aspirin and *COX1* or other relevant platelet receptors. As such, currently, there is no clinical indication for genotyping to optimize aspirin's antiplatelet efficiency. For the platelet P2Y12 receptor inhibitor clopidogrel, additional data suggest that genetics may affect the drug's responsiveness and utility. The responsible genetic variant appears not to be the expected P2Y12 receptor but an enzyme responsible for drug metabolism. Clopidogrel is a prodrug, and liver metabolism by specific cytochrome P450 enzymes is required for activation. The genes encoding the CYP-dependent oxidative steps are polymorphic, and carriers of specific alleles of the CYP2C19 and CYP3A4 loci have increased platelet aggregability. Increased platelet activity has also been specifically associated with the CYP2C19*2 allele, which causes loss of platelet function in select patients. Because these are common genetic variants, this observation has been shown to be clinically relevant in large studies. In summary, although the loss-of-function polymorphisms in CYP2C19 is the strongest individual variable affecting pharmacokinetics and antiplatelet response to clopidogrel, it only

TABLE 142-1 HERITABLE CAUSES OF ARTERIAL AND VENOUS THROMBOSIS

A. Arterial Thrombosis
Platelet Receptors
β3 and α2 integrins
P_I A2 polymorphism
Fc(gamma)RIIA
GPIV T13254C polymorphism
GPIb
Thrombin receptor PAR1-5061 → D
Redox Enzymes
Plasma glutathione peroxidase
H2 promoter haplotype
Endothelial nitric oxide synthase
−786T/C, −922A/G, −1468T/A
Paraoxonase
−107T allele, 192R allele
Homocysteine
Cystathionine β-synthase 833T → C
5,10-Methylene tetrahydrofolate reductase (MTHFR) 677C → T
B. Venous Thrombosis
Procoagulant Proteins
Fibrinogen
455G/A, −854G/A
Prothrombin (20210G → A)
Protein C Anticoagulant Pathway
Factor V Leiden: 1691G → A (Arg506Gln)
Thrombomodulin 1481C → T (Ala455Val)
Fibrinolytic Proteins with Known Polymorphisms
Tissue plasminogen activator (tPA)
7351C/T, 20 099T/C in exon 6, 27 445T/A in intron 10
Plasminogen activator inhibitor (PAI-1)
4G/5G insertion/deletion polymorphism at position −675
Homocysteine
Cystathionine β-synthase 833T → C
5,10-MTHFR 677C → T

accounts for 5–12% of the variability in ADP-induced platelet aggregation on clopidogrel. In addition, genetic variables do not appear to significantly contribute to the clinical outcomes of patients treated with the P2Y12 receptor antagonists prasugrel or ticagrelor.

VENOUS THROMBOSIS

OVERVIEW OF VENOUS THROMBOSIS

Coagulation is the process by which thrombin is activated and soluble plasma fibrinogen is converted into insoluble fibrin. These steps account for both normal hemostasis and the pathophysiologic processes influencing the development of venous thrombosis. The primary forms of venous thrombosis are deep vein thrombosis (DVT) in the extremities and the subsequent embolization to the lungs (pulmonary embolism), referred to together as venous thromboembolic disease. Venous thrombosis occurs due to heritable causes (Table 142-1 *B*) and acquired causes (Table 142-3).

TABLE 142-2 GENETIC VARIATION AND PHARMACOGENETIC RESPONSES TO PLATELET INHIBITORS

Potential Gene Altered	Target Therapeutic Class	Specific Drug
P2Y1 and *P2Y12* *CYP2C19, CYP3A4, CYP3A5*	ADP receptor inhibitors	Clopidogrel, prasugrel
COX1, COX2	Cyclooxygenase inhibitors	Aspirin
PIA1/A2	Receptor inhibitors	Abciximab, eptifibatide, tirofiban
INTB3, GPIbA	Glycoprotein IIb-IIIa receptor inhibitors	

TABLE 142-3 ACQUIRED CAUSES OF VENOUS THROMBOSIS

Surgery
Neurosurgery
Major abdominal surgery
Malignancy
Antiphospholipid syndrome
Other
Trauma
Pregnancy
Long-haul travel
Obesity
Oral contraceptives/hormone replacement
Myeloproliferative disorders
Polycythemia vera

DEEP VENOUS THROMBOSIS AND PULMONARY EMBOLISM

More than 200,000 new cases of venous thromboembolism occur each year. Of these cases, up to 30% of patients die within 30 days and one-fifth suffer sudden death due to pulmonary embolism; 30% go on to develop recurrent venous thromboembolism within 10 years. Data from the Atherosclerosis Risk in Communities (ARIC) study reported a 9% 28-day fatality rate from DVT and a 15% fatality rate from pulmonary embolism. Pulmonary embolism in the setting of cancer has a 25% fatality rate. The mean incidence of first DVT in the general population is 5 per 10,000 person-years; the incidence is similar in males and females when adjusting for factors related to reproduction and birth control and increases dramatically with age from 2 to 3 per 10,000 person-years at 30–49 years of age to 20 at 70–79 years of age.

OVERVIEW OF THE COAGULATION CASCADE AND ITS ROLE IN VENOUS THROMBOSIS

Coagulation is defined as the formation of fibrin by a series of linked enzymatic reactions in which each reaction product converts the subsequent inactive zymogen into an active serine protease (Fig. 142-2). This coordinated sequence is called the coagulation cascade and is a key mechanism for regulating hemostasis. Central to the function of the coagulation cascade is the principle of amplification: due to a series of linked enzymatic reactions, a small stimulus can lead to much greater quantities of fibrin, the end product that prevents hemorrhage at the site of vascular injury. In addition to the known risk factors relevant to hypercoagulopathy, stasis, and vascular dysfunction, newer areas of research have identified contributions from procoagulant microparticles, inflammatory cells, microvesicles, and fibrin structure.

The coagulation cascade is primarily initiated by vascular injury exposing tissue factor to blood components (Fig. 142-2). Tissue factor may also be found in bloodborne cell-derived microparticles and, under pathophysiologic conditions, in leukocytes or platelets. Plasma factor VII (FVII) is the ligand for and is activated (FVIIa) by binding to tissue factor exposed at the site of vessel damage. The binding of FVII/VIIa to tissue factor activates the downstream conversion of factor X (FX) to active FX (FXa). In an alternative reaction, the FVII/FVIIa–tissue factor complex initially converts FIX to FIXa, which then activates FX in conjunction with its cofactor factor VIII (FVIIIa). Factor Xa with its cofactor FVa converts prothrombin to thrombin, which then converts soluble plasma fibrinogen to insoluble fibrin, leading to clot or thrombus formation. Thrombin also activates FXIII to FXIIIa, a transglutaminase that covalently cross-links and stabilizes the fibrin clot. Formation of thrombi is affected by mechanisms governing fibrin structure and stability including specific fibrinogen variants and how they alter fibrin formation, strength and structure.

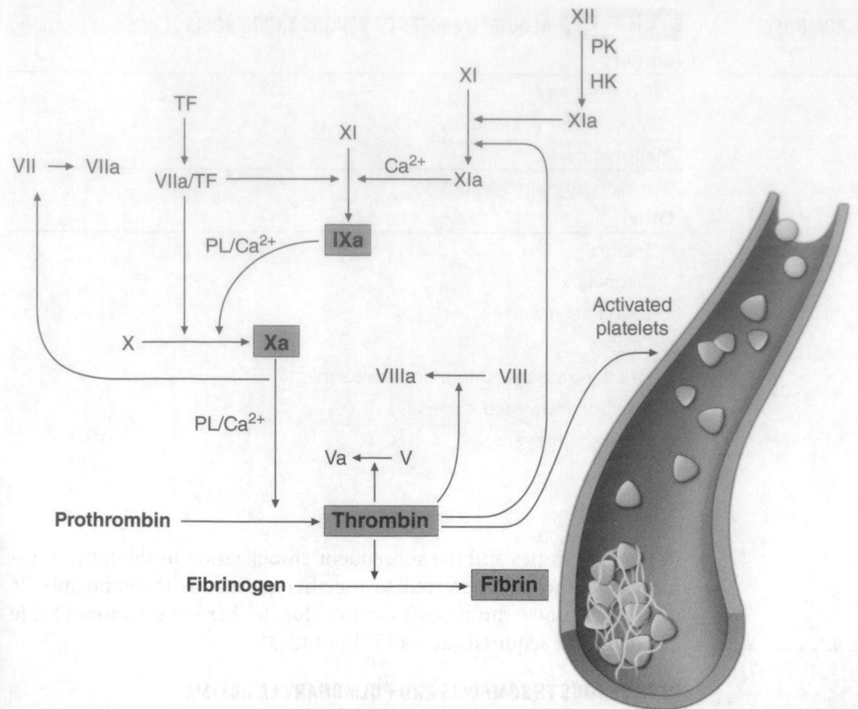

FIGURE 142-2 Summary of the coagulation pathways. Specific coagulation factors ("a" indicates activated form) are responsible for the conversion of soluble plasma fibrinogen into insoluble fibrin. This process occurs via a series of linked reactions in which the enzymatically active product subsequently converts the downstream inactive protein into an active serine protease. In addition, the activation of thrombin leads to stimulation of platelets. HK, high-molecular-weight kininogen; PK, prekallikrein; TF, tissue factor.

Several antithrombotic factors also regulate coagulation; these include antithrombin, tissue factor pathway inhibitor (TFPI), heparin cofactor II, and protein C/protein S. Under normal conditions, these factors limit the production of thrombin to prevent the perpetuation of coagulation and thrombus formation. Typically, after the clot has caused occlusion at the damaged site and begins to expand toward adjacent uninjured vessel segments, the anticoagulant reactions governed by the normal endothelium become pivotal in limiting the extent of this hemostatically protective clot.

RISK FACTORS FOR VENOUS THROMBOSIS

The risk factors for venous thrombosis are primarily related to hypercoagulability, which can be genetic (Table 142-1) or acquired, or due to immobilization and venous stasis. Independent predictors for recurrence include increasing age, obesity, malignant neoplasm, and acute extremity paresis. It is estimated that 5–8% of the U.S. population has a genetic risk factor known to predispose to venous thrombosis. Often, multiple risk factors are present in a single individual. Significant risk is incurred by major orthopedic, abdominal, or neurologic surgeries. Moderate risk is promoted by prolonged bedrest; certain types of cancer, pregnancy, hormone replacement therapy, or oral contraceptive use; and other sedentary conditions such as long-distance plane travel. It has been reported that the risk of developing a venous thromboembolic event doubles after air travel lasting 4 h, although the absolute risk remains low (1 in 6000). The relative risk of venous thromboembolism among pregnant or postpartum women is 4.3, and the overall incidence (absolute risk) is 199.7 per 100,000 woman-years.

GENETICS OF VENOUS THROMBOSIS

(See Table 142-2) Less common causes of venous thrombosis are those due to genetic variants. These abnormalities include loss-of-function mutations of endogenous anticoagulants as well as gain-of-function mutations of procoagulant proteins. Heterozygous antithrombin deficiency and homozygosity of the factor V Leiden mutation significantly increase the risk of venous thrombosis. While homozygous protein C or protein S deficiencies are rare and may lead to fatal purpura fulminans, heterozygous deficiencies are associated with a moderate risk of thrombosis. Activated protein C impairs coagulation by proteolytic degradation of FVa. Patients resistant to the activity of activated protein C may have a point mutation in the FV gene located on chromosome 1, a mutant denoted factor V Leiden. Mildly increased risk has been attributed to elevated levels of procoagulant factors, as well as low levels of tissue factor pathway inhibitor. Polymorphisms of methylene tetrahydrofolate reductase as well as hyperhomocysteinemia have been shown to be independent risk factors for venous thrombosis, as well as arterial vascular disease; however, many of the initial descriptions of genetic variants and their associations with thromboembolism are being questioned in larger, more current studies.

FIBRINOLYSIS AND THROMBOSIS

Specific abnormalities in the fibrinolytic system have been associated with enhanced thrombosis. Factors such as elevated levels of tissue plasminogen activator (tPA) and plasminogen activator inhibitor type 1 (PAI-1) have been associated with decreased fibrinolytic activity and an increased risk of arterial thrombotic disease. Specific genetic variants have been associated with decreased fibrinolytic activity, including the 4G/5G insertion/deletion polymorphism in the (plasminogen activator type 1) *PAI-1* gene. Additionally, the 311-bp Alu insertion/deletion in tPA's intron 8 has been associated with enhanced thrombosis; however, genetic abnormalities have not been associated consistently with altered function or tPA levels, raising questions about the relevant pathophysiologic mechanism. Thrombin-activatable fibrinolysis inhibitor (TAFI) is a carboxypeptidase that regulates fibrinolysis; elevated plasma TAFI levels have been associated with an increased risk of both DVT and cardiovascular disease.

The metabolic syndrome also is accompanied by altered fibrinolytic activity. This syndrome, which comprises abdominal fat (central obesity), altered glucose and insulin metabolism, dyslipidemia, and hypertension, has been associated with atherothrombosis. The mechanism for enhanced thrombosis appears to be due both to altered platelet function and to a procoagulant and hypofibrinolytic state. One of the most frequently documented prothrombotic abnormalities reported in this syndrome is an increase in plasma levels of PAI-1.

In addition to contributing to platelet function, inflammation plays a role in both coagulation-dependent thrombus formation and thrombus resolution. Both polymorphonuclear neutrophils and monocytes/macrophages contribute to multiple overlapping thrombotic functions, including fibrinolysis, chemokine and cytokine production, and phagocytosis.

THE DISTINCTION BETWEEN ARTERIAL AND VENOUS THROMBOSIS

Although there is overlap, venous thrombosis and arterial thrombosis are initiated differently, and clot formation progresses by somewhat distinct pathways. In the setting of stasis or states of hypercoagulability, venous thrombosis is activated with the initiation of the coagulation cascade primarily due to exposure of tissue factor; this leads to the formation of thrombin and the subsequent conversion of fibrinogen to fibrin. In the artery, thrombin formation also occurs, but thrombosis is primarily promoted by the adhesion of platelets to an injured vessel and stimulated by exposed extracellular matrix (Figs. 142-1 and 142-2). There is wide variation in individual responses to vascular injury, an important determinant of which is the predisposition an individual has to arterial or venous thrombosis. This concept has been supported indirectly in prothrombotic animal models in which there is poor correlation between the propensity to develop venous versus arterial thrombosis.

Despite considerable progress in understanding the role of hypercoagulable states in venous thromboembolic disease, the contribution of hypercoagulability to arterial vascular disease is much less well understood. Although specific thrombophilic conditions, such as factor V Leiden and the prothrombin G20210A mutation, are risk factors for DVT, pulmonary embolism, and other venous thromboembolic events, their contribution to arterial thrombosis is less well defined. In fact, to the contrary, many of these thrombophilic factors have not been found to be clinically important risk factors for arterial thrombotic events, such as acute coronary syndromes.

Clinically, although the pathophysiology is distinct, arterial and venous thrombosis do share common risk factors, including age, obesity, cigarette smoking, diabetes mellitus, arterial hypertension, hyperlipidemia, and metabolic syndrome. Select genetic variants, including those of the glutathione peroxidase gene, have also been associated with arterial and venous thrombo occlusive disease. Importantly, arterial and venous thrombosis may both be triggered by pathophysiologic stimuli responsible for activating inflammatory and oxidative pathways.

The diagnosis and treatment of ischemic heart disease are discussed in Chap. 293. Stroke diagnosis and management are discussed in Chap. 330. The diagnosis and management of DVT and pulmonary embolus are discussed in Chap. 300.

143 Antiplatelet, Anticoagulant, and Fibrinolytic Drugs

Jeffrey I. Weitz

Thromboembolic disorders are major causes of morbidity and mortality. Thrombosis can occur in arteries or veins. Arterial thrombosis is the most common cause of acute myocardial infarction (MI), ischemic stroke, and limb gangrene. Venous thromboembolism encompasses deep vein thrombosis (DVT), which can lead to postthrombotic syndrome, and pulmonary embolism (PE), which can be fatal or can result in chronic thromboembolic pulmonary hypertension.

Most arterial thrombi are superimposed on disrupted atherosclerotic plaque because plaque rupture exposes thrombogenic material in the plaque core to the blood. This material then triggers platelet aggregation and fibrin formation, which results in the generation of a platelet-rich thrombus that can temporarily or permanently occlude blood flow. In contrast, venous thrombi rarely form at sites of obvious vascular disruption. Although they can develop after surgical trauma to veins or secondary to indwelling venous catheters, venous thrombi usually originate in the valve cusps of the deep veins of the calf or in the muscular sinuses. Sluggish blood flow reduces the oxygen supply to the avascular valve cusps. Endothelial cells lining these valve cusps become activated and express adhesion molecules on their surface. Tissue factor–bearing leukocytes and microparticles adhere to these activated cells and induce coagulation. DNA extruded from neutrophils forms neutrophil extracelluar traps (NETs) that provide a scaffold that traps red blood cells, promotes platelet adhesion and activation, and augments coagulation. Local thrombus formation is exacerbated by reduced clearance of activated clotting factors as a result of impaired blood flow. If the thrombi extend from the calf veins into the popliteal and more proximal veins of the leg, thrombus fragments can dislodge, travel to the lungs, and produce a PE.

Arterial and venous thrombi are composed of platelets, fibrin, and trapped red blood cells, but the proportions differ. Arterial thrombi

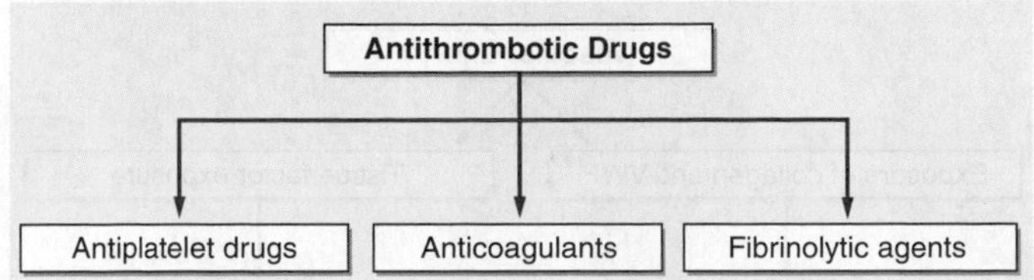

FIGURE 143-1 Classification of antithrombotic drugs.

are rich in platelets because of the high shear in the injured arteries. In contrast, venous thrombi, which form under low shear conditions, contain relatively few platelets and are predominantly composed of fibrin and trapped red cells. Because of the predominance of platelets, arterial thrombi appear white, whereas venous thrombi are red in color, reflecting the trapped red cells.

Antithrombotic drugs are used for prevention and treatment of thrombosis. Targeting the components of thrombi, these agents include (1) antiplatelet drugs, (2) anticoagulants, and (3) fibrinolytic agents (Fig. 143-1). With the predominance of platelets in arterial thrombi, strategies to attenuate arterial thrombosis focus mainly on antiplatelet agents, although, in the acute setting, often include anticoagulants and fibrinolytic agents. Anticoagulants are the mainstay of prevention and treatment of venous thromboembolism because fibrin is the predominant component of venous thrombi. Antiplatelet drugs are less effective than anticoagulants in this setting because of the limited platelet content of venous thrombi. Fibrinolytic therapy is used in selected patients with venous thromboembolism. For example, patients with massive or submassive PE can benefit from systemic or catheter-directed fibrinolytic therapy. Pharmaco mechanical therapy also is used to restore blood flow in patients with extensive DVT involving the iliac and/or femoral veins.

ANTIPLATELET DRUGS

ROLE OF PLATELETS IN ARTERIAL THROMBOSIS

In healthy vasculature, circulating platelets are maintained in an inactive state by nitric oxide (NO) and prostacyclin released by endothelial cells lining the blood vessels. In addition, endothelial cells also express CD39 on their surface, a membrane-associated ecto-adenosine diphosphatase (ADPase) that degrades ADP released from activated platelets. When the vessel wall is damaged, release of these substances is impaired and subendothelial matrix is exposed. Platelets adhere to exposed collagen via $\alpha_2\beta_1$ and glycoprotein (Gp) V1 and to von Willebrand factor (VWF) via Gp Ibα and Gp IIb/IIIa ($\alpha_{IIb}\beta_3$)—receptors that are constitutively expressed on the platelet surface. Adherent platelets undergo a change in shape, secrete ADP from their dense granules, and synthesize and release thromboxane A_2. Released ADP and thromboxane A_2, which are platelet agonists, activate ambient platelets and recruit them to the site of vascular injury (Fig. 143-2).

Disruption of the vessel wall also exposes tissue factor–expressing cells to the blood. Tissue factor binds factor VIIa and initiates coagulation. Activated platelets potentiate coagulation by providing a surface that binds clotting factors and supports the assembly of activation complexes that enhance thrombin generation. In addition to converting fibrinogen to fibrin, thrombin serves as a potent platelet agonist and recruits more platelets to the site of vascular injury. Thrombin also amplifies its own generation by feedback activation of factors V, VIII, and XI and solidifies the fibrin network by activating factor XIII, which then cross-links the fibrin strands.

When platelets are activated, Gp IIb/IIIa, the most abundant receptor on the platelet surface, undergoes a conformational change that enables it to bind fibrinogen and, under high shear conditions, VWF. Divalent fibrinogen or multivalent VWF molecules bridge adjacent platelets together to form platelet aggregates. Fibrin strands, generated through the action of thrombin, then weave these aggregates together to form a platelet/fibrin mesh.

Antiplatelet drugs target various steps in this process. The commonly used drugs include aspirin, ADP receptor inhibitors, which

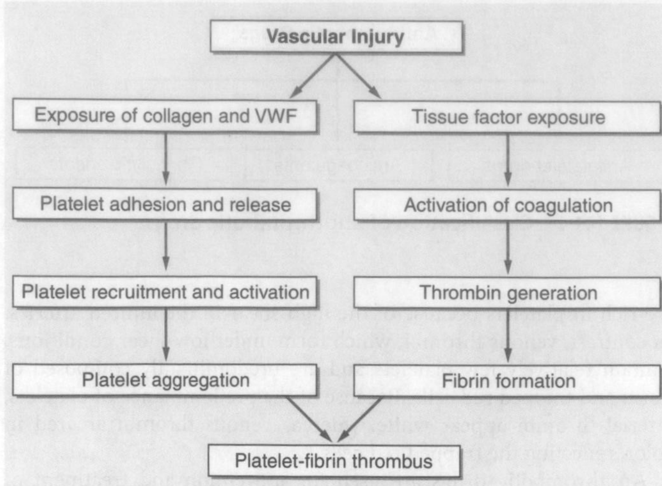

FIGURE 143-2 Coordinated role of platelets and the coagulation system in thrombogenesis. Vascular injury simultaneously triggers platelet activation and aggregation and activation of the coagulation system. Platelet activation is initiated by exposure of subendothelial collagen and von Willebrand factor (VWF), onto which platelets adhere. Adherent platelets become activated and release ADP and thromboxane A_2, platelet agonists that activate ambient platelets and recruit them to the site of injury. When platelets are activated, glycoprotein IIb/IIIa on their surface undergoes a conformational change that enables it to ligate fibrinogen and/or VWF and mediate platelet aggregation. Coagulation is triggered by tissue factor exposed at the site of injury. Tissue factor triggers thrombin generation. As a potent platelet agonist, thrombin amplifies platelet recruitment to the site of injury. Thrombin also converts fibrinogen to fibrin, and the fibrin strands then weave the platelet aggregates together to form a platelet/fibrin thrombus.

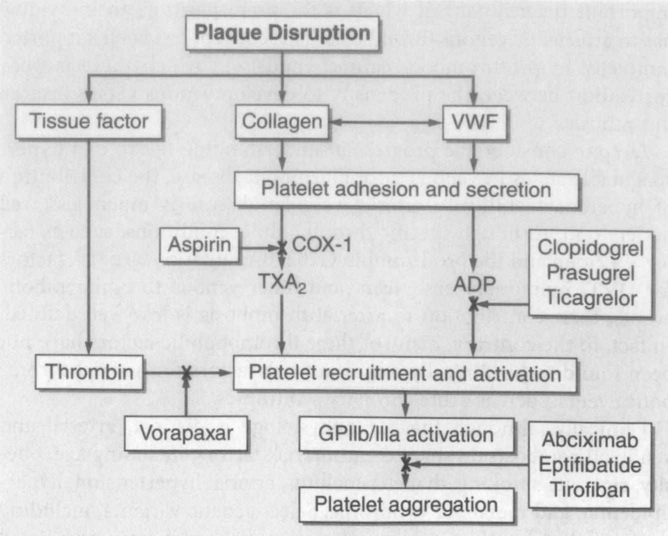

FIGURE 143-3 Site of action of antiplatelet drugs. Aspirin inhibits thromboxane A_2 (TXA_2) synthesis by irreversibly acetylating cyclooxygenase-1 (COX-1). Reduced TXA_2 release attenuates platelet activation and recruitment to the site of vascular injury. Clopidogrel and prasugrel irreversibly block $P2Y_{12}$, a key ADP receptor on the platelet surface; cangrelor and ticagrelor are reversible inhibitors of $P2Y_{12}$. Abciximab, eptifibatide, and tirofiban inhibit the final common pathway of platelet aggregation by blocking fibrinogen and von Willebrand factor binding to activated glycoprotein (Gp) IIb/IIIa. Vorapaxar inhibits thrombin-mediated platelet activation by targeting protease-activated receptor-1 (PAR-1), the major thrombin receptor on human platelets.

include the thienopyridines (clopidogrel and prasugrel) and ticagrelor, dipyridamole, and Gp IIb/IIIa antagonists.

ASPIRIN

The most widely used antiplatelet agent worldwide is aspirin. As a cheap and effective antiplatelet drug, aspirin serves as the foundation of most antiplatelet strategies.

Mechanism of Action Aspirin produces its antithrombotic effect by irreversibly acetylating and inhibiting platelet cyclooxygenase (COX)-1 (Fig. 143-3), a critical enzyme in the biosynthesis of thromboxane A_2. At high doses (~1 g/d), aspirin also inhibits COX-2, an inducible COX isoform found in endothelial cells and inflammatory cells. In endothelial cells, COX-2 initiates the synthesis of prostacyclin, a potent vasodilator and inhibitor of platelet aggregation.

Indications Aspirin is widely used for secondary prevention of cardiovascular events in patients with coronary artery, cerebrovascular, or peripheral vascular disease. Compared with placebo, aspirin produces a 25% reduction in the risk of cardiovascular death, MI, or stroke. Aspirin is also used for primary prevention in patients whose estimated annual risk of MI is >1%, a point where its benefits are likely to outweigh harms. This includes patients older than age 40 years with two or more major risk factors for cardiovascular disease or men older than age 45 years and women over the age of 55 years with one or more such risk factors. Aspirin is equally effective in men and women. In men, aspirin mainly reduces the risk of MI, whereas in women, aspirin lowers the risk of stroke.

Dosages Aspirin is usually administered at doses of 75–325 mg once daily. Higher doses of aspirin are not more effective than lower aspirin doses, and some analyses suggest reduced efficacy with higher doses. Because the side effects of aspirin are dose-related, daily aspirin doses of 75–100 mg are recommended for most indications. When rapid platelet inhibition is required, an initial aspirin dose of at least 160 mg should be given.

Side Effects The most common side effects are gastrointestinal and range from dyspepsia to erosive gastritis or peptic ulcers with bleeding and perforation. These side effects are dose-related. Use of enteric-coated or buffered aspirin in place of plain aspirin does not eliminate gastrointestinal side effects. The overall risk of major bleeding with aspirin is 1–3% per year. The risk of bleeding is increased two- to threefold when aspirin is given in conjunction with other antiplatelet drugs, such as clopidogrel, or with anticoagulants, such as warfarin. When dual or triple therapy is prescribed, low-dose aspirin should be given (75–100 mg daily). Eradication of *Helicobacter pylori* infection and administration of proton pump inhibitors may reduce the risk of aspirin-induced upper gastrointestinal bleeding in patients with peptic ulcer disease.

Aspirin should not be administered to patients with a history of aspirin allergy characterized by bronchospasm. This problem occurs in ~0.3% of the general population but is more common in those with chronic urticaria or asthma, particularly in individuals with nasal polyps or chronic rhinitis. Hepatic and renal toxicity are observed with aspirin overdose.

Aspirin Resistance Clinical aspirin resistance is defined as the failure of aspirin to protect patients from ischemic vascular events. This is not a helpful definition because it is made after the event occurs. Furthermore, it is not realistic to expect aspirin, which only blocks thromboxane A_2–induced platelet activation, to prevent all vascular events.

Aspirin resistance has also been described biochemically as failure of the drug to produce its expected inhibitory effects on tests of platelet function, such as thromboxane A_2 synthesis or arachidonic acid-induced platelet aggregation. Potential causes of aspirin resistance include poor compliance, reduced absorption, drug-drug interaction with ibuprofen, and overexpression of COX-2. Unfortunately, the tests for aspirin resistance have not been well standardized, and there is little evidence that they identify patients at increased risk of recurrent vascular events, or that resistance can be reversed by giving higher doses of aspirin or by adding other antiplatelet drugs. Until such information is available, testing for aspirin resistance remains a research tool.

ADP RECEPTOR ANTAGONISTS

The ADP receptor antagonists include the thienopyridines (clopidogrel and prasugrel) and ticagrelor. All of these drugs target $P2Y_{12}$, the key ADP receptor on platelets.

Thienopyridines • *MECHANISM OF ACTION* The thienopyridines are structurally related drugs that selectively inhibit ADP-induced platelet aggregation by irreversibly blocking $P2Y_{12}$ (Fig. 143-3). Clopidogrel and prasugrel are prodrugs that require metabolic activation by the hepatic cytochrome P450 (CYP) enzyme system. Prasugrel is about 10-fold more potent than clopidogrel and has a more rapid onset of action because of better absorption and more streamlined metabolic activation.

INDICATIONS When compared with aspirin in patients with recent ischemic stroke, recent MI, or a history of peripheral arterial disease, clopidogrel reduced the risk of cardiovascular death, MI, and stroke by 8.7%. Therefore, clopidogrel is more effective than aspirin but is also more expensive. In some patients, clopidogrel and aspirin are combined to capitalize on their capacity to block complementary pathways of platelet activation. For example, the combination of aspirin plus clopidogrel is recommended for at least 4 weeks after implantation of a bare metal stent in a coronary artery and for at least a year in those with a drug-eluting stent. Concerns about late in-stent thrombosis with drug-eluting stents have led some experts to recommend long-term use of clopidogrel plus aspirin for the latter indication. However, these recommendations are likely to change because the risk of late stent thrombosis is decreasing with the newer generation of drug-eluting coronary stents.

The combination of clopidogrel and aspirin is also effective in patients with unstable angina. Thus, in 12,562 such patients, the risk of cardiovascular death, MI, or stroke was 9.3% in those randomized to the combination of clopidogrel and aspirin and 11.4% in those given aspirin alone. This 20% relative risk reduction with combination therapy was highly statistically significant. However, combining clopidogrel with aspirin increases the risk of major bleeding to about 2% per year. This bleeding risk persists even if the daily dose of aspirin is ≤100 mg. Therefore, the combination of clopidogrel and aspirin should only be used when there is a clear benefit. For example, this combination has not proven to be superior to clopidogrel alone in patients with acute ischemic stroke or to aspirin alone for primary prevention in those at risk for cardiovascular events.

Prasugrel was compared with clopidogrel in 13,608 patients with acute coronary syndromes who were scheduled to undergo percutaneous coronary intervention. The incidence of the primary efficacy endpoint, a composite of cardiovascular death, MI, or stroke, was significantly lower with prasugrel than with clopidogrel (9.9% and 12.1%, respectively), mainly reflecting a reduction in the incidence of nonfatal MI. The incidence of stent thrombosis also was significantly lower with prasugrel (1.1% and 2.4%, respectively). However, these advantages were at the expense of significantly higher rates of fatal bleeding (0.4% and 0.1%, respectively) and life-threatening bleeding (1.4% and 0.9%, respectively) with prasugrel. Because patients older than age 75 years and those with a history of prior stroke or transient ischemic attack have a particularly high risk of bleeding, prasugrel should generally be avoided in older patients, and the drug is contraindicated in those with a history of cerebrovascular disease. Caution is required if prasugrel is used in patients weighing less than 60 kg or in those with renal impairment.

When prasugrel was compared with clopidogrel in 7243 patients with unstable angina or MI without ST-segment elevation, prasugrel failed to reduce the rate of the primary efficacy endpoint, which was a composite of cardiovascular death, MI, and stroke. Because of the negative results of this study, prasugrel is reserved for patients undergoing percutaneous coronary intervention. In this setting, prasugrel is usually given in conjunction with aspirin. To reduce the risk of bleeding, the daily aspirin dose should be ≤100 mg.

DOSING Clopidogrel is given once daily at a dose of 75 mg. Loading doses of clopidogrel are given when rapid ADP receptor blockade is desired. For example, patients undergoing coronary stenting are often given a loading dose of 300 mg, which produces inhibition of ADP-induced platelet aggregation in about 6 h; loading doses of 600 or 900 mg produce an even more rapid effect. After a loading dose of 60 mg, prasugrel is given once daily at a dose of 10 mg. Patients older than age 75 years or weighing less than 60 kg should receive a lower daily prasugrel dose of 5 mg.

SIDE EFFECTS The most common side effect of clopidogrel and prasugrel is bleeding. Because of its greater potency, bleeding is more common with prasugrel than clopidogrel. To reduce the risk of bleeding, clopidogrel and prasugrel should be stopped 5–7 days before major surgery. In patients taking clopidogrel or prasugrel who present with serious bleeding, platelet transfusion may be helpful.

Hematologic side effects, including neutropenia, thrombocytopenia, and thrombotic thrombocytopenic purpura, are rare.

THIENOPYRIDINE RESISTANCE The capacity of clopidogrel to inhibit ADP-induced platelet aggregation varies among subjects. This variability reflects, at least in part, genetic polymorphisms in the CYP isoenzymes involved in the metabolic activation of clopidogrel. Most important of these is CYP2C19. Clopidogrel-treated patients with the loss-of-function *CYP2C19*2* allele exhibit reduced platelet inhibition compared with those with the wild-type *CYP2C19*1* allele and experience a higher rate of cardiovascular events. This is important because estimates suggest that up to 25% of whites, 30% of African Americans, and 50% of Asians carry the loss-of-function allele, which would render them resistant to clopidogrel. Even patients with the reduced function *CYP2C19*3*, **4*, or **5* alleles may derive less benefit from clopidogrel than those with the full-function *CYP2C19*1* allele. Concomitant administration of clopidogrel with proton pump inhibitors, which are inhibitors of *CYP2C19*, produces a small reduction in the inhibitory effects of clopidogrel on ADP-induced platelet aggregation. The extent to which this interaction increases the risk of cardiovascular events remains controversial.

In contrast to their effect on the metabolic activation of clopidogrel, *CYP2C19* polymorphisms appear to be less important determinants of the activation of prasugrel. Thus, no association was detected between the loss-of-function allele and decreased platelet inhibition or increased rate of cardiovascular events with prasugrel. The observation that genetic polymorphisms affecting clopidogrel absorption or metabolism influence clinical outcomes raises the possibilities that pharmacogenetic profiling may be useful to identify clopidogrel-resistant patients and that point-of-care assessment of the extent of clopidogrel-induced platelet inhibition may help detect patients at higher risk for subsequent cardiovascular events. Clinical trials designed to evaluate these possibilities have thus far been negative. Although administration of higher doses of clopidogrel can overcome a reduced response to clopidogrel, the clinical benefit of this approach is uncertain. Instead, prasugrel or ticagrelor may be better choices for these patients.

Ticagrelor As an orally active inhibitor of $P2Y_{12}$, ticagrelor differs from the thienopyridines in that ticagrelor does not require metabolic activation and it produces reversible inhibition of the ADP receptor.

MECHANISM OF ACTION Like the thienopyridines, ticagrelor inhibits $P2Y_{12}$. Because it does not require metabolic activation, ticagrelor has a more rapid onset and offset of action than clopidogrel, and it produces greater and more predictable inhibition of ADP-induced platelet aggregation than clopidogrel.

INDICATIONS When compared with clopidogrel in patients with acute coronary syndromes, ticagrelor produced a greater reduction in the primary efficacy endpoint—a composite of cardiovascular death, MI, and stroke at 1 year—than clopidogrel (9.8% and 11.7%, respectively; $p = .001$). This difference reflected a significant reduction in both cardiovascular death (4.0% and 5.1%, respectively; $p = .001$) and MI (5.8% and 6.9%, respectively; $p = .005$) with ticagrelor compared with clopidogrel. Rates of stroke were similar with ticagrelor and clopidogrel (1.5% and 1.3%, respectively), and no difference in rates of major bleeding was noted. When minor bleeding was added to the major bleeding results, however, ticagrelor showed an increase relative to clopidogrel (16.1% and 14.6%, respectively; $p = .008$). Ticagrelor also was superior to clopidogrel in patients with acute coronary syndrome who underwent percutaneous coronary intervention or cardiac surgery. Based on these observations, some guidelines give ticagrelor preference over clopidogrel, particularly in higher risk patients.

DOSING Ticagrelor is initiated with an oral loading dose of 180 mg followed by 90 mg twice daily. The dose does not require adjustment in patients with renal impairment, but the drug should be used with caution in patients with hepatic disease and in those receiving potent inhibitors or inducers of CYP3A4 because ticagrelor is metabolized in the liver via CYP3A4. Ticagrelor is usually administered in conjunction with aspirin; the daily aspirin dose should not exceed 100 mg.

SIDE EFFECTS In addition to bleeding, the most common side effects of ticagrelor are dyspnea, which can occur in up to 15% of patients, and asymptomatic ventricular pauses. The dyspnea, which tends to occur soon after initiating ticagrelor, is usually self-limiting and mild in intensity. The mechanism responsible for this side effect is unknown.

To reduce the risk of bleeding, ticagrelor should be stopped 5–7 days prior to major surgery. Platelet transfusions are unlikely to be of benefit in patients with ticagrelor-related bleeding because the drug will bind to $P2Y_{12}$ on the transfused platelets.

DIPYRIDAMOLE

Dipyridamole is a relatively weak antiplatelet agent on its own, but an extended-release formulation of dipyridamole combined with low-dose aspirin, a preparation known as *Aggrenox*, is used for prevention of stroke in patients with transient ischemic attacks.

Mechanism of Action By inhibiting phosphodiesterase, dipyridamole blocks the breakdown of cyclic adenosine monophosphate (AMP). Increased levels of cyclic AMP reduce intracellular calcium and inhibit platelet activation. Dipyridamole also blocks the uptake of adenosine by platelets and other cells. This produces a further increase in local cyclic AMP levels because the platelet adenosine A_2 receptor is coupled to adenylate cyclase (Fig. 143-4).

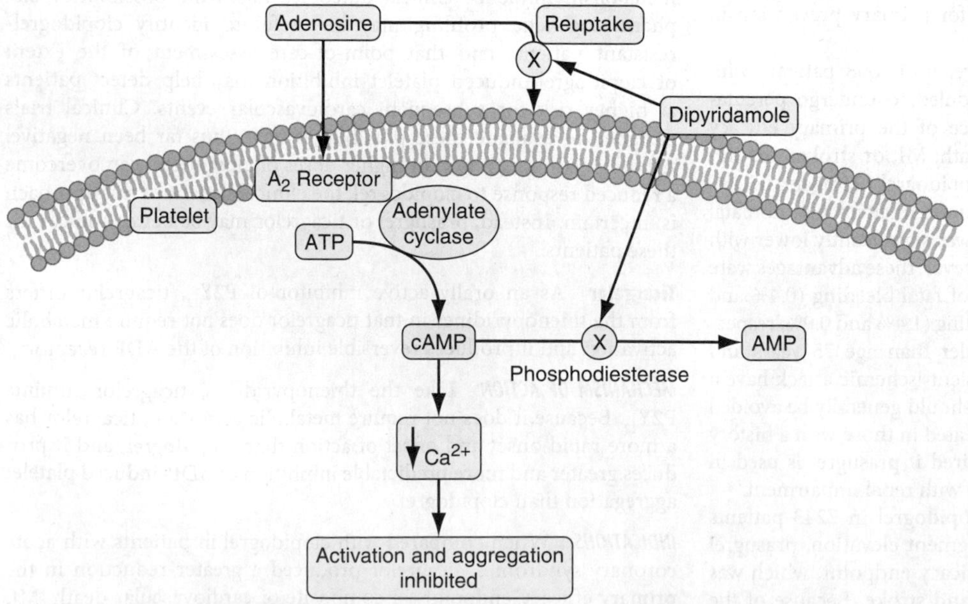

FIGURE 143-4 Mechanism of action of dipyridamole. Dipyridamole increases levels of cyclic AMP (cAMP) in platelets by (1) blocking the reuptake of adenosine and (2) inhibiting phosphodiesterase-mediated cyclic AMP degradation. By promoting calcium uptake, cyclic AMP reduces intracellular levels of calcium. This, in turn, inhibits platelet activation and aggregation.

Indications Dipyridamole plus aspirin was compared with aspirin or dipyridamole alone, or with placebo, in patients with an ischemic stroke or transient ischemic attack. The combination reduced the risk of stroke by 22.1% compared with aspirin and by 24.4% compared with dipyridamole. A second trial compared dipyridamole plus aspirin with aspirin alone for secondary prevention in patients with ischemic stroke. Vascular death, stroke, or MI occurred in 13% of patients given combination therapy and in 16% of those treated with aspirin alone. Another trial randomized 20,332 patients with noncardioembolic ischemic stroke to either Aggrenox or clopidogrel. The primary efficacy endpoint of recurrent stroke occurred in 9.0% of those given Aggrenox and in 8.8% of patients treated with clopidogrel. Although this difference was not statistically significant, the study failed to meet the prespecified margin to claim noninferiority of Aggrenox relative to clopidogrel. These results have dampened enthusiasm for the use of Aggrenox.

Because of its vasodilatory effects and the paucity of data supporting the use of dipyridamole in patients with symptomatic coronary artery disease, Aggrenox should not be used for stroke prevention in such patients. Clopidogrel is a better choice in this setting.

Dosing Aggrenox is given twice daily. Each capsule contains 200 mg of extended-release dipyridamole and 25 mg of aspirin.

Side Effects Because dipyridamole has vasodilatory effects, it must be used with caution in patients with coronary artery disease. Gastrointestinal complaints, headache, facial flushing, dizziness, and hypotension can also occur. These symptoms often subside with continued use of the drug.

GP IIB/IIIA RECEPTOR ANTAGONISTS

As a class, parenteral Gp IIb/IIIa receptor antagonists have an established niche in patients with acute coronary syndromes. The three agents in this class are abciximab, eptifibatide, and tirofiban.

Mechanism of Action A member of the integrin family of adhesion receptors, Gp IIb/IIIa is found on the surface of platelets and megakaryocytes. With about 80,000 copies per platelet, Gp IIb/IIIa is the most abundant receptor. Consisting of a noncovalently linked heterodimer, Gp IIb/IIIa is inactive on resting platelets. When platelets are activated, inside-outside signal transduction pathways trigger a conformational activation of the receptor. Once activated, Gp IIb/IIIa binds adhesive molecules, such as fibrinogen and, under high shear conditions, VWF. Binding is mediated by the Arg-Gly-Asp (RGD) sequence found on the α chains of fibrinogen and on VWF, and by the Lys-Gly-Asp (KGD) sequence located within a unique dodecapeptide domain on the γ chains of fibrinogen. Once bound, fibrinogen and/or VWF bridge adjacent platelets together to induce platelet aggregation.

Although abciximab, eptifibatide, and tirofiban all target the Gp IIb/IIIa receptor, they are structurally and pharmacologically distinct (Table 143-1). Abciximab is a Fab fragment of a humanized murine monoclonal antibody directed against the activated form of Gp IIb/IIIa. Abciximab binds to the activated receptor with high affinity and blocks the binding of adhesive molecules. In contrast, eptifibatide and tirofiban are synthetic small molecules. Eptifibatide is a cyclic heptapeptide that binds Gp IIb/IIIa because it incorporates the KGD motif, whereas tirofiban is a nonpeptidic tyrosine derivative that acts as an RGD mimetic. Abciximab has

TABLE 143-1 FEATURES OF GPIIB/IIIA ANTAGONISTS

Feature	Abciximab	Eptifibatide	Tirofiban
Description	Fab fragment of humanized mouse monoclonal antibody	Cyclical KGD-containing heptapeptide	Nonpeptidic RGD mimetic
Specific for Gp IIb/IIIa	No	Yes	Yes
Plasma half-life	Short (min)	Long (2.5 h)	Long (2.0 h)
Platelet-bound half-life	Long (days)	Short (s)	Short (s)
Renal clearance	No	Yes	Yes

a long half-life and can be detected on the surface of platelets for up to 2 weeks; eptifibatide and tirofiban have short half-lives.

Whereas eptifibatide and tirofiban are specific for Gp IIb/IIIa, abciximab also inhibits the closely related $\alpha_v\beta_3$ receptor, which binds vitronectin, and $\alpha_M\beta_2$, a leukocyte integrin. Inhibition of $\alpha_v\beta_3$ and $\alpha_M\beta_2$ may endow abciximab with anti-inflammatory and/or antiproliferative properties that extend beyond platelet inhibition.

Indications Abciximab and eptifibatide are used in patients undergoing percutaneous coronary interventions, particularly those who have not been pretreated with an ADP receptor antagonist. Tirofiban is used in high-risk patients with unstable angina. Eptifibatide also can be used for this indication.

Dosing All of the Gp IIb/IIIa antagonists are given as an IV bolus followed by an infusion. The recommended dose of abciximab is a bolus of 0.25 mg/kg followed by an infusion of 0.125 μg/kg per minute to a maximum of 10 μg/kg for 12 h. Eptifibatide is given as two 180 μg/kg boluses given 10 min apart, followed by an infusion of 2.0 μg/kg per minute for 18–24 h. Tirofiban is started at a rate of 0.4 μg/kg per minute for 30 min; the drug is then continued at a rate of 0.1 μg/kg per minute for up to 18 h. Because these agents are cleared by the kidneys, the doses of eptifibatide and tirofiban must be reduced in patients with renal insufficiency. Thus, the eptifibatide infusion is reduced to 1 μg/kg per minute in patients with a creatinine clearance below 50 mL/min, whereas the dose of tirofiban is cut in half for patients with a creatinine clearance below 30 mL/min.

Side Effects In addition to bleeding, thrombocytopenia is the most serious complication. Thrombocytopenia is immune-mediated and is caused by antibodies directed against neoantigens on Gp IIb/IIIa that are exposed upon antagonist binding. With abciximab, thrombocytopenia occurs in up to 5% of patients. Thrombocytopenia is severe in ~1% of these individuals. Thrombocytopenia is less common with the other two agents, occurring in ~1% of patients.

NEW ANTIPLATELET AGENTS

New agents in advanced stages of development include cangrelor, a parenteral, rapidly acting, reversible inhibitor of $P2Y_{12}$, and vorapaxar, an orally active inhibitor of protease-activated receptor 1 (PAR-1), the major thrombin receptor on platelets (Fig. 143-3).

Cangrelor An adenosine analogue, cangrelor binds reversibly to $P2Y_{12}$ and inhibits its activity. The drug has a half-life of 3–6 min and is given IV as a bolus followed by an infusion. When stopped, platelet function recovers within 60 min. A trial comparing cangrelor with placebo during percutaneous coronary interventions and a study comparing cangrelor with clopidogrel after such procedures revealed little or no advantage of cangrelor. A third trial compared cangrelor (given as an IV bolus of 30 μg/kg followed by an infusion of 4 μg/kg per minute for at least 2 h, or for the duration of the procedure, whichever was longer) with a loading dose of clopidogrel (300 or 600 mg) in 11,145 patients undergoing urgent or elective percutaneous coronary intervention. The rate of the primary efficacy endpoint, a composite of death, MI, ischemia-driven revascularization, and stent thrombosis, was 4.7% in the cangrelor group and 5.9% in the clopidogrel group ($p = .005$). The rates of severe bleeding, the primary safety endpoint, were 0.16% and 0.11% in the cangrelor and clopidogrel groups, respectively. Using the same efficacy endpoint, a prespecified meta-analysis of the three trials revealed a relative risk reduction of 19% with cangrelor compared with clopidogrel (3.8% and 4.7%, respectively) and a 40% reduction in stent thrombosis (0.5% and 0.8%, respectively) with no significant increase in serious bleeding. Based on these data, cangrelor is currently under regulatory review.

Vorapaxar An orally active PAR-1 antagonist, vorapaxar is slowly eliminated with a half-life of about 200 h. When compared with placebo in 12,944 patients with acute coronary syndrome without ST-segment elevation, vorapaxar failed to significantly reduce the primary efficacy endpoint, a composite of cardiovascular death, MI, stroke, recurrent ischemia requiring rehospitalization, and urgent coronary revascularization. Moreover, vorapaxar was associated with increased rates of bleeding, including intracranial bleeding.

In a second trial, vorapaxar was compared with placebo for secondary prevention in 26,449 patients with prior MI, ischemic stroke, or peripheral arterial disease. Overall, vorapaxar reduced the risk for cardiovascular death, MI, or stroke by 13%, but doubled the risk of intracranial bleeding. In the prespecified subgroup of 17,779 patients with prior MI, however, vorapaxar reduced the risk for cardiovascular death, MI, or stroke by 20% compared with placebo (from 9.7% to 8.1%, respectively). The rate of intracranial hemorrhage was higher with vorapaxar than with placebo (0.6% and 0.4%, respectively; $p = .076$) as was the rate of moderate or severe bleeding (3.4% and 2.1%, respectively; $P < 0.0001$). Based on these data, the drug is under consideration for regulatory approval in MI patients under the age of 75 years who have no history of stroke or transient ischemic attack and have a weight over 60 kg.

ANTICOAGULANTS

There are both parenteral and oral anticoagulants. The parenteral anticoagulants include heparin, low-molecular weight heparin (LMWH), fondaparinux (a synthetic pentasaccharide), lepirudin, desirudin, bivalirudin, and argatroban. Currently available oral anticoagulants include warfarin; dabigatran etexilate, an oral thrombin inhibitor; and rivaroxaban and apixaban, oral factor Xa inhibitors. Edoxaban, a third oral factor Xa inhibitor, is undergoing regulatory review.

PARENTERAL ANTICOAGULANTS

Heparin A sulfated polysaccharide, heparin is isolated from mammalian tissues rich in mast cells. Most commercial heparin is derived from porcine intestinal mucosa and is a polymer of alternating D-glucuronic acid and *N*-acetyl-D-glucosamine residues.

MECHANISM OF ACTION Heparin acts as an anticoagulant by activating antithrombin (previously known as antithrombin III) and accelerating the rate at which antithrombin inhibits clotting enzymes, particularly thrombin and factor Xa. Antithrombin, the obligatory plasma cofactor for heparin, is a member of the serine protease inhibitor (serpin) superfamily. Synthesized in the liver and circulating in plasma at a concentration of 2.6 ± 0.4 μM, antithrombin acts as a suicide substrate for its target enzymes.

To activate antithrombin, heparin binds to the serpin via a unique pentasaccharide sequence that is found on one-third of the chains of commercial heparin (Fig. 143-5). Heparin chains without this pentasaccharide sequence have little or no anticoagulant activity. Once bound to antithrombin, heparin induces a conformational change in the reactive center loop of antithrombin that renders it more readily accessible to its target proteases. This conformational change enhances the rate at which antithrombin inhibits factor Xa by at least two orders of magnitude but has little effect on the rate of thrombin inhibition. To catalyze thrombin inhibition, heparin serves as a template that binds antithrombin and thrombin simultaneously. Formation of this ternary complex brings the enzyme in close apposition to the inhibitor, thereby

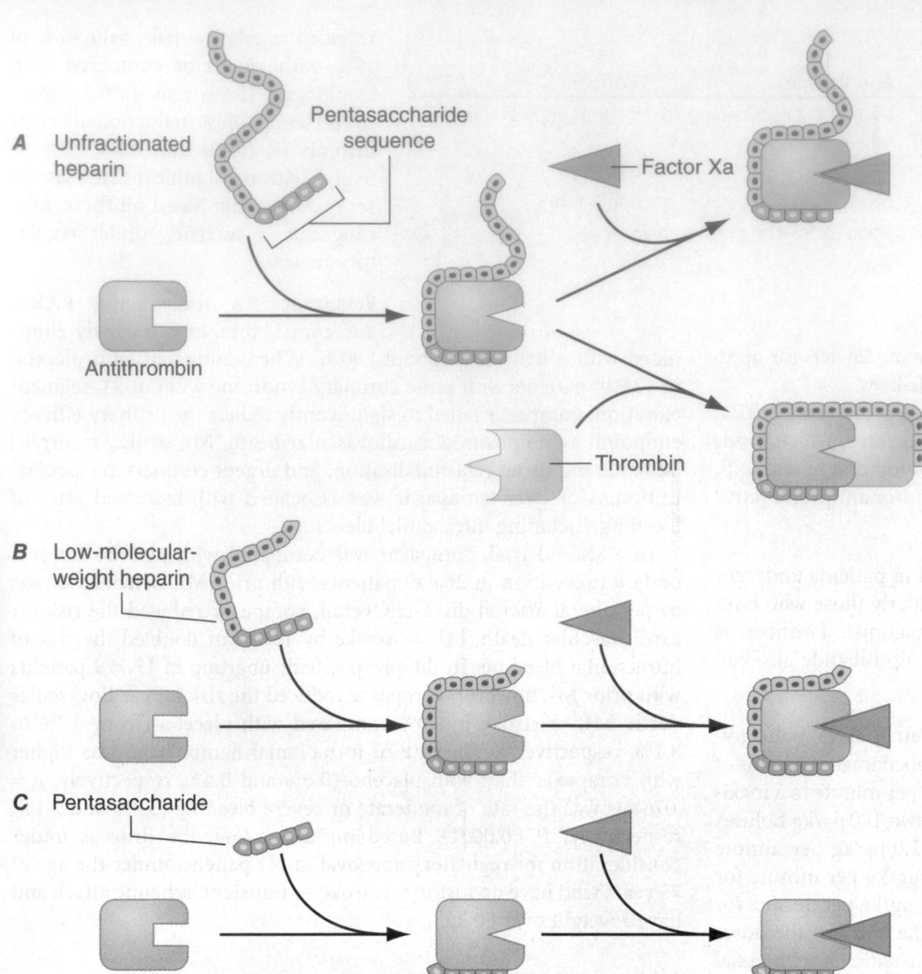

FIGURE 143-5 Mechanism of action of heparin, low-molecular-weight heparin (LMWH), and fondaparinux, a synthetic pentasaccharide. ***A.*** Heparin binds to antithrombin via its pentasaccharide sequence. This induces a conformational change in the reactive center loop of antithrombin that accelerates its interaction with factor Xa. To potentiate thrombin inhibition, heparin must simultaneously bind to antithrombin and thrombin. Only heparin chains composed of at least 18 saccharide units, which corresponds to a molecular weight of 5400, are of sufficient length to perform this bridging function. With a mean molecular weight of 15,000, all of the heparin chains are long enough to do this. ***B.*** LMWH has greater capacity to potentiate factor Xa inhibition by antithrombin than thrombin because, with a mean molecular weight of 4500–5000, at least half of the LMWH chains are too short to bridge antithrombin to thrombin. ***C.*** The pentasaccharide only accelerates factor Xa inhibition by antithrombin because the pentasaccharide is too short to bridge antithrombin to thrombin.

promoting the formation of a stable covalent thrombin-antithrombin complex.

Only pentasaccharide-containing heparin chains composed of at least 18 saccharide units (which correspond to a molecular weight of 5400) are of sufficient length to bridge thrombin and antithrombin together. With a mean molecular weight of 15,000, and a range of 5000–30,000, almost all of the chains of unfractionated heparin are long enough to do so. Consequently, by definition, heparin has equal capacity to promote the inhibition of thrombin and factor Xa by antithrombin and is assigned an anti-factor Xa to anti-factor IIa (thrombin) ratio of 1:1.

Heparin causes the release of tissue factor pathway inhibitor (TFPI) from the endothelium. A factor Xa–dependent inhibitor of tissue factor–bound factor VIIa, TFPI may contribute to the antithrombotic activity of heparin. Longer heparin chains induce the release of more TFPI than shorter ones.

PHARMACOLOGY Heparin must be given parenterally. It is usually administered SC or by continuous IV infusion. When used for therapeutic purposes, the IV route is most often employed. If heparin is given SC for treatment of thrombosis, the dose of heparin must be high enough to overcome the limited bioavailability associated with this method of delivery.

In the circulation, heparin binds to the endothelium and to plasma proteins other than antithrombin. Heparin binding to endothelial cells explains its dose-dependent clearance. At low doses, the half-life of heparin is short because it binds rapidly to the endothelium. With higher doses of heparin, the half-life is longer because heparin is cleared more slowly once the endothelium is saturated. Clearance is mainly extrarenal; heparin binds to macrophages, which internalize and depolymerize the long heparin chains and secrete shorter chains back into the circulation. Because of its dose-dependent clearance mechanism, the plasma half-life of heparin ranges from 30 to 60 min with bolus IV doses of 25 and 100 units/kg, respectively.

Once heparin enters the circulation, it binds to plasma proteins other than antithrombin, a phenomenon that reduces its anticoagulant activity. Some of the heparin-binding proteins found in plasma are acute-phase reactants whose levels are elevated in ill patients. Others, such as high-molecular-weight multimers of VWF, are released from activated platelets or endothelial cells. Activated platelets also release platelet factor 4 (PF4), a highly cationic protein that binds heparin with high affinity. The large amounts of PF4 found in the vicinity of platelet-rich arterial thrombi can neutralize the anticoagulant activity of heparin. This phenomenon may attenuate heparin's capacity to suppress thrombus growth.

Because the levels of heparin-binding proteins in plasma vary from person to person, the anticoagulant response to fixed or weight-adjusted doses of heparin is unpredictable. Consequently, coagulation monitoring is essential to ensure that a therapeutic response is obtained. This is particularly important when heparin is administered for treatment of established thrombosis because a subtherapeutic anticoagulant response may render patients at risk for recurrent thrombosis, whereas excessive anticoagulation increases the risk of bleeding.

MONITORING THE ANTICOAGULANT EFFECT Heparin therapy can be monitored using the activated partial thromboplastin time (aPTT) or anti-factor Xa level. Although the aPTT is the test most often used for this purpose, there are problems with this assay. aPTT reagents vary in their sensitivity to heparin, and the type of coagulometer used for testing can influence the results. Consequently, laboratories must establish a therapeutic aPTT range with each reagent-coagulometer combination by measuring the aPTT and anti-factor Xa level in plasma samples collected from heparin-treated patients. For most of the aPTT reagents and coagulometers in current use, therapeutic heparin levels are achieved with a two- to threefold prolongation of the aPTT.

Anti-factor Xa levels also can be used to monitor heparin therapy. With this test, therapeutic heparin levels range from 0.3 to 0.7 units/mL. Although this test is gaining in popularity, anti-factor Xa assays have yet to be standardized, and results can vary widely between laboratories.

Up to 25% of heparin-treated patients with venous thromboembolism require >35,000 units/d to achieve a therapeutic aPTT. These patients are considered heparin resistant. It is useful to measure anti-factor Xa levels in heparin-resistant patients because many will have a therapeutic anti-factor Xa level despite a subtherapeutic aPTT. This dissociation in test results occurs because elevated plasma levels of fibrinogen and factor VIII, both of which are acute-phase proteins, shorten the aPTT but have no effect on anti-factor Xa levels. Heparin therapy in patients who exhibit this phenomenon is best monitored using anti-factor Xa levels instead of the aPTT. Patients with congenital or acquired antithrombin deficiency and those with elevated levels of heparin-binding proteins may also need high doses of heparin to achieve a therapeutic aPTT or anti-factor Xa level. If there is good correlation between the aPTT and the anti-factor Xa levels, either test can be used to monitor heparin therapy.

DOSING For prophylaxis, heparin is usually given in fixed doses of 5000 units SC two or three times daily. With these low doses, coagulation monitoring is unnecessary. In contrast, monitoring is essential when the drug is given in therapeutic doses. Fixed-dose or weight-based heparin nomograms are used to standardize heparin dosing and to shorten the time required to achieve a therapeutic anticoagulant response. At least two heparin nomograms have been validated in patients with venous thromboembolism and reduce the time required to achieve a therapeutic aPTT. Weight-adjusted heparin nomograms have also been evaluated in patients with acute coronary syndromes. After an IV heparin bolus of 5000 units or 70 units/kg, a heparin infusion rate of 12–15 units/kg per hour is usually administered. In contrast, weight-adjusted heparin nomograms for patients with venous thromboembolism use an initial bolus of 5000 units or 80 units/kg, followed by an infusion of 18 units/kg per h. Thus, patients with venous thromboembolism appear to require higher doses of heparin to achieve a therapeutic aPTT than do patients with acute coronary syndromes. This may reflect differences in the thrombus burden. Heparin binds to fibrin, and the amount of fibrin in patients with extensive DVT is greater than that in those with coronary thrombosis.

Heparin manufacturers in North America have traditionally measured heparin potency in USP units, with a unit defined as the concentration of heparin that prevents 1 mL of citrated sheep plasma from clotting for 1 h after calcium addition. In contrast, manufacturers in Europe measure heparin potency with anti Xa assays using an international heparin standard for comparison. Because of problems with heparin contamination with oversulfated chondroitin sulfate, which the USP assay system does not detect, North American heparin manufacturers now use the anti-Xa assay to assess heparin potency. The use of international units in place of USP units results in a 10% reduction in heparin doses, which is a difference unlikely to affect patient care because monitoring will help to ensure that a therapeutic anticoagulant response has been achieved.

LIMITATIONS Heparin has pharmacokinetic and biophysical limitations (Table 143-2). The pharmacokinetic limitations reflect heparin's propensity to bind in a pentasaccharide-independent fashion to cells and plasma proteins. Heparin binding to endothelial cells explains its dose-dependent clearance, whereas binding to plasma proteins results in a variable anticoagulant response and can lead to heparin resistance.

The biophysical limitations of heparin reflect the inability of the heparin-antithrombin complex to inhibit factor Xa when it is incorporated into the prothrombinase complex, the complex that converts prothrombin to thrombin, and to inhibit thrombin bound to fibrin. Consequently, factor Xa bound to activated platelets within platelet-rich thrombi has the potential to generate thrombin, even in the face of heparin. Once this thrombin binds to fibrin, it too is protected from inhibition by the heparin-antithrombin complex. Clot-associated thrombin can then trigger thrombus growth by locally activating platelets and amplifying its own generation through feedback activation of factors V, VIII, and XI. Further compounding the problem is the potential for heparin neutralization by the high concentrations of PF4 released from activated platelets within the platelet-rich thrombus.

SIDE EFFECTS The most common side effect of heparin is bleeding. Other complications include thrombocytopenia, osteoporosis, and elevated levels of transaminases.

Bleeding The risk of bleeding rises as the dose of heparin is increased. Concomitant administration of drugs that affect hemostasis, such as antiplatelet or fibrinolytic agents, increases the risk of bleeding, as does recent surgery or trauma. Heparin-treated patients with serious bleeding can be given protamine sulfate to neutralize the heparin. Protamine sulfate, a mixture of basic polypeptides isolated from salmon sperm, binds heparin with high affinity, and the resultant protamine-heparin complexes are then cleared. Typically, 1 mg of protamine sulfate neutralizes 100 units of heparin. Protamine sulfate is given IV. Anaphylactoid reactions to protamine sulfate can occur, and drug administration by slow IV infusion is recommended to reduce the risk.

THROMBOCYTOPENIA Heparin can cause thrombocytopenia. Heparin-induced thrombocytopenia (HIT) is an antibody-mediated process that is triggered by antibodies directed against neoantigens on PF4 that are exposed when heparin binds to this protein. These antibodies, which are usually of the IgG isotype, bind simultaneously to the heparin PF4 complex and to platelet Fc receptors. Such binding activates the platelets and generates platelet microparticles. Circulating microparticles are prothrombotic because they express anionic phospholipids on their surface and can bind clotting factors and promote thrombin generation.

The clinical features of HIT are illustrated in Table 143-3. Typically, HIT occurs 5–14 days after initiation of heparin therapy, but it can manifest earlier if the patient has received heparin within the past 3 months. A platelet count below 100,000/μL or a 50% decrease in the platelet count from the pretreatment value should raise the suspicion of HIT in those receiving heparin. HIT is more common in surgical patients than in medical patients and, like many autoimmune disorders, occurs more frequently in females than in males.

HIT can be associated with thrombosis, either arterial or venous. Venous thrombosis, which manifests as DVT and/or PE, is more common than arterial thrombosis. Arterial thrombosis can manifest as ischemic stroke or acute MI. Rarely, platelet-rich thrombi in the distal aorta or iliac arteries can cause critical limb ischemia.

TABLE 143-2 PHARMACOKINETIC AND BIOPHYSICAL LIMITATIONS OF HEPARIN

Limitations	Mechanism
Poor bioavailability at low doses	Binds to endothelial cells and macrophages
Dose-dependent clearance	Binds to macrophages
Variable anticoagulant response	Binds to plasma proteins whose levels vary from patient to patient
Reduced activity in the vicinity of platelet-rich thrombi	Neutralized by platelet factor 4 released from activated platelets
Limited activity against factor Xa incorporated in the prothrombinase complex and thrombin bound to fibrin	Reduced capacity of heparin-antithrombin complex to inhibit factor Xa bound to activated platelets and thrombin bound to fibrin

TABLE 143-3 FEATURES OF HEPARIN-INDUCED THROMBOCYTOPENIA

Features	Details
Thrombocytopenia	Platelet count of ≤100,000/μL or a decrease in platelet count of ≥50%
Timing	Platelet count falls 5–10 days after starting heparin
Type of heparin	More common with unfractionated heparin than low-molecular-weight heparin
Type of patient	More common in surgical patients and patients with cancer than general medical patients; more common in women than in men
Thrombosis	Venous thrombosis more common than arterial thrombosis

TABLE 143-4 MANAGEMENT OF HEPARIN-INDUCED THROMBOCYTOPENIA

Stop all heparin.

Give an alternative anticoagulant, such as lepirudin, argatroban, bivalirudin, or fondaparinux.

Do not give platelet transfusions.

Do not give warfarin until the platelet count returns to its baseline level. If warfarin was administered, give vitamin K to restore the INR to normal.

Evaluate for thrombosis, particularly deep vein thrombosis.

Abbreviation: INR, international normalized ratio.

The diagnosis of HIT is established using enzyme-linked assays to detect antibodies against heparin-PF4 complexes or with platelet activation assays. Enzyme-linked assays are sensitive but can be positive in the absence of any clinical evidence of HIT. The most specific diagnostic test is the serotonin release assay. This test is performed by quantifying serotonin release when washed platelets loaded with labeled serotonin are exposed to patient serum in the absence or presence of varying concentrations of heparin. If the patient serum contains the HIT antibody, heparin addition induces platelet activation and serotonin release.

Management of HIT is outlined in Table 143-4. Heparin should be stopped in patients with suspected or documented HIT, and an alternative anticoagulant should be administered to prevent or treat thrombosis. The agents most often used for this indication are parenteral direct thrombin inhibitors, such as lepirudin, argatroban, or bivalirudin, or factor Xa inhibitors, such as fondaparinux.

Patients with HIT, particularly those with associated thrombosis, often have evidence of increased thrombin generation that can lead to consumption of protein C. If these patients are given warfarin without a concomitant parenteral anticoagulant to inhibit thrombin or thrombin generation, the further decrease in protein C levels induced by the vitamin K antagonist can trigger skin necrosis. To avoid this problem, patients with HIT should be treated with a direct thrombin inhibitor or fondaparinux until the platelet count returns to normal levels. At this point, low-dose warfarin therapy can be introduced, and the thrombin inhibitor can be discontinued when the anticoagulant response to warfarin has been therapeutic for at least 2 days.

Osteoporosis Treatment with therapeutic doses of heparin for >1 month can cause a reduction in bone density. This complication has been reported in up to 30% of patients given long-term heparin therapy, and symptomatic vertebral fractures occur in 2–3% of these individuals.

Heparin causes bone loss both by decreasing bone formation and by enhancing bone resorption. Thus, heparin affects the activity of both osteoblasts and osteoclasts.

Elevated levels of transaminases Therapeutic doses of heparin are frequently associated with modest elevations in the serum levels of hepatic transaminases without a concomitant increase in the level of bilirubin. The levels of transaminases rapidly return to normal when the drug is stopped. The mechanism responsible for this phenomenon is unknown.

Low-Molecular-Weight Heparin Consisting of smaller fragments of heparin, LMWH is prepared from unfractionated heparin by controlled enzymatic or chemical depolymerization. The mean molecular weight of LMWH is about 5000, one-third the mean molecular weight of unfractionated heparin. LMWH has advantages over heparin (Table 143-5) and has replaced heparin for most indications.

MECHANISM OF ACTION Like heparin, LMWH exerts its anticoagulant activity by activating antithrombin. With a mean molecular weight of 5000, which corresponds to about 17 saccharide units, at least half of the pentasaccharide-containing chains of LMWH are too short to bridge thrombin to antithrombin (Fig. 143-5). However, these chains retain the capacity to accelerate factor Xa inhibition by antithrombin because this activity is largely the result of the conformational changes in antithrombin evoked by pentasaccharide binding. Consequently, LMWH catalyzes factor Xa inhibition by antithrombin more than thrombin inhibition. Depending on their unique molecular weight distributions, LMWH preparations have anti-factor Xa to anti-factor IIa ratios ranging from 2:1 to 4:1.

TABLE 143-5 ADVANTAGES OF LMWH OVER HEPARIN

Advantage	Consequence
Better bioavailability and longer half-life after subcutaneous injection	Can be given subcutaneously once or twice daily for both prophylaxis and treatment
Dose-independent clearance	Simplified dosing
Predictable anticoagulant response	Coagulation monitoring is unnecessary in most patients
Lower risk of heparin-induced thrombocytopenia	Safer than heparin for short- or long-term administration
Lower risk of osteoporosis	Safer than heparin for extended administration

Abbreviation: LMWH, low-molecular-weight heparin.

PHARMACOLOGY Although usually given SC, LMWH also can be administered IV if a rapid anticoagulant response is needed. LMWH has pharmacokinetic advantages over heparin. These advantages reflect the fact that shorter heparin chains bind less avidly to endothelial cells, macrophages, and heparin-binding plasma proteins. Reduced binding to endothelial cells and macrophages eliminates the rapid, dose-dependent, and saturable mechanism of clearance that is a characteristic of unfractionated heparin. Instead, the clearance of LMWH is dose-independent and its plasma half-life is longer. Based on measurement of anti-factor Xa levels, LMWH has a plasma half-life of ~4 h. LMWH is cleared almost exclusively by the kidneys, and the drug can accumulate in patients with renal insufficiency.

LMWH exhibits about 90% bioavailability after SC injection. Because LMWH binds less avidly to heparin-binding proteins in plasma than heparin, LMWH produces a more predictable dose response, and resistance to LMWH is rare. With a longer half-life and more predictable anticoagulant response, LMWH can be given SC once or twice daily without coagulation monitoring, even when the drug is given in treatment doses. These properties render LMWH more convenient than unfractionated heparin. Capitalizing on this feature, studies in patients with venous thromboembolism have shown that home treatment with LMWH is as effective and safe as in-hospital treatment with continuous IV infusions of heparin. Outpatient treatment with LMWH streamlines care, reduces health care costs, and increases patient satisfaction.

MONITORING In the majority of patients, LMWH does not require coagulation monitoring. If monitoring is necessary, anti-factor Xa levels must be measured because most LMWH preparations have little effect on the aPTT. Therapeutic anti-factor Xa levels with LMWH range from 0.5 to 1.2 units/mL when measured 3–4 h after drug administration. When LMWH is given in prophylactic doses, peak anti-factor Xa levels of 0.2–0.5 units/mL are desirable.

Indications for LMWH monitoring include renal insufficiency and obesity. LMWH monitoring in patients with a creatinine clearance of ≤50 mL/min is advisable to ensure that there is no drug accumulation. Although weight-adjusted LMWH dosing appears to produce therapeutic anti-factor Xa levels in patients who are overweight, this approach has not been extensively evaluated in those with morbid obesity. It may also be advisable to monitor the anticoagulant activity of LMWH during pregnancy because dose requirements can change, particularly in the third trimester. Monitoring should also be considered in high-risk settings, such as in patients with mechanical heart valves who are given LMWH for prevention of valve thrombosis, and when LMWH is used in treatment doses in infants or children.

DOSING The doses of LMWH recommended for prophylaxis or treatment vary depending on the LMWH preparation. For prophylaxis, once-daily SC doses of 4000–5000 units are often used, whereas doses of 2500–3000 units are given when the drug is administered twice daily. For treatment of venous thromboembolism, a dose of

150–200 units/kg is given if the drug is administered once daily. If a twice-daily regimen is used, a dose of 100 units/kg is given. In patients with unstable angina, LMWH is given SC on a twice-daily basis at a dose of 100–120 units/kg.

SIDE EFFECTS The major complication of LMWH is bleeding. Meta-analyses suggest that the risk of major bleeding is lower with LMWH than with unfractionated heparin. HIT and osteoporosis are less common with LMWH than with unfractionated heparin.

Bleeding Like the situation with heparin, bleeding with LMWH is more common in patients receiving concomitant therapy with antiplatelet or fibrinolytic drugs. Recent surgery, trauma, or underlying hemostatic defects also increase the risk of bleeding with LMWH.

Although protamine sulfate can be used as an antidote for LMWH, protamine sulfate incompletely neutralizes the anticoagulant activity of LMWH because it only binds the longer chains of LMWH. Because longer chains are responsible for catalysis of thrombin inhibition by antithrombin, protamine sulfate completely reverses the anti-factor IIa activity of LMWH. In contrast, protamine sulfate only partially reverses the anti-factor Xa activity of LMWH because the shorter pentasaccharide-containing chains of LMWH do not bind to protamine sulfate. Consequently, patients at high risk for bleeding may be more safely treated with continuous IV unfractionated heparin than with SC LMWH.

Thrombocytopenia The risk of HIT is about fivefold lower with LMWH than with heparin. LMWH binds less avidly to platelets and causes less PF4 release. Furthermore, with lower affinity for PF4 than heparin, LMWH is less likely to induce the conformational changes in PF4 that trigger the formation of HIT antibodies.

LMWH should not be used to treat HIT patients because most HIT antibodies exhibit cross-reactivity with LMWH. This in vitro cross-reactivity is not simply a laboratory phenomenon because there are case reports of thrombosis when HIT patients were switched from heparin to LMWH.

Osteoporosis Because the risk of osteoporosis is lower with LMWH than with heparin, LMWH is the better choice for extended treatment.

Fondaparinux A synthetic analogue of the antithrombin-binding pentasaccharide sequence, fondaparinux differs from LMWH in several ways (Table 143-6). Fondaparinux is licensed for thromboprophylaxis in general medical or surgical patients and in high-risk orthopedic patients and as an alternative to heparin or LMWH for initial treatment of patients with established venous thromboembolism. Although widely used in Europe, as an alternative to heparin or LMWH in patients with acute coronary syndromes, fondaparinux is not licensed for this indication in the United States.

MECHANISM OF ACTION As a synthetic analogue of the antithrombin-binding pentasaccharide sequence found in heparin and LMWH, fondaparinux has a molecular weight of 1728. Fondaparinux binds only to antithrombin (Fig. 143-5) and is too short to bridge thrombin to antithrombin. Consequently, fondaparinux catalyzes factor Xa inhibition by antithrombin and does not enhance the rate of thrombin inhibition.

TABLE 143-6 COMPARISON OF LMWH AND FONDAPARINUX

Features	LMWH	Fondaparinux
Number of saccharide units	15–17	5
Catalysis of factor Xa inhibition	Yes	Yes
Catalysis of thrombin inhibition	Yes	No
Bioavailability after subcutaneous administration (%)	90	100
Plasma half-life (h)	4	17
Renal excretion	Yes	Yes
Induces release of tissue factor pathway inhibitor	Yes	No
Neutralized by protamine sulfate	Partially	No

PHARMACOLOGY Fondaparinux exhibits complete bioavailability after SC injection. With no binding to endothelial cells or plasma proteins, the clearance of fondaparinux is dose independent and its plasma half-life is 17 h. The drug is given SC once daily. Because fondaparinux is cleared unchanged via the kidneys, it is contraindicated in patients with a creatinine clearance <30 mL/min and should be used with caution in those with a creatinine clearance <50 mL/min.

Fondaparinux produces a predictable anticoagulant response after administration in fixed doses because it does not bind to plasma proteins. The drug is given at a dose of 2.5 mg once daily for prevention of venous thromboembolism. For initial treatment of established venous thromboembolism, fondaparinux is given at a dose of 7.5 mg once daily. The dose can be reduced to 5 mg once daily for those weighing <50 kg and increased to 10 mg for those >100 kg. When given in these doses, fondaparinux is as effective as heparin or LMWH for initial treatment of patients with DVT or PE and produces similar rates of bleeding.

Fondaparinux is used at a dose of 2.5 mg once daily in patients with acute coronary syndromes. When this prophylactic dose of fondaparinux was compared with treatment doses of enoxaparin in patients with non-ST-segment elevation acute coronary syndrome, there was no difference in the rate of cardiovascular death, MI, or stroke at 9 days. However, the rate of major bleeding was 50% lower with fondaparinux than with enoxaparin, a difference that likely reflects the fact that the dose of fondaparinux was lower than that of enoxaparin. In acute coronary syndrome patients who require percutaneous coronary intervention, there is a risk of catheter thrombosis with fondaparinux unless adjunctive heparin is given.

SIDE EFFECTS Fondaparinux does not cause HIT because it does not bind to PF4. In contrast to LMWH, there is no cross-reactivity of fondaparinux with HIT antibodies. Consequently, fondaparinux appears to be effective for treatment of HIT patients, although large clinical trials supporting its use are lacking.

The major side effect of fondaparinux is bleeding. There is no antidote for fondaparinux. Protamine sulfate has no effect on the anticoagulant activity of fondaparinux because it fails to bind to the drug. Recombinant activated factor VII reverses the anticoagulant effects of fondaparinux in volunteers, but it is unknown whether this agent controls fondaparinux-induced bleeding.

Parenteral Direct Thrombin Inhibitors Direct thrombin inhibitors bind directly to thrombin and block its interaction with its substrates. Approved parenteral direct thrombin inhibitors include recombinant hirudins (lepirudin and desirudin), argatroban, and bivalirudin (Table 143-7). Lepirudin and argatroban are licensed for treatment of patients with HIT, desirudin is licensed for thromboprophylaxis after elective hip arthroplasty, and bivalirudin is approved as an alternative to heparin in patients undergoing percutaneous coronary intervention, including those with HIT.

LEPIRUDIN AND DESIRUDIN Recombinant forms of hirudin, lepirudin, and desirudin are bivalent direct thrombin inhibitors that interact with the active site and exosite 1, the substrate-binding site on thrombin. For rapid anticoagulation, lepirudin is given by continuous IV infusion, but the drug can be given SC. Lepirudin has a plasma half-life of 60 min after IV infusion and is cleared by the kidneys. Consequently,

TABLE 143-7 COMPARISON OF THE PROPERTIES OF LEPIRUDIN, BIVALIRUDIN, AND ARGATROBAN

	Lepirudin/ Desirudin	Bivalirudin	Argatroban
Molecular mass	7000	1980	527
Site(s) of interaction with thrombin	Active site and exosite 1	Active site and exosite 1	Active site
Renal clearance	Yes	No	No
Hepatic metabolism	No	No	Yes
Plasma half-life (min)	60 (IV) 120–180 (SC)	25	45

lepirudin accumulates in patients with renal insufficiency. For thromboprophylaxis, desirudin is given SC twice daily in fixed doses; the half-life of desirudin is 2–3 h after SC injection.

A high proportion of lepirudin-treated patients develop antibodies against the drug; antibody formation is rare with SC desirudin. Although lepirudin-directed antibodies rarely cause problems, in a small subset of patients, they can delay lepirudin clearance and enhance its anticoagulant activity. Serious bleeding has been reported in some of these patients.

Lepirudin is usually monitored using the aPTT, and the dose is adjusted to maintain an aPTT that is 1.5–2.5 times the control. The aPTT is not an ideal test for monitoring lepirudin therapy because the clotting time plateaus with higher drug concentrations. Although the clotting time with ecarin, a snake venom that converts prothrombin to meizothrombin, provides a better index of lepirudin dose than the aPTT, the ecarin clotting time has yet to be standardized. When used for thromboprophylaxis, desirudin does not require monitoring.

ARGATROBAN A univalent inhibitor that targets the active site of thrombin, argatroban is metabolized in the liver. Consequently, this drug must be used with caution in patients with hepatic insufficiency. Argatroban is not cleared via the kidneys, so this drug is safer than lepirudin for HIT patients with renal insufficiency.

Argatroban is administered by continuous IV infusion and has a plasma half-life of ~45 min. The aPTT is used to monitor its anticoagulant effect, and the dose is adjusted to achieve an aPTT 1.5–3 times the baseline value, but not to exceed 100 s. Argatroban also prolongs the international normalized ratio (INR), a feature that can complicate the transitioning of patients to warfarin. This problem can be circumvented by using the levels of factor X to monitor warfarin in place of the INR. Alternatively, argatroban can be stopped for 2–3 h before INR determination.

BIVALIRUDIN A synthetic 20-amino-acid analogue of hirudin, bivalirudin is a divalent thrombin inhibitor. Thus, the N-terminus of bivalirudin interacts with the active site of thrombin, whereas its C-terminus binds to exosite 1. Bivalirudin has a plasma half-life of 25 min, the shortest half-life of all the parenteral direct thrombin inhibitors. Bivalirudin is degraded by peptidases and is partially excreted via the kidneys. When given in high doses in the cardiac catheterization laboratory, the anticoagulant activity of bivalirudin is monitored using the activated clotting time. With lower doses, its activity can be assessed using the aPTT.

Bivalirudin is licensed as an alternative to heparin in patients undergoing percutaneous coronary intervention. Bivalirudin also has been used successfully in HIT patients who require percutaneous coronary intervention or cardiac bypass surgery.

ORAL ANTICOAGULANTS

Current oral anticoagulant practice dates back almost 60 years to when the vitamin K antagonists were discovered as a result of investigations into the cause of hemorrhagic disease in cattle. Characterized by a decrease in prothrombin levels, this disorder is caused by ingestion of hay containing spoiled sweet clover. Hydroxycoumarin, which was isolated from bacterial contaminants in the hay, interferes with vitamin K metabolism, thereby causing a syndrome similar to vitamin K deficiency. Discovery of this compound provided the impetus for development of other vitamin K antagonists, including warfarin.

For many years, the vitamin K antagonists were the only available oral anticoagulants. This situation changed with the introduction of new oral anticoagulants, including dabigatran, which targets thrombin, and rivaroxaban, apixaban, and edoxaban, which target factor Xa.

Warfarin A water-soluble vitamin K antagonist initially developed as a rodenticide, warfarin is the coumarin derivative most often prescribed in North America. Like other vitamin K antagonists, warfarin interferes with the synthesis of the vitamin K–dependent clotting proteins, which include prothrombin (factor II) and factors VII, IX, and X. The synthesis of the vitamin K–dependent anticoagulant proteins, proteins C and S, is also reduced by vitamin K antagonists.

MECHANISM OF ACTION All of the vitamin K–dependent clotting factors possess glutamic acid residues at their N termini. A posttranslational modification adds a carboxyl group to the γ-carbon of these residues to generate γ-carboxyglutamic acid. This modification is essential for expression of the activity of these clotting factors because it permits their calcium-dependent binding to negatively charged phospholipid surfaces. The γ-carboxylation process is catalyzed by a vitamin K–dependent carboxylase. Thus, vitamin K from the diet is reduced to vitamin K hydroquinone by vitamin K reductase (Fig. 143-6). Vitamin K hydroquinone serves as a cofactor for the carboxylase enzyme, which in the presence of carbon dioxide replaces the hydrogen on the γ-carbon of glutamic acid residues with a carboxyl group. During this process, vitamin K hydroquinone is oxidized to vitamin K epoxide, which is then reduced to vitamin K by vitamin K epoxide reductase.

Warfarin inhibits vitamin K epoxide reductase (VKOR), thereby blocking the γ-carboxylation process. This results in the synthesis of vitamin K–dependent clotting proteins that are only partially γ-carboxylated. Warfarin acts as an anticoagulant because these partially γ-carboxylated proteins have reduced or absent biologic activity. The onset of action of warfarin is delayed until the newly synthesized clotting factors with reduced activity gradually replace their fully active counterparts.

The antithrombotic effect of warfarin depends on a reduction in the functional levels of factor X and prothrombin, clotting factors that have half-lives of 24 and 72 h, respectively. Because the antithrombotic effect of warfarin is delayed, patients with established thrombosis or at high risk for thrombosis require concomitant treatment with a rapidly acting parenteral anticoagulant, such as heparin, LMWH, or fondaparinux, for at least 5 days.

PHARMACOLOGY Warfarin is a racemic mixture of R and S isomers. Warfarin is rapidly and almost completely absorbed from the

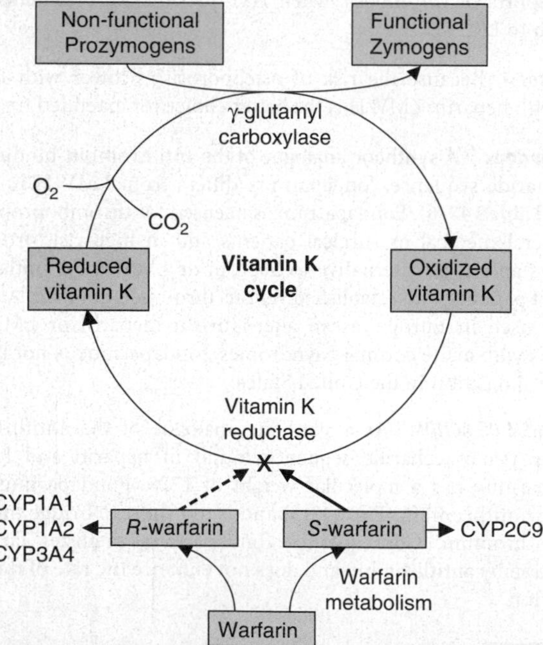

FIGURE 143-6 Mechanism of action of warfarin. A racemic mixture of *S*- and *R*-enantiomers, *S*-warfarin is most active. By blocking vitamin K epoxide reductase, warfarin inhibits the conversion of oxidized vitamin K into its reduced form. This inhibits vitamin K–dependent γ-carboxylation of factors II, VII, IX, and X because reduced vitamin K serves as a cofactor for a γ-glutamyl carboxylase that catalyzes the γ-carboxylation process, thereby converting prozymogens to zymogens capable of binding calcium and interacting with anionic phospholipid surfaces. *S*-warfarin is metabolized by CYP2C9. Common genetic polymorphisms in this enzyme can influence warfarin metabolism. Polymorphisms in the C1 subunit of vitamin K reductase (VKORC1) also can affect the susceptibility of the enzyme to warfarin-induced inhibition, thereby influencing warfarin dosage requirements.

TABLE 143-8 FREQUENCIES OF *CYP2C9* GENOTYPES AND *VKORC1* HAPLOTYPES IN DIFFERENT POPULATIONS AND THEIR EFFECT ON WARFARIN DOSE REQUIREMENTS

	Frequency, %			
Genotype/Haplotype	Caucasians	African Americans (A/A)	Asians (A)	Dose Reduction Compared with Wild-Type
CYP2C9				
*1/*1	70	90	95	–
*1/*2	17	2	0	22
*1/*3	9	3	4	34
*2/*2	2	0	0	43
*2/*3	1	0	0	53
*3/*3	0	0	1	76
VKORC1				
Non-A/non-A	37	82	7	–
Non-A/A	45	12	30	26
A/A	18	6	63	50

gastrointestinal tract. Levels of warfarin in the blood peak about 90 min after drug administration. Racemic warfarin has a plasma half-life of 36–42 h, and more than 97% of circulating warfarin is bound to albumin. Only the small fraction of unbound warfarin is biologically active.

Warfarin accumulates in the liver where the two isomers are metabolized via distinct pathways. *CYP2C9* mediates oxidative metabolism of the more active S isomer (Fig. 143-6). Two relatively common variants, *CYP2C9**2* and *CYP2C9**3*, encode an enzyme with reduced activity. Patients with these variants require lower maintenance doses of warfarin. Approximately 25% of Caucasians have at least one variant allele of *CYP2C9**2* or *CYP2C9**3*, whereas those variant alleles are less common in African Americans and Asians (Table 143-8). Heterozygosity for *CYP2C9**2* or *CYP2C9**3* decreases the warfarin dose requirement by 20–30% relative to that required in subjects with the wild-type *CYP2C9**1/*1* alleles, whereas homozygosity for the *CYP2C9**2* or *CYP2C9**3* alleles reduces the warfarin dose requirement by 50–70%.

Consistent with their decreased warfarin dose requirement, subjects with at least one *CYP2C9* variant allele are at increased risk for bleeding. Compared with individuals with no variant alleles, the relative risks for warfarin-associated bleeding in *CYP2C9**2* or *CYP2C9**3* carriers are 1.9 and 1.8, respectively.

Polymorphisms in *VKORC1* also can influence the anticoagulant response to warfarin. Several genetic variations of *VKORC1* are in strong linkage disequilibrium and have been designated as non-A haplotypes. *VKORC1* variants are more prevalent than variants of *CYP2C9*. Asians have the highest prevalence of *VKORC1* variants, followed by Caucasians and African Americans (Table 143-8). Polymorphisms in *VKORC1* likely explain 30% of the variability in warfarin dose requirements. Compared with *VKORC1* non-A/non-A homozygotes, the warfarin dose requirement decreases by 25 and 50% in A haplotype heterozygotes and homozygotes, respectively. These findings prompted the Food and Drug Administration to amend the prescribing information for warfarin to indicate that lower initiation doses should be considered for patients with *CYP2C9* and *VKORC1* genetic variants. In addition to genotype data, other pertinent patient information has been incorporated into warfarin dosing algorithms. Although such algorithms help predict suitable warfarin doses, it remains unclear whether better dose identification improves patient outcome in terms of reducing hemorrhagic complications or recurrent thrombotic events.

In addition to genetic factors, the anticoagulant effect of warfarin is influenced by diet, drugs, and various disease states. Fluctuations in dietary vitamin K intake affect the activity of warfarin. A wide variety of drugs can alter absorption, clearance, or metabolism of warfarin. Because of the variability in the anticoagulant response to warfarin, coagulation monitoring is essential to ensure that a therapeutic response is obtained.

MONITORING Warfarin therapy is most often monitored using the prothrombin time, a test that is sensitive to reductions in the levels of prothrombin, factor VII, and factor X. The test is performed by adding thromboplastin, a reagent that contains tissue factor, phospholipid, and calcium, to citrated plasma and determining the time to clot formation. Thromboplastins vary in their sensitivity to reductions in the levels of the vitamin K–dependent clotting factors. Thus, less sensitive thromboplastins will trigger the administration of higher doses of warfarin to achieve a target prothrombin time. This is problematic because higher doses of warfarin increase the risk of bleeding.

The INR was developed to circumvent many of the problems associated with the prothrombin time. To calculate the INR, the patient's prothrombin time is divided by the mean normal prothrombin time, and this ratio is then multiplied by the international sensitivity index (ISI), which is an index of the sensitivity of the thromboplastin used for prothrombin time determination to reductions in the levels of the vitamin K–dependent clotting factors. Highly sensitive thromboplastins have an ISI of 1.0. Most current thromboplastins have ISI values that range from 1.0 to 1.4.

Although the INR has helped to standardize anticoagulant practice, problems persist. The precision of INR determination varies depending on reagent-coagulometer combinations. This leads to variability in the INR results. Also complicating INR determination is unreliable reporting of the ISI by thromboplastin manufacturers. Furthermore, every laboratory must establish the mean normal prothrombin time with each new batch of thromboplastin reagent. To accomplish this, the prothrombin time must be measured in fresh plasma samples from at least 20 healthy volunteers using the same coagulometer that is used for patient samples.

For most indications, warfarin is administered in doses that produce a target INR of 2.0–3.0. An exception is patients with mechanical heart valves, particularly those in the mitral position or older ball and cage valves in the aortic position, where a target INR of 2.5–3.5 is recommended. Studies in atrial fibrillation demonstrate an increased risk of cardioembolic stroke when the INR falls to <1.7 and an increase in bleeding with INR values >4.5. These findings highlight the fact that vitamin K antagonists have a narrow therapeutic window. In support of this concept, a study in patients receiving long-term warfarin therapy for unprovoked venous thromboembolism demonstrated a higher rate of recurrent venous thromboembolism with a target INR of 1.5–1.9 compared with a target INR of 2.0–3.0.

DOSING Warfarin is usually started at a dose of 5–10 mg. Lower doses are used for patients with *CYP2C9* or *VKORC1* polymorphisms, which affect the pharmacodynamics or pharmacokinetics of warfarin and render patients more sensitive to the drug. The dose is then titrated to achieve the desired target INR. Because of its delayed onset of action, patients with established thrombosis or those at high risk for thrombosis are given concomitant initial treatment with a rapidly acting parenteral anticoagulant, such as heparin, LMWH, or fondaparinux. Early prolongation of the INR reflects reduction in the functional levels of factor VII. Consequently, concomitant treatment with the parenteral anticoagulant should be continued until the INR has been therapeutic for at least 2 consecutive days. A minimum 5-day course of parenteral anticoagulation is recommended to ensure that the levels of factor Xa and prothrombin have been reduced into the therapeutic range with warfarin.

Because warfarin has a narrow therapeutic window, frequent coagulation monitoring is essential to ensure that a therapeutic anticoagulant response is maintained. Even patients with stable warfarin dose requirements should have their INR determined every 3–4 weeks. More frequent monitoring is necessary when new medications are introduced because so many drugs enhance or reduce the anticoagulant effects of warfarin.

SIDE EFFECTS Like all anticoagulants, the major side effect of warfarin is bleeding. A rare complication is skin necrosis. Warfarin crosses the placenta and can cause fetal abnormalities. Consequently, warfarin should not be used during pregnancy.

Bleeding At least half of the bleeding complications with warfarin occur when the INR exceeds the therapeutic range. Bleeding complications may be mild, such as epistaxis or hematuria, or more severe, such as retroperitoneal or gastrointestinal bleeding. Life-threatening intracranial bleeding can also occur.

To minimize the risk of bleeding, the INR should be maintained in the therapeutic range. In asymptomatic patients whose INR is between 3.5 and 10, warfarin should be withheld until the INR returns to the therapeutic range. If the INR is over 10, oral vitamin K should be administered, at a dose of 2.5–5 mg, although there is no evidence that doing so reduces the bleeding risk. Higher doses of oral vitamin K (5–10 mg) produce more rapid reversal of the INR but may render patients temporarily resistant to warfarin when the drug is restarted. Patients with serious bleeding need more aggressive treatment. These patients should be given 5–10 mg of vitamin K by slow IV infusion. Additional vitamin K should be given until the INR is in the normal range. Treatment with vitamin K should be supplemented with fresh-frozen plasma as a source of the vitamin K–dependent clotting proteins. Four factor prothrombin complex concentrates, which contain all four vitamin K–dependent clotting proteins, are the treatment of choice for (1) life-threatening bleeds, (2) rapid restoration of the INR into the normal range in patients requiring urgent surgery or intervention, and (3) patients who cannot tolerate the volume load of fresh-frozen plasma.

Warfarin-treated patients who experience bleeding when their INR is in the therapeutic range require investigation into the cause of the bleeding. Those with gastrointestinal or genitourinary bleeding often have an underlying lesion.

Skin necrosis A rare complication of warfarin, skin necrosis usually is seen 2–5 days after initiation of therapy. Well-demarcated erythematous lesions form on the thighs, buttocks, breasts, or toes. Typically, the center of the lesion becomes progressively necrotic. Examination of skin biopsies taken from the border of these lesions reveals thrombi in the microvasculature.

Warfarin-induced skin necrosis is seen in patients with congenital or acquired deficiencies of protein C or protein S. Initiation of warfarin therapy in these patients produces a precipitous fall in plasma levels of proteins C or S, thereby eliminating this important anticoagulant pathway before warfarin exerts an antithrombotic effect through lowering of the functional levels of factor X and prothrombin. The resultant procoagulant state triggers thrombosis. Why the thrombosis is localized to the microvasculature of fatty tissues is unclear.

Treatment involves discontinuation of warfarin and reversal with vitamin K, if needed. An alternative anticoagulant, such as heparin or LMWH, should be given in patients with thrombosis. Protein C concentrate can be given to protein C–deficient patients to accelerate healing of the skin lesions; fresh-frozen plasma may be of value if protein C concentrate is unavailable and for those with protein S deficiency. Occasionally, skin grafting is necessary when there is extensive skin loss.

Because of the potential for skin necrosis, patients with known protein C or protein S deficiency require overlapping treatment with a parenteral anticoagulant when initiating warfarin therapy. Warfarin should be started in low doses in these patients, and the parenteral anticoagulant should be continued until the INR is therapeutic for at least 2–3 consecutive days.

Pregnancy Warfarin crosses the placenta and can cause fetal abnormalities or bleeding. The fetal abnormalities include a characteristic embryopathy, which consists of nasal hypoplasia and stippled epiphyses. The risk of embryopathy is highest if warfarin is given in the first trimester of pregnancy. Central nervous system abnormalities can also occur with exposure to warfarin at any time during pregnancy. Finally, maternal administration of warfarin produces an anticoagulant effect in the fetus that can cause bleeding. This is of particular concern at delivery when trauma to the head during passage through the birth canal can lead to intracranial bleeding. Because of these potential problems, warfarin is contraindicated in pregnancy, particularly in the first and third trimesters. Instead, heparin, LMWH, or fondaparinux can be given during pregnancy for prevention or treatment of thrombosis.

Warfarin does not pass into the breast milk. Consequently, warfarin can safely be given to nursing mothers.

Special problems Patients with a lupus anticoagulant and those who need urgent or elective surgery present special challenges. Although observational studies suggested that patients with thrombosis complicating the antiphospholipid antibody syndrome required higher intensity warfarin regimens to prevent recurrent thromboembolic events, two randomized trials showed that targeting an INR of 2.0–3.0 is as effective as higher intensity treatment and produces less bleeding. Monitoring warfarin therapy can be problematic in patients with antiphospholipid antibody syndrome if the lupus anticoagulant prolongs the baseline INR; factor X levels can be used instead of the INR in such patients.

There is no need to stop warfarin before procedures associated with a low risk of bleeding; these include dental cleaning, simple dental extraction, cataract surgery, or skin biopsy. For procedures associated with a moderate or high risk of bleeding, warfarin should be stopped 5 days before the procedure to allow the INR to return to normal levels. Patients at high risk for thrombosis, such as those with mechanical heart valves, can be bridged with once- or twice-daily SC injections of LMWH when the INR falls to <2.0. The last dose of LMWH should be given 12–24 h before the procedure, depending on whether LMWH is administered twice or once daily. After the procedure, treatment with warfarin can be restarted.

New Oral Anticoagulants New oral anticoagulants are now available as alternatives to warfarin. These include dabigatran, which targets thrombin, and rivaroxaban, apixaban, and edoxaban, which target factor Xa. All of these drugs have a rapid onset and offset of action and have half-lives that permit once- or twice-daily administration. Designed to produce a predictable level of anticoagulation, the new oral agents are more convenient to administer than warfarin because they are given in fixed doses without routine coagulation monitoring.

MECHANISM OF ACTION The new oral anticoagulants are small molecules that bind reversibly to the active site of their target enzyme. Table 143-9 summarizes the distinct pharmacologic properties of these agents.

INDICATIONS The new oral anticoagulants have been compared with warfarin for stroke prevention in patients with nonvalvular atrial fibrillation in four randomized trials that enrolled 71,683 patients. A meta-analysis of these data demonstrates that compared with warfarin, the new agents significantly reduce stroke or systemic embolism by 19% (p = .001), primarily driven by a 51% reduction in hemorrhagic stroke (p <.0001), and are associated with a 10% reduction in mortality (p <.0001). New oral anticoagulants reduce intracranial hemorrhage by

TABLE 143-9 COMPARISON OF THE PHARMACOLOGIC PROPERTIES OF THE NEW ORAL ANTICOAGULANTS

Characteristic	Rivaroxaban	Apixaban	Edoxaban	Dabigatran
Target	Factor Xa	Factor Xa	Factor Xa	Thrombin
Prodrug	No	No	No	Yes
Bioavailability	80%	60%	50%	6%
Dosing	qd (bid)	bid	qd	bid (qd)
Half-life	7–11 h	12 h	9–11 h	12–17 h
Renal	33% (66%)	25%	35%	80%
Monitoring	No	No	No	No
Interactions	3A4/P-gp	3A4/P-gp	P-gp	P-gp

Abbreviations: bid, twice a day; P-gp, P-glycoprotein; qd., once a day.

PART 7 Oncology and Hematology

52% compared with warfarin (p <.0001), but increase gastrointestinal bleeding by about 24% (p = .04). Overall, the new agents demonstrate a favorable benefit-to-risk profile compared with warfarin, and their relative efficacy and safety are maintained across a wide spectrum of atrial fibrillation patients, including those over the age of 75 years and those with a prior history of stroke. Based on these findings, dabigatran, rivaroxaban, and apixaban are licensed as alternatives to warfarin for stroke prevention in nonvalvular atrial fibrillation, and edoxaban is under regulatory consideration for this indication. Nonvalvular atrial fibrillation is defined as that occurring in patients without mechanical heart valves or severe rheumatic valvular disease, particularly mitral stenosis and/or regurgitation.

Dabigatran, rivaroxaban, and apixaban have been compared with enoxaparin for thromboprophylaxis after elective hip or knee arthroplasty. Currently, only rivaroxaban and apixaban are licensed for this indication in the United States. Rivaroxaban and dabigatran are also licensed for treatment of DVT or PE. Apixaban and edoxaban have also been investigated for treatment of patients with venous thromboembolism, but have not yet been approved for this indication. Rivaroxaban is licensed in Europe for prevention of recurrent ischemic events in patients who have been stabilized after an acute coronary syndrome. In this setting, rivaroxaban is usually administered in conjunction with dual antiplatelet therapy with aspirin and clopidogrel.

DOSING For stroke prevention in patients with nonvalvular atrial fibrillation, rivaroxaban is given at a dose of 20 mg once daily with a dose reduction to 15 mg once daily in patients with a creatinine clearance of 15–49 mL/min; dabigatran is given at a dose of 150 mg twice daily with a dose reduction to 75 mg twice daily in those with a creatinine clearance of 15–30 mL/min; and apixaban is given at a dose of 5 mg twice daily with a dose reduction to 2.5 mg twice daily for patients with a creatinine >1.5 g/dL, for those 80 years of age or older, or for patients who weigh <60 kg.

For thromboprophylaxis after elective hip or knee replacement surgery, rivaroxaban is given at a dose of 10 mg once daily, whereas apixaban is given at a dose of 2.5 mg twice daily. For treatment of patients with DVT or PE, rivaroxaban is started at a dose of 15 mg twice daily for 3 weeks; the dose is then reduced to 20 mg once daily thereafter. After a minimum of a 5 day course of treatment with heparin or LMWH, dabigatran is given at a dose of 150 mg twice daily.

MONITORING Although designed to be administered without routine monitoring, there are situations where determination of the anticoagulant activity of the new oral anticoagulants can be helpful. These include assessment of adherence, detection of accumulation or overdose, identification of bleeding mechanisms, and determination of activity prior to surgery or intervention. For qualitative assessment of anticoagulant activity, the prothrombin time can be used for factor Xa inhibitors and the aPTT for dabigatran. Rivaroxaban and edoxaban prolong the prothrombin time more than apixaban. In fact, because apixaban has such a limited effect on the prothrombin time, anti-factor Xa assays are needed to assess its activity. The effect of the drugs on tests of coagulation varies depending on the time that the blood is drawn relative to the timing of the last dose of the drug and the reagents used to perform the tests. Chromogenic anti-factor Xa assays and a dilute thrombin clotting time with appropriate calibrators provide quantitative assays to measure the plasma levels of the factor Xa inhibitors and dabigatran, respectively.

SIDE EFFECTS Like all anticoagulants, bleeding is the most common side effect of the new oral anticoagulants. The new agents are associated with less intracranial bleeding than warfarin. The increased risk of intracranial bleeding with warfarin likely reflects the reduction in functional levels of factor VII, which precludes efficient thrombin generation at sites of microvascular bleeding in the brain. Because the new oral anticoagulants target downstream coagulation enzymes, they produce less impairment of hemostatic plug formation at sites of vascular injury.

A downside of the new oral anticoagulants is the increased risk of gastrointestinal bleeding. This likely occurs because unabsorbed active drug in the gut exacerbates bleeding from lesions. Although dabigatran etexilate is a prodrug, only 7% is absorbed. Although the remainder passes through the gut, at least two-thirds is metabolically activated to dabigatran by gut esterases.

Dyspepsia occurs in up to 10% of patients treated with dabigatran; this problem improves with time and can be minimized by administering the drug with food. Dyspepsia is rare with rivaroxaban, apixaban, and edoxaban.

PERIPROCEDURAL MANAGEMENT Like warfarin, the new oral anticoagulants must be stopped before procedures associated with a moderate or high risk of bleeding. The drugs should be held for 1–2 days, or longer if renal function is impaired. Assessment of residual anticoagulant activity before procedures associated with a high bleeding risk is prudent.

MANAGEMENT OF BLEEDING There are no specific antidotes for the new oral anticoagulants. With minor bleeding, holding one or two doses of drug is usually sufficient. The approach to serious bleeding is similar to that with warfarin except that vitamin K administration is of no benefit. Thus, the anticoagulant and antiplatelet drugs should be held, the patient should be resuscitated with fluids and blood products as necessary, and, if possible, the bleeding site should be identified and managed. Coagulation testing will determine the extent of anticoagulation. and renal function should be assessed so that the half-life of the drug can be calculated. Timing of the last dose of anticoagulant is important; administration of oral activated charcoal may help to prevent absorption of drug administered in the past 2–4 h. If bleeding continues or is life-threatening, procoagulants, such as prothrombin complex concentrate (either unactivated or activated) or factor VIIa, can be administered, although the evidence of their effectiveness is limited. Dialysis removes dabigatran from the circulation in patients with renal impairment; dialysis does not remove rivaroxaban, apixaban, or edoxaban because unlike dabigatran, these drugs are highly protein-bound.

PREGNANCY As small molecules, the new oral anticoagulants can all pass through the placenta. Consequently, these agents are contraindicated in pregnancy, and when used by women of childbearing potential, appropriate contraception is important.

ONGOING INVESTIGATIONS Although the lack of antidotes has created concern about the risk of bleeding events in patients taking the new oral anticoagulants, emerging postmarketing data suggest that the rates of bleeding in the real-world setting are similar to those reported in the trials. Nonetheless, specific antidotes are under development. These include a humanized mouse monoclonal antibody fragment against dabigatran and a recombinant variant of factor Xa that serves as a decoy for the oral factor Xa inhibitors. Neither agent is currently available for clinical use.

FIBRINOLYTIC DRUGS

ROLE OF FIBRINOLYTIC THERAPY

Fibrinolytic drugs can be used to degrade thrombi and are administered systemically or can be delivered via catheters directly into the substance of the thrombus. Systemic delivery is used for treatment of acute MI, acute ischemic stroke, and most cases of massive PE. The goal of therapy is to produce rapid thrombus dissolution, thereby restoring antegrade blood flow. In the coronary circulation, restoration of blood flow reduces morbidity and mortality rates by limiting myocardial damage, whereas in the cerebral circulation, rapid thrombus dissolution decreases the neuronal death and brain infarction that produce irreversible brain injury. For patients with massive PE, the goal of thrombolytic therapy is to restore pulmonary artery perfusion.

Peripheral arterial thrombi and thrombi in the proximal deep veins of the leg are most often treated using catheter-directed thrombolytic therapy. Catheters with multiple side holes can be used to enhance drug delivery. In some cases, intravascular devices that fragment and extract the thrombus are used to hasten treatment. These devices can be used alone or in conjunction with fibrinolytic drugs.

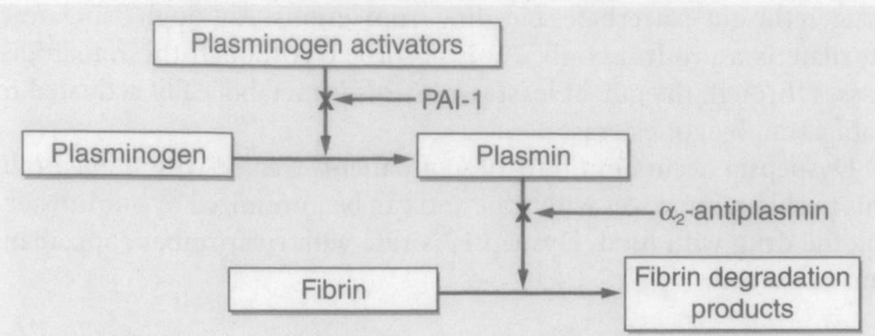

FIGURE 143-7 The fibrinolytic system and its regulation. Plasminogen activators convert plasminogen to plasmin. Plasmin then degrades fibrin into soluble fibrin degradation products. The system is regulated at two levels. Type 1 plasminogen activator inhibitor (PAI-1) regulates the plasminogen activators, whereas α_2-antiplasmin serves as the major inhibitor of plasmin.

MECHANISM OF ACTION

Currently approved fibrinolytic agents include streptokinase; acylated plasminogen streptokinase activator complex (anistreplase); urokinase; recombinant tissue-type plasminogen activator (rtPA), which is also known as alteplase or activase; and two recombinant derivatives of rtPA, tenecteplase and reteplase. All of these agents act by converting plasminogen, the zymogen, to plasmin, the active enzyme (Fig. 143-7). Plasmin then degrades the fibrin matrix of thrombi and produces soluble fibrin degradation products.

Endogenous fibrinolysis is regulated at two levels. Plasminogen activator inhibitors, particularly the type 1 form (PAI-1), prevent excessive plasminogen activation by regulating the activity of tPA and urokinase-type plasminogen activator (uPA). Once plasmin is generated, it is regulated by plasmin inhibitors, the most important of which is α_2-antiplasmin. The plasma concentration of plasminogen is twofold higher than that of α_2-antiplasmin. Consequently, with pharmacologic doses of plasminogen activators, the concentration of plasmin that is generated can exceed that of α_2-antiplasmin. In addition to degrading fibrin, unregulated plasmin can also degrade fibrinogen and other clotting factors. This process, which is known as the *systemic lytic state*, reduces the hemostatic potential of the blood and increases the risk of bleeding.

The endogenous fibrinolytic system is geared to localize plasmin generation to the fibrin surface. Both plasminogen and tPA bind to fibrin to form a ternary complex that promotes efficient plasminogen activation. In contrast to free plasmin, plasmin generated on the fibrin surface is relatively protected from inactivation by α_2-antiplasmin, a feature that promotes fibrin dissolution. Furthermore, C-terminus lysine residues, exposed as plasmin degrades fibrin, serve as binding sites for additional plasminogen and tPA molecules. This creates a positive feedback that enhances plasmin generation. When used pharmacologically, the various plasminogen activators capitalize on these mechanisms to a lesser or greater extent.

Plasminogen activators that preferentially activate fibrin-bound plasminogen are considered fibrin-specific. In contrast, nonspecific plasminogen activators do not discriminate between fibrin-bound and circulating plasminogen. Activation of circulating plasminogen results in the generation of unopposed plasmin that can trigger the systemic lytic state. Alteplase and its derivatives are fibrin-specific plasminogen activators, whereas streptokinase, anistreplase, and urokinase are nonspecific agents.

STREPTOKINASE

Unlike other plasminogen activators, streptokinase is not an enzyme and does not directly convert plasminogen to plasmin. Instead, streptokinase forms a 1:1 stoichiometric complex with plasminogen. Formation of this complex induces a conformational change in plasminogen that exposes its active site (Fig. 143-8). The streptokinase-plasminogen complex then converts additional plasminogen to plasmin.

Streptokinase has no affinity for fibrin, and the streptokinase-plasminogen complex activates both free and fibrin-bound plasminogen. Activation of circulating plasminogen generates sufficient

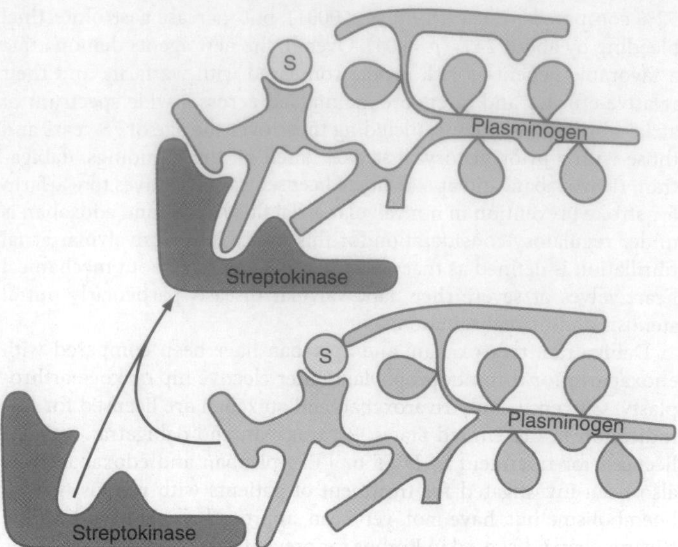

FIGURE 143-8 Mechanism of action of streptokinase. Streptokinase binds to plasminogen and induces a conformational change in plasminogen that exposes its active site. The streptokinase/plasmin(ogen) complex then serves as the activator of additional plasminogen.

amounts of plasmin to overwhelm α_2-antiplasmin. Unopposed plasmin not only degrades fibrin in the occlusive thrombus but also induces a systemic lytic state.

When given systemically to patients with acute MI, streptokinase reduces mortality. For this indication, the drug is usually given as an IV infusion of 1.5 million units over 30–60 min. Patients who receive streptokinase can develop antibodies against the drug, as can patients with prior streptococcal infection. These antibodies can reduce the effectiveness of streptokinase.

Allergic reactions occur in ~5% of patients treated with streptokinase. These may manifest as a rash, fever, chills, and rigors. Although anaphylactic reactions can occur, these are rare. Transient hypotension is common with streptokinase and has been attributed to plasmin-mediated release of bradykinin from kininogen. The hypotension usually responds to leg elevation and administration of IV fluids and low doses of vasopressors, such as dopamine or norepinephrine.

ANISTREPLASE

To generate this drug, streptokinase is combined with equimolar amounts of Lys-plasminogen, a plasmin-cleaved form of plasminogen with a Lys residue at its N terminus. The active site of Lys-plasminogen that is exposed upon combination with streptokinase is then masked with an anisoyl group. After IV infusion, the anisoyl group is slowly removed by deacylation, giving the complex a half-life of ~100 min. This allows drug administration via a single bolus infusion.

Although it is more convenient to administer, anistreplase offers few mechanistic advantages over streptokinase. Like streptokinase, anistreplase does not distinguish between fibrin-bound and circulating plasminogen. Consequently, it too produces a systemic lytic state. Likewise, allergic reactions and hypotension are just as frequent with anistreplase as they are with streptokinase.

When anistreplase was compared with alteplase in patients with acute MI, reperfusion was obtained more rapidly with alteplase than with anistreplase. Improved reperfusion was associated with a trend toward better clinical outcomes and reduced mortality rate with alteplase. These results and the high cost of anistreplase have dampened the enthusiasm for its use.

UROKINASE

Urokinase is a two-chain serine protease derived from cultured fetal kidney cells with a molecular weight of 34,000. Urokinase converts plasminogen to plasmin directly by cleaving the Arg560-Val561 bond. Unlike streptokinase, urokinase is not immunogenic and allergic reactions are rare. Urokinase produces a systemic lytic state because it does not discriminate between fibrin-bound and circulating plasminogen.

Despite many years of use, urokinase has never been systemically evaluated for coronary thrombolysis. Instead, urokinase is often employed for catheter-directed lysis of thrombi in the deep veins or the peripheral arteries. Because of production problems, the availability of urokinase is limited.

ALTEPLASE

A recombinant form of single-chain tPA, alteplase has a molecular weight of 68,000. Alteplase is rapidly converted into its two-chain form by plasmin. Although single- and two-chain forms of tPA have equivalent activity in the presence of fibrin, in its absence, single-chain tPA has tenfold lower activity.

Alteplase consists of five discrete domains (Fig. 143-9); the N-terminus A chain of two-chain alteplase contains four of these domains. Residues 4 through 50 make up the finger domain, a region that resembles the finger domain of fibronectin; residues 50 through 87 are homologous with epidermal growth factor, whereas residues 92 through 173 and 180 through 261, which have homology to the kringle domains of plasminogen, are designated as the first and second kringle, respectively. The fifth alteplase domain is the protease domain; it is located on the C-terminus B chain of two-chain alteplase.

The interaction of alteplase with fibrin is mediated by the finger domain and, to a lesser extent, by the second kringle domain. The affinity of alteplase for fibrin is considerably higher than that for fibrinogen. Consequently, the catalytic efficiency of plasminogen activation by alteplase is two to three orders of magnitude higher in the presence of fibrin than in the presence of fibrinogen. This phenomenon helps to localize plasmin generation to the fibrin surface.

Although alteplase preferentially activates plasminogen in the presence of fibrin, alteplase is not as fibrin-selective as was first predicted. Its fibrin specificity is limited because like fibrin, (DD)E, the major soluble degradation product of cross-linked fibrin, binds alteplase and plasminogen with high affinity. Consequently, (DD)E is as potent as fibrin as a stimulator of plasminogen activation by alteplase. Whereas plasmin generated on the fibrin surface results in thrombolysis, plasmin generated on the surface of circulating (DD)E degrades fibrinogen. Fibrinogen degradation results in the accumulation of fragment X, a high-molecular-weight clottable fibrinogen degradation product. Incorporation of fragment X into hemostatic plugs formed at sites of vascular injury renders them susceptible to lysis. This phenomenon may contribute to alteplase-induced bleeding.

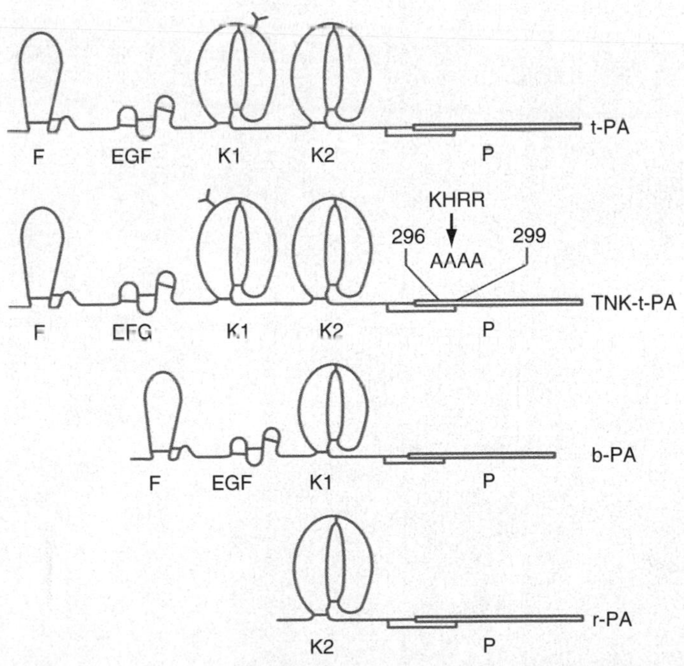

FIGURE 143-9 Domain structures of alteplase (tPA), tenecteplase (TNK-tPA), desmoteplase (b-PA), and reteplase (r-PA). The finger (F), epidermal growth factor (EGF), first and second kringles (K1 and K2, respectively), and protease (P) domains are illustrated. The glycosylation site (Y) on K1 has been repositioned in tenecteplase to endow it with a longer half-life. In addition, a tetra-alanine substitution in the protease domain renders tenecteplase resistant to type 1 plasminogen activator inhibitor (PAI-1) inhibition. Desmoteplase differs from alteplase and tenecteplase in that it lacks a K2 domain. Reteplase is a truncated variant that lacks the F, EGF, and K1 domains.

A trial comparing alteplase with streptokinase for treatment of patients with acute MI demonstrated significantly lower mortality with alteplase than with streptokinase, although the absolute difference was small. The greatest benefit was seen in patients age <75 years with anterior MI who presented <6 h after symptom onset.

For treatment of acute MI or acute ischemic stroke, alteplase is given as an IV infusion over 60–90 min. The total dose of alteplase usually ranges from 90 to 100 mg. Allergic reactions and hypotension are rare, and alteplase is not immunogenic.

TENECTEPLASE

Tenecteplase is a genetically engineered variant of tPA and was designed to have a longer half-life than tPA and to be resistant to inactivation by PAI-1. To prolong its half-life, a new glycosylation site was added to the first kringle domain (Fig. 143-9). Because addition of this extra carbohydrate side chain reduced fibrin affinity, the existing glycosylation site on the first kringle domain was removed. To render the molecule resistant to inhibition by PAI-1, a tetra-alanine substitution was introduced at residues 296–299 in the protease domain, the region responsible for the interaction of tPA with PAI-1.

Tenecteplase is more fibrin-specific than tPA. Although both agents bind to fibrin with similar affinity, the affinity of tenecteplase for (DD)E is significantly lower than that of tPA. Consequently, (DD)E does not stimulate systemic plasminogen activation by tenecteplase to the same extent as tPA. As a result, tenecteplase produces less fibrinogen degradation than tPA.

For coronary thrombolysis, tenecteplase is given as a single IV bolus. In a large phase III trial that enrolled >16,000 patients, the 30-day mortality rate with single-bolus tenecteplase was similar to that with accelerated-dose tPA. Although rates of intracranial hemorrhage were also similar with both treatments, patients given tenecteplase had fewer noncerebral bleeds and a reduced need for blood transfusions than those treated with tPA. The improved safety profile of tenecteplase likely reflects its enhanced fibrin specificity.

RETEPLASE

Reteplase is a is a single-chain, recombinant tPA derivative that lacks the finger, epidermal growth factor, and first kringle domains (Fig. 143-9). This truncated derivative has a molecular weight of 39,000. Reteplase binds fibrin more weakly than tPA because it lacks the finger domain. Because it is produced in *Escherichia coli*, reteplase is not glycosylated. This endows it with a plasma half-life longer than that of tPA. Consequently, reteplase is given as two IV boluses, which are separated by 30 min. Clinical trials have demonstrated that reteplase is at least as effective as streptokinase for treatment of acute MI, but the agent is not superior to tPA.

NEWER FIBRINOLYTIC AGENTS

Two new drugs are under investigation. These include desmoteplase (Fig. 143-9), a recombinant form of the full-length plasminogen activator isolated from the saliva of the vampire bat, and alfimeprase, a truncated form of fibrolase, an enzyme isolated from the venom of the southern copperhead snake. Clinical studies with these agents have been disappointing. Desmoteplase, which is more fibrin-specific than tPA, was investigated for treatment of acute ischemic stroke. Patients presenting 3–9 h after symptom onset were randomized to one of two doses of desmoteplase or to placebo. Overall response rates were low and no different with desmoteplase than with placebo. The mortality rate was higher in the desmoteplase arms.

Alfimeprase is a metalloproteinase that degrades fibrin and fibrinogen in a plasmin-independent fashion. In the circulation, alfimeprase is rapidly inhibited by α_2-macroglobulin. Consequently, the drug must be delivered via a catheter directly into the thrombus. Studies of alfimeprase for treatment of peripheral arterial occlusion or for restoration of flow in blocked central venous catheters were stopped due to lack of efficacy. The disappointing results with desmoteplase and alfimeprase highlight the challenges of introducing new fibrinolytic drugs.

CONCLUSIONS AND FUTURE DIRECTIONS

Thrombosis involves a complex interplay among the vessel wall, platelets, the coagulation system, and the fibrinolytic pathways. Activation of coagulation also triggers inflammatory pathways that may exacerbate thrombosis. A better understanding of the biochemistry of blood coagulation and advances in structure-based drug design have identified new targets and resulted in the development of novel antithrombotic drugs. Well-designed clinical trials have provided detailed information on which drugs to use and when to use them. Despite these advances, however, thromboembolic disorders remain a major cause of morbidity and mortality. Therefore, the search for better targets and more potent antiplatelet, anticoagulant, and fibrinolytic drugs continues.

SECTION 1 BASIC CONSIDERATIONS IN INFECTIOUS DISEASES

144 Approach to the Patient with an Infectious Disease

Neeraj K. Surana, Dennis L. Kasper

HISTORICAL PERSPECTIVE

The origins of the field of infectious diseases are humble. The notion that communicable diseases were due to a *miasma* ("bad air") can be traced back to at least the mid-sixteenth century. Not until the work of Louis Pasteur and Robert Koch in the late nineteenth century was there credible evidence supporting the germ theory of disease—i.e., that microorganisms are the direct cause of infections. In contrast to this relatively slow start, the twentieth century saw remarkable advances in the field of infectious diseases, and the etiologic agents of numerous infectious diseases were soon identified. Furthermore, the discovery of antibiotics and the advent of vaccines against some of the most deadly and debilitating infections greatly altered the landscape of human health. Indeed, the twentieth century saw the elimination of smallpox, one of the great scourges in the history of humanity. These remarkable successes prompted noted scholar Aidan Cockburn to write in a 1963 publication entitled *The Evolution and Eradication of Infectious Diseases*: "It seems reasonable to anticipate that within some measurable time . . . all the major infections will have disappeared." Professor Cockburn was not alone in this view. Robert Petersdorf, a renowned infectious disease expert and former editor of this textbook, wrote in 1978 that "even with my great personal loyalties to infectious diseases, I cannot conceive a need for 309 more [graduating trainees in infectious diseases] unless they spend their time culturing each other." Given the enormous growth of interest in the microbiome in the past 5 years, Dr. Petersdorf's statement might have been ironically clairvoyant, although he could have had no idea what was in store for humanity, with an onslaught of new, emerging, and re-emerging infectious diseases.

Clearly, even with all the advances of the twentieth century, infectious diseases continue to represent a formidable challenge for patients and physicians alike. Furthermore, during the latter half of the century, several chronic diseases were demonstrated to be directly or indirectly caused by infectious microbes, perhaps the most notable examples are the associations of *Helicobacter pylori* with peptic ulcer disease and gastric carcinoma, human papillomavirus with cervical cancer, and hepatitis B and C viruses with liver cancer. In fact, ~16% of all malignancies are now known to be associated with an infectious cause. In addition, numerous emerging and re-emerging infectious diseases continue to have a dire impact on global health: HIV/AIDS, pandemic influenza, and severe acute respiratory syndrome (SARS) are but a few examples. The fear of weaponizing pathogens for bioterrorism is ever present and poses a potentially enormous threat to public health. Moreover, escalating antimicrobial resistance in clinically relevant microbes (e.g., *Mycobacterium tuberculosis*, *Staphylococcus aureus*, *Streptococcus pneumoniae*, *Plasmodium* species, and HIV) signifies that the administration of antimicrobial agents—once thought to be a panacea—requires appropriate stewardship. For all these reasons, infectious diseases continue to exert grim effects on individual patients as well as on international public health. Even with all the successes of the past century, physicians must be as thoughtful about infectious diseases now as they were at the beginning of the twentieth century.

GLOBAL CONSIDERATIONS

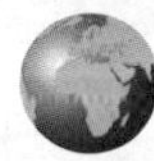

Infectious diseases remain the second leading cause of death worldwide. Although the rate of infectious disease–related deaths has decreased dramatically over the past 20 years, the absolute numbers of such deaths have remained relatively constant, totaling just over 12 million in 2010 (Fig. 144-1A). As shown in Fig. 144-1*B*, these deaths disproportionately affect low- and middle-income countries (Chap. 13e); in 2010, 23% of all deaths worldwide were related to infectious diseases, with rates >60% in most sub-Saharan African countries.

Given that infectious diseases are still a major cause of global mortality, understanding the local epidemiology of disease is critically important in evaluating patients. Diseases such as HIV/AIDS have decimated sub-Saharan Africa, with HIV-infected adults representing 15–26% of the total population in countries like Zimbabwe, Botswana, and Swaziland. Moreover, drug-resistant tuberculosis is rampant throughout the former Soviet-bloc countries, India, China, and South Africa. The ready availability of this type of information allows physicians to develop appropriate differential diagnoses and treatment plans for individual patients. Programs such as the Global Burden of Disease seek to quantify human losses (e.g., deaths, disability-adjusted life years) due to diseases by age, sex, and country over time; these data not only help inform local, national, and international health policy but can also help guide local medical decision-making. Even though some diseases (e.g., pandemic influenza, SARS) are seemingly geographically restricted, the increasing ease of rapid worldwide travel has raised concern about their swift spread around the globe. The world's increasing interconnectedness has profound implications not only for the global economy but also for medicine and the spread of infectious diseases.

UNDERSTANDING THE MICROBIOTA

Normal, healthy humans are colonized with over 100 trillion bacteria as well as countless viruses, fungi, and archaea; taken together, these microorganisms outnumber human cells by 10–100 times (Chap. 86e). The major reservoir of these microbes is the gastrointestinal tract, but very substantial numbers of microbes live in the female genital tract, the oral cavity, and the nasopharynx. There is increasing interest in the skin and even the lungs as sites where microbial colonization might be highly relevant to the biology and disease susceptibility of the host. These commensal organisms provide the host with myriad benefits, from aiding in metabolism to shaping the immune system. With regard to infectious diseases, the vast majority of infections are caused by organisms that are part of the normal flora (e.g., *S. aureus*, *S. pneumoniae*, *Pseudomonas aeruginosa*), with relatively few infections due to organisms that are strictly pathogens (e.g, *Neisseria gonorrhoeae*, rabies virus). Perhaps it is not surprising that a general understanding of the microbiota is essential in the evaluation of infectious diseases. Individuals' microbiotas likely have a major impact on their susceptibility to infectious diseases and even their responses to vaccines. Site-specific knowledge of the indigenous flora may facilitate appropriate interpretation of culture results, aid in selection of empirical antimicrobial therapy based on the likely causative agents, and provide additional impetus for rational antibiotic use to minimize the untoward effects of these drugs on the "beneficial" microbes that inhabit the body.

WHEN TO CONSIDER AN INFECTIOUS ETIOLOGY

The title of this chapter may appear to presuppose that the physician knows when a patient has an infectious disease. In reality, this chapter can serve only as a guide to the evaluation of a patient in whom an

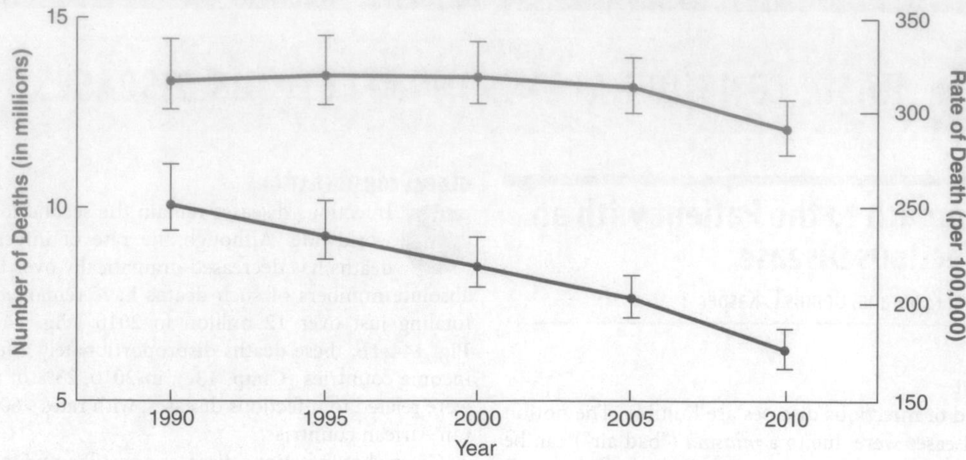

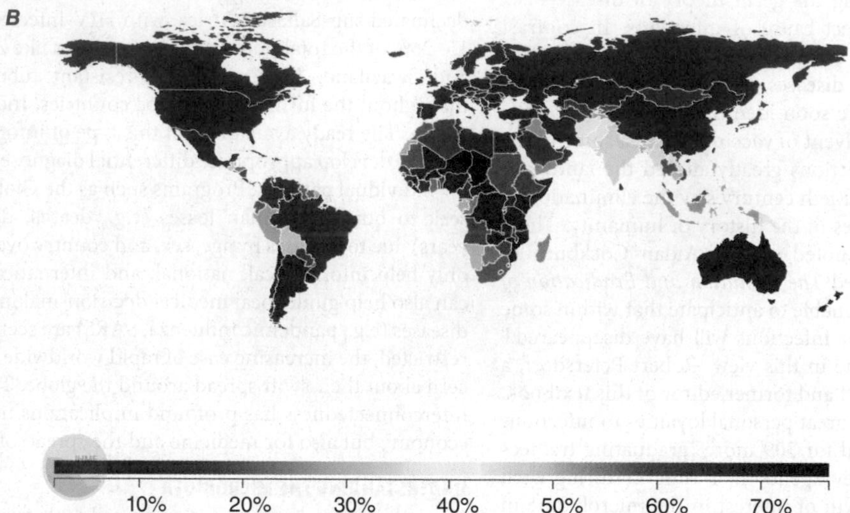

FIGURE 144-1 Magnitude of infectious disease–related deaths globally. ***A.*** The absolute number (*blue line; left axis*) and rate (*red line; right axis*) of infectious disease–related deaths throughout the world since 1990. ***B.*** A map depicting country-specific data for the percentages of total deaths that were attributable to communicable, maternal, neonatal, and nutritional disorders in 2010. *(Source: Global Burden of Disease Study, Institute for Health Metrics and Evaluation.)*

infectious disease is a possibility. Once a specific diagnosis is made, the reader should consult the subsequent chapters that deal with specific microorganisms in detail. The challenge for the physician is to recognize which patients may have an infectious disease as opposed to some other underlying disorder. This task is greatly complicated by the fact that infections have an infinite range of presentations, from acute life-threatening conditions (e.g., meningococcemia) to chronic diseases of varying severity (e.g., *H. pylori*–associated peptic ulcer disease) to no symptoms at all (e.g., latent *M. tuberculosis* infection). While it is impossible to generalize about a presentation that encompasses all infections, common findings in the history, physical examination, and basic laboratory testing often suggest that the patient either has an infectious disease or should be more closely evaluated for one. This chapter focuses on these common findings and how they may direct the ongoing evaluation of the patient.

APPROACH TO THE PATIENT: Infectious Disease

See also Chap. 147.

HISTORY

As in all of medicine, obtaining a complete and thorough history is paramount in the evaluation of a patient with a possible infectious disease. The history is critical for developing a focused differential diagnosis and for guiding the physical exam and initial diagnostic testing. Although detailing all the elements of a history is beyond the scope of this chapter, specific components relevant to infectious diseases require particular attention. In general, these aspects focus on two areas: (1) an exposure history that may identify microorganisms with which the patient may have come into contact and (2) host-specific factors that may predispose to the development of an infection.

Exposure History • ***HISTORY OF INFECTIONS OR EXPOSURE TO DRUG-RESISTANT MICROBES*** Knowledge about a patient's previous infections, with the associated microbial susceptibility profiles, is very helpful in determining possible etiologic agents. Specifically, knowing whether a patient has a history of infection with drug-resistant organisms (e.g., methicillin-resistant *S. aureus,* vancomycin-resistant *Enterococcus* species, enteric organisms that produce an extended-spectrum β-lactamase or carbapenemase) or may have been exposed to drug-resistant microbes (e.g., during a recent stay in a hospital, nursing home, or long-term acute-care facility) may alter the choice of empirical antibiotics. For example, a patient presenting with sepsis who is known to have a history of invasive infection with a multidrug-resistant isolate of *P. aeruginosa* should be treated empirically with an antimicrobial regimen that will cover this strain.

SOCIAL HISTORY Although the social history taken by physicians is often limited to inquiries about a patient's alcohol and tobacco use, a complete social history can offer a number of clues to the underlying diagnosis. Knowing whether the patient has any high-risk behaviors (e.g., unsafe sexual behaviors, IV drug use), potential hobby-associated exposures (e.g., avid gardening, with possible *Sporothrix schenckii* exposure), or occupational exposures (e.g., increased risk for *M. tuberculosis* exposure in funeral service workers) can facilitate diagnosis. The importance of the social history is exemplified by a case in 2009 in which a laboratory researcher died of a *Yersinia pestis* infection acquired during his work; although this patient had visited both an outpatient clinic and an emergency department, his records at both sites failed to include his occupation—information that potentially could have led quickly to appropriate treatment and infection control measures.

DIETARY HABITS As certain pathogens are associated with specific dietary habits, inquiring about a patient's diet can provide insight into possible exposures. For example, Shiga toxin–producing strains of *Escherichia coli* and *Toxoplasma gondii* are associated with the consumption of raw or undercooked meat; *Salmonella typhimurium*, *Listeria monocytogenes*, and *Mycobacterium bovis* with unpasteurized milk; *Leptospira* species, parasites, and enteric bacteria with unpurified water; and *Vibrio* species, norovirus, helminths, and protozoa with raw seafood.

ANIMAL EXPOSURES Because animals are often important vectors of infectious diseases, patients should be asked about exposures to any animals, including contact with their own pets, visits to petting zoos, or random encounters (e.g., home rodent infestation). For example, dogs can carry ticks that serve as agents for the transmission of several infectious diseases, including Lyme disease, Rocky Mountain spotted fever, and ehrlichiosis. Cats are associated with *Bartonella henselae* infection, reptiles with *Salmonella* infection, rodents with leptospirosis, and rabbits with tularemia (Chap. 167e).

TRAVEL HISTORY Attention should be paid to both international and domestic travel. Fever in a patient who has recently returned from abroad significantly broadens the differential diagnosis (Chap. 149); even a remote history of international travel may reflect patients' exposure to infections with pathogens such as *M. tuberculosis* or *Strongyloides stercoralis*. Similarly, domestic travel may have exposed patients to pathogens that are not normally found in their local environment and therefore may not routinely be considered in the differential diagnosis. For example, a patient who has recently visited California or Martha's Vineyard may have been exposed to *Coccidioides immitis* or *Francisella tularensis*, respectively. Beyond simply identifying locations that a patient may have visited, the physician needs to delve deeper to learn what kinds of activities and behaviors the patient engaged in during travel (e.g., the types of food and sources of water consumed, freshwater swimming, animal exposures) and whether the patient had the necessary immunizations and/or took the necessary prophylactic medications prior to travel; these additional exposures, which the patient may not think to report without specific prompting, are as important as exposures during a patient's routine daily living.

Host-Specific Factors Because many opportunistic infections (e.g., with *Pneumocystis jirovecii*, *Aspergillus* species, or JC virus) affect only immunocompromised patients, it is of vital importance to determine the immune status of the patient. Defects in the immune system may be due to an underlying disease (e.g., malignancy, HIV infection, malnutrition), a medication (e.g., chemotherapy, glucocorticoids, monoclonal antibodies to components of the immune system), a treatment modality (e.g., total body irradiation, splenectomy), or a primary immunodeficiency. The type of infection for which the patient is at increased risk varies with the specific type of immune defect (Chap. 375e). In concert with determining whether a patient is immunocompromised for any reason, the physician should review the immunization record to ensure that the patient is adequately protected against vaccine-preventable diseases (Chap. 148).

PHYSICAL EXAMINATION

Similar to the history, a thorough physical examination is crucial in evaluating patients with an infectious disease. Some elements of the physical exam (e.g., skin, lymphatics) that are often performed in a cursory manner as a result of the ever-increasing pace of medical practice may help identify the underlying diagnosis. Moreover, serial exams are critical since new findings may appear as the illness progresses. A description of all the elements of a physical exam is beyond the scope of this chapter, but the following components have particular relevance to infectious diseases.

Vital Signs Given that elevations in temperature are often a hallmark of infection, paying close attention to the temperature may be of value in diagnosing an infectious disease. The idea that 37°C (98.6°F) is the normal human body temperature dates back to the nineteenth century and was initially based on axillary measurements. Rectal temperatures more accurately reflect the core body temperature and are 0.4°C (0.7°F) and 0.8°C (1.4°F) higher than oral and axillary temperatures, respectively. Although the definition of fever varies greatly throughout the medical literature, the most common definition, which is based on studies defining fever of unknown origin (Chap. 26), uses a temperature ≥38.3°C (101°F). Although fever is very commonly associated with infection, it is also documented in many other diseases (Chap. 23). For every 1°C (1.8°F) increase in core temperature, the heart rate typically rises by 15–20 beats/min. Table 144-1 lists infections that are associated with relative bradycardia (*Faget's sign*), where patients have a lower heart rate than might be expected for a given body temperature. Although this pulse-temperature dissociation is not highly sensitive or specific for establishing a diagnosis, it is potentially useful in low-resource settings given its ready availability and simplicity.

Lymphatics There are ~600 lymph nodes throughout the body, and infections are an important cause of lymphadenopathy. A physical examination should include evaluation of lymph nodes in multiple

TABLE 144-1 CAUSES OF RELATIVE BRADYCARDIA

Infectious Causes	
Intracellular organisms	
Gram-negative bacteria	*Salmonella typhi*
	Francisella tularensis
	Brucella spp.
	Coxiella burnetii (Q fever)
	Leptospira interrogans
	Legionella pneumophila
	Mycoplasma pneumoniae
Tick-borne organisms	*Rickettsia* spp.
	Orientia tsutsugamushi (scrub typhus)
	Babesia spp.
Other	*Corynebacterium diphtheriae*
	Plasmodium spp. (malaria)
Viruses/viral infections	Yellow fever virus
	Dengue virus
	Viral hemorrhagic fevers[a]
	Viral myocarditis
Noninfectious Causes	
	Drug fever
	Beta blocker use
	Central nervous system lesions
	Malignant lymphoma
	Factitious fever

[a]Primarily early in the course of infection with Marburg or Ebola virus.

regions (e.g., popliteal, inguinal, epitrochlear, axillary, multiple cervical regions), with notation of the location, size (normal, <1 cm), presence or absence of tenderness, and consistency (soft, firm, or shotty) and of whether the nodes are matted (i.e., connected and moving together). Of note, palpable epitrochlear nodes are always pathologic. Of patients presenting with lymphadenopathy, 75% have localized findings, and the remaining 25% have generalized lymphadenopathy (i.e., that involving more than one anatomic region). Localized lymphadenopathy in the head and neck region is found in 55% of patients, inguinal lymphadenopathy in 14%, and axillary lymphadenopathy in 5%. Determining whether the patient has generalized versus localized lymphadenopathy can help narrow the differential diagnosis, as various infections present differently.

Skin The fact that many infections have cutaneous manifestations gives the skin examination particular importance in the evaluation of patients (Chaps. 24, 25e, 72, and 156). It is important to perform a complete skin exam, with attention to both front and back. Specific rashes are often extremely helpful in narrowing the differential diagnosis of an infection (Chaps. 24 and 25e). In numerous anecdotal instances, patients in the intensive care unit have had "fever of unknown origin" that was actually due to unrecognized pressure ulcers. Moreover, close examination of the distal extremities for splinter hemorrhages, Janeway lesions, or Osler's nodes may yield evidence of endocarditis or other causes of septic emboli.

Foreign Bodies As previously mentioned, many infections are caused by members of the indigenous microbiota. These infections typically occur when these microbes escape their normal habitat and enter a new one. Thus, maintenance of epithelial barriers is one of the most important mechanisms in protection against infection. However, hospitalization of patients is often associated with breaches of these barriers—e.g., due to placement of IV lines, surgical drains, or tubes (such as endotracheal tubes and Foley catheters) that allow microorganisms to localize in sites to which they normally would not have access (Chap. 168). Accordingly, knowing what lines, tubes, and drains are in place is helpful in ascertaining what body sites might be infected.

DIAGNOSTIC TESTING

Laboratory and radiologic testing has advanced greatly over the past few decades and has become an important component in the evaluation of patients. The dramatic increase in the number of serologic diagnostics, antigen tests, and molecular diagnostics available to the physician has, in fact, revolutionized medical care. However, all of these tests should be viewed as adjuncts to the history and physical examination—not a replacement for them. The selection of initial tests should be based directly on the patient's history and physical exam findings. Moreover, diagnostic testing should generally be limited to those conditions that are reasonably likely and treatable, important in terms of public health considerations, and/or capable of providing a definitive diagnosis that will consequently limit other testing.

White Blood Cell (WBC) Count Elevations in the WBC count are often associated with infection, though many viral infections are associated with leukopenia. It is important to assess the WBC differential, given that different classes of microbes are associated with various leukocyte types. For example, bacteria are associated with an increase in polymorphonuclear neutrophils, often with elevated levels of earlier developmental forms such as bands; viruses are associated with an increase in lymphocytes; and certain parasites are associated with an increase in eosinophils. Table 144-2 lists the major infectious causes of eosinophilia.

Inflammatory Markers The erythrocyte sedimentation rate (ESR) and the C-reactive protein (CRP) level are indirect and direct measures of the acute-phase response, respectively, that can be used to assess a patient's general level of inflammation. Moreover, these markers can be followed serially over time to monitor disease progress/resolution. It is noteworthy that the ESR changes relatively slowly, and its measurement more often than weekly usually is not useful; in contrast, CRP concentrations change rapidly, and daily measurements can be useful in the appropriate context. Although these markers are sensitive indicators of inflammation, neither is very specific. An extremely elevated ESR (>100 mm/h) has a 90% predictive value for a serious underlying disease (Table 144-3). Work is ongoing to identify other potentially useful inflammatory markers (e.g., procalcitonin, serum amyloid A protein); however, their clinical utility requires further validation.

Analysis of Cerebrospinal Fluid (CSF) Assessment of CSF is critical for patients with suspected meningitis or encephalitis. An opening pressure should always be recorded, and fluid should routinely be sent for cell counts, Gram's stain and culture, and determination of glucose and protein levels. A CSF Gram's stain typically requires $>10^5$ bacteria/mL for reliable positivity; its specificity approaches 100%. Table 144-4 lists the typical CSF profiles for various infections. In general, CSF with a lymphocytic pleocytosis and a low glucose concentration suggests either infection (e.g., with *Listeria*, *M. tuberculosis*, or a fungus) or a noninfectious disorder (e.g, neoplastic meningitis, sarcoidosis). Bacterial antigen testing of CSF (e.g., latex agglutination tests for *Haemophilus influenzae* type b, group B *Streptococcus*, *S. pneumoniae*, and *Neisseria meningitidis*) is not recommended as a screening assay, given that these tests are no more sensitive than Gram's stain; however, these assays can be helpful in presumptively identifying organisms seen on Gram's stain. In contrast, other antigen tests (e.g., for *Cryptococcus*) and some CSF serologic testing (e.g., for *Treponema pallidum*, *Coccidioides*) are highly sensitive and are useful for select patients. In addition, polymerase chain reaction (PCR) analysis of CSF is increasingly being used for the diagnosis of bacterial (e.g., *N. meningitidis*, *S. pneumoniae*, mycobacteria) and viral (e.g., herpes simplex virus, enterovirus) infections; while these molecular tests permit rapid diagnosis with a high degree of sensitivity and specificity, they often do not allow determination of antimicrobial resistance profiles.

Cultures The mainstays of infectious disease diagnosis include the culture of infected tissue (e.g., surgical specimens) or fluid (e.g., blood, urine, sputum, purulence from a wound). Samples can be sent for culture of bacteria (aerobic or anaerobic), fungi, or viruses. Ideally, specimens are collected before the administration of antimicrobial therapy; in instances where this order of events is not clinically feasible, microscopic examination of the specimen (e.g., Gram-stained or potassium hydroxide [KOH]–treated preparations) is particularly important. Culture of the organism(s) allows identification of the etiologic agent, determination of the antimicrobial susceptibility profile, and—when there is concern about an outbreak—isolate typing. While cultures are extremely useful in the evaluation of patients, determining whether culture results are clinically meaningful or represent contamination (e.g., a non-*aureus*, non-*lugdunensis* staphylococcal species growing in a blood culture) can sometimes be challenging and requires an understanding of the patient's immune status, exposure history, and microbiota. In some cases, serial cultures to demonstrate clearance of the organism may be helpful.

Pathogen-Specific Testing Numerous pathogen-specific tests (e.g., serology, antigen testing, PCR testing) are commercially available, and many hospitals now offer some of these tests in-house to facilitate rapid turnaround that ultimately enhances patient care. The reader is directed to relevant chapters on the pathogens of interest for specific details. Some of these tests (e.g., universal PCRs) identify organisms that currently are not cultivable and have unclear relationships to disease, thereby complicating diagnosis. As these tests become more commonplace and the work of the Human Microbiome Project progresses, the relevance of some of these previously unrecognized bacteria to human health will likely become more apparent.

TABLE 144-2 MAJOR INFECTIOUS CAUSES OF EOSINOPHILIA[a]

Organ Involved	Organism	Exposure	Geographic Distribution	Degree of Eosinophilia[b]
Central nervous system	*Angiostrongylus*	Raw seafood	Asia	Mild
	Gnathostoma	Raw poultry and seafood	Asia	Moderate to extreme
Eye	*Loa loa*	Insect bite	Africa	Moderate (expatriates), mild (patients living in endemic areas)
	Onchocerca	Insect bite	Africa	Mild (expatriates), moderate (patients living in endemic areas)
Lung	*Chlamydia trachomatis*	Sexual transmission	Worldwide	Mild
	Strongyloides	Soil	Tropical	Moderate (acute), mild (chronic)
	Toxocara canis/Toxocara cati[c]	Dogs, soil	Worldwide	Moderate to extreme
	Paragonimus	Crabs and crayfish	Asia	Moderate (acute), mild (chronic)
	Coccidioides immitis	Soil	Southwestern United States	Mild (acute), extreme (disseminated)
	Brugia malayi	Insect bite	Asia	Mild to moderate
	Pneumocystis jirovecii	Air	Worldwide	Mild
Liver	*Schistosoma japonicum*	Freshwater swimming	Asia	Moderate (acute), mild (chronic)
	Schistosoma mansoni	Freshwater swimming	Africa, Middle East, Latin America	Moderate (acute), mild (chronic)
	Fasciola	Watercress	Worldwide	Moderate
	Clonorchis	Raw seafood	Asia	Mild to moderate
	Opisthorchis	Raw seafood	Asia	Mild to moderate
Intestines	*Ascaris*[d]	Raw fruits and vegetables, contaminated water	Worldwide	Mild to extreme
	Hookworm	Soil	Worldwide	Mild to moderate
	Trichuris	Raw fruits and vegetables, contaminated water	Tropical	Mild
	Cystoisospora belli	Contaminated water and food	Worldwide	Mild
	Dientamoeba fragilis	Unclear; spread via fecal-oral route	Worldwide	Mild
	Capillaria	Raw seafood	Asia	Extreme
	Heterophyes	Raw seafood	Asia, Middle East	Mild
	Anisakis	Raw seafood	Worldwide	Mild
	Baylisascaris procyonis[e]	Soil	North America	Moderate to extreme
	Hymenolepis nana	Contaminated water, soil	Worldwide	Mild
Bladder	*Schistosoma haematobium*	Freshwater swimming	Africa, Middle East	Moderate (acute), mild (chronic)
Muscle	*Trichinella*	Pork	Worldwide	Moderate to extreme
Lymphatics	*Wuchereria bancrofti*[d]	Insect bite	Tropical	Moderate to extreme[f]
	Bartonella henselae	Cats	Worldwide	Mild
Other	Recovery from bacterial or viral infections	—	—	Mild
	HIV	Contaminated bodily fluid	Worldwide	Mild
	Cryptococcus neoformans	Soil	Worldwide	Moderate to extreme (disseminated)

[a]There are numerous noninfectious causes of eosinophilia, such as atopic disease, DRESS (drug reaction with eosinophilia and systemic symptoms) syndrome, and pernicious anemia, which can cause mild eosinophilia; drug hypersensitivity and serum sickness, which can cause mild to moderate eosinophilia; collagen vascular disease, which can cause moderate eosinophilia, and malignancy, Churg-Strauss syndrome, and hyper-IgE syndromes, which can cause moderate to extreme eosinophilia. [b]Mild: 500–1500 cells/μL; moderate: 1500–5000 cells/μL; extreme: >5000 cells/μL. [c]Can also affect the liver and the eyes. [d]Can also affect the lungs. [e]Can also affect the eyes and the central nervous system. [f]Levels are typically higher with pulmonary infections.

Radiology Imaging provides an important adjunct to the physical examination, allowing evaluation for lymphadenopathy in regions that are not externally accessible (e.g., mediastinum, intraabdominal sites), assessment of internal organs for evidence of infection, and facilitation of image-guided percutaneous sampling of deep spaces. The choice of imaging modality (e.g., CT, MRI, ultrasound, nuclear medicine, use of contrast) is best made in consultation with a radiologist to ensure that the results will address the physician's specific concerns.

TREATMENT

Physicians often must balance the need for empirical antibiotic treatment with the patient's clinical condition. When clinically feasible, it is best to obtain relevant samples (e.g., blood, CSF, tissue, purulent exudate) for culture prior to the administration of antibiotics, as antibiotic treatment often makes subsequent diagnosis more difficult. Although a general maxim for antibiotic treatment is to use a regimen with as narrow a spectrum as possible (Chap. 170), empirical regimens are necessarily somewhat broad, given that a specific diagnosis has not yet been made. Table 144-5 lists empirical antibiotic treatment regimens for commonly encountered infectious presentations. These regimens should be narrowed as appropriate once a specific diagnosis is made. In addition to antibiotics, there is sometimes a role for adjunctive therapies, such as intravenous immunoglobulin G (IVIG) pooled from healthy adults or hyperimmune globulin prepared from the blood of individuals with high titers of specific antibodies to select pathogens (e.g., cytomegalovirus, hepatitis B virus, rabies virus, vaccinia virus,

TABLE 144-3 CAUSES OF AN EXTREMELY ELEVATED ERYTHROCYTE SEDIMENTATION RATE (>100 mm/h)

Etiologic Category (% of Cases)	Specific Causes
Infectious diseases (35–40)	Subacute bacterial endocarditis
	Abscesses
	Osteomyelitis
	Tuberculosis
	Urinary tract infection
Inflammatory diseases (15–20)	Giant cell arteritis
	Rheumatoid arthritis
	Systemic lupus erythematosus
Malignancies (15–20)	Multiple myeloma
	Leukemias
	Lymphomas
	Carcinomas
Other (20–35)	Drug hypersensitivity reactions (drug fever)
	Ischemic tissue injury/trauma
	Renal diseases

Clostridium tetani, varicella-zoster virus, *Clostridium botulinum* toxin). Although the data suggesting efficacy are limited, IVIG is often used for patients with suspected staphylococcal or streptococcal toxic shock syndrome.

INFECTION CONTROL

When evaluating a patient with a suspected infectious disease, the physician must consider what infection control methods are necessary to prevent transmission of any possible infection to other people. In 2007, the U.S. Centers for Disease Control and Prevention published guidelines for isolation precautions that are available for download at *www.cdc.gov/hicpac/2007IP/2007isolationPrecautions.html*. Persons exposed to certain pathogens (e.g., *N. meningitidis*, HIV, *Bacillus anthracis*) should receive postexposure prophylaxis to prevent disease acquisition. (See relevant chapters for details on specific pathogens.)

WHEN TO OBTAIN AN INFECTIOUS DISEASE CONSULT

At times, primary physicians need assistance with patient management, from a diagnostic and/or therapeutic perspective. Multiple studies have demonstrated that an infectious disease consult is associated with positive outcomes for patients with various diseases. For example, in a prospective cohort study of patients with *S. aureus* bacteremia, infectious disease consultation was independently associated with a 56% reduction in 28-day mortality. In addition, infectious disease specialists provide other services (e.g., infection control, antimicrobial stewardship, management of outpatient antibiotic therapy, occupational exposure programs) that have been shown to benefit patients. Whenever such assistance would be advantageous to a patient with a possible infection, the primary physician should opt for an infectious disease consult. Specific situations that might prompt a consult include (1) difficult-to-diagnose patients with presumed infections, (2) patients who are not responding to treatment as expected, (3) patients with a complicated medical history (e.g., organ transplant recipients, patients immunosuppressed due to autoimmune or inflammatory conditions), and (4) patients with "exotic" diseases (i.e., diseases that are not typically seen within the region).

PERSPECTIVE

The study of infectious diseases is really a study of host-bacterial interactions and represents evolution by both the host and the bacteria—an endless struggle in which microbes have generally been more creative and adaptive. Given that nearly one-quarter of deaths worldwide are still related to infectious diseases, it is clear that the war against infectious diseases has not been won. For example, a cure for HIV infection is still lacking, there have been only marginal improvements in the methods for detection and treatment of tuberculosis after more than a half century of research, new infectious diseases (e.g., pandemic influenza, viral hemorrhagic fevers) continue to emerge, and the threat of microbial bioterrorism remains high. The subsequent chapters in Part 8 detail—on both a syndrome and a microbe-by-microbe basis—the current state of medical knowledge about infectious diseases. At their core, all of these chapters carry a similar message: Despite numerous advances in the diagnosis, treatment, and prevention of infectious diseases, much work and research are required before anyone can confidently claim that "all the major infections have disappeared." In reality, this goal will never be attained, given the rapid adaptability of microbes.

TABLE 144-4 TYPICAL CSF PROFILES FOR MENINGITIS AND ENCEPHALITIS[a]

	Normal	Bacterial Meningitis	Viral Meningitis	Fungal Meningitis[b]	Parasitic Meningitis	Tuberculous Meningitis	Encephalitis
WBC count (per μL)	<5	>1000	25–500	40–600	150–2000	25–100	50–500
Differential of WBC	60–70% lymphocytes, ≤30% monocytes/macrophages	↑↑PMNs (≥80%)	Predominantly lymphocytes[c]	Lymphocytes or PMNs, depending on specific organism	↑↑ Eosinophils (≥50%)[d]	Predominantly lymphocytes[c]	Predominantly lymphocytes[c]
Gram's stain	Negative	Positive (in >60% of cases)	Negative	Rarely positive	Negative	Occasionally positive[e]	Negative
Glucose (mg/dL)	40–85	<40	Normal	↓ to normal	Normal	<50 in 75% of cases	Normal
Protein (mg/dL)	15–45	>100	20–80	150–300	50–200	100–200	50–100
Opening pressure (mmH_2O)	50–180	>300	100–350	160–340	Normal	150–280	Normal to ↑
Common causes	—	*Streptococcus pneumoniae*, *Neisseria meningitidis*	Enteroviruses	*Candida*, *Cryptococcus*, and *Aspergillus* spp.	*Angiostrongylus cantonensis*, *Gnathostoma spinigerum*, *Baylisascaris procyonis*	*Mycobacterium tuberculosis*	Herpesviruses, enteroviruses, influenza virus, rabies virus

[a]Numbers indicate typical results, but actual results may vary. [b]Cerebrospinal fluid characteristics depend greatly on the specific organism. [c]Neutrophils may predominate early in the disease course. [d]Patients typically have striking eosinophilia as well. [e]Sensitivity can be increased by examination of a smear of protein coagulum (pellicle) and the use of acid-fast stains.

Abbreviations: PMNs, polymorphonuclear neutrophils; WBC, white blood cell.

TABLE 144-5 INITIAL EMPIRICAL ANTIBIOTIC THERAPY FOR COMMON INFECTIOUS DISEASE PRESENTATIONS[a]

Clinical Syndrome	Common Etiologies	Antibiotic(s)	Comments	See Chapter(s)
Septic shock	*Staphylococcus aureus, Streptococcus pneumoniae,* enteric gram-negative bacilli	Vancomycin, 15 mg/kg q12h[b]; **plus** A broad-spectrum antipseudomonal β-lactam (piperacillin-tazobactam, 4.5 g q6h; imipenem, 1 g q8h; meropenem, 1 g q8h; or cefepime, 1–2 g q8–12h)	—	**325**
Meningitis	*S. pneumoniae, Neisseria meningitidis*	Vancomycin, 15 mg/kg q12h[b]; **plus** Ceftriaxone, 2 g q12h	Dexamethasone (0.15 mg/kg IV q6h for 2–4 d) should be added for patients with suspected or proven pneumococcal meningitis, with the first dose administered 10–20 min before the first dose of antibiotics.	**164** and pathogen-specific chapters
CNS abscess	*Streptococcus* spp., *Staphylococcus* spp., anaerobes, gram-negative bacilli	Vancomycin, 15 mg/kg q12h[b]; **plus** Ceftriaxone, 2 g q12h; **plus** Metronidazole, 500 mg q8h	—	**164**
Endocarditis	*S. aureus, Streptococcus* spp., coagulase-negative staphylococci	Vancomycin, 15 mg/kg q12h[b]; **plus** Ceftriaxone, 2 g q12h	—	**155**
Pneumonia			If MRSA is a consideration, add vancomycin (15 mg/kg q12h[b]) or linezolid (600 mg q12h); daptomycin should not be used in patients with pneumonia.	**153** and pathogen-specific chapters
Community-acquired, outpatient	*S. pneumoniae, Mycoplasma pneumoniae, Haemophilus influenzae, Chlamydia pneumoniae*	Azithromycin, 500 mg PO × 1, then 250 mg PO qd × 4 days		
Inpatient, non-ICU	Above plus *Legionella* spp.	A respiratory fluoroquinolone (moxifloxacin, 400 mg IV/PO qd; gemifloxacin, 320 mg PO qd; or levofloxacin, 750 mg IV/PO qd); ***or*** A β-lactam (cefotaxime, ceftriaxone, or ampicillin-sulbactam) *plus* azithromycin		
Inpatient, ICU	Above plus *S. aureus*	A β-lactam; **plus** Azithromycin *or* a respiratory fluoroquinolone		
Hospital-acquired pneumonia[d]	*S. pneumoniae, H. influenzae, S. aureus,* gram-negative bacilli (e.g., *Pseudomonas aeruginosa, Klebsiella pneumoniae, Acinetobacter* spp.)	An antipseudomonal β-lactam (cefepime, 1–2 g q8–12 h; ceftazidime, 2 g q8h; imipenem, 1 g q8h; meropenem, 1 g q8h; or piperacillin-tazobactam, 4.5 g q6h); **plus** An antipseudomonal fluoroquinolone (levofloxacin or ciprofloxacin, 400 mg q8h) *or* an aminoglycoside (amikacin, 20 mg/kg q24h[c]; gentamicin, 7 mg/kg q24h[e]; or tobramycin, 7 mg/kg q24h[e])		
Complicated intra-abdominal infection			If MRSA is a consideration, add vancomycin (15 mg/kg q12h[b]).	**159**, **201**, and pathogen-specific chapters
Mild to moderate severity	Anaerobes (*Bacteroides* spp., *Clostridium* spp.), gram-negative bacilli (*Escherichia coli*), *Streptococcus* spp.	Cefoxitin, 2 g q6h; ***or*** A combination of metronidazole (500 mg q8–12h) *plus* cefazolin (1–2 g q8h) *or* cefuroxime (1.5 g q8h) *or* ceftriaxone (1–2 g q12–24h) *or* cefotaxime (1–2 g q6–8h)		
High-risk patient or high degree of severity	Same as above	A carbapenem (imipenem, 1 g q8h; meropenem, 1 g q8h; doripenem, 500 mg q8h); ***or*** Piperacillin-tazobactam, 3.375 g q6h[f]; ***or*** A combination of metronidazole (500 mg q8–12h) *plus* an antipseudomonal cephalosporin (cefepime, 2 g q8–12h; ceftazidime, 2 g q8h) *or* an antipseudomonal fluoroquinolone (ciprofloxacin, 400 mg q12h; levofloxacin, 750 mg q24h)		

(Continued)

TABLE 144-5 INITIAL EMPIRICAL ANTIBIOTIC THERAPY FOR COMMON INFECTIOUS DISEASE PRESENTATIONS[a] (CONTINUED)

Clinical Syndrome	Common Etiologies	Antibiotic(s)	Comments	See Chapter(s)
Skin and soft tissue infection	*S. aureus, Streptococcus pyogenes*	Dicloxacillin, 250–500 mg PO qid; *or* Cephalexin, 250–500 mg PO qid; *or* Clindamycin, 300–450 mg PO tid; *or* Nafcillin/oxacillin, 1–2 g q4h	If MRSA is a consideration, clindamycin, vancomycin (15 mg/kg q12h[b]), linezolid (600 mg IV/PO q12h), or TMP-SMX (1–2 double-strength tablets PO bid[g]) can be used.	**156** and pathogen-specific chapters

[a]This table refers to immunocompetent adults with normal renal and hepatic function. All doses listed are for parenteral administration unless indicated otherwise. Local antimicrobial susceptibility profiles may influence the choice of antibiotic. Therapy should be tailored once a specific etiologic agent and its susceptibilities are identified. [b]Trough levels for vancomycin should be 15–20 μg/mL. [c]Trough levels for amikacin should be <4 μg/mL. [d]In patients with late onset (i.e., after ≥5 days of hospitalization) or risk factors for multidrug-resistant organisms. [e]Trough levels for gentamicin and tobramycin should be <1 μg/mL. [f]If *P. aeruginosa* is a concern, the dosage may be increased to 3.375 g IV q4h or 4.5 g IV q6h. [g]Data on the efficacy of TMP-SMX in skin and soft tissue infections are limited.

Abbreviations: CNS, central nervous system; ICU, intensive care unit; MRSA, methicillin-resistant *S. aureus*; TMP-SMX, trimethoprim-sulfamethoxazole.

145e Molecular Mechanisms of Microbial Pathogenesis

Gerald B. Pier

This is a digital-only chapter. It is available on the DVD that accompanies this book, as well as on Access Medicine/Harrison's Online, and the eBook and "app" editions of HPIM 19e.

Over the past four decades, molecular studies of the pathogenesis of microorganisms have yielded an explosion of information about the various microbial and host molecules that contribute to the processes of infection and disease. These processes can be classified into several stages: microbial encounter with and entry into the host; microbial growth after entry; avoidance of innate host defenses; tissue invasion and tropism; tissue damage; and transmission to new hosts. *Virulence* is the measure of an organism's capacity to cause disease and is a function of the pathogenic factors elaborated by microbes. These factors promote *colonization* (the simple presence of potentially pathogenic microbes in or on a host), *infection* (attachment and growth of pathogens and avoidance of host defenses), and *disease* (often, but not always, the result of activities of secreted toxins or toxic metabolites). In addition, the host's inflammatory response to infection greatly contributes to disease and its attendant clinical signs and symptoms. The recent surge of interest in the role of the microbiota and its associated *microbiome*—the collection of microbial genomes residing in or on mammalian organisms—in the physiology of, susceptibility to, and response to infection and in immune system development has had an enormous impact on our understanding of host-pathogen interaction.

146 Genomics and Infectious Disease

Roby P. Bhattacharyya, Yonatan H. Grad, Deborah T. Hung

Just as microscopy opened up the worlds of microbiology by providing a tool with which to visualize microorganisms, technological advances in genomics are now providing microbiologists with powerful new methods with which to characterize the genetic map underlying all microbes with unprecedented resolution, thereby illuminating their complex and dynamic interactions with one another, the environment, and human health. The field of infectious disease genomics encompasses a vast frontier of active research that has the potential to transform clinical practice in relation to infectious diseases. While genetics has long played a key role in elucidating the process of infection and managing clinical infectious diseases, the ability to extend our thinking and our approaches beyond the study of single genes to an examination of the sequence, structure, and function of entire genomes is identifying new possibilities for research and opportunities to change clinical practice. From the development of diagnostics with unprecedented sensitivity, specificity, and speed to the design of novel public health interventions, technical and statistical genomic innovations are reshaping our understanding of the influence of the microbial world on human health and providing us with new tools to combat infection. This chapter explores the application of genomics methods to microbial pathogens and the infections they cause (Table 146-1). It discusses innovations that are driving the development of diagnostic approaches and the discovery of new pathogens; providing insight into novel therapeutic approaches and paradigms; and advancing methods in infectious disease epidemiology and the study of pathogen evolution that can inform infection control measures, public health responses to outbreaks, and vaccine development. We draw on examples in current practice and from the recent scientific literature as signposts that point toward the ways in which the insights from pathogen genomics may influence infectious diseases in the short and long terms. Table 146-2 provides definitions for a selection of important terms used in genomics.

MICROBIAL DIAGNOSTICS

The basic goals of a clinical microbiology laboratory are to establish the presence of a pathogen in a clinical sample, to identify the pathogen, and, when possible, to provide other information that can help guide clinical management and even prognosis, such as antibiotic susceptibility profiles or the presence of virulence factors. To date, clinical microbiology laboratories have largely approached these goals phenotypically by growth-based assays and biochemical testing. Bacteria, for instance, are algorithmically grouped into species by their characteristic microscopic appearance, nutrient requirements for growth, and ability to catalyze certain reactions. Antibiotic susceptibility is determined in most cases by assessing growth in the presence of antibiotic.

With the sequencing revolution paving the way to easy access of complete pathogen genomes (Fig. 146-1), we are now able to more systematically clarify the genetic basis of these observable phenotypes. Compared with traditional growth-based methods for bacterial diagnostics that dominate the clinical microbiology laboratory, nucleic

TABLE 146-1 CURRENT CLINICAL APPLICATIONS OF INFECTIOUS DISEASE GENOMICS

Application	Technology	Notes/Examples
Organism Identification		
Viral detection	PCR	Identification of HIV, HBV, HCV, respiratory viruses including influenza, and others for diagnosis and response to therapy
TB detection	PCR	Amplification of the *rpoB* gene for species-specific identification of *Mycobacterium tuberculosis*
Bacterial detection	PCR, NAAT	Identification of *Chlamydia, Neisseria gonorrhoeae, Clostridium difficile, Ehrlichia, Anaplasma,* and others
Bacterial detection	16S ribosomal gene PCR	Targeting of highly conserved regions of the 16S rRNA gene for identification of suspected bacterial infections undiagnosed by conventional methods
Pathogen Discovery		
Bacterial pathogens	Sequencing, metagenomic assembly	Unbiased "shotgun" sequencing of isolated nucleic acid from patient samples to identify associated pathogens; proofs-of-concept: new *Bradyrhizobium* species associated with cord colitis, *Escherichia coli* O104:H4 from 2011 diarrheal outbreak in Germany; research use only at this time
Viral pathogens	Microarray, sequencing	Hybridization of clinical samples to microarrays from phylogenetically diverse known viruses identified the SARS coronavirus and others. Direct sequencing has identified West Nile virus and the MERS coronavirus, among others. Use is primarily in research.
Antibiotic Resistance		
MRSA detection	PCR	Detection of the *mecA* gene, the genotypic cause of methicillin resistance in *Staphylococcus aureus*
VRE detection	PCR	Detection of the *vanA* or *vanB* genes, the main genotypic causes of vancomycin resistance in *Enterococcus*
MDR-TB detection	PCR, NAAT	Detection of polymorphisms in the *rpoB* gene from *M. tuberculosis,* which account for 95% of rifampin resistance. Other probes available for *inhA* and *katG* genes can detect up to 85% of isoniazid resistance.
Carbapenemase detection	PCR	Detection of genes encoding one of two enzymes, NDM-1 or KPC, that hydrolyze carbapenems; use in United States currently restricted to CDC
HIV resistance detection	Targeted sequencing	Targeted sequencing of specific genes with known resistance-conferring mutations; now standard of care prior to initial therapy in United States and Europe
Epidemiology		
Outbreak and epidemic tracking	Sequencing	Application to tracking outbreaks and epidemics on local and international scales, including spread of carbapenemase-producing *Klebsiella, S. aureus, M. tuberculosis, E. coli, Vibrio cholerae,* and influenza virus
Evolution and spread of pathogens	Sequencing	Sequencing collections of pathogens to shed light on pathogen dissemination, virulence factors, and antibiotic resistance determinants

Abbreviations: CDC, Centers for Disease Control and Prevention; HBV, hepatitis B virus; HCV, hepatitis C virus; MDR, multidrug-resistant; MERS, Middle East respiratory syndrome; MRSA, methicillin-resistant *Staphylococcus aureus*; NAAT, nucleic acid amplification test; PCR, polymerase chain reaction; SARS, severe acute respiratory syndrome; TB, tuberculosis; VRE, vancomycin-resistant enterococci.

TABLE 146-2 GLOSSARY OF SELECTED TERMS IN GENOMICS

Term	Definition
Contig	A DNA sequence representing a continuous fragment of a genome, assembled from overlapping sequences; relevant for de novo assembly of sequence data that do not align to previously sequenced genomes
Genome	The entire set of heritable genetic material within an organism
Horizontal gene transfer	The transfer of genes between organisms through mechanisms other than by clonal descent, such as through transformation, conjugation, or transduction
Metagenomics	Analysis of genetic material from multiple species directly from primary samples without requiring prior culture steps
Microarray	A collection of DNA oligonucleotides ("oligos") spatially arranged on a solid surface and used to detect or quantify sequences in a sample of interest that are complementary (and therefore bind) to one or more of the arrayed oligos
Mobile genetic element	DNA elements that can move within a genome and can be transferred between genomes through horizontal gene transfer (e.g., plasmids, bacteriophages, and transposons)
Multilocus sequence typing	A methodology for typing organisms based on DNA sequence fragments from a prespecified set of genes
Next-generation sequencing	High-throughput sequencing using a parallelized sequencing process that produces millions of sequences concurrently, far beyond the capacity of prior dye-terminator methods
Nucleic acid amplification test (NAAT)	Biochemical assay that evaluates for the presence of a particular string of nucleic acids through amplification by one of several methods, including polymerase and ligase chain reactions
Polymerase chain reaction (PCR)	A subset of NAAT used to amplify a specific region of DNA with specific oligonucleotide primers and a DNA polymerase
Transcriptome	The catalog of the full set of messenger RNA (mRNA) transcripts from a cell or organism, which are typically measured by microarray or by next-generation sequencing of complementary DNA (cDNA) via a process called RNA-Seq
Whole-genome sequencing	A process that determines the full DNA sequence of an organism's genome; has been greatly facilitated by next-generation sequencing technology

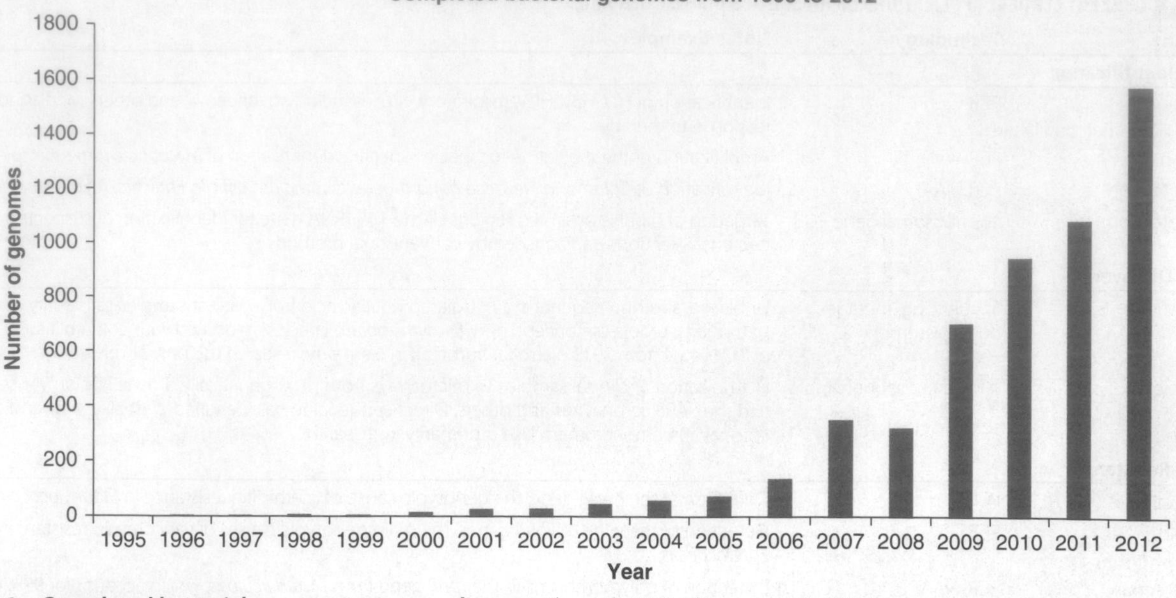

FIGURE 146-1 Completed bacterial genome sequences by year, through 2012. *(Data compiled from www.genomesonline.org.)*

acid–based diagnostics promise improved speed, sensitivity, specificity, and breadth of information. Bridging clinical and research laboratories, adaptations of genomic technologies have begun to deliver on this promise.

HISTORICAL LIMITATIONS AND PROGRESS THROUGH GENETIC APPROACHES

The molecular diagnostics revolution in the clinical microbiology laboratory is well under way, borne of necessity in the effort to identify microbes that are refractory to traditional culture methods. Historically, diagnosis of many so-called unculturable pathogens has relied largely on serology and antigen detection. However, these methods provide only limited clinical information because of their suboptimal sensitivity and specificity as well as the long delays that diminish their utility for real-time patient management. Newer tests to detect pathogens based on nucleic acid content have already offered improvements in the select cases to which they have been applied thus far.

Unlike direct pathogen detection, serologic diagnosis—measurement of the host's response to pathogen exposure—can typically be made only in retrospect, requiring both acute- and convalescent-phase sera. For chronic infections, distinguishing active from latent infection or identifying repeat exposure by serology alone can be difficult or impossible, depending on the syndrome. In addition, the sensitivity of serologic diagnosis varies with the organism and the patient's immune status. For instance, tuberculosis is notoriously difficult to identify by serologic methods; tuberculin skin testing using purified protein derivative (PPD) is especially insensitive in active disease and may be cross-reactive with vaccines or other mycobacteria. Even the newer interferon γ release assays (IGRAs), which measure cytokine release from T lymphocytes in response to *Mycobacterium tuberculosis*–specific antigens in vitro, have limited sensitivity in immunodeficient hosts. Neither PPD testing nor IGRAs can distinguish latent from active infection. Serologic Lyme disease diagnostics suffer similar limitations: in patients from endemic regions, the presence of IgG antibodies to *Borrelia burgdorferi* may reflect prior exposure rather than active disease, while IgM antibodies are imperfectly sensitive and specific (50% and 80%, respectively, in early disease). The complex nature of these tests, particularly in view of the nonspecific symptoms that may accompany Lyme disease, has had substantial implications on public perceptions of Lyme disease and antibiotic misuse in endemic areas. Similarly, syphilis, a chronic infection caused by *Treponema pallidum*, is notoriously difficult to stage by serology alone, requiring the use of multiple different nontreponemal (e.g., rapid protein reagin) and treponemal (e.g., fluorescent treponemal antibody) tests in conjunction with clinical suspicion. Complementing serology, antigen detection can improve sensitivity and specificity in select cases but has been validated only for a limited set of infections. Typically, structural elements of pathogens are detected, including components of viral envelopes (e.g., hepatitis B surface antigen, HIV p24 antigen), cell surface markers in certain bacteria (e.g., *Streptococcus pneumoniae*, *Legionella pneumophila* serotype 1) or fungi (e.g., *Cryptococcus*, *Histoplasma*), and less specific fungal cell-wall components such as galactomannan and β-glucan (e.g., *Aspergillus* and other dimorphic fungi).

Given the impracticality of culture and the lack of sensitivity or sufficient clinical information afforded by serologic and antigenic methods, the push toward nucleic acid–based diagnostics originated in pursuit of viruses and fastidious bacteria, becoming part of the standard of care for select organisms in U.S. hospitals. Such tests, including polymerase chain reaction (PCR) and other nucleic acid amplification tests (NAATs), are now widely used for many viral infections, both chronic (e.g., HIV infection) and acute (e.g., influenza). This technique provides essential information about both the initial diagnosis and the response to therapy and in some cases genotypically predicts drug resistance. Indeed, progression from antigen detection to PCR transformed our understanding of the natural course of HIV infection, with profound implications for treatment (Fig. 146-2). In the early years of the AIDS pandemic, p24 antigenemia was detected in acute HIV infection but then disappeared for years before emerging again with progression to AIDS (Fig. 146-2*B*). Without a marker demonstrating viremia, the role of treatment during HIV infection prior to the development of clinical AIDS was uncertain, and monitoring treatment efficacy was challenging. With the emergence of PCR as a progressively more sensitive test (now able to detect as few as 20 copies of virus per milliliter of blood), viremia was recognized as a near-universal feature of HIV infection. This recognition has been transformative in guiding the initiation of therapy as well as adjustments in therapy and, together with the development of less toxic therapies, has helped to shape guidelines that now favor earlier introduction of antiretroviral therapy for HIV infection.

As they are for viruses, nucleic acid–based tests have become the diagnostic tests of choice for fastidious bacteria, including the common sexually transmitted intracellular bacterial pathogens *Neisseria gonorrhoeae* and *Chlamydia trachomatis* as well as the tick-borne *Ehrlichia chaffeensis* and *Anaplasma phagocytophilum*. More recently, nucleic acid amplification–based detection has offered improved sensitivity for diagnosis of the important nosocomial pathogen *Clostridium difficile*; NAATs can provide clinically relevant information on the presence of cytotoxins A and B as well as molecular markers of hypervirulence such as those characterizing the recently recognized North American pulsotype 1 (NAP1), which is found more frequently in

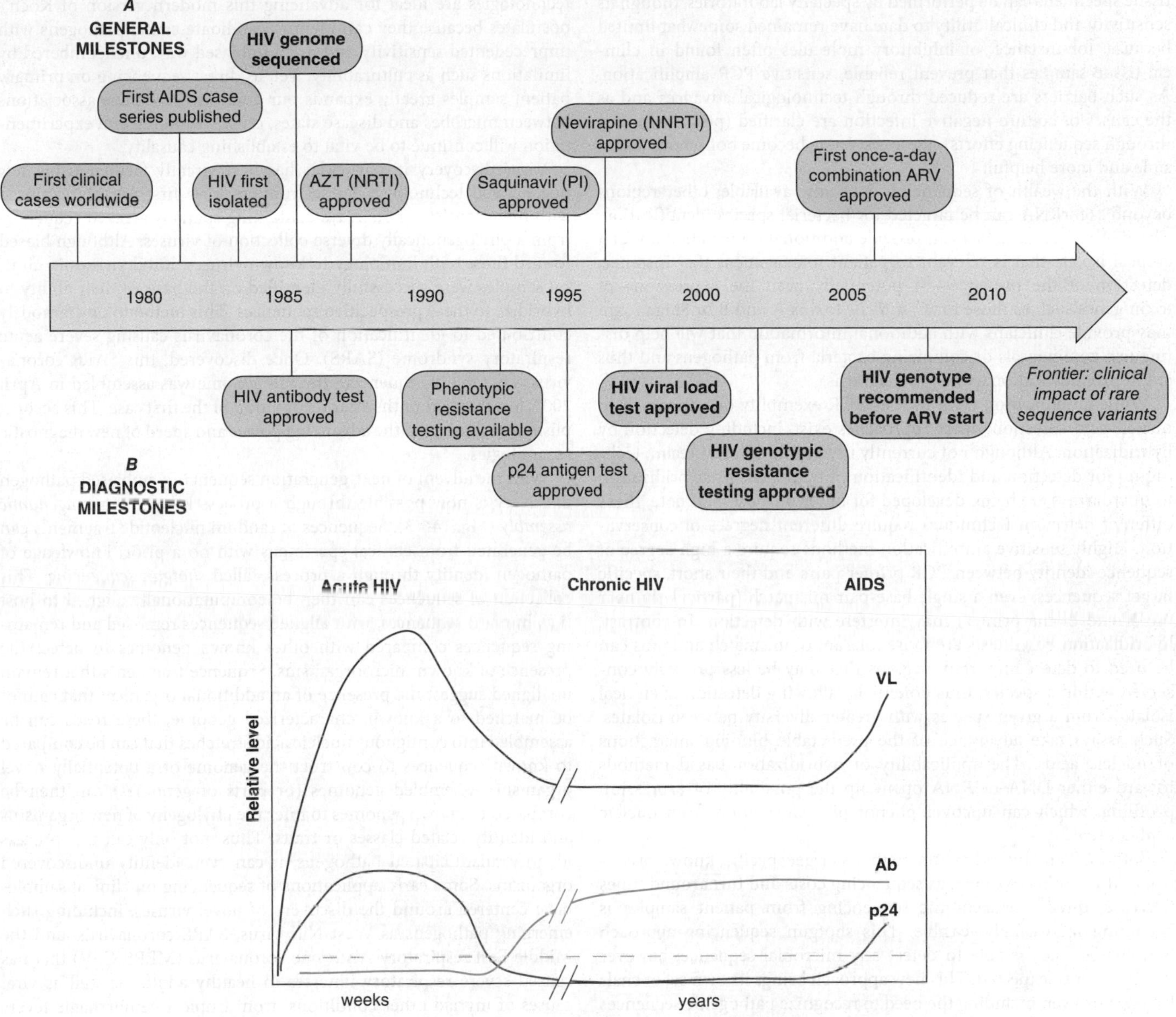

FIGURE 146-2 ***A.*** Timeline of select milestones in HIV management. Genomic advances are shown in bold type. The approvals and recommendations indicated apply to the United States. ARV, antiretroviral; AZT, zidovudine; NRTI, nucleoside reverse transcriptase (RT) inhibitor; NNRTI, non nucleoside RT inhibitor; PI, protease inhibitor. ***B.*** Viral dynamics in the natural history of HIV infection. Three diagnostic markers are shown: HIV antibody (Ab), p24 antigen (p24), and viral load (VL). Dashed gray line represents limit of detection. *(Adapted from data in HH Fiebig et al: Dynamics of HIV viremia and antibody seroconversion in plasma donors: Implications for diagnosis and staging of primary HIV infection. AIDS 17:1871, 2003.)*

cases of severe illness. The importance of genomics in selecting loci for diagnostic assays and in monitoring test sensitivity was recently highlighted by the emergence in Sweden of a new variant of *C. trachomatis* containing a deletion that includes the gene targeted by a set of commercial NAATs. By evading detection through this deletion (which would have prompted the initiation of treatment), this strain came to be highly prevalent in some areas of Sweden. While nucleic acid–based tests remain the diagnostic approach of choice for fastidious bacteria, this example serves as a reminder of the need for careful development and ongoing monitoring of molecular diagnostics.

In contrast, for typical bacterial pathogens for which culture methods are well established, growth-based assays followed by biochemical tests still dominate in the clinical laboratory. Informed by decades of clinical microbiology, these tests have served clinicians well, yet the limitations of growth-based tests—in particular, the delays associated with waiting for growth—have left open opportunities for improvements. Molecular diagnostics, greatly informed by the vast quantity of microbial genome sequences generated in recent years, offers a way forward. First, sequencing studies may identify key genes (or noncoding nucleic acids) that can be developed into targets for clinical assays using PCR or hybridization platforms. Second, sequencing itself may eventually become inexpensive and rapid enough to be performed routinely on clinical specimens, with consequent unbiased detection of pathogens.

ORGANISM IDENTIFICATION

In order to adapt nucleic acid detection to diagnostic tests and thus to identify pathogens on a wide scale, sequences must be identified that are conserved enough within a species to identify the diversity of strains that may be encountered in various clinical settings, yet divergent enough to distinguish one species from another. Until recently, this problem has been solved for bacteria by targeting the element of a bacterial genome that is most highly conserved within a species: the 16S ribosomal RNA (rRNA) subunit. At present, 16S PCR amplification from tissue specimens can be performed by specialty laboratories, though its sensitivity and clinical utility to date have remained somewhat limited because, for instance, of inhibitory molecules often found in clinical tissue samples that prevent reliable, sensitive PCR amplification. As such barriers are reduced through technological advances and as the causes of culture-negative infection are clarified (perhaps in part through sequencing efforts), these tests may become both more accessible and more helpful.

With the wealth of sequencing data now available, other regions beyond 16S rRNA can be targeted for bacterial species identification. These other genomic loci can provide additional information about a clinical isolate that is relevant to patient management. For instance, detection of the presence—or potentially even the expression—of toxin genes such as those for *C. difficile* toxins A and B or Shiga toxin may provide clinicians with additional information that will help distinguish commensals or colonizing bacteria from pathogens and thus aid in prognostication as well as diagnosis.

While amplification tests such as PCR exemplify one approach to nucleic acid detection, other approaches exist, including detection by hybridization. Although not currently used in the clinical realm, techniques for detection and identification of pathogens by hybridization to microarrays are being developed for other purposes. Of note, these different detection techniques require different degrees of conservation. Highly sensitive amplification methods require a high degree of sequence identity between PCR primer pairs and their short, specific target sequences; even a single base-pair mismatch (particularly near the 3′ end of the primer) may interfere with detection. In contrast, hybridization-based tests are more tolerant of mismatch and thus can be used to detect important regions that may be less precisely conserved within a species, thus potentially allowing detection of clinical isolates from a given species with greater diversity between isolates. Such assays take advantage of the predictable binding interactions of nucleic acids. The applicability of hybridization-based methods toward either DNA or RNA opens up the possibility of expression profiling, which can uncover phenotypic information from nucleic acid content.

Both PCR and hybridization methods target specific, known organisms. At the other extreme, as sequencing costs and turnaround times decrease, direct metagenomic sequencing from patient samples is becoming increasingly feasible. This shotgun sequencing approach is unbiased—i.e., is able to detect any microbial sequence, however divergent or unexpected. This new approach brings its own set of challenges, however, including the need to recognize pathogenic sequences against a background of expected host and commensal sequences and to distinguish true pathogens from either colonizers or laboratory contaminants. In a powerful example of this new frontier of sequencing-based clinical diagnosis, investigators diagnosed neuroleptospirosis in a child with an unexplained encephalitis syndrome by finding sequences corresponding to the *Leptospira* genus in cerebrospinal fluid from the patient. Rapid (<48-h) sequencing and analysis informed the patient's care in real time, leading to life-saving targeted antibiotic therapy for an unexpected diagnosis that was impossible to make through standard laboratory testing. The diagnosis was retrospectively confirmed through both convalescent serologies and PCR using primers designed on the basis of sequencing data.

PATHOGEN DISCOVERY

In addition to clinical diagnostic applications, novel genomic technologies, including whole-genome sequencing, are being applied to clinical research specimens with a goal of identifying new pathogens in a variety of circumstances. The tremendous sensitivity and unbiased nature of sequencing is also ideal in searching clinical samples for unknown or unsuspected pathogens.

Causal inference in infectious diseases has progressed since the time of Koch, whose historical postulates provided a rigorous framework for attributing a disease to a microorganism. According to an updated version of Koch's postulates, an organism, whether it can be cultured or not, should induce disease upon introduction into a healthy host if it is to be implicated as a causative pathogen. Current sequencing technologies are ideal for advancing this modern version of Koch's postulates because they can identify candidate causal pathogens with unprecedented sensitivity and in an unbiased way, unencumbered by limitations such as culturability. Yet, as direct sequencing on primary patient samples greatly expands our ability to recognize associations between microbes and disease states, critical thinking and experimentation will continue to be vital to establishing causality.

Virus discovery in particular has been greatly facilitated by new nucleic acid technology. These frontiers were first notably explored with high-density microarrays containing spatially arrayed sequences from a phylogenetically diverse collection of viruses. Although biased toward those with homology to known viruses, novel viruses in clinical samples were successfully identified on the basis of their ability to hybridize to these prespecified sequences. This methodology famously contributed to identification of the coronavirus causing severe acute respiratory syndrome (SARS). Once discovered, this SARS coronavirus was rapidly sequenced: the full genome was assembled in April 2003, less than 6 months after recognition of the first case. This accomplishment illustrated the advancing power and speed of new diagnostic technologies.

With the advent of next-generation sequencing, unbiased pathogen discovery is now possible through a process known as *metagenomic assembly* (Fig. 146-3). Sequences of random nucleotide fragments can be generated from clinical specimens with no a priori knowledge of pathogen identity through a process called *shotgun sequencing*. This collection of sequences can then be computationally aligned to host (i.e., human) sequences, with aligned sequences removed and remaining sequences compared with other known genomes to detect the presence of known microorganisms. Sequence fragments that remain unaligned suggest the presence of an additional organism that cannot be matched to a known, characterized genome; these reads can be assembled into contiguous nucleic acid stretches that can be compared to known sequences to construct the genome of a potentially novel organism. Assembled genomes (or parts of genomes) can then be compared to known genomes to infer the phylogeny of new organisms and identify related classes or traits. Thus, not only can this process identify unanticipated pathogens; it can even identify undiscovered organisms. Some early applications of sequencing on clinical samples have centered around the discovery of novel viruses, including such emerging pathogens as West Nile virus, SARS coronavirus, and the Middle East respiratory syndrome coronavirus (MERS-CoV) that has caused severe respiratory illnesses in healthy adults, as well as viral causes of myriad other conditions, from tropical hemorrhagic fevers to diarrhea in newborns.

More recently, metagenomic assembly has been successfully extended to bacterial pathogen discovery. Investigators identified a new bacterial species associated with "cord colitis"—a rare antibiotic-responsive, culture-negative colitis in recipients of umbilical cord-blood stem cells—by sequencing colon biopsy samples from affected patients and matched controls. A single dominant species emerged from metagenomic assembly in samples from patients that was absent from control samples. The presence of this species was confirmed by PCR and fluorescence in situ hybridization on primary tissue samples. On the basis of its similarity to other known species, the organism was named *Bradyrhizobium enterica*, a novel species from a genus that has proved difficult to culture and thus would have been hard to identify by other means. Correlation versus causation remains an open question; therefore, further efforts will be required to make such links.

As metagenomic sequencing and assembly techniques become more robust, this technology holds great promise for identifying microorganisms that are associated with clinical conditions of unknown etiology. Conventional methods already have unexpectedly linked numerous conditions with specific agents of infection—e.g., cervical and oropharyngeal cancers with human papillomavirus, Kaposi's sarcoma with human herpesvirus 8, and certain lymphomas with Epstein-Barr virus. Sequencing techniques offer unprecedented sensitivity and specificity for identifying foreign nucleic acid sequences that may suggest other conditions—from malignancies to inflammatory conditions to unexplained fevers or other clinical syndromes—associated with organisms

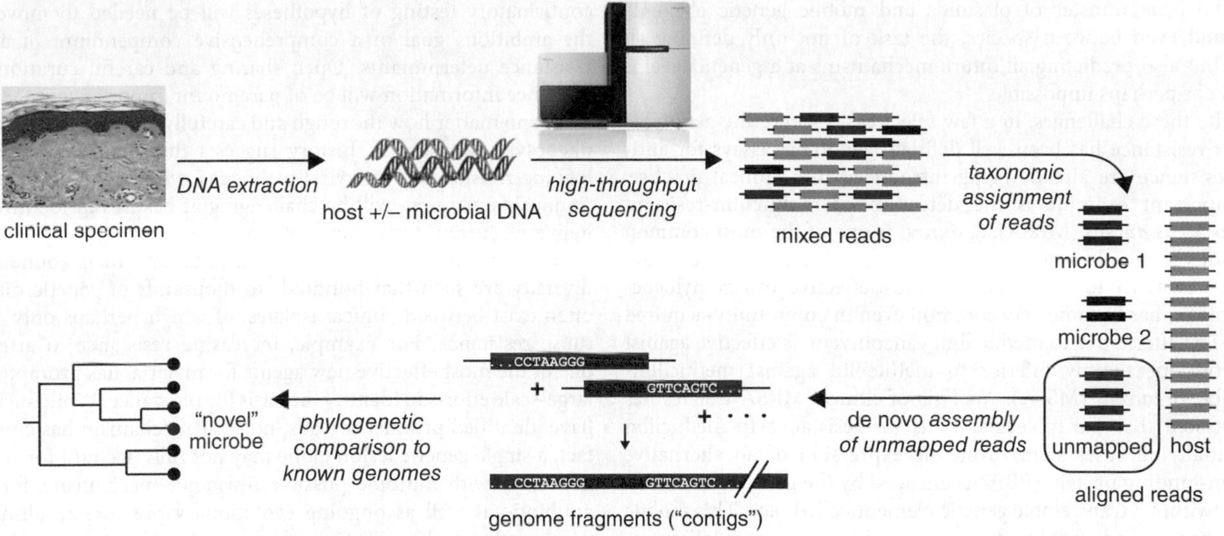

FIGURE 146-3 Workflow of metagenomic assembly for pathogen discovery. DNA is isolated from a specimen of interest (e.g., tissue, body fluid) containing a mixture of host DNA and nucleic acids from coexisting microbes, either commensal or pathogenic. All DNA (and RNA if a reverse transcription step is added) is then sequenced, yielding a mixture of DNA sequence fragments ("reads") from organisms present. These reads are then aligned to existing reference genomes for the host or any known microbes, leaving reads that do not align ("map") to any known sequence. These unmapped reads are then computationally assembled de novo into the largest contiguous stretches of DNA possible ("contigs"), representing fragments of previously unsequenced genomes. These genome fragments (contigs) are then mapped onto a phylogenetic tree based on their sequence. Some may represent known but as yet unsequenced organisms, while others will represent novel species. *(Figure prepared with valuable input from Dr. Ami S. Bhatt, personal communication.)*

from viruses to bacteria to parasites. As sequencing-based discovery expands, microbes may be found to be associated with conditions not classically thought of as infectious. Studies of bowel flora in laboratory animals and even humans are already beginning to suggest correlations between microbe composition and various aspects of metabolic and cardiovascular health. Improved methods for pathogen detection will continue to uncover unexpected correlations between microbes and disease states, but the mere presence of a microbe does not establish causality. Fortunately, once the relatively laborious and computationally intensive metagenomic sequencing and assembly efforts have identified a pathogen, further detection can easily be undertaken with targeted methods such as PCR or hybridization, which are much more straightforward and scalable. This capacity should facilitate the additional careful investigation that will be required to progress beyond correlation and to draw causal inference.

ANTIBIOTIC RESISTANCE

At present, antibiotic resistance in bacteria and fungi is determined by isolating a single colony from a cultured clinical specimen and testing its growth in the presence of a drug. The requirement for multiple growth steps in these conventional assays has several consequences. First, only culturable pathogens can be readily processed. Second, this process requires considerable infrastructure to support the sterile environment required for culture-based testing of diverse organisms. Finally, and perhaps most significantly, even the fastest-growing organisms require 1–2 days of processing for identification and 2–3 days for determination of susceptibilities. Slower-growing organisms take even longer: for instance, weeks must pass before drug-resistant *M. tuberculosis* can be identified by growth phenotype. Given the clinical imperative in serious illness to begin effective therapy early, this inherent delay in susceptibility determination has obvious implications for empirical antibiotic use: broad-spectrum antibiotics often must be chosen up front in situations where it is later shown that preferred narrower-spectrum drugs would have been effective or even that no antibiotics were appropriate (i.e., in viral infections). With this strategy, the empirical choice can be incorrect, often with devastating consequences. Real-time identification of the infecting organism and information on its susceptibility profile would guide initial therapy and support judicious antibiotic use, ideally improving patient outcomes while aiding in the ever-escalating struggle with antibiotic resistance by reserving the use of broad-spectrum agents for cases in which they are truly needed.

Molecular diagnostics and sequencing offer a way to accelerate detection of a pathogen's antibiotic susceptibility profile. If a genotype that confers resistance can be identified, this genotype can be targeted for molecular detection. In infectious disease, this approach has most convincingly come to fruition for HIV (Fig. 146-2*A*). (In a conceptually parallel application of genomic analysis, molecular detection of certain resistance determinants in cancers is beginning to inform chemotherapeutic selection.) Extensive sequencing of HIV strains and correlations drawn between viral genotypes and phenotypic resistance have delineated the majority of mutations in key HIV genes, such as reverse transcriptase, protease, and integrase, that confer resistance to the antiretroviral agents that target these proteins. For instance, the single-amino-acid substitution K103N in the HIV reverse transcriptase gene predicts resistance to the first-line nonnucleoside reverse transcriptase inhibitor efavirenz, and its detection thus informs a clinician to choose a different agent. The effects of these common mutations on HIV susceptibility to various drugs—as well as on viral fitness—are curated in publically available databases. Thus, genotypes are now routinely used to predict drug resistance in HIV, as phenotypic resistance assays are far more cumbersome than targeted sequencing. Indeed, current recommendations in the United States are to sequence virus from a patient's blood before initiating antiretroviral therapy, which is then tailored to the predicted resistance phenotype. As new targeted therapies are introduced, this targeted sequencing–based approach to drug resistance will likely prove important in other viral infections (e.g., hepatitis C).

For several reasons, the challenge of predicting antibiotic susceptibility from genotype has not yet been met in bacteria to the same degree as in HIV. In general, bacteria have evolved diverse resistance mechanisms to most antibiotics; thus, the task cannot be reduced to probing for a single genetic lesion, target, or mechanism. For instance, at least five distinct modes of resistance to fluoroquinolones are known: reduced import, increased efflux, mutated target sites, drug modification, and shielding of the target sites by expression of another protein. Further, we lack a comprehensive compendium of genetic elements conferring resistance, and new mechanisms and genes emerge regularly in the face of antibiotic deployment. As bacteria have far more complex genomes than viruses, with thousands of genes on their chromosomes and the capacity for acquiring many more through horizontal gene transfer of plasmids and mobile genetic elements within and even between species, the task of not only defining all current but also predicting all future mechanisms at a genetic level is daunting or perhaps impossible.

Despite these challenges, in a few select cases where the genotypic basis for resistance has been well defined, genotypic assays for antibiotic resistance are already being introduced into clinical practice. One important example is the detection of methicillin-resistant *Staphylococcus aureus* (MRSA). *S. aureus* is one of the most common and serious bacterial pathogens of humans, particularly in health care settings. Resistance to methicillin, the most effective antistaphylococcal antibiotic, has become very common even in community-acquired strains. The alternative to methicillin, vancomycin, is effective against MRSA but measurably inferior to methicillin against methicillin-susceptible *S. aureus* (MSSA). Analysis of clinical MRSA isolates has demonstrated that the molecular basis for resistance to methicillin in essentially all cases stems from the expression of an alternative penicillin-binding protein (PBP2A) encoded by the gene *mecA*, which is found within a transferable genetic element called *mec*. This mobile cassette has spread rapidly through the *S. aureus* population via horizontal gene transfer and selection from widespread antibiotic use. Because resistance is essentially always due to the presence of the *mec* cassette, MRSA is amenable to molecular detection. In recent years, a PCR test for the presence of the *mec* cassette, which saves hours to days compared with standard culture-based methods, has been approved by the U.S. Food and Drug Administration.

Additional molecular diagnostics are being implemented in the evaluation of bacterial antibiotic resistance. Vancomycin-resistant enterococci (VRE) harbor one of a limited number of *van* genes responsible for resistance to this important antibiotic by altering the mechanism for cell wall cross-linking that vancomycin inhibits. Detection of one of these genes by PCR indicates resistance. Identification of two carbapenemase-encoding plasmids—NDM-1 and KPC—responsible for a significant fraction of carbapenem resistance (though not for all such resistance) has led to the development of a multiplexed PCR assay to detect these important resistance elements. Because carbapenems are broad-spectrum antibiotics frequently reserved for multidrug-resistant bacteria (particularly enteric gram-negative bacilli) and are often used as antibiotics of last resort, the initial appearance of resistance and the subsequent increase in its prevalence have caused considerable concern. Therefore, even though other mechanisms for carbapenem resistance exist, a rapid PCR test for the two plasmids encoding these two carbapenemases has been developed to aid in both diagnostic and infection control efforts. Efforts are under way to extend this multiplexed PCR assay to other plasmid-borne carbapenemases and thus to make it more comprehensive.

The power and application of molecular genetic tests are not limited to high-income settings. With the increasing burden of drug-resistant tuberculosis in the developing world, a molecular diagnostic test has now been developed to detect rifampin-resistant tuberculosis. The genetic basis for rifampin resistance has been well defined by targeted sequencing: characteristic mutations in the molecular target of rifampin, RNA polymerase, account for the vast majority of rifampin-resistant strains of *M. tuberculosis*. A PCR assay that can detect both the *M. tuberculosis* organism and a rifampin-resistant allele of RNA polymerase from clinical samples has recently been approved. Since rifampin resistance frequently accompanies resistance to other antibiotics, this test can suggest the possible presence of multidrug-resistant *M. tuberculosis* within hours instead of weeks.

Despite differences in relative genome complexity, HIV genotypic screening for antiretroviral resistance offers one framework for broadening efforts at genotypic assays for nonviral antibiotic resistance. As whole-genome pathogen sequencing has become increasingly feasible and inexpensive (Fig. 146-1), significant efforts have been launched to sequence hundreds to thousands of antibiotic-sensitive and -resistant isolates of a given pathogen in order to more comprehensively define resistance-conferring genetic elements. In parallel with advancing sequencing technologies, progress in computational techniques, bioinformatics and statistics, and data storage as well as experimental confirmatory testing of hypotheses will be needed to move toward the ambitious goal of a comprehensive compendium of antibiotic resistance determinants. Open sharing and careful curation of new sequence information will be of paramount importance.

Yet no matter how thorough and carefully curated such a genotype-phenotype database is, history suggests that comprehensively cataloguing resistance in nonviral pathogens, with new mechanisms continuously emerging, will be challenging at best. Even identifying and itemizing current resistance mutations is a daunting prospect: nonviral genomes are much larger than viral ones, and their abundance and diversity are such that hundreds to thousands of genetic differences often exist between clinical isolates, of which perhaps only one may cause resistance. For example, increasing resistance to artemisinin, one of the most effective new agents for malaria, has prompted recent large-scale efforts to identify the basis for resistance. While such studies have identified promising leads, no clear mechanism has emerged; in fact, a single genetic lesion alone may not fully account for resistance. Especially with multiple possible resistance mechanisms for a given antibiotic as well as ongoing evolutionary pressure resulting in the development and acquisition of new modes of resistance, a genotypic approach to diagnosing antibiotic resistance is likely to be imperfect.

We have already observed the accumulation of new or unanticipated modes of resistance from ongoing evolutionary pressure caused by the widespread clinical use of antibiotics. Even with MRSA, perhaps the best-studied case of antibiotic resistance and a model of relative simplicity with a single known monogenic resistance determinant (*mecA*), a genotype-based approach to resistance detection proved flawed. One limitation was a recall of the initial commercial genotypic resistance assay that was deployed for the identification of MRSA. A clinical isolate of *S. aureus* emerged in Belgium that expressed a variant of the *mec* cassette not detected by the assay's PCR primers. New primers were added to detect this new variant, and the assay was re-approved for use. More recently, an even more divergent but functionally analogous gene called *mecC*, which confers methicillin resistance but evades PCR detection by this assay, was found. This series of events exemplifies the need for ongoing monitoring of any genotypic resistance assay. A second limitation is that a contradiction can occur between genotypic and phenotypic evidence for resistance. Up to 5% of MSSA strains carry a copy of the *mecA* gene that is either nonfunctional or not expressed. Thus, the erroneous identification of these strains as MRSA by genotypic detection would lead to administration of the inferior antibiotic vancomycin rather than the preferred β-lactam therapy.

These examples illustrate one of the prime challenges of moving beyond growth-based assays: genotype is merely a proxy for the resistance phenotype that directly informs patient care. One alternative approach currently under development attempts to circumvent the limitations of genotypic resistance testing by returning to a phenotypic approach, albeit one informed by genomic methods: transcriptional profiles serve as a rapid phenotypic signature for antibiotic response. Conceptually, since dying cells are transcriptionally distinct from cells fated to survive, susceptible bacteria enact different transcriptional profiles after antibiotic exposure that are different from the profiles of resistant strains, independent of the mechanism of resistance. These differences can be measured and, since transcription is one of the most rapid responses to cell stress (minutes to hours), can be used to determine whether cells are resistant or susceptible much more rapidly than is possible if one waits for growth in the presence of antibiotics (days). Like DNA, RNA can be readily detected through predictable rules governing base pairing via either amplification or hybridization-based methods. Changes in a carefully selected set of transcripts form an expression signature that can represent the total cellular response to antibiotic without requiring full characterization of the entire transcriptome. Preliminary proof-of-concept studies suggest that this approach may identify antibiotic susceptibility on the basis of transcriptional phenotype much more quickly than is possible with growth-based assays.

Because of its sensitivity in detecting even very rare nucleic acid fragments, sequencing is now permitting studies of unprecedented depth into complex populations of cells and tissues. The strength of this depth and sensitivity applies not only to the detection of rare, novel pathogens in a sea of host signal but also to the identification of heterogeneous pathogen subpopulations in a single host that may differ, for example, in drug resistance profiles or pathogenesis determinants. Future studies will be needed to elucidate the clinical significance of these variable subpopulations, even as deep sequencing is now providing unprecedented levels of detail about majority and minority members of this population.

HOST-BASED DIAGNOSTICS

While pathogen-based diagnostics continue to be the mainstay for diagnosing infection, serologic testing has long been the basis of a strategy to diagnose infection by measuring host responses. Here, too, the application of genomics is now being explored to improve upon this approach, given the previously described limitations of serologic testing. Rather than using antibody responses as a retrospective biomarker for infection, recent efforts have focused on transcriptomic analysis of the host response as a new direction with diagnostic implications for human disease. For instance, while pathogen-based diagnostic tests to distinguish active from latent tuberculosis infection have proved elusive, recent work shows that the transcriptional profile of circulating white blood cells exhibits a differential pattern of expression of nearly 400 transcripts that distinguish active from latent tuberculosis; this expression pattern is driven in part by changes in interferon-inducible genes in the myeloid lineage. In a validation cohort, this transcriptional signature was able to distinguish patients with active versus latent disease, to distinguish tuberculosis infection from other pulmonary inflammatory states or infections, and to track responses to treatment in as little as 2 weeks, with normalization of expression toward that of patients without active disease over 6 months of effective therapy. Such a test could play an important role not only in the management of patients but also as a marker of efficacy in clinical trials of new therapeutic agents. Similarly, other investigators have been trying to identify host transcriptional signatures in circulating blood cells that are distinct in influenza A infection from those in upper respiratory infections caused by certain other viruses or bacteria. These signatures also varied with phase of infection and showed promise in distinguishing exposed subjects who will become symptomatic from those who will not. These results suggest that profiling of host transcriptional dynamics could augment the information obtained from studies of pathogens, both enhancing diagnosis and monitoring the progression of illness and the response to therapy.

In this era of genome-wide association studies and attempts to move toward personalized medicine, genomic approaches are also being applied to the identification of host genetic loci and factors that contribute to infection susceptibility. Such loci will have undergone strong selection among populations in which the disease is endemic. By identifying the beneficial genetic alleles among individuals who survive in such settings, markers for susceptibility or resistance are being discovered; these markers can be translated into diagnostic tests to identify susceptible individuals in order to implement preventive or prophylactic interventions. Further, such studies may offer mechanistic insight into the pathogenesis of infection and inform new methods of therapeutic intervention. Such beneficial genetic associations were recognized long before the advent of genomics, as in the protective effects of the negative Duffy blood group or heterozygous hemoglobin abnormalities against *Plasmodium* infection. Genomic methods enable more systematic and widespread investigations of the host to identify not only people with altered susceptibility to numerous diseases (e.g., HIV infection, tuberculosis, and cholera) but also host factors that contribute to and thus might predict the severity of disease.

THERAPEUTICS

Genomics has the potential to impact infectious disease therapeutics in two ways. By transforming the speed of diagnostic information acquisition or the type of diagnostic information that can be attained, it can influence therapeutic decision-making. Alternatively, by opening up new avenues to understanding pathogenesis, providing new ways to disrupt infection, and delineating new approaches to antibiotic discovery, it can facilitate the development of new therapeutic agents.

GENOMIC DIAGNOSTICS INFORMING THERAPEUTICS

Efforts at antibiotic discovery are declining, with few new agents in the pipeline and even fewer entering the market. This phenomenon is due in part to the lack of economic incentives for the private sector; however, it is also attributable in part to the enormous challenges involved in the discovery and development of antibiotics. For obvious market-related reasons, nearly all efforts have focused on broad-spectrum antibiotics; the development of a chemical entity that works across an extremely diverse set of organisms (i.e., more divergent from each other than a human is from an amoeba) is far more challenging than the development of an agent that is designed to target a single bacterial species. Nevertheless, the concept of narrow-spectrum antibiotics has heretofore been rejected because of the lack of early diagnostic information that would guide the selection of such agents. Thus, rapid diagnostics providing antibiotic susceptibility information that can guide antibiotic selection in real time have the potential to alter and simplify antibiotic strategies by allowing a paradigm shift away from broad-spectrum drugs and toward narrow-spectrum agents. Such a paradigm shift clearly would have additional implications for the current escalation of antibiotic resistance.

In yet another diagnostic paradigm with the potential to impact therapeutic interventions, genomics is opening new avenues to a better understanding not only of different host susceptibilities to infection but also of different host responses to therapy. In a sense, the promise of "personalized medicine" has been a tantalizing holy grail. Some signs now point to the realization of this goal. For example, the role of glucocorticoids in tuberculous meningitis has been long debated. Recently, polymorphisms in the human genetic locus *LTA4H*, which encodes a leukotriene-modifying enzyme, were found to modulate the inflammatory response to tuberculosis. Patients with tuberculous meningitis who were homozygous for the proinflammatory *LTA4H* allele were most helped by adjunctive glucocorticoid treatment, while those who were homozygous for the anti-inflammatory allele were negatively affected by steroid treatment. This anti-inflammatory adjunct has become the standard of care in tuberculous meningitis, but this study suggests that perhaps only a subset of patients benefit and further suggests a genetic means of prospectively identifying this subset. Thus, genomic diagnostic tests may eventually inform diagnosis, prognosis, and treatment decisions by revealing the pathogenic potential of the microbe and detecting host responses to both infection and therapy.

GENOMICS IN DRUG AND VACCINE DEVELOPMENT

Genomic technologies are already dramatically changing research on host–pathogen interactions, with a goal of increasingly influencing the process of therapeutic discovery and development. Sequencing offers several possible avenues into antimicrobial therapeutic discovery. First, genomic-scale molecular methods have paved the way for comprehensive identification of all essential genes encoded within a pathogen's genome, with consequent systematic identification of all possible vulnerabilities within a pathogen that could be targeted therapeutically. Second, transcriptional profiling can offer insights into mechanisms of action of new candidate drugs that emerge from screens. For instance, the transcriptional signature of cell wall disruptors (e.g., β-lactams) is distinct from that of DNA-damaging agents (e.g., fluoroquinolones) or protein synthesis inhibitors (e.g., aminoglycosides). Thus, transcriptional analysis of a pathogen's response to a new antibiotic can either suggest a mechanism of action or flag compounds for prioritization because of a potentially novel activity. In an alternative genomic strategy for determining mechanisms of action, an RNA interference approach followed by targeted sequencing has been used to identify genes required for antitrypanosomal drug efficacy. This approach provided new insights into the mechanism of action of drugs that have been in use for decades for human African trypanosomiasis. Third, sequencing can readily identify the most conserved regions of a pathogen's genomes and corresponding gene products; this information is invaluable in narrowing antigen candidates for vaccine development. These surface proteins can be expressed recombinantly and tested for the ability to elicit a serologic response and protective immunity. This process, termed *reverse vaccinology*, has proved particularly useful for pathogens that are difficult to culture or poorly immunogenic, as was the case with the development of a vaccine for *Neisseria meningitidis* serogroup B.

Large-scale gene content analysis from sequencing or expression profiling enables new research directions that provide novel insights into the interplay of pathogen and host during infection or colonization. One important goal of such research is to suggest new therapeutic approaches to disrupt this interaction in favor of the host. Indeed, one of the most immediate applications of next-generation sequencing technology has come from simply characterizing human pathogens and related commensal or environmental strains and then finding genomic correlates for pathogenicity. For instance, as *Escherichia coli* varies from a simple nonpathogenic, lab-adapted strain (K-12) to a Shiga toxin–producing enterohemorrhagic gastrointestinal pathogen (O157:H7), it displays up to a 25% difference in gene content, even though its phylogenetic classification stays the same. Although this is an extreme example, it is not an isolated case. Some isolates of *Enterococcus*—notorious for its increasing incidence of resistance to common antibiotics such as ampicillin, vancomycin, and aminoglycosides—also contain recently acquired genetic material comprising up to 25% of the genome on mobile genetic elements. This fact suggests that horizontal gene transfer may play an important role in the organism's adaptation as a nosocomial pathogen. On closer study, this genome expansion has been demonstrated to be associated with loss of regulatory elements called CRISPRs (*c*lustered, *r*egularly *i*nterspaced *s*hort *p*alindromic *r*epeats). Loss of CRISPR elements, which protect the bacterial genome from invasion by certain foreign genetic materials, may thus facilitate the acquisition of antibiotic resistance–conferring genetic elements. While loss of this regulation appears to impose a competitive disadvantage in antibiotic-free environments, these drug-resistant strains thrive in the presence of even some of the most useful antienterococcal therapies. In addition to insights gained from genome sequencing, extension of unbiased whole-transcriptome sequencing (RNA-Seq) efforts to bacteria is beginning to identify unexpected regulatory, noncoding RNAs in many diverse species. While the functional implications of these new transcripts are as yet largely unknown, the presence of such features—conserved across many bacterial species—implies evolutionary importance and suggests areas for future study and possible new therapeutic avenues.

Thus, genomic studies are already beginning to transform our understanding of infection, offering evidence of virulence factors or toxins and providing insight into ongoing evolution of pathogenicity and drug resistance. One goal of such studies is to identify therapeutic agents that can disrupt the pathogenic process; there is currently much interest in the theoretical concept of antivirulence drugs that inhibit virulence factors rather than killing the pathogen outright as a means to intervene in infection. Further, as sequencing becomes increasingly accessible and efficient, large-scale studies with unprecedented statistical power to associate clinical outcomes with pathogen and host genotypes and thus to further reveal vulnerabilities in the infection process that can be targeted for disruption are being initiated. Although this is just the beginning, such studies point to a tantalizing future in which the clinician is armed with genomic predictors of infection outcome and therapeutic response to guide clinical decision-making.

EPIDEMIOLOGY OF INFECTIOUS DISEASES

Epidemiologic studies of infectious diseases have several main goals: to identify and characterize outbreaks, to describe the pattern and dynamics of an infectious disease as it spreads through populations, and to identify interventions that can limit or reduce the burden of disease. One classic, paradigmatic example is John Snow's elucidation of the origin of the 1854 London cholera outbreak. Snow used careful geographic mapping of cases to determine that the likely source of the outbreak was contaminated water from the Broad Street pump, and, by removing the pump handle, he aborted the outbreak. Whereas that intervention was undertaken without knowledge of the causative agent of cholera, advances in microbiology and genomics have expanded the purview of epidemiology, which now considers not just the disease but also the pathogen, its virulence factors, and the complex relationships between microbial and host populations.

Through the use of novel genomic tools such as high-throughput sequencing, the diversity of a microbial population can now be rapidly described with unprecedented resolution, with discrimination between isolates that have single-nucleotide differences across the entire genome and advancement beyond prior approaches that relied on phenotypes (such as antibiotic resistance testing) or genetic markers (such as multilocus sequence typing). The development of statistical methods grounded in molecular genetics and evolutionary theory has established analytical approaches that translate descriptions of microbial population diversity and structure into insights into the origin and history of pathogen spread. By linking phylogenetic reconstruction with epidemiologic and demographic data, genomic epidemiology provides the opportunity to track transmission from person to person, to infer transmission patterns of both pathogens and sequence elements that confer phenotypes of interest, and to estimate the transmission dynamics of outbreaks.

DECIPHERING PERSON-TO-PERSON TRANSMISSION

The use of comparisons of whole-genome sequencing to infer person-to-person transmission and identify point-source outbreaks of pathogens has proved useful in hospital infection control settings. As reported in a seminal paper in 2010, a study of MRSA in a Thai hospital demonstrated that whole-genome sequencing can be used to infer transmission of a pathogen from patient to patient within a hospital setting through integration of the analysis of accumulation of mutations over time with dates and hospital locations of the infections. Since that time, multiple instances of the use of whole-genome sequencing to define and motivate interventions aimed at interrupting transmission chains have been reported. In another MRSA outbreak in a special-care baby unit in Cambridge, United Kingdom, whole-genome sequencing extended the traditional infection control analysis, which relies on typing organisms by their antibiotic susceptibilities, to sequencing of isolates from clinical samples. This approach identified an otherwise unrecognized outbreak of a specific MRSA strain that was occurring against a background of the usual pattern of infections caused by a diverse circulating population of MRSA strains. The analysis showed evidence of transmission among mothers within the special-care baby unit and in the community and demonstrated the key role of MRSA carriage in a single health care provider in the persistence of the outbreak. MRSA decolonization of the health care provider terminated the outbreak. In yet another example, in response to the observation of 18 cases of infection by carbapenemase-producing *Klebsiella pneumoniae* over 6 months at the National Institutes of Health Clinical Research Center, genome sequencing of the isolates was used to discriminate between the possibilities that these cases represented multiple, independent introductions into the health care system or a single introduction with subsequent transmission. On the basis of network and phylogenetic analysis of genomic and epidemiologic data, the authors reconstructed the likely relationships among the isolates from patient to patient, demonstrating that the spread of resistant *Klebsiella* infection was in fact due to nosocomial transmission of a single strain.

Uncovering of unexpected transmission events by genomic epidemiology studies is motivating renewed questioning of pathogen ecology and modes of transmission. For example, the rise in prevalence of infections with nontuberculous mycobacteria, including *Mycobacterium abscessus*, among patients with cystic fibrosis (CF) has led to speculation about the possible role of patient-to-patient transmission in the CF community; however, conventional typing approaches have lacked the resolution to define population structure accurately, a critical component of inferring transmission. Past infection control guidelines discounted the possibility of acquisition of nontuberculous mycobacteria in health care settings, as no strong evidence for such transmission had been described. In a whole-genome sequencing study of *M. abscessus* isolates from patients with CF, an analytical approach using genome sequencing, epidemiology, and

Bayesian modeling examined the likelihood of transmission between patients within a CF center; the authors found nearly identical isolates in a number of patients and observed that these isolates were less diverse than isolates from a single individual. Because no clear epidemiologic link places the infected patients in the same place at the same time, this finding highlights a need to explore preexisting notions of circumstances required for transmission and a reconsideration of *M. abscessus* infection control guidelines. Similar studies of other pathogens—particularly those that share human, other animal host, and environmental reservoirs—will continue to advance our insight into the relative roles and prominence of sources of infection as well as the modes of spread through populations, thereby establishing evidence-based strategies for prevention and intervention.

As increasing numbers of studies aim to carefully define the origins and spread of infectious agents using the high-resolution lens of whole-genome sequencing, fundamental questions are arising with regard to our understanding of infection in a single individual and the process of a single transmission event. For example, a better understanding of a pathogen population's diversity within a single infected individual is a critical component in interpreting the relationship among isolates from different patients. While we have traditionally thought of individuals as infected with a single bacterial strain, a recent sequencing study of multiple colonies of *S. aureus* from a single individual showed a "cloud" of diversity; this finding raises a number of questions that will be important to address as this field develops: What is the clinical significance of this diversity? What are the processes that generate and limit diversity? What amount of diversity is transmitted under different conditions and routes of transmission? How do the answers to these questions vary by infectious organism, type of infection, and host and in response to treatment? More comprehensive descriptions of diversity, population dynamics, transmission bottlenecks, and the forces that shape and influence the growth and spread of microbial populations will be a critically important focus of future investigations.

RECONSTRUCTING THE ORIGINS AND DYNAMICS OF PATHOGEN SPREAD

In addition to reconstructing the transmission chains of local outbreaks, genomics-based epidemiologic methods are providing insight into broad-scale geographic and temporal spread of pathogens. A classic example has been the study of cholera, the dehydrating diarrheal illness caused by infection with *Vibrio cholerae*. Cholera first spread worldwide from the Indian subcontinent in the 1800s and has since caused seven pandemics; the seventh pandemic has been ongoing since the 1960s. An investigation into the geographic patterns of cholera spread in the seventh pandemic used genome sequences from a global collection of 154 *V. cholerae* strains representing isolates from 1957–2010. This investigation revealed that the seventh pandemic has comprised at least three overlapping waves spreading out from the Indian subcontinent (Fig. 146-4). Further, analysis of the genome of an isolate of *V. cholerae* from the 2010 outbreak of cholera in Haiti showed it to be more closely related to isolates from South Asia than to isolates from neighboring Latin America, a result supporting the hypothesis that the outbreak was derived from *V. cholerae* introduced into Haiti by human travel (likely from Nepal) rather than by environmental or more geographically proximal sources. A subsequent study that dated the time to the most recent common ancestor of a population of *V. cholerae* isolates from Haiti provided further support for a single point-source introduction from Nepal.

Increasing numbers of investigations into the spread of many pathogens—thus far including strains of *S. aureus*, *S. pneumoniae*, *Chlamydia*, *Salmonella*, *Shigella*, *E. coli*, *C. difficile*, West Nile virus, rabies virus, and dengue virus—are contributing to a growing atlas of maps describing routes, patterns, and tempos of microbial diversification and dissemination. Large-scale efforts like the 100K Foodborne Pathogen Genome Project, which aims to sequence the genomes of 100,000 strains of food-borne pathogens collected from sources including food, the environment, and farm animals, are possible because of advances in sequencing technologies. Such studies will yield a vast amount of data that can be used to investigate diversity and microbiologic links within distinct niches and the patterns of spread from one niche to another. The increasingly broad adoption of genome sequencing by health care and public health institutions will ensure that the available catalog of genome sequences and associated epidemiologic data will grow very rapidly. With higher-resolution description of microbial diversity and of the dynamics of that diversity over time and across epidemiologic and demographic boundaries and evolutionary niches, we will gain even greater insights into the relationships of transmission routes and patterns of historic spread.

PREDICTING EPIDEMIC POTENTIAL

Defining pathogen transmissibility is a critical step in the development of public health surveillance and intervention strategies as this information can help predict the epidemic potential of an outbreak. Transmissibility can be estimated by a variety of methods, including inference from the growth rate of an epidemic together with the generation time of an infection (the mean interval between infection of an index case and of the people infected by that index case). Genome

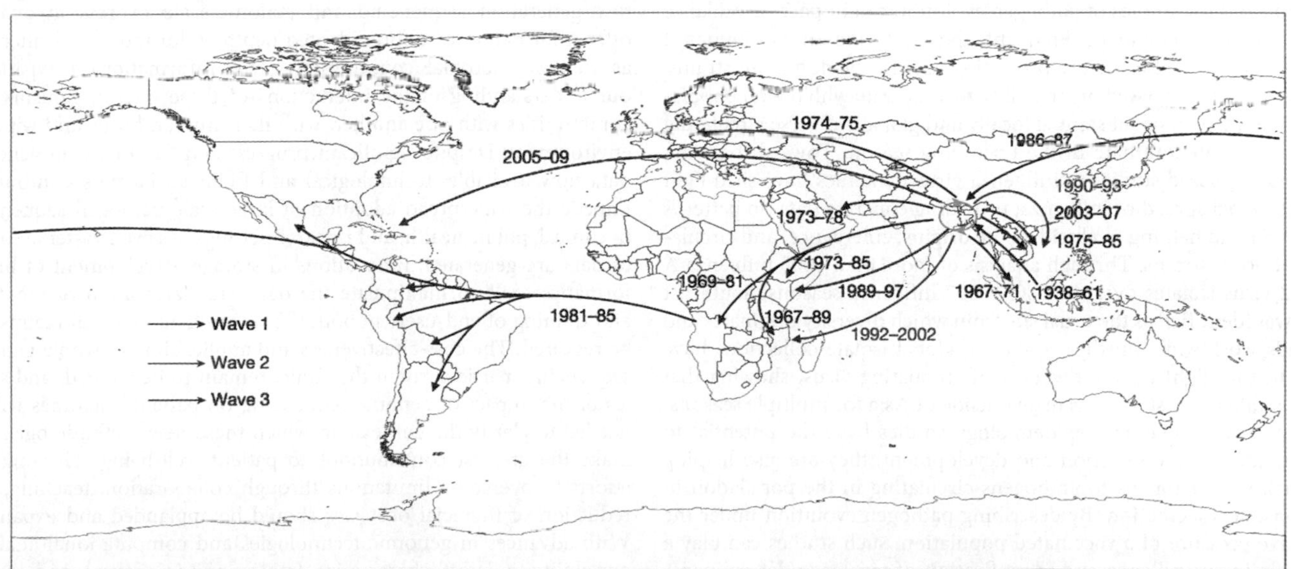

FIGURE 146-4 Transmission events inferred from phylogenetic reconstruction of 154 *Vibrio cholerae* isolates from the seventh cholera pandemic. Date ranges represent estimated time to the most recent common ancestor for strains transmitted from source to destination locations, based on a Bayesian model of the phylogeny. *(Reprinted with permission from A Mutreja et al: Evidence for several waves of global transmission in the seventh cholera pandemic. Nature 477:462, 2011.)*

sequencing and analysis of a well-sampled population provide another method by which to derive similar fundamental epidemiologic parameters. One key measure of transmissibility is the basic reproduction number (R0), defined as the number of secondary infections generated from a single primary infectious case. When the basic reproduction number is greater than 1 (R0 >1), an outbreak has epidemic potential; when it is less than 1 (R0 <1), the outbreak will become extinct. On the basis of sequences from influenza samples obtained from infected patients very early in the 2009 H1N1 influenza pandemic, the basic reproduction number was estimated through a population genomic analysis at 1.2; this compared to estimates of 1.4–1.6 based on several epidemiologic analyses. In addition, with the assumption of a molecular clock model, sequences of H1N1 samples together with information about when and where the samples were obtained have been used to estimate the date and location of the pandemic's origin, providing insight into disease origins and dynamics. Because the magnitude and intensity of the public health response are guided by the predicted size of an outbreak, the ability of genomic methods to elucidate a pathogen's origin and epidemic potential adds an important dimension to the contributions of these methods to infectious disease epidemiology.

PROVIDING INSIGHT INTO PATHOGEN EVOLUTION

Beyond describing transmission and dynamics, pathogen genomics can provide insight into the evolution of pathogens and the interaction of selective pressures, the host, and pathogen populations, which can have implications for vaccine or therapeutic development. From a clinical perspective, this process is central to the acquisition of antibiotic resistance, the generation of increasing pathogenicity or new virulence traits, the evasion of host immunity and clearance (leading to chronic infection), and vaccine efficacy.

Microbial genomes evolve through a variety of mechanisms, including mutation, duplication, insertion, deletion, recombination, and horizontal gene transfer. Segmented viruses (e.g., influenza virus) can reassort gene segments within multiply infected cells. The pandemic 2009 H1N1 influenza A virus, for example, appears to have been generated through reassortment of several avian, swine, and human influenza strains. Such potential for the evolution of novel pandemic strains has precipitated concern about the possible evolution to transmissibility of virulent strains that have been associated with high mortality rates but have not yet exhibited efficient human infectivity. Controversial experiments with H5N1 avian influenza virus, for example, have defined five mutations that render the virus transmissible, at least in ferrets—the animal model system for human influenza.

The continual antigenic evolution of seasonal influenza offers an example of how studies of pathogen evolution can impact surveillance and vaccine development. Frequent updates to the annual influenza vaccine are needed to ensure protection against the dominant strains. These updates are based on an ability to anticipate which viral populations from a pool of substantial locally and globally diverse circulating viruses will predominate in the upcoming season. Toward that end, sequencing-based studies of influenza virus dynamics have shed light on the global spread of influenza, providing concrete data on patterns of spread and helping to elucidate the origins, emergence, and circulation of novel strains. Through analysis of more than 1000 influenza A H3N2 virus isolates over the 2002–2007 influenza seasons, Southeast Asia was identified as the usual site from which diversity originates and spreads worldwide. Further studies of global isolate collections have shed further light on the diversity of circulating virus, showing that some strains persist and circulate outside of Asia for multiple seasons.

Not only do genomic epidemiology studies have the potential to help guide vaccine selection and development; they are also helping to track what happens to pathogens circulating in the population in response to vaccination. By describing pathogen evolution under the selective pressure of a vaccinated population, such studies can play a key role in surveillance and identification of virulence determinants and perhaps may even help to predict the future evolution of escape from vaccine protection. The 7-valent pneumococcal conjugate vaccine (PCV-7) targeted the seven serotypes of *S. pneumoniae* responsible for the majority of cases of invasive disease at the time of its introduction in 2000; since then, PCV-7 has dramatically reduced the incidence of pneumococcal disease and mortality. Population genomic analysis of the sequences of more than 600 Massachusetts pneumococcal isolates from 2001–2007 has shown that preexisting rare nonvaccine serotypes are replacing vaccine serotypes and that some strains have persisted despite vaccination by recombining the vaccine-targeted capsule locus with a cassette of capsule genes from non-vaccine-targeted serotypes.

GLOBAL CONSIDERATIONS

While cutting-edge genomic technologies are largely implemented in the developed world, their application to infectious diseases offers perhaps the biggest potential impact in less developed regions where the burden of these infections is greatest. This globalization of genomic technology and its extensions has already begun in each of the areas of focus highlighted in this chapter; it has occurred both through the application of advanced technologies to samples collected in the developing world and through the adaptation and importation of technologies directly to the developing world for on-site implementation as they become more globally accessible. Genomic characterization of the pathogens responsible for important global illnesses such as tuberculosis, malaria, trypanosomiasis, and cholera has led to insights in diagnosis, treatment, and infection control. For instance, the nucleic acid–based test developed for rapid diagnosis of *M. tuberculosis* infection and detection of rifampin resistance is being priced for implementation in field settings in Africa and Asia where tuberculosis is most prevalent. The potential to diagnose multidrug-resistant tuberculosis in hours instead of weeks or months may truly revolutionize treatment and control of this common and devastating illness. High-resolution genomic tracking of the spread of cholera has yielded insights into which public health measures may prove most effective in controlling local epidemics. Overall, sequencing efforts have become exponentially cheaper with each passing year. As these technologies synergize with efforts to globalize information-technology resources, global implementation of genomic methods promises to spread state-of-the-art methods for diagnosis, treatment, and epidemic tracking of infections to areas that need these capabilities the most.

SUMMARY

By illuminating the genetic information that encodes the most fundamental processes of life, genomic technologies are transforming many aspects of medicine. In infectious diseases, methods such as next-generation sequencing and genome-scale expression analysis offer information of unprecedented depth about individual microbes as well as microbial communities. This information is expanding our understanding of the interactions of these microorganisms and communities with one another, with their human hosts, and with the environment. Despite significant progress and the abundant genomic data now available, technological and financial barriers continue to impede the widespread adoption of large-scale pathogen sequencing in clinical, public health, and research settings. As even vaster amounts of data are generated, innovations in storage, development of bioinformatics tools to manipulate the data, standardization of methods, and training of end-users in both the research and clinical realms will be required. The cost-effectiveness and applicability of whole-genome sequencing, particularly in the clinic, remain to be studied, and studies of the impact of genome sequencing on patient outcomes will be needed to clarify the contexts in which these new methodologies can make the greatest contributions to patient well-being. The ongoing efforts to overcome limitations through collaboration, teaching, and reduction of financial obstacles should be applauded and expanded. With advances in genomic technologies and computational analysis, our ability to detect, characterize, treat, monitor, prevent, and control infections has progressed rapidly in recent years and will continue to do so, with the hope of heralding a new era where the clinician is better armed to combat infection and promote human health.

147 Approach to the Acutely Ill Infected Febrile Patient

Tamar F. Barlam, Dennis L. Kasper

The physician treating the acutely ill febrile patient must be able to recognize infections that require emergent attention. If such infections are not adequately evaluated and treated at initial presentation, the opportunity to alter an adverse outcome may be lost. In this chapter, the clinical presentations of and approach to patients with relatively common infectious disease emergencies are discussed. These infectious processes and their treatments are discussed in detail in other chapters.

APPROACH TO THE PATIENT: Acute Febrile Illness

Before the history is elicited and a physical examination is performed, an immediate assessment of the patient's general appearance can yield valuable information. The perceptive physician's subjective sense that a patient is septic or toxic often proves accurate. Visible agitation or anxiety in a febrile patient can be a harbinger of critical illness.

HISTORY Presenting symptoms are frequently nonspecific. Detailed questions should be asked about the onset and duration of symptoms and about changes in severity or rate of progression over time. Host factors and comorbid conditions may increase the risk of infection with certain organisms or of a more fulminant course than is usually seen. Lack of splenic function, alcoholism with significant liver disease, IV drug use, HIV infection, diabetes, malignancy, organ transplantation, and chemotherapy all predispose to specific infections and frequently to increased severity. The patient should be questioned about factors that might help identify a nidus for invasive infection, such as recent upper respiratory tract infections, influenza, or varicella; prior trauma; disruption of cutaneous barriers due to lacerations, burns, surgery, body piercing, or decubiti; and the presence of foreign bodies, such as nasal packing after rhinoplasty, tampons, or prosthetic joints. Travel, contact with pets or other animals, or activities that might result in tick or mosquito exposure can lead to diagnoses that would not otherwise be considered. Recent dietary intake, medication use, social or occupational contact with ill individuals, vaccination history, recent sexual contacts, and menstrual history may be relevant. A review of systems should focus on any neurologic signs or sensorium alterations, rashes or skin lesions, and focal pain or tenderness and should also include a general review of respiratory, gastrointestinal, or genitourinary symptoms.

PHYSICAL EXAMINATION A complete physical examination should be performed, with special attention to several areas that are sometimes given short shrift in routine examinations. Assessment of the patient's general appearance and vital signs, skin and soft tissue examination, and the neurologic evaluation are of particular importance.

The patient may appear either anxious and agitated or lethargic and apathetic. Fever is usually present, although elderly patients and compromised hosts (e.g., patients who are uremic or cirrhotic and those who are taking glucocorticoids or nonsteroidal anti-inflammatory drugs) may be afebrile despite serious underlying infection. Measurement of blood pressure, heart rate, and respiratory rate helps determine the degree of hemodynamic and metabolic compromise. The patient's airway must be evaluated to rule out the risk of obstruction from an invasive oropharyngeal infection.

The etiologic diagnosis may become evident in the context of a thorough skin examination (Chap. 24). Petechial rashes are typically seen with meningococcemia or Rocky Mountain spotted fever (RMSF; see Fig. 25e-16); erythroderma is associated with toxic shock syndrome (TSS) and drug fever. The soft tissue and muscle examination is critical. Areas of erythema or duskiness, edema, and tenderness may indicate underlying necrotizing fasciitis, myositis, or myonecrosis. The neurologic examination must include a careful assessment of mental status for signs of early encephalopathy. Evidence of nuchal rigidity or focal neurologic findings should be sought.

DIAGNOSTIC WORKUP After a quick clinical assessment, diagnostic material should be obtained rapidly and antibiotic and supportive treatment begun. Blood (for cultures; baseline complete blood count with differential; measurement of serum electrolytes, blood urea nitrogen, serum creatinine, and serum glucose; and liver function tests) can be obtained at the time an IV line is placed and before antibiotics are administered. The blood lactate concentration also should be measured. Three sets of blood cultures should be performed for patients with possible acute endocarditis. Asplenic patients should have a buffy coat examined for bacteria; these patients can have $>10^6$ organisms per milliliter of blood (compared with 10^4/mL in patients with an intact spleen). Blood smears from patients at risk for severe parasitic disease, such as malaria or babesiosis (Chap. 250e), must be examined for the diagnosis and quantitation of parasitemia. Blood smears may also be diagnostic in ehrlichiosis and anaplasmosis.

Patients with possible meningitis should have cerebrospinal fluid (CSF) drawn before the initiation of antibiotic therapy. Focal findings, depressed mental status, or papilledema should be evaluated by brain imaging prior to lumbar puncture, which, in this setting, could initiate herniation. *Antibiotics should be administered before imaging but after blood for cultures has been drawn.* If CSF cultures are negative, blood cultures will provide the diagnosis in 50–70% of cases. Molecular diagnostic techniques (e.g., broad-range 16S rRNA gene polymerase chain reaction testing for bacterial meningitis pathogens) are of increasing importance in the rapid diagnosis of life-threatening infections.

Focal abscesses necessitate immediate CT or MRI as part of an evaluation for surgical intervention. Other diagnostic procedures, such as wound cultures, should not delay the initiation of treatment for more than minutes. Once emergent evaluation, diagnostic procedures, and (if appropriate) surgical consultation (see below) have been completed, other laboratory tests can be conducted. Appropriate radiography, computed axial tomography, MRI, urinalysis, erythrocyte sedimentation rate and C-reactive protein determination, and transthoracic or transesophageal echocardiography all may prove important.

TREATMENT THE ACUTELY ILL PATIENT

In the acutely ill patient, empirical antibiotic therapy is critical and should be administered without undue delay. Increased prevalence of antibiotic resistance in community-acquired bacteria must be considered when antibiotics are selected. Table 147-1 lists first-line empirical regimens for infections considered in this chapter. In addition to the rapid initiation of antibiotic therapy, several of these infections require urgent surgical attention. Neurosurgical evaluation for subdural empyema, otolaryngologic surgery for possible mucormycosis, and cardiothoracic surgery for critically ill patients with acute endocarditis are as important as antibiotic therapy. For infections such as necrotizing fasciitis and clostridial myonecrosis, rapid surgical intervention supersedes other diagnostic or therapeutic maneuvers.

Adjunctive treatments may reduce morbidity and mortality rates and include dexamethasone for bacterial meningitis or IV immunoglobulin for TSS and necrotizing fasciitis caused by group A *Streptococcus*. Adjunctive therapies should usually be initiated within the first hours of treatment; however, dexamethasone for

TABLE 147-1 EMPIRICAL TREATMENT FOR COMMON INFECTIOUS DISEASE EMERGENCIES[a]

Clinical Syndrome	Possible Etiologies	Treatment	Comments	See Chap(s).
Sepsis without a Clear Focus				
Septic shock	*Pseudomonas* spp., gram-negative enteric bacilli, *Staphylococcus* spp., *Streptococcus* spp.	Vancomycin (15/mg/kg q12h)[b] *plus* gentamicin (5 mg/kg per day) ***plus either*** Piperacillin/tazobactam (3.375 g q4h) *or* cefepime (2 g q8h)[c]	Adjust treatment when culture data become available.	172, 173, 186, 189, 325
Overwhelming post-splenectomy sepsis	*Streptococcus pneumoniae, Haemophilus influenzae, Neisseria meningitidis*	Ceftriaxone (2 g q12h) *plus* vancomycin (15 mg/kg q12h)[b]	If a β-lactam-sensitive strain is identified, vancomycin can be discontinued.	325
Babesiosis	*Babesia microti* (U.S.), *B. divergens* (Europe)	Clindamycin (600 mg q8h) *plus* quinine (650 mg q8h)	Atovaquone and azithromycin can be used in less severe disease and are associated with fewer side effects. Treatment with doxycycline (100 mg bid) for potential co-infection with *Borrelia burgdorferi* or *Anaplasma* spp. may be prudent.	246e, 249
Sepsis with Skin Findings				
Meningococcemia	*N. meningitidis*	Penicillin (4 mU q4h) *or* ceftriaxone (2 g q12h)	Consider protein C replacement, if available, in fulminant meningococcemia. Drotrecogin alfa (activated) is no longer produced.	180
Rocky Mountain spotted fever (RMSF)	*Rickettsia rickettsii*	Doxycycline (100 mg bid)	If both meningococcemia and RMSF are being considered, use ceftriaxone (2 g q12h) *plus* doxycycline (100 mg bid). If RMSF is diagnosed, doxycycline is the proven superior agent.	211
Purpura fulminans	*S. pneumoniae, H. influenzae, N. meningitidis*	Ceftriaxone (2 g q12h) *plus* vancomycin (15 mg/kg q12h)[b]	If a β-lactam-sensitive strain is identified, vancomycin can be discontinued.	171, 180, 182, 325
Erythroderma: toxic shock syndrome	Group A *Streptococcus*, *Staphylococcus aureus*	Vancomycin (15 mg/kg q12h)[b] *plus* clindamycin (600 mg q8h	If a penicillin- or oxacillin-sensitive strain is isolated, these agents are superior to vancomycin (penicillin, 2 mU q4h; or oxacillin, 2 g IV q4h). The site of toxigenic bacteria should be debrided; IV immunoglobulin can be used in severe cases.[d]	172, 173
Sepsis with Soft Tissue Findings				
Necrotizing fasciitis	Group A *Streptococcus*, mixed aerobic/anaerobic flora, CA-MRSA[e]	Vancomycin (15 mg/kg q12h)[b] *plus* clindamycin (600 mg q8h) *plus* gentamicin (5 mg/kg q8h)	Urgent surgical evaluation is critical. Adjust treatment when culture data become available.	156, 172, 173
Clostridial myonecrosis	*Clostridium perfringens*	Penicillin (2 mU q4h) *plus* clindamycin (600 mg q8h)	Urgent surgical evaluation is critical.	179
Neurologic Infections				
Bacterial meningitis	*S. pneumoniae, N. meningitidis*	Ceftriaxone (2 g q12h) *plus* vancomycin (15 mg/kg q12h)[b]	If a β-lactam-sensitive strain is identified, vancomycin can be discontinued. If the patient is >50 years old or has comorbid disease, add ampicillin (2 g q4h) for *Listeria* coverage. Dexamethasone (10 mg q6h × 4 days) improves outcome in adults with meningitis (especially pneumococcal) and cloudy CSF, positive CSF Gram's stain, or a CSF leukocyte count >1000/mL.	164
Brain abscess, suppurative intracranial infections	*Streptococcus* spp., *Staphylococcus* spp., anaerobes, gram-negative bacilli	Vancomycin (15 mg/kg q12h)[b] *plus* metronidazole (500 mg q8h) *plus* ceftriaxone (2 g q12h)	Urgent surgical evaluation is critical. If a penicillin- or oxacillin-sensitive strain is isolated, these agents are superior to vancomycin (penicillin, 4 mU q4h; or oxacillin, 2 g q4h).	164
Cerebral malaria	*Plasmodium falciparum*	Artesunate (2.4 mg/kg IV at 0, 12, and 24 h; then once daily)[f] *or* quinine (IV loading dose of 20 mg salt/kg; then 10 mg/kg q8h)	Do not use glucocorticoids. Use IV quinidine if IV quinine is not available. During IV quinidine treatment, blood pressure and cardiac function should be monitored continuously and blood glucose periodically.	246e, 248
Spinal epidural abscess	*Staphylococcus* spp., gram-negative bacilli	Vancomycin (15 mg/kg q12h)[b] *plus* ceftriaxone (2 g q24h)	Surgical evaluation is essential. If a penicillin- or oxacillin-sensitive strain is isolated, these agents are superior to vancomycin (penicillin, 4 mU q4h; or oxacillin, 2 g q4h).	456
Focal Infections				
Acute bacterial endocarditis	*S. aureus*, β-hemolytic streptococci, HACEK group,[g] *Neisseria* spp., *S. pneumoniae*	Ceftriaxone (2 g q12h) *plus* vancomycin (15 mg/kg q12h)[b]	Adjust treatment when culture data become available. Surgical evaluation is essential.	155

[a]These empirical regimens include coverage for gram-positive pathogens that are resistant to β-lactam antibiotics. Local resistance patterns should be considered and may alter the need for empirical vancomycin. [b]A vancomycin loading dose of 20–25 mg/kg can be considered in critically ill patients. [c]β-Lactam antibiotics may exhibit unpredictable pharmacodynamics in sepsis. Prolonged or continuous infusions can be considered. [d]The optimal dose of IV immunoglobulin has not been determined, but the median dose in observational studies is 2 g/kg (total dose administered for 1–5 days). [e]Community-acquired methicillin-resistant *S. aureus*. [f]In the United States, artesunate must be obtained through the Centers for Disease Control and Prevention. For patients diagnosed with severe malaria, full doses of parenteral antimalarial treatment should be started with whichever recommended antimalarial agent is first available. [g]*Haemophilus* species, *Aggregatibacter* species, *Cardiobacterium hominis*, *Eikenella corrodens*, and *Kingella kingae*.

bacterial meningitis must be given before or at the time of the first dose of antibiotic. Glucocorticoids can also be harmful, sometimes resulting in worse outcomes—e.g., when given in the setting of cerebral malaria or viral hepatitis.

SPECIFIC PRESENTATIONS

The infections considered below according to common clinical presentation can have rapidly catastrophic outcomes, and their immediate recognition and treatment can be life-saving. Recommended empirical therapeutic regimens are presented in Table 147-1.

SEPSIS WITHOUT AN OBVIOUS FOCUS OF PRIMARY INFECTION

Patients initially have a brief prodrome of nonspecific symptoms and signs that progresses quickly to hemodynamic instability with hypotension, tachycardia, tachypnea, respiratory distress, and altered mental status. Disseminated intravascular coagulation (DIC) with clinical evidence of a hemorrhagic diathesis is a poor prognostic sign.

Septic Shock (See also Chap. 325) Patients with bacteremia leading to septic shock may have a primary site of infection (e.g., pneumonia, pyelonephritis, or cholangitis) that is not evident initially. Elderly patients with comorbid conditions, hosts compromised by malignancy and neutropenia, and patients who have recently undergone a surgical procedure or hospitalization are at increased risk for an adverse outcome. Gram-negative bacteremia with organisms such as *Pseudomonas aeruginosa* or *Escherichia coli* and gram-positive infection with organisms such as *Staphylococcus aureus* (including methicillin-resistant *S. aureus* [MRSA]) or group A streptococci can present as intractable hypotension and multiorgan failure. Treatment can usually be initiated empirically on the basis of the presentation, host factors (Chap. 325), and local patterns of bacterial resistance. Outcomes are worse when antimicrobial treatment is delayed or when the responsible pathogen ultimately proves not to be susceptible to the initial regimen. Broad-spectrum antimicrobial agents are therefore recommended and should be instituted rapidly, preferably within the first hour after presentation. Risk factors for fungal infection should be assessed, as the incidence of fungal septic shock is increasing. Biomarkers such as C-reactive protein and procalcitonin have not proved reliable diagnostically but, when measured over time, can facilitate appropriate de-escalation of therapy. Glucocorticoids should be considered only for patients with severe sepsis who do not respond to fluid resuscitation and vasopressor therapy.

Overwhelming Infection in Asplenic Patients (See also Chap. 325) Patients without splenic function are at risk for overwhelming bacterial sepsis. Asplenic adult patients succumb to sepsis at 58 times the rate of the general population. Most infections are thought to occur within the first 2 years after splenectomy, with a mortality rate of ~50%, but the increased risk persists throughout life. In asplenia, encapsulated bacteria cause the majority of infections. Adults, who are more likely to have antibody to these organisms, are at lower risk than children. *Streptococcus pneumoniae* is the most common isolate, causing 50–70% of cases, but the risk of infection with *Haemophilus influenzae* or *Neisseria meningitidis* is also high. Severe clinical manifestations of infections due to *E. coli*, *S. aureus*, group B streptococci, *P. aeruginosa*, *Bordetella holmesii*, and *Capnocytophaga*, *Babesia*, and *Plasmodium* species have been described.

Babesiosis (See also Chap. 249) A history of recent travel to endemic areas raises the possibility of infection with *Babesia*. Between 1 and 4 weeks after a tick bite, the patient experiences chills, fatigue, anorexia, myalgia, arthralgia, shortness of breath, nausea, and headache; ecchymosis and/or petechiae are occasionally seen. The tick that most commonly transmits *Babesia*, *Ixodes scapularis*, also transmits *Borrelia burgdorferi* (the agent of Lyme disease) and *Anaplasma*; co-infection can occur, resulting in more severe disease. Infection with the European species *Babesia divergens* is more frequently fulminant than that due to the U.S. species *Babesia microti*. *B. divergens* causes a febrile syndrome with hemolysis, jaundice, hemoglobinemia, and renal failure and is associated with a mortality rate of >40%. Severe babesiosis is especially common in asplenic hosts but does occur in hosts with normal splenic function, particularly those >60 years of age and those with underlying immunosuppressive conditions such as HIV infection or malignancy. Complications include renal failure, acute respiratory failure, and DIC.

Other Sepsis Syndromes Tularemia (Chap. 195) is seen throughout the United States but occurs primarily in Arkansas, Missouri, South Dakota, and Oklahoma. This disease is associated with wild rabbit, tick, and tabanid fly contact. It can be transmitted by arthropod bite, handling of infected animal carcasses, consumption of contaminated food and water, or inhalation. The typhoidal form can be associated with gram-negative septic shock and a mortality rate of >30%, especially in patients with underlying comorbid or immunosuppressive conditions. Plague occurs infrequently in the United States (Chap. 196), primarily after contact with ground squirrels, prairie dogs, or chipmunks, but is endemic in other parts of the world, with >90% of all cases occurring in Africa. The septic form is particularly rare and is associated with shock, multiorgan failure, and a 30% mortality rate. These infections should be considered in the appropriate epidemiologic setting. The Centers for Disease Control and Prevention lists *Francisella tularensis* and *Yersinia pestis* (the agents of tularemia and plague, respectively) along with *Bacillus anthracis* (the agent of anthrax) as important organisms that might be used for bioterrorism (Chap. 261e).

SEPSIS WITH SKIN MANIFESTATIONS

(See also Chap. 24) Maculopapular rashes may reflect early meningococcal or rickettsial disease but are usually associated with nonemergent infections. Exanthems are usually viral. Primary HIV infection commonly presents with a rash that is typically maculopapular and involves the upper part of the body but can spread to the palms and soles. The patient is usually febrile and can have lymphadenopathy, severe headache, dysphagia, diarrhea, myalgias, and arthralgias. Recognition of this syndrome provides an opportunity to prevent transmission and to institute treatment and monitoring early on.

Petechial rashes caused by viruses are seldom associated with hypotension or a toxic appearance, although there can be exceptions (e.g., severe measles or arboviral infection). Petechial rashes limited to the distribution of the superior vena cava are rarely associated with severe disease. In other settings, petechial rashes require more urgent attention.

Meningococcemia (See also Chap. 180) Almost three-quarters of patients with *N. meningitidis* bacteremia have a rash. Meningococcemia most often affects young children (i.e., those 6 months to 5 years old). In sub-Saharan Africa, the high prevalence of serogroup A meningococcal disease has been a threat to public health for more than a century. Thousands of deaths occur annually in this area, which is known as the "meningitis belt," and large epidemic waves occur approximately every 8–12 years. Serogroups W135 and X are also important emerging pathogens in Africa. In the United States, sporadic cases and outbreaks occur in day-care centers, schools (grade school through college, particularly among college freshmen living in residential halls), and army barracks. Household contacts of index cases are at 400–800 times greater risk of disease than the general population. Patients may exhibit fever, headache, nausea, vomiting, myalgias, changes in mental status, and meningismus. However, the rapidly progressive form of disease is not usually associated with meningitis. The rash is initially pink, blanching, and maculopapular, appearing on the trunk and extremities, but then becomes hemorrhagic, forming petechiae. Petechiae are first seen at the ankles, wrists, axillae, mucosal surfaces, and palpebral and bulbar conjunctiva, with subsequent spread on the lower extremities and to the trunk. A cluster of petechiae may be seen at pressure points—e.g., where a blood pressure cuff has been inflated. In rapidly progressive meningococcemia (10–20% of cases), the petechial rash quickly becomes purpuric (see Fig. 70-5), and patients develop DIC, multiorgan failure, and shock; 50–60% of these patients die, and survivors often require extensive debridement or amputation of gangrenous extremities.

Hypotension with petechiae for <12 h is associated with significant mortality. Cyanosis, coma, oliguria, metabolic acidosis, and elevated partial thromboplastin time also are associated with a fatal outcome. Correction of protein C deficiency may improve outcome. Antibiotics given in the office by the primary care provider before hospital evaluation and admission may improve prognosis; this observation suggests that early initiation of treatment may be life-saving. Meningococcal conjugate vaccines are protective against serogroups A, C, Y and W135 and are recommended for children 11–18 years of age and for other high-risk patients.

Rocky Mountain Spotted Fever (See also Chap. 211) RMSF is a tick-borne disease caused by *Rickettsia rickettsii* that occurs throughout North and South America. Up to 40% of patients do not report a history of a tick bite, but a history of travel or outdoor activity (e.g., camping in tick-infested areas) can often be ascertained. For the first 3 days, headache, fever, malaise, myalgias, nausea, vomiting, and anorexia are documented. By day 3, half of patients have skin findings. Blanching macules develop initially on the wrists and ankles and then spread over the legs and trunk. The lesions become hemorrhagic and are frequently petechial. The rash spreads to palms and soles later in the course. The centripetal spread is a classic feature of RMSF but occurs in a minority of patients. Moreover, 10–15% of patients with RMSF never develop a rash. The patient can be hypotensive and develop noncardiogenic pulmonary edema, confusion, lethargy, and encephalitis progressing to coma. The CSF contains 10–100 cells/μL, usually with a predominance of mononuclear cells. The CSF glucose level is often normal; the protein concentration may be slightly elevated. Renal and hepatic injury as well as bleeding secondary to vascular damage are noted. For untreated infections, mortality rates are 20–30%. Delayed recognition and treatment are associated with a greater risk of death; Native Americans, children 5–9 years of age, adults >70 years old, and persons with underlying immunosuppression also are at increased risk of death.

Other rickettsial diseases cause significant morbidity and mortality worldwide. *Mediterranean spotted fever* caused by *Rickettsia conorii* is found in Africa, southwestern and south-central Asia, and southern Europe. Patients have fever, flu-like symptoms, and an inoculation eschar at the site of the tick bite. A maculopapular rash develops within 1–7 days, involving the palms and soles but sparing the face. Elderly patients or those with diabetes, alcoholism, uremia, or congestive heart failure are at risk for severe disease characterized by neurologic involvement, respiratory distress, and gangrene of the digits. Mortality rates associated with this severe form of disease approach 50%. *Epidemic typhus*, caused by *Rickettsia prowazekii*, is transmitted in louse-infested environments and emerges in conditions of extreme poverty, war, and natural disaster. Patients experience a sudden onset of high fevers, severe headache, cough, myalgias, and abdominal pain. A maculopapular rash develops (primarily on the trunk) in more than half of patients and can progress to petechiae and purpura. Serious signs include delirium, coma, seizures, noncardiogenic pulmonary edema, skin necrosis, and peripheral gangrene. Mortality rates approached 60% in the preantibiotic era and continue to exceed 10–15% in contemporary outbreaks. *Scrub typhus*, caused by *Orientia tsutsugamushi* (a separate genus in the family Rickettsiaceae), is transmitted by larval mites or chiggers and is one of the most common infections in southeastern Asia and the western Pacific. The organism is found in areas of heavy scrub vegetation (e.g., along riverbanks). Patients may have an inoculation eschar and may develop a maculopapular rash. Severe cases progress to pneumonia, meningoencephalitis, DIC, and renal failure. Mortality rates range from 1% to 35%.

If recognized in a timely fashion, rickettsial disease is very responsive to treatment. Doxycycline (100 mg twice daily for 3–14 days) is the treatment of choice for both adults and children. The newer macrolides and chloramphenicol may be suitable alternatives, but mortality rates are higher when a tetracycline-based treatment is not given.

Purpura Fulminans (See also Chaps. 180 and 325) Purpura fulminans is the cutaneous manifestation of DIC and presents as large ecchymotic areas and hemorrhagic bullae. Progression of petechiae to purpura, ecchymoses, and gangrene is associated with congestive heart failure, septic shock, acute renal failure, acidosis, hypoxia, hypotension, and death. Purpura fulminans has been associated primarily with *N. meningitidis* but, in splenectomized patients, may be associated with *S. pneumoniae*, *H. influenzae*, and *S. aureus*.

Ecthyma Gangrenosum Septic shock caused by *P. aeruginosa* or *Aeromonas hydrophila* can be associated with ecthyma gangrenosum (see Figs. 189-1 and 25e-35): hemorrhagic vesicles surrounded by a rim of erythema with central necrosis and ulceration. These gram-negative bacteremias are most common among patients with neutropenia, extensive burns, and hypogammaglobulinemia.

Other Emergent Infections Associated with Rash *Vibrio vulnificus* and other noncholera *Vibrio* bacteremic infections (Chap. 193) can cause focal skin lesions and overwhelming sepsis in hosts with chronic liver disease, iron storage disorders, diabetes, renal insufficiency, or other immunocompromising conditions. After ingestion of contaminated raw shellfish, typically oysters from the Gulf Coast, there is a sudden onset of malaise, chills, fever, and hypotension. The patient develops bullous or hemorrhagic skin lesions, usually on the lower extremities, and 75% of patients have leg pain. The mortality rate can be as high as 50–60%, particularly when the patient presents with hypotension. Outcomes are improved when patients are treated with tetracycline-containing regimens. Other infections, caused by agents such as *Aeromonas*, *Klebsiella*, and *E. coli*, can cause hemorrhagic bullae and death due to overwhelming sepsis in cirrhotic patients. *Capnocytophaga canimorsus* can cause septic shock in asplenic patients. Infection typically follows a dog bite. Patients present with fever, chills, myalgia, vomiting, diarrhea, dyspnea, confusion, and headache. Findings can include an exanthem or erythema multiforme (see Figs. 70-9 and 25e-25), cyanotic mottling or peripheral cyanosis, petechiae, and ecchymosis. About 30% of patients with this fulminant form die of overwhelming sepsis and DIC, and survivors may require amputation because of gangrene.

Erythroderma TSS (Chaps. 172 and 173) is usually associated with erythroderma. The patient presents with fever, malaise, myalgias, nausea, vomiting, diarrhea, and confusion. There is a sunburn-type rash that may be subtle and patchy but is usually diffuse and is found on the face, trunk, and extremities. Erythroderma, which desquamates after 1–2 weeks, is more common in *Staphylococcus*-associated than in *Streptococcus*-associated TSS. Hypotension develops rapidly—often within hours—after the onset of symptoms. Multiorgan failure occurs. Early renal failure may precede hypotension and distinguishes this syndrome from other septic shock syndromes. There may be no indication of a primary focal infection, although possible cutaneous or mucosal portals of entry for the organism can be ascertained when a careful history is taken. Colonization rather than overt infection of the vagina or a postoperative wound, for example, is typical with staphylococcal TSS, and the mucosal areas appear hyperemic but not infected. Streptococcal TSS is more often associated with skin or soft tissue infection (including necrotizing fasciitis), and patients are more likely to be bacteremic. TSS caused by *Clostridium sordellii* is associated with childbirth or with skin injection of black-tar heroin. The diagnosis of TSS is defined by the clinical criteria of fever, rash, hypotension, and multiorgan involvement. The mortality rate is 5% for menstruation-associated TSS, 10–15% for nonmenstrual TSS, 30–70% for streptococcal TSS, and up to 90% for obstetric *C. sordellii* TSS.

Viral Hemorrhagic Fevers Viral hemorrhagic fevers (Chaps. 233 and 234) are zoonotic illnesses caused by viruses that reside in either animal reservoirs or arthropod vectors. These diseases occur worldwide and are restricted to areas where the host species live. They are caused by four major groups of viruses: Arenaviridae (e.g., Lassa fever in Africa), Bunyaviridae (e.g., Rift Valley fever in Africa; hantavirus hemorrhagic fever with renal syndrome in Asia; or Crimean-Congo hemorrhagic fever, which has an extensive geographic distribution), Filoviridae (e.g., Ebola and Marburg virus infections in Africa), and Flaviviridae (e.g., yellow fever in Africa and South America and dengue in Asia, Africa, and the Americas). Lassa fever and Ebola and Marburg virus infections are also transmitted from person to person. The vectors for most viral fevers are found in rural areas; dengue and yellow fever are important exceptions. After a prodrome of fever, myalgias, and malaise, patients develop evidence of vascular damage, petechiae, and local hemorrhage. Shock, multifocal hemorrhaging, and neurologic signs (e.g., seizures or coma) predict a poor prognosis. Dengue (Chap. 233) is the most common arboviral disease worldwide. More than half a million cases of dengue hemorrhagic fever occur each year, with at least 12,000 deaths. Patients have a triad of symptoms: hemorrhagic manifestations, evidence of plasma leakage, and platelet counts of <100,000/μL. Mortality rates are 10–20%. If dengue shock syndrome develops, mortality rates can reach 40%. Supportive care to maintain blood pressure and intravascular volume with careful volume-replacement therapy is key to survival. Ribavirin also may be useful against Arenaviridae and Bunyaviridae.

SEPSIS WITH A SOFT TISSUE/MUSCLE PRIMARY FOCUS

See also Chap. 156.

Necrotizing Fasciitis This infection is characterized by extensive necrosis of the subcutaneous tissue and fascia. It may arise at a site of minimal trauma or postoperative incision and may also be associated with recent varicella, childbirth, or muscle strain. The most common causes of necrotizing fasciitis are group A streptococci alone (Chap. 173), the incidence of which has been increasing for the past two decades, and a mixed facultative and anaerobic flora (Chap. 156). Diabetes mellitus, IV drug use, chronic liver or renal disease, and malignancy are associated risk factors. Physical findings are initially minimal compared with the severity of pain and the degree of fever. The examination is often unremarkable except for soft tissue edema and erythema. The infected area is red, hot, shiny, swollen, and exquisitely tender. In untreated infection, the overlying skin develops blue-gray patches after 36 h, and cutaneous bullae and necrosis develop after 3–5 days. Necrotizing fasciitis due to a mixed flora, but not that due to group A streptococci, can be associated with gas production. Without treatment, pain decreases because of thrombosis of the small blood vessels and destruction of the peripheral nerves—an ominous sign. The mortality rate is 15–34% overall, >70% in association with TSS, and nearly 100% without surgical intervention. Necrotizing fasciitis may also be due to *Clostridium perfringens* (Chap. 179); in this condition, the patient is extremely toxic and the mortality rate is high. Within 48 h, rapid tissue invasion and systemic toxicity associated with hemolysis and death ensue. The distinction between this entity and clostridial myonecrosis is made by muscle biopsy. Necrotizing fasciitis caused by community-acquired MRSA also has been reported.

Clostridial Myonecrosis (See also Chap. 179) Myonecrosis is often associated with trauma or surgery but can develop spontaneously. The incubation period is usually 12–24 h long, and massive necrotizing gangrene develops within hours of onset. Systemic toxicity, shock, and death can occur within 12 h. The patient's pain and toxic appearance are out of proportion to physical findings. On examination, the patient is febrile, apathetic, tachycardic, and tachypneic and may express a feeling of impending doom. Hypotension and renal failure develop later, and hyperalertness is evident preterminally. The skin over the affected area is bronze-brown, mottled, and edematous. Bullous lesions with serosanguineous drainage and a mousy or sweet odor can develop. Crepitus can occur secondary to gas production in muscle tissue. The mortality rate is >65% for spontaneous myonecrosis, which is often associated with *Clostridium septicum* or *C. tertium* and underlying malignancy. The mortality rates associated with trunk and limb infection are 63% and 12%, respectively, and any delay in surgical treatment increases the risk of death.

NEUROLOGIC INFECTIONS WITH OR WITHOUT SEPTIC SHOCK

Bacterial Meningitis (See also Chap. 164) Bacterial meningitis is one of the most common infectious disease emergencies involving the central nervous system. Although hosts with cell-mediated immune deficiency (including transplant recipients, diabetic patients, elderly patients, and cancer patients receiving certain chemotherapeutic agents) are at particular risk for *Listeria monocytogenes* meningitis, most cases in adults are due to *S. pneumoniae* (30–60%) and *N. meningitidis* (10–35%). The classic presentation of fever, meningismus, and altered mental status is seen in only one-half to two-thirds of patients. The elderly can present without fever or meningeal signs. Cerebral dysfunction is evidenced by confusion, delirium, and lethargy that can progress to coma. In some cases, the presentation is fulminant, with sepsis and brain edema; papilledema at presentation is unusual and suggests another diagnosis (e.g., an intracranial lesion). Focal signs, including cranial nerve palsies (IV, VI, VII), can be seen in 10–20% of cases; 50–70% of patients have bacteremia. A poor outcome is associated with coma, hypotension, a pneumococcal etiology, respiratory distress, a CSF glucose level of <0.6 mmol/L (<<0 mg/dL), a CSF protein level of >2.5 g/L, a peripheral white blood cell count of <5000/μL, and a serum sodium level of <135 mmol/L. Rapid initiation of treatment is essential; the odds of an unfavorable outcome may increase by 30% for each hour that treatment is delayed. Mortality also increases linearly with age of the patient.

Suppurative Intracranial Infections (See also Chap. 164) In suppurative intracranial infections, rare intracranial lesions present along with sepsis and hemodynamic instability. Rapid recognition of the toxic patient with central neurologic signs is crucial to improvement of the dismal prognosis of these entities. *Subdural empyema* arises from the paranasal sinus in 60–70% of cases. Microaerophilic streptococci and staphylococci are the predominant etiologic organisms. The patient is toxic, with fever, headache, and nuchal rigidity. Of all patients, 75% have focal signs and 6–20% die. Despite improved survival rates, 15–44% of patients are left with permanent neurologic deficits. *Septic cavernous sinus thrombosis* follows a facial or sphenoid sinus infection; 70% of cases are due to staphylococci (including MRSA), and the remainder are due primarily to aerobic or anaerobic streptococci. A unilateral or retroorbital headache progresses to a toxic appearance and fever within days. Three-quarters of patients have unilateral periorbital edema that becomes bilateral and then progresses to ptosis, proptosis, ophthalmoplegia, and papilledema. The mortality rate is as high as 30%. *Septic thrombosis of the superior sagittal sinus* spreads from the ethmoid or maxillary sinuses and is caused by *S. pneumoniae*, other streptococci, and staphylococci. The fulminant course is characterized by headache, nausea, vomiting, rapid progression to confusion and coma, nuchal rigidity, and brainstem signs. If the sinus is totally thrombosed, the mortality rate exceeds 80%.

Brain Abscess (See also Chap. 164) Brain abscess often occurs without systemic signs. Almost half of patients are afebrile, and presentations are more consistent with a space-occupying lesion in the brain; 70% of patients have headache and/or altered mental status, 50% have focal neurologic signs, and 25% have papilledema. Abscesses can present as single or multiple lesions resulting from contiguous foci or hematogenous infection, such as endocarditis. The infection progresses over several days from cerebritis to an abscess with a mature capsule. More than half of infections are polymicrobial, with an etiology consisting of aerobic bacteria (primarily streptococcal species) and anaerobes. Abscesses arising hematogenously are especially apt to rupture into the ventricular space, causing a sudden and severe deterioration in clinical status and a high mortality rate. Otherwise, mortality is low but morbidity is high (30–55%). Patients presenting with stroke and a parameningeal infectious focus, such as sinusitis or otitis, may have a brain abscess, and physicians must maintain a high level of suspicion. Prognosis worsens in patients with a fulminant course, delayed diagnosis, abscess rupture into the ventricles, multiple abscesses, or abnormal neurologic status at presentation.

Cerebral Malaria (See also Chap. 248) This entity should be urgently considered if patients who have recently traveled to areas endemic for malaria present with a febrile illness and lethargy or other neurologic signs. Fulminant malaria is caused by *Plasmodium falciparum* and is associated with temperatures of >40°C (>104°F), hypotension, jaundice, adult respiratory distress syndrome, and bleeding. By definition, any patient with a change in mental status or repeated seizure in the setting of fulminant malaria has cerebral malaria. In adults, this nonspecific febrile illness progresses to coma over several days; occasionally, coma occurs within hours and death within 24 h. Nuchal rigidity and photophobia are rare. On physical examination, symmetric encephalopathy is typical, and upper motor neuron dysfunction with decorticate and decerebrate posturing can be seen in advanced disease. Unrecognized infection results in a 20–30% mortality rate.

Intracranial and Spinal Epidural Abscesses (See also Chap. 456) Spinal and intracranial epidural abscesses (SEAs and ICEAs) can result in permanent neurologic deficits, sepsis, and death. At-risk patients include those with diabetes mellitus; IV drug use; chronic alcohol abuse; recent spinal trauma, surgery, or epidural anesthesia; and other comorbid conditions, such as HIV infection. Fungal epidural abscess and meningitis can follow epidural or paraspinal glucocorticoid infections. In the United States and Canada, where early treatment of otitis and sinusitis is typical, ICEA is rare but the number of cases of SEA is on the rise. In Africa and areas with limited access to health care, SEAs and ICEAs cause significant morbidity and mortality. ICEAs typically present as fever, mental status changes, and neck pain, while SEAs often present as fever, localized spinal tenderness, and back pain. ICEAs are typically polymicrobial, whereas SEAs are most often due to hematogenous seeding, with staphylococci the most common etiologic agent. Early diagnosis and treatment, which may include surgical drainage, minimize rates of mortality and permanent neurologic sequelae. Outcomes are worse for SEA due to MRSA, infection at a higher vertebral-body level, impaired neurologic status on presentation, and dorsal rather than ventral location of the abscess. Elderly patients and persons with renal failure, malignancy, and other comorbidities also have less favorable outcomes.

Other Focal Syndromes with a Fulminant Course Infection at virtually any primary focus (e.g., osteomyelitis, pneumonia, pyelonephritis, or cholangitis) can result in bacteremia and sepsis. Lemierre's disease—jugular septic thrombophlebitis caused by *Fusobacterium necrophorum*—is associated with metastatic infectious emboli (primarily to the lung) and sepsis, with mortality rates of >15%. TSS has been associated with focal infections such as septic arthritis, peritonitis, sinusitis, and wound infection. Rapid clinical deterioration and death can be associated with destruction of the primary site of infection, as is seen in endocarditis and in infections of the oropharynx (e.g., Ludwig's angina or epiglottitis, in which edema suddenly compromises the airway).

Rhinocerebral Mucormycosis (See also Chap. 242) Individuals with diabetes or immunocompromising conditions are at risk for invasive rhinocerebral mucormycosis. Patients present with low-grade fever, dull sinus pain, diplopia, decreased mental status, decreased ocular motion, chemosis, proptosis, dusky or necrotic nasal turbinates, and necrotic hard-palate lesions that respect the midline. Without rapid recognition and intervention, the process continues on an inexorable invasive course, with high mortality rates.

Acute Bacterial Endocarditis (See also Chap. 155) This entity presents with a much more aggressive course than subacute endocarditis. Bacteria such as *S. aureus*, *S. pneumoniae*, *L. monocytogenes*, *Haemophilus* species, and streptococci of groups A, B, and G attack native valves. Native-valve endocarditis caused by *S. aureus* (including MRSA strains) is increasing, particularly in health care settings. Mortality rates range from 10% to 40%. The host may have comorbid conditions such as underlying malignancy, diabetes mellitus, IV drug use, or alcoholism. The patient presents with fever, fatigue, and malaise <2 weeks after onset of infection. On physical examination, a changing murmur and congestive heart failure may be noted. Hemorrhagic macules on palms or soles (*Janeway lesions*) sometimes develop. Petechiae, Roth's spots, splinter hemorrhages, and splenomegaly are unusual. Rapid valvular destruction, particularly of the aortic valve, results in pulmonary edema and hypotension. Myocardial abscesses can form, eroding through the septum or into the conduction system and causing life-threatening arrhythmias or high-degree conduction block. Large friable vegetations can result in major arterial emboli, metastatic infection, or tissue infarction. Older patients with *S. aureus* endocarditis are especially likely to present with nonspecific symptoms—a circumstance that delays diagnosis and worsens prognosis. Rapid intervention is crucial for a successful outcome.

Inhalational Anthrax (See also Chap. 261e) Inhalational anthrax, the most severe form of disease caused by *B. anthracis*, had not been reported in the United States for more than 25 years until the use of this organism as an agent of bioterrorism in 2001. Patients presented with malaise, fever, cough, nausea, drenching sweats, shortness of breath, and headache. Rhinorrhea was unusual. All patients had abnormal chest roentgenograms at presentation. Pulmonary infiltrates, mediastinal widening, and pleural effusions were the most common findings. Hemorrhagic meningitis was seen in 38% of these patients. Survival was more likely when antibiotics were given during the prodromal period and when multidrug regimens were used. In the absence of urgent intervention with antimicrobial agents and supportive care, inhalational anthrax progresses rapidly to hypotension, cyanosis, and death.

Avian and Swine Influenza (See also Chap. 224) Human cases of avian influenza have occurred primarily in Southeast Asia, particularly Vietnam (H5N1) and China (H7N9). Avian influenza should be considered in patients with severe respiratory tract illness, particularly if they have been exposed to poultry. Patients present with high fever, an influenza-like illness, and lower respiratory tract symptoms; this illness can progress rapidly to bilateral pneumonia, acute respiratory distress syndrome, multiorgan failure, and death. Early antiviral treatment with neuraminidase inhibitors should be initiated along with aggressive supportive measures. Unlike avian influenza, for which human-to-human transmission has been rare so far and has not been sustained, a novel swine-associated influenza A/H1N1 virus has spread rapidly throughout the world. Patients most at risk of severe disease are children <5 years of age, elderly persons, patients with underlying chronic conditions, and pregnant women. Obesity also has been identified as a risk factor for severe illness.

Hantavirus Pulmonary Syndrome (See also Chap. 233) Hantavirus pulmonary syndrome has been documented in the United States (primarily the southwestern states), Canada, and South America. Most cases occur in rural areas and are associated with exposure to rodents. Patients present with a nonspecific viral prodrome of fever, malaise, myalgias, nausea, vomiting, and dizziness that may progress to pulmonary edema and respiratory failure. Hantavirus pulmonary syndrome causes myocardial depression and increased pulmonary vascular permeability; therefore, careful fluid resuscitation and use of pressor agents are crucial. Aggressive cardiopulmonary support during the first few hours of illness can be life-saving. The early onset of thrombocytopenia may help distinguish this syndrome from other febrile illnesses in an appropriate epidemiologic setting.

CONCLUSION

Acutely ill febrile patients with the syndromes discussed in this chapter require close observation, aggressive supportive measures, and—in most cases—admission to intensive care units. The most important task of the physician is to distinguish these patients from other infected febrile patients whose illness will not progress to fulminant disease. The alert physician must recognize the acute infectious disease emergency and then proceed with appropriate urgency.

148 Immunization Principles and Vaccine Use

Anne Schuchat, Lisa A. Jackson

Few medical interventions of the past century can rival the effect that immunization has had on longevity, economic savings, and quality of life. Seventeen diseases are now preventable through vaccines routinely administered to children and adults in the United States (Table 148-1), and most vaccine-preventable diseases of childhood are at historically low levels (Table 148-2). Health care providers deliver the vast majority of vaccines in the United States in the course of providing routine health services and therefore play an integral role in the nation's public health system.

VACCINE IMPACT

Direct and Indirect Effects Immunizations against specific infectious diseases protect individuals against infection and thereby prevent symptomatic illnesses. Specific vaccines may blunt the severity of clinical illness (e.g., rotavirus vaccines and severe gastroenteritis) or reduce complications (e.g., zoster vaccines and postherpetic neuralgia). Some immunizations also reduce transmission of infectious disease agents from immunized people to others, thereby reducing the impact of infection spread. This indirect impact is known as *herd immunity*. The level of immunization in a population that is required to achieve indirect protection of unimmunized people varies substantially with the specific vaccine.

Since childhood vaccines have become widely available in the United States, major declines in rates of vaccine preventable diseases among both children and adults have become evident (Table 148-2). For example, vaccination of children <5 years of age against seven types of *Streptococcus pneumoniae* led to a >90% overall reduction in invasive disease caused by those types. A series of childhood vaccines targeting 13 vaccine-preventable diseases in a single birth cohort leads to prevention of 42,000 premature deaths and 20 million illnesses and saves nearly $70 billion (U.S.).

Control, Elimination, and Eradication of Vaccine-Preventable Diseases Immunization programs are associated with the goals of controlling, eliminating, or eradicating a disease. *Control* of a vaccine-preventable disease reduces poor illness outcomes and often limits the disruptive impacts associated with outbreaks of disease in communities, schools, and institutions. Control programs can also reduce absences from work for ill persons and for parents caring for sick children, decrease absences from school, and limit health care utilization associated with treatment visits.

Elimination of a disease is a more demanding goal than control, usually requiring the reduction to zero of cases in a defined geographic area but sometimes defined as reduction in the indigenous sustained transmission of an infection in a geographic area. As of 2013, the United States had eliminated indigenous transmission of measles, rubella, poliomyelitis, and diphtheria. Importation of pathogens from other parts of the world continues to be important, and public health efforts are intended to react promptly to such cases and to limit forward spread of the infectious agent.

Eradication of a disease is achieved when its elimination can be sustained without ongoing interventions. The only vaccine-preventable disease of humans that has been globally eradicated thus far is smallpox. Although smallpox vaccine is no longer given routinely, the disease has not reemerged naturally because all chains of human transmission were interrupted through earlier vaccination efforts and humans were the only natural reservoir of the virus. Currently, a major health initiative is targeting the global eradication of polio. Sustained transmission of polio has been eliminated from most nations but has never been interrupted in three countries—Afghanistan, Nigeria, and Pakistan—while recent outbreaks in Syria and the Horn of Africa underscore that other countries remain at risk for importation until these reservoirs have been addressed. Detection of a case of disease that has been targeted for eradication or elimination is considered a sentinel event that could permit the infectious agent to become reestablished in the community or region. Therefore, such episodes must be promptly reported to public health authorities.

TABLE 148-1 DISEASES PREVENTABLE WITH VACCINES ROUTINELY ADMINISTERED IN THE UNITED STATES TO CHILDREN AND/OR ADULTS

Condition	Target Population(s) for Routine Use
Pertussis	Children, adolescents, adults
Diphtheria	Children, adolescents, adults
Tetanus	Children, adolescents, adults
Poliomyelitis	Children
Measles	Children
Mumps	Children
Rubella, congenital rubella syndrome	Children
Hepatitis B	Children
Haemophilus influenzae type b infection	Children
Hepatitis A	Children
Influenza	Children, adolescents, adults
Varicella	Children
Invasive pneumococcal disease	Children, older adults
Meningococcal disease	Adolescents
Rotavirus infection	Infants
Human papillomavirus infection, cervical and anogenital cancers	Adolescents and young adults
Zoster	Older adults

TABLE 148-2 DECLINE IN VACCINE-PREVENTABLE DISEASES IN THE UNITED STATES FOLLOWING WIDESPREAD IMPLEMENTATION OF NATIONAL VACCINE RECOMMENDATIONS

Condition	Annual No. of Prevaccine Cases (Average)	No. of Cases Reported in 2012[a]	Reduction (%) in Cases After Widespread Vaccination
Smallpox	29,005	0	100
Diphtheria	21,053	1	≥99
Measles	530,217	55	≥99
Mumps	162,344	229	≥99
Pertussis	200,752	48,277	76
Polio (paralytic)	16,316	0	100
Rubella	47,745	9	>99
Congenital rubella syndrome	152	2	99
Tetanus	580	37	94
Haemophilus influenzae type b infection	20,000	30[b]	99
Hepatitis A	117,333	2,890[c]	98
Hepatitis B (acute)	66,232	18,800[c]	72
Invasive pneumococcal infection: all ages	63,067	31,600[d]	50
Invasive pneumococcal infection: <5 years of age	16,069	1,800[d]	89
Varicella	4,085,120	216,511	95

[a]Except for cases of hepatitis A and hepatitis B, for which 2011 figures are shown. [b]An additional 13 type b infections are estimated to have occurred among 210 reports of *H. influenzae* infection caused by unknown types among children <5 years of age. [c]Data are from the CDC's Viral Hepatitis Surveillance, 2011. [d]Data are from the CDC's Active Bacterial Core Surveillance 2012 Provisional Report.

Source: Adapted from SW Roush et al: JAMA 298:2155, 2007; and MMWR 62(33); 669, 2013.

Outbreak Detection and Control Clusters of cases of a vaccine-preventable disease detected in an institution, a medical practice, or a community may signal important changes in the pathogen, vaccine, or environment. Several factors can give rise to increases in vaccine-preventable disease, including (1) low rates of immunization that result in an accumulation of susceptible people (e.g., measles resurgence among vaccination abstainers); (2) changes in the infectious agent that permit it to escape vaccine-induced protection (e.g., non-vaccine-type pneumococci); (3) waning of vaccine-induced immunity (e.g., pertussis among adolescents and adults vaccinated in early childhood); and (4) point-source introductions of large inocula (e.g., food-borne exposure to hepatitis A virus). Reporting episodes of outbreak-prone diseases to public health authorities can facilitate recognition of clusters that require further interventions.

PUBLIC HEALTH REPORTING Recognition of suspected cases of diseases targeted for elimination or eradication—along with other diseases that require urgent public health interventions, such as contact tracing, administration of chemo- or immunoprophylaxis, or epidemiologic investigation for common-source exposure—is typically associated with special reporting requirements. Many diseases against which vaccines are routinely used, including measles, pertussis, *Haemophilus influenzae* type b invasive disease, and varicella, are nationally notifiable. Clinicians and laboratory staff have a responsibility to report some vaccine-preventable disease occurrences to local or state public health authorities according to specific case-definition criteria. All providers should be aware of state or city disease-reporting requirements and the best ways to contact public health authorities. A prompt response to vaccine-preventable disease outbreaks can greatly enhance the effectiveness of control measures.

GLOBAL CONSIDERATIONS Several international health initiatives currently focus on reducing vaccine-preventable diseases in regions throughout the world. These efforts include improving access to new and underutilized vaccines, such as pneumococcal conjugate, rotavirus, human papillomavirus (HPV), and meningococcal A conjugate vaccines. The American Red Cross, the World Health Organization (WHO), the United Nations Foundation, the United Nations Children's Fund (UNICEF), and the Centers for Disease Control and Prevention (CDC) are partners in the Measles & Rubella Initiative, which targets reduction of worldwide measles deaths by 95% from 2000 to 2015. During 2000–2011, global measles mortality rates declined by 71%—i.e., from an estimated 548,000 deaths in 2000 to 158,000 deaths in 2011. Rotary International, UNICEF, the CDC, and the WHO are leading partners in the global eradication of polio, an endeavor that reduced the annual number of paralytic polio cases from 350,000 in 1988 to <250 in 2012. The GAVI Alliance and the Bill and Melinda Gates Foundation have brought substantial momentum to global efforts to reduce vaccine-preventable diseases, expanding on earlier efforts by the WHO, UNICEF, and governments in developed and developing countries.

Enhancing Immunization in Adults Although immunization has become a centerpiece of routine pediatric medical visits, it has not been as well integrated into routine health care visits for adults. This chapter focuses on immunization principles and vaccine use in adults. Accumulating evidence suggests that immunization coverage can be increased through efforts directed at consumer-, provider-, institution-, and system-level factors. The literature suggests that the application of multiple strategies is more effective at raising coverage rates than is the use of any single strategy.

RECOMMENDATIONS FOR ADULT IMMUNIZATIONS The CDC's Advisory Committee on Immunization Practices (ACIP) is the main source of recommendations for administration of vaccines approved by the U.S. Food and Drug Administration (FDA) for use in children and adults in the U.S. civilian population. The ACIP is a federal advisory committee that consists of 15 voting members (experts in fields associated with immunization) appointed by the Secretary of the U.S. Department of Health and Human Services; 8 ex officio members representing federal agencies; and 26 nonvoting representatives of various liaison organizations, including major medical societies and managed-care organizations. The ACIP recommendations are available at *www.cdc.gov/vaccines/hcp/acip-recs/*. These recommendations are harmonized to the greatest extent possible with vaccine recommendations made by other organizations, including the American College of Obstetricians and Gynecologists, the American Academy of Family Physicians, and the American College of Physicians.

ADULT IMMUNIZATION SCHEDULES Immunization schedules for adults in the United States are updated annually and can be found online (*www.cdc.gov/vaccines/schedules/hcp/adult.html*). In January, the schedules are published in *American Family Physician, Annals of Internal Medicine*, and *Morbidity and Mortality Weekly Report* (*www.cdc.gov/mmwr*). The adult immunization schedules for 2013 are summarized in Fig. 148-1. Additional information and specifications are contained in the footnotes to these schedules. In the time between annual publications, additions and changes to schedules are published as Notices to Readers in *Morbidity and Mortality Weekly Report.*

IMMUNIZATION PRACTICE STANDARDS

Administering immunizations to adults involves a number of processes, such as deciding whom to vaccinate, assessing vaccine contraindications and precautions, providing vaccine information statements (VISs), ensuring appropriate storage and handling of vaccines, administering vaccines, and maintaining vaccine records. In addition, provider reporting of adverse events that follow vaccination is an essential component of the vaccine safety monitoring system.

Deciding Whom to Vaccinate Every effort should be made to ensure that adults receive all indicated vaccines as expeditiously as possible. When adults present for care, their immunization history should be assessed and recorded, and this information should be used to identify needed vaccinations according to the most current version of the adult immunization schedule. Decision-support tools incorporated into electronic health records can provide prompts for needed vaccinations. Standing orders, which are often used for routinely indicated vaccines (e.g., influenza and pneumococcal vaccines), permit a nurse or another approved licensed practitioner to administer vaccines without a specific physician order, thus lowering barriers to adult immunization.

Assessing Contraindications and Precautions Before vaccination, all patients should be screened for contraindications and precautions. A *contraindication* is a condition that increases the risk of a serious adverse reaction to vaccination. A vaccine should not be administered when a contraindication is documented. For example, a history of an anaphylactic reaction to a dose of vaccine or to a vaccine component is a contraindication for further doses. A *precaution* is a condition that may increase the risk of an adverse event or that may compromise the ability of the vaccine to evoke immunity (e.g., administering measles vaccine to a person who has recently received a blood transfusion and may consequently have transient passive immunity to measles virus). Normally, a vaccine is not administered when a precaution is noted. However, situations may arise when the benefits of vaccination outweigh the estimated risk of an adverse event, and the provider may decide to vaccinate the patient despite the precaution.

In some cases, contraindications and precautions are temporary and may lead to mere deferral of vaccination until a later time. For example, moderate or severe acute illness with or without fever is generally considered a transient precaution to vaccination and results in postponement of vaccine administration until the acute phase has resolved; thus the superimposition of adverse effects of vaccination on the underlying illness and the mistaken attribution of a manifestation of the underlying illness to the vaccine are avoided. Contraindications and precautions to vaccines licensed in the United States for use in civilian adults are summarized in Table 148-3. It is important to recognize conditions that are *not* contraindications in order not to miss opportunities for vaccination. For example, in most cases, mild acute illness (with or without fever), a history of a mild to moderate local reaction to a previous dose of the vaccine, and breast-feeding are not contraindications to vaccination.

Recommended Immunizations for Adults by Age

If you are this age,

Talk to your healthcare professional about these vaccines:	19–21 years	22–26 years	27–49 years	50–59 years	60–64 years	65+ years
Influenza (Flu)[1]	Get a flu vaccine every year					
Tetanus, diphtheria, pertussis (Td/Tdap)[2]	Get a Tdap vaccine once, then a Td booster vaccine every 10 years					
Varicella (Chickenpox)	2 doses					
HPV Vaccine for Women[3]	3 doses					
HPV Vaccine for Men[3]	3 doses	3 doses				
Zoster (Shingles)					1 dose	
Measles, mumps, rubella (MMR)[4]	1 or 2 doses					
Pneumococcal (Pneumonia)[5]	1-3 doses					1 dose
Meningococcal	1 or more doses					
Hepatitis A	2 doses					
Hepatitis B	3 doses					

Boxes this color show that the vaccine is recommended for all adults unless your healthcare professional tells you that you cannot safely receive the vaccine or that you do not need it.

Boxes this color show when the vaccine is recommended for adults with certain risks related to their health, job or lifestyle that put them at higher risk for serious diseases. Talk to your healthcare professional to see if you are at higher risk.

No recommendation

FOOTNOTES:

(Influenza vaccine)[1] There are several flu vaccines available—talk to your healthcare professional about which flu vaccine is right for you.

(Tdap vaccine)[2] Pregnant women are recommended to get Tdap vaccine with each pregnancy to increase protection for infants who are too young for vaccination but at highest risk for severe illness and death from pertussis (whooping cough).

(HPV vaccine)[3] There are two HPV vaccines but only one HPV vaccine (Gardasil®) should be given to men. Gay men or men who have sex with men who are 22 through 26 years old should get HPV vaccine if they haven't already started or completed the series.

(MMR vaccine)[4] If you were born in 1957 or after, and don't have a record of being vaccinated or having had these infections, talk to your healthcare professional about how many doses you may need.

(Pneumococcal vaccine)[5] There are two different types of pneumococcal vaccine: PCV13 and PPSV23. Talk with your healthcare professional to find out if one or both pneumococcal vaccines are recommended for you.

If you are traveling outside of the United States, you may need additional vaccines. Ask your healthcare professional which vaccines you may need.

For more information, call toll free 1-800-CDC-INFO (1-800-232-4636) or visit http://www.cdc.gov/vaccines

FIGURE 148-1 Recommended adult immunization schedules, United States, 2013. For complete statements by the Advisory Committee on Immunization Practices (ACIP), visit *www.cdc.gov/vaccines/hcp/acip-recs/*.

(Continues)

Recommended Immunizations for Adults by Medical Condition

Talk to your healthcare professional about these vaccines:	If you have this health condition, Pregnancy	Weakened immune system (not human immuno-deficiency virus [HIV])	HIV Infection: CD4 count is less than 200	HIV Infection: CD4 count is 200 or greater	Kidney disease or poor kidney function	Asplenia (if you do not have a spleen or it does not work well)	Heart disease, chronic lung disease, chronic alcoholism	Diabetes (Type 1 and Type 2)	Chronic Liver Disease
Influenza (Flu)[1]	Get a flu vaccine every year								
Tetanus, diphtheria, pertussis (Td/Tdap)	1 dose Tdap each pregnancy	Get a Tdap vaccine once, then a Td booster every 10 years							
Varicella (Chickenpox)	SHOULD NOT GET VACCINE			2 doses					
HPV Vaccine for Women[2]		3 doses through age 26 yrs							
HPV Vaccine for Men[2]		3 doses through age 26 yrs			3 doses through age 21 yrs				
Zoster (Shingles)[3]	SHOULD NOT GET VACCINE				1 dose for those 60 yrs and older				
Measles, mumps, rubella (MMR)[4]	SHOULD NOT GET VACCINE			1 or 2 doses					
Pneumococcal (PPSV23)	1 or 2 doses	1 or 2 doses							
Pneumococcal (PCV13)		1 dose					1 dose		
Meningococcal	1 or more doses					1 or more doses	1 or more doses		
Hepatitis A	2 doses								2 doses
Hepatitis B	3 doses		3 doses			3 doses		3 doses	

- Boxes this color show that the vaccine is recommended for all adults who have not been vaccinated, unless your healthcare professional tells you that you cannot safely receive the vaccine or that you do not need it.
- Boxes this color show when the vaccine is recommended for adults with certain risks related to their health, job or lifestyle that put them at higher risk for serious diseases. Talk to your healthcare professional to see if you are at higher risk.
- Boxes this color indicate the adult should NOT get this vaccine.
- No recommendation

Last updated August 2013 • CS241388-A

FOOTNOTES:

(Influenza vaccine)[1] There are several flu vaccines available—talk to your healthcare professional about which flu vaccine is right for you.

(HPV vaccine)[2] There are two HPV vaccines but only one HPV vaccine (Gardasil®) should be given to men. Gay men or men who have sex with men who are 22 through 26 years old should get HPV vaccine if they haven't already started or completed the series.

(Zoster)[3] You should get zoster vaccine even if you've had shingles before.

(MMR vaccine)[4] If you were born in 1957 or after, and don't have a record of being vaccinated or having had these infections, talk to your healthcare professional about how many doses you may need.

FIGURE 148-1 *(Continued)*

TABLE 148-3 CONTRAINDICATIONS AND PRECAUTIONS FOR COMMONLY USED VACCINES IN ADULTS

Vaccine Formulation	Contraindications and Precautions
All vaccines	**Contraindication**
	Severe allergic reaction (e.g., anaphylaxis) after a previous vaccine dose or to a vaccine component
	Precaution
	Moderate or severe acute illness with or without fever. Defer vaccination until illness resolves.
Td	**Precautions**
	GBS within 6 weeks after a previous dose of TT-containing vaccine
	History of arthus-type hypersensitivity reactions after a previous dose of TD or DT-containing vaccines (including MCV4). Defer vaccination until at least 10 years have elapsed since the last dose.
Tdap	**Contraindication**
	History of encephalopathy (e.g., coma or prolonged seizures) not attributable to another identifiable cause within 7 days of administration of a vaccine with pertussis components, such as DTaP or Tdap
	Precautions
	GBS within 6 weeks after a previous dose of TT-containing vaccine
	Progressive or unstable neurologic disorder, uncontrolled seizures, or progressive encephalopathy. Defer vaccination until a treatment regimen has been established and the condition has stabilized.
	History of arthus-type hypersensitivity reactions after a previous dose of TT- or DT-containing vaccines (including MCV4). Defer vaccination until at least 10 years have elapsed since the last dose.
HPV	**Contraindication**
	History of immediate hypersensitivity to yeast (for Gardasil)
	Precaution
	Pregnancy. If a woman is found to be pregnant after initiation of the vaccination series, the remainder of the 3-dose regimen should be delayed until after completion of the pregnancy. If a vaccine dose has been administered during pregnancy, no intervention is needed. Exposure to Gardasil during pregnancy should be reported to Merck (800 986 8999); exposure to Cervarix during pregnancy should be reported to GlaxoSmithKline (888 452-9622).
MMR	**Contraindications**
	History of immediate hypersensitivity reaction to gelatin[a] or neomycin
	Pregnancy
	Known severe immunodeficiency (e.g., hematologic and solid tumors; chemotherapy; congenital immunodeficiency; long-term immunosuppressive therapy; severe immunocompromise due to HIV infection)
	Precautions
	Recent receipt (within 11 months) of antibody-containing blood product
	History of thrombocytopenia or thrombocytopenic purpura
Varicella	**Contraindications**
	Pregnancy
	Known severe immunodeficiency
	History of immediate hypersensitivity reaction to gelatin[a] or neomycin
	Precaution
	Recent receipt (within 11 months) of antibody-containing blood product
Influenza, inactivated, injectable	**Precautions**
	History of severe allergic reaction (e.g., anaphylaxis) to egg protein[b] (note: not a precaution for Flublok recombinant influenza vaccine, which is approved for persons 18–49 years of age and is manufactured without the use of eggs)
	History of GBS within 6 weeks after a previous influenza vaccine dose
Influenza, live attenuated nasal spray	**Contraindications**
	History of severe allergic reaction (e.g., anaphylaxis) to egg protein[b]
	Age ≥50 years
	Pregnancy
	Immunosuppression, including that caused by medications or by HIV infection; known severe immunodeficiency (e.g., hematologic and solid tumors; chemotherapy; congenital immunodeficiency; long-term immunosuppressive therapy; severe immunocompromise due to HIV infection)
	Certain chronic medical conditions, such as diabetes mellitus; chronic pulmonary disease (including asthma); chronic cardiovascular disease (except hypertension); renal, hepatic, neurologic/neuromuscular, hematologic, or metabolic disorders
	Close contact with severely immunosuppressed persons who require a protected environment, such as isolation in a bone marrow transplantation unit
	Close contact with persons with lesser degrees of immunosuppression (e.g., persons receiving chemotherapy or radiation therapy who are not being cared for in a protective environment; persons with HIV infection) is *not* a contraindication or a precaution. Health care personnel in neonatal intensive care units or oncology clinics may receive live attenuated influenza vaccine.
	Precautions
	History of GBS within 6 weeks of a previous influenza vaccine dose
	Receipt of specific antiviral agents (i.e., amantadine, rimantadine, zanamivir, or oseltamivir) with 48 h before vaccination

(Continued)

TABLE 148-3 CONTRAINDICATIONS AND PRECAUTIONS FOR COMMONLY USED VACCINES IN ADULTS (CONTINUED)

Vaccine Formulation	Contraindications and Precautions
Pneumococcal polysaccharide	None, other than those listed for all vaccines
Pneumococcal conjugate	None, other than those listed for all vaccines
Hepatitis A	**Precaution** Pregnancy
Hepatitis B	**Contraindication** History of immediate hypersensitivity to yeast
Meningococcal conjugate	**Contraindication** History of severe allergic reaction to dry natural rubber (latex) (certain vaccine formulations; see text)
Meningococcal polysaccharide	**Contraindication** History of severe allergic reaction to dry natural rubber (latex)
Zoster	**Contraindications** Age <50 years Pregnancy Known severe immunodeficiency History of immediate hypersensitivity reaction to gelatin[a] or neomycin **Precaution** Receipt of specific antiviral agents (i.e., acyclovir, famciclovir, or valacyclovir) within 24 h before vaccination

[a]Extreme caution must be exercised in administering MMR, varicella, or zoster vaccine to persons with a history of anaphylactic reaction to gelatin or gelatin-containing products. Before administration, skin testing for sensitivity to gelatin can be considered. However, no specific protocols for this purpose have been published. [b]Recommendations for safely administering influenza vaccine to persons with egg allergies are reported in the annual ACIP recommendations for influenza vaccination (*www.cdc.gov/vaccines/hcp/acip-recs/vacc-specific/flu.html*).

Abbreviations: DT, diphtheria toxoid; DTaP, diphtheria, tetanus, and pertussis; GBS, Guillain-Barré syndrome; HPV, human papillomavirus; MCV4, quadrivalent meningococcal conjugate vaccine; MMR, measles, mumps, and rubella; Td, tetanus and diphtheria toxoids; Tdap, tetanus and diphtheria toxoids and acellular pertussis; TT, tetanus toxoid.

HISTORY OF IMMEDIATE HYPERSENSITIVITY TO A VACCINE COMPONENT A severe allergic reaction (e.g., anaphylaxis) to a previous dose of a vaccine or to one of its components is a contraindication to vaccination. While most vaccines have many components, substances to which individuals are most likely to have had a severe allergic reaction include egg protein, gelatin, and yeast. In addition, although natural rubber (latex) is not a vaccine component, some vaccines are supplied in vials or syringes that contain natural rubber latex. These vaccines can be identified by the product insert and should not be administered to persons who report a severe (anaphylactic) allergy to latex unless the benefit of vaccination clearly outweighs the risk for a potential allergic reaction. The much more common local or contact hypersensitivity to latex, such as to medical gloves (which contain synthetic latex that is not linked to allergic reactions), is *not* a contraindication to administration of a vaccine supplied in a vial or syringe that contains natural rubber latex. Vaccines routinely indicated for adults that, as of December 2012, were sometimes supplied in a vial or syringe containing natural rubber include Havrix hepatitis A vaccine (syringe); Vaqta hepatitis A vaccine (vial and syringe); Engerix-B hepatitis B vaccine (syringe); Recombivax HB hepatitis B vaccine (vial); Cervarix HPV vaccine (syringe); Fluarix, Fluvirin, Agriflu, and Flucelvax influenza vaccines (syringe); Adacel and Boostrix Tdap (tetanus and diphtheria toxoids and acellular pertussis) vaccines (syringe); Td (tetanus and diphtheria toxoids) vaccines (syringe); Twinrix hepatitis A and B vaccine (syringe); and Menomune meningococcal polysaccharide vaccine (vial).

PREGNANCY Live-virus vaccines are contraindicated during pregnancy because of the theoretical risk that vaccine virus replication will cause congenital infection or have other adverse effects on the fetus. Most live-virus vaccines, including varicella vaccine, are not secreted in breast milk; therefore, breast-feeding is not a contraindication for live-virus or other vaccines. Pregnancy is not a contraindication to administration of inactivated vaccines, but most are avoided during pregnancy because relevant safety data are limited. Two inactivated vaccines, Tdap vaccine and inactivated influenza vaccine, are routinely recommended for pregnant women in the United States. Tdap vaccine is recommended during each pregnancy, regardless of prior vaccination status, in order to prevent pertussis in neonates. Annual influenza vaccination is recommended for all persons 6 months of age and older, regardless of pregnancy status. Some other vaccines, such as meningococcal vaccines, may be given to pregnant women in certain circumstances.

IMMUNOSUPPRESSION Live-virus vaccines elicit an immune response due to replication of the attenuated (weakened) vaccine virus that is contained by the recipient's immune system. In persons with compromised immune function, enhanced replication of vaccine viruses is possible and could lead to disseminated infection with the vaccine virus. For this reason, live-virus vaccines are contraindicated for persons with severe immunosuppression, the definition of which may vary with the vaccine. Severe immunosuppression may be caused by many disease conditions, including HIV infection and hematologic or generalized malignancy. In some of these conditions, all affected persons are severely immunocompromised. In others (e.g., HIV infection), the degree to which the immune system is compromised depends on the severity of the condition, which in turn depends on the stage of disease or treatment. For example, measles-mumps-rubella (MMR) vaccine may be given to HIV-infected persons who are not severely immunocompromised. Severe immunosuppression may also be due to therapy with immunosuppressive agents, including high-dose glucocorticoids. In this situation, the dose, duration, and route of administration may influence the degree of immunosuppression.

VACCINE INFORMATION STATEMENTS

A VIS is a one-page (two-sided) information sheet produced by the CDC that informs vaccine recipients (or their parents or legal representatives) about the benefits and risks of a vaccine. VISs are mandated by the National Childhood Vaccine Injury Act (NCVIA) of 1986 and—whether the vaccine recipient is a child or an adult—must be provided for any vaccine covered by the Vaccine Injury Compensation Program. As of July 2011, vaccines that are covered by the NCVIA and that are licensed for use in adults include Td, Tdap, hepatitis A, hepatitis B, HPV, trivalent inactivated influenza, trivalent live intranasal influenza, MMR, 13-valent pneumococcal conjugate, meningococcal, polio, and varicella vaccines. When combination vaccines for which no separate VIS exists are given (e.g., hepatitis A and B combination vaccine), all relevant VISs should be provided. VISs also exist for some vaccines not covered by the NCVIA, such as pneumococcal polysaccharide, Japanese encephalitis, rabies, zoster, typhoid, and yellow fever vaccines. The use of these VISs is encouraged but is not mandated.

All current VISs are available on the Internet at two websites: the CDC's Vaccines & Immunizations site *(www.cdc.gov/vaccines/hcp/vis/)* and the Immunization Action Coalition's site *(www.immunize.org/vis/)*. (The latter site also includes translations of the VISs.) VISs from these sites can be downloaded and printed.

STORAGE AND HANDLING

Injectable vaccines are packaged in multidose vials, single-dose vials, or manufacturer-filled single-dose syringes. The live attenuated nasal-spray influenza vaccine is packaged in single-dose sprayers. Oral typhoid vaccine is packaged in capsules. Some vaccines, such as MMR, varicella, zoster, and meningococcal polysaccharide vaccines, come as lyophilized (freeze-dried) powders that must be reconstituted (i.e., mixed with a liquid diluent) before use. The lyophilized powder and the diluent come in separate vials. Diluents are not interchangeable but rather are specifically formulated for each type of vaccine; only the specific diluent provided by the manufacturer for each type of vaccine should be used. Once lyophilized vaccines have been reconstituted, their shelf-life is limited and they must be stored under appropriate temperature and light conditions. For example, varicella and zoster vaccines must be protected from light and administered within 30 min of reconstitution; MMR vaccine likewise must be protected from light but can be used up to 8 h after reconstitution. Single-dose vials of meningococcal polysaccharide vaccine must be used within 30 min of reconstitution, while multidose vials must be used within 35 days.

Vaccines are stored either at refrigerator temperature (2–8°C) or at freezer temperature (–15°C or colder). In general, inactivated vaccines (e.g., inactivated influenza, pneumococcal polysaccharide, and meningococcal conjugate vaccines) are stored at refrigerator temperature, while vials of lyophilized-powder live-virus vaccines (e.g., varicella, zoster, and MMR vaccines) are stored at freezer temperature. Diluents for lyophilized vaccines may be stored at refrigerator or room temperature. Live attenuated influenza vaccine—a live-virus liquid formulation administered by nasal spray—is stored at refrigerator temperature.

Vaccine storage and handling errors can result in the loss of vaccines worth millions of dollars, and administration of improperly stored vaccines may elicit inadequate immune responses in patients. To improve the standard of vaccine storage and handling practices, the CDC has published detailed guidance (available at *www.cdc.gov/vaccines/recs/storage/toolkit/storage-handling-toolkit.pdf*). For vaccine storage, the CDC recommends stand-alone units—i.e., self-contained units that either refrigerate or freeze but do not do both—as these units maintain the required temperatures better than combination refrigerator/freezer units. Dormitory-style combined refrigerator/freezer units should never be used for vaccine storage.

The temperature of refrigerators and freezers used for vaccine storage must be monitored and the temperature recorded at least twice each workday. Ideally, continuous thermometers that measure and record temperature all day and all night are used, and minimum and maximum temperatures are read and documented each workday. The CDC recommends the use of calibrated digital thermometers with a probe in a glycol-filled bottle; more detailed information on specifications of storage units and temperature-monitoring devices is provided at the link given above.

ADMINISTRATION OF VACCINES

Most parenteral vaccines recommended for routine administration to adults in the United States are given by either the IM or the SC route; one influenza vaccine formulation approved for use in adults 18–64 years of age is given intradermally. Live-virus vaccines such as varicella, zoster, and MMR are given SC. Most inactivated vaccines are given IM, except for meningococcal polysaccharide vaccine, which is given SC. The 23-valent pneumococcal polysaccharide vaccine may be given either IM or SC, but IM administration is preferred because it is associated with a lower risk of injection-site reactions.

Vaccines given to adults by the SC route are administered with a 5/8-inch needle into the upper outer-triceps area. Vaccines administered to adults by the IM route are injected into the deltoid muscle (Fig. 148-2) with a needle whose length should be selected on the basis of the recipient's sex and weight to ensure adequate penetration into the muscle. Current guidelines indicate that, for men and women weighing <152 lbs (<70 kg), a 1-inch needle is sufficient; for women weighing 152–200 lbs (70–90 kg) and men weighing 152–260 lbs (70–118 kg), a 1- to 1.5-inch needle is needed; and for women weighing >200 lbs (>90 kg) and men weighing >260 lbs (>118 kg), a 1.5-inch needle is required. Additional illustrations of vaccine injection locations and techniques may be found at *www.immunize.org/catg.d/p2020a.pdf*.

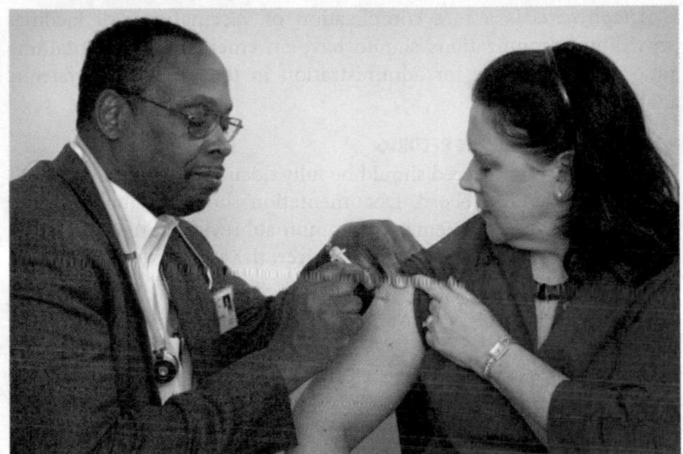

FIGURE 148-2 Technique for IM administration of vaccine. *(Photo credit: James Gathany, Centers for Disease Control and Prevention; accessible at Public Health Image Library, www.cdc.gov. PHIL ID#9420.)*

Aspiration, the process of pulling back on the plunger of the syringe after skin penetration but prior to injection, is not necessary because no large blood vessels are present at the recommended vaccine injection sites.

Multiple vaccines can be administered at the same visit; indeed, administration of all needed vaccines at one visit is encouraged. Studies have shown that vaccines are as effective when administered simultaneously as they are individually, and simultaneous administration of multiple vaccines is not associated with an increased risk of adverse effects. If more than one vaccine must be administered in the same limb, the injection sites should be separated by 1–2 inches so that any local reactions can be differentiated. If a vaccine and an immune globulin preparation are administered simultaneously (e.g., Td vaccine and tetanus immune globulin), a separate anatomic site should be used for each injection.

For certain vaccines (e.g., HPV vaccine and hepatitis B vaccine), multiple doses are required for an adequate and persistent antibody response. The recommended vaccination schedule specifies the interval between doses. Many adults who receive the first dose in a multiple-dose vaccine series do not complete the series or do not receive subsequent doses within the recommended interval. For example, at least one-third of adults who receive the first dose of hepatitis B vaccine in the three-dose series do not complete the series. In these circumstances, vaccine efficacy and/or the duration of protection may be compromised. Providers should implement recall systems that will prompt patients to return for subsequent doses in a vaccination series at the appropriate intervals. With the exception of oral typhoid vaccination, an interruption in the schedule does not require restarting of the entire series or the addition of extra doses.

Syncope may follow vaccination, especially in adolescents and young adults. Serious injuries, including skull fracture and cerebral hemorrhage, have occurred. Adolescents and adults should be seated or lying down during vaccination. The majority of reported syncope episodes after vaccination occur within 15 min. The ACIP recommends that vaccine providers strongly consider observing patients, particularly adolescents, with patients seated or lying down for 15 min after vaccination. If syncope develops, patients should be observed until the symptoms resolve.

Anaphylaxis is a rare complication of vaccination. All facilities providing immunizations should have an emergency kit containing aqueous epinephrine for administration in the event of a systemic anaphylactic reaction.

MAINTENANCE OF VACCINE RECORDS

All vaccines administered should be fully documented in the patient's permanent medical record. Documentation should include the date of administration, the name or common abbreviation of the vaccine, the vaccine lot number and manufacturer, the administration site, the VIS edition, the date the VIS was provided, and the name, address, and title of the person who administered the vaccine. Increasing use of two-dimensional bar codes on vaccine vials and syringes that can be scanned for data entry into compatible electronic medical records and immunization information systems may facilitate more complete and accurate recording of required information.

VACCINE SAFETY MONITORING AND ADVERSE EVENT REPORTING

Prelicensure Evaluations of Vaccine Safety Before vaccines are licensed by the FDA, they are evaluated in clinical trials with volunteers. These trials are conducted in three progressive phases. Phase 1 trials are small, usually involving fewer than 100 volunteers. Their purposes are to provide a basic evaluation of safety and to identify common adverse events. Phase 2 trials, which are larger and may involve several hundred participants, collect additional information on safety and are usually designed to evaluate immunogenicity as well. Data gained from phase 2 trials can be used to determine the composition of the vaccine, the number of doses required, and a profile of common adverse events. Vaccines that appear promising are evaluated in phase 3 trials, which typically involve several hundred to several thousand volunteers and are generally designed to demonstrate vaccine efficacy and provide additional information on vaccine safety.

Postlicensure Monitoring of Vaccine Safety After licensure, a vaccine's safety is assessed by several mechanisms. The NCVIA of 1986 requires health care providers to report certain adverse events that follow vaccination. As a mechanism for that reporting, the Vaccine Adverse Event Reporting System (VAERS) was established in 1990 and is jointly managed by the CDC and the FDA. This safety surveillance system collects reports of adverse events associated with vaccines currently licensed in the United States. *Adverse events* are defined as untoward events that occur after immunization and that might be caused by the vaccine product or vaccination process. While the VAERS was established in response to the NCVIA, any adverse event following vaccination—whether in a child or an adult, and whether or not it is believed to have actually been caused by vaccination—may be reported through the VAERS. The adverse events that health care providers are required to report are listed in the reportable-events table on the VAERS website at *vaers.hhs.gov/reportable.htm*. Approximately 30,000 VAERS reports are filed annually, with ~13% reporting serious events resulting in hospitalization, life-threatening illness, disability, or death.

Anyone can file a VAERS report, including health care providers, manufacturers, and vaccine recipients or their parents or guardians. VAERS reports may be submitted online (*vaers.hhs.gov/esub/step1*) or by completing a paper form requested by email (info@vaers.org), phone (800-822-7967), or fax (877-721-0366). The VAERS form asks for the following information: the type of vaccine received; the timing of vaccination; the time of onset of the adverse event; and the recipient's current illnesses or medications, history of adverse events following vaccination, and demographic characteristics (e.g., age and sex). This information is entered into a database. The individual who reported the adverse event then receives a confirmation letter by mail with a VAERS identification number that can be used if additional information is submitted later. In selected cases of serious adverse reaction, the patient's recovery status may be followed up at 60 days and 1 year after vaccination. The FDA and the CDC have access to VAERS data and use this information to monitor vaccine safety and conduct research studies. VAERS data (minus personal information) are also available to the public.

While the VAERS provides useful information on vaccine safety, this passive reporting system has important limitations. One is that events following vaccination are merely reported; the system cannot assess whether a given type of event occurs more often than expected after vaccination. A second is that event reporting is incomplete and is biased toward events that are believed to be more likely to be due to vaccination and that occur relatively soon after vaccination. To obtain more systematic information on adverse events occurring in both vaccinated and unvaccinated persons, the Vaccine Safety Datalink project was initiated in 1991. Directed by the CDC, this project includes nine managed-care organizations in the United States; member databases include information on immunizations, medical conditions, demographics, laboratory results, and medication prescriptions. The Department of Defense oversees a similar system monitoring the safety of immunizations among active-duty military personnel. In addition, postlicensure evaluations of vaccine safety may be conducted by the vaccine manufacturer. In fact, such evaluations are often required by the FDA as a condition of vaccine licensure.

CONSUMER ACCESS TO AND DEMAND FOR IMMUNIZATION

By removing barriers to the consumer or patient, providers and health care institutions can improve vaccine use. Financial barriers have traditionally been important constraints, particularly among uninsured adults. Even for insured adults, out-of-pocket costs associated with newer, more expensive adult vaccines (e.g., zoster vaccine) are an obstacle to be overcome. After influenza vaccine was included by Medicare for all beneficiaries in 1993, coverage among persons ≥65 years of age doubled (from ~30% in 1989 to >60% in 1997). Other strategies that enhance patients' access to vaccination include extended office hours (e.g., evening and weekend hours) and scheduled vaccination-only clinics where waiting times are reduced. Provision of vaccines outside the "medical home" (e.g., through occupational clinics, universities, pharmacies, and retail settings) can expand access for adults who do not make medical visits frequently. Increasing proportions of adults are being vaccinated in these settings.

Health promotion efforts aimed at increasing the demand for immunization are common. Direct-to-consumer advertising by pharmaceutical companies has been used for some newer adolescent and adult vaccines. Efforts to raise consumer demand for vaccines have not increased immunization rates unless implemented in conjunction with other strategies that target strengthening of provider practices or reduction of consumer barriers. Attitudes and beliefs related to vaccination can be considerable impediments to consumer demand. Many adults view vaccines as important for children but are less familiar with vaccinations targeting disease prevention in adults. Several vaccines are recommended for adults with certain medical risk factors, but self-identification as a high-risk individual is relatively rare. Communication research suggests that many adults with chronic diseases may be more motivated to receive a vaccine by a desire to protect their family members rather than to reduce their own risk. Some vaccines are explicitly recommended for persons at relatively low risk of serious complications, with the goal of reducing the risk of transmission to higher-risk contacts. For example, for protection of newborns, vaccinations against influenza and pertussis are recommended for pregnant women and for others who will be around the infant.

STRATEGIES FOR PROVIDERS AND HEALTH CARE FACILITIES

Recommendation from the Provider Health care providers can have great influence on patients with regard to immunization. A recommendation from a doctor or nurse carries more weight than do recommendations from professional societies or endorsements by celebrities. Providers should be well informed about vaccine risks and benefits so that they can address patients' common concerns. The CDC, the American College of Physicians, and the American Academy of Family Physicians review and update the schedule for adult immunization on an annual basis and also have developed educational materials to facilitate provider–patient discussions about vaccination (*www.cdc.gov/vaccines/hcp.htm*).

System Supports Medical offices can incorporate a variety of methods to ensure that providers consistently offer specific immunizations to patients with indications for specific vaccines. Decision-support tools have been incorporated into some electronic health records to alert the provider when specific vaccines are indicated. Manual or automated reminders and standing orders have been discussed (see "Deciding Whom to Vaccinate," above) and have consistently improved vaccination coverage in both office and hospital settings. Most clinicians' estimates of their own performance diverge from objective measurements of their patients' immunization coverage; quantitative assessment and feedback have been shown in pediatric and adolescent practices to increase immunization performance significantly. Some health plans have instituted incentives for providers with high rates of immunization coverage. Specialty providers, including obstetrician–gynecologists, may be the only providers serving some high-risk patients with indications for selected vaccines (e.g., Tdap, influenza, or pneumococcal polysaccharide vaccine).

Immunization Requirements Vaccination against selected communicable diseases is required for attendance at many universities and colleges as well as for service in the U.S. military or in some occupational settings (e.g., child care, laboratory, veterinary, and health care). Immunizations are recommended and sometimes required for travel to certain countries (Chap. 149).

Vaccination of Health Care Staff A particular area of focus for medical settings is vaccination of health care workers, including those with and without direct patient-care responsibilities. The Joint Commission (which accredits health care organizations), the CDC's Healthcare Infection Control Practices Advisory Committee, and the ACIP all recommend influenza vaccination of all health care personnel; recommendations also focus on requiring documentation of declination for providers who do not accept annual influenza vaccination. As part of their participation in the Centers for Medicare and Medicaid Services' Hospital Inpatient Quality Reporting program, acute-care hospitals are required to report the proportion of their health care personnel who have received seasonal influenza vaccine. Some institutions and jurisdictions have added mandates on influenza vaccination of health care workers and have expanded on earlier requirements related to vaccination or proof of immunity for hepatitis B, measles, mumps, rubella, and varicella.

VACCINATION IN NONMEDICAL SETTINGS

Receipt of vaccination in medical offices is most frequent among young children and adults ≥65 years of age. People in these age groups make more office visits and are more likely to receive care in a consistent "medical home" than are older children, adolescents, and nonelderly adults. Vaccination outside the medical home can expand access to those whose health care visits are limited and reduce the burden on busy clinical practices. In some locations, financial constraints related to inventory and storage requirements have led providers to stock few or no vaccines. Outside private office and hospital settings, vaccination may also occur at health department venues, workplaces, retail sites (including pharmacies and supermarkets), and schools or colleges.

When vaccines are given in nonmedical settings, it remains important for standards of immunization practice to be followed. Consumers should be provided with information on how to report adverse events (e.g., via provision of a VIS), and procedures should ensure that documentation of vaccine administration is forwarded to the primary care provider and the state or city public health immunization registry. Detailed documentation may be required for employment, school attendance, and travel. Personalized health records can help consumers keep track of their immunizations, and some occupational health clinics have incorporated automated immunization reports that help employees stay up-to-date with recommended vaccinations. Some pharmacy chain establishments are using automated systems to report immunization information to the state or local immunization information system.

PERFORMANCE MONITORING

Tracking of immunization coverage at national, state, institution, and practice levels can yield feedback to practitioners and programs and facilitate quality improvement. Healthcare Effectiveness Data and Information Set (HEDIS) measures related to adult immunization facilitate comparison of health plans. The CDC's National Immunization Survey and National Health Interview Survey provide selected information on immunization coverage among adults and track progress toward achievement of Healthy People 2020 targets for immunization coverage. Influenza and pneumococcal vaccine coverage rates have been higher among persons ≥65 years of age (60–70%) than among high-risk 18- to 64-year-olds. Figures on state-specific immunization coverage with pneumococcal polysaccharide and influenza vaccines (as measured through the CDC's Behavioral Risk Factor Surveillance System) reveal substantial geographic variation in coverage. There are persistent disparities in adult immunization coverage rates between whites and racial and ethnic minorities. In contrast, racial and economic disparities in immunization of young children have been dramatically reduced during the past 20 years. Much of this progress is attributed to the Vaccines for Children Program, which since 1994 has entitled uninsured children to receive free vaccines.

FUTURE TRENDS

Although most vaccines developed in the twentieth century targeted common acute infectious diseases of childhood, more recently developed vaccines prevent chronic conditions prevalent among adults. Hepatitis B vaccine prevents hepatitis B–related cirrhosis and hepatocellular carcinoma, zoster vaccine prevents shingles and postherpetic neuralgia, and HPV vaccine prevents some types of cervical cancer, genital warts, and anogenital cancers and may also prevent some oropharyngeal cancers (although this outcome was not studied in prelicensure randomized controlled trials). New targets of vaccine development and research may further broaden the definition of vaccine-preventable disease. Research is ongoing on vaccines to prevent insulin-dependent diabetes mellitus, nicotine addiction, and Alzheimer's disease. Expanding strategies for vaccine development are incorporating molecular approaches such as DNA, vector, and peptide vaccines. New technologies, such as the use of transdermal and other needle-less routes of administration, are being applied to vaccine delivery.

149 Health Recommendations for International Travel

Jay S. Keystone, Phyllis E. Kozarsky

According to the World Tourism Organization, international tourist arrivals grew dramatically from 25 million in 1950 to >1 billion in 2012. Not only are more people traveling; travelers are seeking more exotic and remote destinations. Travel from industrialized to developing regions has been increasing, with Asia and the Pacific, Africa, and the Middle East now emerging destinations. Figure 149-1 summarizes the monthly incidence of health problems during travel in developing countries. Studies continue to show that 50–75% of short-term travelers to the tropics or subtropics report some health impairment. Most of these health problems are minor: only 5% require medical attention, and <1% require hospitalization. Although infectious agents contribute substantially to morbidity among travelers, these pathogens account for only ~1% of deaths in this population. Cardiovascular disease and injuries are the most frequent causes of death among travelers from the United States, accounting for 49% and 22% of deaths, respectively. Age-specific rates of death due to cardiovascular disease are similar among travelers and nontravelers. In contrast, rates of death due to injury (the majority from

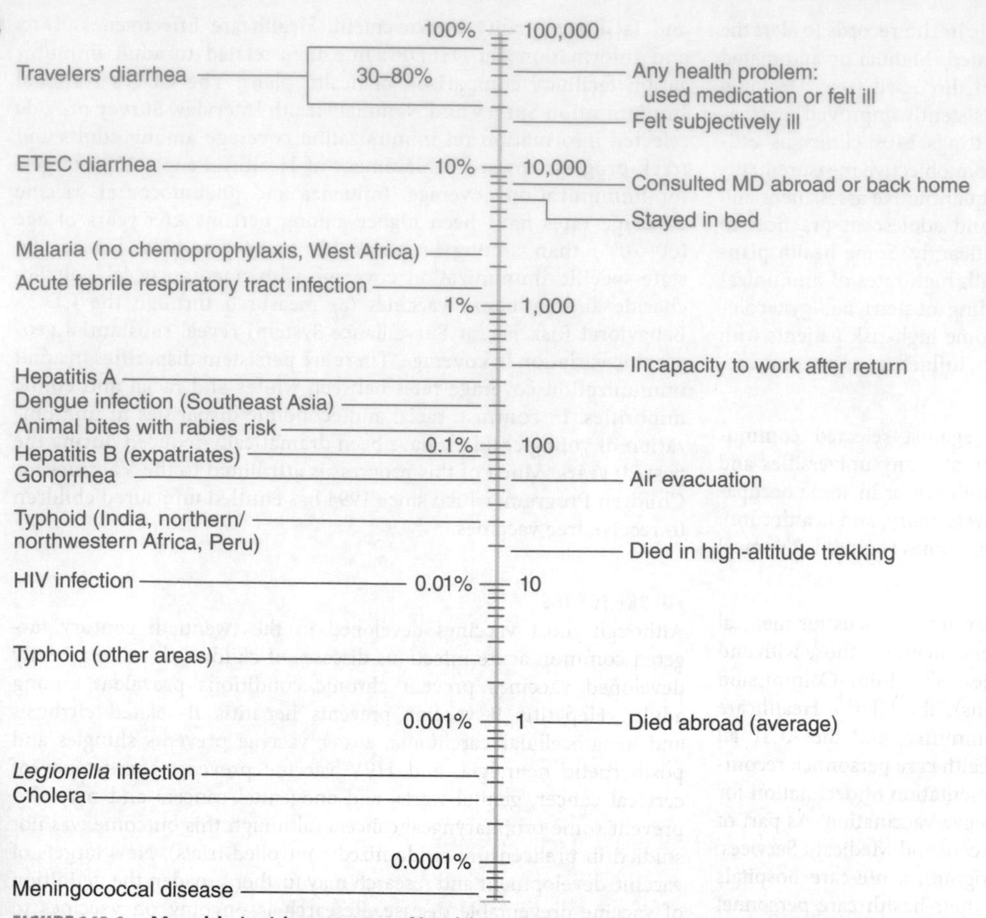

FIGURE 149-1 Monthly incidence rates of health problems during stays in developing countries. ETEC, enterotoxigenic *Escherichia coli*. *(From R Steffen et al: Int J Antimicrob Agents 21:89, 2003.)*

motor vehicle, drowning, or aircraft accidents) are several times higher among travelers. Motor vehicle accidents account for >40% of travelers' deaths that are not due to cardiovascular disease or preexisting illness.

GENERAL ADVICE

Health maintenance recommendations are based not only on the traveler's destination but also on assessment of risk, which is determined by such variables as health status, specific itinerary, purpose of travel, season, and lifestyle during travel. Detailed information regarding country-specific risks and recommendations may be obtained from the Centers for Disease Control and Prevention (CDC) publication *Health Information for International Travel* (available at *www.cdc.gov/travel*).

Fitness for travel is an issue of growing concern in view of the increased numbers of elderly and chronically ill individuals journeying to exotic destinations (see "Travel and Special Hosts," below). Since most commercial aircraft are pressurized to 2500 m (8000 ft) above sea level (corresponding to a Pa_{O_2} of ~55 mmHg), individuals with serious cardiopulmonary problems or anemia should be evaluated before travel. In addition, those who have recently had surgery, a myocardial infarction, a cerebrovascular accident, or a deep-vein thrombosis may be at high risk for adverse events during flight. A summary of current recommendations regarding fitness to fly has been published by the Aerospace Medical Association Air Transport Medicine Committee (*www.asma.org/publications/medical-publications-for-airline-travel*). A pretravel health assessment may be advisable for individuals considering particularly adventurous recreational activities, such as mountain climbing and scuba diving.

IMMUNIZATIONS FOR TRAVEL

Immunizations for travel fall into three broad categories: *routine* (childhood/adult boosters that are necessary regardless of travel), *required* (immunizations that are mandated by international regulations for entry into certain areas or for border crossings), and *recommended* (immunizations that are desirable because of travel-related risks). Required and recommended vaccines commonly given to travelers are listed in Table 149-1.

Routine Immunizations • *DIPHTHERIA, TETANUS, AND POLIO* Diphtheria (Chap. 175) continues to be a problem worldwide. Large outbreaks have occurred in countries that do not have rigorous vaccination programs or that have reduced their public vaccination programs. Serologic surveys show that tetanus (Chap. 177) antibodies are lacking in many North Americans, especially in women over the age of 50. The risk of polio (Chap. 228) to the international traveler is extremely low, and wild-type poliovirus has been eradicated from the Western Hemisphere and Europe. However, studies in the United States suggest that 12% of adult travelers are unprotected against at least one poliovirus serogroup. In addition, challenges continue to be faced by polio eradication programs. Foreign travel offers an ideal opportunity to have these immunizations updated. With the recent increase in pertussis among adults, the diphtheria–tetanus–acellular pertussis (Tdap) combination is now recommended for adults as a once-only replacement for the 10-year tetanus–diphtheria (Td) booster.

MEASLES Measles (rubeola) continues to be a major cause of morbidity and death in the developing world (Chap. 229). Several outbreaks of measles in the United States and Canada have been linked to imported cases, especially from Europe, where large outbreaks have occurred recently. The group at highest risk consists of persons born after 1956 and vaccinated before 1980, in many of whom primary vaccination failed. The measles–mumps–rubella (MMR) vaccine is typically used; its coverage of rubella also addresses a growing concern in some areas of Eastern Europe and Asia.

INFLUENZA Influenza (Chap. 224)—possibly the most common vaccine-preventable infection in travelers—occurs year-round in the tropics and during the summer months in the Southern Hemisphere (coinciding with the winter months in the Northern Hemisphere). One prospective study showed that influenza developed in 1% of travelers to Southeast Asia per month of stay. Annual vaccination should be considered for all travelers who do not have a contraindication. Travel-related influenza continues to occur during summer months in Alaska and the Northwest Territories of Canada among cruise-ship passengers and staff. The speed of global spread of the pandemic H1N1 virus once again illustrates why influenza immunization is so important for travelers.

PNEUMOCOCCAL INFECTION Regardless of travel, pneumococcal vaccine (Chap. 171) should be administered routinely to persons over the age of 65 and to persons at high risk of serious infection, including those with chronic heart, lung, or kidney disease; those who have been splenectomized; and those who have sickle cell disease.

Required Immunizations • *YELLOW FEVER* Documentation of vaccination against yellow fever (Chap. 233) may be required or recommended as a condition for entry into or passage through countries of sub-Saharan Africa and equatorial South America, where the disease is endemic or epidemic, or (by the International Health Regulations) for entry into countries at risk of having the infection introduced. This

TABLE 149-1 VACCINES COMMONLY USED FOR TRAVEL IN ADULTS

Vaccine	Primary Series	Booster Interval
Cholera (Dukoral[a] inactivated whole-cell recombinant subunit; available in Canada and Europe)	1 dose	2 years
Hepatitis A (Havrix), 1440 enzyme immunoassay U/mL	2 doses, 6–12 months apart, IM	None required
Hepatitis A (VAQTA, AVAXIM, EPAXAL)	2 doses, 6–18 months apart, IM	None required
Hepatitis A/B combined (Twinrix)	3 doses at 0, 1, and 6 months 0, 7, and 21–30 days plus booster at 1 year, IM	None required *except* 12 months (once only, for accelerated schedule)
Hepatitis B (Engerix B): accelerated schedule	3 doses at 0, 1, and 2 months 0, 7, and 21 days plus booster at 1 year, IM	12 months, once only
Hepatitis B (Engerix B or Recombivax): standard schedule	3 doses at 0, 1, and 6 months, IM	None required
Immune globulin (hepatitis A prevention)	1 dose IM	Intervals of 3–5 months, depending on initial dose
Japanese encephalitis (Ixiaro)	2 doses at 0 and 28 days, IM	>1 year after primary series (optimal booster schedule not yet determined)
Meningococcus, quadrivalent (Menomune [polysaccharide], Menactra, Menveo [conjugate])	1 dose (Menactra/ Menveo IM; Menomune SC)	>3 years (optimal booster schedule not yet determined)
Rabies human diploid cell vaccine (Imovax), rabies vaccine absorbed (RVA), or purified chick embryo cell vaccine (RabAvert)	3 doses at 0, 7, and 21 or 28 days, IM	None required except with exposure
Typhoid Ty21a, oral live attenuated (Vivotif)	1 capsule every other day × 4 doses	5 years
Typhoid Vi capsular polysaccharide, injectable (Typhim Vi)	1 dose IM	2 years
Yellow fever	1 dose SC	10 years

[a]Cross-protects against enterotoxigenic *Escherichia coli* and provides 30–50% protection against travelers' diarrhea.

vaccine is given only by state authorized yellow fever centers, and its administration must be documented on an official International Certificate of Vaccination. A registry of U.S. clinics that provide the vaccine is available from the CDC (*www.cdc.gov/travel*). Recent data suggest that fewer than 50% of travelers entering areas endemic for yellow fever are immunized; this lack of coverage is a serious problem, as 13 countries in Central and South America and 30 countries in Africa harbor the illness. Severe adverse events associated with this vaccine have recently increased in incidence. First-time vaccine recipients may present with a syndrome characterized as either neurotropic (1 case per 125,000 doses) or viscerotropic (overall, 1 case per 250,000 doses; among persons 60–69 years of age, 1 case per 100,000 doses; and among persons ≥ 70 years of age, 1 case per 40,000 doses). Immunosuppression and thymic disease increase the risk of these adverse events (*www.cdc.gov/vaccines/hcp/vis/vis-statements/yf.pdf*).

MENINGOCOCCAL MENINGITIS Protection against meningitis with one of the quadrivalent (preferably conjugate) vaccines is required for entry into Saudi Arabia during the Hajj (Chap. 180).

INFLUENZA Both seasonal and pandemic H1N1 vaccines (the latter, where available) were required for entry into Saudi Arabia during the Hajj in 2013.

Recommended Immunizations • ***HEPATITIS A AND B*** Hepatitis A (Chap. 360) is one of the most common vaccine-preventable infections of travelers. The risk is six times greater for travelers who stray from the usual tourist routes. The mortality rate for hepatitis A increases with age, reaching almost 2% among individuals over age 50. Of the four hepatitis A vaccines currently available in North America (two in the United States), all are interchangeable and have an efficacy of >95%. Hepatitis A vaccine is currently given to all children in the United States. Since the most frequently identified risk factor for hepatitis A in the United States is international travel, and since morbidity and mortality increase with age, it seems appropriate that all adults be immune prior to travel.

Long-stay overseas workers appear to be at considerable risk for hepatitis B infection (Chap. 360). The recommendation that all travelers be immunized against hepatitis B before departure is supported by two studies showing that 17% of the assessed travelers who received health care abroad had some type of injection; according to the World Health Organization, nonsterile equipment is used for up to 75% of all injections given in parts of the developing world. A 3-week accelerated schedule of the combined hepatitis A and B vaccine has been approved in the United States. Although no data are available on the specific risk of infection with hepatitis B virus among U.S. travelers, ~240 million people in the world have chronic infection. All children and adolescents in the United States are immunized against this illness. Hepatitis B vaccination should be considered for all travelers.

TYPHOID FEVER Most cases of typhoid fever in North America are due to travel, with ~300 cases seen per year in the United States. The attack rate for typhoid fever (Chap. 190) is 1 case per 30,000 travelers per month of travel to the developing world. However, attack rates in India, Senegal, and North Africa are tenfold higher; rates are especially high among travelers to relatively remote destinations and among immigrants and their families who have returned to their homelands to visit friends or relatives (VFRs). Between 1999 and 2006 in the United States, 66% of imported cases involved the latter group. Unfortunately, data show that the causative organism has become increasingly resistant to fluoroquinolone antibiotics (especially in those cases acquired on the Indian subcontinent). Both of the available vaccines—one oral (live) and the other injectable (polysaccharide)—have efficacy rates of ~70%. In some countries, a combined hepatitis A/typhoid vaccine is available.

MENINGOCOCCAL MENINGITIS Although the risk of meningococcal disease among travelers has not been quantified, it is likely to be higher among travelers who live with poor indigenous populations in overcrowded conditions (Chap. 180). Because of its enhanced ability to prevent nasal carriage (compared with the older polysaccharide vaccine), a quadrivalent conjugate vaccine is the product of choice (regardless of age) for immunization of persons traveling to sub-Saharan Africa during the dry season or to areas of the world where there are epidemics. The vaccine, which protects against serogroups A, C, Y, and W-135, has an efficacy rate of >90%.

JAPANESE ENCEPHALITIS The risk of Japanese encephalitis (Chap. 233), an infection transmitted by mosquitoes in rural Asia and Southeast Asia, can be as high as ~1 case per 5000 travelers per month of stay in an endemic area. Most infections are asymptomatic, with a very small proportion of infected persons becoming ill. However, among those who do become ill, severe neurologic sequelae are common. Most symptomatic infections among U.S. residents have involved military personnel or their families. The vaccine efficacy rate is >90%. The vaccine is recommended for persons staying >1 month in rural endemic areas or for shorter periods if their activities (e.g., camping, bicycling, hiking) in these areas will increase exposure risk.

CHOLERA The risk of cholera (Chap. 193) is extremely low, with ~1 case per 500,000 journeys to endemic areas. Cholera vaccine, not currently available in the United States, was rarely recommended but was considered for aid and health care workers in refugee camps or in disaster-stricken/war-torn areas. A more effective oral cholera vaccine is available in other countries.

RABIES Domestic animals, primarily dogs, are the major transmitters of rabies in developing countries (Chap. 232). Several studies have shown that the risk of rabies posed by a dog bite in an endemic area translates into 1–3.6 cases per 1000 travelers per month of stay. Countries where canine rabies is highly endemic include Mexico, the Philippines, Sri Lanka, India, Thailand, China, and Vietnam. The two vaccines available in the United States provide >90% protection. Rabies vaccine is recommended for long-stay travelers, particularly children (who tend to play with animals and may not report bites), and for persons who may be occupationally exposed to rabies in endemic areas; however, in a large-scale study, almost 50% of potential exposures occurred within the first month of travel. Even after receipt of a preexposure rabies vaccine series, two postexposure doses are required. Travelers who have had the preexposure series do not require rabies immune globulin (which is often unavailable in developing countries) if they are exposed to the disease.

PREVENTION OF MALARIA AND OTHER INSECT-BORNE DISEASES

It is estimated that more than 30,000 American and European travelers develop malaria each year (Chap. 248). The risk to travelers is highest in Oceania and sub-Saharan Africa (estimated at 1:5 and 1:50 per month of stay, respectively, among persons not using chemoprophylaxis); intermediate in malarious areas on the Indian subcontinent and in Southeast Asia (1:250–1:1000 per month); and low in South and Central America (1:2500–1:10,000 per month). Of the 1925 cases of malaria reported in 2011 in the United States (the highest figure in 40 years), 90% of those due to *Plasmodium falciparum* occurred in travelers returning or emigrating from Africa and Oceania. VFRs are at the highest risk of acquiring malaria and may die of the disease if their immunity has waned after living outside an endemic area for a number of years. According to data from the CDC, VFRs accounted for 59% of severe malaria cases in the United States in 2011. With the worldwide increase in chloroquine- and multidrug-resistant falciparum malaria, decisions about chemoprophylaxis have become more difficult. The case-fatality rate for falciparum malaria in the United States is 4%; however, *in only one-third of patients who die is the diagnosis of malaria considered before death.*

Several studies indicate that fewer than 50% of travelers adhere to basic recommendations for malaria prevention. Keys to the prevention of malaria include both personal protection measures against mosquito bites (especially between dusk and dawn) and malaria chemoprophylaxis. The former measures entail the use of DEET-containing insect repellents, permethrin-impregnated bed nets and clothing, screened sleeping accommodations, and protective clothing. Thus, in regions where infections such as malaria are transmitted, DEET products (25–50%) are recommended, even for children and infants at birth. Studies suggest that concentrations of DEET above ~50% do not offer a marked increase in protection time against mosquitoes. The CDC also recommends picaridin, oil of lemon eucalyptus (PMD, paramenthane-3,8-diol), and IR3535 (3-[*N*-butyl-*N*-acetyl]-aminopropionic acid, ethyl ester). In general, higher concentrations of any active ingredient provide a longer duration of protection. Personal protection measures also help prevent other insect-transmitted illnesses, such as dengue fever (Chap. 233). Over the past decade, the incidence of dengue has markedly increased, particularly in the Caribbean region, Latin America, Southeast Asia, and (more recently) Africa. Chikungunya, another mosquito-borne infection that clinically resembles dengue fever but with arthralgia and arthritis instead of myalgia, has recently crossed to the Western Hemisphere; many thousands of cases are now occurring in the Caribbean. Both dengue and chikungunya viruses are transmitted by an urban-dwelling mosquito that bites primarily at dawn and dusk.

Table 149-2 lists the currently recommended drugs of choice for prophylaxis of malaria, by destination.

TABLE 149-2 MALARIA CHEMOSUPPRESSIVE REGIMENS, ACCORDING TO GEOGRAPHIC AREA[a]

Geographic Area	Drug of Choice[b]	Alternatives
Central America (north of Panama), Iraq, Turkey, northern Argentina, and Paraguay	Chloroquine	Atovaquone-proguanil[c] Doxycycline Mefloquine Primaquine
South America (but not northern Argentina or Paraguay, where chloroquine may be used); Central America (only Panama east of the Canal); Asia (including Southeast Asia); Africa; and Oceania	Doxycycline Atovaquone-proguanil[c] Mefloquine	
Thai-Myanmar and Thai-Cambodian borders, central Vietnam	Atovaquone-proguanil[c] Doxycycline	

[a]See CDC's *Health Information for International Travel 2014* (www.cdc.gov/travel). [b]In all areas where chloroquine can still be used, the other drugs listed may be used as alternatives. [c]Malarone.

Note: See also **Chap. 248**.

PREVENTION OF GASTROINTESTINAL ILLNESS

Diarrhea, the leading cause of illness in travelers (Chap. 160), is usually a short-lived, self-limited condition. However, 40% of affected individuals need to alter their scheduled activities, and another 20% are confined to bed. The most important determinant of risk is the destination. Incidence rates per 2-week stay have been reported to be as low as 8% in industrialized countries and as high as 55% in parts of Africa, Central and South America, and Southeast Asia. Infants and young adults are at particularly high risk for gastrointestinal illness and for complications such as dehydration. Recent reviews suggest that there is little correlation between dietary indiscretions and the occurrence of travelers' diarrhea. Earlier studies of U.S. students in Mexico showed that eating meals in restaurants and cafeterias or consuming food from street vendors was associated with increased risk. For further discussion, see "Precautions," below.

Etiology (See also Table 160-3) The most frequently identified pathogens causing travelers' diarrhea are enterotoxigenic and enteroaggregative *Escherichia coli* (Chap. 186), although in some parts of the world (notably northern Africa and Southeast Asia) *Campylobacter* infections (Chap. 192) appear to predominate. Other common causative organisms include *Salmonella* (Chap. 190), *Shigella* (Chap. 191), rotavirus (Chap. 227), and norovirus (Chap. 227). The latter virus has caused numerous outbreaks on cruise ships. Except for giardiasis (Chap. 254), parasitic infections are uncommon causes of travelers' diarrhea in short-term travelers. A growing problem for travelers is the development of antibiotic resistance among many bacterial pathogens. Examples include strains of *Campylobacter* resistant to quinolones and strains of *E. coli*, *Shigella*, and *Salmonella* resistant to trimethoprim-sulfamethoxazole *E. coli*. O157 is very rarely a cause of travelers' diarrhea.

Precautions Some experts think that it is not only *what* travelers eat but also where they eat that puts them at risk of illness. Food sold by street vendors can carry a high risk, and restaurant hygiene can be a major problem over which the traveler has no control. In addition to discretion in choosing the source of food and water, general precautions include eating foods piping hot; avoiding foods that are raw or poorly cooked; and drinking only boiled or commercially bottled beverages, particularly those that are carbonated. Heating kills diarrhea-causing organisms, whereas freezing does not; therefore, ice cubes made from unpurified water should be avoided. In spite of these recommendations, the literature has repeatedly documented dietary indiscretions by 98% of travelers within the first 72 h after arrival at their destination. The maxim "Boil it, cook it, peel it, or forget it!" is easy to remember but apparently difficult to follow.

Self-Treatment (See also Table 160-5) As travelers' diarrhea often occurs despite rigorous food and water precautions, travelers should carry medications for self-treatment. An antibiotic is useful in reducing the frequency of bowel movements and the duration of illness in moderate to severe diarrhea. The standard regimen is a 3-day course of a quinolone taken twice daily (or, in the case of some newer formulations, once daily). However, studies have shown that one double dose of a quinolone may be equally effective. For diarrhea acquired in areas such as Thailand, where >90% of *Campylobacter* infections are quinolone resistant, azithromycin may be a better alternative. Rifaximin, a poorly absorbed rifampin derivative, is highly effective against noninvasive bacterial pathogens such as enterotoxigenic and enteroaggregative *E. coli*. The current approach to self-treatment of travelers' diarrhea for the typical short-term traveler is to carry three once-daily doses of an antibiotic and to use as many doses as necessary to resolve the illness. If neither high fever nor blood in the stool accompanies the diarrhea, loperamide should be taken in combination with the antibiotic; studies have shown that this combination is more effective than an antibiotic alone and does not prolong illness.

Prophylaxis Prophylaxis of travelers' diarrhea with bismuth subsalicylate is widely used but only ~60% effective. For certain individuals (e.g., athletes, persons with a repeated history of travelers' diarrhea, and persons with chronic diseases), a single daily dose of a quinolone, azithromycin, or rifaximin during travel of <1 month's duration is 75–90% efficacious in preventing travelers' diarrhea. Probiotics have been only ~20% effective as prophylaxis. In Europe and Canada, an oral subunit cholera vaccine that cross-protects against enterotoxigenic *E. coli* (Dukoral) has been shown to provide 30–50% protection against travelers' diarrhea.

Illness After Return Although extremely common, acute travelers' diarrhea is usually self-limited or amenable to antibiotic therapy. Persistent bowel problems after the traveler returns home have a less well-defined etiology and may require medical attention from a specialist. Infectious agents (e.g., *Giardia lamblia, Cyclospora cayetanensis, Entamoeba histolytica*) appear to be responsible for only a small proportion of cases with persistent bowel symptoms. By far the most common causes of persistent diarrhea after travel are postinfectious sequelae such as lactose intolerance and irritable bowel syndrome. A meta-analysis showed that postinfectious irritable bowel syndrome lasting months to years may occur in as many as 4–13% of cases. When no infectious etiology can be identified, a trial of metronidazole therapy for presumed giardiasis, a strict lactose-free diet for 1 week, or a several-week trial of high-dose hydrophilic mucilloid (plus an osmotic laxative such as lactulose or PEG 3350 for persons with alternating diarrhea and constipation) relieves the symptoms of many patients.

PREVENTION OF OTHER TRAVEL-RELATED PROBLEMS

Travelers are at high risk for *sexually transmitted diseases* (Chap. 163). Surveys have shown that large numbers of travelers engage in casual sex, and there is a reluctance to use condoms consistently. An increasing number of travelers are being diagnosed with illnesses such as *schistosomiasis* (Chap. 259), *dengue* (Chap. 233), *chikungunya* (Chap. 233), and *tick borne rickettsial disease* (Chap. 211). Travelers should be cautioned to avoid bathing, swimming, or wading in freshwater lakes, streams, or rivers in parts of northeastern South America, the Caribbean, Africa, and Southeast Asia. Insect repellents are important for prevention not only of malaria but also of other vector-borne diseases. Prevention of *travel-associated injury* depends mostly on common-sense precautions. Riding on motorcycles (especially without helmets) and in overcrowded public vehicles is not recommended; in developing countries, individuals should *never* travel by road in rural areas after dark. Of persons who die during travel, fewer than 1% die of infection, whereas 40% die in motor vehicle accidents. Excessive alcohol use has been a significant factor in motor vehicle accidents, drownings, assaults, and injuries. Travelers are cautioned to avoid walking barefoot because of the risk of hookworm and *Strongyloides* infections (Chap. 257) and snakebites (Chap. 474).

THE TRAVELER'S MEDICAL KIT

A traveler's medical kit is strongly advisable. The contents may vary widely, depending on the itinerary, duration of stay, style of travel, and local medical facilities. While many medications are available abroad (often over the counter), directions for their use may be nonexistent or in a foreign language, or a product may be outdated or counterfeit. For example, a multicountry study in Southeast Asia showed that a mean of 53% (range, 21–92%) of antimalarial products were counterfeit or contained inadequate amounts of active drug. The sale and marketing of such medications constitute a growing industry. In the medical kit, the short-term traveler should consider carrying an analgesic; an antidiarrheal agent and an antibiotic for self-treatment of travelers' diarrhea; antihistamines; a laxative; oral rehydration salts; a sunscreen with broad-spectrum protection (UVA and UVB, with the latter at a level of at least 30 SPF); a DEET-containing or equivalent insect repellent for the skin; an insecticide for clothing (permethrin); and, if necessary, an antimalarial drug. To these medications, the long-stay traveler might add a broad-spectrum general-purpose antibiotic (levofloxacin or azithromycin), an antibacterial eye and skin ointment, and a topical antifungal cream. Regardless of the duration of travel, a first-aid kit containing such items as scissors, tweezers, and bandages should be considered. A practical approach to self-treatment of infections in the long-stay traveler who carries a once-daily dose of antibiotics (e.g., levofloxacin) is to use 3 tablets "below the waist" (bowel and bladder infections) and 6 tablets "above the waist" (skin and respiratory infections).

TRAVEL AND SPECIAL HOSTS

PREGNANCY AND TRAVEL

(See also Chap. 8) A woman's medical history and itinerary, the quality of medical care at her destinations, and her degree of flexibility determine whether travel is wise during pregnancy. According to the American College of Obstetrics and Gynecology, the safest part of pregnancy in which to travel is between 18 and 24 weeks, when there is the least danger of spontaneous abortion or premature labor. Some obstetricians prefer that women stay within a few hundred miles of home after the 28th week of pregnancy in case problems arise. In general, however, healthy women may be advised that it is acceptable to travel.

Relative contraindications to international travel during pregnancy include a history of miscarriage, premature labor, incompetent cervix, or toxemia. General medical problems such as diabetes, heart failure, severe anemia, or a history of thromboembolic disease also should prompt the pregnant woman to postpone her travels. Finally, regions in which the pregnant woman and her fetus may be at excessive risk (e.g., those at high altitudes, those where live-virus vaccines are required, and those where multidrug-resistant malaria is endemic) are not ideal destinations during any trimester.

Malaria Malaria during pregnancy carries a significant risk of morbidity and death. Levels of parasitemia are highest and failure to clear the parasites after treatment is most frequent among primigravidae. Severe disease, with complications such as cerebral malaria, massive hemolysis, and renal failure, is especially likely in pregnancy. Fetal sequelae include spontaneous abortion, stillbirth, preterm delivery, and congenital infection. Chloroquine and mefloquine are considered to be safe in all trimesters.

Enteric Infections Pregnant travelers must be extremely cautious regarding their food and beverage intake. Dehydration due to travelers' diarrhea can lead to inadequate placental blood flow. Infections such as toxoplasmosis, hepatitis E, and listeriosis also can cause serious sequelae in pregnancy.

The mainstay of therapy for travelers' diarrhea is rehydration. Loperamide may be used if necessary. For self-treatment, azithromycin may be the best option. Although quinolones are increasingly being used safely during pregnancy and rifaximin is poorly absorbed from the gastrointestinal tract, these drugs are not approved for this indication.

Because of the serious problems encountered when infants are given local foods and beverages, women are strongly encouraged to breast-feed when traveling with a neonate. A nursing mother with travelers' diarrhea should not stop breast-feeding but should increase her fluid intake.

Air Travel and High-Altitude Destinations Commercial air travel is not a risk to the healthy pregnant woman or to the fetus. The higher radiation levels reported at altitudes of >10,500 m (>35,000 ft) should pose no problem for the healthy pregnant traveler. Since each airline has a policy regarding pregnancy and flying, it is best to check with the specific carrier when booking reservations. Domestic air travel is usually permitted until the 36th week, whereas international air travel is generally curtailed after the 32nd week.

There are no known risks for pregnant women who travel to high-altitude destinations and stay for short periods. However, there are likewise no data on the safety of pregnant women at altitudes of >4500 m (15,000 ft).

THE HIV-INFECTED TRAVELER

(See also Chap. 226) The HIV-infected traveler is at special risk of serious infections due to a number of pathogens that may be more prevalent at travel destinations than at home. However, the degree of risk depends primarily on the state of the immune system at the time of travel. For persons whose CD4+ T cell counts are normal or >500/μL, data suggest no greater risk during travel than for persons without HIV infection. Individuals with AIDS (CD4+ T cell counts of <200/μL) and others who are symptomatic need special counseling and should visit a travel medicine practitioner before departure, especially when traveling to the developing world.

Several countries routinely deny entry to HIV-positive individuals for prolonged stay, even though these restrictions do not appear to decrease rates of transmission of the virus. In general, HIV testing is required for individuals who wish to stay abroad >3 months or who intend to work or study abroad. Some countries will accept an HIV serologic test done within 6 months of departure, whereas others will not accept a blood test done at any time in the traveler's home country. Border officials often have the authority to make inquiries of individuals entering a country and to check the medications they are carrying. If antiretroviral drugs are identified, the person may be barred from entering the country. Information on testing requirements for specific countries is available from consular offices but is subject to frequent change.

Immunizations All of the HIV-infected traveler's routine immunizations should be up to date (Chap. 148). The response to immunization may be impaired at CD4+ T cell counts of <200/μL and in some cases at even higher counts. Thus HIV-infected persons should be vaccinated as early as possible to ensure adequate immune responses. For patients receiving antiretroviral therapy, at least 3 months must elapse before regenerated CD4+ T cells can be considered fully functional; therefore, vaccination of these patients should be delayed. However, when the risk of illness is high or the sequelae of illness are serious, immunization is recommended. In certain circumstances, it may be prudent to check the adequacy of the serum antibody response before departure.

Because of the increased risk of infections due to Streptococcus pneumoniae and other bacterial pathogens that cause pneumonia after influenza, the conjugate pneumococcal vaccine (Prevnar 13) followed by the 23-valent polysaccharide vaccine (Pneumovax) as well as influenza vaccine should be administered. The estimated rates of response to influenza vaccine are >80% among persons with asymptomatic HIV infection and <50% among those with AIDS.

In general, live attenuated vaccines are contraindicated for persons with immune dysfunction. Because measles (rubeola) can be a severe or lethal infection in HIV-positive patients, these patients should receive the measles vaccine (or the combination MMR vaccine) unless the CD4+ T cell count is <200/μL. Between 18% and 58% of symptomatic HIV-infected vaccinees develop adequate measles antibody titers, and 50–100% of asymptomatic HIV-infected persons seroconvert.

It is recommended that the live yellow fever vaccine not be given to HIV-infected travelers. Although the potential adverse effects of a live vaccine in an HIV-infected individual are always a consideration, there appear to have been no reported cases of illness in those who have inadvertently received this vaccine. Nonetheless, if the CD4+ T cell count is <200/μL, an alternative itinerary that poses no risk of exposure to yellow fever is recommended. If the traveler is passing through or traveling to an area where the vaccine is required but the disease risk is low, a physician's waiver should be issued.

A transient increase in HIV viremia (lasting days to weeks) has been demonstrated in HIV-infected individuals after immunization against influenza, pneumococcal infection, and tetanus (Chap. 226). At this point, however, no evidence indicates that this transient increase is detrimental.

Gastrointestinal Illness Decreased levels of gastric acid, abnormal gastrointestinal mucosal immunity, other complications of HIV infection, and medications taken by HIV-infected patients make travelers' diarrhea especially problematic in these individuals. Travelers' diarrhea is likely to occur more frequently, to be more severe, to be accompanied by bacteremia, and to be more difficult to treat. *Cryptosporidium*, *Isospora belli*, and *Microsporidium* infections, although uncommon, are associated with increased morbidity and mortality rates in AIDS patients.

The HIV-infected traveler must be careful to consume only appropriately prepared foods and beverages and may benefit from antibiotic prophylaxis for travelers' diarrhea. Sulfonamides (as used to prevent pneumocystosis) are ineffective because of widespread resistance.

Other Travel-Related Infections Data are lacking on the severity of many vector-borne diseases in HIV-infected individuals. Malaria is especially severe in asplenic persons and in those with AIDS. The HIV load doubles during malaria, with subsidence in ~8–9 weeks; the significance of this increase in viral load is unknown.

Visceral leishmaniasis (Chap. 251) has been reported in numerous HIV-infected travelers. Diagnosis may be difficult, given that splenomegaly and hyperglobulinemia are often lacking and serologic results are frequently negative. Sandfly bites may be prevented by evening use of insect repellents.

Certain respiratory illnesses, such as histoplasmosis and coccidioidomycosis, cause greater morbidity and mortality among patients with AIDS. Although tuberculosis is common among HIV-infected persons (especially in developing countries), its acquisition by the short-term HIV-infected traveler has not been reported as a major problem. From a prospective study, it is estimated that for travelers not engaged in health care the risk of tuberculosis infection is ~3% per year of travel.

Medications Adverse events due to medications and drug interactions are common and raise complex issues for HIV-infected persons. Rates of cutaneous reaction (e.g., increased cutaneous sensitivity to sulfonamides) are unusually high among patients with AIDS. Since zidovudine is metabolized by hepatic glucuronidation, inhibitors of this process may elevate serum levels of the drug. Concomitant administration of the antimalarial drug mefloquine and the antiretroviral agent ritonavir may result in decreased plasma levels of ritonavir; mefloquine may also interact with many of the other protease inhibitors. In contrast, no significant influence of concomitant mefloquine administration on plasma levels of indinavir or nelfinavir was detected in two HIV-infected travelers. Serum levels of mefloquine may be lowered with the use of efavirenz or nevirapine. There are also potential interactions between atovaquone-proguanil (Malarone) and many of the protease inhibitors as well as between Malarone and the nonnucleoside reverse transcriptase inhibitors (NNRTIs). Because of the increase in antiretroviral agents and the lack of accumulated data on their interactions with antimalarial agents, decisions about malaria chemoprophylaxis continue to be difficult; with a short duration of travel, an interaction may be inconsequential. However, doxycycline appears to have no clinically significant interactions with either the protease inhibitors or the NNRTIs. With regard to malaria treatment, a great hypothetical concern is that the antimalarial drugs lumefantrine (combined with artemisinin in Coartem) and halofantrine may interact with HIV protease inhibitors and NNRTIs since drugs in the latter two categories are known to be potent inhibitors of cytochrome P450. In keeping current with antiretroviral drug interactions, a website from the University of Liverpool (*www.hiv-druginteractions.org*) is helpful.

CHRONIC ILLNESS, DISABILITY, AND TRAVEL

Chronic health problems need not prevent travel, but special measures can make the journey safer and more comfortable.

Heart Disease Cardiovascular events are the main cause of deaths among travelers and of in-flight emergencies on commercial aircraft. Extra supplies of all medications should be kept in carry-on luggage, along with a copy of a recent electrocardiogram and the name and telephone number of the traveler's physician at home. Pacemakers are not affected by airport security devices, although electronic telephone checks of pacemaker function cannot be transmitted by international satellites. Travelers with electronic defibrillators should carry a note to that effect and ask for hand screening. A traveler may benefit from supplemental oxygen; since oxygen delivery systems are not standard, supplementary oxygen should be ordered by the traveler's physician well before flight time. Travelers may benefit from aisle seating and should walk, perform stretching and flexing exercises, consider wearing support hose, and remain hydrated during the flight to prevent venous thrombosis and pulmonary embolism.

Chronic Lung Disease Chronic obstructive pulmonary disease is one of the most common diagnoses in patients who require emergency-department evaluation for symptoms occurring during airline flights. The best predictor of the development of in-flight problems is the sea-level Pa_{O_2}. A Pa_{O_2} of at least 72 mmHg corresponds to an in-flight arterial Pa_{O_2} of ~55 mmHg when the cabin is pressurized to 2500 m (8000 ft). If the traveler's baseline Pa_{O_2} is <72 mmHg, the provision of supplemental oxygen should be considered. Contraindications to flight include active bronchospasm, lower respiratory infection, lower-limb deep-vein phlebitis, pulmonary hypertension, and recent thoracic surgery (within the preceding 3 weeks) or pneumothorax. Decreased outdoor activity at the destination should be considered if air pollution is excessive.

Diabetes Mellitus Alterations in glucose control and changes in insulin requirements are common problems among patients with diabetes who travel. Changes in time zone, in the amount and timing of food intake, and in physical activity demand vigilant assessment of metabolic control. Because of the risk of foot ulcers, travelers should wear closed footwear that has been proven to be comfortable. The traveler with diabetes should pack medication (including a bottle of regular insulin for emergencies), insulin syringes and needles, equipment and supplies for glucose monitoring, and snacks in carry on luggage. Insulin is stable for ~3 months at room temperature but should be kept as cool as possible. The name and telephone number of the home physician and a card and bracelet listing the patient's medical problems and the type and dose of insulin used should accompany the traveler. In order to facilitate international border crossings, travelers should carry a physician's letter authorizing the carriage of needles and syringes. In traveling eastward (e.g., from the United States to Europe), the morning insulin dose on arrival may need to be decreased. The blood glucose can then be checked during the day to determine whether additional insulin is required. For flights westward, with lengthening of the day, an additional dose of regular insulin may be required.

Other Special Groups Other groups for whom special travel measures are encouraged include patients undergoing dialysis, those with transplants, and those with other disabilities. Up to 13% of travelers have some disability, but few advocacy groups and tour companies dedicate themselves to this growing population. Medication interactions are a source of serious concern for these travelers, and appropriate medical information should be carried, along with the home physician's name and telephone number. Some travelers taking glucocorticoids carry stress doses in case they become ill. Immunization of these immunocompromised travelers may result in less than adequate protection. Thus the traveler and the physician must carefully consider which destinations are appropriate.

TRAVEL HEALTH INSURANCE

Today, more elderly or chronically ill individuals travel and more of these individuals journey to remote locations and enjoy adventurous activities. Illness or injury abroad is not uncommon and is best considered before the journey. Persons who develop health problems abroad may incur enormous out-of-pocket expenses. Thus prospective travelers should consider purchasing additional travel health insurance and should check with their health insurance company regarding whether they have coverage for illness or injury overseas. Unfortunately, many insurance companies will not cover pre-existing illness if it is the reason for trip cancellation or illness abroad. Most countries do not accept routine health insurance from other countries unless there is a special traveler supplement. In most circumstances, travelers are asked to pay in cash for services rendered on an emergency basis, whether in a physician's office, in an emergency or urgent care center, or even in a hospital. There are several types of travel insurance. It is wise to purchase *trip cancellation insurance*, especially, for example, if the traveler has an underlying chronic illness and may need to cancel a trip due to an exacerbation of disease. *Travel health insurance* will cover expenses in the event that medical care abroad is needed. *Evacuation insurance* will cover medical evacuation, usually to a medical center in another location where it is deemed that the care is similar to that available in the traveler's home country. The cost of medical evacuation can easily exceed $100,000 US. There are a number of travel insurance providers, and it is very important to read the fine print carefully and to determine exactly what each company provides, thereby ensuring an appropriate fit for the individual's particular circumstances. The U.S. Department of State website lists travel health insurance companies (*http://travel.state.gov/travel/tips/emergencies/emergencies_5981.html*).

MEDICAL TOURISM

Travel for the purpose of obtaining health care abroad has received a great deal of attention in the medical literature and the media. According to the annual U.S. Department of Commerce In-Flight Survey, there were ~500,000 overseas trips during 2006 in which health treatment was at least one purpose of travel. Lower cost is usually cited as the motivation for this type of tourism, and an entire industry has flourished as a result of this phenomenon. However, the quality of facilities, assistance services, and care is neither uniform nor regulated; thus, in most instances, responsibility for assessing the suitability of an individual program or facility lies solely with the traveler. Persons considering this option must recognize that they are almost always at a disadvantage when being treated in a foreign country, particularly if there are complications. Concerns to be addressed include the quality of the health care facility and its staff; language and cultural differences that may impede accurate interpretation of both verbal and nonverbal communication; religious and ethical differences that may be encountered over issues such as efforts to preserve life and limb or the provision of care for the terminally ill; lack of familiarity with the local medical system; limited access of the care provider to the patient's medical history; the use of unfamiliar drugs and medicines; the relative difficulty of arranging follow-up care back in the United States; and the possibility that such follow-up care may be fraught with problems should there be complications. If serious issues arise, legal recourse may be difficult or impossible. Patients planning to travel abroad to obtain health care, particularly when surgery is involved, should be immunized for hepatitis B and should consider having baseline hepatitis C and HIV tests preoperatively. Prevalence rates of hepatitis B and C and HIV infection vary considerably around the world and are generally higher in developing regions than in the United States and Western Europe. The latest information available on the safety of the blood supply outside the United States is the World Health Organization's Global Database on Blood Safety based on data from 2011 (*www.who.int/bloodsafety/global_database/en*). Persons researching the accreditation status of overseas facilities should note that, although these facilities may be part of a chain, they are surveyed and accredited individually. Accreditation resources include (1) the Joint Commission International (*www.jointcommissioninternational.org*), (2) the Australian Council for Healthcare Standards International (*www.achs.org.au/achs-international/*), and (3) the Canadian Council on Health Services (*www.cchsa.ca*). The American Medical Association also offers guidelines for medical tourism (*www.ama-assn.org/ama1/pub/upload/mm/31/medicaltourism.pdf*).

The most common medical problems encountered by travelers after their return home are diarrhea, fever, respiratory illnesses, and skin diseases (Fig. 149-2). Frequently ignored problems are fatigue and emotional stress, especially in long-stay travelers. The approach to diagnosis requires some knowledge of geographic medicine, in particular the epidemiology and clinical presentation of infectious disorders. A geographic history should focus on the traveler's exact itinerary, including dates of arrival and departure; exposure history (food indiscretions, drinking-water sources, freshwater contact, sexual activity, animal contact, insect bites); location and style of travel (urban vs. rural, first-class hotel accommodation vs. camping); immunization history; and use of antimalarial chemosuppression. Recently,

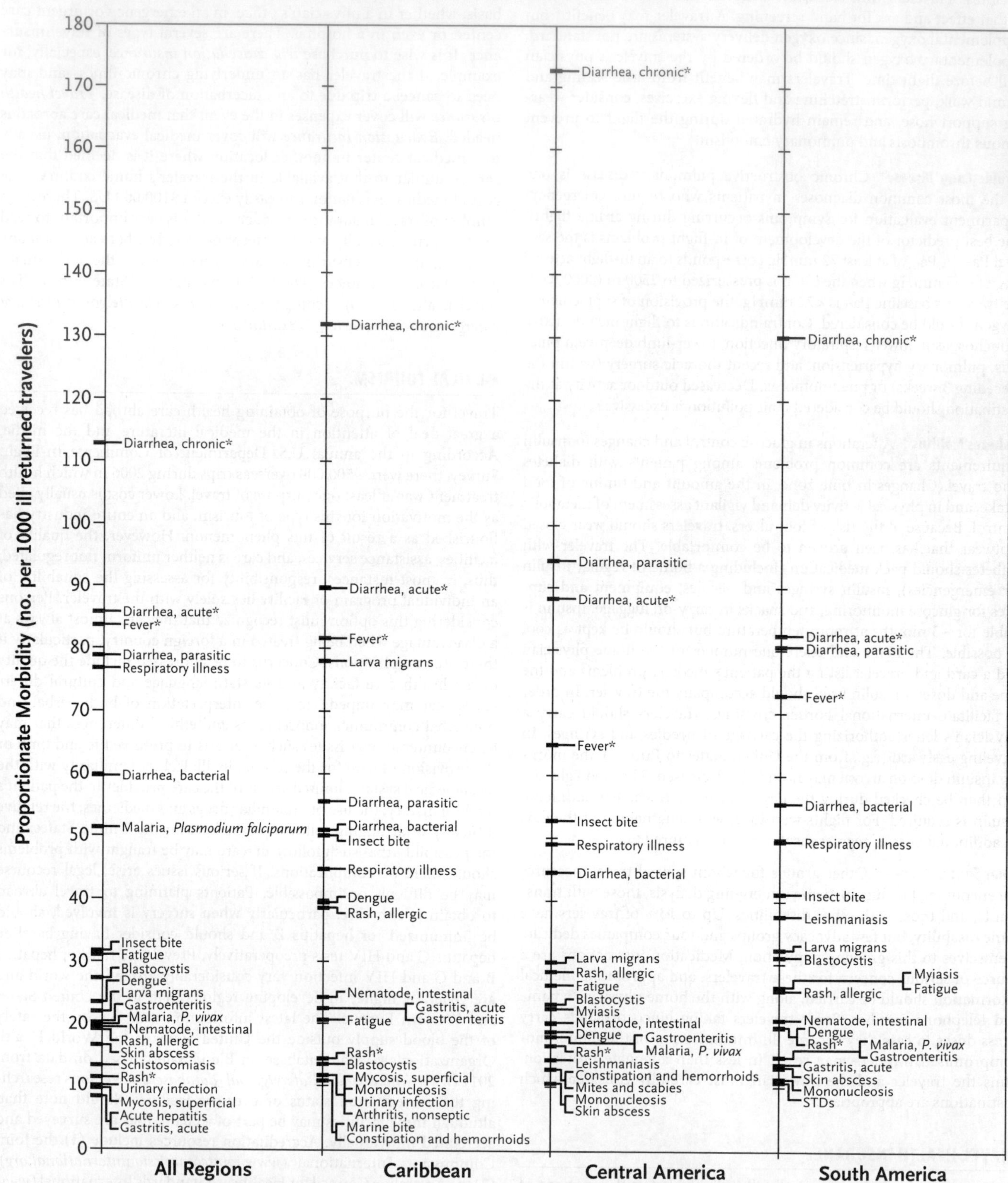

FIGURE 149-2 Proportionate morbidity among ill travelers returning from the developing world, according to region of travel. The proportions (not incidence rates) are shown for each of the top 22 specific diagnoses among all ill returned travelers within each region. STDs, sexually transmitted diseases. Asterisks indicate syndromic diagnoses for which specific etiologies could not be assigned. *(Reprinted from DO Freedman et al: N Engl J Med 354:119, 2006.)*

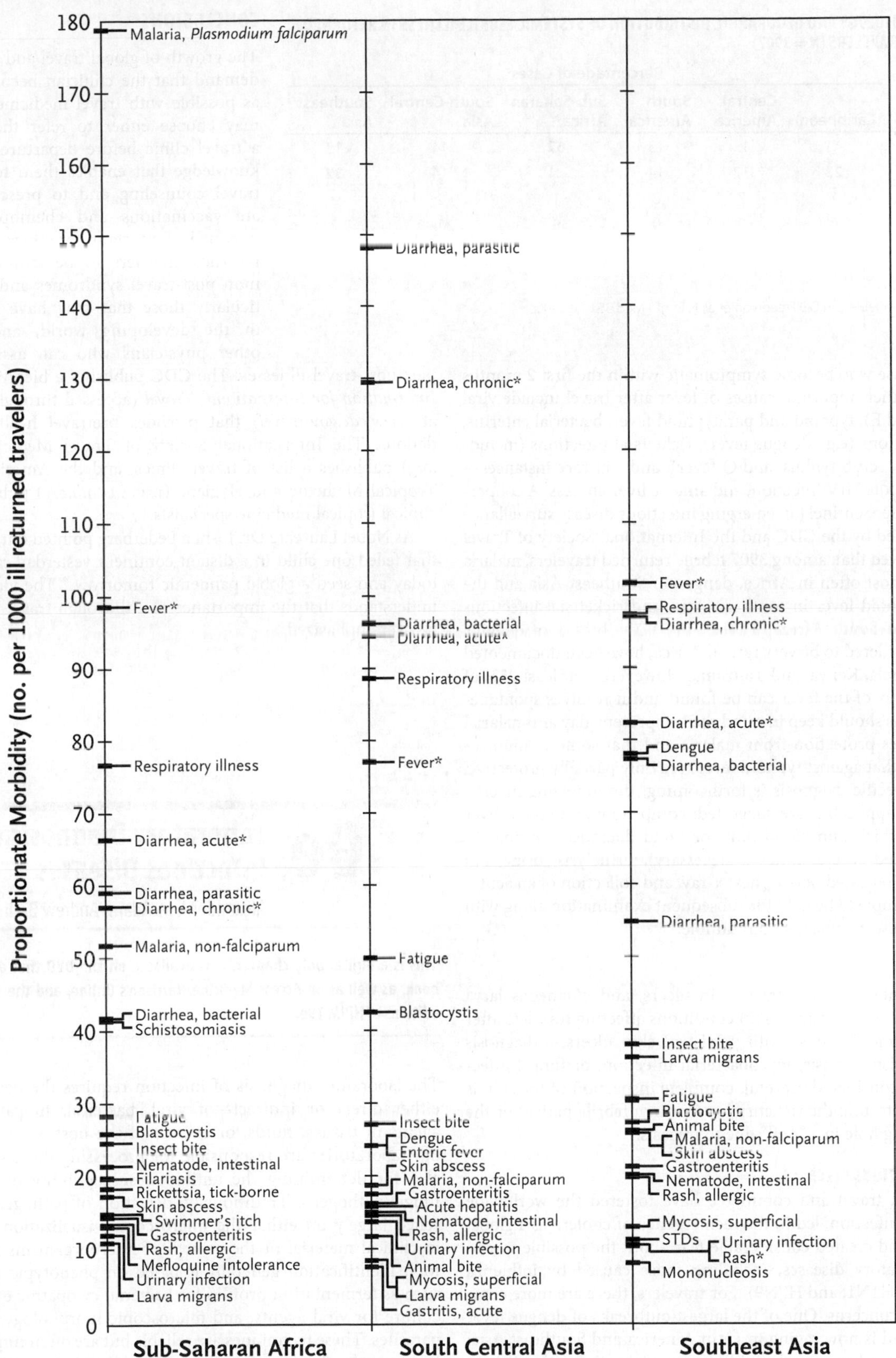

FIGURE 149-2 *(Continued)*

some travelers who have been hospitalized abroad have been shown on return to be colonized with multidrug-resistant bacteria such as Enterobacteriaceae producing extended-spectrum β-lactamases and bacteria producing NDM-1 (New Delhi metallo-β-lactamase 1).

DIARRHEA

See "Prevention of Gastrointestinal Illness," above.

FEVER

Fever in a traveler who has returned from a malarious area should be considered a medical emergency because death from *P. falciparum* malaria can follow an illness of only several days' duration. Although "fever from the tropics" does not always have a tropical cause, malaria should be the first diagnosis considered. The risk of *P. falciparum* malaria is highest among travelers returning from Africa or Oceania

TABLE 149-3 ETIOLOGY AND GEOGRAPHIC DISTRIBUTION OF SYSTEMIC FEBRILE ILLNESS IN RETURNED TRAVELERS (N = 3907)

	Percentage of Cases[a]					
Etiology	Caribbean	Central America	South America	Sub-Saharan Africa	South-Central Asia	Southeast Asia
Malaria	<1	13	13	**62**	14	13
Dengue	**23**	12	14	<1	14	**32**
Mononucleosis	7	7	8	1	2	3
Rickettsia	0	0	0	**6**	1	2
Salmonella	2	3	2	<1	**14**	3

[a]Bold type is for emphasis only.

Source: Revised from Table 2 in DO Freedman et al: N Engl J Med 354:119, 2006.

and among those who become symptomatic within the first 2 months after return. Other important causes of fever after travel include viral hepatitis (A and E), typhoid and paratyphoid fever, bacterial enteritis, arboviral infections (e.g., dengue fever), rickettsial infections (including tick typhus, scrub typhus, and Q fever), and—in rare instances—leptospirosis, acute HIV infection, and amebic liver abscess. A cooperative study by GeoSentinel (an emerging infectious disease surveillance group established by the CDC and the International Society of Travel Medicine) showed that, among 3907 febrile returned travelers, malaria was acquired most often in Africa, dengue in Southeast Asia and the Caribbean, typhoid fever in southern Asia, and rickettsial infections (tick typhus) in South Africa (Table 149-3). Outbreaks of dengue, previously considered to be very rare in Africa, have been documented recently in Angola, Kenya, and Tanzania. However, in at least 25% of cases, no etiology of the fever can be found and it resolves spontaneously. Clinicians should keep in mind that no present-day antimalarial agent guarantees protection from malaria and that some immunizations (notably, that against typhoid fever) are only partially protective.

When no specific diagnosis is forthcoming, the following investigations, where applicable, are suggested: complete blood count, liver function tests, thick/thin blood films or rapid diagnostic testing for malaria (repeated several times if necessary), urinalysis, urine and blood cultures (repeated once), chest x-ray, and collection of an acute-phase serum sample to be held for subsequent examination along with a paired convalescent-phase serum sample.

SKIN DISEASES

Pyodermas, sunburn, insect bites, skin ulcers, and cutaneous larva migrans are the most common skin conditions affecting travelers after their return home. In those with persistent skin ulcers, a diagnosis of cutaneous leishmaniasis, mycobacterial infection, or fungal infection should be considered. Careful, complete inspection of the skin is important in detecting the rickettsial eschar in a febrile patient or the central breathing hole in a "boil" due to myiasis.

EMERGING INFECTIOUS DISEASES

In recent years, travel and commerce have fostered the worldwide spread of HIV infection, led to the reemergence of cholera as a global health threat, and created considerable fear about the possible spread of novel respiratory diseases, including those caused by influenza viruses (H5N1, H1N1, and H7N9). For travelers, there are more common, everyday concerns. One of the largest outbreaks of dengue fever ever documented is now raging in Latin America and Southeast Asia; chikungunya virus has spread rapidly from Africa to southern Asia, southern Europe, and, for the first time in the Western Hemisphere, the Caribbean; schistosomiasis is being described in previously unaffected lakes in Africa; and antibiotic-resistant strains of sexually transmitted and enteric pathogens are emerging at an alarming rate in the developing world. In addition, concerns have been raised about the potential for bioterrorism involving not only standard strains of unusual agents but mutant strains as well.

CONCLUSIONS

The growth of global travel and migration now demand that the clinician become as familiar as possible with travel medicine. Practitioners may choose either to refer their patients to a travel clinic before departure or to acquire knowledge that enables them to provide pretravel counseling and to prescribe appropriate vaccinations and chemoprophylaxis. It is equally important for physicians seeing ill returned travelers to be familiar with common post-travel syndromes and diseases, particularly those that may have been acquired in the developing world, and to identify other physicians who can assist with complex post-travel illnesses. The CDC publishes a biennial text, *Health Information for International Travel* (accessed through their website at *www.cdc.gov/travel*) that provides pretravel health recommendations. The International Society of Travel Medicine (*www.istm.org*) publishes a list of travel clinics, and the American Society of Tropical Medicine and Hygiene (*www.astmh.org*) publishes a list of clinical tropical medicine specialists.

As Nobel Laureate Dr. Joshua Lederberg pointed out, "The microbe that felled one child in a distant continent yesterday can reach yours today and seed a global pandemic tomorrow." The vigilant clinician understands that the importance of a thorough travel history cannot be overemphasized.

150e Laboratory Diagnosis of Infectious Diseases

Alexander J. McAdam, Andrew B. Onderdonk

This is a digital-only chapter. It is available on the DVD that accompanies this book, as well as on Access Medicine/Harrison's Online, and the eBook and "app" editions of HPIM 19e.

The laboratory diagnosis of infection requires the demonstration—either direct or indirect—of viral, bacterial, fungal, or parasitic agents in tissues, fluids, or excreta of the host. Clinical microbiology laboratories are responsible for processing these specimens and also for determining the antibiotic susceptibility of bacterial and fungal pathogens. Traditionally, detection of pathogenic agents has relied largely on either the microscopic visualization of pathogens in clinical material or the growth of microorganisms in the laboratory. Identification generally is based on phenotypic characteristics such as fermentation profiles for bacteria, cytopathic effects in tissue culture for viral agents, and microscopic morphology for fungi and parasites. These techniques are reliable but are often time-consuming. Increasingly, the use of nucleic acid probes is becoming a standard method for detection, quantitation, and/or identification in the clinical microbiology laboratory, gradually replacing phenotypic characterization and microscopic visualization methods. This chapter discusses general concepts of diagnostic testing, with an emphasis on detection of bacteria. Detection of viral, fungal, and parasitic pathogens is discussed in greater detail in separate chapters (see Chaps. 214e, 235, and 245e, respectively).

151e Climate Change and Infectious Disease

Aaron S. Bernstein

This is a digital-only chapter. It is available on the DVD that accompanies this book, as well as on Access Medicine/Harrison's Online, and the eBook and "app" editions of HPIM 19e.

The release of greenhouse gases—principally carbon dioxide—into Earth's atmosphere since the late nineteenth century has contributed to a climate unfamiliar to our species, *Homo sapiens*. This new climate has already altered the epidemiology of some infectious diseases. Continued accumulation of greenhouse gases in the atmosphere will further alter the planet's climate. In some cases climate change may establish conditions favoring the emergence of infectious diseases, while in others it may render areas that are presently suitable for certain diseases unsuitable. This chapter presents the current state of knowledge regarding the known and prospective infectious-disease consequences of climate change.

152e Infections in Veterans Returning from Foreign Wars

Andrew W. Artenstein

This is a digital-only chapter. It is available on the DVD that accompanies this book, as well as on Access Medicine/Harrison's Online, and the eBook and "app" editions of HPIM 19e.

This chapter focuses on infectious diseases that have occurred or have been a source of concern in returning veterans of foreign wars over the past quarter-century. During this period, several pathogens have been associated with disease in this population, as discussed below. Some pathogens have been associated with only rare case reports in war veterans, and some, given their epidemiology, may pose a risk in future conflicts. In general, it is practical to classify infections with delayed signs and symptoms related to prolonged incubation periods or significant clinical latency in terms of their potential to manifest clinically as acute illnesses or chronic/relapsing diseases.

SECTION 2 CLINICAL SYNDROMES: COMMUNITY-ACQUIRED INFECTIONS

153 Pneumonia

Lionel A. Mandell, Richard G. Wunderink

DEFINITION

Pneumonia is an infection of the pulmonary parenchyma. Despite being the cause of significant morbidity and mortality, pneumonia is often misdiagnosed, mistreated, and underestimated. In the past, pneumonia was typically classified as community-acquired (CAP), hospital-acquired (HAP), or ventilator-associated (VAP). Over the past two decades, however, some persons presenting with onset of pneumonia as outpatients have been found to be infected with the multidrug-resistant (MDR) pathogens previously associated with HAP. Factors responsible for this phenomenon include the development and widespread use of potent oral antibiotics, earlier transfer of patients out of acute-care hospitals to their homes or various lower-acuity facilities, increased use of outpatient IV antibiotic therapy, general aging of the population, and more extensive immunomodulatory therapies. The potential involvement of these MDR pathogens has led to a designation for a new category of pneumonia—*health care–associated pneumonia* (HCAP)—that is distinct from CAP. Conditions associated with HCAP and the likely pathogens are listed in Table 153-1.

Although the new classification system has been helpful in designing empirical antibiotic strategies, it is not without its disadvantages. Not all MDR pathogens are associated with all risk factors (Table 153-1). Moreover, HCAP is a distillation of multiple risk factors, and each patient must be considered individually. For example, the risk of infection with MDR pathogens for a nursing home resident who has dementia but can independently dress, ambulate, and eat is quite different from the risk for a patient who is in a chronic vegetative state with a tracheostomy and a percutaneous feeding tube in place. In addition, risk factors for MDR infection do not preclude the development of pneumonia caused by the usual CAP pathogens.

This chapter deals with pneumonia in patients who are not considered to be immunocompromised. **Pneumonia in severely immunocompromised patients, some of whom overlap with the groups**

TABLE 153-1 CLINICAL CONDITIONS ASSOCIATED WITH AND LIKELY PATHOGENS IN HEALTH CARE–ASSOCIATED PNEUMONIA

	Pathogen			
Condition	MRSA	*Pseudomonas aeruginosa*	*Acinetobacter* spp.	MDR Enterobacteriaceae
Hospitalization for ≥48 h	√	√	√	√
Hospitalization for ≥2 days in prior 3 months	√	√	√	√
Nursing home or extended-care-facility residence	√	√	√	√
Antibiotic therapy in preceding 3 months		√		√
Chronic dialysis	√			
Home infusion therapy	√			
Home wound care	√			
Family member with MDR infection	√			√

Abbreviations: MDR, multidrug-resistant; MRSA, methicillin-resistant *Staphylococcus aureus.*

of patients considered in this chapter, warrants separate discussion (see Chaps. 104, 169, and 226).

PATHOPHYSIOLOGY

Pneumonia results from the proliferation of microbial pathogens at the alveolar level and the host's response to those pathogens. Microorganisms gain access to the lower respiratory tract in several ways. The most common is by aspiration from the oropharynx. Small-volume aspiration occurs frequently during sleep (especially in the elderly) and in patients with decreased levels of consciousness. Many pathogens are inhaled as contaminated droplets. Rarely, pneumonia occurs via hematogenous spread (e.g., from tricuspid endocarditis) or by contiguous extension from an infected pleural or mediastinal space.

Mechanical factors are critically important in host defense. The hairs and turbinates of the nares capture larger inhaled particles before they reach the lower respiratory tract. The branching architecture of the tracheobronchial tree traps microbes on the airway lining, where mucociliary clearance and local antibacterial factors either clear or kill the potential pathogen. The gag reflex and the cough mechanism offer critical protection from aspiration. In addition, the normal flora adhering to mucosal cells of the oropharynx, whose components are remarkably constant, prevents pathogenic bacteria from binding and thereby decreases the risk of pneumonia caused by these more virulent bacteria.

When these barriers are overcome or when microorganisms are small enough to be inhaled to the alveolar level, resident alveolar macrophages are extremely efficient at clearing and killing pathogens. Macrophages are assisted by proteins that are produced by the alveolar epithelial cells (e.g., surfactant proteins A and D) and that have intrinsic opsonizing properties or antibacterial or antiviral activity. Once engulfed by the macrophage, the pathogens—even if they are not killed—are eliminated via either the mucociliary elevator or the lymphatics and no longer represent an infectious challenge. Only when the capacity of the alveolar macrophages to ingest or kill the microorganisms is exceeded does clinical pneumonia become manifest. In that situation, the alveolar macrophages initiate the inflammatory response to bolster lower respiratory tract defenses. The host inflammatory response, rather than proliferation of microorganisms, triggers the clinical syndrome of pneumonia. The release of inflammatory mediators, such as interleukin 1 and tumor necrosis factor, results in fever. Chemokines, such as interleukin 8 and granulocyte colony-stimulating factor, stimulate the release of neutrophils and their attraction to the lung, producing both peripheral leukocytosis and increased purulent secretions. Inflammatory mediators released by macrophages and the newly recruited neutrophils create an alveolar capillary leak equivalent to that seen in the acute respiratory distress syndrome, although in pneumonia this leak is localized (at least initially). Even erythrocytes can cross the alveolar-capillary membrane, with consequent hemoptysis. The capillary leak results in a radiographic infiltrate and rales detectable on auscultation, and hypoxemia results from alveolar filling. Moreover, some bacterial pathogens appear to interfere with the hypoxemic vasoconstriction that would normally occur with fluid-filled alveoli, and this interference can result in severe hypoxemia. Increased respiratory drive in the systemic inflammatory response syndrome (Chap. 325) leads to respiratory alkalosis. Decreased compliance due to capillary leak, hypoxemia, increased respiratory drive, increased secretions, and occasionally infection-related bronchospasm all lead to dyspnea. If severe enough, the changes in lung mechanics secondary to reductions in lung volume and compliance and the intrapulmonary shunting of blood may cause respiratory failure and the patient's death.

PATHOLOGY

Classic pneumonia evolves through a series of pathologic changes. The initial phase is one of *edema*, with the presence of a proteinaceous exudate—and often of bacteria—in the alveoli. This phase is rarely evident in clinical or autopsy specimens because of the rapid transition to the *red hepatization* phase. The presence of erythrocytes in the cellular intraalveolar exudate gives this second stage its name, but neutrophil influx is more important with regard to host defense. Bacteria are occasionally seen in pathologic specimens collected during this phase. In the third phase, *gray hepatization*, no new erythrocytes are extravasating, and those already present have been lysed and degraded. The neutrophil is the predominant cell, fibrin deposition is abundant, and bacteria have disappeared. This phase corresponds with successful containment of the infection and improvement in gas exchange. In the final phase, *resolution*, the macrophage reappears as the dominant cell type in the alveolar space, and the debris of neutrophils, bacteria, and fibrin has been cleared, as has the inflammatory response.

This pattern has been described best for lobar pneumococcal pneumonia and may not apply to pneumonia of all etiologies, especially viral or *Pneumocystis* pneumonia. In VAP, respiratory bronchiolitis may precede the development of a radiologically apparent infiltrate. Because of the microaspiration mechanism, a bronchopneumonia pattern is most common in nosocomial pneumonias, whereas a lobar pattern is more common in bacterial CAP. Despite the radiographic appearance, viral and *Pneumocystis* pneumonias represent alveolar rather than interstitial processes.

COMMUNITY-ACQUIRED PNEUMONIA

ETIOLOGY

The extensive list of potential etiologic agents in CAP includes bacteria, fungi, viruses, and protozoa. Newly identified pathogens include metapneumoviruses, the coronaviruses responsible for severe acute respiratory syndrome (SARS) and Middle East respiratory syndrome, and community-acquired strains of methicillin-resistant *Staphylococcus aureus* (MRSA). Most cases of CAP, however, are caused by relatively few pathogens (Table 153-2). Although *Streptococcus pneumoniae* is most common, other organisms also must be considered in light of the patient's risk factors and severity of illness. Separation of potential agents into either "typical" bacterial pathogens or "atypical" organisms may be helpful. The former category includes *S. pneumoniae*, *Haemophilus influenzae*, and (in selected patients) *S. aureus* and gram-negative bacilli such as *Klebsiella pneumoniae* and *Pseudomonas aeruginosa*. The "atypical" organisms include *Mycoplasma pneumoniae*, *Chlamydia pneumoniae*, and *Legionella* species (in inpatients) as well as respiratory viruses such as influenza viruses, adenoviruses, human metapneumovirus, and respiratory syncytial viruses. Viruses may be responsible for a large proportion of CAP cases that require hospital admission, even in adults. Atypical organisms cannot be cultured on standard media or seen on Gram's stain. The frequency and importance of atypical pathogens have significant implications for therapy. These organisms are intrinsically resistant to all β-lactam agents and must be treated with a macrolide, a fluoroquinolone, or a tetracycline. In the ~10–15% of CAP cases that are polymicrobial, the etiology usually includes a combination of typical and atypical pathogens.

Anaerobes play a significant role only when an episode of aspiration has occurred days to weeks before presentation of pneumonia. The

TABLE 153-2 MICROBIAL CAUSES OF COMMUNITY-ACQUIRED PNEUMONIA, BY SITE OF CARE

	Hospitalized Patients	
Outpatients	**Non-ICU**	**ICU**
Streptococcus pneumoniae	*S. pneumoniae*	*S. pneumoniae*
Mycoplasma pneumoniae	*M. pneumoniae*	*Staphylococcus aureus*
Haemophilus influenzae	*Chlamydia pneumoniae*	*Legionella* spp.
C. pneumoniae	*H. influenzae*	Gram-negative bacilli
Respiratory viruses[a]	*Legionella* spp.	*H. influenzae*
	Respiratory viruses[a]	

[a]Influenza A and B viruses, human metapneumovirus, adenoviruses, respiratory syncytial viruses, parainfluenza viruses.

Note: Pathogens are listed in descending order of frequency. ICU, intensive care unit.

combination of an unprotected airway (e.g., in patients with alcohol or drug overdose or a seizure disorder) and significant gingivitis constitutes the major risk factor. Anaerobic pneumonias are often complicated by abscess formation and by significant empyemas or parapneumonic effusions.

S. aureus pneumonia is well known to complicate influenza infection. However, MRSA has been reported as the primary etiologic agent of CAP. While this entity is still relatively uncommon, clinicians must be aware of its potentially serious consequences, such as necrotizing pneumonia. Two important developments have led to this problem: the spread of MRSA from the hospital setting to the community and the emergence of genetically distinct strains of MRSA in the community. The former circumstance is more likely to result in HCAP, whereas the novel community-acquired MRSA (CA-MRSA) strains may infect healthy individuals with no association with health care.

Unfortunately, despite a careful history and physical examination as well as routine radiographic studies, the causative pathogen in a case of CAP is difficult to predict with any degree of certainty; in more than one-half of cases, a specific etiology is never determined. Nevertheless, epidemiologic and risk factors may suggest the involvement of certain pathogens (Table 153-3).

EPIDEMIOLOGY

More than 5 million CAP cases occur annually in the United States; usually, 80% of the affected patients are treated as outpatients and 20% as inpatients. The mortality rate among outpatients is usually ≤1%, whereas among hospitalized patients the rate can range from ~12% to 40%, depending on whether treatment is provided in or outside of the intensive care unit (ICU). CAP results in more than 1.2 million hospitalizations and more than 55,000 deaths annually. The overall yearly cost associated with CAP is estimated at $12 billion. The incidence rates are highest at the extremes of age. The overall annual rate in the United States is 12 cases/1000 persons, but the figure increases to 12–18/1000 among children <4 years of age and to 20/1000 among persons >60 years of age.

TABLE 153-3 EPIDEMIOLOGIC FACTORS SUGGESTING POSSIBLE CAUSES OF COMMUNITY-ACQUIRED PNEUMONIA

Factor	Possible Pathogen(s)
Alcoholism	*Streptococcus pneumoniae*, oral anaerobes, *Klebsiella pneumoniae*, *Acinetobacter* spp., *Mycobacterium tuberculosis*
COPD and/or smoking	*Haemophilus influenzae*, *Pseudomonas aeruginosa*, *Legionella* spp., *S. pneumoniae*, *Moraxella catarrhalis*, *Chlamydia pneumoniae*
Structural lung disease (e.g., bronchiectasis)	*P. aeruginosa*, *Burkholderia cepacia*, *Staphylococcus aureus*
Dementia, stroke, decreased level of consciousness	Oral anaerobes, gram-negative enteric bacteria
Lung abscess	CA-MRSA, oral anaerobes, endemic fungi, *M. tuberculosis*, atypical mycobacteria
Travel to Ohio or St. Lawrence river valleys	*Histoplasma capsulatum*
Travel to southwestern United States	Hantavirus, *Coccidioides* spp.
Travel to Southeast Asia	*Burkholderia pseudomallei*, avian influenza virus
Stay in hotel or on cruise ship in previous 2 weeks	*Legionella* spp.
Local influenza activity	Influenza virus, *S. pneumoniae*, *S. aureus*
Exposure to bats or birds	*H. capsulatum*
Exposure to birds	*Chlamydia psittaci*
Exposure to rabbits	*Francisella tularensis*
Exposure to sheep, goats, parturient cats	*Coxiella burnetii*

Abbreviations: CA-MRSA, community-acquired methicillin-resistant *Staphylococcus aureus*; COPD, chronic obstructive pulmonary disease.

The risk factors for CAP in general and for pneumococcal pneumonia in particular have implications for treatment regimens. Risk factors for CAP include alcoholism, asthma, immunosuppression, institutionalization, and an age of ≥70 years. In the elderly, factors such as decreased cough and gag reflexes as well as reduced antibody and Toll-like receptor responses increase the likelihood of pneumonia. Risk factors for pneumococcal pneumonia include dementia, seizure disorders, heart failure, cerebrovascular disease, alcoholism, tobacco smoking, chronic obstructive pulmonary disease, and HIV infection. CA-MRSA pneumonia is more likely in patients with skin colonization or infection with CA-MRSA. Enterobacteriaceae tend to infect patients who have recently been hospitalized and/or received antibiotic therapy or who have comorbidities such as alcoholism, heart failure, or renal failure. *P. aeruginosa* is a particular problem in patients with severe structural lung disease, such as bronchiectasis, cystic fibrosis, or severe chronic obstructive pulmonary disease. Risk factors for *Legionella* infection include diabetes, hematologic malignancy, cancer, severe renal disease, HIV infection, smoking, male gender, and a recent hotel stay or ship cruise. (Many of these risk factors would now reclassify as HCAP some cases that were previously designated CAP.)

CLINICAL MANIFESTATIONS

CAP can vary from indolent to fulminant in presentation and from mild to fatal in severity. Manifestations of progression and severity include both constitutional findings and those limited to the lung and associated structures. In light of the pathobiology of the disease, many of the findings are to be expected.

The patient is frequently febrile with tachycardia or may have a history of chills and/or sweats. Cough may be either nonproductive or productive of mucoid, purulent, or blood-tinged sputum. Gross hemoptysis is suggestive of CA-MRSA pneumonia. Depending on severity, the patient may be able to speak in full sentences or may be very short of breath. If the pleura is involved, the patient may experience pleuritic chest pain. Up to 20% of patients may have gastrointestinal symptoms such as nausea, vomiting, and/or diarrhea. Other symptoms may include fatigue, headache, myalgias, and arthralgias.

Findings on physical examination vary with the degree of pulmonary consolidation and the presence or absence of a significant pleural effusion. An increased respiratory rate and use of accessory muscles of respiration are common. Palpation may reveal increased or decreased tactile fremitus, and the percussion note can vary from dull to flat, reflecting underlying consolidated lung and pleural fluid, respectively. Crackles, bronchial breath sounds, and possibly a pleural friction rub may be heard on auscultation. The clinical presentation may not be so obvious in the elderly, who may initially display new-onset or worsening confusion and few other manifestations. Severely ill patients may have septic shock and evidence of organ failure.

DIAGNOSIS

When confronted with possible CAP, the physician must ask two questions: Is this pneumonia, and, if so, what is the likely etiology? The former question is typically answered by clinical and radiographic methods, whereas the latter requires the aid of laboratory techniques.

Clinical Diagnosis The differential diagnosis includes both infectious and noninfectious entities such as acute bronchitis, acute exacerbations of chronic bronchitis, heart failure, pulmonary embolism, hypersensitivity pneumonitis, and radiation pneumonitis. The importance of a careful history cannot be overemphasized. For example, known cardiac disease may suggest worsening pulmonary edema, while underlying carcinoma may suggest lung injury secondary to irradiation.

Unfortunately, the sensitivity and specificity of the findings on physical examination are less than ideal, averaging 58% and 67%, respectively. Therefore, chest radiography is often necessary to differentiate CAP from other conditions. Radiographic findings may include risk factors for increased severity (e.g., cavitation or multilobar involvement). Occasionally, radiographic results suggest an etiologic diagnosis. For example, pneumatoceles suggest infection with *S. aureus*, and an upper-lobe cavitating lesion suggests tuberculosis. CT may be of value in a patient with suspected postobstructive pneumonia caused by a tumor or foreign body or suspected cavitary disease. For outpatients, the clinical and radiologic assessments are usually all that is done before treatment for CAP is started since most laboratory results are not available soon enough to influence initial management significantly. In certain cases, the availability of rapid point-of-care outpatient diagnostic tests can be very important; for example, rapid diagnosis of influenza virus infection can prompt specific anti-influenza drug treatment and secondary prevention.

Etiologic Diagnosis The etiology of pneumonia usually cannot be determined solely on the basis of clinical presentation. Except for CAP patients admitted to the ICU, no data exist to show that treatment directed at a specific pathogen is statistically superior to empirical therapy. The benefit of establishing a microbial etiology can therefore be questioned, particularly in light of the cost of diagnostic testing. However, a number of reasons can be advanced for attempting an etiologic diagnosis. Identification of an unexpected pathogen allows narrowing of the initial empirical regimen, thereby decreasing antibiotic selection pressure and lessening the risk of resistance. Pathogens with important public safety implications, such as *Mycobacterium tuberculosis* and influenza virus, may be found in some cases. Finally, without culture and susceptibility data, trends in resistance cannot be followed accurately, and appropriate empirical therapeutic regimens are harder to devise.

GRAM'S STAIN AND CULTURE OF SPUTUM The main purpose of the sputum Gram's stain is to ensure that a sample is suitable for culture. However, Gram's staining may also identify certain pathogens (e.g., *S. pneumoniae, S. aureus*, and gram-negative bacteria) by their characteristic appearance. To be adequate for culture, a sputum sample must have >25 neutrophils and <10 squamous epithelial cells per low-power field. The sensitivity and specificity of the sputum Gram's stain and culture are highly variable. Even in cases of proven bacteremic pneumococcal pneumonia, the yield of positive cultures from sputum samples is ≤50%.

Some patients, particularly elderly individuals, may not be able to produce an appropriate expectorated sputum sample. Others may already have started a course of antibiotics that can interfere with culture results at the time a sample is obtained. Inability to produce sputum can be a consequence of dehydration, and the correction of this condition may result in increased sputum production and a more obvious infiltrate on chest radiography. For patients admitted to the ICU and intubated, a deep-suction aspirate or bronchoalveolar lavage sample (obtained either via bronchoscopy or non-bronchoscopically) has a high yield on culture when sent to the microbiology laboratory as soon as possible. Since the etiologies in severe CAP are somewhat different from those in milder disease (Table 153-2), the greatest benefit of staining and culturing respiratory secretions is to alert the physician of unsuspected and/or resistant pathogens and to permit appropriate modification of therapy. Other stains and cultures (e.g., specific stains for *M. tuberculosis* or fungi) may be useful as well.

BLOOD CULTURES The yield from blood cultures, even when samples are collected before antibiotic therapy, is disappointingly low. Only 5–14% of cultures of blood from patients hospitalized with CAP are positive, and the most frequently isolated pathogen is *S. pneumoniae.* Since recommended empirical regimens all provide pneumococcal coverage, a blood culture positive for this pathogen has little, if any, effect on clinical outcome. However, susceptibility data may allow narrowing of antibiotic therapy in appropriate cases. Because of the low yield and the lack of significant impact on outcome, blood cultures are no longer considered *de rigueur* for all hospitalized CAP patients. Certain high-risk patients—including those with neutropenia secondary to pneumonia, asplenia, complement deficiencies, chronic liver disease, or severe CAP—should have blood cultured.

URINARY ANTIGEN TESTS Two commercially available tests detect pneumococcal and *Legionella* antigen in urine. The test for *Legionella pneumophila* detects only serogroup 1, but this serogroup accounts for most community-acquired cases of Legionnaires' disease in the United States. The sensitivity and specificity of the *Legionella* urine antigen test are as high as 90% and 99%, respectively. The pneumococcal urine antigen test also is quite sensitive and specific (80% and >90%, respectively). Although false-positive results can be obtained with samples from pneumococcus-colonized children, the test is generally reliable. Both tests can detect antigen even after the initiation of appropriate antibiotic therapy.

POLYMERASE CHAIN REACTION Polymerase chain reaction (PCR) tests, which amplify a microorganism's DNA or RNA, are available for a number of pathogens. PCR of nasopharyngeal swabs has become the standard for diagnosis of respiratory viral infection. In addition, PCR can detect the nucleic acid of *Legionella* species, *M. pneumoniae, C. pneumoniae*, and mycobacteria. In patients with pneumococcal pneumonia, an increased bacterial load in whole blood documented by PCR is associated with an increased risk of septic shock, the need for mechanical ventilation, and death. Clinical availability of such a test could conceivably help identify patients suitable for ICU admission.

SEROLOGY A fourfold rise in specific IgM antibody titer between acute- and convalescent-phase serum samples is generally considered diagnostic of infection with the pathogen in question. In the past, serologic tests were used to help identify atypical pathogens as well as selected unusual organisms such as *Coxiella burnetii.* Recently, however, they have fallen out of favor because of the time required to obtain a final result for the convalescent-phase sample.

BIOMARKERS A number of substances can serve as markers of severe inflammation. The two currently in use are C-reactive protein (CRP) and procalcitonin (PCT). Levels of these acute-phase reactants increase in the presence of an inflammatory response, particularly to bacterial pathogens. CRP may be of use in the identification of worsening disease or treatment failure, and PCT may play a role in determining the need for antibacterial therapy. These tests should not be used on their own but, when interpreted in conjunction with other findings from the history, physical examination, radiology, and laboratory tests, may help with antibiotic stewardship and appropriate management of seriously ill patients with CAP.

TREATMENT COMMUNITY-ACQUIRED PNEUMONIA

SITE OF CARE

The cost of inpatient management exceeds that of outpatient treatment by a factor of 20, and hospitalization accounts for most CAP-related expenditures. Thus the decision to admit a patient with CAP to the hospital has considerable implications. Certain patients clearly can be managed at home, and others clearly require treatment in the hospital, but the choice is sometimes difficult. Tools that objectively assess the risk of adverse outcomes, including severe illness and death, can minimize unnecessary hospital admissions. There are currently two sets of criteria: the Pneumonia Severity Index (PSI), a prognostic model used to identify patients at low risk of dying; and the CURB-65 criteria, a severity-of-illness score.

To determine the PSI, points are given for 20 variables, including age, coexisting illness, and abnormal physical and laboratory findings. On the basis of the resulting score, patients are assigned to one of five classes with the following mortality rates: class 1, 0.1%; class 2, 0.6%; class 3, 2.8%; class 4, 8.2%; and class 5, 29.2%. Determination of the PSI is often impractical in a busy emergency-department setting because of the number of variables that must be assessed. However, clinical trials demonstrate that routine use of the PSI results in lower admission rates for class 1 and class 2 patients. Patients in class 3 could ideally be admitted to an observation unit until a further decision can be made.

The CURB-65 criteria include five variables: confusion (C); urea >7 mmol/L (U); respiratory rate ≥30/min (R); blood pressure, systolic ≤90 mmHg or diastolic ≤60 mmHg (B); and age ≥65 years. Patients with a score of 0, among whom the 30-day mortality rate is 1.5%, can be treated outside the hospital. With a score of 2, the 30-day mortality rate is 9.2%, and patients should be admitted to the hospital.

TABLE 153-4 RISK FACTORS FOR EARLY DETERIORATION IN CAP

Multilobar infiltrates	Hypoalbuminemia
Severe hypoxemia (arterial saturation <90%)	Neutropenia
	Thrombocytopenia
Severe acidosis (pH <7.30)	Hyponatremia
Mental confusion	Hypoglycemia
Severe tachypnea (>30 breaths/min)	

Among patients with scores of ≥3, mortality rates are 22% overall; these patients may require ICU admission.

It is not clear which assessment tool is superior. Whichever system is used, these objective criteria must always be tempered by careful consideration of factors relevant to individual patients, including the ability to comply reliably with an oral antibiotic regimen and the resources available to the patient outside the hospital.

Neither PSI nor CURB-65 is accurate in determining the need for ICU admission. Septic shock or respiratory failure in the emergency department is an obvious indication for ICU care. However, mortality rates are higher among less ill patients who are admitted to the floor and then deteriorate than among equally ill patients monitored in the ICU. A variety of scores have been proposed to identify patients most likely to have early deterioration (Table 153-4). Most factors in these scores are similar to the minor severity criteria proposed by the Infectious Diseases Society of America (IDSA) and the American Thoracic Society (ATS) in their guidelines for the management of CAP.

ANTIBIOTIC RESISTANCE

Antimicrobial resistance is a significant problem that threatens to diminish our therapeutic armamentarium. Misuse of antibiotics results in increased antibiotic selection pressure that can affect resistance locally or even globally by clonal dissemination. For CAP, the main resistance issues currently involve *S. pneumoniae* and CA-MRSA.

S. pneumoniae In general, pneumococcal resistance is acquired (1) by direct DNA incorporation and remodeling resulting from contact with closely related oral commensal bacteria, (2) by the process of natural transformation, or (3) by mutation of certain genes.

The minimal inhibitory concentration (MIC) cutoffs for penicillin in pneumonia are ≤2 μg/mL for susceptibility, >2–4 μg/mL for intermediate, and ≥8 μg/mL for resistant. A change in susceptibility thresholds resulted in a dramatic decrease in the proportion of pneumococcal isolates considered nonsusceptible. For meningitis, MIC thresholds remain at the former higher levels. Fortunately, resistance to penicillin appeared to plateau even before the change in MIC thresholds. Pneumococcal resistance to β-lactam drugs is due solely to low-affinity penicillin-binding proteins. Risk factors for penicillin-resistant pneumococcal infection include recent antimicrobial therapy, an age of <2 years or >65 years, attendance at day-care centers, recent hospitalization, and HIV infection.

In contrast to penicillin resistance, resistance to macrolides is increasing through several mechanisms. *Target-site modification* caused by ribosomal methylation in 23S rRNA encoded by the *ermB* gene results in high-level resistance (MICs, ≥64 μg/mL) to macrolides, lincosamides, and streptogramin B–type antibiotics. The *efflux mechanism* encoded by the *mef* gene (*M phenotype*) is usually associated with low-level resistance (MICs, 1–32 μg/mL). These two mechanisms account for ~45% and ~65%, respectively, of resistant pneumococcal isolates in the United States. High-level resistance to macrolides is more common in Europe, whereas lower-level resistance predominates in North America.

Pneumococcal resistance to fluoroquinolones (e.g., ciprofloxacin and levofloxacin) has been reported. Changes can occur in one or both target sites (topoisomerases II and IV) from mutations in the *gyrA* and *parC* genes, respectively. In addition, an efflux pump may play a role in pneumococcal resistance to fluoroquinolones.

Isolates resistant to drugs from three or more antimicrobial classes with different mechanisms of action are considered MDR strains. The propensity for an association of pneumococcal resistance to penicillin with reduced susceptibility to other drugs, such as macrolides, tetracyclines, and trimethoprim-sulfamethoxazole, also is of concern. In the United States, 58.9% of penicillin-resistant pneumococcal isolates from blood are also resistant to macrolides.

The most important risk factor for antibiotic-resistant pneumococcal infection is use of a specific antibiotic within the previous 3 months. Therefore, a patient's history of prior antibiotic treatment is a critical factor in avoiding the use of an inappropriate antibiotic.

CA-MRSA CAP due to MRSA may be caused by the classic hospital-acquired strains or by the more recently identified, genotypically and phenotypically distinct community-acquired strains. Most infections with the former strains have been acquired either directly or indirectly by contact with the health care environment and would now be classified as HCAP. However, in some hospitals, the CA-MRSA strains are displacing the classic hospital-acquired strains—a trend suggesting that the newer strains may be more robust and blurring this distinction.

Methicillin resistance in *S. aureus* is determined by the *mecA* gene, which encodes for resistance to all β-lactam drugs. At least five *staphylococcal chromosomal cassette mec (SCCmec)* types have been described. The typical hospital-acquired strain usually has type II or III, whereas CA-MRSA has a type IV SCC*mec* element. CA-MRSA isolates tend to be less resistant than the older hospital-acquired strains and are often susceptible to trimethoprim-sulfamethoxazole, clindamycin, and tetracycline in addition to vancomycin and linezolid. However, the most important distinction is that CA-MRSA strains also carry genes for superantigens, such as enterotoxins B and C and Panton-Valentine leukocidin, a membrane-tropic toxin that can create cytolytic pores in polymorphonuclear neutrophils, monocytes, and macrophages.

Gram-Negative Bacilli A detailed discussion of resistance among gram-negative bacilli is beyond the scope of this chapter (Chap. 186). Fluoroquinolone resistance among isolates of *Escherichia coli* from the community appears to be increasing. *Enterobacter* species are typically resistant to cephalosporins; the drugs of choice for use against these bacteria are usually fluoroquinolones or carbapenems. Similarly, when infections due to bacteria producing extended-spectrum β-lactamases are documented or suspected, a fluoroquinolone or a carbapenem should be used; these MDR strains are more likely to be involved in HCAP.

INITIAL ANTIBIOTIC MANAGEMENT

Since the etiology of CAP is rarely known at the outset of treatment, initial therapy is usually empirical, designed to cover the most likely pathogens (Table 153-5). In all cases, antibiotic treatment should be initiated as expeditiously as possible. The CAP treatment guidelines in the United States (summarized in Table 153-5) represent joint statements from the IDSA and the ATS; the Canadian guidelines come from the Canadian Infectious Disease Society and the Canadian Thoracic Society. In all these guidelines, coverage is always provided for the pneumococcus and the atypical pathogens. In contrast, guidelines from some European countries do not always include atypical coverage based on local epidemiologic data. The U.S./Canadian approach is supported by retrospective data derived from administrative databases including thousands of patients. Atypical pathogen coverage provided by the addition of a macrolide to a cephalosporin or by the use of a fluoroquinolone alone has been consistently associated with a significant reduction in mortality rates compared with those for β-lactam coverage alone.

Therapy with a macrolide or a fluoroquinolone within the previous 3 months is associated with an increased likelihood of infection with a resistant strain of *S. pneumoniae*. For this reason, a fluoroquinolone-based regimen should be used for patients recently given a macrolide, and vice versa (Table 153-5).

TABLE 153-5 EMPIRICAL ANTIBIOTIC TREATMENT OF COMMUNITY-ACQUIRED PNEUMONIA

Outpatients

1. Previously healthy and no antibiotics in past 3 months
   - A macrolide (clarithromycin [500 mg PO bid] or azithromycin [500 mg PO once, then 250 mg qd]) *or*
   - Doxycycline (100 mg PO bid)
2. Comorbidities or antibiotics in past 3 months: select an alternative from a different class
   - A respiratory fluoroquinolone (moxifloxacin [400 mg PO qd], gemifloxacin [320 mg PO qd], levofloxacin [750 mg PO qd]) *or*
   - A β-lactam (preferred: high-dose amoxicillin [1 g tid] or amoxicillin/clavulanate [2 g bid]; alternatives: ceftriaxone [1–2 g IV qd], cefpodoxime [200 mg PO bid], cefuroxime [500 mg PO bid]) *plus* a macrolide[a]
3. In regions with a high rate of "high-level" pneumococcal macrolide resistance,[b] consider alternatives listed above for patients with comorbidities.

Inpatients, Non-ICU

- A respiratory fluoroquinolone (e.g., moxifloxacin [400 mg PO or IV qd] or levofloxacin [750 mg PO or IV qd])
- A β-lactam[c] (e.g., ceftriaxone [1–2 g IV qd], ampicillin [1–2 g IV q4–6h], cefotaxime [1–2 g IV q8h], ertapenem [1 g IV qd]) *plus* a macrolide[d] (e.g., oral clarithromycin or azithromycin [as listed above] or IV azithromycin [1 g once, then 500 mg qd])

Inpatients, ICU

- A β-lactam[e] (e.g., ceftriaxone [2 g IV qd], ampicillin-sulbactam [2 g IV q8h], or cefotaxime [1–2 g IV q8h]) *plus* either azithromycin or a fluoroquinolone (as listed above for inpatients, non-ICU)

Special Concerns

If Pseudomonas is a consideration:

- An antipseudomonal β-lactam (e.g., piperacillin/tazobactam [4. 5 g IV q6h], cefepime [1–2 g IV q12h], imipenem [500 mg IV q6h], meropenem [1 g IV q8h]) *plus* either ciprofloxacin (400 mg IV q12h) or levofloxacin (750 mg IV qd)
- The above β-lactams *plus* an aminoglycoside (amikacin [15 mg/kg qd] or tobramycin [1. 7 mg/kg qd]) *plus* azithromycin
- The above β-lactams[f] *plus* an aminoglycoside *plus* an antipneumococcal fluoroquinolone

If CA-MRSA is a consideration:

- Add linezolid (600 mg IV q12h) or vancomycin (15 mg/kg q12h initially, with adjusted doses)

[a]Doxycycline (100 mg PO bid) is an alternative to the macrolide. [b]MICs of >16 μg/mL in 25% of isolates. [c]A respiratory fluoroquinolone should be used for penicillin-allergic patients. [d]Doxycycline (100 mg IV q12h) is an alternative to the macrolide. [e]For penicillin-allergic patients, use a respiratory fluoroquinolone and aztreonam (2 g IV q8h). [f]For penicillin-allergic patients, substitute aztreonam.

Abbreviations: CA-MRSA, community-acquired methicillin-resistant *Staphylococcus aureus;* ICU, intensive care unit.

Once the etiologic agent(s) and susceptibilities are known, therapy may be altered to target the specific pathogen(s). However, this decision is not always straightforward. If blood cultures yield *S. pneumoniae* sensitive to penicillin after 2 days of treatment with a macrolide plus a β-lactam or with a fluoroquinolone alone, should therapy be switched to penicillin alone? The concern here is that a β-lactam alone would not be effective in the potential 15% of cases with atypical co-infection. No standard approach exists. In all cases, the individual patient and the various risk factors must be considered.

Management of bacteremic pneumococcal pneumonia also is controversial. Data from nonrandomized studies suggest that combination therapy (especially macrolide/β-lactam) is associated with a lower mortality rate than monotherapy, particularly in severely ill patients. The exact reason is unknown, but possible explanations include an additive or synergistic antibacterial effect, antimicrobial tolerance, atypical co-infection, or the immunomodulatory effects of the macrolides.

For CAP patients admitted to the ICU, the risk of infection with *P. aeruginosa* or CA-MRSA is increased. Empirical coverage should be considered when a patient has risk factors or a Gram's stain suggestive of these pathogens (Table 153–5). If CA-MRSA is suspected, either linezolid or vancomycin can be added to the initial empirical regimen; however, there is increasing concern about vancomycin's loss of potency against MRSA, poor penetration into epithelial lining fluid, and lack of effect on toxin production relative to linezolid.

Although hospitalized patients have traditionally received initial therapy by the IV route, some drugs—particularly the fluoroquinolones—are very well absorbed and can be given orally from the outset to select patients. For patients initially treated IV, a switch to oral treatment is appropriate as long as the patient can ingest and absorb the drugs, is hemodynamically stable, and is showing clinical improvement.

The duration of treatment for CAP has generated considerable interest. Patients were previously treated for 10–14 days, but studies with fluoroquinolones and telithromycin suggest that a 5-day course is sufficient for otherwise uncomplicated CAP. Even a single dose of ceftriaxone has been associated with a significant cure rate. A longer course may be required for patients with bacteremia, metastatic infection, or infection with a virulent pathogen such as *P. aeruginosa* or CA-MRSA.

GENERAL CONSIDERATIONS

In addition to appropriate antimicrobial therapy, certain general considerations apply in dealing with CAP, HCAP, or HAP/VAP. Adequate hydration, oxygen therapy for hypoxemia, and assisted ventilation when necessary are critical to successful treatment. Patients with severe CAP who remain hypotensive despite fluid resuscitation may have adrenal insufficiency and may respond to glucocorticoid treatment. The value of adjunctive therapy, such as glucocorticoids, statins, and angiotensin-converting enzyme inhibitors, remains unproven in the management of CAP.

Failure to Improve Patients slow to respond to therapy should be reevaluated at about day 3 (sooner if their condition is worsening rather than simply not improving), and several possible scenarios should be considered. A number of noninfectious conditions mimic pneumonia, including pulmonary edema, pulmonary embolism, lung carcinoma, radiation and hypersensitivity pneumonitis, and connective tissue disease involving the lungs. If the patient truly has CAP and empirical treatment is aimed at the correct pathogen, lack of response may be explained in a number of ways. The pathogen may be resistant to the drug selected, or a sequestered focus (e.g., lung abscess or empyema) may be blocking access of the antibiotic(s) to the pathogen. The patient may be getting either the wrong drug or the correct drug at the wrong dose or frequency of administration. Another possibility is that CAP is the correct diagnosis but an unsuspected pathogen (e.g., CA-MRSA, *M. tuberculosis*, or a fungus) is the cause. Nosocomial superinfections—both pulmonary and extrapulmonary—are other possible explanations for a patient's failure to improve or deterioration. In all cases of delayed response or deteriorating condition, the patient must be carefully reassessed and appropriate studies initiated, possibly including such diverse procedures as CT or bronchoscopy.

Complications As in other severe infections, common complications of severe CAP include respiratory failure, shock and multiorgan failure, coagulopathy, and exacerbation of comorbid illnesses. Three particularly noteworthy conditions are metastatic infection, lung abscess, and complicated pleural effusion. Metastatic infection (e.g., brain abscess or endocarditis) is very unusual and will require a high degree of suspicion and a detailed workup for proper treatment. Lung abscess may occur in association with aspiration or with infection caused by a single CAP pathogen, such as CA-MRSA, *P. aeruginosa*, or (rarely) *S. pneumoniae*. Aspiration pneumonia is typically a polymicrobial infection involving both aerobes and anaerobes. A significant pleural effusion should be tapped for both diagnostic and therapeutic purposes. If the fluid has a pH of <7, a glucose level of <2. 2 mmol/L, and a lactate dehydrogenase concentration of >1000 U/L or if bacteria are seen or cultured, then it should be completely drained; a chest tube is often required and video-assisted thoracoscopy may be needed for late treatment or difficult cases.

Follow-Up Fever and leukocytosis usually resolve within 2–4 days in otherwise healthy patients with CAP, but physical findings may persist longer. Chest radiographic abnormalities are slowest to resolve (4–12 weeks), with the speed of clearance dependinq on the patient's age and underlying lung disease. Patients may be discharged from the hospital once their clinical conditions, including comorbidities, are stable. The site of residence after discharge (nursing home, home with family, home alone) is an important discharge timing consideration, particularly for elderly patients. For a hospitalized patient, a follow-up radiograph ~4–6 weeks later is recommended. If relapse or recurrence is documented, particularly in the same lung segment, the possibility of an underlying neoplasm must be considered.

PROGNOSIS

The prognosis of CAP depends on the patient's age, comorbidities, and site of treatment (inpatient or outpatient). Young patients without comorbidity do well and usually recover fully after ~2 weeks. Older patients and those with comorbid conditions can take several weeks longer to recover fully. The overall mortality rate for the outpatient group is <1%. For patients requiring hospitalization, the overall mortality rate is estimated at 10%, with ~50% of deaths directly attributable to pneumonia.

PREVENTION

The main preventive measure is vaccination (Chap. 148). Recommendations of the Advisory Committee on Immunization Practices should be followed for influenza and pneumococcal vaccines.

A pneumococcal polysaccharide vaccine (PPV23) and a protein conjugate pneumococcal vaccine (PCV13) are available in the United States. The former product contains capsular material from 23 pneumococcal serotypes; in the latter, capsular polysaccharide from 13 of the most frequent pneumococcal pathogens affecting children is linked to an immunogenic protein. PCV13 produces T cell–dependent antigens that result in long-term immunologic memory. Administration of this vaccine to children has led to an overall decrease in the prevalence of antimicrobial-resistant pneumococci and in the incidence of invasive pneumococcal disease among both children and adults. However, vaccination can be followed by the replacement of vaccine serotypes with nonvaccine serotypes, as was seen with serotypes 19A and 35B after introduction of the original 7-valent conjugate vaccine. PCV13 now is also recommended for the elderly and for younger immunocompromised patients. Because of an increased risk of pneumococcal infection, even among patients without obstructive lung disease, smokers should be strongly encouraged to stop smoking.

Two forms of influenza vaccine are available: intramuscular inactivated vaccine and intranasal live-attenuated cold-adapted vaccine. The latter is contraindicated in immunocompromised patients. In the event of an influenza outbreak, unprotected patients at risk from complications should be vaccinated immediately and given chemoprophylaxis with either oseltamivir or zanamivir for 2 weeks—i.e., until vaccine-induced antibody levels are sufficiently high.

HEALTH CARE–ASSOCIATED PNEUMONIA

HCAP represents a transition between classic CAP and typical HAP. The definition of HCAP is still in some flux because of a lack of consistent large-scale studies. Several early studies were limited to patients with culture-positive pneumonia. In these studies, the incidence of MDR pathogens in HCAP was as high as or higher than in HAP/VAP. MRSA in particular was more common in HCAP than in traditional HAP/VAP. Conversely, prospective studies in nontertiary-care centers have found a low incidence of MDR pathogens in HCAP.

The patients at greatest risk for HCAP are not well defined. Patients from nursing homes are not always at elevated risk for infection with MDR pathogens. Careful evaluation of nursing home residents with pneumonia suggests that their risk of MDR infection is low if they have not recently received antibiotics and are independent in most activities of daily living. Recent hospitalization (i.e., in the preceding 90 days) is also a major risk factor for infection with MDR pathogens. Conversely, nursing home patients are at increased risk of infection with influenza virus and other atypical pneumonia pathogens. Undue concern about MDR pathogens occasionally results in failure to cover atypical pathogens when treating nursing home patients. In addition, patients receiving home infusion therapy or undergoing chronic dialysis are probably at particular risk for MRSA pneumonia but may not be at greater risk for infection with *Pseudomonas* or *Acinetobacter* than are other patients who develop CAP.

In general, the management of HCAP due to MDR pathogens is similar to that of MDR HAP/VAP. This topic will therefore be covered in subsequent sections on HAP and VAP. The prognosis of HCAP is intermediate between that of CAP and VAP and is closer to that of HAP.

VENTILATOR-ASSOCIATED PNEUMONIA

Most hospital-acquired pneumonia research has focused on VAP. However, the information and principles based on this research can be applied to non-ICU HAP and HCAP as well. The greatest difference between VAP and HCAP/HAP studies is the dependence on expectorated sputum for a microbiologic diagnosis of VAP (as for that of CAP), which is further complicated by frequent colonization by pathogens in patients with HAP or HCAP. Therefore, most of the literature has focused on HCAP or HAP resulting in intubation, where, once again, access to the lower respiratory tract facilitates an etiologic diagnosis.

Etiology Potential etiologic agents of VAP include both MDR and non-MDR bacterial pathogens (Table 153-6). The non-MDR group is nearly identical to the pathogens found in severe CAP (Table 153-2); it is not surprising that such pathogens predominate if VAP develops in the first 5–7 days of the hospital stay. However, if patients have other risk factors for HCAP, MDR pathogens are a consideration, even early in the hospital course. The relative frequency of individual MDR pathogens can vary significantly from hospital to hospital and even between different critical care units within the same institution. Most hospitals have problems with *P. aeruginosa* and MRSA, but other MDR pathogens are often institution-specific. Less commonly, fungal and viral pathogens cause VAP, usually affecting severely immunocompromised patients. Rarely, community-associated viruses cause mini-epidemics, usually when introduced by ill health care workers.

TABLE 153-6 MICROBIOLOGIC CAUSES OF VENTILATOR-ASSOCIATED PNEUMONIA

Non-MDR Pathogens	MDR Pathogens
Streptococcus pneumoniae	*Pseudomonas aeruginosa*
Other *Streptococcus* spp.	MRSA
Haemophilus influenzae	*Acinetobacter* spp.
MSSA	Antibiotic-resistant
Antibiotic-sensitive	Enterobacteriaceae
Enterobacteriaceae	*Enterobacter* spp.
Escherichia coli	ESBL-positive strains
Klebsiella pneumoniae	*Klebsiella* spp.
Proteus spp.	*Legionella pneumophila*
Enterobacter spp.	*Burkholderia cepacia*
Serratia marcescens	*Aspergillus* spp.

Abbreviations: ESBL, extended-spectrum β-lactamase; MDR, multidrug-resistant; MRSA, methicillin-resistant *Staphylococcus aureus*; MSSA, methicillin-sensitive *S. aureus*.

Epidemiology Pneumonia is a common complication among patients requiring mechanical ventilation. Prevalence estimates vary between 6 and 52 cases per 100 patients, depending on the population studied. On any given day in the ICU, an average of 10% of patients will have pneumonia—VAP in the overwhelming majority of cases. The frequency of diagnosis is not static but changes with the duration of mechanical ventilation, with the highest hazard ratio in the first 5 days and a plateau in additional cases (1% per day) after ~2 weeks. However, the cumulative rate among patients who remain ventilated for as long as 30 days is as high as 70%. These rates often do not reflect the recurrence of VAP in the same patient. Once a ventilated patient is transferred to a chronic-care facility or to home, the incidence of pneumonia drops significantly, especially in the absence of other risk factors for pneumonia. However, in chronic ventilator units, purulent tracheobronchitis becomes a significant issue, often interfering with efforts to wean patients off mechanical ventilation (Chap. 323).

Three factors are critical in the pathogenesis of VAP: colonization of the oropharynx with pathogenic microorganisms, aspiration of these organisms from the oropharynx into the lower respiratory tract, and compromise of the normal host defense mechanisms. Most risk factors and their corresponding prevention strategies pertain to one of these three factors (Table 153-7).

The most obvious risk factor is the endotracheal tube, which bypasses the normal mechanical factors preventing aspiration. While the presence of an endotracheal tube may prevent large-volume aspiration, microaspiration is actually exacerbated by secretions pooling above the cuff. The endotracheal tube and the concomitant need for suctioning can damage the tracheal mucosa, thereby facilitating tracheal colonization. In addition, pathogenic bacteria can form a glycocalyx biofilm on the tube's surface that protects them from both antibiotics and host defenses. The bacteria can also be dislodged during suctioning and can reinoculate the trachea, or tiny fragments of glycocalyx can embolize to distal airways, carrying bacteria with them.

TABLE 153-7 PATHOGENIC MECHANISMS AND CORRESPONDING PREVENTION STRATEGIES FOR VENTILATOR-ASSOCIATED PNEUMONIA

Pathogenic Mechanism	Prevention Strategy
Oropharyngeal colonization with pathogenic bacteria	
Elimination of normal flora	Avoidance of prolonged antibiotic courses
Large-volume oropharyngeal aspiration around time of intubation	Short course of prophylactic antibiotics for comatose patients[a]
Gastroesophageal reflux	Postpyloric enteral feeding[b]; avoidance of high gastric residuals, prokinetic agents
Bacterial overgrowth of stomach	Avoidance of prophylactic agents that raise gastric pH[b]; selective decontamination of digestive tract with nonabsorbable antibiotics[b]
Cross-infection from other colonized patients	Hand washing, especially with alcohol-based hand rub; intensive infection control education[a]; isolation; proper cleaning of reusable equipment
Large-volume aspiration	Endotracheal intubation; rapid-sequence intubation technique; avoidance of sedation; decompression of small-bowel obstruction
Microaspiration around endotracheal tube	
Endotracheal intubation	Noninvasive ventilation[a]
Prolonged duration of ventilation	Daily awakening from sedation,[a] weaning protocols[a]
Abnormal swallowing function	Early percutaneous tracheostomy[a]
Secretions pooled above endotracheal tube	Head of bed elevated[a]; continuous aspiration of subglottic secretions with specialized endotracheal tube[a]; avoidance of reintubation; minimization of sedation and patient transport
Altered lower respiratory host defenses	Tight glycemic control[b]; lowering of hemoglobin transfusion threshold

[a]Strategies demonstrated to be effective in at least one randomized controlled trial.
[b]Strategies with negative randomized trials or conflicting results.

In a high percentage of critically ill patients, the normal oropharyngeal flora is replaced by pathogenic microorganisms. The most important risk factors are antibiotic selection pressure, cross-infection from other infected/colonized patients or contaminated equipment, and malnutrition. Of these factors, antibiotic exposure poses the greatest risk by far. Pathogens such as *P. aeruginosa* almost never cause infection in patients without prior exposure to antibiotics. The recent emphasis on hand hygiene has lowered the cross-infection rate.

How the lower respiratory tract defenses become overwhelmed remains poorly understood. Almost all intubated patients experience microaspiration and are at least transiently colonized with pathogenic bacteria. However, only around one-third of colonized patients develop VAP. Colony counts increase to high levels, sometimes days before the development of clinical pneumonia; these increases suggest that the final step in VAP development, independent of aspiration and oropharyngeal colonization, is the overwhelming of host defenses. Severely ill patients with sepsis and trauma appear to enter a state of immunoparalysis several days after admission to the ICU—a time that corresponds to the greatest risk of developing VAP. The mechanism of this immunosuppression is not clear, although several factors have been suggested. Hyperglycemia affects neutrophil function, and trials suggest that keeping the blood sugar level close to normal with exogenous insulin may have beneficial effects, including a decreased risk of infection. More frequent transfusions also adversely affect the immune response.

Clinical Manifestations The clinical manifestations are generally the same in VAP as in all other forms of pneumonia: fever, leukocytosis, increase in respiratory secretions, and pulmonary consolidation on physical examination, along with a new or changing radiographic infiltrate. The frequency of abnormal chest radiographs before the onset of pneumonia in intubated patients and the limitations of portable radiographic technique make interpretation of radiographs more difficult than in patients who are not intubated. Other clinical features may include tachypnea, tachycardia, worsening oxygenation, and increased minute ventilation.

Diagnosis No single set of criteria is reliably diagnostic of pneumonia in a ventilated patient. The inability to identify such patients compromises efforts to prevent and treat VAP and even calls into question estimates of the impact of VAP on mortality rates.

Application of clinical criteria consistently results in overdiagnosis of VAP, largely because of three common findings in at-risk patients: (1) tracheal colonization with pathogenic bacteria in patients with endotracheal tubes, (2) multiple alternative causes of radiographic infiltrates in mechanically ventilated patients, and (3) the high frequency of other sources of fever in critically ill patients. The differential diagnosis of VAP includes a number of entities such as atypical pulmonary edema, pulmonary contusion, alveolar hemorrhage, hypersensitivity pneumonitis, acute respiratory distress syndrome, and pulmonary embolism. Clinical findings in ventilated patients with fever and/or leukocytosis may have alternative causes, including antibiotic-associated diarrhea, sinusitis, urinary tract infection, pancreatitis, and drug fever. Conditions mimicking pneumonia are often documented in patients in whom VAP has been ruled out by accurate diagnostic techniques. Most of these alternative diagnoses do not require antibiotic treatment; require antibiotics different from those used to treat VAP; or require some additional intervention, such as surgical drainage or catheter removal, for optimal management.

This diagnostic dilemma has led to debate and controversy. The major question is whether a quantitative-culture approach as a means of eliminating false-positive clinical diagnoses is superior to the clinical approach enhanced by principles learned from quantitative-culture studies. The most recent IDSA/ATS guidelines for HAP/VAP suggest that either approach is clinically valid.

QUANTITATIVE-CULTURE APPROACH The essence of the quantitative-culture approach is to discriminate between colonization and true infection by determining the bacterial burden. The more distal in the respiratory tree the diagnostic sampling, the more specific the results and therefore the lower the threshold of growth necessary to diagnose pneumonia and exclude colonization. For example, a quantitative endotracheal aspirate yields proximate samples, and the diagnostic threshold is 10^6 cfu/mL. The protected specimen brush method, in contrast, obtains distal samples and has a threshold of 10^3 cfu/mL. Conversely, sensitivity declines as more distal secretions are obtained, especially when they are collected blindly (i.e., by a technique other than bronchoscopy). Additional tests that may increase the diagnostic yield include Gram's staining, differential cell counts, staining for intracellular organisms, and detection of local protein levels elevated in response to infection.

The Achilles heel of the quantitative approach is the effect of antibiotic therapy. With sensitive microorganisms, a single antibiotic dose can reduce colony counts below the diagnostic threshold. Recent changes in antibiotic therapy are the most significant. After 3 days, the operating characteristics of the tests are almost the same as if no antibiotic therapy has been given. Conversely, colony counts above the diagnostic threshold during antibiotic therapy suggest that the current antibiotics are ineffective. Even the normal host response may be sufficient to reduce quantitative-culture counts below the diagnostic threshold if sampling is delayed. In short, expertise in quantitative-culture techniques is critical, with a specimen obtained as soon as pneumonia is suspected and before antibiotic therapy is initiated or changed.

In a study comparing the quantitative with the clinical approach, use of bronchoscopic quantitative cultures resulted in significantly less antibiotic use at 14 days after study entry and in lower rates of mortality and severity-adjusted mortality at 28 days. In addition, more alternative sites of infection were found in patients randomized to the quantitative-culture strategy. A critical aspect of this study was that antibiotic treatment was initiated only in patients whose gram-stained respiratory sample was positive or who displayed signs of hemodynamic instability. Fewer than one-half as many patients were treated for pneumonia in the bronchoscopy group, and only one-third as many microorganisms were cultured.

CLINICAL APPROACH The lack of specificity of a clinical diagnosis of VAP has led to efforts to improve the diagnostic criteria. The Clinical Pulmonary Infection Score (CPIS) was developed by weighting of the various clinical criteria usually used for the diagnosis of VAP (Table 153-8). Use of the CPIS allows the selection of low-risk patients who may need only short-course antibiotic therapy or no treatment at all. Moreover, studies have demonstrated that the absence of bacteria in gram-stained endotracheal aspirates makes pneumonia an unlikely cause of fever or pulmonary infiltrates. These findings, coupled with a heightened awareness of the alternative diagnoses possible in patients with suspected VAP, can prevent inappropriate overtreatment for pneumonia. Furthermore, data show that the absence of an MDR pathogen in tracheal aspirate cultures eliminates the need for MDR coverage when empirical antibiotic therapy is narrowed. Since the most likely explanations for the mortality benefit of bronchoscopic quantitative cultures are decreased antibiotic selection pressure (which reduces the risk of subsequent infection with MDR pathogens) and identification of alternative sources of infection, a clinical diagnostic approach that incorporates such principles may result in similar outcomes.

Other large randomized studies that did not demonstrate a similar beneficial impact of quantitative culture on outcomes did not tightly link antibiotic treatment to the results of quantitative culture and other tests. Given the conflicting results only partially explained by methodologic issues, the IDSA/ATS guidelines therefore suggest that the choice depends on availability and local expertise.

TABLE 153-8 CLINICAL PULMONARY INFECTION SCORE (CPIS)

Criterion	Score
Fever (°C)	
≥38.5 but ≤38.9	1
>39 or <36	2
Leukocytosis	
<4000 or >11,000/μL	1
Bands >50%	1 (additional)
Oxygenation (mmHg)	
Pa_{O_2}/FI_{O_2} <250 and no ARDS	2
Chest radiograph	
Localized infiltrate	2
Patchy or diffuse infiltrate	1
Progression of infiltrate (no ARDS or CHF)	2
Tracheal aspirate	
Moderate or heavy growth	1
Same morphology on Gram's stain	1 (additional)
Maximal score[a]	12

[a]At the time of the original diagnosis, the progression of the infiltrate is not known and results of tracheal aspirate culture are often unavailable; thus, the maximal score is initially 8–10.

Abbreviations: ARDS, acute respiratory distress syndrome; CHF, congestive heart failure.

TREATMENT VENTILATOR-ASSOCIATED PNEUMONIA

Many studies have demonstrated higher mortality rates with initially inappropriate empirical antibiotic therapy. The key to appropriate antibiotic management of VAP is an appreciation of the resistance patterns of the most likely pathogens in a given patient.

ANTIBIOTIC RESISTANCE

If not for the higher risk of infection with MDR pathogens (Table 153-1), VAP could be treated with the same antibiotics used for severe CAP. However, antibiotic selection pressure leads to the frequent involvement of MDR pathogens by selecting either for drug-resistant isolates of common pathogens (MRSA and Enterobacteriaceae producing extended-spectrum β-lactamases or carbapenemases) or for intrinsically resistant pathogens (*P. aeruginosa* and *Acinetobacter* species). Frequent use of β-lactam drugs, especially cephalosporins, appears to be the major risk factor for infection with MRSA and extended-spectrum β-lactamase–positive strains.

P. aeruginosa has demonstrated the ability to develop resistance to all routinely used antibiotics. Unfortunately, even if initially sensitive, *P. aeruginosa* isolates also have a propensity to develop resistance during treatment. Either de-repression of resistance genes or selection of resistant clones within the large bacterial inoculum associated with most pneumonias may be the cause. *Acinetobacter* species, *Stenotrophomonas maltophilia*, and *Burkholderia cepacia* are intrinsically resistant to many of the empirical antibiotic regimens employed (see later in this chapter). VAP caused by these pathogens emerges during treatment of other infections, and resistance is always evident at initial diagnosis.

EMPIRICAL THERAPY

Recommended options for empirical therapy are listed in Table 153-9. Treatment should be started once diagnostic specimens have been obtained. The major factor in the selection of agents is the presence of risk factors for MDR pathogens. Choices among the various options listed depend on local patterns of resistance and—a very important factor—the patient's prior antibiotic exposure.

The majority of patients *without* risk factors for MDR infection can be treated with a single agent. The major difference from CAP is the markedly lower incidence of atypical pathogens in VAP; the exception is *Legionella,* which can be a nosocomial pathogen, especially with breakdowns in the treatment of potable water in the hospital.

TABLE 153-9 EMPIRICAL ANTIBIOTIC TREATMENT OF HEALTH CARE–ASSOCIATED PNEUMONIA

Patients without Risk Factors for MDR Pathogens
Ceftriaxone (2 g IV q24h) or cefotaxime (2 g IV q6–8 h) *or*
Moxifloxacin (400 mg IV q24h), ciprofloxacin (400 mg IV q8h), or levofloxacin (750 mg IV q24h) *or*
Ampicillin/sulbactam (3 g IV q6h) *or*
Ertapenem (1 g IV q24h)
Patients with Risk Factors for MDR Pathogens
1. A β-lactam:
Ceftazidime (2 g IV q8h) or cefepime (2 g IV q8–12h) *or*
Piperacillin/tazobactam (4. 5 g IV q6h) *or*
Imipenem (500 mg IV q6h or 1 g IV q8h), or meropenem (1 g IV q8h)
plus
2. A second agent active against gram-negative bacterial pathogens:
Gentamicin or tobramycin (7 mg/kg IV q24h) or amikacin (20 mg/kg IV q24h) *or*
Ciprofloxacin (400 mg IV q8h) or levofloxacin (750 mg IV q24h)
plus
3. An agent active against gram-positive bacterial pathogens:
Linezolid (600 mg IV q12h) *or*
Vancomycin (15 mg/kg q12h initially with adjusted doses)

Abbreviation: MDR, multidrug-resistant.

The standard recommendation for patients *with* risk factors for MDR infection is for three antibiotics: two directed at *P. aeruginosa* and one at MRSA. The choice of a β-lactam agent provides the greatest variability in coverage, yet the use of the broadest-spectrum agent—a carbapenem, even in an antibiotic combination—still represents inappropriate initial therapy in 10–15% of cases.

SPECIFIC TREATMENT

Once an etiologic diagnosis is made, broad-spectrum empirical therapy can be modified to specifically address the known pathogen. For patients with MDR risk factors, antibiotic regimens can be reduced to a single agent in more than one-half of cases and to a two-drug combination in more than one-quarter of cases. Only a minority of cases require a complete course with three drugs. A negative tracheal-aspirate culture or growth below the threshold for quantitative cultures, especially if the sample was obtained before any antibiotic change, strongly suggests that antibiotics should be discontinued. Identification of other confirmed or suspected sites of infection may require ongoing antibiotic therapy, but the spectrum of pathogens (and the corresponding antibiotic choices) may be different from those for VAP. If the CPIS decreases over the first 3 days, antibiotics should be stopped after 8 days. An 8-day course of therapy is just as effective as a 2-week course and is associated with less frequent emergence of antibiotic-resistant strains.

The major controversy regarding specific therapy for VAP concerns the need for ongoing combination treatment of *Pseudomonas* infection. No randomized controlled trials have demonstrated a benefit of combination therapy with a β-lactam and an aminoglycoside, nor have subgroup analyses in other trials found a survival benefit with such a regimen. The unacceptably high rates of clinical failure and death for VAP caused by *P. aeruginosa* despite combination therapy (see "Failure to Improve," later) indicate that better regimens are needed—including, perhaps, aerosolized antibiotics. VAP caused by MRSA is associated with a 40% clinical failure rate when treated with standard-dose vancomycin. One proposed solution is the use of high-dose individualized treatment, although the risk of renal toxicity increases with this strategy. In addition, the MIC of vancomycin has been increasing, and a high percentage of clinical failures occur when the MIC is in the upper range of sensitivity (i.e., 1. 5–2 μg/mL). Linezolid appears to be 15% more efficacious than even adjusted-dose vancomycin and is clearly preferred in patients with renal insufficiency and those infected with high-MIC isolates of MRSA.

FAILURE TO IMPROVE

Treatment failure is not uncommon in VAP, especially that caused by MDR pathogens. In addition to the 40% failure rate for MRSA infection treated with vancomycin, VAP due to *Pseudomonas* has a 50% failure rate, no matter what the regimen. Causes of clinical failure vary with the pathogen(s) and the antibiotic(s). Inappropriate therapy can usually be minimized by use of the recommended triple-drug regimen (Table 153-9). However, the emergence of β-lactam resistance during therapy is an important problem, especially in infection with *Pseudomonas* and *Enterobacter* species. Recurrent VAP caused by the same pathogen is possible because the biofilm on endotracheal tubes allows reintroduction of the microorganism. However, studies of VAP caused by *Pseudomonas* show that approximately half of recurrent cases are caused by a new strain. Inadequate local levels of vancomycin are the likely cause of treatment failure in VAP due to MRSA.

Treatment failure is very difficult to diagnose. Pneumonia due to a new superinfection, the presence of extrapulmonary infection, and drug toxicity must be considered in the differential diagnosis of treatment failure. Serial CPIS calculations appear to track the clinical response accurately, while repeat quantitative cultures may clarify the microbiologic response. A persistently elevated or rising CPIS by day 3 of therapy is likely to indicate treatment failure. The most sensitive component of the CPIS is improvement in oxygenation.

COMPLICATIONS

Apart from death, the major complication of VAP is prolongation of mechanical ventilation, with corresponding increases in length of stay in the ICU and in the hospital. In most studies, an additional week of mechanical ventilation resulting from VAP is common. The additional expense of this complication often warrants costly and aggressive efforts at prevention.

In rare cases, some types of necrotizing pneumonia (e.g., due to *P. aeruginosa*) result in significant pulmonary hemorrhage. More commonly, necrotizing infections result in the long-term complications of bronchiectasis and parenchymal scarring leading to recurrent pneumonias. The long-term complications of pneumonia are underappreciated. Pneumonia results in a catabolic state in a patient already nutritionally at risk. The muscle loss and general debilitation from an episode of VAP often require prolonged rehabilitation and, in the elderly, commonly result in an inability to return to independent function and the need for nursing home placement.

FOLLOW-UP

Clinical improvement, if it occurs, is usually evident within 48–72 h of the initiation of antimicrobial treatment. Because findings on chest radiography often worsen initially during treatment, they are less helpful than clinical criteria as an indicator of clinical response in severe pneumonia. Seriously ill patients with pneumonia often undergo follow-up chest radiography daily, at least until they are being weaned off mechanical ventilation.

Prognosis VAP is associated with significant mortality. Crude mortality rates of 50–70% have been reported, but the real issue is attributable mortality. Many patients with VAP have underlying diseases that would result in death even if VAP did not occur. Attributable mortality exceeded 25% in one matched-cohort study, while more recent studies have suggested much lower rates. Patients who develop VAP are at least twice as likely to die as those who do not. Some of the variability in VAP mortality rates is clearly related to the type of patient and ICU studied. VAP in trauma patients is not associated with attributable mortality, possibly because many of the patients were otherwise healthy before being injured. However, the causative pathogen also plays a major role. Generally, MDR pathogens are associated with significantly greater attributable mortality than non-MDR pathogens. Pneumonia caused by some pathogens (e.g., *S. maltophilia*) is simply a marker for a patient whose immune system is so compromised that death is almost inevitable.

Prevention (Table 153-7) Because of the significance of the endotracheal tube as a risk factor for VAP, the most important preventive intervention is to avoid endotracheal intubation or minimize its duration. Successful use of noninvasive ventilation via a nasal or full-face mask avoids many of the problems associated with endotracheal tubes. Strategies that minimize the duration of ventilation through daily holding of sedation and formal weaning protocols also have been highly effective in preventing VAP.

Unfortunately, a tradeoff in risks is sometimes required. Aggressive attempts to extubate early may result in reintubation(s) and increase aspiration, posing a risk of VAP. Heavy continuous sedation increases the risk, but self-extubation because of insufficient sedation also is a risk. The tradeoffs also apply to antibiotic therapy. Short-course antibiotic prophylaxis can decrease the risk of VAP in comatose patients requiring intubation, and data suggest that antibiotics decrease VAP rates in general. However, the major benefit appears to be a decrease in the incidence of early-onset VAP, which is usually caused by the less pathogenic non-MDR microorganisms. Conversely, prolonged courses of antibiotics consistently increase the risk of VAP caused by the more lethal MDR pathogens. Despite its virulence and associated mortality, VAP caused by *Pseudomonas* is rare among patients who have not recently received antibiotics.

Minimizing the amount of microaspiration around the endotracheal tube cuff also is a strategy for avoidance of VAP. Simply elevating the head of the bed (at least 30° above horizontal but preferably 45°) decreases VAP rates. Specially modified endotracheal tubes that allow removal of the secretions pooled above the cuff also may prevent VAP. The risk-to-benefit ratio of transporting the patient outside the ICU for diagnostic tests or procedures should be carefully considered, since VAP rates are increased among transported patients.

Emphasis on the avoidance of agents that raise gastric pH and on oropharyngeal decontamination has been diminished by the equivocal and conflicting results of recent clinical trials. The role in the pathogenesis of VAP that is played by the overgrowth of bacterial components of the bowel flora in the stomach also has been downplayed. MRSA and the nonfermenters *P. aeruginosa* and *Acinetobacter* species are not normally part of the bowel flora but reside primarily in the nose and on the skin, respectively. Therefore, emphasis on controlling overgrowth of the bowel flora may be relevant only in certain populations, such as liver transplant recipients and patients who have undergone other major intraabdominal procedures or who have bowel obstruction.

In outbreaks of VAP due to specific pathogens, the possibility of a breakdown in infection control measures (particularly contamination of reusable equipment) should be investigated. Even high rates of pathogens that are already common in a particular ICU may be a result of cross-infection. Education and reminders of the need for consistent hand washing and other infection-control practices can minimize this risk.

HOSPITAL-ACQUIRED PNEUMONIA

While significantly less well studied than VAP, HAP in nonintubated patients—both inside and outside the ICU—is similar to VAP. The main differences are the higher frequency of non-MDR pathogens and the better underlying host immunity in nonintubated patients. The lower frequency of MDR pathogens allows monotherapy in a larger proportion of cases of HAP than of VAP.

The only pathogens that may be more common in the non-VAP population are anaerobes. The greater risk of macroaspiration by nonintubated patients and the lower oxygen tensions in the lower respiratory tract of these patients increase the likelihood of a role for anaerobes. While more common in patients with HAP, anaerobes are usually only contributors to polymicrobial pneumonias except in patients with large-volume aspiration or in the setting of bowel obstruction/ileus. As in the management of CAP, specific therapy targeting anaerobes probably is not indicated (unless gross aspiration is a concern) since many of the recommended antibiotics are active against anaerobes.

Diagnosis is even more difficult for HAP in the nonintubated patient than for VAP. Lower respiratory tract samples appropriate for culture are considerably more difficult to obtain from nonintubated patients. Many of the underlying diseases that predispose a patient to HAP are also associated with an inability to cough adequately. Since blood cultures are infrequently positive (<15% of cases), the majority of patients with HAP do not have culture data on which antibiotic modifications can be based. Therefore, de-escalation of therapy is less likely in patients with risk factors for MDR pathogens. Despite these difficulties, the better host defenses in non-ICU patients result in lower mortality rates than are documented for VAP. In addition, the risk of antibiotic failure is lower in HAP.

154 Lung Abscess

Rebecca M. Baron, Miriam Baron Barshak

Lung abscess represents necrosis and cavitation of the lung following microbial infection. Lung abscesses can be single or multiple but usually are marked by a single dominant cavity >2 cm in diameter.

ETIOLOGY

The low prevalence of lung abscesses makes them difficult to study in randomized controlled trials. Although the incidence of lung abscesses has decreased in the postantibiotic era, they are still a source of significant morbidity and mortality.

Lung abscesses are usually characterized as either primary (~80% of cases) or secondary. *Primary* lung abscesses usually arise from aspiration, are often caused principally by anaerobic bacteria, and occur in the absence of an underlying pulmonary or systemic condition. *Secondary* lung abscesses arise in the setting of an underlying condition, such as a postobstructive process (e.g., a bronchial foreign body or tumor) or a systemic process (e.g., HIV infection or another immunocompromising condition). Lung abscesses can also be characterized as acute (<4–6 weeks in duration) or chronic (~40% of cases).

EPIDEMIOLOGY

The majority of the existing epidemiologic information involves primary lung abscesses. In general, middle-aged men are more commonly affected than middle-aged women. The major risk factor for primary lung abscesses is aspiration. Patients at particular risk for aspiration, such as those with altered mental status, alcoholism, drug overdose, seizures, bulbar dysfunction, prior cerebrovascular or cardiovascular events, or neuromuscular disease, are most commonly affected. In addition, patients with esophageal dysmotility or esophageal lesions (strictures or tumors) and those with gastric distention and/or gastroesophageal reflux, especially those who spend substantial time in the recumbent position, are at risk for aspiration.

It is widely thought that colonization of the gingival crevices by anaerobic bacteria or microaerophilic streptococci (especially in patients with gingivitis and periodontal disease), combined with a risk of aspiration, is important in the development of lung abscesses. In fact, many physicians consider it extremely rare for lung abscesses to develop in the absence of teeth as a nidus for bacterial colonization.

The importance of these risk factors in the development of lung abscesses is highlighted by a significant reduction in abscess incidence in the late 1940s that coincided with a change in oral surgical technique: beginning at that time, these operations were no longer performed with the patient in the seated position without a cuffed endotracheal tube, and the frequency of perioperative aspiration events was thus decreased. In addition, the introduction of penicillin around

TABLE 154-1 EXAMPLES OF MICROBIAL PATHOGENS THAT CAN CAUSE LUNG ABSCESSES

Clinical Condition	Pathogens
Primary lung abscess (usually with risk factors for aspiration)	Anaerobes (e.g., *Peptostreptococcus* spp., *Prevotella* spp., *Bacteroides* spp., *Streptococcus milleri*), microaerophilic streptococci
Secondary lung abscess (often with underlying immunocompromise)	*Staphylococcus aureus*, gram-negative rods (e.g., *Pseudomonas aeruginosa*, Enterobacteriaceae), *Nocardia* spp., *Aspergillus* spp., Mucorales, *Cryptococcus* spp., *Legionella* spp., *Rhodococcus equi, Pneumocystis jirovecii*
Embolic lesions	*Staphylococcus aureus* (often from endocarditis), *Fusobacterium necrophorum* (Lemierre's disease; see text for details)
Endemic infections (with or without underlying immunocompromise)	*Mycobacterium tuberculosis* (as well as *Mycobacterium avium* and *Mycobacterium kansasii*), *Coccidioides* spp., *Histoplasma capsulatum*, *Blastomyces* spp., parasites (e.g., *Entamoeba histolytica, Paragonimus westermani, Strongyloides stercoralis*)
Miscellaneous conditions	Bacterial pathogen (often *S. aureus*) after influenza or other viral infection, *Actinomyces* spp.

the same time significantly reduced the incidence of and mortality rate from lung abscess.

PATHOGENESIS

Primary Lung Abscesses The development of primary lung abscesses is thought to originate when chiefly anaerobic bacteria (as well as microaerophilic streptococci) in the gingival crevices are aspirated into the lung parenchyma in a susceptible host (Table 154-1). Thus, patients who develop primary lung abscesses usually carry an overwhelming burden of aspirated material or are unable to clear the bacterial load. Pneumonitis develops initially (exacerbated in part by tissue damage caused by gastric acid); then, over a period of 7–14 days, the anaerobic bacteria produce parenchymal necrosis and cavitation whose extent depends on the host–pathogen interaction (Fig. 154-1). Anaerobes are thought to produce more extensive tissue necrosis in polymicrobial infections in which virulence factors of the various bacteria can act synergistically to cause more significant tissue destruction.

Secondary Lung Abscesses The pathogenesis of secondary abscesses depends on the predisposing factor. For example, in cases of bronchial obstruction from malignancy or a foreign body, the obstructing lesion prevents clearance of oropharyngeal secretions, leading to abscess development. With underlying systemic conditions (e.g., immunosuppression after bone marrow or solid organ transplantation), impaired host defense mechanisms lead to increased susceptibility to development of lung abscesses caused by a broad range of pathogens, including opportunistic organisms (Table 154-1).

Lung abscesses also arise from septic emboli, either in tricuspid valve endocarditis (often involving *Staphylococcus aureus*) or in Lemierre's syndrome, in which an infection begins in the pharynx (classically involving *Fusobacterium necrophorum*) and then spreads to the neck and the carotid sheath (which contains the jugular vein) to cause septic thrombophlebitis.

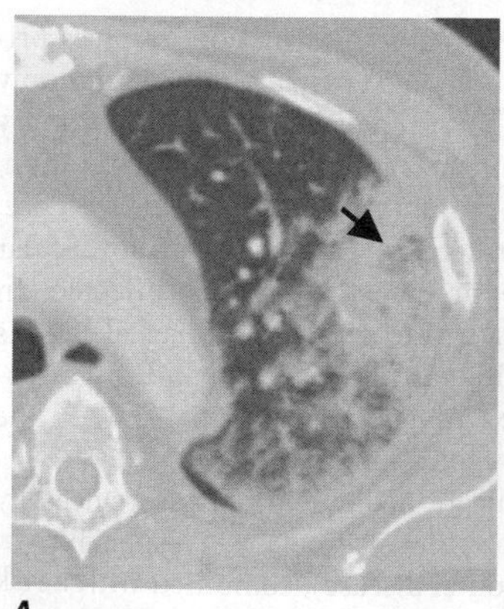

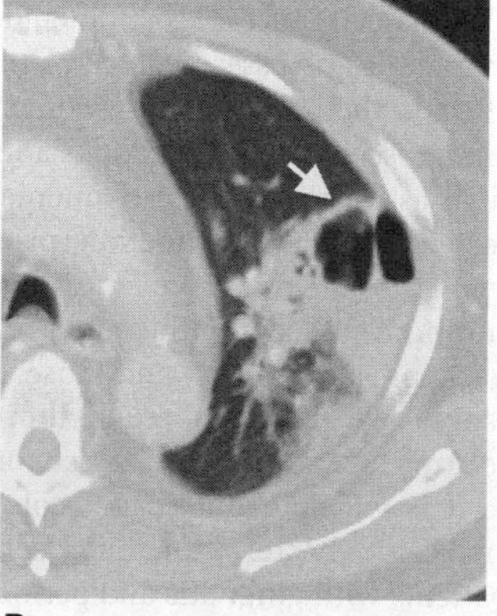

FIGURE 154-1 Representative chest CT scans demonstrating development of lung abscesses. This patient was immunocompromised due to underlying lymphoma and developed severe *Pseudomonas aeruginosa* pneumonia, as represented by a left lung infiltrate with concern for central regions of necrosis (*panel* ***A***, *black arrow*). Two weeks later, areas of cavitation with air fluid levels were visible in this region and were consistent with the development of lung abscesses (*panel* ***B***, *white arrow*). *(Images provided by Dr. Ritu Gill, Division of Chest Radiology, Brigham and Women's Hospital, Boston.)*

PATHOLOGY AND MICROBIOLOGY

Primary Lung Abscesses In primary lung abscesses, the dependent segments (posterior upper lobes and superior lower lobes) are the most common locations, given the predisposition of aspirated materials to be deposited in these areas. Generally, the right lung is affected more commonly than the left because the right mainstem bronchus is less angulated. In secondary abscesses, the location of the abscess may vary with the underlying cause.

The microbiology of primary lung abscesses is often polymicrobial, primarily including anaerobic organisms as well as microaerophilic streptococci (Table 154-1). The retrieval and culture of anaerobes can be complicated by the contamination of samples with microbes from the oral cavity, the need for expeditious transport of the cultures to the laboratory, the need for early plating with special culture techniques, the prolonged time required for culture growth, and the need for collection of specimens prior to administration of antibiotics. When attention is paid to these factors, rates of recovery of specific isolates have been reported to be as high as 78%.

Because it is not clear that knowing the identity of the causative anaerobic isolate alters the response to treatment of a primary lung abscess, practice has shifted away from the use of specialized techniques to obtain material for culture, such as transtracheal aspiration and bronchoalveolar lavage with protected brush specimens that allow recovery of culture material while avoiding contamination from the oral cavity. When no pathogen is isolated from a primary lung abscess (which is the case as often as 40% of the time), the abscess is termed a *nonspecific lung abscess*, and the presence of anaerobes is often presumed. A *putrid lung abscess* refers to foul-smelling breath, sputum, or empyema and is essentially diagnostic of an anaerobic lung abscess.

Secondary Lung Abscesses In contrast, the microbiology of secondary lung abscesses can encompass quite a broad bacterial spectrum, with infection by *Pseudomonas aeruginosa* and other gram-negative rods most common. In addition, a broad array of pathogens can be identified in patients from certain endemic areas and in specific clinical scenarios (e.g., a significant incidence of fungal infections among immunosuppressed patients following bone marrow or solid organ transplantation). Because immunocompromised hosts and patients without the classic presentation of a primary lung abscess can be infected with a wide array of unusual organisms (Table 154-1), it is of special importance to obtain culture material in order to target therapy.

CLINICAL MANIFESTATIONS

Clinical manifestations may initially be similar to those of pneumonia, with fevers, cough, sputum production, and chest pain; a more chronic and indolent presentation that includes night sweats, fatigue, and anemia is often observed with anaerobic lung abscesses. A subset of patients with putrid lung abscesses may report discolored phlegm and foul-tasting or foul-smelling sputum. Patients with lung abscesses due to non-anaerobic organisms, such as *S. aureus*, may present with a more fulminant course characterized by high fevers and rapid progression.

Findings on physical examination may include fevers, poor dentition, and/or gingival disease as well as amphoric and/or cavernous breath sounds on lung auscultation. Additional findings may include digital clubbing and the absence of a gag reflex.

DIFFERENTIAL DIAGNOSIS

The differential diagnosis of lung abscesses includes other noninfectious processes that result in cavitary lung lesions, including lung infarction, malignancy, sequestration, vasculitides (e.g., granulomatosis with polyangiitis), lung cysts or bullae containing fluid, and septic emboli (e.g., from tricuspid valve endocarditis).

DIAGNOSIS

The presence of a lung abscess is determined by chest imaging. Although a chest radiograph usually detects a thick-walled cavity with an air-fluid level, computed tomography (CT) permits better definition and may provide earlier evidence of cavitation. CT may also yield additional information regarding a possible underlying cause of lung abscess, such as malignancy, and may help distinguish a peripheral lung abscess from a pleural infection. This distinction has important implications for treatment, because a pleural space infection, such as an empyema, may require urgent drainage.

As described earlier (see "Pathology and Microbiology," above), more invasive diagnostics (such as transtracheal aspiration) were traditionally undertaken for primary lung abscesses, whereas empirical therapy that includes drugs targeting anaerobic organisms currently is used more often. While sputum can be collected noninvasively for Gram's stain and culture, which may yield a pathogen, it is likely that the infection will be polymicrobial, and culture results may not reflect the presence of anaerobic organisms. Many physicians consider putrid-smelling sputum to be virtually diagnostic of an anaerobic infection.

When a secondary lung abscess is present or empirical therapy fails to elicit a response, sputum and blood cultures are advised in addition to serologic studies for opportunistic pathogens (e.g., viruses and fungi causing infections in immunocompromised hosts). Additional diagnostics, such as bronchoscopy with bronchoalveolar lavage or protected brush specimen collection and CT-guided percutaneous needle aspiration, can be undertaken. Risks posed by these more invasive diagnostics include spillage of abscess contents into the other lung (with bronchoscopy) and pneumothorax and bronchopleural fistula development (with CT-guided needle aspiration). However, early diagnostics in secondary abscesses, especially in immunocompromised hosts, are particularly important, because the patients involved may be especially fragile and at risk for infection with a broad array of pathogens and, therefore, less likely than other patients to respond to empirical therapy.

TREATMENT LUNG ABSCESS

The availability of antibiotics in the 1940s and 1950s established therapy with this drug class as the primary approach to the treatment of lung abscess. Previously, surgery had been relied upon much more frequently. For many decades, penicillin was the antibiotic of choice for primary lung abscesses in light of its anaerobic coverage; however, because oral anaerobes can produce β-lactamases, clindamycin has proved superior to penicillin in clinical trials. For primary lung abscesses, the recommended regimens are (1) clindamycin (600 mg IV three times daily; then, with the disappearance of fever and clinical improvement, 300 mg PO four times daily) or (2) an IV-administered β-lactam/β-lactamase combination, followed—once the patient's condition is stable—by orally administered amoxicillin-clavulanate. This therapy should be continued until imaging demonstrates that the lung abscess has cleared or regressed to a small scar. Treatment duration may range from 3–4 weeks to as long as 14 weeks. One small study suggested that moxifloxacin (400 mg/d PO) is as effective and well tolerated as ampicillin-sulbactam. Notably, metronidazole is not effective as a single agent: it covers anaerobic organisms but not the microaerophilic streptococci that are often components of the mixed flora of primary lung abscesses.

In secondary lung abscesses, antibiotic coverage should be directed at the identified pathogen, and a prolonged course (until resolution of the abscess is documented) is often required. Treatment regimens and courses vary widely, depending on the immune state of the host and the identified pathogen. Other interventions may be necessary as well, such as relief of an obstructing lesion or treatment directed at the underlying condition predisposing the patient to lung abscess. Similarly, if the condition of patients with presumed primary lung abscess fails to improve, additional studies to rule out an underlying predisposing cause for a secondary lung abscess are indicated.

Although it can take as long as 7 days for patients receiving appropriate therapy to defervesce, as many as 10–20% of patients may not respond at all, with continued fevers and progression of the abscess cavity on imaging. An abscess >6–8 cm in diameter is less likely to respond to antibiotic therapy without additional interventions. Options for patients who do not respond to antibiotics and whose additional diagnostic studies fail to identify an additional pathogen that can be treated include surgical resection and percutaneous drainage of the abscess, especially in poor surgical candidates. Possible complications of percutaneous drainage include bacterial contamination of the pleural space as well as pneumothorax and hemothorax.

COMPLICATIONS

Larger cavity size on presentation may correlate with the development of persistent cystic changes (pneumatoceles) or bronchiectasis. Additional possible complications include recurrence of abscesses despite appropriate therapy, extension to the pleural space with development of empyema, life-threatening hemoptysis, and massive aspiration of lung abscess contents.

PROGNOSIS AND PREVENTION

Reported mortality rates for primary abscesses have been as low as 2%, while rates for secondary abscesses are generally higher—as high as 75% in some case series. Other poor prognostic factors include an age >60, the presence of aerobic bacteria, sepsis at presentation, symptom duration of >8 weeks, and abscess size >6 cm.

Mitigation of underlying risk factors may be the best approach to prevention of lung abscesses, with attention directed toward airway protection, oral hygiene, and minimized sedation with elevation of the head of the bed for patients at risk for aspiration. Prophylaxis against certain pathogens in at-risk patients (e.g., recipients of bone marrow or solid organ transplants or patients whose immune systems are significantly compromised by HIV infection) may be undertaken.

APPROACH TO THE PATIENT: Lung Abscess

For patients with a lung abscess and a low likelihood of malignancy (e.g., smokers <45 years old) and with risk factors for aspiration, it is reasonable to administer empirical treatment and then to pursue further evaluation if therapy does not elicit a response. However, some clinicians may opt for up-front cultures, even in primary lung abscesses. In patients with risk factors for malignancy or other underlying conditions (especially immunocompromised hosts) or with an atypical presentation, earlier diagnostics should be considered, such as bronchoscopy with biopsy or CT-guided needle aspiration. Bronchoscopy should be performed early in patients whose history, symptoms, or imaging findings are consistent with possible bronchial obstruction. In patients from areas endemic for tuberculosis or patients with other risk factors for tuberculosis (e.g., underlying HIV infection), induced sputum samples should be examined early in the workup to rule out this disease.

155 Infective Endocarditis

Adolf W. Karchmer

The prototypic lesion of infective endocarditis, the *vegetation* (Fig. 155-1), is a mass of platelets, fibrin, microcolonies of microorganisms, and scant inflammatory cells. Infection most commonly involves heart valves but may also occur on the low-pressure side of a ventricular septal defect, on mural endocardium damaged by aberrant jets of blood or foreign bodies, or on intracardiac devices themselves. The analogous process involving arteriovenous shunts, arterio-arterial shunts (patent ductus arteriosus), or a coarctation of the aorta is called *infective endarteritis*.

Endocarditis can be classified according to the temporal evolution of disease, the site of infection, the cause of infection, or the predisposing risk factor (e.g., injection drug use). While each classification criterion provides therapeutic and prognostic insight, none is sufficient alone. *Acute endocarditis* is a hectically febrile illness that rapidly damages cardiac structures, seeds extracardiac sites, and, if untreated, progresses to death within weeks. *Subacute endocarditis* follows an indolent course; causes structural cardiac damage only slowly, if at all; rarely metastasizes; and is gradually progressive unless complicated by a major embolic event or a ruptured mycotic aneurysm.

In developed countries, the incidence of endocarditis ranges from 4 to 7 cases per 100,000 population per year and has remained relatively stable during recent decades. While congenital heart diseases remain a constant predisposition, predisposing conditions in developed countries have shifted from chronic rheumatic heart disease (still a common predisposition in developing countries) to illicit IV drug use, degenerative valve disease, and intracardiac devices. The incidence of endocarditis is notably increased among the elderly. In developed countries, 25–35% of cases of native valve endocarditis (NVE) are associated with health care, and 16–30% of all cases of endocarditis involve prosthetic valves. The risk of prosthesis infection is greatest during the first 6–12 months after valve replacement; gradually declines to a low, stable rate thereafter; and is similar for mechanical and bioprosthetic devices. The incidence of endocarditis involving cardiovascular implantable electronic devices (CIED), primarily permanent pacemakers and implantable cardioverter-defibrillators, ranges from 0.5 to 1.14 cases per 1000 device recipients and is higher among patients with an implantable cardioverter-defibrillator than among those with a permanent pacemaker.

ETIOLOGY

Although many species of bacteria and fungi cause sporadic episodes of endocarditis, a few bacterial species cause the majority of cases (Table 155-1). The oral cavity, skin, and upper respiratory tract are the respective primary portals for viridans streptococci, staphylococci, and HACEK organisms (*Haemophilus* species, *Aggregatibacter aphrophilus*, *A. actinomycetemcomitans*, *Cardiobacterium* species, *Eikenella* species, and *Kingella* species). *Streptococcus gallolyticus* subspecies *gallolyticus* (formerly *S. bovis* biotype 1) originates from the gastrointestinal tract, where it is associated with polyps and colonic tumors, and enterococci enter the bloodstream from the genitourinary tract. Health care–associated NVE, most commonly caused by *Staphylococcus aureus*, coagulase-negative staphylococci (CoNS), and enterococci, may have either a nosocomial onset (55%) or a community onset (45%); community-onset cases develop in patients who have had extensive contact with the health care system over the preceding 90 days. Endocarditis complicates 6–25% of episodes of catheter-associated *S. aureus* bacteremia; the higher rates are detected in high-risk patients studied by transesophageal echocardiography (TEE) (see "Echocardiography," later).

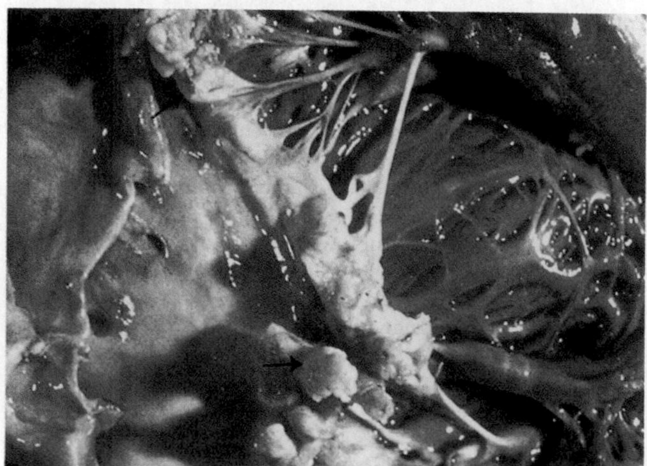

FIGURE 155-1 Vegetations (*arrows*) due to viridans streptococcal endocarditis involving the mitral valve.

Prosthetic valve endocarditis (PVE) arising within 2 months of valve surgery is generally nosocomial, the result of intraoperative contamination of the prosthesis or a bacteremic postoperative complication. This nosocomial origin is reflected in the primary microbial causes: *S. aureus*, CoNS, facultative gram-negative bacilli, diphtheroids, and fungi. The portals of entry and organisms causing cases beginning >12 months after surgery are similar to those in community-acquired NVE. PVE due to CoNS that presents 2–12 months after surgery often represents delayed-onset nosocomial infection. Regardless of the time of onset after surgery, at least 68–85% of CoNS strains that cause PVE are resistant to methicillin.

Endocarditis related to a permanent pacemaker or an implantable cardioverter-defibrillator involves the device or the endothelium at points of device contact. Occasionally, there is concurrent aortic or mitral valve infection. One-third of cases of CIED endocarditis present within 3 months after device implantation or manipulation, one-third present at 4–12 months, and one-third present at >1 year. *S. aureus* and CoNS, both of which are commonly resistant to methicillin, cause the majority of cases.

Injection drug use–associated endocarditis, especially that involving the tricuspid valve, is commonly caused by *S. aureus*, which in many cases is resistant to methicillin. Left-sided valve infections in addicts have a more varied etiology. In addition to the usual causes of endocarditis, these cases can be due to *Pseudomonas aeruginosa* and *Candida* species, and sporadic cases can be caused by unusual organisms such as *Bacillus*, *Lactobacillus*, and *Corynebacterium* species. Polymicrobial endocarditis occurs among injection drug users. HIV infection in drug users does not significantly influence the causes of endocarditis.

From 5% to 15% of patients with endocarditis have negative blood cultures; in one-third to one-half of these cases, cultures are negative because of prior antibiotic exposure. The remainder of these patients are infected by fastidious organisms, such as nutritionally variant bacteria (now designated *Granulicatella* and *Abiotrophia* species), HACEK organisms, *Coxiella burnetii*, and *Bartonella* species. Some fastidious organisms occur in characteristic geographic settings (e.g., *C. burnetii* and *Bartonella* species in Europe, *Brucella* species in the Middle East). *Tropheryma whipplei* causes an indolent, culture-negative, afebrile form of endocarditis.

PATHOGENESIS

The undamaged endothelium is resistant to infection by most bacteria and to thrombus formation. Endothelial injury (e.g., at the site of impact of high-velocity blood jets or on the low-pressure side of a cardiac structural lesion) allows either direct infection by virulent organisms or the development of a platelet-fibrin thrombus—a condition called *nonbacterial thrombotic endocarditis* (NBTE). This thrombus serves as a site of bacterial attachment during transient bacteremia. The cardiac conditions most commonly resulting in NBTE are mitral regurgitation, aortic stenosis, aortic regurgitation, ventricular septal defects, and complex congenital heart disease. NBTE also arises as a result of a hypercoagulable state; this gives rise to *marantic endocarditis* (uninfected vegetations seen in patients with malignancy and chronic diseases) and to bland vegetations

TABLE 155-1 ORGANISMS CAUSING MAJOR CLINICAL FORMS OF ENDOCARDITIS

	Percentage of Cases							
	Native Valve Endocarditis		Prosthetic Valve Endocarditis at Indicated Time of Onset (Months) after Valve Surgery			Endocarditis in Injection Drug Users		
Organism	Community-Acquired (n = 1718)	Health Care–Associated (n = 1110)	<2 (n = 144)	2–12 (n = 31)	>12 (n = 194)	Right-Sided (n = 346)	Left-Sided (n = 204)	Total (n = 675)[a]
Streptococci[b]	40	13	1	9	31	5	15	12
Pneumococci	2	—	—	—	—	—	—	—
Enterococci[c]	9	16	8	12	11	2	24	9
Staphylococcus aureus	28	52[d]	22	12	18	77	23	57
Coagulase-negative staphylococci	5	11	33	32	11	—	—	—
Fastidious gram-negative coccobacilli (HACEK group)[e]	3	—	—	—	6	—	—	—
Gram-negative bacilli	1	1	13	3	6	5	13	7
Candida spp.	<1	1	8	12	1	—	12	4
Polymicrobial/miscellaneous	3	3	3	6	5	8	10	7
Diphtheroids	—	<1	6	—	3	—	—	0.1
Culture-negative	9	3	5	6	8	3	3	3

[a]The total number of cases is larger than the sum of right- and left-sided cases because the location of infection was not specified in some cases. [b]Includes viridans streptococci; *Streptococcus gallolyticus*; other non–group A, groupable streptococci; and *Abiotrophia* and *Granulicatella* spp. (nutritionally variant, pyridoxal-requiring streptococci). [c]Primarily *E. faecalis* or nonspeciated isolates; occasionally *E. faecium* or other, less likely species. [d]Methicillin resistance is common among these *S. aureus* strains. [e]Includes *Haemophilus* spp., *Aggregatibacter aphrophilus, Aggregatibacter actinomycetemcomitans, Cardiobacterium hominis, Eikenella* spp., and *Kingella* spp.

Note: Data are compiled from multiple studies.

complicating systemic lupus erythematosus and the antiphospholipid antibody syndrome.

Organisms that cause endocarditis enter the bloodstream from mucosal surfaces, the skin, or sites of focal infection. Except for more virulent bacteria (e.g., *S. aureus*) that can adhere directly to intact endothelium or exposed subendothelial tissue, microorganisms in the blood adhere at sites of NBTE. The organisms that commonly cause endocarditis have surface adhesin molecules, collectively called microbial surface components recognizing adhesin matrix molecules (MSCRAMMs), that mediate adherence to NBTE sites or injured endothelium. Adherence is facilitated by fibronectin-binding proteins present on many gram-positive bacteria; by clumping factor (a fibrinogen- and fibrin-binding surface protein) on *S. aureus*; by fibrinogen-binding surface proteins (Fss2), collagen-binding surface protein (Ace), and Ebp pili (the latter mediating platelet adherence) in *Enterococcus faecalis*; and by glucans or FimA (a member of the family of oral mucosal adhesins) on streptococci. Fibronectin-binding proteins are required for *S. aureus* invasion of intact endothelium; thus these surface proteins may facilitate infection of previously normal valves. If resistant to the bactericidal activity of serum and the microbicidal peptides released locally by platelets, adherent organisms proliferate to form dense microcolonies. Microorganisms also induce platelet deposition and a localized procoagulant state by eliciting tissue factor from the endothelium or, in the case of *S. aureus*, from monocytes as well. Fibrin deposition combines with platelet aggregation and microorganism proliferation to generate an infected vegetation. Organisms deep in vegetations are metabolically inactive (nongrowing) and relatively resistant to killing by antimicrobial agents. Proliferating surface organisms are shed into the bloodstream continuously.

The clinical manifestations of endocarditis—other than constitutional symptoms, which probably result from cytokine production—arise from damage to intracardiac structures; embolization of vegetation fragments, leading to infection or infarction of remote tissues; hematogenous infection of sites during bacteremia; and tissue injury due to the deposition of circulating immune complexes or immune responses to deposited bacterial antigens.

CLINICAL MANIFESTATIONS

The clinical endocarditis syndrome is highly variable and spans a continuum between acute and subacute presentations. NVE, PVE, and endocarditis due to injection drug use share clinical and laboratory manifestations (Table 155-2). The causative microorganism is primarily responsible for the temporal course of endocarditis. β-Hemolytic streptococci, *S. aureus*, and pneumococci typically result in an acute course, although *S. aureus* occasionally causes subacute disease. Endocarditis caused by *Staphylococcus lugdunensis* (a coagulase-negative species) or by enterococci may present acutely. Subacute endocarditis is typically caused by viridans streptococci, enterococci, CoNS, and the HACEK group. Endocarditis caused by *Bartonella* species, *T. whipplei*, or *C. burnetii* is exceptionally indolent.

TABLE 155-2 CLINICAL AND LABORATORY FEATURES OF INFECTIVE ENDOCARDITIS

Feature	Frequency, %
Fever	80–90
Chills and sweats	40–75
Anorexia, weight loss, malaise	25–50
Myalgias, arthralgias	15–30
Back pain	7–15
Heart murmur	80–85
New/worsened regurgitant murmur	20–50
Arterial emboli	20–50
Splenomegaly	15–50
Clubbing	10–20
Neurologic manifestations	20–40
Peripheral manifestations (Osler's nodes, subungual hemorrhages, Janeway lesions, Roth's spots)	2–15
Petechiae	10–40
Laboratory manifestations	
Anemia	70–90
Leukocytosis	20–30
Microscopic hematuria	30–50
Elevated erythrocyte sedimentation rate	60–90
Elevated C-reactive protein level	>90
Rheumatoid factor	50
Circulating immune complexes	65–100
Decreased serum complement	5–40

In patients with subacute presentations, fever is typically low-grade and rarely exceeds 39.4°C (103°F); in contrast, temperatures of 39.4°–40°C (103°–104°F) are often noted in acute endocarditis. Fever may be blunted in patients who are elderly, are severely debilitated, or have renal failure.

Cardiac Manifestations Although heart murmurs are usually indicative of the predisposing cardiac pathology rather than of endocarditis, valvular damage and ruptured chordae may result in new regurgitant murmurs. In acute endocarditis involving a normal valve, murmurs may be absent initially but ultimately are detected in 85% of cases. Congestive heart failure (CHF) develops in 30–40% of patients as a consequence of valvular dysfunction. Occasionally, CHF is due to endocarditis-associated myocarditis or an intracardiac fistula. Heart failure due to aortic valve dysfunction progresses more rapidly than does that due to mitral valve dysfunction. Extension of infection beyond valve leaflets into adjacent annular or myocardial tissue results in perivalvular abscesses, which in turn may cause intracardiac fistulae with new murmurs. Abscesses may burrow from the aortic valve annulus through the epicardium, causing pericarditis, or into the upper ventricular septum, where they may interrupt the conduction system, leading to varying degrees of heart block. Mitral perivalvular abscesses, which are usually more distant from the conduction system, only rarely cause conduction abnormalities; if such abnormalities occur in this setting, the conduction pathway is most likely disrupted near the atrioventricular node or in the proximal bundle of His. Emboli to a coronary artery occur in 2% of patients and may result in myocardial infarction.

Noncardiac Manifestations The classic nonsuppurative peripheral manifestations of subacute endocarditis (e.g., Janeway lesions; Fig. 155-2A) are related to prolonged infection; with early diagnosis and treatment, these have become infrequent. In contrast, septic embolization mimicking some of these lesions (subungual hemorrhage, Osler's nodes) is common in patients with acute *S. aureus* endocarditis (Fig. 155-2B). Musculoskeletal pain usually remits promptly with treatment but must be distinguished from focal metastatic infections (e.g., spondylodiscitis), which may complicate 10–15% of cases. Hematogenously seeded focal infection occurs most often in the skin, spleen, kidneys, skeletal system, and meninges. Arterial emboli, one-half of which precede the diagnosis, are clinically apparent in up to 50% of patients. Endocarditis caused by *S. aureus*, vegetations >10 mm in diameter (as measured by echocardiography), and infection involving the mitral valve, especially the anterior leaflet, are independently associated with an increased risk of embolization. Symptoms, pain, or ischemia-induced dysfunction relate to the organ or area suffering embolic arterial occlusion (e.g., kidney, spleen, bowel, extremity). Cerebrovascular emboli presenting as strokes or occasionally as encephalopathy complicate 15–35% of cases of endocarditis. Again, one-half of these events precede the diagnosis of endocarditis. The frequency of stroke is 8 per 1000 patient-days during the week prior to diagnosis; the figure falls to 4.8 and 1.7 per 1000 patient-days during the first and second weeks of effective antimicrobial therapy, respectively. This decline exceeds that which can be attributed to change in vegetation size. Only 3% of strokes occur after 1 week of effective therapy. Emboli occurring late during or after effective therapy do not in themselves constitute evidence of failed antimicrobial treatment.

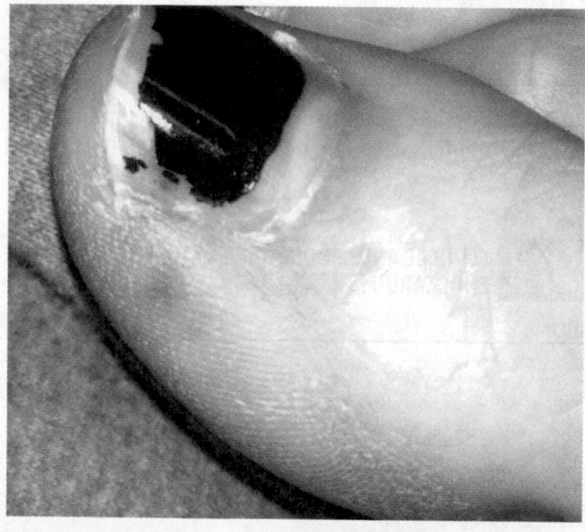

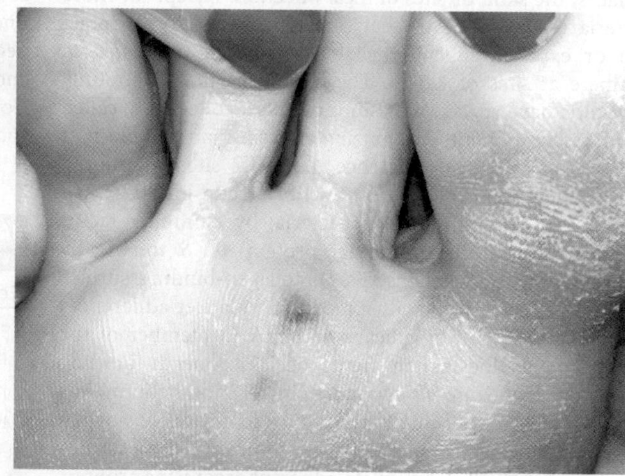

A

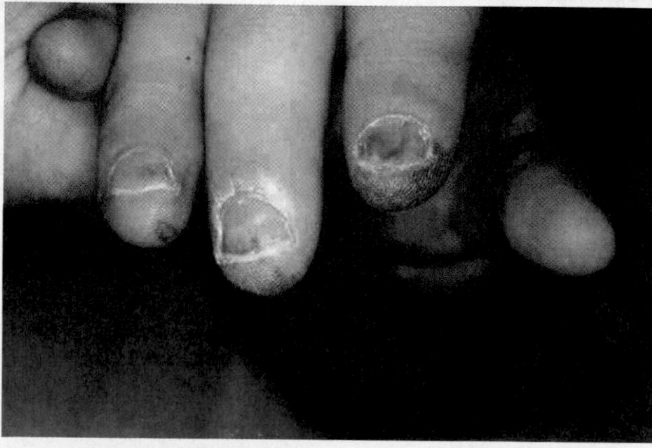

B

FIGURE 155-2 ***A.*** Janeway lesions on toe (*left*) and plantar surface (*right*) of the foot in subacute *Neisseria mucosa* endocarditis. *(Image courtesy of Rachel Baden, MD.)* ***B.*** Septic emboli with hemorrhage and infarction due to acute *Staphylococcus aureus* endocarditis.

Other neurologic complications include aseptic or purulent meningitis, intracranial hemorrhage due to hemorrhagic infarcts or ruptured mycotic aneurysms, and seizures. (*Mycotic aneurysms* are focal dilatations of arteries occurring at points in the artery wall that have been weakened by infection in the vasa vasorum or where septic emboli have lodged.) Microabscesses in brain and meninges occur commonly in *S. aureus* endocarditis; surgically drainable intracerebral abscesses are infrequent.

Immune complex deposition on the glomerular basement membrane causes diffuse hypocomplementemic glomerulonephritis and renal dysfunction, which typically improve with effective antimicrobial therapy. Embolic renal infarcts cause flank pain and hematuria but rarely cause renal dysfunction.

Manifestations of Specific Predisposing Conditions Almost 50% of endocarditis associated with injection drug use is limited to the tricuspid valve and presents with fever but with faint or no murmur and no peripheral manifestations. Septic pulmonary emboli, which are common with tricuspid endocarditis, cause cough, pleuritic chest pain, nodular pulmonary infiltrates, or occasionally pyopneumothorax. Infection of the aortic or mitral valves presents with the typical clinical features of endocarditis, including peripheral manifestations.

If not associated with a retained intracardiac device or masked by the symptoms of concurrent comorbid illness, health care associated endocarditis has typical manifestations. CIED endocarditis may be associated with obvious or cryptic generator pocket infection and results in fever, minimal murmur, and pulmonary symptoms due to septic emboli. Late-onset PVE presents with typical clinical features. In cases arising within 60 days of valve surgery (early onset), typical symptoms may be obscured by comorbidity associated with recent surgery. In both early-onset and more delayed presentations, paravalvular infection is common and often results in partial valve dehiscence, regurgitant murmurs, CHF, or disruption of the conduction system.

DIAGNOSIS

In order to avoid delayed or missed diagnosis, careful clinical, microbiologic, and echocardiographic evaluation should be pursued when febrile patients have endocarditis predispositions, cardiac or noncardiac features of endocarditis, or microbiologic findings consistent with endocarditis (e.g., a stroke or splenic infarct, multiple positive blood cultures for an endocarditis-associated organism).

The Duke Criteria The diagnosis of infective endocarditis is established with certainty only when vegetations are examined histologically and microbiologically. Nevertheless, a highly sensitive and specific diagnostic schema—known as the *modified Duke criteria*—is based on clinical, laboratory, and echocardiographic findings commonly encountered in patients with endocarditis (Table 155-3). While developed as a research tool rather than for patient management, the criteria can be a helpful diagnostic tool. If the criteria are to be maximally helpful in evaluating patients, appropriate data must be collected. Furthermore, clinical judgment must be exercised in order to use the criteria effectively. Documentation of two major criteria, of one major criterion and three minor criteria, or of five minor criteria allows a clinical diagnosis of definite endocarditis. The diagnosis of endocarditis is rejected if an alternative diagnosis is established, if symptoms resolve and do not recur with ≤4 days of antibiotic therapy, or if surgery or autopsy after ≤4 days of antimicrobial therapy yields no histologic evidence of endocarditis. Illnesses not classified as definite endocarditis or rejected as such are considered cases of possible infective endocarditis when either one major and one minor criterion or three minor criteria are fulfilled. Requiring some clinical features of endocarditis for classification as possible infective endocarditis increases the specificity of the schema without significantly reducing its sensitivity. Unless there are extenuating circumstances, patients with definite or possible endocarditis are treated as such.

The criteria emphasize bacteremia and echocardiographic findings typical of endocarditis. The requirement for multiple positive blood cultures over time is consistent with the continuous low-density

TABLE 155-3 THE MODIFIED DUKE CRITERIA FOR THE CLINICAL DIAGNOSIS OF INFECTIVE ENDOCARDITIS[a]

Major Criteria

1. Positive blood culture
   Typical microorganism for infective endocarditis from two separate blood cultures
      Viridans streptococci, *Streptococcus gallolyticus*, HACEK group organisms, *Staphylococcus aureus*, or
      Community-acquired enterococci in the absence of a primary focus,
   or
   Persistently positive blood culture, defined as recovery of a microorganism consistent with infective endocarditis from:
      Blood cultures drawn >12 h apart; *or*
      All of 3 or a majority of ≥4 separate blood cultures, with first and last drawn at least 1 h apart
   or
   Single positive blood culture for *Coxiella burnetii* or phase I IgG antibody titer of >1:800
2. Evidence of endocardial involvement
   Positive echocardiogram[b]
      Oscillating intracardiac mass on valve or supporting structures or in the path of regurgitant jets or in implanted material, in the absence of an alternative anatomic explanation, *or*
      Abscess, *or*
      New partial dehiscence of prosthetic valve,
   or
   New valvular regurgitation (increase or change in preexisting murmur not sufficient)

Minor Criteria

1. Predisposition: predisposing heart conditions[c] or injection drug use
2. Fever >38.0°C (≥100.4°F)
3. Vascular phenomena: major arterial emboli, septic pulmonary infarcts, mycotic aneurysm, intracranial hemorrhage, conjunctival hemorrhages, Janeway lesions
4. Immunologic phenomena: glomerulonephritis, Osler's nodes, Roth's spots, rheumatoid factor
5. Microbiologic evidence: positive blood culture but not meeting major criterion, as noted previously,[d] *or* serologic evidence of active infection with an organism consistent with infective endocarditis

[a]Definite endocarditis is defined by documentation of two major criteria, of one major criterion and three minor criteria, or of five minor criteria. See text for further details. [b]Transesophageal echocardiography is required for optimal assessment of possible prosthetic valve endocarditis or complicated endocarditis. [c]Valvular disease with stenosis or regurgitation, presence of a prosthetic valve, congenital heart disease including corrected or partially corrected conditions (except isolated atrial septal defect, repaired ventricular septal defect, or closed patent ductus arteriosus), prior endocarditis, or hypertrophic cardiomyopathy. [d]Excluding single positive cultures for coagulase-negative staphylococci and diphtheroids, which are common culture contaminants, or for organisms that do not cause endocarditis frequently, such as gram-negative bacilli.

Source: Adapted from JS Li et al: Clin Infect Dis 30:633, 2000. With permission from Oxford University Press.

bacteremia characteristic of endocarditis. Among patients with untreated endocarditis who ultimately have a positive blood culture, 95% of all blood cultures are positive. The diagnostic criteria attach significance to the species of organism isolated from blood cultures. To fulfill a major criterion, the isolation of an organism that causes both endocarditis and bacteremia in the absence of endocarditis (e.g., *S. aureus*, enterococci) must take place repeatedly (i.e., persistent bacteremia) and in the absence of a primary focus of infection. Organisms that rarely cause endocarditis but commonly contaminate blood cultures (e.g., diphtheroids, CoNS) must be isolated repeatedly if their isolation is to serve as a major criterion.

Blood Cultures Isolation of the causative microorganism from blood cultures is critical for diagnosis and for planning treatment. In patients with suspected NVE, PVE, or CIED endocarditis who have not received antibiotics during the prior 2 weeks, three 2-bottle blood culture sets, separated from one another by at least 2 h, should be obtained from different venipuncture sites over 24 h. If the cultures remain negative after 48–72 h, two or three additional blood culture sets should be obtained, and the laboratory should be consulted for advice regarding optimal culture techniques. Pending culture results, empirical antimicrobial therapy should be withheld initially from hemodynamically stable patients with suspected subacute endocarditis, especially those who have received antibiotics within the preceding 2 weeks. Thus, if necessary, additional blood culture sets can be obtained without the confounding effect of empirical treatment. Patients with acute endocarditis or with deteriorating hemodynamics who may require urgent surgery should receive empirical treatment immediately after three sets of blood cultures are obtained over several hours.

Non-Blood-Culture Tests Serologic tests can be used to implicate organisms that are difficult to recover by blood culture: *Brucella*, *Bartonella*, *Legionella*, *Chlamydia psittaci*, and *C. burnetii*. Pathogens can also be identified in vegetations by culture, microscopic examination with special stains (i.e., the periodic acid–Schiff stain for *T. whipplei*), or direct fluorescence antibody techniques and by the use of polymerase chain reaction to recover unique microbial DNA or DNA encoding the 16S or 28S ribosomal unit (16S rRNA or 28S rRNA); sequencing of these DNAs allows identification of bacteria and fungi, respectively.

Echocardiography Echocardiography anatomically confirms and measures vegetations, detects intracardiac complications, and assesses cardiac function (Fig. 155-3). Transthoracic echocardiography (TTE) is noninvasive and exceptionally specific; however, it cannot image vegetations <2 mm in diameter, and in 20% of patients it is technically inadequate because of emphysema or body habitus. TTE detects vegetations in 65–80% of patients with definite clinical endocarditis but is not optimal for evaluating prosthetic valves or detecting intracardiac complications. TEE is safe and detects vegetations in >90% of patients with definite endocarditis; nevertheless, initial studies may yield false-negative results in 6–18% of endocarditis patients. When endocarditis is likely, a negative TEE result does not exclude the diagnosis but rather warrants repetition of the study once or twice in 7–10 days. TEE is the optimal method for the diagnosis of PVE, the detection of myocardial abscess, valve perforation, or intracardiac fistulae and for the detection of vegetations in patients with CIED. In patients with CIED and negative blood cultures, a mass adherent to the lead is likely to be a bland thrombosis rather than an infected vegetation.

Because *S. aureus* bacteremia is associated with a high prevalence of endocarditis, routine echocardiographic evaluation (TTE or preferably TEE) is recommended in these patients. Patients with nosocomial *S. aureus* bacteremia are at increased risk of endocarditis if one or more of the following are present: positive blood cultures for 2–4 days, hemodialysis dependency, a permanent intracardiac device, spine infection, nonvertebral osteomyelitis, or an endocarditis-predisposing valve abnormality. Ideally, these patients should be evaluated with TEE. In patients with none of these findings, the risk of endocarditis is low and evaluation with TTE may suffice.

Experts favor echocardiographic evaluation of all patients with a clinical diagnosis of endocarditis; however, the test should not be used to screen patients with a low probability of endocarditis (e.g., patients with unexplained fever). An American Heart Association approach to the use of echocardiography for evaluation of patients with suspected endocarditis is illustrated in (Fig. 155-4).

Other Studies Many studies that are not diagnostic—i.e., complete blood count, creatinine determination, liver function tests, chest radiography, and electrocardiography—are important in the management of patients with endocarditis. The erythrocyte sedimentation rate, C-reactive protein level, and circulating immune complex titer are commonly increased in endocarditis (Table 155-2). Cardiac catheterization is useful primarily to assess coronary artery patency in older individuals who are to undergo surgery for endocarditis.

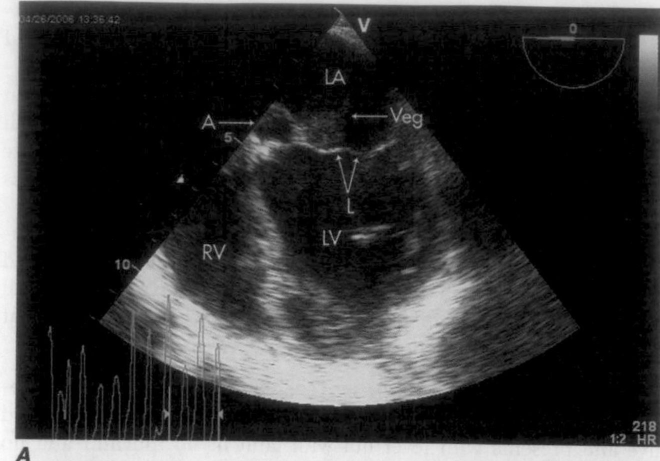

A

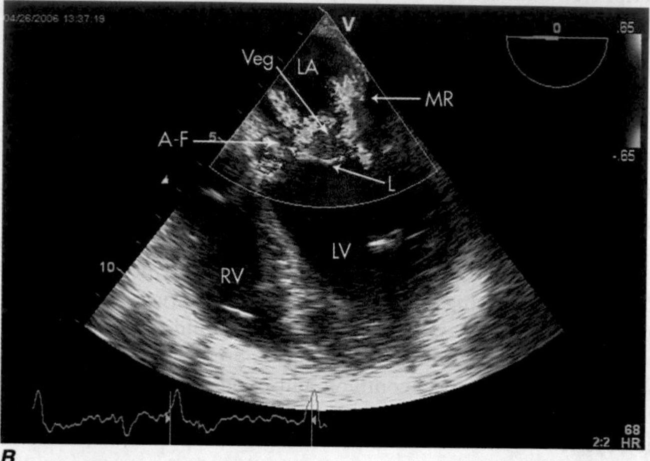

B

FIGURE 155-3 Imaging of a mitral valve infected with *Staphylococcus aureus* by low-esophageal, four-chamber-view, transesophageal echocardiography (TEE). *A.* Two-dimensional echocardiogram showing a large vegetation with an adjacent echolucent abscess cavity. ***B.*** Color-flow Doppler image showing severe mitral regurgitation through both the abscess-fistula and the central valve orifice. A, abscess; A-F, abscess-fistula; L, valve leaflets; LA, left atrium; LV, left ventricle; MR, mitral central valve regurgitation; RV, right ventricle; veg, vegetation. *(With permission of Andrew Burger, MD.)*

TREATMENT INFECTIVE ENDOCARDITIS

ANTIMICROBIAL THERAPY

To cure endocarditis, all bacteria in the vegetation must be killed. However, it is difficult to eradicate these bacteria because local host defenses are deficient and because the bacteria are largely nongrowing and metabolically inactive and thus are less easily killed by antibiotics. Accordingly, therapy must be bactericidal and prolonged. Antibiotics are generally given parenterally to achieve serum concentrations that, through passive diffusion, result in effective concentrations in the depths of the vegetation. To select effective therapy requires knowledge of the susceptibility of the causative microorganisms. The decision to initiate treatment empirically must balance the need to establish a microbiologic diagnosis against the potential progression of disease or the need for urgent surgery (see "Blood Cultures," earlier). Simultaneous infection at other sites (such as the meninges), allergies, end-organ dysfunction, interactions with concomitantly administered medications, and risks of adverse events must be considered in the selection of therapy.

Although given for several weeks longer, the regimens recommended for the treatment of PVE (except that caused by staphylococci) are similar to those used to treat NVE (**Table 155-4**). Recommended doses and durations of therapy should be followed

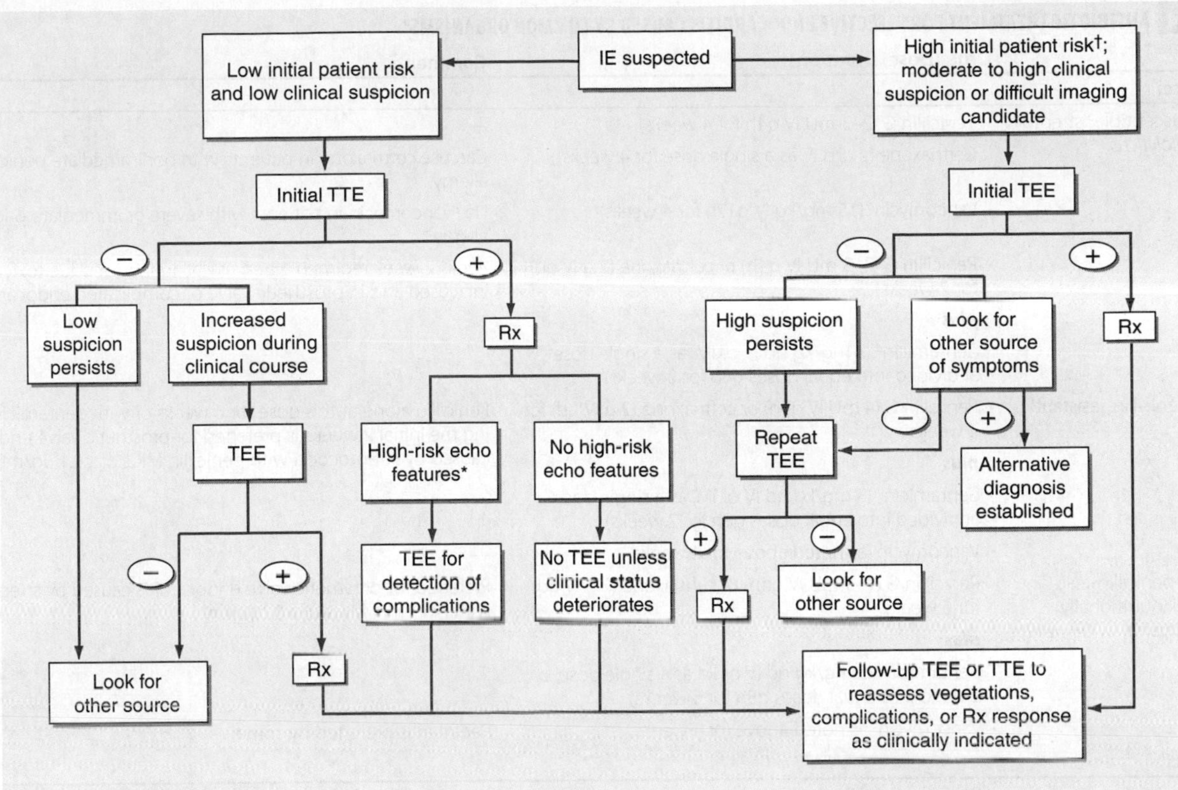

FIGURE 155-4 The diagnostic use of transesophageal and transtracheal echocardiography (TEE and TTE, respectively). †High initial patient risk for infective endocarditis (IE), as listed in Table 155-8, or evidence of intracardiac complications (new regurgitant murmur, new electrocardiographic conduction changes, or congestive heart failure). *High-risk echocardiographic features include large vegetations, valve insufficiency, paravalvular infection, or ventricular dysfunction. Rx indicates initiation of antibiotic therapy. *(Reproduced with permission from Diagnosis and Management of Infective Endocarditis and Its Complications. Circulation 98:2936, 1998. © 1998 American Heart Association.)*

unless alterations are required by end-organ dysfunction or adverse events.

Organism-Specific Therapies • ***STREPTOCOCCI*** Optimal therapy for streptococcal endocarditis is based on the minimal inhibitory concentration (MIC) of penicillin for the causative isolate (Table 155-4). The 2-week penicillin/gentamicin or ceftriaxone/gentamicin regimens should not be used to treat PVE or complicated NVE. Caution should be exercised in considering aminoglycoside-containing regimens for the treatment of patients at increased risk for aminoglycoside toxicity. The regimens recommended for relatively penicillin-resistant streptococci are advocated for treatment of group B, C, or G streptococcal endocarditis. Nutritionally variant organisms (*Granulicatella* or *Abiotrophia* species) and *Gemella* species are treated with the regimens for moderately penicillin-resistant streptococci, as is PVE caused by these organisms or by streptococci with a penicillin MIC of >0.1 μg/mL (Table 155-4).

ENTEROCOCCI Enterococci are resistant to oxacillin, nafcillin, and the cephalosporins and are only inhibited—not killed—by penicillin, ampicillin, teicoplanin (not available in the United States), and vancomycin. To kill enterococci requires the synergistic interaction of a cell wall–active antibiotic that is effective at achievable serum concentrations (penicillin, ampicillin, vancomycin, or teicoplanin) and an aminoglycoside (gentamicin or streptomycin) to which the isolate does not exhibit high-level resistance. An isolate's resistance to cell wall–active agents or its ability to replicate in the presence of gentamicin at ≥500 μg/mL or streptomycin at 1000–2000 μg/mL—a phenomenon called *high-level aminoglycoside resistance*—indicates that the ineffective antimicrobial agent cannot participate in the interaction to produce killing. High-level resistance to gentamicin predicts that tobramycin, netilmicin, amikacin, and kanamycin also will be ineffective. In fact, even when enterococci are not highly resistant to gentamicin, it is difficult to predict the ability of these other aminoglycosides to participate in synergistic killing; consequently, they should not, in general, be used to treat enterococcal endocarditis. High concentrations of ampicillin plus ceftriaxone or cefotaxime, by expanded binding of penicillin-binding proteins, also kill *E. faecalis* in vitro and in animal models of endocarditis.

Enterococci must be tested for high-level resistance to streptomycin and gentamicin, β-lactamase production, and susceptibility to penicillin and ampicillin (MIC, <8 μg/mL) and to vancomycin (MIC, ≤4 μg/mL) and teicoplanin (MIC ≤2 μg/ml). If the isolate produces β-lactamase, ampicillin/sulbactam or vancomycin can be used as the cell wall–active component; if the penicillin/ampicillin MIC is ≥8 μg/mL, vancomycin can be considered; and if the vancomycin MIC is ≥8 μg/mL, penicillin or ampicillin can be considered. In the absence of high-level resistance, gentamicin or streptomycin should be used as the aminoglycoside (Table 155-4). Although the dose of gentamicin used to achieve bactericidal synergy in treating enterococcal endocarditis is smaller than that used in standard therapy, nephrotoxicity (or vestibular toxicity with streptomycin) is not uncommon during treatment lasting 4–6 weeks. Regimens in which the aminoglycoside component is given for only 2–3 weeks have been curative and associated with less nephrotoxicity than those using longer courses of gentamicin. Thus regimens wherein gentamicin is administered for only 2–3 weeks are preferred by some.

If there is high-level resistance to both gentamicin and streptomycin, a synergistic bactericidal effect cannot be achieved by the addition of an aminoglycoside; thus no aminoglycoside should be given. Instead, an 8- to 12-week course of a single cell wall–active agent can be considered; for *E. faecalis* endocarditis, high doses of ampicillin combined with ceftriaxone or cefotaxime are suggested (Table 155-4). Nonrandomized comparative studies suggest that ampicillin-ceftriaxone may be as effective as (and less nephrotoxic than) penicillin or ampicillin plus an aminoglycoside in the treatment of *E. faecalis* endocarditis. Given the reduced risk

TABLE 155-4 ANTIBIOTIC TREATMENT FOR INFECTIVE ENDOCARDITIS CAUSED BY COMMON ORGANISMS[a]

Organism	Drug (Dose, Duration)	Comments
Streptococci		
Penicillin-susceptible[b] streptococci, *S. gallolyticus*	• Penicillin G (2–3 mU IV q4h for 4 weeks)	—
	• Ceftriaxone (2 g/d IV as a single dose for 4 weeks)	Can use ceftriaxone in patients with nonimmediate penicillin allergy.
	• Vancomycin[c] (15 mg/kg IV q12h for 4 weeks)	Use vancomycin in patients with severe or immediate β-lactam allergy.
	• Penicillin G (2–3 mU IV q4h) *or* ceftriaxone (2 g IV qd) for 2 weeks **plus** Gentamicin[d] (3 mg/kg qd IV or IM, as a single dose[e] or divided into equal doses q8h for 2 weeks)	Avoid 2-week regimen when risk of aminoglycoside toxicity is increased and in prosthetic valve or complicated endocarditis.
Relatively penicillin-resistant[f]	• Penicillin G (4 mU IV q4h) *or* ceftriaxone (2 g IV qd) for 4 weeks **plus** Gentamicin[d] (3 mg/kg qd IV or IM, as a single dose[e] or divided into equal doses q8h for 2 weeks)	Penicillin alone at this dose for 6 weeks or with gentamicin during the initial 2 weeks is preferred for prosthetic valve endocarditis caused by streptococci with penicillin MICs of ≤0.1 μg/mL.
	• Vancomycin[c] as noted above for 4 weeks	—
Moderately penicillin-resistant[g] streptococci, nutritionally variant organisms, or *Gemella* species	• Penicillin G (4–5 mU IV q4h) *or* ceftriaxone (2 g IV qd) for 6 weeks **plus** Gentamicin[d] (3 mg/kg qd IV or IM as a single dose[e] *or* divided into equal doses q8h for 6 weeks)	Preferred for prosthetic valve endocarditis caused by streptococci with penicillin MICs of >0.1 μg/mL.
	• Vancomycin[c] as noted above for 4 weeks	Regimen is preferred by some.
Enterococci[h]		
	• Penicillin G (4–5 mU IV q4h) *plus* gentamicin[d] (1 mg/kg IV q8h), both for 4–6 weeks	Can use streptomycin (7.5 mg/kg q12h) in lieu of gentamicin if there is not high-level resistance to streptomycin.
	• Ampicillin (2 g IV q4h) *plus* gentamicin[d] (1 mg/kg IV q8h), both for 4–6 weeks	—
	• Vancomycin[c] (15 mg/kg IV q12h) *plus* gentamicin[d] (1 mg/kg IV q8h), both for 4–6 weeks	Use vancomycin plus gentamicin for penicillin-allergic patients (or desensitize to penicillin) and for isolates resistant to penicillin/ampicillin.
	• Ampicillin (2 g IV q4h) *plus* ceftriaxone (2 g IV q12h), both for 6 weeks	Use for *E. faecalis* isolates with high-level resistance to gentamicin and streptomycin or for patients at high risk for aminoglycoside nephrotoxicity (see text).
Staphylococci		
MSSA infecting native valves (no foreign devices)	• Nafcillin, oxacillin, *or* flucloxacillin (2 g IV q4h for 4–6 weeks)	Can use penicillin (4 mU q4h) if isolate is penicillin-susceptible (does not produce β-lactamase).
	• Cefazolin (2 g IV q8h for 4–6 weeks)	Can use cefazolin regimen for patients with nonimmediate penicillin allergy.
	• Vancomycin[c] (15 mg/kg IV q12h for 4–6 weeks)	Use vancomycin for patients with immediate (urticarial) or severe penicillin allergy; see text regarding addition of gentamicin, fusidic acid, or rifampin.
MRSA infecting native valves (no foreign devices)	• Vancomycin[c] (15 mg/kg IV q8–12h for 4–6 weeks)	No role for routine use of rifampin (see text). Consider alternative treatment (see text) for MRSA with vancomycin MIC >1.0 or persistent bacteremia during vancomycin therapy.
MSSA infecting prosthetic valves	• Nafcillin, oxacillin, *or* flucloxacillin (2 g IV q4h for 6–8 weeks) **plus** Gentamicin[d] (1 mg/kg IM or IV q8h for 2 weeks) **plus** Rifampin[i] (300 mg PO q8h for 6–8 weeks)	Use gentamicin during initial 2 weeks; determine susceptibility to gentamicin before initiating rifampin (see text); if patient is highly allergic to penicillin, use regimen for MRSA; if β-lactam allergy is of the minor nonimmediate type, cefazolin can be substituted for oxacillin/nafcillin.
MRSA infecting prosthetic valves	• Vancomycin[c] (15 mg/kg IV q12h for 6–8 weeks) **plus** Gentamicin[d] (1 mg/kg IM or IV q8h for 2 weeks) **plus** Rifampin[i] (300 mg PO q8h for 6–8 weeks)	Use gentamicin during initial 2 weeks; determine gentamicin susceptibility before initiating rifampin (see text).
HACEK Organisms		
	• Ceftriaxone (2 g/d IV as a single dose for 4 weeks)	Can use another third-generation cephalosporin at comparable dosage.
	• Ampicillin/sulbactam (3 g IV q6h for 4 weeks)	—

(continued)

TABLE 155-4 ANTIBIOTIC TREATMENT FOR INFECTIVE ENDOCARDITIS CAUSED BY COMMON ORGANISMS[a] (CONTINUED)

Organism	Drug (Dose, Duration)	Comments
Coxiella burnetii		
	• Doxycycline (100 mg PO q12h) *plus* hydroxychloroquine (200 mg PO q8h), both for 18 (native valve) or 24 (prosthetic valve) months	Follow serology to monitor response during treatment (antiphase I IgG and IgA decreased 4-fold and IgM antiphase II negative) and thereafter for relapse.
***Bartonella* spp.**		
	• Ceftriaxone (2 g IV q24h) *or* ampicillin (2 g IV q4h) *or* doxycycline (100 mg q12h PO) for 6 weeks ***plus*** Gentamicin (1 mg/kg IV q8h for 3 weeks)	If patient is highly allergic to β-lactams, use doxycycline.

[a]Doses are for adults with normal renal function. Doses of gentamicin, streptomycin, and vancomycin must be adjusted for reduced renal function. Ideal body weight is used to calculate doses of gentamicin and streptomycin per kilogram (men = 50 kg + 2.3 kg per inch over 5 feet; women = 45.5 kg + 2.3 kg per inch over 5 feet). [b]MIC, ≤0.1 µg/mL. [c]Vancomycin dose is based on actual body weight. Adjust for trough level of 10–15 µg/mL for streptococcal and enterococcal infections and 15–20 µg/mL for staphylococcal infections. [d]Aminoglycosides should not be administered as single daily doses for enterococcal endocarditis and should be introduced as part of the initial treatment. Target peak and trough serum concentrations of divided-dose gentamicin 1 h after a 20- to 30-min infusion or IM injection are ~3.5 µg/mL and ≤1 µg/mL, respectively; target peak and trough serum concentrations of streptomycin (timing as with gentamicin) are 20–35 µg/mL and <10 µg/mL, respectively. [e]Netilmicin (4 mg/kg qd, as a single dose) can be used in lieu of gentamicin. [f]MIC, >0.1 µg/mL and <0.5 µg/mL. [g]MIC, ≥0.5 µg/mL and <8 µg/mL. [h]Antimicrobial susceptibility must be evaluated; see text. [i]Rifampin increases warfarin and dicumarol requirements for anticoagulation.

Abbreviations: MIC, minimal inhibitory concentration; MRSA, methicillin-resistant *S. aureus*; MSSA, methicillin-sensitive *S. aureus*.

of nephrotoxicity with ampicillin-ceftriaxone therapy, this regimen may also be preferred in patients who are at increased risk for aminoglycoside nephrotoxicity.

If the enterococcal isolate is resistant to all of the commonly used agents, suppression of bacteremia followed by surgical treatment should be considered. The role of newer agents potentially active against multidrug-resistant enterococci (quinupristin/dalfopristin [*E. faecium* only], linezolid, and daptomycin) in the treatment of endocarditis has not been established.

STAPHYLOCOCCI The regimens used to treat staphylococcal endocarditis (Table 155-4) are based not on coagulase production but rather on the presence or absence of a prosthetic valve or foreign device, the native valve(s) involved, and the susceptibility of the isolate to penicillin, methicillin, and vancomycin. All staphylococci are considered penicillin-resistant until shown not to produce penicillinase. Similarly, methicillin resistance has become so prevalent among staphylococci that empirical therapy should be initiated with a regimen that covers methicillin-resistant organisms and should later be revised if the isolate proves to be susceptible to methicillin. The addition of 3–5 days of gentamicin to a β-lactam antibiotic or vancomycin to enhance therapy for native mitral or aortic valve endocarditis has not improved survival rates and may be associated with nephrotoxicity. Neither this addition nor the addition of fusidic acid or rifampin is recommended.

For treatment of endocarditis caused by *methicillin-resistant S. aureus* (MRSA), vancomycin, dosed to achieve trough concentrations of 15–20 µg/mL, is recommended, with the caveat that this regimen may be associated with nephrotoxicity. Although resistance to vancomycin among staphylococci is rare, reduced vancomycin susceptibility among MRSA strains is increasingly encountered. Isolates with a vancomycin MIC of 4–16 µg/mL have intermediate susceptibility and are referred to as *vancomycin-intermediate S. aureus* (VISA). Isolates with an MIC of 2 µg/mL may harbor subpopulations with higher MICs. These *heteroresistant VISA* (hVISA) isolates are not detectable by routine susceptibility testing. Because of the pharmacokinetics/pharmacodynamics of vancomycin, killing of MRSA with a vancomycin MIC of >1.0 µg/mL is unpredictable, even with aggressive vancomycin dosing. Although not approved by the U.S. Food and Drug Administration for this indication, daptomycin (6 mg/kg [or, as some experts prefer, 8–10 mg/kg] IV once daily) has been recommended as an alternative to vancomycin, particularly for left-sided endocarditis caused by VISA, hVISA, or isolates with a vancomycin MIC of >1.0 µg/mL. These isolates should be tested to document daptomycin susceptibility. Daptomycin activity against MRSA—even against some isolates with reduced daptomycin susceptibility—is enhanced by the addition of nafcillin or ceftaroline. Case reports suggest that either the latter combinations or ceftaroline alone (600 mg IV q8h) may be effective in recalcitrant MRSA endocarditis. Nevertheless, a discussion of treatment of endocarditis in which MRSA bacteremia persists despite therapy is beyond the scope of this chapter and requires consultation with an infectious disease specialist. The efficacy of linezolid for left-sided MRSA endocarditis has not been established. Although not widely adopted by other groups, the recommendation of the British Society for Antimicrobial Chemotherapy is that a second drug be added to vancomycin (rifampin) or to daptomycin (rifampin, gentamicin, or linezolid) for the treatment of NVE due to MRSA.

Methicillin-susceptible *S. aureus* endocarditis that is uncomplicated and limited to the tricuspid or pulmonic valve can often be treated with a 2-week course that combines oxacillin or nafcillin (but not vancomycin) with gentamicin. However, patients with prolonged fever (≥5 days) during therapy or multiple septic pulmonary emboli should receive standard-duration therapy. Vancomycin plus gentamicin for 2 weeks as treatment for right-sided endocarditis caused by MRSA yields suboptimal results; thus this entity is treated for 4 weeks with vancomycin or daptomycin (6 mg/kg as a single daily dose).

Staphylococcal PVE is treated for 6–8 weeks with a multidrug regimen. Rifampin is an essential component because it kills staphylococci that are adherent to foreign material in a biofilm. Two other agents (selected on the basis of susceptibility testing) are combined with rifampin to prevent in vivo emergence of resistance. Because many staphylococci (particularly MRSA and *Staphylococcus epidermidis*) are resistant to gentamicin, the isolate's susceptibility to gentamicin or an alternative agent should be established before rifampin treatment is begun. If the isolate is resistant to gentamicin, then another aminoglycoside, a fluoroquinolone (chosen on the basis of susceptibility), or another active agent should be substituted for gentamicin.

OTHER ORGANISMS In the absence of meningitis, endocarditis caused by *Streptococcus pneumoniae* isolates with a penicillin MIC of ≤1 µg/mL can be treated with IV penicillin (4 million units every 4 h), ceftriaxone (2 g/d as a single dose), or cefotaxime (at a comparable dosage). Infection caused by pneumococcal strains with a penicillin MIC of ≥2 µg/mL should be treated with vancomycin. If meningitis is suspected or present, treatment with vancomycin plus ceftriaxone—at the doses advised for meningitis—should be initiated until susceptibility results are known. Definitive therapy should then be selected on the basis of meningitis breakpoints (penicillin MIC, 0.06 µg/mL; or ceftriaxone MIC, 0.5 µg/mL). *P. aeruginosa* endocarditis is treated with an antipseudomonal penicillin (ticarcillin or piperacillin) and high doses of tobramycin (8 mg/kg per day in three divided doses). Endocarditis caused by Enterobacteriaceae is treated with a potent β-lactam antibiotic plus an aminoglycoside. Corynebacterial endocarditis is treated with a penicillin plus an aminoglycoside (if the organism is susceptible to the aminoglycoside) or with vancomycin, which is highly bactericidal for most strains. Therapy for *Candida* endocarditis consists of amphotericin B plus flucytosine and early surgery; long-term (if not indefinite) suppression with an oral azole is advised. Echinocandin treatment of *Candida* endocarditis has been effective in sporadic cases; nevertheless, the role of echinocandins in this setting has not been established.

Empirical Therapy In designing therapy (largely with antimicrobials and doses from Table 155-4 to target putative microorganisms) to be administered before culture results are known or when cultures are negative, clinical clues (e.g., acute vs. subacute presentation, site of infection, patient's predispositions) as well as epidemiologic clues to etiology must be considered. Thus empirical therapy for acute endocarditis in an injection drug user should cover MRSA and gram-negative bacilli. Treatment with vancomycin plus gentamicin, initiated immediately after blood samples are obtained for culture, covers these organisms as well as many other potential causes. Similarly, treatment of health care–associated endocarditis must cover MRSA. In the treatment of culture-negative episodes, marantic endocarditis must be excluded and fastidious organisms sought by serologic testing. In the absence of prior antibiotic therapy, it is unlikely that *S. aureus*, CoNS, or enterococcal infection will present with negative blood cultures; thus, in this situation, recommended empirical therapy targets not these organisms but rather nutritionally variant organisms, the HACEK group, and *Bartonella* species. Pending the availability of diagnostic data, blood culture–negative subacute NVE is treated with gentamicin plus ampicillin-sulbactam (12 g every 24 h) or ceftriaxone; doxycycline (100 mg twice daily) is added for enhanced *Bartonella* coverage. For culture-negative PVE, vancomycin, gentamicin, cefepime, and rifampin should be used if the prosthetic valve has been in place for ≤1 year. Empirical therapy for infected prosthetic valves in place for >1 year is similar to that for culture-negative NVE. If cultures may be negative because of confounding by prior antibiotic administration, broader empirical therapy may be indicated, with particular attention to pathogens that are likely to be inhibited by the specific prior therapy.

CIED Endocarditis Antimicrobial therapy for CIED endocarditis is adjunctive to complete device removal. The antimicrobial selected is based on the causative organism and should be used as recommended for NVE (Table 155-4). Bacteremic CIED infection may be complicated by coincident NVE or remote-site infection (e.g., osteomyelitis). A 4- to 6-week course of endocarditis-targeted therapy is recommended for patients with CIED endocarditis and for those with bacteremia that continues during ongoing antimicrobial therapy after device removal. Although *S. aureus* bacteremia (and persistent CoNS bacteremia) in patients who have a CIED in place is likely—in the absence of another source—to reflect endocarditis and should be managed accordingly, not all bloodstream infections in these patients indicate endocarditis. If evidence suggesting endocarditis is lacking, bloodstream infection due to gram-negative bacilli, streptococci, enterococci, and *Candida* species may not indicate device infection. However, in the absence of another source, relapse after antimicrobial therapy increases the likelihood of CIED endocarditis and warrants treatment as such.

Outpatient Antimicrobial Therapy Fully compliant, clinically stable patients who are no longer bacteremic, are not febrile, and have no clinical or echocardiographic findings that suggest an impending complication may complete therapy as outpatients. Careful follow-up and a stable home setting are necessary, as are predictable IV access and use of antimicrobial agents that are stable in solution. Recommended regimens should not be compromised to accommodate outpatient therapy.

Monitoring Antimicrobial Therapy Measurement of the serum bactericidal titer—the highest dilution of the patient's serum during therapy that kills 99.9% of the standard inoculum of the infecting organism—is not recommended for assessment of standard regimens but may be useful for assessment of the treatment of endocarditis caused by unusual organisms. Serum concentrations of aminoglycosides and vancomycin should be monitored and doses adjusted to avoid or address toxicity.

Antibiotic toxicities, including allergic reactions, occur in 25–40% of patients and commonly arise after several weeks of therapy. Blood tests to detect renal, hepatic, and hematologic toxicity should be performed periodically.

Blood cultures should be repeated daily until sterile in patients with endocarditis due to *S. aureus* or difficult-to-treat organisms, rechecked if there is recrudescent fever, and performed again 4–6 weeks after therapy to document cure. Blood cultures become sterile within 2 days after the start of appropriate therapy when infection is caused by viridans streptococci, enterococci, or HACEK organisms. In *S. aureus* endocarditis, β-lactam therapy results in sterile cultures in 3–5 days, whereas in MRSA endocarditis, positive cultures may persist for 7–9 days with vancomycin or daptomycin treatment. MRSA bacteremia persisting despite an adequate dosage of vancomycin may indicate infection due to a strain with reduced vancomycin susceptibility and therefore may point to a need for alternative therapy. When fever persists for 7 days despite appropriate antibiotic therapy, patients should be evaluated for paravalvular abscess, extracardiac abscesses (spleen, kidney), or complications (embolic events). Recrudescent fever raises the possibility of these complications but also of drug reactions or complications of hospitalization. Vegetations become smaller with effective therapy; however, 3 months after cure, 50% are unchanged and 25% are slightly larger.

SURGICAL TREATMENT

Intracardiac and central nervous system complications are important causes of morbidity and death due to infective endocarditis. In some cases, effective treatment for these complications requires surgery. The indications for cardiac surgical treatment of endocarditis (**Table 155-5**) have been derived from observational studies and expert opinion. The strength of individual indications varies; thus the risks and benefits as well as the timing of surgery must be individualized (**Table 155-6**). From 25% to 40% of patients with left-sided endocarditis undergo cardiac surgery during active infection, with slightly higher surgery rates for PVE than NVE. Intracardiac complications (which are most reliably detected by TEE) and CHF are the most commonly cited indications for surgery. The benefit of surgery has been assessed primarily in studies comparing populations of medically and surgically treated patients matched for the necessity of

TABLE 155-5 INDICATIONS FOR CARDIAC SURGICAL INTERVENTION IN PATIENTS WITH ENDOCARDITIS

Surgery Required for Optimal Outcome
Moderate to severe congestive heart failure due to valve dysfunction
Partially dehisced unstable prosthetic valve
Persistent bacteremia despite optimal antimicrobial therapy
Lack of effective microbicidal therapy (e.g., fungal or *Brucella* endocarditis)
S. aureus prosthetic valve endocarditis with an intracardiac complication
Relapse of prosthetic valve endocarditis after optimal antimicrobial therapy
Surgery to Be Strongly Considered for Improved Outcome[a]
Perivalvular extension of infection
Poorly responsive *S. aureus* endocarditis involving the aortic or mitral valve
Large (>10 mm in diameter) hypermobile vegetations with increased risk of embolism, particularly with prior embolic event or with significant valve dysfunction
Persistent unexplained fever (≥10 days) in culture-negative native valve endocarditis
Poorly responsive or relapsed endocarditis due to highly antibiotic-resistant enterococci or gram-negative bacilli

[a]Surgery must be carefully considered; findings are often combined with other indications to prompt surgery.

TABLE 155-6 TIMING OF CARDIAC SURGICAL INTERVENTION IN PATIENTS WITH ENDOCARDITIS

Timing	Indication for Surgical Intervention: Strong Supporting Evidence	Indication for Surgical Intervention: Conflicting Evidence, but Majority of Opinions Favor Surgery
Emergent (same day)	Acute aortic regurgitation plus preclosure of mitral valve Sinus of Valsalva abscess ruptured into right heart Rupture into pericardial sac	
Urgent (within 1–2 days)	Valve obstruction by vegetation Unstable (dehisced) prosthesis Acute aortic or mitral regurgitation with heart failure (New York Heart Association class III or IV) Septal perforation Perivalvular extension of infection with or without new electrocardiographic conduction system changes Lack of effective antibiotic therapy	Major embolus plus persisting large vegetation (>10 mm in diameter)
Elective (earlier usually preferred)	Vegetation diameter >10 mm plus severe aortic or mitral valve dysfunction[a] Progressive paravalvular prosthetic regurgitation Valve dysfunction plus persisting infection after ≥7–10 days of antimicrobial therapy Fungal (mold) endocarditis	Staphylococcal prosthetic valve endocarditis Early prosthetic valve endocarditis (≤2 months after valve surgery) Fungal endocarditis (*Candida* spp.) Antibiotic-resistant organisms

[a]Supported by a single-institution randomized trial showing benefit from early surgery. Implementation requires clinical judgment.

Source: Adapted from L Olaison, G Pettersson: Infect Dis Clin North Am 16:453, 2002.

surgery (indications assessed in studies as *propensity*), with adjustments for predictors of death (comorbidities) and timing of the surgical intervention. Although study results vary, surgery for currently advised indications appears to convey a significant survival benefit (27–55%) that becomes apparent only with follow-up for ≥6 months. During the initial weeks after surgery, mortality risk may appear increased (disease + surgery–related mortality).

Indications • ***CONGESTIVE HEART FAILURE*** Moderate to severe refractory CHF caused by new or worsening valve dysfunction is the major indication for cardiac surgery. At 6 months of follow up, patients with left-sided endocarditis and moderate to severe heart failure due to valve dysfunction who are treated medically have a 50% mortality rate, while among matched patients who undergo surgery the mortality rate is 15%. The survival benefit with surgery, which is most predictable among patients with the most weighty indications (propensity), is seen in both NVE and PVE. Surgery can relieve functional stenosis due to large vegetations or restore competence to damaged regurgitant valves by repair or replacement.

PERIVALVULAR INFECTION This complication, which is most common with aortic valve infection, occurs in 10–15% of native valve and 45–60% of prosthetic valve infections. It is suggested by persistent unexplained fever during appropriate therapy, new electrocardiographic conduction disturbances, or pericarditis. TEE with color Doppler is the test of choice to detect perivalvular abscesses (sensitivity, ≥85%). For optimal outcome, surgery is required, especially when fever persists, fistulae develop, prostheses are dehisced and unstable, or infection relapses after appropriate treatment. Cardiac rhythm must be monitored since high-grade heart block may require insertion of a pacemaker.

UNCONTROLLED INFECTION Continued positive blood cultures or otherwise-unexplained persistent fevers (in patients with either blood culture–positive or –negative endocarditis) despite optimal antibiotic therapy may reflect uncontrolled infection and may warrant surgery. Surgical treatment is also advised for endocarditis caused by organisms against which effective antimicrobial therapy is lacking (e.g., yeasts, fungi, *P. aeruginosa*, other highly resistant gram negative bacilli, *Brucella* species).

S. AUREUS ENDOCARDITIS The mortality rate for *S. aureus* PVE exceeds 50% with medical treatment but is reduced to 25% with surgical treatment. In patients with intracardiac complications associated with *S. aureus* PVE, surgical treatment reduces the mortality rate twentyfold. Surgical treatment should be considered for patients with *S. aureus* native aortic or mitral valve infection who have TTE-demonstrable vegetations and remain septic during the initial week of therapy. Isolated tricuspid valve endocarditis, even with persistent fever, rarely requires surgery.

PREVENTION OF SYSTEMIC EMBOLI Death and persisting morbidity may result from cerebral or coronary artery emboli. Predicting a high risk of systemic embolization by echocardiographic determination of vegetation size and anatomy does not by itself identify those patients in whom surgery to prevent emboli will result in increased chances of survival. Net benefits from surgery to prevent emboli are most likely when other surgical benefits can be achieved simultaneously—e.g., repair of a moderately dysfunctional valve or debridement of a paravalvular abscess. Only 3.5% of patients undergo surgery solely to prevent systemic emboli. Valve repair, with the consequent avoidance of prosthesis insertion, improves the benefit-to-risk ratio of surgery performed to address vegetations.

CIED ENDOCARDITIS Removal of all hardware is recommended for patients with established CIED infection (pocket or intracardiac lead) or erosion of the device through the skin. Percutaneous lead extraction is preferred. With lead vegetations of >3 cm and the resulting risk of a pulmonary embolus or with retained hardware after attempted percutaneous extraction, surgical removal should be considered. Removal of the infected CIED during the initial hospitalization is associated with increased 30-day and 1-year survival rates over those attained with antibiotic therapy and device retention. If necessary, the CIED can be reimplanted percutaneously or surgically (epicardial leads) at a new site after at least 10–14 days of effective antimicrobial therapy. CIEDs should be removed and replaced subsequently when patients undergo valve surgery for endocarditis.

Timing of Cardiac Surgery With the more life-threatening indications for surgery (valve dysfunction and severe CHF, paravalvular abscess, major prosthesis dehiscence), early surgery—i.e., during the initial week of therapy—is associated with a greater chance of survival than later surgery. With less compelling indications, surgery may reasonably be delayed to allow further treatment as well as improvement in overall health (Table 155-6). After 14 days of recommended antibiotic therapy, excised valves are culture-negative in 99% and 50% of patients with streptococcal and *S. aureus* endocarditis, respectively. Recrudescent endocarditis on a new implanted prosthetic valve follows surgery for active NVE and PVE in 2% and 6–15% of patients, respectively. These frequencies do not justify the risk of an adverse outcome due to a delay in surgery, particularly in patients with severe heart failure, valve dysfunction, and uncontrolled staphylococcal infections. Delay is justified when infection is controlled and CHF is resolved with medical therapy.

Neurologic complications of endocarditis may be exacerbated as a consequence of cardiac surgery. The risk of neurologic deterioration is related to the type of neurologic complication and the interval between the complication and surgery. Whenever feasible, cardiac surgery should be delayed for 2–3 weeks after a nonhemorrhagic embolic infarction and for 4 weeks after a cerebral hemorrhage. A ruptured mycotic aneurysm should be treated before cardiac surgery.

Antibiotic Therapy after Cardiac Surgery Organisms have been detected on Gram's stain—or their DNA has been detected by polymerase chain reaction—in excised valves from 45% of patients who have successfully completed the recommended therapy for endocarditis. In only 7% of these patients are the organisms, most of which are unusual and antibiotic resistant, cultured from the valve. Detection of organisms or their DNA does not necessarily indicate antibiotic failure; in fact, relapse of endocarditis after surgery is uncommon. Thus, when valve cultures are negative in uncomplicated NVE caused by susceptible organisms, the duration of preoperative plus postoperative treatment should equal the total duration of recommended therapy, with ~2 weeks of treatment administered after surgery. For endocarditis complicated by paravalvular abscess, partially treated PVE, or cases with culture-positive valves, a full course of therapy should be given postoperatively.

Extracardiac Complications Splenic abscess develops in 3–5% of patients with endocarditis. Effective therapy requires either image-guided percutaneous drainage or splenectomy. Mycotic aneurysms occur in 2–15% of endocarditis patients; one-half of these cases involve the cerebral arteries and present as headaches, focal neurologic symptoms, or hemorrhage. Cerebral aneurysms should be monitored by angiography. Some will resolve with effective antimicrobial therapy, but those that persist, enlarge, or leak should be treated surgically if possible. Extracerebral aneurysms present as local pain, a mass, local ischemia, or bleeding; these aneurysms are treated surgically.

OUTCOME

Factors that can adversely affect outcome include older age, severe comorbid conditions and diabetes, delayed diagnosis, involvement of prosthetic valves or the aortic valve, an invasive (*S. aureus*) or antibiotic-resistant (*P. aeruginosa*, yeast) pathogen, intracardiac and major neurologic complications, and an association with health care. Death and poor outcome often are related not to failure of antibiotic therapy but rather to the interactions of comorbidities and endocarditis-related end-organ complications. In developed countries, overall survival rates are 80–85%; however, rates vary considerably among subpopulations of endocarditis patients. Survival rates for patients with NVE caused by viridans streptococci, HACEK organisms, or enterococci (susceptible to synergistic therapy) are 85–90%. For *S. aureus* NVE in patients who do not inject drugs, survival rates are 55–70%, whereas 85–90% of injection drug users survive this infection. PVE beginning within 2 months of valve replacement results in mortality rates of 40–50%, whereas rates are only 10–20% in later-onset cases.

PREVENTION

To prevent endocarditis (long a goal in clinical practice), past expert committees have supported systemic antibiotic administration prior to many bacteremia-inducing procedures. A reappraisal of the evidence for antibiotic prophylaxis for endocarditis by the American Heart Association and the European Society of Cardiology culminated in guidelines advising its more restrictive use. At best, the benefit of antibiotic prophylaxis is minimal. Most endocarditis cases do not follow a procedure. Although dental treatments have been widely considered to predispose to endocarditis, such infection occurs no more frequently in patients who are undergoing dental treatment than in matched controls who are not. Furthermore, the frequency and magnitude of bacteremia associated with dental procedures and a routine day's activities (e.g., tooth brushing and flossing) are similar; because dental procedures are infrequent events, exposure of cardiac structures to bacteremic oral-cavity organisms is notably greater from routine daily activities than from dental care. The relation of gastrointestinal and genitourinary procedures to subsequent endocarditis is even more tenuous than that of dental procedures. In addition, cost-effectiveness and cost-benefit estimates suggest that antibiotic prophylaxis represents a poor use of resources.

Nevertheless, studies in animal models suggest that antibiotic prophylaxis may be effective. Thus it is possible that rare cases of endocarditis are prevented. Weighing the potential benefits, potential adverse events, and costs associated with antibiotic prophylaxis, the American Heart Association and the European Society of Cardiology now recommend prophylactic antibiotics (Table 155-7) only for those patients at highest risk for severe morbidity or death from endocarditis (Table 155-8). Maintaining good dental hygiene is essential. Prophylaxis is recommended only when there is manipulation of gingival tissue or the periapical region of the teeth or perforation of the oral mucosa (including surgery on the respiratory tract). Prophylaxis is not advised for patients undergoing gastrointestinal or genitourinary tract procedures. High-risk patients should be treated before or

TABLE 155-7 ANTIBIOTIC REGIMENS FOR PROPHYLAXIS OF ENDOCARDITIS IN ADULTS WITH HIGH-RISK CARDIAC LESIONS[a,b]

A. Standard oral regimen
   Amoxicillin: 2 g PO 1 h before procedure
B. Inability to take oral medication
   Ampicillin: 2 g IV or IM within 1 h before procedure
C. Penicillin allergy
   1. Clarithromycin or azithromycin: 500 mg PO 1 h before procedure
   2. Cephalexin[c]: 2 g PO 1 h before procedure
   3. Clindamycin: 600 mg PO 1 h before procedure
D. Penicillin allergy, inability to take oral medication
   1. Cefazolin[c] or ceftriaxone[c]: 1 g IV or IM 30 min before procedure
   2. Clindamycin: 600 mg IV or IM 1 h before procedure

[a]Dosing for children: for amoxicillin, ampicillin, cephalexin, or cefadroxil, use 50 mg/kg PO; cefazolin, 25 mg/kg IV; clindamycin, 20 mg/kg PO or 25 mg/kg IV; clarithromycin, 15 mg/kg PO; and vancomycin, 20 mg/kg IV. [b]For high-risk lesions, see Table 155-8. Prophylaxis is not advised for other lesions. [c]Do not use cephalosporins in patients with immediate hypersensitivity (urticaria, angioedema, anaphylaxis) to penicillin.

Source: Table created using the guidelines published by the American Heart Association and the European Society of Cardiology (W Wilson et al: Circulation 116:1736, 2007; and G Habib et al: Eur Heart J 30:2369, 2009).

TABLE 155-8 HIGH-RISK CARDIAC LESIONS FOR WHICH ENDOCARDITIS PROPHYLAXIS IS ADVISED BEFORE DENTAL PROCEDURES

Prosthetic heart valves

Prior endocarditis

Unrepaired cyanotic congenital heart disease, including palliative shunts or conduits

Completely repaired congenital heart defects during the 6 months after repair

Incompletely repaired congenital heart disease with residual defects adjacent to prosthetic material

Valvulopathy developing after cardiac transplantation[a]

[a]Not a target population for prophylaxis according to recommendations of the European Society for Cardiology.

Source: Table created using the guidelines published by the American Heart Association and the European Society of Cardiology (W Wilson et al: Circulation 116:1736, 2007; and G Habib et al: Eur Heart J 30:2369, 2009).

when they undergo procedures on an infected genitourinary tract or on infected skin and soft tissue.

In patients with aortic or mitral valve regurgitation or a prosthetic valve, treatment of acute Q fever with doxycycline plus hydroxychloroquine (for doses, see Table 155-4) for 12 months is highly effective in preventing *C. burnetii* endocarditis.

The National Institute for Health and Clinical Excellence in the United Kingdom has advised discontinuation of all antibiotic prophylaxis for endocarditis. Limited surveillance studies have not detected increased viridans streptococcal endocarditis subsequent to the promulgation of guidelines that are more restrictive or advise no prophylaxis.

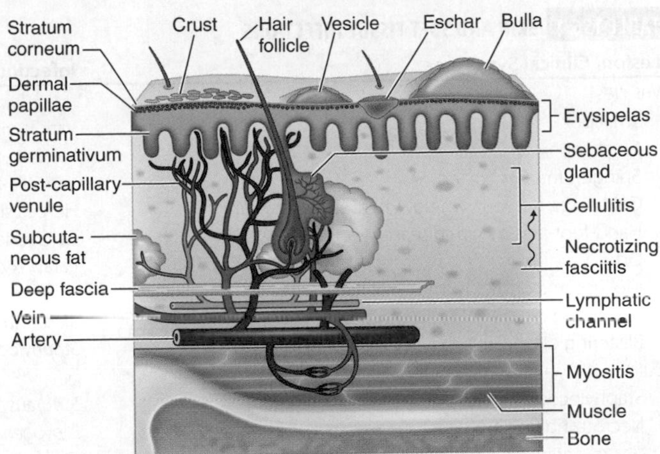

FIGURE 156-1 Structural components of the skin and soft tissue, superficial infections, and infections of the deeper structures. The rich capillary network beneath the dermal papillae plays a key role in the localization of infection and in the development of the acute inflammatory reaction.

156 Infections of the Skin, Muscles, and Soft Tissues

Dennis L. Stevens

Skin and soft tissue infections occur in all races, all ethnic groups, and all geographic locations, although some have unique geographic niches. In modern times, the frequency and severity of some skin and soft tissue infections have increased for several reasons. First, microbes are rapidly disseminated throughout the world via efficient air travel, acquiring genes for virulence factors and antibiotic resistance. Second, natural disasters, such as earthquakes, tsunamis, tornadoes, and hurricanes, appear to be increasing in frequency, and the injuries sustained during these events commonly cause major skin and soft-tissue damage that predisposes to infection. Third, trauma and casualties resulting from combat and terrorist activities can markedly damage or destroy tissues and provide both endogenous and exogenous pathogens with ready access to deeper structures. Unfortunately, because the marvels of modern medicine may not be available during human-instigated and natural disasters, primary treatment may be delayed and the likelihood of severe infection and death increased.

ANATOMIC RELATIONSHIPS: CLUES TO THE DIAGNOSIS OF SOFT TISSUE INFECTIONS

Skin and soft tissue infections have been common human afflictions for centuries. However, between 2000 and 2004, hospital admissions for skin and soft tissue infections rose by 27%, a remarkable increase that was attributable largely to the emergence of the USA300 clone of methicillin-resistant *Staphylococcus aureus* (MRSA). This chapter provides an anatomic approach to understanding the types of soft tissue infections and the diverse microbes responsible.

Protection against infection of the epidermis depends on the mechanical barrier afforded by the stratum corneum, since the epidermis itself is devoid of blood vessels (Fig. 156-1). Disruption of this layer by burns or bites, abrasions, foreign bodies, primary dermatologic disorders (e.g., herpes simplex, varicella, ecthyma gangrenosum), surgery, or vascular or pressure ulcer allows penetration of bacteria to the deeper structures. Similarly, the hair follicle can serve as a portal either for components of the normal flora (e.g., *Staphylococcus*) or for extrinsic bacteria (e.g., *Pseudomonas* in hot-tub folliculitis). Intracellular infection of the squamous epithelium with vesicle formation may arise from cutaneous inoculation, as in infection with herpes simplex virus (HSV) type 1; from the dermal capillary plexus, as in varicella and infections due to other viruses associated with viremia; or from cutaneous nerve roots, as in herpes zoster. Bacteria infecting the epidermis, such as *Streptococcus pyogenes*, may be translocated laterally to deeper structures via lymphatics, an event that results in the rapid superficial spread of erysipelas. Later, engorgement or obstruction of lymphatics causes flaccid edema of the epidermis, another characteristic of erysipelas.

The rich plexus of capillaries beneath the dermal papillae provides nutrition to the stratum germinativum, and physiologic responses of this plexus produce important clinical signs and symptoms. For example, infective vasculitis of the plexus results in petechiae, Osler's nodes, Janeway lesions, and palpable purpura, which, if present, are important clues to the existence of endocarditis (Chap. 155). In addition, metastatic infection within this plexus can result in cutaneous manifestations of disseminated fungal infection (Chap. 240), gonococcal infection (Chap. 181), *Salmonella* infection (Chap. 190), *Pseudomonas* infection (i.e., ecthyma gangrenosum; Chap. 189), meningococcemia (Chap. 180), and staphylococcal infection (Chap. 172). The plexus also provides bacteria with access to the circulation, thereby facilitating local spread or bacteremia. The postcapillary venules of this plexus are a prominent site of polymorphonuclear leukocyte sequestration, diapedesis, and chemotaxis to the site of cutaneous infection.

Amplification of these physiologic mechanisms by excessive levels of cytokines or bacterial toxins causes leukostasis, venous occlusion, and pitting edema. Edema with purple bullae, ecchymosis, and cutaneous anesthesia suggests loss of vascular integrity and necessitates exploration of the deeper structures for evidence of necrotizing fasciitis or myonecrosis. An early diagnosis requires a high level of suspicion in instances of unexplained fever and of pain and tenderness in the soft tissue, even in the absence of acute cutaneous inflammation.

Table 156-1 indicates the chapters in which the infections described below are discussed in greater detail. Many of these infections are illustrated in the chapters cited or in Chap. 25e (Atlas of Rashes Associated with Fever).

INFECTIONS ASSOCIATED WITH VESICLES

(Table 156-1) Vesicle formation due to infection is caused by viral proliferation within the epidermis. In varicella and variola, viremia precedes the onset of a diffuse centripetal rash that progresses from macules to vesicles, then to pustules, and finally to scabs over the course of 1–2 weeks. Vesicles of varicella have a "dewdrop" appearance and develop in crops randomly about the trunk, extremities, and face over 3–4 days. Herpes zoster occurs in a single dermatome; the appearance of vesicles is preceded by pain for several days. Zoster may occur in persons of any age but is most common among immunosuppressed individuals and elderly patients, whereas most cases of varicella occur in young children. Vesicles due to HSV are found on or around the

TABLE 156-1 SKIN AND SOFT TISSUE INFECTIONS

Lesion, Clinical Syndrome	Infectious Agent	See Also Chap(s).
Vesicles		
Smallpox	Variola virus	261e
Chickenpox	Varicella-zoster virus	217
Shingles (herpes zoster)	Varicella-zoster virus	217
Cold sores, herpetic whitlow, herpes gladiatorum	Herpes simplex virus	216
Hand-foot-and-mouth disease	Coxsackievirus A16	228
Orf	Parapoxvirus	220e
Molluscum contagiosum	Molluscum contagiosum poxvirus	220e
Rickettsialpox	*Rickettsia akari*	211
Blistering distal dactylitis	*Staphylococcus aureus* or *Streptococcus pyogenes*	172, 173
Bullae		
Staphylococcal scalded-skin syndrome	*S. aureus*	172
Necrotizing fasciitis	*S. pyogenes, Clostridium* spp., mixed aerobes and anaerobes	173, 179, 201
Gas gangrene	*Clostridium* spp.	179
Halophilic vibrio	*Vibrio vulnificus*	193
Crusted lesions		
Bullous impetigo/ecthyma	*S. aureus*	172
Impetigo contagiosa	*S. pyogenes*	173
Ringworm	Superficial dermatophyte fungi	243
Sporotrichosis	*Sporothrix schenckii*	243
Histoplasmosis	*Histoplasma capsulatum*	236
Coccidioidomycosis	*Coccidioides immitis*	237
Blastomycosis	*Blastomyces dermatitidis*	238
Cutaneous leishmaniasis	*Leishmania* spp.	251
Cutaneous tuberculosis	*Mycobacterium tuberculosis*	202
Nocardiosis	*Nocardia asteroides*	199
Folliculitis		
Furunculosis	*S. aureus*	172
Hot-tub folliculitis	*Pseudomonas aeruginosa*	189
Swimmer's itch	*Schistosoma* spp.	259
Acne vulgaris	*Propionibacterium acnes*	71
Papular and nodular lesions		
Fish-tank or swimming-pool granuloma	*Mycobacterium marinum*	204
Creeping eruption (cutaneous larva migrans)	*Ancylostoma braziliense*	256
Dracunculiasis	*Dracunculus medinensis*	258
Cercarial dermatitis	*Schistosoma mansoni*	259
Verruca vulgaris	Human papillomaviruses 1, 2, 4	222
Condylomata acuminata (anogenital warts)	Human papillomaviruses 6, 11, 16, 18	222
Onchocerciasis nodule	*Onchocerca volvulus*	258
Cutaneous myiasis	*Dermatobia hominis*	475
Verruca peruana	*Bartonella bacilliformis*	197
Cat-scratch disease	*Bartonella henselae*	197
Lepromatous leprosy	*Mycobacterium leprae*	203
Secondary syphilis (papulosquamous and nodular lesions, condylomata lata)	*Treponema pallidum*	206
Tertiary syphilis (nodular gummatous lesions)	*T. pallidum*	206
Ulcers with or without eschars		
Anthrax	*Bacillus anthracis*	261e
Ulceroglandular tularemia	*Francisella tularensis*	195, 261e
Bubonic plague	*Yersinia pestis*	196, 261e
Buruli ulcer	*Mycobacterium ulcerans*	204
Leprosy	*M. leprae*	203
Cutaneous tuberculosis	*M. tuberculosis*	202
Chancroid	*Haemophilus ducreyi*	182
Primary syphilis	*T. pallidum*	206
Erysipelas	*S. pyogenes*	173
Cellulitis	*Staphylococcus* spp., *Streptococcus* spp., various other bacteria	Various
Necrotizing fasciitis		
Streptococcal gangrene	*S. pyogenes*	173
Fournier's gangrene	Mixed aerobic and anaerobic bacteria	201
Staphylococcal necrotizing fasciitis	Methicillin-resistant *S. aureus*	172
Myositis and myonecrosis		
Pyomyositis	*S. aureus*	172
Streptococcal necrotizing myositis	*S. pyogenes*	173
Gas gangrene	*Clostridium* spp.	179
Nonclostridial (crepitant) myositis	Mixed aerobic and anaerobic bacteria	201
Synergistic nonclostridial anaerobic myonecrosis	Mixed aerobic and anaerobic bacteria	201

lips (HSV-1) or genitals (HSV-2) but also may appear on the head and neck of young wrestlers (herpes gladiatorum) or on the digits of health care workers (herpetic whitlow). Recurrent herpes labialis (HSV-1) and herpes genitalis commonly follow primary infection. Coxsackievirus A16 characteristically causes vesicles on the hands, feet, and mouth of children. Orf is caused by a DNA virus related to smallpox virus and infects the fingers of individuals who work around goats and sheep. Molluscum contagiosum virus induces flaccid vesicles on the skin of healthy and immunocompromised individuals. Although variola (smallpox) in nature was eradicated as of 1977, post-millennial terrorist events have renewed interest in this devastating infection (Chap. 261e). Viremia beginning after an incubation period of 12 days is followed by a diffuse maculopapular rash, with rapid evolution to vesicles, pustules, and then scabs. Secondary cases can occur among close contacts.

Rickettsialpox begins after mite-bite inoculation of *Rickettsia akari* into the skin. A papule with a central vesicle evolves to form a 1- to 2.5-cm painless crusted black eschar with an erythematous halo and proximal adenopathy. While more common in the northeastern United States and the Ukraine in 1940–1950, rickettsialpox has recently been described in Ohio, Arizona, and Utah. Blistering dactylitis is a painful, vesicular, localized *S. aureus* or group A streptococcal infection of the pulps of the distal digits of the hands.

INFECTIONS ASSOCIATED WITH BULLAE

(Table 156-1) Staphylococcal scalded-skin syndrome (SSSS) in neonates is caused by a toxin (exfoliatin) from phage group II *S. aureus*. SSSS must be distinguished from toxic epidermal necrolysis (TEN), which occurs primarily in adults, is drug-induced, and is associated with a higher mortality rate. Punch biopsy with frozen section is useful in making this distinction since the cleavage plane is the stratum corneum in SSSS and the stratum germinativum in TEN (Fig. 156-1). Intravenous γ-globulin is a promising treatment for TEN. Necrotizing fasciitis and gas gangrene also induce bulla formation (see "Necrotizing Fasciitis," below). Halophilic vibrio infection can be as aggressive and fulminant as necrotizing fasciitis; a helpful clue in its diagnosis is a history of exposure to waters of the Gulf of Mexico or the Atlantic seaboard or (in a patient with cirrhosis) the ingestion of raw seafood. The etiologic organism (*Vibrio vulnificus*) is highly susceptible to tetracycline.

INFECTIONS ASSOCIATED WITH CRUSTED LESIONS

(Table 156-1) Impetigo contagiosa is caused by *S. pyogenes*, and bullous impetigo is due to *S. aureus*. Both skin lesions may have an early bullous stage but then appear as thick crusts with a golden-brown color. Epidemics of impetigo caused by MRSA have been reported. Streptococcal lesions are most common among children 2–5 years of age, and epidemics may occur in settings of poor hygiene, particularly among children in lower socioeconomic settings in tropical climates. It is important to recognize impetigo contagiosa because of its relationship to poststreptococcal glomerulonephritis. Rheumatic fever is not a complication of skin infection caused by *S. pyogenes*. Superficial dermatophyte infection (ringworm) can occur on any skin surface, and skin scrapings with KOH staining are diagnostic. Primary infections with dimorphic fungi such as *Blastomyces dermatitidis* and *Sporothrix schenckii* can initially present as crusted skin lesions resembling ringworm. Disseminated infection with *Coccidioides immitis* can also involve the skin, and biopsy and culture should be performed on crusted lesions in patients from endemic areas. Crusted nodular lesions caused by *Mycobacterium chelonei* have been described in HIV-seropositive patients. Treatment with clarithromycin looks promising.

FOLLICULITIS

(Table 156-1) Hair follicles serve as portals for a number of bacteria, although *S. aureus* is the most common cause of localized folliculitis. Sebaceous glands empty into hair follicles and ducts and, if these portals are blocked, form sebaceous cysts that may resemble staphylococcal abscesses or may become secondarily infected. Infection of sweat glands (hidradenitis suppurativa) also can mimic infection of hair follicles, particularly in the axillae. Chronic folliculitis is uncommon except in acne vulgaris, where constituents of the normal flora (e.g., *Propionibacterium acnes*) may play a role.

Diffuse folliculitis occurs in two settings. *Hot-tub folliculitis* is caused by *Pseudomonas aeruginosa* in waters that are insufficiently chlorinated and maintained at temperatures of 37–40°C. Infection is usually self-limited, although bacteremia and shock have been reported. *Swimmer's itch* occurs when a skin surface is exposed to water infested with freshwater avian schistosomes. Warm water temperatures and alkaline pH are suitable for mollusks that serve as intermediate hosts between birds and humans. Free-swimming schistosomal cercariae readily penetrate human hair follicles or pores but quickly die and elicit a brisk allergic reaction, causing intense itching and erythema.

PAPULAR AND NODULAR LESIONS

(Table 156-1) Raised lesions of the skin occur in many different forms. *Mycobacterium marinum* infections of the skin may present as cellulitis or as raised erythematous nodules. Similar lesions caused by *Mycobacterium abscessus* and *M. chelonei* have been described among patients undergoing cosmetic laser surgery and tattooing, respectively. Erythematous papules are early manifestations of cat-scratch disease (with lesions developing at the primary site of inoculation of *Bartonella henselae*) and bacillary angiomatosis (also caused by *B. henselae*). Raised serpiginous or linear eruptions are characteristic of cutaneous larva migrans, which is caused by burrowing larvae of dog or cat hookworms (*Ancylostoma braziliense*) and which humans acquire through contact with soil that has been contaminated with dog or cat feces. Similar burrowing raised lesions are present in dracunculiasis caused by migration of the adult female nematode *Dracunculus medinensis*. Nodules caused by *Onchocerca volvulus* measure 1–10 cm in diameter and occur mostly in persons bitten by *Simulium* flies in Africa. The nodules contain the adult worm encased in fibrous tissue. Migration of microfilariae into the eyes may result in blindness. Verruga peruana is caused by *Bartonella bacilliformis*, which is transmitted to humans by the sandfly *Phlebotomus*. This condition can take the form of single gigantic lesions (several centimeters in diameter) or multiple small lesions (several millimeters in diameter). Numerous subcutaneous nodules may also be present in cysticercosis caused by larvae of *Taenia solium*. Multiple erythematous papules develop in schistosomiasis; each represents a cercarial invasion site. Skin nodules as well as thickened subcutaneous tissue are prominent features of lepromatous leprosy. Large nodules or gummas are features of tertiary syphilis, whereas flat papulosquamous lesions are characteristic of secondary syphilis. Human papillomavirus may cause singular warts (verruca vulgaris) or multiple warts in the anogenital area (condylomata acuminata). The latter are major problems in HIV-infected individuals.

ULCERS WITH OR WITHOUT ESCHARS

(Table 156-1) Cutaneous anthrax begins as a pruritic papule, which develops within days into an ulcer with surrounding vesicles and edema and then into an enlarging ulcer with a black eschar. Cutaneous anthrax may cause chronic nonhealing ulcers with an overlying dirty-gray membrane, although lesions may also mimic psoriasis, eczema, or impetigo. Ulceroglandular tularemia may have associated ulcerated skin lesions with painful regional adenopathy. Although buboes are the major cutaneous manifestation of plague, ulcers with eschars, papules, or pustules are also present in 25% of cases.

Mycobacterium ulcerans typically causes chronic skin ulcers on the extremities of individuals living in the tropics. *Mycobacterium leprae* may be associated with cutaneous ulcerations in patients with lepromatous leprosy related to Lucio's phenomenon, in which immune-mediated destruction of tissue bearing high concentrations of *M. leprae* bacilli occurs, usually several months after initiation of effective therapy. *Mycobacterium tuberculosis* also may cause ulcerations, papules, or erythematous macular lesions of the skin in both immunocompetent and immunocompromised patients.

Decubitus ulcers are due to tissue hypoxemia secondary to pressure-induced vascular insufficiency and may become secondarily infected with components of the skin and gastrointestinal flora, including anaerobes. Ulcerative lesions on the anterior shins may be due to pyoderma gangrenosum, which must be distinguished from similar lesions of infectious etiology by histologic evaluation of biopsy sites. Ulcerated lesions on the genitals may be either painful (chancroid) or painless (primary syphilis).

ERYSIPELAS

(Table 156-1) Erysipelas is due to *S. pyogenes* and is characterized by an abrupt onset of fiery-red swelling of the face or extremities. The distinctive features of erysipelas are well-defined indurated margins, particularly along the nasolabial fold; rapid progression; and intense pain. Flaccid bullae may develop during the second or third day of illness, but extension to deeper soft tissues is rare. Treatment with penicillin is effective; swelling may progress despite appropriate treatment, although fever, pain, and the intense red color diminish. Desquamation of the involved skin occurs 5–10 days into the illness. Infants and elderly adults are most commonly afflicted, and the severity of systemic toxicity varies.

CELLULITIS

(Table 156-1) Cellulitis is an acute inflammatory condition of the skin that is characterized by localized pain, erythema, swelling, and heat. It may be caused by indigenous flora colonizing the skin and appendages (e.g., *S. aureus* and *S. pyogenes*) or by a wide variety of exogenous bacteria. Because the exogenous bacteria involved in cellulitis occupy unique niches in nature, a thorough history (including epidemiologic data) provides important clues to etiology. When there is drainage, an open wound, or an obvious portal of entry, Gram's stain and culture provide a definitive diagnosis. In the absence of these findings, the bacterial etiology of cellulitis is difficult to establish, and in some cases staphylococcal and streptococcal cellulitis may have similar features. Even with needle aspiration of the leading edge or a punch biopsy of the cellulitis tissue itself, cultures are positive in only 20% of cases. This observation suggests that relatively low numbers of bacteria may cause cellulitis and that the expanding area of erythema within the skin may be a direct effect of extracellular toxins or of the soluble mediators of inflammation elicited by the host.

Bacteria may gain access to the epidermis through cracks in the skin, abrasions, cuts, burns, insect bites, surgical incisions, and IV catheters. Cellulitis caused by *S. aureus* spreads from a central localized infection, such as an abscess, folliculitis, or an infected foreign body (e.g., a splinter, a prosthetic device, or an IV catheter). MRSA is rapidly replacing methicillin-sensitive *S. aureus* (MSSA) as a cause of cellulitis in both inpatient and outpatient settings. Cellulitis caused by MSSA or MRSA is usually associated with a focal infection, such as a furuncle, a carbuncle, a surgical wound, or an abscess; the U.S. Food and Drug Administration preferentially refers to these types of infection as *purulent cellulitis*. In contrast, cellulitis due to *S. pyogenes* is a more rapidly spreading, diffuse process that is frequently associated with lymphangitis and fever and should be referred to as *nonpurulent cellulitis*. Recurrent streptococcal cellulitis of the lower extremities may be caused by organisms of group A, C, or G in association with chronic venous stasis or with saphenous venectomy for coronary artery bypass surgery. Streptococci also cause recurrent cellulitis among patients with chronic lymphedema resulting from elephantiasis, lymph node dissection, or Milroy's disease. Recurrent staphylococcal cutaneous infections are more common among individuals who have eosinophilia and elevated serum levels of IgE (Job's syndrome) and among nasal carriers of staphylococci. Cellulitis caused by *Streptococcus agalactiae* (group B *Streptococcus*) occurs primarily in elderly patients and those with diabetes mellitus or peripheral vascular disease. *Haemophilus influenzae* typically causes periorbital cellulitis in children in association with sinusitis, otitis media, or epiglottitis. It is unclear whether this form of cellulitis will (like meningitis) become less common as a result of the impressive efficacy of the *H. influenzae* type b vaccine.

Many other bacteria also cause cellulitis. It is fortunate that these organisms occur in such characteristic settings that a good history provides useful clues to the diagnosis. Cellulitis associated with cat bites and, to a lesser degree, with dog bites is commonly caused by *Pasteurella multocida*, although in the latter case *Staphylococcus intermedius* and *Capnocytophaga canimorsus* also must be considered. Sites of cellulitis and abscesses associated with dog bites and human bites also contain a variety of anaerobic organisms, including *Fusobacterium*, *Bacteroides*, aerobic and anaerobic streptococci, and *Eikenella corrodens*. *Pasteurella* is notoriously resistant to dicloxacillin and nafcillin but is sensitive to all other β-lactam antimicrobial agents as well as to quinolones, tetracycline, and erythromycin. Ampicillin/clavulanate, ampicillin/sulbactam, and cefoxitin are good choices for the treatment of animal or human bite infections. *Aeromonas hydrophila* causes aggressive cellulitis in tissues surrounding lacerations sustained in freshwater (lakes, rivers, and streams). This organism remains sensitive to aminoglycosides, fluoroquinolones, chloramphenicol, trimethoprim-sulfamethoxazole, and third-generation cephalosporins; it is resistant to ampicillin, however.

P. aeruginosa causes three types of soft tissue infection: ecthyma gangrenosum in neutropenic patients, hot-tub folliculitis, and cellulitis following penetrating injury. Most commonly, *P. aeruginosa* is introduced into the deep tissues when a person steps on a nail. Treatment includes surgical inspection and drainage, particularly if the injury also involves bone or joint capsule. Choices for empirical treatment while antimicrobial susceptibility data are awaited include an aminoglycoside, a third-generation cephalosporin (ceftazidime, cefoperazone, or cefotaxime), a semisynthetic penicillin (ticarcillin, mezlocillin, or piperacillin), or a fluoroquinolone (although drugs of the last class are not indicated for the treatment of children <13 years old).

Gram-negative bacillary cellulitis, including that due to *P. aeruginosa*, is most common among hospitalized, immunocompromised hosts. Cultures and sensitivity tests are critically important in this setting because of multidrug resistance (Chap. 189).

The gram-positive aerobic rod *Erysipelothrix rhusiopathiae* is most often associated with fish and domestic swine and causes cellulitis primarily in bone renderers and fishmongers. *E. rhusiopathiae* remains susceptible to most β-lactam antibiotics (including penicillin), erythromycin, clindamycin, tetracycline, and cephalosporins but is resistant to sulfonamides, chloramphenicol, and vancomycin. Its resistance to vancomycin, which is unusual among gram-positive bacteria, is of potential clinical significance since this agent is sometimes used in empirical therapy for skin infection. Fish food containing the water flea *Daphnia* is sometimes contaminated with *M. marinum*, which can cause cellulitis or granulomas on skin surfaces exposed to the water in aquariums or injured in swimming pools. Rifampin plus ethambutol has been an effective therapeutic combination in some cases, although no comprehensive studies have been undertaken. In addition, some strains of *M. marinum* are susceptible to tetracycline or to trimethoprim-sulfamethoxazole.

NECROTIZING FASCIITIS

(Table 156-1) Necrotizing fasciitis, formerly called streptococcal gangrene, may be associated with group A *Streptococcus* or mixed aerobic–anaerobic bacteria or may occur as a component of gas gangrene caused by *Clostridium perfringens*. Strains of MRSA that produce the Panton-Valentine leukocidin (PVL) toxin have been reported to cause necrotizing fasciitis. Early diagnosis may be difficult when pain or unexplained fever is the only presenting manifestation. Swelling then develops and is followed by brawny edema and tenderness. With progression, dark-red induration of the epidermis appears, along with bullae filled with blue or purple fluid. Later the skin becomes friable and takes on a bluish, maroon, or black color. By this stage, thrombosis of blood vessels in the dermal papillae (Fig. 156-1) is extensive. Extension of infection to the level of the deep fascia causes this tissue to take on a brownish-gray appearance. Rapid spread occurs along fascial planes, through venous channels and lymphatics. Patients in the later stages are toxic and frequently manifest shock and multiorgan failure.

Necrotizing fasciitis caused by mixed aerobic-anaerobic bacteria begins with a breach in the integrity of a mucous membrane barrier, such as the mucosa of the gastrointestinal or genitourinary tract. The portal can be a malignancy, a diverticulum, a hemorrhoid, an anal fissure, or a urethral tear. Other predisposing factors include peripheral vascular disease, diabetes mellitus, surgery, and penetrating injury to the abdomen. Leakage into the perineal area results in a syndrome called *Fournier's gangrene*, characterized by massive swelling of the scrotum and penis with extension into the perineum or the abdominal wall and the legs.

Necrotizing fasciitis caused by *S. pyogenes* has increased in frequency and severity since 1985. There are two distinct clinical presentations: those with no portal of entry and those with a defined portal of entry. Infections in the first category often begin deep at the site of a nonpenetrating minor trauma, such as a bruise or a muscle strain. Seeding of the site via transient bacteremia is likely, although most patients deny antecedent streptococcal infection. The affected patients present with only severe pain and fever. Late in the course, the classic signs of necrotizing fasciitis, such as purple (violaceous) bullae, skin sloughing, and progressive toxicity, develop. In infections of the second type, *S. pyogenes* may reach the deep fascia from a site of cutaneous infection or penetrating trauma. These patients have early signs of superficial skin infection with progression to necrotizing fasciitis. In either case, toxicity is severe, and renal impairment may precede the development of shock. In 20–40% of cases, myositis occurs concomitantly, and, as in gas gangrene (see below), serum creatine phosphokinase levels may be markedly elevated. Necrotizing fasciitis due to mixed aerobic-anaerobic bacteria may be associated with gas in deep tissue, but gas usually is not present when the cause is *S. pyogenes* or MRSA. Prompt surgical exploration down to the deep fascia and muscle is essential. Necrotic tissue must be surgically removed, and Gram's staining and culture of excised tissue are useful in establishing whether group A streptococci, mixed aerobic-anaerobic bacteria, MRSA, or *Clostridium* species are present (see "Treatment," below).

MYOSITIS AND MYONECROSIS

(Table 156-1) Muscle involvement can occur with viral infection (e.g., influenza, dengue, or coxsackievirus B infection) or parasitic invasion (e.g., trichinellosis, cysticercosis, or toxoplasmosis). Although myalgia develops in most of these infections, severe muscle pain is the hallmark of pleurodynia (coxsackievirus B), trichinellosis, and bacterial infection. Acute rhabdomyolysis predictably occurs with clostridial and streptococcal myositis but may also be associated with influenza virus, echovirus, coxsackievirus, Epstein-Barr virus, and *Legionella* infections.

Pyomyositis is usually due to *S. aureus*, is common in tropical areas, and generally has no known portal of entry. Cases of pyomyositis caused by MRSA producing the PVL toxin have been described among children in the United States. Muscle infection begins at the exact site of blunt trauma or muscle strain. Infection remains localized, and shock does not develop unless organisms produce toxic shock syndrome toxin 1 or certain enterotoxins and the patient lacks antibodies to the toxin produced by the infecting organisms. In contrast, *S. pyogenes* may induce primary myositis (referred to as *streptococcal necrotizing myositis*) in association with severe systemic toxicity. Myonecrosis occurs concomitantly with necrotizing fasciitis in ~50% of cases. Both are part of the streptococcal toxic shock syndrome.

Gas gangrene usually follows severe penetrating injuries that result in interruption of the blood supply and introduction of soil into wounds. Such cases of traumatic gangrene are usually caused by the clostridial species *C. perfringens*, *C. septicum*, and *C. histolyticum*. Rarely, latent or recurrent gangrene can occur years after penetrating trauma; dormant spores that reside at the site of previous injury are most likely responsible. Spontaneous nontraumatic gangrene among patients with neutropenia, gastrointestinal malignancy, diverticulosis, or recent radiation therapy to the abdomen is caused by several clostridial species, of which *C. septicum* is the most commonly involved. The tolerance of this anaerobe to oxygen probably explains why it can initiate infection spontaneously in normal tissue anywhere in the body.

Gas gangrene of the uterus, especially that due to *Clostridium sordellii*, historically occurred as a consequence of illegal or self-induced abortion and nowadays also follows spontaneous abortion, vaginal delivery, and cesarean section. *C. sordellii* has also been implicated in medically induced abortion. Postpartum *C. sordellii* infections in young, previously healthy women present as a unique clinical picture: little or no fever, lack of a purulent discharge, refractory hypotension, extensive peripheral edema and effusions, hemoconcentration, and a markedly elevated white blood cell count. The infection is almost uniformly fatal, with death ensuing rapidly. *C. sordellii* and *C. novyi* have also been associated with cutaneous injection of black tar heroin; mortality rates are lower among the affected individuals, probably because their aggressive injection-site infections are readily apparent and diagnosis is therefore prompt.

Synergistic nonclostridial anaerobic myonecrosis, also known as necrotizing cutaneous myositis and synergistic necrotizing cellulitis, is a variant of necrotizing fasciitis caused by mixed aerobic and anaerobic bacteria with the exclusion of clostridial organisms (see "Necrotizing Fasciitis," above).

DIAGNOSIS

This chapter emphasizes the physical appearance and location of lesions within the soft tissues as important diagnostic clues. Other crucial considerations in narrowing the differential diagnosis are the temporal progression of the lesions as well as the patient's travel history, animal exposure or bite history, age, underlying disease status, and lifestyle. However, even the astute clinician may find it challenging to diagnose all infections of the soft tissues by history and inspection alone. Soft tissue radiography, CT (Fig. 156-2), and MRI may be useful in determining the depth of infection and should be performed when the patient has rapidly progressing lesions or evidence of a systemic inflammatory response syndrome. These tests are particularly valuable for defining a localized abscess or detecting gas in tissue. Unfortunately, they may reveal only soft tissue swelling and thus are not specific for fulminant infections such as necrotizing fasciitis or myonecrosis caused by group A *Streptococcus* (Fig. 156-2), where gas is not found in lesions.

Aspiration of the leading edge or punch biopsy with frozen section may be helpful if the results of imaging tests are positive, but false-negative results occur in ~80% of cases. There is some evidence that aspiration alone may be superior to injection and aspiration with normal saline. Frozen sections are especially useful in distinguishing SSSS from TEN and are quite valuable in cases of necrotizing fasciitis. Open surgical inspection, with debridement as indicated, is clearly the best way to determine the extent and severity of infection and to obtain material for Gram's staining and culture. Such an aggressive approach is important and may be lifesaving if undertaken early in the course of fulminant infections where there is evidence of systemic toxicity.

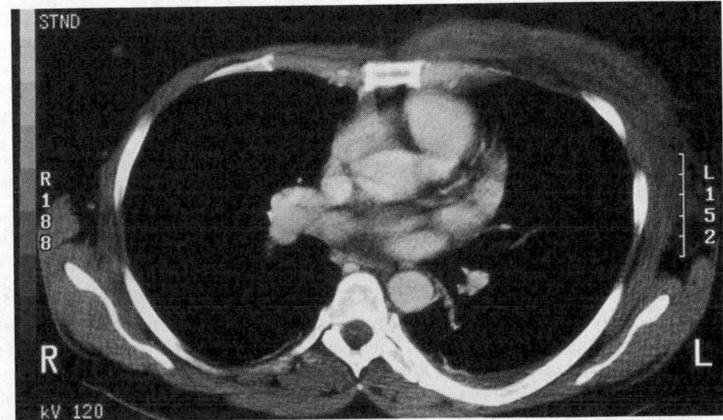

FIGURE 156-2 CT showing edema and inflammation of the left chest wall in a patient with necrotizing fasciitis and myonecrosis caused by group A *Streptococcus*.

TREATMENT INFECTIONS OF THE SKIN, MUSCLES, AND SOFT TISSUES

A full description of the treatment of all the clinical entities described herein is beyond the scope of this chapter. As a guide to the clinician in selecting appropriate treatment, the antimicrobial agents useful in the most common and the most fulminant cutaneous infections are listed in **Table 156-2**.

Furuncles, carbuncles, and abscesses caused by MRSA and MSSA are common, and their treatment depends upon the size of the lesion. Furuncles <2.5 cm in diameter are usually treated with moist heat. Those that are larger (4.5 cm of erythema and induration) require surgical drainage, and the occurrence of these larger lesions in association with fever, chills, or leukocytosis requires both drainage and antibiotic treatment. A study in children demonstrated that surgical drainage of abscesses (mean diameter, 3.8 cm) was as effective when used alone as when combined with trimethoprim-sulfamethoxazole treatment. However, the rate of recurrence of new lesions was lower in the group undergoing both drainage and antibiotic treatment.

Early and aggressive surgical exploration is essential in cases of suspected necrotizing fasciitis, myositis, or gangrene in order to (1) visualize the deep structures, (2) remove necrotic tissue, (3) reduce compartment pressure, and (4) obtain suitable material for Gram's staining and for aerobic and anaerobic cultures. Appropriate empirical antibiotic treatment for mixed aerobic–anaerobic infections could consist of ampicillin/sulbactam, cefoxitin, or the following combination: (1) clindamycin (600–900 mg IV every 8 h) or metronidazole (500 mg every 6 h) plus (2) ampicillin or ampicillin/sulbactam (1.5–3 g IV every 6 h) plus (3) gentamicin (1–1.5 mg/kg every 8 h). Group A streptococcal and clostridial infection of the fascia and/or muscle carries a mortality rate of 20–50% with penicillin treatment. In experimental models of streptococcal and clostridial necrotizing fasciitis/myositis, clindamycin has exhibited markedly superior efficacy, but no comparative clinical trials have been performed. A retrospective study of children with invasive group A streptococcal

TABLE 156-2 TREATMENT OF COMMON INFECTIONS OF THE SKIN

Diagnosis/Condition	Primary Treatment	Alternative Treatment	See Also Chap(s).
Animal bite (prophylaxis or early infection)[a]	Amoxicillin/clavulanate, 875/125 mg PO bid	Doxycycline, 100 mg PO bid	**167e**
Animal bite[a] (established infection)	Ampicillin/sulbactam, 1.5–3 g IV q6h	Clindamycin, 600–900 mg IV q8h, *plus* Ciprofloxacin, 400 mg IV q12h, *or* cefoxitin, 2 g IV q6h	**167e**
Bacillary angiomatosis	Erythromycin, 500 mg PO qid	Doxycycline, 100 mg PO bid	**197**
Herpes simplex (primary genital)	Acyclovir, 400 mg PO tid for 10 days	Famciclovir, 250 mg PO tid for 5–10 days, *or* Valacyclovir, 1000 mg PO bid for 10 days	**216**
Herpes zoster (immunocompetent host >50 years of age)	Acyclovir, 800 mg PO 5 times daily for 7–10 days	Famciclovir, 500 mg PO tid for 7–10 days, *or* Valacyclovir, 1000 mg PO tid for 7 days	**217**
Cellulitis (staphylococcal or streptococcal[b,c])	Nafcillin or oxacillin, 2 g IV q4–6h	Cefazolin, 1–2 g q8h, *or* Ampicillin/sulbactam, 1.5–3 g IV q6h, *or* Erythromycin, 0.5–1 g IV q6h, *or* Clindamycin, 600–900 mg IV q8h	**172, 173**
MRSA skin infection[d]	Vancomycin, 1 g IV q12h	Linezolid, 600 mg IV q12h	**172**
Necrotizing fasciitis (group A streptococcal[b])	Clindamycin, 600–900 mg IV q6–8h, *plus* Penicillin G, 4 million units IV q4h	Clindamycin, 600–900 mg IV q6–8h, *plus* Cephalosporin (first- or second-generation)	**173**
Necrotizing fasciitis (mixed aerobes and anaerobes)	Ampicillin, 2 g IV q4h, *plus* Clindamycin, 600–900 mg IV q6–8h, *plus* Ciprofloxacin, 400 mg IV q6–8h	Vancomycin, 1 g IV q6h, *plus* Metronidazole, 500 mg IV q6h, *plus* Ciprofloxacin, 400 mg IV q6–8h	**201**
Gas gangrene	Clindamycin, 600–900 mg IV q6–8h, *plus* Penicillin G, 4 million units IV q4–6h	Clindamycin, 600–900 mg IV q6–8h, *plus* Cefoxitin, 2 g IV q6h	**179**

[a]*Pasteurella multocida*, a species commonly associated with both dog and cat bites, is resistant to cephalexin, dicloxacillin, clindamycin, and erythromycin. *Eikenella corrodens*, a bacterium commonly associated with human bites, is resistant to clindamycin, penicillinase-resistant penicillins, and metronidazole but is sensitive to trimethoprim-sulfamethoxazole and fluoroquinolones. [b]The frequency of erythromycin resistance in group A *Streptococcus* is currently ~5% in the United States but has reached 70–100% in some other countries. Most, but not all, erythromycin-resistant group A streptococci are susceptible to clindamycin. Approximately 90% of *Staphylococcus aureus* strains are sensitive to clindamycin, but resistance—both intrinsic and inducible—is increasing. [c]Severe hospital-acquired *S. aureus* infections or community-acquired *S. aureus* infections that are not responding to the β-lactam antibiotics recommended in this table may be caused by methicillin-resistant strains, requiring a switch to vancomycin, daptomycin, or linezolid. [d]Some strains of methicillin-resistant *S. aureus* (MRSA) remain sensitive to tetracycline and trimethoprim-sulfamethoxazole. Daptomycin (4 mg/kg IV q24h) or tigecycline (100-mg loading dose followed by 50 mg IV q12h) is an alternative treatment for MRSA.

infection demonstrated higher survival rates with clindamycin treatment than with β-lactam antibiotic therapy. Hyperbaric oxygen treatment also may be useful in gas gangrene due to clostridial species. Antibiotic treatment should be continued until all signs of systemic toxicity have resolved, all devitalized tissue has been removed, and granulation tissue has developed (Chaps. 173, 179, and 201).

In summary, infections of the skin and soft tissues are diverse in presentation and severity and offer a great challenge to the clinician. This chapter provides an approach to diagnosis and understanding of the pathophysiologic mechanisms involved in these infections. More in-depth information is found in chapters on specific infections.

157 Infectious Arthritis

Lawrence C. Madoff

Although *Staphylococcus aureus*, *Neisseria gonorrhoeae*, and other bacteria are the most common causes of infectious arthritis, various mycobacteria, spirochetes, fungi, and viruses also infect joints (Table 157-1). Since acute bacterial infection can destroy articular cartilage rapidly, all inflamed joints must be evaluated without delay to exclude noninfectious processes and determine appropriate antimicrobial therapy and drainage procedures. For more detailed information on infectious arthritis caused by specific organisms, the reader is referred to the chapters on those organisms.

Acute bacterial infection typically involves a single joint or a few joints. Subacute or chronic monarthritis or oligoarthritis suggests mycobacterial or fungal infection; episodic inflammation is seen in syphilis, Lyme disease, and the reactive arthritis that follows enteric infections and chlamydial urethritis. Acute polyarticular inflammation occurs as an immunologic reaction during the course of endocarditis, rheumatic fever, disseminated neisserial infection, and acute hepatitis B. Bacteria and viruses occasionally infect multiple joints, the former most commonly in persons with rheumatoid arthritis.

APPROACH TO THE PATIENT: Infectious Arthritis

Aspiration of synovial fluid—an essential element in the evaluation of potentially infected joints—can be performed without difficulty in most cases by the insertion of a large-bore needle into the site of maximal fluctuance or tenderness or by the route of easiest access. Ultrasonography or fluoroscopy may be used to guide aspiration of difficult-to-localize effusions of the hip and, occasionally, the shoulder and other joints. Normal synovial fluid contains <180 cells (predominantly mononuclear cells) per microliter. Synovial cell counts averaging 100,000/μL (range, 25,000–250,000/μL), with >90% neutrophils, are characteristic of acute bacterial infections. Crystal-induced, rheumatoid, and other noninfectious inflammatory arthritides usually are associated with <30,000–50,000 cells/μL; cell counts of 10,000–30,000/μL, with 50–70% neutrophils and the remainder lymphocytes, are common in mycobacterial and fungal infections. Definitive diagnosis of an infectious process relies on identification of the pathogen in stained smears of synovial fluid, isolation of the pathogen from cultures of synovial fluid and blood, or detection of microbial nucleic acids and proteins by nucleic acid amplification (NAA)–based assays and immunologic techniques.

ACUTE BACTERIAL ARTHRITIS

PATHOGENESIS

Bacteria enter the joint from the bloodstream; from a contiguous site of infection in bone or soft tissue; or by direct inoculation during surgery, injection, animal or human bite, or trauma. In hematogenous infection, bacteria escape from synovial capillaries, which have no limiting basement membrane, and within hours provoke neutrophilic infiltration of the synovium. Neutrophils and bacteria enter the joint space; later, bacteria adhere to articular cartilage. Degradation of cartilage begins within 48 h as a result of increased intraarticular pressure, release of proteases and cytokines from chondrocytes and synovial macrophages, and invasion of the cartilage by bacteria and inflammatory cells. Histologic studies reveal bacteria lining the synovium and

TABLE 157-1 DIFFERENTIAL DIAGNOSIS OF ARTHRITIS SYNDROMES

Acute Monarticular Arthritis	Chronic Monarticular Arthritis	Polyarticular Arthritis
Staphylococcus aureus	*Mycobacterium tuberculosis*	*Neisseria meningitidis*
Streptococcus pneumoniae	Nontuberculous mycobacteria	*N. gonorrhoeae*
β-Hemolytic streptococci	*Borrelia burgdorferi*	Nongonococcal bacterial arthritis
Gram-negative bacilli	*Treponema pallidum*	Bacterial endocarditis
Neisseria gonorrhoeae	*Candida* spp.	*Candida* spp.
Candida spp.	*Sporothrix schenckii*	Poncet's disease (tuberculous rheumatism)
Crystal-induced arthritis	*Coccidioides immitis*	Hepatitis B virus
Fracture	*Blastomyces dermatitidis*	Parvovirus B19
Hemarthrosis	*Aspergillus* spp.	HIV
Foreign body	*Cryptococcus neoformans*	Human T-lymphotropic virus type I
Osteoarthritis	*Nocardia* spp.	Rubella virus
Ischemic necrosis	*Brucella* spp.	Arthropod-borne viruses
Monarticular rheumatoid arthritis	Legg-Calvé-Perthes disease	Sickle cell disease flare
	Osteoarthritis	Reactive arthritis
		Serum sickness
		Acute rheumatic fever
		Inflammatory bowel disease
		Systemic lupus erythematosus
		Rheumatoid arthritis/Still's disease
		Other vasculitides
		Sarcoidosis

cartilage as well as abscesses extending into the synovium, cartilage, and—in severe cases—subchondral bone. Synovial proliferation results in the formation of a pannus over the cartilage, and thrombosis of inflamed synovial vessels develops. Bacterial factors that appear important in the pathogenesis of infective arthritis include various surface-associated adhesins in *S. aureus* that permit adherence to cartilage and endotoxins that promote chondrocyte-mediated breakdown of cartilage.

MICROBIOLOGY

The hematogenous route of infection is the most common route in all age groups, and nearly every bacterial pathogen is capable of causing septic arthritis. In infants, group B streptococci, gram-negative enteric bacilli, and *S. aureus* are the most common pathogens. Since the advent of the *Haemophilus influenzae* vaccine, the predominant causes among children <5 years of age have been *S. aureus*, *Streptococcus pyogenes* (group A *Streptococcus*), and (in some centers) *Kingella kingae*. Among young adults and adolescents, *N. gonorrhoeae* is the most commonly implicated organism. *S. aureus* accounts for most nongonococcal isolates in adults of all ages; gram-negative bacilli, pneumococci, and β-hemolytic streptococci—particularly groups A and B but also groups C, G, and F—are involved in up to one-third of cases in older adults, especially those with underlying comorbid illnesses.

Infections after surgical procedures or penetrating injuries are due most often to *S. aureus* and occasionally to other gram-positive bacteria or gram-negative bacilli. Infections with coagulase-negative staphylococci are unusual except after the implantation of prosthetic joints or arthroscopy. Anaerobic organisms, often in association with aerobic or facultative bacteria, are found after human bites and when decubitus ulcers or intraabdominal abscesses spread into adjacent joints. Polymicrobial infections complicate traumatic injuries with extensive contamination. Bites and scratches from cats and other animals may introduce *Pasteurella multocida* or *Bartonella henselae* into joints either directly or hematogenously, and bites from humans may introduce *Eikenella corrodens* or other components of the oral flora. Penetration of a sharp object through a shoe is associated with *Pseudomonas aeruginosa* arthritis in the foot.

NONGONOCOCCAL BACTERIAL ARTHRITIS

Epidemiology Although hematogenous infections with virulent organisms such as *S. aureus*, *H. influenzae*, and pyogenic streptococci occur in healthy persons, there is an underlying host predisposition in many cases of septic arthritis. Patients with rheumatoid arthritis have the highest incidence of infective arthritis (most often secondary to *S. aureus*) because of chronically inflamed joints; glucocorticoid therapy; and frequent breakdown of rheumatoid nodules, vasculitic ulcers, and skin overlying deformed joints. Diabetes mellitus, glucocorticoid therapy, hemodialysis, and malignancy all carry an increased risk of infection with *S. aureus* and gram-negative bacilli. Tumor necrosis factor inhibitors (e.g., etanercept, infliximab), which increasingly are used for the treatment of rheumatoid arthritis, predispose to mycobacterial infections and possibly to other pyogenic bacterial infections and could be associated with septic arthritis in this population. Pneumococcal infections complicate alcoholism, deficiencies of humoral immunity, and hemoglobinopathies. Pneumococci, *Salmonella* species, and *H. influenzae* cause septic arthritis in persons infected with HIV. Persons with primary immunoglobulin deficiency are at risk for mycoplasmal arthritis, which results in permanent joint damage if tetracycline and replacement therapy with IV immunoglobulin are not administered promptly. IV drug users acquire staphylococcal and streptococcal infections from their own flora and acquire pseudomonal and other gram-negative infections from drugs and injection paraphernalia.

Clinical Manifestations Some 90% of patients present with involvement of a single joint—most commonly the knee; less frequently the hip; and still less often the shoulder, wrist, or elbow. Small joints of the hands and feet are more likely to be affected after direct inoculation or a bite. Among IV drug users, infections of the spine, sacroiliac joints, and sternoclavicular joints (Fig. 157-1) are more common than infections of the appendicular skeleton. Polyarticular infection is most common among patients with rheumatoid arthritis and may resemble a flare of the underlying disease.

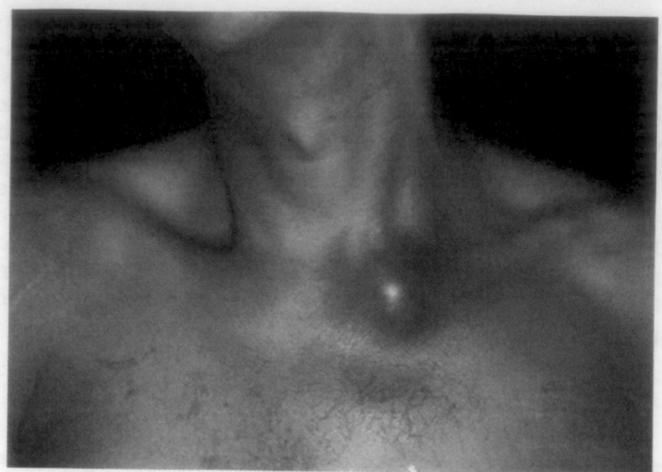

FIGURE 157-1 Acute septic arthritis of the sternoclavicular joint. A man in his forties with a history of cirrhosis presented with a new onset of fever and lower neck pain. He had no history of IV drug use or previous catheter placement. Jaundice and a painful swollen area over his left sternoclavicular joint were evident on physical examination. Cultures of blood drawn at admission grew group B *Streptococcus*. The patient recovered after treatment with IV penicillin. *(Courtesy of Francisco M. Marty, MD, Brigham and Women's Hospital, Boston; with permission.)*

The usual presentation consists of moderate to severe pain that is uniform around the joint, effusion, muscle spasm, and decreased range of motion. Fever in the range of 38.3–38.9°C (101–102°F) and sometimes higher is common but may not be present, especially in persons with rheumatoid arthritis, renal or hepatic insufficiency, or conditions requiring immunosuppressive therapy. The inflamed, swollen joint is usually evident on examination except in the case of a deeply situated joint such as the hip, shoulder, or sacroiliac joint. Cellulitis, bursitis, and acute osteomyelitis, which may produce a similar clinical picture, should be distinguished from septic arthritis by their greater range of motion and less-than-circumferential swelling. A focus of extraarticular infection, such as a boil or pneumonia, should be sought. Peripheral-blood leukocytosis with a left shift and elevation of the erythrocyte sedimentation rate or C-reactive protein level are common.

Plain radiographs show evidence of soft-tissue swelling, joint-space widening, and displacement of tissue planes by the distended capsule. Narrowing of the joint space and bony erosions indicate advanced infection and a poor prognosis. Ultrasound is useful for detecting effusions in the hip, and CT or MRI can demonstrate infections of the sacroiliac joint, the sternoclavicular joint, and the spine very well.

Laboratory Findings Specimens of peripheral blood and synovial fluid should be obtained before antibiotics are administered. Blood cultures are positive in up to 50–70% of *S. aureus* infections but are less frequently positive in infections due to other organisms. The synovial fluid is turbid, serosanguineous, or frankly purulent. Gram-stained smears confirm the presence of large numbers of neutrophils. Levels of total protein and lactate dehydrogenase in synovial fluid are elevated, and the glucose level is depressed; however, these findings are not specific for infection, and measurement of these levels is not necessary for diagnosis. The synovial fluid should be examined for crystals, because gout and pseudogout can resemble septic arthritis clinically, and infection and crystal-induced disease occasionally occur together. Organisms are seen on synovial fluid smears in nearly three-quarters of infections with *S. aureus* and streptococci and in 30–50% of infections due to gram-negative and other bacteria. Cultures of synovial fluid are positive in >90% of cases. Inoculation of synovial fluid into bottles containing liquid media for blood cultures increases the yield of a culture, especially if the pathogen is a fastidious organism or the patient is taking an antibiotic. NAA-based assays for bacterial DNA, when available, can be useful for the diagnosis of partially treated or culture-negative bacterial arthritis.

TREATMENT NONGONOCOCCAL BACTERIAL ARTHRITIS

Prompt administration of systemic antibiotics and drainage of the involved joint can prevent destruction of cartilage, postinfectious degenerative arthritis, joint instability, or deformity. Once samples of blood and synovial fluid have been obtained for culture, empirical antibiotics should be given that are directed against the bacteria visualized on smears or the pathogens that are likely in light of the patient's age and risk factors. Initial therapy should consist of IV administration of bactericidal agents; direct instillation of antibiotics into the joint is not necessary to achieve adequate levels in synovial fluid and tissue. An IV third-generation cephalosporin such as cefotaxime (1 g every 8 h) or ceftriaxone (1–2 g every 24 h) provides adequate empirical coverage for most community-acquired infections in adults when smears show no organisms. IV vancomycin (1 g every 12 h) is used if there are gram-positive cocci on the smear. If methicillin-resistant *S. aureus* is an unlikely pathogen (e.g., when it is not widespread in the community), either oxacillin or nafcillin (2 g every 4 h) should be given. In addition, an aminoglycoside or third-generation cephalosporin should be given to IV drug users and to other patients in whom *P. aeruginosa* may be the responsible agent.

Definitive therapy is based on the identity and antibiotic susceptibility of the bacteria isolated in culture. Infections due to staphylococci are treated with oxacillin, nafcillin, or vancomycin for 4 weeks. Pneumococcal and streptococcal infections due to penicillin-susceptible organisms respond to 2 weeks of therapy with penicillin G (2 million units IV every 4 h); infections caused by *H. influenzae* and by strains of *Streptococcus pneumoniae* that are resistant to penicillin are treated with cefotaxime or ceftriaxone for 2 weeks. Most enteric gram-negative infections can be cured in 3–4 weeks by a second- or third-generation cephalosporin given IV or by a fluoroquinolone such as levofloxacin (500 mg IV or PO every 24 h). *P. aeruginosa* infection should be treated for at least 2 weeks with a combination regimen composed of an aminoglycoside plus either an extended-spectrum penicillin such as mezlocillin (3 g IV every 4 h) or an antipseudomonal cephalosporin such as ceftazidime (1 g IV every 8 h). If tolerated, this regimen is continued for an additional 2 weeks; alternatively, a fluoroquinolone such as ciprofloxacin (750 mg PO twice daily) is given by itself or with the penicillin or cephalosporin in place of the aminoglycoside.

Timely drainage of pus and necrotic debris from the infected joint is required for a favorable outcome. Needle aspiration of readily accessible joints such as the knee may be adequate if loculations or particulate matter in the joint does not prevent its thorough decompression. Arthroscopic drainage and lavage may be employed initially or within several days if repeated needle aspiration fails to relieve symptoms, decrease the volume of the effusion and the synovial white cell count, and clear bacteria from smears and cultures. In some cases, arthrotomy is necessary to remove loculations and debride infected synovium, cartilage, or bone. Septic arthritis of the hip is best managed with arthrotomy, particularly in young children, in whom infection threatens the viability of the femoral head. Septic joints do not require immobilization except for pain control before symptoms are alleviated by treatment. Weight bearing should be avoided until signs of inflammation have subsided, but frequent passive motion of the joint is indicated to maintain full mobility. Although addition of glucocorticoids to antibiotic treatment improves the outcome of *S. aureus* arthritis in experimental animals, no clinical trials have evaluated this approach in humans.

GONOCOCCAL ARTHRITIS

Epidemiology Although its incidence has declined in recent years, gonococcal arthritis (Chap. 181) has accounted for up to 70% of episodes of infectious arthritis in persons <40 years of age in the United States. Arthritis due to *N. gonorrhoeae* is a consequence of bacteremia arising from gonococcal infection or, more frequently, from asymptomatic gonococcal mucosal colonization of the urethra, cervix, or pharynx. Women are at greatest risk during menses and during pregnancy and overall are two to three times more likely than men to develop disseminated gonococcal infection (DGI) and arthritis. Persons with complement deficiencies, especially of the terminal components, are prone to recurrent episodes of gonococcemia. Strains of gonococci that are most likely to cause DGI include those which produce transparent colonies in culture, have the type IA outer-membrane protein, or are of the AUH-auxotroph type.

Clinical Manifestations and Laboratory Findings The most common manifestation of DGI is a syndrome of fever, chills, rash, and articular symptoms. Small numbers of papules that progress to hemorrhagic pustules develop on the trunk and the extensor surfaces of the distal extremities. Migratory arthritis and tenosynovitis of the knees, hands, wrists, feet, and ankles are prominent. The cutaneous lesions and articular findings are believed to be the consequence of an immune reaction to circulating gonococci and immune-complex deposition in tissues. Thus, cultures of synovial fluid are consistently negative, and blood cultures are positive in fewer than 45% of patients. Synovial fluid may be difficult to obtain from inflamed joints and usually contains only 10,000–20,000 leukocytes/μL.

True gonococcal septic arthritis is less common than the DGI syndrome and always follows DGI, which is unrecognized in one-third of patients. A single joint such as the hip, knee, ankle, or wrist is usually involved. Synovial fluid, which contains >50,000 leukocytes/μL, can be obtained with ease; the gonococcus is evident only occasionally in Gram-stained smears, and cultures of synovial fluid are positive in fewer than 40% of cases. Blood cultures are almost always negative.

Because it is difficult to isolate gonococci from synovial fluid and blood, specimens for culture should be obtained from potentially infected mucosal sites. NAA-based urine tests also may be positive. Cultures and Gram-stained smears of skin lesions are occasionally positive. All specimens for culture should be plated onto Thayer-Martin agar directly or in special transport media at the bedside and transferred promptly to the microbiology laboratory in an atmosphere of 5% CO_2, as generated in a candle jar. NAA-based assays are extremely sensitive in detecting gonococcal DNA in synovial fluid. A dramatic alleviation of symptoms within 12–24 h after the initiation of appropriate antibiotic therapy supports a clinical diagnosis of the DGI syndrome if cultures are negative.

TREATMENT GONOCOCCAL ARTHRITIS

Initial treatment consists of ceftriaxone (1 g IV or IM every 24 h) to cover possible penicillin-resistant organisms. Once local and systemic signs are clearly resolving, the 7-day course of therapy can be completed with an oral fluoroquinolone such as ciprofloxacin (500 mg twice daily) if the organism is known to be susceptible. If penicillin-susceptible organisms are isolated, amoxicillin (500 mg three times daily) may be used. Suppurative arthritis usually responds to needle aspiration of involved joints and 7–14 days of antibiotic treatment. Arthroscopic lavage or arthrotomy is rarely required. Patients with DGI should be treated for *Chlamydia trachomatis* infection unless this infection is ruled out by appropriate testing.

It is noteworthy that arthritis symptoms similar to those seen in DGI occur in meningococcemia. A dermatitis-arthritis syndrome, purulent monarthritis, and reactive polyarthritis have been described. All respond to treatment with IV penicillin.

SPIROCHETAL ARTHRITIS

LYME DISEASE

Lyme disease (Chap. 210) due to infection with the spirochete *Borrelia burgdorferi* causes arthritis in up to 60% of persons who are not treated. Intermittent arthralgias and myalgias—but not arthritis—occur within days or weeks of inoculation of the spirochete by the *Ixodes* tick. Later, there are three patterns of joint disease: (1) Fifty percent of untreated persons experience intermittent episodes of monarthritis or oligoarthritis involving the knee and/or other large joints. The symptoms wax and wane without treatment over months, and each year 10–20% of patients report loss of joint symptoms. (2) Twenty percent of untreated persons develop a pattern of waxing and waning arthralgias. (3) Ten percent of untreated patients develop chronic inflammatory synovitis that results in erosive lesions and destruction of the joint. Serologic tests for IgG antibodies to *B. burgdorferi* are positive in more than 90% of persons with Lyme arthritis, and an NAA-based assay detects *Borrelia* DNA in 85%.

TREATMENT LYME ARTHRITIS

Lyme arthritis generally responds well to therapy. A regimen of oral doxycycline (100 mg twice daily for 30 days), oral amoxicillin (500 mg four times daily for 30 days), or parenteral ceftriaxone (2 g/d for 2–4 weeks) is recommended. Patients who do not respond to a total of 2 months of oral therapy or 1 month of parenteral therapy are unlikely to benefit from additional antibiotic therapy and are treated with anti-inflammatory agents or synovectomy. Failure of therapy is associated with host features such as the human leukocyte antigen DR4 (HLA-DR4) genotype, persistent reactivity to OspA (outer-surface protein A), and the presence of hLFA-1 (human leukocyte function–associated antigen 1), which cross-reacts with OspA.

SYPHILITIC ARTHRITIS

Articular manifestations occur in different stages of syphilis (Chap. 206). In early congenital syphilis, periarticular swelling and immobilization of the involved limbs (*Parrot's pseudoparalysis*) complicate osteochondritis of long bones. *Clutton's joint*, a late manifestation of congenital syphilis that typically develops between ages 8 and 15 years, is caused by chronic painless synovitis with effusions of large joints, particularly the knees and elbows. Secondary syphilis may be associated with arthralgias, with symmetric arthritis of the knees and ankles and occasionally of the shoulders and wrists, and with sacroiliitis. The arthritis follows a subacute to chronic course with a mixed mononuclear and neutrophilic synovial-fluid pleocytosis (typical cell counts, 5000–15,000/μL). Immunologic mechanisms may contribute to the arthritis, and symptoms usually improve rapidly with penicillin therapy. In tertiary syphilis, Charcot's joint results from sensory loss due to tabes dorsalis. Penicillin is not helpful in this setting.

MYCOBACTERIAL ARTHRITIS

Tuberculous arthritis (Chap. 202) accounts for ~1% of all cases of tuberculosis and 10% of extrapulmonary cases. The most common presentation is chronic granulomatous monarthritis. An unusual syndrome, *Poncet's disease*, is a reactive symmetric form of polyarthritis that affects persons with visceral or disseminated tuberculosis. No mycobacteria are found in the joints, and symptoms resolve with antituberculous therapy.

Unlike tuberculous osteomyelitis (Chap. 158), which typically involves the thoracic and lumbar spine (50% of cases), tuberculous arthritis primarily involves the large weight-bearing joints, in particular the hips, knees, and ankles, and only occasionally involves smaller non-weight-bearing joints. Progressive monarticular swelling and pain develop over months or years, and systemic symptoms are seen in only half of all cases. Tuberculous arthritis occurs as part of a disseminated primary infection or through late reactivation, often in persons with HIV infection or other immunocompromised hosts. Coexistent active pulmonary tuberculosis is unusual.

Aspiration of the involved joint yields fluid with an average cell count of 20,000/μL, with ~50% neutrophils. Acid-fast staining of the fluid yields positive results in fewer than one-third of cases, and cultures are positive in 80%. Culture of synovial tissue taken at biopsy is positive in ~90% of cases and shows granulomatous inflammation in most. NAA methods can shorten the time to diagnosis to 1 or 2 days. Radiographs reveal peripheral erosions at the points of synovial attachment, periarticular osteopenia, and eventually joint-space narrowing. Therapy for tuberculous arthritis is the same as that for tuberculous pulmonary disease, requiring the administration of multiple agents for 6–9 months. Therapy is more prolonged in immunosuppressed individuals such as those infected with HIV.

Various atypical mycobacteria (Chap. 204) found in water and soil may cause chronic indolent arthritis. Such disease results from trauma and direct inoculation associated with farming, gardening, or aquatic activities. Smaller joints, such as the digits, wrists, and knees, are usually involved. Involvement of tendon sheaths and bursae is typical. The mycobacterial species involved include *Mycobacterium marinum*, *M. avium-intracellulare*, *M. terrae*, *M. kansasii*, *M. fortuitum*, and *M. chelonae*. In persons who have HIV infection or are receiving immunosuppressive therapy, hematogenous spread to the joints has been reported for *M. kansasii*, *M. avium* complex, and *M. haemophilum*. Diagnosis usually requires biopsy and culture, and therapy is based on antimicrobial susceptibility patterns.

FUNGAL ARTHRITIS

Fungi are an unusual cause of chronic monarticular arthritis. Granulomatous articular infection with the endemic dimorphic fungi *Coccidioides immitis*, *Blastomyces dermatitidis*, and (less commonly) *Histoplasma capsulatum* (Fig. 157-2) results from hematogenous seeding or direct extension from bony lesions in persons with disseminated disease. Joint involvement is an unusual complication of sporotrichosis (infection with *Sporothrix schenckii*) among gardeners and other persons who work with soil or sphagnum moss. Articular sporotrichosis is six times more common among men than among women, and alcoholics and other debilitated hosts are at risk for polyarticular infection.

Candida infection involving a single joint—usually the knee, hip, or shoulder—results from surgical procedures, intraarticular injections, or (among critically ill patients with debilitating illnesses such as diabetes mellitus or hepatic or renal insufficiency and patients receiving immunosuppressive therapy) hematogenous spread. *Candida* infections in IV drug users typically involve the spine, sacroiliac joints, or other fibrocartilaginous joints. Unusual cases of arthritis due to *Aspergillus* species, *Cryptococcus neoformans*, *Pseudallescheria boydii*, and the dematiaceous fungi also have resulted from direct inoculation or disseminated hematogenous infection in immunocompromised persons. In the United States, a 2012 national outbreak of fungal arthritis (and meningitis) caused by *Exserohilum rostratum* was linked to intraspinal and intraarticular injection of a contaminated preparation of methylprednisolone acetate.

The synovial fluid in fungal arthritis usually contains 10,000–40,000 cells/μL, with ~70% neutrophils. Stained specimens and cultures of synovial tissue often confirm the diagnosis of fungal arthritis when studies of synovial fluid give negative results. Treatment consists of drainage and lavage of the joint and systemic administration of an antifungal agent directed at a specific pathogen. The doses and duration of therapy are the same as for disseminated disease (see Part 8, Section 16). Intraarticular instillation of amphotericin B has been used in addition to IV therapy.

VIRAL ARTHRITIS

Viruses produce arthritis by infecting synovial tissue during systemic infection or by provoking an immunologic reaction that involves joints. As many as 50% of women report persistent arthralgias, and 10% report frank arthritis within 3 days of the rash that follows natural infection with rubella virus and within 2–6 weeks after receipt of live-virus vaccine. Episodes of symmetric inflammation of fingers, wrists, and knees uncommonly recur for >1 year, but a syndrome of chronic fatigue, low-grade fever, headaches, and myalgias can persist for months or years. IV immunoglobulin has been helpful in selected cases. Self-limited monarticular or migratory polyarthritis may develop within 2 weeks of the parotitis of mumps; this sequela is more common among men than among women. Approximately

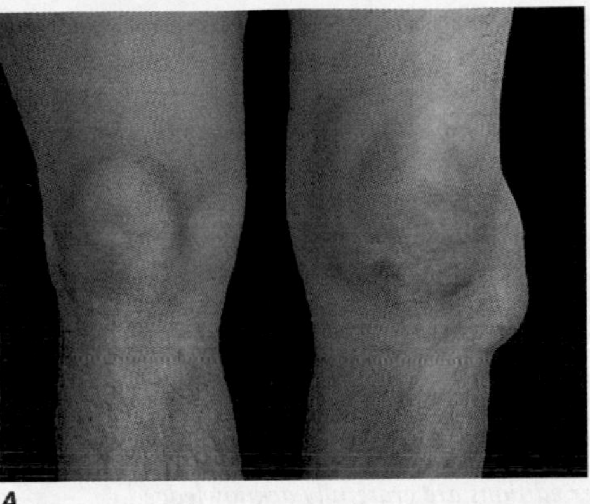

A

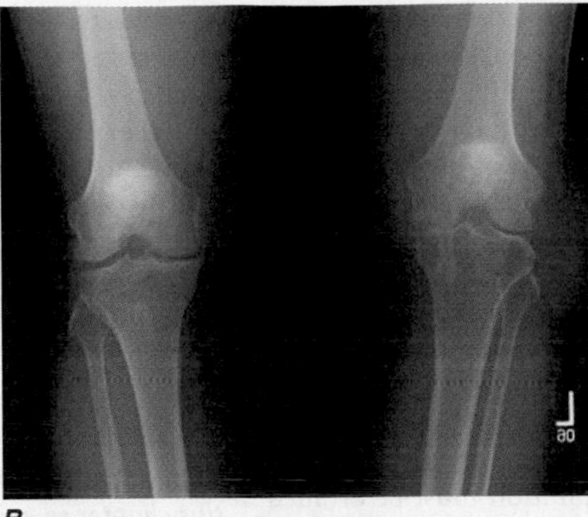

B

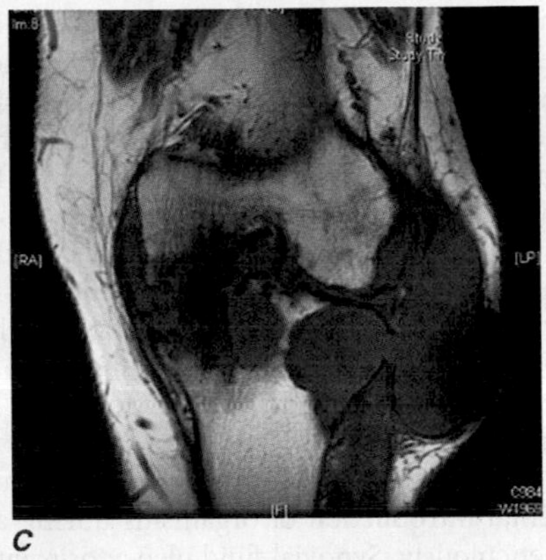

C

FIGURE 157-2 Chronic arthritis caused by *Histoplasma capsulatum* in the left knee. *A.* A man in his sixties from El Salvador presented with a history of progressive knee pain and difficulty walking for several years. He had undergone arthroscopy for a meniscal tear 7 years before presentation (without relief) and had received several intraarticular glucocorticoid injections. The patient developed significant deformity of the knee over time, including a large effusion in the lateral aspect. ***B.*** An x-ray of the knee showed multiple abnormalities, including severe medial femorotibial joint-space narrowing, several large subchondral cysts within the tibia and the patellofemoral compartment, a large suprapatellar joint effusion, and a large soft tissue mass projecting laterally over the knee. ***C.*** MRI further defined these abnormalities and demonstrated the cystic nature of the lateral knee abnormality. Synovial biopsies demonstrated chronic inflammation with giant cells, and cultures grew *H. capsulatum* after 3 weeks of incubation. All clinical cystic lesions and the effusion resolved after 1 year of treatment with itraconazole. The patient underwent a left total knee replacement for definitive treatment. *(Courtesy of Francisco M. Marty, MD, Brigham and Women's Hospital, Boston; with permission.)*

10% of children and 60% of women develop arthritis after infection with parvovirus B19. In adults, arthropathy sometimes occurs without fever or rash. Pain and stiffness, with less prominent swelling (primarily of the hands but also of the knees, wrists, and ankles), usually resolve within weeks, although a small proportion of patients develop chronic arthropathy.

About 2 weeks before the onset of jaundice, up to 10% of persons with acute hepatitis B develop an immune complex–mediated, serum sickness–like reaction with maculopapular rash, urticaria, fever, and arthralgias. Less common developments include symmetric arthritis involving the hands, wrists, elbows, or ankles and morning stiffness that resembles a flare of rheumatoid arthritis. Symptoms resolve at the time jaundice develops. Many persons with chronic hepatitis C infection report persistent arthralgia or arthritis, both in the presence and in the absence of cryoglobulinemia.

Painful arthritis involving larger joints often accompanies the fever and rash of several arthropod-borne viral infections, including those caused by chikungunya, O'nyong-nyong, Ross River, Mayaro, and Barmah Forest viruses (Chap. 233). Symmetric arthritis involving the hands and wrists may occur during the convalescent phase of infection with lymphocytic choriomeningitis virus. Patients infected with an enterovirus frequently report arthralgias, and echovirus has been isolated from patients with acute polyarthritis.

Several arthritis syndromes are associated with HIV infection. Reactive arthritis with painful lower-extremity oligoarthritis often follows an episode of urethritis in HIV-infected persons. HIV-associated reactive arthritis appears to be extremely common among persons with the HLA-B27 haplotype, but sacroiliac joint disease is unusual and is seen mostly in the absence of HLA-B27. Up to one-third of HIV-infected persons with psoriasis develop psoriatic arthritis. Painless monarthropathy and persistent symmetric polyarthropathy occasionally complicate HIV infection. Chronic persistent oligoarthritis of the shoulders, wrists, hands, and knees occurs in women infected with human T-lymphotropic virus type I. Synovial thickening, destruction of articular cartilage, and leukemic-appearing atypical lymphocytes in synovial fluid are characteristic, but progression to T cell leukemia is unusual.

PARASITIC ARTHRITIS

Arthritis due to parasitic infection is rare. The guinea worm *Dracunculus medinensis* may cause destructive joint lesions in the lower extremities as migrating gravid female worms invade joints or cause ulcers in adjacent soft tissues that become secondarily infected. Hydatid cysts infect bones in 1–2% of cases of infection with *Echinococcus granulosus*. The expanding destructive cystic lesions may spread to and destroy adjacent joints, particularly the hip and pelvis. In rare cases, chronic synovitis has been associated with the presence of schistosomal eggs in synovial biopsies. Monarticular arthritis in children with lymphatic filariasis appears to respond to therapy with diethylcarbamazine even in the absence of microfilariae in synovial fluid. Reactive arthritis has been attributed to hookworm, *Strongyloides*, *Cryptosporidium*, and *Giardia* infection in case reports, but confirmation is required.

POSTINFECTIOUS OR REACTIVE ARTHRITIS

Reactive polyarthritis develops several weeks after ~1% of cases of nongonococcal urethritis and 2% of enteric infections, particularly those due to *Yersinia enterocolitica*, *Shigella flexneri*, *Campylobacter jejuni*, and *Salmonella* species. Only a minority of these patients have the other findings of classic reactive arthritis, including urethritis, conjunctivitis, uveitis, oral ulcers, and rash. Studies have identified microbial DNA or antigen in synovial fluid or blood, but the pathogenesis of this condition is poorly understood.

Reactive arthritis is most common among young men (except after *Yersinia* infection) and has been linked to the HLA-B27 locus as a potential genetic predisposing factor. Patients report painful, asymmetric oligoarthritis that affects mainly the knees, ankles, and feet. Low-back pain is common, and radiographic evidence of sacroiliitis is found in patients with long-standing disease. Most patients recover within 6 months, but prolonged recurrent disease is more common in cases that follow chlamydial urethritis. Anti-inflammatory agents help relieve symptoms, but the role of prolonged antibiotic therapy in eliminating microbial antigen from the synovium is controversial.

Migratory polyarthritis and fever constitute the usual presentation of acute rheumatic fever in adults (Chap. 381). This presentation is distinct from that of poststreptococcal reactive arthritis, which also follows infections with group A *Streptococcus* but is not migratory, lasts beyond the typical 3-week maximum of acute rheumatic fever, and responds poorly to aspirin.

INFECTIONS IN PROSTHETIC JOINTS

Infection complicates 1–4% of total joint replacements. The majority of infections are acquired intraoperatively or immediately postoperatively as a result of wound breakdown or infection; less commonly, these joint infections develop later after joint replacement and are the result of hematogenous spread or direct inoculation. The presentation may be acute, with fever, pain, and local signs of inflammation, especially in infections due to *S. aureus*, pyogenic streptococci, and enteric bacilli. Alternatively, infection may persist for months or years without causing constitutional symptoms when less virulent organisms, such as coagulase-negative staphylococci or diphtheroids, are involved. Such indolent infections usually are acquired during joint implantation and are discovered during evaluation of chronic unexplained pain or after a radiograph shows loosening of the prosthesis; the erythrocyte sedimentation rate and C-reactive protein level are usually elevated in such cases.

The diagnosis is best made by needle aspiration of the joint; accidental introduction of organisms during aspiration must be avoided meticulously. Synovial fluid pleocytosis with a predominance of polymorphonuclear leukocytes is highly suggestive of infection, since other inflammatory processes uncommonly affect prosthetic joints. Culture and Gram's stain usually yield the responsible pathogen. Sonication of explanted prosthetic material can improve the yield of culture, presumably by breaking up bacterial biofilms on the surfaces of prostheses. Use of special media for unusual pathogens such as fungi, atypical mycobacteria, and *Mycoplasma* may be necessary if routine and anaerobic cultures are negative.

TREATMENT PROSTHETIC JOINT INFECTIONS

Treatment includes surgery and high doses of parenteral antibiotics, which are given for 4–6 weeks because bone is usually involved. In most cases, the prosthesis must be replaced to cure the infection. Implantation of a new prosthesis is best delayed for several weeks or months because relapses of infection occur most commonly within this time frame. In some cases, reimplantation is not possible, and the patient must manage without a joint, with a fused joint, or even with amputation. Cure of infection without removal of the prosthesis is occasionally possible in cases that are due to streptococci or pneumococci and that lack radiologic evidence of loosening of the prosthesis. In these cases, antibiotic therapy must be initiated within several days of the onset of infection, and the joint should be drained vigorously by open arthrotomy or arthroscopically. In selected patients who prefer to avoid the high morbidity rate associated with joint removal and reimplantation, suppression of the infection with antibiotics may be a reasonable goal. A high cure rate with retention of the prosthesis has been reported when the combination of oral rifampin and ciprofloxacin is given for 3–6 months to persons with staphylococcal prosthetic joint infection of short duration. This approach, which is based on the ability of rifampin to kill organisms adherent to foreign material and in the stationary growth phase, requires confirmation in prospective trials.

PREVENTION

To avoid the disastrous consequences of infection, candidates for joint replacement should be selected with care. Rates of infection are particularly high among patients with rheumatoid arthritis, persons who have undergone previous surgery on the joint, and persons with medical conditions requiring immunosuppressive therapy. Perioperative antibiotic prophylaxis, usually with cefazolin, and measures to decrease intraoperative contamination, such as laminar flow, have lowered the rates of perioperative infection to <1% in many centers. After implantation, measures should be taken to prevent or rapidly treat extra-articular infections that might give rise to hematogenous spread to the prosthesis. The effectiveness of prophylactic antibiotics for the prevention of hematogenous infection after dental procedures has not been demonstrated; in fact, viridans streptococci and other components of the oral flora are extremely unusual causes of prosthetic joint infection. Accordingly, the American Dental Association and the American Academy of Orthopaedic Surgeons do not recommend antibiotic prophylaxis for most dental patients with total joint replacements and have stated that there is no convincing evidence to support its use. Similarly, guidelines issued by the American Urological Association and the American Academy of Orthopaedic Surgeons do not recommend the use of prophylactic antibiotics for most patients with prosthetic joints who are undergoing urologic procedures but state that prophylaxis should be considered in certain situations—e.g., for patients (especially immunocompromised patients) who are undergoing a procedure posing a relatively high risk of bacteremia (such as lithotripsy or surgery involving bowel segments).

Acknowledgments

The contributions of James H. Maguire and the late Scott J. Thaler to this chapter in earlier editions are gratefully acknowledged.

158 Osteomyelitis

Werner Zimmerli

Osteomyelitis, an infection of bone, can be caused by various microorganisms that arrive at bone through different routes. Spontaneous hematogenous osteomyelitis may occur in otherwise healthy individuals, whereas local microbial spread mainly affects either individuals who have underlying disease (e.g., vascular insufficiency) or patients who have compromised skin or other tissue barriers, with consequent exposure of bone. The latter situation typically follows surgery involving bone, such as sternotomy or orthopedic repair.

The manifestations of osteomyelitis are different in children and adults. In children circulating microorganisms seed mainly long bones, whereas in adults the vertebral column is the most commonly affected site.

Management of osteomyelitis differs greatly depending on whether an implant is involved. The most important aim of the management of either type of osteomyelitis is to prevent progression to chronic osteomyelitis by rapid diagnosis and prompt treatment. Device-related bone and joint infection necessitates a multidisciplinary approach requiring antibiotic therapy and, in many cases, surgical removal of the device. The optimal duration of antibiotic treatment has not been established for any type of osteomyelitis in clinical trials. Therefore, the recommendations for therapy in this chapter reflect only expert opinions.

CLASSIFICATION

There is no generally accepted, comprehensive system for classification of osteomyelitis, primarily because of the multifaceted presentation of this infection. Different specialists are confronted with different facets of bone disease. Most often, however, general practitioners or internists are the first to encounter patients with the initial signs and symptoms of osteomyelitis. These primary care physicians should be able to recognize this disease in any of its forms. Osteomyelitis cases can be classified by various criteria, including pathogenesis, duration of infection, location of infection, and presence or absence of foreign material. The widely used Cierny-Mader staging system classifies osteomyelitis according to anatomic site, comorbidity, and radiographic findings, with stratification of long-bone osteomyelitis to optimize surgical management; this system encompasses both systemic and local factors affecting immune status, metabolism, and local vascularity.

Any of three mechanisms can underlie osteomyelitis: (1) hematogenous spread; (2) spread from a contiguous site following surgery; and (3) secondary infection in the setting of vascular insufficiency or concomitant neuropathy. Hematogenous osteomyelitis in adults typically involves the vertebral column. In only about half of patients can a primary focus be detected. The most common primary foci of infection are the urinary tract, skin/soft tissue, intravascular catheterization sites, and the endocardium. Spread from a contiguous source follows either bone trauma or surgical intervention. Wound infection leading to osteomyelitis typically occurs after cardiovascular intervention involving the sternum, orthopedic repair, or prosthetic joint insertion. Osteomyelitis secondary to vascular insufficiency or peripheral neuropathy most often follows chronic, progressively deep skin and soft tissue infection of the foot. The most common underlying condition is diabetes. In diabetes that is poorly controlled, the *diabetic foot syndrome* is caused by skin, soft tissue, and bone ischemia combined with motor, sensory, and autonomic neuropathy.

Classification of osteomyelitis according to the duration of infection, although ill defined (because there is no clear time limit for the transition from acute to chronic osteomyelitis), is useful because the management of acute and chronic osteomyelitis differs. Whereas acute osteomyelitis can generally be treated with antibiotics alone, antibiotic treatment for chronic osteomyelitis should be combined with debridement surgery. Acute hematogenous or contiguous osteomyelitis evolves over a short period—i.e., a few days or weeks. In contrast, subacute or chronic osteomyelitis lasts for weeks or months before treatment is started. Typical examples of a subacute course are vertebral osteomyelitis due to tuberculosis or brucellosis and delayed implant-associated infections caused mainly by low-virulence microorganisms (coagulase-negative staphylococci, *Propionibacterium acnes*). Chronic osteomyelitis develops when insufficient therapy leads to persistence or recurrence, most often after sternal, mandibular, or foot infection.

Classification by location distinguishes among cases in the long bones, the vertebral column, and the periarticular bones. Long bones are generally involved after hematogenous seeding in children or contiguous spread following trauma or surgery. The risk of vertebral osteomyelitis in adults increases with age. Periarticular osteomyelitis, which complicates septic arthritis that has not been adequately treated, is especially common in periprosthetic joint infection.

Osteomyelitis involving a foreign device requires surgical management for cure. Even acute implant-associated infection calls for prolonged antimicrobial therapy. Therefore, identification of this type of disease is of practical importance.

VERTEBRAL OSTEOMYELITIS

PATHOGENESIS

Vertebral osteomyelitis, also referred to as disk-space infection, septic diskitis, spondylodiskitis, or spinal osteomyelitis, is the most common manifestation of hematogenous bone infection in adults. This designation reflects a pathogenic process leading to involvement of the adjacent vertebrae and the corresponding intervertebral disk. In adults, the disk is avascular. Microorganisms invade via the segmental arterial circulation in adjacent endplates and then spread into the disk. Alternative routes of infection are retrograde seeding through the prevertebral venous plexus and direct inoculation during spinal surgery, epidural infiltration, or trauma. In the setting of implant surgery, microorganisms are inoculated either during the procedure or, if wound healing is impaired, in the early postoperative period.

EPIDEMIOLOGY

Vertebral osteomyelitis occurs more often in male than in female patients (ratio, 1.5:1). The overall incidence is 2.4 cases/100,000 population. There is a clear age-dependent increase from 0.3 cases/100,000 at ages <20 years to 6.5 cases/100,000 at ages >70 years. The observed increase in reported cases during the past two decades may reflect improvements in diagnosis resulting from the broad availability of MRI technology. In addition, the fraction of cases of vertebral osteomyelitis acquired in association with health care is certainly increasing as a consequence of the rising number of spinal interventions and local infiltrations.

MICROBIOLOGY

Vertebral osteomyelitis is typically classified as pyogenic or nonpyogenic. However, this distinction is arbitrary because, in "nonpyogenic" cases (tuberculous, brucellar), macroscopic pus formation (caseous necrosis, abscess) is quite common. A more accurate scheme is to classify cases as acute or subacute/chronic. Whereas the microbiologic spectrum of acute cases is similar in different parts of the world, the spectrum of subacute/chronic cases varies according to the geographic region. The great majority of cases are monomicrobial in etiology. Of episodes of acute vertebral osteomyelitis, 40–50% are caused by *Staphylococcus aureus*, 12% by streptococci, and 20% by gram-negative bacilli—mainly *Escherichia coli* (9%) and *Pseudomonas aeruginosa* (6%). Subacute vertebral osteomyelitis is typically caused by *Mycobacterium tuberculosis* or *Brucella* species in regions where these microorganisms are endemic. Osteomyelitis due to viridans streptococci also has a subacute presentation; these infections most often occur as secondary foci in patients with endocarditis. In vertebral osteomyelitis due to *Candida* species, the diagnosis is often delayed by several weeks; this etiology should be suspected in IV drug users who do not use sterile paraphernalia. In implant-associated spinal osteomyelitis, coagulase-negative staphylococci and *P. acnes*—which, in the absence of an implant, are generally considered contaminants—typically cause low-grade (chronic) infections. As an exception, coagulase-negative staphylococci can cause native spinal osteomyelitis in cases of prolonged bacteremia (e.g., in patients with infected pacemaker electrodes or implanted vascular catheters that are not promptly removed).

CLINICAL MANIFESTATIONS

The signs and symptoms of vertebral osteomyelitis are nonspecific. Only about half of patients develop fever >38°C (100.4°F), perhaps because analgesic drugs are frequently used by these patients. Back pain is the leading initial symptom (>85% of cases). The location of the pain corresponds to the site of infection: the cervical spine in ~10% of cases, the thoracic spine in 30%, and the lumbar spine in 60%. One exception is involvement at the thoracic level in two-thirds of cases of tuberculous osteomyelitis and at the lumbar level in only one-third. This difference is due to direct mycobacterial spread via pleural or mediastinal lymph nodes in pulmonary tuberculosis.

Neurologic deficits, such as radiculopathy, weakness, or sensory loss, are observed in about one-third of cases of vertebral osteomyelitis. In brucellar vertebral osteomyelitis, neurologic impairment is less frequent; in tuberculous osteomyelitis, it is about twice as frequent as in cases of other etiologies. Neurologic signs and symptoms are caused mostly by spinal epidural abscess. This complication starts with severe localized back pain and progresses to radicular pain, reflex changes, sensory abnormalities, motor weakness, bowel and bladder dysfunction, and paralysis.

A primary focus should always be sought but is found in only half of cases. Overall, endocarditis is identified in ~10% of patients. In osteomyelitis caused by viridans streptococci, endocarditis is the source in about half of patients.

Implant-associated spinal osteomyelitis can present as either early- or late-onset infection. Early-onset infection is diagnosed within 30 days after implant placement. *S. aureus* is the most common pathogen. Wound healing impairment and fever are the leading findings. Late-onset infection is diagnosed beyond 30 days after surgery, with low-virulence organisms such as coagulase-negative staphylococci or *P. acnes* as typical infecting agents. Fever is rare. One-quarter of patients have a sinus tract. Because of the delayed course and the lack of classic signs of infection, rapid diagnosis requires a high degree of suspicion.

DIAGNOSIS

Leukocytosis and neutrophilia have low levels of diagnostic sensitivity (only 65% and 40%, respectively). In contrast, an increased erythrocyte sedimentation rate or C-reactive protein (CRP) level has been reported in 98% and 100% of cases, respectively; thus, these tests are helpful in excluding vertebral osteomyelitis. The fraction of blood cultures that yield positive results depends heavily on whether the patient has been pretreated with antibiotics; across studies, the range is from 30% to 78%. In view of this low rate of positive blood culture after antibiotic treatment, such therapy should be withheld until microbial growth is proven unless the patient has sepsis syndrome. In patients with negative blood cultures, CT-guided or open biopsy is needed. Whether a CT-guided biopsy with a negative result is repeated or followed by open biopsy depends on the experience of personnel at the specific center. Bone samples should be cultured for aerobic, anaerobic, and fungal agents, with a portion of the sample sent for histopathologic study. In cases with a subacute/chronic presentation, a suggestive history, or a granuloma detected during histopathologic analysis, mycobacteria and brucellae also should be sought. When blood and tissue cultures are negative despite suggestive histopathology, broad-range polymerase chain reaction analysis of biopsy specimens or aspirated pus should be considered. This technique allows detection of unusual pathogens such as *Tropheryma whipplei*.

Given that signs and symptoms of osteomyelitis are nonspecific, the clinical differential diagnosis of febrile back pain is broad, including pyelonephritis, pancreatitis, and viral syndromes. In addition, multiple noninfectious pathologies of the vertebral column, such as osteoporotic fracture, seronegative spondylitis (ankylosing spondylitis, psoriasis, reactive arthritis, enteropathic arthritis), and spinal stenosis must be considered.

Imaging procedures are the most important tools not only for the diagnosis of vertebral osteomyelitis but also for the detection of pyogenic complications and alternative conditions (e.g., bone metastases or osteoporotic fractures). Plain radiography is a reasonable first step in evaluating patients without neurologic symptoms and may reveal an alternative diagnosis. Because of its low sensitivity, plain radiography generally is not helpful in acute osteomyelitis, but it can be useful in subacute or chronic cases. The gold standard is MRI, which should be performed expeditiously in patients with neurologic impairment in order to rule out a herniated disk or to detect pyogenic complications in a timely manner. Even if the pathologic findings on MRI suggest vertebral osteomyelitis, alternative diagnoses should be considered, especially when blood cultures are negative. The most common alternative diagnosis is erosive osteochondrosis. Septic bone necrosis, gouty spondylodiskitis, and erosive diskovertebral lesions (Andersson lesions) in ankylosing spondylitis may likewise mimic vertebral osteomyelitis. CT is less sensitive than MRI but may be helpful in guiding a percutaneous biopsy. In the future, positron-emission tomography (PET) with ^{18}F-fluorodeoxyglucose, which has a high degree of diagnostic accuracy, may be an alternative imaging procedure when MRI is contraindicated. ^{18}F-fluorodeoxyglucose PET should be considered for patients with implants and patients in whom several foci are suspected.

TREATMENT VERTEBRAL OSTEOMYELITIS

The aims of therapy for vertebral osteomyelitis are (1) elimination of the pathogen(s), (2) protection from further bone loss, (3) relief of back pain, (4) prevention of complications, and (5) stabilization, if needed.

ANTIMICROBIAL THERAPY

Table 158-1 summarizes suggested antimicrobial regimens for infections attributable to the most common etiologic agents. For optimal antimicrobial therapy, identification of the infecting agent is required. Therefore, in patients without sepsis syndrome, antibiotics should not be administered until the pathogen is identified in a blood culture, a bone biopsy, or an aspirated pus collection. Traditionally, bone infections are at least initially treated by the IV route. Unfortunately, relevant controlled trials are lacking, and the preference for the IV route is not evidence based. There are no good arguments for the assumption that IV therapy is superior to oral administration if the following requirements are met: (1) optimal antibiotic spectrum, (2) excellent bioavailability of the oral drug, (3) clinical studies confirming efficacy of the oral drug, (4) normal intestinal function, and (5) no vomiting. However, a short initial course of parenteral therapy with a β-lactam antibiotic may lower the risk of emergence of fluoroquinolone resistance, especially if *P. aeruginosa* infection is treated with ciprofloxacin or staphylococcal infection with the combination of a fluoroquinolone plus rifampin. These suggestions are based on observational studies and expert opinion. There are no data from controlled trials on the optimal duration of therapy. Most experts suggest 6 weeks for patients

TABLE 158-1 ANTIBIOTIC THERAPY FOR OSTEOMYELITIS IN ADULTS WITHOUT IMPLANTS[a]

Microorganism	Antimicrobial Agent (Dose,[b] Route)
Staphylococcus spp.	
Methicillin-susceptible	Nafcillin *or* oxacillin[c] (2 g IV q6h)
	followed by
	Rifampin (300–450 mg PO q12h) *plus* levofloxacin (750 mg PO q24h or 500 mg PO q12h)
Methicillin-resistant	Vancomycin[d] (15 mg/kg IV q12h) *or* daptomycin (>6–8 mg/kg IV q24h)
	followed by
	Rifampin (300–450 mg PO q12h)
	plus
	Levofloxacin (750 mg PO q24h or 500 mg PO q12h) *or* TMP-SMX[e] (1 double-strength tablet PO q8h) *or* fusidic acid (500 mg PO q8h)
Streptococcus spp.	Penicillin G[c] (5 million units IV q6h) *or* ceftriaxone (2 g IV q24h)
Enterobacteriaceae	
Quinolone-susceptible	Ciprofloxacin (750 mg PO q24h)
Quinolone-resistant[f]	Imipenem (500 mg IV q6h)
Pseudomonas aeruginosa	Cefepime *or* ceftazidime (2 g IV q8h) *plus* an aminoglycoside[g]
	or
	Piperacillin-tazobactam (4.5 g IV q8h) *plus* an aminoglycoside[g] for 2–4 weeks
	followed by
	Ciprofloxacin[h] (750 mg PO q12h)
Anaerobes	Clindamycin (600 mg IV q6–8h) for 2–4 weeks
	followed by
	Clindamycin[i] (300 mg PO q6h)

[a]Unless otherwise indicated, the total duration of antimicrobial treatment is generally 6 weeks. [b]All dosages are for adults with normal renal function. [c]When the patient has delayed-type penicillin hypersensitivity, cefuroxime (1.5 g IV q6–8h) can be administered. When the patient has immediate-type penicillin hypersensitivity, the penicillin should be replaced by vancomycin (1 g IV q12h). [d]Target vancomycin trough level: 15–20 μg/mL. [e]Trimethoprim-sulfamethoxazole. A double-strength tablet contains 160 mg of trimethoprim and 800 mg of sulfamethoxazole. [f]Including isolates producing extended-spectrum β-lactamase. [g]The need for addition of an aminoglycoside has not yet been proven. However, this addition may decrease the risk of emergence of resistance to the β-lactam. [h]The rationale for starting ciprofloxacin treatment only after pretreatment with a β-lactam is the increased risk of emergence of quinolone resistance in the presence of a heavy bacterial load. [i]Alternatively, penicillin G (5 million units IV q6h) or ceftriaxone (2 g IV q24h) can be used against gram-positive anaerobes (e.g., *Propionibacterium acnes*), and metronidazole (500 mg IV/PO q8h) can be used against gram-negative anaerobes (e.g., *Bacteroides* spp.).

who have acute osteomyelitis without an implant. According to an observational study, prolonging antibiotic therapy beyond 6 weeks does not improve the rate of recovery or lower the risk of recurrence. However, prolonged antibiotic therapy is recommended for patients with abscesses that have not been drained and patients with spinal implants. Treatment efficacy should be regularly monitored through inquiries about signs and symptoms (fever, pain) and assessment for signs of inflammation (elevated CRP concentrations). Follow-up MRI is appropriate only for patients with pyogenic complications, since the correlation between clinical healing and improvement on MRI is very poor.

Surgical treatment generally is not needed in acute hematogenous vertebral osteomyelitis. However, it is always necessary in implant-associated spinal infection. Early infections (those occurring up to 30 days after internal stabilization) can be cured with debridement, implant retention, and a 3-month course of antibiotics (**Table 158-2**). In contrast, in late infection with a duration of >30 days, implant removal and a 6-week-course of antibiotics (Table 158-1)

TABLE 158-2 ANTIBIOTIC THERAPY FOR OSTEOMYELITIS ASSOCIATED WITH ORTHOPEDIC DEVICES

Microorganism	Antimicrobial Agent[a] (Dose, Route)
Staphylococcus spp.	*Recommendation for initial treatment phase (2 weeks with implant)*
Methicillin-susceptible	Rifampin (450 mg PO/IV q12h[b])
	plus
	Nafcillin *or* oxacillin[c] (2 g IV q6h)
Methicillin-resistant	Rifampin (450 mg PO/IV q12h[b])
	plus
	Vancomycin (15 mg/kg IV q12h) *or* daptomycin (6–8 mg/kg IV q24h)
Staphylococcus spp.	*Recommendation after completion of initial treatment phase*
	Rifampin (450 mg PO q12h[b])
	plus
	Levofloxacin (750 mg PO q24h or 500 mg PO q12h *or* ciprofloxacin (750 mg PO q12h) *or* fusidic acid (500 mg PO q8h) *or* TMP-SMX[d] (1 double-strength tablet PO q8h) *or* minocycline (100 mg PO q12h) *or* linezolid (600 mg PO q12h) *or* clindamycin (1200–1350 mg/d PO in 3 or 4 divided doses)
Streptococcus spp.[e]	Penicillin G[c] (18–24 million units/d IV in 6 divided doses) *or* ceftriaxone (2 g IV q24h) for 4 weeks
	followed by
	Amoxicillin (750–1000 mg PO q6–8h) *or* clindamycin (1200–1350 mg/d PO in 3 or 4 divided doses)
Enterococcus spp.[f]	
Penicillin-susceptible	Penicillin G[c] (24 million units/d IV in 6 divided doses) *or* ampicillin or amoxicillin[g] (2 g IV q4–6h)
Penicillin-resistant	Vancomycin (15 mg/kg IV q12h) *or* daptomycin (6–8 mg/kg IV q24h) *or* linezolid (600 mg IV/PO q12h)
Enterobacteriaceae	A β-lactam selected in light of in vitro susceptibility profile for 2 weeks[h]
	followed by
	Ciprofloxacin (750 mg PO q12h)
Enterobacter spp.[i] and nonfermenters[j] (e.g., *Pseudomonas aeruginosa*)	Cefepime or ceftazidime (2 g IV q8h) *or* meropenem (1 g IV q8h[k]) for 2–4 weeks
	followed by
	Ciprofloxacin (750 mg PO q12h)
Propionibacterium spp.	Penicillin G[c] (18–24 million units/d IV in 6 divided doses) *or* clindamycin (600–900 mg IV q8h) for 2–4 weeks
	followed by
	Amoxicillin (750–1000 mg PO q6–8h) *or* clindamycin (1200–1350 mg/d PO in 3 or 4 divided doses)
Gram-negative anaerobes (e.g., *Bacteroides* spp.)	Metronidazole (500 mg IV/PO q8h)
Mixed bacteria (without methicillin-resistant staphylococci)	Ampicillin-sulbactam (3 g IV q6h) *or* amoxicillin-clavulanate[l] (2.2 g IV q6h) *or* piperacillin-tazobactam (4.5 g IV q8h) *or* imipenem (500 mg IV q6h) *or* meropenem (1 g IV q8h[k]) for 2–4 weeks
	followed by
	Individualized oral regimens chosen in light of antimicrobial susceptibility

[a]Antimicrobial agents should be chosen in light of the isolate's in vitro susceptibility, the patient's drug allergies and intolerances, potential drug interactions, and contraindications to specific drugs. All dosages recommended are for adults with normal renal and hepatic function. See text for total durations of antibiotic treatment. [b]Other dosages and intervals of administration with equivalent success rates have been reported. [c]When the patient has delayed-type penicillin hypersensitivity, cefazolin (2 g IV q8h) can be administered. When the patient has immediate-type penicillin hypersensitivity, the penicillin should be replaced by vancomycin (1 g IV q12h). [d]Trimethoprim-sulfamethoxazole. A double-strength tablet contains 160 mg of trimethoprim and 800 mg of sulfamethoxazole. [e]Determination of the minimal inhibitory concentration (MIC) of penicillin is advisable. [f]Combination therapy with an aminoglycoside is optional since its superiority to monotherapy for prosthetic joint infection is unproved. When using combination therapy, monitor signs of aminoglycoside ototoxicity and nephrotoxicity; the latter is potentiated by other nephrotoxic agents (e.g., vancomycin). [g]For patients with hypersensitivity to penicillin, see treatment options for penicillin-resistant enterococci. [h]Ciprofloxacin (PO or IV) can be administered to patients with hypersensitivity to β-lactams. [i]Ceftriaxone and ceftazidime should not be administered for treatment targeting *Enterobacter* species, even strains that test susceptible in the laboratory, but can be used against nonfermenters. Strains producing extended-spectrum β-lactamases should not be treated with any cephalosporin, including cefepime. *Enterobacter* infections can also be treated with ertapenem (1 g IV q24h); however, ertapenem is not effective against *Pseudomonas* spp. and other nonfermenters. [j]Addition of an aminoglycoside is optional. Use of two active drugs can be considered in light of the patient's clinical condition. [k]The recommended dosage is in line with the guidelines of the Infectious Diseases Society of America. In Europe, 2 g IV q8h is suggested for *P. aeruginosa* infections. [l]Not available as an IV formulation in the United States.

Source: Modified from W Zimmerli et al: N Engl J Med 351:1645, 2004. © Massachusetts Medical Society. Reprinted with permission.

are required for complete elimination of the infection. If implants cannot be removed, oral suppressive long-term treatment should follow the initial course of IV antibiotics. The optimal duration of suppressive therapy is unknown. However, if antibiotic therapy is discontinued after, for example, 1 year, close clinical and laboratory (CRP) follow-up is needed.

COMPLICATIONS

Complications include persistent pain, persistently increased CRP levels, and new-onset or persistent neurologic impairment. In cases of persistent pain with or without signs of inflammation, paravertebral, epidural, or psoas abscesses (Fig. 158-1) must be sought. Epidural abscesses occur in 15–20% of cases. This complication is more common in the cervical column (30%) than in the lumbar spine (12%). Persistent pain despite normalization of CRP values indicates mechanical complications such as severe osteonecrosis or spinal instability. These patients require a consult with an experienced orthopedic surgeon.

OSTEOMYELITIS IN LONG BONES

PATHOGENESIS

Osteomyelitis in long bones is a consequence of hematogenous seeding, exogenous contamination during trauma (open fracture), or perioperative contamination during orthopedic repairs. Its presentation is either acute (with a duration of days to a few weeks) or chronic. Hematogenous infection in long bones typically occurs in children. Ineffectively treated hematogenous osteomyelitis during childhood can progress to chronic disease. In adults, the leading pathogenic source is exogenous infection, mainly associated with internal fixation

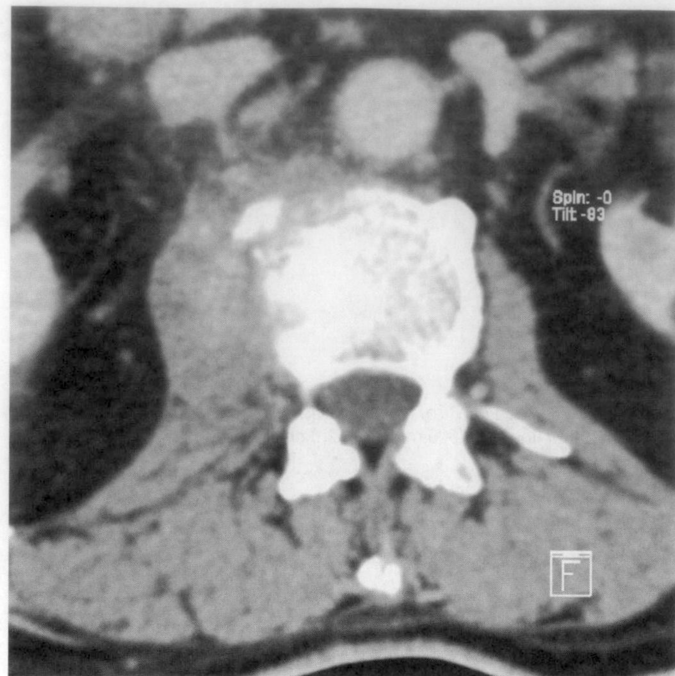

FIGURE 158-1 CT scan of acute vertebral osteomyelitis (L1/L2) due to *Staphylococcus aureus* in a 64-year-old man. Low-grade fever persisted despite appropriate IV antibiotic therapy. The scan revealed a psoas abscess on the right side.

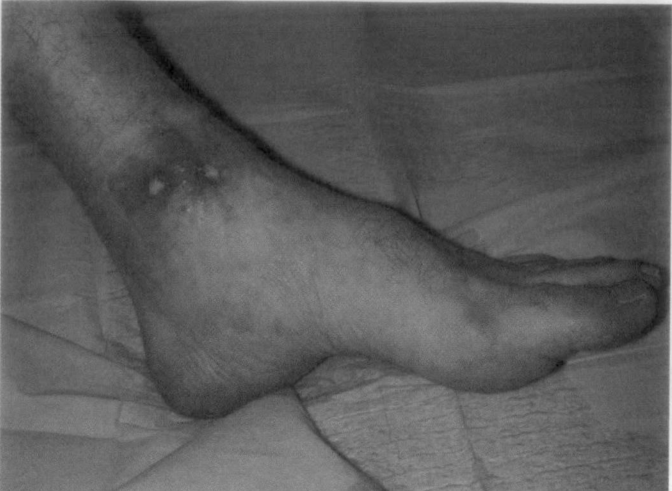

FIGURE 158-2 A 42-year-old man who had had a malleolar fracture 6 weeks previously had persistent pain and slight inflammation after orthopedic repair. His infection was treated with oral antibiotics without debridement surgery. This insufficient management of an implant-associated *Staphylococcus aureus* infection was complicated by a sinus tract.

devices. Chronic osteomyelitis can recur after a symptom-free interval of >50 years. Such recurrences are most common among elderly patients who developed osteomyelitis in the preantibiotic era.

EPIDEMIOLOGY

In adults, most cases of long-bone osteomyelitis are posttraumatic or postsurgical; less frequently, late recurrence arises from hematogenous infections during childhood. The risk of infection depends on the type of fracture. After closed fracture, implant-associated infection occurs in fewer than 1% of patients. In contrast, after open fracture, the risk of osteomyelitis ranges from ~2% up to 16%, with the precise figure depending on the degree of tissue damage during trauma.

MICROBIOLOGY

The spectrum of microorganisms causing hematogenous long-bone osteomyelitis does not differ from that in vertebral osteomyelitis. *S. aureus* is most commonly isolated from adult patients. In rare cases, mycobacteria or fungal agents such as *Cryptococcus* species, *Sporothrix schenckii*, *Blastomyces dermatitidis*, or *Coccidioides* species are found in patients who live or have traveled in endemic regions. Impaired cellular immunity (e.g., in HIV infection or after transplantation) predisposes to these etiologies. Coagulase-negative staphylococci are the second most common etiologic agents (after *S. aureus*) in implant-associated osteomyelitis. After open fracture, contiguous long-bone osteomyelitis is typically caused by gram-negative bacilli or a polymicrobial mixture of organisms.

CLINICAL MANIFESTATIONS

The leading symptoms in adults with primary or recurrent hematogenous long-bone osteomyelitis are pain and low-grade fever. Infection occasionally manifests as clinical sepsis and local signs of inflammation (erythema and swelling). After internal fixation, osteomyelitis can be classified as acute (≤3 weeks) or chronic. Acute long-bone osteomyelitis manifests as signs of surgical site infection, such as erythema and impaired wound healing. Acute implant-associated infection may also follow hematogenous seeding at any time after implantation of a device. Typical symptoms are new-onset pain and signs of sepsis. Chronic infections are usually caused by low-virulence microorganisms or occur after ineffective treatment of early-onset infection. Patients may present with persisting pain, subtle local signs of inflammation, intermittent discharge of pus, or fluctuating erythema over the scar (Fig. 158-2).

DIAGNOSIS

The diagnostic workup for acute hematogenous long-bone osteomyelitis is similar to that for vertebral osteomyelitis. Bone remodeling and thus marker uptake are increased for at least 1 year after surgery. Therefore, the three-phase bone scan is not useful during this interval. However, in late recurrences it allows rapid diagnosis at low cost. If the results are positive, CT is required in order to estimate the extent of inflamed tissue and to detect bone necrosis (sequesters). Implant-associated infection should be suspected if CRP values do not return to the normal range or rise after an initial decrease. Clinical and laboratory suspicion should prompt surgical exploration and sampling.

In chronic osteomyelitis of >1 year's duration, single-photon emission CT plus conventional CT (SPECT/CT) is a good option, either with ^{99m}Tc methylene diphosphonate (^{99m}Tc-MDP)–labeled leukocytes or with labeled monoclonal antibodies to granulocytes. Surgical debridement is needed for diagnostic (biopsy culture, histology) and therapeutic reasons.

TREATMENT OSTEOMYELITIS IN LONG BONES

Treatment for acute hematogenous infection in long bones is identical to that for acute vertebral osteomyelitis (Table 158-1). The suggested duration of antibiotic therapy is 4–6 weeks. In contrast to chronic or implant-associated osteomyelitis, acute hematogenous infection does not require surgical intervention. Initial IV administration of antimicrobial agents is followed by long-term oral treatment. The duration of the initial IV phase of therapy has not been defined. The IV course can be as short as a couple of days if a drug with excellent bioavailability is available. In case of recurrence of chronic osteomyelitis as well as in each type of exogenous osteomyelitis (acute, chronic, with or without an implant), a combination of surgical debridement, obliteration of dead space, and long-term antibiotic therapy is needed.

The therapeutic aims in patients whose infections are associated with internal fixation devices are consolidation of the fracture and prevention of chronic osteomyelitis. Stable implants can be maintained except in patients with uncontrolled sepsis. Appropriate antimicrobial therapies are listed in Table 158-2. The cure rate for early staphylococcal implant-associated infections treated with a fluoroquinolone plus rifampin is >90%. Rifampin is efficacious against staphylococcal biofilms of ≤3 weeks' duration. Similarly, fluoroquinolones are active against biofilms formed by gram-negative bacilli. In these cases, an initial 2-week course of IV therapy with a β-lactam is suggested in order to minimize the risk of emergence of resistance to the oral drugs. The total duration of treatment is 3 months, and the device can be retained even after antibiotics have been discontinued. In contrast, in cases caused by rifampin-resistant staphylococci or fluoroquinolone-resistant gram-negative bacilli, the hardware should be removed after consolidation of the fracture and before discontinuation of antibiotics. These patients are treated with an oral antibiotic (suppressive therapy) as long as retention of the hardware is necessary.

COMPLICATIONS

The main complication of long-bone osteomyelitis is the persistence of infection with progression to chronic osteomyelitis. This risk is especially high after internal fixation of an open fracture and among patients with implant-associated osteomyelitis that is treated without surgical debridement. In chronic osteomyelitis, recurrent sinus tracts result in severe damage to skin and soft tissue (Fig. 158-2). Patients who have chronic open wounds need a therapeutic approach combining orthopedic repair and plastic reconstructive surgery.

PERIPROSTHETIC JOINT INFECTION

PATHOGENESIS

Implanted foreign material is highly susceptible to local infection due to local immunodeficiency around the device. Infection occurs by either the exogenous or the hematogenous route. More rarely, contiguous spread from adjacent sites of osteomyelitis or deep soft-tissue infection may cause periprosthetic joint infection (PJI). The fact that foreign devices are covered with host proteins such as fibronectin favors the adherence of staphylococci and the formation of a biofilm that resists phagocytosis.

EPIDEMIOLOGY

The risk of infection manifesting during the first 2 postoperative years varies according to the joint. It is lowest after hip and knee arthroplasty (0.3–1.5%) and highest after ankle and elbow replacement (4–10%). The risk of hematogenous PJI is highest in the early postoperative period. However, hematogenous seeding occurs throughout life, and most cases therefore develop >2 years after implantation.

MICROBIOLOGY

About 70% of cases of PJI are caused by staphylococci (*S. aureus* and coagulase-negative staphylococci), 10% by streptococci, 10% by gram-negative bacilli, and the rest by various other microorganisms. All microorganisms can cause PJI, including fungi and mycobacteria. *P. acnes* causes up to one-third of episodes of periprosthetic shoulder infection.

CLASSIFICATION AND CLINICAL MANIFESTATIONS

PJI is traditionally classified as early (<3 months after implantation), delayed (3–24 months after surgery), or late (>2 years after implantation). For therapeutic decision-making (see below), it is more useful to classify PJI as (1) acute hematogenous PJI with <3 weeks of symptoms, (2) early postinterventional PJI manifesting within 1 month after surgery, and (3) chronic PJI with symptom duration of >3 weeks.

Acute exogenous PJI typically presents with local signs of infection (Fig. 158-3). In contrast, acute hematogenous PJI, most often caused by *S. aureus*, is characterized by new-onset pain that initially is not accompanied by prominent local inflammatory signs. In most cases, an ongoing sepsis syndrome dominates the clinical picture. Key findings in chronic PJI are joint effusion, local pain, implant loosening, and occasionally a sinus tract. Chronic PJI is most commonly caused by low-virulence microorganisms such as coagulase-negative staphylococci or *P. acnes*. These infections are characterized by nonspecific symptoms, such as chronic pain caused by low-grade inflammation or early loosening.

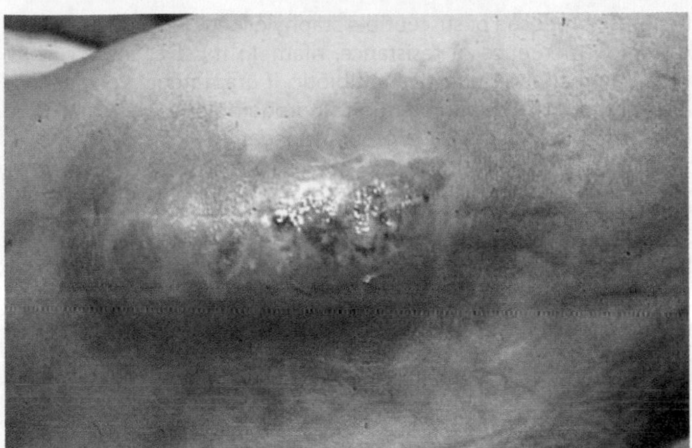

FIGURE 158-3 Early periprosthetic joint infection of the left hip caused by group B streptococci in a 68-year-old woman.

DIAGNOSIS

Blood tests such as the measurement of CRP (elevated levels, ≥10 mg/L) and erythrocyte sedimentation rate (elevated rates, ≥30 mm/h) are sensitive (91–97%) but not specific (70–78%). Synovial fluid cell counts are ~90% sensitive and specific, with threshold values of 1700 leukocytes/μL in periprosthetic knee infection and 4200 leukocytes/μL in periprosthetic hip infection. During debridement surgery, at least three but optimally six tissue samples should be obtained for culture and histopathology. If implant material (modular parts, screws, or the prosthesis) is removed, sonication of this material followed by culture and/or use of molecular methods to examine the sonicate fluid allows the detection of microorganisms in biofilms.

The three-phase bone scan is very sensitive for detecting PJI but is not specific. As mentioned above, this test does not differentiate bone remodeling from infection and therefore is not useful during at least the first year after implantation. CT and MRI detect soft tissue infection, prosthetic loosening, and bone erosion, but imaging artifacts caused by metal implants limit their use. ^{18}F-fluorodeoxyglucose PET is an alternative method with fair sensitivity and specificity for the detection of PJI. However, this technique is not yet an established procedure for this purpose.

TREATMENT PERIPROSTHETIC JOINT INFECTION

Treatment of PJI requires a multidisciplinary approach involving an experienced orthopedic surgeon, an infectious disease specialist, a plastic reconstructive surgeon, and a microbiologist. Therefore, most patients are referred to a specialized center. In general, the goal of treatment is cure—i.e., a pain-free functional joint with complete eradication of the infecting pathogen(s). However, for patients with severe comorbidity, lifelong suppressive antimicrobial therapy may be preferred. As a rule, antimicrobial therapy without surgical intervention is not curative but merely suppressive. There are four curative surgical options: debridement and implant retention, one-stage implant exchange, two-stage implant exchange, and implant removal without replacement. Implant retention offers a good chance of infection-free survival (>80%) only if the following conditions are fulfilled: (1) acute infection, (2) stable implant, (3) pathogen susceptible to a biofilm-active antimicrobial agent (see below), and (4) skin and soft tissue in good condition.

Table 158-2 summarizes pathogen-specific antimicrobial therapy for PJI. Initial IV therapy is followed by long-term oral antibiotics. Efficacious treatment is best defined in staphylococcal implant-associated infections. Rifampin exhibits excellent activity against biofilms composed of susceptible staphylococci. Because of the risk of rapid emergence of resistance, rifampin must always be combined with another effective antibiotic. If gram-negative infections are treated with implant retention, fluoroquinolones should be used because of their activity against gram-negative biofilms.

PREVENTION OF HEMATOGENOUS INFECTION

As mentioned above, hematogenous seeding may occur throughout life. This risk is highest during *S. aureus* bacteremia from a distant focus. Therefore, documented bacterial infections should be promptly treated in patients with prosthetic joints. However, according to a large, prospective, case-control study, the risk of prosthetic hip or knee infection is not increased following dental procedures. Therefore, antibiotic prophylaxis is not needed during dental work.

STERNAL OSTEOMYELITIS

PATHOGENESIS

Sternal osteomyelitis occurs primarily after sternal surgery (with the entry of exogenous organisms) and more rarely by hematogenous seeding or contiguous extension from adjacent sites of sternocostal arthritis. Exogenous sternal osteomyelitis after open sternal surgery is also called *deep sternal wound infection*. Exogenous infection may also follow minor sternal trauma, sternal fracture, and manubriosternal septic arthritis. Tuberculous sternal osteomyelitis typically manifests during hematogenous seeding in children or as reactivated infection in adults. Reactivation is sometimes preceded by blunt trauma. In rare cases, tuberculous sternal osteomyelitis is caused by continuous infection from an infected internal mammary lymph node.

EPIDEMIOLOGY

The incidence of poststernotomy wound infection varies from 0.5% to 5%, but figures are even higher among patients with risk factors such as diabetes, obesity, chronic renal failure, emergency surgery, use of bilateral internal mammary arteries, and reexploration for bleeding. Rapid diagnosis and correct management of superficial sternal wound infection prevent its progression to sternal osteomyelitis. Primary (hematogenous) sternal osteomyelitis accounts for only 0.3% of all cases of osteomyelitis. Risk factors are IV drug use, HIV infection, radiotherapy, blunt trauma, cardiopulmonary resuscitation, alcohol abuse, liver cirrhosis, and hemoglobinopathy.

MICROBIOLOGY

Poststernotomy osteomyelitis is generally caused by *S. aureus* (40–50% of cases), coagulase-negative staphylococci (15–30%), enterococci (5–12%), or gram-negative bacilli (15–25%). Fungal infections caused by *Candida* species also play a role. The fact that ~20% of cases are polymicrobial is indicative of exogenous superinfection during therapy. Hematogenous sternal osteomyelitis is caused most commonly by *S. aureus*. Other microorganisms play a role in special populations—e.g., *P. aeruginosa* in IV drug users, *Salmonella* species in individuals with sickle cell anemia, and *M. tuberculosis* in patients from endemic areas who have previously had tuberculosis.

CLINICAL MANIFESTATIONS

Exogenous sternal osteomyelitis manifests as fever, increased local pain, erythema, wound discharge, and sternal instability (Fig. 158-4). Contiguous mediastinitis is a feared complication, occurring in ~10–30% of patients with sternal osteomyelitis. Hematogenous sternal osteomyelitis is characterized by sternal pain, swelling, and erythema. In addition, most patients have systemic signs and symptoms of sepsis.

The differential diagnosis of hematogenous sternal osteomyelitis includes immunologic processes typically presenting as systemic or multifocal inflammation of the sternum or the sternoclavicular or sternocostal joints (e.g., SAPHO [synovitis, acne, pustulosis, hyperostosis, osteitis], vasculitis, and chronic multifocal relapsing osteomyelitis).

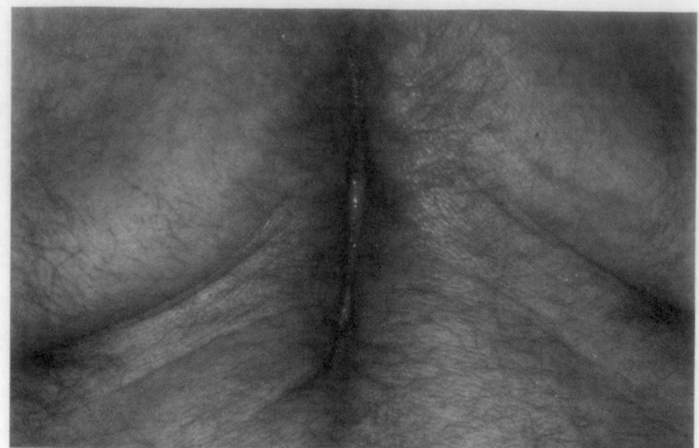

FIGURE 158-4 Sternal osteomyelitis caused by *Staphylococcus epidermidis* 5 weeks after sternotomy for aortocoronary bypass in a 72-year-old man.

DIAGNOSIS

In primary sternal osteomyelitis, the diagnostic workup does not differ from that in other types of hematogenous osteomyelitis (see above). When a patient has grown up in regions where tuberculosis is endemic, a specific workup for mycobacterial infection should be performed, especially if osteomyelitis had its onset after a blunt sternal trauma. In secondary sternal osteomyelitis, leukocyte counts may be normal, but the CRP level is >100 mg/L in most cases. Tissue sampling for microbiologic studies is crucial. In osteomyelitis associated with sternal wires, low-virulence microorganisms, such as coagulase-negative staphylococci, play an important role. In order to differentiate between colonization and infection, samples from at least three deep biopsies should be subjected to microbiologic examination. Superficial swab cultures are not diagnostic and may be misleading. No studies have compared the value of the various imaging modalities in suspected primary sternal osteomyelitis. However, MRI is the current gold standard for detection of each type of osteomyelitis.

TREATMENT STERNAL OSTEOMYELITIS

In cases of deep sternal wound infection, antibiotic therapy should be started immediately after samples have been obtained for microbiologic analyses in order to control clinical sepsis. To protect a newly inserted heart valve, initial treatment should be directed against staphylococci, with consideration of the local susceptibility pattern. In centers with a high prevalence of methicillin-resistant *S. aureus*, vancomycin or daptomycin should be added to a broad-spectrum β-lactam drug. As soon as cultures of blood and/or deep wound biopsies have confirmed the pathogen's identity and susceptibility pattern, treatment should be optimized and narrowed accordingly. Tables 158-1 and 158-2 show appropriate therapeutic choices for the most frequently identified microorganisms causing sternal osteomyelitis in the absence and presence, respectively, of an implanted device. In a recent observational study of patients with staphylococcal deep sternal wound infection, the use of a rifampin-containing regimen was predictive of success. The optimal duration of antibiotic therapy has not been established. In acute sternal osteomyelitis without hardware, a 6-week course is the rule. In patients with remaining sternal wires, treatment duration is generally prolonged to 3 months (Table 158-2). Like other types of tuberculous bone infection, tuberculous sternal osteomyelitis is treated for 6–12 months.

Primary sternal osteomyelitis can generally be treated without surgery. In contrast, in secondary sternal osteomyelitis, debridement is always required. This procedure should be performed by a team of experienced surgeons, since mediastinitis, bone infection, and skin and soft tissue damage may need to be treated during the same intervention.

PROGNOSIS

Primary sternal osteomyelitis poses a minimal mortality risk. In contrast, the in-hospital mortality rates from secondary sternal osteomyelitis are 15–30% after sternal surgery.

FOOT OSTEOMYELITIS

PATHOGENESIS

Osteomyelitis of the foot usually occurs in patients with diabetes, peripheral arterial insufficiency, or peripheral neuropathy and after foot surgery. These entities are often linked to each other, especially in diabetic patients with late complications. However, foot osteomyelitis is also seen in patients with isolated peripheral neuropathy and can manifest as implant-associated osteomyelitis in patients without comorbidity due to a deep wound infection after foot surgery (hallux valgus surgery, arthrodesis, total ankle arthroplasty). Foot osteomyelitis is acquired almost exclusively by the exogenous route. It is a complication of deep pressure ulcers and of impaired wound healing after surgery.

EPIDEMIOLOGY

The incidence of diabetic foot infection is 30–40 cases/1000 persons with diabetes per year. The condition starts with skin and soft tissue lesions and progresses to osteomyelitis, especially in patients with risk factors. About 60–80% of patients with diabetic foot infection have confirmed osteomyelitis. Diabetic foot osteomyelitis increases the risk of amputation. With adequate management of the early stage of diabetic foot infections, the rate of amputation can be lowered.

RISK FACTORS

Risk factors for diabetic foot infection are (1) peripheral motor, sensory, and autonomic neuropathy; (2) neuro-osteoarthropathic deformities (Charcot foot; Fig. 158-5); (3) arterial insufficiency; (4) uncontrolled hyperglycemia; (5) disabilities such as reduced vision; and (6) maladaptive behavior.

MICROBIOLOGY

The correlation between cultures from bone biopsy and those from wound swabs or even deep soft tissue punctures is poor. Consistent results have been found in only 13–43% of cases in various studies. The correlation is better when *S. aureus* is isolated (40–50%) than when anaerobes (20–35%), gram-negative bacilli (20–30%), or coagulase-negative staphylococci (0–20%) are identified. When only bone biopsy samples are considered, the leading pathogens are *S. aureus* (30–40%), anaerobes (10–20%), and various gram-negative bacilli (30–40%). The precise distribution depends on whether the patient already has been treated with antibiotics. Anaerobes are especially prevalent in chronic wounds. Pretreatment typically selects for *P. aeruginosa* or enterococci.

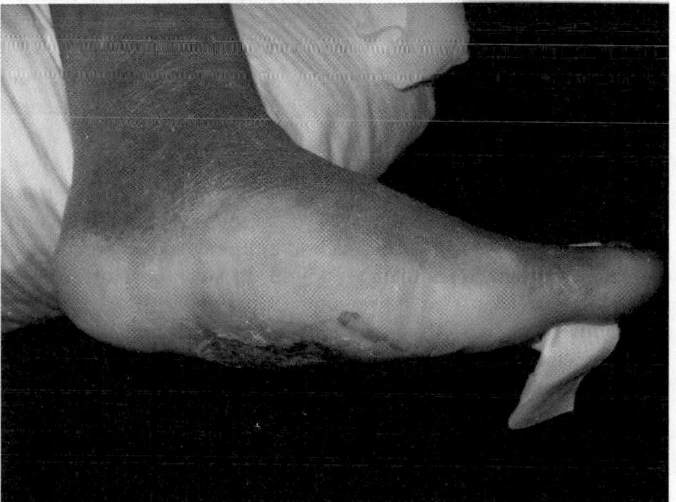

FIGURE 158-5 Neuropathic joint disease (Charcot foot) complicated by chronic foot osteomyelitis in a 78-year old woman with diabetes mellitus complicated by severe neuropathy.

DIAGNOSIS

In many cases, foot osteomyelitis can be diagnosed clinically, without imaging procedures. Most clinicians rely on the "probe-to-bone" test, which has a positive predictive value of ~90% in populations with a high pretest probability. Thus, in a patient with diabetes who is hospitalized for a chronic deep foot ulcer, the diagnosis of foot osteomyelitis is highly probable if bone can be directly touched with a metal instrument. In a patient with a lower pretest probability, MRI should be performed because of its high degree of sensitivity (80–100%) and specificity (80–90%). Plain radiography has a sensitivity of only 30–90% and a specificity of only 50–90%; it may be considered for follow-up of patients with confirmed diabetic foot osteomyelitis.

TREATMENT FOOT OSTEOMYELITIS

As mentioned above, correlation between cultures of bone and those of wound swabs or wound punctures is poor. Antibiotic treatment should be based on bone culture. If no bone biopsy is performed, empirical therapy chosen in light of the most common infecting agents and the type of clinical syndrome should be given. Wound debridement combined with a 4- to 6-week course of antibiotics has been shown to render amputation unnecessary in about two-thirds of patients. According to the 2012 Infectious Diseases Society of America Clinical Practice Guideline for the Diagnosis and Treatment of Diabetic Foot Infections, the following management strategies should be considered. If a foot ulcer is clinically infected, prompt empirical antimicrobial therapy may prevent progression to osteomyelitis. When the risk of methicillin-resistant *S. aureus* is considered high, an agent active against these strains (e.g., vancomycin) should be chosen. If the patient has not recently received antibiotics, the spectrum of the selected antibiotic must include gram-positive cocci (e.g., clindamycin, ampicillin-sulbactam). If the patient has received antibiotics within the past month, the spectrum of empirical antibiotics should include gram-negative bacilli (e.g., clindamycin plus a fluoroquinolone). If the patient has risk factors for *Pseudomonas* infection (previous colonization, residence in a warm climate, frequent exposure of the foot to water), an empirical anti-pseudomonal agent (e.g., piperacillin-tazobactam, cefepime) is indicated. If osteomyelitis is suspected either on clinical grounds (probe to bone) or on the basis of imaging procedures (MRI), bone biopsy should be performed. If not all infected bone is surgically removed, the patient should be treated for 4–6 weeks in line with the identified pathogen(s) and their susceptibility. Treatment should initially be given by the IV route. Whether therapy can later be administered by the oral route depends on the bioavailability of oral drugs that cover the infecting agents. If dead bone cannot be removed, long-term therapy (at least 3 months) should be considered. In such cases, cure of osteomyelitis is usually the exception, and repetitive suppressive treatment may be needed.

159 Intraabdominal Infections and Abscesses

Miriam Baron Barshak, Dennis L. Kasper

Intraperitoneal infections generally arise because a normal anatomic barrier is disrupted. This disruption may occur when the appendix, a diverticulum, or an ulcer ruptures; when the bowel wall is weakened by ischemia, tumor, or inflammation (e.g., in inflammatory bowel disease); or with adjacent inflammatory processes, such as pancreatitis or pelvic inflammatory disease, in which enzymes (in the former case) or organisms (in the latter) may leak into the peritoneal cavity. Whatever the inciting event, once inflammation develops and organisms usually contained within the bowel or another organ enter the normally sterile peritoneal space, a predictable series of events takes place. Intraabdominal infections occur in two stages: peritonitis and—if the patient survives this stage and goes untreated—abscess formation. The types of microorganisms predominating in each stage of infection are responsible for the pathogenesis of disease.

PERITONITIS

Peritonitis is a life-threatening event that is often accompanied by bacteremia and sepsis syndrome (Chap. 325). The peritoneal cavity is large but is divided into compartments. The upper and lower peritoneal cavities are divided by the transverse mesocolon; the greater omentum extends from the transverse mesocolon and from the lower pole of the stomach to line the lower peritoneal cavity. The pancreas, duodenum, and ascending and descending colon are located in the anterior retroperitoneal space; the kidneys, ureters, and adrenals are found in the posterior retroperitoneal space. The other organs, including liver, stomach, gallbladder, spleen, jejunum, ileum, transverse and sigmoid colon, cecum, and appendix, are within the peritoneal cavity. The cavity is lined with a serous membrane that can serve as a conduit for fluids—a property exploited in peritoneal dialysis (Fig. 159-1).

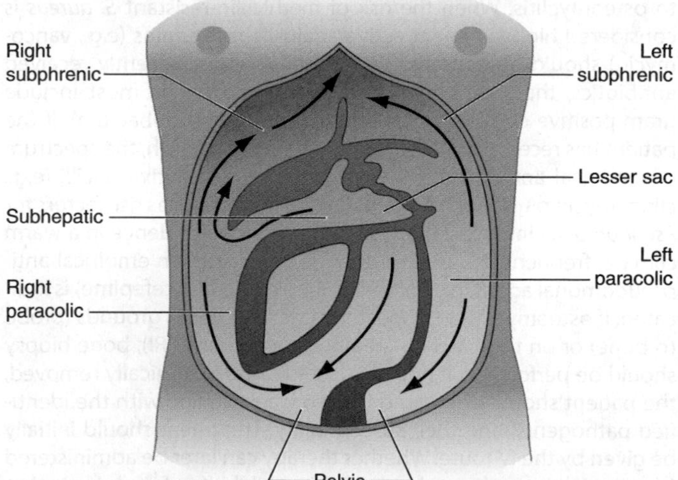

FIGURE 159-1 Diagram of the intraperitoneal spaces, showing the circulation of fluid and potential areas for abscess formation. Some compartments collect fluid or pus more often than others. These compartments include the pelvis (the lowest portion), the subphrenic spaces on the right and left sides, and Morrison's pouch, which is a posterosuperior extension of the subhepatic spaces and is the lowest part of the paravertebral groove when a patient is recumbent. The falciform ligament separating the right and left subphrenic spaces appears to act as a barrier to the spread of infection; consequently, it is unusual to find bilateral subphrenic collections. *(Reprinted with permission from B Lorber [ed]: Atlas of Infectious Diseases, vol VII: Intra-abdominal Infections, Hepatitis, and Gastroenteritis. Philadelphia, Current Medicine, 1996, p 1.13.)*

A small amount of serous fluid is normally present in the peritoneal space, with a protein content (consisting mainly of albumin) of <30 g/L and <300 white blood cells (WBCs, generally mononuclear cells) per microliter. In bacterial infections, leukocyte recruitment into the infected peritoneal cavity consists of an early influx of polymorphonuclear leukocytes (PMNs) and a prolonged subsequent phase of mononuclear cell migration. The phenotype of the infiltrating leukocytes during the course of inflammation is regulated primarily by resident-cell chemokine synthesis.

PRIMARY (SPONTANEOUS) BACTERIAL PERITONITIS

Peritonitis is either primary (without an apparent source of contamination) or secondary. The types of organisms found and the clinical presentations of these two processes are different. In adults, primary bacterial peritonitis (PBP) occurs most commonly in conjunction with cirrhosis of the liver (frequently the result of alcoholism). However, the disease has been reported in adults with metastatic malignant disease, postnecrotic cirrhosis, chronic active hepatitis, acute viral hepatitis, congestive heart failure, systemic lupus erythematosus, and lymphedema as well as in patients with no underlying disease. Although PBP virtually always develops in patients with preexisting ascites, it is, in general, an uncommon event, occurring in ≤10% of cirrhotic patients. The cause of PBP has not been established definitively but is believed to involve hematogenous spread of organisms in a patient in whom a diseased liver and altered portal circulation result in a defect in the usual filtration function. Organisms multiply in ascites, a good medium for growth. The proteins of the complement cascade have been found in peritoneal fluid, with lower levels in cirrhotic patients than in patients with ascites of other etiologies. The opsonic and phagocytic properties of PMNs are diminished in patients with advanced liver disease. Cirrhosis is associated with alterations in the gut microbiota, including an increased prevalence of potentially pathogenic bacteria such as Enterobacteriaceae. Small-intestinal bacterial overgrowth is frequently present in advanced stages of liver cirrhosis and has been linked with pathologic bacterial translocation and PBP. Factors promoting these changes in cirrhosis may include deficiencies in Paneth cell defensins, reduced intestinal motility, decreased pancreatobiliary secretions, and portal-hypertensive enteropathy.

The presentation of PBP differs from that of secondary peritonitis. The most common manifestation is fever, which is reported in up to 80% of patients. Ascites is found but virtually always predates infection. Abdominal pain, an acute onset of symptoms, and peritoneal irritation during physical examination can be helpful diagnostically, but the absence of any of these findings does not exclude this often-subtle diagnosis. Nonlocalizing symptoms (such as malaise, fatigue, or encephalopathy) without another clear etiology should also prompt consideration of PBP in a susceptible patient. It is vital to sample the peritoneal fluid of any cirrhotic patient with ascites and fever. The finding of >250 PMNs/μL is diagnostic for PBP, according to Conn (*http://jac.oxfordjournals.org/cgi/content/full/47/3/369*). This criterion does not apply to secondary peritonitis (see below). The microbiology of PBP is also distinctive. While enteric gram-negative bacilli such as *Escherichia coli* are most commonly encountered, gram-positive organisms such as streptococci, enterococci, or even pneumococci are sometimes found. In an important development, widespread use of quinolones to prevent PBP in high-risk subgroups of patients, frequent hospitalizations, and exposure to broad-spectrum antibiotics have led to a change in flora of infections in patients with cirrhosis, with more gram-positive bacteria and extended-spectrum β-lactamase–producing Enterobacteriaceae in recent years. Risk factors for multiresistant infections include nosocomial origin of infection, long-term norfloxacin prophylaxis, recent infection with multiresistant bacteria, and recent use of β-lactam antibiotics. In PBP, a single organism is typically isolated; anaerobes are found less frequently in PBP than in secondary peritonitis, in which a mixed flora including anaerobes is the rule. In fact, if PBP is suspected and multiple organisms including anaerobes are recovered from the peritoneal fluid, the diagnosis must be reconsidered and a source of secondary peritonitis sought.

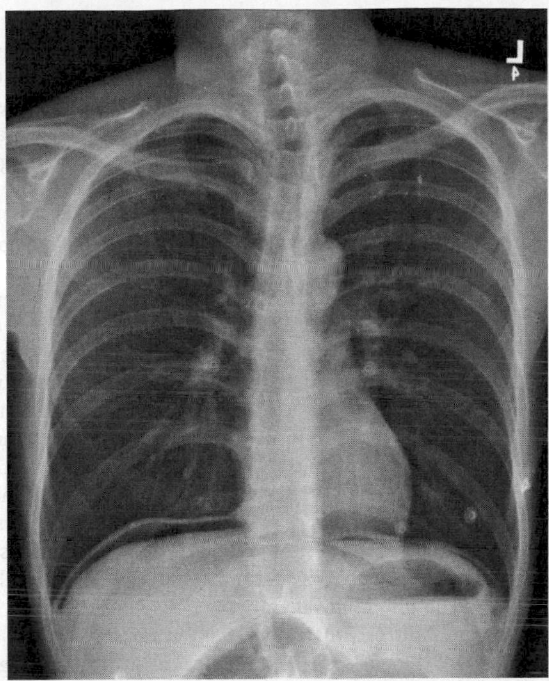

FIGURE 159-2 Pneumoperitoneum. Free air under the diaphragm on an upright chest film suggests the presence of a bowel perforation and associated peritonitis. *(Image courtesy of Dr. John Braver; with permission.)*

The diagnosis of PBP is not easy. It depends on the exclusion of a primary intraabdominal source of infection. Contrast-enhanced CT is useful in identifying an intraabdominal source for infection. It may be difficult to recover organisms from cultures of peritoneal fluid, presumably because the burden of organisms is low. However, the yield can be improved if 10 mL of peritoneal fluid is placed directly into a blood culture bottle. Because bacteremia frequently accompanies PBP, blood should be cultured simultaneously. To maximize the yield, culture samples should be collected prior to administration of antibiotics. No specific radiographic studies are helpful in the diagnosis of PBP. A plain film of the abdomen would be expected to show ascites. Chest and abdominal radiography should be performed in patients with abdominal pain to exclude free air, which signals a perforation (Fig. 159-2).

TREATMENT PRIMARY BACTERIAL PERITONITIS

Treatment for PBP is directed at the isolate from blood or peritoneal fluid. Gram's staining of peritoneal fluid often gives negative results in PBP. Therefore, until culture results become available, therapy should cover gram-negative aerobic bacilli and gram-positive cocci. Third-generation cephalosporins such as cefotaxime (2 g q8h, administered IV) provide reasonable initial coverage in moderately ill patients. Broad-spectrum antibiotics, such as penicillin/β-lactamase inhibitor combinations (e.g., piperacillin/tazobactam, 3.375 g q6h IV for adults with normal renal function) or ceftriaxone (2 g q24h IV), are also options. Broader empirical coverage aimed at resistant hospital-acquired gram-negative bacteria (e.g., treatment with carbapenem) may be appropriate for nosocomially acquired PBP until culture results become available. Empirical coverage for anaerobes is not necessary. A mortality benefit from albumin (1.5 g/kg of body weight within 6 h of detection and 1.0 g/kg on day 3) has been demonstrated for patients who present with serum creatinine levels ≥1 mg/dL, blood urea nitrogen levels ≥30 mg/dL, or total bilirubin levels ≥4 mg/dL but not for patients who do not meet these criteria. After the infecting organism is identified, therapy should be narrowed to target the specific pathogen. Patients with PBP usually respond within 72 h to appropriate antibiotic therapy. Antimicrobial treatment can be administered for as little as 5 days if rapid improvement occurs and blood cultures are negative, but a course of up to 2 weeks may be required for patients with bacteremia and for those whose improvement is slow. Persistence of WBCs in the ascitic fluid after therapy should prompt a search for additional diagnoses.

Prevention • ***PRIMARY PREVENTION*** Several observational studies and a meta-analysis raise the concern that proton pump inhibitor therapy may increase the risk of PBP. No prospective studies have yet addressed whether avoidance of such therapy may prevent PBP. Nonselective beta blockers may prevent secondary bacterial peritonitis. A 2012 guideline from the American Association for the Study of Liver Diseases recommends chronic antibiotic prophylaxis with a regimen described in the next section for patients who are at highest risk for PBP—that is, those with an ascitic-fluid total protein level <1.5 g/dL along with impaired renal function (creatinine, ≥1.2 mg/dL; blood urea nitrogen, ≥25 mg/dL; or serum sodium, ≤130 mg/dL) and/or liver failure (Child-Pugh score, ≥9; and bilirubin, ≥3 mg/dL). A 7-day course of antibiotic prophylaxis is recommended for patients with cirrhosis and gastrointestinal bleeding.

SECONDARY PREVENTION PBP has a high rate of recurrence. Up to 70% of patients experience a recurrence within 1 year. Antibiotic prophylaxis is recommended for patients with a history of PBP to reduce this rate to <20% and improve short-term survival rates. Prophylactic regimens for adults with normal renal function include fluoroquinolones (ciprofloxacin, 750 mg weekly; norfloxacin, 400 mg/d) or trimethoprim-sulfamethoxazole (one double-strength tablet daily). However, long-term administration of broad-spectrum antibiotics in this setting has been shown to increase the risk of severe staphylococcal infections.

SECONDARY PERITONITIS

Secondary peritonitis develops when bacteria contaminate the peritoneum as a result of spillage from an intraabdominal viscus. The organisms found almost always constitute a mixed flora in which facultative gram-negative bacilli and anaerobes predominate, especially when the contaminating source is colonic. Early in the course of infection, when the host response is directed toward containment, exudate containing fibrin and PMNs is found. Early death in this setting is attributable to gram-negative bacillary sepsis and to potent endotoxins circulating in the bloodstream (Chap. 325). Gram-negative bacilli, particularly *E. coli*, are common bloodstream isolates, but *Bacteroides fragilis* bacteremia also occurs. The severity of abdominal pain and the clinical course depend on the inciting process. The organisms isolated from the peritoneum also vary with the source of the initial process and the normal flora at that site. Secondary peritonitis can result primarily from chemical irritation and/or bacterial contamination. For example, as long as the patient is not achlorhydric, a ruptured gastric ulcer will release low-pH gastric contents that will serve as a chemical irritant. The normal flora of the stomach comprises the same organisms found in the oropharynx but in lower numbers. Thus, the bacterial burden in a ruptured ulcer is negligible compared with that in a ruptured appendix. The normal flora of the colon below the ligament of Treitz contains ~10^{11} anaerobic organisms/g of feces but only 10^8 aerobes/g; therefore, anaerobic species account for 99.9% of the bacteria. Leakage of colonic contents (pH 7–8) does not cause significant chemical peritonitis, but infection is intense because of the heavy bacterial load.

Depending on the inciting event, local symptoms may occur in secondary peritonitis—for example, epigastric pain from a ruptured gastric ulcer. In appendicitis (Chap. 356), the initial presenting symptoms are often vague, with periumbilical discomfort and nausea followed in a number of hours by pain more localized to the right lower quadrant. Unusual locations of the appendix (including a retrocecal position) can complicate this presentation further. Once infection has spread to the peritoneal cavity, pain increases, particularly with infection involving the parietal peritoneum, which is innervated extensively. Patients usually lie motionless, often with knees drawn up to avoid stretching the nerve fibers of the peritoneal cavity. Coughing and sneezing, which increase pressure within the peritoneal cavity, are associated with sharp

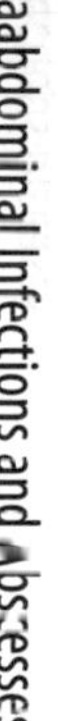

pain. There may or may not be pain localized to the infected or diseased organ from which secondary peritonitis has arisen. Patients with secondary peritonitis generally have abnormal findings on abdominal examination, with marked voluntary and involuntary guarding of the anterior abdominal musculature. Later findings include tenderness, especially rebound tenderness. In addition, there may be localized findings in the area of the inciting event. In general, patients are febrile, with marked leukocytosis and a left shift of the WBCs to band forms.

While recovery of organisms from peritoneal fluid is easier in secondary than in primary peritonitis, a tap of the abdomen is rarely the procedure of choice in secondary peritonitis. An exception is in cases involving trauma, where the possibility of a hemoperitoneum may need to be excluded early. Emergent studies (such as abdominal CT) to find the source of peritoneal contamination should be undertaken if the patient is hemodynamically stable; unstable patients may require surgical intervention without prior imaging.

TREATMENT SECONDARY PERITONITIS

Treatment for secondary peritonitis includes early administration of antibiotics aimed particularly at aerobic gram-negative bacilli and anaerobes (see below). Mild to moderate disease can be treated with many drugs covering these organisms, including broad-spectrum penicillin/β-lactamase inhibitor combinations (e.g., ticarcillin/clavulanate, 3.1 g q4–6h IV), cefoxitin (2 g q4–6h IV), or a combination of either a fluoroquinolone (e.g., levofloxacin, 750 mg q24h IV) or a third-generation cephalosporin (e.g., ceftriaxone, 2 g q24h IV) plus metronidazole (500 mg q8h IV). Patients in intensive care units should receive imipenem (500 mg q6h IV), meropenem (1 g q8h IV), or combinations of drugs, such as ampicillin plus metronidazole plus ciprofloxacin. The role of enterococci and *Candida* species in mixed infections is controversial. Secondary peritonitis usually requires both surgical intervention to address the inciting process and antibiotics to treat early bacteremia, to decrease the incidence of abscess formation and wound infection, and to prevent distant spread of infection. Although surgery is rarely indicated in PBP in adults, it may be life-saving in secondary peritonitis. Recombinant human activated protein C (APC) was considered at one time for treatment of severe sepsis from causes including secondary peritonitis but was withdrawn from the market in 2011 after it was determined that the drug was associated with an increased risk of bleeding and that evidence for its beneficial effects was inadequate. Thus APC should not be used for sepsis or septic shock outside randomized clinical trials.

Peritonitis may develop as a complication of abdominal surgeries. These infections may be accompanied by localizing pain and/or nonlocalizing signs or symptoms such as fever, malaise, anorexia, and toxicity. As a nosocomial infection, postoperative peritonitis may be associated with organisms such as staphylococci, components of the gram-negative hospital microflora, and the microbes that cause PBP and secondary peritonitis, as described above.

PERITONITIS IN PATIENTS UNDERGOING CONTINUOUS AMBULATORY PERITONEAL DIALYSIS

A third type of peritonitis arises in patients who are undergoing continuous ambulatory peritoneal dialysis (CAPD). Unlike PBP and secondary peritonitis, which are caused by endogenous bacteria, CAPD-associated peritonitis usually involves skin organisms. The pathogenesis of infection is similar to that of intravascular device–related infection, in which skin organisms migrate along the catheter, which both serves as an entry point and exerts the effects of a foreign body. Exit-site or tunnel infection may or may not accompany CAPD-associated peritonitis. Like PBP, CAPD-associated peritonitis is usually caused by a single organism. Peritonitis is, in fact, the most common reason for discontinuation of CAPD. Improvements in equipment design, especially the Y-set connector, have resulted in a decrease from one case of peritonitis per 9 months of CAPD to one case per 24 months.

The clinical presentation of CAPD peritonitis resembles that of secondary peritonitis in that diffuse pain and peritoneal signs are common. The dialysate is usually cloudy and contains >100 WBCs/μL, >50% of which are neutrophils. However, the number of cells depends in part on dwell time. According to a guideline from the International Society for Peritoneal Dialysis (2010), for patients undergoing automated peritoneal dialysis who present during their nighttime treatment and whose dwell time is much shorter than with CAPD, the clinician should use the percentage of PMNs rather than the absolute number of WBCs to diagnose peritonitis. As the normal peritoneum has very few PMNs, a proportion above 50% is strong evidence of peritonitis even if the absolute WBC count does not reach 100/μL. Meanwhile, patients undergoing automated peritoneal dialysis without a daytime exchange who present with abdominal pain may have no fluid to withdraw, in which case 1 L of dialysate should be infused and permitted to dwell a minimum of 1–2 h, then drained, examined for turbidity, and sent for cell count with differential and culture. The differential (with a shortened dwell time) may be more useful than the absolute WBC count. In equivocal cases or in patients with systemic or abdominal symptoms in whom the effluent appears clear, a second exchange is performed, with a dwell time of at least 2 h. Clinical judgment should guide initiation of therapy.

The most common organisms are *Staphylococcus* species, which accounted for ~45% of cases in one series. Historically, coagulase-negative staphylococcal species were identified most commonly in these infections, but these isolates have more recently been decreasing in frequency. *Staphylococcus aureus* is more often involved among patients who are nasal carriers of the organism than among those who are not, and this organism is the most common pathogen in overt exit-site infections. Gram-negative bacilli and fungi such as *Candida* species are also found. Vancomycin-resistant enterococci and vancomycin-intermediate *S. aureus* have been reported to produce peritonitis in CAPD patients. The finding of more than one organism in dialysate culture should prompt evaluation for secondary peritonitis. As with PBP, culture of dialysate fluid in blood culture bottles improves the yield. To facilitate diagnosis, several hundred milliliters of removed dialysis fluid should be concentrated by centrifugation before culture.

TREATMENT CAPD PERITONITIS

Empirical therapy for CAPD peritonitis should be directed at *S. aureus*, coagulase-negative *Staphylococcus*, and gram-negative bacilli until the results of cultures become available. Guidelines suggest that agents should be chosen on the basis of local experience with resistant organisms. In some centers, a first-generation cephalosporin such as cefazolin (for gram-positive bacteria) and a fluoroquinolone or a third-generation cephalosporin such as ceftazidime (for gram-negative bacteria) may be reasonable; in areas with high rates of infection with methicillin-resistant *S. aureus*, vancomycin should be used instead of cefazolin, and gram-negative coverage may need to be broadened—e.g., with an aminoglycoside, ceftazidime, cefepime, or carbapenem. Broad coverage including vancomycin should be particularly considered for toxic patients and for those with exit-site infections. Vancomycin should also be included in the regimen if the patient has a history of colonization or infection with methicillin-resistant *S. aureus* or has a history of severe allergy to penicillins and cephalosporins. Loading doses are administered intraperitoneally; doses depend on the dialysis method and the patient's renal function. Antibiotics are given either continuously (i.e., with each exchange) or intermittently (i.e., once daily, with the dose allowed to remain in the peritoneal cavity for at least 6 h). If the patient is severely ill, IV antibiotics should be added at doses appropriate for the patient's degree of renal failure. The clinical response to an empirical treatment regimen should be rapid; if the patient has not responded after 48–96 h of treatment, new samples should be collected for cell counts and cultures, and catheter removal should be considered. For patients who lack exit-site or tunnel infection, the typical duration of antibiotic treatment is 14 days. For patients with exit-site or tunnel infection, catheter removal should be considered, and a longer duration of antibiotic therapy (up to 21 days) may be appropriate. In fungal infections, the catheter should be removed immediately.

TUBERCULOUS PERITONITIS

See Chap. 202.

INTRAABDOMINAL ABSCESSES

INTRAPERITONEAL ABSCESSES

Abscess formation is common in untreated peritonitis if overt gram-negative sepsis either does not develop or develops but is not fatal. In experimental models of abscess formation, mixed aerobic and anaerobic organisms have been implanted intraperitoneally. Without therapy directed at anaerobes, animals develop intraabdominal abscesses. As in humans, these experimental abscesses may stud the peritoneal cavity, lie within the omentum or mesentery, or even develop on the surface of or within viscera such as the liver.

Pathogenesis and Immunity There is often disagreement about whether an abscess represents a disease state or a host response. In a sense, it represents both: while an abscess is an infection in which viable infecting organisms and PMNs are contained in a fibrous capsule, it is also a process by which the host confines microbes to a limited space, thereby preventing further spread of infection. In any event, abscesses do cause significant symptoms, and patients with abscesses can be quite ill. Experimental work has helped to define both the host cells and the bacterial virulence factors responsible—most notably in the case of *B. fragilis*. This organism, although accounting for only 0.5% of the normal colonic flora, is the anaerobe most frequently isolated from intraabdominal infections, is especially prominent in abscesses, and is the most common anaerobic bloodstream isolate. On clinical grounds, therefore, *B. fragilis* appears to be uniquely virulent. Moreover, *B. fragilis* acts alone to cause abscesses in animal models of intraabdominal infection, whereas most other *Bacteroides* species must act synergistically with a facultative organism to induce abscess formation.

Of the several virulence factors identified in *B. fragilis*, one is critical: the capsular polysaccharide complex found on the bacterial surface. This complex comprises at least eight distinct surface polysaccharides. Structural analysis of these polysaccharides has shown an unusual motif of oppositely charged sugars. Polysaccharides having these *zwitterionic* characteristics, such as polysaccharide A, evoke a host response in the peritoneal cavity that localizes bacteria into abscesses. *B. fragilis* and polysaccharide A have been found to adhere to primary mesothelial cells in vitro; this adherence, in turn, stimulates the production of tumor necrosis factor α and intercellular adhesion molecule 1 by peritoneal macrophages. Although abscesses characteristically contain PMNs, the process of abscess induction depends on the stimulation of T lymphocytes by these unique zwitterionic polysaccharides. The stimulated CD4+ T lymphocytes secrete leukoattractant cytokines and chemokines. The alternative pathway of complement and fibrinogen also participate in abscess formation.

While antibodies to the capsular polysaccharide complex enhance bloodstream clearance of *B. fragilis*, CD4+ T cells are critical in immunity to abscesses. When administered subcutaneously, *B. fragilis* polysaccharide A has immunomodulatory characteristics and stimulates CD4+ T regulatory cells via an interleukin 2–dependent mechanism to produce interleukin 10. Interleukin 10 downregulates the inflammatory response, thereby preventing abscess formation.

Clinical Presentation Of all intraabdominal abscesses, 74% are intraperitoneal or retroperitoneal and are not visceral. Most intraperitoneal abscesses result from fecal spillage from a colonic source, such as an inflamed appendix. Abscesses can also arise from other processes. They usually form within weeks of the development of peritonitis and may be found in a variety of locations from omentum to mesentery, pelvis to psoas muscles, and subphrenic space to a visceral organ such as the liver, where they may develop either on the surface of the organ or within it. Periappendiceal and diverticular abscesses occur commonly. Diverticular abscesses are least likely to rupture. Infections of the female genital tract and pancreatitis are also among the more common causative events. When abscesses occur in the female genital tract—either as a primary infection (e.g., tuboovarian abscess) or as an infection extending into the pelvic cavity or peritoneum—*B. fragilis* figures prominently among the organisms isolated. *B. fragilis* is not found in large numbers in the normal vaginal flora. For example, it is encountered less commonly in pelvic inflammatory disease and endometritis without an associated abscess. In pancreatitis with leakage of damaging pancreatic enzymes, inflammation is prominent. Therefore, clinical findings such as fever, leukocytosis, and even abdominal pain do not distinguish pancreatitis itself from complications such as pancreatic pseudocyst, pancreatic abscess (Chap. 371), or intraabdominal collections of pus. Especially in cases of necrotizing pancreatitis, in which the incidence of local pancreatic infection may be as high as 30%, needle aspiration under CT guidance is performed to sample fluid for culture. Many centers prescribe preemptive antibiotics for patients with necrotizing pancreatitis. Imipenem is frequently used for this purpose because it reaches high tissue levels in the pancreas (although it is not unique in this regard). Recent randomized controlled studies have not demonstrated a benefit from this practice, and some guidelines no longer recommend preemptive antibiotics for patients with acute pancreatitis. If needle aspiration yields infected fluid in the setting of acute necrotizing pancreatitis, antibiotic treatment is appropriate in conjunction with surgical and/or percutaneous drainage of infected material. Infected pseudocysts that occur remotely from acute pancreatitis are unlikely to be associated with significant amounts of necrotic tissue and may be treated with either surgical or percutaneous catheter drainage in conjunction with appropriate antibiotic therapy.

Diagnosis Scanning procedures have considerably facilitated the diagnosis of intraabdominal abscesses. Abdominal CT probably has the highest yield, although ultrasonography is particularly useful for the right upper quadrant, kidneys, and pelvis. Both indium-labeled WBCs and gallium tend to localize in abscesses and may be useful in finding a collection. Because gallium is taken up in the bowel, indium-labeled WBCs may have a slightly greater yield for abscesses near the bowel. Neither indium-labeled WBC nor gallium scans serve as a basis for a definitive diagnosis, however; both need to be followed by other, more specific studies, such as CT, if an area of possible abnormality is identified. Abscesses contiguous with or contained within diverticula are particularly difficult to diagnose with scanning procedures. Although barium should not be injected if a perforation is suspected, a barium enema occasionally may detect a diverticular abscess not diagnosed by other procedures. If one study is negative, a second study sometimes reveals a collection. Although exploratory laparotomy has been less commonly used since the advent of CT, this procedure still must be undertaken on occasion if an abscess is strongly suspected on clinical grounds.

TREATMENT INTRAPERITONEAL ABSCESSES

An algorithm for the management of patients with intraabdominal (including intraperitoneal) abscesses by percutaneous drainage is presented in Fig. 159-3. The treatment of intraabdominal infections involves the determination of the initial focus of infection, the administration of broad-spectrum antibiotics targeting the organisms involved, and the performance of a drainage procedure if one or more definitive abscesses have formed. Antimicrobial therapy, in general, is adjunctive to drainage and/or surgical correction of an underlying lesion or process in intraabdominal abscesses. Unlike the intraabdominal abscesses resulting from most causes, for which drainage of some kind is generally required, abscesses associated with diverticulitis usually wall off locally after rupture of a diverticulum, so that surgical intervention is not routinely required.

A number of agents exhibit excellent activity against aerobic gram-negative bacilli. Because death in intraabdominal sepsis is linked to gram-negative bacteremia, empirical therapy for intraabdominal infection always needs to include adequate coverage of gram-negative aerobic, facultative, and anaerobic organisms. Even

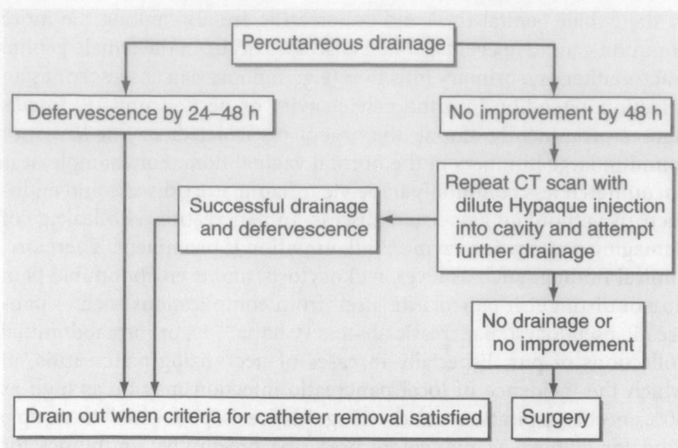

FIGURE 159-3 Algorithm for the management of patients with intraabdominal abscesses using percutaneous drainage. Antimicrobial therapy should be administered concomitantly. *(Reprinted with permission from B Lorber [ed]: Atlas of Infectious Diseases, vol VII: Intra-abdominal Infections, Hepatitis, and Gastroenteritis. Philadelphia, Current Medicine, 1996, p 1.30, as adapted from OD Rotstein, RL Simmons, in SL Gorbach et al [eds]: Infectious Diseases. Philadelphia, Saunders, 1992, p 668.)*

if anaerobes are not cultured from clinical specimens, they still must be covered by the therapeutic regimen. Empirical antibiotic therapy should be the same as that discussed above for secondary peritonitis.

VISCERAL ABSCESSES

Liver Abscesses The liver is the organ most subject to the development of abscesses. In one study of 540 intraabdominal abscesses, 26% were visceral. Liver abscesses made up 13% of the total number, or 48% of all visceral abscesses. Liver abscesses may be solitary or multiple; they may arise from hematogenous spread of bacteria or from local spread from contiguous sites of infection within the peritoneal cavity. In the past, appendicitis with rupture and subsequent spread of infection was the most common source for a liver abscess. Currently, associated disease of the biliary tract is most common. Pylephlebitis (suppurative thrombosis of the portal vein), usually arising from infection in the pelvis but sometimes from infection elsewhere in the peritoneal cavity, is another common source for bacterial seeding of the liver.

Fever is the most common presenting sign of liver abscess. Some patients, particularly those with associated disease of the biliary tract, have symptoms and signs localized to the right upper quadrant, including pain, guarding, punch tenderness, and even rebound tenderness. Nonspecific symptoms, such as chills, anorexia, weight loss, nausea, and vomiting, may also develop. Only 50% of patients with liver abscesses, however, have hepatomegaly, right-upper-quadrant tenderness, or jaundice; thus, one-half of patients have no symptoms or signs to direct attention to the liver. Fever of unknown origin may be the only manifestation of liver abscess, especially in the elderly. Diagnostic studies of the abdomen, especially the right upper quadrant, should be a part of any workup for fever of unknown origin. The single most reliable laboratory finding is an elevated serum concentration of alkaline phosphatase, which is documented in 70% of patients with liver abscesses. Other tests of liver function may yield normal results, but 50% of patients have elevated serum levels of bilirubin, and 48% have elevated concentrations of aspartate aminotransferase. Other laboratory findings include leukocytosis in 77% of patients, anemia (usually normochromic, normocytic) in 50%, and hypoalbuminemia in 33%. Concomitant bacteremia is found in one-third to one-half of patients. A liver abscess is sometimes suggested by chest radiography, especially if a new elevation of the right hemidiaphragm is seen; other suggestive findings include a right basilar infiltrate and a right pleural effusion.

Imaging studies are the most reliable methods for diagnosing liver abscesses. These studies include ultrasonography, CT (Fig. 159-4), indium-labeled WBC or gallium scan, and MRI. More than one such study may be required.

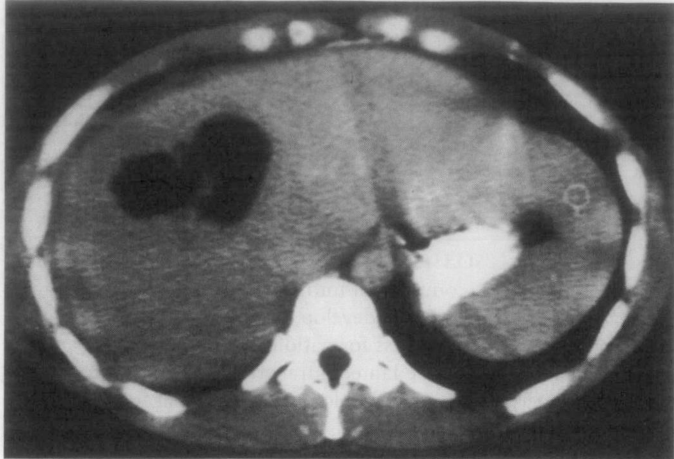

FIGURE 159-4 Multilocular liver abscess on CT scan. Multiple or multilocular abscesses are more common than solitary abscesses. *(Reprinted with permission from B Lorber [ed]: Atlas of Infectious Diseases, vol VII: Intra-abdominal Infections, Hepatitis, and Gastroenteritis. Philadelphia, Current Medicine, 1996, Fig. 1.22.)*

Organisms recovered from liver abscesses vary with the source. In liver infection arising from the biliary tree, enteric gram-negative aerobic bacilli and enterococci are common isolates. *Klebsiella pneumoniae* liver abscess has been well described in Southeast Asia for more than 20 years and has become an emerging syndrome in North America and elsewhere. These community-acquired infections have been linked to a virulent hypermucoviscous *K. pneumoniae* phenotype and to a specific genotype. The typical syndrome includes liver abscess, bacteremia, and metastatic infection. Ampicillin/amoxicillin therapy started within the previous 30 days has been associated with increased risk for this syndrome, presumably because of selection for the causative strain. Unless previous surgery has been performed, anaerobes are not generally involved in liver abscesses arising from biliary infections. In contrast, in liver abscesses arising from pelvic and other intraperitoneal sources, a mixed flora including both aerobic and anaerobic species is common; *B. fragilis* is the species most frequently isolated. With hematogenous spread of infection, usually only a single organism is encountered; this species may be *S. aureus* or a streptococcal species such as one in the *Streptococcus milleri* group. Results of cultures obtained from drain sites are not reliable for defining the etiology of infections. Liver abscesses may also be caused by *Candida* species; such abscesses usually follow fungemia in patients receiving chemotherapy for cancer and often present when PMNs return after a period of neutropenia. Amebic liver abscesses are not an uncommon problem (Chap. 247). Amebic serologic testing gives positive results in >95% of cases. In addition, polymerase chain reaction (PCR) testing has been used in recent years. Negative results from these studies help to exclude this diagnosis.

TREATMENT LIVER ABSCESSES

(Fig. 159-3) Drainage is the mainstay of therapy for intraabdominal abscesses, including liver abscesses; the approach can be either percutaneous (with a pigtail catheter kept in place or possibly with a device that can perform pulse lavage to fragment and evacuate the semisolid contents of a liver abscess) or surgical. However, there is growing interest in medical management alone for pyogenic liver abscesses. The drugs used for empirical therapy include the same ones used in intraabdominal sepsis and secondary bacterial peritonitis. Usually, blood cultures and a diagnostic aspirate of abscess contents should be obtained before the initiation of empirical therapy, with antibiotic choices adjusted when the results of Gram's staining and culture become available. Cases treated without definitive drainage generally require longer courses of antibiotic therapy. When percutaneous drainage was compared with open surgical drainage, the average length of hospital stay for the former was almost twice that for the latter, although both the time required for fever to resolve and the mortality rate were the same for the two procedures. The mortality rate was appreciable despite treatment, averaging 15%. Several factors predict the failure of percutaneous drainage and therefore may favor primary surgical intervention. These factors include the presence of multiple, sizable abscesses; viscous abscess contents that tend to plug the catheter; associated disease (e.g., disease of the biliary tract) requiring surgery; the presence of yeast; communication with an untreated obstructed biliary tree; or the lack of a clinical response to percutaneous drainage in 4–7 days.

Treatment of candidal liver abscesses often entails initial administration of amphotericin B or liposomal amphotericin, with subsequent fluconazole therapy (Chap. 240). In some cases, therapy with fluconazole alone (6 mg/kg daily) may be used—e.g., in clinically stable patients whose infecting isolate is susceptible to this drug.

Splenic Abscesses Splenic abscesses are much less common than liver abscesses. The incidence of splenic abscesses has ranged from 0.14% to 0.7% in various autopsy series. The clinical setting and the organisms isolated usually differ from those for liver abscesses. The degree of clinical suspicion for splenic abscess needs to be high because this condition is frequently fatal if left untreated. Even in the most recently published series, diagnosis was made only at autopsy in 37% of cases. Although splenic abscesses may arise occasionally from contiguous spread of infection or from direct trauma to the spleen, hematogenous spread of infection is more common. Bacterial endocarditis is the most common associated infection (Chap. 155). Splenic abscesses can develop in patients who have received extensive immunosuppressive therapy (particularly those with malignancy involving the spleen) and in patients with hemoglobinopathies or other hematologic disorders (especially sickle cell anemia).

Although ~50% of patients with splenic abscesses have abdominal pain, the pain is localized to the left upper quadrant in only one-half of these cases. Splenomegaly is found in ~50% of cases. Fever and leukocytosis are generally present; the development of fever preceded diagnosis by an average of 20 days in one series. Left-sided chest findings may include abnormalities to auscultation, and chest radiographic findings may include an infiltrate or a left-sided pleural effusion. CT scan of the abdomen has been the most sensitive diagnostic tool. Ultrasonography can yield the diagnosis but is less sensitive. Liver-spleen scan or gallium scan may also be useful. Streptococcal species are the most common bacterial isolates from splenic abscesses, followed by *S. aureus*—presumably reflecting the associated endocarditis. An increase in the prevalence of gram-negative aerobic isolates from splenic abscesses has been reported; these organisms often derive from a urinary tract focus, with associated bacteremia, or from another intraabdominal source. *Salmonella* species are seen fairly commonly, especially in patients with sickle cell hemoglobinopathy. Anaerobic species accounted for only 5% of isolates in the largest collected series, but the reporting of a number of "sterile abscesses" may indicate that optimal techniques for the isolation of anaerobes were not used.

TREATMENT SPLENIC ABSCESSES

Because of the high mortality figures reported for splenic abscesses, splenectomy with adjunctive antibiotics has traditionally been considered standard treatment and remains the best approach for complex, multilocular abscesses or multiple abscesses. However, percutaneous drainage has worked well for single, small (<3-cm) abscesses in some studies and may also be useful for patients with high surgical risk. Patients undergoing splenectomy should be vaccinated against encapsulated organisms (*Streptococcus pneumoniae, Haemophilus influenzae, Neisseria meningitidis*). The most important factor in successful treatment of splenic abscesses is early diagnosis.

Perinephric and Renal Abscesses Perinephric and renal abscesses are not common. The former accounted for only ~0.02% of hospital admissions and the latter for ~0.2% in Altemeier's series of 540 intraabdominal abscesses. Before antibiotics became available, most renal and perinephric abscesses were hematogenous in origin, usually complicating prolonged bacteremia, with *S. aureus* most commonly recovered. Now, in contrast, >75% of perinephric and renal abscesses arise from a urinary tract infection. Infection ascends from the bladder to the kidney, with pyelonephritis preceding abscess development. Bacteria may directly invade the renal parenchyma from medulla to cortex. Local vascular channels within the kidney may also facilitate the transport of organisms. Areas of abscess developing within the parenchyma may rupture into the perinephric space. The kidneys and adrenal glands are surrounded by a layer of perirenal fat that, in turn, is surrounded by Gerota's fascia, which extends superiorly to the diaphragm and inferiorly to the pelvic fat. Abscesses extending into the perinephric space may track through Gerota's fascia into the psoas or transversalis muscles, into the anterior peritoneal cavity, superiorly to the subdiaphragmatic space, or inferiorly to the pelvis. Of the risk factors that have been associated with the development of perinephric abscesses, the most important is concomitant nephrolithiasis obstructing urinary flow. Of patients with perinephric abscess, 20–60% have renal stones. Other structural abnormalities of the urinary tract, prior urologic surgery, trauma, and diabetes mellitus have also been identified as risk factors.

The organisms most frequently encountered in perinephric and renal abscesses are *E. coli*, *Proteus* species, and *Klebsiella* species. *E. coli*, the aerobic species most commonly found in the colonic flora, seems to have unique virulence properties in the urinary tract, including factors promoting adherence to uroepithelial cells. The urease of *Proteus* species splits urea, thereby creating a more alkaline and more hospitable environment for bacterial proliferation. *Proteus* species are frequently found in association with large struvite stones caused by the precipitation of magnesium ammonium sulfate in an alkaline environment. These stones serve as a nidus for recurrent urinary tract infection. Although a single bacterial species is usually recovered from a perinephric or renal abscess, multiple species may also be found. If a urine culture is not contaminated with periurethral flora and is found to contain more than one organism, a perinephric abscess or renal abscess should be considered in the differential diagnosis. Urine cultures may also be polymicrobial in cases of bladder diverticulum.

Candida species can cause renal abscesses. This fungus may spread to the kidney hematogenously or by ascension from the bladder. The hallmark of the latter route of infection is ureteral obstruction with large fungal balls.

The presentation of perinephric and renal abscesses is quite nonspecific. Flank pain and abdominal pain are common. At least 50% of patients are febrile. Pain may be referred to the groin or leg, particularly with extension of infection. The diagnosis of perinephric abscess, like that of splenic abscess, is frequently delayed, and the mortality rate in some series is appreciable, although lower than in the past. Perinephric or renal abscess should be most seriously considered when a patient presents with symptoms and signs of pyelonephritis and remains febrile after 4 or 5 days of treatment. Moreover, when a urine culture yields a polymicrobial flora, when a patient is known to have renal stones, or when fever and pyuria coexist with a sterile urine culture, these diagnoses should be entertained.

Renal ultrasonography and abdominal CT are the most useful diagnostic modalities. If a renal or perinephric abscess is diagnosed, nephrolithiasis should be excluded, especially when a high urinary pH suggests the presence of a urea-splitting organism.

TREATMENT PERINEPHRIC AND RENAL ABSCESSES

Treatment for perinephric and renal abscesses, like that for other intraabdominal abscesses, includes drainage of pus and antibiotic therapy directed at the organism(s) recovered. For perinephric abscesses, percutaneous drainage is usually successful.

Psoas Abscesses The psoas muscle is another location in which abscesses are encountered. Psoas abscesses may arise from a hematogenous source, by contiguous spread from an intraabdominal or pelvic process, or by contiguous spread from nearby bony structures (e.g., vertebral bodies). Associated osteomyelitis due to spread from bone to muscle or from muscle to bone is common in psoas abscesses. When Pott's disease was common, *Mycobacterium tuberculosis* was a frequent cause of psoas abscess. Currently, either *S. aureus* or a mixture of enteric organisms including aerobic and anaerobic gram-negative bacilli is usually isolated from psoas abscesses in the United States. *S. aureus* is most likely to be isolated when a psoas abscess arises from hematogenous spread or a contiguous focus of osteomyelitis; a mixed enteric flora is the most likely etiology when the abscess has an intraabdominal or pelvic source. Patients with psoas abscesses frequently present with fever, lower abdominal or back pain, or pain referred to the hip or knee. CT is the most useful diagnostic technique.

TREATMENT PSOAS ABSCESSES

Treatment includes surgical drainage and the administration of an antibiotic regimen directed at the inciting organism(s).

Pancreatic Abscesses See Chap. 371.

Acknowledgment

The substantial contributions of Dori F. Zaleznik, MD, to this chapter in previous editions are gratefully acknowledged.

160 Acute Infectious Diarrheal Diseases and Bacterial Food Poisoning

Regina C. LaRocque, Edward T. Ryan, Stephen B. Calderwood

Acute diarrheal disease is a leading cause of illness globally and is associated with an estimated 1.4 million deaths per year. Among children <5 years of age, diarrheal disease is second only to lower respiratory infection as the most common infectious cause of death. The incidence rate of diarrheal disease among children in low- and middle-income countries is estimated to be 2.9 episodes per child per year, for a total of 1.7 billion episodes annually. The morbidity from diarrhea is also significant. Recurrent intestinal infections are associated with physical and mental stunting, wasting, micronutrient deficiencies, and malnutrition. In short, diarrheal disease is a driving factor in global morbidity and mortality.

The wide range of clinical manifestations of acute gastrointestinal illnesses is matched by the wide variety of infectious agents involved, including viruses, bacteria, and parasites (Table 160-1). This chapter discusses factors that enable gastrointestinal pathogens to cause disease, reviews host defense mechanisms, and delineates an approach to the evaluation and treatment of patients presenting with acute diarrhea. Individual organisms causing acute gastrointestinal illnesses are discussed in detail in subsequent chapters.

PATHOGENIC MECHANISMS

Enteric pathogens have developed a variety of tactics to overcome host defenses. Understanding the virulence factors employed by these organisms is important in the diagnosis and treatment of clinical disease.

INOCULUM SIZE

The number of microorganisms that must be ingested to cause disease varies considerably from species to species. For *Shigella*, enterohemorrhagic *Escherichia coli*, *Giardia lamblia*, or *Entamoeba*, as few as 10–100 bacteria or cysts can produce infection, while 10^5–10^8 *Vibrio cholerae* organisms must be ingested to cause disease. The infective dose of *Salmonella* varies widely, depending on the species, host, and food vehicle. The ability of organisms to overcome host defenses has important implications for transmission; *Shigella*, enterohemorrhagic *E. coli*, *Entamoeba*, and *Giardia* can spread by person-to-person contact, whereas under some circumstances *Salmonella* may have to grow in food for several hours before reaching an effective infectious dose.

ADHERENCE

Many organisms must adhere to the gastrointestinal mucosa as an initial step in the pathogenic process; thus, organisms that can compete with the normal bowel flora and colonize the mucosa have an important advantage in causing disease. Specific cell-surface proteins involved in attachment of bacteria to intestinal cells are important virulence determinants. *V. cholerae*, for example, adheres to the brush border of small-intestinal enterocytes via specific surface adhesins, including the toxin-coregulated pilus and other accessory colonization factors. Enterotoxigenic *E. coli*, which causes watery diarrhea, produces an adherence protein called *colonization factor antigen* that is necessary for colonization of the upper small intestine by the organism prior to the production of enterotoxin. Enteropathogenic *E. coli*, an agent of diarrhea in young children, and enterohemorrhagic *E. coli*, which causes hemorrhagic colitis and the hemolytic-uremic syndrome, produce virulence determinants that allow these organisms to attach to and efface the brush border of the intestinal epithelium.

TOXIN PRODUCTION

The production of one or more exotoxins is important in the pathogenesis of numerous enteric organisms. Such toxins include *enterotoxins*, which cause watery diarrhea by acting directly on secretory mechanisms

TABLE 160-1 GASTROINTESTINAL PATHOGENS CAUSING ACUTE DIARRHEA

Mechanism	Location	Illness	Stool Findings	Examples of Pathogens Involved
Noninflammatory (enterotoxin)	Proximal small bowel	Watery diarrhea	No fecal leukocytes; mild or no increase in fecal lactoferrin	*Vibrio cholerae*, enterotoxigenic *Escherichia coli* (LT and/or ST), enteroaggregative *E. coli*, *Clostridium perfringens*, *Bacillus cereus*, *Staphylococcus aureus*, *Aeromonas hydrophila*, *Plesiomonas shigelloides*, rotavirus, norovirus, enteric adenoviruses, *Giardia lamblia*, *Cryptosporidium* spp., *Cyclospora* spp., microsporidia
Inflammatory (invasion or cytotoxin)	Colon or distal small bowel	Dysentery or inflammatory diarrhea	Fecal polymorphonuclear leukocytes; substantial increase in fecal lactoferrin	*Shigella* spp., *Salmonella* spp., *Campylobacter jejuni*, enterohemorrhagic *E. coli*, enteroinvasive *E. coli*, *Yersinia enterocolitica*, *Listeria monocytogenes*, *Vibrio parahaemolyticus*, *Clostridium difficile*, *A. hydrophila*, *P. shigelloides*, *Entamoeba histolytica*, *Klebsiella oxytoca*
Penetrating	Distal small bowel	Enteric fever	Fecal mononuclear leukocytes	*Salmonella typhi*, *Y. enterocolitica*

Abbreviations: LT, heat-labile enterotoxin; ST, heat-stable enterotoxin.

in the intestinal mucosa; *cytotoxins*, which cause destruction of mucosal cells and associated inflammatory diarrhea; and *neurotoxins*, which act directly on the central or peripheral nervous system.

The prototypical enterotoxin is cholera toxin, a heterodimeric protein composed of one A and five B subunits. The A subunit contains the enzymatic activity of the toxin, while the B subunit pentamer binds holotoxin to the enterocyte surface receptor, the ganglioside G_{M1}. After the binding of holotoxin, a fragment of the A subunit is translocated across the eukaryotic cell membrane into the cytoplasm, where it catalyzes the adenosine diphosphate ribosylation of a guanosine triphosphate binding protein and causes persistent activation of adenylate cyclase. The end result is an increase of cyclic adenosine monophosphate in the intestinal mucosa, which increases Cl^- secretion and decreases Na^+ absorption, leading to a loss of fluid and the production of diarrhea.

Enterotoxigenic strains of *E. coli* may produce a protein called *heat-labile enterotoxin* (LT) that is similar to cholera toxin and causes secretory diarrhea by the same mechanism. Alternatively, enterotoxigenic strains of *E. coli* may produce *heat-stable enterotoxin* (ST), one form of which causes diarrhea by activation of guanylate cyclase and elevation of intracellular cyclic guanosine monophosphate. Some enterotoxigenic strains of *E. coli* produce both LT and ST.

Bacterial cytotoxins, in contrast, destroy intestinal mucosal cells and produce the syndrome of dysentery, with bloody stools containing inflammatory cells. Enteric pathogens that produce such cytotoxins include *Shigella dysenteriae* type 1, *Vibrio parahaemolyticus*, and *Clostridium difficile*. *S. dysenteriae* type 1 and Shiga toxin–producing strains of *E. coli* produce potent cytotoxins and have been associated with outbreaks of hemorrhagic colitis and hemolytic-uremic syndrome.

Neurotoxins are usually produced by bacteria outside the host and therefore cause symptoms soon after ingestion. Included are the staphylococcal and *Bacillus cereus* toxins, which act on the central nervous system to produce vomiting.

INVASION

Dysentery may result not only from the production of cytotoxins but also from bacterial invasion and destruction of intestinal mucosal cells. Infections due to *Shigella* and enteroinvasive *E. coli* are characterized by the organisms' invasion of mucosal epithelial cells, intraepithelial multiplication, and subsequent spread to adjacent cells. *Salmonella* causes inflammatory diarrhea by invasion of the bowel mucosa but generally is not associated with the destruction of enterocytes or the full clinical syndrome of dysentery. *Salmonella typhi* and *Yersinia enterocolitica* can penetrate intact intestinal mucosa, multiply intracellularly in Peyer's patches and intestinal lymph nodes, and then disseminate through the bloodstream to cause enteric fever, a syndrome characterized by fever, headache, relative bradycardia, abdominal pain, splenomegaly, and leukopenia.

HOST DEFENSES

Given the enormous number of microorganisms ingested with every meal, the normal host must combat a constant influx of potential enteric pathogens. Studies of infections in patients with alterations in defense mechanisms have led to a greater understanding of the variety of ways in which the normal host can protect itself against disease.

INTESTINAL MICROBIOTA

The large numbers of bacteria that normally inhabit the intestine (*the intestinal microbiota*) act as an important host defense mechanism, preventing colonization by potential enteric pathogens. Persons with fewer intestinal bacteria, such as infants who have not yet developed normal enteric colonization or patients receiving antibiotics, are at significantly greater risk of developing infections with enteric pathogens. The composition of the intestinal microbiota is as important as the number of organisms present. More than 99% of the normal colonic microbiota is made up of anaerobic bacteria, and the acidic pH and volatile fatty acids produced by these organisms appear to be critical elements in resistance to colonization.

GASTRIC ACID

The acidic pH of the stomach is an important barrier to enteric pathogens, and an increased frequency of infections due to *Salmonella*, *G. lamblia*, and a variety of helminths has been reported among patients who have undergone gastric surgery or are achlorhydric for some other reason. Neutralization of gastric acid with antacids, proton pump inhibitors, or H_2 blockers—a common practice in the management of hospitalized patients—similarly increases the risk of enteric colonization. In addition, some microorganisms can survive the extreme acidity of the gastric environment; rotavirus, for example, is highly stable to acidity.

INTESTINAL MOTILITY

Normal peristalsis is the major mechanism for clearance of bacteria from the proximal small intestine. When intestinal motility is impaired (e.g., by treatment with opiates or other antimotility drugs, anatomic abnormalities, or hypomotility states), the frequency of bacterial overgrowth and infection of the small bowel with enteric pathogens is increased. Some patients whose treatment for *Shigella* infection consists of diphenoxylate hydrochloride with atropine (Lomotil) experience prolonged fever and shedding of organisms, while patients treated with opiates for mild *Salmonella* gastroenteritis have a higher frequency of bacteremia than those not treated with opiates.

IMMUNITY

Both cellular immune responses and antibody production play important roles in protection from enteric infections. Humoral immunity to enteric pathogens consists of systemic IgG and IgM as well as secretory IgA. The mucosal immune system may be the first line of defense against many gastrointestinal pathogens. The binding of bacterial antigens to the luminal surface of M cells in the distal small bowel and the subsequent presentation of antigens to subepithelial lymphoid tissue lead to the proliferation of sensitized lymphocytes. These lymphocytes circulate and populate all of the mucosal tissues of the body as IgA-secreting plasma cells.

GENETIC DETERMINANTS

Host genetic variation influences susceptibility to diarrheal diseases. People with blood group O show increased susceptibility to disease due to *V. cholerae*, *Shigella*, *E. coli* O157, and norovirus. Polymorphisms in genes encoding inflammatory mediators have been associated with the outcome of infection with enteroaggregative *E. coli*, enterotoxin-producing *E. coli*, *Salmonella*, *C. difficile*, and *V. cholerae*.

APPROACH TO THE PATIENT: Infectious Diarrhea or Bacterial Food Poisoning

The approach to the patient with possible infectious diarrhea or bacterial food poisoning is shown in Fig. 160-1.

HISTORY

The answers to questions with high discriminating value can quickly narrow the range of potential causes of diarrhea and help determine whether treatment is needed. Important elements of the narrative history are detailed in Fig. 160-1.

PHYSICAL EXAMINATION

The examination of patients for signs of dehydration provides essential information about the severity of the diarrheal illness and the need for rapid therapy. Mild dehydration is indicated by thirst, dry mouth, decreased axillary sweat, decreased urine output, and slight weight loss. Signs of moderate dehydration include an orthostatic fall in blood pressure, skin tenting, and sunken eyes (or, in infants, a sunken fontanelle). Signs of severe dehydration include lethargy, obtundation, feeble pulse, hypotension, and frank shock.

DIAGNOSTIC APPROACH

After the severity of illness is assessed, the clinician must distinguish between *inflammatory* and *noninflammatory* disease. Using the history and epidemiologic features of the case as guides, the clinician

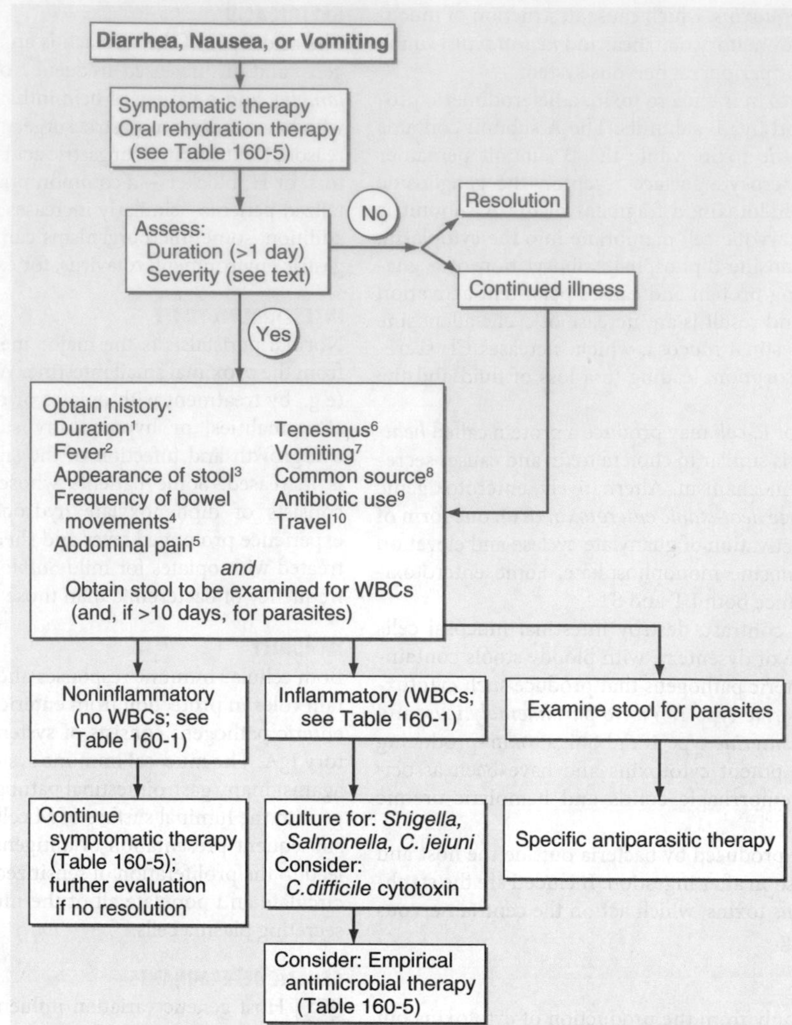

FIGURE 160-1 Clinical algorithm for the approach to patients with community-acquired infectious diarrhea or bacterial food poisoning. Key to superscripts: 1. Diarrhea lasting >2 weeks is generally defined as chronic; in such cases, many of the causes of acute diarrhea are much less likely, and a new spectrum of causes needs to be considered. 2. Fever often implies invasive disease, although fever and diarrhea may also result from infection outside the gastrointestinal tract, as in malaria. 3. Stools that contain blood or mucus indicate ulceration of the large bowel. Bloody stools without fecal leukocytes should alert the laboratory to the possibility of infection with Shiga toxin–producing enterohemorrhagic *Escherichia coli*. Bulky white stools suggest a small-intestinal process that is causing malabsorption. Profuse "rice-water" stools suggest cholera or a similar toxigenic process. 4. Frequent stools over a given period can provide the first warning of impending dehydration. 5. Abdominal pain may be most severe in inflammatory processes like those due to *Shigella*, *Campylobacter*, and necrotizing toxins. Painful abdominal muscle cramps, caused by electrolyte loss, can develop in severe cases of cholera. Bloating is common in giardiasis. An appendicitis-like syndrome should prompt a culture for *Yersinia enterocolitica* with cold enrichment. 6. Tenesmus (painful rectal spasms with a strong urge to defecate but little passage of stool) may be a feature of cases with proctitis, as in shigellosis or amebiasis. 7. Vomiting implies an acute infection (e.g., a toxin-mediated illness or food poisoning) but can also be prominent in a variety of systemic illnesses (e.g., malaria) and in intestinal obstruction. 8. Asking patients whether anyone else they know is sick is a more efficient means of identifying a common source than is constructing a list of recently eaten foods. If a common source seems likely, specific foods can be investigated. See text for a discussion of bacterial food poisoning. 9. Current antibiotic therapy or a recent history of treatment suggests *Clostridium difficile* diarrhea **(Chap. 161)**. Stop antibiotic treatment if possible and consider tests for *C. difficile* toxins. Antibiotic use may increase the risk of chronic intestinal carriage following salmonellosis. 10. See text (and **Chap. 149**) for a discussion of traveler's diarrhea. *(After TS Steiner, RL Guerrant: Principles and syndromes of enteric infection, in Mandell, Douglas, and Bennett's Principles and Practice of Infectious Diseases, 7th ed, GL Mandell et al [eds]. Philadelphia, Churchill Livingstone, 2010, pp 1335–1351; RL Guerrant, DA Bobak: N Engl J Med 325:327, 1991; with permission.)*

can then rapidly evaluate the need for further efforts to define a specific etiology and for therapeutic intervention. Examination of a stool sample may supplement the narrative history. Grossly bloody or mucoid stool suggests an inflammatory process. A test for fecal leukocytes (preparation of a thin smear of stool on a glass slide, addition of a drop of methylene blue, and examination of the wet mount) can suggest inflammatory disease in patients with diarrhea, although the predictive value of this test is still debated. A test for fecal lactoferrin, which is a marker of fecal leukocytes, is more sensitive and is available in latex agglutination and enzyme-linked immunosorbent assay formats. Causes of acute infectious diarrhea, categorized as inflammatory and noninflammatory, are listed in Table 160-1.

POST-DIARRHEA COMPLICATIONS

Chronic complications may follow the resolution of an acute diarrheal episode. The clinician should inquire about prior diarrheal illness if the conditions listed in Table 160-2 are observed.

TABLE 160-2 POST-DIARRHEA COMPLICATIONS OF ACUTE INFECTIOUS DIARRHEAL ILLNESS

Complication	Comments
Chronic diarrhea • Lactase deficiency • Small-bowel bacterial overgrowth • Malabsorption syndromes (tropical and celiac sprue)	Occurs in ~1% of travelers with acute diarrhea • Protozoa account for ~1/3 of cases
Initial presentation or exacerbation of inflammatory bowel disease	May be precipitated by traveler's diarrhea
Irritable bowel syndrome	Occurs in ~10% of travelers with traveler's diarrhea
Reactive arthritis	Particularly likely after infection with invasive organisms (*Shigella, Salmonella, Campylobacter, Yersinia*)
Hemolytic-uremic syndrome (hemolytic anemia, thrombocytopenia, and renal failure)	Follows infection with Shiga toxin–producing bacteria (*Shigella dysenteriae* type 1 and enterohemorrhagic *Escherichia coli*)
Guillain-Barré syndrome	Particularly likely after *Campylobacter* infection

EPIDEMIOLOGY

TRAVEL HISTORY

Of the several million people who travel from temperate industrialized countries to tropical regions of Asia, Africa, and Central and South America each year, 20–50% experience a sudden onset of abdominal cramps, anorexia, and watery diarrhea; thus *traveler's diarrhea* is the most common travel-related infectious illness (Chap. 149). The time of onset is usually 3 days to 2 weeks after the traveler's arrival in a resource-poor area; most cases begin within the first 3–5 days. The illness is generally self-limited, lasting 1–5 days. The high rate of diarrhea among travelers to underdeveloped areas is related to the ingestion of contaminated food or water.

The organisms that cause traveler's diarrhea vary considerably with location (Table 160-3), as does the pattern of antimicrobial resistance. In all areas, enterotoxigenic and enteroaggregative strains of *E. coli* are the most common isolates from persons with the classic secretory traveler's diarrhea syndrome. Infection with *Campylobacter jejuni* is especially common in areas of Asia.

LOCATION

Closed and semi-closed communities, including day-care centers, schools, residential facilities, and cruise ships, are important settings for outbreaks of enteric infections. Norovirus, which is highly contagious and robust in surviving on surfaces, is the most common etiologic agent associated with outbreaks of acute gastroenteritis. Other common organisms, often spread by fecal-oral contact in such communities, are *Shigella*, *C. jejuni*, and *Cryptosporidium*. Rotavirus is rarely a cause of pediatric diarrheal outbreaks in the United States since rotavirus vaccination was broadly recommended in 2006. Similarly, hospitals are sites in which enteric infections are concentrated. Diarrhea is one of the most common manifestations of nosocomial infections. *C. difficile* is the predominant cause of nosocomial diarrhea among adults in the United States, and outbreaks of norovirus infection are common in health care settings. *Klebsiella oxytoca* has been identified as a cause of antibiotic-associated hemorrhagic colitis. Enteropathogenic *E. coli* has been associated with outbreaks of diarrhea in nurseries for newborns. One-third of elderly patients in chronic-care institutions develop a significant diarrheal illness each year; more than one-half of these cases are caused by cytotoxin-producing *C. difficile*. Antimicrobial therapy can predispose to pseudomembranous colitis by altering the normal colonic flora and allowing the multiplication of *C. difficile* (Chap. 161).

TABLE 160-3 CAUSES OF TRAVELER'S DIARRHEA

Etiologic Agent	Approximate Percentage of Cases	Comments
Bacteria	**50–75**	
Enterotoxigenic *Escherichia coli*	10–45	Single most important agent
Enteroaggregative *E. coli*	5–35	Emerging enteric pathogen with worldwide distribution
Campylobacter jejuni	5–25	More common in Asia
Shigella	0–15	Major cause of dysentery
Salmonella	0–15	
Others	0–5	Including *Aeromonas*, *Plesiomonas*, and *Vibrio cholerae*
Viruses	**0–20**	
Norovirus	0–10	Associated with cruise ships
Rotavirus	0–5	Particularly common among children
Parasites	**0–10**	
Giardia lamblia	0–5	Affects hikers and campers who drink from freshwater streams
Cryptosporidium	0–5	Resistant to chlorine treatment
Entamoeba histolytica	<1	
Cyclospora	<1	
Other	**0–10**	
Acute food poisoning[a]	0–5	
No pathogen identified	10–50	

[a]For etiologic agents, see Table 160-4.

Source: After DR Hill et al: The practice of travel medicine: Guidelines by the Infectious Diseases Society of America. Clin Infect Dis 43:1499, 2006.

AGE

Globally, most morbidity and mortality from enteric pathogens involves children <5 years of age. Breast-fed infants are protected from contaminated food and water and derive some protection from maternal antibodies, but their risk of infection rises dramatically when they begin to eat solid foods. Exposure to rotavirus is universal, with most children experiencing their first infection in the first or second year of life if not vaccinated. Older children and adults are more commonly infected with norovirus. Other organisms with higher attack rates among children than among adults include enterotoxigenic, enteropathogenic, and enterohemorrhagic *E. coli*; *Shigella*; *C. jejuni*; and *G. lamblia*.

HOST IMMUNE STATUS

Immunocompromised hosts are at elevated risk of acute and chronic infectious diarrhea. Individuals with defects in cell-mediated immunity (including those with AIDS) are at particularly high risk of invasive enteropathies, including salmonellosis, listeriosis, and cryptosporidiosis. Individuals with hypogammaglobulinemia are at particular risk of *C. difficile* colitis and giardiasis. Patients with cancer are more likely to develop *C. difficile* infection as a result of chemotherapy and frequent hospitalizations. Infectious diarrhea can be life-threatening in immunocompromised hosts, with complications including bacteremia and metastatic seeding of infection. Furthermore, dehydration may compromise renal function and increase the toxicity of immunosuppressive drugs.

BACTERIAL FOOD POISONING

If the history and the stool examination indicate a noninflammatory etiology of diarrhea and there is evidence of a common-source outbreak, questions concerning the ingestion of specific foods and the time of onset of the diarrhea after a meal can provide clues to the bacterial cause of the illness. Potential causes of bacterial food poisoning are shown in Table 160-4.

TABLE 160-4 BACTERIAL FOOD POISONING

Incubation Period, Organism	Symptoms	Common Food Sources
1–6 h		
Staphylococcus aureus	Nausea, vomiting, diarrhea	Ham, poultry, potato or egg salad, mayonnaise, cream pastries
Bacillus cereus	Nausea, vomiting, diarrhea	Fried rice
8–16 h		
Clostridium perfringens	Abdominal cramps, diarrhea (vomiting rare)	Beef, poultry, legumes, gravies
B. cereus	Abdominal cramps, diarrhea (vomiting rare)	Meats, vegetables, dried beans, cereals
>16 h		
Vibrio cholerae	Watery diarrhea	Shellfish, water
Enterotoxigenic *Escherichia coli*	Watery diarrhea	Salads, cheese, meats, water
Enterohemorrhagic *E. coli*	Bloody diarrhea	Ground beef, roast beef, salami, raw milk, raw vegetables, apple juice
Salmonella spp.	Inflammatory diarrhea	Beef, poultry, eggs, dairy products
Campylobacter jejuni	Inflammatory diarrhea	Poultry, raw milk
Shigella spp.	Dysentery	Potato or egg salad, lettuce, raw vegetables
Vibrio parahaemolyticus	Dysentery	Mollusks, crustaceans

Bacterial disease caused by an enterotoxin elaborated outside the host, such as that due to *Staphylococcus aureus* or *B. cereus*, has the shortest incubation period (1–6 h) and generally lasts <12 h. Most cases of staphylococcal food poisoning are caused by contamination from infected human carriers. Staphylococci can multiply at a wide range of temperatures; thus, if food is left to cool slowly and remains at room temperature after cooking, the organisms will have the opportunity to form enterotoxin. Outbreaks following picnics where potato salad, mayonnaise, and cream pastries have been served offer classic examples of staphylococcal food poisoning. Diarrhea, nausea, vomiting, and abdominal cramping are common, while fever is less so.

B. cereus can produce either a syndrome with a short incubation period—the *emetic* form, mediated by a staphylococcal type of enterotoxin—or one with a longer incubation period (8–16 h)—the *diarrheal* form, caused by an enterotoxin resembling *E. coli* LT, in which diarrhea and abdominal cramps are characteristic but vomiting is uncommon. The emetic form of *B. cereus* food poisoning is associated with contaminated fried rice; the organism is common in uncooked rice, and its heat-resistant spores survive boiling. If cooked rice is not refrigerated, the spores can germinate and produce toxin. Frying before serving may not destroy the preformed, heat-stable toxin.

Food poisoning due to *Clostridium perfringens* also has a slightly longer incubation period (8–14 h) and results from the survival of heat-resistant spores in inadequately cooked meat, poultry, or legumes. After ingestion, toxin is produced in the intestinal tract, causing moderately severe abdominal cramps and diarrhea; vomiting is rare, as is fever. The illness is self-limited, rarely lasting >24 h.

Not all food poisoning has a bacterial cause. Nonbacterial agents of short-incubation food poisoning include capsaicin, which is found in hot peppers, and a variety of toxins found in fish and shellfish (Chap. 474).

LABORATORY EVALUATION

Many cases of noninflammatory diarrhea are self-limited or can be treated empirically, and in these instances the clinician may not need to determine a specific etiology. Potentially pathogenic *E. coli* cannot be distinguished from normal fecal flora by routine culture, and tests to detect enterotoxins are not available in most clinical laboratories. In situations in which cholera is a concern, stool should be cultured on selective media such as thiosulfate–citrate–bile salts–sucrose (TCBS) or tellurite-taurocholate-gelatin (TTG) agar. A latex agglutination test has made the rapid detection of rotavirus in stool practical for many laboratories, while reverse-transcriptase polymerase chain reaction (PCR) and specific antigen enzyme immunoassays have been developed for the identification of norovirus. Stool specimens should be examined by immunofluorescence-based rapid assays or (less sensitive) standard microscopy for *Giardia* cysts or *Cryptosporidium* if the level of clinical suspicion regarding the involvement of these organisms is high.

All patients with fever and evidence of inflammatory disease acquired outside the hospital should have stool cultured for *Salmonella*, *Shigella*, and *Campylobacter*. *Salmonella* and *Shigella* can be selected on MacConkey agar as non-lactose-fermenting (colorless) colonies or can be grown on *Salmonella-Shigella* agar or in selenite enrichment broth, both of which inhibit most organisms except these pathogens. Evaluation of nosocomial diarrhea should initially focus on *C. difficile*; stool culture for other pathogens in this setting has an extremely low yield and is not cost-effective. Toxins A and B produced by pathogenic strains of *C. difficile* can be detected by rapid enzyme immunoassays, latex agglutination tests, or PCR (Chap. 161). Isolation of *C. jejuni* requires inoculation of fresh stool onto selective growth medium and incubation at 42°C in a microaerophilic atmosphere. In many laboratories in the United States, *E. coli* O157:H7 is among the most common pathogens isolated from visibly bloody stools. Strains of this enterohemorrhagic serotype can be identified in specialized laboratories by serotyping but also can be identified presumptively in hospital laboratories as lactose-fermenting, indole-positive colonies of sorbitol nonfermenters (white colonies) on sorbitol MacConkey plates. If the clinical presentation suggests the possibility of intestinal amebiasis, stool should be examined by a rapid antigen detection assay or by (less sensitive and less specific) microscopy.

TREATMENT INFECTIOUS DIARRHEA OR BACTERIAL FOOD POISONING

In many cases, a specific diagnosis is not necessary or not available to guide treatment. The clinician can proceed with the information obtained from the history, stool examination, and evaluation of dehydration severity. Empirical regimens for the treatment of traveler's diarrhea are listed in **Table 160-5**.

The mainstay of treatment is adequate rehydration. The treatment of cholera and other dehydrating diarrheal diseases was revolutionized by the promotion of oral rehydration solution (ORS), the efficacy of which depends on the fact that glucose-facilitated absorption of sodium and water in the small intestine remains intact in the presence of cholera toxin. The use of ORS has reduced mortality rates for cholera from >50% (in untreated cases) to <1%. A number of ORS formulas have been used. Initial preparations were based on the treatment of patients with cholera and included a solution containing 3.5 g of sodium chloride, 2.5 g of sodium bicarbonate (or 2.9 g of sodium citrate), 1.5 g of potassium chloride, and 20 g of glucose (or 40 g of sucrose) per liter of water. Such a preparation can still be used for the treatment of severe cholera. Many causes of secretory diarrhea, however, are associated with less electrolyte loss than occurs in cholera. Beginning in 2002, the World Health Organization recommended a "reduced-osmolarity/reduced-salt" ORS that is better tolerated and more effective than classic ORS. This preparation contains 2.6 g of sodium chloride, 2.9 g of trisodium citrate, 1.5 g of potassium chloride, and 13.5 g of glucose (or 27 g of sucrose) per liter of water. ORS formulations containing rice or cereal as the carbohydrate source may be even more effective than glucose-based solutions. Patients who are severely dehydrated or in whom vomiting precludes the use of oral therapy should receive IV solutions such as Ringer's lactate.

Although most secretory forms of traveler's diarrhea (usually due to enterotoxigenic or enteroaggregative *E. coli* or to *Campylobacter*) can be treated effectively with rehydration, bismuth subsalicylate,

TABLE 160-5 TREATMENT OF TRAVELER'S DIARRHEA ON THE BASIS OF CLINICAL FEATURES[a]

Clinical Syndrome	Suggested Therapy
Watery diarrhea (no blood in stool, no fever), 1 or 2 unformed stools per day without distressing enteric symptoms	Oral fluids (oral rehydration solution, Pedialyte, Lytren, or flavored mineral water) and saltine crackers
Watery diarrhea (no blood in stool, no fever), 1 or 2 unformed stools per day with distressing enteric symptoms	Bismuth subsalicylate (for adults): 30 mL or 2 tablets (262 mg/tablet) every 30 min for 8 doses; or loperamide[b]: 4 mg initially followed by 2 mg after passage of each unformed stool, not to exceed 8 tablets (16 mg) per day (prescription dose) or 4 caplets (8 mg) per day (over-the-counter dose); drugs can be taken for 2 days
Watery diarrhea (no blood in stool, no distressing abdominal pain, no fever), >2 unformed stools per day	Antibacterial drug[c] plus (for adults) loperamide[b] (see dose above)
Dysentery (passage of bloody stools) or fever (>37.8°C)	Antibacterial drug[c]
Vomiting, minimal diarrhea	Bismuth subsalicylate (for adults; see dose above)
Diarrhea in infants (<2 years old)	Fluids and electrolytes (oral rehydration solution, Pedialyte, Lytren); continue feeding, especially with breast milk; seek medical attention for moderate dehydration, fever lasting >24 h, bloody stools, or diarrhea lasting more than several days

[a]All patients should take oral fluids (Pedialyte, Lytren, or flavored mineral water) plus saltine crackers. If diarrhea becomes moderate or severe, if fever persists, or if bloody stools or dehydration develops, the patient should seek medical attention. [b]Loperamide should not be used by patients with fever or dysentery; its use may prolong diarrhea in patients with infection due to *Shigella* or other invasive organisms. [c]The recommended antibacterial drugs are as follows:

If the level of suspicion is low for fluoroquinolone-resistant *Campylobacter*:
Adults: (1) A fluoroquinolone such as ciprofloxacin, 750 mg as a single dose or 500 mg bid for 3 days; levofloxacin, 500 mg as a single dose or 500 mg qd for 3 days; or norfloxacin, 800 mg as a single dose or 400 mg bid for 3 days. (2) Azithromycin, 1000 mg as a single dose or 500 mg qd for 3 days. (3) Rifaximin, 200 mg tid or 400 mg bid for 3 days (not recommended for use in dysentery).

Children: Azithromycin, 10 mg/kg on day 1, 5 mg/kg on days 2 and 3 if diarrhea persists.

If fluoroquinolone-resistant *Campylobacter* is suspected (for example, following travel to Southeast Asia):
Adults: Azithromycin (at above dose for adults). *Children:* Same as for children traveling to other areas (see above).

Source: After DR Hill et al: The practice of travel medicine. Guidelines by the Infectious Diseases Society of America. Clin Infect Dis 43:1499, 2006.

or antiperistaltic agents, antimicrobial agents can shorten the duration of illness from 3–4 days to 24–36 h. Changes in diet have not been shown to have an impact on the duration of illness, while the efficacy of probiotics continues to be debated. Most individuals who present with dysentery (bloody diarrhea and fever) should be treated empirically with an antimicrobial agent (e.g., a fluoroquinolone or a macrolide) pending microbiologic analysis of stool. Individuals with shigellosis should receive a 3- to 7-day course. Individuals with *Campylobacter* infection often benefit from antimicrobial treatment as well. Because of widespread resistance of *Campylobacter* to fluoroquinolones, especially in parts of Asia, a macrolide antibiotic such as erythromycin or azithromycin may be preferred for this infection.

Treatment of salmonellosis must be tailored to the individual patient. Since administration of antimicrobial agents often prolongs intestinal colonization with *Salmonella*, these drugs are usually reserved for individuals at high risk of complications from disseminated salmonellosis, such as young children, patients with prosthetic devices, elderly patients, and immunocompromised persons. Antimicrobial agents should not be administered to individuals (especially children) in whom enterohemorrhagic *E. coli* infection is suspected. Laboratory studies of enterohemorrhagic *E. coli* strains have demonstrated that a number of antibiotics induce replication of Shiga toxin–producing lambdoid bacteriophages, thereby significantly increasing toxin production by these strains. Clinical studies have supported these laboratory results, and antibiotics may increase by twentyfold the risk of hemolytic-uremic syndrome and renal failure during enterohemorrhagic *E. coli* infection. A clinical clue in the diagnosis of the latter infection is bloody diarrhea with low fever or none at all.

PROPHYLAXIS

Improvements in hygiene to limit fecal-oral spread of enteric pathogens will be necessary if the prevalence of diarrheal diseases is to be significantly reduced in developing countries. Travelers can reduce their risk of diarrhea by eating only hot, freshly cooked food; by avoiding raw vegetables, salads, and unpeeled fruit; and by drinking only boiled or treated water and avoiding ice. Historically, few travelers to tourist destinations adhere to these dietary restrictions. Bismuth subsalicylate is an inexpensive agent for the prophylaxis of traveler's diarrhea; it is taken at a dosage of 2 tablets (525 mg) four times a day. Treatment appears to be effective and safe for up to 3 weeks, but adverse events such as temporary darkening of the tongue and tinnitus can occur. A meta-analysis suggests that probiotics may lessen the likelihood of traveler's diarrhea by ~15%. Prophylactic antimicrobial agents, although effective, are not generally recommended for the prevention of traveler's diarrhea except when travelers are immunosuppressed or have other underlying illnesses that place them at high risk for morbidity from gastrointestinal infection. The risk of side effects and the possibility of developing an infection with a drug-resistant organism or with more harmful, invasive bacteria make it more reasonable to institute an empirical short course of treatment if symptoms develop. If prophylaxis is indicated, the nonabsorbed antibiotic rifaximin can be considered.

The possibility of exerting a major impact on the worldwide morbidity and mortality associated with diarrheal diseases has led to intense efforts to develop effective vaccines against the common bacterial and viral enteric pathogens. An effective rotavirus vaccine is currently available. Vaccines against *S. typhi* and *V. cholerae* also are available, although the protection they offer is incomplete and/or short lived. At present, there is no effective commercially available vaccine against *Shigella*, enterotoxigenic *E. coli*, *Campylobacter*, nontyphoidal *Salmonella*, norovirus, or intestinal parasites.

161 *Clostridium difficile* Infection, Including Pseudomembranous Colitis

Dale N. Gerding, Stuart Johnson

DEFINITION

Clostridium difficile infection (CDI) is a unique colonic disease that is acquired most often in association with antimicrobial use and the consequent disruption of the normal colonic microbiota. The most commonly diagnosed diarrheal illness acquired in the hospital, CDI results from the ingestion of spores of *C. difficile* that vegetate, multiply, and secrete toxins, causing diarrhea and pseudomembranous colitis (PMC) in the most severe cases.

ETIOLOGY AND EPIDEMIOLOGY

C. difficile is an obligately anaerobic, gram-positive, spore-forming bacillus whose spores are found widely in nature, particularly in the environment of hospitals and chronic-care facilities. CDI occurs frequently in hospitals and nursing homes (or shortly after discharge from these facilities) where the level of antimicrobial use is high and the environment is contaminated by *C. difficile* spores.

Clindamycin, ampicillin, and cephalosporins were the first antibiotics associated with CDI. The second- and third-generation cephalosporins, particularly cefotaxime, ceftriaxone, cefuroxime, and ceftazidime, are frequently responsible for this condition, and the fluoroquinolones (ciprofloxacin, levofloxacin, and moxifloxacin) are the most recent drug class to be implicated in hospital outbreaks. Penicillin/β-lactamase-inhibitor combinations such as ticarcillin/clavulanate and piperacillin/tazobactam pose significantly less risk. However, all antibiotics, including vancomycin and metronidazole (the agents most commonly used to treat CDI), carry a risk of subsequent CDI. Rare cases are reported in patients without prior antibiotic exposure.

C. difficile is acquired exogenously—most frequently in the hospital or nursing home, but also possibly in the outpatient setting—and is carried in the stool of both symptomatic and asymptomatic patients. The rate of fecal colonization is often ≥20% among adult patients hospitalized for >1 week; in contrast, the rate is 1–3% among community residents. Community-onset CDI without recent hospitalization, nursing home residence, or outpatient health-care contact probably accounts for ≤10% of all cases. The risk of *C. difficile* acquisition increases in proportion to the length of hospital stay. Asymptomatic fecal carriage of *C. difficile* in healthy neonates is very common, with repeated colonization by multiple strains in infants (<1 year old), but associated disease in these infants is extremely rare if it occurs at all. Spores of *C. difficile* are found on environmental surfaces (where the organism can persist for months) and on the hands of hospital personnel who fail to practice good hand hygiene. Hospital epidemics of CDI have been attributed to a single *C. difficile* strain and to multiple strains present simultaneously. Other identified risk factors for CDI include older age, greater severity of underlying illness, gastrointestinal surgery, use of electronic rectal thermometers, enteral tube feeding, and antacid treatment. Use of proton pump inhibitors may be a risk factor, but this risk is probably modest, and no firm data have implicated these agents in patients who are not already receiving antibiotics.

PATHOLOGY AND PATHOGENESIS

Spores of toxigenic *C. difficile* are ingested, survive gastric acidity, germinate in the small bowel, and colonize the lower intestinal tract, where they elaborate two large toxins: toxin A (an enterotoxin) and toxin B (a cytotoxin). These toxins initiate processes resulting in the disruption of epithelial-cell barrier function, diarrhea, and pseudomembrane formation. Toxin A is a potent neutrophil chemoattractant, and both toxins glucosylate the guanosine triphosphate (GTP)–binding proteins of the Rho subfamily that regulate the actin cell cytoskeleton. Data from studies using molecular disruption of toxin genes in isogenic mutants suggest that toxin B is the more important virulence factor. This possibility, if confirmed, might account for the occurrence of clinical disease caused by toxin A–negative strains. Disruption of the cytoskeleton results in loss of cell shape, adherence, and tight junctions, with consequent fluid leakage. A third toxin, binary toxin CDT, was previously found in only ~6% of strains but is present in all isolates of the widely recognized epidemic NAP1/BI/027 strain (see "Global Considerations," below); this toxin is related to *C. perfringens* iota toxin. Its role in the pathogenesis of CDI has not yet been defined.

The pseudomembranes of PMC are confined to the colonic mucosa and initially appear as 1- to 2-mm whitish-yellow plaques. The intervening mucosa appears unremarkable, but, as the disease progresses, the pseudomembranes coalesce to form larger plaques and become confluent over the entire colon wall (Fig. 161-1). The whole colon is usually involved, but 10% of patients have rectal sparing. Viewed microscopically, the pseudomembranes have a mucosal attachment point and contain necrotic leukocytes, fibrin, mucus, and cellular debris. The epithelium is eroded and necrotic in focal areas, with neutrophil infiltration of the mucosa.

Patients colonized with *C. difficile* were initially thought to be at high risk for CDI. However, four prospective studies have shown that colonized patients who have not previously had CDI actually have a decreased risk of CDI. At least three events are proposed as essential for the development of CDI (Fig. 161-2). Exposure to antimicrobial agents is the first event and establishes susceptibility to *C. difficile* infection, most likely through disruption of the normal gastrointestinal microbiota. The second event is exposure to toxigenic *C. difficile*. Given that the majority of patients do not develop CDI after the first two events, a third event is clearly essential for its occurrence. Candidate third events include exposure to a *C. difficile* strain of particular virulence, exposure to antimicrobial agents especially likely

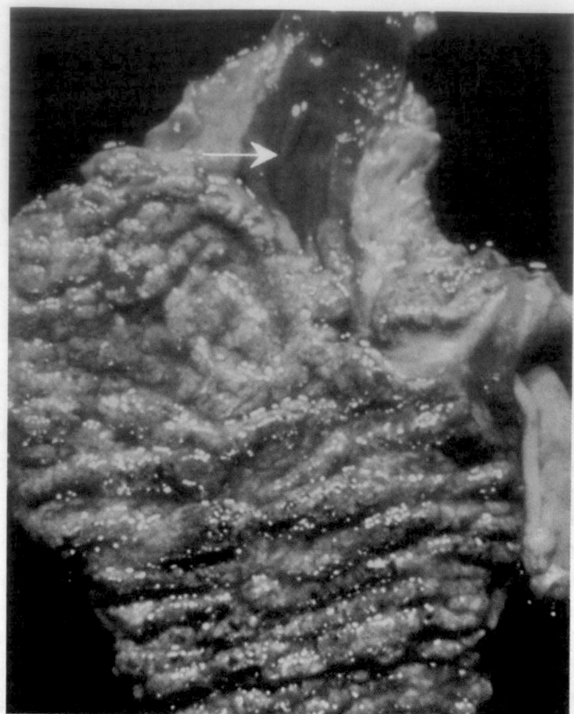

FIGURE 161-1 Autopsy specimen showing confluent pseudomembranes covering the cecum of a patient with pseudomembranous colitis. Note the sparing of the terminal ileum (*arrow*).

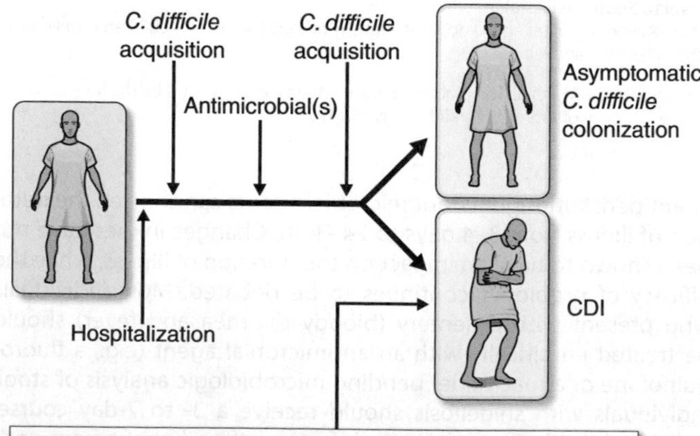

FIGURE 161-2 Pathogenesis model for hospital-acquired *Clostridium difficile* infection (CDI). At least three events are integral to *C. difficile* pathogenesis: (1) Exposure to antibiotics establishes susceptibility to infection. (2) Once susceptible, the patient may acquire nontoxigenic (nonpathogenic) or toxigenic strains of *C. difficile* as a second event. (3) Acquisition of toxigenic *C. difficile* may be followed by asymptomatic colonization or CDI, depending on one or more additional events (e.g., an inadequate host anamnestic IgG response to *C. difficile* toxin A).

to cause CDI, and an inadequate host immune response. The host anamnestic serum IgG antibody response to toxin A of *C. difficile* is the most likely third event that determines which patients develop diarrhea and which patients remain asymptomatic. In all probability, the majority of people first develop antibody to *C. difficile* toxins when colonized asymptomatically during the first year of life or after CDI in childhood. Infants are thought not to develop symptomatic CDI because they lack suitable mucosal toxin receptors that develop later in life. In adulthood, serum levels of IgG antibody to toxin A increase more in response to infection in individuals who become asymptomatic carriers than in those who develop CDI. For persons who develop CDI, development of increasing levels of antitoxin A during treatment correlates with a lower risk of recurrence of CDI. A clinical trial using monoclonal antibodies to both toxin A and toxin B in addition to standard therapy showed rates of recurrence significantly lower than those obtained with placebo plus standard therapy.

GLOBAL CONSIDERATIONS

Rates and severity of CDI in the United States, Canada, and Europe increased markedly after the year 2000. Rates in U.S. hospitals tripled between 2000 and 2005. In 2005, hospitals in Montreal, Quebec, reported rates four times higher than the 1997 baseline, with directly attributable mortality of 6.9% (increased from 1.5%). An epidemic strain, variously known as toxinotype III, REA type BI, polymerase chain reaction (PCR) ribotype 027, and pulsed-field type NAP1 and thus collectively designated NAP1/BI/027, is thought to account for much of the increase in incidence and has been found in North America, Europe, and Asia. It is now recognized that two clones of NAP1/BI/027 originated in the United States and Canada and spread to the United Kingdom, Europe, and Asia. The epidemic organism is characterized by (1) an ability to produce 16–23 times as much toxin A and toxin B as control strains in vitro; (2) the presence of a third toxin (binary toxin CDT); and (3) high-level resistance to all fluoroquinolones. New strains have been and probably will continue to be implicated in outbreaks, including a strain (toxinotype V, ribotype 078) commonly found in food animals that also carries binary toxin and has been associated with high mortality risk in human infections. In the past 5 years, rates of CDI in the United Kingdom have markedly decreased, and the frequency of the NAP1/BI/027 strain in the countries of the European Union has likewise decreased. However, there has been no evidence of decreased rates of CDI or a decreased incidence of NAP1/BI/027 in North America; the latter strain still causes 25–35% of all CDIs in most regions of the United States.

CLINICAL MANIFESTATIONS

Diarrhea is the most common manifestation caused by *C. difficile*. Stools are almost never grossly bloody and range from soft and unformed to watery or mucoid in consistency, with a characteristic odor. Patients may have as many as 20 bowel movements per day. Clinical and laboratory findings include fever in 28% of cases, abdominal pain in 22%, and leukocytosis in 50%. When adynamic ileus (which is seen on x-ray in ~20% of cases) results in cessation of stool passage, the diagnosis of CDI is frequently overlooked. A clue to the presence of unsuspected CDI in these patients is unexplained leukocytosis, with ≥15,000 white blood cells (WBCs)/μL. Such patients are at high risk for complications of *C. difficile* infection, particularly toxic megacolon and sepsis.

C. difficile diarrhea recurs after treatment in ~15–30% of cases, and this figure may be increasing. Recurrences may represent either relapses due to the same strain or reinfections with a new strain. Susceptibility to recurrence of clinical CDI is likely a result of continued fecal-microbiota disruption caused by the antibiotic used to treat CDI.

DIAGNOSIS

The diagnosis of CDI is based on a combination of clinical criteria: (1) diarrhea (≥3 unformed stools per 24 h for ≥2 days) with no other recognized cause plus (2) toxin A or B detected in the stool, toxin-producing *C. difficile* detected in the stool by PCR or culture, or pseudomembranes seen in the colon. PMC is a more advanced form of CDI and is visualized at endoscopy in only ~50% of patients with diarrhea who have a positive stool culture and toxin assay for *C. difficile*. Endoscopy is a rapid diagnostic tool in seriously ill patients with suspected PMC and an acute abdomen, but a negative result in this examination does not rule out CDI.

Despite the array of tests available for *C. difficile* and its toxins (Table 161-1), no single traditional test has high sensitivity, high specificity, and rapid turnaround. Most laboratory tests for toxins, including enzyme immunoassays, lack sensitivity. However, testing of multiple additional stool specimens is not recommended. Nucleic acid amplification tests, including PCR assays, have now been approved for diagnostic purposes and appear to be both rapid and sensitive while retaining high specificity. Testing of asymptomatic patients is not recommended except for epidemiologic study purposes. In particular, so-called tests of cure following treatment are not recommended because >50% of patients continue to harbor the organism and toxin after diarrhea has ceased and test results do not always predict recurrence of CDI. Thus these results should not be used to restrict placement of patients in long-term-care or nursing home facilities.

TREATMENT *CLOSTRIDIUM DIFFICILE* INFECTION

PRIMARY CDI

When possible, discontinuation of any ongoing antimicrobial administration is recommended as the first step in treatment of CDI. Earlier studies indicated that 15–23% of patients respond to this simple measure. However, with the advent of the current epidemic strain and the associated rapid clinical deterioration of some patients,

TABLE 161-1 RELATIVE SENSITIVITY AND SPECIFICITY OF DIAGNOSTIC TESTS FOR *CLOSTRIDIUM DIFFICILE* INFECTION (CDI)

Type of Test	Relative Sensitivity[a]	Relative Specificity[a]	Comment
Stool culture for *C. difficile*	++++	+++	Most sensitive test; specificity of ++++ if the *C. difficile* isolate tests positive for toxin; with clinical data, is diagnostic of CDI; turnaround time too slow for practical use
Cell culture cytotoxin test on stool	+++	++++	With clinical data, is diagnostic of CDI; highly specific but not as sensitive as stool culture; slow turnaround time
Enzyme immunoassay for toxin A or toxins A and B in stool	++ to +++	+++	With clinical data, is diagnostic of CDI; rapid results, but not as sensitive as stool culture or cell culture cytotoxin test
Enzyme immunoassay for *C. difficile* common antigen in stool	+++ to ++++	+++	Detects glutamate dehydrogenase found in toxigenic and nontoxigenic strains of *C. difficile* and other stool organisms; more sensitive and less specific than enzyme immunoassay for toxins; rapid results
Nucleic acid amplification tests for *C. difficile* toxin A or B gene in stool	++++	++++	Detect toxigenic *C. difficile* in stool; newly approved for clinical testing, but appears to be more sensitive than enzyme immunoassay toxin testing and at least as specific
Colonoscopy or sigmoidoscopy	+	++++	Highly specific if pseudomembranes are seen; insensitive compared with other tests

[a]According to both clinical and test-based criteria. ++++, >90%; +++, 71–90%; ++, 51–70%; +, ~50%.

prompt initiation of specific CDI treatment has become the standard. Empirical treatment is appropriate if CDI is strongly suspected on clinical grounds. General treatment guidelines include hydration and the avoidance of antiperistaltic agents and opiates, which may mask symptoms and possibly worsen disease. Nevertheless, antiperistaltic agents have been used safely with vancomycin or metronidazole for mild to moderate CDI.

Oral administration of vancomycin, fidaxomicin, or metronidazole is recommended for CDI treatment. IV vancomycin is ineffective for CDI, and fidaxomicin is available only for oral administration; when IV metronidazole is administered, fecal bactericidal drug concentrations are achieved during acute diarrhea; however, in the presence of adynamic ileus, IV metronidazole treatment of CDI has failed. Two large clinical trials comparing vancomycin and fidaxomicin indicated comparable resolution of diarrhea (~90% of patients) as well as significantly reduced rates of recurrent CDI with fidaxomicin from rates with vancomycin. In previous randomized trials, diarrhea response rates to oral therapy with vancomycin or metronidazole were ≥94%, but four observational studies found that response rates for metronidazole had declined to 62–78%. Although the mean time to resolution of diarrhea is 2–4 days, the response to metronidazole may be much slower. Treatment should not be deemed a failure until a drug has been given for at least 6 days. On the basis of data for shorter courses of vancomycin and the results of two large-scale clinical trials, it is recommended that vancomycin, fidaxomicin, and metronidazole be given for at least 10 days. Metronidazole is not approved for CDI by the U.S. Food and Drug Administration (FDA), but most patients with mild to moderate illness respond to 500 mg given by mouth three times a day for 10 days; extension of the treatment period may be needed for slow responders. In addition to the reports of increases in metronidazole failures, a prospective, randomized, double-blind, placebo-controlled study has demonstrated the superiority of vancomycin over metronidazole for treatment of severe CDI. The severity assessment score in that study included age as well as laboratory parameters (elevated temperature, low albumin level, or elevated WBC count), documentation of PMC by endoscopy, and treatment of CDI in the intensive care unit. Although a validated severity score is not available, it is important to initiate treatment with oral vancomycin for patients who appear seriously ill, particularly if they have a high WBC count (>15,000/μL) or a creatinine level that is ≥1.5 times higher than the premorbid value (Table 161-2). In addition, a randomized blinded trial compared a toxin-binding polymer, tolevamer, with two antibiotic regimens for treatment of CDI and showed that vancomycin was superior to metronidazole for all patients regardless of severity. Small randomized trials of nitazoxanide, bacitracin, rifaximin, and fusidic acid for treatment of CDI have been conducted. These drugs have not been extensively studied, shown to be superior, or approved by the FDA for CDI, but they provide potential alternatives to vancomycin, fidaxomicin, and metronidazole.

RECURRENT CDI

Overall, ~15–30% of successfully treated patients experience recurrences of CDI, either as relapses caused by the original organism or as reinfections following treatment. Rates of CDI recurrence are significantly lower among patients treated with fidaxomicin rather than vancomycin. Rates of recurrence are comparable with vancomycin and metronidazole. Recurrence rates are higher among patients ≥65 years old, those who continue to take antibiotics while being treated for CDI, and those who remain in the hospital after the initial episode of CDI. Patients who have a first recurrence of CDI have a high rate of second recurrence (33–65%). In the first recurrence, re-treatment with metronidazole is comparable to treatment with vancomycin (Table 161-2), and fidaxomicin is superior to vancomycin in reducing the risk of further recurrences in patients who have had one recurrence. Recurrent CDI, once thought to be relatively mild, has now been documented to pose a significant (11%) risk of serious complications (shock, megacolon, perforation, colectomy, or death within 30 days). There is no standard treatment for multiple recurrences, but long or repeated metronidazole courses should be avoided because of potential neurotoxicity. The use of vancomycin in tapering doses or with pulse dosing every other day for 2–8 weeks may be the most practical approach to treatment of patients with multiple recurrences. Other approaches include the administration of vancomycin followed by the yeast *Saccharomyces boulardii*; the administration of vancomycin followed by a fecal microbiota transplant given via nasoduodenal tube, colonoscope, or enema; and the intentional colonization of the patient with a nontoxigenic

TABLE 161-2 RECOMMENDATIONS FOR THE TREATMENT OF *CLOSTRIDIUM DIFFICILE* INFECTION (CDI)[a]

Clinical Setting	Treatment(s)	Comments
Initial episode, mild to moderate	Metronidazole (500 mg tid × 10–14 d)	Vancomycin (125 mg qid × 10–14 d) may be more effective than metronidazole. Fidaxomicin (200 mg bid × 10 d) is another alternative.
Initial episode, severe	Vancomycin (125 mg qid × 10–14 d)	Indicators of severe disease may include leukocytosis (≥15,000 white blood cells/μL) and a creatinine level ≥1.5 times the premorbid value. Fidaxomicin is an alternative.
Initial episode, severe complicated or fulminant	Vancomycin (500 mg PO or via nasogastric tube) ***plus*** metronidazole (500 mg IV q8h) ***plus consider*** Rectal instillation of vancomycin (500 mg in 100 mL of normal saline as a retention enema q6–8h)	Severe complicated or fulminant CDI is defined as severe CDI with the addition of hypotension, shock, ileus, or toxic megacolon. The duration of treatment may need to be >2 weeks and is dictated by response. Consider using tigecycline (50 mg IV q12h after a 100-mg loading dose) in place of metronidazole.
First recurrence	Same as for initial episode	Adjust treatment if severity of CDI has changed with recurrence. Consider fidaxomicin, which significantly decreases the likelihood of additional recurrences.
Second recurrence	Vancomycin in taper/pulse regimen	Typical taper/pulse regimen: 125 mg qid × 10–14 d, then bid × 1 week, then daily × 1 week, then q2–3d for 2–8 weeks.
Multiple recurrences	Consider the following options: • Repeat vancomycin taper/pulse • Vancomycin (500 mg qid × 10 d) plus *Saccharomyces boulardii* (500 mg bid × 28 d) • Vancomycin (125 mg qid × 10–14 d); then stop vancomycin and start rifaximin (400 mg bid × 2 weeks) • Nitazoxanide (500 mg bid × 10 d) • Fecal microbiota transplantation • IV immunoglobulin (400 mg/kg)	The only controlled studies that included patients with one or more recurrent CDI episodes were with vancomycin and *S. boulardii*, which showed borderline significance compared with vancomycin plus placebo, and fecal microbiota transplantation, which was highly significant compared with a high-dose course of vancomycin. (The vancomycin taper was not compared.)

[a]All agents are given orally unless otherwise specified.

strain of *C. difficile*. None of these biotherapeutic approaches has been approved by the FDA for use in the United States. Other non-FDA-approved antibiotic strategies include (1) sequential treatment with vancomycin (125 mg four times daily for 10–14 days) followed by rifaximin (400 mg twice daily for 14 days) and (2) treatment with nitazoxanide (500 mg twice daily for 7 days). IV immunoglobulin, which has also been used with variable success, presumably provides antibodies to *C. difficile* toxins.

SEVERE COMPLICATED OR FULMINANT CDI

Fulminant (rapidly progressive and severe) CDI presents the most difficult treatment challenge. Patients with fulminant disease often do not have diarrhea, and their illness mimics an acute surgical abdomen. Sepsis (hypotension, fever, tachycardia, leukocytosis) may result from severe CDI. An acute abdomen (with or without toxic megacolon) may include signs of obstruction, ileus, colon-wall thickening and ascites on abdominal CT, and peripheral-blood leukocytosis (≥20,000 WBCs/μL). With or without diarrhea, the differential diagnosis of an acute abdomen, sepsis, or toxic megacolon should include CDI if the patient has received antibiotics in the past 2 months. Cautious sigmoidoscopy or colonoscopy to visualize PMC and abdominal CT are the best diagnostic tests in patients without diarrhea.

Medical management of fulminant CDI is suboptimal because of the difficulty of delivering oral fidaxomicin, metronidazole, or vancomycin to the colon in the presence of ileus (Table 161-2). The combination of vancomycin (given via nasogastric tube and by retention enema) plus IV metronidazole has been used with some success in uncontrolled studies, as has IV tigecycline in small-scale uncontrolled studies. Surgical colectomy may be life-saving if there is no response to medical management. If possible, colectomy should be performed before the serum lactate level reaches 5 mmol/L. The incidence of fulminant CDI requiring colectomy appears to be increasing in the evolving epidemic; however, morbidity and death associated with colectomy may be reduced by performing instead a laparoscopic ileostomy followed by colon lavage with polyethylene glycol and vancomycin infusion into the colon via the ileostomy.

PROGNOSIS

The mortality rate attributed to CDI, previously found to be 0.6–3.5%, has reached 6.9% in recent outbreaks and rises progressively with increasing age. Most patients recover, but recurrences are common.

PREVENTION AND CONTROL

Strategies for the prevention of CDI are of two types: those aimed at preventing transmission of the organism to the patient and those aimed at reducing the risk of CDI if the organism is transmitted. Transmission of *C. difficile* in clinical practice has been prevented by gloving of personnel, elimination of the use of contaminated electronic thermometers, and use of hypochlorite (bleach) solution for environmental decontamination of patients' rooms. Hand hygiene is critical; hand washing is recommended in CDI outbreaks because alcohol hand gels are not sporicidal. CDI outbreaks have been best controlled by restricting the use of specific antibiotics, such as clindamycin and second- and third-generation cephalosporins. Outbreaks of CDI due to clindamycin-resistant strains have resolved promptly when clindamycin use is restricted. Future preventive strategies are likely to include use of monoclonal antibodies, vaccines, and biotherapeutics containing live organisms that will restore colonization protection in the microbiota.

162 Urinary Tract Infections, Pyelonephritis, and Prostatitis

Kalpana Gupta, Barbara W. Trautner

Urinary tract infection (UTI) is a common and painful human illness that, fortunately, is rapidly responsive to modern antibiotic therapy. In the preantibiotic era, UTI caused significant morbidity. Hippocrates, writing about a disease that appears to have been acute cystitis, said that the illness could last for a year before either resolving or worsening to involve the kidneys. When chemotherapeutic agents used to treat UTI were introduced in the early twentieth century, they were relatively ineffective, and persistence of infection after 3 weeks of therapy was common. Nitrofurantoin, which became available in the 1950s, was the first tolerable and effective agent for the treatment of UTI.

Since the most common manifestation of UTI is acute cystitis and since acute cystitis is far more prevalent among women than among men, most clinical research on UTI has involved women. Many studies have enrolled women from college campuses or large health maintenance organizations in the United States. Therefore, when reviewing the literature and recommendations concerning UTI, clinicians must consider whether the findings are applicable to their patient populations.

DEFINITIONS

UTI may be asymptomatic (subclinical infection) or symptomatic (disease). Thus, the term *urinary tract infection* encompasses a variety of clinical entities, including asymptomatic bacteriuria (ASB), cystitis, prostatitis, and pyelonephritis. The distinction between symptomatic UTI and ASB has major clinical implications. Both UTI and ASB connote the presence of bacteria in the urinary tract, usually accompanied by white blood cells and inflammatory cytokines in the urine. However, ASB occurs in the absence of symptoms attributable to the bacteria in the urinary tract and does not usually require treatment, while UTI has more typically been assumed to imply symptomatic disease that warrants antimicrobial therapy. Much of the literature concerning UTI, particularly catheter-associated infection, does not differentiate between UTI and ASB. In this chapter, the term *UTI* denotes symptomatic disease; *cystitis*, symptomatic infection of the bladder; and *pyelonephritis*, symptomatic infection of the kidneys. *Uncomplicated UTI* refers to acute cystitis or pyelonephritis in nonpregnant outpatient women without anatomic abnormalities or instrumentation of the urinary tract; the term *complicated UTI* encompasses all other types of UTI. *Recurrent UTI* is not necessarily complicated; individual episodes can be uncomplicated and treated as such. *Catheter-associated bacteriuria* can be either symptomatic (CAUTI) or asymptomatic.

EPIDEMIOLOGY AND RISK FACTORS

Except among infants and the elderly, UTI occurs far more commonly in females than in males. During the neonatal period, the incidence of UTI is slightly higher among males than among females because male infants more commonly have congenital urinary tract anomalies. After 50 years of age, obstruction from prostatic hypertrophy becomes common in men, and the incidence of UTI is almost as high among men as among women. Between 1 year and ~50 years of age, UTI and recurrent UTI are predominantly diseases of females. The prevalence of ASB is ~5% among women between ages 20 and 40 and may be as high as 40–50% among elderly women and men.

As many as 50–80% of women in the general population acquire at least one UTI during their lifetime—uncomplicated cystitis in most cases. Recent use of a diaphragm with spermicide, frequent sexual intercourse, and a history of UTI are independent risk factors for acute cystitis. Cystitis is temporally related to recent sexual intercourse in a dose-response manner, with an increased relative risk ranging from 1.4 with one episode of intercourse to 4.8 with five episodes of intercourse in the preceding week. In healthy postmenopausal women, sexual activity, diabetes mellitus, and incontinence are risk factors for UTI.

Many factors predisposing women to cystitis also increase the risk of pyelonephritis. Factors independently associated with pyelonephritis in young healthy women include frequent sexual intercourse, a new sexual partner, a UTI in the previous 12 months, a maternal history of UTI, diabetes, and incontinence. The common risk factors for cystitis and pyelonephritis are not surprising given that pyelonephritis typically arises through the ascent of bacteria from the bladder to the upper urinary tract. However, pyelonephritis can occur without clear antecedent cystitis.

About 20–30% of women who have had one episode of UTI will have recurrent episodes. Early recurrence (within 2 weeks) is usually regarded as relapse rather than reinfection and may indicate the need to evaluate the patient for a sequestered focus. Intracellular pods of infecting organisms within the bladder epithelium have been demonstrated in animal models of UTI, but the importance of this phenomenon in humans is not yet clear. The rate of recurrence ranges from 0.3 to 7.6 infections per patient per year, with an average of 2.6 infections per year. It is not uncommon for multiple recurrences to follow an initial infection, resulting in clustering of episodes. Clustering may be related temporally to the presence of a new risk factor or to the sloughing of the protective outer bladder epithelial layer in response to bacterial attachment during acute cystitis. The likelihood of a recurrence decreases with increasing time since the last infection. A case-control study of predominantly white premenopausal women with recurrent UTI identified frequent sexual intercourse, use of spermicide, a new sexual partner, a first UTI before 15 years of age, and a maternal history of UTI as independent risk factors for recurrent UTI. The only consistently documented behavioral risk factors for recurrent UTI include frequent sexual intercourse and spermicide use. In postmenopausal women, major risk factors for recurrent UTI include a history of premenopausal UTI and anatomic factors affecting bladder emptying, such as cystoceles, urinary incontinence, and residual urine.

In pregnant women, ASB has clinical consequences, and both screening for and treatment of this condition are indicated. Specifically, ASB during pregnancy is associated with preterm birth and perinatal death of the fetus and with pyelonephritis in the mother. A Cochrane meta-analysis found that treatment of ASB in pregnant women decreased the risk of pyelonephritis by 75%.

The majority of men with UTI have a functional or anatomic abnormality of the urinary tract, most commonly urinary obstruction secondary to prostatic hypertrophy. That said, not all men with UTI have detectable urinary abnormalities; this point is particularly relevant for men ≤45 years of age. Lack of circumcision is also associated with an increased risk of UTI because *Escherichia coli* is more likely to colonize the glans and prepuce and subsequently migrate into the urinary tract.

Women with diabetes have been found to have a two- to threefold higher rate of ASB and UTI than women without diabetes; there is insufficient evidence to make a corresponding statement about men. Increased duration of diabetes and the use of insulin rather than oral medication are also associated with a higher risk of UTI among women with diabetes. Poor bladder function, obstruction in urinary flow, and incomplete voiding are additional factors commonly found in patients with diabetes that increase the risk of UTI. Impaired cytokine secretion may contribute to ASB in diabetic women.

ETIOLOGY

The uropathogens causing UTI vary by clinical syndrome but are usually enteric gram-negative rods that have migrated to the urinary tract. The susceptibility patterns of these organisms vary by clinical syndrome and by geography. In acute uncomplicated cystitis in the United States, the etiologic agents are highly predictable: *E. coli* accounts for 75–90% of isolates; *Staphylococcus saprophyticus* for 5–15% (with particularly frequent isolation from younger women); and *Klebsiella, Proteus, Enterococcus,* and *Citrobacter* species, along with other organisms, for 5–10%. Similar etiologic agents are found in Europe and Brazil. The spectrum of agents causing uncomplicated pyelonephritis is similar, with *E. coli* predominating. In complicated UTI (e.g., CAUTI), *E. coli* remains the predominant organism, but other aerobic gram-negative rods, such as *Pseudomonas aeruginosa* and *Klebsiella, Proteus, Citrobacter, Acinetobacter,* and *Morganella* species, also are frequently isolated. Gram-positive bacteria (e.g., enterococci and *Staphylococcus aureus*) and yeasts are also important pathogens in complicated UTI. Data on etiology and resistance are generally obtained from laboratory surveys and should be understood in the context that organism identification is performed only in cases in which urine is sent for culture—i.e., typically, when complicated UTI or pyelonephritis is suspected. The available data demonstrate a worldwide increase in the resistance of *E. coli* to antibiotics commonly used to treat UTI. North American and European surveys from women with acute cystitis have documented resistance rates of >20% to trimethoprim-sulfamethoxazole (TMP-SMX) and to ciprofloxacin in some regions. In community-acquired infections, the increased prevalence of uropathogens producing extended-spectrum β-lactamases has left few oral options for therapy. Since resistance rates vary by local geographic region, with individual patient characteristics, and over time, it is important to use current and local data when choosing a treatment regimen.

PATHOGENESIS

The urinary tract can be viewed as an anatomic unit united by a continuous column of urine extending from the urethra to the kidneys. In the majority of UTIs, bacteria establish infection by ascending from the urethra to the bladder. Continuing ascent up the ureter to the kidney is the pathway for most renal parenchymal infections. However, introduction of bacteria into the bladder does not inevitably lead to sustained and symptomatic infection. The interplay of host, pathogen, and environmental factors determines whether tissue invasion and symptomatic infection will ensue (Fig. 162-1). For example, bacteria often enter the bladder after sexual intercourse, but normal voiding and innate host defense mechanisms in the bladder eliminate these organisms. Any foreign body in the urinary tract, such as a urinary catheter or stone, provides an inert surface for bacterial colonization. Abnormal micturition and/or significant residual urine volume promotes true infection. In the simplest of terms, anything that increases the likelihood of bacteria entering the bladder and staying there increases the risk of UTI.

Bacteria can also gain access to the urinary tract through the bloodstream. However, hematogenous spread accounts for <2% of documented UTIs and usually results from bacteremia caused by relatively virulent organisms, such as *Salmonella* and *S. aureus*. Indeed, the isolation of either of these pathogens from a patient without a catheter or other instrumentation warrants a search for a bloodstream source. Hematogenous infections may produce focal abscesses or areas of pyelonephritis within a kidney and result in positive urine cultures. The pathogenesis of candiduria is distinct in that the hematogenous route is common. The presence of *Candida* in the urine of a noninstrumented

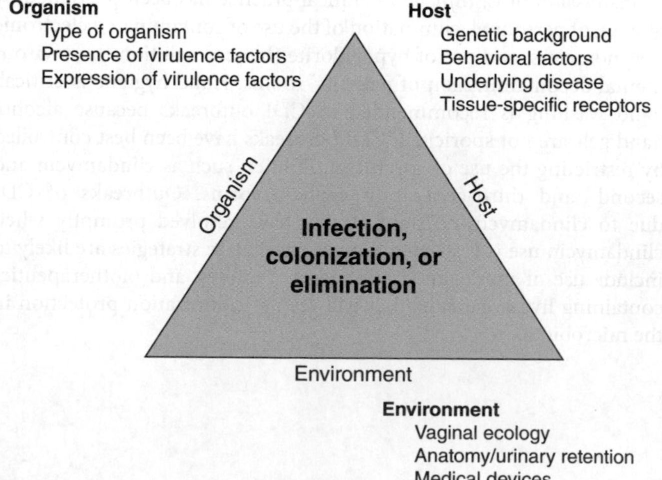

FIGURE 162-1 Pathogenesis of urinary tract infection. The relationship among specific host, pathogen, and environmental factors determines the clinical outcome.

immunocompetent patient implies either genital contamination or potentially widespread visceral dissemination.

Environmental Factors • ***VAGINAL ECOLOGY*** In women, vaginal ecology is an important environmental factor affecting the risk of UTI. Colonization of the vaginal introitus and periurethral area with organisms from the intestinal flora (usually *E. coli*) is the critical initial step in the pathogenesis of UTI. Sexual intercourse is associated with an increased risk of vaginal colonization with *E. coli* and thereby increases the risk of UTI. Nonoxynol-9 in spermicide is toxic to the normal vaginal microflora and thus is likewise associated with an increased risk of *E. coli* vaginal colonization and bacteriuria. In postmenopausal women, the previously predominant vaginal lactobacilli are replaced with colonizing gram-negative bacteria. The use of topical estrogens to prevent UTI in postmenopausal women is controversial; given the side effects of systemic hormone replacement, oral estrogens should not be used to prevent UTI.

ANATOMIC AND FUNCTIONAL ABNORMALITIES Any condition that permits urinary stasis or obstruction predisposes the individual to UTI. Foreign bodies such as stones or urinary catheters provide an inert surface for bacterial colonization and formation of a persistent biofilm. Thus, vesicoureteral reflux, ureteral obstruction secondary to prostatic hypertrophy, neurogenic bladder, and urinary diversion surgery create an environment favorable to UTI. In persons with such conditions, *E. coli* strains lacking typical urinary virulence factors are often the cause of infection. Inhibition of ureteral peristalsis and decreased ureteral tone leading to vesicoureteral reflux are important in the pathogenesis of pyelonephritis in pregnant women. Anatomic factors—specifically, the distance of the urethra from the anus—are considered to be the primary reason why UTI is predominantly an illness of young women rather than of young men.

Host Factors The genetic background of the host influences the individual's susceptibility to recurrent UTI, at least among women. A familial disposition to UTI and to pyelonephritis is well documented. Women with recurrent UTI are more likely to have had their first UTI before the age of 15 years and to have a maternal history of UTI. A component of the underlying pathogenesis of this familial predisposition to recurrent UTI may be persistent vaginal colonization with *E. coli*, even during asymptomatic periods. Vaginal and periurethral mucosal cells from women with recurrent UTI bind threefold more uropathogenic bacteria than do mucosal cells from women without recurrent infection. Epithelial cells from women who are non-secretors of certain blood group antigens may possess specific types of receptors to which *E. coli* can bind, thereby facilitating colonization and invasion. Mutations in host response genes (e.g., those coding for Toll-like receptors and the interleukin 8 receptor) also have been linked to recurrent UTI and pyelonephritis. Polymorphisms in the interleukin 8–specific receptor gene *CXCR1* are associated with increased susceptibility to pyelonephritis. Lower-level expression of *CXCR1* on the surface of neutrophils impairs neutrophil-dependent host defense against bacterial invasion of the renal parenchyma.

Microbial Factors An anatomically normal urinary tract presents a stronger barrier to infection than a compromised urinary tract. Thus, strains of *E. coli* that cause invasive symptomatic infection of the urinary tract in otherwise normal hosts often possess and express genetic virulence factors, including surface adhesins that mediate binding to specific receptors on the surface of uroepithelial cells. The best-studied adhesins are the P fimbriae, hairlike protein structures that interact with a specific receptor on renal epithelial cells. (The letter *P* denotes the ability of these fimbriae to bind to blood group antigen P, which contains a D-galactose-D-galactose residue.) P fimbriae are important in the pathogenesis of pyelonephritis and subsequent bloodstream invasion from the kidney.

Another adhesin is the type 1 pilus (fimbria), which all *E. coli* strains possess but not all *E. coli* strains express. Type 1 pili are thought to play a key role in initiating *E. coli* bladder infection; they mediate binding to uroplakins on the luminal surface of bladder uroepithelial cells. The binding of type 1 fimbriae of *E. coli* to receptors on uroepithelial cells initiates a complex series of signaling events that leads to apoptosis and exfoliation of uroepithelial cells, with the attached *E. coli* organisms carried away in the urine.

APPROACH TO THE PATIENT: Clinical Syndromes

The most important issue to be addressed when a UTI is suspected is the characterization of the clinical syndrome as ASB, uncomplicated cystitis, pyelonephritis, prostatitis, or complicated UTI. This information will shape the diagnostic and therapeutic approach.

ASYMPTOMATIC BACTERIURIA

A diagnosis of ASB can be considered only when the patient does not have local or systemic symptoms referable to the urinary tract. The clinical presentation is usually that of a patient who undergoes a screening urine culture for a reason unrelated to the genitourinary tract and is incidentally found to have bacteriuria. The presence of systemic signs or symptoms such as fever, altered mental status, and leukocytosis in the setting of a positive urine culture does not merit a diagnosis of symptomatic UTI unless other potential etiologies have been considered.

CYSTITIS

The typical symptoms of cystitis are dysuria, urinary frequency, and urgency. Nocturia, hesitancy, suprapubic discomfort, and gross hematuria are often noted as well. Unilateral back or flank pain is generally an indication that the upper urinary tract is involved. Fever also is an indication of invasive infection of either the kidney or the prostate.

PYELONEPHRITIS

Mild pyelonephritis can present as low-grade fever with or without lower-back or costovertebral-angle pain, whereas severe pyelonephritis can manifest as high fever, rigors, nausea, vomiting, and flank and/or loin pain. Symptoms are generally acute in onset, and symptoms of cystitis may not be present. Fever is the main feature distinguishing cystitis and pyelonephritis. The fever of pyelonephritis typically exhibits a high spiking "picket-fence" pattern and resolves over 72 h of therapy. Bacteremia develops in 20–30% of cases of pyelonephritis. Patients with diabetes may present with obstructive uropathy associated with acute papillary necrosis when the sloughed papillae obstruct the ureter. Papillary necrosis may also be evident in some cases of pyelonephritis complicated by obstruction, sickle cell disease, analgesic nephropathy, or combinations of these conditions. In the rare cases of bilateral papillary necrosis, a rapid rise in the serum creatinine level may be the first indication of the condition. *Emphysematous* pyelonephritis is a particularly severe form of the disease that is associated with the production of gas in renal and perinephric tissues and occurs almost exclusively in diabetic patients (Fig. 162-2). *Xanthogranulomatous* pyelonephritis occurs when chronic urinary obstruction (often by staghorn calculi), together with chronic infection, leads to suppurative destruction of renal tissue (Fig. 162-3). On pathologic examination, the residual renal tissue frequently has a yellow coloration, with infiltration by lipid-laden macrophages. Pyelonephritis can also be complicated by intraparenchymal abscess formation; this situation should be suspected when a patient has continued fever and/or bacteremia despite antibacterial therapy.

PROSTATITIS

Prostatitis includes both infectious and noninfectious abnormalities of the prostate gland. Infections can be acute or chronic, are almost always bacterial in nature, and are far less common than the noninfectious entity *chronic pelvic pain syndrome* (formerly known as chronic prostatitis). Acute bacterial prostatitis presents as dysuria, frequency, and pain in the prostatic pelvic or perineal area. Fever and chills are usually present, and symptoms of bladder outlet obstruction are common. Chronic bacterial prostatitis presents

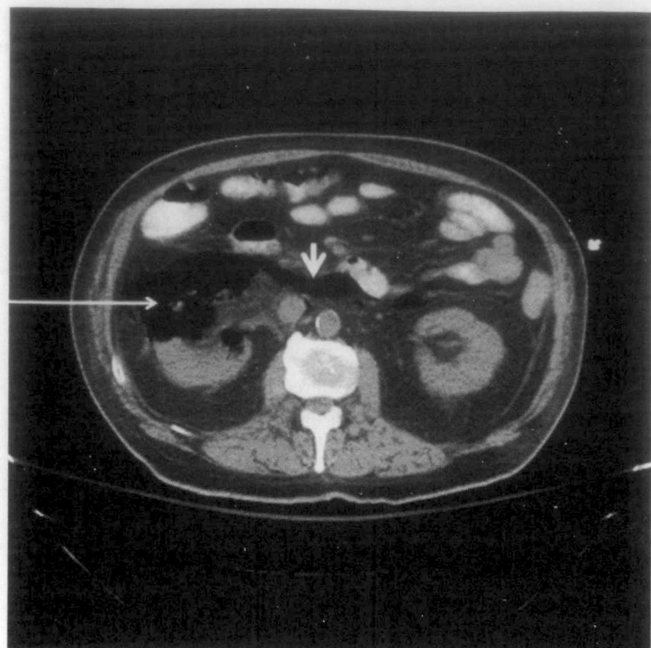

FIGURE 162-2 Emphysematous pyelonephritis. Infection of the right kidney of a diabetic man by *Escherichia coli*, a gas-forming, facultative anaerobic uropathogen, has led to destruction of the renal parenchyma (*arrow*) and tracking of gas through the retroperitoneal space (*arrowhead*).

more insidiously as recurrent episodes of cystitis, sometimes with associated pelvic and perineal pain. Men who present with recurrent cystitis should be evaluated for a prostatic focus.

COMPLICATED UTI

Complicated UTI presents as a symptomatic episode of cystitis or pyelonephritis in a man or woman with an anatomic predisposition to infection, with a foreign body in the urinary tract, or with factors predisposing to a delayed response to therapy.

DIAGNOSTIC TOOLS

History The diagnosis of any of the UTI syndromes or ASB begins with a detailed history (Fig. 162-4). The history given by the patient has a high predictive value in uncomplicated cystitis. A meta-analysis evaluating the probability of acute UTI on the basis of history and physical findings concluded that, in women presenting with at least one symptom of UTI (dysuria, frequency, hematuria, or back pain) and without complicating factors, the probability of acute cystitis or pyelonephritis is 50%. The even higher rates of accuracy of self-diagnosis among women with recurrent UTI probably account for the success of patient-initiated treatment of recurrent cystitis. If vaginal discharge and complicating factors are absent and risk factors for UTI are present, then the probability of UTI is close to 90%, and no laboratory evaluation is needed. Similarly, a combination of dysuria and urinary frequency in the absence of vaginal discharge increases the probability of UTI to 96%. Further laboratory evaluation with dipstick testing or urine culture is not necessary in such patients before the initiation of definitive therapy.

When the patient's history is applied as a diagnostic tool, it is important to recall that the studies included in the meta-analysis cited above did not enroll children, adolescents, pregnant women, men, or patients with complicated UTI. One significant concern is that sexually transmitted disease—that caused by *Chlamydia trachomatis* in particular—may be inappropriately treated as UTI. This concern is particularly relevant for female patients under the age of 25. The differential diagnosis to be considered when women present with dysuria includes cervicitis (*C. trachomatis, Neisseria gonorrhoeae*), vaginitis (*Candida albicans, Trichomonas vaginalis*), herpetic urethritis, interstitial cystitis, and noninfectious vaginal or vulvar irritation. Women with more than one sexual partner and inconsistent use of condoms are at high risk for both UTI and sexually transmitted disease, and symptoms alone do not always distinguish between these conditions.

The Urine Dipstick Test, Urinalysis, and Urine Culture Useful diagnostic tools include the urine dipstick test and urinalysis, both of which provide point-of-care information, and the urine culture, which can retrospectively confirm a prior diagnosis. Understanding the parameters of the dipstick test is important in interpreting its results. Only members of the family Enterobacteriaceae convert nitrate to nitrite, and enough nitrite must accumulate in the urine to reach the threshold of detection. If a woman with acute cystitis is forcing fluids and voiding frequently, the dipstick test for nitrite is less likely to be positive, even when *E. coli* is present. The leukocyte esterase test detects this enzyme in the host's polymorphonuclear leukocytes in the urine, whether the cells are intact or lysed. Many reviews have attempted to describe the diagnostic accuracy of dipstick testing. The bottom line for clinicians is that a urine dipstick test can confirm the diagnosis of uncomplicated cystitis in a patient with a reasonably high pretest probability of this

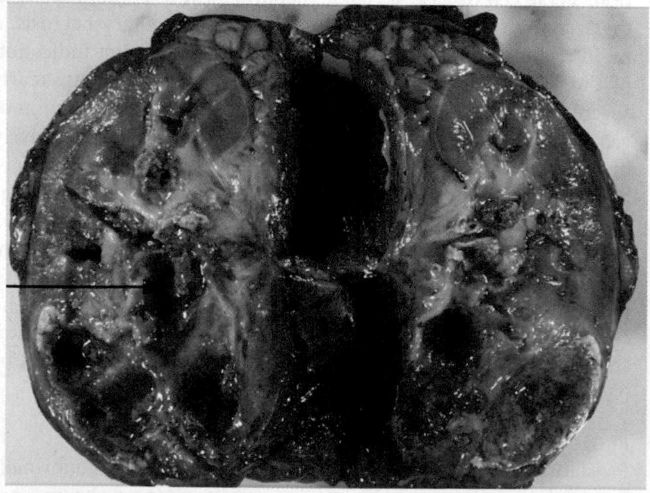

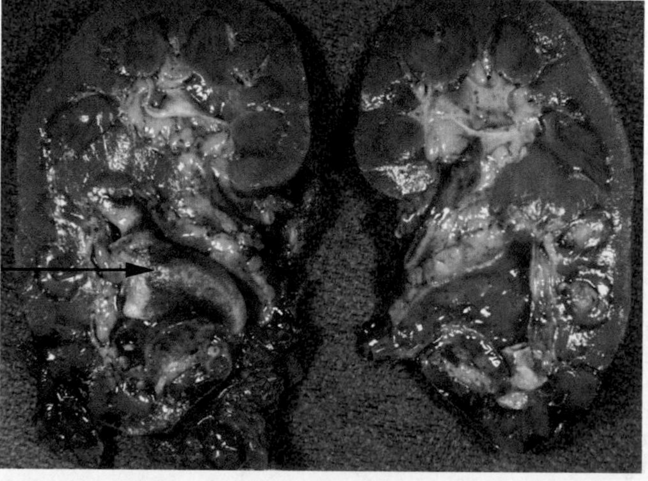

A B

FIGURE 162-3 Xanthogranulomatous pyelonephritis. ***A.*** This photograph shows extensive destruction of renal parenchyma due to long-standing suppurative inflammation. The precipitating factor was obstruction by a staghorn calculus, which has been removed, leaving a depression (*arrow*). The mass effect of xanthogranulomatous pyelonephritis can mimic renal malignancy. ***B.*** A large staghorn calculus (*arrow*) is seen obstructing the renal pelvis and calyceal system. The lower pole of the kidney shows areas of hemorrhage and necrosis with collapse of cortical areas. *(Images courtesy of Dharam M. Ramnani, MD, Virginia Urology Pathology Laboratory, Richmond, VA.)*

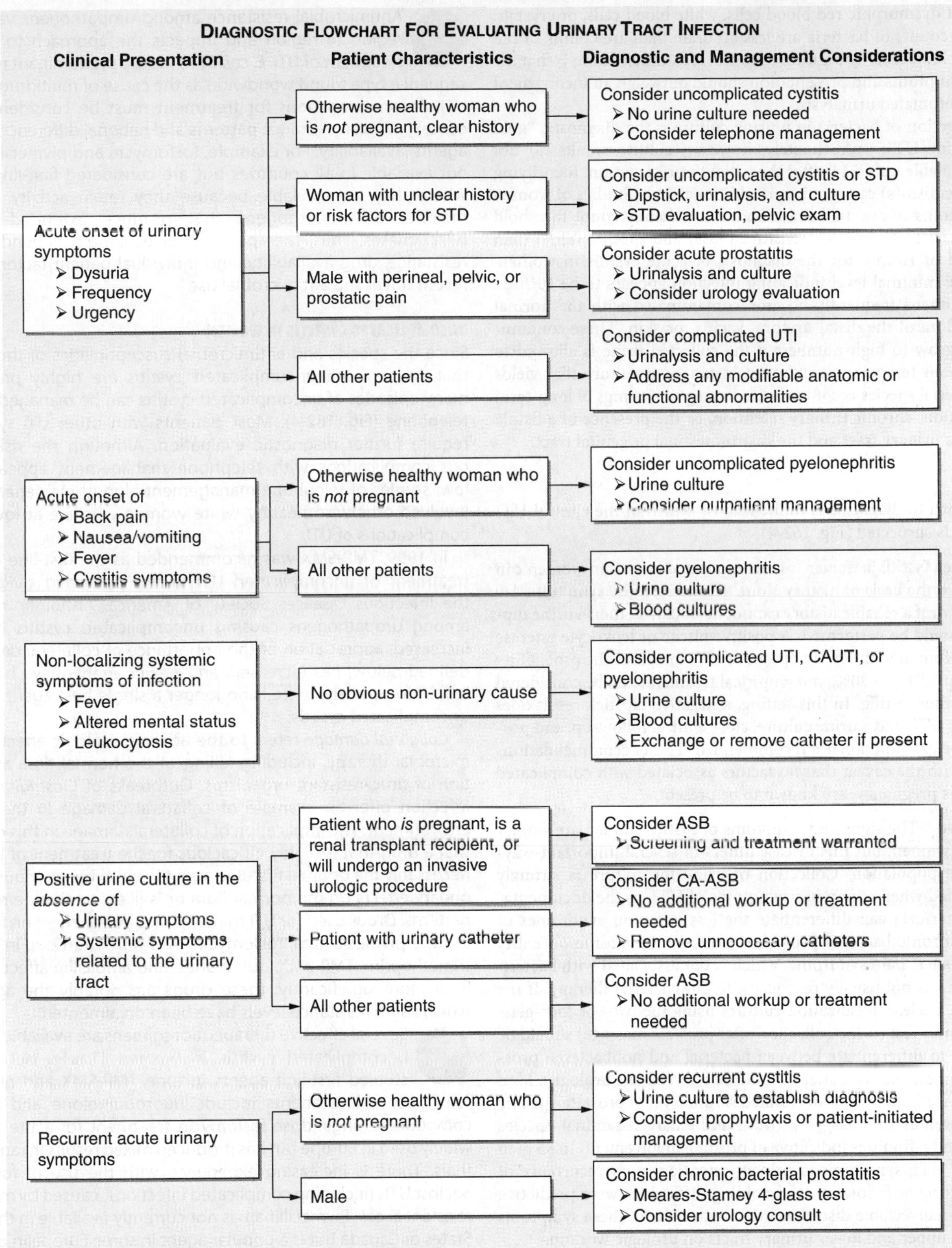

FIGURE 162-4 Diagnostic approach to urinary tract infection (UTI). STD, sexually transmitted disease; CAUTI, catheter-associated UTI; ASB, asymptomatic bacteriuria; CA-ASB, catheter-associated ASB.

disease. Either nitrite or leukocyte esterase positivity can be interpreted as a positive result. Blood in the urine also may suggest a diagnosis of UTI. A dipstick test negative for both nitrite and leukocyte esterase in the same type of patient should prompt consideration of other explanations for the patient's symptoms and collection of urine for culture. A negative dipstick test is not sufficiently sensitive to rule out bacteriuria in pregnant women, in whom it is important to detect all episodes of bacteriuria. Performance characteristics of the dipstick test differ in men (highly specific) and in noncatheterized nursing home residents (highly sensitive).

Urine microscopy reveals pyuria in nearly all cases of cystitis and hematuria in ~30% of cases. In current practice, most hospital laboratories use an automated system rather than manual examination for urine microscopy. A machine aspirates a sample of the urine and then classifies the particles in the urine by size, shape, contrast, light scatter, volume, and other properties. These automated systems can be overwhelmed by high numbers of dysmorphic red blood cells, white blood cells, or crystals; in general, counts of bacteria are less accurate than are counts of red and white blood cells. The authors' clinical recommendation is that the patient's symptoms and presentation should outweigh an incongruent result on automated urinalysis.

The detection of bacteria in a urine culture is the diagnostic "gold standard" for UTI; unfortunately, however, culture results do not become available until 24 h after the patient's presentation. Identifying specific organism(s) can require an additional 24 h. Studies of women with symptoms of cystitis have found that a colony count threshold of >10^2 bacteria/mL is more sensitive (95%) and specific (85%) than a threshold of 10^5/mL for the diagnosis of acute cystitis in women. In men, the minimal level indicating infection appears to be 10^3/mL. Urine specimens frequently become contaminated with the normal microbial flora of the distal urethra, vagina, or skin. These contaminants can grow to high numbers if the collected urine is allowed to stand at room temperature. In most instances, a culture that yields mixed bacterial species is contaminated except in settings of long-term catheterization, chronic urinary retention, or the presence of a fistula between the urinary tract and the gastrointestinal or genital tract.

DIAGNOSIS

The approach to diagnosis is influenced by which of the clinical UTI syndromes is suspected (Fig. 162-4).

Uncomplicated Cystitis in Women Uncomplicated cystitis in women can be treated on the basis of history alone. However, if the symptoms are not specific or if a reliable history cannot be obtained, then a urine dipstick test should be performed. A positive nitrite or leukocyte esterase result in a woman with one symptom of UTI increases the probability of UTI from 50% to ~80%, and empirical treatment can be considered without further testing. In this setting, a negative dipstick result does not rule out UTI, and a urine culture, close clinical follow-up, and possibly a pelvic examination are recommended. These recommendations are made with the caveat that no factors associated with complicated UTI, such as pregnancy, are known to be present.

Cystitis in Men The signs and symptoms of cystitis in men are similar to those in women, but this disease differs in several important ways in the male population. Collection of urine for culture is strongly recommended when a man has symptoms of UTI, as the documentation of bacteriuria can differentiate the less common syndromes of acute and chronic bacterial prostatitis from the very common entity of chronic pelvic pain syndrome, which is not associated with bacteriuria and thus is not usually responsive to antibacterial therapy. If the diagnosis is unclear, localization cultures using the two- or four-glass Meares-Stamey test (urine collection after prostate massage) should be undertaken to differentiate between bacterial and nonbacterial prostatic syndromes, and the patient should be referred to a urologist. Men with febrile UTI often have an elevated serum level of prostate-specific antigen as well as an enlarged prostate and enlarged seminal vesicles on ultrasound—findings indicative of prostate involvement. In 85 men with febrile UTI, symptoms of urinary retention, early recurrence of UTI, hematuria at follow-up, and voiding difficulties were predictive of surgically correctable disorders. Men with none of these symptoms had normal upper and lower urinary tracts on urologic workup.

Asymptomatic Bacteriuria The diagnosis of ASB involves both microbiologic and clinical criteria. The microbiologic criterion is usually ≥10^5 bacterial CFU/mL except in catheter-associated disease, in which ≥10^2 CFU/mL is the cutoff. The clinical criterion is that the person has no signs or symptoms referable to UTI.

TREATMENT URINARY TRACT INFECTIONS

Antimicrobial therapy is warranted for any symptomatic UTI. The choice of antimicrobial agent and the dose and duration of therapy depend on the site of infection and the presence or absence of complicating conditions. Each category of UTI warrants a different approach based on the particular clinical syndrome.

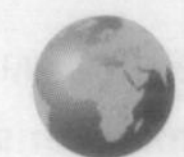

Antimicrobial resistance among uropathogens varies from region to region and impacts the approach to empirical treatment of UTI. *E. coli* ST131 is the predominant multilocus sequence type found worldwide as the cause of multidrug-resistant UTI. Recommendations for treatment must be considered in the context of local resistance patterns and national differences in some agents' availability. For example, fosfomycin and pivmecillinam are not available in all countries but are considered first-line options where they are available because they retain activity against a majority of uropathogens that produce extended-spectrum β-lactamases. Thus, therapeutic choices should depend on local resistance, drug availability, and individual patient factors such as recent travel and antimicrobial use.

UNCOMPLICATED CYSTITIS IN WOMEN

Since the species and antimicrobial susceptibilities of the bacteria that cause acute uncomplicated cystitis are highly predictable, many episodes of uncomplicated cystitis can be managed over the telephone (Fig. 162-4). Most patients with other UTI syndromes require further diagnostic evaluation. Although the risk of serious complications with telephone management appears to be low, studies of telephone management algorithms generally have involved otherwise healthy white women who are at low risk for complications of UTI.

In 1999, TMP-SMX was recommended as the first-line agent for treatment of uncomplicated UTI in the published guidelines of the Infectious Diseases Society of America. Antibiotic resistance among uropathogens causing uncomplicated cystitis has since increased, appreciation of the importance of collateral damage (as defined below) has increased, and newer agents have been studied. Unfortunately, there is no longer a single best agent for acute uncomplicated cystitis.

Collateral damage refers to the adverse ecologic effects of antimicrobial therapy, including killing of the normal flora and selection of drug-resistant organisms. Outbreaks of *Clostridium difficile* infection offer an example of collateral damage in the hospital environment. The implication of collateral damage in this context is that a drug that is highly efficacious for the treatment of UTI is not necessarily the optimal first-line agent if it also has pronounced secondary effects on the normal flora or is likely to change resistance patterns. Drugs used for UTI that have a minimal effect on fecal flora include pivmecillinam, fosfomycin, and nitrofurantoin. In contrast, trimethoprim, TMP-SMX, quinolones, and ampicillin affect the fecal flora more significantly; these drugs are notably the agents for which rising resistance levels have been documented.

Several effective therapeutic regimens are available for acute uncomplicated cystitis in women (Table 162-1). Well-studied first-line agents include TMP-SMX and nitrofurantoin. Second-line agents include fluoroquinolone and β-lactam compounds. Single-dose fosfomycin treatment for acute cystitis is widely used in Europe but has produced mixed results in randomized trials. There is increasing experience with the use of fosfomycin against UTIs (including complicated infections) caused by multidrug-resistant *E. coli*. Pivmecillinam is not currently available in the United States or Canada but is a popular agent in some European countries. The pros and cons of other therapies are discussed briefly below.

Traditionally, TMP-SMX has been recommended as first-line treatment for acute cystitis, and it remains appropriate to consider the use of this drug in regions with resistance rates not exceeding 20%. TMP-SMX resistance has clinical significance: in TMP-SMX-treated patients with resistant isolates, the time to symptom resolution is longer and rates of both clinical and microbiologic failure are higher. Individual host factors associated with an elevated risk of UTI caused by a strain of *E. coli* resistant to TMP-SMX include recent use of TMP-SMX or another antimicrobial agent and recent travel to an area with high rates of TMP-SMX resistance. The optimal setting for empirical use of TMP-SMX is uncomplicated UTI in a female patient who has an established relationship with the practitioner and who can thus seek further care if her symptoms do not respond promptly.

TABLE 162-1 TREATMENT STRATEGIES FOR ACUTE UNCOMPLICATED CYSTITIS

Drug and Dose	Estimated Clinical Efficacy, %	Estimated Bacterial Efficacy,[a] %	Common Side Effects
Nitrofurantoin, 100 mg bid × 5–7 d	84–95	86–92	Nausea, headache
TMP-SMX, 1 DS tablet bid × 3 d	90–100	91–100	Rash, urticaria, nausea, vomiting, hematologic abnormalities
Fosfomycin, 3-g single-dose sachet	70–91	78–83	Diarrhea, nausea, headache
Pivmecillinam, 400 mg bid × 3–7 d	55–82	74–84	Nausea, vomiting, diarrhea
Fluoroquinolones, dose varies by agent; 3-d regimen	85–95	81–98	Nausea, vomiting, diarrhea, headache, drowsiness, insomnia
β-Lactams, dose varies by agent; 5- to 7-d regimen	79–98	74–98	Diarrhea, nausea, vomiting, rash, urticaria

[a]Microbial response as measured by reduction of bacterial counts in the urine.

Note: Efficacy rates are averages or ranges calculated from the data and studies included in the 2010 Infectious Diseases Society of America/European Society of Clinical Microbiology and Infectious Diseases Guideline for Treatment of Uncomplicated UTI. TMP-SMX, trimethoprim-sulfamethoxazole; DS, double-strength.

Resistance to nitrofurantoin remains low despite >60 years of use. Since this drug affects bacterial metabolism in multiple pathways, several mutational steps are required for the development of resistance. Nitrofurantoin remains highly active against *E. coli* and most non–*E. coli* isolates. *Proteus, Pseudomonas, Serratia, Enterobacter*, and yeasts are all intrinsically resistant to this drug. Although nitrofurantoin has traditionally been prescribed as a 7-day regimen, similar microbiologic and clinical efficacies are noted with a 5-day course of nitrofurantoin or a 3-day course of TMP-SMX for treatment of women with acute cystitis; 3-day courses of nitrofurantoin are not recommended for acute cystitis. Nitrofurantoin does not reach significant levels in tissue and cannot be used to treat pyelonephritis.

Most fluoroquinolones are highly effective as short-course therapy for cystitis; the exception is moxifloxacin, which may not reach adequate urinary levels. The fluoroquinolones commonly used for UTI include ofloxacin, ciprofloxacin, and levofloxacin. The main concern about fluoroquinolone use for acute cystitis is the propagation of fluoroquinolone resistance, not only among uropathogens but also among other organisms causing more serious and difficult-to-treat infections at other sites. Fluoroquinolone use is also a factor driving the emergence of *C. difficile* outbreaks in hospital settings. Most experts now call for restricting fluoroquinolones to specific instances of uncomplicated cystitis in which other antimicrobial agents are not suitable. Quinolone use in certain populations, including adults >60 years of age, has been associated with an increased risk of Achilles tendon rupture.

Except for pivmecillinam, β-lactam agents generally have not performed as well as TMP-SMX or fluoroquinolones in acute cystitis. Rates of pathogen eradication are lower and relapse rates are higher with β-lactam drugs. The generally accepted explanation is that β-lactams fail to eradicate uropathogens from the vaginal reservoir. A proposed role for intracellular biofilm communities is intriguing. Many strains of *E. coli* that are resistant to TMP-SMX are also resistant to amoxicillin and cephalexin; thus, these drugs should be used only for patients infected with susceptible strains.

Urinary analgesics are appropriate in certain situations to speed resolution of bladder discomfort. The urinary tract analgesic phenazopyridine is widely used but can cause significant nausea. Combination analgesics containing urinary antiseptics (methenamine, methylene blue), a urine-acidifying agent (sodium phosphate), and an antispasmodic agent (hyoscyamine) also are available.

PYELONEPHRITIS

Since patients with pyelonephritis have tissue-invasive disease, the treatment regimen chosen should have a very high likelihood of eradicating the causative organism and should reach therapeutic blood levels quickly. High rates of TMP-SMX-resistant *E. coli* in patients with pyelonephritis have made fluoroquinolones the first-line therapy for acute uncomplicated pyelonephritis. Whether the fluoroquinolones are given orally or parenterally depends on the patient's tolerance for oral intake. A randomized clinical trial demonstrated that a 7-day course of therapy with oral ciprofloxacin (500 mg twice daily, with or without an initial IV 400-mg dose) was highly effective for the initial management of pyelonephritis in the outpatient setting. Oral TMP-SMX (one double-strength tablet twice daily for 14 days) also is effective for treatment of acute uncomplicated pyelonephritis if the uropathogen is known to be susceptible. If the pathogen's susceptibility is not known and TMP-SMX is used, an initial IV 1-g dose of ceftriaxone is recommended. Oral β-lactam agents are less effective than the fluoroquinolones and should be used with caution and close follow-up. Options for parenteral therapy for uncomplicated pyelonephritis include fluoroquinolones, an extended-spectrum cephalosporin with or without an aminoglycoside, or a carbapenem. Combinations of a β-lactam and a β-lactamase inhibitor (e.g., ampicillin-sulbactam, ticarcillin-clavulanate, piperacillin-tazobactam) or imipenem-cilastatin can be used in patients with more complicated histories, previous episodes of pyelonephritis, or recent urinary tract manipulations; in general, the treatment of such patients should be guided by urine culture results. Once the patient has responded clinically, oral therapy should be substituted for parenteral therapy.

UTI IN PREGNANT WOMEN

Nitrofurantoin, ampicillin, and the cephalosporins are considered relatively safe in early pregnancy. One retrospective case-control study suggesting an association between nitrofurantoin and birth defects has not been confirmed. Sulfonamides should clearly be avoided both in the first trimester (because of possible teratogenic effects) and near term (because of a possible role in the development of kernicterus). Fluoroquinolones are avoided because of possible adverse effects on fetal cartilage development. Ampicillin and the cephalosporins have been used extensively in pregnancy and are the drugs of choice for the treatment of asymptomatic or symptomatic UTI in this group of patients. For pregnant women with overt pyelonephritis, parenteral β-lactam therapy with or without aminoglycosides is the standard of care.

UTI IN MEN

Since the prostate is involved in the majority of cases of febrile UTI in men, the goal in these patients is to eradicate the prostatic infection as well as the bladder infection. A 7- to 14-day course of a fluoroquinolone or TMP-SMX is recommended if the uropathogen is susceptible. If acute bacterial prostatitis is suspected, antimicrobial therapy should be initiated after urine and blood are obtained for cultures. Therapy can be tailored to urine culture results and should be continued for 2–4 weeks. For documented chronic bacterial prostatitis, a 4- to 6-week course of antibiotics is often necessary. Recurrences, which are not uncommon in chronic prostatitis, often warrant a 12-week course of treatment.

COMPLICATED UTI

Complicated UTI (other than that discussed above) occurs in a heterogeneous group of patients with a wide variety of structural and functional abnormalities of the urinary tract and kidneys. The range of species and their susceptibility to antimicrobial agents are likewise heterogeneous. As a consequence, therapy for complicated UTI must be individualized and guided by urine culture results. Frequently, a patient with complicated UTI will have prior urine culture data that can be used to guide empirical therapy while current culture results are awaited. Xanthogranulomatous pyelonephritis is treated with nephrectomy. Percutaneous drainage can be used as the initial therapy in emphysematous pyelonephritis and can be followed by elective nephrectomy as needed. Papillary necrosis with obstruction requires intervention to relieve the obstruction and to preserve renal function.

ASYMPTOMATIC BACTERIURIA

Treatment of ASB does not decrease the frequency of symptomatic infections or complications except in pregnant women, persons undergoing urologic surgery, and perhaps neutropenic patients and renal transplant recipients. Treatment of ASB in pregnant women and patients undergoing urologic procedures should be directed by urine culture results. In all other populations, screening for and treatment of ASB are discouraged. The majority of cases of catheter-associated bacteriuria are asymptomatic and do not warrant antimicrobial therapy.

CATHETER-ASSOCIATED UTI

Multiple institutions have released guidelines for the treatment of CAUTI, which is defined by bacteriuria and symptoms in a catheterized patient. The signs and symptoms either are localized to the urinary tract or can include otherwise unexplained systemic manifestations, such as fever. The accepted threshold for bacteriuria to meet the definition of CAUTI is $\geq 10^3$ CFU/mL, while the threshold for bacteriuria to meet the definition of ASB is $\geq 10^5$ CFU/mL.

The formation of biofilm—a living layer of uropathogens—on the urinary catheter is central to the pathogenesis of CAUTI and affects both therapeutic and preventive strategies. Organisms in a biofilm are relatively resistant to killing by antibiotics, and eradication of a catheter-associated biofilm is difficult without removal of the device itself. Furthermore, because catheters provide a conduit for bacteria to enter the bladder, bacteriuria is inevitable with long-term catheter use.

The typical signs and symptoms of UTI, including pain, urgency, dysuria, fever, peripheral leukocytosis, and pyuria, have less predictive value for the diagnosis of infection in catheterized patients. Furthermore, the presence of bacteria in the urine of a patient who is febrile and catheterized does not necessarily predict CAUTI, and other explanations for the fever should be considered.

The etiology of CAUTI is diverse, and urine culture results are essential to guide treatment. Fairly good evidence supports the practice of catheter change during treatment for CAUTI. The goal is to remove biofilm-associated organisms that could serve as a nidus for reinfection. Pathology studies reveal that many patients with long-term catheters have occult pyelonephritis. A randomized trial in persons with spinal cord injury who were undergoing intermittent catheterization found that relapse was more common after 3 days of therapy than after 14 days. In general, a 7- to 14-day course of antibiotics is recommended, but further studies on the optimal duration of therapy are needed.

In the setting of long-term catheter use, systemic antibiotics, bladder-acidifying agents, antimicrobial bladder washes, topical disinfectants, and antimicrobial drainage-bag solutions have all been ineffective at preventing the onset of bacteriuria and have been associated with the emergence of resistant organisms. The best strategy for prevention of CAUTI is to avoid insertion of unnecessary catheters and to remove catheters once they are no longer necessary. Evidence is insufficient to recommend suprapubic catheters and condom catheters as alternatives to indwelling urinary catheters as a means to prevent CAUTI. However, intermittent catheterization may be preferable to long-term indwelling urethral catheterization in certain populations (e.g., spinal cord–injured persons) to prevent both infectious and anatomic complications. Antimicrobial catheters impregnated with silver or nitrofurazone have not been shown to provide significant clinical benefit in terms of reducing rates of symptomatic UTI.

CANDIDURIA

The appearance of *Candida* in the urine is an increasingly common complication of indwelling catheterization, particularly for patients in the intensive care unit, those taking broad-spectrum antimicrobial drugs, and those with underlying diabetes mellitus. In many studies, >50% of urinary *Candida* isolates have been found to be non-*albicans* species. The clinical presentation varies from an asymptomatic laboratory finding to pyelonephritis and even sepsis. Removal of the urethral catheter results in resolution of candiduria in more than one-third of asymptomatic cases. Treatment of asymptomatic patients does not appear to decrease the frequency of recurrence of candiduria. Treatment is recommended for patients who have symptomatic cystitis or pyelonephritis and for those who are at high risk for disseminated disease. High-risk patients include those with neutropenia, those who are undergoing urologic manipulation, those who are clinically unstable, and low-birth-weight infants. Fluconazole (200–400 mg/d for 14 days) reaches high levels in urine and is the first-line regimen for *Candida* infections of the urinary tract. Although instances of successful eradication of candiduria by some of the newer azoles and echinocandins have been reported, these agents are characterized by only low-level urinary excretion and thus are not recommended. For *Candida* isolates with high levels of resistance to fluconazole, oral flucytosine and/or parenteral amphotericin B are options. Bladder irrigation with amphotericin B generally is not recommended.

PREVENTION OF RECURRENT UTI IN WOMEN

Recurrence of uncomplicated cystitis in reproductive-age women is common, and a preventive strategy is indicated if recurrent UTIs are interfering with a patient's lifestyle. The threshold of two or more symptomatic episodes per year is not absolute; decisions about interventions should take the patient's preferences into account.

Three prophylactic strategies are available: continuous, postcoital, and patient-initiated therapy. Continuous prophylaxis and postcoital prophylaxis usually entail low doses of TMP-SMX, a fluoroquinolone, or nitrofurantoin. These regimens are all highly effective during the period of active antibiotic intake. Typically, a prophylactic regimen is prescribed for 6 months and then discontinued, at which point the rate of recurrent UTI often returns to baseline. If bothersome infections recur, the prophylactic program can be reinstituted for a longer period. Selection of resistant strains in the fecal flora has been documented in studies of women taking prophylactic antibiotics for 12 months.

Patient-initiated therapy involves supplying the patient with materials for urine culture and with a course of antibiotics for self-medication at the first symptoms of infection. The urine culture is refrigerated and delivered to the physician's office for confirmation of the diagnosis. When an established and reliable patient-provider relationship exists, the urine culture can be omitted as long as the symptomatic episodes respond completely to short-course therapy and are not followed by relapse.

PROGNOSIS

Cystitis is a risk factor for recurrent cystitis and pyelonephritis. ASB is common among elderly and catheterized patients but does not in itself increase the risk of death. The relationships among recurrent UTI, chronic pyelonephritis, and renal insufficiency have been widely studied. In the absence of anatomic abnormalities, recurrent infection in children and adults does not lead to chronic pyelonephritis or to renal failure. Moreover, infection does not play a primary role in chronic interstitial nephritis; the primary etiologic factors in this condition are analgesic abuse, obstruction, reflux, and toxin exposure. In the presence of underlying renal abnormalities (particularly obstructing stones), infection as a secondary factor can accelerate renal parenchymal damage. In spinal cord–injured patients, use of a long-term indwelling bladder catheter is a well-documented risk factor for bladder cancer. Chronic bacteriuria resulting in chronic inflammation is one possible explanation for this observation.

163 Sexually Transmitted Infections: Overview and Clinical Approach

Jeanne M. Marrazzo, King K. Holmes

CLASSIFICATION AND EPIDEMIOLOGY

Worldwide, most adults acquire at least one sexually transmitted infection (STI), and many remain at risk for complications. Each year, for example, an estimated 14 million persons in the United States acquire a new genital human papillomavirus (HPV) infection, and many of these individuals are at risk for genital neoplasias. Certain STIs, such as syphilis, gonorrhea, HIV infection, hepatitis B, and chancroid, are most concentrated within "core populations" characterized by high rates of partner change, multiple concurrent partners, or "dense," highly connected sexual networks—e.g., involving sex workers and their clients, some men who have sex with men (MSM), and persons involved in the use of illicit drugs, particularly crack cocaine and methamphetamine. Other STIs are distributed more evenly throughout societies. For example, chlamydial infections, genital infections with HPV, and genital herpes can spread widely, even in relatively low-risk populations.

In general, the product of three factors determines the initial rate of spread of any STI within a population: rate of sexual exposure of susceptible to infectious people, efficiency of transmission per exposure, and duration of infectivity of those infected. Accordingly, efforts to prevent and control STIs aim to decrease the rate of sexual exposure of susceptibles to infected persons (e.g., through individual counseling and efforts to change the norms of sexual behavior and through a variety of STI control efforts aimed at reducing the proportion of the population infected), to decrease the duration of infectivity (through early diagnosis and curative or suppressive treatment), and to decrease the efficiency of transmission (e.g., through promotion of condom use and safer sexual practices, through use of effective vaccines, and recently through male circumcision).

In all societies, STIs rank among the most common of all infectious diseases, with >30 infections now classified as predominantly sexually transmitted or as frequently sexually transmissible (Table 163-1). In developing countries, with three-quarters of the world's population and 90% of the world's STIs, factors such as population growth (especially in adolescent and young-adult age groups), rural-to-urban migration, wars, limited or no provision of reproductive health services for women, and poverty create exceptional vulnerability to disease resulting from unprotected sex. During the 1990s in China, Russia, the other states of the former Soviet Union, and South Africa, internal social structures changed rapidly as borders opened to the West, unleashing enormous new epidemics of HIV infection and other STIs. Despite advances in the provision of highly effective antiretroviral therapy worldwide, HIV remains the leading cause of death in some developing countries, and HPV and hepatitis B virus (HBV) remain important causes of cervical and hepatocellular carcinoma, respectively—two of the most common malignancies in the developing world. Sexually transmitted herpes simplex virus (HSV) infections now cause most genital ulcer disease throughout the world and an increasing proportion of cases of genital herpes in developing countries with generalized HIV epidemics, where the positive-feedback loop between HSV and HIV transmission is a growing, intractable problem. Despite this consistent link, randomized trials evaluating the efficacy of antiviral therapy in suppressing HSV in both HIV-uninfected and HIV-infected persons have not demonstrated a protective effect against acquisition or transmission of HIV. The World Health Organization estimated that 448 million new cases of four curable STIs—gonorrhea, chlamydial infection, syphilis, and trichomoniasis—occurred in 2005. Up to 50% of women of reproductive age in developing countries have bacterial vaginosis (arguably acquired sexually). All of these curable infections have been associated with increased risk of HIV transmission or acquisition.

TABLE 163-1 SEXUALLY TRANSMITTED AND SEXUALLY TRANSMISSIBLE MICROORGANISMS

Bacteria	Viruses	Other[a]
Transmitted in Adults Predominantly by Sexual Intercourse		
Neisseria gonorrhoeae	HIV (types 1 and 2)	*Trichomonas vaginalis*
Chlamydia trachomatis	Human T cell lymphotropic virus type 1	*Pthirus pubis*
Treponema pallidum	Herpes simplex virus type 2	
Haemophilus ducreyi		
Klebsiella (Calymmatobacterium) granulomatis	Human papillomavirus (multiple genital genotypes)	
Ureaplasma urealyticum	Hepatitis B virus[b]	
Mycoplasma genitalium	Molluscum contagiosum virus	
Sexual Transmission Repeatedly Described but Not Well Defined or Not the Predominant Mode		
Mycoplasma hominis	Cytomegalovirus	(?) Epstein-Barr virus
Gardnerella vaginalis and other vaginal bacteria	Human T cell lymphotropic virus type 2	Human herpesvirus type 8
Group B *Streptococcus*	Hepatitis C virus	*Candida albicans*
Mobiluncus spp.	(?) Hepatitis D virus	*Sarcoptes scabiei*
Helicobacter cinaedi	Herpes simplex virus type 1	
Helicobacter fennelliae		
Transmitted by Sexual Contact Involving Oral-Fecal Exposure; of Declining Importance in Men Who Have Sex with Men		
Shigella spp.	Hepatitis A virus	*Giardia lamblia*
Campylobacter spp.		*Entamoeba histolytica*

[a]Includes protozoa, ectoparasites, and fungi. [b]Among U.S. patients for whom a risk factor can be ascertained, most hepatitis B virus infections are transmitted sexually.

In the United States, the prevalence of antibody to HSV-2 began to fall in the late 1990s, especially among adolescents and young adults; the decline is presumably due to delayed sexual debut, increased condom use, and lower rates of multiple (four or more) sex partners, as is well documented by the U.S. Youth Risk Behavior Surveillance System. The estimated annual incidence of HBV infection has also declined dramatically since the mid-1980s; this decrease is probably attributable more to adoption of safer sexual practices and reduced needle sharing among injection drug users than to use of hepatitis B vaccine, for which coverage among young adults (including those at high risk for this infection) initially was very limited. Genital HPV remains the most common sexually transmitted pathogen in this country, infecting 60% of a cohort of initially HPV-negative, sexually active Washington state college women within 5 years in a study conducted from 1990 to 2000. The scale-up of HPV vaccine coverage among young women has already shown promise in reducing the incidence of infection with the HPV types included in the vaccines and of conditions associated with these viruses.

In industrialized countries, fear of HIV infection since the mid-1980s, coupled with widespread behavioral interventions and better-organized systems of care for the curable STIs, initially helped curb the transmission of the latter diseases. However, foci of hyperendemic transmission persist in the southeastern United States and in most large U.S. cities. Rates of gonorrhea and syphilis remain higher in the United States than in any other Western industrialized country.

In the United States, the Centers for Disease Control and Prevention (CDC) has compiled reported rates of STIs since 1941. The incidence of reported gonorrhea peaked at 468 cases per 100,000 population in the mid-1970s and fell to a low of 98 cases per 100,000 in 2012. With increased testing and more sensitive tests, the incidence of reported *Chlamydia trachomatis* infection has been increasing steadily since reporting began in 1984, reaching an all-time peak of 457.6 cases per 100,000 in 2011. The incidence of primary and secondary syphilis per 100,000 peaked at 71 cases in 1946, fell rapidly to 3.9 cases in 1956, ranged from ~10 to 15 cases through 1987 (with markedly increased rates among MSM and African Americans), and then fell to a nadir of 2.1 cases in 2000–2001 (with rates falling most rapidly among heterosexual African Americans). Unfortunately, since 1996, with the introduction of highly active antiretroviral therapy, the increased use of "serosorting" (i.e., the avoidance of unprotected sex with HIV-serodiscordant partners but not with HIV-seroconcordant partners, a strategy that provides no protection against STIs other than HIV infection), and an ongoing epidemic of methamphetamine use, gonorrhea, syphilis, and chlamydial infection have had a remarkable resurgence among MSM in North America and Europe, where outbreaks of a rare type of chlamydial infection (lymphogranuloma venereum [LGV]) that had virtually disappeared during the AIDS era have occurred. In 2012, ~75% of primary and secondary syphilis cases reported to the CDC were in MSM. These developments have resulted in a high degree of co-infection with HIV and other sexually transmitted pathogens (particularly syphilis and LGV), primarily among MSM.

MANAGEMENT OF COMMON SEXUALLY TRANSMITTED DISEASE (STD) SYNDROMES

Although other chapters discuss management of specific STIs, delineating treatment based on diagnosis of a specific infection, most patients are actually managed (at least initially) on the basis of presenting symptoms and signs and associated risk factors, even in industrialized countries. Table 163-2 lists some of the most common clinical STD syndromes and their microbial etiologies. Strategies for their management are outlined below. Chapters 225e and 226 address the management of infections with human retroviruses.

TABLE 163-2 MAJOR SEXUALLY TRANSMITTED DISEASE SYNDROMES AND SEXUALLY TRANSMITTED MICROBIAL ETIOLOGIES

Syndrome	Sexually Transmitted Microbial Etiologies
AIDS	HIV types 1 and 2
Urethritis: males	*Neisseria gonorrhoeae, Chlamydia trachomatis, Mycoplasma genitalium, Ureaplasma urealyticum* (subspecies *urealyticum*), *Trichomonas vaginalis*, HSV
Epididymitis	*C. trachomatis, N. gonorrhoeae*
Lower genital tract infections: females	
Cystitis/urethritis	*C. trachomatis, N. gonorrhoeae*, HSV
Mucopurulent cervicitis	*C. trachomatis, N. gonorrhoeae, M. genitalium*
Vulvitis	*Candida albicans*, HSV
Vulvovaginitis	*C. albicans, T. vaginalis*
BV	BV-associated bacteria (see text)
Acute pelvic inflammatory disease	*N. gonorrhoeae, C. trachomatis*, BV-associated bacteria, *M. genitalium*, group B streptococci
Infertility	*N. gonorrhoeae, C. trachomatis*, BV-associated bacteria
Ulcerative lesions of the genitalia	HSV-1, HSV-2, *Treponema pallidum, Haemophilus ducreyi, C. trachomatis* (LGV strains), *Klebsiella (Calymmatobacterium) granulomatis*
Complications of pregnancy/puerperium	Several agents implicated
Intestinal infections	
Proctitis	*C. trachomatis, N. gonorrhoeae*, HSV, *T. pallidum*
Proctocolitis or enterocolitis	*Campylobacter* spp., *Shigella* spp., *Entamoeba histolytica, Helicobacter* spp., other enteric pathogens
Enteritis	*Giardia lamblia*
Acute arthritis with urogenital infection or viremia	*N. gonorrhoeae* (e.g., DGI), *C. trachomatis* (e.g., reactive arthritis), HBV
Genital and anal warts	HPV (30 genital types)
Mononucleosis syndrome	CMV, HIV, EBV
Hepatitis	Hepatitis viruses, *T. pallidum*, CMV, EBV
Neoplasias	
Squamous cell dysplasias and cancers of the cervix, anus, vulva, vagina, or penis	HPV (especially types 16, 18, 31, 45)
Kaposi's sarcoma, body-cavity lymphomas	HHV-8
T cell leukemia	HTLV-1
Hepatocellular carcinoma	HBV
Tropical spastic paraparesis	HTLV-1
Scabies	*Sarcoptes scabiei*
Pubic lice	*Pthirus pubis*

Abbreviations: BV, bacterial vaginosis; CMV, cytomegalovirus; DGI, disseminated gonococcal infection; EBV, Epstein-Barr virus; HBV, hepatitis B virus; HHV-8, human herpesvirus type 8; HPV, human papillomavirus; HSV, herpes simplex virus; HTLV, human T cell lymphotropic virus; LGV, lymphogranuloma venereum.

STD care and management begin with risk assessment and proceed to clinical assessment, diagnostic testing or screening, treatment, and prevention. Indeed, the routine care of any patient begins with risk assessment (e.g., for risk of heart disease, cancer). STD/HIV risk assessment is important in primary care, urgent care, and emergency care settings as well as in specialty clinics providing adolescent, HIV/AIDS, prenatal, and family planning services. STD/HIV risk assessment guides detection and interpretation of symptoms that could reflect an STD; decisions on screening or prophylactic/preventive treatment; risk reduction counseling and intervention (e.g., hepatitis B vaccination); and treatment of partners of patients with known infections. Consideration of routine demographic data (e.g., gender, age, area of residence) is a simple first step in STD/HIV risk assessment. For example, national guidelines strongly recommend routine screening of sexually active females ≤25 years of age for *C. trachomatis* infection. Table 163-3 provides a set of 11 STD/HIV risk-assessment questions that clinicians can pose verbally or that health care systems can adapt (with yes/no responses) into a routine self-administered questionnaire for use in clinics. The initial framing statement gives permission to discuss topics that may be perceived as sensitive or socially unacceptable by providers and patients alike.

Risk assessment is followed by clinical assessment (elicitation of information on specific current symptoms and signs of STDs). Confirmatory diagnostic tests (for persons with symptoms or signs) or screening tests (for those without symptoms or signs) may involve microscopic examination, culture, antigen detection tests, nucleic acid amplification tests (NAATs), or serology. Initial syndrome-based treatment should cover the most likely causes. For certain syndromes, results of rapid tests can narrow the spectrum of this initial therapy (e.g., saline microscopy of vaginal fluid for women with vaginal discharge, Gram's stain of urethral discharge for men with urethral discharge, rapid plasma reagin test for genital ulcer). After the institution of treatment, STD management proceeds to the "4 Cs" of prevention and control: *c*ontact tracing (see "Prevention and Control of STIs," below), ensuring *c*ompliance with therapy, and *c*ounseling on risk reduction, including *c*ondom promotion and provision.

Consistent with current guidelines, all adults should be screened for infection with HIV-1 at least once and more frequently if they are at elevated risk for acquisition of this infection.

URETHRITIS IN MEN

Urethritis in men produces urethral discharge, dysuria, or both, usually without frequency of urination. Causes include *Neisseria gonorrhoeae, C. trachomatis, Mycoplasma genitalium, Ureaplasma urealyticum, Trichomonas vaginalis*, HSV, and adenovirus.

Until recently, *C. trachomatis* caused ~30–40% of cases of nongonococcal urethritis (NGU), particularly in heterosexual men; however, the proportion of cases due to this organism has probably declined in some populations served by effective chlamydial-control programs, and older men with urethritis appear less likely to have chlamydial infection. HSV and *T. vaginalis* each cause a small proportion of NGU cases in the United States. Recently, multiple studies have consistently implicated *M. genitalium* as a probable cause of many

TABLE 163-3 ELEVEN-QUESTION STD/HIV RISK ASSESSMENT

Framing Statement:
In order to provide the best care for you today and to understand your risk for certain infections, it is necessary for us to talk about your sexual behavior.
Screening Questions:
(1) Do you have any reason to think you might have a sexually transmitted infection? If so, what reason?
(2) For all adolescents <18 years old: Have you begun having any kind of sex yet?
STD History:
(3) Have you ever had any sexually transmitted infections or any genital infections? If so, which ones?
Sexual Preference:
(4) Have you had sex with men, women, or both?
Injection Drug Use:
(5) Have you ever injected yourself ("shot up") with drugs? (If yes, have you ever shared needles or injection equipment?)
(6) Have you ever had sex with a gay or bisexual man or with anyone who had ever injected drugs?
Characteristics of Partner(s):
(7) Has your sex partner had any sexually transmitted infections? If so, which ones?
(8) Has your sex partner had other sex partners during the time you've been together?
STD Symptoms Checklist:
(9) Have you recently developed any of these symptoms?

For Men	For Women
(a) Discharge of pus (drip) from the penis	(a) Abnormal vaginal discharge (increased amount, abnormal odor, abnormal yellow color)
(b) Genital sores (ulcers) or rash	(b) Genital sores (ulcers), rash, or itching

Sexual Practices, Past 2 Months (for patients answering yes to any of the above questions, to guide examination and testing):
(10) Now I'd like to ask what parts of your body may have been sexually exposed to an STD (e.g., your penis, mouth, vagina, anus).
Query about Interest in STD Screening Tests (for patients answering no to all of the above questions):
(11) Would you like to be tested for HIV or any other STDs today? (If yes, clinician can explore which STD and why.)

Source: Adapted from JR Curtis, KK Holmes, in KK Holmes et al (eds): *Sexually Transmitted Diseases*, 4th ed. New York, McGraw-Hill, 2008.

Chlamydia-negative cases. Fewer studies than in the past have implicated *Ureaplasma*; the ureaplasmas have been differentiated into *U. urealyticum* and *Ureaplasma parvum*, and a few studies suggest that *U. urealyticum*—but not *U. parvum* is associated with NGU. Coliform bacteria can cause urethritis in men who practice insertive anal intercourse. The initial diagnosis of urethritis in men currently includes specific tests only for *N. gonorrhoeae* and *C. trachomatis*; it does not yet include testing for *Mycoplasma* or *Ureaplasma* species. The following summarizes the approach to the patient with suspected urethritis:

1. *Establish the presence of urethritis.* If proximal-to-distal "milking" of the urethra does not express a purulent or mucopurulent discharge, even after the patient has not voided for several hours (or preferably overnight), a Gram's-stained smear of an anterior urethral specimen obtained by passage of a small urethrogenital swab 2–3 cm into the urethra usually reveals ≥5 neutrophils per 1000× field in areas containing cells; in gonococcal infection, such a smear usually reveals gram-negative intracellular diplococci as well. Alternatively, the centrifuged sediment of the first 20–30 mL of voided urine—ideally collected as the first morning specimen—can be examined for inflammatory cells, either by microscopy showing ≥10 leukocytes per high-power field or by the leukocyte esterase test. Patients with symptoms who lack objective evidence of urethritis may have functional rather than organic problems and generally do not benefit from repeated courses of antibiotics.
2. *Evaluate for complications or alternative diagnoses.* A brief history and examination will exclude epididymitis and systemic complications, such as disseminated gonococcal infection (DGI) and reactive arthritis. Although digital examination of the prostate gland seldom contributes to the evaluation of sexually active young men with urethritis, men with dysuria who lack evidence of urethritis as well as sexually inactive men with urethritis should undergo prostate palpation, urinalysis, and urine culture to exclude bacterial prostatitis and cystitis.
3. *Evaluate for gonococcal and chlamydial infection.* An absence of typical gram-negative diplococci on Gram's-stained smear of urethral exudate containing inflammatory cells warrants a preliminary diagnosis of NGU, as this test is 98% sensitive for the diagnosis of gonococcal urethral infection. However, an increasing proportion of men with symptoms and/or signs of urethritis are simultaneously assessed for infection with *N. gonorrhoeae* and *C. trachomatis* by "multiplex" NAATs of first-voided urine. The urine specimen tested should consist of the first 10–15 mL of the stream, and, if possible, patients should not have voided for the prior 2 h. Culture or NAAT for *N. gonorrhoeae* may yield positive results when Gram's staining is negative; certain strains of *N. gonorrhoeae* can result in negative urethral Gram's stains in up to 30% of cases of urethral infection. Results of tests for gonococcal and chlamydial infection predict the patient's prognosis (with greater risk for recurrent NGU if neither chlamydiae nor gonococci are found than if either is detected) and can guide both the counseling given to the patient and the management of the patient's sexual partner(s).
4. *Treat urethritis promptly while test results are pending.*

TREATMENT URETHRITIS IN MEN

Table 163-4 summarizes the steps in management of sexually active men with urethral discharge and/or dysuria.

In practice, if Gram's stain does not reveal gonococci, urethritis is treated with a regimen effective for NGU, such as azithromycin or doxycycline. Both are effective, although azithromycin may give better results in *M. genitalium* infection. If gonococci are demonstrated by Gram's stain or if no diagnostic tests are performed to exclude gonorrhea definitively, treatment should include parenteral cephalosporin therapy for gonorrhea **(Chap. 181)** plus oral azithromycin, primarily for additive activity against *N. gonorrhoeae* given concerns about evolving antibiotic resistance. Azithromycin also treats *C. trachomatis*, which often causes urethral co-infection in men with gonococcal urethritis. Ideally, sexual partners should be tested for gonorrhea and chlamydial infection; regardless of whether they are tested for these infections, however, they should receive the same regimen given to the male index case. Patients with confirmed persistence or recurrence of urethritis after treatment should be re-treated with the initial regimen if they did not comply with the original treatment or were reexposed to an untreated partner. Otherwise, an intraurethral swab specimen and a first-voided urine sample should be tested for *T. vaginalis* (currently done by culture, although NAATs are more sensitive and are approved for the diagnosis of trichomoniasis in women). If compliance with initial treatment is confirmed and reexposure to an untreated sex partner is deemed unlikely, the recommended treatment is with metronidazole or tinidazole (2 g by mouth in a single dose) plus azithromycin (1 g by mouth in a single dose); the azithromycin component is especially important if this drug has not been given during initial therapy.

EPIDIDYMITIS

Acute epididymitis, almost always unilateral, produces pain, swelling, and tenderness of the epididymis, with or without symptoms or signs of urethritis. This condition must be differentiated from testicular torsion, tumor, and trauma. Torsion, a surgical emergency, usually occurs in

TABLE 163-4 MANAGEMENT OF URETHRAL DISCHARGE IN MEN

Usual Causes	Usual Initial Evaluation
Chlamydia trachomatis	Demonstration of urethral discharge or pyuria
Neisseria gonorrhoeae	Exclusion of local or systemic complications
Mycoplasma genitalium	Urethral Gram's stain to confirm urethritis, detect gram-negative diplococci
Ureaplasma urealyticum	Test for *N. gonorrhoeae*, *C. trachomatis*
Trichomonas vaginalis	
Herpes simplex virus	

Initial Treatment for Patient and Partners

Treat gonorrhea (unless excluded):

Ceftriaxone, 250 mg IM[a] plus Azithromycin, 1 g PO

Management of Recurrence

Confirm objective evidence of urethritis. If patient was reexposed to untreated or new partner, repeat treatment of patient and partner.

If patient was not reexposed, consider infection with *T. vaginalis*[b] or doxycycline-resistant *M. genitalium*[c] or *Ureaplasma*, and consider treatment with metronidazole, azithromycin, or both.

[a]Neither oral cephalosporins nor fluoroquinolones are recommended for treatment of gonorrhea in the United States because of the emergence of increasing fluoroquinolone resistance in *N. gonorrhoeae*, especially (but not only) among men who have sex with men, and decreasing susceptibility of a still-small proportion of gonococci to ceftriaxone (Fig. 163-1). Updates on the emergence of antimicrobial resistance in *N. gonorrhoeae* can be obtained from the Centers for Disease Control and Prevention at *http://www.cdc.gov/std*. [b]In men, the diagnosis of *T. vaginalis* infection requires culture, DNA testing, or nucleic acid amplification testing (where available) of early-morning first-voided urine sediment or of a urethral swab specimen obtained before voiding. [c]*M. genitalium* is often resistant to doxycycline and azithromycin but is usually susceptible to the fluoroquinolone moxifloxacin. Until nucleic acid amplification testing for *M. genitalium* becomes commercially available, moxifloxacin can be considered for treatment of refractory nongonococcal, nonchlamydial urethritis.

the second or third decade of life and produces a sudden onset of pain, elevation of the testicle within the scrotal sac, rotation of the epididymis from a posterior to an anterior position, and absence of blood flow on Doppler examination or ^{99m}Tc scan. Persistence of symptoms after a course of therapy for epididymitis suggests the possibility of testicular tumor or of a chronic granulomatous disease, such as tuberculosis. In sexually active men under age 35, acute epididymitis is caused most frequently by *C. trachomatis* and less commonly by *N. gonorrhoeae* and is usually associated with overt or subclinical urethritis. Acute epididymitis occurring in older men or following urinary tract instrumentation is usually caused by urinary pathogens. Similarly, epididymitis in men who have practiced insertive rectal intercourse is often caused by Enterobacteriaceae. These older men usually have no urethritis but do have bacteriuria.

TREATMENT EPIDIDYMITIS

Ceftriaxone (250 mg as a single dose IM) followed by doxycycline (100 mg by mouth twice daily for 10 days) constitutes effective treatment for epididymitis caused by *N. gonorrhoeae* or *C. trachomatis*. Neither oral cephalosporins nor fluoroquinolones are recommended for treatment of gonorrhea in the United States because of resistance in *N. gonorrhoeae*, especially (but not only) among MSM (Fig. 163-1). Oral levofloxacin (500 mg once daily for 10 days) is also effective for syndrome-based initial treatment of epididymitis when infection with Enterobacteriaceae is suspected; however, this regimen should be combined with effective therapy for possible gonococcal or chlamydial infection unless bacteriuria with Enterobacteriaceae is confirmed.

URETHRITIS AND THE URETHRAL SYNDROME IN WOMEN

C. trachomatis, *N. gonorrhoeae*, and occasionally HSV cause symptomatic urethritis—known as *the urethral syndrome* in women—that is characterized by "internal" dysuria (usually without urinary urgency or frequency), pyuria, and an absence of *Escherichia coli* and other

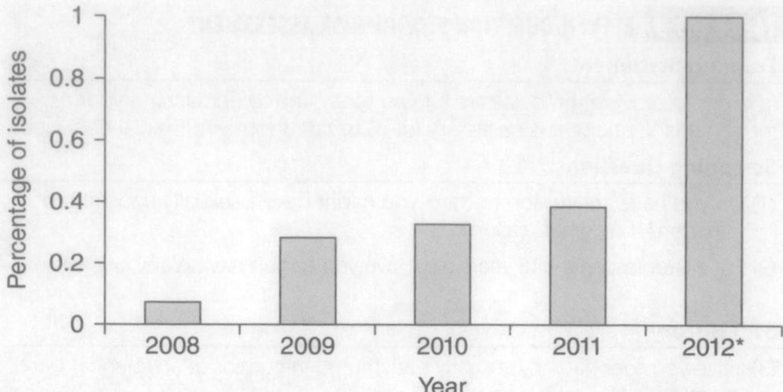

FIGURE 163-1 Proportion of *Neisseria gonorrhoeae* isolates with elevated ceftriaxone minimum inhibitory concentrations (MICs), United States 2008–2012. Elevated resistance is defined by ceftriaxone MICs of ≥0.125 μg/mL. *Preliminary (January–June). *(From the Centers for Disease Control and Prevention: Gonococcal Isolate Surveillance Project [GISP], 2013.)*

uropathogens at counts of $\geq 10^2$/mL in urine. In contrast, the dysuria associated with vulvar herpes or vulvovaginal candidiasis (and perhaps with trichomoniasis) is often described as "external," being caused by painful contact of urine with the inflamed or ulcerated labia or introitus. Acute onset, association with urinary urgency or frequency, hematuria, or suprapubic bladder tenderness suggests bacterial cystitis. Among women with symptoms of acute bacterial cystitis, costovertebral pain and tenderness or fever suggests acute pyelonephritis. The management of bacterial urinary tract infection (UTI) is discussed in Chap. 162.

Signs of vulvovaginitis, coupled with symptoms of external dysuria, suggest vulvar infection (e.g., with HSV or *Candida albicans*). Among dysuric women without signs of vulvovaginitis, bacterial UTI must be differentiated from the urethral syndrome by assessment of risk, evaluation of the pattern of symptoms and signs, and specific microbiologic testing. An STI etiology of the urethral syndrome is suggested by young age, more than one current sexual partner, a new partner within the past month, a partner with urethritis, or coexisting mucopurulent cervicitis (see below). The finding of a single urinary pathogen, such as *E. coli* or *Staphylococcus saprophyticus*, at a concentration of $\geq 10^2$/mL in a properly collected specimen of midstream urine from a dysuric woman with pyuria indicates probable bacterial UTI, whereas pyuria with $<10^2$ conventional uropathogens per milliliter of urine ("sterile" pyuria) suggests acute urethral syndrome due to *C. trachomatis* or *N. gonorrhoeae*. Gonorrhea and chlamydial infection should be sought by specific tests (e.g., NAATs of vaginal secretions collected with a swab). Among dysuric women with sterile pyuria caused by infection with *N. gonorrhoeae* or *C. trachomatis*, appropriate treatment alleviates dysuria. The role of *M. genitalium* in the urethral syndrome in women remains undefined.

VULVOVAGINAL INFECTIONS

Abnormal Vaginal Discharge If directly questioned about vaginal discharge during routine health checkups, many women acknowledge having nonspecific symptoms of vaginal discharge that do not correlate with objective signs of inflammation or with actual infection. However, unsolicited reporting of abnormal vaginal discharge does suggest bacterial vaginosis or trichomoniasis. Specifically, an abnormally increased amount or an abnormal odor of the discharge is associated with one or both of these conditions. Cervical infection with *N. gonorrhoeae* or *C. trachomatis* does not often cause an increased amount or abnormal odor of discharge; however, when these pathogens cause cervicitis, they—like *T. vaginalis*—often result in an increased number of neutrophils in vaginal fluid, which thus takes on a yellow color. Vulvar conditions such as genital herpes or vulvovaginal candidiasis can cause vulvar pruritus, burning, irritation, or lesions as well as external dysuria (as urine passes over the inflamed vulva or areas of epithelial disruption) or vulvar dyspareunia.

Certain vulvovaginal infections may have serious sequelae. Trichomoniasis, bacterial vaginosis, and vulvovaginal candidiasis have all been associated with increased risk of acquisition of HIV infection; bacterial vaginosis may promote HIV transmission from HIV-infected women to their male sex partners. Vaginal trichomoniasis and bacterial vaginosis early in pregnancy independently predict premature onset of labor. Bacterial vaginosis can also lead to anaerobic bacterial infection of the endometrium and salpinges. Vaginitis may be an early and prominent feature of toxic shock syndrome, and recurrent or chronic vulvovaginal candidiasis develops with increased frequency among women who have systemic illnesses, such as diabetes mellitus or HIV-related immunosuppression (although only a very small proportion of women with recurrent vulvovaginal candidiasis in industrialized countries actually have a serious predisposing illness).

Thus vulvovaginal symptoms or signs warrant careful evaluation, including speculum and pelvic examination, simple rapid diagnostic tests, and appropriate therapy specific for the anatomic site and type of infection. Unfortunately, a survey in the United States indicated that clinicians seldom perform the tests required to establish the cause of such symptoms. Further, comparison of telephone and office management of vulvovaginal symptoms has documented the inaccuracy of the former, and comparison of evaluations by nurse-midwives with those by physician-practitioners showed that the practitioners' clinical evaluations correlated poorly both with the nurses' evaluations and with diagnostic tests. The diagnosis and treatment of the three most common types of vaginal infection are summarized in Table 163-5.

Inspection of the vulva and perineum may reveal tender genital ulcerations or fissures (typically due to HSV infection or vulvovaginal candidiasis) or discharge visible at the introitus before insertion of a speculum (suggestive of bacterial vaginosis or trichomoniasis). Speculum examination permits the clinician to discern whether the discharge in fact looks abnormal and whether any abnormal discharge in the vagina emanates from the cervical os (mucoid and, if abnormal, yellow) or from the vagina (not mucoid, since the vaginal epithelium does not produce mucus). Symptoms or signs of abnormal vaginal discharge should prompt testing of vaginal fluid for pH, for a fishy odor when mixed with 10% KOH, and for certain microscopic features when mixed with saline (motile trichomonads and/or "clue cells") and with 10% KOH (pseudohyphae or hyphae indicative of vulvovaginal candidiasis). Additional objective laboratory tests useful for establishing the cause of abnormal vaginal discharge include rapid point-of-care tests for bacterial vaginosis and *T. vaginalis*, as described below; a DNA probe test (the Affirm test) to detect *T. vaginalis* and *C. albicans* as well as the increased concentrations of *Gardnerella vaginalis* associated with bacterial vaginosis; and a NAAT for *T. vaginalis*. Gram's

TABLE 163-5 DIAGNOSTIC FEATURES AND MANAGEMENT OF VAGINAL INFECTION

Feature	Normal Vaginal Examination	Vulvovaginal Candidiasis	Trichomonal Vaginitis	Bacterial Vaginosis
Etiology	Uninfected; lactobacilli predominant	*Candida albicans*	*Trichomonas vaginalis*	Associated with *Gardnerella vaginalis*, various anaerobic and/or noncultured bacteria, and mycoplasmas
Typical symptoms	None	Vulvar itching and/or irritation	Profuse discharge; vulvar itching	Malodorous, slightly increased discharge
Discharge				
Amount	Variable, usually scant	Scant	Often profuse	Moderate
Color[a]	Clear or translucent	White	White or yellow	White or gray
Consistency	Nonhomogeneous, flocculent	Clumped; adherent plaques	Homogeneous	Homogeneous, low viscosity; uniformly coats vaginal walls
Inflammation of vulvar or vaginal epithelium	None	Erythema of vaginal epithelium, introitus; vulvar dermatitis, fissures common	Erythema of vaginal and vulvar epithelium; colpitis macularis	None
pH of vaginal fluid[b]	Usually ≤4.5	Usually ≤4.5	Usually ≥5	Usually >4.5
Amine ("fishy") odor with 10% KOH	None	None	May be present	Present
Microscopy[c]	Normal epithelial cells; lactobacilli predominant	Leukocytes, epithelial cells; mycelia or pseudomycelia in up to 80% of *C. albicans* culture-positive persons with typical symptoms	Leukocytes; motile trichomonads seen in 80–90% of symptomatic patients, less often in the absence of symptoms	Clue cells; few leukocytes; no lactobacilli or only a few outnumbered by profuse mixed microbiota, nearly always including *G. vaginalis* plus anaerobic species on Gram's stain (Nugent's score ≥7)
Other laboratory findings		Isolation of *Candida* spp.	Isolation of *T. vaginalis* or positive NAAT[d]	
Usual treatment	None	Azole cream, tablet, or suppository—e.g., miconazole (100-mg vaginal suppository) or clotrimazole (100-mg vaginal tablet) once daily for 7 days Fluconazole, 150 mg orally (single dose)	Metronidazole or tinidazole, 2 g orally (single dose) Metronidazole, 500 mg PO bid for 7 days	Metronidazole, 500 mg PO bid for 7 days Metronidazole gel, 0.75%, one applicator (5 g) intravaginally once daily for 5 days Clindamycin, 2% cream, one full applicator vaginally each night for 7 days
Usual management of sexual partner	None	None; topical treatment if candidal dermatitis of penis is detected	Examination for sexually transmitted infection; treatment with metronidazole, 2 g PO (single dose)	None

[a]Color of discharge is best determined by examination against the white background of a swab. [b]A pH determination is not useful if blood is present or if the test is performed on endocervical secretions. [c]To detect fungal elements, vaginal fluid is digested with 10% KOH prior to microscopic examination; to examine for other features, fluid is mixed (1:1) with physiologic saline. Gram's stain is also excellent for detecting yeasts (less predictive of vulvovaginitis) and pseudomycelia or mycelia (strongly predictive of vulvovaginitis) and for distinguishing normal flora from the mixed flora seen in bacterial vaginosis, but it is less sensitive than the saline preparation for detection of *T. vaginalis*. [d]NAAT, nucleic acid amplification test (where available).

staining of vaginal fluid can be used to score alterations in the vaginal microbiota but is used primarily for research purposes and requires familiarity with the morphotypes and scale involved.

TREATMENT VAGINAL DISCHARGE

Patterns of treatment for vaginal discharge vary widely. In developing countries, where clinics or pharmacies often dispense treatment based on symptoms alone without examination or testing, oral treatment with metronidazole—particularly with a 7-day regimen—provides reasonable coverage against both trichomoniasis and bacterial vaginosis, the usual causes of symptoms of vaginal discharge. Metronidazole treatment of sex partners prevents reinfection of women with trichomoniasis, even though it does not help prevent the recurrence of bacterial vaginosis. Guidelines for syndromic management promulgated by the World Health Organization suggest consideration of treatment for cervical infection and for trichomoniasis, bacterial vaginosis, and vulvovaginal candidiasis in women with symptoms of abnormal vaginal discharge. However, it is important to note that the majority of chlamydial and gonococcal cervical infections produce no symptoms.

In industrialized countries, clinicians treating symptoms and signs of abnormal vaginal discharge should, at a minimum, differentiate between bacterial vaginosis and trichomoniasis, because optimal management of patients and partners differs for these two conditions (as discussed briefly below).

Vaginal Trichomoniasis (See also Chap. 254) Symptomatic trichomoniasis characteristically produces a profuse, yellow, purulent, homogeneous vaginal discharge and vulvar irritation, sometimes with visible inflammation of the vaginal and vulvar epithelium and petechial lesions on the cervix (the so-called strawberry cervix, usually evident only by colposcopy). The pH of vaginal fluid—normally <4.7—usually rises to ≥5. In women with typical symptoms and signs of trichomoniasis, microscopic examination of vaginal discharge mixed with saline reveals motile trichomonads in most culture-positive cases. However, saline microscopy probably detects only one-half of all cases, and, especially in the absence of symptoms or signs, culture or NAAT is usually required for detection of the organism. NAAT for *T. vaginalis* is as sensitive as or more sensitive than culture, and NAAT of urine has disclosed surprisingly high prevalences of this pathogen among men at several STD clinics in the United States. Treatment of asymptomatic as well as symptomatic cases reduces rates of transmission and prevents later development of symptoms.

TREATMENT VAGINAL TRICHOMONIASIS

Only nitroimidazoles (e.g., metronidazole and tinidazole) consistently cure trichomoniasis. A single 2-g oral dose of metronidazole is effective and much less expensive than the alternatives. Tinidazole has a longer half-life than metronidazole, causes fewer gastrointestinal symptoms, and may be useful in treating trichomoniasis that fails to respond to metronidazole. Treatment of sexual partners—facilitated by dispensing metronidazole to the female patient to give to her partner(s), with a warning about avoiding the concurrent use of alcohol—significantly reduces both the risk of reinfection and the reservoir of infection; treating the partner is the standard of care. Intravaginal treatment with 0.75% metronidazole gel is not reliable for vaginal trichomoniasis. Systemic use of metronidazole is recommended throughout pregnancy. In a large randomized trial, metronidazole treatment of trichomoniasis during pregnancy did not reduce—and in fact actually increased—the frequency of perinatal morbidity; thus routine screening of asymptomatic pregnant women for trichomoniasis is not recommended.

Bacterial Vaginosis Bacterial vaginosis (formerly termed *nonspecific vaginitis, Haemophilus vaginitis, anaerobic vaginitis,* or *Gardnerella-associated vaginal discharge*) is a syndrome of complex etiology that is characterized by symptoms of vaginal malodor and a slightly to moderately increased white discharge, which appears homogeneous, is low in viscosity, and evenly coats the vaginal mucosa. Bacterial vaginosis has been associated with increased risk of acquiring several other genital infections, including those caused by HIV, *C. trachomatis*, and *N. gonorrhoeae*. Other risk factors include recent unprotected vaginal intercourse, having a female sex partner, and vaginal douching. Although bacteria associated with bacterial vaginosis have been detected under the foreskin of uncircumcised men, metronidazole treatment of male partners has not reduced the rate of recurrence among affected women.

Among women with bacterial vaginosis, culture of vaginal fluid has shown markedly increased prevalences and concentrations of *G. vaginalis*, *Mycoplasma hominis*, and several anaerobic bacteria (e.g., *Mobiluncus*, *Prevotella* [formerly *Bacteroides*], and some *Peptostreptococcus* species) as well as an absence of hydrogen peroxide-producing *Lactobacillus* species that constitute most of the normal vaginal microbiota and help protect against certain cervical and vaginal infections. Broad-range polymerase chain reaction (PCR) amplification of 16S rDNA in vaginal fluid, with subsequent identification of specific bacterial species by various methods, has documented an even greater and unexpected bacterial diversity, including several unique species not previously cultivated (e.g., three species in the order Clostridiales that appear to be specific for bacterial vaginosis and are associated with metronidazole treatment failure [Fig. 163-2]). Also detected are DNA sequences related to *Atopobium vaginae*, an organism that is strongly associated with bacterial vaginosis, is resistant to metronidazole, and is also associated with recurrent bacterial vaginosis after metronidazole treatment. Other genera newly implicated in bacterial vaginosis include *Megasphaera*, *Leptotrichia*, *Eggerthella*, and *Dialister*.

Bacterial vaginosis is conventionally diagnosed clinically with the Amsel criteria, which include any three of the following four clinical abnormalities: (1) objective signs of increased white homogeneous vaginal discharge; (2) a vaginal discharge pH of >4.5; (3) liberation of a distinct fishy odor (attributable to volatile amines such as trimethylamine) immediately after vaginal secretions are mixed with a 10% solution of KOH; and (4) microscopic demonstration of "clue cells" (vaginal epithelial cells coated with coccobacillary organisms, which have a granular appearance and indistinct borders; Fig. 163-3) on a wet mount prepared by mixing vaginal secretions with normal saline in a ratio of ~1:1.

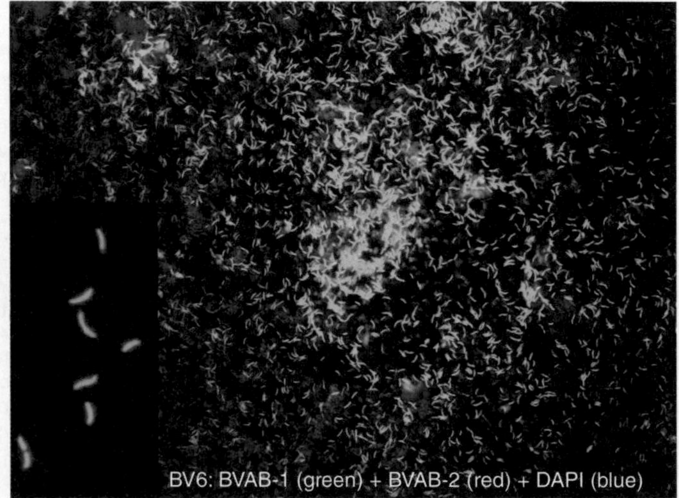

FIGURE 163-2 Broad-range polymerase chain reaction amplification of 16S rDNA in vaginal fluid from a woman with bacterial vaginosis shows a field of bacteria hybridizing with probes for bacterial vaginosis–associated bacterium 1 (BVAB-1, visible as a thin, curved green rod) and for BVAB-2 (red). The *inset* shows that BVAB-1 has a morphology similar to that of *Mobiluncus* (curved rod). *(Reprinted with permission from DN Fredricks et al: N Engl J Med 353:1899, 2005.)*

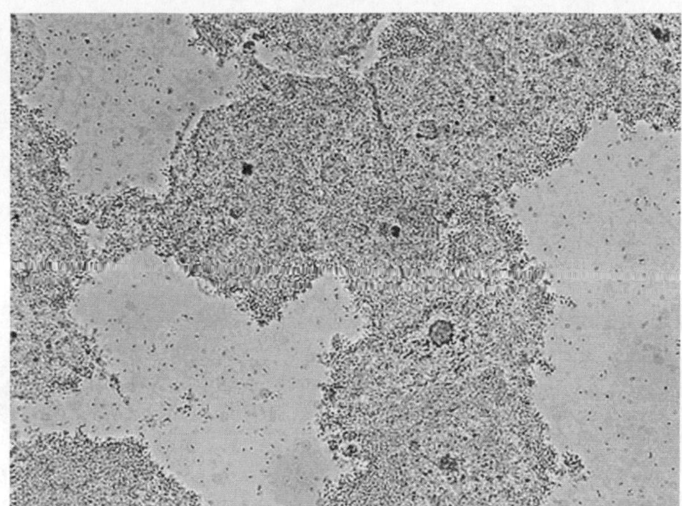

FIGURE 163-3 Wet mount of vaginal fluid showing typical clue cells from a woman with bacterial vaginosis. Note the obscured epithelial cell margins and the granular appearance attributable to many adherent bacteria (×400). *(Photograph provided by Lorna K. Rabe, reprinted with permission from S Hillier et al, in KK Holmes et al [eds]: Sexually Transmitted Diseases, 4th ed. New York, McGraw-Hill, 2008.)*

TREATMENT BACTERIAL VAGINOSIS

The standard dosage of oral metronidazole for the treatment of bacterial vaginosis is 500 mg twice daily for 7 days. The single 2-g oral dose of metronidazole recommended for trichomoniasis produces significantly lower short-term cure rates and should not be used. Intravaginal treatment with 2% clindamycin cream (one full applicator [5 g containing 100 mg of clindamycin phosphate] each night for 7 nights) or with 0.75% metronidazole gel (one full applicator [5 g containing 37.5 mg of metronidazole] twice daily for 5 days) is also approved for use in the United States and does not elicit systemic adverse reactions; the response to both of these treatments is similar to the response to oral metronidazole. Other alternatives include oral clindamycin (300 mg twice daily for 7 days), clindamycin ovules (100 g intravaginally once at bedtime for 3 days), and oral tinidazole (1 g daily for 5 days or 2 g daily for 3 days). Unfortunately, recurrence over the long term (i.e., several months later) is distressingly common after either oral or intravaginal treatment. A randomized trial comparing intravaginal gel containing 37.5 mg of metronidazole with a suppository containing 500 mg of metronidazole plus nystatin (the latter not marketed in the United States) showed significantly higher rates of recurrence with the 37.5-mg regimen; this result suggests that higher metronidazole dosages may be important in topical intravaginal therapy. Recurrences can be significantly lessened with the twice-weekly use of suppressive intravaginal metronidazole gel. As stated above, treatment of male partners with metronidazole does not prevent recurrence of bacterial vaginosis.

Efforts to replenish numbers of vaginal lactobacilli that produce hydrogen peroxide and probably sustain vaginal health have been unsuccessful. While one randomized trial of orally ingested lactobacilli found reduced rates of recurrent bacterial vaginosis, this result has not yet been either confirmed or refuted, and a randomized multicenter trial in the United States found no benefit of repeated intravaginal inoculation of a vaginal peroxide-producing *Lactobacillus* species following treatment of bacterial vaginosis with metronidazole. A meta-analysis of 18 studies concluded that bacterial vaginosis during pregnancy substantially increased the risk of preterm delivery and of spontaneous abortion. However, most studies of topical intravaginal treatment of bacterial vaginosis with clindamycin during pregnancy have not reduced adverse pregnancy outcomes. Numerous trials of oral metronidazole treatment during pregnancy have given inconsistent results, and a 2013 Cochrane review concluded that antenatal treatment of women with bacterial vaginosis—even those with previous preterm delivery—did not reduce the risk of preterm delivery. The U.S. Preventive Services Task Force thus recommends against routine screening of pregnant women for bacterial vaginosis.

Vulvovaginal Pruritus, Burning, or Irritation Vulvovaginal candidiasis produces vulvar pruritus, burning, or irritation, generally without symptoms of increased vaginal discharge or malodor. Genital herpes can produce similar symptoms, with lesions sometimes difficult to distinguish from the fissures and inflammation caused by candidiasis. Signs of vulvovaginal candidiasis include vulvar erythema, edema, fissures, and tenderness. With candidiasis, a white scanty vaginal discharge sometimes takes the form of white thrush-like plaques or cottage cheese–like curds adhering loosely to the vaginal epithelium. *C. albicans* accounts for nearly all cases of symptomatic vulvovaginal candidiasis, which probably arise from endogenous strains of *C. albicans* that have colonized the vagina or the intestinal tract. Complicated vulvovaginal candidiasis includes cases that recur four or more times per year; are unusually severe; are caused by non-*albicans Candida* species; or occur in women with uncontrolled diabetes, debilitation, immunosuppression, or pregnancy.

In addition to compatible clinical symptoms, the diagnosis of vulvovaginal candidiasis usually involves the demonstration of pseudohyphae or hyphae by microscopic examination of vaginal fluid mixed with saline or 10% KOH or subjected to Gram's staining. Microscopic examination is less sensitive than culture but correlates better with symptoms. Culture is typically reserved for cases that do not respond to standard first-line antimycotic agents and is undertaken to rule out imidazole or azole resistance (often associated with *Candida glabrata*) or before the initiation of suppressive antifungal therapy for recurrent disease.

TREATMENT VULVOVAGINAL PRURITUS, BURNING, OR IRRITATION

Symptoms and signs of vulvovaginal candidiasis warrant treatment, usually intravaginal administration of any of several imidazole antibiotics (e.g., miconazole or clotrimazole) for 3–7 days or of a single dose of oral fluconazole (Table 163-5). Over-the-counter marketing of such preparations has reduced the cost of care and made treatment more convenient for many women with recurrent yeast vulvovaginitis. However, most women who purchase these preparations do not have vulvovaginal candidiasis, whereas many do have other vaginal infections that require different treatment. Therefore, only women with classic symptoms of vulvar pruritus and a history of previous episodes of yeast vulvovaginitis documented by an experienced clinician should self-treat. Short-course topical intravaginal azole drugs are effective for the treatment of uncomplicated vulvovaginal candidiasis (e.g., clotrimazole, two 100-mg vaginal tablets daily for 3 days; or miconazole, a 1200-mg vaginal suppository as a single dose). Single-dose oral treatment with fluconazole (150 mg) is also effective and is preferred by many patients. Management of complicated cases (see above) and those that do not respond to the usual intravaginal or single-dose oral therapy often involves prolonged or periodic oral therapy; this situation is discussed extensively in the 2010 CDC STD treatment guidelines (*http://www.cdc.gov/std/treatment*). Treatment of sexual partners is not routinely indicated.

Other Causes of Vaginal Discharge or Vaginitis In the ulcerative vaginitis associated with staphylococcal toxic shock syndrome, *Staphylococcus aureus* should be promptly identified in vaginal fluid by Gram's stain and by culture. In desquamative inflammatory vaginitis, smears of vaginal fluid reveal neutrophils, massive vaginal epithelial-cell exfoliation with increased numbers of parabasal cells, and gram-positive cocci; this syndrome may respond to treatment with 2% clindamycin cream, often given in combination with topical steroid preparations for several weeks. Additional causes of vaginitis and vulvovaginal symptoms include retained foreign bodies (e.g., tampons), cervical caps, vaginal spermicides, vaginal antiseptic preparations or douches, vaginal epithelial atrophy (in postmenopausal women or during prolonged breast-feeding in the postpartum period), allergic reactions to latex condoms, vaginal aphthae associated with HIV infection or Behçet's syndrome, and vestibulitis (a poorly understood syndrome).

MUCOPURULENT CERVICITIS

Mucopurulent cervicitis (MPC) refers to inflammation of the columnar epithelium and subepithelium of the endocervix and of any contiguous columnar epithelium that lies exposed in an ectopic position on the ectocervix. MPC in women represents the "silent partner" of urethritis in men, being equally common and often caused by the same agents (*N. gonorrhoeae*, *C. trachomatis*, or—as shown by case–control studies—*M. genitalium*); however, MPC is more difficult than urethritis to recognize. As the most common manifestation of these serious bacterial infections in women, MPC can be a harbinger or sign of upper genital tract infection, also known as *pelvic inflammatory disease* (PID; see below). In pregnant women, MPC can lead to obstetric complications. In a prospective study in Seattle of 167 consecutive patients with MPC (defined on the basis of yellow endocervical mucopus or ≥30 polymorphonuclear leukocytes [PMNs]/1000× microscopic field) who were seen at STD clinics during the 1980s, slightly more than one-third of cervicovaginal specimens tested for *C. trachomatis*, *N. gonorrhoeae*, *M. genitalium*, HSV, and *T. vaginalis* revealed no identifiable etiology (Fig. 163-4). More recently, a study in Baltimore using NAATs for these pathogens still failed to identify a microbiologic etiology in nearly one-half of the 133 women with MPC.

The diagnosis of MPC rests on the detection of cardinal signs at the cervix, including yellow mucopurulent discharge from the cervical os, endocervical bleeding upon gentle swabbing, and edematous cervical ectopy (see below); the latter two findings are somewhat more common with MPC due to chlamydial infection, but signs alone do not allow a distinction between the causative pathogens. Unlike the endocervicitis produced by gonococcal or chlamydial infection, cervicitis caused by HSV produces ulcerative lesions on the stratified squamous epithelium of the ectocervix as well as on the columnar epithelium. Yellow cervical mucus on a white swab removed from the endocervix indicates the presence of PMNs. Gram's staining may confirm their presence, although it adds relatively little to the diagnostic value of assessment for cervical signs. The presence of ≥20 PMNs/1000× microscopic field within strands of cervical mucus not contaminated by vaginal squamous epithelial cells or vaginal bacteria indicates endocervicitis. Detection of intracellular gram-negative diplococci in carefully collected endocervical mucus is quite specific but ≤50% sensitive for gonorrhea. Therefore, specific and sensitive tests for *N. gonorrhoeae* as well as for *C. trachomatis* (e.g., NAATs) are always indicated in the evaluation of MPC.

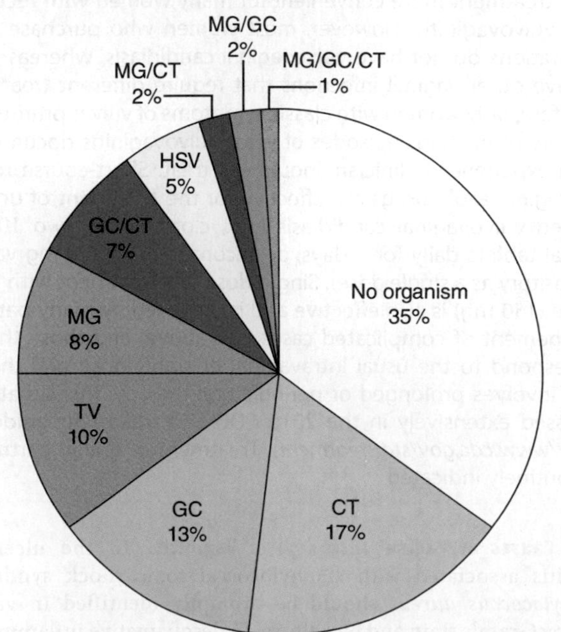

FIGURE 163-4 Organisms detected among female sexually transmitted disease clinic patients with mucopurulent cervicitis (n = 167). CT, *Chlamydia trachomatis*; GC, gonococcus; MG, *Mycoplasma genitalium*; TV, *Trichomonas vaginalis*; HSV, herpes simplex virus. *(Courtesy of Dr. Lisa Manhart; with permission.)*

TREATMENT MUCOPURULENT CERVICITIS

Although the above criteria for MPC are neither highly specific nor highly predictive of gonococcal or chlamydial infection in some settings, the 2010 CDC STD guidelines call for consideration of empirical treatment for MPC, pending test results, in most patients. Presumptive treatment with antibiotics active against *C. trachomatis* should be provided for women at increased risk for this common STI (risk factors: age <25 years, new or multiple sex partners, and unprotected sex), especially if follow-up cannot be ensured. Concurrent therapy for gonorrhea is indicated if the prevalence of this infection is substantial in the relevant patient population (e.g., young adults, a clinic with documented high prevalence). In this situation, therapy should include a single-dose regimen effective for gonorrhea plus treatment for chlamydial infection, as outlined in Table 163-4 for the treatment of urethritis. In settings where gonorrhea is much less common than chlamydial infection, initial therapy for chlamydial infection alone suffices, pending test results for gonorrhea. The etiology and potential benefit of treatment for endocervicitis not associated with gonorrhea or chlamydial infection have not been established. Although the antimicrobial susceptibility of *M. genitalium* is not yet well defined, the organism frequently persists after doxycycline therapy, and it currently seems reasonable to use azithromycin to treat possible *M. genitalium* infection in such cases. With resistance of *M. genitalium* to azithromycin now recognized, moxifloxacin may be a reasonable alternative. The sexual partner(s) of a woman with MPC should be examined and given a regimen similar to that chosen for the woman unless results of tests for gonorrhea or chlamydial infection in either partner warrant different therapy or no therapy.

CERVICAL ECTOPY

Cervical ectopy, often mislabeled "cervical erosion," is easily confused with infectious endocervicitis. Ectopy represents the presence of the one-cell-thick columnar epithelium extending from the endocervix out onto the visible ectocervix. In ectopy, the cervical os may contain clear or slightly cloudy mucus but usually not yellow mucopus. Colposcopy shows intact epithelium. Normally found during adolescence and early adulthood, ectopy gradually recedes through the second and third decades of life, as squamous metaplasia replaces the ectopic columnar epithelium. Oral contraceptive use favors the persistence or reappearance of ectopy, while smoking apparently accelerates squamous metaplasia. Cauterization of ectopy is not warranted. Ectopy may render the cervix more susceptible to infection with *N. gonorrhoeae*, *C. trachomatis*, or HIV.

PELVIC INFLAMMATORY DISEASE

The term *pelvic inflammatory disease* usually refers to infection that ascends from the cervix or vagina to involve the endometrium and/or fallopian tubes. Infection can extend beyond the reproductive tract to cause pelvic peritonitis, generalized peritonitis, perihepatitis, perisplenitis, or pelvic abscess. Rarely, infection not related to specific sexually transmitted pathogens extends secondarily to the pelvic organs (1) from adjacent foci of inflammation (e.g., appendicitis, regional ileitis, or diverticulitis) or bacterial vaginosis, (2) as a result of hematogenous dissemination (e.g., of tuberculosis or staphylococcal bacteremia), or (3) as a complication of certain tropical diseases (e.g., schistosomiasis). Intrauterine infection can be primary (spontaneously occurring and usually sexually transmitted) or secondary to invasive intrauterine surgical procedures (e.g., dilation and curettage, termination of pregnancy, insertion of an intrauterine device [IUD], or hysterosalpingography) or to parturition.

Etiology The agents most often implicated in acute PID include the primary causes of endocervicitis (e.g., *N. gonorrhoeae* and *C. trachomatis*) and organisms that can be regarded as components of an altered vaginal microbiota. In general, PID is most often caused by *N. gonorrhoeae* where there is a high incidence of gonorrhea—e.g., in inner-city populations in the United States. In case–control studies, *M. genitalium* has also been significantly associated with histopathologic diagnoses of endometritis and with salpingitis.

Anaerobic and facultative organisms (especially *Prevotella* species, peptostreptococci, *E. coli, Haemophilus influenzae*, and group B streptococci) as well as genital mycoplasmas have been isolated from the peritoneal fluid or fallopian tubes in a varying proportion (typically one-fourth to one-third) of women with PID studied in the United States. The difficulty of determining the exact microbial etiology of an individual case of PID—short of using invasive procedures for specimen collection—has implications for the approach to empirical antimicrobial treatment of this infection.

Epidemiology In the United States, the estimated annual number of initial visits to physicians' offices for PID by women 15–44 years of age fell from an average of 400,000 during the 1980s to 250,000 in 1999 and then to 90,000 in 2011. Hospitalizations for acute PID in the United States also declined steadily throughout the 1980s and early 1990s but have remained fairly constant at 70,000–100,000 per year since 1995. Important risk factors for acute PID include the presence of endocervical infection or bacterial vaginosis, a history of salpingitis or of recent vaginal douching, and recent insertion of an IUD. Certain other iatrogenic factors, such as dilation and curettage or cesarean section, can increase the risk of PID, especially among women with endocervical gonococcal or chlamydial infection or bacterial vaginosis. Symptoms of *N. gonorrhoeae*–associated and *C. trachomatis*–associated PID often begin during or soon after the menstrual period; this timing suggests that menstruation is a risk factor for ascending infection from the cervix and vagina. Experimental inoculation of the fallopian tubes of nonhuman primates has shown that repeated exposure to *C. trachomatis* leads to the greatest degree of tissue inflammation and damage; thus, immunopathology probably contributes to the pathogenesis of chlamydial salpingitis. Women using oral contraceptives appear to be at decreased risk of symptomatic PID, and tubal sterilization reduces the risk of salpingitis by preventing intraluminal spread of infection into the tubes.

Clinical Manifestations • ***ENDOMETRITIS: A CLINICAL PATHOLOGIC SYNDROME*** A study of women with clinically suspected PID who were undergoing both endometrial biopsy and laparoscopy showed that those with endometritis alone differed from those who also had salpingitis in significantly less often having lower quadrant, adnexal, or cervical motion or abdominal rebound tenderness; fever; or elevated C-reactive protein levels. In addition, women with endometritis alone differed from those with neither endometritis nor salpingitis in more often having gonorrhea, chlamydial infection, and risk factors such as douching or IUD use. Thus, women with endometritis alone were intermediate between those with neither endometritis nor salpingitis and those with salpingitis with respect to risk factors, clinical manifestations, cervical infection prevalence, and elevated C-reactive protein level. Women with endometritis alone are at lower risk of subsequent tubal occlusion and resulting infertility than are those with salpingitis.

SALPINGITIS Symptoms of nontuberculous salpingitis classically evolve from a yellow or malodorous vaginal discharge caused by MPC and/or bacterial vaginosis to midline abdominal pain and abnormal vaginal bleeding caused by endometritis and then to bilateral lower abdominal and pelvic pain caused by salpingitis, with nausea, vomiting, and increased abdominal tenderness if peritonitis develops.

The abdominal pain in nontuberculous salpingitis is usually described as dull or aching. In some cases, pain is lacking or atypical, but active inflammatory changes are found in the course of an unrelated evaluation or procedure, such as a laparoscopic evaluation for infertility. Abnormal uterine bleeding precedes or coincides with the onset of pain in ~40% of women with PID, symptoms of urethritis (dysuria) occur in 20%, and symptoms of proctitis (anorectal pain, tenesmus, and rectal discharge or bleeding) are occasionally seen in women with gonococcal or chlamydial infection.

Speculum examination shows evidence of MPC (yellow endocervical discharge, easily induced endocervical bleeding) in the majority of women with gonococcal or chlamydial PID. Cervical motion tenderness is produced by stretching of the adnexal attachments on the side toward which the cervix is pushed. Bimanual examination reveals uterine fundal tenderness due to endometritis and abnormal adnexal tenderness due to salpingitis that is usually, but not necessarily, bilateral. Adnexal swelling is palpable in about one-half of women with acute salpingitis, but evaluation of the adnexae in a patient with marked tenderness is not reliable. The initial temperature is >38°C in only about one-third of patients with acute salpingitis. Laboratory findings include elevation of the erythrocyte sedimentation rate (ESR) in 75% of patients with acute salpingitis and elevation of the peripheral white blood cell count in up to 60%.

Unlike nontuberculous salpingitis, genital tuberculosis often occurs in older women, many of whom are postmenopausal. Presenting symptoms include abnormal vaginal bleeding, pain (including dysmenorrhea), and infertility. About one-quarter of these women have had adnexal masses. Endometrial biopsy shows tuberculous granulomas and provides optimal specimens for culture.

PERIHEPATITIS AND PERIAPPENDICITIS Pleuritic upper-abdominal pain and tenderness, usually localized to the right upper quadrant (RUQ), develop in 3–10% of women with acute PID. Symptoms of perihepatitis arise during or after the onset of symptoms of PID and may overshadow lower abdominal symptoms, thereby leading to a mistaken diagnosis of cholecystitis. In perhaps 5% of cases of acute salpingitis, early laparoscopy reveals perihepatic inflammation ranging from edema and erythema of the liver capsule to exudate with fibrinous adhesions between the visceral and parietal peritoneum. When treatment is delayed and laparoscopy is performed late, dense "violin-string" adhesions can be seen over the liver; chronic exertional or positional RUQ pain ensues when traction is placed on the adhesions. Although perihepatitis, also known as the *Fitz-Hugh–Curtis syndrome*, was for many years specifically attributed to gonococcal salpingitis, most cases are now attributed to chlamydial salpingitis. In patients with chlamydial salpingitis, serum titers of microimmunofluorescent antibody to *C. trachomatis* are typically much higher when perihepatitis is present than when it is absent.

Physical findings include RUQ tenderness and usually include adnexal tenderness and cervicitis, even in patients whose symptoms do not suggest salpingitis. Results of liver function tests and RUQ ultrasonography are nearly always normal. The presence of MPC and pelvic tenderness in a young woman with subacute pleuritic RUQ pain and normal ultrasonography of the gallbladder points to a diagnosis of perihepatitis.

Periappendicitis (appendiceal serositis without involvement of the intestinal mucosa) has been found in ~5% of patients undergoing appendectomy for suspected appendicitis and can occur as a complication of gonococcal or chlamydial salpingitis.

Among women with salpingitis, HIV infection is associated with increased severity of salpingitis and with tuboovarian abscess requiring hospitalization and surgical drainage. Nonetheless, among women with HIV infection and salpingitis, the clinical response to conventional antimicrobial therapy (coupled with drainage of tuboovarian abscess, when found) has usually been satisfactory.

Diagnosis Treatment appropriate for PID must not be withheld from patients who have an equivocal diagnosis; it is better to err on the side of overdiagnosis and overtreatment. On the other hand, it is essential to differentiate between salpingitis and other pelvic pathology, particularly surgical emergencies such as appendicitis and ectopic pregnancy.

Nothing short of laparoscopy definitively identifies salpingitis, but routine laparoscopy to confirm suspected salpingitis is generally impractical. Most patients with acute PID have lower abdominal pain of <3 weeks' duration, pelvic tenderness on bimanual pelvic examination, and evidence of lower genital tract infection (e.g., MPC). Approximately 60% of such patients have salpingitis at laparoscopy, and perhaps 10–20% have endometritis alone. Among the patients with these findings, a rectal temperature >38°C, a palpable adnexal mass, and elevation of the ESR to >15 mm/h also raise the probability of salpingitis, which has been found at laparoscopy in 68% of patients with one of these additional findings, 90% of patients with two, and 96% of patients with three. However, only 17% of all patients with laparoscopy-confirmed salpingitis have had all three additional findings.

In a woman with pelvic pain and tenderness, increased numbers of PMNs (30 per 1000× microscopic field in strands of cervical mucus) or leukocytes outnumbering epithelial cells in vaginal fluid (in the absence of trichomonal vaginitis, which also produces PMNs in vaginal discharge) increase the predictive value of a clinical diagnosis of acute PID, as do onset with menses, history of recent abnormal menstrual bleeding, presence of an IUD, history of salpingitis, and sexual exposure to a male with urethritis. Appendicitis or another disorder of the gut is favored by the early onset of anorexia, nausea, or vomiting; the onset of pain later than day 14 of the menstrual cycle; or unilateral pain limited to the right or left lower quadrant. Whenever the diagnosis of PID is being considered, serum assays for human β-chorionic gonadotropin should be performed; these tests are usually positive with ectopic pregnancy. Ultrasonography and magnetic resonance imaging (MRI) can be useful for the identification of tuboovarian or pelvic abscess. MRI of the tubes can also show increased tubal diameter, intratubal fluid, or tubal wall thickening in cases of salpingitis.

The primary and uncontested value of laparoscopy in women with lower abdominal pain is for the exclusion of other surgical problems. Some of the most common or serious problems that may be confused with salpingitis (e.g., acute appendicitis, ectopic pregnancy, corpus luteum bleeding, ovarian tumor) are unilateral. Unilateral pain or pelvic mass, although not incompatible with PID, is a strong indication for laparoscopy unless the clinical picture warrants laparotomy instead. Atypical clinical findings such as the absence of lower genital tract infection, a missed menstrual period, a positive pregnancy test, or failure to respond to appropriate therapy are other common indications for laparoscopy. Endometrial biopsy is relatively sensitive and specific for the diagnosis of endometritis, which correlates well with the presence of salpingitis.

Vaginal or endocervical swab specimens should be examined by NAATs for *N. gonorrhoeae* and *C. trachomatis*. At a minimum, vaginal fluid should be evaluated for the presence of PMNs, and endocervical secretions ideally should be assessed by Gram's staining for PMNs and gram-negative diplococci, which indicate gonococcal infection. The clinical diagnosis of PID made by expert gynecologists is confirmed by laparoscopy or endometrial biopsy in ~90% of women who also have cultures positive for *N. gonorrhoeae* or *C. trachomatis*. Even among women with no symptoms suggestive of acute PID who were attending an STD clinic or a gynecology clinic in Pittsburgh, endometritis was significantly associated with endocervical gonorrhea or chlamydial infection or with bacterial vaginosis, being detected in 26%, 27%, and 15% of women with these conditions, respectively.

TREATMENT PELVIC INFLAMMATORY DISEASE

Recommended combination regimens for ambulatory or parenteral management of PID are presented in **Table 163-6**. Women managed as outpatients should receive a combined regimen with broad activity, such as ceftriaxone (to cover possible gonococcal infection) followed by doxycycline (to cover possible chlamydial infection). Metronidazole can be added, if tolerated, to enhance activity against anaerobes; this addition should be strongly considered if bacterial vaginosis is documented. Although few methodologically sound clinical trials (especially with prolonged follow-up) have been conducted, one meta-analysis suggested a benefit of providing good coverage against anaerobes.

TABLE 163-6 COMBINATION ANTIMICROBIAL REGIMENS RECOMMENDED FOR OUTPATIENT TREATMENT OR FOR PARENTERAL TREATMENT OF PELVIC INFLAMMATORY DISEASE

Outpatient Regimens[a]	Parenteral Regimens
Ceftriaxone (250 mg IM once) ***plus*** Doxycycline (100 mg PO bid for 14 days) ***plus***[b] Metronidazole (500 mg PO bid for 14 days)	Initiate parenteral therapy with either of the following regimens; continue parenteral therapy until 48 h after clinical improvement; then change to outpatient therapy, as described in the text **Regimen A** Cefotetan (2 g IV q12h) *or* cefoxitin (2 g IV q6h) ***plus*** Doxycycline (100 mg IV or PO q12h) **Regimen B** Clindamycin (900 mg IV q8h) ***plus*** Gentamicin (loading dose of 2 mg/kg IV or IM, then maintenance dose of 1.5 mg/kg q8h)

[a]See text for discussion of options in the patient who is intolerant of cephalosporins. [b]The addition of metronidazole is recommended by some experts, particularly if bacterial vaginosis is present.

Source: Adapted from Centers for Disease Control and Prevention: MMWR Recomm Rep 59(RR-12):1, 2010.

The CDC STD treatment guidelines recommend initiation of empirical treatment for PID in sexually active young women and other women at risk for PID if they are experiencing pelvic or lower abdominal pain, if no other cause for the pain can be identified, and if pelvic examination reveals one or more of the following criteria for PID: cervical motion tenderness, uterine tenderness, or adnexal tenderness. Women with suspected PID can be treated as either outpatients or inpatients. In the multicenter Pelvic Inflammatory Disease Evaluation and Clinical Health (PEACH) trial, 831 women with mild to moderately severe symptoms and signs of PID were randomized to receive either inpatient treatment with IV cefoxitin and doxycycline or outpatient treatment with a single IM dose of cefoxitin plus oral doxycycline. Short-term clinical and microbiologic outcomes and long-term outcomes were equivalent in the two groups. Nonetheless, hospitalization should be considered when (1) the diagnosis is uncertain and surgical emergencies such as appendicitis and ectopic pregnancy cannot be excluded, (2) the patient is pregnant, (3) pelvic abscess is suspected, (4) severe illness or nausea and vomiting preclude outpatient management, (5) the patient has HIV infection, (6) the patient is assessed as unable to follow or tolerate an outpatient regimen, or (7) the patient has failed to respond to outpatient therapy. Some experts also prefer to hospitalize adolescents with PID for initial therapy, although younger women do as well as older women on outpatient therapy.

Currently, oral cephalosporins, doxycycline, and the fluoroquinolones do not provide reliable coverage for gonococcal infection. Thus, adequate oral treatment of women with serious intolerance to cephalosporins is a challenge. If penicillins are an option, amoxicillin/clavulanic acid combined with doxycycline has elicited a short-term clinical response in one trial. If fluoroquinolones are the only option and if the community prevalence and individual risk of gonorrhea are known to be low, oral levofloxacin (500 mg once daily) or ofloxacin (400 mg twice daily) for 14 days, with or without metronidazole, may be considered; moreover, clinical trials performed outside the United States support the effectiveness of oral moxifloxacin. In this case, it is imperative to perform a sensitive diagnostic test for gonorrhea (ideally, culture to test for antimicrobial susceptibility) before initiation of therapy. For women whose PID involves quinolone-resistant *N. gonorrhoeae*, treatment is uncertain but could include parenteral gentamicin or oral azithromycin, although the latter agent has not been studied for this purpose.

For hospitalized patients, the following two parenteral regimens (Table 163-6) have given nearly identical results in a multicenter randomized trial:

1. Doxycycline plus either cefotetan or cefoxitin: Administration of these drugs should be continued by the IV route for at least 48 h after the patient's condition improves and then followed with oral doxycycline (100 mg twice daily) to complete 14 days of therapy.
2. Clindamycin plus gentamicin in patients with normal renal function: Once-daily administration of gentamicin (with combination of the total daily dose into a single daily dose) has not been evaluated in PID but has been efficacious in other serious infections and could be substituted. Treatment with these drugs should be continued for at least 48 h after the patient's condition improves and then followed with oral doxycycline (100 mg twice daily) or clindamycin (450 mg four times daily) to complete 14 days of therapy. In cases with tuboovarian abscess, clindamycin rather than doxycycline for continued therapy provides better coverage for anaerobic infection.

FOLLOW-UP

Hospitalized patients should show substantial clinical improvement within 3–5 days. Women treated as outpatients should be clinically reevaluated within 72 h. A follow-up telephone survey of women seen in an emergency department and given a prescription for 10 days of oral doxycycline for PID found that 28% never filled the prescription and 41% stopped taking the medication early (after an average of 4.1 days), often because of persistent symptoms, lack of symptoms, or side effects. Women not responding favorably to ambulatory therapy should be hospitalized for parenteral therapy and further diagnostic evaluations, including a consideration of laparoscopy. Male sex partners should be evaluated and treated empirically for gonorrhea and chlamydial infection. After completion of treatment, tests for persistent or recurrent infection with *N. gonorrhoeae* or *C. trachomatis* should be performed if symptoms persist or recur or if the patient has not complied with therapy or has been reexposed to an untreated sex partner.

SURGERY

Surgery is necessary for the treatment of salpingitis only in the face of life-threatening infection (such as rupture or threatened rupture of a tuboovarian abscess) or for drainage of an abscess. Conservative surgical procedures are usually sufficient. Pelvic abscesses can often be drained by posterior colpotomy, and peritoneal lavage can be used for generalized peritonitis.

Prognosis Late sequelae include infertility due to bilateral tubal occlusion, ectopic pregnancy due to tubal scarring without occlusion, chronic pelvic pain, and recurrent salpingitis. The overall post-salpingitis risk of infertility due to tubal occlusion in a large study in Sweden was 11% after one episode of salpingitis, 23% after two episodes, and 54% after three or more episodes. A University of Washington study found a sevenfold increase in the risk of ectopic pregnancy and an eightfold increase in the rate of hysterectomy after PID.

Prevention A randomized controlled trial designed to determine whether selective screening for chlamydial infection reduces the risk of subsequent PID showed that women randomized to undergo screening had a 56% lower rate of PID over the following year than did women receiving the usual care without screening. This report helped prompt U.S. national guidelines for risk-based chlamydial screening of young women to reduce the incidence of PID and the prevalence of post-PID sequelae, while also reducing sexual transmission of *C. trachomatis*. The CDC and the U.S. Preventive Services Task Force recommend that sexually active women ≤25 years of age be screened for genital chlamydial infection annually. Despite this recommendation, screening coverage in many primary care settings remains low.

ULCERATIVE GENITAL OR PERIANAL LESIONS

Genital ulceration reflects a set of important STIs, most of which sharply increase the risk of sexual acquisition and shedding of HIV. In a 1996 study of genital ulcers in 10 of the U.S. cities with the highest rates of primary syphilis, PCR testing of ulcer specimens demonstrated HSV in 62% of patients, *Treponema pallidum* (the cause of syphilis) in 13%, and *Haemophilus ducreyi* (the cause of chancroid) in 12–20%. Today, genital herpes represents an even higher proportion of genital ulcers in the United States and other industrialized countries.

In Asia and Africa, chancroid (Fig. 163-5) was once considered the most common type of genital ulcer, followed in frequency by primary syphilis and then genital herpes (Fig. 163-6). With increased efforts to control chancroid and syphilis and widespread use of broad-spectrum antibiotics to treat STI-related syndromes, together with more frequent recurrences or persistence of genital herpes attributable to HIV infection, PCR testing of genital ulcers now clearly implicates genital herpes as by far the most common cause of genital ulceration in most developing countries. LGV due to *C. trachomatis* (Fig. 163-7) and donovanosis (granuloma inguinale, due to *Klebsiella granulomatis*; see Fig. 198c-1) continue to cause genital ulceration in some developing countries. LGV virtually disappeared in industrialized countries during the first 20 years of the HIV pandemic, but outbreaks are again occurring in Europe (including the United Kingdom), in North America, and in Australia. In these outbreaks, LGV typically presents as proctitis, with or without anal lesions, in men who report unprotected receptive anal intercourse, very often in association with HIV and/or hepatitis C virus infection; the latter may be an acute infection acquired through the same exposure. Other causes of genital ulcers include (1) candidiasis and traumatized genital warts—both readily recognized; (2) lesions due to genital involvement by more widespread dermatoses; (3) cutaneous manifestations of systemic diseases such as genital mucosal ulceration in Stevens-Johnson syndrome or Behçet's disease; (4) superinfections of lesions that may originally have been sexually acquired (for example, methicillin-resistant *S. aureus* complicating a genital ulcer due to HSV-2); and (5) localized drug reactions, such as the ulcers occasionally seen with topical paromomycin cream or boric acid preparations.

Diagnosis Although most genital ulcerations cannot be diagnosed confidently on clinical grounds alone, clinical findings (Table 163-7)

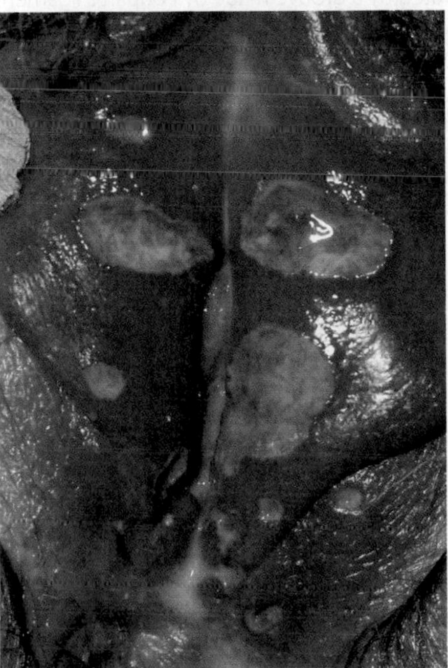

FIGURE 163-5 Chancroid: multiple, painful, punched-out ulcers with undermined borders on the labia occurring after autoinoculation.

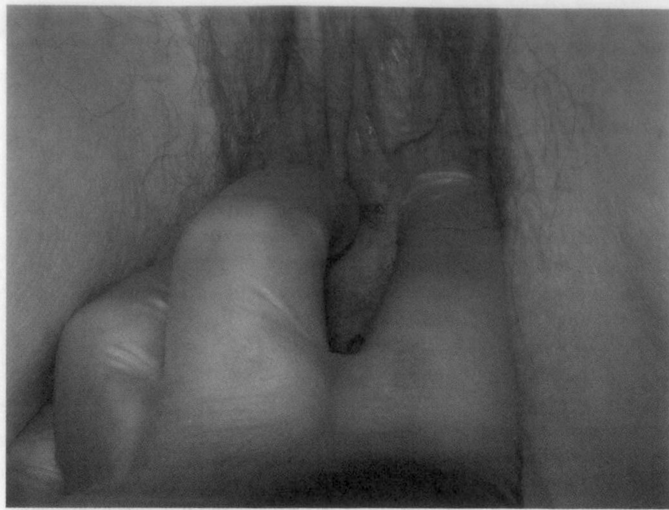

FIGURE 163-6 Genital herpes. A relatively mild, superficial ulcer is typically seen in episodic outbreaks. *(Courtesy of Michael Remington, University of Washington Virology Research Clinic.)*

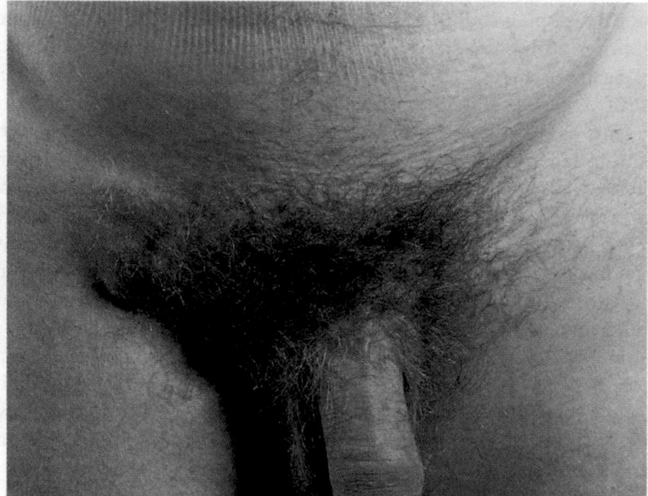

FIGURE 163-7 Lymphogranuloma venereum (LGV): striking tender lymphadenopathy occurring at the femoral and inguinal lymph nodes, separated by a groove made by Poupart's ligament. This "sign-of-the-groove" is not considered specific for LGV; for example, lymphomas may present with this sign.

TABLE 163-8 INITIAL MANAGEMENT OF GENITAL OR PERIANAL ULCER

Causative Pathogens
Herpes simplex virus (HSV)
Treponema pallidum (primary syphilis)
Haemophilus ducreyi (chancroid)
Usual Initial Laboratory Evaluation
Dark-field exam (if available), direct FA, or PCR for *T. pallidum*
RPR, VDRL, or EIA serologic test for syphilis[a]
Culture, direct FA, ELISA, or PCR for HSV
HSV-2-specific serology (consider)
In chancroid-endemic area: PCR or culture for *H. ducreyi*
Initial Treatment
Herpes confirmed or suspected (history or sign of vesicles):
Treat for genital herpes with acyclovir, valacyclovir, or famciclovir.
Syphilis confirmed (dark-field, FA, or PCR showing *T. pallidum*, or RPR reactive):
Benzathine penicillin (2.4 million units IM once to patient, to recent [e.g., within 3 months] seronegative partner[s], and to all seropositive partners)[b]
Chancroid confirmed or suspected (diagnostic test positive, or HSV and syphilis excluded, and persistent lesion):
Ciprofloxacin (500 mg PO as single dose) *or*
Ceftriaxone (250 mg IM as single dose) *or*
Azithromycin (1 g PO as single dose)

[a]If results are negative but primary syphilis is suspected, treat presumptively when indicated by epidemiologic and sexual risk assessment; repeat in 1 week. [b]The same treatment regimen is also effective in HIV-infected persons with early syphilis.

Abbreviations: EIA, enzyme immunoassay; ELISA, enzyme-linked immunosorbent assay; FA, fluorescent antibody; HSV, herpes simplex virus; PCR, polymerase chain reaction; RPR, rapid plasma reagin; VDRL, Venereal Disease Research Laboratory.

and epidemiologic considerations can usually guide initial management (Table 163-8) pending results of specific tests. Clinicians should order a rapid serologic test for syphilis in all cases of genital ulcer. To evaluate lesions except those highly characteristic of infection with HSV (i.e., those with herpetic vesicles), dark-field microscopy, direct immunofluorescence, and PCR for *T. pallidum* can be useful but are rarely available today in most countries. It is important to note that 30% of syphilitic chancres—the primary ulcer of syphilis—are associated with an initially nonreactive syphilis serology. All patients presenting with genital ulceration should be counseled and tested for HIV infection.

Typical vesicles or pustules or a cluster of painful ulcers preceded by vesiculopustular lesions suggests genital herpes. These typical clinical manifestations make detection of the virus optional; however, many patients want confirmation of the diagnosis, and differentiation of

TABLE 163-7 CLINICAL FEATURES OF GENITAL ULCERS

Feature	Syphilis	Herpes	Chancroid	Lymphogranuloma Venereum	Donovanosis
Incubation period	9–90 days	2–7 days	1–14 days	3 days–6 weeks	1–4 weeks (up to 6 months)
Early primary lesions	Papule	Vesicle	Pustule	Papule, pustule, or vesicle	Papule
No. of lesions	Usually one	Multiple	Usually multiple, may coalesce	Usually one; often not detected, despite lymphadenopathy	Variable
Diameter	5–15 mm	1–2 mm	Variable	2–10 mm	Variable
Edges	Sharply demarcated, elevated, round, or oval	Erythematous	Undermined, ragged, irregular	Elevated, round, or oval	Elevated, irregular
Depth	Superficial or deep	Superficial	Excavated	Superficial or deep	Elevated
Base	Smooth, nonpurulent, relatively nonvascular	Serous, erythematous, nonvascular	Purulent, bleeds easily	Variable, nonvascular	Red and velvety, bleeds readily
Induration	Firm	None	Soft	Occasionally firm	Firm
Pain	Uncommon	Frequently tender	Usually very tender	Variable	Uncommon
Lymphadenopathy	Firm, nontender, bilateral	Firm, tender, often bilateral with initial episode	Tender, may suppurate, loculated, usually unilateral	Tender, may suppurate, loculated, usually unilateral	None; pseudobuboes

Source: From RM Ballard, in KK Holmes et al (eds): *Sexually Transmitted Diseases*, 4th ed. New York, McGraw-Hill, 2008.

HSV-1 from HSV-2 has prognostic implications, because the latter causes more frequent genital recurrences.

Painless, nontender, indurated ulcers with firm, nontender inguinal adenopathy suggest primary syphilis. If results of dark-field examination and a rapid serologic test for syphilis are initially negative, presumptive therapy should be provided on the basis of the individual's risk. For example, with increasing rates of syphilis among MSM in the United States, most experts would not withhold therapy for this infection pending watchful waiting and/or subsequent detection of seroconversion. Repeated serologic testing for syphilis 1 or 2 weeks after treatment of seronegative primary syphilis usually demonstrates seroconversion.

"Atypical" or clinically trivial ulcers may be more common manifestations of genital herpes than classic vesiculopustular lesions. Specific tests for HSV in such lesions are therefore indicated (Chap. 216). Commercially available type-specific serologic tests for serum antibody to HSV-2 may give negative results, especially when patients present early with the initial episode of genital herpes or when HSV-1 is the cause of genital herpes (as is often the case today). Furthermore, a positive test for antibody to HSV-2 does not prove that the current lesions are herpetic, because nearly one-fifth of the general population of the United States (and no doubt a higher proportion of those at risk for other STIs) becomes seropositive for HSV-2 during early adulthood. Although even "type-specific" tests for HSV-2 that are commercially available in the United States are not 100% specific, a positive HSV-2 serology does enable the clinician to tell the patient that he or she has probably had genital herpes, should learn to recognize symptoms, and should avoid sex during recurrences. In addition, because genital shedding and sexual transmission of HSV-2 often occur in the absence of symptoms and signs of recurrent herpetic lesions, persons who have a history of genital herpes or who are seropositive for HSV-2 should consider the use of condoms or suppressive antiviral therapy, both of which can reduce the risk of HSV-2 transmission to a sexual partner.

Demonstration of *H. ducreyi* by culture (or by PCR, where available) is most useful when ulcers are painful and purulent, especially if inguinal lymphadenopathy with fluctuance or overlying erythema is noted; if chancroid is prevalent in the community; or if the patient has recently had a sexual exposure elsewhere in a chancroid-endemic area (e.g., a developing country). Enlarged, fluctuant lymph nodes should be aspirated for culture or PCR to detect *H. ducreyi* as well as for Gram's staining and culture to rule out the presence of other pyogenic bacteria.

When genital ulcers persist beyond the natural history of initial episodes of herpes (2–3 weeks) or of chancroid or syphilis (up to 6 weeks) and do not resolve with syndrome-based antimicrobial therapy, then—in addition to the usual tests for herpes, syphilis, and chancroid—biopsy is indicated to exclude donovanosis, carcinoma, and other nonvenereal dermatoses. If not performed previously, HIV serology should be standard because chronic, persistent genital herpes is common in AIDS.

TREATMENT ULCERATIVE GENITAL OR PERIANAL LESIONS

Immediate syndrome-based treatment for acute genital ulcerations (after collection of all necessary diagnostic specimens at the first visit) is often appropriate before all test results become available because patients with typical initial or recurrent episodes of genital or anorectal herpes can benefit from prompt oral antiviral therapy (Chap. 216); because early treatment of sexually transmitted causes of genital ulcers decreases further transmission; and because many patients do not return for test results and treatment. A thorough assessment of the patient's sexual-risk profile and medical history is critical in determining the course of initial management. The patient who has risk factors consistent with exposure to syphilis (e.g., a male patient who reports sex with other men or who has HIV infection) should generally receive initial treatment for syphilis. Empirical therapy for chancroid should be considered if there has been an exposure in an area of the world where chancroid occurs or if regional lymph node suppuration is evident. In resource-poor settings lacking ready access to diagnostic tests, this approach to syndromic treatment for syphilis and chancroid has helped bring these two diseases under control. Finally, empirical antimicrobial therapy may be indicated if ulcers persist and the diagnosis remains unclear after a week of observation despite attempts to diagnose herpes, syphilis, and chancroid.

PROCTITIS, PROCTOCOLITIS, ENTEROCOLITIS, AND ENTERITIS

Sexually acquired *proctitis*, with inflammation limited to the rectal mucosa (the distal 10–12 cm), results from direct rectal inoculation of typical STD pathogens. In contrast, inflammation extending from the rectum to the colon (*proctocolitis*), involving both the small and the large bowel (*enterocolitis*), or involving the small bowel alone (*enteritis*) can result from ingestion of typical intestinal pathogens through oral–anal exposure during sexual contact. Anorectal pain and mucopurulent, bloody rectal discharge suggest proctitis or protocolitis. Proctitis commonly produces tenesmus (causing frequent attempts to defecate, but not true diarrhea) and constipation, whereas proctocolitis and enterocolitis more often cause true diarrhea. In all three conditions, anoscopy usually shows mucosal exudate and easily induced mucosal bleeding (i.e., a positive "wipe test"), sometimes with petechiae or mucosal ulcers. Exudate should be sampled for Gram's staining and other microbiologic studies. Sigmoidoscopy or colonoscopy shows inflammation limited to the rectum in proctitis or disease extending at least up into the sigmoid colon in proctocolitis.

The AIDS era brought an extraordinary shift in the clinical and etiologic spectrum of intestinal infections among MSM. The number of cases of the acute intestinal STIs described above fell as high-risk sexual behaviors became less common in this group. At the same time, the number of AIDS-related opportunistic intestinal infections increased rapidly, many associated with chronic or recurrent symptoms. The incidence of these opportunistic infections has since fallen with increasingly widespread coverage of HIV-infected persons with effective antiretroviral therapy. Two species initially isolated in association with intestinal symptoms in MSM—now known as *Helicobacter cinaedi* and *H. fennelliae*—have both been isolated from the blood of HIV-infected men and other immunosuppressed persons, often in association with a syndrome of multifocal dermatitis and arthritis.

Acquisition of HSV, *N. gonorrhoeae*, or *C. trachomatis* (including LGV strains of *C. trachomatis*) during receptive anorectal intercourse causes most cases of infectious proctitis in women and MSM. Primary and secondary syphilis can also produce anal or anorectal lesions, with or without symptoms. Gonococcal or chlamydial proctitis typically involves the most distal rectal mucosa and the anal crypts and is clinically mild, without systemic manifestations. In contrast, primary proctitis due to HSV and proctocolitis due to the strains of *C. trachomatis* that cause LGV usually produce severe anorectal pain and often cause fever. Perianal ulcers and inguinal lymphadenopathy, most commonly due to HSV, can also occur with LGV or syphilis. Sacral nerve root radiculopathies, usually presenting as urinary retention, laxity of the anal sphincter, or constipation, may complicate primary herpetic proctitis. In LGV, rectal biopsy typically shows crypt abscesses, granulomas, and giant cells—findings resembling those in Crohn's disease; such findings should always prompt rectal culture and serology for LGV, which is a curable infection. Syphilis can also produce rectal granulomas, usually in association with infiltration by plasma cells or other mononuclear cells. Syphilis, LGV, and HSV infection involving the rectum can produce perirectal adenopathy that is sometimes mistaken for malignancy; syphilis, LGV, HSV infection, and chancroid involving the anus can produce inguinal adenopathy because anal lymphatics drain to inguinal lymph nodes.

Diarrhea and abdominal bloating or cramping pain without anorectal symptoms and with normal findings on anoscopy and sigmoidoscopy occur with inflammation of the small intestine (enteritis) or with proximal colitis. In MSM without HIV infection, enteritis is often attributable to *Giardia lamblia*. Sexually acquired proctocolitis is most often due to *Campylobacter* or *Shigella* species.

TREATMENT

PROCTITIS, PROCTOCOLITIS, ENTEROCOLITIS, AND ENTERITIS

Acute proctitis in persons who have practiced receptive anorectal intercourse is usually sexually acquired. Such patients should undergo anoscopy to detect rectal ulcers or vesicles and petechiae after swabbing of the rectal mucosa; to examine rectal exudates for PMNs and gram-negative diplococci; and to obtain rectal swab specimens for testing for rectal gonorrhea, chlamydial infection, herpes, and syphilis. Pending test results, patients with proctitis should receive empirical syndromic treatment—e.g., with ceftriaxone (a single IM dose of 250 mg for gonorrhea) plus doxycycline (100 mg by mouth twice daily for 7 days) for possible chlamydial infection plus treatment for herpes or syphilis if indicated. If LGV proctitis is proven or suspected, the recommended treatment is doxycycline (100 mg by mouth twice daily for 21 days); alternatively, 1 g of azithromycin once a week for 3 weeks is likely to be effective but is little studied.

PREVENTION AND CONTROL OF STIs

Prevention and control of STIs require the following:

1. Reduction of the average rate of sexual exposure to STIs through alteration of sexual risk behaviors and behavioral norms among both susceptible and infected persons in all population groups. The necessary changes include reduction in the total number of sexual partners and the number of concurrent sexual partners.
2. Reduction of the efficiency of transmission through the promotion of safer sexual practices, the use of condoms during casual or commercial sex, vaccination against HBV and HPV infection, male circumcision (which reduces risk of acquisition of HIV infection, chancroid, and perhaps other STIs), and a growing number of other approaches (e.g., early detection and treatment of other STIs to reduce the efficiency of sexual transmission of HIV). Longitudinal studies have shown that consistent condom use is associated with significant protection of both males and females against all STIs that have been examined, including HIV, HPV, and HSV infections as well as gonorrhea and chlamydial infection. The only exceptions are probably sexually transmitted *Pthirus pubis* and *Sarcoptes scabiei* infestations.
3. Shortening of the duration of infectivity of STIs through early detection and curative or suppressive treatment of patients and their sexual partners.

Financial and time constraints imposed by many clinical practices, along with the reluctance of some clinicians to ask questions about stigmatized sexual behaviors, often curtail screening and prevention services. As outlined in Fig. 163-8, the success of clinicians' efforts to detect and treat STIs depends in part on societal efforts to teach young people how to recognize symptoms of STIs; to motivate individuals with symptoms to seek care promptly; to educate persons who are at risk but have no symptoms about what tests they should undergo routinely; and to make high-quality, appropriate care accessible, affordable, and acceptable, especially to the young indigent patients most likely to acquire an STI.

Because many infected individuals develop no symptoms or fail to recognize and report symptoms, clinicians should routinely perform an STI risk assessment for teenagers and young adults as a guide to selective screening. As stated earlier, U.S. Preventive Services Task Force Guidelines recommend screening sexually active female patients ≤25 years of age for *C. trachomatis* whenever they present for health care (at least once a year); older women should be tested if they have more than one sexual partner, have begun a new sexual relationship since the previous test, or have another STI diagnosed. In women 25–29 years of age, chlamydial infection is uncommon but still may reach a prevalence of 3–5% in some settings; information provided by women in this age group on a sex partner's concurrency (whether

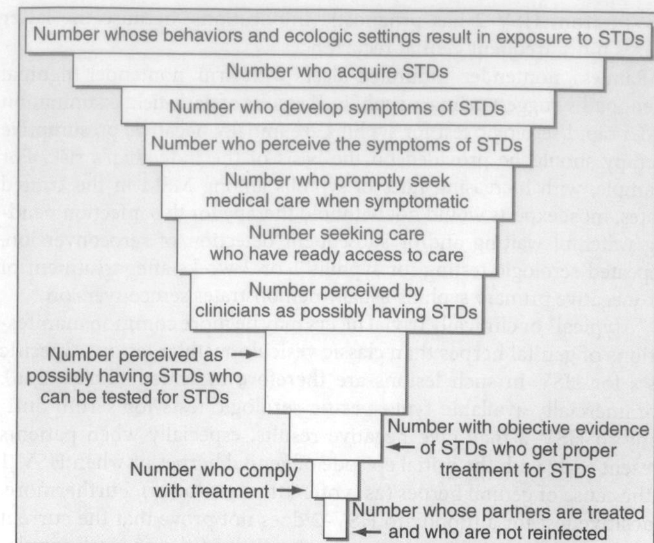

FIGURE 163-8 Critical control points for preventive and clinical interventions against sexually transmitted diseases (STDs). *(Adapted from HT Waller and MA Piot: Bull World Health Organ 41:75, 1969 and 43:1, 1970; and from "Resource allocation model for public health planning—a case study of tuberculosis control," Bull World Health Organ 48 [Suppl], 1973.)*

a male partner has had another sex partner during the time they have been together) is helpful in identifying women at increased risk. In some regions of the United States, widespread selective screening and treatment of young women for cervical *C. trachomatis* infection have been associated with a 50–60% drop in prevalence. Such screening and treatment also protect the individual woman from PID. Sensitive urine-based genetic amplification tests permit expansion of screening to men, teenage boys, and girls in settings where examination is not planned or is impractical (e.g., during preparticipation sports examinations or during initial medical evaluation of adolescent girls). Vaginal swabs—collected either by the health care provider at a pelvic examination or by the woman herself—are highly sensitive and specific for the diagnosis of chlamydial and gonococcal infection; they are now the preferred type of specimen for screening and diagnosis of these infections.

Although gonorrhea is now substantially less common than chlamydial infection in industrialized countries, screening tests for *N. gonorrhoeae* are still appropriate for women and teenage girls attending STD clinics and for sexually active teens and young women from areas of high gonorrhea prevalence. Multiplex NAATs that combine screening for *N. gonorrhoeae* and *C. trachomatis*—and, more recently, for *T. vaginalis*—in a single low-cost assay now facilitate the prevention and control of these infections for populations at high risk.

All patients who have newly detected STIs or are at high risk for STIs according to routine risk assessment as well as all pregnant women should be encouraged to undergo serologic testing for syphilis and HIV infection, with appropriate HIV counseling before and after testing. Randomized trials have shown that risk-reduction counseling of patients with STIs significantly lowers subsequent risk of acquiring an STI; such counseling should now be considered a standard component of STI management. Preimmunization serologic testing for antibody to HBV is indicated for unvaccinated persons who are known to be at high risk, such as MSM and people who use injection drugs. In most young persons, however, it is more cost-effective to vaccinate against HBV without serologic screening. It is important to recognize that, while immunization against HBV has contributed to marked reductions in the incidence of infection with this virus, the majority of new cases that do occur are acquired through sex. In 2006, the Advisory Committee on Immunization Practices (ACIP) of the CDC recommended the following: (1) Universal hepatitis B vaccination should be implemented for all unvaccinated adults in settings in which a high proportion of adults have risk factors for HBV infection (e.g., STD clinics, HIV testing and treatment facilities, drug-abuse treatment and prevention settings, health care settings targeting services to injection drug users or MSM, and correctional facilities). (2) In other primary care and specialty medical settings in which adults at risk for HBV infection receive care, health care providers should inform all patients about the health benefits of vaccination, the risk factors for HBV infection, and the persons for whom vaccination is recommended and should vaccinate adults who report risk factors for HBV infection as well as any adult who requests protection from HBV infection. To promote vaccination in all settings, health care providers should implement standing orders to identify adults recommended for hepatitis B vaccination, should administer hepatitis B vaccine as part of routine clinical services, should not require acknowledgment of an HBV infection risk factor for adult vaccination, and should use available reimbursement mechanisms to remove financial barriers to hepatitis B vaccination.

In 2007, the ACIP recommended routine immunization of 9- to 26-year-old girls and women with the quadrivalent HPV vaccine (against HPV types 6, 11, 16, and 18) approved by the U.S. Food and Drug Administration; the optimal age for recommended vaccination is 11–12 years because of the very high risk of HPV infection after sexual debut. In 2009, the ACIP added bivalent HPV vaccine (against types 6 and 11) as an option and expanded the groups in which immunization (with either quadrivalent or bivalent vaccine) is safe and effective to include boys and men 9–26 years old. HPV vaccines offering broader protection against additional oncogenic HPV types are anticipated. Since 2011, the ACIP has recommended routine administration of quadrivalent HPV vaccine to boys at 11 or 12 years of age and to males 13–21 years of age who have not yet been vaccinated or who have not completed the three-dose vaccine series; men 22–26 years of age may also be vaccinated.

Partner notification is the process of identifying and informing partners of infected patients about possible exposure to an STI and of examining, testing, and treating partners as appropriate. In a series of 22 reports concerning partner notification during the 1990s, index patients with gonorrhea or chlamydial infection named a mean of 0.75–1.6 partners, of whom one-fourth to one-third were infected; those with syphilis named 1.8–6.3 partners, with one-third to one-half infected; and those with HIV infection named 0.76–5.31 partners, with up to one-fourth infected. Persons who transmit infection or who have recently been infected and are still in the incubation period usually have no symptoms or only mild symptoms and seek medical attention only when notified of their exposure. Therefore, the clinician must encourage patients to participate in partner notification, must ensure that exposed persons are notified and treated, and must guarantee confidentiality to all involved. In the United States, local health departments often offer assistance in partner notification, treatment, and/or counseling. It seems both feasible and most useful to notify those partners exposed within the patient's likely period of infectiousness, which is often considered the preceding 1 month for gonorrhea, 1–2 months for chlamydial infection, and up to 3 months for early syphilis.

Persons with a new-onset STI always have a *source* contact who gave them the infection; in addition, they may have a *secondary* (*spread* or *exposed*) contact with whom they had sex after becoming infected. The identification and treatment of these two types of contacts have different objectives. Treatment of the source contact (often a casual contact) benefits the community by preventing further transmission and benefits the source contact; treatment of the recently exposed secondary contact (typically a spouse or another steady sexual partner) prevents the development of serious complications (such as PID) in the partner, reinfection of the index patient, and further spread of infection. A survey of a random sample of U.S. physicians found that most instructed patients to abstain from sex during treatment, to use condoms, and to inform their sex partners after being diagnosed with gonorrhea, chlamydial infection, or syphilis; physicians sometimes gave the patients drugs for their partners. However, follow-up of the partners by physicians was infrequent. A randomized trial compared patients' delivery of therapy to partners exposed to gonorrhea or chlamydial infection with conventional notification and advice to partners to seek evaluation for STD; patients' delivery of partners' therapy, also known as *expedited partner therapy* (EPT), significantly reduced combined rates of reinfection of the index patient with *N. gonorrhoeae* or *C. trachomatis*. State-by-state variations in regulations governing this approach have not been well defined, but the 2010 CDC STD treatment guidelines and the EPT final report of 2006 (*http://www.cdc.gov/std/treatment/EPTFinalReport2006.pdf*) describe its potential use. Currently, EPT is commonly used by many practicing physicians. Its legal status varies by state, but EPT is now permissible in 38 states and potentially allowable in another 9. (Updated information on the legal status of EPT is available at *http://www.cdc.gov/std/ept.*)

In summary, clinicians and public health agencies share responsibility for the prevention and control of STIs. In the current health care environment, the role of primary care clinicians has become increasingly important in STI prevention as well as in diagnosis and treatment, and the resurgence of bacterial STIs like syphilis and LGV among MSM—particularly those co-infected with HIV—emphasizes the need for risk assessment and routine screening.

164 Meningitis, Encephalitis, Brain Abscess, and Empyema

Karen L. Roos, Kenneth L. Tyler

Acute infections of the nervous system are among the most important problems in medicine because early recognition, efficient decision making, and rapid institution of therapy can be lifesaving. These distinct clinical syndromes include acute bacterial meningitis, viral meningitis, encephalitis, focal infections such as brain abscess and subdural empyema, and infectious thrombophlebitis. Each may present with a nonspecific prodrome of fever and headache, which in a previously healthy individual may initially be thought to be benign, until (with the exception of viral meningitis) altered consciousness, focal neurologic signs, or seizures appear. Key goals of early management are to emergently distinguish between these conditions, identify the responsible pathogen, and initiate appropriate antimicrobial therapy.

APPROACH TO THE PATIENT: Meningitis, Encephalitis, Brain Abscess, and Empyema

(Figure 164-1) The first task is to identify whether an infection predominantly involves the subarachnoid space (*meningitis*) or whether there is evidence of either generalized or focal involvement of brain tissue in the cerebral hemispheres, cerebellum, or brainstem. When brain tissue is directly injured by a bacterial or viral infection, the disease is referred to as *encephalitis*, whereas focal infections involving brain tissue are classified as either *cerebritis* or *abscess*, depending on the presence or absence of a capsule.

Nuchal rigidity ("stiff neck") is the pathognomonic sign of meningeal irritation and is present when the neck resists passive flexion. Kernig's and Brudzinski's signs are also classic signs of meningeal irritation. *Kernig's sign* is elicited with the patient in the supine position. The thigh is flexed on the abdomen, with the knee flexed; attempts to passively extend the knee elicit pain when meningeal irritation is present. *Brudzinski's sign* is elicited with the patient in the supine position and is positive when passive flexion of the neck results in spontaneous flexion of the hips and knees. Although commonly tested on physical examinations, the sensitivity and specificity of Kernig's and Brudzinski's signs are uncertain. Both may be absent or reduced in very young or elderly patients, immunocompromised individuals, or patients with a severely depressed mental status. The high prevalence of cervical spine disease in older individuals may result in false-positive tests for nuchal rigidity.

Initial management can be guided by several considerations: (1) Empirical therapy should be initiated promptly whenever bacterial meningitis is a significant diagnostic consideration. (2) All patients who have had recent head trauma, are immunocompromised, have known malignant lesions or central nervous system (CNS) neoplasms, or have focal neurologic findings, papilledema, or a depressed level of consciousness should undergo computed tomography (CT) or magnetic resonance imaging (MRI) of the brain prior to lumbar puncture (LP). In these cases empirical antibiotic therapy should not be delayed pending test results but should be administered prior to neuroimaging and LP. (3) A significantly depressed level of consciousness (e.g., somnolence, coma), seizures, or focal neurologic deficits do not occur in viral meningitis; patients with these symptoms should be hospitalized for further evaluation and treated empirically for bacterial and viral meningoencephalitis. (4) Immunocompetent patients with a normal level of consciousness, no prior antimicrobial treatment, and a cerebrospinal fluid (CSF) profile consistent with viral meningitis (lymphocytic pleocytosis and a normal glucose concentration) can often be treated as outpatients if appropriate contact and monitoring can be ensured. Failure of a patient with suspected viral meningitis to improve within 48 h should prompt a reevaluation including follow-up neurologic and general medical examination and repeat imaging and laboratory studies, often including a second LP.

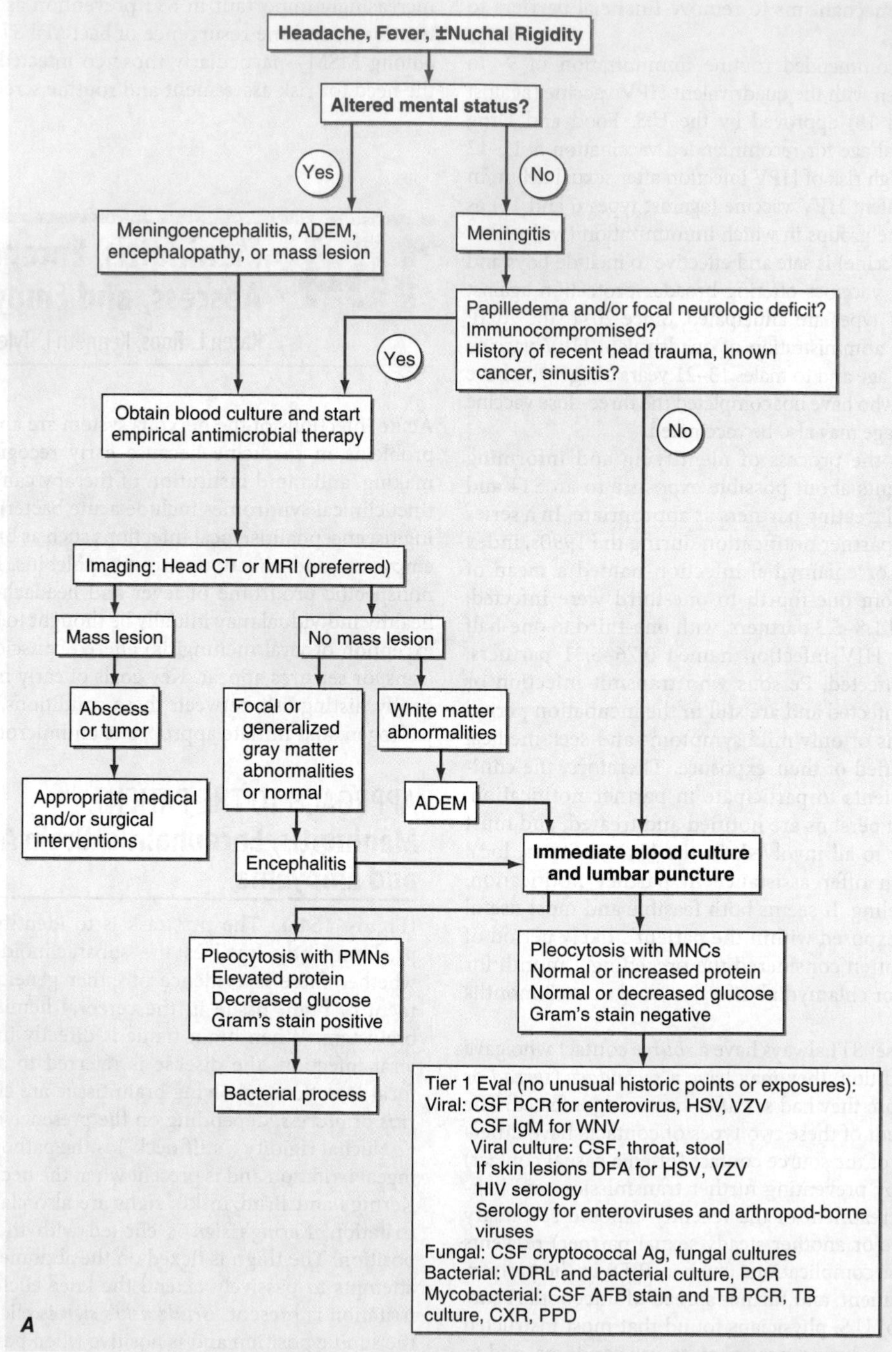

FIGURE 164-1 The management of patients with suspected central nervous system (CNS) infection. ADEM, acute disseminated encephalomyelitis; AFB, acid-fast bacillus; Ag, antigen; CSF, cerebrospinal fluid; CT, computed tomography; CTFV, Colorado tick fever virus; CXR, chest x-ray; DFA, direct fluorescent antibody; EBV, Epstein-Barr virus; HHV, human herpesvirus; HSV, herpes simplex virus; LCMV, lymphocytic choriomeningitis virus; MNCs, mononuclear cells; MRI, magnetic resonance imaging; PCR, polymerase chain reaction; PMNs, polymorphonuclear leukocytes; PPD, purified protein derivative; TB, tuberculosis; VDRL, Venereal Disease Research Laboratory; VZV, varicella-zoster virus; WNV, West Nile virus.

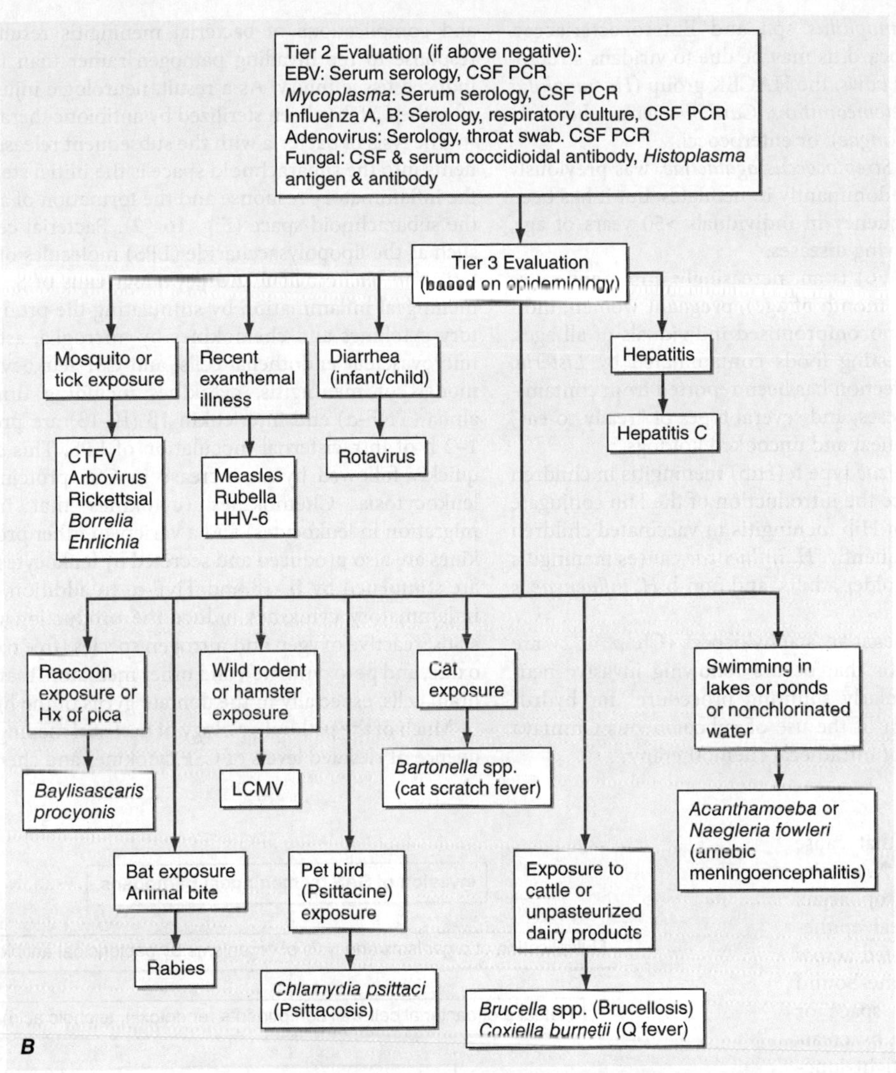

FIGURE 164-1 *(Continued)*

ACUTE BACTERIAL MENINGITIS

DEFINITION

Bacterial meningitis is an acute purulent infection within the subarachnoid space. It is associated with a CNS inflammatory reaction that may result in decreased consciousness, seizures, raised intracranial pressure (ICP), and stroke. The meninges, subarachnoid space, and brain parenchyma are all frequently involved in the inflammatory reaction (*meningoencephalitis*).

EPIDEMIOLOGY

Bacterial meningitis is the most common form of suppurative CNS infection, with an annual incidence in the United States of >2.5 cases/100,000 population. The organisms most often responsible for community-acquired bacterial meningitis are *Streptococcus pneumoniae* (~50%), *Neisseria meningitidis* (~25%), group B streptococci (~15%), and *Listeria monocytogenes* (~10%). *Haemophilus influenzae* type b accounts for <10% of cases of bacterial meningitis in most series. *N. meningitidis* is the causative organism of recurring epidemics of meningitis every 8 to 12 years.

ETIOLOGY

S. pneumoniae (Chap. 173) is the most common cause of meningitis in adults >20 years of age, accounting for nearly half the reported cases (1.1 per 100,000 persons per year). There are a number of predisposing conditions that increase the risk of pneumococcal meningitis, the most important of which is pneumococcal pneumonia. Additional risk factors include coexisting acute or chronic pneumococcal sinusitis or otitis media, alcoholism, diabetes, splenectomy, hypogammaglobulinemia, complement deficiency, and head trauma with basilar skull fracture and CSF rhinorrhea. The mortality rate remains ~20% despite antibiotic therapy.

The incidence of meningitis due to *N. meningitidis* (Chap. 180) has decreased with the routine immunization of 11- to 18-year-olds with the quadrivalent (serogroups A, C, W-135, and Y) meningococcal glycoconjugate vaccine. The vaccine does not contain serogroup B, which is responsible for one-third of cases of meningococcal disease. The presence of petechial or purpuric skin lesions can provide an important clue to the diagnosis of meningococcal infection. In some patients the disease is fulminant, progressing to death within hours of symptom onset. Infection may be initiated by nasopharyngeal colonization, which can result in either an asymptomatic carrier state or invasive meningococcal disease. The risk of invasive disease following nasopharyngeal colonization depends on both bacterial virulence factors and host immune defense mechanisms, including the host's capacity to produce antimeningococcal antibodies and to lyse meningococci by both classic and alternative complement pathways. Individuals with deficiencies of any of the complement components, including properdin, are highly susceptible to meningococcal infections.

Gram-negative bacilli cause meningitis in individuals with chronic and debilitating diseases such as diabetes, cirrhosis, or alcoholism and in those with chronic urinary tract infections. Gram-negative meningitis can also complicate neurosurgical procedures, particularly craniotomy, and head trauma associated with CSF rhinorrhea or otorrhea.

Otitis, mastoiditis, and sinusitis are predisposing and associated conditions for meningitis due to *Streptococci* sp., gram-negative anaerobes,

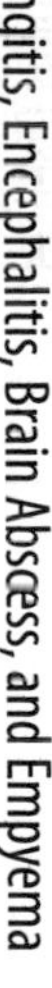

 Staphylococcus aureus, Haemophilus sp., and Enterobacteriaceae. Meningitis complicating endocarditis may be due to viridans streptococci, *S. aureus, Streptococcus bovis*, the HACEK group (*Haemophilus* sp., *Actinobacillus actinomycetemcomitans, Cardiobacterium hominis, Eikenella corrodens, Kingella kingae*), or enterococci.

Group B *Streptococcus*, or *Streptococcus agalactiae*, was previously responsible for meningitis predominantly in neonates, but it has been reported with increasing frequency in individuals >50 years of age, particularly those with underlying diseases.

L. monocytogenes (Chap. 176) is an increasingly important cause of meningitis in neonates (<1 month of age), pregnant women, individuals >60 years, and immunocompromised individuals of all ages. Infection is acquired by ingesting foods contaminated by *Listeria*. Foodborne human listerial infection has been reported from contaminated coleslaw, milk, soft cheeses, and several types of "ready-to-eat" foods, including delicatessen meat and uncooked hotdogs.

The frequency of *H. influenzae* type b (Hib) meningitis in children has declined dramatically since the introduction of the Hib conjugate vaccine, although rare cases of Hib meningitis in vaccinated children have been reported. More frequently, *H. influenzae* causes meningitis in unvaccinated children and older adults, and non-b *H. influenzae* is an emerging pathogen.

S. aureus and coagulase-negative staphylococci (Chap. 172) are important causes of meningitis that occurs following invasive neurosurgical procedures, particularly shunting procedures for hydrocephalus, or as a complication of the use of subcutaneous Ommaya reservoirs for administration of intrathecal chemotherapy.

PATHOPHYSIOLOGY

The most common bacteria that cause meningitis, *S. pneumoniae* and *N. meningitidis*, initially colonize the nasopharynx by attaching to nasopharyngeal epithelial cells. Bacteria are transported across epithelial cells in membrane-bound vacuoles to the intravascular space or invade the intravascular space by creating separations in the apical tight junctions of columnar epithelial cells. Once in the bloodstream, bacteria are able to avoid phagocytosis by neutrophils and classic complement-mediated bactericidal activity because of the presence of a polysaccharide capsule. Bloodborne bacteria can reach the intraventricular choroid plexus, directly infect choroid plexus epithelial cells, and gain access to the CSF. Some bacteria, such as *S. pneumoniae*, can adhere to cerebral capillary endothelial cells and subsequently migrate through or between these cells to reach the CSF. Bacteria are able to multiply rapidly within CSF because of the absence of effective host immune defenses. Normal CSF contains few white blood cells (WBCs) and relatively small amounts of complement proteins and immunoglobulins. The paucity of the latter two prevents effective opsonization of bacteria, an essential prerequisite for bacterial phagocytosis by neutrophils. Phagocytosis of bacteria is further impaired by the fluid nature of CSF, which is less conducive to phagocytosis than a solid tissue substrate.

A critical event in the pathogenesis of bacterial meningitis is the inflammatory reaction induced by the invading bacteria. Many of the neurologic manifestations and complications of bacterial meningitis result from the immune response to the invading pathogen rather than from direct bacteria-induced tissue injury. As a result, neurologic injury can progress even after the CSF has been sterilized by antibiotic therapy.

The lysis of bacteria with the subsequent release of cell-wall components into the subarachnoid space is the initial step in the induction of the inflammatory response and the formation of a purulent exudate in the subarachnoid space (Fig. 164-2). Bacterial cell-wall components, such as the lipopolysaccharide (LPS) molecules of gram-negative bacteria and teichoic acid and peptidoglycans of *S. pneumoniae*, induce meningeal inflammation by stimulating the production of inflammatory cytokines and chemokines by microglia, astrocytes, monocytes, microvascular endothelial cells, and CSF leukocytes. In experimental models of meningitis, cytokines including tumor necrosis factor alpha (TNF-α) and interleukin 1β (IL-1β) are present in CSF within 1–2 h of intracisternal inoculation of LPS. This cytokine response is quickly followed by an increase in CSF protein concentration and leukocytosis. Chemokines (cytokines that induce chemotactic migration in leukocytes) and a variety of other proinflammatory cytokines are also produced and secreted by leukocytes and tissue cells that are stimulated by IL-1β and TNF-α. In addition, bacteremia and the inflammatory cytokines induce the production of excitatory amino acids, reactive oxygen and nitrogen species (free oxygen radicals, nitric oxide, and peroxynitrite), and other mediators that can induce death of brain cells, especially in the dentate gyrus of the hippocampus.

Much of the pathophysiology of bacterial meningitis is a direct consequence of elevated levels of CSF cytokines and chemokines. TNF-α and

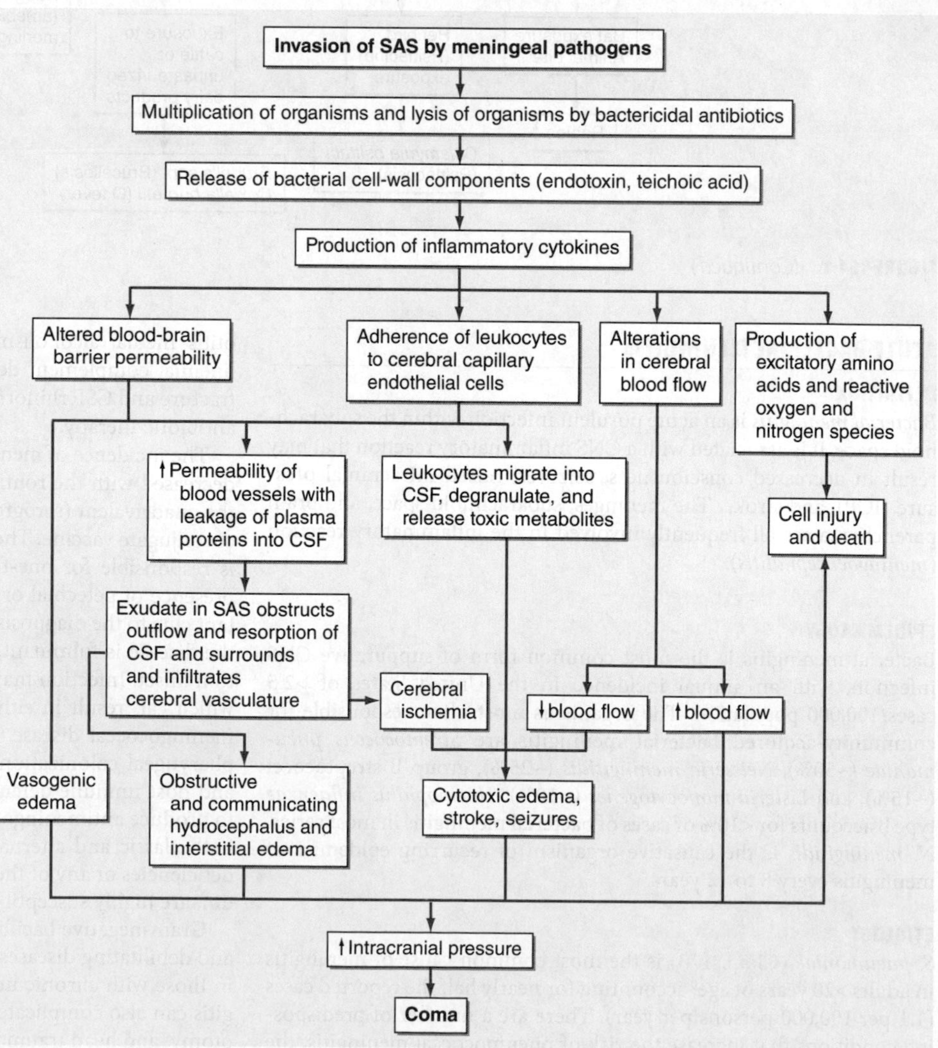

FIGURE 164-2 The pathophysiology of the neurologic complications of bacterial meningitis. CSF, cerebrospinal fluid; SAS, subarachnoid space.

IL-1β act synergistically to increase the permeability of the blood-brain barrier, resulting in induction of vasogenic edema and the leakage of serum proteins into the subarachnoid space (Fig. 164-2). The subarachnoid exudate of proteinaceous material and leukocytes obstructs the flow of CSF through the ventricular system and diminishes the resorptive capacity of the arachnoid granulations in the dural sinuses, leading to obstructive and communicating hydrocephalus and concomitant interstitial edema.

Inflammatory cytokines upregulate the expression of selectins on cerebral capillary endothelial cells and leukocytes, promoting leukocyte adherence to vascular endothelial cells and subsequent migration into the CSF. The adherence of leukocytes to capillary endothelial cells increases the permeability of blood vessels, allowing for the leakage of plasma proteins into the CSF, which adds to the inflammatory exudate. Neutrophil degranulation results in the release of toxic metabolites that contribute to cytotoxic edema, cell injury, and death. Contrary to previous beliefs, CSF leukocytes probably do little to contribute to the clearance of CSF bacterial infection.

During the very early stages of meningitis, there is an increase in cerebral blood flow, soon followed by a decrease in cerebral blood flow and a loss of cerebrovascular autoregulation (Chap. 330). Narrowing of the large arteries at the base of the brain due to encroachment by the purulent exudate in the subarachnoid space and infiltration of the arterial wall by inflammatory cells with intimal thickening (*vasculitis*) also occur and may result in ischemia and infarction, obstruction of branches of the middle cerebral artery by thrombosis, thrombosis of the major cerebral venous sinuses, and thrombophlebitis of the cerebral cortical veins. The combination of interstitial, vasogenic, and cytotoxic edema leads to raised ICP and coma. Cerebral herniation usually results from the effects of cerebral edema, either focal or generalized; hydrocephalus and dural sinus or cortical vein thrombosis may also play a role.

CLINICAL PRESENTATION

Meningitis can present as either an acute fulminant illness that progresses rapidly in a few hours or as a subacute infection that progressively worsens over several days. The classic clinical triad of meningitis is fever, headache, and nuchal rigidity, but the classic triad may not be present. A decreased level of consciousness occurs in >75% of patients and can vary from lethargy to coma. Fever and either headache, stiff neck, or an altered level of consciousness will be present in nearly every patient with bacterial meningitis. Nausea, vomiting, and photophobia are also common complaints.

Seizures occur as part of the initial presentation of bacterial meningitis or during the course of the illness in 20–40% of patients. Focal seizures are usually due to focal arterial ischemia or infarction, cortical venous thrombosis with hemorrhage, or focal edema. Generalized seizure activity and status epilepticus may be due to hyponatremia, cerebral anoxia, or, less commonly, the toxic effects of antimicrobial agents.

Raised ICP is an expected complication of bacterial meningitis and the major cause of obtundation and coma in this disease. More than 90% of patients will have a CSF opening pressure >180 mmH_2O, and 20% have opening pressures >400 mmH_2O. Signs of increased ICP include a deteriorating or reduced level of consciousness, papilledema, dilated poorly reactive pupils, sixth nerve palsies, decerebrate posturing, and the Cushing reflex (bradycardia, hypertension, and irregular respirations). The most disastrous complication of increased ICP is cerebral herniation. The incidence of herniation in patients with bacterial meningitis has been reported to occur in as few as 1% to as many as 8% of cases.

Specific clinical features may provide clues to the diagnosis of individual organisms and are discussed in more detail in specific chapters devoted to individual pathogens. The most important of these clues is the rash of meningococcemia, which begins as a diffuse erythematous maculopapular rash resembling a viral exanthem; however, the skin lesions of meningococcemia rapidly become petechial. Petechiae are found on the trunk and lower extremities, in the mucous membranes and conjunctiva, and occasionally on the palms and soles.

DIAGNOSIS

When bacterial meningitis is suspected, blood cultures should be immediately obtained and empirical antimicrobial and adjunctive dexamethasone therapy initiated without delay (Table 164-1). The diagnosis of bacterial meningitis is made by examination of the CSF (Table 164-2). The need to obtain neuroimaging studies (CT or MRI) prior to LP requires clinical judgment. In an immunocompetent patient with no known history of recent head trauma, a normal level of consciousness, and no evidence of papilledema or focal neurologic deficits, it is considered safe to perform LP without prior neuroimaging studies. If LP is delayed in order to obtain neuroimaging studies, empirical antibiotic therapy should be initiated after blood cultures are obtained. Antibiotic therapy initiated a few hours prior to LP will not significantly alter the CSF WBC count or glucose concentration, nor is it likely to prevent visualization of organisms by Gram's stain or detection of bacterial nucleic acid by polymerase chain reaction (PCR) assay.

The classic CSF abnormalities in bacterial meningitis (Table 164-2) are (1) polymorphonuclear (PMN) leukocytosis (>100 cells/μL in 90%), (2) decreased glucose concentration (<2.2 mmol/L [<40 mg/dL] and/or CSF/serum glucose ratio of <0.4 in ~60%), (3) increased protein concentration (>0.45 g/L [>45 mg/dL] in 90%), and (4) increased opening pressure (>180 mmH_2O in 90%). CSF bacterial cultures are positive in >80% of patients, and CSF Gram's stain demonstrates organisms in >60%.

CSF glucose concentrations <2.2 mmol/L (<40 mg/dL) are abnormal, and a CSF glucose concentration of zero can be seen in bacterial meningitis. Use of the CSF/serum glucose ratio corrects for hyperglycemia

TABLE 164-1 ANTIBIOTICS USED IN EMPIRICAL THERAPY OF BACTERIAL MENINGITIS AND FOCAL CENTRAL NERVOUS SYSTEM INFECTIONS[a]

Indication	Antibiotic
Preterm infants to infants <1 month	Ampicillin + cefotaxime
Infants 1–3 months	Ampicillin + cefotaxime or ceftriaxone
Immunocompetent children >3 months and adults <55	Cefotaxime, ceftriaxone, or cefepime + vancomycin
Adults >55 and adults of any age with alcoholism or other debilitating illnesses	Ampicillin + cefotaxime, ceftriaxone or cefepime + vancomycin
Hospital-acquired meningitis, posttraumatic or postneurosurgery meningitis, neutropenic patients, or patients with impaired cell-mediated immunity	Ampicillin + ceftazidime or meropenem + vancomycin

Antimicrobial Agent	Total Daily Dose and Dosing Interval: Child (>1 month)	Adult
Ampicillin	300 (mg/kg)/d, q6h	12 g/d, q4h
Cefepime	150 (mg/kg)/d, q8h	6 g/d, q8h
Cefotaxime	225-300 (mg/kg)/d, q6h	12 g/d, q4h
Ceftriaxone	100 (mg/kg)/d, q12h	4 g/d, q12h
Ceftazidime	150 (mg/kg)/d, q8h	6 g/d, q8h
Gentamicin	7.5 (mg/kg)/d, q8h[b]	7.5 (mg/kg)/d, q8h
Meropenem	120 (mg/kg)/d, q8h	6 g/d, q8h
Metronidazole	30 (mg/kg)/d, q6h	1500–2000 mg/d, q6h
Nafcillin	100–200 (mg/kg)/d, q6h	9–12 g/d, q4h
Penicillin G	400,000 (U/kg)/d, q4h	20–24 million U/d, q4h
Vancomycin	45-60 (mg/kg)/d, q6h	45-60 (mg/kg)d, q6–12h[b]

[a]All antibiotics are administered intravenously; doses indicated assume normal renal and hepatic function. [b]Doses should be adjusted based on serum peak and trough levels: gentamicin therapeutic level: peak: 5–8 μg/mL; trough: <2 μg/mL; vancomycin therapeutic level: peak: 25–40 μg/mL; trough: 5–15 μg/mL.

TABLE 164-2 CEREBROSPINAL FLUID (CSF) ABNORMALITIES IN BACTERIAL MENINGITIS

Opening pressure	>180 mmH_2O
White blood cells	10/μL to 10,000/μL; neutrophils predominate
Red blood cells	Absent in nontraumatic tap
Glucose	<2.2 mmol/L (<40 mg/dL)
CSF/serum glucose	<0.4
Protein	>0.45 g/L (>45 mg/dL)
Gram's stain	Positive in >60%
Culture	Positive in >80%
Latex agglutination	May be positive in patients with meningitis due to *Streptococcus pneumoniae, Neisseria meningitidis, Haemophilus influenzae* type b, *Escherichia coli*, group B streptococci
Limulus lysate	Positive in cases of gram-negative meningitis
PCR	Detects bacterial DNA

Abbreviation: PCR, polymerase chain reaction

that may mask a relative decrease in the CSF glucose concentration. The CSF glucose concentration is low when the CSF/serum glucose ratio is <0.6. A CSF/serum glucose ratio <0.4 is highly suggestive of bacterial meningitis but may also be seen in other conditions, including fungal, tuberculous, and carcinomatous meningitis. It takes from 30 min to several hours for the concentration of CSF glucose to reach equilibrium with blood glucose levels; therefore, administration of 50 mL of 50% glucose (D50) prior to LP, as commonly occurs in emergency room settings, is unlikely to alter CSF glucose concentration significantly unless more than a few hours have elapsed between glucose administration and LP.

A 16S rRNA conserved sequence broad-based bacterial PCR can detect small numbers of viable and nonviable organisms in CSF and is expected to be useful for making a diagnosis of bacterial meningitis in patients who have been pretreated with oral or parenteral antibiotics and in whom Gram's stain and CSF culture are negative. When the broad-range PCR is positive, a PCR that uses specific bacterial primers to detect the nucleic acid of *S. pneumoniae, N. meningitidis, Escherichia coli, L. monocytogenes, H. influenzae*, and *S. agalactiae* can be obtained based on the clinical suspicion of the meningeal pathogen. The latex agglutination (LA) test for the detection of bacterial antigens of *S. pneumoniae, N. meningitidis, H. influenzae* type b, group B *Streptococcus*, and *E. coli* K1 strains in the CSF has been useful for making a diagnosis of bacterial meningitis but is being replaced by the CSF bacterial PCR assay. The CSF LA test has a *specificity* of 95–100% for *S. pneumoniae* and *N. meningitidis*, so a positive test is virtually diagnostic of bacterial meningitis caused by these organisms. However, the *sensitivity* of the CSF LA test is only 70–100% for detection of *S. pneumoniae* and 33–70% for detection of *N. meningitidis* antigens, so a negative test does not exclude infection by these organisms. The Limulus amebocyte lysate assay is a rapid diagnostic test for the detection of gram-negative endotoxin in CSF and thus for making a diagnosis of gram-negative bacterial meningitis. The test has a specificity of 85–100% and a sensitivity approaching 100%. Thus, a positive Limulus amebocyte lysate assay occurs in virtually all patients with gram-negative bacterial meningitis, but false positives may occur.

Almost all patients with bacterial meningitis will have neuroimaging studies performed during the course of their illness. MRI is preferred over CT because of its superiority in demonstrating areas of cerebral edema and ischemia. In patients with bacterial meningitis, diffuse meningeal enhancement is often seen after the administration of gadolinium. Meningeal enhancement is not diagnostic of meningitis but occurs in any CNS disease associated with increased blood-brain barrier permeability.

Petechial skin lesions, if present, should be biopsied. The rash of meningococcemia results from the dermal seeding of organisms with vascular endothelial damage, and biopsy may reveal the organism on Gram's stain.

DIFFERENTIAL DIAGNOSIS

Viral meningoencephalitis, and particularly herpes simplex virus (HSV) encephalitis, can mimic the clinical presentation of bacterial meningitis (see "Viral Encephalitis," below). HSV encephalitis typically presents with headache, fever, altered consciousness, focal neurologic deficits (e.g., dysphasia, hemiparesis), and focal or generalized seizures. The findings on CSF studies, neuroimaging, and electroencephalogram (EEG) distinguish HSV encephalitis from bacterial meningitis. The typical CSF profile with viral CNS infections is a lymphocytic pleocytosis with a normal glucose concentration, in contrast to the PMN pleocytosis and hypoglycorrhachia characteristic of bacterial meningitis. MRI abnormalities (other than meningeal enhancement) are not seen in uncomplicated bacterial meningitis. By contrast, in HSV encephalitis, on T2-weighted, fluid-attenuated inversion recovery (FLAIR) and diffusion-weighted MRI images, high signal intensity lesions are seen in the orbitofrontal, anterior, and medial temporal lobes in the majority of patients within 48 h of symptom onset. Some patients with HSV encephalitis have a distinctive periodic pattern on EEG (see below).

Rickettsial disease can resemble bacterial meningitis (Chap. 211). Rocky Mountain spotted fever (RMSF) is transmitted by a tick bite and caused by the bacteria *Rickettsia rickettsii*. The disease may present acutely with high fever, prostration, myalgia, headache, nausea, and vomiting. Most patients develop a characteristic rash within 96 h of the onset of symptoms. The rash is initially a diffuse erythematous maculopapular rash that may be difficult to distinguish from that of meningococcemia. It progresses to a petechial rash, then to a purpuric rash, and if untreated, to skin necrosis or gangrene. The color of the lesions changes from bright red to very dark red, then yellowish-green to black. The rash typically begins in the wrist and ankles and then spreads distally and proximally within a matter of a few hours, involving the palms and soles. Diagnosis is made by immunofluorescent staining of skin biopsy specimens. Ehrlichioses are also transmitted by a tick bite. These are small gram-negative coccobacilli of which two species cause human disease. *Anaplasma phagocytophilum* causes human granulocytic ehrlichiosis (anaplasmosis), and *Ehrlichia chaffeensis* causes human monocytic ehrlichiosis. The clinical and laboratory manifestations of the infections are similar. Patients present with fever, headache, confusion, nausea, and vomiting. Twenty percent of patients have a maculopapular or petechial rash. There is laboratory evidence of leukopenia, thrombocytopenia, and anemia, and mild to moderate elevations in alanine aminotransferases, alkaline phosphatase, and lactate dehydrogenase. Patients with RMSF and those with ehrlichial infections may have an altered level of consciousness ranging from mild lethargy to coma, confusion, focal neurologic signs, cranial nerve palsies, hyperreflexia, and seizures.

Focal suppurative CNS infections (see below), including subdural and epidural empyema and brain abscess, should also be considered, especially when focal neurologic findings are present. MRI should be performed promptly in all patients with suspected meningitis who have focal features, both to detect the intracranial infection and to search for associated areas of infection in the sinuses or mastoid bones.

A number of noninfectious CNS disorders can mimic bacterial meningitis. Subarachnoid hemorrhage (SAH; Chap. 330) is generally the major consideration. Other possibilities include chemical meningitis due to rupture of tumor contents into the CSF (e.g., from a cystic glioma or craniopharyngioma epidermoid or dermoid cyst); drug-induced hypersensitivity meningitis; carcinomatous or lymphomatous meningitis; meningitis associated with inflammatory disorders such as sarcoid, systemic lupus erythematosus (SLE), and Behçet's syndrome; pituitary apoplexy; and uveomeningitic syndromes (Vogt-Koyanagi-Harada syndrome).

On occasion, subacutely evolving meningitis (Chap. 165) may be considered in the differential diagnosis of acute meningitis. The principal causes include *Mycobacterium tuberculosis* (Chap. 202), *Cryptococcus neoformans* (Chap. 239), *Histoplasma capsulatum* (Chap. 236), *Coccidioides immitis* (Chap. 237), and *Treponema pallidum* (Chap. 206).

TREATMENT ACUTE BACTERIAL MENINGITIS

EMPIRICAL ANTIMICROBIAL THERAPY

(Table 164-1) Bacterial meningitis is a medical emergency. The goal is to begin antibiotic therapy within 60 min of a patient's arrival in the emergency room. Empirical antimicrobial therapy is initiated in patients with suspected bacterial meningitis before the results of CSF Gram's stain and culture are known. *S. pneumoniae* (Chap. 171) and *N. meningitidis* (Chap. 180) are the most common etiologic organisms of community-acquired bacterial meningitis. Due to the emergence of penicillin- and cephalosporin-resistant *S. pneumoniae*, empirical therapy of community-acquired suspected bacterial meningitis in children and adults should include a combination of dexamethasone, a third- or fourth-generation cephalosporin (e.g., ceftriaxone, cefotaxime, or cefepime), and vancomycin, plus acyclovir, as HSV encephalitis is the leading disease in the differential diagnosis, and doxycycline during tick season to treat tick-borne bacterial infections. Ceftriaxone or cefotaxime provides good coverage for susceptible *S. pneumoniae*, group B streptococci, and *H. influenzae* and adequate coverage for *N. meningitidis*. Cefepime is a broad-spectrum fourth-generation cephalosporin with in vitro activity similar to that of cefotaxime or ceftriaxone against *S. pneumoniae* and *N. meningitidis* and greater activity against *Enterobacter* species and *Pseudomonas aeruginosa*. In clinical trials, cefepime has been demonstrated to be equivalent to cefotaxime in the treatment of penicillin-sensitive pneumococcal and meningococcal meningitis, and it has been used successfully in some patients with meningitis due to *Enterobacter* species and *P. aeruginosa*. Ampicillin should be added to the empirical regimen for coverage of *L. monocytogenes* in individuals <3 months of age, those >55, or those with suspected impaired cell-mediated immunity because of chronic illness, organ transplantation, pregnancy, malignancy, or immunosuppressive therapy. Metronidazole is added to the empirical regimen to cover gram-negative anaerobes in patients with otitis, sinusitis, or mastoiditis. In hospital-acquired meningitis, and particularly meningitis following neurosurgical procedures, staphylococci and gram-negative organisms including *P. aeruginosa* are the most common etiologic organisms. In these patients, empirical therapy should include a combination of vancomycin and ceftazidime, cefepime, or meropenem. Ceftazidime, cefepime, or meropenem should be substituted for ceftriaxone or cefotaxime in neurosurgical patients and in neutropenic patients, because ceftriaxone and cefotaxime do not provide adequate activity against CNS infection with *P. aeruginosa*. Meropenem is a carbapenem antibiotic that is highly active in vitro against *L. monocytogenes*, has been demonstrated to be effective in cases of meningitis caused by *P. aeruginosa*, and shows good activity against penicillin-resistant pneumococci. In experimental pneumococcal meningitis, meropenem was comparable to ceftriaxone and inferior to vancomycin in sterilizing CSF cultures. The number of patients with bacterial meningitis enrolled in clinical trials of meropenem has not been sufficient to definitively assess the efficacy of this antibiotic.

SPECIFIC ANTIMICROBIAL THERAPY

Meningococcal Meningitis (Table 164-3) Although ceftriaxone and cefotaxime provide adequate empirical coverage for *N. meningitidis*, penicillin G remains the antibiotic of choice for meningococcal meningitis caused by susceptible strains. Isolates of *N. meningitidis* with moderate resistance to penicillin have been identified and are increasing in incidence worldwide. CSF isolates of *N. meningitidis* should be tested for penicillin and ampicillin susceptibility, and if resistance is found, cefotaxime or ceftriaxone should be substituted for penicillin. A 7-day course of intravenous antibiotic therapy is adequate for uncomplicated meningococcal meningitis. The index case and all close contacts should receive chemoprophylaxis with a 2-day regimen of rifampin (600 mg every 12 h for 2 days in adults and 10 mg/kg every 12 h for 2 days in children >1 year). Rifampin is not recommended in pregnant women. Alternatively, adults can be treated with one dose of azithromycin (500 mg) or one intramuscular dose of ceftriaxone (250 mg). Close contacts are defined as those individuals who have had contact with oropharyngeal secretions, either through kissing or by sharing toys, beverages, or cigarettes.

TABLE 164-3 ANTIMICROBIAL THERAPY OF CENTRAL NERVOUS SYSTEM BACTERIAL INFECTIONS BASED ON PATHOGEN[a]

Organism	Antibiotic
Neisseria meningitides	
Penicillin-sensitive	Penicillin G or ampicillin
Penicillin-resistant	Ceftriaxone or cefotaxime
Streptococcus pneumoniae	
Penicillin-sensitive	Penicillin G
Penicillin-intermediate	Ceftriaxone or cefotaxime or cefepime
Penicillin-resistant	Ceftriaxone (or cefotaxime or cefepime) + vancomycin
Gram-negative bacilli (except *Pseudomonas* spp.)	Ceftriaxone or cefotaxime
Pseudomonas aeruginosa	Ceftazidime or cefepime or meropenem
Staphylococci spp.	
Methicillin-sensitive	Nafcillin
Methicillin-resistant	Vancomycin
Listeria monocytogenes	Ampicillin + gentamicin
Haemophilus influenzae	Ceftriaxone or cefotaxime or cefepime
Streptococcus agalactiae	Penicillin G or ampicillin
Bacteroides fragilis	Metronidazole
Fusobacterium spp.	Metronidazole

[a]Doses are as indicated in Table 164-1.

Pneumococcal Meningitis Antimicrobial therapy of pneumococcal meningitis is initiated with a cephalosporin (ceftriaxone, cefotaxime, or cefepime) and vancomycin. All CSF isolates of *S. pneumoniae* should be tested for sensitivity to penicillin and the cephalosporins. Once the results of antimicrobial susceptibility tests are known, therapy can be modified accordingly (Table 164-3). For *S. pneumoniae* meningitis, an isolate of *S. pneumoniae* is considered to be susceptible to penicillin with a minimal inhibitory concentration (MIC) <0.06 μg/mL and to be resistant when the MIC is >0.12 μg/mL. Isolates of *S. pneumoniae* that have cephalosporin MICs ≤0.5 μg/mL are considered sensitive to the cephalosporins (cefotaxime, ceftriaxone, cefepime). Those with MICs of 1 μg/mL are considered to have intermediate resistance, and those with MICs ≥2 μg/mL are considered resistant. For meningitis due to pneumococci, with cefotaxime or ceftriaxone MICs ≤0.5 μg/mL, treatment with cefotaxime or ceftriaxone is usually adequate. For MIC >1 μg/mL, vancomycin is the antibiotic of choice. Rifampin can be added to vancomycin for its synergistic effect but is inadequate as monotherapy because resistance develops rapidly when it is used alone.

A 2-week course of intravenous antimicrobial therapy is recommended for pneumococcal meningitis.

Patients with *S. pneumoniae* meningitis should have a repeat LP performed 24–36 h after the initiation of antimicrobial therapy to document sterilization of the CSF. Failure to sterilize the CSF after 24–36 h of antibiotic therapy should be considered presumptive evidence of antibiotic resistance. Patients with penicillin- and cephalosporin-resistant strains of *S. pneumoniae* who do not respond to intravenous vancomycin alone may benefit from the addition of intraventricular vancomycin. The intraventricular route of administration is preferred over the intrathecal route because adequate concentrations of vancomycin in the cerebral ventricles are not always achieved with intrathecal administration.

***Listeria* Meningitis** Meningitis due to *L. monocytogenes* is treated with ampicillin for at least 3 weeks (Table 164-3). Gentamicin is added in critically ill patients (2 mg/kg loading dose, then 7.5 mg/kg per day given every 8 h and adjusted for serum levels and renal function). The combination of trimethoprim (10–20 mg/kg per day) and sulfamethoxazole (50–100 mg/kg per day) given every 6 h may provide an alternative in penicillin-allergic patients.

Staphylococcal Meningitis Meningitis due to susceptible strains of *S. aureus* or coagulase-negative staphylococci is treated with nafcillin (Table 164-3). Vancomycin is the drug of choice for methicillin-resistant staphylococci and for patients allergic to penicillin. In these patients, the CSF should be monitored during therapy. If the CSF is not sterilized after 48 h of intravenous vancomycin therapy, then either intraventricular or intrathecal vancomycin, 20 mg once daily, can be added.

Gram-Negative Bacillary Meningitis The third-generation cephalosporins—cefotaxime, ceftriaxone, and ceftazidime—are equally efficacious for the treatment of gram-negative bacillary meningitis, with the exception of meningitis due to *P. aeruginosa*, which should be treated with ceftazidime, cefepime, or meropenem (Table 164-3). A 3-week course of intravenous antibiotic therapy is recommended for meningitis due to gram-negative bacilli.

ADJUNCTIVE THERAPY

The release of bacterial cell-wall components by bactericidal antibiotics leads to the production of the inflammatory cytokines IL-1β and TNF-α in the subarachnoid space. Dexamethasone exerts its beneficial effect by inhibiting the synthesis of IL-1β and TNF-α at the level of mRNA, decreasing CSF outflow resistance, and stabilizing the blood-brain barrier. The rationale for giving dexamethasone 20 min before antibiotic therapy is that dexamethasone inhibits the production of TNF-α by macrophages and microglia only if it is administered before these cells are activated by endotoxin. Dexamethasone does not alter TNF-α production once it has been induced. The results of clinical trials of dexamethasone therapy in meningitis due to *H. influenzae*, *S. pneumoniae*, and *N. meningitidis* have demonstrated its efficacy in decreasing meningeal inflammation and neurologic sequelae such as the incidence of sensorineural hearing loss.

A prospective European trial of adjunctive therapy for acute bacterial meningitis in 301 adults found that dexamethasone reduced the number of unfavorable outcomes (15 vs. 25%, $p = .03$) including death (7 vs. 15%, $p = .04$). The benefits were most striking in patients with pneumococcal meningitis. Dexamethasone (10 mg intravenously) was administered 15–20 min before the first dose of an antimicrobial agent, and the same dose was repeated every 6 h for 4 days. These results were confirmed in a second trial of dexamethasone in adults with pneumococcal meningitis. Therapy with dexamethasone should ideally be started 20 min before, or not later than concurrent with, the first dose of antibiotics. It is unlikely to be of significant benefit if started >6 h after antimicrobial therapy has been initiated. Dexamethasone may decrease the penetration of vancomycin into CSF, and it delays the sterilization of CSF in experimental models of *S. pneumoniae* meningitis. As a result, to assure reliable penetration of vancomycin into the CSF, children and adults are treated with vancomycin in a dose of 45–60 mg/kg per day. Alternatively, vancomycin can be administered by the intraventricular route.

One of the concerns for using dexamethasone in adults with bacterial meningitis is that in experimental models of meningitis, dexamethasone therapy increased hippocampal cell injury and reduced learning capacity. This has not been the case in clinical series. The efficacy of dexamethasone therapy in preventing neurologic sequelae is different between high- and low-income countries. Three large randomized trials in low-income countries (sub-Saharan Africa, Southeast Asia) failed to show benefit in subgroups of patients. The lack of efficacy of dexamethasone in these trials has been attributed to late presentation to the hospital with more advanced disease, antibiotic pretreatment, malnutrition, infection with HIV, and treatment of patients with probable, but not microbiologically proven, bacterial meningitis. The results of these clinical trials suggest that patients in sub-Saharan Africa and those in low-income countries with negative CSF Gram's stain and culture should not be treated with dexamethasone.

INCREASED INTRACRANIAL PRESSURE

Emergency treatment of increased ICP includes elevation of the patient's head to 30–45°, intubation and hyperventilation (Pa_{CO_2} 25–30 mmHg), and mannitol. Patients with increased ICP should be managed in an intensive care unit; accurate ICP measurements are best obtained with an ICP monitoring device.

Treatment of increased intracranial pressure is discussed in detail in Chap. 330.

PROGNOSIS

Mortality rate is 3–7% for meningitis caused by *H. influenzae*, *N. meningitidis*, or group B streptococci; 15% for that due to *L. monocytogenes*; and 20% for *S. pneumoniae*. In general, the risk of death from bacterial meningitis increases with (1) decreased level of consciousness on admission, (2) onset of seizures within 24 h of admission, (3) signs of increased ICP, (4) young age (infancy) and age >50, (5) the presence of comorbid conditions including shock and/or the need for mechanical ventilation, and (6) delay in the initiation of treatment. Decreased CSF glucose concentration (<2.2 mmol/L [<40 mg/dL]) and markedly increased CSF protein concentration (>3 g/L [> 300 mg/dL]) have been predictive of increased mortality and poorer outcomes in some series. Moderate or severe sequelae occur in ~25% of survivors, although the exact incidence varies with the infecting organism. Common sequelae include decreased intellectual function, memory impairment, seizures, hearing loss and dizziness, and gait disturbances.

ACUTE VIRAL MENINGITIS

CLINICAL MANIFESTATIONS

Immunocompetent adult patients with viral meningitis usually present with headache, fever, and signs of meningeal irritation coupled with an inflammatory CSF profile (see below). Headache is almost invariably present and often characterized as frontal or retroorbital and frequently associated with photophobia and pain on moving the eyes. Nuchal rigidity is present in most cases but may be mild and present only near the limit of neck anteflexion. Constitutional signs can include malaise, myalgia, anorexia, nausea and vomiting, abdominal pain, and/or diarrhea. Patients often have mild lethargy or drowsiness; however, profound alterations in consciousness, such as stupor, coma, or marked confusion, do not occur in viral meningitis and suggest the presence of encephalitis or other alternative diagnoses. Similarly, seizures or focal neurologic signs or symptoms or neuroimaging abnormalities indicative of brain parenchymal involvement are not typical of viral meningitis and suggest the presence of encephalitis or another CNS infectious or inflammatory process.

ETIOLOGY

Using a variety of diagnostic techniques, including CSF PCR, culture, and serology, a specific viral cause can be found in 60–90% of cases of viral meningitis. The most important agents are enteroviruses (including echoviruses and coxsackieviruses in addition to numbered enteroviruses), varicella-zoster virus (VZV), HSV (HSV-2 > HSV-1), HIV, and arboviruses (Table 164-4). CSF cultures are positive in 30–70% of patients, with the frequency of isolation depending on the specific viral agent. Approximately two-thirds of culture-negative cases of "aseptic" meningitis have a specific viral etiology identified by CSF PCR testing (see below).

EPIDEMIOLOGY

Viral meningitis is not a nationally reportable disease; however, it has been estimated that the incidence is ~60,000–75,000 cases per year. In temperate climates, there is a substantial increase in cases during the nonwinter months, reflecting the seasonal predominance of enterovirus and arthropod-borne virus (arbovirus) infections in the summer and fall, with a peak monthly incidence of about 1 reported case per 100,000 population.

TABLE 164-4 VIRUSES CAUSING ACUTE MENINGITIS AND ENCEPHALITIS IN NORTH AMERICA

Acute Meningitis	
Common	**Less Common**
Enteroviruses (coxsackieviruses, echoviruses, and human enteroviruses 68–71)	Herpes simplex virus 1
Varicella-zoster virus	Human herpesvirus 6
Herpes simplex virus 2	Cytomegalovirus
Epstein-Barr virus	Lymphocytic choriomeningitis virus
Arthropod-borne viruses	Mumps
HIV	
Acute Encephalitis	
Common	**Less Common**
Herpesviruses	Rabies
Cytomegalovirus[a]	Eastern equine encephalitis virus
Herpes simplex virus 1[b]	
Herpes simplex virus 2	
Human herpesvirus 6	
Varicella-zoster virus	Powassan virus
Epstein-Barr virus	Cytomegalovirus[a]
Arthropod-borne viruses	Colorado tick fever virus
La Crosse virus	Mumps
West Nile virus[c]	
St. Louis encephalitis virus	
Enteroviruses	

[a]Immunocompromised host. [b]The most common cause of sporadic encephalitis. [c]The most common cause of epidemic encephalitis.

LABORATORY DIAGNOSIS

CSF Examination The most important laboratory test in the diagnosis of viral meningitis is examination of the CSF. The typical profile is a pleocytosis, a normal or slightly elevated protein concentration (0.2–0.8 g/L [20–80 mg/dL]), a normal glucose concentration, and a normal or mildly elevated opening pressure (100–350 mmH_2O). Organisms are *not* seen on Gram's stain of CSF. The total CSF cell count in viral meningitis is typically 25–500/μL, although cell counts of several thousand/μL are occasionally seen, especially with infections due to lymphocytic choriomeningitis virus (LCMV) and mumps virus. Lymphocytes are typically the predominant cell. Rarely, PMNs may predominate in the first 48 h of illness, especially with infections due to echovirus 9, West Nile virus, eastern equine encephalitis (EEE) virus, or mumps. A PMN pleocytosis occurs in 45% of patients with West Nile virus (WNV) meningitis and can persist for a week or longer before shifting to a lymphocytic pleocytosis. PMN pleocytosis with low glucose may also be a feature of cytomegalovirus (CMV) infections in immunocompromised hosts. Despite these exceptions, the presence of a CSF PMN pleocytosis in a patient with suspected viral meningitis in whom a specific diagnosis has not been established should prompt consideration of alternative diagnoses, including bacterial meningitis or parameningeal infections. The CSF glucose concentration is typically normal in viral infections, although it may be decreased in 10–30% of cases due to mumps or LCMV. Rare instances of decreased CSF glucose concentration occur in cases of meningitis due to echoviruses and other enteroviruses, HSV-2, and VZV. As a rule, a lymphocytic pleocytosis with a low glucose concentration should suggest fungal or tuberculous meningitis, *Listeria* meningoencephalitis, or noninfectious disorders (e.g., sarcoid, neoplastic meningitis).

A number of tests measuring levels of various CSF proteins, enzymes, and mediators—including C-reactive protein, lactic acid, lactate dehydrogenase, neopterin, quinolinate, IL-1β, IL-6, soluble IL-2 receptor, β_2-microglobulin, and TNF—have been proposed as potential discriminators between viral and bacterial meningitis or as markers of specific types of viral infection (e.g., infection with HIV), but they remain of uncertain sensitivity and specificity and are not widely used for diagnostic purposes.

Polymerase Chain Reaction Amplification of Viral Nucleic Acid Amplification of viral-specific DNA or RNA from CSF using PCR amplification has become the single most important method for diagnosing CNS viral infections. In both enteroviral and HSV infections of the CNS, CSF PCR has become the diagnostic procedure of choice and is substantially more sensitive than viral cultures. HSV CSF PCR is also an important diagnostic test in patients with recurrent episodes of "aseptic" meningitis, many of whom have amplifiable HSV DNA in CSF despite negative viral cultures. CSF PCR is also used routinely to diagnose CNS viral infections caused by CMV, Epstein-Barr virus (EBV), VZV, and human herpesvirus 6 (HHV-6). CSF PCR tests are available for WNV but are not as sensitive as detection of WNV-specific CSF IgM. PCR is also useful in the diagnosis of CNS infection caused by *Mycoplasma pneumoniae,* which can mimic viral meningitis and encephalitis. PCR of throat washings may assist in diagnosis of enteroviral and mycoplasmal CNS infections. PCR of stool specimens may also assist in diagnosis of enteroviral infections (see below).

Viral Culture The sensitivity of CSF cultures for the diagnosis of viral meningitis and encephalitis, in contrast to its utility in bacterial infections, is generally poor. In addition to CSF, specific viruses may also be isolated from throat swabs, stool, blood, and urine. Enteroviruses and adenoviruses may be found in feces; arboviruses, some enteroviruses, and LCMV in blood; mumps and CMV in urine; and enteroviruses, mumps, and adenoviruses in throat washings. During enteroviral infections, viral shedding in stool may persist for several weeks. The presence of enterovirus in stool is not diagnostic and may result from residual shedding from a previous enteroviral infection; it also occurs in some asymptomatic individuals during enteroviral epidemics.

Serologic Studies For many arboviruses including WNV, serologic studies remain important diagnostic tools. Serum antibody determination is less useful for viruses with high seroprevalence rates in the general population such as HSV, VZV, CMV, and EBV. For viruses with low seroprevalence rates, diagnosis of acute viral infection can be made by documenting seroconversion between acute-phase and convalescent sera (typically obtained after 2–4 weeks) or by demonstrating the presence of virus-specific IgM antibodies. For viruses with high seroprevalence such as VZV and HSV, demonstration of synthesis of virus-specific antibodies in CSF, as shown by an increased IgG index or the presence of CSF IgM antibodies, may be useful and can provide presumptive evidence of CNS infection. Although serum and CSF IgM antibodies generally persist for only a few months after acute infection, there are exceptions to this rule. For example, WNV serum IgM has been shown to persist in some patients for >1 year following acute infection. Unfortunately, the delay between onset of infection and the host's generation of a virus-specific antibody response often means that serologic data are useful mainly for the retrospective establishment of a specific diagnosis, rather than in aiding acute diagnosis or management. In the case of EBV, demonstration of antibody responses consistent with recent/acute infection (e.g., IgM viral capsid antibody, antibody against early antigen, absence of antibody against EBV-associated nuclear antigen) may assist in diagnosis.

CSF oligoclonal gamma globulin bands occur in association with a number of viral infections. The associated antibodies are often directed against viral proteins. Oligoclonal bands also occur commonly in certain noninfectious neurologic diseases (e.g., multiple sclerosis) and may be found in nonviral infections (e.g., neurosyphilis, Lyme neuroborreliosis).

Other Laboratory Studies All patients with suspected viral meningitis should have a complete blood count and differential, liver and renal function tests, erythrocyte sedimentation rate (ESR), and C-reactive protein, electrolytes, glucose, creatine kinase, aldolase, amylase, and lipase. Neuroimaging studies (MRI preferable to CT) are not absolutely necessary in patients with uncomplicated viral meningitis but should be performed in patients with altered consciousness, seizures, focal neurologic signs or symptoms, atypical CSF profiles, or underlying immunocompromising treatments or conditions.

The most important issue in the differential diagnosis of viral meningitis is to consider diseases that can mimic viral meningitis, including (1) untreated or partially treated bacterial meningitis; (2) early stages of meningitis caused by fungi, mycobacteria, or *Treponema pallidum* (neurosyphilis), in which a lymphocytic pleocytosis is common, cultures may be slow growing or negative, and hypoglycorrhachia may not be present early; (3) meningitis caused by agents such as *Mycoplasma, Listeria* spp., *Brucella* spp., *Coxiella* spp., *Leptospira* spp., and *Rickettsia* spp.; (4) parameningeal infections; (5) neoplastic meningitis; and (6) meningitis secondary to noninfectious inflammatory diseases, including autoimmune and hypersensitivity meningitis, SLE and other rheumatologic diseases, sarcoidosis, Behçet's syndrome, and the uveomeningitic syndromes. Studies in children >28 days of age suggest that the presence of CSF protein >0.5 g/L (sensitivity 89%, specificity 78%) and elevated serum procalcitonin levels >0.5 ng/mL (sensitivity 89%, specificity 89%) were clues to the presence of bacterial as opposed to "aseptic" meningitis. A variety of clinical algorithms for differentiating bacterial from aseptic meningitis have been developed. One such prospectively validated system, the *bacterial meningitis score*, suggests that the probability of bacterial meningitis is 0.3% or less (negative predictive value 99.7%, 95% confidence interval 99.6–100%) in children with CSF pleocytosis who have (1) a negative CSF Gram's stain, (2) CSF neutrophil count <1000 cells/μL, (3) CSF protein <80 mg/dL, (4) peripheral absolute neutrophil count of <10,000 cells/μL, and (5) no prior history or current presence of seizures.

SPECIFIC VIRAL ETIOLOGIES

Enteroviruses (EV) (Chap. 228) are the most common cause of viral meningitis, accounting for >85% of cases in which a specific etiology can be identified. Cases may either be sporadic or occur in clusters. EV71 has produced large epidemics of neurologic disease outside the United States, especially in Southeast Asia, but most recently reported cases in the United States have been sporadic. Enteroviruses are the most likely cause of viral meningitis in the summer and fall months, especially in children (<15 years), although cases occur at reduced frequency year round. Although the incidence of enteroviral meningitis declines with increasing age, some outbreaks have preferentially affected older children and adults. Meningitis outside the neonatal period is usually benign. Patients present with sudden onset of fever; headache; nuchal rigidity; and often constitutional signs, including vomiting, anorexia, diarrhea, cough, pharyngitis, and myalgias. The physical examination should include a careful search for stigmata of enterovirus infection, including exanthems, hand-foot-mouth disease, herpangina, pleurodynia, myopericarditis, and hemorrhagic conjunctivitis. The CSF profile is typically a lymphocytic pleocytosis (100–1000 cells/μL) with normal glucose and normal or mildly elevated protein concentration. However, up to 15% of patients, most commonly young infants rather than older children or adults, have a normal CSF leukocyte count. In rare cases, PMNs may predominate during the first 48 h of illness. CSF reverse transcriptase PCR (RT-PCR) is the diagnostic procedure of choice and is both sensitive (>95%) and specific (>100%). CSF PCR has the highest sensitivity if performed within 48 h of symptom onset, with sensitivity declining rapidly after day 5 of symptoms. PCR of throat washings or stool specimens may be positive for several weeks, and positive results can help support the diagnosis of an acute enteroviral infection. The sensitivity of routine enteroviral PCRs for detecting EV71 is low, and specific testing may be required. Treatment is supportive, and patients usually recover without sequelae. Chronic and severe infections can occur in neonates and in individuals with hypo- or agammaglobulinemia.

Arbovirus infections (Chap. 233) occur predominantly in the summer and early fall. Arboviral meningitis should be considered when clusters of meningitis and encephalitis cases occur in a restricted geographic region during the summer or early fall. In the United States, the most important causes of arboviral meningitis and encephalitis are WNV, St. Louis encephalitis virus, and the California encephalitis group of viruses. In WNV epidemics, avian deaths may serve as sentinel infections for subsequent human disease. A history of tick exposure or travel or residence in the appropriate geographic area should suggest the possibility of Colorado tick fever virus or Powassan virus infection, although nonviral tick-borne diseases, including RMSF and Lyme neuroborreliosis, may present similarly. Arbovirus meningoencephalitis is typically associated with a CSF lymphocytic pleocytosis, normal glucose concentration, and normal or mildly elevated protein concentration. However, ~45% of patients with WNV meningoencephalitis have CSF neutrophilia, which can persist for a week or more. The rarity of hypoglycorrhachia in WNV infection, the absence of positive Gram's stains, and the negative cultures help distinguish these patients from those with bacterial meningitis. Definitive diagnosis of arboviral meningoencephalitis is based on demonstration of viral-specific IgM in CSF or seroconversion. The prevalence of CSF IgM increases progressively during the first week after infection, peaking at >80% in patients with neuroinvasive disease; as a result, repeat studies may be needed when disease suspicion is high and an early study is negative. CSF PCR tests are available for some viruses in selected diagnostic laboratories and at the Centers for Disease Control and Prevention (CDC), but in the case of WNV, sensitivity (~70%) of CSF PCR is less than that of CSF serology. WNV CSF PCR may be useful in immunocompromised patients who may have absent or reduced antibody responses.

HSV meningitis (Chap. 216) has been increasingly recognized as a major cause of viral meningitis in adults, and overall, it is probably second in importance to enteroviruses as a cause of viral meningitis, accounting for 5% of total cases overall and undoubtedly a higher frequency of those cases occurring in adults and/or outside of the summer-fall period when enterovirus infections are increasingly common. In adults, the majority of cases of uncomplicated meningitis are due to HSV-2, whereas HSV-1 is responsible for 90% of cases of HSV encephalitis. HSV meningitis occurs in ~25–35% of women and ~10–15% of men at the time of an initial (primary) episode of genital herpes. Of these patients, 20% go on to have recurrent attacks of meningitis. Diagnosis of HSV meningitis is usually by HSV CSF PCR because cultures may be negative, especially in patients with recurrent meningitis. Demonstration of intrathecal synthesis of HSV-specific antibody may also be useful in diagnosis, although antibody tests are less sensitive and less specific than PCR and may not become positive until after the first week of infection. Although a history of or the presence of HSV genital lesions is an important diagnostic clue, many patients with HSV meningitis give no history and have no evidence of active genital herpes at the time of presentation. Most cases of recurrent viral or "aseptic" meningitis, including cases previously diagnosed as Mollaret's meningitis, are due to HSV.

VZV meningitis should be suspected in the presence of concurrent chickenpox or shingles. However, it is important to recognize that VZV is being increasingly identified as an important cause of both meningitis and encephalitis in patients without rash. The frequency of VZV as a cause of meningitis is extremely variable, ranging from as low as 3% to as high as 20% in different series. Diagnosis is usually based on CSF PCR, although the sensitivity of this test may not be as high as for the other herpesviruses. VZV serologic studies complement PCR testing, and the diagnosis of VZV CNS infection can be made by the demonstration of VZV-specific intrathecal antibody synthesis and/or the presence of VZV CSF IgM antibodies, or by positive CSF cultures.

EBV infections may also produce aseptic meningitis, with or without associated infectious mononucleosis. The presence of atypical lymphocytes in the CSF or peripheral blood is suggestive of EBV infection but may occasionally be seen with other viral infections. EBV is almost never cultured from CSF. Serum and CSF serology can help establish the presence of acute infection, which is characterized by IgM viral capsid antibodies (VCAs), antibodies to early antigens (EAs), and the absence of antibodies to EBV-associated nuclear antigen (EBNA). CSF PCR is another important diagnostic test, although false-positive results may reflect viral reactivation associated with other infectious or inflammatory processes or the presence of latent viral DNA in lymphocytes recruited due to other inflammatory conditions.

HIV meningitis should be suspected in any patient presenting with a viral meningitis with known or suspected risk factors for HIV infection.

Meningitis may occur following primary infection with HIV in 5–10% of cases and less commonly at later stages of illness. Cranial nerve palsies, most commonly involving cranial nerves V, VII, or VIII, are more common in HIV meningitis than in other viral infections. Diagnosis can be confirmed by detection of HIV genome in blood or CSF. Seroconversion may be delayed, and patients with negative HIV serologies who are suspected of having HIV meningitis should be monitored for delayed seroconversion. **For further discussion of HIV infection, see Chap. 226.**

Mumps (Chap. 231e) should be considered when meningitis occurs in the late winter or early spring, especially in males (male-to-female ratio 3:1). With the widespread use of the live attenuated mumps vaccine in the United States since 1967, the incidence of mumps meningitis has fallen by >95%; however, mumps remains a potential source of infection in nonimmunized individuals and populations. Rare cases (10–100:100,000 vaccinated individuals) of vaccine-associated mumps meningitis have been described, with onset typically 2–4 weeks after vaccination. The presence of parotitis, orchitis, oophoritis, pancreatitis, or elevations in serum lipase and amylase is suggestive of mumps meningitis; however, their absence does not exclude the diagnosis. Clinical meningitis was previously estimated to occur in 10–30% of patients with mumps parotitis; however, in a recent U.S. outbreak of nearly 2600 cases of mumps, only 11 cases of meningitis were identified, suggesting the incidence may be lower than previously suspected. Mumps infection confers lifelong immunity, so a documented history of previous infection excludes this diagnosis. Patients with meningitis have a CSF pleocytosis that can exceed 1000 cells/μL in 25%. Lymphocytes predominate in 75%, although CSF neutrophilia occurs in 25%. Hypoglycorrhachia, occurs in 10–30% of patients and may be a clue to the diagnosis when present. Diagnosis is typically made by culture of virus from CSF or by detecting IgM antibodies or seroconversion. CSF PCR is available in some diagnostic and research laboratories.

LCMV infection (Chap. 233) should be considered when aseptic meningitis occurs in the late fall or winter and in individuals with a history of exposure to house mice (*Mus musculus*), pet or laboratory rodents (e.g., hamsters, rats, mice), or their excreta. Some patients have an associated rash, pulmonary infiltrates, alopecia, parotitis, orchitis, or myopericarditis. Laboratory clues to the diagnosis of LCMV, in addition to the clinical findings noted above, may include the presence of leukopenia, thrombocytopenia, or abnormal liver function tests. Some cases present with a marked CSF pleocytosis (>1000 cells/μL) and hypoglycorrhachia (<30%). Diagnosis is based on serology and/or culture of virus from CSF.

TREATMENT ACUTE VIRAL MENINGITIS

Treatment of almost all cases of viral meningitis is primarily symptomatic and includes use of analgesics, antipyretics, and antiemetics. Fluid and electrolyte status should be monitored. Patients with suspected bacterial meningitis should receive appropriate empirical therapy pending culture results (see above). Hospitalization may not be required in immunocompetent patients with presumed viral meningitis and no focal signs or symptoms, no significant alteration in consciousness, and a classic CSF profile (lymphocytic pleocytosis, normal glucose, negative Gram's stain) if adequate provision for monitoring at home and medical follow-up can be ensured. Immunocompromised patients; patients with significant alteration in consciousness, seizures, or the presence of focal signs and symptoms suggesting the possibility of encephalitis or parenchymal brain involvement; and patients who have an atypical CSF profile should be hospitalized. Oral or intravenous acyclovir may be of benefit in patients with meningitis caused by HSV-1 or -2 and in cases of severe EBV or VZV infection. Data concerning treatment of HSV, EBV, and VZV meningitis are extremely limited. Seriously ill patients should probably receive intravenous acyclovir (15–30 mg/kg per day in three divided doses), which can be followed by an oral drug such as acyclovir (800 mg five times daily), famciclovir (500 mg tid), or valacyclovir (1000 mg tid) for a total course of 7–14 days. Patients who are less ill can be treated with oral drugs alone. Patients with HIV meningitis should receive highly active antiretroviral therapy (**Chap. 226**). There is no specific therapy of proven benefit for patients with arboviral encephalitis, including that caused by WNV.

Patients with viral meningitis who are known to have deficient humoral immunity (e.g., X-linked agammaglobulinemia) and who are not already receiving either intramuscular gamma globulin or intravenous immunoglobulin (IVIg) should be treated with these agents. Intraventricular administration of immunoglobulin through an Ommaya reservoir has been tried in some patients with chronic enteroviral meningitis who have not responded to intramuscular or intravenous immunoglobulin.

Vaccination is an effective method of preventing the development of meningitis and other neurologic complications associated with poliovirus, mumps, measles, rubella, and varicella infection. A live attenuated VZV vaccine (Varivax) is available in the United States. Clinical studies indicate an effectiveness rate of 70–90% for this vaccine, but a booster may be required after ~10 years to maintain immunity. A related vaccine (Zostavax) is recommended for prevention of herpes zoster (shingles) in adults over the age of 60. An inactivated varicella vaccine is available for transplant recipients and others for whom live viral vaccines are contraindicated

PROGNOSIS

In adults, the prognosis for full recovery from viral meningitis is excellent. Rare patients complain of persisting headache, mild mental impairment, incoordination, or generalized asthenia for weeks to months. The outcome in infants and neonates (<1 year) is less certain; intellectual impairment, learning disabilities, hearing loss, and other lasting sequelae have been reported in some studies.

VIRAL ENCEPHALITIS

DEFINITION

In contrast to viral meningitis, where the infectious process and associated inflammatory response are limited largely to the meninges, in encephalitis the brain parenchyma is also involved. Many patients with encephalitis also have evidence of associated meningitis (meningoencephalitis) and, in some cases, involvement of the spinal cord or nerve roots (encephalomyelitis, encephalomyeloradiculitis).

CLINICAL MANIFESTATIONS

In addition to the acute febrile illness with evidence of meningeal involvement characteristic of meningitis, the patient with encephalitis commonly has an altered level of consciousness (confusion, behavioral abnormalities), or a depressed level of consciousness ranging from mild lethargy to coma, and evidence of either focal or diffuse neurologic signs and symptoms. Patients with encephalitis may have hallucinations, agitation, personality change, behavioral disorders, and, at times, a frankly psychotic state. Focal or generalized seizures occur in many patients with encephalitis. Virtually every possible type of focal neurologic disturbance has been reported in viral encephalitis; the signs and symptoms reflect the sites of infection and inflammation. The most commonly encountered focal findings are aphasia, ataxia, upper or lower motor neuron patterns of weakness, involuntary movements (e.g., myoclonic jerks, tremor), and cranial nerve deficits (e.g., ocular palsies, facial weakness). Involvement of the hypothalamic-pituitary axis may result in temperature dysregulation, diabetes insipidus, or the development of the syndrome of inappropriate secretion of antidiuretic hormone (SIADH). Even though neurotropic viruses typically cause pathologic injury in distinct regions of the CNS, variations in clinical presentations make it impossible to reliably establish the etiology of a specific case of encephalitis on clinical grounds alone (see "Differential Diagnosis," below).

ETIOLOGY

In the United States, there are an estimated ~20,000 cases of encephalitis per year, although the actual number of cases is likely to be significantly larger. Despite comprehensive diagnostic efforts, the majority of cases of acute encephalitis of suspected viral etiology remain of unknown cause. Hundreds of viruses are capable of causing encephalitis, although only a limited subset is responsible for most cases in which a specific cause is identified (Table 164-4). The most commonly identified viruses causing sporadic cases of acute encephalitis in immunocompetent adults are herpesviruses (HSV, VZV, EBV). Epidemics of encephalitis are caused by arboviruses, which belong to several different viral taxonomic groups including *Alphaviruses* (e.g., EEE virus, western equine encephalitis virus), *Flaviviruses* (e.g., WNV, St. Louis encephalitis virus, Japanese encephalitis virus, Powassan virus), and *Bunyaviruses* (e.g., California encephalitis virus serogroup, La Crosse virus). Historically, the largest number of cases of arbovirus encephalitis in the United States has been due to St. Louis encephalitis virus and the California encephalitis virus serogroup. However, since 2002, WNV has been responsible for the majority of arbovirus meningitis and encephalitis cases in the United States. WNV caused 2873 confirmed cases of neuroinvasive disease (encephalitis, meningitis, or myelitis) in 2012 with 286 deaths. States reporting >200 cases included Texas (1868 cases), California (479), Louisiana (335), Illinois (290), Mississippi (249), South Dakota (203), and Michigan (202). In 2013, there were 1140 neuroinvasive cases with 100 deaths. States reporting >100 cases included California (357 cases), Colorado (315), Nebraska (213), Texas (157), South Dakota (148), North Dakota (123), and Illinois (106). It is important to recognize that WNV epidemics are unpredictable and that cases have occurred in every state in the continental United States. New causes of viral CNS infections are constantly appearing, as evidenced by the outbreak of cases of encephalitis in Southeast Asia caused by Nipah virus, a newly identified member of the Paramyxoviridae family; of meningitis in Europe caused by Toscana virus, an arbovirus belonging to the Bunyavirus family; and of neurologic disorders associated with major epidemics of Chikungunya virus, a togavirus, in Africa, India, and Southeast Asia. Parechoviruses including human parechovirus 3 (HPeV3), members of the Picornavirus family, have recently been reported as causes of fever, sepsis, and meningitis in infants (age <3 months) in the United States and abroad.

LABORATORY DIAGNOSIS

CSF Examination CSF examination should be performed in all patients with suspected viral encephalitis unless contraindicated by the presence of severely increased ICP. Ideally at least 20 mL should be collected with 5–10 mL stored frozen for later studies as needed. The characteristic CSF profile is indistinguishable from that of viral meningitis and typically consists of a lymphocytic pleocytosis, a mildly elevated protein concentration, and a normal glucose concentration. A CSF pleocytosis (>5 cells/μL) occurs in >95% of immunocompetent patients with documented viral encephalitis. In rare cases, a pleocytosis may be absent on the initial LP but present on subsequent LPs. Patients who are severely immunocompromised by HIV infection, glucocorticoid or other immunosuppressant drugs, chemotherapy, or lymphoreticular malignancies may fail to mount a CSF inflammatory response. CSF cell counts exceed 500/μL in only about 10% of patients with encephalitis. Infections with certain arboviruses (e.g., EEE virus or California encephalitis virus), mumps, and LCMV may occasionally result in cell counts >1000/μL, but this degree of pleocytosis should suggest the possibility of nonviral infections or other inflammatory processes. Atypical lymphocytes in the CSF may be seen in EBV infection and less commonly with other viruses, including CMV, HSV, and enteroviruses. Increased numbers of plasmacytoid or Mollaret-like large mononuclear cells have been reported in WNV encephalitis. Polymorphonuclear pleocytosis occurs in ~45% of patients with WNV encephalitis and is also a common feature in CMV myeloradiculitis in immunocompromised patients. Large numbers of CSF PMNs may be present in patients with encephalitis due to EEE virus, echovirus 9, and, more rarely, other enteroviruses. However, persisting CSF neutrophilia should prompt consideration of bacterial infection, leptospirosis, amebic infection, and noninfectious processes such as acute hemorrhagic leukoencephalitis. About 20% of patients with encephalitis will have a significant number of red blood cells (>500/μL) in the CSF in a nontraumatic tap. The pathologic correlate of this finding may be a hemorrhagic encephalitis of the type seen with HSV; however, CSF red blood cells occur with similar frequency and in similar numbers in patients with nonherpetic focal encephalitides. A decreased CSF glucose concentration is distinctly unusual in viral encephalitis and should suggest the possibility of bacterial, fungal, tuberculous, parasitic, leptospiral, syphilitic, sarcoid, or neoplastic meningitis. Rare patients with mumps, LCMV, or advanced HSV encephalitis and many patients with CMV myeloradiculitis have low CSF glucose concentrations.

CSF PCR

CSF PCR has become the primary diagnostic test for CNS infections caused by CMV, EBV, HHV-6, and enteroviruses (see "Viral Meningitis," above). In the case of VZV CNS infection, CSF PCR and detection of virus-specific IgM or intrathecal antibody synthesis both provide important aids to diagnosis. The sensitivity and specificity of CSF PCRs vary with the virus being tested. The sensitivity (~96%) and specificity (~99%) of HSV CSF PCR are equivalent to or exceed those of brain biopsy. It is important to recognize that HSV CSF PCR results need to be interpreted after considering the likelihood of disease in the patient being tested, the timing of the test in relationship to onset of symptoms, and the prior use of antiviral therapy. A negative HSV CSF PCR test performed by a qualified laboratory at the appropriate time during illness in a patient with a high likelihood of HSV encephalitis based on clinical and laboratory abnormalities significantly reduces the likelihood of HSV encephalitis but does not exclude it. For example, in a patient with a pretest probability of 35% of having HSV encephalitis, a negative HSV CSF PCR reduces the posttest probability to ~2%, and for a patient with a pretest probability of 60%, a negative test reduces the posttest probability to ~6%. In both situations, a positive test makes the diagnosis almost certain (98–99%). There have been several recent reports of initially negative HSV CSF PCR tests that were obtained early (≤72 h) following symptom onset and that became positive when repeated 1–3 days later. The frequency of positive HSV CSF PCRs in patients with herpes encephalitis also decreases as a function of the duration of illness, with only ~20% of cases remaining positive after ≥14 days. PCR results are generally not affected by ≤1 week of antiviral therapy. In one study, 98% of CSF specimens remained PCR-positive during the first week of initiation of antiviral therapy, but the numbers fell to ~50% by 8–14 days and to ~21% by >15 days after initiation of antiviral therapy.

The sensitivity and specificity of CSF PCR tests for viruses other than HSV have not been definitively characterized. Enteroviral (EV) CSF PCR appears to have a sensitivity and specificity of >95%. EV PCR sensitivity for EV71 may be considerably lower (~30% in some reports). Parechoviruses are also not detected by standard EV RT-PCRs. The specificity of EBV CSF PCR has not been established. Positive EBV CSF PCRs associated with positive tests for other pathogens have been reported and may reflect reactivation of EBV latent in lymphocytes that enter the CNS as a result of an unrelated infectious or inflammatory process. In patients with CNS infection due to VZV, CSF antibody and PCR studies should be considered complementary, because patients may have evidence of intrathecal synthesis of VZV-specific antibodies and negative CSF PCRs. In the case of WNV infection, CSF PCR appears to be less sensitive (~70% sensitivity) than detection of WNV-specific CSF IgM, although PCR testing remains useful in immunocompromised patients who may not mount an effective anti-WNV antibody response.

CSF Culture CSF culture is generally of limited utility in the diagnosis of acute viral encephalitis. Culture may be insensitive (e.g., >95% of patients with HSV encephalitis have negative CSF cultures as do virtually all patients with EBV-associated CNS disease) and often takes too long to significantly affect immediate therapy.

Serologic Studies and Antigen Detection The basic approach to the serodiagnosis of viral encephalitis is identical to that discussed earlier for viral meningitis. Demonstration of WNV IgM antibodies is diagnostic of WNV encephalitis because IgM antibodies do not cross the blood-brain barrier, and their presence in CSF is therefore indicative of intrathecal synthesis. Timing of antibody collection may be important because the rate of CSF WNV IgM seropositivity increases by ~10% per day during the first week after illness onset, reaching 80% or higher on day 7 after symptom onset. In patients with HSV encephalitis, both antibodies to HSV-1 glycoproteins and glycoprotein antigens have been detected in the CSF. Optimal detection of both HSV antibodies and antigen typically occurs after the first week of illness, limiting the utility of these tests in acute diagnosis. Nonetheless, HSV CSF antibody testing is of value in selected patients whose illness is >1 week in duration and who are CSF PCR–negative for HSV. In the case of VZV infection, CSF antibody tests may be positive when PCR fails to detect viral DNA, and both tests should be considered complementary rather than mutually exclusive.

MRI, CT, and EEG Patients with suspected encephalitis almost invariably undergo neuroimaging studies and often EEG. These tests help identify or exclude alternative diagnoses and assist in the differentiation between a focal, as opposed to a diffuse, encephalitic process. Focal findings in a patient with encephalitis should always raise the possibility of HSV encephalitis. Examples of focal findings include: (1) areas of increased signal intensity in the frontotemporal, cingulate, or insular regions of the brain on T2-weighted, FLAIR, or diffusion-weighted MRI (Fig. 164-3); (2) focal areas of low absorption, mass effect, and contrast enhancement on CT; or (3) periodic focal temporal lobe spikes on a background of slow or low-amplitude ("flattened") activity on EEG. Approximately 10% of patients with PCR-documented HSV encephalitis will have a normal MRI, although nearly 80% will have abnormalities in the temporal lobe, and an additional 10% in extratemporal regions. The lesions are typically hyperintense on T2-weighted images. The addition of FLAIR and diffusion-weighted images to the standard MRI sequences enhances sensitivity. Children with HSV encephalitis may have atypical patterns of MRI lesions and often show involvement of brain regions outside the frontotemporal areas. CT is less sensitive than MRI and is normal in up to 20–35% of patients. EEG abnormalities occur in >75% of PCR-documented cases of HSV encephalitis; they typically involve the temporal lobes but are often nonspecific. Some patients with HSV encephalitis have a distinctive EEG pattern consisting of periodic, stereotyped, sharp-and-slow complexes originating in one or both temporal lobes and repeating at regular intervals of 2–3 s. The periodic complexes are typically noted between days 2 and 15 of the illness and are present in two-thirds of pathologically proven cases of HSV encephalitis.

Significant MRI abnormalities are found in only approximately two-thirds of patients with WNV encephalitis, a frequency less than that with HSV encephalitis. When present, abnormalities often involve deep brain structures, including the thalamus, basal ganglia, and brainstem, rather than the cortex and may only be apparent on FLAIR images. EEGs in patients with WNV encephalitis typically show generalized slowing that may be more anteriorly prominent rather than the temporally predominant pattern of sharp or periodic discharges more characteristic of HSV encephalitis. Patients with VZV encephalitis may show multifocal areas of hemorrhagic and ischemic infarction, reflecting the tendency of this virus to produce a CNS vasculopathy rather than a true encephalitis. Immunocompromised adult patients with CMV often have enlarged ventricles with areas of increased T2 signal on MRI outlining the ventricles and subependymal enhancement on T1-weighted postcontrast images. Table 164-5 highlights specific diagnostic test results in encephalitis that can be useful in clinical decision making.

Brain Biopsy Brain biopsy is now generally reserved for patients in whom CSF PCR studies fail to lead to a specific diagnosis, who have focal abnormalities on MRI, and who continue to show progressive clinical deterioration despite treatment with acyclovir and supportive therapy.

DIFFERENTIAL DIAGNOSIS

Infection by a variety of other organisms can mimic viral encephalitis. In studies of biopsy-proven HSV encephalitis, common infectious

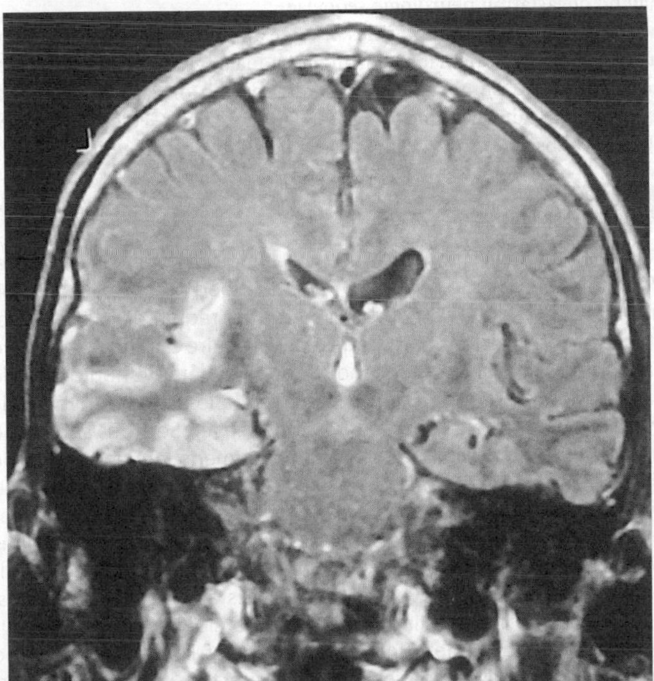

FIGURE 164-3 Coronal fluid-attenuated inversion recovery (FLAIR) magnetic resonance image from a patient with herpes simplex encephalitis. Note the area of increased signal in the right temporal lobe (*left side of image*) confined predominantly to the gray matter. This patient had predominantly unilateral disease; bilateral lesions are more common but may be quite asymmetric in their intensity.

TABLE 164-5 USE OF DIAGNOSTIC TESTS IN ENCEPHALITIS

The best test for WNV encephalitis is the *CSF IgM antibody test*. The prevalence of positive CSF IgM tests increases by about 10% per day after illness onset and reaches 70–80% by the end of the first week. Serum WNV IgM can provide evidence for recent WNV infection, but in the absence of other findings does not establish the diagnosis of neuroinvasive disease (meningitis, encephalitis, acute flaccid paralysis).

Approximately 80% of patients with proven HSV encephalitis have *MRI* abnormalities involving the temporal lobes. This percentage likely increases to >90% when FLAIR and diffusion-weighted MRI sequences are also used. The absence of temporal lobe lesions on MRI reduces the likelihood of HSV encephalitis and should prompt consideration of other diagnostic possibilities.

The *CSF HSV PCR* test may be negative in the first 72 h of symptoms of HSV encephalitis. A repeat study should be considered in patients with an initial early negative PCR in whom diagnostic suspicion of HSV encephalitis remains high and no alternative diagnosis has yet been established.

Detection of *intrathecal synthesis* (increased CSF/serum HSV antibody ratio corrected for breakdown of the blood-brain barrier) of *HSV-specific antibody* may be useful in diagnosis of HSV encephalitis in patients in whom only late (>1 week after onset) CSF specimens are available and PCR studies are negative. Serum serology alone is of no value in diagnosis of HSV encephalitis due to the high seroprevalence rate in the general population.

Negative *CSF viral cultures* are of no value in excluding the diagnosis of HSV or EBV encephalitis.

VZV CSF IgM antibodies may be present in patients with a negative VZV CSF PCR. Both tests should be performed in patients with suspected VZV CNS disease.

The specificity of *EBV CSF PCR* for diagnosis of CNS infection is unknown. Positive tests may occur in patients with a CSF pleocytosis due to other causes. Detection of EBV CSF IgM or intrathecal synthesis of antibody to VCA supports the diagnosis of EBV encephalitis. Serologic studies consistent with acute EBV infection (e.g., IgM VCA, presence of antibodies against EA but not against EBNA) can help support the diagnosis.

Abbreviations: CNS, central nervous system; CSF, cerebrospinal fluid; DWI, diffusion-weighted imaging; EA, early antigen; EBNA, EBV-associated nuclear antigen; EBV, Epstein-Barr virus; FLAIR, fluid-attenuated inversion recovery; HSV, herpes simplex virus; IgM, immunoglobulin M; MRI, magnetic resonance imaging; PCR, polymerase chain reaction; VCA, viral capsid antibody; VZV, varicella-zoster virus; WNV, West Nile virus.

mimics of focal viral encephalitis included mycobacteria, fungi, rickettsiae, *Listeria*, *Mycoplasma*, and other bacteria (including *Bartonella* sp.). Autoimmune causes of encephalitis, including those associated with antibodies against *N*-methyl-D-aspartate (NMDA) receptor, voltage-gated potassium channels (VGKC), α-amino-3-hydroxy-5-methyl-4-isoxazolepropionic acid (AMPA), and γ-aminobutyric acid (GABA) receptors, and GAD-65, have been increasingly recognized as causes of encephalitis that can mimic that caused by viral infection. In most cases, diagnosis is made by detection of the specific autoantibodies in serum and/or CSF. NMDA receptor antibodies have recently been reported in some patients with HSE encephalitis, and their presence should not exclude appropriate testing and treatment for HSV encephalitis. Autoimmune encephalitis may also be associated with specific cancers (paraneoplastic) and onconeuronal antibodies (e.g., anti-Hu, Yo, Ma2, amphiphysin, CRMP5, CV2) (Chap. 122). Subacute or chronic forms of encephalitis may occur in association with autoantibodies against thyroglobulin and thyroperoxidase (Hashimoto's encephalopathy) and with prion diseases.

Infection caused by the ameba *Naegleria fowleri* can also cause acute meningoencephalitis (primary amebic meningoencephalitis), whereas that caused by *Acanthamoeba* and *Balamuthia* more typically produces subacute or chronic granulomatous amebic meningoencephalitis. *Naegleria* thrive in warm, iron-rich pools of water, including those found in drains, canals, and both natural and human-made outdoor pools. Infection has typically occurred in immunocompetent children with a history of swimming in potentially infected water. The CSF, in contrast to the typical profile seen in viral encephalitis, often resembles that of bacterial meningitis with a neutrophilic pleocytosis and hypoglycorrhachia. Motile trophozoites can be seen in a wet mount of warm, fresh CSF. There have been an increasing number of cases of *Balamuthia mandrillaris* amebic encephalitis mimicking acute viral encephalitis in children and immunocompetent adults. This organism has also been associated with encephalitis in recipients of transplanted organs from a donor with unrecognized infection. No effective treatment has been identified, and mortality approaches 100%.

Encephalitis can be caused by the raccoon pinworm *Baylisascaris procyonis*. Clues to the diagnosis include a history of raccoon exposure, especially of playing in or eating dirt potentially contaminated with raccoon feces. Most patients are children, and many have an associated eosinophilia.

Once nonviral causes of encephalitis have been excluded, the major diagnostic challenge is to distinguish HSV from other viruses that cause encephalitis. This distinction is particularly important because in virtually every other instance the therapy is supportive, whereas specific and effective antiviral therapy is available for HSV, and its efficacy is enhanced when it is instituted early in the course of infection. HSV encephalitis should be considered when clinical features suggesting involvement of the inferomedial frontotemporal regions of the brain are present, including prominent olfactory or gustatory hallucinations, anosmia, unusual or bizarre behavior or personality alterations, or memory disturbance. HSV encephalitis should always be suspected in patients with signs and symptoms consistent with acute encephalitis with focal findings on clinical examination, neuroimaging studies, or EEG. The diagnostic procedure of choice in these patients is CSF PCR analysis for HSV. A positive CSF PCR establishes the diagnosis, and a negative test dramatically reduces the likelihood of HSV encephalitis (see above).

The anatomic distribution of lesions may provide an additional clue to diagnosis. Patients with rapidly progressive encephalitis and prominent brainstem signs, symptoms, or neuroimaging abnormalities may be infected by flaviviruses (WNV, St. Louis encephalitis virus, Japanese encephalitis virus), HSV, rabies, or *L. monocytogenes*. Significant involvement of deep gray matter structures, including the basal ganglia and thalamus, should also suggest possible flavivirus infection. These patients may present clinically with prominent movement disorders (tremor, myoclonus) or parkinsonian features. Patients with WNV infection can also present with a poliomyelitis-like acute flaccid paralysis, as can patients infected with EV71 and, less commonly, other enteroviruses. Acute flaccid paralysis is characterized by the acute onset of a lower motor neuron type of weakness with flaccid tone, reduced or absent reflexes, and relatively preserved sensation. The complete eradication of polio remains an ongoing challenge despite a continuing World Health Organization poliovirus elimination campaign. Three hundred forty-one cases of polio (almost all due to serotype 1) have been reported in 2013 from eight countries (Somalia 183 cases, Pakistan 63, Nigeria 51, Kenya 14, Syria 13, Afghanistan 9, Ethiopia 6, and Cameroon 2). There have been small outbreaks of poliomyelitis associated with vaccine strains of virus that have reverted to virulence through mutation or recombination with circulating wild-type enteroviruses in Hispaniola, China, the Philippines, Indonesia, Nigeria, and Madagascar.

Epidemiologic factors may provide important clues to the diagnosis of viral meningitis or encephalitis. Particular attention should be paid to the season of the year; the geographic location and travel history; and possible exposure to animal bites or scratches, rodents, and ticks. Although transmission from the bite of an infected dog remains the most common cause of rabies worldwide, in the United States very few cases of dog rabies occur, and the most common risk factor is exposure to bats—although a clear history of a bite or scratch is often lacking. The classic clinical presentation of encephalitic (furious) rabies is fever, fluctuating consciousness, and autonomic hyperactivity. Phobic spasms of the larynx, pharynx, neck muscles, and diaphragm can be triggered by attempts to swallow water (*hydrophobia*) or by inspiration (*aerophobia*). Patients may also present with paralytic (dumb) rabies characterized by acute ascending paralysis. Rabies due to the bite of a bat has a different clinical presentation than classic rabies due to a dog or wolf bite. Patients present with focal neurologic deficits, myoclonus, seizures, and hallucinations; phobic spasms are not a typical feature. Patients with rabies have a CSF lymphocytic pleocytosis and may show areas of increased T2 signal abnormality in the brainstem, hippocampus, and hypothalamus. Diagnosis can be made by finding rabies virus antigen in brain tissue or in the neural innervation of hair follicles at the nape of the neck. PCR amplification of viral nucleic acid from CSF and saliva or tears may also enable diagnosis. Serology is frequently negative in both serum and CSF in the first week after onset of infection, which limits its acute diagnostic utility. No specific therapy is available, and cases are almost invariably fatal, with isolated survivors having devastating neurologic sequelae.

State public health authorities provide a valuable resource concerning isolation of particular agents in individual regions. Regular updates concerning the number, type, and distribution of cases of arboviral encephalitis can be found on the CDC and U.S. Geological Survey (USGS) websites (*http://www.cdc.gov* and *http://diseasemaps.usgs.gov*).

TREATMENT VIRAL ENCEPHALITIS

Specific antiviral therapy should be initiated when appropriate. Vital functions, including respiration and blood pressure, should be monitored continuously and supported as required. In the initial stages of encephalitis, many patients will require care in an intensive care unit. Basic management and supportive therapy should include careful monitoring of ICP, fluid restriction, avoidance of hypotonic intravenous solutions, and suppression of fever. Seizures should be treated with standard anticonvulsant regimens, and prophylactic therapy should be considered in view of the high frequency of seizures in severe cases of encephalitis. As with all seriously ill, immobilized patients with altered levels of consciousness, encephalitis patients are at risk for aspiration pneumonia, stasis ulcers and decubiti, contractures, deep venous thrombosis and its complications, and infections of indwelling lines and catheters.

Acyclovir is of benefit in the treatment of HSV and should be started empirically in patients with suspected viral encephalitis, especially if focal features are present, while awaiting viral diagnostic studies. Treatment should be discontinued in patients found not to have HSV encephalitis, with the possible exception of patients with severe encephalitis due to VZV or EBV. HSV, VZV, and EBV all encode an enzyme, deoxypyrimidine (thymidine) kinase, that phosphorylates acyclovir to produce acyclovir-5′-monophosphate.

Host cell enzymes then phosphorylate this compound to form a triphosphate derivative. It is the triphosphate that acts as an antiviral agent by inhibiting viral DNA polymerase and by causing premature termination of nascent viral DNA chains. The specificity of action depends on the fact that uninfected cells do not phosphorylate significant amounts of acyclovir to acyclovir-5′-monophosphate. A second level of specificity is provided by the fact that the acyclovir triphosphate is a more potent inhibitor of viral DNA polymerase than of the analogous host cell enzymes.

Adults should receive a dose of 10 mg/kg of acyclovir intravenously every 8 h (30 mg/kg per day total dose) for 14–21 days. CSF PCR can be repeated at the completion of this course, with PCR-positive patients receiving additional treatment, followed by a repeat CSF PCR test. Neonatal HSV CNS infection is less responsive to acyclovir therapy than HSV encephalitis in adults; it is recommended that neonates with HSV encephalitis receive 20 mg/kg of acyclovir every 8 h (60 mg/kg per day total dose) for a minimum of 21 days.

Prior to intravenous administration, acyclovir should be diluted to a concentration ≤7 mg/mL. (A 70-kg person would receive a dose of 700 mg, which would be diluted in a volume of 100 mL.) Each dose should be infused slowly over 1 h, rather than by rapid or bolus infusion, to minimize the risk of renal dysfunction. Care should be taken to avoid extravasation or intramuscular or subcutaneous administration. The alkaline pH of acyclovir can cause local inflammation and phlebitis (9%). Dose adjustment is required in patients with impaired renal glomerular filtration. Penetration into CSF is excellent, with average drug levels ~50% of serum levels. Complications of therapy include elevations in blood urea nitrogen and creatinine levels (5%), thrombocytopenia (6%), gastrointestinal toxicity (nausea, vomiting, diarrhea) (7%), and neurotoxicity (lethargy or obtundation, disorientation, confusion, agitation, hallucinations, tremors, seizures) (1%). Acyclovir resistance may be mediated by changes in either the viral deoxypyrimidine kinase or DNA polymerase. To date, acyclovir-resistant isolates have not been a significant clinical problem in immunocompetent individuals. However, there have been reports of clinically virulent acyclovir-resistant HSV isolates from sites outside the CNS in immunocompromised individuals, including those with AIDS.

Oral antiviral drugs with efficacy against HSV, VZV, and EBV, including acyclovir, famciclovir, and valacyclovir, have not been evaluated in the treatment of encephalitis either as primary therapy or as supplemental therapy following completion of a course of parenteral acyclovir. A recently completed National Institute of Allergy and Infectious Disease (NIAID)/National Institute of Neurological Disorders and Stroke–sponsored phase III trial of supplemental oral valacyclovir therapy (2 g tid for 3 months) following the initial 14- to 21-day course of therapy with parenteral acyclovir (*www.clinicaltrials.gov*, identifier NCT00031486) was terminated early due to low enrollment. Although analysis was compromised due to low numbers, no differences were seen in the 12-month endpoints including dementia rating scale, mini-mental state exam, and Glasgow coma score in patients receiving valacyclovir versus placebo. The role of adjunctive intravenous glucocorticoids in treatment of HSV and VZV infection remains unclear, with most guidelines considering the existing supportive evidence weak and recommendation for possible use based on expert opinion only.

Ganciclovir and foscarnet, either alone or in combination, are often used in the treatment of CMV-related CNS infections, although their efficacy remains unproven. Cidofovir (see below) may provide an alternative in patients who fail to respond to ganciclovir and foscarnet, although data concerning its use in CMV CNS infections are extremely limited.

Ganciclovir is a synthetic nucleoside analogue of 2′-deoxyguanosine. The drug is preferentially phosphorylated by virus-induced cellular kinases. Ganciclovir triphosphate acts as a competitive inhibitor of the CMV DNA polymerase, and its incorporation into nascent viral DNA results in premature chain termination. Following intravenous administration, CSF concentrations of ganciclovir are 25–70% of coincident plasma levels. The usual dose for treatment of severe neurologic illnesses is 5 mg/kg every 12 h given intravenously at a constant rate over 1 h. Induction therapy is followed by maintenance therapy of 5 mg/kg every day for an indefinite period. Induction therapy should be continued until patients show a decline in CSF pleocytosis and a reduction in CSF CMV DNA copy number on quantitative PCR testing (where available). Doses should be adjusted in patients with renal insufficiency. Treatment is often limited by the development of granulocytopenia and thrombocytopenia (20–25%), which may require reduction in or discontinuation of therapy. Gastrointestinal side effects, including nausea, vomiting, diarrhea, and abdominal pain, occur in ~20% of patients. Some patients treated with ganciclovir for CMV retinitis have developed retinal detachment, but the causal relationship to ganciclovir treatment is unclear. Valganciclovir is an orally bioavailable prodrug that can generate high serum levels of ganciclovir, although studies of its efficacy in treating CMV CNS infections are limited.

Foscarnet is a pyrophosphate analogue that inhibits viral DNA polymerases by binding to the pyrophosphate-binding site. Following intravenous infusion, CSF concentrations range from 15 to 100% of coincident plasma levels. The usual dose for serious CMV-related neurologic illness is 60 mg/kg every 8 h administered by constant infusion over 1 h. Induction therapy for 14–21 days is followed by maintenance therapy (60–120 mg/kg per day). Induction therapy may need to be extended in patients who fail to show a decline in CSF pleocytosis and a reduction in CSF CMV DNA copy number on quantitative PCR tests (where available). Approximately one-third of patients develop renal impairment during treatment, which is reversible following discontinuation of therapy in most, but not all, cases. This is often associated with elevations in serum creatinine and proteinuria and is less frequent in patients who are adequately hydrated. Many patients experience fatigue and nausea. Reductions in serum calcium, magnesium, and potassium occur in ~15% of patients and may be associated with tetany, cardiac rhythm disturbances, or seizures.

Cidofovir is a nucleotide analogue that is effective in treating CMV retinitis and equivalent to or better than ganciclovir in some experimental models of murine CMV encephalitis, although data concerning its efficacy in human CMV CNS disease are limited. The usual dose is 5 mg/kg intravenously once weekly for 2 weeks, then biweekly for two or more additional doses, depending on clinical response. Patients must be prehydrated with normal saline (e.g., 1 L over 1–2 h) prior to each dose and treated with probenecid (e.g., 1 g 3 h before cidofovir and 1 g 2 and 8 h after cidofovir). Nephrotoxicity is common; the dose should be reduced if renal function deteriorates.

Intravenous ribavirin (15–25 mg/kg per day in divided doses given every 8 h) has been reported to be of benefit in isolated cases of severe encephalitis due to California encephalitis (La Crosse) virus. Ribavirin might be of benefit for the rare patients, typically infants or young children, with severe adenovirus or rotavirus encephalitis and in patients with encephalitis due to LCMV or other arenaviruses. However, clinical trials are lacking. Hemolysis, with resulting anemia, has been the major side effect limiting therapy.

No specific antiviral therapy of proven efficacy is currently available for treatment of WNV encephalitis. Patients have been treated with a-interferon, ribavirin, an Israeli IVIg preparation that contains high-titer anti-WNV antibody (Omr-IgG-am) (*www.clinicaltrials.gov*, identifier NCT00069316 and 0068055), and humanized monoclonal antibodies directed against the viral envelope glycoprotein (*www.clinicaltrials.gov*, identifier NCT00927953 and 00515385). WNV chimeric vaccines, in which WNV envelope and premembrane proteins are inserted into the background of another flavivirus, are already undergoing human clinical testing and have been found to be both safe and immunogenic in healthy adults but have not yet been tested for disease prevention in humans (*www.clinicaltrials.gov*, identifier NCT00746798, 00442169, 00094718, and 00537147). Both chimeric and killed inactivated WNV vaccines have been found to be safe and effective in preventing equine WNV infection, and several effective flavivirus vaccines are already in human use, creating optimism that a safe and effective human WNV vaccine can also be developed.

SEQUELAE

There is considerable variation in the incidence and severity of sequelae in patients surviving viral encephalitis. In the case of EEE virus infection, nearly 80% of survivors have severe neurologic sequelae. At the other extreme are infections due to EBV, California encephalitis virus, and Venezuelan equine encephalitis virus, where severe sequelae are unusual. For example, approximately 5–15% of children infected with La Crosse virus have a residual seizure disorder, and 1% have persistent hemiparesis. Detailed information about sequelae in patients with HSV encephalitis treated with acyclovir is available from the NIAID-Collaborative Antiviral Study Group (CASG) trials. Of 32 acyclovir-treated patients, 26 survived (81%). Of the 26 survivors, 12 (46%) had no or only minor sequelae, 3 (12%) were moderately impaired (gainfully employed but not functioning at their previous level), and 11 (42%) were severely impaired (requiring continuous supportive care). The incidence and severity of sequelae were directly related to the age of the patient and the level of consciousness at the time of initiation of therapy. Patients with severe neurologic impairment (Glasgow coma score 6) at initiation of therapy either died or survived with severe sequelae. Young patients (<30 years) with good neurologic function at initiation of therapy did substantially better (100% survival, 62% with no or mild sequelae) compared with their older counterparts (>30 years; 64% survival, 57% no or mild sequelae). Some recent studies using quantitative HSV CSF PCR tests indicate that clinical outcome following treatment also correlates with the amount of HSV DNA present in CSF at the time of presentation. Many patients with WNV infection have sequelae, including cognitive impairment; weakness; and hyper- or hypokinetic movement disorders, including tremor, myoclonus, and parkinsonism. In a large longitudinal study of prognosis in 156 patients with WNV infection, the mean time to achieve recovery (defined as 95% of maximal predicted score on specific validated tests) was 112–148 days for fatigue, 121–175 days for physical function, 131–139 days for mood, and 302–455 days for mental function (the longer interval in each case representing patients with neuroinvasive disease).

SUBACUTE MENINGITIS

CLINICAL MANIFESTATIONS

Patients with subacute meningitis typically have an unrelenting headache, stiff neck, low-grade fever, and lethargy for days to several weeks before they present for evaluation. Cranial nerve abnormalities and night sweats may be present. This syndrome overlaps that of chronic meningitis, discussed in detail in Chap. 165.

ETIOLOGY

Common causative organisms include *M. tuberculosis, C. neoformans, H. capsulatum, C. immitis*, and *T. pallidum*. Initial infection with *M. tuberculosis* is acquired by inhalation of aerosolized droplet nuclei. Tuberculous meningitis in adults does not develop acutely from hematogenous spread of tubercle bacilli to the meninges. Rather, millet seed–sized (miliary) tubercles form in the parenchyma of the brain during hematogenous dissemination of tubercle bacilli in the course of primary infection. These tubercles enlarge and are usually caseating. The propensity for a caseous lesion to produce meningitis is determined by its proximity to the subarachnoid space (SAS) and the rate at which fibrous encapsulation develops. Subependymal caseous foci cause meningitis via discharge of bacilli and tuberculous antigens into the SAS. Mycobacterial antigens produce an intense inflammatory reaction that leads to the production of a thick exudate that fills the basilar cisterns and surrounds the cranial nerves and major blood vessels at the base of the brain.

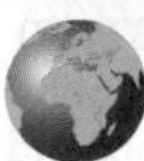

Fungal infections are typically acquired by the inhalation of airborne fungal spores. The initial pulmonary infection may be asymptomatic or present with fever, cough, sputum production, and chest pain. The pulmonary infection is often self-limited. A localized pulmonary fungal infection can then remain dormant in the lungs until there is an abnormality in cell-mediated immunity that allows the fungus to reactivate and disseminate to the CNS. The most common pathogen causing fungal meningitis is *C. neoformans*. This fungus is found worldwide in soil and bird excreta. *H. capsulatum* is endemic to the Ohio and Mississippi River valleys of the central United States and to parts of Central and South America. *C. immitis* is endemic to the desert areas of the southwest United States, northern Mexico, and Argentina.

Syphilis is a sexually transmitted disease that is manifest by the appearance of a painless chancre at the site of inoculation. *T. pallidum* invades the CNS early in the course of syphilis. Cranial nerves VII and VIII are most frequently involved.

LABORATORY DIAGNOSIS

The classic CSF abnormalities in tuberculous meningitis are as follows: (1) elevated opening pressure, (2) lymphocytic pleocytosis (10–500 cells/μL), (3) elevated protein concentration in the range of 1–5 g/L, and (4) decreased glucose concentration in the range of 1.1–2.2 mmol/L (20–40 mg/dL). *The combination of unrelenting headache, stiff neck, fatigue, night sweats, and fever with a CSF lymphocytic pleocytosis and a mildly decreased glucose concentration is highly suspicious for tuberculous meningitis.* The last tube of fluid collected at LP is the best tube to send for a smear for acid-fast bacilli (AFB). If there is a pellicle in the CSF or a cobweb-like clot on the surface of the fluid, AFB can best be demonstrated in a smear of the clot or pellicle. Positive smears are typically reported in only 10–40% of cases of tuberculous meningitis in adults. Cultures of CSF take 4–8 weeks to identify the organism and are positive in ~50% of adults. Culture remains the gold standard to make the diagnosis of tuberculous meningitis. PCR for the detection of *M. tuberculosis* DNA should be sent on CSF if available, but the sensitivity and specificity on CSF have not been defined. The CDC recommends the use of nucleic acid amplification tests for the diagnosis of pulmonary tuberculosis.

The characteristic CSF abnormalities in fungal meningitis are a mononuclear or lymphocytic pleocytosis, an increased protein concentration, and a decreased glucose concentration. There may be eosinophils in the CSF in *C. immitis* meningitis. Large volumes of CSF are often required to demonstrate the organism on India ink smear or grow the organism in culture. If spinal fluid examined by LP on two separate occasions fails to yield an organism, CSF should be obtained by high-cervical or cisternal puncture.

The cryptococcal polysaccharide antigen test is a highly sensitive and specific test for cryptococcal meningitis. A reactive CSF cryptococcal antigen test establishes the diagnosis. The detection of the *Histoplasma* polysaccharide antigen in CSF establishes the diagnosis of a fungal meningitis but is not specific for meningitis due to *H. capsulatum*. It may be falsely positive in coccidioidal meningitis. The CSF complement fixation antibody test is reported to have a specificity of 100% and a sensitivity of 75% for coccidioidal meningitis.

The diagnosis of syphilitic meningitis is made when a reactive serum treponemal test (fluorescent treponemal antibody absorption test [FTA-ABS] or microhemagglutination assay–*T. pallidum* [MHA-TP]) is associated with a CSF lymphocytic or mononuclear pleocytosis and an elevated protein concentration, or when the CSF Venereal Disease Research Laboratory (VDRL) test is positive. A reactive CSF FTA-ABS is not definitive evidence of neurosyphilis. The CSF FTA-ABS can be falsely positive from blood contamination. A negative CSF VDRL does not rule out neurosyphilis. A negative CSF FTA-ABS or MHA-TP rules out neurosyphilis.

TREATMENT SUBACUTE MENINGITIS

Empirical therapy of tuberculous meningitis is often initiated on the basis of a high index of suspicion without adequate laboratory support. Initial therapy is a combination of isoniazid (300 mg/d), rifampin (10 mg/kg per day), pyrazinamide (30 mg/kg per day in divided doses), ethambutol (15–25 mg/kg per day in divided doses), and pyridoxine (50 mg/d). When the antimicrobial sensitivity of the *M. tuberculosis* isolate is known, ethambutol can be discontinued. If the clinical response is good, pyrazinamide can be discontinued after 8 weeks and isoniazid and rifampin continued alone for the next 6–12 months. A 6-month course of therapy is acceptable, but therapy should be prolonged for 9–12 months in patients who have an inadequate resolution of symptoms of meningitis or who have positive mycobacterial cultures of CSF during the course of therapy. Dexamethasone therapy is recommended for HIV-negative patients with tuberculous meningitis. The dose is 12–16 mg/d for 3 weeks, and then tapered over 3 weeks.

Meningitis due to *C. neoformans* in non-HIV, nontransplant patients is treated with induction therapy with amphotericin B (AmB) (0.7 mg/kg IV per day) plus flucytosine (100 mg/kg per day in four divided doses) for at least 4 weeks if CSF culture results are negative after 2 weeks of treatment. Therapy should be extended for a total of 6 weeks in the patient with neurologic complications. Induction therapy is followed by consolidation therapy with fluconazole 400 mg/d for 8 weeks. Organ transplant recipients are treated with liposomal AmB (3–4 mg/kg per day) or AmB lipid complex (ABLC) 5 mg/kg per day plus flucytosine (100 mg/kg per day in four divided doses) for at least 2 weeks or until CSF culture is sterile. Follow CSF yeast cultures for sterilization rather than the cryptococcal antigen titer. This treatment is followed by an 8- to 10-week course of fluconazole (400–800 mg/d [6–12 mg/kg] PO). If the CSF culture is sterile after 10 weeks of acute therapy, the dose of fluconazole is decreased to 200 mg/d for 6 months to a year. Patients with HIV infection are treated with AmB or a lipid formulation plus flucytosine for at least 2 weeks, followed by fluconazole for a minimum of 8 weeks. HIV-infected patients may require indefinite maintenance therapy with fluconazole 200 mg/d. Meningitis due to *H. capsulatum* is treated with AmB (0.7–1.0 mg/kg per day) for 4–12 weeks. A total dose of 30 mg/kg is recommended. Therapy with AmB is not discontinued until fungal cultures are sterile. After completing a course of AmB, maintenance therapy with itraconazole 200 mg two or three times daily is initiated and continued for at least 9 months to a year. *C. immitis* meningitis is treated with either high-dose fluconazole (1000 mg daily) as monotherapy or intravenous AmB (0.5–0.7 mg/kg per day) for >4 weeks. Intrathecal AmB (0.25–0.75 mg/d three times weekly) may be required to eradicate the infection. Lifelong therapy with fluconazole (200–400 mg daily) is recommended to prevent relapse. AmBisome (5 mg/kg per day) or AmB lipid complex (5 mg/kg per day) can be substituted for AmB in patients who have or who develop significant renal dysfunction. The most common complication of fungal meningitis is hydrocephalus. Patients who develop hydrocephalus should receive a CSF diversion device. A ventriculostomy can be used until CSF fungal cultures are sterile, at which time the ventriculostomy is replaced by a ventriculoperitoneal shunt.

Syphilitic meningitis is treated with aqueous penicillin G in a dose of 3–4 million units intravenously every 4 h for 10–14 days. An alternative regimen is 2.4 million units of procaine penicillin G intramuscularly daily with 500 mg of oral probenecid four times daily for 10–14 days. Either regimen is followed with 2.4 million units of benzathine penicillin G intramuscularly once a week for 3 weeks. The standard criterion for treatment success is reexamination of the CSF. The CSF should be reexamined at 6-month intervals for 2 years. The cell count is expected to normalize within 12 months, and the VDRL titer to decrease by two dilutions or revert to nonreactive within 2 years of completion of therapy. Failure of the CSF pleocytosis to resolve or an increase in the CSF VDRL titer by two or more dilutions requires retreatment.

CHRONIC ENCEPHALITIS

PROGRESSIVE MULTIFOCAL LEUKOENCEPHALOPATHY

Clinical Features and Pathology Progressive multifocal leukoencephalopathy (PML) is characterized pathologically by multifocal areas of demyelination of varying size distributed throughout the brain but sparing the spinal cord and optic nerves. In addition to demyelination, there are characteristic cytologic alterations in both astrocytes and oligodendrocytes. Astrocytes are enlarged and contain hyperchromatic, deformed, and bizarre nuclei and frequent mitotic figures. Oligodendrocytes have enlarged, densely staining nuclei that contain viral inclusions formed by crystalline arrays of JC virus (JCV) particles. Patients often present with visual deficits (45%), typically a homonymous hemianopia; mental impairment (38%) (dementia, confusion, personality change); weakness, including hemi- or monoparesis; and ataxia. Seizures occur in ~20% of patients, predominantly in those with lesions abutting the cortex.

Almost all patients have an underlying immunosuppressive disorder or are receiving immunomodulatory therapy. In recent series, the most common associated conditions were AIDS (80%), hematologic malignancies (13%), transplant recipients (5%), and chronic inflammatory diseases (2%). It has been estimated that up to 5% of AIDS patients will develop PML. There have been over 400 reported cases of PML occurring in patients being treated for multiple sclerosis and inflammatory bowel disease with natalizumab, a humanized monoclonal antibody that inhibits lymphocyte trafficking into CNS and bowel mucosa by binding to α_4 integrins. Overall risk in these patients has been estimated at ~3.4 PML cases per 1000 treated patients, but the risk depends on a variety of factors including anti-JCV antibody serostatus, prior immunosuppressive therapy use, and duration of natalizumab therapy. Patients who lack detectable JCV antibody have a risk of developing PML of <0.1 case/1000 patients, whereas those who are JCV seropositive and have been exposed to prior immunosuppressive therapy and have received >24 months of natalizumab therapy have a risk of >1 case/100 treated patients. PML cases have also been reported in patients receiving other humanized monoclonal antibodies with immunomodulatory activity including efalizumab and rituximab, although the relative risks have not been clearly established. The basic clinical and diagnostic features appear to be similar in HIV-associated PML and PML associated with immunomodulatory drugs with the exception of an increased likelihood of peripheral enhancement in MRIs of PML lesions in immunomodulatory cases. In natalizumab-associated PML, patients will also almost invariably develop clinical and radiographic worsening of lesions with discontinuation of therapy, attributed to development of immune reconstitution inflammatory syndrome (IRIS).

Diagnostic Studies The diagnosis of PML is frequently suggested by MRI. MRI reveals multifocal asymmetric, coalescing white matter lesions located periventricularly, in the centrum semiovale, in the parietal-occipital region, and in the cerebellum. These lesions have increased signal on T2 and FLAIR images and decreased signal on T1-weighted images. HIV-PML lesions are classically nonenhancing (90%), but patients with immunomodulatory drug associated PML may have peripheral ring enhancement. PML lesions are not typically associated with edema or mass effect. CT scans, which are less sensitive than MRI for the diagnosis of PML, often show hypodense nonenhancing white matter lesions.

The CSF is typically normal, although mild elevation in protein and/or IgG may be found. Pleocytosis occurs in <25% of cases, is predominantly mononuclear, and rarely exceeds 25 cells/μL. PCR amplification of JCV DNA from CSF has become an important diagnostic tool. The presence of a positive CSF PCR for JCV DNA in association with typical MRI lesions in the appropriate clinical setting is diagnostic of PML, reflecting the assay's relatively high specificity (92–100%); however, sensitivity is variable, and a negative CSF PCR does not exclude the diagnosis. In HIV-negative patients and HIV-positive patients not receiving highly active antiviral therapy (HAART), sensitivity is likely 70–90%. In HAART-treated patients, sensitivity may be closer to 60%, reflecting the lower JCV CSF viral load in this relatively more immunocompetent group. Studies with quantitative JCV CSF PCR indicate that patients with low JCV loads (<100 copies/μL) have a generally better prognosis than those with higher viral loads. Patients with negative CSF PCR studies may require brain biopsy for definitive diagnosis. In biopsy or necropsy specimens of brain, JCV antigen and nucleic acid can be detected by immunocytochemistry, in situ hybridization, or PCR amplification.

Serologic studies are of no utility in diagnosis due to high basal seroprevalence level, but may contribute to risk stratification in patients contemplating therapy with immunomodulatory drugs such as natalizumab.

TREATMENT PROGRESSIVE MULTIFOCAL LEUKOENCEPHALOPATHY

No effective therapy for PML is available. There are case reports of potential beneficial effects of the 5-HT_{2a} receptor antagonist mirtazapine, which may inhibit binding of JCV to its receptor on oligodendrocytes. Retrospective noncontrolled studies have also suggested a possible beneficial effect of treatment with interferon-α. Neither of these agents has been tested in randomized controlled clinical trials. A prospective multicenter clinical trial to evaluate the efficacy of the antimalarial drug mefloquine failed to show benefit. Intravenous and/or intrathecal cytarabine were not shown to be of benefit in a randomized controlled trial in HIV-associated PML, although some experts suggest that cytarabine may have therapeutic efficacy in situations where breakdown of the blood-brain barrier allows sufficient CSF penetration. A randomized controlled trial of cidofovir in HIV-associated PML also failed to show significant benefit. Because PML almost invariably occurs in immunocompromised individuals, any therapeutic interventions designed to enhance or restore immunocompetence should be considered. Perhaps the most dramatic demonstration of this is disease stabilization and, in rare cases, improvement associated with the improvement in the immune status of HIV-positive patients with AIDS following institution of HAART. In HIV-positive PML patients treated with HAART, 1-year survival is ~50%, although up to 80% of survivors may have significant neurologic sequelae. HIV-positive PML patients with higher CD4 counts (>300/μL) and low or nondetectable HIV viral loads have a better prognosis than those with lower CD4 counts and higher viral loads. Although institution of HAART enhances survival in HIV-positive PML patients, the associated immune reconstitution in patients with an underlying opportunistic infection such as PML may also result in a severe CNS inflammatory syndrome (IRIS) associated with clinical worsening, CSF pleocytosis, and the appearance of new enhancing MRI lesions. Patients receiving natalizumab or other immunomodulatory antibodies, who are suspected of having PML, should have therapy immediately halted and circulating antibodies removed by plasma exchange. Patients should be closely monitored for development of IRIS, which is generally treated with intravenous glucocorticoids, although controlled clinical trials of efficacy remain lacking.

SUBACUTE SCLEROSING PANENCEPHALITIS (SSPE)

SSPE is a rare chronic, progressive demyelinating disease of the CNS associated with a chronic nonpermissive infection of brain tissue with measles virus. The frequency has been estimated at 1 in 100,000–500,000 measles cases. An average of five cases per year are reported in the United States. The incidence has declined dramatically since the introduction of a measles vaccine. Most patients give a history of primary measles infection at an early age (2 years), which is followed after a latent interval of 6–8 years by the development of a progressive neurologic disorder. Some 85% of patients are between 5 and 15 years old at diagnosis. Initial manifestations include poor school performance and mood and personality changes. Typical signs of a CNS viral infection, including fever and headache, do not occur. As the disease progresses, patients develop progressive intellectual deterioration, focal and/or generalized seizures, myoclonus, ataxia, and visual disturbances. In the late stage of the illness, patients are unresponsive, quadriparetic, and spastic, with hyperactive tendon reflexes and extensor plantar responses.

Diagnostic Studies MRI is often normal early, although areas of increased T2 signal develop in the white matter of the brain and brainstem as disease progresses. The EEG may initially show only nonspecific slowing, but with disease progression, patients develop a characteristic periodic pattern with bursts of high-voltage, sharp, slow waves every 3–8 s, followed by periods of attenuated ("flat") background. The CSF is acellular with a normal or mildly elevated protein concentration and a markedly elevated gamma globulin level (>20% of total CSF protein). CSF antimeasles antibody levels are invariably elevated, and oligoclonal antimeasles antibodies are often present. Measles virus can be cultured from brain tissue using special cocultivation techniques. Viral antigen can be identified immunocytochemically, and viral genome can be detected by in situ hybridization or PCR amplification.

TREATMENT SUBACUTE SCLEROSING PANENCEPHALITIS

No definitive therapy for SSPE is available. Treatment with isoprinosine (Inosiplex, 100 mg/kg per day), alone or in combination with intrathecal or intraventricular interferon-α, has been reported to prolong survival and produce clinical improvement in some patients but has never been subjected to a controlled clinical trial.

PROGRESSIVE RUBELLA PANENCEPHALITIS

This is an extremely rare disorder that primarily affects males with congenital rubella syndrome, although isolated cases have been reported following childhood rubella. After a latent period of 8–19 years, patients develop progressive neurologic deterioration. The manifestations are similar to those seen in SSPE. CSF shows a mild lymphocytic pleocytosis, slightly elevated protein concentration, markedly increased gamma globulin, and rubella virus–specific oligoclonal bands. No therapy is available. Universal prevention of both congenital and childhood rubella through the use of the available live attenuated rubella vaccine would be expected to eliminate the disease.

BRAIN ABSCESS

DEFINITION

A brain abscess is a focal, suppurative infection within the brain parenchyma, typically surrounded by a vascularized capsule. The term *cerebritis* is often employed to describe a nonencapsulated brain abscess.

EPIDEMIOLOGY

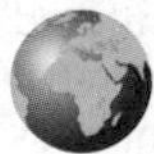

A bacterial brain abscess is a relatively uncommon intracranial infection, with an incidence of ~0.3–1.3:100,000 persons per year. Predisposing conditions include otitis media and mastoiditis, paranasal sinusitis, pyogenic infections in the chest or other body sites, penetrating head trauma or neurosurgical procedures, and dental infections. In immunocompetent individuals the most important pathogens are *Streptococcus* spp. (anaerobic, aerobic, and viridans [40%]), Enterobacteriaceae (*Proteus* spp., *E. coli* sp., *Klebsiella* spp. [25%]), anaerobes (e.g., *Bacteroides* spp., *Fusobacterium* spp. [30%]), and staphylococci (10%). In immunocompromised hosts with underlying HIV infection, organ transplantation, cancer, or immunosuppressive therapy, most brain abscesses are caused by *Nocardia* spp., *Toxoplasma gondii*, *Aspergillus* spp., *Candida* spp., and *C. neoformans*. In Latin America and in immigrants from Latin America, the most common cause of brain abscess is *Taenia solium* (neurocysticercosis). In India and East Asia, mycobacterial infection (tuberculoma) remains a major cause of focal CNS mass lesions.

ETIOLOGY

A brain abscess may develop (1) by direct spread from a contiguous cranial site of infection, such as paranasal sinusitis, otitis media, mastoiditis, or dental infection; (2) following head trauma or a neurosurgical procedure; or (3) as a result of hematogenous spread from a remote site of infection. In up to 25% of cases, no obvious primary source of infection is apparent (cryptogenic brain abscess).

Approximately one-third of brain abscesses are associated with otitis media and mastoiditis, often with an associated cholesteatoma.

Otogenic abscesses occur predominantly in the temporal lobe (55–75%) and cerebellum (20–30%). In some series, up to 90% of cerebellar abscesses are otogenic. Common organisms include streptococci, *Bacteroides* spp., *Pseudomonas* spp., *Haemophilus* spp., and Enterobacteriaceae. Abscesses that develop as a result of direct spread of infection from the frontal, ethmoidal, or sphenoidal sinuses and those that occur due to dental infections are usually located in the frontal lobes. Approximately 10% of brain abscesses are associated with paranasal sinusitis, and this association is particularly strong in young males in their second and third decades of life. The most common pathogens in brain abscesses associated with paranasal sinusitis are streptococci (especially *Streptococcus milleri*), *Haemophilus* spp., *Bacteroides* spp., *Pseudomonas* spp., and *S. aureus*. Dental infections are associated with ~2% of brain abscesses, although it is often suggested that many "cryptogenic" abscesses are in fact due to dental infections. The most common pathogens in this setting are streptococci, staphylococci, *Bacteroides* spp., and *Fusobacterium* spp.

Hematogenous abscesses account for ~25% of brain abscesses. Hematogenous abscesses are often multiple, and multiple abscesses often (50%) have a hematogenous origin. These abscesses show a predilection for the territory of the middle cerebral artery (i.e., posterior frontal or parietal lobes). Hematogenous abscesses are often located at the junction of the gray and white matter and are often poorly encapsulated. The microbiology of hematogenous abscesses is dependent on the primary source of infection. For example, brain abscesses that develop as a complication of infective endocarditis are often due to viridans streptococci or *S. aureus*. Abscesses associated with pyogenic lung infections such as lung abscess or bronchiectasis are often due to streptococci, staphylococci, *Bacteroides* spp., *Fusobacterium* spp., or Enterobacteriaceae. Abscesses that follow penetrating head trauma or neurosurgical procedures are frequently due to methicillin-resistant *S. aureus* (MRSA), *S. epidermidis*, Enterobacteriaceae, *Pseudomonas* spp., and *Clostridium* spp. Enterobacteriaceae and *P. aeruginosa* are important causes of abscesses associated with urinary sepsis. Congenital cardiac malformations that produce a right-to-left shunt, such as tetralogy of Fallot, patent ductus arteriosus, and atrial and ventricular septal defects, allow bloodborne bacteria to bypass the pulmonary capillary bed and reach the brain. Similar phenomena can occur with pulmonary arteriovenous malformations. The decreased arterial oxygenation and saturation from the right-to-left shunt and polycythemia may cause focal areas of cerebral ischemia, thus providing a nidus for microorganisms that bypassed the pulmonary circulation to multiply and form an abscess. Streptococci are the most common pathogens in this setting.

PATHOGENESIS AND HISTOPATHOLOGY

Results of experimental models of brain abscess formation suggest that for bacterial invasion of brain parenchyma to occur, there must be preexisting or concomitant areas of ischemia, necrosis, or hypoxemia in brain tissue. The intact brain parenchyma is relatively resistant to infection. Once bacteria have established infection, brain abscess frequently evolves through a series of stages, influenced by the nature of the infecting organism and by the immunocompetence of the host. The early cerebritis stage (days 1–3) is characterized by a perivascular infiltration of inflammatory cells, which surround a central core of coagulative necrosis. Marked edema surrounds the lesion at this stage. In the late cerebritis stage (days 4–9), pus formation leads to enlargement of the necrotic center, which is surrounded at its border by an inflammatory infiltrate of macrophages and fibroblasts. A thin capsule of fibroblasts and reticular fibers gradually develops, and the surrounding area of cerebral edema becomes more distinct than in the previous stage. The third stage, early capsule formation (days 10–13), is characterized by the formation of a capsule that is better developed on the cortical than on the ventricular side of the lesion. This stage correlates with the appearance of a ring-enhancing capsule on neuroimaging studies. The final stage, late capsule formation (day 14 and beyond), is defined by a well-formed necrotic center surrounded by a dense collagenous capsule. The surrounding area of cerebral edema has regressed, but marked gliosis with large numbers of reactive astrocytes has developed outside the capsule. This gliotic process may contribute to the development of seizures as a sequela of brain abscess.

CLINICAL PRESENTATION

A brain abscess typically presents as an expanding intracranial mass lesion rather than as an infectious process. Although the evolution of signs and symptoms is extremely variable, ranging from hours to weeks or even months, most patients present to the hospital 11–12 days following onset of symptoms. The classic clinical triad of headache, fever, and a focal neurologic deficit is present in <50% of cases. The most common symptom in patients with a brain abscess is headache, occurring in >75% of patients. The headache is often characterized as a constant, dull, aching sensation, either hemicranial or generalized, and it becomes progressively more severe and refractory to therapy. Fever is present in only 50% of patients at the time of diagnosis, and its absence should not exclude the diagnosis. The new onset of focal or generalized seizure activity is a presenting sign in 15–35% of patients. Focal neurologic deficits including hemiparesis, aphasia, or visual field defects are part of the initial presentation in >60% of patients.

The clinical presentation of a brain abscess depends on its location, the nature of the primary infection if present, and the level of the ICP. Hemiparesis is the most common localizing sign of a frontal lobe abscess. A temporal lobe abscess may present with a disturbance of language (dysphasia) or an upper homonymous quadrantanopia. Nystagmus and ataxia are signs of a cerebellar abscess. Signs of raised ICP—papilledema, nausea and vomiting, and drowsiness or confusion—can be the dominant presentation of some abscesses, particularly those in the cerebellum. Meningismus is not present unless the abscess has ruptured into the ventricle or the infection has spread to the subarachnoid space.

DIAGNOSIS

Diagnosis is made by neuroimaging studies. MRI (Fig. 164-4) is better than CT for demonstrating abscesses in the early (cerebritis) stages and is superior to CT for identifying abscesses in the posterior fossa. Cerebritis appears on MRI as an area of low-signal intensity on T1-weighted images with irregular postgadolinium enhancement and as an area of increased signal intensity on T2-weighted images. Cerebritis is often not visualized by CT scan, but when present, appears as an area of hypodensity. On a contrast-enhanced CT scan, a mature brain abscess appears as a focal area of hypodensity surrounded by ring enhancement with surrounding edema (hypodensity). On contrast-enhanced T1-weighted MRI, a mature brain abscess has a capsule that enhances surrounding a hypodense center and surrounded by a hypodense area of edema. On T2-weighted MRI, there is a hyperintense central area of pus surrounded by a well-defined hypointense capsule and a hyperintense surrounding area of edema. It is important to recognize that the CT and MRI appearance, particularly of the capsule, may be altered by treatment with glucocorticoids. The distinction between a brain abscess and other focal CNS lesions such as primary or metastatic tumors may be facilitated by the use of diffusion-weighted imaging sequences on which a brain abscess typically shows increased signal due to restricted diffusion of the abscess cavity with corresponding low signal on apparent diffusion coefficient images.

Microbiologic diagnosis of the etiologic agent is most accurately determined by Gram's stain and culture of abscess material obtained by CT-guided stereotactic needle aspiration. Aerobic and anaerobic bacterial cultures and mycobacterial and fungal cultures should be obtained. Up to 10% of patients will also have positive blood cultures. LP should not be performed in patients with known or suspected focal intracranial infections such as abscess or empyema; CSF analysis contributes nothing to diagnosis or therapy, and LP increases the risk of herniation.

Additional laboratory studies may provide clues to the diagnosis of brain abscess in patients with a CNS mass lesion. About 50% of patients have a peripheral leukocytosis, 60% an elevated ESR, and 80% an elevated C-reactive protein. Blood cultures are positive in ~10% of cases overall but may be positive in >85% of patients with abscesses due to *Listeria*.

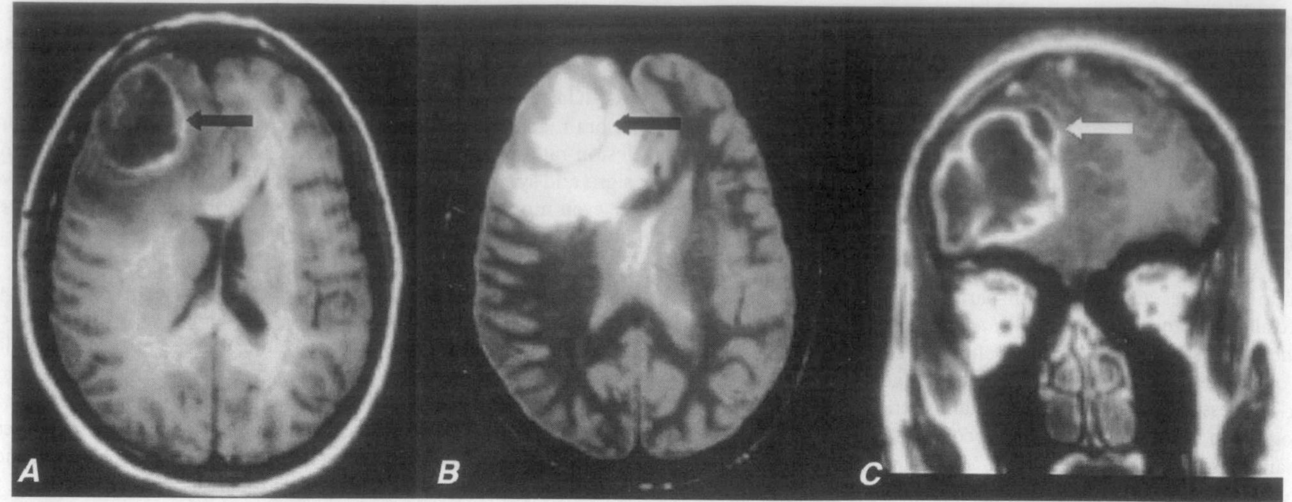

FIGURE 164-4 Pneumococcal brain abscess. Note that the abscess wall has hyperintense signal on the axial T1-weighted magnetic resonance imaging (MRI) (***A***, *black arrow*), hypointense signal on the axial proton density images (***B***, *black arrow*), and enhances prominently after gadolinium administration on the coronal T1-weighted image (***C***). The abscess is surrounded by a large amount of vasogenic edema and has a small "daughter" abscess (***C***, *white arrow*). (*Courtesy of Joseph Lurito, MD; with permission.*)

DIFFERENTIAL DIAGNOSIS

Conditions that can cause headache, fever, focal neurologic signs, and seizure activity include brain abscess, subdural empyema, bacterial meningitis, viral meningoencephalitis, superior sagittal sinus thrombosis, and acute disseminated encephalomyelitis. When fever is absent, primary and metastatic brain tumors become the major differential diagnosis. Less commonly, cerebral infarction or hematoma can have an MRI or CT appearance resembling brain abscess.

TREATMENT BRAIN ABSCESS

Optimal therapy of brain abscesses involves a combination of high-dose parenteral antibiotics and neurosurgical drainage. Empirical therapy of community-acquired brain abscess in an immunocompetent patient typically includes a third- or fourth-generation cephalosporin (e.g., cefotaxime, ceftriaxone, or cefepime) and metronidazole (see Table 164-1 for antibiotic dosages). In patients with penetrating head trauma or recent neurosurgical procedures, treatment should include ceftazidime as the third-generation cephalosporin to enhance coverage of *Pseudomonas* spp. and vancomycin for coverage of staphylococci. Meropenem plus vancomycin also provides good coverage in this setting.

Aspiration and drainage of the abscess under stereotactic guidance are beneficial for both diagnosis and therapy. Empirical antibiotic coverage should be modified based on the results of Gram's stain and culture of the abscess contents. Complete excision of a bacterial abscess via craniotomy or craniectomy is generally reserved for multiloculated abscesses or those in which stereotactic aspiration is unsuccessful.

Medical therapy alone is not optimal for treatment of brain abscess and should be reserved for patients whose abscesses are neurosurgically inaccessible, for patients with small (<2–3 cm) or nonencapsulated abscesses (cerebritis), and for patients whose condition is too tenuous to allow performance of a neurosurgical procedure. All patients should receive a minimum of 6–8 weeks of parenteral antibiotic therapy. The role, if any, of supplemental oral antibiotic therapy following completion of a standard course of parenteral therapy has never been adequately studied.

In addition to surgical drainage and antibiotic therapy, patients should receive prophylactic anticonvulsant therapy because of the high risk (~35%) of focal or generalized seizures. Anticonvulsant therapy is continued for at least 3 months after resolution of the abscess, and decisions regarding withdrawal are then based on the EEG. If the EEG is abnormal, anticonvulsant therapy should be continued. If the EEG is normal, anticonvulsant therapy can be slowly withdrawn, with close follow-up and repeat EEG after the medication has been discontinued.

Glucocorticoids should not be given routinely to patients with brain abscesses. Intravenous dexamethasone therapy (10 mg every 6 h) is usually reserved for patients with substantial periabscess edema and associated mass effect and increased ICP. Dexamethasone should be tapered as rapidly as possible to avoid delaying the natural process of encapsulation of the abscess.

Serial MRI or CT scans should be obtained on a monthly or twice-monthly basis to document resolution of the abscess. More frequent studies (e.g., weekly) are probably warranted in the subset of patients who are receiving antibiotic therapy alone. A small amount of enhancement may remain for months after the abscess has been successfully treated.

PROGNOSIS

The mortality rate of brain abscess has declined in parallel with the development of enhanced neuroimaging techniques, improved neurosurgical procedures for stereotactic aspiration, and improved antibiotics. In modern series, the mortality rate is typically <15%. Significant sequelae, including seizures, persisting weakness, aphasia, or mental impairment, occur in ≥20% of survivors.

NONBACTERIAL CAUSES OF INFECTIOUS FOCAL CNS LESIONS

ETIOLOGY

Neurocysticercosis is the most common parasitic disease of the CNS worldwide. Humans acquire cysticercosis by the ingestion of food contaminated with the eggs of the parasite *T. solium*. Toxoplasmosis is a parasitic disease caused by *T. gondii* and acquired from the ingestion of undercooked meat and from handling cat feces.

CLINICAL PRESENTATION

The most common manifestation of neurocysticercosis is new-onset partial seizures with or without secondary generalization. Cysticerci may develop in the brain parenchyma and cause seizures or focal neurologic deficits. When present in the subarachnoid or ventricular spaces, cysticerci can produce increased ICP by interference with CSF flow. Spinal cysticerci can mimic the presentation of intraspinal tumors. When the cysticerci first lodge in the brain, they frequently cause little in the way of an inflammatory response. As the cysticercal cyst degenerates, it elicits an inflammatory response that may present clinically as a seizure. Eventually the cyst dies, a process that may take several years and is typically associated with resolution of the inflammatory response and, often, abatement of seizures.

Primary *Toxoplasma* infection is often asymptomatic. However, during this phase parasites may spread to the CNS, where they become latent. Reactivation of CNS infection is almost exclusively associated with immunocompromised hosts, particularly those with HIV infection. During this phase patients present with headache, fever, seizures, and focal neurologic deficits.

DIAGNOSIS

The lesions of neurocysticercosis are readily visualized by MRI or CT scans. Lesions with viable parasites appear as cystic lesions. The scolex can often be visualized on MRI. Lesions may appear as contrast-enhancing lesions surrounded by edema. A very early sign of cyst death is hypointensity of the vesicular fluid on T2-weighted images when compared with CSF. Parenchymal brain calcifications are the most common finding and evidence that the parasite is no longer viable. MRI findings of toxoplasmosis consist of multiple lesions in the deep white matter, the thalamus, and basal ganglia and at the gray-white junction in the cerebral hemispheres. With contrast administration, the majority of the lesions enhance in a ringed, nodular, or homogeneous pattern and are surrounded by edema. In the presence of the characteristic neuroimaging abnormalities of *T. gondii* infection, serum IgG antibody to *T. gondii* should be obtained and, when positive, the patient should be treated.

TREATMENT INFECTIOUS FOCAL CNS LESIONS

Anticonvulsant therapy is initiated when the patient with neurocysticercosis presents with a seizure. There is controversy about whether or not anthelmintic therapy should be given to all patients, and recommendations are based on the stage of the lesion. Cysticerci appearing as cystic lesions in the brain parenchyma with or without pericystic edema or in the subarachnoid space at the convexity of the cerebral hemispheres should be treated with anticysticidal therapy. Cysticidal drugs accelerate the destruction of the parasites, resulting in a faster resolution of the infection. Albendazole and praziquantel are used in the treatment of neurocysticercosis. Approximately 85% of parenchymal cysts are destroyed by a single course of albendazole, and ~75% are destroyed by a single course of praziquantel. The dose of albendazole is 15 mg/kg per day in two doses for 8 days. The dose of praziquantel is 50 mg/kg per day for 15 days, although a number of other dosage regimens are also frequently cited. Prednisone or dexamethasone is given with anticysticidal therapy to reduce the host inflammatory response to degenerating parasites. Many, but not all, experts recommend anticysticidal therapy for lesions that are surrounded by a contrast-enhancing ring. There is universal agreement that calcified lesions do not need to be treated with anticysticidal therapy. Antiepileptic therapy can be stopped once the follow-up CT scan shows resolution of the lesion. Long-term antiepileptic therapy is recommended when seizures occur after resolution of edema and resorption or calcification of the degenerating cyst.

CNS toxoplasmosis is treated with a combination of sulfadiazine, 1.5–2.0 g orally qid, plus pyrimethamine, 100 mg orally to load, then 75–100 mg orally qd, plus folinic acid, 10–15 mg orally qd. Folinic acid is added to the regimen to prevent megaloblastic anemia. Therapy is continued until there is no evidence of active disease on neuroimaging studies, which typically takes at least 6 weeks, and then the dose of sulfadiazine is reduced to 2–4 g/d and pyrimethamine to 50 mg/d. Clindamycin plus pyrimethamine is an alternative therapy for patients who cannot tolerate sulfadiazine, but the combination of pyrimethamine and sulfadiazine is more effective.

SUBDURAL EMPYEMA

A subdural empyema (SDE) is a collection of pus between the dura and arachnoid membranes (Fig. 164-5).

EPIDEMIOLOGY

SDE is a rare disorder that accounts for 15–25% of focal suppurative CNS infections. Sinusitis is the most common predisposing condition and typically involves the frontal sinuses, either alone or in combination with the ethmoid and maxillary sinuses. Sinusitis-associated empyema has a striking predilection for young males, possibly reflecting sex-related differences in sinus anatomy and development. It has been suggested that SDE may complicate 1–2% of cases of frontal sinusitis severe enough to require hospitalization. As a consequence of this epidemiology, SDE shows an ~3:1 male/female predominance, with 70% of cases occurring in the second and third decades of life. SDE may also develop as a complication of head trauma or neurosurgery. Secondary infection of a subdural effusion may also result in empyema, although secondary infection of hematomas, in the absence of a prior neurosurgical procedure, is rare.

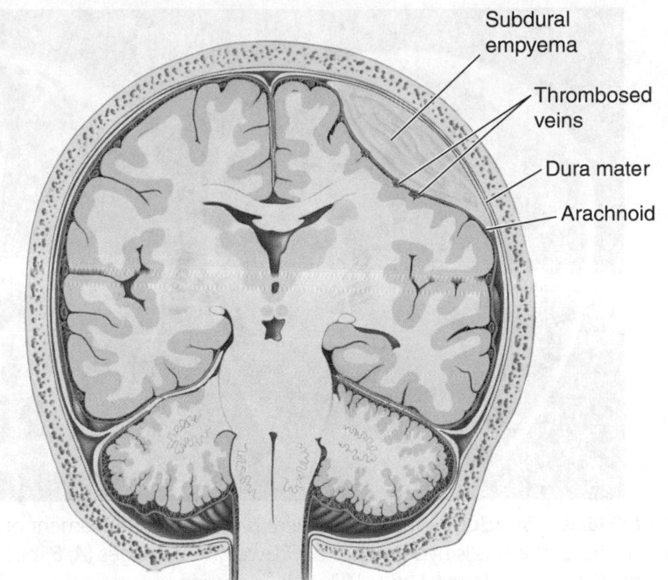

FIGURE 164-5 Subdural empyema.

ETIOLOGY

Aerobic and anaerobic streptococci, staphylococci, Enterobacteriaceae, and anaerobic bacteria are the most common causative organisms of sinusitis-associated SDE. Staphylococci and gram-negative bacilli are often the etiologic organisms when SDE follows neurosurgical procedures or head trauma. Up to one-third of cases are culture-negative, possibly reflecting difficulty in obtaining adequate anaerobic cultures.

PATHOPHYSIOLOGY

Sinusitis-associated SDE develops as a result of either retrograde spread of infection from septic thrombophlebitis of the mucosal veins draining the sinuses or contiguous spread of infection to the brain from osteomyelitis in the posterior wall of the frontal or other sinuses. SDE may also develop from direct introduction of bacteria into the subdural space as a complication of a neurosurgical procedure. The evolution of SDE can be extremely rapid because the subdural space is a large compartment that offers few mechanical barriers to the spread of infection. In patients with sinusitis-associated SDE, suppuration typically begins in the upper and anterior portions of one cerebral hemisphere and then extends posteriorly. SDE is often associated with other intracranial infections, including epidural empyema (40%), cortical thrombophlebitis (35%), and intracranial abscess or cerebritis (>25%). Cortical venous infarction produces necrosis of underlying cerebral cortex and subcortical white matter, with focal neurologic deficits and seizures (see below).

CLINICAL PRESENTATION

A patient with SDE typically presents with fever and a progressively worsening headache. The diagnosis of SDE should always be suspected in a patient with known sinusitis who presents with new CNS signs or symptoms. Patients with underlying sinusitis frequently have symptoms related to this infection. As the infection progresses, focal

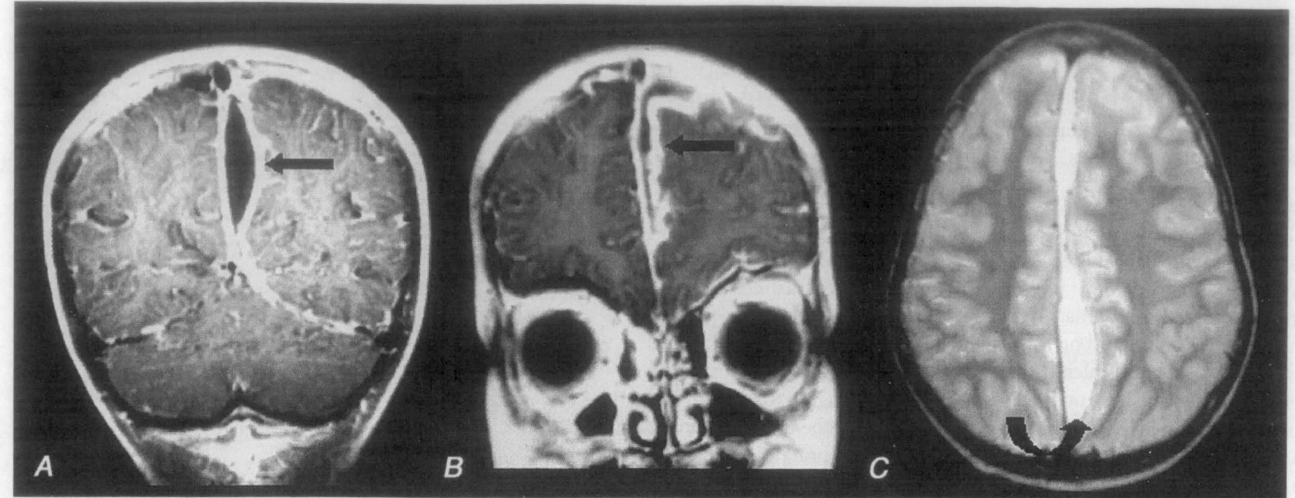

FIGURE 164-6 **Subdural empyema.** There is marked enhancement of the dura and leptomeninges (***A, B***, *straight arrows*) along the left medial hemisphere. The pus is hypointense on T1-weighted images (***A, B***) but markedly hyperintense on the proton density–weighted (***C***, *curved arrow*) image. *(Courtesy of Joseph Lurito, MD; with permission.)*

neurologic deficits, seizures, nuchal rigidity, and signs of increased ICP commonly occur. Headache is the most common complaint at the time of presentation; initially it is localized to the side of the subdural infection, but then it becomes more severe and generalized. Contralateral hemiparesis or hemiplegia is the most common focal neurologic deficit and can occur from the direct effects of the SDE on the cortex or as a consequence of venous infarction. Seizures begin as partial motor seizures that then become secondarily generalized. Seizures may be due to the direct irritative effect of the SDE on the underlying cortex or result from cortical venous infarction (see above). In untreated SDE, the increasing mass effect and increase in ICP cause progressive deterioration in consciousness, leading ultimately to coma.

DIAGNOSIS

MRI (Fig. 164-6) is superior to CT in identifying SDE and any associated intracranial infections. The administration of gadolinium greatly improves diagnosis by enhancing the rim of the empyema and allowing the empyema to be clearly delineated from the underlying brain parenchyma. Cranial MRI is also extremely valuable in identifying sinusitis, other focal CNS infections, cortical venous infarction, cerebral edema, and cerebritis. CT may show a crescent-shaped hypodense lesion over one or both hemispheres or in the interhemispheric fissure. Frequently the degree of mass effect, exemplified by midline shift, ventricular compression, and sulcal effacement, is far out of proportion to the mass of the SDE.

CSF examination should be avoided in patients with known or suspected SDE because it adds no useful information and is associated with the risk of cerebral herniation.

DIFFERENTIAL DIAGNOSIS

The differential diagnosis of the combination of headache, fever, focal neurologic signs, and seizure activity that progresses rapidly to an altered level of consciousness includes subdural hematoma, bacterial meningitis, viral encephalitis, brain abscess, superior sagittal sinus thrombosis, and acute disseminated encephalomyelitis. The presence of nuchal rigidity is unusual with brain abscess or epidural empyema and should suggest the possibility of SDE when associated with significant focal neurologic signs and fever. Patients with bacterial meningitis also have nuchal rigidity but do not typically have focal deficits of the severity seen with SDE.

TREATMENT SUBDURAL EMPYEMA

SDE is a medical emergency. Emergent neurosurgical evacuation of the empyema, either through craniotomy, craniectomy, or burr-hole drainage, is the definitive step in the management of this infection. Empirical antimicrobial therapy for community-acquired SDE should include a combination of a third-generation cephalosporin (e.g., cefotaxime or ceftriaxone), vancomycin, and metronidazole (see Table 164-1 for dosages). Patients with hospital-acquired SDE may have infections due to *Pseudomonas* spp. or MRSA and should receive coverage with a carbapenem (e.g., meropenem) and vancomycin. Metronidazole is not necessary for antianaerobic therapy when meropenem is being used. Parenteral antibiotic therapy should be continued for a minimum of 3–4 weeks after SDE drainage. Patients with associated cranial osteomyelitis may require longer therapy. Specific diagnosis of the etiologic organisms is made based on Gram's stain and culture of fluid obtained via either burr holes or craniotomy; the initial empirical antibiotic coverage can be modified accordingly.

PROGNOSIS

Prognosis is influenced by the level of consciousness of the patient at the time of hospital presentation, the size of the empyema, and the speed with which therapy is instituted. Long-term neurologic sequelae, which include seizures and hemiparesis, occur in up to 50% of cases.

CRANIAL EPIDURAL ABSCESS

Cranial epidural abscess is a suppurative infection occurring in the potential space between the inner skull table and dura (Fig. 164-7).

ETIOLOGY AND PATHOPHYSIOLOGY

Cranial epidural abscess is less common than either brain abscess or SDE and accounts for <2% of focal suppurative CNS infections. A

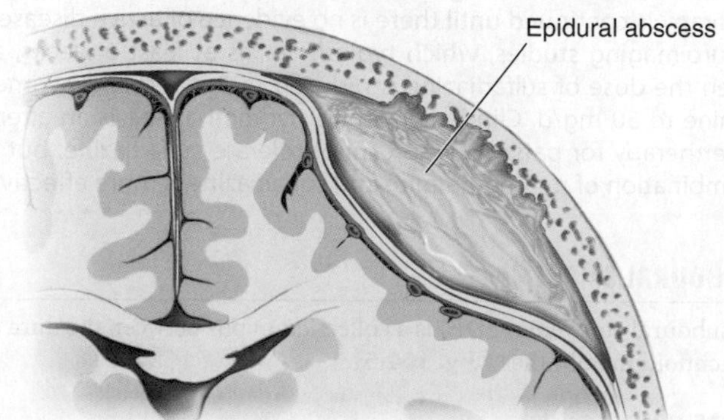

FIGURE 164-7 **Cranial epidural abscess** is a collection of pus between the dura and the inner table of the skull.

cranial epidural abscess develops as a complication of a craniotomy or compound skull fracture or as a result of spread of infection from the frontal sinuses, middle ear, mastoid, or orbit. An epidural abscess may develop contiguous to an area of osteomyelitis, when craniotomy is complicated by infection of the wound or bone flap, or as a result of direct infection of the epidural space. Infection in the frontal sinus, middle ear, mastoid, or orbit can reach the epidural space through retrograde spread of infection from septic thrombophlebitis in the emissary veins that drain these areas or by way of direct spread of infection through areas of osteomyelitis. Unlike the subdural space, the epidural space is really a potential rather than an actual compartment. The dura is normally tightly adherent to the inner skull table, and infection must dissect the dura away from the skull table as it spreads. As a result, epidural abscesses are often smaller than SDEs. Cranial epidural abscesses, unlike brain abscesses, only rarely result from hematogenous spread of infection from extracranial primary sites. The bacteriology of a cranial epidural abscess is similar to that of SDE (see above). The etiologic organisms of an epidural abscess that arises from frontal sinusitis, middle-ear infections, or mastoiditis are usually streptococci or anaerobic organisms. Staphylococci or gram-negative organisms are the usual cause of an epidural abscess that develops as a complication of craniotomy or compound skull fracture.

CLINICAL PRESENTATION

Patients present with fever (60%), headache (40%), nuchal rigidity (35%), seizures (10%), and focal deficits (5%). Development of symptoms may be insidious, as the empyema usually enlarges slowly in the confined anatomic space between the dura and the inner table of the skull. Periorbital edema and Pott's puffy tumor, reflecting underlying associated frontal bone osteomyelitis, are present in ~40%. In patients with a recent neurosurgical procedure, wound infection is invariably present, but other symptoms may be subtle and can include altered mental status (45%), fever (35%), and headache (20%). The diagnosis should be considered when fever and headache follow recent head trauma or occur in the setting of frontal sinusitis, mastoiditis, or otitis media.

DIAGNOSIS

Cranial MRI with gadolinium enhancement is the procedure of choice to demonstrate a cranial epidural abscess. The sensitivity of CT is limited by the presence of signal artifacts arising from the bone of the inner skull table. The CT appearance of an epidural empyema is that of a lens or crescent-shaped hypodense extraaxial lesion. On MRI, an epidural empyema appears as a lentiform or crescent-shaped fluid collection that is hyperintense compared to CSF on T2-weighted images. On T1-weighted images, the fluid collection may be either isointense or hypointense compared to brain. Following the administration of gadolinium, there is linear enhancement of the dura on T1-weighted images. In distinction to subdural empyema, signs of mass effect or other parenchymal abnormalities are uncommon.

TREATMENT EPIDURAL ABSCESS

Immediate neurosurgical drainage is indicated. Empirical antimicrobial therapy, pending the results of Gram's stain and culture of the purulent material obtained at surgery, should include a combination of a third-generation cephalosporin, vancomycin, and metronidazole (Table 164-1). Ceftazidime or meropenem should be substituted for ceftriaxone or cefotaxime in neurosurgical patients. Metronidazole is not necessary for antianaerobic coverage in patients receiving meropenem. When the organism has been identified, antimicrobial therapy can be modified accordingly. Antibiotics should be continued for 3–6 weeks after surgical drainage. Patients with associated osteomyelitis may require additional therapy.

PROGNOSIS

The mortality rate is <5% in modern series, and full recovery is the rule in most survivors.

SUPPURATIVE THROMBOPHLEBITIS

DEFINITION

Suppurative intracranial thrombophlebitis is septic venous thrombosis of cortical veins and sinuses. This may occur as a complication of bacterial meningitis; SDE; epidural abscess; or infection in the skin of the face, paranasal sinuses, middle ear, or mastoid.

ANATOMY AND PATHOPHYSIOLOGY

The cerebral veins and venous sinuses have no valves; therefore, blood within them can flow in either direction. The superior sagittal sinus is the largest of the venous sinuses (Fig. 164-8). It receives blood from the frontal, parietal, and occipital superior cerebral veins and the diploic veins, which communicate with the meningeal veins. Bacterial meningitis is a common predisposing condition for septic thrombosis of the superior sagittal sinus. The diploic veins, which drain into the superior sagittal sinus, provide a route for the spread of infection from the meninges, especially in cases where there is purulent exudate near areas of the superior sagittal sinus. Infection can also spread to the superior sagittal sinus from nearby SDE or epidural abscess. Dehydration from vomiting, hypercoagulable states, and immunologic abnormalities, including the presence of circulating antiphospholipid antibodies, also contribute to cerebral venous sinus thrombosis. Thrombosis may extend from one sinus to another, and at autopsy, thrombi of different histologic ages can often be detected in several sinuses. Thrombosis of the superior sagittal sinus is often associated with thrombosis of superior cortical veins and small parenchymal hemorrhages.

The superior sagittal sinus drains into the transverse sinuses (Fig. 164-8). The transverse sinuses also receive venous drainage from small veins from both the middle ear and mastoid cells. The transverse sinus becomes the sigmoid sinus before draining into the internal jugular vein. Septic transverse/sigmoid sinus thrombosis can be a complication of acute and chronic otitis media or mastoiditis. Infection spreads from the mastoid air cells to the transverse sinus via the emissary veins or by direct invasion. The cavernous sinuses are inferior to the superior sagittal sinus at the base of the skull. The cavernous sinuses receive blood from the facial veins via the superior and inferior ophthalmic veins. Bacteria in the facial veins enter the cavernous sinus via these veins. Bacteria in the sphenoid and ethmoid sinuses can spread to the cavernous sinuses via the small emissary veins. The sphenoid and ethmoid sinuses are the most common sites of primary infection resulting in septic cavernous sinus thrombosis.

CLINICAL MANIFESTATIONS

Septic thrombosis of the superior sagittal sinus presents with headache, fever, nausea and vomiting, confusion, and focal or generalized seizures. There may be a rapid development of stupor and coma.

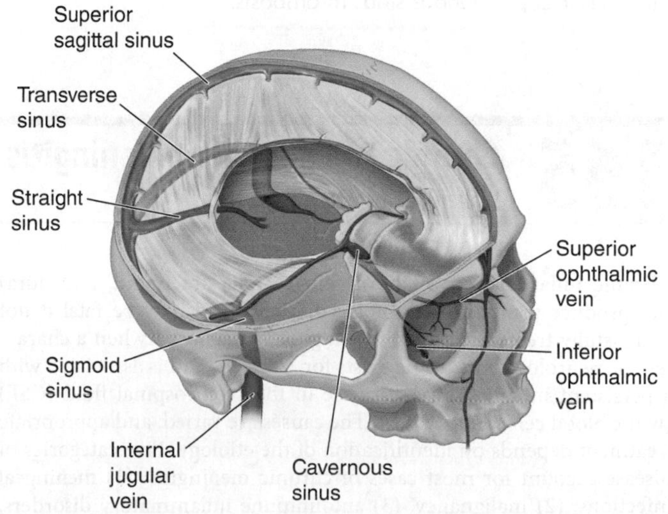

FIGURE 164-8 Anatomy of the cerebral venous sinuses.

Weakness of the lower extremities with bilateral Babinski's signs or hemiparesis is often present. When superior sagittal sinus thrombosis occurs as a complication of bacterial meningitis, nuchal rigidity and Kernig's and Brudzinski's signs may be present.

The oculomotor nerve, the trochlear nerve, the abducens nerve, the ophthalmic and maxillary branches of the trigeminal nerve, and the internal carotid artery all pass through the cavernous sinus (see Fig. 455-4). The symptoms of *septic cavernous sinus thrombosis* are fever, headache, frontal and retroorbital pain, and diplopia. The classic signs are ptosis, proptosis, chemosis, and extraocular dysmotility due to deficits of cranial nerves III, IV, and VI; hyperesthesia of the ophthalmic and maxillary divisions of the fifth cranial nerve and a decreased corneal reflex may be detected. There may be evidence of dilated, tortuous retinal veins and papilledema.

Headache and earache are the most frequent symptoms of *transverse sinus thrombosis*. A transverse sinus thrombosis may also present with otitis media, sixth nerve palsy, and retroorbital or facial pain (*Gradenigo's syndrome*). Sigmoid sinus and internal jugular vein thrombosis may present with neck pain.

DIAGNOSIS

The diagnosis of septic venous sinus thrombosis is suggested by an absent flow void within the affected venous sinus on MRI and confirmed by magnetic resonance venography, CT angiogram, or the venous phase of cerebral angiography. The diagnosis of thrombophlebitis of intracerebral and meningeal veins is suggested by the presence of intracerebral hemorrhage but requires cerebral angiography for definitive diagnosis.

TREATMENT SUPPURATIVE THROMBOPHLEBITIS

Septic venous sinus thrombosis is treated with antibiotics, hydration, and removal of infected tissue and thrombus in septic lateral or cavernous sinus thrombosis. The choice of antimicrobial therapy is based on the bacteria responsible for the predisposing or associated condition. Optimal duration of therapy is unknown, but antibiotics are usually continued for 6 weeks or until there is radiographic evidence of resolution of thrombosis. Anticoagulation with dose-adjusted intravenous heparin is recommended for aseptic venous sinus thrombosis and in the treatment of septic venous sinus thrombosis complicating bacterial meningitis in patients who have progressive neurologic deterioration despite antimicrobial therapy and intravenous fluids. The presence of a small intracerebral hemorrhage from septic thrombophlebitis is not an absolute contraindication to heparin therapy. Successful management of aseptic venous sinus thrombosis has been reported with surgical thrombectomy, catheter-directed urokinase therapy, and a combination of intrathrombus recombinant tissue plasminogen activator (rtPA) and intravenous heparin, but there are not enough data to recommend these therapies in septic venous sinus thrombosis.

165 Chronic and Recurrent Meningitis

Walter J. Koroshetz, Avindra Nath

Chronic inflammation of the meninges (pia, arachnoid, and dura) can produce profound neurologic disability and may be fatal if not successfully treated. Chronic meningitis is diagnosed when a characteristic neurologic syndrome exists for >4 weeks and is associated with a persistent inflammatory response in the cerebrospinal fluid (CSF) (white blood cell count >5/μL). The causes are varied, and appropriate treatment depends on identification of the etiology. Five categories of disease account for most cases of chronic meningitis: (1) meningeal infections, (2) malignancy, (3) autoimmune inflammatory disorders, (4) chemical meningitis, and (5) parameningeal infections.

TABLE 165-1 SYMPTOMS AND SIGNS OF CHRONIC MENINGITIS

Symptom	Sign
Chronic headache	± Papilledema
Neck or back pain/stiffness	Brudzinski's or Kernig's sign of meningeal irritation
Change in personality	Altered mental status—drowsiness, inattention, disorientation, memory loss, frontal release signs (grasp, suck, snout), perseveration
Facial weakness	Peripheral seventh CN paresis
Double vision	Paresis of CNs III, IV, VI
Diminished Vision	Papilledema, optic atrophy
Hearing loss	Eighth CN paresis
Arm or leg weakness	Myelopathy or radiculopathy
Numbness in arms or legs	Myelopathy or radiculopathy
Urinary retention/incontinence	Myelopathy or radiculopathy Frontal lobe dysfunction (hydrocephalus)
Clumsiness	Ataxia

Abbreviation: CN, cranial nerve.

CLINICAL PATHOPHYSIOLOGY

Neurologic manifestations of chronic meningitis (Table 165-1) are determined by the anatomic location of the inflammation and its consequences. Persistent headache with or without a stiff neck, hydrocephalus, cranial neuropathies, radiculopathies, and cognitive or personality changes are the cardinal features. These can occur alone or in combination. When they appear in combination, widespread dissemination of the inflammatory process along CSF pathways has occurred. In some cases, the presence of an underlying systemic illness points to a specific agent or class of agents as the probable cause. The diagnosis of chronic meningitis is usually made when the clinical presentation prompts the physician to examine the CSF for signs of inflammation. CSF is produced by the choroid plexus of the cerebral ventricles, exits through narrow foramina into the subarachnoid space surrounding the brain and spinal cord, circulates around the base of the brain and over the cerebral hemispheres, and is resorbed by arachnoid villi projecting into the superior sagittal sinus. CSF flow provides a pathway for rapid spread of infectious and other infiltrative processes over the brain, spinal cord, and cranial and spinal nerve roots. Spread from the subarachnoid space into brain parenchyma may occur via the arachnoid cuffs that surround blood vessels that penetrate brain tissue (Virchow-Robin spaces).

Intracranial Meningitis Nociceptive nerve fibers of the meninges are stimulated by the inflammatory process, resulting in headache, neck pain, or back pain. Obstruction of CSF pathways at the foramina or arachnoid villi may produce *hydrocephalus* and symptoms of raised intracranial pressure (ICP), including headache, vomiting, apathy or drowsiness, gait instability, papilledema, visual loss, impaired upgaze, or palsy of the sixth cranial nerve (CN) (Chap. 455). Cognitive and behavioral changes during the course of chronic meningitis may also result from vascular damage, which may similarly produce seizures, stroke, or myelopathy. Inflammatory deposits seeded via the CSF circulation are often prominent around the brainstem and cranial nerves and along the undersurface of the frontal and temporal lobes. Such cases, termed *basal meningitis*, often present as multiple cranial neuropathies, with decreased vision (CN II), facial weakness (CN VII), decreased hearing (CN VIII), diplopia (CNs III, IV, and VI), sensory or motor abnormalities of the oropharynx (CNs IX, X, and XII), decreased olfaction (CN I), or decreased facial sensation and masseter weakness (CN V).

Spinal Meningitis Injury may occur to motor and sensory roots as they traverse the subarachnoid space and penetrate the meninges. These cases present as multiple radiculopathies with combinations of radicular pain, sensory loss, motor weakness, and urinary or fecal incontinence. Meningeal inflammation can encircle the cord, resulting in a myelopathy. Patients with slowly progressive involvement of multiple cranial nerves and/or spinal nerve roots are likely to have chronic meningitis. Electrophysiologic testing (electromyography, nerve conduction studies, and evoked response testing) may be helpful in determining whether there is involvement of cranial and spinal nerve roots.

Systemic Manifestations In some patients, evidence of systemic disease provides clues to the underlying cause of chronic meningitis. A complete history of travel, sexual practice, and exposure to infectious agents should be sought. Infectious causes are often associated with fever, malaise, anorexia, and signs of localized or disseminated infection outside the nervous system. Infectious causes are of major concern in the immunosuppressed patient, especially in patients with AIDS, in whom chronic meningitis may present without headache or fever. Noninfectious inflammatory disorders often produce systemic manifestations, but meningitis may be the initial manifestation. Carcinomatous meningitis may or may not be accompanied by clinical evidence of the primary neoplasm.

APPROACH TO THE PATIENT: Chronic Meningitis

The occurrence of chronic headache, hydrocephalus, cranial neuropathy, radiculopathy, and/or cognitive decline in a patient should prompt consideration of a lumbar puncture for evidence of meningeal inflammation. On occasion, the diagnosis is made when an imaging study (CT or MRI) shows contrast enhancement of the meninges, which is always concerning with the exception of dural enhancement after lumbar puncture, neurosurgical procedures, or spontaneous CSF leakage. Once chronic meningitis is confirmed by CSF examination, effort is focused on identifying the cause (Tables 165-2 and 165-3) by (1) further analysis of the CSF, (2) diagnosis of an underlying systemic infection or noninfectious inflammatory condition, or (3) pathologic examination of meningeal biopsy specimens.

Two clinical forms of chronic meningitis exist. In the first, the symptoms are chronic and persistent, whereas in the second there are recurrent, discrete episodes of illness. In the latter group, all symptoms, signs, and CSF parameters of meningeal inflammation resolve completely between episodes without specific therapy. In such patients, the likely etiologies include herpes simplex virus (HSV) type 2; chemical meningitis due to episodic leakage from an epidermoid tumor, craniopharyngioma, or cholesteatoma into CSF; primary autoimmune inflammatory conditions, including Vogt-Koyanagi-Harada syndrome, Behçet's syndrome, systemic lupus erythematosus (SLE), and Mollaret's meningitis; and drug hypersensitivity with repeated administration of the offending agent.

The epidemiologic history is of considerable importance and may provide direction for selection of laboratory studies. Pertinent features include a history of tuberculosis or exposure to a likely case; past travel to areas endemic for fungal infections (the San Joaquin Valley in California and southwestern states for coccidioidomycosis, midwestern states for histoplasmosis, southeastern states for blastomycosis); travel to the Mediterranean region or ingestion of imported unpasteurized dairy products (*Brucella*); time spent in wooded areas endemic for Lyme disease; exposure to sexually transmitted disease (syphilis); exposure of an immunocompromised host to pigeons and their droppings (*Cryptococcus*); gardening (*Sporothrix schenckii*); ingestion of poorly cooked meat or contact with a household cat (*Toxoplasma gondii*); residence in Thailand or Japan (*Gnathostoma spinigerum*), Latin America (*Paracoccidioides brasiliensis*), or the South Pacific (*Angiostrongylus cantonensis*); rural residence and raccoon exposure (*Baylisascaris procyonis*); and residence in Latin America, the Philippines, or Southeast Asia (*Taenia solium/cysticercosis*).

The presence of focal cerebral signs in a patient with chronic meningitis suggests the possibility of a brain abscess or other

TABLE 165-2 INFECTIOUS CAUSES OF CHRONIC MENINGITIS

Causative Agent	CSF Formula	Helpful Diagnostic Tests	Risk Factors and Systemic Manifestations
Common Bacterial Causes			
Partially treated suppurative meningitis	Mononuclear or mixed mononuclear-polymorphonuclear cells	CSF culture and Gram's stain	History consistent with acute bacterial meningitis and incomplete treatment
Parameningeal infection	Mononuclear or mixed polymorphonuclear-mononuclear cells	Contrast-enhanced CT or MRI to detect parenchymal, subdural, epidural, or sinus infection	Otitis media, pleuropulmonary infection, right-to-left cardiopulmonary shunt for brain abscess; focal neurologic signs; neck, back, ear, or sinus tenderness
Mycobacterium tuberculosis	Mononuclear cells except polymorphonuclear cells in early infection (commonly <500 WBC/μL); low CSF glucose, high protein	Tuberculin skin test may be negative; AFB culture of CSF (sputum, urine, gastric contents if indicated); tuberculostearic acid detection in CSF; identify tubercle bacillus on acid-fast stain of CSF or protein pellicle; PCR	Exposure history; previous tuberculous illness; immunosuppressed, anti-TNF therapy or AIDS; young children; fever, meningismus, night sweats, miliary TB on x-ray or liver biopsy; stroke due to arteritis
Lyme disease (Bannwarth's syndrome) *Borrelia burgdorferi*	Mononuclear cells, elevated protein	Serum Lyme antibody titer; Western blot confirmation; (patients with syphilis may have false-positive Lyme titer)	History of tick bite or appropriate exposure history; erythema chronicum migrans skin rash; arthritis, radiculopathy, Bell's palsy, meningoencephalitis–multiple sclerosis-like syndrome
Syphilis (secondary, tertiary) *Treponema pallidum*	Mononuclear cells; elevated protein	CSF VDRL; serum VDRL (or RPR); fluorescent treponemal antibody-absorbed (FTA) or MHA-TP; serum VDRL may be negative in tertiary syphilis	Appropriate exposure history; HIV-seropositive individuals at increased risk of aggressive infection; "dementia"; cerebral infarction due to endarteritis
Uncommon Bacterial Causes			
Actinomyces	Polymorphonuclear cells	Anaerobic culture	Parameningeal abscess or sinus tract (oral or dental focus); pneumonitis
Nocardia	Polymorphonuclear; occasionally mononuclear cells; often low glucose	Isolation may require weeks; weakly acid fast	Associated brain abscess may be present
Brucella	Mononuclear cells (rarely polymorphonuclear); elevated protein; often low glucose	CSF antibody detection; serum antibody detection	Intake of unpasteurized dairy products; exposure to goats, sheep, cows; fever, arthralgia, myalgia, vertebral osteomyelitis
Whipple's disease *Tropheryma whipplei*	Mononuclear cells	Biopsy of small bowel or lymph node; CSF PCR for *T. whipplei*; brain and meningeal biopsy (with PAS stain and EM examination)	Diarrhea, weight loss, arthralgias, fever; dementia, ataxia, paresis, ophthalmoplegia, oculomasticatory myoclonus

(Continued)

TABLE 165-2 INFECTIOUS CAUSES OF CHRONIC MENINGITIS (*CONTINUED*)

Causative Agent	CSF Formula	Helpful Diagnostic Tests	Risk Factors and Systemic Manifestations
Rare Bacterial Causes			
Leptospirosis (occasionally if left untreated may last 3–4 weeks)			
Fungal Causes			
Cryptococcus neoformans	Mononuclear cells; count not elevated in some patients with AIDS	India ink or fungal wet mount of CSF (budding yeast); blood and urine cultures; antigen detection in CSF	AIDS and immune suppression; pigeon exposure; skin and other organ involvement due to disseminated infection
Coccidioides immitis	Mononuclear cells (sometimes 10–20% eosinophils); often low glucose	Antibody detection in CSF and serum	Exposure history—southwestern U.S.; increased virulence in dark-skinned races
Candida sp.	Polymorphonuclear or mononuclear	Fungal stain and culture of CSF	IV drug abuse; post surgery; prolonged IV therapy; disseminated candidiasis
Histoplasma capsulatum	Mononuclear cells; low glucose	Fungal stain and culture of large volumes of CSF; antigen detection in CSF, serum, and urine; antibody detection in serum, CSF	Exposure history—Ohio and central Mississippi River Valley; AIDS; mucosal lesions
Blastomyces dermatitidis	Mononuclear cells	Fungal stain and culture of CSF; biopsy and culture of skin, lung lesions; antibody detection in serum	Midwestern and southeastern U.S.; usually systemic infection; abscesses, draining sinus, ulcers
Aspergillus sp.	Mononuclear or polymorphonuclear	CSF culture	Sinusitis; granulocytopenia or immunosuppression
Sporothrix schenckii	Mononuclear cells	Antibody detection in CSF and serum; CSF culture	Traumatic inoculation; IV drug use; ulcerated skin lesion
Rare Fungal Causes			
Xylohypha (formerly *Cladosporium*) *trichoides* and other dark-walled (dematiaceous) fungi such as *Curvularia, Drechslera; Mucor*, and, after water aspiration, *Pseudallescheria boydii*, iatrogenic *Exserohilum rostratum* infection following spinal blocks			
Protozoal Causes			
Toxoplasma gondii	Mononuclear cells	Biopsy or response to empirical therapy in clinically appropriate context (including presence of antibody in serum)	Usually with intracerebral abscesses; common in HIV-seropositive patients
Trypanosomiasis *Trypanosoma gambiense, T. rhodesiense*	Mononuclear cells, elevated protein	Elevated CSF IgM; identification of trypanosomes in CSF and blood smear	Endemic in Africa; chancre, lymphadenopathy; prominent sleep disorder
Rare Protozoal Causes			
Acanthamoeba sp. causing granulomatous amebic encephalitis and meningoencephalitis in immunocompromised and debilitated individuals. *Balamuthia mandrillaris* causing chronic meningoencephalitis in immunocompetent hosts.			
Helminthic Causes			
Cysticercosis (infection with cysts of *Taenia solium*)	Mononuclear cells; may have eosinophils; glucose level may be low	Indirect hemagglutination assay in CSF; ELISA immunoblotting in serum	Usually with multiple cysts in basal meninges and hydrocephalus; cerebral cysts, muscle calcification
Gnathostoma spinigerum	Eosinophils, mononuclear cells	Peripheral eosinophilia	History of eating raw fish; common in Thailand and Japan; subarachnoid hemorrhage; painful radiculopathy
Angiostrongylus cantonensis	Eosinophils, mononuclear cells	Recovery of worms from CSF	History of eating raw shellfish; common in tropical Pacific regions; often benign
Baylisascaris procyonis (raccoon ascarid)	Eosinophils, mononuclear cells		Infection follows accidental ingestion of *B. procyonis* eggs from raccoon feces; fatal meningoencephalitis
Rare Helminthic Causes			
Trichinella spiralis (trichinosis); *Fasciola hepatica* (liver fluke), *Echinococcus* cysts; *Schistosoma* sp. The former may produce a lymphocytic pleocytosis whereas the latter two may produce an eosinophilic response in CSF associated with cerebral cysts (*Echinococcus*) or granulomatous lesions of brain or spinal cord			
Viral Causes			
Mumps	Mononuclear cells	Antibody in serum	No prior mumps or immunization; may produce meningoencephalitis; may persist for 3–4 weeks
Lymphocytic choriomeningitis	Mononuclear cells	Antibody in serum	Contact with rodents or their excreta; may persist for 3–4 weeks
Echovirus	Mononuclear cells; may have low glucose	Virus isolation from CSF	Congenital hypogammaglobulinemia; history of recurrent meningitis
HIV (acute retroviral syndrome)	Mononuclear cells	p24 antigen in serum and CSF; high level of HIV viremia.	HIV risk factors; rash, fever, lymphadenopathy; lymphopenia in peripheral blood; syndrome may persist long enough to be considered as "chronic meningitis"; or chronic meningitis may develop in later stages (AIDS) due to HIV
Herpes simplex (HSV)	Mononuclear cells	PCR for HSV, CMV DNA; CSF antibody for HSV, EBV	Recurrent meningitis due to HSV-2 (rarely HSV-1) often associated with genital recurrences; EBV associated with myeloradiculopathy, CMV with polyradiculopathy

Abbreviations: AFB, acid-fast bacillus; CMV, cytomegalovirus; CSF, cerebrospinal fluid; CT, computed tomography; EBV, Epstein-Barr virus; ELISA, enzyme-linked immunosorbent assay; EM, electron microscopy; FTA, fluorescent treponemal antibody absorption test; HSV, herpes simplex virus; MHA-TP, microhemagglutination assay–*T. pallidum;* MRI, magnetic resonance imaging; PAS, periodic acid–Schiff; PCR, polymerase chain reaction; RPR, rapid plasma reagin test; TB, tuberculosis; VDRL, Venereal Disease Research Laboratories test.

TABLE 165-3 NONINFECTIOUS CAUSES OF CHRONIC MENINGITIS

Causative Agents	CSF Formula	Helpful Diagnostic Tests	Risk Factors and Systemic Manifestations
Malignancy	Mononuclear cells, elevated protein, low glucose	Repeated cytologic examination of large volumes of CSF; CSF exam by polarizing microscopy; clonal lymphocyte markers; deposits on nerve roots or meninges seen on myelogram or contrast-enhanced MRI; meningeal biopsy	Metastatic cancer of breast, lung, stomach, or pancreas; melanoma, lymphoma, leukemia; meningeal gliomatosis; meningeal sarcoma; cerebral dysgerminoma; meningeal melanoma or B cell lymphoma
Chemical compounds (may cause recurrent meningitis)	Mononuclear or PMNs, low glucose, elevated protein; xanthochromia from subarachnoid hemorrhage in week prior to presentation with "meningitis"	Contrast-enhanced CT scan or MRI; cerebral angiogram to detect aneurysm	History of recent injection into the subarachnoid space; history of sudden onset of headache; recent resection of acoustic neuroma or craniopharyngioma; epidermoid tumor of brain or spine, sometimes with dermoid sinus tract; pituitary apoplexy
Primary inflammation			
CNS sarcoidosis	Mononuclear cells; elevated protein; often low glucose	Serum and CSF angiotensin-converting enzyme levels; biopsy of extraneural affected tissues or brain lesion/meningeal biopsy	CN palsy, especially of CN VII; hypothalamic dysfunction, especially diabetes insipidus; abnormal chest radiograph; peripheral neuropathy or myopathy
Vogt-Koyanagi-Harada syndrome (recurrent meningitis)	Mononuclear cells		Recurrent meningoencephalitis with uveitis, retinal detachment, alopecia, lightening of eyebrows and lashes, dysacousia, cataracts, glaucoma
Isolated granulomatous angiitis of the nervous system	Mononuclear cells, elevated protein	Angiography or meningeal biopsy	Subacute dementia; multiple cerebral infarctions; recent zoster ophthalmicus
Systemic lupus erythematosus	Mononuclear or PMNs	Anti-DNA antibody, antinuclear antibodies	Encephalopathy; seizures; stroke; transverse myelopathy; rash; arthritis
Behçet's syndrome (recurrent meningitis)	Mononuclear or PMNs, elevated protein		Oral and genital aphthous ulcers; iridocyclitis; retinal hemorrhages; pathergic lesions at site of skin puncture
Chronic benign lymphocytic meningitis	Mononuclear cells		Recovery in 2–6 months, diagnosis by exclusion
Mollaret's meningitis (recurrent meningitis)	Large endothelial cells and PMNs in first hours, followed by mononuclear cells	PCR for herpes; MRI/CT to rule out epidermoid tumor or dural cyst	Recurrent meningitis; exclude HSV-2; rare cases due to HSV-1; occasional case associated with dural cyst
Drug hypersensitivity	PMNs; occasionally mononuclear cells or eosinophils	Complete blood count (eosinophilia)	Exposure to nonsteroidal anti-inflammatory agents, sulfonamides, isoniazid, tolmetin, ciprofloxacin, penicillin, carbamazepine, lamotrigine, IV immunoglobulin, OKT3 antibodies, phenazopyridine; improvement after discontinuation of drug; recurrence with repeat exposure
Granulomatosis with polyangiitis (Wegener's)	Mononuclear cells	Chest and sinus radiographs; urinalysis; ANCA antibodies in serum	Associated sinus, pulmonary, or renal lesions; CN palsies; skin lesions; peripheral neuropathy
Other: multiple sclerosis, Sjögren's syndrome, monogenic autoinflammatory disorders, and rarer forms of vasculitis (e.g., Cogan's syndrome)			

Abbreviations: ANCA, antineutrophil cytoplasmic antibodies, CN, cranial nerve; CSF, cerebrospinal fluid; CT, computed tomography; HSV, herpes simplex virus; MRI, magnetic resonance imaging; PCR, polymerase chain reaction; PMNs, polymorphonuclear cells.

parameningeal infection; identification of a potential source of infection (chronic draining ear, sinusitis, right-to-left cardiac or pulmonary shunt, chronic pleuropulmonary infection) supports this diagnosis. In some cases, diagnosis may be established by recognition and biopsy of unusual skin lesions (Behçet's syndrome, SLE, cryptococcosis, blastomycosis, Lyme disease, sporotrichosis, trypanosomiasis, IV drug use) or enlarged lymph nodes (lymphoma, sarcoid, tuberculosis, HIV, secondary syphilis, or Whipple's disease). A careful ophthalmologic examination may reveal uveitis (Vogt-Koyanagi-Harada syndrome, sarcoid, or central nervous system [CNS] lymphoma), keratoconjunctivitis sicca (Sjögren's syndrome), or iridocyclitis (Behçet's syndrome) and is essential to assess visual loss from papilledema. Aphthous oral lesions, genital ulcers, and hypopyon suggest Behçet's syndrome. Hepatosplenomegaly suggests lymphoma, sarcoid, tuberculosis, or brucellosis. Herpetic lesions in the genital area or on the thighs suggest HSV-2 infection. A breast nodule, a suspicious pigmented skin lesion, focal bone pain, or an abdominal mass directs attention to possible carcinomatous meningitis.

IMAGING

Once the clinical syndrome is recognized as a potential manifestation of chronic meningitis, proper analysis of the CSF is essential. However, if the possibility of raised ICP exists, a brain imaging study should be performed before lumbar puncture. If ICP is elevated because of a mass lesion, brain swelling, or a block in ventricular CSF outflow (obstructive hydrocephalus), then lumbar puncture carries the potential risk of brain herniation. Obstructive hydrocephalus usually requires direct ventricular drainage. In patients with open CSF flow pathways, elevated ICP can still occur due to impaired resorption of CSF by arachnoid villi. In such patients, lumbar puncture is usually safe, but repetitive or continuous lumbar drainage may be necessary to prevent abrupt deterioration and death from raised ICP. In some patients, especially those with cryptococcal meningitis, fatal levels of raised ICP can occur without enlarged ventricles.

Contrast-enhanced MRI or CT studies of the brain and spinal cord can identify meningeal enhancement, parameningeal infections (including brain abscess), encasement of the spinal cord (malignancy, inflammation or infection), or nodular deposits on the meninges or nerve roots (malignancy or sarcoidosis) (Fig. 165-1). Imaging studies are also useful to localize areas of meningeal disease prior to meningeal biopsy.

Angiographic studies can identify evidence of cerebral arteritis in patients with chronic meningitis and stroke.

CEREBROSPINAL FLUID ANALYSIS

The CSF pressure should be measured and samples sent for bacterial, fungal, and tuberculous culture; Venereal Disease Research Laboratories (VDRL) test; cell count and differential; Gram's stain; and measurement of glucose and protein. Wet mount for fungus and parasites, india ink preparation and culture, culture

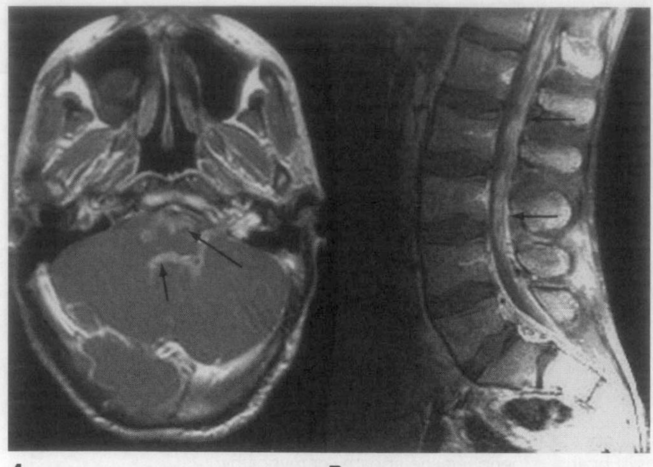

FIGURE 165-1 Primary central nervous system lymphoma. A 24-year-old man, immunosuppressed due to intestinal lymphangiectasia, developed multiple cranial neuropathies. CSF findings consisted of 100 lymphocytes/μL and a protein of 2.5 g/L (250 mg/dL); cytology and cultures were negative. Gadolinium-enhanced T1 MRI revealed diffuse, multifocal meningeal enhancement surrounding the brainstem (***A***), spinal cord, and cauda equina (***B***).

for fastidious bacteria and fungi, assays for cryptococcal antigen and oligoclonal immunoglobulin bands, and cytology should be performed. Other specific CSF tests (Tables 165-2 and 165-3) or blood tests and cultures should be ordered as indicated on the basis of the history, physical examination, or preliminary CSF results (i.e., eosinophilic, mononuclear, or polymorphonuclear meningitis). Rapid diagnosis may be facilitated by serologic tests and polymerase chain reaction (PCR) testing to identify DNA sequences in the CSF that are specific for the suspected pathogen. In patients with suspected fungal infections, when other tests are negative, assays for beta-glucans may be a useful adjunct in establishing the diagnosis.

In most categories of chronic (not recurrent) meningitis, mononuclear cells predominate in the CSF. When neutrophils predominate after 3 weeks of illness, the principal etiologic considerations are *Nocardia asteroides*, *Actinomyces israelii*, *Brucella*, *Mycobacterium tuberculosis* (5–10% of early cases only), various fungi (*Blastomyces dermatitidis*, *Candida albicans*, *Histoplasma capsulatum*, *Aspergillus* spp., *Pseudallescheria boydii*, *Cladophialophora bantiana*), and noninfectious causes (SLE, exogenous chemical meningitis). When eosinophils predominate or are present in limited numbers in a primarily mononuclear cell response in the CSF, the differential diagnosis includes parasitic diseases (*A. cantonensis*, *G. spinigerum*, *B. procyonis*, or *Toxocara canis* infection, cysticercosis, schistosomiasis, echinococcal disease, *T. gondii* infection), fungal infections (6–20% eosinophils along with a predominantly lymphocyte pleocytosis, particularly with coccidioidal meningitis), neoplastic disease (lymphoma, leukemia, metastatic carcinoma), or other inflammatory processes (sarcoidosis, hypereosinophilic syndrome).

It is often necessary to broaden the number of diagnostic tests if the initial workup does not reveal the cause. In addition, repeated samples of large volumes of CSF may be required to diagnose certain infectious and malignant causes of chronic meningitis. Flow cytometry for malignant cells may be useful in patients with suspected carcinomatous meningitis. Lymphomatous or carcinomatous meningitis may be diagnosed by examination of sections cut from a cell block formed by spinning down the sediment from a large volume of CSF. The diagnosis of fungal meningitis may require large volumes of CSF for culture of sediment. If standard lumbar puncture is unrewarding, a cervical cisternal tap to sample CSF near to the basal meninges may be fruitful.

LABORATORY INVESTIGATION

In addition to the CSF examination, an attempt should be made to uncover pertinent underlying illnesses. Tuberculin skin test, chest radiograph, urine analysis and culture, blood count and differential, renal and liver function tests, alkaline phosphatase, sedimentation rate, antinuclear antibody, anti-Ro antibody, anti-La antibody, and serum angiotensin-converting enzyme level are often indicated. In some cases, a thorough search for a systemic site of infection is indicated. Pulmonary foci of infection may be present, particularly with fungal or tuberculous disease. Hence a CT or MRI of the chest and a sputum examination may be helpful. Abnormalities can be pursued by bronchoscopy or transthoracic needle biopsy. A tuberculin skin test is often placed, although the test has limited specificity and sensitivity for diagnosis of active disease. Liver or bone marrow biopsy may be diagnostic in some cases of miliary tuberculosis, disseminated fungal infection, sarcoidosis, or metastatic malignancy. Positron emission tomography with fluorodeoxyglucose may be useful in identifying a systemic site for biopsy in patients with suspected carcinomatous meningitis or sarcoidosis when other tests are unrevealing. Genetic testing can identify mutations that cause rare monogenic autoinflammatory disorders.

MENINGEAL BIOPSY

If CSF is not diagnostic then a meningeal biopsy should be strongly considered in patients who are severely disabled, who need chronic ventricular decompression, or whose illness is progressing rapidly. The activities of the surgeon, pathologist, microbiologist, and cytologist should be coordinated so that a large enough sample is obtained and the appropriate cultures and histologic and molecular studies, including electron-microscopic and PCR studies, are performed. The diagnostic yield of meningeal biopsy can be increased by targeting regions that enhance with contrast on MRI or CT. With current microsurgical techniques, most areas of the basal meninges can be accessed for biopsy via a limited craniotomy. In a series from the Mayo Clinic reported by TM Cheng et al. (*Neurosurgery* 34:590, 1994), MRI demonstrated meningeal enhancement in 47% of patients undergoing meningeal biopsy. Biopsy of an enhancing region was diagnostic in 80% of cases; biopsy of nonenhancing regions was diagnostic in only 9%; sarcoid (31%) and metastatic adenocarcinoma (25%) were the most common conditions identified. Tuberculosis is the most common condition identified in many reports from outside the United States.

APPROACH TO THE ENIGMATIC CASE

In approximately one-third of cases, the diagnosis is not known despite careful evaluation of CSF and potential extraneural sites of disease. A number of the organisms that cause chronic meningitis may take weeks to be identified by cultures. In enigmatic cases, several options are available, determined by the extent of the clinical deficits and rate of progression. It is prudent to wait until cultures are finalized if the patient is asymptomatic or symptoms are mild and not progressive. Unfortunately, in many cases progressive neurologic deterioration occurs, and rapid treatment is required. Ventricular-peritoneal shunts may be placed to relieve hydrocephalus, but the risk of disseminating the undiagnosed inflammatory process into the abdomen must be considered.

Empirical Treatment Diagnosis of the causative agent is essential because effective therapies exist for many etiologies of chronic meningitis, but if the condition is left untreated, progressive damage to the CNS and cranial nerves and roots is likely to occur. Occasionally, empirical therapy must be initiated when all attempts at diagnosis fail. In general, empirical therapy in the United States consists of antimycobacterial agents, amphotericin for fungal infection, or glucocorticoids for noninfectious inflammatory causes. It is important to direct empirical therapy of lymphocytic meningitis at tuberculosis, particularly if the condition is associated with low CSF glucose and sixth and other CN palsies, since untreated disease can be devastating within weeks. Patients on prolonged anti–tumor necrosis factor therapy who develop chronic meningitis also should be treated empirically with antituberculous therapy if the etiology is uncertain. In the Mayo Clinic series, the most useful empirical therapy was administration of glucocorticoids rather than antituberculous therapy. Carcinomatous or lymphomatous meningitis may be difficult to diagnose initially, but the diagnosis becomes evident with time.

THE IMMUNOSUPPRESSED PATIENT

Chronic meningitis is not uncommon in the course of HIV infection. Pleocytosis and mild meningeal signs often occur at the onset of HIV infection, and occasionally low-grade meningitis persists. Toxoplasmosis commonly presents as intracranial abscesses and also may be associated with meningitis. Other important causes of chronic meningitis in AIDS include infection with *Cryptococcus, Nocardia, Candida*, or other fungi; syphilis; and lymphoma (Fig. 165-1). Toxoplasmosis, cryptococcosis, nocardiosis, and other fungal infections are important etiologic considerations in individuals with immunodeficiency states other than AIDS, including those due to immunosuppressive medications. Because of the increased risk of chronic meningitis and the attenuation of clinical signs of meningeal irritation in immunosuppressed individuals, CSF examination should be performed for any persistent headache or unexplained change in mental state.

ACKNOWLEDGMENT
Morton N. Swartz contributed to earlier editions of this chapter.

166e Infectious Complications of Burns

Lawrence C. Madoff, Florencia Pereyra

This is a digital-only chapter. It is available on the DVD that accompanies this book, as well as on Access Medicine/Harrison's Online, and the eBook and "app" editions of HPIM 19e.

The skin is an essential component of immunity, protecting the host from potential pathogens in the environment. Breaches in this protective barrier thus represent a form of immunocompromise that predisposes the patient to infection. Thermal burns may cause massive destruction of the integument as well as derangements in humoral and cellular immunity, permitting the development of infection caused by environmental opportunists and components of the host's skin flora.

167e Infectious Complications of Bites

Lawrence C. Madoff, Florencia Pereyra

This is a digital-only chapter. It is available on the DVD that accompanies this book, as well as on Access Medicine/Harrison's Online, and the eBook and "app" editions of HPIM 19e.

The skin is an essential component of nonspecific immunity, protecting the host from potential pathogens in the environment. Breaches in this protective barrier thus represent a form of immunocompromise that predisposes the patient to infection. Bites and scratches from animals and humans allow the inoculation of microorganisms past the skin's protective barrier into deeper, susceptible host tissues.

Each year in the United States, millions of animal-bite wounds are sustained. The vast majority are inflicted by pet dogs and cats, which number >100 million; the annual incidence of dog and cat bites has been reported as 300 bites per 100,000 population. Other bite wounds are a consequence of encounters with animals in the wild or in occupational settings. While many of these wounds require minimal or no therapy, a significant number result in infection, which may be life threatening. The microbiology of bite-wound infections in general reflects the oropharyngeal flora of the biting animal, although organisms from the soil, the skin of the animal and the victim, and the animal's feces may also be involved.

SECTION 3 CLINICAL SYNDROMES: HEALTH CARE–ASSOCIATED INFECTIONS

168 Infections Acquired in Health Care Facilities

Robert A. Weinstein

The costs of hospital-acquired (nosocomial) and other health care–associated infections are great. These infections have affected as many as 1.7 million patients at a cost of ~$28–33 billion and 99,000 lives in U.S. hospitals annually. Although efforts to lower infection risks have been challenged by the numbers of immunocompromised patients, antibiotic-resistant bacteria, fungal and viral superinfections, and invasive devices and procedures, a prevailing viewpoint—often termed "zero tolerance"—is that almost all health care–associated infections should be avoidable with strict application of evidence-based prevention guidelines (Table 168-1). In fact, rates of device-related infections—historically, the largest drivers of risk—have fallen steadily over the past few years. Unfortunately, at the same time, antimicrobial-resistant pathogens have risen in number and are estimated to contribute to ~23,000 deaths in and outside of hospitals annually. This chapter reviews health care–associated and device-related infections as well as basic surveillance, prevention, control, and treatment activities.

ORGANIZATION, RESPONSIBILITIES, AND INCREASING SCRUTINY OF HEALTH CARE–ASSOCIATED INFECTION PROGRAMS

The standards of the Joint Commission require all accredited hospitals to have active programs for surveillance, prevention, and control of nosocomial infections. Education of physicians in infection control and health care epidemiology is required in infectious disease fellowship programs and is available in online courses. Concerns over "patient safety" have led to federal legislation that prevents U.S. hospitals from upgrading Medicare charges to pay for hospital costs resulting from at least 14 specific nosocomial events (Table 168-2) and have prompted national efforts to publicly

TABLE 168-1 SOURCES OF INFECTION CONTROL GUIDELINES AND OVERSIGHT

Organization	Role	Major Constituents	Website
Joint Commission	Regulatory	Hospitals, long-term-care facilities, laboratories	*www.jointcommission.org*
CAP	Regulatory	Laboratories	*www.cap.org*
OSHA	Regulatory	Workers	*www.osha.gov*
CMS	Regulatory	Medicare/Medicaid providers	*www.cms.hhs.gov*
PQRI	Regulatory and advisory	Eligible professionals	*www.cms.hhs.gov/pqri/*
HHS Action Plan	Regulatory and advisory	Health care and infection prevention personnel	*www.hhs.gov/ash/initiatives/hai/actionplan/*
CDC			
DHQP	Advisory	Health care facilities and personnel	*www.cdc.gov/ncezid/dhqp/*
HICPAC	Advisory	Health care facilities and personnel	*www.cdc.gov/hicpac/*
NIOSH	Advisory	Workers	*www.cdc.gov/niosh/*
AHRQ	Advisory	Broad (e.g., health care personnel)	*www.ahrq.gov*
NQF	Advisory	Broad (e.g., health care personnel)	*www.qualityforum.org*
IOM	Advisory	Broad (e.g., health care personnel)	*www.iom.edu*
Federal Influenza Planning	Advisory	Health care and public health personnel	*www.flu.gov/planning-preparedness/hospital#*
Trust for America's Health	Advisory	Broad (e.g., the public)	*healthyamericans.org*
CSTE	Advisory and professional society	Public health personnel	*www.cste.org*
IDSA	Professional society	Infectious disease physicians/researchers	*www.idsociety.org*
SHEA	Professional society	Health care epidemiologists	*www.shea-online.org*
HIS	Professional society	Health care epidemiologists	*www.his.org.uk*
APIC	Professional society	Infection preventionists	*www.apic.org*
MedQIC	Quality improvement	Broad (e.g., health care personnel)	*www.qualitynet.org*
IHI	Quality improvement	Broad (e.g., health care personnel)	*www.ihi.org*
Leapfrog Group	Quality improvement	Broad (payers, consumers, employers, and health care personnel)	*www.leapfroggroup.org*
NSQIP	Quality improvement	Surgery services	*www.acsnsqip.org*

Abbreviations: AHRQ, Agency for Healthcare Research and Quality; APIC, Association for Professionals in Infection Control and Epidemiology; CAP, College of American Pathologists; CDC, Centers for Disease Control and Prevention; CMS, Centers for Medicare & Medicaid Services; CSTE, Council of State and Territorial Epidemiologists; DHQP, Division of Healthcare Quality Promotion; HHS, Health and Human Services; HICPAC, Healthcare Infection Control Practices Advisory Committee; HIS, Hospital Infection Society; IDSA, Infectious Diseases Society of America; IHI, Institute for Healthcare Improvement; IOM, Institute of Medicine; MedQIC, Medicare Quality Improvement Community; NIOSH, National Institute for Occupational Safety and Health; NQF, National Quality Forum; NSQIP, National Surgical Quality Improvement Program; OSHA, Occupational Safety & Health Administration; PQRI, Physician Quality Reporting Initiative; SHEA, Society for Healthcare Epidemiology of America.

report on processes of patient care (e.g., timely administration and appropriateness of perioperative antibiotic prophylaxis) and patient outcomes (e.g., surgical wound infection rates). Neither the carrot (pay-for-performance) nor the stick (nonpayment for preventable infections) appears to have impacted infection rates. The effect of public attention may be more positive; in 2009, the U.S. Department of Health and Human Services released a major interagency Action Plan to Prevent Healthcare-Associated Infections, including a list of 5-year national prevention targets that are mostly on track (Table 168-3).

TABLE 168-2 HEALTH CARE–ACQUIRED CONDITIONS NOT ELIGIBLE FOR ADDITIONAL FEDERAL PAYMENT[a]

Foreign objects retained after surgery
Air embolism
Blood incompatibilities
Decubitus ulcers (stages III and IV)
Fractures/other injuries from falls or trauma
Catheter-associated urinary tract infections
Vascular catheter–associated infections
Manifestations of poor glycemic control
Surgical-site infection or mediastinitis following coronary artery bypass graft
Surgical-site infection following certain orthopedic procedures
Surgical-site infection following bariatric surgery for obesity
Surgical-site infection following cardiac electronic device implantation
Venous thromboembolism (after hip or knee replacement)
Iatrogenic pneumothorax with venous catheterization

[a]Based on the U.S. Federal Deficit Reduction Act of 2005. As of October 2012, Medicare stopped paying additional money to hospitals for these 14 health care–acquired conditions. See *www.cms.gov/HospitalAcqCond/* (last accessed November 13, 2014).

SURVEILLANCE

Traditionally, infection preventionists have surveyed inpatients for infections acquired in hospitals (defined as those neither present nor incubating at the time of admission). Surveillance most often requires review of microbiology laboratory results, "shoe-leather" epidemiology on nursing wards, and application of standardized definitions of infection. Progressively more infection-control programs use computerized hospital databases for algorithm-driven electronic surveillance (e.g., of vascular catheter and surgical wound infections) that removes observer bias and, by so doing, provides data that are more reliable for interfacility comparisons. Although infection surveillance in nursing homes and some long-term acute-care hospitals (LTACHs) is still in its formative stage, the role of these facilities in the transmission of antimicrobial-resistant pathogens will require their increased attention to infection surveillance and control.

Most hospitals aim surveillance at infections associated with high-level morbidity or expense. Quality-improvement activities in infection control have led to increased surveillance of personnel compliance with infection control policies (e.g., adherence to influenza vaccination recommendations). In the spirit of "what is measured improves," the majority of states now require public reporting of processes for prevention of health care–associated infection and/or patient outcomes. As a result, in some locales, the surveillance pendulum is swinging

TABLE 168-3 SUMMARY OF PROGRESS TOWARD THE NINE NATIONAL TARGETS FOR ELIMINATION OF HEALTH CARE–ASSOCIATED INFECTIONS, U.S. DEPARTMENT OF HEALTH AND HUMAN SERVICES: MIDPOINT EVALUATION

Metric	Source	National 5-Year Prevention Target	On Track to Meet 2013 Targets?
Bloodstream infections	NHSN	50% reduction	Yes[a]
Adherence to central-line insertion practices	NHSN	100% adherence	Retired
Clostridium difficile diagnosed in hospital	HCUP	30% reduction	No
C. difficile infections	NHSN	30% reduction	No[a]
Urinary tract infections	NHSN	25% reduction	Yes[a]
MRSA invasive infections (population)	EIP	50% reduction	Yes[a]
MRSA bacteremia (hospital)	NHSN	25% reduction	Yes
Surgical-site infections	NHSN	25% reduction	Yes
Surgical Care Improvement Project Measures	SCIP	95% adherence	Yes

[a]Examples of changes: Catheter-related bloodstream infections decreased to ~1.7/1000 catheter days; *C. difficile* infections increased to ~11.2 cases/10,000 discharges; catheter-related urinary tract infections decreased to ~3.1/1000 catheter-days; and hospital-onset MRSA invasive infections decreased to ~4.5/100,000 persons.

Abbreviations: EIP, CDC's Emerging Infections Program; HCUP, Agency for Healthcare Research and Quality's Healthcare Cost and Utilization Project; MRSA, methicillin-resistant *Staphylococcus aureus*; NHSN, CDC's National Healthcare Safety Network; SCIP, Surgical Care Improvement Project.

Source: Adapted from *www.hhs.gov/ash/initiatives/hai/nationaltargets/* (last accessed November 13, 2014).

back to use of "house-wide" surveillance, and many states now require that hospitals use the Centers for Disease Control and Prevention's (CDC's) National Healthcare Safety Network (NHSN) reporting system to provide uniform definitions and to facilitate transmission of data. Increasing reliance on the NHSN by states to facilitate public reporting has led to participation by more than 12,000 facilities (~4700 of the ~5700 acute-care hospitals in the United States, ~540 LTACHs, ~270 inpatient rehabilitation facilities, ~6000 outpatient dialysis facilities, ~300 ambulatory surgery centers, ~150 long-term-care facilities). This level of participation provides a nationwide view of health care–associated infections and represents a watershed in potential access to national rates of antimicrobial use and resistance.

Results of surveillance are expressed as rates. In general, for example, 5–10% of patients develop nosocomial infections. However, such broad statistics have little value unless qualified by duration of risk, by site of infection, by patient population, and by exposure to risk factors. To account for some of these variables, the CDC now uses a Standardized Infection Ratio (SIR; *www.cdc.gov/hai/national-annual-sir/*) as part of NHSN rate reporting. Meaningful denominators for infection rates include the number of patients exposed to a specific risk (e.g., patients using mechanical ventilators) or the number of intervention days (e.g., 1000 patient-days on a ventilator). As use of invasive devices such as indwelling bladder catheters has purposely been decreased, the denominators have become smaller, but the fact that patients who still require such devices may be those at intrinsically higher risk (potential numerators) may paradoxically increase rates when device-days account for the denominator. Temporal trends in rates should be reviewed, and rates should be compared with regional and national benchmarks that incorporate the SIR. Interhospital comparisons still may be misleading because of the wide range in risk factors and severity of underlying illnesses. Process measures (e.g., adherence to hand hygiene) do not usually require risk adjustment, and outcome measures (e.g., cardiac surgery wound-infection rates) can identify hospitals with outlier infection rates (e.g., in the top deciles) for further evaluation. Moreover, temporal analysis of a hospital's infection rates can help to determine whether control measures are succeeding and where increased efforts should be focused.

EPIDEMIOLOGIC BASIS AND GENERAL MEASURES FOR PREVENTION AND CONTROL

Nosocomial infections follow basic epidemiologic patterns that can help to direct prevention and control measures. Nosocomial pathogens have reservoirs, are transmitted by largely predictable routes, and require susceptible hosts. Reservoirs and sources exist in the inanimate environment (e.g., residual *Clostridium difficile* spores on frequently touched surfaces in patients' rooms) and in the animate environment (e.g., infected or colonized health care workers, patients, and hospital visitors). The mode of transmission usually is either cross-infection (e.g., indirect spread of pathogens from one patient to another on the inadequately cleaned hands of hospital personnel) or autoinoculation (e.g., aspiration of oropharyngeal flora into the lungs along an endotracheal tube). Occasionally, pathogens (e.g., group A streptococci and many respiratory viruses) are spread from person to person via large infectious droplets released by coughing or sneezing. Much less common—but often devastating in terms of epidemic risk—is true airborne spread of small or droplet nuclei (as in nosocomial chickenpox) or common-source spread (e.g., by contaminated IV fluids). Factors that increase host susceptibility include underlying conditions, abnormalities of innate defense (e.g., due to genetic polymorphisms; see Chap. 82), and medical-surgical interventions and procedures that compromise host defenses.

Hospitals' infection-control programs must determine general and specific control measures. Given the prominence of cross-infection, hand hygiene is cited traditionally as the most important preventive measure. Health care workers' rates of adherence to hand-hygiene recommendations are abysmally low (often <50%). Reasons cited include inconvenience, time pressures, and skin damage from frequent washing. Sinkless alcohol rubs are quick and highly effective and actually improve hand condition since they contain emollients and allow the retention of natural protective oils that would be removed with repeated rinsing. Use of alcohol hand rubs between patient contacts is recommended for all health care workers except when hands are visibly soiled or after care of a patient who is part of a health care facility outbreak of infection with *C. difficile*, whose spores resist killing by alcohol and require mechanical removal. In these cases, washing with soap and running water is recommended. A number of innovative systems have been developed to track hand-hygiene adherence in real time and to provide feedback; although this approach is exciting, sustained improvements in rates remain to be seen.

NOSOCOMIAL AND DEVICE-RELATED INFECTIONS

The fact that >25–50% of nosocomial infections are due to the combined effect of the patient's own flora and invasive devices highlights the importance of improvements in the use and design of such devices. Intensive education, "bundling" of evidence-based interventions (Table 168-4), and use of checklists to facilitate adherence have reduced infection rates (Table 168-3) through improved asepsis in handling and earlier removal of invasive devices. It is especially noteworthy that turnover or shortages of trained personnel jeopardize safe and effective patient care and have been associated with increased infection rates.

URINARY TRACT INFECTIONS

Urinary tract infections (UTIs) account for ~30–40% of nosocomial infections; up to 3% of bacteriuric patients develop bacteremia. Although UTIs contribute at most 15% to prolongation of hospital stay and may have an attributable cost in the range of only $1300, these infections are reservoirs and sources for spread of antibiotic-resistant bacteria. Most nosocomial UTIs are associated with preceding instrumentation or indwelling bladder catheters, which create a 3–7% risk of infection each day. UTIs generally are caused by pathogens that spread up the periurethral space from the patient's perineum or gastrointestinal tract—the most common pathogenesis in women—or via intraluminal contamination of urinary catheters, usually due to cross-infection by caregivers who are irrigating catheters or emptying drainage bags. Pathogens come occasionally from

TABLE 168-4 EXAMPLES OF EVIDENCE-BASED "BUNDLED INTERVENTIONS" TO PREVENT COMMON HEALTH CARE–ASSOCIATED INFECTIONS AND OTHER ADVERSE EVENTS

Prevention of Central Venous Catheter Infections
Catheter insertion bundle:
Educate personnel about catheter insertion and care.
Use chlorhexidine to prepare the insertion site.
Use maximal barrier precautions and asepsis during catheter insertion.
Consolidate insertion supplies (e.g., in an insertion kit or cart).
Use a checklist to enhance adherence to the "insertion bundle."
Empower nurses to halt insertion if asepsis is breached.
Catheter maintenance bundle:
Cleanse patients daily with chlorhexidine.
Maintain clean, dry dressings.
Enforce hand hygiene among health care workers.
Ask daily: Is the catheter needed? Remove catheter if not needed or used.
Prevention of Ventilator-Associated Events
Elevate head of bed to 30–45 degrees.
Decontaminate oropharynx regularly with chlorhexidine (controversial).
Give "sedation vacation" and assess readiness to extubate daily.
Use peptic ulcer disease prophylaxis.
Use deep-vein thrombosis prophylaxis (unless contraindicated).
Prevention of Surgical-Site Infections
Choose a surgeon wisely.
Administer prophylactic antibiotics within 1 h before surgery; discontinue within 24 h.
Limit any hair removal to the time of surgery; use clippers or do not remove hair at all.
Prepare surgical site with chlorhexidine-alcohol.
Maintain normal perioperative glucose levels (cardiac surgery patients).[a]
Maintain perioperative normothermia (colorectal surgery patients).[a]
Prevention of Urinary Tract Infections
Place bladder catheters only when absolutely needed (e.g., to relieve obstruction), not solely for the provider's convenience.
Use aseptic technique for catheter insertion and urinary tract instrumentation.
Minimize manipulation or opening of drainage systems.
Ask daily: Is the bladder catheter needed? Remove catheter if not needed.
Prevention of Pathogen Cross-Transmission
Cleanse hands with alcohol hand rub before and after all contacts with patients or their environments.

[a]These components of care are supported by clinical trials and experimental evidence in the specified populations; they may prove valuable for other surgical patients as well.

Source: Adapted from information presented at the following websites: *www.cdc.gov/hicpac/pubs.html; www.cdc.gov/HAI/prevent/prevention.html; www.ihi.org.*

inadequately disinfected urologic equipment and rarely from contaminated supplies.

Hospitals should monitor essential performance measures for preventing nosocomial UTIs (Table 168-4). Prompts to clinicians to assess a patient's need for continued use of an indwelling bladder catheter can improve removal rates and lessen the risk of UTI. Guidelines for managing postoperative urinary retention (e.g., with bladder scanners) also may limit the use or duration of catheterization. Other approaches to the prevention of UTIs have included the use of topical meatal antimicrobial agents, drainage bag disinfectants, and anti-infective catheters. None of the latter three measures is considered routine.

Administration of systemic antimicrobial agents for other purposes decreases the risk of UTI during the first 4 days of catheterization, after which resistant bacteria or yeasts emerge as pathogens. Prophylactic antibiotic administration at the time of catheter removal has been reported to decrease the risk of UTI. Selective decontamination of the gut also is associated with a reduced risk. Again, however, none of these approaches is routine.

Irrigation of catheters, with or without antimicrobial agents, may actually increase the risk of infection. A condom catheter for men without bladder obstruction may be more acceptable than an indwelling catheter and may lessen the risk of UTI if maintained carefully. The role of suprapubic catheters in preventing infection is not well defined.

Treatment of UTIs is based on the results of quantitative urine cultures (Chap. 162). The most common pathogens are *Escherichia coli*, nosocomial gram-negative bacilli, enterococci, and *Candida*. Several caveats apply in the treatment of institutionally acquired infection. First, in patients with chronic indwelling bladder catheters, especially those in long-term-care facilities, "catheter flora"—microorganisms living on encrustations within the catheter lumen—may differ from actual urinary tract pathogens. Therefore, for suspected UTI in the setting of chronic catheterization (especially in women), it is useful to replace the bladder catheter and to obtain a freshly voided urine specimen. Second, as in all nosocomial infections, at the time treatment is initiated on the basis of a positive culture, it is useful to repeat the culture to verify the persistence of infection. Third, the frequency with which UTIs occur may lead to the erroneous assumption that the urinary tract alone is the source of infection in a febrile hospitalized patient. Fourth, recovery of *Staphylococcus aureus* from urine cultures may result from hematogenous seeding and may indicate an occult systemic infection. Finally, although *Candida* is now the most common pathogen in nosocomial UTIs among patients on intensive care units (ICUs), treatment of candiduria is often unsuccessful and is recommended only when there is upper-pole or bladder-wall invasion, obstruction, neutropenia, or immunosuppression.

PNEUMONIA

Historically, pneumonia has accounted for ~10–15% of nosocomial infections; ventilator-associated pneumonia (VAP) occurred in 1 to >4 patients per 1000 ventilator-days, and these infections were reported as responsible for a mean of 10 extra hospital days and $23,000 in extra costs per episode. Most cases of bacterial nosocomial pneumonia are caused by aspiration of endogenous or hospital-acquired oropharyngeal (and occasionally gastric) flora. Nosocomial pneumonias are associated with more deaths than are infections at any other body site. However, attributable mortality rates suggest that the risk of dying from nosocomial pneumonia is affected greatly by other factors, including comorbidities, inadequate antibiotic treatment, and the involvement of specific pathogens (particularly *Pseudomonas aeruginosa* or *Acinetobacter*). Surveillance and accurate diagnosis of pneumonia have been problematic in hospitals because many patients, especially those in the ICU, have abnormal chest roentgenographs, fever, and leukocytosis potentially attributable to multiple causes. This diagnostic uncertainty has led to a refocus from VAP to "ventilator-associated events" (VAEs), conditions, and complications, for which worsening physiologic parameters, such as oxygenation, are key metrics. Early data suggest that ~5–10% of patients using mechanical ventilators develop VAEs. Viral pneumonias, which are particularly important in pediatric and immunocompromised patients, are discussed in the virology section and in Chap. 153.

Risk factors for nosocomial pneumonia include those events that increase colonization by potential pathogens (e.g., prior antimicrobial therapy, contaminated ventilator circuits or equipment, or decreased gastric acidity); those that facilitate aspiration of oropharyngeal contents into the lower respiratory tract (e.g., intubation, decreased levels of consciousness, or presence of a nasogastric tube); and those that reduce host defense mechanisms in the lung and permit overgrowth of aspirated pathogens (e.g., chronic obstructive pulmonary disease, extremes of age, or upper abdominal surgery).

Control measures for pneumonia (Table 168-4) are aimed at frequent testing of readiness for extubation, remediation of risk factors in patient care (e.g., minimizing aspiration-prone supine positioning), and aseptic care of respirator equipment (e.g., disinfecting or sterilizing all inline reusable components such as nebulizers, replacing tubing/breathing circuits only if required because of malfunction or visible soiling—rather than on the basis of duration of use—to lessen the number of breaks in the system, and teaching aseptic technique for suctioning). Although the benefits of selective decontamination of the oropharynx and gut with nonabsorbable antimicrobial agents and/or use of short-course postintubation systemic antibiotics have been controversial, a randomized multicenter trial demonstrated lowered ICU mortality rates among patients on mechanical ventilation who underwent oropharyngeal decontamination.

Among the logical preventive measures that require further investigation are placement of endotracheal tubes that provide channels for subglottic drainage of secretions, which has been associated with reduced infection risks during short-term postoperative use, and noninvasive mechanical ventilation whenever feasible. Use of silver-coated endotracheal tubes may lessen risk of VAP but is not considered routine. It is noteworthy that reducing the rate of VAP often has not reduced overall ICU mortality; this fact suggests that this infection is a marker for patients with an otherwise-heightened risk of death.

The most likely pathogens for nosocomial pneumonia and treatment options are discussed in Chap. 153. Several considerations regarding diagnosis and treatment are worth emphasizing. First, clinical criteria for diagnosis (e.g., fever, leukocytosis, development of purulent secretions, new or changing radiographic infiltrates, changes in oxygen requirement or ventilator settings) have high sensitivity but relatively low specificity. These criteria are most useful for selecting patients for bronchoscopic or nonbronchoscopic procedures that yield lower respiratory tract samples protected from upper-tract contamination; quantitative cultures of such specimens have diagnostic sensitivities in the range of 80%. Second, early-onset nosocomial pneumonia, which manifests within the first 4 days of hospitalization, is most often caused by community-acquired pathogens such as *Streptococcus pneumoniae* and *Haemophilus* species, although some studies have challenged this view. Late-onset pneumonias most commonly are due to *S. aureus*, *P. aeruginosa*, *Enterobacter* species, *Klebsiella pneumoniae*, or *Acinetobacter*. When invasive techniques are used to diagnose VAP, the proportion of isolates accounted for by gram-negative bacilli decreases from 50–70% to 35–45%. Infection is polymicrobial in as many as 20–40% of cases. The role of anaerobic bacteria in VAP is not well defined. Third, one multicenter study suggested that 8 days is an appropriate duration of therapy for nosocomial pneumonia, with a longer duration (15 days in that study) when the pathogen is *Acinetobacter* or *P. aeruginosa*. Finally, in febrile patients (particularly those who have endotracheal or gastric tubes inserted through the nares), occult respiratory tract infections, especially bacterial sinusitis and otitis media, should be considered.

SURGICAL WOUND INFECTIONS

Wound infections occur in ~500,000 patients each year, account for ~15–20% of nosocomial infections, contribute up to 7–10 extra postoperative hospital days, and result in $3000 to $29,000 in extra costs, depending on the operative procedure and pathogen(s). The average wound infection has an incubation period of 5–7 days—longer than many postoperative stays. For this reason and because many procedures are now performed on an outpatient basis, the incidence of wound infections has become more difficult to assess. These infections usually are caused by the patient's endogenous or hospital-acquired skin and mucosal flora and occasionally are due to airborne spread of skin squames that may be shed into the wound from members of the operating-room team. True airborne spread of infection through droplet nuclei is rare in operating rooms unless there is a "disseminator" (e.g., of group A streptococci or staphylococci) among the staff. In general, the common risks for postoperative wound infection are related to the surgeon's technical skill, the patient's underlying conditions (e.g., diabetes mellitus, obesity) or advanced age, and inappropriate timing of antibiotic prophylaxis. Additional risks include the presence of drains, prolonged preoperative hospital stays, shaving of operative sites by razor the day before surgery, long duration of surgery, and infection at remote sites (e.g., untreated UTI).

The substantial literature related to risk factors for surgical-site infections and the recognized morbidity and cost of these infections have led to national prevention efforts and to recommendations for "bundling" preventive measures (Table 168-4). Additional measures include attention to technical surgical issues (e.g., avoiding open or prophylactic drains), operating-room asepsis, and preoperative therapy for active infection. Reporting surveillance results to surgeons has been associated with reductions in infection rates. Preoperative administration of intranasal mupirocin to patients colonized with *S. aureus*, preoperative antiseptic bathing, and intra- and postoperative oxygen supplementation have been controversial because of conflicting study results, but evidence seems mostly to favor these interventions.

The process of diagnosing and treating wound infections begins with a careful assessment of the surgical site in the febrile postoperative patient. Diagnosis of deeper organ-space infections or subphrenic abscesses requires a high index of suspicion and the use of CT or MRI. Diagnosis of infections of prosthetic devices, such as orthopedic implants, may be particularly difficult and often requires the use of interventional radiographic techniques to obtain periprosthetic specimens for culture. Cultures of periprosthetic joint tissue obtained at surgery may miss pathogens that are cloistered in prosthesis-adherent biofilms; cultures of sonicates from explanted prosthetic joints have been more sensitive, particularly for patients who have received antimicrobial agents within 2 weeks of surgery.

The most common pathogens in postoperative wound infections are *S. aureus*, coagulase-negative staphylococci, and enteric and anaerobic bacteria. In rapidly progressing postoperative infections manifesting within 24–48 h of a surgical procedure, the level of suspicion regarding group A streptococcal or clostridial infection (Chaps. 173 and 179) should be high. Treatment of postoperative wound infections requires drainage or surgical excision of infected or necrotic material and antibiotic therapy aimed at the most likely or laboratory-confirmed pathogens.

INFECTIONS RELATED TO VASCULAR ACCESS AND MONITORING

Intravascular device–related bacteremias cause ~10–15% of nosocomial infections; central vascular catheters (CVCs) account for most of these bloodstream infections. Past national estimates indicated that as many as 200,000 bloodstream infections associated with CVCs occurred each year in the United States, with attributable mortality rates of 12–25%, an excess mean length of hospital stay of 12 days, and an estimated cost of $3700 to $29,000 per episode; one-third to one-half of these episodes occurred in ICUs. However, infection rates have dropped steadily (Table 168-3) since the publication of guidelines by the Healthcare Infection Control Practices Advisory Committee (HICPAC) in 2002. With increasing care of seriously ill patients in the community, vascular catheter–associated bloodstream infections acquired in outpatient settings are becoming more frequent. Broader surveillance for infections—outside ICUs and even outside hospitals—will be needed.

Catheter-related bloodstream infections derive largely from the cutaneous microflora of the insertion site, with pathogens migrating extraluminally to the catheter tip, usually during the first week after insertion. In addition, contamination of the hubs of CVCs or of the ports of "needle-less" systems may lead to intraluminal infection over longer periods, particularly with surgically implanted or cuffed catheters. Intrinsic (during the manufacturing process) or extrinsic (on-site in a health care facility) contamination of infusate, although rare, is the most common cause of epidemic device-related bloodstream infection; extrinsic contamination may cause up to half of endemic bacteremias related to arterial infusions used for hemodynamic monitoring. The most common pathogens isolated from vascular device–associated bacteremias include coagulase-negative staphylococci, *S. aureus* (with ≥50% of isolates in the United States resistant to methicillin), enterococci, nosocomial gram-negative bacilli, and *Candida*. Many pathogens, especially staphylococci, produce extracellular polysaccharide biofilms that facilitate attachment to catheters and provide sanctuary from antimicrobial agents. "Quorum-sensing" proteins, a target for future interventions, help bacterial cells communicate during biofilm development.

Evidence-based bundles of control measures (Table 168-4) have been strikingly effective, eliminating almost all CVC-associated infections in one ICU study. Additional control measures for infections associated with vascular access include use of a chlorhexidine-impregnated patch at the skin-catheter junction; daily bathing of ICU patients with chlorhexidine; application of semitransparent access-site dressings (for ease of bathing and site inspection and protection of the site from secretions); avoidance of the femoral site for catheterization because of a higher risk of infection (most likely related to the density of the skin flora); rotation of peripheral catheters to a new site at specified intervals (e.g., every 72–96 h), which may be facilitated by use of an IV therapy team; and application of aseptic technique when accessing pressure transducers or other vascular ports.

Unresolved issues include the role of gut translocation rather than vascular access sites as a cause of primary bacteremia in immunocompromised patients and the implications for surveillance definitions; the best frequency for rotation of CVC sites (given that guidewire-assisted catheter changes at the same site do not lessen and can even increase infection risk); the appropriate role of mupirocin ointment, a topical antibiotic with excellent antistaphylococcal activity, in site care; the relative degrees of risk posed by peripherally inserted central catheters (PICC lines); and the risk-benefit of prophylactic use of heparin (to avoid catheter thrombi, which may be associated with increased risk of infection) or of vancomycin or alcohol (as catheter flushes or "locks"—i.e., concentrated anti-infective solutions instilled into the catheter lumen) for high-risk patients.

Vascular device–related infection is suspected on the basis of the appearance of the catheter site or the presence of fever or bacteremia without another source in patients with vascular catheters. The diagnosis is confirmed by the recovery of the same species of microorganism from peripheral-blood cultures (preferably two samples drawn from peripheral veins by separate venipunctures) and from semiquantitative or quantitative cultures of the vascular catheter tip. Less commonly used diagnostic measures include (1) differential (faster) time to positivity (>2 h) for blood drawn through the vascular access device than for a sample from a peripheral vein and (2) differences in quantitative cultures (a threefold or greater "step-up") for blood samples drawn simultaneously from a peripheral vein and from a CVC, which should show the step-up if infected. When infusion-related sepsis is considered (e.g., because of the abrupt onset of fever or shock temporally related to infusion therapy), a sample of the infusate or blood product should be retained for culture.

Therapy for vascular access–related infection is directed at the pathogen recovered from the blood and/or infected site. Important considerations in treatment are the need for an echocardiogram (to evaluate the patient for endocarditis), the duration of therapy, and the need to remove potentially infected catheters. In one report, approximately one-fourth of patients with intravascular catheter-associated *S. aureus* bacteremia who were studied by transesophageal echocardiography had evidence of endocarditis; this test may be useful in determining the appropriate duration of treatment.

Detailed consensus guidelines for the management of intravascular catheter–related infections have been published and recommend catheter removal in most cases of bacteremia or fungemia due to nontunneled CVCs. When attempting to salvage a potentially infected catheter, some clinicians use the "antibiotic lock" technique, which may facilitate penetration of infected biofilms, in addition to systemic antimicrobial therapy (see *www.idsociety.org/Other_Guidelines/*).

The authors of the consensus treatment guidelines advise that the decision to remove a tunneled catheter or implanted device suspected of being the source of bacteremia or fungemia should be based on the severity of the patient's illness, the strength of evidence that the device is infected, the presence of local or systemic complications, an assessment of the specific pathogens, and the patient's response to antimicrobial therapy if the catheter or device is initially retained. For patients with track-site infection, successful therapy without catheter removal is unusual. For patients with suppurative venous thrombophlebitis, excision of affected veins is usually required.

ISOLATION TECHNIQUES

Written policies for the isolation of infectious patients are a standard component of infection control programs. To replace its prior pathogen-specific guidelines, the CDC published recommendations in 2006 for the control of multidrug-resistant organisms in health care settings; in 2007, the CDC published a revised edition of its basic isolation guidelines to provide updated recommendations for all components of health care, including acute-care hospitals and long-term, ambulatory, and home-care settings (see *www.cdc.gov/hicpac/pdf/isolation/Isolation2007.pdf*).

Standard precautions are designed for the care of all patients in hospitals and aim to reduce the risk of transmission of microorganisms from both recognized and unrecognized sources. These precautions include gloving as well as hand cleansing for potential contact with (1) blood; (2) all other body fluids, secretions, and excretions, whether or not they contain visible blood; (3) nonintact skin; and (4) mucous membranes. Depending on exposure risks, standard precautions also include use of masks, eye protection, and gowns.

Precautions for the care of patients with potentially contagious clinical syndromes (e.g., acute diarrhea) or with suspected or diagnosed colonization or infection by transmissible pathogens are based on probable routes of transmission: *airborne*, *droplet*, or *contact*, for which personnel don, at a minimum, N95 respirators, surgical face masks, or glove and gown, respectively. Sets of precautions may be combined for diseases that have more than one route of transmission (e.g., contact and airborne isolation for varicella).

Some prevalent antibiotic-resistant pathogens, particularly those that colonize the gastrointestinal tract (e.g., vancomycin-resistant enterococci [VRE] and even multidrug-resistant gram-negative bacilli such as carbapenemase-producing strains of *K. pneumoniae* [KPCs]), may be present on *intact* skin of patients in hospitals (the "fecal patina"). This issue has led some experts to recommend gloving for all contact with patients who are acutely ill and/or in high-risk units, such as ICUs or LTACHs. Wearing gloves does not replace the need for hand hygiene because hands sometimes (in up to 20% of interactions) become contaminated during wearing or removal of gloves.

EPIDEMIC AND EMERGING PROBLEMS

Outbreaks are always big news but probably account for <5% of nosocomial infections. The investigation and control of nosocomial epidemics require that infection control personnel (1) develop a case definition, (2) confirm that an outbreak really exists (since apparent epidemics may actually be pseudo-outbreaks due to surveillance or laboratory artifacts), (3) review aseptic practices and disinfectant use, (4) determine the extent of the outbreak, (5) perform an epidemiologic investigation to determine modes of transmission, (6) work closely with microbiology personnel to culture for common sources or personnel carriers as appropriate and to type epidemiologically important isolates, and (7) heighten surveillance to judge the effect of control measures. Control measures generally include reinforcing routine aseptic practices and hand hygiene, ensuring appropriate isolation of cases (and instituting cohort isolation and nursing if needed), and implementing further controls on the basis of the investigation's findings. Examples of some emerging and potential epidemic problems follow.

VIRAL RESPIRATORY INFECTIONS: PANDEMIC INFLUENZA

Infections caused by the severe acute respiratory syndrome (SARS)–associated coronavirus challenged health care systems globally in 2003 (Chap. 223), and in 2012 Middle East respiratory syndrome coronavirus (MERS-CoV) emerged as a more geographically localized problem (Chap. 223). For SARS, basic infection-control measures helped to keep the worldwide case and death counts at ~8000 and ~800, respectively, although the virus was unforgiving of lapses in protocol adherence or laboratory biosafety. The epidemiology of SARS—spread largely in households once patients were ill or in hospitals—contrasts markedly with that of influenza (Chap. 224), which is often contagious a day before symptom onset; can spread rapidly in the community among nonimmune persons; and, even in its seasonal variety, kills as many as 35,000 persons each year in the United States.

Control of seasonal influenza has depended on (1) the use of effective vaccines, with increasingly broad evidence-based recommendations for vaccination of children, the general public, and health care workers; (2) the use of antiviral medications for early treatment and for prophylaxis as part of outbreak control, especially for high-risk patients and in high-risk settings like nursing homes or hospitals; and (3) infection control (surveillance and droplet precautions) for symptomatic patients. Controversial infection-control issues have been the questionable role of airborne spread of influenza and the need to mandate influenza vaccination of health care workers because of the embarrassingly low rates of vaccination in this high-risk group.

With the occurrence of localized outbreaks of avian (H5N1) influenza in Asia over the past few years, concerns about potential pandemic influenza led to (1) recommendations for universal "respiratory hygiene and cough etiquette" (basically, "cover your cough"), as described and promoted in the CDC's 2007 *Guideline for Isolation Precautions*, and for "source containment" (e.g., use of face masks and spatial separation) for outpatients with potentially infectious respiratory illnesses; (2) re-examinations of the value in the 1918–1919 influenza pandemic of nonpharmacologic interventions, such as "social distancing" (e.g., closing of schools and community venues); and (3) debate about the level of respiratory protection required for health care workers (i.e., whether to use the higher-efficiency N95 respirators recommended for airborne isolation rather than the surgical masks used for droplet precautions).

In the spring of 2009, a novel strain of influenza virus—H1N1 or "swine flu" virus—caused the first influenza pandemic in four decades. Recombinant events that create new strains (e.g., H7N9) continue to challenge global efforts at infection control and vaccine development (Chap. 224).

NOSOCOMIAL DIARRHEA

A new, more virulent strain of *C. difficile*—NAP1/BI/027—emerged in North America, and overall rates of *C. difficile*-associated diarrhea (Chap. 161) have increased, especially among older patients, in U.S. hospitals during the past few years. *C. difficile* control measures include judicious use of all antibiotics, especially fluoroquinolone antibiotics that have been implicated in driving these changes; heightened suspicion for "atypical" presentations (e.g., toxic megacolon or leukemoid reaction without diarrhea); and early diagnosis, treatment, and contact precautions. To improve diagnosis, use of more sensitive polymerase chain reaction–based rather than enzyme immunoassay–based testing of diarrheal stool is now recommended, with resultant artificial doubling of infection rates in some hospitals. Preliminary data suggest a role for probiotics in the prevention of *C. difficile*-associated diarrhea in patients in whom systemic antibiotic therapy is being initiated. Fecal transplantation has had dramatic results in the treatment of relapsing cases of *C. difficile*-associated diarrhea (Chap. 161). Successes with fecal transplants and probiotics have called attention to the potential role of manipulation of the intestinal microbiome as a broader infection-control strategy.

Outbreaks of norovirus infection (Chap. 227) in U.S. and European health care facilities appear to continue to increase in frequency or at least in reporting, with the virus often introduced by ill visitors or staff. This pathogen should be suspected when nausea and vomiting are prominent aspects of bacterial culture–negative diarrheal syndromes. Contact precautions may need to be augmented by aggressive environmental cleaning (given the persistence of norovirus on inanimate objects), prevention of secondary cases in cleaning staff through an emphasis on the use of personal protective equipment and hand hygiene, and active exclusion of ill staff and visitors.

CHICKENPOX

Infection control practitioners institute a varicella exposure investigation and control plan whenever health care workers have been exposed to chickenpox (Chap. 217) or have worked while having or during the 24 h before developing chickenpox. The names of exposed workers and patients are obtained; medical histories are reviewed, and (if necessary) serologic tests for immunity are conducted; physicians are notified of susceptible exposed patients; postexposure prophylaxis with a preparation of varicella-zoster immune globulin (VZIG) is considered for immunocompromised or pregnant contacts, with administration as soon as possible (but as long as 10 days after exposure) (Table 217-1); varicella vaccine is recommended or preemptive use of acyclovir is considered as an alternative strategy in other susceptible persons; and susceptible exposed employees are furloughed during the at-risk period for disease (8–21 days or, if VZIG has been administered, 28 days). Routine varicella vaccination of children and susceptible employees has made nosocomial spread less common and less problematic.

TUBERCULOSIS

Important measures for the control of tuberculosis (Chap. 202) include prompt recognition, isolation, and treatment of cases; recognition of atypical presentations (e.g., lower-lobe infiltrates without cavitation); use of negative-pressure, 100% exhaust, private isolation rooms with closed doors and at least 6–12 air changes per hour; use of N95 respirators by caregivers entering isolation rooms; possible use of high-efficiency particulate air filter units and/or ultraviolet lights for disinfecting air when other engineering controls are not feasible or reliable; and follow-up testing of susceptible personnel who have been exposed to infectious patients before isolation. The use of serologic tests, rather than skin tests, in the diagnosis of latent tuberculosis for infection control purposes has become common, mostly for logistic reasons. As tuberculosis once again is on the decline in the United States, we need to remember that the price of freedom—in this instance, from a communicable disease—is eternal vigilance.

GROUP A STREPTOCOCCAL INFECTIONS

The potential for an outbreak of group A streptococcal infection (Chap. 173) should be considered when even one or two nosocomial cases occur. Most outbreaks involve surgical wounds and are due to the presence of an asymptomatic carrier in the operating room. Investigation can be confounded by carriage at extrapharyngeal sites such as the rectum and vagina. Health care workers in whom carriage has been linked to nosocomial transmission of group A streptococci are removed from the patient-care setting and are not permitted to return until carriage has been eliminated by antimicrobial therapy.

FUNGAL INFECTIONS

Fungal spores are common in the environment, particularly on dusty surfaces. When dusty areas are disturbed during hospital repairs or renovation, the spores become airborne. Inhalation of spores by immunosuppressed (especially neutropenic) patients creates a risk of pulmonary and/or paranasal sinus infection and disseminated aspergillosis (Chap. 241). Routine surveillance among neutropenic patients for infections with filamentous fungi, such as *Aspergillus* and *Fusarium*, helps hospitals to determine whether they are facing environmental risks. As a matter of routine, hospitals should inspect and clean air-handling equipment, review all planned renovations with infection control personnel and subsequently construct appropriate barriers, remove immunosuppressed patients from renovation sites, and consider the use of high-efficiency particulate air intake filters for rooms housing immunosuppressed patients.

A major multistate iatrogenic outbreak of meningitis, localized spinal or paraspinal infection, and arthritis due to *Exserohilum rostratum* was recognized in 2012 and traced to contamination of an injectable preservative-free steroid product produced by a single compounding pharmacy (Chap. 241).

LEGIONELLOSIS

Nosocomial *Legionella* pneumonia (Chap. 184) is most often due to contamination of potable water and predominantly affects immunosuppressed patients, particularly those receiving glucocorticoid medications. The risk varies greatly within and among geographic regions, depending on the extent of hospital water contamination and on specific hospital practices (e.g., inappropriate use of nonsterile water in respiratory therapy equipment). Laboratory-based surveillance for nosocomial *Legionella* should be performed, and a diagnosis of legionellosis should probably be considered more often than it is. If nosocomial cases are detected, environmental samples (e.g., tap water) should be cultured. If cultures yield *Legionella* and if typing of clinical and environmental isolates reveals a correlation, eradication measures should be pursued. An alternative approach is to periodically culture tap water in wards housing high-risk patients. If *Legionella* is found, a concerted effort should be made to culture samples from all patients with nosocomial pneumonia for *Legionella*.

ANTIBIOTIC-RESISTANT BACTERIA

Emerging multidrug-resistant bacteria like KPCs are harbingers of a potential "postantibiotic" era. Control of antibiotic resistance depends on close laboratory surveillance, with early detection of problems; on aggressive reinforcement of routine asepsis; on implementation of barrier precautions for all colonized and/or infected patients; on use of patient-surveillance cultures to more fully ascertain the extent of patient colonization; on antimicrobial stewardship to lessen ecologic pressures; and on timely initiation of an epidemiologic investigation when rates increase. Molecular typing (e.g., pulsed-field gel electrophoresis and, most recently, whole-genome sequencing) can help differentiate an outbreak due to a single strain (which necessitates an emphasis on hand hygiene and an evaluation of potential common-source exposures) from a polyclonal outbreak (which requires an emphasis on antibiotic prudence and device bundles; Table 168-4). Continuing emergence of multidrug-resistant organisms suggests that control efforts have been insufficient and that regional or broader (national and global) strategies and interventions are urgently needed (see *www.cdc.gov/drugresistance/threat-report-2013/* and *www.gov.uk/government/publications/uk-5-year-antimicrobial-resistance-strategy-2013-to-2018/*).

Currently, several antibiotic resistance problems are of particular concern. First, over the past decade or so, the emergence of community-associated methicillin-resistant *S. aureus* (CA-MRSA) has been dramatic in many countries, with as many as 50% of community-acquired "staph infections" in some U.S. cities now caused by strains resistant to β-lactam antibiotics (Chap. 172). The incursion of CA-MRSA into hospitals is well documented and has impacted surveillance and control of nosocomial MRSA infections.

Second, in the ongoing global reemergence of nosocomial multidrug-resistant gram-negative bacilli, new problems include plasmid-mediated resistance to fluoroquinolones, metallo-β-lactamase-mediated resistance to carbapenems, KPCs, and panresistant strains of *Acinetobacter*. The problematic New Delhi metallo-β-lactamase (NDM) is plasmid-mediated, has been highly successful in inter-genus transmission, and has quickly become a global threat (see *wwwnc.cdc.gov/eid/article/17/10/11-0655_article.htm*). For several years, KPCs were a very focal problem in the United States (predominantly in Brooklyn, NY), but more recently these strains have become a national threat. Many multidrug-resistant gram-negative bacilli are susceptible only to colistin, a drug that is consequently being "rediscovered," or to no available agents.

Third, there has been renewed recognition of the role of nursing homes, and now LTACHs, in the spread of resistant gram-negative bacilli such as KPCs. In some LTACHs, as many as 30–50% of patients may be colonized with KPCs.

Fourth, there has been increasing community-based spread of *E. coli* strains harboring an enzyme, CTX-M, that renders them broadly resistant to β-lactam antibiotics. Given the community focus of spread, these strains may be seen as a gram-negative version of CA-MRSA.

Finally, clinical infections with MRSA strains exhibiting high-level vancomycin resistance due to VRE-derived plasmids have been reported in a few patients—almost all in the United States and most in Michigan—in the setting of prolonged or repeated treatment with vancomycin and/or VRE colonization. Much more common is vancomycin "MIC creep": an increasing prevalence of MRSA strains that exhibit upper-limit susceptibility to vancomycin.

Colonized personnel who are implicated in nosocomial transmission of multidrug-resistant pathogens and patients who pose a threat can be decontaminated, depending on the pathogen. In a few ICUs, nonabsorbed antimicrobial agents for gastrointestinal decontamination of patients have been used successfully as a temporary emergency control measure for outbreaks of infection due to gram-negative bacilli. Potentially, manipulation of patients' intestinal microbiome could be a more durable strategy to control outbreaks of multidrug-resistant pathogens that have a gastrointestinal reservoir.

In several trials over the past 10 years, source control—i.e., removal of patients' fecal patina—by daily bathing with chlorhexidine has reduced the risk of bacteremia in ICU patients. "Search-and-destroy" methods—i.e., active surveillance cultures to detect and isolate the "resistance iceberg" of patients colonized with MRSA—in nonoutbreak settings are credited with elimination of nosocomial MRSA in the Netherlands and Denmark. In a recent multicenter trial in the United States, universal source control with chlorhexidine and nasal mupirocin was significantly more effective for controlling MRSA than was a search-and-destroy approach and led to control of other pathogens as well, providing a broad ("horizontal") rather than a narrower ("vertical") intervention (see *www.ahrq.gov/professionals/systems/hospital/universal_icu_decolonization/*). For some pathogens, such as VRE, enforcement of environmental cleaning also reduces cross-transmission risk.

Because the excessive use of broad-spectrum antibiotics underlies many resistance problems, "antibiotic stewardship" has been promulgated actively. The main tenets are to restrict the use of particular agents to narrowly defined indications in order to limit selective pressure on the nosocomial flora and, when broad-spectrum therapy is begun empirically in critically ill patients, to "de-escalate" treatment as soon as possible on the basis of the results of culture and susceptibility tests.

BIOTERRORISM AND OTHER "SURGE-EVENT" PREPAREDNESS

The horrific attack on the World Trade Center in New York City on September 11, 2001; the subsequent mailings of anthrax spores in the United States; the Boston Marathon bombing in 2013; and ongoing revelations of terrorist plans and activities in many other countries as well as the United States have made bioterrorism a prominent source of concern to hospital infection-control programs. The essentials for hospital preparedness entail education, internal and external communication, and risk assessment. Up-to-date information is available from the CDC (see *www.bt.cdc.gov*).

EMPLOYEE HEALTH SERVICE ISSUES

An institution's employee health service is a critical component of its infection control efforts. New employees should be processed through the service, where a contagious-disease history can be taken; evidence of immunity to a variety of diseases, such as hepatitis B, chickenpox, measles, mumps, and rubella, can be sought; immunizations for hepatitis B, measles, mumps, rubella, varicella, and pertussis (the only vaccine-preventable childhood disease that is on the rise again in the United States) can be given as needed; baseline tuberculosis testing can be performed; and education about personal responsibility for infection control can be initiated. Evaluations of employees should be codified to meet the requirements of accrediting and regulatory agencies.

The employee health service must have protocols for dealing with workers exposed to contagious diseases (e.g., influenza) and those percutaneously or mucosally exposed to the blood of patients infected with HIV or hepatitis B or C virus. For example, postexposure HIV prophylaxis (PEP) with combination antiretroviral agents is recommended, as indicated; free consultation is available from the CDC-funded PEPLine (888-HIV-4911). Protocols are also needed for dealing with caregivers who have common contagious diseases (such as chickenpox, group A streptococcal infection, influenza or another respiratory infection, or infectious diarrhea) and for those who have less common but high-visibility public health problems (such as chronic hepatitis B or C or HIV infection) for which exposure-control guidelines have been published by the CDC and by the Society for Healthcare Epidemiology of America.

169 Infections in Transplant Recipients

Robert W. Finberg, Joyce Fingeroth

This chapter considers aspects of infection unique to patients receiving transplanted tissue. The evaluation of infections in transplant recipients involves consideration of both the donor and the recipient of the transplanted cells or organ. Two central issues are of paramount importance: (1) infectious agents (particularly viruses, but also bacteria, fungi, and parasites) can be introduced into the recipient by the donor; and (2) treatment of the recipient with medicine to prevent rejection can suppress normal immune responses, greatly increasing susceptibility to infection. Thus, what might have been a latent or asymptomatic infection in an immunocompetent donor or in the recipient prior to therapy can become a life-threatening problem when the recipient becomes immunosuppressed. The pretransplantation evaluation of each patient should be guided by an analysis of both (1) what infections the recipient is currently harboring, since organisms that exist in a state of latency or dormancy before the procedure may cause fatal disease when the patient receives immunosuppressive treatment; and (2) what organisms are likely to be transmitted by the donor, particularly those to which the recipient may be naïve.

PRETRANSPLANTATION EVALUATION

The Donor A variety of organisms have been transmitted by organ transplantation. Transmission of infections that may have been latent or not clinically apparent in the donor has resulted in the development of specific donor-screening protocols. Results from routine blood bank studies, including those for antibodies to *Treponema pallidum* (syphilis), *Trypanosoma cruzi*, hepatitis B and C viruses, HIV-1 and -2, human T-lymphotropic virus types 1 and 2 (HTLV-1 and -2), and West Nile virus (WNV), should be documented. Serologic studies should be ordered to identify latent infection with viruses such as herpes simplex virus types 1 and 2 (HSV-1, HSV-2), varicella-zoster virus (VZV), cytomegalovirus (CMV), Epstein-Barr virus (EBV), Kaposi's sarcoma–associated herpesvirus (KSHV); acute infection with hepatitis A virus; and infection with the common parasite *Toxoplasma gondii*. Donors should be screened, when relevant, for viruses such as rabies virus and lymphocytic choriomeningitis virus as well as for parasites such as *Strongyloides stercoralis* and *Schistosoma* species. Clinicians caring for prospective organ donors should examine chest radiographs for evidence of granulomatous disease (e.g., caused by mycobacteria or fungi) and should perform skin testing or obtain blood for immune cell–based assays that detect active or latent *Mycobacterium tuberculosis* infection. An investigation of the donor's dietary habits (e.g., consumption of raw meat or fish or of unpasteurized dairy products), occupations or avocations (e.g., gardening or spelunking), and travel history (e.g., travel to areas with endemic fungi) also is indicated and may mandate additional testing. Creutzfeldt-Jakob disease has been transmitted through corneal transplants. Whether it can be transmitted by transfused blood is not known. Variant Creutzfeldt-Jakob disease can be transmitted with transfused non-leukodepleted blood, posing a theoretical risk to transplant recipients.

The Recipient It is expected that the recipient will have been even more comprehensively assessed than the donor. Additional studies recommended for the recipient include evaluation for acute respiratory viruses and gastrointestinal pathogens in the immediate pretransplantation period. An important caveat is that, because of immune dysfunction resulting from chemotherapy or underlying chronic disease, serologic testing of the recipient may prove less reliable than usual.

The Donor Cells/Organ Careful attention to the sterility of the medium used to process the donor organ, combined with meticulous microbiologic evaluation, reduces rates of transmission of bacteria (or, rarely, yeasts) that may be present or grow in the organ culture medium. From 2% to >20% of donor kidneys are estimated to be contaminated with bacteria—in most cases, with the organisms that colonize the skin or grow in the tissue culture medium used to bathe the donor organ while it awaits implantation. The reported rate of bacterial contamination of transplanted stem cells (bone marrow, peripheral blood, cord blood) is as high as 17% but most commonly is ~1%. The use of enrichment columns and monoclonal antibody depletion procedures results in a higher incidence of contamination. In one series of patients receiving contaminated stem cells, 14% had fever or bacteremia, but none died. Results of cultures performed at the time of cryopreservation and at the time of thawing were helpful in guiding therapy for the recipient.

INFECTIONS IN HEMATOPOIETIC STEM CELL TRANSPLANT RECIPIENTS

Transplantation of hematopoietic stem cells (HSCs) from bone marrow or from peripheral or cord blood for cancer, immunodeficiency, or autoimmune disease most often results in a transient state of complete immunologic incompetence. Immediately after myeloablative chemotherapy and transplantation, both innate immune cells (phagocytes, dendritic cells, natural killer cells) and adaptive immune cells (T and B cells) are absent, and the host is extremely susceptible to infection. The reconstitution that follows transplantation has been likened to maturation of the immune system in neonates. The analogy does not entirely predict infections seen in HSC transplant recipients, however, because the stem cells mature in an old host who has several latent infections already. The choice among the current variety of methods for obtaining stem cells is determined by availability and by the need to optimize the chances of a cure for an individual recipient. One strategy is autologous HSC transplantation, in which the donor and the recipient are the same. After chemotherapy, stem cells are collected and are purged (ex vivo) of residual neoplastic populations. Allogeneic HSC transplantation has the advantage of providing a graft-versus-tumor effect. In this case, the recipient is matched to varying degrees for human leukocyte antigens (HLAs) with a donor who may be related or unrelated. In some individuals, nonmyeloablative therapy (mini-allo transplantation) is used and permits recipient cells to persist for some time after transplantation while preserving the graft-versus-tumor effect and sparing the recipient myeloablative therapy. Cord blood transplantation is increasingly utilized in adults; two independent cord-blood units are typically required for suitable neutrophil engraftment early after transplantation, even though only one of the units is likely to provide long-term engraftment. In each circumstance, a different balance is struck among the toxicity of conditioning therapy, the need for a maximal graft-versus-target effect, short-term and long-term infectious complications, and the risk of graft-versus-host disease (GVHD; acute versus chronic). The various approaches differ in terms of reconstitution speed, cell lineages introduced, and likelihood of GVHD—all factors that can produce distinct effects on the risk of infection after transplantation (Table 169-1). Despite these caveats, most infections occur in a predictable time frame after transplantation (Table 169-2).

BACTERIAL INFECTIONS

In the first month after HSC transplantation, infectious complications are similar to those in granulocytopenic patients receiving chemotherapy for acute leukemia (Chap. 104). Because of the anticipated 1- to 4-week duration of neutropenia and the high rate of bacterial infection in this population, many centers give prophylactic antibiotics to patients upon initiation of myeloablative therapy. Quinolones decrease the incidence of gram-negative bacteremia among these patients. Bacterial infections are common in the first few days after HSC transplantation. The organisms involved are predominantly those found on skin, mucosa, or IV catheters (*Staphylococcus aureus*, coagulase-negative staphylococci, streptococci) or aerobic bacteria that colonize the bowel (*Escherichia coli*, *Klebsiella*, *Pseudomonas*). *Bacillus cereus*, although rare, has emerged as a pathogen early after transplantation and can cause meningitis, which is unusual in these patients. Chemotherapy, use of broad-spectrum antibiotics, and delayed reconstitution of humoral immunity place HSC transplant patients at risk for diarrhea and colitis caused by *Clostridium difficile* overgrowth and toxin production.

TABLE 169-1 RISK OF INFECTION, BY TYPE OF HEMATOPOIETIC STEM CELL TRANSPLANT

Type of Hematopoietic Stem Cell Transplant	Source of Stem Cells	Risk of Early Infection: Neutrophil Depletion	Risk of Late Infection: Impaired T and B Cell Function	Risk of Ongoing Infection: GVHD and Iatrogenic Immunosuppression	Graft vs. Tumor Effect
Autologous	Recipient (self)	High risk; neutrophil recovery sometimes prolonged	~1 year	Minimal to no risk of GVHD and late-onset severe infection	None (–)
Syngeneic (genetic twin)	Identical twin	Low risk; 1–2 weeks for neutrophil recovery	~1 year	Minimal risk of GVHD and late-onset severe infection	+/–
Allogeneic related	Sibling	Low risk; 1–2 weeks for neutrophil recovery	~1 year	Minimal to moderate risk of GVHD and late-onset severe infection	++
Allogeneic related	Child/parent (haploidentical)	Intermediate risk; 2–3 weeks for neutrophil recovery	1–2 years	Moderate risk of GVHD and late-onset severe infection	++++
Allogeneic unrelated adult	Unrelated donor	Intermediate risk; 2–3 weeks for neutrophil recovery	1–2 years	High risk of GVHD and late-onset severe infection	++++
Allogeneic unrelated cord blood	Unrelated cord-blood units (×2)	Intermediate to high risk; neutrophil recovery sometimes prolonged	Prolonged	Minimal to moderate risk of GVHD and late-onset severe infection	++++
Allogeneic mini (nonmyeloablative)	Donor (transiently coexisting with recipient cells)	Low risk; neutrophil counts close to normal	1–2+ years	Variable risk of GVHD and late-onset severe infection[a]	++++ (but develops slowly)

[a]Depending on the disparity of the match (major and minor histocompatibility antigens), GVHD may be severe or mild, the requirement for immunosuppression intense or minimal, and the risk of severe late infections coordinate with the degree of immunosuppression.

Abbreviation: GVHD, graft-versus-host disease.

Beyond the first few days of neutropenia, infections with nosocomial pathogens (e.g., vancomycin-resistant enterococci, *Stenotrophomonas maltophilia*, *Acinetobacter* species, and extended-spectrum β-lactamase–producing gram-negative bacteria) as well as with filamentous bacteria (e.g., *Nocardia* species) become more common. Vigilance is indicated, particularly for patients with a history of active or known latent tuberculosis, even when they have been appropriately pretreated. A form of bacterial colitis among cord-blood recipients has occurred 90–300 days after transplantation, responds to antimicrobial agents such as metronidazole, and—as determined by polymerase chain reaction (PCR) of biopsy specimens—may be attributed to the bacterium *Bradyrhizobium enterica* (related to *B. japonicum*). Episodes of bacteremia due to encapsulated organisms mark the late posttransplantation period (>6 months after HSC reconstitution); patients who have undergone splenectomy and those with persistent hypogammaglobulinemia are at particular risk.

FUNGAL INFECTIONS

Beyond the first week after transplantation, fungal infections become increasingly common, particularly among patients who have received broad-spectrum antibiotics. As in most granulocytopenic patients, *Candida* infections are most commonly seen in this setting. However, with increased use of prophylactic fluconazole, infections with resistant fungi—in particular, *Aspergillus* and other non-*Aspergillus* molds (*Rhizopus*, *Fusarium*, *Scedosporium*, *Penicillium*)—have become more common, prompting some centers to replace fluconazole with agents such as micafungin, voriconazole, or posaconazole. The role of antifungal prophylaxis with these different agents, in contrast to empirical treatment for suspected infection that is based on a positive β-D-glucan assay or galactomannan antigen test, remains controversial (**Chap. 104**). Documented infection should be aggressively treated, ideally with agents of proven activity. In patients with GVHD who require prolonged or indefinite courses of glucocorticoids and other immunosuppressive agents (e.g., cyclosporine, tacrolimus [FK 506, Prograf], mycophenolate mofetil [Cellcept], rapamycin [sirolimus, Rapamune], antithymocyte globulin, or anti-CD52 antibody [alemtuzumab, Campath—an antilymphocyte and antimonocyte monoclonal antibody]), there is a high risk of fungal infection (usually with *Candida* or *Aspergillus*) even after engraftment and resolution of neutropenia. These patients are also at high risk for reactivation of latent fungal infection (histoplasmosis, coccidioidomycosis, or blastomycosis) in areas where endemic fungi reside and after involvement

TABLE 169-2 COMMON SOURCES OF INFECTIONS AFTER HEMATOPOIETIC STEM CELL TRANSPLANTATION

	Period after Transplantation		
Infection Site	**Early (<1 Month)**	**Middle (1–4 Months)**	**Late (>6 Months)**
Disseminated	Aerobic bacteria (gram-negative, gram-positive)	*Candida*, *Aspergillus*, EBV	Encapsulated bacteria (*Streptococcus pneumoniae*, *Haemophilus influenzae*, *Neisseria meningitidis*)
Skin and mucous membranes	HSV	HHV-6	VZV, HPV (warts)
Lungs	Aerobic bacteria (gram-negative, gram-positive), *Candida*, *Aspergillus*, other molds, HSV	CMV, seasonal respiratory viruses, *Pneumocystis*, *Toxoplasma*	*Pneumocystis*, *Nocardia*, *S. pneumoniae*
Gastrointestinal tract	*Clostridium difficile*	CMV, adenovirus, *Bradyrhizobium enterica* (cord blood cells)	EBV, CMV, *B. enterica* (cord blood cells)
Kidney		BK virus, adenovirus	
Brain		HHV-6, *Toxoplasma*	*Toxoplasma*, JC virus (rare)
Bone marrow		CMV, HHV-6	CMV, HHV-6

Abbreviations: CMV, cytomegalovirus; EBV, Epstein-Barr virus; HHV-6, human herpesvirus type 6; HPV, human papillomavirus; HSV, herpes simplex virus; VZV, varicella-zoster virus.

in activities such as gardening or caving. Prolonged use of central venous catheters for parenteral nutrition (lipids) increases the risk of fungemia with *Malassezia*. Some centers administer prophylactic antifungal agents to these patients. Because of the high and prolonged risk of *Pneumocystis jirovecii* pneumonia (especially among patients being treated for hematologic malignancies), most patients receive maintenance prophylaxis with trimethoprim-sulfamethoxazole (TMP-SMX) starting 1 month after engraftment and continuing for at least 1 year.

PARASITIC INFECTIONS

The regimen just described for the fungal pathogen *Pneumocystis* may also protect patients seropositive for the parasite *T. gondii*, which can cause pneumonia, visceral disease (occasionally), and central nervous system (CNS) lesions (more commonly). The advantages of maintaining HSC transplant recipients on daily TMP-SMX for 1 year after transplantation include some protection against *Listeria monocytogenes* and nocardial disease as well as late infections with *Streptococcus pneumoniae* and *Haemophilus influenzae*, which stem from the inability of the immature immune system to respond to polysaccharide antigens.

With increasing international travel, parasitic diseases typically restricted to particular environmental niches may pose a risk of reactivation in certain patients after HSC transplantation. Thus, in recipients with an appropriate history who were not screened and/or treated before transplantation or in patients with recent exposures, evaluation for infection with *Strongyloides*, *Leishmania*, schistosomes, trypanosomes, or various parasitic causes of diarrheal illness (*Giardia*, *Entamoeba*, *Cryptosporidium*, microsporidia) may be warranted.

VIRAL INFECTIONS

HSC transplant recipients are susceptible to infection with a variety of viruses, including primary and reactivation syndromes caused by most human herpesviruses (Table 169-3) and acute infections caused by viruses that circulate in the community.

TABLE 169-3 HERPESVIRUS SYNDROMES OF TRANSPLANT RECIPIENTS

Virus	Reactivation Disease
Herpes simplex virus type 1	Oral lesions
	Esophageal lesions
	Pneumonia (primarily HSC transplant recipients)
	Hepatitis (rare)
Herpes simplex virus type 2	Anogenital lesions
	Hepatitis (rare)
Varicella-zoster virus	Zoster (can disseminate)
Cytomegalovirus	Associated with graft rejection
	Fever and malaise
	Bone marrow failure
	Pneumonitis
	Gastrointestinal disease
Epstein-Barr virus	B cell lymphoproliferative disease/lymphoma
	Oral hairy leukoplakia (rare)
Human herpesvirus type 6	Fever
	Delayed monocyte/platelet engraftment
	Encephalitis (rare)
Human herpesvirus type 7	Undefined
Kaposi's sarcoma–associated virus	Kaposi's sarcoma
	Primary effusion lymphoma (rare)
	Multicentric Castleman's disease (rare)
	Marrow aplasia (rare)

Abbreviation: HSC, hematopoietic stem cell.

Herpes Simplex Virus Within the first 2 weeks after transplantation, most patients who are seropositive for HSV-1 excrete the virus from the oropharynx. The ability to isolate HSV declines with time. Administration of prophylactic acyclovir (or valacyclovir) to seropositive HSC transplant recipients has been shown to reduce mucositis and prevent HSV pneumonia (a rare condition reported almost exclusively in allogeneic HSC transplant recipients). Both esophagitis (usually due to HSV-1) and anogenital disease (commonly caused by HSV-2) may be prevented with acyclovir prophylaxis. For further discussion, see Chap. 216.

Varicella-Zoster Virus Reactivation of VZV manifests as herpes zoster and may occur within the first month but more commonly occurs several months after transplantation. Reactivation rates are ~40% for allogeneic HSC transplant recipients and 25% for autologous recipients. Localized zoster can spread rapidly in an immunosuppressed patient. Fortunately, disseminated disease can usually be controlled with high doses of acyclovir. Because of frequent dissemination among patients with skin lesions, acyclovir is given prophylactically in some centers to prevent severe disease. Low doses of acyclovir appear to be effective in preventing reactivation of VZV. However, acyclovir can also suppress the development of VZV-specific immunity. Thus, its administration for only 6 months after transplantation does not prevent zoster from occurring when treatment is stopped. Administration of low doses of acyclovir for an entire year after transplantation is effective and may eliminate most cases of posttransplantation zoster, even among cord-blood recipients. For further discussion, see Chap. 217.

Cytomegalovirus The onset of CMV disease (interstitial pneumonia, bone marrow suppression, graft failure, hepatitis/colitis) usually begins 30–90 days after HSC transplantation, when the granulocyte count is adequate but immunologic reconstitution has not occurred. CMV disease rarely develops earlier than 14 days after transplantation and may become evident as late as 4 months after the procedure. It is of greatest concern in the second month after transplantation, particularly in allogeneic HSC transplant recipients. In cases in which the donor marrow is depleted of T cells (to prevent GVHD or eliminate a T cell tumor) and in cord-blood recipients, the disease may manifest earlier. The use of alemtuzumab to prevent GVHD in nonmyeloablative transplantation has been associated with an increase in CMV disease. Patients who receive ganciclovir for prophylaxis, preemptive treatment, or treatment (see below) may develop recurrent CMV infection even later than 4 months after transplantation, as treatment appears to delay the development of the normal immune response to CMV infection. Although CMV disease may present as isolated fever, granulocytopenia, thrombocytopenia, or gastrointestinal disease, the foremost cause of death from CMV infection in the setting of HSC transplantation is pneumonia.

With the standard use of CMV-negative or filtered blood products, CMV infection should be a major risk in allogeneic transplantation only when the recipient is CMV seropositive and the donor is CMV-seronegative. This situation is the reverse of that in solid organ transplant recipients. CMV reactivates from latent reservoirs present in the recipient at a time when donor T cells (especially cord-blood T cells) are too immature to control CMV replication. If the T cells from the donor have never encountered CMV and the recipient carries the virus, the patient is at maximal risk of severe disease. Reactivation disease or superinfection with another strain from the donor also can occur in CMV-positive recipients, but clinical manifestations are typically less severe, presumably because of CMV-specific memory in transplanted donor T cells. Most patients infected with CMV who undergo HSC transplantation excrete virus, with or without clinical findings. Serious CMV disease is much more common among allogeneic than autologous recipients and is often associated with GVHD. In addition to pneumonia and marrow suppression (and, less often, graft failure), manifestations of CMV disease in HSC transplant recipients include fever with or without arthralgias, myalgias, hepatitis, and esophagitis. CMV ulcerations occur in both the lower and the upper gastrointestinal tract, and it may be difficult to distinguish diarrhea due to GVHD from that due to CMV infection. The finding of CMV in the liver of a patient with GVHD does not necessarily mean that CMV is responsible for hepatic enzyme abnormalities. It is interesting that the ocular and neurologic manifestations of CMV infections, which are common in patients with AIDS, are uncommon in patients who develop disease after transplantation.

Management of CMV disease in HSC transplant recipients includes strategies directed at prophylaxis, preemptive therapy (suppression of silent replication), and treatment of disease. Prophylaxis results in a lower incidence of disease at the cost of treating many patients who otherwise would not require therapy. Because of the high fatality rate associated with CMV pneumonia in these patients and the difficulty of early diagnosis of CMV infection, prophylactic IV ganciclovir (or oral valganciclovir) has been used in some centers and has been shown to prevent CMV disease during the period of maximal vulnerability (from engraftment to day 120 after transplantation). Ganciclovir also prevents HSV reactivation and reduces the risk of VZV reactivation; thus acyclovir prophylaxis should be discontinued when ganciclovir is administered. The foremost problem with the administration of ganciclovir relates to adverse effects, which include dose-related bone marrow suppression (thrombocytopenia, leukopenia, anemia, and pancytopenia). Because the frequency of CMV pneumonia is lower among autologous HSC transplant recipients (2–7%) than among allogeneic HSC transplant recipients (10–40%), prophylaxis in the former group will not become the rule until a less toxic oral antiviral agent becomes available. Several are under study.

Preemptive treatment of CMV—that is, initiation of therapy with drugs only after CMV is detected in blood by a nucleic acid amplification test (NAAT)—is used at most centers. To limit variability between tests, the World Health Organization (WHO) has developed an international reference standard for measurement of CMV load by NAAT-based assays. Because of toxic drug side effects (e.g., neutropenia and bone marrow suppression), the preemptive approach has supplanted prophylactic therapy; it has also replaced treatment of all seropositive (recipient and/or donor) HSC transplants with an antiviral agent (typically ganciclovir). A positive test (or increasing viral load) prompts the initiation of preemptive therapy with ganciclovir. Preemptive approaches that target patients who have quantitative NAAT evidence of CMV infection can still lead to unnecessary treatment of many individuals with drugs that have adverse effects on the basis of a laboratory test that is not highly predictive of disease; however, invasive disease, particularly in the form of pulmonary infection, is difficult to treat and is associated with high mortality rates. When prophylaxis or preemptive therapy is stopped, late manifestations of CMV replication may occur, although by then the HSC transplant patient is often equipped with improved graft function and is better able to combat disease. Cord-blood transplant recipients are especially vulnerable to disease caused by members of the human herpesvirus family, including CMV. Implementation of the WHO standard for CMV load measurement will facilitate large-scale comparative studies and thus the establishment of optimal guidelines for distinct patient subsets.

CMV pneumonia in HSC transplant recipients (unlike that in other clinical settings) is often treated with both IV immunoglobulin (IVIg) and ganciclovir. In patients who cannot tolerate ganciclovir, foscarnet is a useful alternative, although it may produce nephrotoxicity and electrolyte imbalance. When neither ganciclovir nor foscarnet is clinically tolerated, cidofovir can be used; however, its efficacy is less well established, and its side effects include nephrotoxicity. A lipid-conjugate form of cidofovir and an oral antiviral agent, maribavir, are in clinical trials. Case reports have suggested that the immunosuppressive agent leflunomide may be active in this setting, but controlled studies are lacking. Transfusion of CMV-specific T cells from the donor has decreased viral load in a small series of patients; this result suggests that immunotherapy (e.g., banked T cells) may play a role in the management of this disease in the future. **For further discussion, see Chap. 219.**

Human Herpesviruses 6 and 7 Human herpesvirus type 6 (HHV-6), the cause of roseola in children, is a ubiquitous herpesvirus that is reactivated (as determined by quantitative plasma PCR) in ~50% of HSC transplant recipients 2–4 weeks after transplantation. Reactivation is more common among patients requiring glucocorticoids for GVHD and among those receiving second transplants. Reactivation of HHV-6, primarily type B, may be associated with delayed monocyte and platelet engraftment. Limbic encephalitis developing after transplantation has been associated with HHV-6 in cerebrospinal fluid (CSF). The causality of the association is not well defined; in several cases, plasma viremia was detected long before the onset of encephalitis. Nevertheless, most patients with encephalitis had very high viral loads in plasma at the time of CNS illness, and viral antigen has been detected in hippocampal astrocytes. HHV-6 DNA is sometimes found in lung samples after transplantation. However, its role in pneumonitis is unclear, as co-pathogens are frequently present. While HHV-6 is susceptible to foscarnet or cidofovir (and possibly to ganciclovir) in vitro, the efficacy of antiviral treatment has not been well studied. Little is known about the related herpesvirus HHV-7 or its role in posttransplantation infection. **For further discussion, see Chap. 219.**

Epstein-Barr Virus Primary EBV infection can be fatal to HSC transplant recipients; EBV reactivation can cause EBV–B cell lymphoproliferative disease (EBV-LPD), which may also be fatal to patients taking immunosuppressive drugs. Latent EBV infection of B cells leads to several interesting phenomena in HSC transplant recipients. The marrow ablation that occurs as part of the HSC transplantation procedure may sometimes eliminate latent EBV from the host. Infection can then be reacquired immediately after transplantation by transfer of infected donor B cells. Rarely, transplantation from a seronegative donor may result in a cure. The recipient is then at risk for a second primary infection.

EBV-LPD can develop in the recipient's B cells (if any survive marrow ablation) but is more likely to be a consequence of outgrowth of infected donor cells. Both lytic replication and latent replication of EBV are more likely during immunosuppression (e.g., they are associated with GVHD and the use of antibodies to T cells). Although less likely in autologous transplantation, reactivation can occur in T cell–depleted autologous recipients (e.g., patients being given antibodies to T cells for the treatment of a T cell lymphoma with marrow depletion). EBV-LPD, which can become apparent as early as 1–3 months after engraftment, can cause high fevers and cervical adenopathy resembling the symptoms of infectious mononucleosis but more commonly presents as an extranodal mass. The incidence of EBV-LPD among allogeneic HSC transplant recipients is 0.6–1%, which contrasts with figures of ~5% for renal transplant recipients and up to 20% for cardiac transplant patients. In all cases, EBV-LPD is more likely to occur with high-dose, prolonged immunosuppression, especially that caused by the use of antibodies to T cells, glucocorticoids, and calcineurin inhibitors (e.g., cyclosporine, tacrolimus). Cord-blood recipients constitute another high-risk group because of delayed T cell function. Ganciclovir, administered to preempt CMV disease, may reduce EBV lytic replication and thereby diminish the pool of B cells that can become newly infected and give rise to LPD. Increasing evidence indicates that replacement of calcineurin inhibitors with mTor inhibitors (e.g., rapamycin) exerts an antiproliferative effect on EBV-infected B cells that decreases the likelihood of development of LPD or unrelated proliferative disorders associated with transplant-related immunosuppression.

PCR can be used to monitor EBV production after HSC transplantation. High or increasing viral loads predict an enhanced likelihood of EBV-LPD development and should prompt rapid reduction of immunosuppression and a search for nodal or extranodal disease. If reduction of immunosuppression does not have the desired effect, administration of a monoclonal antibody to CD20 (e.g., rituximab) for the treatment of B cell lymphomas that express this surface protein has elicited dramatic responses and currently constitutes first-line therapy for CD20-positive EBV-LPD. However, long-term suppression of new antibody responses accompanies therapy, and recurrences are not infrequent. Additional B cell–directed antibodies, including anti-CD22, are under study. The role of antiviral drugs is uncertain because no available agents have been documented to have activity against the different forms of latent EBV infection. Diminishing lytic replication and virion production in these patients would theoretically produce a statistical decrease in the frequency of latent disease by decreasing the number of virions available to cause additional infection. In case reports and animal studies, ganciclovir and/or high-dose zidovudine, together with other agents, has been used to eradicate EBV-LPD and CNS lymphomas, another EBV-associated complication of transplantation. Both interferon and retinoic acid have been employed in the treatment of EBV-LPD, as has IVIg, but no large-scale prospective studies have assessed the efficacy of any of these agents. Several additional drugs are undergoing preclinical evaluation. Standard chemotherapeutic regimens are used if disease persists after reduction of immunosuppressive agents and administration of antibodies. EBV-specific T cells generated from the donor have been used experimentally to prevent and treat EBV-LPD in allogeneic recipients, and efforts are under way to increase the activity and specificity of ex vivo–generated T cells. For further discussion, see Chap. 218.

Human Herpesvirus 8 (KSHV) The EBV-related gammaherpesvirus KSHV, which is causally associated with Kaposi's sarcoma, primary effusion lymphoma, and multicentric Castleman's disease, has rarely resulted in disease in HSC transplant recipients, although some cases of virus-associated marrow aplasia have been reported in the peri transplantation period. The relatively low seroprevalence of KSHV in the population and the limited duration of profound T cell suppression after HSC transplantation provide a plausible explanation for the currently low incidence of KSHV disease compared with that in recipients of solid organ transplants and patients with HIV infection. For further discussion, see Chap. 219.

Other (Non-Herpes) Viruses The diagnosis of pneumonia in HSC transplant recipients poses special problems. Because patients have undergone treatment with multiple chemotherapeutic agents and sometimes irradiation, their differential diagnosis should include—in addition to bacterial and fungal pneumonia—CMV pneumonitis, pneumonia of other viral etiologies, parasitic pneumonia, diffuse alveolar hemorrhage, and chemical- or radiation-associated pneumonitis. Since fungi and viruses (e.g., influenza A and B viruses, respiratory syncytial virus [RSV], parainfluenza virus [types 1–4], adenovirus, enterovirus, bocavirus, human metapneumovirus, coronavirus, and rhinovirus [increasingly detected by multiplex PCR]) also can cause pneumonia in this setting, it is important to obtain a specific diagnosis. Diagnostic modalities include Gram's stain, microbiologic culture, antigen testing, and—increasingly—multipathogen PCR and mass spectrometry assays. *M. tuberculosis* has been an uncommon cause of pneumonia among HSC transplant recipients in Western countries (accounting for <0.1–0.2% of cases) but is common in Hong Kong (5.5%) and in countries where the prevalence of tuberculosis is high. The recipient's exposure history is clearly critical in an assessment of posttransplantation infections.

Both RSV and parainfluenza viruses, particularly type 3, can cause severe or even fatal pneumonia in HSC transplant recipients. Infections with both of these agents sometimes occur as disastrous nosocomial epidemics. Therapy with palivizumab or ribavirin for RSV infection remains controversial. New agents, some host-directed, are under study. Influenza also occurs in HSC transplant recipients and generally mirrors the presence of infection in the community. Progression to pneumonia is more common when infection occurs early after transplantation and when the recipient is lymphopenic. The neuraminidase inhibitors oseltamivir (oral) and zanamivir (aerosolized) are active against both influenza A virus and influenza B virus and are a reasonable treatment option. Parenteral forms of neuraminidase inhibitors such as peramivir (intravenous) and several new oral agents remain in trial status. An important preventive measure is immunization of household members, hospital staff members, and other frequent contacts. Adenoviruses can be isolated from HSC transplant recipients at rates varying from 5% to ≥18%. Like CMV infection, adenovirus infection usually occurs in the first to third month after transplantation and is often asymptomatic, although pneumonia, hemorrhagic cystitis/nephritis, severe gastroenteritis with hemorrhage, and fatal disseminated infection have been reported and may be strain-specific. A role for cidofovir therapy has been suggested, but the efficacy of this agent in adenovirus infection remains to be determined. Banked virus-specific T cell therapy is under study for adenovirus infection (as well as for CMV and EBV infections).

Although diverse respiratory viruses can sometimes cause severe pneumonia and respiratory failure in HSC transplant recipients, mild or even asymptomatic infection may be more common. For example, rhinoviruses and coronaviruses are frequent co-pathogens in HSC transplant recipients; however, whether they independently contribute to significant pulmonary infection is not known. At present, the overall contribution of these viral respiratory pathogens to the burden of lower respiratory tract disease in HSC transplant recipients requires further study. Infections with parvovirus B19 (presenting as anemia or occasionally as pancytopenia) and disseminated enteroviruses (sometimes fatal) can occur. Parvovirus B19 infection can be treated with IVIg (Chap. 221).

Rotaviruses are a cause of gastroenteritis in HSC transplant recipients, more frequently in children. Norovirus is a common cause of vomiting and diarrhea, and symptoms can be prolonged in HSC recipients. The polyomavirus BK virus is found at high titers in the urine of patients who are profoundly immunosuppressed. BK viruria may be associated with hemorrhagic cystitis in these patients. In contrast to its incidence among patients with impaired T cell function due to AIDS (4–5%), progressive multifocal leukoencephalopathy caused by the related JC virus is relatively rare among HSC transplant recipients (Chap. 164). When transmitted by mosquitoes or by blood transfusion, WNV can cause encephalitis and death after HSC transplantation.

INFECTIONS IN SOLID ORGAN TRANSPLANT RECIPIENTS

Rates of morbidity and mortality among recipients of solid organ transplants (SOTs) are reduced by the use of effective antibiotics. The organisms that cause acute infections in recipients of SOTs are different from those that infect HSC transplant recipients because SOT recipients do not go through a period of neutropenia. As the transplantation procedure involves major surgery, however, SOT recipients are subject to infections at anastomotic sites and to wound infections. Compared with HSC transplant recipients, SOT patients are immunosuppressed for longer periods (often permanently). Thus they are susceptible to many of the same organisms as patients with chronically impaired T cell immunity (Chap. 104, especially Table 104-1). Moreover, the persistent HLA mismatch between recipient immune cells (e.g., effector T cells) and the donor organ (allograft) places the organ at permanently increased risk of infection.

During the early period (<1 month after transplantation; Table 169-4), infections are most commonly caused by extracellular bacteria (staphylococci, streptococci, enterococci, and *E. coli* and other gram-negative organisms, including nosocomial organisms with broad antibiotic resistance), which often originate in surgical wound or anastomotic sites. The type of transplant largely determines the spectrum of infection. In subsequent weeks, the consequences of the administration of agents that suppress cell-mediated immunity become apparent, and acquisition—or, more commonly, reactivation—of viruses, mycobacteria, endemic fungi, and parasites (from the recipient or from the transplanted organ) can occur. CMV infection is often a problem, particularly in the first 6 months after transplantation, and may present as severe systemic disease or as infection of the transplanted organ. HHV-6 reactivation (assessed by plasma PCR) occurs within the first 2–4 weeks after transplantation and may be associated with fever, leukopenia, and very rare cases of encephalitis. Data suggest that replication of HHV-6 and HHV-7 may exacerbate CMV-induced disease. CMV is associated not only with generalized immunosuppression but also with organ-specific, rejection-related syndromes: glomerulopathy in kidney transplant recipients, bronchiolitis obliterans in lung transplant recipients, vasculopathy in heart transplant recipients, and the vanishing bile duct syndrome in liver transplant recipients. A complex interplay between increased CMV

TABLE 169-4 COMMON INFECTIONS AFTER SOLID ORGAN TRANSPLANTATION, BY SITE OF INFECTION

Infected Site	Period after Transplantation		
	Early (<1 Month)	Middle (1–4 Months)	Late (>6 Months)
Donor organ	Bacterial and fungal infections of the graft, anastomotic site, and surgical wound	CMV infection	EBV infection (may present in allograft organ)
Systemic	Bacteremia and candidemia (often resulting from central venous catheter colonization)	CMV infection (fever, bone marrow suppression)	CMV infection, especially in patients given early posttransplantation prophylaxis; EBV proliferative syndromes (may occur in donor organs)
Lung	Bacterial aspiration pneumonia with prevalent nosocomial organisms associated with intubation and sedation (highest risk in lung transplantation)	*Pneumocystis* infection; CMV pneumonia (highest risk in lung transplantation); *Aspergillus* infection (highest risk in lung transplantation)	*Pneumocystis* infection; granulomatous lung diseases (nocardial and reactivated fungal and mycobacterial diseases)
Kidney	Bacterial and fungal (*Candida*) infections (cystitis, pyelonephritis) associated with urinary tract catheters (highest risk in kidney transplantation)	Kidney transplantation: BK virus infection (associated with nephropathy); JC virus infection	Kidney transplantation: bacterial infections (late urinary tract infections, usually not associated with bacteremia); BK virus infection (nephropathy, graft failure, generalized vasculopathy)
Liver and biliary tract	Cholangitis	CMV hepatitis	CMV hepatitis
Heart		*Toxoplasma gondii* infection (highest risk in heart transplantation); endocarditis (*Aspergillus* and gram-negative organisms more common than in general population)	*T. gondii* (highest risk in heart transplantation)
Gastrointestinal tract	Peritonitis, especially after liver transplantation	Colitis secondary to *Clostridium difficile* infection (risk can persist)	Colitis secondary to *C. difficile* infection (risk can persist)
Central nervous system		*Listeria* infection (meningitis); *T. gondii* infection; CMV infection	Listerial meningitis; cryptococcal meningitis; nocardial abscess; JC virus–associated PML

Abbreviations: CMV, cytomegalovirus; EBV, Epstein-Barr virus; PML, progressive multifocal leukoencephalopathy.

replication and enhanced graft rejection is well established: elevated immunosuppression leads to increased CMV replication, which is associated with graft rejection. For this reason, considerable attention has been focused on the diagnosis, prophylaxis, and treatment of CMV infection in SOT recipients. Early transmission of WNV to transplant recipients from a donated organ or transfused blood has been reported; however, the risk of WNV acquisition has been reduced by implementation of screening procedures. In rare instances, rabies virus and lymphocytic choriomeningitis virus also have been acutely transmitted in this setting; although accompanied by distinct clinical syndromes, both viral infections have resulted in fatal encephalitis. As screening for unusual viruses is not routine, only vigilant assessment of the prospective donor is likely to prevent the use of an infected organ.

Beyond 6 months after transplantation, infections characteristic of patients with defects in cell-mediated immunity—e.g., infections with *Listeria*, *Nocardia*, *Rhodococcus*, mycobacteria, various fungi, and other intracellular pathogens—may be a problem. International patients and global travelers may experience reactivation of dormant infections with trypanosomes, *Leishmania*, *Plasmodium*, *Strongyloides*, and other parasites. Reactivation of latent *M. tuberculosis* infection, while rare in Western nations, is far more common among persons from developing countries. The recipient is typically the source, although reactivation and spread from the donor organ can occur. While pulmonary disease remains most common, atypical sites can be involved and mortality rates can be high (up to 30%). Vigilance, prophylaxis/preemptive therapy (when indicated), and rapid diagnosis and treatment of infections can be lifesaving in SOT recipients, who, unlike most HSC transplant recipients, continue to be immunosuppressed.

SOT recipients are susceptible to EBV-LPD from as early as 2 months to many years after transplantation. The prevalence of this complication is increased by potent and prolonged use of T cell–suppressive drugs. Decreasing the degree of immunosuppression may in some cases reverse the condition. Among SOT patients, those with heart and lung transplants—who receive the most intensive immunosuppressive regimens—are most likely to develop EBV-LPD, particularly in the lungs. Although the disease usually originates in recipient B cells, several cases of donor origin, particularly in the transplanted organ, have been noted. High organ-specific content of B lymphoid tissues (e.g., bronchus-associated lymphoid tissue in the lung), anatomic factors (e.g., lack of access of host T cells to the transplanted organ because of disturbed lymphatics), and differences in major histocompatibility loci between the host T cells and the organ (e.g., lack of cell migration or lack of effective T cell/macrophage/dendritic cell cooperation) may result in defective elimination of EBV-infected B cells. SOT recipients are also highly susceptible to the development of Kaposi's sarcoma and, less frequently, to the B cell–proliferative disorders associated with KSHV, such as primary effusion lymphoma and multicentric Castleman's disease. Kaposi's sarcoma is 550–1000 times more common among SOT recipients than in the general population, can develop very rapidly after transplantation, and can also occur in the allograft. However, because the seroprevalence of KSHV is very low in Western countries, Kaposi's sarcoma is not common. Recipients (or donors) from Iceland, the Middle East, Mediterranean countries, and Africa are at highest risk of disease. Data suggest that a switch of immunosuppressive agents—from calcineurin inhibitors (cyclosporine, tacrolimus) to mTor pathway–active agents (sirolimus, everolimus)—after adequate wound healing may significantly reduce the likelihood of development of Kaposi's sarcoma and perhaps of EBV-LPD and certain other posttransplantation malignancies.

KIDNEY TRANSPLANTATION

See Table 169-4.

Early Infections Bacteria often cause infections that develop in the period immediately after kidney transplantation. There is a role for perioperative antibiotic prophylaxis, and many centers give cephalosporins to decrease the risk of postoperative complications. Urinary tract infections developing soon after transplantation are usually related to anatomic alterations resulting from surgery. Such early infections may require prolonged treatment (e.g., 6 weeks of antibiotic administration for pyelonephritis). Urinary tract infections that occur >6 months after transplantation may be treated for shorter periods because they do not seem to be associated with the high rate of pyelonephritis or relapse seen with infections that occur during the first 3 months.

TABLE 169-5 PROPHYLACTIC REGIMENS COMMONLY USED TO DECREASE RISK OF INFECTION IN TRANSPLANT RECIPIENTS[a]

Risk Factor	Organism	Prophylactic Drug	Examination(s)[b]
Travel to or residence in area with known risk of endemic fungal infection	*Histoplasma, Blastomyces, Coccidioides*	Triazoles considered in context of clinical and laboratory assessment	Chest radiography, antigen testing, serology
Latent herpesviruses	HSV, VZV, CMV, EBV	Acyclovir after HSC transplantation to prevent HSV and VZV infection or reactivation; ganciclovir to prevent CMV infection, with possible effect on EBV/KSHV/HHV-6 infections in some settings	Serologic tests for HSV, VZV, CMV, HHV-6, EBV, KSHV; PCR
Latent fungi and parasites	*Pneumocystis jirovecii, Toxoplasma gondii*	Trimethoprim-sulfamethoxazole (or alternatives)	Serologic test for *Toxoplasma*
History of exposure to active or latent tuberculosis	*Mycobacterium tuberculosis*	Isoniazid in patients with recent sero-conversion or positive chest imaging and/or no previous treatment	Chest imaging; TST and/or cell-based assay

[a]For information on latent infection with hepatitis B or C virus, see **Chap. 362**. [b]Serologic examination, tuberculin skin test, and interferon assays may be less reliable after transplantation.

Abbreviations: CMV, cytomegalovirus; EBV, Epstein-Barr virus; HHV-6, human herpesvirus type 6; HSC, hematopoietic stem cell; HSV, herpes simplex virus; KSHV, Kaposi's sarcoma–associated herpesvirus; PCR, polymerase chain reaction; TST, tuberculin skin test; VZV, varicella-zoster virus.

Prophylaxis with TMP-SMX for the first 4–6 months after transplantation decreases the incidence of early and middle-period infections (see below, Table 169-4, and Table 169-5).

Middle-Period Infections Because of continuing immunosuppression, kidney transplant recipients are predisposed to lung infections characteristic of those in patients with T cell deficiency (i.e., infections with intracellular bacteria, mycobacteria, nocardiae, fungi, viruses, and parasites). A high mortality rate associated with *Legionella pneumophila* infection (Chap. 184) led to the closing of renal transplant units in hospitals with endemic legionellosis.

About 50% of all renal transplant recipients presenting with fever 1–4 months after transplantation have evidence of CMV disease; CMV itself accounts for the fever in more than two-thirds of cases and thus is the predominant pathogen during this period. CMV infection (Chap. 219) may also present as arthralgias, myalgias, or organ-specific symptoms. During this period, this infection may represent primary disease (in the case of a seronegative recipient of a kidney from a seropositive donor) or may represent reactivation disease or superinfection. Patients may have atypical lymphocytosis. Unlike immunocompetent patients, however, they rarely have lymphadenopathy or splenomegaly. Therefore, clinical suspicion and laboratory confirmation are necessary for diagnosis. The clinical syndrome may be accompanied by bone marrow suppression (particularly leukopenia). CMV also causes glomerulopathy and is associated with an increased incidence of other opportunistic infections. Because of the frequency and severity of disease, a considerable effort has been made to prevent and treat CMV infection in renal transplant recipients. An immune globulin preparation enriched with antibodies to CMV was used by many centers in the past in an effort to protect the group at highest risk for severe infection (seronegative recipients of seropositive kidneys). However, with the development of effective oral antiviral agents, CMV immune globulin is no longer used. Ganciclovir (or valganciclovir) is beneficial for prophylaxis (when indicated) and for the treatment of serious CMV disease. The availability of valganciclovir has allowed most centers to move to oral prophylaxis for transplant recipients. Infection with the other herpesviruses may become evident within 6 months after transplantation or later. Early after transplantation, HSV may cause either oral or anogenital lesions that are usually responsive to acyclovir. Large ulcerating lesions in the anogenital area may lead to bladder and rectal dysfunction and may predispose the patient to bacterial infection. VZV may cause fatal disseminated infection in nonimmune kidney transplant recipients, but in immune patients reactivation zoster usually does not disseminate outside the dermatome; thus disseminated VZV infection is a less fearsome complication in kidney transplantation than in HSC transplantation. HHV-6 reactivation may take place and (although usually asymptomatic) may be associated with fever, rash, marrow suppression, or rare instances of renal impairment, hepatitis, colitis, or encephalitis.

EBV disease is more serious; it may present as an extranodal proliferation of B cells that invade the CNS, nasopharynx, liver, small bowel, heart, and other organs, including the transplanted kidney. The disease is diagnosed by the finding of a mass of proliferating EBV-positive B cells. The incidence of EBV-LPD is elevated among patients who acquire EBV infection from the donor and among patients given high doses of cyclosporine, tacrolimus, glucocorticoids, and anti T cell antibodies. Disease may regress once immunocompetence is restored. KSHV infection can be transmitted with the donor kidney and result in development of Kaposi's sarcoma, although it more often represents reactivation of latent infection of the recipient. Kaposi's sarcoma often appears within 1 year after transplantation, although the time of onset ranges widely (1 month to ~20 years). Avoidance of immunosuppressive agents that inhibit calcineurin has been associated with less Kaposi's sarcoma, less EBV disease, and even less CMV replication. The use of rapamycin (sirolimus) has independently led to regression of Kaposi's sarcoma.

The papovaviruses BK virus and JC virus (polyomavirus hominis types 1 and 2) have been cultured from the urine of kidney transplant recipients (as they have from that of HSC transplant recipients) in the setting of profound immunosuppression. High levels of BK virus replication detected by PCR in urine and blood are predictive of pathology, especially in the setting of renal transplantation. JC virus may rarely cause similar disease in kidney transplantation. Urinary excretion of BK virus and BK viremia are associated with the development of ureteral strictures, polyomavirus-associated nephropathy (1–10% of renal transplant recipients), and (less commonly) generalized vasculopathy. Timely detection and early reduction of immunosuppression are critical and can reduce rates of graft loss related to polyomavirus-associated nephropathy from 90% to 10–30%. Therapeutic responses to IVIg, quinolones, leflunomide, and cidofovir have been reported, but the efficacy of these agents has not been substantiated through adequate clinical study. Most centers approach the problem by reducing immunosuppression in an effort to enhance host immunity and decrease viral titers. JC virus is associated with rare cases of progressive multifocal leukoencephalopathy. Adenoviruses may persist and cause hemorrhagic nephritis/cystitis with continued immunosuppression in these patients, but disseminated disease like that seen in HSC transplant recipients is much less common.

Kidney transplant recipients are also subject to infections with other intracellular organisms. These patients may develop pulmonary infections with *Mycobacterium*, *Aspergillus*, and *Mucor* species as well as infections with other pathogens in which the T cell/macrophage axis plays an important role. *L. monocytogenes* is a common cause of bacteremia ≥1 month after renal transplantation and should be seriously considered in renal transplant recipients presenting with fever and headache. Kidney transplant recipients may develop *Salmonella* bacteremia, which can lead to endovascular infections and require prolonged therapy. Pulmonary infections with *Pneumocystis* are common unless the patient is maintained on TMP-SMX prophylaxis.

Acute interstitial nephritis caused by TMP-SMX is rare. However, because transient increases in creatinine (artifactual) and hyperkalemia (manageable) can occur, early discontinuation of prophylaxis, especially after kidney transplantation, is recommended by some groups. Although additional monitoring is indicated, the benefits of TMP-SMX in kidney transplant recipients may outweigh the risks; otherwise, second-line prophylactic agents should be used. *Nocardia* infection (Chap. 199) may present in the skin, bones, and lungs or in the CNS, where it usually takes the form of single or multiple brain abscesses. Nocardiosis generally occurs ≥1 month after transplantation and may follow immunosuppressive treatment for an episode of rejection. Pulmonary manifestations most commonly consist of localized disease with or without cavities, but the disease may be disseminated. The diagnosis is made by culture of the organism from sputum or from the involved nodule. As it is for *P. jirovecii* infection, prophylaxis with TMP-SMX is often efficacious in the prevention of nocardiosis.

Toxoplasmosis can occur in seropositive patients but is less common than in other transplantation settings, usually developing in the first few months after kidney transplantation. Again, TMP-SMX is helpful in prevention. In endemic areas, histoplasmosis, coccidioidomycosis, and blastomycosis may cause pulmonary infiltrates or disseminated disease.

Late Infections Late infections (>6 months after kidney transplantation) may involve the CNS and include CMV retinitis as well as other CNS manifestations of CMV disease. Patients (particularly those whose immunosuppression has been increased) are at risk for subacute meningitis due to *Cryptococcus neoformans*. Cryptococcal disease may present in an insidious manner (sometimes as a skin infection before the development of clear CNS findings). *Listeria* meningitis may have an acute presentation and requires prompt therapy to avoid a fatal outcome. TMP-SMX prophylaxis may reduce the frequency of *Listeria* infections.

Patients who continue to take glucocorticoids are predisposed to ongoing infection. "Transplant elbow," a recurrent bacterial infection in and around the elbow that is thought to result from a combination of poor tensile strength of the skin of steroid-treated patients and steroid-induced proximal myopathy, requires patients to push themselves up with their elbows to get out of chairs. Bouts of cellulitis (usually caused by *S. aureus*) recur until patients are provided with elbow protection.

Kidney transplant recipients are susceptible to invasive fungal infections, including those due to *Aspergillus* and *Rhizopus*, which may present as superficial lesions before dissemination. Mycobacterial infection (particularly that with *Mycobacterium marinum*) can be diagnosed by skin examination. Infection with *Prototheca wickerhamii* (an achlorophyllic alga) has been diagnosed by skin biopsy. Warts caused by human papillomaviruses (HPVs) are a late consequence of persistent immunosuppression; imiquimod or other forms of local therapy are usually satisfactory. Merkel cell carcinoma, a rare and aggressive neuroendocrine skin tumor whose frequency is increased fivefold in elderly SOT (especially kidney) recipients, is causally linked to a novel polyomavirus, Merkel cell polyomavirus.

Notably, although BK virus replication and virus-associated disease can be detected far earlier, polyomavirus-associated nephropathy is clinically diagnosed in a median of ~300 days and thus qualifies as a late-onset disease. With the establishment of better screening procedures (e.g., urine cytology, urine nucleic acid load, plasma PCR), disease onset is being detected earlier (see "Middle-Period Infections," above) and preemptive strategies (decrease or modification of immunosuppression) are being instituted more promptly, as the efficacy of antiviral therapy is not well established.

HEART TRANSPLANTATION

Early Infections Sternal wound infection and mediastinitis are early complications of heart transplantation. An indolent course is common, with fever or a mildly elevated white blood cell count preceding the development of site tenderness or drainage. Clinical suspicion based on evidence of sternal instability and failure to heal may lead to the diagnosis. Common microbial residents of the skin (e.g., *S. aureus*, including methicillin-resistant strains, and *Staphylococcus epidermidis*) as well as gram-negative organisms (e.g., *Pseudomonas aeruginosa*) and fungi (e.g., *Candida*) are often involved. In rare cases, mediastinitis in heart transplant recipients can also be due to *Mycoplasma hominis* (Chap. 212); since this organism requires an anaerobic environment for growth and may be difficult to see on conventional medium, the laboratory should be alerted that its involvement is suspected. *M. hominis* mediastinitis has been cured with a combination of surgical debridement (sometimes requiring muscle-flap placement) and the administration of clindamycin and tetracycline. Organisms associated with mediastinitis may sometimes be cultured from pericardial fluid.

Middle-Period Infections *T. gondii* (Chap. 253) residing in the heart of a seropositive donor may be transmitted to a seronegative recipient. Thus serologic screening for *T. gondii* infection is important before and in the months after cardiac transplantation. Rarely, active disease can be introduced at the time of transplantation. The overall incidence of toxoplasmosis is so high in the setting of heart transplantation that some prophylaxis is always warranted. Although alternatives are available, the most frequently used agent is TMP-SMX, which prevents infection with *Pneumocystis* as well as with *Nocardia* and several other bacterial pathogens. CMV also has been transmitted by heart transplantation. *Toxoplasma*, *Nocardia*, and *Aspergillus* can cause CNS infections. *L. monocytogenes* meningitis should be considered in heart transplant recipients with fever and headache.

CMV infection is associated with poor outcomes after heart transplantation. The virus is usually detected 1–2 months after transplantation, causes early signs and laboratory abnormalities (usually fever and atypical lymphocytosis or leukopenia and thrombocytopenia) at 2–3 months, and can produce severe disease (e.g., pneumonia) at 3–4 months. An interesting observation is that seropositive recipients usually develop viremia faster than patients whose primary CMV infection is a consequence of transplantation. Between 40% and 70% of patients develop symptomatic CMV disease in the form of (1) CMV pneumonia, the form most likely to be fatal; (2) CMV esophagitis and gastritis, sometimes accompanied by abdominal pain with or without ulcerations and bleeding; and (3) the CMV syndrome, consisting of CMV in the bloodstream along with fever, leukopenia, thrombocytopenia, and hepatic enzyme abnormalities. Ganciclovir is efficacious in the treatment of CMV infection; prophylaxis with ganciclovir or possibly with other antiviral agents, as described for renal transplantation, may reduce the overall incidence of CMV-related disease.

Late Infections EBV infection usually presents as a lymphoma-like proliferation of B cells late after heart transplantation, particularly in patients maintained on intense immunosuppressive therapy. A subset of heart and heart-lung transplant recipients may develop early fulminant EBV-LPD (within 2 months). Treatment includes the reduction of immunosuppression (if possible), the use of glucocorticoid and calcineurin inhibitor–sparing regimens, and the consideration of therapy with anti–B cell antibodies (rituximab and possibly others). Immunomodulatory and antiviral agents continue to be studied. Ganciclovir prophylaxis for CMV disease may indirectly reduce the risk of EBV-LPD through reduced spread of replicating EBV to naïve B cells. Aggressive chemotherapy is a last resort, as discussed earlier for HSC transplant recipients. KSHV-associated disease, including Kaposi's sarcoma and primary effusion lymphoma, has been reported in heart transplant recipients. GVHD prophylaxis with sirolimus may decrease the risk of both rejection and outgrowth of KSHV-infected cells. Antitumor therapy is discussed in Chap. 103e. Prophylaxis for *Pneumocystis* infection is required for these patients (see "Lung Transplantation, Late Infections," below).

LUNG TRANSPLANTATION

Early Infections It is not surprising that lung transplant recipients are predisposed to the development of pneumonia. The combination of ischemia and the resulting mucosal damage, together with accompanying denervation and lack of lymphatic drainage, probably contributes to the high rate of pneumonia (66% in one series). The prophylactic use of high doses of broad-spectrum antibiotics for the first 3–4 days after surgery may decrease the incidence of pneumonia. Gram-negative pathogens (Enterobacteriaceae and *Pseudomonas* species) are troublesome in the first 2 weeks after surgery (the period of maximal vulnerability). Pneumonia can also be caused by *Candida* (possibly as a result of colonization of the donor lung), *Aspergillus*, and *Cryptococcus*. Many centers use antifungal prophylaxis (typically fluconazole or liposomal amphotericin B) for the first 1–2 weeks.

Mediastinitis may occur at an even higher rate among lung transplant recipients than among heart transplant recipients and most commonly develops within 2 weeks of surgery. In the absence of prophylaxis, pneumonitis due to CMV (which may be transmitted as a consequence of transplantation) usually presents between 2 weeks and 3 months after surgery, with primary disease occurring later than reactivation disease.

Middle-Period Infections The incidence of CMV infection, either reactivated or primary, is 75–100% if either the donor or the recipient is seropositive for CMV. CMV-induced disease after solid organ transplantation appears to be most severe in recipients of lung and heart-lung transplants. Whether this severity relates to the mismatch in lung antigen presentation and host immune cells or is attributable to nonimmunologic factors is not known. More than half of lung transplant recipients with symptomatic CMV disease have pneumonia. Difficulty in distinguishing the radiographic picture of CMV infection from that of other infections or from organ rejection further complicates therapy. CMV can also cause bronchiolitis obliterans in lung transplants. The development of pneumonitis related to HSV has led to the prophylactic use of acyclovir. Such prophylaxis may also decrease rates of CMV disease, but ganciclovir is more active against CMV and is also active against HSV. The prophylaxis of CMV infection with IV ganciclovir—or increasingly with valganciclovir, the oral alternative—is recommended for lung transplant recipients. Antiviral alternatives are discussed in the earlier section on HSC transplantation. Although the overall incidence of serious disease is decreased during prophylaxis, late disease may occur when prophylaxis is stopped—a pattern observed increasingly in recent years. With recovery from peritransplantation complications and, in many cases, a decrease in immunosuppression, the recipient is often better equipped to combat late infection.

Late Infections The incidence of *Pneumocystis* infection (which may present with a paucity of findings) is high among lung and heart-lung transplant recipients. Some form of prophylaxis for *Pneumocystis* pneumonia is indicated in all organ transplant situations (Table 169-5). Prophylaxis with TMP-SMX for 12 months after transplantation may be sufficient to prevent *Pneumocystis* disease in patients whose immunosuppression is not increased.

As in other transplant recipients, EBV infection in lung and heart-lung recipients may cause either a mononucleosis-like syndrome or EBV-LPD. The tendency of the B cell blasts to present in the lung appears to be greater after lung transplantation than after the transplantation of other organs, possibly because of a rich source of B cells in bronchus-associated lymphoid tissue. Reduction of immunosuppression and switching of regimens, as discussed in earlier sections, cause remission in some cases, but mTor inhibitors such as rapamycin may contribute to lung toxicity. Airway compression can be fatal, and rapid intervention may therefore become necessary. The approach to EBV-LPD is similar to that described in other sections.

LIVER TRANSPLANTATION

Early Infections As in other transplantation settings, early bacterial infections are a major problem after liver transplantation. Many centers administer systemic broad-spectrum antibiotics for the first 24 h or sometimes longer after surgery, even in the absence of documented infection. However, despite prophylaxis, infectious complications are common and correlate with the duration of the surgical procedure and the type of biliary drainage. An operation lasting >12 h is associated with an increased likelihood of infection. Patients who have a choledochojejunostomy with drainage of the biliary duct to a Roux-en-Y jejunal bowel loop have more fungal infections than those whose bile is drained via anastomosis of the donor common bile duct to the recipient common bile duct. Overall, liver transplant patients have a high incidence of fungal infections, and the occurrence of fungal (often candidal) infection in the setting of choledochojejunostomy correlates with retransplantation, elevated creatinine levels, long procedures, transfusion of >40 units of blood, reoperation, preoperative use of glucocorticoids, prolonged treatment with antibacterial agents, and fungal colonization 2 days before and 3 days after surgery. Many centers give antifungal agents prophylactically in this setting.

Peritonitis and intraabdominal abscesses are common complications of liver transplantation. Bacterial peritonitis or localized abscesses may result from biliary leaks. Early leaks are especially common with live-donor liver transplants. Peritonitis in liver transplant recipients is often polymicrobial, frequently involving enterococci, aerobic gram-negative bacteria, staphylococci, anaerobes, or *Candida* and sometimes involving other invasive fungi. Only one-third of patients with intraabdominal abscesses have bacteremia. Abscesses within the first month after surgery may occur not only in and around the liver but also in the spleen, pericolic area, and pelvis. Treatment includes antibiotic administration and drainage as necessary.

Middle-Period Infections The development of postsurgical biliary stricture predisposes patients to cholangitis. The incidence of strictures is increased in live-donor liver transplantation. Transplant recipients who develop cholangitis may have high spiking fevers and rigors but often lack the characteristic signs and symptoms of classic cholangitis, including abdominal pain and jaundice. Although these findings may suggest graft rejection, rejection is typically accompanied by marked elevation of liver function enzymes. In contrast, in cholangitis in transplant recipients, results of liver function tests (with the possible exception of alkaline phosphatase levels) are often within the normal range. Definitive diagnosis of cholangitis in liver transplant recipients requires demonstration of aggregated neutrophils in bile duct biopsy specimens. Unfortunately, invasive studies of the biliary tract (either T-tube cholangiography or endoscopic retrograde cholangiopancreatography) may themselves lead to cholangitis. For this reason, many clinicians recommend an empirical trial of therapy with antibiotics covering gram-negative organisms and anaerobes before these procedures are undertaken as well as antibiotic coverage if procedures are eventually performed.

Reactivation of viral hepatitis is a common complication of liver transplantation (Chap. 360). Recurrent hepatitis B and C infections, for which transplantation may be performed, are problematic. To prevent hepatitis B virus reinfection, prophylaxis with an optimal antiviral agent or combination of agents (lamivudine, adefovir, entecavir) and hepatitis B immune globulin is currently recommended, although the optimal dose, route, and duration of therapy remain controversial. Success in preventing reinfection with hepatitis B virus has increased in recent years. Complications related to hepatitis C infection are the most common reason for liver transplantation in the United States. Reinfection of the graft with hepatitis C virus occurs in all patients, with a variable time frame. Studies of aggressive pretransplantation treatment of selected recipients with antiviral agents and prophylactic/preemptive regimens are ongoing. However, early posttransplantation initiation of treatment for histologically documented disease with the classic combination of ribavirin and pegylated interferon has produced sustained responses at rates in the range of 25–40%. Several protease and polymerase inhibitors that block production of hepatitis C virus as well as regimens that spare interferon and a monoclonal antibody to the virus are undergoing preclinical and clinical trials for prevention and or control of infection after transplantation (Chap. 360).

As in other transplantation settings, reactivation disease with herpesviruses is common (Table 169-3). Herpesviruses can be transmitted in donor organs. Although CMV hepatitis occurs in ~4% of liver transplant recipients, it is usually not so severe as to require retransplantation. Without prophylaxis, CMV disease develops in the majority of seronegative recipients of organs from CMV-positive donors, but fatality rates are lower among liver transplant recipients than among lung or heart-lung transplant recipients. Disease due to CMV can also be associated with the vanishing bile duct syndrome after liver transplantation. Patients respond to treatment with ganciclovir; prophylaxis with oral forms of ganciclovir or high-dose acyclovir may decrease the frequency of disease. A role for HHV-6 reactivation in early posttransplantation fever and leukopenia has been proposed, although the more severe sequelae described in HSC transplantation are unusual. HHV-6 and HHV-7 appear to exacerbate CMV disease in this setting. EBV-LPD after liver transplantation shows a propensity for involvement of the liver, and such disease may be of donor origin. See previous sections for discussion of EBV infections in solid organ transplantation.

PANCREAS TRANSPLANTATION

Pancreas transplantation is most frequently performed together with or after kidney transplantation, although it may be performed alone. Transplantation of the pancreas can be complicated by early bacterial and yeast infections. Most pancreatic transplants are drained into the bowel, and the rest are drained into the bladder. A cuff of duodenum is used in the anastomosis between the pancreatic graft and either the gut or the bladder. Bowel drainage poses a risk of early intraabdominal and allograft infections with enteric bacteria and yeasts. These infections can result in loss of the graft. Bladder drainage causes a high rate of urinary tract infection and sterile cystitis; however, such infection can usually be cured with appropriate antimicrobial agents. In both procedures, prophylactic antimicrobial agents are commonly used at the time of surgery. Aggressive immunosuppression, especially when the patient receives a kidney and a pancreas from different donors, is associated with late-onset systemic fungal and viral infections; thus many centers administer an antifungal drug and an antiviral agent (ganciclovir or a congener) for extended prophylaxis.

Issues related to the development of CMV infection, EBV-LPD, and infections with opportunistic pathogens in patients receiving a pancreatic transplant are similar to those in other SOT recipients.

COMPOSITE TISSUE TRANSPLANTATION

Composite tissue allotransplantation (CTA) is a new field in which, rather than a single organ, multiple tissue types composing a major body part are transplanted. The sites involved have included an upper extremity, the face, the trachea, the knee, and the abdominal wall. The numbers of recipients are limited. The different procedures and the associated infectious complications vary. Nevertheless, some early trends related to infectious complications have become apparent, as very intense and prolonged immunosuppression is typically required to prevent rejection. For example, in the early postoperative period, bacterial infections are especially frequent in facial transplant recipients. Perioperative prophylaxis is tailored to the organisms likely to complicate the different procedures. As in SOT recipients, complicated CMV infections have been observed in several CTA settings, particularly when the recipient is seronegative and the donor is seropositive. In some patients, anti-CMV immune globulin in addition to ganciclovir (as used in HSC transplant recipients with CMV pneumonia) was needed to control disease, and ganciclovir resistance requiring alternative therapies developed in several patients. Infectious complications from reactivation of other members of the human herpesvirus family and other latent viruses also caused significant morbidity, as discussed for SOT recipients. Prophylaxis for CMV infection, *P. jirovecii* infection, toxoplasmosis, and fungal infection is administered for several months on the basis of the limited studies available.

MISCELLANEOUS INFECTIONS IN SOLID ORGAN TRANSPLANTATION

Indwelling IV Catheter Infections The prolonged use of indwelling IV catheters for administration of medications, blood products, and nutrition is common in diverse transplantation settings and poses a risk of local and bloodstream infections. Exit-site infection is most commonly caused by staphylococcal species. Bloodstream infection most frequently develops within 1 week of catheter placement or in patients who become neutropenic. Coagulase-negative staphylococci are the most common isolates from blood. Although infective endocarditis in HSC transplant recipients is uncommon, the incidence of endocarditis in SOT recipients has been estimated to be as high as 1%, and this infection is associated with excessive high mortality in this population. Although staphylococci predominate, the involvement of fungal and gram-negative organisms may be more common than in the general population.

For further discussion of differential diagnosis and therapeutic options, see Chap. 104.

Tuberculosis The incidence of tuberculosis within the first 12 months after solid organ transplantation is greater than that observed after HSC transplantation (0.23–0.79%) and ranges broadly worldwide (1.2–15%), reflecting the prevalence of tuberculosis in local populations. Lesions suggesting prior tuberculosis on chest radiography, older age, diabetes, chronic liver disease, GVHD, and intense immunosuppression are predictive of tuberculosis reactivation and development of disseminated disease in a host with latent disease. Tuberculosis has rarely been transmitted from the donor organ. In contrast to the low mortality rate among HSC transplant recipients, mortality rates among SOT recipients are reported to be as high as 30%. Vigilance is indicated, as the presentation of disease is often extrapulmonary (gastrointestinal, genitourinary, central nervous, endocrine, musculoskeletal, laryngeal) and atypical; tuberculosis in this setting sometimes manifests as fever of unknown origin. Careful elicitation of a history and direct evaluation of both the recipient and the donor prior to transplantation are optimal. Skin testing of the recipient with purified protein derivative may be unreliable because of chronic disease and/or immunosuppression. Cell-based assays that measure interferon γ and/or cytokine production may prove more sensitive in the future. Isoniazid toxicity has not been a significant problem except in the setting of liver transplantation. Therefore, appropriate prophylaxis should be used (see recommendations from the Centers for Disease Control and Prevention [CDC] at *www.cdc.gov/tb/topic/treatment/ltbi.htm*). An assessment of the need to treat latent disease should include careful consideration of the possibility of a false-negative test result. Pending final confirmation of suspected tuberculosis, aggressive multidrug treatment in accordance with the guidelines of the CDC, the Infectious Diseases Society of America, and the American Thoracic Society is indicated because of the high mortality rates among these patients. Altered drug metabolism (e.g., upon coadministration of antituberculous medications and certain immunosuppressive agents) can be managed with careful monitoring of drug levels and appropriate dose adjustment. Close follow-up of hepatic enzymes is warranted. Drug-resistant tuberculosis is especially problematic in these individuals (Chap. 202).

Virus-Associated Malignancies In addition to malignancy associated with gammaherpesvirus infection (EBV, KSHV) and simple warts (HPV), other tumors that are virus-associated or suspected of being virus-associated are more likely to develop in transplant recipients, particularly those who require long-term immunosuppression, than in the general population. The interval to tumor development is usually >1 year. Transplant recipients develop nonmelanoma skin or lip cancers that, in contrast to de novo skin cancers, have a high ratio of squamous cells to basal cells. HPV may play a major role in these lesions. Cervical and vulvar carcinomas, which are quite clearly associated with HPV, develop with increased frequency in female transplant recipients. The frequency of Merkel cell carcinoma associated with Merkel cell polyomavirus is also increased in transplant recipients; however, it is unclear whether recipients infected with HTLV-1 are at increased risk of leukemia. Among renal transplant recipients, rates of melanoma are modestly increased and rates of cancers of the kidney and bladder are increased.

VACCINATION OF TRANSPLANT RECIPIENTS

(See also Chap. 148) In addition to receiving antibiotic prophylaxis, transplant recipients should be vaccinated against likely pathogens (Table 169-6). In the case of HSC transplant recipients, optimal responses cannot be achieved until after immune reconstitution, despite previous immunization of both donor and recipient. Recipients of an allogeneic HSC transplant must be reimmunized if they are to be protected against pathogens. The situation is less clear-cut in the case of autologous transplantation. T and B cells in the peripheral blood may reconstitute the immune response if they are transferred

TABLE 169-6 VACCINATION OF HEMATOPOIETIC STEM CELL TRANSPLANT (HSCT) AND SOLID ORGAN TRANSPLANT (SOT) RECIPIENTS

	Type of Transplantation	
Vaccine	**HSCT**	**SOT**[a]
Streptococcus pneumoniae, Haemophilus influenzae, Neisseria meningitidis	Immunize after transplantation. See CDC-ACIP recommendations. (For *S. pneumoniae*, a new primary series may be indicated.)	Immunize before transplantation. See CDC-ACIP recommendations. (For *S. pneumoniae*, a booster dose of polysaccharide vaccine after 5 years is recommended.)
Influenza	Vaccinate in the fall. Vaccinate close contacts.	Vaccinate in the fall. Vaccinate close contacts.
Polio	Administer inactivated vaccine.	Administer inactivated vaccine.
Measles/mumps/rubella	Immunize 24 months after transplantation if GVHD is absent.	Immunize before transplantation.
Diphtheria, pertussis, tetanus	Reimmunize after transplantation with primary series, DTaP. See IDSA 2013 recommendations (*www.idsociety.org/Other_Guidelines/#immunizationFortheCompromisedHost*).	Immunize or boost before transplantation with Tdap; give boosters at 10-year intervals or as required
Hepatitis B and A	Reimmunize after transplantation. See recommendations.	Immunize before transplantation.
Human papillomavirus	Recommendations are pending (*www.cdc.gov/std/hpv/stdfact-hpv-vaccine-hcp.htm*).	Recommendations are pending.

[a]Immunizations should be given before solid organ transplantation whenever possible.

Abbreviations: CDC, Centers for Disease Control and Prevention; ACIP, Advisory Committee on Immunization Practices; DTaP, full-level diphtheria and tetanus toxoids and acellular pertussis, adsorbed; GVHD, graft-versus-host disease; Tdap, tetanus toxoid, reduced diphtheria toxoid, and acellular pertussis; IDSA, Infectious Diseases Society of America.

Note: Recommendations from the CDC should be checked regularly as they frequently change upon receipt of new clinical information and new formulations of specific vaccines.

in adequate numbers. However, cancer patients (particularly those with Hodgkin's disease, in whom vaccination has been extensively studied) who are undergoing chemotherapy do not respond normally to immunization, and titers of antibodies to infectious agents fall more rapidly than in healthy individuals. Therefore, even immunosuppressed patients who have not undergone HSC transplantation may need booster vaccine injections. If memory cells are specifically eliminated as part of a stem cell "cleanup" procedure, it will be necessary to reimmunize the recipient with a new primary series. Optimal times for immunizations of different transplant populations are being evaluated. Yearly immunization of household and other contacts (including health care personnel) against influenza benefits the patient by preventing local spread.

In the absence of compelling data as to optimal timing, it is reasonable to administer the pneumococcal and *H. influenzae* type b conjugate vaccines to both autologous and allogeneic HSC transplant recipients beginning 12 months after transplantation. A series that includes both the 13-valent pneumococcal conjugate vaccine (Prevnar) and the 23-valent pneumococcal polysaccharide vaccine (Pneumovax) is now recommended (according to CDC guidelines). The pneumococcal and *H. influenzae* type b vaccines are particularly important for patients who have undergone splenectomy. The *Neisseria meningitidis* polysaccharide conjugate vaccine (Menactra or Menveo) also is recommended. In addition, diphtheria, tetanus, acellular pertussis, and inactivated polio vaccines can all be given at these same intervals (12 months and, as required, 24 months after transplantation). Some authorities recommend a new primary series for tetanus/diphtheria/pertussis and inactivated poliovirus vaccines beginning 12 months after transplantation. Vaccination to prevent hepatitis B and hepatitis A (both killed vaccines) also seems advisable. A formal recommendation regarding immunization with the tetravalent HPV virus-like particle vaccine (Gardasil) after HSC transplantation has not been issued. However, HPV vaccination, which can prevent genital warts as well as specific cancers, is recommended through age 26 for healthy young adults who previously have not been vaccinated or have not received the full series. Live-virus measles/mumps/rubella (MMR) vaccine can be given to autologous HSC transplant recipients 24 months after transplantation and to most allogeneic HSC transplant recipients at the same point if they are not receiving maintenance therapy with immunosuppressive drugs and do not have ongoing GVHD. The risk of spread from a household contact is low for MMR vaccine. In parts of the world where live poliovirus vaccine is used, patients as well as contacts should be advised to receive only the killed vaccine. In the rare setting where both donor and recipient are VZV naïve and the recipient is no longer receiving acyclovir or ganciclovir prophylaxis, the patient should be counseled to receive varicella-zoster immune globulin (VariZIG) up to 10 days after an exposure to a person with chickenpox or uncovered zoster; such patients should avoid close contact with persons recently vaccinated with Varivax. A formal recommendation regarding Varivax immunization of such patients is not currently available. Neither patients nor their household contacts should receive vaccinia vaccine unless they have been exposed to smallpox virus. Among patients who have active GVHD and/or are taking high maintenance doses of glucocorticoids, it may be prudent to avoid all live-virus vaccines.

In the case of SOT recipients, administration of all the usual vaccines and of the indicated booster doses should be completed before immunosuppression, if possible, to maximize responses. For patients taking immunosuppressive agents, the administration of pneumococcal vaccine should be repeated every 5 years. No data are available for the meningococcal vaccine, but it is probably reasonable to administer it along with the pneumococcal vaccine. *H. influenzae* conjugate vaccine is safe and should be efficacious in this population; therefore, its administration before transplantation is recommended. Booster doses of this vaccine are not recommended for adults. SOT recipients who continue to receive immunosuppressive drugs should not receive live-virus vaccines. A person in this group who is exposed to measles should be given measles immune globulin. Similarly, an immunocompromised patient who is seronegative for varicella and who comes into contact with a person who has chickenpox should be given varicella-zoster immune globulin as soon as possible (optimally within 96 h; up to 10 days after contact); if this is not possible, a 10- to 14-day course of acyclovir therapy should be started immediately. Upon the discontinuation of treatment, clinical disease may still occur in a small number of patients; thus vigilance is indicated. Rapid re-treatment with acyclovir should limit the symptoms of disease. Household contacts of transplant recipients can receive live attenuated VZV vaccine, but vaccinees should avoid direct contact with the patient if a rash develops. Virus-like particle vaccines have been licensed for the prevention of infection with several HPV serotypes most commonly implicated in cervical and anal carcinomas and in anogenital and laryngeal warts. These vaccines are not live; however, no information is yet available about their immunogenicity or efficacy in transplant recipients.

Immunocompromised patients who travel may benefit from some but not all vaccines (Chaps. 148 and 149). In general, these patients should receive any killed or inactivated vaccine preparation appropriate to the area they are visiting; this recommendation includes the vaccines for Japanese encephalitis, hepatitis A and B, poliomyelitis, meningococcal infection, and typhoid. The live typhoid vaccines are not recommended for use in most immunocompromised patients, but an inactivated or purified polysaccharide typhoid vaccine can be used. Live yellow fever vaccine should not be administered. On the other hand, primary immunization or boosting with the purified-protein hepatitis B vaccine is indicated. Inactivated hepatitis A vaccine should also be used in the appropriate setting (Chap. 148). A vaccine is now available that provides dual protection against hepatitis A and hepatitis B. If hepatitis A vaccine is not administered, travelers should consider receiving passive protection with immune globulin (the dose depending on the duration of travel in the high-risk area).

170 Treatment and Prophylaxis of Bacterial Infections

David C. Hooper, Erica S. Shenoy, Christy A. Varughese

Antimicrobial agents have had a major impact on human health. Together with vaccines, they have contributed to reduced mortality, extended lifespan, and enhanced quality of life. Among drugs used in human medicine, however, they are distinctive in that their use promotes the occurrence of drug resistance in the pathogens they are designed to treat as well as in other "bystander" organisms. Indeed, the history of antimicrobial development has been driven in large part by the medical need engendered by the emergence of resistance to each generation of agents. Thus, the careful and appropriate use of antimicrobial drugs is particularly important not only for optimizing efficacy and minimizing adverse effects but also for minimizing the risk of resistance and preserving the value of existing agents. Although this chapter focuses on antibacterial agents, the optimal use of all antimicrobials depends on an understanding of each drug's mechanism of action, spectrum of activity, mechanisms of resistance, pharmacology, and adverse effect profile. This information is then applied in the context of the patient's clinical presentation, underlying conditions, and epidemiology to define the site and likely nature of the infection or other condition and thus to choose the best therapy. Gathering of microbiologic information is important for refining therapeutic choices on the basis of documented pathogen and susceptibility data whenever possible; this information also makes it possible to choose more targeted therapy, thereby reducing the risk of selection of resistant bacteria. Durations of therapy are chosen according to the nature of the infection and the patient's response to treatment and are informed by clinical studies when they are available, with the understanding that shorter courses are less likely than longer ones to promote the emergence of resistance. This chapter provides specific information that is necessary for making informed choices among antibacterial agents.

MECHANISMS OF ACTION AND RESISTANCE

The mechanisms of action of and resistance to antibacterial agents are discussed in detail in the text and are summarized for the most commonly used groups of agents in Table 170-1. A schematic of antibacterial targets is provided in Fig. 170-1.

MECHANISMS OF ACTION

Multiple essential components of bacterial cell structures and metabolism have been the targets of antibacterial agents used in clinical medicine, and the interaction of an agent with its target results in either inhibition of bacterial growth and replication (*bacteriostatic effect*) or bacterial killing (*bactericidal effect*). In general, targets have been chosen because they either do not exist in mammalian cells and physiology or are sufficiently different from their bacterial counterparts to allow selective bacterial targeting. Treatment with bacteriostatic agents is effective when the patient's host defenses are sufficient to contribute to eradication of the infecting pathogen. In patients with impaired host defenses (e.g., neutropenia) or infections at body sites with impaired or limited host defenses (e.g., meningitis and endocarditis), bactericidal agents are generally preferred.

Inhibition of Cell Wall Synthesis The bacterial cell wall, which is external to the cytoplasmic membrane and has no counterpart in mammalian cells, protects bacterial cells from lysis under low osmotic conditions. The cell wall is a cross-linked peptidoglycan composed of a polymer of alternating units of *N*-acetylglucosamine (NAG) and *N*-acetylmuramic acid (NAM), four-amino-acid stem peptides linked to each NAM, and a peptide cross-bridge that links adjacent stem peptides to form a net-like structure. Several steps in peptidoglycan synthesis are targets of antibacterial agents. Inhibition of cell wall synthesis generally results in a bactericidal effect that is linked to cell lysis. This effect results not only from the blocking of new cell-wall formation but from the uninhibited action of cell wall–remodeling enzymes called *autolysins*, which cleave peptidoglycan as part of normal cell-wall growth.

In gram-positive bacteria the peptidoglycan is the most external cell structure, but in gram-negative bacteria an asymmetric lipid outer membrane is external to the peptidoglycan and contains diffusion channels called *porins*. The space between the cytoplasmic membrane peptidoglycan and the outer membrane is referred to as the *periplasmic space*. Most antibacterial drugs enter the gram-negative bacterial cell through a porin channel, since the outer membrane is a major diffusion barrier. Although the peptidoglycan layer is thicker in gram-positive (20–80 nm) than in gram-negative (1 nm) bacteria, peptidoglycan itself constitutes only a limited diffusion barrier for antibacterial agents.

β-LACTAMS The β-lactam drugs, including penicillins, cephalosporins, monobactams, and carbapenems, target transpeptidase enzymes (also called *penicillin-binding proteins*, or PBPs) involved in the stem-peptide cross-linking step.

GLYCOPEPTIDES The glycopeptides, including vancomycin, teicoplanin, telavancin, dalbavancin, and oritavancin, bind the two terminal D-alanine residues of the stem peptide, hindering the glycosyltransferase involved in polymerizing NAG–NAM units. Telavancin also binds to the lipid II intermediate that delivers cell-wall precursor subunits. Likewise, dalbavancin and oritavancin interact with the cell membrane, and oritavancin may also inhibit transpeptidases. Both β-lactams and glycopeptides interact with their targets external to the cytoplasmic membrane.

BACITRACIN (TOPICAL) AND FOSFOMYCIN These agents interrupt enzymatic steps in the production of peptidoglycan precursors in the cytoplasm.

Inhibition of Protein Synthesis Most inhibitors of bacterial protein synthesis target bacterial ribosomes, whose difference from eukaryotic ribosomes allows selective antibacterial action. Some inhibitors bind to the 30S ribosomal subunit and others to the 50S subunit. Most protein synthesis–inhibiting agents are bacteriostatic; aminoglycosides are an exception and are bactericidal.

AMINOGLYCOSIDES Aminoglycosides (amikacin, gentamicin, kanamycin, netilmicin, streptomycin, tobramycin) bind irreversibly to 16S ribosomal RNA (rRNA) of the 30S ribosomal subunit, blocking the translocation of peptidyl transfer RNA (tRNA) from the A (aminoacyl) to the P (peptidyl) site and, at low concentrations, causing misreading of messenger RNA (mRNA) codons and thus causing the introduction of incorrect amino acids into the peptide chain; at higher concentrations, translocation of the peptide chain is blocked. Cellular uptake of aminoglycosides is dependent on the electrochemical gradient across the bacterial membrane. Under anaerobic conditions, this gradient is reduced, with a consequent reduction in the uptake and activity of the aminoglycosides. Spectinomycin is a related aminocyclitol antibiotic that also binds to 16S rRNA of the 30S ribosomal subunit but at a different site. This drug inhibits translocation of the growing peptide chain but does not trigger codon misreading and produces only a bacteriostatic effect.

TETRACYCLINES AND GLYCYLCYCLINES Tetracyclines (doxycycline, minocycline, tetracycline) bind reversibly to the 16S rRNA of the 30S ribosomal subunit and block the binding of aminoacyl tRNA to the ribosomal A site, thereby inhibiting peptide elongation. Active transport of tetracyclines into bacterial but not mammalian cells contributes to the selectivity of these agents. Tigecycline, a derivative of minocycline and

TABLE 170-1 MECHANISMS OF ACTION OF AND RESISTANCE TO ANTIBACTERIAL AGENTS

Antibacterial Agent(s)	Major Target	Mechanism(s) of Action	Mechanism(s) of Resistance
β-Lactams (penicillins, cephalosporins, monobactams, carbapenems)	Cell wall synthesis	Bind cell wall cross-linking enzymes (PBPs, transpeptidases)	1. Drug inactivation by β-lactamases 2. Altered PBP targets 3. Reduced diffusion through porin channels
Glycopeptides (vancomycin, teicoplanin, telavancin, dalbavancin, oritavancin)	Cell wall synthesis	Block cell wall glycosyltransferases by binding D-Ala-D-Ala stem-peptide terminus Telavancin, dalbavancin, and oritavancin: affect membrane function Oritavancin: inhibits transpeptidases	1. Altered D-Ala-D-Ala target (D-Ala-D-Lac) 2. Increased D-Ala-D-Ala target binding at sites distant from cell wall synthesis enzymes
Bacitracin	Cell wall synthesis	Blocks lipid carrier of cell wall precursors	Active drug efflux
Fosfomycin	Cell wall synthesis	Blocks linkage of stem peptide to NAG by enoyltransferase	1. Target enzyme overexpression 2. Drug-modifying enzymes
Aminoglycosides (gentamicin, tobramycin, amikacin)	Protein synthesis	Bind 30S ribosomal subunit Block translocation of peptide chain Cause misreading of mRNA	1. Drug-modifying enzymes 2. Methylation at ribosome binding site 3. Decreased permeation to target due to active efflux
Tetracyclines (tetracycline, doxycycline, minocycline)	Protein synthesis	Bind 30S ribosomal subunit Inhibit peptide elongation	1. Active drug efflux 2. Ribosomal protection proteins
Tigecycline	Protein synthesis	Same as tetracyclines	Active drug efflux (pumps different from those affecting tetracyclines)
Macrolides (erythromycin, clarithromycin, azithromycin) and ketolide (telithromycin)	Protein synthesis	Bind 50S ribosomal subunit Block peptide chain exit	1. Methylation at ribosome binding site 2. Active drug efflux
Lincosamides (clindamycin)	Protein synthesis	Bind 50S ribosomal subunit Block peptide bond formation	Methylation at ribosome binding site
Streptogramins (quinupristin, dalfopristin)	Protein synthesis	Same as macrolides	1. Same as macrolides 2. Drug-modifying enzymes
Chloramphenicol	Protein synthesis	Binds 50S ribosomal subunit Blocks aminoacyl tRNA positioning	Drug-modifying enzymes
Oxazolidinones (linezolid, tedizolid)	Protein synthesis	Bind 50S ribosomal subunit Inhibit initiation of peptide synthesis	1. Altered rRNA binding site 2. Methylation of ribosome binding site
Mupirocin	Protein synthesis	Blocks isoleucyl tRNA synthetase	1. Acquired resistant tRNA synthetase (drug bypass) 2. Altered native tRNA synthetase target
Sulfonamides (sulfadiazine, sulfisoxazole, and sulfamethoxazole)	Folate synthesis	Inhibit dihydropteroate synthetase	Acquired resistant dihydropteroate synthetase (drug bypass)
Trimethoprim	Folate synthesis	Inhibits dihydrofolate reductase	Acquired resistant dihydrofolate reductase (drug bypass)
Quinolones (norfloxacin, ciprofloxacin, ofloxacin, levofloxacin, moxifloxacin, gemifloxacin)	DNA synthesis	Inhibit DNA gyrase and DNA topoisomerase IV Enzyme–DNA–drug complex: blocks DNA replication apparatus	1. Altered target(s) 2. Active efflux 3. Protection of target from drug 4. Drug-modifying enzyme (ciprofloxacin)
Rifamycins (rifampin, rifabutin, rifapentine)	RNA synthesis	Inhibit RNA polymerase	Altered target
Nitrofurantoin	Nucleic acid synthesis	Reduce reactive drug derivatives that damage DNA	Altered drug-activating enzymes
Metronidazole	Nucleic acid synthesis	Reduce reactive drug derivatives that damage DNA	1. Altered drug-activating enzyme 2. Acquired detoxifying enzymes 3. Active efflux
Polymyxins (polymyxin B and polymyxin E [colistin])	Cell membrane	Bind LPS and disrupt both outer and cytoplasmic membranes	Altered cell membrane charge with reduced drug binding
Daptomycin	Cell membrane	Produces membrane channel and membrane leakage	Altered cell membrane with reduced drug binding

Abbreviations: LPS, lipopolysaccharide; NAG, *N*-acetylglucosamine; PBP, penicillin-binding protein.

the only available glycylcycline, acts similarly to the tetracyclines but is distinctive for its ability to circumvent the most common mechanisms of resistance to the tetracyclines.

MACROLIDES AND KETOLIDES In contrast to the aminoglycosides and tetracyclines, the macrolides (azithromycin, clarithromycin, erythromycin) and ketolides (telithromycin) bind to the 23S rRNA of the 50S ribosomal subunit. These agents block translocation of the growing peptide chain by binding to the tunnel from which the chain exits the ribosome.

LINCOSAMIDES Clindamycin is the only lincosamide in clinical use. It binds to the 23S rRNA of the 50S ribosomal subunit, interacting with both the ribosomal A and P sites and blocking peptide bond formation.

STREPTOGRAMINS The only streptogramin in clinical use is a combination of quinupristin, a group B streptogramin, and dalfopristin, a group A streptogramin. Both components bind to 23S rRNA of the 50S ribosome: dalfopristin binds to both the A and P sites of the peptidyl transferase center, and quinupristin binds to a site that overlaps the macrolide-binding site, blocking the emergence of nascent peptide

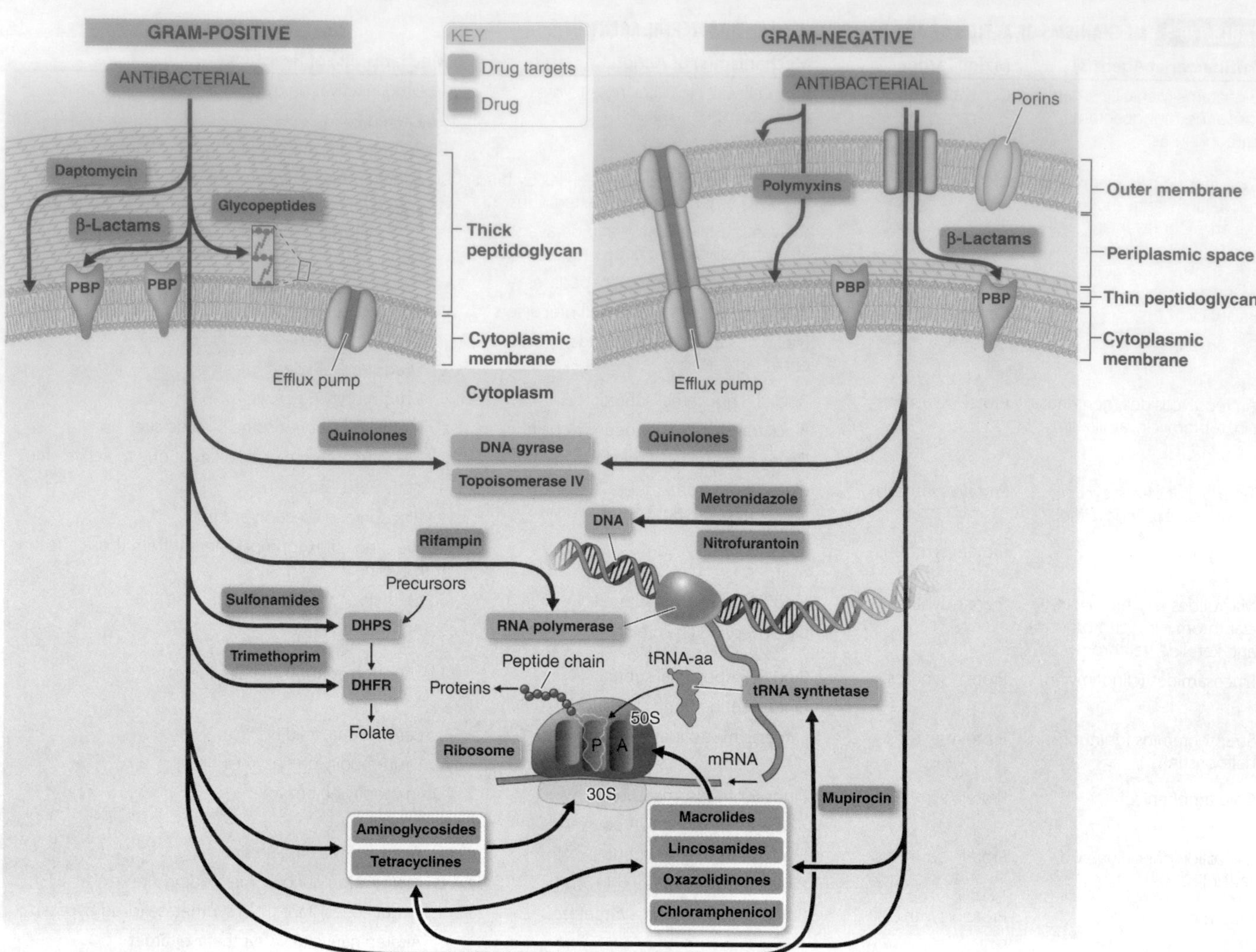

FIGURE 170-1 Antibacterial targets. A, aminoacyl site; DHFR, dihydrofolate reductase; DHPS, dihydropteroate synthetase; P, peptidyl site; PBP, penicillin-binding protein; tRNA-aa, aminoacyl tRNA.

from the ribosome. The combination is bactericidal, but macrolide-resistant bacteria exhibit cross-resistance to quinupristin, and the remaining activity of dalfopristin alone is bacteriostatic.

CHLORAMPHENICOL Chloramphenicol binds reversibly to the 23S rRNA of the 50S subunit in a manner that interferes with the proper positioning of the aminoacyl component of tRNA in the A site. This site of binding is near those of the macrolides and lincosamides.

OXAZOLIDINONES Linezolid and tedizolid are the only oxazolidinones in clinical use. They bind directly to the A site in the 23S rRNA of the 50S ribosomal subunit and block binding of aminoacyl tRNA, inhibiting the initiation of protein synthesis.

MUPIROCIN Mupirocin (pseudomonic acid) is used topically. It competes with isoleucine for binding to isoleucyl tRNA synthetase, depleting stores of isoleucyl tRNA and thereby inhibiting protein synthesis.

Inhibition of Bacterial Metabolism Available inhibitors (antimetabolites) target the pathway for synthesis of folate, which is a cofactor in a number of one-carbon transfer reactions involved in the synthesis of some nucleic acids, including pyrimidine, thymidine, and all purines (adenine and guanine), as well as some amino acids (methionine and serine) and acetyl coenzyme A (CoA). Two sequential steps in folate synthesis are targeted. The selective antibacterial effect stems from the inability of mammalian cells to synthesize folate; they depend instead on exogenous sources. Antibacterial activity, however, may be reduced in the presence of high exogenous concentrations of the end products of the folate pathway (e.g., thymidine and purines) that may occur in some infections, resulting from local breakdown of leukocytes and host tissues.

SULFONAMIDES Sulfonamides, including sulfadiazine, sulfisoxazole, and sulfamethoxazole, inhibit dihydropteroate synthetase, which adds *p*-aminobenzoic acid (PABA) to pteridine, producing dihydropteroate. Sulfonamides are structural analogues of PABA and act as competing enzyme substrates.

TRIMETHOPRIM Subsequent steps in folate synthesis are catalyzed by dihydrofolate synthase, which adds glutamate to dihydropteroate, and dihydrofolate reductase, which then generates the final product, tetrahydrofolate. Trimethoprim is a structural analogue of pteridine and inhibits dihydrofolate reductase. Trimethoprim is available alone but is most often used in combination products that also contain sulfamethoxazole and thus block two sequential steps in folate synthesis.

Inhibition of DNA and RNA Synthesis or Activity A variety of antibacterial agents act on these processes.

QUINOLONES The quinolones include nalidixic acid, the first agent in the class, and newer, more widely used fluorinated derivatives (fluoroquinolones), including norfloxacin, ciprofloxacin, levofloxacin, moxifloxacin, and gemifloxacin. The quinolones are synthetic compounds that inhibit bacterial DNA synthesis by interacting with the DNA complexes of two essential enzymes, DNA gyrase and DNA topoisomerase IV, which alter DNA topology. Quinolones trap enzyme–DNA complexes in such a way that they block movement of the DNA replication apparatus and can generate lethal double-strand breaks in DNA, resulting in bactericidal activity. Although mammalian cells also have type II DNA topoisomerases like gyrase and topoisomerase IV, the structures of the mammalian enzymes are sufficiently different from those of the bacterial enzymes that quinolones have substantially selective antibacterial activity.

RIFAMYCINS Rifampin, rifabutin, and rifapentine are semisynthetic derivatives of rifamycin B and bind the β subunit of bacterial RNA polymerase, thereby blocking elongation of mRNA. Their action is highly selective for the bacterial enzyme over mammalian RNA polymerases.

NITROFURANTOIN The reduction of nitrofurantoin, a nitrofuran compound, by bacterial enzymes produces highly reactive derivatives that are thought to cause DNA strand breakage. Nitrofurantoin is used only for the treatment of lower urinary tract infections.

METRONIDAZOLE Metronidazole is a synthetic nitroimidazole with activity limited to anaerobic bacteria and certain anaerobic protozoa. Reduction of its nitro group by the electron-transport system in anaerobic bacteria produces reactive intermediates that damage DNA and result in bactericidal activity. Both nitrofurantoin and metronidazole have selective antibacterial activity because the reducing activity needed to generate active derivatives is generated only by bacterial and not mammalian enzymes.

Disruption of Membrane Integrity The integrity of the bacterial cytoplasmic membrane—and, in gram-negative bacteria, the outer membrane is important for bacterial viability. Two bactericidal drugs have membrane targets.

POLYMYXINS The polymyxins, including polymyxin B and polymyxin E (colistin), are cationic cyclic polypeptides that disrupt the cytoplasmic membrane and the outer membrane (the latter by binding lipopolysaccharide).

DAPTOMYCIN Daptomycin is a lipopeptide that binds the cytoplasmic membrane of gram-positive bacteria in the presence of calcium, generating a channel that leads to leakage of cytoplasmic potassium ions and membrane depolarization.

MECHANISMS OF RESISTANCE

Bacteria use a wide variety of mechanisms to block or circumvent the activity of antibacterial agents. Although myriad, these mechanisms can generally be grouped into three categories: (1) altered or bypass targets that exhibit reduced binding of the drug, (2) altered access of the drug to its target by reductions in uptake or increases in active efflux, and (3) a modification of the drug that reduces its activity. These mechanisms result from either mutations in bacterial chromosomal genes occurring spontaneously during bacterial DNA replication or the acquisition of new genes by DNA transfer from other bacteria or uptake of exogenous DNA. New genes are most often acquired on self-replicating plasmids or other DNA elements transferred from other bacteria. However, some bacteria, such as *Streptococcus pneumoniae* and *Neisseria gonorrhoeae*, can also take up fragments of environmental DNA from related species and recombine that DNA directly into their own chromosomes, a process called *transformation*. Not uncommonly, resistant bacteria have combinations of resistance mechanisms either within one category or among categories, and many plasmids contain more than one resistance gene. Thus, plasmid acquisition itself can in many cases confer resistance to multiple antibacterial agents.

Many antibacterial drugs are derived from natural products of microbial species. Some genes encoding resistance to these drugs may have evolved and been mobilized onto plasmids from a protection mechanism in the producer organism or in other surviving bacteria in the exposed environment. Exposure to antibacterial agents either in nature or from human or animal use results in the selection of resistant strains within an otherwise susceptible bacterial population. Because the patterns and extent of resistance may differ among settings, initial choices of antibacterial drugs should be based, whenever possible, on local susceptibility data and should be modified as needed as soon as specific microbiology susceptibility data become available.

β-Lactams The most common mechanism of resistance to β-lactams is their degradation by β-lactamases, enzymes that break down the core β-lactam ring and destroy drug activity. Different β-lactamases degrade different β-lactams. Some β-lactamases are encoded on the bacterial chromosome, and their activity contributes to the susceptibility profile of a particular species. Because other β-lactamases are encoded by acquired plasmids, their resistance profiles may be present in some strains of a species but not others. In gram-positive bacteria β-lactamases are secreted into the extracellular environment, whereas in gram-negative bacteria these enzymes are secreted into the periplasmic space between the cytoplasmic and outer membranes. Thus, in gram-negative bacteria, access of β-lactams both to their target PBPs and to β-lactamases requires diffusion across the outer membrane, generally through the porin channels.

Most strains of *Staphylococcus aureus* produce a plasmid-encoded β-lactamase that degrades penicillin but not semisynthetic penicillins, such as oxacillin and nafcillin. The most common plasmid-encoded β-lactamases of gram-negative bacteria are able to inactivate all penicillins and most earlier-generation cephalosporins. Extended-spectrum β-lactamase (ESBL) variants of these early enzymes that can degrade later-generation cephalosporins (ceftriaxone, cefotaxime, ceftazidime) as well as the monobactam aztreonam have now emerged and are widely disseminated. Some ESBLs also degrade the fourth-generation cephalosporin cefepime. Carbapenems (imipenem, meropenem, ertapenem, doripenem) are not degraded by ESBLs, but additional β-lactamases, called *carbapenemases*, that degrade carbapenems and most if not all other β-lactams have begun to emerge.

The chromosomal β-lactamase of *Klebsiella pneumoniae* preferentially degrades penicillins but not cephalosporins. In contrast, the chromosomal β-lactamase of *Enterobacter* and related genera, AmpC, can degrade almost all cephalosporins but is normally expressed in small amounts. Mutations that cause increased amounts of AmpC to be produced confer full resistance to penicillins and cephalosporins; the exceptions are cefoxitin and cefepime, which are relatively stable to AmpC. Resistance to cefepime can develop, however, through the combined effects of increased AmpC production and decreased porin diffusion channels. Genes encoding AmpC have also been found on plasmids but are less common than plasmid-encoded ESBLs.

Inhibitors of β-lactamases such as clavulanate, sulbactam, and tazobactam have been developed and paired with amoxicillin and ticarcillin, ampicillin, and piperacillin, respectively. These inhibitors have little or no antibacterial activity of their own but inhibit plasmid-mediated β-lactamases, including ESBLs but not AmpC enzymes.

Resistance to β-lactams also occurs through alterations in their target PBPs. In *S. pneumoniae*, *N. gonorrhoeae*, and *Neisseria meningitidis*, resistance to penicillin occurs by recombination of transformed DNA from related species. In staphylococci, resistance to methicillin and other β-lactams occurs by the acquisition of the *mec* gene, which encodes PBP2a with reduced drug affinity. Ceftaroline is the only β-lactam that has affinity for PBP2a and is thus active against methicillin-resistant staphylococcal strains.

Glycopeptides Resistance to vancomycin in enterococci is due to the acquisition of a set of *van* genes that result in (1) the production of D-alanine-D-lactate—instead of the normal D-alanine-D-alanine—at the end of the peptidoglycan stem peptide and (2) the reduction of existing D-alanine-D-alanine terminated peptides. Vancomycin binds D-alanine-D-lactate with a thousandfold lower affinity than D-alanine-D-alanine. In a small number of cases, the *van* gene cassettes have been transferred from enterococci to *S. aureus*, with the consequent generation of full vancomycin resistance. Particularly in patients receiving prolonged courses of vancomycin, intermediate resistance to this drug has developed in *S. aureus* by a different mechanism: multiple chromosomal mutations that result in a thickened and poorly cross-linked cell wall in which multiple distant D-alanine-D-alanine stem peptide termini exist and bind vancomycin, impeding its access to the binding sites proximal to the cell membrane where new cell-wall synthesis occurs and where binding would block transpeptidase and transglycosylase enzymes. Susceptibility to telavancin, dalbavancin, and oritavancin is also reduced in strains that exhibit resistance or intermediate susceptibility to vancomycin, although in some cases strains may still be classified as susceptible on the basis of clinical interpretive criteria.

Aminoglycosides The most common mechanism of resistance is due to acquisition of plasmid genes encoding transferase enzymes that modify aminoglycosides by the addition of acetyl, adenyl, or phosphate groups; these added groups decrease the drugs' binding affinity to their ribosomal target site. Transferases differ in which aminoglycosides they modify, and amikacin resistance occurs less often than resistance to gentamicin or tobramycin. More recently, plasmids encoding methyltransferases that modify the ribosomal site of aminoglycoside binding and confer resistance to all aminoglycosides have been found in enteric gram-negative bacteria. For streptomycin, a ribosomal protein mutation may cause resistance. In *Pseudomonas aeruginosa*, resistance may also occur through mutations causing increased expression of a chromosomally encoded efflux pump, MexXY.

Tetracyclines and Glycylcyclines For tetracyclines, resistance is most often plasmid mediated and attributable either to active efflux pumps, which are generally specific for tetracyclines, or to proteins that protect the ribosome from tetracycline action. Resistance to the glycylcycline tigecycline, which is not affected by the usual tetracycline resistance mechanisms, can occur through mutations that cause overexpression of certain broad-spectrum efflux pumps in *Proteus* species.

Macrolides, Ketolides, Lincosamides, and Streptogramins Resistance to macrolides, clindamycin, and quinupristin is most often due to plasmid-acquired methylases that modify the drug binding site on the ribosome. Resistance to quinupristin by this mechanism renders the quinupristin-dalfopristin combination bacteriostatic rather than bactericidal. Telithromycin, a ketolide, has an additional binding site on the ribosome and remains active in the presence of these methylases. Acquired genes encoding active efflux pumps can also contribute to resistance to macrolides in streptococci and resistance to macrolides, clindamycin, and dalfopristin in staphylococci. Plasmid-acquired drug-modifying enzymes in staphylococci can also cause resistance to quinupristin and dalfopristin. Macrolide resistance due to 23S rRNA mutations is uncommon in staphylococci and streptococci because of the multiple copies of the rRNA genes on the chromosomes of these species; such resistance may occur more frequently, however, in mycobacteria and *Helicobacter pylori*, which have only single chromosomal copies of these rRNA genes.

Chloramphenicol Resistance to chloramphenicol is most often due to a plasmid-encoded drug-modifying acetyltransferase.

Oxazolidinones Linezolid resistance has been seen in enterococci more often than in staphylococci and, in both organisms, is due to mutations in multiple copies of the 23S rRNA genes that reduce drug binding to the ribosome. A plasmid-acquired ribosomal methylase gene that confers resistance to both chloramphenicol and linezolid has also been found in some strains of staphylococci but is not yet widespread. Tedizolid may still be active against some but not all linezolid-resistant strains.

Mupirocin Resistance to mupirocin occurs by either mutation in the target leucyl-tRNA synthetase (low-level resistance) or the acquisition of a plasmid-encoded resistant tRNA synthetase (high-level resistance).

Sulfonamides and Trimethoprim Resistance to both of these antimetabolites is due to plasmid-acquired genes encoding resistant enzymes that bypass the inhibition of the native sensitive enzymes—a resistant dihydropteroate synthetase in the case of sulfonamides and a resistant dihydrofolate reductase in the case of trimethoprim.

Quinolones Resistance to quinolones is most often due either to chromosomal mutations altering the target enzymes DNA gyrase and DNA topoisomerase IV, with consequent reduction in drug binding, or to mutations that increase the expression of native broad-spectrum efflux pumps for which quinolones (among other compounds) are substrates. In addition, three types of genes can confer reduced susceptibility or low-level resistance by protecting target enzymes, modifying some quinolones, or pumping quinolones out of the cell (efflux). These genes are located on multidrug resistance plasmids that have spread worldwide. Their presence can promote the selection of higher levels of quinolone resistance linked to resistance to other antibacterial drugs that is encoded on the same plasmid.

Rifampin and Rifabutin Single mutations in the β subunit of RNA polymerase can cause high-level resistance to rifampin. Thus rifampin and other rifamycins are used for treatment of infections only in combination with other antibacterial drugs in order to prevent resistance.

Metronidazole Acquired resistance to metronidazole in *Bacteroides* species is rare. Such resistance has been reported in strains that lack endogenous nitroreductase activity or that have acquired *nim* genes responsible for further reduction of DNA-damaging nitroso intermediates to an inactive derivative. Active efflux and enhanced DNA repair mechanisms also have been associated with resistance.

Nitrofurantoin Resistance to nitrofurantoin in *Escherichia coli* can emerge through a series of mutations that progressively decrease the nitroreductase activity necessary for generating active nitrofuran metabolites.

Polymyxins Because of emerging multidrug resistance in gram-negative bacteria, colistin and polymyxin B are being used increasingly for infections due to resistant Enterobacteriaceae, *P. aeruginosa*, and *Acinetobacter* species. Rates of resistance vary. Resistance can emerge during therapy through mutations that cause reductions in the negative charge of the gram-negative bacterial cell surface, thereby reducing binding of the positively charged colistin.

Daptomycin The mechanisms of resistance to daptomycin are complex and involve mutations in several genes that can alter cell membrane charge and reduce daptomycin binding. Resistance to daptomycin is relatively infrequent but has emerged in some *S. aureus* strains with intermediate vancomycin susceptibility from patients treated with vancomycin but not with daptomycin. In some methicillin-resistant *S. aureus* (MRSA) strains, daptomycin resistance has been linked to acquired susceptibility to β-lactams; combinations of daptomycin and nafcillin have been successful for treatment of patients infected with resistant strains when daptomycin alone or in combination with other agents has failed. The mechanism of this effect is not yet clear.

PHARMACOKINETICS AND PHARMACODYNAMICS

The term *pharmacokinetics* describes the disposition of a drug in the body, whereas *pharmacodynamics* describes the determinants of drug action on the pathogen in relation to pharmacokinetic factors. An understanding of the principles governing these two areas is required for effective drug selection, dosing, and prevention of toxicities.

PHARMACOKINETICS

The process of drug disposition has four principal phases: absorption, distribution, metabolism, and excretion. These components determine the time course of drug concentrations in serum and subsequently the concentrations in other tissues and body fluids.

Absorption When a drug is given by a particular route, *absorption* is defined as the percentage of the dose that reaches the systemic circulation. For example, since IV administration provides direct access to the systemic circulation, 100% of a drug dose given IV is usually absorbed. The level of absorption becomes more relevant when non-IV routes are used—e.g., the oral, IM, SC, and topical routes. The percentage of a drug that is absorbed is termed its *bioavailability*. Examples of antibacterial agents with a high oral bioavailability include metronidazole, levofloxacin, and linezolid. IV administration and oral dosing for highly bioavailable agents usually give equivalent results. Many factors can affect a drug's oral bioavailability, including the timing of food consumption relative to drug administration, drug-metabolizing enzymes, efflux transporters, concentration-dependent solubility, and acid degradation. Underlying conditions such as diarrhea or ileus can also affect the site of drug absorption and thereby alter bioavailability. Certain orally administered drugs have lower bioavailability because of the *first-pass effect*—the process by which drugs are absorbed in the small intestine through the portal circulation and then directly transported to the liver for metabolism.

Distribution *Distribution* describes the process by which a drug transfers reversibly between the general circulation and the tissues. After absorption into the general circulation and the central compartment (the extensively perfused organs), the drug will also distribute into the peripheral compartment (less well-perfused tissues). The volume of distribution (Vd) is a pharmacokinetic parameter that describes the amount of drug in the body at a given time relative to the measured serum concentration. Properties such as the drug's lipophilicity, partition coefficient within different body tissues, and protein binding; blood flow; and pH can affect the volume of distribution. Drugs with a small volume of distribution are limited to certain areas within the body (typically extracellular fluid), whereas those with a higher volume of distribution penetrate extensively into tissues throughout the body. Antibacterial drugs can bind to serum proteins, and a given drug is usually described as either poorly or highly protein bound. Only the unbound (free) drug is active and available to exert antibacterial effects. For example, because tigecycline is highly protein bound and also has a large volume of distribution, concentrations of free drug in the serum are low.

Metabolism *Metabolism* is the chemical transformation of a drug by the body. This modification can occur within several areas; the liver is the organ most commonly involved. Drugs are metabolized by enzymes, but enzyme systems have a finite capacity to metabolize a substrate drug. If a drug is given in a dose at which the concentration does not exceed the rate of metabolism, then the metabolic process is generally linear. If the dose exceeds the amount that can be metabolized, drug accumulation and potential toxicity may occur. Drugs are metabolized through phase I or phase II reactions. In phase I reactions, the drug is made more polar through dealkylation, hydroxylation, oxidation, and deamination. Polarity facilitates drug removal from the body. Phase II reactions, which include glucuronidation, sulfation, and acetylation, result in compounds larger and more polar than the parent drug. Both phases usually inactivate the parent drug, but some drugs are rendered more active. The cytochrome P450 (CYP) enzyme system is responsible for phase I reactions and is generally found in the liver. CYP3A4 is a common subfamily within this system that is responsible for the majority of drug metabolism. Antibacterial drugs can be substrates, inhibitors, or inducers of a particular CYP enzyme. Inducers, such as rifampin, can increase the production of CYP enzymes and consequently increase the metabolism of other drugs. Inhibitors, such as quinupristin-dalfopristin, cause a decrease in enzyme activity (or competition for CYP substrate) and therefore an increase in the concentration of the interacting drug.

Excretion *Excretion* describes the body's mechanisms of drug elimination. Drugs can be eliminated through more than one mechanism. Renal clearance is the most common route and includes elimination through glomerular filtration, tubular secretion, and/or passive diffusion. Some agents have nonrenal clearance and rely on the biliary tree or the intestine for excretion. Excretion affects the half-life of a drug—i.e., the time it takes for the blood concentration of a drug to decrease by one-half. This value can range from minutes to days. Approximately five to seven half-lives are required for a drug to reach steady state when multiple doses are given in a time frame shorter than the half-life itself. Drug half-life and overall clearance can be extended if the organ responsible for clearance is impaired. Patients with renal or hepatic impairment may require dose adjustments that take delayed clearance into account and prevent toxicities from drug accumulation. For example, imipenem is cleared predominantly through glomerular filtration, and in the presence of renal impairment the dosing interval is typically increased to account for the increased half-life.

PHARMACODYNAMICS

The term *pharmacodynamics* describes the relationship between the serum concentrations that determine the efficacy of the drug and the serum concentrations that produce the toxic effects of the drug. For an antibacterial agent, the pharmacodynamic focus is the type of drug

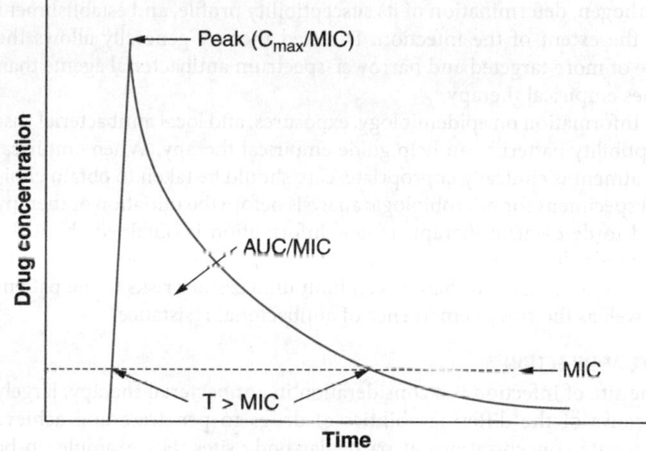

FIGURE 170-2 Pharmacokinetic and pharmacodynamic model predicting efficacy of antibacterial drugs. AUC, area under the time–concentration curve; C_{max}, peak serum concentration of drug; MIC, minimal inhibitory concentration; T>MIC, duration of drug concentrations above the MIC.

exposure needed for optimal antibacterial effect in relation to the minimal inhibitory concentration (MIC)—the lowest drug concentration that inhibits the visible growth of a microorganism under standardized laboratory conditions. Antibacterial effect usually correlates with one of the following parameters: (1) ratio of peak serum concentration to the MIC (C_{max}/MIC), (2) ratio of the area under the concentration–time curve to the MIC (AUC/MIC), or (3) duration of concentrations above the MIC (T>MIC) (Fig. 170-2).

For *concentration dependent* killing agents, as the designation implies, the higher the drug concentration, the higher the rate and extent of bacterial killing. Aminoglycosides fit into the C_{max}/MIC model of pharmacodynamics activity, and a particular peak serum concentration is often targeted to achieve optimal killing. Fluoroquinolones exemplify antibacterial agents for which the AUC/MIC is a predictor of efficacy. For example, studies have found that an AUC/MIC ratio of >30 will maximize killing of *S. pneumoniae* by fluoroquinolones. In contrast, *time-dependent* killing agents reach a ceiling at which higher concentrations do not result in increased effect. Instead, these agents are active against bacteria only when the drug concentration is above the MIC. The T>MIC predicts clinical efficacy for all β-lactams. The longer the concentration of the β-lactam remains above the MIC for an infecting pathogen during the dosing interval, the greater the killing effect. For some drug classes, such as aminoglycosides, a *postantibiotic effect*—the delayed regrowth of surviving bacteria after exposure to an antibiotic—supports less frequent dosing.

APPROACH TO THERAPY

The approach to antibiotic therapy is driven by host factors, site of infection, and local resistance profiles of suspected or known pathogens. Further, national and local drug shortages and formulary restrictions can affect available therapies. Regular monitoring of the patient and collection of laboratory data should be undertaken to streamline antibacterial therapy as appropriate and to investigate the possibility of treatment failure if the patient fails to respond appropriately.

EMPIRICAL AND DIRECTED THERAPY

Therapy is considered *empirical* when the causative agent has yet to be determined and therapeutic decisions are based on the severity of illness and the clinician's assessment of likely pathogens in light of the clinical syndrome, the patient's medical conditions and prior therapy, and relevant epidemiologic factors. For patients with severe illness, empirical therapy often takes the form of an antibacterial combination that provides broad coverage of diverse agents and thus ensures adequate treatment of possible pathogens while additional data are being collected. *Directed* therapy is predicated on identification of the pathogen, determination of its susceptibility profile, and establishment of the extent of the infection. Directed therapy generally allows the use of more targeted and narrower-spectrum antibacterial agents than does empirical therapy.

Information on epidemiology, exposures, and local antibacterial susceptibility patterns can help guide empirical therapy. When empirical treatment is clinically appropriate, care should be taken to obtain clinical specimens for microbiologic analysis before the initiation of therapy and to de-escalate therapy as new information is obtained about the patient's clinical condition and the causal pathogens. De-escalation to the point of directed therapy can limit unnecessary risks to the patient as well as the risk of emergence of antibacterial resistance.

SITE OF INFECTION

The site of infection is a consideration in antibacterial therapy, largely because of the differing abilities of drugs to penetrate and achieve adequate concentrations at particular body sites. For example, to be effective in the treatment of meningitis, an agent must (1) be able to cross the blood–brain barrier and reach adequate concentrations in the cerebrospinal fluid (CSF) and (2) be active against the relevant pathogen(s). Dexamethasone, administered with or 15–20 min before the first dose of an antibacterial drug, has been shown to improve outcomes in patients with acute bacterial meningitis, but its use may reduce penetration of some antibacterial agents, such as vancomycin, into the CSF. In this case, rifampin is added because its penetration is not reduced by dexamethasone. Infections at other sites where either pathogens are protected from normal host defenses or penetration of an antibacterial drug is suboptimal include osteomyelitis, prostatitis, intraocular infections, and abscesses. In such cases, consideration must be given to the mechanism of drug delivery (e.g., intravitreal injections) as well as to the role of interventions to drain, debride, or otherwise reduce the barriers to effective antibacterial therapy.

HOST FACTORS

Host factors, including immune function, pregnancy, allergies, age, renal and hepatic function, drug–drug interactions, comorbid conditions, and occupational or social exposures, should be considered.

Immune Dysfunction Patients with deficits in immune function that blunt the response to bacterial infection, including neutropenia, deficient humoral immunity, and asplenia (either surgical or functional), are all at increased risk of severe bacterial infection. Such patients should be treated aggressively and often broadly in the early stages of suspected infection pending results of microbiologic tests. For asplenic patients, treatment should include coverage of encapsulated organisms, particularly *S. pneumoniae*, that may cause rapidly life-threatening infection.

Pregnancy Pregnancy affects decisions regarding antibacterial therapy in two respects. First, pregnancy is associated with an increased risk of particular infections (e.g., those caused by *Listeria*). Second, the potential risks to the fetus that are posed by specific drugs must be considered. As for other drugs, the safety of the vast majority of antibacterial agents in pregnancy has not been established, and such agents are grouped in categories B and C by the U.S. Food and Drug Administration. Drugs in categories D and X are contraindicated in pregnancy or lactation due to established risks. The risks associated with antibacterial use in pregnancy and during lactation are summarized in Table 170-2.

Allergies Allergies to antibiotics are among the most common allergies reported, and an allergy history should be obtained whenever possible before therapy is chosen. A detailed allergy history can shed light on the type of reaction experienced previously and on whether rechallenge with the same or a related medication is advisable (and, if so, under what circumstances). Allergies to the penicillins are most common. Although as many as 10% of patients may report an allergy to penicillin, studies suggest that up to 90% of these patients could tolerate a penicillin or cephalosporin. Adverse effects (Table 170-3) should be distinguished from true allergies to ensure appropriate selection of antibacterial therapy.

Drug–Drug Interactions Patients commonly receive other drugs that may interact with antibacterial agents. A summary of the most common drug–drug interactions, by antibacterial class, is provided in Table 170-4.

Exposures Exposures, both occupational and social, may provide clues to likely pathogens. When relevant, inquiries about exposure to ill contacts, animals, insects, and water should be included in the history, along with sites of residence and travel.

Other Host Factors Age, renal and hepatic function, and comorbid conditions are all considerations in the choice of and schedule for therapy. Dose adjustments should be made accordingly. In patients with decreased or unreliable oral absorption, IV therapy may be preferred to ensure adequate blood levels of drug and delivery of the antibacterial agent to the site of infection.

DURATION OF THERAPY

Whether empirical or directed, the duration of therapy should be planned in most clinical situations. Guidelines that synthesize available literature and expert opinion provide recommendations on therapy duration that are based on infecting organism, organ system, and patient factors. For example, the American Heart Association has published guidelines endorsed by the Infectious Diseases Society of America (IDSA) on diagnosis, antibacterial therapy, and management of complications of infective endocarditis. Similar guidelines from the IDSA exist for bacterial meningitis, catheter-associated urinary tract infections, intraabdominal infections, community- and hospital-acquired pneumonia, and other infections.

FAILURE OF THERAPY

If a patient does not respond to therapy, investigations often should include the collection of additional specimens for microbiologic testing and imaging as indicated. Failure to respond can be the result of an antibacterial regimen that does not address the underlying causative organism, the development of resistance during therapy, or the existence of a focus of infection at a site poorly penetrated by systemic therapy. Some infections may also require surgical interventions for cure (e.g., large abscesses, myonecrosis). Fever due to allergic drug reactions can sometimes complicate assessment of the patient's response to antibacterial treatment.

EXPERT GUIDANCE

Selected websites with the most up-to-date information and guidance for the clinician include the following:

- Johns Hopkins ABX Guide (*www.hopkins-abxguide.org*)
- IDSA Practice Guidelines (*www.idsociety.org/IDSA_Practice_Guidelines/*)
- Center for Disease Dynamics, Economics and Policy Resistance Map (*www.cddep.org/map*)
- CDC Antibiotic/Antimicrobial Resistance (*www.cdc.gov/drugresistance/*)

CLINICAL USE OF ANTIBACTERIAL AGENTS

The clinical application of antibacterial therapy is guided by the spectrum of the agent and the suspected or known target pathogen. Infections for which specific antibacterial agents are among the drugs of choice are listed, along with associated pathogens and susceptibility data, in Table 170-5. Resistance rates of specific organisms are dynamic and should be taken into account in the approach to antibacterial therapy. While national resistance rates can serve as a reference, the most useful reference for the clinician is the most recent local laboratory antibiogram, which provides details on local resistance patterns, often on an annual or semiannual basis.

β-LACTAMS

The β-lactam class of antibiotics consists of penicillins, cephalosporins, carbapenems, and monobactams. The term *β-lactam* reflects the drugs' four-membered lactam ring, which is their core structure. The differing

TABLE 170-2 RISKS ASSOCIATED WITH USE OF ANTIBACTERIAL DRUGS IN PREGNANCY AND LACTATION

Pregnancy Category[a]	Antibacterial Drug	Fetal Risk Recommendation[b]	Breast-Feeding Risk Recommendation[b]
B	Azithromycin	Limited human data. Animal data suggest low risk.	Limited human data; probably compatible
	Cephalosporins (including cephalexin, cefuroxime, cefixime, cefpodoxime, cefotaxime, ceftriaxone)	Compatible	Compatible
	Clindamycin	Compatible	Compatible
	Ertapenem	No human data; probably compatible	Limited human data; probably compatible
	Erythromycin	Compatible (excluding estolate salt)	Compatible
	Meropenem	No human data. Animal data suggest low risk.	No human data; probably compatible
	Metronidazole	Human data suggest low risk.	Interrupt breast-feeding for 12–24 h after single 2-g dose. Limited human data; potential toxicity in divided doses
	Nitrofurantoin	Human data suggest risk in third trimester.	Limited human data; probably compatible. Higher risk associated with younger infants and those with G6PD deficiency
	Penicillins (Including amoxicillin, ampicillin, cloxacillin)	Compatible	Compatible
	Quinupristin-dalfopristin	Compatible. Maternal benefit must far outweigh risk to embryo/fetus.	No human data; potential toxicity
	Vancomycin	Compatible	Limited human data; probably compatible
C	Chloramphenicol	Compatible	Limited human data; potential toxicity
	Fluoroquinolones	Human data suggest low risk.	Limited human data; probably compatible
	Clarithromycin	Limited human data. Animal data suggest high risk.	No human data; probably compatible
	Imipenem/cilastatin	Limited human data. Animal data suggest low risk.	Limited human data; probably compatible
	Linezolid	Compatible. Maternal benefit must far outweigh risk to embryo/fetus.	No human data; potential toxicity
	Telavancin	No human data. Animal studies have revealed evidence of teratogenicity.[c]	No human data. Animal studies have revealed evidence of teratogenicity.[c]
	Tedizolid	Limited data. Embryo-fetal studies in mice, rats, and rabbits have demonstrated fetal developmental toxicities. Use only if benefit outweighs risk.	Excreted in the breastmilk of rats; unknown in humans; caution use
	Dalbavancin	Limited human data. At high doses in animal studies, delayed fetal maturation, increased embryo and offspring death. Use only if benefit outweighs risk.	Excreted in the breastmilk of animals; unknown in humans; caution use
	Oritavancin	Limited human data. Studies in rats and rabbits demonstrated no harm at 25% of recommended human dose. Use only if benefit outweighs risk.	Excreted in the breastmilk of rats; unknown in humans; caution use
C/D	Amikacin	Human data suggest low risk.	Compatible
	Gentamicin	Human data suggest low risk.	Compatible
D	Kanamycin	Human data suggest risk.	Limited human data; probably compatible
	Streptomycin	Human data suggest risk.	Compatible
	Sulfonamides	Human data suggest risk in third trimester.	Limited human data; potential toxicity. Avoid in ill, stressed, premature infants and in infants with hyperbilirubinemia or G6PD deficiency.
	Tetracyclines	Contraindicated in second and third trimesters	Compatible
	Tigecycline	Human data suggest risk in second and third trimesters.	No human data; potential toxicity

[a]***Category B:*** *Either* animal reproduction studies have failed to demonstrate a risk to the fetus, and there are no adequate and well-controlled studies in pregnant women; *or* animal studies have shown an adverse effect, but adequate and well-controlled studies in pregnant women have failed to demonstrate a risk to the fetus in any trimester. ***Category C:*** Animal reproduction studies have shown an adverse effect on the fetus, and there are no adequate and well-controlled studies in humans, but potential benefits may warrant use of the drug in pregnant women despite potential risks. ***Category D:*** There is positive evidence of human fetal risk based on adverse reaction data from investigational or marketing experience or studies in humans, but potential benefits may warrant use of the drug in pregnant women despite potential risks. [b]Fetal risk recommendation and breast-feeding risk recommendation adapted from GG Briggs et al, eds: *Drugs in Pregnancy and Lactation*, 9th ed. Philadelphia, Lippincott Williams and Wilkins, 2011; and the U.S. Food and Drug Administration (Drugs@FDA).
[c]A registry has been established to monitor pregnancy outcomes of pregnant women exposed to telavancin. Physicians are encouraged to register pregnant patients, or pregnant women may enroll themselves by calling 1-855-633-8479.

Abbreviation: G6PD, glucose-6-phosphate dehydrogenase.

side chains among the agents of this family determine the spectrum of activity. All β-lactams exert a bactericidal effect by inhibiting bacterial cell-wall synthesis. The β-lactams are classified as time-dependent killing agents; therefore, their clinical efficacy is best correlated with the proportion of the dosing interval during which the drug levels remain above the MIC for the pathogenic organism.

Penicillins and β-Lactamase Inhibitors Penicillin, the first β-lactam, was discovered in 1928 by Alexander Fleming. Natural penicillins, such as penicillin G, are active against non-β-lactamase-producing gram-positive and gram-negative bacteria, anaerobes, and some gram-negative cocci. Penicillin G is used for penicillin-susceptible streptococcal infections, pneumococcal and meningococcal meningitis, enterococcal endocarditis, and syphilis. The antistaphyloccocal penicillins, which have potent activity against methicillin-susceptible *S. aureus* (MSSA), include nafcillin, oxacillin, dicloxacillin, and flucloxacillin. Aminopenicillins, such as ampicillin and amoxicillin, provide added coverage beyond penicillin against gram-negative cocci, such as *Haemophilus influenzae*,

TABLE 170-3 COMMON ADVERSE REACTIONS TO ANTIBACTERIAL AGENTS

Antibacterial(s)	Potential Adverse Effects	Comments
β-Lactams	Hypersensitivity reactions	Range from rash to anaphylaxis. Cross-reactivity among β-lactams is related to chemical structure and side chain similarity.
	Neurotoxicity	More commonly described with cefepime and imipenem, but likely a class effect. Risk is increased in patients with history of seizures, renal impairment, and advanced age.
	Neutropenia/hematologic reactions	May be related to high doses and prolonged duration
Vancomycin	Nephrotoxicity	Risk increases with vancomycin trough levels >20 μg/mL or concomitant administration with other potentially nephrotoxic agents. The effect is usually reversible.
	"Red man syndrome"	Can be managed with a slower vancomycin infusion and pretreatment with antihistamine
Telavancin	QT prolongation	
	Interference with coagulation tests	May falsely affect INR, PT, aPTT. Perform these tests before the next dose of telavancin (when serum drug levels are at their nadir).
	Taste disturbances	
	Nephrotoxicity	
Oritavancin	Interference with coagulation tests	May falsely affect INR, PT, aPTT. Perform these tests at least 24 h after the dose was administered
Dalbavancin, oritivancin	Similar to vancomycin without "red man syndrome"	
Daptomycin	Myopathy	Monitor CPK levels during therapy. Rhabdomyolysis has been reported but appears to be rare.
	Eosinophilic pneumonia	
Aminoglycosides	Nephrotoxicity	Associated with prolonged use; usually reversible
	Ototoxicity	Can cause both vestibular and cochlear toxicity. Ototoxicity may be irreversible.
Fluoroquinolones	QTc prolongation	Moxifloxacin appears more likely than other quinolones to exert this effect. Risk of arrhythmia increases when these drugs are given concomitantly with other QTc-prolonging agents.
	Tendinitis	Risk is greater among elderly and patients receiving steroids.
	Dysglycemia	
	Exacerbation of myasthenia gravis	
Rifampin	Hepatotoxicity	Risk is greater when drug is given with other antituberculosis agents. When rifampin is given alone, LFT values may be transiently elevated without symptoms.
	Orange discoloration of body fluids	
Tetracyclines and glycylcyclines	Photosensitivity	
	Gastrointestinal distress	High incidence of diarrhea, nausea, vomiting
Macrolides	Gastrointestinal distress	Erythromycin is occasionally used as a therapeutic agent for some gastric motility disorders.
	QTc prolongation	Azithromycin use is associated with an increased risk of death from cardiovascular causes among patients at high baseline risk.
Metronidazole	Peripheral neuropathy	Associated with prolonged use
Clindamycin	Diarrhea and pseudomembranous colitis	
Linezolid, tedizolid	Myelosuppression	Associated with prolonged use
	Optic and peripheral neuropathy	Associated with prolonged use
TMP-SMX	Hypersensitivity reactions	Allergy usually associated with sulfonamide moiety
	Nephrotoxicity	Associated with high doses
	Hematologic effects	Associated with prolonged use
Nitrofurantoin	Pneumonitis and other pulmonary reactions	Associated with prolonged use
	Peripheral neuropathy	Associated with accumulation of nitrofurantoin in renal failure. Avoid use in renal impairment.
Fosfomycin	Gastrointestinal effects	
Polymyxins	Nephrotoxicity	Associated with high dose
	Neurotoxicity	Neuromuscular blockade and muscle weakness are well described and usually reversible.
Quinupristin-dalfopristin	Arthralgias and myalgias	
Chloramphenicol	Bone marrow suppression	Aplastic anemia or hematopoietic toxicity

Note: All systemic antibiotics have the potential to alter abdominal flora and induce *Clostridium difficile* infection.

Abbreviations: aPTT, activated partial thromboplastin time; CPK, creatine phosphokinase; INR, international normalized ratio; LFT, liver function test; PT, prothrombin time; TMP-SMX, trimethoprim-sulfamethoxazole.

and some Enterobacteriaceae, including *E. coli*, *Proteus mirabilis*, *Salmonella*, and *Shigella*. The aminopenicillins are hydrolyzed by many common β-lactamases. These drugs are commonly used for otitis media, respiratory tract infections, intraabdominal infections, endocarditis, meningitis, and urinary tract infections. The antipseudomonal penicillins include ticarcillin and piperacillin. These penicillin groups generally offer adequate anaerobic coverage; the exceptions are *Bacteroides* species (such as *Bacteroides fragilis*), which produce β-lactamases and are generally resistant. The rising prevalence of β-lactamase-producing bacteria has led to the increased use of β-lactam/β-lactamase inhibitor combinations, such as ampicillin-sulbactam, amoxicillin-clavulanate, ticarcillin-clavulanate, and piperacillin-tazobactam. The β-lactamase inhibitors themselves do not have antibacterial activity (with the exception of sulbactam, which has activity against *Acinetobacter baumannii*)

TABLE 170-4 SIGNIFICANT ANTIBACTERIAL DRUG INTERACTIONS

Antibacterial(s)	Interacting Agent(s)	Potential Effect and Management
Nafcillin	Warfarin, cyclosporine, tacrolimus	Decreased levels of warfarin, cyclosporine via CYP3A4 induction. Monitor levels of affected drug closely if drugs are given concomitantly.
Ceftriaxone	Calcium-containing IV solutions	Concomitant use is contraindicated in neonates (<28 days); the combination can lead to precipitation of ceftriaxone-calcium particulate.
		Ceftriaxone and calcium-containing solutions can be given to infants >28 days of age provided they are given sequentially and the lines are thoroughly flushed between infusions.
Carbapenems	Valproic acid	Decreased levels of valproic acid. Monitor valproic acid levels closely if drugs are given concomitantly.
Linezolid, tedizolid	Serotonergic and adrenergic agents (e.g., SSRIs, vasopressors)	Increased levels of serotonergic and adrenergic agents. Monitor for serotonin syndrome. Tedizolid may have less potential than linezolid to cause this drug interaction.
Quinupristin dalfopristin	Substrates of cytochrome CYP3A4 (e.g., warfarin, ritonavir, cyclosporine, diazepam, verapamil)	Can result in increased levels of interacting drug. Erythromycin and clarithromycin are more potent CYP3A4 inhibitors than azithromycin. Avoid concomitant administration if possible.
Fluoroquinolones	Theophylline[a]	Can result in theophylline toxicity
	Sucralfate; antacids containing aluminum, calcium, or magnesium; ferrous sulfate and zinc-containing multivitamins	Can result in subtherapeutic fluoroquinolone levels. Administer fluoroquinolone 2 h before or 6 h after interacting drug.
	Tizanidine[a]	Can result in increased levels of tizanidine and hypotensive, sedative effects. Monitor for side effects if drugs are given concomitantly.
Rifampin	Substrates of cytochrome CYP3A4 (e.g., warfarin, ritonavir, cyclosporine, diazepam, verapamil, protease inhibitors, voriconazole)	Can result in decreased levels of interacting drug. Avoid concomitant use if possible. If giving drugs concomitantly, monitor drug levels if possible.
	Substrates of cytochrome CYP2C19 (e.g., omeprazole, lansoprazole)	
	Substrates of cytochrome CYP2C9 (e.g., warfarin, tolbutamide)	
	Substrates of cytochrome CYP2C8 (e.g., repaglinide, rosiglitazone)	
	Substrates of cytochrome CYP2B6 (e.g., efavirenz)	
	Hormone therapy (e.g., norethindrone)	Can result in decreased levels of hormone. If oral contraceptive and rifampin are given concomitantly, use alternative form of birth control.
Tetracyclines	Antacids or drugs containing calcium, magnesium, iron, or aluminum	Can result in decreased absorption of tetracyclines. Administer tetracycline 2 h before or 6 h after interacting drug.
Macrolides[b]	Substrates of cytochrome CYP3A4 (e.g., warfarin, ritonavir, cyclosporine, diazepam, verapamil)	Avoid concomitant administration if possible.
	QTc-prolonging agents (e.g., fluoroquinolones, sotalol)	Increased risk of cardiotoxicity and arrhythmias. Monitor QTc.
	Protease inhibitors (e.g., ritonavir)	Can result in increased levels of both macrolides and protease inhibitors. Avoid concomitant use if possible.
	Cimetidine	Cimetidine can increase levels of macrolides.
Metronidazole	Ethanol	Can result in disulfiram-like reaction. Ethanol may be present in some formulations of oral drug suspensions (e.g., ritonavir).
	Warfarin	Can increase warfarin levels. Monitor INR closely if drugs are given concomitantly
TMP-SMX	Warfarin	Increased effect of warfarin. Monitor levels closely if drugs are given concomitantly.
	Phenytoin	Increased levels of phenytoin. Monitor levels closely if drugs are given concomitantly.
	Methotrexate	Increased levels of methotrexate. Monitor levels closely if drugs are given concomitantly.
Oritavancin	Substrates of cytochrome CYP3A4 (e.g., cyclosporine, warfarin) and CYP2D6 (e.g., aripiprazole)	Can result in decreased levels of interacting drug. Avoid concomitant use if possible. If giving drugs concomitantly, monitor drug levels if possible.
	Substrates of cytochrome CYP2C19 (e.g., omeprazole) and CYP2C9 (e.g., warfarin)	Can result in increased levels of interacting drug. Avoid concomitant use if possible. If giving drugs concomitantly, monitor drug levels if possible.

[a]Drug reaction described with ciprofloxacin only. [b]Clarithromycin and erythromycin are potent CYP3A4 inhibitors; the probability of a drug interaction with azithromycin is lower.

Abbreviations: INR, international normalized ratio; SSRI, selective serotonin-reuptake inhibitor; TMP-SMX, trimethoprim-sulfamethoxazole.

but typically inhibit the *S. aureus* class A β-lactamase, β-lactamases of *H. influenzae* and *Bacteroides* species, and a number of plasmid-encoded β-lactamases. These combination agents are typically used when broader-spectrum coverage is needed—e.g., in pneumonia and intraabdominal infections. Piperacillin-tazobactam is a useful agent for broad coverage in febrile neutropenic patients. The combination agents, however, are not effective against organisms that produce AmpC β-lactamases or carbapenemases.

Cephalosporins The cephalosporin drug class encompasses five generations determined by spectrum of antibacterial activity. The first generation (cefazolin, cefadroxil, cephalexin) largely has activity

TABLE 170-5 DRUG INDICATIONS FOR SPECIFIC INFECTIONS, ASSOCIATED PATHOGENS, AND SAMPLE SUSCEPTIBILITY RATES

Antimicrobial(s)	Infections	Common Pathogens (% Susceptible); Resistance as Noted[a]
Penicillin G	Syphilis; yaws; leptospirosis; streptococcal infections; pneumococcal infections; actinomycosis; oral and periodontal infections; meningococcal meningitis and meningococcemia; viridans streptococcal endocarditis; clostridial myonecrosis; tetanus; rat-bite fever; *Pasteurella multocida* infections; erysipeloid (*Erysipelothrix rhusiopathiae*)	*Neisseria meningitidis*; viridans streptococci (73%); *Streptococcus pneumoniae* (92% nonmeningitis; 65% meningitis)
Ampicillin, amoxicillin	Salmonellosis; acute otitis media; *Haemophilus influenzae* meningitis and epiglottitis; *Listeria monocytogenes* meningitis; *Enterococcus faecalis* UTI	*Escherichia coli* (52%); *H. influenzae* (70%); *Salmonella* spp. (91%)
Nafcillin, oxacillin	MSSA bacteremia and endocarditis	*Staphylococcus aureus* (68%); coagulase-negative staphylococci (47%)
Piperacillin-tazobactam	Intraabdominal infections (facultative enteric gram-negative bacilli and obligate anaerobes); infections caused by mixed flora (aspiration pneumonia, diabetic foot ulcers); infections caused by *Pseudomonas aeruginosa*	*P. aeruginosa* (88%)[b]
Cefazolin	*E. coli* UTI; surgical prophylaxis; MSSA bacteremia and endocarditis	*E. coli* (85%)
Cefoxitin, cefotetan	Intraabdominal infections and pelvic inflammatory disease	*Bacteroides fragilis* (60%)[c]
Ceftriaxone	Gonococcal infections; pneumococcal meningitis; viridans streptococcal endocarditis; salmonellosis and typhoid fever; hospital-acquired infections caused by nonpseudomonal facultative gram-negative enteric bacilli	*S. pneumoniae* (93%);[d] *E. coli* (93%); *Klebsiella pneumoniae* (89%)
Ceftazidime, cefepime	Hospital-acquired infections caused by facultative gram-negative bacilli and *Pseudomonas* spp.	*P. aeruginosa* (89%)
Ceftaroline	CAP caused by *S. pneumoniae*, MSSA, *H. influenzae*, *K. pneumoniae*, *Klebsiella oxytoca*, and *E. coli*; acute bacterial skin and skin-structure infections caused by MSSA, MRSA, *Streptococcus pyogenes*, *Streptococcus agalactiae*, *E. coli*, *K. pneumoniae*, and *K. oxytoca*	Mostly susceptible; four strains of MRSA with ceftaroline MICs >4 μg/mL reported in isolates from a single Greek hospital[e]
Imipenem, meropenem	Intraabdominal infections, infections caused by *Enterobacter* spp. and ESBL-producing gram-negative bacilli	*P. aeruginosa* (76% and 83%); *Acinetobacter calcoaceticus-baumannii* complex (81% and 82%)
Ertapenem	CAP; complicated UTIs, including pyelonephritis; acute pelvic infections; complicated intraabdominal infections; complicated skin and skin-structure infections, excluding diabetic foot infections accompanied by osteomyelitis or caused by *P. aeruginosa*	*Enterobacter cloacae* (87%); *K. pneumoniae* (97%)
Aztreonam	HAIs caused by facultative gram-negative bacilli and *Pseudomonas* in penicillin-allergic patients	*P. aeruginosa* (76%)
Vancomycin	Bacteremia, endocarditis, and other invasive disease caused by MRSA; pneumococcal meningitis; oral formulation for CDAD	*S. aureus* (100%); *E. faecalis* (89%); *E. faecium* (24%)
Telavancin	Hospital- and ventilator-associated pneumonia or skin and soft tissue infections caused by MRSA	*S. aureus* (100%)
Dalbavancin, oritavancin	Complicated skin and soft tissue infections	*S. aureus* (100%)
Daptomycin	VRE infections; MRSA bacteremia	*E. faecalis* (99.9%);[f] *E. faecium* (99.7%);[f] *S. aureus* (99.9%)[f]
Gentamicin, tobramycin, amikacin	Combined with penicillin for staphylococcal, enterococcal, or streptococcal endocarditis; combined with β-lactam for gram-negative bacteremia; pyelonephritis	*E. coli* (gentamicin, 91%); *P. aeruginosa* (amikacin, 87%; gentamicin, 81%); *A. calcoaceticus-baumannii* complex (amikacin, 68%; gentamicin, 83%)
Azithromycin, clarithromycin, erythromycin	*Legionella*, *Campylobacter*, and *Mycoplasma* infections; CAP; GAS pharyngitis in penicillin-allergic patients; bacillary angiomatosis; gastric infections due to *Helicobacter pylori*; MAI infections	*S. pneumoniae* (59%); group A streptococci (78%); *H. pylori* (75%)[g]
Clindamycin	Severe, invasive GAS infections (with β-lactam); infections caused by obligate anaerobes; infections caused by susceptible staphylococci	*S. aureus* (67%)
Doxycycline, minocycline	Acute bacterial exacerbations of chronic bronchitis; granuloma inguinale; brucellosis (with streptomycin); tularemia; glanders; melioidosis; spirochetal infections caused by *Borrelia* (Lyme disease and relapsing fever; doxycycline); infections caused by *Vibrio vulnificus*; some *Aeromonas* infections; infections due to *Stenotrophomonas* (minocycline); plague; ehrlichiosis; chlamydial infections (doxycycline); granulomatous infections due to *Mycobacterium marinum* (minocycline); rickettsial infections; mild CAP; skin and soft tissue infections caused by gram-positive cocci (e.g., CA-MRSA infections); leptospirosis; syphilis; and actinomycosis in the penicillin-allergic patient	*S. pneumoniae* (75%); *S. aureus* (94%)
Tigecycline	CAP caused by *S. pneumoniae*, *H. influenzae*, or *Legionella pneumophila*; complicated skin infections caused by *E. coli*, MRSA, MSSA, *S. pyogenes*, *Streptococcus anginosus*, *S. agalactiae*, *B. fragilis*; complicated intraabdominal infections caused by *E. coli*, vancomycin-susceptible *E. faecalis*, *Citrobacter freundii*, *Enterobacter cloacae*, *K. pneumoniae*, *K. oxytoca*, *Bacteroides* spp., *Clostridium perfringens*, and *Peptostreptococcus* spp.	Mostly susceptible, though case reports of resistance in *A. baumannii* and *K. pneumoniae*

(Continued)

TABLE 170-5 DRUG INDICATIONS FOR SPECIFIC INFECTIONS, ASSOCIATED PATHOGENS, AND SAMPLE SUSCEPTIBILITY RATES (*CONTINUED*)

Antimicrobial(s)	Infections	Common Pathogens (% Susceptible); Resistance as Noted[a]
TMP-SMX	Community-acquired UTI; CA-MRSA skin and soft tissue infections	*E. coli* (73%); *S. aureus* (96%)
Sulfonamides	Nocardial infections; leprosy (dapsone); toxoplasmosis (sulfadiazine)	Unknown
Ciprofloxacin, levofloxacin, moxifloxacin	CAP (levofloxacin and moxifloxacin); UTI; bacterial gastroenteritis; hospital-acquired gram-negative enteric infections; *Pseudomonas* infections (ciprofloxacin and levofloxacin)	*S. pneumoniae* (99%); *E. coli* (80%); *P. aeruginosa* (ciprofloxacin, 72%; levofloxacin, 69%); *Salmonella* spp. (ciprofloxacin, 98%; levofloxacin, 100%)
Rifampin	Staphylococcal foreign body infections in combination with other antistaphylococcal agents, *Legionella* pneumonia; *Mycobacterium tuberculosis*; atypical nontuberculous mycobacterial infection; pneumococcal meningitis when organisms are susceptible or response is delayed	*S. aureus* (99%), although staphylococci rapidly develop resistance with monotherapy
Metronidazole	Obligate anaerobic gram-negative bacteria (e.g., *Bacteroides* spp); abscess in lung, brain, or abdomen; bacterial vaginosis; CDAD	Mostly susceptible; resistance very rare
Linezolid, tedizolid	VRE; uncomplicated and complicated skin and soft tissue infections caused by MSSA and MRSA; CAP with concurrent bacteremia; hospital-acquired pneumonia	Mostly susceptible; resistance occasionally seen in VRE
Chloramphenicol	HAI due to gram-positive and gram-negative organisms resistant to standard alternatives (e.g., *Burkholderia*)	Unknown
Colistin	HAI due to gram-negative bacilli resistant to all other chemotherapy (e.g., *P. aeruginosa*, *Acinetobacter* spp., and *Stenotrophomonas maltophilia*)	*P. aeruginosa* (case reports, outbreaks)
Quinupristin-dalfopristin	VRE; complicated skin and skin structure infections due to MSSA and *S. pyogenes*	*E. faecalis* (<20%);[h] *E. faecium* (>90%)[h]
Mupirocin	Topical application to nares for *S. aureus* decolonization	*S. aureus* (74–100%)[i]
Nitrofurantoin	UTI caused by most gram-negative bacilli and some gram-positive organisms; prophylaxis in recurrent cystitis	*E. coli* (92%); *E. faecalis* (99%)
Fosfomycin	UTI caused by most gram-negative bacilli and some gram-positive organisms; prophylaxis in recurrent cystitis	Unknown

[a]Unless otherwise noted, susceptibility rates are based on isolates from the Massachusetts General Hospital Clinical Microbiology Laboratory collected between January and December 2012. Local rates will vary. [b]The Center for Disease Dynamics, Economics and Policy Resistance Map, Washington, DC. [c]S Sepehri et al: Prevalence of antimicrobial resistance among clinical isolates of *Bacteroides fragilis* group in Canada in 2010–2011: CANWARD Surveillance Study. Abstract C2-1814, presented at the 51st Interscience Conference on Antimicrobial Agents and Chemotherapy, 2011. Available at *www.can-r.com/posters/ICAAC2011/Sepehri%20Prevalence%20Bfragilis%20ICAAC2011.pdf*. [d]GV Doern et al: Clin Infect Dis 41:139, 2005. [e]RE Mendes et al: J Antimicrob Chemother 67:1321, 2012. [f]HS Sader et al: J Chemother 23:200, 2011. [g]J Torres et al: J Clin Microbiol 39:2677, 2001. [h]WS Oh et al: Antimicrob Agents Chemother 49:5176, 2005. [i]AE Simor et al: Antimicrob Agents Chemother 51:3880, 2007.

Abbreviations: CA-MRSA, community-acquired MRSA; CAP, community-acquired pneumonia; CA-UTI, community-acquired UTI; CDAD, *Clostridium difficile*–associated diarrhea; ESBL, extended-spectrum β-lactamase; GAS, group A streptococcal; HAI, hospital-acquired infection; MAI, *Mycobacterium avium-intracellulare*; MIC, minimal inhibitory concentration; MRSA, methicillin-resistant *Staphylococcus aureus*; MSSA, methicillin-susceptible *S. aureus*; TMP-SMX, trimethoprim-sulfamethoxazole; UTI, urinary tract infection; VRE, vancomycin-resistant *Enterococcus*.

against gram positive bacteria, with some additional activity against *E. coli*, *P. mirabilis*, and *K. pneumoniae*. First-generation cephalosporins are commonly used for infections caused by MSSA and streptococci (e.g., skin and soft tissue infections). Cefazolin is a popular choice for surgical prophylaxis against skin organisms. The second generation (cefamandole, cefuroxime, cefaclor, cefprozil, cefuroxime axetil, cefoxitin, cefotetan) has additional activity against *H. influenzae* and *Moraxella catarrhalis*. Cefoxitin and cefotetan have potent activity against anaerobes as well. Second-generation cephalosporins are used to treat community-acquired pneumonia because of their activity against *S. pneumoniae*, *H. influenzae*, and *M. catarrhalis*. They are also used for other mild or moderate infections, such as acute otitis media and sinusitis. The third-generation cephalosporins are characterized by greater potency against gram-negative bacilli and reduced potency against gram-positive cocci. These cephalosporins, which include cefoperazone, cefotaxime, ceftazidime, ceftriaxone, cefdinir, cefixime, and cefpodoxime, are used for infections caused by Enterobacteriaceae, although resistance is an increasing concern. It is noteworthy that ceftazidime is the only third-generation cephalosporin with activity against *P. aeruginosa* but lacks activity against gram-positive bacteria. This drug is frequently used for pulmonary infections in cystic fibrosis and febrile neutropenia. Ceftriaxone penetrates the CSF and can be used to treat meningitis caused by *H. influenzae*, *N. meningitidis*, and susceptible strains of *S. pneumoniae*. It is also used for the treatment of later-stage Lyme disease. The fourth generation includes cefepime and cefpirome, broad-coverage agents that provide potent activity against both gram-negative bacilli, including *P. aeruginosa*, and gram-positive cocci. The fourth generation has clinical applications similar to those of the third generation and can be used in bacteremia, pneumonia, skin and soft tissue infections, and urinary tract infections caused by susceptible bacteria. Cefepime is also commonly used in febrile neutropenia. Ceftaroline, a fifth-generation cephalosporin, differs from the other cephalosporins in its added activity against MRSA, which is resistant to all other β-lactams. Ceftaroline's gram-negative activity is similar to that of the third-generation cephalosporins but does not include *P. aeruginosa*. Ceftaroline is efficacious in community-acquired pneumonia and skin infections, but few data are available on its use for more serious infections, such as bacteremia.

Carbapenems With a few exceptions for cefepime, all penicillins and cephalosporins are ineffective in the presence of ESBLs. Carbapenems, including doripenem, imipenem, meropenem, and ertapenem, offer the most reliable coverage for strains containing ESBLs. All carbapenems have broad activity against gram-positive cocci, gram-negative bacilli, and anaerobes. None is active against MRSA, but all are active against MSSA, *Streptococcus* species, and Enterobacteriaceae. Ertapenem is the only carbapenem that has poor activity against *P. aeruginosa* and *Acinetobacter*. Imipenem is active against penicillin-susceptible *Enterococcus faecalis* but not *Enterococcus faecium*. Carbapenems are not active against Enterobacteriaceae containing carbapenemases. *Stenotrophomonas maltophilia* and some *Bacillus* species are intrinsically resistant to carbapenems because of a zinc-dependent carbapenemase.

Monobactams Aztreonam is the sole monobactam. Its activity is limited to gram-negative bacteria and includes *P. aeruginosa* and most other Enterobacteriaceae. This drug is inactivated by ESBLs and carbapenemases. The principal use for aztreonam is as an alternative to penicillins, cephalosporins, or carbapenems in patients with serious β-lactam allergy. Aztreonam is structurally related to ceftazidime and should be used cautiously in individuals with a serious ceftazidime allergy. It is commonly used in febrile neutropenia and intraabdominal infections. Aztreonam does not penetrate the CSF and should not be used for treatment of meningitis.

Adverse Reactions to β-Lactam Drugs Agents within the β-lactam class are known for several adverse effects. Gastrointestinal side effects, mainly diarrhea, are common, but hypersensitivity reactions constitute the most common adverse effect of β-lactams. The reactions' severity can range from rash to anaphylaxis, but the rate of true anaphylactic reactions is only 0.05%. An individual with an accelerated IgE-mediated reaction to one β-lactam agent may still receive another agent within the class, but caution should be taken to choose a β-lactam that has a dissimilar side chain and a low level of cross-reactivity. For example, the second-, third-, and fourth-generation cephalosporins and the carbapenems display very low cross-reactivity in patients with penicillin allergy. Aztreonam is the only β-lactam that has no cross-reactivity with the penicillin group. In cases of severe allergy, desensitization (a graded challenge) to the indicated β-lactam, with close monitoring, may be warranted if other antibacterial options are not suitable.

β-Lactams can rarely cause serum sickness, Stevens-Johnson syndrome, nephropathy, hematologic reactions, and neurotoxicity. Neutropenia appears to be related to high doses or prolonged use. Neutropenia and interstitial nephritis caused by β-lactams generally resolve upon discontinuation of the agent. Imipenem and cefepime are associated with an increased risk of seizure, but this risk is likely a class effect and related to high doses or doses that are not adjusted in renal impairment.

GLYCOPEPTIDES

The glycopeptide antibiotics include vancomycin and telavancin. Vancomycin has activity against staphylococci (including MRSA and coagulase-negative staphylococci), streptococci (including *S. pneumoniae*), and enterococci. It is not active against gram-negative organisms. Vancomycin also displays activity against *Bacillus* species, *Corynebacterium jeikeium*, *Listeria monocytogenes*, and gram-positive anaerobes such as *Peptostreptococcus*, *Actinomyces*, *Clostridium*, and *Propionibacterium* species. Vancomycin has several important clinical uses. It is used for serious infections caused by MRSA, including health care–associated pneumonia, bacteremia, osteomyelitis, and endocarditis. It is also commonly used for skin and soft tissue infections. Oral vancomycin is not absorbed systemically and is reserved for the treatment of *Clostridium difficile* infection. Vancomycin is also an alternative for the treatment of infections caused by MSSA in patients who cannot tolerate β-lactams. Resistance to vancomycin is a rising concern. Strains of vancomycin-intermediate *S. aureus* (VISA) and vancomycin-resistant enterococci (VRE) are not uncommon. Vancomycin appears to be a concentration-dependent killer, with AUC/MIC ratio being the best predictor of efficacy (Fig. 170-2). Guidelines recommend targeting a vancomycin trough level of 15–20 μg/mL in MRSA infections in order to maintain an AUC/MIC ratio >400. When using vancomycin, clinicians should monitor for nephrotoxicity. The risk increases when trough levels are >20 μg/mL. Concomitant therapy with other nephrotoxic agents, such as aminoglycosides, also increases the risk of nephrotoxicity. Ototoxicity was reported with early formulations of vancomycin but is currently uncommon because purer formulations are available. Both of these adverse effects are reversible upon discontinuation of vancomycin. Clinicians should be aware of the "red man syndrome," a common reaction that presents as a rapid onset of erythematous rash or pruritus on the head, face, neck, and upper trunk. This reaction is caused by histamine release from basophils and mast cells and can be treated with diphenhydramine and slowing of the vancomycin infusion.

Telavancin, dalbavancin, and oritavancin are structurally similar to vancomycin and are referred to as *lipoglycopeptides*. They have antibacterial activity against *S. aureus* (including MRSA and some strains of VISA and vancomycin-resistant *S. aureus* [VRSA]), streptococci, and enterococci. They also have good activity against anaerobic gram-positive organisms except for *Lactobacillus* and some *Clostridium* species. The clinical efficacy of telavancin has been demonstrated in both skin and soft tissue infections and nosocomial pneumonia, and the efficacy of dalbavancin and oritivancin has been shown in skin and soft tissue infections. The vancomycin resistance phenotype may reduce the potency of all three lipoglycopeptides, but the rate of resistance to these drugs among *S. aureus* and enterococci has been low. Adverse effects of telavancin include insomnia, a metallic taste, nephrotoxicity, and gastrointestinal side effects. Clinicians should be aware of the potential for electrocardiographic QTc prolongation that can increase the risk of cardiac arrhythmias when telavancin is used concomitantly with other QTc-prolonging agents. Telavancin may interfere with certain coagulation tests (e.g., causing false elevations in prothrombin time). Dalbavancin and oritavancin have safety profiles similar to that of vancomycin.

LIPOPEPTIDES

Daptomycin is a lipopeptide antibiotic with activity against a broad range of gram-positive organisms. This drug is active against staphylococci (including MRSA and coagulase-negative staphylococci), streptococci, and enterococci. Daptomycin remains active against enterococci that are resistant to vancomycin. In addition, it exhibits activity against *Bacillus*, *Corynebacterium*, *Peptostreptococcus*, and *Clostridium* species. Daptomycin's pharmacodynamic parameter for efficacy is concentration-dependent killing. Resistance to daptomycin is rare, but MICs may be higher for VISA strains. Daptomycin is efficacious in skin and soft tissue infections, bacteremia, endocarditis, and osteomyelitis. It is an important alternative for MRSA and other gram-positive infections when bactericidal therapy is needed and vancomycin cannot be used. Daptomycin is generally well tolerated, and its main toxicity consists of elevation of creatinine phosphokinase (CPK) levels and myopathy. CPK should be monitored during daptomycin treatment, and the drug should be discontinued if muscular toxicities occur. There have also been case reports of reversible eosinophilic pneumonia associated with daptomycin use.

AMINOGLYCOSIDES

The aminoglycosides are a class of antibacterial agents with concentration-dependent activity against most gram-negative organisms. The most commonly used aminoglycosides are gentamicin, tobramycin, and amikacin, although others, such as streptomycin, kanamycin, neomycin, and paromomycin, may be used in special circumstances. Aminoglycosides have a significant dose-dependent postantibiotic effect, meaning that they have an antibacterial effect even after serum drug levels are undetectable. The postantibiotic effect and concentration-dependent killing form the rationale behind extended-interval aminoglycoside dosing, in which a larger dose is given once daily rather than smaller doses multiple times daily. Aminoglycosides are active against gram-negative bacilli, such as Enterobacteriaceae, *P. aeruginosa*, and *Acinetobacter*. They also enhance the activity of cell wall–active agents such as β-lactams or vancomycin in some gram-positive bacteria, including staphylococci and enterococci. This combination therapy is termed *synergistic* because the effect of both agents provides a killing effect greater than would be predicted from the effects of either agent alone. Amikacin and streptomycin have activity against *Mycobacterium tuberculosis*, and amikacin has activity against *Mycobacterium avium-intracellulare*. The aminoglycosides do not have activity against anaerobes, *S. maltophilia*, or *Burkholderia cepacia*. Aminoglycosides are used in clinical practice in a variety of infections caused by gram-negative organisms, including bacteremia and urinary tract infections. They are frequently used alone or in combination for the treatment of *P. aeruginosa* infection. When used in combination with a cell wall–active agent, gentamicin and streptomycin are also important for the treatment of gram-positive bacterial endocarditis. All aminoglycosides can cause nephrotoxicity and ototoxicity. The risk of nephrotoxicity is related to the dose and duration of therapy as well as the concomitant use of other nephrotoxic agents. Nephrotoxicity is usually reversible, but ototoxicity can be irreversible.

MACROLIDES AND KETOLIDES

The macrolides (azithromycin, clarithromycin, erythromycin) and ketolides (telithromycin) are classes of antibiotics that inhibit protein synthesis. Compared with erythromycin (the older antibiotic), azithromycin and clarithromycin have better oral absorption and tolerability.

Azithromycin, clarithromycin, and telithromycin all have broader spectra of activity than erythromycin, which is less frequently used. These agents are commonly used in the treatment of upper and lower respiratory tract infections caused by *S. pneumoniae*, *H. influenzae*, *M. catarrhalis*, and atypical organisms (e.g., *Chlamydia pneumoniae*, *Legionella pneumophila*, and *Mycoplasma pneumoniae*); group A streptococcal pharyngitis in penicillin-allergic patients; and nontuberculous mycobacterial infections (e.g., caused by *M. marinum* and *M. chelonae*) as well as in the prophylaxis and treatment of *M. avium-intracellulare* infection in patients with HIV/AIDS and in combination therapy for *H. pylori* infection and bartonellosis. Enterobacteriaceae, *Pseudomonas* species, and *Acinetobacter* species are intrinsically resistant to macrolides as a result of decreased membrane permeability, although azithromycin is active against gram-negative diarrheal pathogens. The major adverse effects of this drug class include nausea, vomiting, diarrhea and abdominal pain, prolongation of QT_c interval, exacerbation of myasthenia gravis, and tinnitus. Azithromycin specifically has been associated with an increased risk of death, especially among patients with underlying heart disease, because of the risk of QT_c interval prolongation and torsades de pointes. Erythromycin, clarithromycin, and telithromycin inhibit the CYP3A4 hepatic drug-metabolizing enzyme and can result in increased levels of coadministered drugs, including benzodiazepines, statins, warfarin, cyclosporine, and tacrolimus. Azithromycin does not inhibit CYP3A4 and lacks these drug–drug interactions.

CLINDAMYCIN

Clindamycin is a lincosamide antibiotic and is bacteriostatic against some organisms and bactericidal against others. It is used most often to treat bacterial infections caused by anaerobes (e.g., *B. fragilis*, *Clostridium perfringens*, *Fusobacterium* species, *Prevotella melaninogenicus*, and *Peptostreptococcus* species) and susceptible staphylococci and streptococci. Clindamycin is used for treatment of dental infections, anaerobic lung abscess, and skin and soft tissue infections. It is used together with bactericidal agents (penicillins or vancomycin) to inhibit new toxin synthesis in the treatment of streptococcal or staphylococcal toxic shock syndrome. Other uses include treatment of infections caused by *Capnocytophaga canimorsus*, a component of combination therapy for malaria and babesiosis, and therapy for toxoplasmosis. Clindamycin has excellent oral bioavailability. Adverse effects include nausea, vomiting, diarrhea, *C. difficile*–associated diarrhea and pseudomembranous colitis, maculopapular rash, and (rarely) Stevens-Johnson syndrome.

TETRACYCLINES AND GLYCYLCYCLINES

The tetracyclines (doxycycline, minocycline, and tetracycline) and the glycylcyclines (tigecycline) inhibit protein synthesis and are bacteriostatic. These drugs have wide clinical uses. They are used in the treatment of skin and soft tissue infections caused by gram-positive cocci (including MRSA), spirochetal infections (e.g., Lyme disease, syphilis, leptospirosis, and relapsing fever), rickettsial infections (e.g., Rocky Mountain spotted fever), atypical pneumonia, sexually transmitted infections (e.g., *Chlamydia trachomatis* infection, lymphogranuloma venereum, and granuloma inguinale), infections with *Nocardia* and *Actinomyces*, brucellosis, tularemia, Whipple's disease, and malaria. Tigecycline, the only approved agent in the glycylcycline class, is a derivative of minocycline and is indicated in the treatment of infections due to MRSA, vancomycin-sensitive enterococci, many Enterobacteriaceae, and *Bacteroides* species. Tigecycline has no activity against *P. aeruginosa*. It has been used in combination with colistin for the treatment of serious infections with multidrug-resistant gram-negative organisms. A pooled analysis of 13 clinical trials found an increased risk of death and treatment failure among patients treated with tigecycline alone. Tetracyclines have reduced absorption when coadministered with calcium- and iron-containing compounds, including milk, and doses should be spaced at least 2 h apart. The major adverse reactions to both of these classes are nausea, vomiting, diarrhea, and photosensitivity. Tetracyclines have been associated with fetal bone-growth abnormalities and should be avoided during pregnancy and in the treatment of children <8 years old.

TRIMETHOPRIM-SULFAMETHOXAZOLE

Trimethoprim-sulfamethoxazole (TMP-SMX) is an antibiotic whose two components both inhibit folate synthesis and produce antibacterial activity. TMP-SMX is active against gram-positive bacteria such as staphylococci and streptococci; however, its use against MRSA is usually limited to community-acquired infections, and its activity against *Streptococcus pyogenes* may not be reliable. TMP-SMX is also active against many gram-negative bacteria, including *H. influenzae*, *E. coli*, *P. mirabilis*, *N. gonorrhoeae*, and *S. maltophilia*. TMP-SMX does not have activity against anaerobes or *P. aeruginosa*. It has many uses because of its wide spectrum of activity and high oral bioavailability. Urinary tract infections, skin and soft tissue infections, and respiratory tract infections are among the common uses. Another important indication is for both prophylaxis and treatment of *Pneumocystis jirovecii* infections in immunocompromised patients. Resistance to TMP-SMX has limited its use against many Enterobacteriaceae. Resistance rates among urinary isolates of *E. coli* are almost 25% in the United States. The most common adverse reactions associated with TMP-SMX are gastrointestinal effects such as nausea, vomiting, and diarrhea. In addition, rash is a common allergic reaction and may preclude the subsequent use of other sulfonamides. With prolonged use, leukopenia, thrombocytopenia, and granulocytopenia can develop. TMP-SMX can also cause nephrotoxicity, hyperkalemia, and hyponatremia, which are more common at high doses. TMP-SMX has several important interactions with other drugs (Table 170-4), including warfarin, phenytoin, and methotrexate.

FLUOROQUINOLONES

The fluoroquinolones include norfloxacin, ciprofloxacin, ofloxacin, levofloxacin, moxifloxacin, and gemifloxacin. Ciprofloxacin and levofloxacin have the broadest spectrum of activity against gram-negative bacteria, including *P. aeruginosa* (similar to that of third-generation cephalosporins). Because of the risk of selection of resistance during fluoroquinolone treatment of serious pseudomonal infections, these agents are usually used in combination with an antipseudomonal β-lactam. Levofloxacin, moxifloxacin, and gemifloxacin have additional gram-positive activity, including that against *S. pneumoniae* and some strains of MSSA, and are used for treatment of community-acquired pneumonia. Strains of MRSA are commonly resistant to all fluoroquinolones. Moxifloxacin is used as one component of second-line regimens for multidrug-resistant tuberculosis. Fluoroquinolones exhibit concentration-dependent killing, are well absorbed orally, and have elimination half-lives that usually support once- or twice-daily dosing. Oral coadministration with compounds containing high concentrations of aluminum, magnesium, or calcium can reduce fluoroquinolone absorption. Their penetration into prostate tissue supports their use for bacterial prostatitis. Fluoroquinolones are generally well tolerated but can cause CNS stimulatory effects, including seizures; glucose dysregulation; and tendinopathy associated with Achilles tendon rupture, particularly in older patients, organ transplant recipients, and patients taking glucocorticoids. Worsening of myasthenia gravis also has been associated with quinolone use. Moxifloxacin causes modest prolongation of the QT_c interval and should be used with caution in patients receiving other QT_c-prolonging drugs.

RIFAMYCINS

The rifamycins include rifampin, rifabutin, and rifapentine. Rifampin is the most commonly used rifamycin. For almost all therapeutic indications, it is used in combination with other agents to reduce the likelihood of selection of high-level rifampin resistance. Rifampin is used foremost in the treatment of mycobacterial infections—specifically, as a mainstay of combination therapy for *M. tuberculosis* infection or as a single agent in the treatment of latent *M. tuberculosis* infection. In addition, it is often used in the treatment of nontuberculous mycobacterial infection. Rifampin is used in combination regimens for the treatment of staphylococcal infections, particularly prosthetic valve endocarditis and bone infections with retained hardware. It is a component of combination therapy for brucellosis (with doxycycline) and leprosy (with dapsone for tuberculoid leprosy and with dapsone and clofazimine for lepromatous disease). Rifampin can be used alone for prophylaxis in close contacts of patients with *H. influenzae* or *N. meningitidis* meningitis. The drug has high oral bioavailability, which is further enhanced when it is taken on an empty stomach. Rifampin has several adverse effects, including elevated aminotransferase levels (14%), rash (1–5%), and gastrointestinal events such as nausea, vomiting, and diarrhea (1–2%). Its many clinically relevant interactions with other drugs mandate the clinician's careful review of the patient's medications before rifampin initiation to assess safety and the need for additional monitoring.

METRONIDAZOLE

Metronidazole is used in the treatment of anaerobic bacterial infections as well as infections caused by protozoa (e.g., amebiasis, giardiasis, trichomoniasis). It is the agent of choice as a component of combination therapy for polymicrobial abscesses in the lung, brain, or abdomen, the etiology of which often includes anaerobic bacteria, and for bacterial vaginosis, pelvic inflammatory disease, mild to moderate *C. difficile*–associated diarrhea, and anaerobic infections, such as those due to *Bacteroides*, *Fusobacterium*, and *Prevotella* species. Metronidazole is bactericidal against anaerobic bacteria and exhibits concentration-dependent killing. It has high oral bioavailability and tissue penetration, including penetration of the blood–brain barrier. The majority of *Actinomyces*, *Propionibacterium*, and *Lactobacillus* species are intrinsically resistant to metronidazole. The major adverse effects include nausea, diarrhea, and a metallic taste. Concomitant ingestion of alcohol may result in a disulfiram-like reaction, and patients are usually instructed to avoid alcohol during treatment. Long-term treatment carries the risk of leukopenia, neutropenia, peripheral neuropathy, and central nervous system toxicity manifesting as confusion, dysarthria, ataxia, nystagmus, and ophthalmoparesis. Through metronidazole's effect on the CYP2C9 drug-metabolizing enzyme, its coadministration with warfarin can result in decreased metabolism and enhanced anticoagulant effects that require close monitoring. Concomitant administration of metronidazole with lithium can result in increased serum levels of lithium and associated toxicity; coadministration with phenytoin can result in phenytoin toxicity and possibly decreased levels of metronidazole.

OXAZOLIDINONES

Linezolid is a bacteriostatic agent and is indicated for serious infections due to resistant gram-positive bacteria, such as MRSA and VRE. The intrinsic resistance of gram-negative bacteria is mediated primarily by endogenous efflux pumps. Linezolid has excellent oral bioavailability. Adverse effects include myelosuppression and ocular and peripheral neuropathy with prolonged therapy. Peripheral neuropathy may be irreversible. Linezolid is a weak, reversible monoamine oxidase inhibitor, and coadministration with sympathomimetics and foods rich in tyramine should be avoided. Linezolid has been associated with serotonin syndrome when coadministered with selective serotonin-reuptake inhibitors. Tedizolid has properties similar to those of linezolid, but with lower dosing it may be less likely to cause adverse hematologic and neuropathic effects.

NITROFURANTOIN

Nitrofurantoin's antibacterial activity results from the drug's conversion to highly reactive intermediates that can damage DNA and other macromolecules. Nitrofurantoin is bactericidal, and its action is concentration dependent. It displays activity against a range of gram-positive bacteria, including *S. aureus*, *Staphylococcus epidermidis*, *Staphylococcus saprophyticus*, *E. faecalis*, *Streptococcus agalactiae*, group D streptococci, viridans streptococci, and corynebacteria, as well as gram-negative organisms, including *E. coli* and *Enterobacter*, *Neisseria*, *Salmonella*, and *Shigella* species. Nitrofurantoin is used primarily in the treatment of urinary tract infections and is preferred in the treatment of such infections in pregnancy. It may be used for the prevention of recurrent cystitis. Recently, there has been interest in the use of nitrofurantoin for treatment of urinary tract infections caused by ESBL-producing Enterobacteriaceae such as *E. coli*, although resistance has been growing in Latin America and parts of Europe. Coadministration with magnesium should be avoided because of decreased absorption, and patients should be encouraged to take the drug with food to increase its bioavailability and decrease the risk of adverse effects, which include nausea, vomiting, and diarrhea. Nitrofurantoin may also cause pulmonary fibrosis and drug-induced hepatitis. Because the risk of adverse reactions increases with age, the use of nitrofurantoin in elderly patients is not recommended. Patients with glucose-6-phosphate dehydrogenase (G6PD) deficiency are at elevated risk for nitrofurantoin-associated hemolytic anemia.

POLYMYXINS

Colistin and polymyxin B act by disrupting cell membrane integrity and are active against the nonenteric pathogens *P. aeruginosa* and *A. baumannii* but not against *Burkholderia*. These drugs also exhibit activity against many Enterobacteriaceae,with the exceptions of *Proteus*, *Providencia*, and *Serratia* species. They lack activity against gram-positive bacteria. Polymyxins are bactericidal and are available in IV formulations. Colistimethate is converted to the active form (colistin) in plasma. Polymyxins are most often used for infections due to pathogens resistant to multiple other antibacterial agents, including urinary tract infections, hospital-acquired pneumonia, and bloodstream infections. Nebulized formulations have been used for adjunctive treatment of refractory ventilator-associated pneumonia. The most important adverse effect is dose-dependent reversible nephrotoxicity. Neurotoxicity, including paresthesias, muscle weakness, and confusion, is reversible and less common than nephrotoxicity.

QUINUPRISTIN-DALFOPRISTIN

Quinupristin-dalfopristin is a member of the streptogramin class of antibiotics and kills bacteria by inhibiting protein synthesis. The antibacterial spectrum of quinupristin-dalfopristin includes staphylococci (including MRSA), streptococci, and *E. faecium* (but not *E. faecalis*). This drug is also active against *Corynebacterium* species and *L. monocytogenes*. Quinupristin-dalfopristin is not reliably active against gram-negative organisms. It exhibits concentration-dependent killing, with an AUC/MIC ratio predicting efficacy. The clinical use of quinupristin-dalfopristin is largely for infections due to vancomycin-resistant *E. faecium* and other gram-positive bacterial infections. The drug has demonstrated efficacy in a variety of infections, including urinary tract infections, bone and joint infections, and bacteremia. Adverse effects associated with quinupristin-dalfopristin include infusion-related reactions, arthralgias, and myalgias. The arthralgias and myalgias may be severe enough to warrant drug discontinuation. Quinupristin-dalfopristin inhibits the CYP3A4 drug-metabolizing enzyme, with consequent drug interactions (Table 170-4).

FOSFOMYCIN

Fosfomycin is a phosphonic acid antibiotic that has greater activity in acidic environments and is excreted in its active form in the urine. Thus, its use is primarily for prophylaxis and treatment of uncomplicated cystitis. The drug is administered as a single 3-g dose that results in high urine concentrations for up to 48 h. Fosfomycin is active against *S. aureus*, vancomycin-susceptible and vancomycin-resistant enterococci, and a wide range of gram-negative organisms, including *E. coli*, *Enterobacter* species, *S. marcescens*, *P. aeruginosa*, and *K. pneumoniae*. Notably, the vast majority of ESBL-producing Enterobacteriaceae are susceptible to fosfomycin. *A. baumannii* and *Burkholderia* species are resistant. The emergence of resistance to fosfomycin has not been observed during treatment of cystitis but has been documented during treatment of respiratory tract infections and osteomyelitis. The few adverse effects that have been reported include nausea and diarrhea.

CHLORAMPHENICOL

The use of chloramphenicol is limited by its potentially serious toxicities. When other agents are contraindicated or ineffective, chloramphenicol represents an alternative treatment for infections, including meningitis caused by susceptible bacteria such as *N. meningitidis*,

H. influenzae, and *S. pneumoniae*. It has also been used for the treatment of anthrax, brucellosis, *Burkholderia* infections, chlamydial infections, clostridial infections, erlichiosis, rickettsial infections, and typhoid fever. Adverse reactions include aplastic anemia, myelosuppression, and gray baby syndrome. Chloramphenicol inhibits the CYP2C19 and CYP3A4 drug-metabolizing enzymes and consequently increases levels of many classes of drugs.

APPROACH TO PROPHYLAXIS OF INFECTION

Antibacterial prophylaxis is indicated only in selected circumstances (Table 170-6) and should be supported by well-designed studies or expert panel recommendations. In all cases the risk or severity of the infection to be prevented should be greater than the adverse consequences of antibacterial therapy, including the potential for selection of resistance. In addition, the timing and duration of antibacterial treatment should be targeted for maximal effect and minimal required exposure. Prophylaxis of surgical site infections targets bacteria that may contaminate the wound during the surgical procedure, including the skin flora of the patient or operating team and the air in the operating room. Delivery of the antibacterial drug within 1 h before the surgical incision is most effective. For prolonged procedures, redosing may be necessary to maintain effective blood and tissue levels until the wound is closed. In patients with nasal carriage of *S. aureus*, preoperative decolonization with nasal mupirocin reduces the rate of *S. aureus* surgical site infections and is generally recommended for high-risk procedures such as cardiac surgery and orthopedic implantation of prosthetic devices. For dental procedures, preprocedure antibacterial drugs are given to prevent transient bacteremia and the seeding of certain high-risk cardiac lesions. Prophylaxis is also used in nonprocedural settings in certain patients who have recurrent infections or who are at risk of serious infection from a specific exposure (e.g., close contact with a patient with meningococcal meningitis). Extension of prophylaxis beyond the period of infection risk (24 h in the case of surgical procedures) does not add further benefit and may increase the risk of resistance selection or *C. difficile* disease.

ANTIMICROBIAL STEWARDSHIP

In an era of increasing prevalence of multidrug-resistant bacteria and with a substantial amount of inappropriate antimicrobial use, the need for rational antimicrobial prescribing has never been greater. *Antimicrobial stewardship* describes the practice of promoting the selection of the appropriate drug, dosage, route, and duration of antimicrobial therapy. Antimicrobial stewardship programs implement a variety of strategies to (1) improve patient care through appropriate

TABLE 170-6 PROPHYLAXIS OF BACTERIAL INFECTIONS IN ADULTS

Condition	Antibacterial Agents[a]	Timing or Duration of Prophylaxis
Surgical		
Clean (cardiac, thoracic, neurologic, orthopedic, vascular, plastic)	Cefazolin (vancomycin,[b] clindamycin)	1 h before incision; redose with long procedures
Clean (ophthalmic)	Topical neomycin–polymyxin B–gramicidin, topical moxifloxacin	Every 5–15 min for 5 doses immediately prior to procedure
Clean-contaminated (head and neck)	Cefazolin + metronidazole, ampicillin-sulbactam[c] (clindamycin)	1 h before incision; redose with long procedures
Clean-contaminated (hysterectomy, gastroduodenal, biliary, unobstructed small intestine, urologic)	Cefazolin, ampicillin-sulbactam[c] (clindamycin + aminoglycoside, aztreonam, or fluoroquinolone)	1 h before incision; redose with long procedures
Clean-contaminated (colorectal, appendectomy)	Cefazolin + metronidazole, ampicillin-sulbactam,[c] ertapenem (clindamycin + aminoglycoside, aztreonam, or fluoroquinolone)	1 h before incision; redose with long procedures
Dirty (ruptured viscus)	Therapeutic regimen directed at anaerobes and gram-negative bacteria (e.g., ceftriaxone + metronidazole)	1 h before incision; redose with long procedures; continue for 3–5 days after procedure
Dirty (traumatic wound)	Therapeutic regimen: cefazolin (clindamycin ± aminoglycoside, aztreonam, or fluoroquinolone)	1 h before incision; redose with long procedures; continue for 3–5 days after procedure
Nonsurgical		
Dental, oral, or upper respiratory procedures in patients with high-risk cardiac lesions (prosthetic valves, congenital heart defects, prior endocarditis)	Amoxicillin PO, ampicillin IM (clindamycin PO, IV)	Oral agents 1 h before procedure; injection 30 min before procedure
Recurrent *S. aureus* skin infections[d]	Mupirocin[e]	Intranasal application for 5 days
Recurrent cellulitis associated with lymphatic disruption[d]	Benzathine penicillin IM monthly, oral penicillin or erythromycin twice daily	Undefined
Recurrent cystitis in women[d]	Nitrofurantoin, TMP-SMX, fluoroquinolone	After sexual intercourse *or* 3 times weekly for up to 1 year
Bite wounds	Amoxicillin-clavulanate (doxycycline, moxifloxacin)	3–5 days
Recurrent spontaneous bacterial peritonitis in cirrhotic patients[d]	Fluoroquinolone[f]	Undefined
Recurrent pneumococcal meningitis in patient with CSF leak or humoral immune defect[d]	Penicillin	Undefined
Exposure to patient with meningococcal meningitis	Rifampin, ciprofloxacin	2 days (rifampin), single dose (ciprofloxacin)
High-risk neutropenia (ANC, ≤100/μL for >7 days)[d]	Levofloxacin or ciprofloxacin[f]	Until neutropenia resolves or fever dictates use of other antibacterials

[a]Regimens in parentheses are alternatives for patients allergic to β-lactams. [b]Vancomycin may be given together with cefazolin to patients known to be colonized with methicillin-resistant *Staphylococcus aureus*. [c]Cefoxitin or cefotetan may also be considered. [d]Not considered routine for all patients, but an acceptable consideration among alternative approaches. [e]Usually coupled with bathing with chlorhexidine-containing skin antiseptic. [f]Choice of fluoroquinolone prophylaxis must be balanced against the risk of selection of resistance.

Abbreviations: ANC, absolute neutrophil count; CSF, cerebrospinal fluid; TMP-SMX, trimethoprim-sulfamethoxazole.

antimicrobial use; (2) decrease the development of resistance within patients and populations; (3) reduce the incidence of adverse effects; and (4) control costs.

Infections caused by resistant pathogens result in significant morbidity and mortality as well as increased health care costs. Antimicrobial stewardship programs are typically multidisciplinary and often include infectious disease physicians, clinical pharmacists (usually with special training in infectious disease), clinical microbiologists, information systems specialists, infection prevention and control practitioners, and epidemiologists. These teams employ a variety of approaches to achieving the program's goals.

Established strategies of antimicrobial stewardship programs include (1) prospective audit of antimicrobial use, with intervention and feedback; (2) formulary restriction; and (3) preauthorization. *Prospective audit and feedback* are usually undertaken by an infectious disease physician or a pharmacist. In this process, orders for broad-spectrum antimicrobials (e.g., carbapenems) or high-impact agents (e.g., linezolid, daptomycin) are reviewed on a regular basis for appropriateness. In circumstances in which an antimicrobial is used in the absence of an appropriate indication, the stewardship program team intervenes and recommends an alternative to the primary team caring for the patient. This process has been successful in several quasi-experimental studies, resulting in declines in use of broad-spectrum drugs and decreases in adverse events, such as *C. difficile* infection. *Formulary restriction* is the inclusion of a limited set of antimicrobial agents in a hospital formulary for the purpose of limiting indiscriminant use of antimicrobials in the absence of demonstrated benefit. Such restriction coincidentally serves to reduce costs. *Preauthorization* is the practice of requiring clinicians to obtain approval before using selected antimicrobials. Approval may be provided electronically with sophisticated Computerized Provider Order Entry (CPOE) software, after specific criteria for use are met, or after communication with an infectious disease specialist as designated by the stewardship program. These strategies have led to a decrease in *C. difficile* infections and to improvements in drug susceptibility patterns.

Additional strategies used in specific health-care settings are guidelines and pathways, dose optimization, parenteral-to-oral conversion, and de-escalation of therapy. Antimicrobial stewardship is an evolving area and an increasingly active area of research aimed at identifying the best practices. The IDSA, in collaboration with several other professional organizations, has published guidelines for developing institutional antimicrobial stewardship programs (*www.idsociety.org/Antimicrobial_Agents/*).

SECTION 5 DISEASES CAUSED BY GRAM-POSITIVE BACTERIA

171 Pneumococcal Infections

David Goldblatt, Katherine L. O'Brien

In the late nineteenth century, pairs of micrococci were first recognized in the blood of rabbits injected with human saliva by both Louis Pasteur, working in France, and George Sternberg, an American army physician. The important role of these micrococci in human disease was not appreciated at that time. By 1886, when the organism was designated "pneumokokkus" and *Diplococcus pneumoniae*, the pneumococcus had been isolated by many independent investigators, and its role in the etiology of pneumonia was well known. In the 1930s, pneumonia was the third leading cause of death in the United States (after heart disease and cancer) and was responsible for ~7% of all deaths both in the United States and in Europe. While pneumonia was caused by a host of pathogens, lobar pneumonia—a pattern more likely to be caused by the pneumococcus—accounted for approximately one-half of all pneumonia deaths in the United States in 1929. In 1974, the organism was reclassified as *Streptococcus pneumoniae*.

MICROBIOLOGY

Etiologic Agent Pneumococci are spherical gram-positive bacteria of the genus *Streptococcus*. Within this genus, cell division occurs along a single axis, and bacteria grow in chains or pairs—hence the name *Streptococcus*, from the Greek *streptos*, meaning "twisted," and *kokkos*, meaning "berry." At least 22 streptococcal species are recognized and are divided further into groups based on their hemolytic properties. *S. pneumoniae* belongs to the α-hemolytic group that characteristically produces a greenish color on blood agar because of the reduction of iron in hemoglobin (Fig. 171-1). The bacteria are fastidious and grow best in 5% CO_2 but require a source of catalase (e.g., blood) for growth on agar plates, where they develop mucoid (smooth/shiny) colonies. Pneumococci without a capsule produce colonies with a rough surface. Unlike that of other α-hemolytic streptococci, their growth is inhibited in the presence of optochin (ethylhydrocupreine hydrochloride), and they are bile soluble.

In common with other gram-positive bacteria, pneumococci have a cell membrane beneath a cell wall, which in turn is covered by a polysaccharide capsule. Pneumococci are divided into serogroups or serotypes based on capsular polysaccharide structure, as distinguished with rabbit polyclonal antisera; capsules swell in the presence of specific antiserum (the Quellung reaction). The most recently discovered serotypes, 6C, 6D, and 11E, have been identified with monoclonal antibodies and by serologic, genetic, and biochemical means, respectively. The currently recognized 93 serotypes fall into 21 serogroups, and each serogroup contains two to five serotypes with closely related capsules. The capsule protects the bacteria from phagocytosis by host cells in the absence of type-specific antibody and is arguably the most

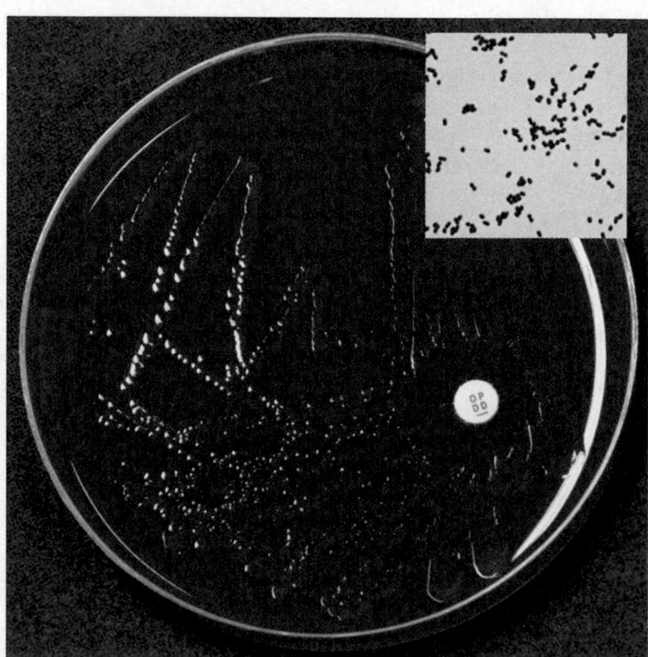

FIGURE 171-1 Pneumococci growing on blood agar, illustrating α hemolysis and optochin sensitivity (zone around optochin disk). *Inset:* Gram's stain, illustrating gram-positive diplococci. *(Photographs courtesy of Paul Turner, Shoklo Malaria Research Unit, Thailand.)*

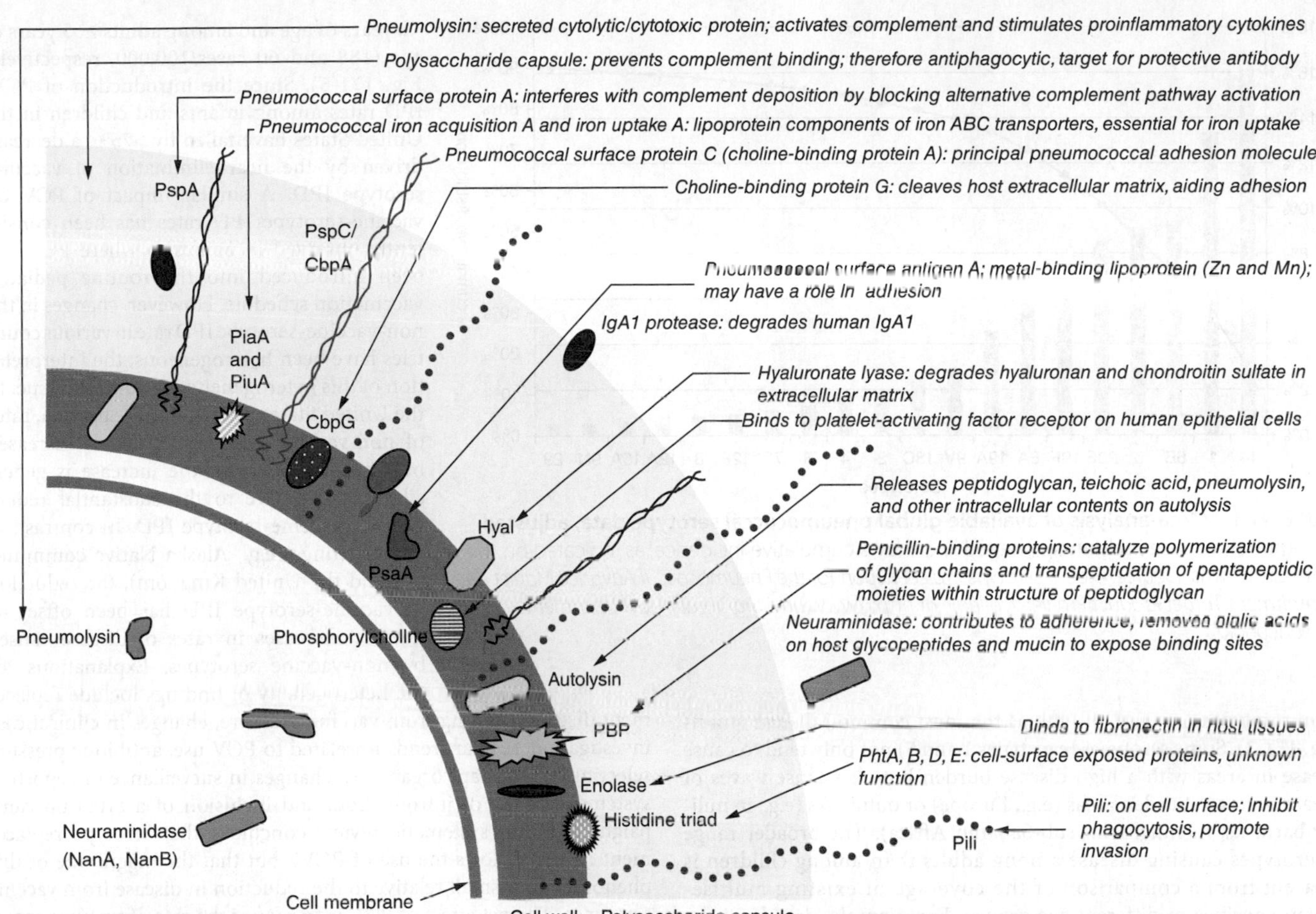
Pneumolysin: secreted cytolytic/cytotoxic protein; activates complement and stimulates proinflammatory cytokines
Polysaccharide capsule: prevents complement binding; therefore antiphagocytic, target for protective antibody
Pneumococcal surface protein A: interferes with complement deposition by blocking alternative complement pathway activation
Pneumococcal iron acquisition A and iron uptake A: lipoprotein components of iron ABC transporters, essential for iron uptake
Pneumococcal surface protein C (choline-binding protein A): principal pneumococcal adhesion molecule
Choline-binding protein G: cleaves host extracellular matrix, aiding adhesion
PspA
PspC/
CbpA
Pneumococcal surface antigen A: metal-binding lipoprotein (Zn and Mn); may have a role in adhesion
IgA1 protease: degrades human IgA1
PiaA
and
PiuA
CbpG
Hyaluronate lyase: degrades hyaluronan and chondroitin sulfate in extracellular matrix
Binds to platelet-activating factor receptor on human epithelial cells
Releases peptidoglycan, teichoic acid, pneumolysin, and other intracellular contents on autolysis
Hyal
Penicillin-binding proteins: catalyze polymerization of glycan chains and transpeptidation of pentapeptidic moieties within structure of peptidoglycan
PsaA
Neuraminidase: contributes to adherence, removes sialic acids on host glycopeptides and mucin to expose binding sites
Pneumolysin
Phosphorylcholine
Autolysin
Binds to fibronectin in host tissues
PBP
PhtA, B, D, E: cell-surface exposed proteins, unknown function
Enolase
Pili: on cell surface; inhibit phagocytosis, promote invasion
Histidine triad
Neuraminidase
(NanA, NanB)
Pili
Cell membrane
Cell wall
Polysaccharide capsule

FIGURE 171-2 Schematic diagram of the pneumococcal cell surface, with key antigens and their roles highlighted.

important determinant of pneumococcal virulence. Unencapsulated variants tend not to cause invasive disease.

Virulence Factors Within the cytoplasm, cell membrane, and cell wall, many molecules that may play a role in pneumococcal pathogenesis and virulence have been identified (Fig. 171-2). These proteins are often involved in direct interactions with host tissues or in concealment of the bacterial surface from host defense mechanisms. Pneumolysin is a secreted cytotoxin thought to result in cytolysis of cells and tissues, and LytA enhances pathogenesis. A number of cell wall proteins interfere with the complement pathway, thus inhibiting complement deposition and preventing lysis and/or opsonophagocytosis. The pneumococcal H inhibitor (Hic) impedes the formation of C3 convertase, while pneumococcal surface protein C (PspC), also known as choline-binding protein A (CbpA), binds factor H and is thought to accelerate the breakdown of C3. PspA and CbpA inhibit the deposition of or degrade C3b. The numerous pneumococcal proteins thought to be involved in adhesion include the ubiquitous surface-anchored sialidase (neuraminidase) NanA, which cleaves sialic acid on host cells and proteins, and pneumococcal surface adhesin A (PsaA). Pili recently recognized by electron microscopy also may play an important role in binding to cells. Some of the antigens mentioned above are potential vaccine candidates (see "Prevention," below).

Although the capsule surrounding the cell wall of *S. pneumoniae* is the basis for categorization by serotype, the behavior and pathogenic potential of a serotype may also be related to the genetic origin of the strain. Molecular typing is therefore of considerable interest. Initially, techniques such as pulsed-field gel electrophoresis were used to determine genetic relatedness; such techniques have been superseded by sequencing of housekeeping genes to define a clone (multilocus sequence typing, MLST). For *S. pneumoniae*, alleles at each of the loci *aroE*, *gdh*, *gki*, *recP*, *spi*, *xpt*, and *ddl* are sequenced and compared with all of the known alleles at that locus. Sequences identical to a known allele are assigned the same allele number, whereas those differing from any known allele—even at a single nucleotide site—are assigned new numbers. Software for assignment of alleles at each locus is available on the pneumococcal MLST website (*spneumoniae.mlst.net*), and the allelic profile of each isolate and its consequent sequence type are generated. With the advent of high-throughput and relatively inexpensive sequencing techniques, whole-genome sequencing will soon supersede MLST.

EPIDEMIOLOGY

Pneumococcal infections remain a significant global cause of morbidity and death, particularly among children and the elderly. Rapid and dramatic changes in the epidemiology of this disease during the past decade in several developed countries followed the licensure and routine childhood administration of pneumococcal polysaccharide–protein conjugate vaccine (PCV). With PCV introduction in developing and middle-income countries, additional profound changes in pneumococcal ecology and disease epidemiology are likely. The disease burden and serotype distribution in the PCV era may be different than expected because of concomitant secular trends in pneumococcal disease, the impact of antibiotic use on pneumococcal strain ecology, and surveillance system attributes that can themselves affect analysis of epidemiologic features.

Serotype Distribution Not all pneumococcal serotypes are equally likely to cause disease; serotype distribution varies by age, disease syndrome, and geography. Geographic differences may be driven by variation in the burden of disease rather than by true serotype distribution differences. Most data on serotype distribution are related to pediatric invasive pneumococcal disease (IPD, defined as infection of a normally sterile site); much less information on global distribution is available for disease in adults. Among children <5 years of age, five to seven serotypes cause >60% of IPD cases in most parts of the world, seven serotypes (1, 5, 6A, 6B, 14, 19F, and 23F) account for ~60% of cases in all areas of the world, but in any given region these

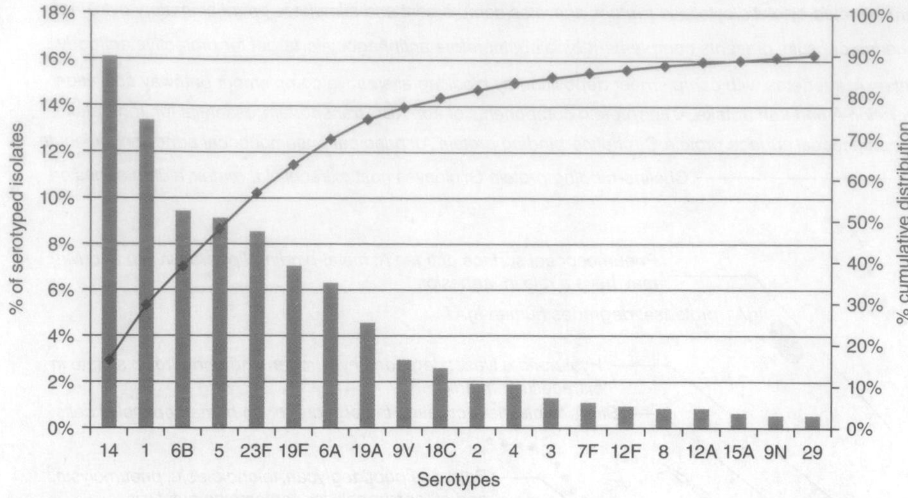

FIGURE 171-3 Meta-analysis of available global pneumococcal serotype data, adjusted for regional disease incidence. The red line shows cumulative incidence, as indicated on the right-hand Y axis. *(Source: Global Serotype Project Report for the Pneumococcal Advance Market Commitment Target Product Profile; available at http://www.gavi.org/library/gavi-documents/amc/tpp-codebook/.)*

seven serotypes may not all rank as the most common disease strains (Fig. 171-3). Some serotypes (e.g., types 1 and 5) not only tend to cause disease in areas with a high disease burden but also cause waves of disease in lower-burden areas (e.g., Europe) or outbreaks (e.g., in military barracks; meningitis in sub-Saharan Africa). The broader range of serotypes causing disease among adults than among children is apparent from a comparison of the coverage of existing multiserotype vaccines in different age groups. For example, data from the United States for 2006–2007 on the serotypes causing IPD indicated that a polysaccharide vaccine containing 23 serotypes (PPSV23) would cover 84% of cases among children <5 years of age and 76% of those among persons 18–64 years of age but only 65% of those among persons ≥65 years of age.

Nasopharyngeal Carriage Pneumococci are intermittent inhabitants of the healthy human nasopharynx and are transmitted by respiratory droplets. In children, pneumococcal nasopharyngeal ecology varies by geographic region, socioeconomic status, climate, degree of crowding, and particularly intensity of exposure to other children, with children in day-care settings having higher rates of colonization. In developed-world settings, children serve as the major vectors of pneumococcal transmission. By 1 year of age, ~50% of children have had at least one episode of pneumococcal colonization. Cross-sectional prevalence data show rates of pneumococcal carriage ranging from 20% to 50% among children <5 years of age and from 5% to 15% among young and middle-aged adults; Fig. 171-4 shows relevant data from the United Kingdom. Data on colonization rates among healthy elderly individuals are limited. In developing-world settings, pneumococcal acquisition occurs much earlier, sometimes within the first few days after birth, and nearly all infants have had at least one episode of colonization by 2 months of age. Cross-sectional studies show that up to the age of 5 years, 70–90% of children carry *S. pneumoniae* in the nasopharynx, and a significant proportion of adults (sometimes >40%) also are colonized. Their high rates of colonization make adults an important source of transmission and may affect community transmission dynamics.

Invasive Disease and Pneumonia IPD develops when *S. pneumoniae* invades the bloodstream and seeds other organs or directly reaches the cerebrospinal fluid (CSF) by local extension. Pneumonia may follow aspiration of pneumococci, although only 10–30% of such cases are associated with a positive blood culture (and thus contribute to the measured burden of IPD). The dramatic variation of IPD rates with age is illustrated by data from the United States for 1998–1999, a period prior to PCV introduction. Rates of IPD were highest among children <2 years of age and among adults ≥65 years of age (188 and 60 cases/100,000, respectively; Fig. 171-5). Since the introduction of PCV, IPD rates among infants and children in the United States have fallen by >75%, a decrease driven by the near elimination of vaccine-serotype IPD. A similar impact of PCV on vaccine-serotype IPD rates has been consistently observed in countries where PCV has been introduced into the routine pediatric vaccination schedule. However, changes in the non-vaccine-serotype IPD rate in various countries have been heterogeneous; the interpretation of this heterogeneity is a complex issue. In the United States, Canada, and Australia, rates of non-vaccine-serotype IPD have increased but the magnitude of the increase is generally small relative to the substantial reductions in vaccine-serotype IPD. In contrast, in other settings (e.g., Alaska Native communities and the United Kingdom), the reduction in vaccine-serotype IPD has been offset by notable increases in rates of disease caused by non-vaccine serotypes. Explanations for the heterogeneity of findings include replacement disease resulting from vaccine pressure, changes in clinical case investigation, secular trends unrelated to PCV use, antibiotic pressure selecting for resistant organisms, changes in surveillance or reporting systems, rapidity of introduction, and inclusion of a catch-up campaign. A recent systematic review concludes that serotype replacement in IPD follows the use of PCV7 but that the magnitude of this phenomenon is small relative to the reduction in disease from vaccine serotypes. The net effect of PCV is to reduce the rate of pneumococcal disease both in the age group targeted for vaccination and in unvaccinated age groups.

Pneumonia is the most common of the serious pneumococcal disease syndromes and poses special challenges from a clinical and public health perspective. Most cases of pneumococcal pneumonia are not associated with bacteremia, and in these cases a definitive etiologic diagnosis is difficult. As a result, estimates of disease burden focus primarily on IPD rates and fail to include the major portion of the burden of serious pneumococcal disease. Among children, PCV trials designed to collect efficacy data on syndrome-based outcomes (e.g., radiographically confirmed pneumonia, clinically diagnosed pneumonia) have revealed the burden of culture-negative pneumococcal pneumonia.

The case-fatality ratios (CFRs) for pneumococcal pneumonia and IPD vary by age, underlying medical condition, and access to care. In addition, the CFR for pneumococcal pneumonia varies with the

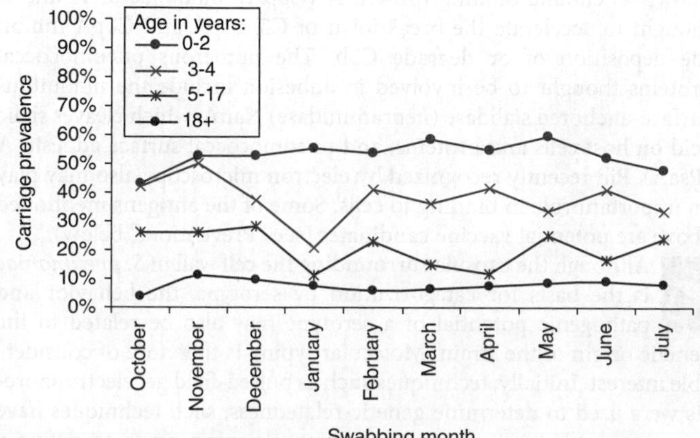

FIGURE 171-4 Prevalence of pneumococcal carriage in adults and children resident in the United Kingdom who had nasopharyngeal swabs collected monthly for 10 months (no seasonal trend; *t* test trend, >.05). *(Data adapted from D Goldblatt et al: J Infect Dis 192:387, 2005.)*

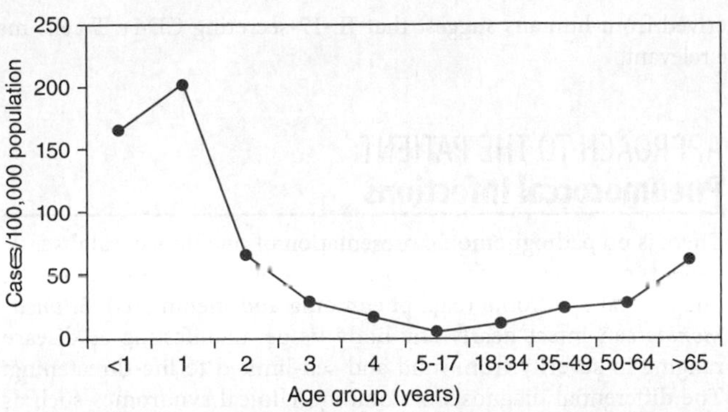

FIGURE 171-5 Rates of invasive pneumococcal disease before the introduction of pneumococcal conjugate vaccine, by age group: United States, 1998. *(Source: CDC, Active Bacterial Core Surveillance/Emerging Infectious Program Network, 2000. Data adapted from MMWR 49[RR-9], 2000.)*

severity of disease at presentation (rather than according to whether the pneumonia episode is associated with bacteremia) and with the patient's age (from <5% among hospitalized patients 18–44 years old to >12% among those >65 years old, even when appropriate and timely management is available). Notably, the likelihood of death in the first 24 h of hospitalization did not change substantially with the introduction of antibiotics; this surprising observation highlights the fact that the pathophysiology of severe pneumococcal pneumonia among adults reflects a rapidly progressive cascade of events that often unfolds irrespective of antibiotic administration. Management in an intensive care unit can provide critical support for the patient through the acute period, with lower CFRs.

Rates of pneumococcal disease vary by season, with higher rates in colder than in warmer months in temperate climates; by sex, with males more often affected than females; and by risk group, with risk factors including underlying medical conditions, behavioral issues, and ethnic group. In the United States, some Native American populations (including Alaska natives) and African Americans have higher rates of disease than the general population; the increased risk is probably attributable to socioeconomic conditions and the prevalence of underlying risk factors for pneumococcal disease. Medical conditions that increase the risk of pneumococcal infection are listed in Table 171-1. Outbreaks of disease are well recognized in crowded settings with susceptible individuals, such as infant day-care facilities, military barracks, and nursing homes. Furthermore, there is a clear association between preceding viral respiratory disease (especially but not exclusively influenza) and risk of secondary pneumococcal infections. The significant role of pneumococcal pneumonia in the morbidity and mortality associated with seasonal and pandemic influenza is increasingly recognized.

Antibiotic Resistance Reduced pneumococcal susceptibility to penicillin was first noted in 1967, but not until the 1990s did reduced antibiotic susceptibility emerge as a significant clinical and public health issue, with an increasing prevalence of pneumococcal isolates resistant to single or multiple classes of antibiotics and a rising absolute magnitude of minimal inhibitory concentrations (MICs). Strains with reduced susceptibility to penicillin G, cefotaxime, ceftriaxone, macrolides, and other antibiotics are now found worldwide and account for a significant proportion of disease-causing strains in many locations, especially among children. Vancomycin resistance has not yet been observed in clinical pneumococcal strains. Lack of antimicrobial susceptibility is clearly related to a subset of serotypes, many of which disproportionately cause disease among children. The vicious cycle of antibiotic exposure, selection of resistant organisms in the nasopharynx, and transmission of these organisms within the community, leading to difficult-to-treat infections and increased antibiotic exposure, has been interrupted to some extent by the introduction and routine use of PCV. The clinical implications of pneumococcal antimicrobial nonsusceptibility are addressed below in the section on treatment.

TABLE 171-1 CLINICAL RISK GROUPS FOR PNEUMOCOCCAL INFECTION

Clinical Risk Group	Examples
Asplenia or splenic dysfunction	Sickle cell disease, celiac disease
Chronic respiratory disease	Chronic obstructive pulmonary disease, bronchiectasis, cystic fibrosis, interstitial lung fibrosis, pneumoconiosis, bronchopulmonary dysplasia, aspiration risk, neuromuscular disease (e.g., cerebral palsy), severe asthma
Chronic heart disease	Ischemic heart disease, congenital heart disease, hypertension with cardiac complications, chronic heart failure
Chronic kidney disease	Nephrotic syndrome, chronic renal failure, renal transplantation
Chronic liver disease	Cirrhosis, biliary atresia, chronic hepatitis
Diabetes mellitus	Diabetes mellitus requiring insulin or oral hypoglycemic drugs
Immunocompromise/immunosuppression	HIV infection, common variable immunodeficiency, leukemia, lymphoma, Hodgkin's disease, multiple myeloma, generalized malignancy, chemotherapy, organ or bone marrow transplantation, systemic glucocorticoid treatment for >1 month at a dose equivalent to ≥20 mg/d (children, ≥1 mg/kg per day)
Cochlear implants	...
Cerebrospinal fluid leaks	...
Miscellaneous	Infancy and old age; prior hospitalization; alcoholism; malnutrition; cigarette smoking; day-care center attendance; residence in military training camps, prisons, homeless shelters

Note: Groups for whom pneumococcal vaccines are recommended by the Advisory Committee on Immunization Practices can be found at *www.cdc.gov/vaccines/schedules/*.

PATHOGENESIS

Pneumococci colonize the human nasopharynx from an early age; colonization acquisition events are generally described as asymptomatic, but evidence exists to associate acquisition with mild respiratory symptoms, especially in the very young. From the nasopharynx, the bacteria spread either via the bloodstream to distant sites (e.g., brain, joint, bones, peritoneal cavity) or locally to mucosal surfaces where they can cause otitis media or pneumonia. Direct spread from the nasopharynx to the central nervous system (CNS) can occur in rare cases of skull base fracture, although most cases of pneumococcal meningitis are secondary to hematogenous spread. Pneumococci can cause disease in almost any organ or part of the body; however, otitis media, pneumonia, bacteremia, and meningitis are most common. Colonization is a relatively frequent event, yet disease is rare. In the nasopharynx, pneumococci survive in mucus secreted by epithelial cells, where they can avoid local immune factors such as leukocytes and complement. The mucus itself is a component of local defense mechanisms, and the flow of mucus (driven in part by cilia in what is known as the *mucociliary escalator*) effects mechanical clearance of pneumococci. While many colonization episodes are of short duration, longitudinal studies in adults and children have revealed persistent colonization with a specific serotype over many months. Colonization eventually results in the development of capsule-specific serum IgG, which is thought to play a role in mediating clearance of bacteria from the nasopharynx. IgG antibodies to surface-exposed cell wall or secreted proteins also appear in the circulation in an age-dependent fashion or after colonization; the biologic role of these antibodies is less clear. Recent acquisition of a new colonizing serotype is more likely to be associated with subsequent invasion, presumably as a result of the absence of type-specific immunity. Intercurrent viral infections make the host more susceptible to pneumococcal colonization, and pneumococcal disease in a colonized individual often follows perturbation of the nasopharyngeal mucosa by such infections. Local cytokine production after a viral infection is thought to upregulate adhesion factors in the respiratory epithelium, allowing pneumococci to adhere via a variety of surface adhesin molecules, including PsaA, PspA,

CbpA, PspC, Hyl, pneumolysin, and the neuraminidases (Fig. 171-2). Adhesion coupled with inflammation induced by pneumococcal factors such as peptidoglycans and teichoic acids results in invasion. It is the inflammation induced by various bacterium-derived factors that is responsible for the pathology associated with pneumococcal infection. Cell wall–derived teichoic acids and peptidoglycans induce a variety of cytokines, including the proinflammatory cytokines interleukin (IL) 1, IL-6, and tumor necrosis factor, and activate complement via the alternative pathway. Polymorphonuclear leukocytes are thus attracted, and an intense inflammatory response is initiated. Pneumolysin also is important in local pathology, inducing proinflammatory cytokine production by local monocytes.

The pneumococcal capsule, consisting of polysaccharides with antiphagocytic properties due to resistance to the deposition of complement, plays an important role in pathogenesis. While most capsular types can cause human disease, certain capsular types are more commonly isolated from sites of infection. The reason for the dominance of some serotypes over others in IPD, as depicted in Fig. 171-3, is unclear.

HOST DEFENSE MECHANISMS

Innate Immunity As described above, intact respiratory epithelium and a host of nonspecific or innate immune factors (e.g., mucus, splenic function, complement, neutrophils, and macrophages) constitute the first line of defense against pneumococci. Physical factors such as the cough reflex and the mucociliary escalator are important in clearing bacteria from the lungs. Immunologic factors are critical as well: C-reactive protein (CRP) binds phosphorylcholine in the pneumococcal cell wall, inducing complement activation and leading to bacterial clearance; Toll-like receptor 2 (TLR2) recognizes both pneumococcal lipoteichoic acid and cell wall peptidoglycan; and in animal models, the absence of host TLR2 leads to more severe infection and impaired clearance of nasopharyngeal colonization. TLR4 appears to be necessary for the proinflammatory effect of pneumolysin on macrophages. The importance of TLR recognition is underlined by descriptions of an inherited deficiency of human IL-1 receptor–associated kinase 4 (IRAK-4) that manifests as an unusual susceptibility to infection with bacteria, including *S. pneumoniae*. IRAK-4 is essential for the normal functioning of several TLRs. Other factors that interfere with these nonspecific mechanisms (e.g., viral infections, cystic fibrosis, bronchiectasis, complement deficiency, and chronic obstructive pulmonary disease) all predispose to the development of pneumococcal pneumonia. Patients who lack a spleen or have abnormal splenic function (e.g., persons with sickle cell disease) are at high risk of developing overwhelming pneumococcal disease.

Acquired Immunity Acquired immunity induced via contact following colonization or through cross-reactive antigens rests largely on the development of serum IgG antibody specific for the pneumococcal capsular polysaccharide. Nearly all polysaccharides are T cell–independent antigens; B cells can make antibodies to such antigens without T cell help. However, in children <1–2 years old, such B cell responses are poorly developed. This delayed ontogeny of capsule-specific IgG in young children is associated with susceptibility to pneumococcal infection (Fig. 171-5). The extremely high risk of pneumococcal infection in the absence of serum immunoglobulin (i.e., in conditions such as agammaglobulinemia) highlights the important role of capsular antibody in protection against disease. Each serotype's capsule is chemically distinct; thus immunity tends to be serotype specific, although some cross-immunity exists. For example, conjugate vaccine–induced antibodies to serotype 6B prevent infection due to serotype 6A. However, cross-protection against serotypes within serogroups is not universal; for instance, antibodies to serotype 19F do not appear to confer protection against disease caused by serotype 19A. Antibodies to surface-exposed or secreted pneumococcal proteins (such as pneumolysin, PsaA, and PspA) also appear in the circulation with increasing age of the host, but their functional significance remains unclear. Data from murine models suggest that CD4+ T cells may play a role in preventing pneumococcal colonization and disease, and recent experimental data derived from humans suggest that IL-17-secreting CD4+ T cells may be relevant.

APPROACH TO THE PATIENT: Pneumococcal Infections

There is no pathognomonic presentation of pneumococcal disease; patients may present with a range of syndromes and with more than one clinical syndrome (e.g., pneumonia and meningitis). *S. pneumoniae* can infect nearly any body tissue, manifesting as disease ranging in severity from mild and self-limited to life-threatening. The differential diagnosis of common clinical syndromes such as pneumonia, otitis media, fever of unknown origin, and meningitis should always include pneumococcal infection. A microbiologically confirmed diagnosis is made in only a minority of pneumococcal cases since, in most circumstances (and especially in pneumonia and otitis media), fluid from the site of infection is not available for etiologic determination. Empirical therapy that includes appropriate treatment for *S. pneumoniae* is often indicated.

Algorithms for assessment and management of ill children have been developed for use in the developing world or in other settings where evaluation by a trained physician may not be feasible. Children who present with ominous signs such as an inability to drink, convulsions, lethargy, and severe malnutrition are categorized as having very severe disease without further evaluation by the community health care worker, are given antibiotics, and are immediately referred to a hospital for diagnosis and management. Children who present with cough and tachypnea (the latter defined according to specific age strata) are further stratified into severity categories based on the presence or absence of lower chest wall indrawing and are managed accordingly with either antibiotics alone or antibiotics and referral to a hospital facility. Children with cough but no tachypnea are categorized as having a nonpneumonia respiratory illness.

CLINICAL MANIFESTATIONS

The clinical manifestations of pneumococcal disease depend on the site of infection and the duration of illness. Clinical syndromes are classified as noninvasive (e.g., otitis media and nonbacteremic pneumonia) or invasive (e.g., bacteremic pneumonia). The pathogenesis of noninvasive illness involves contiguous spread from the nasopharynx or skin; invasive disease involves infection of a normally sterile body fluid or follows bacteremia.

Pneumonia Pneumonia is the most common serious pneumococcal syndrome and is considered invasive when associated with a positive blood culture. Pneumococcal pneumonia can present as a mild community-acquired infection at one extreme and as a life-threatening disease requiring intubation and intensive support at the other.

PRESENTING MANIFESTATIONS The presentation of pneumococcal pneumonia does not reliably distinguish it from pneumonia of other etiologies. In a subset of cases, pneumococcal pneumonia is recognized at the outset as associated with a viral upper respiratory infection and is characterized by the abrupt onset of cough and dyspnea accompanied by fever, shaking chills, and myalgias. The cough evolves from nonpurulent to productive of sputum that is purulent and sometimes tinged with blood. Patients may describe stabbing pleuritic chest pain and significant dyspnea indicating involvement of the parietal pleura. Among the elderly, the presenting clinical symptoms may be less specific, with confusion or malaise but without fever or cough. In such cases, a high index of suspicion is required because failure to treat pneumococcal pneumonia promptly in an elderly patient is likely to result in rapid evolution of the infection, with increased severity, morbidity, and risk of death.

FINDINGS ON PHYSICAL EXAMINATION The clinical signs associated with pneumococcal pneumonia among adults include tachypnea

(>30 breaths/min) and tachycardia, hypotension in severe cases, and fever in most cases (although not in all elderly patients). Respiratory signs are varied, including dullness to percussion in areas of the chest with significant consolidation, crackles on auscultation, reduced expansion of the chest in some cases as a result of splinting to reduce pain, bronchial breathing in a minority of cases, pleural rub in occasional cases, and cyanosis in cases with significant hypoxemia. Among infants with severe pneumonia, chest wall indrawing and nasal flaring are common. Nonrespiratory findings can include upper abdominal pain if the diaphragmatic pleura is involved as well as mental status changes, particularly confusion in elderly patients.

DIFFERENTIAL DIAGNOSIS The differential diagnosis of pneumococcal pneumonia includes cardiac conditions such as myocardial infarction and heart failure with atypical pulmonary edema; pulmonary conditions such as atelectasis; and pneumonia caused by viral pathogens, mycoplasmas, *Haemophilus influenzae, Klebsiella pneumoniae, Staphylococcus aureus, Legionella*, or (in HIV-infected and otherwise immunocompromised hosts) *Pneumocystis*. In cases with abdominal symptoms, the differential diagnosis includes cholecystitis, appendicitis, perforated peptic ulcer disease, and subphrenic abscesses. The challenge in cases with abdominal symptoms is to remember to include pneumococcal pneumonia—a nonabdominal process—in the differential diagnosis.

DIAGNOSIS Some authorities advocate treating uncomplicated, nonsevere, community-acquired pneumonia without determining the microbiologic etiology, given that this information is unlikely to alter clinical management. However, efforts to identify the cause of pneumonia are important when the disease is more severe and when the diagnosis of pneumonia is not clearly established. The gold standard for etiologic diagnosis of pneumococcal pneumonia is pathologic examination of lung tissue. In lieu of that procedure, evidence of an infiltrate on chest radiography warrants a diagnosis of pneumonia. However, cases of pneumonia without radiographic evidence do occur. An infiltrate can be absent either early in the course of the illness or with dehydration; upon rehydration, an infiltrate usually appears. The radiographic appearance of pneumococcal pneumonia is varied; it classically consists of lobar or segmental consolidation (Fig. 171-6) but in some cases is patchy. More than one lobe is involved in ~30% of cases. Consolidation may be associated with a small pleural effusion or empyema in complicated cases. In children, "round pneumonia," a distinctly spherical consolidation on chest radiography, is associated with a pneumococcal etiology. Round pneumonia is uncommon in adults. *S. pneumoniae* is not the only cause of such lesions; other causes, especially cancer, should be considered.

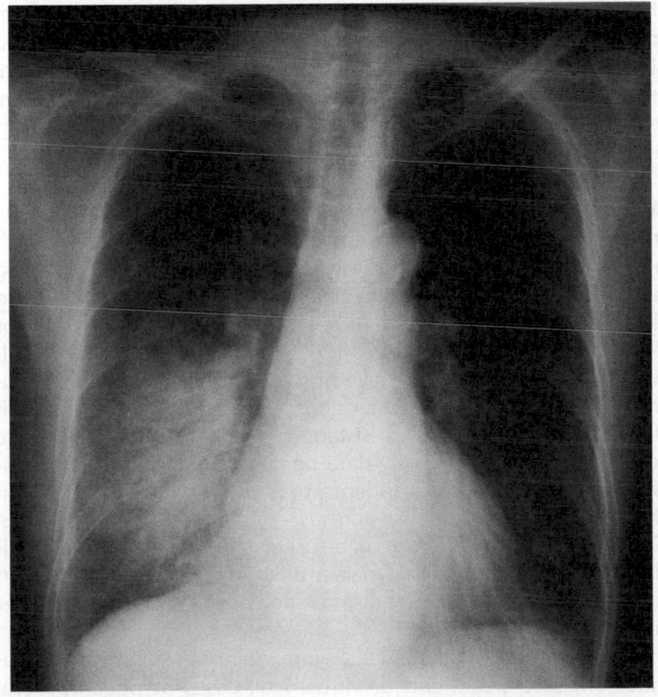

FIGURE 171-6 Chest radiograph depicting classic lobar pneumococcal pneumonia in the right lower lobe of an elderly patient's lung.

Blood drawn from patients with suspected pneumococcal pneumonia can be used for supportive or definitive diagnostic tests. Blood cultures are positive for pneumococci in a minority (<30%) of cases of pneumococcal pneumonia. Nonspecific findings include an elevated polymorphonuclear leukocyte count (>15,000/μL in most cases and upward of 40,000/μL in some), leukopenia in <10% of cases (a poor prognostic sign associated with a fatal outcome), and elevated values in liver function tests (e.g., both conjugated and unconjugated hyperbilirubinemia). Anemia, low serum albumin levels, hyponatremia, and elevated serum creatinine levels are all found in ~20–30% of patients.

Urinary pneumococcal antigen assays have facilitated etiologic diagnosis. In adults, among whom the prevalence of pneumococcal nasopharyngeal colonization is relatively low, a positive pneumococcal urinary antigen test has a high predictive value. The same is not true for children, in whom a positive urinary antigen test can reflect the mere presence of *S. pneumoniae* in the nasopharynx.

Most cases of pneumococcal pneumonia are diagnosed by Gram's staining and culture of sputum. The utility of a sputum specimen is directly related to its quality and the patient's antibiotic treatment status.

COMPLICATIONS Empyema is the most common focal complication of pneumococcal pneumonia, occurring in <5% of cases. When fluid in the pleural space is accompanied by fever and leukocytosis (even low-grade) after 4–5 days of appropriate antibiotic treatment for pneumococcal pneumonia, empyema should be considered. Parapneumonic effusions are more common than empyema, representing a self-limited inflammatory response to pneumonia. Pleural fluid with frank pus, bacteria (detected by microscopic examination), or a pH of ≤7.1 indicates empyema and demands aggressive and complete drainage, usually through chest tube insertion.

Meningitis Pneumococcal meningitis typically presents as a pyogenic condition that is clinically indistinguishable from meningitis of other bacterial etiologies. Meningitis can be the primary presenting pneumococcal syndrome or a complication of other conditions such as skull fracture, otitis media, bacteremia, or mastoiditis. Now that *H. influenzae* type b vaccine is routinely used, *S. pneumoniae* and *Neisseria meningitidis* are the most common bacterial causes of meningitis in both adults and children. Pyogenic meningitis, including that due to *S. pneumoniae*, is associated clinically with findings that include severe, generalized, gradual-onset headache, fever, and nausea as well as specific CNS manifestations such as stiff neck, photophobia, seizures, and confusion. Clinical signs include a toxic appearance, altered consciousness, bradycardia, and hypertension indicative of increased intracranial pressure. A small proportion of adult patients have Kernig's or Brudzinski's sign or cranial nerve palsies (particularly of the third and sixth cranial nerves).

A definitive diagnosis of pneumococcal meningitis rests on the examination of CSF for (1) evidence of turbidity (visual inspection); (2) elevated protein level, elevated white blood cell count, and reduced glucose concentration (quantitative measurement); and (3) specific identification of the etiologic agent (culture, Gram's staining, antigen testing, or polymerase chain reaction [PCR]). A blood culture positive for *S. pneumoniae* in conjunction with clinical manifestations of meningitis also is considered confirmatory. Among adults, detection of pneumococcal antigen in urine is considered highly specific because of the low prevalence of nasopharyngeal colonization in this age group.

The mortality rate for pneumococcal meningitis is ~20%. In addition, up to 50% of survivors experience acute or chronic complications, including deafness, hydrocephalus, and mental retardation in children and diffuse brain swelling, subarachnoid bleeding, hydrocephalus, cerebrovascular complications, and hearing loss in adults.

Other Invasive Syndromes *S. pneumoniae* can cause other invasive syndromes involving virtually any body site. These syndromes include primary bacteremia without other sites of infection (bacteremia without a source; occult bacteremia), osteomyelitis, septic arthritis, endocarditis, pericarditis, and peritonitis. The essential diagnostic approach is collection of fluid from the site of infection by sterile technique and examination by Gram's staining, culture, and—when relevant—capsular antigen assay or PCR. Hemolytic-uremic syndrome can complicate invasive pneumococcal disease.

Noninvasive Syndromes The two major noninvasive syndromes caused by *S. pneumoniae* are sinusitis and otitis media; the latter is the most common pneumococcal syndrome and most often affects young children. The manifestations of otitis media include the acute onset of severe pain, fever, deafness, and tinnitus, most frequently in the setting of a recent upper respiratory tract infection. Clinical signs include a red, swollen, often bulging tympanic membrane with reduced movement on insufflation or tympanography. Redness of the tympanic membrane is not sufficient for the diagnosis of otitis media.

Pneumococcal sinusitis is also a complication of upper respiratory tract infections and presents with facial pain, congestion, fever, and—in many cases—persistent nighttime cough. A definitive diagnosis is made by aspiration and culture of sinus material; however, presumptive treatment is most commonly initiated after application of a strict set of clinical diagnostic criteria.

TREATMENT PNEUMOCOCCAL INFECTIONS

Historically, the activity of penicillin against pneumococci made parenteral penicillin G the drug of choice for disease caused by susceptible organisms, including community-acquired pneumonia. For susceptible strains, penicillin G remains the most commonly used agent, with daily doses ranging from 50,000 U/kg for minor infections to 300,000 U/kg for meningitis. Other parenteral β-lactam drugs, such as ampicillin, cefotaxime, ceftriaxone, and cefuroxime, can be used against penicillin-susceptible strains but offer little advantage over penicillin. Macrolides and cephalosporins are alternatives for penicillin-allergic patients. While agents such as clindamycin, tetracycline, and trimethoprim-sulfamethoxazole exhibit some activity against pneumococci, resistance to these agents is frequently encountered in different parts of the world.

Penicillin-resistant pneumococci were first described in the mid-1960s, at which point tetracycline- and macrolide-resistant strains had already been reported. Multidrug-resistant strains were first described in the 1970s, but it was during the 1990s that pneumococcal drug resistance reached pandemic proportions. The use of antibiotics selects for resistant pneumococci, and strains resistant to β-lactam agents and to multiple drugs are now found all over the world. The emergence of high rates of macrolide and fluoroquinolone resistance also has been described.

The molecular basis of penicillin resistance in *S. pneumoniae* is the alteration of penicillin-binding protein (PBP) genes by transformation and horizontal transfer of DNA from related streptococcal species. Such alteration of PBPs results in lower affinity for penicillins. Depending on the specific PBP(s) and the number of PBPs altered, the level of resistance ranges from intermediate to high. For many years, penicillin susceptibility breakpoints have been defined by MICs as follows: susceptible, ≤0.06 μg/mL; intermediate, 0.12–1.0 μg/mL; and resistant, ≥2.0 μg/mL. However, in vitro results often were not predictive of the response of a patient to treatment for pneumococcal diseases other than meningitis. New recommendations have been based on the revised penicillin G breakpoints established in 2008 by the Clinical and Laboratory Standards Institute. For IV treatment of meningitis with at least 24 million units per day in 8 divided doses, the susceptibility breakpoint remains ≤0.06 μg/mL, and MICs of ≥0.12 μg/mL indicate resistance. For IV treatment of nonmeningeal infections with 12 million units per day in 6 divided doses, the breakpoints are ≤2 μg/mL for susceptible organisms, 4 μg/mL for intermediate organisms, and ≥8 μg/mL for resistant organisms; a dosage of 18–24 million units per day is recommended for strains with MICs in the intermediate category. The original breakpoints remain the same for oral treatment of nonmeningeal infections with penicillin V.

Although guidelines for antibiotic therapy should be driven in part by local patterns of resistance, guidelines from national organizations in many countries (e.g., the Infectious Diseases Society of America/American Thoracic Society, the British Thoracic Society, and the European Respiratory Society) lay out evidence-based approaches. The following guidelines for the treatment of individual sepsis syndromes are based on those advocated by the American Academy of Pediatrics and published in the 2012 *Red Book*.

MENINGITIS LIKELY OR PROVEN TO BE DUE TO *S. PNEUMONIAE*

As a result of the increased prevalence of resistant pneumococci, first-line therapy for persons ≥1 month of age is a combination of vancomycin (adults, 30–60 mg/kg per day; infants and children, 60 mg/kg per day) and cefotaxime (adults, 8–12 g/d in 4–6 divided doses; children, 225–300 mg/kg per day in 1 dose or 2 divided doses) or ceftriaxone (adults, 4 g/d in 1 dose or 2 divided doses; children, 100 mg/kg per day in 1 dose or 2 divided doses). If children are hypersensitive to β-lactam agents (penicillins and cephalosporins), rifampin (adults, 600 mg/d; children, 20 mg/d in 1 dose or 2 divided doses) can be substituted for cefotaxime or ceftriaxone. A repeat lumbar puncture should be considered after 48 h if the organism is not susceptible to penicillin and information on cephalosporin sensitivity is not yet available, if the patient's clinical condition does not improve or deteriorates, or if dexamethasone has been administered and may be compromising clinical evaluation. When antibiotic sensitivity data become available, treatment should be modified accordingly. If the isolate is sensitive to penicillin, vancomycin can be discontinued and penicillin can replace the cephalosporin, or cefotaxime or ceftriaxone can be continued alone. If the isolate displays any resistance to penicillin but is susceptible to the cephalosporins, vancomycin can be discontinued and cefotaxime or ceftriaxone continued. If the isolate exhibits any resistance to penicillin and is not susceptible to cefotaxime and ceftriaxone, vancomycin and high-dose cefotaxime or ceftriaxone can be continued; rifampin may be added as well if the isolate is susceptible and the patient's clinical condition is worsening, if the CSF remains positive for bacteria, or if the MIC of the cephalosporin in question against the infecting strain is high. Some physicians advocate the use of glucocorticoids in children >6 months old, but this recommendation remains controversial and is not universally considered the standard of care. Glucocorticoids significantly reduce rates of mortality, severe hearing loss, and neurologic sequelae in adults and should be administered to those with community-acquired bacterial meningitis. If dexamethasone is given to either adults or children, it should be administered before or in conjunction with the first antibiotic dose.

INVASIVE INFECTIONS (EXCLUDING MENINGITIS)

In previously well children with noncritical illness, therapy with a recommended antibiotic should be instigated at the following dosages: penicillin G, 250,000–400,000 units/kg per day (in divided doses 4–6 h apart); cefotaxime, 75–100 mg/d (doses 8 h apart); or ceftriaxone, 50–75 mg/d (doses 12–24 h apart). For critically ill children, including those who have myocarditis or multilobular pneumonia with hypoxia or hypotension, vancomycin may be added if the isolate may possibly be resistant to β-lactam drugs, with its use reviewed once susceptibility data become available. If the organism is resistant to β-lactam agents, therapy should be modified on the basis of clinical response and susceptibility to other antibiotics. Clindamycin or vancomycin can be used as a first-line agent for children with severe β-lactam hypersensitivity, but vancomycin should not be continued if the organism is shown to be sensitive to other non-β-lactam antibiotics.

For outpatient management, amoxicillin (1 g every 8 h) provides effective treatment for virtually all cases of pneumococcal pneumonia. Neither cephalosporins nor quinolones, which are far more expensive, offer any advantage over amoxicillin. Levofloxacin

(500–750 mg/d as a single dose) and moxifloxacin (400 mg/d as a single dose) also are highly likely to be effective in the United States except in patients who come from closed populations where these drugs are used widely or who have themselves been treated recently with a quinolone. Clindamycin (600–1200 mg/d every 6 h) is effective in 90% of cases and azithromycin (500 mg on day 1 followed by 250–500 mg/d) or clarithromycin (500–750 mg/d as a single dose) in 80% of cases. Treatment failure resulting in bacteremic disease due to macrolide-resistant isolates has been amply documented in patients given azithromycin empirically. As noted above, rates of resistance to all these antibiotics are relatively low in some countries and much higher in others; high-dose amoxicillin remains the best option worldwide.

The optimal duration of treatment for pneumococcal pneumonia is uncertain, but its continuation for at least 5 days once the patient becomes afebrile appears to be a prudent approach. Cases with a second focus of infection (e.g., empyema or septic arthritis) require longer therapy.

ACUTE OTITIS MEDIA

Amoxicillin (80–90 mg/kg per day) is recommended for children with acute otitis media except in situations where observation and symptom-based treatment without antibiotics are advocated. These situations include nonsevere illness and an uncertain diagnosis in children 6 months to 2 years of age and nonsevere illness (even if the diagnosis seems certain) in children >2 years of age. Although the optimal duration of therapy has not been conclusively established, a 10-day course is recommended for younger children and for children with severe disease at any age. For children >6 years old who have mild or moderate disease, a course of 5–7 days is considered adequate. Patients whose illness fails to respond should be reassessed at 48–72 h. If acute otitis media is confirmed and antibiotic treatment has not been started, administration of amoxicillin should be commenced. If antibiotic therapy fails, a change is indicated. Failure to respond to second-line antibiotics as well indicates that myringotomy or tympanocentesis may need to be undertaken in order to obtain samples for culture.

The above recommendations can also be followed for the treatment of sinusitis. Detailed information on the further management of these conditions in children has been published by the American Academy of Pediatrics and the American Academy of Family Physicians.

PREVENTION

Measures to prevent pneumococcal disease include vaccination against *S. pneumoniae* and influenza viruses, reduction of comorbidities that increase the risk of pneumococcal disease, and prevention of antibiotic overuse, which fuels pneumococcal resistance.

Capsular Polysaccharide Vaccines The 23-valent pneumococcal polysaccharide vaccine (PPSV23), containing 25 μg of each capsular polysaccharide, has been licensed for use since 1983. Recommendations for its use vary by country. The U.S. Advisory Committee on Immunization Practices recommends PPSV23 for all persons ≥65 years of age and for those 2–64 years of age who have underlying medical conditions that put them at increased risk for pneumococcal disease or, if infected, disease of increased severity (Table 171-1; see also *www.cdc.gov/vaccines/schedules/*). The committee recently updated their recommendations to include the combined use of PPSV23 and a conjugate vaccine in at-risk individuals (see "Polysaccharide–Protein Conjugate Vaccines," below). Revaccination 5 years after the first dose is recommended for persons >2 years of age who have underlying medical conditions but not routinely for those whose only indication is an age of ≥65 years. PPSV23 does not induce an anamnestic response, and antibody concentrations wane over time; thus revaccination is particularly important for individuals with conditions resulting in loss of antibody. Concerns about repeated revaccination have focused on safety (i.e., local reactions) and the induction of immune hyporesponsiveness. Neither the clinical relevance nor the biologic basis of hyporesponsiveness is clear, but, given the possibility of its occurrence, more than one revaccination has not been recommended.

The effectiveness of PPSV23 against IPD, pneumococcal pneumonia, all-cause pneumonia, and death is controversial, with wide variation in observations. The many published meta-analyses of PPSV efficacy have often reached opposing conclusions with regard to a given clinical entity. Generally, observational studies cite greater effectiveness than do controlled clinical trials. The consensus is that PPSV is effective against IPD but is less effective or ineffective against nonbacteremic pneumococcal pneumonia. However, published trials, observational studies, and meta-analyses contradict this view. Efficacy is often lower in the elderly and in immunodeficient patients whose condition is associated with reduced antibody responses to vaccines than in younger, healthier populations. When PPSV is effective, the duration of protection following a single dose of vaccine is estimated to be ~5 years.

What is not disputed is that improved pneumococcal vaccines are needed for adults. Even in the setting of routine pneumococcal conjugate vaccination of infants (which indirectly protects adults from vaccine-serotype strains), disease caused by serotypes not represented in the conjugate vaccine continues to be a significant burden among adults.

Polysaccharide–Protein Conjugate Vaccines Infants and young children respond poorly to PPSV, which contains T cell–independent antigens. Consequently, another class of pneumococcal vaccines, the PCVs, were developed specifically for infants and young children. The first product, a 7-valent PCV, was licensed in 2000 in the United States. Three PCV products—containing 7, 10, and 13 serotypes, respectively—are currently (2014) commercially available. The serotypes included in these PCV formulations are important causes of IPD and antibiotic resistance among young children. Randomized controlled trials have demonstrated a high degree of efficacy of PCVs against vaccine-serotype IPD as well as efficacy against pneumonia, otitis media, nasopharyngeal colonization, and all-cause mortality. PCVs are recommended by the World Health Organization for inclusion in routine childhood immunization schedules worldwide, especially in countries with high infant mortality rates.

The United States was the first country to introduce PCV and therefore has the longest experience with its community-wide effects. The introduction of PCV in the United States has resulted in a >90% reduction in vaccine-serotype IPD among the whole population (Fig. 171-7). This decline has been noted not only in those age groups immunized but also in adults and is attributable to the near elimination of vaccine-serotype nasopharyngeal colonization in immunized infants, which reduces spread to adults. This protection of unimmunized community members through vaccination of a subset of the community is termed *the indirect effect*. Increases in colonization with—and concomitantly in disease due to—non-vaccine-serotype strains (i.e., replacement colonization and disease) have been seen; however, the absolute rate increases in IPD caused by non-vaccine serotypes are generally small, especially relative to decreases in vaccine-serotype IPD (see "Epidemiology," above). Since vaccine-serotype strains are more commonly resistant to antibiotics than are non-vaccine serotypes, use of PCV has also resulted in dramatic declines in the proportion and absolute rates of drug-resistant pneumococcal disease. The recommendations of the Advisory Committee on Immunization Practices for the use of conjugate vaccines can be found at *www.cdc.gov/MMWR/pdf/wk/mm5909.pdf*. Recently, PCV has been shown to prevent pneumococcal infection in HIV-infected adults. In the United States, PCV13 followed by a dose of PPSV23 is now recommended for all immunocompromised children and adults.

Other Prevention Strategies Pneumococcal disease can also be averted through the prevention of illnesses that predispose individuals to pneumococcal infections. Relevant measures include influenza vaccination and improved management and control of diabetes, HIV infection, heart disease, and lung disease. Finally, the reduction of antibiotic misuse is a strategy for the prevention of pneumococcal disease in that

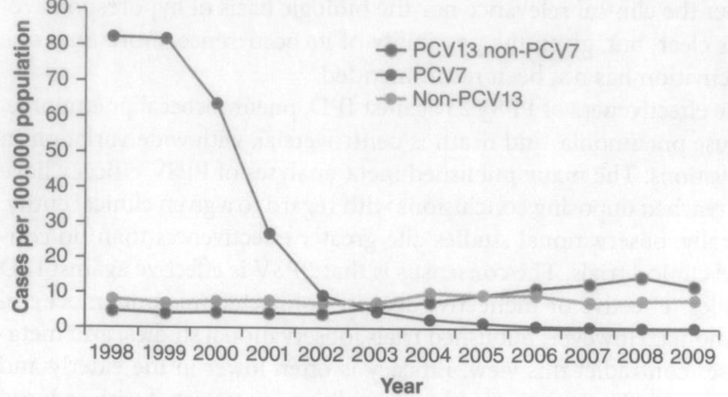

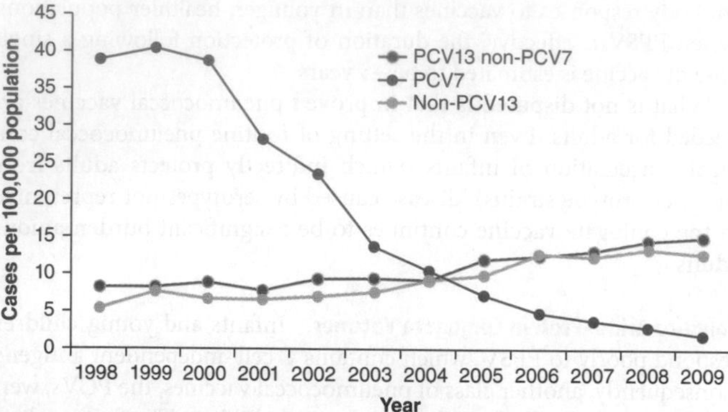

FIGURE 171-7 Changes in invasive pneumococcal disease (IPD) incidence, by serotype group, among children <5 years old (*top*) and adults >65 years old (*bottom*), 1998–2009. 7-Valent pneumococcal conjugate vaccine (PCV7) was introduced in the United States for routine administration to infants and young children during the second half of 2000, while PCV13 was introduced in 2010, the year following this surveillance period. PCV7 serotypes include serotypes 4, 6B, 9V, 14, 18C, 19F, and 23F as well as cross-reactive serotype 6A. PCV13 serotypes include the PCV7 serotypes as well as serotypes 1, 3, 5, 6A, 7F, and 19A. *(Reprinted with permission from Dr. M. Moore, Centers for Disease Control and Prevention.)*

antimicrobial resistance directly and indirectly perpetuates organism transmission and disease in the community.

WEBSITES

American Academy of Pediatrics RED BOOK. The report of the Committee on Infectious Diseases: *aapredbook.aappublications.org*; Pneumococcal Regional Serotype Distribution for Pneumococcal AMC TPP: *www.gavialliance.org/library/documents/amc/tpp-codebook/*

172 Staphylococcal Infections

Franklin D. Lowy

Staphylococcus aureus, the most virulent of the many staphylococcal species, has demonstrated its versatility by remaining a major cause of morbidity and mortality worldwide despite the availability of numerous effective antistaphylococcal antibiotics. *S. aureus* is a pluripotent pathogen, causing disease through both toxin- and non-toxin-mediated mechanisms. This organism is responsible for numerous nosocomial and community-based infections that range from relatively minor skin and soft tissue infections to life-threatening systemic infections.

The "other" staphylococci, collectively designated *coagulase-negative staphylococci* (CoNS), are considerably less virulent than *S. aureus* but remain important pathogens in infections that are primarily associated with prosthetic devices.

MICROBIOLOGY AND TAXONOMY

Staphylococci, gram-positive cocci in the family Micrococcaceae, form grapelike clusters on Gram's stain (Fig. 172-1). These organisms (~1 μm in diameter) are catalase-positive (unlike streptococcal species), nonmotile, aerobic, and facultatively anaerobic. They are capable of prolonged survival on environmental surfaces under varying conditions. Some species have a relatively broad host range, including mammals and birds, whereas for others the host range is quite narrow—i.e., limited to one or two closely related animals.

More than 30 staphylococcal species are pathogenic. Identification of the more clinically important species has generally relied on a series of biochemical tests. Automated diagnostic systems, kits for biochemical characterization, and DNA-based assays are available for species identification. With few exceptions, *S. aureus* is distinguished from other staphylococcal species by its production of coagulase, a surface enzyme that converts fibrinogen to fibrin. Latex kits that detect both protein A and clumping factor also distinguish *S. aureus* from most other staphylococcal species. *S. aureus* ferments mannitol, is positive for protein A, and produces DNAse. On blood agar plates, *S. aureus* tends to form golden β-hemolytic colonies; in contrast, CoNS produce small white nonhemolytic colonies. Increasingly, sequence-based methods (e.g., 16S rRNA) are being used to identify different staphylococcal species.

Determining whether multiple staphylococcal isolates from different patients are the same or different is often relevant when there is concern that a nosocomial outbreak is due to a common point source (e.g., a contaminated medical instrument). Molecular typing methods, such as pulsed-field gel electrophoresis and sequence-based techniques (e.g., staphylococcal protein A [SpA] typing), have increasingly been used for this purpose. More recently, whole-genome sequencing has enhanced the ability to discriminate among clinical isolates.

S. AUREUS INFECTIONS

EPIDEMIOLOGY

S. aureus is both a commensal and an opportunistic pathogen. Approximately 30% of healthy persons are colonized with *S. aureus*, with a smaller percentage (~10%) persistently colonized. The rate of colonization is elevated among insulin-dependent diabetics, HIV-infected patients, patients undergoing hemodialysis, injection drug users, and individuals with skin damage. The anterior nares and oropharynx are frequent sites of human colonization, although the skin (especially when damaged), vagina, axilla, and perineum may also be colonized. These colonization sites serve as a reservoir for future infections.

Transmission of *S. aureus* most frequently results from direct personal contact. Colonization of different body sites allows transfer from one person to another during contact. Spread of staphylococci in aerosols of respiratory or nasal secretions from heavily colonized individuals has also been reported. Most individuals who develop

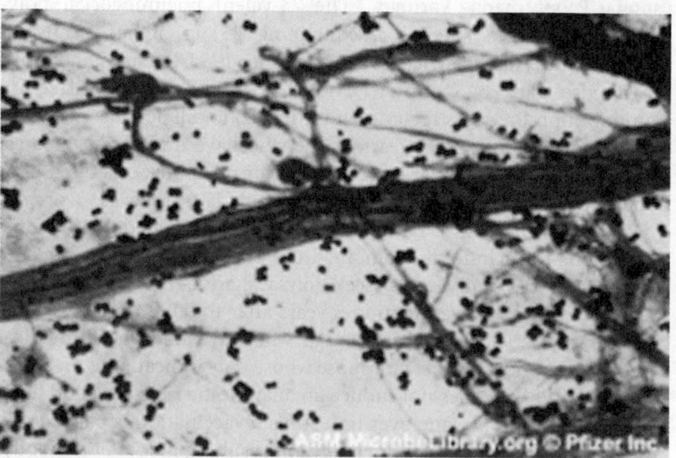

FIGURE 172-1 Gram's stain of *S. aureus* in a sputum sample. *(From ASM MicrobeLibrary.org.© Pfizer, Inc.)*

S. aureus infections become infected with a strain that is already a part of their own commensal flora. Breaches of the skin or mucosal membrane allow *S. aureus* to initiate infection.

Some diseases increase the risk of *S. aureus* infection; diabetes, for example, combines an increased rate of *S. aureus* colonization and the use of injectable insulin with the possibility of impaired leukocyte function. Individuals with congenital or acquired qualitative or quantitative defects of polymorphonuclear leukocytes (PMNs) are at increased risk of *S. aureus* infections; this group includes neutropenic patients (e.g., those receiving chemotherapeutic agents), those with chronic granulomatous disease, and those with Job's or Chédiak-Higashi syndrome. Other groups at risk include individuals with end-stage renal disease, HIV infection, skin abnormalities, or prosthetic devices.

S. aureus is a leading cause of health care–associated infections (Chap. 168). It is the most common cause of surgical wound infections and is second only to CoNS as a cause of primary bacteremia. These isolates are generally resistant to multiple antibiotics; thus available therapeutic options are limited. In the community, *S. aureus* remains an important cause of skin and soft tissue infections, respiratory infections, and (among injection drug users) infective endocarditis. The increasing use of home infusion therapy is another cause of community-acquired staphylococcal infections.

In the past two decades, there has been a dramatic change in the epidemiology of infections due to methicillin-resistant *S. aureus* (MRSA). In addition to its major role as a nosocomial pathogen, MRSA has become an established community-based pathogen. Numerous outbreaks of community-associated MRSA (CA-MRSA) infections have been reported in both rural and urban settings in widely separated regions throughout the world. The outbreaks have occurred among such diverse groups as children, prisoners, athletes, Native Americans, and drug users. Risk factors common to these outbreaks include poor hygienic conditions, close contact, contaminated material, and damaged skin. These infections have been caused by a limited number of MRSA strains. In the United States, strain USA300 (defined by pulsed-field gel electrophoresis) has been the predominant clone. In other geographic regions of the world, different strains of CA-MRSA have been responsible for these community-based outbreaks. Although the majority of infections caused by these strains have involved the skin and soft tissue, 5–10% have been invasive and potentially life-threatening. CA-MRSA strains have also been responsible for an increasing number of nosocomial infections. Of concern has been the apparent capacity of CA-MRSA to cause disease in immunocompetent individuals.

PATHOGENESIS

General Concepts *S. aureus* is a pyogenic pathogen known for its capacity to induce abscess formation at sites of both local and metastatic infections. This classic pathologic response to *S. aureus* defines the framework within which the infection will progress. The bacteria elicit an inflammatory response characterized by an initial intense infiltration of PMNs and a subsequent infiltration of macrophages and fibroblasts. Either the host cellular response (including the deposition of fibrin and collagen) contains the infection, or infection spreads to the adjoining tissue or the bloodstream.

In toxin-mediated staphylococcal disease, infection is not invariably present. For example, once toxin has been elaborated into food, staphylococcal food poisoning can develop in the absence of viable bacteria. In staphylococcal toxic shock syndrome (TSS), conditions allowing toxin elaboration at colonization sites (e.g., the presence of a superabsorbent tampon) suffice for initiation of clinical illness.

The *S. aureus* Genome The complete genomes of numerous strains of *S. aureus* have now been fully sequenced. Among the interesting revelations are (1) the high degree of nucleotide sequence similarity of the core genomes of different strains; (2) acquisition of a relatively large amount of genetic information by horizontal transfer from other bacterial species; and (3) the presence of unique "pathogenicity" or "genomic" islands—mobile genetic elements that contain clusters of enterotoxin and exotoxin genes and/or antimicrobial resistance determinants. Among the genes in these islands are those carrying *mecA*, the gene responsible for methicillin resistance. Methicillin resistance–containing islands have been designated staphylococcal cassette chromosome *mec* (SCC*mec*) types and range in size from ~20 to 60 kb. To date, 11 SCC*mec* types have been identified. Among the more common types, types 1–3 are traditionally associated with nosocomial MRSA isolates, whereas types 4–6 have been associated with the epidemic CA-MRSA strains.

A limited number of MRSA clones have been responsible for most community- and hospital-associated infections worldwide. A comparison of these strains with those from earlier outbreaks (e.g., the phage 80/81 strains from the 1950s) has revealed preservation of the nucleotide sequence over time. This observation suggests that these strains possess determinants that facilitate survival and spread.

Regulation of Virulence Gene Expression In both toxin-mediated and non-toxin-mediated diseases due to *S. aureus*, the expression of virulence determinants associated with infection depends on a series of regulatory genes (e.g., accessory gene regulator [*agr*] and staphylococcal accessory regulator [*sar*]) that coordinately control the expression of many virulence genes. The regulatory gene *agr* is part of a quorum-sensing signal transduction pathway that senses and responds to bacterial density. Staphylococcal surface proteins are synthesized during the bacterial exponential growth phase in vitro. In contrast, many secreted proteins, such as α toxin, the enterotoxins, and assorted enzymes, are released during the postexponential growth phase in response to transcription of the effector molecule of *agr*, RNAIII.

It has been hypothesized that these regulatory genes serve a similar function in vivo. Successful invasion requires the sequential expression of these different bacterial elements. Bacterial adhesins are needed to initiate colonization of host tissue surfaces. The subsequent release of various enzymes enables the colony to obtain nutritional support and permits bacteria to spread to adjacent tissues. Studies with strains in which these regulatory genes are inactivated show reduced virulence in several animal models of *S. aureus* infection.

Pathogenesis of Invasive *S. aureus* Infection Staphylococci are opportunists. For these organisms to invade the host and cause infection, some or all of the following steps are necessary: contamination and colonization of host tissue surfaces, breach of cutaneous or mucosal barriers, establishment of a localized infection, invasion, evasion of the host response, and metastatic spread. Colonizing strains or strains transferred from other individuals are introduced into damaged skin, a wound, or the bloodstream. Recurrences of *S. aureus* infections are common, apparently because of the capacity of these pathogens to survive, to persist in a quiescent state in various tissues, and then to cause recrudescent infections when suitable conditions arise.

***S. AUREUS* COLONIZATION OF BODY SURFACES** The anterior nares is one of the primary sites of staphylococcal colonization in humans. Colonization appears to involve the attachment of *S. aureus* to keratinized epithelial cells of the anterior nares. Other factors that may contribute to colonization include the influence of other resident nasal flora and their bacterial density, host factors, and nasal mucosal damage (e.g., that resulting from inhalational drug use). Other colonized body sites, such as damaged skin, the groin, and the oropharynx, may be particularly important reservoirs for CA-MRSA strains.

INOCULATION AND COLONIZATION OF TISSUE SURFACES Staphylococci may be introduced into tissue as a result of minor abrasions, administration of medications such as insulin, or establishment of IV access with catheters. After their introduction into a tissue site, bacteria replicate and colonize the host tissue surface. A family of structurally related *S. aureus* surface proteins referred to as MSCRAMMs (microbial surface components recognizing adhesive matrix molecules) plays an important role in mediating adherence to these sites. By adhering to exposed matrix molecules (e.g., fibrinogen, fibronectin), MSCRAMMs such as clumping factor and collagen-binding protein enable the bacteria to colonize different tissue surfaces; these proteins contribute to the pathogenesis of invasive infections such as endocarditis and septic arthritis by facilitating the adherence of *S. aureus* to surfaces with exposed fibrinogen or collagen.

Although CoNS are classically known for their ability to elaborate biofilms and to colonize prosthetic devices, *S. aureus* also possesses the genes responsible for biofilm formation, such as the intercellular adhesion (*ica*) locus. Binding to these devices occurs in a stepwise fashion, involving staphylococcal adherence to serum constituents that have coated the device surface and subsequent biofilm elaboration. *S. aureus* is thus a frequent cause of biomedical-device infections.

INVASION After colonization, staphylococci replicate at the initial site of infection, elaborating enzymes that include serine proteases, hyaluronidases, thermonucleases, and lipases. These enzymes facilitate bacterial survival and local spread across tissue surfaces, although their precise role in infections is not well defined. The lipases may facilitate survival in lipid-rich areas such as the hair follicles, where *S. aureus* infections are often initiated. The *S. aureus* toxin Panton-Valentine leukocidin is cytolytic to PMNs, macrophages, and monocytes. Strains elaborating this toxin have been epidemiologically linked with cutaneous and more serious infections caused by strains of CA-MRSA. MSCRAMMs also appear to play an important role in the ability of *S. aureus* to spread and cause disease at other tissue sites.

Constitutional findings may result from either localized or systemic infections. The staphylococcal cell wall—consisting of alternating N-acetyl muramic acid and N-acetyl glucosamine units in combination with an additional cell wall component, lipoteichoic acid—can initiate an inflammatory response that includes the sepsis syndrome. Staphylococcal α toxin, which causes pore formation in various eukaryotic cells, can also initiate an inflammatory response with findings suggestive of sepsis.

EVASION OF HOST DEFENSE MECHANISMS Staphylococci have a multitude of immune evasion strategies that are critical to their success as invasive pathogens. They possess an antiphagocytic polysaccharide microcapsule. Most human *S. aureus* infections are due to capsular types 5 and 8. The zwitterionic (both negatively and positively charged) *S. aureus* capsule plays a critical role in the induction of abscess formation. Protein A, an MSCRAMM unique to *S. aureus*, acts as an Fc receptor, binding the Fc portion of IgG subclasses 1, 2, and 4 and preventing opsonophagocytosis by PMNs. Both chemotaxis inhibitory protein of staphylococci (CHIPS, a secreted protein) and extracellular adherence protein (EAP, a surface protein) interfere with PMN migration to sites of infection.

An additional potential mechanism of *S. aureus* evasion is its capacity for intracellular survival. Both professional and nonprofessional phagocytes internalize staphylococci. Internalization by these cells may provide a sanctuary that protects bacteria against the host's defenses. The intracellular environment favors the phenotypic expression of *S. aureus* small-colony variants. Small-colony variants are found in patients receiving antimicrobial therapy (e.g., with aminoglycosides) and in those with cystic fibrosis or osteomyelitis. These variants, whether intra- or extracellular, may facilitate prolonged staphylococcal survival in different tissue sites and enhance the likelihood of recurrences. Finally, *S. aureus* can survive within PMNs and may use these cells to spread and to seed other tissue sites.

PATHOGENESIS OF COMMUNITY-ACQUIRED MRSA INFECTIONS A number of virulence determinants have been identified as contributing to the pathogenesis of CA-MRSA infections. There is a strong epidemiologic association linking the presence of the gene for the Panton-Valentine leukocidin with skin and soft tissue infections as well as with necrotizing postinfluenza pneumonia. Other determinants that play a role in the pathogenesis of these infections include the arginine catabolic mobile element (ACME), a cluster of unique genes that may facilitate evasion of host defense mechanisms; phenol-soluble modulins, a family of cytolytic peptides; and α toxin.

Host Response to *S. aureus* Infection The primary host response to *S. aureus* infection is the recruitment of PMNs. These cells are attracted to infection sites by bacterial components such as formylated peptides or peptidoglycan as well as by the cytokines tumor necrosis factor (TNF) and interleukins (ILs) 1 and 6, which are released by activated macrophages and endothelial cells.

Although most individuals have antibodies to staphylococci, it is not clear that antibody levels are qualitatively or quantitatively sufficient to protect against infection. Although anticapsular and anti-MSCRAMM antibodies facilitate opsonization in vitro and have been protective against infection in several animal models, they have not yet successfully prevented staphylococcal infections in clinical trials.

Pathogenesis of Toxin-Mediated Disease *S. aureus* produces three types of toxin: cytotoxins, pyrogenic toxin superantigens, and exfoliative toxins. Both epidemiologic data and studies in animals suggest that antitoxin antibodies are protective against illness in TSS, staphylococcal food poisoning, and staphylococcal scalded-skin syndrome (SSSS). Illness develops after toxin synthesis and absorption and the subsequent toxin-initiated host response.

ENTEROTOXIN AND TOXIC SHOCK SYNDROME TOXIN 1 (TSST-1) The pyrogenic toxin superantigens are a family of small-molecular-size, structurally similar proteins that are responsible for two diseases: TSS and food poisoning. TSS results from the ability of enterotoxins and TSST-1 to function as T cell mitogens. In the normal process of antigen presentation, the antigen is first processed within the cell, and peptides are then presented in the major histocompatibility complex (MHC) class II groove, initiating a measured T cell response. In contrast, enterotoxins bind directly to the invariant region of MHC—outside the MHC class II groove. The enterotoxins can then bind T cell receptors via the vβ chain; this binding results in a dramatic overexpansion of T cell clones (up to 20% of the total T cell population). The consequence of this T cell expansion is a "cytokine storm," with the release of inflammatory mediators that include interferon γ, IL-1, IL-6, TNF-α, and TNF-β. The resulting multisystem disease produces a constellation of findings that mimic those in endotoxin shock; however, the pathogenic mechanisms differ. The release of endotoxin from the gastrointestinal tract may synergistically enhance the toxin's effects.

A different region of the enterotoxin molecule is responsible for the symptoms of food poisoning. The enterotoxins are heat stable and can survive conditions that kill the bacteria. Illness results from the ingestion of preformed toxin. As a result, the incubation period is short (1–6 h). The toxin stimulates the vagus nerve and the vomiting center of the brain. It also appears to stimulate intestinal peristaltic activity.

EXFOLIATIVE TOXINS AND SSSS The exfoliative toxins are responsible for SSSS. The toxins that produce disease in humans are of two serotypes: ETA and ETB. These toxins are serine proteases, which cleave desmosomal cadherins in the superficial layer of the skin, triggering exfoliation. The result is a split in the epidermis at the granular level, which is responsible for the superficial desquamation of the skin that typifies this illness.

DIAGNOSIS

Staphylococcal infections are readily diagnosed by Gram's stain (Fig. 172-1) and microscopic examination of abscess contents or of infected tissue. Routine culture of infected material usually yields positive results, and blood cultures are sometimes positive even when infections are localized to extravascular sites. *S. aureus* is rarely a blood culture contaminant. Polymerase chain reaction (PCR)–based assays have been applied to the rapid diagnosis of *S. aureus* infection and are increasingly used in clinical microbiology laboratories. A number of point-of-care tests are now available to screen patients for colonization with MRSA. Determining whether patients with documented *S. aureus* bacteremia also have infective endocarditis or a metastatic focus of infection remains a diagnostic challenge. Uniformly positive blood cultures suggest an endovascular infection such as endocarditis (see "Bacteremia, Sepsis, and Infective Endocarditis," below).

CLINICAL SYNDROMES

(Table 172-1)

Skin and Soft Tissue Infections *S. aureus* causes a variety of cutaneous infections, many of which can also be caused by group A streptococci

TABLE 172-1 COMMON ILLNESSES CAUSED BY *STAPHYLOCOCCUS AUREUS*
Skin and Soft Tissue Infections
Folliculitis
Abscess, furuncle, carbuncle
Cellulitis
Impetigo
Mastitis
Surgical wound infections
Musculoskeletal Infections
Septic arthritis
Osteomyelitis (hematogenous or contiguous spread)
Pyomyositis
Psoas abscess
Respiratory Tract Infections
Ventilator-associated or nosocomial pneumonia
Septic pulmonary emboli
Postviral pneumonia (e.g., influenza)
Empyema
Bacteremia and its Complications
Sepsis, septic shock
Metastatic foci of infection (kidney, joints, bone, lung)
Infective endocarditis
Infective Endocarditis
Injection drug use–associated
Native-valve
Prosthetic-valve
Nosocomial
Device-Related Infections (e.g., intravascular catheters, prosthetic joints)
Toxin-Mediated Illnesses
Toxic shock syndrome
Food poisoning
Staphylococcal scalded-skin syndrome
Invasive Infections Associated with Community-Acquired Methicillin-Resistant *S. aureus*
Necrotizing fasciitis
Waterhouse-Friderichsen syndrome
Necrotizing pneumonia
Purpura fulminans

or (less commonly) other streptococcal species. Common factors predisposing to *S. aureus* cutaneous infection include chronic skin conditions (e.g., eczema), skin damage (e.g., insect bites, minor trauma), injections (e.g., in diabetes, injection drug use), and poor personal hygiene. These infections are characterized by the formation of pus-containing blisters, which often begin in hair follicles and spread to adjoining tissues. *Folliculitis* is a superficial infection that involves the hair follicle, with a central area of purulence (pus) surrounded by induration and erythema. *Furuncles* (boils) are more extensive, painful lesions that tend to occur in hairy, moist regions of the body and extend from the hair follicle to become a true abscess with an area of central purulence. *Carbuncles* are most often located in the lower neck and are even more severe and painful, resulting from the coalescence of other lesions that extend to a deeper layer of the subcutaneous tissue. In general, furuncles and carbuncles are readily apparent, with pus often expressible or discharging from the abscess. Other cutaneous *S. aureus* infections include impetigo and cellulitis. *S. aureus* is one of the most common causes of surgical wound infection.

Mastitis develops in 1–3% of nursing mothers. This infection of the breast, which generally presents within 2–3 weeks after delivery, is characterized by findings that range from cellulitis to abscess formation. Systemic signs, such as fever and chills, are often present in more severe cases.

Musculoskeletal Infections *S. aureus* is among the most common causes of bone infections—both those resulting from hematogenous dissemination and those arising from contiguous spread from a soft tissue site. *Hematogenous osteomyelitis* in children most often involves the long bones. Infections present as fever and bone pain or with a child's reluctance to bear weight. The white blood cell count and erythrocyte sedimentation rate are often elevated. Blood cultures are positive in ~50% of cases. When necessary, bone biopsies for culture and histopathologic examination are usually diagnostic. Routine x-rays may be normal for up to 14 days after the onset of symptoms. ^{99m}Tc-phosphonate scanning often detects early evidence of infection. MRI is more sensitive than other techniques in establishing a radiologic diagnosis.

In adults, hematogenous osteomyelitis involving the long bones is less common. However, *vertebral osteomyelitis* is among the more common clinical presentations. Vertebral bone infections are most often seen in patients with endocarditis, those undergoing hemodialysis, diabetics, and injection drug users. These infections may present as intense back pain and fever but may also be clinically occult, presenting as chronic back pain and low-grade fever. *S. aureus* is the most common cause of epidural abscess, a complication that can result in neurologic compromise. Patients complain of difficulty voiding or walking and of radicular pain in addition to the symptoms associated with their osteomyelitis. Surgical intervention in this setting often constitutes a medical emergency. MRI most reliably establishes the diagnosis (Fig. 172-2).

Bone infections that result from contiguous spread tend to develop from soft tissue infections, such as those associated with diabetic or vascular ulcers, surgery, or trauma. Exposure of bone, a draining fistulous tract, failure to heal, or continued drainage suggests involvement of underlying bone. Bone involvement is established by bone culture and histopathologic examination (revealing evidence of PMN infiltration). Contamination of culture material from adjacent tissue can make the diagnosis of osteomyelitis difficult in the absence of pathologic confirmation. In addition, it is sometimes hard to distinguish radiologically between osteomyelitis and overlying soft tissue infection with underlying osteitis.

In both children and adults, *S. aureus* is the most common cause of *septic arthritis* in native joints. This infection is rapidly progressive and may be associated with extensive joint destruction if left untreated. It presents as intense pain on motion of the affected joint, swelling, and fever. Aspiration of the joint reveals turbid fluid, with >50,000 PMNs/μL and gram-positive cocci in clusters on Gram's stain (Fig. 172-1). In

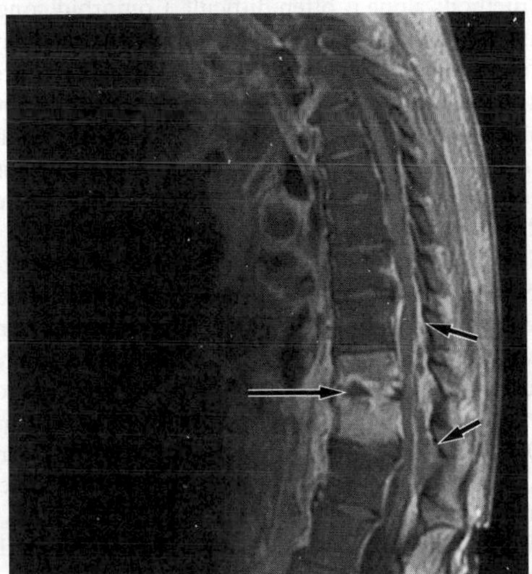

FIGURE 172-2 *S. aureus* vertebral osteomyelitis and epidural abscess involving the thoracic disk between T9 and T10. Sagittal postcontrast MRI of the spine illustrates destruction of the T9–T10 intervertebral space with enhancement (*arrow*). There is impingement on the thoracic cord and an epidural collection extending from T9 through T11 (*short arrows*).

adults, septic arthritis may result from trauma, surgery, or hematogenous dissemination. The most commonly involved joints include the knees, shoulders, hips, and phalanges. Infection frequently develops in joints previously damaged by osteoarthritis or rheumatoid arthritis. Iatrogenic infections resulting from aspiration or injection of agents into the joint also occur. In these settings, the patient experiences increased pain and swelling in the involved joint in association with fever.

Pyomyositis is an unusual infection of skeletal muscles that is seen primarily in tropical climates but also occurs in immunocompromised and HIV-infected patients. It is believed to arise from occult bacteremia. Pyomyositis presents as fever, swelling, and pain overlying the involved muscle. Aspiration of fluid from the involved tissue yields pus. Although a history of trauma may be associated with the infection, its pathogenesis is poorly understood.

Respiratory Tract Infections Respiratory tract infections caused by *S. aureus* occur in selected clinical settings. *S. aureus* is a cause of serious respiratory tract infections in newborns and infants; these infections present with shortness of breath, fever, and respiratory failure. Chest x-ray may reveal pneumatoceles (shaggy, thin-walled cavities). Pneumothorax and empyema are recognized complications.

In adults, nosocomial *S. aureus* pulmonary infections are common among intubated patients in intensive care units. Nasally colonized patients are at increased risk of these infections. The clinical presentation is no different from that encountered in pulmonary infections of other bacterial etiologies. Patients produce increased volumes of purulent sputum and develop respiratory distress, fever, and new pulmonary infiltrates. Distinguishing bacterial pneumonia from respiratory failure or other causes of new pulmonary infiltrates in critically ill patients is often difficult and relies on a constellation of clinical, radiologic, and laboratory findings.

Community-acquired respiratory tract infections due to *S. aureus* usually follow viral infections—most commonly influenza. Patients may present with fever, bloody sputum production, and midlung-field pneumatoceles or multiple, patchy pulmonary infiltrates. Diagnosis is made by sputum Gram's stain and culture. Blood cultures, although useful, are usually negative.

Bacteremia, Sepsis, and Infective Endocarditis *S. aureus* bacteremia may be complicated by sepsis, endocarditis, vasculitis, or metastatic seeding (establishment of suppurative collections at other tissue sites). The frequency of metastatic seeding during bacteremia has been estimated to be as high as 31%. Among the more commonly seeded tissue sites are bones, joints, kidneys, and lungs.

Recognition of these complications by clinical and laboratory diagnostic methods alone is often difficult. Comorbid conditions that are frequently seen in association with *S. aureus* bacteremia and that increase the risk of complications include diabetes, HIV infection, and renal insufficiency. Other host factors associated with an increased risk of complications include presentation with community-acquired *S. aureus* bacteremia (except in injection drug users), lack of an identifiable primary focus of infection, and the presence of prosthetic devices or material.

Clinically, *S. aureus* sepsis presents in a manner similar to that documented for sepsis due to other bacteria. The well-described progression of hemodynamic changes—beginning with respiratory alkalosis and clinical findings of hypotension and fever—is commonly seen. The microbiologic diagnosis is established by positive blood cultures.

The overall incidence of *S. aureus* endocarditis has increased over the past 20 years. *S. aureus* is now the leading cause of endocarditis worldwide, accounting for 25–35% of cases. This increase is due, at least in part, to the increased use of intravascular devices. Studies of patients with *S. aureus* bacteremia and intravascular catheters that used transesophageal echocardiography found an infective endocarditis incidence of ~25%. Other factors associated with an increased risk of endocarditis are injection drug use, hemodialysis, the presence of intravascular prosthetic devices at the time of bacteremia, and immunosuppression. Patients with implantable cardiac devices (e.g., permanent pacemakers) are at increased risk of endocarditis or device-related infections. Despite the availability of effective antibiotics, mortality rates from these infections continue to range from 20% to 40%, depending on both the host and the nature of the infection. Complications of *S. aureus* endocarditis include cardiac valvular insufficiency, peripheral emboli, metastatic seeding, and central nervous system (CNS) involvement (e.g., mycotic aneurysms, embolic strokes).

S. aureus endocarditis is encountered in four clinical settings: (1) right-sided endocarditis in association with injection drug use, (2) left-sided native-valve endocarditis, (3) prosthetic-valve endocarditis, and (4) nosocomial endocarditis. In each of these settings, the diagnosis is suspected by recognition of clinical stigmata suggestive of endocarditis. These findings include cardiac manifestations, such as new or changing cardiac valvular murmurs; cutaneous evidence, such as vasculitic lesions, Osler's nodes, or Janeway lesions; evidence of right- or left-sided embolic disease; and a history suggesting a risk for *S. aureus* bacteremia. In the absence of antecedent antibiotic therapy, blood cultures are almost uniformly positive. Transthoracic echocardiography, while less sensitive than transesophageal echocardiography, is less invasive and may establish the presence of valvular vegetations. The Duke criteria (see Table 155-3) are now commonly used to help establish the likelihood of this diagnosis.

Acute right-sided tricuspid valvular *S. aureus* endocarditis is most often seen in injection drug users. The classic presentation includes a high fever, a toxic clinical appearance, pleuritic chest pain, and the production of purulent (sometimes bloody) sputum. Chest x-rays or CT scans reveal evidence of septic pulmonary emboli (small, peripheral, circular lesions that may cavitate with time) (Fig. 172-3). A high percentage of affected patients have no history of antecedent valvular damage. At the outset of their illness, patients may present with fever alone, without cardiac or other localizing findings. As a result, a high index of clinical suspicion is essential for diagnosis.

Individuals with antecedent cardiac valvular damage more commonly present with left-sided native-valve endocarditis involving the damaged valve. These patients tend to be older than those with right-sided endocarditis, their prognosis is worse, and their incidence of complications (including peripheral emboli, cardiac decompensation, and metastatic seeding) is higher.

S. aureus is one of the more common causes of prosthetic-valve endocarditis. This infection is especially fulminant in the early postoperative period and is associated with a high mortality rate. In most instances, medical therapy alone is not sufficient and urgent valve replacement is necessary. Patients are prone to develop valvular insufficiency or myocardial abscesses originating from the region of valve implantation.

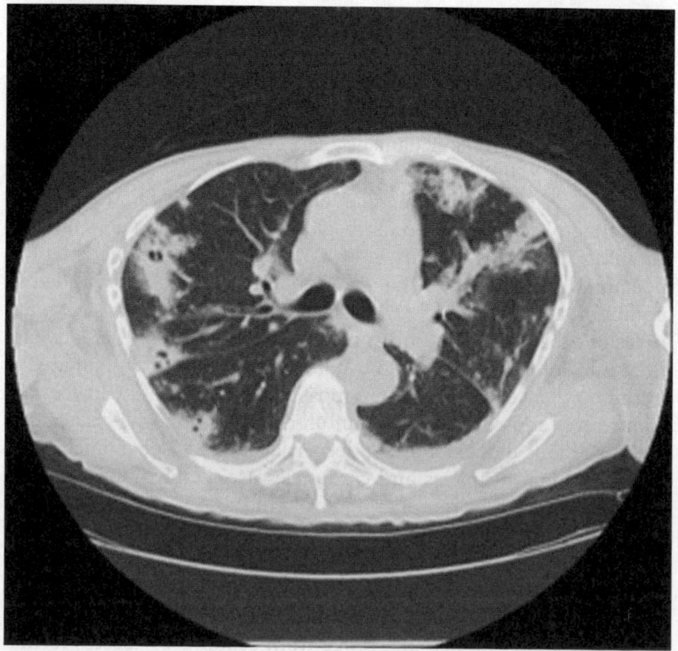

FIGURE 172-3 CT scan illustrating septic pulmonary emboli in a patient with methicillin-resistant *Staphylococcus aureus* bacteremia.

The increased frequency of nosocomial endocarditis (15–30% of cases, depending on the series) reflects in part the increased use of intravascular devices. This form of endocarditis is most commonly caused by *S. aureus*. Because patients often are critically ill, are receiving antibiotics for various other indications, and have comorbid conditions, the diagnosis is often missed.

Urinary Tract Infections Urinary tract infections (UTIs) are infrequently caused by *S. aureus*. The presence of *S. aureus* in the urine generally suggests hematogenous dissemination. Ascending *S. aureus* infections occasionally result from instrumentation of the genitourinary tract.

Prosthetic Device–Related Infections *S. aureus* accounts for a large proportion of prosthetic device–related infections. These infections often involve intravascular catheters, prosthetic valves, orthopedic devices, peritoneal catheters, pacemakers, left-ventricular-assist devices, and vascular grafts. In contrast with the more indolent presentation of CoNS infections, *S. aureus* device-related infections are often more acute, with both localized and systemic manifestations. The latter infections also tend to progress more rapidly. It is relatively common for a pyogenic collection to be present at the device site. Aspiration of these collections and performance of blood cultures are important components in establishing a diagnosis. *S. aureus* infections tend to occur more commonly soon after implantation unless the device is used for access (e.g., intravascular or hemodialysis catheters). In the latter instance, infections can occur at any time. As in most prosthetic-device infections, successful therapy usually involves removal of the device. Left in place, the device is a potential nidus for either persistent or recurrent infections.

Infections Associated with Community-Acquired MRSA Although the skin and soft tissues are the most common sites of infection associated with CA-MRSA, 5–10% of these infections are invasive and can even be life-threatening. The latter unique infections, including necrotizing fasciitis, necrotizing pneumonia, and sepsis with Waterhouse-Friderichsen syndrome or purpura fulminans, were rarely associated with *S. aureus* prior to the emergence of CA-MRSA. These life-threatening infections reflect the increased virulence of CA-MRSA strains.

Toxin-Mediated Diseases • ***FOOD POISONING*** *S. aureus* is among the most common causes of foodborne outbreaks of infection in the United States. Staphylococcal food poisoning results from the inoculation of toxin-producing *S. aureus* into food by colonized food handlers. Toxin is then elaborated in such growth-promoting food as custards, potato salad, or processed meats. Even if the bacteria are killed by warming, the heat-stable toxin is not destroyed. The onset of illness is rapid, occurring within 1–6 h of ingestion. The illness is characterized by nausea and vomiting, although diarrhea, hypotension, and dehydration may also occur. The differential diagnosis includes diarrhea of other etiologies, especially that caused by similar toxins (e.g., the toxins elaborated by *Bacillus cereus*). The rapidity of onset, the absence of fever, and the epidemic nature of the presentation (without second-degree spread) arouse suspicion of staphylococcal food poisoning. Symptoms generally resolve within 8–10 h. The diagnosis can be established by the demonstration of bacteria or the documentation of enterotoxin in the implicated food. Treatment is entirely supportive.

TOXIC SHOCK SYNDROME TSS gained attention in the early 1980s, when a nationwide outbreak occurred in the United States among young, otherwise healthy, menstruating women. Epidemiologic investigation demonstrated that these cases were associated with the use of a highly absorbent tampon that had recently been introduced to the market. Subsequent studies established the role of TSST-1 in these illnesses. Withdrawal of the tampon from the market resulted in a rapid decline in the incidence of this disease. However, menstrual and nonmenstrual cases continue to be reported. Nonmenstrual cases are frequently seen in patients with surgical or postpartum wound infections.

The clinical presentation is similar in menstrual and nonmenstrual TSS. Evidence of clinical *S. aureus* infection is not a prerequisite.

TABLE 172-2 CASE DEFINITION OF *S. AUREUS* TOXIC SHOCK SYNDROME

1. Fever: temperature of ≥38.9°C (≥102°F)
2. Hypotension: systolic blood pressure of ≤90 mmHg or orthostatic hypotension (orthostatic drop in diastolic blood pressure by ≥15 mmHg, orthostatic syncope, or orthostatic dizziness)
3. Diffuse macular rash, with desquamation 1–2 weeks after onset (including the palms and soles)
4. Multisystem involvement
    a. Hepatic: bilirubin or aminotransferase levels ≥2 times normal
    b. Hematologic: platelet count ≤100,000/μL
    c. Renal: blood urea nitrogen or serum creatinine level ≥2 times the normal upper limit
    d. Mucous membranes: vaginal, oropharyngeal, or conjunctival hyperemia
    e. Gastrointestinal: vomiting or diarrhea at onset of illness
    f. Muscular: severe myalgias or serum creatine phosphokinase level ≥2 times the normal upper limit
    g. Central nervous system: disorientation or alteration in consciousness without focal neurologic signs and in the absence of fever and hypotension
5. Negative serologic or other tests for measles, leptospirosis, and Rocky Mountain spotted fever as well as negative blood or cerebrospinal fluid cultures for organisms other than *S. aureus*

Source: M Wharton et al: Case definitions for public health surveillance. MMWR 39:1, 1990; with permission.

TSS results from the elaboration of an enterotoxin or the structurally related enterotoxin-like TSST-1. More than 90% of menstrual cases are caused by TSST-1, whereas a high percentage of nonmenstrual cases are caused by enterotoxins. TSS begins with relatively nonspecific flu-like symptoms. In menstrual cases, the onset usually comes 2 or 3 days after the start of menstruation. Patients present with fever, hypotension, and erythroderma of variable intensity. Mucosal involvement is common (e.g., conjunctival hyperemia). The illness can rapidly progress to symptoms that include vomiting, diarrhea, confusion, myalgias, and abdominal pain. These symptoms reflect the multisystemic nature of the disease, with involvement of the liver, kidneys, gastrointestinal tract, and/or CNS. Desquamation of the skin occurs during convalescence, usually 1–2 weeks after the onset of illness. Laboratory findings may include azotemia, leukocytosis, hypoalbuminemia, thrombocytopenia, and liver function abnormalities.

Diagnosis of TSS still depends on a constellation of findings rather than one specific finding and on a lack of evidence of other possible infections (Table 172-2). Other diagnoses to be considered are drug toxicities, viral exanthems, Rocky Mountain spotted fever, sepsis, and Kawasaki disease. Illness occurs only in persons who lack antibody to TSST-1. Recurrences are possible if antibody fails to develop after the illness.

STAPHYLOCOCCAL SCALDED-SKIN SYNDROME SSSS primarily affects newborns and children. The illness may vary from a localized blister to exfoliation of much of the skin surface. The skin is usually fragile and often tender, with thin-walled, fluid-filled bullae. Gentle pressure results in rupture of the lesions, leaving denuded underlying skin (*Nikolsky's sign*; Fig. 172-4). The mucous membranes are usually spared. In more generalized infection, there are often constitutional symptoms, including fever, lethargy, and irritability with poor feeding. Significant amounts of fluid can be lost in more extensive cases. Illness usually follows localized infection at one of a number of possible sites. SSSS is much less common among adults but can follow infections caused by exfoliative toxin–producing strains.

PREVENTION

Primary prevention of *S. aureus* infections in the hospital setting involves hand washing and careful attention to appropriate isolation procedures. Through careful screening for MRSA carriage and strict isolation practices, several Scandinavian countries have been remarkably

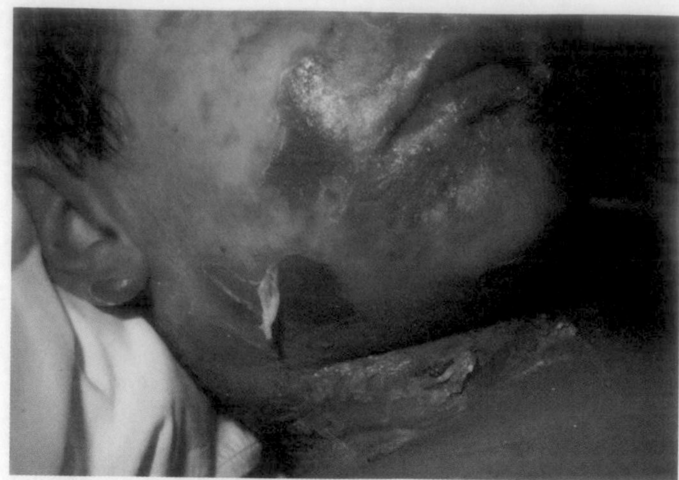

FIGURE 172-4 Evidence of staphylococcal scalded-skin syndrome in a 6-year-old boy. Nikolsky's sign, with separation of the superficial layer of the outer epidermal layer, is visible. *(Reprinted with permission from LA Schenfeld et al: N Engl J Med 342:1178, 2000. © 2000 Massachusetts Medical Society. All rights reserved.)*

successful at preventing the introduction and dissemination of MRSA in hospitals.

Decolonization strategies, using both universal and targeted approaches with topical agents (e.g., mupirocin) to eliminate nasal colonization and/or chlorhexidine to eliminate cutaneous colonization with *S. aureus*, have been successful in some clinical settings (e.g., intensive care units) where the risk of infection is high. An analysis of clinical trials suggests that there may also be a reduction in the incidence of postsurgical infections among persons who are nasally colonized with *S. aureus*.

"Bundling" (the application of selected medical interventions in a sequence of prescribed steps) has reduced rates of nosocomial infections related to such procedures as the insertion of intravenous catheters, in which staphylococci are among the most common pathogens (see Table 168-4). A number of immunization strategies to prevent *S. aureus* infections—both active (e.g., capsular polysaccharide–protein conjugate vaccine) and passive (e.g., clumping factor antibody)—have been investigated. However, none has been successful for either prophylaxis or therapy in clinical trials.

COAGULASE-NEGATIVE STAPHYLOCOCCAL INFECTIONS

Although considerably less virulent than *S. aureus*, CoNS are among the most common causes of prosthetic-device infections. Approximately half of the identified CoNS species have been associated with human infections. Of these species, *Staphylococcus epidermidis* is the most common human pathogen. This component of the normal human flora is found on the skin (where it is the most abundant bacterial species) as well as in the oropharynx and vagina. *Staphylococcus saprophyticus*, a novobiocin-resistant species, is a common pathogen in UTIs.

PATHOGENESIS

S. epidermidis is the CoNS species most often associated with prosthetic-device infections. Infection is a two-step process, with initial adhesion to the device followed by colonization. *S. epidermidis* is uniquely adapted to colonize these devices by its capacity to elaborate the extracellular polysaccharide (glycocalyx or slime) that facilitates formation of a protective biofilm on the device surface.

Implanted prosthetic material is rapidly coated with host serum or tissue constituents such as fibrinogen or fibronectin. These molecules serve as potential bridging ligands, facilitating initial bacterial attachment to the device surface. A number of staphylococcal surface-associated proteins, such as autolysin (AtlE), fibrinogen-binding protein, and accumulation-associated protein (AAP), may play a role in attachment to either modified or unmodified prosthetic surfaces. The polysaccharide intercellular adhesin facilitates subsequent staphylococcal colonization and accumulation on the device surface. In *S. epidermidis*, intercellular adhesin (*ica*) genes are more commonly found in strains associated with device infections than in strains associated with colonization of mucosal surfaces. Biofilm appears to act as a barrier protecting bacteria from host defense mechanisms as well as from antibiotics, while providing a suitable environment for bacterial survival. Poly-γ-DL-glutamic acid is secreted by *S. epidermidis* and provides protection against neutrophil phagocytosis.

Two additional staphylococcal species, *Staphylococcus lugdunensis* and *Staphylococcus schleiferi*, produce more serious infections (native-valve endocarditis and osteomyelitis) than do other CoNS. The basis for this enhanced virulence is not known, although both species appear to share more virulence determinants with *S. aureus* (e.g., clumping factor and lipase) than do other CoNS.

The capacity of *S. saprophyticus* to cause UTIs in young women appears to be related to its enhanced capacity to adhere to uroepithelial cells. A 160-kDa hemagglutinin/adhesin may contribute to this affinity.

DIAGNOSIS

Although the detection of CoNS at sites of infection or in the bloodstream is not difficult by standard microbiologic culture methods, interpretation of these results is frequently problematic. Because these organisms are present in large numbers on the skin, they often contaminate cultures. It has been estimated that only 10–25% of blood cultures positive for CoNS reflect true bacteremia. Similar problems arise with cultures obtained from other sites. Among the clinical findings suggestive of true bacteremia are fever, evidence of local infection (e.g., erythema or purulent drainage at the IV catheter site), leukocytosis, and systemic signs of sepsis. Laboratory findings suggestive of true bacteremia include multiple isolations of the same strain (i.e., the same species with the same antibiogram or a closely related DNA fingerprint) from separate cultures, growth of the strain within 48 h, and bacterial growth in both aerobic and anaerobic bottles.

CLINICAL SYNDROMES

CoNS cause a diverse array of prosthetic device–related infections, including those that involve prosthetic cardiac valves and joints, vascular grafts, intravascular devices, and CNS shunts. In all of these settings, the clinical presentation is similar. The signs of localized infection are often subtle, the rate of disease progression is slow, and the systemic findings are often limited. Signs of infection, such as purulent drainage, pain at the site, or loosening of prosthetic implants, are sometimes evident. Fever is frequently but not always present, and there may be mild leukocytosis. Acute-phase reactant levels, the erythrocyte sedimentation rate, and the C-reactive protein concentration may be elevated.

Infections that are not associated with prosthetic devices are infrequent, although native-valve endocarditis due to CoNS has accounted for ~5% of cases in some reviews. *S. lugdunensis* appears to be a more aggressive pathogen in this setting, causing greater mortality and rapid valvular destruction with abscess formation.

TREATMENT STAPHYLOCOCCAL INFECTIONS

GENERAL PRINCIPLES OF THERAPY

Surgical incision and drainage of all suppurative collections constitute the most important therapeutic intervention for staphylococcal infections. The emergence of MRSA in the community has increased the importance of culturing all collections in order to identify pathogens and to determine antimicrobial susceptibility. Successful therapy for prosthetic-device infections generally requires device removal. In situations in which removal is not possible or the infection is due to CoNS, an initial attempt at medical therapy without device removal may be warranted. Because of the well-recognized risk of complications associated with *S. aureus* bacteremia (e.g., endocarditis, metastatic foci of infection), therapy is generally prolonged (4–6 weeks) unless the patient is identified as being among those individuals who are at low risk for complications.

DURATION OF ANTIMICROBIAL THERAPY

Debate continues regarding the duration of therapy for bacteremic *S. aureus* infections. Patients with "complicated" bacteremia are at increased risk of endocarditis and metastatic infections. Among the findings associated with an increased risk of complicated bacteremia are persistently positive blood cultures 96 h after institution of therapy, acquisition of the infection in the community, failure to remove a removable focus of infection (i.e., an intravascular catheter), and infection with cutaneous or embolic manifestations. For immunocompetent patients in whom short-course therapy is planned, transesophageal echocardiography to rule out endocarditis is warranted because neither clinical nor laboratory findings can reliably detect cardiac involvement. In addition, an aggressive radiologic investigation to identify potential metastatic collections is indicated. All symptomatic body sites must be carefully evaluated.

CHOICE OF ANTIMICROBIAL AGENTS

The choice of antimicrobial agents to treat both coagulase-positive and coagulase-negative staphylococcal infections has become increasingly problematic because of the prevalence of multidrug-resistant strains. Staphylococcal resistance to most antibiotic families, including β-lactams, aminoglycosides, fluoroquinolones, and (to a lesser extent) glycopeptides, has increased. This trend is more apparent with CoNS: >80% of nosocomial isolates are resistant to methicillin, and these methicillin-resistant strains are usually resistant to most other antibiotics as well. Because the selection of antimicrobial agents for *S. aureus* infections is similar to that for CoNS infections, treatment options for these pathogens are discussed together and are summarized in Table 172-3.

As a result of the widespread dissemination of plasmids containing the enzyme penicillinase, few strains of staphylococci (≤5%) remain susceptible to penicillin. However, penicillin remains the drug of choice against susceptible strains if the laboratory can reliably test for penicillin susceptibility. Penicillin-resistant isolates are treated with semisynthetic penicillinase-resistant penicillins (SPRPs), such as oxacillin or nafcillin. Methicillin, the first of the SPRPs, is now used infrequently. Cephalosporins are alternative therapeutic agents for these infections. Second- and third-generation cephalosporins do not offer a therapeutic advantage over first-generation cephalosporins for the treatment of staphylococcal infections. The carbapenems have excellent activity against methicillin-sensitive *S. aureus* but not against MRSA.

The isolation of MRSA was reported within 1 year of the introduction of methicillin. Since then, the prevalence of MRSA has steadily increased. In many hospitals, 40–50% of *S. aureus* isolates are now resistant to methicillin. Resistance to methicillin indicates resistance to all SPRPs as well as to all cephalosporins (except ceftaroline). Production of a novel penicillin-binding protein (PBP2a) is responsible for methicillin resistance. This protein is synthesized by the *mecA* gene, which (as stated above) is part of a large mobile genetic element—a pathogenicity or genomic island—called SCC*mec*. It is hypothesized that this genetic material was acquired via horizontal transfer from a related staphylococcal species, such as *Staphylococcus sciuri*. Phenotypic expression of methicillin resistance may be constitutive (i.e., expressed in all organisms in a population) or heterogeneous (i.e., displayed by only a proportion of the total organism population). Detection of methicillin resistance in the clinical microbiology laboratory can be difficult if the strain expresses heterogeneous resistance. Therefore, susceptibility studies are routinely performed at reduced temperatures (≤35°C for 24 h), with increased concentrations of salt in the medium to enhance the expression of resistance. In addition to PCR-based techniques, a number of rapid methods for the detection of methicillin resistance have been developed.

In light of decreasing susceptibility of MRSA isolates to vancomycin, both vancomycin and daptomycin are now recommended as the drugs of choice for the treatment of MRSA infections. Vancomycin is less effective than SPRPs for the treatment of infections due to methicillin-susceptible strains. Alternatives to SPRPs should be used only after careful consideration in patients with a history of serious β-lactam allergies.

Three types of staphylococcal resistance to vancomycin have emerged. (1) Minimal inhibitory concentration (MIC) "creep" refers to the incremental increase in vancomycin MICs that has been detected in various geographic areas. Studies suggest that infections due to *S. aureus* strains with vancomycin MICs of >1 μg/mL may not respond as well to vancomycin therapy as those due to strains with MICs of <1 μg/mL. Some authorities (e.g., *The Medical Letter*) have recommended choosing an alternative agent in this setting. (2) In 1997, an *S. aureus* strain with reduced susceptibility to vancomycin (vancomycin-intermediate *S. aureus* [VISA]) was reported from Japan. Subsequently, additional VISA clinical isolates were reported. These strains were all resistant to methicillin and many other antimicrobial agents. The VISA strains appear to evolve (under vancomycin selective pressure) from strains that are susceptible to vancomycin but are heterogeneous, with a small proportion of the bacterial population expressing the resistance phenotype. The mechanism of VISA resistance is in part due to an abnormally thick cell wall. Vancomycin is trapped by the abnormal peptidoglycan cross-linking and is unable to gain access to its target site. (3) In 2002, the first clinical isolate of fully vancomycin-resistant *S. aureus* was reported. Resistance in this and several additional clinical isolates was due to the presence of *vanA*, the gene responsible for expression of vancomycin resistance in enterococci. This observation suggested that resistance was acquired as a result of horizontal conjugal transfer from a vancomycin-resistant strain of *Enterococcus faecalis*. Several patients had both MRSA and vancomycin-resistant enterococci cultured from infection sites. The *vanA* gene is responsible for the synthesis of the dipeptide D-Ala-D-Lac in place of D-Ala-D-Ala. Vancomycin cannot bind to the altered peptide.

Daptomycin, a parenteral bactericidal agent with antistaphylococcal activity, is approved for the treatment of bacteremia (including right-sided endocarditis) and complicated skin infections. It is not effective in respiratory infections. This drug has a novel mechanism of action: it disrupts the cytoplasmic membrane. Staphylococcal resistance to daptomycin, sometimes developing during therapy, has been reported.

Linezolid—the first oxazolidinone—is bacteriostatic against staphylococci and offers the advantage of comparable bioavailability after oral or parenteral administration. Cross-resistance with other inhibitors of protein synthesis has not been detected. However, resistance to linezolid has been reported. Serious adverse reactions to linezolid include thrombocytopenia, occasional cases of neutropenia, and rare instances of peripheral and optic neuropathy.

Tedizolid, a second oxazolidinone released in 2014, is available as both oral and parenteral preparations. It has enhanced in vitro activity against antibiotic-resistant gram-positive bacteria, including staphylococci. Tedizolid is administered once a day.

Ceftaroline is a fifth-generation cephalosporin with bactericidal activity against MRSA (including strains with reduced susceptibility to vancomycin and daptomycin). It is approved for use in nosocomial pneumonias and for skin and soft tissue infections.

The parenteral streptogramin antibiotic quinupristin/dalfopristin displays bactericidal activity against all staphylococci, including VISA strains. This drug has been used successfully to treat serious MRSA infections. In cases of resistance to erythromycin or clindamycin, quinupristin/dalfopristin is bacteriostatic against staphylococci. There are limited data on the efficacy of either quinupristin/dalfopristin or linezolid for the treatment of infective endocarditis.

Telavancin is a parenteral lipoglycopeptide derivative of vancomycin that is approved for the treatment of complicated skin and soft tissue infections and for nosocomial pneumonia. The drug has two targets: the cell wall and the cell membrane. It remains active against VISA strains. Because of its nephrotoxicity, it should be avoided in patients with renal disease.

Dalbavancin is a long-acting, parenterally administered lipoglycopeptide that has been used to treat skin and soft tissue infections. Because of its long half-life, it can be administered on a weekly basis. There are limited data on its use in the treatment of invasive staphylococcal infections.

TABLE 172-3 ANTIMICROBIAL THERAPY FOR STAPHYLOCOCCAL INFECTIONS[a]

Sensitivity/Resistance of Isolate	Drug of Choice	Alternative(s)	Comments
Parenteral Therapy for Serious Infections			
Sensitive to penicillin	Penicillin G (4 mU q4h)	Nafcillin or oxacillin (2 g q4h), cefazolin (2 g q8h), vancomycin (1 g q12h[b])	Fewer than 5% of isolates are sensitive to penicillin. The clinical microbiology laboratory must verify that the strain is not a β-lactamase producer.
Sensitive to methicillin	Nafcillin or oxacillin (2 g q4h)	Cefazolin (2 g q8h), vancomycin (15–20 mg/kg q8–12h[b])	Patients with penicillin allergy can be treated with a cephalosporin if the allergy does not involve an anaphylactic or accelerated reaction; desensitization to β-lactams may be indicated in selected cases of serious infection when maximal bactericidal activity is needed (e.g., prosthetic-valve endocarditis[c]). Type A β-lactamase may rapidly hydrolyze cefazolin and reduce its efficacy in endocarditis. Vancomycin is a less effective option.
Resistant to methicillin	Vancomycin (15–20 mg/kg q8–12h[b]), daptomycin (6 mg/kg IV q24h[b,d]) for bacteremia, endocarditis, and complicated skin infections	Linezolid (600 mg q12h PO or IV), ceftaroline (600 mg IV q12h)	Sensitivity testing is necessary before an alternative drug is selected. For some serious infections, higher doses of daptomycin have been used. Quinupristin/dalfopristin is bactericidal against methicillin-resistant isolates unless the strain is resistant to erythromycin or clindamycin. The efficacy of adjunctive therapy is not well established in many settings. Both linezolid and quinupristin/dalfopristin have had in vitro activity against most VISA and VRSA strains. See footnote for treatment of prosthetic-valve endocarditis.[c]
Resistant to methicillin with intermediate or complete resistance to vancomycin[e]	Daptomycin (6 mg/kg q24h[b,d]) for bacteremia, endocarditis, and complicated skin infections	Same as for methicillin-resistant strains; check antibiotic susceptibilities *or* Ceftaroline (600 mg IV q12h) Newer agents include tedizolid (200 mg administered once daily either IV or orally) or dalbavancin (two IV doses: 1000 mg followed in 1 week by 500 mg). Both drugs are approved only for the treatment of skin and soft tissue infections.	Same as for methicillin-resistant strains; check antibiotic susceptibilities. Ceftaroline is used either alone or in combination with daptomycin.
Not yet known (i.e., empirical therapy)	Vancomycin (15–20 mg/kg q8–12h[b]), daptomycin (6 mg/kg q24h[b,d]) for bacteremia, endocarditis, and complicated skin infections	—	Empirical therapy is given when the susceptibility of the isolate is not known. Vancomycin is recommended for suspected community- or hospital-acquired *Staphylococcus aureus* infections because of the increased frequency of methicillin-resistant strains in the community.
Oral Therapy for Skin and Soft Tissue Infections			
Sensitive to methicillin	Dicloxacillin (500 mg qid), cephalexin (500 mg qid)	Minocycline or doxycycline (100 mg q12h[b]), TMP-SMX (1 or 2 ds tablets bid), clindamycin (300–450 mg/kg tid), linezolid (600 mg PO q12h), tedizolid (200 mg PO q24h)	It is important to know the antibiotic susceptibility of isolates in the specific geographic region. All drainage should be cultured.
Resistant to methicillin	Clindamycin (300–450 mg/kg tid), TMP-SMX (1 or 2 ds tablets bid), minocycline or doxycycline (100 mg q12h[b]), linezolid (600 mg bid) or tedizolid (200 mg once daily)	Same options as under "Drug of Choice"	It is important to know the antibiotic susceptibility of isolates in the specific geographic region. All drainage should be cultured.

[a]Recommended dosages are for adults with normal renal and hepatic function. [b]The dosage must be adjusted for patients with reduced creatinine clearance. [c]For the treatment of prosthetic-valve endocarditis, the addition of gentamicin (1 mg/kg q8h) and rifampin (300 mg PO q8h) is recommended, with adjustment of the gentamicin dosage if the creatinine clearance rate is reduced. [d]Daptomycin cannot be used for the treatment of pneumonia. [e]Vancomycin-resistant *S. aureus* isolates from clinical infections have been reported.

Abbreviations: ds, double-strength; TMP-SMX, trimethoprim-sulfamethoxazole; VISA, vancomycin-intermediate *S. aureus*; VRSA, vancomycin-resistant *S. aureus*.

Source: Modified with permission from FD Lowy: N Engl J Med 339:520, 1998 (© 1998 Massachusetts Medical Society. All rights reserved.); C Liu et al: Clin Infect Dis 52:285, 2011; DL Stevens et al: Clin Infect Dis 59:148, 2014; and Med Lett Drugs Ther 56:39, 2014.

Although the quinolones are active against staphylococci in vitro, the frequency of staphylococcal resistance to these agents has increased progressively, especially among methicillin-resistant isolates. Of particular concern in MRSA is the possible emergence of quinolone resistance during therapy. Therefore, quinolones are not recommended for the treatment of MRSA infections. Resistance to the quinolones is most commonly chromosomal and results from mutations of the topoisomerase IV or DNA gyrase genes, although multidrug efflux pumps may also contribute. Although the newer quinolones exhibit increased in vitro activity against staphylococci, it is uncertain whether this increase translates into enhanced in vivo activity.

Tigecycline, a broad-spectrum minocycline analogue, has bacteriostatic activity against MRSA and is approved for use in skin and soft tissue infections as well as intraabdominal infections caused by *S. aureus*. Other antibiotics, such as minocycline and trimethoprim-sulfamethoxazole, have been used successfully to treat MRSA infections in cases of vancomycin toxicity or intolerance.

Combinations of antistaphylococcal agents have been used to enhance bactericidal activity in the treatment of serious infections such as endocarditis or osteomyelitis. In selected instances (e.g., right-sided endocarditis), drug combinations are also used to shorten the duration of therapy. Among the antimicrobial agents used in combinations are rifampin, aminoglycosides (e.g., gentamicin), and fusidic acid (not readily available in the United States). To date, clinical studies have not documented a therapeutic benefit; recent reports have raised concern about the potential nephrotoxicity of gentamicin and about adverse drug reactions from the addition of rifampin. As a result, the use of gentamicin in combination with β-lactams or other antimicrobial agents is no longer routinely recommended for the treatment of endocarditis. Rifampin continues to be used for the treatment of prosthetic device–related infections and for osteomyelitis.

The combination of daptomycin with a β-lactam antibiotic has been successfully used to treat patients with persistent MRSA bacteremia, even those infected with isolates that exhibit reduced susceptibility to daptomycin. The combination appears to enhance the bactericidal activity of daptomycin, perhaps by reducing the bacterial cell surface charge and thus allowing more daptomycin binding.

ANTIMICROBIAL THERAPY FOR SELECTED SETTINGS

When necessary, the use of oral antistaphylococcal agents for uncomplicated skin and soft tissue infections is usually successful. For other infections, parenteral therapy is indicated.

S. aureus endocarditis is usually an acute, life-threatening infection. Thus, prompt collection of blood for cultures must be followed immediately by empirical antimicrobial therapy. For life-threatening *S. aureus* native-valve endocarditis, therapy with a β-lactam is recommended. If a MRSA strain is isolated, vancomycin (15–20 mg/kg every 8–12 h, given in equal doses up to a total of 2 g) or daptomycin (6 mg/kg every 24 h) is recommended. The vancomycin dose should be adjusted on the basis of trough vancomycin levels. Patients are generally treated for 4–6 weeks, with duration depending on whether there are complications. For prosthetic-valve endocarditis, surgery in addition to antibiotic therapy is often necessary. The combination of a β-lactam agent—or, if the isolate is β-lactam-resistant, vancomycin (30 mg/kg every 24 h, given in doses up to a total of 2 g) or daptomycin (6 mg/kg every 24 h)—with an aminoglycoside (gentamicin, 1 mg/kg IV every 8 h) and rifampin (300 mg orally or IV every 8 h) for ≥6 weeks is recommended.

For hematogenous osteomyelitis or septic arthritis in children, a 4-week course of therapy is usually adequate. In adults, treatment is often more prolonged. For chronic forms of osteomyelitis, surgical debridement is necessary in combination with antimicrobial therapy. For joint infections, a critical component of therapy is the repeated aspiration or arthroscopy of the affected joint to prevent damage from leukocytes. The combination of rifampin with ciprofloxacin has been used successfully to treat prosthetic joint infections, especially when the device cannot be removed. The efficacy of this combination may reflect enhanced activity against staphylococci in biofilms as well as the attainment of effective intracellular concentrations.

The choice of empirical therapy for staphylococcal infections depends in part on susceptibility data for the local geographic area. Increasingly, vancomycin and daptomycin are the drugs of choice for both community- and hospital-acquired infections. The increase in CA-MRSA skin and soft tissue infections has drawn attention to the need for initiation of appropriate empirical therapy. Oral agents that have been effective against these isolates include clindamycin, trimethoprim-sulfamethoxazole, doxycycline, linezolid, and tedizolid.

THERAPY FOR TOXIC SHOCK SYNDROME

Supportive therapy with reversal of hypotension is the mainstay of therapy for TSS. Both fluids and pressors may be necessary. Tampons or other packing material should be promptly removed. The role of antibiotics is less clear. Some investigators recommend a combination of clindamycin and a semisynthetic penicillin or vancomycin (if the isolate is resistant to methicillin). Clindamycin is advocated because, as a protein synthesis inhibitor, it reduces toxin synthesis in vitro. Linezolid also appears to be effective. A semisynthetic penicillin or glycopeptide is suggested to eliminate any potential focus of infection as well as to eradicate persistent carriage that might increase the likelihood of recurrent illness. Anecdotal reports document the successful use of IV immunoglobulin to treat TSS. The role of glucocorticoids in the treatment of this disease is uncertain.

THERAPY FOR OTHER TOXIN-MEDIATED DISEASES

Therapy for staphylococcal food poisoning is entirely supportive. For SSSS, antistaphylococcal therapy targets the primary site of infection.

173 Streptococcal Infections

Michael R. Wessels

Many varieties of streptococci are found as part of the normal flora colonizing the human respiratory, gastrointestinal, and genitourinary tracts. Several species are important causes of human disease. Group A *Streptococcus* (GAS, *Streptococcus pyogenes*) is responsible for streptococcal pharyngitis, one of the most common bacterial infections of school-age children, and for the postinfectious syndromes of acute rheumatic fever (ARF) and poststreptococcal glomerulonephritis (PSGN). Group B *Streptococcus* (GBS, *Streptococcus agalactiae*) is the leading cause of bacterial sepsis and meningitis in newborns and a major cause of endometritis and fever in parturient women. Viridans streptococci are the most common cause of bacterial endocarditis. Enterococci, which are morphologically similar to streptococci, are now considered a separate genus on the basis of DNA homology studies. Thus, the species previously designated as *Streptococcus faecalis* and *Streptococcus faecium* have been renamed *Enterococcus faecalis* and *Enterococcus faecium*, respectively. The enterococci are discussed in Chap. 174.

Streptococci are gram-positive, spherical to ovoid bacteria that characteristically form chains when grown in liquid media. Most streptococci that cause human infections are facultative anaerobes, although some are strict anaerobes. Streptococci are relatively fastidious organisms, requiring enriched media for growth in the laboratory. Clinicians and clinical microbiologists identify streptococci by several classification systems, including hemolytic pattern, Lancefield group, species name, and common or trivial name. Many streptococci associated with human infection produce a zone of complete (β) hemolysis around the bacterial colony when cultured on blood agar. The β-hemolytic streptococci can be classified by the Lancefield system, a serologic grouping based on the reaction of specific antisera with bacterial cell-wall carbohydrate antigens. With rare exceptions, organisms belonging to Lancefield groups A, B, C, and G are all β hemolytic, and each is associated with characteristic patterns of human infection. Other streptococci produce a zone of partial (α) hemolysis, often imparting a greenish appearance to the agar. These α-hemolytic streptococci are further identified by biochemical testing and include *Streptococcus pneumoniae* (Chap. 171), an important cause of pneumonia, meningitis, and other infections, and the several species referred to collectively as the *viridans streptococci*, which are part of the normal oral flora and are important agents of subacute bacterial endocarditis. Finally, some streptococci are nonhemolytic, a pattern sometimes called γ *hemolysis*. Among the organisms classified serologically as group D streptococci, the enterococci are classified as a distinct genus (Chap. 174). The classification of the major streptococcal groups causing human infections is outlined in Table 173-1.

GROUP A STREPTOCOCCI

Lancefield's group A consists of a single species, *S. pyogenes*. As its species name implies, this organism is associated with a variety of suppurative infections. In addition, GAS can trigger the postinfectious syndromes of ARF (which is uniquely associated with *S. pyogenes* infection; Chap. 381) and PSGN (Chap. 338).

TABLE 173-1 CLASSIFICATION OF STREPTOCOCCI

Lancefield Group	Representative Species	Hemolytic Pattern	Typical Infections
A	*S. pyogenes*	β	Pharyngitis, impetigo, cellulitis, scarlet fever
B	*S. agalactiae*	β	Neonatal sepsis and meningitis, puerperal infection, urinary tract infection, diabetic ulcer infection, endocarditis
C, G	*S. dysgalactiae* subsp. *equisimilis*	β	Cellulitis, bacteremia, endocarditis
D	Enterococci[a]: *E. faecalis, E. faecium*	Usually nonhemolytic	Urinary tract infection, nosocomial bacteremia, endocarditis
	Nonenterococci: *S. gallolyticus* (formerly *S. bovis*)	Usually nonhemolytic	Bacteremia, endocarditis
Variable or nongroupable	Viridans streptococci: *S. sanguis, S. mitis*	α	Endocarditis, dental abscess, brain abscess
	Intermedius or *milleri* group: *S. intermedius, S. anginosus, S. constellatus*	Variable	Brain abscess, visceral abscess
	Anaerobic streptococci[b]: *Peptostreptococcus magnus*	Usually nonhemolytic	Sinusitis, pneumonia, empyema, brain abscess, liver abscess

[a]See Chap. 174. [b]See Chap. 201.

Worldwide, GAS infections and their postinfectious sequelae (primarily ARF and rheumatic heart disease) account for an estimated 500,000 deaths per year. Although data are incomplete, the incidence of all forms of GAS infection and that of rheumatic heart disease are thought to be tenfold higher in resource-limited countries than in developed countries (Fig. 173-1).

PATHOGENESIS

GAS elaborates a number of cell-surface components and extracellular products important in both the pathogenesis of infection and the human immune response. The cell wall contains a carbohydrate antigen that may be released by acid treatment. The reaction of such acid extracts with group A–specific antiserum is the basis for definitive identification of a streptococcal strain as *S. pyogenes*. The major surface protein of GAS is M protein, which occurs in more than 100 antigenically distinct types and is the basis for the serotyping of strains with specific antisera. The M protein molecules are fibrillar structures anchored in the cell wall of the organism that extend as hairlike projections away from the cell surface. The amino acid sequence of the distal or amino-terminal portion of the M protein molecule is quite variable, accounting for the antigenic variation of the different M types, while more proximal regions of the protein are relatively conserved. A newer technique for assignment of M type to GAS isolates uses the polymerase chain reaction to amplify the variable region of the *emm* gene, which encodes M protein. DNA sequence analysis of the amplified gene segment can be compared with an extensive database (developed at the Centers for Disease Control and Prevention [CDC]) for assignment of *emm* type. This method eliminates the need for typing sera, which are available in only a few reference laboratories. The presence of M protein on a GAS isolate correlates with its capacity to resist phagocytic killing in fresh human blood. This phenomenon appears to be due, at least in part, to the binding of plasma fibrinogen to M protein molecules on the streptococcal surface, which interferes with complement activation and deposition of opsonic complement fragments on the bacterial cell. This resistance to phagocytosis may be overcome by M protein–specific antibodies; thus individuals with antibodies to a given M type acquired as a result of prior infection are protected against subsequent infection with organisms of the same M type but not against that with different M types.

GAS also elaborates, to varying degrees, a polysaccharide capsule composed of hyaluronic acid. The production of large amounts of capsule by certain strains imparts a characteristic mucoid appearance to the colonies. The capsular polysaccharide plays an important role in protecting GAS from ingestion and killing by phagocytes. In contrast to M protein, the hyaluronic acid capsule is a weak immunogen, and antibodies to hyaluronate have not been shown to be important in protective immunity. The presumed explanation is the apparent structural identity between streptococcal hyaluronic acid and the hyaluronic

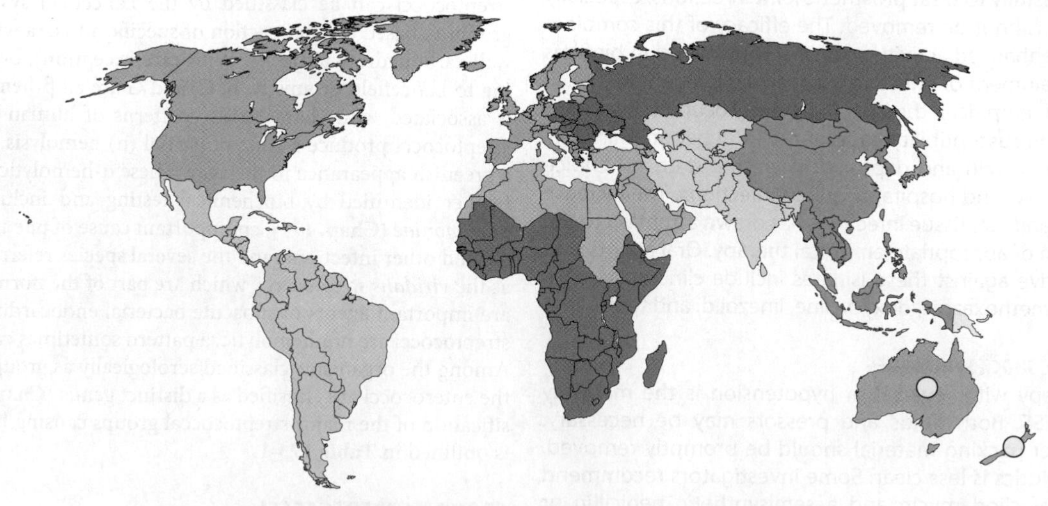

FIGURE 173-1 Prevalence of rheumatic heart disease in children 5–14 years old. The *circles* within Australia and New Zealand represent indigenous populations (and also Pacific Islanders in New Zealand). *(From JR Carapetis et al: Lancet Infect Dis 5:685, 2005, with permission.)*

acid of mammalian connective tissues. The capsular polysaccharide may also play a role in GAS colonization of the pharynx by binding to CD44, a hyaluronic acid–binding protein expressed on human pharyngeal epithelial cells.

GAS produces a large number of extracellular products that may be important in local and systemic toxicity and in the spread of infection through tissues. These products include streptolysins S and O, toxins that damage cell membranes and account for the hemolysis produced by the organisms; streptokinase; DNAses; SpyCEP, a serine protease that cleaves and inactivates the chemoattractant cytokine interleukin 8, thereby inhibiting neutrophil recruitment to the site of infection; and several pyrogenic exotoxins. Previously known as erythrogenic toxins, the pyrogenic exotoxins cause the rash of scarlet fever. Since the mid-1980s, pyrogenic exotoxin–producing strains of GAS have been linked to unusually severe invasive infections, including necrotizing fasciitis and the streptococcal toxic shock syndrome (TSS). Several extracellular products stimulate specific antibody responses useful for serodiagnosis of recent streptococcal infection. Tests for these antibodies are used primarily for detection of preceding streptococcal infection in cases of suspected ARF or PSGN.

CLINICAL MANIFESTATIONS

Pharyngitis Although seen in patients of all ages, GAS pharyngitis is one of the most common bacterial infections of childhood, accounting for 20–40% of all cases of exudative pharyngitis in children; it is rare among those under the age of 3. Younger children may manifest streptococcal infection with a syndrome of fever, malaise, and lymphadenopathy without exudative pharyngitis. Infection is acquired through contact with another individual carrying the organism. Respiratory droplets are the usual mechanism of spread, although other routes, including food-borne outbreaks, have been well described. The incubation period is 1–4 days. Symptoms include sore throat, fever and chills, malaise, and sometimes abdominal complaints and vomiting, particularly in children. Both symptoms and signs are quite variable, ranging from mild throat discomfort with minimal physical findings to high fever and severe sore throat associated with intense erythema and swelling of the pharyngeal mucosa and the presence of purulent exudate over the posterior pharyngeal wall and tonsillar pillars. Enlarged, tender anterior cervical lymph nodes commonly accompany exudative pharyngitis.

The differential diagnosis of streptococcal pharyngitis includes the many other bacterial and viral etiologies (Table 173-2). Streptococcal infection is an unlikely cause when symptoms and signs suggestive of viral infection are prominent (conjunctivitis, coryza, cough, hoarseness, or discrete ulcerative lesions of the buccal or pharyngeal mucosa). Because of the range of clinical presentations of streptococcal pharyngitis and the large number of other agents that can produce the same clinical picture, diagnosis of streptococcal pharyngitis on clinical grounds alone is not reliable. The throat culture remains the diagnostic gold standard. Culture of a throat specimen that is properly collected (i.e., by vigorous rubbing of a sterile swab over both tonsillar pillars) and properly processed is the most sensitive and specific means of definitive diagnosis. A rapid diagnostic kit for latex agglutination or enzyme immunoassay of swab specimens is a useful adjunct to throat culture. While precise figures on sensitivity and specificity vary, rapid diagnostic kits generally are >95% specific. Thus a positive result can be relied upon for definitive diagnosis and eliminates the need for throat culture. However, because rapid diagnostic tests are less sensitive than throat culture (relative sensitivity in comparative studies, 55–90%), a negative result should be confirmed by throat culture.

TREATMENT GAS PHARYNGITIS

In the usual course of uncomplicated streptococcal pharyngitis, symptoms resolve after 3–5 days. The course is shortened little by treatment, which is given primarily to prevent suppurative complications and ARF. Prevention of ARF depends on eradication of the organism from the pharynx, not simply on resolution of symptoms, and requires 10 days of penicillin treatment (Table 173-3). A first-generation cephalosporin, such as cephalexin or cefadroxil, may be substituted for penicillin in cases of penicillin allergy if the nature of the allergy is not an immediate hypersensitivity reaction (anaphylaxis or urticaria) or another potentially life-threatening manifestation (e.g., severe rash and fever).

TABLE 173-2 INFECTIOUS ETIOLOGIES OF ACUTE PHARYNGITIS

Organism	Associated Clinical Syndrome(s)
Viruses	
Rhinovirus	Common cold
Coronavirus	Common cold
Adenovirus	Pharyngoconjunctival fever
Influenza virus	Influenza
Parainfluenza virus	Cold, croup
Coxsackievirus	Herpangina, hand-foot-and-mouth disease
Herpes simplex virus	Gingivostomatitis (primary infection)
Epstein-Barr virus	Infectious mononucleosis
Cytomegalovirus	Mononucleosis-like syndrome
HIV	Acute (primary) infection syndrome
Bacteria	
Group A streptococci	Pharyngitis, scarlet fever
Group C or G streptococci	Pharyngitis
Mixed anaerobes	Vincent's angina
Arcanobacterium haemolyticum	Pharyngitis, scarlatiniform rash
Neisseria gonorrhoeae	Pharyngitis
Treponema pallidum	Secondary syphilis
Francisella tularensis	Pharyngeal tularemia
Corynebacterium diphtheriae	Diphtheria
Yersinia enterocolitica	Pharyngitis, enterocolitis
Yersinia pestis	Plague
Chlamydiae	
Chlamydia pneumoniae	Bronchitis, pneumonia
Chlamydia psittaci	Psittacosis
Mycoplasmas	
Mycoplasma pneumoniae	Bronchitis, pneumonia

TABLE 173-3 TREATMENT OF GROUP A STREPTOCOCCAL INFECTIONS

Infection	Treatment[a]
Pharyngitis	Benzathine penicillin G (1.2 mU IM) *or* penicillin V (250 mg PO tid or 500 mg PO bid) × 10 days
	(Children <27 kg: Benzathine penicillin G [600,000 units IM] *or* penicillin V [250 mg PO bid or tid] × 10 days)
Impetigo	Same as pharyngitis
Erysipelas/cellulitis	Severe: Penicillin G (1–2 mU IV q4h)
	Mild to moderate: Procaine penicillin (1.2 mU IM bid)
Necrotizing fasciitis/ myositis	Surgical debridement *plus* penicillin G (2–4 mU IV q4h) *plus* clindamycin[b] (600–900 mg IV q8h)
Pneumonia/empyema	Penicillin G (2–4 mU IV q4h) *plus* drainage of empyema
Streptococcal toxic shock syndrome	Penicillin G (2–4 mU IV q4h) *plus* clindamycin[b] (600–900 mg IV q8h) *plus* IV immunoglobulin[b] (2 g/kg as a single dose)

[a]Penicillin allergy: A first-generation cephalosporin, such as cephalexin or cefadroxil, may be substituted for penicillin in cases of penicillin allergy if the nature of the allergy is not an immediate hypersensitivity reaction (anaphylaxis or urticaria) or another potentially life-threatening manifestation (e.g., severe rash and fever). Alternative agents for oral therapy are erythromycin (10 mg/kg PO qid, up to a maximum of 250 mg per dose) and azithromycin (a 5-day course at a dose of 12 mg/kg once daily, up to a maximum of 500 mg/d). Vancomycin is an alternative for parenteral therapy. [b]Efficacy unproven, but recommended by several experts. See text for discussion.

Alternative agents are erythromycin and azithromycin. Azithromycin is more expensive but offers the advantages of better gastrointestinal tolerability, once-daily dosing, and a 5-day treatment course. Resistance to erythromycin and other macrolides is common among isolates from several countries, including Spain, Italy, Finland, Japan, and Korea. Macrolide resistance may be becoming more prevalent elsewhere with the increasing use of this class of antibiotics. In areas with resistance rates exceeding 5–10%, macrolides should be avoided unless results of susceptibility testing are known.

Follow-up culture after treatment is no longer routinely recommended but may be warranted in selected cases, such as those involving patients or families with frequent streptococcal infections or those occurring in situations in which the risk of ARF is thought to be high (e.g., when cases of ARF have recently been reported in the community).

COMPLICATIONS Suppurative complications of streptococcal pharyngitis have become uncommon with the widespread use of antibiotics for most symptomatic cases. These complications result from the spread of infection from the pharyngeal mucosa to deeper tissues by direct extension or by the hematogenous or lymphatic route and may include cervical lymphadenitis, peritonsillar or retropharyngeal abscess, sinusitis, otitis media, meningitis, bacteremia, endocarditis, and pneumonia. Local complications, such as peritonsillar or parapharyngeal abscess formation, should be considered in a patient with unusually severe or prolonged symptoms or localized pain associated with high fever and a toxic appearance. Nonsuppurative complications include ARF (Chap. 381) and PSGN (Chap. 338), both of which are thought to result from immune responses to streptococcal infection. Penicillin treatment of streptococcal pharyngitis has been shown to reduce the likelihood of ARF but not that of PSGN.

BACTERIOLOGIC TREATMENT FAILURE AND THE ASYMPTOMATIC CARRIER STATE Surveillance cultures have shown that up to 20% of individuals in certain populations may have asymptomatic pharyngeal colonization with GAS. There are no definitive guidelines for management of these asymptomatic carriers or of asymptomatic patients who still have a positive throat culture after a full course of treatment for symptomatic pharyngitis. A reasonable course of action is to give a single 10-day course of penicillin for symptomatic pharyngitis and, if positive cultures persist, not to re-treat unless symptoms recur. Studies of the natural history of streptococcal carriage and infection have shown that the risk both of developing ARF and of transmitting infection to others is substantially lower among asymptomatic carriers than among individuals with symptomatic pharyngitis. Therefore, overly aggressive attempts to eradicate carriage probably are not justified under most circumstances. An exception is the situation in which an asymptomatic carrier is a potential source of infection to others. Outbreaks of food-borne infection and nosocomial puerperal infection have been traced to asymptomatic carriers who may harbor the organisms in the throat, vagina, or anus or on the skin.

TREATMENT ASYMPTOMATIC PHARYNGEAL COLONIZATION WITH GAS

When a carrier is transmitting infection to others, attempts to eradicate carriage are warranted. Data are limited on the best regimen to clear GAS after penicillin alone has failed. Regimens reported to have efficacy superior to that of penicillin alone for eradication of carriage include (1) oral clindamycin (7 mg/kg; 300 mg maximum) three times daily for 10 days or (2) penicillin (as recommended for treatment of pharyngitis in Table 173-3) plus oral rifampin (10 mg/kg; 300 mg maximum) twice daily for the first 4 days of treatment. A 10-day course of oral vancomycin (250 mg four times daily) and rifampin (600 mg twice daily) has eradicated rectal colonization.

Scarlet Fever Scarlet fever consists of streptococcal infection, usually pharyngitis, accompanied by a characteristic rash (Fig. 173-2).

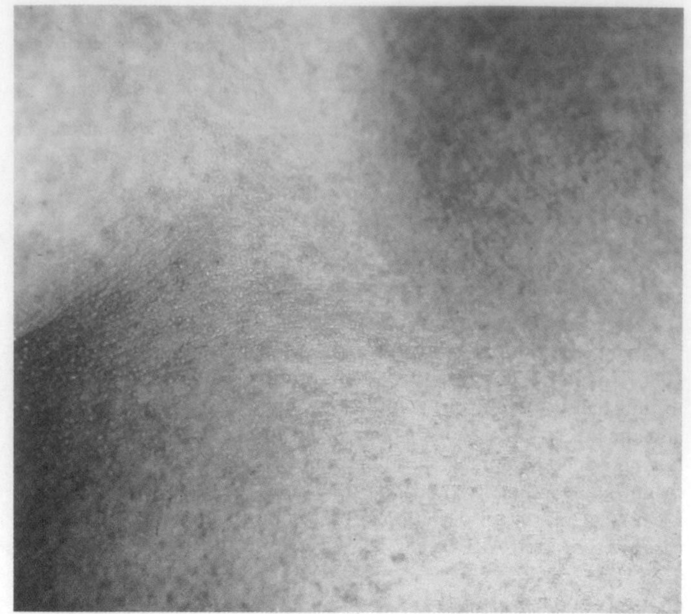

FIGURE 173-2 Scarlet fever exanthem. Finely punctate erythema has become confluent (scarlatiniform); petechiae can occur and have a linear configuration within the exanthem in body folds (Pastia's lines). *(From Fitzpatrick, Johnson, Wolff: Color Atlas and Synopsis of Clinical Dermatology, 4th ed, New York, McGraw-Hill, 2001, with permission.)*

The rash arises from the effects of one of several toxins, currently designated *streptococcal pyrogenic exotoxins* and previously known as *erythrogenic* or *scarlet fever toxins.* In the past, scarlet fever was thought to reflect infection of an individual lacking toxin-specific immunity with a toxin-producing strain of GAS. Susceptibility to scarlet fever was correlated with results of the Dick test, in which a small amount of erythrogenic toxin injected intradermally produced local erythema in susceptible individuals but elicited no reaction in those with specific immunity. Subsequent studies have suggested that development of the scarlet fever rash may reflect a hypersensitivity reaction requiring prior exposure to the toxin. For reasons that are not clear, scarlet fever has become less common in recent years, although strains of GAS that produce pyrogenic exotoxins continue to be prevalent in the population. The symptoms of scarlet fever are the same as those of pharyngitis alone. The rash typically begins on the first or second day of illness over the upper trunk, spreading to involve the extremities but sparing the palms and soles. The rash is made up of minute papules, giving a characteristic "sandpaper" feel to the skin. Associated findings include circumoral pallor, "strawberry tongue" (enlarged papillae on a coated tongue, which later may become denuded), and accentuation of the rash in skinfolds (*Pastia's lines*). Subsidence of the rash in 6–9 days is followed after several days by desquamation of the palms and soles. The differential diagnosis of scarlet fever includes other causes of fever and generalized rash, such as measles and other viral exanthems, Kawasaki disease, TSS, and systemic allergic reactions (e.g., drug eruptions).

Skin and Soft Tissue Infections GAS—and occasionally other streptococcal species—can cause a variety of infections involving the skin, subcutaneous tissues, muscles, and fascia. While several clinical syndromes offer a useful means for classification of these infections, not all cases fit exactly into one category. The classic syndromes are general guides to predicting the level of tissue involvement in a particular patient, the probable clinical course, and the likelihood that surgical intervention or aggressive life support will be required.

IMPETIGO (PYODERMA) Impetigo, a superficial infection of the skin, is caused primarily by GAS and occasionally by other streptococci or *Staphylococcus aureus.* Impetigo is seen most often in young children, tends to occur during warmer months, and is more common in semitropical or tropical climates than in cooler regions. Infection is more

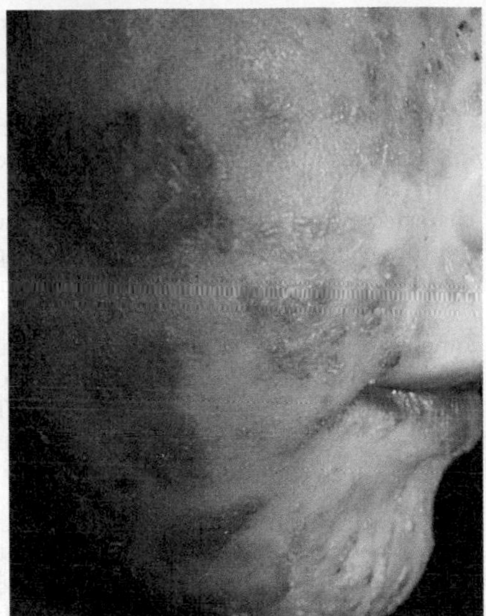

FIGURE 173-3 Impetigo contagiosa is a superficial streptococcal or *Staphylococcus aureus* infection consisting of honey-colored crusts and erythematous weeping erosions. Occasionally, bullous lesions may be seen. *(Courtesy of Mary Spraker, MD; with permission.)*

common among children living under conditions of poor hygiene. Prospective studies have shown that colonization of unbroken skin with GAS precedes clinical infection. Minor trauma, such as a scratch or an insect bite, may then serve to inoculate organisms into the skin. Impetigo is best prevented, therefore, by attention to adequate hygiene. The usual sites of involvement are the face (particularly around the nose and mouth) and the legs, although lesions may occur at other locations. Individual lesions begin as red papules, which evolve quickly into vesicular and then pustular lesions that break down and coalesce to form characteristic honeycomb-like crusts (Fig. 173-3). Lesions generally are not painful, and patients do not appear ill. Fever is not a feature of impetigo and, if present, suggests either infection extending to deeper tissues or another diagnosis. The classic presentation of impetigo usually poses little diagnostic difficulty. Cultures of impetiginous lesions often yield *S. aureus* as well as GAS. In almost all cases, streptococci are isolated initially and staphylococci appear later, presumably as secondary colonizing flora. In the past, penicillin was nearly always effective against these infections. However, an increasing frequency of penicillin treatment failure suggests that *S. aureus* may have become more prominent as a cause of impetigo. *Bullous impetigo* due to *S. aureus* is distinguished from typical streptococcal infection by more extensive, bullous lesions that break down and leave thin paper-like crusts instead of the thick amber crusts of streptococcal impetigo. Other skin lesions that may be confused with impetigo include herpetic lesions—either those of orolabial herpes simplex or those of chickenpox or zoster. Herpetic lesions can generally be distinguished by their appearance as more discrete, grouped vesicles and by a positive Tzanck test. In difficult cases, cultures of vesicular fluid should yield GAS in impetigo and the responsible virus in herpesvirus infections.

TREATMENT STREPTOCOCCAL IMPETIGO

Treatment of streptococcal impetigo is the same as that for streptococcal pharyngitis. In view of evidence that *S. aureus* has become a relatively frequent cause of impetigo, empirical regimens should cover both streptococci and *S. aureus*. For example, either dicloxacillin or cephalexin can be given at a dose of 250 mg four times daily for 10 days. Topical mupirocin ointment is also effective. Culture may be indicated to rule out methicillin-resistant *S. aureus*, especially if the response to empirical treatment is unsatisfactory. ARF is not a sequela to streptococcal skin infections, although PSGN may follow either skin or throat infection. The reason for this difference is not known. One hypothesis is that the immune response necessary for development of ARF occurs only after infection of the pharyngeal mucosa. In addition, the strains of GAS that cause pharyngitis are generally of different M protein types than those associated with skin infections; thus the strains that cause pharyngitis may have rheumatogenic potential, while the skin-infecting strains may not.

CELLULITIS Inoculation of organisms into the skin may lead to *cellulitis*: infection involving the skin and subcutaneous tissues. The portal of entry may be a traumatic or surgical wound, an insect bite, or any other break in skin integrity. Often, no entry site is apparent. One form of streptococcal cellulitis, *erysipelas*, is characterized by a bright red appearance of the involved skin, which forms a plateau sharply demarcated from surrounding normal skin (Fig. 173-4). The lesion is warm to the touch, may be tender, and appears shiny and swollen. The skin often has a *peau d'orange* texture, which is thought to reflect involvement of superficial lymphatics; superficial blebs or bullae may form, usually 2–3 days after onset. The lesion typically develops over a few hours and is associated with fever and chills. Erysipelas tends to occur on the malar area of the face (often with extension over the bridge of the nose to the contralateral malar region) and the lower extremities. After one episode, recurrence at the same site—sometimes years later—is not uncommon. Classic cases of erysipelas, with typical features, are almost always due to β-hemolytic streptococci, usually GAS and occasionally group C or G. Often, however, the appearance of streptococcal cellulitis is not sufficiently distinctive to permit a specific diagnosis on clinical grounds. The area involved may not be typical for erysipelas, the lesion may be less intensely red than usual and may fade into surrounding skin, and/or the patient may appear only mildly ill. In such cases, it is prudent to broaden the spectrum of empirical antimicrobial therapy to include other pathogens, particularly *S. aureus*, that can produce cellulitis with the same appearance. Staphylococcal infection should be suspected if cellulitis develops around a wound or an ulcer.

Streptococcal cellulitis tends to develop at anatomic sites in which normal lymphatic drainage has been disrupted, such as sites of prior cellulitis, the arm ipsilateral to a mastectomy and axillary lymph node dissection, a lower extremity previously involved in deep venous thrombosis or chronic lymphedema, or the leg from which a saphenous vein has been harvested for coronary artery bypass grafting. The organism may enter via a dermal breach some distance from the eventual site of clinical cellulitis. For example, some patients with recurrent leg cellulitis following saphenous vein removal stop having recurrent episodes only after treatment of tinea pedis on the affected

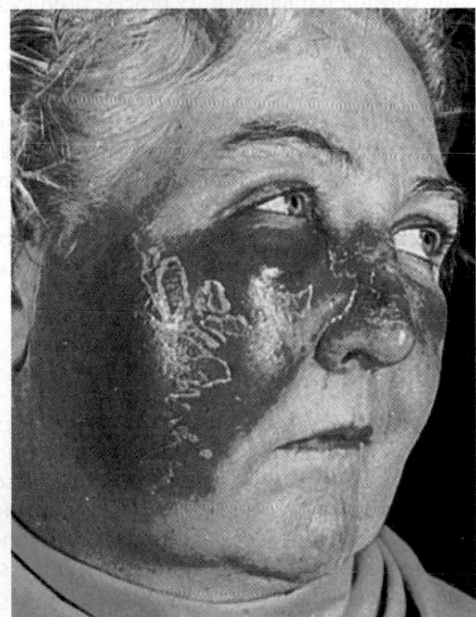

FIGURE 173-4 Erysipelas is a streptococcal infection of the superficial dermis and consists of well-demarcated, erythematous, edematous, warm plaques.

extremity. Fissures in the skin presumably serve as a portal of entry for streptococci, which then produce infection more proximally in the leg at the site of previous injury. Streptococcal cellulitis may also involve recent surgical wounds. GAS is among the few bacterial pathogens that typically produce signs of wound infection and surrounding cellulitis within the first 24 h after surgery. These wound infections are usually associated with a thin exudate and may spread rapidly, either as cellulitis in the skin and subcutaneous tissue or as a deeper tissue infection (see below). Streptococcal wound infection or localized cellulitis may also be associated with *lymphangitis*, manifested by red streaks extending proximally along superficial lymphatics from the infection site.

TREATMENT STREPTOCOCCAL CELLULITIS

See Table 173-3 and **Chap. 156.**

DEEP SOFT-TISSUE INFECTIONS *Necrotizing fasciitis* (*hemolytic streptococcal gangrene*) involves the superficial and/or deep fascia investing the muscles of an extremity or the trunk. The source of the infection is either the skin, with organisms introduced into tissue through trauma (sometimes trivial), or the bowel flora, with organisms released during abdominal surgery or from an occult enteric source, such as a diverticular or appendiceal abscess. The inoculation site may be inapparent and is often some distance from the site of clinical involvement; e.g., the introduction of organisms via minor trauma to the hand may be associated with clinical infection of the tissues overlying the shoulder or chest. Cases associated with the bowel flora are usually polymicrobial, involving a mixture of anaerobic bacteria (such as *Bacteroides fragilis* or anaerobic streptococci) and facultative organisms (usually gram-negative bacilli). Cases unrelated to contamination from bowel organisms are most commonly caused by GAS alone or in combination with other organisms (most often *S. aureus*). Overall, GAS is implicated in ~60% of cases of necrotizing fasciitis. The onset of symptoms is usually quite acute and is marked by severe pain at the site of involvement, malaise, fever, chills, and a toxic appearance. The physical findings, particularly early on, may not be striking, with only minimal erythema of the overlying skin. Pain and tenderness are usually severe. In contrast, in more superficial cellulitis, the skin appearance is more abnormal, but pain and tenderness are only mild or moderate. As the infection progresses (often over several hours), the severity and extent of symptoms worsen, and skin changes become more evident, with the appearance of dusky or mottled erythema and edema. The marked tenderness of the involved area may evolve into anesthesia as the spreading inflammatory process produces infarction of cutaneous nerves.

Although myositis is more commonly due to *S. aureus* infection, GAS occasionally produces abscesses in skeletal muscles (*streptococcal myositis*), with little or no involvement of the surrounding fascia or overlying skin. The presentation is usually subacute, but a fulminant form has been described in association with severe systemic toxicity, bacteremia, and a high mortality rate. The fulminant form may reflect the same basic disease process seen in necrotizing fasciitis, but with the necrotizing inflammatory process extending into the muscles themselves rather than remaining limited to the fascial layers.

TREATMENT DEEP SOFT-TISSUE INFECTIONS

Once necrotizing fasciitis is suspected, early surgical exploration is both diagnostically and therapeutically indicated. Surgery reveals necrosis and inflammatory fluid tracking along the fascial planes above and between muscle groups, without involvement of the muscles themselves. The process usually extends beyond the area of clinical involvement, and extensive debridement is required. Drainage and debridement are central to the management of necrotizing fasciitis; antibiotic treatment is a useful adjunct (Table 173-3), but surgery is life-saving. Treatment for streptococcal myositis consists of surgical drainage—usually by an open procedure that permits evaluation of the extent of infection and ensures adequate debridement of involved tissues—and high-dose penicillin (Table 173-3).

Pneumonia and Empyema GAS is an occasional cause of pneumonia, generally in previously healthy individuals. The onset of symptoms may be abrupt or gradual. Pleuritic chest pain, fever, chills, and dyspnea are the characteristic manifestations. Cough is usually present but may not be prominent. Approximately one-half of patients with GAS pneumonia have an accompanying pleural effusion. In contrast to the sterile parapneumonic effusions typical of pneumococcal pneumonia, those complicating streptococcal pneumonia are almost always infected. The empyema fluid is usually visible by chest radiography on initial presentation, and its volume may increase rapidly. These pleural collections should be drained early, as they tend to become loculated rapidly, resulting in a chronic fibrotic reaction that may require thoracotomy for removal.

Bacteremia, Puerperal Sepsis, and Streptococcal Toxic Shock Syndrome GAS bacteremia is usually associated with an identifiable local infection. Bacteremia occurs rarely with otherwise uncomplicated pharyngitis, occasionally with cellulitis or pneumonia, and relatively frequently with necrotizing fasciitis. Bacteremia without an identified source raises the possibility of endocarditis, an occult abscess, or osteomyelitis. A variety of focal infections may arise secondarily from streptococcal bacteremia, including endocarditis, meningitis, septic arthritis, osteomyelitis, peritonitis, and visceral abscesses. GAS is occasionally implicated in infectious complications of childbirth, usually endometritis and associated bacteremia. In the preantibiotic era, puerperal sepsis was commonly caused by GAS; currently, it is more often caused by GBS. Several nosocomial outbreaks of puerperal GAS infection have been traced to an asymptomatic carrier, usually someone present at delivery. The site of carriage may be the skin, throat, anus, or vagina.

Beginning in the late 1980s, several reports described patients with GAS infections associated with shock and multisystem organ failure. This syndrome was called *streptococcal TSS* because it shares certain features with staphylococcal TSS. In 1993, a case definition for streptococcal TSS was formulated (Table 173-4). The general features of the illness include fever, hypotension, renal impairment, and respiratory distress syndrome. Various types of rash have been described, but rash usually does not develop. Laboratory abnormalities include a marked shift to the left in the white blood cell differential, with many immature granulocytes; hypocalcemia; hypoalbuminemia; and thrombocytopenia, which usually becomes more pronounced on the second or third day of illness. In contrast to patients with staphylococcal TSS, the majority with streptococcal TSS are bacteremic. The most common associated infection is a soft tissue infection—necrotizing

TABLE 173-4 PROPOSED CASE DEFINITION FOR THE STREPTOCOCCAL TOXIC SHOCK SYNDROME[a]

I. Isolation of group A streptococci (*Streptococcus pyogenes*)
   A. From a normally sterile site
   B. From a nonsterile site
II. Clinical signs of severity
   A. Hypotension *and*
   B. ≥2 of the following signs
      1. Renal impairment
      2. Coagulopathy
      3. Liver function impairment
      4. Adult respiratory distress syndrome
      5. A generalized erythematous macular rash that may desquamate
      6. Soft tissue necrosis, including necrotizing fasciitis or myositis; *or* gangrene

[a]An illness fulfilling criteria IA, IIA, and IIB is defined as a *definite* case. An illness fulfilling criteria IB, IIA, and IIB is defined as a *probable* case if no other etiology for the illness is identified.

Source: Modified from Working Group on Severe Streptococcal Infections: JAMA 269:390, 1993.

fasciitis, myositis, or cellulitis—although a variety of other associated local infections have been described, including pneumonia, peritonitis, osteomyelitis, and myometritis. Streptococcal TSS is associated with a mortality rate of ≥30%, with most deaths secondary to shock and respiratory failure. Because of its rapidly progressive and lethal course, early recognition of the syndrome is essential. Patients should receive aggressive supportive care (fluid resuscitation, pressors, and mechanical ventilation) in addition to antimicrobial therapy and, in cases associated with necrotizing fasciitis, surgical debridement. Exactly why certain patients develop this fulminant syndrome is not known. Early studies of the streptococcal strains isolated from these patients demonstrated a strong association with the production of pyrogenic exotoxin A. This association has been inconsistent in subsequent case series. Pyrogenic exotoxin A and several other streptococcal exotoxins act as superantigens to trigger release of inflammatory cytokines from T lymphocytes. Fever, shock, and organ dysfunction in streptococcal TSS may reflect, in part, the systemic effects of superantigen-mediated cytokine release.

TREATMENT STREPTOCOCCAL TOXIC SHOCK SYNDROME

In light of the possible role of pyrogenic exotoxins or other streptococcal toxins in streptococcal TSS, treatment with clindamycin has been advocated by some authorities (Table 173-3), who argue that, through its direct action on protein synthesis, clindamycin is more effective in rapidly terminating toxin production than is penicillin—a cell wall agent. Support for this view comes from studies of an experimental model of streptococcal myositis, in which mice given clindamycin had a higher rate of survival than those given penicillin. Comparable data on the treatment of human infections are not available, although retrospective analysis has suggested a better outcome when patients with invasive soft-tissue infection are treated with clindamycin rather than with cell wall-active antibiotics. Although clindamycin resistance in GAS is uncommon (<2% among U.S. isolates), it has been documented. Thus, if clindamycin is used for initial treatment of a critically ill patient, penicillin should be given as well until the antibiotic susceptibility of the streptococcal isolate is known. IV immunoglobulin has been used as adjunctive therapy for streptococcal TSS (Table 173-3). Pooled immunoglobulin preparations contain antibodies capable of neutralizing the effects of streptococcal toxins. Anecdotal reports and case series have suggested favorable clinical responses to IV immunoglobulin, but no adequately powered, prospective, controlled trials have been reported.

PREVENTION

No vaccine against GAS is commercially available. A formulation that consists of recombinant peptides containing epitopes of 26 M-protein types has undergone phase 1 and 2 testing in volunteers. Early results indicate that the vaccine is well tolerated and elicits type-specific antibody responses. Vaccines based on a conserved region of M protein or on a mixture of other conserved GAS protein antigens are in earlier stages of development.

Household contacts of individuals with invasive GAS infection (e.g., bacteremia, necrotizing fasciitis, or streptococcal TSS) are at greater risk of invasive infection than the general population. Asymptomatic pharyngeal colonization with GAS has been detected in up to 25% of persons with >4 h/d of same-room exposure to an index case. However, antibiotic prophylaxis is not routinely recommended for contacts of patients with invasive disease because such an approach (if effective) would require treatment of hundreds of contacts to prevent a single case.

STREPTOCOCCI OF GROUPS C AND G

Group C and group G streptococci are β-hemolytic bacteria that occasionally cause human infections similar to those caused by GAS. Strains that form small colonies on blood agar (<0.5 mm) are generally members of the *Streptococcus milleri (Streptococcus intermedius, Streptococcus anginosus)* group (see "Viridans Streptococci," below). Large-colony group C and G streptococci of human origin are now considered a single species, *Streptococcus dysgalactiae* subspecies *equisimilis*. These organisms have been associated with pharyngitis, cellulitis and soft tissue infections, pneumonia, bacteremia, endocarditis, and septic arthritis. Puerperal sepsis, meningitis, epidural abscess, intraabdominal abscess, urinary tract infection, and neonatal sepsis have also been reported. Group C or G streptococcal bacteremia most often affects elderly or chronically ill patients and, in the absence of obvious local infection, is likely to reflect endocarditis. Septic arthritis, sometimes involving multiple joints, may complicate endocarditis or develop in its absence. Distinct streptococcal species of Lancefield group C cause infections in domesticated animals, especially horses and cattle; some human infections are acquired through contact with animals or consumption of unpasteurized milk. These zoonotic organisms include *Streptococcus equi* subspecies *zooepidemicus* and *S. equi* subspecies *equi*.

TREATMENT GROUP C OR G STREPTOCOCCAL INFECTION

Penicillin is the drug of choice for treatment of group C or G streptococcal infections. Antibiotic treatment is the same as for similar syndromes due to GAS (Table 173-3). Patients with bacteremia or septic arthritis should receive IV penicillin (2–4 mU every 4 h). All group C and G streptococci are sensitive to penicillin; nearly all are inhibited in vitro by concentrations of ≤0.03 μg/mL. Occasional isolates exhibit tolerance: although inhibited by low concentrations of penicillin, they are killed only by significantly higher concentrations. The clinical significance of tolerance is unknown. Because of the poor clinical response of some patients to penicillin alone, the addition of gentamicin (1 mg/kg every 8 h for patients with normal renal function) is recommended by some authorities for treatment of endocarditis or septic arthritis due to group C or G streptococci; however, combination therapy has not been shown to be superior to penicillin treatment alone. Patients with joint infections often require repeated aspiration or open drainage and debridement for cure; the response to treatment may be slow, particularly in debilitated patients and those with involvement of multiple joints. Infection of prosthetic joints almost always requires prosthesis removal in addition to antibiotic therapy.

GROUP B STREPTOCOCCI

Identified first as a cause of mastitis in cows, streptococci belonging to Lancefield's group B have since been recognized as a major cause of sepsis and meningitis in human neonates. GBS is also a frequent cause of peripartum fever in women and an occasional cause of serious infection in nonpregnant adults. Since the widespread institution of prenatal screening for GBS in the 1990s, the incidence of neonatal infection per 1000 live births has fallen from ~2–3 cases to ~0.6 case. During the same period, GBS infection in adults with underlying chronic illnesses has become more common; adults now account for a larger proportion of invasive GBS infections than do newborns. Lancefield group B consists of a single species, *S. agalactiae*, which is definitively identified with specific antiserum to the group B cell wall–associated carbohydrate antigen. A streptococcal isolate can be classified presumptively as GBS on the basis of biochemical tests, including hydrolysis of sodium hippurate (in which 99% of isolates are positive), hydrolysis of bile esculin (in which 99–100% are negative), bacitracin susceptibility (in which 92% are resistant), and production of CAMP factor (in which 98–100% are positive). CAMP factor is a phospholipase produced by GBS that causes synergistic hemolysis with β lysin produced by certain strains of *S. aureus*. Its presence can be demonstrated by cross-streaking of the test isolate and an appropriate staphylococcal strain on a blood agar plate. GBS organisms causing human infections are encapsulated by one of ten antigenically distinct polysaccharides. The capsular polysaccharide is an important virulence factor. Antibodies to the capsular polysaccharide afford protection against GBS of the same (but not of a different) capsular type.

Two general types of GBS infection in infants are defined by the age of the patient at presentation. *Early-onset infections* occur within the first week of life, with a median age of 20 h at onset. Approximately half of these infants have signs of GBS disease at birth. The infection is acquired during or shortly before birth from the colonized maternal genital tract. Surveillance studies have shown that 5–40% of women are vaginal or rectal carriers of GBS. Approximately 50% of infants delivered vaginally by carrier mothers become colonized, although only 1–2% develop clinically evident infection. Prematurity, prolonged labor, obstetric complications, and maternal fever are risk factors for early-onset infection. The presentation of early-onset infection is the same as that of other forms of neonatal sepsis. Typical findings include respiratory distress, lethargy, and hypotension. Essentially all infants with early-onset disease are bacteremic, one-third to one-half have pneumonia and/or respiratory distress syndrome, and one-third have meningitis.

Late-onset infections occur in infants 1 week to 3 months old and, in rare instances, in older infants (mean age at onset, 3–4 weeks). The infecting organism may be acquired during delivery (as in early-onset cases) or during later contact with a colonized mother, nursery personnel, or another source. Meningitis is the most common manifestation of late-onset infection and in most cases is associated with a strain of capsular type III. Infants present with fever, lethargy or irritability, poor feeding, and seizures. The various other types of late-onset infection include bacteremia without an identified source, osteomyelitis, septic arthritis, and facial cellulitis associated with submandibular or preauricular adenitis.

TREATMENT GROUP B STREPTOCOCCAL INFECTION IN NEONATES

Penicillin is the agent of choice for all GBS infections. Empirical broad-spectrum therapy for suspected bacterial sepsis, consisting of ampicillin and gentamicin, is generally administered until culture results become available. If cultures yield GBS, many pediatricians continue to administer gentamicin, along with ampicillin or penicillin, for a few days until clinical improvement becomes evident. Infants with bacteremia or soft tissue infection should receive penicillin at a dosage of 200,000 units/kg per day in divided doses. For meningitis, infants ≤7 days of age should receive 250,000–450,000 units/kg per day in three divided doses; infants >7 days of age should receive 450,000–500,000 units/kg per day in four divided doses. Meningitis should be treated for at least 14 days because of the risk of relapse with shorter courses.

PREVENTION

The incidence of GBS infection is unusually high among infants of women with risk factors: preterm delivery, early rupture of membranes (>24 h before delivery), prolonged labor, fever, or chorioamnionitis. Because the usual source of the organisms infecting a neonate is the mother's birth canal, efforts have been made to prevent GBS infections by the identification of high-risk carrier mothers and their treatment with various forms of antibiotic prophylaxis or immunoprophylaxis. Prophylactic administration of ampicillin or penicillin to such patients during delivery reduces the risk of infection in the newborn. This approach has been hampered by logistical difficulties in identifying colonized women before delivery; the results of vaginal cultures early in pregnancy are poor predictors of carrier status at delivery. The CDC recommends screening for anogenital colonization at 35–37 weeks of pregnancy by a swab culture of the lower vagina and anorectum; intrapartum chemoprophylaxis is recommended for culture-positive women and for women who, regardless of culture status, have previously given birth to an infant with GBS infection or have a history of GBS bacteriuria during pregnancy. Women whose culture status is unknown and who develop premature labor (<37 weeks), prolonged rupture of membranes (>18 h), or intrapartum fever or who have a positive intrapartum nucleic acid amplification test for GBS should also receive intrapartum chemoprophylaxis. The recommended regimen for chemoprophylaxis is a loading dose of 5 million units of penicillin G followed by 2.5 million units every 4 h until delivery. Cefazolin is an alternative for women with a history of penicillin allergy who are thought not to be at high risk for anaphylaxis. For women with a history of immediate hypersensitivity, clindamycin may be substituted, but only if the colonizing isolate has been demonstrated to be susceptible. If susceptibility testing results are not available or indicate resistance, vancomycin should be used in this situation.

Treatment of all pregnant women who are colonized or have risk factors for neonatal infection will result in exposure of up to one-third of pregnant women and newborns to antibiotics, with the attendant risks of allergic reactions and selection for resistant organisms. Although still in the developmental stages, a GBS vaccine may ultimately offer a better solution to prevention. Because transplacental passage of maternal antibodies produces protective antibody levels in newborns, efforts are under way to develop a vaccine against GBS that can be given to childbearing-age women before or during pregnancy. Results of phase 1 clinical trials of GBS capsular polysaccharide–protein conjugate vaccines suggest that a multivalent conjugate vaccine would be safe and highly immunogenic.

INFECTION IN ADULTS

The majority of GBS infections in otherwise healthy adults are related to pregnancy and parturition. Peripartum fever, the most common manifestation, is sometimes accompanied by symptoms and signs of endometritis or chorioamnionitis (abdominal distention and uterine or adnexal tenderness). Blood and vaginal swab cultures are often positive. Bacteremia is usually transitory but occasionally results in meningitis or endocarditis. Infections in adults that are not associated with the peripartum period generally involve individuals who are elderly or have an underlying chronic illness, such as diabetes mellitus or a malignancy. Among the infections that develop with some frequency in adults are cellulitis and soft tissue infection (including infected diabetic skin ulcers), urinary tract infection, pneumonia, endocarditis, and septic arthritis. Other reported infections include meningitis, osteomyelitis, and intraabdominal or pelvic abscesses. Relapse or recurrence of invasive infection weeks to months after a first episode is documented in ~4% of cases.

TREATMENT GROUP B STREPTOCOCCAL INFECTION IN ADULTS

GBS is less sensitive to penicillin than GAS, requiring somewhat higher doses. Adults with serious localized infections (pneumonia, pyelonephritis, abscess) should receive doses of ~12 million units of penicillin G daily; patients with endocarditis or meningitis should receive 18–24 million units per day in divided doses. Vancomycin is an acceptable alternative for penicillin-allergic patients.

NONENTEROCOCCAL GROUP D STREPTOCOCCI

The main nonenterococcal group D streptococci that cause human infections were previously considered a single species, *Streptococcus bovis*. The organisms encompassed by *S. bovis* have been reclassified into two species, each of which has two subspecies: *Streptococcus gallolyticus* subspecies *gallolyticus*, *S. gallolyticus* subspecies *pasteurianus*, *Streptococcus infantarius* subspecies *infantarius*, and *S. infantarius* subspecies *coli*. Endocarditis caused by these organisms is often associated with neoplasms of the gastrointestinal tract—most frequently, a colon carcinoma or polyp—but is also reported in association with other bowel lesions. When occult gastrointestinal lesions are carefully sought, abnormalities are found in >60% of patients with endocarditis due to *S. gallolyticus* or *S. infantarius*. In contrast to the enterococci, nonenterococcal group D streptococci like these organisms are reliably killed by penicillin as a single agent, and penicillin is the agent of choice for the infections they cause.

VIRIDANS STREPTOCOCCI

Consisting of multiple species of α-hemolytic streptococci, the viridans streptococci are a heterogeneous group of organisms that are important agents of bacterial endocarditis (Chap. 155). Several species of viridans streptococci, including *Streptococcus salivarius, Streptococcus mitis, Streptococcus sanguis,* and *Streptococcus mutans,* are part of the normal flora of the mouth, where they live in close association with the teeth and gingiva. Some species contribute to the development of dental caries.

Previously known as *Streptococcus morbillorum, Gemella morbillorum* has been placed in a separate genus, along with *Gemella haemolysans,* on the basis of genetic-relatedness studies. These species resemble viridans streptococci with respect to habitat in the human host and associated infections.

The transient viridans streptococcal bacteremia induced by eating, toothbrushing, flossing, and other sources of minor trauma, together with adherence to biologic surfaces, is thought to account for the predilection of these organisms to cause endocarditis (see Fig. 155-1). Viridans streptococci are also isolated, often as part of a mixed flora, from sites of sinusitis, brain abscess, and liver abscess.

Viridans streptococcal bacteremia occurs relatively frequently in neutropenic patients, particularly after bone marrow transplantation or high-dose chemotherapy for cancer. Some of these patients develop a sepsis syndrome with high fever and shock. Risk factors for viridans streptococcal bacteremia include chemotherapy with high-dose cytosine arabinoside, prior treatment with trimethoprim-sulfamethoxazole or a fluoroquinolone, treatment with antacids or histamine antagonists, mucositis, and profound neutropenia.

The *S. milleri* group (also referred to as the *S. intermedius* or *S. anginosus* group) includes three species that cause human disease: *S. intermedius, S. anginosus,* and *Streptococcus constellatus.* These organisms are often considered viridans streptococci, although they differ somewhat from other viridans streptococci in both their hemolytic pattern (they may be α-, β-, or nonhemolytic) and the disease syndromes they cause. This group commonly produces suppurative infections, particularly abscesses of brain and abdominal viscera, and infections related to the oral cavity or respiratory tract, such as peritonsillar abscess, lung abscess, and empyema.

TREATMENT INFECTION WITH VIRIDANS STREPTOCOCCI

Isolates from neutropenic patients with bacteremia are often resistant to penicillin; thus these patients should be treated presumptively with vancomycin until the results of susceptibility testing become available. Viridans streptococci isolated in other clinical settings usually are sensitive to penicillin.

ABIOTROPHIA AND *GRANULICATELLA* SPECIES (NUTRITIONALLY VARIANT STREPTOCOCCI)

Occasional isolates cultured from the blood of patients with endocarditis fail to grow when subcultured on solid media. These *nutritionally variant streptococci* require supplemental thiol compounds or active forms of vitamin B_6 (pyridoxal or pyridoxamine) for growth in the laboratory. The nutritionally variant streptococci are generally grouped with the viridans streptococci because they cause similar types of infections. However, they have been reclassified on the basis of 16S ribosomal RNA sequence comparisons into two separate genera: *Abiotrophia,* with a single species (*Abiotrophia defectiva*), and *Granulicatella,* with three species associated with human infection (*Granulicatella adiacens, Granulicatella para-adiacens,* and *Granulicatella elegans*).

TREATMENT INFECTION WITH NUTRITIONALLY VARIANT STREPTOCOCCI

Treatment failure and relapse appear to be more common in cases of endocarditis due to nutritionally variant streptococci than in those due to the usual viridans streptococci. Thus the addition of gentamicin (1 mg/kg every 8 h for patients with normal renal function) to the penicillin regimen is recommended for endocarditis due to the nutritionally variant organisms.

OTHER STREPTOCOCCI

Streptococcus suis is an important pathogen in swine and has been reported to cause meningitis in humans, usually in individuals with occupational exposure to pigs. Strains of *S. suis* associated with human infections have generally reacted with Lancefield group R typing serum and sometimes with group D typing serum as well. Isolates may be α- or β-hemolytic and are sensitive to penicillin. *Streptococcus iniae,* a pathogen of fish, has been associated with infections in humans who have handled live or freshly killed fish. Cellulitis of the hand is the most common form of human infection, although bacteremia and endocarditis have been reported. *Anaerobic streptococci,* or *peptostreptococci,* are part of the normal flora of the oral cavity, bowel, and vagina. Infections caused by the anaerobic streptococci are discussed in Chap. 201.

174 Enterococcal Infections

Cesar A. Arias, Barbara E. Murray

Enterococci have been recognized as potential human pathogens for more than a century, but only in recent years have these organisms acquired prominence as important causes of nosocomial infections. The ability of enterococci to survive and/or disseminate in the hospital environment and to acquire antibiotic resistance determinants makes the treatment of some enterococcal infections in critically ill patients a difficult challenge. Enterococci were first mentioned in the French literature in 1899; the "entérocoque" was found in the human gastrointestinal tract and was noted to have the potential to produce significant disease. Indeed, the first pathologic description of an enterococcal infection dates to the same year. A clinical isolate from a patient who died as a consequence of endocarditis was initially designated *Micrococcus zymogenes,* was later named *Streptococcus faecalis* subspecies *zymogenes,* and would now be classified as *Enterococcus faecalis.* The ability of this isolate to cause severe disease in both rabbits and mice illustrated its potential lethality in the appropriate settings.

ETIOLOGY

Enterococci are gram-positive organisms. In clinical specimens, they are usually observed as single cells, diplococci, or short chains (Fig. 174-1), although long chains are noted with some strains. Enterococci were originally classified as streptococci because organisms of the two genera share many morphologic and phenotypic characteristics, including a generally negative catalase reaction. Only DNA hybridization studies and later 16S rRNA sequencing clearly demonstrated that enterococci should be grouped as a genus distinct from the streptococci. Nonetheless, unlike the majority of streptococci, enterococci hydrolyze esculin in the presence of 40% bile salts and grow at high salt concentrations (e.g., 6.5%) and at high temperatures (46°C). Enterococci are usually reported by the clinical laboratory to be nonhemolytic on the basis of their inability to lyse the ovine or bovine red blood cells (RBCs) commonly used in agar plates; however, some strains of *E. faecalis* do lyse RBCs from humans, horses, and rabbits. The majority of clinically relevant enterococcal species hydrolyze pyrrolidonyl-β-naphthylamide (PYR); this characteristic is helpful in differentiating enterococci from organisms of the *Streptococcus gallolyticus* group (formerly known as *S. bovis*), which includes *S. gallolyticus, Streptococcus pasteurianus,* and *Streptococcus infantarius,* and from *Leuconostoc* species. Although at least 18 species of enterococci have been isolated from human infections, the overwhelming

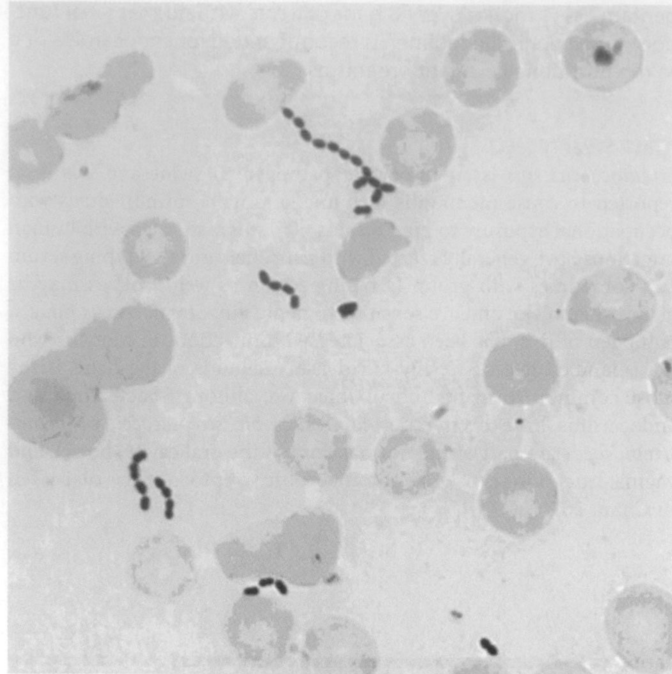

FIGURE 174-1 Gram's stain of cultured blood from a patient with enterococcal bacteremia. Oval gram-positive bacterial cells are arranged as diplococci and short chains. *(Courtesy of Audrey Wanger, PhD.)*

majority of cases are caused by two species, *E. faecalis* and *Enterococcus faecium*. Less frequently isolated species include *Enterococcus gallinarum, Enterococcus durans, Enterococcus hirae*, and *Enterococcus avium*.

PATHOGENESIS

Enterococci are normal inhabitants of the large bowel of human adults, although they usually make up <1% of the culturable intestinal microflora. In the healthy human gastrointestinal tract, enterococci are typical symbionts that coexist with other gastrointestinal bacteria; in fact, the utility of certain enterococcal strains as probiotics in the treatment of diarrhea suggests their possible role in maintaining the homeostatic equilibrium of the bowel. Enterococci are intrinsically resistant to a variety of commonly used antibacterial drugs. One of the most important factors that disrupts this equilibrium and promotes increased gastrointestinal colonization by enterococci is the administration of antimicrobial agents. In particular, antibiotics that are excreted in the bile and have broad-spectrum activity (e.g., certain cephalosporins that target anaerobes and gram-negative bacteria) are usually associated with the recovery of higher numbers of enterococci from feces. This increased colonization appears to be due not only to the simple enterococcal replacement in a "biologic niche" after the eradication of competing components of the flora, but also (at least in mice) to the suppression—upon reduction of the gram-negative microflora by antibiotics—of important immunologic signals (e.g., by the lectin RegIIIγ) that help keep enterococcal counts low in the normal human bowel. Several studies have shown that higher levels of gastrointestinal colonization are a critical factor in the pathogenesis of enterococcal infections. However, the mechanisms by which enterococci successfully colonize the bowel and gain access to the lymphatics and/or bloodstream remain incompletely understood.

Several vertebrate, worm, and insect models have been developed to study the role of possible pathogenic determinants in both *E. faecalis* and *E. faecium*. Three main groups of virulence factors may increase the ability of enterococci to colonize the gastrointestinal tract and/or cause disease. The first group, *enterococcal secreted factors*, are molecules released outside the bacterial cell that contribute to the process of infection. The best-studied of these molecules include enterococcal hemolysin/cytolysin and two enterococcal proteases (gelatinase and serine protease). Enterococcal cytolysin is a heterodimeric toxin produced by some strains of *E. faecalis* that is capable of lysing human RBCs as well as polymorphonuclear leukocytes and macrophages. *E. faecalis* gelatinase and serine protease are thought to mediate virulence by several mechanisms, including the degradation of host tissues and the modification of critical components of the immune system. Mutants lacking the genes corresponding to these proteins are highly attenuated in experimental peritonitis, endocarditis, and endophthalmitis.

A second group of virulence factors, *enterococcal surface components*, are thought to contribute to bacterial attachment to extracellular matrix molecules in the human host. Several molecules on the surface of enterococci have been characterized and shown to play a role in the pathogenesis of enterococcal infections. Among the characterized adhesins is aggregation substance of *E. faecalis*, which mediates the attachment of bacterial cells to each other, thereby facilitating conjugative plasmid exchange. Several lines of evidence indicate that aggregation substance and enterococcal cytolysin act synergistically to increase the virulence potential of *E. faecalis* strains in experimental endocarditis. The surface protein adhesin of collagen of *E. faecalis* (Ace) and its *E. faecium* homologue (Acm) recognize adhesive matrix molecules (MSCRAMMs) involved in bacterial attachment to host proteins such as collagen, fibronectin, and fibrinogen; both Ace and Acm are important in the pathogenesis of experimental endocarditis. Pili of gram-positive bacteria have been shown to be important mediators of attachment to and invasion of host tissues and are considered potential targets for immunotherapy. Both *E. faecalis* and *E. faecium* have surface pili. Mutants of *E. faecalis* lacking pili are attenuated in biofilm production, experimental endocarditis, and urinary tract infections (UTIs). Other surface proteins that share structural homology with MSCRAMMs and appear to play a role in enterococcal attachment to the host and in virulence include the *E. faecalis* surface protein Esp and its *E. faecium* homologue Esp_{fm}, the second collagen adhesin of *E. faecium* (Scm), the surface proteins of *E. faecium* (Fms), SgrA (which binds to components of the basal lamina), and EcbA (which binds to collagen type V). Additional surface components apparently associated with pathogenicity include the Elr protein (a protein from the WxL family) and polysaccharides, which are thought to interfere with phagocytosis of the organism by host immune cells. Some *E. faecalis* strains appear to harbor at least three distinct classes of capsular polysaccharide; some of these polysaccharides play a role in virulence and are potential targets for immunotherapy.

The third group of virulence factors has not been well characterized but consists of the *E. faecalis* stress protein Gls24, which has been associated with enterococcal resistance to bile salts and appears to be important in the pathogenesis of endocarditis, and the hyl_{Efm}-containing plasmids of *E. faecium*, which are transferable between strains and increase gastrointestinal colonization by *E. faecium*. In mouse peritonitis, acquisition of these plasmids increased the lethality of a commensal strain of *E. faecium*. Recently, a gene encoding a regulator of oxidative stress (AsrR) has been identified as an important virulence factor of *E. faecium*.

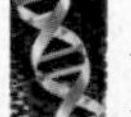

The ability to sequence bacterial genomes has increased our understanding of bacterial diversity, evolution, pathogenesis, and mechanisms of antibiotic resistance. The genome sequences of more than 560 enterococcal strains are currently available, and some have been entirely closed and annotated. Sequence analysis has shown that the genetic diversity of enterococci is related in large part to the acquisition of exogenous DNA and the mobilization of large chromosomal regions, resulting in recombination of the "core" genomes. In addition, analyses indicate that *E. faecium* harbors a malleable *accessory genome* incorporating a substantial content of exogenous elements, including DNA from phages. Indeed, a hospital-associated *E. faecium* clade that contains most clinical and outbreak-associated strains is the predominant genetic lineage circulating in hospitals around the world. This clade appears to be evolving rapidly, and genomic comparisons suggest that this lineage emerged 75 years ago—a time point that coincides with the introduction of antimicrobial drugs—and evolved from animal strains, not from human commensal isolates. An initial genomic separation within *E. faecium* appears to have occurred ~3000 years ago, simultaneous with urbanization and domestication of animals. This genomic information provides new clues with regard to the evolution of enterococci from commensal organisms to important nosocomial pathogens.

EPIDEMIOLOGY

According to the National Healthcare Safety Network of the Centers for Disease Control and Prevention, enterococci are the second most common organisms (after staphylococci) isolated from hospital-associated infections in the United States. Although *E. faecalis* remains the predominant species recovered from nosocomial infections, the isolation of *E. faecium* has increased substantially in the past 20 years. In fact, *E. faecium* is now almost as common as *E. faecalis* as an etiologic agent of hospital-associated infections. This point is important, because *E. faecium* is by far the most resistant and challenging enterococcal species to treat; indeed, more than 80% of *E. faecium* isolates recovered in U.S. hospitals are resistant to vancomycin, and more than 90% are resistant to ampicillin (historically the most effective β-lactam agent against enterococci). Resistance to vancomycin and ampicillin in *E. faecalis* isolates is much less common (~7% and ~4%, respectively).

The dynamics of enterococcal transmission and dissemination in the hospital environment have been extensively studied, with a focus on vancomycin-resistant enterococci (VRE). These studies have revealed that VRE colonization of the gastrointestinal tract is a critical step in the natural history of enterococcal disease and that a substantial proportion of patients colonized with VRE remain colonized for prolonged periods (sometimes >1 year) and are more likely to develop an *Enterococcus*-related illness (e.g., bacteremia). The most important factors associated with VRE colonization and persistence in the gut include prolonged hospitalization; long courses of antibiotic therapy; hospitalization in long-term-care facilities, surgical units, and/or intensive care units; organ transplantation; renal failure (particularly in patients undergoing hemodialysis) and/or diabetes; high Acute Physiology and Chronic Health Evaluation (APACHE) scores; and physical proximity to patients infected or colonized with VRE or these patients' rooms. Once a patient becomes colonized with VRE, several key factors are involved in the organisms' dissemination in the hospital environment. VRE can survive exposure to heat and certain disinfectants and have been found on numerous inanimate objects in the hospital, including bed rails, medical equipment, doorknobs, gloves, telephones, and computer keyboards. Thus health care workers and the environment play pivotal roles in enterococcal transmission from patient to patient, and infection control measures are crucial in breaking the chain of transmission. Moreover, two meta-analyses have found that, independent of the patient's clinical status, VRE infection increases the risk of death over that among individuals infected with a glycopeptide-susceptible enterococcal strain.

The epidemiology of enterococcal disease and the emergence of VRE have followed slightly different trends in other parts of the world than in the United States. In Europe, the emergence of VRE in the mid-1980s was seen primarily in isolates recovered from animals and healthy humans rather than from hospitalized patients. The presence of VRE was associated with the use of the glycopeptide avoparcin as a growth promoter in animal feeds; this association prompted the European Union to ban the use of this compound in animal husbandry in 1996. However, after an initial decrease in the isolation of VRE from animals and humans, the prevalence of hospital-associated VRE infections has slowly increased in certain European countries, with important regional differences. For example, rates of vancomycin resistance among *E. faecium* clinical isolates in Europe are highest in Greece, the United Kingdom, and Portugal (10–30%), whereas rates in the Scandinavian countries and the Netherlands are <1%. These regional differences have been attributed in part to the implementation of aggressive "search-and-destroy" policies of infection control in countries such as the Netherlands; these policies have kept the frequency of nosocomial methicillin-resistant *Staphylococcus aureus* (MRSA) and VRE very low. Despite regional differences, rates of VRE continue to be much lower in Europe than in the United States. The reasons are not totally understood, although it has been postulated that this difference is related to the higher levels of human antibiotic use in the United States. Rates of enterococcal resistance to vancomycin in some Latin American countries are also lower (~4%) than those in the United States. Conversely, in Asia, rates of vancomycin resistance among enterococci appear to be similar to those in U.S. hospitals.

As mentioned above, genomic analyses of vancomycin-resistant *E. faecium* in different parts of the world suggest that the emergence and dissemination of these organisms in the hospital environment worldwide are due to the success of a unique hospital-associated genetic clade that acquired the genes responsible for vancomycin resistance as well as other antibiotic resistance determinants.

CLINICAL SYNDROMES

URINARY TRACT INFECTION AND PROSTATITIS

Enterococci are well-known causes of nosocomial UTI—the most common infection caused by these organisms (Chap. 162). Enterococcal UTIs are usually associated with indwelling catheters, instrumentation, or anatomic abnormalities of the genitourinary tract, and it is often challenging to differentiate between true infection and colonization (particularly in patients with chronic indwelling catheters). The presence of leukocytes in the urine in conjunction with systemic manifestations (e.g., fever) or local signs and symptoms of infection with no other explanation and a positive urine culture ($\geq 10^5$ colony forming units [CFU]/mL) suggests the diagnosis. Moreover, enterococcal UTIs often occur in critically ill patients whose comorbidities may obscure the diagnosis. In many cases, removal of the indwelling catheter may suffice to eradicate the organism without specific antimicrobial therapy. In rare circumstances, UTIs caused by enterococci may run a complicated course, with the development of pyelonephritis and perinephric abscesses that may be a portal of entry for bloodstream infections (see below). Enterococci are also known causes of chronic prostatitis, particularly in patients whose urinary tract has been manipulated surgically or endoscopically. These infections can be difficult to treat because the agents most potent against enterococci (i.e., aminopenicillins and glycopeptides) penetrate prostatic tissue poorly. Chronic prostatic infection can be a source of recurrent enterococcal bacteremia.

BACTEREMIA AND ENDOCARDITIS

Bacteremia without endocarditis is one of the most common presentations of enterococcal disease. Intravascular catheters and other devices are commonly associated with these bacteremic episodes (Chap. 168). Other well-known sources of enterococcal bacteremia include the gastrointestinal and hepatobiliary tracts; pelvic and intraabdominal foci; and, less frequently, wound infections, UTIs, and bone infections. In the United States, enterococci are ranked second (after coagulase-negative staphylococci) as etiologic agents of central line–associated bacteremia. Patients with enterococcal bacteremia usually have comorbidities and have been in the hospital for prolonged periods; they commonly have received several courses of antibiotics. Several studies indicate that the isolation of *E. faecium* from the blood may lead to worse outcomes and higher mortality rates than when other enterococcal species are isolated; this finding may be related to the higher prevalence of vancomycin and ampicillin resistance in *E. faecium* than in other enterococcal species, with the consequent reduction of therapeutic options. In many cases (usually when the gastrointestinal tract is the source), enterococcal bacteremia may be polymicrobial, with gram-negative organisms isolated at the same time. In addition, several cases have now been documented in which enterococcal bacteremia was associated with *Strongyloides stercoralis* hyperinfection syndrome in immunocompromised patients.

Enterococci are important causes of community- and health care–associated endocarditis, ranking second after staphylococci in the latter infections. The presumed initial source of bacteremia leading to endocarditis is the gastrointestinal or genitourinary tract—e.g., in patients who have malignant and inflammatory conditions of the gut or have undergone procedures in which these tracts are manipulated. The affected patients tend to be male and elderly and to have other debilitating diseases and heart conditions. Both prosthetic and native valves can be involved; mitral and aortic valves are affected most often. Community-associated endocarditis (usually caused by *E. faecalis*) also occurs in patients with no apparent risk factors or cardiac abnormalities. Endocarditis in women of childbearing age has been well described. The typical presentation of enterococcal endocarditis is a subacute course of fever, weight loss, malaise, and cardiac murmur; typical stigmata of endocarditis (e.g., petechiae, Osler's nodes, Roth's spots) are found in only a minority of patients. Atypical manifestations include arthralgias and manifestations of metastatic disease (splenic abscesses, hiccups, pain in the left flank, pleural effusion, and spondylodiscitis). Embolic complications are variable and can affect the brain. Heart failure is a common complication of enterococcal endocarditis, and valve replacement may be critical in curing this infection, particularly when multidrug-resistant organisms or major complications are involved. The duration of therapy is usually 4–6 weeks, with more prolonged courses suggested for multidrug-resistant isolates in the absence of valvular replacement.

MENINGITIS

Enterococcal meningitis is an uncommon disease (accounting for only ~4% of meningitis cases) that is usually associated with neurosurgical interventions and conditions such as shunts, central nervous system (CNS) trauma, and cerebrospinal fluid (CSF) leakage. In some instances—usually in patients with a debilitating condition, such as cardiovascular or congenital heart disease, chronic renal failure, malignancy, receipt of immunosuppressive therapy, or HIV/AIDS—presumed hematogenous seeding of the meninges is seen in infections such as endocarditis or bacteremia. Fever and changes in mental status are common, whereas overt meningeal signs are less so. CSF findings are consistent with bacterial infection—i.e., pleocytosis with a predominance of polymorphonuclear leukocytes (average, ~500/μL), an elevated serum protein level (usually >100 mg/dL), and a decreased glucose concentration (average, 28 mg/dL). Gram's staining yields a positive result in about half of cases, with a high rate of organism recovery from CSF cultures; the most common species isolated are *E. faecalis* and *E. faecium*. Complications include hydrocephalus, brain abscesses, and stroke. As mentioned before for bacteremia, an association with *Strongyloides* hyperinfection has also been documented.

INTRAABDOMINAL, PELVIC, AND SOFT TISSUE INFECTIONS

As mentioned earlier, enterococci are part of the commensal flora of the gastrointestinal tract and can produce spontaneous peritonitis in cirrhotic individuals and in patients undergoing chronic ambulatory peritoneal dialysis (Chap. 159). These organisms are commonly found (usually along with other bacteria, including enteric gram-negative species and anaerobes) in clinical samples from intraabdominal and pelvic collections. The presence of enterococci in intraabdominal infections is sometimes considered to be of little clinical relevance. Several studies have shown that the role of enterococci in intraabdominal infections originating in the community and involving previously healthy patients is minor, because surgery and broad-spectrum antimicrobial drugs that do not target enterococci are often sufficient to treat these infections successfully. In the last few decades, however, these organisms have become prominent as a cause of intraabdominal infections in hospitalized patients because of the emergence and spread of vancomycin resistance among enterococci and the increase in rates of nosocomial infections due to multidrug-resistant *E. faecium* isolates. In fact, several studies have now documented treatment failures due to enterococci, with consequently increased rates of postoperative complications and death among patients with intraabdominal infections. Thus, anti-enterococcal therapy is recommended for nosocomial peritonitis in immunocompromised and severely ill patients who have had a prolonged hospital stay, have undergone multiple procedures, have persistent abdominal sepsis and collections, or have risk factors for the development of endocarditis (e.g., prosthetic or damaged heart valves). Conversely, specific treatment for enterococci in the first episode of intraabdominal infections originating in the community and affecting previously healthy patients with no important cardiac risk factors for endocarditis does not appear to be beneficial.

Enterococci are commonly isolated from soft tissue infections (Chap. 156), particularly those involving surgical wounds (Chap. 168). In fact, these organisms rank third as agents of nosocomial surgical-site infections, with *E. faecalis* the most frequently isolated species. The clinical relevance of enterococci in some of these infections—as in intraabdominal infections—is a matter of debate; differentiating between colonization and true infection is sometimes challenging, although in some cases enterococci have been recovered from lung, liver, and skin abscesses. Diabetic foot and decubitus ulcers are often colonized with enterococci and may be the portal of entry for bone infections.

OTHER INFECTIONS

Enterococci are well-known causes of neonatal infections, including sepsis (mostly late-onset), bacteremia, meningitis, pneumonia, and UTI. Outbreaks of enterococcal sepsis in neonatal units have been well documented. Risk factors for enterococcal disease in newborns include prematurity, low birth weight, indwelling devices, and abdominal surgery. Enterococci have also been described as etiologic agents of bone and joint infections, including vertebral osteomyelitis, usually in patients with underlying conditions such as diabetes or endocarditis. Similarly, enterococci have been isolated from bone infections in patients who have undergone arthroplasty or reconstruction of fractures with the placement of hardware. Because enterococci can produce a biofilm that is likely to alter the efficacy of otherwise active anti-enterococcal agents, treatment of infections that involve foreign material is challenging, and removal of the hardware may be necessary to eradicate the infection. Rare cases of enterococcal pneumonia, lung abscess, and spontaneous empyema have been described.

TREATMENT ENTEROCOCCAL INFECTIONS

GENERAL PRINCIPLES

Enterococci are intrinsically resistant and/or tolerant to several antimicrobial agents (with *tolerance* defined as lack of killing by drug concentrations 32 times higher than the minimal inhibitory concentration [MIC]). Monotherapy for endocarditis with a β-lactam antibiotic (to which many enterococci are tolerant) has produced disappointing results, with low cure rates at the end of therapy. However, the addition of an aminoglycoside to a cell wall–active agent (a β-lactam or a glycopeptide) increases cure rates and eradicates the organisms; moreover, this combination is synergistic and bactericidal in vitro. Therefore, for many decades, combination therapy with a cell wall–active agent and an aminoglycoside has been the standard of care for endovascular infections caused by enterococci. This synergistic effect can be explained, at least in part, by the increased penetration of the aminoglycoside into the bacterial cell, presumably as a result of cell wall alterations produced by the β-lactam (or glycopeptide). Nonetheless, attaining synergistic bactericidal activity in the treatment of severe enterococcal infections has become increasingly difficult because of the development of resistance to virtually all antibiotics available for this purpose.

The treatment of *E. faecalis* differs substantially from that of *E. faecium* (Tables 174-1 and 174-2), mainly because of differences in resistance profiles (see below). For example, resistance to ampicillin and vancomycin is rare in *E. faecalis*, whereas these antibiotics are only infrequently useful against current isolates of *E. faecium*. Moreover, as a consequence of the challenges and therapeutic limitations posed by the emergence of drug resistance in enterococci,

TABLE 174-1 SUGGESTED REGIMENS FOR THE MANAGEMENT OF INFECTIONS CAUSED BY *ENTEROCOCCUS FAECALIS*

Clinical Syndrome	Suggested Therapeutic Options[a]
Endovascular infections (including endocarditis)	• Ampicillin[b] (12 g/d IV in divided doses q4h or by continuous infusion) *or* penicillin (18–30 million units/d IV in divided doses q4h or by continuous infusion) ***plus*** an aminoglycoside[c] • Ampicillin[b] (12 g/d IV in divided doses q4h) *plus* ceftriaxone (2 g IV q12h) • Vancomycin[d] (15 mg/kg IV per dose) *plus* an aminoglycoside[c] • High-dose daptomycin[e] ± another active agent[f] • Ampicillin[b] *plus* imipenem
Nonendovascular bacteremia[g]	• Ampicillin (12 g/d IV in divided doses q4h) *or* penicillin (18 million units/d IV in divided doses q4h) ± an aminoglycoside[c] or ceftriaxone • Vancomycin[d] (15 mg/kg IV per dose) • High-dose daptomycin[e] ± another active agent[f] • Linezolid (600 mg IV/PO q12h)
Meningitis	• Ampicillin (20–24 g/d IV in divided doses q4h) *or* penicillin (24 million units/d IV in divided doses q4h) ***plus*** an aminoglycoside[c,h] or ceftriaxone • Vancomycin (500–750 mg IV q6h)[d] ***plus*** an aminoglycoside[c] *or* rifampin • Linezolid • High-dose daptomycin[e] (*plus* intrathecal daptomycin) ± another active agent[f]
Urinary tract infections (uncomplicated)	• Fosfomycin (3 g PO, one dose)[i] • Ampicillin (500 mg IV or PO q6h) • Nitrofurantoin (100 mg PO q6h)

[a]Authors' preferences are underlined for each category; many of these regimens are off-label. [b]In rare cases, β-lactamase-producing isolates may be found. Because these isolates are not detected by conventional minimal inhibitory concentration determination, additional tests (e.g., the nitrocefin disk) are recommended for isolates from endocarditis. The use of ampicillin/sulbactam (12–24 g/d) is suggested in these cases. [c]Only if the organism does not exhibit high-level resistance (HLR) to aminoglycosides. HLR is assessed by the clinical microbiology laboratory only for gentamicin or streptomycin, because gentamicin (1–1.5 mg/kg IV q8h) and streptomycin (15 mg/kg per day IV/IM, in two divided doses) are the only two recommended aminoglycosides. The test used to detect HLR is the growth of enterococci on agar containing gentamicin (500 μg/mL) or streptomycin (2000 μg/mL). If HLR is documented, the aminoglycoside will not act synergistically with the other agent in the combination. HLR to gentamicin implies lack of synergism with tobramycin and with amikacin. [d]Vancomycin is recommended only as an alternative to β-lactam agents in cases of allergy, toxicity, and inability to desensitize. Cerebrospinal fluid (CSF) concentrations should be determined in meningitis. Vancomycin-resistant strains of *E. faecalis* have been reported. [e]Consider doses of 8–10 mg/kg per day if used in combination and 10–12 mg/kg per day if used alone. Close monitoring of creatine phosphokinase levels is recommended throughout therapy because of possible rhabdomyolysis. [f]Potentially active agents may include an aminoglycoside (if HLR is not detected), ampicillin, ceftaroline, tigecycline, or a fluoroquinolone (which, if the isolate is susceptible, may be favored in meningitis). [g]In selected cases of catheter-associated bacteremia, removal of the catheter and a short course of therapy (~5–7 days) may be sufficient. A single positive blood culture that is likely to be associated with a catheter in a patient who is otherwise doing well may not require therapy after removal of the catheter. Patients at high risk for endovascular infections or with severe disease may benefit from synergistic combination therapy. [h]The addition of intrathecal or intraventricular therapy with gentamicin (2–10 mg/d if the organism does not exhibit HLR) or vancomycin (10–20 mg/d when the isolate is susceptible) has been suggested by some authorities. The addition of systemic rifampin (a good CSF-penetrating agent) may be considered. The combination of ampicillin and ceftriaxone may have clinical benefit (by analogy with endocarditis), but no cases treated with this combination have been reported. [i]Approved by the Food and Drug Administration only for uncomplicated urinary tract infections caused by vancomycin-susceptible *E. faecalis*.

TABLE 174-2 SUGGESTED REGIMENS FOR THE MANAGEMENT OF INFECTIONS CAUSED BY VANCOMYCIN- AND AMPICILLIN-RESISTANT *ENTEROCOCCUS FAECIUM*

Clinical Syndrome	Suggested Therapeutic Options[a]
Endovascular infections (including endocarditis)	• High-dose daptomycin[b] ***plus*** another agent[c] ± an aminoglycoside[d] • Q/D[e] (22.5 mg/kg per day in divided doses q8h) ± another active agent[f] • Linezolid[e] (600 mg IV q12h) • High-dose ampicillin (if MIC is ≤64 μg/mL) ± an aminoglycoside[d]
Nonendovascular bacteremia[g]	• High-dose daptomycin[b] ± another agent[c] ± an aminoglycoside[d] • Q/D (22.5 mg/kg per day in divided doses q8h) ± another active agent[f] • Linezolid (600 mg IV q12h)
Meningitis	• Linezolid (600 mg IV q12h) ± another CSF-penetrating active agent[h] • Q/D (22.5 mg/kg per day in divided doses q8h *plus* intraventricular Q/D)[i] ± another active agent[h] • High-dose daptomycin[b] (*plus* intraventricular daptomycin) ± another CSF-penetrating active agent[h,j]
Urinary tract infections	• Fosfomycin (3 g PO, one dose)[k] • Nitrofurantoin (100 mg PO q6h) • Ampicillin or amoxicillin (2 g IV/PO q4–6h)[l]

[a]Authors' preferences are underlined for each category; many of these regimens are off-label. [b]Consider doses of 8–10 mg/kg per day if used in combination and 10–12 mg/kg per day if used alone (off-label). Close monitoring of creatine phosphokinase levels is recommended throughout therapy because of possible rhabdomyolysis. [c]Potentially active agents may include ampicillin or ceftaroline (even if the infecting strain is resistant in vitro) or tigecycline. In vitro synergism of daptomycin with some β-lactam agents is observed against some isolates that subsequently become nonsusceptible to daptomycin during therapy. Consider combination therapy if the daptomycin minimal inhibitory concentration (MIC) is ≥3 μg/mL. [d]Only if the organism does not exhibit high-level resistance to aminoglycosides (see Table 174–1, footnote c). [e]Quinupristin-dalfopristin (Q/D) and linezolid are listed in the American Heart Association's recommendations for the treatment of endocarditis caused by vancomycin- and ampicillin resistant *E. faecium*. [f]Agents that may be useful in combination with Q/D (if the isolate is susceptible to each agent) include doxycycline with rifampin (one reported case) and fluoroquinolones (one reported case). [g]In selected cases of catheter-associated bacteremia, removal of the catheter and a short course of therapy (~5–7 days) may be sufficient. A single positive blood culture that is likely to be associated with a catheter in a patient who is otherwise doing well may not require therapy after removal of the catheter. [h]Fluoroquinolone antibiotics (e.g., moxifloxacin) and rifampin (if the isolate is susceptible to each agent) reach therapeutic levels in the cerebrospinal fluid (CSF). [i]Intrathecal Q/D (1–5 mg/d) has been used in combination with Q/D systemic therapy in meningitis. If Q/D is chosen, simultaneous use of both systemic and intrathecal therapy is suggested. [j]Intrathecal gentamicin (2–10 mg/d) if high-level resistance is not detected. Intraventricular daptomycin has been used in two cases of meningitis. [k]Approved by the Food and Drug Administration only for uncomplicated urinary tract infections caused by vancomycin-susceptible *E. faecalis*. [l]Concentrations of amoxicillin and ampicillin in urine far exceed those in serum and may be potentially effective even against isolates with high MICs. Doses up to 12 g/d are suggested for isolates with MICs of ≥64 μg/mL.

valve replacement may need to be considered in the treatment of endocarditis caused by multidrug-resistant enterococci. Less severe infections are often related to indwelling intravascular catheters; removal of the catheter increases the likelihood of enterococcal eradication by a subsequent short course of appropriate antimicrobial therapy.

CHOICE OF ANTIMICROBIAL AGENTS

Among the β-lactams, the most active are the aminopenicillins (ampicillin, amoxicillin) and ureidopenicillins (i.e., piperacillin); next most active are penicillin G and imipenem. For *E. faecium*, a combination of high-dose ampicillin (up to 30 g/d) plus an aminoglycoside has been suggested—even for ampicillin-resistant strains if the MIC is ≤64 μg/mL—because a plasma ampicillin concentration of >100 μg/mL can be achieved at high doses. The only two aminoglycosides recommended for synergistic therapy in severe enterococcal infections are gentamicin and streptomycin. The use of amikacin is discouraged, tobramycin should never be used against *E. faecium*, and aminoglycoside monotherapy is not effective. Vancomycin is an alternative to β-lactam drugs for the treatment of *E. faecalis* infections but is less useful against *E. faecium* because resistance is common.

As mentioned above, use of the aminoglycoside–ampicillin combination for *E. faecalis* infections has become increasingly problematic because of toxicity in critically ill patients and increased rates of high-level resistance to aminoglycosides. A recent observational, nonrandomized, comparative study encompassing a multicenter cohort was conducted in 17 Spanish hospitals and 1 Italian hospital; this study found that the combination of ampicillin and ceftriaxone is as effective as ampicillin plus gentamicin in the treatment of *E. faecalis* endocarditis, with less risk of toxicity. Therefore, this regimen should be considered in patients at risk for aminoglycoside toxicity and could be considered for all patients.

Linezolid and quinupristin/dalfopristin (Q/D) are two agents approved by the U.S. Food and Drug Administration (FDA) for the treatment of some VRE infections (Table 174–2). Linezolid is not bactericidal, and its use in severe endovascular infections has produced mixed results; therefore, it is recommended only as an alternative to other agents. In addition, linezolid may cause significant toxicities (thrombocytopenia, peripheral neuropathy, and optic neuritis) when used in regimens given for >2 weeks. Nonetheless, linezolid may play a role in the treatment of enterococcal meningitis and other CNS infections, although clinical data are limited. Q/D is not active against most *E. faecalis* isolates, and its in vivo efficacy against *E. faecium* may often be compromised by resistance (see below). Adverse reactions to Q/D are common, including pain and inflammation at the infusion site and severe arthralgias and myalgias leading to discontinuation of treatment. Thus, Q/D should be used with caution and probably combined with other agents (Table 174–2).

The lipopeptide daptomycin is a bactericidal antibiotic with potent in vitro activity against all enterococci. Although daptomycin is not approved by the FDA for the treatment of VRE or *E. faecium* infections, it has been used alone (at high dosage) or in combination with other agents (ampicillin, ceftaroline, and tigecycline) with apparent success against multidrug-resistant enterococcal infections (Tables 174–1 and 174–2). The main adverse reactions to daptomycin are elevated creatine phosphokinase levels and eosinophilic pneumonitis (rare). Daptomycin is not useful against pulmonary infections because the pulmonary surfactant inhibits its antibacterial activity. Although the glycylcycline drug tigecycline is active in vitro against all enterococci (regardless of the isolates' vancomycin susceptibility), its use as monotherapy for endovascular or severe enterococcal infections is not recommended because of low attainable blood levels. Telavancin, a lipoglycopeptide approved by the FDA for the treatment of skin and soft tissue infections as well as hospital-associated pneumonia, is active against vancomycin-susceptible enterococci but not VRE. Oritavancin, a compound of the same class that is active against VRE, has recently been approved by the FDA for the treatment of bacterial skin and soft tissue infections and may offer promise for the treatment of VRE in the future.

ANTIMICROBIAL RESISTANCE

As mentioned above, resistance to β-lactam agents continues to be observed only infrequently in *E. faecalis*, although rare outbreaks caused by β-lactamase-producing isolates have occurred in the United States and Argentina. However, ampicillin resistance is common in *E. faecium*. The mechanism of this resistance is related to a penicillin-binding protein (PBP) designated PBP5, which is the target of β-lactam antibiotics. PBP5 exhibits lower affinity for ampicillin and can synthesize cell wall in the presence of this antibiotic, even when other PBPs are inhibited. Two common mechanisms of high-level ampicillin resistance (MIC, >64 μg/mL) in clinical strains are (1) mutations in the PBP5-encoding gene that further decrease the protein's affinity for ampicillin and (2) hyperproduction of PBP5. These factors preclude the use of all β-lactam agents in the treatment of *E. faecium* infections.

Vancomycin is a glycopeptide antibiotic that inhibits cell wall peptidoglycan synthesis in susceptible enterococci and has been widely used against enterococcal infections in clinical practice when the utility of β-lactams is limited by resistance, allergy, or adverse reactions. This effect is mediated by binding of the antibiotic to peptidoglycan precursors (UDP-MurNAc-pentapeptides) upon their exit from the bacterial cell cytoplasm. The interaction of vancomycin with the peptidoglycan is specific and involves the last two D-alanine residues of the precursor. The first isolates of VRE were documented in 1986, and vancomycin resistance (particularly in *E. faecium*) has since increased considerably around the world. The mechanism involves the replacement of the last D-alanine residue of peptidoglycan precursors with D-lactate or D-serine, with consequent high- and low-level resistance, respectively. There is significant heterogeneity among isolates, but either substitution substantially decreases the affinity of vancomycin for the peptidoglycan; with the D-lactate substitution, the MIC is increased by up to 1000-fold. Vancomycin-resistant organisms also produce enzymes that destroy the D-alanine-D-alanine ending precursors, ensuring that additional binding sites for vancomycin are not available.

High-level resistance to aminoglycosides (of which gentamicin and streptomycin are the only two tested by clinical laboratories) abolishes the synergism observed between cell wall–active agents and the aminoglycoside. This important phenotype is routinely sought in isolates from serious infections (Tables 174–1 and 174–2). The laboratory reports high-level resistance as gentamicin and streptomycin MICs of >500 μg/mL and >2000 μg/mL, respectively (agar dilution method) or as "SYN-R" (resistance to synergism). Genes encoding aminoglycoside-modifying enzymes are usually the cause of high-level resistance to these compounds and are widely disseminated among enterococci, decreasing the options for the treatment of severe enterococcal infections. The aforementioned enterococcal resistance to newer antibiotics such as linezolid (usually due to mutations in the 23S rRNA genes and the presence of an rRNA methylase), Q/D, daptomycin (involving major changes in cell membrane homeostasis), and tigecycline further reduces therapeutic alternatives.

175 Diphtheria and Other Corynebacterial Infections

William R. Bishai, John R. Murphy

DIPHTHERIA

Diphtheria is a nasopharyngeal and skin infection caused by *Corynebacterium diphtheriae*. Toxigenic strains of *C. diphtheriae* produce a protein toxin that causes systemic toxicity, myocarditis, and polyneuropathy. The toxin is associated with the formation of pseudomembranes in the pharynx during respiratory diphtheria. While toxigenic strains most frequently cause pharyngeal diphtheria, nontoxigenic strains commonly cause cutaneous disease.

ETIOLOGY

C. diphtheriae is a gram-positive bacillus that is unencapsulated, nonmotile, and nonsporulating. The organism was first identified microscopically in 1883 by Klebs and a year later was isolated in pure culture by Löffler in Robert Koch's laboratory. The bacteria have a characteristic club-shaped bacillary appearance and typically form clusters of parallel rays, or *palisades*, that are referred to as "Chinese characters." The specific laboratory media recommended for the cultivation of *C. diphtheriae* rely upon tellurite, colistin, or nalidixic acid for the organism's selective isolation from other autochthonous pharyngeal microbes. *C. diphtheriae* may be isolated from individuals with both nontoxigenic (*tox*$^-$) and toxigenic (*tox*$^+$) phenotypes. Uchida and Pappenheimer demonstrated that corynebacteriophage beta carries the structural gene *tox*, which encodes diphtheria toxin, and that a family of closely related corynebacteriophages are responsible for toxigenic conversion of *tox*$^-$ *C. diphtheriae* to the *tox*$^+$ phenotype. Moreover, lysogenic conversion from a nontoxigenic to a toxigenic phenotype has been shown to occur in situ. Growth of toxigenic strains of *C. diphtheriae* under iron-limiting conditions leads to the optimal expression of diphtheria toxin and is believed to be a pathogenic mechanism during human infection.

EPIDEMIOLOGY

While in many regions diphtheria has been controlled in recent years with effective vaccination, there have been sporadic outbreaks in the United States and Europe. Diphtheria is still common in the Caribbean, Latin America, and the Indian subcontinent, where mass immunization programs are not enforced. Large-scale epidemics of diphtheria have occurred in the post-Soviet independent states. Additional outbreaks have been reported in Algeria, China, and Ecuador.

C. diphtheriae is transmitted via the aerosol route, usually during close contact with an infected person. There are no significant reservoirs other than humans. The incubation period for respiratory diphtheria is 2–5 days, but disease onset has occurred as late as 10 days after exposure. Prior to the vaccination era, most individuals over the age of 10 were immune to *C. diphtheriae*; infants were protected by maternal IgG antibodies but became susceptible after ~6 months of age. Thus, the disease primarily affected children and nonimmune young adults. In temperate regions, respiratory diphtheria occurs year-round but is most common during winter months.

The development of diphtheria antitoxin in 1898 by von Behring and of the diphtheria toxoid vaccine in 1924 by Ramon led to the near-elimination of diphtheria in Western countries. The annual incidence rate in the United States peaked in 1921 at 191 cases per 100,000 population. In contrast, since 1980, the annual figure in the United States has been <5 cases per 100,000. Nevertheless, pockets of colonization persist in North America, particularly in South Dakota, Ontario, and recently the state of Washington. Immunity to diphtheria induced by childhood vaccination gradually decreases in adulthood. An estimated 30% of men 60–69 years old have antitoxin titers below the protective level. In addition to older age and lack of vaccination, risk factors for diphtheria outbreaks include alcoholism, low socioeconomic status, crowded living conditions, and Native American ethnic background. An outbreak of diphtheria in Seattle, Washington, between 1972 and 1982 comprised 1100 cases, most of which were cutaneous. During the 1990s in the states of the former Soviet Union, a much larger diphtheria epidemic included more than 150,000 cases and more than 5000 deaths. Clonally related toxigenic *C. diphtheriae* strains of the ET8 complex were associated with this outbreak. Given that the ET8 complex expressed a toxin against which the prevalent diphtheria toxoid vaccine was effective, the epidemic was attributed to failure of the public health infrastructure to effectively vaccinate the population. Beginning in 1998, this epidemic was controlled by mass vaccination programs. During the epidemic, the incidence rate was high among individuals between 16 and 50 years of age. Socioeconomic instability, migration, deteriorating public health programs, frequent vaccine shortages, delayed implementation of vaccination and treatment in response to cases, and lack of public education and awareness were contributing factors.

Significant outbreaks of diphtheria and diphtheria-related mortality continue to be reported from many developing countries, particularly in Africa and Asia. Statistics collected by the World Health Organization indicated the occurrence of ~7000 reported diphtheria cases in 2008 and ~5000 diphtheria deaths in 2004. Although ~82% of the global population has been adequately vaccinated, only 26% of countries have successfully vaccinated >80% of individuals in all districts.

Cutaneous diphtheria is usually a secondary infection that follows a primary skin lesion due to trauma, allergy, or autoimmunity. Most often, these isolates lack the *tox* gene and thus do not express diphtheria toxin. In tropical latitudes, cutaneous diphtheria is more common than respiratory diphtheria. In contrast to respiratory disease, cutaneous diphtheria is not reportable in the United States. Nontoxigenic strains of *C. diphtheriae* have also been associated with pharyngitis in Europe, causing outbreaks among men who have sex with men and persons who use illicit IV drugs.

PATHOGENESIS AND IMMUNOLOGY

Diphtheria toxin produced by *tox*$^+$ strains of *C. diphtheriae* is the primary virulence factor in clinical disease. The toxin is synthesized in precursor form; is released as a 535-amino-acid, single-chain protein; and, in sensitive species (e.g., guinea pigs and humans, but not mice or rats), has a 50% lethal dose of ~100 ng/kg of body weight. The toxin is produced in the pseudomembranous lesion and is taken up in the bloodstream, from which it is distributed to all organ systems in the body. Once bound to its cell surface receptor (a heparin-binding epidermal growth factor–like precursor), the toxin is internalized by receptor-mediated endocytosis and enters the cytosol from an acidified early endosomal compartment. In vitro, the toxin may be separated into two chains by digestion with serine proteases: the N-terminal A fragment and the C-terminal B fragment. Delivery of the A fragment into the eukaryotic cell cytosol results in irreversible inhibition of protein synthesis by NAD$^+$-dependent ADP-ribosylation of elongation factor 2. The eventual result is the death of the cell.

In 1926, Ramon at the Institut Pasteur found that formalinization of diphtheria toxin resulted in the production of a nontoxic but highly immunogenic diphtheria toxoid. Subsequent studies showed that immunization with diphtheria toxoid elicited antibodies that neutralized the toxin and prevented most disease manifestations. In the 1930s, mass immunization of children and susceptible adults with diphtheria toxoid commenced in the United States and Europe.

Individuals with a diphtheria antitoxin titer of >0.01 U/mL are at low risk of disease. In populations where a majority of individuals have protective antitoxin titers, the carrier rate for toxigenic strains of *C. diphtheriae* decreases and the overall risk of diphtheria among susceptible individuals is reduced. Nevertheless, individuals with nonprotective titers may contract diphtheria through either travel or exposure to individuals who have recently returned from regions where the disease is endemic.

Characteristic pathologic findings of diphtheria include mucosal ulcers with a pseudomembranous coating composed of an inner band of fibrin and a luminal band of neutrophils. Initially white and firmly adherent, in advanced diphtheria the pseudomembranes turn gray or even green or black as necrosis progresses. Mucosal ulcers result from toxin-induced necrosis of the epithelium accompanied by edema, hyperemia, and vascular congestion of the submucosal base. A significant fibrinosuppurative exudate from the ulcer develops into the pseudomembrane. Ulcers and pseudomembranes in severe respiratory diphtheria may extend from the pharynx into medium-sized bronchial airways. Expanding and sloughing membranes may result in fatal airway obstruction.

APPROACH TO THE PATIENT: Diphtheria

Diphtheria, though rare in the United States and other developed countries, should be considered when a patient has severe pharyngitis, particularly when there is difficulty swallowing, respiratory compromise, or signs of systemic disease (e.g., myocarditis or generalized weakness). The leading causes of pharyngitis are respiratory viruses (rhinoviruses, influenza viruses, parainfluenza viruses, coronaviruses, adenoviruses; ~25% of cases), group A streptococci (15–30%), group C streptococci (~5%), atypical bacteria such as *Mycoplasma pneumoniae* and *Chlamydia pneumoniae* (15–20% in some series), and other viruses such as herpes simplex virus (~4%) and Epstein-Barr virus (<1% in infectious mononucleosis). Less common causes are acute HIV infection, gonorrhea, fusobacterial infection (e.g., Lemierre's syndrome), thrush due to *Candida albicans* or other *Candida* species, and diphtheria. The presence of a pharyngeal pseudomembrane or an extensive exudate should prompt consideration of diphtheria (Figure 175-1).

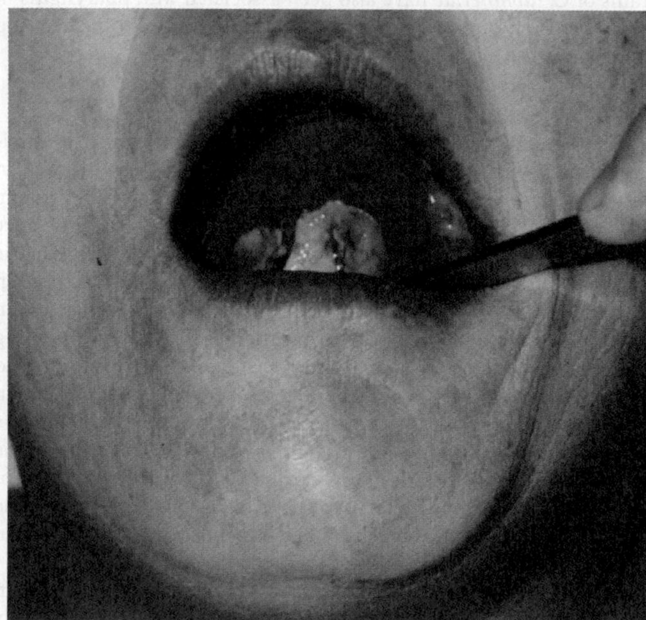

FIGURE 175-1 Respiratory diphtheria due to toxigenic *C. diphtheriae* producing exudative pharyngitis in a 47-year-old female patient displaying neck edema and a pseudomembrane extending from the uvula to the pharyngeal wall. The characteristic white pseudomembrane is caused by diphtheria toxin–mediated necrosis of the respiratory epithelial layer, producing a fibrinous coagulative exudate. Submucosal edema adds to airway narrowing. The pharyngitis is acute in onset, and respiratory obstruction from the pseudomembrane may occur in severe cases. Inoculation of pseudomembrane fragments or submembranous swabs onto Löffler's or tellurite selective medium reveals *C. diphtheriae*. *(Photograph by P. Strebel, MD, used by permission. From R. Kadirova et al: J Infect Dis 181:S110, 2000. With permission of Oxford University Press.)*

CLINICAL MANIFESTATIONS

Respiratory Diphtheria The clinical diagnosis of diphtheria is based on the constellation of sore throat; adherent tonsillar, pharyngeal, or nasal pseudomembranous lesions; and low-grade fever. In addition, diagnosis requires the isolation of *C. diphtheriae* or histopathologic isolation of compatible gram-positive organisms. The Centers for Disease Control and Prevention (CDC) recognizes *confirmed* respiratory diphtheria (laboratory proven or epidemiologically linked to a culture-confirmed case) and *probable* respiratory diphtheria (clinically compatible but not laboratory proven or epidemiologically linked). Carriers are defined as individuals who have positive cultures for *C. diphtheriae* and who either are asymptomatic or have symptoms but lack pseudomembranes. Most patients seek medical care for sore throat and fever several days into the illness. Occasionally, weakness, dysphagia, headache, and voice change are the initial manifestations. Neck edema and difficulty breathing are evident in more advanced cases and carry a poor prognosis.

The systemic manifestations of diphtheria stem from the effects of diphtheria toxin and include weakness as a result of neurotoxicity and cardiac arrhythmias or congestive heart failure due to myocarditis. Most commonly, the pseudomembranous lesion is located in the tonsillopharyngeal region. Less commonly, the lesions are located in the larynx, nares, and trachea or bronchial passages. Large pseudomembranes are associated with severe disease and a poor prognosis. A few patients develop massive swelling of the tonsils and present with "bull-neck" diphtheria, which results from massive edema of the submandibular and paratracheal region and is further characterized by foul breath, thick speech, and stridorous breathing. The diphtheritic pseudomembrane is gray or whitish and sharply demarcated. Unlike the exudative lesion associated with streptococcal pharyngitis, the pseudomembrane in diphtheria is tightly adherent to the underlying tissues. Attempts to dislodge the membrane may cause bleeding. Hoarseness suggests laryngeal diphtheria, in which laryngoscopy may be diagnostically helpful.

Cutaneous Diphtheria This dermatosis is characterized by punched-out ulcerative lesions with necrotic sloughing or pseudomembrane formation (Figure 175-2). The diagnosis requires cultivation of *C. diphtheriae* from lesions, which most commonly occur on the lower and upper extremities, head, and trunk.

Infections Due to Non-*diphtheriae Corynebacterium* Species and Nontoxigenic *C. diphtheriae* Non-*diphtheriae* species of *Corynebacterium* and related genera (discussed below) as well as nontoxigenic strains of *C. diphtheriae* itself have been found in bloodstream and respiratory infections, often in individuals with immunosuppression or chronic respiratory disease. These organisms can cause disease manifestations and should not necessarily be dismissed as colonizers.

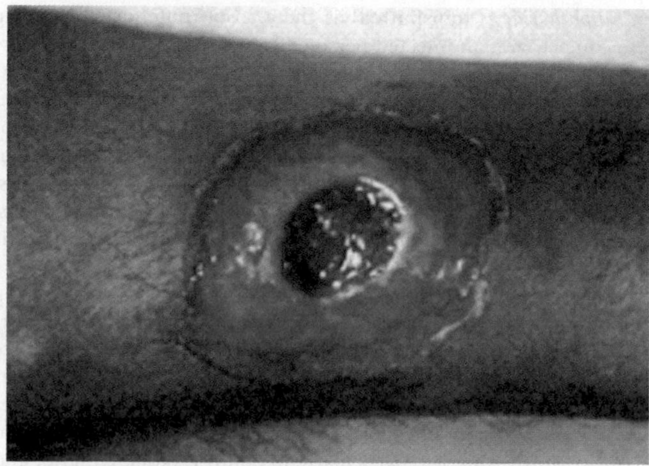

FIGURE 175-2 Cutaneous diphtheria due to nontoxigenic *C. diphtheriae* on the lower extremity. *(From the Centers for Disease Control and Prevention.)*

Other Clinical Manifestations *C. diphtheriae* causes rare cases of endocarditis and septic arthritis, most often in patients with preexisting risk factors, such as abnormal cardiac valves, injection drug use, or cirrhosis.

COMPLICATIONS

Airway obstruction poses a significant early risk in patients presenting with advanced diphtheria. Pseudomembranes may slough and obstruct the airway or may advance to the larynx or into the tracheobronchial tree. Children are particularly prone to obstruction because of their small airways.

Polyneuropathy and myocarditis are late toxic manifestations of diphtheria. During a diphtheria outbreak in the Kyrgyz Republic in 1999, myocarditis was found in 22% and neuropathy in 5% of 656 hospitalized patients. The mortality rate was 7% among patients with myocarditis as opposed to 2% among those without myocardial manifestations. The median time to death in hospitalized patients was 4.5 days. Myocarditis is typically associated with dysrhythmia of the conduction tract and dilated cardiomyopathy.

Polyneuropathy is seen 3–5 weeks after the onset of diphtheria and has a slow indolent course. However, patients may develop severe and prolonged neurologic abnormalities. The disorders typically occur in the mouth and neck, with lingual or facial numbness as well as dysphonia, dysphagia, and cranial nerve paresthesias. More ominous signs include weakness of respiratory and abdominal muscles and paresis of the extremities. Sensory manifestations and sensory ataxia also are observed. Cranial nerve dysfunction typically precedes disturbances of the trunk and extremities because of proximity to the site of infection. Autonomic dysfunction also is associated with polyneuropathy and can lead to hypotension. Polyneuropathy is typically reversible in patients who survive the acute phase.

Other complications of diphtheria include pneumonia, renal failure, encephalitis, cerebral infarction, pulmonary embolism, and serum sickness from antitoxin therapy.

DIAGNOSIS

The diagnosis of diphtheria is based on clinical signs and symptoms plus laboratory confirmation. Respiratory diphtheria should be considered in patients with sore throat, pharyngeal exudates, and fever. Other symptoms may include hoarseness, stridor, or palatal paralysis. The presence of a pseudomembrane should prompt strong consideration of diphtheria. Once a clinical diagnosis of diphtheria is made, diphtheria antitoxin should be obtained and administered as rapidly as possible.

Laboratory diagnosis of diphtheria is based either on cultivation of *C. diphtheriae* or toxigenic *Corynebacterium ulcerans* from the site of infection or on the demonstration of local lesions with characteristic histopathology. *Corynebacterium pseudodiphtheriticum*, a nontoxigenic organism, is a common component of the normal throat flora and does not pose a significant risk. Throat samples should be submitted to the laboratory for culture with the notation that diphtheria is being considered. This information should prompt cultivation on special selective medium and subsequent biochemical testing to differentiate *C. diphtheriae* from other nasopharyngeal commensal corynebacteria. All laboratory isolates of *C. diphtheriae*, including nontoxigenic strains, should be submitted to the CDC.

A diagnosis of cutaneous diphtheria requires laboratory confirmation since the lesions are not characteristic and are indistinguishable from other dermatoses. Diphtheritic ulcers occasionally—but not consistently—have a punched-out appearance (Fig. 175-2). Patients in whom cutaneous diphtheria is identified should have the nasopharynx cultured for *C. diphtheriae*. The laboratory medium for cutaneous diphtheria specimens is the same as that used for respiratory diphtheria: Löffler's or Tinsdale's selective medium in addition to nonselective medium such as blood agar. As has been mentioned, respiratory diphtheria remains a notifiable disease in the United States, whereas cutaneous diphtheria is not.

TREATMENT DIPHTHERIA

DIPHTHERIA ANTITOXIN

Prompt administration of diphtheria antitoxin is critical in the management of respiratory diphtheria. Diphtheria antitoxin, a horse antiserum, is effective in reducing the extent of local disease as well as the risk of complications of myocarditis and neuropathy. Rapid institution of antitoxin therapy is also associated with a significant reduction in mortality risk. Because diphtheria antitoxin cannot neutralize cell-bound toxin, prompt initiation is important. This product, which is no longer commercially available in the United States, can be obtained from the CDC by calling the Bacterial Vaccine Preventable Disease Branch of the National Immunization Program at 404-639-8257 (8:00 A.M. to 4:30 P.M., U.S. Eastern time) or, at other hours, the Emergency Operations Center at 770-488-7100; the relevant website is *www.cdc.gov/diphtheria/dat.html*. The current protocol for the use of diphtheria antitoxin involves a test dose to rule out immediate hypersensitivity. Patients who demonstrate hypersensitivity require desensitization before a full therapeutic dose of antitoxin is administered.

ANTIMICROBIAL THERAPY

Antibiotics are used in the management of diphtheria primarily to prevent transmission to susceptible contacts. Antibiotics also prevent further toxin production and reduce the severity of local infection. Recommended treatment options for patients with respiratory diphtheria are as follows:

- Procaine penicillin G, 600,000 U IM q12h (for children: 12,500–25,000 U/kg IM q12h) until the patient can swallow comfortably; then oral penicillin V, 125–250 mg qid to complete a 14-day course
- Erythromycin, 500 mg IV q6h (for children: 40–50 mg/kg per day IV in two or four divided doses) until the patient can swallow comfortably; then 500 mg PO qid to complete a 14-day course

A clinical study in Vietnam found that penicillin was associated with a more rapid resolution of fever and a lower rate of bacterial resistance than erythromycin; however, relapses were more common in the penicillin group. Erythromycin therapy targets protein synthesis and thus offers the presumed benefit of stopping toxin synthesis more quickly than a cell wall–active β-lactam agent. Alternative therapeutic agents for patients who are allergic to penicillin or cannot take erythromycin include rifampin and clindamycin. Eradication of *C. diphtheriae* should be documented after antimicrobial therapy is complete. A repeat throat culture 2 weeks later is recommended. For patients in whom the organism is not eradicated after a 14-day course of erythromycin or penicillin, an additional 10-day course followed by repeat culture is recommended. Drug-resistant strains of *C. diphtheriae* exist, and several reports have described multidrug resistant strains, predominantly in Southeast Asia. Drug resistance should be considered when efforts at pathogen eradication fail.

Cutaneous diphtheria should be treated as described above for respiratory disease. Individuals infected with toxigenic strains should receive antitoxin. It is important to treat the underlying cause of the dermatoses in addition to the superinfection with *C. diphtheriae*.

Patients who recover from respiratory or cutaneous diphtheria should have antitoxin levels measured. If diphtheria antitoxin has been administered, this test should be performed 6 months later. Patients who recover from respiratory or cutaneous diphtheria should receive the appropriate vaccine to ensure the development of protective antibody titers.

MANAGEMENT STRATEGIES

Patients in whom diphtheria is suspected should be hospitalized in respiratory isolation rooms, with close monitoring of cardiac and respiratory function. A cardiac workup is recommended to assess the possibility of myocarditis. In patients with extensive pseudomembranes, an anesthesiology or an ear, nose, and throat consultation is recommended because of the possible need for tracheostomy or intubation. In some settings, pseudomembranes can be removed surgically. Treatment with glucocorticoids has not been shown to reduce the risk of myocarditis or polyneuropathy.

PROGNOSIS

Fatal pseudomembranous diphtheria typically occurs in patients with nonprotective antibody titers and in unimmunized patients. The pseudomembrane may actually increase in size from the time it is first noted. Risk factors for death include bullneck diphtheria; myocarditis with ventricular tachycardia; atrial fibrillation; complete heart block; an age of >60 years or <6 months; alcoholism; extensive pseudomembrane elongation; and laryngeal, tracheal, or bronchial involvement. Another important predictor of fatal outcome is the interval between the onset of local disease and the administration of antitoxin. Cutaneous diphtheria has a low mortality rate and is rarely associated with myocarditis or peripheral neuropathy.

PREVENTION

Vaccination Sustained campaigns for vaccination of children and adequate boosting vaccination of adults are responsible for the exceedingly low incidence of diphtheria in most developed nations. Currently, diphtheria toxoid vaccine is coadministered with tetanus vaccine (with or without acellular pertussis). DTaP (a full-level diphtheria and tetanus toxoids and acellular pertussis vaccine) is currently recommended for children up to the age of 7; DTaP replaced the earlier whole-cell pertussis vaccine DTP in 1997. Tdap is a tetanus toxoid, reduced diphtheria toxoid, and acellular pertussis vaccine formulated for adolescents and adults. Tdap was licensed for use in the United States in 2005 and is the recommended booster vaccine for children 11–12 years old and the recommended catch-up vaccine for children 7–10 and 13–18 years of age. It is recommended that all adults (i.e., persons >19 years old) receive a single dose of Tdap if they have not received it previously, regardless of the interval since the last dose of Td (tetanus and reduced-dose diphtheria toxoids, adsorbed). Tdap vaccination is a priority for health care workers, pregnant women, adults anticipating contact with infants, and adults not previously vaccinated for pertussis. Adults who have received acellular pertussis vaccine should continue to receive decennial Td booster vaccinations. The vaccine schedule is detailed in Chap. 148.

Prophylaxis Administration to Contacts Close contacts of diphtheria patients should undergo throat culture to determine whether they are carriers. After samples for throat culture are obtained, antimicrobial prophylaxis should be considered for all contacts, even those whose cultures are negative. The options are 7–10 days of oral erythromycin or one dose of IM benzathine penicillin G (1.2 million units for persons ≥6 years of age or 600,000 units for children <6 years of age).

Contacts of diphtheria patients whose immunization status is uncertain should receive the appropriate diphtheria toxoid–containing vaccine. The Tdap vaccine (rather than Td) is now the booster vaccine of choice for adults who have not recently received an acellular pertussis–containing vaccine. Carriers of *C. diphtheriae* in the community should be treated and vaccinated when identified.

OTHER CORYNEBACTERIAL AND *RHODOCOCCUS* INFECTIONS

Nondiphtherial corynebacteria, referred to as *diphtheroids* or *coryneforms*, are frequently considered colonizers or contaminants; however, they have been associated with invasive disease, particularly in immunocompromised patients. These organisms have been isolated from the bloodstream, particularly in association with catheter infection, endocarditis, prosthetic valve infection, meningitis, neurosurgical shunt infection, brain abscess, and peritonitis and often in the setting of chronic ambulatory peritoneal dialysis, osteomyelitis, septic arthritis, urinary tract infection, empyema, and pneumonia, among other infections. Patients infected with these organisms usually have significant medical comorbidity or are immunosuppressed. The nondiphtherial coryneforms are a diverse collection of bacteria that are taxonomically grouped together in the genus *Corynebacterium* on the basis of their 16S rDNA signature nucleotides. Despite the shared rDNA signatures, these isolates are quite diverse. For example, their guanine-cytosine content ranges from 45% to 70%. Several nondiphtheroid corynebacteria, including *Corynebacterium jeikeium* and *Corynebacterium urealyticum*, are associated with resistance to multiple antibiotics. *Rhodococcus equi* is associated with necrotizing pneumonia and granulomatous infection, particularly in immunocompromised individuals.

MICROBIOLOGY AND LABORATORY DIAGNOSIS

These organisms are non-acid-fast, catalase-positive, aerobic or facultatively anaerobic rods. Their colonial morphologies vary widely; some species are small and α-hemolytic (similar to lactobacilli), whereas others form large white colonies (similar to yeasts). Many nondiphtherial coryneforms require special media, such as Löffler's, Tinsdale's, or telluride medium. These cultivation idiosyncrasies have led to a complex taxonomic categorization of the organisms.

EPIDEMIOLOGY

Humans are the natural reservoirs for several nondiphtherial coryneforms, including *C. xerosis, C. pseudodiphtheriticum, C. striatum, C. minutissimum, C. jeikeium, C. urealyticum*, and *Arcanobacterium haemolyticum*. Animal reservoirs are responsible for carriage of *Arcanobacterium pyogenes, C. ulcerans*, and *C. pseudotuberculosis*. Soil is the natural reservoir for *R. equi*.

C. pseudodiphtheriticum is a component of the normal flora of the human pharynx and skin. *C. xerosis* is found on the skin, nasopharynx, and conjunctiva; *C. auris* in the external auditory canal; and *C. striatum* in the anterior nares and on the skin. *C. jeikeium* and *C. urealyticum* are found in the axilla, groin, and perineum, particularly in hospitalized patients. Infections with *C. ulcerans* and *C. pseudotuberculosis* have been associated with the consumption of raw milk from infected cattle.

C. ulcerans This organism causes a diphtheria-like illness and produces both diphtheria toxin and a dermonecrotic toxin. The organism is a commensal in horses and cattle and has been isolated from cow's milk. *C. ulcerans* causes exudative pharyngitis, primarily during summer months, in rural areas, and among individuals exposed to cattle. In contrast to diphtheria, this infection is considered a zoonosis whose person-to-person transmission has not been documented. Nevertheless, treatment with antitoxin and antibiotics should be initiated when respiratory *C. ulcerans* is identified, and a contact investigation (including throat cultures to determine the need for antimicrobial prophylaxis and, in unimmunized contacts, administration of the appropriate diphtheria toxoid–containing vaccine) should be conducted. The organism grows on Löffler's, Tinsdale's, and telluride agars as well as blood agar. In addition to exudative pharyngitis, cutaneous disease due to *C. ulcerans* has been reported. *C. ulcerans* is susceptible to a wide panel of antibiotics. Erythromycin and macrolides appear to be the first-line agents.

C. pseudotuberculosis (ovis) Infection caused by *C. pseudotuberculosis* is rare and is reported almost exclusively from Australia. *C. pseudotuberculosis* causes suppurative granulomatous lymphadenitis and an eosinophilic pneumonia syndrome among individuals who handle horses, cattle, goats, and deer or who drink raw milk. The organism is an important veterinary pathogen, causing suppurative lymphadenitis, abscesses, and pneumonia, but is rarely a human pathogen. Successful treatment with erythromycin or tetracycline has been reported, with surgery also performed when indicated.

***C. jeikeium* (Group JK)** Originally described in American hospitals, *C. jeikeium* infection was subsequently reported in Europe. After a 1976 survey of diseases caused by nondiphtherial corynebacteria, CDC group JK emerged as an important opportunistic pathogen among neutropenic and HIV-infected patients. The organism has now been designated a separate species. *C. jeikeium* forms small, gray to white, glistening, nonhemolytic colonies on blood agar. It lacks urease and nitrate reductase and does not ferment most carbohydrates. The predominant syndrome associated with *C. jeikeium* is sepsis with pneumonia, endocarditis, meningitis, osteomyelitis, and epidural abscess. Risk factors for *C. jeikeium* infection include hematologic malignancy, neutropenia from comorbid conditions, prolonged hospitalization, exposure to multiple antibiotics, and skin disruption. There is evidence that *C. jeikeium* is part of the inguinal, axillary, genital, and perirectal flora of hospitalized patients.

Broad-spectrum antimicrobial therapy appears to select for colonization. Gram's staining shows gram-positive coccobacillary forms slightly resembling streptococci. Moreover, *C. jeikeium* is resistant to all antibiotics tested except vancomycin. Effective therapy involves removal of the infectious source, whether a catheter, prosthetic joint, or prosthetic valve. Efforts have been made to prevent *C. jeikeium* infection by improving hygienic conditions for high-risk patients in intensive care settings with antibacterial soap.

C. urealyticum (Group D2) Identified as a urease-positive nondiphtherial *Corynebacterium* in 1972, *C. urealyticum* is an opportunistic pathogen causing sepsis and urinary tract infection. *C. urealyticum* appears to be the etiologic agent of a severe urinary tract syndrome known as *alkaline-encrusted cystitis*, a chronic inflammatory bladder infection associated with deposition of ammonium magnesium phosphate on the surface and walls of ulcerating lesions in the bladder. In addition, *C. urealyticum* has been associated with pneumonia, peritonitis, endocarditis, osteomyelitis, and wound infection. It is similar to *C. jeikeium* in its resistance to most antibiotics except vancomycin. Vancomycin therapy has been used successfully in severe infections.

C. minutissimum (Erythrasma) Erythrasma is a cutaneous infection producing reddish-brown, macular, scaly, pruritic intertriginous patches. The dermatologic presentation under the Wood's lamp is of coral red fluorescence. *C. minutissimum* appears to be a common cause of erythrasma, although there is evidence for a polymicrobial etiology in certain settings. This microbe has also been associated with bacteremia in patients with hematologic malignancy. Erythrasma responds to topical erythromycin, clarithromycin, clindamycin, or fusidic acid, although more severe infections may require oral macrolide therapy.

Other Nondiphtherial Corynebacterial Infections *C. xerosis* is a human commensal found in the conjunctiva, nasopharynx, and skin. This nontoxigenic organism is occasionally identified as a source of invasive infection in immunocompromised or postoperative patients and prosthetic joint recipients. *C. striatum* is found in the anterior nares, skin, face, and upper torso of healthy individuals. Also nontoxigenic, this organism has been associated with invasive opportunistic infections in severely ill or immunocompromised patients. *C. amycolatum* is isolated from human skin and is identified on the basis of a unique 16S ribosomal RNA sequence associated with opportunistic infection. *C. glucuronolyticum* is a nonlipophilic species that causes male genitourinary tract infections such as prostatitis and urethritis. These infections may be successfully treated with a wide variety of antibacterial agents, including β-lactams, rifampin, aminoglycosides, or vancomycin; however, the organism appears to be resistant to fluoroquinolones, macrolides, and tetracyclines. *C. imitans* has been identified in eastern Europe as a nontoxigenic cause of pharyngitis. *C. auris* has been identified in children with otitis media; it is susceptible to fluoroquinolones, rifampin, tetracycline, and vancomycin but resistant to penicillin G and variably susceptible to macrolides. *C. pseudodiphtheriticum* (*C. hoffmanii*) is a nontoxigenic species that is part of the normal human flora. Human infections—particularly endocarditis of either prosthetic or natural valves and invasive pneumonia—have been reported only rarely. Although *C. pseudodiphtheriticum* may be isolated from the nasopharynx of patients with suspected diphtheria, it is part of the normal flora and does not produce diphtheria toxin. *C. propinquum*, a close relative of *C. pseudodiphtheriticum*, is part of CDC group ANF-3 and is isolated from the human respiratory tract and blood. *C. afermentans* subspecies *lipophilum* belongs to CDC group ANF-1 and has been isolated from human blood and abscesses. *C. accolens* has been isolated from wound drainage, throat swabs, and sputum and is typically identified as a satellite of staphylococcal organisms; this species has been associated with endocarditis. *C. bovis* is a veterinary commensal that has not been clearly associated with human disease. *C. aquaticum* is a water-dwelling organism that is occasionally isolated from patients using medical devices (e.g., for chronic ambulatory peritoneal dialysis or venous access).

Rhodococcus *Rhodococcus* species are phylogenetically related to the corynebacteria. These gram-positive coccobacilli have been associated with tuberculosis-like infections in humans with granulomatous pathology. While *R. equi* is best known, other species have been identified, including *R. (Gordonia) bronchialis, R. (Tsukamurella) aurantiacus, R. luteus, R. erythropolis, R. rhodochrous*, and *R. rubropertinctus*.

R. equi has been recognized as a cause of pneumonia in horses since the 1920s and as a cause of related infections in cattle, sheep, and swine. It is found in soil as an environmental microbe. The organisms vary in length; appear as spherical to long, curved, clubbed rods; and produce large irregular mucoid colonies. *R. equi* cannot ferment carbohydrates or liquefy gelatin and is often acid fast. An intracellular pathogen of macrophages, *R. equi* can cause granulomatous necrosis and caseation. This organism has most commonly been identified in pulmonary infection, but infections of brain, bone, and skin also have been reported. Most commonly, *R. equi* disease manifests as nodular cavitary pneumonia of the upper lobe—a picture similar to that seen in tuberculosis or nocardiosis. Most patients are immunocompromised, often by HIV infection. Subcutaneous nodular lesions have also been identified. The involvement of *R. equi* should be considered when any patient presents with a tuberculosis-like syndrome.

Infection due to *R. equi* has been treated successfully with antibiotics that penetrate intracellularly, including macrolides, clindamycin, rifampin, and trimethoprim-sulfamethoxazole. β-Lactam antibiotics have not been useful. The organism is routinely susceptible to vancomycin, which is considered the drug of choice.

Other Related Species • ***ACTINOMYCES PYOGENES*** This organism, a well-known pathogen of cattle, sheep, goats, and pigs, causes seasonal leg ulcers in rural Thailand. A few human cases of sepsis, endocarditis, septic arthritis, pneumonia, meningitis, and empyema have been reported. This species is susceptible to β-lactams, tetracyclines, aminoglycosides, and fluoroquinolones.

ARCANOBACTERIUM HAEMOLYTICUM *A. haemolyticum* was identified as an agent of wound infections in U.S. soldiers in the South Pacific during World War II. It appears to be a human commensal of the nasopharynx and skin, but has also been implicated in pharyngitis and chronic skin ulcers. In contrast to the much more common pharyngitis caused by *Streptococcus pyogenes*, *A. haemolyticum* pharyngitis is associated with a scarlatiniform rash on the trunk and proximal extremities in about half of cases; this illness is occasionally confused with toxic shock syndrome. Because *A. haemolyticum* pharyngitis primarily affects teenagers, it has been postulated that the rash-pharyngitis syndrome may represent copathogenicity, synergy, or opportunistic secondary infection with Epstein-Barr virus. *A. haemolyticum* has also been reported as a cause of bacteremia, soft tissue infections, osteomyelitis, and cavitary pneumonia, predominantly in the setting of underlying diabetes mellitus. The organism is susceptible to β-lactams, macrolides, fluoroquinolones, clindamycin, vancomycin, and doxycycline. Penicillin resistance has been reported.

176 *Listeria monocytogenes* Infections

Elizabeth L. Hohmann, Daniel A. Portnoy

Listeria monocytogenes is a food-borne pathogen that can cause serious infections, particularly in pregnant women and immunocompromised individuals. A ubiquitous saprophytic environmental bacterium, *L. monocytogenes* is also a facultative intracellular pathogen with a broad host range. Humans are probably accidental hosts for this microorganism. *L. monocytogenes* is of interest not only to clinicians but also to basic scientists as a model intracellular pathogen that is used to study basic mechanisms of microbial pathogenesis and host immunity.

MICROBIOLOGY

L. monocytogenes is a facultatively anaerobic, nonsporulating, gram-positive rod that grows over a broad temperature range, including refrigeration temperatures. This organism is motile during growth at low temperatures but much less so at 37°C. The vast majority of cases of human listerial disease can be traced to serotypes 1/2a, 1/2b, and 4. *L. monocytogenes* is weakly β-hemolytic on blood agar, and (as detailed below) its β-hemolysin is an essential determinant of its pathogenicity.

PATHOGENESIS

Infections with *L. monocytogenes* follow ingestion of contaminated food that contains the bacteria at high concentrations. The conversion from environmental saprophyte to pathogen involves the coordinate regulation of bacterial determinants of pathogenesis that mediate entry into cells, intracellular growth, and cell-to-cell spread. Many of the organism's pathogenic strategies can be examined experimentally in tissue culture models of infection (Fig. 176-1). Like other enteric pathogens, *L. monocytogenes* induces its own internalization by cells that are not normally phagocytic. Its entry into cells is mediated by host surface proteins classified as internalins. Internalin-mediated entry is important in the crossing of intestinal, blood-brain, and feto-placental barriers, although how *L. monocytogenes* traffics from the intestine to the brain or fetus is only beginning to be investigated. In a pregnant guinea pig model of infection, *L. monocytogenes* was shown to traffic from maternal organs to the placenta; surprisingly, however, it also trafficked from the placenta back to maternal organs. These data are consistent with a model in which miscarriage can be viewed as a host defense strategy to eliminate a nidus of infection.

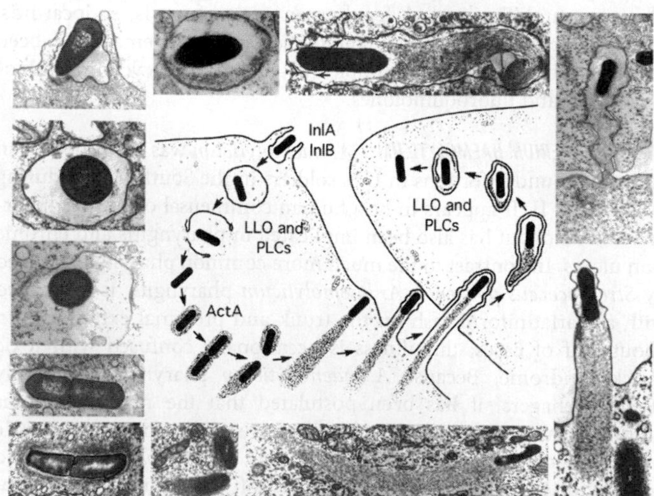

FIGURE 176-1 Stages in the intracellular life cycle of *Listeria monocytogenes*. The central diagram depicts cell entry, escape from a vacuole, actin nucleation, actin-based motility, and cell-to-cell spread. Surrounding the diagram are representative electron micrographs from which it was derived. ActA, surface protein mediating nucleation of host actin filaments to propel bacteria intra- and intercellularly; LLO, listeriolysin O; PLCs, phospholipases C; Inl, internalin. See text for further details. *(Adapted with permission from LG Tilney, DA Portnoy: J Cell Biol 109:1597, 1989. © Rockefeller University Press.)*

An essential determinant of the pathogenesis of *L. monocytogenes* is its β-hemolysin, listeriolysin O (LLO). LLO is a pore-forming, cholesterol-dependent cytolysin. (Related cytolysins include streptolysin O, pneumolysin, and perfringolysin O, all of which are produced by extracellular pathogens.) LLO is largely responsible for mediating the rupture of the phagosomal membrane that forms after phagocytosis of *L. monocytogenes*. LLO probably acts by insertion into an acidifying phagosome, which prevents the vesicle's maturation. In addition, LLO acts as a translocation pore for one or both of the *L. monocytogenes* phospholipases that also contribute to vacuolar lysis. LLO synthesis and activity are controlled at multiple levels to ensure that its lytic activity is limited to acidic vacuoles and does not affect the cytosol. Mutations in LLO that influence its synthesis, cytosolic half-life, or pH optimum cause premature toxicity to infected cells. There is an inverse relationship between toxicity and virulence—i.e., the more cytotoxic the strain, the less virulent it is in animals. This relationship may seem paradoxical, but, as an intracellular pathogen, *L. monocytogenes* benefits from leaving its host cell unharmed.

Shortly after exposure to the mammalian-cell cytosol, *L. monocytogenes* expresses a surface protein, ActA, that mediates the nucleation of host actin filaments to propel the bacteria intra- and intercellularly. ActA mimics host proteins of the Wiskott-Aldrich syndrome protein (WASP) family by promoting the actin nucleation properties of the Arp2/3 complex. Thus, *L. monocytogenes* can enter the cytosol of almost any eukaryotic cell or cell extract and can exploit a conserved and essential actin-based motility system. Other pathogens as diverse as certain *Shigella, Mycobacterium, Rickettsia,* and *Burkholderia* species use a related pathogenic strategy that allows cell-to-cell spread without exposure to the extracellular milieu.

IMMUNE RESPONSE

The innate and acquired immune responses to *L. monocytogenes* have been studied extensively in mice. Shortly after IV injection, most bacteria are found in Kupffer cells in the liver, with some organisms in splenic dendritic cells and macrophages. Listeriae that survive the bactericidal activity of initially infected macrophages grow in the cytosol and spread from cell to cell. *L. monocytogenes* triggers three innate immune pathways: a MyD88-dependent pathway leading to inflammatory cytokines, a STING/IRF3 pathway leading to a type I interferon response; and low-level inflammasome activation. Neutrophils are crucial to host defense during the first 24 h of infection, whereas an influx of activated macrophages from the bone marrow is critical subsequently. Mice that survive sublethal infection clear the organisms within a week, with consequent sterile immunity. Studies with knockout mice have been instrumental in dissecting the roles played by chemokines and cytokines during infection. For example, interferon γ, tumor necrosis factor, and CCR2 are essential in controlling infection. While innate immunity is sufficient to control infection, the acquired immune response is required for sterile immunity. Immunity is cell mediated; antibody plays no measurable role. The critical effector cells are cytotoxic (CD8+) T cells that recognize and lyse infected cells; the resulting extracellular bacteria are killed by circulating activated phagocytes.

A hallmark of the *L. monocytogenes* model is that killed vaccines do not provide protective immunity. The explanation for this fundamental observation is multifactorial, involving the generation of appropriate cytokines and the compartmentalization of bacterial proteins for antigen processing and presentation. Because the organism has the capacity to induce a robust cell-mediated immune response, attenuated strains have been engineered to express foreign antigens and are undergoing clinical studies as therapeutic vaccines for cancer.

EPIDEMIOLOGY

L. monocytogenes usually enters the body via the gastrointestinal tract in foods. Listeriosis is most often sporadic, although outbreaks do occur. No epidemiologic or clinical evidence supports person-to-person transmission (other than vertical transmission from mother to fetus) or waterborne infection. In line with its survival and multiplication at refrigeration temperatures, *L. monocytogenes* is commonly found in processed and unprocessed foods of animal and plant origin, especially soft cheeses, delicatessen meats, hot dogs, milk, and cold salads; fresh fruits and vegetables can also transmit the organism. Because food supplies are increasingly centralized and normal hosts tolerate the organism well, outbreaks may not be immediately apparent. The U.S. Food and Drug Administration has a zero-tolerance policy for *L. monocytogenes* in ready-to-eat foods.

DIAGNOSIS

Symptoms of listerial infection overlap greatly with those of other infectious diseases. Timely diagnosis requires that the illness be considered in groups at risk: pregnant women; elderly persons; neonates; individuals immunocompromised by organ transplantation, cancer, or treatment with tumor necrosis factor antagonists or glucocorticoids; and patients with a variety of chronic medical conditions, including alcoholism, diabetes, renal disease, and rheumatologic and hepatic illnesses. Meningitis in older adults (especially with parenchymal brain involvement or subcortical brain abscess) should trigger consideration of *L. monocytogenes* infection and treatment. Listeriosis occasionally affects healthy, young, nonpregnant individuals. HIV-infected patients are at risk; however, listeriosis seems to be prevented by trimethoprim-sulfamethoxazole (TMP-SMX) prophylaxis targeting other AIDS-related infections. The diagnosis is typically made by culture of blood, cerebrospinal fluid (CSF), or amniotic fluid. *L. monocytogenes* may be confused with "diphtheroids" or pneumococci in Gram-stained CSF or may be gram-variable and confused with *Haemophilus* species. Polymerase chain reaction diagnostics have been described but are not widely available, and serology is not clinically useful.

CLINICAL MANIFESTATIONS

Listerial infections present as several clinical syndromes, of which meningitis and septicemia are most common. Monocytosis is seen in infected rabbits but is not a hallmark of human infection.

Gastroenteritis Appreciated only since the outbreaks of the late 1980s, listerial gastroenteritis typically develops within 48 h of ingestion of a large inoculum of bacteria in contaminated foods. Attack rates are high (50–100%). *L. monocytogenes* is neither sought nor found in routine fecal cultures, but its involvement should be considered in outbreaks when cultures for other likely pathogens are negative. Sporadic intestinal illness appears to be uncommon. Manifestations include fever, diarrhea, headache, and constitutional symptoms. The largest reported outbreak occurred in an Italian school system and included 1566 individuals; ~20% of patients were hospitalized, but only one person had a positive blood culture. Isolated gastrointestinal illness does not require antibiotic treatment. Surveillance studies show that 0.1–5% of healthy asymptomatic adults may have stool cultures positive for the organism.

Bacteremia *L. monocytogenes* septicemia presents with fever, chills, and myalgias/arthralgias and cannot be differentiated from septicemia involving other organisms. Meningeal symptoms, focal neurologic findings, or mental status changes may suggest the diagnosis. Bacteremia is documented in 70–90% of cancer patients with listeriosis. A nonspecific flulike illness with fever is a common presentation in pregnant women. Endocarditis of prosthetic and native valves is an uncommon complication, with reported fatality rates of 35–50% in case series. A lumbar puncture is often prudent, although not necessary, in pregnant women without central nervous system (CNS) symptoms.

Meningitis *L. monocytogenes* causes ~5–10% of all cases of community-acquired bacterial meningitis in adults in the United States. Case-fatality rates are reported to be 15–26% and do not appear to have changed over time. This diagnosis should be considered in all older or chronically ill adults with "aseptic" meningitis. The presentation is more frequently subacute (with illness developing over several days) than in meningitis of other bacterial etiologies, and nuchal rigidity and meningeal signs are less common. Photophobia is infrequent. Focal findings and seizures are common in some but not all series. The CSF profile in listerial meningitis most often shows white blood cell counts in the range of 100–5000/μL (rarely higher); 75% of patients have counts below 1000/μL, usually with a neutrophil predominance more modest than that in other bacterial meningitides. Low glucose levels and positive results on Gram's staining are found ~30–40% of the time. Hydrocephalus can occur.

Meningoencephalitis and Focal CNS Infection *L. monocytogenes* can directly invade the brain parenchyma, producing either cerebritis or focal abscess. Approximately 10% of cases of CNS infection are macroscopic abscesses resulting from bacteremic seeding; the affected patients often have positive blood cultures. Concurrent meningitis can exist, but the CSF may appear normal. Abscesses can be misdiagnosed as metastatic or primary tumors and, in rare instances, occur in the cerebellum and the spinal cord. Invasion of the brainstem results in a characteristic severe rhombencephalitis, usually in otherwise healthy older adults (although there are numerous other infectious and noninfectious causes of this syndrome). The presentation may be biphasic, with a prodrome of fever and headache followed by asymmetric cranial nerve deficits, cerebellar signs, and hemiparetic and hemisensory deficits. Respiratory failure can occur. The subacute course and the often minimally abnormal CSF findings may delay the diagnosis, which may be suggested by MRI showing ring-enhancing lesions after gadolinium contrast and hyperintense lesions on diffusion-weighted imaging. MRI is superior to CT for the diagnosis of these infections.

Infection in Pregnant Women and Neonates Listeriosis in pregnancy is a severe and important infection. The usual presentation is a nonspecific acute or subacute febrile illness with myalgias, arthralgias, backache, and headache. Pregnant women with listeriosis are usually bacteremic. This syndrome should prompt blood cultures, especially if there is no other reasonable explanation. Involvement of the CNS is rare in the absence of other risk factors. Preterm delivery is a common complication, and the diagnosis may be made only post-partum. As many as 70–90% of fetuses from infected women can become infected. Prepartum treatment of bacteremic women enhances the chances of delivery of a healthy infant. Women usually do well after delivery: maternal deaths are very rare, even when the diagnosis is made late in pregnancy or post-partum. Overall mortality rates for fetuses infected in utero approach 50% in some series; among live-born neonates treated with antibiotics, mortality rates are much lower (~20%). *Granulomatosis infantiseptica* is an overwhelming listerial fetal infection with miliary microabscesses and granulomas, most often in the skin, liver, and spleen. Less severe neonatal infection acquired in utero presents at birth. "Late-onset" neonatal illness typically develops ~10–30 days post-partum. Mothers of infants with late-onset disease are not ill.

TREATMENT INFECTIONS CAUSED BY *LISTERIA MONOCYTOGENES*

ANTIBIOTICS

No clinical trials have compared antimicrobial agents for the treatment of *L. monocytogenes* infections. Data from studies conducted in vitro and in animals as well as observational clinical data indicate that ampicillin is the drug of choice, although penicillin also is highly active. Adults should receive IV ampicillin at high doses (2 g every 6 h). Many experts recommend the addition of gentamicin for synergy (1.0–1.7 mg/kg every 8 h); retrospective uncontrolled trials are not conclusive, but one study suggests that gentamicin may not help. TMP-SMX, given IV, is the best alternative for the penicillin-allergic patient (15–20 mg of TMP/kg per day in divided doses every 6–8 h). The dosages recommended cover CNS infection and bacteremia (see below for duration); dosages must be reduced for patients with renal insufficiency. One small nonrandomized study supports a combination of ampicillin and TMP-SMX. Case reports document success with vancomycin, imipenem, meropenem, linezolid, tetracycline, and macrolides, although there are also reports of clinical failure or disease development with some of these agents. Acquired resistance to antimicrobial agents has been sought but not found in large strain collections. Cephalosporins are *not* effective and should not be used. Neonates should receive ampicillin and gentamicin at doses based on weight.

DURATION

The duration of therapy depends on the syndrome: 2 weeks for bacteremia, 3 weeks for meningitis, 6–8 weeks for brain abscess/encephalitis, and 4–6 weeks for endocarditis in both neonates and adults. Early-onset neonatal disease may be more severe and should be treated for >2 weeks.

COMPLICATIONS AND PROGNOSIS

Many individuals who are promptly diagnosed and treated recover fully, but permanent neurologic sequelae are common in patients with brain abscess or rhombencephalitis. Focal infections of visceral organs; the eye; the pleural, peritoneal, and pericardial spaces; the bones; and both native and prosthetic joints have all been reported. Of 100 live-born, treated neonates in one series, 60% recovered fully, 24% died, and 13% had long-term neurologic or other complications.

PREVENTION

Healthy persons should take standard precautions to prevent food-borne illness: fully cooking meats, washing fresh vegetables, carefully cleaning utensils, and avoiding unpasteurized dairy products. In addition, persons at risk for listeriosis, including pregnant women, should avoid soft cheeses (hard cheeses and yogurt are not problematic) and should avoid or thoroughly reheat ready-to-eat and delicatessen foods.

177 Tetanus

C. Louise Thwaites, Lam Minh Yen

Tetanus is an acute disease manifested by skeletal muscle spasm and autonomic nervous system disturbance. It is caused by a powerful neurotoxin produced by the bacterium *Clostridium tetani* and is completely preventable by vaccination. *C. tetani* is found throughout the world, and tetanus commonly occurs where the vaccination coverage rate is low. In developed countries, the disease is seen occasionally in individuals who are incompletely vaccinated. In any setting, established tetanus is a severe disease with a high mortality rate.

DEFINITION

Tetanus is diagnosed on clinical grounds (sometimes with supportive laboratory confirmation of the presence of *C. tetani*; see "Diagnosis," below), and case definitions are often used to facilitate clinical and epidemiologic assessments. The Centers for Disease Control and Prevention (CDC) defines tetanus as "the acute onset of hypertonia or … painful muscular contractions (usually of the muscles of the jaw and neck) and generalized muscle spasms without other apparent medical cause." *Neonatal* tetanus is defined by the World Health Organization (WHO) as "an illness occurring in a child who has the normal ability to suck and cry in the first 2 days of life but who loses this ability between days 3 and 28 of life and becomes rigid and has spasms." Given the unique presentation of neonatal tetanus, the history generally permits accurate classification of the illness with a high degree of probability.

Maternal tetanus is defined by the WHO as tetanus occurring during pregnancy or within 6 weeks after the conclusion of pregnancy (whether with birth, miscarriage, or abortion).

ETIOLOGY

C. tetani is an anaerobic, gram-positive, spore-forming rod whose spores are highly resilient and can survive readily in the environment throughout the world. Spores resist boiling and many disinfectants. In addition, *C. tetani* spores and bacilli survive in the intestinal systems of many animals, and fecal carriage is common. The spores or bacteria enter the body through abrasions, wounds, or (in the case of neonates) the umbilical stump. Once in a suitable anaerobic environment, the organisms grow, multiply, and release tetanus toxin, an exotoxin that enters the nervous system and causes disease. Very low concentrations of this highly potent toxin can result in tetanus (minimum lethal human dose, 2.5 ng/kg).

In 20–30% of cases of tetanus, no puncture entry wound is found. Superficial abrasions to the limbs are the commonest infection sites in adults. Deeper infections (e.g., attributable to open fracture, abortion, or drug injection) are associated with more severe disease and worse outcomes. In neonates, infection of the umbilical stump can result from inadequate umbilical cord care; in some cultures, for example, the cord is cut with grass or animal dung is applied to the stump. Circumcision or ear-piercing also can result in neonatal tetanus.

EPIDEMIOLOGY

Tetanus is a rare disease in the developed world. Two cases of neonatal tetanus have occurred in the United States since 1989. Between 2001 and 2008, a total of 231 cases of tetanus were reported to the U.S. national surveillance system. Most cases occur in incompletely vaccinated or unvaccinated individuals. Vaccination status is known in 50% of cases reported in the United States between 1972 and 2009; among these cases, only 16% of patients had had three or more doses of tetanus toxoid.

Persons >60 years of age are at greater risk of tetanus because antibody levels decrease over time. One-third of recent cases in the United States were in persons >65 years old. Injection drug users—particularly those injecting heroin subcutaneously ("skin-popping")—are increasingly recognized as a high-risk group (15% of all cases in 2001–2008). In 2004, an outbreak of tetanus occurred in the United Kingdom, which had previously reported low rates among drug users. The reasons for this outbreak remain unclear but are thought to involve a combination of heroin contamination, skin-popping, and incomplete vaccination. Since then, only seven sporadic cases have been reported in the United Kingdom.

PATHOGENESIS

Genome sequencing of *C. tetani* has allowed identification of several exotoxins and virulence factors. Only those bacteria producing tetanus toxin (*tetanospasmin*) can cause tetanus. Although closely related to the botulinum toxins in structure and mode of action, tetanus toxin undergoes retrograde transport into the central nervous system and thus produces clinical effects different from those caused by the botulinum toxins, which remain at the neuromuscular junction.

Toxin is transported by intra-axonal transport to motor nuclei of the cranial nerves or ventral horns of the spinal cord. Tetanus toxin is produced as a single 150-kDa protein that is cleaved to produce heavy (100-kDa) and light (50-kDa) chains linked by a disulfide bond and noncovalent forces. The carboxy terminal of the heavy chain binds to specific membrane components in presynaptic α-motor nerve terminals; evidence suggests binding to both polysialogangliosides and membrane proteins. This binding results in toxin internalization and uptake into the nerves. Once inside the neuron, the toxin enters a retrograde transport pathway, whereby it is transported proximally to the motor neuron body in what appears to be a highly specific process. Unlike other components of the endosomal contents, which undergo acidification following internalization, tetanus toxin is transported in a carefully regulated pH-neutral environment that prevents an acid-induced conformational change that would result in light-chain expulsion into the surrounding cytosol.

The next stage in toxin trafficking is less clearly understood but involves tetanus toxin's escaping normal lysosomal degradation processes and undergoing translocation across the synapse to the GABA-ergic presynaptic inhibitory interneuron terminals. Here the light chain, which is a zinc-dependent endopeptidase, cleaves vesicle-associated membrane protein 2 (VAMP2, also known as *synaptobrevin*). This molecule is necessary for presynaptic binding and release of neurotransmitter; thus tetanus toxin prevents transmitter release and effectively blocks inhibitory interneuron discharge. The result is unregulated activity in the motor nervous system. Similar activity in the autonomic system accounts for the characteristic features of skeletal muscle spasm and autonomic system disturbance. The increased circulating catecholamine levels in severe tetanus are associated with cardiovascular complications.

Relatively little is known about the processes of recovery from tetanus. Recovery can take several weeks. Peripheral nerve sprouting is involved in recovery from botulism, and similar central nervous system sprouting may occur in tetanus. Other evidence suggests toxin degradation as a mechanism of recovery.

APPROACH TO THE PATIENT: Tetanus

The clinical manifestations of tetanus occur only after tetanus toxin has reached presynaptic inhibitory nerves. Once these effects become apparent, there may be little that can be done to affect disease progression. Treatment should not be delayed while the results of laboratory tests are awaited. Management strategies aim to neutralize remaining unbound toxin and support vital functions until the effects of the toxin have worn off. Recent interest has focused on intrathecal methods of antitoxin administration to neutralize toxin within the central nervous system and limit disease progression (see "Treatment," below).

CLINICAL MANIFESTATIONS

Tetanus produces a wide spectrum of clinical features that are broadly divided into generalized (including neonatal) and local. In the usually mild form of local tetanus, only isolated areas of the body are affected and only small areas of local muscle spasm may be apparent. If the cranial nerves are involved in localized cephalic tetanus, the pharyngeal or laryngeal muscles may spasm, with consequent aspiration or airway obstruction, and the prognosis may be poor. In the typical progression of generalized tetanus (Fig. 177-1), muscles of the face and jaw often are affected first, presumably because of the shorter distances toxin must travel up motor nerves to reach presynaptic terminals. Neonates typically present with inability to suck.

In assessing prognosis, the speed at which tetanus develops is important. The incubation period (time from wound to first symptom) and the period of onset (time from first symptom to first generalized spasm) are of particular significance; shorter times are associated with worse outcome. In neonatal tetanus, the younger the infant is when symptoms occur, the worse the prognosis.

The commonest initial symptoms are trismus (lockjaw), muscle pain and stiffness, back pain, and difficulty swallowing. In neonates, difficulty in feeding is the usual presentation. As the disease progresses, muscle spasm develops. Generalized muscle spasm can be very painful. Commonly, the laryngeal muscles are involved early or even in isolation. This is a life-threatening event as complete airway obstruction may ensue. Spasm of the respiratory muscles results in respiratory failure. Without ventilatory support, respiratory failure is the commonest cause of death in tetanus. Spasms strong enough to produce tendon avulsions and crush fractures have been reported, but this outcome is rare.

Autonomic disturbance is maximal during the second week of severe tetanus, and death due to cardiovascular events becomes the major risk. Blood pressure is usually labile, with rapid fluctuations from high to low accompanied by tachycardia. Episodes of bradycardia and heart block can also occur. Autonomic involvement is evidenced by gastrointestinal stasis, sweating, increased tracheal secretions, and acute (often high-output) renal failure.

DIAGNOSIS

The diagnosis of tetanus is based on clinical findings. As stated above, treatment should not be delayed while laboratory tests are conducted. Culture of *C. tetani* from a wound provides supportive evidence. Serum anti-tetanus immunoglobulin G may also be measured in a sample taken before the administration of antitoxin or immunoglobulin. Serum levels >0.1 IU/mL are deemed protective and do not support the diagnosis of tetanus. If levels are below this threshold, a

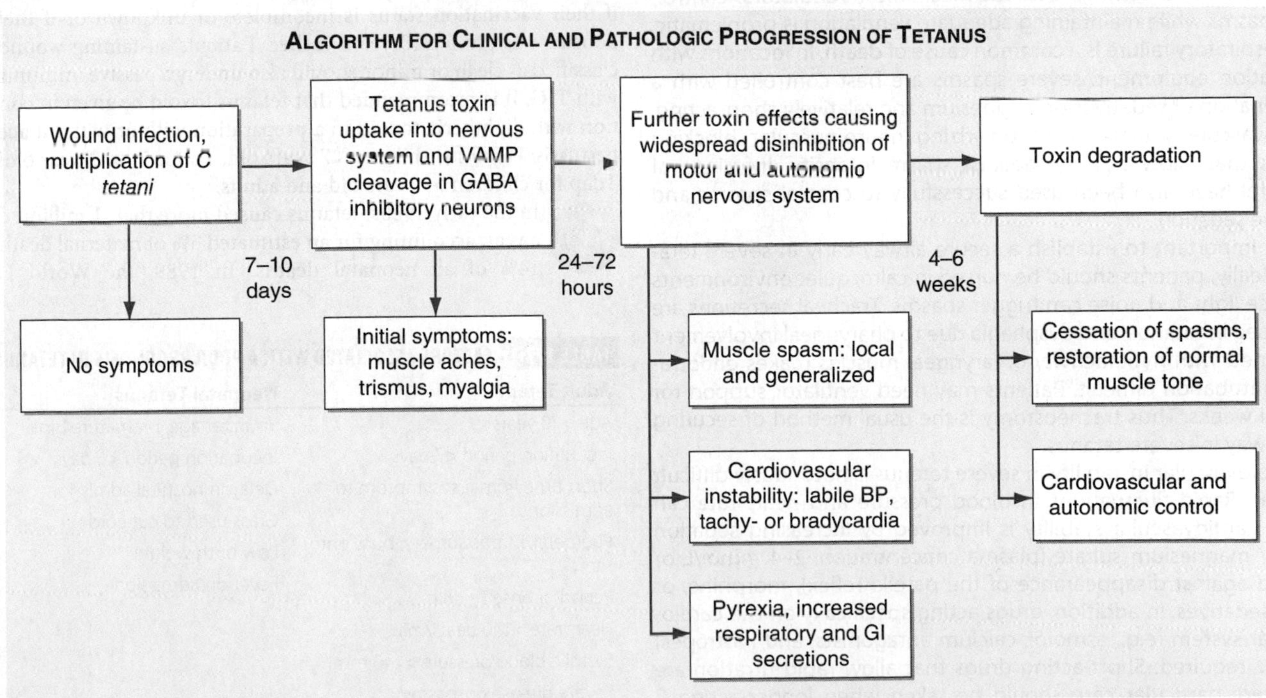

FIGURE 177-1 Clinical and pathologic progression of tetanus. BP, blood pressure; GABA, γ-aminobutyric acid; GI, gastrointestinal; VAMP, vesicle-associated membrane protein (synaptobrevin).

 bioassay for serum tetanus toxin may be helpful, but a negative result does not exclude the diagnosis. Polymerase chain reaction also has been used for detection of tetanus toxin, but its sensitivity is unknown.

The few conditions that mimic generalized tetanus include strychnine poisoning and dystonic reactions to antidopaminergic drugs. Abdominal muscle rigidity is characteristically continuous in tetanus but is episodic in the latter two conditions. Cephalic tetanus can be confused with other causes of trismus, such as oropharyngeal infection. Hypocalcemia and meningoencephalitis are included in the differential diagnosis of neonatal tetanus.

TREATMENT TETANUS

If possible, the entry wound should be identified, cleaned, and debrided of necrotic material in order to remove anaerobic foci of infection and prevent further toxin production. Metronidazole (400 mg rectally or 500 mg IV every 6 h for 7 days) is the preferred antibiotic. An alternative is penicillin (100,000–200,000 IU/kg per day), although this drug theoretically may exacerbate spasms. Failure to remove pockets of ongoing infection may result in recurrent or prolonged tetanus.

Antitoxin should be given early in an attempt to deactivate any circulating tetanus toxin and prevent its uptake into the nervous system. Two preparations are available: human tetanus immune globulin (TIG) and equine antitoxin. TIG is the preparation of choice, as it is less likely to be associated with anaphylactoid reactions. Recommended therapy is 3000–5000 IU of TIG as a single IM dose, a portion of which should be injected around the wound. Equine-derived antitoxin is available widely and is used in low-income countries at a dosage of 10,000–20,000 U administered IM as a single dose or as divided doses after testing for hypersensitivity. Some evidence indicates that intrathecal administration of TIG inhibits disease progression and leads to a better outcome. The results of relevant studies have been supported by a meta-analysis of trials involving both adults and neonates, with TIG doses of 50–1500 IU administered intrathecally.

Spasms are controlled by heavy sedation with benzodiazepines. Chlorpromazine and phenobarbital are commonly used worldwide, and IV magnesium sulfate has been used as a muscle relaxant. A significant problem with all these treatments is that the doses necessary to control spasms also cause respiratory depression; thus, in resource-limited settings without mechanical ventilators, controlling spasms while maintaining adequate ventilation is problematic, and respiratory failure is a common cause of death. In locations with ventilation equipment, severe spasms are best controlled with a combination of sedatives or magnesium and relatively short-acting, cardiovascularly inert, nondepolarizing neuromuscular blocking agents that allow titration against spasm intensity. Infusions of propofol have also been used successfully to control spasms and provide sedation.

It is important to establish a secure airway early in severe tetanus. Ideally, patients should be nursed in calm, quiet environments because light and noise can trigger spasms. Tracheal secretions are increased in tetanus, and dysphagia due to pharyngeal involvement combined with hyperactivity of laryngeal muscles makes endotracheal intubation difficult. Patients may need ventilator support for several weeks. Thus tracheostomy is the usual method of securing the airway in severe tetanus.

Cardiovascular instability in severe tetanus is notoriously difficult to treat. Rapid fluctuations in blood pressure and heart rate can occur. Cardiovascular stability is improved by increasing sedation with IV magnesium sulfate (plasma concentration, 2–4 mmol/L or titrated against disappearance of the patella reflex), morphine, or other sedatives. In addition, drugs acting specifically on the cardiovascular system (e.g., esmolol, calcium antagonists, and inotropes) may be required. Short-acting drugs that allow rapid titration are preferred; particular care should be taken when longer-acting β antagonists are administered, as their use has been associated with hypotensive cardiac arrest.

Complications arising from treatment are common and include thrombophlebitis associated with diazepam injection, ventilator-associated pneumonia, central-line infections, and septicemia. In some centers, prophylaxis against deep-vein thrombosis and thromboembolism is routine.

Recovery from tetanus may take 4–6 weeks. Patients must be given a full primary course of immunization, as tetanus toxin is poorly immunogenic and the immune response following natural infection is inadequate.

PROGNOSIS

Rapid development of tetanus is associated with more severe disease and poorer outcome; it is important to note time of onset and length of incubation period. More sophisticated modeling has revealed other important predictors of prognosis (Table 177-1). Few studies have formally addressed long-term outcomes of tetanus. However, it is generally accepted that recovery is typically complete unless periods of hypoventilation have been prolonged or other complications have ensued. Studies of children and neonates have suggested a higher incidence of neurologic sequelae. Neonates may be at increased risk of learning disabilities, behavioral problems, cerebral palsy, and deafness.

PREVENTION

Tetanus is prevented by good wound care and immunization (Chap. 148). In neonates, use of safe, clean delivery and cord-care practices as well as maternal vaccination are essential. The WHO guidelines for tetanus vaccination consist of a primary course of three doses in infancy, boosters at 4–7 and 12–15 years of age, and one booster in adulthood. In the United States, the CDC suggests an additional dose at 14–16 months and boosters every 10 years. "Catch-up" schedules recommend a three-dose primary course for unimmunized adolescents followed by two further doses. For persons who have received a complete primary course in childhood but no further boosters, two doses at least 4 weeks apart are recommended.

Standard WHO recommendations for prevention of maternal and neonatal tetanus call for administration of two doses of tetanus toxoid at least 4 weeks apart to previously unimmunized pregnant women. However, in high-risk areas, a more intensive approach has been successful, with all women of childbearing age receiving a primary course along with education on safe delivery and postnatal practices.

Individuals sustaining tetanus-prone wounds should be immunized if their vaccination status is incomplete or unknown or if their last booster was given >10 years earlier. Patients sustaining wounds not classified as clean or minor should also undergo passive immunization with TIG. It is recommended that tetanus toxoid be given in conjunction with diphtheria toxoid in a preparation with or without acellular pertussis: DTaP for children <7 years old, Td for 7- to 9-year olds, and Tdap for children >9 years old and adults.

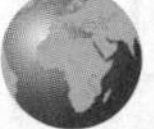

In the early 1980s, tetanus caused more than 1 million deaths a year, accounting for an estimated 5% of maternal deaths and 14% of all neonatal deaths. In 1989, the World Health

TABLE 177-1 FACTORS ASSOCIATED WITH A POOR PROGNOSIS IN TETANUS

Adult Tetanus	Neonatal Tetanus
Age >70 years	Younger age, premature birth
Incubation period <7 days	Incubation period <6 days
Short time from first symptom to admission	Delay in hospital admission
Puerperal, IV, postsurgery, burn entry site	Grass used to cut cord
Period of onset[a] <48 h	Low birth weight
Heart rate >140 beats/min[b]	Fever on admission
Systolic blood pressure >140 mmHg[b]	
Severe disease or spasms[b]	
Temperature >38.5°C[b]	

[a]Time from first symptom to first generalized spasm. [b]At hospital admission.

Assembly adopted a resolution to eliminate neonatal tetanus by the year 2000; elimination was defined as <1 case/1000 live births in every district in every country. By 1999, elimination was still to be achieved in 57 countries and the deadline was extended until 2005, with the additional target of eliminating maternal tetanus (tetanus occurring during pregnancy or within 6 weeks of its end). Ratification of the Millennium Development Goals, in particular goal 4 (achieving a two-thirds reduction in the mortality rate among children under 5 by 2015), has further focused attention on reducing deaths from vaccine-preventable disease, particularly in the first 4 weeks of life.

Because vaccination reduces the incidence of neonatal tetanus by an estimated 94%, immunization of pregnant women with two doses of tetanus toxoid at least 4 weeks apart has been the primary method of maternal and neonatal tetanus elimination. In some areas, all women of childbearing age have been targeted as a means of increasing vaccination coverage. In addition, educational programs have focused on improving hygiene during the birth process, an intervention that in itself is estimated to reduce neonatal tetanus deaths by up to 40%.

The latest available data show that 34 countries have yet to eliminate maternal and neonatal tetanus, although incidence has declined significantly. Worldwide, deaths from neonatal tetanus fell by 92% between 1990 and 2008; in the latter year, with 81% of newborns protected from the disease by maternal vaccination, there were an estimated 59,000 neonatal tetanus deaths. Despite this relative success, immunization programs need to be ongoing as there is no tetanus herd immunity effect and *C. tetani* contamination of soil and feces is widespread.

178 Botulism

Susan Maslanka, Agam K. Rao

Botulism, recognized at least since the eighteenth century, is a neuroparalytic disease caused by botulinum toxin, one of the most toxic substances known. While initially thought to be caused only by the ingestion of botulinum toxin in contaminated food (food-borne botulism), three additional forms caused by in situ toxin production after germination of spores in either a wound or the intestine are now recognized worldwide: wound botulism, infant botulism, and adult intestinal colonization botulism. In addition to occurring in these recognized natural forms of the disease, botulism symptoms have been reported in patients receiving injections of botulinum toxin for cosmetic or therapeutic purposes (iatrogenic botulism). Moreover, botulism was reported after inhalation of botulinum toxin in a laboratory setting. All forms of botulism manifest as a relatively distinct clinical syndrome of symmetric cranial-nerve palsies followed by descending bilateral flaccid paralysis of voluntary muscles, which may progress to respiratory compromise and death. The mainstays of therapy are meticulous intensive care and treatment with antitoxin as soon as botulism is suspected and before other illnesses have been ruled out.

ETIOLOGY AND PATHOGENESIS

Seven serologically distinct confirmed serotypes of botulinum toxin (A through G) have been confirmed. Botulinum toxin is produced by four recognized species of clostridia: *Clostridium botulinum, Clostridium argentinense, Clostridium baratii,* and *Clostridium butyricum*. Certain strains may produce more than one serotype. All are anaerobic gram-positive organisms that form subterminal spores; *C. botulinum* and *C. argentinense* spores have been recovered from the environment. The spores survive environmental conditions and ordinary cooking procedures. Toxin production, however, requires a rare confluence of product storage conditions: an anaerobic environment, a pH of >4.6, low salt and sugar concentrations, and temperatures of >4°C. Although commonly ingested, spores do not normally germinate and produce toxin in the adult human intestine.

Food-borne botulism is caused by consumption of foods contaminated with botulinum toxin; no confirmed host-specific factors are involved in the disease. *Wound botulism* is caused by contamination of wounds with *C. botulinum* spores, subsequent spore germination, and toxin production in the anaerobic milieu of an abscess or a wound. *Infant botulism* results from absorption of toxin produced in situ by toxigenic clostridia colonizing the intestine of children ≤1 year of age. Colonization is thought to occur because the normal bowel microbiota is not yet fully established; this theory is supported by studies in animals. *Adult intestinal colonization botulism,* a very rare form that is poorly understood, has a pathology similar to that of infant botulism but occurs in adults; typically, patients have some anatomic or functional bowel abnormality or have recently used antibiotics that may help toxigenic clostridia compete more successfully against the normal bowel microbiota. Despite antitoxin treatment, relapse due to intermittent intraluminal production of toxin may be observed in patients with adult intestinal colonization botulism.

Regardless of how exposure occurs, botulinum neurotoxin enters the vascular system and is transported to peripheral cholinergic nerve terminals, including neuromuscular junctions, postganglionic parasympathetic nerve endings, and peripheral ganglia. Botulinum toxin is a zinc-endopeptidase protein of ~150 kDa, consisting of a 100-kDa heavy chain and a 50-kDa light chain. Steps in neurotoxin activity include (1) heavy-chain binding to nerve terminals, (2) internalization in endocytic vesicles, (3) translocation of the light chain to cytosol, and (4) light-chain serotype-specific cleavage of one of several proteins involved in the release of the neurotransmitter acetylcholine. Inhibition of acetylcholine release by any of the seven toxin serotypes results in characteristic flaccid paralysis. Recovery follows sprouting of new nerve terminals.

All botulinum toxin serotypes have been demonstrated to cause botulism in nonhuman primates. Human cases associated with serotypes A, B, E, and F are reported each year. Serotype A produces the most severe syndrome, with the greatest proportion of patients requiring mechanical ventilation. Serotype B appears to cause milder disease than type A in both food-borne and infant botulism. Serotype E, most often associated with foods of aquatic origin, produces a syndrome of variable severity. The rare cases of illness caused by toxin serotype F, whether in infants or adults, are characterized by rapid progression to quadriplegia and respiratory failure but also by relatively rapid recovery. Recent studies have shown that at least some serotypes can be differentiated into subtypes through neurotoxin gene sequencing; however, the impact of these subtype differences on clinical illness is not yet known.

EPIDEMIOLOGY

Botulism occurs worldwide, but the number of cases reported varies among countries and regions. The variation may be due not only to actual differences in incidence but also to (1) availability of resources to identify botulism, a rare disease; (2) differences in reporting requirements; and (3) limited external access to data collections. There is no universal surveillance system to capture worldwide botulism incidence. However, 30 countries currently participate in voluntary reporting of botulism cases to the European Union through an established surveillance system that includes standardized case definitions similar to those used in the United States and Canada. Other countries (e.g., Argentina, China, Thailand, Japan) maintain independent botulism surveillance.

Food-Borne Botulism From 1899 to 2011, 1225 food-borne botulism events (single cases or outbreaks) were reported in the United States; from 1990 to 2000, a median of 23 cases were reported annually. Most such events (~80%) involve vegetables or fish/aquatic animals, usually home-preserved (canned, jarred). Native communities in both the United States (Alaska) and Canada have a high incidence of food-borne botulism due to traditional food-preparation practices; 85% of all cases in Canada occur in Native communities. Outbreaks typically involve two or three cases; however, one restaurant-associated outbreak in 1977 affected 59 persons. Worldwide, the highest incidence rate is reported from Georgia and Armenia in the southern Caucasus region, where illness is also associated with home-canning practices. Outbreaks in Asia are attributable to consumption of home-preserved fish or vegetable products such as bean curd and bamboo shoots. In parts of Europe, including Poland, France, and Germany, illness is often associated with home-preserved meat such as ham or sausage. Since 1950, commercial products have rarely been implicated in botulism in the United States, and botulism from commercial products is most often attributed to consumer error in storage or cooking. However, manufacturer deficiencies do occur. In 2007, botulism developed in eight persons in the United States who consumed a commercially canned hot-dog chili sauce. Significant deficiencies discovered by regulatory authorities involved 91 different products and resulted in the recall of 111 million cans of food.

Wound Botulism This form of disease was first recognized in 1951 as a result of a review of the clinical records on an accidental injury in 1943. Between 1943 and 2011, 491 cases of wound botulism were reported in the United States; 97% of cases reported after 1990 were associated with injection drug use. The typical patient was a 30- to 50-year-old resident of the western United States with a long history of black-tar heroin injection. In the early 2000s, wound botulism associated with drug use emerged in Europe, and at least two case clusters have been reported.

Infant Botulism More than 3900 infant botulism cases have been reported worldwide (84% in the United States alone) since this form of the disease was first recognized in 1976; ~80–100 cases (commonly caused by serotypes A and B) are reported annually in the United States.

Adult Intestinal Colonization Botulism This form of botulism is difficult to confirm because it is poorly understood and because no clear guidelines are available to help differentiate it from other adult botulism cases. Often these cases are caused by *C. baratii* type F, but the involvement of both *C. botulinum* type A and *C. butyricum* type E has been reported.

Iatrogenic Botulism Paralysis of variable severity has followed injection of licensed botulinum toxin products for treatment of conditions involving hypertonicity of large muscle groups. The U.S. Food and Drug Administration received 658 reports of adverse events related to botulinum toxin use—some very serious—between 1997 and 2006. Although some patients had symptoms consistent with botulism, no cases were laboratory confirmed. Injection of approved doses of licensed products for cosmetic purposes has not been associated with botulism. However, four cases of laboratory-confirmed botulism resulted from illegal injection of research-grade toxin for cosmetic purposes in a U.S. medical facility in 2004.

Inhalational Botulism Inhalational botulism does not occur naturally. One report from Germany has described botulism resulting from possible inhalational exposure to botulinum toxin in a laboratory incident.

Intentional Botulism Botulinum toxin has been "weaponized" by governments and terrorist organizations. An attack might use aerosolization of toxin or contamination of foods or beverages ranging in scope from small-scale tampering to contamination of a widely distributed food item. An unnatural event may be suggested by unusual relationships between patients (e.g., a visit to the same building), atypical exposure vehicles, or atypical toxin serotypes.

CLINICAL MANIFESTATIONS

The distinctive clinical syndrome of botulism consists of symmetric cranial-nerve palsies followed by bilateral descending flaccid paralysis that may progress to respiratory failure and death. The incubation period from ingestion of contaminated food to onset of symptoms in food-borne botulism is usually 8–36 h but can be as long as 10 days and is dose dependent. Incubation periods of 4–17 days have been documented in wound botulism associated with accidental injury. However, estimation is difficult in cases involving injection drug users because most of these patients inject drugs several times daily. Similarly, the incubation period for infant botulism has not been established, but the fact that the illness has affected infants <3 days old suggests that this interval may be very short.

Cranial nerve deficits may include some of the following: diplopia, dysarthria, dysphonia, ptosis, ophthalmoplegia, facial paralysis, and impaired gag reflex. Pupillary reflexes may be depressed, and fixed or dilated pupils are sometimes noted. Autonomic symptoms such as dizziness, dry mouth, and very dry, occasionally sore throat are common. Constipation due to paralytic ileus is nearly universal, and urinary retention is also common. Patients are afebrile and remain alert and oriented. Respiratory failure may occur due to either paralysis of the diaphragm and accessory breathing muscles or pharyngeal collapse secondary to cranial nerve paralysis. Weakness descends, often rapidly, from the head to involve the neck, arms, thorax, and legs; occasionally, weakness is asymmetric. Deep tendon reflexes may be normal or may progressively disappear. Paresthesias, while rare, have been reported and may represent secondary nerve compression from immobility due to paralysis. Absence of cranial nerve palsies or their onset after the appearance of other true neurologic symptoms makes botulism highly unlikely. Nausea, vomiting, and abdominal pain may precede or follow the onset of paralysis in food-borne botulism. Infants with botulism typically present with reduced ability to suck and swallow, constipation, weakened voice, ptosis, sluggish pupils, hypotonia, and floppy neck; as in adults, illness can progress to generalized flaccidity and respiratory compromise.

Even when intubated, patients can respond to questions by moving their fingers or toes unless paralysis has affected the digits. In some instances, unfortunately, the severe ptosis, expressionless face, and weak phonation of patients with botulism have been interpreted as signs of mental status changes due to alcohol intoxication, drug overdose, encephalitis, or meningitis—a conclusion that delays an accurate diagnosis. Because of skeletal muscle paralysis, patients experiencing respiratory distress may appear placid and detached even as they near respiratory arrest. Death in untreated botulism is usually due to airway obstruction from pharyngeal muscle paralysis and inadequate tidal volume resulting from paralysis of diaphragmatic and accessory respiratory muscles. Death can also result from hospital-associated infections and other sequelae of long-term paralysis, hospitalization, and mechanical ventilation.

A history of preparing home-canned foods may assist with the diagnosis. Patients with wound botulism may or may not have a discernible wound or abscess. A history of injection drug use or the presence of track marks may raise suspicion of the diagnosis. Clinical improvement follows sprouting of new nerve terminals and may take weeks to months. Patients often require outpatient rehabilitation therapy and may experience residual deficits.

DIAGNOSIS

Botulism is diagnosed primarily on clinical grounds, with laboratory confirmation by specific tests that identify botulinum toxin in clinical and food samples. In the setting of an outbreak with multiple patients presenting to the same treatment facility, the diagnosis is apparent as long as physicians recognize that cases within a cluster may have varied signs and symptoms. The temporal occurrence of two or more cases with symptoms compatible with botulism is essentially pathognomonic because other illnesses that resemble botulism do not usually occur in clusters. In lone (sporadic) cases, the diagnosis is often missed. The rarity of this disease prevents many physicians from gaining experience with its clinical diagnosis, and some patients present with signs and symptoms that do not fit the classic pattern. Assessing clinical characteristics of other paralytic illnesses in single cases is sometimes critical to rule in or rule out the diagnosis of botulism.

In adults, a food history and the names of contacts who may have shared foods should be obtained before illness progresses to respiratory failure; specific questions should include information about the consumption of home-preserved and/or exotic foods and of products requiring refrigeration that have been left at room temperature in sealed plastic containers or bags. A history of recent consumption of home-canned food substantially enhances the probability of food-borne botulism.

Ascertainment of the patient's behavioral history related to injection drug use is critical to the diagnosis of wound botulism unless an accidental wound is evident. Caretakers' observations up to and including the onset of symptoms are vital to the diagnosis of infant botulism. A history of recent abdominal surgery or antibiotic use may be important in the diagnosis of adult intestinal colonization botulism.

Differential Diagnosis The illnesses most commonly considered in the differential diagnosis of adult botulism cases include Guillain-Barré syndrome (GBS), myasthenia gravis, stroke syndromes, Eaton-Lambert syndrome, and tick paralysis. Less likely possibilities are poisoning by tetrodotoxin, shellfish, or a host of rarer agents and antimicrobial drug–associated paralysis. A thorough history and a meticulous physical examination can effectively eliminate most alternative diagnoses, but a workup for other diagnoses should not delay treatment with botulinum antitoxin.

GBS, a rare autoimmune demyelinating polyneuropathy that often follows an acute infection, presents most often as an ascending paralysis. Case clusters are rare. Occasional GBS cases present as the Miller Fisher variant, whose characteristic triad of ophthalmoplegia, ataxia, and areflexia is easily mistaken for the early descending paralysis of botulism. Protein levels in cerebrospinal fluid (CSF) are elevated in GBS; because this increase may be delayed until several days after symptom onset, an early lumbar puncture with a negative result may need to be repeated. In contrast, CSF findings are generally normal in botulism, although marginally elevated CSF protein concentrations have been reported. In experienced hands, electromyography may differentiate GBS from botulism.

The edrophonium (Tensilon) test is sometimes of value in distinguishing botulism (usually a negative result) from myasthenia gravis (usually a positive result).

In most cerebrovascular accidents, physical examination reveals asymmetry of paralysis and upper motor neuron signs. Brain imaging can reveal the rare basilar stroke that produces symmetric bulbar palsies. Eaton-Lambert syndrome usually manifests as proximal limb weakness in a patient already debilitated by cancer. Tick paralysis is a rare flaccid condition closely resembling botulism and caused by neurotoxins of certain ticks.

Botulism-Specific Laboratory Tests Botulism is confirmed in the laboratory by demonstration of toxin in clinical specimens (e.g., serum, stool, gastric aspirate, and sterile-water enema samples) or in samples of ingested foods. Isolation of toxigenic clostridia from stool also provides evidence of botulism. Wound cultures yielding the organism are highly suggestive in symptomatic cases. The universally accepted method for confirmation of botulism is the mouse bioassay, which is available only in specialized laboratories. Specific guidance about what specimens to collect should be obtained from the testing laboratory because the requirements vary with the form of botulism suspected. Clinical specimens collected early in the hospital admission process should be submitted for testing; toxin results may be negative if specimens are collected >7 days after symptom onset. Because of the extreme potency of botulinum toxin, a test may yield a negative result even when a patient has botulism; thus, a negative result does not exclude this diagnosis. In suspected wound botulism, material from abscesses should be collected in anaerobic culture tubes. New laboratory tests for botulism are being developed but remain experimental. Nerve conduction studies showing reduced amplitude of motor potentials—with or without potentiation by rapid repetitive stimulation in weak muscles—and needle electromyography showing small-motor-unit action potentials are consistent with botulism; these results and those that make alternative diagnoses more likely may be useful. Standard blood work and radiologic studies are not useful in diagnosing botulism.

TREATMENT BOTULISM

The cornerstones of treatment for botulism are meticulous intensive care and immediate administration of botulinum antitoxin. Because antitoxin is most beneficial early in the course of clinical illness, it should be administered as soon as botulism is suspected and before the time-consuming workup for other illnesses is complete. Persons of all ages (including infants) in whom botulism is suspected should be hospitalized immediately so that respiratory failure—the usual cause of death—can be detected and managed promptly. Vital capacity should be monitored frequently and mechanical ventilation provided as needed. Botulinum antitoxin can limit the progression of illness because it neutralizes toxin molecules in the circulation that have not yet bound to nerve endings. However, antitoxin does not reverse existing paralysis, which may take weeks to improve. In the United States, there are two licensed antitoxin products: Botulism Antitoxin Heptavalent® (BAT; Emergent Biosolutions, Rockville, MD), an equine-derived heptavalent (A through G) product enzymatically de-speciated for treatment of all forms of adult botulism and infant cases not involving serotypes A and B; and Botulism Immune Globulin Intravenous (BabyBIG®; California Department of Public Health, Sacramento, CA), a human-derived product for treating infant botulism caused by serotype A and/or B only. Antitoxin is also available in some other countries. Aminoglycosides and other medications that block the neuromuscular junction may potentiate botulism and should be avoided.

In wound botulism, suspect wounds and abscesses should be cleaned, debrided, and drained promptly. The role of penicillin and metronidazole in treatment and decolonization is unclear. It has been hypothesized that antimicrobial agents may increase circulating botulinum toxin from lysis of bacterial cells.

Person-to-person transmission of botulism does not occur. Universal precautions are the only infection-control measures required during inpatient care.

NOTIFICATION, EXPERT CONSULTATION, AND ANTITOXIN PROVISION

Every botulism case is a public health emergency. Antitoxin is not universally available. Some countries maintain stockpiles of antitoxin for immediate response, whereas others must access supplies from other nations when an outbreak occurs.

In the United States, clinicians must report every suspected case, regardless of form, on an emergency basis to their state health department. The state health department may put the physician in contact with the 24/7 botulism consultation service at the Centers for Disease Control and Prevention (CDC) through the CDC Emergency Operations Center (770-488-7100) or a locally available service. The botulism consultant will review the case and determine whether botulism is likely. If indicated, the consultant will coordinate laboratory confirmation at appropriate testing facilities and facilitate emergency shipment of antitoxin for all adult cases and for infant cases not involving serotypes A and B. In this country, botulinum antitoxin for noninfant cases is available exclusively from the CDC. Physicians who see suspected infant botulism cases should contact the California Department of Public Health Infant Botulism Treatment and Prevention Program (510-231-7600), which provides 24-h consultation and distributes antitoxin (BabyBIG) for the treatment of infant botulism nationwide. Except in cases involving infants who reside in California, laboratory testing requests must still be authorized by the state health department where the infant is located or by the CDC.

PREVENTION

No prophylaxis or licensed vaccine is available against botulism. Home-canning instructions and equipment have changed over the years. Up-to-date canning instructions from reliable sources (e.g., the U.S. Department of Agriculture or the U.S. Food and Drug Administration) should be followed to ensure food safety. Processed food should be stored properly and heated thoroughly prior to consumption. Because of the possible presence of spores, honey should not be given to infants (≤12 months of age). Injection of illicit drugs should be avoided. All wounds should be meticulously cleaned to eliminate possible contamination with bacterial spores. Clinicians should educate individuals or family members of at-risk individuals, including infants, illegal drug users, and preparers of home-preserved foods.

ACKNOWLEDGMENT

The authors thank Dr. Jeremy Sobel for his valued contributions to the previous version of this chapter.

179 Gas Gangrene and Other Clostridial Infections

Amy E. Bryant, Dennis L. Stevens

The genus *Clostridium* encompasses more than 60 species that may be commensals of the gut microflora or may cause a variety of infections in humans and animals through the production of a plethora of proteinaceous exotoxins. *C. tetani* and *C. botulinum*, for example, cause specific clinical disease by elaborating single but highly potent toxins. In contrast, *C. perfringens* and *C. septicum* cause aggressive necrotizing infections that are attributable to multiple toxins, including bacterial proteases, phospholipases, and cytotoxins.

ETIOLOGIC AGENT

Vegetative cells of *Clostridium* species are pleomorphic, rod-shaped, and arranged singly or in short chains (Fig. 179-1); the cells have rounded or sometimes pointed ends. Although clostridia stain gram-positive in the early stages of growth, they may appear to be gram-negative or gram-variable later in the growth cycle or in infected tissue specimens. Most strains are motile by means of peritrichous flagella; *C. septicum* swarms on solid media. Nonmotile species include *C. perfringens*, *C. ramosum*, and *C. innocuum*. Most species are obligately anaerobic, although clostridial tolerance to oxygen varies widely; some species (e.g., *C. septicum*, *C. tertium*) will grow but will not sporulate in air.

Clostridia produce more protein toxins than any other bacterial genus, and more than 25 clostridial toxins lethal to mice have been identified. These proteins include neurotoxins, enterotoxins, cytotoxins, collagenases, permeases, necrotizing toxins, lipases, lecithinases, hemolysins, proteinases, hyaluronidases, DNases, ADP-ribosyltransferases, and neuraminidases. Botulinum and tetanus neurotoxins are the most potent toxins known, with lethal doses of 0.2–10 ng/kg for humans. Epsilon toxin, a 33-kDa protein produced by *C. perfringens* types B and D, causes edema and hemorrhage in the brain, heart, spinal cord, and kidneys of animals. It is among the most lethal of the clostridial toxins and is considered a potential agent of bioterrorism (Chap. 261e). The genomic sequences of some pathogenic clostridia are now available and are likely to facilitate a comprehensive approach to understanding the virulence factors involved in clostridial pathogenesis.

EPIDEMIOLOGY AND TRANSMISSION

Clostridium species are widespread in nature, forming endospores that are commonly found in soil, feces, sewage, and marine sediments. The ecology of *C. perfringens* in soil is greatly influenced by the degree and duration of animal husbandry in a given location and is relevant to the incidence of gas gangrene caused by contamination of war wounds with soil. For example, the incidence of clostridial gas gangrene is higher in agricultural regions of Europe than in the Sahara Desert of Africa. Similarly, the incidences of tetanus and food-borne botulism are clearly related to the presence of clostridial spores in soil, water, and many foods. Clostridia are present in large numbers in the indigenous microbiota of the intestinal tract of humans and animals, in the female genital tract, and on the oral mucosa. It should be noted that not all commensal clostridia are toxigenic.

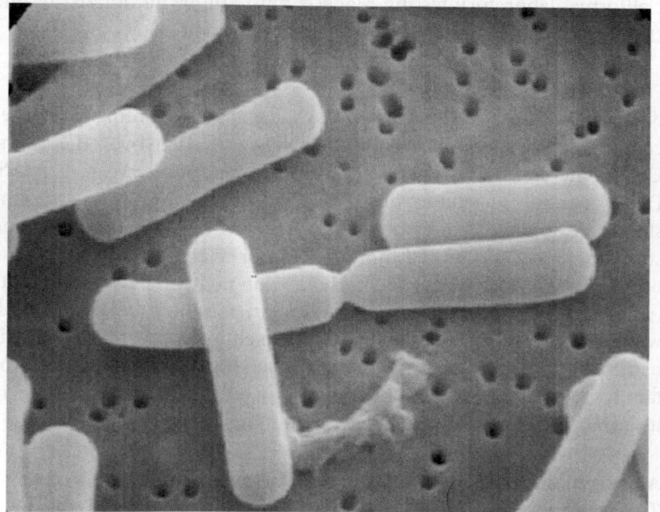

FIGURE 179-1 Scanning electron micrograph of *C. perfringens*.

Clostridial infections remain a serious public health concern worldwide. In developing nations, food poisoning, necrotizing enterocolitis, and gas gangrene are common because large portions of the population are poor and have little or no immediate access to health care. These infections remain prevalent in developed countries as well. Gas gangrene commonly follows knife or gunshot wounds or vehicular accidents or develops as a complication of surgery or gastrointestinal carcinoma. Severe clostridial infections have emerged as a health threat to injection drug users and to women undergoing childbirth or abortion. Historically, clostridial gas gangrene has been the scourge of the battlefield. The global political situation portends another possible scenario involving mass casualties of war or terrorism, with extensive injuries conducive to gas gangrene. Thus there is an ongoing need to develop novel strategies to prevent or attenuate the course of clostridial infections in both civilians and military personnel. Vaccination against exotoxins important in pathogenesis would be of great benefit in developing nations and could also be used safely in at-risk populations such as the elderly, patients with diabetes who may require lower-limb surgery due to trauma or poor circulation, and those undergoing intestinal surgery. Moreover, a hyperimmune globulin would be a valuable tool for prophylaxis in victims of acute traumatic injury or for attenuation of the spread of infection in patients with established gas gangrene.

CLINICAL SYNDROMES

Life-threatening clostridial infections range from intoxications (e.g., food poisoning, tetanus) to necrotizing enteritis/colitis, bacteremia, myonecrosis, and toxic shock syndrome (TSS). Tetanus and botulism are discussed in Chaps. 177 and 178, respectively. Colitis due to *C. difficile* is discussed in Chap. 161.

CLOSTRIDIAL WOUND CONTAMINATION

Of open traumatic wounds, 30–80% reportedly are contaminated with clostridial species. In the absence of devitalized tissue, the presence of clostridia does not necessarily lead to infection. In traumatic injuries, clostridia are isolated with equal frequency from both suppurative and well-healing wounds. Thus, diagnosis and treatment of clostridial infection should be based on clinical signs and symptoms and not solely on bacteriologic findings.

POLYMICROBIAL INFECTIONS INVOLVING CLOSTRIDIA

Clostridial species may be found in polymicrobial infections also involving microbial components of the indigenous flora. In these infections, clostridia often appear in association with non-spore-forming anaerobes and facultative or aerobic organisms. Head and neck infections, conjunctivitis, brain abscess, sinusitis, otitis, aspiration pneumonia, lung abscess, pleural empyema, cholecystitis, septic arthritis, and bone infections all may involve clostridia. These conditions are often associated with severe local inflammation but may lack the characteristic systemic signs of toxicity and rapid progression seen in other clostridial infections. In addition, clostridia are isolated from ~66% of intraabdominal infections in which the mucosal integrity of the bowel or respiratory system has been compromised. In this setting, *C. ramosum*, *C. perfringens*, and *C. bifermentans* are the most commonly isolated species. Their presence does not invariably lead to a poor outcome. Clostridia have been isolated from suppurative infections of the female genital tract (e.g., ovarian or pelvic abscess) and from diseased gallbladders. Although the most frequently isolated species is *C. perfringens*, gangrene is not typically observed; however, gas formation in the biliary system can lead to emphysematous cholecystitis, especially in diabetic patients. *C. perfringens* in association with mixed aerobic and anaerobic microbes can cause aggressive life-threatening type I necrotizing fasciitis or Fournier's gangrene.

The treatment of mixed aerobic/anaerobic infection of the abdomen, perineum, or gynecologic organs should be based on Gram's staining, culture, and antibiotic sensitivity information. Reasonable empirical treatment consists of ampicillin or ampicillin/sulbactam combined with either clindamycin or metronidazole (Table 179-1). Broader gram-negative coverage may be necessary if the patient has recently been hospitalized or treated with antibiotics. Such coverage can be obtained by substituting ticarcillin/clavulanic acid, piperacillin/sulbactam, or a penem antibiotic for ampicillin or by adding a fluoroquinolone or an aminoglycoside to the regimen. Empirical treatment should be given for 10–14 days or until the patient's clinical condition improves.

ENTERIC CLOSTRIDIAL INFECTIONS

C. perfringens type A is one of the most common bacterial causes of food-borne illness in the United States and Canada. The foods typically implicated include improperly cooked meat and meat products (e.g., gravy) in which residual spores germinate and proliferate during slow cooling or insufficient reheating. Illness results from the ingestion of food containing at least ~10^8 viable vegetative cells, which sporulate in the alkaline environment of the small intestine, producing *C. perfringens* enterotoxin in the process. The diarrhea that develops within 7–30 h of ingestion of contaminated food is generally mild and self-limiting; however, in the very young, the elderly, and the immunocompromised, symptoms are more severe and occasionally fatal. Enterotoxin-producing *C. perfringens* has been implicated as an etiologic agent of persistent diarrhea in elderly patients in nursing homes and tertiary-care institutions and has been considered to play a role in antibiotic-associated diarrhea without pseudomembranous colitis.

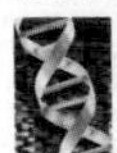

C. perfringens strains associated with food poisoning possess the gene (*cpe*) coding for enterotoxin, which acts by forming pores in host cell membranes. *C. perfringens* strains isolated from non-food-borne diseases, such as antibiotic-associated and sporadic diarrhea, carry *cpe* on a plasmid that may be transmitted to other strains. Several methods have been described for the detection of *C. perfringens* enterotoxin in feces, including cell culture assay (Vero cells), enzyme-linked immunosorbent assay, reversed-phase latex agglutination, and polymerase chain reaction (PCR) amplification of *cpe*. Each method has its advantages and limitations.

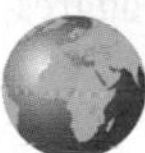

Enteritis necroticans (gas gangrene of the bowel) is a fulminating clinical illness characterized by extensive necrosis of the intestinal mucosa and wall. Cases can occur sporadically in adults or as epidemics in people of all ages. Enteritis necroticans is caused by α toxin– and β toxin–producing strains of *C. perfringens* type C; β toxin is located on a plasmid and is mainly responsible for pathogenesis. This life-threatening infection causes ischemic necrosis of the jejunum. In Papua New Guinea during the 1960s, enteritis necroticans (known in that locale as *pigbel*) was found to be the most common cause of death in childhood; it was associated with pig feasts and occurred both sporadically and in outbreaks. Intramuscular immunization against the β toxin resulted in a decreased incidence of the disease in Papua New Guinea, although the condition remains common. Enteritis necroticans has also been recognized in the United States, the United Kingdom, Germany (where it is known as *darmbrand*), and other developed nations; especially affected are adults who are malnourished or who have diabetes, alcoholic liver disease, or neutropenia.

Necrotizing enterocolitis, a disease resembling enteritis necroticans but associated with *C. perfringens* type A, has been found in North America in previously healthy adults. It is also a serious gastrointestinal disease of low-birth-weight (premature) infants hospitalized in neonatal intensive care units. The etiology and pathogenesis of this disease have remained enigmatic for more than four decades. Pathologic similarities between necrotizing enterocolitis and enteritis necroticans include the pattern of small-bowel necrosis involving the submucosa, mucosa, and muscularis; the presence of gas dissecting the tissue planes; and the degree of inflammation. In contrast to enteritis necroticans, which most commonly involves the jejunum, necrotizing enterocolitis affects the ileum and frequently the ileocecal valve. Both diseases may manifest as intestinal gas cysts, although this feature is more common in necrotizing enterocolitis. The sources of the gas, which contains hydrogen, methane, and carbon dioxide, are probably the fermentative activities of intestinal bacteria, including clostridia. Epidemiologic data support an important role for *C. perfringens* or other gas-producing microorganisms (e.g., *C. neonatale*, certain other clostridia, or *Klebsiella* species) in the pathogenesis of necrotizing enterocolitis.

Patients with suspected clostridial enteric infection should undergo nasogastric suction and receive IV fluids. Pyrantel is given by mouth, and the bowel is rested by fasting. Benzylpenicillin (1 mU) is given IV every 4 h, and the patient is observed for complications requiring surgery. Patients with mild cases recover without surgical intervention. If surgical indications are present (gas in the peritoneal cavity, absent bowel sounds, rebound tenderness, abdominal rigidity), however, the mortality rate ranges from 35% to 100%; a fatal outcome is due in part to perforation of the intestine.

As pigbel continues to be a common disease in Papua New Guinea, consideration should be given to the use of a *C. perfringens*

TABLE 179-1 TREATMENT OF CLOSTRIDIAL INFECTIONS

Condition	Antibiotic Treatment	Penicillin Allergy	Adjunctive Treatment/Note
Wound contamination	None	—	Treatment should be based on clinical signs and symptoms as listed below and not solely on bacteriologic findings.
Polymicrobial anaerobic infections involving clostridia (e.g., abdominal wall, gynecologic)	Ampicillin (2 g IV q4h) ***plus*** Clindamycin (600–900 mg IV q6–8h) ***plus*** Ciprofloxacin (400 mg IV q6–8 h)	Vancomycin (1 g IV q12h) ***plus*** Metronidazole (500 mg IV q6h) ***plus*** Ciprofloxacin (400 mg IV q6–8h)	Empirical therapy should be initiated. Therapy should be based on Gram's stain and culture results and on sensitivity data when available. Add gram-negative coverage if indicated (see text).
Clostridial sepsis	Penicillin, 3–4 mU IV q4–6h ***plus*** Clindamycin (600–900 mg IV q6–8h)	Clindamycin alone ***or*** Metronidazole (as above) ***or*** Vancomycin (as above)	Transient bacteremia without signs of systemic toxicity may be clinically insignificant.
Gas gangrene	Penicillin G (4 mU IV q4–6 h) ***plus*** Clindamycin (600–900 mg IV q6–8h)	Cefoxitin (2 g IV q6h) ***plus*** Clindamycin (600–900 mg IV q6–8h)	Emergent surgical exploration and thorough debridement are extremely important. Hyperbaric oxygen therapy may be considered after surgery and antibiotic initiation.

type C β toxoid vaccine in local areas. Two doses given 3–4 months apart are preventive.

CLOSTRIDIAL BACTEREMIA

Clostridium species are important causes of bloodstream infections. Molecular epidemiologic studies of anaerobic bacteremia have identified *C. perfringens* and *C. tertium* as the two most frequently isolated species; these organisms cause up to 79% and 5%, respectively, of clostridial bacteremias. Occasionally, *C. perfringens* bacteremia occurs in the absence of an identifiable infection at another site. When associated with myonecrosis, bacteremia has a grave prognosis.

C. septicum is also commonly associated with bacteremia. This species is isolated only rarely from the feces of healthy individuals but may be found in the normal appendix. More than 50% of patients whose blood cultures are positive for this organism have some gastrointestinal anomaly (e.g., diverticular disease) or underlying malignancy (e.g., carcinoma of the colon). In addition, a clinically important association of *C. septicum* bacteremia with neutropenia of any origin—and, more specifically, with neutropenic enterocolitis involving the terminal ileum or cecum—has been observed. Patients with diabetes mellitus, severe atherosclerotic cardiovascular disease, or anaerobic myonecrosis (gas gangrene) also may develop *C. septicum* bacteremia. *C. septicum* has been recovered from the bloodstream of cirrhotic patients, as have *C. perfringens*, *C. bifermentans*, and other clostridia. Infections of the bloodstream by *C. sordellii* and *C. perfringens* have been associated with TSS.

Bloodstream infection by *C. tertium*, either alone or in combination with *C. septicum* or *C. perfringens*, can be found in patients with serious underlying disease such as malignancy or acute pancreatitis, with or without neutropenic enterocolitis; the frequency has not been systematically studied. *C. tertium* may present special problems in terms of both identification and treatment. This organism may stain gram-negative; is aerotolerant; and is resistant to metronidazole, clindamycin, and cephalosporins.

Other clostridia from the *C. clostridioforme* group (including *C. clostridioforme*, *C. hathewayi*, and *C. bolteae*) can cause bacteremia.

The clinical importance of recognizing clostridial bacteremia—especially that due to *C. septicum*—and starting appropriate treatment immediately (Table 179-1) cannot be overemphasized. Patients with this condition usually are gravely ill, and infection may metastasize to distant anatomic sites, resulting in spontaneous myonecrosis (see next section). Alternative methods to identify bacteremia-causing clostridial species, such as PCR or other rapid diagnostic tests, are not currently available. Anaerobic blood cultures and Gram's stain interpretation remain the best diagnostic tests at this point.

CLOSTRIDIAL SKIN AND SOFT-TISSUE INFECTIONS

Histotoxic clostridial species such as *C. perfringens*, *C. histolyticum*, *C. septicum*, *C. novyi*, and *C. sordellii* cause aggressive necrotizing infections of the skin and soft tissues. These infections are attributable in part to the elaboration of bacterial proteases, phospholipases, and cytotoxins. Necrotizing clostridial soft-tissue infections are rapidly progressive and are characterized by marked tissue destruction, gas in the tissues, and shock; they frequently end in death. Severe pain, crepitus, brawny induration with rapid progression to skin sloughing, violaceous bullae, and marked tachycardia are characteristics found in the majority of patients.

Clostridial Myonecrosis (Gas Gangrene) • ***TRAUMATIC GAS GANGRENE*** *C. perfringens* myonecrosis (gas gangrene) is one of the most fulminant gram-positive bacterial infections of humans. Even with appropriate antibiotic therapy and management in an intensive care unit, tissue destruction can progress rapidly. Gas gangrene is accompanied by bacteremia, hypotension, and multiorgan failure and is invariably fatal if untreated. Gas gangrene is a true emergency and requires immediate surgical debridement.

The development of gas gangrene requires an anaerobic environment and contamination of a wound with spores or vegetative organisms. Devitalized tissue, foreign bodies, and ischemia reduce locally available oxygen levels and favor outgrowth of vegetative cells and spores. Thus conditions predisposing to traumatic gas gangrene include crush-type injury, laceration of large or medium-sized arteries, and open fractures of long bones that are contaminated with soil or bits of clothing containing the bacterial spores. Gas gangrene of the abdominal wall and flanks follows penetrating injuries such as knife or gunshot wounds that are sufficient to compromise intestinal integrity, with resultant leakage of the bowel contents into the soft tissues. Proximity to fecal sources of bacteria is a risk factor for cases following hip surgery, adrenaline injections into the buttocks, or amputation of the leg for ischemic vascular disease. In the last decade, cutaneous gas gangrene caused by *C. perfringens*, *C. novyi*, and *C. sordellii* has been described in the United States and northern Europe among persons injecting black-tar heroin subcutaneously.

The incubation period for traumatic gas gangrene can be as short as 6 h and is usually <4 days. The infection is characterized by the sudden onset of excruciating pain at the affected site and the rapid development of a foul-smelling wound containing a thin serosanguineous discharge and gas bubbles. Brawny edema and induration develop and give way to cutaneous blisters containing bluish to maroon-colored fluid. Such tissue later may become liquefied and slough. The margin between healthy and necrotic tissue often advances several inches per hour despite appropriate antibiotic therapy, and radical amputation remains the single best life-saving intervention. Shock and organ failure frequently accompany gas gangrene; when patients become bacteremic, the mortality rate exceeds 50%.

Diagnosis of traumatic gas gangrene is not difficult because the infection always begins at the site of significant trauma, is associated with gas in the tissue, and is rapidly progressive. Gram's staining of drainage or tissue biopsy is usually definitive, demonstrating large gram-positive (or gram-variable) rods, an absence of inflammatory cells, and widespread soft-tissue necrosis.

SPONTANEOUS (NONTRAUMATIC) GAS GANGRENE Spontaneous gas gangrene generally occurs via hematogenous seeding of normal muscle with histotoxic clostridia—principally *C. perfringens*, *C. septicum*, and *C. novyi* and occasionally *C. tertium*—from a gastrointestinal tract portal of entry (as in colonic malignancy, inflammatory bowel disease, diverticulitis, necrotizing enterocolitis, cecitis, or distal ileitis or after gastrointestinal surgery). These gastrointestinal pathologies permit bacterial access to the bloodstream; consequently, aerotolerant *C. septicum* can proliferate in normal tissues. Patients surviving bacteremia or spontaneous gangrene due to *C. septicum* should undergo aggressive diagnostic studies to rule out gastrointestinal pathology.

Additional predisposing host factors include leukemia, lymphoproliferative disorders, cancer chemotherapy, radiation therapy, and AIDS. Cyclic, congenital, or acquired neutropenia also is strongly associated with an increased incidence of spontaneous gas gangrene due to *C. septicum*; in such cases, necrotizing enterocolitis, cecitis, or distal ileitis is common, particularly among children.

The first symptom of spontaneous gas gangrene may be confusion followed by the abrupt onset of excruciating pain in the absence of trauma. These findings, along with fever, should heighten suspicion of spontaneous gas gangrene. However, because of the lack of an obvious portal of entry, the correct diagnosis is frequently delayed or missed. The infection is characterized by rapid progression of tissue destruction with demonstrable gas in the tissue (Fig. 179-2). Swelling increases, and bullae filled with clear, cloudy, hemorrhagic, or purplish fluid appear. The surrounding skin has a purple hue, which may reflect vascular compromise resulting from the diffusion of bacterial toxins into surrounding tissues. Invasion of healthy tissue rapidly ensues, with quick progression to shock and multiple-organ failure. Mortality rates in this setting range from 67 to 100% among adults; among children, the mortality rate is 59%, with the majority of deaths occurring within 24 h of onset.

PATHOGENESIS OF GAS GANGRENE In traumatic gas gangrene, organisms are introduced into devitalized tissue. It is important to recognize that for *C. perfringens* and *C. novyi*, trauma must be sufficient to interrupt the blood supply and thereby to establish an optimal anaerobic

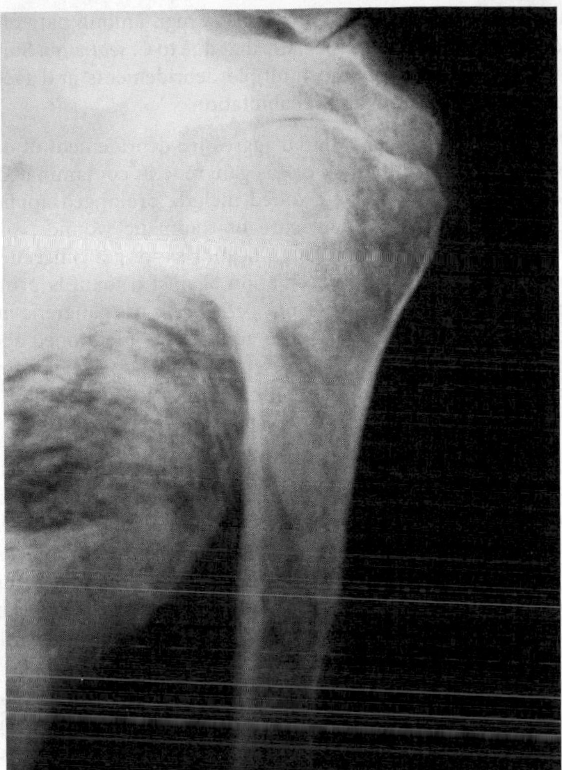

FIGURE 179-2 Radiograph of patient with spontaneous gas gangrene due to *C. septicum*, demonstrating gas in the affected arm and shoulder.

environment for growth of these species. These conditions are not strictly required for the more aerotolerant species such as *C. septicum* and *C. tertium*, which can seed normal tissues from gastrointestinal lesions. Once introduced into an appropriate niche, the organisms proliferate locally and elaborate exotoxins.

The major *C. perfringens* extracellular toxins implicated in gas gangrene are α toxin and θ toxin. A lethal hemolysin that has both phospholipase C and sphingomyelinase activities, α toxin has been implicated as the major virulence factor of *C. perfringens*: immunization of mice with the C-terminal domain of α toxin provides protection against lethal challenge with *C. perfringens*, and isogenic α toxin–deficient mutant strains of *C. perfringens* are not lethal in a murine model of gas gangrene. It has been shown in experimental models that the severe pain, rapid progression, marked tissue destruction, and absence of neutrophils in *C. perfringens* gas gangrene are attributable in large part to α toxin–induced occlusion of blood vessels by heterotypic aggregates of platelets and neutrophils. The formation of these aggregates, which occurs within minutes, is largely mediated by α toxin's ability to activate the platelet adhesion molecule gpIIb/IIIa (Fig. 179-3); the implication is that platelet glycoprotein inhibitors (e.g., eptifibatide, abciximab) may be therapeutic for maintaining tissue blood flow.

C. perfringens θ toxin (*perfringolysin*) is a member of the thiol-activated cytolysin family known as cholesterol-dependent cytolysins, which includes streptolysin O from group A *Streptococcus*, pneumolysin from *Streptococcus pneumoniae*, and several other toxins. Cholesterol-dependent cytolysins bind as oligomers to cholesterol in host cell membranes. At high concentrations, these toxins form ring-like pores resulting in cell lysis. At sublytic concentrations, θ toxin hyperactivates phagocytes and vascular endothelial cells.

Cardiovascular collapse and end-organ failure occur late in the course of *C. perfringens* gas gangrene and are largely attributable to both direct and indirect effects of α and θ toxins. In experimental models, θ toxin causes markedly reduced systemic vascular resistance but increased cardiac output (i.e., "warm shock"), probably via induction of endogenous mediators (e.g., prostacyclin, platelet-activating factor)

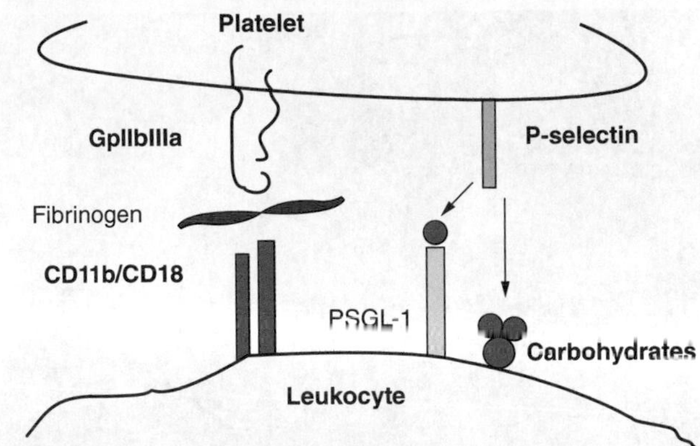

FIGURE 179-3 Schematic illustration of the molecular mechanisms of *C. perfringens* α toxin–induced platelet/neutrophil aggregates. Homotypic aggregates of platelets (not shown) and heterotypic aggregates of platelets and leukocytes are due to α toxin–induced activation of the platelet fibrinogen receptor gpIIb/IIIa and upregulation of leukocyte CD11b/CD18. Binding of fibrinogen (*red*) bridges the connection between these adhesion molecules on adjacent cells. An auxiliary role for α toxin–induced upregulation of platelet P-selectin and its binding to leukocyte P-selectin glycoprotein ligand 1 (PSGL-1) or other leukocyte surface carbohydrates also has been demonstrated.

that cause vasodilation. This effect is similar to that observed in gram-negative sepsis. In sharp contrast, α toxin directly suppresses myocardial contractility; the consequence is profound hypotension due to a sudden reduction in cardiac output. The roles of other endogenous mediators, such as cytokines (e.g., tumor necrosis factor, interleukin 1, interleukin 6) and vasodilators (e.g., bradykinin) have not been fully elucidated.

C. septicum produces four main toxins—α toxin (lethal, hemolytic, necrotizing activity), β toxin (DNase), γ toxin (hyaluronidase), and Δ toxin (septicolysin, an oxygen-labile hemolysin)—as well as a protease and a neuraminidase. Unlike the α toxin of *C. perfringens*, that of *C. septicum* does not possess phospholipase activity. The mechanisms remain to be fully elucidated, but it is likely that each of these toxins contributes uniquely to *C. septicum* gas gangrene.

TREATMENT GAS GANGRENE

Patients with suspected gas gangrene (either traumatic or spontaneous) should undergo prompt surgical inspection of the infected site. Direct examination of a Gram-stained smear of the involved tissues is of major importance. Characteristic histologic findings in clostridial gas gangrene include widespread tissue destruction, a paucity of leukocytes in infected tissues in conjunction with an accumulation of leukocytes in adjacent vessels (Fig. 179-4), and the presence of gram-positive rods (with or without spores). CT and MRI are invaluable for determining whether the infection is localized or is spreading along fascial planes, and needle aspiration or punch biopsy may provide an etiologic diagnosis in at least 20% of cases. However, these techniques should not replace surgical exploration, Gram's staining, and histopathologic examination. When spontaneous gas gangrene is suspected, blood should be cultured since bacteremia usually precedes cutaneous manifestations by several hours.

For patients with evidence of clostridial gas gangrene, thorough emergent surgical debridement is of extreme importance. All devitalized tissue should be widely resected back to healthy viable muscle and skin so as to remove conditions that allow anaerobic organisms to continue proliferating. Closure of traumatic wounds or compound fractures should be delayed for 5–6 days until it is certain that these sites are free of infection.

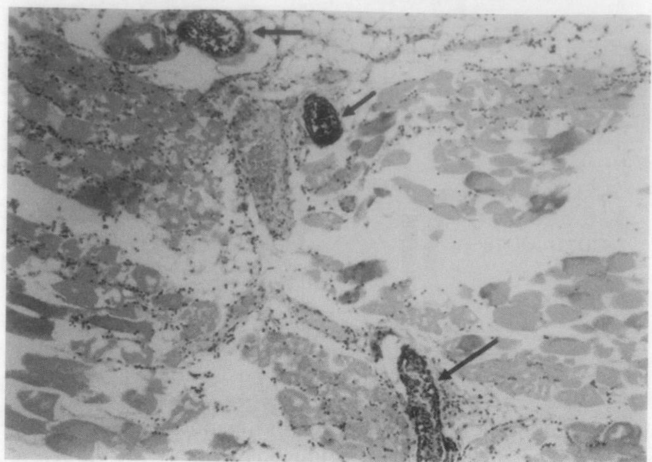

FIGURE 179-4 Histopathology of experimental gas gangrene due to *C. perfringens*, demonstrating widespread muscle necrosis, a paucity of leukocytes in infected tissues, and accumulation of leukocytes in adjacent vessels (*arrows*). These features are due to the effects of α and θ toxins on muscle cells, platelets, leukocytes, and endothelial cells.

Antibiotic treatment of traumatic or spontaneous gas gangrene (Table 179-1) consists of the administration of penicillin and clindamycin for 10–14 days. Penicillin is recommended on the basis of in vitro sensitivity data; clindamycin is recommended because of its superior efficacy over penicillin in animal models of *C. perfringens* gas gangrene and in some clinical reports. Controlled clinical trials comparing the efficacy of these agents in humans have not been performed. In the penicillin-allergic patient, clindamycin may be used alone. The superior efficacy of clindamycin is probably due to its ability to inhibit bacterial protein toxin production, its insensitivity to the size of the bacterial load or the stage of bacterial growth, and its ability to modulate the host's immune response.

C. tertium is resistant to penicillin, cephalosporins, and clindamycin. Appropriate antibiotic therapy for *C. tertium* infection is vancomycin (1 g every 12 h IV) or metronidazole (500 mg every 8 h IV).

The value of adjunctive treatment with hyperbaric oxygen (HBO) for gas gangrene remains controversial. Basic science studies suggest that HBO can inhibit the growth of *C. perfringens* but not that of the more aerotolerant *C. septicum*. In vitro, blood and macerated muscle inhibit the bactericidal potential of HBO. Numerous studies in animals demonstrate little efficacy of HBO alone, whereas antibiotics alone—especially those that inhibit bacterial protein synthesis—confer marked benefits. Addition of HBO to the therapeutic regimen provides some additional benefit, but only if surgery and antibiotic administration precede HBO treatment.

In conclusion, gas gangrene is a rapidly progressive infection whose outcome depends on prompt recognition, emergent surgery, and timely administration of antibiotics that inhibit toxin production. Gas gangrene associated with bacteremia probably represents a later stage of illness and is associated with the worst outcomes. Emergent surgical debridement is crucial to ensure survival, and ancillary procedures (e.g., CT or MRI) or transport to HBO units should not delay this intervention. Some trauma centers associated with HBO units may have special expertise in managing these aggressive infections, but proximity and speed of transfer must be carefully weighed against the need for haste.

PROGNOSIS OF GAS GANGRENE The prognosis for patients with gas gangrene is more favorable when the infection involves an extremity rather than the trunk or visceral organs, since debridement of the latter sites is more difficult. Gas gangrene is most likely to progress to shock and death in patients with associated bacteremia and intravascular hemolysis. Mortality rates are highest for patients in shock at the time of diagnosis. Mortality rates are relatively high among patients with spontaneous gas gangrene, especially that due to *C. septicum*. Survivors of gas gangrene may undergo multiple debridements and face long periods of hospitalization and rehabilitation.

PREVENTION OF GAS GANGRENE Initial aggressive debridement of devitalized tissue can reduce the risk of gas gangrene in contaminated deep wounds. Interventions to be avoided include prolonged application of tourniquets and surgical closure of traumatic wounds; patients with compound fractures are at significant risk for gas gangrene if the wound is closed surgically. Vaccination against α toxin is protective in experimental animal models of *C. perfringens* gas gangrene but has not been investigated in humans. In addition, as mentioned above, a hyperimmune globulin would represent a significant advance for prophylaxis in victims of acute traumatic injury or for attenuation of the spread of infection in patients with established gas gangrene.

Toxic Shock Syndrome Clostridial infection of the endometrium, particularly that due to *C. sordellii*, can develop after gynecologic procedures, childbirth, or abortion (spontaneous or elective, surgical or medical) and, once established, proceeds rapidly to TSS and death. Systemic manifestations, including edema, effusions, profound leukocytosis, and hemoconcentration, are followed by the rapid onset of hypotension and multiple-organ failure. Elevation of the hematocrit to 75–80% and leukocytosis of 50,000–200,000 cells/μL, with a left shift, are characteristic of *C. sordellii* infection. Pain may not be a prominent feature, and fever is typically absent. In one series, 18% of 45 cases of *C. sordellii* infection were associated with normal childbirth, 11% with medically induced abortion, and 0.4% with spontaneous abortion; the case-fatality rate was 100% in these groups. Of the infections in this series that were not related to gynecologic procedures or childbirth, 22% occurred in injection drug users, and 50% of these patients died. Other infections followed trauma or surgery (42%), mostly in healthy persons, and 53% of these patients died. Overall, the mortality rate was 69% (31 of 45 cases). Of patients who succumbed, 85% died within 2–6 days after infection onset or following procedures.

Early diagnosis of *C. sordellii* infections often proves difficult for several reasons. First, the prevalence of these infections is low. Second, the initial symptoms are nonspecific and frankly misleading. Early in the course, the illness resembles any number of infectious diseases, including viral syndromes. Given these vague symptoms and an absence of fever, physicians usually do not aggressively pursue additional diagnostic tests. The absence of local evidence of infection and the lack of fever make early diagnosis of *C. sordellii* infection particularly problematic in patients who develop deep-seated infection following childbirth, therapeutic abortion, gastrointestinal surgery, or trauma. Such patients are frequently evaluated for pulmonary embolization, gastrointestinal bleeding, pyelonephritis, or cholecystitis. Unfortunately, such delays in diagnosis increase the risk of death, and, as in most necrotizing soft-tissue infections, patients are hypotensive with evidence of organ dysfunction by the time local signs and symptoms become apparent. In contrast, infection is more readily suspected in injection drug users presenting with local swelling, pain, and redness at injection sites; early recognition probably contributes to the lower mortality rates in this group.

Physicians should suspect *C. sordellii* infection in patients who present within 2–7 days after injury, surgery, drug injection, childbirth, or abortion and who report pain, nausea, vomiting, and diarrhea but are afebrile. There is little information regarding appropriate treatment for *C. sordellii* infections. In fact, the interval between onset of symptoms and death is often so short that there is little time to initiate empirical antimicrobial therapy. Indeed, anaerobic cultures of blood and wound aspirates are time-consuming, and many hospital laboratories do not routinely perform antimicrobial sensitivity testing on anaerobes. Antibiotic susceptibility data from older studies suggest that *C. sordellii*, like most clostridia, is susceptible to β-lactam antibiotics, clindamycin, tetracycline, and chloramphenicol but is resistant to aminoglycosides and sulfonamides. Antibiotics that suppress toxin synthesis (e.g., clindamycin) may possibly prove useful as therapeutic adjuncts since they are effective in necrotizing infections due to other toxin-producing gram-positive organisms.

Other Clostridial Skin and Soft-Tissue Infections *Crepitant cellulitis* (also called *anaerobic cellulitis*) occurs principally in diabetic patients and characteristically involves subcutaneous tissues or retroperitoneal tissues, whereas the muscle and fascia are not involved. This infection can progress to fulminant systemic disease.

Cases of *C. histolyticum* infection with cellulitis, abscess formation, or endocarditis have also been documented in injection drug users. Endophthalmitis due to *C. sordellii* or *C. perfringens* has been described. *C. ramosum* is also isolated frequently from clinical specimens, including blood and both intraabdominal and soft tissues. This species may be resistant to clindamycin and multiple cephalosporins.

SECTION 6 DISEASES CAUSED BY GRAM-NEGATIVE BACTERIA

180 Meningococcal Infections

Andrew J. Pollard

DEFINITION

Infection with *Neisseria meningitidis* most commonly manifests as asymptomatic colonization in the nasopharynx of healthy adolescents and adults. Invasive disease occurs rarely, usually presenting as either bacterial meningitis or meningococcal septicemia. Patients may also present with occult bacteremia, pneumonia, septic arthritis, conjunctivitis, and chronic meningococcemia.

ETIOLOGY AND MICROBIOLOGY

N. meningitidis is a gram-negative aerobic diplococcus that colonizes humans only and that causes disease after transmission to a susceptible individual. Several related organisms have been recognized, including the pathogen *N. gonorrhoeae* and the commensals *N. lactamica*, *N. flavescens*, *N. mucosa*, *N. sicca*, and *N. subflava*. *N. meningitidis* is a catalase- and oxidase-positive organism that utilizes glucose and maltose to produce acid

Meningococci associated with invasive disease are usually encapsulated with polysaccharide, and the antigenic nature of the capsule determines an organism's serogroup (Table 180-1). In total, 13 serogroups have been identified (A–D, X–Z, 29E, W, H–J, and L), but just 6 serogroups—A, B, C, X, Y, and W (formerly W135)—account for the majority of cases of invasive disease. Acapsular meningococci are commonly isolated from the nasopharynx in studies of carriage; the lack of capsule often is a result of phase variation of capsule expression, but as many as 16% of isolates lack the genes for capsule synthesis and assembly. These "capsule-null" meningococci and those that express capsules other than A, B, C, X, Y, and W are only rarely associated with invasive disease and are most commonly identified in the nasopharynx of asymptomatic carriers.

Beneath the capsule, meningococci are surrounded by an outer phospholipid membrane containing lipopolysaccharide (LPS, endotoxin) and multiple outer-membrane proteins (Figs. 180-1 and 180-2). Antigenic variability in porins expressed in the outer membrane defines the serotype (PorB) and serosubtype (PorA) of the organism, and structural differences in LPS determine the immunotype. Serologic methods for typing of meningococci are restricted by the limited availability of serologic reagents that can distinguish among the organisms' highly variable surface proteins. Where available, high-throughput antigen gene sequencing has superseded serology for meningococcal typing. A large database of antigen gene sequences for the outer-membrane proteins PorA, PorB, FetA, Opa, and factor H–binding protein is available online (*www.neisseria.org*). The number of specialized iron-regulated proteins found in the meningococcal outer membrane (e.g., FetA and transferrin-binding proteins) highlights the organisms' dependence on iron from human sources. A thin peptidoglycan cell wall separates the outer membrane from the cytoplasmic membrane.

The structure of meningococcal populations involved in local and global spread has been studied with multilocus enzyme electrophoresis (MLEE), which characterizes isolates according to differences in the electrophoretic mobility of cytoplasmic enzymes. However, this technique has mostly been replaced by multilocus sequence typing (MLST), in which meningococci are characterized by sequence types assigned on the basis of sequences of internal fragments of seven housekeeping genes. The online MLST database currently includes more than 27,000 meningococcal isolates and 10,500 unique sequence types (*pubmlst.org/neisseria/*). A limited number of hyperinvasive lineages of *N. meningitidis* have been recognized

TABLE 180-1 STRUCTURE OF THE POLYSACCHARIDE CAPSULE OF COMMON DISEASE-CAUSING MENINGOCOCCI

Meningococcal Serogroup	Chemical Structure of Oligosaccharide	Current Disease Epidemiology
A	2-Acetamido-2-deoxy-D-mannopyranosyl phosphate	Epidemic disease mainly in sub-Saharan Africa; sporadic cases worldwide
B	α-2,8-*N*-acetylneuraminic acid	Sporadic cases worldwide; propensity to cause hyperendemic disease
C	α-2,9-*O*-acetylneuraminic acid	Small outbreaks and sporadic disease
Y	4-*O*-α-D-glucopyranosyl-*N*-acetylneuraminic acid	Sporadic disease and occasional small institutional outbreaks
W	4-*O*-α-D-galactopyranosyl-*N*-acetylneuraminic acid	Sporadic disease; outbreaks of disease associated with mass gatherings; epidemics in sub-Saharan Africa
X	(α1→4) N-acetyl-D-glucosamine-1-phosphate	Sporadic disease and large outbreaks in the meningitis belt of Africa

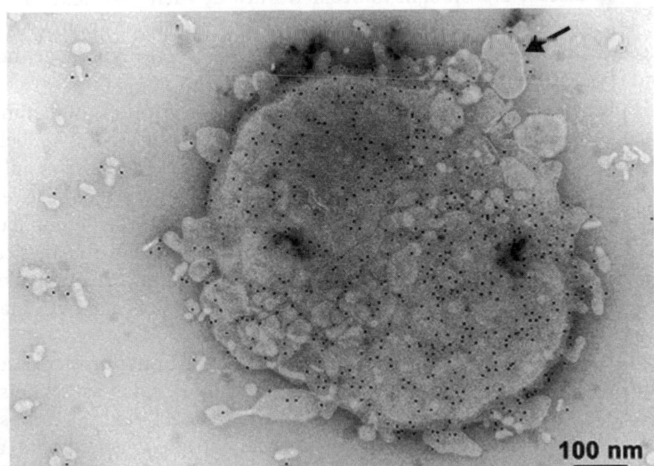

FIGURE 180-1 Electron micrograph of *Neisseria meningitidis*. Black dots are gold-labeled polyclonal antibodies binding surface opacity proteins. Blebs of outer membrane can be seen being released from the bacterial surface (*arrow*). *(Photo courtesy of D. Ferguson, Oxford University.)*

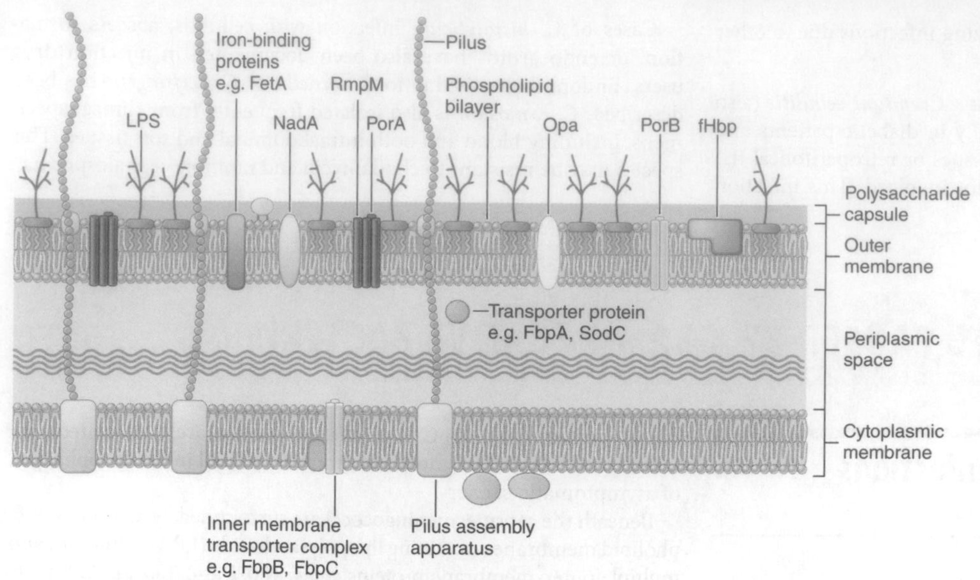

FIGURE 180-2 Cross-section through surface structures of *Neisseria meningitidis*. LPS, lipopolysaccharide. *(Reprinted with permission from M Sadarangani, AJ Pollard: Lancet Infect Dis 10:112, 2010.)*

and are responsible for the majority of cases of invasive meningococcal disease worldwide. The apparent genetic stability of these meningococcal clones over decades and during wide geographic spread indicates that they are well adapted to the nasopharyngeal environment of the host and to efficient transmission. While MLST has become established as the main method of genotyping meningococci in many reference laboratories over the past decade, whole-genome sequencing is set to replace this approach in the decade ahead, with almost 1000 genomes already available in the United Kingdom's national library (*www.meningitis.org/genome-library*).

The group B meningococcal genome is >2 megabases in length and contains 2158 coding regions. Many genes undergo phase variation that makes it possible to control their expression; this capacity is likely to be important in meningococcal adaptation to the host environment and evasion of the immune response. Meningococci can obtain DNA from their environment and can acquire new genes—including the capsular operon—such that *capsule switching* from one serogroup to another can occur.

EPIDEMIOLOGY

Patterns of Disease Up to 500,000 cases of meningococcal disease are thought to occur worldwide each year, and ~10% of the individuals affected die. There are several patterns of disease: epidemic, outbreak (small clusters of cases), hyperendemic, and sporadic or endemic.

Epidemics have continued since the original descriptions of meningococcal disease, especially affecting the sub-Saharan meningitis belt of Africa, where tens to hundreds of thousands of cases (caused mainly by serogroup A but also by serogroups W and X) may be reported over a season and rates may be as high as 1000 cases per 100,000 population. Serogroup A epidemics took place in Europe and North America after the First and Second World Wars, and serogroup A outbreaks have been documented over the past 30 years in New Zealand, China, Nepal, Mongolia, India, Pakistan, Poland, and Russia.

Clusters of cases occur where there is an opportunity for increased transmission—i.e., in (semi-)closed communities such as schools, colleges, universities, military training centers, and refugee camps. Recently, such clusters have been especially strongly linked with a particular clone (sequence type 11) that is mainly associated with the serogroup C or W capsule but was first described in association with serogroup B. Wider and more prolonged community outbreaks (hyperendemic disease) due to single clones of serogroup B meningococci account for ≥10 cases per 100,000. Regions affected in the past decade include the U.S. Pacific Northwest, New Zealand (both islands), and the province of Normandy in France.

Most countries now experience predominantly sporadic cases (0.3–5 cases per 100,000 population), with many different disease-causing clones involved and usually no clear epidemiologic link between one case and another. The disease rate and the distribution of meningococcal strains vary in different regions of the world and also in any one location over time. For example, in the United States, the rate of meningococcal disease fell from 1.2 cases per 100,000 population in 1997 to <0.15 case per 100,000 in 2012 (Fig. 180-3). Meningococcal disease in the United States was previously dominated by serogroups B and C; however, serogroup Y emerged during the 1990s and became more common than serogroup C in 2007. In contrast, rates of disease in England and Wales rose to >5 cases per 100,000 during the 1990s because of an increase in cases caused by the ST11 serogroup C clone. As a result of a mass immunization program against serogroup C in 1999, almost all cases in the United Kingdom are now attributed to serogroup B (Fig. 180-4). Over the last decade, most industrialized nations have seen a general decrease in meningococcal disease; this decrease is linked to immunization against serogroup C meningococci in Europe, Canada, and Australia and to adolescent immunization programs for A, C, Y and W in the United States. However, other factors, including changes in population immunity (probably the explanation for the cyclic nature of meningococcal disease rates) as well as a reduction in smoking and passive exposure to tobacco smoke (driven by bans on smoking in buildings and public spaces) across wealthy countries are likely to have contributed to the fall in cases.

Factors Associated with Disease Risk and Susceptibility The principal determinant of disease susceptibility is age, with the peak incidence in the first year of life (Fig. 180-5). The susceptibility of the very young presumably results from an absence of specific adaptive immunity in combination with very close contact with colonized individuals, including parents. Compared with other age groups, infants appear to be particularly susceptible to serogroup B disease: >30% of serogroup B cases in the United States occur during the first year of life. In the early

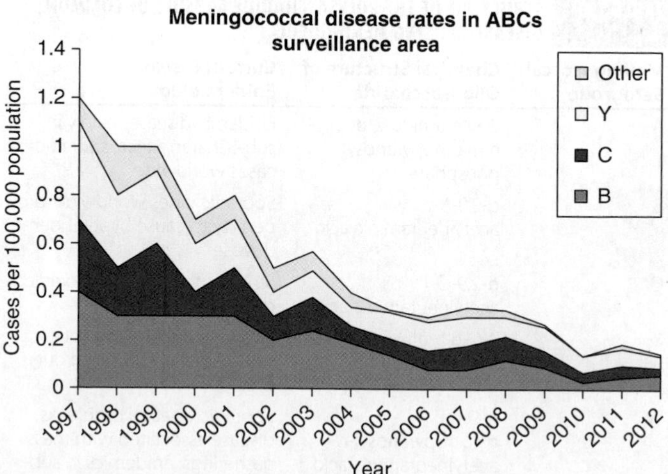

FIGURE 180-3 Meningococcal disease in the United States over time. ABCs, active bacterial cores. *(Adapted from ABC Surveillance data, Centers for Disease Control and Prevention; www.cdc.gov.)*

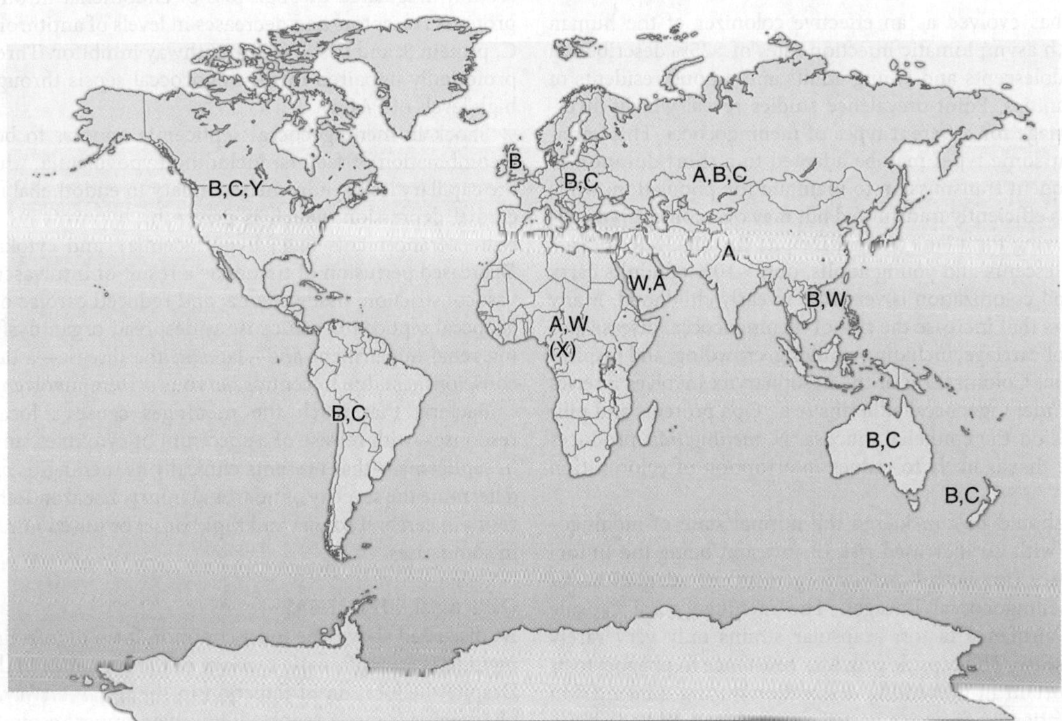

FIGURE 180-4 Global distribution of meningococcal serogroups, 1999–2009.

1990s in North America, the median ages for patients with disease due to serogroups B, C, Y, and W were 6, 17, 24, and 33 years, respectively.

After early childhood, a second peak of disease occurs among adolescents and young adults (15–25 years of age) in Europe and North America. It is thought that this peak relates to social behaviors and environmental exposures in this age group, as discussed below. Most cases of infection with *N. meningitidis* in developed countries today are sporadic, and the rarity of the disease suggests that individual susceptibility may be important. A number of factors probably contribute to individual susceptibility, including the host's genetic constitution, environment, and contact with a carrier or a case.

The best-documented genetic association with meningococcal disease is complement deficiency, chiefly of the terminal complement components (C5–9), properdin, or factor D; such a deficiency increases the risk of disease by up to 600-fold and may result in recurrent attacks. Complement components are believed to be important for the bactericidal activity of serum, which is considered the principal mechanism of immunity against invasive meningococcal disease. However, when investigated, complement deficiency is found in only a very small proportion of individuals with meningococcal disease (0.3%). Conversely, 7–20% of persons whose disease is caused by the less common serogroups (W, X, Y, Z, 29E) have a complement deficiency. Complement deficiency appears to be associated with serogroup B disease only rarely. Individuals with recurrences of meningococcal disease, particularly those caused by non-B serogroups, should be assessed for complement deficiency by measurement of total hemolytic complement activity. There is also limited evidence that hyposplenism (through reduction in phagocytic capacity) and hypogammaglobulinemia (through absence of specific antibody) increase the risk of meningococcal disease. Genetic studies have revealed various associations with disease susceptibility, including complement and mannose-binding lectin deficiency, single-nucleotide polymorphisms in Toll-like receptor (TLR) 4 and complement factor H, and variants of Fc gamma receptors.

Factors that increase the chance of a susceptible individual's acquiring *N. meningitidis* via the respiratory route also increase the risk of meningococcal disease. Acquisition occurs through close contact with carriers as a result of overcrowding (e.g., in poor socioeconomic settings, in refugee camps, during the Hajj pilgrimage to Mecca, and during freshman-year residence in college dormitories) and certain social behaviors (e.g., attendance at bars and nightclubs, kissing). Secondary cases may occur in close contacts of an index case (e.g., household members and persons kissing the infected individual); the risk to these contacts may be as high as 1000 times the background rate in the population. Factors that damage the nasopharyngeal epithelium also increase the risk of both colonization with *N. meningitidis* and invasive disease. The most important of these factors are cigarette smoking (odds ratio, 4.1) and passive exposure to cigarette smoke. In addition, recent viral respiratory tract infection, infection with *Mycoplasma* species, and winter or the dry season have been associated with meningococcal disease; all of these factors presumably either increase the expression of adhesion molecules in the nasopharynx, thus enhancing meningococcal adhesion, or facilitate meningococcal invasion of the bloodstream.

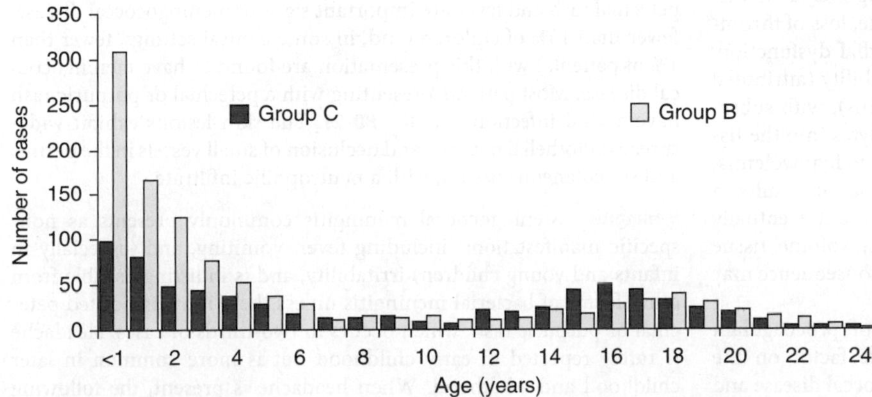

FIGURE 180-5 Age distribution of serogroups B and C meningococcal disease in England and Wales, 1998–1999. *(Health Protection Agency, UK; www.hpa.org.uk.)*

PATHOGENESIS

N. meningitidis has evolved as an effective colonizer of the human nasopharynx, with asymptomatic infection rates of >25% described in some series of adolescents and young adults and among residents of crowded communities. Point-prevalence studies reveal widely divergent rates of carriage for different types of meningococci. This variation suggests that some types may be adapted to a short duration of carriage with frequent transmission to maintain the population, while others may be less efficiently transmitted but may overcome this disadvantage by colonizing for a long period. Despite the high rates of carriage among adolescents and young adults, only ~10% of adults carry meningococci, and colonization is very rare in early childhood. Many of the same factors that increase the risk of meningococcal disease also increase the risk of carriage, including smoking, crowding, and respiratory viral infection. Colonization of the nasopharynx involves a series of interactions of meningococcal adhesins (e.g., Opa proteins and pili) with their ligands on the epithelial mucosa. *N. meningitidis* produces an IgA1 protease that is likely to reduce interruption of colonization by mucosal IgA.

Colonization should be considered the normal state of meningococcal infection, with an increased risk of invasion being the unfortunate consequence (for both host and organism) of adaptations of hyperinvasive meningococcal lineages. The meningococcal capsule is an important virulence factor: acapsular strains only very rarely cause invasive disease. The capsule provides resistance to phagocytosis and may be important in preventing desiccation during transmission between hosts. Antigenic diversity in surface structures and an ability to vary levels of their expression have probably evolved as important factors in maintaining meningococcal populations within and between individual hosts.

Invasion through the mucosa into the blood occurs rarely, usually within a few days of acquisition of an invasive strain by a susceptible individual. Only occasional cases of prolonged colonization prior to invasion have been documented. Once the organism is in the bloodstream, its growth may be limited if the individual is partially immune, although bacteremia may allow seeding of another site, such as the meninges or the joints. Alternatively, unchecked proliferation may continue, resulting in high bacterial counts in the circulation. During growth, meningococci release blebs of outer membrane (Fig. 180-1) containing outer-membrane proteins and LPS. Endotoxin binds cell-bound CD14 in association with TLR4 to initiate an inflammatory cascade with the release of high levels of various mediators, including tumor necrosis factor (TNF) α, soluble TNF receptor, interleukin (IL) 1, IL-1 receptor antagonist, IL-1β, IL-6, IL-8, IL-10, plasminogen-activator inhibitor 1 (PAI-1), and leukemia inhibitory factor. Soluble CD14-bound endotoxin acts as a mediator of endothelial activation. The severity of meningococcal disease is related both to the levels of endotoxin in the blood and to the magnitude of the inflammatory response. The latter is determined to some extent by polymorphisms in the inflammatory response genes (and their inhibitors), and the release of the inflammatory cascade heralds the development of meningococcal septicemia (meningococcemia). Endothelial injury is central to many clinical features of meningococcemia, including increased vascular permeability, pathologic changes in vascular tone, loss of thromboresistance, intravascular coagulation, and myocardial dysfunction. Endothelial injury leads to increased vascular permeability (attributed to loss of glycosaminoglycans and endothelial proteins), with subsequent gross proteinuria. Leakage of fluid and electrolytes into the tissues from capillaries ("capillary leak syndrome") leads to hypovolemia, tissue edema, and pulmonary edema. Initial compensation results in vasoconstriction and tachycardia, although cardiac output eventually falls. While resuscitation fluids may restore circulating volume, tissue edema will continue to increase, and, in the lung, the consequence may be respiratory failure.

Intravascular thrombosis (caused by activation of procoagulant pathways in association with upregulation of tissue factor on the endothelium) occurs in some patients with meningococcal disease and results in purpura fulminans and infarction of areas of skin or even of whole limbs. At the same time, multiple anticoagulant pathways are downregulated through loss of endothelial thrombomodulin and protein C receptors and decreases in levels of antithrombin III, protein C, protein S, and tissue factor pathway inhibitor. Thrombolysis is also profoundly impaired in meningococcal sepsis through the release of high levels of PAI-1.

Shock in meningococcal septicemia appears to be attributable to a combination of factors, including hypovolemia, which results from the capillary leak syndrome secondary to endothelial injury, and myocardial depression, which is driven by hypovolemia, hypoxia, metabolic derangements (e.g., hypocalcemia), and cytokines (e.g., IL-6). Decreased perfusion of tissues as a result of intravascular thrombosis, vasoconstriction, tissue edema, and reduced cardiac output in meningococcal septicemia can cause widespread organ dysfunction, including renal impairment and—later in the disease—a decreased level of consciousness due to central nervous system involvement.

Bacteria that reach the meninges cause a local inflammatory response—with release of a spectrum of cytokines similar to that seen in septicemia—that presents clinically as meningitis and is thought to determine the severity of neuronal injury. Local endothelial injury may result in cerebral edema and rapid onset of raised intracranial pressure in some cases.

CLINICAL MANIFESTATIONS

As discussed above, the most common form of infection with *N. meningitidis* is asymptomatic carriage of the organism in the nasopharynx. Despite the location of infection in the upper airway, meningococcal pharyngitis is rarely reported; however, upper respiratory tract symptoms are common prior to presentation with invasive disease. It is not clear whether these symptoms relate to preceding viral infection (which may promote meningococcal acquisition) or to meningococcal acquisition itself. After acquiring the organism, susceptible individuals develop disease manifestations in 1–10 days (usually <4 days, although colonization for 11 weeks has been documented).

Along the spectrum of presentations of meningococcal disease, the most common clinical syndromes are meningitis and meningococcal septicemia. In fulminant cases, death may occur within hours of the first symptoms. Occult bacteremia is also recognized and, if untreated, progresses in two-thirds of cases to focal infection, including meningitis or septicemia. Meningococcal disease may also present as pneumonia, pyogenic arthritis or osteomyelitis, purulent pericarditis, endophthalmitis, conjunctivitis, primary peritonitis, or (rarely) urethritis. Perhaps because it is difficult to diagnose, pneumococcal pneumonia is not commonly reported but is associated with serogroups Y, W, and Z and appears most often to affect individuals >10 years of age.

Rash A nonblanching rash (petechial or purpuric) develops in >80% of cases of meningococcal disease; however, the rash is often absent early in the illness. Usually initially blanching in nature (macules, maculopapules, or urticaria) and indistinguishable from more common viral rashes, the rash of meningococcal infection becomes petechial or frankly purpuric over the hours after onset. In the most severe cases, large purpuric lesions develop (purpura fulminans). Some patients (including those with overwhelming sepsis) may have no rash. While petechial rash and fever are important signs of meningococcal disease, fewer than 10% of children (and, in some clinical settings, fewer than 1% of patients) with this presentation are found to have meningococcal disease. Most patients presenting with a petechial or purpuric rash have a viral infection (Table 180-2). The skin lesions exhibit widespread endothelial necrosis and occlusion of small vessels in the dermis and subcutaneous tissues, with a neutrophilic infiltrate.

Meningitis Meningococcal meningitis commonly presents as nonspecific manifestations, including fever, vomiting, and (especially in infants and young children) irritability, and is indistinguishable from other forms of bacterial meningitis unless there is an associated petechial or purpuric rash, which occurs in two-thirds of cases. Headache is rarely reported in early childhood but is more common in later childhood and adulthood. When headache is present, the following features, in association with fever or a history of fever, are suggestive of bacterial meningitis: neck stiffness, photophobia, decreased

TABLE 180-2 COMMON CAUSES OF PETECHIAL OR PURPURIC RASHES
Enteroviruses
Influenza and other respiratory viruses
Measles virus
Epstein-Barr virus
Cytomegalovirus
Parvovirus
Deficiency of protein C or S (including postvaricella protein S deficiency)
Platelet disorders (e.g., idiopathic thrombocytopenic purpura, drug effects, bone marrow infiltration)
Henoch-Schönlein purpura, connective tissue disorders, trauma (including nonaccidental injuries in children)
Pneumococcal, streptococcal, staphylococcal, or gram-negative bacterial sepsis

level of consciousness, seizures or status epilepticus, and focal neurologic signs. Classic signs of meningitis, such as neck stiffness and photophobia, are often absent in infants and young children with bacterial meningitis, who more usually present with fever and irritability and may have a bulging fontanelle.

While 30–50% of patients present with a meningitis syndrome alone, up to 40% of meningitis patients also present with some features of septicemia. Most deaths from meningococcal meningitis alone (i.e., without septicemia) are associated with raised intracranial pressure presenting as a reduced level of consciousness, relative bradycardia and hypertension, focal neurologic signs, abnormal posturing, and signs of brainstem involvement—e.g., unequal, dilated, or poorly reactive pupils; abnormal eye movement; and impaired corneal responses (Chap. 328).

Septicemia Meningococcal septicemia alone accounts for up to 20% of cases of meningococcal disease. The condition may progress from early nonspecific symptoms to death within hours. Mortality rates among children with this syndrome have been high (25–40%), but early aggressive management (as discussed below) may reduce the figure to <10%. Early symptoms are nonspecific and suggest an influenza-like illness with fever, headache, and myalgia accompanied by vomiting and abdominal pain. As discussed above, the rash, if present, may appear to be viral early in the course until petechiae or purpuric lesions develop. Purpura fulminans occurs in severe cases, with multiple large purpuric lesions and signs of peripheral ischemia. Surveys of patients have indicated that limb pain, pallor (including a mottled appearance and cyanosis), and cold hands and feet may be prominent. Shock is manifested by tachycardia, poor peripheral perfusion, tachypnea, and oliguria. Decreased cerebral perfusion leads to confusion, agitation, or decreased level of consciousness. With progressive shock, multiorgan failure ensues; hypotension is a late sign in children, who more commonly present with compensated shock (tachycardia, poor peripheral perfusion, and normal blood pressure). Poor outcome is associated with an absence of meningism, hypotension, young age, coma, relatively low temperature (<38°C), leukopenia, and thrombocytopenia. Spontaneous hemorrhage (pulmonary, gastric, or cerebral) may result from consumption of coagulation factors and thrombocytopenia.

Chronic Meningococcemia Chronic meningococcemia, which is rarely recognized, presents as repeated episodes of petechial rash associated with fever, joint pain, features of arthritis, and splenomegaly that may progress to acute meningococcal septicemia if untreated. During the relapsing course, bacteremia characteristically clears without treatment and then recurs. The differential diagnosis includes bacterial endocarditis, acute rheumatic fever, Henoch-Schönlein purpura, infectious mononucleosis, disseminated gonococcal infection, and immune-mediated vasculitis. This condition has been associated with complement deficiencies in some cases and with inadequate sulfonamide therapy in others.

A study from the Netherlands found that half of isolates from patients with chronic meningococcemia had an underacylated lipid A (part of the surface LPS molecule) due to an lpxL1 gene mutation, which markedly reduces the inflammatory response to endotoxin.

Postmeningococcal Reactive Disease In a small proportion of patients, an immune complex disease develops ~4–10 days after the onset of meningococcal disease, with manifestations that include a maculopapular or vasculitic rash (2% of cases), arthritis (up to 8% of cases), iritis (1%), pericarditis, and/or polyserositis associated with fever. The immune complexes involve meningococcal polysaccharide antigen and result in immunoglobulin and complement deposition with an inflammatory infiltrate. These features resolve spontaneously without sequelae. It is important to recognize this condition since a new onset of fever and rash can lead to concerns about relapse of meningococcal disease and unnecessarily prolonged antibiotic treatment.

DIAGNOSIS

Like other invasive bacterial infections, meningococcal disease may produce elevations of the white blood cell (WBC) count and of values for inflammatory markers (e.g., C-reactive protein and procalcitonin levels or the erythrocyte sedimentation rate). Values may be normal or low in rapidly progressive disease, and a lack of rise in these laboratory test values does not exclude the diagnosis. However, in the presence of fever and a petechial rash, these elevations are suggestive of meningococcal disease. In patients with severe meningococcal septicemia, common laboratory findings include hypoglycemia, acidosis, hypokalemia, hypocalcemia, hypomagnesemia, hypophosphatemia, anemia, and coagulopathy.

Although meningococcal disease is often diagnosed on clinical grounds, in suspected meningococcal meningitis or meningococcemia, blood should routinely be sent for culture to confirm the diagnosis and to facilitate public health investigations; blood cultures are positive in up to 75% of cases. Culture media containing sodium polyanethol sulfonate, which may inhibit meningococcal growth, should be avoided. Meningococcal viability is reduced if there is a delay in transport of the specimen to the microbiology laboratory for culture or in plating of cerebrospinal fluid (CSF) samples. In countries where treatment with antibiotics before hospitalization is recommended for meningococcal disease, the majority of clinically suspected cases are culture negative. Real-time polymerase chain reaction (PCR) analysis of whole-blood samples increases the diagnostic yield by >40%, and results obtained with this method may remain positive for several days after administration of antibiotics. Indeed, in the United Kingdom, more than half of clinically suspected cases are currently identified by PCR.

Unless contraindications exist (raised intracranial pressure, uncorrected shock, disordered coagulation, thrombocytopenia, respiratory insufficiency, local infection, ongoing convulsions), lumbar puncture should be undertaken to identify and confirm the etiology of suspected meningococcal meningitis, whose presentation cannot be distinguished from that of meningitis of other bacterial causes. Some authorities have recommended a CT brain scan prior to lumbar puncture because of the risk of cerebral herniation in patients with raised intracranial pressure. However, a normal CT scan is not uncommon in the presence of raised intracranial pressure in meningococcal meningitis, and the decision to perform a lumbar puncture should be made on clinical grounds. CSF features of meningococcal meningitis (elevated protein level and WBC count, decreased glucose level) are indistinguishable from those of other types of bacterial meningitis unless a gram-negative diplococcus is identified. (Gram's staining is up to 80% sensitive for meningococcal meningitis.) CSF should be submitted for culture (sensitivity, 90%) and (where available) PCR analysis. CSF antigen testing with latex agglutination is insensitive and should be replaced by molecular diagnosis when possible.

Lumbar puncture should generally be avoided in meningococcal septicemia, as positioning for the procedure may critically compromise the patient's circulation in the context of hypovolemic shock. Delayed lumbar puncture may still be useful when the diagnosis is uncertain, particularly if molecular diagnostic technology is available.

In other types of focal infection, culture and PCR analysis of normally sterile body fluids (e.g., synovial fluid) may aid in the diagnosis. Although some authorities have recommended cultures of scrapings or aspirates from skin lesions, this procedure adds little to the diagnostic yield when compared with a combination of blood culture and PCR analysis. Urinary antigen testing also is insensitive, and serologic testing for meningococcal infection has not been adequately studied. Because *N. meningitidis* is a component of the normal human nasopharyngeal flora, identification of the organism on throat swabs has no diagnostic value.

TREATMENT MENINGOCOCCAL INFECTIONS

Death from meningococcal disease is associated most commonly with hypovolemic shock (meningococcemia) and occasionally with raised intracranial pressure (meningococcal meningitis). Therefore, management should focus on the treatment of these urgent clinical issues in addition to the administration of specific antibiotic therapy. Delayed recognition of meningococcal disease or its associated physiologic derangements, together with inadequate emergency management, is associated with poor outcome. Since the disease is rare, protocols for emergency management have been developed (see *www.meningitis.org*).

Airway patency may be compromised if the level of consciousness is depressed as a result of shock (impaired cerebral perfusion) or raised intracranial pressure; this situation may require intervention. In meningococcemia, pulmonary edema and pulmonary oligemia (presenting as hypoxia) require oxygen therapy or elective endotracheal intubation. In cases with shock, aggressive fluid resuscitation (with replacement of the circulating volume several times in severe cases) and inotropic support may be necessary to maintain cardiac output. If shock persists after volume resuscitation at 40 mL/kg, the risk of pulmonary edema is high, and elective intubation is recommended to improve oxygenation and decrease the work of breathing. Metabolic derangements, including hypoglycemia, acidosis, hypokalemia, hypocalcemia, hypomagnesemia, hypophosphatemia, anemia, and coagulopathy, should be anticipated and corrected. In the presence of raised intracranial pressure, management includes correction of coexistent shock and neurointensive care to maintain cerebral perfusion.

Empirical antibiotic therapy for suspected meningococcal disease consists of a third-generation cephalosporin such as ceftriaxone (75–100 mg/kg per day [maximum, 4 g/d] in one or two divided IV doses) or cefotaxime (200 mg/kg per day [maximum, 8 g/d] in four divided IV doses) to cover the various other (potentially penicillin-resistant) bacteria that may produce an indistinguishable clinical syndrome. Although unusual in most isolates, reduced meningococcal sensitivity to penicillin (a minimal inhibitory concentration of 0.12–1.0 μg/mL) has been reported widely.

Both meningococcal meningitis and meningococcal septicemia are conventionally treated for 7 days, although courses of 3–5 days may be equally effective. Furthermore, a single dose of ceftriaxone or an oily suspension of chloramphenicol has been used successfully in resource-poor settings. No data are available to guide the duration of treatment for meningococcal infection at other foci (e.g., pneumonia, arthritis); antimicrobial therapy is usually continued until clinical and laboratory evidence of infection has resolved. Cultures usually become sterile within 24 h of initiation of appropriate antibiotic chemotherapy.

The use of glucocorticoids for adjunctive treatment of meningococcal meningitis remains controversial since no relevant studies have had sufficient power to determine true efficacy. One large study in adults did indicate a trend toward benefit, and in clinical practice a decision to use glucocorticoids usually must precede a definite microbiologic diagnosis. Therapeutic doses of glucocorticoids are not recommended in meningococcal septicemia, but many intensivists recommend replacement glucocorticoid doses for patients who have refractory shock in association with impaired adrenal gland responsiveness.

Various other adjunctive therapies for meningococcal disease have been considered, but few have been subjected to clinical trials and none can currently be recommended. An antibody to LPS (HA1A) failed to confer a demonstrable benefit. Recombinant bactericidal/permeability-increasing protein (which is not currently available) was tested in a study that had inadequate power to show an effect on mortality rates; however, there were trends toward lower mortality rates among patients who received a complete infusion, and this group also had fewer amputations, fewer blood-product transfusions, and a significantly improved functional outcome. Given that protein C concentrations are reduced in meningococcal disease, the use of activated protein C has been considered since a survival benefit was demonstrated in adult sepsis trials; however, trials in pediatric sepsis (of particular relevance for meningococcal disease) found no benefit and indicated a potential risk of bleeding complications with use of activated protein C.

The postmeningococcal immune-complex inflammatory syndrome has been treated with nonsteroidal anti-inflammatory agents until spontaneous resolution occurs.

COMPLICATIONS

About 10% of patients with meningococcal disease die despite the availability of antimicrobial therapy and other intensive medical interventions. The most common complication of meningococcal disease (10% of cases) is scarring after necrosis of purpuric skin lesions, for which skin grafting may be necessary. The lower limbs are most often affected; next in frequency are the upper limbs, the trunk, and the face. On average, 13% of the skin surface area is involved. Amputations are necessary in 1–2% of survivors of meningococcal disease because of a loss of tissue viability after peripheral ischemia or compartment syndromes. Unless there is local infection, amputation should usually be delayed to allow the demarcation between viable and nonviable tissue to become apparent. Approximately 5% of patients with meningococcal disease suffer hearing loss, and 7% have neurologic complications. In one study pain was reported by 21% of survivors, and in a recent analysis of serogroup B meningococcal disease (the MOSAIC study) as many as one-quarter of survivors had psychological disorders. In some investigations, the rate of complications is higher for serogroup C disease (mostly associated with the ST11 clone) than for serogroup B disease. In patients with severe hypovolemic shock, renal perfusion may be impaired and prerenal failure is common, but permanent renal replacement therapy is rarely needed.

Several studies suggest adverse psychosocial outcomes after meningococcal disease, with reduced quality of life, lowered self-esteem, and poorer neurologic development, including increased rates of attention deficit/hyperactivity disorder and special educational needs. Other studies have not found evidence of such outcomes.

PROGNOSIS

Several prognostic scoring systems have been developed to identify patients with meningococcal disease who are least likely to survive. Factors associated with a poorer prognosis are shock; young age (infancy), old age, and adolescence; coma; purpura fulminans; disseminated intravascular coagulation; thrombocytopenia; leukopenia; absence of meningitis; metabolic acidosis; low plasma concentrations of antithrombin and proteins S and C; high blood levels of PAI-1; and a low erythrocyte sedimentation rate or C-reactive protein level. The Glasgow Meningococcal Septicaemia Prognostic Score (GMSPS) is probably the best-performing scoring system studied so far and may be clinically useful for severity assessment in meningococcal disease. However, scoring systems do not direct the clinician to specific interventions, and the priority in management should be recognition of compromised airways, breathing, or circulation and direct, urgent intervention. Most patients improve rapidly with appropriate antibiotics and supportive therapy. Fulminant meningococcemia is more likely to result in death or ischemic skin loss than is meningitis; optimal emergency management may reduce mortality rates among the most severely affected patients.

PREVENTION

Since mortality rates in meningococcal disease remain high despite improvements in intensive care management, immunization is the only rational approach to prevention at a population level. Secondary cases are common among household and "kissing" contacts of cases, and secondary prophylaxis with antibiotic therapy is widely recommended for these contacts (see below).

Polysaccharide Vaccines Purified meningococcal capsular polysaccharide has been used for immunization since the 1960s. Meningococcal polysaccharide vaccines are currently formulated as either bivalent (serogroups A and C) or quadrivalent (serogroups A, C, Y, and W), with 50 μg of each polysaccharide per dose. Local reactions (erythema, induration, and tenderness) may occur in up to 40% of vaccinees, but serious adverse events (including febrile convulsions in young children) are very rarely reported. In adults, the vaccines are immunogenic, but immunity appears to be relatively short-lived (with antibody levels above baseline for only 2–10 years), and booster doses do not induce a further rise in antibody concentration. Indeed, a state of immunologic hyporesponsiveness has been widely reported to follow booster doses of plain polysaccharide vaccines. The repeating units of these vaccines cross-link B cell receptors to drive specific memory B cells to become plasma cells and produce antibody. Because meningococcal polysaccharides are T cell–independent antigens, no memory B cells are produced after immunization, and the memory B-cell pool is depleted such that fewer polysaccharide-specific cells are available to respond to a subsequent dose of vaccine (Fig. 180-6). The clinical relevance of hyporesponsiveness is unknown. Plain polysaccharide vaccines generally are not immunogenic in early childhood, possibly because marginal-zone B cells are involved in polysaccharide responses and maturation of the splenic marginal zone is not complete until 18 months to 2 years of age. The efficacy of the meningococcal serogroup C component is >90% in young adults; no efficacy data are available for the serogroup Y and W polysaccharides in this age group.

Group A meningococcal polysaccharides are exceptional in that they have been found to be effective in preventing disease at all ages. Two doses administered 2–3 months apart to children 3–18 months of age or a single dose administered to older children or adults has a protective efficacy rate of >95%. The vaccine has been widely used in the control of meningococcal disease in the African meningitis belt. The duration of protection appears to be only 3–5 years.

There is no meningococcal serogroup B plain polysaccharide vaccine because α-2,8-*N*-acetylneuraminic acid is expressed on the surface of neural cells in the fetus such that the B polysaccharide is perceived as "self" and therefore is not immunogenic in humans.

Conjugate Vaccines The poor immunogenicity of plain polysaccharide vaccines in infancy has been overcome by chemical conjugation of the polysaccharides to a carrier protein (CRM_{197}, tetanus toxoid, or diphtheria toxoid). Conjugates that contain monovalent serogroup C polysaccharide and quadrivalent vaccines with A, C, Y, and W polysaccharides have been developed, as have vaccines including various other antigen combinations (e.g., tetanus conjugates with serogroup C

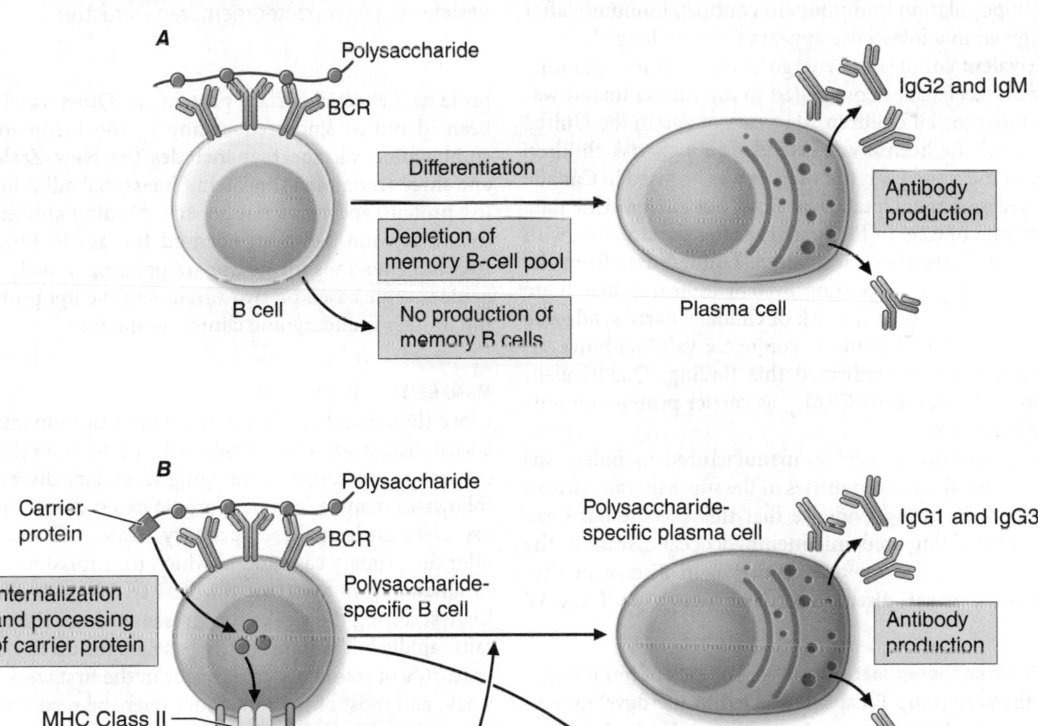

FIGURE 180-6 ***A.*** Polysaccharides from the encapsulated bacteria that cause disease in early childhood stimulate B cells by cross-linking the BCR and driving the production of immunoglobulins. There is no production of memory B cells, and the B-cell pool may be depleted by this process such that subsequent immune responses are decreased. ***B.*** The carrier protein from protein-polysaccharide conjugate vaccines is processed by the polysaccharide-specific B cell, and peptides are presented to carrier peptide–specific T cells, with the consequent production of both plasma cells and memory B cells. BCR, B-cell receptor; MHC, major histocompatibility complex; TCR, T-cell receptor. *(Reprinted from AJ Pollard et al: Nat Rev Immunol 9:213, 2009.)*

and/or Y polysaccharide with *Haemophilus influenzae* type b polysaccharide). After immunization, peptides from the carrier protein are conventionally thought to be presented to peptide-specific T cells in association with major histocompatibility complex (MHC) class II molecules (some recent data suggesting that carrier protein peptide may actually be presented in association with an oligosaccharide and MHCII) by polysaccharide-specific B cells; the result is a T cell–dependent immune response that allows production of antibody and generation of an expanded B-cell memory pool. Unlike responses to booster doses of plain polysaccharides, responses to booster doses of conjugate vaccines have the characteristics of memory responses. Indeed, conjugate vaccines overcome the hyporesponsiveness induced by plain polysaccharides by replenishing the memory pool. The reactogenicity of conjugate vaccines is similar to that of plain polysaccharide vaccines.

The first widespread use of serogroup C meningococcal conjugate vaccine (MenC) came in 1999 in the United Kingdom after a rise in serogroup C disease. A mass vaccination campaign involving all individuals <19 years of age was undertaken, and the number of laboratory-confirmed serogroup C cases fell from 955 in 1998–1999 to just 29 in 2011–2012. The effectiveness of the immunization program was attributed both to direct protection of immunized persons and to reduced transmission of the organism in the population as a result of decreased rates of colonization among the immunized (herd immunity). Data on immunogenicity and effectiveness have shown that the duration of protection is short when the vaccine is administered in early childhood; thus booster doses are needed to maintain population immunity. In contrast, immunity after a dose of vaccine given in adolescence appears to be prolonged.

The first quadrivalent conjugate meningococcal vaccine containing A, C, Y, and W polysaccharides conjugated to diphtheria toxoid was initially recommended for all children >11 years of age in the United States in 2005. In 2007 the license was extended to high-risk children 2–10 years of age. In the same year, the vaccine was licensed in Canada for persons 2–55 years of age. Uptake was slow, but current U.S. data suggest an efficacy rate of 82% in the first year after vaccination, with waning to 59% at 3–6 years after vaccination. Limited data from the U.S. Vaccine Adverse Events Reporting System indicated that there might be a short-term increase in the risk of Guillain-Barré syndrome after immunization with the diphtheria conjugate vaccine; however, further investigation has not confirmed this finding. Quadrivalent conjugate vaccines with tetanus or CRM_{197} as carrier protein are now available in many countries.

A monovalent serogroup A vaccine, manufactured in India, was licensed in 2010 and rolled out to countries in the sub-Saharan African meningitis belt. There is strong evidence that this vaccine has been highly effective in controlling epidemic meningococcal disease in the region, with some evidence of a >90% reduction in disease in vaccinated populations. However, disease caused by serogroup X and W persists.

Vaccines Based on Subcapsular Antigens The lack of immunogenicity of the serogroup B capsule has led to the development of vaccines based on subcapsular antigens. Various surface components have been studied in early-phase clinical trials. Outer-membrane vesicles (OMVs) containing outer-membrane proteins, phospholipid, and LPS can be extracted from cultures of *N. meningitidis* by detergent treatment (Fig. 180-7). OMVs prepared in this way were used in efficacy trials with a Norwegian outbreak strain and reduced the incidence of group B disease among 14- to 16-year-old schoolchildren by 53%. Similarly, OMV vaccines constructed from local outbreak strains in Cuba and New Zealand have had reported efficacy rates of >70%. These OMV vaccines appear to produce strain-specific immune responses, with only limited cross-protection, and are therefore best suited to clonal outbreaks (e.g., those in Cuba and New Zealand as well as others in Norway and the province of Normandy in France).

Several purified surface proteins have been evaluated in phase 1 clinical trials but have not yet been developed further because of antigenic variability or poor immunogenicity (e.g., transferrin-binding

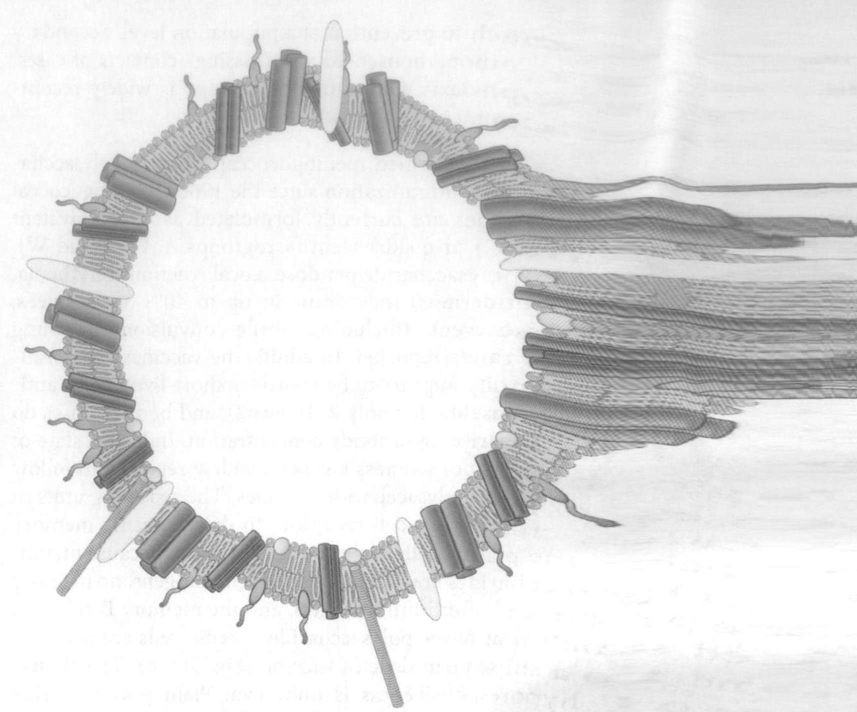

FIGURE 180-7 Illustration of meningococcal outer-membrane vesicle containing outer-membrane structures.

proteins, neisserial surface protein A). Other vaccine candidates [illegible] been identified since sequencing of the meningococcal geno[illegible] combination vaccine that includes the New Zealand OMV va[illegible] and three recombinant proteins (neisserial adhesin A, factor H [illegible] ing protein, and neisserial heparin-binding antigen) is immun[illegible] in infancy and has been licensed for use in Europe and Au[illegible] Recommendations for its use are pending. Finally, a highly im[illegible] genic vaccine based on two variants of the lipoprotein factor H [illegible] ing protein is undergoing clinical evaluation

MANAGEMENT OF CONTACTS

Close (household and kissing) contacts of individuals with me[illegible] coccal disease are at increased risk (up to 1000 times the rate [illegible] general population) of developing secondary disease; a second[illegible] follows as many as 3% of sporadic cases. About one-fifth of [illegible] ary cases are actually co-primary cases—i.e., cases that [illegible] after the primary case and in which transmission is presumed [illegible] originated from the same third party. The rate of secondary [illegible] highest during the week after presentation of the index case [illegible] falls rapidly but remains above baseline for up to 1 year after [illegible] case; 30% of secondary cases occur in the first week, 20% in t[illegible] week, and most of the remainder over the next 6 weeks. In [illegible] of meningococcal disease, mass prophylaxis has been use[illegible] limited data support population intervention, and signifi[illegible] have arisen about adverse events and the development o[illegible] For these reasons, prophylaxis is usually restricted to (1 [illegible] greatest risk who are intimate and/or household contacts [illegible] case and (2) health care workers who have been direct[illegible] respiratory secretions. In most cases, members of wider [illegible] (e.g., at schools or colleges) are not offered prophylaxis[illegible]

The aim of prophylaxis is to eradicate colon[illegible] contacts with the strain that has caused invasi[illegible] index case. Prophylaxis should be given to [illegible] same time to avoid recolonization by meningococci [illegible] untreated contacts and should also be used as soon a[illegible] early disease in secondary cases. If the index patient [illegible] antibiotic that does not reliably clear colonization (e[illegible] or she should be given a prophylactic agent at the e[illegible] prevent relapse or onward transmission. Although most widely used and studied, it is not the optimal agent because it fails to eradicate carriage in 15–20% of cases, rates of adverse events have been high, compliance is affected by the need for four doses, and emerging resistance has been reported. Ceftriaxone as a single IM or IV injection is highly (97%) effective in carriage eradication and can be used at all ages and in pregnancy. Reduced susceptibility of isolates to ceftriaxone has occasionally been reported. Ciprofloxacin or ofloxacin is preferred in some countries; these agents are highly effective and can be administered by mouth but are not recommended in pregnancy. Resistance to fluoroquinolones has been reported in some meningococci in North America, Europe, and Asia.

In documented serogroup A, C, Y, or W disease, contacts may be offered immunization (preferably with a conjugate vaccine) in addition to chemoprophylaxis to provide protection beyond the duration of antibiotic therapy. Mass vaccination has been used successfully to control disease during outbreaks in closed communities (educational and military establishments) as well as during epidemics in open communities.

181 Gonococcal Infections

Sanjay Ram, Peter A. Rice

DEFINITION

Gonorrhea is a sexually transmitted infection (STI) of epithelium and commonly manifests as cervicitis, urethritis, proctitis, and conjunctivitis. If untreated, infections at these sites can lead to local complications such as endometritis, salpingitis, tuboovarian abscess, bartholinitis, peritonitis, and perihepatitis in female patients; periurethritis and epididymitis in male patients; and ophthalmia neonatorum in newborns. Disseminated gonococcemia is an uncommon event whose manifestations include skin lesions, tenosynovitis, arthritis, and (in rare cases) endocarditis or meningitis.

MICROBIOLOGY

Neisseria gonorrhoeae is a gram-negative, nonmotile, non-spore-forming organism that grows singly and in pairs (i.e., as monococci and diplococci, respectively). Exclusively a human pathogen, the gonococcus contains, on average, three genome copies per coccal unit; this polyploidy permits a high level of antigenic variation and the survival of the organism in its host. Gonococci, like all other *Neisseria* species, are oxidase positive. They are distinguished from other neisseriae by their ability to grow on selective media and to use glucose but not maltose, sucrose, or lactose.

EPIDEMIOLOGY

The incidence of gonorrhea has declined significantly in the United States, but there were still ~311,000 newly reported cases in 2012. Gonorrhea remains a major public health problem worldwide, is a significant cause of morbidity in developing countries, and may play a role in enhancing transmission of HIV.

Gonorrhea predominantly affects young, nonwhite, unmarried, less educated members of urban populations. The number of reported cases probably represents half of the true number of cases—a discrepancy resulting from underreporting, self-treatment, and nonspecific treatment without a laboratory-proven diagnosis. The number of reported new cases of gonorrhea in the United States rose from ~250,000 in the early 1960s to a high of 1.01 million in 1978. The recorded incidence of gonorrhea in modern times peaked in 1975, with 468 reported new cases per 100,000 population in the United States. This peak was attributable to the interaction of several variables, including improved accuracy of diagnosis, changes in patterns of contraceptive use, and changes in sexual behavior. The incidence of the disease has since declined gradually and is currently estimated at 120 cases per 100,000, a figure that is still the highest among industrialized countries. A further decline in the overall incidence of gonorrhea in the United States over the past quarter-century may reflect increased condom use resulting from public health efforts to curtail HIV transmission. At present, the attack rate in the United States is highest among 15- to 19-year-old women and 20- to 24-year-old men; 60% of all reported cases occur in the preceding two groups together. From the standpoint of ethnicity, rates are highest among African Americans and lowest among persons of Asian or Pacific Island descent.

The incidence of gonorrhea is higher in developing countries than in industrialized nations. The exact incidence of any STI is difficult to ascertain in developing countries because of limited surveillance and variable diagnostic criteria. Studies in Africa have clearly demonstrated that nonulcerative STIs such as gonorrhea (in addition to ulcerative STIs) are an independent risk factor for the transmission of HIV (Chap. 226).

Gonorrhea is transmitted from males to females more efficiently than in the opposite direction. The rate of transmission to a woman during a single unprotected sexual encounter with an infected man is ~50–70%. Oropharyngeal gonorrhea occurs in ~20% of women who practice fellatio with infected partners. Transmission in either direction by cunnilingus is rare.

In any population, there exists a small minority of individuals who have high rates of new-partner acquisition. These "core-group members" or "high-frequency transmitters" are vital in sustaining STI transmission at the population level. Another instrumental factor in sustaining gonorrhea in the population is the large number of infected individuals who are asymptomatic or have minor symptoms that are ignored. These persons, unlike symptomatic individuals, may not cease sexual activity and therefore continue to transmit the infection. This situation underscores the importance of contact tracing and empirical treatment of the sex partners of index cases.

PATHOGENESIS, IMMUNOLOGY, AND ANTIMICROBIAL RESISTANCE

Outer-Membrane Proteins • *PILI* Fresh clinical isolates of *N. gonorrhoeae* initially form piliated (fimbriated) colonies distinguishable on translucent agar. Pilus expression is rapidly switched off with unselected subculture because of rearrangements in pilus genes. This change is a basis for antigenic variation of gonococci. Piliated strains adhere better to cells derived from human mucosal surfaces and are more virulent in organ culture models and human inoculation experiments than nonpiliated variants. In a fallopian tube explant model, pili mediate gonococcal attachment to nonciliated columnar epithelial cells. This event initiates gonococcal phagocytosis and transport through these cells to intercellular spaces near the basement membrane or directly into the subepithelial tissue. Pili are also essential for genetic competence and transformation of *N. gonorrhoeae*, which permit horizontal transfer of genetic material between different gonococcal lineages in vivo.

OPACITY-ASSOCIATED PROTEIN Another gonococcal surface protein that is important in adherence to epithelial cells is opacity-associated protein (Opa, formerly called protein II). Opa contributes to intergonococcal adhesion, which is responsible for the opaque nature of gonococcal colonies on translucent agar and the organism's adherence to a variety of eukaryotic cells, including polymorphonuclear leukocytes (PMNs). Certain Opa variants promote invasion of epithelial cells, and this effect has been linked with the ability of Opa to bind vitronectin, glycosaminoglycans, and several members of the carcinoembryonic antigen–related cell adhesion molecule (CEACAM) receptor family. *N. gonorrhoeae* Opa proteins that bind CEACAM1, which is expressed by primary CD4+ T lymphocytes, suppress the activation and proliferation of these lymphocytes. This phenomenon may serve to explain the transient decrease in CD4+ T lymphocyte counts associated with gonococcal infection. Select Opa proteins can engage CEACAM3, which is expressed on neutrophils, with consequent nonopsonic phagocytosis (i.e., phagocytosis independent of antibody and complement) and killing of bacteria.

PORIN Porin (previously designated protein I) is the most abundant gonococcal surface protein, accounting for >50% of the organism's total outer-membrane protein. Porin molecules exist as trimers that provide anion-transporting aqueous channels through the otherwise hydrophobic outer membrane. Porin exhibits stable interstrain antigenic variation and forms the basis for gonococcal serotyping. Two main serotypes have been identified: PorB.1A strains are often associated with disseminated gonococcal infection (DGI), whereas PorB.1B strains usually cause local genital infections only. DGI strains are generally resistant to the killing action of normal human serum and do not incite a significant local inflammatory response; therefore, they may not cause symptoms at genital sites. These characteristics may be related to the ability of PorB.1A strains to bind to complement-inhibitory molecules, resulting in a diminished inflammatory response. Porin can translocate to the cytoplasmic membrane of host cells—a process that could initiate gonococcal endocytosis and invasion.

OTHER OUTER-MEMBRANE PROTEINS Other notable outer-membrane proteins include H.8, a lipoprotein that is present in high concentration on the surface of all gonococcal strains and is an excellent target for antibody-based diagnostic testing. Transferrin-binding proteins (Tbp1 and Tbp2) and lactoferrin-binding protein are required for scavenging iron from transferrin and lactoferrin in vivo. Transferrin and iron have been shown to enhance the attachment of iron-deprived *N. gonorrhoeae* to human endometrial cells. IgA1 protease is produced by *N. gonorrhoeae* and may protect the organism from the action of mucosal IgA.

Lipooligosaccharide Gonococcal lipooligosaccharide (LOS) consists of a lipid A and a core oligosaccharide that lacks the repeating O-carbohydrate antigenic side chain seen in other gram-negative bacteria (Chap. 145e). Gonococcal LOS possesses marked endotoxic activity and contributes to the local cytotoxic effect in a fallopian tube model. LOS core sugars undergo a high degree of phase variation under different conditions of growth; this variation reflects genetic regulation and expression of glycotransferase genes that dictate the carbohydrate structure of LOS. These phenotypic changes may affect interactions of *N. gonorrhoeae* with elements of the humoral immune system (antibodies and complement) and may also influence direct binding of organisms to both professional phagocytes and nonprofessional phagocytes (epithelial cells). For example, gonococci that are sialylated at their LOS sites bind complement factor H and inhibit the alternative pathway of complement. LOS sialylation may also decrease nonopsonic Opa-mediated association with neutrophils and inhibit the oxidative burst in PMNs. The binding of the unsialylated terminal lactosamine residue of LOS to an asialoglycoprotein receptor on male epithelial cells facilitates adherence and subsequent gonococcal invasion of these cells. Moreover, oligosaccharide structures in LOS can modulate host immune responses. For example, the terminal monosaccharide expressed by LOS determines the C-type lectin receptor on dendritic cells that is targeted by the bacteria. In turn, the specific C-type lectin receptor engaged influences whether a T_H1- or T_H2-type response is elicited; the latter response may be less favorable for clearance of gonococcal infection.

Host Factors In addition to gonococcal structures that interact with epithelial cells, host factors seem to be important in mediating entry of gonococci into nonphagocytic cells. Activation of phosphatidylcholine-specific phospholipase C and acidic sphingomyelinase by *N. gonorrhoeae*, which results in the release of diacylglycerol and ceramide, is a requirement for the entry of *N. gonorrhoeae* into epithelial cells. Ceramide accumulation within cells leads to apoptosis, which may disrupt epithelial integrity and facilitate entry of gonococci into subepithelial tissue. Release of chemotactic factors as a result of complement activation contributes to inflammation, as does the toxic effect of LOS in provoking the release of inflammatory cytokines.

The importance of humoral immunity in host defenses against neisserial infections is best illustrated by the predisposition of persons deficient in terminal complement components (C5 through C9) to recurrent bacteremic gonococcal infections and to recurrent meningococcal meningitis or meningococcemia. Gonococcal porin induces T cell–proliferative responses in persons with urogenital gonococcal disease. A significant increase in porin-specific interleukin (IL) 4–producing CD4+ as well as CD8+ T lymphocytes is seen in individuals with mucosal gonococcal disease. A portion of these lymphocytes that show a porin-specific T_H2-type response could traffic to mucosal surfaces and play a role in immune protection against the disease. Few data clearly indicate that protective immunity is acquired from a previous gonococcal infection, although bactericidal and opsonophagocytic antibodies to porin and LOS may offer partial protection. On the other hand, women who are infected and acquire high levels of antibody to another outer-membrane protein, Rmp (reduction modifiable protein, formerly called protein III), may be especially likely to become reinfected with *N. gonorrhoeae* because Rmp antibodies block the effect of bactericidal antibodies to porin and LOS. Rmp shows little, if any, interstrain antigenic variation; therefore, Rmp antibodies potentially may block antibody-mediated killing of all gonococci. The mechanism of blocking has not been fully characterized, but Rmp antibodies may noncompetitively inhibit binding of porin and LOS antibodies because of the proximity of these structures in the gonococcal outer membrane. In male volunteers who have no history of gonorrhea, the net effect of these events may influence the outcome of experimental challenge with *N. gonorrhoeae*. Because Rmp bears extensive homology to enterobacterial OmpA and meningococcal class 4 proteins, it is possible that these blocking antibodies result from prior exposure to cross-reacting proteins from these species and also play a role in first-time infection with *N. gonorrhoeae*.

Gonococcal Resistance to Antimicrobial Agents It is no surprise that *N. gonorrhoeae*, with its remarkable capacity to alter its antigenic structure and adapt to changes in the microenvironment, has become resistant to numerous antibiotics. The first effective agents against gonorrhea were the sulfonamides, which were introduced in the 1930s and became ineffective within a decade. Penicillin was then used as the drug of choice for the treatment of gonorrhea. By 1965, 42% of gonococcal isolates had developed low-level resistance to penicillin G. Resistance due to the production of penicillinase arose later.

Gonococci become fully resistant to antibiotics either by chromosomal mutations or by acquisition of R factors (plasmids). Two types of chromosomal mutations have been described. The first type, which is drug specific, is a single-step mutation leading to high-level resistance. The second type involves mutations at several chromosomal loci that combine to determine the level as well as the pattern of resistance. Strains with mutations in chromosomal genes were first observed in the late 1950s. As recently as 2007, chromosomal mutations accounted for resistance to penicillin, tetracycline, or both in ~16% of strains surveyed in the United States.

β-Lactamase (penicillinase)–producing strains of *N. gonorrhoeae* (PPNG) carrying plasmids with the Pc^r determinant had rapidly spread worldwide by the early 1980s. *N. gonorrhoeae* strains with plasmid-borne tetracycline resistance (TRNG) can mobilize some β-lactamase plasmids, and PPNG and TRNG occur together, sometimes along with strains exhibiting chromosomally mediated resistance (CMRNG). Penicillin, ampicillin, and tetracycline are no longer reliable for the treatment of gonorrhea and should not be used.

Quinolone-containing regimens were also recommended for treatment of gonococcal infections; the fluoroquinolones offered the advantage of antichlamydial activity when administered for 7 days. However, quinolone-resistant *N. gonorrhoeae* (QRNG) appeared soon after these agents were first used to treat gonorrhea. QRNG is particularly common in the Pacific Islands (including Hawaii) and Asia, where, in certain areas, all gonococcal strains are now resistant to quinolones. At present, QRNG is also common in parts of Europe and the Middle East. In the United States, QRNG has been identified in midwestern and eastern areas as well as in states on the Pacific coast, where resistant strains were first seen. Alterations in DNA gyrase and topoisomerase IV have been implicated as mechanisms of fluoroquinolone resistance.

Resistance to spectinomycin, which has been used in the past as an alternative agent, has been reported. Because this agent usually is not associated with resistance to other antibiotics, spectinomycin can be reserved for use against multidrug-resistant strains of *N. gonorrhoeae.* Nevertheless, outbreaks caused by strains resistant to spectinomycin have been documented in Korea and England when the drug has been used for primary treatment of gonorrhea.

Third-generation cephalosporins have remained highly effective as single-dose therapy for gonorrhea, but the recent isolation of strains highly resistant to ceftriaxone (minimal inhibitory concentrations [MICs], 2 μg/mL) in Japan and some European countries is cause for concern. Even though the MICs of ceftriaxone against certain strains may reach 0.015–0.125 μg/mL (higher than the MICs of 0.0001–0.008 μg/mL for fully susceptible strains), these levels are greatly exceeded in the blood, the urethra, and the cervix when the routinely recommended parenteral dose of ceftriaxone is administered. The rising MICs of oral cefixime (the previously recommended alternative oral third-generation cephalosporin) against *N. gonorrhoeae,* combined with this drug's limited capacity to reach levels sufficiently higher than MICs in the blood, the urethra, the cervix, and especially the pharynx, have resulted in the removal of cefixime from the list of first-line agents for treatment of uncomplicated gonorrhea. All *N. gonorrhoeae* strains with reduced susceptibility to ceftriaxone and cefixime (i.e., cephalosporin-intermediate/resistant strains) contain (1) a mosaic *penA* allele, which is the principal resistance determinant and encodes a penicillin-binding protein (PBP2) whose sequence differs in 60 amino acids from that of wild-type PBP2, and (2) additional genetic resistance determinants that are also required for high-level penicillin resistance.

CLINICAL MANIFESTATIONS

Gonococcal Infections in Men Acute urethritis is the most common clinical manifestation of gonorrhea in male patients. The usual incubation period after exposure is 2–7 days, although the interval can be longer and some men remain asymptomatic. Strains of the PorB.1A serotype tend to cause a greater proportion of cases of mild and asymptomatic urethritis than do PorB.1B strains. Urethral discharge and dysuria, usually without urinary frequency or urgency, are the major symptoms. The discharge initially is scant and mucoid but becomes profuse and purulent within a day or two. Gram's staining of the urethral discharge may reveal PMNs and gram-negative intracellular monococci and diplococci (Fig. 181-1). The clinical manifestations of gonococcal urethritis are usually more severe and overt than those of nongonococcal urethritis, including urethritis caused by *Chlamydia trachomatis* (Chap. 213); however, exceptions are common, and it is often impossible to differentiate the causes of urethritis on clinical grounds alone. The majority of cases of urethritis seen in the United States today are not caused by *N. gonorrhoeae* and/or *C. trachomatis.* Although a number of other organisms may be responsible, many cases do not have a specific etiologic agent identified.

Most symptomatic men with gonorrhea seek treatment and cease to be infectious. The remaining men, who are largely asymptomatic, accumulate in number over time and constitute about two-thirds of all infected men at any point in time; together with men incubating the organism (who shed the organism but are asymptomatic), they serve as the source of spread of infection. Before the antibiotic era, symptoms of urethritis persisted for ~8 weeks. Epididymitis is now an uncommon complication, and gonococcal prostatitis occurs rarely, if at all. Other unusual local complications of gonococcal urethritis include edema of the penis due to dorsal lymphangitis or thrombophlebitis, submucous inflammatory "soft" infiltration of the urethral wall, periurethral abscess or fistula, inflammation or abscess of Cowper's gland, and seminal vesiculitis. Balanitis may develop in uncircumcised men.

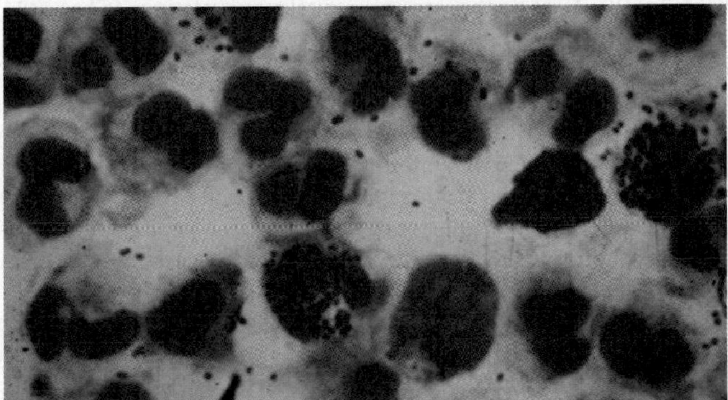

FIGURE 181-1 Gram's stain of urethral discharge from a male patient with gonorrhea shows gram-negative intracellular monococci and diplococci. *(From the Public Health Agency of Canada.)*

Gonococcal Infections in Women • ***GONOCOCCAL CERVICITIS*** Mucopurulent cervicitis is a common STI diagnosis in American women and may be caused by *N. gonorrhoeae, C. trachomatis,* and other organisms, including *Mycoplasma genitalium* (Chap. 212). Cervicitis may coexist with candidal or trichomonal vaginitis. *N. gonorrhoeae* primarily infects the columnar epithelium of the cervical os. Bartholin's glands occasionally become infected.

Women infected with *N. gonorrhoeae* usually develop symptoms. However, the women who either remain asymptomatic or have only minor symptoms may delay in seeking medical attention. These minor symptoms may include scant vaginal discharge issuing from the inflamed cervix (without vaginitis or vaginosis per se) and dysuria (often without urgency or frequency) that may be associated with gonococcal urethritis. Although the incubation period of gonorrhea is less well defined in women than in men, symptoms usually develop within 10 days of infection and are more acute and intense than those of chlamydial cervicitis.

The physical examination may reveal a mucopurulent discharge (mucopus) issuing from the cervical os. Because Gram's stain is not sensitive for the diagnosis of gonorrhea in women, specimens should be submitted for culture or a nonculture assay (see "Laboratory Diagnosis," below). Edematous and friable cervical ectopy and endocervical bleeding induced by gentle swabbing are more often seen in chlamydial infection. Gonococcal infection may extend deep enough to produce dyspareunia and lower abdominal or back pain. In such cases, it is imperative to consider a diagnosis of pelvic inflammatory disease (PID) and to administer treatment for that disease (Chaps. 163 and 213).

N. gonorrhoeae may also be recovered from the urethra and rectum of women with cervicitis, but these are rarely the only infected sites. Urethritis in women may produce symptoms of internal dysuria, which is often attributed to "cystitis." Pyuria in the absence of bacteriuria seen on Gram's stain of unspun urine, accompanied by urine cultures that fail to yield >10^2 colonies of bacteria usually associated with urinary tract infection, signifies the possibility of urethritis due to *C. trachomatis.* Urethral infection with *N. gonorrhoeae* may also occur in this context, but in this instance urethral cultures are usually positive.

GONOCOCCAL VAGINITIS The vaginal mucosa of healthy women is lined by stratified squamous epithelium and is rarely infected by *N. gonorrhoeae.* However, gonococcal vaginitis can occur in anestrogenic women (e.g., prepubertal girls and postmenopausal women), in whom the vaginal stratified squamous epithelium is often thinned down to the basilar layer, which can be infected by *N. gonorrhoeae.* The intense inflammation of the vagina makes the physical (speculum and bimanual) examination extremely painful. The vaginal mucosa is red and edematous, and an abundant purulent discharge is often present. Infection in the urethra and in Skene's and Bartholin's glands often accompanies gonococcal vaginitis. Inflamed cervical erosion or abscesses in nabothian cysts may also occur. Coexisting cervicitis may result in pus in the cervical os.

Anorectal Gonorrhea Because the female anatomy permits the spread of cervical exudate to the rectum, *N. gonorrhoeae* is sometimes recovered from the rectum of women with uncomplicated gonococcal cervicitis. The rectum is the sole site of infection in only 5% of women with gonorrhea. Such women are usually asymptomatic but occasionally have acute proctitis manifested by anorectal pain or pruritus, tenesmus, purulent rectal discharge, and rectal bleeding. Among men who have sex with men (MSM), the frequency of gonococcal infection, including rectal infection, fell by ≥90% throughout the United States in the early 1980s, but a resurgence of gonorrhea among MSM has been documented in several cities since the 1990s. Gonococcal isolates from the rectum of MSM tend to be more resistant to antimicrobial agents than are gonococcal isolates from other sites. Gonococcal isolates with a mutation in *mtrR* (multiple transferable resistance repressor) or in the promoter region of the gene that encodes for this transcriptional repressor develop increased resistance to antimicrobial hydrophobic agents such as bile acids and fatty acids in feces and thus are found with increased frequency in MSM. This situation may have been responsible for higher rates of failure of treatment for rectal gonorrhea with older regimens consisting of penicillin or tetracyclines.

Pharyngeal Gonorrhea Pharyngeal gonorrhea is usually mild or asymptomatic, although symptomatic pharyngitis does occasionally occur with cervical lymphadenitis. The mode of acquisition is oral-genital sexual exposure, with fellatio being a more efficient means of transmission than cunnilingus. In certain female adolescent populations in the United States, pharyngeal gonorrhea has become as common as genital gonorrhea. Most cases resolve spontaneously, and transmission from the pharynx to sexual contacts is rare. Pharyngeal infection almost always coexists with genital infection. Swabs from the pharynx should be plated directly onto gonococcal selective media. Pharyngeal colonization with *Neisseria meningitidis* needs to be differentiated from that with other *Neisseria* species.

Ocular Gonorrhea in Adults Ocular gonorrhea in an adult usually results from autoinoculation of *N. gonorrhoeae* from an infected genital site. As in genital infection, the manifestations range from severe to occasionally mild or asymptomatic disease. The variability in clinical manifestations may be attributable to differences in the ability of the infecting strain to elicit an inflammatory response. Infection may result in a markedly swollen eyelid, severe hyperemia and chemosis, and a profuse purulent discharge. The massively inflamed conjunctiva may be draped over the cornea and limbus. Lytic enzymes from the infiltrating PMNs occasionally cause corneal ulceration and rarely cause perforation.

Prompt recognition and treatment of this condition are of paramount importance. Gram's stain and culture of the purulent discharge establish the diagnosis. Genital cultures should also be performed.

Gonorrhea in Pregnant Women, Neonates, and Children Gonorrhea in pregnancy can have serious consequences for both the mother and the infant. Recognition of gonorrhea early in pregnancy also identifies a population at risk for other STIs, particularly chlamydial infection, syphilis, and trichomoniasis. The risks of salpingitis and PID—conditions associated with a high rate of fetal loss—are highest during the first trimester. Pharyngeal infection, most often asymptomatic, may be more common during pregnancy because of altered sexual practices. Prolonged rupture of the membranes, premature delivery, chorioamnionitis, funisitis (infection of the umbilical cord stump), and sepsis in the infant (with *N. gonorrhoeae* detected in the newborn's gastric aspirate during delivery) are common complications of maternal gonococcal infection at term. Other conditions and microorganisms, including *Mycoplasma hominis, Ureaplasma urealyticum, C. trachomatis*, and bacterial vaginosis (often accompanied by infection with *Trichomonas vaginalis*), have been associated with similar complications.

The most common form of gonorrhea in neonates is ophthalmia neonatorum, which results from exposure to infected cervical secretions during parturition. Ocular neonatal instillation of a prophylactic agent (e.g., 1% silver nitrate eye drops or ophthalmic preparations containing erythromycin or tetracycline) prevents ophthalmia neonatorum but is not effective for its treatment, which requires systemic antibiotics. The clinical manifestations are acute and usually begin 2–5 days after birth. An initial nonspecific conjunctivitis with a serosanguineous discharge is followed by tense edema of the eyelids, chemosis, and a profuse, thick, purulent discharge. Corneal ulcerations that result in nebulae or perforation may lead to anterior synechiae, anterior staphyloma, panophthalmitis, and blindness. Infections described at other mucosal sites in infants, including vaginitis, rhinitis, and anorectal infection, are likely to be asymptomatic. Pharyngeal colonization has been demonstrated in 35% of infants with gonococcal ophthalmia, and coughing is the most prominent symptom in these cases. Septic arthritis (see below) is the most common manifestation of systemic infection or DGI in the newborn. The onset usually comes at 3–21 days of age, and polyarticular involvement is common. Sepsis, meningitis, and pneumonia are seen in rare instances.

Any STI in children beyond the neonatal period raises the possibility of sexual abuse. Gonococcal vulvovaginitis is the most common manifestation of gonococcal infection in children beyond infancy. Anorectal and pharyngeal infections are common in these children and are frequently asymptomatic. The urethra, Bartholin's and Skene's glands, and the upper genital tract are rarely involved. All children with gonococcal infection should also be evaluated for chlamydial infection, syphilis, and possibly HIV infection.

Gonococcal Arthritis (DGI) DGI (gonococcal arthritis) results from gonococcal bacteremia. In the 1970s, DGI occurred in ~0.5–3% of persons with untreated gonococcal mucosal infection. The lower incidence of DGI at present is probably attributable to a decline in the prevalence of particular strains that are likely to disseminate. DGI strains resist the bactericidal action of human serum and generally do not incite inflammation at genital sites, probably because of limited generation of chemotactic factors. Strains recovered from DGI cases in the 1970s were often of the PorB.1A serotype, were highly susceptible to penicillin, and had special growth requirements—including arginine, hypoxanthine, and uracil—that made the organism more fastidious and more difficult to isolate.

Menstruation is a risk factor for dissemination, and approximately two-thirds of cases of DGI are in women. In about half of affected women, symptoms of DGI begin within 7 days of onset of menses. Complement deficiencies, especially of the components involved in the assembly of the membrane attack complex (C5 through C9), predispose to neisserial bacteremia, and persons with more than one episode of DGI should be screened with an assay for total hemolytic complement activity.

The clinical manifestations of DGI have sometimes been classified into two stages: a bacteremic stage, which is less common today, and a joint-localized stage with suppurative arthritis. A clear-cut progression usually is not evident. Patients in the bacteremic stage have higher temperatures, and chills more frequently accompany their fever. Painful joints are common and often occur together with tenosynovitis and skin lesions. Polyarthralgias usually include the knees, elbows, and more distal joints; the axial skeleton is generally spared. Skin lesions are seen in ~75% of patients and include papules and pustules, often with a hemorrhagic component (**Fig. 181-2; see also Fig. 25e-44**). Other manifestations of noninfectious dermatitis, such as nodular lesions, urticaria, and erythema multiforme, have been described. These lesions are usually on the extremities and number between 5 and 40. The differential diagnosis of the bacteremic stage of DGI includes reactive arthritis, acute rheumatoid arthritis, sarcoidosis, erythema nodosum, drug-induced arthritis, and viral infections (e.g., hepatitis B and acute HIV infection). The distribution of joint symptoms in reactive arthritis differs from that in DGI (**Fig. 181-3**), as do the skin and genital manifestations (**Chap. 384**).

Suppurative arthritis involves one or two joints, most often the knees, wrists, ankles, and elbows (in decreasing order of frequency); other joints occasionally are involved. Most patients who develop gonococcal septic arthritis do so without prior polyarthralgias or skin lesions; in the absence of symptomatic genital infection, this disease cannot be distinguished from septic arthritis caused by other pathogens. The differential diagnosis of acute arthritis in young adults is discussed in **Chap. 157**. Rarely, osteomyelitis complicates septic arthritis involving small joints of the hand.

Gonococcal endocarditis, although rare today, was a relatively common complication of DGI in the preantibiotic era, accounting for about one-quarter of reported cases of endocarditis. Another unusual complication of DGI is meningitis.

Gonococcal Infections in HIV-Infected Persons The association between gonorrhea and the acquisition of HIV has been demonstrated in

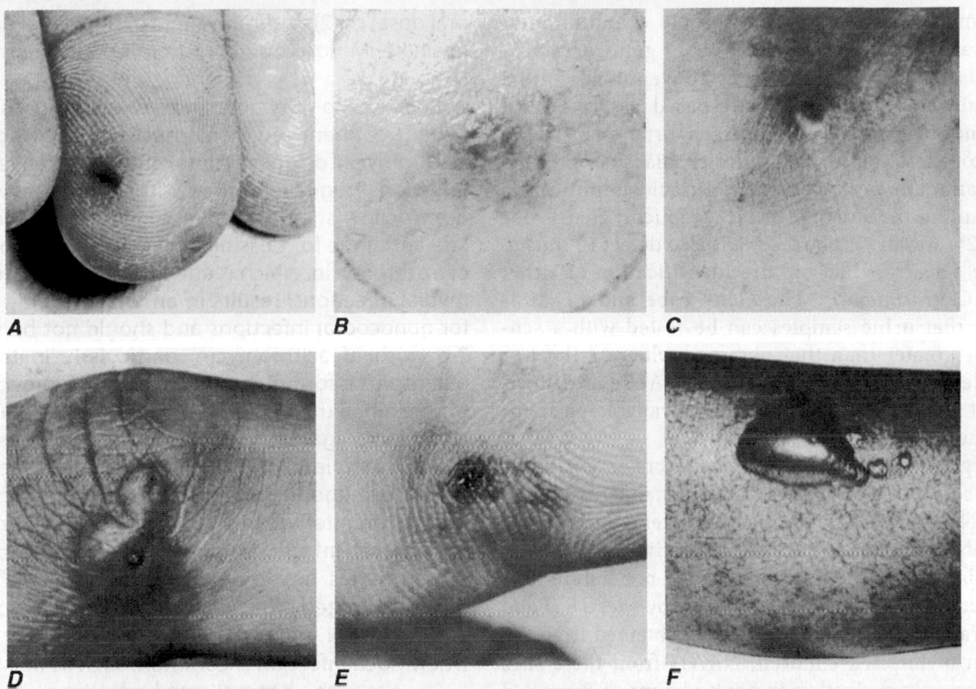

FIGURE 181-2 Characteristic skin lesions in patients with proven gonococcal bacteremia. The lesions are in various stages of evolution. ***A.*** Very early petechia on finger. ***B.*** Early papular lesion, 7 mm in diameter, on lower leg. ***C.*** Pustule with central eschar resulting from early petechial lesion. ***D.*** Pustular lesion on finger. ***E.*** Mature lesion with central necrosis (black) on hemorrhagic base. ***F.*** Bullae on anterior tibial surface. *(Reprinted with permission from KK Holmes et al: Disseminated gonococcal infection. Ann Intern Med 74:979, 1971.)*

several well-controlled studies, mainly in Kenya and Zaire. The nonulcerative STIs enhance the transmission of HIV by three- to fivefold; transmission of HIV-infected immune cells and increased viral shedding by persons with urethritis or cervicitis may contribute (Chap. 226). HIV has been detected by polymerase chain reaction (PCR) more commonly in ejaculates from HIV-positive men with gonococcal urethritis than in those from HIV-positive men with nongonococcal urethritis. PCR positivity diminishes by twofold after appropriate therapy for urethritis. Not only does gonorrhea enhance the transmission of HIV, but it may also increase the individual's risk for acquisition of HIV. A proposed mechanism is the significantly greater number of CD4+ T lymphocytes and dendritic cells that can be infected by HIV in endocervical secretions from women with nonulcerative STIs than in those from women with ulcerative STIs.

Disseminated gonococcal infection (*N* = 102) | Reactive arthritis (*N* = 173)

Hand and fingers
Wrist
Elbow
Shoulder
Sternal*
Spine and SI†
Hip
Knee
Ankle
Foot and toes

60 50 40 30 20 10 0 10 20 30 40 50 60
Percent of patients

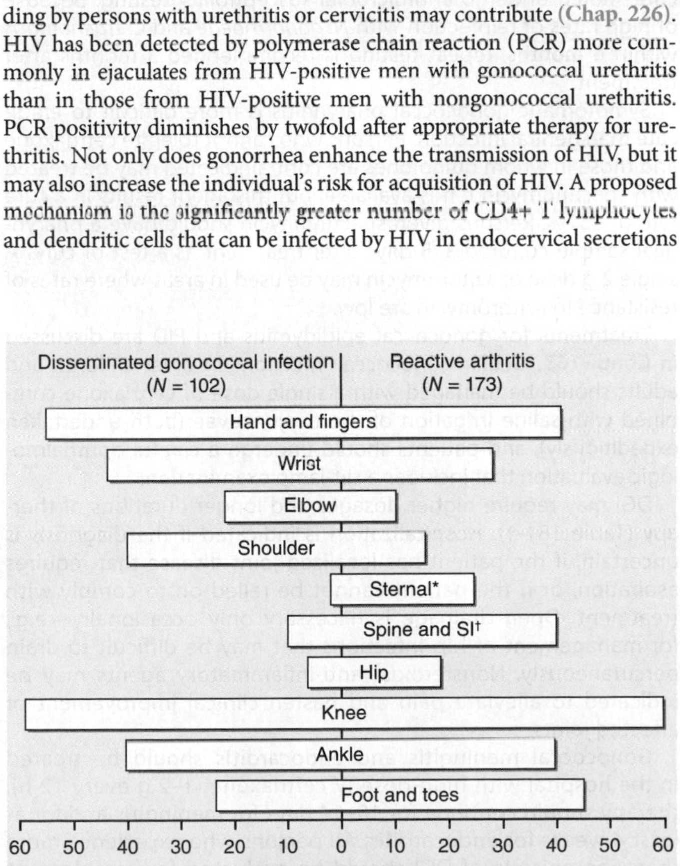

FIGURE 181-3 Distribution of joints with arthritis in 102 patients with disseminated gonococcal infection and 173 patients with reactive arthritis. *Includes the sternoclavicular joints. †SI, sacroiliac joint.

LABORATORY DIAGNOSIS

A rapid diagnosis of gonococcal infection in men may be obtained by Gram's staining of urethral exudates (Fig. 181-1). The detection of gram-negative intracellular monococci and diplococci is usually highly specific and sensitive in diagnosing gonococcal urethritis in symptomatic males but is only ~50% sensitive in diagnosing gonococcal cervicitis. Samples should be collected with Dacron or rayon swabs. Part of the sample should be inoculated onto a plate of modified Thayer-Martin or other gonococcal selective medium for culture. It is important to process all samples immediately because gonococci do not tolerate drying. If plates cannot be incubated immediately, they can be held safely for several hours at room temperature in candle extinction jars prior to incubation. If processing is to occur within 6 h, transport of specimens may be facilitated by the use of nonnutritive swab transport systems such as Stuart or Amies medium. For longer holding periods (e.g., when specimens for culture are to be mailed), culture media with self-contained CO_2-generating systems (such as the JEMBEC or Gono-Pak systems) may be used. Specimens should also be obtained for the diagnosis of chlamydial infection (Chap. 213).

PMNs are often seen in the endocervix on a Gram's stain, and an abnormally increased number (≥30 PMNs per field in five 1000× oil-immersion microscopic fields) establishes the presence of an inflammatory discharge. Unfortunately, the presence or absence of gram-negative intracellular monococci or diplococci in cervical smears does not accurately predict which patients have gonorrhea, and the diagnosis in this setting should be made by culture or another suitable nonculture diagnostic method. The sensitivity of a single endocervical culture is ~80–90%. If a history of rectal sex is elicited, a rectal wall swab (uncontaminated with feces) should be cultured. A presumptive diagnosis of gonorrhea cannot be made on the basis of gram-negative diplococci in smears from the pharynx, where other *Neisseria* species are components of the normal flora.

Increasingly, nucleic acid probe tests are being substituted for culture for the direct detection of *N. gonorrhoeae* in urogenital specimens. A common assay uses a nonisotopic chemiluminescent DNA probe that hybridizes specifically with gonococcal 16S ribosomal RNA; this assay is as sensitive as conventional culture techniques. A disadvantage of non-culture-based assays is that *N. gonorrhoeae* cannot be grown from the transport systems. Thus a culture-confirmatory test and formal antimicrobial susceptibility testing, if needed, cannot be performed. Nucleic acid amplification tests (NAATs), including the Roche Cobas® Amplicor, Gen-Probe APTIMA COMBO 2®, and BD ProbeTec™ ET, also detect *C. trachomatis* and are more sensitive than culture identification of either *N. gonorrhoeae* or *C. trachomatis*. The Gen-Probe and BD tests offer the advantage that urine samples can be tested with a sensitivity similar to or greater than that obtained when urethral or cervical swab samples are assessed by other non-NAATs or culture, respectively. Several amplification tests are now available on semiautomated or fully automated platforms.

Because of the legal implications, the preferred method for the diagnosis of gonococcal infection in children is a standardized culture. Two positive NAATs, each targeting a different nucleic acid sequence, may be substituted for culture of the cervix or the urethra as legal evidence of infection in children. Although nonculture tests for gonococcal infection have not been approved by the U.S. Food and Drug Administration for use with specimens obtained from the pharynx and rectum of infected children, NAATs from these sites are preferred for diagnostic evaluation in adult victims of suspected sexual abuse, especially if the NAATs have been evaluated by the local laboratory and found to be superior. Cultures should be obtained from the pharynx and anus of both girls and boys, the urethra of boys, and the vagina of girls; cervical specimens are not recommended for prepubertal girls. For boys with a urethral discharge, a meatal specimen of the discharge is adequate for culture. Presumptive colonies of *N. gonorrhoeae* should be identified definitively by at least two independent methods.

Blood should be cultured in suspected cases of DGI. The use of Isolator blood culture tubes may enhance the yield. The probability of positive blood cultures decreases after 48 h of illness. Synovial fluid should be inoculated into blood culture broth medium and plated onto chocolate agar rather than selective medium because this fluid is not likely to be contaminated with commensal bacteria. Gonococci are infrequently recovered from early joint effusions containing <20,000 leukocytes/μL but may be recovered from effusions containing >80,000 leukocytes/μL. The organisms are seldom recovered from blood and synovial fluid of the same patient.

TREATMENT GONOCOCCAL INFECTIONS

Treatment failure can lead to continued transmission and the emergence of antibiotic resistance. The importance of adequate treatment with a regimen that the patient will adhere to cannot be overemphasized. Thus highly effective single-dose regimens have been developed for uncomplicated gonococcal infections. The modified 2010 treatment guidelines for gonococcal infections from the Centers for Disease Control and Prevention (CDC) are summarized in **Table 181-1**. Rising MICs of cefixime worldwide have led the CDC to discontinue its recommendation of this agent as first-line treatment for uncomplicated gonorrhea. The recommendations for uncomplicated gonorrhea apply to HIV-infected as well as HIV-uninfected patients.

Currently, a single IM dose of the third-generation cephalosporin ceftriaxone is the mainstay of therapy for uncomplicated gonococcal infection of the urethra, cervix, rectum, or pharynx and almost always results in an effective cure. Quinolone-containing regimens are no longer recommended in the United States as first-line treatment because of widespread resistance. A recent multicenter trial of treatment for uncomplicated gonorrhea in the United States showed ≥99.5% efficacy of two combination regimens: (1) gemifloxacin (320 mg, single oral dose) plus azithromycin (2 g, single oral dose) or (2) azithromycin (2 g, single oral dose) plus gentamicin (a single IM dose of 240 mg or, in individuals who weigh ≤45 kg, 5 mg/kg).

Because co-infection with *C. trachomatis* occurs frequently, initial treatment regimens must also incorporate an agent (e.g., azithromycin or doxycycline) that is effective against chlamydial infection. Pregnant women with gonorrhea, who should not take doxycycline, should receive concurrent treatment with a macrolide antibiotic for possible chlamydial infection. A single 1-g dose of azithromycin, which is effective therapy for uncomplicated chlamydial infections, results in an unacceptably low cure rate (93%) for gonococcal infections and should not be used alone. A single 2-g dose of azithromycin, particularly in the extended-release microsphere formulation, delivers azithromycin to the lower gastrointestinal tract, thereby improving tolerability. Azithromycin is effective against sensitive strains, but this drug is expensive, causes gastrointestinal distress, and is not recommended for routine or first-line treatment of gonorrhea. Spectinomycin has been used as an alternative agent for the treatment of uncomplicated gonococcal infections in penicillin-allergic persons outside the United States but is not currently available in this country. Of note, the limited effectiveness of spectinomycin for the treatment of pharyngeal infection reduces its utility in populations among whom such infection is common, such as MSM.

Persons with uncomplicated infections who receive ceftriaxone do not need a test of cure; however, cultures for *N. gonorrhoeae* should be performed if symptoms persist after therapy with an established regimen, and any gonococci isolated should be tested for antimicrobial susceptibility. Persons given an alternative regimen should return for a test of cure targeting the infected anatomic site. This test ideally should be a culture. If culture is not readily available and a NAAT is positive, every effort should be made to perform a confirmatory culture. All positive cultures for test of cure should undergo antimicrobial susceptibility testing. Because of high rates of reinfection with *N. gonorrhoeae* and *C. trachomatis* within 6 months, repeat testing is recommended 3 months after treatment.

Symptomatic gonococcal pharyngitis is more difficult to eradicate than genital infection. Persons who cannot tolerate ceftriaxone and those in whom quinolones are contraindicated may be treated with spectinomycin if it is available, but this agent results in a cure rate of ≤52%. Persons given spectinomycin should have a pharyngeal sample cultured 3–5 days after treatment as a test of cure. A single 2-g dose of azithromycin may be used in areas where rates of resistance to azithromycin are low.

Treatments for gonococcal epididymitis and PID are discussed in **Chap. 163**. Ocular gonococcal infections in older children and adults should be managed with a single dose of ceftriaxone combined with saline irrigation of the conjunctivae (both undertaken expeditiously), and patients should undergo a careful ophthalmologic evaluation that includes a slit-lamp examination.

DGI may require higher dosages and longer durations of therapy (Table 181-1). Hospitalization is indicated if the diagnosis is uncertain, if the patient has localized joint disease that requires aspiration, or if the patient cannot be relied on to comply with treatment. Open drainage is necessary only occasionally—e.g., for management of hip infections that may be difficult to drain percutaneously. Nonsteroidal anti-inflammatory agents may be indicated to alleviate pain and hasten clinical improvement of affected joints.

Gonococcal meningitis and endocarditis should be treated in the hospital with high-dose IV ceftriaxone (1–2 g every 12 h); therapy should continue for 10–14 days for meningitis and for at least 4 weeks for endocarditis. All persons who experience more than one episode of DGI should be evaluated for complement deficiency.

TABLE 181-1 RECOMMENDED TREATMENT FOR GONOCOCCAL INFECTIONS: ADAPTED FROM THE 2010 GUIDELINES OF THE CENTERS FOR DISEASE CONTROL AND PREVENTION

Diagnosis	Treatment of Choice[a]
Uncomplicated gonococcal infection of the cervix, urethra, pharynx[b], or rectum	
First-line regimen	Ceftriaxone (250 mg IM, single dose)
	plus
	Treatment for *Chlamydia* if chlamydial infection is not ruled out:
	Azithromycin (1 g PO, single dose)
	or
	Doxycycline (100 mg PO bid for 7 days)
Alternative regimens[c]	Cefixime (400 mg PO, single dose)
	or
	Ceftizoxime (500 mg IM, single dose)
	or
	Cefotaxime (500 mg IM, single dose)
	or
	Spectinomycin (2 g IM, single dose)[d,e]
	or
	Cefotetan (1 g IM, single dose) *plus* probenecid (1 g PO, single dose)[d]
	or
	Cefoxitin (2 g IM, single dose) ***plus*** probenecid (1 g PO, single dose)[d]
Epididymitis	See **Chap. 163**
Pelvic inflammatory disease	See **Chap. 163**
Gonococcal conjunctivitis in an adult	Ceftriaxone (1 g IM, single dose)[f]
Ophthalmia neonatorum[g]	Ceftriaxone (25–50 mg/kg IV, single dose, not to exceed 125 mg)
Disseminated gonococcal infection[h]	
Initial therapy[i]	
Patient tolerant of β-lactam drugs	Ceftriaxone (1 g IM or IV q24h; recommended)
	or
	Cefotaxime (1 g IV q8h)
	or
	Ceftizoxime (1 g IV q8h)
Patients allergic to β-lactam drugs	Spectinomycin (2 g IM q12h)[d]
Continuation therapy[i]	Cefixime (400 mg PO bid)
Meningitis or endocarditis	See text[j]

[a]True failure of treatment with a recommended regimen is rare and should prompt an evaluation for reinfection, infection with a drug-resistant strain, or an alternative diagnosis. [b]Ceftriaxone is the only agent recommended for treatment of pharyngeal infection. [c]See text for follow-up of persons with infection who are treated with alternative regimens. [d]Spectinomycin, cefotetan, and cefoxitin, which are alternative agents, currently are unavailable or in short supply in the United States. [e]Spectinomycin may be ineffective for the treatment of pharyngeal gonorrhea. [f]Plus lavage of the infected eye with saline solution (once). [g]Prophylactic regimens are discussed in the text. [h]Hospitalization is indicated if the diagnosis is uncertain, if the patient has frank arthritis with an effusion, or if the patient cannot be relied on to adhere to treatment. [i]All initial regimens should be continued for 24–48 h after clinical improvement begins, at which time the switch may be made to an oral agent (e.g., cefixime or a quinolone) if antimicrobial susceptibility can be documented by culture of the causative organism. If no organism is isolated and the diagnosis is secure, then treatment with ceftriaxone should be continued for at least 1 week. Treatment for chlamydial infection (as above) should be given if this infection has not been ruled out. [j]Hospitalization is indicated to exclude suspected meningitis or endocarditis.

PREVENTION AND CONTROL

Condoms, if properly used, provide effective protection against the transmission and acquisition of gonorrhea as well as other infections that are transmitted to and from genital mucosal surfaces. Spermicidal preparations used with a diaphragm or cervical sponges impregnated with nonoxynol 9 offer some protection against gonorrhea and chlamydial infection. However, the frequent use of preparations that contain nonoxynol 9 is associated with mucosal disruption that paradoxically may enhance the risk of HIV infection in the event of exposure. All patients should be instructed to refer sex partners for evaluation and treatment. All sex partners of persons with gonorrhea should be evaluated and treated for *N. gonorrhoeae* and *C. trachomatis* infections if their last contact with the patient took place within 60 days before the onset of symptoms or the diagnosis of infection in the patient. If the patient's last sexual encounter was >60 days before onset of symptoms or diagnosis, the patient's most recent sex partner should be treated. Partner-delivered medications or prescriptions for medications to treat gonorrhea and chlamydial infection diminish the likelihood of reinfection (or relapse) in the infected patient. In states where it is legal, this approach is an option for partner management. Patients should be instructed to abstain from sexual intercourse until therapy is completed and until they and their sex partners no longer have symptoms. Greater emphasis must be placed on prevention by public health education, individual patient counseling, and behavior modification. Sexually active persons, especially adolescents, should be offered screening for STIs. For male patients, a NAAT on urine or a urethral swab may be used for screening. Preventing the spread of gonorrhea may help reduce the transmission of HIV. No effective vaccine for gonorrhea is yet available, but efforts to test several candidates are under way.

Acknowledgment

The authors acknowledge the contributions of Dr. King K. Holmes and Dr. Stephen A. Morse to the chapter on this subject in earlier editions.

182 Haemophilus and Moraxella Infections

Timothy F. Murphy

HAEMOPHILUS INFLUENZAE

MICROBIOLOGY

Haemophilus influenzae was first recognized in 1892 by Pfeiffer, who erroneously concluded that the bacterium was the cause of influenza. *H. influenzae* is a small (1- × 0.3-μm) gram-negative organism of variable shape; thus, it is often described as a pleomorphic coccobacillus. In clinical specimens such as cerebrospinal fluid (CSF) and sputum, *H. influenzae* frequently stains only faintly with safranin and therefore can easily be overlooked.

H. influenzae grows both aerobically and anaerobically. Its aerobic growth requires two factors: hemin (X factor) and nicotinamide adenine dinucleotide (V factor). These requirements are used in the clinical laboratory to identify the bacterium. Caution must be used to distinguish *H. influenzae* from *H. haemolyticus*, a respiratory tract commensal that has identical growth requirements. *H. haemolyticus* has classically been distinguished from *H. influenzae* by the hemolysis of the former species on horse blood agar. However, a significant proportion of isolates of *H. haemolyticus* have now been recognized as nonhemolytic. Analysis of various genotypic and phenotypic markers, including16S ribosomal sequences, superoxide dismutase, outer-membrane protein P6, protein D, and fuculose kinase, can be used to distinguish these two species.

Six major serotypes of *H. influenzae* have been identified; designated *a* through *f*, they are based on antigenically distinct polysaccharide capsules. In addition, some strains lack a polysaccharide capsule and are referred to as *nontypable* strains. Type b and nontypable strains are the most relevant strains clinically (**Table 182-1**), although encapsulated strains other than type b can cause disease. *H. influenzae* was the first free-living organism to have its entire genome sequenced.

The antigenically distinct type b capsule is a linear polymer composed of ribosyl-ribitol phosphate. Strains of *H. influenzae* type b (Hib) cause disease primarily in infants and children <6 years of age. Nontypable strains are primarily mucosal pathogens but occasionally cause invasive disease.

EPIDEMIOLOGY AND TRANSMISSION

H. influenzae, an exclusively human pathogen, is spread by airborne droplets or by direct contact with secretions or fomites. Colonization with nontypable *H. influenzae* is a dynamic process; new strains are acquired and other strains are replaced periodically.

The widespread use of Hib conjugate vaccines in many industrialized countries has resulted in striking decreases in the rate of nasopharyngeal colonization by Hib and in the incidence of Hib infection (**Fig. 182-1**). However, the majority of the world's children remain unimmunized. Worldwide, invasive Hib disease occurs predominantly in unimmunized children and in those who have not completed the primary immunization series. Certain groups have a higher incidence of invasive Hib disease than the general population, including African-American children and Native American groups. Although this increased incidence has not yet been accounted for, several factors may be relevant, including age at exposure to the bacterium, socioeconomic conditions, and genetic differences.

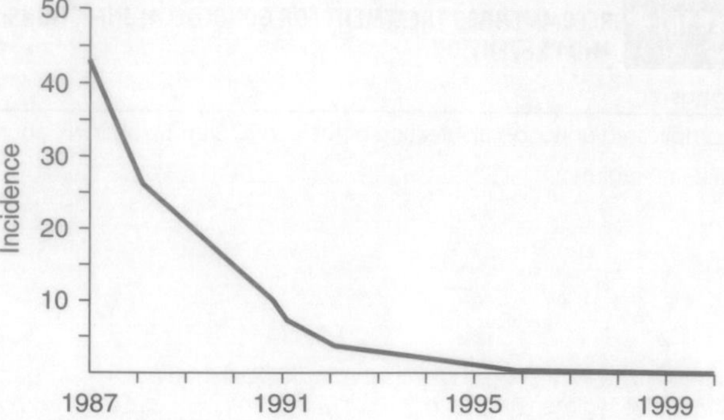

FIGURE 182-1 Estimated incidence (rate per 100,000) of invasive disease due to *Haemophilus influenzae* type b among children <5 years of age: 1987–2000. Fewer than 40 cases per year have been reported since 2000. *(Data from the Centers for Disease Control and Prevention.)*

TABLE 182-1 CHARACTERISTICS OF TYPE b AND NONTYPABLE STRAINS OF *HAEMOPHILUS INFLUENZAE*

Feature	Type b Strains	Nontypable Strains
Capsule	Ribosyl-ribitol phosphate	Unencapsulated
Pathogenesis	Invasive infections due to hematogenous spread	Mucosal infections due to contiguous spread
Clinical manifestations	Meningitis and invasive infections in incompletely immunized infants and children	Otitis media in infants and children; lower respiratory tract infections in adults with chronic bronchitis
Evolutionary history	Basically clonal	Genetically diverse
Vaccine	Highly effective conjugate vaccines	None available; under development

PATHOGENESIS

Hib strains cause systemic disease by invasion and hematogenous spread from the respiratory tract to distant sites such as the meninges, bones, and joints. The type b polysaccharide capsule is an important virulence factor affecting the bacterium's ability to avoid opsonization and cause systemic disease.

Nontypable strains cause disease by local invasion of mucosal surfaces. Otitis media results when bacteria reach the middle ear by way of the eustachian tube. Adults with chronic bronchitis experience recurrent lower respiratory tract infection due to nontypable strains. In addition, persistent nontypable *H. influenzae* colonization of the lower airways of adults with chronic obstructive pulmonary disease (COPD) contributes to the airway inflammation that is a hallmark of the disease. Nontypable strains that cause infection in adults with COPD differ in pathogenic potential and genome content from strains that cause otitis media. In the middle ear, nontypable strains form biofilms. More resistant to host clearance mechanisms and to antibiotics than are planktonic bacteria, biofilms are associated with chronic and recurrent otitis media. The incidence of invasive disease caused by nontypable strains is low. Strains that cause invasive disease are genetically and phenotypically diverse.

IMMUNE RESPONSE

Antibody to the capsule is important in protection from infection by Hib strains. The level of (maternally acquired) serum antibody to the capsular polysaccharide, which is a polymer of polyribitol ribose phosphate (PRP), declines from birth to 6 months of age and, in the absence of vaccination, remains low until ~2 or 3 years of age. The age at the antibody nadir correlates with that of the peak incidence of type b disease. Antibody to PRP then appears partly as a result of exposure to Hib or cross-reacting antigens. Systemic Hib disease is unusual after the age of 6 years because of the presence of protective antibody. Vaccines in which PRP is conjugated to protein carrier molecules have been developed and are now used widely. These vaccines generate an antibody response to PRP in infants and effectively prevent invasive infections in infants and children.

Since nontypable strains lack a capsule, the immune response to infection is directed at noncapsular antigens. These antigens have generated considerable interest as immune targets and potential vaccine components. The human immune response to nontypable strains appears to be strain-specific, a characteristic that accounts in part for the propensity of these strains to cause recurrent otitis media and recurrent exacerbations of chronic bronchitis in immunocompetent hosts.

CLINICAL MANIFESTATIONS

Hib The most serious manifestation of infection with Hib is *meningitis* (Chap. 164), which primarily affects children <2 years of age. The clinical manifestations of Hib meningitis are similar to those of meningitis caused by other bacterial pathogens. Fever and altered central nervous system function are the most common features at presentation. Nuchal rigidity may or may not be evident. Subdural effusion, the most common complication, is suspected when, despite 2 or 3 days of appropriate antibiotic therapy, the infant has seizures, hemiparesis, or continued obtundation. The overall mortality rate from Hib meningitis is ~5%, and the morbidity rate is high. Of survivors, 6% have permanent sensorineural hearing loss, and about one-fourth have a significant handicap of some type. If more subtle handicaps are sought, up to half of survivors are found to have some neurologic sequelae, such as partial hearing loss and delayed language development.

Epiglottitis (Chap. 44) is a life-threatening Hib infection involving cellulitis of the epiglottis and supraglottic tissues. It can lead to acute upper airway obstruction. Its unique epidemiologic features are its occurrence in an older age group (2–7 years old) than other Hib infections and its absence among Navajo Indians and Alaskan Eskimos. Sore throat and fever rapidly progress to dysphagia, drooling, and airway obstruction. Epiglottitis also occurs in adults.

Cellulitis (Chap. 156) due to Hib occurs in young children. The most common location is on the head or neck, and the involved area sometimes takes on a characteristic bluish-red color. Most patients have bacteremia, and 10% have an additional focus of infection.

Hib causes *pneumonia* in infants. The infection is clinically indistinguishable from other types of bacterial pneumonia (e.g., pneumococcal pneumonia) except that Hib is more likely to involve the pleura. Several less common invasive conditions can be important clinical manifestations of Hib infection in children. These include osteomyelitis, septic arthritis, pericarditis, orbital cellulitis, endophthalmitis, urinary tract infection, abscesses, and bacteremia without an identifiable focus.

Non–type b encapsulated strains of *H. influenzae* (types a, c, d, e, and f) are unusual causes of invasive infection manifested predominantly by bacteremia and pneumonia. Most such infections occur in the setting of underlying conditions.

Nontypable *H. influenzae* Nontypable *H. influenzae* is the most common bacterial cause of exacerbations of COPD; these exacerbations are characterized by increased cough, sputum production, and shortness of breath. Fever is low grade, and no infiltrates are evident on chest x-ray. Nontypable strains also cause community-acquired bacterial pneumonia in adults, especially among patients with COPD or AIDS. The clinical features of *H. influenzae* pneumonia are similar to those of other types of bacterial pneumonia, including pneumococcal pneumonia.

Nontypable *H. influenzae* is one of the three most common causes of childhood otitis media (the other two being *Streptococcus pneumoniae* and *Moraxella catarrhalis*) (Chap. 44). Infants are febrile and irritable, while older children report ear pain. Symptoms of viral upper respiratory infection often precede otitis media. The diagnosis is made by pneumatic otoscopy. An etiologic diagnosis, although not routinely sought, can be established by tympanocentesis and culture of middle-ear fluid. Clinical features associated with *H. influenzae* otitis media include a history of recurrent episodes, treatment failure, concomitant conjunctivitis, bilateral otitis media, and recent antimicrobial therapy. The increasing use of pneumococcal polysaccharide conjugate vaccines in infants is resulting in a relative increase in the proportion of otitis media cases that are caused by *H. influenzae.*

Nontypable *H. influenzae* also causes puerperal sepsis and is an important cause of neonatal bacteremia. These nontypable strains, which are closely related to *H. haemolyticus*, tend to be of biotype IV and cause invasive disease after colonizing the female genital tract.

Nontypable *H. influenzae* causes sinusitis (Chap. 44) in adults and children. In addition, the bacterium is a less common cause of various invasive infections. These infections include empyema, adult epiglottitis, pericarditis, cellulitis, septic arthritis, osteomyelitis, endocarditis, cholecystitis, intraabdominal infections, urinary tract infections, mastoiditis, aortic graft infection, and bacteremia without a detectable focus. While most *H. influenzae* invasive infections in countries where Hib vaccines are used widely are caused by nontypable strains, there is no convincing evidence of an increased incidence of infection by nontypable *H. influenzae* as a result of use of Hib vaccines. Continued monitoring will be important. Many patients with *H. influenzae* bacteremia have an underlying condition, such as HIV infection, cardiopulmonary disease, alcoholism, or cancer.

DIAGNOSIS

The most reliable method for establishing a diagnosis of Hib infection is recovery of the organism in culture. The presence of gram-negative coccobacilli in Gram-stained CSF is strong evidence for Hib meningitis. Recovery of the organism from CSF confirms the diagnosis. Cultures of other normally sterile body fluids, such as blood, joint fluid, pleural fluid, pericardial fluid, and subdural effusion, are confirmatory in other infections.

Detection of PRP is an important adjunct to culture in rapid diagnosis of Hib meningitis. Immunoelectrophoresis, latex agglutination, coagglutination, and enzyme-linked immunosorbent assay are effective in detecting PRP. These assays are particularly helpful when patients have received prior antimicrobial therapy and thus are especially likely to have negative cultures.

Because nontypable *H. influenzae* is primarily a mucosal pathogen, it is a component of a mixed flora; thus etiologic diagnosis is challenging. Nontypable *H. influenzae* infection is strongly suggested by the predominance of gram-negative coccobacilli among abundant polymorphonuclear leukocytes in a Gram-stained sputum specimen from a patient in whom pneumonia is suspected. Although bacteremia is detectable in a small proportion of patients with pneumonia due to nontypable *H. influenzae*, most such patients have negative blood cultures.

A diagnosis of otitis media is based on the detection by pneumatic otoscopy of fluid in the middle ear. An etiologic diagnosis requires tympanocentesis but is not routinely sought. An invasive procedure is also required to determine the etiology of sinusitis; thus, treatment is often empirical once the diagnosis is suspected in light of clinical symptoms and sinus radiographs.

TREATMENT HAEMOPHILUS INFLUENZAE

Initial therapy for meningitis due to Hib should consist of a cephalosporin such as ceftriaxone or cefotaxime. For children, the dosage of ceftriaxone is 75–100 mg/kg daily given in two doses 12 h apart. The pediatric dosage of cefotaxime is 200 mg/kg daily given in four doses 6 h apart. Adult dosages are 2 g every 12 h for ceftriaxone and 2 g every 4–6 h for cefotaxime. An alternative regimen for initial therapy is ampicillin (200–300 mg/kg daily in four divided doses) plus chloramphenicol (75–100 mg/kg daily in four divided doses). Therapy should continue for a total of 1–2 weeks.

Administration of glucocorticoids to patients with Hib meningitis reduces the incidence of neurologic sequelae. The presumed mechanism is reduction of the inflammation induced by bacterial cell-wall mediators of inflammation when cells are killed by antimicrobial agents. Dexamethasone (0.6 mg/kg per day intravenously in four divided doses for 2 days) is recommended for the treatment of Hib meningitis in children >2 months of age.

Invasive infections other than meningitis are treated with the same antimicrobial agents. For epiglottitis, the dosage of ceftriaxone is 50 mg/kg daily, and the dosage of cefotaxime is 150 mg/kg daily, given in three divided doses 8 h apart. Epiglottitis constitutes a medical emergency, and maintenance of an airway is critical. The duration of therapy is determined by the clinical response. A course of 1–2 weeks is usually appropriate.

Many infections caused by nontypable strains of *H. influenzae*, such as otitis media, sinusitis, and exacerbations of COPD, can be treated with oral antimicrobial agents. Approximately 20–35% of nontypable strains produce β-lactamase (with the exact proportion depending on geographic location), and these strains are resistant to ampicillin. Several agents have excellent activity against nontypable *H. influenzae*, including amoxicillin/clavulanic acid, various extended-spectrum cephalosporins, and the macrolides azithromycin and clarithromycin. Fluoroquinolones are highly active against *H. influenzae* and are useful in adults with exacerbations of COPD. However, fluoroquinolones are not currently recommended for the treatment of children or pregnant women because of possible effects on articular cartilage.

In addition to β-lactamase production, alteration of penicillin-binding proteins—a second mechanism of ampicillin resistance—has been detected in isolates of *H. influenzae*. Although rare in the United States, these β-lactamase-negative ampicillin-resistant strains are common in Japan and are increasing in prevalence in Europe. Continued monitoring of the evolving antimicrobial susceptibility patterns of *H. influenzae* will be important.

PREVENTION

Vaccination (See also Chap. 148) Two conjugate vaccines that prevent invasive infections with Hib in infants and children are licensed in the United States. In addition to eliciting protective antibody, these vaccines prevent disease by reducing rates of pharyngeal colonization with Hib. The widespread use of conjugate vaccines has dramatically reduced the incidence of Hib disease in developed countries. Even though the manufacture of Hib vaccines is costly, vaccination is cost-effective. The Global Alliance for Vaccines and Immunizations has recognized the underuse of Hib conjugate vaccines.

The disease burden has been reduced in developing countries that have implemented routine vaccination (e.g., The Gambia, Chile). An important obstacle to more widespread vaccination is the lack of data on the epidemiology and burden of Hib disease in many developing countries.

All children should be immunized with an Hib conjugate vaccine, receiving the first dose at ~2 months of age, the rest of the primary series at 2–6 months of age, and a booster dose at 12–15 months of age. Specific recommendations vary for the different conjugate vaccines. The reader is referred to the recommendations of the American Academy of Pediatrics (Chap. 148 and *www.cispimmunize.org*).

Currently, no vaccines are available specifically for the prevention of disease caused by nontypable *H. influenzae*. However, a vaccine that contains protein D—a surface protein of *H. influenzae*—conjugated to pneumococcal polysaccharides is licensed in other countries and is used widely in Europe. The vaccine has shown partial efficacy in preventing *H. influenzae* otitis media in clinical trials. Additional progress in the development of vaccines against nontypable *H. influenzae* is anticipated.

Chemoprophylaxis The risk of secondary disease is greater than normal among household contacts of patients with Hib disease. Therefore, all children and adults (except pregnant women) in households with an index case and at least one incompletely immunized contact <4 years of age should receive prophylaxis with oral rifampin. When two or more cases of invasive Hib disease have occurred within 60 days at a child-care facility attended by incompletely vaccinated children, administration of rifampin to all attendees and personnel is indicated, as is recommended for household contacts. Chemoprophylaxis is not indicated in nursery and child-care contacts of a single index case. The reader is referred to the recommendations of the American Academy of Pediatrics.

HAEMOPHILUS DUCREYI

Haemophilus ducreyi is the etiologic agent of chancroid (Chap. 163), a sexually transmitted disease characterized by genital ulceration and inguinal adenitis. In addition to being a cause of morbidity in itself, chancroid is associated with HIV infection because of the role played by genital ulceration in HIV transmission. Chancroid increases the efficiency of transmission of and the degree of susceptibility to HIV infection.

MICROBIOLOGY

H. ducreyi is a highly fastidious coccobacillary gram-negative bacterium whose growth requires X factor (hemin). Although, in light of this requirement, the bacterium has been classified in the genus *Haemophilus*, DNA homology and chemotaxonomic studies have established substantial differences between *H. ducreyi* and other *Haemophilus* species. Taxonomic reclassification of the organism is likely in the future but awaits further study. Ulcers contain predominantly T cells. The fact that patients who have had chancroid may have repeated infections indicates that infection does not confer protection.

EPIDEMIOLOGY AND PREVALENCE

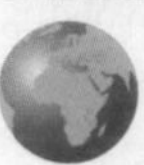

The prevalence of chancroid has declined in the United States and worldwide. However, prevalence data must be interpreted with caution because of the difficulty of establishing a diagnosis. The infection appears to be more common in developing countries. Transmission is predominantly heterosexual, and cases in males have outnumbered those in females by ratios of 3:1 to 25:1 during outbreaks. Contact with commercial sex workers and illicit drug use are strongly associated with chancroid.

CLINICAL MANIFESTATIONS AND DIFFERENTIAL DIAGNOSIS

Infection is acquired as the result of a break in the epithelium during sexual contact with an infected individual. After an incubation period of 4–7 days, the initial lesion—a papule with surrounding erythema—appears. In 2 or 3 days, the papule evolves into a pustule, which spontaneously ruptures and forms a sharply circumscribed ulcer that generally is not indurated (Fig. 182-2). The ulcers are painful and bleed easily; little or no inflammation of the surrounding skin is evident. Approximately half of patients develop enlarged, tender inguinal lymph nodes, which frequently become fluctuant and spontaneously rupture. Patients usually seek medical care after 1–3 weeks of painful symptoms.

The presentation of chancroid does not usually include all of the typical clinical features and is sometimes atypical. Multiple ulcers can coalesce to form giant ulcers. Ulcers can appear and then resolve, with inguinal adenitis (Fig. 182-2) and suppuration following 1–3 weeks later; this clinical picture can be confused with that of lymphogranuloma venereum (Chap. 213). Multiple small ulcers can resemble

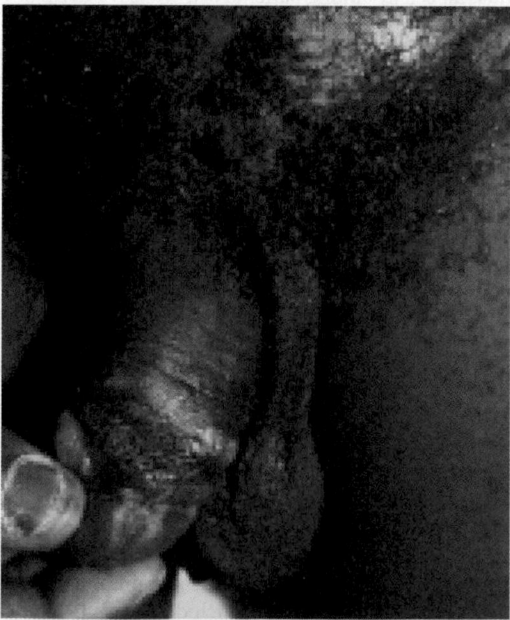

FIGURE 182-2 Chancroid with characteristic penile ulcers and associated left inguinal adenitis (bubo).

folliculitis. Other differential diagnostic considerations include the various infections causing genital ulceration, such as primary syphilis, secondary syphilis (condyloma latum), genital herpes, and donovanosis. In rare cases, chancroid lesions become secondarily infected with bacteria; the result is extensive inflammation.

DIAGNOSIS

Clinical diagnosis of chancroid is often inaccurate, and laboratory confirmation should be attempted in suspected cases. An accurate diagnosis of chancroid relies on culture of *H. ducreyi* from the lesion or from an aspirate of suppurative lymph nodes. Since the organism can be difficult to grow, the use of selective and supplemented media is necessary. No polymerase chain reaction assay for *H. ducreyi* is commercially available; such tests can be performed by Clinical Laboratory Improvement Amendment (CLIA)–certified clinical laboratories that have developed their own assays.

A probable diagnosis of chancroid can be made when the following criteria are met: (1) one or more painful genital ulcers; (2) no evidence of *Treponema pallidum* infection by dark-field examination of ulcer exudate or by a negative serologic test for syphilis performed at least 7 days after ulcer onset; (3) a typical clinical presentation for chancroid; and (4) a negative test for herpes simplex virus in the ulcer exudate.

TREATMENT *HAEMOPHILUS DUCREYI*

Treatment regimens recommended by the Centers for Disease Control and Prevention include (1) a single 1-g oral dose of azithromycin; (2) ceftriaxone (250 mg intramuscularly in a single dose); (3) ciprofloxacin (500 mg by mouth twice a day for 3 days); and (4) erythromycin base (500 mg by mouth three times a day for 7 days). Isolates from patients who do not respond promptly to treatment should be tested for antimicrobial resistance. In patients with HIV infection, healing may be slow and longer courses of treatment may be necessary. Clinical treatment failure in HIV-seropositive patients may reflect co-infection, especially with herpes simplex virus. Contacts of patients with chancroid should be identified and treated, whether or not symptoms are present, if they have had sexual contact with the patient during the 10 days preceding the patient's onset of symptoms.

MORAXELLA CATARRHALIS

MICROBIOLOGY

M. catarrhalis is an unencapsulated gram-negative diplococcus whose ecologic niche is the human respiratory tract. The organism was initially designated *Micrococcus catarrhalis*. Its name was changed to *Neisseria catarrhalis* in 1970 because of phenotypic similarities to commensal *Neisseria* species. On the basis of more rigorous analysis of genetic relatedness, *Moraxella catarrhalis* is now the widely accepted name for this species.

EPIDEMIOLOGY

Nasopharyngeal colonization by *M. catarrhalis* is common in infancy, with colonization rates ranging between 33% and 100% and depending on geographic location. Several factors probably account for this geographic variation, including living conditions, day-care attendance, hygiene, household smoking, and population genetics. The prevalence of colonization decreases steadily with age.

The widespread use of pneumococcal conjugate vaccines in some countries has resulted in alterations in patterns of nasopharyngeal colonization in resident populations. A relative increase in colonization by nonvaccine pneumococcal serotypes, nontypable *H. influenzae*, and *M. catarrhalis* has occurred. These changes in colonization patterns may be altering the distribution of pathogens of both otitis media and sinusitis in children.

PATHOGENESIS

M. catarrhalis causes mucosal infections of the respiratory tract by contiguous spread from its colonizing site in the upper airway. A preceding viral upper respiratory tract infection is a common inciting event for otitis media. In exacerbations of COPD, the acquisition of new strains is critical for pathogenesis. Strains exhibit substantial genetic diversity and differences in virulence properties.

The expression of several adhesin molecules with differing specificities for various host cell receptors reflects the importance of adherence to the respiratory epithelial surface in the pathogenesis of infection. *M. catarrhalis* invades multiple cell types. Its intracellular residence in lymphoid tissue provides a potential reservoir for persistence in the human respiratory tract. Like many gram-negative bacteria, *M. catarrhalis* sheds vesicles into the surrounding environment. The vesicles are internalized by host cells and mediate several virulence mechanisms, including induction of inflammation and delivery of β-lactamase, that can promote the survival of co-pathogens.

CLINICAL MANIFESTATIONS

In children, *M. catarrhalis* causes predominantly mucosal infections when the bacterium migrates from the nasopharynx to the middle ear or the sinuses (Chap. 44). The inciting event for both otitis media and sinusitis is often a preceding viral infection. Overall, cultures of middle-ear fluid obtained by tympanocentesis indicate that *M. catarrhalis* causes 15–20% of cases of acute otitis media. Acute otitis media caused by *M. catarrhalis* or nontypable *H. influenzae* is clinically milder than otitis media caused by *S. pneumoniae*, with less fever and a lower prevalence of a red bulging tympanic membrane. However, substantial overlap makes it impossible to predict etiology in an individual child on the basis of clinical features.

A small proportion of viral upper respiratory tract infections are complicated by bacterial sinusitis. Cultures of sinus puncture aspirates show that *M. catarrhalis* accounts for ~20% of cases of acute bacterial sinusitis in children and for a smaller proportion in adults.

M. catarrhalis is a common cause of exacerbations in adults with COPD. The bacterium has been overlooked in this clinical setting because it has long been considered to be a commensal and because it is easily mistaken for commensal *Neisseria* species in cultures of respiratory secretions (see "Diagnosis," below). Several independent lines of evidence have established *M. catarrhalis* as a pathogen in COPD. These include (1) the demonstration of *M. catarrhalis* in the lower airways during exacerbations, (2) the association of exacerbation with acquisition of new strains, (3) elevations of inflammatory markers in association with *M. catarrhalis*, and (4) the development of specific immune responses following infection. *M. catarrhalis* is the second most common bacterial cause of COPD exacerbations (after *H. influenzae*), as shown in a 10-year prospective study; the distribution of exacerbations associated with new-strain acquisitions is shown in Fig. 182-3. Not included are culture-negative cases or cases from which a pathogen had been previously isolated. With the application of rigorous clinical criteria for defining the etiology of exacerbations (both culture-positive and culture-negative), ~10% of all exacerbations in the same study were caused by *M. catarrhalis*. The clinical features of an exacerbation due to *M. catarrhalis* are similar to those of exacerbations due to other bacterial pathogens, including *H. influenzae* and *S. pneumoniae*. The cardinal symptoms are cough with increased sputum production, sputum purulence, and dyspnea in comparison with baseline symptoms.

Pneumonia due to *M. catarrhalis* occurs in the elderly, particularly in the setting of underlying cardiopulmonary disease, but is infrequent. Invasive infections, such as bacteremia, endocarditis, neonatal meningitis, and septic arthritis, are rare.

DIAGNOSIS

Tympanocentesis is required for etiologic diagnosis of otitis media, but this procedure is not performed routinely. Therefore, treatment of otitis media is generally empirical. Similarly, an etiologic diagnosis of sinusitis requires an invasive procedure and thus is usually not available to the clinician. Isolation of *M. catarrhalis* from an expectorated sputum sample from an adult experiencing clinical symptoms of an exacerbation is suggestive, but not diagnostic, of *M. catarrhalis* as the cause.

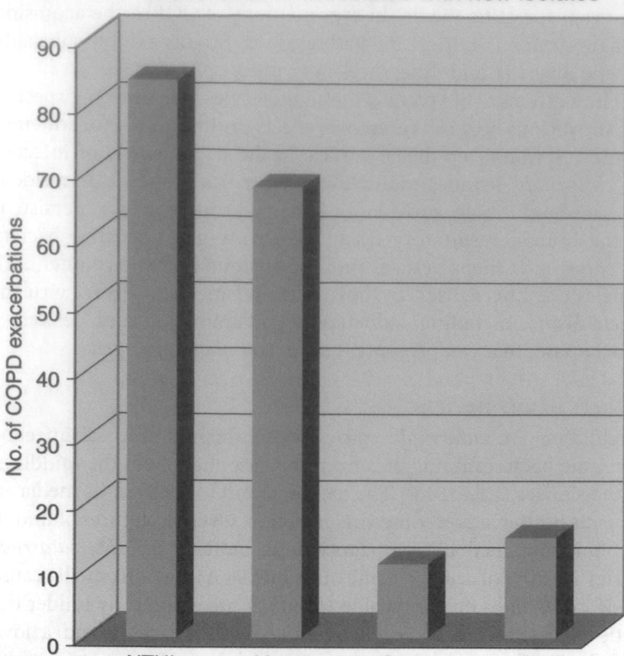

FIGURE 182-3 Cumulative results of a prospective study (1994–2004) of bacterial infection in chronic obstructive pulmonary disease (COPD) showing etiology of exacerbations. The numbers of exacerbations shown indicate the acquisition of a new strain simultaneous with clinical symptoms of an exacerbation. NTHI, nontypable *H. influenzae*; M.cat, *M. catarrhalis*; S.pn, *Streptococcus pneumoniae*; PA, *Pseudomonas aeruginosa*. *(Adapted from TF Murphy, GI Parameswaran: Clin Infect Dis 49:124, 2009, with permission. © 2009 Infectious Diseases Society of America.)*

Upon culture, colonies of *M. catarrhalis* resemble commensal neisseriae that are part of the normal upper airway flora. As mentioned above, the difficulty in distinguishing colonies of *M. catarrhalis* from neisserial colonies in cultures of respiratory secretions explains in part why *M. catarrhalis* has been overlooked as a pathogen. In contrast to these *Neisseria* species, *M. catarrhalis* colonies can be slid across the agar surface without disruption (the "hockey puck sign"). In addition, after 48 h of growth, *M. catarrhalis* colonies take on a pink color and tend to be larger than neisserial colonies. A variety of biochemical tests can distinguish *M. catarrhalis* from neisseriae. Kits that rely on these biochemical reactions are commercially available.

TREATMENT *MORAXELLA CATARRHALIS*

M. catarrhalis rapidly acquired β-lactamases during the 1970s and 1980s; antimicrobial susceptibility patterns have remained relatively stable since that time, with >90% of strains now producing β-lactamase and thus resistant to amoxicillin. Otitis media in children and exacerbations of COPD in adults are generally managed empirically with antimicrobial agents that are active against *S. pneumoniae*, *H. influenzae*, and *M. catarrhalis*. Most strains of *M. catarrhalis* are susceptible to amoxicillin/clavulanic acid, extended-spectrum cephalosporins, newer macrolides (azithromycin, clarithromycin), trimethoprim-sulfamethoxazole, and fluoroquinolones.

183e Infections Due to the HACEK Group and Miscellaneous Gram-Negative Bacteria

Tamar F. Barlam, Dennis L. Kasper

This is a digital-only chapter. It is available on the DVD that accompanies this book, as well as on Access Medicine/Harrison's Online, and the eBook and "app" editions of HPIM 19e.

THE HACEK GROUP

HACEK organisms are a group of fastidious, slow-growing, gram-negative bacteria whose growth requires an atmosphere of carbon dioxide. Species belonging to this group include several *Haemophilus* species, *Aggregatibacter* (formerly *Actinobacillus*) species, *Cardiobacterium hominis*, *Eikenella corrodens*, and *Kingella kingae*. HACEK bacteria normally reside in the oral cavity and have been associated with local infections in the mouth. They are also known to cause severe systemic infections—most often bacterial endocarditis, which can develop on either native or prosthetic valves (Chap. 155).

184 *Legionella* Infections

Victor L. Yu, M. Luisa Pedro-Botet, Yusen E. Lin

Legionellosis refers to the two clinical syndromes caused by bacteria of the genus *Legionella*. *Pontiac fever* is an acute, febrile, self-limited illness that has been serologically linked to *Legionella* species, whereas *Legionnaires' disease* is the designation for pneumonia caused by these species. Legionnaires' disease was first recognized in 1976, when an outbreak of pneumonia took place at a Philadelphia hotel during an American Legion convention.

MICROBIOLOGY

The family Legionellaceae comprises more than 50 species with more than 70 serogroups. The species *L. pneumophila* causes 80–90% of human infections and includes at least 16 serogroups; serogroups 1, 4, and 6 are most commonly implicated in human infections. To date, 18 species other than *L. pneumophila* have been associated with human infections, among which *L. micdadei* (Pittsburgh pneumonia agent), *L. bozemanii*, *L. dumoffii*, and *L. longbeachae* are the most common. Members of the Legionellaceae are aerobic gram-negative bacilli that do not grow on routine microbiologic media. Buffered charcoal yeast extract (BCYE) agar is the medium used to grow *Legionella*.

ECOLOGY AND TRANSMISSION

The natural habitats for *L. pneumophila* are aquatic bodies, including lakes and streams. *L. longbeachae* has been isolated from natural soil. Commercial potting soil has been suggested as the reservoir for *L. longbeachae* infections in Australia and New Zealand. *Legionella* can survive under a wide range of environmental conditions; for example, the organisms can live for years in refrigerated water samples. Natural bodies of water contain only small numbers of legionellae. However, once the organisms enter human-constructed aquatic reservoirs (such as drinking-water systems), they can grow and proliferate. Factors known to enhance colonization by and amplification of legionellae include warm temperatures (25°–42°C) and the presence of scale and sediment. *L. pneumophila* can form microcolonies within biofilms; its eradication from drinking-water systems requires disinfectants that can penetrate the biofilm. The presence of symbiotic microorganisms, including algae, amebas, ciliated protozoa, and other water-dwelling bacteria, promotes the growth of *Legionella*. The organisms can invade and multiply within free-living protozoa.

Heavy rainfall and flooding can result in the entry of high numbers of legionellae into water-distribution systems, leading to an upsurge of cases. Large buildings over three stories high are commonly colonized with *Legionella*. Sporadic community-acquired Legionnaires' disease has been linked to colonization of hotels, office buildings, factories, and even private homes. Drinking-water systems in hospitals and extended-care facilities have been the source for health care–associated Legionnaires' disease.

In contrast, cooling towers and evaporative condensers have been overestimated as sources of *Legionella* causing human illness. Early investigations that implicated cooling towers antedated the discovery that the organism could also exist in drinking water. In many outbreaks attributed to cooling towers, cases of Legionnaires' disease continued to occur despite disinfection of the towers; drinking water was found to be the actual source. Koch's postulates have never been fulfilled for *Legionella* links to cooling tower–associated outbreaks as they have been for hospital-acquired Legionnaires' disease. Nevertheless, cooling towers have, in rare instances, been implicated in community-acquired outbreaks, including an outbreak in Murcia, Spain. As mentioned above, *L. longbeachae* infections have been linked to potting soil, but the mode of transmission remains to be clarified.

Multiple modes of transmission of *Legionella* to humans exist, including aerosolization, aspiration, and direct instillation into the lungs during respiratory tract manipulations. Aspiration is now known to be the predominant mode of transmission, but it is unclear whether *Legionella* enters the lungs via oropharyngeal colonization or directly via the drinking of contaminated water. Oropharyngeal colonization with *Legionella* has been demonstrated in patients undergoing transplantation. Nasogastric tubes have been linked to hospital-acquired Legionnaires' disease; microaspiration of contaminated water was the hypothesized mode of transmission. Surgery with general anesthesia is a known risk factor that is consistent with aspiration. Especially compelling is the reported 30% incidence of postoperative Legionnaires' disease among patients undergoing head and neck surgery at a hospital with a contaminated water supply; aspiration is a recognized postoperative complication in such cases. One observational study showed that patients with hospital-acquired Legionnaires' disease underwent endotracheal intubation significantly more often and for a significantly longer duration than patients with hospital-acquired pneumonias of other etiologies.

Aerosolization of *Legionella* by devices filled with tap water, including whirlpools, nebulizers, and humidifiers, has been linked to cases in patients. An ultrasonic mist machine in the produce section of a grocery store has been the source in community outbreaks. Pontiac fever has been linked to *Legionella*-containing aerosols from water-using machinery, a cooling tower, air conditioners, and whirlpools.

EPIDEMIOLOGY

Community-Acquired Pneumonia The incidence of Legionnaires' disease depends on the degree of contamination of the aquatic reservoir, the immune status of the persons exposed to water from that reservoir, the intensity of exposure, and the availability of specialized laboratory tests on which the correct diagnosis can be based. Numerous prospective studies have ranked *Legionella* among the top four microbial causes of community acquired pneumonia, finding that it accounts for 2–13% of cases. (*Streptococcus pneumoniae*, *Haemophilus influenzae*, and *Chlamydia pneumoniae* are usually ranked first, second, and third, respectively.) On the basis of a multihospital study of community-acquired pneumonia in Ohio, the Centers for Disease Control and Prevention (CDC) estimated that only 3% of community-acquired cases of Legionnaires' disease are diagnosed as such. Observational studies of community-acquired pneumonia showed that Legionnaires' disease was largely unrecognized unless *Legionella* diagnostic testing was routinely applied to all patients with pneumonia; such studies in Spain and Germany resulted in detection of increased numbers of cases throughout Europe. It is likely that observational studies in Taiwan and Australia will have a similar result, with more cases identified throughout Asia as the index of suspicion rises.

Hospital-Acquired Pneumonia *Legionella* is responsible for 10–50% of cases of nosocomial pneumonia when a hospital's water system is colonized with the organism. The incidence of hospital-acquired Legionnaires' disease depends on the degree of contamination of drinking water, as defined by the rate of positivity of distal water sites; in contrast, the use of quantitative criteria of the number of colony-forming units per milliliter has proven useless.

Proactive culture of the hospital water supply has increased the detection of hospital-acquired Legionnaires' disease and simultaneously allowed expeditious diagnosis resulting in early administration of antibiotic therapy. In the early years after its recognition, Legionnaires' disease was documented primarily in the United States. As diagnostic modalities (especially the urinary antigen test) became more widely used, cases were documented in European hospitals. Likewise, following the enactment of public health guidelines in Taiwan, cases attributable to hospital tap water were found in Taiwanese hospitals. Risk factors for Legionnaires' disease include cigarette smoking, chronic lung disease, advanced age, prior hospitalization with discharge within 10 days before onset of pneumonia symptoms, and immunosuppression. Immunosuppressive conditions that predispose to Legionnaires' disease include transplantation, HIV infection, and treatment with glucocorticoids or tumor necrosis factor α antagonists. However, in a large prospective study of community-acquired pneumonia, 28% of patients with Legionnaires' disease did not have these classic risk factors. Hospital-acquired cases are now being recognized among neonates and immunosuppressed children.

Pneumonia in Transplant Recipients Transplant recipients appear to be at unusually high risk of *Legionella* pneumonia. This elevated risk may be due to diagnostic bias, given the extensive workup for opportunistic pathogens with pneumonic symptoms as well as the long-standing immunosuppression in this population of patients. Legionnaires' disease usually occurs in the 3 months after transplantation. Cavitation is seen on chest radiograph more frequently in transplant recipients, and mortality rates are higher.

Pontiac Fever Pontiac fever occurs in epidemics. The high attack rate (>90%) reflects airborne transmission.

PATHOGENESIS AND IMMUNITY

Legionella enters the lungs through aspiration or direct inhalation. Attachment to host cells is mediated by bacterial type IV pili, heat-shock proteins, a major outer-membrane protein, and complement. Because the organism possesses pili that mediate adherence to respiratory tract epithelial cells, conditions that impair mucociliary clearance, including cigarette smoking, lung disease, or alcoholism, predispose to Legionnaires' disease.

Both innate and adaptive immune responses play a role in host defense. Toll-like receptors mediate recognition of *L. pneumophila* in alveolar macrophages and enhance early neutrophil recruitment to the site of infection. Alveolar macrophages phagocytose legionellae by a conventional or a coiling mechanism. After phagocytosis, *L. pneumophila* evades intracellular killing by inhibiting phagosome–lysosome fusion. Although many legionellae are killed, some proliferate intracellularly until the cells rupture; the bacteria are then phagocytosed again by newly recruited phagocytes, and the cycle begins anew. The role of neutrophils in immunity appears to be minimal: neutropenic patients are not predisposed to Legionnaires' disease. Although *L. pneumophila* is susceptible to oxygen-dependent microbiologic systems in vitro, it resists killing by neutrophils. The humoral immune system is active against *Legionella*. Type-specific IgM and IgG antibodies are measurable within weeks of infection. In vitro, antibodies promote killing of *Legionella* by phagocytes (neutrophils, monocytes, and alveolar macrophages). Immunized animals develop a specific antibody response, with subsequent resistance to *Legionella* challenge. However, antibodies neither enhance lysis by complement nor inhibit intracellular multiplication within phagocytes.

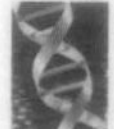

The genome of *L. pneumophila* has been sequenced. A broad range of membrane transporters within the genome are thought to optimize the use of nutrients in water and soil.

Some *L. pneumophila* strains are clearly more virulent than others, although the precise factors mediating virulence remain uncertain. For example, although multiple strains may colonize water-distribution systems, only a few cause disease in patients exposed to water from these systems. At least one surface epitope of *L. pneumophila* serogroup 1 is associated with virulence. Monoclonal antibody subtype mAb2 has been linked to virulence. *L. pneumophila* serogroup 6 is more commonly involved in hospital-acquired Legionnaires' disease and is especially likely to be associated with a poor outcome.

CLINICAL AND LABORATORY FEATURES

Pontiac Fever Pontiac fever is an acute, self-limiting, flu-like illness with an incubation period of 24–48 h. Pneumonia does not develop. Malaise, fatigue, and myalgias are the most common symptoms, occurring in 97% of cases. Fever (usually with chills) develops in 80–90% of cases and headache in 80%. Other symptoms (seen in fewer than 50% of cases) include arthralgias, nausea, cough, abdominal pain, and diarrhea. Modest leukocytosis with a neutrophilic predominance is sometimes detected. Complete recovery occurs within a few days; antibiotic therapy is unnecessary. A few patients may experience lassitude for some weeks after recovery. The diagnosis is established by antibody seroconversion. Pontiac fever due to *L. longbeachae* has been reported in individuals exposed to potting soil.

Legionnaires' Disease (Pneumonia) Legionnaires' disease is often included in the differential diagnosis of "atypical pneumonia," along with pneumonia due to *C. pneumoniae*, *Chlamydia psittaci*, *Mycoplasma pneumoniae*, *Coxiella burnetii*, and some viruses. The clinical similarities among "atypical" pneumonias include a nonproductive cough with a low frequency of grossly purulent sputum. The clinical manifestations of Legionnaires' disease are usually more severe than those of most "atypical" pneumonias. The course and prognosis of *Legionella* pneumonia more closely resemble those of bacteremic pneumococcal pneumonia than those of pneumonia due to other "atypical" pathogens. Patients with community-acquired Legionnaires' disease are significantly more likely than patients with pneumonia of other etiologies to be admitted to an intensive care unit (ICU) on presentation.

The incubation period for Legionnaires' disease is usually 2–10 days, although slightly longer incubation periods have been documented. Fever is almost universal. In one observational study, 20% of patients had temperatures in excess of 40°C (104°F). The symptoms and signs may range from a mild cough and a slight fever to stupor with widespread pulmonary infiltrates and multisystem failure. The mild cough of Legionnaires' disease is only slightly productive. Sometimes the sputum is streaked with blood. Chest pain—either pleuritic or nonpleuritic—can be a prominent feature and, when coupled with hemoptysis, can lead to an incorrect diagnosis of pulmonary embolism. Shortness of breath is reported by one-third to one-half of patients. Gastrointestinal difficulties are often pronounced; abdominal pain, nausea, and vomiting affect 10–20% of patients. Diarrhea (watery rather than bloody) is reported in 25–50% of cases. The most common neurologic abnormalities are confusion or changes in mental status; however, the multitudinous neurologic symptoms reported range from headache and lethargy to encephalopathy. Nonspecific symptoms—malaise, fatigue, anorexia, and headache—are reported early in the illness. Myalgias and arthralgias are uncommon but are prominent in a few patients. Upper respiratory symptoms, including coryza, are rare.

Relative bradycardia has been overemphasized as a useful diagnostic finding; it occurs primarily in older patients with severe pneumonia. Rales are detected by chest examination early in the course, and evidence of consolidation is found as the disease progresses. Abdominal examination may reveal generalized or local tenderness.

TABLE 184-1 CLINICAL CLUES SUGGESTIVE OF LEGIONNAIRES' DISEASE

Diarrhea
High fever (>40°C; >104°F)
Numerous neutrophils but no organisms revealed by Gram's staining of respiratory secretions
Hyponatremia (serum sodium level <131 mg/dL)
Failure to respond to β-lactam drugs (penicillins or cephalosporins) and aminoglycoside antibiotics
Occurrence of illness in an environment in which the potable water supply is known to be contaminated with *Legionella*
Onset of symptoms within 10 days after discharge from the hospital (hospital-acquired legionellosis manifesting after discharge or transfer)

Although the clinical manifestations often considered classic for Legionnaires' disease may suggest the diagnosis (Table 184-1), prospective comparative studies have shown that clinical manifestations are generally nonspecific and that Legionnaires' disease is not readily distinguishable from pneumonia of other etiologies. In a review of 13 studies of community-acquired pneumonia, clinical manifestations that occurred significantly more often in Legionnaires' disease included diarrhea, neurologic findings (including confusion), and a temperature of >39°C. Hyponatremia, elevated values in liver function tests, and hematuria also occurred more frequently in Legionnaires' disease. Other laboratory abnormalities include creatine phosphokinase elevation, hypophosphatemia, serum creatinine elevation, and proteinuria.

Sporadic cases of Legionnaires' disease appear to be more severe than outbreak-associated and hospital-acquired cases, presumably because their diagnosis is delayed. Results of the German CAPNETZ Study showed that, among cases of community-acquired *Legionella* pneumonia, ambulatory patients were as common as hospitalized patients.

Extrapulmonary Legionellosis Because the portal of entry for *Legionella* is the lung in virtually all cases, extrapulmonary manifestations usually result from bloodborne dissemination from the lung. *Legionella* has been identified in lymph nodes, spleen, liver, or kidneys in autopsied cases. Sinusitis, peritonitis, pyelonephritis, skin and soft tissue infection, septic arthritis, and pancreatitis have developed predominantly in immunosuppressed patients. The most severe sequela, neurologic dysfunction, is rare but can be debilitating. The most common neurologic deficits in the long term—ataxia and speech difficulties—result from cerebellar dysfunction.

We speculate that cardiac abnormalities in patients without pneumonia are caused by *Legionella*-contaminated water entering through an intravenous site, chest tube, or surgical wound, with subsequent seeding of a prosthetic valve, the myocardium, or the pericardium. This scenario is supported by cases occurring at Stanford University Hospital in which sternal wound infections and prosthetic valve endocarditis due to *L. pneumophila* were observed. The source was a sink in the postoperative surgical recovery ward.

Chest Radiography Virtually all patients with Legionnaires' disease have abnormal chest radiographs showing pulmonary infiltrates at the time of clinical presentation. In a few cases of hospital-acquired disease, fever and respiratory tract symptoms have preceded the radiographic appearance of the infiltrate. Radiologic findings are nonspecific. Pleural effusion is evident in 28–63% of patients on hospital admission. In immunosuppressed patients, especially those receiving glucocorticoids, distinctive rounded nodular opacities may be seen; these lesions may expand and cavitate (Fig. 184-1). Likewise, abscesses can occur in immunosuppressed hosts. The progression of infiltrates and pleural effusion on chest radiography despite appropriate antibiotic therapy within the first week is common, and radiographic improvement lags behind clinical improvement by several days. Complete clearing of infiltrates requires 1–4 months. Computed tomography (CT) is more sensitive than chest radiography, may show more extensive disease, and should be performed if fever persists during treatment with presumably effective antibiotics (Fig. 184-2).

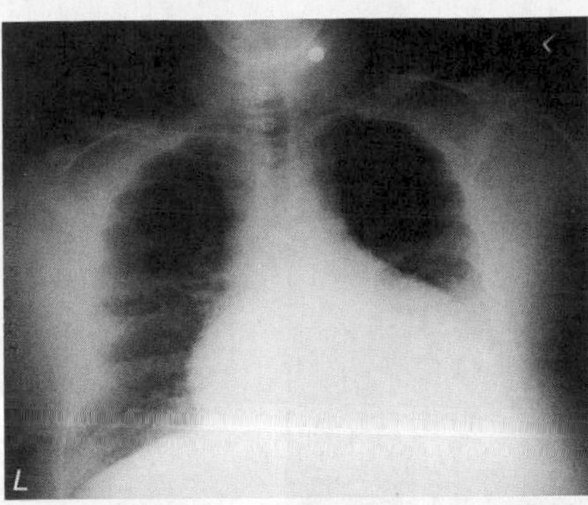

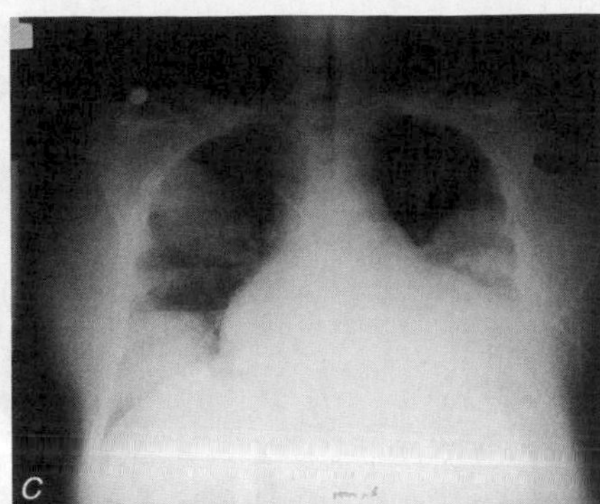

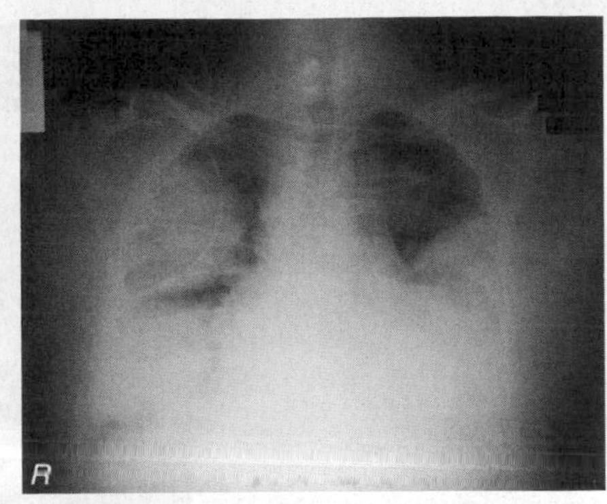

FIGURE 184-1 Chest radiographic findings in a 52-year-old man who presented with pneumonia subsequently diagnosed as Legionnaires' disease. The patient was a cigarette smoker with chronic obstructive pulmonary disease and alcoholic cardiomyopathy; he had received glucocorticoids. *Legionella pneumophila* was identified by direct fluorescent antibody staining and culture of sputum. ***Left:*** Baseline chest radiograph showing long-standing cardiomegaly. ***Center:*** Admission chest radiograph showing new rounded opacities. ***Right:*** Chest radiograph taken 3 days after admission, during treatment with erythromycin.

DIAGNOSIS

Given the nonspecific clinical manifestations of Legionnaires' disease and the high mortality rates for untreated Legionnaires' disease, *Legionella* testing—especially the *Legionella* urinary antigen test—is recommended for all patients with pneumonia, including patients with ambulatory pneumonia and hospitalized children. *Legionella* cultures should be made more widely available because the urinary antigen test can diagnose only *L. pneumophila* serogroup 1. Hospitals in which the drinking water is known to be colonized with *Legionella* species should have *Legionella* cultures routinely available.

The diagnosis of Legionnaires' disease requires special microbiologic tests (Table 184-2). The sensitivity of bronchoscopy specimens is similar to that of sputum samples for culture on selective media; if sputum is not available, bronchoscopy specimens may yield the organism. Bronchoalveolar lavage fluid gives higher yields than bronchial wash specimens. Thoracentesis should be performed if pleural effusion is found, and the fluid should be evaluated by direct fluorescent antibody (DFA) staining, culture, and the antigen assay designed for use with urine.

Stains Gram's staining of material from normally sterile sites, such as pleural fluid or lung tissue, occasionally suggests the diagnosis; efforts to detect *Legionella* in sputum by Gram's staining typically reveal numerous leukocytes but no organisms. When they are visualized, the organisms appear as small, pleomorphic, faint, gram-negative bacilli. *L. micdadei* organisms can be detected as weakly or partially acid-fast bacilli in clinical specimens.

The DFA stain is rapid and highly specific but is less sensitive than culture because large numbers of organisms are required for microscopic visualization. This test is more likely to be positive in advanced than in early disease.

Culture The definitive method for diagnosis of *Legionella* infection is isolation of the organism from respiratory secretions, although culture for 3–5 days is required. Antibiotics added to the medium suppress the growth of competing flora from nonsterile sites, and dyes color the colonies and assist in identification. The use of multiple selective BCYE media is necessary for maximal sensitivity. When culture plates are overgrown with other microflora, pretreatment of the specimen with acid or heat can markedly improve the yield. *L. pneumophila* is often isolated from sputum that is not grossly or microscopically purulent; sputum containing more than 25 epithelial cells per high-power field (a finding that classically suggests contamination) may still yield *L. pneumophila*.

Antibody Detection Antibody testing of both acute- and convalescent-phase sera is necessary. A fourfold rise in titer is diagnostic; 12 weeks are often required for the detection of an antibody response. A single titer of 1:128 in a patient with pneumonia constitutes circumstantial evidence for Legionnaires' disease. The CDC uses a titer of 1:256 as presumptive evidence for Legionnaires' disease. Serology is of use primarily in epidemiologic studies. The specificity of serology for *Legionella* species other than *L. pneumophila* is uncertain; there is cross-reactivity within *Legionella* species and with some gram-negative bacilli. Serology is used as the criterion for the diagnosis of Pontiac fever.

Urinary Antigen The assay for *Legionella* soluble antigen in urine is second only to culture in terms of sensitivity and is highly specific. A rapid immunochromatographic assay is commercially available (BinaxNOW; Alere, Waltham, MA). This assay is relatively inexpensive and easy to perform. Its drawback is that the urinary antigen test is reliable only for *L. pneumophila* serogroup 1, which causes ~80% of *Legionella* infections. Cross-reactivity with other *L. pneumophila* serogroups and other *Legionella* species has been detected in up to 22% of urine samples from patients with culture-proven cases. Antigen in urine is detectable 3 days after the onset of clinical disease and disappears over 2 months; positivity can be prolonged when patients receive glucocorticoids. The test is not affected by antibiotic administration.

Molecular Methods DFA stains can identify a number of *Legionella* species. Both polyclonal and monoclonal antibody stains are commercially available. Polymerase chain reaction (PCR) with DNA probes is being applied in-house in selected hospitals but is not yet commercially available. PCR has proven somewhat useful in the identification of *Legionella* from environmental water specimens. Epidemiologic links cannot easily be made with PCR because the infecting pathogen is not available for molecular subtyping.

Procalcitonin can be used as an indicator of severity of illness in patients in ICUs. Clinical response to antibiotics can be monitored by procalcitonin levels.

TREATMENT *LEGIONELLA* INFECTION

Because *Legionella* is an intracellular pathogen, antibiotics that can attain high intracellular concentrations are most likely to be effective. The dosages for various drugs used in the treatment of *Legionella* infection are listed in Table 184-3.

The macrolides (especially azithromycin) and the respiratory quinolones are now the antibiotics of choice and are effective as monotherapy. Compared with erythromycin, the newer macrolides have superior in vitro activity, display greater intracellular activity, reach higher concentrations in respiratory secretions and lung tissue, and have fewer adverse effects. The pharmacokinetics of the newer macrolides and quinolones also allow once- or twice-daily dosing. Quinolones are the preferred antibiotics for transplant recipients because both macrolides and rifampin interact pharmacologically with cyclosporine and tacrolimus. Retrospective uncontrolled studies have shown that complications of pneumonia are fewer and clinical response is more rapid in patients receiving quinolones than in those receiving macrolides. Initial therapy should be given by the

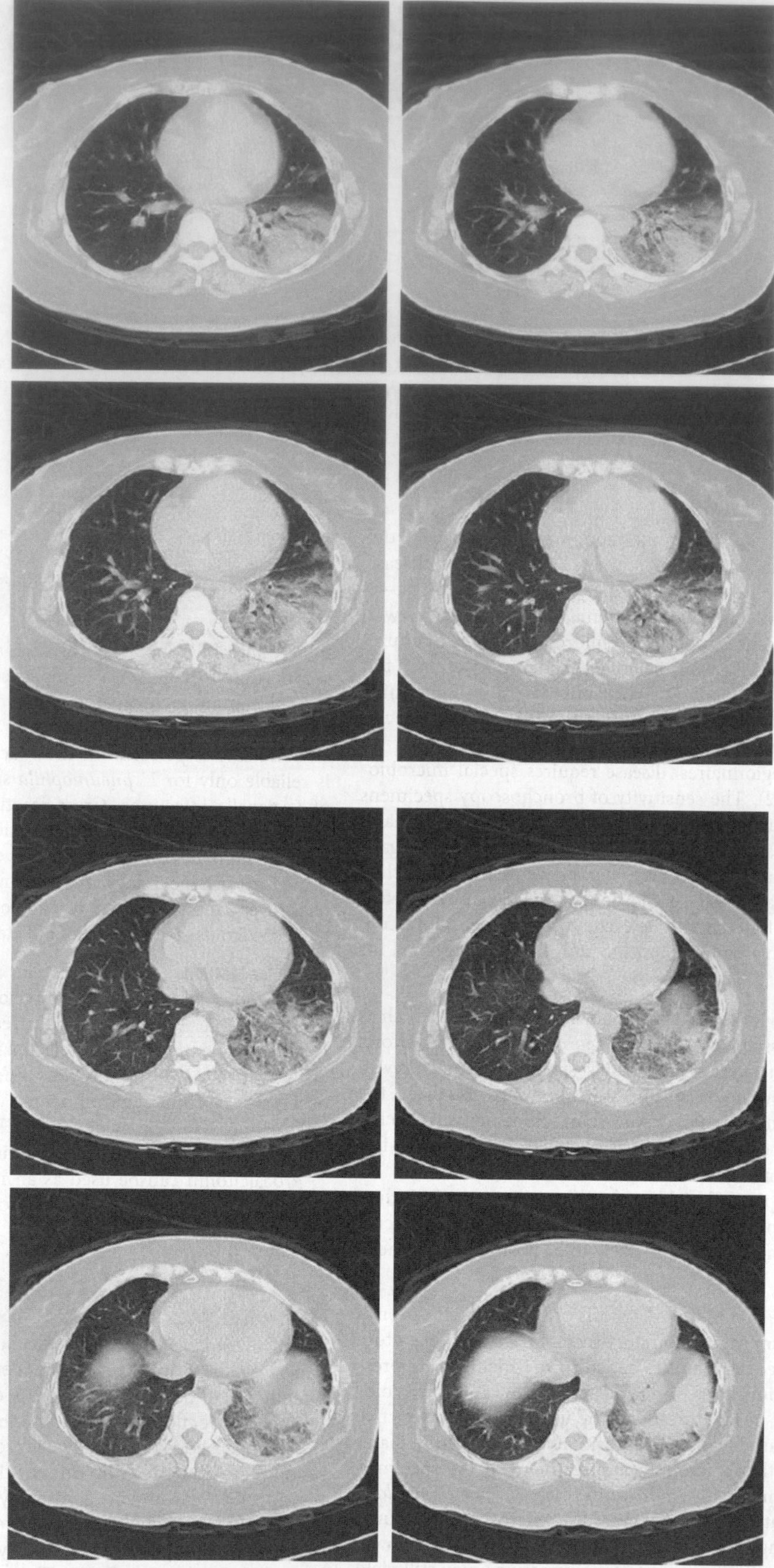

FIGURE 184-2 Computed tomography (CT) scans of a 49-year-old woman with no underlying conditions who presented with community-acquired pneumonia. CT revealed multilobar infiltrates, some of which were not as prominent on chest x-ray. Cultures of both the patient's sputum and her home water supply yielded *Legionella pneumophila* serogroup 1. *(Images courtesy of Dr. Wen-Chien Ko, National Cheng Kung University Hospital, Tainan, Taiwan.)*

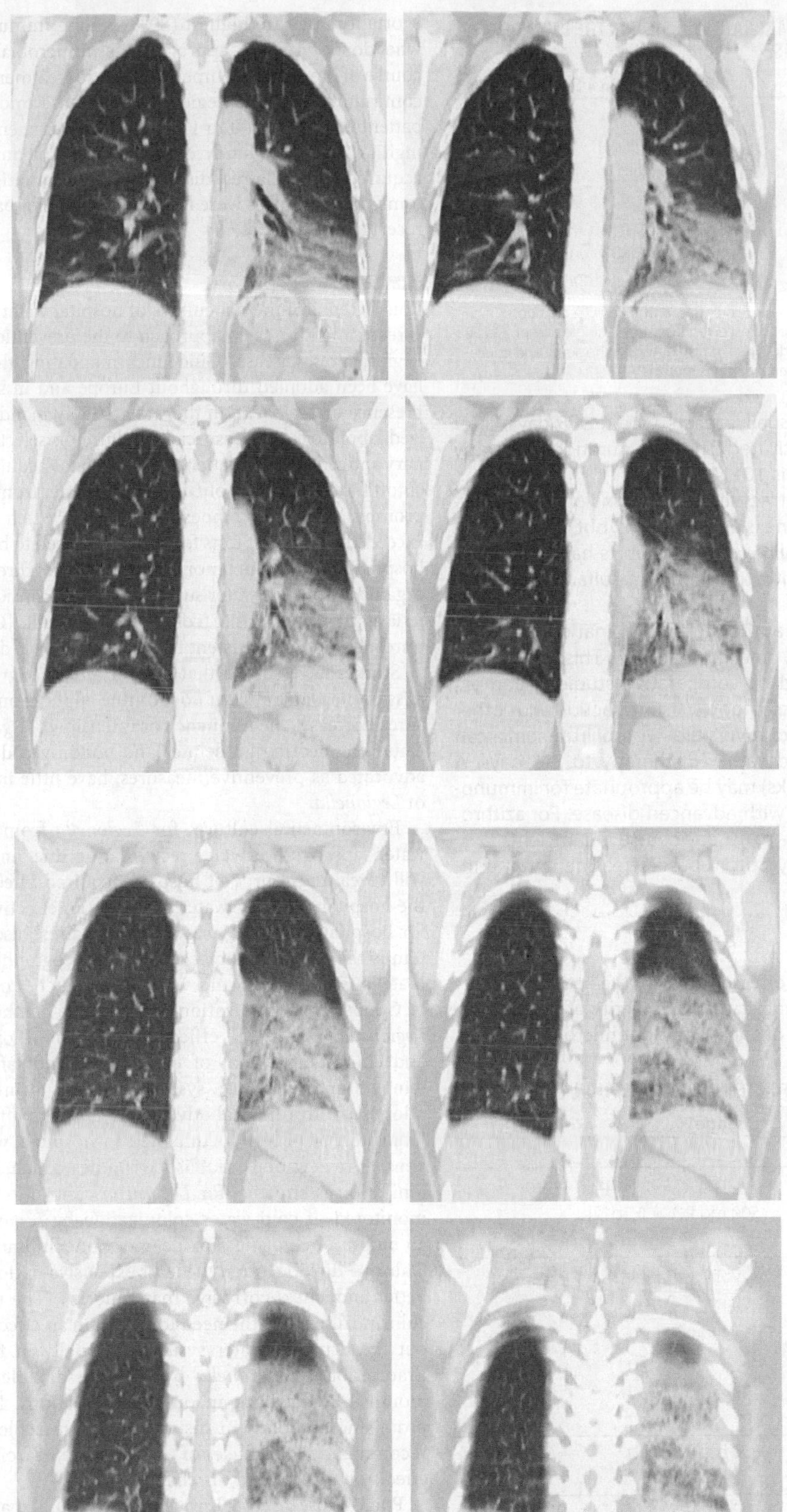

FIGURE 184-2 *(Continued)*

TABLE 184-2 UTILITY OF SPECIAL LABORATORY TESTS FOR THE DIAGNOSIS OF LEGIONNAIRES' DISEASE

Test	Sensitivity, %	Specificity, %
Culture		
Sputum[a]	80	100
Transtracheal aspirate	90	100
Direct fluorescent antibody staining of sputum	50–70	96–99
Urinary antigen testing[b]	70	100
Antibody serology[c]	40–60	96–99

[a]Use of multiple selective media with dyes. [b]Reliable only for *L. pneumophila* serogroup 1. [c]IgG and IgM testing of both acute- and convalescent-phase sera. A single titer of ≥1:256 is considered presumptive, whereas a fourfold rise in titer between the acute and convalescent phases is considered definitive. Titers peak at 3 months.

IV route. A clinical response usually occurs within 3–5 days, after which oral therapy can be substituted. The total duration of therapy in the immunocompetent host is 10–14 days.

Alternative agents include tetracycline and its analogues doxycycline and minocycline. Tigecycline is active in vitro, but clinical experience with this drug is minimal. Anecdotal reports have described both successes and failures with trimethoprim-sulfamethoxazole, imipenem, and clindamycin.

For critically ill patients, the authors use combination regimens of azithromycin, a quinolone, and/or rifampin. This practice is empirical and is not supported by comparative studies. Rifampin is highly active in vitro and in cell models. Its interaction with other medications and its side effect of reversible hyperbilirubinemia can be minimized by limiting the duration of therapy to 3–5 days. A longer course of therapy (3 weeks) may be appropriate for immunosuppressed patients and those with advanced disease. For azithromycin, with its long half-life, a 5- to 10-day course is sufficient.

Pontiac fever requires only symptom-based treatment, not antimicrobial therapy.

PROGNOSIS

Mortality rates for Legionnaires' disease vary with the patient's underlying disease, the patient's immune status, the severity of pneumonia, and the timing of administration of appropriate antimicrobial therapy.

TABLE 184-3 ANTIBIOTIC THERAPY FOR *LEGIONELLA* INFECTION

Antimicrobial Agent	Dosage[a]
Macrolides	
Azithromycin	500 mg[b] PO or IV[c] q24h
Clarithromycin	500 mg PO or IV[c] q12h
Quinolones	
Levofloxacin	750 mg IV q24h
	500 mg[b] PO q24h
Ciprofloxacin	400 mg IV q8h
	750 mg PO q12h
Moxifloxacin	400 mg[b] PO q24h
Ketolide	
Telithromycin	800 mg PO q24h
Tetracyclines	
Doxycycline	100 mg[b] PO or IV q12h
Minocycline	100 mg[b] PO or IV q12h
Tetracycline	500 mg PO or IV q6h
Tigecycline	100-mg IV load, then 50 mg IV q12h
Others	
Trimethoprim-sulfamethoxazole	160/800 mg IV q8h
	160/800 mg PO q12h
Rifampin[d]	300–600 mg PO or IV q12h

[a]Dosages are derived from clinical experience. [b]The authors recommend doubling the first dose. [c]The IV formulation is not available in some countries. [d]Rifampin should be used only in combination with a macrolide or a quinolone.

Mortality rates are highest (80%) among immunosuppressed patients who do not receive appropriate antimicrobial therapy early in the course of illness. With timely antibiotic treatment, mortality rates from community-acquired Legionnaires' disease among immunocompetent patients range from 0 to 11%; without treatment, the figure may be as high as 31%. In a study of survivors of an outbreak of community-acquired Legionnaires' disease, sequelae of fatigue, neurologic symptoms, and weakness were found in 63–75% of patients 17 months after receipt of antibiotics.

PREVENTION

Routine environmental culture of hospital water supplies for *Legionella* is recommended as an approach to the prevention of hospital-acquired Legionnaires' disease. Guidelines mandating this proactive approach have been adopted throughout Europe and in several U.S. states. The presence of *Legionella* in the water supply mandates the use of specialized laboratory tests (especially culture on selective media and the urinary antigen test) for patients with hospital-acquired pneumonia. A 30% cutoff for the presence of *Legionella* in water from multiple hospital sites prompts an increased index of suspicion. When the 30% cutoff point is exceeded, diagnostic tests for *Legionella* need to be applied in all cases of hospital-acquired pneumonia, and measures directed at eliminating the organism from the water supply should be considered. Quantitative criteria at a given water site (colony-forming units [CFU]/mL) have proven unreliable and inconsistent in the prediction of disease.

Studies have shown that neither a high degree of outward cleanliness of the water system nor routine application of maintenance measures decreases the frequency or intensity of *Legionella* contamination. Thus, engineering guidelines and building codes, although routinely advocated as preventive measures, have little impact on the presence of *Legionella*.

Environmental cultures for *Legionella* from cold-water taps, hot-water taps, the hot-water recirculating line, and water-storage tanks will reveal the source of hospital-acquired infections. Disinfection of the hospital drinking-water system is an effective preventive measure for hospital-acquired cases of Legionnaires' diseases because this system is the reservoir for *Legionella*. In geographic areas where the climate is semitropical, cold-water lines may be colonized by *Legionella*.

Copper-silver ionization is a reliable method for eradication of *Legionella*. Unlike the efficacy of chlorine dioxide decontamination and chlorination, that of ionization is not affected by high water temperature. Ionization systems are easy to install, and the ions are odorless, with minimal adverse effects. The efficacy of copper-silver ionization has been documented in hospitals worldwide. A comprehensive review of 10 published studies concluded that copper-silver ionization is effective for *Legionella* control as long as ion levels are monitored. If cold-water colonization by *Legionella* is the source of an outbreak, chlorine dioxide and monochloramine offer advantages. Chlorine dioxide, often the least expensive option, penetrates biofilms better and is less corrosive than chlorine. The major disadvantage of chlorine dioxide is the need to maintain an effective residual throughout the drinking-water system, especially in the hot-water system. Eradication of *Legionella* by chlorine dioxide may require several months—a drawback in outbreak situations. Monochloramine is a promising approach in disinfection. Hyperchlorination is no longer recommended because of its expense, carcinogenicity, corrosive effects on piping, and unreliable efficacy.

Point-of-use disposable water filters (0.2 μm) may be an economical and effective option in high-risk areas (e.g., ICUs and transplantation units). These filters can be used in an outbreak situation for a limited period.

Ineffective yet expensive methods that are often promulgated include removal of stagnation ("dead legs") in the water-distribution system and replacement or disinfection/cleaning of distal outlets. Infection control personnel should oversee the selection of disinfection technology and should apply evidence-based criteria when making their choice. Managers of health care facilities should not be given the primary responsibility for selection and subsequent monitoring of measures to eliminate and control *Legionella*.

185 Pertussis and Other *Bordetella* Infections

Karina A. Top, Scott A. Halperin

Pertussis is an acute infection of the respiratory tract caused by *Bordetella pertussis*. The name *pertussis* means "violent cough," which aptly describes the most consistent and prominent feature of the illness. The inspiratory sound made at the end of an episode of paroxysmal coughing gives rise to the common name for the illness, "whooping cough." However, this feature is variable: it is uncommon among infants ≤6 months of age and is frequently absent in older children and adults. The Chinese name for pertussis is "the 100-day cough," which accurately describes the clinical course of the illness. The identification of *B. pertussis* was first reported by Bordet and Gengou in 1906, and vaccines were produced over the following two decades.

MICROBIOLOGY

Of the 10 identified species in the genus *Bordetella*, only four are of major medical significance. *B. pertussis* infects only humans and is the most important *Bordetella* species causing human disease. *B. parapertussis* causes an illness in humans that is similar to pertussis but is typically milder; co-infections with *B. parapertussis* and *B. pertussis* have been documented. With improved polymerase chain reaction (PCR) diagnostic methodology, up to 20% of patients with a pertussis-like syndrome have been found to be infected with *B. holmesii*, formerly thought to be an unusual cause of bacteremia. *B. bronchiseptica* is an important pathogen of domestic animals that causes kennel cough in dogs, atrophic rhinitis and pneumonia in pigs, and pneumonia in cats. Both respiratory infection and opportunistic infection due to *B. bronchiseptica* are occasionally reported in humans. *B. petrii*, *B. hinzii*, and *B. ansorpii* have been isolated from patients who are immunocompromised.

Bordetella species are gram-negative pleomorphic aerobic bacilli that share common genotypic characteristics. *B. pertussis* and *B. parapertussis* are the most similar of the species, but *B. parapertussis* does not express the gene coding for pertussis toxin. *B. pertussis* is a slow-growing fastidious organism that requires selective medium and forms small, glistening, bifurcated colonies. Suspicious colonies are presumptively identified as *B. pertussis* by direct fluorescent antibody testing or by agglutination with species-specific antiserum. *B. pertussis* is further differentiated from other *Bordetella* species by biochemical and motility characteristics.

B. pertussis produces a wide array of toxins and biologically active products that are important in its pathogenesis and in immunity. Most of these virulence factors are under the control of a single genetic locus that regulates their production, resulting in antigenic modulation and phase variation. Although these processes occur both in vitro and in vivo, their importance in the pathobiology of the organism is unknown; they may play a role in intracellular persistence and person-to-person spread. The organism's most important virulence factor is *pertussis toxin*, which is composed of a B oligomer–binding subunit and an enzymatically active A protomer that ADP-ribosylates a guanine nucleotide-binding regulatory protein (G protein) in target cells, producing a variety of biologic effects. Pertussis toxin has important mitogenic activity, affects the circulation of lymphocytes, and serves as an adhesin for bacterial binding to respiratory ciliated cells. Other important virulence factors and adhesins are *filamentous hemagglutinin*, a component of the cell wall, and *pertactin*, an outer membrane protein. *Fimbriae*, bacterial appendages that play a role in bacterial attachment, are the major antigens against which agglutinating antibodies are directed. These agglutinating antibodies have historically been the primary means of serotyping *B. pertussis* strains. Other virulence factors include tracheal cytotoxin, which causes respiratory epithelial damage; adenylate cyclase toxin, which impairs host immune-cell function; dermonecrotic toxin, which may contribute to respiratory mucosal damage; and lipooligosaccharide, which has properties similar to those of other gram-negative bacterial endotoxins.

EPIDEMIOLOGY

Pertussis is a highly communicable disease, with attack rates of 80–100% among unimmunized household contacts and 20% within households in well-immunized populations. The infection has a worldwide distribution, with cyclical outbreaks every 3–5 years (a pattern that has persisted despite widespread immunization). Pertussis occurs in all months; however, in North America, its activity peaks in summer and autumn.

In developing countries, pertussis remains an important cause of infant morbidity and death. The reported incidence of pertussis worldwide has decreased as a result of improved vaccine coverage (Fig. 185-1). However, coverage rates are still <50% in many developing nations; the World Health Organization (WHO) estimates that 90% of the burden of pertussis is in developing regions. In addition, overreporting of immunization coverage and underreporting of disease result in substantial underestimation of the global burden of pertussis. The WHO estimates that there were 195,000 deaths from pertussis among children in 2008.

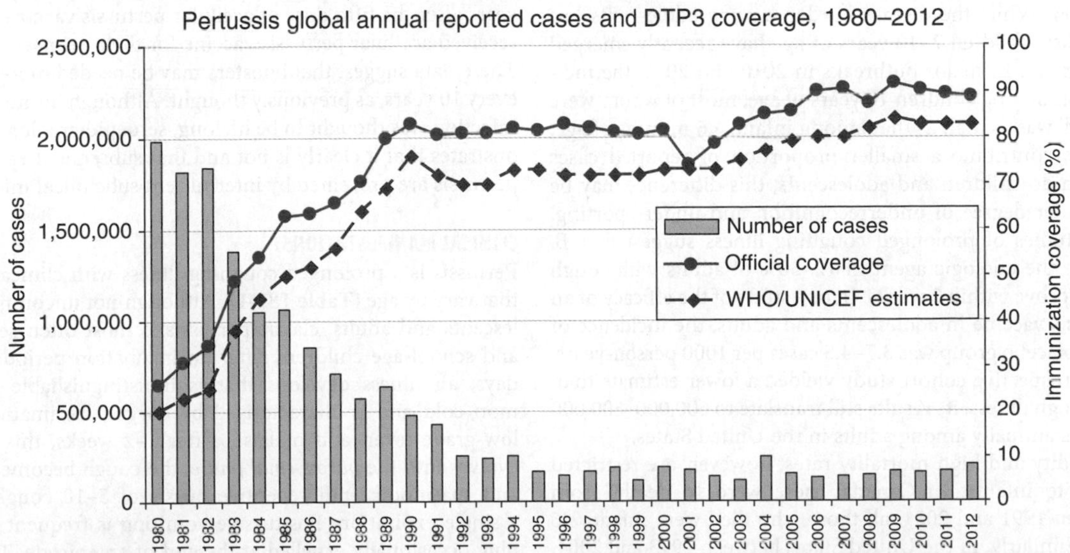

FIGURE 185-1 Global annual reported cases of pertussis and rate of coverage with DTP3 (diphtheria toxoid, tetanus toxoid, and pertussis vaccine; 3 doses), 1980–2012. *(© World Health Organization, 2013. All rights reserved. From www.who.int/immunization/monitoring_surveillance/burden/vpd/surveillance_type/passive/Pertussis_coverage.JPG. Source: WHO/IVB database, 2013.)*

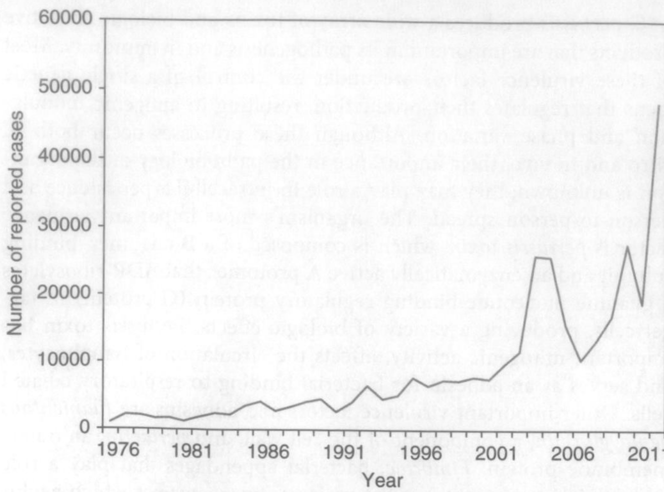

FIGURE 185-2 Reported cases of pertussis by year—United States, 1976–2012. *(From the Centers for Disease Control and Prevention, www.cdc.gov/pertussis/surv-reporting/cases-by-year.html. Accessed December 17, 2013.)*

Before the institution of widespread immunization programs in the developed world, pertussis was one of the most common infectious causes of morbidity and death. In the United States before the 1940s, between 115,000 and 270,000 cases of pertussis were reported annually, with an average yearly rate of 150 cases per 100,000 population. With universal childhood immunization, the number of reported cases fell by >95%, and mortality rates decreased even more dramatically. Only 1010 cases of pertussis were reported in 1976 (**Fig. 185-2**). After that historic low, rates of pertussis slowly increased. In recent years, pertussis epidemics have been reported with increasing frequency worldwide. The United States experienced widespread outbreaks of pertussis in 2005, 2010, and 2012 at levels not seen in 40–50 years (>40,000 reported cases in 2012).

Although thought of as a disease of childhood, pertussis can affect people of all ages and is increasingly being identified as a cause of prolonged coughing illness in adolescents and adults. In unimmunized populations, pertussis incidence peaks during the preschool years, and well over half of children have the disease before reaching adulthood. In highly immunized populations such as those in North America, the peak incidence is among infants <1 year of age who have not completed the three-dose primary immunization series. An increase in pertussis incidence among adolescents and adults began in the late 1990s and led to the introduction of an adolescent booster across North America by 2006. While the disease burden among adolescents has started to decrease, children 7–10 years of age have recently emerged as a high-risk group. In major outbreaks in 2010 and 2012, the incidence of pertussis among children 10 years of age, most of whom were fully immunized, was as high as that among infants <6 months of age. Although adults contribute a smaller proportion of reported cases of pertussis than do children and adolescents, this difference may be related to a greater degree of underrecognition and underreporting. A number of studies of prolonged coughing illness suggest that *B. pertussis* may be the etiologic agent in 12–30% of adults with cough that does not improve within 2 weeks. In one study of the efficacy of an acellular pertussis vaccine in adolescents and adults, the incidence of pertussis in the placebo group was 3.7–4.5 cases per 1000 person-years. Although this prospective cohort study yielded a lower estimate than the studies of cough illness, its results still translate to 600,000–800,000 cases of pertussis annually among adults in the United States.

Severe morbidity and high mortality rates, however, are restricted almost entirely to infants. In Canada, there were 16 deaths from pertussis between 1991 and 2001; all those who died were infants ≤6 months of age. Similarly, in the United States between 1993 and 2004, all pertussis deaths and 86% of hospitalizations for pertussis involved infants ≤3 months of age. Although school-age children are the source of infection for most households, adults are the likely source for cases in high-risk infants and may serve as the reservoir of infection between epidemic years.

PATHOGENESIS

Infection with *B. pertussis* is initiated by attachment of the organism to the ciliated epithelial cells of the nasopharynx. Attachment is mediated by surface adhesins (e.g., pertactin and filamentous hemagglutinin), which bind to the integrin family of cell-surface proteins, probably in conjunction with pertussis toxin. The role of fimbriae in adhesion and in maintenance of infection has not been fully delineated. At the site of attachment, the organism multiplies, producing a variety of other toxins that cause local mucosal damage (tracheal cytotoxin, dermonecrotic toxin). Impairment of host defense by *B. pertussis* is mediated by pertussis toxin and adenylate cyclase toxin. There is local cellular invasion, with intracellular bacterial persistence; however, systemic dissemination does not occur. Systemic manifestations (lymphocytosis) result from the effects of the toxins.

The pathogenesis of the clinical manifestations of pertussis is poorly understood. It is not known what causes the hallmark paroxysmal cough. A pivotal role for pertussis toxin has been proposed. Proponents of this position point to the efficacy of preventing clinical symptoms with a vaccine containing only pertussis toxoid. Detractors counter that pertussis toxin is not the critical factor because paroxysmal cough also occurs in patients infected with *B. parapertussis*, which does not produce pertussis toxin. It is thought that neurologic events in pertussis, such as seizures and encephalopathy, are due to hypoxia from coughing paroxysms or apnea rather than to the effects of specific bacterial products. *B. pertussis* pneumonia, which occurs in up to 10% of infants with pertussis, is usually a diffuse bilateral primary infection. In older children and adults with pertussis, pneumonia is often due to secondary bacterial infection with streptococci or staphylococci. Deaths from pertussis among young infants are frequently associated with very high levels of leukocytosis and pulmonary hypertension.

IMMUNITY

Both humoral and cell-mediated immunity are thought to be important in pertussis. Antibodies to pertussis toxin, filamentous hemagglutinin, pertactin, and fimbriae are all protective in animal models. Pertussis agglutinins were correlated with protection in early studies of whole-cell pertussis vaccines. Serologic correlates of protection conferred by acellular pertussis vaccines have not been established, although antibody to pertactin, fimbriae, and (to a lesser degree) pertussis toxin correlated best with protection in two efficacy trials. The duration of immunity after whole-cell pertussis vaccination is short-lived, with little protection remaining after 10–12 years. Recent studies have demonstrated early waning of immunity—i.e., within 2–4 years after the fifth dose of acellular pertussis vaccine in children who received acellular pertussis vaccine for their primary series in infancy. These data suggest that boosters may be needed more frequently than every 10 years, as previously thought. Although immunity after natural infection was thought to be lifelong, seroepidemiologic evidence demonstrates that it clearly is not and that subsequent episodes of clinical pertussis are prevented by intermittent subclinical infection.

CLINICAL MANIFESTATIONS

Pertussis is a prolonged coughing illness with clinical manifestations that vary by age (**Table 185-1**). Although not uncommon among adolescents and adults, classic pertussis is most often seen in preschool and school-age children. After an incubation period averaging 7–10 days, an illness develops that is indistinguishable from the common cold and is characterized by coryza, lacrimation, mild cough, low-grade fever, and malaise. After 1–2 weeks, this *catarrhal phase* evolves into the *paroxysmal phase*: the cough becomes more frequent and spasmodic with repetitive bursts of 5–10 coughs, often within a single expiration. Posttussive vomiting is frequent, with a mucous plug occasionally expelled at the end of an episode. The episode may be terminated by an audible whoop, which occurs upon rapid inspiration against a closed glottis at the end of a paroxysm. During a spasm, there may be impressive neck-vein distension, bulging eyes, tongue

TABLE 185-1 CLINICAL FEATURES OF PERTUSSIS, BY AGE GROUP AND DIAGNOSTIC STATUS

	Percentage of Patients		
	Adolescents and Adults		
Feature	Laboratory Confirmation	No Laboratory Confirmation	Children
Cough	95–100	95–100	95–100
Prolonged	60–80	60–80	60–95
Paroxysmal	60–90	50–90	80–95
Sleep-disturbing	50–80	50–80	90–100
Whoop	10–40	5–30	40–80
Posttussive vomiting	20–50	5–30	80–90

protrusion, and cyanosis. Paroxysms may be precipitated by noise, eating, or physical contact. Between attacks, the patient's appearance is normal but increasing fatigue is evident. The frequency of paroxysmal episodes varies widely, from several per hour to 5–10 per day. Episodes are often worse at night and interfere with sleep. Weight loss is not uncommon as a result of the illness's interference with eating. Most complications occur during the paroxysmal stage. Fever is uncommon and suggests bacterial superinfection.

After 2–4 weeks, the coughing episodes become less frequent and less severe—changes heralding the onset of the *convalescent phase.* This phase can last 1–3 months and is characterized by gradual resolution of coughing episodes. For 6–12 months, intercurrent viral infections may be associated with a recrudescence of paroxysmal cough.

Not all individuals who develop pertussis have classic disease. The clinical manifestations in adolescents and adults are more often atypical. In a German study of pertussis in adults, more than two-thirds had paroxysmal cough and more than one-third had whoop. Adult illness in North America differs from this experience: the cough may be severe and prolonged but is less frequently paroxysmal, and a whoop is uncommon. Vomiting with cough is the best predictor of pertussis as the cause of prolonged cough in adults. Other predictive features are a cough at night, sweating episodes between paroxysms of coughing, and exposure to other individuals with a prolonged coughing illness.

COMPLICATIONS

Complications are frequently associated with pertussis and are more common among infants than among older children or adults. Subconjunctival hemorrhages, abdominal and inguinal hernias, pneumothoraces, and facial and truncal petechiae can result from increased intrathoracic pressure generated by severe fits of coughing. Weight loss can follow decreased caloric intake. In a series of more than 1100 children <2 years of age who were hospitalized with pertussis, 27.1% had apnea, 9.4% had pneumonia, 2.6% had seizures, and 0.4% had encephalopathy; 10 children (0.9%) died. Pneumonia is reported in <5% of adolescents and adults and increases in frequency after 50 years of age. In contrast to the primary *B. pertussis* pneumonia that develops in infants, pneumonia in adolescents and adults with pertussis is usually caused by a secondary infection with encapsulated organisms such as *Streptococcus pneumoniae* or *Haemophilus influenzae.* Pneumothorax, severe weight loss, inguinal hernia, rib fracture, carotid artery aneurysm, and cough syncope have all been reported in adolescents and adults with pertussis.

DIAGNOSIS

If the classic symptoms of pertussis are present, clinical diagnosis is not difficult. However, particularly in older children and adults, it is difficult to differentiate infections caused by *B. pertussis* and *B. parapertussis* from other respiratory tract infections on clinical grounds. Therefore, laboratory confirmation should be attempted in all cases. Lymphocytosis (an absolute lymphocyte count of $>10^8$–10^9/L) is common among young children, in whom it is unusual with other infections, but not among adolescents and adults. Culture of nasopharyngeal secretions remains the gold standard of diagnosis, although DNA detection by PCR has replaced culture in many laboratories because of increased sensitivity and quicker results. Appropriate PCR methodology must include primers to differentiate among *B. pertussis, B. parapertussis,* and *B. holmesii.* The best specimen is collected by nasopharyngeal aspiration, in which a fine flexible plastic catheter attached to a 10-mL syringe is passed into the nasopharynx and withdrawn while gentle suction is applied. Since *B. pertussis* is highly sensitive to drying, secretions for culture should be inoculated without delay onto appropriate medium (Bordet-Gengou or Regan-Lowe), or the catheter should be flushed with a phosphate-buffered saline solution for culture and/or PCR. An alternative to the aspirate is a Dacron or rayon nasopharyngeal swab; again, inoculation of culture plates should be immediate or an appropriate transport medium (e.g., Regan-Lowe charcoal medium) should be used. Results of PCR can be available within hours; cultures become positive by day 5 of incubation. *B. pertussis* and *B. parapertussis* can be differentiated by agglutination with specific antisera or by direct immunofluorescence.

Nasopharyngeal cultures in untreated pertussis remain positive for a mean of 3 weeks after the onset of illness; these cultures become negative within 5 days of the institution of appropriate antimicrobial therapy. The duration of a positive PCR in untreated pertussis or after therapy is not known but exceeds that of positive cultures. Since much of the period during which the organism can be recovered from the nasopharynx falls into the catarrhal phase, when the etiology of the infection is not suspected, there is only a small window of opportunity for culture-proven diagnosis. Cultures from infants and young children are more frequently positive than those from older children and adults; this difference may reflect earlier presentation of the former age group for medical care. Direct fluorescent antibody tests of nasopharyngeal secretions for direct diagnosis may still be available in some laboratories but should not be used because of poor sensitivity and specificity. Pseudo-outbreaks of pertussis have been reported as a result of false-positive PCR results. Greater standardization of PCR methodology can alleviate this problem.

As a result of the difficulties with laboratory diagnosis of pertussis in adolescents, adults, and patients who have been symptomatic for >4 weeks, increasing attention is being given to serologic diagnosis. Enzyme immunoassays detecting IgA and IgG antibodies to pertussis toxin, filamentous hemagglutinin, pertactin, and fimbriae have been developed and assessed for reproducibility. Two- or fourfold increases in antibody titer are suggestive of pertussis, although cross-reactivity of some antigens (such as filamentous hemagglutinin and pertactin) among *Bordetella* species makes it difficult to depend diagnostically on seroconversion involving a single type of antibody. Late presentation for medical care and prior immunization also complicate serologic diagnosis because the first sample obtained may in fact be a convalescent-phase specimen. Criteria for serologic diagnosis based on comparison of results for a single serum specimen with established population values are gaining acceptance, and serologic measurement of antibody to pertussis toxin is becoming more widely standardized and available for diagnostic purposes, particularly in outbreak settings and for surveillance.

DIFFERENTIAL DIAGNOSIS

A child presenting with paroxysmal cough, posttussive vomiting, and whoop is likely to have an infection caused by *B. pertussis* or *B. parapertussis*; lymphocytosis increases the likelihood of a *B. pertussis* etiology. Viruses such as respiratory syncytial virus and adenovirus have been isolated from patients with clinical pertussis but probably represent co-infection.

In adolescents and adults, who often do not have paroxysmal cough or whoop, the differential diagnosis of a prolonged coughing illness is more extensive. Pertussis should be suspected when any patient has a cough that does not improve within 14 days, a paroxysmal cough of any duration, a cough followed by vomiting (adolescents and adults), or any respiratory symptoms after contact with a laboratory-confirmed case of pertussis. Other etiologies to consider include infections caused by *Mycoplasma pneumoniae, Chlamydia pneumoniae,* adenovirus, influenza virus, and other respiratory viruses. Use of angiotensin-converting

TABLE 185-2 ANTIMICROBIAL THERAPY FOR PERTUSSIS

Drug	Adult Daily Dose	Frequency	Duration, Days	Comments
Erythromycin estolate	1–2 g	3 divided doses	7–14	Frequent gastrointestinal side effects
Clarithromycin	500 mg	2 divided doses	7	—
Azithromycin	500 mg on day 1, 250 mg subsequently	1 daily dose	5	—
Trimethoprim-sulfamethoxazole	160 mg of trimethoprim, 800 mg of sulfamethoxazole	2 divided doses	14	For patients allergic to macrolides; data on effectiveness limited

enzyme (ACE) inhibitors, reactive airway disease, and gastroesophageal reflux disease are well-described noninfectious causes of prolonged cough in adults.

TREATMENT PERTUSSIS

ANTIBIOTICS

The purpose of antibiotic therapy for pertussis is to eradicate the infecting bacteria from the nasopharynx; therapy does not substantially alter the clinical course unless given early in the catarrhal phase. Macrolide antibiotics are the drugs of choice for treatment of pertussis (**Table 185-2**); macrolide-resistant *B. pertussis* strains have been reported but are rare. Trimethoprim-sulfamethoxazole is recommended as an alternative for individuals allergic to macrolides.

SUPPORTIVE CARE

Young infants have the highest rates of complication and death from pertussis; therefore, most infants (and older children with severe disease) should be hospitalized. A quiet environment may decrease the stimulation that can trigger paroxysmal episodes. Use of β-adrenergic agonists and/or glucocorticoids has been advocated by some authorities but has not been proven to be effective. Cough suppressants are not effective and play no role in the management of pertussis.

INFECTION CONTROL MEASURES

Hospitalized patients with pertussis should be placed in respiratory isolation, with the use of precautions appropriate for pathogens spread by large respiratory droplets. Isolation should continue for 5 days after initiation of macrolide therapy or, in untreated patients, for 3 weeks (i.e., until nasopharyngeal cultures are consistently negative).

PREVENTION

Chemoprophylaxis Because the risk of transmission of *B. pertussis* within households is high, chemoprophylaxis is widely recommended for household contacts of pertussis cases. The effectiveness of chemoprophylaxis, although unproven, is supported by several epidemiologic studies of institutional and community outbreaks. In the only randomized placebo-controlled study, erythromycin estolate (50 mg/kg per day in three divided doses; maximum dose, 1 g/d) was effective in reducing the incidence of bacteriologically confirmed pertussis by 67%; however, there was no decrease in the incidence of clinical disease. Despite these disappointing results, many authorities continue to recommend chemoprophylaxis, particularly in households with members at high risk of severe disease (children <1 year of age, pregnant women). Data are not available on use of the newer macrolides for chemoprophylaxis, but these drugs are commonly used because of their increased tolerability and their effectiveness.

Immunization (See also Chap. 148) The mainstay of pertussis prevention is active immunization. Pertussis vaccine became widely used in North America after 1940; the reported number of pertussis cases subsequently fell by >90%. Whole-cell pertussis vaccines are prepared through the heating, chemical inactivation, and purification of whole *B. pertussis* organisms. Despite their efficacy (average estimate, 85%; range for different products, 30–100%), whole-cell pertussis vaccines are associated with adverse events—both common (fever; injection-site pain, erythema, and swelling; irritability) and uncommon (febrile seizures, hypotonic hyporesponsive episodes). Alleged associations of whole-cell pertussis vaccine with encephalopathy, sudden infant death syndrome, and autism, although not substantiated, have spawned an active anti-immunization lobby. The development of acellular pertussis vaccines, which are effective and less reactogenic, has greatly alleviated concerns about the inclusion of pertussis vaccine in the combined infant immunization series.

Although whole-cell vaccines are still used extensively in developing regions of the world, acellular pertussis vaccines are used exclusively for childhood immunization in much of the developed world. In North America, acellular pertussis vaccines for children are given as a three-dose primary series at 2, 4, and 6 months of age, with a reinforcing dose at 15–18 months of age and a booster dose at 4–6 years of age.

Although a wide variety of acellular pertussis vaccines were developed, only a few are still widely marketed; all contain pertussis toxoid and filamentous hemagglutinin. One acellular pertussis vaccine also contains pertactin, and another contains pertactin and two types of fimbriae. In light of phase 3 efficacy studies, most experts have concluded that two-component acellular pertussis vaccines are more effective than monocomponent vaccines and that the addition of pertactin increases efficacy still more. The further addition of fimbriae appears to enhance protective efficacy against milder disease. In two studies, protection conferred by pertussis vaccines correlated best with the production of antibody to pertactin, fimbriae, and pertussis toxin.

Adult formulations of acellular pertussis vaccines have been shown to be safe, immunogenic, and efficacious in clinical trials in adolescents and adults and are now recommended for routine immunization of these groups in several countries, including the United States. In this country, adolescents should receive a dose of the adult-formulation diphtheria–tetanus–acellular pertussis vaccine at the preadolescence physician's visit, and all unvaccinated adults should receive a single dose of this combined vaccine. In addition, in the United States, pertussis immunization is specifically recommended for health care workers and for women during each pregnancy to increase passive transfer of maternal antibodies to the fetus. Pertussis vaccine coverage among U.S. adolescents was 78.2% in 2011, but coverage among adults is low (2.1% as of 2007). Further improvements in adult vaccine coverage may permit better control of pertussis across the age spectrum, with collateral protection of infants too young to be immunized. However, more effective vaccines with longer-lasting protection will ultimately be needed to control this disease.

186 Diseases Caused by Gram-Negative Enteric Bacilli

Thomas A. Russo, James R. Johnson

GENERAL FEATURES AND PRINCIPLES

Escherichia coli, *Klebsiella*, *Proteus*, *Enterobacter*, *Serratia*, *Citrobacter*, *Morganella*, *Providencia*, *Cronobacter*, and *Edwardsiella* are gram-negative enteric bacilli that are members of the family Enterobacteriaceae. *Salmonella*, *Shigella*, and *Yersinia*, also in the family Enterobacteriaceae, are discussed in Chaps. 190, 191, and 196, respectively. These pathogens cause a wide variety of infections involving diverse anatomic sites in both healthy and compromised hosts. Increasing antimicrobial resistance in this group has put them at the forefront of an evolving public health crisis. In addition, new infectious syndromes have emerged. Therefore, a thorough knowledge of clinical presentations and appropriate therapeutic choices is necessary for optimal outcomes.

EPIDEMIOLOGY

E. coli, *Klebsiella*, *Proteus*, *Enterobacter*, *Serratia*, *Citrobacter*, *Morganella*, *Providencia*, *Cronobacter*, and *Edwardsiella* are components of the normal animal and human colonic microbiota and/or the microbiota of a variety of environmental habitats, including long-term-care facilities (LTCFs) and hospitals. As a result, except for certain pathotypes of intestinal pathogenic *E. coli*, these genera are global pathogens. The incidence of infection due to these agents is increasing because of the combination of an aging population and increasing antimicrobial resistance. In healthy humans, *E. coli* is the predominant species of gram-negative bacilli (GNB) in the colonic flora; *Klebsiella* and *Proteus* are less prevalent. GNB (primarily *E. coli*, *Klebsiella*, and *Proteus*) only transiently colonize the oropharynx and skin of healthy individuals. In contrast, in LTCFs and hospital settings, a variety of GNB emerge as the dominant microbiota of both mucosal and skin surfaces, particularly in association with antimicrobial use, severe illness, and extended length of stay. LTCFs are emerging as an important reservoir for resistant GNB. This colonization may lead to subsequent infection; for example, oropharyngeal colonization may lead to pneumonia. Interestingly, the use of ampicillin or amoxicillin was associated with an increased risk of subsequent infection due to the hypervirulent variant of *Klebsiella pneumoniae* in Taiwan; this association suggests that changes in the quantity or prevalence of colonizing bacteria may be important. *Serratia* and *Enterobacter* infection may be acquired through a variety of infusates (e.g., medications, blood products). *Edwardsiella* infections are acquired through freshwater and marine environment exposures and are most common in Southeast Asia.

STRUCTURE AND FUNCTION

Enteric GNB possess an extracytoplasmic outer membrane, which consists of a lipid bilayer with associated proteins, lipoproteins, and polysaccharides (capsule, lipopolysaccharide). The outer membrane interfaces with the external environment, including the human host. A variety of components of the outer membrane are critical determinants in pathogenesis (e.g., capsule) and antimicrobial resistance (e.g., permeability barrier, efflux pumps).

PATHOGENESIS

Multiple bacterial virulence factors are required for the pathogenesis of infections caused by GNB. Possession of specialized virulence genes defines pathogens and enables them to infect the host efficiently. Hosts and their cognate pathogens have been co-adapting throughout evolutionary history. During the host-pathogen "chess match" over time, various and redundant strategies have emerged in both the pathogens and their hosts (Table 186-1).

Intestinal pathogenic mechanisms are discussed below. The members of the Enterobacteriaceae family that cause extraintestinal infections are primarily extracellular pathogens and therefore share certain pathogenic features. Innate immunity (including the activities of complement, antimicrobial peptides, and professional phagocytes) and humoral immunity are the principal host defense components. Both susceptibility to and severity of infection are increased with dysfunction or deficiencies of these components. By contrast, the virulence traits of intestinal pathogenic *E. coli*—i.e., the distinctive strains that can cause diarrheal disease—are for the most part different from those of extraintestinal pathogenic *E. coli* (ExPEC) and other GNB that cause extraintestinal infections. This distinction reflects site-specific differences in host environments and defense mechanisms.

A given strain usually possesses multiple adhesins for binding to a variety of host cells (e.g., in *E. coli*: type 1, S, and F1C fimbriae; P pili). Nutrient acquisition (e.g., of iron via siderophores) requires many genes that are necessary but not sufficient for pathogenesis. The ability to resist the bactericidal activity of complement and phagocytes in the absence of antibody (e.g., as conferred by capsule or O antigen of lipopolysaccharide) is one of the defining traits of an extracellular pathogen. Tissue damage (e.g., as mediated by hemolysin in the case of *E. coli*) may facilitate spread within the host. Without doubt, many important virulence genes await identification (Chap. 145e).

The ability to induce septic shock is another defining feature of these genera. GNB are the most common causes of this potentially lethal syndrome. Pathogen-associated molecular pattern molecules (PAMPs; e.g., the lipid A moiety of lipopolysaccharide) stimulate a proinflammatory host response via pattern recognition receptors (e.g., Toll-like or C-type lectin receptors) that activate host defense signaling pathways; if overly exuberant, this response results in shock (Chap. 325). Direct bacterial damage of host tissue (e.g., by toxins) or collateral damage from the host response can result in the release of damage-associated molecular pattern molecules (DAMPs; e.g., HMGB1) that can propagate a detrimental proinflammatory host response.

Many antigenic variants (serotypes) exist in most genera of GNB. For example, *E. coli* has more than 150 O-specific antigens and more than 80 capsular antigens. This antigenic variability, which permits immune evasion and allows recurrent infection by different strains of the same species, has impeded vaccine development (Chap. 148).

TABLE 186-1 INTERACTIONS OF EXTRAINTESTINAL PATHOGENIC *ESCHERICHIA COLI* WITH THE HUMAN HOST: A PARADIGM FOR EXTRACELLULAR, EXTRAINTESTINAL GRAM-NEGATIVE BACTERIAL PATHOGENS

Bacterial Goal	Host Obstacle	Bacterial Solution
Extraintestinal attachment	Flow of urine, mucociliary blanket	Multiple adhesins (e.g., type 1, S, and F1C fimbriae; P pili)
Nutrient acquisition for growth	Nutrient sequestration (e.g., iron via intracellular storage and extracellular scavenging via lactoferrin and transferrin)	Cellular lysis (e.g., hemolysin), multiple mechanisms for competing for iron (e.g., siderophores) and other nutrients
Initial avoidance of host bactericidal activity	Complement, phagocytic cells, antimicrobial peptides	Capsular polysaccharide, lipopolysaccharide
Dissemination (within host and between hosts)	?	Irritant tissue damage resulting in increased excretion (e.g., toxins such as hemolysin)
Late avoidance of host bactericidal activity	Acquired immunity (e.g., specific antibodies), treatment with antibiotics	?Cell entry, acquisition of antimicrobial resistance

E. coli can cause either intestinal or extraintestinal infection, depending on the particular pathotype, and *Edwardsiella tarda* can cause both intestinal and extraintestinal infection. *Klebsiella* primarily causes extraintestinal infection, but hemorrhagic colitis has been associated with a toxin-producing variant of *Klebsiella oxytoca*. Depending on both the host and the pathogen, nearly every organ or body cavity can be infected with GNB. *E. coli* and—to a lesser degree—*Klebsiella* account for most extraintestinal infections due to GNB and are the most virulent pathogens within this group; this virulence is demonstrated by the ability of *E. coli* and *Klebsiella pneumoniae* (primarily the hypervirulent variant) to cause severe infections in healthy, ambulatory hosts from the community. However, the other genera are also important, especially among LTCF residents and hospitalized patients, in large part because of the intrinsic or acquired antimicrobial resistance of these organisms and the increasing number of individuals with compromised host defenses. The mortality rate is substantial in many GNB infections and correlates with the severity of illness. Especially problematic are pneumonia and bacteremia (arising from any source), particularly when complicated by organ failure (severe sepsis) and/or shock, for which the associated mortality rates are 20–50%.

DIAGNOSIS

Isolation of GNB from sterile sites almost always implies infection, whereas their isolation from nonsterile sites, particularly from open soft-tissue wounds and the respiratory tract, requires clinical correlation to differentiate colonization from infection. Tentative laboratory identification based on lactose fermentation and indole production (described for each genus below), which usually is possible before final identification of the organism and determination of its antimicrobial susceptibilities, may help to guide empirical antimicrobial therapy.

TREATMENT INFECTIONS CAUSED BY GRAM-NEGATIVE ENTERIC BACILLI

(See also Chap. 170) Evidence indicates that initiation of appropriate empirical antimicrobial therapy early in the course of GNB infections (particularly serious infections) leads to improved outcomes. The ever-increasing prevalence of multidrug-resistant (MDR) and extensively drug-resistant (XDR) GNB; the lag between published (historical) and current resistance rates; and variations by species, geographic location, regional antimicrobial use, and hospital site (e.g., intensive care units [ICUs] versus wards) necessitate familiarity with evolving patterns of antimicrobial resistance for the selection of appropriate empirical therapy. Factors predictive of isolate resistance include recent antimicrobial use, a health care association (e.g., recent or ongoing hospitalization, dialysis, residence in an LTCF), or international travel (e.g., to Asia, Latin America, Africa, southern Europe). For appropriately selected patients, it may be prudent initially, while susceptibility results are awaited, to use two potentially active agents with the rationale that at least one agent will be active. If broad-spectrum treatment has been initiated, it is critical to switch to the most appropriate narrower-spectrum agent when information on antimicrobial susceptibility becomes available. Such responsible antimicrobial stewardship will slow down the ever-escalating cycle of selection for increasingly resistant bacteria, decrease the likelihood of *Clostridium difficile* infection, decrease costs, and maximize the useful longevity of available antimicrobial agents. Likewise, it is important to avoid treatment of patients who are colonized but not infected (e.g., who have a positive sputum culture without evidence of pneumonia). At present, the most reliably active agents against enteric GNB are the carbapenems (e.g., imipenem), the aminoglycoside amikacin, the fourth-generation cephalosporin cefepime, the β-lactam/β-lactamase inhibitor combination piperacillin-tazobactam, and the polymyxins (e.g., colistin or polymyxin B). The number of antimicrobials effective against certain Enterobacteriaceae is shrinking. Truly pan-resistant GNB exist, and it is unlikely that new agents will come to market in the short term. Accordingly, the presently available antimicrobials must be used judiciously.

β-Lactamases, which inactivate β-lactam agents, are the most important mediators of resistance to these drugs in GNB. Decreased permeability and/or active efflux of β-lactam agents, although less common, may occur alone or in combination with β-lactamase-mediated resistance.

Broad-spectrum β-lactamases (e.g., TEM, SHV), which mediate resistance to many penicillins and first-generation cephalosporins, are frequently expressed in enteric GNB. These enzymes are inhibited by β-lactamase inhibitors (e.g., clavulanate, sulbactam, tazobactam). They usually do not hydrolyze third- and fourth-generation cephalosporins or cephamycins (e.g., cefoxitin).

Extended-spectrum β-lactamases (ESBLs; e.g., CTX-M, SHV, TEM) are modified broad-spectrum enzymes that confer resistance to the same drugs as well as to third-generation cephalosporins, aztreonam, and (in some instances) fourth-generation cephalosporins. GNB that express ESBLs may also possess porin mutations that result in decreased uptake of cephalosporins and β-lactam/β-lactamase inhibitor combinations. The prevalence of acquired ESBL production, particularly of CTX-M-type enzymes, is increasing in GNB worldwide, in large part due to the presence of the responsible genes on large transferable plasmids with linked or associated resistance to fluoroquinolones, trimethoprim-sulfamethoxazole (TMP-SMX), aminoglycosides, and tetracyclines. To date, ESBLs are most prevalent in *K. pneumoniae*, *K. oxytoca*, and *E. coli* but also occur (and are probably underrecognized) in *Enterobacter*, *Citrobacter*, *Proteus*, *Serratia*, and other enteric GNB. At present, the rough regional prevalence of ESBL-producing GNB is India > China > rest of Asia, Latin America, Africa, southern Europe > northern Europe > United States, Canada, and Australia. International travel to high-prevalence regions increases the likelihood of colonization with these strains. ESBL-producing GNB were initially described in hospitals (ICUs > wards) and LTCFs, where outbreaks occurred in association with extensive use of third-generation cephalosporins. However, over the last decade, the incidence of uncomplicated cystitis due to CTX-M ESBL-containing *E. coli* has increased worldwide (including in the United States) among healthy ambulatory women without health care or antimicrobial exposure. Antimicrobial use in food animals has also been implicated in the rise of ESBLs.

The carbapenems are the most reliably active β-lactam agents against ESBL-expressing strains. Clinical experience with alternatives is more limited, but, for organisms susceptible to piperacillin-tazobactam (minimal inhibitory concentration [MIC], ≤4 μg/mL), this agent—at a dosage of 4.5 g q6h—may offer a carbapenem-sparing alternative, at least for *E. coli*. The role of tigecycline is unclear despite its excellent in vitro activity; *Proteus*, *Morganella*, and *Providencia* are inherently resistant, and attainable serum and urine levels are low. Therefore, caution appears to be prudent, especially with serious infections, until more clinical data become available. Oral options for the treatment of strains expressing CTX-M ESBLs are limited, with fosfomycin being the most reliably active agent (see section below on the treatment of extraintestinal *E. coli* infections).

AmpC β-lactamases, when induced or stably derepressed to high levels of expression, confer resistance to the same substrates as ESBLs plus the cephamycins (e.g., cefoxitin and cefotetan). The genes encoding these enzymes are primarily chromosomally located and therefore may not exhibit the linked or associated resistance to fluoroquinolones, TMP-SMX, aminoglycosides, and tetracyclines that is common with ESBLs. These enzymes are problematic for the clinician: resistance may develop during therapy with third-generation cephalosporins, resulting in clinical failure, particularly in the setting of bacteremia. Although chromosomal AmpC β-lactamases are present in nearly all members of the Enterobacteriaceae family, the risk of clinically significant induction of high expression levels or selection of stably derepressed mutants with cephalosporin treatment is greatest with *Enterobacter cloacae* and *Enterobacter aerogenes*, lower with *Serratia marcescens* and *Citrobacter freundii*, and lowest with *Providencia* and *Morganella morganii*. In addition, rare strains of *E. coli*, *K. pneumoniae*, and other Enterobacteriaceae have acquired plasmids containing inducible AmpC β-lactamase genes. Carbapenems are a viable treatment option. The fourth-generation cephalosporin cefepime may be an appropriate option if the concomitant presence of an ESBL can be excluded and source control is achieved. Other carbapenem-sparing alternatives to consider if isolates are susceptible in vitro are fluoroquinolones, piperacillin-tazobactam, TMP-SMX, tigecycline, and aminoglycosides, although clinical data are limited.

Carbapenemases (e.g., KPC [class A]; NDM-1, VIM, and IMP [class B]; and OXA-48 [class D]) confer resistance to the same drugs as ESBLs and also to cephamycins and carbapenems. Similar to ESBLs, carbapenemases are usually encoded on large transferable plasmids, which often encode linked resistance to fluoroquinolones, TMP-SMX, tetracyclines, and aminoglycosides. Unfortunately, carbapenemase-producing Enterobacteriaceae are becoming increasingly common, particularly in Asia, and infection with these strains is associated with elevated mortality rates. This reality has prompted the Centers for Disease Control and Prevention (CDC) to categorize carbapenem-resistant Enterobacteriaceae as an "urgent threat" to health care. Carbapenemase production by Enterobacteriaceae is most prevalent in *K. pneumoniae* and *E. coli* but has been described in nearly all members of the family. Automated susceptibility systems may be unreliable for detection of carbapenemases. An elevated MIC or a diminished zone diameter for meropenem or imipenem should prompt genotypic confirmation, if available. Alternatively, the phenotype can be confirmed with a modified Hodge test (which detects classes A, B, and D, although results can be false positive) and/or inhibition tests with boronic acid (class A), EDTA (class B), or dipicolinic acid (class B). Carbapenem resistance may also occur in the absence of carbapenemase production and can be mediated by AmpC β-lactamase and ESBL production coupled with modifications in permeability/efflux.

For treatment of carbapenem-resistant Enterobacteriaceae, tigecycline and colistin are the parenteral agents with the most reliable in vitro activity. However, because tigecycline reaches only low serum and urine concentrations, caution is warranted in using it to treat bacteremia and perhaps urinary tract infection (UTI), although a few case reports describe some success with tigecycline therapy for UTI. Colistin has nephrotoxic and neurotoxic potential. Furthermore, increasing resistance has been described to both of these agents. Thus the clinician is left with few or no therapeutic options. Aminoglycosides may have some utility if active. Fosfomycin is often active in vitro, but clinical data are limited, concerns exist about the development of resistance with monotherapy, and no parenteral formulation is available in the United States. Although control data are lacking, combination therapy is being used in this setting with the goals of increasing efficacy and decreasing the emergence of resistance.

Resistance to fluoroquinolones usually is due to alterations of the target site (DNA gyrase and/or topoisomerase IV), with or without decreased permeability, active efflux, or protection of the target site. Resistance to this drug class is increasingly prevalent among GNB and is associated with resistance to other antimicrobial classes; for example, 20–80% of ESBL-producing enteric GNB are also resistant to fluoroquinolones. At present, quinolones should be considered unreliable as empirical therapy for infections due to GNB in critically ill patients.

In this era of increasing antimicrobial resistance, it is critical to culture the local site of infection before the initiation of antimicrobial therapy and, for systemically ill patients, to obtain blood samples for culture. Antimicrobial resistance may not always be identified by in vitro testing; therefore, it is important to assess the clinical response to treatment. Moreover, as discussed above, resistance may emerge during therapy through the induction or stable derepression of AmpC β-lactamases. In addition, drainage of abscesses, resection of necrotic tissue, and removal of infected foreign bodies are often required for cure. GNB are commonly involved in polymicrobial infections, in which the role of each individual pathogen is uncertain (Chap. 201). Although some GNB are more pathogenic than others, it is usually prudent, if possible, to design an antimicrobial regimen active against all of the GNB identified, because each is capable of pathogenicity in its own right. Lastly, for patients treated initially with a broad-spectrum empirical regimen, the regimen should be de-escalated as expeditiously as possible once susceptibility results are known and the patient has responded to therapy.

PREVENTION

(See also Chap. 168) Avoidance of inappropriate antimicrobial use is a key measure in preventing infections due to antimicrobial-resistant strains and the further development of antimicrobial resistance. Antimicrobial stewardship programs should be adopted to facilitate achievement of this goal. Diligent adherence to hand-hygiene protocols by health care personnel, cleaning/disinfection of objects that come into contact with patients (e.g., stethoscopes and blood pressure cuffs), and contact precautions should be implemented for patients colonized or infected with carbapenem-resistant (and perhaps other XDR) GNB. Avoidance of the use of indwelling devices (e.g., urinary and intravascular catheters, endotracheal tubes) and, when such devices are necessary, placement according to an appropriate protocol decrease infection risk. Likewise, protocols for daily use evaluation and removal as soon as possible should be implemented. Patient positioning (e.g., head of bed at ≥30°) and good oral hygiene decrease the incidence of pneumonia among ventilated patients. Increasing data support the implementation of universal decolonization to prevent infection in ICU patients.

ESCHERICHIA COLI INFECTIONS

Strains of *E. coli* are united by a core genome of ~2000 genes. A strain's ability to cause infections and the nature of such infections are defined by ancillary genes that encode various virulence factors. This experiment of nature is fluid and ongoing, as demonstrated by the recent evolution of Shiga toxin–producing enteroaggregative *E. coli*.

COMMENSAL STRAINS

For the most part, commensal *E. coli* variants, which constitute the bulk of the normal facultative intestinal flora in most humans, confer benefits to the host (e.g., resistance to colonization with pathogenic organisms). These strains generally lack the specialized virulence traits that enable extraintestinal and intestinal pathogenic *E. coli* strains to cause disease outside and within the gastrointestinal tract, respectively. However, even commensal *E. coli* strains can be involved in extraintestinal infections in the presence of an aggravating factor, such as a foreign body (e.g., a urinary catheter), host compromise (e.g., local anatomic or functional abnormalities, such as urinary or biliary tract obstruction or systemic immunocompromise), or an inoculum that is large or contains a mixture of bacterial species (e.g., fecal contamination of the peritoneal cavity).

EXTRAINTESTINAL PATHOGENIC STRAINS

ExPEC strains are the most common enteric GNB to cause community-acquired and health care–associated bacterial infections. The emerging propensity of these strains to acquire new antimicrobial resistance mechanisms (e.g., ESBL and carbapenemase production) has posed challenges in managing ExPEC infection. One clonal group—ST131, the members of which are usually resistant to fluoroquinolones and increasingly express an ESBL (CTX-M)—has undergone global dissemination.

Like commensal *E. coli* (but in contrast to intestinal pathogenic *E. coli*), ExPEC strains are often found in the intestinal flora of healthy individuals and do not cause gastroenteritis in humans. Entry from their site of colonization (e.g., the colon, vagina, or oropharynx) into a normally sterile extraintestinal site (e.g., the urinary tract, peritoneal cavity, or lungs) is the rate-limiting step for infection. ExPEC strains have acquired genes encoding diverse extraintestinal virulence factors that enable the bacteria to cause infections outside the gastrointestinal tract in both normal and compromised hosts (Table 186-1). These virulence genes define ExPEC and, for the most part, are distinct from those that enable intestinal pathogenic strains to cause diarrheal disease (Table 186-2). All age groups, all types of hosts, and nearly all organs and anatomic sites are susceptible to infection by ExPEC. Even previously healthy hosts can become severely ill or die when infected with ExPEC; however, adverse outcomes are more common among hosts with comorbid illnesses and host defense abnormalities. The diversity and the medical and economic impact of ExPEC infections are evident from consideration of the following specific syndromes.

Extraintestinal Infectious Syndromes • ***URINARY TRACT INFECTION*** The urinary tract is the site most frequently infected by ExPEC. An exceedingly common infection among ambulatory patients, UTI accounts for 1% of ambulatory care visits in the United States and is second only to lower respiratory tract infection among infections responsible for hospitalization. UTIs are best considered by clinical syndrome (e.g., uncomplicated cystitis, pyelonephritis, and catheter-associated UTIs) and within the context of specific hosts (e.g., premenopausal women, compromised hosts; Chap. 162). *E. coli* is the single most common pathogen for all UTI syndrome/host group combinations. Each year in the United States, *E. coli* causes 80–90% of an estimated 6–8 million episodes of uncomplicated cystitis in premenopausal women. Furthermore, 20% of women with an initial cystitis episode develop frequent recurrences.

Uncomplicated cystitis, the most common acute UTI syndrome, is characterized by dysuria, urinary frequency, and suprapubic pain. Fever and/or back pain suggests progression to pyelonephritis. Even with appropriate treatment of pyelonephritis, fever may take 5–7 days to resolve completely. Persistently elevated or increasing fever and neutrophil counts should prompt evaluation for intrarenal or perinephric abscess and/or obstruction. Renal parenchymal damage and loss of renal function during pyelonephritis occur primarily with urinary obstruction, which can be preexisting or, rarely, occurs de novo in diabetic patients who develop renal papillary necrosis as a result of kidney infection. Pregnant women are at unusually high risk for developing pyelonephritis, which can adversely affect the outcome of pregnancy. As a result, prenatal screening for and treatment of asymptomatic bacteriuria are standard. Prostatic infection is a potential complication of UTI in men. The diagnosis and treatment of UTI, as detailed in Chap. 162, should be tailored to the individual host, the nature and site of infection, and local patterns of antimicrobial susceptibility.

ABDOMINAL AND PELVIC INFECTION The abdomen/pelvis is the second most common site of extraintestinal infection due to *E. coli*. A wide variety of clinical syndromes occur in this location, including acute peritonitis secondary to fecal contamination, spontaneous bacterial peritonitis, dialysis-associated peritonitis, diverticulitis, appendicitis, intraperitoneal or visceral abscesses (hepatic, pancreatic, splenic), infected pancreatic pseudocysts, and septic cholangitis and/or cholecystitis. In intraabdominal infections, *E. coli* can be isolated either alone or (as often occurs) in combination with other facultative and/or anaerobic members of the intestinal flora (Chap. 159).

PNEUMONIA *E. coli* is not usually considered a cause of pneumonia (Chap. 153). Indeed, enteric GNB account for only 1–3% of cases of community-acquired pneumonia, in part because these organisms only transiently colonize the oropharynx in a minority of healthy individuals. However, rates of oral colonization with *E. coli* and other GNB increase with severity of illness and antibiotic use. Consequently, GNB are a more common cause of pneumonia among residents of LTCFs and are the most common cause (60–70% of cases) of hospital-acquired pneumonia (Chap. 168), particularly among postoperative and ICU patients (e.g., ventilator-associated pneumonia). Pulmonary infection is usually acquired by small-volume aspiration but occasionally occurs via hematogenous spread, in which case multifocal nodular infiltrates can be seen. Tissue necrosis, probably due to bacterial cytotoxins, is common. Despite significant institutional variation, *E. coli* is generally the third or fourth most commonly isolated GNB in hospital-acquired pneumonia, accounting for 5–8% of episodes in both U.S.-based and Europe-based studies. Regardless of the host, pneumonia due to ExPEC is a serious disease, with high crude and attributable mortality rates (20–60% and 10–20%, respectively).

MENINGITIS (See also Chap. 164) *E. coli* is one of the two leading causes of neonatal meningitis, the other being group B *Streptococcus*. Most *E. coli* strains that cause neonatal meningitis possess the K1 capsular antigen and derive from a limited number of meningitis-associated clonal groups. Ventriculomegaly commonly occurs. After the first month of life, *E. coli* meningitis is uncommon, occurring predominantly in the setting of surgical or traumatic disruption of the meninges or in the presence of cirrhosis. In patients with cirrhosis who develop meningitis, the meninges are presumably seeded as a result of poor hepatic clearance of portal vein bacteremia.

CELLULITIS/MUSCULOSKELETAL INFECTION *E. coli* contributes frequently to infections of decubitus ulcers and occasionally to infections of ulcers and wounds of the lower extremity in diabetic patients and other hosts with neurovascular compromise. Osteomyelitis secondary to contiguous spread can occur in these settings. *E. coli* also causes cellulitis or infections of burn sites and surgical wounds (accounting for ~10% of surgical site infections), particularly when the infection originates

TABLE 186-2 INTESTINAL PATHOGENIC *E. COLI*

Pathotype	Epidemiology	Clinical Syndrome[a]	Defining Molecular Trait	Responsible Genetic Element[b]
STEC/EHEC/STEAEC	Food, water, person-to-person; all ages, industrialized countries	Hemorrhagic colitis, hemolytic-uremic syndrome	Shiga toxin	Lambda-like Stx1- or Stx2-encoding bacteriophage
ETEC	Food, water; young children in and travelers to developing countries	Traveler's diarrhea	Heat-stable and labile enterotoxins, colonization factors	Virulence plasmid(s)
EPEC	Person-to-person; young children and neonates in developing countries	Watery diarrhea, persistent diarrhea	Localized adherence, attaching and effacing lesion on intestinal epithelium	EPEC adherence factor plasmid pathogenicity island (locus for enterocyte effacement [LEE])
EIEC	Food, water; children in and travelers to developing countries	Dysentery	Invasion of colonic epithelial cells, intracellular multiplication, cell-to-cell spread	Multiple genes contained primarily in a large virulence plasmid
EAEC	?Food, water; children in and travelers to developing countries; all ages, industrialized countries	Traveler's diarrhea, acute diarrhea, persistent diarrhea	Aggregative/diffuse adherence, virulence factors regulated by AggR	Chromosomal or plasmid-associated adherence and toxin genes

Abbreviations: EAEC, enteroaggregative *E. coli*; EHEC, enterohemorrhagic *E. coli*; EIEC, enteroinvasive *E. coli*; EPEC, enteropathogenic *E. coli*; ETEC, enterotoxigenic *E. coli*; STEAEC, Shiga toxin–producing enteroaggregative *E. coli*; STEC, Shiga toxin–producing *E. coli*. [a] Classic syndromes; see text for details on disease spectrum. [b] Pathogenesis involves multiple genes, including genes in addition to those listed.

close to the perineum. Hematogenously acquired osteomyelitis, especially of vertebral bodies, is more commonly caused by *E. coli* than is generally appreciated; this organism accounts for up to 10% of cases in some series (Chap. 158). *E. coli* occasionally causes orthopedic device–associated infection or septic arthritis and rarely causes hematogenous myositis. Upper-leg myositis or fasciitis due to *E. coli* should prompt an evaluation for an abdominal source with contiguous spread.

ENDOVASCULAR INFECTION Despite being one of the most common causes of bacteremia, *E. coli* rarely seeds native heart valves. When the organism does seed native valves, it usually does so in the setting of prior valvular disease. *E. coli* infections of aneurysms, the portal vein (*pylephlebitis*), and vascular grafts are quite uncommon.

MISCELLANEOUS INFECTIONS *E. coli* can cause infection in nearly every organ and anatomic site. It occasionally causes postoperative mediastinitis or complicated sinusitis and uncommonly causes endophthalmitis, ecthyma gangrenosum, or brain abscess.

BACTEREMIA *E. coli* bacteremia can arise from primary infection at any extraintestinal site. In addition, primary *E. coli* bacteremia can arise from percutaneous intravascular devices or transrectal prostate biopsy or from the increased intestinal mucosal permeability seen in neonates and in the settings of neutropenia and chemotherapy-induced mucositis, trauma, and burns. Roughly equal proportions of *E. coli* bacteremia cases originate in the community and in health care settings. In most studies, *E. coli* and *Staphylococcus aureus* are the two most common blood isolates of clinical significance. Isolation of *E. coli* from the blood is almost always clinically significant and is typically accompanied by the sepsis syndrome, severe sepsis (sepsis-induced dysfunction of at least one organ or system), or septic shock (Chap. 325).

The urinary tract is the most common source of *E. coli* bacteremia, accounting for one-half to two-thirds of episodes. Bacteremia from a urinary tract source is particularly common among patients with pyelonephritis, urinary tract obstruction, or urinary instrumentation in the presence of infected urine. The abdomen is the second most common source, accounting for 25% of episodes. Although biliary obstruction (stones, tumor) and overt bowel disruption, which typically are readily apparent, are responsible for many of these cases, some abdominal sources (e.g., abscesses) are remarkably silent clinically and require identification via imaging studies (e.g., CT). Therefore, the physician should be cautious in designating the urinary tract as the source of *E. coli* bacteremia in the absence of characteristic signs and symptoms of UTI. Soft tissue, bone, pulmonary, and intravascular catheter infections are other sources of *E. coli* bacteremia

Diagnosis Strains of *E. coli* that cause extraintestinal infections usually grow both aerobically and anaerobically within 24 h on standard diagnostic media and are easily identified by the clinical microbiology laboratory according to routine biochemical criteria. More than 90% of ExPEC strains are rapid lactose fermenters and are indole positive.

TREATMENT EXTRAINTESTINAL *E. COLI* INFECTIONS

In the past, most *E. coli* isolates were highly susceptible to a broad range of antimicrobial agents. Unfortunately, this situation has changed. In general, the high prevalence of resistance precludes empirical use of ampicillin and amoxicillin-clavulanate, even for community-acquired infections. The prevalence of resistance to first-generation cephalosporins and TMP-SMX is increasing among community-acquired strains in the United States (with current rates of 10–40%) and is even higher outside North America. Until recently, TMP-SMX was the drug of choice for the treatment of uncomplicated cystitis in many locales. Although continued empirical use of TMP-SMX will predictably result in ever-diminishing cure rates, a wholesale switch to alternative agents (e.g., fluoroquinolones) will just as predictably accelerate the widespread emergence of resistance to these antimicrobial classes, as has already occurred in some areas. More than 90% of isolates that cause uncomplicated cystitis remain susceptible to nitrofurantoin and fosfomycin.

The prevalence of resistance to fluoroquinolones among *E. coli* isolates from U.S. outpatients has increased steadily over the last decade (i.e., from 3% in 2000 to 17.1% in 2010, according to one survey). Resistance rates are generally higher in the ambulatory setting outside the United States and are even higher in populations for which fluoroquinolone prophylaxis is used extensively (e.g., patients with leukemia, transplant recipients, and patients with cirrhosis) and among isolates from LTCFs and hospitals. For example, the National Healthcare Safety Network (NHSN) reported fluoroquinolone resistance in 41.8% of central line–associated bloodstream infection (CLABSI) *E. coli* isolates in 2009–2010, and the International Nosocomial Infection Control Consortium (INICC) reported that 33.4% of ICU *E. coli* isolates were resistant to quinolones in 2004–2009. Furthermore, the NHSN reported 19% resistance to third- and fourth-generation cephalosporins in CLABSI *E. coli* isolates, and the INICC found that 66.6% of ICU *E. coli* isolates were resistant to third-generation cephalosporins.

ESBL-producing strains are increasingly prevalent among both health care–associated (5–10%) and ambulatory isolates (region-dependent figures). An increasing number of reports describe community-acquired UTIs caused by *E. coli* strains that produce CTX-M ESBLs. Data suggest that acquisition of CTX-M-producing, fluoroquinolone-resistant strains may result from consumption of meat products from food animals treated with third- and fourth-generation cephalosporins and fluoroquinolones. Oral treatment options for such strains are limited; however, in vitro and limited clinical data indicate that, for cystitis, fosfomycin and nitrofurantoin appear to be useful options. Carbapenems and amikacin are the most predictably active agents overall, but carbapenemase-producing strains are on the rise (1–5% among health care–associated isolates in the United States and higher rates in many other countries). Tigecycline and the polymyxins, with or without a second agent, have been used most frequently against these extremely resistant isolates.

This evolving antimicrobial resistance—a source of serious concern—necessitates not only the increasing use of broad-spectrum agents but also the use of the most appropriate narrower-spectrum agent whenever possible and the avoidance of treatment of colonized but uninfected patients.

INTESTINAL PATHOGENIC STRAINS

Pathotypes Certain strains of *E. coli* are capable of causing diarrheal disease. Other important intestinal pathogens are discussed in Chaps. 160, 161, and 190–193. At least in the industrialized world, intestinal pathogenic strains of *E. coli* are rarely encountered in the fecal flora of healthy persons and instead appear to be essentially obligate pathogens. These strains have evolved a special ability to cause enteritis, enterocolitis, and colitis when ingested in sufficient quantities by a naive host. At least five distinct pathotypes of intestinal pathogenic *E. coli* exist: (1) Shiga toxin–producing *E. coli* (STEC), which includes the subsets of enterohemorrhagic *E. coli* (EHEC) and the recently evolved Shiga toxin–producing enteroaggregative *E. coli* (STEAEC); (2) enterotoxigenic *E. coli* (ETEC); (3) enteropathogenic *E. coli* (EPEC); (4) enteroinvasive *E. coli* (EIEC); and (5) enteroaggregative *E. coli* (EAEC). Diffusely adherent *E. coli* (DAEC) and cytodetaching *E. coli* are additional putative pathotypes. Lastly, a variant termed adherent invasive *E. coli* (AIEC) has been associated with Crohn's disease (although a causal role remains unproven) but does not cause acute diarrheal disease. Transmission occurs predominantly via contaminated food and water for ETEC, STEC/EHEC/STEAEC, EIEC, and EAEC and by person-to-person spread for EPEC (and occasionally STEC/EHEC/STEAEC). Gastric acidity confers some protection against infection; therefore, persons with decreased stomach acid levels are especially susceptible. Humans are the major reservoir (except for STEC/EHEC, with regard to which bovines are the main concern); host range appears to be dictated by species-specific attachment factors. Although there is some overlap, each pathotype possesses a largely unique combination of virulence traits that results in a distinctive intestinal pathogenic mechanism (Table 186-2). These strains are largely incapable of causing disease outside the intestinal tract. Except in the cases of STEC/EHEC/STEAEC and EAEC, disease due to this group of pathogens occurs primarily in developing countries.

ENTEROHEMORRHAGIC E. COLI/SHIGA TOXIN–PRODUCING ENTEROAGGREGATIVE E. COLI STEC/EHEC/STEAEC strains constitute an emerging group of pathogens that can cause hemorrhagic colitis and the hemolytic-uremic syndrome (HUS). Several large outbreaks resulting from the consumption of fresh produce (e.g., lettuce, spinach, sprouts) and of undercooked ground beef have received significant attention in the media. An outbreak in central Europe in 2011 due to STEAEC (O104:H4) that was probably transmitted by sprouts, with some subsequent human-to-human transmission, resulted in more than 800 cases of HUS and 54 deaths. Within this group of organisms, O157:H7 is the most prominent serotype, but many other serotypes have also been associated with these syndromes, including O6, O26, O45, O55, O91, O103, O111, O113, O121, O145, and OX3.

The ability of STEC/EHEC/STEAEC to produce Shiga toxin (Stx2 and/or Stx1) or related toxins is a critical factor in the occurrence of clinical disease. *Shigella dysenteriae* strains that produce the closely related Shiga toxin Stx can cause the same syndrome. Stx2 and its Stx2C variant (which may be variably present in combination with Stx2 and/or Stx1) appear to be more important than Stx1 in the development of HUS. All Shiga toxins studied to date are multimers comprising one enzymatically active A subunit and five identical B subunits that mediate binding to globosyl ceramides, which are membrane-associated glycolipids expressed on certain host cells. As in ricin, the A subunit cleaves an adenine from the host cell's 28S rRNA, thereby irreversibly inhibiting ribosomal function and potentially leading to apoptosis. Stx2-mediated activation of complement may also play a role in the development of HUS.

Additional properties, such as acid tolerance and epithelial cell adherence, are necessary for full pathogenicity among STEC strains. Most disease-causing isolates possess the chromosomal locus for enterocyte effacement (LEE). This pathogenicity island was first described in EPEC strains and contains genes that mediate adherence to intestinal epithelial cells and a system that subverts host cells by the translocation of bacterial proteins (type III secretion system). EHEC strains make up the subgroup of STEC strains that possess stx_1 and/or stx_2 as well as LEE. STEAEC (LEE-negative) evolved from EAEC via the acquisition of a number of genes, including those that encode Stx2, the Iha adhesin, tellurite resistance, a type VI secretion system, and the CTX-M-15 ESBL.

Domesticated ruminant animals, particularly cattle and young calves, serve as the major reservoir for STEC/EHEC. Ground beef—the most common food source of STEC/EHEC strains—is often contaminated during processing. Furthermore, manure from cattle or other animals (including that in the form of fertilizer) can contaminate produce (potatoes, lettuce, spinach, sprouts, fallen fruits, nuts, strawberries), and fecal runoff from this source can contaminate water systems. Dairy products and petting zoos are additional sources of infection. By contrast, humans appear to be the reservoir for STEAEC. It is estimated that $<10^2$ colony-forming units (CFU) of STEC/EHEC/STEAEC can cause disease. Therefore, not only can low levels of food or environmental contamination (e.g., in water swallowed while swimming) result in disease, but person-to-person transmission (e.g., at day-care centers and in institutions) is an important route for secondary spread. Laboratory-associated infections also occur. Illness due to this group of pathogens occurs both as outbreaks and as sporadic cases, with a peak incidence in the summer months.

In contrast to other intestinal pathotypes, STEC/EHEC/STEAEC causes infections more frequently in industrialized countries than in developing regions. O157:H7 strains are the fourth most commonly reported cause of bacterial diarrhea in the United States (after *Campylobacter*, *Salmonella*, and *Shigella*). Colonization of the colon and perhaps the ileum results in symptoms after an incubation period of 3 or 4 days. Colonic edema and an initial nonbloody secretory diarrhea may develop into the STEC/EHEC/STEAEC hallmark syndrome of grossly bloody diarrhea (identified by history or examination) in >90% of cases. Significant abdominal pain and fecal leukocytes are common (70% of cases), whereas fever is not; absence of fever can incorrectly lead to consideration of noninfectious conditions (e.g., intussusception and inflammatory or ischemic bowel disease). Occasionally, infections caused by *C. difficile*, *K. oxytoca* (see "*Klebsiella* Infections," below), *Campylobacter*, and *Salmonella* present in a similar fashion. STEC/EHEC disease is usually self-limited, lasting 5–10 days. An uncommon but feared complication of this infection is HUS, which occurs 2–14 days after diarrhea in 2–8% of cases, most often affecting very young or elderly patients. Distinctive features of STEAEC infection, as compared with classical STEC/EHEC disease, include a higher incidence among adults, especially young women, and a higher rate of HUS (~20%). It is estimated that >50% of all cases of HUS in the United States and 90% of HUS cases in children are caused by STEC/EHEC. This complication is mediated by the systemic translocation of Shiga toxins. Erythrocytes may serve as carriers of Stx to endothelial cells located in the small vessels of the kidney and brain. The subsequent development of thrombotic microangiopathy (perhaps with direct toxin-mediated effects on various nonendothelial cells) commonly produces some combination of fever, thrombocytopenia, renal failure, and encephalopathy. Although the mortality rate with dialysis support is <10%, residual renal and neurologic dysfunction may persist.

ENTEROTOXIGENIC E. COLI In tropical or developing countries, ETEC is a major cause of endemic diarrhea. After weaning, children in these locales commonly experience several episodes of ETEC infection during the first 3 years of life. The incidence of disease diminishes with age, a pattern that correlates with the development of mucosal immunity to colonization factors (i.e., adhesins). In industrialized countries, infection usually follows travel to endemic areas, although occasional food-borne outbreaks occur. ETEC is the most common agent of traveler's diarrhea, causing 25–75% of cases. The incidence of infection may be decreased by prudent avoidance of potentially contaminated fluids and foods, particularly items that are poorly cooked, unpeeled, or unrefrigerated (Chap. 149). ETEC infection is uncommon in the United States, but outbreaks secondary to consumption of food products imported from endemic areas have occurred. A large inoculum (10^6–10^{10} CFU) is needed to produce disease, which usually develops after an incubation period of 12–72 h.

After adherence of ETEC via colonization factors (e.g., CFA/I, CS1-6), disease is mediated primarily by a heat-labile toxin (LT-1) and/or a heat-stable toxin (STa) that causes net fluid secretion via activation of adenylate cyclase (LT-1) and/or guanylate cyclase (STa) in the jejunum and ileum. The result is watery diarrhea accompanied by cramps. LT-1 consists of an A and a B subunit and is structurally and functionally similar to cholera toxin. Strong binding of the B subunit to the GM_1 ganglioside on intestinal epithelial cells leads to the intracellular translocation of the A subunit, which functions as an ADP-ribosyltransferase. Mature STa is an 18- or 19-amino-acid secreted peptide whose biologic activity is mediated by binding to the guanylate cyclase C found in the brush-border membrane of enterocytes and results in increased intracellular concentrations of cyclic GMP. Characteristically absent in ETEC-mediated disease are histopathologic changes within the small bowel; mucus, blood, and inflammatory cells in stool; and fever. The disease spectrum ranges from a mild illness to a life-threatening cholera-like syndrome. Although symptoms are usually self-limited (typically lasting for 3 days), infection may result in significant morbidity and mortality (mostly from profound volume depletion) when access to health care or suitable rehydration fluids is limited and when small and/or undernourished children are affected.

ENTEROPATHOGENIC E. COLI EPEC causes disease primarily in young children, including neonates. The first *E. coli* pathotype recognized as an agent of diarrheal disease, EPEC was responsible for outbreaks of infantile diarrhea (including some outbreaks in hospital nurseries) in industrialized countries in the 1940s and 1950s. At present, EPEC infection is an uncommon cause of diarrhea in developed countries but is an important cause of diarrhea (both sporadic and epidemic) among infants in developing countries. Breast-feeding diminishes the incidence of EPEC infection. Rapid person-to-person spread may occur. Upon colonization of the small bowel, symptoms develop after a brief incubation period (1 or 2 days). Initial localized adherence via bundle-forming pili leads to a characteristic effacement of microvilli, with the formation of cuplike, actin-rich pedestals mediated by factors in the LEE. Diarrhea production is a complex and regulated process in which host cell modulation by a type III secretion system plays an important role. Strains lacking bundle-forming pili have been categorized as atypical EPEC (aEPEC); increasing data support a role for these strains as intestinal pathogens. Diarrheal stool often contains mucus but not blood. Although EPEC diarrhea is usually self-limited (lasting 5–15 days), it may persist for weeks.

ENTEROINVASIVE E. COLI EIEC, a relatively uncommon cause of diarrhea, is rarely identified in the United States, although a few food-related outbreaks have been described. In developing countries, sporadic disease is infrequently recognized in children and travelers. EIEC shares many genetic and clinical features with *Shigella*, both of which evolved from a common ancestor. However, unlike *Shigella*, EIEC produces disease only with a large inoculum (10^8–10^{10} CFU), with onset generally following an incubation period of 1–3 days. Initially, enterotoxins are believed to induce secretory small-bowel diarrhea. Subsequently, colonization and invasion of the colonic mucosa, followed by replication therein and cell-to-cell spread, result in the development of inflammatory colitis characterized by fever, abdominal pain, tenesmus, and scant stool containing mucus, blood, and inflammatory cells. Symptoms are usually self-limited (7–10 days).

ENTEROAGGREGATIVE AND DIFFUSELY ADHERENT E. COLI EAEC has been described primarily in developing countries and in young children. However, recent studies indicate that it may be a relatively common cause of diarrhea in all age groups in industrialized countries. EAEC has also been recognized increasingly as an important cause of traveler's diarrhea. It is highly adapted to humans, the probable reservoir. A large inoculum is required for infection, which usually manifests as watery and sometimes persistent diarrhea in healthy, malnourished, and HIV-infected hosts. In vitro, the organisms exhibit a diffuse or "stacked-brick" pattern of adherence to small-intestine epithelial cells. Virulence factors that probably are necessary for disease are regulated in part by the transcriptional activator AggR and include the aggregative adherence fimbriae (AAF/I-III); the Hda adhesin; the mucinase Pic; the enterotoxins Pet, EAST-1, ShET1, and HlyE; and dispersin, an antiaggregation protein that promotes mucosal spread. Some strains of DAEC are capable of causing diarrheal disease, primarily in children 2–6 years of age in some developing countries, and may perhaps cause traveler's diarrhea. The Afa/Dr adhesins may contribute to the pathogenesis of such infections.

Diagnosis A practical approach to the evaluation of diarrhea is to distinguish noninflammatory from inflammatory cases; the latter is suggested by grossly bloody or mucoid stool or a positive test for fecal leukocytes (Chap. 160). ETEC, EPEC, and DAEC cause noninflammatory diarrhea and are uncommon in the United States; in this country, the incidence of EAEC infection, which also causes noninflammatory diarrhea, may be underrecognized. The diagnosis of these infections requires specialized assays (e.g., polymerase chain reaction–based tests for pathotype-specific genes) that are not routinely available and are rarely needed because the diseases are self-limited. ETEC causes the majority and EAEC a minority of cases of noninflammatory traveler's diarrhea. Definitive diagnosis generally is not necessary. Empirical antimicrobial (or symptom-based) treatment, along with rehydration therapy, is a reasonable approach. If diarrhea persists for >10 days despite treatment, *Giardia* or *Cryptosporidium* (or, in immunocompromised hosts, certain other microbial agents) should be sought. The diagnosis of infection with EIEC, a rare cause of inflammatory diarrhea in the United States, also requires specialized assays. The CDC now recommends that all patients with community-acquired diarrhea, whether inflammatory or not, be evaluated for STEC/EHEC/STEAEC infection by simultaneous culture (which is important for outbreak detection and control) and assay for the detection of Shiga toxin or its associated genes. The reasons for this recommendation are that bloody stool is not always present and detection of fecal white blood cells is not optimally sensitive for the diagnosis of STEC/EHEC/STEAEC infection. The use of both tests increases the rate of identification of infection over rates obtained with either test alone. O157 STEC/EHEC may be identified via culture by screening for *E. coli* strains that do not ferment sorbitol, with subsequent serotyping and testing for Shiga toxin. Selective or screening media are not available for the culture of non-O157 strains. Detection of Shiga toxins or toxin genes via DNA-based, enzyme-linked immunosorbent, and cytotoxicity assays offers the advantages of rapidity plus detection of non-O157 STEC/EHEC/STEAEC strains. Specimens positive for toxin but culture-negative for O157 should be forwarded to the local or state public health laboratory.

TREATMENT INTESTINAL *E. COLI* INFECTIONS

(See also Chap. 128) The mainstay of treatment for all diarrheal syndromes is replacement of water and electrolytes. This measure is especially important for STEC/EHEC/STEAEC infection because appropriate volume expansion may decrease renal damage and improve outcome. The use of prophylactic antibiotics to prevent traveler's diarrhea generally should be discouraged, especially in light of high rates of antimicrobial resistance. However, in selected patients (e.g., those who cannot afford a brief illness or are predisposed to infection), the use of rifaximin, which is nonabsorbable and is well tolerated, is reasonable. When stools are free of mucus and blood, early patient-initiated treatment of traveler's diarrhea with a fluoroquinolone or azithromycin decreases the duration of illness, and the use of loperamide may halt symptoms within a few hours. Although dysentery caused by EIEC is self-limited, treatment hastens the resolution of symptoms, particularly in severe cases. In contrast, antimicrobial therapy for STEC/EHEC/STEAEC infection (the presence of which is suggested by grossly bloody diarrhea without fever) should be avoided because antibiotics may increase the incidence of HUS (possibly via increased production/release of Stx). The role of plasmapheresis and inhibition of C5 (eculizumab) in the treatment of HUS is unresolved.

KLEBSIELLA INFECTIONS

K. pneumoniae is the most important *Klebsiella* species from a medical standpoint, causing community-acquired, LTCF-acquired, and nosocomial infections. *K. oxytoca* is primarily a pathogen in LTCF and hospital settings. *Klebsiella* species are broadly prevalent in the environment and colonize mucosal surfaces of mammals. In healthy humans, the prevalence of *K. pneumoniae* colonization is 5–35% in the colon and 1–5% in the oropharynx; the skin is usually colonized only transiently. Person-to-person spread is the predominant mode of acquisition. Most *Klebsiella* infections in Western countries are caused by "classic" *K. pneumoniae* (cKP) and occur in hospitals and LTCFs. The most common clinical syndromes due to cKP are pneumonia, UTI, abdominal infection, intravascular device infection, surgical site infection, soft tissue infection, and subsequent bacteremia. cKP strains have gained notoriety because their propensity for acquiring antimicrobial resistance determinants makes treatment challenging. Clonal group ST258, many members of which produce the KPC carbapenemase, is undergoing international dissemination. The spread of NDM-1 carbapenemase-producing strains from India in association with medical tourism has captured the attention of physicians and the lay press.

cKP strains appear to be phenotypically and clinically distinct from hypervirulent *K. pneumoniae* (hvKP), an emerging variant that was first recognized in Taiwan in 1986. Although hvKP infections have occurred globally in all ethnic groups, the majority have been reported in the Asian Pacific Rim. This concentration of cases raises the question of whether a geo-specific distribution of the organism or increased susceptibility of Asian hosts is responsible. In contrast to the usual health care–associated venue for cKP infections in the West, hvKP causes serious life- and organ-threatening infections in younger, healthy individuals from the community and can spread metastatically from primary sites of infection. hvKP infection initially was characterized and distinguished from traditional infections due to cKP by (1) presentation as community-acquired pyogenic liver abscess (Fig. 186-1, *top*), (2) occurrence in patients lacking a history of hepatobiliary disease, and (3) a propensity for metastatic spread to distant sites (e.g., eyes, central nervous system, lungs), which occurred in 11–80% of cases. More recently, this variant has been recognized as the cause of a variety of serious community-acquired extrahepatic abscesses/infections in the absence of liver involvement, including pneumonia, meningitis, endophthalmitis (Fig. 186-1, *middle*), splenic abscess, and necrotizing fasciitis. The affected individuals often have diabetes mellitus and are of Asian ethnicity; however, nondiabetics and all ethnic groups can be affected. Survivors often suffer catastrophic morbidity, such as loss of vision and neurologic sequelae.

K. pneumoniae subspecies *rhinoscleromatis* is the causative agent of rhinoscleroma, a granulomatous mucosal upper respiratory infection that progresses slowly (over months or years) and causes necrosis and occasionally obstruction of the nasal passages. *K. pneumoniae* subspecies *ozaenae* has been implicated as a cause of chronic atrophic rhinitis and rarely of invasive disease in compromised hosts. These two *K. pneumoniae* subspecies are usually isolated from patients in tropical climates and are genomically distinct from both cKP and hvKP.

INFECTIOUS SYNDROMES

Pneumonia Although cKP accounts for only a small proportion of cases of community-acquired pneumonia in Western countries (Chap. 153), cKP and *K. oxytoca* are common causes of pneumonia among LTCF residents and hospitalized patients because of increased rates of oropharyngeal colonization. Mechanical ventilation is an important risk factor. In Asia and South Africa, community-acquired pneumonia due to hvKP is becoming increasingly common and often occurs in younger patients with no underlying disease. *Klebsiella* is also a common cause of pneumonia in severely malnourished children in developing countries.

As in all pneumonias due to enteric GNB, production of purulent sputum and evidence of airspace disease are typical. Presentation with earlier, less extensive infection is now more common than that with the classically described lobar infiltrate and bulging fissure. Pulmonary infection due to hvKP that has spread metastatically (e.g., from a hepatic abscess) usually includes nodular bilateral densities, more commonly in the lower lobes. Pulmonary necrosis, pleural effusion, and empyema can occur with disease progression.

UTI cKP accounts for only 1–2% of UTI episodes among otherwise healthy adults but for 5–17% of episodes of complicated UTI, including infections associated with indwelling urinary catheters. UTI due to hvKP presents more commonly as renal or prostatic abscess due to bacteremic spread than as ascending infection.

Abdominal Infection cKP causes a spectrum of abdominal infections similar to that caused by *E. coli* but is less frequently isolated from these infections. hvKP is a common cause of monomicrobial community-acquired pyogenic liver abscess and in the Asian Pacific Rim has been recovered with steadily increasing frequency over the past two decades, replacing *E. coli* as the most common pathogen causing this syndrome. hvKP is increasingly described as a cause of spontaneous bacterial peritonitis and splenic abscess.

Other Infections cKP- and *K. oxytoca*–mediated cellulitis or soft tissue infection most frequently affects devitalized tissue (e.g., decubitus and diabetic ulcers, burn sites) and immunocompromised hosts. cKP and *K. oxytoca* cause some cases of surgical site infection and nosocomial sinusitis in addition to occasional cases of osteomyelitis contiguous to soft tissue infection, nontropical myositis, and meningitis (both during the neonatal period and after neurosurgery). By contrast, hvKP has become an important cause of community-acquired

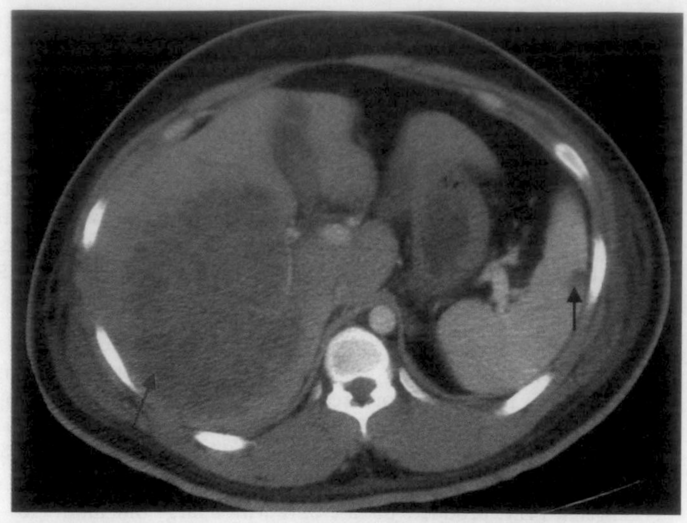

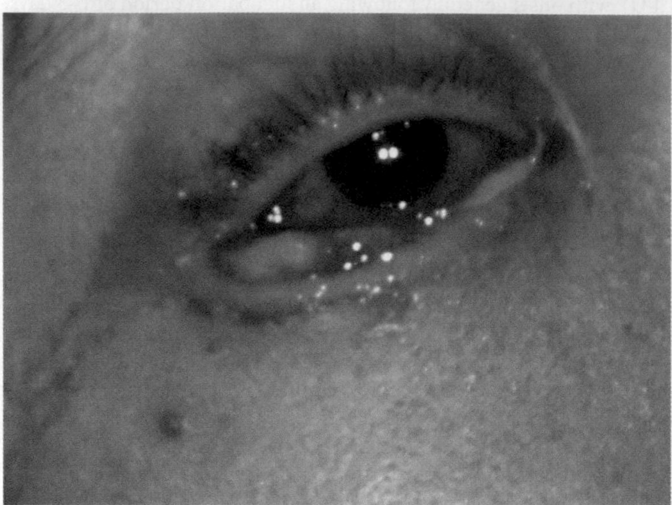

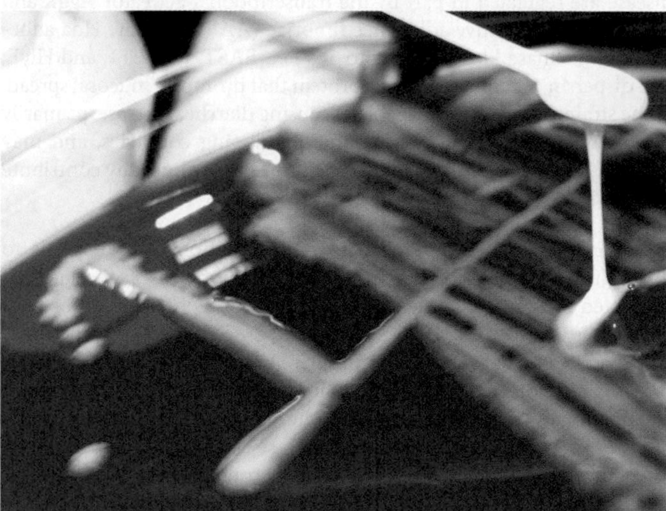

FIGURE 186-1 New hypervirulent variant of *K. pneumoniae* (hvKP). ***Top:*** Abdominal CT scan of a previously healthy 24-year-old Vietnamese man shows a primary liver abscess (*red arrow*) with metastatic spread to the spleen (*black arrow*). *(Courtesy of Drs. Chiu-Bin Hsaio and Diana Pomakova.)* ***Middle:*** A previously healthy 33-year-old Chinese man presented with endophthalmitis. *(From Virulence 4:2, 1-12 Feb. 15, 2013.)* ***Bottom:*** A hypermucoviscous phenotype (which does not necessarily equate with a mucoid phenotype) has been associated with hvKP strains. This phenotype has been semiquantitatively defined by a positive "string test" (formation of a viscous string >5 mm long when bacterial colonies on an agar plate are stretched by an inoculation loop). *(Courtesy of Dr. Russo.)*

monomicrobial necrotizing fasciitis; meningitis; brain, subdural, and epidural abscess; and endophthalmitis (Fig. 186-1, *middle*), particularly in the Asian Pacific Rim but also globally. Cytotoxin-producing strains of *K. oxytoca* have been implicated as a cause of hemorrhagic antibiotic-associated non–*C. difficile* colitis.

Bacteremia *Klebsiella* infection at any site can produce bacteremia. Infections of the urinary tract, respiratory tract, and abdomen (especially hepatic abscess) each account for 15–30% of episodes of *Klebsiella* bacteremia. Intravascular device–related infections account for another 5–15% of episodes, and surgical site and miscellaneous infections account for the rest. *Klebsiella* is a cause of sepsis in neonates and of bacteremia in neutropenic patients. Like enteric GNB in general, *Klebsiella* rarely causes endocarditis or endovascular infection.

DIAGNOSIS

Klebsiellae are readily isolated and identified in the laboratory. These organisms usually ferment lactose, although the subspecies *rhinoscleromatis* and *ozaenae* are nonfermenters and are indole negative. hvKP usually possesses a hypermucoviscous phenotype (Fig. 186-1, *bottom*), although the sensitivity and specificity of this test are undefined and probably less than optimal. A better diagnostic test for hvKP is desirable.

TREATMENT *KLEBSIELLA* INFECTIONS

cKP and *K. oxytoca* have similar antibiotic resistance profiles. These species are intrinsically resistant to ampicillin and ticarcillin, and nitrofurantoin is inconsistently active against them. NHSN data for 2009–2010 documented resistance to third- and fourth-generation cephalosporins in 28.9% of CLABSI isolates of cKP and *K. oxytoca*, and INICC data for 2004–2009 identified resistance to third-generation cephalosporins in 76.3% of ICU isolates of *K. pneumoniae*. This increasing resistance is mediated primarily by plasmid-encoded ESBLs. In addition, such plasmids usually encode resistance to aminoglycosides, tetracyclines, and TMP-SMX. Furthermore, isolates of cKP that produce CTX-M ESBLs have been obtained from ambulatory patients with no recent health care contact (see the section on the treatment of extraintestinal *E. coli* infections for treatment considerations). Resistance to β-lactam/β-lactamase inhibitor combinations and cephamycins independent of ESBL-encoding plasmids has also been described with increasing frequency, particularly in Latin America. The prevalence of fluoroquinolone resistance is 15–20% overall and is 50% among ESBL-containing strains. Given both the undesirability of treating the latter strains with penicillins or cephalosporins and the fluoroquinolone resistance often associated with ESBLs, empirical treatment of serious or health care–associated cKP and *K. oxytoca* infections with amikacin or carbapenems is prudent, as dictated by local susceptibilities. Predictably, however, the ESBL-driven use of carbapenems has selected for strains of cKP and *K. oxytoca* that express carbapenemases. NHSN data for 2009–2010 documented resistance to carbapenems in 12.8% of CLABSI isolates of cKP and *K. oxytoca*. Treatment of infections due to strains that produce carbapenemases is highly challenging; increasingly, these strains are nearly pan-resistant. The optimal choice for therapy is unclear. Tigecycline and the polymyxins (e.g., colistin) are the most active agents in vitro and are used most frequently. However, resistance to these agents is already emerging, and strains of cKP resistant to all known antimicrobial agents have been described in the United States and globally. Combination therapy is often used in this setting.

PROTEUS INFECTIONS

Proteus mirabilis causes 90% of *Proteus* infections, which occur in the community, LTCFs, and hospitals. *Proteus vulgaris* and *Proteus penneri* are associated primarily with infections acquired in LTCFs or hospitals. *Proteus* species are part of the colonic flora of a wide variety of mammals, birds, fish, and reptiles. The ability of these GNB to generate histamine from contaminated fish has implicated them in the pathogenesis of scombroid (fish) poisoning (Chap. 474). *P. mirabilis* colonizes healthy humans (prevalence, 50%), whereas *P. vulgaris* and *P. penneri* are isolated primarily from individuals with underlying disease. The urinary tract is by far the most common site of *Proteus* infection, with adhesins, flagella, IgA-IgG protease, iron acquisition systems, and urease representing the principal known urovirulence factors. *Proteus* less commonly causes infection at a variety of other extraintestinal sites.

INFECTIOUS SYNDROMES

UTI Most *Proteus* infections arise from the urinary tract. *P. mirabilis* causes only 1–2% of UTIs in healthy women, and *Proteus* species collectively cause only 5% of hospital-acquired UTIs. However, *Proteus* is responsible for 10–15% of cases of complicated UTI, primarily those associated with catheterization; indeed, among UTI isolates from chronically catheterized patients, the prevalence of *Proteus* is 20–45%. This high prevalence is due in part to bacterial production of urease, which hydrolyzes urea to ammonia and results in alkalization of the urine. Alkalization of urine, in turn, leads to precipitation of organic and inorganic compounds, which contributes to formation of struvite and carbonate-apatite crystals, formation of biofilms on catheters, and/or development of frank calculi. *Proteus* becomes associated with the stones and biofilms; thereafter, it usually can be eradicated only by removal of the stones or the catheter. Over time, staghorn calculi may form within the renal pelvis and lead to obstruction and renal failure. Thus, urine samples with unexplained alkalinity should be cultured for *Proteus*, and identification of a *Proteus* species in urine should prompt consideration of an evaluation for urolithiasis.

Other Infections *Proteus* occasionally causes pneumonia (primarily in LTCF residents or hospitalized patients), nosocomial sinusitis, intraabdominal abscesses, biliary tract infection, surgical site infection, soft tissue infection (especially decubitus and diabetic ulcers), and osteomyelitis (primarily contiguous); in rare cases, it causes nontropical myositis. In addition, *Proteus* uncommonly causes neonatal meningitis, with the umbilicus frequently implicated as the source; this disease is often complicated by development of a cerebral abscess. Otogenic brain abscess also occurs.

Bacteremia The majority of *Proteus* bacteremia episodes originate from the urinary tract; however, any of the less common sites of infection as well as intravascular devices are also potential sources. Endovascular infection is rare. *Proteus* species are occasional agents of sepsis in neonates and of bacteremia in neutropenic patients.

DIAGNOSIS

Proteus is readily isolated and identified in the laboratory. Most strains are lactose negative, produce H_2S, and demonstrate characteristic swarming motility on agar plates. *P. mirabilis* and *P. penneri* are indole negative, whereas *P. vulgaris* is indole positive. The inability to produce ornithine decarboxylase differentiates *P. penneri* from *P. mirabilis*.

TREATMENT *PROTEUS* INFECTIONS

P. mirabilis is usually susceptible to most antimicrobial agents except tetracycline, nitrofurantoin, the polymyxins, and tigecycline. Resistance to ampicillin and first-generation cephalosporins has been acquired by 10–50% of strains. Overall, 10–15% of *P. mirabilis* isolates are resistant to fluoroquinolones; 5% of isolates in the United States now produce ESBLs. Furthermore, isolates of *P. mirabilis* that produce CTX-M ESBLs have been recovered from ambulatory patients with no recent health care contact (see the section on the treatment of extraintestinal *E. coli* infections for treatment considerations). *P. vulgaris* and *P. penneri* exhibit more extensive drug resistance than does *P. mirabilis*. Resistance to ampicillin and first-generation cephalosporins is the rule, and 30–40% of isolates are resistant to fluoroquinolones. Induction or selection of variants with stable derepression of chromosomal AmpC β-lactamase may occur with *P. vulgaris* isolates. Carbapenems, fourth-generation cephalosporins (e.g., cefepime), amikacin, TMP-SMX, and fosfomycin display excellent activity against *Proteus* species (90–100% of isolates susceptible).

ENTEROBACTER AND *CRONOBACTER* INFECTIONS

E. cloacae and *E. aerogenes* are responsible for most *Enterobacter* infections (65–75% and 15–25%, respectively); *Cronobacter sakazakii* (formerly *Enterobacter sakazakii*) and *Enterobacter gergoviae* are less commonly isolated (1% for each). *Enterobacter* species cause primarily health care–related infections. The organisms are widely prevalent in foods, environmental sources (including equipment at health care facilities), and a variety of animals. Few healthy humans are colonized, but the percentage increases significantly with LTCF residence or hospitalization. Although colonization is an important prelude to infection, direct introduction via IV lines (e.g., contaminated IV fluids or pressure monitors) also occurs. Extensive antibiotic resistance has developed in *Enterobacter* species and probably has contributed to the emergence of the organisms as prominent nosocomial pathogens. Individuals who have previously received antibiotic treatment, have comorbid disease, and are ICU residents are at greatest risk for infection. *Enterobacter* causes a spectrum of extraintestinal infections similar to that described for other GNB.

INFECTIOUS SYNDROMES

Pneumonia, UTI (particularly catheter-related), intravascular device–related infection, surgical site infection, and abdominal infection (primarily postoperative or related to devices such as biliary stents) are the most common syndromes encountered. Nosocomial sinusitis, meningitis related to neurosurgical procedures (including use of intracranial pressure monitors), osteomyelitis, and endophthalmitis after eye surgery are less frequent. *C. sakazakii* is associated with neonatal bacteremia, necrotizing enterocolitis, and meningitis (which is often complicated by brain abscess or ventriculitis); contaminated formula has been implicated as a source for such infections. *Enterobacter* bacteremia can result from infection at any anatomic site. In bacteremia of unclear origin, the contamination of IV fluids or medications, blood components or plasma derivatives, catheter-flushing fluids, pressure monitors, and dialysis equipment should be considered, particularly in an outbreak setting. *Enterobacter* can also cause bacteremia in neutropenic patients. *Enterobacter* endocarditis is rare, occurring primarily in association with illicit IV drug use or prosthetic valves.

DIAGNOSIS

Enterobacter is readily isolated and identified in the laboratory. Most strains are lactose positive and indole negative.

TREATMENT *ENTEROBACTER* INFECTIONS

Significant antimicrobial resistance exists among *Enterobacter* strains. Ampicillin and first- and second-generation cephalosporins have little or no activity. Extensive use of third-generation cephalosporins can induce or select for variants with stable derepression of AmpC β-lactamase, which confers resistance to these agents as well as monobactams (e.g., aztreonam) and—in many cases—β-lactam/β-lactamase inhibitor combinations. Resistance may emerge during therapy; in one study, this phenomenon was documented in 20% of clinical isolates. De novo resistance should be considered when clinical deterioration follows initial improvement, and third-generation cephalosporins should be avoided in the treatment of serious *Enterobacter* infections. Cefepime is stable in the presence of AmpC β-lactamases; thus, it is a suitable option for treatment of *Enterobacter* infections so long as no coexistent ESBL is present. Detection of ESBLs in *Enterobacter* is difficult because of the presence of AmpC β-lactamase; nonetheless, their prevalence (particularly in *E. cloacae*) is known to be variable worldwide but is generally increasing and is now 5–50% overall. This increase is evidenced by NHSN data, which documented resistance to third- and fourth-generation cephalosporins in 37.4% of CLABSI *Enterobacter* isolates in the United States; fortunately, carbapenems, amikacin, and tigecycline have generally retained excellent activity (90–99% susceptibility) and fluoroquinolones have good activity (85–95% susceptibility). Once susceptibility data become available, it is critical to de-escalate the antimicrobial regimen whenever possible.

SERRATIA INFECTIONS

S. marcescens causes the majority (>90%) of *Serratia* infections; *Serratia liquefaciens*, *Serratia rubidaea*, *Serratia fonticola*, *Serratia grimesii*, *Serratia plymuthica*, and *Serratia odorifera* are isolated occasionally. Serratiae are found primarily in the environment (including in health care institutions), particularly in moist settings. Serratiae have been isolated from a variety of animals, insects, and plants, but healthy humans are rarely colonized. In LTCFs or hospitals, reservoirs for the organisms include the hands and fingernails of health care personnel, food, milk (on neonatal units), sinks, respiratory and other medical equipment or devices, pressure monitors, IV solutions or parenteral medications (particularly those generated by compounding pharmacies), prefilled syringes and multiple-access medication vials (e.g., heparin, saline), blood products (e.g., platelets), hand soaps and lotions, irrigation solutions, and even disinfectants. Infection results from either direct inoculation (e.g., via IV fluid) or colonization (primarily of the respiratory tract). Sporadic infection is most common, but epidemics (often involving MDR strains in adult and neonatal ICUs) and common-source outbreaks also occur. The spectrum of extraintestinal infections caused by *Serratia* is similar to that for other GNB. *Serratia* species are usually considered causative agents of health care–associated infection and account for 1–3% of hospital-acquired infections. However, population-based laboratory surveillance studies in Canada and Australia demonstrated that community-acquired infections occur more commonly than was previously appreciated.

INFECTIOUS SYNDROMES

The respiratory tract, the genitourinary tract, intravascular devices, the eye (contact lens–associated keratitis and other ocular infections), surgical wounds, and the bloodstream (from contaminated infusions) are the most common sites of *Serratia* infection; the former five sites are the most common sources of *Serratia* bacteremia. Soft tissue infections (including myositis, fasciitis, mastitis), osteomyelitis, abdominal and biliary tract infection (postprocedural), and septic arthritis (primarily from intraarticular injections) occur less commonly. Serratiae are uncommon causes of neonatal or postsurgical meningitis and of bacteremia in neutropenic patients. Endocarditis is rare.

DIAGNOSIS

Serratiae are readily cultured and identified by the laboratory and are usually lactose and indole negative. Some *S. marcescens* strains and *S. rubidaea* are red pigmented.

TREATMENT *SERRATIA* INFECTIONS

Most *Serratia* strains (>80%) are resistant to ampicillin, amoxicillin-clavulanate, ampicillin-sulbactam, first-generation cephalosporins, cephamycins, nitrofurantoin, and colistin. In general, >90% of *Serratia* isolates are susceptible to other antibiotics appropriate for use against GNB. Induction or selection of variants with stable derepression of chromosomal AmpC β-lactamases may develop during therapy. Both in the United States and globally, the prevalence of ESBL-producing isolates is generally low (<5%), but rates of 20–30% have been reported in Asia and Latin America. Acquisition of carbapenemase-encoding genes is uncommon but increasing.

CITROBACTER INFECTIONS

C. freundii and *Citrobacter koseri* cause most human *Citrobacter* infections, which are epidemiologically and clinically similar to *Enterobacter* infections. *Citrobacter* species are commonly present in water, food, soil, and certain animals. *Citrobacter* is part of the normal fecal flora in a minority of healthy humans, but colonization rates are higher in LTCFs and hospitals—the settings in which nearly all *Citrobacter* infections occur. *Citrobacter* species account for 1–2% of nosocomial infections. The affected hosts are usually immunocompromised or have comorbid disease. *Citrobacter* causes extraintestinal infections similar to those described for other GNB.

INFECTIOUS SYNDROMES

The urinary tract accounts for 40–50% of *Citrobacter* infections. Less commonly involved sites include the biliary tree (particularly with stones or obstruction), the respiratory tract, surgical sites, soft tissue (e.g., decubitus ulcers), the peritoneum, and intravascular devices. Osteomyelitis (usually from a contiguous focus), adult central nervous system infection (from neurosurgical or other types of meningeal disruption), and myositis occur rarely. *Citrobacter* (primarily *C. koseri*) also causes 1–2% of neonatal meningitis cases, of which 50–80% are complicated by brain abscess. Further, case reports in adults suggest that *C. koseri* infection has a predilection for abscess formation. Bacteremia is most often due to UTI, biliary/abdominal infection, or intravascular device infection. *Citrobacter* occasionally causes bacteremia in neutropenic patients. Endocarditis and endovascular infections are rare.

DIAGNOSIS

Citrobacter species are readily isolated and identified; 35–50% of isolates are lactose positive, and 100% are oxidase negative. *C. freundii* is indole negative, whereas *C. koseri* is indole positive.

TREATMENT *CITROBACTER* INFECTIONS

C. freundii is more extensively resistant to antibiotics than is *C. koseri*. More than 90% of isolates are resistant to ampicillin and first- and second-generation cephalosporins. *Citrobacter* species (except *C. koseri*) possess AmpC β-lactamases; induction or selection of variants with stable derepression may develop during therapy. Resistance to antipseudomonal penicillins, aztreonam, fluoroquinolones, gentamicin, and third-generation cephalosporins is variable but increasing. The prevalence of ESBL-producing isolates is <5%. Carbapenems, amikacin, cefepime, tigecycline (with which clinical experience is limited), fosfomycin (which is available in the United States only as an oral formulation), and colistin (which is an agent of last resort because of potential toxicities) are most active, with >90% of strains susceptible.

MORGANELLA AND *PROVIDENCIA* INFECTIONS

M. morganii, *Providencia stuartii*, and (less frequently) *Providencia rettgeri* are the members of their respective genera that cause human infections. The epidemiologic associations, pathogenic properties, and clinical manifestations of these organisms resemble those of *Proteus* species. However, *Morganella* and *Providencia* occur more commonly among LTCF residents; to a lesser degree, they affect hospitalized patients. In settings with extensive use of polymyxins and tigecycline, these organisms may become increasingly common because of their intrinsic resistance to these agents.

INFECTIOUS SYNDROMES

These species are primarily urinary tract pathogens, causing UTIs that are most often associated with long-term (>30-day) catheterization. Such infections commonly lead to biofilm formation and catheter encrustation (sometimes causing catheter obstruction) or to the development of struvite bladder or renal stones (sometimes causing renal obstruction and serving as foci for relapse). *Morganella* is also commonly isolated from snakebite infection. Other, less common infectious syndromes include surgical site infection, soft tissue infection (primarily involving decubitus and diabetic ulcers), burn site infection, pneumonia (particularly ventilator-associated), intravascular device infection, and intraabdominal infection. Rarely, the other extraintestinal infections described for GNB also occur. Bacteremia is uncommon; any infected site can serve as the source, but the urinary tract accounts for most cases, with the next most common sources being surgical site, soft tissue, and hepatobiliary infections.

DIAGNOSIS

M. morganii and *Providencia* are readily isolated and identified. Nearly all isolates are lactose negative and indole positive.

TREATMENT *MORGANELLA AND PROVIDENCIA* INFECTIONS

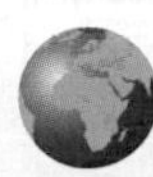

Morganella and *Providencia* may be extensively resistant to antibiotics. Most isolates are resistant to ampicillin, first-generation cephalosporins, nitrofurantoin, fosfomycin, tigecycline, and the polymyxins; 40% are resistant to fluoroquinolones. *Morganella* and *Providencia* possess inducible AmpC β-lactamases; clinically significant induction or selection of stably derepressed mutants may develop during therapy. Resistance to antipseudomonal penicillins, aztreonam, gentamicin, TMP-SMX, and second- and third-generation cephalosporins is emerging but is still variably prevalent. The β-lactamase inhibitor tazobactam increases susceptibility to β-lactam agents, but sulbactam and clavulanic acid do not. Carbapenems, amikacin, and cefepime are the most active agents (>90% of isolates susceptible); however, resistance to the carbapenems, when present, is a concern because of the inherent resistance of *Morganella* and *Providencia* to the polymyxins and tigecycline. Removal of a colonized catheter or stone is critical for eradication of UTI.

EDWARDSIELLA INFECTIONS

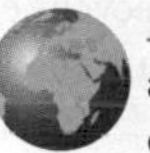

E. tarda is the only member of the genus *Edwardsiella* that is associated with human disease. This organism is found predominantly in freshwater and marine environments and in the associated aquatic animal species. Human acquisition occurs primarily during interaction with these reservoirs and ingestion of inadequately cooked aquatic animals. *E. tarda* infection is rare in the United States; recently reported cases are mostly from Southeast Asia. This pathogen shares clinical features with *Salmonella* species (as an intestinal pathogen; **Chap. 190**), *Vibrio vulnificus* (as an extraintestinal pathogen; **Chap. 193**) and *Aeromonas hydrophila* (as both an intestinal and extraintestinal pathogen; **Chap. 183e**).

INFECTIOUS SYNDROMES

Gastroenteritis is the predominant infectious syndrome (50–80% of infections). Self-limiting watery diarrhea is most common, but severe colitis also occurs. The most common extraintestinal infection is wound infection due to direct inoculation, which is often associated with freshwater, marine, or snake-related injuries. Other infectious syndromes result from invasion of the gastrointestinal tract and subsequent bacteremia. Most afflicted hosts have comorbidities (e.g., hepatobiliary disease, iron overload, cancer, or diabetes mellitus). A primary bacteremic syndrome, sometimes complicated by meningitis, has a 40% case-fatality rate. Visceral (primarily hepatic) and intraperitoneal abscesses also occur. Endocarditis and empyema have been described.

DIAGNOSIS

Although *E. tarda* can readily be isolated and identified, most laboratories do not routinely seek to identify it in stool samples. Production of hydrogen sulfide is a characteristic biochemical property.

TREATMENT *EDWARDSIELLA* INFECTIONS

E. tarda is susceptible to most antimicrobial agents appropriate for use against GNB. Gastroenteritis is generally self-limiting, but treatment with a fluoroquinolone may hasten resolution. In the setting of severe sepsis, fluoroquinolones, third- and fourth-generation cephalosporins, carbapenems, and amikacin—either alone or in combination—are the safest choices pending susceptibility data.

INFECTIONS CAUSED BY MISCELLANEOUS GENERA

Species of *Hafnia, Kluyvera, Cedecea, Pantoea, Ewingella, Leclercia,* and *Photorhabdus* are occasionally isolated from diverse clinical specimens, including blood, sputum, urine, cerebrospinal fluid, joint fluid, bile, and wounds. These organisms are rare and usually cause infection in a compromised host or in the setting of an invasive procedure or a foreign body. Cephalosporinases from *Kluyvera* have been implicated as the progenitors of CTX-M ESBLs.

187 *Acinetobacter* Infections

David L. Paterson, Anton Y. Peleg

Infections with bacteria of the genus *Acinetobacter* are established as a significant problem worldwide. *Acinetobacter baumannii* is particularly formidable because of its propensity to acquire antibiotic resistance determinants. Endemic infections caused by strains of *A. baumannii* resistant to multiple antibiotic classes, including carbapenems, are a serious concern in many specialized hospital units, especially intensive care units (ICUs). The foremost implication of infection with carbapenem-resistant *A. baumannii* is the need to use "last-line" antibiotics such as colistin, polymyxin B, or tigecycline; these options have the potential to render these bacteria resistant to all available antibiotics.

DEFINITION

Acinetobacter species are oxidase-negative, nonfermenting, short, gram-negative bacilli. They were traditionally thought of as nonmotile—a characteristic from which the genus name was derived (from the Greek *akineto*, meaning "nonmotile"). However, recent work has shown that *Acinetobacter* organisms demonstrate motility under certain growth conditions. The bacteria grow well at 37°C in aerobic conditions on a range of laboratory media (e.g., blood agar). Some species may not grow on MacConkey agar. Differentiation of *Acinetobacter* species is difficult with the means typically available to most clinical microbiology laboratories, including commercial semiautomated identification systems. The commonly used matrix-assisted laser desorption ionization–time of flight mass spectrometry (MALDI-TOF MS) systems are undergoing evaluation for species-level identification of *Acinetobacter.* DNA–DNA hybridization is a method used for speciation in reference laboratories. Naturally occurring oxacillinase genes (bla_{OXA}) have been identified in several *Acinetobacter* species, and their detection by polymerase chain reaction can aid in species identification.

ETIOLOGY

Widely distributed in nature, *Acinetobacter* species can be found in water, in soil, and on vegetables. *Acinetobacter* is a component of the human skin flora and is sometimes identified as a contaminant in blood samples collected for culture. Fecal carriage can be detected in both healthy and hospitalized individuals. However, despite the ubiquity of some *Acinetobacter* species, the natural habitat of the most clinically important species, *A. baumannii,* remains to be fully defined.

EPIDEMIOLOGY

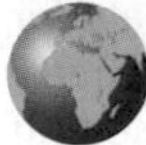

A. baumannii infections have been diagnosed in patients on all inhabited continents. The vast majority of infections occur in hospitalized patients and other patients with significant health-care contact. Outbreaks of carbapenem-resistant *A. baumannii* are particularly problematic. A significant issue is the introduction of carbapenem-resistant *A. baumannii* into hospitals as a result of medical transfers, especially from hospitals where the organism is highly endemic.

The Americas In 1991 and 1992, outbreaks of carbapenem-resistant *A. baumannii* infection occurred in a hospital in New York City. Subsequently, numerous other hospitals in the United States and South America have had outbreaks of carbapenem-resistant *A. baumannii.* Infections with *A. baumannii* among military personnel from the United States and Canada injured in Iraq or Afghanistan were widely observed beginning in 2002. *Acinetobacter* was one of the most common causes of bloodstream infections and bone and soft tissue infections after war-related injury. An epidemiologic investigation revealed that *A. baumannii* could be grown from environmental sites in field hospitals and that the environmental strains were closely related genotypically to clinical isolates.

Europe *A. baumannii* infections have posed a substantial clinical challenge in many parts of Europe since the early 1980s. Three clones (European clones I, II, and III) have been the predominant causes of *A. baumannii* infection in hospitals in Europe. Carbapenem resistance in *A. baumannii* is a significant issue in many European countries, most notably the United Kingdom, Greece, Italy, Spain, and Turkey.

Asia, Australia, the Middle East, and Africa Although surveillance data are sparse from many countries in these regions, problems with carbapenem-resistant *A. baumannii* abound. Community-acquired infections are well described in northern Australia and some parts of Asia. These infections may be more likely in men >45 years of age who have histories of cigarette smoking, alcoholism, diabetes mellitus, or chronic obstructive airway disease. Community-acquired strains are more susceptible to antimicrobial agents than are hospital-acquired strains, but the clinical presentation of community-acquired disease is quite distinct and is characterized by overwhelming infection with severe pneumonia, septic shock, and multiorgan failure.

PATHOGENESIS

A. baumannii colonizes patients exposed to heavily contaminated hospital environments or to the hands of health care workers in these locations. Emerging data suggest that the organism can be found in the air in rooms of patients infected with *Acinetobacter.* Colonization of the upper airways in mechanically ventilated patients may lead to nosocomial pneumonia. Colonization of the skin may lead to central line–associated bloodstream infection, catheter-associated urinary tract infection (UTI), wound infection, or postneurosurgical meningitis. Throat carriage and microaspiration may be involved in the pathogenesis of community-acquired pneumonia due to *A. baumannii.*

Much less is known about the virulence mechanisms of and host responses to *A. baumannii* than about these aspects of other pathogenic gram-negative bacteria. Because of the emergence of multidrug-resistant strains, including those resistant to all available antibiotics, the impetus to study *A. baumannii* pathogenesis has grown. Novel targets for antibacterial drug development are desperately required, and drugs that have antivirulence mechanisms may provide new therapeutic options. Specific virulence mechanisms in *A. baumannii* include iron acquisition and transport systems; outer-membrane protein A (OmpA), which mediates mammalian cell adhesion, invasion, and cytotoxicity through mitochondrial damage and initiation of caspase-dependent apoptosis; lipopolysaccharide (LPS); and proteins important in the formation of biofilm on abiotic and biotic surfaces. Biofilm formation on abiotic surfaces is dependent on a pilus assembly system, which in turn is controlled by a traditional two-component regulatory system mediated by *bfmR.* Also important in biofilm formation are a gene that encodes a biofilm-associated protein (Bap); OmpA; the quorum-sensing gene *abaI,* which controls the secretion of 3-hydroxy-C_{12}-homoserine lactone; and the *pga* locus, which is essential for the production of the polysaccharide poly-β-1,6-*N*-acetylglucosamine. Most recently, a global virulence regulator known as GacSA was described as important in regulating *A. baumannii* biofilms, motility, growth in human serum, and virulence in a mammalian infection model.

New model systems for the study of *A. baumannii* infection, including both nonmammalian (invertebrate) and mammalian models, have been described. Furthermore, the use of *A. baumannii* transposon-generated mutant libraries to screen for mutants with attenuated growth in human biologic fluids (serum and ascites fluid) has allowed the identification of new virulence mechanisms. These include phospholipase D; capsule production mediated by *ptk* and *epsA*; penicillin-binding protein 7/8 encoded by the *pbpG* gene; and a glycosyltransferase important for LPS biosynthesis encoded by the *lpsB* gene.

The LPS of *A. baumannii* appears to play a significant role in eliciting host responses. In studies with knockout mice, Toll-like receptor 4 and CD14 were shown to be important in host recognition, signaling, and cytokine production in response to *A. baumannii*. Humoral responses targeting iron-regulated outer-membrane proteins and the O-polysaccharide component of LPS also have been described.

APPROACH TO THE PATIENT: *Acinetobacter* Infection

Acinetobacter must be considered in the differential diagnosis of hospital-acquired pneumonia, central line–associated bloodstream infection, posttraumatic wound infection in military personnel, and postneurosurgical meningitis.

CLINICAL MANIFESTATIONS

Pneumonia It may be difficult to distinguish between upper-airway colonization with *A. baumannii* and hospital-acquired pneumonia. An estimated 5–10% of cases of ventilator-associated pneumonia are due to *A. baumannii*, although much regional variation exists. Typically, patients with *A. baumannii* ventilator-associated pneumonia have had a prolonged stay in an ICU; in outbreak situations, however, patients may acquire the infection within days of arrival in an ICU.

Community-acquired pneumonia due to *A. baumannii* has been described in tropical regions of Australia and Asia. The disease typically occurs during the "wet" season among people with a history of alcohol abuse. Infection may result in fulminant pneumonia requiring admission to an ICU, with a mortality rate of ~50%.

Bloodstream Infection Although *A. baumannii* accounts for only ~1–2% of nosocomial bloodstream infections, crude mortality rates from these infections may be as high as 40%. Sources of bloodstream infection are typically a central line or underlying pneumonia, UTI, or wound infection.

Traumatic Battlefield and Other Wounds *A. baumannii* is a well-known pathogen in burn units. This organism is commonly isolated from wounds of combat casualties; it was the most commonly isolated organism in one assessment of combat victims with open tibial fractures but did not appear to contribute directly to persistent nonunion or the need for amputation.

Meningitis *A. baumannii* may cause meningitis following neurosurgical procedures. Patients typically have an external ventricular drain in situ.

Urinary Tract Infection *A. baumannii* is an occasional cause of catheter-associated UTI. It is highly unusual for this organism to cause uncomplicated UTI in healthy women.

Other Clinical Manifestations A small number of case reports describe *Acinetobacter* prosthetic-valve endocarditis and endophthalmitis/keratitis. The latter is sometimes related to contact lens use or eye surgery.

DIAGNOSIS

Acinetobacter infection should be suspected when plump coccobacilli are seen in Gram's-stained respiratory tract secretions, blood cultures, or cerebrospinal fluid. Sometimes the organisms are difficult to de-stain. Given their small size, they may be misidentified as either gram-negative or gram-positive cocci.

TREATMENT *ACINETOBACTER* INFECTION (TABLE 187-1)

Treatment is hampered by the remarkable ability of *A. baumannii* to upregulate or acquire antibiotic resistance determinants. The most prominent example is that of β-lactamases, including those capable of inactivating carbapenems, cephalosporins, and penicillins. These enzymes, which include the OXA-type β-lactamases (e.g., OXA-23), the metallo-β-lactamases (e.g., NDM), and rarely KPC-type carbapenemases, are typically resistant to currently available β-lactamase inhibitors such as clavulanate or tazobactam. Plasmids that harbor genes encoding these β-lactamases may also harbor genes encoding resistance to aminoglycosides and sulfur antibiotics. The end result is that carbapenem-resistant *A. baumannii* may become truly multidrug resistant.

Selection of empirical antibiotic therapy when *A. baumannii* is suspected is challenging and must rely on a knowledge of local epidemiology. Receipt of prompt, effective antibiotic therapy is the goal. Given the diversity of resistance mechanisms in *A. baumannii*, definitive therapy should be based on the results of antimicrobial susceptibility testing. Carbapenems (imipenem, meropenem, and doripenem but not ertapenem) have long been thought of as the agents of choice for serious *A. baumannii* infections. However, the clinical utility of carbapenems is now widely jeopardized by the production of carbapenemases, as described above. Sulbactam may be an alternative to carbapenems. Unlike other β-lactamase inhibitors (e.g., clavulanic acid and tazobactam), sulbactam has intrinsic activity against *Acinetobacter*; this activity is mediated by the drug's binding to penicillin-binding protein 2 rather than by its ability to inhibit β-lactamases. Sulbactam is commercially available in a combined formulation with either ampicillin or cefoperazone and may also be available as a single agent in some countries. Despite the absence of randomized clinical trials, sulbactam seems to be equivalent to carbapenems in clinical effectiveness against susceptible strains.

Therapy for carbapenem-resistant *A. baumannii* is particularly problematic. The only currently available choices are polymyxins (colistin and polymyxin B) and tigecycline. Neither option is perfect. Polymyxins may be nephrotoxic and neurotoxic. Definition of the optimal dose and schedule for administration of polymyxins to patients in vulnerable groups (e.g., those requiring renal replacement therapy) remains challenging, and emergence of resistance in association with monotherapy is a concern. Conventional doses of tigecycline may not result in serum concentrations adequate to treat bloodstream infections. Resistance of *A. baumannii* to tigecycline may develop during treatment with this drug.

As a consequence of these issues with the polymyxins and tigecycline, combination therapy is now favored for carbapenem-resistant *Acinetobacter*. However, in a randomized controlled trial, 30-day mortality was not reduced by the addition of rifampin to colistin. Nevertheless, a significant increase in microbiologic eradication was observed in the colistin plus rifampin arm over that attained with

TABLE 187-1 TREATMENT OPTIONS FOR *ACINETOBACTER* INFECTIONS

Antibiotic	Comments
Sulbactam	Intrinsic activity against *Acinetobacter*, not linked to β-lactamase inhibition
Trimethoprim-sulfamethoxazole	May be an option for urinary tract infection or wound infection
Meropenem	Carbapenem resistance now widespread
Amikacin	May be an option for carbapenem-resistant strains
Tigecycline	May be an option for carbapenem-resistant strains but inappropriate for urinary tract infection, bloodstream infection, or meningitis
Colistin or polymyxin B	May be an option for carbapenem-resistant strains, but pharmacokinetics not yet well understood

colistin alone. Combinations of polymyxins with a carbapenem look more promising and are being evaluated in prospective clinical trials. Fosfomycin has poor activity against *Acinetobacter* and should not be relied upon for treatment. Clearly, new treatment options are needed for serious *Acinetobacter* infections.

COMPLICATIONS AND PROGNOSIS

Given the propensity of *A. baumannii* to cause infections in seriously ill patients in ICUs, it is not surprising that *A. baumannii* infections are associated with high mortality rates. Thus a pertinent question is whether *A. baumannii* infections are associated with high attributable mortality rates after the severity of illness is controlled for. A number of studies have addressed this issue but have had disparate results. Whether the discrepant results can be explained purely by methodologic differences is unknown at present.

PREVENTION

Multidrug-resistant *A. baumannii* clearly causes outbreaks of infection and then establishes endemicity. In endemic situations, a small number of strain types predominate. In the 1991–1992 outbreaks in New York City, for example, two strain types accounted for more than 80% of carbapenem-resistant isolates. This "oligoclonality" plainly demonstrates the potential importance of infection control interventions in response to outbreaks of multidrug-resistant *A. baumannii* infection.

The hospital environment is an important reservoir of organisms capable of colonizing patients and causing infection. Environmental sources of *A. baumannii* include computer keyboards, glucometers, multidose medication vials, IV nutrition, inadequately sterilized reusable arterial pressure transducers, ventilator tubing, suction catheters, humidifiers, containers of distilled water, urine collection jugs, and moist bedding articles. Pulsatile-lavage wound treatment—a high-pressure irrigation system used to debride wounds—has been associated with an outbreak of *A. baumannii* infection.

Contaminated inanimate objects should be removed from the patient-care environment or subjected to enhanced environmental cleaning. Although contact-isolation procedures (use of gloves and gowns when dealing with colonized patients or their environment), accommodation of patients in single rooms, and improved hand hygiene are critical, attention to the patient-care environment may be the only measure that leads to control of outbreaks of *A. baumannii* infection. One study found that *Acinetobacter* can be cultured from the air in rooms of patients with *A. baumannii* infection; the infection-control implications are not yet clear.

188 *Helicobacter pylori* Infections

John C. Atherton, Martin J. Blaser

DEFINITION

Helicobacter pylori colonizes the stomach in ~50% of the world's human population, essentially for life unless eradicated by antibiotic treatment. Colonization with this organism is the main risk factor for peptic ulceration (Chap. 348) as well as for gastric adenocarcinoma and gastric mucosa-associated lymphoid tissue (MALT) lymphoma (Chap. 109). Treatment for *H. pylori* has revolutionized the management of peptic ulcer disease, providing a permanent cure in most cases. Such treatment also represents first-line therapy for patients with low-grade gastric MALT lymphoma. Treatment of *H. pylori* is of no benefit in the treatment of gastric adenocarcinoma, but prevention of *H. pylori* colonization could potentially prevent gastric malignancy and peptic ulceration. In contrast, increasing evidence indicates that lifelong *H. pylori* colonization may offer some protection against complications of gastroesophageal reflux disease (GERD), including esophageal adenocarcinoma. Recent research has focused on whether *H. pylori* colonization is also a risk factor for some extragastric diseases and whether it is protective against some recently emergent medical problems, such as childhood-onset asthma and obesity.

ETIOLOGIC AGENT

Helicobacter pylori *H. pylori* is a gram-negative bacillus that has naturally colonized humans for at least 100,000 years, and probably throughout human evolution. It lives in gastric mucus, with a small proportion of the bacteria adherent to the mucosa and possibly a very small number of the organisms entering cells or penetrating the mucosa; the organism's distribution is never systemic. Its spiral shape and flagella render *H. pylori* motile in the mucus environment. The organism has several acid-resistance mechanisms, most notably a highly expressed urease that catalyzes urea hydrolysis to produce buffering ammonia. *H. pylori* is microaerophilic (i.e., requires low levels of oxygen), is slow-growing, and requires complex growth media in vitro.

Other Helicobacter Species A very small proportion of gastric *Helicobacter* infections are due to species other than *H. pylori*, possibly acquired as zoonoses. These non-*pylori* gastric helicobacters are associated with low-level inflammation and occasionally with disease. In immunocompromised hosts, several nongastric (intestinal) *Helicobacter* species can cause disease with clinical features resembling those of *Campylobacter* infections; these species are covered in Chap. 192.

EPIDEMIOLOGY

Prevalence and Risk Factors The prevalence of *H. pylori* among adults is <30% in most parts of the United States and in other developed countries as opposed to >80% in most developing countries. In the United States, prevalence varies with age: up to 50% of 60-year-old persons, ~20% of 30-year-old persons, and fewer than 10% of children are colonized. *H. pylori* is usually acquired in childhood. The age association is due mostly to a birth-cohort effect whereby current 60-year-olds were more commonly colonized as children than are current children. Spontaneous acquisition or loss of *H. pylori* in adulthood is uncommon. Childhood acquisition explains why the main risk factors for infection are markers of crowding and social deprivation in childhood.

Transmission Humans are the only important reservoir of *H. pylori*. Children may acquire the organism from their parents (most often the primary caregiver) or from other children. The former is more common in developed countries and the latter in less developed countries. Whether transmission takes place more often by the fecal-oral or the oral-oral route is unknown, but *H. pylori* is easily cultured from vomitus and gastroesophageal refluxate and is less easily cultured from stool.

PATHOLOGY AND PATHOGENESIS

H. pylori colonization induces *chronic superficial gastritis*, a tissue response in the stomach that includes infiltration of the mucosa by both mononuclear and polymorphonuclear cells. (The term *gastritis* should be used specifically to describe histologic features; it has also been used to describe endoscopic appearances and even symptoms, but these features do not correlate with microscopic findings or even with the presence of *H. pylori*.) Although *H. pylori* is capable of numerous adaptations that prevent excessive stimulation of the immune system, colonization is accompanied by a considerable persistent local and systemic immune response, including the production of antibodies and cell-mediated responses. However, these responses are ineffective in clearing the bacterium. This inefficient clearing appears to be due in part to *H. pylori*'s downregulation of the immune system, which fosters its own persistence.

Most *H. pylori*–colonized persons do not develop clinical sequelae. That some persons develop overt disease whereas others do not is related to a combination of factors: bacterial strain differences, host susceptibility to disease, and environmental factors.

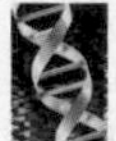

Bacterial Virulence Factors Several *H. pylori* virulence factors are more common among strains that are associated with disease than among those that are not. The *cag* island is a group of genes that encodes a bacterial type IV secretion system. Through this system, an effector protein, CagA, is translocated into epithelial cells, where it may be transformed by phosphorylation and induces host cell signal transduction; proliferative, cytoskeletal, and inflammatory changes in the cell result. The protein at the tip of the secretory apparatus, CagL, binds to integrins on the cell surface, transducing further signaling. Finally, soluble components of the peptidoglycan cell wall enter the cell, mediated by the same secretory system. These components are recognized by the emergency intracellular bacterial receptor Nod1, which stimulates a proinflammatory cytokine response resulting in enhanced gastric inflammation. Carriage of *cag*-positive strains increases the risk of peptic ulcer or gastric adenocarcinoma. A second major virulence factor is the vacuolating cytotoxin VacA, which forms pores in cell membranes. VacA is polymorphic, and carriage of more active forms also increases the risk of disease. Other bacterial factors that are associated with increased disease risk include adhesins, such as BabA (which binds to blood group antigens on epithelial cells), and incompletely characterized factors, such as another recently described bacterial type 4 secretion system.

Host Genetic and Environmental Factors The best-characterized host determinants of disease are genetic polymorphisms leading to enhanced activation of the innate immune response, including polymorphisms in cytokine genes or in genes encoding bacterial recognition proteins such as Toll-like receptors. For example, colonized people with polymorphisms in the interleukin 1 gene that increase the production of this cytokine in response to *H. pylori* infection are at increased risk of gastric adenocarcinoma. In addition, environmental cofactors are important in pathogenesis. Smoking increases the risks of duodenal ulcers and gastric cancer in *H. pylori*–positive individuals. Diets high in salt and preserved foods increase cancer risk, whereas diets high in antioxidants and vitamin C are modestly protective.

Distribution of Gastritis and Differential Disease Risk The pattern of gastric inflammation is associated with disease risk: antral-predominant gastritis is most closely linked with duodenal ulceration, whereas pan-gastritis is linked with gastric ulceration and adenocarcinoma. This difference probably explains why patients with duodenal ulceration are not at high risk of developing gastric adenocarcinoma later in life, despite being colonized by *H. pylori*.

PATHOGENESIS OF DUODENAL ULCERATION How gastric colonization causes duodenal ulceration is now becoming more clear. *H. pylori*–induced inflammation of the gastric antrum diminishes the number of somatostatin-producing D cells. Because somatostatin inhibits gastrin release, gastrin levels are higher than in *H. pylori*–negative persons, and these higher levels lead to increased meal-stimulated acid secretion from the relatively spared gastric corpus. How this situation increases duodenal ulcer risk remains controversial, but the increased acid secretion may contribute to the formation of the potentially protective gastric metaplasia found in the duodenum of duodenal ulcer patients. Gastric metaplasia in the duodenum may become colonized by *H. pylori* and subsequently inflamed and ulcerated.

PATHOGENESIS OF GASTRIC ULCERATION AND GASTRIC ADENOCARCINOMA The pathogenesis of these conditions is less well understood, although both arise in association with pan- or corpus-predominant gastritis. The hormonal changes described above still occur, but the inflammation in the gastric corpus means that it produces less acid (hypochlorhydria) despite hypergastrinemia. Gastric ulcers usually occur at the junction of antral and corpus-type mucosa, an area that is often particularly inflamed. Gastric cancer probably stems from progressive DNA damage and the survival of abnormal epithelial cell clones. The DNA damage is thought to be due principally to reactive oxygen and nitrogen species arising from inflammatory cells, perhaps in relation to other bacteria that survive in a hypochlorhydric stomach. Longitudinal analyses of gastric biopsy specimens taken years apart from the same patient show that the common *intestinal* type of gastric adenocarcinoma follows stepwise changes from simple gastritis to gastric atrophy, intestinal metaplasia, and dysplasia. A second, *diffuse* type of gastric adenocarcinoma found more commonly in younger adults may arise directly from chronic gastritis without atrophic changes.

CLINICAL MANIFESTATIONS

Essentially all *H. pylori*–colonized persons have histologic gastritis, but only ~10–15% develop associated illnesses such as peptic ulceration, gastric adenocarcinoma, or gastric lymphoma (Fig. 188-1). Rates among women are less than half of those among men for both diseases.

Peptic Ulcer Disease Worldwide, >80% of duodenal ulcers and >60% of gastric ulcers are related to *H. pylori* colonization (Chap. 348). However, in particular, the proportion of gastric ulcers caused by aspirin and nonsteroidal anti-inflammatory drugs (NSAIDs) is increasing, and in many developed countries these drugs have overtaken *H. pylori* as a cause of gastric ulceration. The main lines of evidence supporting an ulcer-promoting role for *H. pylori* are that (1) the presence of the organism is a risk factor for the development of ulcers, (2) non-NSAID-induced ulcers rarely develop in the absence of *H. pylori*, (3) eradication of *H. pylori* virtually abolishes long-term ulcer relapse, and (4) experimental *H. pylori* infection of gerbils can cause gastric ulceration.

Gastric Adenocarcinoma and Lymphoma Prospective nested case-control studies have shown that *H. pylori* colonization is a risk factor for adenocarcinomas of the distal (noncardia) stomach (Chap. 109). Long-term experimental infection of gerbils also may result in gastric adenocarcinoma. Moreover, *H. pylori* may induce primary gastric

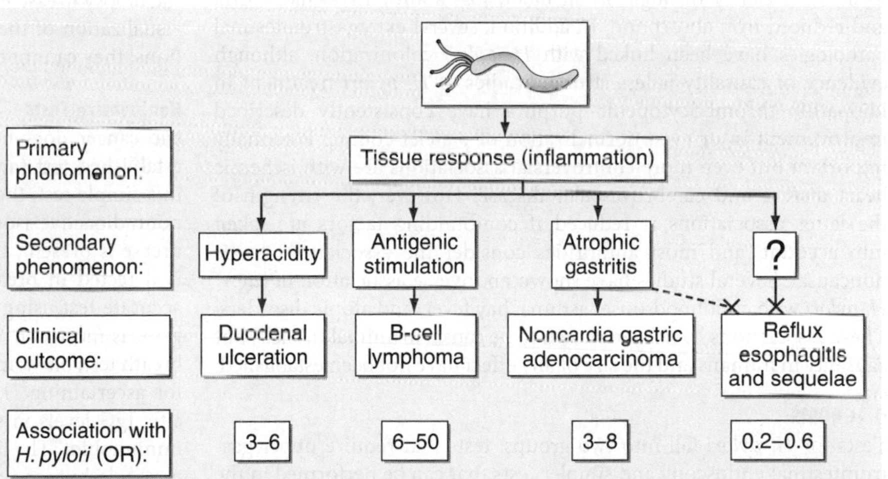

FIGURE 188-1 Schematic of the relationships between colonization with *Helicobacter pylori* and diseases of the upper gastrointestinal tract. Essentially all persons colonized with *H. pylori* develop a host response, which is generally termed *chronic gastritis*. The nature of the host's interaction with the particular bacterial population determines the clinical outcome. *H. pylori* colonization increases the lifetime risk of peptic ulcer disease, noncardia gastric cancer, and B-cell non-Hodgkin's gastric lymphoma (odds ratios [ORs] for all, >3). In contrast, a growing body of evidence indicates that *H. pylori* colonization (especially with *cagA*$^+$ strains) protects against adenocarcinoma of the esophagus (and the sometimes related gastric cardia) and premalignant lesions such as Barrett's esophagus (OR, <1). Although the incidences of peptic ulcer disease (cases not due to nonsteroidal anti-inflammatory drugs) and noncardia gastric cancer are declining in developed countries, the incidence of adenocarcinoma of the esophagus is increasing. *(Adapted from MJ Blaser: Hypothesis: The changing relationships of Helicobacter pylori and humans: Implications for health and disease. J Infect Dis 179:1523, 1999, with permission.)*

lymphoma, although this condition is much less common. Many low-grade gastric B-cell lymphomas are dependent on *H. pylori* for continuing growth and proliferation, and these tumors may regress either fully or partially after *H. pylori* eradication. However, they require careful short- and long-term monitoring, and some necessitate additional treatment with chemotherapeutic agents.

Functional Dyspepsia Many patients have upper gastrointestinal symptoms but have normal results on upper gastrointestinal endoscopy (so-called functional or nonulcer dyspepsia; Chap. 348). Because *H. pylori* is common, some of these patients will be colonized with the organism. *H. pylori* eradication leads to symptom resolution a little more commonly (from 0 to 7% in different studies) than does placebo treatment. Whether such patients have peptic ulcers in remission at the time of endoscopy or whether a small subgroup of patients with "true" functional dyspepsia respond to *H. pylori* treatment is unclear.

Protection Against Peptic Esophageal Disease, Including Esophageal Adenocarcinoma Much interest has focused on a protective role for *H. pylori* against GERD (Chap. 347), Barrett's esophagus (Chap. 347), and adenocarcinoma of the esophagus and gastric cardia (Chap. 109). The main lines of evidence for this role are (1) that there is a temporal relationship between a falling prevalence of gastric *H. pylori* colonization and a rising incidence of these conditions; (2) that, in most studies, the prevalence of *H. pylori* colonization (especially with proinflammatory *cagA*$^+$ strains) is significantly lower among patients with these esophageal diseases than among control participants; and (3) that, in prospective nested studies (see above), the presence of *H. pylori* is inversely related to these cancers. The mechanism underlying this protective effect is likely *H. pylori*–induced hypochlorhydria. Because, at the individual level, GERD symptoms may decrease, worsen, or remain unchanged after *H. pylori* treatment, concerns about GERD should not affect decisions about whether to treat *H. pylori* when an indication exists.

Other Pathologies *H. pylori* has an increasingly recognized role in other gastric pathologies. It may be one initial precipitant of autoimmune gastritis and pernicious anemia and also may predispose some patients to iron deficiency through occult blood loss and/or hypochlorhydria and reduced iron absorption. In addition, several extragastrointestinal pathologies have been linked with *H. pylori* colonization, although evidence of causality is less strong. Studies of *H. pylori* treatment in idiopathic thrombocytopenic purpura have consistently described improvement in or even normalization of platelet counts. Potentially important but even more controversial associations are with ischemic heart disease and cerebrovascular disease. However, the strength of the latter associations is reduced if confounding factors are taken into account, and most authorities consider the associations to be noncausal. Several studies have shown an inverse association of *cagA*$^+$ *H. pylori* with childhood-onset asthma, hay fever, and atopic disorders. These associations have been shown to be causal in animal models, but causality in humans and the size of any effect have not been established.

DIAGNOSIS

Tests for *H. pylori* fall into two groups: tests that require upper gastrointestinal endoscopy and simpler tests that can be performed in the clinic (Table 188-1).

Endoscopy-Based Tests Endoscopy is usually unnecessary in the initial management of young patients with simple dyspepsia but is commonly used to exclude malignancy and make a positive diagnosis in older patients or those with "alarm" symptoms. If endoscopy is performed, the most convenient biopsy-based test is the biopsy urease test, in which one large or two small gastric biopsy specimens are placed into a gel containing urea and an indicator. The presence of *H. pylori* urease leads to a pH alteration and therefore to a color change, which often occurs within minutes but can require up to 24 h. Histologic examination of biopsy specimens for *H. pylori* also is accurate, provided that a special stain (e.g., a modified Giemsa or silver stain) permitting optimal visualization of the organism is used. If biopsy specimens are obtained from both antrum and corpus, histologic study yields additional information, including the degree and pattern of inflammation and the presence of any atrophy, metaplasia, or dysplasia. Microbiologic culture is most specific but may be insensitive because of difficulty with *H. pylori* isolation. Once the organism is cultured, its identity as *H. pylori* can be confirmed by its typical appearance on Gram's stain and its positive reactions in oxidase, catalase, and urease tests. Moreover, the organism's susceptibility to antibiotics can be determined, and this information can be clinically useful in difficult cases. The occasional biopsy specimens containing the less common non-*pylori* gastric helicobacters give only weakly positive results in the biopsy urease test. Positive identification of these bacteria requires visualization of the characteristic long, tight spirals in histologic sections; they cannot easily be cultured.

TABLE 188-1 TESTS COMMONLY USED TO DETECT *HELICOBACTER PYLORI*

Test	Advantages	Disadvantages
Tests Based on Endoscopic Biopsy		
Biopsy urease test	Quick, simple	Some commercial tests not fully sensitive before 24 h
Histology	May give additional histologic information	Sensitivity dependent on experience and use of special stains
Culture	Permits determination of antibiotic susceptibility	Sensitivity dependent on experience
Noninvasive Tests		
Serology	Inexpensive and convenient; not affected by recent antibiotics or proton pump inhibitors to the same extent as breath and stool tests	Cannot be used for early follow-up after treatment; some commercial kits inaccurate, and most less accurate than urea breath test
^{13}C urea breath test	Inexpensive and simpler than endoscopy; useful for follow-up after treatment	Requires fasting; not as convenient as blood or stool tests
Stool antigen test	Inexpensive and convenient; useful for follow-up after treatment; may be useful in children	Stool-based tests are disliked by people from some cultures

Noninvasive Tests Noninvasive *H. pylori* testing is the norm if gastric cancer does not need to be excluded by endoscopy. The best-established test (and a very accurate one) is the *urea breath test.* In this simple test, the patient drinks a solution of urea labeled with the nonradioactive isotope ^{13}C and then blows into a tube. If *H. pylori* urease is present, the urea is hydrolyzed, and labeled carbon dioxide is detected in breath samples. The *stool antigen test,* a simple and accurate test using monoclonal antibodies specific for *H. pylori* antigens, is more convenient and potentially less expensive than the urea breath test, but some patients dislike sampling stool. The simplest tests for ascertaining *H. pylori* status are *serologic assays* measuring specific IgG levels in serum by enzyme-linked immunosorbent assay or immunoblot. The best of these tests are as accurate as other diagnostic methods, but many commercial tests—especially rapid office tests—do not perform well.

Use of Tests to Assess Treatment Success The urea breath test, the stool antigen test, and biopsy-based tests can all be used to assess the success of treatment (Fig. 188-2). However, because these tests are dependent on *H. pylori* load, their use <4 weeks after treatment may yield false-negative results. Furthermore, these tests are unreliable if performed within 4 weeks of intercurrent treatment with antibiotics or bismuth compounds or within 2 weeks of the discontinuation of proton pump inhibitor (PPI) treatment. In the assessment of treatment success, noninvasive tests are normally preferred; however, after gastric ulceration, endoscopy should be repeated to ensure healing and to exclude gastric carcinoma by further histologic sampling. Serologic tests are not used to monitor treatment success, as the gradual drop in titer of *H. pylori*–specific antibodies is too slow to be of practical use.

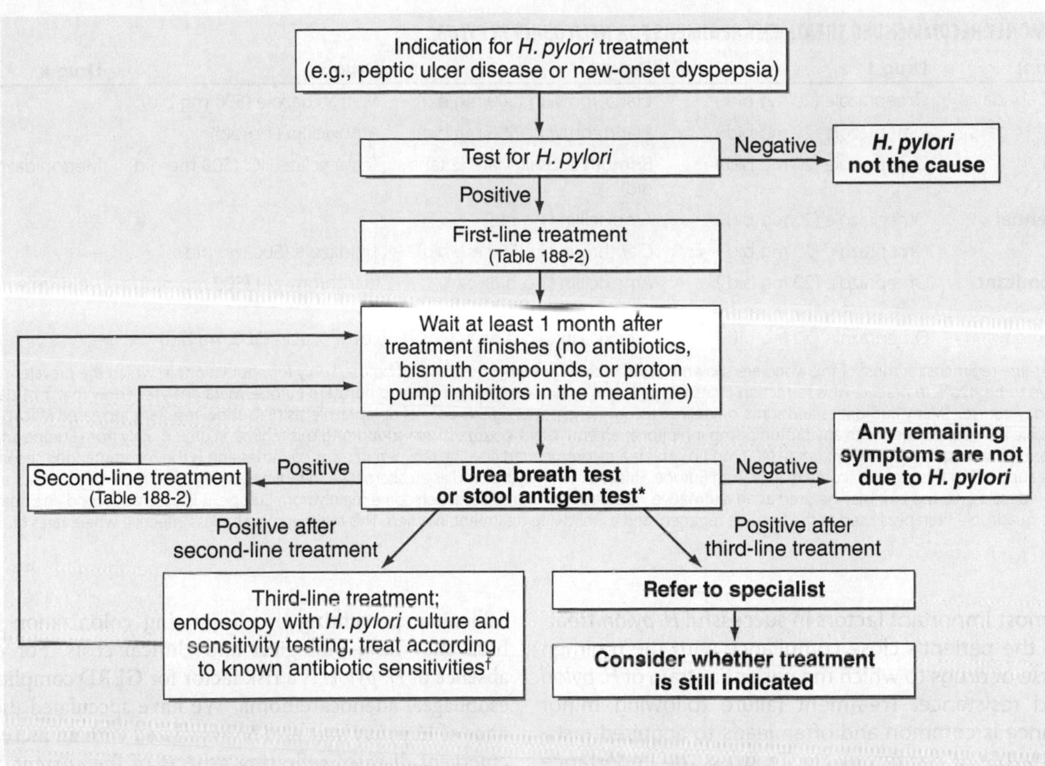

FIGURE 188-2 Algorithm for the management of *Helicobacter pylori* infection. *Note that either the urea breath test or the stool antigen test can be used in this algorithm. Occasionally, endoscopy and a biopsy-based test are used instead of either of these tests in follow-up after treatment. The main indication for these invasive tests is gastric ulceration; in this condition, as opposed to duodenal ulceration, it is important to check healing and to exclude underlying gastric adenocarcinoma. However, even in this situation, patients undergoing endoscopy may still be receiving proton pump inhibitor therapy, which precludes *H. pylori* testing. Thus a urea breath test or a stool antigen test is still required at a suitable interval after the end of therapy to determine whether treatment has been successful (see text). †Some authorities use empirical third-line regimens, of which several have been described.

TREATMENT *HELICOBACTER PYLORI* INFECTION

INDICATIONS

The most clear-cut indications for treatment are *H. pylori*–related duodenal or gastric ulceration or low-grade gastric B-cell lymphoma. Whether or not the ulcers are currently active, *H. pylori* should be eradicated in patients with documented ulcer disease to prevent relapse (Fig. 188-2). Testing for *H. pylori* and treatment if the results are positive also have been advocated in uninvestigated simple dyspepsia, but only when the prevalence of *H. pylori* in the community is >20% are these measures more cost-effective than simply treating the dyspepsia with PPIs. Guidelines have recommended *H. pylori* treatment in functional dyspepsia in case the patient is one of the perhaps 0–7% who will benefit from such treatment (beyond placebo effects). Some guidelines also recommend treatment of conditions not definitively known to respond to *H. pylori* eradication, including idiopathic thrombocytopenic purpura, vitamin B12 deficiency, and iron-deficiency anemia (in the last instance, only when other causes have been carefully excluded). Test-and-treat has emerged as a common clinical practice in recent years despite the lack of direct evidence that it is advantageous; whether this practice will survive the scrutiny of time and further study remains to be determined. For individuals with a strong family history of gastric cancer, treatment to eradicate *H. pylori* in the hope of reducing their cancer risk is reasonable but of unproven value. Currently, widespread community screening for and treatment of *H. pylori* as primary prophylaxis for gastric cancer and peptic ulcers are not recommended in most countries, mainly because the extent of the consequent reduction in cancer risk is not known. Several studies have found a modestly reduced cancer risk after treatment, but the period of follow-up is still fairly short and the size of the effect in different populations remains unclear. Other reasons not to treat *H. pylori* in asymptomatic populations at present include (1) the adverse side effects (which are common and can be severe in rare cases) of the multiple-antibiotic regimens used; (2) antibiotic resistance, which may emerge in *H. pylori* or other incidentally carried bacteria; (3) the anxiety that may arise in otherwise healthy people, especially if treatment is unsuccessful; and (4) the existence of a subset of people who will develop GERD symptoms after treatment, although, on average, *H. pylori* treatment does not affect GERD symptoms or severity. Despite the absence of screening strategies, many doctors treat *H. pylori* if it is known to be present (particularly in children and younger adults), even when the patient is asymptomatic. The rationale is that it reduces patient concern and may reduce future gastric cancer risk and that any reduction in risk is likely to be greater in younger patients. However, such practices do not factor in any potential benefits of *H. pylori* colonization. Overall, despite widespread clinical activity in this area, most treatment of asymptomatic *H. pylori* carriage is given without a firm evidence base.

REGIMENS

Although *H. pylori* is susceptible to a wide range of antibiotics in vitro, monotherapy is not usually successful, probably because of inadequate antibiotic delivery to the colonization niche. Failure of monotherapy prompted the development of multidrug regimens, the most successful of which are triple and quadruple combinations. Current regimens consist of a PPI and two or three antimicrobial agents given for 7–14 days (Table 188-2). Research on optimizing drug combinations to increase efficacy continues, and guidelines are likely to change as the field develops and as countries increasingly tailor treatment to suit local antibiotic resistance patterns and economic needs.

TABLE 188-2 COMMONLY RECOMMENDED TREATMENT REGIMENS FOR *HELICOBACTER PYLORI*

Regimen[a] (Duration)	Drug 1	Drug 2	Drug 3	Drug 4
Regimen 1: OCM (7–14 days)[b]	Omeprazole (20 mg bid[c])	Clarithromycin (500 mg bid)	Metronidazole (500 mg bid)	—
Regimen 2: OCA (7–14 days)[b]	Omeprazole (20 mg bid[c])	Clarithromycin (500 mg bid)	Amoxicillin (1 g bid)	—
Regimen 3: OBTM (14 days)[d]	Omeprazole (20 mg bid[c])	Bismuth subsalicylate (2 tabs qid)	Tetracycline HCl (500 mg qid)	Metronidazole (500 mg tid)
Regimen 4[e]: sequential (5 days + 5 days)	Omeprazole (20 mg bid[c])	Amoxicillin (1 g bid)	—	—
	Omeprazole (20 mg bid[c])	Clarithromycin (500 mg bid)	Tinidazole (500 mg bid[g])	—
Regimen 5[f]: concomitant (14 days)	Omeprazole (20 mg bid[c])	Amoxicillin (1 g bid)	Clarithromycin (500 mg bid)	Tinidazole (500 mg bid[g])
Regimen 6[h]: OAL (10 days)	Omeprazole (20 mg bid[c])	Amoxicillin (1 g bid)	Levofloxacin (500 mg bid)	—

[a]The recommended first-line regimens for most of the world are shown in **bold** type. [b]These regimens should be used only for populations in which the prevalence of clarithromycin-resistant strains is known to be <20%. In practice, this restriction limits the regimens' appropriate range mainly to northern Europe. Meta-analyses show that a 14-day course of therapy is slightly superior to a 7-day course. [c]Many authorities and some guidelines recommend doubling this dose of omeprazole, as trials show resultant increased efficacy with some antibiotic combinations. Omeprazole may be replaced with any proton pump inhibitor at an equivalent dosage. [d]Data supporting this regimen come mainly from Europe and are based on the use of bismuth subcitrate (1 tablet qid) and metronidazole (400 mg tid). This is a recommended first-line regimen in most countries and is the recommended second-line regimen in northern Europe. [e]Data supporting this regimen come mainly from Europe. This regimen may be used as an alternative to regimen 3. [f]This regimen may be used as an alternative to regimen 3 or 4. [g]Metronidazole (500 mg bid) may be used as an alternative. [h]Data supporting this regimen come mainly from Europe. It is used as second-line treatment in many countries (particularly where quadruple therapy is used as the first-line regimen) and as third-line treatment in others. This regimen may be less effective where rates of quinolone use are high.

The two most important factors in successful *H. pylori* treatment are the patient's close compliance with the regimen and the use of drugs to which the patient's strain of *H. pylori* has not acquired resistance. Treatment failure following minor lapses in compliance is common and often leads to acquired resistance to metronidazole or clarithromycin. To stress the importance of compliance, written instructions should be given to the patient, and minor side effects of the regimen should be explained. Increasing levels of *H. pylori* resistance to clarithromycin, quinolones, and—to a lesser extent—metronidazole are of growing concern and are thought to be responsible for the reduced efficacy of previously popular clarithromycin-based triple-therapy regimens worldwide. Treatment with these regimens is now virtually confined to certain northern European countries where the use of clarithromycin (or azithromycin) for respiratory infections has not been widespread and resistance rates in *H. pylori* are still low. Strains of *H. pylori* with some degree of in vitro resistance to metronidazole are common but still may be eradicated with metronidazole-containing regimens, which have only slightly reduced efficacy in vivo. Assessment of antibiotic susceptibilities before treatment would be optimal but is not usually undertaken because endoscopy and mucosal biopsy are necessary to obtain *H. pylori* for culture and because most microbiology laboratories are inexperienced in *H. pylori* culture. In the absence of susceptibility information, the patient's history of (even distant) antibiotic use for other conditions should be ascertained; use of the previously administered agent(s) should then be avoided if possible, particularly in the case of clarithromycin (e.g., previous use for upper respiratory infection) and quinolones. If initial *H. pylori* treatment fails, the usual approach is empirical re-treatment with another drug regimen (Table 188-2). The third-line approach should ideally be endoscopy, biopsy, and culture plus treatment based on documented antibiotic sensitivities. However, empirical third-line therapies are often used.

Non-*pylori* gastric helicobacters are treated in the same way as *H. pylori*. However, in the absence of trials, it is unclear whether a positive outcome always represents successful treatment or whether it is sometimes due to natural clearance of the bacteria.

PREVENTION

Carriage of *H. pylori* has considerable public health significance in developed countries, where it is associated with peptic ulcer disease and gastric adenocarcinoma, and in developing countries, where gastric adenocarcinoma may be an even more common cause of cancer death late in life. If mass prevention were contemplated, vaccination would be the most obvious method, and experimental immunization of animals has given promising results. However, given that *H. pylori* has co-evolved with its human host over millennia, preventing or eliminating colonization on a population basis may have biological and clinical costs. For example, lifelong absence of *H. pylori* is a risk factor for GERD complications, including esophageal adenocarcinoma. We have speculated that the disappearance of *H. pylori* may also be associated with an increased risk of other emergent diseases reflecting aspects of the current Western lifestyle, such as childhood-onset asthma and allergy.

189 Infections Due to *Pseudomonas* Species and Related Organisms

Reuben Ramphal

The pseudomonads are a heterogeneous group of gram-negative bacteria that have in common an inability to ferment lactose. Formerly classified in the genus *Pseudomonas*, the members of this group have been assigned to three medically important genera—*Pseudomonas, Burkholderia,* and *Stenotrophomonas*—whose biologic behaviors encompass both similarities and marked differences and whose genetic repertoires differ in many respects. The pathogenicity of most pseudomonads is based on opportunism; the exceptions are the organisms that cause melioidosis (*Burkholderia pseudomallei*) and glanders (*Burkholderia mallei*), which can be considered as primary pathogens.

Pseudomonas aeruginosa, the major pathogen of the group, is a significant cause of infections in hospitalized patients and in patients with cystic fibrosis (CF; Chap. 313). Cytotoxic chemotherapy, mechanical ventilation, and broad-spectrum antibiotic therapy probably paved the way for colonization and infection of increasing numbers of hospitalized patients by this organism. Thus most conditions predisposing to *P. aeruginosa* infections have involved host compromise and/or broad-spectrum antibiotic use. The other members of the genus *Pseudomonas*—*Pseudomonas putida, Pseudomonas fluorescens,* and *Pseudomonas stutzeri*—infect humans infrequently.

The genus *Burkholderia* comprises more than 40 species, of which *Burkholderia cepacia* is most frequently encountered in Western countries. Like *P. aeruginosa, B. cepacia* is both a nosocomial pathogen and a cause of infection in CF. The other medically important members of this genus are *B. pseudomallei* and *B. mallei,* the etiologic agents of melioidosis and glanders, respectively.

The genus *Stenotrophomonas* contains one species of medical significance, *Stenotrophomonas maltophilia* (previously classified in the genera *Pseudomonas* and *Xanthomonas*). This organism is strictly an opportunist that "overgrows" in the setting of potent broad-spectrum antibiotic use.

PSEUDOMONAS AERUGINOSA

EPIDEMIOLOGY

P. aeruginosa is found in most moist environments. Soil, plants, vegetables, tap water, and countertops are all potential reservoirs for this microbe, as it has simple nutritional needs. Given the ubiquity of *P. aeruginosa*, simple contact with the organism is not sufficient for colonization or infection. Clinical and experimental observations suggest that *P. aeruginosa* infection often occurs concomitantly with host defense compromise, mucosal trauma, physiologic derangement, and antibiotic-mediated suppression of normal flora. Thus, it comes as no surprise that the majority of *P. aeruginosa* infections occur in intensive care units (ICUs), where these factors frequently converge. The organism is initially acquired from environmental sources, but patient-to-patient spread also occurs in clinics and families.

In the past, burned patients appeared to be unusually susceptible to *P. aeruginosa*. For example, in 1959–1963, *Pseudomonas* burn-wound sepsis was the principal cause of death in 60% of burned patients dying at the U.S. Army Institute of Surgical Research. For reasons that are unclear, *P. aeruginosa* infection in burns is no longer the major problem that it was during the 1950s and 1960s. Similarly, in the 1960s, *P. aeruginosa* appeared as a common pathogen in patients receiving cytotoxic chemotherapy at many institutions in the United States, but it subsequently diminished in importance. Despite this subsidence, *P. aeruginosa* remains one of the most feared pathogens in this population because of its high attributable mortality rate.

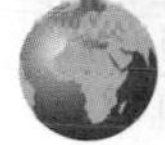

In some parts of Asia and Latin America, *P. aeruginosa* continues to be the most common cause of gram-negative bacteremia in neutropenic patients.

In contrast to the trends for burned patients and neutropenic patients in the United States, the incidence of *P. aeruginosa* infections among patients with CF has not changed. *P. aeruginosa* remains the most common contributing factor to respiratory failure in CF and is responsible for the majority of deaths among CF patients.

LABORATORY FEATURES

P. aeruginosa is a nonfastidious, motile, gram-negative rod that grows on most common laboratory media, including blood and MacConkey agars. It is easily identified in the laboratory on primary-isolation agar plates by pigment production that confers a yellow to dark green or even bluish appearance. Colonies have a shiny "gun-metal" appearance and a characteristic fruity odor. Two of the identifying biochemical characteristics of *P. aeruginosa* are an inability to ferment lactose on MacConkey agar and a positive reaction in the oxidase test. Most strains are identified on the basis of these readily detectable laboratory features even before extensive biochemical testing is done. Some isolates from CF patients are easily identified by their mucoid appearance, which is due to the production of large amounts of the mucoid exopolysaccharide or alginate.

PATHOGENESIS

Unraveling the mechanisms that underlie disease caused by *P. aeruginosa* has proved challenging. Of the common gram-negative bacteria, no other species produces such a large number of putative virulence factors (Table 189-1). Yet *P. aeruginosa* rarely initiates an infectious process in the absence of host injury or compromise, and few of its putative virulence factors have been shown definitively to be involved in disease in humans. Despite its metabolic versatility and possession of multiple colonizing factors, *P. aeruginosa* exhibits no competitive advantage over enteric bacteria in the human gut; neither is it a normal inhabitant of the human gastrointestinal tract, despite the host's continuous environmental exposure to the organism.

Virulence Attributes Involved in Acute *P. aeruginosa* Infections • ***MOTILITY AND COLONIZATION*** A general tenet of bacterial pathogenesis is that most bacteria must adhere to surfaces or colonize a host niche in order to initiate disease. Most pathogens examined thus far possess adherence factors called *adhesins*. *P. aeruginosa* is no exception. Among its many adhesins are its pili, which demonstrate adhesive properties for a variety of cells and adhere best to injured cell surfaces. In the organism's flagellum, the flagellin molecule binds to cells, and the flagellar cap attaches to mucins through the recognition of glycan chains. Other *P. aeruginosa* adhesins include the outer core of the lipopolysaccharide (LPS) molecule, which binds to the cystic fibrosis transmembrane conductance regulator (CFTR) and aids in internalization of the organism, and the alginate coat of mucoid strains, which enhances adhesion to cells and mucins. In addition, membrane proteins and lectins have been proposed as colonization factors. The deletion of any given adhesin is not sufficient to abrogate the ability of *P. aeruginosa* to colonize surfaces. Motility is important in host invasion via mucosal surfaces in some animal models; however, nonmotile strains are not uniformly avirulent.

TABLE 189-1 MAIN PUTATIVE VIRULENCE FACTORS OF *PSEUDOMONAS AERUGINOSA*

Substance/Organelle	Function	Virulence in Animal Disease
Pili	Adhesion to cells	?
Flagella	Adhesion, motility, inflammation	Yes
Lipopolysaccharide	Antiphagocytic activity, inflammation	Yes
Type III secretion system	Toxic activity (ExoU, ExoS)	Yes
Type II secretion system	Toxic activity	Yes
Proteases	Proteolytic activity	?
Phospholipases	Cytotoxicity	?
Exotoxin A	Cytotoxicity	?

EVASION OF HOST DEFENSES The transition from bacterial colonization to disease requires the evasion of host defenses followed by invasion of the microorganism. *P. aeruginosa* appears to be well equipped for evasion. Attached bacteria inject four known toxins (ExoS or ExoU, ExoT, and ExoY) via a type III secretion system that allows the bacteria to evade phagocytic cells either by direct cytotoxicity or by inhibition of phagocytosis. Mutants with defects in this system fail to disseminate in some animal models of infection. The type II secretion system as a whole secretes toxins that can kill animals, and some of its secreted toxins, such as exotoxin A, have the potential to kill phagocytic cells. Multiple proteases secreted by this system may degrade host effector molecules, such as cytokines and chemokines, that are released in response to infection. Thus this system may also contribute to host evasion.

TISSUE INJURY Among gram-negative bacteria, *P. aeruginosa* probably produces the largest number of substances that are toxic to cells and thus may injure tissues. The toxins secreted by its type III secretion system are capable of tissue injury. However, their delivery requires the adherence of the organism to cells. Thus, the effects of these toxins are likely to be local or to depend on the presence of vast numbers of bacteria. On the other hand, diffusible toxins, secreted by the organism's type II secretion system, can act freely wherever they come into contact with cells. Possible effectors include exotoxin A, four different proteases, and at least two phospholipases; in addition to these secreted toxins, rhamnolipids, pyocyanin, and hydrocyanic acid are produced by *P. aeruginosa* and are all capable of inducing host injury.

INFLAMMATORY COMPONENTS The inflammatory components of *P. aeruginosa*—e.g., the inflammatory responses to the lipid A component of LPSs and to flagellin, mediated through the Toll-like receptor (TLR) system (principally TLR4 and TLR5)—have been thought to represent important factors in disease causation. Although these inflammatory responses are required for successful defense against *P. aeruginosa* (i.e., in their absence, animals are defenseless against *P. aeruginosa* infection), florid responses are likely to result in disease. When the sepsis syndrome and septic shock develop in *P. aeruginosa* infection, they are probably the result of the host response to one or both of these substances, but injury to the lung by *Pseudomonas* toxins may also result in sepsis syndromes, possibly by causing cell death and the release of cellular components (e.g., heat-shock proteins) that may activate the TLR or another proinflammatory system.

Chronic *P. aeruginosa* Infections Chronic infection due to *P. aeruginosa* occurs mainly in the lungs in the setting of structural pulmonary diseases. The classic example is CF; others include bronchiectasis and chronic relapsing panbronchiolitis, a disease seen in Japan and some Pacific Islands. Hallmarks of these illnesses are altered mucociliary clearance leading to mucus stasis and mucus accumulation in the lungs. There is probably a common factor that selects for *P. aeruginosa* colonization in these lung diseases—perhaps the adhesiveness of *P. aeruginosa* for mucus, a phenomenon that is not noted for most other common gram-negative bacteria, and/or the ability of *P. aeruginosa* to evade host defenses in mucus. Furthermore, *P. aeruginosa* seems to evolve in ways that allow its prolonged survival in the lung without an early fatal outcome for the host. The strains found in CF patients exhibit minimal production of virulence factors. Some strains even lose the ability to produce pili and flagella, and most become complement-sensitive because of the loss of the O side chain of their LPS molecules. An example of the impact of these changes is found in the organism's discontinuation of the production of flagellin (probably its most strongly proinflammatory molecule) when it encounters purulent mucus. This response probably dampens the host's response, allowing the organism to survive in mucus. *P. aeruginosa* is also believed to lose the ability to secrete many of its injectable toxins during growth in mucus. Although the alginate coat is thought to play a role in the organism's survival, alginate is not essential, as nonmucoid strains may also predominate for long periods. In short, virulence in chronic infections may be mediated by the chronic but attenuated host inflammatory response, which injures the lungs over decades.

CLINICAL MANIFESTATIONS

P. aeruginosa causes infections at almost all sites in the body but shows a rather strong predilection for the lungs. The infections encountered most commonly in hospitalized patients are described below.

Bacteremia Crude mortality rates exceeding 50% have been reported among patients with *P. aeruginosa* bacteremia. Consequently, this clinical entity has been much feared, and its management has been attempted with the use of multiple antibiotics. Recent publications report attributable mortality rates of 28–44%, with the precise figure depending on the adequacy of treatment and the seriousness of the underlying disease. In the past, the patient with *P. aeruginosa* bacteremia classically was neutropenic or had a burn injury. Today, however, a minority of such patients have bacteremic *P. aeruginosa* infections. Rather, *P. aeruginosa* bacteremia is seen most often in patients in ICUs.

The clinical presentation of *P. aeruginosa* bacteremia rarely differs from that of sepsis in general (Chap. 324). Patients are usually febrile, but those who are most severely ill may be in shock or even hypothermic. The only point differentiating this entity from gram-negative sepsis of other causes may be the distinctive skin lesions (ecthyma gangrenosum) of *Pseudomonas* infection, which occur almost exclusively in markedly neutropenic patients and patients with AIDS. These small or large, painful, reddish, maculopapular lesions have a geographic margin; they are initially pink, then darken to purple, and finally become black and necrotic (Fig. 189-1). Histopathologic studies indicate that the lesions are due to vascular invasion and are teeming with bacteria. Although similar lesions may occur in aspergillosis and mucormycosis, their presence suggests *P. aeruginosa* bacteremia as the most likely diagnosis.

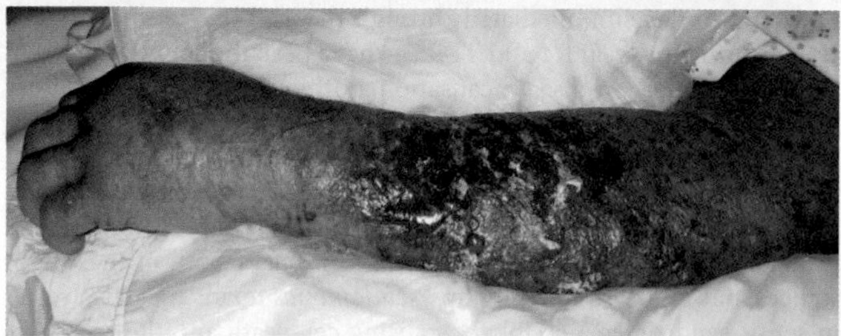

FIGURE 189-1 Ecthyma gangrenosum in a neutropenic patient 3 days after onset.

TREATMENT *P. AERUGINOSA* BACTEREMIA

(Table 189-2) Antimicrobial treatment of *P. aeruginosa* bacteremia has been controversial. Before 1971, the outcome of *Pseudomonas* bacteremia in febrile neutropenic patients treated with the available agents—gentamicin and the polymyxins—was dismal. However, treatment with carbenicillin, with or without an aminoglycoside, significantly improved outcomes. Concurrently, several retrospective analyses suggested that the use of two agents that were synergistic against gram-negative pathogens in vitro resulted in better outcomes in neutropenic patients. Thus, combination therapy became the standard of care—first for *P. aeruginosa* bacteremia in febrile neutropenic patients and then for all *P. aeruginosa* infections in neutropenic or nonneutropenic patients.

With the introduction of newer antipseudomonal drugs, a number of studies have revisited the choice between combination treatment and monotherapy for *Pseudomonas* bacteremia. Although the majority of experts still favor combination therapy, most of these observational studies indicate that a single modern antipseudomonal β-lactam agent to which the isolate is sensitive is as efficacious as a combination. Even in patients at greatest risk of early death from *P. aeruginosa* bacteremia (i.e., those with fever and neutropenia), empirical antipseudomonal monotherapy is deemed to be as efficacious as empirical combination therapy by the practice guidelines of the Infectious Diseases Society of America. One firm conclusion is that monotherapy with an aminoglycoside is not optimal.

There are, of course, institutions and countries where rates of susceptibility of *P. aeruginosa* to first-line antibiotics are <80%. Thus, when a septic patient with a high probability of *P. aeruginosa* infection is encountered in such settings, empirical combination therapy should be administered until the pathogen is identified and susceptibility data become available. Thereafter, whether one or two agents should be continued remains a matter of individual preference. Recent studies suggest that extended infusions of β-lactams such as cefepime or piperacillin-tazobactam may result in better outcomes of *Pseudomonas* bacteremia and possibly *Pseudomonas* pneumonia.

Acute Pneumonia Respiratory infections are the most common of all infections caused by *P. aeruginosa*. This organism appears first or second among the causes of ventilator-associated pneumonia (VAP). However, much debate centers on the actual role of *P. aeruginosa* in VAP. Many of the relevant data are based on cultures of sputum or endotracheal tube aspirates and may represent nonpathogenic colonization of the tracheobronchial tree, biofilms on the endotracheal tube, or simple tracheobronchitis.

Older reports of *P. aeruginosa* pneumonia described patients with an acute clinical syndrome of fever, chills, cough, and necrotizing pneumonia indistinguishable from other gram-negative bacterial pneumonias. The traditional accounts described a fulminant infection. Chest radiographs demonstrated bilateral pneumonia, often with nodular densities with or without cavities. This picture is now remarkably rare. Today, the typical patient is on a ventilator, has a slowly progressive infiltrate, and has been colonized with *P. aeruginosa* for days. While some cases may progress rapidly over 48–72 h, they are the exceptions. Nodular densities are not commonly seen. However, infiltrates may go on to necrosis. Necrotizing pneumonia has also been seen in the community (e.g., after inhalation of hot-tub water contaminated with *P. aeruginosa*). The typical patient has fever, leukocytosis, and purulent sputum, and the chest radiograph shows a new infiltrate or the expansion of a preexisting infiltrate. Chest examination generally detects rales or dullness. Of course, such findings are quite common among ventilated patients in the ICU. A sputum Gram's stain showing mainly polymorphonuclear leukocytes (PMNs) in conjunction with a culture positive for *P. aeruginosa* in this setting suggests a diagnosis of acute *P. aeruginosa* pneumonia. There is no consensus about whether

TABLE 189-2 ANTIBIOTIC TREATMENT OF INFECTIONS DUE TO *PSEUDOMONAS AERUGINOSA* AND RELATED SPECIES

Infection	Antibiotics and Dosages	Other Considerations
Bacteremia		
Nonneutropenic host	Monotherapy: Ceftazidime (2 g q8h IV) *or* cefepime (2 g q12h IV) Combination therapy: Piperacillin/tazobactam (3.375 g q4h IV) *or* imipenem (500 mg q6h IV) *or* meropenem (1 g q8h IV) *or* doripenem (500 mg q8h IV) ***plus*** Amikacin (7.5 mg/kg q12h or 15 mg/kg q24h IV)	Add an aminoglycoside for patients in shock and in regions or hospitals where rates of resistance to the primary β-lactam agents are high. Tobramycin may be used instead of amikacin (susceptibility permitting). The duration of therapy is 7 days for nonneutropenic patients. Neutropenic patients should be treated until no longer neutropenic.
Neutropenic host	Cefepime (2 g q8h IV) or all other agents (except doripenem) in above dosages	
Endocarditis	Antibiotic regimens as for bacteremia for 6–8 weeks	Resistance during therapy is common. Surgery is required for relapse.
Pneumonia	Drugs and dosages as for bacteremia, except that the available carbapenems should not be the sole primary drugs because of high rates of resistance during therapy	IDSA guidelines recommend the addition of an aminoglycoside or ciprofloxacin. The duration of therapy is 10–14 days.
Bone infection, malignant otitis externa	Cefepime or ceftazidime at the same dosages as for bacteremia; aminoglycosides not a necessary component of therapy; ciprofloxacin (500–750 mg q12h PO) may be used	Duration of therapy varies with the drug used (e.g., 6 weeks for a β-lactam agent; at least 3 months for oral therapy except in puncture-wound osteomyelitis, for which the duration should be 2–4 weeks).
Central nervous system infection	Ceftazidime or cefepime (2 g q8h IV) or meropenem (1 g q8h IV)	Abscesses or other closed-space infections may require drainage. The duration of therapy is ≥2 weeks.
Eye infection		
Keratitis/ulcer	Topical therapy with tobramycin/ciprofloxacin/levofloxacin eyedrops	Use maximal strengths available or compounded by pharmacy. Therapy should be administered for 2 weeks or until the resolution of eye lesions, whichever is shorter.
Endophthalmitis	Ceftazidime or cefepime as for central nervous system infection ***plus*** Topical therapy	
Urinary tract infection	Ciprofloxacin (500 mg q12h PO) *or* levofloxacin (750 mg q24h) *or* any aminoglycoside (total daily dose given once daily)	Relapse may occur if an obstruction or a foreign body is present. The duration of therapy for complicated UTI is 7–10 days (up to 2 weeks for pyelonephritis).
Multidrug-resistant *P. aeruginosa* infection	Colistin (100 mg q12h IV) for the shortest possible period to obtain a clinical response	Doses used have varied. Dosage adjustment is required in renal failure. Inhaled colistin may be added for pneumonia (100 mg q12h).
Stenotrophomonas maltophilia infection	TMP-SMX (1600/320 mg q12h IV) *plus* ticarcillin/clavulanate (3.1 g q4h IV) for 14 days	Resistance to all agents is increasing. Levofloxacin or tigecycline may be alternatives, but there is little published clinical experience with these agents.
Burkholderia cepacia infection	Meropenem (1 g q8h IV) *or* TMP-SMX (1600/320 mg q12h IV) for 14 days	Resistance to both agents is increasing. Do not use them in combination because of possible antagonism.
Melioidosis, glanders	Ceftazidime (2 g q6h) *or* meropenem (1 g q8h) *or* imipenem (500 mg q6h) for 2 weeks ***followed by*** TMP-SMX (1600/320 mg q12h PO) for 3 months	

Abbreviations: IDSA, Infectious Diseases Society of America; TMP-SMX, trimethoprim-sulfamethoxazole.

an invasive procedure (e.g., bronchoalveolar lavage or protected-brush sampling of the distal airways) is superior to tracheal aspiration to obtain samples for lung cultures in order to substantiate the occurrence of *P. aeruginosa* pneumonia and prevent antibiotic overuse.

TREATMENT ACUTE PNEUMONIA

(Table 189-2) Therapy for *P. aeruginosa* pneumonia has been unsatisfactory. Reports suggest mortality rates of 40–80%, but how many of these deaths are attributable to underlying disease remains unknown. The drugs of choice for *P. aeruginosa* pneumonia are similar to those given for bacteremia. A potent antipseudomonal β-lactam drug is the mainstay of therapy. Failure rates were high when aminoglycosides were used as single agents, possibly because of their poor penetration into the airways and their binding to airway secretions. Thus a strong case cannot be made for the inclusion of the aminoglycoside component in regimens used against fully susceptible organisms, especially given the evidence that aminoglycosides are not optimally active in the lungs at concentrations normally reached after IV administration. Nonetheless, aminoglycosides are commonly used in clinical practice. Some experts suggest the combination of a β-lactam agent and an antipseudomonal fluoroquinolone instead when combination therapy is desired.

Chronic Respiratory Tract Infections *P. aeruginosa* is responsible for chronic infections of the airways associated with a number of underlying or predisposing conditions—most commonly CF (Chap. 313). A state of chronic colonization beginning early in childhood is seen in some Asian populations with chronic or diffuse panbronchiolitis, a disease of unknown etiology. *P. aeruginosa* is one of the organisms that colonizes damaged bronchi in bronchiectasis, a disease secondary to multiple causes in which profound structural abnormalities of the airways result in mucus stasis.

TREATMENT CHRONIC RESPIRATORY TRACT INFECTIONS

Optimal management of chronic *P. aeruginosa* lung infection has not been determined. Patients respond clinically to antipseudomonal therapy, but the organism is rarely eradicated. Because eradication is unlikely, the aim of treatment for chronic infection is to quell exacerbations of inflammation. The regimens used are similar to those used for pneumonia, but an aminoglycoside is almost always added because resistance is common in chronic disease. However, it may be appropriate to use an inhaled aminoglycoside preparation in order to maximize airway drug levels.

Endovascular Infections Infective endocarditis due to *P. aeruginosa* is a disease of IV drug users whose native valves are involved. This organism has also been reported to cause prosthetic valve endocarditis. Sites of prior native-valve injury due to the injection of foreign material such as talc or fibers probably serve as niduses for bacterial attachment to the heart valve. The manifestations of *P. aeruginosa* endocarditis resemble those of other forms of endocarditis in IV drug users except that the disease is more indolent than *Staphylococcus aureus* endocarditis. While most disease involves the right side of the heart, left-sided involvement is not rare and multivalvular disease is common. Fever is a common manifestation, as is pulmonary involvement (due to septic emboli to the lungs). Hence, patients may also experience chest pain and hemoptysis. Involvement of the left side of the heart may lead to signs of cardiac failure, systemic emboli, and local cardiac involvement with sinus of Valsalva abscesses and conduction defects. Skin manifestations are rare in this disease, and ecthyma gangrenosum is not seen. The diagnosis is based on positive blood cultures along with clinical signs of endocarditis.

TREATMENT ENDOVASCULAR INFECTIONS

(Table 189-2) It has been customary to use synergistic antibiotic combinations in treating *P. aeruginosa* endocarditis because of the development of resistance during therapy with a single antipseudomonal β-lactam agent. Which combination therapy is preferable is unclear, as all combinations have failed. Cases of *P. aeruginosa* endocarditis that relapse during or fail to respond to therapy are often caused by resistant organisms and may require surgical therapy. Other considerations for valve replacement are similar to those in other forms of endocarditis (Chap. 155).

Bone and Joint Infections *P. aeruginosa* is an infrequent cause of bone and joint infections. However, *Pseudomonas* bacteremia or infective endocarditis caused by the injection of contaminated illicit drugs has been documented to result in vertebral osteomyelitis and sternoclavicular joint arthritis. The clinical presentation of vertebral *P. aeruginosa* osteomyelitis is more indolent than that of staphylococcal osteomyelitis. The duration of symptoms in IV drug users with vertebral osteomyelitis due to *P. aeruginosa* varies from weeks to months. Fever is not uniformly present; when present, it tends to be low grade. There may be mild tenderness at the site of involvement. Blood cultures are usually negative unless there is concomitant endocarditis. The erythrocyte sedimentation rate (ESR) is generally elevated. Vertebral osteomyelitis due to *P. aeruginosa* has also been reported in the elderly, in whom it originates from urinary tract infections (UTIs). The infection generally involves the lumbosacral area because of a shared venous drainage (Batson's plexus) between the lumbosacral spine and the pelvis. Sternoclavicular septic arthritis due to *P. aeruginosa* is seen almost exclusively in IV drug users. This disease may occur with or without endocarditis, and a primary site of infection often is not found. Plain radiographs show joint or bone involvement. Treatment of these forms of disease is generally successful.

Pseudomonas osteomyelitis of the foot most often follows puncture wounds through sneakers and mostly affects children. The main manifestation is pain in the foot, sometimes with superficial cellulitis around the puncture wound and tenderness on deep palpation of the wound. Multiple joints or bones of the foot may be involved. Systemic symptoms are generally absent, and blood cultures are usually negative. Radiographs may or may not be abnormal, but the bone scan is usually positive, as are magnetic resonance imaging (MRI) studies. Needle aspiration usually yields a diagnosis. Prompt surgery, with exploration of the nail puncture tract and debridement of the involved bones and cartilage, is generally recommended in addition to antibiotic therapy.

Central Nervous System (CNS) Infections CNS infections due to *P. aeruginosa* are relatively rare. Involvement of the CNS is almost always secondary to a surgical procedure or head trauma. The entity seen most often is postoperative or posttraumatic meningitis. Subdural or epidural infection occasionally results from contamination of these areas. Embolic disease arising from endocarditis in IV drug users and leading to brain abscesses has also been described. The cerebrospinal fluid (CSF) profile of *P. aeruginosa* meningitis is no different from that of pyogenic meningitis of any other etiology.

TREATMENT CENTRAL NERVOUS SYSTEM INFECTIONS

(Table 189-2) Treatment of *Pseudomonas* meningitis is difficult; little information has been published, and no controlled trials in humans have been undertaken. However, the general principles involved in the treatment of meningitis apply, including the need for high doses of bactericidal antibiotics to attain high drug levels in the CSF. The agent with which there is the most published experience in *P. aeruginosa* meningitis is ceftazidime, but other antipseudomonal β-lactam drugs that reach high CSF concentrations, such as cefepime and meropenem, have also been used successfully. Other forms of *P. aeruginosa* CNS infection, such as brain abscesses and epidural and subdural empyema, generally require surgical drainage in addition to antibiotic therapy.

Eye Infections Eye infections due to *P. aeruginosa* occur mainly as a result of direct inoculation into the tissue during trauma or surface injury by contact lenses. Keratitis and corneal ulcers are the most common types of eye disease and are often associated with contact lenses (especially the extended-wear variety). Keratitis can be slowly or rapidly progressive, but the classic description is disease progressing over 48 h to involve the entire cornea, with opacification and sometimes perforation. *P. aeruginosa* keratitis should be considered a medical emergency because of the rapidity with which it can progress to loss of sight. *P. aeruginosa* endophthalmitis secondary to bacteremia is the most devastating of *P. aeruginosa* eye infections. The disease is fulminant, with severe pain, chemosis, decreased visual acuity, anterior uveitis, vitreous involvement, and panophthalmitis.

TREATMENT EYE INFECTIONS

(Table 189-2) The usual therapy for keratitis is the administration of topical antibiotics. Therapy for endophthalmitis includes the use of high-dose local and systemic antibiotics (to achieve higher drug concentrations in the eye) and vitrectomy.

Ear Infections *P. aeruginosa* infections of the ears vary from mild swimmer's ear to serious life-threatening infections with neurologic sequelae. Swimmer's ear is common among children and results from infection of moist macerated skin of the external ear canal. Most cases resolve with treatment, but some patients develop chronic drainage. Swimmer's ear is managed with topical antibiotic agents (otic solutions). The most serious form of *Pseudomonas* infection involving the ear has been given various names: two of these designations, *malignant otitis externa* and *necrotizing otitis externa*, are now used for the same entity. This disease was originally described in elderly diabetic patients, in whom the majority of cases still occur. However, it has also been described in patients with AIDS and in elderly patients without underlying diabetes or immunocompromise. The usual presenting symptoms are decreased hearing and ear pain, which may be severe and lancinating. The pinna is usually painful, and the external canal may be tender. The ear canal almost always shows signs of inflammation, with granulation tissue and exudate. Tenderness anterior to the tragus may extend as far as the temporomandibular joint and mastoid process. A small minority of patients have systemic symptoms. Patients in whom the diagnosis is made late may present with cranial nerve palsies or even with cavernous venous sinus thrombosis. The ESR is invariably elevated (≥100 mm/h). The diagnosis is made on clinical grounds in severe cases; however, the "gold standard" is a positive technetium-99 bone scan in a patient with otitis externa due to *P. aeruginosa*. In diabetic patients, a positive bone scan constitutes presumptive evidence for this diagnosis and should prompt biopsy or empirical therapy.

TREATMENT EAR INFECTIONS

(Table 189-2) Given the infection of the ear cartilage, sometimes with mastoid or petrous ridge involvement, patients with malignant (necrotizing) otitis externa are treated as for osteomyelitis.

Urinary Tract Infections UTIs due to *P. aeruginosa* generally occur as a complication of a foreign body in the urinary tract, an obstruction in the genitourinary system, or urinary tract instrumentation or surgery. However, UTIs caused by *P. aeruginosa* have been described in pediatric outpatients without stones or evident obstruction.

TREATMENT URINARY TRACT INFECTIONS

(Table 189-2) Most *P. aeruginosa* UTIs are considered complicated infections that must be treated longer than uncomplicated cystitis. In general, a 7- to 10-day course of treatment suffices, with up to 2 weeks of therapy in cases of pyelonephritis. Urinary catheters, stents, or stones should be removed to prevent relapse, which is common and may be due not to resistance but rather to factors such as a foreign body that has been left in place or an ongoing obstruction.

Skin and Soft Tissue Infections Besides pyoderma gangrenosum in neutropenic patients, folliculitis and other papular or vesicular lesions due to *P. aeruginosa* have been extensively described and are collectively referred to as *dermatitis*. Multiple outbreaks have been linked to whirlpools, spas, and swimming pools. To prevent such outbreaks, the growth of *P. aeruginosa* in the home and in recreational environments must be controlled by proper chlorination of water. Most cases of hot-tub folliculitis are self-limited, requiring only the avoidance of exposure to the contaminated source of water.

Toe-web infections occur especially often in the tropics, and the "green nail syndrome" is caused by *P. aeruginosa* paronychia, which results from frequent submersion of the hands in water. In the latter entity, the green discoloration results from diffusion of pyocyanin into the nail bed. *P. aeruginosa* remains a prominent cause of burn wound infections in some parts of the world. The management of these infections is best left to specialists in burn wound care.

Infections in Febrile Neutropenic Patients In febrile neutropenia, *P. aeruginosa* has historically been the organism against which empirical coverage is always essential. Although in Western countries these infections are now less common, their importance has not diminished because of persistently high mortality rates. In other parts of the world as well, *P. aeruginosa* continues to be a significant problem in febrile neutropenia, causing a larger proportion of infections in febrile neutropenic patients than any other single organism. For example, *P. aeruginosa* was responsible for 28% of documented infections in 499 febrile neutropenic patients in one study from the Indian subcontinent and for 31% of such infections in another. In a large study of infections in leukemia patients from Japan, *P. aeruginosa* was the most frequently documented cause of bacterial infection. In studies performed in North America, northern Europe, and Australia, the incidence of *P. aeruginosa* bacteremia in febrile neutropenia was quite variable. In a review of 97 reports published in 1987–1994, the incidence was reported to be 1–2.5% among febrile neutropenic patients given empirical therapy and 5–12% among microbiologically documented infections. The most common clinical syndromes encountered were bacteremia, pneumonia, and soft tissue infections manifesting mainly as ecthyma gangrenosum.

TREATMENT INFECTIONS IN FEBRILE NEUTROPENIC PATIENTS

(Table 189-2) Compared with rates three decades ago, improved rates of response to antibiotic therapy have been reported in many studies. A study of 127 patients demonstrated a reduction in the mortality rate from 71% to 25% with the introduction of ceftazidime and imipenem. Because neutrophils—the normal host defenses against this organism—are absent in febrile neutropenic patients, maximal doses of antipseudomonal β-lactam antibiotics should be used for the management of *P. aeruginosa* bacteremia in this setting.

Infections in Patients with AIDS Both community- and hospital-acquired *P. aeruginosa* infections were documented in patients with AIDS before the advent of antiretroviral therapy. Since the introduction of protease inhibitors, *P. aeruginosa* infections in AIDS patients have been seen less frequently but still occur, particularly in the form of sinusitis. The clinical presentation of *Pseudomonas* infection (especially pneumonia and bacteremia) in AIDS patients is remarkable in that, although the illness may appear not to be severe, the infection may nonetheless be fatal. Patients with bacteremia may have only a low-grade fever and may present with ecthyma gangrenosum. Pneumonia, with or without bacteremia, is perhaps the most common type of *P. aeruginosa* infection in AIDS patients. Patients with AIDS and *P. aeruginosa* pneumonia exhibit the classic clinical signs and symptoms of pneumonia, such as fever, productive cough, and chest pain. The infection may be lobar or multilobar and shows no predisposition for any particular location. The most striking feature is the high frequency of cavitary disease.

TREATMENT INFECTIONS IN PATIENTS WITH AIDS

Therapy for any of these conditions in AIDS patients is no different from that in other patients. However, relapse is the rule unless the patient's CD4+ T cell count rises to >50/μL or suppressive antibiotic therapy is given. In attempts to achieve cures and prevent relapses, therapy tends to be more prolonged than in the case of an immunocompetent patient.

Multidrug-Resistant Infections (Table 189-2) *P. aeruginosa* has a notorious propensity to develop antibiotic resistance. During three decades, the impact of resistance was minimized by the rapid development of potent antipseudomonal agents. However, the situation has recently changed, with the worldwide selection of strains carrying determinants that mediate resistance to β-lactams, fluoroquinolones, and aminoglycosides. This situation has been compounded by the lack of development of new classes of antipseudomonal drugs for nearly two decades. Physicians now resort to drugs such as colistin and polymyxin, which were discarded decades ago. These alternative approaches to the management of multiresistant *P. aeruginosa* infections were first used some time ago in CF patients, who receive colistin (polymyxin E) IV and by aerosol despite its renal toxicity. Colistin is rapidly becoming the last-resort agent of choice, even in non-CF patients infected with multiresistant *P. aeruginosa*.

The clinical outcome of multidrug-resistant *P. aeruginosa* infections treated with colistin is difficult to judge from case reports, especially given the many drugs used in the complicated management of these patients. Although earlier reports described marginal efficacy and serious nephrotoxicity and neurotoxicity, recent reports have been more encouraging. Because colistin shows synergy with other antimicrobial agents in vitro, it may be possible to reduce the dosage—and thus the toxicity—of this drug when it is combined with drugs such as rifampin and β-lactams; however, no studies in humans or animals support this approach at this time.

OTHER PSEUDOMONADS

STENOTROPHOMONAS MALTOPHILIA

S. maltophilia is the only potential human pathogen among a genus of ubiquitous organisms found in the rhizosphere (i.e., the soil that surrounds the roots of plants). The organism is an opportunist that is acquired from the environment but is even more limited than *P. aeruginosa* in its ability to colonize patients or cause infections. Immunocompromise is not sufficient to permit these events; rather, major perturbations of the human flora are usually necessary for the establishment of *S. maltophilia*. Accordingly, most cases of human infection occur in the setting of very broad-spectrum antibiotic therapy with agents such as advanced cephalosporins and carbapenems, which eradicate the normal flora and other pathogens. The remarkable ability of *S. maltophilia* to resist virtually all classes of antibiotics is attributable to the possession of antibiotic efflux pumps and of two β-lactamases (L1 and L2) that mediate β-lactam resistance, including that to carbapenems. It is fortunate that the virulence of *S. maltophilia* appears to be limited. Although a serine protease is present in some strains, virulence is probably a result of the host's inflammatory response to components of the organism such as LPS and flagellin. *S. maltophilia* is most commonly found in the respiratory tract of ventilated patients, where the distinction between its roles as a colonizer and as a pathogen is often difficult to make. However, *S. maltophilia* does cause pneumonia and bacteremia in such patients, and these infections have led to septic shock. Also common is central venous line–associated infection (with or without bacteremia), which has been reported most often in patients with cancer. *S. maltophilia* is a rare cause of ecthyma gangrenosum in neutropenic patients. It has been isolated from ~5% of CF patients but is not believed to be a significant pathogen in this setting.

TREATMENT *S. MALTOPHILIA* INFECTIONS

The intrinsic resistance of *S. maltophilia* to most antibiotics renders infection difficult to treat. The antibiotics to which it is most often (although not uniformly) susceptible are trimethoprim-sulfamethoxazole (TMP-SMX), ticarcillin/clavulanate, levofloxacin, and tigecycline (Table 189-2). Consequently, a combination of TMP-SMX and ticarcillin/clavulanate is recommended for initial therapy. Catheters must be removed in the treatment of bacteremia to hasten cure and prevent relapses. The treatment of VAP due to *S. maltophilia* is much more difficult than that of bacteremia, with the frequent development of resistance during therapy.

BURKHOLDERIA CEPACIA

B. cepacia gained notoriety as the cause of a rapidly fatal syndrome of respiratory distress and septicemia (the "cepacia syndrome") in CF patients. Previously, it had been recognized as an antibiotic-resistant nosocomial pathogen (then designated *P. cepacia*) in ICU patients. Patients with chronic granulomatous disease are also predisposed to *B. cepacia* lung disease. The organism has been reclassified into nine subgroups, only some of which are common in CF. *B. cepacia* is an environmental organism that inhabits moist environments and is found in the rhizosphere. This organism possesses multiple virulence factors that may play roles in disease as well as colonizing factors that are capable of binding to lung mucus—an ability that may explain the predilection of *B. cepacia* for the lungs in CF. *B. cepacia* secretes elastase and possesses components of an injectable toxin-secretion system like that of *P. aeruginosa*; its LPS is among the most potent of all LPSs in stimulating an inflammatory response in the lungs. Inflammation may be the major cause of the lung disease seen in the cepacia syndrome. The organism can penetrate epithelial surfaces by virtue of motility and inhibition of host innate immune defenses. Besides infecting the lungs in CF, *B. cepacia* appears as an airway colonizer during broad-spectrum antibiotic therapy and is a cause of VAP, catheter-associated infections, and wound infections.

TREATMENT *B. CEPACIA* INFECTIONS

B. cepacia is intrinsically resistant to many antibiotics. Therefore, treatment must be tailored according to sensitivities. TMP-SMX, meropenem, and doxycycline are the most effective agents in vitro and may be started as first-line agents (Table 189-2). Some strains are susceptible to third-generation cephalosporins and fluoroquinolones, and these agents may be used against isolates known to be susceptible. Combination therapy for serious pulmonary infection (e.g., in CF) is suggested when multidrug-resistant strains are implicated; the combination of meropenem and TMP-SMX may be antagonistic, however. Resistance to all agents used has been reported during therapy.

BURKHOLDERIA PSEUDOMALLEI

B. pseudomallei is the causative agent of melioidosis, a disease of humans and animals that is geographically restricted to Southeast Asia and northern Australia, with occasional cases in countries such as India and China. This organism may be isolated from individuals returning directly from these endemic regions and from military personnel who have served in endemic regions and then returned home after stops in Europe. Symptoms of this illness may develop only at a later date because of the organism's ability to cause latent infections. *B. pseudomallei* is found in soil and water. Humans and animals are infected by inoculation, inhalation, or ingestion; only rarely is the organism transmitted from person to person. Humans are not colonized without being infected. Among the pseudomonads, *B. pseudomallei* is perhaps the most virulent. Host compromise is not an essential prerequisite for disease, although many patients have common underlying medical diseases (e.g., diabetes or renal failure). *B. pseudomallei* is a facultative intracellular organism whose replication in PMNs and macrophages may be aided by the possession of a polysaccharide capsule. The organism also possesses elements of a type III secretion system that plays a role in its intracellular survival. During infection, there is a florid inflammatory response whose role in disease is unclear.

B. pseudomallei causes a wide spectrum of disease, ranging from asymptomatic infection to abscesses, pneumonia, and disseminated disease. It is a significant cause of fatal community-acquired pneumonia and septicemia in endemic areas, with mortality rates as high as 44% reported in Thailand. Acute pulmonary infection is the most commonly diagnosed form of melioidosis. Pneumonia may be asymptomatic (with routine chest radiographs showing mainly upper-lobe infiltrates) or may present as severe necrotizing disease. *B. pseudomallei* also causes chronic pulmonary infections with systemic manifestations that mimic those of tuberculosis, including chronic cough, fever, hemoptysis, night sweats, and cavitary lung disease. Besides pneumonia, the other principal form of *B. pseudomallei* disease is skin ulceration with associated lymphangitis and regional lymphadenopathy. Spread from the lungs or skin, which is most often documented in debilitated individuals, gives rise to septicemic forms of melioidosis that carry a high mortality rate.

TREATMENT *B. PSEUDOMALLEI* INFECTIONS

B. pseudomallei is susceptible to advanced penicillins and cephalosporins and to carbapenems (Table 189-2). Treatment is divided into two stages: an intensive 2-week phase of therapy with ceftazidime or a carbapenem followed by at least 12 weeks of oral TMP-SMX to eradicate the organism and prevent relapse. The recognition of this bacterium as a potential agent of biologic warfare has stimulated interest in the development of a vaccine.

BURKHOLDERIA MALLEI

B. mallei causes the equine disease glanders in Africa, Asia, and South America. The organism was eradicated from Europe and North America decades ago. The last case seen in the United States occurred in 2001 in a laboratory worker; before that, *B. mallei* had last been seen in this country in 1949. In contrast to the other organisms discussed in this chapter, *B. mallei* is not an environmental organism and does not persist outside its equine hosts. Consequently, *B. mallei* infection is an occupational risk for handlers of horses, equine butchers, and veterinarians in areas of the world where it still exists. The polysaccharide capsule is a critical virulence determinant; diabetics are thought to be especially susceptible to infection by this organism. The organism is transmitted from animals to humans by inoculation into the skin, where it causes local infection with nodules and lymphadenitis. Regional lymphadenopathy is common. Respiratory secretions from infected horses are extremely infectious. Inhalation results in clinical signs of typical pneumonia but may also cause an acute febrile illness with ulceration of the trachea. The organism may disseminate from the skin or lungs to cause septicemia with signs of sepsis. The septicemic form is frequently associated with shock and a high mortality rate. The infection may also enter a chronic phase and present as disseminated abscesses. *B. mallei* infection may present as early as 1–2 days after inhalation or (in cutaneous disease) may not become evident for months.

TREATMENT *B. MALLEI* INFECTIONS

The antibiotic susceptibility pattern of *B. mallei* is similar to that of *B. pseudomallei*; in addition, the organism is susceptible to the newer macrolides azithromycin and clarithromycin. *B. mallei* infection should be treated with the same drugs and for the same duration as melioidosis.

190 Salmonellosis

David A. Pegues, Samuel I. Miller

Bacteria of the genus *Salmonella* are highly adapted for growth in both humans and animals and cause a wide spectrum of disease. The growth of serotypes *Salmonella typhi* and *Salmonella paratyphi* is restricted to human hosts, in whom these organisms cause enteric (typhoid) fever. The remaining serotypes (nontyphoidal *Salmonella*, or NTS) can colonize the gastrointestinal tracts of a broad range of animals, including mammals, reptiles, birds, and insects. More than 200 serotypes of *Salmonella* are pathogenic to humans, in whom they often cause gastroenteritis and can be associated with localized infections and/or bacteremia.

ETIOLOGY

This large genus of gram-negative bacilli within the family Enterobacteriaceae consists of two species: *Salmonella enterica*, which contains six subspecies, and *Salmonella bongori*. *S. enterica* subspecies I includes almost all the serotypes pathogenic for humans. Members of the seven *Salmonella* subspecies are classified into >2500 serotypes (serovars); for simplicity, *Salmonella* serotypes (most of which are named for the city where they were identified) are often used as the species designation. For example, the full taxonomic designation *S. enterica* subspecies *enterica* serotype Typhimurium can be shortened to *Salmonella* serotype Typhimurium or simply *S. typhimurium*. Serotyping is based on the somatic O antigen (lipopolysaccharide cell-wall components), the surface Vi antigen (restricted to *S. typhi* and *S. paratyphi* C), and the flagellar H antigen.

Salmonellae are gram-negative, non-spore-forming, facultatively anaerobic bacilli that measure 2–3 μm by 0.4–0.6 μm. The initial identification of salmonellae in the clinical microbiology laboratory is based on growth characteristics. Salmonellae, like other Enterobacteriaceae, produce acid on glucose fermentation, reduce nitrates, and do not produce cytochrome oxidase. In addition, all salmonellae except *Salmonella gallinarum-pullorum* are motile by means of peritrichous flagella, and all but *S. typhi* produce gas (H_2S) on sugar fermentation. Notably, only 1% of clinical isolates ferment lactose; a high level of suspicion must be maintained to detect these rare clinical lactose-fermenting isolates.

Although serotyping of all surface antigens can be used for formal identification, most laboratories perform a few simple agglutination reactions that define specific O-antigen serogroups, designated A, B, C_1, C_2, D, and E. Strains in these six serogroups cause ~99% of *Salmonella* infections in humans and other warm-blooded animals. Molecular typing methods, including pulsed-field gel electrophoresis, polymerase chain reaction fingerprinting, and genomic DNA microarray analysis, are used in epidemiologic investigations to differentiate *Salmonella* strains of a common serotype.

PATHOGENESIS

All *Salmonella* infections begin with ingestion of organisms, most commonly in contaminated food or water. The infectious dose ranges from 200 colony-forming units (CFU) to 10^6 CFU, and the ingested dose is an important determinant of incubation period and disease severity. Conditions that decrease either stomach acidity (an age of <1 year, antacid ingestion, or achlorhydric disease) or intestinal integrity (inflammatory bowel disease, prior gastrointestinal surgery, or alteration of the intestinal flora by antibiotic administration) increase susceptibility to *Salmonella* infection.

Once *S. typhi* and *S. paratyphi* reach the small intestine, they penetrate the mucus layer of the gut and traverse the intestinal layer through phagocytic microfold (M) cells that reside within Peyer's patches. Salmonellae can trigger the formation of membrane ruffles in normally nonphagocytic epithelial cells. These ruffles reach out and enclose adherent bacteria within large vesicles by *bacterial-mediated endocytosis*. This process is dependent on the direct delivery of *Salmonella* proteins into the cytoplasm of epithelial cells by the specialized bacterial type III secretion system. These bacterial proteins mediate alterations in the actin cytoskeleton that are required for *Salmonella* uptake.

After crossing the epithelial layer of the small intestine, *S. typhi* and *S. paratyphi*, which cause enteric (typhoid) fever, are phagocytosed by macrophages. These salmonellae survive the antimicrobial environment of the macrophage by sensing environmental signals that trigger alterations in regulatory systems of the phagocytosed bacteria. For example, PhoP/PhoQ (the best-characterized regulatory system) triggers the expression of outer-membrane proteins and mediates modifications in lipopolysaccharide so that the altered bacterial surface can resist microbicidal activities and potentially alter host cell signaling. In addition, salmonellae encode a second type III secretion system that directly delivers bacterial proteins across the phagosome membrane into the macrophage cytoplasm. This secretion system functions to remodel the *Salmonella*-containing vacuole, promoting bacterial survival and replication.

Once phagocytosed, typhoidal salmonellae disseminate throughout the body in macrophages via the lymphatics and colonize reticuloendothelial tissues (liver, spleen, lymph nodes, and bone marrow). Patients have relatively few or no signs and symptoms during this initial incubation stage. Signs and symptoms, including fever and abdominal pain, probably result from secretion of cytokines by macrophages and epithelial cells in response to bacterial products that are recognized by innate immune receptors when a critical number of organisms have replicated. Over time, the development of hepatosplenomegaly is likely to be related to the recruitment of mononuclear cells and the development of a specific acquired cell-mediated immune response to *S. typhi* colonization. The recruitment of additional mononuclear cells and lymphocytes to Peyer's patches during the several weeks after initial colonization/infection can result in marked enlargement and necrosis of the Peyer's patches, which may be mediated by bacterial products that promote cell death as well as the inflammatory response.

In contrast to enteric fever, which is characterized by an infiltration of mononuclear cells into the small-bowel mucosa, NTS gastroenteritis is characterized by massive polymorphonuclear leukocyte infiltration into both the large- and small-bowel mucosa. This response appears to depend on the induction of interleukin 8, a strong neutrophil chemotactic factor, which is secreted by intestinal cells as a result of *Salmonella* colonization and translocation of bacterial proteins into host cell cytoplasm. The degranulation and release of toxic substances by neutrophils may result in damage to the intestinal mucosa, causing the inflammatory diarrhea observed with nontyphoidal gastroenteritis. An additional important factor in the persistence of nontyphoidal salmonellae in the intestinal tract and the organisms' capacity to compete with endogenous flora is the ability to utilize the sulfur-containing compound tetrathionate for metabolism in a microaerophilic environment. In the presence of intestinal inflammation, tetrathionate is generated from thiosulfate produced by epithelial cells through inflammatory cell production of reactive oxygen species.

ENTERIC (TYPHOID) FEVER

Enteric (typhoid) fever is a systemic disease characterized by fever and abdominal pain and caused by dissemination of *S. typhi* or *S. paratyphi*. The disease was initially called *typhoid fever* because of its clinical similarity to typhus. In the early 1800s, typhoid fever was clearly defined pathologically as a unique illness on the basis of its association with enlarged Peyer's patches and mesenteric lymph nodes. In 1869, given the anatomic site of infection, the term *enteric fever* was proposed as an alternative designation to distinguish typhoid fever from typhus. However, to this day, the two designations are used interchangeably.

EPIDEMIOLOGY

In contrast to other *Salmonella* serotypes, the etiologic agents of enteric fever—*S. typhi* and *S. paratyphi* serotypes A, B, and C—have no known hosts other than humans. Most commonly, food-borne or waterborne transmission results from fecal contamination by ill or asymptomatic chronic carriers. Sexual transmission between male partners has been described. Health care workers occasionally acquire enteric fever after exposure to infected patients or during processing of clinical specimens and cultures.

With improvements in food handling and water/sewage treatment, enteric fever has become rare in developed nations. Worldwide, however, there are an estimated 27 million cases of enteric fever, with 200,000–600,000 deaths annually. The annual incidence is highest (>100 cases/100,000 population) in south-central and Southeast Asia; medium (10–100 cases/100,000) in the rest of Asia, Africa, Latin America, and Oceania (excluding Australia and New Zealand); and low in other parts of the world (Fig. 190-1). A high incidence of enteric fever correlates with poor sanitation and lack of access to clean drinking water. In endemic regions, enteric fever is more common in urban than rural areas and among young children and adolescents than among other age groups. Risk factors include contaminated water or ice, flooding, food and drinks purchased from street vendors, raw fruits and vegetables grown in fields fertilized with sewage, ill household contacts, lack of hand washing and toilet access, and evidence of prior *Helicobacter pylori* infection (an association probably related to chronically reduced gastric acidity). It is estimated that there is one case of paratyphoid fever for every four cases of typhoid fever, but the incidence of infection associated with *S. paratyphi* A appears to be increasing, especially in India; this increase may be a result of vaccination for *S. typhi*.

Multidrug-resistant (MDR) strains of *S. typhi* emerged in the 1980s in China and Southeast Asia and have since disseminated widely. These strains contain plasmids encoding resistance to chloramphenicol, ampicillin, and trimethoprim—antibiotics long used to treat enteric fever. With the increased use of fluoroquinolones to treat MDR enteric fever in the 1990s, strains of *S. typhi* and *S. paratyphi* with decreased ciprofloxacin susceptibility (DCS; minimal inhibitory concentration [MIC], 0.125–0.5 μg/mL) or ciprofloxacin resistance (MIC, ≥1 μg/mL) have emerged on the Indian subcontinent, in southern Asia, and (most recently) in sub-Saharan Africa and have been associated with clinical treatment failure. Testing of isolates for resistance to the first-generation quinolone nalidixic acid detects many but not all strains with reduced susceptibility to ciprofloxacin and is no longer recommended. Strains of *S. typhi* and *S. paratyphi* producing extended-spectrum β-lactamases have emerged recently, primarily in India and Nepal.

Approximately 300 cases of typhoid and 150 cases of paratyphoid fever are reported annually in the United States. Of 1902 cases of *S. typhi*–associated enteric fever reported to the Centers for Disease Control and Prevention in 1999–2006, 79% were associated with recent international travel, most commonly to India (47%), Pakistan (10%), Bangladesh (10%), Mexico (7%), and the Philippines (4%). Only 5% of travelers diagnosed with enteric fever had received *S. typhi* vaccine. Overall, 13% of *S. typhi* isolates in the United States were resistant to ampicillin, chloramphenicol, and trimethoprim-sulfamethoxazole (TMP-SMX), and the proportion of DCS isolates increased from 19% in 1999 to 58% in 2006. Infection with DCS *S. typhi* was associated with travel to the Indian subcontinent. Of the 25–30% of reported cases of enteric fever in the United States that are domestically acquired, the majority are sporadic, but outbreaks linked to contaminated food products and previously unrecognized chronic carriers continue to occur.

CLINICAL COURSE

Enteric fever is a misnomer, in that the hallmark features of this disease—fever and abdominal pain—are variable. While fever is documented at presentation in >75% of cases, abdominal pain is reported in only 30–40%. Thus, a high index of suspicion for this potentially fatal systemic illness is necessary when a person presents with fever and a history of recent travel to a developing country.

The incubation period for *S. typhi* averages 10–14 days but ranges from 5 to 21 days, depending on the inoculum size and the host's health and immune status. The most prominent symptom is prolonged fever (38.8°–40.5°C; 101.8°–104.9°F), which can continue for

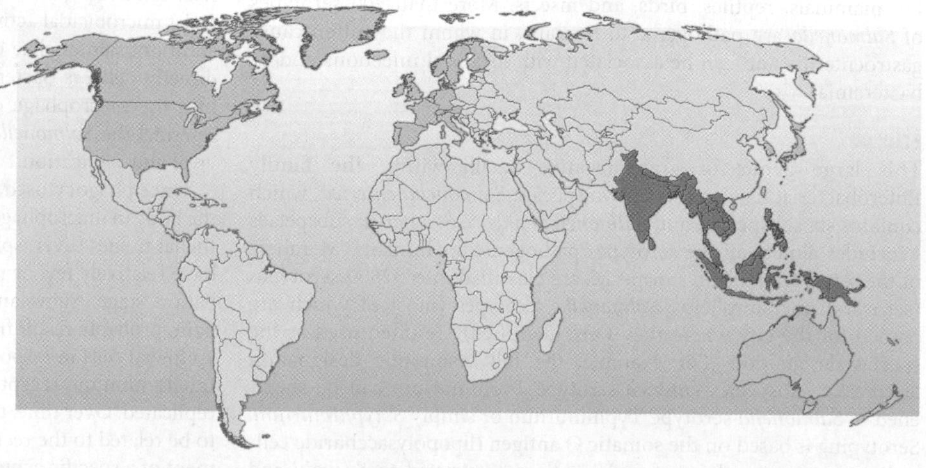

High (>100/100,000/year) Medium (10–100/100,000/year) Low (<10/100,000/year)

FIGURE 190-1 Annual incidence of typhoid fever per 100,000 population. *(Adapted from JA Crump et al: The global burden of typhoid fever. Bull World Health Organ 82:346, 2004.)*

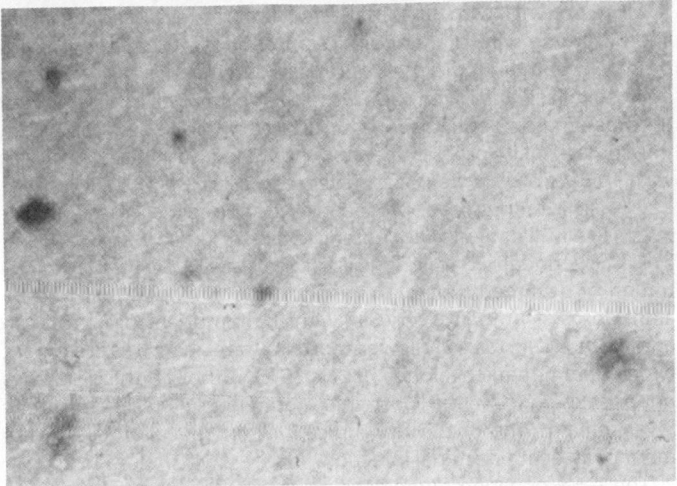

FIGURE 190-2 **"Rose spots,"** the rash of enteric fever due to *Salmonella typhi* or *Salmonella paratyphi*.

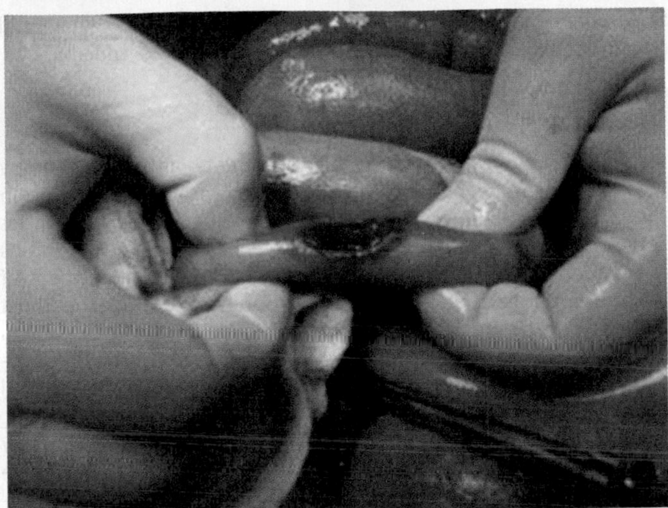

FIGURE 190-3 **Typical ileal perforation associated with *Salmonella typhi* infection.** *(From JM Saxe, R Cropsey: Is operative management effective in treatment of perforated typhoid? Am J Surg 189:342, 2005.)*

up to 4 weeks if untreated. *S. paratyphi* A is thought to cause milder disease than *S. typhi*, with predominantly gastrointestinal symptoms. However, a prospective study of 669 consecutive cases of enteric fever in Kathmandu, Nepal, found that the infections caused by these organisms were clinically indistinguishable. In this series, symptoms reported on initial medical evaluation included headache (80%), chills (35–45%), cough (30%), sweating (20–25%), myalgias (20%), malaise (10%), and arthralgia (2–4%). Gastrointestinal manifestations included anorexia (55%), abdominal pain (30–40%), nausea (18–24%), vomiting (18%), and diarrhea (22–28%) more commonly than constipation (13–16%). Physical findings included coated tongue (51–56%), splenomegaly (5–6%), and abdominal tenderness (4–5%).

Early physical findings of enteric fever include rash ("rose spots"; 30%), hepatosplenomegaly (3–6%), epistaxis, and relative bradycardia at the peak of high fever (<50%). Rose spots (Fig. 190-2; see also Fig. 25e-9) make up a faint, salmon-colored, blanching, maculopapular rash located primarily on the trunk and chest. The rash is evident in ~30% of patients at the end of the first week and resolves without a trace after 2–5 days. Patients can have two or three crops of lesions, and *Salmonella* can be cultured from punch biopsies of these lesions. The faintness of the rash makes it difficult to detect in highly pigmented patients.

The development of severe disease (which occurs in ~10–15% of patients) depends on host factors (immunosuppression, antacid therapy, previous exposure, and vaccination), strain virulence and inoculum, and choice of antibiotic therapy. Gastrointestinal bleeding (10–20%) and intestinal perforation (1–3%) most commonly occur in the third and fourth weeks of illness and result from hyperplasia, ulceration, and necrosis of the ileocecal Peyer's patches at the initial site of *Salmonella* infiltration (Fig. 190-3). Both complications are life-threatening and require immediate fluid resuscitation and surgical intervention, with broadened antibiotic coverage for polymicrobial peritonitis (Chap. 159) and treatment of gastrointestinal hemorrhages, including bowel resection. Neurologic manifestations occur in 2–40% of patients and include meningitis, Guillain-Barré syndrome, neuritis, and neuropsychiatric symptoms (described as "muttering delirium" or "coma vigil"), with picking at bedclothes or imaginary objects.

Rare complications whose incidences are reduced by prompt antibiotic treatment include disseminated intravascular coagulation, hematophagocytic syndrome, pancreatitis, hepatic and splenic abscesses and granulomas, endocarditis, pericarditis, myocarditis, orchitis, hepatitis, glomerulonephritis, pyelonephritis and hemolytic-uremic syndrome, severe pneumonia, arthritis, osteomyelitis, endophthalmitis, and parotitis. Up to 10% of patients develop mild relapse, usually within 2–3 weeks of fever resolution and in association with the same strain type and susceptibility profile.

Up to 10% of untreated patients with typhoid fever excrete *S. typhi* in the feces for up to 3 months, and 1–4% develop chronic asymptomatic carriage, shedding *S. typhi* in either urine or stool for >1 year. Chronic carriage is more common among women, infants, and persons who have biliary abnormalities or concurrent bladder infection with *Schistosoma haematobium*. The anatomic abnormalities associated with the latter conditions presumably allow prolonged colonization.

DIAGNOSIS

Because the clinical presentation of enteric fever is relatively nonspecific, the diagnosis needs to be considered in any febrile traveler returning from a developing region, especially the Indian subcontinent, the Philippines, or Latin America. Other diagnoses that should be considered in these travelers include malaria, hepatitis, bacterial enteritis, dengue fever, rickettsial infections, leptospirosis, amebic liver abscesses, and acute HIV infection (Chap. 149). Other than a positive culture, no specific laboratory test is diagnostic for enteric fever. In 15–25% of cases, leukopenia and neutropenia are detectable. Leukocytosis is more common among children, during the first 10 days of illness, and in cases complicated by intestinal perforation or secondary infection. Other nonspecific laboratory findings include moderately elevated values in liver function tests and muscle enzyme levels.

The definitive diagnosis of enteric fever requires the isolation of *S. typhi* or *S. paratyphi* from blood, bone marrow, other sterile sites, rose spots, stool, or intestinal secretions. The sensitivity of blood culture is only 40–80%, probably because of high rates of antibiotic use in endemic areas and the small number of *S. typhi* organisms (i.e., <15/mL) typically present in the blood. Because almost all *S. typhi* organisms in blood are associated with the mononuclear cell/platelet fraction, centrifugation of blood and culture of the buffy coat can substantially reduce the time to isolation of the organism but do not increase sensitivity.

Bone marrow culture is 55–90% sensitive, and, unlike that of blood culture, its yield is not reduced by up to 5 days of prior antibiotic therapy. Culture of intestinal secretions (best obtained by a noninvasive duodenal string test) can be positive despite a negative bone marrow culture. If blood, bone marrow, and intestinal secretions are all cultured, the yield is >90%. Stool cultures, although negative in 60–70% of cases during the first week, can become positive during the third week of infection in untreated patients.

Serologic tests, including the classic Widal test for "febrile agglutinins," and rapid tests to detect antibodies to outer-membrane proteins or O:9 antigen are available for detection of *S. typhi* in developing countries but have lower positive predictive values than blood culture. More sensitive antigen and nucleic acid amplification tests have been developed to detect *S. typhi* and

 S. paratyphi in blood but are not yet commercially available and remain impractical in many areas where enteric fever is endemic.

TREATMENT ENTERIC (TYPHOID) FEVER

Prompt administration of appropriate antibiotic therapy prevents severe complications of enteric fever and results in a case-fatality rate of <1%. The initial choice of antibiotics depends on the susceptibility of the *S. typhi* and *S. paratyphi* strains in the area of residence or travel (**Table 190-1**). For treatment of drug-susceptible typhoid fever, fluoroquinolones are the most effective class of agents, with cure rates of ~98% and relapse and fecal carriage rates of <2%. Experience is most extensive with ciprofloxacin. Short-course ofloxacin therapy is similarly successful against infection caused by quinolone-susceptible strains. However, the increased incidence of DCS *S. typhi* in Asia, which is probably related to the widespread availability of fluoroquinolones over the counter, is now limiting the use of this drug class for empirical therapy. Patients infected with DCS *S. typhi* strains should be treated with ceftriaxone, azithromycin, or high-dose ciprofloxacin. A 7-day course of high-dose fluoroquinolone therapy for DCS enteric fever has been associated with delayed resolution of fever and high rates of fecal carriage during convalescence. Thus, for DCS strains, a 10- to 14-day course of high-dose ciprofloxacin is preferred.

Ceftriaxone, cefotaxime, and (oral) cefixime are effective for treatment of MDR enteric fever, including that caused by DCS and fluoroquinolone-resistant strains. These agents clear fever in ~1 week, with failure rates of ~5–10%, fecal carriage rates of <3%, and relapse rates of 3–6%. Oral azithromycin results in defervescence in 4–6 days, with rates of relapse and convalescent stool carriage of <3%. Against DCS strains, azithromycin is associated with lower rates of treatment failure and shorter durations of hospitalization than are fluoroquinolones. Despite efficient in vitro killing of *Salmonella*, first- and second-generation cephalosporins as well as aminoglycosides are ineffective in the treatment of clinical infections.

TABLE 190-1 ANTIBIOTIC THERAPY FOR ENTERIC FEVER IN ADULTS

Indication	Agent	Dosage (Route)	Duration, Days
Empirical Treatment			
	Ceftriaxone[a]	2 g/d (IV)	10–14
	Azithromycin[b]	1 g/d (PO)	5
Fully Susceptible			
Optimal treatment	Ciprofloxacin[c]	500 mg bid (PO) or 400 mg q12h (IV)	5–7
	Azithromycin	1 g/d (PO)	5
Alternative treatment	Amoxicillin	1 g tid (PO) or 2 g q6h (IV)	14
	Chloramphenicol	25 mg/kg tid (PO or IV)	14–21
	Trimethoprim-sulfamethoxazole	160/800 mg bid (PO)	7–14
Multidrug-Resistant			
Optimal treatment	Ceftriaxone[a]	2 g/d (IV)	10–14
	Azithromycin	1 g/d (PO)	5
Alternative treatment	Ciprofloxacin	500 mg bid (PO) or 400 mg q12h (IV)	5–14
Quinolone-Resistant			
Optimal treatment	Ceftriaxone	2 g/d (IV)	10–14
	Azithromycin	1 g/d (PO)	5
Alternative treatment	High-dose ciprofloxacin	750 mg bid (PO) or 400 mg q8h (IV)	10–14

[a]Or another third-generation cephalosporin (e.g., cefotaxime, 2 g q8h IV; or cefixime, 400 mg bid PO). [b]Or 1 g on day 1 followed by 500 mg/d PO for 6 days. [c]Or ofloxacin, 400 mg bid PO for 2–5 days.

Most patients with uncomplicated enteric fever can be managed at home with oral antibiotics and antipyretics. Patients with persistent vomiting, diarrhea, and/or abdominal distension should be hospitalized and given supportive therapy as well as a parenteral third-generation cephalosporin or fluoroquinolone, depending on the susceptibility profile. Therapy should be administered for at least 10 days or for 5 days after fever resolution.

In a randomized, prospective, double-blind study of critically ill patients with enteric fever (i.e., those with shock and obtundation) in Indonesia in the early 1980s, the administration of dexamethasone (an initial dose of 3 mg/kg followed by eight doses of 1 mg/kg every 6 h) with chloramphenicol was associated with a substantially lower mortality rate than was treatment with chloramphenicol alone (10% vs 55%). Although this study has not been repeated in the "post-chloramphenicol era," severe enteric fever remains one of the few indications for glucocorticoid treatment of an acute bacterial infection.

The 1–5% of patients who develop chronic carriage of *Salmonella* can be treated for 4–6 weeks with an appropriate oral antibiotic. Treatment with oral amoxicillin, TMP-SMX, ciprofloxacin, or norfloxacin is ~80% effective in eradicating chronic carriage of susceptible organisms. However, in cases of anatomic abnormality (e.g., biliary or kidney stones), eradication often requires both antibiotic therapy and surgical correction.

PREVENTION AND CONTROL

Theoretically, it is possible to eliminate the salmonellae that cause enteric fever because they survive only in human hosts and are spread by contaminated food and water. However, given the high prevalence of the disease in developing countries that lack adequate sewage disposal and water treatment, this goal is currently unrealistic. Thus, travelers to developing countries should be advised to monitor their food and water intake carefully and to strongly consider immunization against *S. typhi*.

Two typhoid vaccines are commercially available: (1) Ty21a, an oral live attenuated *S. typhi* vaccine (given on days 1, 3, 5, and 7, with a booster every 5 years); and (2) Vi CPS, a parenteral vaccine consisting of purified Vi polysaccharide from the bacterial capsule (given in a single dose, with a booster every 2 years). The old parenteral whole-cell typhoid/paratyphoid A and B vaccine is no longer licensed, largely because of significant side effects, especially fever. An acetone-killed whole-cell vaccine is available only for use by the U.S. military. The minimal age for vaccination is 6 years for Ty21a and 2 years for Vi CPS. In a recent meta-analysis of vaccines for preventing typhoid fever in populations in endemic areas, the cumulative efficacy was 48% for Ty21a at 2.5–3.5 years and 55% for Vi CPS at 3 years. Although data on typhoid vaccines in travelers are limited, some evidence suggests that efficacy rates may be substantially lower than those for local populations in endemic areas. Currently, there is no licensed vaccine for paratyphoid fever.

Vi CPS typhoid vaccine is poorly immunogenic in children <5 years of age because of T cell–independent properties. In the more recently developed Vi-rEPA vaccine, Vi is bound to a nontoxic recombinant protein that is identical to *Pseudomonas aeruginosa* exotoxin A. In 2- to 4-year-olds, two injections of Vi-rEPA induced higher T cell responses and higher levels of serum IgG antibody to Vi than did Vi CPS in 5- to 14-year-olds. In a two-dose trial in 2- to 5-year-old children in Vietnam, Vi-rEPA provided 91% efficacy at 27 months and 89% efficacy at 46 months and was very well tolerated. This vaccine is not yet commercially available in the United States. Efforts to improve the immunogenicity and reduce the number of doses of live attenuated oral vaccines are ongoing.

Typhoid vaccine is not required for international travel, but it is recommended for travelers to areas where there is a moderate to high risk of exposure to *S. typhi*, especially those who are traveling to southern Asia and other developing regions of Asia, Africa, the Caribbean, and Central and South America and who will be exposed to potentially contaminated food and drink. Typhoid vaccine should be considered even for persons planning <2 weeks of travel to high-risk areas. In addition, laboratory workers who deal with *S. typhi* and household contacts of known *S. typhi* carriers should be vaccinated. Because the protective efficacy of vaccine can be overcome by the high inocula that are commonly encountered in food-borne exposures, immunization is an adjunct and not a substitute for the avoidance of high-risk foods and beverages. Immunization is not recommended for adults residing in typhoid-endemic areas or for the management of persons who may have been exposed in a common-source outbreak.

Enteric fever is a notifiable disease in the United States. Individual health departments have their own guidelines for allowing ill or colonized food handlers or health care workers to return to their jobs. The reporting system enables public health departments to identify potential source patients and to treat chronic carriers in order to prevent further outbreaks. In addition, because 1–4% of patients with *S. typhi* infection become chronic carriers, it is important to monitor patients (especially child-care providers and food handlers) for chronic carriage and to treat this condition if indicated.

NONTYPHOIDAL SALMONELLOSIS

EPIDEMIOLOGY

In the United States, NTS causes ~12 million illnesses annually, and the incidence has remained relatively unchanged during the past two decades. In 2011, the incidence of NTS infection in this country was 16.5/100,000 persons—the highest rate among the 10 food-borne enteric pathogens under active surveillance. Five serotypes accounted for more than half of U.S. infections during the period 1996–2006: *typhimurium* (23%), *enteritidis* (16%), *newport* (10%), *heidelberg* (6%), and *javiana* (5%).

The incidence of nontyphoidal salmonellosis is highest during the rainy season in tropical climates and during the warmer months in temperate climates—a pattern coinciding with the peak in food-borne outbreaks. Rates of morbidity and mortality associated with NTS are highest among the elderly, infants, and immunocompromised individuals, including those with hemoglobinopathies, HIV infection, or infections that cause blockade of the reticuloendothelial system (e.g., bartonellosis, malaria, schistosomiasis, histoplasmosis).

Unlike *S. typhi* and *S. paratyphi*, whose only reservoir is humans, NTS can be acquired from multiple animal reservoirs. Transmission is most commonly associated with food products of animal origin (especially eggs, poultry, undercooked ground meat, and dairy products), fresh produce contaminated with animal waste, and contact with animals or their environments.

S. enteritidis infection associated with chicken eggs emerged as a major cause of food-borne disease during the 1980s and 1990s. *S. enteritidis* infection of the ovaries and upper oviduct tissue of hens results in contamination of egg contents before shell deposition. Infection is spread to egg-laying hens from breeding flocks and through contact with rodents and manure. The percentage of *Salmonella* outbreaks attributed to eggs has declined significantly in the United States, from 33% during 1998–1999 to 15% during 2006–2008. This decrease probably reflects the impact of the coordinated public health response to *S. enteritidis* infection attributed to eggs, including improved on-farm control measures, refrigeration, and education of consumers and food-service workers. Transmission via contaminated eggs can be prevented by cooking eggs until the yolk is solidified and pasteurizing egg products. Despite these control efforts, outbreaks of *S. enteritidis* infection associated with shell eggs continue to occur. In 2010, a national outbreak of *S. enteritidis* infection resulted in more than 1900 reported illnesses and the recall of 500 million eggs.

Centralization of food processing and widespread food distribution have contributed to the increased incidence of NTS in developed countries. Manufactured foods to which recent *Salmonella* outbreaks have been traced include peanut butter; milk products, including infant formula; and various processed foods, including packaged breakfast cereal, salsa, frozen prepared meals, and snack foods. Large outbreaks have also been linked to fresh produce, including alfalfa sprouts, cantaloupe, mangoes, papayas, and tomatoes; these items become contaminated by manure or water at a single site and then are widely distributed.

An estimated 6% of sporadic *Salmonella* infections in the United States are attributed to contact with reptiles or amphibians, especially iguanas, snakes, turtles, and lizards. Reptile-associated *Salmonella* infection more commonly leads to hospitalization and more frequently involves children, including infants, than do other *Salmonella* infections. Other pets, including African hedgehogs, birds, rodents, baby chicks, ducklings, dogs, and cats, are also potential sources of NTS.

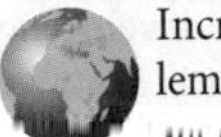

Increasing antibiotic resistance in NTS species is a global problem and has been linked to the widespread use of antimicrobial agents in food animals and especially in animal feed. In the early 1990s, *S. typhimurium* definitive phage type 104 (DT104), characterized by resistance to at least five antibiotics (ampicillin, chloramphenicol, streptomycin, sulfonamides, and tetracyclines; R-type ACSSuT), emerged worldwide. In 2010, resistance to at least ACSSuT was reported in 4.3% of NTS isolates, including 18.6% of *S. typhimurium* isolates. Acquisition is associated with exposure to ill farm animals and to various meat products, including uncooked or undercooked ground beef. Although probably no more virulent than susceptible *S. typhimurium* strains, DT104 strains are associated with an increased risk of bloodstream infection and hospitalization. DCS and trimethoprim-resistant DT104 strains are emerging, especially in the United Kingdom.

Because of increased resistance to conventional antibiotics such as ampicillin and TMP-SMX, extended-spectrum cephalosporins and fluoroquinolones have emerged as the agents of choice for the treatment of MDR NTS infections. In 2010, 2.8% of all NTS strains were resistant to ceftriaxone. Most ceftriaxone-resistant isolates were from children <18 years of age, in whom ceftriaxone is the antibiotic of choice for treatment of invasive NTS infection. These strains contained plasmid-encoded AmpC β-lactamases that were probably acquired by horizontal genetic transfer from *Escherichia coli* strains in food-producing animals—an event linked to the widespread use of the veterinary cephalosporin ceftiofur.

Over the last decade, strains of DCS NTS (MIC, 0.125–1 μg/mL) have emerged and have been associated with delayed response and treatment failure. In 2009, 2.4% of NTS isolates in the United States were DCS or resistant to ciprofloxacin. These strains have diverse resistance mechanisms, including single and multiple mutations in the DNA gyrase genes *gyrA* and *gyrB* and plasmid-encoded quinolone resistance determinants that may not be reliably detected by nalidixic acid susceptibility testing. In 2012, the U.S. Clinical Laboratory Standards Institute proposed a lower ciprofloxacin susceptibility breakpoint (≥0.06 μg/mL) for all *Salmonella* species to address this issue. Currently, because commercial test systems do not contain ciprofloxacin concentrations low enough to allow use of these breakpoints, laboratories need to determine the ciprofloxacin MIC by Etest or another alternative method.

CLINICAL MANIFESTATIONS

Gastroenteritis Infection with NTS most often results in gastroenteritis indistinguishable from that caused by other enteric pathogens. Nausea, vomiting, and diarrhea occur 6–48 h after the ingestion of contaminated food or water. Patients often experience abdominal cramping and fever (38–39°C; 100.5–102.2°F). Diarrheal stools are usually loose, nonbloody, and of moderate volume. However, large-volume watery stools, bloody stools, or symptoms of dysentery may occur. Rarely, NTS causes pseudoappendicitis or an illness that mimics inflammatory bowel disease.

Gastroenteritis caused by NTS is usually self-limited. Diarrhea resolves within 3–7 days and fever within 72 h. Stool cultures remain positive for 4–5 weeks after infection and—in rare cases of chronic carriage (<1%)—for >1 year. Antibiotic treatment usually is not recommended and may prolong fecal carriage. Neonates, the elderly, and immunosuppressed patients (e.g., transplant recipients, HIV-infected persons) with NTS gastroenteritis are especially susceptible to dehydration and dissemination and may require hospitalization and antibiotic therapy. Acute NTS gastroenteritis was associated with a threefold increased risk of dyspepsia and irritable bowel syndrome at 1 year in a study from Spain.

Bacteremia and Endovascular Infections Up to 8% of patients with NTS gastroenteritis develop bacteremia; of these, 5–10% develop localized infections. Bacteremia and metastatic infection are most common with *Salmonella choleraesuis* and *Salmonella dublin* and among infants, the elderly, and immunocompromised patients, especially those with HIV infection. NTS endovascular infection should be suspected in high-grade or persistent bacteremia, especially with preexisting valvular heart disease, atherosclerotic vascular disease, prosthetic vascular graft, or aortic aneurysm. Arteritis should be suspected in elderly patients with prolonged fever and back, chest, or abdominal pain developing after an episode of gastroenteritis. Endocarditis and arteritis are rare (<1% of cases) but are associated with potentially fatal complications, including valve perforation, endomyocardial abscess, infected mural thrombus, pericarditis, mycotic aneurysms, aneurysm rupture, aorto-enteric fistula, and vertebral osteomyelitis.

In some areas of sub-Saharan Africa, NTS may be among the most common causes—or even the most common cause—of bacteremia in children. NTS bacteremia among these children is not associated with diarrhea and has been associated with nutritional status and HIV infection.

Localized Infections • ***INTRAABDOMINAL INFECTIONS*** Intraabdominal infections due to NTS are rare and usually manifest as hepatic or splenic abscesses or as cholecystitis. Risk factors include hepatobiliary anatomic abnormalities (e.g., gallstones), abdominal malignancy, and sickle cell disease (especially with splenic abscesses). Eradication of the infection often requires surgical correction of abnormalities and percutaneous drainage of abscesses.

CENTRAL NERVOUS SYSTEM INFECTIONS NTS meningitis most commonly develops in infants 1–4 months of age. It often results in severe sequelae (including seizures, hydrocephalus, brain infarction, and mental retardation), with death in up to 60% of cases. Other rare central nervous system infections include ventriculitis, subdural empyema, and brain abscesses.

PULMONARY INFECTIONS NTS pulmonary infections usually present as lobar pneumonia, and complications include lung abscess, empyema, and bronchopleural fistula formation. The majority of cases occur in patients with lung cancer, structural lung disease, sickle cell disease, or glucocorticoid use.

URINARY AND GENITAL TRACT INFECTIONS Urinary tract infections caused by NTS present as either cystitis or pyelonephritis. Risk factors include malignancy, urolithiasis, structural abnormalities, HIV infection, and renal transplantation. NTS genital infections are rare and include ovarian and testicular abscesses, prostatitis, and epididymitis. Like other focal infections, both genital and urinary tract infections can be complicated by abscess formation.

BONE, JOINT, AND SOFT TISSUE INFECTIONS *Salmonella* osteomyelitis most commonly affects the femur, tibia, humerus, or lumbar vertebrae and is most often seen in association with sickle cell disease, hemoglobinopathies, or preexisting bone disease (e.g., fractures). Prolonged antibiotic treatment is recommended to decrease the risk of relapse and chronic osteomyelitis. Septic arthritis occurs in the same patient population as osteomyelitis and usually involves the knee, hip, or shoulder joints. Reactive arthritis can follow NTS gastroenteritis and is seen most frequently in persons with the HLA-B27 histocompatibility antigen. NTS rarely can cause soft tissue infections, usually at sites of local trauma in immunosuppressed patients.

DIAGNOSIS

The diagnosis of NTS infection is based on isolation of the organism from freshly passed stool or from blood or another ordinarily sterile body fluid. All salmonellae isolated in clinical laboratories should be sent to local public health departments for serotyping. Blood cultures should be done whenever a patient has prolonged or recurrent fever. Endovascular infection should be suspected if there is high-grade bacteremia (>50% of three or more positive blood cultures). Echocardiography, computed tomography (CT), and indium-labeled white cell scanning are used to identify localized infection. When another localized infection is suspected, joint fluid, abscess drainage, or cerebrospinal fluid should be cultured, as clinically indicated.

TREATMENT NONTYPHOIDAL SALMONELLOSIS

Antibiotics should not be used routinely to treat uncomplicated NTS gastroenteritis. The symptoms are usually self-limited, and the duration of fever and diarrhea is not significantly decreased by antibiotic therapy. In addition, antibiotic treatment has been associated with increased rates of relapse, prolonged gastrointestinal carriage, and adverse drug reactions. Dehydration secondary to diarrhea should be treated with fluid and electrolyte replacement.

Preemptive antibiotic treatment (Table 190-2) should be considered for patients at increased risk for invasive NTS infection, including neonates (probably up to 3 months of age); persons >50 years of age with suspected atherosclerosis; and patients with immunosuppression, cardiac valvular or endovascular abnormalities, or significant joint disease. Treatment should consist of an oral or IV antibiotic administered for 48–72 h or until the patient becomes afebrile. Immunocompromised persons may require up to 7–14 days of therapy. The <1% of persons who develop chronic carriage of NTS should receive a prolonged antibiotic course, as described above for chronic carriage of *S. typhi*.

Because of the increasing prevalence of antibiotic resistance, empirical therapy for life-threatening NTS bacteremia or focal NTS infection should include a third-generation cephalosporin or a fluoroquinolone (Table 190-2). If the bacteremia is low-grade (<50% of positive blood cultures), the patient should be treated for 7–14 days. Patients with HIV/AIDS and NTS bacteremia should receive 1–2 weeks of IV antibiotic therapy followed by 4 weeks of oral therapy with a

TABLE 190-2 ANTIBIOTIC THERAPY FOR NONTYPHOIDAL *SALMONELLA* INFECTION IN ADULTS

Indication	Agent	Dosage (Route)	Duration, Days
Preemptive Treatment[a]			
	Ciprofloxacin[b]	500 mg bid (PO)	2–3
Severe Gastroenteritis[c]			
	Ciprofloxacin	500 mg bid (PO) or 400 mg q12h (IV)	3–7
	Trimethoprim-sulfamethoxazole	160/800 mg bid (PO)	
	Amoxicillin	1 g tid (PO)	
	Ceftriaxone	1–2 g/d (IV)	
Bacteremia			
	Ceftriaxone[d]	2 g/d (IV)	7–14
	Ciprofloxacin	400 mg q12h (IV), then 500 mg bid (PO)	
Endocarditis or Arteritis			
	Ceftriaxone	2 g/d (IV)	42
	Ciprofloxacin	400 mg q8h (IV), then 750 mg bid (PO)	
	Ampicillin	2 g q4h (IV)	
Meningitis			
	Ceftriaxone	2 g q12 h (IV)	14–21
	Ampicillin	2 g q4h (IV)	
Other Localized Infection			
	Ceftriaxone	2 g/d (IV)	14–28
	Ciprofloxacin	500 mg bid (PO) or 400 mg q12h (IV)	
	Ampicillin	2 g q6h (IV)	

[a]Consider for neonates; persons >50 years of age with possible atherosclerotic vascular disease; and patients with immunosuppression, endovascular graft, or joint prosthesis. [b]Or ofloxacin, 400 mg bid (PO). [c]Consider on an individualized basis for patients with severe diarrhea and high fever who require hospitalization. [d]Or cefotaxime, 2 g q8h (IV).

fluoroquinolone. Patients whose infections relapse after this regimen should receive long-term suppressive therapy with a fluoroquinolone or TMP-SMX, as indicated by bacterial sensitivities.

If the patient has endocarditis or arteritis, treatment for 6 weeks with an IV β-lactam antibiotic (such as ceftriaxone or ampicillin) is indicated. IV ciprofloxacin followed by prolonged oral therapy is an option, but published experience is limited. Early surgical resection of infected aneurysms or other infected endovascular sites is recommended. Patients with infected prosthetic vascular grafts that cannot be resected have been maintained successfully on chronic suppressive oral therapy. For extraintestinal nonvascular infections, a 2- to 4-week course of antibiotic therapy (depending on the infection site) is usually recommended. In chronic osteomyelitis, abscess, or urinary or hepatobiliary infection associated with anatomic abnormalities, surgical resection or drainage may be required in addition to prolonged antibiotic therapy for eradication of infection.

PREVENTION AND CONTROL

Despite widespread efforts to prevent or reduce bacterial contamination of animal-derived food products and to improve food-safety education and training, recent declines in the incidence of NTS in the United States have been modest compared with those of other food-borne pathogens. This observation probably reflects the complex epidemiology of NTS. Identifying effective risk-reduction strategies requires monitoring of every step of food production, from handling of raw animal or plant products to preparation of finished foods. Contaminated food can be made safe for consumption by pasteurization, irradiation, or proper cooking. All cases of NTS infection should be reported to local public health departments because tracking and monitoring of these cases can identify the source(s) of infection and help authorities anticipate large outbreaks. Lastly, the prudent use of antimicrobial agents in both humans and animals is needed to limit the emergence of MDR *Salmonella*.

191 Shigellosis

Philippe J. Sansonetti, Jean Bergounioux

The discovery of *Shigella* as the etiologic agent of dysentery—a clinical syndrome of fever, intestinal cramps, and frequent passage of small, bloody, mucopurulent stools—is attributed to the Japanese microbiologist Kiyoshi Shiga, who isolated the Shiga bacillus (now known as *Shigella dysenteriae* type 1) from patients' stools in 1897 during a large and devastating dysentery epidemic. *Shigella* cannot be distinguished from *Escherichia coli* by DNA hybridization and remains a separate species only on historical and clinical grounds.

DEFINITION

Shigella is a non-spore-forming, gram-negative bacterium that, unlike *E. coli*, is nonmotile and does not produce gas from sugars, decarboxylate lysine, or hydrolyze arginine. Some serovars produce indole, and occasional strains utilize sodium acetate. *Shigella dysenteriae*, *Shigella flexneri*, *Shigella boydii*, and *Shigella sonnei* (serogroups A, B, C, and D, respectively) can be differentiated on the basis of biochemical and serologic characteristics. Genome sequencing of *E. coli* K12, *S. flexneri* 2a, *S. sonnei*, *S. dysenteriae* type 1, and *S. boydii* has revealed that these species have ~93% of genes in common. The three major genomic "signatures" of *Shigella* are (1) a 215-kb virulence plasmid that carries most of the genes required for pathogenicity (particularly invasive capacity); (2) the lack or alteration of genetic sequences encoding products (e.g., lysine decarboxylase) that, if expressed, would attenuate pathogenicity; and (3) in *S. dysenteriae* type 1, the presence of genes encoding Shiga toxin, a potent cytotoxin.

EPIDEMIOLOGY

The human intestinal tract represents the major reservoir of *Shigella*, which is also found (albeit rarely) in the higher primates. Because excretion of shigellae is greatest in the acute phase of disease, the bacteria are transmitted most efficiently by the fecal-oral route via hand carriage; however, some outbreaks reflect foodborne or waterborne transmission. In impoverished areas, *Shigella* can be transmitted by flies. The high-level infectivity of *Shigella* is reflected by the very small inoculum required for experimental infection of volunteers (100 colony-forming units [CFU]), by the very high attack rates during outbreaks in day-care centers (33–73%), and by the high rates of secondary cases among family members of sick children (26–33%). Shigellosis can also be transmitted sexually.

Throughout history, *Shigella* epidemics have often occurred in settings of human crowding under conditions of poor hygiene—e.g., among soldiers in campaigning armies, inhabitants of besieged cities, groups on pilgrimages, and refugees in camps. Epidemics follow a cyclical pattern in areas such as the Indian subcontinent and sub-Saharan Africa. These devastating epidemics, which are most often caused by *S. dysenteriae* type 1, are characterized by high attack and mortality rates. In Bangladesh, for instance, an epidemic caused by *S. dysenteriae* type 1 was associated with a 42% increase in mortality rate among children 1–4 years of age. Apart from these epidemics, shigellosis is mostly an endemic disease, with 99% of cases occurring in the developing world and the highest prevalences in the most impoverished areas, where personal and general hygiene is below standard. *S. flexneri* isolates predominate in the least developed areas, whereas *S. sonnei* is more prevalent in economically emerging countries and in the industrialized world.

Prevalence in the Developing World In a review published under the auspices of the World Health Organization (WHO), the total annual number of cases in 1966–1997 was estimated at 165 million, and 69% of these cases occurred in children <5 years of age. In this review, the annual number of deaths was calculated to range between 500,000 and 1.1 million. More recent data (2000–2004) from six Asian countries indicate that, even though the incidence of shigellosis remains stable, mortality rates associated with this disease may have decreased significantly, possibly as a result of improved nutritional status. However, extensive and essentially uncontrolled use of antibiotics, which may also account for declining mortality rates, has increased the rate of emergence of multidrug-resistant *Shigella* strains. A 2013 prospective matched case-control study of children <5 years of age emphasizes the importance of *Shigella* in the burden and etiology of diarrheal diseases in developing countries. *Shigella* is one of the top four pathogens associated with moderate to severe diarrhea and is now ranked first among children 12–59 months of age. These moderate to severe cases account for an 8.5-fold increase in mortality incidence over the average diarrheal disease-related mortality. The study's authors conclude that *Shigella* remains a major pathogen to be targeted by health care programs.

An often-overlooked complication of shigellosis is the short- and long-term impairment of the nutritional status of infected children in endemic areas. Combined with anorexia, the exudative enteropathy resulting from mucosal abrasions contributes to rapid deterioration of the patient's nutritional status. Shigellosis is thus a major contributor to stunted growth among children in developing countries.

Peaking in incidence in the pediatric population, endemic shigellosis is rare among young and middle-aged adults, probably because of naturally acquired immunity. Incidence then increases again in the elderly population.

Prevalence in the Industrialized World In pediatric populations, local outbreaks occur when proper and adapted hygiene policies are not implemented in group facilities like day-care centers and institutions for the mentally retarded. In adults, as in children, sporadic cases occur among travelers returning from endemic areas, and rare outbreaks of varying size can follow waterborne or food-borne infections.

Shigella infection occurs essentially through oral contamination via direct fecal-oral transmission, the organism being poorly adapted to survive in the environment. Resistance to low-pH conditions allows shigellae to survive passage through the gastric barrier, an ability that may explain in part why a small inoculum (as few as 100 CFU) is sufficient to cause infection.

The watery diarrhea that usually precedes the dysenteric syndrome is attributable to active secretion and abnormal water reabsorption—a secretory effect at the jejunal level described in experimentally infected rhesus monkeys. This initial purge is probably due to the combined action of an enterotoxin (ShET-1) and mucosal inflammation. The dysenteric syndrome, manifested by bloody and mucopurulent stools, reflects invasion of the mucosa.

The pathogenesis of *Shigella* is essentially determined by a large virulence plasmid of 214 kb comprising ~100 genes, of which 25 encode a type III secretion system that inserts into the membrane of the host cell to allow effectors to transit from the bacterial cytoplasm to the host cell cytoplasm (Fig. 191-1). Bacteria are thereby able to invade intestinal epithelial cells by inducing their own uptake after the initial crossing of the epithelial barrier through M cells (the specialized translocating epithelial cells in the follicle-associated epithelium that covers mucosal lymphoid nodules). The organisms induce apoptosis of subepithelial resident macrophages. Once inside the cytoplasm of intestinal epithelial cells, *Shigella* effectors trigger the cytoskeletal rearrangements necessary to direct uptake of the organism into the epithelial cell. The *Shigella*-containing vacuole is then quickly lysed, releasing bacteria into the cytosol.

Intracellular shigellae next use cytoskeletal components to propel themselves inside the infected cell; when the moving organism and the host cell membrane come into contact, cellular protrusions form and are engulfed by neighboring cells. This series of events permits bacterial cell-to-cell spread.

Cytokines released by a growing number of infected intestinal epithelial cells attract increased numbers of immune cells (particularly polymorphonuclear leukocytes [PMNs]) to the infected site, thus further destabilizing the epithelial barrier, exacerbating inflammation, and leading to the acute colitis that characterizes shigellosis. Evidence indicates that some type III secretion system–injected effectors can control the extent of inflammation, thus facilitating bacterial survival.

Shiga toxin produced by *S. dysenteriae* type 1 increases disease severity. This toxin belongs to a group of A1-B5 protein toxins whose B subunit binds to the receptor globotriaosylceramide on the target cell surface and whose catalytic A subunit is internalized by receptor-mediated endocytosis and interacts with the subcellular machinery to inhibit protein synthesis by expressing RNA N-glycosidase activity on 28S ribosomal RNA. This process leads to inhibition of binding of the amino-acyl-tRNA to the 60S ribosomal subunit and thus to a general shutoff of cell protein biosynthesis. Shiga toxins are translocated from the bowel into the circulation. After binding of the toxins to target cells in the kidney, pathophysiologic alterations may result in hemolytic-uremic syndrome (HUS; see below).

CLINICAL MANIFESTATIONS

The presentation and severity of shigellosis depend to some extent on the infecting serotype but even more on the age and the immunologic and nutritional status of the host. Poverty and poor standards of hygiene are strongly related to the number and severity of diarrheal episodes, especially in children <5 years old who have been weaned.

Shigellosis typically evolves through four phases: incubation, watery diarrhea, dysentery, and the postinfectious phase. The incubation period usually lasts 1–4 days but may be as long as 8 days. Typical initial manifestations are transient fever, limited watery diarrhea, malaise, and anorexia. Signs and symptoms may range from mild abdominal discomfort to severe cramps, diarrhea, fever, vomiting, and tenesmus. The manifestations are usually exacerbated in children, with temperatures up to 40°–41°C (104.0°–105.8°F) and more severe anorexia and watery diarrhea. This initial phase may represent the only clinical manifestation of shigellosis, especially in developed countries. Otherwise, dysentery follows within hours or days and is characterized by uninterrupted excretion of small volumes of bloody mucopurulent stools with increased tenesmus and abdominal cramps. At this stage, *Shigella* produces acute colitis involving mainly the distal colon and the rectum. Unlike most diarrheal syndromes, dysenteric syndromes rarely present with dehydration as a major feature. Endoscopy shows an edematous and hemorrhagic mucosa, with ulcerations and possibly overlying exudates resembling pseudomembranes. The extent of the lesions correlates with the number and frequency of stools and with the degree of protein loss by exudative mechanisms. Most episodes are self-limited and resolve without treatment in 1 week. With appropriate treatment, recovery takes place within a few days to a week, with no sequelae.

Acute life-threatening complications are seen most often in children <5 years of age (particularly those who are malnourished) and in elderly patients. Risk factors for death in a clinically severe case include nonbloody diarrhea, moderate to severe dehydration, bacteremia, absence of fever, abdominal tenderness, and rectal prolapse. Major complications are predominantly intestinal (e.g., toxic megacolon, intestinal perforations, rectal prolapse) or metabolic (e.g., hypoglycemia, hyponatremia, dehydration). Bacteremia is rare and is reported most frequently in severely malnourished and HIV-infected patients. Alterations of consciousness, including seizures, delirium, and coma, may occur, especially in children <5 years old, and are associated with a poor prognosis; fever and severe metabolic alterations are more often the major causes of altered consciousness than is meningitis or the Ekiri syndrome (toxic encephalopathy associated with bizarre posturing, cerebral edema, and fatty degeneration of viscera), which has been reported mostly in Japanese children. Pneumonia, vaginitis, and keratoconjunctivitis due to *Shigella* are rarely reported. In the absence of serious malnutrition, severe and very unusual clinical manifestations, such as meningitis, may be linked to genetic defects in innate immune functions (i.e., deficiency in interleukin 1 receptor–associated kinase 4 [IRAK-4]) and may require genetic investigation.

Two complications of particular importance are toxic megacolon and HUS. Toxic megacolon is a consequence of severe inflammation extending to the colonic smooth-muscle layer and causing paralysis and dilation. The patient presents with abdominal distention and tenderness, with or without signs of localized or generalized peritonitis. The abdominal x-ray characteristically shows

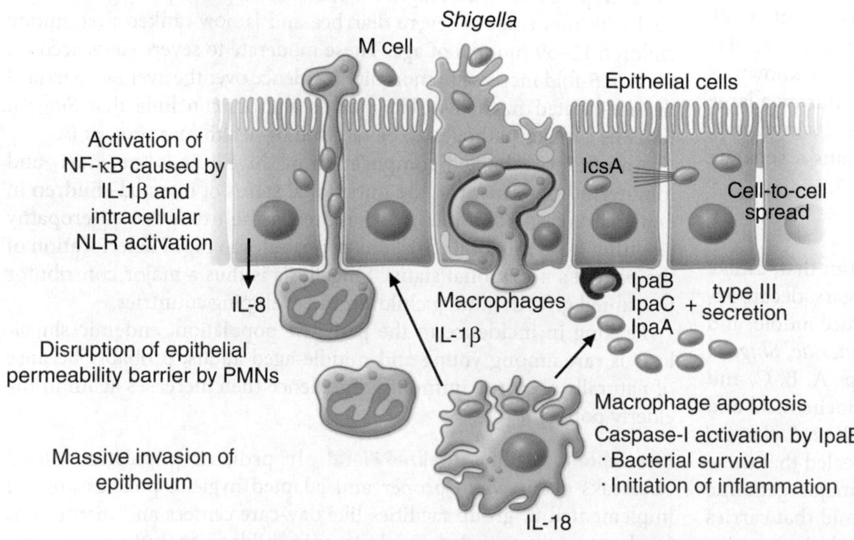

FIGURE 191-1 Invasive strategy of *Shigella flexneri*. IL, interleukin; NF-κB, nuclear factor κB; NLR, NOD-like receptor; PMN, polymorphonuclear leukocyte.

marked dilation of the transverse colon (with the greatest distention in the ascending and descending segments); thumbprinting caused by mucosal inflammatory edema; and loss of the normal haustral pattern associated with pseudopolyps, often extending into the lumen. Pneumatosis coli is an occasional finding. If perforation occurs, radiographic signs of pneumoperitoneum may be apparent. Predisposing factors (e.g., hypokalemia and use of opioids, anticholinergics, loperamide, psyllium seeds, and antidepressants) should be investigated.

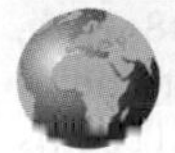

Shiga toxin produced by *S. dysenteriae* type 1 has been linked to HUS in developing countries but rarely in industrialized countries, where enterohemorrhagic *E. coli* (EHEC) predominates as the etiologic agent of this syndrome. HUS is an early complication that most often develops after several days of diarrhea. Clinical examination shows pallor, asthenia, and irritability and, in some cases, bleeding of the nose and gums, oliguria, and increasing edema. HUS is a nonimmune (Coombs test–negative) hemolytic anemia defined by a diagnostic triad: microangiopathic hemolytic anemia (hemoglobin level typically <80 g/L [<8 g/dL]), thrombocytopenia (mild to moderate in severity; typically <60,000 platelets/μL), and acute renal failure due to thrombosis of the glomerular capillaries (with markedly elevated creatinine levels). Anemia is severe, with fragmented red blood cells (*schizocytes*) in the peripheral smear, high serum concentrations of lactate dehydrogenase and free circulating hemoglobin, and elevated reticulocyte counts. Acute renal failure occurs in 55–70% of cases; however, renal function recovers in most of these cases (up to 70% in various series). Leukemoid reactions, with leukocyte counts of 50,000/μL, are sometimes noted in association with HUS.

The postinfectious immunologic complication known as *reactive arthritis* can develop weeks or months after shigellosis, especially in patients expressing the histocompatibility antigen HLA-B27. About 3% of patients infected with *S. flexneri* later develop this syndrome, with arthritis, ocular inflammation, and urethritis—a condition that can last for months or years and can progress to difficult-to-treat chronic arthritis. Postinfectious arthropathy occurs only after infection with *S. flexneri* and not after infection with the other *Shigella* serotypes.

LABORATORY DIAGNOSIS

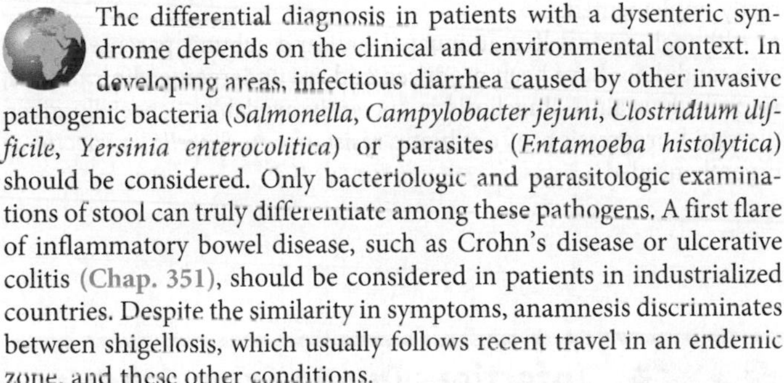

The differential diagnosis in patients with a dysenteric syndrome depends on the clinical and environmental context. In developing areas, infectious diarrhea caused by other invasive pathogenic bacteria (*Salmonella, Campylobacter jejuni, Clostridium difficile, Yersinia enterocolitica*) or parasites (*Entamoeba histolytica*) should be considered. Only bacteriologic and parasitologic examinations of stool can truly differentiate among these pathogens. A first flare of inflammatory bowel disease, such as Crohn's disease or ulcerative colitis (Chap. 351), should be considered in patients in industrialized countries. Despite the similarity in symptoms, anamnesis discriminates between shigellosis, which usually follows recent travel in an endemic zone, and these other conditions.

Microscopic examination of stool smears shows erythrophagocytic trophozoites with very few PMNs in *E. histolytica* infection, whereas bacterial enteroinvasive infections (particularly shigellosis) are characterized by high PMN counts in each microscopic field. However, because shigellosis often manifests only as watery diarrhea, systematic attempts to isolate *Shigella* are necessary.

The "gold standard" for the diagnosis of *Shigella* infection remains the isolation and identification of the pathogen from fecal material. One major difficulty, particularly in endemic areas where laboratory facilities are not immediately available, is the fragility of *Shigella* and its common disappearance during transport, especially with rapid changes in temperature and pH. In the absence of a reliable enrichment medium, buffered glycerol saline or Cary-Blair medium can be used as a holding medium, but prompt inoculation onto isolation medium is essential. The probability of isolation is higher if the portion of stools that contains bloody and/or mucopurulent material is directly sampled. Rectal swabs can be used, as they offer the highest rate of successful isolation during the acute phase of disease. Blood cultures are positive in fewer than 5% of cases but should be done when a patient presents with a clinical picture of severe sepsis.

In addition to quick processing, the use of several media increases the likelihood of successful isolation: a nonselective medium such as bromocresol-purple agar lactose; a low-selectivity medium such as MacConkey or eosin-methylene blue; and a high-selectivity medium such as Hektoen, *Salmonella-Shigella*, or xylose-lysine-deoxycholate agar. After incubation on these media for 12–18 h at 37°C (98.6°F), shigellae appear as non-lactose-fermenting colonies that measure 0.5–1 mm in diameter and have a convex, translucent, smooth surface. Suspected colonies on nonselective or low-selectivity medium can be subcultured on a high-selectivity medium before being specifically identified or can be identified directly by standard commercial systems on the basis of four major characteristics: glucose positivity (usually without production of gas), lactose negativity, H_2S negativity, and lack of motility. The four *Shigella* serogroups (A–D) can then be differentiated by additional characteristics. This approach adds time and difficulty to the identification process; however, after presumptive diagnosis, the use of serologic methods (e.g., slide agglutination, with group- and then type-specific antisera) should be considered. Group-specific antisera are widely available; in contrast, because of the large number of serotypes and subserotypes, type-specific antisera are rare and more expensive and thus are often restricted to reference laboratories.

TREATMENT SHIGELLOSIS

ANTIBIOTIC SUSCEPTIBILITY OF *SHIGELLA*

As an enteroinvasive disease, shigellosis requires antibiotic treatment. Since the mid-1960s, however, increasing resistance to multiple drugs has been a dominant factor in treatment decisions. Resistance rates are highly dependent on the geographic area. Clonal spread of particular strains and horizontal transfer of resistance determinants, particularly via plasmids and transposons, contribute to multidrug resistance. The current global status—i.e., high rates of resistance to classic first-line antibiotics such as amoxicillin—has led to a rapid switch to quinolones such as nalidixic acid. However, resistance to such early-generation quinolones has also emerged and spread quickly as a result of chromosomal mutations affecting DNA gyrase and topoisomerase IV; this resistance has necessitated the use of later-generation quinolones as first-line antibiotics in many areas. For instance, a review of the antibiotic resistance history of *Shigella* in India found that, after their introduction in the late 1980s, the second-generation quinolones norfloxacin, ciprofloxacin, and ofloxacin were highly effective in the treatment of shigellosis, including cases caused by multidrug-resistant strains of *S. dysenteriae* type 1. However, investigations of subsequent outbreaks in India and Bangladesh detected resistance to norfloxacin, ciprofloxacin, and ofloxacin in 5% of isolates. The incidence of multidrug resistance parallels the widespread, uncontrolled use of antibiotics and calls for the rational use of effective drugs.

ANTIBIOTIC TREATMENT OF SHIGELLOSIS (TABLE 191-1)

Because of the ready transmissibility of *Shigella*, current public health recommendations in the United States are that every case be treated with antibiotics. Ciprofloxacin is recommended as first-line treatment. A number of other drugs have been tested and shown to be effective, including ceftriaxone, azithromycin, pivmecillinam, and some fifth-generation quinolones. Whereas infections caused by non-*dysenteriae Shigella* in immunocompetent individuals are routinely treated with a 3-day course of antibiotics, it is recommended that *S. dysenteriae* type 1 infections be treated for 5 days and that *Shigella* infections in immunocompromised patients be treated for 7–10 days.

Treatment for shigellosis must be adapted to the clinical context, with the recognition that the most fragile patients are children <5 years old, who represent two-thirds of all cases worldwide. There are few data on the use of quinolones in children, but *Shigella*-induced dysentery is a well-recognized indication

TABLE 191-1 RECOMMENDED ANTIMICROBIAL THERAPY FOR SHIGELLOSIS

Antimicrobial Agent	Treatment Schedule: Children	Adults	Limitations
First Line			
Ciprofloxacin	15 mg/kg	500 mg	
	2 times per day for 3 days, PO		
Second Line			
Pivmecillinam	20 mg/kg	100 mg	Cost
	4 times per day for 5 days PO		No pediatric formulation
			Frequent administration
			Emerging resistance
Ceftriaxone	50–100 mg/kg	–	Efficacy not validated
	Once a day IM for 2–5 days		Must be injected
Azithromycin	6–20 mg/kg	1–1.5 g	Cost
	Once a day for 1–5 days PO		Efficacy not validated
			Minimum inhibitory concentration near serum concentration
			Rapid emergence of resistance and spread to other bacteria

Source: WHO Library Cataloguing-in-Publication Data: Guidelines for the control of shigellosis, including epidemics due to *Shigella dysenteriae* type 1 (*www.who.int/cholera/publications/shigellosis/en/*).

for their use. The half-life of ciprofloxacin is longer in infants than in older individuals. The ciprofloxacin dose generally recommended for children is 30 mg/kg per day in two divided doses. Adults living in areas with high standards of hygiene are likely to develop milder, shorter-duration disease, whereas infants in endemic areas can develop severe, sometimes fatal, dysentery. In the former setting, treatment will remain minimal and bacteriologic proof of infection will often come after symptoms have resolved; in the latter setting, antibiotic treatment and more aggressive measures, possibly including resuscitation, are often required.

REHYDRATION AND NUTRITION

Shigella infection rarely causes significant dehydration. Cases requiring aggressive rehydration (particularly in industrialized countries) are uncommon. In developing countries, malnutrition remains the primary indicator for diarrhea-related death, highlighting the importance of nutrition in early management. Rehydration should be oral unless the patient is comatose or presents in shock. Because of the improved effectiveness of reduced-osmolarity oral rehydration solution (especially for children with acute noncholera diarrhea), the WHO and UNICEF now recommend a standard solution of 245 mOsm/L (sodium, 75 mmol/L; chloride, 65 mmol/L; glucose [anhydrous], 75 mmol/L; potassium, 20 mmol/L; citrate, 10 mmol/L). In shigellosis, the coupled transport of sodium to glucose may be variably affected, but oral rehydration therapy remains the easiest and most efficient form of rehydration, especially in severe cases.

Nutrition should be started as soon as possible after completion of initial rehydration. Early refeeding is safe, well tolerated, and clinically beneficial. Because breast-feeding reduces diarrheal losses and the need for oral rehydration in infants, it should be maintained in the absence of contraindications (e.g., maternal HIV infection).

NONSPECIFIC, SYMPTOM-BASED THERAPY

Antimotility agents have been implicated in prolonged fever in volunteers with shigellosis. These agents are suspected of increasing the risk of toxic megacolon and are thought to have been responsible for HUS in children infected by EHEC strains. For safety reasons, it is better to avoid antimotility agents in bloody diarrhea.

TREATMENT OF COMPLICATIONS

There is no consensus regarding the best treatment for toxic megacolon. The patient should be assessed frequently by both medical and surgical teams. Anemia, dehydration, and electrolyte deficits (particularly hypokalemia) may aggravate colonic atony and should be actively treated. Nasogastric aspiration helps to deflate the colon. Parenteral nutrition has not been proven to be beneficial. Fever persisting beyond 48–72 h raises the possibility of local perforation or abscess. Most studies recommend colectomy if, after 48–72 h, colonic distention persists. However, some physicians recommend continuation of medical therapy for up to 7 days if the patient seems to be improving clinically despite persistent megacolon without free perforation. Intestinal perforation, either isolated or complicating toxic megacolon, requires surgical treatment and intensive medical support.

Rectal prolapse must be treated as soon as possible. With the health care provider using surgical gloves or a soft warm wet cloth and the patient in the knee-chest position, the prolapsed rectum is gently pushed back into place. If edema of the rectal mucosa is evident (rendering reintegration difficult), it can be osmotically reduced by the application of gauze impregnated with a warm solution of saturated magnesium sulfate. Rectal prolapse often relapses but usually resolves along with the resolution of dysentery.

HUS must be treated by water restriction, including discontinuation of oral rehydration solution and potassium-rich alimentation. Hemofiltration is usually required.

PREVENTION

Hand washing after defecation or handling of children's feces and before handling of food is recommended. Stool decontamination (e.g., with sodium hypochlorite), together with a cleaning protocol for medical staff as well as for patients, has proven useful in limiting the spread of infection during *Shigella* outbreaks. Ideally, patients should have a negative stool culture before their infection is considered cured. Recurrences are rare if therapeutic and preventive measures are correctly implemented.

Although several live attenuated oral and subunit parenteral vaccine candidates have been produced and are undergoing clinical trials, no vaccine against shigellosis is currently available. Especially given the rapid progression of antibiotic resistance in *Shigella*, a vaccine is urgently needed.

192 Infections Due to *Campylobacter* and Related Organisms

Martin J. Blaser

DEFINITION

Bacteria of the genus *Campylobacter* and of the related genera *Arcobacter* and *Helicobacter* (Chap. 188) cause a variety of inflammatory conditions. Although acute diarrheal illnesses are most common, these organisms may cause infections in virtually all parts of the body, especially in compromised hosts, and these infections may have late nonsuppurative sequelae. The designation *Campylobacter* comes from the Greek for "curved rod" and refers to the organism's vibrio-like morphology.

ETIOLOGY

Campylobacters are motile, non-spore-forming, curved, gram-negative rods. Originally known as *Vibrio fetus*, these bacilli were reclassified as a new genus in 1973 after their dissimilarity to other vibrios was recognized. More than 15 species have since been identified. These species are currently divided into three genera: *Campylobacter*, *Arcobacter*, and *Helicobacter*. Not all of the species are pathogens of humans. The human pathogens fall into two major groups: those that primarily cause diarrheal disease and those that cause extraintestinal infection. The principal diarrheal pathogen is *Campylobacter jejuni*, which accounts for 80–90% of all cases of recognized illness due to campylobacters and related genera. Other organisms that cause diarrheal disease include *Campylobacter coli, Campylobacter upsaliensis, Campylobacter lari, Campylobacter hyointestinalis, Campylobacter fetus, Arcobacter butzleri, Arcobacter cryaerophilus, Helicobacter cinaedi*, and *Helicobacter fennelliae*. The two *Helicobacter* species causing diarrheal disease, *H. cinaedi* and *H. fennelliae*, are intestinal rather than gastric organisms; in terms of the clinical features of the illnesses they cause, these species most closely resemble *Campylobacter* rather than *Helicobacter pylori* (Chap. 188) and thus are considered in this chapter. The pathogenic roles of *Campylobacter concisus, Campylobacter ureolyticus, Campylobacter troglodytis*, and *Campylobacter pyloridis* are uncertain. A new subspecies—*C. fetus* subspecies *testudinum*—has been described, chiefly in Asian patients; its close resemblance to strains isolated from reptiles suggests a food source.

The major species causing extraintestinal illnesses is *C. fetus*. However, any of the diarrheal agents listed above may cause systemic or localized infection as well, especially in compromised hosts. Neither aerobes nor strict anaerobes, these microaerophilic organisms are adapted for survival in the gastrointestinal mucous layer. This chapter focuses on *C. jejuni* and *C. fetus* as the major pathogens in and prototypes for their groups. The key features of infection are listed by species (excluding *C. jejuni*, described in detail in the text below) in Table 192-1.

EPIDEMIOLOGY

Campylobacters are found in the gastrointestinal tract of many animals used for food (including poultry, cattle, sheep, and swine) and many household pets (including birds, dogs, and cats). These microorganisms usually do not cause illness in their animal hosts. In most cases, campylobacters are transmitted to humans in raw or undercooked food products or through direct contact with infected animals. In the United States and other developed countries, ingestion of contaminated poultry that has not been sufficiently cooked is the most common mode of acquisition (30–70% of cases). Other modes include ingestion of raw (unpasteurized) milk or untreated water, contact with infected household pets, travel to developing countries (campylobacters being among the leading causes of traveler's diarrhea; Chaps. 149 and 160), oral-anal sexual contact, and (occasionally) contact with an index case who is incontinent of stool (e.g., a baby).

Campylobacter infections are common. Several studies indicate that, in the United States, diarrheal disease due to campylobacters is more common than that due to *Salmonella* and *Shigella* combined. Infections occur throughout the year, but their incidence peaks during summer and early autumn. Persons of all ages are affected; however, attack rates for *C. jejuni* are highest among young children and young adults, whereas those for *C. fetus* are highest at the extremes of age. Systemic infections due to *C. fetus* (and to other *Campylobacter* and related species) are most common among compromised hosts. Persons at increased risk include those with AIDS, hypogammaglobulinemia, neoplasia, liver disease, diabetes mellitus, and generalized atherosclerosis as well as neonates and pregnant women. However, apparently healthy nonpregnant persons occasionally develop transient *Campylobacter* bacteremia as part of a gastrointestinal illness.

In contrast, in many developing countries, *C. jejuni* infections are hyperendemic, with the highest rates among children <2 years old. Infection rates fall with age, as does the illness-to-infection ratio. These observations suggest that frequent exposure to *C. jejuni* leads to the acquisition of immunity.

PATHOLOGY AND PATHOGENESIS

C. jejuni infections may be subclinical, especially in hosts in developing countries who have had multiple prior infections and thus are partially immune. Symptomatic infections mostly occur within 2–4 days (range, 1–7 days) of exposure to the organism in food or water. The sites of tissue injury include the jejunum, ileum, and colon. Biopsies show an acute nonspecific inflammatory reaction, with neutrophils, monocytes, and eosinophils in the lamina propria, as well as damage to the epithelium, including loss of mucus, glandular degeneration, and crypt abscesses. Biopsy findings may be consistent with Crohn's disease or ulcerative colitis, but these "idiopathic"

TABLE 192-1 CLINICAL FEATURES ASSOCIATED WITH INFECTION DUE TO "ATYPICAL" *CAMPYLOBACTER* AND RELATED SPECIES IMPLICATED AS CAUSES OF HUMAN ILLNESS

Species	Common Clinical Features	Less Common Clinical Features	Additional Information
Campylobacter coli	Fever, diarrhea, abdominal pain	Bacteremia[a]	Clinically indistinguishable from *C. jejuni*
Campylobacter fetus	Bacteremia,[a] sepsis, meningitis, vascular infections	Diarrhea, relapsing fevers	Not usually isolated from media containing cephalothin or incubated at 42°C
Campylobacter upsaliensis	Watery diarrhea, low-grade fever, abdominal pain	Bacteremia, abscesses	Difficult to isolate because of cephalothin susceptibility
Campylobacter lari	Abdominal pain, diarrhea	Colitis, appendicitis	Seagulls frequently colonized; organism often transmitted to humans via contaminated water
Campylobacter hyointestinalis	Watery or bloody diarrhea, vomiting, abdominal pain	Bacteremia	Causes proliferative enteritis in swine
Helicobacter fennelliae	Chronic mild diarrhea, abdominal cramps, proctitis	Bacteremia[a]	Best treated with fluoroquinolones
Helicobacter cinaedi	Chronic mild diarrhea, abdominal cramps, proctitis	Bacteremia[a]	Best treated with fluoroquinolones; identified in healthy hamsters
Campylobacter jejuni subspecies *doylei*	Diarrhea	Chronic gastritis, bacteremia[b]	Uncertain role as human pathogen
Arcobacter cryaerophilus	Diarrhea	Bacteremia	Cultured under aerobic conditions
Arcobacter butzleri	Fever, diarrhea, abdominal pain, nausea	Bacteremia, appendicitis	Cultured under aerobic conditions; enzootic in nonhuman primates
Campylobacter sputorum	Pulmonary, perianal, groin, and axillary abscesses; diarrhea	Bacteremia	Three clinically relevant biovars: *sputorum, faecalis*, and *paraureolyticus*

[a]In immunocompromised hosts, especially HIV-infected persons. [b]In children.

Source: Adapted from BM Allos, MJ Blaser: Clin Infect Dis 20:1092, 1995.

chronic inflammatory diseases should not be diagnosed unless infectious colitis, *specifically including* that due to infection with *Campylobacter* species and related organisms, has been ruled out.

The high frequency of *C. jejuni* infections and their severity and recurrence among hypogammaglobulinemic patients suggest that antibodies are important in protective immunity. The pathogenesis of infection is uncertain. Both the motility of the strain and its capacity to adhere to host tissues appear to favor disease, but classic enterotoxins and cytotoxins (although they have been described and include cytolethal distending toxin, or CDT) appear not to play substantial roles in tissue injury or disease production. The organisms have been visualized within the epithelium, albeit in low numbers. The documentation of a significant tissue response and occasionally of *C. jejuni* bacteremia further suggests that tissue invasion is clinically significant, and in vitro studies are consistent with this pathogenetic feature.

The pathogenesis of *C. fetus* infections is better defined. Virtually all clinical isolates of *C. fetus* possess a proteinaceous capsule-like structure (an S-layer) that renders the organisms resistant to complement-mediated killing and opsonization. As a result, *C. fetus* can cause bacteremia and can seed sites beyond the intestinal tract. The ability of the organism to switch the S-layer proteins expressed—a phenomenon that results in antigenic variability—may contribute to the chronicity and high rate of recurrence of *C. fetus* infections in compromised hosts.

CLINICAL MANIFESTATIONS

The clinical features of infections due to *Campylobacter* and the related *Arcobacter* and intestinal *Helicobacter* species causing enteric disease appear to be highly similar. *C. jejuni* can be considered the prototype, in part because it is by far the most common enteric pathogen in the group. A prodrome of fever, headache, myalgia, and/or malaise often occurs 12–48 h before the onset of diarrheal symptoms. The most common signs and symptoms of the intestinal phase are diarrhea, abdominal pain, and fever. The degree of diarrhea varies from several loose stools to grossly bloody stools; most patients presenting for medical attention have ≥10 bowel movements on the worst day of illness. Abdominal pain usually consists of cramping and may be the most prominent symptom. Pain is usually generalized but may become localized; *C. jejuni* infection may cause pseudoappendicitis. Fever may be the only initial manifestation of *C. jejuni* infection, a situation mimicking the early stages of typhoid fever. Febrile young children may develop convulsions. *Campylobacter* enteritis is generally self-limited; however, symptoms persist for >1 week in 10–20% of patients seeking medical attention, and clinical relapses occur in 5–10% of such untreated patients. Studies of common-source epidemics indicate that milder illnesses or asymptomatic infections may commonly occur.

C. fetus may cause a diarrheal illness similar to that due to *C. jejuni*, especially in normal hosts. This organism also may cause either intermittent diarrhea or nonspecific abdominal pain without localizing signs. Sequelae are uncommon, and the outcome is benign. *C. fetus* may also cause a prolonged relapsing systemic illness (with fever, chills, and myalgias) that has no obvious primary source; this manifestation is especially common among compromised hosts. Secondary seeding of an organ (e.g., meninges, brain, bone, urinary tract, or soft tissue) complicates the course, which may be fulminant. *C. fetus* infections have a tropism for vascular sites: endocarditis, mycotic aneurysm, and septic thrombophlebitis may all occur. Infection during pregnancy often leads to fetal death. A variety of *Campylobacter* species and *H. cinaedi* can cause recurrent cellulitis with fever and bacteremia in immunocompromised hosts.

COMPLICATIONS

Except in infection with *C. fetus*, bacteremia is uncommon, developing most often in immunocompromised hosts and at the extremes of age. Three patterns of extraintestinal infection have been noted: (1) transient bacteremia in a normal host with enteritis (benign course, no specific treatment needed); (2) sustained bacteremia or focal infection in a normal host (bacteremia originating from enteritis, with patients responding well to antimicrobial therapy); and (3) sustained bacteremia or focal infection in a compromised host. Enteritis may not be clinically apparent. Antimicrobial therapy, possibly prolonged, is necessary for suppression or cure of the infection.

Campylobacter, Arcobacter, and intestinal *Helicobacter* infections in patients with AIDS or hypogammaglobulinemia may be severe, persistent, and extraintestinal; relapse after cessation of therapy is common. Hypogammaglobulinemic patients also may develop osteomyelitis and an erysipelas-like rash or cellulitis.

Local suppurative complications of infection include cholecystitis, pancreatitis, and cystitis; distant complications include meningitis, endocarditis, arthritis, peritonitis, cellulitis, and septic abortion. All these complications are rare, except in immunocompromised hosts. Hepatitis, interstitial nephritis, and the hemolytic-uremic syndrome occasionally complicate acute infection. Reactive arthritis and other rheumatologic complaints may develop several weeks after infection, especially in persons with the HLA-B27 phenotype. Guillain-Barré syndrome or its Miller Fisher (cranial polyneuropathy) variant follows *Campylobacter* infections uncommonly—i.e., in 1 of every 1000–2000 cases or, for certain *C. jejuni* serotypes (such as O19), in 1 of every 100–200 cases. Despite the low frequency of this complication, it is now estimated that *Campylobacter* infections, because of their high incidence, may trigger 20–40% of all cases of Guillain-Barré syndrome. The presence of sialylated lipopolysaccharides on *C. jejuni* strains is a form of molecular mimicry that promotes autoimmune recognition of sialylated cell surface molecules on axons. Asymptomatic *Campylobacter* infection also may trigger Guillain-Barré syndrome. Immunoproliferative small-intestinal disease (*alpha chain disease*), a form of lymphoma that originates in small-intestinal mucosa-associated lymphoid tissue, has been associated with *C. jejuni*; antimicrobial therapy has led to marked clinical improvement.

DIAGNOSIS

In patients with *Campylobacter* enteritis, peripheral leukocyte counts reflect the severity of the inflammatory process. However, stools from nearly all *Campylobacter*-infected patients presenting for medical attention in the United States contain leukocytes or erythrocytes. Gram- or Wright-stained fecal smears should be examined in all suspected cases. When the diagnosis of *Campylobacter* enteritis is suspected on the basis of findings indicating inflammatory diarrhea (fever, fecal leukocytes), clinicians can ask the microbiology laboratory to attempt the visualization of organisms with characteristic vibrioid morphology by direct microscopic examination of stools with Gram's staining or to use phase-contrast or dark-field microscopy to identify the organisms' characteristic "darting" motility. Confirmation of the diagnosis of *Campylobacter* infection is based on identification of an isolate from cultures of stool, blood, or another site. *Campylobacter*-specific media should be used to culture stools from all patients with inflammatory or bloody diarrhea. Because all *Campylobacter* species are fastidious, they will not be isolated unless selective media or other selective techniques are used. Not all media are equally useful for isolation of the broad array of campylobacters; therefore, failure to isolate campylobacters from stool does not entirely rule out their presence. Species-specific polymerase chain reaction techniques have been developed to facilitate exact diagnoses. The detection of the organisms in stool almost always implies infection; there is a brief period of post-convalescent fecal carriage and no obvious commensalism in humans. In contrast, *Campylobacter sputorum* and related organisms found in the oral cavity are commensals that only rarely have pathogenic significance. Because of the low levels of metabolic activity of *Campylobacter* species in standard blood culture media, *Campylobacter* bacteremia may be difficult to detect unless laboratorians check for low-positive results in quantitative assays.

DIFFERENTIAL DIAGNOSIS

The symptoms of *Campylobacter* enteritis are not sufficiently unusual to distinguish this illness from that due to *Salmonella, Shigella, Yersinia*, and other pathogens. The combination of fever and fecal leukocytes or erythrocytes is indicative of inflammatory diarrhea, and definitive diagnosis is based on culture or demonstration of the characteristic organisms on stained fecal smears. Similarly, extraintestinal *Campylobacter* illness is diagnosed by culture. Infection due to *Campylobacter* should be suspected in the setting of septic abortion, and that due to *C. fetus* should be suspected specifically in the setting of septic thrombophlebitis. It is important to reiterate that (1) the presentation of *Campylobacter* enteritis may mimic that of ulcerative colitis or Crohn's disease, (2) *Campylobacter* enteritis is much more common than either of the latter (especially among young adults), and (3) biopsy may not distinguish among these entities. Thus a diagnosis of inflammatory bowel disease should not be made until *Campylobacter* infection has been ruled out, especially in persons with a history of foreign travel, significant animal contact, immunodeficiency, or exposure incurring a high risk of transmission.

TREATMENT *CAMPYLOBACTER* INFECTION

Fluid and electrolyte replacement is central to the treatment of diarrheal illnesses (Chap. 160). Even among patients presenting for medical attention with *Campylobacter* enteritis, not all clearly benefit from specific antimicrobial therapy. Indications for therapy include high fever, bloody diarrhea, severe diarrhea, persistence for >1 week, and worsening of symptoms. A 5- to 7-day course of erythromycin (250 mg orally four times daily or—for children—30–50 mg/kg per day, in divided doses) is the regimen of choice. Both clinical trials and in vitro susceptibility testing indicate that other macrolides, including azithromycin (a 1- or 3-day regimen), also are useful therapeutic agents. An alternative regimen for adults is ciprofloxacin (500 mg orally twice daily) or another fluoroquinolone for 5–7 days, but resistance to this class of agents as well as to tetracyclines is substantial; ~22% of U.S. isolates in 2010 were resistant to ciprofloxacin. Because macrolide resistance usually is much less common (<10%), these drugs are the empirical agents of choice. Patients infected with antibiotic-resistant strains are at increased risk of adverse outcomes. Use of antimotility agents, which may prolong the duration of symptoms and have been associated with toxic megacolon and with death, is not recommended.

For systemic infections, treatment with gentamicin (1.7 mg/kg IV every 8 h after a loading dose of 2 mg/kg), imipenem (500 mg IV every 6 h), or chloramphenicol (50 mg/kg IV each day in three or four divided doses) should be started empirically, but susceptibility testing should then be performed. Ciprofloxacin and amoxicillin-clavulanate are alternative agents for susceptible strains. In the absence of immunocompromise or endovascular infections, therapy should be administered for 14 days. For immunocompromised patients with systemic infections due to *C. fetus* and for patients with endovascular infections, prolonged therapy (for up to 4 weeks) is usually necessary. For recurrent infections in immunocompromised hosts, lifelong therapy/prophylaxis is sometimes necessary.

PROGNOSIS

Nearly all patients recover fully from *Campylobacter* enteritis, either spontaneously or after antimicrobial therapy. Volume depletion probably contributes to the few deaths that are reported. As stated above, occasional patients develop reactive arthritis or Guillain-Barré syndrome or its variants. Systemic infection with *C. fetus* is much more often fatal than that due to related species; this higher mortality rate reflects in part the population affected. Prognosis depends on the rapidity with which appropriate therapy is begun. Otherwise healthy hosts usually survive *C. fetus* infections without sequelae. Compromised hosts often have recurrent and/or life-threatening infections due to a variety of *Campylobacter* species.

193 Cholera and Other Vibrioses

Matthew K. Waldor, Edward T. Ryan

Members of the genus *Vibrio* cause a number of important infectious syndromes. Classic among them is cholera, a devastating diarrheal disease caused by *Vibrio cholerae* that has been responsible for seven global pandemics and much suffering over the past two centuries. Epidemic cholera remains a significant public health concern in the developing world today. Other vibrioses caused by other *Vibrio* species include syndromes of diarrhea, soft tissue infection, or primary sepsis. All *Vibrio* species are highly motile, facultatively anaerobic, curved gram-negative rods with one or more flagella. In nature, vibrios most commonly reside in tidal rivers and bays under conditions of moderate salinity. They proliferate in the summer months when water temperatures exceed 20°C. As might be expected, the illnesses they cause also increase in frequency during the warm months.

CHOLERA

DEFINITION

Cholera is an acute diarrheal disease that can, in a matter of hours, result in profound, rapidly progressive dehydration and death. Accordingly, *cholera gravis* (the severe form) is a much-feared disease, particularly in its epidemic presentation. Fortunately, prompt aggressive fluid repletion and supportive care can obviate the high mortality that is historically associated with cholera. Although the term *cholera* has occasionally been applied to any severely dehydrating secretory diarrheal illness, whether infectious in etiology or not, it now refers to disease caused by *V. cholerae* serogroup O1 or O139—i.e., the serogroups with epidemic potential.

MICROBIOLOGY AND EPIDEMIOLOGY

The species *V. cholerae* is classified into more than 200 serogroups based on the carbohydrate determinants of their lipopolysaccharide (LPS) O antigens. Although some non-O1 *V. cholerae* serogroups (strains that do not agglutinate in antisera to the O1 group antigen) have occasionally caused sporadic outbreaks of diarrhea, serogroup O1 was, until the emergence of serogroup O139 in 1992, the exclusive cause of epidemic cholera. Two biotypes of *V. cholerae* O1, classical and El Tor, are distinguished. Each biotype is further subdivided into two serotypes, termed *Inaba* and *Ogawa*.

The natural habitat of *V. cholerae* is coastal salt water and brackish estuaries, where the organism lives in close relation to plankton. *V. cholerae* can also exist in freshwater in the presence of adequate nutrients and warmth. Humans become infected incidentally but, once infected, can act as vehicles for spread. Ingestion of water contaminated by human feces is the most common means of acquisition of *V. cholerae*. Consumption of contaminated food also can contribute to spread. There is no known animal reservoir. Although the infectious dose is relatively high, it is markedly reduced in hypochlorhydric persons, in those using antacids, and when gastric acidity is buffered by a meal. Cholera is predominantly a pediatric disease in endemic areas, but it affects adults and children equally when newly introduced into a population. In endemic areas, the burden of disease is often greatest during "cholera seasons" associated with high temperatures, heavy rainfall, and flooding, but cholera can occur year-round. For unexplained reasons, susceptibility to cholera is significantly influenced by ABO blood group status; persons with type O blood are at greatest risk of severe disease if infected, whereas those with type AB are at least risk.

Cholera is native to the Ganges delta in the Indian subcontinent. Since 1817, seven global pandemics have occurred. The current (seventh) pandemic—the first due to the El Tor biotype—began in Indonesia in 1961 and spread in serial waves throughout Asia as *V. cholerae* El Tor displaced the endemic classical biotype, which is thought to have caused the previous six pandemics. In the early 1970s, El Tor cholera erupted in Africa, causing major epidemics

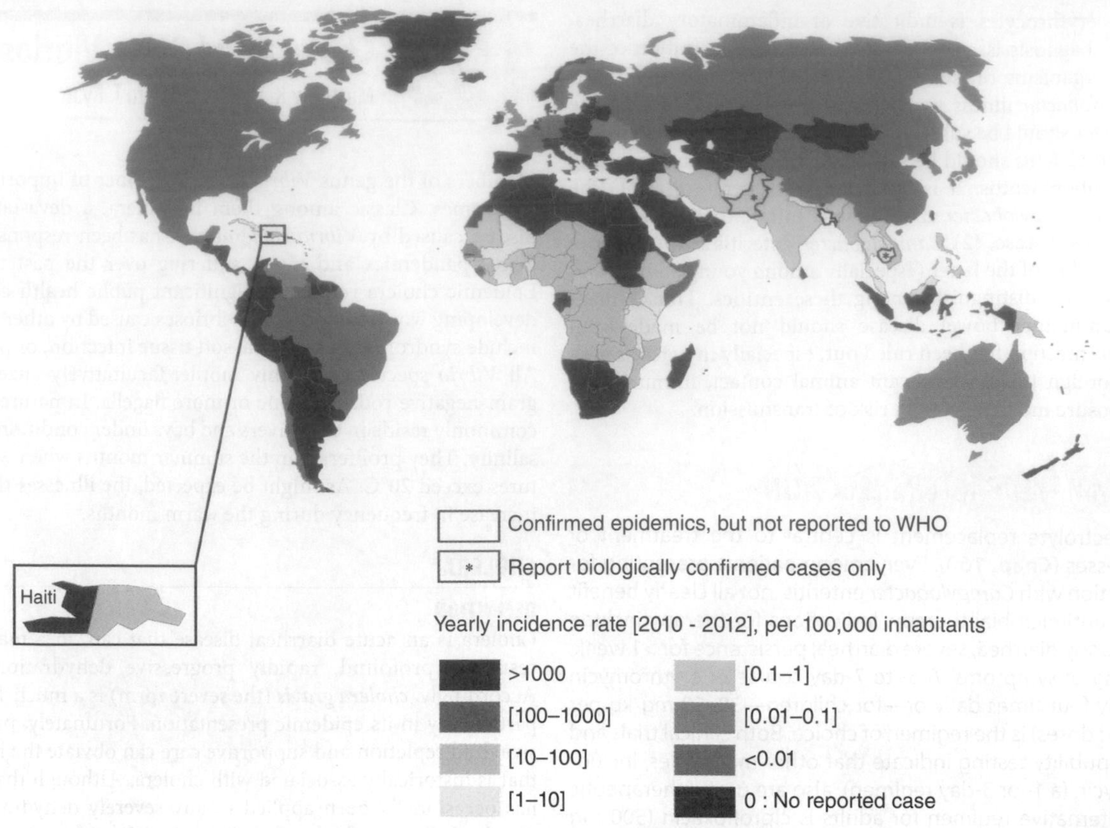

FIGURE 193-1 World distribution of cholera in 2010–2012. WHO, World Health Organization. *(Courtesy of Drs. M. and R. Piarroux, Université de la Méditerranée, France; with permission.)*

before becoming a persistent endemic problem. Currently, >90% of cholera cases reported annually to the World Health Organization (WHO) are from Africa (Fig. 193-1), but the true burden in Africa as well as in Asia is unknown because diagnosis is often syndromic and because many countries with endemic cholera do not report cholera to the WHO. It is possible that >3 million cases of cholera occur yearly (of which only ~200,000 are reported to the WHO), resulting in >100,000 deaths annually (of which <5000 are reported to the WHO).

After a century without cholera in Latin America, the current cholera pandemic reached Central and South America in 1991. Following an initial explosive spread that affected millions, the burden of disease has markedly decreased in Latin America. In 2010, a severe cholera outbreak began in Haiti, a country with no recorded history of this disease. Several lines of evidence indicate that cholera was likely introduced into Haiti by United Nations security forces from Asia, raising the possibility that asymptomatic carriers of *V. cholerae* play an important role in transmitting cholera over long distances. To date, the outbreak has involved more than 700,000 individuals, resulting in thousands of deaths. The recent history of cholera has been punctuated by such severe outbreaks, especially among impoverished or displaced persons. These outbreaks are often precipitated by war or other circumstances that lead to the breakdown of public health measures. Such was the case in the camps for Rwandan refugees set up in 1994 around Goma, Zaire, and in 2008–2009 in Zimbabwe.

Sporadic endemic infections due to *V. cholerae* O1 strains related to the seventh-pandemic strain have been recognized along the U.S. Gulf Coast of Louisiana and Texas. These infections are typically associated with the consumption of contaminated, locally harvested shellfish. Occasionally, cases in U.S. locations remote from the Gulf Coast have been linked to shipped-in Gulf Coast seafood.

In October 1992, a large-scale outbreak of clinical cholera caused by a new serogroup, O139, occurred in southeastern India. The organism appears to be a derivative of El Tor O1 but has a distinct LPS and an immunologically related O-antigen polysaccharide capsule. (O1 organisms are not encapsulated.) After an initial spread across 11 Asian countries, *V. cholerae* O139 has once again been almost entirely replaced by O1 strains. The clinical manifestations of disease caused by *V. cholerae* O139 are indistinguishable from those of O1 cholera. Immunity to one, however, is not protective against the other.

PATHOGENESIS

In the final analysis, cholera is a toxin-mediated disease. The watery diarrhea characteristic of cholera is due to the action of cholera toxin, a potent protein enterotoxin elaborated by the organism in the small intestine. The toxin-coregulated pilus (TCP), so named because its synthesis is regulated in parallel with that of cholera toxin, is essential for *V. cholerae* to survive and multiply in (colonize) the small intestine. Cholera toxin, TCP, and several other virulence factors are coordinately regulated by ToxR. This protein modulates the expression of genes coding for virulence factors in response to environmental signals via a cascade of regulatory proteins. Additional regulatory processes, including bacterial responses to the density of the bacterial population (in a phenomenon known as *quorum sensing*), modulate the virulence of *V. cholerae*.

Once established in the human small bowel, the organism produces cholera toxin, which consists of a monomeric enzymatic moiety (the A subunit) and a pentameric binding moiety (the B subunit). The B pentamer binds to GM_1 ganglioside, a glycolipid on the surface of epithelial cells that serves as the toxin receptor and makes possible the delivery of the A subunit to its cytosolic target. The activated A subunit (A_1) irreversibly transfers ADP-ribose from nicotinamide adenine dinucleotide to its specific target protein, the GTP-binding regulatory component of adenylate cyclase. The ADP-ribosylated G protein upregulates the activity of adenylate cyclase; the result is the intracellular accumulation of high levels of cyclic AMP. In intestinal epithelial cells, cyclic AMP inhibits the absorptive sodium transport system in villus cells and activates the secretory chloride transport system in crypt cells, and these events lead to the accumulation of sodium chloride in the intestinal lumen. Because water moves passively to maintain osmolality, isotonic fluid accumulates in the lumen. When the volume of that fluid exceeds the capacity of the rest of the gut to resorb it, watery diarrhea results. Unless the wasted fluid and electrolytes are adequately replaced, shock (due to profound dehydration) and acidosis (due to loss of bicarbonate) follow. Although perturbation of the adenylate cyclase pathway is the primary mechanism by which cholera toxin causes excess fluid secretion, cholera toxin also enhances intestinal secretion via prostaglandins and/or neural histamine receptors.

The *V. cholerae* genome comprises two circular chromosomes. Lateral gene transfer has played a key role in the evolution of epidemic *V. cholerae*. The genes encoding cholera toxin (*ctxAB*) are part of the genome of a bacteriophage, CTXΦ. The receptor for this phage on the *V. cholerae* surface is the intestinal colonization factor TCP. Because *ctxAB* is part of a mobile genetic element (CTXΦ), horizontal transfer of this bacteriophage may account for the emergence of new toxigenic *V. cholerae* serogroups. Many of the other genes important for *V. cholerae* pathogenicity, including the genes encoding the biosynthesis of TCP, those encoding accessory colonization factors, and those regulating virulence gene expression, are clustered together in the *V. cholerae* pathogenicity island. Similar clustering of virulence genes is found in other bacterial pathogens. It is believed that pathogenicity islands are acquired by horizontal gene transfer. *V. cholerae* O139 is probably derived from an El Tor O1 strain that acquired the genes for O139 O-antigen synthesis by horizontal gene transfer.

CLINICAL MANIFESTATIONS

Individuals infected with *V. cholerae* O1 or O139 exhibit a range of clinical manifestations. Some individuals are asymptomatic or have only mild diarrhea; others present with the sudden onset of explosive and life-threatening diarrhea (*cholera gravis*). The reasons for the range in signs and symptoms of disease are incompletely understood but include the level of preexisting immunity, blood type, and nutritional status. In a nonimmune individual, after a 24- to 48-h incubation period, cholera characteristically begins with the sudden onset of painless watery diarrhea that may quickly become voluminous. Patients often vomit. In severe cases, volume loss can exceed 250 mL/kg in the first 24 h. If fluids and electrolytes are not replaced, hypovolemic shock and death may ensue. Fever is usually absent. Muscle cramps due to electrolyte disturbances are common. The stool has a characteristic appearance: a nonbilious, gray, slightly cloudy fluid with flecks of mucus, no blood, and a somewhat fishy, inoffensive odor. It has been called "rice-water" stool because of its resemblance to the water in which rice has been washed (Fig. 193-2). Clinical symptoms parallel volume contraction: at losses of <5% of normal body weight, thirst develops; at 5–10%, postural hypotension, weakness, tachycardia, and decreased skin turgor are documented; and at >10%, oliguria, weak or absent pulses, sunken eyes (and, in infants, sunken fontanelles), wrinkled ("washerwoman") skin, somnolence, and coma are characteristic. Complications derive exclusively from the effects of volume and electrolyte depletion and include renal failure due to acute tubular necrosis. Thus, if the patient is adequately treated with fluid and electrolytes, complications are averted and the process is self-limited, resolving in a few days.

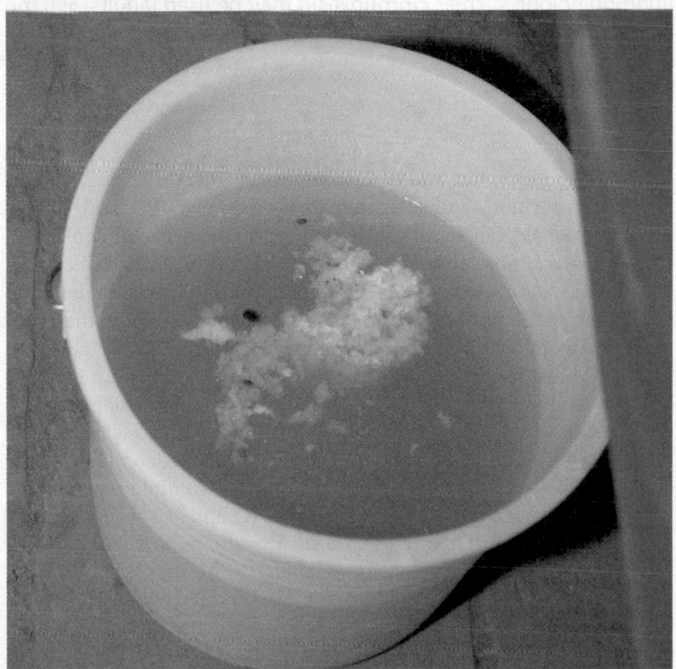

FIGURE 193-2 Rice water cholera stool. Note floating mucus and gray watery appearance. *(Courtesy of Dr. A. S. G. Faruque, International Centre for Diarrhoeal Disease Research, Dhaka; with permission.)*

Laboratory data usually reveal an elevated hematocrit (due to hemoconcentration) in nonanemic patients; mild neutrophilic leukocytosis; elevated levels of blood urea nitrogen and creatinine consistent with prerenal azotemia; normal sodium, potassium, and chloride levels; a markedly reduced bicarbonate level (<15 mmol/L); and an elevated anion gap (due to increases in serum lactate, protein, and phosphate). Arterial pH is usually low (~7.2).

DIAGNOSIS

Cholera should be suspected when a patient ≥2 years of age develops acute watery diarrhea in an area known to have cholera or when a patient ≥5 years of age develops severe dehydration or dies from acute watery diarrhea, even in an area where cholera is not known to be present. The clinical suspicion of cholera can be confirmed by the identification of *V. cholerae* in stool; however, the organism must be specifically sought. With experience, it can be detected directly by dark-field microscopy on a wet mount of fresh stool, and its serotype can be discerned by immobilization with specific antiserum. Laboratory isolation of the organism requires the use of a selective medium such as taurocholate-tellurite-gelatin (TTG) agar or thiosulfate-citrate-bile salts-sucrose (TCBS) agar. If a delay in sample processing is expected, Carey-Blair transport medium and/or alkaline-peptone water-enrichment medium may be used as well. In endemic areas, there is little need for biochemical confirmation and characterization, although these tasks may be worthwhile in places where *V. cholerae* is an uncommon isolate. Standard microbiologic biochemical testing for Enterobacteriaceae will suffice for identification of *V. cholerae*. All vibrios are oxidase-positive. A point-of-care antigen-detection cholera dipstick assay is now commercially available for use in the field or where laboratory facilities are lacking.

TREATMENT CHOLERA

Death from cholera is due to hypovolemic shock; thus treatment of individuals with cholera first and foremost requires fluid resuscitation and management. In light of the level of dehydration (Table 193-1) and the patient's age and weight, euvolemia should first be rapidly restored, and adequate hydration should then be maintained to replace ongoing fluid losses (Table 193-2). Administration of oral rehydration solution (ORS) takes advantage of the hexose-Na^+ co-transport mechanism to move Na^+ across the gut mucosa together with an actively transported molecule such as glucose (or galactose). Cl^- and water follow. This transport mechanism remains intact even when cholera toxin is active. ORS may be made by adding safe water to prepackaged sachets containing salts and sugar or by adding 0.5 teaspoon of table salt and 6 teaspoons of table sugar to 1 L of safe water. Potassium intake in bananas or green coconut water should be encouraged. A number of ORS formulations are available, and the WHO now recommends "low-osmolarity" ORS for treatment of individuals with dehydrating diarrhea of any cause (Table 193-3). If available, rice-based ORS is considered superior to standard ORS in the treatment of cholera. ORS can be administered via a nasogastric tube to individuals who cannot ingest fluid; however, optimal management of individuals with severe dehydration includes the administration of IV fluid and electrolytes. Because profound acidosis (pH <7.2) is common in this group, Ringer's lactate is the best choice among commercial products (Table 193-4); it must be used with additional potassium supplements, preferably given by mouth.

TABLE 193-1 ASSESSING THE DEGREE OF DEHYDRATION IN PATIENTS WITH CHOLERA

Degree of Dehydration	Clinical Findings
None or mild, but diarrhea	Thirst in some cases; <5% loss of total body weight
Moderate	Thirst, postural hypotension, weakness, tachycardia, decreased skin turgor, dry mouth/tongue, no tears; 5–10% loss of total body weight
Severe	Unconsciousness, lethargy, or "floppiness"; weak or absent pulse; inability to drink; sunken eyes (and, in infants, sunken fontanelles); >10% loss of total body weight

TABLE 193-2 TREATMENT OF CHOLERA, BASED ON DEGREE OF DEHYDRATION[a]

Degree of Dehydration, Patient's Age (Weight)	Treatment[b]
None or Mild, But Diarrhea[c]	
<2 years	1/4–1/2 cup (50–100 mL) of ORS, to a maximum of 0.5 L/d
2–9 years	1/2–1 cup (100–200 mL) of ORS, to a maximum of 1 L/d
≥10 years	As much ORS as desired, to a maximum of 2 L/d
Moderate[c,d]	
<4 months (<5 kg)	200–400 mL of ORS
4–11 months (5–<8 kg)	400–600 mL of ORS
12–23 months (8–<11 kg)	600–800 mL of ORS
2–4 years (11–<16 kg)	800–1200 mL of ORS
5–14 years (16–<30 kg)	1200–2200 mL of ORS
≥15 years (≥30 kg)	2200–4000 mL of ORS
Severe[c]	
All ages and weights	Undertake IV fluid replacement with Ringer's lactate (or, if not available, normal saline). Give 100 mL/kg in the first 3-h period (or the first 6-h period for children <12 months old); start rapidly, then slow down. Give a total of 200 mL/kg in the first 24 h. Continue until the patient is awake, can ingest ORS, and no longer has a weak pulse.

[a]Adapted from World Health Organization: First steps for managing an outbreak of acute diarrhoea. Global Task Force on Cholera Control, 2009 (*www.who.int/topics/cholera*). [b]Continue normal feeding during treatment. [c]Reassess regularly; monitor stool and vomit output. [d]Volumes of ORS listed should be given within the first 4 h.

Abbreviation: ORS, oral rehydration solution.

TABLE 193-3 COMPOSITION OF WORLD HEALTH ORGANIZATION REDUCED-OSMOLARITY ORAL REHYDRATION SOLUTION (ORS)[a,b]

Constituent	Concentration, mmol/L
Na^+	75
K^+	20
Cl^-	65
Citrate[c]	10
Glucose	75
Total osmolarity	245

[a]Contains (per package, to be added to 1 L of drinking water): NaCl, 2.6 g; $Na_3C_6H_5O_7$·$2H_2O$, 2.9 g; KCl, 1.5 g; and glucose (anhydrous), 13.5 g. [b]If prepackaged ORS is unavailable, a simple homemade alternative can be prepared by combining 3.5 g (~1/2 teaspoon) of NaCl with either 50 g of precooked rice cereal or 6 teaspoons of table sugar (sucrose) in 1 L of drinking water. In that case, potassium must be supplied separately (e.g., in orange juice or coconut water). [c]10 mmol of citrate per liter, which supplies 30 mmol HCO_3/L.

TABLE 193-4 ELECTROLYTE COMPOSITION OF CHOLERA STOOL AND OF INTRAVENOUS REHYDRATION SOLUTION

	Concentration, mmol/L			
Substance	Na^+	K^+	Cl^-	Base
Stool				
Adult	135	15	100	45
Child	100	25	90	30
Ringer's lactate	130	4[a]	109	28

[a]Potassium supplements, preferably administered by mouth, are required to replace the usual potassium losses from stool.

The total fluid deficit in severely dehydrated patients (>10% of body weight) can be replaced safely within the first 3–4 h of therapy, half within the first hour. Transient muscle cramps and tetany are common. Thereafter, oral therapy can usually be initiated, with the goal of maintaining fluid intake equal to fluid output. However, patients with continued large-volume diarrhea may require prolonged IV treatment to match gastrointestinal fluid losses. Severe hypokalemia can develop but will respond to potassium given either IV or orally. In the absence of adequate staff to monitor the patient's progress, the oral route of rehydration and potassium replacement is safer than the IV route.

Although not necessary for cure, the use of an antibiotic to which the organism is susceptible diminishes the duration and volume of fluid loss and hastens clearance of the organism from the stool. Adjunctive antibiotics should therefore be administered to patients with moderate or severe dehydration due to cholera. In many areas, macrolides such as erythromycin (adults, 250 mg orally four times a day for 3 days; children, 12.5 mg/kg per dose four times a day for 3 days) or azithromycin (adults, a single 1-g dose; children, a single 20-mg/kg dose) are the agents of choice. Increasing resistance to tetracyclines is widespread; however, in areas with confirmed susceptibility, tetracycline (nonpregnant adults, 500 mg orally four times a day for 3 days; children >8 years old, 12.5 mg/kg per dose four times a day for 3 days) or doxycycline (nonpregnant adults, a 300-mg single dose; children >8 years old, a single dose of 4–6 mg/kg) may be used. Similarly, increasing resistance to fluoroquinolones is being reported, but in areas with confirmed susceptibility, a fluoroquinolone such as ciprofloxacin may be used (adults, 500 mg twice a day for 3 days; children, 15 mg/kg twice a day for 3 days).

PREVENTION

Provision of safe water and of facilities for sanitary disposal of feces, improved nutrition, and attention to food preparation and storage in the household can significantly reduce the incidence of cholera. In addition, precautions should be taken to prevent the spread of cholera via infected and potentially asymptomatic persons from endemic to nonendemic regions of the world (as was probably the case in the ongoing outbreak in Haiti; see "Microbiology and Epidemiology," above).

Much effort has been devoted to the development of an effective cholera vaccine over the past few decades, with a particular focus on oral vaccine strains. In an attempt to maximize mucosal responses, two types of oral cholera vaccine have been developed: oral killed vaccines and live attenuated vaccines. Currently, two oral killed cholera vaccines have been prequalified by the WHO and are available internationally. WC-rBS (Dukoral®; Crucell, Stockholm, Sweden) contains several biotypes and serotypes of *V. cholerae* O1 supplemented with 1 mg of recombinant cholera toxin B subunit per dose. BivWC (Shanchol™; Shantha Biotechnics–Sanofi Pasteur, Mumbai, India) contains several biotypes and serotypes of *V. cholerae* O1 and *V. cholerae* O139 without supplemental cholera toxin B subunit. The vaccines are administered as a two- or three-dose regimen, with

PART 8 Infectious Diseases

doses usually separated by 14 days. They provide ~60–85% protection for the first few months. Booster immunizations of WC-rBS are recommended after 2 years for individuals ≥6 years of age and after 6 months for children 2–5 years of age. For BivWC, which was developed more recently, no formal recommendation regarding booster immunizations exists. However, BivWC was associated with ~60% protection over 5 years among recipients of all ages in a study in Kolkata, India; the rate of protection among children ≤5 years of age approximated 40%. Models predict significant herd immunity when vaccination coverage rates exceed 50%. The killed vaccines have been safely administered among populations with high rates of HIV.

Oral live attenuated vaccines for *V. cholerae* are also in development. These strains have in common the fact that they lack the genes encoding cholera toxin. One such vaccine, CVD 103-HgR, was safe and immunogenic in phase 1 and 2 studies but afforded minimal protection in a large field trial in Indonesia. Other live attenuated vaccine candidate strains have been prepared from El Tor and O139 *V. cholerae* and have been tested in studies of volunteers. A possible advantage of live attenuated cholera vaccines is that they may induce protection after a single oral dose. Conjugate and subunit cholera vaccines are also being developed. Recognizing that it may be decades before safe water and adequate sanitation become a reality for those most at risk of cholera, the WHO has now recommended incorporation of cholera vaccination into comprehensive control strategies and has established an international stockpile of oral killed cholera vaccine to assist in outbreak responses. No cholera vaccine is commercially available in the United States.

OTHER *VIBRIO* SPECIES

The genus *Vibrio* includes several human pathogens that do not cause cholera. Abundant in coastal waters throughout the world, noncholera vibrios can reach high concentrations in the tissues of filter-feeding mollusks. As a result, human infection commonly follows the ingestion of seawater or of raw or undercooked shellfish (Table 193-5). Most noncholera vibrios can be cultured on blood or MacConkey agar, which contains enough salt to support the growth of these halophilic species. In the microbiology laboratory, the species of noncholera vibrios are distinguished by standard biochemical tests. The most important of these organisms are *Vibrio parahaemolyticus* and *Vibrio vulnificus*.

The two major types of syndromes for which these species are responsible are gastrointestinal illness (due to *V. parahaemolyticus*, non-O1/O139 *V. cholerae*, *Vibrio mimicus*, *Vibrio fluvialis*, *Vibrio hollisae*, and *Vibrio furnissii*) and soft tissue infections (due to *V. vulnificus*, *Vibrio alginolyticus*, and *Vibrio damselae*). *V. vulnificus* is also a cause of primary sepsis in some compromised individuals.

SPECIES ASSOCIATED PRIMARILY WITH GASTROINTESTINAL ILLNESS

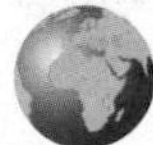

V. parahaemolyticus Widespread in marine environments, the halophilic *V. parahaemolyticus* causes food-borne enteritis worldwide. This species was originally implicated in enteritis in Japan in 1953, accounting for 24% of reported cases in one study—a rate that presumably was due to the common practice of eating raw seafood in that country. In the United States, common-source outbreaks of diarrhea caused by this organism have been linked to the consumption of undercooked or improperly handled seafood or of other foods contaminated by seawater. Since the mid-1990s, the incidence of *V. parahaemolyticus* infections has increased in several countries, including the United States. Serotypes O3:K6, O4:K68, and O1:K-untypable, which are genetically related to one another, account in part for this increase. Serotypes O4:K12 and O4:KUT were initially unique to the Pacific Northwest but caused recent outbreaks in the eastern United States and Spain. The enteropathogenicity of *V. parahaemolyticus* is linked to its ability to cause hemolysis on Wagatsuma agar (i.e., the *Kanagawa phenomenon*). Although the mechanisms by which the organism causes diarrhea are not fully defined, the genome sequence of *V. parahaemolyticus* contains two type III secretion systems, which directly inject toxic bacterial proteins into host cells. The activity of one of these secretion systems is required for intestinal colonization and virulence in animal models. *V. parahaemolyticus* should be considered a possible etiologic agent in all cases of diarrhea that can be linked epidemiologically to seafood consumption or to the sea itself.

Infections with *V. parahaemolyticus* can result in two distinct gastrointestinal presentations. The more common of the two presentations (including nearly all cases in North America) is characterized by watery diarrhea, usually occurring in conjunction with abdominal cramps, nausea, and vomiting and accompanied in ~25% of cases by fever and chills. After an incubation period of 4 h to 4 days, symptoms develop and persist for a median of 3 days. Dysentery, the less common presentation, is characterized by severe abdominal cramps, nausea, vomiting, and bloody or mucoid stools. *V. parahaemolyticus* also causes rare cases of wound infection and otitis and very rare cases of sepsis.

Most cases of *V. parahaemolyticus*–associated gastrointestinal illness, regardless of the presentation, are self-limited. Fluid replacement should be stressed. The role of antimicrobials is uncertain, but they may be of benefit in moderate or severe disease. Doxycycline, fluoroquinolones, or macrolides are usually used. Deaths are extremely rare among immunocompetent individuals. Severe infections are associated with underlying diseases, including diabetes, preexisting liver disease, iron-overload states, or immunosuppression.

Non-O1/O139 (Noncholera) *V. cholerae* The heterogeneous non-O1/O139 *V. cholerae* organisms cannot be distinguished from *V. cholerae* O1 or O139 by routine biochemical tests but do not agglutinate in O1 or O139 antiserum. Non-O1/O139 strains have caused several well-studied food-borne outbreaks of gastroenteritis and have also been responsible for sporadic cases of otitis media, wound infection, and bacteremia; although gastroenteritis outbreaks can occur, non-O1/O139 *V. cholerae* strains do not cause epidemics of cholera. Like other vibrios, non-O1/O139 *V. cholerae* organisms are widely distributed in marine environments. In most instances, recognized cases in the United States have been associated with the consumption of raw oysters or with recent travel. The broad clinical spectrum of diarrheal illness caused by these

TABLE 193-5 FEATURES OF SELECTED NONCHOLERA VIBRIOSES

Organism	Vehicle or Activity	Host at Risk	Syndrome
Vibrio parahaemolyticus	Shellfish, seawater	Normal	Gastroenteritis
	Seawater	Normal	Wound infection
Non-O1/O139 *Vibrio cholerae*	Shellfish, travel	Normal	Gastroenteritis
	Seawater	Normal	Wound infection, otitis media
Vibrio vulnificus	Shellfish	Immunosuppressed[a]	Sepsis, secondary cellulitis
	Seawater	Normal, immunosuppressed[a]	Wound infection, cellulitis
Vibrio alginolyticus	Seawater	Normal	Wound infection, cellulitis, otitis
	Seawater	Burned, other immunosuppressed	Sepsis

[a]Especially with liver disease or hemochromatosis.

Source: Table 161-3 in *Harrisons Principles of Internal Medicine*, 14th edition.

organisms is probably due to the group's heterogeneous virulence attributes.

In the United States, about half of all non-O1/O139 *V. cholerae* isolates are from stool samples. The typical incubation period for gastroenteritis due to these organisms is <2 days, and the illness lasts for ~2–7 days. Patients' stools may be copious and watery or may be partly formed, less voluminous, and bloody or mucoid. Diarrhea can result in severe dehydration. Many cases include abdominal cramps, nausea, vomiting, and fever. Like those with cholera, patients who are seriously dehydrated should receive oral or IV fluids; the value of antibiotics is not clear.

Extraintestinal infections due to non-O1/O139 *V. cholerae* commonly follow occupational or recreational exposure to seawater. Around 10% of non-O1/O139 *V. cholerae* isolates come from cases of wound infection, 10% from cases of otitis media, and 20% from cases of bacteremia (which is particularly likely to develop in patients with liver disease). Extraintestinal infections should be treated with antibiotics. Information to guide antibiotic selection and dosing is limited, but most strains are sensitive in vitro to tetracycline, ciprofloxacin, and third-generation cephalosporins.

SPECIES ASSOCIATED PRIMARILY WITH SOFT TISSUE INFECTION OR BACTEREMIA

(See also Chap. 156)

V. vulnificus Infection with *V. vulnificus* is rare, but this organism is the most common cause of severe *Vibrio* infections in the United States. Like most vibrios, *V. vulnificus* proliferates in the warm summer months and requires a saline environment for growth. In the United States, infections in humans typically occur in coastal states between May and October and most commonly affect men >40 years of age. *V. vulnificus* has been linked to two distinct syndromes: primary sepsis, which usually occurs in patients with underlying liver disease, and primary wound infection, which generally affects people without underlying disease. (*Vulnificus* is Latin for "wound maker.") Some authors have suggested that *V. vulnificus* also causes gastroenteritis independent of other clinical manifestations. *V. vulnificus* is endowed with a number of virulence attributes, including a capsule that confers resistance to phagocytosis and to the bactericidal activity of human serum as well as a cytolysin. Measured as the 50% lethal dose in mice, the organism's virulence is considerably increased under conditions of iron overload; this observation is consistent with the propensity of *V. vulnificus* to infect patients who have hemochromatosis.

Primary sepsis most often develops in patients who have cirrhosis or hemochromatosis. However, *V. vulnificus* bacteremia can also affect individuals who have hematopoietic disorders or chronic renal insufficiency, those who are using immunosuppressive medications or alcohol, or (in rare instances) those who have no known underlying disease. After a median incubation period of 16 h, the patient develops malaise, chills, fever, and prostration. One-third of patients develop hypotension, which is often apparent at admission. Cutaneous manifestations develop in most cases (usually within 36 h of onset) and characteristically involve the extremities (the lower more often than the upper). In a common sequence, erythematous patches are followed by ecchymoses, vesicles, and bullae. In fact, sepsis and hemorrhagic bullous skin lesions suggest the diagnosis in appropriate settings. Necrosis and sloughing may also be evident. Laboratory studies reveal leukopenia more often than leukocytosis, thrombocytopenia, or elevated levels of fibrin split products. *V. vulnificus* can be cultured from blood or cutaneous lesions. The mortality rate approaches 50%, with most deaths due to uncontrolled sepsis (Chap. 325). Accordingly, prompt treatment is critical and should include empirical antibiotic administration, aggressive debridement, and general supportive care. *V. vulnificus* is sensitive in vitro to a number of antibiotics, including tetracycline, fluoroquinolones, and third-generation cephalosporins. Data from animal models suggest that either a fluoroquinolone or the combination of a tetracycline and a third-generation cephalosporin should be used in the treatment of *V. vulnificus* septicemia.

V. vulnificus–associated soft tissue infection can complicate either a fresh or an old wound that comes into contact with seawater; the patient may or may not have underlying disease. After a short incubation period (4 h to 4 days; mean, 12 h), the disease begins with swelling, erythema, and (in many cases) intense pain around the wound. These signs and symptoms are followed by cellulitis, which spreads rapidly and is sometimes accompanied by vesicular, bullous, or necrotic lesions. Metastatic events are uncommon. Most patients have fever and leukocytosis. *V. vulnificus* can be cultured from skin lesions and occasionally from the blood. Prompt antibiotic therapy and debridement are usually curative.

V. alginolyticus First identified as a pathogen of humans in 1973, *V. alginolyticus* occasionally causes eye, ear, and wound infections. This species is the most salt-tolerant of the vibrios and can grow in salt concentrations of >10%. Most clinical isolates come from superinfected wounds that presumably become contaminated at the beach. Although its severity varies, *V. alginolyticus* infection tends not to be serious and generally responds well to antibiotic therapy and drainage. A few cases of otitis externa, otitis media, and conjunctivitis due to this pathogen have been described. Tetracycline treatment usually results in cure. *V. alginolyticus* is a rare cause of bacteremia in immunocompromised hosts.

Acknowledgment

The authors gratefully acknowledge the valuable contributions of Drs. Robert Deresiewicz and Gerald T. Keusch, coauthors of this chapter for previous editions.

194e Brucellosis

Nicholas J. Beeching, Michael J. Corbel

This is a digital-only chapter. It is available on the DVD that accompanies this book, as well as on Access Medicine/Harrison's Online, and the eBook and "app" editions of HPIM 19e. The authors thank Dr. Adrian M. Whatmore for his review of the manuscript.

DEFINITION

Brucellosis is a bacterial zoonosis transmitted directly or indirectly to humans from infected animals, predominantly domesticated ruminants and swine. The disease is known colloquially as *undulant fever* because of its remittent character. Although brucellosis commonly presents as an acute febrile illness, its clinical manifestations vary widely, and definitive signs indicative of the diagnosis may be lacking. Thus the clinical diagnosis usually must be supported by the results of bacteriologic and/or serologic tests.

195 Tularemia

Richard F. Jacobs, Gordon E. Schutze

Tularemia is a zoonosis caused by *Francisella tularensis.* Humans of any age, sex, or race are universally susceptible to this systemic infection. Tularemia is primarily a disease of wild animals and persists in contaminated environments, ectoparasites, and animal carriers. Human infection is incidental and usually results from interaction with biting or blood-sucking insects, contact with wild or domestic animals, ingestion of contaminated water or food, or inhalation of infective aerosols. The illness is characterized by various clinical syndromes, the most common of which consists of an ulcerative lesion at the site of inoculation, with regional lymphadenopathy and lymphadenitis. Systemic manifestations, including pneumonia, typhoidal tularemia, meningitis, and fever without localizing findings, pose a greater diagnostic challenge.

ETIOLOGY AND EPIDEMIOLOGY

F. tularensis is a class A bioterrorism agent (Chap. 261e). With rare exceptions, tularemia is the only disease produced by *F. tularensis*—a small (0.2 μm by 0.2–0.7 μm), gram-negative, pleomorphic, nonmotile, non-spore-forming bacillus. Bipolar staining results in a coccoid appearance. The organism is a thinly encapsulated, nonpiliated strict aerobe that invades host cells. In nature, *F. tularensis* is a hardy organism that persists for weeks or months in mud, water, and decaying animal carcasses. Dozens of biting and blood-sucking insects, especially ticks and tabanid flies, serve as vectors. Ticks and wild rabbits are the source for most human cases in endemic areas of the southeastern United States. In Utah, Nevada, and California, tabanid flies are the most common vectors. Animal reservoirs include wild rabbits, squirrels, birds, sheep, beavers, muskrats, and domestic dogs and cats. Person-to-person transmission is rare or nonexistent.

The four subspecies of *F. tularensis* are *tularensis*, *holarctica*, *novicida*, and *mediasiatica*. The first three of these subspecies are found in North America; in fact, subspecies *tularensis* has been isolated only in North America, where it accounts for >70% of cases of tularemia and produces more serious human disease than other subspecies (although, with treatment, the associated fatality rate is <2%). The progression of illness depends on the infecting strain's virulence, the inoculum size, the portal of entry, and the host's immune status.

Ticks pass *F. tularensis* to their offspring transovarially. The organism is found in tick feces but not in large quantities in tick salivary glands. In the United States, the disease is carried by *Dermacentor andersoni* (Rocky Mountain wood tick), *Dermacentor variabilis* (American dog tick), *Dermacentor occidentalis* (Pacific Coast dog tick), and *Amblyomma americanum* (Lone Star tick). *F. tularensis* is transmitted frequently during blood meals taken by embedded ticks after hours of attachment. It is the taking of a blood meal through a fecally contaminated field that transmits the organism. Transmission by ticks and tabanid flies takes place mainly in the spring and summer. However, continued transmission in the winter by trapped or hunted animals has been documented.

Tularemia is most common in the southeastern United States; Arkansas, Missouri, and Oklahoma account for more than half of all reported cases in this country. Small outbreaks in higher-risk populations (e.g., professional landscapers cutting up brush, mowing, and using a leaf blower) have been reported. Although the irregular distribution of cases of tularemia makes worldwide estimates difficult, increasing numbers of cases have been reported between latitudes 30° and 71°N (the Holarctic region) in the Northern Hemisphere. Cases of tularemia have been reported from Europe, Turkey, Canada, Mexico, and Asia. If the disease is caused by subspecies *tularensis*, the clinical manifestations are similar to those in the United States. However, in areas where tularemia is due largely to subspecies *holarctica*, oropharyngeal disease is common. Disease acquisition results from the consumption of water contaminated by live organisms shed by animals (e.g., muskrats, beavers). Subspecies *holarctica* is known to cause milder disease than other subspecies and responds well to fluoroquinolones, especially ciprofloxacin.

PATHOGENESIS AND PATHOLOGY

The most common portal of entry for human infection is through skin or mucous membranes, either directly—through the bite of ticks, other arthropods, or other animals—or via inapparent abrasions. Inhalation or ingestion of *F. tularensis* also can result in infection. *F. tularensis* is extremely infectious: Although $>10^8$ organisms are usually required to produce infection via the oral route (oropharyngeal or gastrointestinal tularemia), as few as 10 organisms can result in infection when injected into the skin (ulceroglandular/glandular tularemia) or inhaled (pulmonary tularemia). After inoculation into the skin, the organism multiplies locally; within 2–5 days (range, 1–10 days), it produces an erythematous, tender, or pruritic papule. The papule rapidly enlarges and forms an ulcer with a black base (chancriform lesion). The bacteria spread to regional lymph nodes, producing lymphadenopathy (buboes). All forms can lead to bacteremia with spread to distant organs, including the central nervous system.

Tularemia is characterized by mononuclear cell infiltration with pyogranulomatous pathology. The histopathologic findings can be quite similar to those in tuberculosis, although tularemia develops more rapidly. As a facultatively intracellular bacterium, *F. tularensis* can parasitize both phagocytic and nonphagocytic host cells and can survive intracellularly for prolonged periods. In the acute phase of infection, the primary organs affected (skin, lymph nodes, liver, and spleen) include areas of focal necrosis, which are initially surrounded by polymorphonuclear leukocytes (PMNs). Subsequently, granulomas form, with epithelioid cells, lymphocytes, and multinucleated giant cells surrounded by areas of necrosis. These areas may resemble caseation necrosis but later coalesce to form abscesses.

Conjunctival inoculation can result in infection of the eye, with regional lymph node enlargement (preauricular lymphadenopathy, Parinaud's complex). Aerosolization and inhalation or hematogenous spread of organisms can result in pneumonia. In the lung, an inflammatory reaction develops, including foci of alveolar necrosis and cell infiltration (initially polymorphonuclear and later mononuclear) with granulomas. Chest roentgenograms usually reveal bilateral patchy infiltrates rather than large areas of consolidation. Pleural effusions are common and may contain blood. Lymphadenopathy occurs in regions draining infected organs. Therefore, in pulmonary infection, mediastinal adenopathy may be evident, whereas patients with oropharyngeal tularemia develop cervical lymphadenopathy. In gastrointestinal or typhoidal tularemia, mesenteric lymphadenopathy may follow the ingestion of large numbers of organisms. (The term *typhoidal tularemia* may be used to describe severe bacteremic disease, irrespective of the mode of transmission or portal of entry.) Meningitis has been reported as a primary or secondary manifestation of bacteremia. Patients may also present with fever and no localizing signs.

IMMUNOLOGY

Although a complete and widely accepted understanding of the protective immune response to *F. tularensis* is lacking, significant advances in the study of natural and protective immunity have been made in recent years and may ultimately result in a vaccine candidate. Complete genomic sequencing and the availability of attenuated *F. tularensis* strains developed through genetic manipulation are facilitating research that will expand our knowledge in this area.

A number of investigators have studied various models and proposed various hypotheses regarding the induction of protective immunity to *F. tularensis*. Although further research is needed, synergy between humoral and cell-mediated immune (CMI) responses appears to be critical in inducing effective immune protection. Elucidation of the molecular mechanisms for the organism's evasion of the host response, pathogen-associated molecular patterns, and effective host immune protection has led to novel vaccination strategies tested in animal models. Antibodies to Fc receptors on antigen-presenting cells have been shown to be protective in animal models of pulmonary tularemia, resulting in both mucosal and CMI responses. This enhanced understanding of mucosal and serum antibodies in combination with a targeted CMI response holds great promise for future vaccine development.

CLINICAL MANIFESTATIONS

Tularemia often starts with a sudden onset of fever, chills, headache, and generalized myalgias and arthralgias (Table 195-1). This onset takes place when the organism penetrates the skin, is ingested, or is inhaled. An incubation period of 2–10 days is followed by the formation of an ulcer at the site of penetration, with local inflammation. The ulcer may persist for several months as organisms are transported via the lymphatics to the regional lymph nodes. These nodes enlarge and may become necrotic and suppurative. If the organism enters the bloodstream, widespread dissemination can result.

TABLE 195-1 CLINICAL PRESENTATION OF TULAREMIA

	Rate of Occurrence, %	
Sign or Symptom	Children	Adults
Lymphadenopathy	96	65
Fever (≥38.3°C or ≥101°F)	87	21
Ulcer/eschar/papule	45	51
Myalgias/arthralgias	39	2
Headache	9	5
Cough	9	5
Pharyngitis	43	—
Diarrhea	43	—

Source: Adapted from RF Jacobs, JP Narain: Pediatrics 76:818, 1985; with permission.

In the United States, most patients with tularemia (75–85%) acquire the infection by inoculation of the skin. In adults, the most common localized form is inguinal/femoral lymphadenopathy; in children, it is cervical lymphadenopathy. About 20% of patients develop a generalized maculopapular rash, which occasionally becomes pustular. Erythema nodosum occurs infrequently. The clinical manifestations of tularemia have been divided into various syndromes, which are listed in Table 195-2.

Ulceroglandular/Glandular Tularemia These two forms of tularemia account for ~75–85% of cases. The predominant form in children involves cervical or posterior auricular lymphadenopathy and is usually related to tick bites on the head and neck. In adults, the most common form is inguinal/femoral lymphadenopathy resulting from insect and tick exposures on the lower limbs. In cases related to wild game, the usual portal of entry for *F. tularensis* is either an injury sustained while skinning or cleaning an animal carcass or a bite (usually on the hand). Epitrochlear lymphadenopathy/lymphadenitis is common in patients with bite-related injuries.

In ulceroglandular tularemia, the ulcer is erythematous, indurated, and nonhealing, with a punched-out appearance that lasts 1–3 weeks. The papule may begin as an erythematous lesion that is tender or pruritic; it evolves over several days into an ulcer with sharply demarcated edges and a yellow exudate. The ulcer gradually develops a black base, and simultaneously the regional lymph nodes become tender and severely enlarged (Fig. 195-1). The affected lymph nodes may become fluctuant and drain spontaneously, but the condition usually resolves with effective treatment. Late suppuration of lymph nodes has been described in up to 25% of patients with ulceroglandular/glandular tularemia. Examination of material taken from these late fluctuant nodes after successful antimicrobial treatment reveals sterile necrotic tissue. In 5–10% of patients, the skin lesion may be inapparent, with lymphadenopathy plus systemic signs and symptoms the only physical findings (*glandular tularemia*). Conversely, a tick or deerfly bite on the trunk may result in an ulcer without evident lymphadenopathy.

Oculoglandular Tularemia In ~1% of patients, the portal of entry for *F. tularensis* is the conjunctiva, which the organism usually reaches through contact with contaminated fingers. The inflamed conjunctiva is painful, with numerous yellowish nodules and pinpoint ulcers.

TABLE 195-2 CLINICAL SYNDROMES OF TULAREMIA

	Rate of Occurrence, %	
Syndrome	Children	Adults
Ulceroglandular	45	51
Glandular	25	12
Pulmonary (pneumonia)	14	18
Oropharyngeal	4	—
Oculoglandular	2	—
Typhoidal	2	12
Unclassified	6	11

Source: Adapted from RF Jacobs, JP Narain: Pediatrics 76:818, 1985; with permission.

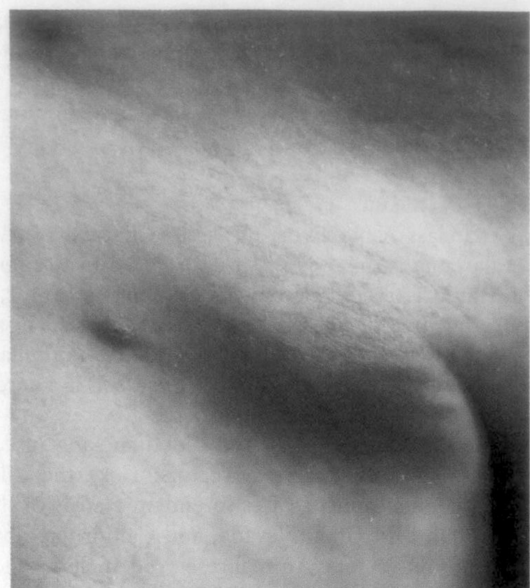

FIGURE 195-1 An 8-year-old boy with inguinal lymphadenitis and associated tick-bite site characteristic of ulceroglandular tularemia.

Purulent conjunctivitis with regional lymphadenopathy (preauricular, submandibular, or cervical) is evident. Because of debilitating pain, the patient may seek medical attention before regional lymphadenopathy develops. Painful preauricular lymphadenopathy is unique to tularemia and distinguishes it from tuberculosis, sporotrichosis, and syphilis. Corneal perforation may occur.

Oropharyngeal and Gastrointestinal Tularemia Rarely, tularemia follows ingestion of contaminated undercooked meat, oral inoculation of *F. tularensis* from the hands in association with the skinning and cleaning of animal carcasses, or consumption of contaminated food or water. Oral inoculation may result in acute, exudative, or membranous pharyngitis associated with cervical lymphadenopathy or in ulcerative intestinal lesions associated with mesenteric lymphadenopathy, diarrhea, abdominal pain, nausea, vomiting, and gastrointestinal bleeding. Infected tonsils become enlarged and develop a yellowish-white pseudomembrane, which can be confused with that of diphtheria. The clinical severity of gastrointestinal tularemia varies from mild, unexplained, persistent diarrhea with no other symptoms to a fulminant, fatal disease. In fatal cases, the extensive intestinal ulceration found at autopsy suggests an enormous inoculum.

Pulmonary Tularemia Pneumonia due to *F. tularensis* presents as variable parenchymal infiltrates that are unresponsive to treatment with β-lactam antibiotics. Tularemia must be considered in the differential diagnosis of atypical pneumonia in a patient with a history of travel to an endemic area. The disease can result from inhalation of an infectious aerosol or can spread to the lungs and pleura via bacteremia. Inhalation-related pneumonia has been described in laboratory workers after exposure to contaminated materials and, if untreated, can be associated with a relatively high mortality rate. Exposure to *F. tularensis* in aerosols from live domestic animals or dead wildlife (including birds) has been reported to cause pneumonia. Hematogenous dissemination to the lungs occurs in 10–15% of cases of ulceroglandular tularemia and in about half of cases of typhoidal tularemia. Previously, tularemia pneumonia was thought to be a disease of older patients, but as many as 10–15% of children with clinical manifestations of tularemia have parenchymal infiltrates detected by chest roentgenography. Patients with pneumonia usually have a nonproductive cough and may have dyspnea or pleuritic chest pain. Roentgenograms of the chest usually reveal bilateral patchy infiltrates (described as ovoid or lobar densities), lobar parenchymal infiltrates, and cavitary lesions. Pleural effusions may have a predominance of mononuclear leukocytes or PMNs and sometimes red blood cells. Empyema may develop. Blood cultures may be positive for *F. tularensis*.

Typhoidal Tularemia The typhoidal presentation is now considered rare in the United States. The source of infection in typhoidal tularemia is usually associated with pharyngeal and/or gastrointestinal inoculation or bacteremic disease. Fever usually develops without apparent skin lesions or lymphadenopathy. Some patients have cervical and mesenteric lymphadenopathy. In the absence of a history of possible contact with a vector, diagnosis can be extremely difficult. Blood cultures may be positive and patients may present with classic sepsis or septic shock in this acute systemic form of the infection. Typhoidal tularemia is usually associated with a huge inoculum or with a preexisting compromising condition. High continuous fevers, signs of sepsis, and severe headache are common. The patient may be delirious and may develop prostration and shock. If presumptive antibiotic therapy in culture-negative cases does not include an aminoglycoside, the estimated mortality rate is relatively high.

Other Manifestations *F. tularensis* infection has been associated with meningitis, pericarditis, hepatitis, peritonitis, endocarditis, osteomyelitis, and sepsis and septic shock with rhabdomyolysis and acute renal failure. In cases of tularemia meningitis, a mean white blood cell count of 1788/μL, a predominantly mononuclear cell response (70–100%), a depressed glucose level, an elevated protein concentration, and a negative Gram's stain are typically found on examination of cerebrospinal fluid.

DIFFERENTIAL DIAGNOSIS

When patients in endemic areas present with fever, chronic ulcerative skin lesions, and large tender lymph nodes (Fig. 195-1), a diagnosis of tularemia should be made presumptively, and confirmatory diagnostic testing and appropriate therapy should be undertaken. When the possibility of tularemia is considered in a nonendemic area, an attempt should be made to identify contact with a potential animal vector. The level of suspicion should be especially high in hunters, trappers, game wardens, professional landscapers, veterinarians, laboratory workers, and individuals exposed to an insect or another animal vector. However, up to 40% of patients with tularemia have no known history of epidemiologic contact with an animal vector.

The characteristic presentation of ulceroglandular tularemia does not pose a diagnostic problem, but a less classic progression of regional lymphadenopathy or glandular tularemia must be differentiated from other diseases (Table 195-3). The skin lesion of tularemia may resemble those seen in various other diseases but is generally accompanied by more impressive regional lymphadenopathy. In children, the differentiation of tularemia from cat-scratch disease is made more difficult by the chronic papulovesicular lesion associated with *Bartonella henselae* infection (Chap. 197). Oropharyngeal tularemia can resemble and must be differentiated from pharyngitis due to other bacteria or viruses. Pulmonary tularemia may resemble any atypical pneumonia. Typhoidal tularemia and tularemia meningitis may resemble a variety of other infections.

LABORATORY DIAGNOSIS

The diagnosis of tularemia is most frequently confirmed by agglutination testing. Microagglutination and tube agglutination are the techniques most commonly used to detect antibody to *F. tularensis*. In the standard tube agglutination test, a single titer of ≥1:160 is interpreted as a presumptive positive result. A fourfold increase in titer between paired serum samples collected 2–3 weeks apart is considered diagnostic. False-negative serologic responses are obtained early in infection; up to 30% of patients infected for 3 weeks have sera that test negative. Late in infection, titers into the thousands are common, and titers of 1:20–1:80 may persist for years. Enzyme-linked immunosorbent assays have proved useful for the detection of both antibodies and antigens.

Culture and isolation of *F. tularensis* are difficult. In one study, the organism was isolated in only 10% of more than 1000 human cases, 84% of which were confirmed by serology. The medium of choice is cysteine-glucose-blood agar. *F. tularensis* can be isolated directly from infected ulcer scrapings, lymph node biopsy specimens, gastric washings, sputum, and blood cultures. Colonies are blue-gray, round, smooth, and slightly mucoid. On media containing blood, a small zone of α hemolysis usually surrounds the colony. Slide agglutination tests or direct fluorescent antibody tests with commercially available antisera can be applied directly to culture suspensions for identification. Most clinical laboratories will not attempt to culture *F. tularensis* because of the infectivity of the organism from the culture media and the consequent risk of a laboratory-acquired infection. Although tularemia is not spread from person to person, the organism can be inhaled from culture plates and infect unsuspecting laboratory workers. In most clinical laboratories, biosafety level 2 practices are recommended to handle clinical specimens thought to contain *F. tularensis*; however, biosafety level 3 conditions are required for procedures that produce aerosols or droplets during manipulation of cultures containing or possibly containing this organism.

A variety of polymerase chain reaction (PCR) methods have been used to detect *F. tularensis* DNA in many clinical specimens but mostly in ulceroglandular disease. The majority of these methods target the genes encoding outer membrane proteins (e.g., *fopA* or *tul4*). A 16S rDNA sequence identification PCR may be helpful when the patient's clinical information does not lead the clinician to suspect a diagnosis of tularemia.

TREATMENT TULAREMIA

Only aminoglycosides, tetracyclines, chloramphenicol, and rifampin are currently approved by the U.S. Food and Drug Administration for the treatment of tularemia. Gentamicin is considered the drug of choice for both adults and children. The dosage for adults and children is 5 mg/kg daily in two divided doses. Gentamicin therapy is typically continued for 7–10 days; however, in mild to moderate

TABLE 195-3 TULAREMIA: DIFFERENTIAL DIAGNOSIS, BY CLINICAL DISEASE CATEGORY

Glandular	Oropharyngeal	Typhoidal	Pulmonary
Pyogenic bacterial infection[a]	Group A streptococcal pharyngitis	Typhoid fever	*Mycoplasma pneumoniae* pneumonia
Nontuberculous mycobacterial infection	*Arcanobacterium haemolyticum* pharyngitis	Other *Salmonella* bacteremias	*Chlamydia pneumoniae* pneumonia
Sporotrichosis	Diphtheria	Rocky Mountain spotted fever	Psittacosis
Tuberculosis	Infectious mononucleosis	Human monocytotropic ehrlichiosis	*Legionella pneumophila* pneumonia
Syphilis	Various viral infections[b]	Human granulocytotropic anaplasmosis	Q fever
Anthrax		Infectious mononucleosis	Histoplasmosis
Rat-bite fever		Brucellosis	Blastomycosis
Scrub typhus		Toxoplasmosis	Coccidioidomycosis
Plague		Tuberculosis	Various viral infections[d]
Lymphogranuloma venereum		Sarcoidosis	
Cat-scratch disease		Malignancy[c]	

[a]*Staphylococcus aureus, Streptococcus pyogenes.* [b]Adenovirus, enteroviruses, parainfluenza virus, influenza viruses A and B, respiratory syncytial virus. [c]Hematologic and reticuloendothelial malignancies. [d]Influenza viruses A and B, parainfluenza virus, respiratory syncytial virus, adenovirus, enteroviruses, hantavirus.

cases of tularemia in which the patient becomes afebrile within the first 48–72 h of gentamicin treatment, a 5- to 7-day course has been successful.

If available, streptomycin given intramuscularly is also effective. The dosage for adults is 2 g/d in two divided doses. For children, the dosage is 30 mg/kg daily in two divided doses (maximal daily dose, 2 g). After a clinical response is demonstrated at 3–5 days, the dosage for children can be reduced to 10–15 mg/kg daily in two divided doses. The total duration of streptomycin therapy in both adults and children is usually 10 days. Unlike streptomycin and gentamicin, tobramycin is ineffective in the treatment of tularemia and should not be used.

Because doxycycline is bacteriostatic against *F. tularensis*, there is a risk of relapse if the patient is not treated for a long enough period. Therefore, if doxycycline is used, it should be given for at least 14 days. The lack of availability of chloramphenicol limits the utility of this agent as a viable treatment option. Fluoroquinolones—specifically, ciprofloxacin and levofloxacin—have been used with good outcomes to treat infections caused by subspecies *holarctica*, which is most often found in Europe. The lack of data on the efficacy of these agents against subspecies *tularensis* limits their use in North America at this time.

F. tularensis cannot be subjected to standardized antimicrobial susceptibility testing because the organism will not grow on the media used. A wide variety of antibiotics, including all β-lactam antibiotics and the cephalosporins, are ineffective for the treatment of tularemia. Several studies indicated that third-generation cephalosporins were active against *F. tularensis* in vitro, but clinical case reports suggested nearly universal failure of ceftriaxone in pediatric patients with tularemia. Although in vitro data indicate that imipenem may be active, therapy with imipenem, sulfanilamides, and macrolides is not presently recommended because of the lack of relevant clinical data.

Virtually all strains of *F. tularensis* are susceptible to streptomycin and gentamicin. Hearing screening should be considered before initiation of streptomycin or gentamicin therapy. In successfully treated patients, defervescence usually occurs within 2 days, but skin lesions and lymph nodes may take 1–2 weeks to heal. When therapy is not initiated within the first several days of illness, defervescence may be delayed. Relapses are uncommon with streptomycin or gentamicin therapy. Late lymph-node suppuration, however, occurs in ~40% of children, regardless of the treatment received. These nodes have typically been found to contain sterile necrotic tissue without evidence of active infection. Patients with fluctuant nodes should receive several days of antibiotic therapy before drainage to minimize the risk to hospital personnel.

PROGNOSIS

If tularemia goes untreated, symptoms usually last 1–4 weeks but may continue for months. The mortality rate from severe untreated infection (including all cases of untreated pulmonary and typhoidal tularemia) can be as high as 30%. However, the overall mortality rate for untreated tularemia is <8%. With appropriate treatment, the mortality rate is <1%. Poor outcomes are often associated with long delays in diagnosis and treatment. Lifelong immunity usually follows tularemia.

PREVENTION

The prevention of tularemia is based on avoidance of exposure to biting and blood-sucking insects, especially ticks and deerflies. A wide range of approaches to vaccine development are being evaluated, but no vaccine against tularemia is yet licensed. Prophylaxis of tularemia has not proved effective in patients with embedded ticks or insect bites. However, in patients who are known to have been exposed to large quantities of organisms (e.g., in the laboratory) and who have incubating infection with *F. tularensis*, early treatment can prevent the development of significant clinical disease.

196 Plague and Other *Yersinia* Infections

Michael B. Prentice

PLAGUE

Plague is a systemic zoonosis caused by *Yersinia pestis*. It predominantly affects small rodents in rural areas of Africa, Asia, and the Americas and is usually transmitted to humans by an arthropod vector (the flea). Less often, infection follows contact with animal tissues or respiratory droplets. Plague is an acute febrile illness that is treatable with antimicrobial agents, but mortality rates among untreated patients are high. Ancient DNA studies have confirmed that the fourteenth-century "Black Death" in Europe was *Y. pestis* infection. Patients can present with the bubonic, septicemic, or pneumonic form of the disease. Although there is concern among the general public about epidemic spread of plague by the respiratory route, this is not the usual route of plague transmission, and established infection-control measures for respiratory plague exist. However, the fatalities associated with plague and the capacity for infection via the respiratory tract mean that *Y. pestis* fits the profile of a potential agent of bioterrorism. Consequently, measures have been taken to restrict access to the organism, including legislation affecting diagnostic and research procedures in some countries (e.g., the United States).

ETIOLOGY

The genus *Yersinia* comprises gram-negative bacteria of the family Enterobacteriaceae (gamma proteobacteria). Overwhelming taxonomic evidence showing *Y. pestis* strains as a clonal group within *Yersinia pseudotuberculosis* suggests recent evolution from the latter organism—an enteric pathogen of mammals that is spread by the fecal-oral route and thus has a phenotype distinctly different from that of *Y. pestis*. When grown in vivo or at 37°C, *Y. pestis* forms an amorphous capsule made from a plasmid-specified fimbrial protein, Caf or fraction 1 (F1) antigen, which is an immunodiagnostic marker of infection.

EPIDEMIOLOGY

Human plague generally follows an outbreak in a host rodent population (epizootic). Mass deaths among the rodent primary hosts lead to a search by fleas for new hosts, with consequent incidental infection of other mammals. The precipitating cause for an epizootic may ultimately be related to climate or other environmental factors. The reservoir for *Y. pestis* causing enzootic plague in natural endemic foci between epizootics (i.e., when the organism may be difficult to detect in rodents or fleas) is a topic of ongoing research and may not be the same in all regions. The enzootic/epizootic pattern may be the result of complex dynamic interactions of host rodents that have different plague susceptibilities and different flea vectors; alternatively, an environmental reservoir may be important.

In general, the enzootic areas for plague are lightly populated regions of Africa, Asia, and the Americas (Fig. 196-1). Between 2004 and 2009, 12,503 cases of plague, with a global case-fatality rate of 6.7%, were recorded by the World Health Organization (WHO); these figures were obtained by combining cases notified under the International Health Regulations with data from national surveillance programs and publications. More than 97% of these cases were in Africa; the majority of cases were reported from the Democratic Republic of the Congo and the island of Madagascar. The period covered spans a change in the International Health Regulations from a requirement for nations to notify the WHO of all cases of plague to a requirement to report pneumonic plague or any suspected case of plague in an area not known to be endemic for plague. In the past decade, outbreaks of pneumonic plague have been recorded in the Democratic Republic of the Congo, Uganda, Algeria, Madagascar, China, and Peru.

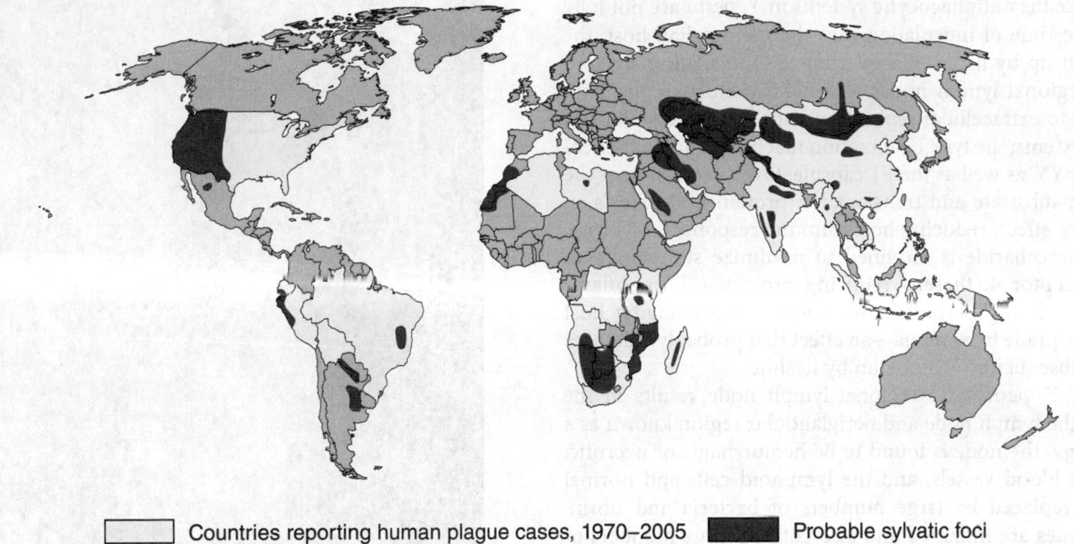

FIGURE 196-1 Approximate global distribution of *Yersinia pestis*. *(Compiled from WHO, CDC, and country sources. Reprinted with permission from DT Dennis, GL Campbell: Plague and other Yersinia infections, in Harrison's Principles of Internal Medicine, 17th ed, AS Fauci et al [eds]. New York, McGraw-Hill, Chap. 152, 2008.)*

Plague was introduced into North America via the port of San Francisco in 1900 as part of the Third Pandemic, which spread around the world from Hong Kong. The disease is presently enzootic on the western side of the continent from southwestern Canada to Mexico. Most human cases in the United States occur in two regions: "Four Corners" (the junction point of New Mexico, Arizona, Colorado, and Utah), especially northern New Mexico, northern Arizona, and southern Colorado; and further west in California, southern Oregon, and western Nevada (*http://www.cdc.gov/plague/maps/index.html*). From 1990 to 2011, 151 cases of plague were reported in the United States, a mean of seven cases per year. Most cases occurred from May to October—the time of year when people are outdoors and rodents and their fleas are most plentiful. The infection is most often acquired by fleabite in peridomestic environments; it can also be acquired through the handling of living or dead small mammals (e.g., rabbits, hares, and prairie dogs) or wild carnivores (e.g., wildcats, coyotes, or mountain lions). Dogs and cats may bring plague-infected fleas into the home, and infected cats may transmit plague directly to humans by the respiratory route. The last recorded case of person-to-person transmission in the United States occurred in 1925.

Plague most often develops in areas with poor sanitary conditions and infestations of rats—in particular, the widely distributed roof rat *Rattus rattus* and the brown rat *Rattus norvegicus* (which serves as a laboratory model of plague). Rat control in warehouses and shipping facilities has been recognized as important in preventing the spread of plague since the early twentieth century and features in the current WHO International Health Regulations. Urban rodents acquire infection from wild rodents, and the proximity of the former to humans increases the risk of transmission. The oriental rat flea *Xenopsylla cheopis* is the most efficient vector for transmission of plague among rats and onward to humans in Asia, Africa, and South America.

Worldwide, bubonic plague is the predominant form reported (80–95% of suspected cases), with mortality rates of 10–20%. The mortality rate is higher (22%) in the small proportion of patients (10–20%) with primary septicemic plague (i.e., systemic *Y. pestis* sepsis with no bubo; see "Clinical Manifestations," below) and is highest with primary pulmonary plague; in this, the least common of the main plague presentations, the mortality rate approaches 100% without antimicrobial treatment and is >50% even with such treatment. Rare outbreaks of pharyngeal plague following consumption of raw or undercooked camel or goat meat have been reported.

A total of 81 (76%) of the 107 plague cases reported in the United States from 1990 to 2005 were primary bubonic disease, 19 (18%) were primary septicemic disease, and 5 (5%) were primary pneumonic disease; 2 cases (2%) were not classified. Eleven cases (10%) were fatal.

PATHOGENESIS

As mentioned earlier, genetic evidence suggests that *Y. pestis* is a clone derived from the enteric pathogen *Y. pseudotuberculosis* in the recent evolutionary past (9000–40,000 years ago). The change from infection by the fecal-oral route to a two-stage life cycle, with alternate parasitization of arthropod and mammalian hosts, followed the acquisition of two plasmids (pFra and pPst) and the inactivation of remarkably few *Y. pseudotuberculosis* genes in conjunction with preexisting properties of the *Y. pseudotuberculosis* ancestor (e.g., the presence of a third plasmid, pYV, and the capacity to cause septicemia). In the arthropod-parasitizing portion of its life cycle, *Y. pestis* multiplies and forms biofilm-embedded aggregates in the flea midgut after ingestion of a blood meal containing bacteria. In some fleas, biofilm-embedded bacteria eventually fill the proventriculus (a valve connecting the esophagus to the midgut) and block normal blood feeding. Both "blocked" fleas and those containing masses of biofilm-embedded *Y. pestis* without complete blockage inoculate *Y. pestis* into each bite site. The ability of *Y. pestis* to colonize and multiply in the flea requires phospholipase D encoded by the *ymt* gene on the pFra plasmid, and biofilm synthesis requires the chromosomal *hms* locus shared with *Y. pseudotuberculosis*. However, three *Y. pseudotuberculosis* genes inhibiting biofilm formation or promoting its degradation are inactivated in *Y. pestis*, together with urease, which causes acute flea gastrointestinal toxicity. Blockage takes days or weeks to come about after initial infection of the flea and is followed by the flea's death. In addition, many flea vectors (including *X. cheopis*) are able to transmit plague in an early-phase unblocked state for up to 1 week after feeding, but 10 fleas in this state are required to infect a mammalian host (mass transmission).

Y. pestis disseminates from the site of inoculation in the mammalian host in a process initially dependent on plasminogen activator Pla, which is encoded by the small pPst plasmid. This surface protease activates mammalian plasminogen, degrades complement, and adheres to the extracellular matrix component laminin. Pla is essential for the high-level virulence of *Y. pestis* in mice by subcutaneous or intradermal injection (laboratory proxies for fleabites) and for the development of primary pneumonic plague. When actual fleabite inoculation is used in mouse models, the fimbrial capsule-forming protein (Ca1 or fraction 1; F1 antigen) encoded on pFra increases the efficiency of transmission, and plasminogen activator is required for the formation of buboes. Because the antiphagocytic systems in *Y. pestis* are not fully operational at the time of inoculation into the mammalian host, the organism is taken up by macrophages from the inoculation site and transported to regional lymph nodes. After intracellular replication, *Y. pestis* switches to extracellular replication with full expression of its antiphagocytic systems: the type III secretion machines and their effectors encoded by pYV as well as the F1 capsule. Overproduction of the type III secretion substrate and translocation protein LcrV exerts an anti-inflammatory effect, reducing host immune responses. Likewise, *Y. pestis* lipopolysaccharide is modified to minimize stimulation of host Toll-like receptor 4, thereby reducing protective host inflammatory responses during peripheral infection and prolonging host survival with high-grade bacteremia—an effect that probably enhances the pathogen's subsequent transmission by fleabite.

Replication of *Y. pestis* in a regional lymph node results in the local swelling of the lymph node and periglandular region known as a *bubo*. On histology, the node is found to be hemorrhagic or necrotic, with thrombosed blood vessels, and the lymphoid cells and normal architecture are replaced by large numbers of bacteria and fibrin. Periglandular tissues are inflamed and also contain large numbers of bacteria in a serosanguineous, gelatinous exudate.

Continued spread through the lymphatic vessels to contiguous lymph nodes produces second-order primary buboes. Infection is initially contained in the infected regional lymph nodes, although transient bacteremia can be detected. As the infection progresses, spread via efferent lymphatics to the thoracic duct produces high-grade bacteremia. Hematogenous spread to the spleen, liver, and secondary buboes follows, with subsequent uncontrolled septicemia, endotoxic shock, and disseminated intravascular coagulation leading to death. In some patients, this septicemic phase occurs without obvious prior bubo development or lung disease (*septicemic plague*). Hematogenous spread to the lungs results in *secondary plague pneumonia*, with bacteria initially more prominent in the interstitium than in the air spaces (the reverse being the case in *primary plague pneumonia*). Hematogenous spread to other organs, including the meninges, can occur.

CLINICAL MANIFESTATIONS

Bubonic Plague After an incubation period of 2–6 days, the onset of bubonic plague is sudden and is characterized by fever (>38°C), malaise, myalgia, dizziness, and increasing pain due to progressive lymphadenitis in the regional lymph nodes near the fleabite or other inoculation site. Lymphadenitis manifests as a tense, tender swelling (bubo) that, when palpated, has a boggy consistency with an underlying hard core. Generally, there is one painful and erythematous bubo with surrounding periganglionic edema. The bubo is most commonly inguinal but can also be crural, axillary (Fig. 196-2), cervical, or submaxillary, depending on the site of the bite. Abdominal pain from intraabdominal node involvement can occur without other visible signs. Children are most likely to present with cervical or axillary buboes.

The differential diagnosis includes acute focal lymphadenopathy of other etiologies, such as streptococcal or staphylococcal infection, tularemia, cat-scratch disease, tick typhus, infectious mononucleosis, or lymphatic filariasis. These infections do not progress as rapidly, are not as painful, and are associated with visible cellulitis or ascending lymphangitis—both of which are absent in plague.

Without treatment, *Y. pestis* dissemination occurs and causes serious illness, including pneumonia (*secondary pneumonic plague*) and meningitis. Secondary pneumonic plague can be the source of person-to-person transmission of respiratory infection by productive cough (droplet infection), with the consequent development of primary plague pneumonia. Appropriate treatment of bubonic plague results in fever resolution within 2–5 days, but buboes may remain enlarged for >1 week after initial treatment and can become fluctuant.

Primary Septicemic Plague A minority (10–25%) of infections with *Y. pestis* present as gram-negative septicemia (hypotension, shock) without preceding lymphadenopathy. Septicemic plague occurs in all age groups, but persons older than age 40 years are at elevated risk. Some chronic conditions may predispose to septicemic plague: in

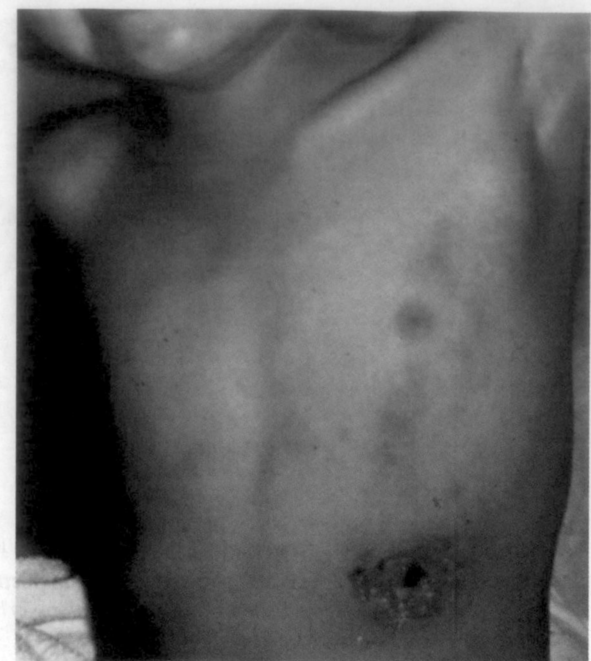

FIGURE 196-2 Plague patient in the southwestern United States with a left axillary bubo and an unusual plague ulcer and eschar at the site of the infective flea bite. *(Reprinted with permission from DT Dennis, GL Campbell: Plague and other Yersinia infections, in Harrison's Principles of Internal Medicine, 17th ed, AS Fauci et al [eds]. New York, McGraw-Hill, Chap. 152, 2008.)*

2009 in the United States, a fatal laboratory-acquired infection with an attenuated *Y. pestis* strain manifested as septicemic plague in a 60-year-old researcher with diabetes mellitus and undiagnosed hemochromatosis. These conditions also carry an increased risk of septicemia with other pathogenic *Yersinia* species. The term *septicemic plague* can be confusing since most patients with buboes have detectable bacteremia at some stage, with or without systemic signs of sepsis. In laboratory experiments, however, septicemic disease without histologic changes in lymph nodes is seen in a minority of mice infected via fleabites.

Pneumonic Plague Primary pneumonic plague results from inhalation of infectious bacteria in droplets expelled from another person or an animal with primary or secondary plague pneumonia. This syndrome has a short incubation period, averaging from a few hours to 2–3 days (range, 1–7 days), and is characterized by a sudden onset of fever, headache, myalgia, weakness, nausea, vomiting, and dizziness. Respiratory signs—cough, dyspnea, chest pain, and sputum production with hemoptysis—typically arise after 24 h. Progression of initial segmental pneumonitis to lobar pneumonia and then to bilateral lung involvement may occur (Fig. 196-3). The possible release of aerosolized *Y. pestis* bacteria in a bioterrorist attack, manifesting as an outbreak of primary pneumonic plague in nonendemic regions or in an urban setting where plague is rarely seen, has been a source of public health concern. Secondary pneumonic plague is a consequence of bacteremia occurring in ~10–15% of patients with bubonic plague. Bilateral alveolar infiltrates are seen on chest x-ray, and diffuse interstitial pneumonitis with scanty sputum production is typical.

Meningitis *Meningeal plague* is uncommon, occurring in ≤6% of plague cases reported in the United States. Presentation with headache and fever typically occurs >1 week after the onset of bubonic or septicemic plague and may be associated with suboptimal antimicrobial therapy (delayed therapy, penicillin administration, or low-dose tetracycline treatment) and cervical or axillary buboes.

Pharyngitis Symptomatic *plague pharyngitis* can follow the consumption of contaminated meat from an animal dying of plague or contact with persons or animals with pneumonic plague. This condition can resemble tonsillitis, with peritonsillar abscess and cervical

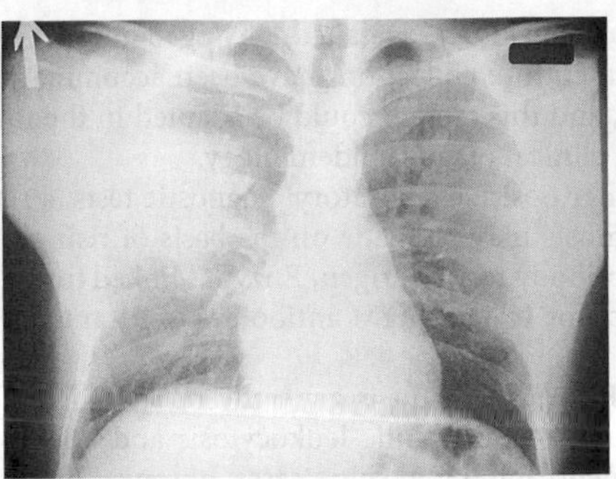

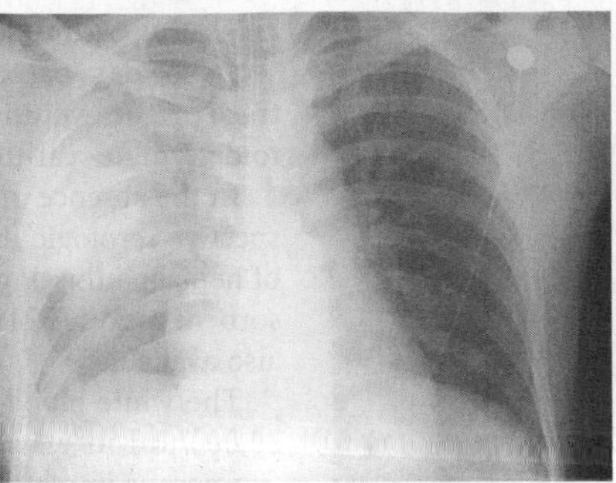

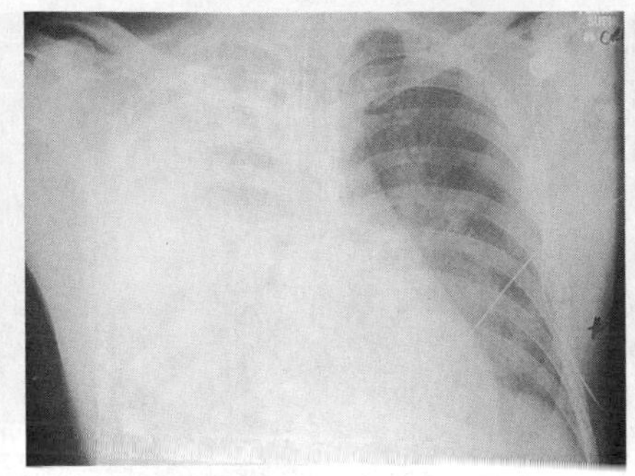

FIGURE 196-3 Sequential chest radiographs of a patient with fatal primary plague pneumonia. ***Left:*** Upright posteroanterior film taken at admission to the hospital emergency department on the third day of illness, showing segmental consolidation of the right upper lobe. ***Center:*** Portable anteroposterior film taken 8 h after admission, showing extension of pneumonia to the right middle and right lower lobes. ***Right:*** Portable anteroposterior film taken 13 h after admission (when the patient had clinical adult respiratory distress syndrome), showing diffuse infiltration throughout the right lung and patchy infiltration of the left lower lung. A cavity later developed at the site of the initial right-upper-lobe consolidation. *(Reprinted with permission from DT Dennis, GL Campbell: Plague and other Yersinia infections, in Harrison's Principles of Internal Medicine, 17th ed., AS Fauci et al [eds]. New York, McGraw-Hill, Chap. 152, 2008.)*

lymphadenopathy. Asymptomatic pharyngeal carriage of *Y. pestis* can also occur in close contacts of patients with pneumonic plague.

LABORATORY DIAGNOSIS

Because of the scarcity of laboratory facilities in regions where human *Y. pestis* infection is most common, and because of the potential significance of *Y. pestis* isolation in a nonendemic area or an area from which human plague has been absent for many years, the WHO recommends an initial presumptive diagnosis followed by reference laboratory confirmation (Table 196-1). In the United States, comprehensive national diagnostic facilities for plague have been in place since a federal Laboratory Response Network (LRN; *www.bt.cdc.gov/lrn/*) was set up in 1999 to detect possible use of biological terrorism agents, including *Y. pestis*. Routine diagnostic clinical microbiology laboratories that are included in this network as sentinel-level laboratories use joint protocols from the Centers for Disease Control and Prevention (CDC) and the American Society for Microbiology to identify suspected *Y. pestis* isolates and to refer these specimens to LRN reference laboratories for confirmatory tests (*http://www.asm.org/index.php/issues/sentinel-laboratory-guidelines*). *Y. pestis* is designated a "Tier 1 select agent" under the Public Health Security and Bioterrorism Preparedness and Response Act of 2002 and subsequent executive orders; the provisions of this act, the Patriot Act of 2001, and related executive orders apply to all U.S. laboratories and individuals working with *Y. pestis*. Details of the applicable regulations are available from the CDC.

Yersinia species are gram-negative coccobacilli (short rods with rounded ends) 1–3 μm in length and 0.5–0.8 μm in diameter. *Y. pestis* in particular appears bipolar (with a "closed safety pin" appearance) and pleomorphic when stained with a polychromatic stain (Wayson or Wright-Giemsa; Fig. 196-4). Its lack of motility distinguishes *Y. pestis* from other *Yersinia* species, which are motile at 25°C and nonmotile at 37°C. Transport medium (e.g., Cary-Blair medium) preserves the viability of *Y. pestis* if transport is delayed.

TABLE 196-1 WORLD HEALTH ORGANIZATION CASE DEFINITIONS OF PLAGUE

Suspected case	Compatible clinical presentation ***and*** Consistent epidemiologic features, such as exposure to infected animals or humans and/or evidence of fleabites and/or residence in or travel to a known endemic focus within the previous 10 days
Presumptive case	Meeting the definition of a suspected case ***plus*** **Putative new or reemerging focus:** ≥2 of the following tests positive • Microscopy: gram-negative coccobacilli in material from bubo, blood, or sputum; bipolar appearance on Wayson or Wright-Giemsa staining • F1 antigen detected in bubo aspirate, blood, or sputum • A single anti-F1 serology without evidence of previous *Y. pestis* infection or immunization • Polymerase chain reaction (PCR) detection of *Y. pestis* in bubo aspirate, blood, or sputum **Known endemic focus:** ≥1 of the following tests positive • Microscopic evidence of gram-negative or bipolar (Wayson, Wright-Giemsa) coccobacilli from bubo, blood, or sputum sample • A single anti-F1 serology without evidence of previous plague infection or immunization • F1 antigen detected in bubo aspirate, blood, or sputum
Confirmed case	Meeting the definition of a suspected case ***plus*** • Identification of an isolate from a clinical sample as *Y. pestis* (colonial morphology and 2 of the 4 following tests positive: phage lysis of cultures at 20–25°C and 37°C; F1 antigen detection; PCR; *Y. pestis* biochemical profile) ***or*** • A fourfold rise in anti-F1 antibody titer in paired serum samples ***or*** • In endemic areas when no other confirmatory test can be performed, a positive rapid diagnostic test with immunochromatography to detect F1 antigen

Source: Interregional Meeting on Prevention and Control of Plague, Antananarivo, Madagascar, 7–11 April 2006 *(www.who.int/entity/csr/resources/publications/WHO_HSE_EPR_2008_3w.pdf)*.

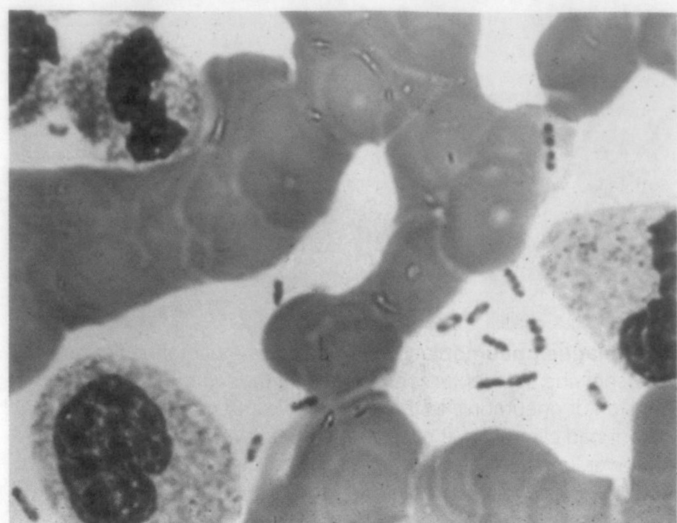

FIGURE 196-4 Peripheral blood smear from a patient with fatal plague septicemia and shock, showing characteristic bipolar-staining *Yersinia pestis* bacilli (Wright's stain, oil immersion). *(Reprinted with permission from DT Dennis, GL Campbell: Plague and other Yersinia infections, in Harrison's Principles of Internal Medicine, 17th ed, AS Fauci et al [eds]. New York, McGraw-Hill, Chap. 152, 2008.)*

The appropriate specimens for diagnosis of bubonic, pneumonic, and septicemic plague are bubo aspirate, bronchoalveolar lavage fluid or sputum, and blood, respectively. Culture of postmortem organ biopsy samples can also be diagnostic. A bubo aspirate is obtained by injection of 1 mL of sterile normal saline into a bubo under local anesthetic and aspiration of a small amount of (usually blood-stained) fluid. Gram's staining of these specimens may reveal gram-negative rods, which are shown by Wayson or Wright-Giemsa staining to be bipolar. These bacteria may even be visible in direct blood smears in septicemic plague (Fig. 196-4); this finding indicates very high numbers of circulating bacteria and a poor prognosis.

Y. pestis grows on nutrient agar and other standard laboratory media but forms smaller colonies than do other Enterobacteriaceae. Specimens should be inoculated onto nutrient-rich media such as sheep blood agar (SBA), into nutrient-rich broth such as brain-heart infusion broth, and onto selective agar such as MacConkey or eosin methylene blue (EMB) agar. *Yersinia*-specific CIN (cefsulodin, triclosan [Irgasan], novobiocin) agar can be useful for culture of contaminated specimens, such as sputum. Blood should be cultured in a standard blood culture system. The optimal growth temperature is <37°C (25–29°C), with pinpoint colonies only on SBA at 24 h. Slower growth occurs at 37°C. *Y. pestis* is oxidase-negative, catalase-positive, urea-negative, indole-negative, and lactose-negative. Automated biochemical identification systems can misidentify *Y. pestis* as *Y. pseudotuberculosis* or other bacterial species.

Reference laboratory tests for definitive identification of isolates include direct immunofluorescence for F1 antigen; specific polymerase chain reaction (PCR) for targets such as F1 antigen, the pesticin gene, and the plasminogen activator gene; and specific bacteriophage lysis. PCR can also be applied to diagnostic specimens, as can direct immunofluorescence for F1 antigen (produced in large amounts by *Y. pestis*) by slide microscopy. An immunochromatographic test strip for F1 antigen detection by monoclonal antibodies in clinical specimens has been devised in Madagascar. This method is effective for both laboratory and near-patient use and is now widely used in endemic countries. A similar test strip for Pla antigen has recently been developed and could be used to detect wild-type or engineered F1-negative virulent strains. Many other rapid diagnostic kits for possible bioterrorism pathogens, including *Y. pestis*, have been described in recent years, but none is widely used for primary or reference laboratory identification, and only one (a field real-time PCR for a range of potential bioterrorism agents) is approved by the U.S. Food and Drug Administration (FDA). Detailed phylogeographic DNA sequence data based on culture collections have been accumulated to trace plague evolution, and this system could be adapted in the future to determine real-time clinical plague epidemiology.

In the absence of other positive laboratory diagnostic tests, a retrospective serologic diagnosis may be made on the basis of rising titers of hemagglutinating antibody to F1 antigen. Enzyme-linked immunosorbent assays (ELISAs) for IgG and IgM antibodies to F1 antigen are also available.

The white blood cell (WBC) count is generally raised (to 10,000–20,000/μL) in plague, with neutrophilic leukocytosis and a left shift (numerous immature neutrophils); in some cases, however, the WBC count is normal or leukopenia develops. WBC counts are occasionally very high, especially in children (>100,000/μL). Levels of fibrinogen degradation products are elevated in a majority of patients, but platelet counts are usually normal or low-normal. However, disseminated intravascular coagulation, with low platelet counts, prolonged prothrombin times, reduced fibrinogen, and elevated fibrinogen degradation product levels, occurs in a significant minority of patients.

TREATMENT PLAGUE

Guidelines for the treatment of plague are given in Table 196-2. A 10-day course of antimicrobial therapy is recommended. Streptomycin has historically been the parenteral treatment of choice for plague and is approved for this indication by the FDA. Although not yet approved by the FDA for plague, gentamicin has proven safe and effective in clinical trials in Tanzania and Madagascar

TABLE 196-2 GUIDELINES FOR THE TREATMENT OF PLAGUE

Drug	Daily Dose	Interval, h	Route
Gentamicin			
Adult	5 mg/kg[a]	24	IM/IV
	3–5 mg/kg	8 (2 mg/kg loading dose followed by 1.7 mg/kg tid, reduced)	IM/IV
Child	5 mg/kg[a]	24	IM/IV
	7.5 mg/kg	8 (2.5 mg/kg tid)	IM/IV
Streptomycin			
Adult	2 g	12	IM
Child	30 mg/kg	12	IM
Levofloxacin			
Adult and child >50 kg	500 mg	24	PO/IV
Child <50 kg and ≥6 months	8 mg/kg (not to exceed 250 mg/dose)	12	PO/IV
Doxycycline			
Adult	200 mg	12 or 24	PO/IV
Child >8 y	4.4. mg/kg	12 or 24	PO/IV
Tetracycline			
Adult	2 g	6	PO/IV
Child >8 y	25–50 mg/kg	6	PO/IV
Chloramphenicol			
Adult	50 mg/kg	6	PO/IV
Child >1 y	50 mg/kg	6	PO/IV

[a]Aminoglycoside dose should be adjusted in light of renal function. There are no published trial data for once-daily gentamicin as plague therapy in adults or children, but this regimen is efficacious in gram-negative sepsis of other causes and was successful in a recent outbreak of pneumonic plague in the Democratic Republic of the Congo. Neonates up to 1 week of age and premature infants should receive gentamicin (2.5 mg/kg IV bid).

Source: Dennis DT, Campbell GL: Plague and other *Yersinia* infections, in AS Fauci et al (eds): *Harrison's Principles of Internal Medicine*, 17th ed. 2008, p. 980; Inglesby TV et al: Plague as a biological weapon: medical and public health management. Working Group on Civilian Biodefense. JAMA 283:2281, 2000; and FDA Product Label Reference ID 3123374 *(www.accessdata.fda.gov/drugsatfda_docs/label/2012/020634s061,020635s067,021721s028lbl.pdf).*

and in retrospectively reviewed cases in the United States. In view of streptomycin's adverse-reaction profile and limited availability, some experts now recommend gentamicin over streptomycin. In 2012, the FDA approved levofloxacin for prophylaxis and treatment of plague (including septicemic and pneumonic disease), making it the first antibiotic approved for a new indication under a regulatory approach based on animal studies alone, known as the Animal Rule. An FDA decision on ciprofloxacin is pending. Levofloxacin is more efficacious than ciprofloxacin for postexposure prophylaxis of inhalational anthrax in animal models and also received FDA approval for this indication (Chap. 261e); thus it is approved for multiagent prophylaxis in possible bioterrorism exposures.

While systemic chloramphenicol therapy is available in the resource-poor countries primarily affected by plague, it is less likely to be available or used in high-income countries because of its adverse effect profile. Tetracyclines are also effective and can be given by mouth but are not recommended for children under the age of 7 years because of tooth discoloration. Doxycycline is the tetracycline of choice; at an oral dosage of 100 mg twice daily, this drug was as effective as IM gentamicin (2.5 mg/kg twice daily) in a trial in Tanzania.

Although *Y. pestis* is sensitive to β-lactam drugs in vitro and these drugs have been efficacious against plague in some animal models, the response to penicillins has been poor in some clinical cases; thus β-lactams and macrolides are not generally recommended as first-line therapy. Chloramphenicol, alone or in combination, is recommended for some focal complications of plague (e.g., meningitis, endophthalmitis, myocarditis) because of its tissue penetration properties. Fluoroquinolones, effective in vitro and in animal models, are recommended in guidelines for possible bioterrorism-associated pneumonic plague and are increasingly used in therapy, although the only human efficacy data available so far are from a case report. Animal and in vitro studies suggest that fluoroquinolones other than levofloxacin, at doses used in systemic gram-negative sepsis, should be effective as therapy for plague: e.g., ciprofloxacin (400 mg twice daily IV, 500 mg twice daily by mouth), ofloxacin (400 mg twice daily IV or by mouth), or moxifloxacin (400 mg/d IV or by mouth).

PREVENTION

In endemic areas, the control of plague in humans is based on reduction of the likelihood of being bitten by infected fleas or exposed to infected droplets from either humans or animals with plague pneumonia. In the United States, residence and outdoor activity in rural areas of western states where epizootics occur are the main risk factors for infection. To assess potential risks to humans in specific areas, surveillance for *Y. pestis* infection among animal plague hosts and vectors is carried out regularly as well as in response to observed animal die-offs. Personal protective measures include avoidance of areas where a plague epizootic has been identified and publicized (e.g., by warning signs or closure of campsites). Sick or dead animals should not be handled by the general public. Hunters and zoologists should wear gloves when handling wild-animal carcasses in endemic areas. General measures to avoid rodent fleabite during outdoor activity are appropriate and include the use of insect repellant, insecticide, and protective clothing. General measures to reduce peridomestic and occupational human contact with rodents are advised and include rodent-proofing of buildings and food-waste stores and removal of potential rodent habitats (e.g., woodpiles and junk heaps). Flea control by insecticide treatment of wild rodents is an effective means of minimizing human contact with plague if an epizootic is identified in an area close to human habitation. Any attempt to reduce rodent numbers must be preceded by flea suppression to reduce the migration of infected fleas to human hosts. An oral F1-V subunit vaccine using raccoon poxvirus (RCN) as a vector protects prairie dogs against *Y. pestis* injections and is being investigated for efficacy in preventing disease in wild animals, thus potentially reducing human exposure.

Patients in whom pneumonic plague is suspected should be managed in isolation, with droplet precautions observed until pneumonia is excluded or effective antimicrobial therapy has been given for 48 h. Review of the literature published before the advent of antimicrobial agents suggests that the main infective risk is posed by patients in the final stages of disease who are coughing up sputum with plentiful visible blood and/or pus. Cotton and gauze masks were protective in these circumstances. Current surgical masks capable of barrier protection against droplets, including large respiratory particles, are considered protective; a particulate respirator (e.g., N95 or greater) is not required.

Antimicrobial Prophylaxis Postexposure antimicrobial prophylaxis lasting 7 days is recommended following household, hospital, or other close contact with persons with untreated pneumonic plague. (*Close contact* is defined as contact with a patient at <2 m.) In animal aerosol-infection studies, levofloxacin and ciprofloxacin are associated with higher survival rates than doxycycline (Table 196-3).

Immunization Studies with candidate plague vaccines in animal models show that neutralizing antibody provides protection against exposure but that cell-mediated immunity is critical for protection and clearance of *Y. pestis* from the host. A killed whole-cell vaccine used in humans required multiple doses, caused significant local and systemic reactions, and was not protective against pneumonic plague; this vaccine is not currently available in the United States. A live attenuated vaccine based on strain EV76 is still used in countries of the former Soviet Union but has significant side effects. The vaccines closest to licensure are subunit vaccines comprising recombinant F1 (rF1) and various recombinant V (rV) proteins produced in *Escherichia coli*, which are combined either as a fusion protein or as a mixture, purified, and adsorbed to aluminum hydroxide for injection. This combination protects mice and various nonhuman primates in laboratory models of bubonic and pneumonic plague and has been evaluated in phase 2 clinical trials. Special ethical considerations with controlled clinical studies involving plague in humans make prelicensure field efficacy studies unlikely. In the United States, the FDA is therefore prepared to assess plague vaccines for human use under the Animal Rule, using efficacy data and other results from animal studies as well as antibodies and other correlates of immunity from human vaccine recipients (*www.fda.gov/BiologicsBloodVaccines/ScienceResearch/BiologicsResearchAreas/ucm127288.htm*). Live attenuated

TABLE 196-3 GUIDELINES FOR PLAGUE PROPHYLAXIS

Drug	Daily Dose	Interval, h	Route
Doxycycline			
Adult	200 mg	12 or 24	PO
Child ≥8 y	If ≥45 kg, give adult dosage; If <45 kg, give 2.2 mg/kg PO bid (maximum, 200 mg)	12	PO
Tetracycline			
Adult	1–2 g	6 or 12	PO
Child ≥8 y	25–50 mg/kg	6 or 12	PO
Levofloxacin			
Adult and child >50 kg	500 mg	24	PO
Child <50 kg and ≥6 months	8 mg/kg (not to exceed 250 mg/dose)	12	PO
Ciprofloxacin			
Adult	1 g	12	PO
Child	40 mg/kg	12	PO
Trimethoprim-Sulfamethoxazole			
Adult	320 mg	12	PO
Child	40 mg/kg	12	PO

Source: Dennis DT, Campbell GL: Plague and other *Yersinia* infections, in AS Fauci et al (eds): *Harrison's Principles of Internal Medicine*. 2008, p. 980; Inglesby TV et al: Plague as a biological weapon: medical and public health management. Working Group on Civilian Biodefense. JAMA 283:2281, 2000; and FDA Drug Product Label Reference ID 3123374 (*www.accessdata.fda.gov/drugsatfda_docs/label/2012/020634s061,020635s067,021721s028lbl.pdf*).

Y. pseudotuberculosis and *Salmonella* strains expressing *Y. pestis*–specific antigens have been shown to be protective in laboratory animal models of bubonic and pneumonic plague and could be delivered by the oral route. A wide variety of other delivery mechanisms for *Y. pestis* antigens are being explored. Antigens other than F1 and V that could be added to subunit vaccines are being investigated. Advances providing impetus for exploration of these antigens are (1) the recovery of F1-negative *Y. pestis* strains from natural sources and (2) the observation that F1 antigen is not required for virulence in primate models of pneumonic plague.

YERSINIOSIS

Yersiniosis is a zoonotic infection with an enteropathogenic *Yersinia* species, usually *Yersinia enterocolitica* or *Y. pseudotuberculosis*. The usual hosts for these organisms are pigs and other wild and domestic animals; humans are usually infected by the oral route, and outbreaks from contaminated food occur. Yersiniosis is most common in childhood and in colder climates. Patients present with abdominal pain and sometimes with diarrhea (which may not occur in up to 50% of cases). *Y. enterocolitica* is more closely associated with terminal ileitis and *Y. pseudotuberculosis* with mesenteric adenitis, but both organisms may cause mesenteric adenitis and symptoms of abdominal pain and tenderness that result in pseudoappendicitis, with the surgical removal of a normal appendix. Diagnosis is based on culture of the organism or convalescent serology. *Y. pseudotuberculosis* and some rarer strains of *Y. enterocolitica* are especially likely to cause systemic infection, which is also particularly common among patients with diabetes or iron overload. Systemic sepsis is treatable with antimicrobial agents, but postinfective arthropathy responds poorly to such therapy. Fourteen other *Yersinia* species are now recognized, but all lack the virulence plasmid pYV common to *Y. pestis, Y. pseudotuberculosis*, and *Y. enterocolitica* and are generally considered to be, at most, opportunistic pathogens of humans (*Y. aldovae, Y. aleksiciae, Y. bercovieri, Y. entomophaga, Y. frederiksenii, Y. intermedia, Y. kristensenii, Y. massiliensis, Y. mollaretii, Y. nurmii, Y. pekkanenii, Y. rohdei, Y. similis*, and *Y. ruckeri*). Molecular phylogeny shows that *Y. enterocolitica* is more distantly related to *Y. pseudotuberculosis* than these other *Yersinia* species, and the similar virulence plasmid they share has probably been acquired independently by at least one of the two since the species diverged.

EPIDEMIOLOGY

Y. enterocolitica *Y. enterocolitica* is found worldwide and has been isolated from a wide variety of wild and domestic animals and environmental samples, including samples of food and water. In vitro, *Y. enterocolitica* is resistant to predation by the protozoon *Acanthamoeba castellanii* and can survive inside it, suggesting a possible mode of environmental persistence. Strains are differentiated by combined biochemical reactions (biovar) and serogroup. Most clinical infections are associated with serogroups O:3, O:9, and O:5,27, with a declining number of O:8 infections in North America. Some O:8 infections, previously confined to North America, have been reported from Europe and Japan in recent years, and serogroup O:8 now causes a high percentage of yersiniosis cases in Poland. Yersiniosis, mostly due to *Y. enterocolitica*, is the third commonest zoonosis reported in Europe; most reports come from northern Europe, especially Germany and Scandinavia. The incidence is highest among children; children under the age of 4 years are more likely to present with diarrhea than are older children. Abdominal pain with mesenteric adenitis and terminal ileitis is more prominent among older children and adults. Septicemia is more likely in patients with preexisting conditions such as diabetes mellitus, liver disease, any condition involving iron overload (including thalassemia and hemochromatosis), advanced age, malignancy, or HIV/AIDS. As in enteritis of other bacterial etiologies, postinfective complications such as reactive arthritis occur mainly in individuals who are HLA-B27 positive. Erythema nodosum (see Fig. 25e-40) following *Yersinia* infection is not associated with HLA-B27 and is more common among women than among men.

Consumption or preparation of raw pork products (such as chitterlings) and some processed pork products is strongly linked with infection because a high percentage of pigs carry pathogenic *Y. enterocolitica* strains. Outbreaks of *Y. enterocolitica* infection have been associated with consumption of milk (pasteurized, unpasteurized, and chocolate-flavored) and various foods contaminated with springwater. Person-to-person transmission is suspected in a few cases (e.g., in nosocomial and familial outbreaks) but is much less likely with *Y. enterocolitica* than with other causes of gastrointestinal infection, such as *Salmonella*. A multivariate analysis indicates that contact with companion animals is a risk factor for *Y. enterocolitica* infection among children in Sweden, and low-level colonization of dogs and cats with *Y. enterocolitica* has been reported. Transfusion-associated septicemia due to *Y. enterocolitica*, while recognized as a very rare but frequently fatal event for over 30 years, has been difficult to eradicate.

Y. pseudotuberculosis *Y. pseudotuberculosis* is less frequently reported as a cause of human disease than *Y. enterocolitica*, and infection with *Y. pseudotuberculosis* is more likely to present as fever and abdominal pain due to mesenteric lymphadenitis. This organism is associated with wild mammals (rodents, rabbits, and deer), birds, and domestic pigs. Strains are differentiated by combined biochemical reactions (biovar) and serogroup. Although outbreaks are generally rare, several have recently occurred in Finland in association with consumption of lettuce and raw carrots.

PATHOGENESIS

The usual route of infection is oral. Studies with both *Y. enterocolitica* and *Y. pseudotuberculosis* in animal models suggest that initial replication in the small intestine is followed by invasion of Peyer's patches of the distal ileum via M cells, with onward spread to mesenteric lymph nodes. The liver and spleen can also be involved after oral infection. The characteristic histologic appearance of enteropathogenic yersiniae after invasion of host tissues is as extracellular microabscesses surrounded by an epithelioid granulomatous lesion.

Experiments involving oral infection of mice with tagged *Y. enterocolitica* show that only a very small proportion of bacteria in the gut invade tissues. Individual bacterial clones from an orally inoculated pool give rise to each microabscess in a Peyer's patch, and the host restricts the invasion of previously infected Peyer's patches. A prior model positing progressive bacterial spread from Peyer's patches and mesenteric lymph nodes to the liver and spleen appears to be inaccurate: spread of individually tagged clones of *Y. pseudotuberculosis* to the liver and spleen of mice occurs independently of regional lymph node colonization and in mice lacking Peyer's patches.

Invasion requires the expression of several nonfimbrial adhesins, such as invasin (Inv) and—in *Y. pseudotuberculosis*—*Yersinia* adhesin A (YadA). Inv interacts directly with β1 integrins, which are expressed on the apical surfaces of M cells but not enterocytes. YadA of *Y. pseudotuberculosis* interacts with extracellular matrix proteins such as collagen and fibronectin to facilitate host cell integrin association and invasion. YadA of *Y. enterocolitica* lacks a crucial N-terminal region and binds collagen and laminin but not fibronectin and does not cause invasion. Inv is chromosomally encoded, whereas YadA is encoded on the virulence plasmid pYV. YadA helps to confer serum resistance by binding host complement regulators such as factor H and C4-binding protein. Another chromosomal gene, *ail* (attachment and invasion locus), encodes the extracellular protein Ail, which also confers serum resistance by binding these complement regulators.

By binding to host cell surfaces, YadA allows targeting of immune effector cells by the pYV plasmid–encoded type III secretion system (*injectisome*). As a consequence, the host's innate immune response is altered; toxins (*Yersinia* outer proteins, or Yops) are injected into host macrophages, neutrophils, and dendritic cells, affecting signal transduction pathways, resulting in reduced phagocytosis and inhibited production of reactive oxygen species by neutrophils, and triggering apoptosis of macrophages. Other factors functional in invasive disease include yersiniabactin (Ybt), a siderophore produced by some strains of *Y. pseudotuberculosis* and *Y. enterocolitica* as well as other Enterobacteriaceae. Yersiniabactin allows bacteria to access iron from saturated lactoferrin during infection and reduces the production of reactive oxygen species by innate immune effector cells, thereby decreasing bacterial killing. *Y. pseudotuberculosis* and *Y. pestis* make other siderophores in addition to yersiniabactin.

CLINICAL MANIFESTATIONS

Self-limiting diarrhea is the most common reported presentation in infection with pathogenic *Y. enterocolitica*, especially in children under the age of 4, who form the single largest group in most case series. Blood may be detected in diarrheal stool. Older children and adults are more likely than younger children to present with abdominal pain, which can be localized to the right iliac fossa—a situation that often leads to laparotomy for presumed appendicitis (pseudoappendicitis). Appendectomy is not indicated for *Yersinia* infection causing pseudoappendicitis. Thickening of the terminal ileum and cecum is seen on endoscopy and ultrasound, with elevated round or oval lesions that may overlie Peyer's patches. Mesenteric lymph nodes are enlarged. Ulcerations of the mucosa are noted on endoscopy. Gastrointestinal complications include granulomatous appendicitis, a chronic inflammatory condition affecting the appendix that is responsible for ≤2% of cases of appendicitis; *Yersinia* is involved in a minority of cases. *Y. enterocolitica* infection can present as acute pharyngitis with or without other gastrointestinal symptoms. Fatal *Y. enterocolitica* pharyngitis has been recorded. Mycotic aneurysm can follow *Y. enterocolitica* bacteremia, as can focal infection (abscess) in many other sites and body compartments (liver, spleen, kidney, bone, meninges, endocardium).

In all age groups, *Y. pseudotuberculosis* infection is more likely to present as abdominal pain and fever than as diarrhea. A superantigenic toxin—*Y. pseudotuberculosis* mitogen (YPM)—is produced by strains seen in eastern Russia in association with Far Eastern scarlet-like fever, a childhood illness with desquamating rash, arthralgia, and toxic shock. A similar illness is recognized in Japan (Izumi fever) and Korea. Similarities have been noted with Kawasaki disease, the idiopathic acute systematic vasculitis of childhood. There is an epidemiologic link between exposure of populations to superantigen-positive *Y. pseudotuberculosis* and an elevated incidence of Kawasaki disease.

Y. enterocolitica or *Y. pseudotuberculosis* septicemia presents as a severe illness with fever and leukocytosis, often without localizing features, and is significantly associated with predisposing conditions such as diabetes mellitus, liver disease, and iron overload. Hemochromatosis combines several of these risk factors. Administration of iron chelators like desferrioxamine, which provide iron accessible to *Yersinia* (and have an inhibitory effect on neutrophil function), may result in *Yersinia* septicemia in patients with iron overload who presumably have an otherwise mild gastrointestinal infection. HIV/AIDS has been associated with *Y. pseudotuberculosis* septicemia. The unusual phenomenon of transfusion-associated septicemia is linked to the ability of *Y. enterocolitica* to multiply at refrigerator temperature (*psychrotrophy*). Typically, the transfused unit has been stored for >20 days, and it is believed that small numbers of yersiniae from an apparently healthy donor with subclinical bacteremia are amplified to very high numbers by growth inside the bag at ≤4°C, with consequent septic shock after transfusion. A method for preventing this very rare event (i.e., a range of 1 case in 500,000 to 1 case in several million transfused units in countries such as the United States and France) without unacceptable restriction in the blood supply has not yet been devised.

POSTINFECTIVE PHENOMENA

Like other invasive infections of intestinal origin (salmonellosis, shigellosis), reactive arthritis (articular arthritis of multiple joints developing within 2–4 weeks of a preceding infection) results from autoimmune activity initiated by the deposition of bacterial components (not viable bacteria) in joints in combination with the immune response to invading bacteria. The majority of individuals affected by reactive arthritis due to *Yersinia* are HLA-B27 positive. Myocarditis with electrocardiographic ST-segment abnormalities may occur with *Yersinia*-associated reactive arthritis. Most *Yersinia*-associated cases follow *Y. enterocolitica* infection (presumably because it is more common than infection with other species), but *Y. pseudotuberculosis*-associated reactive arthritis is also well documented in Finland, where sporadic and outbreak infections with *Y. pseudotuberculosis* are more common than in other countries. Of infected individuals identified in a recent *Y. pseudotuberculosis* serotype O:3 outbreak in Finland, 12% developed reactive arthritis affecting the small joints of the hands and feet, knees, ankles, and shoulders and lasting >6 months in most cases. Erythema nodosum (see Fig. 25e-40) occurs after *Yersinia* infection (more commonly in women) with no evidence of HLA-B27 linkage.

There is a long-standing association between antithyroid and anti-*Yersinia* antibodies. Antibody evidence of prior *Y. enterocolitica* infection in Graves' disease and increased levels of antithyroid antibody in patients with *Y. enterocolitica* antibodies were first noted in the 1970s. *Y. enterocolitica* contains a thyroid-stimulating hormone (TSH)–binding site that is recognized by anti-TSH antibodies from Graves' disease patients. Raised titers of antibodies to *Y. enterocolitica* whole cells and Yops have been found in some series of Graves' disease patients but not in others. One Danish study of twins found no evidence of an association between asymptomatic *Yersinia* infection (as evidenced by anti-Yop antibody titers) and antithyroid antibodies in euthyroid individuals, while another Danish study of twins with and without Graves' disease found that increased anti-Yop antibody titers were associated with Graves' disease. It remains unclear whether this cross-reactivity is significant in the etiology of Graves' disease.

LABORATORY DIAGNOSIS

Standard laboratory culture methods can be used to isolate enteropathogenic *Yersinia* species from sterile samples, including blood and cerebrospinal fluid. Culture on specific selective media (CIN agar), with or without pre-enrichment in broth or phosphate-buffered saline at either 4°C or 16°C, is the basis of most schema for isolation of yersiniae from stool or other nonsterile samples. Outside known high-incidence areas, specific culture may be carried out by laboratories only upon request. Virulence plasmid–negative strains of *Y. enterocolitica* can be isolated from cultures of stool from asymptomatic individuals, especially after cold enrichment. These strains usually differ in biotype (typically biovar 1a) from virulence plasmid–possessing strains; although some display apparent pathogenicity in a mouse model, virulence plasmid–negative strains are not commonly accepted as human pathogens. Because of the frequency with which the virulence plasmid is lost on laboratory subculture, combined biochemical identification (with biotyping according to a standard schema) and serologic identification are usually required to interpret the significance of an isolate of *Y. enterocolitica* from a nonsterile site. Most pathogenic *Y. enterocolitica* strains currently isolated from humans are of serogroup O:3/biovar 4 or serogroup O:9/biovar 2; this pattern holds even in the United States, where serogroup O:8/biovar 1B strains were previously predominant. Many self-validated multiplex PCR screens for detection of *Y. enterocolitica* in clinical samples—and rather more for its detection in food—have been described, but none of these assays is widely used outside its originating laboratory. Some CE-marked real-time PCR kits are now available in Europe for the diagnosis of yersiniosis in animals; as molecular diagnosis of enteric infection becomes more routine in human disease, it is likely that *Y. enterocolitica* will be included in diagnostic multiplex PCR screens of feces. Because of the presence of Ail in biovar 1a strains, this antigen cannot be used alone in diagnostic assays. A standard for PCR detection in food samples is being prepared by the International Organization for Standardization.

Agglutinating or ELISA antibody titers to specific O-antigen types are used in the retrospective diagnosis of both *Y. enterocolitica* and *Y. pseudotuberculosis* infections. IgA and IgG antibodies persist in patients with reactive arthritis. Serologic cross-reactions between *Y. enterocolitica* serogroup O:9 and *Brucella* are due to the similarity of their lipopolysaccharide structures. Multiple assays are required to cover even the predominant serogroups (*Y. enterocolitica* O:3, O:5,27, and O:9; *Y. pseudotuberculosis* O:1a, O:1b, and O:3), and these assays are generally available only in reference laboratories. ELISA and western blot tests for antibodies to Yops, which are expressed by all pathogenic strains of *Y. enterocolitica* and *Y. pseudotuberculosis*, are also available; most of the positivity in these assays probably relates to previous infection with *Y. enterocolitica*.

TREATMENT YERSINIOSIS

Most cases of diarrhea caused by enteropathogenic *Yersinia* are self-limiting. Data from clinical trials do not support antimicrobial treatment for adults or children with *Y. enterocolitica* diarrhea. Systemic infections with bacteremia or focal infections outside the gastrointestinal tract generally require antimicrobial therapy. Infants <3 months of age with documented *Y. enterocolitica* infection may require antimicrobial treatment because of the increased likelihood of bacteremia in this age group. *Y. enterocolitica* strains nearly always express β-lactamases. Because of the relative rarity of systemic *Y. enterocolitica* infection, there are no clinical trial data to guide antimicrobial choice or to suggest the optimal dose and duration of therapy. On the basis of retrospective case series and in vitro sensitivity data, fluoroquinolone therapy is effective for bacteremia in adults; for example, ciprofloxacin is given at a typical dose of 500 mg twice daily by mouth or 400 mg twice daily IV for at least 2 weeks (longer if positive blood cultures persist). A third-generation cephalosporin is an alternative—e.g., cefotaxime (typical dose, 6–8 g/d in three or four divided doses). In children, third-generation cephalosporins are effective; for example, cefotaxime is given to children ≥1 month of age at a typical dose of 75–100 mg/kg per day in three or four divided doses, with an increase to 150–200 mg/kg per day in severe cases (maximal daily dose, 8–10 g). Amoxicillin and amoxicillin/clavulanate have shown poor efficacy in case series. Trimethoprim-sulfamethoxazole, gentamicin, and imipenem are all active in vitro. *Y. pseudotuberculosis* strains do not express β-lactamase but are intrinsically resistant to polymyxin. Because human infection with *Y. pseudotuberculosis* is less common than that with *Y. enterocolitica*, less case information is available; however, studies in mice suggest that ampicillin is ineffective. Drugs similar to those used against *Y. enterocolitica* should be used. The best results have been obtained with a quinolone.

Some trials of treatment for reactive arthritis (with a large proportion of cases due to *Yersinia*) found that 3 months of oral ciprofloxacin therapy did not affect outcome. One trial in which the same therapy was given specifically for *Y. enterocolitica*–reactive arthritis found that, while outcome indeed was not affected, there was a trend toward faster remission of symptoms in the treated group. Follow-up 4–7 years after initial antibiotic treatment of reactive arthritis (predominantly following *Salmonella* and *Yersinia* infections) demonstrated apparent efficacy in the prevention of chronic arthritis in HLA-B27-positive individuals. A trial showing that azithromycin therapy did not affect outcome in reactive arthritis included cases believed to follow yersiniosis, although no breakdown of cases was provided. A Cochrane review evaluating the use of antibiotics for reactive arthritis is in progress.

PREVENTION AND CONTROL

Current control measures are similar to those used against other enteric pathogens like *Salmonella* and *Campylobacter*, which colonize the intestine of food animals. The focus is on safe handling and processing of food. No vaccine is effective in preventing intestinal colonization of food animals by enteropathogenic *Yersinia*. Consumption of food made from raw pork (which is popular in Germany and Belgium) should be discouraged at present because it is not possible to eliminate contamination with the enteropathogenic *Yersinia* strains found worldwide in pigs. Exposure of infants to raw pig intestine during domestic preparation of chitterlings is inadvisable. Modification of abattoir technique in Scandinavian countries from the 1990s onward included the removal of pig intestines in a closed plastic bag; levels of carcass contamination with *Y. enterocolitica* were reduced, but such contamination was not eliminated. Experimental pig herds free of pathogenic *Y. enterocolitica* O:3 (and also of *Salmonella*, *Toxoplasma*, and *Trichinella*) have been established in Norway and may be commercialized in the future because of their enhanced safety. In the food industry, vigilance is required because of the potential for large outbreaks if small numbers of enteropathogenic yersiniae contaminate any ready-to-eat food whose safe preservation is based on refrigeration before consumption.

The rare phenomenon of contamination of blood for transfusion has proved impossible to eradicate. However, leukodepletion is now practiced in most blood transfusion centers, primarily to prevent nonhemolytic febrile transfusion reactions and alloimmunization against HLA antigens. This measure reduces but does not eliminate the risk of *Yersinia* blood contamination.

Notification of yersiniosis is now obligatory in some countries.

197 *Bartonella* Infections, Including Cat-Scratch Disease

Michael Giladi, Moshe Ephros

Bartonella species are fastidious, facultative intracellular, slow-growing, gram-negative bacteria that cause a broad spectrum of diseases in humans. This genus includes more than 30 distinct species or subspecies, of which at least 16 have been recognized as confirmed or potential human pathogens; *Bartonella bacilliformis*, *Bartonella quintana*, and *Bartonella henselae* are most commonly identified (Table 197-1). Most *Bartonella* species have successfully adapted to survival in specific domestic or wild mammals. Prolonged intraerythrocytic infection in these animals creates a niche where the bacteria are protected from both innate and adaptive immunity and which serves as a reservoir for human infections. *Bartonella* characteristically evades the host immune system by modification of its virulence factors (e.g., lipopolysaccharides or flagella) and by attenuation of the immune response. *B. bacilliformis* and *B. quintana*, which are not zoonotic, are exceptions. Arthropod vectors are often involved. Isolation and characterization of *Bartonella* species are difficult and require special techniques. Clinical presentation generally depends on both the infecting *Bartonella* species and the immune status of the infected individual. *Bartonella* species are susceptible to many antibiotics in vitro; however, clinical responses to therapy and studies in animal models suggest that the minimal inhibitory concentrations of many antimicrobial agents correlate poorly with the drugs' in vivo efficacies in patients with *Bartonella* infections.

CAT-SCRATCH DISEASE

DEFINITION AND ETIOLOGY

Usually a self-limited illness, cat-scratch disease (CSD) has two general clinical presentations. *Typical* CSD, the more common, is characterized by subacute regional lymphadenopathy; *atypical* CSD is the collective designation for numerous extranodal manifestations involving various organs. *B. henselae* is the principal etiologic agent of CSD. Rare cases have been associated with *Afipia felis* and other *Bartonella* species.

EPIDEMIOLOGY

CSD occurs worldwide, favoring warm and humid climates. In temperate climates, incidence peaks during fall and winter; in the tropics, disease occurs year-round. Adults are affected nearly as frequently as children. Intrafamilial clustering is rare, and person-to-person transmission does not occur. Apparently healthy cats constitute the major reservoir of *B. henselae*, and cat fleas (*Ctenocephalides felis*) may be responsible for cat-to-cat transmission. CSD usually follows contact with cats (especially kittens), but other animals (e.g., dogs) have been implicated as possible reservoirs in rare instances. In the United States, the estimated disease incidence is ~10 cases per 100,000 population. About 10% of patients are hospitalized.

TABLE 197-1 *BARTONELLA* SPECIES KNOWN OR SUSPECTED TO BE HUMAN PATHOGENS

Bartonella Species[a]	Disease[b]	Reservoir Host[c]	Arthropod Vector
B. henselae	Cat-scratch disease, bacillary angiomatosis, bacillary peliosis, bacteremia, endocarditis	Cats, other felines	Cat fleas (*Ctenocephalides felis*): associated with cat-to-cat, but not with cat-to-human, transmission
B. quintana	Trench fever, chronic bacteremia, bacillary angiomatosis, endocarditis	Humans	Human body lice (*Pediculus humanus corporis*)
B. bacilliformis	Carrión's disease	Humans	Sandflies (*Lutzomyia verrucarum*)
B. elizabethae	Endocarditis	Rats, dogs	Unknown
B. grahamii[d]	Lymphadenopathy	Mice, voles	Fleas
B. vinsonii subsp. *arupensis*	Endocarditis, febrile illness	Mice, dogs	Ticks
B. vinsonii subsp. *berkhoffii*	Endocarditis	Domestic dogs, coyotes, gray foxes	Ticks
B. washoensis	Myocarditis, meningitis	Squirrels, possibly other rodents	Fleas
B. alsatica	Endocarditis	Rabbits	Unknown
B. koehlerae	Endocarditis	Cats	Unknown
B. clarridgeiae	Possibly cat-scratch disease	Cats	Unknown
B. rochalimae	Bacteremia, fever, splenomegaly	Unknown	Possibly fleas
B. tamiae	Bacteremia, fever, myalgia, rash	Unknown	Unknown
Candidatus B. melophagi[e]	Various clinical manifestations	Unknown	Unknown
Candidatus B. mayotimonensis[e]	Endocarditis	Unknown	Unknown
Candidatus B. ancashi[e]	Verruga peruana–like illness	Unknown	Unknown

[a]Many other *Bartonella* species exist but are not recognized as human pathogens. [b]*B. henselae*, *B. vinsonii* subsp. *berkhoffii*, *B. koehlerae*, *Candidatus B. melophagi*, or more than one *Bartonella* spp. (co-infection) were detected in blood samples from patients with extensive arthropod and other animal exposure who presented with various chronic neurologic or neurocognitive syndromes. The role of these pathogens in these patients needs further study. [c]Animals are implicated when existing evidence supports their infection with *Bartonella* species. Data supporting animal-to-human transmission may be lacking. [d]Retinitis may also be associated with *B. grahamii*. [e]*Candidatus* is a taxonomic status for bacteria that cannot be described in sufficient detail to warrant establishment of a novel taxon or cannot be cultured or propagated in culture media. The phylogenetic relatedness of these bacteria has been determined by gene amplification and sequence analysis.

PATHOGENESIS

Inoculation of *B. henselae*, possibly via contaminated flea feces, usually results from a cat scratch or bite. Infection of mucous membranes or conjunctivae via droplets or licking may occur as well. With lymphatic drainage to one or more regional lymph nodes in immunocompetent hosts, a T_H1 response can result in necrotizing granulomatous lymphadenitis. Dendritic cells, along with their associated chemokines, play a role in the host inflammatory response and granuloma formation.

CLINICAL MANIFESTATIONS AND PROGNOSIS

Of patients with CSD, 85–90% have typical disease. The primary lesion, a small (0.3- to 1-cm) painless erythematous papule or pustule, develops at the inoculation site (usually the site of a scratch or a bite) within days to 2 weeks in about one-third to two-thirds of patients (Fig. 197–1*A*, *B*). Lymphadenopathy develops 1–3 weeks or longer after cat contact. The affected lymph node(s) are enlarged and usually painful, sometimes have overlying erythema, and suppurate in 10–15% of cases (Fig. 197–1*C*, *D*, and *E*). Axillary/epitrochlear nodes are most commonly involved; next in frequency are head/neck nodes and then inguinal/femoral nodes. Approximately 50% of patients have fever, malaise, and anorexia. A smaller proportion experience weight loss and night sweats mimicking the presentation of lymphoma. Fever is usually low-grade but infrequently rises to ≥39°C. Resolution is slow, requiring weeks (for fever, pain, and accompanying signs and symptoms) to months (for node shrinkage).

Atypical CSD occurs in 10–15% of patients as extranodal or complicated disease in the absence or presence of lymphadenopathy. Atypical disease includes Parinaud's oculoglandular syndrome (granulomatous conjunctivitis with ipsilateral preauricular lymphadenitis; Fig. 197–1*E*), granulomatous hepatitis/splenitis, neuroretinitis (often presenting as unilateral deterioration of vision; Fig. 197–1*F*), and other ophthalmologic manifestations. In addition, neurologic involvement (encephalopathy, seizures, myelitis, radiculitis, cerebellitis, facial and other cranial or peripheral palsies), fever of unknown origin, debilitating myalgia, arthritis or arthralgia (affecting mostly women >20 years old), osteomyelitis (including multifocal disease), tendinitis, neuralgia, and dermatologic manifestations (including erythema nodosum [see Fig. 25e-40], sometimes accompanying arthropathy) occur. Other manifestations and syndromes (pneumonitis, pleural effusion, idiopathic thrombocytopenic purpura, Henoch-Schönlein purpura, erythema multiforme [see Fig. 25e-25], hypercalcemia, glomerulonephritis, myocarditis) have also been associated with CSD. In elderly patients (>60 years old), lymphadenopathy is more often absent but encephalitis and fever of unknown origin are more common than in younger patients. In immunocompetent individuals, CSD—whether typical or atypical—usually resolves without treatment and without sequelae. Lifelong immunity is the rule.

DIAGNOSIS

Routine laboratory tests usually yield normal or nonspecific results. Histopathology initially shows lymphoid hyperplasia and later demonstrates stellate granulomata with necrosis, coalescing microabscesses, and occasional multinucleated giant cells—findings that, although nonspecific, may narrow the differential diagnosis. Serologic testing (immunofluorescence or enzyme immunoassay) is the most commonly used laboratory diagnostic approach, with variable sensitivity and specificity. Seroconversion may take a few weeks. Other tests are of low sensitivity (culture, Warthin-Starry silver staining), of low specificity (cytology, histopathology), or of limited availability in routine diagnostic laboratories (polymerase chain reaction [PCR], immunohistochemistry). PCR of lymph node tissue, pus, or the primary inoculation lesion is highly sensitive and specific and is particularly useful for definitive and rapid diagnosis in seronegative patients.

APPROACH TO THE PATIENT: Cat-Scratch Disease

A history of cat contact, a primary inoculation lesion, and regional lymphadenopathy are highly suggestive of CSD. A characteristic clinical course and corroborative laboratory tests make the diagnosis very likely. Conversely, when acute- and convalescent-phase sera are negative (as is the case in 10–20% of CSD patients), when spontaneous regression of lymph node size does not occur, and particularly when constitutional symptoms persist, malignancy must be ruled out. Pyogenic lymphadenitis, mycobacterial infection, brucellosis, syphilis, tularemia, plague, toxoplasmosis, sporotrichosis, and histoplasmosis should also be considered. In clinically suspected CSD in a seronegative individual, fine-needle aspiration may be adequate and PCR can confirm the diagnosis. When data are less supportive of CSD, lymph node biopsy rather than fine-needle aspiration is preferred. In seronegative CSD patients with lymphadenopathy and severe complications (e.g., encephalitis or neuroretinitis), early biopsy is important to establish a specific diagnosis.

TREATMENT CAT-SCRATCH DISEASE

(Table 197-2) Treatment regimens are based on only minimal data. Suppurative nodes should be drained by large-bore needle aspiration and not by incision and drainage in order to avoid chronic draining tracts. Immunocompromised patients must always be treated with systemic antimicrobials.

PREVENTION

Avoiding cats (especially kittens) and instituting flea control are options for immunocompromised patients and for patients with valvular heart disease.

TRENCH FEVER AND CHRONIC BACTEREMIA

DEFINITION AND ETIOLOGY

Trench fever, also known as *5-day fever* or *quintan fever*, is a febrile illness caused by *B. quintana*. It was first described as an epidemic in the trenches of World War I and recently reemerged as chronic bacteremia seen most often in homeless people (also referred to in the latter setting as *urban* or *contemporary trench fever*).

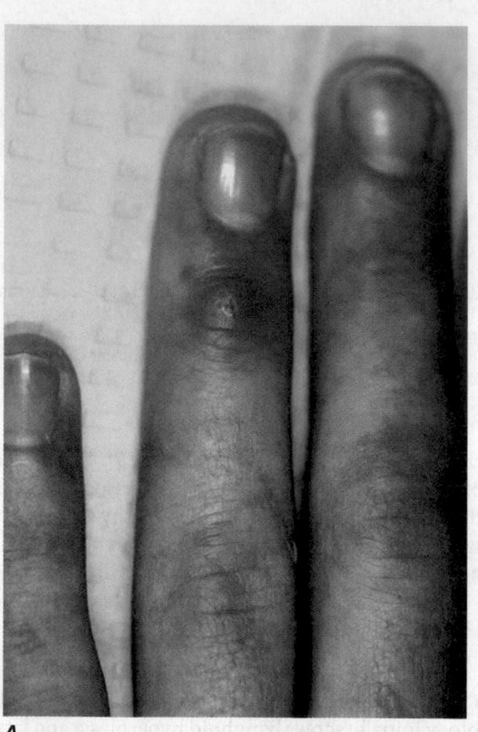

A

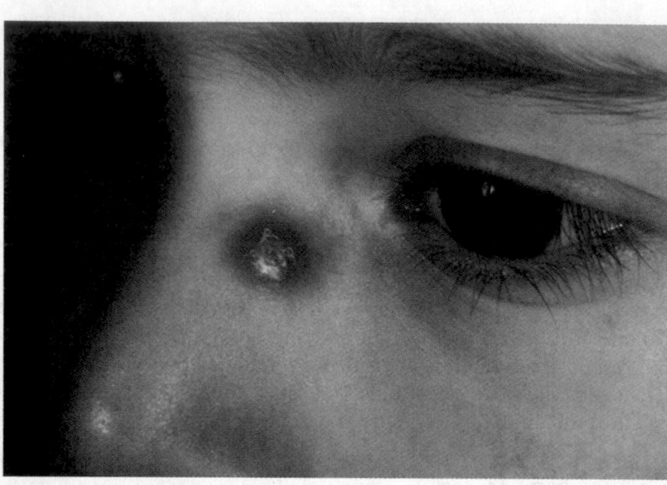

B

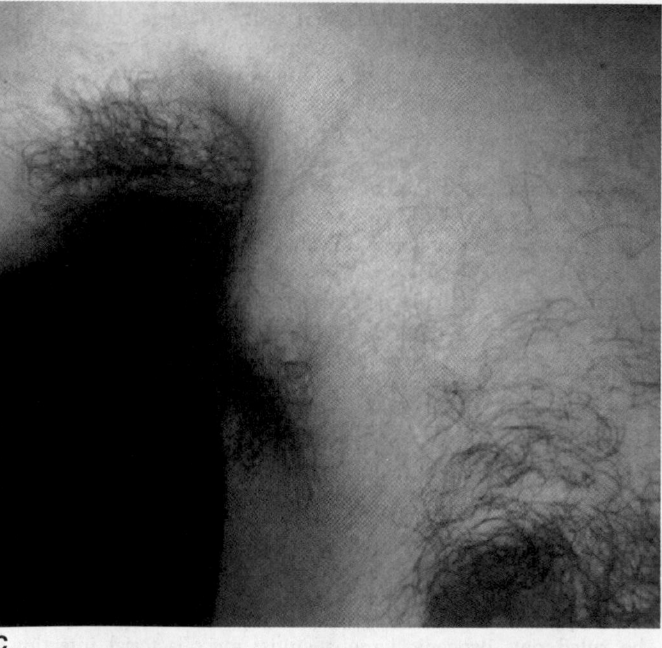

C

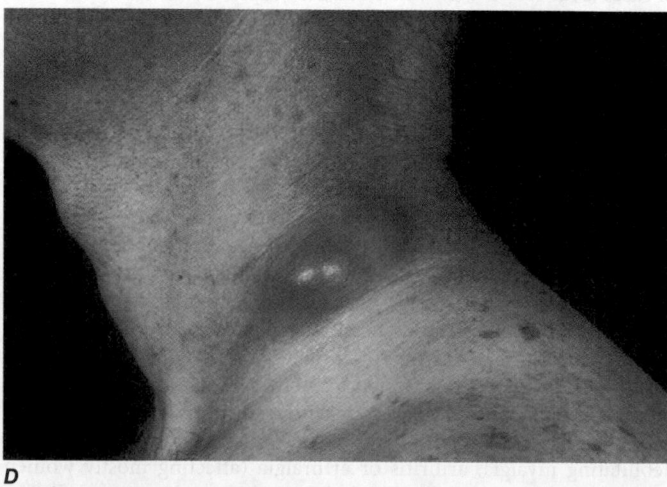

D

FIGURE 197-1 Manifestations of cat-scratch disease. *A.* Primary inoculation lesion. Axillary and epitrochlear lymphadenitis appeared 2 weeks later. ***B.*** Primary inoculation lesion. Submental lymphadenitis appeared 10 days later. ***C.*** Axillary lymphadenopathy of 2 weeks' duration. The overlying skin appears normal. ***D.*** Cervical lymphadenopathy of 6 weeks' duration. The overlying skin is red. Thick, odorless pus (12 mL) was aspirated. ***E.*** Preauricular lymphadenopathy. ***F.*** Left-eye neuroretinitis. Note papilledema and stellate macular exudates ("macular star").

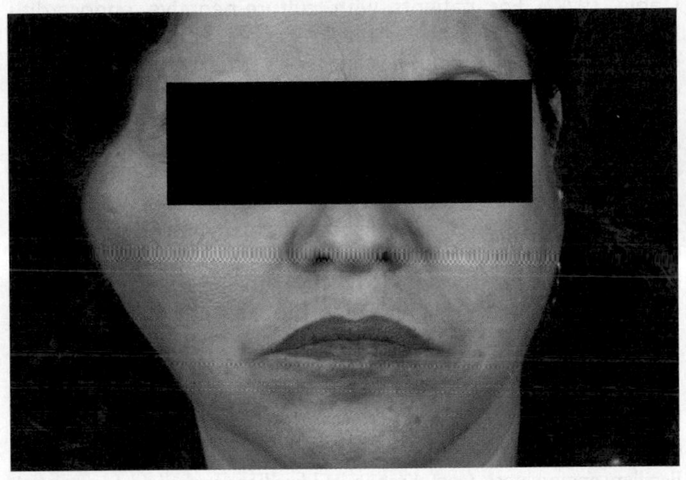

E

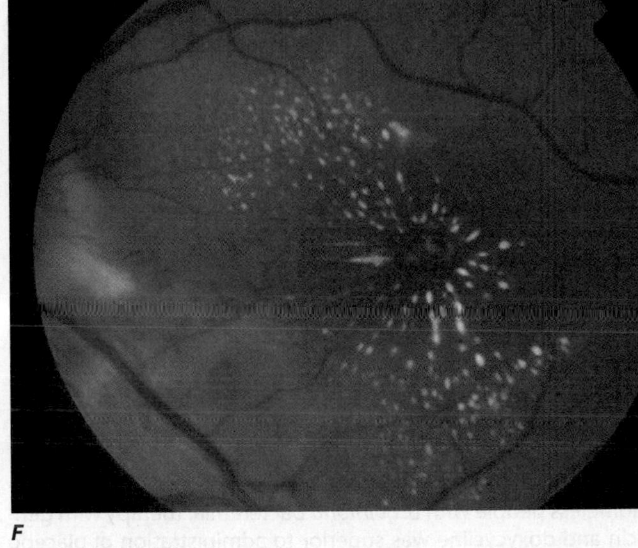

F

FIGURE 197-1 *(Continued)*

EPIDEMIOLOGY

In addition to epidemics during World Wars I and II, sporadic outbreaks of trench fever have been reported in many regions of the world. The human body louse has been identified as the vector and humans as the only known reservoir. After a hiatus of several decades during which trench fever was almost forgotten, small clusters of cases of *B. quintana* chronic bacteremia were reported sporadically, primarily from the United States and France, in HIV-uninfected homeless people. Alcoholism and louse infestation were identified as risk factors.

CLINICAL MANIFESTATIONS

The typical incubation period is 15–25 days (range, 3–38 days). "Classical" trench fever, as described in 1919, ranges from a mild febrile illness to a recurrent or protracted and debilitating disease. Onset may be abrupt or preceded by a prodrome of several days. Fever is often periodic, lasting 4–5 days with 5-day (range, 3- to 8-day) intervals between episodes. Other symptoms and signs include headache, back and limb pain, profuse sweating, shivering, myalgia, arthralgia, splenomegaly, a maculopapular rash in occasional cases, and nuchal rigidity in some cases. Untreated, the disease usually lasts

TABLE 197-2 ANTIMICROBIAL THERAPY FOR DISEASE CAUSED BY *BARTONELLA* SPECIES IN ADULTS

Disease	Antimicrobial Therapy
Typical cat-scratch disease	Not routinely indicated; for patients with extensive lymphadenopathy, consider azithromycin (500 mg PO on day 1, then 250 mg PO qd for 4 days)
Cat-scratch disease retinitis	Doxycycline (100 mg PO bid) *plus* rifampin (300 mg PO bid) for 4–6 weeks
Other atypical cat-scratch disease manifestations[a]	As per retinitis; treatment duration should be individualized
Trench fever or chronic bacteremia with *B. quintana*	Gentamicin (3 mg/kg IV qd for 14 days) *plus* doxycycline (200 mg PO qd or 100 mg PO bid for 6 weeks)
Suspected *Bartonella* endocarditis	Gentamicin[b] (1 mg/kg IV q8h for ≥14 days) *plus* doxycycline (100 mg PO/IV bid for 6 weeks[c]) *plus* ceftriaxone (2 g IV qd for 6 weeks)
Confirmed *Bartonella* endocarditis	As for suspected *Bartonella* endocarditis *minus* ceftriaxone
Bacillary angiomatosis	Erythromycin[d] (500 mg PO qid for 3 months) *or* Doxycycline (100 mg PO bid for 3 months)
Bacillary peliosis	Erythromycin[d] (500 mg PO qid for 4 months) *or* Doxycycline (100 mg PO bid for 4 months)
Carrión's disease	
Oroya fever	Chloramphenicol (500 mg PO/IV qid for 14 days) *plus* another antibiotic (β-lactam preferred) *or* Ciprofloxacin (500 mg PO bid for 10 days)
Verruga peruana	Rifampin (10 mg/kg PO qd, to a maximum of 600 mg, for 14 days) *or* Streptomycin (15–20 mg/kg IM qd for 10 days)

[a]Data on treatment efficacy for encephalitis and hepatosplenic CSD are lacking. Therapy similar to that given for retinitis is reasonable. [b]Some experts recommend gentamicin at 3 mg/kg IV qd. If gentamicin is contraindicated, rifampin (300 mg PO bid) can be added to doxycycline for documented *Bartonella* endocarditis. [c]Some experts recommend extending oral doxycycline therapy for 3–6 months. [d]Other macrolides are probably effective and may be substituted for erythromycin or doxycycline.

Source: Recommendations are modified from JM Rolain et al: Antimicrob Agents Chemother 48:1921, 2004.

4–6 weeks. Death is rare. The clinical spectrum of *B. quintana* bacteremia in homeless people ranges from asymptomatic infection to a febrile illness with headache, severe leg pain, and thrombocytopenia. Endocarditis sometimes develops.

DIAGNOSIS

Definitive diagnosis requires isolation of *B. quintana* by blood culture. Some patients have positive blood cultures for several weeks. Patients with acute trench fever typically develop significant titers of antibody to *Bartonella*, whereas those with chronic *B. quintana* bacteremia may be seronegative. Patients with high titers of IgG antibodies should be evaluated for endocarditis. In epidemics, trench fever should be differentiated from epidemic louse-borne typhus and relapsing fever, which occur under similar conditions and share many features.

TREATMENT *B. QUINTANA* BACTEREMIA

(Table 197–2) In a small, randomized, placebo-controlled trial involving homeless people with *B. quintana* bacteremia, therapy with gentamicin and doxycycline was superior to administration of placebo in eradicating bacteremia. Treatment of bacteremia is important even in clinically mild cases to prevent endocarditis. Optimal therapy for trench fever without documented bacteremia is uncertain.

BARTONELLA ENDOCARDITIS

DEFINITION AND ETIOLOGY

Coxiella burnetii (Chap. 211) and *Bartonella* species are the most common pathogens in culture-negative endocarditis (Chap. 155). In France, for example, *Bartonella* species were identified as the etiologic agents in 28% of 348 cases of culture-negative endocarditis. Prevalence, however, varies by geographic location and epidemiologic setting. In addition to *B. quintana* and *B. henselae* (the most common *Bartonella* species implicated in endocarditis, the former more commonly than the latter), other *Bartonella* species have reportedly caused rare cases (Table 197-1).

EPIDEMIOLOGY

Bartonella endocarditis has been reported worldwide. Most patients are adults; more are male than female. Risk factors associated with *B. quintana* endocarditis include homelessness, alcoholism, and body louse infestation; however, individuals with no risk factors have had *Bartonella* endocarditis diagnosed as well. *B. henselae* endocarditis is associated with exposure to cats. Most cases involve native rather than prosthetic valves; the aortic valve accounts for ~60% of cases. Patients with *B. henselae* endocarditis usually have preexisting valvulopathy, whereas *B. quintana* often infects normal valves.

CLINICAL MANIFESTATIONS

Clinical manifestations are usually characteristic of subacute endocarditis of any etiology. However, a substantial number of patients have a prolonged, minimally febrile or even afebrile indolent illness, with mild nonspecific symptoms lasting weeks or months before the diagnosis is made. Initial echocardiography may not show vegetations. Acute, aggressive disease is rare.

DIAGNOSIS

Blood cultures, even with use of special techniques (lysis centrifugation or EDTA-containing tubes), are positive in only ~25% of cases—mostly those caused by *B. quintana* and only rarely those caused by *B. henselae*. Prolonged incubation of cultures (up to 6 weeks) is required. Serologic tests—either immunofluorescence or enzyme immunoassay—usually demonstrate high-titer IgG antibodies to *Bartonella*. Because of cross-antigenicity, serology does not distinguish between *B. quintana* and *B. henselae* and may also be low-titer cross-reactive with other pathogens, such as *C. burnetii* and *Chlamydia* species. Identification of *Bartonella* to the species level is usually accomplished by application of PCR-based methods to valve tissue.

TREATMENT *BARTONELLA* ENDOCARDITIS

(Table 197-2) For patients with culture-negative endocarditis suspected to be due to *Bartonella* species, empirical treatment consists of gentamicin, doxycycline, and ceftriaxone; the major role of ceftriaxone in this regimen is to adequately treat other potential causes of culture-negative endocarditis, including members of the HACEK group (Chap. 183e). Once a diagnosis of *Bartonella* endocarditis has been established, ceftriaxone is discontinued. Aminoglycosides, the only antibiotics known to be bactericidal against *Bartonella*, should be included in the regimen for ≥2 weeks. Indications for valvular surgery are the same as in subacute endocarditis due to other pathogens; however, the proportion of patients who undergo surgery (~60%) is high, probably as a consequence of delayed diagnosis.

BACILLARY ANGIOMATOSIS AND PELIOSIS

DEFINITION AND ETIOLOGY

Bacillary angiomatosis (sometimes called *bacillary epithelioid angiomatosis* or *epithelioid angiomatosis*) is a disease of severely immunocompromised patients, is caused by *B. henselae* or *B. quintana*, and is characterized by neovascular proliferative lesions involving the skin and other organs. Both species cause cutaneous lesions; hepatosplenic lesions are caused only by *B. henselae*, whereas subcutaneous and lytic bone lesions are more frequently associated with *B. quintana*. Bacillary peliosis is a closely related angioproliferative disorder caused by *B. henselae* and involving primarily the liver (peliosis hepatis) but also the spleen and lymph nodes. Bacillary peliosis is characterized by blood-filled cystic structures whose size ranges from microscopic to several millimeters.

EPIDEMIOLOGY

Bacillary angiomatosis and bacillary peliosis occur primarily in HIV-infected persons (Chap. 226) with CD4+ T cell counts <100/μL but also affect other immunosuppressed patients and, in rare instances, immunocompetent patients. The previously reported incidence of ~1 case per 1000 HIV-infected persons is now lower; the decrease is most likely attributable to effective antiretroviral therapy and the routine use of rifabutin and macrolides to prevent *Mycobacterium avium* complex infection in AIDS patients. Contact with cats or cat fleas increases the risk of *B. henselae* infection. Risk factors for *B. quintana* infection are low income, homelessness, and body louse infestation.

CLINICAL MANIFESTATIONS

Bacillary angiomatosis presents most commonly as one or more cutaneous lesions that are not painful and that may be tan, red, or purple in color. Subcutaneous masses or nodules, superficial ulcerated plaques (Fig. 197-2), and verrucous growths are also seen. Nodular forms resemble those seen in fungal or mycobacterial infections. Subcutaneous nodules are often tender. Painful osseous lesions, most often involving long bones, may underlie cutaneous lesions and occasionally develop in their absence. In rare cases, other organs are involved in bacillary angiomatosis. Patients usually have constitutional symptoms, including fever, chills, malaise, headache, anorexia, weight loss, and night sweats. In osseous disease, lytic lesions are generally seen on radiography, and technetium scan shows focal uptake. The differential diagnosis of cutaneous bacillary angiomatosis includes Kaposi's sarcoma, pyogenic granuloma, subcutaneous tumors, and verruga peruana. In bacillary peliosis, hypodense hepatic areas are usually evident on imaging. In patients with advanced immunodeficiency, *B. henselae* and *B. quintana* are important causes of fever of unknown origin. Intermittent bacteremia with positive blood cultures can occur with or without endocarditis.

PATHOLOGY

Bacillary angiomatosis consists of lobular proliferations of small blood vessels lined by enlarged endothelial cells interspersed with mixed infiltrates of neutrophils and lymphocytes, with predominance of the former. Histologic examination of organs with bacillary peliosis reveals small blood-filled cystic lesions partially lined by endothelial

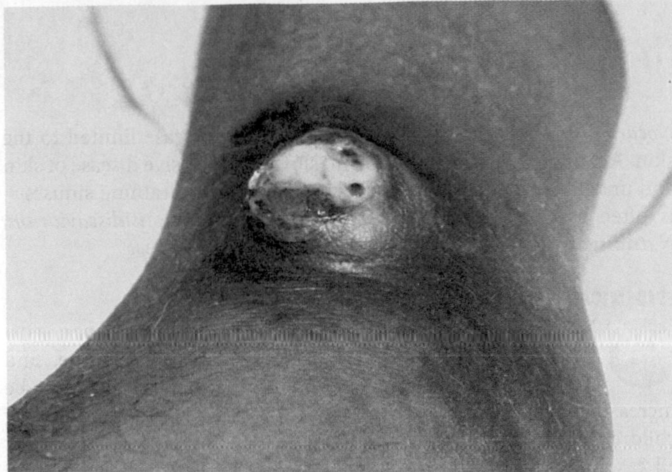

FIGURE 197-2 Nodular lesion of bacillary angiomatosis with superficial ulceration in an AIDS patient with advanced immunodeficiency. *(Reprinted with permission from DH Spach and E Darby: Bartonella Infections, Including Cat-Scratch Disease, in Harrison's Principles of Internal Medicine, 17th ed, AF Fauci et al [eds]. New York, McGraw-Hill, 2008, p 989.)*

cells that can be several millimeters in size. Peliotic lesions are surrounded by fibromyxoid stroma containing inflammatory cells, dilated capillaries, and clumps of granular material. Warthin-Starry silver staining of bacillary angiomatosis and peliosis lesions reveals clusters of bacilli. Cultures are usually negative.

DIAGNOSIS

Bacillary angiomatosis and bacillary peliosis are diagnosed on histologic grounds. Blood cultures may be positive.

TREATMENT BACILLARY ANGIOMATOSIS AND PELIOSIS

(Table 197-2) Prolonged therapy with a macrolide or doxycycline is recommended for both bacillary angiomatosis and bacillary peliosis.

PREVENTION

Control of cat-flea infestation and avoidance of cat scratches (for prevention of *B. henselae*) and avoidance and treatment of body louse infestation (for prevention of *B. quintana*) are reasonable strategies for HIV-infected persons. Primary prophylaxis is not recommended, but suppressive therapy with a macrolide or doxycycline is indicated in HIV-infected patients with bacillary angiomatosis or bacillary peliosis until CD4+ T cell counts are >200/μL. Relapse may necessitate lifelong suppressive therapy in individual cases.

CARRIÓN'S DISEASE (OROYA FEVER AND VERRUGA PERUANA)

DEFINITION AND ETIOLOGY

Carrión's disease is a biphasic disease caused by *B. bacilliformis*. *Oroya fever* is the initial, bacteremic, systemic form, and *verruga peruana* is its late-onset, eruptive manifestation.

EPIDEMIOLOGY AND PREVENTION

Infection is endemic to the geographically restricted Andes valleys of Peru, Ecuador, and Colombia (~500–3200 m above sea level). Sporadic epidemics occur. The disease is transmitted by the phlebotomine sandfly *Lutzomyia verrucarum*. Humans are the only known reservoir of *B. bacilliformis*. Sandfly control measures (e.g., insecticides) and personal protection measures (e.g., repellents, screening, bed nets) may decrease the risk of infection.

PATHOGENESIS

After inoculation by the sandfly, bacteria invade the blood vessel endothelium and proliferate; the reticuloendothelial system and various organs may also be involved. Upon reentry into blood vessels, *B. bacilliformis* invades, replicates, and ultimately destroys erythrocytes, with consequent massive hemolysis and sudden, severe anemia. Microvascular thrombosis results in end-organ ischemia. Survivors sometimes develop cutaneous hemangiomatous lesions characterized by various inflammatory cells, endothelial proliferation, and the presence of *B. bacilliformis*.

CLINICAL MANIFESTATIONS

The incubation period is 3 weeks (range, 2–14 weeks). Oroya fever may present as a nonspecific bacteremic febrile illness without anemia or as an acute, severe hemolytic anemia with hepatomegaly and jaundice of rapid onset leading to vascular collapse and clouded sensorium. Myalgia, arthralgia, lymphadenopathy, and abdominal pain may develop. Temperature is elevated but not extremely so; high fever may suggest intercurrent infection. Subclinical asymptomatic infection also occurs. In verruga peruana, red, hemangioma-like, cutaneous vascular lesions of various sizes appear either weeks to months after systemic illness or with no previous suggestive history. These lesions persist for months up to 1 year. Mucosal and internal lesions may also develop.

DIAGNOSIS AND APPROACH TO THE PATIENT

Systemic illness (with or without anemia) or the development of cutaneous lesions in a person who has been to an endemic area raises the possibility of *B. bacilliformis* infection. Severe anemia with exuberant reticulocytosis—and sometimes thrombocytopenia—can occur. In systemic illness, Giemsa-stained blood films show typical intraerythrocytic bacilli, and blood and bone marrow cultures are positive. Serologic assays may be helpful. Biopsy may be required to confirm the diagnosis of verruga peruana. Differential diagnosis includes the spectrum of coendemic systemic febrile illnesses (e.g., typhoid fever, malaria, brucellosis) as well as diseases producing cutaneous vascular lesions (e.g., hemangiomata, bacillary angiomatosis, Kaposi's sarcoma).

TREATMENT CARRIÓN'S DISEASE

(Table 197-2) Antibiotic therapy for systemic *B. bacilliformis* infection usually results in rapid defervescence. Additional antibiotic treatment of intercurrent infection (particularly salmonellosis) is often required. Blood transfusion may be necessary. Treatment of verruga peruana usually is not required, although large lesions or those interfering with function may require excision. Patients with numerous lesions, especially lesions that have been present for only a short period, may respond well to antibiotic therapy.

COMPLICATIONS AND PROGNOSIS

Mortality rates associated with Oroya fever have been reported to be as high as 40% without treatment but are considerably lower (~10%) with treatment. Complications such as bacterial superinfection and neurologic and cardiac manifestations occur frequently. Generalized massive edema (anasarca) and petechiae are associated with poor outcome. Permanent immunity usually develops.

198e Donovanosis

Nigel O'Farrell

This is a digital-only chapter. It is available on the DVD that accompanies this book, as well as on Access Medicine/Harrison's Online, and the eBook and "app" editions of HPIM 19e.

Donovanosis is a chronic, progressive bacterial infection that usually involves the genital region. The condition is generally regarded as a sexually transmitted infection of low infectivity. This infection has been known by many other names, the most common being *granuloma inguinale*.

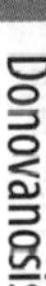

199 Nocardiosis

Gregory A. Filice

Nocardia, a genus of saprophytic aerobic actinomycetes that are common worldwide, resides in soil, contributing to the decay of organic matter. Nearly 100 species have been identified, mostly on the basis of 16S rRNA gene sequences. Nocardiae are relatively inactive in standard biochemical tests, and speciation is difficult without molecular phylogenetic techniques. Historically, the majority of isolates associated with pneumonia and systemic disease were identified as *Nocardia asteroides*, but the lineage of the type strain was muddled, and it is now clear that human disease is associated with several species. Most clinical laboratories cannot speciate isolates accurately and may identify them simply as *N. asteroides* or *Nocardia* species.

Nine species or species complexes are commonly associated with human disease (Table 199-1). Most systemic disease involves *Nocardia cyriacigeorgica, Nocardia farcinica, Nocardia pseudobrasiliensis*, and species in the *Nocardia transvalensis* and *Nocardia nova* complexes.

TABLE 199-1 *NOCARDIA* SPECIES MOST COMMONLY ASSOCIATED WITH HUMAN DISEASE AND THEIR IN VITRO SUSCEPTIBILITY PATTERNS

Species	Susceptible to	Resistant to
N. abscessus	Amikacin, amoxicillin/clavulanic acid, ampicillin, ceftriaxone, gentamicin, linezolid, minocycline, TMP-SMX	Ciprofloxacin, clarithromycin, erythromycin, imipenem (v)[a]
N. brevicatena/paucivorans complex (*N. brevicatena, N. paucivorans, N. carnea*, others)	Amikacin, amoxicillin/clavulanic acid, ampicillin, ceftriaxone, ciprofloxacin, linezolid, minocycline (v), moxifloxacin, tobramycin, TMP-SMX	Ciprofloxacin, clarithromycin, erythromycin, gentamicin, imipenem (v)
N. nova complex (*N. nova, N. veterana, N. africana, N. kruczakiae, N. elegans*, others)	Amikacin, ampicillin, ceftriaxone, clarithromycin, erythromycin, imipenem, linezolid, minocycline, TMP-SMX	Amoxicillin/clavulanic acid, ciprofloxacin, gentamicin, tobramycin
N. transvalensis complex (*N. blacklockiae, N. wallacei*, others)	Amoxicillin/clavulanic acid (v), ceftriaxone (v), ciprofloxacin, linezolid, minocycline (v), TMP-SMX	Amikacin, ampicillin, clarithromycin, erythromycin, gentamicin, imipenem (v)
N. farcinica	Amikacin, amoxicillin/clavulanic acid, imipenem (v), linezolid, minocycline (v), TMP-SMX	Ampicillin, ceftriaxone, ciprofloxacin, clarithromycin, erythromycin, gentamicin, tobramycin
N. cyriacigeorgica	Amikacin, ceftriaxone (v), imipenem, linezolid, minocycline (v), TMP-SMX	Amoxicillin/clavulanic acid, ampicillin (v), ciprofloxacin, erythromycin, gentamicin
N. brasiliensis	Amikacin, amoxicillin/clavulanic acid, minocycline, moxifloxacin, TMP-SMX	Ampicillin, ceftriaxone, ciprofloxacin, clarithromycin, imipenem
N. pseudobrasiliensis	Amikacin, ceftriaxone (v), ciprofloxacin, clarithromycin, TMP-SMX	Amoxicillin/clavulanic acid, ampicillin, imipenem, minocycline
N. otitidiscaviarum complex	Amikacin, ciprofloxacin, gentamicin, TMP-SMX	Amoxicillin/clavulanic acid, ampicillin, ceftriaxone, imipenem

[a]Variable.

Abbreviation: TMP-SMX, trimethoprim-sulfamethoxazole.

Source: Adapted from multiple sources.

Nocardia brasiliensis is usually associated with disease limited to the skin. Actinomycetoma—an indolent, slowly progressive disease of skin and underlying tissues with nodular swellings and draining sinuses—is often associated with *N. brasiliensis, Nocardia otitidiscaviarum, N. transvalensis* complex strains, or other actinomycetes.

EPIDEMIOLOGY

Nocardiosis occurs worldwide. The annual incidence, estimated on three continents (North America, Europe, and Australia), is ~0.375 cases per 100,000 persons and may be increasing. The disease is more common among adults than among children and more common among males than among females. Nearly all cases are sporadic, but outbreaks have been associated with contamination of the hospital environment, cosmetic procedures, and parenteral illicit drug use. Person-to-person spread is not well documented. There is no known seasonality.

The majority of cases of pulmonary or disseminated disease occur in people with a host defense defect. Most have deficient cell-mediated immunity, especially that associated with lymphoma, transplantation, glucocorticoid therapy, or AIDS. The incidence is ~140-fold greater among patients with AIDS and ~340-fold greater among bone marrow transplant recipients than in general populations. In AIDS, nocardiosis usually affects persons with <250 CD4+ T lymphocytes/μL. Nocardiosis has also been associated with pulmonary alveolar proteinosis, tuberculosis and other mycobacterial diseases, chronic granulomatous disease, interleukin 12 deficiency, and treatment with monoclonal antibodies that interfere with tumor necrosis factor. Any child with nocardiosis and no known cause of immunosuppression should undergo tests to determine the adequacy of the phagocytic respiratory burst.

Cases of actinomycetoma occur mainly in tropical and subtropical regions, especially those of Mexico, Central and South America, Africa, and India. The most important risk factor is frequent contact with soil or vegetable matter, especially in laborers.

PATHOLOGY AND PATHOGENESIS

Pneumonia and disseminated disease are both thought to follow inhalation of fragmented bacterial mycelia. The characteristic histologic feature of nocardiosis is an abscess with extensive neutrophil infiltration and prominent necrosis. Granulation tissue usually surrounds the lesions, but extensive fibrosis or encapsulation is uncommon.

Actinomycetoma is characterized by suppurative inflammation with sinus tract formation. Granules—microcolonies composed of dense masses of bacterial filaments extending radially from a central core—are occasionally observed in histologic preparations. The granules are frequently found in discharges from lesions of actinomycetoma but almost never in discharges from lesions in other forms of nocardiosis.

Nocardiae have evolved a number of properties that enable them to survive within phagocytes, including neutralization of oxidants, prevention of phagosome-lysosome fusion, and prevention of phagosome acidification. Neutrophils phagocytose the organisms and limit their growth but do not kill them efficiently. Cell-mediated immunity is important for definitive control and elimination of nocardiae.

CLINICAL MANIFESTATIONS

Respiratory Tract Disease Pneumonia, the most common form of nocardial disease in the respiratory tract, is typically subacute; symptoms have usually been present for days or weeks at presentation. The onset is occasionally more acute in immunosuppressed patients. Cough is prominent and produces small amounts of thick, purulent sputum that is not malodorous. Fever, anorexia, weight loss, and malaise are common; dyspnea, pleuritic pain, and hemoptysis are less common. Remissions and exacerbations over several weeks are frequent. Roentgenographic patterns vary, but some are highly suggestive of

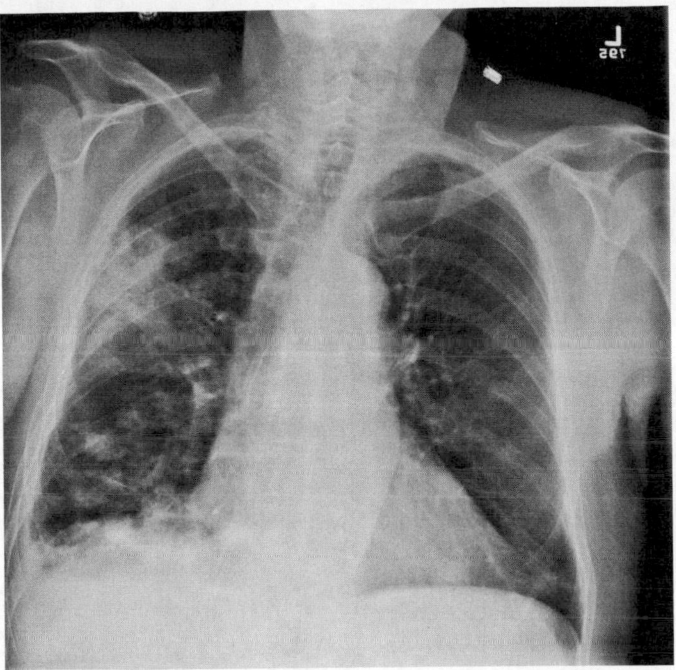

FIGURE 199-1 **Nocardial pneumonia.** A dense infiltrate with a possible cavity and several nodules are apparent in the right lung.

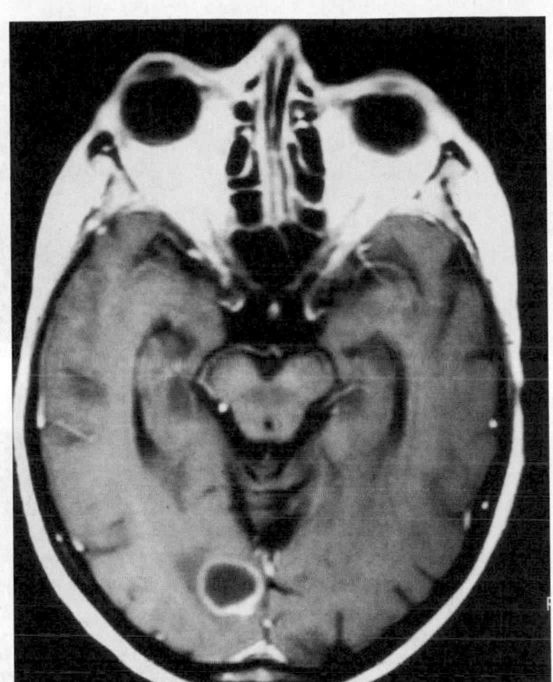

FIGURE 199-3 **Nocardial abscesses** in the right occipital lobe.

nocardial pneumonia. Infiltrates vary in size and are typically dense. Single or multiple nodules are common (Figs. 199-1 and 199-2), sometimes suggesting tumors or metastases. Infiltrates and nodules tend to cavitate (Fig. 199-2). Empyema is present in one-quarter of cases. Co-infection with *Nocardia* and *Mycobacterium tuberculosis* has been reported from regions where tuberculosis is common.

Nocardiosis may spread directly from the lungs to adjacent tissues. Pericarditis, mediastinitis, and the superior vena cava syndrome have all been reported. Nocardial laryngitis, tracheitis, bronchitis, and sinusitis are much less common than pneumonia. In the major airways, disease often presents as a nodular or granulomatous mass. Nocardiae are sometimes isolated from respiratory secretions of persons without apparent nocardial disease, usually individuals who have underlying lung or airway abnormalities.

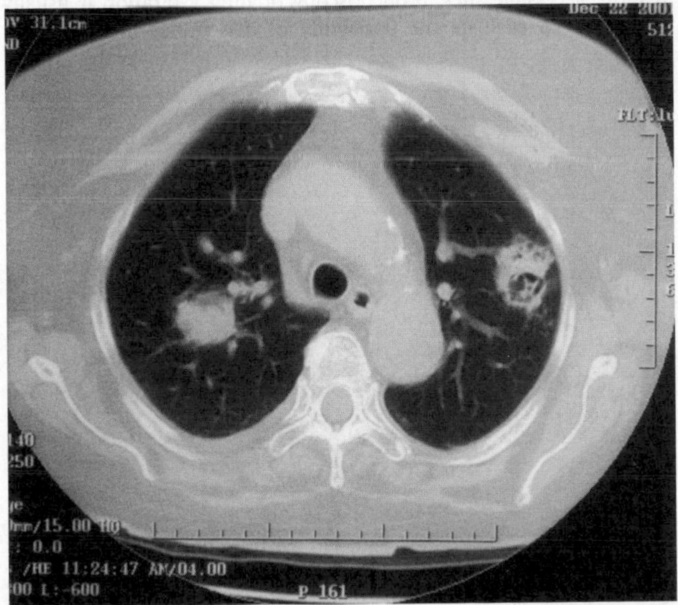

FIGURE 199-2 **Nocardial pneumonia.** A computed tomography scan shows bilateral nodules, with cavitation in the nodule in the left lung.

Extrapulmonary Disease In half of all cases of pulmonary nocardiosis, disease appears outside the lungs. In one-fifth of cases of disseminated disease, lung disease is not apparent. The most common site of dissemination is the brain. Other common sites include the skin and supporting structures, kidneys, bone, muscle, and eye, but almost any organ can be involved. Peritonitis has been reported in patients undergoing peritoneal dialysis. Nocardiae have been recovered from blood in a few cases of pneumonia, disseminated disease, or central venous catheter infection. Nocardial endocarditis occurs rarely and can affect either native or prosthetic valves.

The typical manifestation of extrapulmonary dissemination is a subacute abscess. A minority of abscesses outside the lungs or central nervous system (CNS) form fistulas and discharge small amounts of pus. In CNS infections, brain abscesses are usually supratentorial, are often multiloculated, and may be single or multiple (Fig. 199-3). Brain abscesses tend to burrow into the ventricles or extend out into the subarachnoid space. The symptoms and signs are somewhat more indolent than those of other types of bacterial brain abscess. Meningitis is uncommon and is usually due to spread from a nearby brain abscess. Nocardiae are not easily recovered from cerebrospinal fluid (CSF).

Disease Following Transcutaneous Inoculation Disease that follows transcutaneous nocardial inoculation usually takes one of three forms: cellulitis, lymphocutaneous syndrome, or actinomycetoma.

Cellulitis generally begins 1–3 weeks after a recognized breach of the skin, often with soil contamination. Subacute cellulitis, with pain, swelling, erythema, and warmth, develops over days to weeks. The lesions are usually firm and not fluctuant. Disease may progress to involve underlying muscles, tendons, bones, or joints. Dissemination is rare. *N. brasiliensis* and species in the *N. otitidiscaviarum* complex are most common in cellulitis cases.

Lymphocutaneous disease usually begins as a pyodermatous nodule at the site of inoculation, with central ulceration and purulent or honey-colored drainage. Subcutaneous nodules often appear along lymphatics that drain the primary lesion. Most cases of nocardial lymphocutaneous syndrome are associated with *N. brasiliensis*. Similar disease occurs with other pathogens, most notably *Sporothrix schenckii* (Chap. 243) and *Mycobacterium marinum* (Chap. 204).

Actinomycetoma usually begins with a nodular swelling, sometimes at a site of local trauma. Lesions (Fig. 199-4A) typically develop on the feet or hands but may involve the posterior part of the neck, the upper back, the head, and other sites. The nodule eventually breaks down,

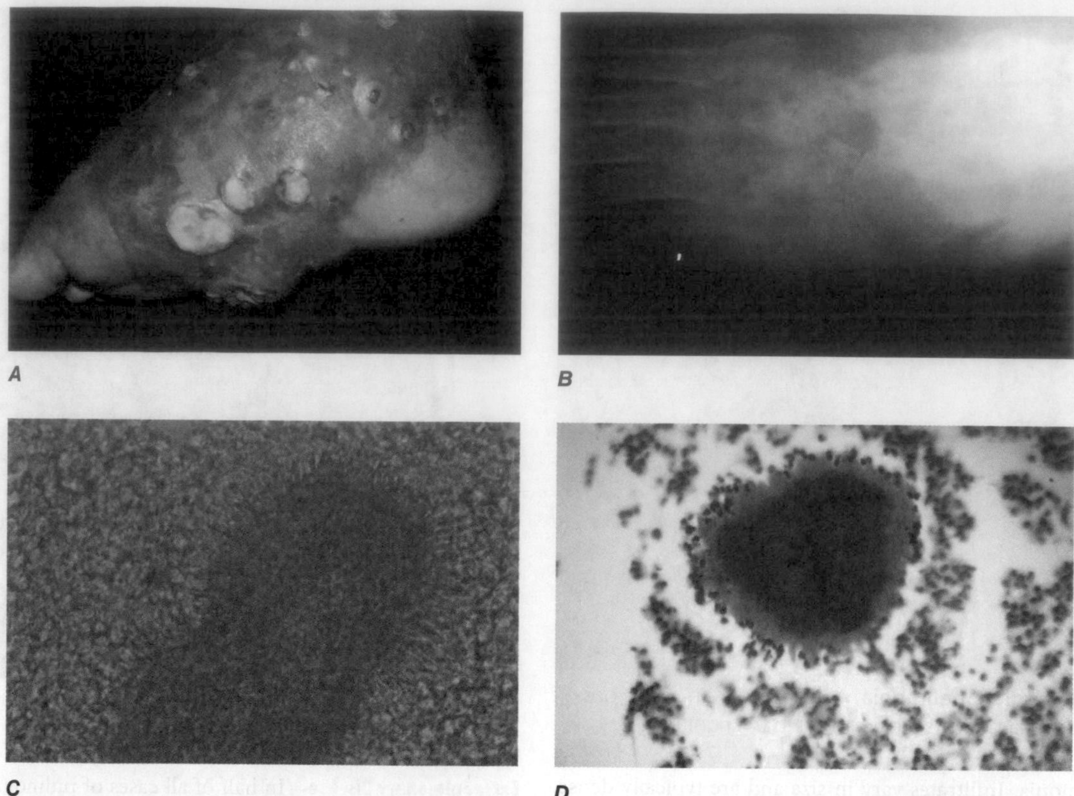

FIGURE 199-4 ***Nocardia brasiliensis* mycetoma. *A.*** Draining sinuses and giant white grains with a seropurulent discharge. ***B.*** Radiography of the foot showing marked soft tissue enlargement and bony lytic lesions. ***C.*** Direct microscopy of grains stained with Lugol's iodine (×40). ***D.*** Periodic acid–Schiff stain of skin biopsy (×40). *(Image provided by Roberto Arenas and Mahreen Ameen, St. John's Institute of Dermatology, Guy's & St Thomas' NHS Trust, London, UK. Reprinted with permission from R Arenas, M Ameen: Lancet Infect Dis 10:66, 2010.)*

and a fistula appears, typically followed by others. The fistulas tend to come and go, with new ones forming as old ones disappear. The discharge is serous or purulent, may be bloody, and often contains 0.1- to 2-mm white granules consisting of masses of mycelia (Figs. 199-4C and 199-4D). The lesions spread slowly along fascial planes to involve adjacent areas of skin, subcutaneous tissue, and bone. Over months or years, there may be extensive deformation of the affected part. Lesions involving soft tissues are only mildly painful; those affecting bones or joints are more so (Fig. 199-4B). Systemic symptoms are absent or minimal. Infection rarely disseminates from actinomycetoma, and lesions on the hands and feet usually cause only local disability. Lesions on the head, neck, and trunk can invade locally to involve deep organs, with consequent severe disability or death.

Eye Infections Nocardia species are uncommon causes of subacute keratitis, usually following eye trauma. Nocardial endophthalmitis can develop after eye surgery. In one series, nocardiae accounted for more than half of culture-proved cases of endophthalmitis after cataract surgery. Endophthalmitis can also occur during disseminated disease. Nocardial infection of lachrymal glands has been reported.

DIAGNOSIS

The first step in diagnosis is examination of sputum or pus for crooked, branching, beaded, gram-positive filaments 1 μm wide and up to 50 μm long (Fig. 199-5). Most nocardiae are acid-fast in direct smears if a weak acid is used for decolorization (e.g., in the modified Kinyoun, Ziehl-Neelsen, and Fite-Faraco methods). The organisms often take up silver stains. Recovery from specimens containing a mixed flora can be improved with selective media (colistin–nalidixic acid agar, modified Thayer-Martin agar, or buffered charcoal–yeast extract agar). Nocardiae grow well on most fungal and mycobacterial media, but procedures used for decontamination of specimens for mycobacterial culture can kill nocardiae and thus should not be used when nocardiae are suspected. Nocardiae grow relatively slowly; colonies may take up to 2 weeks to appear and may not develop their characteristic appearance—white, yellow, or orange, with aerial mycelia and delicate, dichotomously branched substrate mycelia—for up to 4 weeks. Several blood culture systems support nocardial growth, although nocardiae may not be detected for up to 2 weeks. The growth of nocardiae is so different from that of more common pathogens that the laboratory should be alerted when nocardiosis is suspected in order to maximize the likelihood of isolation.

In nocardial pneumonia, sputum smears are often negative. Unless the diagnosis can be made in smear-negative cases by sampling lesions in more accessible sites, bronchoscopy or lung aspiration is usually necessary. To evaluate the possibility of dissemination in patients

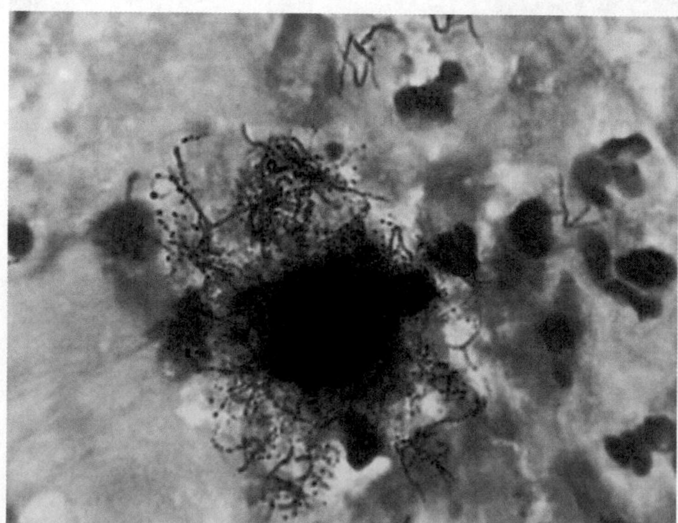

FIGURE 199-5 Gram-stained sputum from a patient with nocardial pneumonia. *(Image provided by Charles Cartwright and Susan Nelson, Hennepin County Medical Center, Minneapolis, MN.)*

with nocardial pneumonia, a careful history should be obtained and a thorough physical examination performed. Suggestive symptoms or signs should be pursued with further diagnostic tests. Computed tomography (CT) or magnetic resonance imaging (MRI) of the head, with and without contrast material, should be undertaken if signs or symptoms suggest brain involvement. Some authorities recommend brain imaging in all cases of pulmonary or disseminated disease. When clinically indicated, CSF or urine should be concentrated and then cultured. Actinomycetoma, eumycetoma (cases involving fungi; Chap. 243), and botryomycosis (cases involving cocci or bacilli, often *Staphylococcus aureus*) are difficult to distinguish clinically but are readily distinguished with microbiologic testing or biopsy. Granules should be sought in any discharge. Suspect particles should be washed in saline, examined microscopically, and cultured. Granules in actinomycetoma cases are usually white, pale yellow, pink, or red. Viewed microscopically, they consist of tight masses of fine filaments (0.5–1 μm wide) radiating outward from a central core (Fig. 199-5). Granules from eumycetoma cases are white, yellow, brown, black, or green. Under the microscope, they appear as masses of broader filaments (2–5 μm wide) encased in a matrix. Granules of botryomycosis consist of loose masses of cocci or bacilli. Organisms can also be seen in wound discharge or histologic specimens. The most reliable way to differentiate among the various organisms associated with mycetoma is by culture.

Isolation of nocardiae from sputum or blood occasionally represents colonization, transient infection, or contamination. In typical cases of respiratory tract colonization, Gram-stained specimens are negative and cultures are only intermittently positive. A positive sputum culture in an immunosuppressed patient usually reflects disease. When nocardiae are isolated from sputum of an immunocompetent patient without apparent nocardial disease, the patient should be observed carefully without treatment. A patient with a host-defense defect that increases the risk of nocardiosis should usually receive antimicrobial treatment.

TREATMENT NOCARDIOSIS

For mild or moderate cases, therapy with drugs known to be effective against most isolates is usually adequate. For severe cases or cases that do not respond promptly to antimicrobial therapy, isolates should be sent to a laboratory experienced with *Nocardia* for identification and susceptibility testing. Identification of an isolate to the species level is accomplished with molecular testing, and susceptibility is assessed with a Clinical Laboratory Standards Institute (CLSI)–approved broth dilution test. Nocardial growth is slower than the growth of most clinically important bacteria, and nocardiae tend to clump in suspension so that susceptibility test endpoints are unusual; thus experience is necessary for reliable results. Because nocardiosis is uncommon, data on the relation between susceptibility test results for specific drugs and clinical outcomes in patients treated with these drugs are meager. Careful clinical monitoring is essential, and consultation with clinicians who have experience with nocardiosis is often needed.

Sulfonamides are the drugs of choice (Tables 199-1 and 199-2). The combination of sulfamethoxazole (SMX) and trimethoprim (TMP) is at least equivalent to a sulfonamide alone and may be slightly more effective, but the combination also poses a modestly greater risk of hematologic toxicity. At the outset, 10–20 mg/kg of TMP and 50–100 mg/kg of SMX are given each day in two divided doses. Later, daily doses can be decreased to as little as 5 mg/kg and 25 mg/kg, respectively. In persons with sulfonamide allergies, desensitization usually allows continuation of therapy with these effective and inexpensive drugs.

Sulfonamide susceptibility testing is difficult. The CLSI standard methodology includes a technique for TMP-SMX but not for a sulfonamide alone. Reported rates of sulfonamide susceptibility have varied widely, and controversy has ensued about the reliability of sulfonamides for therapy. However, clinical responses to appropriate sulfonamide treatment are nearly always satisfactory. Sulfonamides remain the drugs of choice in nearly all cases.

TABLE 199-2 TREATMENT DURATION FOR NOCARDIOSIS

Disease	Duration
Pulmonary or systemic	
Intact host defenses	6–12 months
Deficient host defenses	12 months[a]
CNS disease	12 months[b]
Cellulitis, lymphocutaneous syndrome	2 months
Osteomyelitis, arthritis, laryngitis, sinusitis	4 months
Actinomycetoma	6–12 months after clinical cure
Keratitis	Topical: until apparent cure
	Systemic: until 2–4 months after apparent cure

[a]In some patients with AIDS and CD4+ T lymphocyte counts of <200/μL or with chronic granulomatous disease, therapy for pulmonary or systemic disease must be continued indefinitely. [b]If all apparent CNS disease has been excised, the duration of therapy may be reduced to 6 months.

Clinical experience with other oral drugs is limited. Minocycline (100–200 mg twice a day) is often effective; other tetracyclines are usually less effective. Linezolid is active against all species in vitro and in vivo, but adverse effects are common with long-term use. Tigecycline appears to be active in vitro against some species, but little clinical experience has been reported. Amoxicillin (875 mg) combined with clavulanic acid (125 mg), given twice a day, has been effective but should be avoided in cases involving strains of the *N. nova* complex, in which clavulanate induces β-lactamase production. Among the quinolones, moxifloxacin and gemifloxacin appear to be most active.

Amikacin, the best-established parenteral drug except in cases involving the *N. transvalensis* complex, is given in doses of 5–7.5 mg/kg every 12 h or 15 mg/kg every 24 h. Serum drug levels should be monitored during prolonged therapy in patients with diminished renal function and in the elderly. Ceftriaxone and imipenem are usually effective except as indicated in Table 199-1.

Patients with severe disease are initially treated with a combination including TMP-SMX, amikacin, and ceftriaxone or imipenem. Clinical improvement is usually noticeable after 1–2 weeks of therapy but may take longer, especially with CNS disease. After definite clinical improvement, therapy can be continued with a single oral drug, usually TMP-SMX. Some experts use two or more drugs for the entire course of therapy, but whether multiple drugs are better than a single agent is not known, and additional drugs increase the risk of toxicity. In patients with nocardiosis who need immunosuppressive therapy for an underlying disease or prevention of transplant rejection, immunosuppressive therapy should be continued.

Use of SMX and TMP in high-risk populations to prevent *Pneumocystis* disease or urinary tract infections appears to reduce but not eliminate the risk of nocardiosis. The incidence of nocardiosis is low enough that prophylaxis solely to prevent this disease is not recommended.

Surgical management of nocardial disease is similar to that of other bacterial diseases. Brain abscesses should be aspirated, drained, or excised if the diagnosis is unclear, if an abscess is large and accessible, or if an abscess fails to respond to chemotherapy. Small or inaccessible brain abscesses should be treated medically; clinical improvement should be noticeable within 1–2 weeks. Brain imaging should be repeated to document the resolution of lesions, although abatement on images often lags behind clinical improvement.

Antimicrobial therapy usually suffices for nocardial actinomycetoma. In deep or extensive cases, drainage or excision of heavily involved tissue may facilitate healing, but structure and function should be preserved whenever possible. Keratitis is treated with topical sulfonamide or amikacin drops plus a sulfonamide or an alternative drug given by mouth.

Nocardial infections tend to relapse (particularly in patients with chronic granulomatous disease), and long courses of antimicrobial therapy are necessary (Table 199-2). If disease is unusually extensive or if the response to therapy is slow, the recommendations in Table 199-2 should be exceeded.

With appropriate treatment, the mortality rate for pulmonary or disseminated nocardiosis outside the CNS should be <5%. CNS disease carries a higher mortality rate. Patients should be followed carefully for at least 6 months after therapy has ended.

200 Actinomycosis and Whipple's Disease

Thomas A. Russo

Actinomycosis and Whipple's disease share characteristics that confound even the skilled diagnostician. Because both diseases are uncommon, the physician's personal experience with their clinical presentations is limited. The laboratory identification of the etiologic agents from the order Actinomycetales is not routine. Thus they remain a diagnostic challenge. However, both of these chronic infections are curable, usually with medical therapy alone. Therefore, an awareness of the full spectrum of these diseases, prompting clinical suspicion, can expedite their diagnosis and treatment and minimize unnecessary surgical interventions (especially with actinomycosis), morbidity, and mortality risk.

ACTINOMYCOSIS

Actinomycosis is an indolent, slowly progressive infection caused by anaerobic or microaerophilic bacteria, primarily of the genus *Actinomyces*, that colonize the mouth, colon, and vagina. Mucosal disruption may lead to infection at virtually any site in the body. In vivo growth of actinomycetes usually results in the formation of characteristic clumps called *grains* or *sulfur granules*. The clinical presentations of actinomycosis are myriad. Common in the preantibiotic era, actinomycosis has diminished in incidence, as has its timely recognition. Actinomycosis has been called the most misdiagnosed disease, and it has been said that no disease is so often missed by experienced clinicians.

Three "classic" clinical presentations that should prompt consideration of this unique infection are (1) the combination of chronicity, progression across tissue boundaries, and mass-like features (mimicking malignancy, with which it is often confused); (2) the development of a sinus tract, which may spontaneously resolve and recur; and (3) a refractory or relapsing infection after a short course of therapy, since cure of established actinomycosis requires prolonged treatment.

ETIOLOGIC AGENTS

Actinomycosis is most commonly caused by *A. israelii, A. naeslundii, A. odontolyticus, A. viscosus, A. meyeri, and A. gerencseriae*. Most if not all actinomycotic infections are polymicrobial. *Aggregatibacter (Actinobacillus) actinomycetemcomitans, Eikenella corrodens*, Enterobacteriaceae, and species of *Fusobacterium, Bacteroides, Capnocytophaga, Staphylococcus*, and *Streptococcus* are commonly isolated with actinomycetes in various combinations, depending on the site of infection. Their contribution to the pathogenesis of actinomycosis is uncertain.

Comparative 16S rRNA gene sequencing has led to the identification of an ever-expanding list of *Actinomyces* species and a reclassification of some species to other genera. At present, 46 species and 2 subspecies have been recognized (*www.bacterio.cict.fr/a/actinomyces.html*). *A. europaeus, A. neuii, A. radingae, A. graevenitzii, A. turicensis, A. cardiffensis, A. houstonensis, A. hongkongensis, A. lingnae, A. massiliensis, A. timonensis*, and *A. funkei* as well as two former *Actinomyces* species—*Arcanobacterium pyogenes* and *Arcanobacterium bernardiae*—are additional causes of human actinomycosis, albeit not always with a "classic" presentation.

EPIDEMIOLOGY

Actinomycosis has no geographic boundaries and occurs throughout life, with a peak incidence in the middle decades. Males have a threefold higher incidence than females, possibly because of poorer dental hygiene and/or more frequent trauma. Improved dental hygiene and the initiation of antimicrobial treatment before actinomycosis fully develops have probably contributed to a decrease in incidence since the advent of antibiotics. Individuals who do not seek or have access to health care, those who have an intrauterine contraceptive device (IUCD) in place for a prolonged period (see "Pelvic Disease," below), and those who receive bisphosphonate treatment (see "Oral-Cervicofacial Disease," below) are probably at higher risk.

PATHOGENESIS AND PATHOLOGY

The etiologic agents of actinomycosis are members of the normal oral flora and are often cultured from the bronchi, the gastrointestinal tract, and the female genital tract. The critical step in the development of actinomycosis is disruption of the mucosal barrier. Local infection may ensue. Once established, actinomycosis spreads contiguously in a slow, progressive manner, ignoring tissue planes. Although acute inflammation may initially develop at the infection site, the hallmark of actinomycosis is the characteristic chronic, indolent phase manifested by lesions that usually appear as single or multiple indurations. Central necrosis consisting of neutrophils and sulfur granules develops and is virtually diagnostic. The fibrotic walls of the mass are typically described as "wooden." The responsible bacterial and/or host factors have not been identified. Over time, sinus tracts to the skin, adjacent organs, or bone may develop. In rare instances, distant hematogenous seeding may occur. As mentioned above, these unique features of actinomycosis mimic malignancy, with which it is often confused.

Foreign bodies appear to facilitate infection. This association most frequently involves IUCDs. Reports have described an association of actinomycosis with HIV infection; transplantation; common variable immunodeficiency; chronic granulomatous disease; treatment with infliximab, glucocorticoids, or bisphosphonates; and radio- or chemotherapy. Ulcerative mucosal infections (e.g., by herpes simplex virus or cytomegalovirus) may facilitate disease development.

CLINICAL MANIFESTATIONS

Oral-Cervicofacial Disease Actinomycosis occurs most frequently at an oral, cervical, or facial site, usually as a soft tissue swelling, abscess, or mass lesion that is often mistaken for a neoplasm. The angle of the jaw is generally involved, but a diagnosis of actinomycosis should be considered with any mass lesion or relapsing infection in the head and neck (Chap. 44). Radiation therapy and especially bisphosphonate treatment have been recognized as contributing to an increasing incidence of actinomycotic infection of the mandible and maxilla (Fig. 200-1). Canaliculitis (also commonly due to *Propionibacterium propionicum*), otitis, and sinusitis also can develop. Pain, fever, and leukocytosis are variably reported. Contiguous extension to the cranium, cervical spine, or thorax is a potential sequela.

Thoracic Disease Thoracic actinomycosis, which may be facilitated by foreign material, usually follows an indolent progressive course, with involvement of the pulmonary parenchyma and/or the pleural space. Chest pain, fever, and weight loss are common. A cough, when present, is variably productive. The usual radiographic finding is either a mass lesion or pneumonia. On CT, central areas of low attenuation and ring-like rim enhancement may be seen. Cavitary disease or mediastinal or hilar adenopathy may develop. More than 50% of cases include pleural thickening, effusion, or empyema (Fig. 200-2). Rarely, pulmonary nodules or endobronchial lesions occur. Lesions suggestive of actinomycosis include those that cross fissures or pleura; extend into the mediastinum, contiguous bone, or chest wall; or are associated with a sinus tract. In the absence of these findings, thoracic actinomycosis is usually mistaken for a neoplasm or pneumonia due to more usual causes.

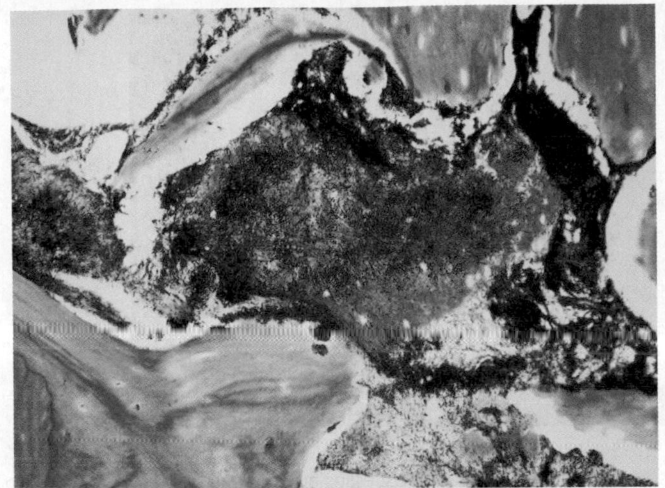

FIGURE 200-1 Bisphosphonate-associated maxillary osteomyelitis due to *A. viscosus*. A sulfur granule is seen within the bone. *(Reprinted with permission from NH Naik, TA Russo: Bisphosphonate related osteonecrosis of the jaw: The role of Actinomyces. Clin Infect Dis 49:1729, 2009. © 2009 University of Chicago Press.)*

Mediastinal infection is uncommon, usually arising from thoracic extension but rarely from perforation of the esophagus, trauma, or extension of head and neck or abdominal disease. The structures within the mediastinum and the heart can be involved in various combinations; consequently, the possible presentations are diverse. Primary endocarditis (in which *A. neuii* has been increasingly described) and isolated disease of the breast occur.

Abdominal Disease Abdominal actinomycosis poses a great diagnostic challenge. Months or years usually pass from the inciting event (e.g., appendicitis, diverticulitis, peptic ulcer disease, spillage of gall stones or bile during laparoscopic cholecystectomy, foreign-body perforation, bowel surgery, or ascension from IUCD-associated pelvic disease) to clinical recognition. Because of the flow of peritoneal fluid and/or the direct extension of primary disease, virtually any abdominal organ, region, or space can be involved. The disease usually presents as an abscess, a mass, or a mixed lesion that is often fixed to underlying tissue and mistaken for a tumor. On CT, enhancement is most often heterogeneous and adjacent bowel is thickened. Sinus tracts to the abdominal wall, to the perianal region, or between the bowel and other organs may develop and mimic inflammatory bowel disease (Chap. 351). Recurrent disease or a wound or fistula that fails to heal suggests actinomycosis.

Hepatic infection usually presents as one or more abscesses or masses (Fig. 200-3). Isolated disease presumably develops via hematogenous seeding from cryptic foci. Imaging and percutaneous techniques have resulted in improved diagnosis and treatment.

All levels of the urogenital tract can be infected. Renal disease usually presents as pyelonephritis and/or renal and perinephric abscess. Bladder involvement, usually due to extension of pelvic disease, may result in ureteral obstruction or fistulas to bowel, skin, or uterus. *Actinomyces* can be detected in urine with appropriate stains and cultures.

Pelvic Disease Actinomycotic involvement of the pelvis occurs most commonly in association with an IUCD. When an IUCD is in place or has recently been removed, pelvic symptoms should prompt consideration of actinomycosis. The risk, although not quantified, appears small. The disease rarely develops when the IUCD has been in place for <1 year, but the risk increases with time. Actinomycosis can also present months after IUCD removal. Symptoms are typically indolent; fever, weight loss, abdominal pain, and abnormal vaginal bleeding or discharge are the most common. The earliest stage of disease—often endometritis—commonly progresses to pelvic masses or a tuboovarian abscess (Fig. 200-4). Unfortunately, because the diagnosis is often delayed, a "frozen pelvis" mimicking malignancy or endometriosis can develop by the time of recognition. Ca125 levels may be elevated, further contributing to misdiagnosis.

Actinomyces-like organisms (ALOs), which are identified in Papanicolaou-stained specimens in (on average) 7% of women using an IUCD, have a low positive predictive value for diagnosis. Nonetheless, although the risk appears small, the consequences of infection are significant. Therefore, until more quantitative data become available, it seems prudent to remove the IUCD in the presence of symptoms that cannot be accounted for, regardless of whether ALOs are detected, and—if advanced disease is excluded—to initiate a 14-day course of empirical treatment for possible early endometritis. The detection of ALOs in the asymptomatic patient warrants education and close follow-up but not removal of the IUCD unless a suitable contraceptive alternative is agreed on.

Central Nervous System Disease Actinomycosis of the central nervous system (CNS) is rare. Single or multiple brain abscesses are most common. An abscess usually appears on CT as a ring-enhancing lesion with a thick wall that may be irregular or nodular. Magnetic resonance perfusion and spectroscopy findings have also been described, as have primary meningitis, epidural or subdural space infection, and cavernous sinus syndrome.

Musculoskeletal and Soft Tissue Infection Actinomycotic infection of bone and joints is usually due to adjacent soft-tissue infection but may be associated with trauma (e.g., fracture of the mandible), injections,

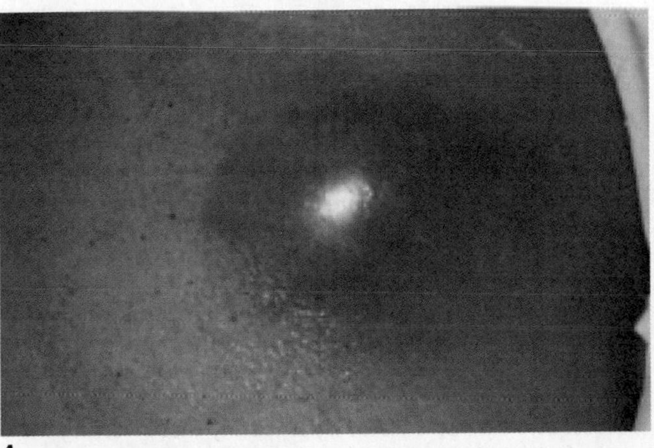

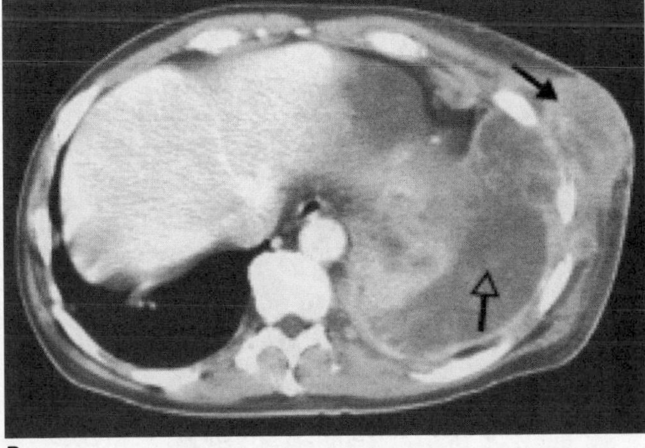

FIGURE 200-2 Thoracic actinomycosis. *A.* A chest wall mass from extension of pulmonary infection. ***B.*** Pulmonary infection is complicated by empyema (*open arrow*) and extension to the chest wall (*closed arrow*). *(Courtesy of Dr. C. B. Hsiao, Division of Infectious Diseases, Department of Medicine, State University of New York at Buffalo.)*

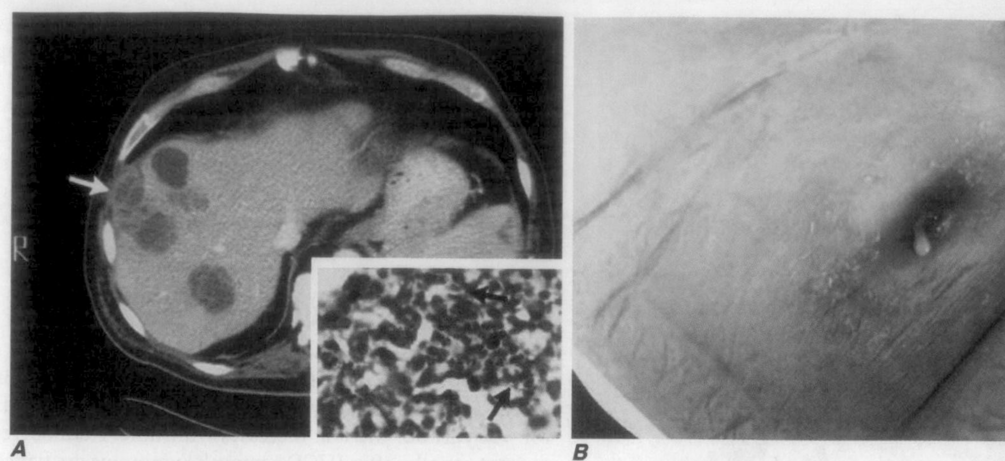

FIGURE 200-3 Hepatic-splenic actinomycosis. ***A.*** Computed tomogram showing multiple hepatic abscesses and a small splenic lesion due to *A. israelii.* Arrow indicates extension outside the liver. *Inset:* Gram's stain of abscess fluid demonstrating beaded filamentous gram-positive rods. ***B.*** Subsequent formation of a sinus tract. *(Reprinted with permission from Saad M: Actinomyces hepatic abscess with cutaneous fistula. N Engl J Med 353:e16, 2005. © 2005 Massachusetts Medical Society. All rights reserved.)*

surgery, osteoradionecrosis and bisphosphonate osteonecrosis (limited to mandibular and maxillary bones), or hematogenous spread. Because of slow disease progression, new bone formation and bone destruction are seen concomitantly. Infection of an extremity is uncommon and is usually a result of trauma. Skin, subcutaneous tissue, muscle, and bone (with periostitis or acute or chronic osteomyelitis) are involved alone or in various combinations. Cutaneous sinus tracts frequently develop.

Disseminated Disease Hematogenous dissemination of disease from any location rarely results in multiple-organ involvement. *A. meyeri* is most commonly involved. The lungs and liver are most commonly affected, with the presentation of multiple nodules mimicking disseminated malignancy. The clinical presentation may be surprisingly indolent given the extent of disease.

DIAGNOSIS

The diagnosis of actinomycosis is rarely considered. All too often, actinomycosis is first mentioned by the pathologist after extensive surgery. Since medical therapy alone is frequently sufficient for cure, the challenge for the clinician is to consider the possibility of actinomycosis, to diagnose it in the least invasive fashion, and to avoid unnecessary surgery. The clinical and radiographic presentations that suggest actinomycosis are discussed above. Of note, hypermetabolism has been demonstrated by ^{18}F-fluorodeoxyglucose positron emission tomography (FDG-PET) in actinomycotic disease. Aspirations and biopsies (with or without CT or ultrasound guidance) are being used successfully to obtain clinical material for diagnosis, although surgery may be required. The diagnosis is most commonly made by microscopic identification of sulfur granules (an in vivo matrix of bacteria, calcium phosphate, and host material) in pus or tissues. Occasionally, these granules are identified grossly from draining sinus tracts or pus. Although sulfur granules are a defining characteristic of actinomycosis, granules also are found in mycetoma (Chaps. 199 and 243) and botryomycosis (a chronic suppurative bacterial infection of soft tissue or, in rare cases, visceral tissue that produces clumps of bacteria resembling granules). These entities can easily be differentiated from actinomycosis with appropriate histopathologic and microbiologic studies. Microbiologic identification of actinomycetes is often precluded by prior antimicrobial therapy or failure to perform appropriate microbiologic cultures. For optimal yield, the avoidance of even a single dose of antibiotics is mandatory. Primary isolation usually requires 5–7 days under anaerobic conditions but may take as long as 2–4 weeks. Although not routinely used, 16S rRNA gene amplification and sequencing have been successfully applied to increase diagnostic sensitivity and specificity. Because actinomycetes are components of the normal oral and genital-tract flora, their identification in the absence of sulfur granules in sputum, bronchial washings, and cervicovaginal secretions is of little significance.

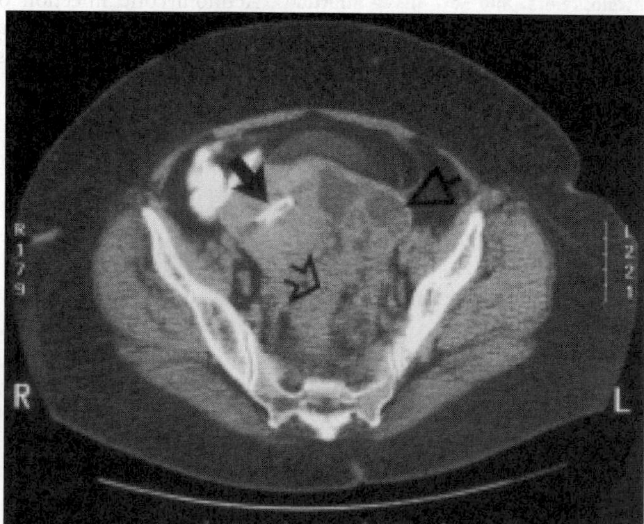

FIGURE 200-4 Computed tomogram showing pelvic actinomycosis associated with an intrauterine contraceptive device. The device is encased by endometrial fibrosis (*solid arrow*); also visible are paraendometrial fibrosis (*open triangular arrowhead*) and an area of suppuration (*open arrow*).

TREATMENT ACTINOMYCOSIS

Decisions about treatment are based on the collective clinical experience of the past 65 years. Actinomycosis requires prolonged treatment with high doses of antimicrobial agents; suitable antimicrobial agents and those deemed unreliable are listed in Table 200-1. The need for intensive treatment is presumably due to the drugs' poor penetration of the thick-walled masses common in this infection and/or the sulfur granules themselves, which may represent a biofilm. Although therapy must be individualized, the IV administration of 18–24 million units of penicillin daily for 2–6 weeks, followed by oral therapy with penicillin or amoxicillin (total duration, 6–12 months), is a reasonable guideline for serious infections and bulky disease. Less extensive disease, particularly that involving the oral-cervicofacial region, may be cured with a shorter course. If therapy is extended beyond the resolution of measurable disease, the risk of relapse—a clinical hallmark of this infection—will be minimized; CT and MRI are generally the most sensitive and objective techniques

TABLE 200-1 APPROPRIATE AND INAPPROPRIATE ANTIBIOTIC THERAPY FOR ACTINOMYCOSIS[a]

Category	Agent
Extensive successful clinical experience[b]	Penicillin: 3–4 million units IV q4h[c]
	Amoxicillin: 500 mg PO q6h
	Erythromycin: 500–1000 mg IV q6h or 500 mg PO q6h
	Tetracycline: 500 mg PO q6h
	Doxycycline: 100 mg IV or PO q12h
	Minocycline: 100 mg IV or PO q12h
	Clindamycin: 900 mg IV q8h or 300–450 mg PO q6h
Anecdotal successful clinical experience	Ceftriaxone[c]
	Ceftizoxime
	Imipenem-cilastatin
	Piperacillin-tazobactam
Agents that should be avoided	Metronidazole
	Aminoglycosides
	Oxacillin
	Dicloxacillin
	Cephalexin
Agents predicted to be efficacious on the basis of in vitro activity	Moxifloxacin
	Vancomycin
	Linezolid
	Quinupristin-dalfopristin
	Ertapenem[c]
	Azithromycin[c]

[a]Additional coverage for concomitant "companion" bacteria may be required. [b]Controlled evaluations have not been performed. Dose and duration require individualization depending on the host, site, and extent of infection. As a general rule, a maximal parenteral antimicrobial dose for 2–6 weeks followed by oral therapy, for a total duration of 6–12 months, is required for serious infections and bulky disease, whereas a shorter course may suffice for less extensive disease, particularly in the oral-cervicofacial region. Monitoring the impact of therapy with CT or MRI is advisable when appropriate. [c]These agents can be considered for at-home parenteral therapy; penicillin requires a continuous infusion pump.

by which to accomplish this goal. A similar approach is reasonable for immunocompromised patients, although refractory disease has been described in HIV-infected individuals. Although the role played by "companion" microbes in actinomycosis is unclear, many isolates are pathogens in their own right, and a regimen covering these organisms during the initial treatment course is reasonable.

Combined medical-surgical therapy is still advocated in some reports. However, an increasing body of literature now supports an initial attempt at cure with medical therapy alone, even in extensive disease. CT and MRI should be used to monitor the response to therapy. In most cases, either surgery can be avoided or a less extensive procedure can be used. This approach is particularly valuable in sparing critical organs, such as the bladder or the reproductive organs in women of childbearing age. For a well-defined abscess, percutaneous drainage in combination with medical therapy is a reasonable approach. When a critical location is involved (e.g., the epidural space, the CNS), when there is significant hemoptysis, or when suitable medical therapy fails, surgical intervention may be appropriate. In the absence of optimal data, the combination of a prolonged course of antimicrobial therapy and resection—at least of necrotic bone for bisphosphonate-related osteonecrosis of the jaw (BRONJ)—is a reasonable approach.

WHIPPLE'S DISEASE

Whipple's disease, a chronic multiorgan infection caused by *Tropheryma whipplei*, was first described in 1907. The long-held belief that Whipple's disease is an infection was supported by observations on its responsiveness to antimicrobial therapy in the 1950s and the identification of bacilli via electron microscopy in small-bowel biopsy specimens in the 1960s. This hypothesis was finally confirmed by amplification and sequencing of a partial 16S rRNA polymerase chain reaction (PCR)–generated amplicon from duodenal tissue in 1991. The subsequent successful cultivation of *T. whipplei* enabled whole-genome sequencing and the development of additional diagnostic tests. The development of PCR-based diagnostics has broadened our understanding of both the epidemiology and the clinical syndromes attributable to *T. whipplei*. Exposure to *T. whipplei*, which appears to be much more common than has been appreciated, can be followed by asymptomatic carriage, acute disease, or chronic infection. Chronic infection (Whipple's disease) is a rare development after exposure. "Classic" Whipple's disease is manifested variably by a combination of arthralgias/arthritis, weight loss, chronic diarrhea, abdominal pain, and fever; less commonly, involvement at sites other than the gastrointestinal tract is documented. Acute infection and chronic organ disease in the absence of intestinal involvement (see "Isolated Infection," below) are described with increasing frequency. Since untreated Whipple's disease is often fatal and delayed diagnosis may lead to irreparable organ damage (e.g., in the CNS), knowledge of the clinical scenarios in which Whipple's should be considered and of an appropriate diagnostic strategy is mandatory.

ETIOLOGIC AGENT

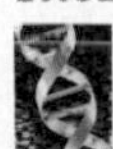

T. whipplei is a weakly staining gram-positive bacillus. Genomic sequence data have revealed that the organism has a small (<1-megabase) chromosome, with many biosynthetic pathways absent or incomplete. This finding is consistent with a host-dependent intracellular pathogen or a pathogen that requires a nutritionally rich extracellular environment. A genotyping scheme based on a variable region has disclosed more than 70 genotypes (GTs) to date. GTs 1 and 3 are most commonly reported, but all GTs appear to be capable of causing similar clinical syndromes.

EPIDEMIOLOGY

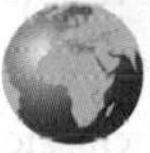

Whipple's disease is rare but has been increasingly recognized since the advent of PCR-based diagnostic tools. It occurs in all parts of the globe, with an incidence presently estimated at 1 case per 1 million patient-years. Seroprevalence studies indicate that ~50% of Western Europeans and ~75% of Africans from rural Senegal have been exposed to *T. whipplei*. A predilection for chronic disease has been observed in middle-aged Caucasian men. Males are infected five to eight times more frequently than females. To date, no clear animal or environmental reservoir has been demonstrated. However, the organism has been identified by PCR in sewage water and human feces. Workers with direct exposure to sewage are more likely to be asymptomatically colonized than controls, a pattern suggesting fecal-oral spread. Recent data support oral-oral or fecal-oral spread among family members. Further, the development of acute *T. whipplei* pneumonia in children raises the possibility of droplet or airborne transmission.

PATHOGENESIS AND PATHOLOGY

Since rates of exposure to *T. whipplei* appear to be much higher (e.g., ~50% in Western Europe, as stated above) than rates of chronic disease development (0.00001%), it has been hypothesized that chronically infected individuals possess a subtle host-defense abnormality that does not place them at risk for non–*T. whipplei* infection. The HLA alleles DRB1*13 and DQB1*06 may be associated with an increased risk of infection. Chronic infection results in a general state of immunosuppression characterized by low CD4+ T cell counts, high levels of interleukin 10 production, increased activity of regulatory T cells, alternative activation of macrophages with diminished antimicrobial activity (M2 polarization) and ensuing apoptosis, and blunted development of *T. whipplei*–specific T cells. Immunosuppressive glucocorticoid treatment or anti–tumor necrosis factor α therapy appears to accelerate progression of disease. Recently, asymptomatic HIV-infected individuals were found to have significantly higher levels of *T. whipplei* sequence in bronchoalveolar lavage fluid (BALF) than did non-HIV-infected individuals, and these levels decreased with antiretroviral therapy. A weak humoral response, perhaps due to bacterial glycosylation in patients with chronic disease, appears to differentiate persons who clear the bacillus from asymptomatic carriers. In the initiation of chronic infection, the relative importance of the host's genetic background versus the modulation of the host response by *T. whipplei* is unknown.

T. whipplei has a tropism for myeloid cells, which it invades and in which it can avoid being killed. Infiltration of infected tissue by large numbers of foamy macrophages is a characteristic finding. In the intestine, villi are flat and wide with dilated lacteals. Involvement of lymphatic or hepatic tissue may manifest as noncaseating granulomas that can mimic sarcoid.

CLINICAL MANIFESTATIONS

Asymptomatic Colonization/Carriage Studies using primarily PCR have detected *T. whipplei* sequence in stool, saliva, duodenal tissue, and (rarely) blood in the absence of symptoms. Although prevalence rates are still being defined, in Western European countries, detection in saliva (0.2%) is less common than that in stool (1–11%) and appears to occur only with concomitant fecal carriage. The prevalence of fecal carriage is elevated in individuals with exposure to waste water or sewage (12–26%). However, in rural Senegal, 44% of children age 2–10 had *T. whipplei* detected in fecal samples. The duration of carriage at these sites is still being examined but can be at least 1 year. It is not known how often the carrier state is associated with acute infection, but evolution into chronic disease is uncommon. Bacterial loads are lighter in asymptomatic carriage than in active disease.

Acute Infection *T. whipplei* has been implicated as a cause of acute gastroenteritis in children. It was also detected via PCR in the blood of 6.4% of febrile patients (primarily children) from two villages in Senegal, often with concomitant cough and rhinorrhea. Further, *T. whipplei* has been implicated as a cause of acute pneumonia in the United States and France. These data suggest that primary acquisition can result in symptomatic pulmonary or intestinal infection, which may be more common than has been thought, and only rarely results in chronic disease.

Chronic Infection • *"CLASSIC" WHIPPLE'S DISEASE* So-called classic Whipple's disease was the initial clinical syndrome recognized, with consequent identification of *T. whipplei*. This chronic infection is defined by involvement of the duodenum and/or jejunum that develops over years. In most individuals, the initial phase of disease manifests primarily as intermittent, occasionally chronic and destructive migratory oligo- or polyarthralgias/seronegative arthritis. Spondylitis, sacroiliitis, and prosthetic hip infection also have been described. This initial stage is often confused with a variety of rheumatologic disorders and, on average, lasts 6–8 years before gastrointestinal symptoms commence. Treatment of presumed inflammatory arthritis with immunosuppressive agents (e.g., glucocorticoids, tumor necrosis factor α antagonists) can accelerate progression of the disease process. Alternatively, antimicrobial therapy used for another indication may reduce symptoms. In fact, the modulation of symptoms in these settings should prompt consideration of Whipple's disease. The intestinal symptoms that develop in the majority of cases are characterized by diarrhea with accompanying weight loss and may be associated with fever and abdominal pain. Diagnostic misdirection can be caused by co-infection with *Giardia lamblia*, which is occasionally identified. Occult gastrointestinal blood loss, hepatosplenomegaly, and ascites are less common. Anemia and hypereosinophilia may be detected. Rheumatoid factor and antinuclear antibody tests are usually negative. The most common finding on abdominal CT is mesenteric and/or retroperitoneal lymphadenopathy. The endoscopic or video capsule observation of pale, yellow, or shaggy mucosa with erythema or ulceration past the first portion of the duodenum suggests Whipple's disease (Fig. 200-5). In addition to rheumatologic and proximal intestinal disease, neurologic (6–63%), cardiac (17–55%), pulmonary (10–40%), lymphatic (10%), ocular (5–10%), dermal (1–5%), and (in rare instances) other sites are variably involved in classic Whipple's disease.

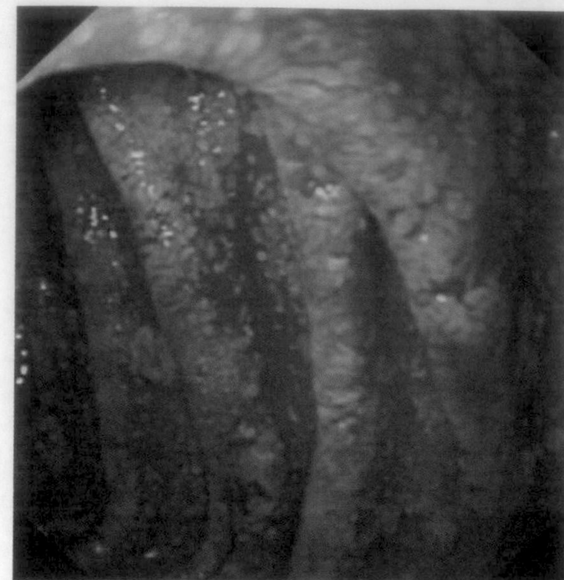

FIGURE 200-5 Endoscopic view of the jejunal mucosa demonstrating a thickened, granular mucosa and "white spots" due to dilated lacteals. *(Reprinted with permission from J Bureš et al: Whipple's disease: Our own experience and review of the literature. Gastroenterol Res Pract, 2013. http://dx.doi.org/10.1155/2013/478349.)*

Neurologic disease Asymptomatic neurologic involvement in Whipple's disease has been documented by PCR-based detection in cerebrospinal fluid (CSF). A variety of neurologic manifestations have been reported, the most common of which are cognitive changes progressing to dementia; personality, mood, and sleep-cycle disorders; hypothalamic involvement; and supranuclear ophthalmoplegia. In addition to the latter, neuro-ophthalmologic manifestations of Whipple's disease include supranuclear gaze palsy, oculomasticatory and oculofacial myorhythmia (highly suggestive of Whipple's), nystagmus, and retrobulbar neuritis. Focal neurologic presentations (dependent on lesion location), seizures, ataxia, meningitis, encephalitis, hydrocephalus, myelopathy, and distal polyneuropathy also have been described. Neurologic sequelae occur with CNS disease, and the mortality risk is significant.

MRI results may be normal. Identified lesions (solitary or multifocal) are usually T2 and fluid-attenuated inversion recovery (FLAIR) hyperintense and may enhance with gadolinium. Findings are myriad and not diagnostic, but the limbic system is commonly involved. FDG-PET may reveal increased uptake. CSF analysis may be abnormal; leukocytosis (generally lymphocyte-predominant) and an elevated protein concentration are common. A low CSF glucose level has been reported.

Cardiac disease Endocarditis, which is increasingly recognized in Whipple's disease, presents as culture-negative infection and/or congestive heart failure; hypotension occurs rarely. Embolic events or various arrhythmias may also be noted. Fever is often absent, and Duke clinical criteria are rarely met. Vegetations are identified by echocardiography in 50–75% of cases. All valves, alone or in combination, can be affected; most commonly involved are the aortic and mitral valves. Preexisting valvular disease is found in only a minority of cases, although infection of bioprosthetic valves has been described. Mural, myocardial, or pericardial disease also occurs alone or in combination with valvular involvement. Constrictive pericarditis develops infrequently.

Pulmonary disease Some combination of interstitial disease, nodules, parenchymal infiltrate, and pleural effusion is observed. The clinical significance of *T. whipplei* dominating sequence reads in BALF from HIV-infected individuals is unresolved.

Lymphatic disease Mesenteric and retroperitoneal lymphadenopathy are common with intestinal disease, and mediastinal adenopathy may be associated with pulmonary infection. Peripheral adenopathy is less common.

Ocular disease (non-neuro-ophthalmologic) Uveitis is the most common form of ocular disease, usually presenting as a change in vision or "floaters." Anterior (anterior chamber), intermediate (vitreous), and posterior (retina/choroid) uveitis can occur alone or in combination. Postoperative acute or chronic ocular Whipple's disease has been described in association with local or systemic glucocorticoid use; its detection in this setting raises the possibility that asymptomatic or subclinical disease has been unmasked. Keratitis and crystalline keratopathy also have been reported. Patients may be misdiagnosed with sarcoid or Behçet's disease prior to the recognition of Whipple's.

Dermatologic disease Skin hyperpigmentation, particularly in light-exposed areas in the absence of adrenal dysfunction, should be suggestive of Whipple's disease. A variety of other cutaneous manifestations have been described, including erythematous macular lesions, nonthrombocytopenic purpura, subcutaneous nodules, and hyperkeratosis.

Miscellaneous sites Thyroid, renal, testicular, epididymal, gallbladder, skeletal muscle, and bone marrow involvement have all been described. In fact, almost any organ can be involved in classic Whipple's disease, with varying frequency, variable combinations, and myriad signs and symptoms. As a result, Whipple's disease should be considered in the setting of a chronic multisystemic process. Despite its rarity, the combination of rheumatologic and intestinal disease with weight loss, with or without neurologic and cardiac involvement, warrants heightened suspicion.

ISOLATED INFECTION This entity has been defined as infection in the absence of intestinal symptoms, although an occasional small-bowel biopsy may be PCR-positive in this setting. "Isolated infection" is something of a misnomer since multiple nonintestinal sites of *T. whipplei* infection are not uncommon. Infection at the same nonintestinal sites (single or multiple) that are variably involved in classic Whipple's disease may also present as "isolated infection." Endocarditis, neurologic disease, uveitis, rheumatologic manifestations, and pulmonary involvement are most commonly described. Signs and symptoms are similar to those described for *T. whipplei* infection of these sites in classic Whipple's disease. With enhanced PCR-based diagnostic capabilities, *T. whipplei* infection without concomitant intestinal involvement (of which endocarditis is the best example) will probably be diagnosed increasingly often.

REINFECTION/RELAPSING DISEASE/IMMUNE RECONSTITUTION INFLAMMATORY SYNDROME (IRIS) It has been suggested that, if an underlying host immune defect places an individual at risk for chronic infection, then that person may be at risk for reinfection due to occupational exposure or contact with family members who are asymptomatically colonized. One case of apparent relapse that was due to a different genotype supports this contention.

Optimal treatment regimens and durations are still being defined. However, it is clear, especially in the setting of occult or overt CNS disease, that treatment with oral tetracycline or trimethoprim-sulfamethoxazole (TMP-SMX) alone may result in disease relapse.

As in patients treated for HIV or mycobacterial disease, IRIS has been described in patients treated for *T. whipplei* infection. Prior immunosuppressive therapy increases the likelihood of IRIS, in which inflammation recurs after an initial clinical response to treatment and loss of PCR detection of *T. whipplei*. Manifestations include fever, arthritis, skin lesions, pleuritis, uveitis, and orbital and periorbital inflammation.

DIAGNOSIS

Considering *T. whipplei* infection and ensuring that the appropriate tests are performed are the critical steps in making the diagnosis, which otherwise will likely be missed. The clinical presentation will in part dictate which clinical specimens are most likely to enable the diagnosis. In the presence (and perhaps the absence) of gastrointestinal symptoms, postbulbar duodenal biopsies should be performed. As a general rule, diagnostic yield is greater for tissue specimens than for body fluids. Biopsy of normal-appearing skin may detect *T. whipplei* in the setting of classic Whipple's disease and serve as a minimally invasive means to establish the diagnosis. It is unclear whether CSF should be obtained in the absence of CNS symptoms, but its collection should be considered: the CNS is the most common site for relapse, and thus the information gained by CSF examination could influence the design of the treatment regimen.

The development and implementation of PCR-based diagnostics have significantly increased the sensitivity and specificity of *T. whipplei* identification. PCR can be applied to affected tissues (fixed and nonfixed) and various body fluids (e.g., CSF; aqueous or vitreous humor; joint, pericardial, or pleural fluid; BALF; blood; feces). In some clinical scenarios, a generic 16S rRNA bacterial assay combined with amplicon sequencing can be used to detect and identify *T. whipplei* sequence. Delineation of the *T. whipplei* genomic sequence has enabled the development and broad availability of more sensitive and specific PCR-based assays. The interpretation of a PCR-based diagnostic approach must take into account limitations such as false-positive results due to sample contamination and false-negative results due to organism load, sample quality, and inadequate DNA extraction.

The diagnosis of classic Whipple's disease was originally based on histologic findings in intestinal biopsy specimens, and this diagnostic procedure remains important. Infiltration of the lamina propria with macrophages containing inclusions (representing ingested bacteria) that are positive on periodic acid–Schiff (PAS) staining and resistant to diastase is observed. However, PAS is nonspecific, also yielding positive results with mycobacteria (which can be differentiated with Ziehl-Neelsen stain), *Rhodococcus equi*, *Bacillus cereus*, *Corynebacterium* species, and *Histoplasma* species. *T. whipplei* can also be detected by silver stain, Brown-Brenn (weakly positive), or acridine orange and is not stained by calcofluor. Staining of other tissues or fluids (e.g., ocular aspirations) for PAS-positive inclusions in macrophages can be performed to support the diagnosis. Electron microscopy can be used to identify the trilaminar cell wall of *T. whipplei*.

When available, immunohistochemistry has greater specificity and sensitivity than PAS staining and can be performed on archived fixed tissue. *T. whipplei* has been successfully cultured from blood, CSF, synovial fluid, BALF, valve tissue, duodenal tissue, skeletal muscle, and lymph nodes, but culture is not practical since it takes months to obtain a positive result. Likewise, serology is of limited value for the diagnosis of Whipple's disease because the prevalence of exposure is much higher than that of chronic disease development and the antibody response to *T. whipplei* appears to be blunted in the disease state.

Although histologic or cytologic detection of *T. whipplei* is less specific and sensitive than PCR, a positive result is strongly supportive within the appropriate clinical context and is definitive when combined with a more specific test (e.g., PCR, immunohistochemistry).

TREATMENT WHIPPLE'S DISEASE

Data on treatment are emerging, but questions persist regarding the optimal regimen and duration, which may depend on the site of infection (e.g., CNS and heart valve). Appropriate treatment usually results in a rapid and at times remarkable clinical response (e.g., in CNS disease). Maintenance of a durable response has been more challenging.

Rates of relapse, particularly of CNS disease, were unacceptable with oral tetracycline or TMP-SMX monotherapy. Sequence data now indicate that TMP is not active against *T. whipplei* due to the absence of dihydrofolate reductase, but this drug was used extensively before this fact was known. This information prompted a randomized controlled trial in 40 patients, who received either ceftriaxone (2 g IV q24h) or meropenem (1 g IV q8h) for 2 weeks followed by oral TMP-SMX (160/800 mg) twice a day for 1 year. The efficacy of these regimens was outstanding. The only instance of therapy failure—in a case of asymptomatic CNS infection that was not eradicated by either regimen—was subsequently cured with oral minocycline and chloroquine (250 mg/d after a loading dose). A follow-up trial reported similar efficacy with a regimen of ceftriaxone (2 g IV q24h) for 2 weeks followed by oral TMP-SMX for 3 months. One issue in these trials was that the CNS doses—and perhaps the duration of ceftriaxone and meropenem treatment as well—were not optimal. Further, investigators have speculated that oral regimens with greater CNS penetrance, such as sulfadiazine (2–4 g/d in 3 or 4 divided doses) and/or doxycycline or minocycline (200 mg/d in 2 divided doses) plus hydroxychloroquine (200 mg three times a day, to raise phagosome pH and increase drug activity in vitro), might render the parenteral phase of treatment unnecessary, given that the one failure of therapy for CNS disease was cured with a similar regimen. Another issue is concern about the potential development of resistance to sulfa drugs. Lastly, it is unclear whether oral sulfa- or tetracycline-based regimens will suffice in endocarditis. Until more data become available, it seems prudent—at least in asymptomatic/symptomatic CNS disease or cardiac infection—to administer CNS-optimized doses of IV ceftriaxone (2 g q12h) or meropenem (2 g q8h) for at least 2 weeks followed by oral doxycycline or minocycline plus hydroxychloroquine or chloroquine for at least 1 year, if tolerated. Although data on the use of PCR to guide therapy do not exist, it seems reasonable that continued *T. whipplei* detection by PCR, especially in the CSF, should dictate at least continuation of therapy and perhaps consideration of an alternative regimen.

The occurrence of a Jarisch-Herxheimer reaction within 24 h of treatment initiation has been described, with rapid resolution. The addition of glucocorticoids may be beneficial in the management of clearly documented IRIS.

Data on certain site-specific treatment issues are even more limited. Anecdotal reports describe successful treatment of uveitis with oral TMP-SMX with or without rifampin, whereas treatment with tetracycline alone has resulted in relapse. Although a role for adjunctive intraocular therapy has been reported, the data are unclear on this point. Surgery may be needed in the setting of endocarditis with significant valve dysfunction; however, timely recognition can result in cure with medical management alone. Although data on the treatment of foreign body–associated infection are virtually nonexistent, medical treatment for a prosthetic hip infection was apparently successful; however, follow-up was limited.

Regardless of the therapeutic regimen chosen, an effort to ensure compliance and close follow-up for potential relapse (or perhaps reinfection), which can occur many years after an apparent cure, will maximize the chances for a good outcome.

201 Infections Due to Mixed Anaerobic Organisms

Ronit Cohen-Poradosu, Dennis L. Kasper

Anaerobes comprise the predominant class of bacteria of the normal human microbiota (formerly termed "the normal human flora") that reside on mucous membranes and predominate in many infectious processes, particularly those arising from mucosal surfaces. These organisms generally cause disease subsequent to the breakdown of mucosal barriers and the leakage of the microbiota into normally sterile sites. Infections resulting from contamination by the microbiota are usually polymicrobial and involve both aerobic and anaerobic bacteria. However, the difficulties encountered in handling specimens in which anaerobes may be important and the technical challenges entailed in cultivating and identifying these organisms in clinical microbiology laboratories continue to leave the anaerobic etiology of an infectious process unproven in many cases. Therefore, an understanding of the types of infections in which anaerobes can play a role is crucial in selecting appropriate microbiologic tools to identify the organisms in clinical specimens and in choosing the most appropriate treatment, including antibiotics and surgical drainage or debridement of the infected site.

This chapter focuses on infections caused by nonsporulating anaerobic bacteria. It does not address clostridial infections and syndromes, which are covered elsewhere (Chaps. 161 and 179).

DEFINITIONS

Anaerobic bacteria are organisms that require reduced oxygen tension for growth, failing to grow on the surface of solid media in 10% CO_2 in air. (In contrast, *microaerophilic bacteria* can grow in an atmosphere of 10% CO_2 in air or under anaerobic or aerobic conditions, although they grow best in the presence of only a small amount of atmospheric oxygen, and *facultative bacteria* can grow in the presence or absence of air). Most clinically relevant anaerobes, such as *Bacteroides fragilis, Prevotella melaninogenica,* and *Fusobacterium nucleatum,* are relatively aerotolerant. Although they can survive for sustained periods in the presence of up to 2–8% oxygen, they generally do not multiply in this environment. A smaller number of pathogenic anaerobic bacteria (which are also part of the microbiota) die after brief contact with oxygen, even in low concentrations.

ANAEROBES OF THE HUMAN MICROBIOTA

Most human mucocutaneous surfaces harbor a rich indigenous normal microbiota composed of aerobic and anaerobic bacteria. These surfaces are dominated by anaerobic bacteria, which often account for 99.0–99.9% of the culturable microbiota and range in concentration from 10^9/mL in saliva to 10^{12}/mL in gingival scrapings and the colon. It is interesting that anaerobes inhabit many areas of the body that are exposed to air: skin, nose, mouth, and throat. Anaerobes are thought to reside in the portions of these sites that are relatively well protected from oxygen, such as gingival crevices. New technologies based on analyses of microbial DNA have expanded our knowledge of these bacterial populations. For example, in an analysis of 13,555 prokaryotic ribosomal RNA gene sequences from the colon, most bacteria identified were considered uncultivated and novel microorganisms. Two immense projects based on these new technologies, the Human Microbiome Project funded by the U.S. National Institutes of Health and MetaHIT financed by the European Commission, aim to characterize the normal microbiota of healthy individuals.

The major reservoirs of anaerobic bacteria are the mouth, lower gastrointestinal tract, skin, and female genital tract (Table 201-1). In the oral cavity, the ratio of anaerobic to aerobic bacteria ranges from 1:1 on the surface of a tooth to 1000:1 in the gingival crevices. *Prevotella* and *Porphyromonas* species comprise much of the indigenous oral anaerobic microbiota. *Fusobacterium* and *Bacteroides* (non–*B. fragilis* group) are present in lower numbers. Anaerobic bacteria are not found in appreciable numbers in the normal stomach and upper small intestine. In the distal ileum, the microbiota begins to resemble that of the colon. In the colon, the ratio of anaerobes to facultative species is high; for example, there are 10^{11}–10^{12} organisms/g of stool, and >99% of these organisms are anaerobic, with an anaerobe-to-aerobe ratio of ~1000:1. The predominant anaerobes in the human intestine belong to the phyla Bacteroidetes and Firmicutes and include a number of *Bacteroides* species (e.g., members of the *B. fragilis* group, such as *B. fragilis, B. thetaiotaomicron, B. ovatus, B. vulgatus, B. uniformis,* and *Parabacteroides distasonis*) as well as various clostridial, peptostreptococcal, and fusobacterial species. In the female genital tract, there are ~10^9 organisms/mL of secretions, with an anaerobe-to-aerobe ratio of 1:1 to 10:1. The predominant anaerobes in the female genital tract are *Prevotella, Bacteroides, Fusobacterium, Clostridium,* and the anaerobic *Lactobacillus* species.

TABLE 201-1 ANAEROBIC HUMAN MICROBIOTA: AN OVERVIEW

Anatomic Site	Total Bacteria[a]	Anaerobic/Aerobic Ratio	Potential Pathogens
Oral cavity			
Saliva	10^8–10^9	1:1	*Fusobacterium nucleatum, Prevotella melaninogenica, Prevotella oralis* group, *Bacteroides ureolyticus* group, *Peptostreptococcus* spp.
Tooth surface	10^{10}–10^{11}	1:1	
Gingival crevices	10^{11}–10^{12}	10^3:1	
Gastrointestinal tract			
Stomach	0–10^5	1:1	*Bacteroides* spp. (principally members of the *B. fragilis* group), *Prevotella* spp., *Clostridium* spp., *Peptostreptococcus* spp.
Jejunum/ileum	10^4–10^7	1:1	
Terminal ileum and colon	10^{11}–10^{12}	10^3:1	
Female genital tract	10^7–10^9	10:1	*Peptostreptococcus* spp., *Bacteroides* spp., *Prevotella bivia*

[a]Per gram or milliliter.

The skin microbiota contains anaerobes as well, the predominant species being *Propionibacterium acnes* and, in lower numbers, other species of propionibacteria and peptostreptococci.

Commensal bacteria in general and commensal anaerobes in particular have been implicated as crucial mediators of physiologic, metabolic, and immunologic functions in the mammalian host. One of the most important roles that anaerobes serve as components of the normal colonic microbiota is the promotion of resistance to colonization; the presence of anaerobic bacteria effectively interferes with colonization by potentially pathogenic bacterial species through the depletion of oxygen and nutrients, the production of enzymes and toxic end products, and the modulation of the host's intestinal innate immune response. For example, *B. thetaiotaomicron* stimulates Paneth cells to produce RegIIIγ, a bactericidal lectin that can result in killing of gram-positive bacteria. The normal colonic microbiota plays an important role in protection against *Clostridium difficile*–associated diarrhea or colitis—a toxin-mediated, potentially life-threatening disease that results when *C. difficile* spores in the colon transform into toxin-producing vegetative forms after antibiotic elimination of critical components of the competing colonic microbiota.

Bacteroides and other intestinal bacteria ferment carbohydrates and produce volatile fatty acids that are reabsorbed and used by the host as an energy source. The anaerobic intestinal microbiota is also responsible for the production of secreted products that promote human health (e.g., vitamin K and bile acids useful in fat absorption and cholesterol regulation).

Moreover, the anaerobic intestinal microbiota influences the development of an intact mucosa and of mucosa-associated lymphoid tissue. Colonization of germ-free mice with a single species, *B. thetaiotaomicron*, affects the expression of various host genes and corrects deficiencies of nutrient uptake, metabolism, angiogenesis, mucosal barrier function, and enteric nervous system development. The symbiosis factor polysaccharide A (PSA) of *B. fragilis* influences the normal development and function of the mammalian immune system and protects mice against colitis in a model of inflammatory bowel disease. It has also been shown that PSA can confer protection both prophylactically and therapeutically, restraining inflammatory processes at an extraintestinal site (the central nervous system [CNS]) and ameliorating disease in a mouse model of multiple sclerosis. Anaerobes can stimulate specific lymphocyte populations of the small and large intestine and can influence immunologic balance (including T_H1/T_H2 balance) as well as the number of T_H17 and regulatory T cells in gut tissues.

Clearly, the gut microbiota confers many benefits, and its dysregulation may play a role in the pathogenesis of diseases characterized by inflammation and aberrant immune responses, such as inflammatory bowel disease, rheumatoid arthritis, multiple sclerosis, asthma, and type 1 diabetes. Furthermore, the gut microbiota has been associated with obesity and metabolic syndrome. An interesting association between certain microbes found in the microbiota and testosterone production has been suggested as well.

ETIOLOGY

Thousands of species of anaerobic bacteria have been identified as components of the complete human microbiota, with each individual colonized by hundreds of these species. Despite the complex array of bacteria in the normal microbiota, relatively few species are isolated commonly from human infections. Anaerobic infections occur when the harmonious relationship between the host and the host's microbiota is disrupted. Any site in the body is susceptible to infection with these indigenous organisms when a mucosal barrier or the skin is compromised by surgery, trauma, tumor, ischemia, or necrosis, all of which can reduce local tissue redox potentials. Because the sites that are colonized by anaerobes contain many species of bacteria, disruption of anatomic barriers allows contamination of normally sterile sites by many organisms, resulting in mixed infections involving multiple species of anaerobes in combination with synergistically acting facultative or microaerophilic organisms.

Severe mixed infections of the head and neck may arise from an abscessed tooth infected with commensal microbiota of the mouth. Examples of infections arising from an oral source are chronic sinusitis, chronic otitis media, Ludwig's angina, and periodontal abscesses. Brain abscesses and subdural empyema are also commonly associated with the oral microbiota. Oral anaerobes are usually responsible for pleuropulmonary diseases such as aspiration pneumonia, necrotizing pneumonia, lung abscess, and empyema.

Anaerobes from the intestine play an important role in various intraabdominal infections, such as peritonitis and intraabdominal abscesses (Chap. 159). Colonic contents are the source of microorganisms in the case of these infections, which usually follow disruption of intestinal continuity and contamination of the peritoneal cavity. Anaerobic bacteria are isolated frequently in female genital tract infections, such as salpingitis, pelvic peritonitis, tuboovarian abscess, vulvovaginal abscess, septic abortion, and endometritis (Chap. 163). In addition, these bacteria are often found in bacteremia and in infections of the skin, soft tissues, and bones.

Predominant among the anaerobic gram-positive cocci that produce disease are the peptostreptococci; the species of this genus that are most commonly involved in infections are *P. micros*, *P. magnus*, *P. asaccharolyticus*, *P. anaerobius*, and *P. prevotii*. Clostridia (Chap. 179) are anaerobic spore-forming gram-positive rods that are isolated from wounds, abscesses, sites of abdominal infection, and blood. Gram-positive anaerobic non-spore-forming bacilli are uncommon as etiologic agents of human infection. *P. acnes*, a component of the skin microbiota and a rare cause of foreign-body infections, is one of the few nonclostridial gram-positive rods associated with infections. The principal anaerobic gram-negative bacilli found in human infections belong to the *B. fragilis* group and to *Fusobacterium*, *Prevotella*, and *Porphyromonas* species.

The most important potential anaerobic pathogens found in the upper airways and isolated from clinical specimens of oral and pleuropulmonary infections are the *Fusobacterium* species *F. necrophorum*, *F. nucleatum*, and *F. varium*; *P. melaninogenica*; the *Prevotella oralis* group; *Porphyromonas gingivalis*; *Porphyromonas asaccharolytica*; *Peptostreptococcus* species; and the *Bacteroides ureolyticus* group.

The *B. fragilis* group contains the anaerobic pathogens most frequently isolated from clinical infections. Members of this group are part of the normal bowel microbiota; they include several distinct species, such as *B. fragilis*, *B. thetaiotaomicron*, *B. vulgatus*, *B. uniformis*, *B. ovatus*, and *P. distasonis*. *B. fragilis* is the most important clinical isolate, although it is isolated in lower numbers than some other *Bacteroides* species from cultures of the commensal fecal microbiota.

In female genital tract infections, organisms normally colonizing the vagina (e.g., *Prevotella bivia* and *Prevotella disiens*) are the most common isolates. However, *B. fragilis* is not uncommon.

PATHOGENESIS

Anaerobic bacterial infections usually occur when an anatomic barrier is disrupted and constituents of the local microbiota enter a site that was previously sterile. Because of the specific growth requirements of anaerobic organisms and their presence as commensals on mucosal surfaces, conditions must arise that allow these organisms to penetrate mucosal barriers and enter tissue with a lowered oxidation-reduction potential. Therefore, tissue ischemia, trauma, surgery, perforated viscus, shock, and aspiration provide environments conducive to the proliferation of anaerobes. The introduction of many bacterial species into otherwise sterile sites leads to a polymicrobial infection in which certain organisms predominate. Three major factors are involved in the pathogenesis of anaerobic infections: bacterial synergy, bacterial virulence factors, and mechanisms of abscess formation. The ability of different anaerobic bacteria to act synergistically during polymicrobial infection contributes to the pathogenesis of anaerobic infections. It has been postulated that facultative organisms function in part to lower the oxidation-reduction potential in the microenvironment, allowing the propagation of obligate anaerobes. Anaerobes can produce compounds such as succinic acid and short-chain fatty acids that inhibit the ability of phagocytes to clear facultative organisms. In experimental models, facultative and obligate anaerobes synergistically potentiate abscess formation.

Virulence factors associated with anaerobes typically confer the ability to evade host defenses, adhere to cell surfaces, produce toxins and/or enzymes, or display surface structures such as capsular polysaccharides and lipopolysaccharide (LPS) that contribute to pathogenic potential. The ability of an organism to adhere to host tissues is important to the establishment of infection. Some oral species adhere to the epithelium in the oral cavity. *P. melaninogenica* actually attaches to other microorganisms. *P. gingivalis*, a common isolate in periodontal disease, has fimbriae that facilitate attachment. Some *Bacteroides* strains appear to be piliated, a characteristic that may account for their ability to adhere.

The most extensively studied virulence factor of the nonsporulating anaerobes is the capsular polysaccharide complex of *B. fragilis*. This organism is unique among anaerobes in its potential for virulence during growth at normally sterile sites. Although it constitutes only 0.5–1% of the normal colonic microbiota, *B. fragilis* is the anaerobe most commonly isolated from intraabdominal infections and bacteremia. In an animal model of intraabdominal sepsis, the capsular polysaccharide was identified as the major virulence factor of *B. fragilis;* this polymer plays a specific, central role in the induction of abscesses. A series of detailed biologic and molecular studies of this virulence factor showed that *B. fragilis* produces at least eight distinct capsular polysaccharides, far more than the number reported for any other encapsulated bacterium. *B. fragilis* can exhibit distinct surface polysaccharides either alone or in combination by regulating the expression of these different capsules in an on–off manner through a reversible inversion of DNA segments within the promoters for operons containing the genes required for polysaccharide synthesis. Structural analysis of two of these polysaccharides, PSA and PSB, revealed that each polymer consists of repeating units with positively charged free amino groups and negatively charged groups. This structural feature is rare among bacterial polysaccharides, and the ability of PSA—and, to a lesser extent, PSB—to induce abscesses in animals depends on this zwitterionic charge motif. Intraabdominal abscess induction is related to the capacity of this polysaccharide to stimulate macrophages to release cytokines and chemokines—in particular, interleukin (IL) 8, IL-17, and tumor necrosis factor α (TNF-α)—from resident peritoneal cells through a Toll-like receptor 2–dependent mechanism. The release of cytokines and chemokines results in the chemotaxis of polymorphonuclear neutrophils (PMNs) into the peritoneum, where they adhere to mesothelial cells induced by TNF-α to upregulate their expression of intercellular adhesion molecule 1 (ICAM-1). PMNs adherent to ICAM-1-expressing cells probably represent the nidus for an abscess. PSA also activates T cells to produce certain cytokines, including IL-17 and interferon γ, that are necessary for abscess formation.

B. fragilis produces other virulence factors that allow it to predominate in disease. This organism synthesizes pili, fimbriae, and hemagglutinins that aid in attachment to host cell surfaces. In addition, *Bacteroides* species produce many enzymes and toxins that contribute to pathogenicity. Enzymes such as neuraminidase, protease, glycoside hydrolases, and superoxide dismutases are all produced by *B. fragilis.* Anaerobic bacteria produce a number of exoproteins that can enhance the organisms' virulence. The collagenase produced by *P. gingivalis* may enhance tissue destruction. An association of *B. fragilis* strains positive for the enterotoxin BFT with clinical episodes of diarrhea in children and adults has been suggested. BFT is a metalloprotease that is cytopathic for intestinal epithelial cells and induces fluid secretion and tissue damage in ligated intestinal loops of experimental animals. Recent evidence from mouse models indicates that enterotoxin-producing strains of *B. fragilis* may play a role in colon carcinoma.

Exotoxins produced by clostridial species, including botulinum toxins, tetanus toxin, *C. difficile* toxins A and B, and five toxins produced by *Clostridium perfringens*, are among the most virulent bacterial toxins in mouse lethality assays. Anaerobic gram-negative bacteria such as *B. fragilis* possess LPSs (endotoxins) that are 100–1000 times less biologically potent than endotoxins associated with aerobic gram-negative bacteria. This relative biologic inactivity may account for the lower frequency of disseminated intravascular coagulation and purpura in *Bacteroides* bacteremia than in facultative and aerobic gram-negative bacillary bacteremia. An exception is the LPS from *Fusobacterium*, which may account for the severity of Lemierre's syndrome (see "Complications of Anaerobic Head and Neck Infections," below).

APPROACH TO THE PATIENT: **Infection Due to Anaerobic Bacteria**

The physician must consider several points when approaching the patient with possible infection due to anaerobic bacteria.

1. Most of the organisms colonizing mucosal sites are commensals; very few cause disease. When these organisms do cause disease, it often occurs in proximity to the mucosal site they colonize.
2. For anaerobes to cause tissue infection, they must spread beyond the normal mucosal barriers.
3. Conditions favoring the propagation of anaerobic bacteria, particularly a lowered oxidation-reduction potential, are necessary. These conditions exist at sites of trauma, tissue destruction, compromised vascular supply, and complications of preexisting infection, which produce necrosis.
4. Frequently, a complex array of infecting microbes can be found. For example, as many as 12 species of organisms can be isolated from a suppurative site.
5. Anaerobic organisms tend to be found in abscess cavities or in necrotic tissue. The failure of an abscess to yield organisms

on routine culture is a clue that the abscess is likely to contain anaerobic bacteria. Often smears of this "sterile pus" are found to be teeming with bacteria when Gram's stain is applied. Although some facultative organisms (e.g., *Staphylococcus aureus*) are also capable of causing abscesses, abscesses in organs or deeper body tissues should call anaerobic infection to mind.

6. Gas is found in many anaerobic infections of deep tissues but is not diagnostic because it can be produced by aerobic bacteria as well.
7. Although a putrid-smelling infection site or discharge is considered diagnostic for anaerobic infection, this manifestation usually develops late in the course and is present in only 30–50% of cases.
8. Some species (the best example being the *B. fragilis* group) require specific therapy. However, many synergistic infections can be cured with antibiotics directed at some but not all of the organisms involved. Antibiotic therapy, combined with debridement and drainage, disrupts the interdependent relationship among the bacteria, and some species that are resistant to the antibiotic do not survive without the co-infecting organisms.
9. Manifestations of severe sepsis and disseminated intravascular coagulation are unusual in patients with purely anaerobic infection.

EPIDEMIOLOGY

Difficulties in the performance of appropriate cultures, contamination of cultures by components of the normal microbiota, and the lack of readily available, reliable culture techniques have made it impossible to obtain accurate data on incidence or prevalence. However, anaerobic infections are encountered frequently in hospitals with active surgical, trauma, and obstetric and gynecologic services. Depending on the institution, anaerobic bacteria account for 0.5–12% of all cases of bacteremia.

CLINICAL MANIFESTATIONS

Anaerobic Infections of the Mouth, Head, and Neck Anaerobic bacteria are commonly involved in infections of the mouth, head, and neck (Chap. 44). The predominant isolates are components of the normal microbiota of the upper airways—mainly the *Bacteroides oralis* group, pigmented *Prevotella* species, *P. asaccharolytica*, *Fusobacterium* species, peptostreptococci, and microaerophilic streptococci.

Soft tissue infections of the oral-facial area may or may not be odontogenic. Odontogenic infections—primarily dental caries and periodontal disease (gingivitis and periodontitis)—are common and have both local consequences (especially tooth loss) and the potential for life-threatening spread to the deep fascial spaces of the head and neck. Infections of the mouth can arise from either supragingival or subgingival dental plaque composed of bacteria colonizing the tooth surface. Supragingival plaque formation begins with the adherence of gram-positive bacteria to the tooth surface. This form of plaque is influenced by salivary and dietary components, oral hygiene, and local host factors. Supragingival plaque can lead to dental caries and, with further invasion, to pulpitis (endodontic infection) that can further perforate the alveolar bone, causing periapical abscess. Subgingival plaque is associated with periodontal infections (e.g., gingivitis, periodontitis, and periodontal abscess) that can further disseminate to adjacent structures such as the mandible, causing osteomyelitis of the maxillary sinuses. Periodontitis may also result in spreading infection that can involve adjacent bone or soft tissues. In the healthy periodontium, the sparse microbiota consists mainly of gram-positive organisms such as *Streptococcus sanguinis* and *Actinomyces* species. In the presence of gingivitis, there is a shift to a greater proportion of anaerobic gram-negative bacilli in the subgingival microbiota, with predominance of *Prevotella intermedia*. In well-established periodontitis, the complexity of the microbiota increases further. The predominant isolates are *P. gingivalis*, *P. intermedia*, *Aggregatibacter actinomycetemcomitans*, *Treponema denticola*, and *Tannerella forsythensis*.

Necrotizing Ulcerative Gingivitis Gingivitis may become a necrotizing infection (*trench mouth, Vincent's stomatitis*) (Chap. 44). The onset of disease is usually sudden and is associated with tender bleeding gums, foul breath, and a bad taste. The gingival mucosa, especially the papillae between the teeth, becomes ulcerated and may be covered by a gray exudate, which is removable with gentle pressure. Patients may become systemically ill, developing fever, cervical lymphadenopathy, and leukocytosis.

Noma (*cancrum oris*) is a necrotizing infection of the oral mucous membranes. It is characterized by destruction of soft tissue and bone and evolves rapidly from gingival inflammation to orofacial gangrene. Noma occurs most frequently in young children (1–4 years of age) with malnutrition or systemic disease. This infection occurs worldwide but is most common in sub-Saharan Africa.

Acute Necrotizing Infections of the Pharynx These infections usually occur in association with ulcerative gingivitis. Symptoms include an extremely sore throat, foul breath, and a bad taste accompanied by fever and a sensation of choking. Examination of the pharynx demonstrates that the tonsillar pillars are swollen, red, ulcerated, and covered with a grayish membrane that peels easily. Lymphadenopathy and leukocytosis are common. The disease may last for only a few days or, if not treated, may persist for weeks. Lesions begin unilaterally but may spread to the other side of the pharynx or the larynx. Aspiration of the infected material by the patient can result in lung abscesses.

Peripharyngeal Space Infections These infections arise from the spread of organisms from the upper airways to potential spaces formed by the fascial planes of the head and neck. The etiology is typically polymicrobial and represents the normal microbiota of the mucosa of the originating site.

Peritonsillar abscess (*quinsy*) is a complication of acute tonsillitis caused mainly by a mixed flora containing anaerobes (e.g., *F. necrophorum* and *Peptostreptococcus* species) and the facultative anaerobe group A *Streptococcus* (Chap. 44). Of cases of submandibular space infection (*Ludwig's angina*), 80% are caused by infection of the tissues surrounding the second and third molar teeth. This infection results in marked local swelling of tissues, with pain, trismus, and superior and posterior displacement of the tongue. Submandibular swelling of the neck can impair swallowing and cause respiratory obstruction. In some cases, tracheotomy is life-saving. Cervicofacial actinomycosis (Chap. 200) is caused by a branching, gram-positive, non-spore-forming, strict/facultative anaerobe that is a part of the normal oral microbiota. This chronic disease is characterized by abscesses, draining sinus tracts, fistula, bone destruction, and fibrosis. It can easily be mistaken for malignancy or granulomatous disease. Actinomycosis less frequently involves the thorax, abdomen, pelvis, and CNS.

Sinusitis and Otitis Anaerobic bacteria have been implicated in chronic sinusitis but play little role in acute sinusitis. In several studies on chronic sinusitis, anaerobic bacteria were found in 0–52% of cases, depending on the method used to collect specimens. Polymicrobial infection is common, and the predominant anaerobic isolates are pigmented *Prevotella*, *Fusobacterium*, *Peptostreptococcus*, and *P. acnes*. Aerobic gram-negative bacilli and *S. aureus* have also been implicated in chronic sinusitis. Anaerobic bacteria have been isolated in a large percentage of cases of chronic suppurative otitis media in children. The role of anaerobes in acute otitis media is less clear.

Complications of Anaerobic Head and Neck Infections Contiguous cranial spread of these infections can result in osteomyelitis of the skull or mandible or in intracranial infections such as brain abscess and subdural empyema. Caudal spread can produce mediastinitis or pleuropulmonary infection. Hematogenous complications can also result from anaerobic infections of the head and neck. Bacteremia, which occasionally is polymicrobial, can lead to endocarditis or other distant infections. Lemierre's syndrome (Chap. 44), which has been uncommon in the antimicrobial era, is an acute oropharyngeal infection with secondary septic thrombophlebitis of the internal jugular vein and frequent metastasis, most commonly to the lung. *F. necrophorum* is the usual cause. This infection typically begins with pharyngitis, which is followed by local invasion in the lateral pharyngeal space, with resultant internal jugular vein thrombophlebitis. A typical clinical triad includes pharyngitis, a tender/swollen neck, and noncavitating pulmonary infiltrates.

CNS Infections CNS infections associated with anaerobic bacteria are brain abscess, epidural abscess, and subdural empyema. Anaerobic meningitis is rare and is usually related to parameningeal collection or shunt infection. If optimal bacteriologic techniques are used, as many as 85% of brain abscesses yield anaerobic bacteria. Most anaerobic brain abscesses arise by direct extension from a site of otorhinolaryngeal infection such as otitis, sinusitis, or tooth infection. Hematogenous dissemination from a distant infected site, usually intraabdominal or pelvic, can occur. Common isolates are *Peptostreptococcus, Fusobacterium, Bacteroides, Prevotella, Propionibacterium, Eubacterium, Veillonella,* and *Actinomyces* species. Facultative or microaerophilic streptococci and coliforms are often part of a mixed infecting flora in brain abscesses.

Pleuropulmonary Infections Anaerobic pleuropulmonary infections result from the aspiration of oropharyngeal contents by patients with predisposing conditions such as dysphagia due to neurologic or esophageal disorders or transiently impaired consciousness due to conditions such as alcohol or drug abuse, seizures, head trauma, and cerebrovascular accidents. Clinical syndromes that are associated with anaerobic pleuropulmonary infection produced by aspiration include aspiration pneumonitis, which can be complicated by necrotizing pneumonia, lung abscess, and empyema. Many of these infections have an indolent course that may serve as a clinical clue differentiating them, for example, from pneumococcal pneumonia, which often presents with abrupt onset, shaking chills, and rapid progression.

The anaerobes most common in pleuropulmonary infections are indigenous to the oral cavity, especially the gingival crevice, and include pigmented and nonpigmented *Prevotella, Peptostreptococcus,* and *Bacteroides* species and *F. nucleatum*. Many of these infections are of mixed aerobic-anaerobic etiology, and the predominant aerobes isolated from community-acquired aspiration pneumonias are microaerophilic streptococci such as *Streptococcus milleri*. Studies using in-depth culture techniques in patients with community-acquired lung abscess showed aerobic and microaerophilic streptococci to be the most common pathogens (60% of patients) and anaerobes to be the second most common (26%). In a study on aspiration pneumonia from a long-term care facility, the most common isolates were gram-negative bacilli (49%), anaerobes (16%), and *S. aureus* (12%). Nosocomial aspiration pneumonia commonly involves a mixture of anaerobes and gram-negative bacilli or *S. aureus*.

ASPIRATION PNEUMONITIS Bacterial aspiration pneumonitis must be distinguished from two other clinical syndromes associated with aspiration that are not of bacterial etiology. One syndrome results from aspiration of solids, usually food. Obstruction of major airways typically results in atelectasis and moderate nonspecific inflammation. Therapy consists of removal of the foreign body. The second aspiration syndrome is more easily confused with bacterial aspiration. *Mendelson's syndrome,* a chemical pneumonitis, results from regurgitation of stomach contents and aspiration of chemical material, usually acidic gastric juices. Pulmonary inflammation—including the destruction of the alveolar lining, with transudation of fluid into the alveolar space—occurs with remarkable rapidity. Typically this syndrome develops within hours, often following anesthesia when the gag reflex is depressed. The patient becomes tachypneic, hypoxic, and febrile. The leukocyte count may rise, and the chest x-ray may evolve from normal to a complete bilateral "whiteout" within 8–24 h. Sputum production is minimal. The pulmonary signs and symptoms can resolve quickly with symptom-based therapy or can culminate in respiratory failure, with the subsequent development of bacterial superinfection over a period of days. Antibiotic therapy is not indicated unless bacterial infection supervenes.

In contrast to these syndromes, bacterial aspiration pneumonitis develops over a period of several days or weeks rather than hours. Patients who enter the hospital with this syndrome typically have been ill for several days and generally report low-grade fever, malaise, and sputum production. In some patients, weight loss and anemia reflect a more chronic process. Usually the history reveals factors predisposing to aspiration, such as alcohol overdose or residence in a nursing home. Examination sometimes yields evidence of periodontal disease. Sputum characteristically is not malodorous unless the process has been under way for at least a week. A mixed bacterial flora with many PMNs is evident on Gram's staining of sputum. Expectorated sputum is unreliable for anaerobic cultures because of inevitable contamination by the normal oral microbiota. Reliable specimens for culture can be obtained by transtracheal or transthoracic aspiration—techniques that are rarely used at present. Culture of protected-brush specimens or bronchoalveolar lavage fluid obtained by bronchoscopy is controversial.

Chest x-rays show consolidation in dependent pulmonary segments: in the basilar segments of the lower lobes if the patient has aspirated while upright and in either the posterior segment of the upper lobe (usually on the right side) or the superior segment of the lower lobe if the patient has aspirated while supine.

NECROTIZING PNEUMONITIS This form of anaerobic pneumonitis is characterized by numerous small abscesses that spread to involve several pulmonary segments. The process can be indolent or fulminating. This syndrome is less common than either aspiration pneumonitis or lung abscess and includes features of both types of infection.

ANAEROBIC LUNG ABSCESSES (See also Chap. 154) These abscesses result from subacute anaerobic pulmonary infection. The clinical syndrome typically involves a history of constitutional signs and symptoms (including malaise, weight loss, fever, night sweats, and foul-smelling sputum), perhaps over a period of weeks (Chap. 153). Patients who develop lung abscesses characteristically have dental infection and periodontitis, but lung abscesses in edentulous patients have been reported. Abscess cavities may be single or multiple and generally occur in dependent pulmonary segments (Fig. 201-1). Anaerobic abscesses must be distinguished from lesions associated with tuberculosis, neoplasia, and other conditions.

Septic pulmonary emboli may originate from intraabdominal or female genital tract infections and can produce anaerobic pneumonia and abscess.

EMPYEMA Empyema is a manifestation of long-standing anaerobic pulmonary infection complicated by bronchopleural fistula. The clinical presentation, which includes foul-smelling sputum, resembles that

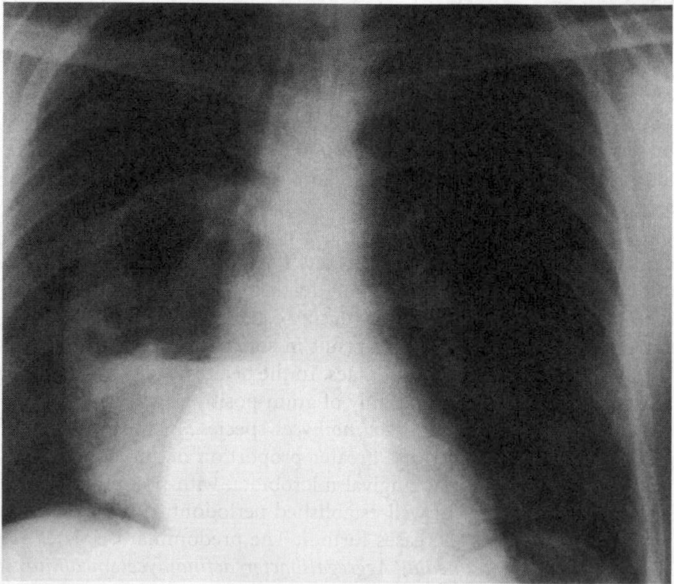

FIGURE 201-1 Chest radiograph of right-lower-lobe lung abscess in a 60-year-old alcoholic patient. *(From GL Mandell [ed]: Atlas of Infectious Diseases, Vol VI. Philadelphia, Current Medicine Inc, Churchill Livingstone, 1996; with permission.)*

of other anaerobic pulmonary infections. Patients may report pleuritic chest pain and marked chest-wall tenderness.

Empyema may be masked by overlying pneumonitis and should be considered especially in cases of persistent fever despite antibiotic therapy. Diligent physical examination and the use of ultrasound to localize a loculated empyema are important diagnostic tools. The collection of a foul-smelling exudate by thoracentesis is typical. Cultures of infected pleural fluid yield an average of 3.5 anaerobic and 0.6 facultative or aerobic bacterial species. Drainage is required. Defervescence, a return to a feeling of well-being, and resolution of the process may require several months.

Extension from a subdiaphragmatic infection may also result in anaerobic empyema.

Intraabdominal Infections Intraabdominal infections—mainly peritonitis and abscesses—are usually polymicrobial and represent the normal intestinal (especially colonic) microbiota. These infections most often follow a breach in the mucosal barrier resulting from appendicitis, diverticulitis, neoplasm, inflammatory bowel disease, surgery, or trauma. On average, four to six bacterial species are isolated per specimen submitted to the microbiology laboratory, with a predominance of enteric aerobic/facultative gram-negative bacilli, anaerobes, and streptococci/enterococci. The most common isolates are *Escherichia coli* (found in ≥50% of patients) and *B. fragilis* (30–50%). Other anaerobes commonly isolated from this type of infection include *Peptostreptococcus, Prevotella*, and *Fusobacterium* species. The involvement of clostridia can lead to severe infections. The dominance of four to six bacterial species out of the more than 500 colonic mucosal species is related both to the virulence factors of these species and to the inability of clinical laboratories to culture many other species residing in the colonic mucosa.

Disease originating from proximal-bowel perforation reflects the microbiota of this site, with a predominance of aerobic and anaerobic gram-positive bacteria and *Candida*.

Neutropenic enterocolitis (typhlitis) has been associated with anaerobic infection of the cecum but—in the setting of neutropenia (Chap. 104)—may involve the entire bowel. Patients usually present with fever; abdominal pain, tenderness, and distention; and watery diarrhea. The bowel wall is edematous with hemorrhage and necrosis. The primary pathogen is thought by some authorities to be *Clostridium septicum*, but other clostridia and mixed anaerobes have also been implicated. More than 50% of patients developing early clinical signs can benefit from antibiotic therapy and bowel rest. Surgery is sometimes required to remove gangrenous bowel. See Chap. 159 for a complete discussion of intraabdominal infections.

Enterotoxigenic *B. fragilis* has been associated with watery diarrhea in a few young children and adults. In case–control studies of children with undiagnosed diarrheal disease, enterotoxigenic *B. fragilis* was isolated from significantly more children with diarrhea than children in the control group.

Pelvic Infections The vagina of a healthy woman is a major reservoir of anaerobic and aerobic bacteria. In the normal microbiota of the female genital tract, anaerobes outnumber aerobes by a ratio of ~10:1 and include anaerobic gram-positive cocci and *Bacteroides* species (Table 201-1). Anaerobes are isolated from most women with genital tract infections that are not caused by a sexually transmitted pathogen. The major anaerobic pathogens are *B. fragilis, P. bivia, P. disiens, P. melaninogenica*, anaerobic cocci, and *Clostridium* species. Anaerobes are frequently encountered in pelvic inflammatory disease, pelvic abscess, endometritis, tubo-ovarian abscess, septic abortion, and postoperative or postpartum infections. These infections are often of mixed etiology, involving both anaerobes and coliforms; pure anaerobic infections without coliform or other facultative bacterial species occur more often in pelvic than in intraabdominal sites. Septic pelvic thrombophlebitis may complicate the infections and lead to repeated episodes of septic pulmonary emboli. See Chap. 163 for a complete discussion of pelvic inflammatory disease.

Anaerobic bacteria have been thought to be contributing factors in the etiology of bacterial vaginosis. This syndrome of unknown etiology is characterized by a profuse malodorous discharge and a change in the bacterial ecology that results in replacement of the *Lactobacillus*-dominated normal microbiota with an overgrowth of bacterial species including *Gardnerella vaginalis, Prevotella* species, *Mobiluncus* species, peptostreptococci, and genital mycoplasmas. A study based on 16S rRNA identification found other anaerobes that were predominant in cases but not in controls: *Atopobium, Leptotrichia, Megasphaera*, and *Eggerthella*. Pelvic infections due to *Actinomyces* species have been associated with the use of intrauterine devices (Chap. 200).

Skin and Soft Tissue Infections Injury to skin, bone, or soft tissue by trauma, ischemia, or surgery creates a suitable environment for anaerobic infections. These infections are most frequently found in sites prone to contamination with feces or with upper airway secretions—e.g., wounds associated with intestinal surgery, decubitus ulcers, or human bites. Moreover, anaerobes have been isolated from cutaneous abscesses, rectal abscesses, and axillary sweat gland infections (*hidradenitis suppurativa*). Anaerobes also are often cultured from foot ulcers of diabetic patients. The deep soft-tissue infections associated with anaerobic bacteria are crepitant cellulitis, synergistic cellulitis, gangrene, and necrotizing fasciitis (Chaps. 156 and 179).

These soft tissue or skin infections are usually polymicrobial. A mean of 4.8 bacterial species are isolated, with an anaerobe-to-aerobe ratio of ~3:2. The most frequently isolated organisms include *Bacteroides, Peptostreptococcus, Clostridium, Enterococcus*, and *Proteus* species. The involvement of anaerobes in these types of infections is associated with a higher frequency of fever, foul-smelling lesions, gas in the tissues, and visible foot ulcer.

Anaerobic bacterial synergistic gangrene (*Meleney's gangrene*), a rare infection of the superficial fascia, is characterized by exquisite pain, redness, and swelling followed by induration. Erythema surrounds a central zone of necrosis. A granulating ulcer forms at the original center as necrosis and erythema extend outward. Symptoms are limited to pain; fever is not typical. These infections usually involve a combination of *Peptostreptococcus* species and *S. aureus*; the usual site of infection is an abdominal surgical wound or the area surrounding an ulcer on an extremity. Treatment includes surgical removal of necrotic tissue and antimicrobial administration.

Necrotizing fasciitis, a rapidly spreading destructive disease of the fascia, is usually attributed to group A streptococci (Chap. 173) but can also be a mixed infection involving anaerobes and aerobes, usually occurring after surgeries and in patients with diabetes or peripheral vascular disease. The most frequently isolated anaerobes in these infections are *Peptostreptococcus* and *Bacteroides* species. Gas may be found in the tissues. Similarly, myonecrosis can be associated with mixed anaerobic infection. *Fournier's gangrene* consists of cellulitis involving the scrotum, perineum, and anterior abdominal wall, with mixed anaerobic organisms spreading along deep external fascial planes and causing extensive loss of skin.

Bone and Joint Infections Although actinomycosis (Chap. 200) accounts on a worldwide basis for most anaerobic infections in bone, organisms including peptostreptococci or microaerophilic cocci, *Bacteroides* species, *Fusobacterium* species, and *Clostridium* species can also be involved in osteomyelitis (Chap. 158). These infections frequently arise adjacent to soft tissue infections. Many patients with osteomyelitis due to anaerobic bacteria have evidence of an anaerobic infection elsewhere in the body; most commonly, infected adjacent soft-tissue sites are the source of the organisms involved. Examples are diabetic foot ulcers and decubitus ulcers that may be complicated by mixed aerobic-anaerobic osteomyelitis. Hematogenous seeding of bone is uncommon. *Prevotella* and *Porphyromonas* species are detected in infections involving the maxilla and mandible, whereas *Clostridium* species have been reported as anaerobic pathogens in cases of osteomyelitis of the long bones following fracture or trauma. Fusobacteria have been isolated in pure culture from sites of osteomyelitis adjacent to the perinasal sinuses. Peptostreptococci and microaerophilic cocci have been reported as significant pathogens in infections involving the skull, mastoid, and prosthetic implants placed in bone. In patients with osteomyelitis, the most reliable culture specimen is a bone biopsy sample free of normal uninfected skin and subcutaneous tissue.

In contrast to anaerobic osteomyelitis, most cases of anaerobic arthritis (Chap. 157) involve a single isolate, and most cases are secondary to hematogenous spread. The most common isolates are *Fusobacterium* species. Most of the patients involved have uncontrolled peritonsillar infections progressing to septic cervical venous thrombophlebitis (Lemierre's syndrome) and resulting in hematogenous dissemination with a predilection for the joints. Unlike anaerobic osteomyelitis, anaerobic pyoarthritis in most cases is not polymicrobial and may be acquired hematogenously. Anaerobes are important pathogens in infections involving prosthetic joints; in these infections, the causative organisms (such as *Peptostreptococcus* species and *P. acnes*) are part of the normal skin microbiota.

Bacteremia Transient bacteremia is a well-known event in healthy individuals whose anatomic mucosal barriers have been injured (e.g., during dental extractions or dental scaling). These bacteremic episodes, which are often due to anaerobes, have no pathologic consequences. However, anaerobic bacteria are found in cultures of blood from clinically ill patients when proper culture techniques are used. Anaerobes have accounted for 5% (range at various institutions, 0.5–12%) of cases of clinically significant bacteremia. The incidence of anaerobic bacteremia decreased from the 1970s through the early 1990s. This change may have been related to the administration of antibiotic prophylaxis before intestinal surgery, the earlier recognition of localized infections, and the empirical use of broad-spectrum antibiotics for presumed infection. Recent reports present conflicting data regarding rates of anaerobic bacteremia. A study from the Mayo Clinic compared three periods (1993–1996, 1997–2000, and 2001–2004) and found a 74% increase in the mean incidence of anaerobic bacteremia; this finding contrasts with a 45% decrease in incidence from 1977 to 1988 at the same institution. In contrast, a report from Switzerland compared two periods (1997–2001 and 2002–2006) and found decreases in both the number of anaerobe-positive blood cultures and the proportion of all blood culture isolates that were anaerobes.

The majority of anaerobic bacteremias are due to gram-negative bacilli—mainly the *B. fragilis group*, with *B. fragilis* most commonly isolated (60–80% of cases). Other organisms causing bacteremia include *Clostridium* species (10%), *Peptostreptococcus* species (10%), and *Fusobacterium* species (5%).

Once the organism in the blood has been identified, both the portal of bloodstream entry and the underlying problem that probably led to seeding of the bloodstream can often be deduced from an understanding of the organism's normal site of residence. For example, mixed anaerobic bacteremia including *B. fragilis* usually implies a colonic pathology with mucosal disruption from neoplasia, diverticulitis, or some other inflammatory lesion. Debilitating diseases such as malignancies, diabetes, organ transplantation, and abdominal and pelvic surgeries are among the predisposing factors for anaerobic bacteremia. In a retrospective nested case–control study, diabetes was identified as a risk factor for anaerobic bacteremia when the source of bacteremia was unknown. The initial manifestations are determined by the portal of entry and reflect the localized condition. When bloodstream invasion occurs, patients can become extremely ill, with rigors and hectic fevers. The clinical picture may be quite similar to that seen in sepsis involving aerobic gram-negative bacilli. Although complications of anaerobic bacteremia (e.g., septic thrombophlebitis and septic shock) have been reported, their incidence in association with anaerobic bacteremia is low. Anaerobic bacteremia is potentially fatal and requires rapid diagnosis and appropriate therapy. Reported case–fatality rates are high, ranging from 25% to 44%, and appear to increase with the age of the patient (with reported rates of >66% among patients >60 years old), with the isolation of multiple species from the bloodstream, and with the failure to surgically remove a focus of infection. The attributable mortality rate for bacteremia associated with the *B. fragilis* group was examined in a matched case–control study. Patients with *B. fragilis*–group bacteremia had a significantly higher mortality rate (28% vs 8%), with an attributable mortality rate of 19.3% and a mortality risk ratio of 3.2.

Endocarditis and Pericarditis (See also Chap. 155) Endocarditis due to anaerobes is uncommon. However, anaerobic streptococci, which are often classified incorrectly, are responsible for this disease more frequently than is generally appreciated. Gram-negative anaerobes are unusual causes of endocarditis. Signs and symptoms of anaerobic endocarditis are similar to those of endocarditis due to facultative organisms. Mortality rates of 21–43% have been reported for anaerobic endocarditis.

Anaerobes, particularly *B. fragilis* and *Peptostreptococcus* species, are uncommonly found in infected pericardial fluids. Anaerobic pericarditis is associated with a mortality rate of >50%. Anaerobes can reach the pericardial space by hematogenous spread, by spread from a contiguous site of infection (e.g., heart or esophagus), or by direct inoculation arising from trauma or surgery.

DIAGNOSIS

There are three critical steps in the diagnosis of anaerobic infection: (1) proper collection of specimens; (2) rapid transport of the specimens to the microbiology laboratory, preferably in anaerobic transport media; and (3) proper handling of the specimens by the laboratory. Specimens must be collected by meticulous sampling of infected sites, with avoidance of contamination by the normal microbiota. When such contamination is likely, the specimen is unacceptable. Examples of specimens unacceptable for anaerobic culture include sputum collected by expectoration or nasal tracheal suction, bronchoscopy specimens, samples collected directly through the vaginal vault, urine collected by voiding, and feces. Specimens appropriate for anaerobic culture include sterile body fluids such as blood, pleural fluid, peritoneal fluid, cerebrospinal fluid, and aspirates or biopsy samples from normally sterile sites. As a general rule, liquid or tissue specimens are preferred; swab specimens should be avoided.

Because even brief exposure to oxygen may kill some anaerobic organisms and result in failure to isolate them in the laboratory, air must be expelled from the syringe used to aspirate the abscess cavity, and the needle must be capped with a sterile rubber stopper. It is also important to remember that prior antibiotic therapy reduces the cultivability of these bacteria. Specimens can be injected into transport bottles containing a reduced medium or taken immediately in syringes to the laboratory for direct culture on anaerobic media. Delays in transport may lead to a failure to isolate anaerobes due to exposure to oxygen or overgrowth of facultative organisms, which may eliminate or obscure any anaerobes that are present. All clinical specimens from suspected anaerobic infections should be subjected to Gram's staining and examined for organisms with characteristic morphology. It is not unusual for organisms to be observed on Gram's staining but not isolated in culture.

Because of the time and difficulty involved in the isolation of anaerobic bacteria, diagnosis of anaerobic infections must frequently be based on presumptive evidence. There are few clinical clues to the probable presence of anaerobic bacteria at infected sites. The involvement of certain sites with lowered oxidation-reduction potential (e.g., avascular necrotic tissues) and the presence of an abscess favor the diagnosis of an anaerobic infection. When infections occur in proximity to mucosal surfaces normally harboring an anaerobic microbiota, such as the gastrointestinal tract, female genital tract, or oropharynx, anaerobes should be considered as potential etiologic agents. A foul odor is often indicative of anaerobes, which produce certain organic acids as they proliferate in necrotic tissue. Although these odors are nearly pathognomonic for anaerobic infection, the absence of odor does not exclude an anaerobic etiology. The presence of gas in tissues is highly suggestive, but not diagnostic, of anaerobic infection. Because anaerobes often coexist with other bacteria and cause mixed or synergistic infection, Gram's staining of exudate frequently reveals multiple morphotypes suggestive of anaerobes. Sometimes these organisms have morphologic characteristics associated with specific species.

When cultures of obviously infected sites or purulent material yield no growth, streptococci only, or a single aerobic species (such as *E. coli*) and Gram's staining reveals a mixed flora, the involvement of anaerobes should be suspected; the implication is that the anaerobic microorganisms have failed to grow because of inadequate transport and/or culture techniques. Failure of an infection to respond to antibiotics that are not active against anaerobes (e.g., aminoglycosides and—in some circumstances—penicillin, cephalosporins, or tetracyclines) suggests an anaerobic etiology.

TREATMENT ANAEROBIC INFECTIONS

Successful therapy for anaerobic infections requires the administration of a combination of appropriate antibiotics, surgical resection, debridement of devitalized tissues, and drainage either surgically or percutaneously (guided by an imaging technique such as CT, MRI, or ultrasound). Any anatomic breach must be closed promptly, closed spaces drained, tissue compartments decompressed, and an adequate blood supply established. Abscess cavities should be drained as soon as fluctuation or localization occurs.

ANTIBIOTIC THERAPY AND RESISTANCE

The antibiotics used to treat anaerobic infections should be active against both aerobic and anaerobic organisms because many of these infections are of mixed etiology. Antibiotic regimens can usually be selected empirically on the basis of the type of infection, the species of the organisms usually present in such cases, the results of Gram's staining, and a knowledge of antimicrobial resistance patterns (Chap. 170 and Table 201-2). Other factors influencing the selection of antibiotics include need for bactericidal activity and for penetration into certain organs (such as the brain), toxicity, and impact on the normal microbiota. Antibiotics active against clinically relevant anaerobes can be grouped into four categories based on their predicted activity (Table 201-2). Nearly all the drugs listed have toxic side effects, which are described in detail in Chap. 170.

Antibiotic susceptibility testing of anaerobic bacteria has been difficult and controversial. Because of the slow growth rate of many anaerobes, the lack of standardized testing methods and of clinically relevant standards for resistance, and the generally good results obtained with empirical therapy, there has been limited interest in testing these organisms for antibiotic susceptibility. However, one study of antibiotic-treated patients with *Bacteroides* isolates from blood found mortality rates of 45% among those whose isolates were deemed resistant to the agent used and 16% among those whose isolates were deemed sensitive. It is accepted that testing is important for patients with serious or prolonged infections or in cases in which antibiotics have not had an impact. Testing is also helpful in monitoring the activity of new drugs and recording current resistance patterns among anaerobic pathogens. The antibiotics with the greatest activity against nearly all anaerobic bacteria include carbapenems, β-lactam/β-lactamase inhibitor combinations, metronidazole, and chloramphenicol.

Antibiotic resistance in anaerobic bacteria is an increasing problem. Resistance rates vary with the institution and the geographic region. In recent years, the activity of clindamycin, cefoxitin, cefotetan, and moxifloxacin has decreased against *B. fragilis* and related strains (*B. distasonis, B. ovatus, B. thetaiotaomicron, B. uniformis, B. vulgatus*). Multidrug-resistant *B. fragilis* has recently been reported. Nearly all organisms in the *B. fragilis* group (>97%) are resistant to penicillin G. The cephamycins cefoxitin and cefotetan display greater activity against this group, but rates of resistance have increased, with current figures at ~10% in the United States and higher in Argentina (28%) and Europe (17%). Rates of resistance to β-lactam agents among anaerobes other than *Bacteroides* are lower but are highly variable. β-Lactam/β-lactamase inhibitor combinations such as ampicillin/sulbactam, ticarcillin/clavulanic acid, and piperacillin/tazobactam are usually good therapeutic options against β-lactamase-producing anaerobes, including the *B. fragilis* group. Although resistance rates reported from most countries are still low, several studies have documented nonsusceptibility to ampicillin/sulbactam in 0.5–3% of isolates in the United States, 3–10% in Europe, and 1–8% in Argentina. Recently, up to 48% of *B. fragilis* isolates in Taiwan were found to be nonsusceptible to ampicillin/sulbactam, and a significant increase in resistance to this combination was also identified among other *Bacteroides, Prevotella,* and *Fusobacterium* species.

Carbapenems (ertapenem, doripenem, meropenem, and imipenem) are equally active against anaerobes, with <1% of *B. fragilis* strains showing resistance in the United States and Europe. Higher rates of carbapenem nonsusceptibility are being reported from some countries (5% in Germany, 8% [to doripenem] in Canada, and 7–12% in Taiwan).

Metronidazole is active against gram-negative anaerobes, including the *B. fragilis* group; resistance, although rare (<1%), has been reported in both Europe and the United States. Resistance to metronidazole is more common among gram-positive anaerobes, including *P. acnes, Actinomyces* species, lactobacilli, and anaerobic streptococci. Clindamycin is active against many anaerobes. However, rates of resistance to clindamycin among the *B. fragilis* group have increased in the United States from 3% in 1982 to 16% in 1996 and 26% in 2000, with rates as high as 40–50% in some series. Resistance to clindamycin among non-*Bacteroides* anaerobes is much less common (<10%).

Tigecycline is active against some anaerobic bacteria, including *Peptostreptococcus, Propionibacterium, Prevotella, Fusobacterium,* and most *Bacteroides* species. Its efficacy for treatment of intraabdominal infections was comparable to that of imipenem in two phase 3 double-blind clinical trials. This drug is therefore recommended as single-agent treatment for complicated intraabdominal infections, but resistance (~6%) among *Bacteroides* and non-*Bacteroides* species has been reported.

Fluoroquinolones such as moxifloxacin have shown potential in the treatment of mixed aerobic-anaerobic infections. A survey in the United States found a 38% rate of resistance to moxifloxacin among the *B. fragilis* group; in Europe 14–30% of isolates were nonsusceptible to this drug, as were 7–25% of anaerobes isolated from blood cultures in Taiwan. Despite excellent in vitro activity against all clinically important anaerobes, chloramphenicol is less desirable than other active drugs for the treatment of anaerobic infection because of documented clinical failures.

TABLE 201-2 ANTIMICROBIAL THERAPY FOR INFECTIONS INVOLVING COMMONLY ENCOUNTERED ANAEROBIC GRAM-NEGATIVE RODS

Category 1 (Nearly Always Active)	Category 2 (Usually Active)	Category 3 (Variable Resistance)	Category 4 (Resistance)
Carbapenems (imipenem, meropenem, doripenem)	Tigecycline	Cephamycins (cefoxitin, cefotetan)	Aminoglycosides
Metronidazole[a]	High-dose antipseudomonal penicillins	Clindamycin	Monobactams
β-Lactam/β-lactamase inhibitor combination (ampicillin/sulbactam, ticarcillin/clavulanic acid, piperacillin/tazobactam)		Penicillins	Trimethoprim-sulfamethoxazole
Chloramphenicol[b]		Cephalosporins	
		Tetracycline	
		Vancomycin	
		Erythromycin	
		Moxifloxacin	

[a]Usually needs to be given in combination with aerobic bacterial coverage. For infections originating below the diaphragm, aerobic gram-negative coverage is essential. For infections from an oral source, aerobic gram-positive coverage is added. Metronidazole also is not active against *Actinomyces, Propionibacterium,* or other gram-positive non-spore-forming bacilli (e.g., *Eubacterium, Bifidobacterium*) and is unreliable against peptostreptococci. [b]Despite excellent in vitro activity against all clinically important anaerobes, this drug is less desirable than other active drugs because of documented clinical failures.

If a patient fails to respond to one of the category 1 or category 2 drugs (Table 201-2), consideration should be given to alternative therapy and to determination of the resistance patterns among *Bacteroides* isolates.

INFECTIONS AT SPECIFIC SITES

In clinical situations, specific regimens must be tailored to the initial site of infection. The duration of therapy also depends on the infection site; the reader is referred to specific chapters on sites of infection for recommendations.

Infections above the diaphragm usually reflect the orodental microbiota, which does not include the *B. fragilis* group. β-Lactamase production has been reported in anaerobic strains that are usually isolated from infections originating above the diaphragm. Up to 60% of clinical isolates classified as *Prevotella* or *Porphyromonas* species, non–*B. fragilis* species of *Bacteroides*, or *Fusobacterium* species reportedly produce β-lactamase; thus all β-lactam drugs (penicillins and cephalosporins) are poor options. Because most of these infections have a mixed etiology that includes microaerophilic and aerobic streptococci, antibiotics that cover both aerobic and anaerobic bacteria are recommended. The recommended regimens include clindamycin, a β-lactam/β-lactamase inhibitor combination, or metronidazole in combination with a drug active against microaerophilic and aerobic streptococci.

Bronchoscopy in lung abscess is indicated only to rule out airway obstruction and does not enhance drainage; in any event, it should be delayed until the antimicrobial regimen has begun to affect the disease process so that the procedure does not spread the infection. Surgery is almost never indicated because of the danger of spilling the abscess contents into the lungs.

Chloramphenicol has been used successfully against anaerobic CNS infections at doses of 30–60 mg/kg per day, with the exact dose depending on the severity of illness. However, penicillin G and metronidazole also cross the blood–brain barrier and are bactericidal for many anaerobic organisms.

Anaerobic infections arising below the diaphragm (e.g., colonic and intraabdominal infections) must be treated specifically with agents active against *Bacteroides* species (Table 201-2). In intraabdominal sepsis (**Chap. 159**), the use of antibiotics effective against penicillin-resistant anaerobes has clearly reduced the incidence of postoperative infections and serious infectious complications. Specifically, a drug from category 1 (Table 201-2) must be included for broad-spectrum coverage. Single agents suitable for this purpose include the carbapenems, cefoxitin, and β-lactam/β-lactamase inhibitor combinations. A two-drug regimen is an alternative, with one drug active against coliforms and the other against anaerobes (e.g., a third-generation cephalosporin or a quinolone with metronidazole). In addition, if the clinician suspects that gram-positive facultative organisms such as enterococci are involved, therapeutic regimens should include ampicillin or vancomycin. Although clindamycin and cefotetan were previously considered acceptable options for intraabdominal infections involving anaerobes, these drugs are no longer recommended because of escalating rates of resistance in the *B. fragilis* group. Ampicillin/sulbactam is not recommended because of high rates of resistance among community-acquired strains of *E. coli* rather than because of resistance in anaerobic bacteria.

A meta-analysis of 40 randomized or quasi-randomized controlled trials of 16 antibiotic regimens for secondary peritonitis showed equivalent clinical success for all regimens.

Cases of anaerobic osteomyelitis in which a mixed flora is isolated from a bone biopsy specimen should be treated with a regimen that covers all isolates. When an anaerobic organism is recognized as a major or sole pathogen infecting a joint, the duration of treatment should be similar to that used for arthritis caused by aerobic bacteria (**Chap. 157**). Therapy includes the management of underlying disease states, the administration of appropriate antimicrobial agents, temporary joint immobilization, percutaneous drainage of effusions, and (usually) the removal of infected prostheses or internal fixation devices. Surgical drainage and debridement procedures such as sequestrectomy are essential for the removal of necrotic tissue that can sustain anaerobic infections.

The outcome of anaerobic bacteremia is significantly better in patients either initially given or switched to appropriate therapy on the basis of known antibiotic susceptibilities.

FAILURE OF THERAPY

Anaerobic infections that fail to respond to treatment or that relapse should be reassessed. Consideration should be given to additional surgical drainage or debridement. Superinfections with resistant gram-negative facultative or aerobic bacteria should be ruled out. The possibility of drug resistance must be entertained; if resistance is involved, repeat cultures may yield the pathogen.

SUPPORTIVE MEASURES

Other supportive measures in the management of anaerobic infections include careful attention to fluid and electrolyte balance (since extensive local edema may lead to hypoalbuminemia), hemodynamic support for septic shock, immobilization of infected extremities, maintenance of adequate nutrition during chronic infections by parenteral hyperalimentation, relief of pain, and anticoagulation for thrombophlebitis. For patients with severe anaerobic infections of soft tissues, hyperbaric oxygen therapy is advocated by some experts, but its value has not been proven in controlled trials.

SECTION 8 MYCOBACTERIAL DISEASES

202 Tuberculosis

Mario C. Raviglione

Tuberculosis (TB), which is caused by bacteria of the *Mycobacterium tuberculosis* complex, is one of the oldest diseases known to affect humans and a major cause of death worldwide. Recent population genomic studies suggest that *M. tuberculosis* may have emerged ~70,000 years ago in Africa and subsequently disseminated along with anatomically modern humans, expanding globally during the Neolithic Age as human density started to increase. Progenitors of *M. tuberculosis* are likely to have affected prehominids. This disease most often affects the lungs, although other organs are involved in up to one-third of cases. If properly treated, TB caused by drug-susceptible strains is curable in the vast majority of cases. If untreated, the disease may be fatal within 5 years in 50–65% of cases. Transmission usually takes place through the airborne spread of droplet nuclei produced by patients with infectious pulmonary TB.

ETIOLOGIC AGENT

Mycobacteria belong to the family Mycobacteriaceae and the order Actinomycetales. Of the pathogenic species belonging to the *M. tuberculosis* complex, which comprises eight distinct subgroups, the most common and important agent of human disease is *M. tuberculosis*. The

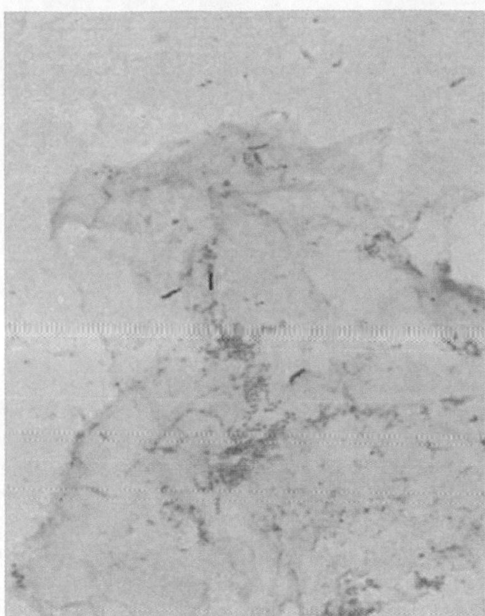

FIGURE 202-1 Acid-fast bacillus smear showing *M. tuberculosis* bacilli. *(Courtesy of the Centers for Disease Control and Prevention, Atlanta.)*

complex includes *M. bovis* (the bovine tubercle bacillus—characteristically resistant to pyrazinamide, once an important cause of TB transmitted by unpasteurized milk, and currently the cause of a small percentage of human cases worldwide), *M. caprae* (related to *M. bovis*), *M. africanum* (isolated from cases in West, Central, and East Africa), *M. microti* (the "vole" bacillus, a less virulent and rarely encountered organism), *M. pinnipedii* (a bacillus infecting seals and sea lions in the Southern Hemisphere and recently isolated from humans), *M. mungi* (isolated from banded mongooses in southern Africa), *M. orygis* (described recently in oryxes and other Bovidae in Africa and Asia and a potential cause of infection in humans), and *M. canetti* (a rare isolate from East African cases that produces unusual smooth colonies on solid media and is considered closely related to a supposed progenitor type).

M. tuberculosis is a rod-shaped, non-spore-forming, thin aerobic bacterium measuring 0.5 μm by 3 μm. Mycobacteria, including *M. tuberculosis*, are often neutral on Gram's staining. However, once stained, the bacilli cannot be decolorized by acid alcohol; this characteristic justifies their classification as acid-fast bacilli (AFB; Fig. 202-1). Acid fastness is due mainly to the organisms' high content of mycolic acids, long-chain cross-linked fatty acids, and other cell-wall lipids. Microorganisms other than mycobacteria that display some acid fastness include species of *Nocardia* and *Rhodococcus*, *Legionella micdadei*, and the protozoa *Isospora* and *Cryptosporidium*. In the mycobacterial cell wall, lipids (e.g., mycolic acids) are linked to underlying arabinogalactan and peptidoglycan. This structure results in very low permeability of the cell wall, thus reducing the effectiveness of most antibiotics. Another molecule in the mycobacterial cell wall, lipoarabinomannan, is involved in the pathogen–host interaction and facilitates the survival of *M. tuberculosis* within macrophages. The complete genome sequence of *M. tuberculosis* comprises 4043 genes encoding 3993 proteins and 50 genes encoding RNAs; its high guanine-plus-cytosine content (65.6%) is indicative of an aerobic "lifestyle." A large proportion of genes are devoted to the production of enzymes involved in cell wall metabolism.

EPIDEMIOLOGY

More than 5.7 million new cases of TB (all forms, both pulmonary and extrapulmonary) were reported to the World Health Organization (WHO) in 2013; 95% of cases were reported from developing countries. However, because of insufficient case detection and incomplete notification, reported cases may represent only about two-thirds of the total estimated cases. The WHO estimated that 9 million (range, 8.6–9.4 million) new cases of TB occurred worldwide in 2013, 95% of them in developing countries of Asia (5 million), Africa (2.6 million), the Middle East (0.7 million), and Latin America (0.3 million). It is further estimated that 1.49 million (range, 1.32–1.67 million) deaths from TB, including 0.36 million among people living with HIV infection, occurred in 2013, 96% of them in developing countries. Estimates of TB incidence rates (per 100,000 population) and numbers of TB-related deaths in 2013 are depicted in Figs. 202-2 and 202-3, respectively. During the late 1980s and early 1990s, numbers of reported cases of TB increased in industrialized countries. These increases were related largely to immigration from countries with a high incidence of TB; the spread of the HIV epidemic; social problems, such as increased urban poverty, homelessness, and drug abuse; and dismantling of TB services. During the past few years, numbers of reported cases have begun to decline again or have stabilized in most industrialized nations. In the United States, with the re-establishment of stronger control programs, the decline resumed in 1993 and has since been maintained. In 2013, 9582 cases of TB (3.0 cases/100,000 population) were reported to the Centers for Disease Control and Prevention (CDC).

In the United States, TB is uncommon among young adults of European descent, who have only rarely been exposed to *M. tuberculosis* infection during recent decades. In contrast, because of a high risk of transmission in the past, the prevalence of latent *M. tuberculosis* infection (LTBI) is relatively high among elderly whites. In general, adults ≥65 years of age have the highest incidence rate per capita (4.9 cases/100,000 population in 2013) and children <14 years of age the lowest (0.8 case/100,000 population). Blacks account for the highest proportion of cases (37%; 1257 cases in 2013) among U.S.-born persons. TB in the United States is also a disease of adult members of the HIV-infected population, the foreign-born population (64.6% of all cases in 2013), and disadvantaged/marginalized populations. Of the 6193 cases reported among foreign-born persons in 2013, 37% occurred in persons from the Americas and 32% occurred in persons born in the Western Pacific region. Overall, the highest rates per capita were among Asian Americans (18.7 cases/100,000 population). A total of 536 deaths were caused by TB in the United States in 2011. In Canada in 2013, 1638 TB cases were reported (4.7 cases/100,000 population); 70% (1145) of these cases occurred in foreign-born persons and 19% (309 cases) occurred in members of the Canadian aboriginal peoples, whose per capita rate is disproportionately high (23.4 cases/100,000 population) with a peak in the Nunavut territory of 143 cases/100,000 population—a rate similar to that in many highly endemic countries. Similarly, in Europe, TB has reemerged as an important public health problem, mainly as a result of cases among immigrants from high-incidence countries and among marginalized populations, often in large urban settings like London; in 2013, 41% of all cases reported from the United Kingdom occurred in London, and the rate per capita (36 cases/100,000 population) was similar to that in some middle-income countries. In most Western European countries, there are more cases annually among foreign-born than native populations.

Recent data on global trends indicate that in 2013 the TB incidence was stable or falling in most regions; this trend began in the early 2000s and appears to have continued, with an average annual decline of 2% globally. This global decrease is explained largely by the simultaneous reduction in TB incidence in sub-Saharan Africa, where rates had risen steeply since the 1980s as a result of the HIV epidemic and the lack of capacity of health systems and services to deal with the problem effectively, and in Eastern Europe, where incidence increased rapidly during the 1990s because of a deterioration in socioeconomic conditions and the health care infrastructure (although, after peaking in 2001, incidence in Eastern Europe has since declined slowly).

Of the estimated 9 million new cases of TB in 2013, 13% (1.1 million) were associated with HIV infection, and 78% of these HIV-associated cases occurred in Africa. An estimated 0.36 million persons with HIV-associated TB died in 2013. Furthermore, an estimated 480,000 cases (range, 350,000–610,000) of multidrug-resistant TB (MDR-TB)—a form of the disease caused by bacilli resistant at least to isoniazid and rifampin—occurred in 2013. Only 28% of these

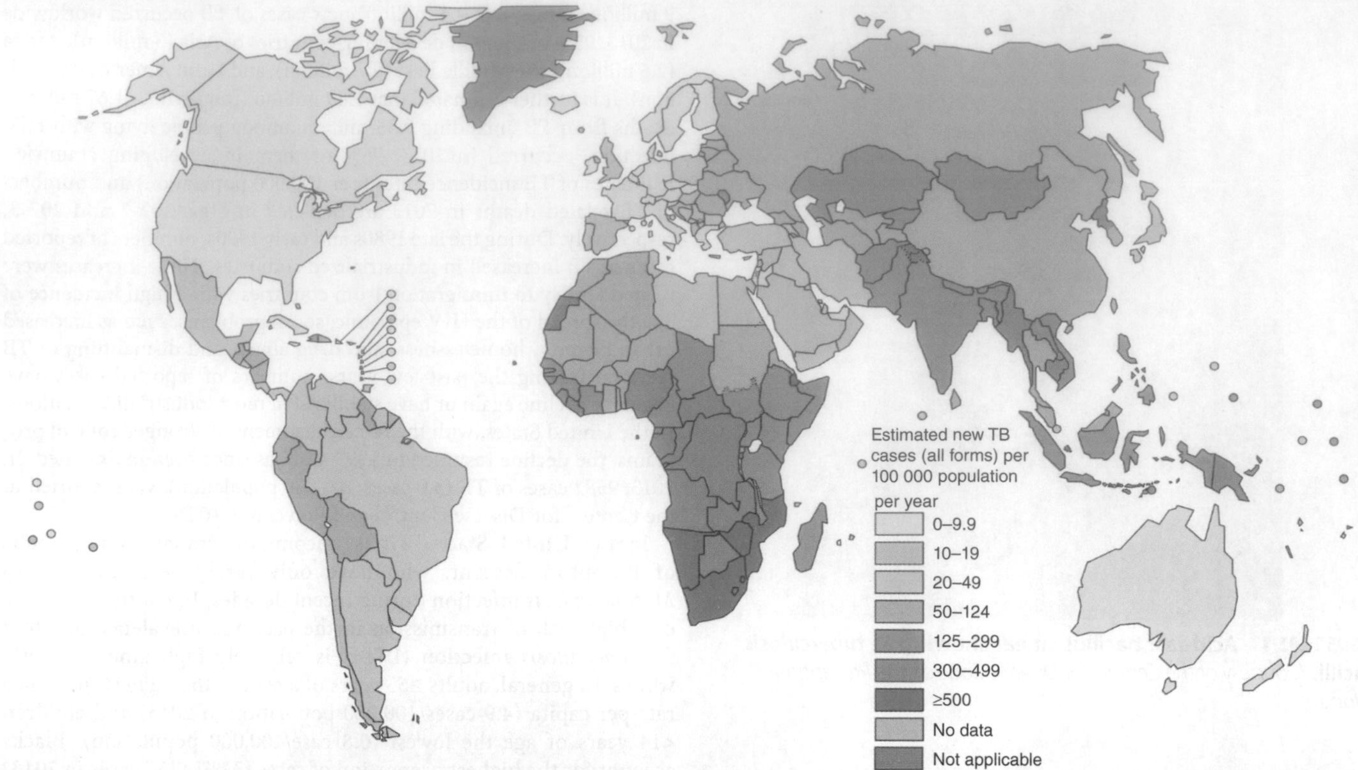

FIGURE 202-2 Estimated tuberculosis (TB) incidence rates (per 100,000 population) in 2013. The designations used and the presentation of material on this map do not imply the expression of any opinion whatsoever on the part of the World Health Organization (WHO) concerning the legal status of any country, territory, city, or area or of its authorities or concerning the delimitation of its frontiers or boundaries. *Dotted*, *dashed*, and *white lines* represent approximate border lines for which there may not yet be full agreement. *(Courtesy of the Global TB Programme, WHO; with permission.)*

cases were diagnosed because of a lack of culture and drug-susceptibility testing capacity in most settings worldwide. The countries of the former Soviet Union have reported the highest proportions of MDR disease among new TB cases (up to 35–40% in some regions of Russia and Belarus). Overall, 60% of all MDR-TB cases occur in China, India, the Russian Federation, Pakistan, and Ukraine. Since 2006, 100 countries, including the United States, have reported cases of extensively drug-resistant TB (XDR-TB), in which MDR-TB is compounded by additional resistance to the most powerful second-line anti-TB drugs (fluoroquinolones and at least one of the injectable

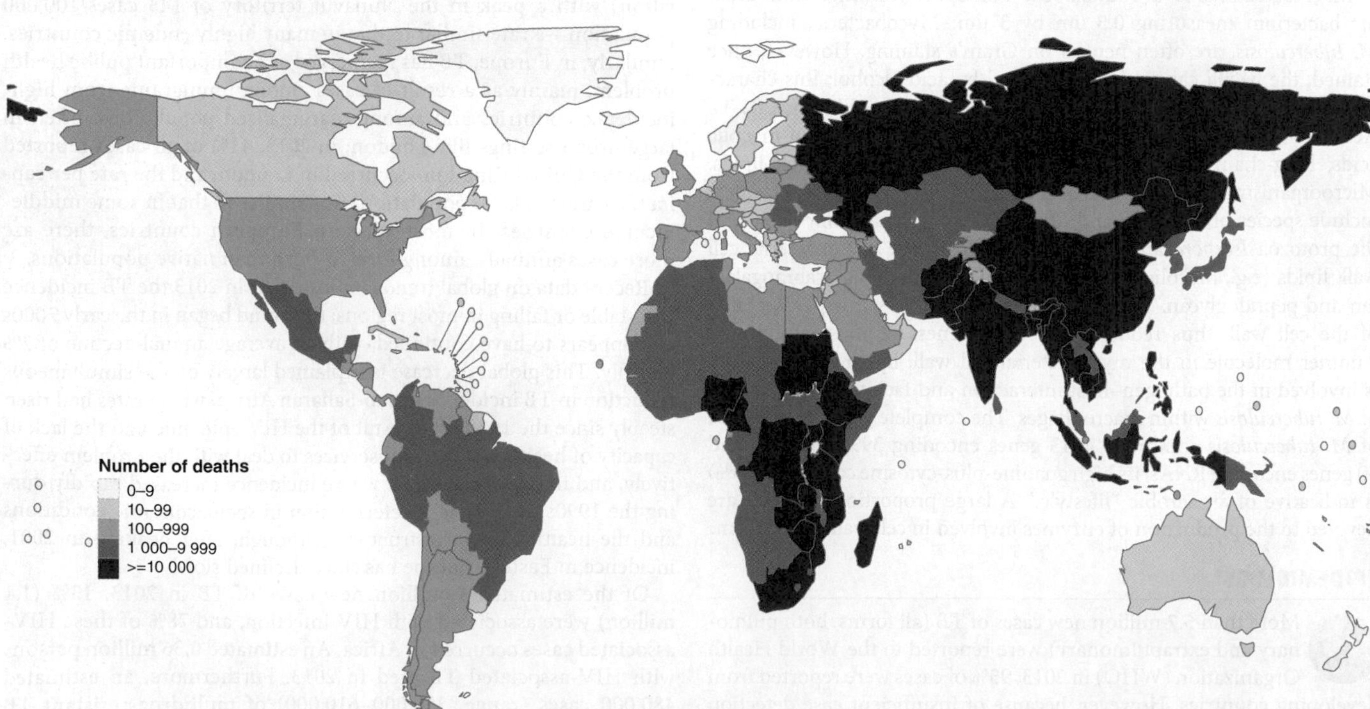

FIGURE 202-3 Estimated numbers of tuberculosis-related deaths in 2013. *(See disclaimer in Fig. 202-2. Courtesy of the Global TB Programme, WHO; with permission.)*

drugs amikacin, kanamycin, and capreomycin). Up to 10% of the MDR-TB cases worldwide may actually be XDR-TB, but the vast majority of XDR-TB cases remain undiagnosed because reliable methods for drug susceptibility testing are lacking and laboratory capacity is limited. Lately, cases deemed resistant to all anti-TB drugs have been reported from countries such as India, Italy, and Iran; however, this information must be interpreted with caution because drug susceptibility testing for several second-line drugs is neither accurate nor reproducible.

FROM EXPOSURE TO INFECTION

M. tuberculosis is most commonly transmitted from a person with infectious pulmonary TB by droplet nuclei, which are aerosolized by coughing, sneezing, or speaking. The tiny droplets dry rapidly; the smallest (<5–10 μm in diameter) may remain suspended in the air for several hours and may reach the terminal air passages when inhaled. There may be as many as 3000 infectious nuclei per cough. Other routes of transmission of tubercle bacilli (e.g., through the skin or the placenta) are uncommon and of no epidemiologic significance. The probability of contact with a person who has an infectious form of TB, the intimacy and duration of that contact, the degree of infectiousness of the case, and the shared environment in which the contact takes place are all important determinants of the likelihood of transmission. Several studies of close-contact situations have clearly demonstrated that TB patients whose sputum contains AFB visible by microscopy (sputum smear–positive cases) are the most likely to transmit the infection. The most infectious patients have cavitary pulmonary disease or, much less commonly, laryngeal TB and produce sputum containing as many as 10^5–10^7 AFB/mL. Patients with sputum smear–negative/culture-positive TB are less infectious, although they have been responsible for up to 20% of transmission in some studies in the United States. Those with culture-negative pulmonary TB and extrapulmonary TB are essentially noninfectious. Because persons with both HIV infection and TB are less likely to have cavitations, they may be less infectious than persons without HIV co-infection. Crowding in poorly ventilated rooms is one of the most important factors in the transmission of tubercle bacilli because it increases the intensity of contact with a case.

The risk of acquiring *M. tuberculosis* infection is determined mainly by exogenous factors. Because of delays in seeking care and in making a diagnosis, it is generally estimated that, in high-prevalence settings, up to 20 contacts may be infected by each AFB positive case before the index case is diagnosed.

FROM INFECTION TO DISEASE

Unlike the risk of acquiring infection with *M. tuberculosis*, the risk of developing disease after being infected depends largely on endogenous factors, such as the individual's innate immunologic and nonimmunologic defenses and the level at which the individual's cell-mediated immunity (CMI) is functioning. Clinical illness directly following infection is classified as *primary TB* and is common among children in the first few years of life and among immunocompromised persons. Although primary TB may be severe and disseminated, it generally is not associated with high-level transmissibility. When infection is acquired later in life, the chance is greater that the mature immune system will contain it at least temporarily. Bacilli, however, may persist for years before reactivating to produce *secondary* (or *postprimary*) *TB*, which, because of frequent cavitation, is more often infectious than is primary disease. Overall, it is estimated that up to 10% of infected persons will eventually develop active TB in their lifetime—half of them during the first 18 months after infection. The risk is much higher among HIV-infected persons. Reinfection of a previously infected individual, which is common in areas with high rates of TB transmission, may also favor the development of disease. At the height of the TB resurgence in the United States in the early 1990s, molecular typing and comparison of strains of *M. tuberculosis* suggested that up to one-third of cases of active TB in some inner-city communities were due to recent transmission rather than to reactivation of old latent infection. Age is an important determinant of the risk of disease after infection. Among infected persons, the incidence of TB is highest

TABLE 202-1 RISK FACTORS FOR ACTIVE TUBERCULOSIS IN PERSONS WHO HAVE BEEN INFECTED WITH TUBERCLE BACILLI

Factor	Relative Risk/Odds[a]
Recent infection (<1 year)	12.9
Fibrotic lesions (spontaneously healed)	2–20
Comorbidities and iatrogenic causes	
HIV infection	21–>30
Silicosis	30
Chronic renal failure/hemodialysis	10–25
Diabetes	2–4
IV drug use	10–30
Immunosuppressive treatment	10
Tumor necrosis factor α inhibitors	4–5
Gastrectomy	2–5
Jejunoileal bypass	30–60
Posttransplantation period (renal, cardiac)	20–70
Tobacco smoking	2–3
Malnutrition and severe underweight	2

[a]Old infection = 1.

during late adolescence and early adulthood; the reasons are unclear. The incidence among women peaks at 25–34 years of age. In this age group, rates among women may be higher than those among men, whereas at older ages the opposite is true. The risk increases in the elderly, possibly because of waning immunity and comorbidity.

A variety of diseases and conditions favor the development of active TB (Table 202-1). In absolute terms, the most potent risk factor for TB among infected individuals is clearly HIV co-infection, which suppresses cellular immunity. The risk that LTBI will proceed to active disease is directly related to the patient's degree of immunosuppression. In a study of HIV-infected, tuberculin skin test (TST)–positive persons, this risk varied from 2.6 to 13.3 cases/100 person years and increased as the CD4+ T cell count decreased.

NATURAL HISTORY OF DISEASE

Studies conducted in various countries before the advent of chemotherapy showed that untreated TB is often fatal. About one-third of patients died within 1 year after diagnosis, and more than 50% died within 5 years. The 5-year mortality rate among sputum smear–positive cases was 65%. Of the survivors at 5 years, ~60% had undergone spontaneous remission, while the remainder were still excreting tubercle bacilli. With effective, timely, and proper chemotherapy, patients have a very high chance of being cured. However, improper use of anti-TB drugs, while reducing mortality rates, may also result in large numbers of chronic infectious cases, often with drug-resistant bacilli.

PATHOGENESIS AND IMMUNITY

INFECTION AND MACROPHAGE INVASION

The interaction of *M. tuberculosis* with the human host begins when droplet nuclei containing viable microorganisms propelled into the air by infectious patients are inhaled by a close bystander. Although the majority of inhaled bacilli are trapped in the upper airways and expelled by ciliated mucosal cells, a fraction (usually <10%) reach the alveoli, a unique immunoregulatory environment. There, alveolar macrophages that have not yet been activated (prototypic alternatively activated macrophages) phagocytose the bacilli. Adhesion of mycobacteria to macrophages results largely from binding of the bacterial cell wall to a variety of macrophage cell-surface molecules, including complement receptors, the mannose receptor, the immunoglobulin GFcγ receptor, and type A scavenger receptors. Phagocytosis is enhanced by complement activation leading to opsonization of bacilli with C3 activation products such as C3b and C3bi. (Bacilli are resistant to complement-mediated lysis.) Binding of certain receptors, such as the mannose receptor, regulates postphagocytic events such as phagosome–lysosome fusion and inflammatory cytokine production. After a phagosome forms, the survival of *M. tuberculosis* within it seems to depend in part on reduced acidification due to lack of assembly of a complete vesicular proton-adenosine triphosphatase. A complex series of events is generated by the bacterial cell-wall lipoglycan lipoarabinomannan (ManLAM). ManLAM inhibits the intracellular increase of Ca^{2+}. Thus, the Ca^{2+}/calmodulin pathway (leading to phagosome–lysosome fusion) is impaired, and the bacilli survive within the phagosomes. The *M. tuberculosis* phagosome has been found to inhibit the production of phosphatidylinositol 3-phosphate (PI3P). Normally, PI3P earmarks phagosomes for membrane sorting and maturation, including phagolysosome formation, which would destroy the bacteria. Bacterial factors have also been found to block the host defense of autophagy, in which the cell sequesters the phagosome in a double-membrane vesicle (*autophagosome*) that is destined to fuse with lysosomes. If the bacilli are successful in arresting phagosome maturation, then replication begins and the macrophage eventually ruptures and releases its bacillary contents. Other uninfected phagocytic cells are then recruited to continue the infection cycle by ingesting dying macrophages and their bacillary content, thus in turn becoming infected themselves and expanding the infection.

VIRULENCE OF TUBERCLE BACILLI

M. tuberculosis must be viewed as a complex formed by a multitude of strains that differ in virulence and are capable of producing a variety of manifestations of disease. Since the elucidation of the *M. tuberculosis* genome in 1998, large mutant collections have been generated, and many bacterial genes that contribute to *M. tuberculosis* virulence have been found. Different patterns of virulence defects have been defined in various animal models—predominantly mice but also guinea pigs, rabbits, and nonhuman primates. The *katG* gene encodes for a catalase/peroxidase enzyme that protects against oxidative stress and is required for isoniazid activation and subsequent bactericidal activity. Region of difference 1 (RD1) is a 9.5-kb locus that encodes two key small protein antigens—early secretory antigen-6 (ESAT-6) and culture filtrate protein-10 (CFP-10)—as well as a putative secretion apparatus that may facilitate their egress; the absence of this locus in the vaccine strain *M. bovis* bacille Calmette-Guérin (BCG) has been shown to be a key attenuating mutation. The validity of a recent observation in *M. marinum* needs to be confirmed in *M. tuberculosis*; in *M. marinum*, a mutation in the RD1 virulence locus encoding the ESX1 secretion system impairs the capacity of apoptotic macrophages to recruit uninfected cells for further rounds of infection. The results are less replication and fewer new granulomas. Mutants lacking key enzymes of bacterial biosynthesis become auxotrophic for the missing substrate and often are totally unable to proliferate in animals; these include the *leuCD* and *panCD* mutants, which require leucine and pantothenic acid, respectively. The isocitrate lyase gene *icl1* encodes a key step in the glyoxylate shunt that facilitates bacterial growth on fatty acid substrates; this gene is required for long-term persistence of *M. tuberculosis* infection in mice with chronic TB. *M. tuberculosis* mutants in regulatory genes such as sigma factor C and sigma factor H (*sigC* and *sigH*) are associated with normal bacterial growth in mice, but they fail to elicit full tissue pathology. Finally, the mycobacterial protein CarD (expressed by the *carD* gene) seems essential for the control of rRNA transcription that is required for replication and persistence in the host cell. Its loss exposes mycobacteria to oxidative stress, starvation, DNA damage, and ultimately sensitivity to killing by a variety of host mutagens and defensive mechanisms.

INNATE RESISTANCE TO INFECTION

Several observations suggest that genetic factors play a key role in innate nonimmune resistance to infection with *M. tuberculosis* and the development of disease. The existence of this resistance, which is polygenic in nature, is suggested by the differing degrees of susceptibility to TB in different populations. In mice, a gene called *Nramp1* (natural resistance–associated macrophage protein 1) plays a regulatory role in resistance/susceptibility to mycobacteria. The human homologue NRAMP1, which maps to chromosome 2q, may play a role in determining susceptibility to TB, as is suggested by a study among West Africans. Studies of mouse genetics identified a novel host resistance gene, *ipr1*, which is encoded within the *sst1* locus; *ipr1* encodes an interferon (IFN)–inducible nuclear protein that interacts with other nuclear proteins in macrophages primed with IFNs or infected by *M. tuberculosis*. In addition, polymorphisms in multiple genes, such as those encoding for various major histocompatibility complex (MHC) alleles, IFN-γ, T cell growth factor β, interleukin (IL) 10, mannose-binding protein, IFN-γ receptor, Toll-like receptor 2, vitamin D receptor, and IL-1, have been associated with susceptibility to TB.

THE HOST RESPONSE, GRANULOMA FORMATION, AND "LATENCY"

In the initial stage of host–bacterium interaction, prior to the onset of an acquired CMI response, *M. tuberculosis* disseminates widely through the lymph vessels, spreading to other sites in the lungs and other organs, and undergoes a period of extensive growth within naïve unactivated macrophages; additional naïve macrophages are recruited to the early granuloma. Studies suggest that *M. tuberculosis* uses specific virulence mechanisms to subvert host cellular signaling and to elicit an early regulated proinflammatory response that promotes granuloma expansion and bacterial growth during this key early phase. A study of *M. marinum* infection in zebrafish has delineated one molecular mechanism by which mycobacteria induce granuloma formation. The mycobacterial protein ESAT-6 induces secretion of matrix metalloproteinase 9 (MMP9) by nearby epithelial cells that are in contact with infected macrophages. MMP9 in turn stimulates recruitment of naïve macrophages, thus inducing granuloma maturation and bacterial growth. Disruption of MMP9 function results in reduced bacterial growth. Another study has shown that *M. tuberculosis*–derived cyclic AMP is secreted from the phagosome into host macrophages, subverting the cell's signal transduction pathways and stimulating an elevation in the secretion of tumor necrosis factor α (TNF-α) as well as further proinflammatory cell recruitment. Ultimately, the chemoattractants and bacterial products released during the repeated rounds of cell lysis and infection of newly arriving macrophages enable dendritic cells to access bacilli; these cells migrate to the draining lymph nodes and present mycobacterial antigens to T lymphocytes. At this point, the development of CMI and humoral immunity begins. These initial stages of infection are usually asymptomatic.

About 2–4 weeks after infection, two host responses to *M. tuberculosis* develop: a macrophage-activating CMI response and a tissue-damaging response. The *macrophage-activating response* is a T cell–mediated phenomenon resulting in the activation of macrophages that are capable of killing and digesting tubercle bacilli. The *tissue-damaging response* is the result of a delayed-type hypersensitivity (DTH) reaction to various bacillary antigens; it destroys unactivated macrophages that contain multiplying bacilli but also causes caseous necrosis of the involved tissues (see below). Although both of these responses can inhibit mycobacterial growth, it is the balance between the two that determines the forms of TB that will develop subsequently. With the development of specific immunity and the accumulation of large numbers of activated macrophages at the site of the primary lesion, granulomatous lesions (tubercles) are formed. These lesions consist of accumulations of lymphocytes and activated macrophages that evolve toward epithelioid and giant cell morphologies. Initially, the tissue-damaging response can limit mycobacterial growth within macrophages. As stated above, this response, mediated by various bacterial products, not only destroys macrophages but also produces early solid necrosis in the center of the tubercle. Although *M. tuberculosis* can survive, its growth is inhibited within this necrotic environment by low oxygen tension and low pH. At this point, some lesions may heal by fibrosis, with subsequent calcification, whereas inflammation and necrosis occur in other lesions. Some observations have challenged the traditional view that any encounter between mycobacteria and macrophages results in chronic infection. It is possible that an immune response capable of eradicating early infection may sometimes develop as a consequence, for instance, of disabling mutations in mycobacterial genomes rendering their replication ineffective. Individual granulomas that are formed during this phase of infection can vary in size and cell composition; some can contain the spread of mycobacteria, while others cannot. LTBI ensues as a result of this dynamic balance between the microorganism and the host. According to recent developments, *latency* may not be an accurate term because bacilli may remain active during this "latent" stage, forming biofilms in necrotic areas within which they temporarily hide. Thus, the term *persister* is probably more accurate to indicate the behavior of the bacilli in this phase. It is important to recognize that latent infection and disease represent not a binary state but rather a continuum along which infection will eventually move in the direction of full containment or disease. The ability to predict, through systemic biomarkers, which affected individuals will progress toward disease would be of immense value in devising prophylactic interventions.

MACROPHAGE-ACTIVATING RESPONSE

CMI is critical at this early stage. In the majority of infected individuals, local macrophages are activated when bacillary antigens processed by macrophages stimulate T lymphocytes to release a variety of lymphokines. These activated macrophages aggregate around the lesion's center and effectively neutralize tubercle bacilli without causing further tissue destruction. In the central part of the lesion, the necrotic material resembles soft cheese (*caseous necrosis*)—a phenomenon that may also be observed in other conditions, such as neoplasms. Even when healing takes place, viable bacilli may remain dormant within macrophages or in the necrotic material for many years. These "healed" lesions in the lung parenchyma and hilar lymph nodes may later undergo calcification.

DELAYED-TYPE HYPERSENSITIVITY

In a minority of cases, the macrophage-activating response is weak, and mycobacterial growth can be inhibited only by intensified DTH reactions, which lead to lung tissue destruction. The lesion tends to enlarge further, and the surrounding tissue is progressively damaged. At the center of the lesion, the caseous material liquefies. Bronchial walls and blood vessels are invaded and destroyed, and cavities are formed. The liquefied caseous material, containing large numbers of bacilli, is drained through bronchi. Within the cavity, tubercle bacilli multiply, spill into the airways, and are discharged into the environment through expiratory maneuvers such as coughing and talking. In the early stages of infection, bacilli are usually transported by macrophages to regional lymph nodes, from which they gain access to the central venous return; from there they reseed the lungs and may also disseminate beyond the pulmonary vasculature throughout the body via the systemic circulation. The resulting extrapulmonary lesions may undergo the same evolution as those in the lungs, although most tend to heal. In young children with poor natural immunity, hematogenous dissemination may result in highly fatal miliary TB or tuberculous meningitis.

ROLE OF MACROPHAGES AND MONOCYTES

While CMI confers partial protection against *M. tuberculosis*, humoral immunity plays a less well-defined role in protection (although evidence is accumulating on the existence of antibodies to lipoarabinomannan, which may prevent dissemination of infection in children). In the case of CMI, two types of cells are essential: macrophages, which directly phagocytose tubercle bacilli, and T cells (mainly CD4+ T lymphocytes), which induce protection through the production of cytokines, especially IFN-γ. After infection with *M. tuberculosis*, alveolar macrophages secrete various cytokines responsible for a number of events (e.g., the formation of granulomas) as well as systemic effects (e.g., fever and weight loss). However, alternatively activated alveolar macrophages may be particularly susceptible to *M. tuberculosis* growth early on, given their more limited proinflammatory and bactericidal activity, which is related in part to being bathed in surfactant. New monocytes and macrophages attracted to the site are key components of the immune response. Their primary mechanism is probably related to production of oxidants (such as reactive oxygen intermediates or nitric oxide) that have antimycobacterial activity and increase the synthesis of cytokines such as TNF-α and IL-1, which in turn regulate the release of reactive oxygen intermediates and reactive nitrogen intermediates. In addition, macrophages can undergo apoptosis—a defensive mechanism to prevent release of cytokines and bacilli via their sequestration in the apoptotic cell. Recent work also describes the involvement of neutrophils in the host response, although the timing of their appearance and their effectiveness remain uncertain.

ROLE OF T LYMPHOCYTES

Alveolar macrophages, monocytes, and dendritic cells are also critical in processing and presenting antigens to T lymphocytes, primarily CD4+ and CD8+ T cells; the result is the activation and proliferation of CD4+ T lymphocytes, which are crucial to the host's defense against *M. tuberculosis*. Qualitative and quantitative defects of CD4+ T cells explain the inability of HIV-infected individuals to contain mycobacterial proliferation. Activated CD4+ T lymphocytes can differentiate into cytokine-producing T_H1 or T_H2 cells. T_H1 cells produce IFN-γ—an activator of macrophages and monocytes—and IL-2. T_H2 cells produce IL-4, IL-5, IL-10, and IL-13 and may also promote humoral immunity. The interplay of these various cytokines and their cross-regulation determine the host's response. The role of cytokines in promoting intracellular killing of mycobacteria, however, has not been entirely elucidated. IFN-γ may induce the generation of reactive nitrogen intermediates and regulate genes involved in bactericidal effects. TNF-α also seems to be important. Observations made originally in transgenic knockout mice and more recently in humans suggest that other T cell subsets, especially CD8+ T cells, may play an important role. CD8+ T cells have been associated with protective activities via cytotoxic responses and lysis of infected cells as well as with production of IFN-γ and TNF-α. Finally, natural killer cells act as co-regulators of CD8+ T cell lytic activities, and γδ T cells are increasingly thought to be involved in protective responses in humans.

MYCOBACTERIAL LIPIDS AND PROTEINS

Lipids have been involved in mycobacterial recognition by the innate immune system, and lipoproteins (such as 19-kDa lipoprotein) have been proven to trigger potent signals through Toll-like receptors present in blood dendritic cells. *M. tuberculosis* possesses various protein antigens. Some are present in the cytoplasm and cell wall; others are secreted. That the latter are more important in eliciting a T lymphocyte response is suggested by experiments documenting the appearance of protective immunity in animals after immunization with live, protein-secreting mycobacteria. Among the antigens that may play a protective role are the 30-kDa (or 85B) and ESAT-6 antigens. Protective immunity is probably the result of reactivity to many different mycobacterial antigens. These antigens are being incorporated into newly designed vaccines on various platforms.

SKIN TEST REACTIVITY

Coincident with the appearance of immunity, DTH to *M. tuberculosis* develops. This reactivity is the basis of the TST, which is used primarily for the detection of *M. tuberculosis* infection in persons without symptoms. The cellular mechanisms responsible for TST reactivity are related mainly to previously sensitized CD4+ T lymphocytes, which are attracted to the skin-test site. There, they proliferate and produce cytokines. Although DTH is associated with protective immunity (TST-positive persons are less susceptible to a new *M. tuberculosis* infection than TST-negative persons), it by no means guarantees protection against reactivation. In fact, cases of active TB are often accompanied by strongly positive skin-test reactions. There is also evidence of reinfection with a new strain of *M. tuberculosis* in patients previously treated for active disease. This evidence underscores the fact that previous latent or active TB may not confer fully protective immunity.

CLINICAL MANIFESTATIONS

TB is classified as pulmonary, extrapulmonary, or both. Depending on several factors linked to different populations and bacterial strains, extrapulmonary TB may occur in 10–40% of patients. Furthermore, up to two-thirds of HIV-infected patients with TB may have both pulmonary and extrapulmonary TB or extrapulmonary TB alone.

PULMONARY TB

Pulmonary TB is conventionally categorized as primary or postprimary (adult-type, secondary). This distinction has been challenged by molecular evidence from TB-endemic areas indicating that a large percentage of cases of adult pulmonary TB result from recent infection (either primary infection or reinfection) and not from reactivation.

Primary Disease Primary pulmonary TB occurs soon after the initial infection with tubercle bacilli. It may be asymptomatic or may present with fever and occasionally pleuritic chest pain. In areas of high TB transmission, this form of disease is often seen in children. Because most inspired air is distributed to the middle and lower lung zones, these areas are most commonly involved in primary TB. The lesion forming after initial infection (*Ghon focus*) is usually peripheral and accompanied by transient hilar or paratracheal lymphadenopathy, which may or may not be visible on standard chest radiography (Fig. 202-4). Some patients develop erythema nodosum on the legs (see Fig. 25e-40) or phlyctenular conjunctivitis. In the majority of cases, the lesion heals spontaneously and becomes evident only as a small calcified nodule. Pleural reaction overlying a subpleural focus is also common. The Ghon focus, with or without overlying pleural reaction, thickening, and regional lymphadenopathy, is referred to as the *Ghon complex*.

In young children with immature CMI and in persons with impaired immunity (e.g., those with malnutrition or HIV infection), primary pulmonary TB may progress rapidly to clinical illness. The initial lesion increases in size and can evolve in different ways. Pleural effusion, which is found in up to two-thirds of cases, results from the penetration of bacilli into the pleural space from an adjacent subpleural focus. In severe cases, the primary site rapidly enlarges, its central portion undergoes necrosis, and cavitation develops (*progressive primary TB*). TB in young children is almost invariably accompanied by hilar or paratracheal lymphadenopathy due to the spread of bacilli from the lung parenchyma through lymphatic vessels. Enlarged lymph nodes may compress bronchi, causing total obstruction with distal collapse, partial obstruction with large-airway wheezing, or a ball-valve effect with segmental/lobar hyperinflation. Lymph nodes may also rupture into the airway with development of pneumonia, often including areas of necrosis and cavitation, distal to the obstruction. Bronchiectasis (Chap. 312) may develop in any segment/lobe damaged by progressive caseating pneumonia. Occult hematogenous dissemination commonly follows primary infection. However, in the absence of a sufficient acquired immune response, which usually contains the infection, disseminated or miliary disease may result (Fig. 202-5). Small granulomatous lesions develop in multiple organs and may cause

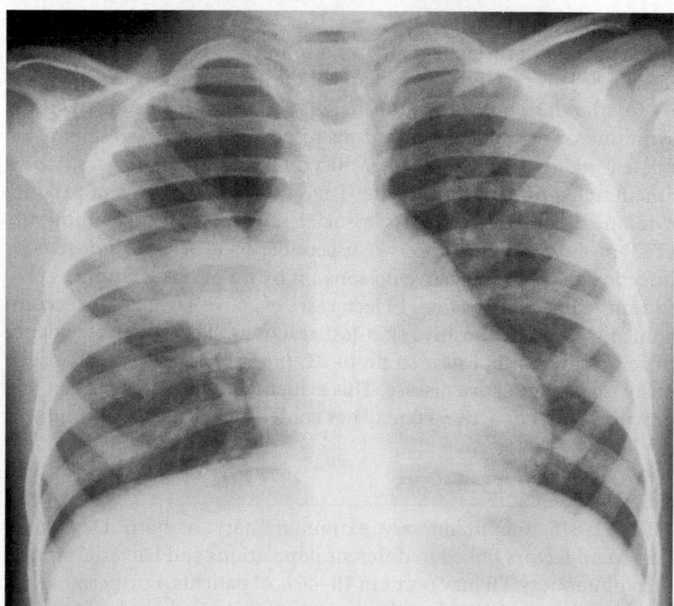

FIGURE 202-4 Chest radiograph showing right hilar lymph node enlargement with infiltration into the surrounding lung tissue in a child with primary tuberculosis. *(Courtesy of Prof. Robert Gie, Department of Paediatrics and Child Health, Stellenbosch University, South Africa; with permission.)*

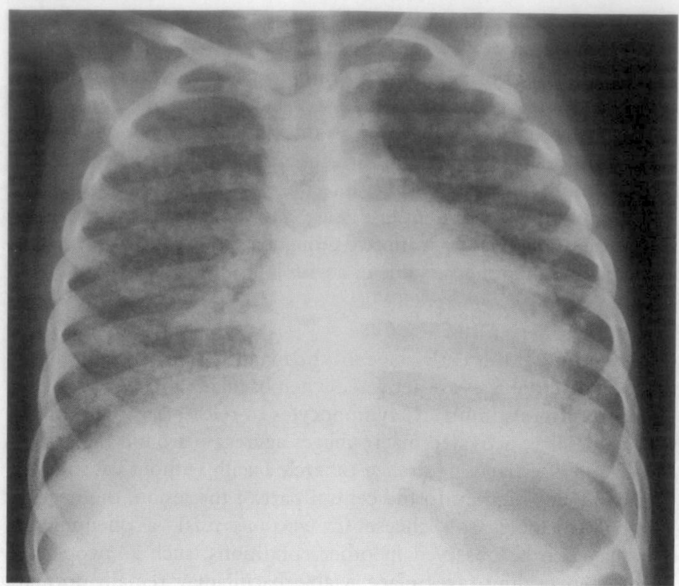

FIGURE 202-5 Chest radiograph showing bilateral miliary (millet-sized) infiltrates in a child. *(Courtesy of Prof. Robert Gie, Department of Paediatrics and Child Health, Stellenbosch University, South Africa; with permission.)*

locally progressive disease or result in tuberculous meningitis; this is a particular concern in very young children and immunocompromised persons (e.g., patients with HIV infection).

Postprimary (Adult-Type) Disease Also referred to as *reactivation* or *secondary TB*, postprimary TB is probably most accurately termed *adult-type TB* because it may result from endogenous reactivation of distant LTBI or recent infection (primary infection or reinfection). It is usually localized to the apical and posterior segments of the upper lobes, where the substantially higher mean oxygen tension (compared with that in the lower zones) favors mycobacterial growth. The superior segments of the lower lobes are also more frequently involved. The extent of lung parenchymal involvement varies greatly, from small infiltrates to extensive cavitary disease. With cavity formation, liquefied necrotic contents are ultimately discharged into the airways and may undergo bronchogenic spread, resulting in satellite lesions within the lungs that may in turn undergo cavitation (Figs. 202-6 and 202-7). Massive involvement of pulmonary segments or lobes, with coalescence of lesions, produces caseating pneumonia. While up to one-third of untreated patients reportedly succumb to severe pulmonary TB within a few months after onset (the classic "galloping consumption" of the past), others may undergo a process of spontaneous remission or proceed along a chronic, progressively debilitating course ("consumption" or *phthisis*). Under these circumstances, some pulmonary lesions become fibrotic and may later calcify, but cavities persist in other parts of the lungs. Individuals with such chronic disease continue to discharge tubercle bacilli into the environment. Most patients respond to treatment, with defervescence, decreasing cough, weight gain, and a general improvement in well-being within several weeks.

Early in the course of disease, symptoms and signs are often nonspecific and insidious, consisting mainly of diurnal fever and night sweats due to defervescence, weight loss, anorexia, general malaise, and weakness. However, in up to 90% of cases, cough eventually develops—often initially nonproductive and limited to the morning and subsequently accompanied by the production of purulent sputum, sometimes with blood streaking. Hemoptysis develops in 20–30% of cases, and massive hemoptysis may ensue as a consequence of the erosion of a blood vessel in the wall of a cavity. Hemoptysis, however, may also result from rupture of a dilated vessel in a cavity (*Rasmussen's aneurysm*) or from aspergilloma formation in an old cavity. Pleuritic chest pain sometimes develops in patients with subpleural parenchymal lesions or pleural disease. Extensive disease may produce dyspnea

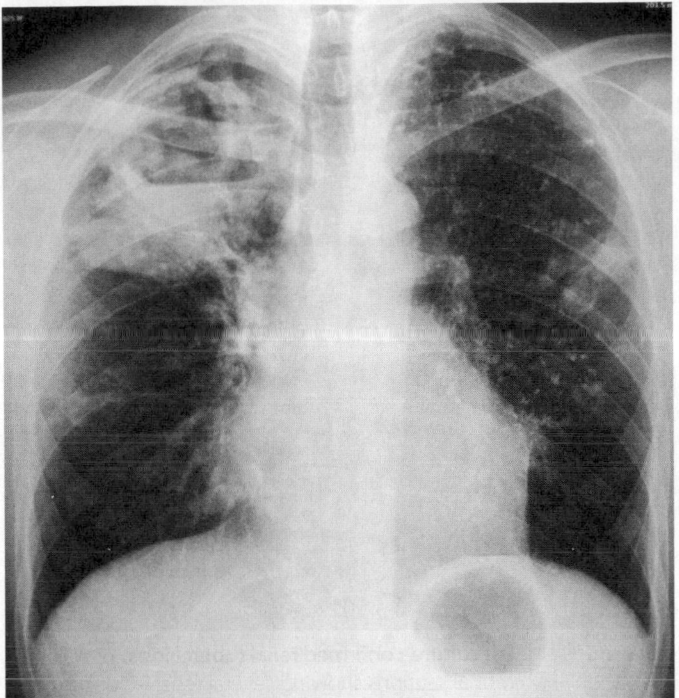

FIGURE 202-6 Chest radiograph showing a right-upper-lobe infiltrate and a cavity with an air-fluid level in a patient with active tuberculosis. *(Courtesy of Dr. Andrea Gori, Department of Infectious Diseases, S. Paolo University Hospital, Milan, Italy; with permission.)*

and, in rare instances, adult respiratory distress syndrome. Physical findings are of limited use in pulmonary TB. Many patients have no abnormalities detectable by chest examination, whereas others have detectable rales in the involved areas during inspiration, especially after coughing. Occasionally, rhonchi due to partial bronchial obstruction and classic amphoric breath sounds in areas with large cavities may be heard. Systemic features include fever (often low-grade and intermittent) in up to 80% of cases and wasting. Absence of fever, however, does not exclude TB. In some cases, pallor and finger clubbing develop. The most common hematologic findings are mild anemia, leukocytosis, and thrombocytosis with a slightly elevated erythrocyte sedimentation rate and/or C-reactive protein level. None of these findings is consistent or sufficiently accurate for diagnostic purposes. Hyponatremia due to the syndrome of inappropriate secretion of antidiuretic hormone has also been reported.

EXTRAPULMONARY TB

In order of frequency, the extrapulmonary sites most commonly involved in TB are the lymph nodes, pleura, genitourinary tract, bones and joints, meninges, peritoneum, and pericardium. However, virtually all organ systems may be affected. As a result of hematogenous dissemination in HIV-infected individuals, extrapulmonary TB is seen more commonly today than in the past in settings of high HIV prevalence.

Lymph Node TB (Tuberculous Lymphadenitis) The most common presentation of extrapulmonary TB in both HIV-seronegative and HIV-infected patients (35% of cases worldwide and more than 40% of cases in the United States in recent series), lymph node disease is particularly frequent among HIV-infected patients and among children (Fig. 202-8). In the United States, besides children, women (particularly non-Caucasians) seem to be especially susceptible. Once caused mainly by *M. bovis*, tuberculous lymphadenitis today is due largely to *M. tuberculosis*. Lymph node TB presents as painless swelling of the lymph nodes, most commonly at posterior cervical and supraclavicular sites (a condition historically referred to as *scrofula*). Lymph nodes are usually discrete in early disease but develop into a matted nontender mass over time and may result in a fistulous tract draining caseous material. Associated pulmonary disease is present in fewer than 50% of cases, and systemic symptoms are uncommon except in HIV-infected patients. The diagnosis is established by fine-needle aspiration biopsy (with a yield of up to 80%) or surgical excision biopsy. Bacteriologic confirmation is achieved in the vast majority of cases, granulomatous lesions with or without visible AFBs are typically seen, and cultures are positive in 70–80% of cases. Among HIV-infected patients, granulomas are less well organized and are frequently absent entirely, but bacterial loads are heavier than in HIV-seronegative patients, with higher yields from microscopy and culture. Differential diagnosis includes a variety of infectious conditions, neoplastic diseases such as lymphomas or metastatic carcinomas, and rare disorders like Kikuchi's disease (necrotizing histiocytic lymphadenitis), Kimura's disease, and Castleman's disease.

Pleural TB Involvement of the pleura accounts for ~20% of extrapulmonary cases in the United States and elsewhere. Isolated pleural effusion usually reflects recent primary infection, and the collection of fluid in the pleural space represents a hypersensitivity response to mycobacterial antigens. Pleural disease may also result from contiguous parenchymal spread, as in many cases of pleurisy accompanying

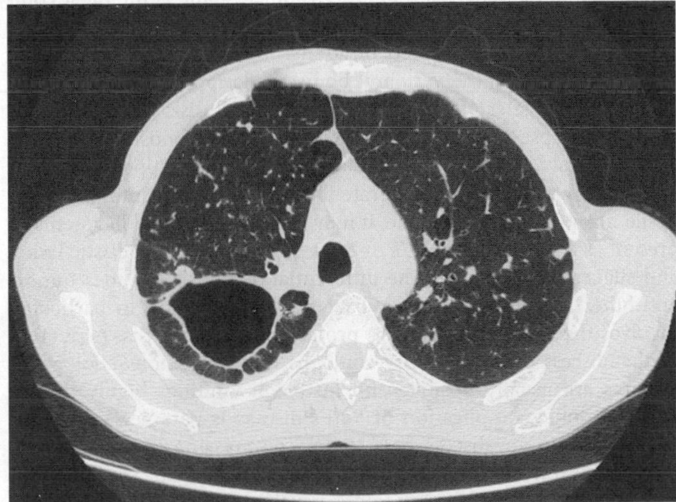

FIGURE 202-7 CT scan showing a large cavity in the right lung of a patient with active tuberculosis. *(Courtesy of Dr. Elisa Busi Rizzi, National Institute for Infectious Diseases, Spallanzani Hospital, Rome, Italy; with permission.)*

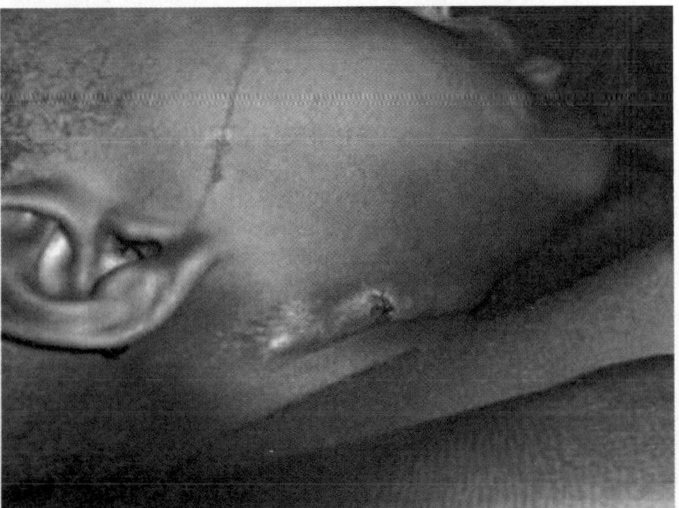

FIGURE 202-8 Tuberculous lymphadenitis affecting the cervical lymph nodes in a 2-year-old child from Malawi. *(Courtesy of Prof. S. Graham, Centre for International Child Health, University of Melbourne, Australia; with permission.)*

postprimary disease. Depending on the extent of reactivity, the effusion may be small, remain unnoticed, and resolve spontaneously or may be sufficiently large to cause symptoms such as fever, pleuritic chest pain, and dyspnea. Physical findings are those of pleural effusion: dullness to percussion and absence of breath sounds. A chest radiograph reveals the effusion and, in up to one-third of cases, also shows a parenchymal lesion. Thoracentesis is required to ascertain the nature of the effusion and to differentiate it from manifestations of other etiologies. The fluid is straw colored and at times hemorrhagic; it is an exudate with a protein concentration >50% of that in serum (usually ~4–6 g/dL), a normal to low glucose concentration, a pH of ~7.3 (occasionally <7.2), and detectable white blood cells (usually 500–6000/μL). Neutrophils may predominate in the early stage, but lymphocyte predominance is the typical finding later. Mesothelial cells are generally rare or absent. AFB are rarely seen on direct smear, and cultures often may be falsely negative for *M. tuberculosis*; positive cultures are more common among postprimary cases. Determination of the pleural concentration of adenosine deaminase (ADA) may be a useful screening test, and TB may be excluded if the value is very low. Lysozyme is also present in the pleural effusion. Measurement of IFN-γ, either directly or through stimulation of sensitized T cells with mycobacterial antigens, can be helpful. Needle biopsy of the pleura is often required for diagnosis and is recommended over pleural fluid; it reveals granulomas and/or yields a positive culture in up to 80% of cases. Pleural biopsy can yield a positive result in ~75% of cases when real-time automated nucleic acid amplification is used (the Xpert® MTB/RIF assay [Cepheid, Sunnyvale, CA]; see "Nucleic Acid Amplification Technology," below), although pleural fluid testing with this assay is not recommended because of low sensitivity. This form of pleural TB responds rapidly to chemotherapy and may resolve spontaneously. Concurrent glucocorticoid administration may reduce the duration of fever and/or chest pain but is not of proven benefit.

Tuberculous empyema is a less common complication of pulmonary TB. It is usually the result of the rupture of a cavity, with spillage of a large number of organisms into the pleural space. This process may create a bronchopleural fistula with evident air in the pleural space. A chest radiograph shows hydropneumothorax with an air-fluid level. The pleural fluid is purulent and thick and contains large numbers of lymphocytes. Acid-fast smears and mycobacterial cultures are often positive. Surgical drainage is usually required as an adjunct to chemotherapy. Tuberculous empyema may result in severe pleural fibrosis and restrictive lung disease. Removal of the thickened visceral pleura (*decortication*) is occasionally necessary to improve lung function.

TB of the Upper Airways Nearly always a complication of advanced cavitary pulmonary TB, TB of the upper airways may involve the larynx, pharynx, and epiglottis. Symptoms include hoarseness, dysphonia, and dysphagia in addition to chronic productive cough. Findings depend on the site of involvement, and ulcerations may be seen on laryngoscopy. Acid-fast smear of the sputum is often positive, but biopsy may be necessary in some cases to establish the diagnosis. Carcinoma of the larynx may have similar features but is usually painless.

Genitourinary TB Genitourinary TB, which accounts for ~10–15% of all extrapulmonary cases in the United States and elsewhere, may involve any portion of the genitourinary tract. Local symptoms predominate, and up to 75% of patients have chest radiographic abnormalities suggesting previous or concomitant pulmonary disease. Urinary frequency, dysuria, nocturia, hematuria, and flank or abdominal pain are common presentations. However, patients may be asymptomatic and their disease discovered only after severe destructive lesions of the kidneys have developed. Urinalysis gives abnormal results in 90% of cases, revealing pyuria and hematuria. The documentation of culture-negative pyuria in acidic urine should raise the suspicion of TB. IV pyelography, abdominal computed tomography (CT), or magnetic resonance imaging (MRI) (Fig. 202-9) may show deformities and obstructions; calcifications and ureteral strictures are suggestive findings. Culture of three morning urine specimens yields a definitive diagnosis in nearly 90% of cases. Severe ureteral strictures may lead to hydronephrosis and renal damage. Genital TB is diagnosed more commonly in female than in male patients. In female patients, it affects the fallopian tubes and the endometrium and may cause infertility, pelvic pain, and menstrual abnormalities. Diagnosis requires biopsy or culture of specimens obtained by dilation and curettage. In male patients, genital TB preferentially affects the epididymis, producing a slightly tender mass that may drain externally through a fistulous tract; orchitis and prostatitis may also develop. In almost half of cases of genitourinary TB, urinary tract disease is also present. Genitourinary TB responds well to chemotherapy.

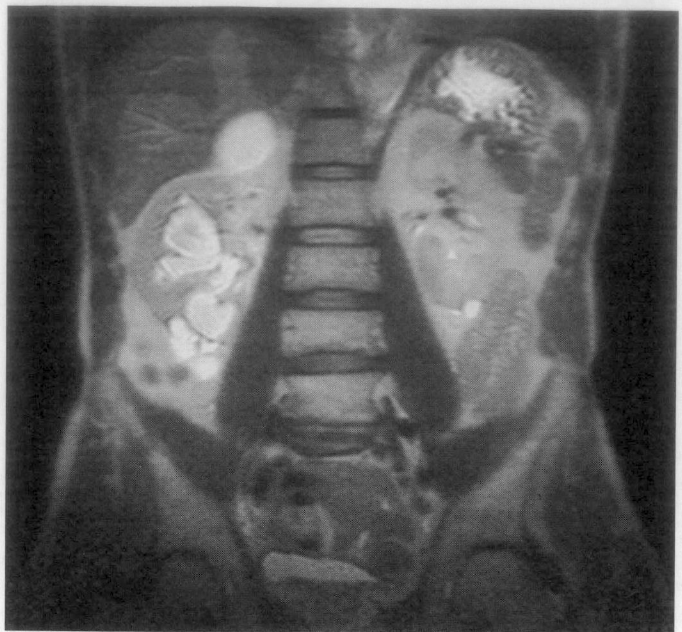

FIGURE 202-9 MRI of culture-confirmed renal tuberculosis. T2-weighted coronary plane: coronal sections showing several renal lesions in both the cortical and the medullary tissues of the right kidney. *(Courtesy of Dr. Alberto Matteelli, Department of Infectious Diseases, University of Brescia, Italy; with permission.)*

Skeletal TB In the United States, TB of the bones and joints is responsible for ~10% of extrapulmonary cases. In bone and joint disease, pathogenesis is related to reactivation of hematogenous foci or to spread from adjacent paravertebral lymph nodes. Weight-bearing joints (the spine in 40% of cases, the hips in 13%, and the knees in 10%) are most commonly affected. Spinal TB (Pott's disease or tuberculous spondylitis; Fig. 202-10) often involves two or more adjacent vertebral bodies. Whereas the upper thoracic spine is the most common site of spinal TB in children, the lower thoracic and upper lumbar vertebrae are usually affected in adults. From the anterior superior or inferior angle of the vertebral body, the lesion slowly reaches the adjacent body, later affecting the intervertebral disk. With advanced disease, collapse of vertebral bodies results in kyphosis (*gibbus*). A paravertebral "cold" abscess may also form. In the upper spine, this abscess may track to and penetrate the chest wall, presenting as a soft tissue mass; in the lower spine, it may reach the inguinal ligaments or present as a psoas abscess. CT or MRI reveals the characteristic lesion and suggests its etiology. The differential diagnosis includes tumors and other infections. Pyogenic bacterial osteomyelitis, in particular, involves the disk very early and produces rapid sclerosis. Aspiration of the abscess or bone biopsy confirms the tuberculous etiology, as cultures are usually positive and histologic findings highly typical. A catastrophic complication of Pott's disease is paraplegia, which is usually due to an abscess or a lesion compressing the spinal cord. Paraparesis due to a large abscess is a medical emergency and requires rapid drainage. TB of the hip joints, usually involving the head of the femur, causes pain; TB of the knee produces pain and swelling. If the disease goes unrecognized, the joints may be destroyed. Diagnosis requires examination of the synovial fluid, which is thick in appearance, with a high protein concentration and a variable cell count.

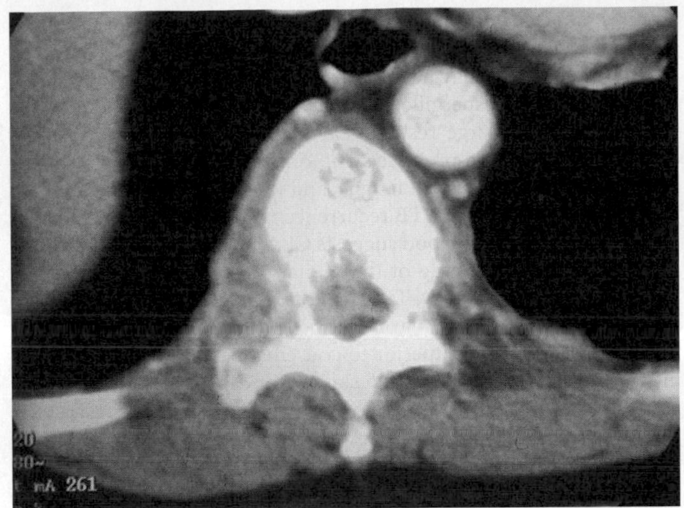

FIGURE 202-10 CT scan demonstrating destruction of the right pedicle of T10 due to Pott's disease. The patient, a 70-year-old Asian woman, presented with back pain and weight loss and had biopsy-proven tuberculosis. *(Courtesy of Charles L. Daley, MD, University of California, San Francisco; with permission.)*

Although synovial fluid culture is positive in a high percentage of cases, synovial biopsy and tissue culture may be necessary to establish the diagnosis. Skeletal TB responds to chemotherapy, but severe cases may require surgery.

Tuberculous Meningitis and Tuberculoma TB of the central nervous system accounts for ~5% of extrapulmonary cases in the United States. It is seen most often in young children but also develops in adults, especially those infected with HIV. Tuberculous meningitis results from the hematogenous spread of primary or postprimary pulmonary TB or from the rupture of a subependymal tubercle into the subarachnoid space. In more than half of cases, evidence of old pulmonary lesions or a miliary pattern is found on chest radiography. The disease often presents subtly as headache and slight mental changes after a prodrome of weeks of low-grade fever, malaise, anorexia, and irritability. If not recognized, tuberculous meningitis may evolve acutely with severe headache, confusion, lethargy, altered sensorium, and neck rigidity. Typically, the disease evolves over 1–2 weeks, a course longer than that of bacterial meningitis. Because meningeal involvement is pronounced at the base of the brain, paresis of cranial nerves (ocular nerves in particular) is a frequent finding, and the involvement of cerebral arteries may produce focal ischemia. The ultimate evolution is toward coma, with hydrocephalus and intracranial hypertension.

Lumbar puncture is the cornerstone of diagnosis. In general, examination of cerebrospinal fluid (CSF) reveals a high leukocyte count (up to 1000/μL), usually with a predominance of lymphocytes but sometimes with a predominance of neutrophils in the early stage; a protein content of 1–8 g/L (100–800 mg/dL); and a low glucose concentration. However, any of these three parameters can be within the normal range. AFBs are infrequently seen on direct smear of CSF sediment, and repeated lumbar punctures increase the yield. Culture of CSF is diagnostic in up to 80% of cases and remains the gold standard. Real-time automated nucleic acid amplification (the Xpert MTB/RIF assay; see "Nucleic Acid Amplification Technology," below) has a sensitivity of up to 80% and is the preferred initial diagnostic option. Treatment should be initiated immediately upon a positive Xpert MTB/RIF result. A negative result does not exclude a diagnosis of TB and requires further diagnostic workup. Imaging studies (CT and MRI) may show hydrocephalus and abnormal enhancement of basal cisterns or ependyma. If unrecognized, tuberculous meningitis is uniformly fatal. This disease responds to chemotherapy; however, neurologic sequelae are documented in 25% of treated cases, in most of which the diagnosis has been delayed. Clinical trials have demonstrated that patients given adjunctive glucocorticoids may experience faster resolution of CSF abnormalities and elevated CSF pressure. In one study, adjunctive dexamethasone significantly enhanced the chances of survival among persons >14 years of age but did not reduce the frequency of neurologic sequelae. The dexamethasone schedule was (1) 0.4 mg/kg per day given IV with tapering by 0.1 mg/kg per week until the fourth week, when 0.1 mg/kg per day was administered; followed by (2) 4 mg/d given by mouth with tapering by 1 mg per week until the fourth week, when 1 mg/d was administered.

Tuberculoma, an uncommon manifestation of central nervous system TB, presents as one or more space-occupying lesions and usually causes seizures and focal signs. CT or MRI reveals contrast-enhanced ring lesions, but biopsy is necessary to establish the diagnosis.

Gastrointestinal TB Gastrointestinal TB is uncommon, making up 3.5% of extrapulmonary cases in the United States. Various pathogenetic mechanisms are involved: swallowing of sputum with direct seeding, hematogenous spread, or (largely in developing areas) ingestion of milk from cows affected by bovine TB. Although any portion of the gastrointestinal tract may be affected, the terminal ileum and the cecum are the sites most commonly involved. Abdominal pain (at times similar to that associated with appendicitis) and swelling, obstruction, hematochezia, and a palpable mass in the abdomen are common findings at presentation. Fever, weight loss, anorexia, and night sweats are also common. With intestinal-wall involvement, ulcerations and fistulae may simulate Crohn's disease; the differential diagnosis of this entity is always difficult. Anal fistulae should prompt an evaluation for rectal TB. Because surgery is required in most cases, the diagnosis can be established by histologic examination and culture of specimens obtained intraoperatively.

Tuberculous peritonitis follows either the direct spread of tubercle bacilli from ruptured lymph nodes and intraabdominal organs (e.g., genital TB in women) or hematogenous seeding. Nonspecific abdominal pain, fever, and ascites should raise the suspicion of tuberculous peritonitis. The coexistence of cirrhosis (Chap. 363) in patients with tuberculous peritonitis complicates the diagnosis. In tuberculous peritonitis, paracentesis reveals an exudative fluid with a high protein content and leukocytosis that is usually lymphocytic (although neutrophils occasionally predominate). The yield of direct smear and culture is relatively low; culture of a large volume of ascitic fluid can increase the yield, but peritoneal biopsy (with a specimen best obtained by laparoscopy) is often needed to establish the diagnosis.

Pericardial TB (Tuberculous Pericarditis) Due either to direct extension from adjacent mediastinal or hilar lymph nodes or to hematogenous spread, pericardial TB has often been a disease of the elderly in countries with low TB prevalence. However, it also develops frequently in HIV-infected patients. Case-fatality rates are as high as 40% in some series. The onset may be subacute, although an acute presentation, with dyspnea, fever, dull retrosternal pain, and a pericardial friction rub, is possible. An effusion eventually develops in many cases; cardiovascular symptoms and signs of cardiac tamponade may ultimately appear (Chap. 288). In the presence of effusion, TB must be suspected if the patient belongs to a high-risk population (HIV-infected, originating in a high-prevalence country); if there is evidence of previous TB in other organs; or if echocardiography, CT, or MRI shows effusion and thickness across the pericardial space. A definitive diagnosis can be obtained by pericardiocentesis under echocardiographic guidance. The pericardial fluid must be submitted for biochemical, cytologic, and microbiologic evaluation. The effusion is exudative in nature, with a high count of lymphocytes and monocytes. Hemorrhagic effusion is common. Direct smear examination is very rarely positive. Culture of pericardial fluid reveals *M. tuberculosis* in up to two-thirds of cases, whereas pericardial biopsy has a higher yield. High levels of ADA, lysozyme, and IFN-γ may suggest a tuberculous etiology.

Without treatment, pericardial TB is usually fatal. Even with treatment, complications may develop, including chronic constrictive pericarditis with thickening of the pericardium, fibrosis, and sometimes calcification, which may be visible on a chest radiograph. Systematic reviews and meta-analyses show that adjunctive glucocorticoid treatment remains controversial, with no conclusive evidence of benefits for all principal outcomes of pericarditis—i.e., no significant impact on resolution of effusion, no significant difference in functional status after treatment, and no significant reduction in the frequency of development of constriction or death. However, in HIV-infected patients, glucocorticoids do improve functional status after treatment.

Caused by direct extension from the pericardium or by retrograde lymphatic extension from affected mediastinal lymph nodes, tuberculous myocarditis is an extremely rare disease. Usually it is fatal and is diagnosed postmortem.

Miliary or Disseminated TB Miliary TB is due to hematogenous spread of tubercle bacilli. Although in children it is often the consequence of primary infection, in adults it may be due to either recent infection or reactivation of old disseminated foci. The lesions are usually yellowish granulomas 1–2 mm in diameter that resemble millet seeds (thus the term *miliary*, coined by nineteenth-century pathologists). Clinical manifestations are nonspecific and protean, depending on the predominant site of involvement. Fever, night sweats, anorexia, weakness, and weight loss are presenting symptoms in the majority of cases. At times, patients have a cough and other respiratory symptoms due to pulmonary involvement as well as abdominal symptoms. Physical findings include hepatomegaly, splenomegaly, and lymphadenopathy. Eye examination may reveal choroidal tubercles, which are pathognomonic of miliary TB, in up to 30% of cases. Meningismus occurs in fewer than 10% of cases.

A high index of suspicion is required for the diagnosis of miliary TB. Frequently, chest radiography (Fig. 202-5) reveals a miliary reticulonodular pattern (more easily seen on underpenetrated film), although no radiographic abnormality may be evident early in the course and among HIV-infected patients. Other radiologic findings include large infiltrates, interstitial infiltrates (especially in HIV-infected patients), and pleural effusion. Sputum-smear microscopy is negative in most cases. Various hematologic abnormalities may be seen, including anemia with leukopenia, lymphopenia, neutrophilic leukocytosis and leukemoid reactions, and polycythemia. Disseminated intravascular coagulation has been reported. Elevation of alkaline phosphatase levels and other abnormal values in liver function tests are detected in patients with severe hepatic involvement. The TST may be negative in up to half of cases, but reactivity may be restored during chemotherapy. Bronchoalveolar lavage and transbronchial biopsy are more likely to provide bacteriologic confirmation, and granulomas are evident in liver or bone-marrow biopsy specimens from many patients. If it goes unrecognized, miliary TB is lethal; with proper early treatment, however, it is amenable to cure. Glucocorticoid therapy has not proved beneficial.

A rare presentation seen in the elderly, *cryptic miliary TB* has a chronic course characterized by mild intermittent fever, anemia, and—ultimately—meningeal involvement preceding death. An acute septicemic form, *nonreactive miliary TB*, occurs very rarely and is due to massive hematogenous dissemination of tubercle bacilli. Pancytopenia is common in this form of disease, which is rapidly fatal. At postmortem examination, multiple necrotic but nongranulomatous ("nonreactive") lesions are detected.

Less Common Extrapulmonary Forms TB may cause chorioretinitis, uveitis, panophthalmitis, and painful hypersensitivity-related phlyctenular conjunctivitis. Tuberculous otitis is rare and presents as hearing loss, otorrhea, and tympanic membrane perforation. In the nasopharynx, TB may simulate granulomatosis with polyangiitis. Cutaneous manifestations of TB include primary infection due to direct inoculation, abscesses and chronic ulcers, scrofuloderma, lupus vulgaris (a smoldering disease with nodules, plaques, and fissures), miliary lesions, and erythema nodosum. Tuberculous mastitis results from retrograde lymphatic spread, often from the axillary lymph nodes. Adrenal TB is a manifestation of disseminated disease presenting rarely as adrenal insufficiency. Finally, congenital TB results from transplacental spread of tubercle bacilli to the fetus or from ingestion of contaminated amniotic fluid. This rare disease affects the liver, spleen, lymph nodes, and various other organs.

Post-TB Complications TB may cause persisting pulmonary damage in patients whose infection has been considered cured on clinical grounds. Chronic impairment of lung functions, bronchiectasis, aspergillomas, and chronic pulmonary aspergillosis (CPA) have been associated with TB. CPA may manifest as simple aspergilloma (fungal ball) or chronic cavitary aspergillosis. Early studies revealed that, especially in the presence of large residual cavities, *Aspergillus fumigatus* may colonize the lesion and produce symptoms such as respiratory impairment, hemoptysis, persistent fatigue, and weight loss, often resulting in the erroneous diagnosis of TB recurrence. The detection of *Aspergillus* precipitins (IgG) in the blood suggests CPA, as do radiographic abnormalities such as thickening of the cavitary walls or the presence of a fungal ball inside the cavity. Treatment is difficult. Recent preliminary studies on the use of itraconazole for 6 months suggest that treatment with this agent may be superior to conservative treatment in improving radiologic and clinical manifestations of CPA. Surgical removal of lesions is risky.

HIV-Associated TB (See also Chap. 226) TB is one of the most common diseases among HIV-infected persons worldwide and a major cause of death in this population; more specifically, it is responsible for an estimated 24% of all HIV-related mortality. In certain urban settings in some African countries, the rate of HIV infection among TB patients reaches 70–80%. A person with a positive TST who acquires HIV infection has a 3–13% annual risk of developing active TB. A new TB infection acquired by an HIV-infected individual may evolve to active disease in a matter of weeks rather than months or years. TB can appear at any stage of HIV infection, and its presentation varies with the stage. When CMI is only partially compromised, pulmonary TB presents in a typical manner (Figs. 202-6 and 202-7), with upper-lobe infiltrates and cavitation and without significant lymphadenopathy or pleural effusion. In late stages of HIV infection, when the CD4+ T cell count is <200/μL, a primary TB–like pattern, with diffuse interstitial and subtle infiltrates, little or no cavitation, pleural effusion, and intrathoracic lymphadenopathy, is more common. However, these forms are becoming less common because of the expanded use of antiretroviral treatment (ART). Overall, sputum smears are less frequently positive among TB patients with HIV infection than among those without; thus, the diagnosis of TB may be difficult, especially in view of the variety of HIV-related pulmonary conditions mimicking TB. Extrapulmonary TB is common among HIV-infected patients. In various series, extrapulmonary TB—alone or in association with pulmonary disease—has been documented in 40–60% of all cases in HIV-co-infected individuals. The most common forms are lymphatic, disseminated, pleural, and pericardial. Mycobacteremia and meningitis are also common, particularly in advanced HIV disease. The diagnosis of TB in HIV-infected patients may be complicated not only by the increased frequency of sputum-smear negativity (up to 40% in culture-proven pulmonary cases) but also by atypical radiographic findings, a lack of classic granuloma formation in the late stages, and a negative TST. The Xpert MTB/RIF assay (see "Nucleic Acid Amplification Technology," below) is the preferred initial diagnostic option, and therapy should be started on the basis of a positive result because treatment delays may be fatal. A negative Xpert MTB/RIF result does not exclude a diagnosis of TB, and culture remains the gold standard.

Exacerbations in systemic (lymphadenopathy) or respiratory symptoms, signs, and laboratory or radiographic manifestations of TB—termed the *immune reconstitution inflammatory syndrome* (IRIS) or *TB immune reconstitution disease* (TB-IRD)—have been associated with the administration of ART and occur in ~10% of HIV-infected TB patients. Usually developing 1–3 months after initiation of ART, IRIS is more common among patients with advanced immunosuppression and extrapulmonary TB. "Unmasking IRIS" may also develop after the initiation of ART in patients with undiagnosed subclinical TB. The earlier ART is started and the lower the baseline CD4+ T cell count, the greater the risk of IRIS. Death due to IRIS is relatively infrequent and occurs mainly among patients who have a high preexisting mortality risk. The presumed pathogenesis of IRIS consists of an immune response that is elicited by antigens released as bacilli are killed during effective chemotherapy and that is temporally associated with improving immune function. There is no diagnostic test for IRIS, and its confirmation relies heavily upon case definitions incorporating clinical and laboratory data; a variety of case definitions have been suggested. The first priority in the management of a possible case of IRIS is to ensure that the clinical syndrome does not represent a failure of TB treatment or the development of another infection. Mild paradoxical reactions can be managed with symptom-based treatment. Glucocorticoids have been used for more severe reactions, and prednisolone given for 4 weeks at a low dosage (1.5 mg/kg per day for 2 weeks and half that dose for the remaining 2 weeks) has reduced the need for hospitalization and therapeutic procedures and hastened alleviation of symptoms, as reflected by Karnofsky performance scores, quality-of-life assessments, radiographic response, and C-reactive protein levels. The effectiveness of glucocorticoids in alleviating the symptoms of IRIS is probably linked to suppression of proinflammatory cytokine concentrations, as these medications reduce serum concentrations of IL-6, IL-10, IL-12p40, TNF-α, IFN-γ, and IFN-γ-inducible protein 10 (IP-10). Recommendations for the prevention and treatment of TB in HIV-infected individuals are provided below.

DIAGNOSIS

The key to the diagnosis of TB remains a high index of suspicion. Diagnosis is not difficult in persons belonging to high-risk populations who present with typical symptoms and a classic chest radiograph showing upper-lobe infiltrates with cavities (Fig. 202-6). On the other hand, the diagnosis can easily be missed in an elderly nursing-home resident or a teenager with a focal infiltrate. Often, the diagnosis is first entertained when the chest radiograph of a patient being evaluated for respiratory symptoms is abnormal. If the patient has no complicating medical conditions that cause immunosuppression, the chest radiograph may show typical upper-lobe infiltrates with cavitation (Fig. 202-6). The longer the delay between the onset of symptoms and the diagnosis, the more likely is the finding of cavitary disease. In contrast, immunosuppressed patients, including those with HIV infection, may have "atypical" findings on chest radiography—e.g., lower-zone infiltrates without cavity formation.

The several approaches to the diagnosis of TB require, above all, a well-organized laboratory network with an appropriate distribution of tasks at different levels of the health care system. At the peripheral and community levels, screening and referral are the principal tasks—besides clinical assessment and radiography—that can be accomplished through AFB microscopy and/or real-time automated nucleic acid amplification technology (the Xpert MTB/RIF assay; see below). At a secondary level (e.g., a traditional district hospital in a high-incidence setting), additional technology can be adopted, including rapid culture and drug susceptibility testing.

AFB MICROSCOPY

A presumptive diagnosis is commonly based on the finding of AFB on microscopic examination of a diagnostic specimen, such as a smear of expectorated sputum or of tissue (e.g., a lymph node biopsy). Although inexpensive, AFB microscopy has relatively low sensitivity (40–60%) in culture-confirmed cases of pulmonary TB. The traditional method—light microscopy of specimens stained with Ziehl-Neelsen basic fuchsin dyes—is nevertheless satisfactory, although time-consuming. Most modern laboratories processing large numbers of diagnostic specimens use auramine-rhodamine staining and fluorescence microscopy; this approach is more sensitive than the Ziehl-Neelsen method. However, it is expensive because it requires high-cost mercury vapor light sources and a dark room. Less expensive light-emitting diode (LED) fluorescence microscopes are now available. They are as sensitive as—or more sensitive than—traditional fluorescence microscopes. As a result, conventional light and fluorescence microscopes are being replaced with this more recent technology, especially in developing countries. For patients with suspected pulmonary TB, it has been recommended that two or three sputum specimens, preferably collected early in the morning, should be submitted to the laboratory for AFB smear and mycobacterial culture. Two specimens collected on the same visit may be as effective as three. If tissue is obtained, it is critical that the portion of the specimen intended for culture not be put in formaldehyde. The use of AFB microscopy in examining urine or gastric lavage fluid is limited by the presence of commensal mycobacteria that can cause false-positive results.

NUCLEIC ACID AMPLIFICATION TECHNOLOGY

Several test systems based on amplification of mycobacterial nucleic acid have become available in the past few years. These tests are most useful for the rapid confirmation of TB in persons with AFB-positive specimens, but some also have utility for the diagnosis of AFB-negative pulmonary and extrapulmonary TB. One system that permits rapid diagnosis of TB with high specificity and sensitivity (approaching that of culture) is the fully automated, real-time nucleic acid amplification technology known as the Xpert MTB/RIF assay. Xpert MTB/RIF can simultaneously detect TB and rifampin resistance in <2 h and has minimal biosafety and training requirements. Therefore, it can be housed in nonconventional laboratory settings. The WHO recommends its use worldwide as the initial diagnostic test in adults and children presumed to have MDR-TB or HIV-associated TB. Taking into account the availability of resources, the test may also be used in any adult or child presumed to have TB or as a follow-up test after microscopy in adults presumed to have TB but not at risk of MDR-TB or HIV-associated TB. Xpert MTB/RIF should be the initial test applied to CSF from patients in whom TB meningitis is suspected as well as a replacement test (over conventional microscopy, culture, and histopathology) for selected nonrespiratory specimens—obtained by gastric lavage, fine-needle aspiration, or pleural or other biopsies—from patients in whom extrapulmonary TB is suspected. This test has a sensitivity of 98% among AFB-positive cases and ~70% among AFB-negative specimens. Other tests, such as those based on manual amplification platforms, have not yet been deemed satisfactory for introduction into clinical practice as replacements for existing tests.

MYCOBACTERIAL CULTURE

Definitive diagnosis depends on the isolation and identification of *M. tuberculosis* from a clinical specimen or the identification of specific DNA sequences in a nucleic acid amplification test. Specimens may be inoculated onto egg- or agar-based medium (e.g., Löwenstein-Jensen or Middlebrook 7H10) and incubated at 37°C (under 5% CO_2 for Middlebrook medium). Because most species of mycobacteria, including *M. tuberculosis*, grow slowly, 4–8 weeks may be required before growth is detected. Although *M. tuberculosis* may be identified presumptively on the basis of growth time and colony pigmentation and morphology, a variety of biochemical tests have traditionally been used to speciate mycobacterial isolates. In modern, well-equipped laboratories, liquid culture for isolation and species identification by molecular methods or high-pressure liquid chromatography of mycolic acids has replaced isolation on solid media and identification by biochemical tests. A widely used technology is the mycobacterial growth indicator tube (BBL™ MGIT™; BD, Franklin Lakes, NJ), which uses a fluorescent compound sensitive to the presence of oxygen dissolved in the liquid medium. The appearance of fluorescence detected by fluorometric technology indicates active growth of mycobacteria. A low-cost, rapid immunochromatographic lateral-flow assay based on detection of MTP64 antigen may also be used for species identification of the *M. tuberculosis* complex in culture isolates. These new methods, which are also being introduced in low-income countries, have decreased the time required for bacteriologic confirmation of TB to 2–3 weeks.

DRUG SUSCEPTIBILITY TESTING

Any initial isolate of *M. tuberculosis* should be tested for susceptibility to isoniazid and rifampin in order to detect drug resistance and/or MDR-TB, particularly if one or more risk factors for drug resistance are identified or if the patient either fails to respond to initial therapy or has a relapse after the completion of treatment (see "Treatment Failure and Relapse," below). In addition, expanded susceptibility testing for second-line anti-TB drugs (especially the fluoroquinolones and the injectable drugs) is mandatory when MDR-TB is found. Susceptibility testing may be conducted directly (with the clinical specimen) or indirectly (with mycobacterial cultures) on solid or liquid medium. Results are obtained rapidly by direct susceptibility testing on liquid medium, with an average reporting time of 3 weeks. With indirect testing on solid medium, results may be unavailable for ≥8 weeks. Highly reliable genotypic methods for the rapid identification of genetic mutations in gene regions known to be associated with resistance to rifampin (such as those in *rpo*B) and isoniazid (such as those in *kat*G and *inh*A) have been developed and are being widely implemented for screening of patients at increased risk of drug-resistant TB. Apart from the Xpert MTB/RIF assay, which, as mentioned above, detects rifampin resistance, the most widely used are molecular line probe assays. After extraction of DNA from *M. tuberculosis* isolates or from clinical specimens, the resistance gene regions are amplified by polymerase chain reaction (PCR), and labeled and probe-hybridized PCR products are detected by colorimetric development. This assay reveals the presence of *M. tuberculosis* as well as mutations in target resistance gene regions. A similar approach has been developed for second-line anti-TB drugs such as the fluoroquinolones, the aminoglycosides kanamycin and amikacin, and capreomycin, but the diagnostic accuracy of the current technology is not yet sufficient to recommend its use in clinical practice. Finally, a few noncommercial, inexpensive culture and drug-susceptibility testing methods (e.g., microscopically observed drug susceptibility, or MODS; nitrate reductase assays; and colorimetric redox indicator assays) may be useful in resource-limited settings. Their use is restricted to national reference laboratories with proven proficiency and adequate external quality control as an interim solution while genotypic or automated liquid culture technology is introduced.

RADIOGRAPHIC PROCEDURES

As noted above, the initial suspicion of pulmonary TB is often based on abnormal chest radiographic findings in a patient with respiratory symptoms. Although the "classic" picture is that of upper-lobe disease with infiltrates and cavities (Fig. 202-6), virtually any radiographic pattern—from a normal film or a solitary pulmonary nodule to diffuse alveolar infiltrates in a patient with adult respiratory distress syndrome—may be seen. In the era of AIDS, no radiographic pattern can be considered pathognomonic. CT (Fig. 202-7) may be useful in interpreting questionable findings on plain chest radiography and may be helpful in diagnosing some forms of extrapulmonary TB (e.g., Pott's disease; Fig. 202-10). MRI is useful in the diagnosis of intracranial TB.

ADDITIONAL DIAGNOSTIC PROCEDURES

Other diagnostic tests may be used when pulmonary TB is suspected. Sputum induction by ultrasonic nebulization of hypertonic saline may be useful for patients who cannot produce a sputum specimen spontaneously. Frequently, patients with radiographic abnormalities that are consistent with other diagnoses (e.g., bronchogenic carcinoma) undergo fiberoptic bronchoscopy with bronchial brushings and endobronchial or transbronchial biopsy of the lesion. Bronchoalveolar lavage of a lung segment containing an abnormality may also be performed. In all cases, it is essential that specimens be submitted for AFB smear, mycobacterial culture, and molecular testing with the Xpert MTB/RIF assay. For the diagnosis of primary pulmonary TB in children, who often do not expectorate sputum, induced sputum specimens and specimens from early-morning gastric lavage may yield positive cultures and/or Xpert MTB/RIF assay results.

Invasive diagnostic procedures are indicated for patients with suspected extrapulmonary TB. In addition to testing of specimens from involved sites (e.g., CSF for tuberculous meningitis, pleural fluid and biopsy samples for pleural disease), biopsy and culture of bone marrow and liver tissue have a good diagnostic yield in disseminated (miliary) TB, particularly in HIV-infected patients, who also have a high frequency of positive blood cultures. In some cases, culture or Xpert MTB/RIF assay results are negative but a clinical diagnosis of TB is supported by consistent epidemiologic evidence (e.g., a history of close contact with an infectious patient) and a compatible clinical and radiographic response to treatment. In the United States and other industrialized countries with low rates of TB, some patients with limited abnormalities on chest radiographs and sputum positive for AFB are infected with nontuberculous mycobacteria, most commonly organisms of the *M. avium* complex or *M. kansasii* (Chap. 204). Factors favoring the diagnosis of nontuberculous mycobacterial disease over TB include an absence of risk factors for TB and the presence of underlying chronic pulmonary disease.

Patients with HIV-associated TB pose several diagnostic problems (see "HIV-Associated TB," above). Moreover, HIV-infected patients with sputum culture–positive, AFB-positive TB may present with a normal chest radiograph. The Xpert MTB/RIF assay is the preferred rapid diagnostic test in this population of patients because of simplicity of use and a sensitivity of ~60% among AFB-negative culture-positive cases and of 97% among AFB-positive cases. With the advent of ART, the occurrence of disseminated *M. avium* complex disease that can be confused with TB has become much less common.

SEROLOGIC AND OTHER DIAGNOSTIC TESTS FOR ACTIVE TB

A number of serologic tests based on detection of antibodies to a variety of mycobacterial antigens are marketed in developing countries but not in the United States. Careful independent assessments of these tests suggest that they are not useful as diagnostic aids—especially in persons with a low probability of TB—because of their low sensitivity and specificity and their poor reproducibility. After a rigorous evaluation of the tests, the WHO issued a "negative" recommendation in 2011 in order to prevent their abuse in the private sector of many resource-limited countries. Various methods aimed at detection of mycobacterial antigens in diagnostic specimens are being investigated but are limited at present by low sensitivity. Determinations of ADA and IFN-γ levels in pleural fluid may be useful adjunctive tests in the diagnosis of pleural TB; their utility in the diagnosis of other forms of extrapulmonary TB (e.g., pericardial, peritoneal, and meningeal) is less clear.

DIAGNOSIS OF LATENT *M. TUBERCULOSIS* INFECTION

Tuberculin Skin Testing In 1891, Robert Koch discovered that components of *M. tuberculosis* in a concentrated liquid culture medium, subsequently named "old tuberculin," were capable of eliciting a skin reaction when injected subcutaneously into patients with TB. In 1932, Seibert and Munday purified this product by ammonium sulfate precipitation to produce an active protein fraction known as *tuberculin purified protein derivative* (PPD). In 1941, PPD-S, developed by Seibert and Glenn, was chosen as the international standard. Later, the WHO and UNICEF sponsored large-scale production of a master batch of PPD (RT23) and made it available for general use. The greatest limitation of PPD is its lack of mycobacterial species specificity, a property due to the large number of proteins in this product that are highly conserved in the various species. In addition, subjectivity of the skin-reaction interpretation, deterioration of the product, and batch-to-batch variations limit the usefulness of PPD.

The skin test with tuberculin PPD (TST) is most widely used in screening for LTBI. It probably measures the response to antigenic stimulation by T cells that reside in the skin rather than the response of recirculating memory T cells. The test is of limited value in the diagnosis of active TB because of its relatively low sensitivity and specificity and its inability to discriminate between LTBI and active disease. False-negative reactions are common in immunosuppressed patients and in those with overwhelming TB. False-positive reactions may be caused by infections with nontuberculous mycobacteria (Chap. 204) and by BCG vaccination. Repeated TST can produce larger reaction sizes due to either boosting or true conversion. The "boosting phenomenon" is a spurious TST conversion resulting from boosting of reactivity on subsequent TST 1–5 weeks after the initial test. Distinguishing boosting from true conversion is difficult yet important and can be based on clinical and epidemiologic considerations. For instance, true conversions are likely after BCG vaccination in a previously TST-negative person or in a close contact of an infectious patient.

IFN-γ Release Assays Two in vitro assays that measure T cell release of IFN-γ in response to stimulation with the highly TB-specific antigens ESAT-6 and CFP-10 are available. The T-SPOT®.TB test (Oxford Immunotec, Oxford, United Kingdom) is an enzyme-linked immunospot (ELISpot) assay, and the QuantiFERON®-TB Gold test (Qiagen GmbH, Hilden, Germany) is a whole-blood enzyme-linked immunosorbent assay (ELISA) for measurement of IFN-γ. The QuantiFERON®-TB Gold In-Tube assay, which facilitates blood collection and initial incubation, also contains another specific antigen, TB7.7. These tests likely measure the response of recirculating memory T cells—normally part of a reservoir in the spleen, bone marrow, and lymph nodes—to persisting bacilli producing antigenic signals.

In settings or population groups with low TB and HIV burdens, IFN-γ release assays (IGRAs) have previously been reported to be more specific than the TST as a result of less cross-reactivity due to BCG vaccination and sensitization by nontuberculous mycobacteria. Recent studies, however, suggest that IGRAs may not perform well in serial testing (e.g., among health care workers) and that interpretation of test results is dependent on cutoff values used to define positivity. Potential advantages of IGRAs include logistical convenience, the need for fewer patient visits to complete testing, and the avoidance of somewhat subjective measurements such as skin induration. However, IGRAs require that blood be drawn from the individual and then delivered to the laboratory in a timely fashion. IGRAs also require that testing be performed in a laboratory setting. These requirements pose challenges similar to those faced with the TST, including cold-chain requirements and batch-to-batch variations. Because of higher specificity and other potential advantages, IGRAs have usually replaced the TST for LTBI diagnosis in low-incidence, high income settings. However, in high-incidence TB and HIV settings and population groups, there is limited and inconclusive evidence about the performance and usefulness of IGRAs. In view of higher costs and increased technical requirements, the WHO does not recommend the replacement of the TST by IGRAs in low- and middle-income countries.

A number of national guidelines on the use of IGRAs for LTBI testing have been issued. In the United States, an IGRA is preferred to the TST for most persons over the age of 5 years who are being screened for LTBI. However, for those at high risk of progression to active TB (e.g., HIV-infected persons), either test—or, to optimize sensitivity, both tests—may be used. Because of the paucity of data on the use of IGRAs in children, the TST is preferred for LTBI testing of children under age 5. In Canada and some European countries, a two-step approach for those with positive TSTs—i.e., initial TST followed by an IGRA—is recommended. However, a TST may boost an IGRA response if the interval between the two tests exceeds 3 days. Similar to the TST, current IGRAs have only modest predictive value for incident active TB, are not useful in identifying patients with the highest risk of progression toward disease, and cannot be used for diagnosis of active TB.

TREATMENT TUBERCULOSIS

The two aims of TB treatment are (1) to prevent morbidity and death by curing TB while preventing the emergence of drug resistance and (2) to interrupt transmission by rendering patients noninfectious. Chemotherapy for TB became possible with the discovery of streptomycin in 1943. Randomized clinical trials clearly indicated that the administration of streptomycin to patients with chronic TB reduced mortality rates and led to cure in the majority of cases. However, monotherapy with streptomycin eventually was associated with the development of resistance to this drug and the resulting failure of treatment. With the introduction into clinical practice of para-aminosalicylic acid (PAS) and isoniazid, it became axiomatic in the early 1950s that cure of TB required the concomitant administration of at least two agents to which the organism was susceptible. Furthermore, early clinical trials demonstrated that a long period of treatment—i.e., 12–24 months—was required to prevent recurrence. The introduction of rifampin (rifampicin) in the early 1970s heralded the era of effective short-course chemotherapy, with a treatment duration of <12 months. The discovery that pyrazinamide, which was first used in the 1950s, augmented the potency of isoniazid/rifampin regimens led to the use of a 6-month course of this triple-drug regimen as standard therapy.

DRUGS

Four major drugs are considered first-line agents for the treatment of TB: isoniazid, rifampin, pyrazinamide, and ethambutol (Table 202-2). These drugs are well absorbed after oral administration, with peak serum levels at 2–4 h and nearly complete elimination within 24 h. These agents are recommended on the basis of their bactericidal activity (i.e., their ability to rapidly reduce the number of viable organisms and render patients noninfectious), their sterilizing activity (i.e., their ability to kill all bacilli and thus sterilize the affected tissues, measured in terms of the ability to prevent relapses), and their low rate of induction of drug resistance by selection of mutant bacilli. Two additional rifamycins, rifapentine and rifabutin, are also available in the United States; however, the level of cross-resistance with rifampin is high. For a detailed discussion of the drugs used for the treatment of TB, see Chap. 205e.

Because of a lower degree of efficacy and a higher degree of intolerability and toxicity, six classes of second-line drugs are generally used only for the treatment of patients with TB resistant to first-line drugs: (1) the fluoroquinolone antibiotics; (2) the injectable aminoglycosides kanamycin, amikacin, and streptomycin; (3) the injectable polypeptide capreomycin; and the oral agents (4) ethionamide and prothionamide, (5) cycloserine and terizidone (therizidone), and (6) PAS. Streptomycin, formerly a first-line agent, is now rarely used for drug-resistant TB because resistance levels worldwide are high and it is more toxic than the other drugs in the same class; however, the level of cross-resistance with the other injectables is low. Of the quinolones, later-generation agents such as levofloxacin and moxifloxacin are preferred. Gatifloxacin (no longer marketed in several countries, including the United States, because of previously observed dysglycemia) has recently been tested in a 4-month regimen that produced no detectable major side effects; thus, this drug could be reconsidered as a good alternative. Other drugs (referred to by the WHO as "group 5") whose efficacy is not clearly defined are used in the treatment of patients with TB resistant to most of the first- and second-line agents; these drugs include clofazimine, linezolid, amoxicillin/clavulanic acid, clarithromycin, and carbapenems such as imipenem/cilastatin and meropenem. Today amithiozone (thiacetazone) is used very rarely because it has been associated with severe and at times fatal skin reactions among HIV-infected patients. Two novel drugs belonging to two new antibiotic classes—the diarylquinoline bedaquiline and the nitroimidazole delamanid—have recently been approved for use in severe cases of MDR-TB by stringent regulatory authorities (the U.S. Food and Drug Administration

TABLE 202-2 RECOMMENDED DOSAGE[a] FOR INITIAL TREATMENT OF TUBERCULOSIS IN ADULTS[b]

	Dosage	
Drug	**Daily Dose**	**Thrice-Weekly Dose**
Isoniazid	5 mg/kg, max 300 mg	10 mg/kg, max 900 mg
Rifampin	10 mg/kg, max 600 mg	10 mg/kg, max 600 mg
Pyrazinamide	25 mg/kg, max 2 g	35 mg/kg, max 3 g
Ethambutol[c]	15 mg/kg	30 mg/kg

[a]The duration of treatment with individual drugs varies by regimen, as detailed in Table 202-3. [b]The World Health Organization recommends the following dosages for children: isoniazid,10–15 mg/kg daily, max 300 mg/d; rifampin, 15 (range, 10–20) mg/kg daily, max 600 mg/d; pyrazinamide, 35 (range, 30–40) mg/kg daily; ethambutol, 20 (range, 15–25) mg/kg daily. [c]In certain settings, streptomycin (15 mg/kg daily, with a maximum dose of 1 g; or 25–30 mg/kg thrice weekly, with a maximum dose of 1.5 g) can replace ethambutol in the initial phase of treatment. However, streptomycin generally is no longer considered a first-line drug.

Source: Based on recommendations of the American Thoracic Society/Infectious Diseases Society of America/Centers for Disease Control and Prevention and the World Health Organization.

[FDA] and the European Medicine Agency [EMA] in the case of bedaquiline; the EMA and the Pharmaceuticals and Medical Devices Agency of Japan in the case of delamanid).

REGIMENS

Standard short-course regimens are divided into an initial, or bactericidal, phase and a continuation, or sterilizing, phase. During the initial phase, the majority of the tubercle bacilli are killed, symptoms resolve, and usually the patient becomes noninfectious. The continuation phase is required to eliminate persisting mycobacteria and prevent relapse. The treatment regimen of choice for virtually all forms of drug-susceptible TB in adults consists of a 2-month initial (or intensive) phase of isoniazid, rifampin, pyrazinamide, and ethambutol followed by a 4-month continuation phase of isoniazid and rifampin (Table 202-3). This regimen can cure TB in more than 90% of patients. In children, most forms of TB in the absence of HIV infection or suspected isoniazid resistance can be safely treated without ethambutol in the intensive phase. Treatment should be given daily throughout the course. However, daily treatment during the intensive phase and intermittently (three times weekly) during the continuation phase is an alternative for patients who can be directly supervised and properly supported. A fully supervised, three-times-weekly regimen throughout the course also can be offered in the absence of HIV infection, although the risk of acquired drug resistance is higher than that among patients treated daily for the full course. In addition, if the infecting strain is resistant to isoniazid, the risks of both acquired resistance and treatment failure are higher with three-times-weekly intensive therapy than with daily treatment in the intensive phase. HIV-infected patients should always receive their initial-phase regimen daily (see below). A continuation phase of once-weekly rifapentine and isoniazid has been shown to be equally effective for HIV-seronegative patients with noncavitary pulmonary TB who have negative sputum cultures at 2 months. Patients with cavitary pulmonary TB and delayed sputum-culture conversion (i.e., those who remain culture-positive at 2 months) should be tested immediately for drug-resistant TB, and a change of regimen should be considered. To prevent isoniazid-related neuropathy, pyridoxine (10–25 mg/d) should be added to the regimen given to persons at high risk of vitamin B_6 deficiency (e.g., alcoholics; malnourished persons; pregnant and lactating women; and patients with conditions such as chronic renal failure, diabetes, and HIV infection, which are also associated with neuropathy). A full course of therapy (completion of treatment) is defined more accurately by the total number of doses taken than by the duration of treatment, although the course should not include interruptions of longer than 4 weeks. Specific recommendations on the required number of doses for each of the various treatment regimens have been published jointly by the American Thoracic Society, the Infectious Diseases Society of America, and the CDC. In some developing countries where the ability to ensure adherence to treatment is limited, a continuation-phase regimen of daily isoniazid and ethambutol for 6 months was used in the past. However, this regimen is associated with a higher rate of relapse, failure, and death, especially among HIV-infected patients, and is no longer recommended by the WHO.

Lack of adherence to treatment is recognized worldwide as the most important impediment to cure. Moreover, the tubercle bacilli infecting patients who do not fully adhere to the prescribed regimen are likely to become drug resistant. Both patient- and provider-related factors may affect adherence. Patient-related factors include a lack of belief that the illness is significant and/or that treatment will have a beneficial effect; the existence of concomitant medical conditions (notably alcohol or substance abuse); lack of social support; fear of stigma and discrimination associated with TB; and poverty, with attendant joblessness and homelessness. Provider-related factors that may promote adherence include the support, education, and encouragement of patients and the offering of convenient clinic hours. In addition to specific measures promoting adherence, two other strategic approaches are used: direct supervision of treatment with support to the patient, consisting of incentives and enablers such as meals, travel vouchers, cash transfers, and grants to replace income loss; and provision of fixed-drug-combination products that reduce the number of tablets the patient needs to swallow. Because it is difficult to predict which patients will adhere to the recommended treatment for a disease that has important public as well as individual health implications, all patients should have their therapy directly supervised, especially during the initial phase, with

TABLE 202-3 RECOMMENDED ANTITUBERCULOSIS TREATMENT REGIMENS

Indication	Initial Phase		Continuation Phase	
	Duration, Months	Drugs	Duration, Months	Drugs
New smear- or culture-positive cases	2	HRZE[a,b]	4	HR[a,c,d]
New culture-negative cases	2	HRZE[a]	4	HR[a]
Pregnancy	2	HRE[e]	7	HR
Relapses and treatment default (pending susceptibility testing)	3	HRZES[f]	5	HRE
Failures[g]	← Tailored according to drug susceptibility testing →			
Resistance (or intolerance) to H	Throughout (6–9)	RZE[h]		
Resistance (or intolerance) to R	← Same as for MDR-TB; see below[i] →			
MDR-TB (resistance to at least H + R)	Throughout (20 months in most cases)	Q, Inj[j], Eto/Pto, Z, Cs/PAS		
XDR-TB	← See Table 202-4 →			
Intolerance to Z	2	HRE	7	HR

[a]All drugs can be given daily or intermittently (three times weekly throughout). A twice-weekly regimen after 2–8 weeks of daily therapy during the initial phase is sometimes used, although it is not recommended by the WHO. [b]Streptomycin can be used in place of ethambutol but is no longer considered a first-line drug. [c]Some experts suggest extending the continuation phase to 7 months for patients with cavitary pulmonary tuberculosis who remain sputum culture–positive after the initial phase of treatment. However, treatment in such patients must be guided by drug susceptibility testing to rule out drug-resistant TB. [d]A clinical trial showed that HIV-negative patients with noncavitary pulmonary tuberculosis who have negative sputum AFB smears after the initial phase of treatment can be given once-weekly rifapentine/isoniazid in the continuation phase. [e]The 6-month regimen with pyrazinamide can probably be used safely during pregnancy and is recommended by the WHO and the International Union Against Tuberculosis and Lung Disease. If pyrazinamide is not included in the initial treatment regimen, the minimal duration of therapy is 9 months. [f]Streptomycin should be discontinued after 2 months. Drug susceptibility results will determine the best regimen option. [g]The availability of rapid molecular methods to identify drug resistance allows initiation of a proper regimen at the start of treatment. [h]Although normally not recommended, a fluoroquinolone may strengthen the regimen for patients with extensive disease. A later-generation agent (such as levofloxacin, moxifloxacin, or possibly gatifloxacin; see text) is preferred. [i]Isoniazid is added if susceptibility to this agent is confirmed or presumed. [j]Amikacin and kanamycin (aminoglycosides) or capreomycin (polypeptide). Any of these injectable agents is recommended for the first 8 months in most patients, but the duration may be modified according to the clinical response to therapy. Continuation of treatment with the injectable drug for at least 4 months after culture conversion is advised.

Abbreviations: Cs/PAS, cycloserine or para-aminosalicylic acid; E, ethambutol; Eto/Pto, ethionamide or prothionamide; H, isoniazid; Inj, an injectable agent (the aminoglycosides amikacin and kanamycin or the polypeptide capreomycin); MDR-TB, multidrug-resistant tuberculosis; Q, a quinolone antibiotic; R, rifampin; S, streptomycin; WHO, World Health Organization; XDR-TB, extensively drug-resistant tuberculosis; Z, pyrazinamide.

proper social support including education, psychosocial counseling, and material sustainment. In an increasing number of countries, personnel to supervise therapy are usually available through TB control programs of local public health departments and from members of the community who are accepted by the patient to undertake that role and who have been properly educated by health workers. Direct supervision with patient support usually increases the proportion of patients completing treatment in all settings and greatly lessens the chances of failure, relapse, and acquired drug resistance. Fixed-drug-combination products (e.g., isoniazid/rifampin, isoniazid/rifampin/pyrazinamide, and isoniazid/rifampin/pyrazinamide/ethambutol) are available and are strongly recommended as a means of minimizing the likelihood of prescription error and of the development of drug resistance as the result of monotherapy. In some formulations of these combination products, the bioavailability of rifampin has been found to be substandard. Stringent regulatory authorities ensure that combination products are of good quality; however, this type of quality assurance is not always operative in low-income countries. Alternative regimens for patients who exhibit drug intolerance or adverse reactions are listed in Table 202-3. However, severe side effects prompting discontinuation of any of the first-line drugs and use of these alternative regimens are uncommon. The fluoroquinolones moxifloxacin and gatifloxacin have been tested as 4-month treatment-shortening regimens for drug-susceptible TB. Recently published results from these clinical trials failed to show that a 4 month regimen substituting gatifloxacin for ethambutol or moxifloxacin for either ethambutol or isoniazid is noninferior to the standard 6-month regimen. Thus, currently there is no 4-month regimen available for TB treatment.

MONITORING TREATMENT RESPONSE AND DRUG TOXICITY

Bacteriologic evaluation through culture and/or smear microscopy is essential in monitoring the response to treatment for TB. In addition, the patient's weight should be monitored regularly and the drug dosage adjusted with any significant weight change. Patients with pulmonary disease should have their sputum examined monthly until cultures become negative to allow early detection of treatment failure. With the recommended regimen, more than 80% of patients will have negative sputum cultures at the end of the second month of treatment. By the end of the third month, the sputum of virtually all patients should be culture negative. In some patients, especially those with extensive cavitary disease and large numbers of organisms, AFB smear conversion may lag behind culture conversion. This phenomenon is presumably due to the expectoration and microscopic visualization of dead bacilli. As noted above, patients with cavitary disease in whom sputum culture conversion does not occur by 2 months require immediate testing for drug resistance. When a patient's sputum cultures remain positive at ≥3 months, treatment failure and drug resistance or poor adherence to the regimen are likely, and testing of drug resistance should guide the choice of the best treatment option (see below). A sputum specimen should be collected by the end of treatment to document cure. If mycobacterial cultures are not practical, then monitoring by AFB smear examination should be undertaken at 2, 5, and 6 months. Smears that are positive after 3 months of treatment when the patient is known to be adherent are indicative of treatment failure and possible drug resistance. Therefore, if not done at the start of treatment, drug susceptibility testing is mandatory at this stage. Bacteriologic monitoring of patients with extrapulmonary TB is more difficult and often is not feasible. In these cases, the response to treatment must be assessed clinically and radiographically.

Monitoring of the response during chemotherapy by nucleic acid amplification technology has not been shown to be suitable. Thus Xpert MTB/RIF should not be used to monitor treatment. Likewise, serial chest radiographs are not recommended because radiographic changes may lag behind bacteriologic response and are not highly sensitive. After the completion of treatment, neither sputum examination nor chest radiography is recommended for routine follow-up purposes. However, a chest radiograph obtained at the end of treatment may be useful for comparative purposes should the patient develop symptoms of recurrent TB months or years later. Patients should be instructed to report promptly for medical assessment if they develop any such symptoms. In addition, an end-of-treatment chest radiograph may reveal earlier the post-TB complications described above.

During treatment, patients should be monitored for drug toxicity. The most common adverse reaction of significance is hepatitis. Patients should be carefully educated about the signs and symptoms of drug-induced hepatitis (e.g., dark urine, loss of appetite) and should be instructed to discontinue treatment promptly and see their health care provider should these symptoms occur. Although biochemical monitoring is not routinely recommended, all adult patients should undergo baseline assessment of liver function (e.g., measurement of serum levels of hepatic aminotransferases and bilirubin). Older patients, those with concomitant diseases, those with a history of hepatic disease (especially hepatitis C), and those using alcohol daily should be monitored especially closely (i.e., monthly), with repeated measurements of aminotransferases, during the initial phase of treatment. Up to 20% of patients have small increases in aspartate aminotransferase (up to three times the upper limit of normal) that are not accompanied by symptoms and are of no consequence. For patients with symptomatic hepatitis and those with marked (five- to sixfold) elevations in serum levels of aspartate aminotransferase, treatment should be stopped and drugs reintroduced one at a time after liver function has returned to normal. Hypersensitivity reactions usually require the discontinuation of all drugs and rechallenge to determine which agent is the culprit. Because of the variety of regimens available, it usually is not necessary—although it is possible—to desensitize patients. Hyperuricemia and arthralgia caused by pyrazinamide can usually be managed by the administration of acetylsalicylic acid; however, pyrazinamide treatment should be stopped if the patient develops gouty arthritis. Individuals who develop autoimmune thrombocytopenia secondary to rifampin therapy should not receive the drug thereafter. Similarly, the occurrence of optic neuritis with ethambutol is an indication for permanent discontinuation of this drug. Other common manifestations of drug intolerance, such as pruritus and gastrointestinal upset, can generally be managed without the interruption of therapy.

TREATMENT FAILURE AND RELAPSE

As stated above, treatment failure should be suspected when a patient's sputum smears and/or cultures remain positive after 3 months of treatment. In the management of such patients, it is imperative that the current isolate be urgently tested for susceptibility to first- and second-line agents. Initial molecular testing for rifampin resistance should be done if the technology is available. When the results of susceptibility testing are based on molecular methods and are expected to become available within a few days, changes in the regimen can be postponed until that time. However, if the patient's clinical condition is deteriorating, an earlier change in regimen may be indicated. A cardinal rule in the latter situation is always to add more than one drug at a time to a failing regimen: at least two and preferably three drugs that have never been used and to which the bacilli are likely to be susceptible should be added. The patient may continue to take isoniazid and rifampin along with these new agents pending the results of susceptibility tests.

Patients who experience a recurrence after apparently successful treatment (relapse) are less likely to harbor drug-resistant strains (see below) than are patients in whom treatment has failed. Acquired resistance is uncommon among strains from patients in whom relapse follows the completion of a standard short-course regimen. However, pending the results of susceptibility testing, it is prudent to begin the treatment of all patients whose infections have relapsed with a standard regimen containing all four first-line drugs plus streptomycin. In less affluent countries and other settings where facilities for culture and drug susceptibility testing are not yet routinely available and where the prevalence of MDR-TB is low, the WHO recommends that a standard regimen with all four first-line drugs plus streptomycin be used in all instances of relapse and treatment default. Patients with treatment failure and those relapsing or defaulting with a high likelihood of MDR-TB should receive a regimen that includes second-line agents and is based on their history of anti-TB treatment and the drug resistance patterns in the population (Table 202-3). Once drug susceptibility test results are available, the regimen can be adjusted accordingly.

DRUG-RESISTANT TB

Strains of *M. tuberculosis* resistant to individual drugs arise by spontaneous point mutations in the mycobacterial genome that occur at low but predictable rates (10^{-7}–10^{-10} for the key drugs). Resistance to rifampin is associated with mutations in the *rpo*B gene in 95% of cases; that to isoniazid with mutations mainly in the *kat*G (50–95% of cases) and *inh*A (up to 45%) genes; that to pyrazinamide in the *pnc*A gene (up to 98%); that to ethambutol in the *emb*B gene (50–65%); that to the fluoroquinolones in the *gyr*A–*gyr*B genes (75–95%); and that to the aminoglycosides mainly in the *rrs* gene (up to 80%). Because there is no cross-resistance among the commonly used drugs, the probability that a strain will be resistant to two drugs is the product of the probabilities of resistance to each drug and thus is low. The development of drug-resistant TB is almost invariably the result of monotherapy—i.e., the failure of the health care provider to prescribe at least two drugs to which tubercle bacilli are susceptible or of the patient to take properly prescribed therapy. In addition, the use of drugs of substandard quality may cause the emergence of drug resistance. Drug-resistant TB may be either primary or acquired. Primary drug resistance is that which develops in a patient infected from the start by a drug-resistant strain. Acquired resistance is that which develops during treatment with an inappropriate regimen. In North America, Western Europe, most of Latin America, and the Persian Gulf States, rates of primary resistance are generally low and isoniazid resistance is most common. In the United States, although rates of primary isoniazid resistance have been stable at ~7–8%, the rate of primary MDR-TB has declined from 2.5% in 1993 to 1% since 2000. As described above, MDR-TB is an increasingly serious problem in some regions, especially in the states of the former Soviet Union and some countries of Asia (**Fig. 202-11**). Even more serious is the recently described occurrence of XDR-TB due to MDR strains that are also resistant to any fluoroquinolones and to any of three second-line injectable agents (amikacin, kanamycin, and capreomycin). Creation of drug-resistant TB can be prevented by adherence to the principles of sound treatment: inclusion of at least two quality-assured, bactericidal drugs to which the organism is susceptible; use of fixed-drug-combination products; supervision of treatment with patient support; and verification that patients complete the prescribed course. Transmission of drug-resistant strains can be prevented by implementation of respiratory infection-control measures (see below).

Although the 6-month regimen described in Table 202-3 is generally effective for patients with initial isoniazid-resistant disease, it is prudent to include at least ethambutol and possibly pyrazinamide for the full 6 months and to consider extending the treatment course to 9 months. In such cases, isoniazid probably does not contribute to a successful outcome and could be omitted. In case of documented resistance to both isoniazid and ethambutol, a 9- to 12-month regimen of rifampin, pyrazinamide, and a fluoroquinolone can be used. Any patients whose isolates exhibit resistance to rifampin should be managed as if they had MDR-TB (see below), with the addition of isoniazid if susceptibility to this agent is confirmed via rapid testing or is presumed. MDR-TB, in which bacilli are resistant to (at least) isoniazid and rifampin, is more difficult to manage than is disease caused by drug-susceptible organisms because these two bactericidal drugs are the most potent agents available and because associated resistance to other first-line drugs as well (e.g., ethambutol) is not uncommon. For treatment of MDR-TB, the WHO recommends that in most patients five drugs be used in the initial phase of at least 8 months: a later-generation fluoroquinolone, an injectable agent (the aminoglycosides amikacin or kanamycin or the polypeptide capreomycin), ethionamide (or prothionamide), either cycloserine or PAS, and pyrazinamide. Ethambutol can be added (Table 202-3). Although the optimal duration of treatment is not known, a course of at least 20 months is recommended for previously untreated patients, including the initial phase with an injectable agent, which is usually discontinued at 4 months after culture conversion.

In late 2012, the FDA granted accelerated approval of bedaquiline, a diarylquinoline antibiotic. This new drug, when given for the first 24 weeks (400 mg daily for 2 weeks followed by 200 mg thrice weekly for 22 weeks), has been shown to increase the efficacy of the WHO standard regimen for MDR-TB with faster sputum conversion.

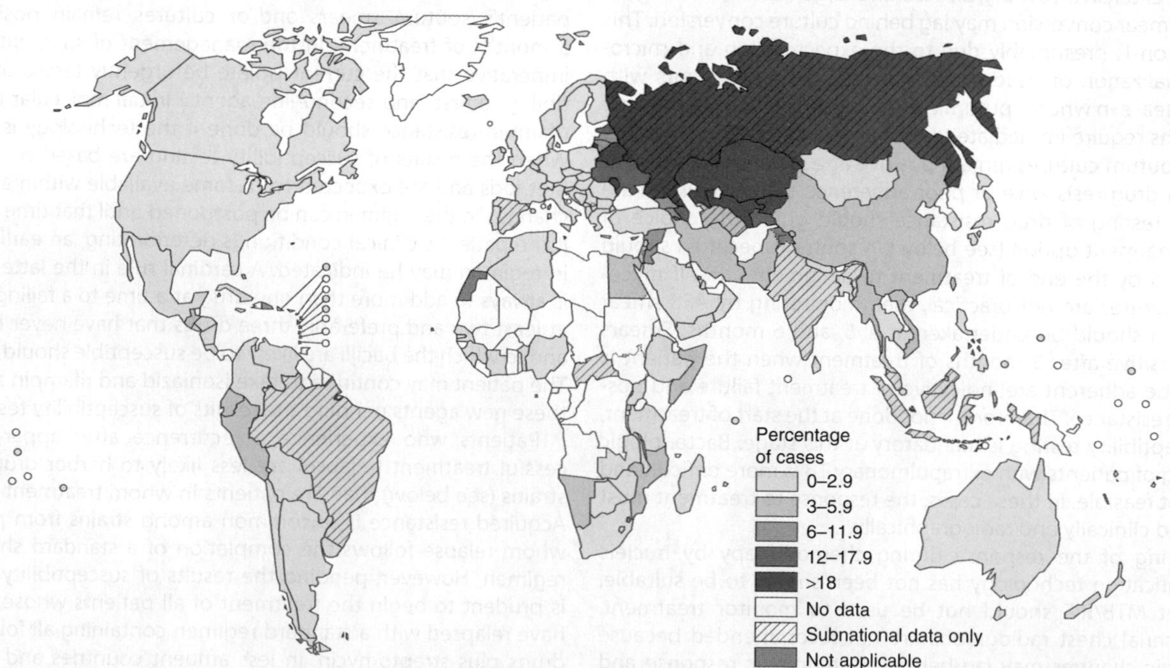

FIGURE 202-11 Percentage of new tuberculosis cases with multidrug resistance in all countries surveyed by the World Health Organization (WHO) Global Drug Resistance Surveillance Project during 1994–2013. *(See disclaimer in Fig. 202-2. Courtesy of the Global TB Programme, WHO; with permission.)*

Bedaquiline should be used with caution in people >65 years of age and in HIV-infected patients; its use is not advised in children and pregnant women. In early 2014, the European Medical Agency granted accelerated approval of another new agent, the nitroimidazole compound delamanid. Data from a phase 2B clinical trial in which delamanid was added to the WHO-recommended standard MDR-TB regimen have shown increased culture conversion at 2 months. Pending phase 3 trial results and in view of potential side effects of both new drugs (including QT interval prolongation in both cases and hepatotoxicity in the case of bedaquiline), the WHO recommends limiting the use of bedaquiline and delamanid to cases of MDR-TB when an effective WHO-recommended standard MDR-TB regimen cannot be designed because of known resistance, intolerance, or nonavailability of any second-line drugs in the regimen. Patients treated with bedaquiline or delamanid should be counseled, should give informed consent, and should be closely monitored during treatment. In particular, patients with cardiac anomalies such as prolonged QT interval or a history of ventricular arrhythmias should not be given these drugs. Currently, there is no information about simultaneous use of these two agents; therefore, combining them is not recommended.

Finally, a shorter (9-month) regimen consisting of gatifloxacin or moxifloxacin, clofazimine, ethambutol, and pyrazinamide given throughout the treatment period and supplemented by prothionamide, kanamycin, and high-dose isoniazid during an intensive phase of at least 4 months is reportedly effective for MDR-TB in certain settings. Further investigations are necessary to elucidate the role of this shorter regimen in MDR-TB treatment.

Patients with XDR-TB have fewer treatment options and a much poorer prognosis. However, observational studies have shown that aggressive management of cases comprising early drug-susceptibility testing, rational combination of at least five drugs, readjustment of the regimen, strict directly observed therapy, monthly bacteriologic monitoring, and intensive patient support may result in cure and avert death. Table 202-4 summarizes the management of patients with XDR-TB. Some recently published studies regarding the use of linezolid in patients with XDR-TB suggest that, although it carries a high level of toxicity, this drug increases culture conversion.

For patients with localized disease and sufficient pulmonary reserve, lobectomy or pneumonectomy may be considered. Because the management of patients with MDR- and XDR-TB is complicated by both social and medical factors, care of these patients is ideally provided in specialized centers or, in their absence, in the context of programs with adequate resources and capacity, including community support.

TABLE 202-4 MANAGEMENT GUIDELINES FOR PATIENTS WITH DOCUMENTED OR STRONGLY SUSPECTED EXTENSIVELY DRUG-RESISTANT TUBERCULOSIS (XDR-TB)

1. Use pyrazinamide and any first-line oral agents that may be effective.
2. Use an injectable agent to which the strain is susceptible, and consider an extended duration of use (12 months or possibly the whole treatment period). If the strain is resistant to all injectable agents, use of one that the patient has not previously received is recommended.[a]
3. Use a later-generation fluoroquinolone, such as moxifloxacin, high-dose levofloxacin, or possibly gatifloxacin.[b]
4. Use all second-line oral bacteriostatic agents (para-aminosalicylic acid, cycloserine, and ethionamide or prothionamide) that have not been used extensively in a previous regimen or any such agents that are likely to be effective.
5. Add bedaquiline or delamanid and one or more of the following drugs[c]: clofazimine, linezolid, amoxicillin/clavulanic acid, clarithromycin, and carbapenems such as imipenem/cilastatin and meropenem.
6. The simultaneous use of bedaquiline and delamanid is not recommended at the moment in view of the current lack of information on the potential of adverse reactions when these drugs are administered together.
7. Consider treatment with high-dose isoniazid if low-level resistance to this drug is documented.
8. Consider adjuvant surgery if there is localized disease.
9. Enforce strong infection-control measures.
10. Implement strict directly observed therapy and full adherence support as well as comprehensive bacteriologic and clinical monitoring.

[a]This recommendation is made because, although the reproducibility and reliability of susceptibility testing with injectable agents are good, few data are available on the correlation of clinical efficacy with test results. Options with XDR-TB are very limited, and some strains may be affected in vivo by an injectable agent even though they test resistant in vitro. [b]Gatifloxacin (no longer marketed in several countries, including the United States, because of previously observed dysglycemia) has recently been tested in a 4-month regimen that produced no detectable major side effects; thus, this drug could be reconsidered as a good alternative. [c]The number of drugs added is based on how many oral bacteriostatic drugs (see point 4 above) are believed to be effective: the advice is to add one drug if there is confidence in all three bacteriostatic drugs; two if there is confidence in only two bacteriostatic drugs; and three or more if there is confidence in only one bacteriostatic drug or none.

HIV-ASSOCIATED TB

Several observational studies and randomized controlled trials have shown that treatment of HIV-associated TB with anti-TB drugs and simultaneous use of ART are associated with significant reductions in mortality risk and AIDS-related events. Evidence from randomized controlled trials shows that early initiation of ART during anti-TB treatment is associated with a 34–68% reduction in mortality rates, with especially good results in patients with CD4+ T cell counts of <50/μL. Therefore, the main aim in the management of HIV-associated TB is to initiate anti-TB treatment and to immediately consider initiating or continuing ART. All HIV-infected TB patients, regardless of CD4+ T cell count, are candidates for ART, which optimally is initiated as soon as possible after the diagnosis of TB and within the first 8 weeks of anti-TB therapy. However, ART should be started within the first 2 weeks of TB treatment for patients with CD4+ T cell counts of <50/μL. In general, the standard 6-month daily regimen is equally efficacious in HIV-negative and HIV-positive patients for treatment of drug-susceptible TB. As for any other adult living with HIV (Chap. 226), first-line ART for TB patients should consist of two nucleoside reverse transcriptase inhibitors (NRTIs) plus a nonnucleoside reverse transcriptase inhibitor (NNRTI). Although TB treatment modalities are similar to those in HIV-negative patients, adverse drug effects may be more pronounced in HIV-infected patients. In this regard, three important considerations are relevant: an increased frequency of paradoxical reactions, interactions between ART components and rifamycins, and development of rifampin monoresistance with intermittent treatment. IRIS—i.e., the exacerbation of symptoms and signs of TB—has been described above. Rifampin, a potent inducer of enzymes of the cytochrome P450 system, lowers serum levels of many HIV protease inhibitors and some NNRTIs—essential drugs used in ART. In such cases, rifabutin, which has much less enzyme-inducing activity, has been used in place of rifampin. However, dosage adjustments for rifabutin and protease inhibitors are still being assessed. Several clinical trials have found that patients with HIV-associated TB whose degree of immunosuppression is advanced (e.g., CD4+ T cell counts of <100/μL) are prone to treatment failure and relapse with rifampin-resistant organisms when treated with "highly intermittent" (i.e., once- or twice-weekly) rifamycin-containing regimens. Consequently, it is recommended that all TB patients who are infected with HIV receive a rifampin-containing regimen on a daily basis. Because recommendations are frequently updated, consultation of the following websites is advised: *www.who.int/hiv*, *www.who.int/tb*, *www.cdc.gov/hiv*, and *www.cdc.gov/tb*.

SPECIAL CLINICAL SITUATIONS

Although comparative clinical trials of treatment for extrapulmonary TB are limited, the available evidence indicates that most forms of disease can be treated with the 6-month regimen recommended for patients with pulmonary disease. The WHO and the American Academy of Pediatrics recommend that children with bone and joint TB, tuberculous meningitis, or miliary TB receive up to 12 months of treatment. Treatment for TB may be complicated by underlying medical problems that require special consideration. As a rule, patients with chronic renal failure should not receive aminoglycosides and should receive ethambutol only if serum drug levels can be monitored. Isoniazid, rifampin, and pyrazinamide may be given in the usual doses in cases of mild to moderate renal failure, but the dosages of isoniazid and pyrazinamide should be reduced for all patients with severe renal failure except those undergoing hemodialysis. Patients with hepatic disease pose a special problem because of the hepatotoxicity of isoniazid, rifampin, and pyrazinamide. Patients with severe hepatic disease may be treated with ethambutol, streptomycin, and possibly another drug (e.g., a fluoroquinolone); if required, isoniazid and rifampin may be administered under close supervision. The use of pyrazinamide by patients with liver failure should be avoided. Silicotuberculosis necessitates the extension of therapy by at least 2 months.

The regimen of choice for pregnant women (Table 202-3) is 9 months of treatment with isoniazid and rifampin supplemented by ethambutol for the first 2 months. Although the WHO has recommended routine use of pyrazinamide for pregnant women, this drug has not been recommended in the United States because of insufficient data documenting its safety in pregnancy. Streptomycin is contraindicated because it is known to cause eighth-cranial-nerve damage in the fetus. Treatment for TB is not a contraindication to breast-feeding; most of the drugs administered will be present in small quantities in breast milk, albeit at concentrations far too low to provide any therapeutic or prophylactic benefit to the child.

Medical consultation on difficult-to-manage cases is provided by the U.S. CDC Regional Training and Medical Consultation Centers (*www.cdc.gov/tb/education/rtmc/*).

PREVENTION

The best way to prevent TB is to diagnose and isolate infectious cases rapidly and to administer appropriate treatment until patients are rendered noninfectious (usually 2–4 weeks after the start of proper treatment) and the disease is cured. Additional strategies include BCG vaccination and treatment of persons with LTBI who are at high risk of developing active disease.

BCG VACCINATION

BCG was derived from an attenuated strain of *M. bovis* and was first administered to humans in 1921. Many BCG vaccines are available worldwide; all are derived from the original strain, but the vaccines vary in efficacy, ranging from 80% to nil in randomized, placebo-controlled trials. A similar range of efficacy was found in recent observational studies (case–control, historic cohort, and cross-sectional) in areas where infants are vaccinated at birth. These studies and a meta-analysis also found higher rates of efficacy in the protection of infants and young children from serious disseminated forms of childhood TB, such as tuberculous meningitis and miliary TB. BCG vaccine is safe and rarely causes serious complications. The local tissue response begins 2–3 weeks after vaccination, with scar formation and healing within 3 months. Side effects—most commonly, ulceration at the vaccination site and regional lymphadenitis—occur in 1–10% of vaccinated persons. Some vaccine strains have caused osteomyelitis in ~1 case per million doses administered. Disseminated BCG infection ("BCGitis") and death have occurred in 1–10 cases per 10 million doses administered, although this problem is restricted almost exclusively to persons with impaired immunity, such as children with severe combined immunodeficiency syndrome or adults with HIV infection. BCG vaccination induces TST reactivity, which tends to wane with time. The presence or size of TST reactions after vaccination does not predict the degree of protection afforded.

BCG vaccine is recommended for routine use at birth in countries with high TB prevalence. However, because of the low risk of transmission of TB in the United States and other high-income countries, the unreliable protection afforded by BCG, and its impact on the TST, the vaccine is not recommended for general use. HIV-infected adults and children should not receive BCG vaccine. Moreover, infants whose HIV status is unknown but who have signs and symptoms consistent with HIV infection or who are born to HIV-infected mothers should not receive BCG.

Over the past decade, renewed research and development efforts have been made toward a new TB vaccine. In mid-2014, 16 candidates were in clinical trials and 12 were being field tested. The first new vaccine, for which results of a clinical trial became available in early 2013, is MVA85A/AERAS-485; unfortunately, this viral-vectored vaccine did not show clinical benefit as a booster to BCG.

TREATMENT LATENT TUBERCULOSIS INFECTION

It is estimated that about 2 billion people, or nearly one-third of the human population, have been infected with *M. tuberculosis*. Although only a small fraction of these infections will progress toward active disease, new active cases will continue to emerge from this pool of "latently" infected individuals. Unfortunately, there is no diagnostic test at present that can predict which individuals with LTBI will develop active TB. Treatment of selected persons with LTBI aims at preventing active disease. This intervention (also called *preventive chemotherapy* or *chemoprophylaxis*) is based on the results of a large number of randomized, placebo-controlled clinical trials demonstrating that a 6- to 9-month course of isoniazid reduces the risk of active TB in infected people by up to 90%. Analysis of available data indicates that the optimal duration of treatment is ~9 months. In the absence of reinfection, the protective effect is believed to be lifelong. Clinical trials have shown that isoniazid reduces rates of TB among TST-positive persons with HIV infection. Studies in HIV-infected patients have also demonstrated the effectiveness of shorter courses of rifampin-based treatment.

Candidates for treatment of LTBI are listed in **Table 202-5**. They can be identified by TST or IGRA of persons in defined high-risk groups. For skin testing, 5 tuberculin units of polysorbate-stabilized PPD should be injected intradermally into the volar surface of the forearm (i.e., the Mantoux method). Multipuncture tests are not recommended. Reactions are read at 48–72 h as the transverse

TABLE 202-5 TUBERCULIN REACTION SIZE AND TREATMENT OF LATENT *MYCOBACTERIUM TUBERCULOSIS* INFECTION

Risk Group	Tuberculin Reaction Size, mm
HIV-infected persons	≥5
Recent contacts of a patient with TB	≥5[a]
Organ transplant recipients	≥5
Persons with fibrotic lesions consistent with old TB on chest radiography	≥5
Persons who are immunosuppressed, e.g., due to the use of glucocorticoids or tumor necrosis factor α inhibitors	≥5
Persons with high-risk medical conditions[b]	≥5
Recent immigrants (≤5 years) from high-prevalence countries	≥10
Injection drug users	≥10
Mycobacteriology laboratory personnel; residents and employees of high-risk congregate settings[c]	≥10
Children <5 years of age; children and adolescents exposed to adults in high-risk categories	≥10
Low-risk persons[d]	≥15

[a]Tuberculin-negative contacts, especially children, should receive prophylaxis for 2–3 months after contact ends and should then undergo repeat TST. Those whose results remain negative should discontinue prophylaxis. HIV-infected contacts should receive a full course of treatment regardless of TST results. [b]These conditions include silicosis and end-stage renal disease managed by hemodialysis [c]These settings include correctional facilities, nursing homes, homeless shelters, and hospitals and other health care facilities. [d]Except for employment purposes where longitudinal TST screening is anticipated, TST is not indicated for these low-risk persons. A decision to treat should be based on individual risk/benefit considerations.

Source: Adapted from Centers for Disease Control and Prevention: TB elimination—treatment options for latent tuberculosis infection (2011). Available at *http://www.cdc.gov/tb/publications/factsheets/testing/skintestresults.pdf.*

diameter (in millimeters) of induration; the diameter of erythema is not considered. In some persons, TST reactivity wanes with time but can be recalled by a second skin test administered ≥1 week after the first (i.e., two-step testing). For persons periodically undergoing the TST, such as health care workers and individuals admitted to long-term-care institutions, initial two-step testing may preclude subsequent misclassification of those who have boosted reactions as TST converters. The cutoff for a positive TST (and thus for treatment) is related both to the probability that the reaction represents true infection and to the likelihood that the individual, if truly infected, will develop TB. Table 202-5 suggests possible cutoff by risk group. Thus, positive reactions for persons with HIV infection, recent close contacts of infectious cases, organ transplant recipients, previously untreated persons whose chest radiograph shows fibrotic lesions consistent with old TB, and persons receiving drugs that suppress the immune system are defined as an area of induration >5 mm in diameter. A 10-mm cutoff is used to define positive reactions in most other at-risk persons. For persons with a very low risk of developing TB if infected, a cutoff of 15 mm is used. (Except for employment purposes where longitudinal screening is anticipated, the TST is not indicated for these low-risk persons.) A positive IGRA is based on the manufacturers' recommendations; however, good clinical practice requires that epidemiologic and clinical factors also guide the decision to implement treatment for LTBI and that active TB be definitively excluded before the initiation of chemoprophylaxis.

Some TST- and IGRA-negative individuals are also candidates for treatment. Once an appropriate clinical evaluation has excluded active TB, infants and children who have come into contact with infectious cases should be treated for presumed LTBI. HIV-infected persons who have been exposed to an infectious TB patient should receive treatment regardless of the TST result. Any HIV-infected candidate for LTBI treatment must be screened carefully to exclude active TB, which would necessitate full treatment. The use of a clinical algorithm based on four symptoms (current cough, fever, weight loss, and night sweats) helps to define which HIV-infected person is a candidate for LTBI treatment. The absence of all four symptoms tends to exclude active TB. The presence of one of the four symptoms, on the other hand, warrants further investigation for active TB before treatment of LTBI is started. Although administering a TST is prudent, this test is not an absolute requirement—given the logistical challenges—among people living with HIV in high-TB-incidence and low-resource settings.

Before treatment of LTBI begins, it is mandatory to carefully exclude active TB. Several regimens can be used to treat LTBI. The most widely used is that based on isoniazid alone at a daily dose of 5 mg/kg (up to 300 mg/d) for 9 months. On the basis of cost-benefit analyses and concerns about feasibility, a 6-month period of treatment is currently recommended by the WHO, especially in highly TB-endemic countries. Isoniazid can be administered intermittently (twice weekly) at a dose of 15 mg/kg (up to 900 mg) but only as directly observed therapy. An alternative regimen for adults is 4 months of daily rifampin. A 3-month regimen of daily isoniazid and rifampin is used in some countries (e.g., the United Kingdom) for both adults and children who are known not to have HIV infection. A previously recommended regimen of 2 months of rifampin and pyrazinamide has been associated with serious or even fatal hepatotoxicity and now is generally not recommended. The rifampin-containing regimens should be considered for persons who are likely to have been infected with an isoniazid-resistant strain. A recent clinical trial showed that a regimen of isoniazid (900 mg) and rifapentine (900 mg) given once weekly for 12 weeks is as effective as the standard 9-month isoniazid regimen. This regimen was associated with higher treatment completion (82% vs 69%) and less hepatotoxicity (0.4% vs 2.7%) than isoniazid alone, although the rate of permanent discontinuation due to an adverse event was higher (4.9% vs 3.7%).

Currently, the isoniazid–rifapentine regimen is not recommended for children <2 years of age, people living with HIV infection who are receiving ART, or pregnant women. Rifampin and rifapentine are contraindicated in HIV-infected individuals receiving protease inhibitors and most NNRTIs. (Efavirenz is the safest agent in this class of antiretrovirals for simultaneous administration with a rifamycin.) Clinical trials to assess the efficacy of long-term isoniazid administration (i.e., for at least 3 years) among people living with HIV in high-TB-transmission settings have shown that this regimen can be more effective than 9 months of isoniazid and is therefore recommended under those circumstances. Isoniazid should not be given to persons with active liver disease. All persons at increased risk of hepatotoxicity (e.g., those abusing alcohol daily and those with a history of liver disease) should undergo baseline and then monthly assessment of liver function. All patients should be carefully educated about hepatitis and instructed to discontinue use of the drug immediately should any symptoms develop. Moreover, patients should be seen and questioned monthly during therapy about adverse reactions and should be given no more than a 1-month supply of drug at each visit. Treatment of LTBI among persons likely to have been infected by a multidrug-resistant strain is a challenge because no regimens have yet been tested in clinical trials. Close observation for early signs of disease is one option; consultation with a TB expert is advised.

It may be more difficult to ensure compliance when treating persons with LTBI than when treating those with active TB. If family members of active cases are being treated, compliance and monitoring may be easier. When feasible, supervised therapy may increase the likelihood of completion. As in active cases, the provision of incentives may also be helpful.

PRINCIPLES OF TB CONTROL

The highest priority in any TB control program is the prompt detection of cases and the provision of short-course chemotherapy to all TB patients under proper case-management conditions, including directly observed therapy. In addition, screening of high-risk groups, including immigrants from high-prevalence countries, migratory workers, prisoners, homeless individuals, substance abusers, and HIV-seropositive persons, is recommended. TST-positive high-risk persons should be treated for LTBI as described above. Contact investigation is an important component of efficient TB control. In the United States and other countries worldwide, a great deal of attention has been given to the transmission of TB (particularly in association with HIV infection) in institutional settings such as hospitals, homeless shelters, and prisons. Measures to limit such transmission include respiratory isolation of persons with suspected TB until they are proven to be noninfectious (at least by sputum AFB smear negativity), proper ventilation in rooms of patients with infectious TB, use of ultraviolet irradiation in areas of increased risk of TB transmission, and periodic screening of personnel who may come into contact with known or unsuspected cases of TB. In the past, radiographic surveys, especially those conducted with portable equipment and miniature films, were advocated for case finding. Today, however, the prevalence of TB in industrialized countries is sufficiently low that "mass miniature radiography" is not cost-effective.

In high-prevalence countries, most TB control programs have made remarkable progress in reducing morbidity and mortality since the mid-1990s by adopting and implementing the strategy promoted by the WHO. Between 2000 and 2013, 37 million lives were saved, and since 1995, 61 million TB cases have been successfully treated. The essential elements of good TB care and control (the DOTS strategy) are (1) political commitment with increased and sustained financing; (2) case detection through quality-assured bacteriology (starting with examination of sputum from patients with cough of >2–3 weeks' duration); (3) administration of standardized short-course chemotherapy, with direct supervision and patient support; (4) an effective drug supply and management system; and (5) a monitoring and evaluation system, with impact measurement (including assessment of treatment outcomes—e.g., cure, completion of treatment without bacteriologic proof of cure, death, treatment failure, and default—in all cases registered and notified). In 2006, the WHO indicated that, although these essential elements remain the fundamental components of any control strategy, additional steps must be undertaken to reach the 2015 international TB control targets set within the United Nations Millennium Development Goals. Thus, a new "Stop TB Strategy" with six components has been promoted since 2006: (1) Pursue high-quality DOTS expansion and enhancement. (2) Address HIV-associated TB, MDR-TB, and the needs of poor and vulnerable populations. (3) Contribute to health system strengthening. (4) Engage all care providers. (5) Empower people with TB and their communities. (6) Enable and promote research. As part of the fourth component, evidence-based International Standards for Tuberculosis Care—focused on diagnosis, treatment, and public health responsibilities—have been introduced for wide adoption by medical and professional societies, academic institutions, and all practitioners worldwide (*http://www.who.int/tb/publications/ISTC_3rdEd.pdf?ua=1*).

Care and control of HIV-associated TB are particularly challenging in developing countries because existing interventions require collaboration between HIV/AIDS and TB programs as well as standard services. While TB programs must test every patient for HIV in order to provide access to trimethoprim-sulfamethoxazole prophylaxis against common infections and ART, HIV/AIDS programs must regularly screen persons living with HIV/AIDS for active TB, provide treatment for LTBI, and ensure infection control in settings where people living with HIV congregate.

Early and active case detection is considered an important intervention not only among persons living with HIV/AIDS but also among other vulnerable populations, as it reduces transmission in a community and provides early effective care. For TB control efforts to succeed and for elimination to become a realistic target, programs must optimize their performance and include additional interventions as described. Moreover, the approach to TB control and care needs to become holistic and engage beyond dedicated programs. Therefore, the WHO's "End TB" strategy has been designed and builds on three pillars for the post-2015 era of increased efforts by governments and national programs worldwide: (1) integrated, patient-centered care and prevention; (2) bold policies and supportive systems; and (3) intensified research and innovation. The first pillar incorporates all technological innovations, such as early diagnostic approaches (including universal drug-susceptibility testing and systematic screening of identified, setting-specific, high-risk groups); well-designed treatment regimens for all forms of TB; proper management of HIV-associated TB and other comorbidities; and preventive treatment of persons at high risk. The second pillar is fundamental and is normally beyond the control of dedicated programs, relying on policies forged by the highest-level health and governmental authorities: availability of adequate and well-identified human and financial resources; engagement of civil society organizations and all relevant public and private providers to facilitate care and prevention of all patients; a policy of universal health coverage (which implies avoidance of catastrophic expenditures caused by TB among the poorest); regulatory frameworks for case notifications, vital registration, quality and rational use of medicines, and infection control; social protection mechanisms; poverty alleviation strategies; and interventions on the broader determinants of TB. Finally, the third pillar of the new strategy emphasizes intensification of engagement in research and development of new tools and interventions as well as optimization of implementation and rapid adoption of new tools in endemic countries. In the end, besides specific clinical care and control interventions as described in this chapter, elimination of TB ultimately will require control and attenuation of the multitude of risk factors (e.g., HIV, smoking, and diabetes) and socioeconomic determinants (e.g., extreme poverty, inadequate living conditions and bad housing, alcoholism, malnutrition, and indoor air pollution) with clearly implemented policies within the health sector and other sectors linked to human development and welfare.

ACKNOWLEDGMENT

The contributions of Richard J. O'Brien to this chapter in previous editions are gratefully acknowledged.

203 Leprosy

Robert H. Gelber

Leprosy, first described in ancient Indian texts from the sixth century B.C., is a nonfatal, chronic infectious disease caused by *Mycobacterium leprae*, the clinical manifestations of which are largely confined to the skin, peripheral nervous system, upper respiratory tract, eyes, and testes. The unique tropism of *M. leprae* for peripheral nerves (from large nerve trunks to microscopic dermal nerves) and certain immunologically mediated reactional states are the major causes of morbidity in leprosy. The propensity of the disease, when untreated, to result in characteristic deformities and the recognition in most cultures that the disease is communicable from person to person have resulted historically in a profound social stigma. Today, with early diagnosis and the institution of appropriate and effective antimicrobial therapy, patients can lead productive lives in the community, and deformities and other visible manifestations can largely be prevented.

ETIOLOGY

M. leprae is an obligate intracellular bacillus (0.3–1 μm wide and 1–8 μm long) that is confined to humans, armadillos in certain locales, and sphagnum moss. The organism is acid-fast, indistinguishable microscopically from other mycobacteria, and ideally detected in tissue sections by a modified Fite stain. Strain variability has been documented in this organism. *M. leprae* produces no known toxins and is well adapted to penetrate and reside within macrophages, yet it may survive outside the body for months. In untreated patients, only ~1% of *M. leprae* organisms are viable. The morphologic index (MI), a measure of the number of acid-fast bacilli (AFB) in skin scrapings that stain uniformly bright, correlates with viability. The bacteriologic index (BI), a logarithmic-scaled measure of the density of *M. leprae* in the dermis, may be as high as 4–6+ in untreated patients and falls by 1 unit per year during effective antimicrobial therapy; the rate of decrease is independent of the relative potency of therapy. A rising MI or BI suggests relapse and perhaps—if the patient is being treated—drug resistance. Drug resistance can be confirmed or excluded in the mouse model of leprosy, and resistance to dapsone and rifampin can be documented by the recognition of mutant genes. However, the availability of these technologies is extremely limited.

As a result of reductive evolution, almost half of the *M. leprae* genome contains nonfunctional genes; only 1605 genes encode for proteins, and 1439 genes are shared with *Mycobacterium tuberculosis*. In contrast, *M. tuberculosis* uses 91% of its genome to encode for 4000 proteins. Among the lost genes in *M. leprae* are those for catabolic and respiratory pathways; transport systems; purine, methionine, and glutamine synthesis; and nitrogen regulation. The genome of *M. leprae* provides a metabolic rationale for its obligate intracellular existence and reliance on host biochemical support, a template for targets of drug development, and ultimately a pathway to cultivation. The finding of strain variability among *M. leprae* isolates has provided a powerful tool with which to address anew the organism's epidemiology and pathobiology and to determine whether relapse represents reactivation or reinfection. The bacterium's complex cell wall contains large amounts of an *M. leprae*–specific phenolic glycolipid (PGL-1), which is detected in serologic tests. The unique trisaccharide of *M. leprae* binds to the basal lamina of Schwann cells; this interaction is probably relevant to the fact that *M. leprae* is the only bacterium to invade peripheral nerves.

Although it was the first bacterium to be etiologically associated with human disease, *M. leprae* remains one of the few bacterial species that still has not been cultivated on artificial medium or tissue culture. The multiplication of *M. leprae* in mouse footpads (albeit limited, with a doubling time of ~2 weeks) has provided a means to evaluate antimicrobial agents, monitor clinical trials, and screen vaccines. *M. leprae* grows best in cooler tissues (the skin, peripheral nerves, anterior chamber of the eye, upper respiratory tract, and testes), sparing warmer areas of the skin (the axilla, groin, scalp, and midline of the back).

EPIDEMIOLOGY

Demographics Leprosy is almost exclusively a disease of the developing world, affecting areas of Asia, Africa, Latin America, and the Pacific. While Africa has the highest disease prevalence, Asia has the most cases. More than 80% of the world's cases occur in a few countries: India, China, Myanmar, Indonesia, Brazil, Nigeria, Madagascar, and Nepal. Within endemic locales, the distribution of leprosy is quite uneven, with areas of high prevalence bordering on areas with little or no disease. In Brazil the majority of cases occur in the Amazon basin and two western states, while in Mexico leprosy is mostly confined to the Pacific coast. Except as imported cases, leprosy is largely absent from the United States, Canada, and northwestern Europe. In the United States, ~4000 persons have leprosy and 100–200 new cases are reported annually, most of them in California, Texas, New York, and Hawaii among immigrants from Mexico, Southeast Asia, the Philippines, and the Caribbean.

The comparative genomics of single-nucleotide polymorphisms support the likelihood that four distinct strains exist, having originated in East Africa or Central Asia. A mutation spread to Europe and subsequently underwent two separate mutations that were then followed by spread to West Africa and the Americas.

The global prevalence of leprosy is difficult to assess, given that many of the locales with high prevalence lack a significant medical or public health infrastructure. Estimates range from 0.6 to 8 million affected individuals. The lower estimate includes only persons who have not completed chemotherapy, excluding those who may be physically or psychologically damaged from leprosy and who may yet relapse or develop immune-mediated reactions. The higher figure includes patients whose infections probably are already cured and many who have no leprosy-related deformity or disability. Although the figures on the worldwide prevalence of leprosy are debatable, incidence is not falling; there are still an estimated 500,000 new cases annually.

Leprosy is associated with poverty and rural residence. It appears not to be associated with AIDS, perhaps because of leprosy's long incubation period. Most individuals appear to be naturally immune to leprosy and do not develop disease manifestations after exposure. The time of peak onset is in the second and third decades of life.

The most severe lepromatous form of leprosy is twice as common among men as among women and is rarely encountered in children. The frequency of the polar forms of leprosy in different countries varies widely and may in part be genetically determined; certain human leukocyte antigen (HLA) associations are known for both polar forms of leprosy (see below). Furthermore, variations in immunoregulatory genes are associated with an increased susceptibility to leprosy, particularly the multibacillary form. In India and Africa, 90% of cases are tuberculoid; in Southeast Asia, 50% are tuberculoid and 50% lepromatous; and in Mexico, 90% are lepromatous. (For definitions of disease types, see Table 203-1 and "Clinical, Histologic, and Immunologic Spectrum," below.)

Transmission The route of transmission of leprosy remains uncertain, and transmission routes may in fact be multiple. Nasal droplet infection, contact with infected soil, and even insect vectors have been considered the prime candidates. Aerosolized *M. leprae* can cause infection in immunosuppressed mice, and a sneeze from an untreated lepromatous patient may contain $>10^{10}$ AFB. Furthermore, both IgA antibody to *M. leprae* and genes of *M. leprae*—demonstrable by polymerase chain reaction (PCR)—have been found in the nose of individuals from endemic areas who have no signs of leprosy and in 19% of occupational contacts of lepromatous patients. Several lines of evidence implicate soil transmission. (1) In endemic countries such as India, leprosy is primarily a rural and not an urban disease. (2) *M. leprae* products reside in soil in endemic locales. (3) Direct dermal inoculation (e.g., during tattooing) may transmit *M. leprae*, and common sites of leprosy in children are the buttocks and thighs, suggesting that microinoculation of infected soil may transmit the disease. Evidence for insect vectors of leprosy includes the demonstration that bedbugs and mosquitoes in the vicinity of leprosaria regularly harbor *M. leprae* and that experimentally infected mosquitoes can transmit the infection to mice. Skin-to-skin contact generally is not considered an important route of transmission.

In endemic countries, ~50% of leprosy patients have a history of intimate contact with an infected person (often a household member), while, for unknown reasons, leprosy patients in nonendemic locales can identify such contact only 10% of the time. Moreover, household contact with an infected lepromatous case carries an eventual risk of disease acquisition of ~10% in endemic areas as opposed to only 1% in nonendemic locales. Contact with a tuberculoid case carries a very low risk. Physicians and nurses caring for leprosy patients and the coworkers of these patients are not at risk for leprosy.

Although multilocus variable-number short-nucleotide tandem-repeat (VNTR) analyses have generally demonstrated considerable variability among isolates, highly similar and even identical VNTR results have been obtained with isolates from a limited number

TABLE 203-1 CLINICAL, BACTERIOLOGIC, PATHOLOGIC, AND IMMUNOLOGIC SPECTRUM OF LEPROSY

Feature	Tuberculoid (TT, BT) Leprosy	Borderline (BB, BL) Leprosy	Lepromatous (LL) Leprosy
Skin lesions	One or a few sharply defined annular asymmetric macules or plaques with a tendency toward central clearing, elevated borders	Intermediate between BT- and LL-type lesions; ill-defined plaques with an occasional sharp margin; few or many in number	Symmetric, poorly marginated, multiple infiltrated nodules and plaques or diffuse infiltration; xanthoma-like or dermatofibroma papules; leonine facies and eyebrow alopecia
Nerve lesions	Skin lesions anesthetic early; nerve near lesions sometimes enlarged; nerve abscesses most common in BT	Hypesthetic or anesthetic skin lesions; nerve trunk palsies, at times symmetric	Hypesthesia a late sign; nerve palsies variable; acral, distal, symmetric anesthesia common
Acid-fast bacilli (BI[a])	0–1+	3–5+	4–6+
Lymphocytes	2+	1+	0–1+
Macrophage differentiation	Epithelioid	Epithelioid in BB; usually undifferentiated but may have foamy changes in BL	Foamy change the rule; may be undifferentiated in early lesions
Langerhans giant cells	1–3+	—	—
Lepromin skin test	+++	—	—
Lymphocyte transformation test	Generally positive	1–10%	1–2%
CD4+/CD8+ T cell ratio in lesions	1.2	BB: NT; BL: 0.48	0.50
M. leprae PGL-1 antibodies	60%	85%	95%

[a]See text.

Abbreviations: BB, mid-borderline; BL, borderline lepromatous; BT, borderline tuberculoid; TT, polar tuberculoid; LL, polar lepromatous; BI, bacteriologic index; NT, not tested; PGL-1, phenolic glycolipid 1.

of families with multiple cases. Moreover, VNTR results have been similar for isolates within certain geographic locales and divergent for isolates within others. These findings suggest that genomic analyses may prove useful in the future for defining *M. leprae* transmission patterns.

M. leprae causes disease primarily in humans. However, in Texas and Louisiana, 15% of nine-banded armadillos are infected, and armadillo contact occasionally results in human disease. Armadillos develop disseminated infection after IV inoculation of live *M. leprae*.

CLINICAL, HISTOLOGIC, AND IMMUNOLOGIC SPECTRUM

The incubation period prior to manifestation of clinical disease can vary between 2 and 40 years, although it is generally 5–7 years in duration. This long incubation period is probably, at least in part, a consequence of the extremely long doubling time for *M. leprae* (14 days in mice versus in vitro doubling times of 1 day and 20 min for *M. tuberculosis* and *Escherichia coli*, respectively). Leprosy presents as a spectrum of clinical manifestations that have bacteriologic, pathologic, and immunologic counterparts. The spectrum from polar tuberculoid (TT) to borderline tuberculoid (BT) to mid-borderline (BB, which is rarely encountered) to borderline lepromatous (BL) to polar lepromatous (LL) disease is associated with an evolution from asymmetric localized macules and plaques to nodular and indurated symmetric generalized skin manifestations, an increasing bacterial load, and loss of *M. leprae*–specific cellular immunity (Table 203-1). Distinguishing dermatopathologic characteristics include the number of lymphocytes, giant cells, and AFB as well as the nature of epithelioid cell differentiation. Where a patient presents on the clinical spectrum largely determines prognosis, complications, reactional states, and the intensity of antimicrobial therapy required.

Tuberculoid Leprosy At the less severe end of the spectrum is tuberculoid leprosy, which encompasses TT and BT disease. In general, these forms of leprosy result in symptoms confined to the skin and peripheral nerves. TT leprosy is the most common form of the disease encountered in India and Africa but is virtually absent in Southeast Asia, where BT leprosy is frequent.

The skin lesions of tuberculoid leprosy consist of one or a few hypopigmented macules or plaques (Fig. 203-1) that are sharply demarcated and hypesthetic, often have erythematous or raised borders, and are devoid of the normal skin organs (sweat glands and hair follicles) and thus are dry, scaly, and anhidrotic. AFB are generally absent or few in number. Tuberculoid leprosy patients may have asymmetric enlargement of one or a few peripheral nerves. Indeed, leprosy and certain rare hereditary neuropathies are the only human diseases associated with peripheral-nerve enlargement. Although any peripheral nerve may be enlarged (including small digital and supraclavicular nerves), those most commonly affected are the ulnar, posterior auricular, peroneal, and posterior tibial nerves, with associated hypesthesia and myopathy.

In tuberculoid leprosy, T cells breach the perineurium, and destruction of Schwann cells and axons may be evident, resulting in fibrosis of the epineurium, replacement of the endoneurium with epithelial granulomas, and occasionally caseous necrosis. Such invasion and destruction of nerves in the dermis by T cells are pathognomonic for leprosy.

Circulating lymphocytes from patients with tuberculoid leprosy readily recognize *M. leprae* and its constituent proteins, patients have positive lepromin skin tests (see "Diagnosis," below), and—owing to a type 1 cytokine pattern in tuberculoid tissues—strong T cell and macrophage activation results in a localized infection. In tuberculoid leprosy tissue, there is a 2:1 predominance of helper CD4+ over CD8+ T lymphocytes. Tuberculoid tissues are rich in the mRNAs of the proinflammatory T_H1 family of cytokines: interleukin (IL) 2, interferon γ (IFN-γ), and IL-12; in contrast, IL-4, IL-5, and IL-10 mRNAs are scarce.

Lepromatous Leprosy Lepromatous leprosy patients present with symmetrically distributed skin nodules (Fig. 203-2), raised plaques, or diffuse dermal infiltration, which, when on the face, results in *leonine facies*. Late manifestations include loss of eyebrows (initially the lateral margins only) and eyelashes, pendulous earlobes, and dry scaling skin, particularly on the feet. In LL leprosy, bacilli are numerous in the skin (as many as 10^9/g), where they are often found in large clumps (*globi*), and in peripheral nerves, where they initially invade Schwann cells, resulting in foamy degenerative myelination and axonal degeneration and later in Wallerian degeneration. In addition, bacilli are plentiful in circulating blood and in all organ systems except the lungs and the central nervous system. Nevertheless, patients are afebrile, and there is no evidence of major organ system dysfunction.

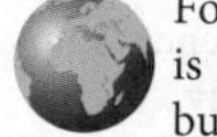

Found almost exclusively in western Mexico and the Caribbean is a form of lepromatous leprosy without visible skin lesions but with diffuse dermal infiltration and a demonstrably thickened dermis, termed *diffuse lepromatosis*.

In lepromatous leprosy, nerve enlargement and damage tend to be symmetric, result from actual bacillary invasion, and are more insidious but ultimately more extensive than in tuberculoid leprosy. Patients with LL leprosy have acral, distal, symmetric peripheral neuropathy and a tendency toward symmetric nerve-trunk enlargement. They may also have signs and symptoms related to involvement of the upper respiratory tract, the anterior chamber of the eye, and the testes.

In untreated LL patients, lymphocytes regularly fail to recognize either *M. leprae* or its protein constituents, and lepromin skin tests are negative (see "Diagnosis," below). This loss of protective cellular immunity appears to be antigen-specific, as patients are not unusually

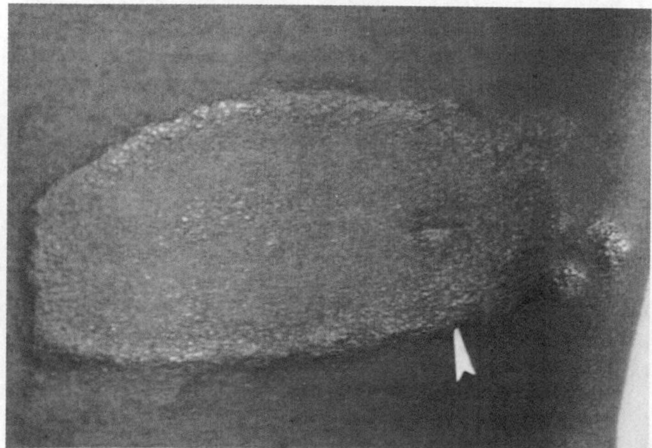

FIGURE 203-1 Tuberculoid (TT) leprosy: a well-defined, hypopigmented, anesthetic macule with anhidrosis and a raised granular margin *(arrowhead)*.

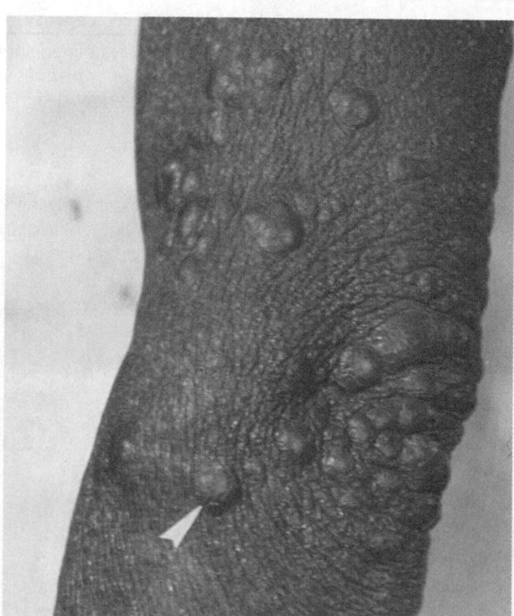

FIGURE 203-2 Lepromatous (LL) leprosy: advanced nodular lesions.

susceptible to opportunistic infections, cancer, or AIDS and maintain delayed-type hypersensitivity to *Candida*, *Trichophyton*, mumps virus, tetanus toxoid, and even purified protein derivative of tuberculin. At times, *M. leprae*–specific anergy is reversible with effective chemotherapy. In LL tissues, there is a 2:1 ratio of CD8+ to CD4+ T lymphocytes. LL patients have a predominant T_H2 response and hyperglobulinemia, and LL tissues demonstrate a T_H2 cytokine profile, being rich in mRNAs for IL-4, IL-5, and IL-10 and poor in those for IL-2, IFN-γ, and IL-12. It appears that cytokines mediate a protective tissue response in leprosy, as injection of IFN-γ or IL-2 into lepromatous lesions causes a loss of AFB and histopathologic conversion toward a tuberculoid pattern. Macrophages of lepromatous leprosy patients appear to be functionally intact; circulating monocytes exhibit normal microbicidal function and responsiveness to IFN-γ.

Reactional States Lepra reactions comprise several common immunologically mediated inflammatory states that cause considerable morbidity. Some of these reactions precede diagnosis and the institution of effective antimicrobial therapy; indeed, these reactions may precipitate presentation for medical attention and diagnosis. Other reactions follow the initiation of appropriate chemotherapy; these reactions may cause patients to perceive that their leprosy is worsening and to lose confidence in conventional therapy. Only by warning patients of the potential for these reactions and describing their manifestations can physicians treating leprosy patients ensure continued credibility.

TYPE 1 LEPRA REACTIONS (DOWNGRADING AND REVERSAL REACTIONS) Type 1 lepra reactions occur in almost half of patients with borderline forms of leprosy but not in patients with pure lepromatous disease. Manifestations include classic signs of inflammation within previously involved macules, papules, and plaques and, on occasion, the appearance of new skin lesions, neuritis, and (less commonly) fever—generally low-grade. The nerve trunk most frequently involved in this process is the ulnar nerve at the elbow, which may be painful and exquisitely tender. If patients with affected nerves are not treated promptly with glucocorticoids (see below), irreversible nerve damage may result in as little as 24 h. The most dramatic manifestation is footdrop, which occurs when the peroneal nerve is involved.

When type 1 lepra reactions precede the initiation of appropriate antimicrobial therapy, they are termed *downgrading reactions*, and the case becomes histologically more lepromatous; when they occur after the initiation of therapy, they are termed *reversal reactions*, and the case becomes more tuberculoid. Reversal reactions often occur in the first months or years after the initiation of therapy but may also develop several years thereafter.

Edema is the most characteristic microscopic feature of type 1 lepra lesions, whose diagnosis is primarily clinical. Reversal reactions are typified by a T_H1 cytokine profile, with an influx of CD4+ T helper cells and increased levels of IFN-γ and IL-2. In addition, type 1 reactions are associated with large numbers of T cells bearing γ/δ receptors—a unique feature of leprosy.

TYPE 2 LEPRA REACTIONS: ERYTHEMA NODOSUM LEPROSUM Erythema nodosum leprosum (ENL) (Fig. 203-3) occurs exclusively in patients near the lepromatous end of the leprosy spectrum (BL/LL), affecting nearly 50% of this group. Although ENL may precede leprosy diagnosis and the initiation of therapy (sometimes, in fact, prompting the diagnosis), in 90% of cases it follows the institution of chemotherapy, generally within 2 years. The most common features of ENL are crops of painful erythematous papules that resolve spontaneously in a few days to a week but may recur; malaise; and fever that can be profound. However, patients may also experience symptoms of neuritis, lymphadenitis, uveitis, orchitis, and glomerulonephritis and may develop anemia, leukocytosis, and abnormal liver function tests (particularly increased aminotransferase levels). Individual patients may have either a single bout of ENL or chronic recurrent manifestations. Bouts may be either mild or severe and generalized; in rare instances, ENL results in death. Skin biopsy of ENL papules reveals vasculitis or panniculitis, sometimes with many lymphocytes but characteristically with polymorphonuclear leukocytes as well.

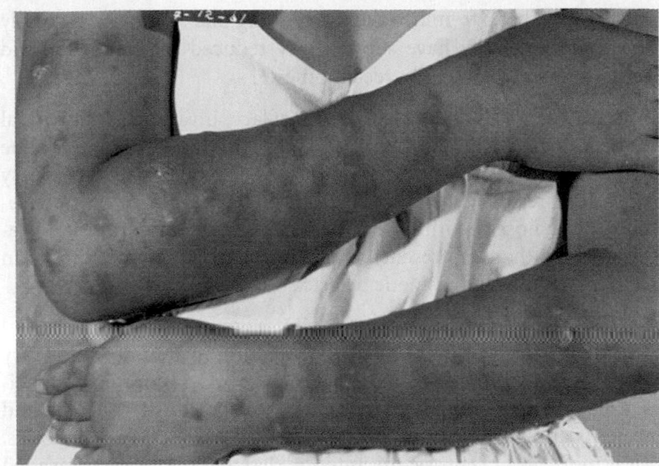

FIGURE 203-3 Moderately severe skin lesions of erythema nodosum leprosum, some with pustulation and ulceration.

Elevated levels of circulating tumor necrosis factor (TNF) have been demonstrated in ENL; thus, TNF may play a central role in the pathobiology of this syndrome. ENL is thought to be a consequence of immune complex deposition, given its T_H2 cytokine profile and its high levels of IL-6 and IL-8. However, in ENL tissue, the presence of HLA-DR framework antigen of epidermal cells—considered a marker for a delayed-type hypersensitivity response—and evidence of higher levels of IL-2 and IFN-γ than are usually seen in polar lepromatous disease suggest an alternative mechanism.

LUCIO'S PHENOMENON Lucio's phenomenon is an unusual reaction seen exclusively in patients from the Caribbean and Mexico who have the diffuse lepromatosis form of lepromatous leprosy, most often those who are untreated. Patients with this reaction develop recurrent crops of large, sharply marginated, ulcerative lesions—particularly on the lower extremities—that may be generalized and, when so, are frequently fatal as a result of secondary infection and consequent septic bacteremia. Histologically, the lesions are characterized by ischemic necrosis of the epidermis and superficial dermis, heavy parasitism of endothelial cells with AFB, and endothelial proliferation and thrombus formation in the larger vessels of the deeper dermis. Like ENL, Lucio's phenomenon is probably mediated by immune complexes.

Complications • ***THE EXTREMITIES*** Complications of the extremities in leprosy patients are primarily a consequence of neuropathy leading to insensitivity and myopathy. Insensitivity affects fine touch, pain, and heat receptors but generally spares position and vibration appreciation. The most commonly affected nerve trunk is the ulnar nerve at the elbow, whose involvement results in clawing of the fourth and fifth fingers, loss of dorsal interosseous musculature in the affected hand, and loss of sensation in these distributions. Median nerve involvement in leprosy impairs thumb opposition and grasp; radial nerve dysfunction, although rare in leprosy, leads to wristdrop. Tendon transfers can restore hand function but should not be performed until 6 months after the initiation of antimicrobial therapy and the conclusion of episodes of acute neuritis.

Plantar ulceration, particularly at the metatarsal heads, is probably the most common complication of leprous neuropathy. Therapy requires careful debridement; administration of appropriate antibiotics; avoidance of weight-bearing until ulcerations are healed, with slowly progressive ambulation thereafter; and wearing of special shoes to prevent recurrence.

Footdrop as a result of peroneal nerve palsy should be treated with a simple nonmetallic brace in the shoe or with surgical correction attained by tendon transfers. Although uncommon, Charcot's joints, particularly of the foot and ankle, may result from leprosy.

The loss of distal digits in leprosy is a consequence of insensitivity, trauma, secondary infection, and—in lepromatous disease—a poorly understood and sometimes profound osteolytic process. Conscientious protection of the extremities during cooking and work and the early institution of therapy have substantially reduced the frequency and severity of distal digit loss in recent times.

THE NOSE In lepromatous leprosy, bacillary invasion of the nasal mucosa can result in chronic nasal congestion and epistaxis. Saline nose drops may relieve these symptoms. Long-untreated LL leprosy may further result in destruction of the nasal cartilage, with consequent saddle-nose deformity or anosmia (more common in the preantibiotic era than at present). Nasal reconstructive procedures can ameliorate significant cosmetic defects.

THE EYE Owing to cranial nerve palsies, lagophthalmos and corneal insensitivity may complicate leprosy, resulting in trauma, secondary infection, and (without treatment) corneal ulcerations and opacities. For patients with these conditions, eyedrops during the day and ointments at night provide some protection from such consequences. Furthermore, in LL leprosy, the anterior chamber of the eye is invaded by bacilli, and ENL may result in uveitis, with consequent cataracts and glaucoma. Thus leprosy is a major cause of blindness in the developing world. Slit-lamp evaluation of LL patients often reveals "corneal beading," representing globi of *M. leprae.*

THE TESTES *M. leprae* invades the testes, while ENL may cause orchitis. Thus males with lepromatous leprosy often manifest mild to severe testicular dysfunction, with an elevation of luteinizing and follicle-stimulating hormones, decreased testosterone, and aspermia or hypospermia in 85% of LL patients but in only 25% of BL patients. LL patients may become impotent and infertile. Impotence is sometimes responsive to testosterone replacement.

AMYLOIDOSIS Secondary amyloidosis is a complication of LL leprosy and ENL that is encountered infrequently in the antibiotic era. This complication may result in abnormalities of hepatic and particularly renal function.

NERVE ABSCESSES Patients with various forms of leprosy, but particularly those with the BT form, may develop abscesses of nerves (most commonly the ulnar), with a cellulitic appearance of adjacent skin. In such conditions, the affected nerve is swollen and exquisitely tender. Although glucocorticoids may reduce signs of inflammation, rapid surgical decompression is necessary to prevent irreversible sequelae.

DIAGNOSIS

Leprosy most commonly presents with both characteristic skin lesions and skin histopathology. Thus the disease should be suspected when a patient from an endemic area has suggestive skin lesions or peripheral neuropathy. The diagnosis should be confirmed by histopathology. In tuberculoid leprosy, lesional areas—preferably the advancing edge—must be biopsied because normal-appearing skin does not have pathologic features. In lepromatous leprosy, nodules, plaques, and indurated areas are optimal biopsy sites, but biopsies of normal-appearing skin also are generally diagnostic. Lepromatous leprosy is associated with diffuse hyperglobulinemia, which may result in false-positive serologic tests (e.g., Venereal Disease Research Laboratory, rheumatoid arthritis, and antinuclear antibody tests) and therefore may cause diagnostic confusion. On occasion, tuberculoid lesions may not (1) appear typical, (2) be hypesthetic, and (3) contain granulomas (instead containing only nonspecific lymphocytic infiltrates). In such instances, two of these three characteristics are considered sufficient for a diagnosis. It is preferable to overdiagnose leprosy rather than to allow a patient to remain untreated.

IgM antibodies to PGL-1 are found in 95% of patients with untreated lepromatous leprosy; the titer decreases with effective therapy. However, in tuberculoid leprosy—the form of disease most often associated with diagnostic uncertainty owing to the absence or paucity of AFB—patients have significant antibodies to PGL-1 only 60% of the time; moreover, in endemic locales, exposed individuals without clinical leprosy may harbor antibodies to PGL-1. Thus PGL-1 serology is of little diagnostic utility in tuberculoid leprosy. Heat-killed *M. leprae* (lepromin) has been used as a skin test reagent. It generally elicits a reaction in tuberculoid leprosy patients, may do so in individuals without leprosy, and gives negative results in lepromatous leprosy patients; consequently, it is likewise of little diagnostic value. Unfortunately, PCR of the skin for *M. leprae,* although positive in LL and BL disease, yields negative results in 50% of tuberculoid cases, again offering little diagnostic assistance.

DIFFERENTIAL DIAGNOSIS

Included in the differential diagnosis of lesions that resemble leprosy are sarcoidosis, leishmaniasis, lupus vulgaris, dermatofibroma, histiocytoma, lymphoma, syphilis, yaws, granuloma annulare, and various other disorders causing hypopigmentation (notably pityriasis alba, tinea, and vitiligo). Sarcoidosis may result in perineural inflammation, but actual granuloma formation within dermal nerves is pathognomonic for leprosy. In lepromatous leprosy, sputum specimens may be loaded with AFB—a finding that can be incorrectly interpreted as representing pulmonary tuberculosis.

TREATMENT LEPROSY

ANTIMICROBIAL THERAPY

Active Agents Established agents used to treat leprosy include dapsone (50–100 mg/d), clofazimine (50–100 mg/d, 100 mg three times weekly, or 300 mg monthly), and rifampin (600 mg daily or monthly; see "Choice of Regimens," below). Of these drugs, only rifampin is bactericidal. The sulfones (folate antagonists), the foremost of which is dapsone, were the first antimicrobial agents found to be effective for the treatment of leprosy and are still the mainstays of therapy. With sulfone treatment, skin lesions resolve and numbers of viable bacilli in the skin are reduced. Although primarily bacteriostatic, dapsone monotherapy results in a resistance-related relapse rate of only 2.5%; after ≥18 years of therapy and subsequent discontinuation, only another 10% of patients relapse, developing new, usually asymptomatic, shiny, "histoid" nodules. Dapsone is generally safe and inexpensive. Individuals with glucose-6-phosphate dehydrogenase deficiency who are treated with dapsone may develop severe hemolysis; those without this deficiency also have reduced red cell survival and a hemoglobin decrease averaging 1 g/dL. Dapsone's usefulness is limited occasionally by allergic dermatitis and rarely by the sulfone syndrome (including high fever, anemia, exfoliative dermatitis, and a mononucleosis-type blood picture). It must be remembered that rifampin induces microsomal enzymes, necessitating increased doses of medications such as glucocorticoids and oral birth control regimens. Clofazimine is often cosmetically unacceptable to light-skinned leprosy patients because it causes a red-black skin discoloration that accumulates, particularly in lesional areas, and makes the patient's diagnosis obvious to members of the community.

Other antimicrobial agents active against *M. leprae* in animal models and at the usual daily doses used in clinical trials include ethionamide/prothionamide; the aminoglycosides streptomycin, kanamycin, and amikacin (but not gentamicin or tobramycin); minocycline; clarithromycin; and several fluoroquinolones, particularly ofloxacin. Next to rifampin, minocycline, clarithromycin, and ofloxacin appear to be most bactericidal for *M. leprae,* but these drugs have not been used extensively in leprosy control programs. Most recently, rifapentine and moxifloxacin have been found to be especially potent against *M. leprae* in mice. In a clinical trial in lepromatous leprosy, moxifloxacin was profoundly bactericidal, matched in potency only by rifampin.

Choice of Regimens Antimicrobial therapy for leprosy must be individualized, depending on the clinical/pathologic form of the disease encountered. Tuberculoid leprosy, which is associated with a low bacterial burden and a protective cellular immune response, is the easiest form to treat and can be cured reliably with a finite course of chemotherapy. In contrast, lepromatous leprosy may have a higher bacillary load than any other human bacterial disease, and the absence of a salutary T cell repertoire requires prolonged or even lifelong chemotherapy. Hence, careful classification of disease prior to therapy is important.

In developed countries, clinical experience with leprosy classification is limited; fortunately, however, the resources needed for skin biopsy are highly accessible, and those for pathologic interpretation are readily available. In developing countries, clinical expertise is greater but is now waning substantially as the care of leprosy patients is integrated into general health services. In addition, access to dermatopathology services is often limited. In such instances, skin smears may prove useful, but in many locales access to the resources needed for their preparation and interpretation also may be unavailable. Use of skin smears is no longer encouraged by the World Health Organization (WHO) and is often replaced by mere counting of lesions, which, together with a lack of capacity for histopathologic assessment, may negatively affect decisions about chemotherapy, increase the potential for reactions, and worsen the ultimate prognosis. A reasoned approach to the treatment of leprosy is confounded by these and several other issues:

1. Even without therapy, TT leprosy may heal spontaneously, and prolonged dapsone monotherapy (even for LL leprosy) is generally curative in 80% of cases.
2. In tuberculoid disease, it is common for no bacilli to be found in the skin prior to therapy, and thus there is no objective measure of therapeutic success. Furthermore, despite adequate treatment, TT and particularly BT lesions often resolve minimally or incompletely, while relapse and late type 1 lepra reactions can be difficult to distinguish.
3. LL leprosy patients commonly harbor viable persistent *M. leprae* organisms after prolonged intensive therapy; the propensity of these organisms to initiate clinical relapse is unclear. Because relapse in LL patients after discontinuation of rifampin-containing regimens usually begins only after 7–10 years, follow-up over the very long term is necessary to assess ultimate clinical outcomes.
4. Even though primary dapsone resistance is exceedingly rare and multidrug therapy is generally recommended (at least for lepromatous leprosy), there is a paucity of information from experimental animals and clinical trials on the optimal combination of antimicrobial agents, dosing schedule, and duration of therapy.

In 1982, the WHO made recommendations for leprosy chemotherapy administered in control programs. These recommendations came on the heels of the demonstration of the relative success of long-term dapsone monotherapy and in the context of concerns about dapsone resistance. Other complicating considerations included the limited resources available for leprosy care in the very areas where it is most prevalent and the frustration and discouragement of patients and program managers with the previous requirement for lifelong therapy for many leprosy patients. Thus, for the first time, the WHO advocated a finite duration of therapy for all forms of leprosy and—given the prohibitive cost of daily rifampin treatment in developing countries—encouraged the monthly administration of this agent as part of a multidrug regimen. Over the ensuing years, the WHO recommendations have been broadly implemented, and the duration of therapy required, particularly for lepromatous leprosy, has been progressively shortened. For treatment purposes, the WHO classifies patients as *paucibacillary* or *multibacillary*. Previously, patients without demonstrable AFB in the dermis were classified as paucibacillary and those with AFB as multibacillary. Currently, in light of the perceived unreliability of skin smears in the field, patients are classified as multibacillary if they have six or more skin lesions and as paucibacillary if they have fewer. (Unfortunately, this classification method has been found wanting, as some patients near the lepromatous pole have only one or a few skin lesions.) The WHO recommends that paucibacillary adults be treated with 100 mg of dapsone daily and 600 mg of rifampin monthly (supervised) for 6 months **(Table 203-2)**. For patients with single-lesion paucibacillary leprosy, the WHO recommends as an alternative a single dose of rifampin (600 mg), ofloxacin (400 mg), and minocycline (100 mg). Multibacillary adults should be treated with 100 mg of dapsone plus 50 mg of clofazimine daily (unsupervised)

TABLE 203-2 ANTIMICROBIAL REGIMENS RECOMMENDED FOR THE TREATMENT OF LEPROSY IN ADULTS

Form of Leprosy	More Intensive Regimen	WHO-Recommended Regimen (1982)
Tuberculoid (paucibacillary)	Dapsone (100 mg/d) for 5 years	Dapsone (100 mg/d, unsupervised) *plus* rifampin (600 mg/month, supervised) for 6 months
Lepromatous (multibacillary)	Rifampin (600 mg/d) for 3 years *plus* dapsone (100 mg/d) indefinitely	Dapsone (100 mg/d) *plus* clofazimine (50 mg/d), unsupervised; *and* rifampin (600 mg) *plus* clofazimine (300 mg) monthly (supervised) for 1–2 years

Note: See text for discussion and comparison of the WHO recommendations with the more intensive approach as well as the alternative WHO regimen for single-lesion paucibacillary leprosy.

and with 600 mg of rifampin plus 300 mg of clofazimine monthly (supervised). Originally, the WHO recommended that lepromatous patients be treated for 2 years or until smears became negative (generally in ~5 years); subsequently, the acceptable course was reduced to 1 year—a change that remains especially controversial in the absence of supporting clinical trials.

Several factors have caused many authorities to question the WHO recommendations and to favor a more intensive approach. Among these factors are—for multibacillary patients—a high (double-digit) relapse rate in several locales (reaching 20–40% in one locale, with the rate directly related to the initial bacterial burden) and—for paucibacillary patients—demonstrable lesional activity for years in fully half of patients after the completion of therapy. The more intensive approach (Table 203-2) calls for tuberculoid leprosy to be treated with dapsone (100 mg/d) for 5 years and for lepromatous leprosy to be treated with rifampin (600 mg/d) for 3 years and with dapsone (100 mg/d) throughout life.

With effective antimicrobial therapy, new skin lesions and signs and symptoms of peripheral neuropathy cease appearing. Nodules and plaques of lepromatous leprosy noticeably flatten in 1–2 months and resolve in 1 year or a few years, while tuberculoid skin lesions may disappear, ameliorate, or remain relatively unchanged. Although the peripheral neuropathy of leprosy may improve somewhat in the first few months of therapy, rarely is it significantly alleviated by treatment.

Despite the drawbacks of the WHO's recommendations for multidrug therapy, these regimens have been used almost exclusively worldwide. Although two of the three recommended drugs (dapsone and clofazimine) are only bacteriostatic against *M. leprae* and bactericidal agents have been identified since the WHO formulated its recommendations, significant studies employing the available alternatives in newly designed regimens have not been initiated. Given the recent findings that moxifloxacin, like rifampin, is profoundly bactericidal in leprosy patients and that short-course chemotherapy for tuberculosis is possible only when two or more bactericidal agents are used, a moxifloxacin/rifamycin-based regimen including either minocycline or clarithromycin appears promising; such a regimen may prove to be more reliably curative than WHO-recommended multidrug therapy for lepromatous leprosy and may allow a considerably shorter course of treatment.

THERAPY FOR REACTIONS

Type 1 Type 1 lepra reactions are best treated with glucocorticoids (e.g., prednisone, initially at doses of 40–60 mg/d). As inflammation subsides, the glucocorticoid dose can be tapered, but steroid therapy must be continued for at least 3–6 months lest recurrence supervene. Because of the myriad toxicities of prolonged glucocorticoid therapy, the indications for its initiation are strictly limited to lesions whose intense inflammation poses a threat of ulceration; lesions at cosmetically important sites, such as the face; and cases in which neuritis is present. Mild to moderate lepra reactions that do not meet these criteria should be tolerated and glucocorticoid treatment withheld. Thalidomide is ineffective against type 1 lepra reactions. Clofazimine (200–300 mg/d) is of questionable benefit but in any event is far less efficacious than glucocorticoids.

Type 2 Treatment of ENL must be individualized. If ENL is mild (i.e., if it occurs without fever or other organ involvement and with occasional crops of only a few skin papules), it may be treated with antipyretics alone. However, in cases with many skin lesions, fever, malaise, and other tissue involvement, brief courses (1–2 weeks) of glucocorticoid treatment (initially 40–60 mg/d) are often effective. With or without therapy, individual inflamed papules last for <1 week. Successful therapy is defined by the cessation of skin lesion development and the disappearance of other systemic signs and symptoms. If, despite two courses of glucocorticoid therapy, ENL appears to be recurring and persisting, treatment with thalidomide (100–300 mg nightly) should be initiated, with the dose depending on the initial severity of the reaction. Because even a single dose of thalidomide administered early in pregnancy may result in severe birth defects, including phocomelia, the use of this drug in the United States for the treatment of fertile female patients is tightly regulated and requires informed consent, prior pregnancy testing, and maintenance of birth control measures. Although the mechanism of thalidomide's dramatic action against ENL is not entirely clear, the drug's efficacy is probably attributable to its reduction of TNF levels and IgM synthesis and its slowing of polymorphonuclear leukocyte migration. After the reaction is controlled, lower doses of thalidomide (50–200 mg nightly) are effective in preventing relapses of ENL. Clofazimine in high doses (300 mg nightly) has some efficacy against ENL, but its use permits only a modest reduction of the glucocorticoid dose necessary for ENL control.

Lucio's Phenomenon Neither glucocorticoids nor thalidomide is effective against this syndrome. Optimal wound care and therapy for bacteremia are indicated. Ulcers tend to be chronic and heal poorly. In severe cases, exchange transfusion may prove useful.

PREVENTION AND CONTROL

Vaccination at birth with bacille Calmette-Guérin (BCG) has proved variably effective in preventing leprosy: the results have ranged from total inefficacy to 80% efficacy. The addition of heat-killed *M. leprae* to BCG does not increase the effectiveness of the vaccine. Because whole mycobacteria contain large amounts of lipids and carbohydrates that have proved in vitro to be immunosuppressive for lymphocytes and macrophages, *M. leprae* proteins may prove to be superior vaccines. Data from a mouse model support this possibility.

Chemoprophylaxis with dapsone may reduce the number of tuberculoid leprosy cases but not the number of lepromatous cases and hence is not recommended, even for household contacts. In addition, single-dose rifampin prophylaxis is of doubtful efficacy. Because leprosy transmission appears to require close prolonged household contact, hospitalized patients need not be isolated.

In 1992, the WHO—on the basis of that organization's treatment recommendations—launched a landmark campaign to eliminate leprosy as a public health problem by the year 2000 (goal, <1 case per 10,000 population). The campaign mobilized and energized nongovernmental organizations and national health services to treat leprosy with multiple drugs and to clean up outdated registries. In these respects, the effort has proved hugely successful, with >6 million patients completing therapy. However, the target of leprosy elimination has not yet been reached. In fact, the success of the WHO campaign in reducing the number of cases worldwide has been largely attributable to the redefinition of what constitutes a case of leprosy. Formerly calculated by disease prevalence, the count is now limited to cases not yet treated with multiple drugs. Worldwide, the annual incidence of leprosy has not fallen. Furthermore, after the completion of therapy, when a patient is no longer considered to represent a "case," half of all patients continue to manifest disease activity for years; relapse rates (at least for multibacillary patients) are unacceptably high; disabilities and deformities go unchecked; and the social stigma of the disease persists.

During most of the twentieth century, nongovernmental organizations, particularly Christian missionaries, provided a medical infrastructure devoted to the care and treatment of leprosy patients—the envy of those with other medical priorities in the developing world. With the public perception that leprosy is near eradication, resources for patient care are rapidly being diverted, and the burden of patient care is being transferred to nonexistent or overloaded national health services and to health workers who lack the tools and skills needed for the disease's diagnosis and classification and for the selection of nuanced therapy (particularly in cases of reactional neuritis). Thus the prerequisites for a salutary outcome increasingly go unmet.

204 Nontuberculous Mycobacterial Infections

Steven M. Holland

Several terms—nontuberculous mycobacteria (NTM), atypical mycobacteria, mycobacteria other than tuberculosis, and environmental mycobacteria—all refer to mycobacteria other than *Mycobacterium tuberculosis*, its close relatives (*M. bovis, M. caprae, M. africanum, M. pinnipedii, M. canetti*), and *M. leprae*. The number of identified species of NTM is growing and will continue to do so because of the use of DNA sequence typing for speciation. The number of known species currently exceeds 150. NTM are highly adaptable and can inhabit hostile environments, including industrial solvents.

EPIDEMIOLOGY

NTM are ubiquitous in soil and water. Specific organisms have recurring niches, such as *M. simiae* in certain aquifers, *M. fortuitum* in pedicure baths, and *M. immunogenum* in metalworking fluids. Most NTM cause disease in humans only rarely unless some aspect of host defense is impaired, as in bronchiectasis, or breached, as by inoculation (e.g., liposuction, trauma). There are few instances of human-to-human transmission of NTM, which occurs almost exclusively in cystic fibrosis. Because infections due to NTM are rarely reported to health agencies and because their identification is sometimes problematic, reliable data on incidence and prevalence are lacking. Disseminated disease denotes significant immune dysfunction (e.g., advanced HIV infection), whereas pulmonary disease, which is much more common, is highly associated with pulmonary epithelial defects but not with systemic immunodeficiency.

In the United States, the incidence and prevalence of pulmonary infection with NTM, mostly in association with bronchiectasis (**Chap. 312**), have for many years been several-fold higher than the corresponding figures for tuberculosis, and rates of the former are increasing among the elderly. Among patients with cystic fibrosis, who often have bronchiectasis, rates of clinical infection with NTM range from 3% to 15%, with even higher rates among older patients. Although NTM may be recovered from the sputa of many individuals, it is critical to differentiate active disease from commensal harboring of the organisms. A scheme to help with the proper diagnosis of pulmonary infection caused by NTM has been developed by the American Thoracic Society and is widely used. The bulk of nontuberculous mycobacterial disease in North America is due to *M. kansasii*, organisms of the *M. avium* complex (MAC), and *M. abscessus*.

In Europe, Asia, and Australia, the distribution of NTM in clinical specimens is roughly similar to that in North America, with MAC species and rapidly growing organisms such as *M. abscessus* encountered frequently. *M. xenopi* and *M. malmoense* are especially prominent in northern Europe. *M. ulcerans* causes the distinct clinical entity Buruli ulcer, which occurs throughout tropical zones, especially in western Africa. *M. marinum* is a common cause of cutaneous and tendon infections in coastal regions and among individuals exposed to fish tanks or swimming pools.

The true international epidemiology of infections due to NTM is hard to determine because the isolation of these organisms often is not reported and speciation often is not performed for *M. tuberculosis* and NTM. The increasing ease of identification and speciation of these organisms is likely to have a major impact on the description of their international epidemiology in the next few years.

PATHOBIOLOGY

Because exposure to NTM is essentially universal and disease is rare, it can be assumed that normal host defenses against these organisms must be strong and that otherwise healthy individuals in whom significant disease develops are highly likely to have specific susceptibility factors that permit NTM to become established, multiply, and cause disease. At the advent of HIV infection, CD4+ T lymphocytes were recognized as key effector cells against NTM; the development of disseminated MAC disease was highly correlated with a decline in CD4+ T lymphocyte numbers. Such a decrease has also been implicated in disseminated MAC infection in patients with idiopathic CD4+ T lymphocytopenia. Potent inhibitors of tumor necrosis factor α (TNF-α), such as infliximab, adalimumab, certolizumab, golimumab, and etanercept, can neutralize this critical cytokine. The occasional result is severe mycobacterial or fungal infection; these associations indicate that TNF-α is a crucial element in mycobacterial control. However, in cases without the above risk factors, much of the genetic basis of susceptibility to disseminated infection with NTM is accounted for by specific mutations in the interferon γ (IFN-γ)/interleukin 12 (IL-12) synthesis and response pathways.

Mycobacteria are typically phagocytosed by macrophages, which respond with the production of IL-12, a heterodimer composed of IL-12p35 and IL-12p40 moieties that together make up IL-12p70. IL-12 activates T lymphocytes and natural killer cells through binding to its receptor (composed of IL-12Rβ1 and IL-12Rβ2/IL-23R), with consequent phosphorylation of STAT4. IL-12 stimulation of STAT4 leads to secretion of IFN-γ, which activates neutrophils and macrophages to produce reactive oxidants, to increase expression of the major histocompatibility complex and Fc receptors, and to concentrate certain antibiotics intracellularly. Signaling by IFN-γ through its receptor (composed of IFN-γR1 and IFN-γR2) leads to phosphorylation of STAT1, which in turn regulates IFN-γ-responsive genes, such as those coding for IL-12 and TNF-α. TNF-α signals through its own receptor via a downstream complex containing the nuclear factor κB (NF-κB) essential modulator (NEMO). Therefore, the positive feedback loop between IFN-γ and IL-12/IL-23 drives the immune response to mycobacteria and other intracellular infections. These genes are known to be the critical ones in the pathway of mycobacterial control: specific Mendelian mutations have been identified in *IFN-γR1, IFN-γR2, STAT1, GATA2, ISG15, IRF8, IL-12A, IL-12Rβ1, IL-12Rβ2, CYBB*, and *NEMO* (Fig. 204-1). Despite the identification of genes associated with disseminated disease, only ~70% of cases of disseminated nontuberculous mycobacterial infections that are not associated with HIV infection have a genetic diagnosis; the implication is that more mycobacterial susceptibility genes and pathways remain to be identified.

In contrast to the recognized genes and mechanisms associated with disseminated nontuberculous mycobacterial infection, the best-recognized underlying condition for pulmonary infection with NTM is bronchiectasis (Chap. 312). Most of the well-characterized forms of bronchiectasis, including cystic fibrosis, primary ciliary dyskinesia, STAT3-deficient hyper-IgE syndrome, and idiopathic bronchiectasis, have high rates of association with nontuberculous mycobacterial infection. The precise mechanism by which bronchiectasis predisposes to locally destructive but not systemic involvement is unknown.

Unlike disseminated or pulmonary infection, "hot-tub lung" represents pulmonary hypersensitivity to NTM—most commonly MAC organisms—growing in underchlorinated, often indoor hot tubs.

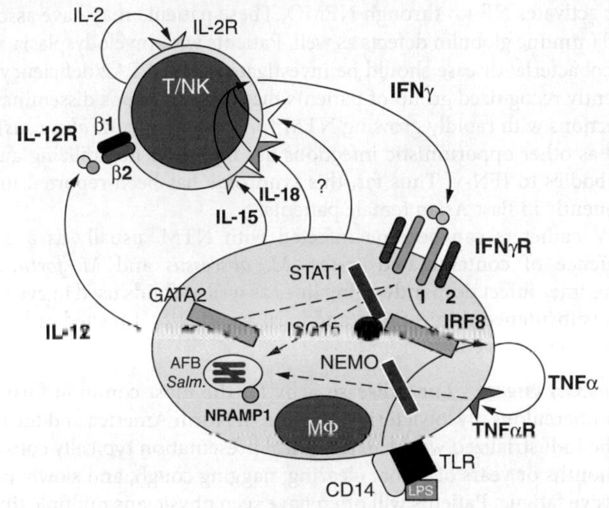

FIGURE 204-1 Cytokine interactions of infected macrophages (Mϕ) with T and natural killer (NK) lymphocytes. Infection of macrophages by mycobacteria (AFB) leads to the release of heterodimeric interleukin 12 (IL-12). IL-12 acts on its receptor complex (IL-12R), with consequent STAT4 activation and production of homodimeric interferon γ (IFNγ). Through its receptor (IFNγR), IFNγ activates STAT1, stimulating the production of tumor necrosis factor α (TNFα) and leading to the killing of intracellular organisms such as mycobacteria, salmonellae (Salm), and some fungi. Homotrimeric TNFα acts through its receptor (TNFαR) and requires nuclear factor κB essential modulator (NEMO) to activate nuclear factor κB, which also contributes to the killing of intracellular bacteria. Both IFNγ and TNFα lead to upregulation of IL-12. TNFα-blocking antibodies work either by blocking the ligand (infliximab, adalimumab, certolizumab, golimumab) or by providing soluble receptor (etanercept). Mutations in *IFNγR1, IFNγR2, IL-12p40, IL-12Rβ1, IL-12Rβ2, STAT1, GATA2, ISG15, IRF8, CYBB*, and *NEMO* have been associated with a predisposition to mycobacterial infections. Other cytokines, such as IL-15 and IL-18, also contribute to IFNγ production. Signaling through the Toll-like receptor (TLR) complex and CD14 also upregulates TNFα production. LPS, lipopolysaccharide; NRAMP1, natural resistance-associated macrophage protein 1.

CLINICAL MANIFESTATIONS

Disseminated Disease Disseminated MAC or *M. kansasii* infections in patients with advanced HIV infection are now uncommon in North America because of effective antimycobacterial prophylaxis and improved treatment of HIV infection. When such mycobacterial disease was common, the portal of entry was the bowel, with spread to bone marrow and the bloodstream. Surprisingly, disseminated infections with rapidly growing NTM (e.g., *M. abscessus, M. fortuitum*) are very rare in HIV-infected patients, even those with very advanced HIV infection. Because these organisms are of low intrinsic virulence and disseminate only in conjunction with impaired immunity, disseminated disease can be indolent and progressive over weeks to months. Typical manifestations of malaise, fever, and weight loss are often accompanied by organomegaly, lymphadenopathy, and anemia. Because special cultures or stains are required to identify the organisms, the most critical step in diagnosis is to suspect infection with NTM. Blood cultures may be negative, but involved organs typically have significant organism burdens, sometimes with a grossly impaired granulomatous response. In a child, disseminated involvement (i.e., involvement of two or more organs) without an underlying iatrogenic cause should prompt an investigation of the IFN-γ/IL-12 pathway. Recessive mutations in *IFN-γR1* and *IFN-γR2* typically lead to severe infection with NTM. In contrast, dominant negative mutations in *IFN-γR1*, which lead to overaccumulation of a defective interfering mutant receptor on the cell surface, inhibit normal IFN-γ signaling and thus lead to nontuberculous mycobacterial osteomyelitis. Dominant negative mutations in *STAT1* and recessive mutations in *IL-12Rβ1* can produce variable phenotypes consistent with their residual capacities for IFN-γ synthesis and response. Male patients who have disseminated nontuberculous mycobacterial infections along with conical, peg, or missing teeth and an abnormal hair pattern should be evaluated for defects in the pathway that activates NF-κB through NEMO. These patients may have associated immune globulin defects as well. Patients with myelodysplasia and mycobacterial disease should be investigated for GATA2 deficiency. A recently recognized group of patients that often develops disseminated infections with rapidly growing NTM (predominantly *M. abscessus*) as well as other opportunistic infections has high-titer neutralizing autoantibodies to IFN-γ. Thus far, this syndrome has been reported most frequently in East Asian female patients.

IV catheters can become infected with NTM, usually as a consequence of contaminated water. *M. abscessus* and *M. fortuitum* sometimes infect deep indwelling lines as well as fluids used in eye surgery, subcutaneous injections, and local anesthetics. Infected catheters should be removed.

Pulmonary Disease Lung disease is by far the most common form of nontuberculous mycobacterial infection in North America and the rest of the industrialized world. The clinical presentation typically consists of months or years of throat clearing, nagging cough, and slowly progressive fatigue. Patients will often have seen physicians multiple times and received symptom-based or transient therapy before the diagnosis is entertained and samples are sent for mycobacterial stains and cultures. Because not all patients can produce sputum, bronchoscopy may be required for diagnosis. The typical lag between onset of symptoms and diagnosis is ~5 years in older women. Predisposing factors include underlying lung diseases such as bronchiectasis (Chap. 312), pneumoconiosis (Chap. 311), chronic obstructive pulmonary disease (Chap. 314), primary ciliary dyskinesia (Chap. 312), α_1 antitrypsin deficiency (Chap. 367e), and cystic fibrosis (Chap. 313). Bronchiectasis and nontuberculous mycobacterial infection often coexist and progress in tandem. This situation makes causality difficult to determine in a given index case, but bronchiectasis is certainly among the most critical predisposing factors that are exacerbated by infection.

MAC organisms are the most common causes of pulmonary nontuberculous mycobacterial infection in North America, but rates vary somewhat by region. MAC infection most commonly develops during the sixth or seventh decade of life in women who have had months or years of nagging intermittent cough and fatigue, with or without sputum production or chest pain. The constellation of pulmonary disease due to NTM in a tall and thin woman who may have chest wall abnormalities is often referred to as Lady Windermere syndrome, after an Oscar Wilde character of the same name. In fact, pulmonary MAC infection does afflict older nonsmoking white women more than men, with onset at ~60 years. Patients tend to be taller and thinner than the general population, with high rates of scoliosis, mitral valve prolapse, and pectus anomalies. Whereas male smokers with upper-lobe cavitary disease tend to carry the same single strain of MAC indefinitely, nonsmoking females with nodular bronchiectasis tend to carry several strains of MAC simultaneously, with changes over the course of their disease.

M. kansasii can cause a clinical syndrome that strongly resembles tuberculosis, consisting of hemoptysis, chest pain, and cavitary lung disease. The rapidly growing NTM, such as *M. abscessus*, have been associated with esophageal motility disorders such as achalasia. Patients with pulmonary alveolar proteinosis are prone to pulmonary nontuberculous mycobacterial and *Nocardia* infections; the underlying mechanism may be inhibition of alveolar macrophage function due to the autoantibodies to granulocyte-macrophage colony-stimulating factor found in these patients.

Cervical Lymph Nodes The most common form of nontuberculous mycobacterial infection among young children in North America is isolated cervical lymphadenopathy, caused most frequently by MAC organisms but also by other NTM. The cervical swelling is typically firm and relatively painless, with a paucity of systemic signs. Because the differential diagnosis of painless adenopathy includes malignancy, many children have infection with NTM diagnosed inadvertently at biopsy; cultures and special stains may not have been requested because mycobacterial disease was not ranked high in the differential. Local fistulae usually resolve completely with resection and/or antibiotic therapy. Likewise, the entity of isolated pediatric intrathoracic nontuberculous mycobacterial infection, which is probably related to cervical lymph node infection, is usually mistaken for cancer. In neither isolated cervical nor isolated intrathoracic infections with NTM have children with underlying immune defects been identified, nor do the affected children go on to develop other opportunistic infections.

Skin and Soft Tissue Disease Cutaneous involvement with NTM usually requires a break in the skin for introduction of the bacteria. Pedicure bath–associated infection with *M. fortuitum* is more likely if skin abrasion (e.g., during leg shaving) has occurred just before the pedicure. Outbreaks of skin infection are often caused by rapidly growing NTM (especially *M. abscessus, M. fortuitum*, and *M. chelonae*) acquired via skin contamination from surgical instruments (especially in cosmetic surgery), injections, and other procedures. These infections are typically accompanied by painful, erythematous, draining subcutaneous nodules, usually without associated fever or systemic symptoms.

M. marinum lives in many water sources and can be acquired from fish tanks, swimming pools, barnacles, and fish scales. This organism typically causes papules or ulcers ("fish-tank granuloma"), but the infection can progress to tendinitis with significant impairment of manual dexterity. Lesions appear days to weeks after inoculation of organisms by a typically minor trauma (e.g., incurred during the cleaning of boats or the handling of fish). Tender nodules due to *M. marinum* can advance up the arm in a pattern also seen with *Sporothrix schenckii* (*sporotricoid spread*). The typical carpal tendon involvement may be the first presenting manifestation and may lead to surgical exploration or steroid injection. The index of suspicion for *M. marinum* infections must be high to ensure that proper specimens obtained during procedures are sent for culture.

M. ulcerans, another waterborne skin pathogen, is found mainly in the tropics, especially in tropical areas of Africa. Infection follows skin trauma or insect bites that allow admission to contaminated water. The skin lesions are typically painless, clean ulcers that slough and can cause osteomyelitis. The toxin mycolactone accounts for the modest host inflammatory response and the painless ulcerations.

DIAGNOSIS

NTM can be detected on acid-fast or fluorochrome smears of sputum or other body fluids. When the organism burden is high, the organisms may appear as gram-positive beaded rods, but this finding is unreliable. (In contrast, nocardiae may appear as gram-positive and beaded but filamentous bacteria.) Again, the requisite and most sensitive step in the diagnosis of any mycobacterial disease is to think of including it in the differential. In almost all laboratories, mycobacterial sample processing, staining, and culture are conducted separately from routine bacteriologic tests; thus many infections go undiagnosed because of the physician's failure to request the appropriate test. In addition, mycobacteria usually require separate blood culture media. NTM are broadly differentiated into rapidly growing (<7 days) and slowly growing (≥7 days) forms. Because *M. tuberculosis* typically takes ≥2 weeks to grow, many laboratories refuse to consider culture results final until 6 weeks have elapsed. Newer techniques using liquid culture media permit more rapid isolation of mycobacteria from specimens than is possible with traditional media. Species more readily detected with incubation at 30°C include *M. marinum, M. haemophilum*, and *M. ulcerans*. *M. haemophilum* prefers iron supplementation or blood, whereas *M. genavense* requires supplemented medium with the additive mycobactin J. Bacterial formation of pigment in light conditions (*photochromogenicity*) or dark conditions (*scotochromogenicity*) or a lack of bacterial pigment formation (*nonchromogenicity*) has been used to help categorize NTM. In contrast to NTM colonies, *M. tuberculosis* colonies are beige, rough, dry, and flat. Current identification schemes can reliably use biochemical, nucleic acid, or cell wall composition, as assessed by high-performance liquid chromatography or mass spectrometry, for speciation. With the remarkable decline in U.S. cases of tuberculosis over recent decades, NTM have become the mycobacteria most commonly isolated from humans in North America. However, not all isolations of NTM, especially from the lung, reflect pathology and require treatment. Whereas identification of an organism in a blood or organ biopsy specimen in a compatible clinical setting is diagnostic, the

American Thoracic Society recommends that pulmonary infection due to NTM be diagnosed only when disease is clearly demonstrable—i.e., in an appropriate clinical and radiographic setting (nodules, bronchiectasis, cavities) and with repeated isolation of NTM from expectorated sputum or recovery of NTM from bronchoscopy or biopsy specimens. Given the large number of species of NTM and the importance of accurate diagnosis for the implementation of proper therapy, identification of these organisms is ideally taken to the species level.

The purified protein derivative (PPD) of tuberculin is delivered intradermally to evoke a memory T cell response to mycobacterial antigens. This test is variously referred to as the PPD test, the tuberculin skin test, and the Mantoux test, among other designations. Unfortunately, the cutaneous immune response to these tuberculosis-derived filtrate proteins does not differentiate well between infection with NTM and that with *M. tuberculosis*. Because intermediate reactions (~10 mm) to PPD in latent tuberculosis and nontuberculous mycobacterial infections can overlap significantly, the progressive decline in active tuberculosis in the United States means that NTM probably account for increasing proportions of PPD reactivity. In addition, bacille Calmette-Guérin (BCG) can cause some degree of cross-reactivity, posing problems of interpretation for patients who have received BCG vaccine. Assays to measure the elaboration of IFN-γ in response to the relatively tuberculosis-specific proteins ESAT6 and CFP10 form the basis for IFN-γ-release assays (IGRAs). These assays can be performed with whole blood or on membranes. It is important to note that *M. marinum*, *M. kansasii*, and *M. szulgai* also have ESAT6 and CFP10 and may cause false-positive reactions in IGRAs. Despite cross-reactivity with NTM, large PPD reactions (>15 mm) most commonly signify tuberculosis.

Isolation of NTM from blood specimens is clear evidence of disease. Whereas rapidly growing mycobacteria may proliferate in routine blood culture media, slow-growing NTM typically do not; thus it is imperative to suspect the diagnosis and to use the correct bottles for cultures. Isolation of NTM from a biopsy specimen constitutes strong evidence for infection, but cases of laboratory contamination do occur. Identification of organisms on stained sections of biopsy material confirms the authenticity of the culture. Certain NTM require lower incubation temperatures (*M. genavense*) or special additives (*M. haemophilum*) for growth. Some NTM (e.g., *M. tilburgii*) remain noncultivable but can be identified molecularly in clinical samples.

The radiographic appearance of nontuberculous mycobacterial disease in the lung depends on the underlying disease, the severity of the infection, and the imaging modality used. The advent and increase in the use of computed tomography (CT) has allowed the identification of characteristic changes that are highly consistent with nontuberculous mycobacterial infection, such as the "tree-in-bud" pattern of bronchiolar inflammation (Fig. 204-2). Involvement of the lingual and right-middle lobes is commonly seen on chest CT but is difficult to appreciate on plain film. Severe bronchiectasis and cavity formation are common in more advanced disease. Isolation of NTM from respiratory samples can be confusing. *M. gordonae* is often recovered from respiratory samples but is not usually seen on smear and is almost never a pathogen. Patients with bronchiectasis occasionally have NTM recovered from sputum culture with a negative smear. The American Thoracic Society has developed guidelines for the diagnosis of infection with MAC, *M. abscessus*, and *M. kansasii*. A positive diagnosis requires the growth of NTM from two of three sputum samples, regardless of smear findings; a positive bronchoscopic alveolar sample, regardless of smear findings; or a pulmonary parenchyma biopsy sample with granulomatous inflammation or mycobacteria found on section and NTM found on culture. These guidelines probably apply to other NTM as well.

Although many laboratories use DNA probes to identify *M. tuberculosis*, MAC, *M. gordonae*, and *M. kansasii*, speciation of NTM helps determine the antimycobacterial therapy to be used. Only testing of MAC organisms for susceptibility to clarithromycin and of *M. kansasii* for susceptibility to rifampin is indicated; few data support other in vitro susceptibility tests, attractive though they appear. MAC isolates that have not been exposed to macrolides are almost always

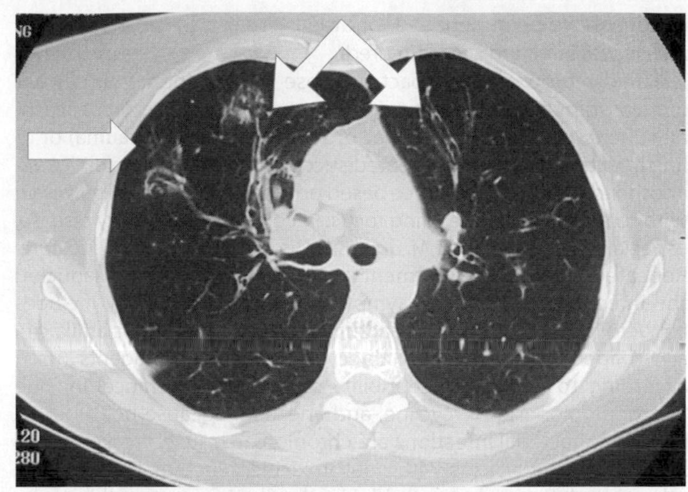

FIGURE 204-2 Chest computed tomography of a patient with pulmonary *Mycobacterium avium* complex infection. *Arrows* indicate the "tree-in-bud" pattern of bronchiolar inflammation (peripheral right lung) and bronchiectasis (central right and left lungs).

susceptible. NTM that have persisted beyond a course of antimicrobial therapy are often tested for antibiotic susceptibility, but the value and meaning of these tests are undetermined.

PREVENTION

Prophylaxis of MAC disease in patients infected with HIV is started when the CD4+ T lymphocyte count falls to <50/μL. Azithromycin (1200 mg weekly), clarithromycin (1000 mg daily), or rifabutin (300 mg daily) is effective. Macrolide prophylaxis in immunodeficient patients who are susceptible to NTM (e.g., those with defects in the IFN-γ/IL-12 axis) has not been prospectively validated but seems prudent.

TREATMENT NONTUBERCULOUS MYCOBACTERIA

NTM cause chronic infections that evolve relatively slowly over a period of weeks to years. Therefore, it is rarely necessary to initiate treatment on an emergent basis before the diagnosis is clear and the infecting species is known. Treatment of NTM is complex, often poorly tolerated, and potentially toxic. Just as in tuberculosis, inadequate single-drug therapy is almost always associated with the emergence of antimicrobial resistance and relapse.

MAC infection often requires multidrug therapy, the foundation of which is a macrolide (clarithromycin or azithromycin), ethambutol, and a rifamycin (rifampin or rifabutin). For disseminated nontuberculous mycobacterial disease in HIV-infected patients, the use of rifamycins poses special problems—i.e., rifamycin interactions with protease inhibitors. For pulmonary MAC disease, thrice-weekly administration of a macrolide, a rifamycin, and ethambutol has been successful. Therapy is prolonged, generally continuing for 12 months after culture conversion; typically, a course lasts for at least 18 months. Other drugs with activity against MAC organisms include IV and aerosolized aminoglycosides, fluoroquinolones, and clofazimine. In elderly patients, rifabutin can exert significant toxicity. However, with only modest efforts, most antimycobacterial regimens are well tolerated by most patients. Resection of cavitary lesions or severely bronchiectatic segments has been advocated for some patients, especially those with macrolide-resistant infections. The success of therapy for pulmonary MAC infections depends on whether disease is nodular or cavitary and on whether it is early or advanced, ranging from 20% to 80%.

M. kansasii lung disease is similar to tuberculosis in many ways and is also effectively treated with isoniazid (300 mg/d), rifampin (600 mg/d), and ethambutol (15 mg/kg per day). Other drugs with very high-level activity against *M. kansasii* include clarithromycin, fluoroquinolones, and aminoglycosides. Treatment should continue until cultures have been negative for at least 1 year. In most instances, *M. kansasii* infection is easily cured.

Rapidly growing mycobacteria pose special therapeutic problems. Extrapulmonary disease in an immunocompetent host is usually due to inoculation (e.g., via surgery, injections, or trauma) or to line infection and is often treated successfully with a macrolide and another drug (with the choice based on in vitro susceptibility), along with removal of the offending focus. In contrast, pulmonary disease, especially that caused by *M. abscessus*, is extremely difficult to cure. Repeated courses of treatment are usually effective in reducing the infectious burden and symptoms. Therapy generally includes a macrolide along with an IV-administered agent such as amikacin, a carbapenem, cefoxitin, or tigecycline. Other oral agents (used according to in vitro susceptibility testing and tolerance) include fluoroquinolones, doxycycline, and linezolid. Because nontuberculous mycobacterial infections are chronic, care must be taken in the long-term use of drugs with neurotoxicities, such as linezolid and ethambutol. Prophylactic pyridoxine has been suggested in these cases. Durations of therapy for *M. abscessus* lung disease are difficult to predict because so many cases are chronic and require intermittent therapy. Expert consultation and management are strongly recommended.

Once recognized, *M. marinum* infection is highly responsive to antimicrobial therapy and is cured relatively easily with any combination of a macrolide, ethambutol, and a rifamycin. Therapy should be continued for 1–2 months after clinical resolution of isolated soft tissue disease; tendon and bone involvement may require longer courses in light of clinical evolution. Other drugs with activity against *M. marinum* include sulfonamides, trimethoprim-sulfamethoxazole, doxycycline, and minocycline.

Treatment of the other NTM is less well defined, but macrolides and aminoglycosides are usually effective, with other agents added as indicated. Expert consultation is strongly encouraged for difficult or unusual infections due to NTM.

PROGNOSIS

The outcomes of nontuberculous mycobacterial infections are closely tied to the underlying condition (e.g., IFN-γ/IL-12 pathway defect, cystic fibrosis) and can range from recovery to death. With no or inadequate treatment, symptoms and signs can be debilitating, including persistent cough, fever, anorexia, and severe lung destruction. With treatment, patients typically regain strength and energy. The optimal duration of therapy when NTM persist in sputum is unknown, but treatment in this situation can be prolonged.

GLOBAL CONSIDERATIONS

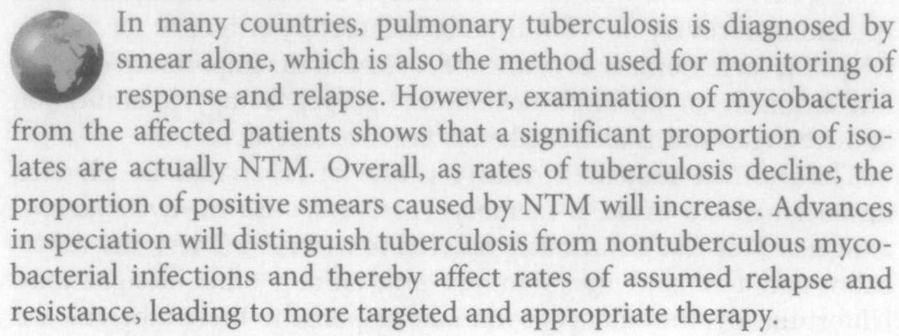

In many countries, pulmonary tuberculosis is diagnosed by smear alone, which is also the method used for monitoring of response and relapse. However, examination of mycobacteria from the affected patients shows that a significant proportion of isolates are actually NTM. Overall, as rates of tuberculosis decline, the proportion of positive smears caused by NTM will increase. Advances in speciation will distinguish tuberculosis from nontuberculous mycobacterial infections and thereby affect rates of assumed relapse and resistance, leading to more targeted and appropriate therapy.

205e Antimycobacterial Agents

Max R. O'Donnell, Divya Reddy, Jussi J. Saukkonen

This is a digital-only chapter. It is available on the DVD that accompanies this book, as well as on Access Medicine/Harrison's Online, and the eBook and "app" editions of HPIM 19e.

Agents used for the treatment of mycobacterial infections, including tuberculosis (TB), leprosy, and infections due to nontuberculous mycobacteria (NTM), are administered in multiple-drug regimens for prolonged courses. Currently, more than 160 species of mycobacteria have been identified, the majority of which do not cause disease in humans. While the incidence of disease caused by *Mycobacterium tuberculosis* has been declining in the United States, TB remains a leading cause of morbidity and mortality in developing countries—particularly in sub-Saharan Africa, where the HIV epidemic rages. Effective drug regimens are not all that is needed; without a well-organized infrastructure for diagnosis and treatment of TB, therapeutic and control efforts are severely hampered (Chaps. 2 and 13e). Infections with NTM have gained in clinical prominence in the United States and other developed countries. These largely environmental organisms often establish infection in immunocompromised patients or in persons with structural lung disease.

SECTION 9 SPIROCHETAL DISEASES

206 Syphilis

Sheila A. Lukehart

DEFINITION

Syphilis, a chronic systemic infection caused by *Treponema pallidum* subspecies *pallidum*, is usually sexually transmitted and is characterized by episodes of active disease interrupted by periods of latency. After an incubation period averaging 2–6 weeks, a primary lesion appears—often associated with regional lymphadenopathy—that resolves without treatment. The secondary stage, associated with generalized mucocutaneous lesions and generalized lymphadenopathy, is followed by a latent period of subclinical infection lasting years or decades. Central nervous system (CNS) involvement may occur early in infection and may be symptomatic or asymptomatic. In the preantibiotic era, about one-third of patients with untreated cases developed the tertiary stage, characterized by progressive destructive mucocutaneous, musculoskeletal, or parenchymal lesions; aortitis; or late CNS manifestations.

ETIOLOGY

The Spirochaetales include four genera that are pathogenic for humans and for a variety of other animals: *Leptospira* species, which cause leptospirosis (Chap. 208); *Borrelia* species, which cause relapsing fever and Lyme disease (Chaps. 209 and 210); *Brachyspira* species, which cause intestinal infections; and *Treponema* species, which cause the diseases known collectively as *treponematoses* (see also Chap. 207e). The *Treponema* species include *T. pallidum* subspecies *pallidum*, which causes venereal syphilis; *T. pallidum* subspecies *pertenue*, which causes yaws; *T. pallidum* subspecies *endemicum*, which causes endemic syphilis or bejel; and *T. carateum*, which causes pinta. Until recently, the subspecies were distinguished primarily by the clinical syndromes they produce. Researchers have now identified molecular signatures that can differentiate the three subspecies of *T. pallidum* by culture-independent methods based on polymerase chain reaction (PCR), but other sequence signatures cross subspecies boundaries in certain strains. Other *Treponema* species found in the human mouth, genital mucosa, and gastrointestinal tract have been associated with disease (e.g., periodontitis), but their role as primary etiologic agents is unclear.

T. pallidum subspecies *pallidum* (referred to hereafter as *T. pallidum*), a thin spiral organism, has a cell body surrounded by a trilaminar cytoplasmic membrane, a delicate peptidoglycan layer providing some structural rigidity, and a lipid-rich outer membrane containing relatively few integral membrane proteins. Endoflagella wind around the cell body in the periplasmic space and are responsible for motility. *T. pallidum* cannot be cultured in vitro, and little was known about its metabolism until the genome was sequenced in 1998. This spirochete possesses severely limited metabolic capabilities, lacking the genes required for de novo synthesis of most amino acids, nucleotides, and lipids. In addition, *T. pallidum* lacks genes encoding the enzymes of the Krebs cycle and oxidative phosphorylation. The organism contains numerous compensatory genes predicted to encode transporters of amino acids, carbohydrates, and lipids. In addition, genome analyses and other studies have revealed the existence of a 12-member gene family (*tpr*) that bears similarities to variable outer-membrane antigens of other spirochetes. One member, TprK, has discrete variable (V) regions that undergo antigenic variation during infection, providing a mechanism for immune evasion.

The only known natural host for *T. pallidum* is the human. *T. pallidum* can infect many mammals, but only humans, higher apes, and a few laboratory animals regularly develop syphilitic lesions. Rabbits are used to propagate virulent strains of *T. pallidum* and serve as the animal model that best reflects human disease and immunopathology.

TRANSMISSION AND EPIDEMIOLOGY

Nearly all cases of syphilis are acquired by sexual contact with infectious lesions (i.e., the chancre, mucous patch, skin rash, or condylomata lata; see Fig. 25e-20). Less common modes of transmission include nonsexual personal contact, infection in utero, blood transfusion, and organ transplantation.

SYPHILIS IN THE UNITED STATES

With the advent of penicillin therapy, the total number of cases of syphilis reported annually in the United States declined significantly to a low of 31,575 cases in 2000—a 95% decrease from 1943—with <6000 reported cases of infectious primary and secondary syphilis (the latter being a better indicator of disease activity than total syphilis cases). Since 2000, the number of cases of primary and secondary syphilis has more than doubled, with more than 14,000 cases reported in 2012 (Fig. 206-1). Approximately 70% of these cases were in men who have sex with men (MSM), 20–70% of whom are co-infected with HIV (depending on geographic location). The number of primary and secondary cases among women in the United States increased from 2004 to 2008 but has since been declining in conjunction with a decline in congenital syphilis. Surveillance of the number of new cases of primary and secondary syphilis has revealed multiple 7- to 10-year cycles, which may be attributed to herd immunity in at-risk populations, changing sexual behaviors, and changes in control efforts.

The populations at highest risk for acquiring syphilis have changed over time, with outbreaks among MSM in the pre-HIV era of the late 1970s and early 1980s as well as at present. It is speculated that recent increases in syphilis and other sexually transmitted infections in MSM may be due to unprotected sex between persons who are HIV concordant and to disinhibition caused by highly effective antiretroviral therapies. The syphilis epidemic that peaked in 1990 predominantly affected African-American heterosexual men and women and occurred largely in urban areas, where infectious syphilis was correlated with the exchange of sex for crack cocaine. The rate of primary and secondary syphilis among African Americans nearly doubled between 2003 and 2009, remains higher than rates for other racial/ethnic groups, but has since declined somewhat (Fig. 206-1).

The incidence of congenital syphilis roughly parallels that of infectious syphilis in women. In 2011, 360 cases in infants <1 year of age were reported, for a decline of 20% since 2008. The case definition for congenital syphilis was broadened in 1989 and now includes all live or stillborn infants delivered to women with untreated or inadequately treated syphilis.

One-third to one-half of individuals named as sexual contacts of persons with infectious syphilis become infected. Many have already developed manifestations of syphilis when they are first seen, and ~30% of asymptomatic contacts examined within 30 days of exposure actually have incubating infection and will later develop infectious syphilis if not treated. Thus, identification and treatment of all recently exposed sexual contacts continue to be important aspects of syphilis control.

GLOBAL SYPHILIS

Syphilis remains a significant health problem globally; the number of new infections is estimated at 11 million per year. The regions that are most affected include sub-Saharan Africa, South America, China, and Southeast Asia. During the past decade, the incidence rate in China has increased by approximately eightfold, and higher rates of infectious syphilis have been reported among MSM in many European countries. Worldwide, there are estimated to be 1.4 million cases of syphilis among pregnant women, with 500,000 adverse pregnancy outcomes annually (e.g., stillbirth, neonatal and early fetal death, prematurity/low birth weight, and infection in newborns). Congenital syphilis rates in China are ~150 cases per 100,000 live births.

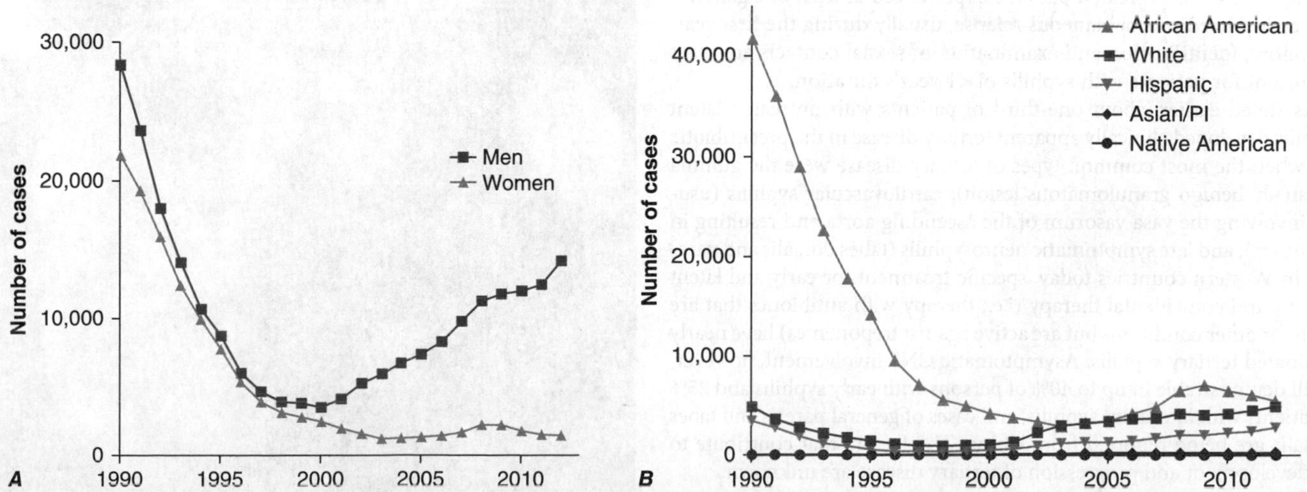

FIGURE 206-1 Primary and secondary syphilis in the United States, 1990–2012, by sex (*A*) and by race or ethnicity (*B*). *(Data from the Centers for Disease Control and Prevention.)*

T. pallidum rapidly penetrates intact mucous membranes or microscopic abrasions in skin and, within a few hours, enters the lymphatics and blood to produce systemic infection and metastatic foci long before the appearance of a primary lesion. Blood from a patient with incubating or early syphilis is infectious. The generation time of *T. pallidum* during early active disease in vivo is estimated to be ~30 h, and the incubation period of syphilis is inversely proportional to the number of organisms inoculated. The 50% infectious dose for intradermal inoculation in humans has been calculated to be 57 organisms, and the treponeme concentration generally reaches 10^7/g of tissue before a clinical lesion appears. The median incubation period in humans (~21 days) suggests an average inoculum of 500–1000 infectious organisms for naturally acquired disease; the incubation period rarely exceeds 6 weeks.

The primary lesion appears at the site of inoculation, usually persists for 4–6 weeks, and then heals spontaneously. Histopathologic examination shows perivascular infiltration, chiefly by CD4+ and CD8+ T lymphocytes, plasma cells, and macrophages, with capillary endothelial proliferation and subsequent obliteration of small blood vessels. The cellular infiltration displays a T_H1-type cytokine profile consistent with the activation of macrophages. Phagocytosis of opsonized organisms by activated macrophages ultimately causes their destruction, resulting in spontaneous resolution of the chancre.

The generalized parenchymal, constitutional, and mucocutaneous manifestations of secondary syphilis usually appear ~6–8 weeks after the chancre heals, although primary and secondary manifestations may overlap. In contrast, some patients may enter the latent stage without ever recognizing secondary lesions. The histopathologic features of secondary maculopapular skin lesions include hyperkeratosis of the epidermis, capillary proliferation with endothelial swelling in the superficial dermis, dermal papillae with transmigration of polymorphonuclear leukocytes, and—in the deeper dermis—perivascular infiltration by CD8+ T lymphocytes, CD4+ T lymphocytes, macrophages, and plasma cells. Treponemes are found in many tissues, including the aqueous humor of the eye and the cerebrospinal fluid (CSF). *T. pallidum* invades the CNS during the first weeks or months of infection, and CSF abnormalities are detected in as many as 40% of patients during the secondary stage. Clinical hepatitis and immune complex–induced glomerulonephritis are relatively rare but recognized manifestations of secondary syphilis; liver function tests may yield abnormal results in up to one-quarter of patients with early syphilis. Generalized nontender lymphadenopathy is noted in 85% of patients with secondary syphilis. The paradoxical appearance of secondary manifestations despite high titers of antibody (including immobilizing antibody) to *T. pallidum* may result from immune evasion due to antigenic variation or changes in expression of surface antigens. Secondary lesions generally subside within 2–6 weeks, and the infection enters the latent stage, which is detectable only by serologic testing. In the preantibiotic era, up to 25% of untreated patients experienced at least one generalized or localized mucocutaneous relapse, usually during the first year. Therefore, identification and examination of sexual contacts are most important for patients with syphilis of <1 year's duration.

As stated earlier, about one-third of patients with untreated latent syphilis developed clinically apparent tertiary disease in the preantibiotic era, when the most common types of tertiary disease were the gumma (a usually benign granulomatous lesion); cardiovascular syphilis (usually involving the vasa vasorum of the ascending aorta and resulting in aneurysm); and late symptomatic neurosyphilis (tabes dorsalis and paresis). In Western countries today, specific treatment for early and latent syphilis and coincidental therapy (i.e., therapy with antibiotics that are given for other conditions but are active against treponemes) have nearly eliminated tertiary syphilis. Asymptomatic CNS involvement, however, is still demonstrable in up to 40% of persons with early syphilis and 25% of patients with late latent syphilis, and cases of general paresis and tabes dorsalis are being reported from China. The factors that contribute to the development and progression of tertiary disease are unknown.

The course of untreated syphilis was studied retrospectively in a group of nearly 2000 patients with primary or secondary disease diagnosed clinically (the Oslo Study, 1891–1951) and was assessed prospectively in 431 African-American men with seropositive latent syphilis of ≥3 years' duration (the notorious Tuskegee Study, 1932–1972). In the Oslo Study, 24% of patients developed relapsing secondary lesions within 4 years, and 28% eventually developed one or more manifestations of tertiary syphilis. Cardiovascular syphilis, including aortitis, was detected in 10% of patients; 7% of patients developed symptomatic neurosyphilis, and 16% developed benign tertiary gummatous syphilis. Syphilis was the primary cause of death in 15% of men and 8% of women. Cardiovascular syphilis was documented in 35% of men and 22% of women who eventually came to autopsy. In general, serious late complications were nearly twice as common among men as among women.

The Tuskegee Study showed that the death rate among untreated African-American men with syphilis (25–50 years old) was 17% higher than the rate among uninfected subjects and that 30% of all deaths were attributable to cardiovascular or, to a lesser extent, CNS syphilis. Anatomic evidence of aortitis was found in 40–60% of autopsied subjects with syphilis (vs 15% of control subjects), whereas CNS syphilis was found in only 4%. Rates of hypertension were also higher among the infected subjects. The ethical issues eventually raised by this study, begun in the preantibiotic era but continuing into the early 1970s, had a major influence on the development of current guidelines for human medical experimentation, and the history of the study may still contribute to a reluctance of some African Americans to participate as subjects in clinical research.

CLINICAL MANIFESTATIONS

Primary Syphilis The typical primary chancre usually begins as a single painless papule that rapidly becomes eroded and usually becomes indurated, with a characteristic cartilaginous consistency on palpation of the edge and base of the ulcer. Multiple primary lesions are seen in a minority of patients. In heterosexual men the chancre is usually located on the penis (Fig. 206-2; see also Fig. 25e-17), whereas in MSM it may be found in the anal canal or rectum, in the mouth, or on the external genitalia. Oral sex has been identified as the source of infection in some MSM. In women, common primary sites are the cervix and labia. Consequently, primary syphilis goes unrecognized in women and homosexual men more often than in heterosexual men.

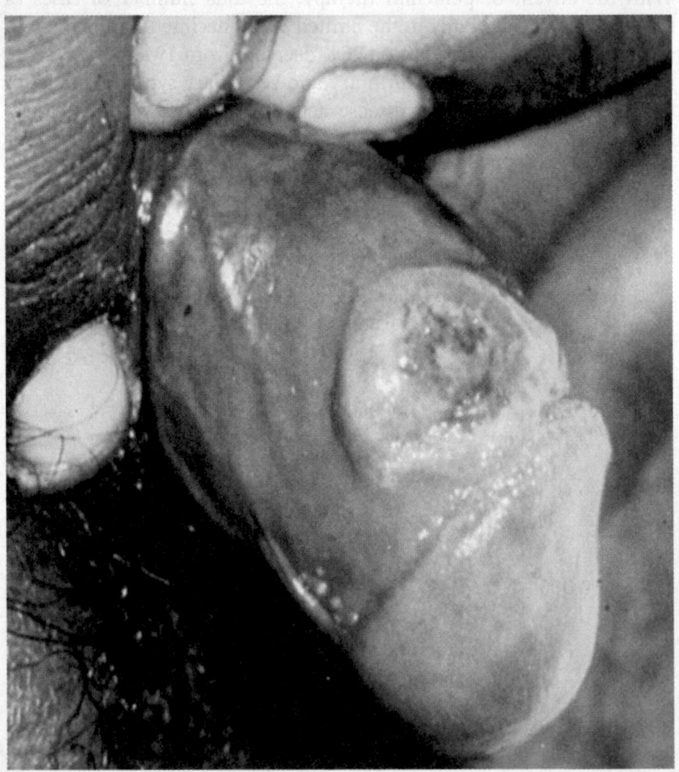

FIGURE 206-2 **Primary syphilis** with a firm, nontender chancre.

Atypical primary lesions are common. The clinical appearance depends on the number of treponemes inoculated and on the immunologic status of the patient. A large inoculum produces a dark-field-positive ulcerative lesion in nonimmune volunteers but may produce a small dark-field-negative papule, an asymptomatic but seropositive latent infection, or no response at all in some individuals with a history of syphilis. A small inoculum may produce only a papular lesion, even in nonimmune individuals. Therefore, syphilis should be considered even in the evaluation of trivial or atypical dark-field-negative genital lesions. The genital lesions that most commonly must be differentiated from those of primary syphilis include those caused by herpes simplex virus infection (Chap. 216), chancroid (Chap. 182), traumatic injury, and donovanosis (Chap. 198e). Regional (usually inguinal) lymphadenopathy accompanies the primary syphilitic lesion, appearing within 1 week of lesion onset. The nodes are firm, nonsuppurative, and painless. Inguinal lymphadenopathy is bilateral and may occur with anal as well as with external genital chancres. The chancre generally heals within 4–6 weeks (range, 2–12 weeks), but lymphadenopathy may persist for months.

Secondary Syphilis The protean manifestations of the secondary stage usually include mucocutaneous lesions and generalized nontender lymphadenopathy. The healing primary chancre may still be present in ~15% of cases, and the stages may overlap more frequently in persons with concurrent HIV infection. The skin rash consists of macular, papular, papulosquamous, and occasionally pustular syphilides; often more than one form is present simultaneously. The eruption may be very subtle, and 25% of patients with a discernible rash may be unaware that they have dermatologic manifestations. Initial lesions are pale red or pink, nonpruritic, discrete macules distributed on the trunk and proximal extremities; these macules progress to papular lesions that are distributed widely and that frequently involve the palms and soles (Fig. 206-3; see also Figs. 25e-18 and 25e-19). Rarely, severe necrotic lesions (*lues maligna*) may appear; they are more commonly reported in HIV-infected individuals. Involvement of the hair follicles may result in patchy alopecia of the scalp hair, eyebrows, or beard in up to 5% of cases.

In warm, moist, intertriginous areas (commonly the perianal region, vulva, and scrotum), papules can enlarge to produce broad, moist, pink or gray-white, highly infectious lesions (*condylomata lata*; see Fig. 25e-20) in 10% of patients with secondary syphilis. Superficial mucosal erosions (*mucous patches*) occur in 10–15% of patients and commonly involve the oral or genital mucosa (see Fig. 25e-21). The typical mucous patch is a painless silver-gray erosion surrounded by a red periphery.

Constitutional signs and symptoms that may accompany or precede secondary syphilis include sore throat (15–30%), fever (5–8%), weight loss (2–20%), malaise (25%), anorexia (2–10%), headache (10%), and meningismus (5%). *Acute meningitis* occurs in only 1–2% of cases, but CSF cell and protein concentrations are increased in up to 40% of cases, and viable *T. pallidum* organisms have been recovered from CSF during primary and secondary syphilis in 30% of cases; the latter finding is often but not always associated with other CSF abnormalities.

Less common complications of secondary syphilis include hepatitis, nephropathy, gastrointestinal involvement (hypertrophic gastritis, patchy proctitis, or a rectosigmoid mass), arthritis, and periostitis. Ocular findings associated with secondary syphilis include pupillary abnormalities and optic neuritis as well as the classic iritis or uveitis. The diagnosis of ocular syphilis is often considered in affected patients only after they fail to respond to steroid therapy. Anterior uveitis has been reported in 5–10% of patients with secondary syphilis, and *T. pallidum* has been demonstrated in aqueous humor from such patients. Hepatic involvement is common in syphilis; although it is usually asymptomatic, up to 25% of patients may have abnormal liver function tests. Frank syphilitic hepatitis may be seen. Renal involvement usually results from immune complex deposition and produces proteinuria associated with an acute nephrotic syndrome. Like those of primary syphilis, the manifestations of the secondary stage resolve spontaneously, usually within 1–6 months.

Latent Syphilis Positive serologic tests for syphilis, together with a normal CSF examination and the absence of clinical manifestations of syphilis, indicate a diagnosis of latent syphilis in an untreated person. The diagnosis is often suspected on the basis of a history of primary or secondary lesions, a history of exposure to syphilis, or the delivery of an infant with congenital syphilis. A previous negative serologic test or a history of lesions or exposure may help establish the duration of latent infection, which is an important factor in the selection of appropriate therapy. *Early latent* syphilis is limited to the first year after infection, whereas *late latent* syphilis is defined as that of ≥1 year's duration (or of unknown duration). *T. pallidum* may still seed the bloodstream intermittently during the latent stage, and pregnant women with latent syphilis may infect the fetus in utero. Moreover, syphilis has been transmitted through blood transfusion or organ donation from patients with latent syphilis. It was previously thought that untreated late latent syphilis had three possible outcomes: (1) persistent lifelong infection; (2) development of late syphilis; or (3) spontaneous cure, with reversion of serologic tests to negative. It is now apparent, however, that the more sensitive treponemal antibody tests rarely, if ever, become nonreactive without treatment. Although progression to clinically evident late syphilis is very rare today, the occurrence of spontaneous cure is in doubt.

Involvement of the CNS Traditionally, neurosyphilis has been considered a late manifestation of syphilis, but this view is inaccurate. CNS syphilis represents a continuum encompassing early invasion (usually within the first weeks or months of infection), months to years of asymptomatic involvement, and, in some cases, development of early or late neurologic manifestations.

ASYMPTOMATIC NEUROSYPHILIS The diagnosis of asymptomatic neurosyphilis is made in patients who lack neurologic symptoms and signs but who have CSF abnormalities including mononuclear pleocytosis, increased protein concentrations, or CSF reactivity in the Venereal Disease Research Laboratory (VDRL) test. CSF abnormalities are demonstrated in up to 40% of cases of primary or secondary syphilis and in 25% of cases of latent syphilis. *T. pallidum* has been recovered by inoculation into rabbits of CSF from up to 30% of patients with primary or secondary syphilis but less frequently by inoculation of CSF from patients with latent syphilis. The presence of *T. pallidum* in CSF is often associated with other CSF abnormalities, but organisms can be recovered from patients with otherwise normal CSF. Although the prognostic implications of these findings in early syphilis are uncertain, it may be appropriate to conclude that even patients with

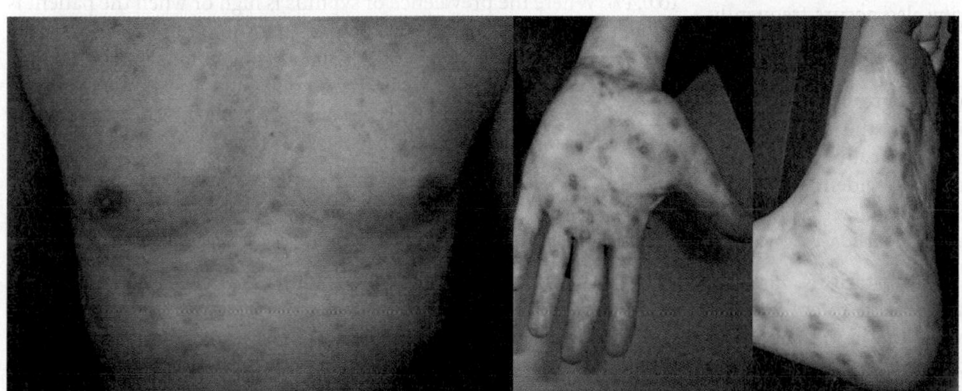

FIGURE 206-3 Secondary syphilis. ***Left:*** Maculopapular truncal eruption. ***Middle:*** Papules on the palms. ***Right:*** Papules on the soles. *(Courtesy of Jill McKenzie and Christina Marra.)*

early syphilis who have such findings do indeed have asymptomatic neurosyphilis and should be treated for neurosyphilis; such treatment is particularly important in patients with concurrent HIV infection. Before the advent of penicillin, the risk of development of clinical neurosyphilis in untreated asymptomatic persons was roughly proportional to the intensity of CSF changes, with the overall cumulative probability of progression to clinical neurosyphilis ~20% in the first 10 years but increasing with time. Most experts agree that neurosyphilis is more common in HIV-infected persons, while immunocompetent patients with untreated latent syphilis and normal CSF probably run a very low risk of subsequent neurosyphilis. In several recent studies, neurosyphilis was associated with a rapid plasma reagin (RPR) titer of ≥1:32, regardless of clinical stage or HIV infection status.

SYMPTOMATIC NEUROSYPHILIS The major clinical categories of symptomatic neurosyphilis include meningeal, meningovascular, and parenchymatous syphilis. The last category includes general paresis and tabes dorsalis. The onset of symptoms usually occurs <1 year after infection for meningeal syphilis, up to 10 years after infection for meningovascular syphilis, at ~20 years for general paresis, and at 25–30 years for tabes dorsalis. Neurosyphilis is more frequently symptomatic in patients who are co-infected with HIV, particularly in the setting of a low CD4+ T lymphocyte count. In addition, recent evidence suggests that syphilis infection worsens the cognitive impairment seen in HIV-infected persons and that this effect persists even after treatment for syphilis.

Meningeal syphilis may present as headache, nausea, vomiting, neck stiffness, cranial nerve involvement, seizures, and changes in mental status. This condition may be concurrent with or may follow the secondary stage. Patients presenting with uveitis, iritis, or hearing loss often have meningeal syphilis, but these clinical findings can also be seen in patients with normal CSF.

Meningovascular syphilis reflects meningitis together with inflammatory vasculitis of small, medium, or large vessels. The most common presentation is a stroke syndrome involving the middle cerebral artery of a relatively young adult. However, unlike the usual thrombotic or embolic stroke syndrome of sudden onset, meningovascular syphilis often becomes manifest after a subacute encephalitic prodrome (with headaches, vertigo, insomnia, and psychological abnormalities), which is followed by a gradually progressive vascular syndrome.

The manifestations of *general paresis* reflect widespread late parenchymal damage and include abnormalities corresponding to the mnemonic *paresis: p*ersonality, *a*ffect, *r*eflexes (hyperactive), *e*ye (e.g., Argyll Robertson pupils), *s*ensorium (illusions, delusions, hallucinations), *i*ntellect (a decrease in recent memory and in the capacity for orientation, calculations, judgment, and insight), and *s*peech. *Tabes dorsalis* is a late manifestation of syphilis that presents as symptoms and signs of demyelination of the posterior columns, dorsal roots, and dorsal root ganglia. Symptoms include ataxic wide-based gait and foot drop; paresthesia; bladder disturbances; impotence; areflexia; and loss of positional, deep-pain, and temperature sensations. Trophic joint degeneration (Charcot's joints) and perforating ulceration of the feet can result from loss of pain sensation. The small, irregular Argyll Robertson pupil, a feature of both tabes dorsalis and paresis, reacts to accommodation but not to light. *Optic atrophy* also occurs frequently in association with tabes.

Other Manifestations of Late Syphilis The slowly progressive inflammatory process leading to tertiary disease begins early during infection, although these manifestations may not become clinically apparent for years or decades. Early syphilitic aortitis becomes evident soon after secondary lesions subside, and treponemes that trigger the development of gummas may have seeded the tissue years earlier.

CARDIOVASCULAR SYPHILIS Cardiovascular manifestations, usually appearing 10–40 years after infection, are attributable to endarteritis obliterans of the vasa vasorum, which provide the blood supply to large vessels; *T. pallidum* DNA has been detected by PCR in aortic tissue. Cardiovascular involvement results in uncomplicated aortitis, aortic regurgitation, saccular aneurysm (usually of the ascending aorta), or coronary ostial stenosis. In the preantibiotic era, symptomatic cardiovascular complications developed in ~10% of persons with late untreated syphilis. Today, this form of late syphilis is rarely seen in the developed world. Linear calcification of the ascending aorta on chest x-ray films suggests asymptomatic syphilitic aortitis, as arteriosclerosis seldom produces this sign. Only 1 in 10 aortic aneurysms of syphilitic origin involves the abdominal aorta.

LATE BENIGN SYPHILIS (GUMMA) Gummas are usually solitary lesions ranging from microscopic to several centimeters in diameter. Histologic examination shows a granulomatous inflammation, with a central area of necrosis due to endarteritis obliterans. Although rarely demonstrated microscopically, *T. pallidum* has been detected by PCR or recovered from these lesions, and penicillin treatment results in rapid resolution, confirming the treponemal stimulus for the inflammation. Common sites include the skin and skeletal system; however, any organ (including the brain) may be involved. Gummas of the skin produce indolent, painless, indurated nodular or ulcerative lesions that may resemble other chronic granulomatous conditions, including tuberculosis, sarcoidosis, leprosy, and deep fungal infections. Skeletal gummas most frequently involve the long bones, although any bone may be affected. Upper respiratory gummas can lead to perforation of the nasal septum or palate.

Congenital Syphilis Transmission of *T. pallidum* across the placenta from a syphilitic woman to her fetus may occur at any stage of pregnancy, but fetal damage generally does not occur until after the fourth month of gestation, when fetal immunologic competence begins to develop. This timing suggests that the pathogenesis of congenital syphilis, like that of adult syphilis, depends on the host immune response rather than on a direct toxic effect of *T. pallidum*. The risk of fetal infection during untreated early maternal syphilis is ~75–95%, decreasing to ~35% for maternal syphilis of >2 years' duration. Adequate treatment of the woman before the 16th week of pregnancy should prevent fetal damage, and treatment before the third trimester should adequately treat the infected fetus. Untreated maternal infection may result in a rate of fetal loss of up to 40% (with stillbirth more common than abortion because of the late onset of fetal pathology), prematurity, neonatal death, or nonfatal congenital syphilis. Among infants born alive, only fulminant congenital syphilis is clinically apparent at birth, and these babies have a very poor prognosis. The most common clinical problem is the healthy-appearing baby born to a mother with a positive serologic test

Routine serologic testing in early pregnancy is considered cost-effective in virtually all populations, even in areas with a low prenatal prevalence of syphilis. Low-tech point-of-care tests have been developed and are being widely implemented to facilitate antenatal testing in resource-poor settings. A recent study demonstrated the high cost-effectiveness of using these tests for screening (with subsequent treatment) in sub-Saharan Africa. Adverse outcomes were reduced, with 64,000 fewer stillbirths, 25,000 fewer neonatal deaths, and up to 25,000 fewer live births of infants with syphilis. The intervention would remain cost-effective even if the current syphilis seroprevalence among pregnant women declined from its present 3.1% to 0.4%. Where the prevalence of syphilis is high or when the patient is at high risk of reinfection, serologic testing should be repeated in the third trimester and at delivery. Neonatal congenital syphilis must be differentiated from other generalized congenital infections, including rubella, cytomegalovirus or herpes simplex virus infection, and toxoplasmosis, as well as from erythroblastosis fetalis.

The manifestations of congenital syphilis include (1) early manifestations, which appear within the first 2 years of life (often at 2–10 weeks of age), are infectious, and resemble the manifestations of secondary syphilis in the adult; (2) late manifestations, which appear after 2 years and are noninfectious; and (3) residual stigmata. The earliest manifestations of congenital syphilis include rhinitis, or "snuffles" (23%); mucocutaneous lesions (35–41%); bone changes (61%), including osteochondritis, osteitis, and periostitis detectable by x-ray examination of long bones; hepatosplenomegaly (50%); lymphadenopathy (32%); anemia (34%); jaundice (30%); thrombocytopenia; and leukocytosis. CNS invasion by *T. pallidum* is detectable in 22% of infected neonates. Neonatal death is usually due to pulmonary hemorrhage, secondary bacterial infection, or severe hepatitis.

Late congenital syphilis (untreated after 2 years of age) is subclinical in 60% of cases; the clinical spectrum in the remainder of cases may include interstitial keratitis (which occurs at 5–25 years of age), eighth-nerve deafness, and recurrent arthropathy. Bilateral knee effusions are known as *Clutton's joints*. Neurosyphilis was present in about one-quarter of untreated patients with late congenital syphilis in the preantibiotic era. Gummatous periostitis occurs at 5–20 years of age and, as in nonvenereal endemic syphilis, tends to cause destructive lesions of the palate and nasal septum.

Classic stigmata include *Hutchinson's teeth* (centrally notched, widely spaced, peg-shaped upper central incisors), "mulberry" molars (sixth-year molars with multiple, poorly developed cusps), saddle nose, and saber shins.

LABORATORY EXAMINATIONS

Demonstration of the Organism *T. pallidum* cannot be detected by culture. Historically, dark-field microscopy and immunofluorescence antibody staining have been used to identify this spirochete in samples from moist lesions such as chancres or condylomata lata, but these tests are rarely available outside of research laboratories. Sensitive and specific PCR tests have been developed but are not commercially available, although a number of laboratories perform in-house validated PCR testing.

T. pallidum can be found in tissue with appropriate silver stains, but these results should be interpreted with caution because artifacts resembling *T. pallidum* are often seen. Tissue treponemes can be demonstrated more reliably in research laboratories by PCR or by immunofluorescence or immunohistochemical methods using specific monoclonal or polyclonal antibodies to *T. pallidum*.

Serologic Tests for Syphilis There are two types of serologic test for syphilis: nontreponemal and treponemal. Both are reactive in persons with any treponemal infection, including yaws, pinta, and endemic syphilis.

The most widely used nontreponemal antibody tests for syphilis are the RPR and VDRL tests, which measure IgG and IgM directed against a cardiolipin-lecithin-cholesterol antigen complex. The RPR test is easier to perform and uses unheated serum or plasma; it is the test of choice for rapid serologic diagnosis in a clinical setting. The VDRL test remains the standard for examining CSF and is superior to the RPR for this purpose. The RPR and VDRL tests are recommended for screening or for quantitation of serum antibody. The titer reflects disease activity, rising during the evolution of early syphilis, often exceeding 1:32 in secondary syphilis, and declining thereafter without therapy. After treatment for early syphilis, a persistent fall by fourfold or more (e.g., a decline from 1:32 to 1:8) is considered an adequate response. VDRL titers do not correspond directly to RPR titers, and sequential quantitative testing (as for response to therapy) must employ a single test. As will be discussed (see "Evaluation for Neurosyphilis," below), the RPR titer may be useful in determining which patients will benefit from CSF examination.

Treponemal tests measure antibodies to native or recombinant *T. pallidum* antigens and include the fluorescent treponemal antibody–absorbed (FTA-ABS) test and the *T. pallidum* particle agglutination (TPPA) test, both of which are more sensitive for primary syphilis than the previously used hemagglutination tests. The *T. pallidum* hemagglutination (TPHA) test is widely used in Europe but is not available in the United States. When used to confirm positive nontreponemal test results, treponemal tests have a very high positive predictive value for diagnosis of syphilis. Treponemal enzyme or chemiluminescence immunoassays (EIAs/CIAs), based largely on reactivity to recombinant antigens, have also been developed and are now widely used as screening tests by large laboratories. In a screening setting, however, treponemal tests give false-positive results at rates as high as 1–2%, and the rate is higher with the EIA/CIA tests. Treponemal tests are likely to remain reactive even after adequate treatment and cannot differentiate

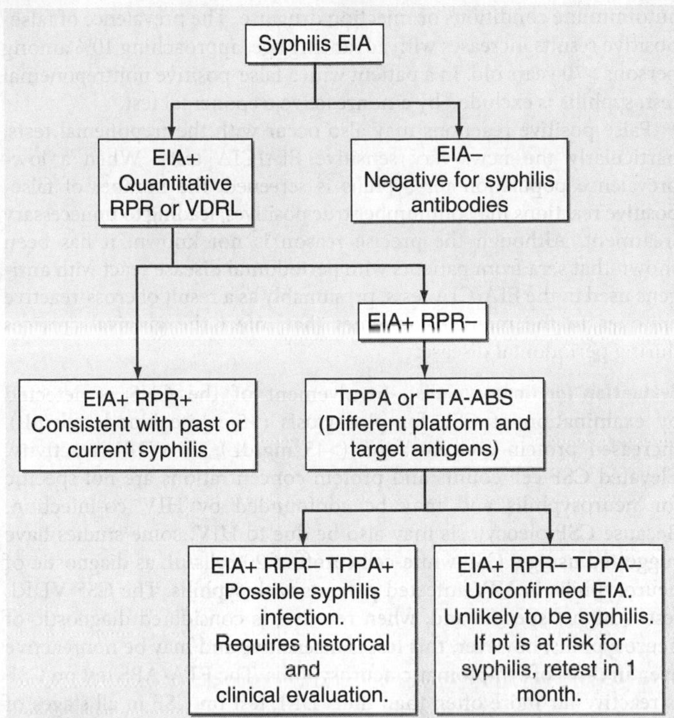

FIGURE 206-4 Algorithm for interpretation of results from syphilis enzyme immunoassays (EIAs) used for screening. FTA-ABS, fluorescent treponemal antibody–absorbed; RPR, rapid plasma reagin; TPPA, *Treponema pallidum* particle agglutination; VDRL, Venereal Disease Research Laboratory. *(Based on the 2010 Sexually Transmitted Diseases Treatment Guidelines from the Centers for Disease Control and Prevention.)*

past from current *T. pallidum* infection. Figure 206-4 provides a suggested algorithm for management of such cases.

Both nontreponemal and treponemal tests may be nonreactive in early primary syphilis, although treponemal tests are slightly more sensitive (85–90%) during this stage than nontreponemal tests (~80%). All tests are reactive during secondary syphilis. (Fewer than 1% of patients with high titers have a nontreponemal test that is nonreactive or weakly reactive with undiluted serum but is reactive with diluted serum—the *prozone phenomenon.*) VDRL and RPR sensitivity and titers may decline in untreated persons with late latent syphilis, but treponemal tests remain sensitive in these stages. After treatment for early syphilis, nontreponemal test titers will generally decline or the tests will become nonreactive, whereas treponemal tests often remain reactive after therapy and are not helpful in determining the infection status of persons with past syphilis.

For practical purposes, most clinicians need to be familiar with three uses of serologic tests for syphilis recommended by the Centers for Disease Control and Prevention (CDC): (1) screening or diagnosis (RPR or VDRL), (2) quantitative measurement of antibody to assess clinical syphilis activity or to monitor response to therapy (RPR or VDRL), and (3) confirmation of a syphilis diagnosis in a patient with a reactive RPR or VDRL test (FTA-ABS, TPPA, EIA/CIA). Studies have not demonstrated the utility of IgM testing for adult syphilis. Whereas IgM titers appear to decline after therapy, the presence or absence of specific IgM does not strictly correlate with *T. pallidum* infection. Moreover, no commercially available IgM test is recommended, even for evaluation of infants with suspected congenital syphilis.

False-Positive Serologic Tests for Syphilis The lipid antigens of nontreponemal tests are similar to those found in human tissues, and the tests may be reactive (usually with titers ≤1:8) in persons without treponemal infection. Among patients being screened for syphilis because of risk factors, clinical suspicion, or history of exposure, ~1% of reactive tests are falsely positive. Modern VDRL and RPR tests are highly specific, and false-positive reactions are largely limited to persons with autoimmune conditions or injection drug use. The prevalence of false-positive results increases with advancing age, approaching 10% among persons >70 years old. In a patient with a false-positive nontreponemal test, syphilis is excluded by a nonreactive treponemal test.

False-positive reactions may also occur with the treponemal tests, particularly the new, very sensitive EIA/CIA tests. When a low-prevalence population for syphilis is screened, the number of false-positive reactions may outnumber true positives, leading to unnecessary treatment. Although the precise reason is not known, it has been shown that sera from patients with periodontal disease react with antigens used in the EIA/CIA tests, presumably as a result of cross-reactive epitopes in the many treponemes that infect the gingival crevices during periodontal disease.

Evaluation for Neurosyphilis Involvement of the CNS is detected by examination of CSF for pleocytosis (>5 white blood cells/μL), increased protein concentration (>45 mg/dL), or VDRL reactivity. Elevated CSF cell counts and protein concentrations are not specific for neurosyphilis and may be confounded by HIV co-infection. Because CSF pleocytosis may also be due to HIV, some studies have suggested using a CSF white-cell cutoff of 20 cells/μL as diagnostic of neurosyphilis in HIV-infected patients with syphilis. The CSF VDRL test is highly specific and, when reactive, is considered diagnostic of neurosyphilis; however, this test is insensitive and may be nonreactive even in cases of symptomatic neurosyphilis. The FTA-ABS test on CSF is reactive far more often than the VDRL test on CSF in all stages of syphilis, but reactivity may reflect passive transfer of serum antibody into the CSF. A nonreactive FTA-ABS test on CSF, however, may be used to rule out asymptomatic neurosyphilis. The utility of measuring CXCL13 in CSF to distinguish between neurosyphilis and HIV-related CSF abnormalities has been demonstrated.

Clearly, all *T. pallidum*–infected patients who have signs or symptoms consistent with neurologic disease (e.g., meningitis, hearing loss) or ophthalmic disease (e.g., uveitis, iritis) should have a CSF examination, regardless of disease stage. The appropriate management of asymptomatic persons is less clear. Lumbar puncture on all asymptomatic patients with untreated syphilis is impractical and unnecessary. Because standard therapy with penicillin G benzathine fails to result in treponemicidal drug levels in CSF, however, it is important to identify those persons at higher risk for having or developing neurosyphilis so that appropriate therapy may be given. Viable *T. pallidum* has been isolated from the CSF of several patients (with and without concurrent HIV infection) after penicillin G benzathine therapy for early syphilis. Large-scale prospective studies have now provided evidence-based guidelines for determining which syphilis patients may benefit most from CSF examination for evidence of neurosyphilis. Specifically, patients with RPR titers of ≥1:32 are at higher risk of having neurosyphilis (11-fold and 6-fold higher in HIV-infected and HIV-uninfected persons, respectively), as are HIV-infected patients with CD4+ T cell counts of ≤350/μL. Guidelines for CSF examination are shown in Table 206-1.

Evaluation of HIV-Infected Patients for Syphilis Because persons at highest risk for syphilis are also at increased risk for HIV infection, these two infections frequently coexist. There is evidence that syphilis and other genital ulcer diseases are important risk factors for acquisition and transmission of HIV infection. Some manifestations of syphilis may be altered in patients with concurrent HIV infection, and multiple cases of neurologic relapse after standard therapy have been reported in these patients.

Persons with newly diagnosed HIV infection should be tested for syphilis; conversely, all patients with newly diagnosed syphilis should be tested for HIV infection. Some authorities, persuaded by reports of persistent *T. pallidum* in CSF of HIV-infected persons after standard therapy for early syphilis, recommend CSF examination for evidence of neurosyphilis for all co-infected patients, regardless of the stage of syphilis, with treatment for neurosyphilis if CSF abnormalities are found. Others, on the basis of their own clinical experience, believe that standard therapy—without CSF examination—is sufficient for all cases of early syphilis in HIV-infected patients without neurologic signs or symptoms. As described above, RPR titer and CD4+ T cell count can be used to identify patients at higher risk of neurosyphilis for lumbar puncture, although some cases of neurosyphilis will be missed, even when these criteria are used. Table 206-1 summarizes guidelines suggested by published studies. Serologic testing after treatment is important for all patients with syphilis, particularly for those also infected with HIV.

TABLE 206-1 INDICATIONS FOR CEREBROSPINAL FLUID EXAMINATION IN ADULTS WITH ALL STAGES OF SYPHILIS

All Patients
Signs or symptoms of nervous system involvement (e.g., meningitis, hearing loss, cranial nerve dysfunction, altered mental status, ophthalmic disease [e.g., uveitis, iritis, pupillary abnormalities], ataxia, loss of vibration sense), *or*
RPR or VDRL titer ≥1:32, *or*
Active tertiary syphilis, *or*
Suspected treatment failure
Additional Indications in HIV-Infected Persons
CD4+ T cell count ≤350/μL, *or*
All HIV-infected persons (recommended by some experts)

Source: Adapted from the 2010 Sexually Transmitted Diseases Treatment Guidelines from the Centers for Disease Control and Prevention.

TREATMENT SYPHILIS

TREATMENT OF ACQUIRED SYPHILIS

The CDC's 2010 guidelines for the treatment of syphilis are summarized in Table 206-2 and are discussed below. Penicillin G is the drug of choice for all stages of syphilis. *T. pallidum* is killed by very low concentrations of penicillin G, although a long period of exposure to penicillin is required because of the unusually slow rate of multiplication of the organism. The efficacy of penicillin against syphilis remains undiminished after 60 years of use, and there is no evidence of penicillin resistance in *T. pallidum*. Other antibiotics effective in syphilis include the tetracyclines and the cephalosporins. Aminoglycosides and spectinomycin inhibit *T. pallidum* only in very large doses, and the sulfonamides and the quinolones are inactive. Azithromycin has shown significant promise as an effective oral agent against *T. pallidum*; however, strains harboring 23S rRNA mutations that confer macrolide resistance are widespread; such strains represent >80% of recent isolates from Seattle and San Francisco and have now been identified in multiple North American and European sites. Macrolide resistance mutations have been identified in nearly all samples reported from some regions of China. In contrast, a study based in Madagascar documented the equivalence of benzathine penicillin and azithromycin for treatment of early syphilis, although a sample from one azithromycin clinical failure in that study showed the presence of a 23S rRNA resistance mutation. A more recent survey from South Africa showed a very low (1%) frequency of known 23s rRNA resistance mutations. In short, the prevalence of resistant strains varies widely by geographic location, and routine treatment of syphilis with azithromycin is not recommended. In all cases, careful follow-up of any patient treated for syphilis with azithromycin must be ensured.

Early Syphilis Patients and Their Contacts Penicillin G benzathine is the most widely used agent for the treatment of early syphilis; a single dose of 2.4 million units is recommended. Preventive treatment is also recommended for individuals who have been exposed to infectious syphilis within the previous 3 months. *The regimens recommended for prevention are the same as those recommended for early syphilis.* Penicillin G benzathine cures >95% of cases of early syphilis, although clinical relapse can follow treatment, particularly in patients with concurrent HIV infection. Because the risk of neurologic relapse may be higher in HIV-infected patients, CSF examination is recommended in HIV-seropositive individuals with syphilis of any stage, particularly those with a serum RPR titer of ≥1:32 or a

TABLE 206-2 RECOMMENDATIONS FOR THE TREATMENT OF SYPHILIS[a]

Stage of Syphilis	Patients without Penicillin Allergy	Patients with Confirmed Penicillin Allergy[b]
Primary, secondary, or early latent	*CSF normal or not examined:* Penicillin G benzathine (single dose of 2.4 mU IM) *CSF abnormal:* Treat as neurosyphilis	*CSF normal or not examined:* Tetracycline HCl (500 mg PO qid) or doxycycline (100 mg PO bid) for 2 weeks *CSF abnormal:* Treat as neurosyphilis
Late latent (or latent of uncertain duration), cardiovascular, or benign tertiary	*CSF normal or not examined:* Penicillin G benzathine (2.4 mU IM weekly for 3 weeks) *CSF abnormal:* Treat as neurosyphilis	*CSF normal and patient not infected with HIV:* Tetracycline HCl (500 mg PO qid) or doxycycline (100 mg PO bid) for 4 weeks *CSF normal and patient infected with HIV:* Desensitization and treatment with penicillin if compliance cannot be ensured *CSF abnormal:* Treat as neurosyphilis
Neurosyphilis (asymptomatic or symptomatic)	Aqueous crystalline penicillin G (18–24 mU/d IV, given as 3–4 mU q4h or continuous infusion) for 10–14 days *or* Aqueous procaine penicillin G (2.4 mU/d IM) plus oral probenecid (500 mg qid), both for 10–14 days	Desensitization and treatment with penicillin[c]
Syphilis in pregnancy	According to stage	Desensitization and treatment with penicillin

[a]See Table 206-1 and text for indications for CSF examination. [b]Because of the documented presence of macrolide resistance in many *T. pallidum* strains in North America, Europe, and China, azithromycin or other macrolides should be used with caution only when treatment with penicillin or doxycycline is not feasible. Azithromycin should not be used for men who have sex with men or for pregnant women. [c]Limited data suggest that ceftriaxone (2 g/d either IM or IV for 10–14 days) can be used; however, cross-reactivity between penicillin and ceftriaxone is possible.

Abbreviations: CSF, cerebrospinal fluid; mU, million units.

Source: Adapted from the 2010 Sexually Transmitted Diseases Treatment Guidelines from the Centers for Disease Control and Prevention.

CD4+ T cell count of ≤350/μL. Therapy appropriate for neurosyphilis should be given if there is any evidence of CNS infection.

Late Latent Syphilis or Syphilis of Unknown Duration If the CSF is normal or is not examined, the recommended treatment is penicillin G benzathine (7.2 million units total; Table 206-2). If CSF abnormalities are found, the patient should be treated for neurosyphilis.

Tertiary Syphilis CSF examination should be performed. If the CSF is normal, the recommended treatment is penicillin G benzathine (7.2 million units total; Table 206-2). If CSF abnormalities are found, the patient should be treated for neurosyphilis. The clinical response to treatment for benign tertiary syphilis is usually impressive. However, responses to therapy for cardiovascular syphilis are not dramatic because aortic aneurysm and aortic regurgitation cannot be reversed by antibiotics.

Syphilis in Penicillin-Allergic Patients For penicillin-allergic patients with syphilis, a 2-week (early syphilis) or 4-week (late or late latent syphilis) course of therapy with doxycycline or tetracycline is recommended (Table 206-2). These regimens appear to be effective in early syphilis but have not been tested for late or late latent syphilis, and compliance may be problematic. Limited studies suggest that ceftriaxone (1 g/d, given IM or IV for 8–10 days) is effective for early syphilis. These nonpenicillin regimens have not been carefully evaluated in HIV-infected individuals and should be used with caution. If compliance and follow-up cannot be ensured, penicillin-allergic HIV-infected persons with late latent or late syphilis should be desensitized and treated with penicillin.

Neurosyphilis Penicillin G benzathine, given in total doses of up to 7.2 million units, does not produce detectable concentrations of penicillin G in CSF and should not be used for treatment of neurosyphilis. Asymptomatic neurosyphilis may relapse as symptomatic disease after treatment with benzathine penicillin, and the risk of relapse may be higher in HIV-infected patients. Both symptomatic and asymptomatic neurosyphilis should be treated with aqueous penicillin (Table 206-2). Administration either of IV aqueous crystalline penicillin G or of IM aqueous procaine penicillin G plus oral probenecid in recommended doses is thought to ensure treponemicidal concentrations of penicillin G in CSF. The clinical response to penicillin therapy for meningeal syphilis is dramatic, but treatment of neurosyphilis with existing parenchymal damage may only arrest disease progression. No data suggest that additional therapy (e.g., penicillin G benzathine for 3 weeks) is beneficial after treatment for neurosyphilis.

The use of antibiotics other than penicillin G for the treatment of neurosyphilis has not been studied, although very limited data suggest that ceftriaxone may be used. In patients with penicillin allergy demonstrated by skin testing, desensitization and treatment with penicillin are recommended.

Management of Syphilis in Pregnancy Every pregnant woman should undergo a nontreponemal test at her first prenatal visit and, if at high risk of exposure, again in the third trimester and at delivery. In the untreated pregnant patient with presumed syphilis, expeditious treatment appropriate to the stage of the disease is essential. Patients should be warned of the risk of a Jarisch-Herxheimer reaction, which may be associated with mild premature contractions but rarely results in premature delivery.

Penicillin is the only recommended agent for the treatment of syphilis in pregnancy. If the patient has a documented penicillin allergy, desensitization and penicillin therapy should be undertaken according to the CDC's 2010 guidelines. After treatment, a quantitative nontreponemal test should be repeated monthly throughout pregnancy to assess therapeutic efficacy. Treated women whose antibody titers rise by fourfold or whose titers do not decrease by fourfold over a 3-month period should be re-treated.

EVALUATION AND MANAGEMENT OF CONGENITAL SYPHILIS

Whether or not they are infected, newborn infants of mothers with reactive serologic tests may themselves have reactive tests because of transplacental transfer of maternal IgG antibody. For asymptomatic infants born to women treated adequately with penicillin during the first or second trimester of pregnancy, monthly quantitative nontreponemal tests may be performed to monitor for appropriate reduction in antibody titers. Rising or persistent titers indicate infection, and the infant should be treated. Detection of neonatal IgM antibody may be useful, but no commercially available test is currently recommended.

An infant should be treated at birth if the treatment status of the seropositive mother is unknown; if the mother has received inadequate or nonpenicillin therapy; if the mother received penicillin therapy in the third trimester; or if the infant may be difficult to follow. The CSF should be examined to obtain baseline values before treatment. Penicillin is the only recommended drug for the treatment of syphilis in infants. Specific recommendations for the treatment of infants and older children are included in the CDC's 2010 treatment guidelines.

JARISCH-HERXHEIMER REACTION

A dramatic although usually mild reaction consisting of fever, chills, myalgias, headache, tachycardia, increased respiratory rate, increased circulating neutrophil count, and vasodilation with mild hypotension may follow the initiation of treatment for syphilis. This reaction is thought to be a response to lipoproteins released by dying *T. pallidum* organisms. The Jarisch-Herxheimer reaction occurs in ~50% of patients with primary syphilis, 90% of those with secondary syphilis, and a lower proportion of persons with later-stage disease. Defervescence takes place within 12–24 h. In patients with secondary syphilis, erythema and edema of the mucocutaneous lesions may increase. Patients should be warned to expect such symptoms, which can be managed with symptom-based treatment. Steroid or other anti-inflammatory therapy is not required for this mild transient reaction.

FOLLOW-UP EVALUATION OF RESPONSES TO THERAPY

Efficacy of treatment should be assessed by clinical evaluation and monitoring of the quantitative VDRL or RPR titer for a fourfold decline (e.g., from 1:32 to 1:8). Patients with primary or secondary syphilis should be examined 6 and 12 months after treatment and persons with latent or late syphilis at 6, 12, and 24 months. More frequent clinical and serologic examination (3, 6, 9, 12, and 24 months) is recommended for patients concurrently infected with HIV, regardless of the stage of syphilis.

After successful treatment of seropositive first-episode primary or secondary syphilis, the VDRL or RPR titer progressively declines, becoming negative by 12 months in 40–75% of seropositive primary cases and in 20–40% of secondary cases. Patients with HIV infection or a history of prior syphilis are less likely to become nonreactive in the VDRL or RPR test. Rates of decline of serologic titers appear to be slower, and serologically defined treatment failures more common, among HIV-infected patients than among those without HIV co-infection; however, effective antiretroviral therapy may reduce these differences. Re-treatment should be considered if serologic responses are not adequate or if clinical signs persist or recur. Because it is difficult to differentiate treatment failure from reinfection, the CSF should be examined, with treatment for neurosyphilis if CSF is abnormal and treatment for late latent syphilis if CSF is normal. A minority of patients treated for early syphilis may experience a one-dilution titer increase within 14 days after treatment; however, this early elevation does not significantly affect the serologic outcome at 6 months after treatment. Patients treated for late latent syphilis frequently have low initial VDRL or RPR titers and may not have a fourfold decline after therapy with penicillin. In such patients, re-treatment is not warranted unless the titer rises or signs and symptoms of syphilis appear. Because treponemal tests may remain reactive despite treatment for seropositive syphilis, these tests are not useful in following the response to therapy.

The activity of neurosyphilis (symptomatic or asymptomatic) correlates best with CSF pleocytosis, and this measure provides the most sensitive index of response to treatment. Repeat CSF examinations should be performed every 6 months until the cell count is normal. An elevated CSF cell count falls to normal in 3–12 months in adequately treated HIV-uninfected patients. The persistence of mild pleocytosis in HIV-infected patients may be due to the presence of HIV in CSF; this scenario may be difficult to distinguish from treatment failure. Elevated levels of CSF protein fall more slowly, and the CSF VDRL titer declines gradually over several years. In patients treated for neurosyphilis, a fourfold reduction in serum RPR titer has been positively correlated with normalization of CSF abnormalities; this correlation is stronger in HIV-uninfected patients and in HIV-infected patients receiving effective antiretroviral therapy.

IMMUNITY TO SYPHILIS

The rate of development of acquired resistance to *T. pallidum* after natural or experimental infection is related to the size of the antigenic stimulus, which depends on both the size of the infecting inoculum and the duration of infection before treatment. Both humoral and cellular responses are considered to be of major importance in immunity and in the healing of early lesions. Cellular infiltration, predominantly by T lymphocytes and macrophages, produces a T_H1 cytokine milieu consistent with the clearance of organisms by activated macrophages. Specific antibody enhances phagocytosis and is required for macrophage-mediated killing of *T. pallidum*. Recent studies demonstrate antigenic variation of the TprK protein, which may lead to persistence of infection and determine susceptibility to reinfection with another strain. Comparative genomic studies have revealed some sequence variations among *T. pallidum* strains, which can be differentiated by molecular typing methods. Possible correlations between molecular type and clinical manifestations are being examined.

207e Endemic Treponematoses

Sheila A. Lukehart

This is a digital-only chapter. It is available on the DVD that accompanies this book, as well as on Access Medicine/Harrison's Online, and the eBook and "app" editions of HPIM 19e.

The endemic treponematoses are chronic diseases that are transmitted by direct contact, usually during childhood, and, like syphilis, can cause severe late manifestations years after initial infection. These diseases are caused by very close relatives of *Treponema pallidum* subspecies *pallidum*, the etiologic agent of venereal syphilis (Chap. 206). Yaws, pinta, and endemic syphilis are traditionally distinguished from venereal syphilis by mode of transmission, age of acquisition, geographic distribution, and clinical features; however, there is some overlap for each of these factors. Generally, yaws flourishes in moist tropical areas of several regions, endemic syphilis is found primarily in arid climates, and pinta is found in temperate foci in the Americas. These infections are usually limited to rural areas of developing nations and are seen in developed countries only among recent immigrants from endemic regions.

208 Leptospirosis

Rudy A. Hartskeerl, Jiří F. P. Wagenaar

Leptospirosis is a globally important zoonotic disease whose apparent reemergence is illustrated by recent outbreaks on virtually all continents. The disease is caused by pathogenic *Leptospira* species and is characterized by a broad spectrum of clinical manifestations, varying from asymptomatic infection to fulminant, fatal disease. In its mild form, leptospirosis may present as nonspecific symptoms such as fever, headache, and myalgia. Severe leptospirosis, characterized by jaundice, renal dysfunction, and hemorrhagic diathesis, is often referred to as *Weil's syndrome*. With or without jaundice, severe pulmonary hemorrhage is increasingly recognized as an important presentation of severe disease.

ETIOLOGIC AGENT

Leptospira species are spirochetes belonging to the order Spirochaetales and the family Leptospiraceae. Traditionally, the genus *Leptospira* comprised two species: the pathogenic *L. interrogans* and the free-living *L. biflexa*, now designated *L. interrogans* sensu lato and *L. biflexa* sensu lato, respectively. Twenty-two *Leptospira* species with pathogenic (10 species), intermediate (5 species), and nonpathogenic (7 species) status have now been described on the basis of phylogenetic and virulence

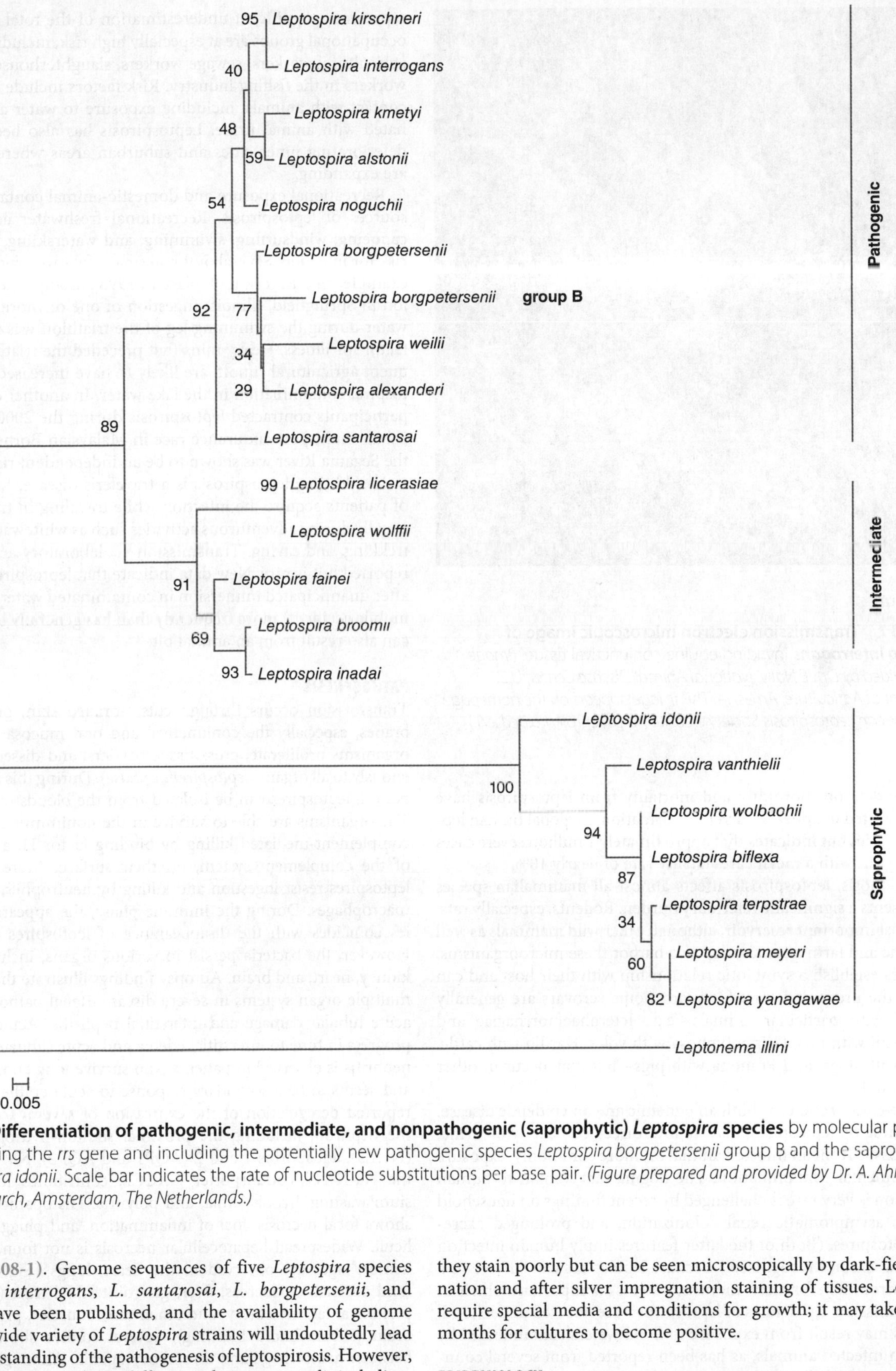

95 Leptospira kirschneri
40 Leptospira interrogans
48 Leptospira kmetyi
59 Leptospira alstonii
54 Leptospira noguchii
Leptospira borgpetersenii
92 77 Leptospira borgpetersenii group B
34 Leptospira weilii
29 Leptospira alexanderi
89 Leptospira santarosai
99 Leptospira licerasiae
Leptospira wolffii
91 Leptospira fainei
69 Leptospira broomii
93 Leptospira inadai
Leptospira idonii
100 Leptospira vanthielii
94 Leptospira wolbachii
87 Leptospira biflexa
34 Leptospira terpstrae
60 Leptospira meyeri
82 Leptospira yanagawae
Leptonema illini
0.005
Pathogenic
Intermediate
Saprophytic

FIGURE 208-1 Differentiation of pathogenic, intermediate, and nonpathogenic (saprophytic) *Leptospira* species by molecular phylogenetic analysis using the *rrs* gene and including the potentially new pathogenic species *Leptospira borgpetersenii* group B and the saprophytic species *Leptospira idonii*. Scale bar indicates the rate of nucleotide substitutions per base pair. *(Figure prepared and provided by Dr. A. Ahmed, KIT Biomedical Research, Amsterdam, The Netherlands.)*

analyses (Fig. 208-1). Genome sequences of five *Leptospira* species (*L. biflexa*, *L. interrogans*, *L. santarosai*, *L. borgpetersenii*, and *L. licerasiae*) have been published, and the availability of genome sequences of a wide variety of *Leptospira* strains will undoubtedly lead to a better understanding of the pathogenesis of leptospirosis. However, classification based on serologic differences better serves clinical, diagnostic, and epidemiologic purposes. Pathogenic *Leptospira* species are divided into serovars according to their antigenic composition. More than 250 serovars make up the 26 serogroups.

Leptospires are coiled, thin, highly motile organisms that have hooked ends and two periplasmic flagella, with polar extrusions from the cytoplasmic membrane that are responsible for motility (Fig. 208-2). These organisms are 6–20 μm long and ~0.1 μm wide; they stain poorly but can be seen microscopically by dark-field examination and after silver impregnation staining of tissues. Leptospires require special media and conditions for growth; it may take weeks to months for cultures to become positive.

EPIDEMIOLOGY

Leptospirosis has a worldwide distribution but occurs most commonly in the tropics and subtropics because the climate and occasionally poor hygienic conditions favor the pathogen's survival and distribution. In most countries, leptospirosis is an underappreciated problem. Most cases occur in men, with a peak incidence during the summer and fall in both the Northern and Southern Hemispheres and during the rainy season in the tropics.

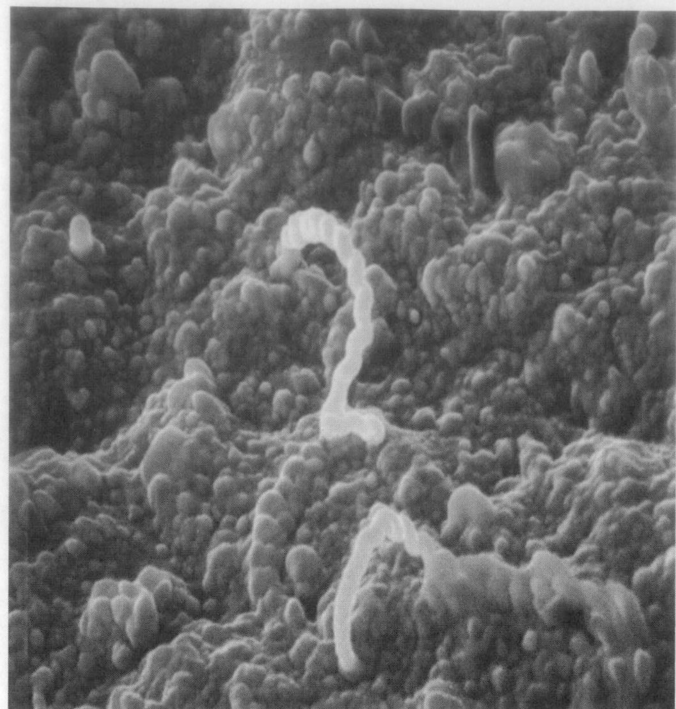

FIGURE 208-2 Transmission electron microscopic image of *Leptospira interrogans* invading equine conjunctival tissue. *(Image kindly provided by Dr. JE Nally, National Animal Disease Center, U.S. Department of Agriculture, Ames, IA. This image appears on the homepage of the European Leptospirosis Society website [http://eurolepto.ucd.ie/].)*

Reliable data on morbidity and mortality from leptospirosis have gradually started to appear. Current information on global human leptospirosis varies but indicates that approximately 1 million severe cases occur per year, with a mean case–fatality rate of nearly 10%.

As a zoonosis, leptospirosis affects almost all mammalian species and represents a significant veterinary burden. Rodents, especially rats, are the most important reservoir, although other wild mammals as well as domestic and farm animals may also harbor these microorganisms. Leptospires establish a symbiotic relationship with their host and can persist in the urogenital tract for years. Some serovars are generally associated with particular animals—e.g., Icterohaemorrhagiae and Copenhageni with rats, Grippotyphosa with voles, Hardjo with cattle, Canicola with dogs, and Pomona with pigs—but may occur in other animals as well.

Leptospirosis presents as both an endemic and an epidemic disease. Transmission of leptospires may follow direct contact with urine, blood, or tissue from an infected animal or, more commonly, exposure to environmental contamination. The dogma that human-to-human transmission is very rare is challenged by recent findings on household clustering, asymptomatic renal colonization, and prolonged excretion of leptospires. (Both of the latter features imply human infection sources that are not recognized.) Because leptospires can survive in a humid environment for many months, water is an important vehicle in their transmission. Epidemics of leptospirosis are not well understood. Outbreaks may result from exposure to flood waters contaminated by urine from infected animals, as has been reported from several countries. However, it is also true that outbreaks may occur without floods, and floods often occur without outbreaks.

The vast majority of infections with *Leptospira* cause no or only mild disease in humans. A small percentage of infections (~1%) lead to severe, potentially fatal complications. The proportion of leptospirosis cases that are mild is unknown because patients either do not seek or do not have access to medical care or because the nonspecific symptoms are interpreted as an influenza-like illness. Reported cases surely represent a significant underestimation of the total number. Certain occupational groups are at especially high risk, including veterinarians, agricultural workers, sewage workers, slaughterhouse employees, and workers in the fishing industry. Risk factors include direct or indirect contact with animals, including exposure to water and soil contaminated with animal urine. Leptospirosis has also been recognized in deteriorating inner cities and suburban areas where rat populations are expanding.

Recreational exposure and domestic-animal contact are prominent sources of leptospirosis. Recreational freshwater activities, such as canoeing, windsurfing, swimming, and waterskiing, place persons at risk for infection. Several outbreaks have followed sporting events. For example, an outbreak took place in 1998 among athletes after a triathlon in Springfield, Illinois. Ingestion of one or more swallows of lake water during the swimming leg of the triathlon was a prominent risk factor for illness. Heavy rains that preceded the triathlon, with consequent agricultural runoff, are likely to have increased the level of leptospiral contamination in the lake water. In another outbreak, 42% of participants contracted leptospirosis during the 2000 Eco-Challenge-Sabah multisport endurance race in Malaysian Borneo. Swimming in the Segama River was shown to be an independent risk factor.

In addition, leptospirosis is a traveler's disease. Large proportions of patients acquire the infection while traveling in tropical countries, usually during adventurous activities such as whitewater rafting, jungle trekking, and caving. Transmission via laboratory accidents has been reported but is rare. New data indicate that leptospirosis may develop after unanticipated immersion in contaminated water (e.g., in an automobile accident) more frequently than has generally been thought and can also result from an animal bite.

PATHOGENESIS

Transmission occurs through cuts, abraded skin, or mucous membranes, especially the conjunctival and oral mucosa. After entry, the organisms proliferate, cross tissue barriers, and disseminate hematogenously to all organs (*leptospiremic phase*). During this initial incubation period, leptospires can be isolated from the bloodstream (Fig. 208-3). The organisms are able to survive in the nonimmune host: they evade complement-mediated killing by binding factor H, a strong inhibitor of the complement system, on their surface. Moreover, pathogenic leptospires resist ingestion and killing by neutrophils, monocytes, and macrophages. During the immune phase, the appearance of antibodies coincides with the disappearance of leptospires from the blood. However, the bacteria persist in various organs, including liver, lung, kidney, heart, and brain. Autopsy findings illustrate the involvement of multiple organ systems in severe disease. Renal pathology shows both acute tubular damage and interstitial nephritis. Acute tubular lesions progress in time to interstitial edema and acute tubular necrosis. Severe nephritis is observed in patients who survive long enough to develop it and seems to be a secondary response to acute epithelial damage. The reported deregulation of the expression of several transporters along the nephron, including the proximal sodium-hydrogen exchanger 3 (NHE3), aquaporins 1 and 2 (AQP1 and AQP2), Na^+-K^+ ATPase, and the Na-K-2Cl cotransporter NKCC2, contributes to tubular potassium wasting, hypokalemia, and polyuria. Histopathology of the liver shows focal necrosis, foci of inflammation, and plugging of bile canaliculi. Widespread hepatocellular necrosis is not found. Petechiae and hemorrhages are observed in the heart, lungs (Fig. 208-4), kidneys (and adrenals), pancreas, liver, gastrointestinal tract (including retroperitoneal fat, mesentery, and omentum), muscles, prostate, testis, and brain (subarachnoid bleeding). Several studies show an association between hemorrhage and thrombocytopenia. Although the underlying mechanisms of thrombocytopenia have not been elucidated, it seems likely that platelet consumption plays an important role. A consumptive coagulopathy may occur, with elevated markers of coagulation activation (thrombin–antithrombin complexes, prothrombin fragments 1 and 2, D-dimer), diminished anticoagulant markers (antithrombin, protein C), and deregulated fibrinolytic activity. Overt disseminated intravascular coagulation (DIC) has been documented in patients from Thailand and Indonesia. Elevated plasma levels of soluble E-selectin and

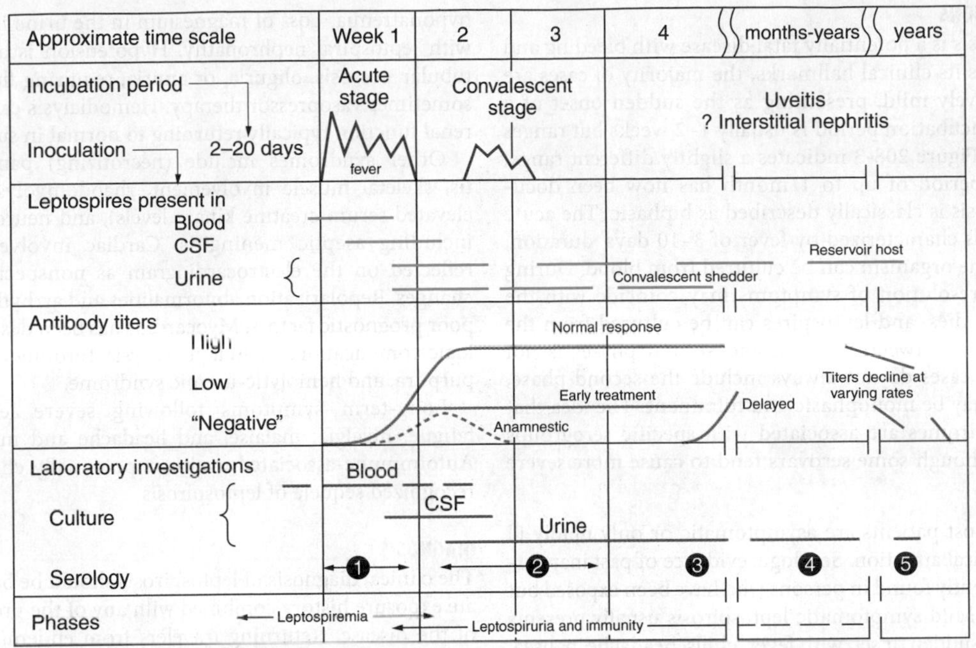

FIGURE 208-3 Biphasic nature of leptospirosis and relevant investigations at different stages of disease. *Note that an incubation period of up to 1 month has now been documented.* Specimens 1 and 2 for serology are acute-phase serum samples, specimen 3 is a convalescent-phase serum sample that may facilitate detection of a delayed immune response; and specimens 4 and 5 are follow-up serum samples that can provide epidemiologic information, such as the presumptive infecting serogroup. CSF, cerebrospinal fluid. *(Reprinted as adapted by PN Levett: Clin Microbiol Rev 14:296, 2001 [from LH Turner: Leptospirosis. BMJ 1:231, 1969] with permission from the American Society for Microbiology and the BMJ Publishing Group.)*

von Willebrand factor in patients with leptospirosis reflect endothelial cell activation. Experimental models show that pathogenic leptospires or leptospiral proteins are able to activate endothelial cells in vitro and to disrupt endothelial-cell barrier function, promoting dissemination. Platelets have been shown to aggregate on activated endothelium in the human lung, whereas histology reveals swelling of activated endothelial cells but no evident vasculitis or necrosis. Immunoglobulin and complement deposition have been demonstrated in lung tissue involved in pulmonary hemorrhage.

Leptospira species have a typical double-membrane cell wall structure harboring a variety of membrane associated proteins, including an unusually high number of lipoproteins. The peptidoglycan layer is located close to the cytoplasmic membrane. The lipopolysaccharide (LPS) in the outer membrane has an unusual structure with a relatively low endotoxic potency. Pathogenic leptospires contain a variety of genes coding for proteins involved in motility and in cell and tissue adhesion and invasion that represent potential virulence factors. Many of these are surface-exposed outer-membrane proteins (OMPs). To date, the only leptospiral virulence factor shown to satisfy Koch's molecular postulates is *loa22* encoding a surface-exposed protein with an unknown function. However, the gene is not confined to pathogenic *Leptospira* species.

Immunity to *Leptospira* depends on the production of circulating antibodies to serovar-specific LPS. It is unclear whether other antigens play a significant role in protective humoral immunity. Moreover, immunity may not be confined to antibody responses; involvement of the innate-immune Toll-like receptor 2 (TLR2) and TLR4 activation pathways in controlling infection has been demonstrated, whereas in vaccinated cattle a cell-mediated immune response is correlated with protection.

It is likely that several surface-exposed proteins mediate leptospire–host cell interactions, and these proteins may represent candidate vaccine components. Although animal-model studies have shown various degrees of vaccine efficacy for various putative virulence-associated OMPs, it is not yet clear whether such proteins elicit acceptable levels of sterilizing immunity.

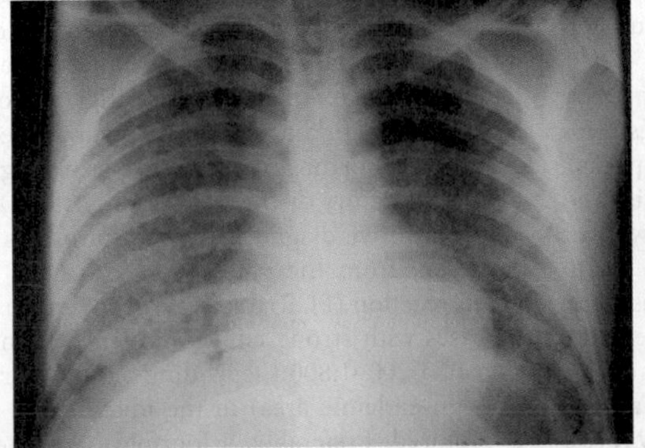

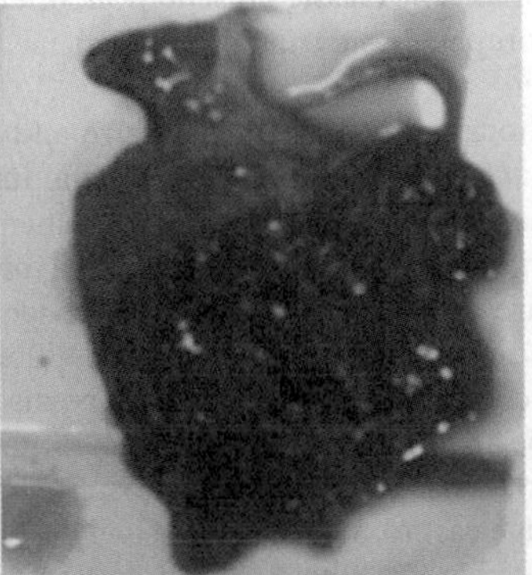

FIGURE 208-4 Severe pulmonary hemorrhage in leptospirosis. ***Left panel:*** Chest x-ray. ***Right panel:*** Gross appearance of right lower lobes of lung at autopsy. This patient, a 15-year-old from the Peruvian Amazonian city of Iquitos, died several days after presentation with acute illness, jaundice, and hemoptysis. Blood culture yielded *Leptospira interrogans* serovar Copenhageni/Icterohaemorrhagiae. *(Adapted with permission from E Segura et al: Clin Infect Dis 40:343, 2005. © 2005 by the Infectious Diseases Society of America.)*

Although leptospirosis is a potentially fatal disease with bleeding and multiorgan failure as its clinical hallmarks, the majority of cases are thought to be relatively mild, presenting as the sudden onset of a febrile illness. The incubation period is usually 1–2 weeks but ranges from 1 to 30 days. (Figure 208-3 indicates a slightly different range, but an incubation period of up to 1 month has now been documented.) Leptospirosis is classically described as biphasic. The acute *leptospiremic phase* is characterized by fever of 3–10 days' duration, during which time the organism can be cultured from blood. During the *immune phase*, resolution of symptoms may coincide with the appearance of antibodies, and leptospires can be cultured from the urine. The distinction between the first and second phases is not always clear: milder cases do not always include the second phase, and severe disease may be monophasic and fulminant. The idea that distinct clinical syndromes are associated with specific serogroups has been refuted, although some serovars tend to cause more severe disease than others.

Mild Leptospirosis Most patients are asymptomatic or only mildly ill and do not seek medical attention. Serologic evidence of past inapparent infection is frequently found in persons who have been exposed but have not become ill. Mild symptomatic leptospirosis usually presents as a flu-like illness of sudden onset, with fever, chills, headache, nausea, vomiting, abdominal pain, conjunctival suffusion (redness without exudate), and myalgia. Muscle pain is intense and especially affects the calves, back, and abdomen. The headache is intense, localized to the frontal or retroorbital region (resembling that occurring in dengue), and sometimes accompanied by photophobia. Aseptic meningitis may be present and is more common among children than among adults. Although *Leptospira* can be cultured from the cerebrospinal fluid (CSF) in the early phase, the majority of cases follow a benign course with regard to the central nervous system; symptoms disappear within a few days but may persist for weeks.

Physical examination may include any of the following findings, none of which is pathognomonic for leptospirosis: fever, conjunctival suffusion, pharyngeal injection, muscle tenderness, lymphadenopathy, rash, meningismus, hepatomegaly, and splenomegaly. If present, the rash is often transient; may be macular, maculopapular, erythematous, or hemorrhagic (petechial or ecchymotic); and may be misdiagnosed as due to scrub typhus or viral infection. Lung auscultation may reveal crackles, and mild jaundice may be present.

The natural course of mild leptospirosis usually involves spontaneous resolution within 7–10 days, but persistent symptoms have been documented. In the absence of a clinical diagnosis and antimicrobial therapy, the mortality rate in mild leptospirosis is low.

Severe Leptospirosis Although the onset of severe leptospirosis may be no different from that of mild leptospirosis, severe disease is often rapidly progressive and is associated with a case–fatality rate ranging from 1 to 50%. Higher mortality rates are associated with an age >40, altered mental status, acute renal failure, respiratory insufficiency, hypotension, and arrhythmias. The classic presentation, often referred to as *Weil's syndrome*, encompasses the triad of hemorrhage, jaundice, and acute kidney injury.

Patients die of septic shock with multiorgan failure and/or severe bleeding complications that most commonly involve the lungs (pulmonary hemorrhage), gastrointestinal tract (melena, hemoptysis), urogenital tract (hematuria), and skin (petechiae, ecchymosis, and bleeding from venipuncture sites). Pulmonary hemorrhage (with or without jaundice) is now recognized as a widespread public health problem, presenting with cough, chest pain, respiratory distress, and hemoptysis that may not be apparent until patients are intubated.

Jaundice occurs in 5–10% of all patients with leptospirosis; it can be profound and give an orange cast to the skin but usually is not associated with fulminant hepatic necrosis. Physical examination may reveal an enlarged and tender liver.

Acute kidney injury is common in severe disease, presenting after several days of illness, and can be either nonoliguric or oliguric. Typical electrolyte abnormalities include hypokalemia and hyponatremia. Loss of magnesium in the urine is uniquely associated with leptospiral nephropathy. Hypotension is associated with acute tubular necrosis, oliguria, or anuria, requiring fluid resuscitation and sometimes vasopressor therapy. Hemodialysis can be life-saving, with renal function typically returning to normal in survivors.

Other syndromes include (necrotizing) pancreatitis, cholecystitis, skeletal muscle involvement, rhabdomyolysis (with moderately elevated serum creatine kinase levels), and neurologic manifestations including aseptic meningitis. Cardiac involvement is commonly reflected on the electrocardiogram as nonspecific ST- and T-wave changes. Repolarization abnormalities and arrhythmias are considered poor prognostic factors. Myocarditis has been described. Rare hematologic complications include hemolysis, thrombotic thrombocytopenic purpura, and hemolytic-uremic syndrome.

Long-term symptoms following severe leptospirosis include fatigue, myalgia, malaise, and headache and may persist for years. Autoimmune-associated uveitis, a potentially chronic condition, is a recognized sequela of leptospirosis.

DIAGNOSIS

The clinical diagnosis of leptospirosis should be based on an appropriate exposure history combined with any of the protean manifestations of the disease. Returning travelers from endemic areas usually have a history of recreational freshwater activities or other mucosal or percutaneous contact with contaminated surface waters or soil. For nontravelers, recreational water contact and occupational hazards that involve direct or indirect animal contact should be explored (see "Epidemiology," above).

Although biochemical, hematologic, and urinalysis findings in acute leptospirosis are nonspecific, certain patterns may suggest the diagnosis. Laboratory results usually show signs of a bacterial infection, including leukocytosis with a left shift and elevated markers of inflammation (C-reactive protein level and erythrocyte sedimentation rate). Thrombocytopenia (platelet count $\leq 100 \times 10^9$/L) is common and is associated with bleeding and renal failure. In severe disease, signs of coagulation activation may be present, varying from borderline abnormalities to a serious derangement compatible with DIC as defined by international criteria. The kidneys are invariably involved in leptospirosis. Related findings range from urinary sediment changes (leukocytes, erythrocytes, and hyaline or granular casts) and mild proteinuria in mild disease to renal failure and azotemia in severe leptospirosis. Nonoliguric hypokalemic renal insufficiency (see "Clinical Manifestations," above) is characteristic of early leptospirosis. Serum bilirubin levels may be high, whereas rises in aminotransferase and alkaline phosphatase levels are usually moderate. Although clinical symptoms of pancreatitis are not a common finding, amylase levels are often elevated. When symptoms of aseptic meningitis develop, examination of the CSF shows pleocytosis that can range from a few cells to >1000 cells/μL, with a polymorphonuclear cell predominance. The protein concentration in the CSF may be elevated; CSF glucose levels are normal.

In severe leptospirosis, pulmonary radiographic abnormalities are more common than would be expected on the basis of physical examination (Fig. 208-4). The most common radiographic finding is a patchy bilateral alveolar pattern that corresponds to scattered alveolar hemorrhage. These abnormalities predominantly affect the lower lobes. Other findings include pleura-based densities (representing areas of hemorrhage) and diffuse ground-glass attenuation typical of acute respiratory distress syndrome (ARDS).

A definitive diagnosis of leptospirosis is based on isolation of the organism from the patient, on a positive result in the polymerase chain reaction (PCR), or on seroconversion or a rise in antibody titer. In cases with strong clinical evidence of infection, a single antibody titer of 1:200–1:800 (depending on whether the case occurs in a low- or high-endemic area) in the microscopic agglutination test (MAT) is required. Preferably, a fourfold or greater rise in titer is detected between acute- and convalescent-phase serum specimens. Antibodies generally do not reach detectable levels until the second week of illness. The antibody response can be affected by early treatment with antibiotics.

The MAT, which uses a battery of live leptospiral strains, and the enzyme-linked immunosorbent assay (ELISA), which uses a broadly reacting antigen, are the standard serologic procedures. The MAT usually is available only in specialized laboratories and is used for determination of the antibody titer and for tentative identification of the involved leptospiral serogroup—and, when epidemiologic background information is available, the putative serovar. This point underscores the importance of testing antigens representative of the serovars prevalent in the particular geographic area. However, cross-reactions occur frequently, and thus definitive identification of the infecting serovar or serogroup is not possible without isolation of the causative organism. Because serologic testing lacks sensitivity in the early acute phase of the disease (up to day 5), it cannot be used as the basis for a timely decision about whether to start treatment.

In addition to the MAT and the ELISA, various rapid tests with diagnostic value have been developed, and some of these are commercially available. These rapid tests mainly apply lateral flow, (latex) agglutination, or ELISA methodology and are reasonably sensitive and specific, although results reported in the literature vary, probably as a consequence of differences in test interpretation, (re)exposure risks, serovar distribution, and the use of biased serum panels. These methods do not require culture or MAT facilities and are useful in settings that lack a strong medical infrastructure. PCR methodologies, notably real-time PCR, have become increasingly widely implemented. Compared with serology, PCR offers a great advantage: the capacity to confirm the diagnosis of leptospirosis with a high degree of accuracy during the first 5 days of illness.

DIFFERENTIAL DIAGNOSIS

The differential diagnosis of leptospirosis is broad, reflecting the diverse clinical presentations of the disease. Although leptospirosis transmission is more common in tropical and subtropical regions, the absence of a travel history does not exclude the diagnosis. When fever, headache, and myalgia predominate, influenza and other common and less common (e.g., dengue and chikungunya) viral infections should be considered. Malaria, typhoid fever, ehrlichiosis, viral hepatitis, and acute HIV infection may mimic the early stages of leptospirosis and are important to recognize. Rickettsial diseases, hantavirus infections (hemorrhagic fever with renal syndrome or hantavirus cardiopulmonary syndrome), and dengue share epidemiologic and clinical features with leptospirosis. Dual infections have been reported. In this light, it is advisable to conduct serologic testing for hantavirus, rickettsiae, and dengue virus when leptospirosis is suspected. When bleeding is detected, dengue hemorrhagic fever and other viral hemorrhagic fevers, including hantavirus infection, yellow fever, Rift Valley fever, filovirus infections, and Lassa fever, should be considered.

TREATMENT LEPTOSPIROSIS

Severe leptospirosis should be treated with IV penicillin (Table 208-1) as soon as the diagnosis is considered. Leptospires are highly susceptible to a broad range of antibiotics, and early intervention may prevent the development of major organ system failure or lessen its severity. Although studies supporting antibiotic therapy have produced conflicting results, clinical trials are difficult to perform in settings where patients frequently present for medical care with late stages of disease. Antibiotics are less likely to benefit patients in whom organ damage has already occurred. Two open-label randomized studies comparing penicillin with parenteral cefotaxime, parenteral ceftriaxone, and doxycycline showed no significant differences among the antibiotics with regard to complications and mortality risk. Thus ceftriaxone, cefotaxime, or doxycycline is a satisfactory alternative to penicillin for the treatment of severe leptospirosis.

In mild cases, oral treatment with doxycycline, azithromycin, ampicillin, or amoxicillin is recommended. In regions where rickettsial diseases are coendemic, doxycycline or azithromycin is the drug of choice. In rare instances, a Jarisch-Herxheimer reaction develops within hours after the initiation of antimicrobial therapy.

TABLE 208-1 TREATMENT AND CHEMOPROPHYLAXIS OF LEPTOSPIROSIS IN ADULTS[a]

Indication	Regimen
Treatment	
Mild leptospirosis	Doxycycline[b] (100 mg PO bid) *or*
	Amoxicillin (500 mg PO tid) *or*
	Ampicillin (500 mg PO tid)
Moderate/severe leptospirosis	Penicillin (1.5 million units IV or IM q6h) *or*
	Ceftriaxone (2 g/d IV) *or*
	Cefotaxime (1 g IV q6h) *or*
	Doxycycline (loading dose of 200 mg IV, then 100 mg IV q12h)
Chemoprophylaxis[c]	
	Doxycycline[b] (200 mg PO once a week) *or*
	Azithromycin (250 mg PO once or twice a week)

[a]All regimens are given for 7 days. [b]Doxycycline should not be given to pregnant women or children. [c]The efficacy of doxycycline prophylaxis in endemic or epidemic settings remains unclear. Experiments in animal models and a cost-effectiveness model indicate that azithromycin has a number of characteristics that may make it efficacious in treatment and prophylaxis.

Aggressive supportive care for leptospirosis is essential and can be life-saving. Patients with nonoliguric renal dysfunction require aggressive fluid and electrolyte resuscitation to prevent dehydration and precipitation of oliguric renal failure. Peritoneal dialysis or hemodialysis should be provided to patients with oliguric renal failure. Rapid initiation of hemodialysis has been shown to reduce mortality risk and typically is necessary only for short periods. Patients with pulmonary hemorrhage may have reduced pulmonary compliance (as seen in ARDS) and may benefit from mechanical ventilation with low tidal volumes to avoid high ventilation pressures. Evidence is contradictory for the use of glucocorticoids and desmopressin as adjunct therapy for pulmonary involvement associated with severe leptospirosis.

PROGNOSIS

Most patients with leptospirosis recover. However, post-leptospirosis symptoms, mainly of a depression-like nature, may occur and persist for years after the acute disease. Mortality rates are highest among patients who are elderly and those who have severe disease (pulmonary hemorrhage, Weil's syndrome). Leptospirosis during pregnancy is associated with high fetal mortality rates. Long-term follow-up of patients with renal failure and hepatic dysfunction has documented good recovery of renal and hepatic function.

PREVENTION

Individuals who may be exposed to *Leptospira* through their occupations or their involvement in recreational freshwater activities should be informed about the risks. Measures for controlling leptospirosis include avoidance of exposure to urine and tissues from infected animals through proper eyewear, footwear, and other protective equipment. Targeted rodent control strategies could be considered.

Vaccines for agricultural and companion animals are generally available, and their use should be encouraged. The veterinary vaccine used in a given area should contain the serovars known to be present in that area. Unfortunately, some vaccinated animals still excrete leptospires in their urine. Vaccination of humans against a specific serovar prevalent in an area has been undertaken in some European and Asian countries and has proved effective. Although a large-scale trial of vaccine in humans has been reported from Cuba, no conclusions can be drawn about efficacy and adverse reactions because of insufficient details on study design. The efficacy of chemoprophylaxis with doxycycline (200 mg once a week) or azithromycin (in pregnant women and children) is being disputed, but focused pre- and postexposure administration is indicated in instances of well-defined short-term exposure (Table 208-1).

209 Relapsing Fever

Alan G. Barbour

Relapsing fever is caused by infection with any of several species of *Borrelia* spirochetes. Physicians in ancient Greece distinguished relapsing fever from other febrile disorders by its characteristic clinical presentation: two or more fever episodes separated by varying periods of well-being. In the nineteenth century, relapsing fever was one of the first diseases to be associated with a specific microbe by virtue of its characteristic laboratory finding: the presence of large numbers of spirochetes of the genus *Borrelia* in the blood.

The host responds with systemic inflammation that results in an illness ranging from a flulike syndrome to sepsis. Other manifestations are the consequences of central nervous system (CNS) involvement and coagulopathy. Antigenic variation of the spirochetes' surface proteins accounts for the infection's relapsing course. Acquired immunity follows the serial development of antibodies to each of the several variants appearing during an infection. Treatment with antibiotics results in rapid cure but at the risk of a moderate to severe Jarisch-Herxheimer reaction.

Louse-borne relapsing fever caused large epidemics well into the twentieth century and currently occurs in northeastern Africa. At present, however, most cases of relapsing fever are tick-borne in origin. Sporadic cases and small outbreaks are focally distributed on most continents, with Africa most affected. In North America, the majority of reports of relapsing fever have been from the western United States and Canada. Nevertheless, the recent discovery that another species in the relapsing fever group causes human disease in the same geographic distribution as Lyme disease (Chap. 210) confounds epidemiologic distinctions between the two major types of *Borrelia* infection.

ETIOLOGIC AGENT

Coiled, thin microscopic filaments that swim in one direction and then coil up before heading in another were first observed in the blood of patients with relapsing fever in the 1880s (*www.youtube.com/watch?v=VxDPV2lBd9U*). These microbes were categorized as spirochetes and grouped as several species in the genus *Borrelia*. It was not until the 1960s that the organisms were isolated in pure culture. The breakthrough cultivation medium and its derivatives are rich in their ingredients, ranging from simple (e.g., amino acids and *N*-acetylglucosamine) to more complex (e.g., serum and protein hydrolysates). The limited biosynthetic capacity of *Borrelia* cells is accounted for by a genome content one-quarter that of *Escherichia coli*.

Like other spirochetes, the helix-shaped *Borrelia* cells have two membranes, the outer of which is more loosely secured than in other double-membrane bacteria, such as *E. coli*. As a consequence, fixed organisms with damaged membranes can assume a variety of morphologies in smears and histologic preparations. The flagella of spirochetes run between the two membranes and are not on the cell surface. Although technically gram-negative in their staining properties, the 10- to 20-μm-long *Borrelia* cells, with a diameter of 0.1–0.2 μm, are too narrow to be seen by bright-field microscopy of Gram-stained specimens.

EPIDEMIOLOGY

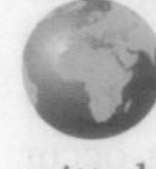

The several species of *Borrelia* that cause relapsing fever have restricted geographic distributions (Table 209-1). The exception is *Borrelia recurrentis*, which is also the only species transmitted by the louse. Louse-borne relapsing fever (LBRF) is usually acquired from a body louse (*Pediculus humanus corporis*), with humans serving as the reservoir. Acquisition occurs not from the bite itself but from either rubbing the insect's feces into the bite site with the fingers in response to irritation or inoculation of feces into the conjunctivae or an open wound. Although LBRF transmission is currently limited to Ethiopia and adjacent countries, the disease has had a global distribution in the past, and that potential remains. Epidemics with thousands of cases of LBRF can occur under circumstances of famine, natural disaster, refugee migration, and war.

All other known species of relapsing fever agents are tick-borne—in most cases, by soft ticks of the genus *Ornithodoros* (Fig. 209-1). Tick-borne relapsing fever (TBRF) is found on most continents but is absent or rare in tropical, low-desert, arctic, or alpine environments. For most species, the reservoirs of infection are small to medium-sized mammals, usually rodents but sometimes pigs and other domestic animals living in or around human habitats. However, one species, *Borrelia duttonii* in sub-Saharan Africa, is largely maintained by tick transmission between human hosts. In North America, TBRF occurs as single cases or small case clusters through transient exposure of persons to infested buildings or caves in less populated areas where the rodent reservoirs have nests. The two main *Borrelia* species involved in North America are *Borrelia hermsii* (in the mountainous west) and *Borrelia turicatae* (in the southwestern and south-central regions). The soft tick vectors typically feed for no more than 30 min, usually without being noticed, while the victim is sleeping. Transovarial transmission from one generation of ticks to the next means that infection risk may persist in an area long after incriminated mammalian reservoirs have been eradicated.

A newly recognized pathogen, *Borrelia miyamotoi*, belongs to the clade of relapsing fever species but is transmitted to humans from other mammals by hard ticks (e.g., *Ixodes scapularis* in the eastern United States) that also transmit Lyme disease, babesiosis, anaplasmosis, ehrlichiosis, and arboviral encephalitis. *B. miyamotoi* is acquired through outdoor activities and through contact with ticks in forested and shrubby areas during recreation, work, or activities around the home. In residents of areas where *B. miyamotoi* and *Borrelia burgdorferi* coexist, the prevalence of antibodies to the former is about one-third of that to the latter.

PATHOGENESIS AND IMMUNITY

Unlike LBRF spirochetes, TBRF spirochetes enter the body in the tick's saliva with the onset of feeding. From an inoculum of a few cells, the spirochetes proliferate in the blood, doubling every 6 h to numbers of 10^6–10^7/mL or more. *Borrelia* species are extracellular pathogens; their

TABLE 209-1 RELAPSING FEVER *BORRELIA* SPECIES, BY GEOGRAPHIC REGION, VECTOR, AND PRIMARY RESERVOIR

Species	Region(s)	Arthropod Vector(s)	Primary Reservoir
B. crocidurae	Africa	*Ornithodoros erraticus, O. sonrai* (soft ticks)	Mammals
B. duttonii	Africa	*O. moubata*	Humans
B. hermsii	North America	*O. hermsi*	Mammals
B. hispanica	Europe, North Africa	*O. erraticus* complex	Mammals
B. miyamotoi	Eurasia, North America	*Ixodes* species (hard ticks)	Mammals
B. persica	Eurasia	*O. tholozani*	Mammals
B. recurrentis	Africa, global[a]	*Pediculus humanus corporis* (human body louse)	Humans
B. turicatae	North America	*O. turicata*	Mammals
B. venezuelensis	Central and South America	*O. rudis*	Mammals

[a]Although transmission is currently limited to Ethiopia and adjacent countries, *B. recurrentis* infection has had a global distribution in the past, and that potential remains.

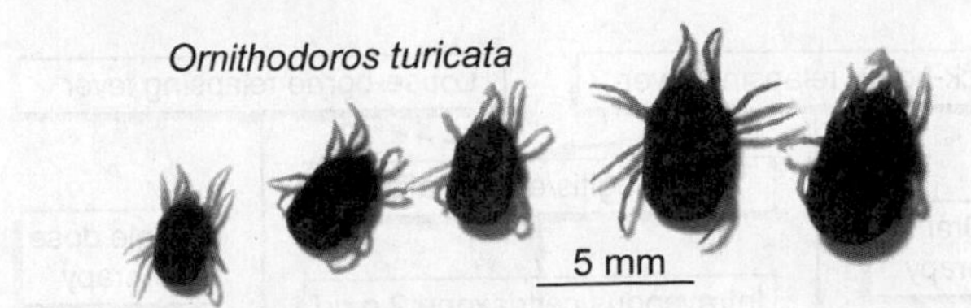

FIGURE 209-1 ***Ornithodoros turicata*** **soft ticks** of different ages.

presence inside cells likely represents a dead end for the bacteria after phagocytosis. Binding of the spirochetes to erythrocytes leads to aggregation of red blood cells, their sequestration in the spleen and liver, and hepatosplenomegaly and anemia. A bleeding disorder is probably the consequence of thrombocytopenia, impaired hepatic production of clotting factors, and/or blockage of small vessels by aggregates of spirochetes, erythrocytes, and platelets. Some species are neurotropic and frequently enter the brain, where they are comparatively sheltered from host immunity. Relapsing fever spirochetes can cross the maternal-fetal barrier and cause placental damage and inflammation, leading to intrauterine growth retardation and congenital infection.

Although *Borrelia* species do not have potent exotoxins or a lipopolysaccharide endotoxin, they have abundant membrane-associated lipoproteins whose recognition and binding by Toll-like receptors on host cells can lead to a proinflammatory process similar to that in endotoxemia, with elevations of tumor necrosis factor α, interleukin 6, and interleukin 8 concentrations.

IgM antibodies specific for the serotype-defining surface lipoprotein appear after a few days of infection and soon reach a concentration that causes lysis of bacteria in the blood through either direct bactericidal action or opsonization. The release of large amounts of lipoproteins and other bacterial products from dying bacteria provokes a "crisis," during which there can be an increase in temperature, hypotension, and other signs of shock. A similar phenomenon occurring in some patients soon after the initiation of antibiotic treatment is characterized by the abrupt worsening of the condition, which is called a Jarisch-Herxheimer reaction (JHR).

CLINICAL MANIFESTATIONS

Relapsing fever presents with the sudden onset of fever. Febrile periods are punctuated by intervening afebrile periods of a few days; this pattern occurs at least twice. The patient's temperature is ≥39°C and may be as high as 43°C. The first fever episode often ends in a crisis lasting ~15–30 min and consisting of rigors, a further elevation in temperature, and increases in pulse and blood pressure. The crisis phase is followed by profuse diaphoresis, falling temperature, and hypotension, which usually persist for several hours. In LBRF, the first episode of fever is unremitting for 3–6 days; it is usually followed by a single milder episode. In TBRF, multiple febrile periods last 1–3 days each. In both forms, the interval between fevers ranges from 4 to 14 days, sometimes with symptoms of malaise and fatigue.

The symptoms that accompany the fevers are usually nonspecific. Headache, neck stiffness, arthralgia, myalgia, and nausea may accompany the first and subsequent febrile episodes. An enlarging spleen and liver cause abdominal pain. A nonproductive cough is common during LBRF and—in combination with fever and myalgias—may suggest influenza. Acute respiratory distress syndrome may occur during TBRF.

On physical examination, the patient may be delirious or apathetic. There may be body lice in the patient's clothes or signs of insect bites. In regions with *B. miyamotoi* infection, a hard tick may be embedded in the skin. Epistaxis, petechiae, and ecchymoses are common during LBRF but not in TBRF. Splenomegaly or spleen tenderness is common in both forms of relapsing fever. The majority of patients with LBRF and ~10% of patients with TBRF have discernible hepatomegaly.

Localizing neurologic findings are more common in TBRF than in LBRF. In North America, *B. turicatae* infection has neurologic manifestations more often than *B. hermsii* infection. Meningoencephalitis can result in residual hemiplegia or aphasia. Myelitis and radiculopathy may develop. Unilateral or bilateral Bell's palsy and deafness from seventh or eighth cranial nerve involvement are the most common forms of cranial neuritis and typically present in the second or third febrile episode, not the first. Visual impairment from unilateral or bilateral iridocyclitis or panophthalmitis may be permanent. In LBRF, neurologic manifestations such as altered mental state or stiff neck are thought to be secondary to spirochetemia and systemic inflammation rather than to direct invasion of the nervous system.

Myocarditis appears to be common in both forms of relapsing fever and accounts for some deaths. Most commonly, myocarditis is evidenced by gallops on cardiac auscultation, a prolonged QT_c interval, and cardiomegaly and pulmonary edema on chest radiography.

General laboratory studies are not specific. Mild to moderate normocytic anemia is common, but frank hemolysis and hemoglobinuria do not develop. Leukocyte counts are usually in the normal range or only slightly elevated, and leukopenia can occur during the crisis. Platelet counts can fall below 50,000/μL. Laboratory evidence of hepatitis can be found, with elevated serum concentrations of unconjugated bilirubin and aminotransferases; the prothrombin and partial thromboplastin times may be moderately prolonged.

Analysis of the cerebrospinal fluid (CSF) is indicated in cases of suspected relapsing fever with signs of meningitis or meningoencephalitis. The presence of mononuclear pleocytosis and mildly to moderately elevated protein levels justifies intravenous antibiotic therapy in TBRF.

The manifestations and course of *B. miyamotoi* infection remain incompletely characterized, but reports to date indicate that the sign most often reported by patients at presentation is fever without respiratory symptoms starting 1–2 weeks after a tick bite and recurring once or twice in some cases. Meningoencephalitis with spirochetes in the CSF was documented in one immunodeficient adult.

DIAGNOSIS

Relapsing fever should be considered in a patient with the characteristic fever pattern and a history of recent exposure—i.e., within 1–2 weeks before illness onset—to body lice or soft-bodied ticks in geographic areas with documented current or past transmission. Because of the longevity of the ticks and the transovarial transmission of the pathogen in the ticks, a case of relapsing fever may be diagnosed many years after the last case reported in that locale.

The bedrock for laboratory diagnosis remains the same as it has been for a century: direct detection of the spirochetes by microscopy of the blood. Manual differential counts of white blood cells by Wright or Giemsa stain usually reveal spirochetes in thin blood smears if their concentration is $\geq 10^5$/mL and several oil-immersion fields are examined (Fig. 209-2). The preferred time to obtain a blood specimen is between the fever's onset and its peak. Lower concentrations of spirochetes may be revealed by a thick blood smear that is either directly stained with acridine orange and then examined by fluorescence microscopy or treated with 0.5% acetic acid before Giemsa or Wright staining. An alternative to a fixed blood smear is a wet mount of anticoagulated blood mixed with saline and examined by phase-contrast or dark-field microscopy for motile spirochetes.

Polymerase chain reaction (PCR) and similar DNA amplification procedures are increasingly used for examination of an extract of blood. PCR may reveal spirochetes between febrile episodes, since there are already escape variants in the population when the first wave of bacteria is neutralized.

Culture of blood or CSF in Barbour-Stoenner-Kelly broth medium is an option for isolation of *Borrelia* species except for *B. miyamotoi*, which is noncultivable or poorly cultivable. However, few laboratories offer this service. An alternative for tick-borne *Borrelia* species, including *B. miyamotoi*, is inoculation of blood or CSF into immunodeficient mice and examination of the animal's blood after a few days.

Options for serologic confirmation of infection are limited. Most assays that are available commercially or in reference laboratories are based on whole cells of a single *Borrelia* species. These assays may not detect the major variant antigens to which the patient is mainly responding or may yield false-positive results due to antibodies to cross-reactive antigens of related bacteria, including *B. burgdorferi*. The most

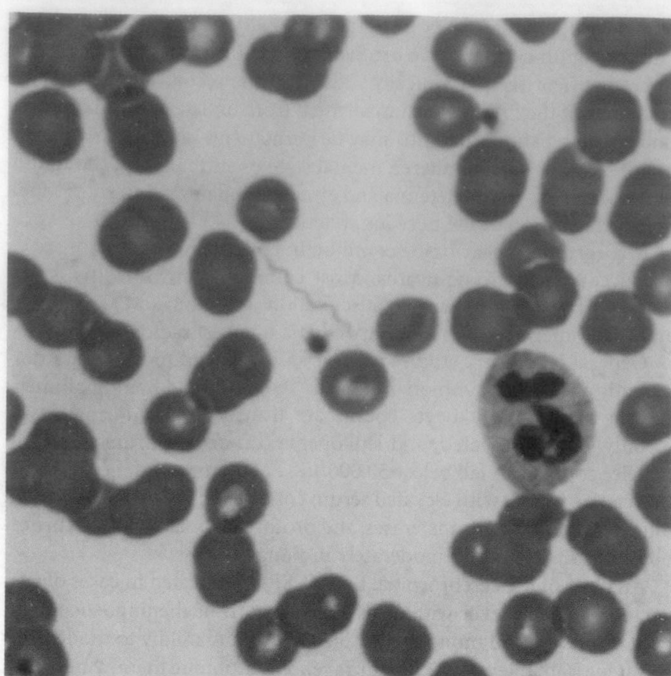

FIGURE 209-2 **Photomicrograph of tick-borne relapsing fever spirochete (*Borrelia turicatae*)** in a Wright-Giemsa-stained thin blood smear. Included in the figure are a polymorphonuclear leukocyte and two platelets.

promising new assays under development are based on recombinant antigens such as GlpQ, a protein antigen of all relapsing fever *Borrelia* species (including *B. miyamotoi*) but not of any Lyme disease species.

DIFFERENTIAL DIAGNOSIS

Depending on the patient's history of residential, occupational, travel, and recreational exposures, the differential diagnosis of relapsing fever includes one or more of the following infections that feature either periodicity in the fever pattern or an extended single febrile period with nonspecific constitutional symptoms: Colorado tick fever (which, along with dengue, can have a "saddleback" fever course), Rocky Mountain spotted fever and other rickettsioses, ehrlichiosis, anaplasmosis, tick-borne arbovirus infection, and babesiosis in North America, Europe, Russia, and northeastern Asia. Elsewhere in the Americas and Asia and in most of Africa, malaria, typhoid fever, typhus and other rickettsioses, dengue, brucellosis, and leptospirosis may also be considered. Depending on the geographic area and types of exposure, malaria, louse-borne typhus, typhoid fever, or Lyme disease may complicate relapsing fever.

TREATMENT RELAPSING FEVER

Penicillins and tetracyclines have been the antibiotics of choice for relapsing fever for several decades. Erythromycin has been a longstanding second choice. There is no evidence of acquired resistance to these antibiotics. *Borrelia* species are also susceptible to most cephalosporins and chloramphenicol, but there is less clinical experience with these drugs. Borreliae are relatively resistant to rifampin, sulfonamides, fluoroquinolones, and aminoglycosides. Spirochetes are no longer detectable in the blood within a few hours after the first dose of an effective antibiotic.

A single dose of antibiotic is usually sufficient for the treatment of LBRF (Fig. 209-3). The recurrence rate after antibiotic treatment is ≤5%. For adults, a single dose of oral tetracycline (500 mg), oral doxycycline (200 mg), or intramuscular penicillin G procaine (400,000–800,000 units) is effective. The corresponding doses for children are oral tetracycline at 12.5 mg/kg, oral doxycycline at 5 mg/kg, and intramuscular penicillin G procaine at 200,000–400,000 units.

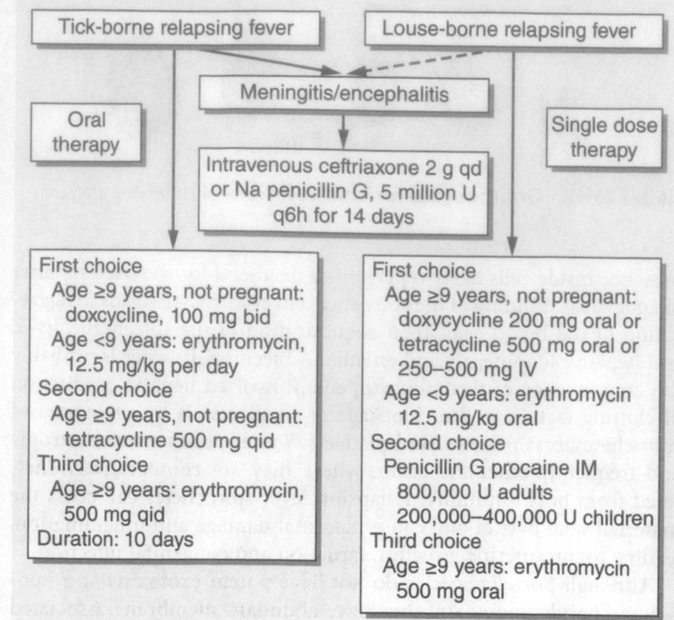

FIGURE 209-3 **Algorithm for treatment of relapsing fever.** If it is not known whether the patient has tick-borne or louse-borne relapsing fever, the patient should be treated for the tick-borne form. The *dashed line* indicates that central nervous system invasion in louse-borne relapsing fever is uncommon.

When an adult patient is stuporous or nauseated, the intravenous dose is 250–500 mg. Tetracycline is contraindicated in pregnant and nursing women and in children <9 years old; for individuals in these groups who are allergic to penicillin, oral erythromycin (500 mg for adults and 12.5 mg/kg for children) is an alternative. Tetracycline is marginally superior to penicillin G in terms of time to fever clearance and relapse rate.

The accumulated anecdotal reports on TBRF therapy indicate a recurrence rate of ≥20% after single-dose treatment. This high rate of recurrence plausibly is due to the greater propensity of tick-borne species than of *B. recurrentis* to invade the CNS, from which they can reinvade the bloodstream after antibiotic levels decline. Accordingly, multiple antibiotic doses are recommended. The preferred treatment for adults is a 10-day course of tetracycline (500 mg or 12.5 mg/kg orally every 6 h) or doxycycline (100 mg twice daily). When tetracyclines are contraindicated, the alternative is erythromycin (500 mg or 12.5 mg/kg orally every 6 h) for 10 days. If a β-lactam antibiotic is given, it should be administered intravenously rather than orally, especially if CNS involvement is confirmed or suspected. For adults, the regimen is penicillin G (5 million units IV every 6 h) or ceftriaxone (2 g IV daily) for 10–14 days.

Experience with the treatment of *B. miyamotoi* infection is limited, but this organism likely has the same antibiotic susceptibilities as other *Borrelia* species. Until more is known about treatment efficacy, therapy for *B. miyamotoi* infection can follow the guidelines for Lyme disease—including parenteral therapy for CNS involvement—because it may be difficult to rule out co-infection.

The JHR during treatment of relapsing fever can be severe and can even end in death if precautions are not in place for close monitoring and provision of cardiovascular and volume support as needed. Rigors, fever, and hypotension occur within 2–3 h of initiation of antibiotic treatment. The incidence of the JHR is ~80% in LBRF and ~50% in TBRF. Both penicillin and tetracycline can elicit the JHR.

PROGNOSIS

The mortality rates for untreated LBRF and TBRF are in the ranges of 10–70% and 4–10%, respectively, and are largely determined by coexisting conditions, such as malnutrition and dehydration.

Death from untreated relapsing fever is most common during the first fever episode. With prompt antibiotic treatment, the mortality rate is 2–5% for LBRF and <2% for TBRF. Features associated with a poor prognosis include concurrence with malaria, typhus, or typhoid; pregnancy; stupor or coma on admission; diffuse bleeding; poor liver function; myocarditis; and bronchopneumonia. The mortality rate from the JHR in LBRF, in the absence of adequate monitoring and resuscitation measures, is ~5%. Some patients have survived the crisis or the JHR only to die suddenly either later that day or on the next day. Relapsing fever during pregnancy frequently leads to abortion or stillbirth, but congenital malformations have not been reported. Although it is possible that spirochetes may persist in the CNS or other sequestered sites after bacteremia has resolved, chronic disease or disability from a persistent infection has not been attributed to relapsing fever. Partial immunity against reinfection seems to develop in residents of endemic areas.

PREVENTION

There is no vaccine for either LBRF or TBRF. Reduction of exposure to lice and ticks is the key strategy for prevention. LBRF can be prevented through improved personal hygiene, reduction of crowding, better access to washing facilities, and selected use of pesticides. Infested clothing is an important factor in maintaining body lice. The risk of TBRF can be reduced by construction of houses with concrete or sealed plank floors and without thatched roofs or mud walls. Log cabins pose a particular risk in North America when rodents nest in the roof or beneath the house or porch. Interiors of buildings infested with *Ornithodoros* ticks can be treated with pesticides. If residing in a high-risk environment, individuals should not sleep on the floor, and beds should be moved away from the wall. With an exposure to TBRF, postexposure treatment with doxycycline (200 mg on day 1 followed by 100 mg/d for 4 days) was efficacious in preventing infection in a placebo-controlled trial.

210 Lyme Borreliosis

Allen C. Steere

DEFINITION

Lyme borreliosis is caused by a spirochete, *Borrelia burgdorferi sensu lato*, that is transmitted by ticks of the *Ixodes ricinus* complex. The infection usually begins with a characteristic expanding skin lesion, erythema migrans (EM; stage 1, localized infection). After several days or weeks, the spirochete may spread to many different sites (stage 2, disseminated infection). Possible manifestations of disseminated infection include secondary annular skin lesions, meningitis, cranial neuritis, radiculoneuritis, peripheral neuritis, carditis, atrioventricular nodal block, or migratory musculoskeletal pain. Months or years later (usually after periods of latent infection), intermittent or persistent arthritis, chronic encephalopathy or polyneuropathy, or acrodermatitis may develop (stage 3, persistent infection). Most patients experience early symptoms of the illness during the summer, but the infection may not become symptomatic until it progresses to stage 2 or 3.

Lyme disease was recognized as a separate entity in 1976 because of a geographic cluster of children in Lyme, Connecticut, who were thought to have juvenile rheumatoid arthritis. It became apparent that Lyme disease was a multisystemic illness that affected primarily the skin, nervous system, heart, and joints. Epidemiologic studies of patients with EM implicated certain *Ixodes* ticks as vectors of the disease. Early in the twentieth century, EM had been described in Europe and attributed to *I. ricinus* tick bites. In 1982, a previously unrecognized spirochete, now called *Borrelia burgdorferi*, was recovered from *Ixodes scapularis* ticks and then from patients with Lyme disease. The entity is now called Lyme disease or Lyme borreliosis.

ETIOLOGIC AGENT

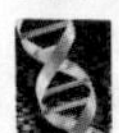

B. burgdorferi, the causative agent of Lyme disease, is a fastidious microaerophilic bacterium. The spirochete's genome is quite small (~1.5 Mb) and consists of a highly unusual linear chromosome of 950 kb as well as 17–21 linear and circular plasmids. The most remarkable aspect of the *B. burgdorferi* genome is that there are sequences for more than 100 known or predicted lipoproteins—a larger number than in any other organism. The spirochete has few proteins with biosynthetic activity and depends on its host for most of its nutritional requirements. It has no sequences for recognizable toxins.

Currently, 13 closely related borrelial species are collectively referred to as *Borrelia burgdorferi sensu lato* (i.e., "*B. burgdorferi* in the general sense"). The human infection Lyme borreliosis is caused primarily by three pathogenic genospecies: *B. burgdorferi sensu stricto* ("*B. burgdorferi* in the strict sense," hereafter referred to simply as *B. burgdorferi*), *Borrelia garinii*, and *Borrelia afzelii*. *B. burgdorferi* is the sole cause of the infection in the United States; all three genospecies are found in Europe, and the latter two species occur in Asia.

Strains of *B. burgdorferi* have been subdivided according to several typing schemes: one based on sequence variation of outer-surface protein C (OspC), a second based on differences in the 16S–23S rRNA intergenic spacer region (RST or IGS), and a third called *multilocus sequence typing*. From these typing systems, it is apparent that strains of *B. burgdorferi* differ in pathogenicity. OspC type A (RST1) strains seem to be particularly virulent and may have played a role in the emergence of Lyme disease in epidemic form in the northeastern United States in the late twentieth century.

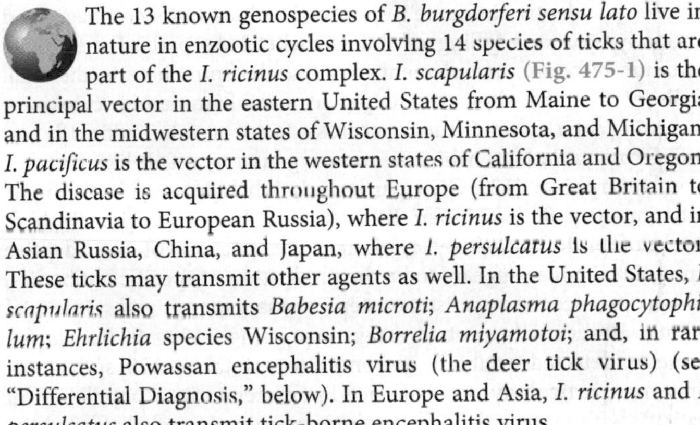

EPIDEMIOLOGY

The 13 known genospecies of *B. burgdorferi sensu lato* live in nature in enzootic cycles involving 14 species of ticks that are part of the *I. ricinus* complex. *I. scapularis* (Fig. 475-1) is the principal vector in the eastern United States from Maine to Georgia and in the midwestern states of Wisconsin, Minnesota, and Michigan. *I. pacificus* is the vector in the western states of California and Oregon. The disease is acquired throughout Europe (from Great Britain to Scandinavia to European Russia), where *I. ricinus* is the vector, and in Asian Russia, China, and Japan, where *I. persulcatus* is the vector. These ticks may transmit other agents as well. In the United States, *I. scapularis* also transmits *Babesia microti*; *Anaplasma phagocytophilum*; *Ehrlichia* species Wisconsin; *Borrelia miyamotoi*; and, in rare instances, Powassan encephalitis virus (the deer tick virus) (see "Differential Diagnosis," below). In Europe and Asia, *I. ricinus* and *I. persulcatus* also transmit tick-borne encephalitis virus.

Ticks of the *I. ricinus* complex have larval, nymphal, and adult stages. They require a blood meal at each stage. The risk of infection in a given area depends largely on the density of these ticks as well as their feeding habits and animal hosts, which have evolved differently in different locations. For *I. scapularis* in the northeastern United States, the white-footed mouse and certain other rodents are the preferred hosts of the immature larvae and nymphs. It is critical that both of the tick's immature stages feed on the same host because the life cycle of the spirochete depends on horizontal transmission: in early summer from infected nymphs to mice and in late summer from infected mice to larvae, which then molt to become the infected nymphs that will begin the cycle again the following year. It is the tiny nymphal tick that is primarily responsible for transmission of the disease to humans during the early summer months. White-tailed deer, which are not involved in the life cycle of the spirochete, are the preferred host for the adult stage of *I. scapularis* and seem to be critical to the tick's survival.

Lyme disease is now the most common vector-borne infection in the United States and Europe. Since surveillance was begun by the Centers for Disease Control and Prevention (CDC) in 1982, the number of cases in the United States has increased dramatically. More than 30,000 new cases are now reported each summer, but the actual number of new cases is probably closer to 300,000 annually. In Europe, reported frequencies of the disease are highest in the middle of the continent and in Scandinavia.

To maintain its complex enzootic cycle, *B. burgdorferi* must adapt to two markedly different environments: the tick and the mammalian host. The spirochete expresses outer-surface protein A (OspA) in the midgut of the tick, whereas OspC is upregulated as the organism travels to the tick's salivary gland. There, OspC binds a tick salivary-gland protein (Salp15), which is required for infection of the mammalian host. The tick usually must be attached for at least 24 h for transmission of *B. burgdorferi*.

After injection into the human skin, the spirochete downregulates OspC and upregulates the VlsE lipoprotein. This protein undergoes extensive antigenic variation, which is necessary for spirochetal survival. After several days to weeks, *B. burgdorferi* may migrate outward in the skin, producing EM, and may spread hematogenously or in the lymph to other organs. The only known virulence factors of *B. burgdorferi* are surface proteins that allow the spirochete to attach to mammalian proteins, integrins, glycosaminoglycans, or glycoproteins. For example, spread through the skin and other tissue matrices may be facilitated by the binding of human plasminogen and its activators to the surface of the spirochete. Some *Borrelia* strains bind complement regulator–acquiring surface proteins (FHL-1/reconectin, or factor H), which help to protect spirochetes from complement-mediated lysis. Dissemination of the organism in the blood is facilitated by binding to the fibrinogen receptor on activated platelets ($\alpha_{IIb}\beta_3$) and the vitronectin receptor ($\alpha_v\beta_3$) on endothelial cells. As the name indicates, spirochetal decorin-binding proteins A and B bind decorin, a glycosaminoglycan on collagen fibrils; this binding may explain why the organism is commonly aligned with collagen fibrils in the extracellular matrix in the heart, nervous system, or joints.

To control and eradicate *B. burgdorferi*, the host mounts both innate and adaptive immune responses, resulting in macrophage- and antibody-mediated killing of the spirochete. As part of the innate immune response, complement may lyse the spirochete in the skin. Cells at affected sites release potent proinflammatory cytokines, including interleukin 6, tumor necrosis factor α, interleukin 1β, and interferon γ. Patients who are homozygous for a Toll-like receptor 1 polymorphism (1805GG), particularly when infected with highly inflammatory *B. burgdorferi* RST1 strains, have exceptionally high levels of proinflammatory cytokines. The purpose of the adaptive immune response appears to be the production of specific antibodies, which opsonize the organism—a step necessary for optimal spirochetal killing. Studies with protein arrays expressing ~1200 *B. burgdorferi* proteins detected antibody responses to a total of 120 spirochetal proteins (particularly outer-surface lipoproteins) in a population of patients with Lyme arthritis. Histologic examination of all affected tissues reveals an infiltration of lymphocytes, macrophages, and plasma cells with some degree of vascular damage, including mild vasculitis or hypervascular occlusion. These findings suggest that the spirochete may have been present in or around blood vessels.

In enzootic infection, *B. burgdorferi* spirochetes must survive this immune assault only during the summer months before returning to larval ticks to begin the cycle again the following year. In contrast, infection of humans is a dead-end event for the spirochete. Within several weeks or months, innate and adaptive immune mechanisms—even without antibiotic treatment—control widely disseminated infection, and generalized systemic symptoms wane. However, without antibiotic therapy, spirochetes may survive in localized niches for several more years. For example, *B. burgdorferi* infection in the United States may cause persistent arthritis or, in rare cases, subtle encephalopathy or polyneuropathy. Thus, immune mechanisms seem to succeed eventually in the near or total eradication of *B. burgdorferi* from selected niches, including the joints or nervous system, and symptoms resolve in most patients.

CLINICAL MANIFESTATIONS

Early Infection: Stage 1 (Localized Infection) Because of the small size of nymphal ixodid ticks, most patients do not remember the preceding tick bite. After an incubation period of 3–32 days, EM usually begins as a red macule or papule at the site of the tick bite that expands slowly to form a large annular lesion (Fig. 210-1). As the lesion increases in size, it often develops a bright red outer border and partial central clearing. The center of the lesion sometimes becomes intensely erythematous and indurated, vesicular, or necrotic. In other instances, the expanding lesion remains an even, intense red; several red rings are found within an outside ring; or the central area turns blue before the lesion clears. Although EM can be located anywhere, the thigh, groin, and axilla are particularly common sites. The lesion is warm but not often painful. Approximately 20% of patients do not exhibit this characteristic skin manifestation.

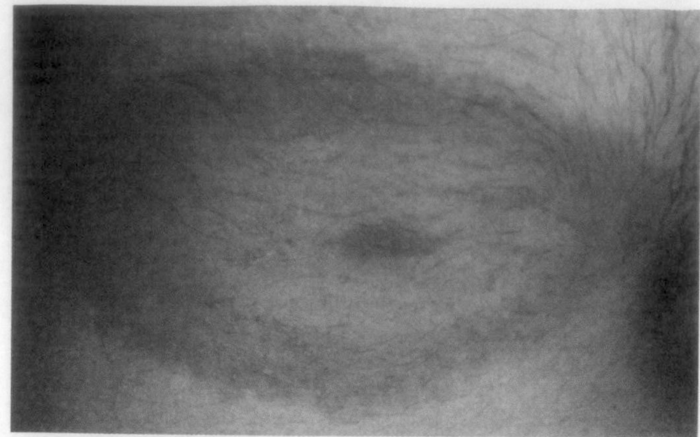

FIGURE 210-1 A classic erythema migrans lesion (9 cm in diameter) is shown near the right axilla. The lesion has partial central clearing, a bright red outer border, and a target center. *(Courtesy of Vijay K. Sikand, MD; with permission.)*

Early Infection: Stage 2 (Disseminated Infection) In cases in the United States, *B. burgdorferi* often spreads hematogenously to many sites within days or weeks after the onset of EM. In these cases, patients may develop secondary annular skin lesions similar in appearance to the initial lesion. Skin involvement is commonly accompanied by severe headache, mild stiffness of the neck, fever, chills, migratory musculoskeletal pain, arthralgias, and profound malaise and fatigue. Less common manifestations include generalized lymphadenopathy or splenomegaly, hepatitis, sore throat, nonproductive cough, conjunctivitis, iritis, or testicular swelling. Except for fatigue and lethargy, which are often constant, the early signs and symptoms of Lyme disease are typically intermittent and changing. Even in untreated patients, the early symptoms usually become less severe or disappear within several weeks. In ~15% of patients, the infection presents with these nonspecific systemic symptoms.

Symptoms suggestive of meningeal irritation may develop early in Lyme disease when EM is present but usually are not associated with cerebrospinal fluid (CSF) pleocytosis or an objective neurologic deficit. After several weeks or months, ~15% of untreated patients develop frank neurologic abnormalities, including meningitis, subtle encephalitic signs, cranial neuritis (including bilateral facial palsy), motor or sensory radiculoneuropathy, peripheral neuropathy, mononeuritis multiplex, cerebellar ataxia, or myelitis—alone or in various combinations. In children, the optic nerve may be affected because of inflammation or increased intracranial pressure, and these effects may lead to blindness. In the United States, the usual pattern consists of fluctuating symptoms of meningitis accompanied by facial palsy and peripheral radiculoneuropathy. Lymphocytic pleocytosis (~100 cells/μL) is found in CSF, often along with elevated protein levels and normal or slightly low glucose concentrations. In Europe and Asia, the first neurologic sign is characteristically radicular pain, which is followed by the development of CSF pleocytosis (meningopolyneuritis or *Bannwarth's syndrome*); meningeal or encephalitic signs are frequently absent. These early neurologic abnormalities usually resolve completely within months, but in rare cases chronic neurologic disease may occur later.

Within several weeks after the onset of illness, ~8% of patients develop cardiac involvement. The most common abnormality is a fluctuating degree of atrioventricular block (first-degree, Wenckebach, or complete heart block). Some patients have more diffuse cardiac involvement, including electrocardiographic changes indicative of acute myopericarditis, left ventricular dysfunction evident on radionuclide scans, or (in rare cases) cardiomegaly or fatal pancarditis. Cardiac involvement lasts for only a few weeks in most patients but may recur in untreated patients. Chronic cardiomyopathy caused by *B. burgdorferi* has been reported in Europe.

During this stage, musculoskeletal pain is common. The typical pattern consists of migratory pain in joints, tendons, bursae, muscles, or bones (usually without joint swelling) lasting for hours or days and affecting one or two locations at a time.

Late Infection: Stage 3 (Persistent Infection) Months after the onset of infection, ~60% of patients in the United States who have received no antibiotic treatment develop frank arthritis. The typical pattern comprises intermittent attacks of oligoarticular arthritis in large joints (especially the knees), lasting for weeks or months in a given joint. A few small joints or periarticular sites also may be affected, primarily during early attacks. The number of patients who continue to have recurrent attacks decreases each year. However, in a small percentage of cases, involvement of large joints—usually one or both knees—is persistent and may lead to erosion of cartilage and bone.

White cell counts in joint fluid range from 500 to 110,000/μL (average, 25,000/μL); most of these cells are polymorphonuclear leukocytes. Tests for rheumatoid factor or antinuclear antibodies usually give negative results. Examination of synovial biopsy samples reveals fibrin deposits, villous hypertrophy, vascular proliferation, microangiopathic lesions, and a heavy infiltration of lymphocytes and plasma cells.

Although most patients with Lyme arthritis respond well to antibiotic therapy, a small percentage in the northeastern United States have persistent (*antibiotic-refractory*) arthritis for months or even for several years after receiving oral and IV antibiotic therapy for 2 or 3 months. Although more often these patients are initially infected with RST1 strains of *B. burgdorferi*, this complication is not thought to result from persistent infection. Results of culture and polymerase chain reaction (PCR) for *B. burgdorferi* in synovial tissue obtained in the postantibiotic period have been uniformly negative. Rather, infection-induced autoimmunity, retained spirochetal antigens, or both may play a role in this outcome. Antibiotic-refractory arthritis is associated with a higher frequency of certain class II major histocompatibility complex molecules (particularly HLA-DRBI*0401 or -*0101 molecules); the Toll-like receptor 1 polymorphism 1805GG, which leads to exceptionally high levels of cytokines and chemokines in affected joints; and low frequencies of FoxP3+ T regulatory cells in synovial fluid, which correlate with longer posttreatment durations of arthritis. The recent identification of a novel human autoantigen, endothelial cell growth factor, as a target of T and B cell responses in patients with Lyme disease provided the first direct evidence of autoimmune T and B cell responses in this illness. However, multiple spirochetal or additional yet-to-be identified autoantigens may have a role in antibiotic-refractory arthritis.

Although rare, chronic neurologic involvement also may become apparent from months to several years after the onset of infection, sometimes after long periods of latent infection. The most common form of chronic central nervous system involvement is subtle encephalopathy affecting memory, mood, or sleep, and the most common form of peripheral neuropathy is an axonal polyneuropathy manifested as either distal paresthesia or spinal radicular pain. Patients with encephalopathy frequently have evidence of memory impairment in neuropsychological tests and abnormal results in CSF analyses. In cases of polyneuropathy, electromyography generally shows extensive abnormalities of proximal and distal nerve segments. Encephalomyelitis or leukoencephalitis, a rare manifestation of Lyme borreliosis associated primarily with *B. garinii* infection in Europe, is a severe neurologic disorder that may include spastic paraparesis, upper motor-neuron bladder dysfunction, and, rarely, lesions in the periventricular white matter.

Acrodermatitis chronica atrophicans, the late skin manifestation of Lyme borreliosis, has been associated primarily with *B. afzelii* infection in Europe and Asia. It has been observed especially often in elderly women. The skin lesions, which are usually found on the acral surface of an arm or leg, begin insidiously with reddish-violaceous discoloration; they become sclerotic or atrophic over a period of years.

The basic patterns of Lyme borreliosis are similar worldwide, but there are regional variations, primarily between the illness found in North America, which is caused exclusively by *B. burgdorferi*, and that found in Europe, which is caused primarily by *B. afzelii* and *B. garinii*. With each of the *Borrelia* species, the infection usually begins with EM. However, *B. burgdorferi* strains in the eastern United States often disseminate widely; they are particularly arthritogenic, and they may cause antibiotic refractory arthritis. *B. garinii* typically disseminates less widely, but it is especially neurotropic and may cause borrelial encephalomyelitis. *B. afzelii* often infects only the skin but may persist in that site, where it may cause several different dermatoborislioses, including acrodermatitis chronica atrophicans.

Post–Lyme Syndrome (Chronic Lyme Disease) Despite resolution of the objective manifestations of the infection with antibiotic therapy, ~10% of patients (although the reported percentages vary widely) continue to have subjective pain, neurocognitive manifestations, or fatigue symptoms. These symptoms usually improve and resolve within months but may last for years. At the far end of the spectrum, the symptoms may be similar to or indistinguishable from chronic fatigue syndrome (Chap. 464e) and fibromyalgia (Chap. 396). Compared with symptoms of active Lyme disease, post-Lyme symptoms tend to be more generalized or disabling. They include marked fatigue, severe headache, diffuse musculoskeletal pain, multiple symmetric tender points in characteristic locations, pain and stiffness in many joints, diffuse paresthesias, difficulty with concentration, and sleep disturbances. Patients with this condition lack evidence of joint inflammation, have normal neurologic test results, and may exhibit anxiety and depression. In contrast, late manifestations of Lyme disease, including arthritis, encephalopathy, and neuropathy, are usually associated with minimal systemic symptoms. Currently, no evidence indicates that persistent subjective symptoms after recommended courses of antibiotic therapy are caused by active infection.

DIAGNOSIS

The culture of *B. burgdorferi* in Barbour-Stoenner-Kelly (BSK) medium permits definitive diagnosis, but this method has been used primarily in research studies. Moreover, with a few exceptions, positive cultures have been obtained only early in the illness—particularly from biopsy samples of EM skin lesions, less often from plasma samples, and occasionally from CSF samples. Later in the infection, PCR is greatly superior to culture for the detection of *B. burgdorferi* DNA in joint fluid; this is the major use for PCR testing in Lyme disease. However, because *B. burgdorferi* DNA may persist for at least weeks after spirochetal killing with antibiotics, detection of spirochetal DNA in joint fluid is not an accurate test of active joint infection in Lyme disease and cannot be used reliably to determine the adequacy of antibiotic therapy. The sensitivity of PCR determinations in CSF from patients with neuroborreliosis has been much lower than that in joint fluid. There seems to be little if any role for PCR in the detection of *B. burgdorferi* DNA in blood or urine samples. Moreover, this procedure must be carefully controlled to prevent contamination.

Because of the problems associated with direct detection of *B. burgdorferi*, Lyme disease is usually diagnosed by the recognition of a characteristic clinical picture accompanied by serologic confirmation. Although serologic testing may yield negative results during the first several weeks of infection, almost all patients have a positive antibody response to *B. burgdorferi* after that time. The limitation of serologic tests is that they do not clearly distinguish between active and inactive infection. Patients with previous Lyme disease—particularly in cases progressing to late stages—often remain seropositive for years, even after adequate antibiotic treatment. In addition, ~10% of patients are seropositive because of asymptomatic infection. If these individuals subsequently develop another illness, the positive serologic test for

TABLE 210-1 ALGORITHM FOR TESTING FOR AND TREATING LYME DISEASE

Pretest Probability	Example	Recommendation
High	Patients with erythema migrans	Empirical antibiotic treatment without serologic testing
Intermediate	Patients with oligoarticular arthritis	Serologic testing and antibiotic treatment if test results are positive
Low	Patients with nonspecific symptoms (myalgias, arthralgias, fatigue)	Neither serologic testing nor antibiotic treatment

Source: Adapted from the recommendations of the American College of Physicians (G Nichol et al: Ann Intern Med 128:37, 1998, with permission).

Lyme disease may cause diagnostic confusion. According to an algorithm published by the American College of Physicians (Table 210-1), serologic testing for Lyme disease is recommended only for patients with at least an intermediate pretest probability of Lyme disease, such as those with oligoarticular arthritis. It should not be used as a screening procedure in patients with pain or fatigue syndromes. In such patients, the probability of a false-positive serologic result is higher than that of a true-positive result.

For serologic analysis of Lyme disease in the United States, the CDC recommends a two-step approach in which samples are first tested by enzyme-linked immunosorbent assay (ELISA) and equivocal or positive results are then tested by western blotting. During the first weeks of infection, both IgM and IgG responses to the spirochete should be determined, preferably in both acute- and convalescent-phase serum samples. Approximately 20–30% of patients have a positive response detectable in acute-phase samples, whereas ~70–80% have a positive response during convalescence (2–4 weeks later). After 4–8 weeks of infection (by which time most patients with active Lyme disease have disseminated infection), the sensitivity and specificity of the IgG response to the spirochete are both very high—in the range of 99%—as determined by the two-test approach of ELISA and western blot. At this point and thereafter, a single test (that for IgG) is usually sufficient. In persons with illness of >2 months' duration, a positive IgM test result alone is likely to be false-positive and therefore should not be used to support the diagnosis.

According to current criteria adopted by the CDC, an IgM western blot is considered positive if two of the following three bands are present: 23, 39, and 41 kDa. However, the combination of two such bands may still represent a false-positive result. Misuse or misinterpretation of IgM blots has been a factor in the incorrect diagnosis of Lyme disease in patients with other illnesses. An IgG blot is considered positive if 5 of the following 10 bands are present: 18, 23, 28, 30, 39, 41, 45, 58, 66, and 93 kDa. In European cases, no single set of criteria for the interpretation of immunoblots results in high levels of sensitivity and specificity in all countries.

The most promising second-generation serologic test is the VlsE C6 peptide IgG ELISA, which employs a 26-mer of the sixth invariant region of the VlsE lipoprotein of *B. burgdorferi*. The results achieved with this test are similar to those obtained with the standard two-test approach (sonicate IgM and IgG ELISA and western blot). The principal advantage of the C6 peptide ELISA is the early detection of an IgG response, which renders an IgM test unnecessary. However, not all patients with late Lyme disease have a response to the C6 peptide, and this test is not quite as specific as sonicate western blot. Thus, at present, a two-test approach that includes western blot is still recommended. Blotting can also be helpful in assessing the duration of current or past disease.

After successful antibiotic treatment, antibody titers decline slowly but responses (including that to the VlsE C6 peptide) may persist for years. Moreover, not only the IgG but also the IgM response may persist for years after therapy. Therefore, even a positive IgM response cannot be interpreted as confirmation of recent infection or reinfection unless the clinical picture is appropriate.

DIFFERENTIAL DIAGNOSIS

Classic EM is a slowly expanding erythema, often with partial central clearing. If the lesion expands little, it may represent the red papule of an uninfected tick bite. If the lesion expands rapidly, it may represent cellulitis (e.g., streptococcal cellulitis) or an allergic reaction, perhaps to tick saliva. Patients with secondary annular lesions may be thought to have erythema multiforme, but neither the development of blistering mucosal lesions nor the involvement of the palms or soles is a feature of *B. burgdorferi* infection. In the eastern United States, an EM-like skin lesion, sometimes with mild systemic symptoms, may be associated with *Amblyomma americanum* tick bites. However, the cause of this Southern tick-associated rash illness (STARI) has not yet been identified. This tick may also transmit *Ehrlichia chaffeensis*, a rickettsial agent (Chap. 211).

As stated above, *I. scapularis* ticks in the United States may transmit not only *B. burgdorferi* but also *B. microti*, a red blood cell parasite (Chap. 249); *A. phagocytophilum*, the agent of human granulocytotropic anaplasmosis (Chap. 211); *Ehrlichia* species Wisconsin; *B. miyamotoi*, a relapsing fever spirochete (Chap. 209); or (rarely) Powassan encephalitis virus (the deer tick virus, which is closely related to European tick-borne encephalitis virus) (Chap. 233). Although babesiosis and anaplasmosis are most often asymptomatic, infection with any of these agents may cause nonspecific systemic symptoms, particularly in the young or elderly, and co-infected patients may have more severe or persistent symptoms than patients infected with a single agent. Standard blood counts may yield clues regarding the presence of co-infection with *Anaplasma* or *Babesia*. Anaplasmosis may cause leukopenia or thrombocytopenia, and babesiosis may cause thrombocytopenia or (in severe cases) hemolytic anemia. IgM serologic responses may confuse the diagnosis. For example, *A. phagocytophilum* may elicit a positive IgM response to *B. burgdorferi*. The frequency of co-infection in different studies has been variable. In one prospective study, 4% of patients with EM had evidence of co-infection.

Facial palsy caused by *B. burgdorferi*, which occurs in the early disseminated phase of the infection (often in July, August, or September), is usually recognized by its association with EM. However, in rare cases, facial palsy without EM may be the presenting manifestation of Lyme disease. In such cases, both the IgM and the IgG responses to the spirochete are usually positive. The most common infectious agents that cause facial palsy are herpes simplex virus type 1 (Bell's palsy; Chap. 216) and varicella-zoster virus (Ramsay Hunt syndrome; Chap. 217).

Later in the infection, oligoarticular Lyme arthritis most resembles reactive arthritis in an adult or the pauciarticular form of juvenile idiopathic arthritis in a child. Patients with Lyme arthritis usually have the strongest IgG antibody responses seen in Lyme borreliosis, with reactivity to many spirochetal proteins.

The most common problem in diagnosis is to mistake Lyme disease for chronic fatigue syndrome (Chap. 464e) or fibromyalgia (Chap. 396). This difficulty is compounded by the fact that a small percentage of patients do in fact develop these chronic pain or fatigue syndromes in association with or soon after Lyme disease. Moreover, a counterculture has emerged that ascribes pain and fatigue syndromes to chronic Lyme disease when there is little or no evidence of *B. burgdorferi* infection. In such cases, the term *chronic Lyme disease*, which is equated with chronic *B. burgdorferi* infection, is a misnomer, and the use of prolonged, dangerous, and expensive antibiotic treatment is not warranted.

TREATMENT LYME BORRELIOSIS

ANTIBIOTIC TREATMENT

As outlined in the algorithm in Fig. 210-2, the various manifestations of Lyme disease can usually be treated successfully with orally administered antibiotics; the exceptions are objective neurologic abnormalities and third-degree atrioventricular heart block, which are generally treated with IV antibiotics, and arthritis that does not

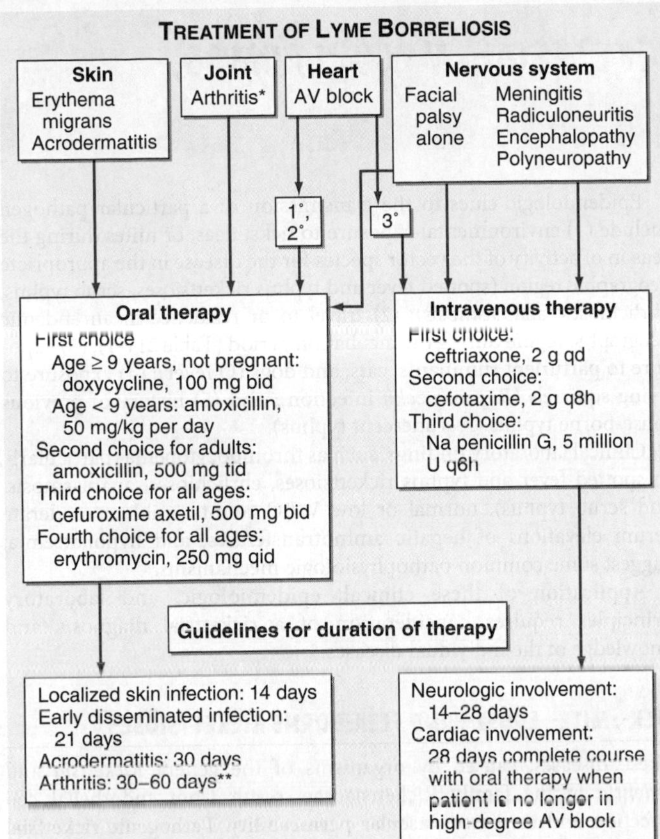

FIGURE 210-2 Algorithm for the treatment of the various early or late manifestations of Lyme borreliosis. AV, atrioventricular. *For arthritis, oral therapy should be tried first; if arthritis is unresponsive, IV therapy should be administered. **For Lyme arthritis, IV ceftriaxone (2 g given once a day for 14–28 days) also is effective and is necessary for a small percentage of patients; however, compared with oral treatment, this regimen is less convenient to administer, has more side effects, and is more expensive.

respond to therapy. For early Lyme disease, doxycycline is effective and can be administered to men and nonpregnant women. An advantage of this regimen is that it is also effective against *A. phagocytophilum*, which is transmitted by the same tick that transmits the Lyme disease agent. Amoxicillin, cefuroxime axetil, and erythromycin or its congeners are second-, third-, and fourth-choice alternatives, respectively. In children, amoxicillin is effective (not more than 2 g/d); in cases of penicillin allergy, cefuroxime axetil or erythromycin may be used. In contrast to second- or third-generation cephalosporin antibiotics, first-generation cephalosporins, such as cephalexin, are not effective. For patients with infection localized to the skin, a 14-day course of therapy is generally sufficient; in contrast, for patients with disseminated infection, a 21-day course is recommended. Approximately 15% of patients experience a Jarisch-Herxheimer-like reaction during the first 24 h of therapy. In multicenter studies, more than 90% of patients whose early Lyme disease was treated with these regimens had satisfactory outcomes. Although some patients reported symptoms after treatment, objective evidence of persistent infection or relapse was rare, and re-treatment was usually unnecessary.

Oral administration of doxycycline or amoxicillin for 30 days is recommended for the initial treatment of Lyme arthritis in patients who do not have concomitant neurologic involvement. Among patients with arthritis who do not respond to oral antibiotics, re-treatment with IV ceftriaxone for 28 days is appropriate. In patients with arthritis in whom joint inflammation persists for months or even several years after both oral and IV antibiotics, treatment with nonsteroidal anti-inflammatory agents, therapy with disease-modifying antirheumatic drugs, or synovectomy may be successful.

In the United States, parenteral antibiotic therapy is usually used for objective neurologic abnormalities (with the exception of facial palsy alone). Patients with neurologic involvement are most commonly treated with IV ceftriaxone for 14–28 days, but IV cefotaxime or IV penicillin G for the same duration also may be effective. In Europe, similar results have been obtained with oral doxycycline and IV antibiotics in the treatment of acute neuroborreliosis. In patients with high-degree atrioventricular block or a PR interval of >0.3 s, IV therapy for at least part of the course and cardiac monitoring are recommended, but the insertion of a permanent pacemaker is not necessary.

It is unclear how and whether asymptomatic infection should be treated, but patients with such infection are often given a course of oral antibiotics. Because maternal-fetal transmission of *B. burgdorferi* seems to occur rarely (if at all), standard therapy for the manifestations of the illness is recommended for pregnant women. Long-term persistence of *B. burgdorferi* has not been documented in any large series of patients after treatment with currently recommended regimens. Although an occasional patient requires a second course of antibiotics, there is no indication for multiple, repeated antibiotic courses in the treatment of Lyme disease.

CHRONIC LYME DISEASE

After appropriately treated Lyme disease, a small percentage of patients continue to have subjective symptoms, primarily musculoskeletal pain, neurocognitive difficulties, or fatigue. This *chronic Lyme disease* or *post–Lyme syndrome* is sometimes a disabling condition that is similar to chronic fatigue syndrome or fibromyalgia. In a large study, one group of patients with post–Lyme syndrome received IV ceftriaxone for 30 days followed by oral doxycycline for 60 days, while another group received IV and oral placebo preparations for the same durations. No significant differences were found between groups in the numbers of patients reporting that their symptoms had improved, become worse, or stayed the same. Such patients are best treated for the relief of symptoms rather than with prolonged courses of antibiotics.

PROPHYLAXIS AFTER A TICK BITE

The risk of infection with *B. burgdorferi* after a recognized tick bite is so low that antibiotic prophylaxis is not routinely indicated. However, if an attached, engorged *I. scapularis* nymph is found or if follow-up is anticipated to be difficult, a single 200-mg dose of doxycycline, which usually prevents Lyme disease when given within 72 h after the tick bite, may be administered.

PROGNOSIS

The response to treatment is best early in the disease. Later treatment of Lyme borreliosis is still effective, but the period of convalescence may be longer. Eventually, most patients recover with minimal or no residual deficits.

REINFECTION

Reinfection may occur after EM when patients are treated with antimicrobial agents. In such cases, the immune response is not adequate to provide protection from subsequent infection. However, patients who develop an expanded immune response to the spirochete over a period of months (e.g., those with Lyme arthritis) have protective immunity for a period of years and rarely, if ever, acquire the infection again.

PREVENTION

Protective measures for the prevention of Lyme disease may include the avoidance of tick-infested areas, the use of repellents and acaricides, tick checks, and modification of landscapes in or near residential areas. Although a vaccine for Lyme disease used to be available, the manufacturer has discontinued its production. Therefore, no vaccine is now commercially available for the prevention of this infection.

SECTION 10 DISEASES CAUSED BY RICKETTSIAE, MYCOPLASMAS, AND CHLAMYDIAE

211 Rickettsial Diseases

David H. Walker, J. Stephen Dumler, Thomas Marrie

The rickettsiae are a heterogeneous group of small, obligately intracellular, gram-negative coccobacilli and short bacilli, most of which are transmitted by a tick, mite, flea, or louse vector. Except in the case of louse-borne typhus, humans are incidental hosts. Among rickettsiae, *Coxiella burnetii*, *Rickettsia prowazekii*, and *R. typhi* have the well-documented ability to survive for an extended period outside the reservoir or vector and to be extremely infectious: inhalation of a single *Coxiella* microorganism can cause pneumonia. High-level infectivity and severe illness after inhalation make *R. prowazekii*, *R. rickettsii*, *R. typhi*, *R. conorii*, and *C. burnetii* bioterrorism threats.

Clinical infections with rickettsiae can be classified according to (1) the taxonomy and diverse microbial characteristics of the agents, which belong to seven genera (*Rickettsia*, *Orientia*, *Ehrlichia*, *Anaplasma*, *Neorickettsia*, *Candidatus* Neoehrlichia, and *Coxiella*); (2) epidemiology; or (3) clinical manifestations. The clinical manifestations of all the acute presentations are similar during the first 5 days: fever, headache, and myalgias with or without nausea, vomiting, and cough. As the course progresses, clinical manifestations—including occurrence of a macular, maculopapular, or vesicular rash; eschar; pneumonitis; and meningoencephalitis—vary from one disease to another. Given the 15 etiologic agents with varied mechanisms of transmission, geographic distributions, and associated disease manifestations, the consideration of rickettsial diseases as a single entity poses complex challenges (Table 211-1).

Establishing the etiologic diagnosis of rickettsioses is very difficult during the acute stage of illness, and definitive diagnosis usually requires the examination of paired serum samples after convalescence. Heightened clinical suspicion is based on epidemiologic data, history of exposure to vectors or reservoir animals, travel to endemic locations, clinical manifestations (sometimes including rash or eschar), and characteristic laboratory findings (including thrombocytopenia, normal or low white blood cell [WBC] counts, elevated hepatic enzyme levels, and hyponatremia). Such suspicion should prompt empirical treatment. Doxycycline is the drug of choice for most of these infections. Only one agent, *C. burnetii*, has been documented to cause chronic illness. One other species, *R. prowazekii*, causes recrudescent illness (Brill-Zinsser disease) when latent infection is reactivated years after resolution of the acute illness.

Rickettsial infections dominated by fever may resolve without further clinical evolution. However, after nonspecific early manifestations, the illnesses can also evolve along one or more of several principal clinical lines: (1) development of a macular or maculopapular rash; (2) development of an eschar at the site of tick or mite feeding; (3) development of a vesicular rash (often in rickettsialpox and African tick-bite fever); (4) development of pneumonitis with chest radiographic opacities and/or rales (Q fever and severe cases of Rocky Mountain spotted fever [RMSF], Mediterranean spotted fever [MSF], louse-borne typhus, human monocytotropic ehrlichiosis [HME], human granulocytotropic anaplasmosis [HGA], scrub typhus, and murine typhus); (5) development of meningoencephalitis (louse-borne typhus and severe cases of RMSF, scrub typhus, HME, murine typhus, MSF, and [rarely] Q fever); and (6) progressive hypotension and multiorgan failure as seen with sepsis or toxic shock syndromes (RMSF, MSF, louse-borne typhus, murine typhus, scrub typhus, HME, HGA, and neoehrlichiosis).

Epidemiologic clues to the transmission of a particular pathogen include (1) environmental exposure to ticks, fleas, or mites during the season of activity of the vector species for the disease in the appropriate geographic region (spotted fever and typhus rickettsioses, scrub typhus, ehrlichioses, anaplasmosis); (2) travel to or residence in an endemic geographic region during the incubation period (Table 211-1); (3) exposure to parturient ruminants, cats, and dogs (Q fever); (4) exposure to flying squirrels (*R. prowazekii* infection); and (5) history of previous louse-borne typhus (recrudescent typhus).

Clinical laboratory findings, such as thrombocytopenia (particularly in spotted fever and typhus rickettsioses, ehrlichioses, anaplasmosis, and scrub typhus), normal or low WBC counts, mild to moderate serum elevations of hepatic aminotransferases, and hyponatremia, suggest some common pathophysiologic mechanisms.

Application of these clinical, epidemiologic, and laboratory principles requires consideration of a rickettsial diagnosis and knowledge of the individual diseases.

TICK-, MITE-, LOUSE-, AND FLEA-BORNE RICKETTSIOSES

These diseases, caused by organisms of the genera *Rickettsia* and *Orientia* in the family Rickettsiaceae, result from endothelial cell infection and increased vascular permeability. Pathogenic rickettsial species are very closely related, have small genomes (as a result of reductive evolution, which eliminated many genes for biosynthesis of intracellularly available molecules), and are traditionally separated into typhus and spotted fever groups on the basis of lipopolysaccharide antigens. Some diseases and their agents (e.g., *R. africae*, *R. parkeri*, and *R. sibirica*) are too similar to require separate descriptions. Indeed, the similarities among MSF (*R. conorii* [all strains] and *R. massiliae*), North Asian tick typhus (*R. sibirica*), Japanese spotted fever (*R. japonica*), and Flinders Island spotted fever (*R. honei*) far outweigh the minor variations. The Rickettsiaceae that cause life-threatening infections are, in order of decreasing case-fatality rate, *R. rickettsii* (RMSF); *R. prowazekii* (louse-borne typhus); *Orientia tsutsugamushi* (scrub typhus); *R. conorii* (MSF); *R. typhi* (murine typhus); and, in rare cases, other spotted fever–group organisms. Some agents (e.g., *R. parkeri*, *R. africae*, *R. akari*, *R. slovaca*, *R. honei*, *R. felis*, *R. massiliae*, *R. helvetica*, *R. heilongjiangensis*, *R. aeschlimannii*, and *R. monacensis*) have never been documented to cause a fatal illness.

ROCKY MOUNTAIN SPOTTED FEVER

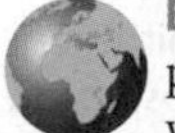

Epidemiology RMSF occurs in 47 states (with the highest prevalence in the south-central and southeastern states) as well as in Canada, Mexico, and Central and South America. The infection is transmitted by *Dermacentor variabilis*, the American dog tick, in the eastern two-thirds of the United States and California; by *D. andersoni*, the Rocky Mountain wood tick, in the western United States; by *Rhipicephalus sanguineus* in Mexico, Arizona, and probably Brazil; and by *Amblyomma cajennense* and *A. aureolatum* in Central and/or South America. Maintained principally by transovarian transmission from one generation of ticks to the next, *R. rickettsii* can be acquired by uninfected ticks through the ingestion of a blood meal from rickettsemic small mammals.

Humans become infected during tick season (in the Northern Hemisphere, from May to September), although some cases occur in winter. The mortality rate was 20–25% in the preantibiotic era and remains at ~3–5%, principally because of delayed diagnosis and treatment. The case-fatality ratio increases with each decade of life above age 20.

Pathogenesis *R. rickettsii* organisms are inoculated into the dermis along with secretions of the tick's salivary glands after ≥6 h of feeding.

PART 8 Infectious Diseases

TABLE 211-1 FEATURES OF SELECTED RICKETTSIAL INFECTIONS

Disease	Organism	Transmission	Geographic Range	Incubation Period, Days	Duration, Days	Rash, %	Eschar, %	Lymphadenopathy[a]
Rocky Mountain spotted fever	*Rickettsia rickettsii*	Tick bite: *Dermacentor andersoni, D. variabilis*	United States	2–14	10–20	90	<1	+
		Amblyomma cajennense, A. aureolatum	Central/South America					
		Rhipicephalus sanguineus	Mexico, Brazil, United States					
Mediterranean spotted fever	*R. conorii*	Tick bite: *R. sanguineus, Rhipicephalus pumilio*	Southern Europe, Africa, Middle East, Central Asia	5–7	7–14	97	50	+
African tick-bite fever	*R. africae*	Tick bite: *A. hebraeum, A. variegatum*	Sub-Saharan Africa, West Indies	4–10	4–19	50	90	++++
Maculatum disease	*R. parkeri*	Tick bite: *A. maculatum*	United States, South America	2–10	6–16	88	94	++
Rickettsialpox	*R. akari*	Mite bite: *Liponyssoides sanguineus*	United States, Ukraine, Turkey, Mexico, Croatia	10–17	3–11	100	90	+++
Tick-borne lymphadenopathy	*R. slovaca*	Tick bite: *D. marginatus, D. reticularis*	Europe	7–9	17–180	5	100	++++
Flea-borne spotted fever	*R. felis*	Flea (mechanism undetermined): *Ctenocephalides felis*	Worldwide	8–16	8–16	80	15	—
Epidemic typhus	*R. prowazekii*	Louse feces: *Pediculus humanus corporis*, fleas and lice of flying squirrels, or recrudescence	Worldwide	7–14	10–18	80	None	—
Murine typhus	*R. typhi*	Flea feces: *Xenopsylla cheopis, C. felis*, others	Worldwide	8–16	9–18	80	None	—
Human monocytotropic ehrlichiosis	*Ehrlichia chaffeensis*	Tick bite: *A. americanum, D. variabilis*	United States	1–21	3–21	26	None	++
Ewingii ehrlichiosis	*E. ewingii*	Tick bite: *A. americanum*	United States	1–21	4–21	0	None	
Unnamed ehrlichiosis	*E. muris*–like agent	Tick bite: *Ixodes scapularis*	United States	Unknown	3–14	None	None	
Human granulocytotropic anaplasmosis	*Anaplasma phagocytophilum*	Tick bite: *I. scapularis, I. ricinus, I. pacificus, I. persulcatus*	United States, Europe, Asia	4–8	3–14	Rare	None	—
Unnamed disease	*Candidatus* Neoehrlichia mikurensis	Tick bite: *I. ricinus, I. persulcatus, Haemaphysalis concinna*	Europe, China	≥8	11–75	10	None	
Scrub typhus	*Orientia tsutsugamushi*	Mite bite: *Leptotrombidium deliense*, others	Asia, Australia, Pacific and Indian Ocean islands	9–18	6–21	50	35	+++
Q fever	*Coxiella burnetii*	Inhalation of aerosols of infected parturition material (goats, sheep, cattle, cats, others), ingestion of infected milk or milk products	Worldwide except New Zealand, Antarctica	3–30	5–57	<1	None	—

[a]++++, severe; +++, marked; ++, moderate; +, present in a small proportion of cases; —, not a noted feature.

The rickettsiae spread lymphohematogenously throughout the body and infect numerous foci of contiguous endothelial cells. The dose-dependent incubation period is ~1 week (range, 2–14 days). Occlusive thrombosis and ischemic necrosis are not the fundamental pathologic bases for tissue and organ injury. Instead, increased vascular permeability, with resulting edema, hypovolemia, and ischemia, is responsible. Consumption of platelets results in thrombocytopenia in 32–52% of patients, but disseminated intravascular coagulation with hypofibrinogenemia is rare. Activation of platelets, generation of thrombin, and activation of the fibrinolytic system all appear to be homeostatic physiologic responses to endothelial injury.

Clinical Manifestations Early in the illness, when medical attention usually is first sought, RMSF is difficult to distinguish from many self-limiting viral illnesses. Fever, headache, malaise, myalgia, nausea, vomiting, and anorexia are the most common symptoms during the first 3 days. The patient becomes progressively more ill as vascular infection and injury advance. In one large series, only one-third of patients were diagnosed with presumptive RMSF early in the clinical course and treated appropriately as outpatients. In the tertiary-care setting, RMSF is all too often recognized only when late severe manifestations, developing at the end of the first week or during the second week of illness in patients without appropriate treatment, prompt return to a physician or hospital and admission to an intensive care unit.

The progressive nature of the infection is clearly manifested in the skin. Rash is evident in only 14% of patients on the first day of illness and in only 49% during the first 3 days. Macules (1–5 mm) appear first on the wrists and ankles and then on the remainder of the extremities and the trunk. Later, more severe vascular damage results in frank hemorrhage at the center of the maculopapule, producing a petechia that does not disappear upon compression (Fig. 211-1). This sequence of events is sometimes delayed or aborted by effective treatment. However, the rash is a variable manifestation, appearing on day 6 or later in 20% of cases and not appearing at all in 9–16% of cases. Petechiae occur in 41–59% of cases, appearing on or after day 6 in 74% of cases that manifest a rash. Involvement of the palms and soles, often considered diagnostically important, usually develops relatively late in

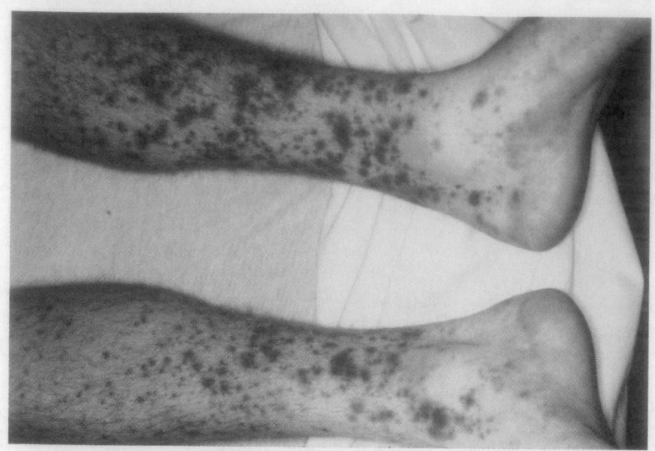

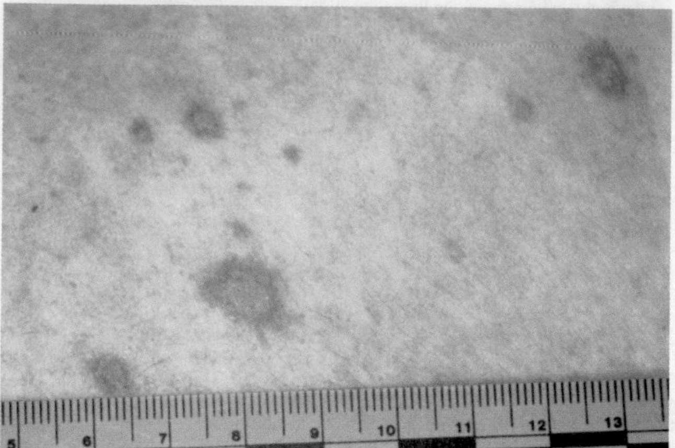

FIGURE 211-1 ***Top:*** Petechial lesions of Rocky Mountain spotted fever on the lower legs and soles of a young, previously healthy patient. ***Bottom:*** Close-up of lesions from the same patient. *(Photos courtesy of Dr. Lindsey Baden; with permission.)*

the course (after day 5 in 43% of cases) and does not develop at all in 18–64% of cases.

Hypovolemia leads to prerenal azotemia and (in 17% of cases) hypotension. Infection of the pulmonary microcirculation leads to noncardiogenic pulmonary edema; 12% of patients have severe respiratory disease, and 8% require mechanical ventilation. Cardiac involvement manifests as dysrhythmia in 7–16% of cases.

Besides respiratory failure, central nervous system (CNS) involvement is the other important determinant of the outcome of RMSF. Encephalitis, presenting as confusion or lethargy, is apparent in 26–28% of cases. Progressively severe encephalitis manifests as stupor or delirium in 21–26% of cases, ataxia in 18%, coma in 10%, and seizures in 8%. Numerous focal neurologic deficits have been reported. Meningoencephalitis results in cerebrospinal fluid (CSF) pleocytosis in 34–38% of cases; usually there are 10–100 cells/μL and a mononuclear predominance, but occasionally there are >100 cells/μL and a polymorphonuclear predominance. The CSF protein concentration is increased in 30–35% of cases, but the CSF glucose concentration is usually normal.

Renal failure, often reversible with rehydration, is caused by acute tubular necrosis in severe cases with shock. Hepatic injury with increased serum aminotransferase concentrations (38% of cases) is due to focal death of individual hepatocytes without hepatic failure. Jaundice is recognized in 9% of cases and an elevated serum bilirubin concentration in 18–30%.

Life-threatening bleeding is rare. Anemia develops in 30% of cases and is severe enough to require transfusions in 11%. Blood is detected in the stool or vomitus of 10% of patients, and death has followed massive upper-gastrointestinal hemorrhage.

Other characteristic clinical laboratory findings include increased plasma levels of proteins of the acute-phase response (C-reactive protein, fibrinogen, ferritin, and others), hypoalbuminemia, and hyponatremia (in 56% of cases) due to the appropriate secretion of antidiuretic hormone in response to the hypovolemic state. Myositis occurs occasionally, with marked elevations in serum creatine kinase levels and multifocal rhabdomyonecrosis. Ocular involvement includes conjunctivitis in 30% of cases and retinal vein engorgement, flame hemorrhages, arterial occlusion, and papilledema with normal CSF pressure in some instances.

In untreated cases, the patient usually dies 8–15 days after onset. A rare presentation, fulminant RMSF, is fatal within 5 days after onset. This fulminant presentation is seen most often in male black patients with glucose-6-phosphate dehydrogenase (G6PD) deficiency and may be related to an undefined effect of hemolysis on the rickettsial infection. Although survivors of RMSF usually return to their previous state of health, permanent sequelae, including neurologic deficits and gangrene necessitating amputation of extremities, may follow severe illness.

Diagnosis The diagnosis of RMSF during the acute stage is more difficult than is generally appreciated. The most important epidemiologic factor is a history of exposure to a potentially tick-infested environment within the 14 days preceding disease onset during a season of possible tick activity. However, only 60% of patients actually recall being bitten by a tick during the incubation period.

The differential diagnosis for early clinical manifestations of RMSF (fever, headache, and myalgia without a rash) includes influenza, enteroviral infection, infectious mononucleosis, viral hepatitis, leptospirosis, typhoid fever, gram-negative or gram-positive bacterial sepsis, HME, HGA, murine typhus, sylvatic flying-squirrel typhus, and rickettsialpox. Enterocolitis may be suggested by nausea, vomiting, and abdominal pain; prominence of abdominal tenderness has resulted in exploratory laparotomy. CNS involvement can masquerade as bacterial or viral meningoencephalitis. Cough, pulmonary signs, and chest radiographic opacities can lead to a diagnostic consideration of bronchitis or pneumonia.

At presentation during the first 3 days of illness, only 3% of patients exhibit the classic triad of fever, rash, and history of tick exposure. When a rash appears, a diagnosis of RMSF should be considered. However, many illnesses considered in the differential diagnosis also can be associated with a rash, including rubeola, rubella, meningococcemia, disseminated gonococcal infection, secondary syphilis, toxic shock syndrome, drug hypersensitivity, idiopathic thrombocytopenic purpura, thrombotic thrombocytopenic purpura, Kawasaki syndrome, and immune complex vasculitis. Conversely, any person in an endemic area with a provisional diagnosis of one of the above illnesses could have RMSF. Thus, if a viral infection is suspected during RMSF season in an endemic area, it should always be kept in mind that RMSF can mimic viral infection early in the course; if the illness worsens over the next couple of days after initial presentation, the patient should return for reevaluation.

The most common serologic test for confirmation of the diagnosis is the indirect immunofluorescence assay. Not until 7–10 days after onset is a diagnostic titer of ≥64 usually detectable. The sensitivity and specificity of the indirect immunofluorescence IgG assay are 89–100% and 99–100%, respectively. It is important to understand that serologic tests for RMSF are usually negative at the time of presentation for medical care and that treatment should not be delayed while a positive serologic result is awaited.

The only diagnostic test that has proven useful during the acute illness is immunohistologic examination of a cutaneous biopsy sample from a rash lesion for *R. rickettsii*. Examination of a 3-mm punch biopsy from such a lesion is 70% sensitive and 100% specific. The sensitivity of polymerase chain reaction (PCR) amplification and detection of *R. rickettsii* DNA in peripheral blood is improving. However, although rickettsiae are present in large quantities in heavily infected foci of endothelial cells, there are relatively low quantities in the circulation. Cultivation of rickettsiae in cell culture is feasible but is seldom undertaken because of biohazard concerns. The recent dramatic increase in the reported incidence of RMSF correlates with the use of single-titer spotted fever–group cross-reactive enzyme immunoassay serology. Few cases are specifically determined to be caused by *R. rickettsii*. Currently, many febrile persons who do not have RMSF present with cross-reactive antibodies, possibly because of previous exposure to the highly prevalent spotted fever–group rickettsia *R. amblyommii*.

TREATMENT ROCKY MOUNTAIN SPOTTED FEVER

The drug of choice for the treatment of both children and adults with RMSF is doxycycline, except when the patient is pregnant or allergic to this drug (see below). Because of the severity of RMSF, immediate empirical administration of doxycycline should be strongly considered for any patient with a consistent clinical presentation in the appropriate epidemiologic setting. Doxycycline is administered orally (or, in the presence of coma or vomiting, intravenously) at 200 mg/d in two divided doses. For children with suspected RMSF, up to five courses of doxycycline may be administered with minimal risk of dental staining. Other regimens include oral tetracycline (25–50 mg/kg per day) in four divided doses. Treatment with chloramphenicol, a less effective drug, is advised only for patients who are pregnant or allergic to doxycycline. The antirickettsial drug should be administered until the patient has been afebrile and improving clinically for 2–3 days. β-Lactam antibiotics, erythromycin, and aminoglycosides have no role in the treatment of RMSF, and sulfa-containing drugs are associated with more adverse outcomes than no treatment at all. There is little clinical experience with fluoroquinolones, clarithromycin, and azithromycin, which are not recommended. The most seriously ill patients are managed in intensive care units, with careful administration of fluids to achieve optimal tissue perfusion without precipitating noncardiogenic pulmonary edema. In some severely ill patients, hypoxemia requires intubation and mechanical ventilation; oliguric or anuric acute renal failure requires hemodialysis; seizures necessitate the use of antiseizure medication; anemia or severe hemorrhage necessitates transfusions of packed red blood cells; or bleeding with severe thrombocytopenia requires platelet transfusions. Heparin is not a useful component of treatment, and there is no evidence that glucocorticoids affect outcome.

Prevention Avoidance of tick bites is the only available preventive approach. Use of protective clothing and tick repellents, inspection of the body once or twice a day, and removal of ticks before they inoculate rickettsiae reduce the risk of infection. Prophylactic doxycycline treatment of tick bites has no proven role in preventing RMSF.

MEDITERRANEAN SPOTTED FEVER (BOUTONNEUSE FEVER), AFRICAN TICK-BITE FEVER, AND OTHER TICK-BORNE SPOTTED FEVERS

Epidemiology *R. conorii* is prevalent in southern Europe, Africa, and southwestern and south-central Asia. Regional names for the disease caused by this organism include Mediterranean spotted fever, Kenya tick typhus, Indian tick typhus, Israeli spotted fever, and Astrakhan spotted fever. The disease is characterized by high fever, rash, and—in most geographic locales—an inoculation eschar (*tâche noire*) at the site of the tick bite. A severe form of the disease (mortality rate, 50%) occurs in patients with diabetes, alcoholism, or heart failure.

African tick-bite fever, caused by *R. africae*, occurs in rural areas of sub-Saharan Africa and in the Caribbean islands and is transmitted by *Amblyomma hebraeum* and *A. variegatum* ticks. The average incubation period is 4–10 days. The mild illness consists of headache, fever, eschar, and regional lymphadenopathy. *Amblyomma* ticks often feed in groups, with the consequent development of multiple eschars. Rash may be vesicular, sparse, or absent altogether. Because of tourism in sub-Saharan Africa, African tick-bite fever is the rickettsiosis most frequently imported into Europe and North America. A similar disease caused by the closely related species *R. parkeri* is transmitted by *A. maculatum* in the United States and by *A. triste* in South America.

R. japonica causes Japanese spotted fever, which also occurs in Korea. Similar diseases in northern Asia are caused by *R. sibirica* and *R. heilongjiangensis*. Queensland tick typhus due to *R. australis* is transmitted by *Ixodes holocyclus* ticks. Flinders Island spotted fever, found on the island for which it is named as well as in Tasmania, mainland Australia, and Asia, is caused by *R. honei*. In Europe, patients infected with *R. slovaca* after a wintertime *Dermacentor* tick bite manifest an afebrile illness with an eschar (usually on the scalp) and painful regional lymphadenopathy.

Diagnosis Diagnosis of these tick-borne spotted fevers is based on clinical and epidemiologic findings and is confirmed by serology, immunohistochemical demonstration of rickettsiae in skin biopsy specimens, cell-culture isolation of rickettsiae, or PCR of skin biopsy, eschar, or blood samples. Serologic diagnosis detects antibodies to antigens shared among spotted fever–group rickettsiae, hindering identification of the etiologic species. In an endemic area, a possible diagnosis of rickettsial spotted fevers should be considered when patients present with fever, rash, and/or a skin lesion consisting of a black necrotic area or a crust surrounded by erythema.

TREATMENT TICK-BORNE SPOTTED FEVERS

Successful therapeutic agents include doxycycline (100 mg bid orally for 1–5 days) and chloramphenicol (500 mg qid orally for 7–10 days). Pregnant patients may be treated with josamycin (3 g/d orally for 5 days). Data on the efficacy of treatment of mildly ill children with clarithromycin or azithromycin should not be extrapolated to adults or to patients with moderate or severe illness.

RICKETTSIALPOX

R. akari infects mice and their mites (*Liponyssoides sanguineus*), which maintain the organisms by transovarial transmission.

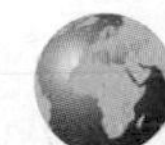

Epidemiology Rickettsialpox is recognized principally in New York City, but cases have also been reported in other urban and rural locations in the United States and in Ukraine, Croatia, Mexico, and Turkey. Investigation of eschars suspected of representing bioterrorism-associated cutaneous anthrax revealed that rickettsialpox occurs more frequently than previously realized.

Clinical Manifestations A papule forms at the site of the mite's feeding, develops a central vesicle, and becomes a 1- to 2.5-cm painless black crusted eschar surrounded by an erythematous halo (Fig. 211-2). Enlargement of the regional lymph nodes draining the eschar suggests initial lymphogenous spread. After an incubation period of

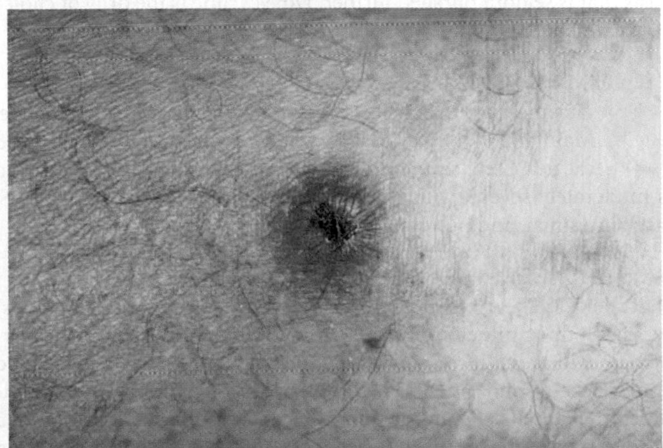

FIGURE 211-2 Eschar at the site of the mite bite in a patient with rickettsialpox. *(Reprinted from A Krusell et al: Emerg Infect Dis 8:727, 2002. Photo obtained by Dr. Kenneth Kaye.)*

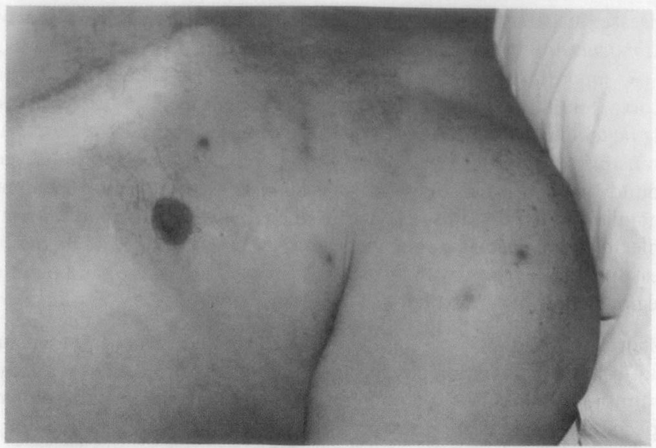

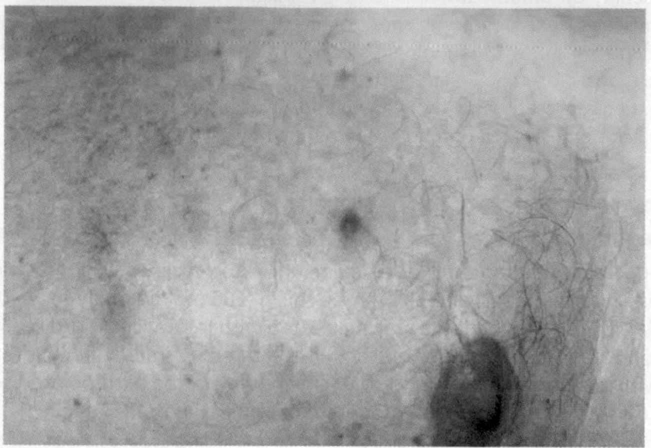

FIGURE 211-3 ***Top:*** Papulovesicular lesions on the trunk of the patient with rickettsialpox shown in Fig. 211-2. ***Bottom:*** Close-up of lesions from the same patient. *(Reprinted from A Krusell et al: Emerg Infect Dis 8:727, 2002. Photos obtained by Dr. Kenneth Kaye.)*

10–17 days, during which the eschar and regional lymphadenopathy frequently go unnoticed, disease onset is marked by malaise, chills, fever, headache, and myalgia. A macular rash appears 2–6 days after onset and usually evolves sequentially into papules, vesicles, and crusts that heal without scarring (Fig. 211-3); in some cases, the rash remains macular or maculopapular. Some patients develop nausea, vomiting, abdominal pain, cough, conjunctivitis, or photophobia. Without treatment, fever lasts 6–10 days.

Diagnosis and Treatment Clinical, epidemiologic, and convalescent serologic data establish the diagnosis of a spotted fever–group rickettsiosis that is seldom pursued further. Doxycycline is the drug of choice for treatment.

FLEA-BORNE SPOTTED FEVER

An emerging rickettsiosis caused by *R. felis* occurs worldwide. Maintained transovarially in the geographically widespread cat flea *Ctenocephalides felis*, the infection has been described as moderately severe, with fever, rash, and headache as well as CNS, gastrointestinal, and pulmonary symptoms.

EPIDEMIC (LOUSE-BORNE) TYPHUS

Epidemiology The human body louse (*Pediculus humanus corporis*) lives in clothing under poor hygienic conditions and usually in impoverished cold areas. Lice acquire *R. prowazekii* when they ingest blood from a rickettsemic patient. The rickettsiae multiply in the louse's midgut epithelial cells and are shed in its feces. The infected louse leaves a febrile person and deposits infected feces on its subsequent host during its blood meal; the patient autoinoculates the organisms by scratching. The louse is killed by the rickettsiae and does not pass *R. prowazekii* to its offspring.

Epidemic typhus haunts regions afflicted by wars and disasters. An outbreak involved 100,000 people in refugee camps in Burundi in 1997. A small focus was documented in Russia in 1998; sporadic cases were reported from Algeria, and frequent outbreaks occurred in Peru. Eastern flying squirrels (*Glaucomys volans*) and their lice and fleas maintain *R. prowazekii* in a zoonotic cycle.

Brill-Zinsser disease is a recrudescent illness occurring years after acute epidemic typhus, probably as a result of waning immunity. *R. prowazekii* remains latent for years; its reactivation results in sporadic cases of disease in louse-free populations or in epidemics in louse-infested populations.

Rickettsiae are potential agents of bioterrorism (Chap. 261e). Infections with *R. prowazekii* and *R. rickettsii* have high case–fatality ratios. These organisms cause difficult-to-diagnose diseases and are highly infectious when inhaled as aerosols. Organisms resistant to tetracycline or chloramphenicol have been developed in the laboratory.

Clinical Manifestations After an incubation period of ~1–2 weeks, the onset of illness is abrupt, with prostration, severe headache, and fever rising rapidly to 38.8°–40.0°C (102°–104°F). Cough is prominent, developing in 70% of patients. Myalgias are usually severe. A rash begins on the upper trunk, usually on the fifth day, and then becomes generalized, involving the entire body except the face, palms, and soles. Initially, this rash is macular; without treatment, it becomes maculopapular, petechial, and confluent. The rash often goes undetected in black skin; 60% of African patients have spotless epidemic typhus. Photophobia, with considerable conjunctival injection and eye pain, is common. The tongue may be dry, brown, and furred. Confusion and coma are common. Skin necrosis and gangrene of the digits as well as interstitial pneumonia may occur in severe cases. Untreated disease is fatal in 7–40% of cases, with outcome depending primarily on the condition of the host. Patients with untreated infections develop renal insufficiency and multiorgan involvement in which neurologic manifestations are frequently prominent. Overall, 12% of patients with epidemic typhus have neurologic involvement. Infection associated with North American flying squirrels is a milder illness; whether this milder disease is due to host factors (e.g., better health status) or attenuated virulence is unknown.

Diagnosis and Treatment Epidemic typhus is sometimes misdiagnosed as typhoid fever in tropical countries (Chap. 190). The means even for serologic studies are often unavailable in settings of louse-borne typhus. Epidemics can be recognized by the serologic or immunohistochemical diagnosis of a single case or by detection of *R. prowazekii* in a louse found on a patient. Doxycycline (200 mg/d, given in two divided doses) is administered orally or—if the patient is comatose or vomiting—intravenously. Although under epidemic conditions a single 200-mg oral dose is effective, treatment is generally continued until 2–3 days after defervescence. Pregnant patients should be evaluated individually and treated with chloramphenicol early in pregnancy or, if necessary, with doxycycline late in pregnancy.

Prevention Prevention of epidemic typhus involves control of body lice. Clothes should be changed regularly, and insecticides should be used every 6 weeks to control the louse population.

ENDEMIC MURINE TYPHUS

Epidemiology *R. typhi* is maintained in mammalian host/flea cycles, with rats (*Rattus rattus* and *R. norvegicus*) and the Oriental rat flea (*Xenopsylla cheopis*) as the classic zoonotic niche. Fleas acquire *R. typhi* from rickettsemic rats and carry the organism throughout their life span. Nonimmune rats and humans are infected when rickettsia-laden flea feces contaminate pruritic bite lesions; less frequently, the flea bite transmits the organisms. Transmission can also occur via inhalation of aerosolized rickettsiae from flea feces. Infected rats appear healthy, although they are rickettsemic for ~2 weeks.

Murine typhus occurs mainly in Texas and southern California, where the classic rat/flea cycle is absent and an opossum/cat flea (*C. felis*) cycle is prominent. Globally, endemic typhus occurs mainly in warm (often coastal) areas throughout the tropics and subtropics, where it is highly prevalent though often unrecognized. The incidence peaks from April through June in southern Texas and during the warm months of summer and early fall in other geographic locations. Patients seldom recall exposure to fleas, although exposure to animals such as cats, opossums, and rats is reported in nearly 40% of cases.

Clinical Manifestations The incubation period of experimental murine typhus averages 11 days (range, 8–16 days). Headache, myalgia, arthralgia, nausea, and malaise develop 1–3 days before onset of chills and fever. Nearly all patients experience nausea and vomiting early in the illness.

The duration of untreated illness averages 12 days (range, 9–18 days). Rash is present in only 13% of patients at presentation for medical care (usually ~4 days after onset of fever), appearing an average of 2 days later in half of the remaining patients and never appearing in the others. The initial macular rash is often detected by careful inspection of the axilla or the inner surface of the arm. Subsequently, the rash becomes maculopapular, involving the trunk more often than the extremities; it is seldom petechial and rarely involves the face, palms, or soles. A rash is detected in only 20% of patients with darkly pigmented skin.

Pulmonary involvement is frequently prominent; 35% of patients have a hacking, nonproductive cough, and 23% of patients who undergo chest radiography have pulmonary densities due to interstitial pneumonia, pulmonary edema, and pleural effusions. Bibasilar rales are the most common pulmonary sign. Less common clinical manifestations include abdominal pain, confusion, stupor, seizures, ataxia, coma, and jaundice. Clinical laboratory studies frequently reveal anemia and leukopenia early in the course, leukocytosis late in the course, thrombocytopenia, hyponatremia, hypoalbuminemia, mildly increased serum hepatic aminotransferases, and prerenal azotemia. Complications can include respiratory failure, hematemesis, cerebral hemorrhage, and hemolysis. Severe illness necessitates the admission of 10% of hospitalized patients to an intensive care unit. Greater severity is generally associated with old age, underlying disease, and treatment with a sulfonamide; the case-fatality rate is 1%. In a study of children with murine typhus, 50% suffered only nocturnal fevers, feeling well enough for active daytime play.

Diagnosis and Treatment Serologic studies of acute- and convalescent-phase sera can provide a diagnosis, and an immunohistochemical method for identification of typhus group-specific antigens in biopsy samples has been developed. Cultivation and PCR are used only infrequently and are not widely available. Nevertheless, most patients are treated empirically with doxycycline (100 mg bid orally for 7–15 days) on the basis of clinical suspicion. Ciprofloxacin provides an alternative if doxycycline is contraindicated.

SCRUB TYPHUS

Epidemiology *O. tsutsugamushi* differs substantially from *Rickettsia* species both genetically and in cell wall composition (i.e., it lacks lipopolysaccharide). *O. tsutsugamushi* is maintained by transovarial transmission in trombiculid mites. After hatching, infected larval mites (chiggers, the only stage that feeds on a host) inoculate organisms into the skin. Infected chiggers are particularly likely to be found in areas of heavy scrub vegetation during the wet season, when mites lay eggs.

Scrub typhus is endemic and reemerging in eastern and southern Asia, northern Australia, and islands of the western Pacific and Indian Oceans. Infections are prevalent in these regions; in some areas, >3% of the population is infected or reinfected each month. Immunity wanes over 1–3 years, and the organism exhibits remarkable antigenic diversity.

Clinical Manifestations Illness varies from mild and self-limiting to fatal. After an incubation period of 6–21 days, onset is characterized by fever, headache, myalgia, cough, and gastrointestinal symptoms. Some patients recover spontaneously after a few days. The classic case description includes an eschar where the chigger has fed, regional lymphadenopathy, and a maculopapular rash—signs that are seldom seen in indigenous patients. Fewer than 50% of Westerners develop an eschar, and fewer than 40% develop a rash (on day 4–6 of illness). Severe cases typically manifest with encephalitis and interstitial pneumonia due to vascular injury. The case-fatality rate for untreated classic cases is 7% but would probably be lower if all mild cases were diagnosed.

Diagnosis and Treatment Serologic assays (indirect fluorescent antibody, indirect immunoperoxidase, and enzyme immunoassays) are the mainstays of laboratory diagnosis. PCR amplification of *Orientia* genes from eschars and blood also is effective. Patients are treated with doxycycline (100 mg bid orally for 7–15 days), azithromycin (500 mg orally for 3 days), or chloramphenicol (500 mg qid orally for 7–15 days). Some cases of scrub typhus in Thailand are caused by strains that have high doxycycline or chloramphenicol minimal inhibitory concentrations (MICs) but that are susceptible to azithromycin and rifampin.

EHRLICHIOSES AND ANAPLASMOSIS

Ehrlichioses are acute febrile infections caused by members of the family Anaplasmataceae, which is made up of obligately intracellular organisms of five genera: *Ehrlichia*, *Anaplasma*, *Wolbachia*, *Candidatus* Neoehrlichia, and *Neorickettsia*. The bacteria reside in vertebrate reservoirs and target vacuoles of hematopoietic cells (Fig. 211-4). Three *Ehrlichia* species and one *Anaplasma* species are transmitted by ticks to humans and cause infection that can be severe and prevalent. *E. chaffeensis*, the agent of HME, and an *E. muris*-like agent (EMLA) infect predominantly mononuclear phagocytes; *E. ewingii* and *A. phagocytophilum* infect neutrophils. Infection with *Candidatus* Neoehrlichia mikurensis is less well characterized, but the agent has been identified in human blood neutrophils.

Ehrlichia, *Candidatus* Neoehrlichia, and *Anaplasma* are maintained by horizontal tick-mammal-tick transmission, and humans are only inadvertently infected. Wolbachiae are associated with human filariasis, since they are important for filarial viability and pathogenicity; antibiotic treatment targeting wolbachiae is a strategy for filariasis control. Neorickettsiae parasitize flukes (trematodes) that in turn parasitize aquatic snails, fish, and insects. Only a single human neorickettsiosis has been described: sennetsu fever, an infectious mononucleosis–like illness that was first identified in 1953 and is associated with the ingestion of raw fish containing *N. sennetsu*–infected flukes.

HUMAN MONOCYTOTROPIC EHRLICHIOSIS

Epidemiology More than 8404 cases of *E. chaffeensis* infection had been reported to the Centers for Disease Control and Prevention (CDC) as of April 2013. However, active prospective surveillance has documented an incidence as high as 414 cases per 100,000 population

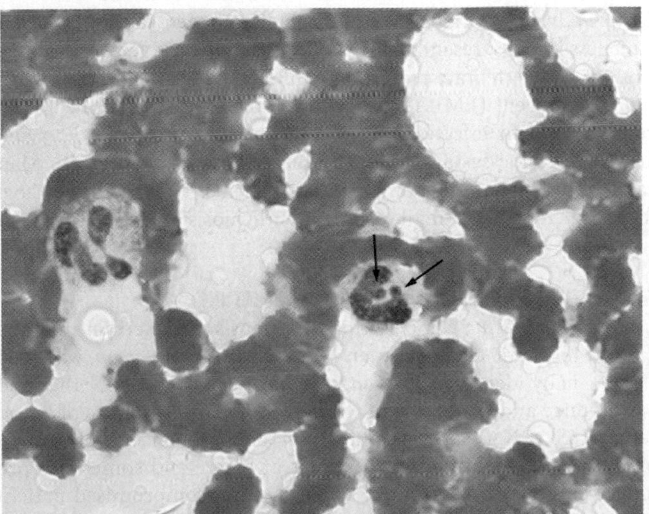

FIGURE 211-4 Peripheral-blood smear from a patient with human granulocytotropic anaplasmosis. A neutrophil contains two morulae (vacuoles filled with *A. phagocytophilum*). *(Photo courtesy of Dr. J. Stephen Dumler.)*

in some U.S. regions. Most *E. chaffeensis* infections are identified in the south-central, southeastern, and mid-Atlantic states, but cases have also been recognized in California and New York. All stages of the Lone Star tick (*A. americanum*) feed on white-tailed deer—a major reservoir. Dogs and coyotes also serve as reservoirs and often lack clinical signs. Tick bites and exposures are frequently reported by patients in rural areas, especially in May through July. The median age of HME patients is 52 years; however, severe and fatal infections in children also are well recognized. Of patients with HME, 60% are male.

E. chaffeensis has been detected in South America, Africa, and Asia.

Clinical Manifestations *E. chaffeensis* disseminates hematogenously from the dermal blood pool created by the feeding tick. After a median incubation period of 8 days, illness develops. Clinical manifestations are undifferentiated and include fever (96% of cases), headache (72%), myalgia (68%), and malaise (77%). Less frequently observed are nausea, vomiting, and diarrhea (25–57%); cough (28%); rash (26% overall, 6% at presentation); and confusion (20%). HME can be severe: 49% of patients with documented cases are hospitalized, and ~2% die. Severe manifestations include a toxic shock–like or septic shock–like syndrome, adult respiratory distress syndrome, cardiac failure, hepatitis, meningoencephalitis, hemorrhage, and—in immunocompromised patients—overwhelming ehrlichial infection. Laboratory findings are valuable in the differential diagnosis of HME; 61% of patients have leukopenia (initially lymphopenia, later neutropenia), 73% have thrombocytopenia, and 84% have elevated serum levels of hepatic aminotransferases. Despite low blood cell counts, the bone marrow is hypercellular, and noncaseating granulomas can be present. Vasculitis is not a component of HME.

Diagnosis HME can be fatal. Early empirical antibiotic therapy based on clinical diagnosis diminishes adverse outcomes. This diagnosis is suggested by fever with a known tick exposure during the preceding 3 weeks, thrombocytopenia and/or leukopenia, and increased serum aminotransferase levels. Morulae are demonstrated in <10% of peripheral-blood smears. HME can be confirmed during active infection by PCR amplification of *E. chaffeensis* nucleic acids in blood obtained before the start of doxycycline therapy. Retrospective serodiagnosis requires a consistent clinical picture and a fourfold increase in *E. chaffeensis* antibody titer to ≥64 in paired sera obtained ~3 weeks apart. Separate specific diagnostic tests are necessary for HME and HGA.

EWINGII EHRLICHIOSIS AND *EHRLICHIA MURIS*–LIKE INFECTIONS

Ehrlichia ewingii, originally a neutrophil pathogen causing fever and lameness in dogs, resembles *E. chaffeensis* in its tick vector (*A. americanum*) and vertebrate reservoirs (white-tailed deer and dogs). An *E. muris*–like agent (EMLA) has been discovered and identified as the cause of human infections in Wisconsin and Minnesota. *E. ewingii* and EMLA illnesses are similar to but less severe than HME. Many cases occur in immunocompromised patients. No specific serologic diagnostic tests for ewingii or EMLA ehrlichiosis are readily available.

CANDIDATUS NEOEHRLICHIA MIKURENSIS INFECTION

Candidatus Neoehrlichia mikurensis, a bacterium in a phylogenetic clade between *Ehrlichia* and *Anaplasma*, was originally identified in *Ixodes ricinus* ticks from the Netherlands and in mice and *Ixodes ovatus* ticks from Japan. By means of broad-range 16S rRNA gene amplification and sequence analysis, this organism was identified as the cause of severe and sometimes prolonged febrile illnesses in European immunocompromised patients with tick bites or exposures and in Chinese patients with a mild febrile illness after being bitten by *Ixodes persulcatus* and *Haemaphysalis concinna* ticks. The clinical presentation is similar to those of HME and HGA. Specific diagnostic methods have been developed but are not widely available.

TREATMENT EHRLICHIOSES

Doxycycline is effective for HME as well as for ewingii and EMLA ehrlichioses; the use of this drug in *Candidatus* N. mikurensis infection is associated with disease resolution. Therapy with doxycycline (100 mg given PO or IV twice daily) or tetracycline (250–500 mg given PO every 6 h) lowers hospitalization rates and shortens fever duration. *E. chaffeensis* is not susceptible to chloramphenicol in vitro, and the use of this drug is controversial. While a few reports document *E. chaffeensis* persistence in humans, this finding is rare; most infections are cured by short courses of doxycycline (continuing for 3–5 days after defervescence). Although poorly studied, rifampin may be suitable when doxycycline is contraindicated.

PREVENTION

HME, ewingii ehrlichiosis, EMLA infection, and *Candidatus* N. mikurensis infection can be prevented by the avoidance of ticks in endemic areas. The use of protective clothing and tick repellents, careful post-exposure tick searches, and prompt removal of attached ticks probably diminish infection risk.

HUMAN GRANULOCYTOTROPIC ANAPLASMOSIS

Epidemiology As of April 2013, 10,181 cases of HGA had been reported to the CDC, most in the upper midwestern and northeastern United States; the geographic distribution is similar to that for Lyme disease because of the shared *I. scapularis* tick vector. White-footed mice, squirrels, and white-tailed deer in the United States and red deer in Europe are natural reservoirs for *A. phagocytophilum*. HGA incidence peaks in May through July, but the disease can occur throughout the year with exposure to *Ixodes* ticks. HGA often affects males (59%) and older persons (median age, 51 years).

Clinical Manifestations Seroprevalence rates are high in endemic regions; thus it seems likely that most individuals develop subclinical infections. The incubation period for HGA is 4–8 days, after which the disease manifests as fever (75–100% of cases), myalgia (77%), headache (82%), and malaise (97%). A minority of patients develop nausea, vomiting, or diarrhea (22–39%); cough (27%); or confusion (17%). Rash (6%) is almost invariably concurrent erythema migrans attributable to Lyme disease. Most patients develop thrombocytopenia (75%) and/or leukopenia (55%) with increased serum hepatic aminotransferase levels (83%).

Severe complications occur most often in the elderly and include adult respiratory distress syndrome, a toxic shock–like syndrome, and life-threatening opportunistic infections. Meningoencephalitis is rarely documented with HGA, but brachial plexopathy, cranial nerve involvement, and demyelinating polyneuropathy are reported. For HGA, 7% of patients require intensive care, and the case-fatality rate is 0.6%. Neither vasculitis nor granulomas are components of HGA. While co-infections with *Borrelia burgdorferi* and *Babesia microti* (transmitted by the same tick vector[s]) occur, there is little evidence of comorbidity or persistence. HGA is rarely acquired via transfusion.

Diagnosis HGA should be included in the differential diagnosis of influenza-like illnesses during seasons with *Ixodes* tick activity (May through December), especially with known tick bite or exposure. Concurrent thrombocytopenia, leukopenia, or elevated serum levels of alanine or aspartate aminotransferase further increase the likelihood of HGA. Many HGA patients develop Lyme disease antibodies in the absence of clinical findings consistent with that diagnosis. Thus, HGA should be considered in the differential diagnosis of atypical severe Lyme disease presentations. Peripheral-blood film examination for neutrophil morulae can yield a diagnosis in 20–75% of infections. PCR testing of blood from patients with active disease before doxycycline therapy is sensitive and specific. Serodiagnosis is retrospective, requiring a fourfold increase in *A. phagocytophilum* antibody titer (to ≥160) in paired serum samples obtained 1 month apart. Since seroprevalence is high in some regions, a single acute-phase titer should not be used for diagnosis.

TREATMENT HUMAN GRANULOCYTOTROPIC ANAPLASMOSIS

No prospective studies of therapy for HGA have been conducted. However, doxycycline (100 mg PO twice daily) is effective. Rifampin therapy is associated with improvement of HGA in pregnant women and children. Most treated patients defervesce within 24–48 h.

Prevention HGA prevention requires tick avoidance. Transmission can be documented as few as 4 h after a tick bite.

Q FEVER

The agent of Q fever is *Coxiella burnetii*, a small intracellular prokaryote that only recently was grown in cell-free medium. *C. burnetii*, a pleomorphic coccobacillus with a gram-negative cell wall, survives in harsh environments; it escapes intracellular killing in macrophages by inhibiting the final step in phagosome maturation (cathepsin fusion) and has adapted to the acidic phagolysosome by producing superoxide dismutase. Infection with *C. burnetii* induces a range of immunomodulatory responses, from immunosuppression in chronic Q fever to the production of autoantibodies, particularly those to smooth muscle and cardiac muscle.

Q fever encompasses two broad clinical syndromes: acute and chronic infection. The host's immune response (rather than the particular strain) most likely determines whether chronic Q fever develops. *C. burnetii* survives in monocytes from patients with chronic Q fever but not in monocytes from patients with acute Q fever or from uninfected subjects. Impairment of the bactericidal activity of the *C. burnetii*–infected monocyte is associated with overproduction of interleukin 10. The CD4+/CD8+ ratio is decreased in Q fever endocarditis. Very few organisms and a strong cellular response are observed in patients with acute Q fever, while many organisms and a moderate cellular response occur in chronic Q fever. Immune control of *C. burnetii* is T cell–dependent, but 80–90% of bone marrow aspirates obtained years after recovery from Q fever contain *C. burnetii* DNA. *C. burnetii*'s ready multiplication within trophoblasts accounts for the high concentrations it can reach in the placenta.

Epidemiology Q fever is a zoonosis. The primary sources of human infection are infected cattle, sheep, and goats. However, cats, rabbits, pigeons, and dogs also serve as sources for transmission of *C. burnetii* to humans. The wildlife reservoir is extensive and includes ticks, coyotes, gray foxes, skunks, raccoons, rabbits, deer, mice, bears, birds, and opossums. In female animals *C. burnetii* localizes to the uterus and mammary glands. Infection is reactivated during pregnancy and after radiotherapy in mouse models. High concentrations of *C. burnetii* are found in the placenta. At the time of parturition, the bacteria are released into the air, and infection follows inhalation of aerosolized organisms by a susceptible host. Windstorms can generate *C. burnetii* aerosols months after soil contamination during parturition. Individuals up to 18 km from the source have been infected. Because it is easily dispersed as an aerosol, *C. burnetii* is a potential agent of bioterrorism (Chap. 261e), with a high infectivity rate and pneumonia as the major manifestation.

Determining the source of an outbreak of Q fever can be challenging. An outbreak of Q fever at a horse-boarding ranch in Colorado in 2005 was due to spread of infection from two herds of goats that had been acquired by the owners. PCR testing confirmed the presence of *C. burnetii* in the soil and among the goats. Of 138 persons who lived within 1 mile of the ranch and who were also tested, 11 (8%) had evidence of *C. burnetii* infection, and 8 of these 11 individuals had no direct contact with the ranch.

Persons at risk for Q fever include abattoir workers, veterinarians, farmers, and other individuals who have contact with infected animals (particularly newborn animals) or products of conception. The organism is shed in milk for weeks to months after parturition. The ingestion of contaminated milk in some geographic areas probably represents a major route of transmission to humans. A recent outbreak of Q fever associated with ingestion of raw milk confirms the oral route of transmission. In rare instances, person-to-person transmission follows labor and childbirth in an infected woman, autopsy of an infected individual, or blood transfusion. Some evidence suggests that *C. burnetii* can be sexually transmitted among humans. Crushing an infected tick between the fingers has resulted in Q fever; the implication is that percutaneous transmission can occur.

Infections due to *C. burnetii* occur in most geographic locations except New Zealand and Antarctica. Thus Q fever can be associated with travel. The number of reported cases of Q fever in the United States ranges from 28 to 54 per year. More than 70% of these cases occur in males, and April, May, and June are the most common months for acquisition. Q fever continues to be common in Australia, with 30 cases per 1 million population per year. Cases among abattoir workers in Australia declined dramatically as a result of a vaccination program. An outbreak of Q fever began in the Netherlands in 2007, and by 2010 more than 4000 cases had been reported. Pneumonia was a common manifestation in this outbreak. The outbreak was due to a combination of high-density goat farming in areas abutting large urban populations and environmental factors. Farms where spread did not occur had high vegetation densities and lower groundwater concentrations.

The primary manifestations of acute Q fever differ geographically (e.g., pneumonia in Nova Scotia and granulomatous hepatitis in Marseille). These differences could reflect the route of infection (i.e., ingestion of contaminated milk for hepatitis and inhalation of contaminated aerosols for pneumonia) or strain differences. In the Netherlands outbreak, sequelae of infection in pregnant women were rare; this was not the case among pregnant women elsewhere.

Young age seems to be protective against disease caused by *C. burnetii*. In a large outbreak in Switzerland, symptomatic infection occurred five times more often among persons >15 years of age than among younger individuals. In many outbreaks, men are affected more commonly than women; the proposed explanation is that female hormones are partially protective.

Clinical Manifestations • ***ACUTE Q FEVER*** The symptoms of acute Q fever are nonspecific; common among them are fever, extreme fatigue, photophobia, and severe headache that is frequently retro-orbital. Other symptoms include chills, sweats, nausea, vomiting, and diarrhea, each occurring in 5–20% of cases. Cough develops in about half of patients with Q fever pneumonia. Neurologic manifestations of acute Q fever are uncommon; however, in one outbreak in the United Kingdom, 23% of 102 patients had neurologic signs and symptoms as the major manifestation. A nonspecific rash may be evident in 4–18% of patients. The WBC count is usually normal. Thrombocytopenia occurs in ~25% of patients, and reactive thrombocytosis (with platelet counts exceeding 10^6/μL) frequently develops during recovery. Chest radiography can show opacities similar to those seen in pneumonia caused by other pathogens, but multiple rounded opacities in patients in endemic areas suggest a diagnosis of Q fever pneumonia.

Acute Q fever occasionally complicates pregnancy. In one series, it resulted in premature birth in 35% of cases and in abortion or neonatal death in 43%. Neonatal death (previous or current) and lower infant birth weight are three times more likely among women seropositive for *C. burnetii*.

After the usual incubation period of 3–30 days, 1070 patients with acute Q fever in southern France presented with hepatitis (40%), both pneumonia and hepatitis (20%), pneumonia (17%), isolated fever (14%), CNS involvement (2%), and pericarditis or myocarditis (1%). Acalculous cholecystitis, pancreatitis, lymphadenopathy, spontaneous rupture of the spleen, transient hypoplastic anemia, bone marrow necrosis, hemolytic anemia, histiocytic hemophagocytosis, optic neuritis, and erythema nodosum were less common manifestations.

POST–Q FEVER FATIGUE SYNDROME Prolonged fatigue can follow Q fever and can be accompanied by a constellation of symptoms including headaches, sweats, arthralgia, myalgias, blurred vision, muscle fasciculations, and enlarged and painful lymph nodes. Long-term persistence of a noninfective, nonbiodegraded complex of *Coxiella* cell components, with its antigens and specific lipopolysaccharide, has been detected in the affected persons. Patients who develop this syndrome have a higher frequency of carriage of HLA-DRB1*11 and of the 2/2 genotype of the interferon γ intron 1 microsatellite.

CHRONIC Q FEVER Chronic Q fever almost always implies endocarditis and usually occurs in patients with previous valvular heart disease, immunosuppression, or chronic renal insufficiency. Fever is usually absent or low grade. Valvular vegetations are detected in only 12% of patients by transthoracic echocardiography, but the rate of detection is higher (21–50%) with transesophageal echocardiography. The vegetations in chronic Q fever endocarditis differ from those in bacterial endocarditis, manifesting as endothelium-covered nodules on the valves. A high index of suspicion is necessary for timely diagnosis. Patients with chronic Q fever are often ill for >1 year before the diagnosis is made. The disease should be suspected in all patients with culture-negative endocarditis. In addition, all patients with valvular heart disease and an unexplained purpuric eruption, renal insufficiency, stroke, and/or progressive heart failure should be tested for *C. burnetii* infection. Patients with chronic Q fever have hepatomegaly and/or splenomegaly, which—in combination with rheumatoid factor, elevated erythrocyte sedimentation rate, high C-reactive protein level, and/or increased γ-globulin concentrations (up to 60–70 g/L)—suggests this diagnosis. Other manifestations of chronic Q fever include infection of vascular prostheses, aneurysms, and bone as well as chronic sternal wound infection. Unusual manifestations include chronic thrombocytopenia, mixed cryoglobulinemia, and livedo reticularis.

Diagnosis Isolation of *C. burnetii* from buffy-coat blood samples or tissue specimens by a shell-vial technique is easy but requires a biosafety level 3 laboratory. PCR detects *C. burnetii* DNA in tissue specimens, including paraffin-embedded samples. Serology is the most commonly used diagnostic tool. Indirect immunofluorescence is sensitive and specific and is the method of choice. Rheumatoid factor should be adsorbed from the specimen before testing. With chronic infection, the titer to phase I antigen is usually much higher than that to phase II antigen (i.e., *C. burnetii* that has truncated lipopolysaccharide associated with gene deletions during laboratory passages), and the diagnosis should not be based on serology alone. Rather, the entire clinical setting must be taken into consideration. An anti–phase I IgG titer of ≥6400 would be considered a major criterion for the diagnosis of chronic Q fever, while a titer of ≥800 but ≤6400 would be a minor criterion. In acute Q fever, a fourfold rise in titer can be demonstrated between acute- and convalescent-phase serum samples.

Fluorodeoxyglucose positron emission tomography combined with CT (FDG-PET/CT) can be useful because it can detect not only valvular infection but also intravascular infection elsewhere as well as osteomyelitis.

TREATMENT Q FEVER

ANTIBIOTICS

Treatment of acute Q fever with doxycycline (100 mg twice daily for 14 days) is usually successful. Quinolones also are effective. When Q fever is diagnosed during pregnancy, treatment with trimethoprim-sulfamethoxazole (TMP-SMX) is recommended for the duration of the pregnancy. One study showed no intrauterine fetal deaths and substantial reduction of obstetric complications in a group of Q fever patients treated with TMP-SMX.

The treatment of chronic Q fever is difficult and requires careful follow-up. Addition of hydroxychloroquine (to alkalinize the phagolysosome) renders doxycycline bactericidal against *C. burnetii*, and this combination is currently the favored regimen. Treatment with doxycycline (100 mg bid) and hydroxychloroquine (200 mg tid; plasma concentration maintained at 0.8–1.2 μg/mL) for 18 months is superior to a regimen of doxycycline and ofloxacin. Among 21 patients who received doxycycline and hydroxychloroquine, 1 died of a surgical complication, 2 were still being treated at the end of the study, 1 was still being evaluated, and 17 were cured. The mean duration of treatment was 31 months. In the ofloxacin and doxycycline group of 14 patients, 1 had died, 1 was still being treated, 7 had relapsed, and 5 had been cured by the end of the study. Optimal management of Q fever endocarditis entails determining the MIC of doxycycline for the patient's isolate and measuring serum doxycycline levels. A serum level–to–doxycycline MIC ratio of ≥1 is associated with a rapid decline in phase I antibodies with the doxycycline-hydroxychloroquine regimen. Patients treated with this regimen must be advised about photosensitivity and retinal toxicity risks. The doxycycline-hydroxychloroquine regimen was successful in one patient with HIV infection and Q fever endocarditis. The Jarisch-Herxheimer reaction occasionally complicates the treatment of chronic Q fever. Treatment of *C. burnetii*–infected aortic aneurysms is the same as that for Q fever endocarditis. Surgical intervention is often required.

If doxycycline-hydroxychloroquine cannot be used, the regimen chosen should include at least two antibiotics active against *C. burnetii*. Rifampin (300 mg once daily) combined with doxycycline (100 mg twice daily) or ciprofloxacin (750 mg twice daily) has been used successfully. The management of patients with Q fever endocarditis is complex and should preferably be undertaken by individuals with experience in managing this illness. Monitoring of antibody titers on a quarterly basis is an essential part of the management of these patients. Thus the laboratory should be contacted and asked to save all serum samples from such patients so that the current sample can be run with the previous one. There is incomplete agreement on the antibody titer at which therapy can be stopped. However, it is reasonable to discontinue treatment if IgG antibody levels have decreased by fourfold at 1 year, if IgM antibody to phase II has disappeared, and if the patient is clinically stable.

Patients with acute Q fever and lesions of native heart valves (e.g., bicuspid aortic valve), prosthetic valves, or prosthetic intravascular material should undergo serologic monitoring every 4 months for 2 years. If the phase I IgG titer is >800, further investigation is warranted. Some authorities recommend that patients with valvulopathy and acute Q fever receive doxycycline and hydroxychloroquine to prevent chronic Q fever. For women who exhibit a serologic profile of chronic Q fever after childbirth, hydroxychloroquine and doxycycline should be given for 1 year.

BIOLOGIC MODIFYING AGENTS

Interferon γ was successful in the treatment of a 3-year-old boy with prolonged fever, abdominal pain, and thrombocytopenia due to *C. burnetii* that had not been eradicated with conventional antibiotic therapy. Many patients with granulomatous hepatitis due to Q fever have a prolonged febrile illness that is unresponsive to antibiotics. For these individuals, treatment with prednisone (0.5 mg/kg) has resulted in defervescence within 2–15 days. After defervescence, the glucocorticoid dose is tapered over the next month.

Prevention A whole-cell vaccine (Q-Vax) licensed in Australia effectively prevents Q fever in abattoir workers. Before administration of the vaccine, skin testing with intradermal diluted *C. burnetii* vaccine is performed, serologic testing is undertaken, and a history of possible Q fever is sought. Vaccine is given only to patients with no history of Q fever and negative results in serologic and skin testing.

Good animal-husbandry practices are important in preventing widespread contamination of the environment by *C. burnetii*. These practices include isolating aborting animals for up to 14 days, raising feed bunks to prevent contamination of feed by excreta, destroying aborted materials (by burning and burying fetal membranes and stillborn animals), and wearing masks and gloves when handling aborted materials. Vaccination of sheep and goats and a culling program were effective in the Netherlands outbreak. Only seronegative pregnant animals should be used in research settings, and only seronegative animals should be permitted in petting zoos.

During an outbreak of Q fever and for 4 weeks after it ceases, blood donations should not be accepted from individuals who live in the affected area.

ACKNOWLEDGMENT

The contributions of Didier Raoult, MD, to this chapter in previous editions are gratefully acknowledged.

212 Infections Due to Mycoplasmas

R. Doug Hardy

Mycoplasmas are prokaryotes of the class Mollicutes. Their size (150–350 nm) is closer to that of viruses than to that of bacteria. Unlike viruses, however, mycoplasmas grow in cell-free culture media; in fact, they are the smallest organisms capable of independent replication.

The entire genomes of many *Mycoplasma* species have been sequenced and have been found to be among the smallest of all prokaryotic genomes. Sequencing information for these genomes has helped define the minimal set of genes necessary for cellular life. The absence of genes related to the synthesis of amino acids, fatty acid metabolism, and cholesterol dictates the mycoplasmas' parasitic or saprophytic dependence on a host for exogenous nutrients and necessitates the use of complex fastidious media to culture these organisms. Mycoplasmas lack a cell wall and are bound only by a cell membrane. The absence of a cell wall explains the inactivity of β-lactam antibiotics (penicillins and cephalosporins) against infections caused by these organisms.

At least 13 *Mycoplasma* species, two *Acholeplasma* species, and two *Ureaplasma* species have been isolated from humans. Most of these species are thought to be normal inhabitants of oral and urogenital mucous membranes. Only four species—*M. pneumoniae*, *M. hominis*, *U. urealyticum*, and *U. parvum*—have been shown conclusively to be pathogenic in immunocompetent humans. *M. pneumoniae* primarily infects the respiratory tract, while *M. hominis*, *U. urealyticum*, and *U. parvum* are associated with a variety of genitourinary tract disorders and neonatal infections. Some data indicate that *M. genitalium* may be a cause of disease in humans. Other mycoplasmas may cause disease in immunocompromised persons.

MYCOPLASMA PNEUMONIAE

PATHOGENESIS

M. pneumoniae is generally thought to act as an extracellular pathogen. Although the organism has been shown to exist and replicate within human cells, it is not known whether these intracellular events contribute to the pathogenesis of disease. *M. pneumoniae* attaches to ciliated respiratory epithelial cells by means of a complex terminal organelle at the tip of one end of the organism. Cytoadherence is mediated by interactive adhesins and accessory proteins clustered on this organelle. After extracellular attachment, *M. pneumoniae* causes injury to host respiratory tissue. The mechanism of injury is thought to be mediated by the production of hydrogen peroxide and of a recently identified ADP-ribosylating and vacuolating cytotoxin of *M. pneumoniae* that has many similarities to pertussis toxin. Because mycoplasmas lack a cell wall, they also lack cell wall–derived stimulators of the innate immune system, such as lipopolysaccharide, lipoteichoic acid, and murein (peptidoglycan) fragments. However, lipoproteins from the mycoplasmal cell membrane appear to have inflammatory properties, probably acting through Toll-like receptors (primarily TLR2) on macrophages and other cells. Lung biopsy specimens from patients with *M. pneumoniae* respiratory tract infection reveal an inflammatory process involving the trachea, bronchioles, and peribronchial tissue, with a monocytic infiltrate coinciding with a luminal exudate of polymorphonuclear leukocytes.

Experimental evidence indicates that innate immunity provides most of the host's defense against mycoplasmal infection in the lungs, whereas cellular immunity may actually play an immunopathogenic role, exacerbating mycoplasmal lung disease. Humoral immunity appears to provide protection against dissemination of *M. pneumoniae* infection; patients with humoral immunodeficiencies do not have more severe lung disease than do immunocompetent patients in the early stages of infection but more often develop disseminated infection resulting in syndromes such as arthritis, meningitis, and osteomyelitis. The immunity that follows severe *M. pneumoniae* infections is more protective and longer-lasting than that following mild infections. Genuine second attacks of *M. pneumoniae* pneumonia have been reported infrequently.

EPIDEMIOLOGY

M. pneumoniae infection occurs worldwide. It is likely that the incidence of upper respiratory illness due to *M. pneumoniae* is up to 20 times that of pneumonia caused by this organism. Infection is spread from one person to another by respiratory droplets expectorated during coughing and results in clinically apparent disease in an estimated 80% of cases. The incubation period for *M. pneumoniae* is 2–4 weeks; therefore, the time-course of infection in a specific population may be several weeks long. Intrafamilial attack rates are as high as 84% among children and 41% among adults. Outbreaks of *M. pneumoniae* illness often occur in institutional settings such as military bases, boarding schools, and summer camps. Infections tend to be endemic, with sporadic epidemics every 4–7 years. There is no seasonal pattern.

Most significantly, *M. pneumoniae* is a major cause of community-acquired respiratory illness in both children and adults and is often grouped with *Chlamydia pneumoniae* and *Legionella* species as being among the most important bacterial causes of "atypical" community-acquired pneumonia. For community-acquired pneumonia in adults, *M. pneumoniae* is the most frequently detected "atypical" organism. Analysis of 13 studies of community-acquired pneumonia published since 1995 (which included 6207 ambulatory and hospitalized adults) showed that the overall prevalence of *M. pneumoniae* was 22.7%; by comparison, the prevalence of *C. pneumoniae* was 11.7%, and that of *Legionella* species was 4.6%. *M. pneumoniae* pneumonia is also referred to as Eaton agent pneumonia (the organism having first been isolated in the early 1940s by Monroe Eaton), primary atypical pneumonia, and "walking" pneumonia.

CLINICAL MANIFESTATIONS

Upper Respiratory Tract Infections and Pneumonia Acute *M. pneumoniae* infections generally manifest as pharyngitis, tracheobronchitis, reactive airway disease/wheezing, or a nonspecific upper respiratory syndrome. Little evidence supports the commonly held belief that this organism is an important cause of otitis media, with or without bullous myringitis. Pneumonia develops in 3–13% of infected individuals; its onset is usually gradual, occurring over several days, but may be more abrupt. Although *Mycoplasma* pneumonia may begin with a sore throat, the most common presenting symptom is cough. The cough is typically nonproductive, but some patients produce sputum. Headache, malaise, chills, and fever are noted in the majority of patients.

On physical examination, wheezes or rales are detected in ~80% of patients with *M. pneumoniae* pneumonia. In many patients, however, pneumonia can be diagnosed only by chest radiography. The most common radiographic pattern is that of peribronchial pneumonia with thickened bronchial markings, streaks of interstitial infiltration, and areas of subsegmental atelectasis. Segmental or lobar consolidation is not uncommon. While clinically evident pleural effusions are infrequent, lateral decubitus views reveal that up to 20% of patients have pleural effusions.

Overall, the clinical presentation of pneumonia in an individual patient is not useful for differentiating *M. pneumoniae* pneumonia from other types of community-acquired pneumonia. The possibility of *M. pneumoniae* infection deserves particular consideration when community-acquired pneumonia fails to respond to treatment with a penicillin or a cephalosporin—antibiotics that are ineffective against mycoplasmas. Symptoms usually resolve within 2–3 weeks after the onset of illness. Although *M. pneumoniae* pneumonia is generally self-limited, appropriate antimicrobial therapy significantly shortens the duration of clinical illness. Infection uncommonly results in critical illness and only rarely in death. In some patients, long-term recurrent wheezing or reactive airway disease may follow the resolution of acute pneumonia. The significance of chronic infection, especially as it relates to asthma, is an area of active investigation.

Extrapulmonary Manifestations An array of extrapulmonary manifestations may develop during *M. pneumoniae* infection. The most significant are neurologic, dermatologic, cardiac, rheumatologic, and hematologic in nature. Extrapulmonary manifestations can be a result of disseminated infection, especially in patients with humoral immunodeficiencies (e.g., septic arthritis); postinfectious autoimmune phenomena (e.g., Guillain-Barré syndrome); or possibly ADP-ribosylating toxin. Overall, these manifestations are uncommon, given the frequency of *M. pneumoniae* infection. Notably, many patients with extrapulmonary *M. pneumoniae* disease do not have respiratory disease.

Skin eruptions described with *M. pneumoniae* infection include erythematous (macular or maculopapular), vesicular, bullous, petechial, and urticarial rashes. In some reports, 17% of patients with *M. pneumoniae* pneumonia have had an exanthem. Erythema multiforme major (Stevens-Johnson syndrome) is the most clinically significant skin eruption associated with *M. pneumoniae* infection; it appears to occur more commonly with *M. pneumoniae* than with other infectious agents.

A wide spectrum of neurologic manifestations has been reported with *M. pneumoniae* infection. The most common are meningoencephalitis, encephalitis, Guillain-Barré syndrome, and aseptic meningitis. *M. pneumoniae* has been implicated as a likely etiologic agent in 5–7% of cases of encephalitis. Other neurologic manifestations may include cranial neuropathy, acute psychosis, cerebellar ataxia, acute demyelinating encephalomyelitis, cerebrovascular thromboembolic events, and transverse myelitis.

Hematologic manifestations of *M. pneumoniae* infection include hemolytic anemia, aplastic anemia, cold agglutinins, disseminated intravascular coagulation, and hypercoagulopathy. When anemia does occur, it generally develops in the second or third week of illness.

In addition, hepatitis, glomerulonephritis, pancreatitis, myocarditis, pericarditis, rhabdomyolysis, and arthritis (septic and reactive) have been convincingly ascribed to *M. pneumoniae* infection. Septic arthritis has been described most commonly in hypogammaglobulinemic patients.

DIAGNOSIS

Clinical findings, nonmicrobiologic laboratory tests, and chest radiography are not useful for differentiating *M. pneumoniae* pneumonia from other types of community-acquired pneumonia. In addition, since *M. pneumoniae* lacks a cell wall, it is not visible on Gram's stain. Although of historical interest, the measurement of cold agglutinin titers is no longer recommended for the diagnosis of *M. pneumoniae* infection because the findings are nonspecific and assays specific for *M. pneumoniae* are now available.

Acute *M. pneumoniae* infection can be diagnosed by polymerase chain reaction (PCR) detection of the organism in respiratory tract secretions or by isolation of the organism in culture (Table 212-1). Oropharyngeal, nasopharyngeal, and pulmonary specimens are all acceptable for diagnosing *M. pneumoniae* pneumonia. Other bodily fluids, such cerebrospinal fluid, are acceptable for extrapulmonary infection. *M. pneumoniae* culture (which requires special media) is not recommended for routine diagnosis because the organism may take weeks to grow and is often difficult to isolate from clinical specimens. In contrast, PCR allows rapid, specific diagnosis earlier in the course of clinical illness.

The diagnosis can also be established by serologic tests for IgM and IgG antibodies to *M. pneumoniae* in paired (acute- and convalescent-phase) serum samples; enzyme-linked immunoassay is the recommended serologic method. An acute-phase sample alone is not adequate for diagnosis, as antibodies to *M. pneumoniae* may not develop until 2 weeks into the illness; therefore, it is important to test paired samples. In addition, IgM antibody to *M. pneumoniae* can persist for up to 1 year after acute infection. Thus its presence may indicate recent rather than acute infection.

The combination of PCR of respiratory tract secretions and serologic testing constitutes the most sensitive and rapid approach to the diagnosis of *M. pneumoniae* infection.

TABLE 212-1 DIAGNOSTIC TESTS FOR RESPIRATORY *MYCOPLASMA PNEUMONIAE* INFECTION[a]

Test	Sensitivity, %	Specificity, %
Respiratory culture	≤60	100
Respiratory PCR	65–90	90–100
Serologic studies[b]	55–100	55–100

[a]A combination of PCR and serology is suggested for routine diagnosis. If macrolide resistance is suspected, *M. pneumoniae* culture may prove useful, providing an isolate for susceptibility testing. [b]Acute- and convalescent-phase serum samples are recommended.

Abbreviation: PCR, polymerase chain reaction.

TREATMENT *MYCOPLASMA PNEUMONIAE* INFECTIONS

Although in the majority of untreated cases symptoms resolve within 2–3 weeks without significant associated morbidity, *M. pneumoniae* pneumonia can be a serious illness that responds to appropriate antimicrobial therapy (Table 212-2). Randomized, double-blind, placebo-controlled trials in adults have demonstrated that antimicrobial treatment significantly decreases the duration of fever, cough, malaise, hospitalization, and radiologic abnormalities in *M. pneumoniae* pneumonia. Treatment options for acute *M. pneumoniae* infection include macrolides (e.g., oral azithromycin, 500 mg on day 1, then 250 mg/d on days 2–5), tetracyclines (e.g., oral doxycycline, 100 mg twice daily for 10–14 days), and respiratory fluoroquinolones. However, ciprofloxacin and ofloxacin are *not* recommended because of their high minimal inhibitory concentrations against *M. pneumoniae* isolates and their poor performance in experimental studies. A 10- to 14-day course of quinolone therapy appears adequate.

In Japan and China, very high levels (up to ≥90%) of *M. pneumoniae* resistance to macrolides have been reported. In Europe and to a lesser degree in the United States, macrolide-resistant *M. pneumoniae* is emerging. In investigated outbreaks of respiratory illness due to *M. pneumoniae* in the United States, macrolide resistance has been reported in 8–27% of isolates. Clinical studies have demonstrated that, when treated with macrolides, patients with community-acquired pneumonia due to macrolide-resistant *M. pneumoniae* experience a significantly longer duration of symptoms than do patients infected with macrolide-sensitive organisms; thus macrolide resistance in *M. pneumoniae* does appear to have clinical significance. If macrolide resistance is prominent in a particular geographic locale or is suspected, then a nonmacrolide antibiotic should be considered for treatment; in addition, culture of *M. pneumoniae* may prove useful in these instances, providing an isolate for susceptibility testing.

Clinical observations and experimental data suggest that the addition of glucocorticoids to an antibiotic regimen may be of value for the treatment of severe or refractory *M. pneumoniae* pneumonia. However, relevant clinical experience is limited. Even though appropriate antibiotic therapy significantly reduces the duration of respiratory illness, it does not appear to shorten the duration of detection of *M. pneumoniae* by culture or PCR; therefore, a test of cure or eradication is not suggested.

The roles of antimicrobial drugs, glucocorticoids, and IV immunoglobulin in the treatment of neurologic disease due to *M. pneumoniae* remain unknown.

TABLE 212-2 ANTIMICROBIAL AGENTS OF CHOICE FOR *MYCOPLASMA* INFECTIONS[a]

Organism	Drug(s)
M. pneumoniae	Azithromycin, clarithromycin, erythromycin, doxycycline, levofloxacin, moxifloxacin, gemifloxacin (*not* ciprofloxacin or ofloxacin)
U. urealyticum, U. parvum	Azithromycin, clarithromycin, erythromycin, doxycycline
M. hominis	Doxycycline, clindamycin
M. genitalium	Azithromycin

[a]Antimicrobial resistance has been reported in mycoplasmas, as described in the text.

UROGENITAL MYCOPLASMAS (SEE ALSO CHAP. 163)

EPIDEMIOLOGY

M. hominis, *M. genitalium*, *U. urealyticum*, and *U. parvum* can cause urogenital tract disease. The significance of isolation of these organisms in a variety of other syndromes is unknown and in some cases is being investigated. *M. fermentans* has not been shown convincingly to cause human disease.

While urogenital mycoplasmas may be transmitted to a fetus during passage through a colonized birth canal, sexual contact is the major mode of transmission, and the risk of colonization increases dramatically with increasing numbers of sexual partners. In asymptomatic women, these mycoplasmas may be found throughout the lower urogenital tract. The vagina yields the largest number of organisms; next most densely colonized are the periurethral area and the cervix. Ureaplasmas are isolated less often from urine than from the cervix, but *M. hominis* is found with approximately the same frequency at these two sites. Ureaplasmas are isolated from the vagina of 40–80% of sexually active, asymptomatic women and *M. hominis* from 21–70%. The two microorganisms are found concurrently in 31–60% of women. In men, colonization with each organism is less prevalent. Mycoplasmas have been isolated from urine, semen, and the distal urethra of asymptomatic men.

CLINICAL MANIFESTATIONS

Urethritis, Pyelonephritis, and Urinary Calculi In many episodes of *Chlamydia*-negative nongonococcal urethritis, ureaplasmas may be the causative agent. These organisms may also cause chronic voiding symptoms in women. The common presence of ureaplasmas in the urethra of asymptomatic men suggests either that only certain serovars are pathogenic or that predisposing factors, such as lack of immunity, must exist in persons who develop symptomatic infection. Alternatively, disease may develop only upon initial exposure to ureaplasmas. Ureaplasmas have been implicated in epididymitis. *M. genitalium* also appears to cause urethritis. *M. genitalium* and ureaplasmas do not have a known role in prostatitis. *M. hominis* does not appear to play a primary etiologic role in urethritis, epididymitis, or prostatitis.

Evidence suggests that *M. hominis* causes up to 5% of cases of acute pyelonephritis. Ureaplasmas have not been associated with this disease.

Ureaplasmas play a limited role in the production of urinary calculi. The frequency with which ureaplasmas reach the kidney, the predisposing factors that allow them to do so, and the relative frequency of urinary tract calculi induced by this organism (compared with other organisms) are not known.

Pelvic Inflammatory Disease *M. hominis* can cause pelvic inflammatory disease. In most episodes, *M. hominis* occurs as part of a polymicrobial infection, but the organism may play an independent role in a limited number of cases. Some data also support an association of *M. genitalium* with pelvic inflammatory disease. Ureaplasmas are not thought to cause pelvic inflammatory disease.

Postpartum and Postabortal Infection Studies implicate *M. hominis* as the primary pathogen in ~5–10% of women who have postpartum or postabortal fever; ureaplasmas have been implicated to a lesser degree. These infections are generally self-limited; however, if symptoms persist, specific antimicrobial therapy should be given. Ureaplasmas also appear to play a role in occasional postcesarean wound infections.

Non-urogenital Infection In rare instances, *M. hominis* causes non-urogenital infections, such as brain abscess, wound infection, poststernotomy mediastinitis, endocarditis, and neonatal meningitis. These infections are most common among immunocompromised and hypogammaglobulinemic patients. Ureaplasmas and *M. hominis* can cause septic arthritis in immunodeficient patients. Ureaplasmas probably cause neonatal pneumonitis; their significant role in the development of bronchopulmonary dysplasia—the chronic lung disease of premature infants—has been documented in a number of studies. It is unclear whether ureaplasmas and *M. hominis* cause infertility, spontaneous abortion, premature labor, low birth weight, or chorioamnionitis.

DIAGNOSIS

Culture and PCR are both appropriate methods for the isolation of urogenital mycoplasmas. Culture of these organisms, however, requires special techniques and media that generally are available only at larger medical centers and reference laboratories. Serologic testing is not recommended for the clinical diagnosis of urogenital *Mycoplasma* infections.

TREATMENT UROGENITAL *MYCOPLASMA* INFECTIONS

Because colonization with urogenital mycoplasmas is common, it appears at present that their isolation from the urogenital tract in the absence of disease generally does not warrant treatment. Macrolides and doxycycline are considered the antimicrobial agents of choice for *Ureaplasma* infections (Table 212-2). *Ureaplasma* resistance to macrolides, doxycycline, quinolones, and chloramphenicol has been reported. *M. hominis* is resistant to macrolides. Doxycycline is generally the drug of choice for *M. hominis* infections, although resistance has been reported. Clindamycin is generally active against *M. hominis*. Quinolones are active in vitro against *M. hominis*. For *M. genitalium*, the agent of choice appears to be azithromycin; treatment failures have been reported with other macrolides as well as with quinolones.

213 Chlamydial Infections

Charlotte A. Gaydos, Thomas C. Quinn

Chlamydiae are obligate intracellular bacteria that cause a wide variety of diseases in humans and animals.

ETIOLOGIC AGENTS

The chlamydiae were originally classified as four species in the genus *Chlamydia*: *C. trachomatis*, *C. pneumoniae*, *C. psittaci*, and *C. pecorum* (the last species being found in ruminants). The *C. psittaci* group has been separated into three species: *C. psittaci*, *C. felis*, and *C. abortus*. The mouse pneumonitis strain (MoPn) is now classified as *C. muridarum*, and the guinea pig inclusion conjunctivitis strain (GPIC) is now designated *C. caviae*.

C. trachomatis is divided into two biovars: trachoma and LGV (lymphogranuloma venereum). The trachoma biovar causes two major types of disease in humans: ocular trachoma, the leading infectious cause of preventable blindness in the developing world; and urogenital infections, which are sexually or neonatally transmitted. The 18 serovars of *C. trachomatis* fall into three groups: the trachoma serovars A, B, Ba, and C; the oculogenital serovars D–K; and the LGV serovars L_1–L_3. Serovars can be distinguished by serologic typing with monoclonal antibodies or by molecular gene typing. However, serovar identification usually is not important clinically since the antibiotic susceptibility pattern is the same for all three groups. The one exception applies when LGV is suspected on clinical grounds; in this situation, serovar determination is important because a longer treatment duration is required for LGV strains.

BIOLOGY, GROWTH CYCLE, AND PATHOGENESIS

BIOLOGY

During their intracellular growth, chlamydiae produce characteristic intracytoplasmic inclusions that can be visualized by direct fluorescent antibody (DFA) or Giemsa staining of infected clinical material, such as conjunctival scrapings or cervical or urethral epithelial cells. Chlamydiae are nonmotile, gram-negative, obligate intracellular bacteria that replicate within the cytoplasm of host cells, forming the characteristic membrane-bound inclusions that are the basis for some diagnostic tests. Originally considered to be large viruses, chlamydiae differ from viruses in possessing RNA and DNA as well as a cell wall that is quite similar in structure to the cell wall of typical gram-negative bacteria. However, chlamydiae lack peptidoglycan; their structural integrity depends on disulfide binding of outer-membrane proteins.

GROWTH CYCLE

Among the defining characteristics of chlamydiae is a unique growth cycle that involves alternation between two highly specialized morphologic forms (Figs. 213-1 and 213-2): the elementary body (EB), which is the infectious form and is specifically adapted for extracellular survival, and the metabolically active and replicating reticulate body (RB), which is not infectious, is adapted for an intracellular environment, and does not survive well outside the host cell. The biphasic growth cycle begins with attachment of the EB (diameter, 0.25–0.35 μm) at specific sites on the surface of the host cell. The EB enters the cell through a process similar to receptor-mediated endocytosis and resides in an inclusion, where the entire growth cycle is completed. The chlamydiae prevent phagosome-lysosome fusion. The inclusion membrane is modified by insertion of chlamydial antigens. Once the EB has entered the cell, it reorganizes into an RB, which is larger (0.5–1 μm) and contains more RNA. After ~8 h, the RB starts to divide by binary fission. The intracytoplasmic, membrane-bound inclusion body containing the RBs increases in size as the RBs multiply. Approximately 18–24 h after infection of the cell, these RBs begin to become EBs by a reorganization or condensation process that is poorly understood. After rupture of the inclusion body, the EBs are released to initiate another cycle of infection.

Chlamydiae are susceptible to many broad-spectrum antibiotics and possess a number of enzymes, but they have a very restricted metabolic capacity. None of these metabolic reactions results in the production of energy. Chlamydiae have thus been considered to be energy parasites that use the ATP produced by the host cell for their own metabolic functions. Many aspects of chlamydial molecular biology are not well understood, but the sequencing of several chlamydial genomes and new proteomics research have provided researchers with many relevant tools for elucidating the biology of the life cycle.

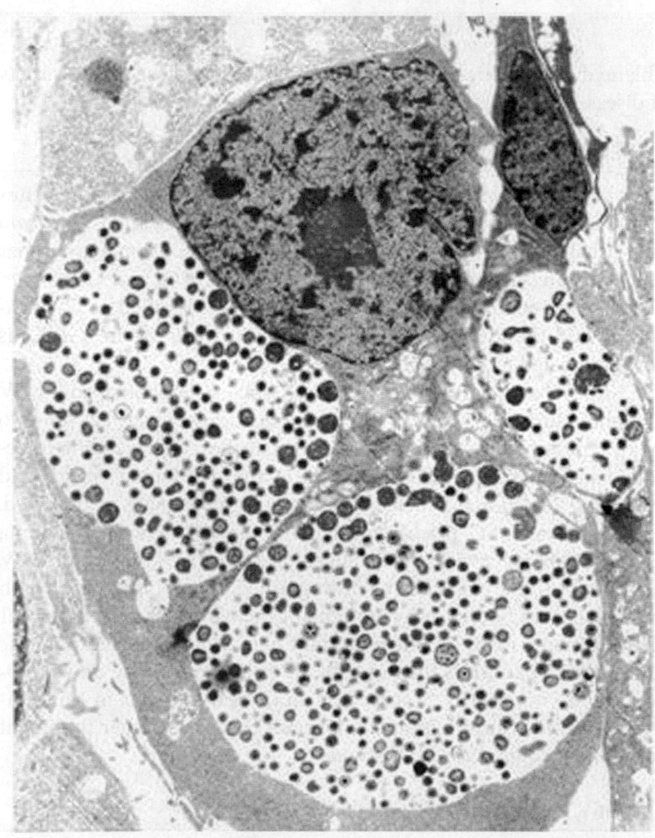

FIGURE 213-1 Chlamydial intracellular inclusions filled with smaller dense elementary bodies and larger reticulate bodies. *(Reprinted with permission from WE Stamm: Chlamydial infections, in Harrison's Principles of Internal Medicine, 17th ed, AS Fauci et al [eds]. New York, McGraw-Hill, 2008, p 1070.)*

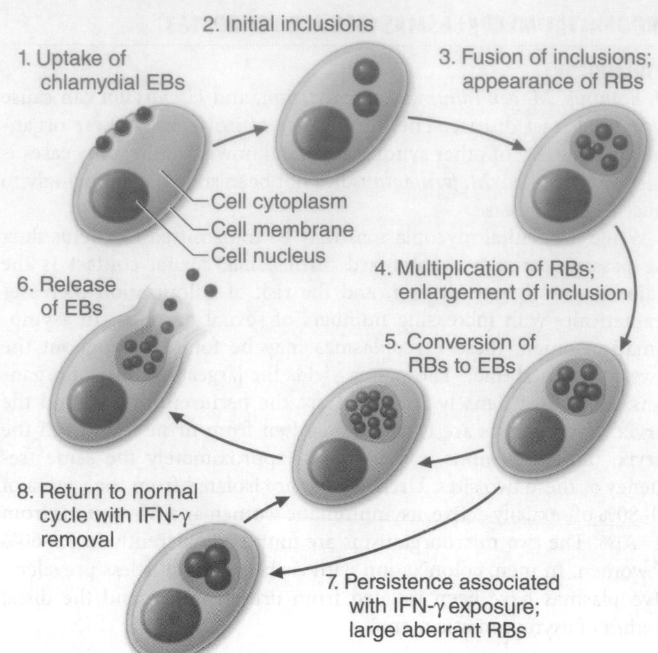

FIGURE 213-2 Chlamydial life cycle. EBs, elementary bodies; RBs, reticulate bodies; IFN-γ, interferon γ. *(Reprinted with permission from WE Stamm: Chlamydial infections, in Harrison's Principles of Internal Medicine, 17th ed, AS Fauci et al [eds]. New York, McGraw-Hill, 2008, p 1071.)*

PATHOGENESIS

Genital infections are mostly caused by *C. trachomatis* serovars D–K, with serovars D, E, and F involved most often. Molecular typing of the major outer-membrane protein gene (*omp1*) from which serovar differences arise has been used to demonstrate that polymorphisms can occur in isolates from patients who are exposed frequently to multiple infections, while less variation is observed in isolates from less sexually active populations. Polymorphisms in the major outer-membrane protein may provide antigenic variation, and the different forms allow persistence in the community because immunity to one is not protective against the others.

The trachoma biovar is essentially a parasite of squamocolumnar epithelial cells; the LGV biovar is more invasive and involves lymphoid cells. As is typical of chlamydiae, *C. trachomatis* strains are capable of causing chronic, clinically inapparent, asymptomatic infections. Because the duration of the chlamydial growth cycle is ~48–72 h, the incubation period of sexually transmitted chlamydial infections is relatively long—generally 1–3 weeks. *C. trachomatis* causes cell death as a result of its replicative cycle and can induce cell damage whenever it persists. However, few toxic effects are demonstrated, and cell death because of chlamydial replication is not sufficient to account for disease manifestations, the majority of which are due to immunopathologic mechanisms or nonspecific host responses to the organism or its byproducts.

In recent years, the entire genomes of various chlamydial species have been sequenced, the field of proteomics has become established, host innate immunity has been more precisely delineated, and innovative host cell–chlamydial interaction studies have been conducted. As a result, many insights have been gained into how chlamydiae adapt and replicate in their intracellular environment and produce disease. These insights into pathogenesis include information on the regulation of gene expression, protein localization, the type III secretion system, the roles of CD4+ and CD8+ T lymphocytes in the host response, and T lymphocyte trafficking.

The chlamydial heat-shock protein, which shares antigenic epitopes with similar proteins of other bacteria and with human heat-shock protein, may sensitize the host, and repeated infections may cause host cell damage. Persistent or recurrent chlamydial infections are associated with fibrosis, scarring, and complications following simple epithelial infections. A common endpoint of these late consequences is scarring of mucous membranes. Genital complications can lead to pelvic inflammatory disease (PID) and its late consequences of infertility, ectopic pregnancy, and chronic pelvic pain, while ocular infections may lead to blinding trachoma. High levels of antibody to human heat-shock protein have been associated with tubal factor infertility and ectopic pregnancy. Without adequate therapy, chlamydial infections may persist for several years, although symptoms—if present—usually abate.

The pathogenic mechanisms of *C. pneumoniae* have yet to be completely elucidated. The same is true for *C. psittaci*, except that this agent infects cells very efficiently and causes disease that may reflect direct cytopathic effects.

CHLAMYDIA TRACHOMATIS INFECTIONS

GENITAL INFECTIONS

Spectrum Although chlamydiae cause a number of human diseases, localized lower genital tract infections caused by *C. trachomatis* and the sequelae of such infections are the most important in terms of medical and economic impact. Oculogenital infections due to *C. trachomatis* serovars D–K are transmitted during sexual contact or from mother to baby during childbirth and are associated with many syndromes, including cervicitis, salpingitis, acute urethral syndrome, endometritis, ectopic pregnancy, infertility, and PID in female patients; urethritis, proctitis, and epididymitis in male patients; and conjunctivitis and pneumonia in infants. Women bear the greatest burden of morbidity because of the serious sequelae of these infections. Untreated infections lead to PID, and multiple episodes of PID can lead to tubal factor infertility and chronic pelvic pain. Studies estimate that up to 80–90% of women and >50% of men with *C. trachomatis* genital infections lack symptoms; other patients have very mild symptoms. Thus a large reservoir of infected persons continues to transmit infection to sexual partners.

As their designations reflect, the LGV serovars (L_1, L_2, and L_3) cause LGV, an invasive sexually transmitted disease (STD) characterized by acute lymphadenitis with bubo formation and/or acute hemorrhagic proctitis (see "Lymphogranuloma Venereum," below).

Epidemiology *C. trachomatis* genital infections are global in distribution. The World Health Organization (WHO) estimated in 2008 that >106.4 million cases occur annually worldwide. This figure makes chlamydial infection the most prevalent sexually transmitted bacterial infection in the world. The associated morbidity is substantial, and economic costs are high.

In the United States, chlamydial infections are the most commonly reported of all infectious diseases. In 2012, 1.3 million cases were reported to the U.S. Centers for Disease Control and Prevention (CDC); however, the CDC estimates that 2–3 million new cases occur per year, with substantial underreporting due to lack of screening in some populations. Rates of infection have increased every year; higher rates among women than among men reflect the focus on expansion of screening programs for women during the past 20 years, the use of increasingly sensitive diagnostic tests, an increased emphasis on case reporting, and improvements in the information systems used for reporting. The CDC and other professional organizations recommend annual screening of all sexually active women ≤25 years of age as well as rescreening of previously infected individuals at 3 months. Young women have the highest infection rates; in 2012, the figures were 3416.5 and 3722.5 cases per 100,000 population at 15–19 and 20–24 years of age, respectively. Age-specific rates among men, while much lower than those among women, were highest in the 20- to 24-year-old age group, at 1343.3 cases per 100,000. In 2012, rates increased for all racial and ethnic groups, with the highest rates among African Americans. For example, the rate of chlamydial infection among African-American girls 15–19 years of age was 7507.1 cases per 100,000—almost six times the rate among Caucasian girls in the same age group (1301.5/100,000). The rate among African-American women 20–24 years old was 4.8 times the rate among Caucasian women in the same age group. Similar racial disparities in reported rates of chlamydial infection exist among men. For boys 15–19 years of age, the rate among African Americans was 11.1 times the rate among Caucasians. The rate among Native Americans/Alaska Natives was more than four times the rate among Caucasians (648.3), and the rate among Latinos (383.6) was two times higher than that among Caucasians. These disparities are important reflections of health inequities in the United States.

The above statistics are based on case reporting. Studies based on screening surveys estimate that the U.S. prevalence of *C. trachomatis* cervical infection is 5% among asymptomatic female college students and prenatal patients, >10% among women seen in family planning clinics, and >20% among women seen in STD clinics. The prevalence of genital *C. trachomatis* infections varies substantially by geographic locale, with the highest rates in the southeastern United States. However, asymptomatic infections have been detected in >8–10% of young female military recruits from all parts of the country. The prevalence of *C. trachomatis* in the cervix of pregnant women is 5–10 times higher than that of *Neisseria gonorrhoeae*. The prevalence of genital infection with either agent is highest among women who are between the ages of 18 and 24, single, and non-Caucasian (e.g., African-American, Latina, Asian, Pacific Islander). Infections recur frequently in these same risk groups and are often acquired from untreated sexual partners. The use of oral contraception and the presence of cervical ectopy also confer an increased risk. The proportion of infections that are asymptomatic appears to be higher for *C. trachomatis* than for *N. gonorrhoeae*, and symptomatic *C. trachomatis* infections are clinically less severe. Mild or asymptomatic *C. trachomatis* infections of the fallopian tubes nonetheless cause ongoing tubal damage and infertility. The costs of *C. trachomatis* infections and their complications to the U.S. health care system have recently been estimated to exceed $516.7 million annually.

Clinical Manifestations • *NONGONOCOCCAL AND POSTGONOCOCCAL URETHRITIS* *C. trachomatis* is the most common cause of nongonococcal urethritis (NGU) and postgonococcal urethritis (PGU). The designation *PGU* refers to NGU developing in men 2–3 weeks after treatment of gonococcal urethritis with single doses of agents such as penicillin or cephalosporins, which lack antimicrobial activity against chlamydiae. Since current treatment regimens for gonorrhea have evolved and now include combination therapy with tetracycline, doxycycline, or azithromycin—all of which are effective against concomitant chlamydial infection—both the incidence of PGU and the causative role of *C. trachomatis* in this syndrome have declined.

In the United States, most of the estimated 2 million cases of acute urethritis are NGU, and *C. trachomatis* is implicated in 30–50% of these cases. The cause of most of the remaining cases of NGU is uncertain, but recent evidence suggests that *Ureaplasma urealyticum, Mycoplasma genitalium, Trichomonas vaginalis*, and herpes simplex virus (HSV) cause some cases. The rate of involvement of *C. trachomatis* in urethral infection ranges from 3–7% among asymptomatic men to 15–20% among symptomatic men attending STD clinics. A multisite study of men in Baltimore, Seattle, Denver, and San Francisco reported an overall chlamydial prevalence of 7% in urine samples assessed by nucleic acid amplification tests (NAATs). As in women, infection in men is age related, with young age as the greatest risk factor for chlamydial urethritis. The prevalence among men is highest at 20–24 years of age. In STD clinics, urethritis is usually less prevalent among men who have sex with men (MSM) than among heterosexual men and is almost always much more common among African-American men than among Caucasian men. One study reported prevalences of 19% and 9% among nonwhite and white heterosexual men, respectively.

NGU is diagnosed by documentation of a leukocytic urethral exudate and by exclusion of gonorrhea by Gram's staining or culture. *C. trachomatis* urethritis is generally less severe than gonococcal urethritis, although in any individual patient these two forms of urethritis cannot reliably be differentiated solely on clinical grounds. Symptoms include urethral discharge (often whitish and mucoid rather than frankly purulent), dysuria, and urethral itching. Physical examination may reveal meatal erythema and tenderness as well as a urethral exudate that is often demonstrable only by stripping of the urethra.

At least one-third of male patients with *C. trachomatis* urethral infection have no evident signs or symptoms of urethritis. The availability of NAATs for first-void urine specimens has facilitated broader-based testing for asymptomatic infection in male patients. As a result, asymptomatic chlamydial urethritis has been demonstrated in 5–10% of sexually active male adolescents screened at school-based clinics or community centers. Such patients generally have pyuria (≥15 leukocytes per 400× microscopic field in the sediment of first-void urine), a positive leukocyte esterase test, or an increased number of leukocytes on a Gram-stained smear prepared from a urogenital swab inserted 1–2 cm into the anterior urethra. To differentiate between true urethritis and functional symptoms in symptomatic patients or to make a presumptive diagnosis of *C. trachomatis* infection in high-risk but asymptomatic men (e.g., male patients in STD clinics, sex partners of women with nongonococcal salpingitis or mucopurulent cervicitis, fathers of children with inclusion conjunctivitis), the examination of an endourethral specimen for increased leukocytes is useful if specific diagnostic tests for chlamydiae are not available. Alternatively, urethritis can be assayed noninvasively by examination of a first-void urine sample for pyuria, either by microscopy or by the leukocyte esterase test. Urine (or a urethral swab) can also be tested directly for chlamydiae by DNA amplification methods, as described below (see "Detection Methods").

EPIDIDYMITIS Chlamydial urethritis may be followed by acute epididymitis, but this condition is rare, generally occurring in sexually active patients <35 years of age; in older men, epididymitis is usually associated with gram-negative bacterial infection and/or instrumentation procedures. It is estimated that 50–70% of cases of acute epididymitis are caused by *C. trachomatis*. The condition usually presents as unilateral scrotal pain with tenderness, swelling, and fever in a young man, often occurring in association with chlamydial urethritis. The illness may be mild enough to treat with oral antibiotics on an outpatient basis or severe enough to require hospitalization and parenteral therapy. Testicular torsion should be excluded promptly by radionuclide scan, Doppler flow study, or surgical exploration in a teenager or young adult who presents with acute unilateral testicular pain without urethritis. The possibility of testicular tumor or chronic infection (e.g., tuberculosis) should be excluded when a patient with unilateral intrascrotal pain and swelling does not respond to appropriate antimicrobial therapy.

REACTIVE ARTHRITIS Reactive arthritis consists of conjunctivitis, urethritis (or, in female patients, cervicitis), arthritis, and characteristic mucocutaneous lesions. It may develop in 1–2% of cases of NGU and is thought to be the most common type of peripheral inflammatory arthritis in young men. *C. trachomatis* has been recovered from the urethra of 16–44% of patients with reactive arthritis and from 69% of men who have signs of urogenital inflammation at the time of examination. Antibodies to *C. trachomatis* have also been detected in 46–67% of patients with reactive arthritis, and *Chlamydia*-specific cell-mediated immunity has been documented in 72%. In addition, *C. trachomatis* has been isolated from synovial biopsy samples from 15 of 29 patients in a number of small series and from a smaller proportion of synovial fluid specimens. Chlamydial nucleic acids have been identified in synovial membranes and chlamydial EBs in joint fluid. The pathogenesis of reactive arthritis is unclear, but this condition probably represents an abnormal host response to a number of infectious agents, including those associated with bacterial gastroenteritis (e.g., *Salmonella, Shigella, Yersinia*, or *Campylobacter*), or to infection with *C. trachomatis* or *N. gonorrhoeae*. Since >80% of affected patients have the HLA-B27 phenotype and since other mucosal infections produce an identical syndrome, chlamydial infection is thought to initiate an aberrant hyperactive immune response that produces inflammation of the involved target organs in these genetically predisposed individuals. Evidence of exaggerated cell-mediated and humoral immune responses to chlamydial antigens in reactive arthritis supports this hypothesis. The finding of chlamydial EBs and DNA in joint fluid and synovial tissue from patients with reactive arthritis suggests that chlamydiae may actually spread from genital to joint tissues in these patients—perhaps in macrophages.

NGU is the initial manifestation of reactive arthritis in 80% of patients, typically occurring within 14 days after sexual exposure. The urethritis may be mild and may even go unnoticed by the patient. Similarly, gonococcal urethritis may precede reactive arthritis, but co-infection with an agent of NGU is difficult to rule out. The urethral discharge may be purulent or mucopurulent, and patients may or may not report dysuria. Accompanying prostatitis, usually asymptomatic, has been described. Arthritis usually begins ~4 weeks after the onset of urethritis but may develop sooner or, in a small percentage of cases, may actually precede urethritis. The knees are most frequently involved; next most commonly affected are the ankles and small joints of the feet. Sacroiliitis, either symmetrical or asymmetrical, is documented in two-thirds of patients. Mild bilateral conjunctivitis, iritis, keratitis, or uveitis is sometimes present but lasts for only a few days. Finally, dermatologic manifestations occur in up to 50% of patients. The initial lesions—usually papules with a central yellow spot—most often involve the soles and palms and, in ~25% of patients, eventually epithelialize and thicken to produce keratoderma blenorrhagicum. Circinate balanitis is usually painless and occurs in fewer than half of patients. The initial episode of reactive arthritis usually lasts 2–6 months.

PROCTITIS Primary anal or rectal infections with *C. trachomatis* have been described in women and MSM who practice anal intercourse. In these infections, rectal involvement is initially characterized by severe anorectal pain, a bloody mucopurulent discharge, and tenesmus. Oculogenital serovars D–K and LGV serovars L_1, L_2, and L_3 have been found to cause proctitis. The LGV serovars are far more invasive and cause much more severely symptomatic disease, including severe ulcerative proctocolitis that can be clinically confused with HSV proctitis. Histologically, LGV proctitis may resemble Crohn's disease in that giant cell formation and granulomas are detected. In the United States and Europe, cases of LGV proctitis occur almost exclusively in MSM, many of whom are positive for HIV infection.

The less invasive non-LGV serovars of *C. trachomatis* cause mild proctitis. Many infected individuals are asymptomatic, and in these cases infection is diagnosed only by routine culture or NAAT of rectal swabs. The number of fecal leukocytes is usually abnormal in both asymptomatic and symptomatic cases. Sigmoidoscopy may yield normal findings or may reveal mild inflammatory changes or small erosions or follicles in the lower 10 cm of the rectum. Histologic examination of rectal biopsies generally shows anal crypts and prominent follicles as well as neutrophilic infiltration of the lamina propria. Chlamydial proctitis is best diagnosed by isolation of *C. trachomatis* from the rectum and documentation of a response to appropriate therapy. NAATs are reportedly more sensitive than culture for diagnosis and are also specific.

MUCOPURULENT CERVICITIS Although many women with chlamydial infections of the cervix have no symptoms, almost half generally have local signs of infection on examination. Cervicitis is usually characterized by the presence of a mucopurulent discharge, with >20 neutrophils per microscopic field visible in strands of cervical mucus in a thinly smeared, gram-stained preparation of endocervical exudate. Hypertrophic ectopy of the cervix may also be evident as an edematous area near the cervical os that is congested and bleeds easily on minor trauma (e.g., when a specimen is collected with a swab). A Papanicolaou smear shows increased numbers of neutrophils as well as a characteristic pattern of mononuclear inflammatory cells including plasma cells, transformed lymphocytes, and histiocytes. Cervical biopsy shows a predominantly mononuclear cell infiltrate of the subepithelial stroma. Clinical experience and collaborative studies indicate that a cutoff of >30 polymorphonuclear neutrophils (PMNs) per 1000× field in a gram-stained smear of cervical mucus correlates best with chlamydial or gonococcal cervicitis.

Clinical recognition of chlamydial cervicitis depends on a high index of suspicion and careful cervical examination. No genital symptoms are specifically correlated with chlamydial cervical infection. The differential diagnosis of a mucopurulent discharge from the endocervical canal in a young, sexually active woman includes gonococcal endocervicitis, salpingitis, endometritis, and intrauterine contraceptive device–induced inflammation. Diagnosis of cervicitis is based on the presence of PMNs on a cervical swab as noted above; the presence of chlamydiae is confirmed by either culture or NAAT.

PELVIC INFLAMMATORY DISEASE Inflammation of sections of the fallopian tube is often referred to as salpingitis or PID. The proportion of acute salpingitis cases caused by *C. trachomatis* varies geographically and with the population studied. It has been estimated that *C. trachomatis* causes up to 50% of PID cases in the United States. PID occurs via ascending intraluminal spread of *C. trachomatis* or *N. gonorrhoeae* from the lower genital tract. Mucopurulent cervicitis is often followed by endometritis, endosalpingitis, and finally pelvic peritonitis. Evidence of mucopurulent cervicitis is often found in women with laparoscopically verified salpingitis. Similarly, endometritis, demonstrated by an endometrial biopsy showing plasma cell infiltration of the endometrial epithelium, is documented in most women with laparoscopy-verified chlamydial (or gonococcal) salpingitis. Chlamydial endometritis can also occur in the absence of clinical evidence of salpingitis. Histologic evidence of endometritis has been correlated with a syndrome consisting of vaginal bleeding, lower abdominal pain, and uterine tenderness in the absence of adnexal tenderness. Chlamydial salpingitis produces milder symptoms than gonococcal salpingitis and may be associated with less marked adnexal tenderness. Thus, mild adnexal or uterine tenderness in a sexually active woman with cervicitis suggests chlamydial PID.

Chronic untreated endometrial and tubal inflammation can result in tubal scarring, impaired tubal function, tubal occlusion, and infertility, even among women who report no prior treatment for PID. *C. trachomatis* has been implicated particularly often in "subclinical" PID on the basis of (1) a lack of history of PID among *Chlamydia*-seropositive women with tubal damage or (2) detection of chlamydial DNA or antigen among asymptomatic women with tubal infertility. These data suggest that the best method to prevent PID and its sequelae is surveillance and control of lower genital tract infections along with diagnosis and treatment of sex partners and prevention of reinfections. Promotion of early symptom recognition and health care presentation may reduce the frequency and severity of sequelae of PID.

PERIHEPATITIS The Fitz-Hugh–Curtis syndrome was originally described as a complication of gonococcal PID. However, studies over the past several decades have suggested that chlamydial infection is more commonly associated with perihepatitis than is *N. gonorrhoeae*. Perihepatitis should be suspected in young, sexually active women who develop right-upper-quadrant pain, fever, or nausea. Evidence of salpingitis may or may not be found on examination. Frequently, perihepatitis is strongly associated with extensive tubal scarring, adhesions, and inflammation observed at laparoscopy, and high titers of antibody to the 57-kDa chlamydial heat-shock protein have been documented. Culture and/or serologic evidence of *C. trachomatis* is found in three-fourths of women with this syndrome.

URETHRAL SYNDROME IN WOMEN In the absence of infection with uropathogens such as coliforms or *Staphylococcus saprophyticus*, *C. trachomatis* is the pathogen most commonly isolated from college women with dysuria, frequency, and pyuria. Screening studies can recover *C. trachomatis* from both the cervix and the urethra; in up to 25% of infected women, the organism is isolated only from the urethra. The urethral syndrome in women consists of dysuria and frequency in conjunction with chlamydial urethritis, pyuria, and no bacteriuria or urinary pathogens. Although symptoms of the urethral syndrome may develop in some women with chlamydial infection, the majority of women attending STD clinics for urethral chlamydial infection do not have dysuria or frequency. Even in women with chlamydial urethritis causing the acute urethral syndrome, signs of urethritis such as urethral discharge, meatal redness, and swelling are uncommon. However, mucopurulent cervicitis in a woman presenting with dysuria and frequency strongly suggests *C. trachomatis* urethritis. Other correlates of chlamydial urethral syndrome include a duration of dysuria of >7–10 days, lack of hematuria, and lack of suprapubic tenderness. Abnormal urethral Gram's stains showing >10 PMNs per 1000× field in women with dysuria but without coliform bacteriuria support the diagnosis of chlamydial urethritis. Other possible diagnoses include gonococcal or trichomonal infection of the urethra.

INFECTION IN PREGNANCY AND THE NEONATAL PERIOD Infections during pregnancy can be transmitted to infants during delivery. Approximately 20–30% of infants exposed to *C. trachomatis* in the birth canal develop conjunctivitis, and 10–15% subsequently develop pneumonia. Consequently, all newborn infants receive ocular prophylaxis at birth to prevent ophthalmia neonatorum. Without treatment, conjunctivitis usually develops at 5–19 days of life and often results in a profuse mucopurulent discharge. Roughly half of infected infants develop clinical evidence of inclusion conjunctivitis. However, it is impossible to differentiate chlamydial conjunctivitis from other forms of neonatal conjunctivitis (e.g., that due to *N. gonorrhoeae, Haemophilus influenzae, Streptococcus pneumoniae*, or HSV) on clinical grounds; thus laboratory diagnosis is required. Inclusions within epithelial cells are often detected in Giemsa-stained conjunctival smears, but these smears are considerably less sensitive than cultures or NAATs for chlamydiae. Gram-stained smears may show gonococci or occasional small gram-negative coccobacilli in *Haemophilus* conjunctivitis, but smears should be accompanied by cultures or NAATs for these agents.

C. trachomatis has also been isolated frequently and persistently from the nasopharynx, rectum, and vagina of infected infants—occasionally for >1 year in the absence of treatment. In some cases, otitis media results from perinatally acquired chlamydial infection. Pneumonia may develop in infants from 2 weeks to 4 months of age. *C. trachomatis* is estimated to cause 20–30% of pneumonia cases in infants <6 months of age. Epidemiologic studies have linked chlamydial pulmonary infection in infants with increased occurrence of subacute lung disease (bronchitis, asthma, wheezing) in later childhood.

LYMPHOGRANULOMA VENEREUM *C. trachomatis* serovars L_1, L_2, and L_3 cause LGV, an invasive systemic STD. The peak incidence of LGV corresponds with the age of greatest sexual activity: the second and third decades of life. The worldwide incidence of LGV is falling, but the disease is still endemic and a major cause of morbidity in parts of Asia, Africa, South America, and the Caribbean. LGV is rare in industrialized countries; for more than a decade, the reported incidence in the United States has been only 0.1 case per 100,000 population. In the Bahamas, an apparent outbreak of LGV was described in association with a concurrent increase in heterosexual infection with HIV. Reports of outbreaks with the newly identified variant L_{2b} in Europe, Australia, and the United States indicate that LGV is becoming more prevalent among MSM. These cases have usually presented as hemorrhagic proctocolitis in HIV-positive men. More widespread use of NAATs for identification of rectal infections may have enhanced case recognition.

LGV begins as a small painless papule that tends to ulcerate at the site of inoculation, often escaping attention. This primary lesion heals in a few days without scarring and is usually recognized as LGV only in retrospect. LGV strains of *C. trachomatis* have occasionally been recovered from genital ulcers and from the urethra of men and the endocervix of women who present with inguinal adenopathy; these areas may be the primary sites of infection in some cases. Proctitis is more common among people who practice receptive anal intercourse, and an elevated white blood cell count in anorectal smears may predict LGV in these patients. Ulcer formation may facilitate transmission of HIV infection and other sexually transmitted and blood-borne diseases.

As NAATs for *C. trachomatis* are being used more often, increasing numbers of cases of LGV proctitis are being recognized in MSM. Such patients present with anorectal pain and mucopurulent, bloody rectal discharge. Sigmoidoscopy reveals ulcerative proctitis or proctocolitis, with purulent exudate and mucosal bleeding. Histopathologic findings in the rectal mucosa include granulomas with giant cells, crypt abscesses, and extensive inflammation. These clinical, sigmoidoscopic, and histopathologic findings may closely resemble those of Crohn's disease of the rectum.

The most common presenting picture in heterosexual men and women is the *inguinal syndrome*, which is characterized by painful inguinal lymphadenopathy beginning 2–6 weeks after presumed exposure; in rare instances, the onset comes after a few months. The inguinal adenopathy is unilateral in two-thirds of cases, and palpable enlargement of the iliac and femoral nodes is often evident on the same side as the enlarged inguinal nodes. The nodes are initially discrete, but progressive periadenitis results in a matted mass of nodes that becomes fluctuant and suppurative. The overlying skin becomes fixed, inflamed, and thin, and multiple draining fistulas finally develop. Extensive enlargement of chains of inguinal nodes above and below the inguinal ligament ("the sign of the groove") is not specific and, although not uncommon, is documented in only a minority of cases. Spontaneous healing usually takes place after several months; inguinal scars or granulomatous masses of various sizes persist for life. Massive pelvic lymphadenopathy may lead to exploratory laparotomy.

Constitutional symptoms are common during the stage of regional lymphadenopathy and, in cases of proctitis, may include fever, chills, headache, meningismus, anorexia, myalgias, and arthralgias. Other systemic complications are infrequent but include arthritis with sterile effusion, aseptic meningitis, meningoencephalitis, conjunctivitis, hepatitis, and erythema nodosum (Fig. 25e-40). Complications of untreated anorectal infection include perirectal abscess; anal fistulas; and rectovaginal, rectovesical, and ischiorectal fistulas. Secondary bacterial infection probably contributes to these complications. Rectal stricture is a late complication of anorectal infection and usually develops 2–6 cm from the anal orifice—i.e., at a site within reach on digital rectal examination. A small percentage of cases of LGV in men present as chronic progressive infiltrative, ulcerative, or fistular lesions of the penis, urethra, or scrotum. Associated lymphatic obstruction may produce elephantiasis. When urethral stricture occurs, it usually involves the posterior urethra and causes incontinence or difficulty with urination.

Diagnosis • ***DETECTION METHODS*** Historically, chlamydiae were cultivated in the yolk sac of embryonated eggs. The organisms can be grown more easily in tissue culture, but cell culture—once considered the diagnostic gold standard—has been replaced by nonculture assays (Table 213-1). In general, culture for chlamydiae in clinical specimens is now performed only in specialized laboratories. The first nonculture assays, such as DFA staining of clinical material and enzyme immunoassay (EIA), have been replaced by NAATS, which are molecular

TABLE 213-1 DIAGNOSTIC TESTS FOR SEXUALLY TRANSMITTED AND PERINATAL *CHLAMYDIA TRACHOMATIS* INFECTION

Infection	Suggestive Signs/Symptoms	Presumptive Diagnosis[a]	Confirmatory Test of Choice
Men			
NGU, PGU	Discharge, dysuria	Gram's stain with >4 neutrophils per oil-immersion field; no gonococci	Urine or urethral NAAT for *C. trachomatis*
Epididymitis	Unilateral intrascrotal swelling, pain, tenderness; fever; NGU	Gram's stain with >4 neutrophils per oil-immersion field; no gonococci; urinalysis with pyuria	Urine or urethral NAAT for *C. trachomatis*
Women			
Cervicitis	Mucopurulent cervical discharge, bleeding and edema of the zone of cervical ectopy	Cervical Gram's stain with ≥20 neutrophils per oil-immersion field in cervical mucus	Urine, cervical, or vaginal NAAT for *C. trachomatis*
Salpingitis	Lower abdominal pain, cervical motion tenderness, adnexal tenderness or masses	*C. trachomatis* always potentially present in salpingitis	Urine, cervical, or vaginal NAAT for *C. trachomatis*
Urethritis	Dysuria and frequency without hematuria	MPC; sterile pyuria; negative routine urine culture	Urine or urethral NAAT for *C. trachomatis*
Adults of Either Sex			
Proctitis	Rectal pain, discharge, tenesmus, bleeding; history of receptive anorectal intercourse	Negative gonococcal culture and Gram's stain; at least 1 neutrophil per oil-immersion field in rectal Gram's stain	Rectal NAAT for *C. trachomatis* or culture
Reactive arthritis	NGU, arthritis, conjunctivitis, typical skin lesions	Gram's stain with >4 neutrophils per oil-immersion field; lack of gonococci indicative of NGU	Urine or urethral NAAT for *C. trachomatis*
LGV	Regional adenopathy, primary lesion, proctitis, systemic symptoms	None	Culture of LGV strain from node or rectum, occasionally from urethra or cervix; NAAT for *C. trachomatis* from these sites; LGV CF titer, ≥1:64; micro-IF titer, ≥1:512
Neonates			
Conjunctivitis	Purulent conjunctival discharge 6–18 days after delivery	Negative culture and Gram's stain for gonococci, *Haemophilus* spp., pneumococci, staphylococci	Conjunctival NAAT for *C. trachomatis*; FA-stained scraping of conjunctival material
Infant pneumonia	Afebrile; staccato cough, diffuse rales, bilateral hyperinflation, interstitial infiltrates	None	Chlamydial culture or NAAT of sputum, pharynx, eye, rectum; micro-IF antibody to *C. trachomatis*—fourfold change in IgG or IgM antibody titer

[a]A presumptive diagnosis of chlamydial infection is often made in the syndromes listed when gonococci are not found. A positive test for *Neisseria gonorrhoeae* does not exclude the involvement of *C. trachomatis*, which often is present in patients with gonorrhea.

Abbreviations: CF, complement-fixing; FA, fluorescent antibody; LGV, lymphogranuloma venereum; micro-IF, microimmunofluorescence; MPC, mucopurulent cervicitis; NAAT, nucleic acid amplification test; NGU, nongonococcal urethritis; PGU, postgonococcal urethritis.

Source: Reprinted with permission from WE Stamm: Chlamydial infections, in *Harrison's Principles of Internal Medicine*, 17th ed, AS Fauci et al (eds). New York, McGraw-Hill, 2008, p 1075.

tests that amplify the nucleic acids in clinical specimens. NAATS are currently recommended by the CDC as the diagnostic assays of choice; four or five NAAT assays approved by the U.S. Food and Drug Administration (FDA) are commercially available, some as high-throughput robotic platforms. Point-of-care diagnostic assays (including NAATs), by which patients can be treated before leaving the clinic, are of increasing interest and are becoming available.

CHOICE OF SPECIMEN Cervical and urethral swabs have traditionally been used for the diagnosis of STDs in female and male patients, respectively. However, given the greatly increased sensitivity and specificity of NAATs, less invasive samples (e.g., urine for both sexes and vaginal swabs for women) can be used. For screening of asymptomatic women, the CDC now recommends that self-collected or clinician-collected vaginal swabs, which are slightly more sensitive than urine, be used. Urine screening tests are often used in outreach screening programs, however. For symptomatic women undergoing a pelvic examination, cervical swab samples are desirable because they have slightly higher chlamydial counts. For male patients, a urine specimen is the sample of choice, but self-collected penile-meatal swabs have been explored.

ALTERNATIVE SPECIMEN TYPES Ocular samples from babies and adults can be assessed by NAATs. However, since commercial NAATs for this purpose have not yet been approved by the FDA, laboratories must perform their own verification studies. Samples from rectal and pharyngeal sites have been used successfully to detect chlamydiae, but laboratories must verify test performance.

OTHER DIAGNOSTIC ISSUES Because NAATs detect nucleic acids instead of live organisms, they should be used with caution as test-of-cure assays. Residual nucleic acid from cells rendered noninfective by antibiotics may continue to yield a positive result in NAATs until as long as 3 weeks after therapy, when viable organisms have actually been eradicated. Therefore, clinicians should not use NAATs for test of cure until after 3 weeks. The CDC currently does not recommend a test of cure after treatment for infection with *C. trachomatis*. However, because incidence studies have demonstrated that previous chlamydial infection increases the probability of becoming reinfected, the CDC does recommend that previously infected individuals be rescreened 3 months after treatment.

SEROLOGY Serologic testing may be helpful in the diagnosis of LGV and neonatal pneumonia caused by *C. trachomatis.* The serologic test of choice is the microimmunofluorescence (MIF) test, in which high-titer purified EBs mixed with embryonated chicken yolk-sac material are affixed to a glass microscope slide to which dilutions of serum are applied. After incubation and washing, fluorescein-conjugated IgG or IgM antibody is applied. The test is read with an epifluorescence microscope, with the highest dilution of serum producing visible fluorescence designated as the titer. The MIF test is not widely available and is highly labor intensive. Although the complement fixation (CF) test also can be used, it employs only lipopolysaccharide (LPS) as the antigen and therefore identifies the pathogen only to the genus level. Single-point titers of >1:64 support a diagnosis of LGV, in which it is difficult to demonstrate rising antibody titers; i.e., paired serum samples are difficult to obtain since, by its very nature, the disease results in the patient's being seen by the physician after the acute stage. Any antibody titer of >1:16 is considered significant evidence of exposure to chlamydiae. However, serologic testing is never recommended for diagnosis of uncomplicated genital infections of the cervix, urethra, and lower genital tract or for *C. trachomatis* screening of asymptomatic individuals.

TREATMENT *C. TRACHOMATIS* GENITAL INFECTIONS

A 7-day course of tetracycline (500 mg four times daily), doxycycline (100 mg twice daily), erythromycin (500 mg four times daily), or a fluoroquinolone (ofloxacin, 300 mg twice daily; or levofloxacin, 500 mg/d) can be used for treatment of uncomplicated chlamydial infections. A single 1-g oral dose of azithromycin is as effective as a 7-day course of doxycycline for the treatment of uncomplicated genital *C. trachomatis* infections in adults. Azithromycin causes fewer adverse gastrointestinal reactions than do older macrolides such as erythromycin. The single-dose regimen of azithromycin has great appeal for the treatment of patients with uncomplicated chlamydial infection (especially those without symptoms and those with a likelihood of poor compliance) and of the sexual partners of infected patients. These advantages must be weighed against the considerably greater cost of azithromycin. Whenever possible, the single 1-g dose should be given as directly observed therapy. Although not approved by the FDA for use in pregnancy, this regimen appears to be safe and effective for this purpose. However, amoxicillin (500 mg three times daily for 7 days) also can be given to pregnant women. The fluoroquinolones are contraindicated in pregnancy. A 2-week course of treatment is recommended for complicated chlamydial infections (e.g., PID, epididymitis) and at least a 3-week course of doxycycline (100 mg orally twice daily) or erythromycin base (500 mg orally four times daily) for LGV. Failure of treatment with a tetracycline in genital infections usually indicates poor compliance or reinfection rather than involvement of a drug-resistant strain. To date, clinically significant drug resistance has not been observed in *C. trachomatis*.

Treatment or testing for chlamydiae should be considered among *N. gonorrhoeae*–infected patients because of the frequency of co-infection. Systemic treatment with erythromycin has been recommended for ophthalmia neonatorum and for *C. trachomatis* pneumonia in infants. For the treatment of adult inclusion conjunctivitis, a single 1-g dose of azithromycin is as effective as standard 10-day treatment with doxycycline. Recommended treatment regimens for both bubonic and anogenital LGV include tetracycline, doxycycline, or erythromycin for 21 days.

SEX PARTNERS

The continued high prevalence of chlamydial infections in most parts of the United States is due primarily to the failure to diagnose—and therefore treat—patients with symptomatic or asymptomatic infection and their sex partners. Urethral or cervical infection with *C. trachomatis* has been well documented in a high proportion of the sex partners of patients with NGU, epididymitis, reactive arthritis, salpingitis, and endocervicitis. If possible, confirmatory laboratory tests for chlamydiae should be undertaken in these individuals, but even those without positive tests or evidence of clinical disease who have recently been exposed to proven or possible chlamydial infection (e.g., NGU) should be offered therapy. A novel approach is partner-delivered therapy, in which infected patients receive treatment and are also provided with single-dose azithromycin to give to their sex partner(s).

NEONATES AND INFANTS

In neonates with conjunctivitis or infants with pneumonia, erythromycin ethylsuccinate or estolate can be given orally at a dosage of 50 mg/kg per day, preferably in four divided doses, for 2 weeks. Careful attention must be given to compliance with therapy—a frequent problem. Relapses of eye infection are common after topical treatment with erythromycin or tetracycline ophthalmic ointment and may also follow oral erythromycin therapy. Thus follow-up cultures should be performed after treatment. Both parents should be examined for *C. trachomatis* infection and, if diagnostic testing is not readily available, should be treated with doxycycline or azithromycin.

Prevention Since many chlamydial infections are asymptomatic, effective control and prevention must involve periodic screening of individuals at risk. Selective cost-effective screening criteria have been developed. Among women, young age (generally <25 years) is a critical risk factor for chlamydial infections in nearly all studies. Other risk factors include mucopurulent cervicitis; multiple, new, or symptomatic male sex partners; and lack of barrier contraceptive use. In some settings, screening based on young age may be as sensitive as criteria that incorporate behavioral and clinical measures. Another strategy is universal testing of all patients in high-prevalence clinic populations (e.g., STD clinics, juvenile detention facilities, and family planning clinics).

The effectiveness of selective screening in reducing the prevalence of chlamydial infection among women has been demonstrated in several studies. In the Pacific Northwest, where extensive screening began in family planning clinics in 1998 and in STD clinics in 1993, the prevalence declined from 10% in the 1980s to <5% in 2000. Similar trends have occurred in association with screening programs elsewhere. In addition, screening can effect a reduction in upper genital tract disease. In Seattle, women at a large health maintenance organization who were screened for chlamydial infection on a routine basis had a lower incidence of symptomatic PID than did women who received standard care and underwent more selective screening.

In settings with low to moderate prevalence, the prevalence at which selective screening becomes more cost-effective than universal screening must be defined. Most studies have concluded that universal screening is preferable in settings with a chlamydial prevalence of >3–7%. Depending on the criteria used, selective screening is likely to be more cost-effective when prevalence falls below 3%. Nearly all regions of the United States have now initiated screening programs, particularly in family planning and STD clinics. Along with single-dose therapy, the availability of highly sensitive and specific diagnostic NAATs using urine specimens and self-obtained vaginal swabs makes it feasible to mount an effective nationwide *Chlamydia* control program, with screening of high-risk individuals in traditional health-care settings and in novel outreach and community-based settings. The U.S. Preventive Services Task Force has given *C. trachomatis* screening a Grade A recommendation, which means that private insurance and Medicare will cover its cost under the Affordable Care Act.

TRACHOMA

Epidemiology Trachoma—a sequela of ocular disease in developing countries—continues to be a leading cause of preventable infectious blindness worldwide. The WHO estimates that ~6 million people have been blinded by trachoma and that ~1.3 million people in developing countries still suffer from preventable blindness due to trachoma; certainly hundreds of millions live in trachoma-endemic areas. Foci of trachoma persist in Australia, the South Pacific, and Latin America. Serovars A, B, Ba, and C are isolated from patients with clinical trachoma in areas of endemicity in developing countries in Africa, the Middle East, Asia, and South America.

The trachoma-hyperendemic areas of the world are in northern and sub-Saharan Africa, the Middle East, drier regions of the Indian subcontinent, and Southeast Asia. In hyperendemic areas, the prevalence of trachoma is essentially 100% by the second or third year of life. Active disease is most common among young children, who are the reservoir for trachoma. By adulthood, active infection is infrequent but sequelae result in blindness. In such areas, trachoma constitutes the major cause of blindness.

Trachoma is transmitted through contact with discharges from the eyes of infected patients. Transmission is most common under poor hygienic conditions and most often takes place between family members or between families with shared facilities. Flies can also transfer the mucopurulent ocular discharges, carrying the organisms on their legs from one person to another. The International Trachoma Initiative founded by the WHO in 1998 aims to eliminate blinding trachoma globally by 2020.

Clinical Manifestations Both endemic trachoma and adult inclusion conjunctivitis present initially as conjunctivitis characterized by small lymphoid follicles in the conjunctiva. In regions with hyperendemic classic blinding trachoma, the disease usually starts insidiously before the age of 2 years. Reinfection is common and probably contributes to the pathogenesis of trachoma. Studies using polymerase chain reaction (PCR) or other NAATs indicate that chlamydial DNA is often present in the ocular secretions of patients with trachoma, even in the absence of positive cultures. Thus persistent infection may be more common than was previously thought.

The cornea becomes involved, with inflammatory leukocytic infiltrations and superficial vascularization (*pannus formation*). As the inflammation continues, conjunctival scarring eventually distorts the eyelids, causing them to turn inward so that the lashes constantly abrade the eyeball (*trichiasis and entropion*); eventually the corneal epithelium is abraded and may ulcerate, with subsequent corneal scarring and blindness. Destruction of the conjunctival goblet cells, lacrimal ducts, and lacrimal gland may produce a "dry-eye" syndrome, with resultant corneal opacity due to drying (*xerosis*) or secondary bacterial corneal ulcers.

Communities with blinding trachoma often experience seasonal epidemics of conjunctivitis due to *H. influenzae* that contribute to the intensity of the inflammatory process. In such areas, the active infectious process usually resolves spontaneously in affected persons at 10–15 years of age, but conjunctival scars continue to shrink, producing trichiasis and entropion with subsequent corneal scarring in adults. In areas with milder and less prevalent disease, the process may be much slower, with active disease continuing into adulthood; blindness is rare in these cases.

Eye infection with oculogenital *C. trachomatis* strains in sexually active young adults presents as an acute onset of unilateral follicular conjunctivitis and preauricular lymphadenopathy similar to that seen in acute conjunctivitis caused by adenovirus or HSV. If untreated, the disease may persist for 6 weeks to 2 years. It is frequently associated with corneal inflammation in the form of discrete opacities ("infiltrates"), punctate epithelial erosions, and minor degrees of superficial corneal vascularization. Very rarely, conjunctival scarring and eyelid distortion occur, particularly in patients treated for many months with topical glucocorticoids. Recurrent eye infections develop most often in patients whose sexual partners are not treated with antimicrobial agents.

Diagnosis

The clinical diagnosis of classic trachoma can be made if two of the following signs are present: (1) lymphoid follicles on the upper tarsal conjunctiva; (2) typical conjunctival scarring; (3) vascular pannus; or (4) limbal follicles or their sequelae, Herbert's pits. The clinical diagnosis of endemic trachoma should be confirmed by laboratory tests in children with relatively marked degrees of inflammation. Intracytoplasmic chlamydial inclusions are found in 10–60% of Giemsa-stained conjunctival smears in such populations, but chlamydial NAATs are more sensitive and are often positive when smears or cultures are negative. Follicular conjunctivitis in European or American adults living in trachomatous regions is rarely due to trachoma.

TREATMENT TRACHOMA

Adult inclusion conjunctivitis responds well to treatment with the same regimens used in uncomplicated genital infections—namely, azithromycin (a 1-g single oral dose) or doxycycline (100 mg twice daily for 7 days). Simultaneous treatment of all sexual partners is necessary to prevent ocular reinfection and chlamydial genital disease. Topical antibiotic treatment is not required for patients who receive systemic antibiotics.

PSITTACOSIS

Psittacine birds and many other avian species act as natural reservoirs for *C. psittaci*–type organisms, which are common pathogens in domestic mammals and birds. The species *C. psittaci,* which now includes only avian strains, affects humans only as a zoonosis. (The other strains previously included in this species have been placed into different species that generally reflect the animals they infect: *C. abortus, C. muridarum, C. suis, C. felis,* and *C. caviae.*) Although all birds are susceptible, pet birds (parrots, parakeets, macaws, and cockatiels) and poultry (turkeys and ducks) are most frequently involved in transmission of *C. psittaci* to humans. Exposure is greatest among poultry-processing workers and owners of pet birds. Infectious forms of the organisms are shed from both symptomatic and apparently healthy birds and may remain viable for several months. *C. psittaci* can be transmitted to humans by direct contact with infected birds or by inhalation of aerosols from avian nasal discharges and from infectious avian fecal or feather dust. Transmission from person to person has never been demonstrated.

The diagnosis is usually established serologically. Psittacosis in humans may present as acute primary atypical pneumonia (which can be fatal in up to 10% of untreated cases); as severe chronic pneumonia; or as a mild illness or asymptomatic infection in persons exposed to infected birds.

EPIDEMIOLOGY

Fewer than 50 confirmed cases of psittacosis are reported in the United States each year, although many more cases probably occur than are reported. Control of psittacosis depends on control of avian sources of infection. A pandemic of psittacosis was once stopped by banning shipment or importation of psittacine birds. Birds can receive prophylaxis in the form of a tetracycline-containing feed. Imported birds are currently quarantined for 30 days of treatment.

CLINICAL MANIFESTATIONS

Typical symptoms include fever, chills, muscular aches and pains, severe headache, hepato- and/or splenomegaly, and gastrointestinal symptoms. Cardiac complications may involve endocarditis and myocarditis. Fatal cases were common in the preantibiotic era. As a result of quarantine of imported birds and improved veterinary-hygienic measures, outbreaks and sporadic cases of psittacosis are now rare. Severe pneumonia requiring management in an intensive care unit may develop. Endocarditis, hepatitis, and neurologic complications may occur, and fatal cases have been reported. The incubation period is usually 5–19 days but can last as long as 28 days.

DIAGNOSIS

Previously, the most widely used serologic test for diagnosing chlamydial infections was the genus-specific CF test, in which assay of paired serum specimens often shows fourfold or greater increases in antibody titer. The CF test remains useful, but the gold standard of serologic tests is now the MIF test, which is not widely available (see section on diagnosis of *C. trachomatis* genital infection, above). Any antibody titer above 1:16 is considered significant evidence of exposure to chlamydiae, and a fourfold titer rise in paired sera in combination with a clinically compatible syndrome can be used to diagnose psittacosis. Some commercially available serologic tests based on measurement of antibodies to LPS can be useful when the clinical diagnosis is consistent with bird exposure; however, since these tests are reactive for all chlamydiae (i.e., all chlamydiae contain LPS), caution must be used in their interpretation.

TREATMENT PSITTACOSIS

The antibiotic of choice is tetracycline; the dosage for adults is 250 mg four times a day, continued for at least 3 weeks to avoid relapse. Severely ill patients may need cardiovascular and respiratory support. Erythromycin (500 mg four times a day by mouth) is an alternative therapy.

CHLAMYDIA PNEUMONIAE INFECTIONS

C. pneumoniae is a common cause of human respiratory diseases, such as pneumonia and bronchitis. This organism has been reported to account for as many as 10% of cases of community-acquired pneumonia, most of which are diagnosed by serology. Serologic studies have linked *C. pneumoniae* to atherosclerosis; isolation and PCR detection in cardiovascular tissues have also been reported. These findings suggest an expanded range of diseases and syndromes for *C. pneumoniae*. The role of *C. pneumoniae* in the etiology of atherosclerosis has been discussed since 1988, when Finnish researchers presented serologic evidence of an association of this organism with coronary heart disease and acute myocardial infarction. Subsequently, the organism was identified in atherosclerotic lesions by culture, PCR, immunohistochemistry, and transmission electron microscopy; however, discrepant study results (including those of animal studies) and failure of large-scale treatment studies have raised doubts as to the etiologic role of *C. pneumoniae* in atherosclerosis. Large-scale case cohort studies have demonstrated some association of *C. pneumoniae* with lung cancer, as evaluated by serology.

EPIDEMIOLOGY

Primary infection occurs mainly in school-aged children and reinfection in adults. Seroprevalence rates of 40–70% show that *C. pneumoniae* is widespread in both industrialized and developing countries. Seropositivity usually is first detected at school age, and rates generally increase by ~10% per decade. About 50% of individuals have detectable antibody at 30 years of age, and most have detectable antibody by the eighth decade of life. Although serologic evidence suggests that *C. pneumoniae* may be associated with up to 10% of cases of community-acquired pneumonia, most of this evidence is based not on paired serum samples but rather on a single high IgG titer. Some doubt exists about the true prevalence and etiologic role of *C. pneumoniae* in atypical pneumonia, especially since reports of cross-reactivity have raised questions about the specificity of serology when only a single serum sample is used for diagnosis.

PATHOGENESIS

Little is known about the pathogenesis of *C. pneumoniae* infection. It begins in the upper respiratory tract and, in many persons, persists as a prolonged asymptomatic condition of the upper respiratory mucosal surfaces. However, evidence of replication within vascular endothelium and synovial membranes of joints shows that, in at least some individuals, the organism is transported to distant sites, perhaps within macrophages. A *C. pneumoniae* outer-membrane protein may induce host immune responses whose cross-reactivity with human proteins results in an autoimmune reaction.

As mentioned above, epidemiologic studies have demonstrated an association between serologic evidence of *C. pneumoniae* infection and atherosclerotic disease of the coronary and other arteries. In addition, *C. pneumoniae* has been identified in atherosclerotic plaques by electron microscopy, DNA hybridization, and immunocytochemistry. The organism has been recovered in culture from atheromatous plaque—a result indicating the presence of viable replicating bacteria in vessels. Evidence from animal models supports the hypothesis that *C. pneumoniae* infection of the upper respiratory tract is followed by recovery of the organism from atheromatous lesions in the aorta and that the infection accelerates the process of atherosclerosis, especially in hypercholesterolemic animals. Antimicrobial treatment of the infected animals reverses the increased risk of atherosclerosis. In humans, two small trials in patients with unstable angina or recent myocardial infarction suggested that antibiotics reduce the likelihood of subsequent untoward cardiac events. However, larger-scale trials have not documented an effect of various antichlamydial regimens on the risk of these events.

CLINICAL MANIFESTATIONS

C. pneumoniae was first reported as the etiologic agent of mild atypical pneumonia in military recruits and college students. The clinical spectrum of *C. pneumoniae* infection includes acute pharyngitis, sinusitis, bronchitis, and pneumonitis, primarily in young adults. The clinical manifestations of primary infection appear to be more severe and prolonged than those of reinfection. The pneumonitis of *C. pneumoniae* pneumonia resembles that of *Mycoplasma* pneumonia in that leukocytosis is frequently lacking and patients often have prominent antecedent upper respiratory tract symptoms, fever, nonproductive cough, mild to moderate illness, minimal findings on chest auscultation, and small segmental infiltrates on chest x-ray. In elderly patients, pneumonia due to *C. pneumoniae* can be especially severe and may necessitate hospitalization and respiratory support.

Chronic infection with *C. pneumoniae* has been reported among patients with chronic obstructive pulmonary disease and may also play a role in the natural history of asthma, including exacerbations. The clinical symptoms of respiratory infections caused by *C. pneumoniae* are nonspecific and do not differ from those caused by other agents of atypical pneumonia, such as *Mycoplasma pneumoniae*.

DIAGNOSIS

Serology, PCR amplification, and culture can be used to diagnose *C. pneumoniae* infection. Serology has been the traditional method of diagnosing infection by *C. pneumoniae*. The gold standard serologic test is the MIF test (see section on diagnosis of *C. trachomatis* genital infection, above). Any antibody titer above 1:16 is considered significant evidence of exposure to chlamydiae. According to a CDC-sponsored expert working group, the diagnosis of acute *C. pneumoniae* infection requires demonstration of a fourfold rise in titer in paired serum samples. There are no official recommendations for diagnosis of chronic infections, although many research studies have used high titers of IgA as an indicator. The older CF tests and EIAs for LPS are not recommended, as they are not specific for *C. pneumoniae* but identify the chlamydiae only to the genus level. The organism is very difficult to grow in tissue culture but has been cultivated in HeLa cells, HEp-2 cells, and HL cells. Although NAATs are commercially available for *C. trachomatis*, only research-based PCR assays are available for *C. pneumoniae*.

TREATMENT *C. PNEUMONIAE* INFECTIONS

Although few controlled trials of treatment have been reported, *C. pneumoniae* is inhibited in vitro by erythromycin, tetracycline, azithromycin, clarithromycin, gatifloxacin, and gemifloxacin. Recommended therapy consists of 2 g/d of either tetracycline or erythromycin for 10–14 days. Other macrolides (e.g., azithromycin) and some fluoroquinolones (e.g., levofloxacin and gatifloxacin) also appear to be effective.

ACKNOWLEDGMENT

The authors wish to acknowledge the late Walter E. Stamm, MD, for his significant contributions to the field of Chlamydia research. Dr. Stamm wrote the chapters on chlamydiae for previous editions of Harrison's Principles of Internal Medicine, and we thank the editors for permission to reproduce Figs. 213-1 and 213-2 as well as Table 213-1 from his chapter in the 17th edition. Dr. Stamm died on December 14, 2009, and this chapter is dedicated to him.

SECTION 11 VIRAL DISEASES: GENERAL CONSIDERATIONS

214e Medical Virology

Fred Wang, Elliott Kieff

This is a digital-only chapter. It is available on the DVD that accompanies this book, as well as on Access Medicine/Harrison's Online, and the eBook and "app" editions of HPIM 19e.

DEFINING A VIRUS

Viruses are obligate intracellular parasites. They consist of a DNA or RNA genome surrounded by protein. They may also have an outer-membrane lipoprotein envelope. Viruses can replicate only within cells, because their nucleic acid does not encode many enzymes necessary for the metabolism of proteins, carbohydrates, or lipids or for the generation of high-energy phosphates. Typically, viral nucleic acids encode messenger RNA (mRNA) and proteins necessary for replicating, packaging, and releasing progeny virus from infected cells.

Viruses differ from virusoids, viroids, and prions. Virusoids are nucleic acids that depend on cells and helper viruses for packaging their nucleic acids into virus-like particles. Viroids are naked, cyclical, mostly double-strand small RNAs that appear to be restricted to plants, spread from cell to cell, and are replicated by cellular RNA polymerase II. Prions (Chap. 453e) are abnormal proteins that propagate and cause disease by altering the structure of a normal cell protein. Prions cause neurodegenerative diseases such as Creutzfeldt-Jakob disease, Gerstmann-Straüssler disease, kuru, and human or bovine spongiform encephalopathy ("mad cow disease").

215e Antiviral Chemotherapy, Excluding Antiretroviral Drugs

Lindsey R. Baden, Raphael Dolin

This is a digital-only chapter. It is available on the DVD that accompanies this book, as well as on Access Medicine/Harrison's Online, and the eBook and "app" editions of HPIM 19e.

The field of antiviral therapy—both the number of antiviral drugs and our understanding of their optimal use—historically has lagged behind that of antibacterial treatment, but significant progress has been made in recent years on new drugs for several viral infections. The development of antiviral drugs poses several challenges. Viruses replicate intracellularly and often use host cell enzymes, macromolecules, and organelles for synthesis of viral particles. Therefore, useful antiviral compounds must discriminate between host and viral functions with a high degree of specificity; agents without such selectivity are likely to be too toxic for clinical use.

SECTION 12 INFECTIONS DUE TO DNA VIRUSES

216 Herpes Simplex Virus Infections

Lawrence Corey

DEFINITION

Herpes simplex viruses (HSV-1, HSV-2; *Herpesvirus hominis*) produce a variety of infections involving mucocutaneous surfaces, the central nervous system (CNS), and—on occasion—visceral organs. Prompt recognition and treatment reduce the morbidity and mortality rates associated with HSV infections.

ETIOLOGIC AGENT

The genome of HSV is a linear, double-strand DNA molecule (molecular weight, ~100 × 10^6) that encodes >90 transcription units with 84 identified proteins. The genomic structures of the two HSV subtypes are similar. The overall genomic sequence homology between HSV-1 and HSV-2 is ~50%, whereas the proteome homology is >80%. The homologous sequences are distributed over the entire genome map, and most of the polypeptides specified by one viral type are antigenically related to polypeptides of the other viral type. Many type-specific regions unique to HSV-1 and HSV-2 proteins do exist, however, and a number of them appear to be important in host immunity. These type-specific regions have been used to develop serologic assays that distinguish between the two viral subtypes. Either restriction endonuclease analysis or sequencing of viral DNA can be used to distinguish between the two subtypes and among strains of each subtype. The variability of nucleotide sequences from clinical strains of HSV-1 and HSV-2 is such that HSV isolates obtained from two individuals can be differentiated by restriction enzyme patterns or genomic sequences. Moreover, epidemiologically related sources, such as sexual partners, mother-infant pairs, or persons involved in a common-source outbreak, can be inferred from such patterns.

The viral genome is packaged in a regular icosahedral protein shell (capsid) composed of 162 capsomeres (see Fig. 214e-1). The outer covering of the virus is a lipid-containing membrane (envelope) acquired as the DNA-containing capsid buds through the inner nuclear membrane of the host cell. Between the capsid and lipid bilayer of the envelope is the tegument. Viral replication has both nuclear and cytoplasmic phases. Initial attachment to the cell membrane involves interactions of viral glycoproteins C and B with several cellular heparan sulfate–like surface receptors. Subsequently, viral glycoprotein D binds to cellular co-receptors that belong to the tumor necrosis factor receptor family of proteins, the immunoglobulin superfamily (nectin family), or both. The ubiquity of these receptors contributes to the wide host range of herpesviruses. HSV replication is highly regulated. After fusion and entry, the nucleocapsid enters the cytoplasm and several viral proteins are released from the virion. Some of these viral proteins shut off host protein synthesis (by increasing cellular RNA degradation), whereas others "turn on" the transcription of early genes of HSV replication. These early gene products, designated *α genes*, are required for synthesis of the subsequent polypeptide group, the β polypeptides, many of which are regulatory proteins and enzymes required for DNA replication. Most current antiviral drugs interfere with β proteins, such as viral DNA polymerase. The third (γ) class of HSV genes requires viral DNA replication for expression and encodes most structural proteins specified by the virus.

After viral genome replication and structural protein synthesis, nucleocapsids are assembled in the cell's nucleus. Envelopment occurs as the nucleocapsids bud through the inner nuclear membrane into the perinuclear space. In some cells, viral replication in the nucleus forms two types of inclusion bodies: type A basophilic Feulgen-positive bodies that contain viral DNA and eosinophilic inclusion bodies that are devoid of viral nucleic acid or protein and represent a "scar" of viral infection. Enveloped virions are then transported via the endoplasmic reticulum and the Golgi apparatus to the cell surface.

Viral genomes are maintained by some neuronal cells in a repressed state called *latency*. Latency, which is associated with transcription of only a limited number of virus-encoded RNAs, accounts for the presence of viral DNA and RNA in neural tissue at times when infectious virus cannot be isolated. Maintenance and growth of neural cells from latently infected ganglia in tissue culture result in production of infectious virions (*explantation*) and in subsequent permissive infection of susceptible cells (*co-cultivation*). Activation of the viral genome may then occur, resulting in *reactivation*—the normal pattern of regulated viral gene expression and replication and HSV release. The release of virions from the neuron follows a complex process of anterograde transport down the length of neuronal axons. In experimental animals, ultraviolet light, systemic and local immunosuppression, and trauma to the skin or ganglia are associated with reactivation.

Three noncoding RNA latency-associated transcripts (LATs) are found in the nuclei of latently infected neurons. Deletion mutants of the LAT region exhibit reduced efficiency in their later reactivation. Substitution of HSV-1 LATs for HSV-2 LATs induces an HSV-1 reactivation pattern. These data indicate that LATs apparently maintain—rather than establish—latency. HSV-1 LATs promote the survival of acutely infected neurons, perhaps by inhibiting apoptotic pathways. LAT transcript abundance and low genome-copy number correlate with subnuclear positioning of HSV genomes around the centromere. Indeed, chromatization of HSV DNA appears to play a vital role in silencing expression of lytic replication genes. Highly expressed during latency, LAT-derived micro-RNA appears to silence expression of the key neurovirulence factor infected-cell protein 34.5 (ICP34.5) and to bind in an antisense configuration to the immediate early protein ICP0 messenger RNA to prevent expression, which is vital to HSV reactivation. Although certain viral transcripts are known to be necessary for reactivation from latency, the molecular mechanisms of HSV latency are not fully understood, and strategies to interrupt or maintain latency in neurons are in developmental stages.

While latency is the predominant state of virus on a per-neuron basis, the high frequency of oral and genital tract reactivation for HSV-1 and HSV-2 suggests that the viruses are rarely quiescent within the entire biomass of ganglionic tissue. Recent data indicate that HSV-2 antigen is often shed: most persons infected with HSV-2 have frequent subclinical bursts of reactivation lasting 2–4 h, and the host mucosal immune system can contain viral reactivation in the mucosa before the development of clinical reactivation. Supporting this clinical observation, recent work using microdissection plus real-time polymerase chain reaction (PCR) of individual neurons from cadaveric trigeminal ganglia explants revealed that many more neurons (2–10%) harbor HSV than would be predicted by in situ hybridization studies for LATs. Viral copy number is highly variable between neurons, with extremely high levels in certain neurons, and HSV DNA copy numbers are similar in LAT-positive and LAT-negative neurons; these findings add to the uncertainty about the role that LATs play in preventing reactivation.

PATHOGENESIS

Exposure to HSV at mucosal surfaces or abraded skin sites permits entry of the virus into cells of the epidermis and dermis and initiation of viral replication therein. HSV infections are usually acquired subclinically. Whether clinical or subclinical, HSV acquisition is associated with sufficient viral replication to permit infection of either sensory or autonomic nerve endings. On entry into the neuronal cell, the virus—or, more likely, the nucleocapsid—is transported intra-axonally to the nerve cell bodies in ganglia. In humans, the transit interval of spread to the ganglia after virus inoculation into peripheral tissue is unknown. During the initial phase of infection, viral replication occurs in ganglia and contiguous neural tissue. Virus then spreads to other mucocutaneous surfaces through centrifugal migration of infectious virions via peripheral sensory nerves. This mode of spread helps explain the large surface area involved, the high frequency of new lesions distant from the initial crop of vesicles that is characteristic in patients with primary genital or oral-labial HSV infection, and the ability to recover virus from neural tissue distant from neurons innervating the inoculation site. Contiguous spread of locally inoculated virus also may take place and allow further mucosal extension of disease. Recent studies have demonstrated HSV viremia—another mechanism for extension of infection throughout the body—in ~30–40% of persons with primary HSV-2 infection. Latent infection with both viral subtypes in both sensory and autonomic ganglia has been demonstrated. For HSV-1 infection, trigeminal ganglia are most commonly infected, although extension to the inferior and superior cervical ganglia also occurs. With genital infection, sacral nerve root ganglia (S2–S5) are most commonly affected.

After resolution of primary disease, infectious HSV can no longer be cultured from the ganglia; however, latent infection, as defined by the presence of viral DNA, persists in 2–11% of ganglionic cells in the anatomic region of the initial infection. The mechanism of reactivation from latency is unknown. Increasingly, studies indicate that host T cell responses at the ganglionic and peripheral mucosal levels influence the frequency and severity of HSV reactivation. HSV-specific T cells have been recovered from peripheral-nerve root ganglia. Many of these resident CD8+ T cells are juxtaposed with latently HSV-1-infected neurons in the trigeminal ganglia and can block reactivation with both interferon (IFN) γ release and granzyme B degradation of the immediate-early protein ICP4. In addition, there appears to be a latent viral load in the ganglia that correlates positively with the number of neurons infected and the rate of reactivation but inversely with the number of CD8+ cells present. It is not known whether reactivating stimuli transiently suppress these immune cells, independently upregulate transcription of lytic genes, or both. Moreover, host containment in the mucosa has been demonstrated. Once virus reaches the dermal-epidermal junction, there are three possible outcomes: rapid host containment of infection near the site of reactivation; spread of virus into the epidermis, with a micro-ulceration associated with low-titer subclinical shedding; and subsequent rapid (within hours) containment of virus with widespread replication and necrosis of epithelial cells and subsequent clinical recurrence (the latter defined clinically by a skin blister and ulceration). Histologically, herpetic lesions involve a thin-walled vesicle or ulceration in the basal region, multinucleated cells that may include intranuclear inclusions, necrosis, and an acute inflammatory infection. Re-epithelialization occurs once viral replication is restricted, almost always in the absence of a scar.

Analysis of the DNA from sequential isolates of HSV or from isolates from multiple infected ganglia in any one individual has revealed similar, if not identical, restriction endonuclease or DNA sequence patterns in most persons. As more sensitive genomic technologies are developed, evidence of multiple strains of the same subtype is increasingly being reported. For example, infection of individual neurons with multiple strains of drug-susceptible and drug-resistant virus in severely immunosuppressed patients indicates that ganglia can be reseeded during chronic infection. Because exposure to mucosal shedding is relatively common during a person's lifetime, current data suggest that exogenous infection with different strains of the same subtype, while possible, is uncommon.

IMMUNITY

Host responses influence the acquisition of HSV disease, the severity of infection, resistance to the development of latency, the maintenance of latency, and the frequency of recurrences. Both antibody-mediated and cell-mediated reactions are clinically important. Immunocompromised patients with defects in cell-mediated immunity experience more severe and more extensive HSV infections than those with deficits in humoral immunity, such as agammaglobulinemia. Experimental ablation of lymphocytes indicates that T cells play a major role in preventing lethal disseminated disease, although antibodies help reduce titers of virus in neural tissue. Some clinical manifestations of HSV appear to be related to the host immune response (e.g., stromal opacities associated with recurrent herpetic keratitis). The surface viral glycoproteins have been shown to be targets of antibodies that mediate neutralization and immune-mediated cytolysis (antibody-dependent cell-mediated cytotoxicity). Monoclonal antibodies specific for each of the known viral glycoproteins have, in experimental infections, conferred protection against subsequent neurologic disease or ganglionic latency. In humans, however, subunit glycoprotein vaccines have been largely ineffective in reducing acquisition of infection. Multiple cell populations, including natural killer cells, macrophages, and a variety of T lymphocytes, play a role in host defenses against HSV infections, as do lymphokines generated by T lymphocytes. In animals, passive transfer of primed lymphocytes confers protection from subsequent HSV challenge. Maximal protection usually requires the activation of multiple T cell subpopulations, including cytotoxic T cells and T cells responsible for delayed hypersensitivity. The latter may confer protection by the antigen-stimulated release of lymphokines (e.g., IFNs), which in turn have a direct antiviral effect and both activate and enhance a variety of specific and nonspecific effector cells. The HSV virion contains a variety of genes that are directed at the inhibition of host responses. These include gene no. 12 (*US-12*), which can bind to the cellular transporter-activating protein TAP-1 and reduce the ability of this protein to bind HSV peptides to human leukocyte antigen (HLA) class I, thereby reducing recognition of viral proteins by cytotoxic T cells of the host. This effect can be overcome by the addition of IFN-γ, but this reversal requires 24–48 h; thus, the virus has time to replicate and invade other host cells. Entry of infectious HSV-1 and HSV-2 inhibits several signaling pathways of both CD4+ and CD8+ T cells, leading to their functional impairment in killing and influencing the spectrum of their cytokine secretion.

Increasing evidence suggests that HSV-specific CD8+ T cell responses are critical for clearance of virus from lesions. Immunosuppressed patients with frequent and prolonged HSV lesions have fewer functional CD8+ T cells directed at HSV. HSV-specific CD8+ T cells have been shown to persist in the genital skin at the dermal–epidermal junction contiguous to neuronal endings. Even during clinical quiescence, these CD8+ T cells make both antiviral and cytotoxic proteins indicative of immune surveillance. These resident memory CD8+ T cells appear to be "first responders" capable of controlling viral reactivation at the site of viral release into the dermis. This rapid "on and off" interplay between the virus and host helps explain the variability in clinical disease severity between episodes in any single individual. Differences of 30–60 min in host responses can result in 100- to 1000-fold differences in viral levels and can determine whether an episode of disease is subclinical or clinical.

There is a strong association between the magnitude of the CD8+ T lymphocyte response and the clearance of virus from genital lesions. The location, effectiveness, and longevity of the T lymphocytes (and perhaps of other immune effector cells) may be important in the expression of disease and the likelihood of transmission over time.

EPIDEMIOLOGY

Seroepidemiologic studies have documented HSV infections worldwide. The past 15 years have shown that the prevalence of HSV-2 is even higher in the developing than in the developed world. In sub-Saharan Africa, HSV-2 seroprevalence among pregnant women may approach 60%, and annual acquisition rates among teenage girls may verge on 20%. The global incidence has been estimated at ~23.6 million infections per year. As in the developed world, the rate of HSV-2 coital acquisition as well as the serologic prevalence is higher among women than among men. Most of this HSV-2 acquisition is preceded by acquisition of HSV-1; the frequency of genital HSV-1 in the developing world is low at present.

Infection with HSV-1 is acquired more frequently and earlier than infection with HSV-2. More than 90% of adults have antibodies to HSV-1 by the fifth decade of life. In populations of low socioeconomic status, most persons acquire HSV-1 infection before the third decade of life. Antibodies to HSV-2 are not detected routinely until puberty.

Antibody prevalence rates correlate with past sexual activity and vary greatly among different population groups. There is evidence that the prevalence of HSV-2 has decreased slightly over the past decade in the United States. Serosurveys indicate that 15–20% of the U.S. population has antibodies to HSV-2. In most routine obstetric and family planning clinics, 25% of women have HSV-2 antibodies, although only 10% of those who are seropositive for HSV-2 report a history of genital lesions. As many as 50% of heterosexual adults attending sexually transmitted disease clinics have antibodies to HSV-2.

Many studies continue to show that both incident and—more important—prevalent HSV-2 infection enhances the acquisition rate of HIV-1. More specifically, HSV-2 infection is associated with a two- to fourfold increase in HIV-1 acquisition. This association has been amply demonstrated in heterosexual men and women in both the developed and the developing worlds. Epidemiologically, regions of the world with high HSV-2 prevalence and selected populations within such regions have a higher population-based incidence of HIV-1. One study indicated that approximately one-quarter of HIV infections in the high-prevalence city of Kisumu, Kenya, were directly attributable to HSV-2.

In addition, HSV-2 facilitates the spread of HIV into low-risk populations on a per-coital basis, and prevalent HSV-2 appears to increase the risk of HIV infection by seven- to ninefold. Mathematical models suggest that ~33–50% of HIV-1 infections may be attributable to HSV-2 both in men who have sex with men (MSM) and in sub-Saharan Africa. In addition, HSV-2 is more frequently reactivated in and transmitted by persons co-infected with HIV-1 as opposed to persons not co-infected. Thus, most areas of the world with a high HIV-1 prevalence also have a high HSV-2 prevalence. A wide variety of serologic surveys have indicated a similar or even higher seroprevalence of HSV-2 in most parts of Central America, South America, and Africa. In Africa, HSV-2 seroprevalence has ranged from 40% to 70% in obstetric and other sexually experienced populations. Antibody prevalence rates average ~5–10% higher among women than among men.

Several studies suggest that many cases of "asymptomatic" genital HSV-2 infection are, in fact, simply unrecognized or confined to anatomic regions of the genital tract that are not easily visualized. Asymptomatic seropositive persons shed virus on mucosal surfaces almost as frequently as do those with symptomatic disease. This large reservoir of unidentified carriers of HSV-2 and the frequent asymptomatic reactivation of the virus from the genital tract have fostered the continued spread of genital herpes throughout the world. HSV-2 infection is an independent risk factor for the acquisition and transmission of infection with HIV-1. Among co-infected persons, HIV-1 virions can be shed from herpetic lesions of the genital region. This shedding may facilitate the spread of HIV through sexual contact. HSV-2 reactivation is associated with a localized persistent inflammatory response consisting of high concentrations of CCR5-enriched CD4+ T cells as well as inflammatory dendritic cells in the submucosa of the genital skin. These cells can support HIV infection and replication and hence are likely to account for the almost threefold increase in HIV acquisition among persons with genital herpes. Unfortunately, antiviral therapy does not reduce this subclinical postreactivation inflammation, probably because of the inability of current antiviral agents to prevent the release of small amounts of HSV antigen into the genital mucosa.

HSV infections occur throughout the year. Transmission can result from contact with persons who have active ulcerative lesions or with persons who have no clinical manifestations of infection but who are shedding HSV from mucocutaneous surfaces. HSV reactivation on genital skin and mucosal surfaces is common. The frequency of sampling influences the frequency of detection. Recent studies indicate that most HSV-1 and HSV-2 episodes last <4–6 h; thus, replication of virus and clearance by the host are rapid. Even with once-daily sampling, HSV DNA can be detected on 20–30% of days by PCR. Corresponding figures for HSV-1 in oral secretions are similar. Rates of shedding are highest during the initial years after acquisition, with viral shedding occurring on as many as 30–50% of days during this period. Immunosuppressed patients shed HSV from mucosal sites at an even higher frequency (20–80% of days). These high rates of mucocutaneous reactivation suggest that exposure to HSV from sexual or other close contact (kissing, sharing of glasses or silverware) is common and help explain the continuing spread and high seroprevalence of HSV infections worldwide. Reactivation rates vary widely among individuals. Among HIV-positive patients, a low CD4+ T cell count and a high HIV-1 load are associated with increased rates of HSV reactivation. Daily antiviral chemotherapy for HSV-2 infection can reduce shedding rates but does not eliminate shedding, as measured by PCR or culture.

CLINICAL SPECTRUM

HSV has been isolated from nearly all visceral and mucocutaneous sites. The clinical manifestations and course of HSV infection depend on the anatomic site involved, the age and immune status of the host, and the antigenic type of the virus. Primary HSV infections (i.e., first infections with either HSV-1 or HSV-2 in which the host lacks HSV antibodies in acute-phase serum) are frequently accompanied by systemic signs and symptoms. Compared with recurrent episodes, primary infections, which involve both mucosal and extramucosal sites, are characterized by a longer duration of symptoms and virus isolation from lesions. The incubation period ranges from 1 to 26 days (median, 6–8 days). Both viral subtypes can cause genital and oral-facial infections, and the infections caused by the two subtypes are clinically indistinguishable. However, the frequency of reactivation of infection is influenced by anatomic site and virus type. Genital HSV-2 infection is twice as likely to reactivate and recurs 8–10 times more frequently than genital HSV-1 infection. Conversely, oral-labial HSV-1 infection recurs more frequently than oral-labial HSV-2 infection. Asymptomatic shedding rates follow the same pattern.

Oral-Facial Infections Gingivostomatitis and pharyngitis are the most common clinical manifestations of first-episode HSV-1 infection, whereas recurrent herpes labialis is the most common clinical manifestation of reactivation HSV-1 infection. HSV pharyngitis and gingivostomatitis usually result from primary infection and are most common among children and young adults. Clinical symptoms and signs, which include fever, malaise, myalgias, inability to eat, irritability, and cervical adenopathy, may last 3–14 days. Lesions may involve the hard and soft palate, gingiva, tongue, lip, and facial area. HSV-1 or HSV-2 infection of the pharynx usually results in exudative or ulcerative lesions of the posterior pharynx and/or tonsillar pillars. Lesions of the tongue, buccal mucosa, or gingiva may occur later in the course in one-third of cases. Fever lasting 2–7 days and cervical adenopathy are common. It can be difficult to differentiate HSV pharyngitis clinically from bacterial pharyngitis, *Mycoplasma pneumoniae* infections, and pharyngeal ulcerations of noninfectious etiologies (e.g., Stevens-Johnson syndrome). No substantial evidence suggests that reactivation of oral-labial HSV infection is associated with symptomatic recurrent pharyngitis.

Reactivation of HSV from the trigeminal ganglia may be associated with asymptomatic virus excretion in the saliva, development of intraoral mucosal ulcerations, or herpetic ulcerations on the vermilion border of the lip or external facial skin. About 50–70% of seropositive patients undergoing trigeminal nerve-root decompression and 10–15% of those undergoing dental extraction develop oral-labial HSV infection a median of 3 days after these procedures. Clinical differentiation of intraoral mucosal ulcerations due to HSV from aphthous, traumatic, or drug-induced ulcerations is difficult.

In immunosuppressed patients, HSV infection may extend into mucosal and deep cutaneous layers. Friability, necrosis, bleeding, severe pain, and inability to eat or drink may result. The lesions of HSV mucositis are clinically similar to mucosal lesions caused by cytotoxic drug therapy, trauma, or fungal or bacterial infections. Persistent ulcerative HSV infections are among the most common infections in patients with AIDS. HSV and *Candida* infections often occur concurrently. Systemic antiviral therapy speeds the rate of healing and relieves the pain of mucosal HSV infections in immunosuppressed patients. The frequency of HSV reactivation during the early phases of transplantation or induction chemotherapy is high (50–90%), and prophylactic systemic antiviral agents such as IV acyclovir and penciclovir or the oral congeners of these drugs are used to reduce reactivation rates. Patients with atopic eczema may also develop severe oral-facial HSV infections (*eczema herpeticum*), which may rapidly involve extensive areas of skin and occasionally disseminate to visceral organs. Extensive eczema herpeticum has resolved promptly with the administration of IV acyclovir. Erythema multiforme may also be associated with HSV infections (see Figs. 70-9 and 25e-25); some evidence suggests that HSV infection is the precipitating event in ~75% of cases of cutaneous erythema multiforme. HSV antigen has been demonstrated both in circulatory immune complexes and in skin lesion biopsy samples from these cases. Patients with severe HSV-associated erythema multiforme are candidates for chronic suppressive oral antiviral therapy.

HSV-1 and varicella-zoster virus (VZV) have been implicated in the etiology of Bell's palsy (flaccid paralysis of the mandibular portion of the facial nerve). Some but not all trials have documented quicker resolution of facial paralysis with the prompt initiation of antiviral therapy, with or without glucocorticoids. However, other trials have shown little benefit. Thus there is no consensus on the relative value of antiviral drugs alone, glucocorticoids alone, and the two modalities combined for the treatment of Bell's palsy.

Genital Infections First-episode primary genital herpes is characterized by fever, headache, malaise, and myalgias. Pain, itching, dysuria, vaginal and urethral discharge, and tender inguinal lymphadenopathy are the predominant local symptoms. Widely spaced bilateral lesions of the external genitalia are characteristic (Fig. 216-1). Lesions may be present in varying stages, including vesicles, pustules, or painful erythematous ulcers. The cervix and urethra are involved in >80% of women with first-episode infections. First episodes of genital herpes in patients who have had prior HSV-1 infection are associated with systemic symptoms in a few patients and with faster healing than primary genital herpes. Subclinical DNAemia has been found in ~30% of cases of true primary genital herpes. The clinical courses of acute first-episode genital herpes are similar for HSV-1 and HSV-2 infection. However, the recurrence rates of genital disease differ with the viral subtype: the 12-month recurrence rates among patients with first-episode HSV-2 and HSV-1 infections are ~90% and ~55%, respectively (median number of recurrences, 4 and <1, respectively). Recurrence rates for genital HSV-2 infections vary greatly among individuals and

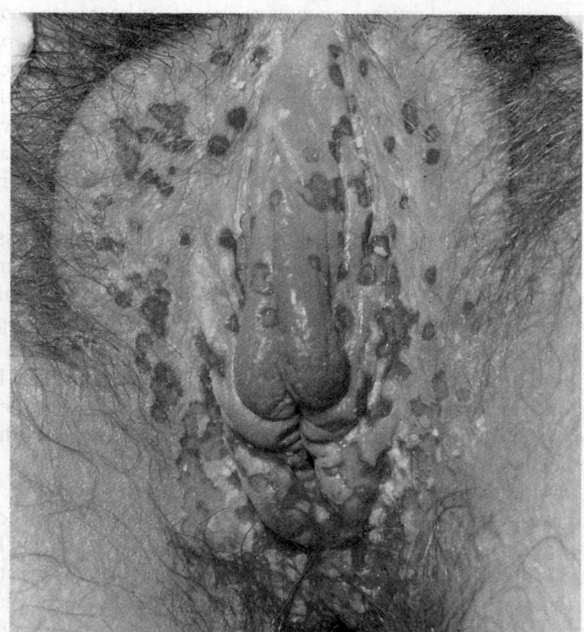

FIGURE 216-1 Genital herpes: primary vulvar infection, with multiple, extremely painful, punched-out, confluent, shallow ulcers on the edematous vulva and perineum. Micturition is often very painful. Associated inguinal lymphadenopathy is common. *(Reprinted with permission from K Wolff et al: Fitzpatrick's Color Atlas & Synopsis of Clinical Dermatology, 5th ed. New York, McGraw-Hill, 2005.)*

over time within the same individual. HSV has been isolated from the urethra and urine of men and women without external genital lesions. A clear mucoid discharge and dysuria are characteristics of symptomatic HSV urethritis. HSV has been isolated from the urethra of 5% of women with the dysuria-frequency syndrome. Occasionally, HSV genital tract disease is manifested by endometritis and salpingitis in women and by prostatitis in men. About 15% of cases of HSV-2 acquisition are associated with nonlesional clinical syndromes, such as aseptic meningitis, cervicitis, or urethritis. A more complete discussion of the differential diagnosis of genital herpes is presented in Chap. 163.

Both HSV-1 and HSV-2 can cause symptomatic or asymptomatic rectal and perianal infections. HSV proctitis is usually associated with rectal intercourse. However, subclinical perianal shedding of HSV is detected in women and men who report no rectal intercourse. This phenomenon is due to the establishment of latency in the sacral dermatome from prior genital tract infection, with subsequent reactivation in epithelial cells in the perianal region. Such reactivations are often subclinical. Symptoms of HSV proctitis include anorectal pain, anorectal discharge, tenesmus, and constipation. Sigmoidoscopy reveals ulcerative lesions of the distal 10 cm of the rectal mucosa. Rectal biopsies show mucosal ulceration, necrosis, polymorphonuclear and lymphocytic infiltration of the lamina propria, and (in occasional cases) multinucleated intranuclear inclusion-bearing cells. Perianal herpetic lesions are also found in immunosuppressed patients receiving cytotoxic therapy. Extensive perianal herpetic lesions and/or HSV proctitis is common among patients with HIV infection.

Herpetic Whitlow Herpetic whitlow—HSV infection of the finger—may occur as a complication of primary oral or genital herpes by inoculation of virus through a break in the epidermal surface or by direct introduction of virus into the hand through occupational or some other type of exposure. Clinical signs and symptoms include abrupt-onset edema, erythema, and localized tenderness of the infected finger. Vesicular or pustular lesions of the fingertip that are indistinguishable from lesions of pyogenic bacterial infection are seen. Fever, lymphadenitis, and epitrochlear and axillary lymphadenopathy are common. The infection may recur. Prompt diagnosis (to avoid unnecessary and potentially exacerbating surgical therapy and/or transmission) is essential. Antiviral chemotherapy is usually recommended (see below).

Herpes Gladiatorum HSV may infect almost any area of skin. Mucocutaneous HSV infections of the thorax, ears, face, and hands have been described among wrestlers. Transmission of these infections is facilitated by trauma to the skin sustained during wrestling. Several recent outbreaks have illustrated the importance of prompt diagnosis and therapy to contain the spread of this infection.

Eye Infections HSV infection of the eye is the most common cause of corneal blindness in the United States. HSV keratitis presents as an acute onset of pain, blurred vision, chemosis, conjunctivitis, and characteristic dendritic lesions of the cornea. Use of topical glucocorticoids may exacerbate symptoms and lead to involvement of deep structures of the eye. Debridement, topical antiviral treatment, and/or IFN therapy hastens healing. However, recurrences are common, and the deeper structures of the eye may sustain immunopathologic injury. Stromal keratitis due to HSV appears to be related to T cell–dependent destruction of deep corneal tissue. An HSV-1 epitope that is autoreactive with T cell–targeting corneal antigens has been postulated to be a factor in this infection. Chorioretinitis, usually a manifestation of disseminated HSV infection, may occur in neonates or in patients with HIV infection. HSV and VZV can cause acute necrotizing retinitis as an uncommon but severe manifestation.

Central and Peripheral Nervous System Infections HSV accounts for 10–20% of all cases of sporadic viral encephalitis in the United States. The estimated incidence is ~2.3 cases per 1 million persons per year. Cases are distributed throughout the year, and the age distribution appears to be biphasic, with peaks at 5–30 and >50 years of age. HSV-1 causes >95% of cases.

The pathogenesis of HSV encephalitis varies. In children and young adults, primary HSV infection may result in encephalitis; presumably, exogenously acquired virus enters the CNS by neurotropic spread from the periphery via the olfactory bulb. However, most adults with HSV encephalitis have clinical or serologic evidence of mucocutaneous HSV-1 infection before the onset of CNS symptoms. In ~25% of the cases examined, the HSV-1 strains from the oropharynx and brain tissue of the same patient differ; thus some cases may result from reinfection with another strain of HSV-1 that reaches the CNS. Two theories have been proposed to explain the development of actively replicating HSV in localized areas of the CNS in persons whose ganglionic and CNS isolates are similar. Reactivation of latent HSV-1 infection in trigeminal or autonomic nerve roots may be associated with extension of virus into the CNS via nerves innervating the middle cranial fossa. HSV DNA has been demonstrated by DNA hybridization in brain tissue obtained at autopsy—even from healthy adults. Thus, reactivation of long-standing latent CNS infection may be another mechanism for the development of HSV encephalitis.

Recent studies have identified genetic polymorphisms in two separate genes among families with a high frequency of HSV encephalitis. Peripheral-blood mononuclear cells from these patients (predominantly children) appear to secrete reduced levels of IFN in response to HSV. These observations suggest that some cases of sporadic HSV encephalitis may be related to host genetic determinants.

The clinical hallmark of HSV encephalitis has been the acute onset of fever and focal neurologic symptoms and signs, especially in the temporal lobe (Fig. 216-2). Clinical differentiation of HSV encephalitis from other viral encephalitides, focal infections, or noninfectious processes is difficult. Elevated cerebrospinal fluid (CSF) protein levels, leukocytosis (predominantly lymphocytes), and red blood cell counts due to hemorrhagic necrosis are common. While brain biopsy has been the gold standard for defining HSV encephalitis, a highly sensitive and specific PCR for detection of HSV DNA in CSF has largely replaced biopsy for defining CNS infection. Although titers of antibody to HSV in CSF and serum increase in most cases of HSV encephalitis, they rarely do so earlier than 10 days into the illness and therefore, although useful in retrospect, generally are not helpful in establishing an early clinical diagnosis. In rare cases, demonstration of HSV antigen, HSV DNA, or HSV replication in brain tissue obtained by biopsy is highly sensitive; examination of such tissue also provides the opportunity to identify alternative, potentially treatable causes of encephalitis. Antiviral chemotherapy with acyclovir reduces the rate of death from HSV encephalitis. Most authorities recommend the administration of IV acyclovir to patients with presumed HSV encephalitis until the diagnosis is confirmed or an alternative diagnosis is made. All confirmed cases should be treated with IV acyclovir (30 mg/kg per day in three divided doses for 14–21 days). After the completion of therapy, the clinical recurrence of encephalitis requiring more treatment has been reported. For this reason, some authorities prefer to treat initially for 21 days, and many continue therapy until HSV DNA has been eliminated from the CSF. Even with therapy, neurologic sequelae are common, especially among persons >50 years of age.

HSV DNA has been detected in CSF from 3–15% of persons presenting to the hospital with aseptic meningitis. HSV meningitis, which is usually seen in association with primary genital HSV infection, is an acute, self-limited disease manifested by headache, fever, and mild photophobia and lasting 2–7 days. Lymphocytic pleocytosis in the CSF is characteristic. Neurologic sequelae of HSV meningitis are rare. HSV is the most commonly identified cause of recurrent lymphocytic meningitis (*Mollaret's meningitis*). Demonstration of HSV antibodies in CSF or persistence of HSV DNA in CSF can establish the diagnosis. For persons with frequent recurrences of HSV meningitis, daily antiviral therapy has reduced the occurrence of such episodes.

Autonomic nervous system dysfunction, especially of the sacral region, has been reported in association with both HSV and VZV infections. Numbness, tingling of the buttocks or perineal areas, urinary retention, constipation, CSF pleocytosis, and (in males) impotence may occur. Symptoms appear to resolve slowly over days or weeks. Occasionally, hypoesthesia and/or weakness of the lower extremities persists for many months. Transitory hypoesthesia of the area of skin innervated by the trigeminal nerve and vestibular system dysfunction (as measured by electronystagmography) are the predominant signs of disease. Whether antiviral chemotherapy can abort these signs or reduce their frequency and severity is not yet known. Rarely, transverse myelitis, manifested by a rapidly progressive symmetric paralysis of the lower extremities or Guillain-Barré syndrome, follows HSV infection. Similarly, peripheral nervous system involvement (Bell's palsy) or cranial polyneuritis may be related to reactivation of HSV-1 infection.

Visceral Infections HSV infection of visceral organs usually results from viremia, and multiple-organ involvement is common. Occasionally, however, the clinical manifestations of HSV infection involve only the esophagus, lung, or liver. HSV esophagitis may result from direct extension of oral-pharyngeal HSV infection into the esophagus or may occur de novo by reactivation and spread of HSV to the esophageal mucosa via the vagus nerve. The predominant symptoms of HSV esophagitis are odynophagia, dysphagia, substernal pain, and weight loss. Multiple oval ulcerations appear on an erythematous base with or without a patchy white pseudomembrane. The distal esophagus is most commonly involved. With extensive disease, diffuse friability may spread to the entire esophagus. Neither endoscopic nor barium examination can reliably differentiate HSV esophagitis from *Candida* esophagitis or from esophageal ulcerations due to thermal injury, radiation, or corrosives. Endoscopically obtained secretions for cytologic examination and culture or DNA detection by PCR provide the most useful material for diagnosis. Systemic antiviral chemotherapy usually reduces the severity and duration of symptoms and heals esophageal ulcerations.

HSV pneumonitis is uncommon except in severely immunosuppressed patients and may result from extension of herpetic tracheobronchitis into lung parenchyma. Focal necrotizing pneumonitis usually ensues. Hematogenous dissemination of virus from sites of oral or genital mucocutaneous

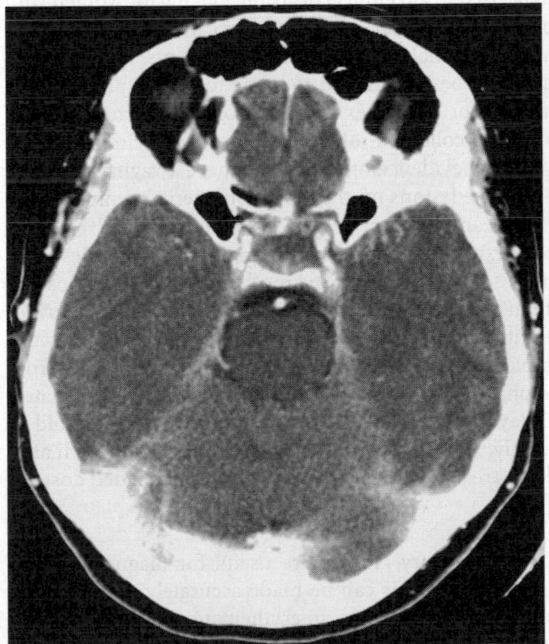

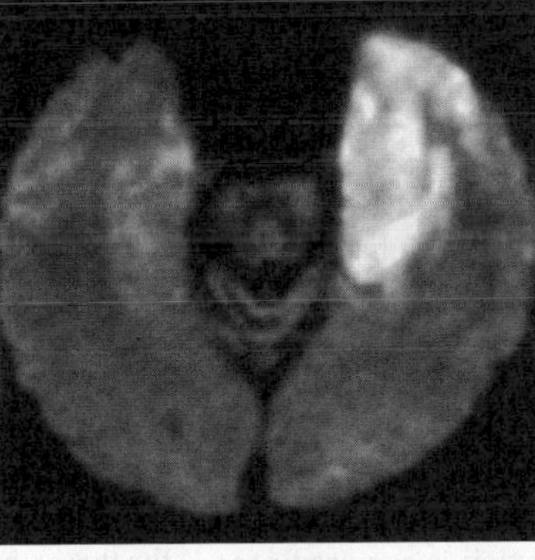

FIGURE 216-2 Computed tomography and diffusion-weighted magnetic resonance imaging scans of the brain of a patient with left-temporal-lobe herpes simplex virus encephalitis.

disease may also occur, producing bilateral interstitial pneumonitis. Bacterial, fungal, and parasitic pathogens are commonly present in HSV pneumonitis. The mortality rate from untreated HSV pneumonia in immunosuppressed patients is high (>80%). HSV has also been isolated from the lower respiratory tract of persons with acute respiratory distress syndrome and prolonged intubation. Most authorities believe that the presence of HSV in tracheal aspirates in such settings is due to reactivation of HSV in the tracheal region and localized tracheitis in persons with long-term intubation. Such patients should be evaluated for extension of HSV infection into the lung parenchyma. Controlled trials assessing the role of antiviral agents used against HSV in morbidity and mortality associated with acute respiratory distress syndrome have not been conducted. The role of lower respiratory tract HSV infection in overall rates of morbidity and mortality associated with these conditions is unclear. HSV is an uncommon cause of hepatitis in immunocompetent patients. HSV infection of the liver is associated with fever, abrupt elevations of bilirubin and serum aminotransferase levels, and leukopenia (<4000 white blood cells/μL). Disseminated intravascular coagulation may also develop.

Other reported complications of HSV infection include monarticular arthritis, adrenal necrosis, idiopathic thrombocytopenia, and glomerulonephritis. Disseminated HSV infection in immunocompetent patients is rare. In immunocompromised patients, burn patients, or malnourished individuals, HSV occasionally disseminates to other visceral organs, such as the adrenal glands, pancreas, small and large intestines, and bone marrow. Rarely, primary HSV infection in pregnancy disseminates and may be associated with the death of both mother and fetus. This uncommon event is usually related to the acquisition of primary infection in the third trimester. Disseminated HSV infection is best detected by the presence of HSV DNA in plasma or blood.

Neonatal HSV Infections Of all HSV-infected populations, neonates (infants younger than 6 weeks) have the highest frequency of visceral and/or CNS infection. Without therapy, the overall rate of death from neonatal herpes is 65%; <10% of neonates with CNS infection develop normally. Although skin lesions are the most commonly recognized features of disease, many infants do not develop lesions at all or do so only well into the course of disease. Neonatal infection is usually acquired perinatally from contact with infected genital secretions at delivery. Congenitally infected infants have been reported. Of neonatal HSV infections, 30–50% are due to HSV-1 and 50–70% to HSV-2. The risk of developing neonatal HSV infection is 10 times higher for an infant born to a mother who has recently acquired HSV than for other infants. Neonatal HSV-1 infections may also be acquired through postnatal contact with immediate family members who have symptomatic or asymptomatic oral-labial HSV-1 infection or through nosocomial transmission within the hospital. All neonates with presumed herpes should be treated with IV acyclovir and then placed on maintenance oral antiviral therapy for the first 6–12 months of life. Antiviral chemotherapy with high-dose IV acyclovir (60 mg/kg per day) has reduced the mortality rate from neonatal herpes to ~15%. However, rates of morbidity, especially among infants with HSV-2 infection involving the CNS, are still very high.

HSV in Pregnancy In the United States, 22% of all pregnant women and 55% of non-Hispanic black pregnant women are seropositive for HSV-2. However, the risk of mother-to-child transmission of HSV in the perinatal period is highest when the infection is acquired near the time of labor—that is, in previously HSV-seronegative women. The clinical manifestations of recurrent genital herpes—including the frequency of subclinical versus clinical infection, duration of lesions, pain, and constitutional symptoms—are similar in pregnant and nonpregnant women. Recurrences increase in frequency over the course of pregnancy. However, when women are seropositive for HSV-2 at the outset of pregnancy, no effect on neonatal outcomes (including birth weight and gestational age) is seen. First-episode infections in pregnancy have more severe consequences for mother and infant. Maternal visceral dissemination during the third trimester occasionally occurs, as does premature birth or intrauterine growth retardation. The acquisition of primary disease in pregnancy, whether related to HSV-1 or HSV-2, carries the risk of transplacental transmission of virus to the neonate and can result in spontaneous abortion, although this outcome is relatively uncommon. For newly acquired genital HSV infection during pregnancy, most authorities recommend treatment with acyclovir (400 mg three times daily) or valacyclovir (500–1000 mg twice daily) for 7–10 days. However, the impact of this intervention on transmission is unknown. The high HSV-2 prevalence rate in pregnancy and the low incidence of neonatal disease (1 case per 6000–20,000 live births) indicate that only a few infants are at risk of acquiring HSV. Therefore, cesarean section is not warranted for all women with recurrent genital disease. Because intrapartum transmission of infection accounts for the majority of cases, abdominal delivery need be considered only for women who are shedding HSV at delivery. Several studies have shown no correlation between recurrence of viral shedding before delivery and viral shedding at term. Hence, weekly virologic monitoring and amniocentesis are not recommended.

The frequency of transmission from mother to infant is markedly higher among women who acquire HSV near term (30–50%) than among those in whom HSV-2 infection is reactivated at delivery (<1%). Although maternal antibody to HSV-2 is protective, antibody to HSV-1 offers little or no protection against neonatal HSV-2 infection. Primary genital infection with HSV-1 leads to a particularly high risk of transmission during pregnancy and accounts for an increasing proportion of neonatal HSV cases. Moreover, during reactivation, HSV-1 appears more transmissible to the neonate than HSV-2. Only 2% of women who are seropositive for HSV-2 have HSV-2 isolated from cervical secretions at delivery, and only 1% of infants exposed in this manner develop infection, presumably because of the protective effects of maternally transferred antibodies and perhaps lower viral titers during reactivation. Despite the low frequency of transmission of HSV in this setting, 30–50% of infants with neonatal HSV are born to mothers with established genital herpes.

Isolation of HSV by cervicovaginal swab at the time of delivery is the greatest risk factor for intrapartum HSV transmission (relative risk = 346); however, culture-negative, PCR-positive cases of intrapartum transmission are well described. New acquisition of HSV (odds ratio [OR] = 49), isolation of HSV-1 versus HSV-2 (OR = 35), cervical versus vulvar HSV detection (OR = 15), use of fetal scalp electrodes (OR = 3.5), and young age confer further risk of transmission, whereas abdominal delivery is protective (OR = 0.14). Physical examination poorly predicts the absence of shedding, and PCR far exceeds culture in terms of sensitivity and speed. Therefore, PCR detection at the onset of labor should be used to aid clinical decision-making for women with HSV-2 antibody. Because cesarean section appears to be an effective means of reducing maternal-fetal transmission, patients with recurrent genital herpes should be encouraged to come to the hospital early at the time of delivery for careful examination of the external genitalia and cervix as well as collection of a swab sample for viral isolation. Women who have no evidence of lesions can have a vaginal delivery. The presence of active lesions on the cervix or external genitalia is an indication for cesarean delivery.

If first-episode exposure has occurred (e.g., if HSV serologies show that the mother is seronegative or if the mother is HSV-1-seropositive and the isolate at delivery is found to be HSV-2), many authorities would initiate antiviral therapy for the infant with IV acyclovir. At a minimum, samples for viral cultures and PCR should be obtained from the throat, nasopharynx, eyes, and rectum of these infants immediately and at 5- to 10-day intervals. Lethargy, skin lesions, or fever should be evaluated promptly. All infants from whom HSV is isolated 24 h after delivery should be treated with IV acyclovir at recommended doses.

DIAGNOSIS

Both clinical and laboratory criteria are useful for diagnosing HSV infections. A clinical diagnosis can be made accurately when characteristic multiple vesicular lesions on an erythematous base are present. However, herpetic ulcerations may resemble skin ulcerations of other etiologies. Mucosal HSV infections may also present as urethritis or pharyngitis without cutaneous lesions. Thus, laboratory studies to confirm the diagnosis and to guide therapy are recommended. While staining of scrapings from the base of the lesions with Wright's, Giemsa's (Tzanck preparation), or Papanicolaou's stain to detect giant cells or intranuclear inclusions of *Herpesvirus* infection is a well-described procedure, few clinicians are skilled in this technique, the sensitivity of staining is low (<30% for mucosal swabs), and these cytologic methods do not differentiate between HSV and VZV infections.

HSV infection is best confirmed in the laboratory by detection of virus, viral antigen, or viral DNA in scrapings from lesions. HSV DNA detection by PCR is the most sensitive laboratory technique for detecting mucosal or visceral HSV infections and should be used when available. HSV causes a discernible cytopathic effect in a variety of cell culture systems, and this effect can be identified within 48–96 h after inoculation. Spin-amplified culture with subsequent staining for HSV antigen has shortened the time needed to identify HSV to <24 h. The sensitivity of all detection methods depends on the stage of the lesions (with higher sensitivity for vesicular than for ulcerative lesions), on whether the patient has a first or a recurrent episode of the disease (with higher sensitivity in first than in recurrent episodes), and on whether the sample is from an immunosuppressed or an immunocompetent patient (with more antigen or DNA in immunosuppressed patients). Laboratory confirmation permits subtyping of the virus; information on subtype may be useful epidemiologically and may help to predict the frequency of reactivation after first-episode oral-labial or genital HSV infection.

Serologic assays with whole-virus antigen preparations, such as complement fixation, neutralization, indirect immunofluorescence, passive hemagglutination, radioimmunoassay, and enzyme-linked immunosorbent assay, are useful for differentiating uninfected (seronegative) persons from those with past HSV-1 or HSV-2 infection, but they do not reliably distinguish between the two viral subtypes. Serologic assays that identify antibodies to type-specific surface proteins (epitopes) of the two viral subtypes have been developed and can distinguish reliably between the human antibody responses to HSV-1 and HSV-2. The most commonly used assays are those that measure antibodies to glycoprotein G of HSV-1 (gG1) and HSV-2 (gG2). A western blot assay that can detect several HSV type-specific proteins can also be used.

Acute- and convalescent-phase serum samples can be useful in demonstrating seroconversion during primary HSV-1 or HSV-2 infection. However, few available tests report titers, and increases in index values do not reflect first episodes in all patients. Serologic assays based on type-specific proteins should be used to identify asymptomatic carriers of HSV-1 or HSV-2. No reliable IgM method for defining acute HSV infection is available.

Several studies have shown that persons with previously unrecognized HSV-2 infection can be taught to identify symptomatic reactivations. Individuals seropositive for HSV-2 should be told about the high frequency of subclinical reactivation on mucosal surfaces that are not visible to the eye (e.g., cervix, urethra, perianal skin) or in microscopic ulcerations that may not be clinically symptomatic. Transmission of infection during such episodes is well established. HSV-2-seropositive persons should be educated about the high likelihood of subclinical shedding and the role condoms (male or female) may play in reducing transmission. Antiviral therapy with valacyclovir (500 mg once daily) has been shown to reduce the transmission of HSV-2 between sexual partners.

TREATMENT HERPES SIMPLEX VIRUS INFECTIONS

Many aspects of mucocutaneous and visceral HSV infections are amenable to antiviral chemotherapy. For mucocutaneous infections, acyclovir and its congeners famciclovir and valacyclovir have been the mainstays of therapy. Several antiviral agents are available for topical use in HSV eye infections: idoxuridine, trifluorothymidine, topical vidarabine, and cidofovir. For HSV encephalitis and neonatal herpes, IV acyclovir is the treatment of choice.

All licensed antiviral agents for use against HSV inhibit the viral DNA polymerase. One class of drugs, typified by the drug acyclovir, is made up of substrates for the HSV enzyme thymidine kinase (TK). Acyclovir, ganciclovir, famciclovir, and valacyclovir are all selectively phosphorylated to the monophosphate form in virus-infected cells. Cellular enzymes convert the monophosphate form of the drug to the triphosphate, which is then incorporated into the viral DNA chain. Acyclovir is the agent most frequently used for the treatment of HSV infections and is available in IV, oral, and topical formulations. Valacyclovir, the valyl ester of acyclovir, offers greater bioavailability than acyclovir and thus can be administered less frequently. Famciclovir, the oral formulation of penciclovir, is clinically effective in the treatment of a variety of HSV-1 and HSV-2 infections. Ganciclovir is active against both HSV-1 and HSV-2; however, it is more toxic than acyclovir, valacyclovir, and famciclovir and generally is not recommended for the treatment of HSV infections. Anecdotal case reports suggest that ganciclovir may also be less effective than acyclovir for treatment of HSV infections. All three recommended compounds—acyclovir, valacyclovir, and famciclovir—have proved effective in shortening the duration of symptoms and lesions of mucocutaneous HSV infections in both immunocompromised and immunocompetent patients (Table 216-1). IV and oral formulations prevent reactivation of HSV in seropositive immunocompromised patients during induction chemotherapy or in the period immediately after bone marrow or solid organ transplantation. Chronic daily suppressive therapy reduces the frequency of reactivation disease among patients with frequent genital or oral-labial herpes. Only valacyclovir has been subjected to clinical trials that demonstrated reduced transmission of HSV-2 infection between sexual partners. IV acyclovir (30 mg/kg per day, given as a 10-mg/kg infusion over 1 h at 8-h intervals) is effective in reducing rates of death and morbidity from HSV encephalitis. Early initiation of therapy is a critical factor in outcome. The major side effect associated with IV acyclovir is transient renal insufficiency, usually due to crystallization of the compound in the renal parenchyma. This adverse reaction can be avoided if the medication is given slowly over 1 h and the patient is well hydrated. Because CSF levels of acyclovir average only 30–50% of plasma levels, the dosage of acyclovir used for treatment of CNS infection (30 mg/kg per day) is double that used for treatment of mucocutaneous or visceral disease (15 mg/kg per day). Even higher doses of IV acyclovir are used for neonatal HSV infection (60 mg/kg per day in three divided doses).

Increasingly, shorter courses of therapy are being used for recurrent mucocutaneous infection with HSV-1 or HSV-2 in immunocompetent patients. One-day courses of famciclovir and valacyclovir are clinically effective, more convenient, and generally less costly than longer courses of therapy (Table 216-1). These short-course regimens should be reserved for immunocompetent hosts.

SUPPRESSION OF MUCOCUTANEOUS HERPES

Recognition of the high frequency of subclinical reactivation provides a well-accepted rationale for the use of daily antiviral therapy to suppress reactivations of HSV, especially in persons with frequent clinical reactivations (e.g., those with recently acquired genital HSV infection). Immunosuppressed persons, including those with HIV infection, may also benefit from daily antiviral therapy. Recent studies have shown the efficacy of daily acyclovir and valacyclovir in reducing the frequency of HSV reactivations among HIV-positive persons. Regimens used include acyclovir (400–800 mg twice daily), famciclovir (500 mg twice daily), and valacyclovir (500 mg twice daily); valacyclovir at a dose of 4 g/d was associated with thrombotic thrombocytopenic purpura in one study of HIV-infected persons. In addition, daily treatment of HSV-2 reduces the titer of HIV RNA in plasma (0.5-log reduction) and in genital mucosa (0.33-log reduction).

REDUCED HSV TRANSMISSION TO SEXUAL PARTNERS

Once-daily valacyclovir (500 mg) has been shown to reduce transmission of HSV-2 between sexual partners. Transmission rates are higher from males to females and among persons with frequent HSV-2 reactivation. Serologic screening can be used to identify at-risk couples. Daily valacyclovir appears to be more effective at reducing subclinical shedding than daily famciclovir.

TABLE 216-1 ANTIVIRAL CHEMOTHERAPY FOR HERPES SIMPLEX VIRUS (HSV) INFECTION

I. Mucocutaneous HSV infections

A. *Infections in immunosuppressed patients*

1. *Acute symptomatic first or recurrent episodes:* IV acyclovir (5 mg/kg q8h) or oral acyclovir (400 mg qid), famciclovir (500 mg bid or tid), or valacyclovir (500 mg bid) is effective. Treatment duration may vary from 7 to 14 days.
2. *Suppression of reactivation disease (genital or oral-labial):* IV acyclovir (5 mg/kg q8h) or oral valacyclovir (500 mg bid) or acyclovir (400–800 mg 3–5 times per day) prevents recurrences during the 30-day period immediately after transplantation. Longer-term HSV suppression is often used for persons with continued immunosuppression. In bone marrow and renal transplant recipients, oral valacyclovir (2 g/d) is also effective in reducing cytomegalovirus infection. Oral valacyclovir at a dose of 4 g/d has been associated with thrombotic thrombocytopenic purpura after extended use in HIV-positive persons. In HIV-infected persons, oral acyclovir (400–800 mg bid), valacyclovir (500 mg bid), or famciclovir (500 mg bid) is effective in reducing clinical and subclinical reactivations of HSV-1 and HSV-2.

B. *Infections in immunocompetent patients*

1. *Genital herpes*
   a. *First episodes:* Oral acyclovir (200 mg 5 times per day or 400 mg tid), valacyclovir (1 g bid), or famciclovir (250 mg bid) for 7–14 days is effective. IV acyclovir (5 mg/kg q8h for 5 days) is given for severe disease or neurologic complications such as aseptic meningitis.
   b. *Symptomatic recurrent genital herpes:* Short-course (1- to 3-day) regimens are preferred because of low cost, likelihood of adherence, and convenience. Oral acyclovir (800 mg tid for 2 days), valacyclovir (500 mg bid for 3 days), or famciclovir (750 or 1000 mg bid for 1 day, a 1500-mg single dose, or 500 mg stat followed by 250 mg q12h for 3 days) effectively shortens lesion duration. Other options include oral acyclovir (200 mg 5 times per day), valacyclovir (500 mg bid), and famciclovir (125 mg bid for 5 days).
   c. *Suppression of recurrent genital herpes:* Oral acyclovir (400–800 mg bid) or valacyclovir (500 mg daily) is given. Patients with >9 episodes per year should take oral valacyclovir (1 g daily or 500 mg bid) or famciclovir (250 mg bid or 500 mg bid).
2. *Oral-labial HSV infections*
   a. *First episode:* Oral acyclovir is given (200 mg 5 times per day or 400 mg tid); an oral acyclovir suspension can be used (600 mg/m² qid). Oral famciclovir (250 mg bid) or valacyclovir (1 g bid) has been used clinically. The duration of therapy is 5–10 days.
   b. *Recurrent episodes:* If initiated at the onset of the prodrome, single-dose or 1-day therapy effectively reduces pain and speeds healing. Regimens include oral famciclovir (a 1500-mg single dose or 750 mg bid for 1 day) or valacyclovir (a 2-g single dose or 2 g bid for 1 day). Self-initiated therapy with 6-times-daily topical penciclovir cream effectively speeds healing of oral-labial HSV. Topical acyclovir cream has also been shown to speed healing.
   c. *Suppression of reactivation of oral-labial HSV:* If started before exposure and continued for the duration of exposure (usually 5–10 days), oral acyclovir (400 mg bid) prevents reactivation of recurrent oral-labial HSV infection associated with severe sun exposure.
3. *Surgical prophylaxis of oral or genital HSV infection:* Several surgical procedures, such as laser skin resurfacing, trigeminal nerve-root decompression, and lumbar disk surgery, have been associated with HSV reactivation. IV acyclovir (3–5 mg/kg q8h) or oral acyclovir (800 mg bid), valacyclovir (500 mg bid), or famciclovir (250 mg bid) effectively reduces reactivation. Therapy should be initiated 48 h before surgery and continued for 3–7 days.
4. *Herpetic whitlow:* Oral acyclovir (200 mg) is given 5 times daily (alternative: 400 mg tid) for 7–10 days.
5. *HSV proctitis:* Oral acyclovir (400 mg 5 times per day) is useful in shortening the course of infection. In immunosuppressed patients or in patients with severe infection, IV acyclovir (5 mg/kg q8h) may be useful.
6. *Herpetic eye infections:* In acute keratitis, topical trifluorothymidine, vidarabine, idoxuridine, acyclovir, penciclovir, and interferon are all beneficial. Debridement may be required. Topical steroids may worsen disease.

II. Central nervous system HSV infections

A. *HSV encephalitis:* IV acyclovir (10 mg/kg q8h; 30 mg/kg per day) is given for 10 days or until HSV DNA is no longer detected in cerebrospinal fluid.

B. *HSV aseptic meningitis:* No studies of systemic antiviral chemotherapy exist. If therapy is to be given, IV acyclovir (15–30 mg/kg per day) should be used.

C. *Autonomic radiculopathy:* No studies are available. Most authorities recommend a trial of IV acyclovir.

III. Neonatal HSV infections: Oral acyclovir (60 mg/kg per day, divided into 3 doses) is given. The recommended duration of IV treatment is 21 days. Monitoring for relapse should be undertaken. Continued suppression with oral acyclovir suspension should be given for 3–4 months.

IV. Visceral HSV infections

A. *HSV esophagitis:* IV acyclovir (15 mg/kg per day) is given. In some patients with milder forms of immunosuppression, oral therapy with valacyclovir or famciclovir is effective.

B. *HSV pneumonitis:* No controlled studies exist. IV acyclovir (15 mg/kg per day) should be considered.

V. Disseminated HSV infections: No controlled studies exist. IV acyclovir (5 mg/kg q8h) should be tried. Adjustments for renal insufficiency may be needed. No definite evidence indicates that therapy will decrease the risk of death.

VI. Erythema multiforme associated with HSV: Anecdotal observations suggest that oral acyclovir (400 mg bid or tid) or valacyclovir (500 mg bid) will suppress erythema multiforme.

VII. Infections due to acyclovir-resistant HSV: IV foscarnet (40 mg/kg IV q8h) should be given until lesions heal. The optimal duration of therapy and the usefulness of its continuation to suppress lesions are unclear. Some patients may benefit from cutaneous application of trifluorothymidine or 5% cidofovir gel.

ACYCLOVIR RESISTANCE

Acyclovir-resistant strains of HSV have been identified. Most of these strains have an altered substrate specificity for phosphorylating acyclovir. Thus, cross-resistance to famciclovir and valacyclovir is usually found. Occasionally, an isolate with altered TK specificity arises and is sensitive to famciclovir but not to acyclovir. In some patients infected with TK-deficient virus, higher doses of acyclovir are associated with clearing of lesions. In others, clinical disease progresses despite high-dose therapy. Almost all clinically significant acyclovir resistance has been seen in immunocompromised patients, and HSV-2 isolates are more often resistant than HSV-1 strains. A study by the Centers for Disease Control and Prevention indicated that ~5% of HSV-2 isolates from HIV-positive persons exhibit some degree of in vitro resistance to acyclovir. Of HSV-2 isolates from immunocompetent patients attending sexually transmitted disease clinics, <0.5% show reduced in vitro sensitivity to acyclovir. The lack of appreciable change in the frequency of detection of such isolates in the past 20 years probably reflects the reduced transmission of TK-deficient mutants. Isolation of HSV from lesions persisting despite adequate dosages and blood levels of acyclovir should raise the suspicion of acyclovir resistance. Therapy with the antiviral drug foscarnet is useful in acyclovir-resistant cases (Chap. 215e). Because of its toxicity and cost, this drug is usually reserved for patients with extensive mucocutaneous infections. Cidofovir is a nucleotide analogue and exists as a phosphonate or monophosphate form. Most TK-deficient strains of HSV are sensitive to cidofovir. Cidofovir ointment speeds healing of acyclovir-resistant lesions. No well-controlled trials of systemic cidofovir have been reported. True TK-negative variants of HSV appear to have a reduced capacity to spread because of altered neurovirulence—a feature important in the relatively infrequent presence of such strains in immunocompetent populations, even with increasing use of antiviral drugs.

ACYCLOVIR EFFICACY IN THE DEVELOPING WORLD

Early studies of acyclovir-like drugs were performed solely in the developed world. Recent studies have shown that, although acyclovir-like drugs are effective in the developing world, their clinical and virologic benefits seem reduced from those in European and U.S. populations. The mechanism of this phenomenon is uncertain. Acyclovir therapy does not reduce the rate of HIV acquisition; however, HIV load among MSM in the United States decreased by 1.3 $\log_{10}$ in contrast to 0.9 $\log_{10}$ among Peruvian MSM and 0.5 $\log_{10}$ among African women.

PREVENTION

The success of efforts to control HSV disease on a population basis through suppressive antiviral chemotherapy and/or educational programs will be limited. Barrier forms of contraception (especially condoms) decrease the likelihood of transmission of HSV infection, particularly during periods of asymptomatic viral excretion. When lesions are present, HSV infection may be transmitted by skin-to-skin contact despite the use of a condom. Nevertheless, the available data suggest that consistent condom use is an effective means of reducing the risk of genital HSV-2 transmission. Chronic daily antiviral therapy with valacyclovir can also be partially effective in reducing acquisition of HSV-2, especially among susceptible women. There are no comparative efficacy studies of valacyclovir versus condom use. Most authorities suggest both approaches. The need for a vaccine to prevent acquisition of HSV infection is great, especially in light of the role HSV-2 plays in enhancing the acquisition and transmission of HIV-1.

A substantial portion of neonatal HSV cases could be prevented by reducing the acquisition of HSV by women in the third trimester of pregnancy. Neonatal HSV infection can result from either the acquisition of maternal infection near term or the reactivation of infection at delivery in the already-infected mother. Thus strategies for reducing neonatal HSV are complex. Some authorities have recommended that antiviral therapy with acyclovir or valacyclovir be given to HSV-2-infected women in late pregnancy as a means of reducing reactivation of HSV-2 at term. Data are not available to support the efficacy of this approach. Moreover, the high treatment-to-prevention ratio makes this a dubious public health approach, even though it can reduce the frequency of HSV-associated cesarean delivery.

217 Varicella-Zoster Virus Infections

Richard J. Whitley

DEFINITION

Varicella-zoster virus (VZV) causes two distinct clinical entities: varicella (chickenpox) and herpes zoster (shingles). Chickenpox, a ubiquitous and extremely contagious infection, is usually a benign illness of childhood characterized by an exanthematous vesicular rash. With reactivation of latent VZV (which is most common after the sixth decade of life), herpes zoster presents as a dermatomal vesicular rash, usually associated with severe pain.

ETIOLOGY

Early in the twentieth century, similarities in the histopathologic features of skin lesions resulting from varicella and herpes zoster were demonstrated. Viral isolates from patients with chickenpox and herpes zoster produced similar alterations in tissue culture—specifically, the appearance of eosinophilic intranuclear inclusions and multinucleated giant cells. These results suggested that the viruses were biologically similar. Restriction endonuclease analyses of viral DNA from a patient with chickenpox who subsequently developed herpes zoster verified the molecular identity of the two viruses responsible for these different clinical presentations.

VZV is a member of the family Herpesviridae, sharing with other members such structural characteristics as a lipid envelope surrounding a nucleocapsid with icosahedral symmetry, a total diameter of ~180–200 nm, and centrally located double-stranded DNA that is ~125,000 bp in length.

PATHOGENESIS AND PATHOLOGY

Primary Infection Transmission occurs readily by the respiratory route; the subsequent localized replication of the virus at an undefined site (presumably the nasopharynx) leads to seeding of the lymphatic/reticuloendothelial system and ultimately to the development of viremia. Viremia in patients with chickenpox is reflected in the diffuse and scattered nature of the skin lesions and can be confirmed in selected cases by the recovery of VZV from the blood or routinely by the detection of viral DNA in either blood or lesions by polymerase chain reaction (PCR). Vesicles involve the corium and dermis, with degenerative changes characterized by ballooning, the presence of multinucleated giant cells, and eosinophilic intranuclear inclusions. Infection may involve localized blood vessels of the skin, resulting in necrosis and epidermal hemorrhage. With the evolution of disease, the vesicular fluid becomes cloudy because of the recruitment of polymorphonuclear leukocytes and the presence of degenerated cells and fibrin. Ultimately, the vesicles either rupture and release their fluid (which includes infectious virus) or are gradually reabsorbed.

Recurrent Infection The mechanism of reactivation of VZV that results in herpes zoster is unknown. Presumably, the virus infects dorsal root ganglia during chickenpox, where it remains latent until reactivated. Histopathologic examination of representative dorsal root ganglia during active herpes zoster demonstrates hemorrhage, edema, and lymphocytic infiltration.

Active replication of VZV in other organs, such as the lung or the brain, can occur during either chickenpox or herpes zoster but is uncommon in the immunocompetent host. Pulmonary involvement is characterized by interstitial pneumonitis, multinucleated giant cell formation, intranuclear inclusions, and pulmonary hemorrhage. Central nervous system (CNS) infection leads to histopathologic evidence of perivascular cuffing similar to that encountered in measles and other viral encephalitides. Focal hemorrhagic necrosis of the brain, characteristic of herpes simplex virus (HSV) encephalitis, develops infrequently in VZV infection.

EPIDEMIOLOGY AND CLINICAL MANIFESTATIONS

Chickenpox Humans are the only known reservoir for VZV. Chickenpox is highly contagious, with an attack rate of at least 90% among susceptible (seronegative) individuals. Persons of both sexes and all races are infected equally. The virus is endemic in the population at large; however, it becomes epidemic among susceptible individuals during seasonal peaks—namely, late winter and early spring in the temperate zone. Much of our knowledge of the disease's natural history and incidence predates the licensure of the chickenpox vaccine in 1995. Historically, children 5–9 years old are most commonly affected and account for 50% of all cases. Most other cases involve children 1–4 and 10–14 years old. Approximately 10% of the population of the United States over the age of 15 is susceptible to infection. VZV vaccination during the second year of life has dramatically changed the epidemiology of infection, causing a significant decrease in the annualized incidence of chickenpox.

The incubation period of chickenpox ranges from 10 to 21 days but is usually 14–17 days. Secondary attack rates in susceptible siblings

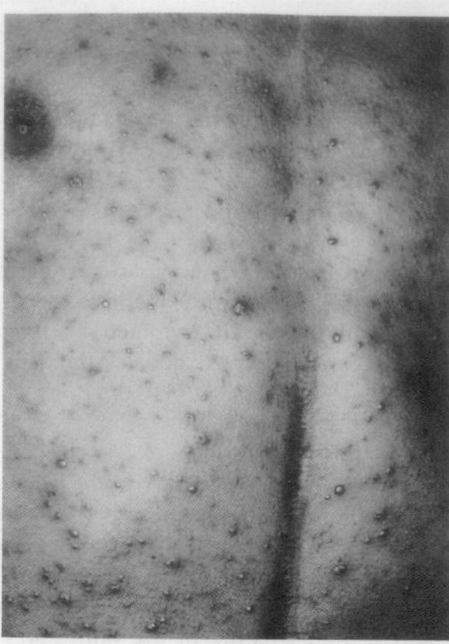

FIGURE 217-1 Varicella lesions at various stages of evolution: vesicles on an erythematous base, umbilical vesicles, and crusts.

within a household are 70–90%. Patients are infectious ~48 h before onset of the vesicular rash, during the period of vesicle formation (which generally lasts 4–5 days), and until all vesicles are crusted.

Clinically, chickenpox presents as a rash, low-grade fever, and malaise, although a few patients develop a prodrome 1–2 days before onset of the exanthem. In the immunocompetent patient, chickenpox is usually a benign illness associated with lassitude and with body temperatures of 37.8°–39.4°C (100°–103°F) of 3–5 days' duration. The skin lesions—the hallmark of the infection—include maculopapules, vesicles, and scabs in various stages of evolution (Fig. 217-1). These lesions, which evolve from maculopapules to vesicles over hours to days, appear on the trunk and face and rapidly spread to involve other areas of the body. Most are small and have an erythematous base with a diameter of 5–10 mm. Successive crops appear over a 2- to 4-day period. Lesions can also be found on the mucosa of the pharynx and/or the vagina. Their severity varies from one person to another. Some individuals have very few lesions, while others have as many as 2000. Younger children tend to have fewer vesicles than older individuals. Secondary and tertiary cases within families are associated with a relatively large number of vesicles. Immunocompromised patients—both children and adults, particularly those with leukemia—have lesions (often with a hemorrhagic base) that are more numerous and take longer to heal than those of immunocompetent patients. Immunocompromised individuals are also at greater risk for visceral complications, which occur in 30–50% of cases and are fatal 15% of the time in the absence of antiviral therapy.

The most common infectious complication of varicella is secondary bacterial superinfection of the skin, which is usually caused by *Streptococcus pyogenes* or *Staphylococcus aureus,* including strains that are methicillin-resistant. Skin infection results from excoriation of lesions after scratching. Gram's staining of skin lesions should help clarify the etiology of unusually erythematous and pustulated lesions.

The most common extracutaneous site of involvement in children is the CNS. The syndrome of acute cerebellar ataxia and meningeal inflammation generally appears ~21 days after onset of the rash and rarely develops in the pre-eruptive phase. The cerebrospinal fluid (CSF) contains lymphocytes and elevated levels of protein. CNS involvement is a benign complication of VZV infection in children and generally does not require hospitalization. Aseptic meningitis, encephalitis, transverse myelitis, and Guillain-Barré syndrome can also occur. Reye's syndrome has been reported in children concomitantly treated with aspirin. Encephalitis is reported in 0.1–0.2% of children with chickenpox. Other than supportive care, no specific therapy (e.g., acyclovir administration) has proved efficacious for patients with CNS involvement.

Varicella pneumonia, the most serious complication following chickenpox, develops more often in adults (up to 20% of cases) than in children and is particularly severe in pregnant women. Pneumonia due to VZV usually has its onset 3–5 days into the illness and is associated with tachypnea, cough, dyspnea, and fever. Cyanosis, pleuritic chest pain, and hemoptysis are frequently noted. Roentgenographic evidence of disease consists of nodular infiltrates and interstitial pneumonitis. Resolution of pneumonitis parallels improvement of the skin rash; however, patients may have persistent fever and compromised pulmonary function for weeks.

Other complications of chickenpox include myocarditis, corneal lesions, nephritis, arthritis, bleeding diatheses, acute glomerulonephritis, and hepatitis. Hepatic involvement, distinct from Reye's syndrome and usually asymptomatic, is common in chickenpox and is generally characterized by elevated levels of liver enzymes, particularly aspartate and alanine aminotransferases.

Perinatal varicella is associated with mortality rates as high as 30% when maternal disease develops within 5 days before delivery or within 48 h thereafter. Illness in this setting is unusually severe because the newborn does not receive protective transplacental antibodies and has an immature immune system. *Congenital varicella,* with clinical manifestations of limb hypoplasia, cicatricial skin lesions, and microcephaly at birth, is extremely uncommon.

Herpes Zoster Herpes zoster (shingles) is a sporadic disease that results from reactivation of latent VZV from dorsal root ganglia. Most patients with shingles have no history of recent exposure to other individuals with VZV infection. Herpes zoster occurs at all ages, but its incidence is highest (5–10 cases per 1000 persons) among individuals in the sixth decade of life and beyond. Data suggest that 1.2 million cases occur annually in the United States. Recurrent herpes zoster is exceedingly rare except in immunocompromised hosts, especially those with AIDS.

Herpes zoster is characterized by a unilateral vesicular dermatomal eruption, often associated with severe pain. The dermatomes from T3 to L3 are most frequently involved. If the ophthalmic branch of the trigeminal nerve is involved, *zoster ophthalmicus* results. The factors responsible for the reactivation of VZV are not known. In children, reactivation is usually benign; in adults, it can be debilitating because of pain. The onset of disease is heralded by pain within the dermatome, which may precede lesions by 48–72 h; an erythematous maculopapular rash evolves rapidly into vesicular lesions (Fig. 217-2). In the normal host, these lesions may remain few in number and continue to form for

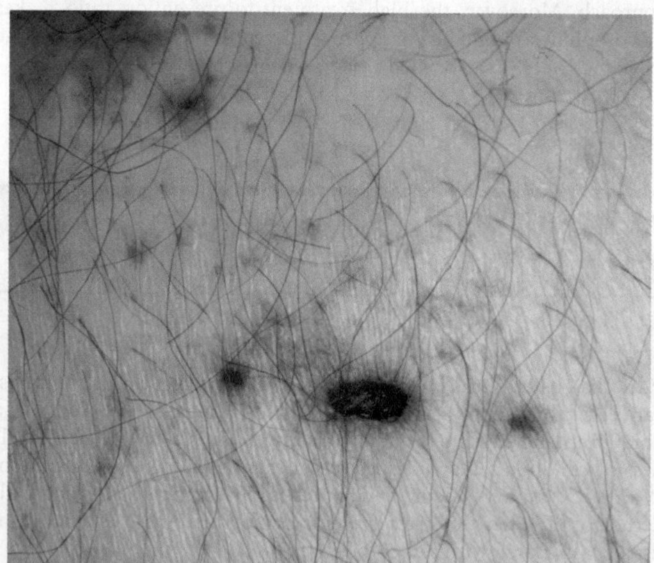

FIGURE 217-2 Close-up of lesions of disseminated zoster. Note lesions at different stages of evolution, including pustules and crusting. *(Photo courtesy of Lindsey Baden; with permission.)*

only 3–5 days. The total duration of disease is generally 7–10 days; however, it may take as long as 2–4 weeks for the skin to return to normal. Patients with herpes zoster can transmit infection to seronegative individuals, with consequent chickenpox. In a few patients, characteristic localization of pain to a dermatome with serologic evidence of herpes zoster has been reported in the absence of skin lesions, an entity known as *zoster sine herpetica*. When branches of the trigeminal nerve are involved, lesions may appear on the face, in the mouth, in the eye, or on the tongue. *Zoster ophthalmicus* is usually a debilitating condition that can result in blindness in the absence of antiviral therapy. In *Ramsay Hunt syndrome*, pain and vesicles appear in the external auditory canal, and patients lose their sense of taste in the anterior two-thirds of the tongue while developing ipsilateral facial palsy. The geniculate ganglion of the sensory branch of the facial nerve is involved.

In both normal and immunocompromised hosts, the most debilitating complication of herpes zoster is pain associated with acute neuritis and postherpetic neuralgia. Postherpetic neuralgia is uncommon in young individuals; however, at least 50% of zoster patients over age 50 report some degree of pain in the involved dermatome for months after the resolution of cutaneous disease. Changes in sensation in the dermatome, resulting in either hypo- or hyperesthesia, are common.

CNS involvement may follow localized herpes zoster. Many patients without signs of meningeal irritation have CSF pleocytosis and moderately elevated levels of CSF protein. Symptomatic meningoencephalitis is characterized by headache, fever, photophobia, meningitis, and vomiting. A rare manifestation of CNS involvement is granulomatous angiitis with contralateral hemiplegia, which can be diagnosed by cerebral arteriography. Other neurologic manifestations include transverse myelitis with or without motor paralysis.

Like chickenpox, herpes zoster is more severe in immunocompromised than immunocompetent individuals. Lesions continue to form for >1 week, and scabbing is not complete in most cases until 3 weeks into the illness. Patients with Hodgkin's disease and non-Hodgkin's lymphoma are at greatest risk for progressive herpes zoster. Cutaneous dissemination (Fig. 217-3) develops in ~40% of these patients. Among patients with cutaneous dissemination, the risk of pneumonitis, meningoencephalitis, hepatitis, and other serious complications is increased by 5–10%. However, even in immunocompromised patients, disseminated zoster is rarely fatal.

Recipients of hematopoietic stem cell transplants are at particularly high risk of VZV infection. Of all cases of posttransplantation VZV infection, 30% occur within 1 year (50% of these within 9 months); 45% of the patients involved have cutaneous or visceral dissemination. The mortality rate in this situation is 10%. Postherpetic neuralgia, scarring, and bacterial superinfection are especially common in VZV infections occurring within 9 months of transplantation. Among infected patients, concomitant graft-versus-host disease increases the chance of dissemination and/or death.

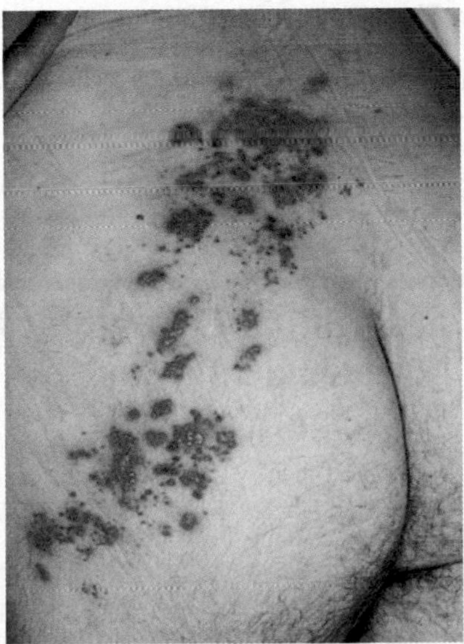

FIGURE 217-3 Herpes zoster in an HIV-infected patient is seen as hemorrhagic vesicles and pustules on an erythematous base grouped in a dermatomal distribution.

DIFFERENTIAL DIAGNOSIS

(See also Chap. 25e) The diagnosis of chickenpox is not difficult. The characteristic rash and a history of recent exposure should lead to a prompt diagnosis. Other viral infections that can mimic chickenpox include disseminated HSV infection in patients with atopic dermatitis and the disseminated vesiculopapular lesions sometimes associated with coxsackievirus infection, echovirus infection, or atypical measles. However, these rashes are more commonly morbilliform with a hemorrhagic component rather than vesicular or vesiculopustular. Rickettsialpox (Chap. 211) is sometimes confused with chickenpox; however, rickettsialpox can be distinguished easily by detection of the "herald spot" at the site of the mite bite and the development of a more pronounced headache. Serologic testing is also useful in differentiating rickettsialpox from varicella and can confirm susceptibility in adults unsure of their chickenpox history. Concern about smallpox has recently increased because of the threat of bioterrorism (Chap. 261e). The lesions of smallpox are larger than those of chickenpox and are all at the same stage of evolution at any given time.

Unilateral vesicular lesions in a dermatomal pattern should lead rapidly to the diagnosis of herpes zoster, although the occurrence of shingles without a rash has been reported. Both HSV and coxsackievirus infections can cause dermatomal vesicular lesions. Supportive diagnostic virology and fluorescent staining of skin scrapings with monoclonal antibodies are helpful in ensuring the proper diagnosis. In the prodromal stage of herpes zoster, the diagnosis can be exceedingly difficult and may be made only after lesions have appeared or by retrospective serologic assessment.

LABORATORY FINDINGS

Unequivocal confirmation of the diagnosis is possible only through the isolation of VZV in susceptible tissue culture cell lines, the demonstration of either seroconversion or a fourfold or greater rise in antibody titer between acute-phase and convalescent-phase serum specimens, or the detection of VZV DNA by PCR. A rapid impression can be obtained by a Tzanck smear, with scraping of the base of the lesions in an attempt to demonstrate multinucleated giant cells; however, the sensitivity of this method is low (~60%). PCR technology for the detection of viral DNA in vesicular fluid is available in a limited number of diagnostic laboratories. Direct immunofluorescent staining of cells from the lesion base or detection of viral antigens by other assays (such as the immunoperoxidase assay) is also useful, although these tests are not commercially available. The most frequently employed serologic tools for assessing host response are the immunofluorescent detection of antibodies to VZV membrane antigens, the fluorescent antibody to membrane antigen (FAMA) test, immune adherence hemagglutination, and enzyme-linked immunosorbent assay (ELISA). The FAMA test and the ELISA appear to be most sensitive.

TREATMENT VARICELLA-ZOSTER VIRUS INFECTIONS

Medical management of chickenpox in the immunologically normal host is directed toward the prevention of avoidable complications. Obviously, good hygiene includes daily bathing and soaks. Secondary bacterial infection of the skin can be avoided by meticulous skin care, particularly with close cropping of fingernails. Pruritus can be decreased with topical dressings or the administration of antipruritic drugs. Tepid water baths and wet compresses are better than drying lotions for the relief of itching. Administration of aspirin to children with chickenpox should be avoided because of the association of aspirin derivatives with the development of Reye's syndrome. Acyclovir (800 mg by mouth five times daily), valacyclovir (1 g three times daily), or famciclovir (250 mg three times daily) for 5–7 days is recommended for adolescents and adults with chickenpox of

≤24 h duration. (Valacyclovir is licensed for use in children and adolescents. Famciclovir is recommended but not licensed for varicella.) Likewise, acyclovir therapy may be of benefit to children <12 years of age if initiated early in the disease (<24 h) at a dose of 20 mg/kg every 6 h. The advantages (i.e., pharmacokinetics) of the second-generation agents valacyclovir and famciclovir are described in **Chap. 215e**.

Aluminum acetate soaks for the management of herpes zoster can be both soothing and cleansing. Patients with herpes zoster benefit from oral antiviral therapy, as evidenced by accelerated healing of lesions and resolution of zoster-associated pain with acyclovir, valacyclovir, or famciclovir. Acyclovir is administered at a dosage of 800 mg five times daily for 7–10 days. However, valacyclovir and famciclovir are superior in terms of pharmacokinetics and pharmacodynamics and should be used preferentially. Famciclovir, the prodrug of penciclovir, is at least as effective as acyclovir and perhaps more so; the dose is 500 mg by mouth three times daily for 7 days. Valacyclovir, the prodrug of acyclovir, accelerates healing and resolution of zoster-associated pain more promptly than acyclovir. The dose is 1 g by mouth three times daily for 5–7 days. Compared with acyclovir, both famciclovir and valacyclovir offer the advantage of less frequent administration. All three of these drugs are now off patent.

In severely immunocompromised hosts (e.g., transplant recipients, patients with lymphoproliferative malignancies), both chickenpox and herpes zoster (including disseminated disease) should be treated, at least at the outset, with IV acyclovir, which reduces the occurrence of visceral complications but has no effect on healing of skin lesions or pain. The dose is 10 mg/kg every 8 h for 7 days. For low-risk immunocompromised hosts, oral therapy with valacyclovir or famciclovir appears beneficial. If medically feasible, it is desirable to decrease immunosuppressive treatment concomitant with the administration of IV acyclovir.

Patients with varicella pneumonia often require ventilatory support. Persons with zoster ophthalmicus should be referred immediately to an ophthalmologist. Therapy for this condition consists of the administration of analgesics for severe pain and the use of atropine. Acyclovir, valacyclovir, and famciclovir all accelerate healing. Decisions about the use of glucocorticoids should be made by the ophthalmologist.

The management of acute neuritis and/or postherpetic neuralgia can be particularly difficult. In addition to the judicious use of analgesics ranging from nonnarcotics to narcotic derivatives, drugs such as gabapentin, pregabalin, amitriptyline hydrochloride, lidocaine (patches), and fluphenazine hydrochloride are reportedly beneficial for pain relief. In one study, glucocorticoid therapy administered early in the course of localized herpes zoster significantly accelerated such quality-of-life improvements as a return to usual activity and termination of analgesic medications. The dose of prednisone administered orally was 60 mg/d on days 1–7, 30 mg/d on days 8–14, and 15 mg/d on days 15–21. This regimen is appropriate only for relatively healthy elderly persons with moderate or severe pain at presentation. Patients with osteoporosis, diabetes mellitus, glycosuria, or hypertension may not be appropriate candidates. Glucocorticoids should not be used without concomitant antiviral therapy.

PREVENTION

Three methods are used for the prevention of VZV infections. First, a live attenuated varicella vaccine (Oka) is recommended for all children >1 year of age (up to 12 years of age) who have not had chickenpox and for adults known to be seronegative for VZV. Two doses are recommended for all children: the first at 12–15 months of age and the second at ~4–6 years of age. VZV-seronegative persons >13 years of age should receive two doses of vaccine at least 1 month apart. The vaccine is both safe and efficacious. Breakthrough cases are mild and may result in spread of the vaccine virus to susceptible contacts. The universal vaccination of children is resulting in a decreased incidence of chickenpox in sentinel communities. Furthermore, inactivation of the vaccine virus significantly decreases the occurrence of herpes zoster after hematopoietic stem-cell transplantation.

TABLE 217-1 RECOMMENDATIONS FOR VZIG ADMINISTRATION

Exposure Criteria
1. Exposure to a person with chickenpox or zoster
a. Household: residence in the same household
b. Playmate: face-to-face indoor play
c. Hospital
Varicella: same 2- to 4-bed room or adjacent beds in large ward, face-to-face contact with infectious staff member or patient, visit by a person deemed contagious
Zoster: intimate contact (e.g., touching or hugging) with a person deemed contagious
d. Newborn infant: onset of varicella in the mother ≤5 days before delivery or ≤48 h after delivery; VZIG not indicated if the mother has zoster
2. Patient should receive VZIG as soon as possible but not >96 h after exposure
Candidates (Provided They Have Significant Exposure) Include:
1. Immunocompromised susceptible children without a history of varicella or varicella immunization
2. Susceptible pregnant women
3. Newborn infants whose mother had onset of chickenpox within 5 days before or within 48 h after delivery
4. Hospitalized premature infant (≥28 weeks of gestation) whose mother lacks a reliable history of chickenpox or serologic evidence of protection against varicella
5. Hospitalized premature infant (<28 weeks of gestation or ≤1000-g birth weight), regardless of maternal history of varicella or VZV serologic status

In individuals >50 years of age, a VZV vaccine with 18 times the viral content of the Oka vaccine decreased the incidence of shingles by 51%, the burden of illness by 61%, and the incidence of postherpetic neuralgia by 66%. The Advisory Committee on Immunization Practices has therefore recommended that persons in this age group be offered this vaccine in order to reduce the frequency of shingles and the severity of postherpetic neuralgia.

A second approach is to administer varicella-zoster immune globulin (VZIG) to individuals who are susceptible, are at high risk for developing complications of varicella, and have had a significant exposure. This product should be given within 96 h (preferably within 72 h) of the exposure. Indications for administration of VZIG appear in **Table 217-1**.

Lastly, antiviral therapy can be given as prophylaxis to individuals at high risk who are ineligible for vaccine or who are beyond the 96-h window after direct contact. While the initial studies have used acyclovir, similar benefit can be anticipated with either valacyclovir or famciclovir. Therapy is instituted 7 days after intense exposure. At this time, the host is midway into the incubation period. This approach significantly decreases disease severity, if not totally preventing disease.

218 Epstein-Barr Virus Infections, Including Infectious Mononucleosis

Jeffrey I. Cohen

DEFINITION

Epstein-Barr virus (EBV) is the cause of heterophile-positive infectious mononucleosis (IM), which is characterized by fever, sore throat, lymphadenopathy, and atypical lymphocytosis. EBV is also associated with several tumors, including nasopharyngeal and gastric carcinoma, Burkitt's lymphoma, Hodgkin's disease, and (in patients with immunodeficiencies) B cell lymphoma. The virus is a member of the family Herpesviridae. The two types of EBV that are widely prevalent in nature are not distinguishable by conventional serologic tests.

EPIDEMIOLOGY

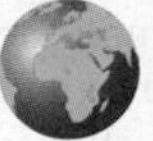

EBV infections occur worldwide. These infections are most common in early childhood, with a second peak during late adolescence. By adulthood, more than 90% of individuals have been infected and have antibodies to the virus. IM is usually a disease of young adults. In lower socioeconomic groups and in areas of the world with deficient standards of hygiene (e.g., developing regions), EBV tends to infect children at an early age, and IM is uncommon. In areas with higher standards of hygiene, infection with EBV is often delayed until adulthood, and IM is more prevalent.

EBV is spread by contact with oral secretions. The virus is frequently transmitted from asymptomatic adults to infants and among young adults by transfer of saliva during kissing. Transmission by less intimate contact is rare. EBV has been transmitted by blood transfusion and by bone marrow transplantation. More than 90% of asymptomatic seropositive individuals shed the virus in oropharyngeal secretions. Shedding is increased in immunocompromised patients and those with IM.

PATHOGENESIS

EBV is transmitted by salivary secretions. The virus infects the epithelium of the oropharynx and the salivary glands and is shed from these cells. While B cells may become infected after contact with epithelial cells, studies suggest that lymphocytes in the tonsillar crypts can be infected directly. The virus then spreads through the bloodstream. The proliferation and expansion of EBV-infected B cells along with reactive T cells during IM result in enlargement of lymphoid tissue. Polyclonal activation of B cells leads to the production of antibodies to host-cell and viral proteins. During the acute phase of IM, up to 1 in every 100 B cells in the peripheral blood is infected by EBV; after recovery, 1–50 in every 1 million B cells is infected. During IM, there is an inverted CD4+/CD8+ T cell ratio. The percentage of CD4+ T cells decreases, while there are large clonal expansions of CD8+ T cells; up to 40% of CD8+ T cells are directed against EBV antigens during acute infection. Memory B cells, not epithelial cells, are the reservoir for EBV in the body. When patients are treated with acyclovir, shedding of EBV from the oropharynx stops but the virus persists in B cells.

The EBV receptor (CD21) on the surface of B cells is also the receptor for the C3d component of complement. EBV infection of epithelial cells results in viral replication and production of virions. When B cells are infected by EBV in vitro, they become transformed and can proliferate indefinitely. During latent infection of B cells, only the EBV nuclear antigens (EBNAs), latent membrane proteins (LMPs), and small EBV RNAs (EBERs) are expressed in vitro. EBV-transformed B cells secrete immunoglobulin; only a small fraction of these cells produce virus.

Cellular immunity is more important than humoral immunity in controlling EBV infection. In the initial phase of infection, suppressor T cells, natural killer cells, and nonspecific cytotoxic T cells are important in controlling the proliferation of EBV-infected B cells. Levels of markers of T cell activation and serum interferon γ are elevated. Later in infection, human leukocyte antigen–restricted cytotoxic T cells that recognize EBNAs and LMPs and destroy EBV-infected cells are generated.

If T cell immunity is compromised, EBV-infected B cells may begin to proliferate. When EBV is associated with lymphoma in immunocompetent persons, virus-induced proliferation is but one step in a multistep process of neoplastic transformation. In many EBV-containing tumors, LMP-1 mimics members of the tumor necrosis factor receptor family (e.g., CD40), transmitting growth-proliferating signals.

CLINICAL MANIFESTATIONS

Signs and Symptoms Most EBV infections in infants and young children either are asymptomatic or present as mild pharyngitis with or without tonsillitis. In contrast, ~75% of infections in adolescents present as IM. IM in the elderly often presents with nonspecific symptoms, including prolonged fever, fatigue, myalgia, and malaise. In contrast, pharyngitis, lymphadenopathy, splenomegaly, and atypical lymphocytes are relatively rare in elderly patients.

TABLE 218-1 SIGNS AND SYMPTOMS OF INFECTIOUS MONONUCLEOSIS

Manifestation	Median Percentage of Patients (Range)
Symptoms	
Sore throat	75 (50–87)
Malaise	47 (42–76)
Headache	38 (22–67)
Abdominal pain, nausea, or vomiting	17 (5–25)
Chills	10 (9–11)
Signs	
Lymphadenopathy	95 (83–100)
Fever	93 (60–100)
Pharyngitis or tonsillitis	82 (68–90)
Splenomegaly	51 (43–64)
Hepatomegaly	11 (6–15)
Rash	10 (0–25)
Periorbital edema	13 (2–34)
Palatal enanthem	7 (3–13)
Jaundice	5 (2–10)

The incubation period for IM in young adults is ~4–6 weeks. A prodrome of fatigue, malaise, and myalgia may last for 1–2 weeks before the onset of fever, sore throat, and lymphadenopathy. Fever is usually low-grade and is most common in the first 2 weeks of the illness; however, it may persist for >1 month. Common signs and symptoms are listed along with their frequencies in Table 218-1. Lymphadenopathy and pharyngitis are most prominent during the first 2 weeks of the illness, while splenomegaly is more prominent during the second and third weeks. Lymphadenopathy most often affects the posterior cervical nodes but may be generalized. Enlarged lymph nodes are frequently tender and symmetric but are not fixed in place. Pharyngitis, often the most prominent sign, can be accompanied by enlargement of the tonsils with an exudate resembling that of streptococcal pharyngitis. A morbilliform or papular rash, usually on the arms or trunk, develops in ~5% of cases (Fig. 218-1). Many patients treated with ampicillin develop a macular rash; this rash is not predictive of future adverse reactions to penicillins. Erythema nodosum and erythema multiforme also have been described (Chap. 72). The severity of the disease correlates with the levels of CD8+ T cells and EBV DNA in the blood. Most patients have symptoms for 2–4 weeks, but nearly 10% have fatigue that persists for ≥6 months.

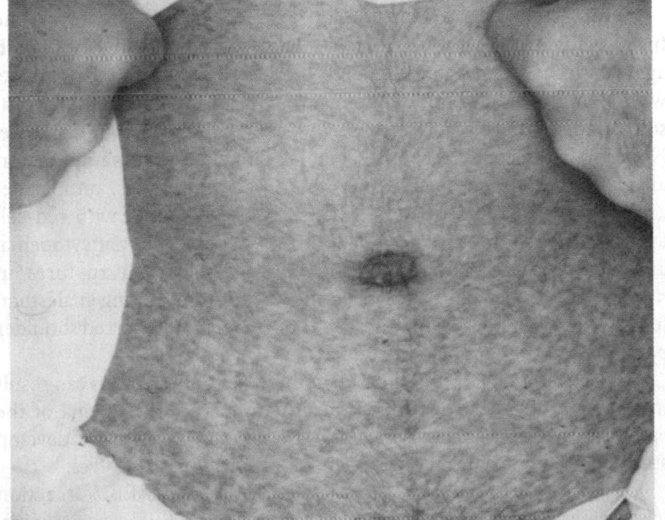

FIGURE 218-1 Rash in a patient with infectious mononucleosis due to Epstein-Barr virus. *(Courtesy of Maria Turner, MD; with permission.)*

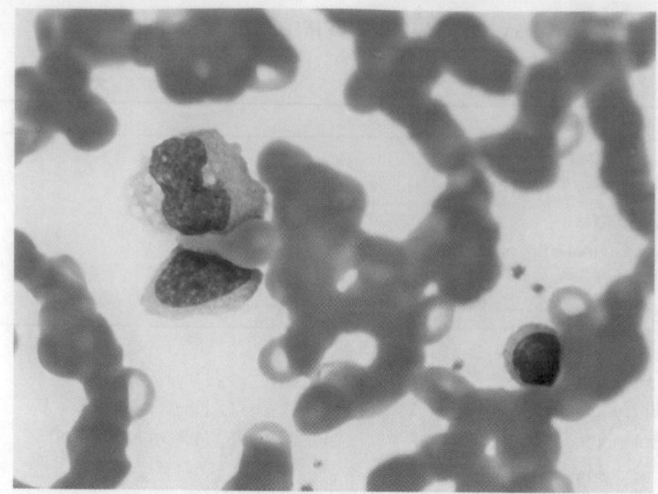

FIGURE 218-2 Atypical lymphocytes from a patient with infectious mononucleosis due to Epstein-Barr virus.

Laboratory Findings The white blood cell count is usually elevated and peaks at 10,000–20,000/μL during the second or third week of illness. Lymphocytosis is usually demonstrable, with >10% atypical lymphocytes. The latter cells are enlarged lymphocytes that have abundant cytoplasm, vacuoles, and indentations of the cell membrane (Fig. 218-2). CD8+ cells predominate among the atypical lymphocytes. Low-grade neutropenia and thrombocytopenia are common during the first month of illness. Liver function is abnormal in >90% of cases. Serum levels of aminotransferases and alkaline phosphatase are usually mildly elevated. The serum concentration of bilirubin is elevated in ~40% of cases.

Complications Most cases of IM are self-limited. Deaths are very rare and are most often due to central nervous system (CNS) complications, splenic rupture, upper airway obstruction, or bacterial superinfection.

When CNS complications develop, they usually do so during the first 2 weeks of EBV infection; in some patients, especially children, they are the only clinical manifestations of IM. Heterophile antibodies and atypical lymphocytes may be absent. Meningitis and encephalitis are the most common neurologic abnormalities, and patients may present with headache, meningismus, or cerebellar ataxia. Acute hemiplegia and psychosis also have been described. The cerebrospinal fluid contains mainly lymphocytes, with occasional atypical lymphocytes. Most cases resolve without neurologic sequelae. Acute EBV infection has also been associated with cranial nerve palsies (especially those involving cranial nerve VII), Guillain-Barré syndrome, acute transverse myelitis, and peripheral neuritis.

Autoimmune hemolytic anemia occurs in ~2% of cases during the first 2 weeks. In most cases, the anemia is Coombs-positive, with cold agglutinins directed against the red blood cell antigen. Most patients with hemolysis have mild anemia that lasts for 1–2 months, but some patients have severe disease with hemoglobinuria and jaundice. Nonspecific antibody responses may also include rheumatoid factor, antinuclear antibodies, anti–smooth muscle antibodies, antiplatelet antibodies, and cryoglobulins. IM has been associated with red-cell aplasia, severe granulocytopenia, thrombocytopenia, pancytopenia, and hemophagocytic lymphohistiocytosis. The spleen ruptures in <0.5% of cases. Splenic rupture is more common among male than female patients and may manifest as abdominal pain, referred shoulder pain, or hemodynamic compromise.

Hypertrophy of lymphoid tissue in the tonsils or adenoids can result in upper airway obstruction, as can inflammation and edema of the epiglottis, pharynx, or uvula. About 10% of patients with IM develop streptococcal pharyngitis after their initial sore throat resolves.

Other rare complications associated with acute EBV infection include hepatitis (which can be fulminant), myocarditis or pericarditis, pneumonia with pleural effusion, interstitial nephritis, genital ulcerations, and vasculitis.

EBV-Associated Diseases Other Than IM EBV-associated lymphoproliferative disease has been described in patients with congenital or acquired immunodeficiency, including those with severe combined immunodeficiency, patients with AIDS, and recipients of bone marrow or organ transplants who are receiving immunosuppressive drugs (especially cyclosporine). Proliferating EBV-infected B cells infiltrate lymph nodes and multiple organs, and patients present with fever and lymphadenopathy or gastrointestinal symptoms. Pathologic studies show B cell hyperplasia or poly- or monoclonal lymphoma.

X-linked lymphoproliferative disease is a recessive disorder of young boys who have a normal response to childhood infections but develop fatal lymphoproliferative disorders after infection with EBV. The protein associated with most cases of this syndrome (SAP) binds to a protein that mediates interactions of B and T cells. Most patients with this syndrome die of acute IM. Others develop hypogammaglobulinemia, malignant B cell lymphomas, aplastic anemia, or agranulocytosis. Disease resembling X-linked lymphoproliferative disease has also been associated with mutations in XIAP. Mutations in ITK, MagT1, or CD27 are associated with inability to control EBV and lymphoma. Moreover, IM has proved fatal to some patients with no obvious preexisting immune abnormality.

Oral hairy leukoplakia (Fig. 218-3) is an early manifestation of infection with HIV in adults (Chap. 226). Most patients present with raised, white corrugated lesions on the tongue (and occasionally on the buccal mucosa) that contain EBV DNA. Children infected with HIV can develop lymphoid interstitial pneumonitis; EBV DNA is often found in lung tissue from these patients.

Patients with chronic fatigue syndrome may have titers of antibody to EBV that are elevated but are not significantly different from those in healthy EBV-seropositive adults. While some patients have malaise and fatigue that persist for weeks or months after IM, persistent EBV infection is not a cause of chronic fatigue syndrome. Chronic active EBV infection is very rare and is distinct from chronic fatigue syndrome. The affected patients have an illness lasting >6 months, with elevated levels of EBV DNA in the blood, high titers of antibody to EBV, and evidence of organ involvement, including hepatosplenomegaly, lymphadenopathy, and pneumonitis, uveitis, or neurologic disease.

EBV is associated with several malignancies. About 15% of cases of Burkitt's lymphoma in the United States and ~90% of those in Africa are associated with EBV (Chap. 134). African patients with Burkitt's lymphoma have high levels of antibody to EBV, and their tumor tissue usually contains viral DNA. Malaria in African patients may impair cellular immunity to EBV and induce polyclonal B cell activation with an expansion of EBV-infected B cells. These changes may enhance the proliferation of B cells with elevated EBV DNA in the bloodstream, thereby increasing the likelihood of a *c-myc* translocation—the hallmark of Burkitt's lymphoma. EBV-containing Burkitt's lymphoma also occurs in patients with AIDS.

Anaplastic nasopharyngeal carcinoma is common in southern China and is uniformly associated with EBV; the affected tissues

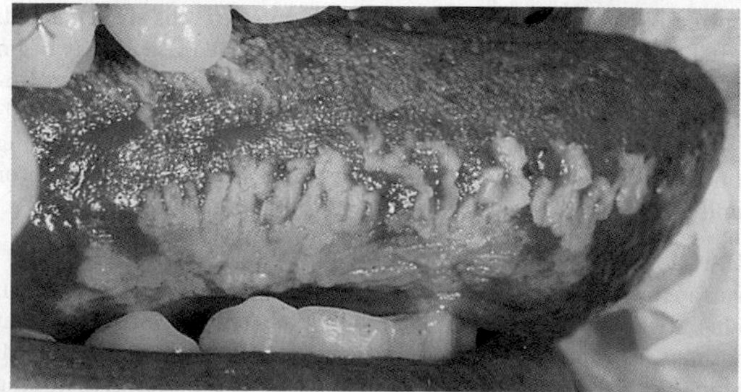

FIGURE 218-3 Oral hairy leukoplakia often presents as white plaques on the lateral surface of the tongue and is associated with Epstein-Barr virus infection.

contain viral DNA and antigens. Patients with nasopharyngeal carcinoma often have elevated titers of antibody to EBV (Chap. 106). High levels of EBV plasma DNA before treatment or detectable levels of EBV DNA after radiation therapy correlate with lower rates of overall survival and relapse-free survival among patients with nasopharyngeal carcinoma.

Worldwide, the most common EBV-associated malignancy is gastric carcinoma. About 9% of these tumors are EBV-positive.

EBV has been associated with Hodgkin's disease, especially the mixed-cellularity type (Chap. 134). Patients with Hodgkin's disease often have elevated titers of antibody to EBV. In about half of cases in the United States, viral DNA and antigens are found in Reed-Sternberg cells. The risk of EBV-positive Hodgkin's disease is significantly increased in young adults for several years after EBV-seropositive IM. About 50% of non-Hodgkin's lymphomas in patients with AIDS are EBV-positive.

EBV is present in B cells of lesions from patients with lymphomatoid granulomatosis. In some cases, EBV DNA has been detected in tumors from immunocompetent patients with angiocentric nasal NK/T cell lymphoma, T cell lymphoma, and CNS lymphoma. Studies have demonstrated viral DNA in leiomyosarcomas from AIDS patients and in smooth-muscle tumors from organ transplant recipients. Virtually all CNS lymphomas in AIDS patients are associated with EBV. Studies have found that a history of IM and higher levels of antibodies to EBV before the onset of disease is more common in persons with multiple sclerosis than in the general population; additional research on a possible causal relationship is needed.

DIAGNOSIS

Serologic Testing (Fig. 218-4) The heterophile test is used for the diagnosis of IM in children and adults. In the test for this antibody, human serum is absorbed with guinea pig kidney, and the heterophile titer is defined as the greatest serum dilution that agglutinates sheep, horse, or cow erythrocytes. The heterophile antibody does not interact with EBV proteins. A titer of ≥40 is diagnostic of acute EBV infection in a patient who has symptoms compatible with IM and atypical lymphocytes. Tests for heterophile antibodies are positive in 40% of patients with IM during the first week of illness and in 80–90% during the third week. Therefore, repeated testing may be necessary, especially if the initial test is performed early. Tests usually remain positive for 3 months after the onset of illness, but heterophile antibodies can persist for up to 1 year. These antibodies usually are not detectable in children <5 years of age, in the elderly, or in patients presenting with symptoms not typical of IM. The commercially available monospot test for heterophile antibodies is somewhat more sensitive than the classic heterophile test. The monospot test is ~75% sensitive and ~90% specific compared with EBV-specific serologies (see below). False-positive monospot results are more common among persons with connective tissue disease, lymphoma, viral hepatitis, and malaria.

EBV-specific antibody testing is used for patients with suspected acute EBV infection who lack heterophile antibodies and for patients with atypical infections. Titers of IgM and IgG antibodies to viral capsid antigen (VCA) are elevated in the serum of more than 90% of patients at the onset of disease. IgM antibody to VCA is most useful for the diagnosis of acute IM because it is present at elevated titers only during the first 2–3 months of the disease; in contrast, IgG antibody to VCA is usually not useful for diagnosis of IM but is often used to assess past exposure to EBV because it persists for life. Seroconversion to EBNA positivity also is useful for the diagnosis of acute infection with EBV. Antibodies to EBNA become detectable relatively late (3–6 weeks after the onset of symptoms) in nearly all cases of acute EBV infection and persist for the lifetime of the patient. These antibodies may be lacking in immunodeficient patients and in those with chronic active EBV infection.

Titers of other antibodies also may be elevated in IM; however, these elevations are less useful for diagnosis. Antibodies to early antigens are detectable 3–4 weeks after the onset of symptoms in patients with IM. About 70% of individuals with IM have early antigen diffuse (EA-D) antibodies during the illness; the presence of EA-D antibodies is especially likely in patients with relatively severe disease. These antibodies usually persist for only 3–6 months. Levels of EA-D antibodies are also elevated in patients with nasopharyngeal carcinoma or chronic active EBV infection. Early antigen restricted (EA-R) antibodies are only occasionally detected in patients with IM but are often found at elevated titers in patients with African Burkitt's lymphoma or chronic active EBV infection. IgA antibodies to EBV antigens have proved useful for the identification of patients with nasopharyngeal carcinoma and of persons at high risk for the disease.

Other Studies Detection of EBV DNA, RNA, or proteins has been valuable in demonstrating the association of the virus with various malignancies. The polymerase chain reaction has been used to detect EBV DNA in the cerebrospinal fluid of some AIDS patients with lymphomas and to monitor the amount of EBV DNA in the blood of patients with lymphoproliferative disease. Detection of high levels of EBV DNA in blood for a few days to several weeks after the onset of IM may be useful if serologic studies yield equivocal results. Culture of EBV from throat washings or blood is not helpful in the diagnosis of acute infection, since EBV persists in the oropharynx and in B cells for the lifetime of the infected individual.

Differential Diagnosis Whereas ~90% of cases of IM are due to EBV, 5–10% of cases are due to cytomegalovirus (CMV) (Chap. 219). CMV is the most common cause of heterophile-negative mononucleosis; less common causes of IM and differences from IM due to EBV are shown in Table 218-2.

TREATMENT EBV-ASSOCIATED DISEASE

Therapy for IM consists of supportive measures, with rest and analgesia. Excessive physical activity during the first month should be avoided to reduce the possibility of splenic rupture, which often necessitates splenectomy. Glucocorticoid therapy is not indicated for uncomplicated IM and in fact may predispose to bacterial superinfection. Prednisone (40–60 mg/d for 2–3 days, with subsequent tapering of the dose over 1–2 weeks) has been used for the prevention of airway obstruction in patients with severe tonsillar hypertrophy, for

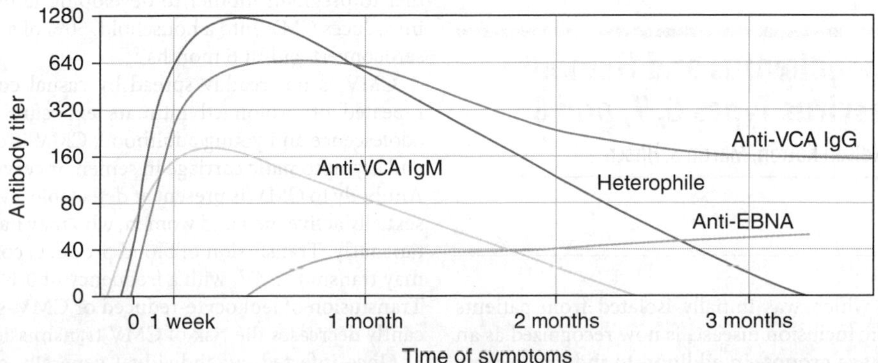

FIGURE 218-4 Pattern of Epstein-Barr virus (EBV) serology during acute infection. EBNA, Epstein-Barr nuclear antigen; VCA, viral capsid antigen. *(From JI Cohen, in NS Young et al [eds]: Clinical Hematology. Philadelphia, Mosby, 2006.)*

TABLE 218-2 DIFFERENTIAL DIAGNOSIS OF INFECTIOUS MONONUCLEOSIS

Etiology	Sign or Symptom: Fever	Adenopathy	Sore Throat	Atypical Lymphocytes	Differences from EBV Mononucleosis
EBV infection	+	+	+	+	—
CMV infection	+	±	±	+	Older age at presentation, longer duration of fever
HIV infection	+	+	+	±	Diffuse rash, oral/genital ulcers, aseptic meningitis
Toxoplasmosis	+	+	±	±	Less splenomegaly, exposure to cats or raw meat
HHV-6	+	+	+	+	Older age at presentation
Streptococcal pharyngitis	+	+	+	–	No splenomegaly, less fatigue
Viral hepatitis	+	±	–	±	Higher aminotransferase levels
Rubella	+	+	±	±	Maculopapular rash, no splenomegaly
Lymphoma	+	+	+	+	Fixed, nontender lymph nodes
Drugs[a]	+	+	–	±	Occurs at any age

[a]Most commonly phenytoin, carbamazepine, sulfonamides, or minocycline.

Abbreviations: CMV, cytomegalovirus; EBV, Epstein-Barr virus; HHV, human herpesvirus.

autoimmune hemolytic anemia, for hemophagocytic lymphohistiocytosis, and for severe thrombocytopenia. Glucocorticoids have also been administered to rare patients with severe malaise and fever and to patients with severe CNS or cardiac disease.

Acyclovir has had no significant clinical impact on IM in controlled trials. In one study, the combination of acyclovir and prednisolone had no significant effect on the duration of symptoms of IM.

Acyclovir, at a dosage of 400–800 mg five times daily, has been effective for the treatment of oral hairy leukoplakia (despite common relapses). The posttransplantation EBV lymphoproliferative syndrome **(Chap. 169)** generally does not respond to antiviral therapy. When possible, therapy should be directed toward reduction of immunosuppression. Antibody to CD20 (rituximab) has been effective in some cases. Infusions of donor lymphocytes are often effective for stem cell transplant recipients, although graft-versus-host disease can occur. Infusions of EBV-specific cytotoxic T cells have been used to prevent EBV lymphoproliferative disease in high-risk settings as well as to treat the disease. Interferon α administration, cytotoxic chemotherapy, and radiation therapy (especially for CNS lesions) also have been used. Infusion of autologous EBV-specific cytotoxic T lymphocytes has shown promise in small studies of patients with nasopharyngeal carcinoma and Hodgkin's disease. Treatment of several cases of X-linked lymphoproliferative disease with antibody to CD20 resulted in a successful outcome of what otherwise would probably have been fatal acute EBV infection.

PREVENTION

The isolation of patients with IM is unnecessary. A vaccine directed against the major EBV glycoprotein reduced the frequency of IM but did not affect the rate of asymptomatic infection in a phase 2 trial.

219 Cytomegalovirus and Human Herpesvirus Types 6, 7, and 8

Camille Nelson Kotton, Martin S. Hirsch

CYTOMEGALOVIRUS

DEFINITION

Cytomegalovirus (CMV), which was initially isolated from patients with congenital cytomegalic inclusion disease, is now recognized as an important pathogen in all age groups. In addition to inducing severe birth defects, CMV causes a wide spectrum of disorders in older children and adults, ranging from an asymptomatic subclinical infection to a mononucleosis syndrome in healthy individuals to disseminated disease in immunocompromised patients. Human CMV is one of several related species-specific viruses that cause similar diseases in various animals. All are associated with the production of characteristic enlarged cells—hence the name *cytomegalovirus*.

CMV, a β-herpesvirus, has double-stranded DNA, four species of mRNA, a protein capsid, and a lipoprotein envelope. Like other herpesviruses, CMV demonstrates icosahedral symmetry, replicates in the cell nucleus, and can cause either a lytic and productive or a latent infection. CMV can be distinguished from other herpesviruses by certain biologic properties, such as host range and type of cytopathology. Viral replication is associated with the production of large intranuclear inclusions and smaller cytoplasmic inclusions. CMV appears to replicate in a variety of cell types in vivo; in tissue culture it grows preferentially in fibroblasts. Although there is little evidence that CMV is oncogenic in vivo, it does transform fibroblasts in rare instances, and genomic transforming fragments have been identified.

EPIDEMIOLOGY

CMV has a worldwide distribution. In many regions of the world, the vast majority of adults are seropositive for CMV, whereas only half of adults in the United States and Canada are seropositive. In regions where the prevalence of CMV antibody is high, immunocompromised adults are more likely to undergo reactivation disease rather than primary infection. Data generated in specific regions should be considered in the context of local seropositivity rates, when appropriate.

Of newborns in the United States, ~1% are infected with CMV; the percentages are higher in many less-developed countries. Communal living and poor personal hygiene facilitate spread. Perinatal and early childhood infections are common. CMV may be present in breast milk, saliva, feces, and urine. Transmission has occurred among young children in day-care centers and has been traced from infected toddler to pregnant mother to developing fetus. When an infected child introduces CMV into a household, 50% of susceptible family members seroconvert within 6 months.

CMV is not readily spread by casual contact but rather requires repeated or prolonged intimate exposure for transmission. In late adolescence and young adulthood, CMV is often transmitted sexually, and asymptomatic carriage in semen or cervical secretions is common. Antibody to CMV is present at detectable levels in a high proportion of sexually active men and women, who may harbor several strains simultaneously. Transfusion of blood products containing viable leukocytes may transmit CMV, with a frequency of 0.14–10% per unit transfused. Transfusion of leukocyte-reduced or CMV-seronegative blood significantly decreases the risk of CMV transmission.

Once infected, an individual generally carries CMV for life. The infection usually remains silent. CMV reactivation syndromes develop more frequently, however, when T lymphocyte–mediated immunity is compromised—for example, after organ transplantation, with lymphoid neoplasms and certain acquired immunodeficiencies (in particular, HIV infection; Chap. 226), or during critical illness in intensive care units. Most primary CMV infections in organ transplant recipients (Chap. 169) result from transmission via the graft. In CMV-seropositive transplant recipients, infection results from reactivation of latent virus or from infection by a new strain. CMV infection may also be associated with diseases as diverse as coronary artery stenosis and malignant gliomas, but these associations require further validation.

PATHOGENESIS

Congenital CMV infection can result from either primary or reactivation infection of the mother. However, clinical disease in the fetus or newborn is related almost exclusively to primary maternal infection (Table 219-1). The factors determining the severity of congenital infection are unknown; a deficient capacity to produce precipitating antibodies and to mount T cell responses to CMV is associated with relatively severe disease.

Primary infection with CMV in late childhood or adulthood is often associated with a vigorous T lymphocyte response that may contribute to the development of a mononucleosis syndrome similar to that which follows infection with Epstein-Barr virus (Chap. 218). The hallmark of such infection is the appearance of atypical lymphocytes in the peripheral blood; these cells are predominantly activated CD8+ T lymphocytes. Polyclonal activation of B cells by CMV contributes to the development of rheumatoid factors and other autoantibodies during mononucleosis.

Once acquired, CMV persists indefinitely in host tissues. The sites of persistent infection probably include multiple cell types and various organs. Transmission via blood transfusion or organ transplantation is due primarily to latent infections in these tissues. If the host's T cell responses become compromised by disease or by iatrogenic immunosuppression, latent virus can reactivate to cause a variety of syndromes. Chronic antigenic stimulation in the presence of immunosuppression (for example, after organ transplantation) appears to be an ideal setting for CMV activation and CMV disease. Certain particularly potent suppressants of T cell immunity (e.g., antithymocyte globulin, alemtuzumab) are associated with a high rate of clinical CMV syndromes. CMV may itself contribute to further T lymphocyte hyporesponsiveness, which often precedes superinfection with other opportunistic pathogens such as bacteria, molds, and *Pneumocystis*.

PATHOLOGY

Cytomegalic cells in vivo (presumed to be infected epithelial cells) are two to four times larger than surrounding cells and often contain an 8- to 10-μm intranuclear inclusion that is eccentrically placed and is surrounded by a clear halo, producing an "owl's eye" appearance. Smaller granular cytoplasmic inclusions are demonstrated occasionally. Cytomegalic cells are found in a wide variety of organs, including the salivary gland, lung, liver, kidney, intestine, pancreas, adrenal gland, and central nervous system.

The cellular inflammatory response to infection consists of plasma cells, lymphocytes, and monocyte-macrophages. Granulomatous reactions occasionally develop, particularly in the liver. Immunopathologic reactions may contribute to CMV disease. Immune complexes have been detected in infected infants, sometimes in association with CMV-related glomerulopathies. Immune-complex glomerulopathy has also been observed in some CMV-infected patients after renal transplantation.

CLINICAL MANIFESTATIONS

Congenital CMV Infection Fetal infections range from subclinical to severe and disseminated. Cytomegalic inclusion disease develops in ~5% of infected fetuses and is seen almost exclusively in infants born to mothers who develop primary infections during pregnancy. Petechiae, hepatosplenomegaly, and jaundice are the most common presenting features (60–80% of cases). Microcephaly with or without cerebral calcifications, intrauterine growth retardation, and prematurity are reported in 30–50% of cases. Inguinal hernias and chorioretinitis are less common. Laboratory abnormalities include elevated alanine aminotransferase levels in serum, thrombocytopenia, conjugated hyperbilirubinemia, hemolysis, and elevated protein levels in cerebrospinal fluid. The prognosis for severely infected infants is poor; the mortality rate is 20–30%, and few survivors escape intellectual or hearing difficulties later in childhood. The differential diagnosis of cytomegalic inclusion disease in infants includes syphilis, rubella, toxoplasmosis, infection with herpes simplex virus or enterovirus, and bacterial sepsis.

Most congenital CMV infections are clinically inapparent at birth. Of asymptomatically infected infants, 5–25% develop significant psychomotor, hearing, ocular, or dental abnormalities over the next several years.

Perinatal CMV Infection The newborn may acquire CMV at delivery by passage through an infected birth canal or by postnatal contact with infected breast milk or other maternal secretions. Of infants who are breast-fed for >1 month by seropositive mothers, 40–60% become infected. Iatrogenic transmission can result from blood transfusion; use of leukocyte-reduced or CMV-seronegative blood products for transfusion into low-birth-weight seronegative infants or seronegative pregnant women decreases risk.

The great majority of infants infected at or after delivery remain asymptomatic. However, protracted interstitial pneumonitis has been associated with perinatally acquired CMV infection, particularly in premature infants, and occasionally has been accompanied by infection with *Chlamydia trachomatis*, *Pneumocystis*, or *Ureaplasma urealyticum*. Poor weight gain, adenopathy, rash, hepatitis, anemia, and atypical lymphocytosis may also be found, and CMV excretion often persists for months or years.

CMV Mononucleosis The most common clinical manifestation of CMV infection in immunocompetent hosts beyond the neonatal period is a heterophile antibody–negative mononucleosis syndrome, which may develop spontaneously or follow transfusion of leukocyte-containing blood products. Although the syndrome occurs at all ages, it most

TABLE 219-1 CMV DISEASE IN THE IMMUNOCOMPROMISED HOST

Population	Risk Factors	Principal Syndromes	Treatment	Prevention
Fetus	Primary maternal infection/early pregnancy	Cytomegalic inclusion disease	Ganciclovir for symptomatic neonates	Avoidance of exposure; possibly, maternal treatment with CMV immunoglobulin during pregnancy
Organ transplant recipient	Seropositivity of donor and/or recipient; potent immunosuppressive regimen; treatment of rejection	Febrile leukopenia; gastrointestinal disease; pneumonia	Ganciclovir or valganciclovir	Prophylaxis or preemptive therapy with ganciclovir or valganciclovir
Hematopoietic stem cell transplant recipient	Graft-vs.-host disease; older age of recipient; seropositive recipient; viremia	Pneumonia; gastrointestinal disease	Ganciclovir or valganciclovir or foscarnet, ± CMV immunoglobulin	Prophylaxis or preemptive therapy with ganciclovir or valganciclovir
Person with AIDS	<100 CD4+ T cells/μL; CMV seropositivity	Retinitis; gastrointestinal disease; neurologic disease	Ganciclovir, valganciclovir, foscarnet, or cidofovir	Oral valganciclovir

often involves sexually active young adults. With incubation periods of 20–60 days, the illness generally lasts for 2–6 weeks. Prolonged high fevers, sometimes with chills, profound fatigue, and malaise, characterize this disorder. Myalgias, headache, and splenomegaly are common, but in CMV (as opposed to Epstein-Barr virus) mononucleosis, exudative pharyngitis and cervical lymphadenopathy are rare. Occasional patients develop rubelliform rashes, often after exposure to ampicillin or certain other antibiotics. Less common are interstitial or segmental pneumonia, myocarditis, pleuritis, arthritis, and encephalitis. In rare cases, Guillain-Barré syndrome complicates CMV mononucleosis. The characteristic laboratory abnormality is relative lymphocytosis in peripheral blood, with >10% atypical lymphocytes. Total leukocyte counts may be low, normal, or markedly elevated. Although significant jaundice is uncommon, serum aminotransferase and alkaline phosphatase levels are often moderately elevated. Heterophile antibodies are absent; however, transient immunologic abnormalities are common and may include the presence of cryoglobulins, rheumatoid factors, cold agglutinins, and antinuclear antibodies. Hemolytic anemia, thrombocytopenia, and granulocytopenia complicate recovery in rare instances.

Most patients recover without sequelae, although postviral asthenia may persist for months. The excretion of CMV in urine, genital secretions, and/or saliva often continues for months or years. Rarely, CMV infection is fatal in immunocompetent hosts; survivors can have recurrent episodes of fever and malaise, sometimes associated with autonomic nervous system dysfunction (e.g., attacks of sweating or flushing).

CMV Infection in the Immunocompromised Host (Table 219-1) CMV is the viral pathogen most commonly complicating organ transplantation (Chap. 169). In recipients of kidney, heart, lung, liver, pancreas, and vascularized composite (hand, face, other) transplants, CMV induces a variety of syndromes, including fever and leukopenia, hepatitis, colitis, pneumonitis, esophagitis, gastritis, and retinitis. CMV disease is an independent risk factor for both graft loss and death. Without prophylaxis, the period of maximal risk is between 1 and 4 months after transplantation. Disease likelihood and viral replication levels generally are greater after primary infection than after reactivation. Molecular studies indicate that seropositive transplant recipients are susceptible to infection with donor-derived, genotypically variant CMV, and such infection often results in disease. Reactivation infection, although common, is less likely than primary infection to be important clinically. The risk of clinical disease is related to various factors, such as degree of immunosuppression, use of antilymphocyte antibodies, lack of anti-CMV prophylaxis, and co-infection with other pathogens. The transplanted organ is particularly vulnerable as a target for CMV infection; thus there is a tendency for CMV hepatitis to follow liver transplantation and for CMV pneumonitis to follow lung transplantation.

CMV viremia occurs in roughly one-third of hematopoietic stem cell transplant recipients; the risk of severe disease may be reduced by prophylaxis or preemptive therapy with antiviral drugs. The risk is greatest 5–13 weeks after transplantation, and identified risk factors include certain types of immunosuppressive therapy, an allogeneic (rather than an autologous) graft, acute graft-versus-host disease, older age, and pretransplantation recipient seropositivity.

CMV is an important pathogen in patients with advanced HIV infection (Chap. 226), in whom it may cause retinitis or disseminated disease, particularly when peripheral-blood CD4+ T cell counts fall below 50–100/μL. As treatment for underlying HIV infection has improved, the incidence of serious CMV infections (e.g., retinitis) has decreased. However, during the first few weeks after institution of highly active antiretroviral therapy, acute flare-ups of CMV retinitis may occur secondary to an immune reconstitution inflammatory syndrome.

Syndromes produced by CMV in immunocompromised hosts often begin with prolonged fatigue, fever, malaise, anorexia, night sweats, and arthralgias or myalgias. Liver function abnormalities, leukopenia, thrombocytopenia, and atypical lymphocytosis may be observed during these episodes. The development of tachypnea, hypoxemia, and unproductive cough signals respiratory involvement. Radiologic examination of the lung often shows bilateral interstitial or reticulonodular infiltrates that begin in the periphery of the lower lobes and spread centrally and superiorly; localized segmental, nodular, or alveolar patterns are less common. The differential diagnosis includes *Pneumocystis* infection; other viral, bacterial, or fungal infections; pulmonary hemorrhage; and injury secondary to irradiation or to treatment with cytotoxic drugs.

Gastrointestinal CMV involvement may be localized or extensive and almost exclusively affects immunocompromised hosts. Colitis is the most common clinical manifestation in organ transplant recipients. Ulcers of the esophagus, stomach, small intestine, or colon may result in bleeding or perforation. CMV infection may lead to exacerbations of underlying ulcerative colitis. Hepatitis occurs frequently, particularly after liver transplantation. Acalculous cholecystitis and adrenalitis also have been described.

CMV rarely causes meningoencephalitis in otherwise healthy individuals. Two forms of CMV encephalitis are seen in patients with AIDS. One resembles HIV encephalitis and presents as progressive dementia; the other is a ventriculoencephalitis characterized by cranial-nerve deficits, nystagmus, disorientation, lethargy, and ventriculomegaly. In immunocompromised patients, CMV can also cause subacute progressive polyradiculopathy, which is often reversible if recognized and treated promptly.

CMV retinitis is an important cause of blindness in immunocompromised patients, particularly patients with advanced AIDS (Chap. 226). Early lesions consist of small, opaque, white areas of granular retinal necrosis that spread in a centrifugal manner and are later accompanied by hemorrhages, vessel sheathing, and retinal edema (Fig. 219-1). CMV retinopathy must be distinguished from that due to other conditions, including toxoplasmosis, candidiasis, and herpes simplex virus infection.

Fatal CMV infections are often associated with persistent viremia and the involvement of multiple organ systems. Progressive pulmonary infiltrates, pancytopenia, hyperamylasemia, and hypotension are characteristic features that are frequently found in conjunction with a terminal bacterial, fungal, or protozoan superinfection. Extensive adrenal necrosis with CMV inclusions is often documented at autopsy, as is CMV involvement of many other organs.

DIAGNOSIS

CMV infection usually cannot be diagnosed reliably on clinical grounds alone. Isolation of CMV or detection of its antigens or DNA in appropriate clinical specimens is the preferred approach. The most common method of detection is quantitative nucleic acid testing (QNAT) for CMV by polymerase chain reaction (PCR) technology,

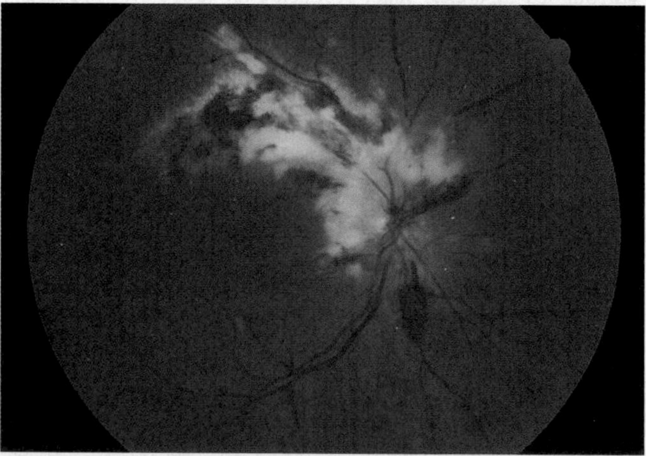

FIGURE 219-1 Cytomegalovirus infection in a patient with AIDS may appear as an arcuate zone of retinitis with hemorrhages and optic disk swelling. Often CMV is confined to the retinal periphery, beyond view of the direct ophthalmoscope.

for which blood or other specimens can be used; some centers use a CMV antigenemia test, an immunofluorescence assay that detects CMV antigens (pp65) in peripheral-blood leukocytes. Such assays may yield a positive result several days earlier than culture methods. QNAT may predict the risk for disease progression, particularly in immunocompromised hosts. CMV DNA in cerebrospinal fluid is useful in the diagnosis of CMV encephalitis or polyradiculopathy. Considerable variation exists among assays and laboratories; a recently introduced international testing standard should help reduce variation in PCR test results.

Virus excretion or viremia is readily detected by culture of appropriate specimens on human fibroblast monolayers. If CMV titers are high, as is common in congenital disseminated infection and in AIDS, characteristic cytopathic effects may be detected within a few days. However, in some situations (e.g., CMV mononucleosis), viral titers are low, and cytopathic effects may take several weeks to appear. Many laboratories expedite diagnosis with an overnight tissue-culture method (shell vial assay) involving centrifugation and an immunocytochemical detection technique employing monoclonal antibodies to an immediate-early CMV antigen. Isolation of virus from urine or saliva does not, by itself, constitute proof of acute infection, since excretion from these sites may continue for months or years after illness. Detection of viremia is a better predictor of acute infection.

A variety of serologic assays detect antibody to CMV. An increased level of IgG antibody to CMV may not be detectable for up to 4 weeks after primary infection. Detection of CMV-specific IgM is sometimes useful in the diagnosis of recent or active infection; however, circulating rheumatoid factors may result in occasional false-positive IgM tests. Serology is especially helpful when used to predict risk of CMV infection and disease in transplant recipients.

PREVENTION

Prevention of CMV in organ and hematopoietic stem cell transplant recipients is usually based on one of two methods: universal prophylaxis or preemptive therapy. With universal prophylaxis, antiviral drugs are used for a defined period, often 3 or 6 months. One clinical trial demonstrated that, in CMV-seronegative recipients with seropositive donors, prophylaxis was more effective at prevention when given for 200 days rather than 100 days. With preemptive therapy, patients are monitored weekly for CMV viremia, and antiviral treatment is initiated once viremia is detected. Because of the bone marrow–suppressive effects of universal prophylaxis, preemptive therapy is more commonly employed in hematopoietic stem cell transplant recipients. For patients with advanced HIV infection (CD4+ T cell counts of <50/μL), some experts have advocated prophylaxis with valganciclovir (see below). However, side effects, lack of proven benefit, possible induction of viral resistance, and high cost have precluded the wide acceptance of this practice. Preemptive therapy is under study in HIV-infected patients.

Several additional measures are useful for the prevention of CMV transmission to CMV-naïve, high-risk patients. The use of CMV-seronegative or leukocyte-depleted blood greatly decreases the rate of transfusion-associated transmission. In a placebo-controlled trial, a CMV glycoprotein B vaccine reduced infection rates among 464 CMV-seronegative women; this outcome raises the possibility that this experimental vaccine will reduce rates of congenital infection, but further studies must validate this approach. A CMV glycoprotein B vaccine with MF59 adjuvant appeared effective in reducing the risk and duration of viremia in both seropositive and seronegative renal transplant recipients at risk for CMV infection. CMV immune globulin has been reported to prevent congenital CMV infection in infants of women with primary infection during pregnancy. Studies in hematopoietic stem cell transplant recipients have produced conflicting results.

Prophylactic acyclovir or valacyclovir may reduce rates of CMV infection and disease in renal transplant recipients, although neither drug is effective in the treatment of active CMV disease.

TREATMENT CYTOMEGALOVIRUS INFECTION

Ganciclovir is a guanosine derivative that has considerably more activity against CMV than its congener acyclovir. After intracellular conversion by a viral phosphotransferase encoded by CMV gene region UL97, ganciclovir triphosphate is a selective inhibitor of CMV DNA polymerase. Several clinical studies have indicated response rates of 70–90% among patients with AIDS who are given ganciclovir for the treatment of CMV retinitis or colitis. In severe infections (e.g., CMV pneumonia in hematopoietic stem cell transplant recipients), ganciclovir is often combined with CMV immune globulin. Prophylactic or suppressive ganciclovir may be useful in high-risk hematopoietic stem cell or organ transplant recipients (e.g., those who are CMV-seropositive before transplantation). In many patients with AIDS, persistently low CD4+ T cell counts, and CMV disease, clinical and virologic relapses occur promptly if treatment with ganciclovir is discontinued. Therefore, prolonged maintenance regimens are recommended for such patients. Resistance to ganciclovir is more common among patients treated for >3 months and is usually related to mutations in the CMV UL97 gene (or, less commonly, the UL54 gene).

Valganciclovir is an orally bioavailable prodrug that is rapidly metabolized to ganciclovir in intestinal tissues and the liver. Approximately 60–70% of an oral dose of valganciclovir is absorbed. An oral valganciclovir dose of 900 mg results in ganciclovir blood levels similar to those obtained with an IV ganciclovir dose of 5 mg/kg. Valganciclovir appears to be as effective as IV ganciclovir for both CMV induction (treatment) and maintenance regimens, while providing the ease of oral dosing. Furthermore, the adverse-event profiles and rates of resistance for the two drugs are similar.

Ganciclovir or valganciclovir therapy for CMV disease consists of a 14- to 21-day induction course (5 mg/kg IV twice daily for ganciclovir or 900 mg PO twice daily for valganciclovir), sometimes followed by maintenance therapy (e.g., valganciclovir, 900 mg/d). Peripheral-blood neutropenia develops in roughly one-quarter of treated patients but may be ameliorated by granulocyte colony-stimulating factor or granulocyte-macrophage colony-stimulating factor. Whether to use maintenance therapy should depend on the overall level of immunocompromise and the risk of recurrent disease. Discontinuation of maintenance therapy should be considered in patients with AIDS who, while receiving antiretroviral therapy, have a sustained (3- to 6-month) increase in CD4+ T cell counts to >100/μL.

For treatment of CMV retinitis, ganciclovir may also be administered via a slow-release pellet sutured into the eye. Although this intraocular device provides good local protection, contralateral eye disease and disseminated disease are not affected, and early retinal detachment is possible. A combination of intraocular and systemic therapy may be better than the intraocular implant alone.

Foscarnet (sodium phosphonoformate) inhibits CMV DNA polymerase. Because this agent does not require phosphorylation to be active, it is also effective against most ganciclovir-resistant isolates. Foscarnet is less well tolerated than ganciclovir and causes considerable toxicity, including renal dysfunction, hypomagnesemia, hypokalemia, hypocalcemia, genital ulcers, dysuria, nausea, and paresthesia. Moreover, foscarnet administration requires the use of an infusion pump and close clinical monitoring. With aggressive hydration and dose adjustments for renal dysfunction, the toxicity of foscarnet can be reduced. The use of foscarnet should be avoided when a saline load cannot be tolerated (e.g., in cardiomyopathy). The approved induction regimen is 60 mg/kg every 8 h for 2 weeks, although 90 mg/kg every 12 h is equally effective and no more toxic. Maintenance infusions should deliver 90–120 mg/kg once daily. No oral preparation is available. Foscarnet-resistant virus may emerge during extended therapy. This drug is used more frequently after hematopoietic stem cell transplantation than in other situations to avoid the myelosuppressive effects of ganciclovir; in general, foscarnet is also the first choice for infections with ganciclovir-resistant CMV.

Cidofovir is a nucleotide analogue with a long intracellular half-life that allows intermittent IV administration. Induction regimens of 5 mg/kg weekly for 2 weeks are followed by maintenance regimens of 3–5 mg/kg every 2 weeks. Cidofovir can cause severe nephrotoxicity through dose-dependent proximal tubular cell injury; however, this adverse effect can be tempered somewhat by saline hydration and probenecid. Cidofovir is used primarily for ganciclovir-resistant virus.

HUMAN HERPESVIRUS (HHV) TYPES 6, 7, AND 8

HHV-6 AND HHV-7

HHV-6 and -7 seropositivity rates are generally high throughout the world. HHV-6 was first isolated in 1986 from peripheral-blood leukocytes of six persons with various lymphoproliferative disorders. Two genetically distinct variants (HHV-6A and HHV-6B) are now recognized. HHV-6 appears to be transmitted by saliva and possibly by genital secretions.

Infection with HHV-6 frequently occurs during infancy as maternal antibody wanes. The peak age of acquisition is 9–21 months; by 24 months, seropositivity rates approach 80%. Older siblings appear to serve as a source of transmission. Congenital infection also may occur, and ~1% of newborns are infected with HHV-6; placental infection with HHV-6 has been described. Most postnatally infected children develop symptoms (fever, fussiness, and diarrhea). A minority develop exanthem subitum (roseola infantum; see Fig. 25e-5), a common illness characterized by fever with subsequent rash. In addition, ~10–20% of febrile seizures without rash during infancy are caused by HHV-6. After initial infection, HHV-6 persists in peripheral-blood mononuclear cells as well as in the central nervous system, salivary glands, and female genital tract.

In older age groups, HHV-6 has been associated with mononucleosis syndromes; in immunocompromised hosts, encephalitis, pneumonitis, syncytial giant-cell hepatitis, and disseminated disease are seen. In transplant recipients, HHV-6 infection may also be associated with graft dysfunction. Acute HHV-6-associated limbic encephalitis has been reported in hematopoietic stem cell transplant recipients and is characterized by memory loss, confusion, seizures, hyponatremia, and abnormal electroencephalographic and MRI results. High plasma loads of HHV-6 DNA in hematopoietic stem cell transplant recipients are associated with allelic-mismatched donors, use of glucocorticoids, delayed monocyte and platelet engraftment, development of limbic encephalitis, and increased all-cause mortality rates. Like many other viruses, HHV-6 has been implicated in the pathogenesis of multiple sclerosis, although further study is needed to distinguish between association and etiology.

HHV-7 was isolated in 1990 from T lymphocytes from the peripheral blood of a healthy 26-year-old man. The virus is frequently acquired during childhood, albeit at a later age than HHV-6. HHV-7 is commonly present in saliva, which is presumed to be the principal source of infection; breast milk also can carry the virus. Viremia can be associated with either primary or reactivation infection. The most common clinical manifestations of childhood HHV-7 infections are fever and seizures. Some children present with respiratory or gastrointestinal signs and symptoms. An association has been made between HHV-7 and pityriasis rosea, but evidence is insufficient to indicate a causal relationship.

Clustering of HHV-6, HHV-7, and CMV infections in transplant recipients can make it difficult to sort out the roles of the various agents in individual clinical syndromes. HHV-6 and HHV-7 appear to be susceptible to ganciclovir and foscarnet, although definitive evidence of clinical response is lacking.

HHV-8

Unique herpesvirus-like DNA sequences were reported during 1994 and 1995 in tissues derived from Kaposi's sarcoma (KS) and body cavity–based lymphoma occurring in patients with AIDS. The virus from which these sequences were derived is designated HHV-8 or Kaposi's sarcoma–associated herpesvirus (KSHV). HHV-8, which infects B lymphocytes, macrophages, and both endothelial and epithelial cells, appears to be causally related not only to KS and a subgroup of AIDS-related B cell body cavity–based lymphomas (primary effusion lymphomas) but also to multicentric Castleman's disease, a lymphoproliferative disorder of B cells. The association of HHV-8 with several other diseases has been reported but not confirmed.

HHV-8 seropositivity occurs worldwide, with areas of high endemicity influencing rates of disease. Unlike other herpesvirus infections, HHV-8 infection is much more common in some geographic areas (e.g., central and southern Africa) than in others (North America, Asia, northern Europe). In high-prevalence areas, infection occurs in childhood, seropositivity is associated with having a seropositive mother or (to a lesser extent) older sibling, and HHV-8 may be transmitted in saliva. In low-prevalence areas, infections typically occur in adults, probably with sexual transmission. Concurrent epidemics of HIV-1 and HHV-8 infections among certain populations (e.g., men who have sex with men) in the late 1970s and early 1980s appear to have resulted in the frequent association of AIDS and KS. Transmission of HHV-8 may also be associated with organ transplantation, injection drug use, and blood transfusion; however, transmission via blood transfusion in the United States appears to be quite rare.

Primary HHV-8 infection in immunocompetent children may manifest as fever and maculopapular rash. Among individuals with intact immunity, chronic asymptomatic infection is the rule, and neoplastic disorders generally develop only after subsequent immunocompromise. Immunocompromised persons with primary infection may present with fever, splenomegaly, lymphoid hyperplasia, pancytopenia, or rapid-onset KS. Quantitative analysis of HHV-8 DNA suggests a predominance of latently infected cells in KS lesions and frequent lytic replication in multicentric Castleman's disease.

Effective antiretroviral therapy for HIV-infected individuals has led to a marked reduction in rates of KS among persons dually infected with HHV-8 and HIV in resource-rich areas. HHV-8 itself is susceptible in vitro to ganciclovir, foscarnet, and cidofovir. A small, randomized, double-blind, placebo-controlled, crossover trial suggested that oral valganciclovir administered once daily reduced HHV-8 replication. However, clinical benefits of valganciclovir or other drugs in HHV-8 infection have not yet been demonstrated. Sirolimus has been shown to inhibit the progression of dermal KS in kidney transplant recipients while providing effective immunosuppression.

220e Molluscum Contagiosum, Monkeypox, and Other Poxvirus Infections

Fred Wang

This is a digital-only chapter. It is available on the DVD that accompanies this book, as well as on Access Medicine/Harrison's Online, and the eBook and "app" editions of HPIM 19e.

The poxvirus family includes a large number of related DNA viruses that infect various vertebrate hosts. The poxviruses responsible for infections in humans, the geographic locations in which these infections are found, the host reservoirs, and the main manifestations are described in this chapter. Infections with orthopoxviruses—e.g., smallpox (variola major) virus (Chap. 261e) or the zoonotic monkeypox virus—can result in systemic, potentially lethal human disease. Other poxvirus infections cause primarily localized skin disease in humans.

221 Parvovirus Infections

Kevin E. Brown

Parvoviruses, members of the family Parvoviridae, are small (diameter, ~22 nm), nonenveloped, icosahedral viruses with a linear single-strand DNA genome of ~5000 nucleotides. These viruses are dependent on either rapidly dividing host cells or helper viruses for replication. At least four groups of parvoviruses infect humans: parvovirus B19 (B19V), dependoparvoviruses (adeno-associated viruses; AAVs), PARV4/5 virus, and human bocaviruses (HBoVs). Human dependoparvoviruses are nonpathogenic and will not be considered further in this chapter.

PARVOVIRUS B19

DEFINITION

B19V is the type member of the genus *Erythroparvovirus*. On the basis of viral sequence, B19V is divided into three genotypes (designated 1, 2, and 3), but only a single B19V antigenic type has been described. Genotype 1 is predominant in most parts of the world; genotype 2 is rarely associated with active infection; and genotype 3 appears to predominate in parts of western Africa.

EPIDEMIOLOGY

B19V exclusively infects humans, and infection is endemic in virtually all parts of the world. Transmission occurs predominantly via the respiratory route and is followed by the onset of rash and arthralgia. By the age of 15 years, ~ 50% of children have detectable IgG; this figure rises to >90% among the elderly. In pregnant women, the estimated annual seroconversion rate is ~1%. Within households, secondary infection rates approach 50%.

Detection of high-titer B19V in blood is not unusual (see "Pathogenesis," below). Transmission can occur as a result of transfusion, most commonly of pooled components. To reduce the risk of transmission, plasma pools are screened by nucleic acid amplification technology, and high-titer pools are discarded. B19V is resistant to both heat and solvent-detergent inactivation.

PATHOGENESIS

B19V replicates primarily in erythroid progenitors. This specificity is due in part to the limited tissue distribution of the primary B19V receptor, blood group P antigen (globoside). Infection leads to high-titer viremia, with $>10^{12}$ virus particles (or IU)/mL detectable in the blood at the apex (Fig. 221-1), and virus-induced cytotoxicity results in cessation of red cell production. In immunocompetent individuals, viremia and arrest of erythropoiesis are transient and resolve as the IgM and IgG antibody response is mounted. In individuals with normal erythropoiesis, there is only a minimal drop in hemoglobin levels; however, in those with increased erythropoiesis (especially with hemolytic anemia), this cessation of red cell production can induce a transient crisis with severe anemia (Fig. 221-1). Similarly, if an individual (or, after maternal infection, a fetus) does not mount a neutralizing antibody response and halt the lytic infection, erythroid production is compromised and chronic anemia develops (Fig. 221-1).

The immune-mediated phase of illness, which begins 2–3 weeks after infection as the IgM response peaks, manifests as the rash of fifth disease together with arthralgia and/or frank arthritis. Low-level B19V DNA can be detected by polymerase chain reaction (PCR) in blood and tissues for months to years after acute infection. The B19V

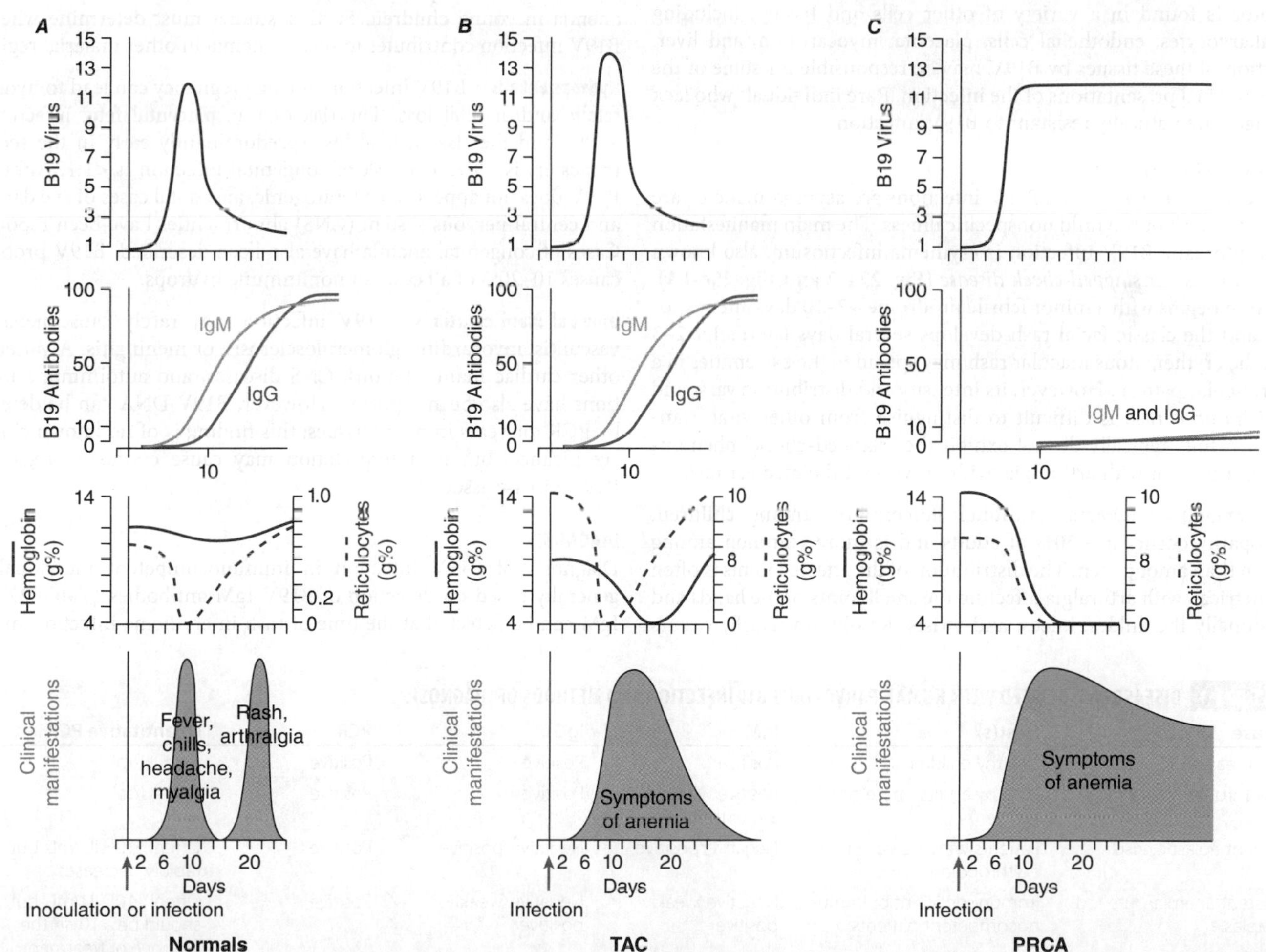

FIGURE 221-1 Schematic of the time course of parvovirus B19V infection in (*A*) normals (erythema infectiosum), (*B*) transient aplastic crisis (TAC), and (*C*) chronic anemia/pure red-cell aplasia (PRCA). *(Reprinted with permission from NS Young, KE Brown: N Engl J Med 350:586, 2004. © 2004 Massachusetts Medical Society. All rights reserved.)*

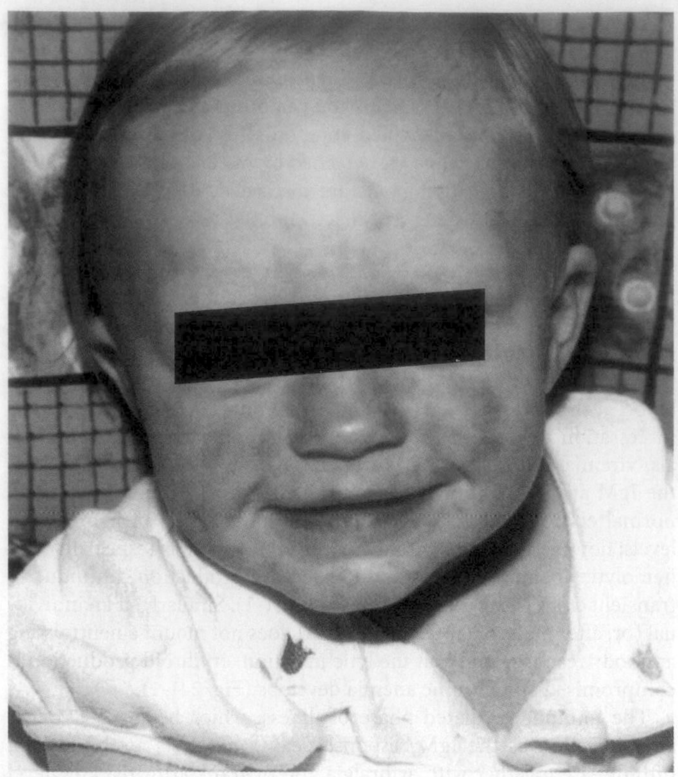

FIGURE 221-2 Young child with erythema infectiosum, or fifth disease, showing typical "slapped-cheek" appearance.

receptor is found in a variety of other cells and tissues, including megakaryocytes, endothelial cells, placenta, myocardium, and liver. Infection of these tissues by B19V may be responsible for some of the more unusual presentations of the infection. Rare individuals who lack P antigen are naturally resistant to B19V infection.

CLINICAL MANIFESTATIONS

Erythema Infectiosum Most B19V infections are asymptomatic or are associated with only a mild nonspecific illness. The main manifestation of symptomatic B19V infection is erythema infectiosum, also known as *fifth disease* or *slapped-cheek disease* (Fig. 221-2 and Fig. 25e-1A). Infection begins with a minor febrile prodrome ~7–10 days after exposure, and the classic facial rash develops several days later; after 2–3 days, the erythematous macular rash may spread to the extremities in a lacy reticular pattern. However, its intensity and distribution vary, and B19V-induced rash is difficult to distinguish from other viral exanthems. Adults typically do not exhibit the "slapped-cheek" phenomenon but present with arthralgia, with or without the macular rash.

Polyarthropathy Syndrome Although uncommon among children, arthropathy occurs in ~50% of adults and is more common among women than among men. The distribution of the affected joints is often symmetrical, with arthralgia affecting the small joints of the hands and occasionally the ankles, knees, and wrists. Resolution usually occurs within a few weeks, but recurring symptoms can continue for months. The illness may mimic rheumatoid arthritis, and rheumatoid factor can often be detected in serum. B19V infection may trigger rheumatoid disease in some patients and has been associated with juvenile idiopathic arthritis.

Transient Aplastic Crisis Asymptomatic transient reticulocytopenia occurs in most individuals with B19V infection. However, in patients who depend on continual rapid production of red cells, infection can cause transient aplastic crisis (TAC). Affected individuals include those with hemolytic disorders, hemoglobinopathies, red cell enzymopathies, and autoimmune hemolytic anemias. Patients present with symptoms of severe anemia (sometimes life-threatening) and a low reticulocyte count, and bone marrow examination reveals an absence of erythroid precursors and characteristic giant pronormoblasts. As its name indicates, the illness is transient, and anemia resolves with the cessation of cytopathic infection in the erythroid progenitors.

Pure Red-Cell Aplasia/Chronic Anemia Chronic B19V infection has been reported in a wide range of immunosuppressed patients, including those with congenital immunodeficiency, AIDS (Chap. 226), lymphoproliferative disorders (especially acute lymphocytic leukemia), and transplantation (Chap. 169). Patients have persistent anemia with reticulocytopenia, absent or low levels of B19V IgG, high titers of B19V DNA in serum, and—in many cases—scattered giant pronormoblasts in bone marrow. Rarely, nonerythroid hematologic lineages are also affected. Transient neutropenia, lymphopenia, and thrombocytopenia (including idiopathic thrombocytopenic purpura) have been observed. B19V occasionally causes a hemophagocytic syndrome.

Recent studies in Papua New Guinea and Ghana, where malaria is endemic, suggest that co-infection with *Plasmodium* and B19V plays a major role in the development of severe anemia in young children. Further studies must determine whether B19V infection contributes to severe anemia in other malarial regions.

Hydrops Fetalis B19V infection during pregnancy can lead to hydrops fetalis and/or fetal loss. The risk of transplacental fetal infection is ~30%, and the risk of fetal loss (predominantly early in the second trimester) is ~9%. The risk of congenital infection is <1%. Although B19V does not appear to be teratogenic, anecdotal cases of eye damage and central nervous system (CNS) abnormalities have been reported. Cases of congenital anemia have also been described. B19V probably causes 10–20% of all cases of nonimmune hydrops.

Unusual Manifestations B19V infection may rarely cause hepatitis, vasculitis, myocarditis, glomerulosclerosis, or meningitis. A variety of other cardiac manifestations, CNS diseases, and autoimmune infections have also been reported. However, B19V DNA can be detected by PCR for years in many tissues; this finding is of no known clinical significance, but its interpretation may cause confusion regarding B19V disease association.

DIAGNOSIS

Diagnosis of B19V infection in immunocompetent individuals is generally based on detection of B19V IgM antibodies (Table 221-1). IgM can be detected at the time of rash in erythema infectiosum and

TABLE 221-1 DISEASES ASSOCIATED WITH HUMAN PARVOVIRUS B19 INFECTION AND METHODS OF DIAGNOSIS

Disease	Host(s)	IgM	IgG	PCR	Quantitative PCR
Fifth disease	Healthy children	Positive	Positive	Positive	>10^4 IU/mL
Polyarthropathy syndrome	Healthy adults (more often women)	Positive within 3 months of onset	Positive	Positive	>10^4 IU/mL
Transient aplastic crisis	Patients with increased erythropoiesis	Negative/positive	Negative/positive	Positive	Often >10^{12} IU/mL, but rapidly decreases
Persistent anemia/pure red-cell aplasia	Immunodeficient or immunocompetent patients	Negative/weakly positive	Negative/weakly positive	Positive	Often >10^{12} IU/mL, but should be >10^6 in the absence of treatment
Hydrops fetalis/congenital anemia	Fetus (<20 weeks)	Negative/positive	Positive	Positive amniotic fluid or tissue	n/a

Abbreviations: IU, international units (1 IU equals ~1 genome); n/a, not applicable; PCR, polymerase chain reaction.

by the third day of TAC in patients with hematologic disorders; these antibodies remain detectable for ~3 months. B19V IgG is detectable by the seventh day of illness and persists throughout life. Quantitative detection of B19V DNA should be used for the diagnosis of early TAC or chronic anemia. Although B19V levels fall rapidly with the development of the immune response, DNA can be detectable by PCR for months or even years after infection, even in healthy individuals; therefore, quantitative PCR should be used. In acute infection at the height of viremia, $>10^{12}$ B19V DNA IU/mL of serum can be detected; however, titers fall rapidly within 2 days. Patients with aplastic crisis or B19V-induced chronic anemia generally have $>10^5$ B19V DNA IU/mL.

TREATMENT PARVOVIRUS B19 INFECTION

No antiviral drug effective against B19V is available, and treatment of B19V infection often targets symptoms only. TAC precipitated by B19V infection frequently necessitates symptom-based treatment with blood transfusions. In patients receiving chemotherapy, temporary cessation of treatment may result in an immune response and resolution. If this approach is unsuccessful or not applicable, commercial immune globulin (IVIg; Gammagard, Sandoglobulin) from healthy blood donors can cure or ameliorate persistent B19V infection in immunosuppressed patients. Generally, the dose used is 400 mg/kg daily for 5–10 days. Like patients with TAC, immunosuppressed patients with persistent B19V infection should be considered infectious. Administration of IVIg is not beneficial for erythema infectiosum or B19V-associated polyarthropathy. Intrauterine blood transfusion can prevent fetal loss in some cases of fetal hydrops.

PREVENTION

No vaccine has been approved for the prevention of B19V infection, although vaccines based on B19V virus-like particles expressed in insect cells are known to be highly immunogenic. Phase 1 trials of a putative vaccine were discontinued because of adverse side effects.

PARV4/5

DEFINITION

The PARV4 viral sequence was initially detected in a patient with an acute viral syndrome. Similar sequences, including the related PARV5 sequence, have been detected in pooled plasma collections. The DNA sequence of PARV4/5 is distinctly different from that of all other parvoviruses, and this virus is now classified as a member of the newly described genus *Tetraparvovirus.*

EPIDEMIOLOGY

PARV4 DNA is commonly found in plasma pools but at lower concentrations than levels of B19V DNA found before in plasma pools prior to screening. The higher levels of PARV4 DNA and IgG antibody in tissues (bone marrow and lymphoid tissue) and sera from IV drug users than in the corresponding specimens from control patients suggest that the virus is transmitted predominantly by parenteral means in the United States and Europe. Evidence for nonparenteral transmission in other parts of the world is limited.

CLINICAL MANIFESTATIONS

To date, PARV4/5 infection has been associated only with mild clinical disease (rash and/or transient aminotransferase elevation).

HUMAN BOCAVIRUSES

DEFINITION

Animal bocaviruses are associated with mild respiratory symptoms and enteritis in young animals. HBoV1 was originally identified in the respiratory tract of young children with lower respiratory tract infections. More recently, HBoV1 and the related viruses HBoV2, HBoV3, and HBoV4 have all been identified in human fecal samples.

EPIDEMIOLOGY

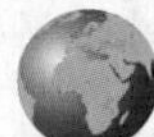

Seroepidemiologic studies with HBoV virus-like particles suggest that human bocavirus infection is common. Worldwide, most individuals are infected before the age of 5 years.

CLINICAL MANIFESTATIONS

HBoV1 DNA is found in respiratory secretions from 2–20% of children with acute respiratory infection, often in the presence of other pathogens; in these circumstances, the role of HBoV1 in disease pathogenesis is unknown. Clinical disease due to HBoV1 is associated with evidence of primary infection (IgG seroconversion or the presence of IgM), HBoV1 DNA in serum, or high titer HBoV1 DNA ($>10^4$ genome copies/mL) in respiratory secretions. Symptoms are not dissimilar from those of other viral respiratory infections, and cough and wheezing are commonly reported. There is no specific treatment for bocavirus infection. The role of human bocaviruses in childhood gastroenteritis remains to be established.

222 Human Papillomavirus Infections

Aaron C. Ermel, Darron R. Brown

Investigation of human papillomavirus (HPV) infection began in earnest in the 1980s after Harold zur Hausen postulated that infection with these viruses was associated with cervical cancer. It is now recognized that HPV infection of the human genital tract is extremely common and causes clinical states ranging from asymptomatic infection to genital warts (*condylomata acuminata*); dysplastic lesions or invasive cancers of the anus, penis, vulva, vagina, and cervix; and a subset of oropharyngeal cancers. This chapter describes the epidemiology of HPV in general and as a pathogen, the natural history of HPV infections and associated cancers, strategies to prevent HPV infection and HPV-associated disease, and treatment modalities.

PATHOGENESIS

Molecular Overview HPV is an icosahedral, nonenveloped, 8000-base-pair, double-stranded DNA virus with a diameter of 55 nm. Like those of other papillomaviruses, HPV's genome consists of an early (E) gene region, a late (L) gene region, and a noncoding region that contains regulatory elements. The E1, E2, E5, E6, and E7 proteins are expressed early in the growth cycle and are necessary for viral replication and cellular transformation. The E6 and E7 proteins cause malignant transformation by targeting the human cell cycle–regulatory molecules p53 and Rb (retinoblastoma protein), respectively, for degradation. Translation of the L1 and L2 transcripts and splicing of an E1^E4 transcript occur later. The L1 gene encodes the 54-kDa major capsid protein that makes up the majority of the virus shell; the 77-kDa L2 minor protein constitutes a smaller percentage of the capsid mass.

More than 125 HPV types have been identified and are numerically designated according to a unique L1 gene sequence. Approximately 40 HPV types are regularly found in the anogenital tract and are subdivided into high-risk and low-risk categories on the basis of the associated risk of cervical cancer. For example, HPV-6 and HPV-11 cause genital warts and ~10% of low-grade cervical lesions and are thus designated low risk. HPV-16 and HPV-18 cause dysplastic lesions and invasive cancers of the cervix and are considered high risk.

HPV targets basal keratinocytes after microtrauma has exposed these cells to the virus. The HPV replication cycle is completed as keratinocytes undergo differentiation. Virions are assembled in the nuclei of differentiated keratinocytes and can be detected by electron microscopy. Infection is transmitted by contact with virus contained in these desquamated keratinocytes (or with free virus) from an infected individual.

Immune Response to HPV Infection A cell-mediated immune response plays an important role in controlling the progression of natural HPV infection. Histologic examination of lesions in individuals who experience regression of genital warts demonstrates infiltration of T cells and macrophages. CD4+ T cell regulation is particularly important in controlling HPV infections, as evidenced by the higher rates of infection and disease among immunosuppressed individuals, particularly those who are infected with HIV. Specific T-cell responses may be measured against HPV proteins, the most important of which appear to be the E2 and E6 proteins. In women with HPV-16 cervical infection, a strong T-cell response to HPV-16-derived E2 protein is associated with a lack of progression of cervical disease.

Natural HPV infection of the genital tract gives rise to a serum antibody response in only 60–70% of individuals because there is no viremic phase during infection. Significant, although incomplete, protection against type-specific reinfection is associated with the presence of neutralizing antibodies. Serum antibodies likely reach the cervical epithelium and secretions by transudation and exudation. Therefore, protection against infection is related to the amount of neutralizing antibody at the site of infection and lasts as long as levels of neutralizing antibodies are sufficient.

EPIDEMIOLOGY AND NATURAL HISTORY OF HPV-ASSOCIATED MALIGNANCY

General Population HPV is transmitted by sexual intercourse, by oral sex, and possibly by touching of a partner's genitalia. In cross-sectional and longitudinal studies, ~40% of young women have evidence of HPV infection, with peaks during the teens and early twenties—soon after first coitus. The number of lifetime sexual partners correlates with the likelihood of HPV infection and the subsequent risk of HPV-associated malignancy. HPV infection may develop in a monogamous person whose partner is infected. Most HPV infections become undetectable after 6–9 months. However, with prolonged follow-up and frequent sampling, the same HPV types may again be detected weeks or months after becoming undetectable. Whether such episodic detection indicates viral latency followed by reactivation or reinfection with an identical HPV type is still debated.

Although HPV is the causative agent of several cancers, most attention has focused on cervical cancer—the second most common cancer among women worldwide, which affects more than 500,000 women and kills more than 275,000 women annually. More than 85% of all cervical cancer cases and deaths occur in women living in low-income countries, especially in sub-Saharan Africa, Asia, and South and Central America. A quarter-century of evidence shows that HPV causes nearly 100% of cervical cancers. HPV infection is the most significant risk factor for cervical cancer; relative risks range from 10 to 20 and exceed 100 in prospective and case-control studies, respectively. The time from HPV infection to cervical cancer diagnosis may exceed 20 years. Cervical cancer peaks in the fifth and sixth decades of life among women living in developed countries but as much as a decade earlier among women living in resource-poor countries. Persistent carriers of oncogenic HPV types are at greatest risk for high-grade cervical dysplasia and cancer. Why only certain HPV infections eventually lead to malignancy is not clear. Biomarkers that can predict which women will develop cervical cancer are not available. Immunosuppression in general plays a significant role in re-detection/reactivation of HPV infections, while other factors such as smoking, hormonal changes, *Chlamydia* infection, and nutritional deficits promote viral persistence and cancer.

The International Agency for Research on Cancer concludes that HPV types 16, 18, 31, 33, 35, 39, 45, 51, 52, 56, 58, and 59 are carcinogenic in the uterine cervix. HPV-16 is particularly virulent and causes 50% of cervical cancers. Worldwide, HPV-16 and HPV-18 cause 70% of cervical squamous cell carcinomas and 85% of cervical adenocarcinomas. Oncogenic types other than HPV-16 and HPV-18 cause the remaining 30% of cervical cancers. HPV-16 and HPV-18 also cause nearly 90% of anal cancers worldwide. Although oncogenic HPV infection is necessary for the development of cervical malignancy, only ~3–5% of infected women will ever develop this cancer, even in the absence of cytologic screening.

In addition to cervical and anal cancer, other HPV-associated cancers include vulvar and vaginal cancer, which are associated with HPV in 50–70% of cases; penile cancer, which is caused by HPV in 50% of cases; and oropharyngeal squamous cell carcinoma (OPSCC). Over the past two decades, an epidemic of OPSCC related to oncogenic infection with HPV (primarily HPV-16) has developed. Annual rates of OPSCC among men in the United States have been increasing from a low of 0.27 case/100,000 in 1973 to 0.57 case/100,000 as of 2004; rates in women have remained relatively stable at ~0.17 case/100,000 per year. The increase in the incidence of OPSCC is greatest among white men 40–50 years of age. Nearly 14,000 new cases were diagnosed in the United States in 2013. Annual rates of OPSCCs of the base of the tongue and the tonsil have increased dramatically—i.e., by 1.3% and 0.6%, respectively. Fewer data are available from developing countries about OPSCCs.

Effects of HIV on HPV-Associated Disease HIV infection accelerates the natural progression of HPV infections. HIV-infected persons are more likely than other individuals to develop genital warts and to have lesions that are more recalcitrant to treatment. HIV infection has been consistently associated with precancerous cervical lesions, including low-grade cervical intraepithelial neoplasia (CIN) and CIN 3, the immediate precursor to cervical cancer. Women with HIV/AIDS have significantly higher rates of cervical cancer and of subsets of some vulvar, vaginal, and oropharyngeal tumors than women in the general population. Studies indicate a direct relation between low CD4+ T lymphocyte counts and the risk of cervical cancer. Some studies show a reduced likelihood of HPV infection and precancerous lesions of the cervix in HIV-infected women receiving antiretroviral therapy (ART). The incidence of cervical cancer among HIV-infected women has not changed significantly since ART was introduced, possibly because of preexisting oncogenic HPV infections.

The burden of HPV-related cancers is expected to increase in HIV-infected patients, given the prolonged life expectancies made possible by ART. For women living in developing countries where cervical cancer screening is not widely available, this situation may have significant consequences. Thus, elucidating the interactions of HIV infection and cervical cancer with cofactors such as diet, other sexually transmitted infections, and environmental exposures is a research focus with potentially enormous implications for women living in low- and middle-income countries.

Similar to that of cervical cancer, the incidence of anal cancer is strongly influenced by HIV infection. HIV-infected men who have sex with men (MSM) and HIV-infected women have much higher rates of anal cancer than HIV-uninfected populations. Specifically, the incidence has been found to be as high as 130 cases/100,000 among HIV-positive MSM as opposed to only 5 cases/100,000 among HIV-negative MSM. The advent of ART has not impacted the incidence of anal cancer and high-grade anal intraepithelial neoplasia in the HIV-infected population.

More information on screening, prevention, and treatment in the HIV-infected population can be found at the Department of Health and Human Services website (*aidsinfo.nih.gov/guidelines*).

CLINICAL MANIFESTATIONS OF HPV INFECTION

HPV infects the female vulva, vagina, and cervix and the male urethra, penis, and scrotum. Perianal, anal, and oropharyngeal infections occur in both genders. Figures 222-1, 222-2, and 222-3 show vulvar, penile, and perianal warts, respectively. Genital warts are caused primarily by HPV-6 or HPV-11; their surface is either smooth or rough. Penile genital warts are usually 2–5 mm in diameter and often occur in groups. A second type of penile lesion, keratotic plaques, is slightly raised above the normal epithelium and has a rough, often pigmented surface. Vulvar warts are soft, whitish papules that either are sessile or have multiple fine, finger-like projections. These lesions are most often located in the introitus and on the labia. In nonmucosal areas, lesions

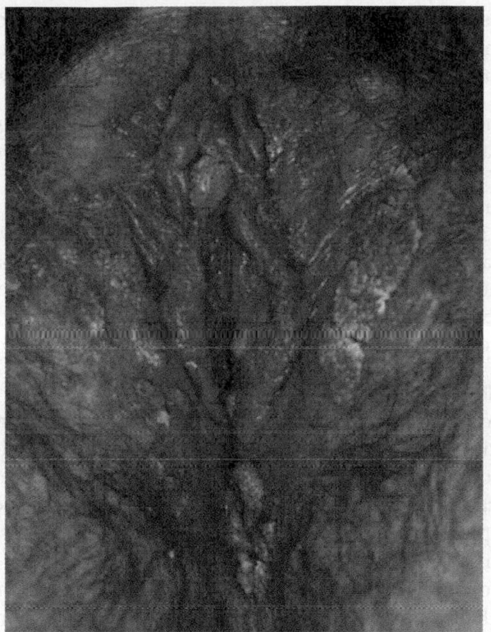

FIGURE 222-1 Vulvar warts. *(Downloaded from http://www2a.cdc.gov/stdtraining/ready-to-use/Manuals/HPV/hpv-slides-2013.pdf.)*

are similar in appearance to those in men: dry and keratotic. Vulvar lesions can appear as smooth, sometimes pigmented papules that may coalesce. Vaginal lesions appear as multiple areas of elongated papillae. Biopsy of vulvar or vaginal lesions may reveal malignancy, which is not always reliably identified by clinical examination.

Subclinical cervical HPV infections are common, and the cervix may appear normal on examination. Cervical lesions often appear as papillary proliferations near the transformation zone. Irregular vascular loops are present beneath the surface epithelium. Patients who develop cervical cancer arising from HPV infection may present with a variety of symptoms. Early carcinomas appear eroded and bleed easily. More advanced carcinomas present as ulcerated lesions or as an exophytic cervical mass. Some cervical carcinomas are located in the cervical canal and may be difficult to see. Bleeding, symptoms of a mass lesion in late stages, and metastatic disease that may manifest as bowel or bladder obstruction due to direct extension of the tumor have also been described.

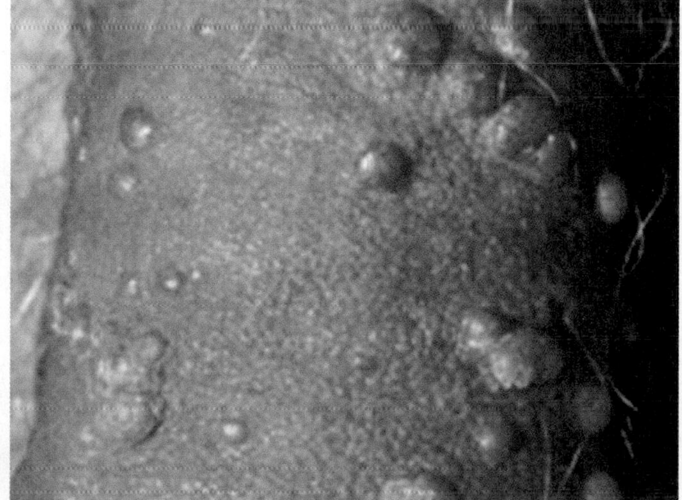

FIGURE 222-2 Condyloma acuminata of the shaft of the penis.

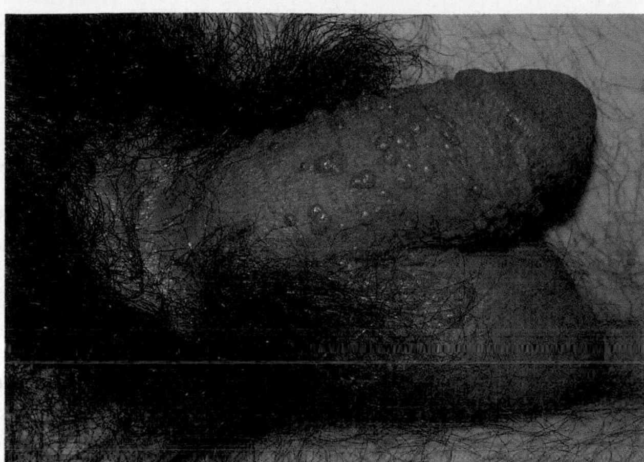

FIGURE 222-3 Perianal warts. *(Reprinted from K Wolff, RA Johnson, AP Saavedra: Fitzpatrick's Color Atlas & Synopsis of Clinical Dermatology, 7th ed. New York, McGraw-Hill, 2013.)*

Patients with squamous cell cancer of the anus have more variable presentations. The most common presentations include rectal bleeding and pain or a mass sensation. Of patients who are diagnosed with anal cancer, 20% may present with no specific symptoms at the time of diagnosis; rather, the lesion is found fortuitously.

PREVENTION OF HPV INFECTION: HPV VACCINES

Vaccines effective in preventing HPV infection and HPV-associated disease represent a major development in the last decade. The vaccines use virus-like particles (VLPs) that consist of the HPV L1 major capsid protein. The L1 protein self-assembles into VLPs when expressed in eukaryotic cells (i.e., yeast for the Merck vaccine or insect cells for the GlaxoSmithKline vaccine; see below). These VLPs contain the same epitopes as the HPV virion. However, they do not contain genetic material and cannot transmit infection. The immunogenicity of HPV vaccines relies on the development of conformational neutralizing antibodies to epitopes displayed on viral capsids.

Several large trials have demonstrated the high degree of safety and efficacy of HPV vaccines. The evidence to date has shown high and sustained efficacy against disease caused by those HPV types represented in the vaccines (HPV-6, -11, -16, and -18 in the Merck vaccine and HPV-16 and -18 in the GlaxoSmithKline vaccine). However, no therapeutic effect against active infection or disease has been found for either vaccine.

Bivalent Vaccine (Cervarix) A bivalent L1 VLP vaccine (HPV-16 and -18), marketed under the name Cervarix (GlaxoSmithKline), is administered by IM injection at months 0, 1, and 6. This vaccine was tested in 18,644 women 15–25 years of age who were residing in the United States, South America, Europe, and Asia. The primary endpoints of the study included vaccine efficacy against persistent infections with HPV-16 and -18. Investigators also assessed the vaccine's efficacy against CIN of grade 2 or higher due to HPV-16 and -18 in women who had no evidence of infection with these HPV types at baseline; in these women, vaccine efficacy was 94.9% (95% confidence interval [CI], 87.7 to 98.4) against CIN ≥2 related to HPV-16 or HPV-18, 91.7% (95% CI, 66.6 to 99.1) against CIN ≥3, and 100% (95% CI, –8.6 to 100) against adenocarcinoma in situ.

Adverse events were evaluated in phase 3 trials in a subset of 3077 women who received the bivalent vaccine and 3080 women (controls) who received hepatitis A vaccine. Injection-site adverse events (pain, redness, and swelling) and systemic adverse events (fatigue, headache, and myalgia) were reported more frequently in the HPV vaccine group than in the control group. Serious adverse events (mainly injection-site reactions), new-onset chronic disease, or medically significant conditions occurred in 3.5% of HPV vaccine recipients and in 3.5% of women receiving the control vaccine.

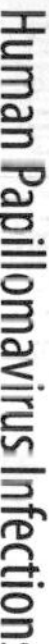

The bivalent vaccine is approved in the United States for prevention of cervical cancer, CIN ≥2, adenocarcinoma in situ, and CIN 1 caused by HPV-16 and -18. This vaccine is approved for administration to girls and women 9–25 years of age.

Quadrivalent Vaccine (Gardasil) A quadrivalent L1 VLP (HPV-6, -11, -16, and -18) vaccine, marketed under the name Gardasil (Merck), is administered IM at months 0, 2, and 6. A combined efficacy analysis based on data from four randomized double-blind clinical studies including more than 20,000 participants demonstrated that the vaccine's efficacy against external genital warts was 98.9% (95% CI, 93.7 to 100). Its efficacy was 95.2% (95% CI, 87.2 to 98.7) in protecting against CIN, 100% (95% CI, 92.9 to 100) against HPV-16- or HPV-18-related CIN 2/3 or adenocarcinoma in situ, and 100% (95% CI, 55.5 to 100.0) against HPV-16- or HPV-18-related vulvar intraepithelial neoplasia grades 2 and 3 (VIN 2/3) and vaginal intraepithelial neoplasia grades 2 and 3 (VaIN 2/3).

Safety data on the quadrivalent HPV vaccine are available from seven clinical trials including nearly 12,000 girls and women 9–26 years of age who received the vaccine and ~10,000 who received placebo. A larger proportion of young women reported injection-site adverse events in the vaccine groups than in the aluminum-containing or saline placebo groups. Systemic adverse events were reported by similar proportions of vaccine and placebo recipients and were described as mild or moderate by most participants. The types of serious adverse events reported were similar for the two groups. Ten persons who received the quadrivalent vaccine and seven persons who received placebo died during the course of the trials; no deaths were considered to be vaccine related.

During the course of the quadrivalent vaccine trials, surveillance data on the development of new medical conditions were collected for up to 4 years after vaccination. No statistically significant differences in the incidence of any medical conditions between vaccine and placebo recipients were found; this result indicated a very good safety profile. A recent safety review by the U.S. Food and Drug Administration and the Centers for Disease Control and Prevention (CDC) examined events related to Gardasil that had been reported to the Vaccine Adverse Events Reporting System. Adverse events were consistent with those seen in previous safety studies of the vaccine. It is noteworthy that rates of syncope and venous thrombotic events were higher with Gardasil than those that have usually been documented for other vaccines.

The quadrivalent vaccine is approved for (1) vaccination of girls and women 9–26 years of age to prevent genital warts and cervical cancer caused by HPV-6, -11, -16, and -18; (2) vaccination of the same population to prevent precancerous or dysplastic lesions, including cervical adenocarcinoma in situ, CIN 2/3, VIN 2/3, VaIN 2/3, and CIN 1; (3) vaccination of boys and men 9–26 years of age to prevent genital warts caused by HPV-6 and -11; and (4) vaccination of individuals 9–26 years of age to prevent anal cancer and associated precancerous lesions due to HPV-6, -11, -16, and -18.

Cross-Protection of HPV Vaccines Women vaccinated with either of the available vaccines produce neutralizing antibodies against types related to HPV-16 or -18. Analyses of data from clinical trials suggest that both vaccines may offer cross-protection against nonvaccine types. The bivalent vaccine appears more efficacious against HPV-31, -33, and -45 than the quadrivalent vaccine, but differences in study design make direct comparisons difficult. In addition, vaccine efficacy against persistent infections with HPV-31 and -45 appeared to wane over time in the bivalent vaccine trials, whereas efficacy against persistent infection with HPV-16 or -18 remained stable.

Second-Generation Vaccines While HPV-16 and -18 cause the majority of cervical cancers worldwide, global data have shown that HPV-31, -33, -35, -45, -52, and -58 are the next most frequently detected types in invasive cervical cancers. Second-generation vaccines that are in development incorporate VLPs of additional oncogenic HPV types (other than HPV-16 and -18), including HPV-31, -33, -45, -52, and -58; efficacy studies are ongoing. If vaccines with these five additional oncogenic types prove to be effective, mathematical models estimate that the level of protection could be raised to 90% of all squamous cell cervical cancers worldwide.

Recommendations for Vaccination The CDC's Advisory Committee for Immunization Practice recommends administration of the quadrivalent HPV vaccine—with the schedule used in the vaccine trials—to all boys and girls 11–12 years of age as well as to boys/men and girls/women 13–26 years of age who have not previously been vaccinated or who have not completed the full series. For women, Papanicolaou (Pap) smear testing and screening for HPV DNA are not recommended before vaccination. After vaccination, Pap testing is recommended to detect disease caused by other oncogenic HPV types.

PREVENTION OF HPV-ASSOCIATED DISEASE

After HPV infection occurs, prevention of HPV-associated disease relies on screening. Women residing in developing countries who lack access to cervical screening programs have a higher rate of cervical cancer and a lower rate of cancer-specific survival. Approximately 75% of women living in developed countries have been screened in the past 5 years, whereas the figure is only ~5% among women living in developing countries. Economic and logistic obstacles likely impede routine screening of these populations for cervical cancer.

The primary method used for cancer screening is cervical cytology via Pap smear. The guidelines of the American Society of Colposcopy and Cervical Pathology recommend initiation of cervical cancer screening at age 21, regardless of the age of sexual debut. Women 21–29 years old with a normal Pap smear should have the test repeated every 3 years. Although adolescent and young women often test positive for HPV DNA, they are at very low risk of cervical cancer. Co-testing, or testing for HPV DNA at the time of the Pap smear, is not recommended for women in this age group because the presence of HPV DNA does not correlate with the presence of high-grade squamous intraepithelial neoplasia. Women 30–65 years of age should have a Pap smear every 3 years if testing for HPV DNA is not performed. The screening interval for women in this age group can be extended to every 5 years if co-testing results are negative. HPV testing is not recommended for partners of women with HPV or for screening for conditions other than cervical cancer.

Currently, there is no clear consensus regarding screening for anal cancer and its precursors, including high-grade anal intraepithelial lesions. This lack of clarity is due to an inadequate understanding of optimal treatment for low- or high-grade anal dysplasia found during cytologic screening. The current HIV treatment guidelines suggest that there may be a benefit to screening, but an effect on the associated morbidity and mortality of anal squamous cell cancer has not been consistently demonstrated.

TREATMENT HPV-ASSOCIATED LESIONS

OVERVIEW AND GENERAL RECOMMENDATIONS

A variety of treatment modalities are available for various HPV infections, but none has been proven to eliminate HPV from tissue adjacent to the destroyed and infected tissue. Treatment efficacies are limited by frequent recurrences (presumably due to reinfection acquired from an infected partner), reactivation of latent virus, or autoinoculation from nearby infected cells. The goals of treatment include prevention of virus transmission, eradication of premalignant lesions, and reduction of symptoms.

Treatment is generally successful in eliminating visible lesions and grossly diseased tissue. Different therapies are indicated for genital warts, vaginal and cervical disease, and perianal and anal disease.

An optimal therapy for HPV-related genital tract disease that combines high efficacy, low toxicity, low cost, and low recurrence rate is not available. For genital warts of the penis or vulva, cryotherapy (see below) is safest, least expensive, and most effective. Guidelines for the treatment of genital warts can be found on the CDC website (*www.cdc.gov/std/treatment/2010/genital-warts.htm*). Women with vaginal lesions should be referred to a gynecologist experienced in colposcopy and treatment of these lesions. Treatment of cervical disease involves careful inspection, biopsy, and histopathologic grading to determine the severity and extent of disease. Women with evidence of cervical HPV infection should be referred to a gynecologist familiar with HPV and experienced in colposcopy. Optimal follow-up of these patients includes colposcopic examination of the cervix and vagina on a yearly basis. Guidelines from the American College of Gynecology and Obstetrics are available for the treatment of cervical dysplasia and cancer.

For anal or perianal lesions, cryotherapy or surgical removal is safest and most effective. Anoscopy and/or sigmoidoscopy should be performed when patients have perianal lesions, and suspicious lesions should be biopsied to rule out malignancy.

THERAPEUTIC OPTIONS

Tables 222-1 and 222-2 list the available patient-administered and physician-administered treatments, respectively.

Podophyllotoxin Podophyllotoxin (0.05% solution or gel and 0.15% cream) induces necrosis of genital wart tissue that heals within a few days. It is relatively effective and can be self-administered. Podophyllotoxin is applied twice daily on three consecutive days of the week for a maximum of 4 weeks. Adverse effects are common and include pain, inflammation, erosion, and burning or itching. Podophyllotoxin should not be used to treat vaginal, cervical, or anal lesions. The safety of podophyllotoxin during pregnancy has not been established.

Sinecatechins Sinecatechins (15% ointment) is used to treat genital warts but should not be used to treat vaginal, cervical, or anal lesions. Sinecatechins causes an inflammatory response when applied topically three times a day for up to 4 months. Clearance rates approach 60% in some studies, and recurrence rates are 6–9%. Adverse effects (redness, burning, itching, and pain at the site of application) are generally mild. The safety of sinecatechins during pregnancy is unknown.

Imiquimod Imiquimod (5% or 3.75% cream) is a patient-applied topical immunomodulatory agent thought to activate immune cells by binding to a Toll-like receptor—an event that leads to an inflammatory response. Imiquimod 5% cream is applied to genital warts at bedtime three times per week for up to 16 weeks. Warts are cleared in ~56% of patients, more often in women than in men; recurrence rates approach 13%. Local inflammatory side effects are common. Rates of clearance of genital warts with the 3.75% formulation are not as high, but the duration of treatment is shorter (i.e., daily application for a maximum of 8 weeks), and fewer local and systemic adverse reactions occur. Imiquimod should not be used to treat vaginal, cervical, or anal lesions. The safety of imiquimod during pregnancy has not been established.

Cryotherapy Cryotherapy (liquid nitrogen) for HPV-associated lesions causes cellular death. Genital warts usually disappear after two or three weekly sessions but often recur. Cryotherapy, which is nontoxic and is not associated with significant adverse reactions, can also be used for diseased cervical tissue. Local pain occurs frequently.

Surgical Methods Exophytic lesions can be surgically removed after intradermal injection of 1% lidocaine. This treatment is well tolerated but can cause scarring and requires hemostasis. Genital warts can also be destroyed by electrocautery, in which no additional hemostasis is required.

Laser Therapy Laser treatment affords destruction of exophytic lesions and other HPV-infected tissue while preserving normal tissue. Local anesthetics are generally adequate. Efficacy for genital lesions is at least equal to that of other therapies (60–90%), with low recurrence rates (5–10%). Complications include local pain, vaginal discharge, periurethral swelling, and penile or vulvar swelling. Laser therapy has also been used successfully to treat cervical dysplasia and anal disease caused by HPV.

Interferon (IFN) Recombinant IFN-α is used for intralesional treatment of genital warts, including perianal lesions. The recommended dosage is 1.0×10^6 IU of IFN injected into each lesion three times weekly for 3 weeks. IFN therapy causes clearance of infected cells by immune-boosting effects. Adverse events include headache, nausea, vomiting, fatigue, and myalgia. IFN therapy is costly and should be reserved for severe cases that do not respond to cheaper treatments. IFN should not be used to treat vaginal, cervical, or anal lesions.

Other Therapies Both trichloroacetic acid and bichloroacetic acid are caustic agents that destroy warts by coagulation of proteins. Neither of these agents is recommended for treatment.

TABLE 222-1 RECOMMENDED TREATMENTS THAT CAN BE SELF-ADMINISTERED FOR GENITAL WARTS

Variable	Podophyllotoxin	Sinecatechins	Imiquimod
Effectiveness	Good	Good	Good
Recurrence	Frequent	Frequent	Frequent
Adverse effects	Frequent, can be severe	Frequent, mild	Frequent, mild to moderate
Availability	Good	Fair	Fair
Cost	Inexpensive	Inexpensive	Expensive

TABLE 222-2 RECOMMENDED TREATMENTS THAT MUST BE ADMINISTERED BY A CLINICIAN FOR GENITAL WARTS AND OTHER HUMAN PAPILLOMAVIRUS–ASSOCIATED LESIONS

Variable	Cryotherapy	Surgical Removal	Laser	Interferon
Effectiveness	Good	Excellent	Excellent	Good
Recurrence	Frequent	Frequent	Frequent	Frequent
Adverse effects	Mild, well tolerated	Mild, well tolerated	Mild to moderate, well tolerated	Frequent, moderately severe
Availability	Good	Good	Fair	Fair
Cost	Inexpensive	Moderately expensive	Very expensive	Very expensive

COUNSELING

Most sexually active adults will be infected with HPV during their lives. For all patients (vaccinated or unvaccinated), certain behavioral interventions can reduce the risk of acquiring HPV. Physicians can provide their patients with measures that can reduce this risk. The only way to avoid acquiring an HPV infection is to abstain from sexual activity, including intimate touching and oral sex. Practicing safe sex (partner reduction, condom use) may lower the likelihood of HPV transmission. Most HPV infections are controlled by the immune system and cause no symptoms or disease. Some infections lead to genital warts and cervical precancers. Genital warts can be treated for cosmetic reasons and to prevent spread of infection to others. Even after resolution of genital warts, latent virus can persist in normal-appearing skin or mucosa and thus theoretically can be transmitted to uninfected partners. Precancerous cervical lesions should be treated to prevent progression to cancer.

223 Common Viral Respiratory Infections

Raphael Dolin

GENERAL CONSIDERATIONS

Acute viral respiratory illnesses are among the most common of human diseases, accounting for one-half or more of all acute illnesses. The incidence of acute respiratory disease in the United States is 3–5.6 cases per person per year. The rates are highest among children <1 year old (6.1–8.3 cases per year) and remain high until age 6, when a progressive decrease begins. Adults have 3–4 cases per person per year. Morbidity from acute respiratory illnesses accounts for 30–50% of time lost from work by adults and for 60–80% of time lost from school by children. The use of antibacterial agents to treat viral respiratory infections represents a major source of abuse of that category of drugs.

It has been estimated that two-thirds to three-fourths of cases of acute respiratory illness are caused by viruses. More than 200 antigenically distinct viruses from 10 genera have been reported to cause acute respiratory illness, and it is likely that additional agents will be described in the future. The vast majority of these viral infections involve the upper respiratory tract, but lower respiratory tract disease can also develop, particularly in younger age groups, in the elderly, and in certain epidemiologic settings.

The illnesses caused by respiratory viruses traditionally have been divided into multiple distinct syndromes, such as the "common cold," pharyngitis, croup (laryngotracheobronchitis), tracheitis, bronchiolitis, bronchitis, and pneumonia. Each of these general categories of illness has a certain epidemiologic and clinical profile; for example, croup occurs exclusively in very young children and has a characteristic clinical course. Some types of respiratory illness are more likely to be associated with certain viruses (e.g., the common cold with rhinoviruses), whereas others occupy characteristic epidemiologic niches (e.g., adenovirus infections in military recruits). The syndromes most commonly associated with infections with the major respiratory virus groups are summarized in Table 223-1. Most respiratory viruses clearly have the potential to cause more than one type of respiratory illness, and features of several types of illness may be found in the same patient. Moreover, the clinical illnesses induced by these viruses are rarely sufficiently distinctive to permit an etiologic diagnosis on clinical grounds alone, although the epidemiologic setting increases the likelihood that one group of viruses rather than another is involved. In general, laboratory methods must be relied on to establish a specific viral diagnosis.

This chapter reviews viral infections caused by six of the major groups of respiratory viruses: rhinoviruses, coronaviruses, respiratory syncytial viruses, metapneumoviruses, parainfluenza viruses, and adenoviruses. The extraordinary outbreaks of lower respiratory tract disease associated with coronaviruses (severe acute respiratory syndrome [SARS] in 2002–2003 and Middle East respiratory syndrome [MERS] in 2012–2013) are also discussed. Influenza viruses, which are a major cause of death as well as morbidity, are reviewed in Chap. 224. Herpesviruses, which occasionally cause pharyngitis and which also cause lower respiratory tract disease in immunosuppressed patients, are reviewed in Chap. 216. Enteroviruses, which account for occasional respiratory illnesses during the summer months, are reviewed in Chap. 228.

RHINOVIRUS INFECTIONS

ETIOLOGIC AGENT

Rhinoviruses are members of the Picornaviridae family—small (15- to 30-nm) nonenveloped viruses that contain a single-stranded RNA genome. Human rhinoviruses were first classified by immunologic serotype and are now divided into three genetic species: HRV-A, HRV-B, and HRV-C. The 102 serotypes described initially are encompassed by HRV-A and HRV-B species, whereas HRV-C encompasses more than 60 previously unrecognized serotypes. In contrast to other members of the picornavirus family, such as enteroviruses, rhinoviruses are acid-labile and are almost completely inactivated at pH ≤3. HRV-A and HRV-B species grow preferentially at 33°–34°C (the temperature of the human nasal passages) rather

TABLE 223-1 ILLNESSES ASSOCIATED WITH RESPIRATORY VIRUSES

	Frequency of Respiratory Syndromes		
Virus	**Most Frequent**	**Occasional**	**Infrequent**
Rhinoviruses	Common cold	Exacerbation of chronic bronchitis and asthma	Pneumonia in children
Coronaviruses[a,b]	Common cold	Exacerbation of chronic bronchitis and asthma	Pneumonia and bronchiolitis
Human respiratory syncytial virus	Pneumonia and bronchiolitis in young children	Common cold in adults	Pneumonia in elderly and immunosuppressed patients
Parainfluenza viruses	Croup and lower respiratory tract disease in young children	Pharyngitis and common cold	Tracheobronchitis in adults; lower respiratory tract disease in immunosuppressed patients
Adenoviruses	Common cold and pharyngitis in children	Outbreaks of acute respiratory disease in military recruits[c]	Pneumonia in children; lower respiratory tract and disseminated disease in immunosuppressed patients
Influenza A viruses	Influenza[d]	Pneumonia and excess mortality in high-risk patients	Pneumonia in healthy individuals
Influenza B viruses	Influenza[d]	Rhinitis or pharyngitis alone	Pneumonia
Enteroviruses	Acute undifferentiated febrile illnesses[e]	Rhinitis or pharyngitis alone	Pneumonia
Herpes simplex viruses	Gingivostomatitis in children; pharyngotonsillitis in adults	Tracheitis and pneumonia in immunocompromised patients	Disseminated infection in immunocompromised patients
Human metapneumoviruses	Upper and lower respiratory tract disease in children	Upper respiratory tract illness in adults	Pneumonia in elderly and immunosuppressed patients

[a]Severe acute respiratory syndrome–associated coronavirus (SARS-CoV) caused epidemics of pneumonia from November 2002 to July 2003 (see text). [b]Middle East respiratory syndrome coronavirus (MERS-CoV) has caused severe respiratory illnesses from 2012 to the time of this writing (2014); see text. [c]Serotypes 4 and 7 most commonly; also serotypes 14 and 21. [d]Fever, cough, myalgia, malaise. [e]May or may not have a respiratory component.

than at 37°C (the temperature of the lower respiratory tract), whereas HRV-C viruses replicate well at either temperature. Of the 101 initially recognized serotypes of rhinovirus, 88 use intercellular adhesion molecule 1 (ICAM-1) as a cellular receptor and constitute the "major" receptor group, 12 use the low-density lipoprotein receptor (LDLR) and constitute the "minor" receptor group, and 1 uses decay-accelerating factor.

EPIDEMIOLOGY

Rhinovirus infections are worldwide in distribution. They are a prominent cause of the common cold and have been detected in up to 50% of common cold–like illnesses by tissue culture and polymerase chain reaction (PCR) techniques. Overall rates of rhinovirus infection are higher among infants and young children and decrease with increasing age. Rhinovirus infections occur throughout the year, with seasonal peaks in early fall and spring in temperate climates. These infections are most often introduced into families by preschool or grade-school children <6 years old. Of initial illnesses in family settings, 25–70% are followed by secondary cases, with the highest attack rates among the youngest siblings at home. Attack rates also increase with family size.

Rhinoviruses appear to spread through direct contact with infected secretions, usually respiratory droplets. In some studies of volunteers, transmission was most efficient by hand-to-hand contact, with subsequent self-inoculation of the conjunctival or nasal mucosa. Other studies demonstrated transmission by large- or small-particle aerosol. Virus can be recovered from plastic surfaces inoculated 1–3 h previously; this observation suggests that environmental surfaces contribute to transmission. In studies of married couples in which neither partner had detectable serum antibody, transmission was associated with prolonged contact (≥122 h) during a 7-day period. Transmission was infrequent unless (1) virus was recoverable from the donor's hands and nasal mucosa, (2) at least 1000 $TCID_{50}$ (50% tissue culture infectious dose) of virus was present in nasal washes from the donor, and (3) the donor was at least moderately symptomatic with the "cold." Despite anecdotal observations, exposure to cold temperatures, fatigue, and sleep deprivation have not been associated with increased rates of rhinovirus-induced illness in volunteers, although some studies have suggested that psychologically defined "stress" may contribute to development of symptoms.

By adulthood, nearly all individuals have neutralizing antibodies to multiple rhinovirus serotypes, although the prevalence of antibody to any one serotype varies widely. Multiple serotypes circulate simultaneously, and generally no single serotype or group of serotypes has been more prevalent than the others.

PATHOGENESIS

Rhinoviruses infect cells through attachment to specific cellular receptors; as mentioned above, most serotypes attach to ICAM-1, while a few use LDLR. Relatively limited information is available on the histopathology and pathogenesis of acute rhinovirus infections in humans. Examination of biopsy specimens obtained during experimentally induced and naturally occurring illness indicates that the nasal mucosa is edematous, is often hyperemic, and—during acute illness—is covered by a mucoid discharge. There is a mild infiltrate with inflammatory cells, including neutrophils, lymphocytes, plasma cells, and eosinophils. Mucus-secreting glands in the submucosa appear hyperactive; the nasal turbinates are engorged, a condition that may lead to obstruction of nearby openings of sinus cavities. Several mediators—e.g., bradykinin; lysylbradykinin; prostaglandins; histamine; interleukins 1β, 6, and 8; interferon γ-induced protein 10; and tumor necrosis factor α—have been linked to the development of signs and symptoms in rhinovirus-induced colds.

The incubation period for rhinovirus illness is short, generally 1–2 days. Virus shedding coincides with the onset of illness or may begin shortly before symptoms develop. The mechanisms of immunity to rhinovirus infection are not well worked out. In some studies, the presence of homotypic antibody has been associated with significantly reduced rates of subsequent infection and illness, but data conflict regarding the relative importance of serum and local antibody in protection from rhinovirus infection.

CLINICAL MANIFESTATIONS

The most common clinical manifestations of rhinovirus infections are those of the common cold. Illness usually begins with rhinorrhea and sneezing accompanied by nasal congestion. The throat is frequently sore, and in some cases sore throat is the initial complaint. Systemic signs and symptoms, such as malaise and headache, are mild or absent, and fever is unusual in adults but may occur in up to one-third of children. Illness generally lasts for 4–9 days and resolves spontaneously without sequelae. In children, bronchitis, bronchiolitis, and bronchopneumonia have been reported; nevertheless, it appears that rhinoviruses are not major causes of lower respiratory tract disease in children. Rhinoviruses may cause exacerbations of asthma and chronic pulmonary disease in adults. The vast majority of rhinovirus infections resolve without sequelae, but complications related to obstruction of the eustachian tubes or sinus ostia, including otitis media or acute sinusitis, can develop. In immunosuppressed patients, particularly bone marrow transplant recipients, severe and even fatal pneumonias have been associated with rhinovirus infections.

DIAGNOSIS

Although rhinoviruses are the most frequently recognized cause of the common cold, similar illnesses are caused by a variety of other viruses, and a specific viral etiologic diagnosis cannot be made on clinical grounds alone. Rather, rhinovirus infection is diagnosed by isolation of the virus from nasal washes or nasal secretions in tissue culture. In practice, this procedure is rarely undertaken because of the benign, self-limited nature of the illness. In most settings, detection of rhinovirus RNA is more sensitive and easier by PCR than by tissue culture. Accordingly, PCR has generally become the standard for detection of rhinoviruses in clinical specimens. Given the many serotypes of rhinovirus, diagnosis by serum antibody tests is currently impractical. Likewise, common laboratory tests, such as white blood cell count and erythrocyte sedimentation rate, are not helpful.

TREATMENT RHINOVIRUS INFECTIONS

Because rhinovirus infections are generally mild and self-limited, treatment is not usually necessary. Therapy in the form of first-generation antihistamines and nonsteroidal anti-inflammatory drugs may be beneficial in patients with particularly pronounced symptoms, and an oral decongestant may be added if nasal obstruction is particularly troublesome. Reduction of activity is prudent in instances of significant discomfort or fatigability. Antibacterial agents should be used only if bacterial complications such as otitis media or sinusitis develop. Specific antiviral therapy is not available.

PREVENTION

Intranasal application of interferon sprays has been effective in the prophylaxis of rhinovirus infections but is also associated with local irritation of the nasal mucosa. Studies of prevention of rhinovirus infection by blocking of ICAM-1 or by binding of drug (pleconaril) to parts of the viral capsid have yielded mixed results. Experimental vaccines to certain rhinovirus serotypes have been generated, but their usefulness is questionable because of the myriad serotypes involved and the uncertainty about mechanisms of immunity. Thorough hand washing, environmental decontamination, and protection against autoinoculation may help to reduce rates of transmission of infection.

CORONAVIRUS INFECTIONS

ETIOLOGIC AGENT

Coronaviruses are pleomorphic, single-stranded RNA viruses that measure 100–160 nm in diameter. The name derives from the crown-like appearance produced by the club-shaped projections that stud the viral envelope. Coronaviruses infect a wide variety of animal species and have been divided into four genera. Coronaviruses that infect humans (HCoVs) fall into two genera: *Alphacoronavirus* and *Betacoronavirus*. Severe acute respiratory syndrome coronavirus (SARS-CoV) and Middle East respiratory syndrome coronavirus (MERS-CoV) are betacoronaviruses.

In general, human coronaviruses have been difficult to cultivate in vitro, and some strains grow only in human tracheal organ cultures rather than in tissue culture. SARS-CoV and MERS-CoV are exceptions whose ready growth in African green monkey kidney (Vero E6) cells greatly facilitates their study.

EPIDEMIOLOGY

Human coronavirus infections are present throughout the world. Seroprevalence studies of strains HCoV-229E and HCoV-OC43 have demonstrated that serum antibodies are acquired early in life and increase in prevalence with advancing age, so that >80% of adult populations have antibodies detectable by enzyme-linked immunosorbent assay (ELISA). Overall, coronaviruses account for 10–35% of common colds, depending on the season. Coronavirus infections appear to be particularly prevalent in late fall, winter, and early spring—times when rhinovirus infections are less common.

An extraordinary outbreak of the coronavirus-associated illness known as SARS occurred in 2002–2003. The outbreak apparently began in southern China and eventually resulted in 8096 recognized cases in 28 countries in Asia, Europe, and North and South America; ~90% of cases occurred in China and Hong Kong. The natural reservoir of SARS-CoV appeared to be the horseshoe bat, and the outbreak may have originated from human contact with infected semidomesticated animals such as the palm civet. In most cases, however, the infection was transmitted from human to human. Case–fatality rates varied among outbreaks, with an overall figure of ~9.5%. The disease appeared to be somewhat milder in cases in the United States and was clearly less severe among children. The outbreak ceased in 2003; 17 cases were detected in 2004, mostly in laboratory-associated settings, and no cases have been reported subsequently.

The mechanisms of transmission of SARS are incompletely understood. Clusters of cases suggest that spread may occur via both large- and small-droplet aerosols and perhaps via the fecal–oral route as well. The outbreak of illness in a large apartment complex in Hong Kong suggested that environmental sources, such as sewage or water, may also play a role in transmission. Some ill individuals ("super-spreaders") appeared to be hyperinfectious and were capable of transmitting infection to 10–40 contacts, although most infections resulted in spread either to no one or to three or fewer individuals.

Since it began in June 2012, another extraordinary outbreak of serious respiratory illness, MERS, has been linked with a coronavirus (MERS-CoV). Through May 2014, a total of 536 cases and 145 deaths (27%) have been reported. All cases have been associated with contact or travel to six countries in or near the Arabian Peninsula: Jordan, Kuwait, Oman, Qatar, Saudi Arabia, and the United Arab Emirates. Cases have also been reported in France, Italy, Tunisia, Germany, Spain, and the United Kingdom. Person-to-person transmission has been documented, but sustained spread in communities has not. The source of MERS-CoV has not been established, but it is suspected that bats may be the animal reservoir and that camels serve as an intermediate host.

PATHOGENESIS

Coronaviruses that cause the common cold (e.g., strains HCoV-229E and HCoV-OC43) infect ciliated epithelial cells in the nasopharynx via the aminopeptidase N receptor (group 1) or a sialic acid receptor (group 2). Viral replication leads to damage of ciliated cells and induction of chemokines and interleukins, with consequent common-cold symptoms similar to those induced by rhinoviruses.

SARS-CoV infects cells of the respiratory tract via the angiotensin-converting enzyme 2 receptor. The result is a systemic illness in which virus is also found in the bloodstream, in the urine, and (for up to 2 months) in the stool. Virus persists in the respiratory tract for 2–3 weeks, and titers peak ~10 days after the onset of systemic illness. Pulmonary pathology consists of hyaline membrane formation, desquamation of pneumocytes in alveolar spaces, and an interstitial infiltrate made up of lymphocytes and mononuclear cells. Giant cells are frequently seen, and coronavirus particles have been detected in type II pneumocytes. Elevated levels of proinflammatory cytokines and chemokines have been detected in sera from patients with SARS.

Because MERS-CoV was so recently detected, little is known at present about its pathogenesis. However, it may well be similar to that of SARS-CoV.

CLINICAL MANIFESTATIONS

After an incubation period that generally lasts 2–7 days (range, 1–14 days), SARS usually begins as a systemic illness marked by the onset of fever, which is often accompanied by malaise, headache, and myalgias and is followed in 1–2 days by a nonproductive cough and dyspnea. Approximately 25% of patients have diarrhea. Chest x-rays can show a variety of infiltrates, including patchy areas of consolidation—most frequently in peripheral and lower lung fields—or interstitial infiltrates, which can progress to diffuse involvement. In severe cases, respiratory function may worsen during the second week of illness and progress to frank adult respiratory distress syndrome accompanied by multiorgan dysfunction. Risk factors for severe disease include an age of >50 years and comorbidities such as cardiovascular disease, diabetes, and hepatitis. Illness in pregnant women may be particularly severe, but SARS-CoV infection appears to be milder in children than in adults.

Information regarding the clinical manifestations of MERS-CoV is limited. The case–fatality rate has been high in the initial cases, but this may represent an ascertainment bias, and it is clear that mild cases occur as well. The median incubation period has been estimated to be 5.2 days, and a secondary case was estimated to have an incubation period of 9–12 days. Cases have been reported that begin with cough and fever and progress to acute respiratory distress and respiratory failure within a week. Other cases have manifested as mild upper respiratory symptoms only. Renal failure has been noted, and DPP-4, the host cell receptor for MERS-CoV, is expressed at high levels in the kidney; these findings suggest that direct viral infection of the kidney may lead to renal dysfunction. Diarrhea and vomiting are also common in MERS, and pericarditis has been reported.

The clinical features of common colds caused by human coronaviruses are similar to those of illness caused by rhinoviruses. In studies of volunteers, the mean incubation period of colds induced by coronaviruses (3 days) is somewhat longer than that of illness caused by rhinoviruses, and the duration of illness is somewhat shorter (mean, 6–7 days). In some studies, the amount of nasal discharge was greater in colds induced by coronaviruses than in those induced by rhinoviruses. Coronaviruses other than SARS-CoV have been recovered occasionally from infants with pneumonia and from military recruits with lower respiratory tract disease and have been associated with worsening of chronic bronchitis. Two novel coronaviruses, HCoV-NL63 and HCoV-HKU1, have been isolated from patients hospitalized with acute respiratory illness. Their overall role as causes of human respiratory disease remains to be determined.

LABORATORY FINDINGS AND DIAGNOSIS

Laboratory abnormalities in SARS include lymphopenia, which is documented in ~50% of cases and which mostly affects CD4+ T cells but also involves CD8+ T cells and natural killer cells. Total white blood cell counts are normal or slightly low, and thrombocytopenia may develop as the illness progresses. Elevated serum levels of aminotransferases, creatine kinase, and lactate dehydrogenase have been reported.

A rapid diagnosis of SARS-CoV infection can be made by reverse-transcription PCR (RT-PCR) of respiratory tract samples and plasma early in the illness and of urine and stool later on. SARS-CoV can also be grown from respiratory tract samples by inoculation into Vero E6 tissue culture cells, in which a cytopathic effect is seen within days. RT-PCR appears to be more sensitive than tissue culture, but only around one-third of cases are positive by PCR at initial presentation. Serum antibodies can be detected by ELISA or immunofluorescence, and nearly all patients develop detectable serum antibodies within 28 days after the onset of illness.

Laboratory abnormalities in MERS-CoV infection include lymphopenia with or without neutropenia, thrombocytopenia, and elevated levels of lactate dehydrogenase. MERS-CoV can be isolated in tissue culture in Vero and LLC-MK2 cells, but PCR techniques are more sensitive and rapid and are the standard for laboratory diagnosis. Serologic tests using ELISA and immunofluorescence techniques have also been developed.

Laboratory diagnosis of coronavirus-induced colds is rarely required. Coronaviruses that cause those illnesses are frequently difficult to cultivate in vitro but can be detected in clinical samples by ELISA or immunofluorescence assays or by RT-PCR for viral RNA. These research procedures can be used to detect coronaviruses in unusual clinical settings.

TREATMENT CORONAVIRUS INFECTIONS

There is no specific therapy for SARS with established efficacy. Although ribavirin has frequently been used, it has little if any activity against SARS-CoV in vitro, and no beneficial effect on the course of illness has been demonstrated. Because of suggestions that immunopathology may contribute to the disease, glucocorticoids have also been widely used, but their benefit, if any, likewise remains to be established. Supportive care to maintain pulmonary and other organ-system functions remains the mainstay of therapy. Similarly, there is no established antiviral therapy for MERS. Interferon α2b and ribavirin have displayed activity against MERS-CoV in vitro and in a rhesus macaque model, but data are not available on its use in human cases of MERS. The approach to the treatment of common colds caused by coronaviruses is similar to that discussed above for rhinovirus-induced illnesses.

PREVENTION

The recognition of SARS led to a worldwide mobilization of public health resources to apply infection control practices to contain the disease. Case definitions were established, travel advisories were proposed, and quarantines were imposed in certain locales. As of this writing, no additional cases of SARS have been reported since 2004. However, it remains unknown whether the disappearance of cases is a result of control measures, whether it is part of a seasonal or otherwise unexplained epidemiologic pattern of SARS, or when or whether SARS might reemerge. The U.S. Centers for Disease Control and Prevention (CDC) and the World Health Organization (WHO) maintain recommendations for surveillance and assessment of potential cases of SARS (*www.cdc.gov/sars/*). The frequent transmission of the disease to health care workers makes it mandatory that strict infection-control practices be employed by health care facilities to prevent airborne, droplet, and contact transmission from any suspected cases of SARS. Health care workers who enter areas in which patients with SARS may be present should don gowns, gloves, and eye and respiratory protective equipment (e.g., an N95 filtering facepiece respirator certified by the National Institute for Occupational Safety and Health).

Similarly, the WHO and the CDC have issued recommendations for identification, prevention, and control of MERS-CoV infections (*www.cdc.gov/coronavirus/mers/index.html*). Isolation precautions against airborne spread of infection should be instituted for patients hospitalized for suspected MERS, as described above for SARS.

Vaccines have been developed against several animal coronaviruses but not against known human coronaviruses. The emergence of SARS-CoV and MERS-CoV has stimulated interest in the development of vaccines against such agents.

HUMAN RESPIRATORY SYNCYTIAL VIRUS INFECTIONS

ETIOLOGIC AGENT

Human respiratory syncytial virus (HRSV) is a member of the Paramyxoviridae family (genus *Pneumovirus*). It is an enveloped virus ~150–350 nm in diameter and is so named because its replication in vitro leads to the fusion of neighboring cells into large multinucleated syncytia. The single-stranded RNA genome codes for 11 virus-specific proteins. Viral RNA is contained in a helical nucleocapsid surrounded by a lipid envelope bearing two glycoproteins: the G protein, by which the virus attaches to cells, and the F (fusion) protein, which facilitates entry of the virus into the cell by fusing host and viral membranes. HRSV is considered to be of a single antigenic type, but two distinct subgroups (A and B) and multiple subtypes within each subgroup have now been described. Antigenic diversity is reflected by differences in the G protein, whereas the F protein is relatively conserved. Both antigenic groups can circulate simultaneously in outbreaks, although there are typically alternating patterns in which one subgroup predominates over 1- to 2-year periods.

EPIDEMIOLOGY

HRSV is a major respiratory pathogen of young children and the foremost cause of lower respiratory disease in infants. Infection with HRSV is seen throughout the world in annual epidemics that occur in late fall, winter, or spring and last up to 5 months. The virus is rarely encountered during the summer. Rates of illness are highest among infants 1–6 months of age, peaking at 2–3 months of age. The attack rates among susceptible infants and children are extraordinarily high, approaching 100% in settings such as day-care centers where large numbers of susceptible infants are present. By age 2, virtually all children will have been infected with HRSV. HRSV accounts for 20–25% of hospital admissions of young infants and children for pneumonia and for up to 75% of cases of bronchiolitis in this age group. It has been estimated that more than half of infants who are at risk will become infected during an HRSV epidemic.

In older children and adults, reinfection with HRSV is frequent, but disease is milder than in infancy. A common cold–like syndrome is the illness most commonly associated with HRSV infection in adults. It has been increasingly appreciated that severe lower respiratory tract disease with pneumonitis can occur in elderly (often institutionalized) adults, in individuals with cardiopulmonary disease, and in patients with immunocompromising disorders or treatment, including recipients of hematopoietic stem cell transplants (HSCTs) and solid-organ transplants (SOTs). HRSV is also an important nosocomial pathogen; during an outbreak, it can infect pediatric patients and up to 25–50% of the staff on pediatric wards. The spread of HRSV among families is efficient: up to 40% of siblings may become infected when the virus is introduced into the family setting.

HRSV is transmitted primarily by close contact with contaminated fingers or fomites and by self-inoculation of the conjunctiva or anterior nares. Virus may also be spread by coarse aerosols produced by coughing or sneezing, but it is inefficiently spread by fine-particle aerosols. The incubation period is ~4–6 days, and virus shedding may last for ≥2 weeks in children and for shorter periods in adults. In immunosuppressed patients, shedding can continue for weeks.

PATHOGENESIS

Little is known about the histopathology of minor HRSV infection. Severe bronchiolitis or pneumonia is characterized by necrosis of the bronchiolar epithelium and a peribronchiolar infiltrate of lymphocytes and mononuclear cells. Interalveolar thickening and filling of alveolar spaces with fluid can also be found. The correlates of protective immunity to HRSV are incompletely understood. Because reinfection occurs frequently and is often associated with illness, the immunity that develops after single episodes of infection clearly is not complete or long-lasting. However, the cumulative effect of multiple reinfections is to temper subsequent disease and to provide some temporary measure of protection against infection. Studies of experimentally induced disease in healthy volunteers indicate that the presence of nasal IgA neutralizing antibody correlates more closely with protection than does the presence of serum antibody. Studies in infants, however, suggest that maternally acquired antibody provides some protection from lower respiratory tract disease, although illness can be severe even in infants who have moderate levels of maternally derived serum antibody. The relatively severe disease observed in immunosuppressed patients and experimental animal models indicates that cell-mediated immunity is an important mechanism of host defense against HRSV. Evidence suggests that major histocompatibility class I–restricted cytotoxic T cells may be particularly important in this regard.

CLINICAL MANIFESTATIONS

HRSV infection leads to a wide spectrum of respiratory illnesses. In infants, 25–40% of infections result in lower respiratory tract involvement, including pneumonia, bronchiolitis, and tracheobronchitis. In this age group, illness begins most frequently with rhinorrhea, low-grade fever, and mild systemic symptoms, often accompanied by cough and wheezing. Most patients recover gradually over 1–2 weeks. In more severe illness, tachypnea and dyspnea develop, and eventually frank hypoxia, cyanosis, and apnea can ensue. Physical examination may reveal diffuse wheezing, rhonchi, and rales. Chest radiography shows hyperexpansion, peribronchial thickening, and variable infiltrates ranging from diffuse interstitial infiltrates to segmental or lobar consolidation. Illness may be particularly severe in children born prematurely and in those with congenital cardiac disease, bronchopulmonary dysplasia, nephrotic syndrome, or immunosuppression. One study documented a 37% mortality rate among infants with HRSV pneumonia and congenital cardiac disease.

In adults, the most common symptoms of HRSV infection are those of the common cold, with rhinorrhea, sore throat, and cough. Illness is occasionally associated with moderate systemic symptoms such as malaise, headache, and fever. HRSV has also been reported to cause lower respiratory tract disease with fever in adults, including severe pneumonia in the elderly—particularly in nursing-home residents, among whom its impact can rival that of influenza. HRSV pneumonia can be a significant cause of morbidity and death among patients undergoing stem cell and solid organ transplantation, in whom case-fatality rates of 20–80% have been reported. Sinusitis, otitis media, and worsening of chronic obstructive and reactive airway disease have also been associated with HRSV infection.

LABORATORY FINDINGS AND DIAGNOSIS

The diagnosis of HRSV infection can be suspected on the basis of a suggestive epidemiologic setting—that is, severe illness among infants during an outbreak of HRSV in the community. Infections in older children and adults cannot be differentiated with certainty from those caused by other respiratory viruses. The specific diagnosis is established by detection of HRSV in respiratory secretions, such as sputum, throat swabs, or nasopharyngeal washes. Virus can be isolated in tissue culture, but this method has been largely supplanted by rapid viral diagnostic techniques consisting of immunofluorescence or ELISA of nasopharyngeal washes, aspirates, and (less satisfactorily) nasopharyngeal swabs. With specimens from children, these techniques have sensitivities and specificities of 80–95%; they are somewhat less sensitive with specimens from adults. RT-PCR detection techniques have shown even higher rates of sensitivity and specificity, particularly in adults. Serologic diagnosis may be made by comparison of acute- and convalescent-phase serum specimens by ELISA or by neutralization or complement-fixation tests. These tests may be useful in older children and adults but are less sensitive in children <4 months of age.

TREATMENT HUMAN RESPIRATORY SYNCYTIAL VIRUS INFECTIONS

Treatment of upper respiratory tract HRSV infection is aimed primarily at the alleviation of symptoms and is similar to that for other viral infections of the upper respiratory tract. For lower respiratory tract infections, respiratory therapy, including hydration, suctioning of secretions, and administration of humidified oxygen and antibronchospastic agents, is given as needed. In severe hypoxia, intubation and ventilatory assistance may be required. Studies of infants with HRSV infection who were given aerosolized ribavirin, a nucleoside analogue active in vitro against HRSV, demonstrated a modest beneficial effect on the resolution of lower respiratory tract illness, including alleviation of blood-gas abnormalities, in some studies. The American Academy of Pediatrics does not recommend routine use of ribavirin but states that treatment with aerosolized ribavirin "may be considered" for infants who are severely ill or who are at high risk for complications of HRSV infection; included are premature infants and those with bronchopulmonary dysplasia, congenital heart disease, or immunosuppression. The efficacy of ribavirin against HRSV pneumonia in older children and adults, including those with immunosuppression, has not been established. No benefit has been found in the treatment of HRSV pneumonia with standard immunoglobulin; immunoglobulin with high titers of antibody to HRSV (RSVIg), which is no longer available; or chimeric mouse–human monoclonal IgG antibody to HRSV (palivizumab). Combined therapy with aerosolized ribavirin and palivizumab is being evaluated in immunosuppressed patients with HRSV pneumonia.

PREVENTION

Monthly administration of RSVIg (no longer available) or palivizumab has been approved as prophylaxis against HRSV for children <2 years of age who have bronchopulmonary dysplasia or cyanotic heart disease or who were born prematurely. Considerable interest exists in the development of vaccines against HRSV. Inactivated whole-virus vaccines have been ineffective; in one study, they actually potentiated disease in infants. Other approaches include immunization with purified F and G surface glycoproteins of HRSV or generation of stable live attenuated virus vaccines. In settings where rates of transmission are high (e.g., pediatric wards), barrier methods for the protection of hands and conjunctivae may be useful in reducing the spread of virus.

HUMAN METAPNEUMOVIRUS INFECTIONS

ETIOLOGIC AGENT

Human metapneumovirus (HMPV) is a viral respiratory pathogen that has been assigned to the Paramyxoviridae family (genus *Metapneumovirus*). Its morphology and genomic organization are similar to those of avian metapneumoviruses, which are recognized respiratory pathogens of turkeys. HMPV particles may be spherical, filamentous, or pleomorphic in shape and measure 150–600 nm in diameter. Particles contain 15-nm projections from the surface that are similar in appearance to those of other Paramyxoviridae. The single-stranded RNA genome codes for nine proteins that, except for the absence of nonstructural proteins, generally correspond to those of HRSV. HMPV is of only one antigenic type; two closely related genotypes (A and B), four subgroups, and two sublineages have been described.

EPIDEMIOLOGY

HMPV infections are worldwide in distribution, are most frequent during the winter in temperate climates, and occur early in life, so that serum antibodies to the virus are present in 50% of children by age 2 and in nearly all children by age 5. HMPV infections have been detected in older age groups, including elderly adults, and in both immunocompetent and immunosuppressed hosts. This virus accounts for 1–5% of childhood upper respiratory tract infections and for 10–15% of respiratory tract illnesses requiring hospitalization of children. In addition, HMPV causes 2–4% of acute respiratory illnesses in ambulatory adults and elderly patients. HMPV has been detected in a few cases of SARS, but its role (if any) in these illnesses has not been established.

CLINICAL MANIFESTATIONS

The spectrum of clinical illnesses associated with HMPV is similar to that associated with HRSV and includes both upper and lower respiratory tract illnesses, such as bronchiolitis, croup, and pneumonia. Reinfection with HMPV is common among older children and adults and has manifestations ranging from subclinical infections to common cold syndromes and occasionally pneumonia, which is seen primarily in elderly patients and those with cardiopulmonary diseases. Serious HMPV infections occur in immunocompromised patients, including those with neoplasia, recipients of HSCTs, and children with HIV infection.

DIAGNOSIS

HMPV can be detected in nasal aspirates and respiratory secretions by immunofluorescence, by PCR (the most sensitive technique), or by growth in rhesus monkey kidney (LLC-MK2) tissue cultures. A serologic diagnosis can be made by ELISA, which uses HMPV-infected tissue culture lysates as sources of antigens.

TREATMENT HUMAN METAPNEUMOVIRUS INFECTIONS

Treatment for HMPV infections is primarily supportive and symptom-based. Ribavirin is active against HMPV in vitro, but its efficacy in vivo is unknown.

PREVENTION

Vaccines against HMPV are in the early stages of development.

PARAINFLUENZA VIRUS INFECTIONS

ETIOLOGIC AGENT

Parainfluenza viruses belong to the Paramyxoviridae family (genera *Respirovirus* and *Rubulavirus*). They are 150–200 nm in diameter, are enveloped, and contain a single-stranded RNA genome. The envelope is studded with two glycoproteins: one possesses both hemagglutinin and neuraminidase activity, and the other contains fusion activity. The viral RNA genome is enclosed in a helical nucleocapsid and codes for six structural and several accessory proteins. All types of parainfluenza virus (1, 2, 3, 4A, and 4B) share certain antigens with other members of the Paramyxoviridae family, including mumps and Newcastle disease viruses.

EPIDEMIOLOGY

Parainfluenza viruses are distributed throughout the world; infection with serotypes 4A and 4B has been reported less widely, probably because these types are more difficult than the other three to grow in tissue culture. Infection is acquired in early childhood; by 5 years of age, most children have antibodies to serotypes 1, 2, and 3. Types 1 and 2 cause epidemics during the fall, often occurring in an alternate-year pattern. Type 3 infection has been detected during all seasons, but epidemics have occurred annually in the spring.

The contribution of parainfluenza infections to respiratory disease varies with both the location and the year. In studies conducted in the United States, parainfluenza virus infections have accounted for 4.3–22% of respiratory illnesses in children. The major importance of these viruses is as a cause of lower respiratory illness in young children, in whom they rank second only to HRSV in that regard. Parainfluenza virus type 1 is the most common cause of croup (laryngotracheobronchitis) in children, whereas serotype 2 causes similar, although generally less severe, disease. Type 3 is an important cause of bronchiolitis and pneumonia in infants, whereas illnesses associated with types 4A and 4B have generally been mild. Unlike types 1 and 2, type 3 frequently causes illness during the first month of life, when passively acquired maternal antibody is still present. Parainfluenza viruses are spread through infected respiratory secretions, primarily by person-to-person contact and/or by large droplets, and by contact with fomites contaminated with respiratory secretions. The incubation period has varied from 3 to 6 days in experimental infections but may be somewhat shorter for naturally occurring disease in children.

In adults, parainfluenza virus infections are generally mild and account for fewer than 10% of respiratory illnesses. The advent of contemporary laboratory methods for diagnosis has increased awareness of the impact of parainfluenza infections in adults. In a recent study, parainfluenza virus was the third most common viral isolate from patients 16–64 years old who required hospitalization (0.7 isolate/1000 population). In the 2009 influenza pandemic, parainfluenza virus type 3 was the second most common cause of illness after influenza virus.

PATHOGENESIS

Immunity to parainfluenza viruses is incompletely understood, but evidence suggests that immunity to infections with serotypes 1 and 2 is mediated by local IgA antibodies in the respiratory tract. Passively acquired serum neutralizing antibodies also confer some protection against infection with types 1, 2, and (to a lesser degree) 3. Studies in experimental animal models and in immunosuppressed patients suggest that T cell–mediated immunity may also be important in parainfluenza virus infections. Lack of cellular immune responses is associated with an increased risk of progressive and fatal disease in HSCT recipients.

CLINICAL MANIFESTATIONS

Parainfluenza virus infections occur most frequently among children, in whom initial infection with serotype 1, 2, or 3 is associated with an acute febrile illness in 50–80% of cases. Children may present with coryza, sore throat, hoarseness, and cough that may or may not be croupy. In severe croup, fever persists, with worsening coryza and sore throat. A brassy or barking cough may progress to frank stridor. Most children recover over the next 1 or 2 days, although progressive airway obstruction and hypoxia ensue occasionally. If bronchiolitis or pneumonia develops, progressive cough accompanied by wheezing, tachypnea, and intercostal retractions may occur. In this setting, sputum production increases modestly. Physical examination documents nasopharyngeal discharge and oropharyngeal injection, along with rhonchi, wheezes, or coarse breath sounds. Chest x-rays can show air trapping and occasionally interstitial infiltrates.

In older children and adults, parainfluenza infections tend to be milder, presenting most frequently as a common cold or as hoarseness, with or without cough. Lower respiratory tract involvement in older children and adults is uncommon, although tracheobronchitis and community-acquired pneumonia have been reported in adults.

Parainfluenza viruses, most frequently type 3, are important pathogens in immunosuppressed patients—particularly in HSCT recipients but also in SOT recipients (especially recipients of lung transplants). Patients receiving cancer chemotherapy are also at risk for severe parainfluenza infection. Severe, prolonged, and even fatal parainfluenza-associated respiratory illnesses have been reported in children and adults with severe immunosuppression.

LABORATORY FINDINGS AND DIAGNOSIS

The clinical syndromes caused by parainfluenza viruses (with the possible exception of croup in young children) are not sufficiently distinctive to be diagnosed on clinical grounds alone. A specific diagnosis is established by detection of virus in respiratory tract secretions, throat swabs, or nasopharyngeal washings. Growth of the virus in tissue culture is detected either by hemagglutination or by a cytopathic effect. A rapid diagnosis may be made by identification of parainfluenza antigens in exfoliated cells from the respiratory tract with immunofluorescence or ELISA, although these techniques appear to be less sensitive than tissue culture. Highly specific and sensitive PCR assays have also been developed and have now become the standard for viral diagnosis. Serologic diagnosis can be established by hemagglutination-inhibition, complement-fixation, or neutralization testing of acute- and convalescent-phase specimens. However, because frequent heterotypic responses occur among the parainfluenza serotypes, the serotype causing illness often cannot be identified by serologic techniques alone.

Acute epiglottitis caused by *Haemophilus influenzae* type b must be differentiated from viral croup. Influenza A virus is also a common cause of croup during epidemic periods.

TREATMENT PARAINFLUENZA VIRUS INFECTIONS

For upper respiratory tract illness, symptoms can be treated as discussed for other viral respiratory tract illnesses. If complications such as sinusitis, otitis, or superimposed bacterial bronchitis develop, appropriate antibacterial drugs should be administered. Mild cases of croup should be treated with bed rest and moist air generated by vaporizers. More severe cases require hospitalization and close observation for the development of respiratory distress. If acute respiratory distress develops, humidified oxygen and intermittent racemic epinephrine are usually administered. Aerosolized or systemically administered glucocorticoids are beneficial; systemic administration has a more profound effect. No specific antiviral therapy has been established. Ribavirin is active against parainfluenza viruses in vitro, and anecdotal reports describe its use clinically, particularly in immunosuppressed patients, but its efficacy, if any, is unclear. DAS181, a sialidase with activity against parainfluenza viruses, is undergoing evaluation in immunosuppressed patients.

PREVENTION

Vaccines against parainfluenza viruses are under development.

ADENOVIRUS INFECTIONS

ETIOLOGIC AGENT

Adenoviruses are complex DNA viruses that measure 70–80 nm in diameter. Human adenoviruses belong to the genus *Mastadenovirus*, which includes 51 serotypes. Adenoviruses have a characteristic morphology consisting of an icosahedral shell composed of 20 equilateral triangular faces and 12 vertices. The protein coat (capsid) consists of hexon subunits with group-specific and type-specific antigenic determinants and penton subunits at each vertex primarily containing group-specific antigens. A fiber with a knob at the end projects from each penton; this fiber contains type-specific and some group-specific antigens. Human adenoviruses have been divided into seven subgroups (A through G) on the basis of the homology of DNA genomes and other properties. Revised criteria for classifying human adenoviruses have been proposed; reflecting recent approaches to the characterization of novel adenoviruses, the revised criteria include genome sequence and computational analysis in addition to traditional serologic criteria. The adenovirus genome is a linear double-stranded DNA that codes for structural and nonstructural polypeptides. The replicative cycle of adenovirus may result either in lytic infection of cells or in the establishment of a latent infection (primarily involving lymphoid cells). Some adenovirus types can induce oncogenic transformation, and tumor formation has been observed in rodents; however, despite intensive investigation, adenoviruses have not been associated with tumors in humans.

EPIDEMIOLOGY

Adenovirus infections most frequently affect infants and children. Infections occur throughout the year but are most common from fall to spring. In the United States, adenoviruses account for ~10% of acute respiratory infections in children but for <2% of respiratory illnesses in civilian adults. Nearly 100% of adults have serum antibody to multiple serotypes—a finding indicating that infection is common in childhood. Types 1, 2, 3, and 5 are the most common isolates from children. Certain adenovirus serotypes—particularly 4 and 7 but also 3, 14, and 21—are associated with outbreaks of acute respiratory disease in military recruits. Clusters of particularly severe disease have been seen with adenovirus 14.

Adenovirus infection can be transmitted by inhalation of aerosolized virus, by inoculation of virus into conjunctival sacs, and probably by the fecal-oral route as well. Type-specific antibody generally develops after infection and is associated with protection—albeit incomplete—against infection with the same serotype.

CLINICAL MANIFESTATIONS

In children, adenoviruses cause a variety of clinical syndromes. The most common is an acute upper respiratory tract infection, with prominent rhinitis. On occasion, lower respiratory tract disease, including bronchiolitis and pneumonia, also develops. Adenoviruses, particularly types 3 and 7, cause pharyngoconjunctival fever, a characteristic acute febrile illness of children that occurs in outbreaks, most often in summer camps. The syndrome is marked by bilateral conjunctivitis in which the bulbar and palpebral conjunctivae have a granular appearance. Low-grade fever is frequently present for the first 3–5 days, and rhinitis, sore throat, and cervical adenopathy develop. The illness generally lasts for 1–2 weeks and resolves spontaneously. Febrile pharyngitis without conjunctivitis has also been associated with adenovirus infection. Adenoviruses have been isolated from cases of whooping cough with or without *Bordetella pertussis*; the significance of adenovirus in that disease is unknown.

In adults, the most frequently reported illness has been acute respiratory disease caused by adenovirus types 4 and 7 in military recruits. This illness is marked by a prominent sore throat and the gradual onset of fever, which often reaches 39°C (102.2°F) on the second or third day of illness. Cough is almost always present, and coryza and regional lymphadenopathy are frequently seen. Physical examination may show pharyngeal edema, injection, and tonsillar enlargement with little or no exudate. If pneumonia has developed, auscultation and x-ray of the chest may indicate areas of patchy infiltration.

Adenoviruses have been associated with a number of non–respiratory tract diseases, including acute diarrheal illness caused by types 40 and 41 in young children and hemorrhagic cystitis caused by types 11 and 21. Epidemic keratoconjunctivitis, caused most frequently by types 8, 19, and 37, has been associated with contaminated common sources such as ophthalmic solutions and roller towels. Adenoviruses have also been implicated in disseminated disease and pneumonia in immunosuppressed patients, including recipients of SOTs or HSCTs. In HSCT recipients, adenovirus infections have manifested as pneumonia, hepatitis, nephritis, colitis, encephalitis, and hemorrhagic cystitis. In SOT recipients, adenovirus infection may involve the organ transplanted (e.g., hepatitis in liver transplants, nephritis in renal transplants) but can disseminate to other organs as well. In patients with AIDS, high-numbered and intermediate adenovirus serotypes have been isolated, usually in the setting of low CD4+ T cell counts, but their isolation often has not been clearly linked to disease manifestations. Adenovirus nucleic acids have been detected in myocardial cells from patients with "idiopathic" myocardiopathies, and adenoviruses have been suggested as causative agents in some cases.

LABORATORY FINDINGS AND DIAGNOSIS

Adenovirus infection should be suspected in the epidemiologic setting of acute respiratory disease in military recruits and in certain clinical syndromes (such as pharyngoconjunctival fever or epidemic keratoconjunctivitis) in which outbreaks of characteristic illnesses occur. In most cases, however, illnesses caused by adenovirus infection cannot be differentiated from those caused by a number of other viral respiratory agents and *Mycoplasma pneumoniae*. A definitive diagnosis of adenovirus infection is established by detection of the virus in tissue culture (as evidenced by cytopathic changes) and by specific identification with immunofluorescence or other immunologic techniques. Rapid viral diagnosis can be established by immunofluorescence or ELISA of nasopharyngeal aspirates, conjunctival or respiratory secretions, urine, or stool. Highly sensitive and specific PCR assays and nucleic acid hybridization are available and have become the standard for diagnosis based on clinical specimens. Adenovirus types 40 and 41, which have been associated with diarrheal disease in children, require special tissue-culture cells for isolation, and these serotypes are most commonly detected by direct ELISA of stool or by PCR. Serum antibody rises can be demonstrated by complement-fixation or neutralization tests, ELISA, radioimmunoassay, or (for those adenoviruses that hemagglutinate red cells) hemagglutination-inhibition tests.

TREATMENT ADENOVIRUS INFECTIONS

Only symptom-based treatment and supportive therapy are available for adenovirus infections, and clinically useful antiviral therapy has not been established. Ribavirin and cidofovir are active in vitro against certain adenoviruses. Retrospective studies and anecdotes describe the use of these agents in disseminated adenovirus infections, but definitive efficacy data from controlled studies are not available. An oral liposomal form of cidofovir (CMX001) is being evaluated for adenovirus infections in immunosuppressed patients.

PREVENTION

Live vaccines have been developed against adenovirus types 4 and 7 and have been highly efficacious in control of acute respiratory disease among military recruits. These vaccines consist of live, unattenuated virus administered in enteric-coated capsules. Infection of the gastrointestinal tract with types 4 and 7 does not cause disease but stimulates local and systemic antibodies that are protective against subsequent acute respiratory disease due to those serotypes. These vaccines were not produced from 1999 to 2011 but are now available again and are being used effectively in military recruits. Adenoviruses are also being studied as live-virus vectors for the delivery of vaccine antigens and for gene therapy.

224 Influenza

Yehuda Z. Cohen, Raphael Dolin

DEFINITION

Influenza is an acute respiratory illness caused by infection with influenza viruses. The illness affects the upper and/or lower respiratory tract and is often accompanied by systemic signs and symptoms such as fever, headache, myalgia, and weakness. Outbreaks of illness of variable extent and severity occur nearly every year. Such outbreaks result in significant morbidity rates in the general population and in increased mortality rates among certain high-risk patients, mainly as a result of pulmonary complications.

ETIOLOGIC AGENT

Influenza viruses are members of the Orthomyxoviridae family, of which influenza A, B, and C viruses constitute three separate genera. The designation of influenza viruses as type A, B, or C is based on antigenic characteristics of the nucleoprotein (NP) and matrix (M) protein antigens. Influenza A viruses are further subdivided (subtyped) on the basis of the surface hemagglutinin (H) and neuraminidase (N) antigens; individual strains are designated according to the site of origin, isolate number, year of isolation, and subtype—for example, influenza A/California/07/2009 (H1N1). Influenza A has 18 distinct H subtypes and 11 distinct N subtypes, of which only H1, H2, H3, N1, and N2 have been associated with epidemics of disease in humans. Avian influenza A viruses have been associated with small outbreaks and sporadic cases in humans (see below). Influenza B and C viruses are designated similarly to influenza A viruses, but H and N antigens from these viruses do not receive subtype designations because intratypic variations in influenza B antigens are less extensive than those in influenza A viruses and may not occur with influenza C virus.

Influenza A and B viruses are major human pathogens and the most extensively studied of the Orthomyxoviridae. Type A and type B viruses are morphologically similar. The virions are irregularly shaped spherical particles, measure 80–120 nm in diameter, and have a lipid envelope from the surface of which the H and N glycoproteins project (Fig. 224-1). The hemagglutinin is the site by which the virus binds to sialic acid cell receptors, whereas the neuraminidase degrades the receptor and plays a role in the release of the virus from infected cells after replication has taken place. Influenza viruses enter cells by receptor-mediated endocytosis, forming a virus-containing endosome. The viral hemagglutinin mediates fusion of the endosomal membrane with the virus envelope, and viral nucleocapsids are subsequently released into the cytoplasm. Immune responses to the H antigen are the major determinants of protection against infection with influenza virus, whereas those to the N antigen limit viral spread and contribute to reduction of the infection. The lipid envelope of influenza A virus also contains the M proteins M1 and M2, which are involved in stabilization of the lipid envelope and in virus assembly. The virion also contains the NP antigen, which is associated with the viral genome, as well as three polymerase (P) proteins that are essential for transcription and synthesis of viral RNA. Two nonstructural proteins function as an interferon antagonist and posttranscriptional regulator (NS1) and a nuclear export factor (NS2 or NEP).

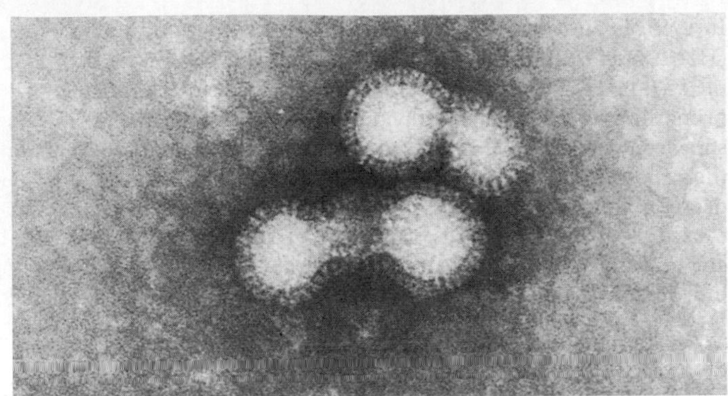

FIGURE 224-1 An electron micrograph of influenza A virus (×40,000).

The genomes of influenza A and B viruses consist of eight single-strand RNA segments, which code for the structural and nonstructural proteins. Because the genome is segmented, the opportunity for gene reassortment during infection is high; reassortment often takes place during infection of cells with more than one influenza A virus.

EPIDEMIOLOGY

Influenza outbreaks occur virtually every year, although their extent and severity vary widely. Localized outbreaks take place at variable intervals, usually every 1–3 years. Global pandemics have occurred at variable intervals, but much less frequently than interpandemic outbreaks (Table 224-1). The most recent pandemic emerged in March of 2009 and was caused by an influenza A/H1N1 virus that rapidly spread worldwide over the next several months.

Influenza A Virus • *ANTIGENIC VARIATION AND INFLUENZA OUTBREAKS AND PANDEMICS* The most extensive and severe outbreaks of influenza are caused by influenza A viruses, in part because of the remarkable propensity of the H and N antigens of these viruses to undergo periodic antigenic variation. Major antigenic variations, called *antigenic shifts*, are seen only with influenza A viruses and may be associated with pandemics. Minor variations are called *antigenic drifts*. Antigenic variation may involve the hemagglutinin alone or both the hemagglutinin and the neuraminidase. An example of an antigenic shift involving both the hemagglutinin and the neuraminidase is that of 1957, when the predominant influenza A virus subtype shifted from H1N1 to H2N2; this shift resulted in a severe pandemic, with an estimated 70,000 excess deaths (i.e., deaths in excess of the number expected without an influenza epidemic) in the United States alone. This excess mortality was significantly greater than that during interpandemic influenza seasons.

TABLE 224-1 EMERGENCE OF ANTIGENIC SUBTYPES OF INFLUENZA A VIRUS ASSOCIATED WITH PANDEMIC OR EPIDEMIC DISEASE

Years	Subtype	Extent of Outbreak
1889–1890	H2N8[a]	Severe pandemic
1900–1903	H3N8[a]	?Moderate epidemic
1918–1919	H1N1[b] (formerly HswN1)	Severe pandemic
1933–1935	H1N1[b] (formerly H0N1)	Mild epidemic
1946–1947	H1N1	Mild epidemic
1957–1958	H2N2	Severe pandemic
1968–1969	H3N2	Moderate pandemic
1977–1978[c]	H1N1	Mild pandemic
2009–2010[d]	H1N1	Pandemic

[a] As determined by retrospective serologic survey of individuals alive during those years ("seroarchaeology"). [b] Hemagglutinins formerly designated as Hsw and H0 are now classified as variants of H1. [c] From this time until 2008–2009, viruses of the H1N1 and H3N2 subtypes circulated either in alternating years or concurrently. [d] A novel influenza A/H1N1 virus emerged to cause this pandemic.

In 1968, an antigenic shift involving only the hemagglutinin occurred (H2N2 to H3N2); the subsequent pandemic was less severe than that of 1957. In 1977, an H1N1 virus emerged and caused a pandemic that primarily affected younger individuals (i.e., those born after 1957). As shown in Table 224-1, H1N1 viruses circulated from 1918 to 1956; thus, individuals born prior to 1957 would be expected to have some degree of immunity to H1N1 viruses. The pandemic of 2009–2010 was caused by an A/H1N1 virus against which little immunity was present in the general population, although approximately one-third of individuals born before 1950 had some apparent immunity to related H1N1 strains.

During most outbreaks of influenza A, a single subtype has circulated at a time. However, since 1977, H1N1 and H3N2 viruses have circulated simultaneously, resulting in outbreaks of varying severity. In some outbreaks, influenza B viruses have also circulated simultaneously with influenza A viruses. In 2009–2010, the pandemic A/H1N1 virus appeared to circulate nearly exclusively.

FEATURES OF PANDEMIC AND INTERPANDEMIC INFLUENZA A Pandemics provide the most dramatic evidence of the impact of influenza A. However, illnesses occurring between pandemics (interpandemic disease) also account for extensive mortality and morbidity, albeit over a longer period. In the United States, influenza was associated with an average of 23,000 excess deaths per season in 1976–2007 and with a maximum of 48,600 excess deaths during the 2003–2004 season.

Influenza A viruses that circulate between pandemics demonstrate antigenic drifts in the H antigen. These antigenic drifts result from point mutations in the RNA segment that codes for the hemagglutinin and occur most frequently in five hypervariable regions. Epidemiologically significant strains—that is, those with the potential to cause widespread outbreaks—exhibit changes in amino acids in at least two of the major antigenic sites in the hemagglutinin molecule. Because two point mutations are unlikely to occur simultaneously, it is believed that antigenic drifts result from point mutations occurring sequentially during the spread of virus from person to person. Antigenic drifts have been reported nearly annually since 1977 for H1N1 viruses and since 1968 for H3N2 viruses.

Interpandemic influenza A outbreaks usually begin abruptly, peak over a 2- to 3-week period, generally last for 2–3 months, and often subside almost as rapidly as they began. In contrast, pandemic influenza may begin with rapid transmission at multiple locations, have high attack rates, and extend beyond the usual seasonality, with multiple waves of attack before or after the main outbreak. In interpandemic outbreaks, the first indication of influenza activity is an increase in the number of children with febrile respiratory illnesses who present for medical attention. This increase is followed by increases in rates of influenza-like illnesses among adults and eventually by an increase in hospital admissions for patients with pneumonia, worsening of congestive heart failure, and exacerbations of chronic pulmonary disease. Rates of absence from work and school also rise at this time. An increase in the number of deaths caused by pneumonia and influenza is generally a late observation in an outbreak. Attack rates have been highly variable from outbreak to outbreak in interpandemic influenza but most commonly are in the range of 10–20% of the general population.

Although pandemic influenza may occur throughout the year, interpandemic influenza occurs almost exclusively during the winter months in the temperate zones of the Northern and Southern hemispheres. In those locations, it is highly unusual to detect influenza A virus at other times, although rises in serum antibody titer or even outbreaks have been noted rarely during warm-weather months. In contrast, influenza virus infections occur throughout the year in the tropics. Where or how influenza A viruses persist between outbreaks in temperate zones is unknown. It is possible that the viruses are maintained in the human population on a worldwide basis by person-to-person transmission and that large population clusters support a low level of interepidemic transmission. Alternatively, human strains may persist in animal reservoirs. Convincing evidence to support either explanation is not available. In the modern era, rapid transportation may contribute to the transmission of viruses among widespread geographic locales.

The factors that result in the inception and termination of outbreaks of influenza A are incompletely understood. A major determinant of the extent and severity of an outbreak is the level of immunity in the population at risk. With the emergence of an antigenically novel influenza virus to which little or no immunity is present in a community, extensive outbreaks may occur. When the absence of immunity is worldwide, epidemic disease may spread around the globe, resulting in a pandemic. Such pandemic waves can continue for several years, until immunity in the population reaches a high level. In the years following pandemic influenza, antigenic drifts among influenza viruses result in outbreaks of variable severity in populations with high levels of immunity to the pandemic strain that circulated earlier. This situation persists until another antigenically novel pandemic strain emerges. On the other hand, outbreaks sometimes end despite the persistence of a large pool of susceptible individuals in the population. It has been suggested that certain influenza A viruses may be intrinsically less virulent and cause less severe disease than other variants, even in immunologically virgin subjects. If so, then other (undefined) factors besides the level of preexisting immunity must play a role in the epidemiology of influenza.

Avian and Swine Influenza Viruses Aquatic birds are the largest reservoir of influenza A viruses, harboring 16 hemagglutinin (H1–H16) and nine neuraminidase (N1–N9) subtypes. (In addition, H17N10 and H18N11 viruses are found in bats.) Influenza A pandemic strains in 1957 (A/H2N2) and in 1968 (A/H3N2) resulted from reassortment of gene segments between human and avian viruses. The influenza A/H1N1 virus that caused the most severe pandemic of modern times (1918–1919) appears to have been an adaptation of an avian virus to human infection. Thus, there is concern that avian influenza viruses with novel hemagglutinin and neuraminidase antigens have the potential to emerge as pandemic strains.

Avian influenza A viruses have been reported to cause sporadic cases and small outbreaks in humans, usually after direct contact with birds (most commonly poultry). Sustained person-to-person transmission in the community has not been observed. Avian influenza A/H5N1 virus has been noted to cause illness in humans since 1997, with 648 cases reported to the World Health Organization as of January 2014. It is not clear whether the high observed case–fatality rate (59%) reflects preferential detection of severe cases. A/H7N7 infections have been noted in poultry industry workers; conjunctivitis was the most prominent feature, although a minority of individuals also had respiratory illness. More than 333 cases of avian A/H7N9 infection have been reported in China, with case–fatality rates of 36% among the infected patients admitted to the hospital. Most H7N9 isolates are sensitive to neuraminidase inhibitors, but a few isolates have exhibited high-level resistance to oseltamivir and diminished sensitivity to zanamivir. Infections with avian H9N2 viruses have been reported primarily among children in Hong Kong and have consisted largely of mild respiratory illnesses. Mild cases of illness due to influenza H10N7 virus in Egypt and Australia have also been reported. In 2013, the first cases of human infection with avian A/H10N8 and H6N1 viruses were described.

Influenza A viruses also circulate in swine but rarely infect humans. Whereas humans primarily have α-2,6-galactose receptors for hemagglutinins and birds primarily have α-2,3-galactose receptors, swine have both types of receptors. Thus, swine hosts efficiently sustain simultaneous infection with both human and avian viruses, thereby facilitating reassortment of genetic segments between viruses of both species. The pandemic A/H1N1 strain of 2009–2010 was a quadruple reassortant among swine, avian, and human influenza viruses. The influenza A virus subtypes that circulate most commonly in swine are H1N1, H1N2, and H3N2. When a predominantly swine virus causes infections in humans, it is designated a variant virus by the addition of "v" after the subtype. For example, influenza A/H3N2v virus was responsible for 321 cases of human infection reported in the United States in 2011 and 2012 and for 18 cases in 2013. Almost all of the affected patients had had close contact with swine. Only limited person-to-person transmission of swine influenza virus has been noted. Since 2005, 16 human cases caused by A/H1N1v virus and 5 caused by A/H1N2v virus have been detected in the United States.

Influenza B and C Viruses Influenza B virus causes outbreaks that are generally less extensive and are associated with less severe disease than those caused by influenza A virus, although the disease may occasionally be severe. The hemagglutinin and neuraminidase of influenza B viruses undergo less frequent and less extensive variation than those of influenza A viruses; this characteristic may account, in part, for the lesser severity of influenza B. Outbreaks of influenza B occur most frequently in schools and military camps, although outbreaks in institutions in which elderly individuals reside have also been noted on occasion. Since the 1980s, two antigenically distinct "lineages" of influenza B virus have circulated: Victoria and Yamagata.

In contrast to influenza A and B viruses, influenza C virus appears to be a relatively minor cause of disease in humans. It has been associated with common cold–like symptoms and occasionally with lower respiratory tract illness. The widespread prevalence of serum antibody to this virus indicates that asymptomatic infection may be common.

Influenza-Associated Morbidity and Mortality Rates Rates of morbidity and mortality caused by influenza outbreaks continue to be substantial. Most individuals who die in this setting have underlying diseases that place them at high risk for complications of influenza (Table 224-2). On average, there were 226,000 influenza-associated hospitalizations per year in the United States in 1979–2001. Recently, the moderately severe influenza season in 2012–2013 was associated with 381,500 hospitalizations (42 per 100,000 persons). Excess annual hospitalizations for groups of adults and children with high-risk medical conditions ranged from 40 to 1900 per 100,000 during outbreaks of influenza in 1973–2004. The most prominent high-risk conditions are chronic cardiac and pulmonary diseases and old age. Mortality rates among individuals with chronic metabolic or renal diseases or certain immunosuppressive diseases have also been elevated, although they remain lower than mortality rates among patients with chronic cardiopulmonary diseases. In the pandemic of 2009–2010, increased risk of severe disease was noted in children from birth to 4 years of age and in pregnant women. The morbidity rate attributable to influenza in the general population is considerable. It is estimated that interpandemic outbreaks of influenza currently incur annual economic costs of more than $87 billion in the United States. For pandemics, it is estimated that annual economic costs would range from $89.7 to $209.4 billion for attack rates of 15–35%.

PATHOGENESIS AND IMMUNITY

The initial event in influenza is infection of the respiratory epithelium with influenza virus acquired from respiratory secretions of acutely infected individuals. In all likelihood, the virus is transmitted via aerosols generated by coughs and sneezes, although transmission through hand-to-hand contact, other personal contact, and even fomites may take place. Experimental evidence suggests that infection by a small-particle aerosol (particle diameter <10 μm) is more efficient than that by larger droplets. Initially, viral infection involves the ciliated columnar epithelial cells, but it may also involve other respiratory tract cells, including alveolar cells, mucous gland cells, and macrophages. In infected cells, virus replicates within 4–6 h, after which infectious virus is released to infect adjacent or nearby cells. In this way, infection spreads from a few foci to a large number of respiratory cells over several hours. In experimentally induced infection, the incubation period of illness has ranged from 18 to 72 h, depending on the size of the viral inoculum. Histopathologic study reveals degenerative changes, including granulation, vacuolization, swelling, and pyknotic nuclei in infected ciliated cells. The cells eventually become necrotic and desquamate; in some areas, previously columnar epithelium is replaced by flattened and metaplastic epithelial cells. The severity of illness is correlated with the quantity of virus shed in secretions; thus, the degree of viral replication itself may be an important factor in pathogenesis. Despite the frequent development of systemic signs and symptoms such as fever, headache, and myalgias, influenza virus has only rarely been detected in extrapulmonary sites (including the bloodstream). Evidence suggests that the pathogenesis of systemic symptoms in influenza may be related to the induction of certain cytokines, particularly tumor necrosis factor α, interferon α, interleukin 6, and interleukin 8, in respiratory secretions and in the bloodstream.

The host response to influenza infections involves a complex interplay of humoral antibody, local antibody, cell-mediated immunity, interferon, and other host defenses. Serum antibody responses, which can be detected by the second week after primary infection, are measured by a variety of techniques: hemagglutination inhibition (HI), complement fixation (CF), neutralization, enzyme-linked immunosorbent assay (ELISA), and antineuraminidase antibody assay. Antibodies to the hemagglutinin appear to be the most important mediators of immunity; in several studies, HI titers of ≥40 have been associated with protection from infection. Secretory antibodies produced in the respiratory tract are predominantly of the IgA class, and secretory antibody neutralization titers of ≥4 have also been associated with protection. A variety of cell-mediated immune responses, both antigen-specific and antigen-nonspecific, can be detected early after infection and depend on the prior immune status of the host. These responses include T cell proliferative, T cell cytotoxic, and natural killer cell activity. In humans, CD8+ as well as CD4+ T lymphocytes are directed at conserved regions of internal proteins (NP, M, and P) as well as at the surface proteins H and N. Interferons can be detected in respiratory secretions shortly after the shedding of virus has begun, and rises in interferon titers coincide with decreases in virus shedding.

The host defense factors responsible for cessation of virus shedding and resolution of illness have not been defined specifically. Virus shedding generally stops within 2–5 days after symptoms first appear, at a time when serum and local antibody responses often are not detectable by conventional techniques, although antibody rises may be detected earlier by use of highly sensitive techniques, particularly in individuals with previous immunity to the virus. It has been suggested that interferon, cell-mediated immune responses, and/or nonspecific inflammatory responses all contribute to the resolution of illness. CD8+ cytotoxic T lymphocyte responses may be particularly important in this regard.

TABLE 224-2 PERSONS AT HIGHER RISK FOR COMPLICATIONS OF INFLUENZA OR FOR INFLUENZA-RELATED VISITS TO HEALTH CARE FACILITIES

All children from birth to <5 years, especially <2 years
All persons ≥50 years old
Pregnant women
Adults and children who have chronic pulmonary (including asthma) or cardiovascular (except isolated hypertension), renal, hepatic, neurologic, hematologic, or metabolic disorders (including diabetes mellitus)
Persons who have immunosuppression (including that caused by medications or by HIV infection)
Children and adolescents (6 months to 18 years old) who are receiving long-term aspirin therapy and who might be at risk for Reye's syndrome after influenza virus infection
Residents of nursing homes and other long-term care facilities
Native Americans/Alaska Natives
Persons who are morbidly obese (body mass index ≥40 kg/m^2)

CLINICAL MANIFESTATIONS

Influenza is most frequently described as a respiratory illness characterized by systemic symptoms, such as headache, feverishness, chills, myalgia, and malaise, as well as accompanying respiratory tract signs and symptoms, particularly cough and sore throat. In some cases, the onset is so abrupt that patients can recall the precise time they became ill. However, the spectrum of clinical presentations is wide, ranging from a mild, afebrile respiratory illness similar to the common cold (with either a gradual or an abrupt onset) to severe prostration with relatively few respiratory signs and symptoms. In most of the cases that come to a physician's attention, the patient has a fever, with temperatures of 38°–41°C (100.4°–105.8°F). A rapid temperature rise within the first 24 h of illness is generally followed by gradual defervescence over 2–3 days, although, on occasion, fever may last as long as 1 week.

Patients report a feverish feeling and chilliness, but true rigors are rare. Headache, either generalized or frontal, is often particularly troublesome. Myalgias may involve any part of the body but are most common in the legs and lumbosacral area. Arthralgias may also develop.

Respiratory symptoms often become more prominent as systemic symptoms subside. Many patients have a sore throat or persistent cough, which may last for ≥1 week and which is often accompanied by substernal discomfort. Ocular signs and symptoms include pain on motion of the eyes, photophobia, and burning of the eyes.

In the elderly, influenza may have a relatively subtle presentation. Typical features such as sore throat, myalgia, and even fever may be absent, and general symptoms such as anorexia, malaise, weakness, and dizziness may predominate.

Physical findings are usually minimal in uncomplicated influenza. Early in the illness, the patient appears flushed, and the skin is hot and dry, although diaphoresis and mottled extremities are sometimes evident, particularly in older patients. Examination of the pharynx may yield surprisingly unremarkable results despite a severe sore throat, but injection of the mucous membranes and postnasal discharge are apparent in some cases. Mild cervical lymphadenopathy may be noted, especially in younger individuals. The results of chest examination are largely negative in uncomplicated influenza, although rhonchi, wheezes, and scattered rales have been reported with variable frequency in different outbreaks. Frank dyspnea, hyperpnea, cyanosis, diffuse rales, and signs of consolidation are indicative of pulmonary complications. Patients with apparently uncomplicated influenza have been reported to have a variety of mild ventilatory defects and increased alveolar-capillary diffusion gradients; thus, subclinical pulmonary involvement may be more common than is appreciated.

In uncomplicated influenza, the acute illness generally resolves over 2–5 days, and most patients have largely recovered in 1 week, although cough may persist 1–2 weeks longer. In a significant minority (particularly the elderly), however, symptoms of weakness or lassitude (postinfluenza asthenia) may persist for several weeks and may prove troublesome for persons who wish to resume their full level of activity promptly. The pathogenetic basis for this asthenia is unknown, although pulmonary function abnormalities may persist for several weeks after uncomplicated influenza.

COMPLICATIONS

Complications of influenza occur most frequently in patients >65 years old and in those with certain chronic disorders, including cardiac or pulmonary diseases, diabetes mellitus, hemoglobinopathies, renal dysfunction, and immunosuppression. Pregnancy in the second or third trimester predisposes to complications with influenza. Children <5 years old (especially infants) are also at high risk for complications (Table 224-2).

Pulmonary Complications • *PNEUMONIA* The most significant complication of influenza is pneumonia: "primary" influenza viral pneumonia, secondary bacterial pneumonia, or mixed viral and bacterial pneumonia (discussed below).

Primary influenza viral pneumonia Primary influenza viral pneumonia is the least common but most severe of the pneumonic complications. It presents as acute influenza that does not resolve but instead progresses relentlessly, with persistent fever, dyspnea, and eventual cyanosis. Sputum production is generally scanty, but the sputum can contain blood. Few physical signs may be evident early in the illness. In more advanced cases, diffuse rales may be noted, and imaging findings consistent with diffuse interstitial infiltrates and/or acute respiratory distress syndrome may be present. In such cases, arterial blood-gas determinations show marked hypoxia. Viral cultures of respiratory secretions and lung parenchyma, especially if samples are taken early in illness, yield high titers of virus. In fatal cases of primary viral pneumonia, histopathologic examination reveals a marked inflammatory reaction in the alveolar septa, with edema and infiltration by lymphocytes, macrophages, occasional plasma cells, and variable numbers of neutrophils. Fibrin thrombi in alveolar capillaries, along with necrosis and hemorrhage, have also been noted. Eosinophilic hyaline membranes can be found lining alveoli and alveolar ducts.

Primary influenza viral pneumonia has a predilection for individuals with cardiac disease, particularly those with mitral stenosis, but has also been reported in otherwise-healthy young adults as well as in older individuals with chronic pulmonary disorders. In some pandemics of influenza (notably those of 1918 and 1957), pregnancy increased the risk of primary influenza pneumonia. Subsequent epidemics of influenza have been associated with increased rates of hospitalization among pregnant women, which were also noted in the pandemic of 2009–2010.

Secondary bacterial pneumonia Secondary bacterial pneumonia follows acute influenza. Improvement of the patient's condition over 2–3 days is followed by a reappearance of fever along with clinical signs and symptoms of bacterial pneumonia, including cough, production of purulent sputum, and physical and x-ray signs of consolidation. The most common bacterial pathogens in this setting are *Streptococcus pneumoniae*, *Staphylococcus aureus*, and *Haemophilus influenzae*—organisms that can colonize the nasopharynx and that cause infection in the wake of changes in bronchopulmonary defenses. Secondary bacterial pneumonia occurs most frequently in high-risk individuals with chronic pulmonary and cardiac disease and in elderly individuals. Patients with secondary bacterial pneumonia often respond to appropriate antibiotic therapy when it is instituted promptly.

Mixed viral and bacterial pneumonia Perhaps the most common pneumonic complications during outbreaks of influenza have mixed features of viral and bacterial pneumonia. Patients may experience a gradual progression of their acute illness or may show transient improvement followed by clinical exacerbation, with eventual manifestation of the clinical features of bacterial pneumonia. Sputum cultures may contain both influenza A virus and one of the bacterial pathogens described above. Patchy infiltrates or areas of consolidation may be detected by physical examination and chest x-ray. Patients with mixed viral and bacterial pneumonia generally have less widespread involvement of the lung than those with primary viral pneumonia, and their bacterial infections may respond to appropriate antibacterial drugs. Mixed viral and bacterial pneumonia occurs primarily in patients with chronic cardiovascular and pulmonary diseases.

OTHER PULMONARY COMPLICATIONS Other pulmonary complications associated with influenza include worsening of chronic obstructive pulmonary disease and exacerbation of chronic bronchitis and asthma. In children, influenza infection may present as croup. Sinusitis and otitis media (the latter occurring particularly often in children) may also be associated with influenza.

Extrapulmonary Complications Myositis, rhabdomyolysis, and myoglobinuria are occasional complications of influenza infection. Although myalgias are exceedingly common in influenza, true myositis is rare. Patients with acute myositis have exquisite tenderness of the affected muscles, most commonly in the legs, and may not be able to tolerate even the slightest pressure, such as the touch of bedsheets. In the most severe cases, there is frank swelling and bogginess of muscles. Serum levels of creatine phosphokinase and aldolase are markedly elevated, and an occasional patient develops renal failure from myoglobinuria. The pathogenesis of influenza-associated myositis is also unclear, although the presence of influenza virus in affected muscles has been reported.

Myocarditis and pericarditis were reported in association with influenza virus infection during the 1918–1919 pandemic; these reports were based largely on histopathologic findings, and these complications have been reported only infrequently since that time. Electrocardiographic changes during acute influenza are common among patients who have cardiac disease but have been ascribed most often to exacerbations of the underlying cardiac disease rather than to direct involvement of the myocardium with influenza virus. Epidemiologic data have shown an association between influenza outbreaks and increased cardiovascular-associated hospitalizations.

Central nervous system (CNS) complications such as encephalitis and transverse myelitis have been associated with influenza. Encephalitis is a rare but potentially serious complication that has been reported with influenza A and B virus infections. Children <5 years of age appear to be at greatest risk. The pathogenetic mechanisms by which influenza causes CNS disease are unclear. Guillain-Barré syndrome has been reported following influenza infection and, uncommonly, after influenza vaccination (see "Prophylaxis," below).

Toxic shock syndrome associated with *S. aureus* or group A streptococcal infection following acute influenza infection has been described (Chaps. 172 and 173).

Reye's syndrome is a serious complication in children that is associated with influenza B and—to a lesser extent—influenza A virus infection as well as with varicella-zoster virus and other viral infections. An epidemiologic association between Reye's syndrome and aspirin therapy for the antecedent viral infection has been noted; the syndrome's incidence has decreased markedly with widespread warnings regarding aspirin use by children with acute viral respiratory infections.

In addition to complications involving the specific organ systems described above, influenza outbreaks include cases in which elderly and other high-risk individuals develop influenza and subsequently experience a gradual deterioration of underlying cardiovascular, pulmonary, or renal function—changes that occasionally are irreversible and lead to death. These deaths contribute to the overall excess mortality associated with influenza outbreaks.

LABORATORY FINDINGS AND DIAGNOSIS

During acute influenza, virus may be detected in throat swabs, nasopharyngeal swabs or washes, or sputum. Reverse-transcriptase polymerase chain reaction (RT-PCR) is the most sensitive and specific technique for detection of influenza viruses. RT-PCR can differentiate among influenza subtypes and is used for detection of avian influenza viruses. Rapid influenza diagnostic tests (RIDTs) detect influenza virus antigens by immunologic or enzymatic techniques. RIDTs yield results quickly, and some tests can distinguish between influenza A and B viruses. Although relatively specific, RIDTs vary in sensitivity with the technique and the virus to be detected.

Influenza virus may be isolated from tissue culture or chick embryos, but these labor-intensive procedures generally are no longer used for diagnostic purposes. Serologic methods for diagnosis require comparison of antibody titers in sera obtained during the acute illness with those in sera obtained 10–14 days after the onset of illness and are useful primarily in retrospect and for epidemiologic studies.

Other laboratory tests generally are not helpful in the specific diagnosis of influenza virus infection. Leukocyte counts are variable, frequently being low early in illness and normal or slightly elevated later. Severe leukopenia has been described in overwhelming viral or bacterial infection, whereas leukocytosis with >15,000 cells/μL raises the suspicion of secondary bacterial infection.

DIFFERENTIAL DIAGNOSIS

During a community-wide outbreak, a clinical diagnosis of influenza can be made with a high degree of certainty in patients who present to a physician's office with the typical febrile respiratory illness described above. In the absence of an outbreak (i.e., in sporadic or isolated cases), influenza may be difficult to differentiate on clinical grounds alone from an acute respiratory illness caused by any of a variety of respiratory viruses or by *Mycoplasma pneumoniae*. Severe streptococcal pharyngitis or early bacterial pneumonia may mimic acute influenza, although bacterial pneumonias generally do not run a self-limited course. Purulent sputum in which a bacterial pathogen can be detected by Gram's staining is an important diagnostic feature in bacterial pneumonia.

TREATMENT INFLUENZA

(See also Chap. 215e) Specific antiviral therapy is available for influenza (Table 224-3): the neuraminidase inhibitors zanamivir and oseltamivir for both influenza A and influenza B and the adamantane agents amantadine and rimantadine for influenza A. The epidemiologic patterns of resistance to the influenza antiviral drugs are crucial elements in the selection of treatment. Up-to-date information on patterns of resistance to influenza antiviral drugs is available through *www.cdc.gov/flu*.

A 5-day course of oseltamivir or zanamivir reduces the duration of signs and symptoms of uncomplicated influenza by 1–1.5 days if treatment is started within 2 days of the onset of illness and may be effective if started up to 5 days after onset of symptoms. Zanamivir is administered via an oral inhalation device and may exacerbate bronchospasm in asthmatic patients. Oseltamivir has been associated with nausea and vomiting, whose frequency can be reduced by administration of the drug with food. Oseltamivir has also been associated with neuropsychiatric side effects in children. Peramivir, an investigational neuraminidase inhibitor that can be administered intravenously, is being evaluated in clinical trials, as is an intravenous form of zanamivir.

Amantadine and rimantadine are active only against influenza A, and widespread resistance exists among influenza A/H1N1 and A/H3N2 viruses that are circulating currently; thus, the use of these drugs is not recommended unless influenza isolates are known to be sensitive. Amantadine or rimantadine treatment of illness caused by sensitive strains of influenza A virus reduces the duration of symptoms of uncomplicated influenza by ~50% if begun within 48 h after onset of illness—an effect similar to that of the neuraminidase inhibitors. Of amantadine recipients, 5–10% experience mild

TABLE 224-3 ANTIVIRAL MEDICATIONS FOR TREATMENT AND PROPHYLAXIS OF INFLUENZA

		Age Group (Years)	
Antiviral Drug	**Children (≤12)**	**13–64**	**≥65**
Oseltamivir			
Treatment, influenza A and B	Age 1–12, dose varies by weight[a]	75 mg PO bid	75 mg PO bid
Prophylaxis, influenza A and B	Age 1–12, dose varies by weight[b]	75 mg PO qd	75 mg PO qd
Zanamivir			
Treatment, influenza A and B	Age 7–12, 10 mg bid by inhalation	10 mg bid by inhalation	10 mg bid by inhalation
Prophylaxis, influenza A and B	Age 5–12, 10 mg qd by inhalation	10 mg qd by inhalation	10 mg qd by inhalation
Amantadine[c]			
Treatment, influenza A	Age 1–9, 5 mg/kg in 2 divided doses, up to 150 mg/d	Age ≥10, 100 mg PO bid	≤100 mg/d
Prophylaxis, influenza A	Age 1–9, 5 mg/kg in 2 divided doses, up to 150 mg/d	Age ≥10, 100 mg PO bid	≤100 mg/d
Rimantadine[c]			
Treatment, influenza A	Not approved	100 mg PO bid	100–200 mg/d
Prophylaxis, influenza A	Age 1–9, 5 mg/kg in 2 divided doses, up to 150 mg/d	Age ≥10, 100 mg PO bid	100–200 mg/d

[a]<15 kg: 30 mg bid; >15–23 kg: 45 mg bid; >23–40 kg: 60 mg bid; >40 kg: 75 mg bid. For children <1 year of age, see *www.cdc.gov/h1n1flu/recommendations.htm*. [b]<15 kg: 30 mg qd; >15–23 kg: 45 mg qd; >23–40 kg: 60 mg qd; >40 kg: 75 mg qd. For children <1 year of age, see *www.cdc.gov/h1n1flu/recommendations.htm*. [c]Amantadine and rimantadine are not currently recommended (2013–2014) because of widespread resistance in influenza A viruses. Their use may be reconsidered if viral susceptibility is reestablished.

CNS side effects, primarily jitteriness, anxiety, insomnia, or difficulty concentrating. These side effects disappear promptly upon cessation of therapy. Rimantadine appears to be equally efficacious and is associated with less frequent CNS side effects than is amantadine.

Ribavirin is a nucleoside analogue with activity against influenza A and B viruses in vitro. Its efficacy against influenza when administered as an aerosol is reportedly variable, and it is ineffective when administered orally. Its efficacy in the treatment of influenza A or B has not been established.

The therapeutic efficacy of antiviral compounds in influenza has been demonstrated primarily in studies of young adults with uncomplicated disease. The effectiveness of these drugs in the treatment or prevention of complications of influenza is unclear. Pooled analyses of observational investigations and some efficacy studies have suggested that treatment with oseltamivir may reduce the frequency of lower respiratory complications and hospitalization. Therapy for primary influenza pneumonia is directed at maintaining oxygenation and is most appropriately undertaken in an intensive care unit, with aggressive respiratory and hemodynamic support as needed.

Antibacterial drugs should be reserved for the treatment of bacterial complications of acute influenza, such as secondary bacterial pneumonia. The choice of antibiotics should be guided by Gram's staining and culture of appropriate specimens of respiratory secretions, such as sputum. If the etiology of a case of bacterial pneumonia is unclear from an examination of respiratory secretions, empirical antibiotics effective against the most common bacterial pathogens in this setting (*S. pneumoniae*, *S. aureus*, and *H. influenzae*) should be selected (Chaps. 171, 172, and 182).

For uncomplicated influenza in individuals at low risk of complications, symptom-based rather than antiviral therapy may be considered. Acetaminophen or nonsteroidal anti-inflammatory agents can be used for relief of headache, myalgia, and fever, but salicylates should be avoided in children <18 years of age because of the possible association with Reye's syndrome (see "Extrapulmonary Complications," above). Because cough is ordinarily self-limited, treatment with cough suppressants generally is not indicated; codeine-containing compounds may be used if the cough is particularly troublesome. Patients should be advised to rest and maintain hydration during acute illness and to return to full activity only gradually after illness has resolved, especially if it has been severe.

PROPHYLAXIS

The major public health measure for prevention of influenza is vaccination. Both inactivated (killed) and live attenuated vaccines are available and are generated from isolates of influenza A and B viruses that circulated in the previous influenza seasons and are anticipated to circulate in the upcoming season. For inactivated vaccines, 50–80% protection against influenza is expected if the vaccine virus and the currently circulating viruses are closely related. Available inactivated vaccines have been highly purified and are associated with few reactions. Up to 5% of individuals experience low-grade fever and mild systemic symptoms 8–24 h after vaccination, and up to one-third develop mild redness or tenderness at the vaccination site. Although the 1976 swine influenza vaccine appears to have been associated with an increased frequency of Guillain-Barré syndrome, influenza vaccines administered since 1976 generally have not been. Possible exceptions were noted during the 1992–1993 and 1993–1994 influenza seasons, when there may have been an excess risk of this syndrome (slightly more than 1 case per 1 million vaccine recipients). Large-scale studies of vaccination with the 2009 pandemic H1N1 vaccine also suggested a possible increased risk of Guillain-Barré syndrome (1 case per 1 million vaccinees). However, the overall health risk following influenza substantially outweighs the potential risk associated with vaccination.

A live attenuated influenza vaccine administered by intranasal spray is available. The vaccine is generated by reassortment between currently circulating strains of influenza A and B viruses and a cold-adapted, attenuated master strain. The cold-adapted vaccine is well tolerated and highly efficacious (>90% protective) in young children; in one study, it provided protection against a circulating influenza virus that had drifted antigenically away from the vaccine strain. Live attenuated vaccine is approved for use in healthy nonpregnant persons 2–49 years of age.

Since 1975, influenza vaccines have been trivalent—i.e., they have contained two influenza A subtypes (H3N2 and H1N1) and one influenza B component. However, two antigenically distinct lineages of influenza B virus have circulated since the 1980s, and a quadrivalent vaccine that includes both B lineages is now available (2013–2014) as well. Quadrivalent vaccines are available in both inactivated and live-attenuated vaccine formulations.

Inactivated influenza vaccines have been noted to be less immunogenic in the elderly. A higher-dose trivalent vaccine containing 60 μg of each antigen and a lower-dose, intradermally administered trivalent vaccine containing 9 μg of each antigen have been approved for use in individuals ≥65 years of age and individuals 18–64 years of age, respectively.

The influenza vaccines discussed above are manufactured in eggs and should not be administered to persons with true hypersensitivity to eggs. For use in this situation, an egg-free vaccine manufactured in cells through recombinant DNA techniques (Flublok®; Protein Sciences Corporation, Meriden, CT) has been approved. Active research is under way to develop vaccines with broad activity against antigenically distinct subtypes ("universal influenza vaccines").

Historically, the U.S. Public Health Service has recommended influenza vaccination for certain groups at high risk for complications of influenza on the basis of age or underlying disease (Table 224-2) or for their close contacts. Although such individuals will continue to be the focus of vaccination programs, the recommendations have been progressively expanded, and immunization of the entire population above the age of 6 months has been recommended since 2010–2011. (Approved influenza vaccines are not available for infants <6 months of age.) This expanded recommendation reflects increased recognition of previously unappreciated risk factors (e.g., obesity, postpartum conditions, and racial or ethnic influences) as well as an appreciation that more widespread use of vaccine is required for influenza control. Inactivated vaccines may be administered safely to immunocompromised patients. Influenza vaccination is not associated with exacerbations of chronic nervous system diseases such as multiple sclerosis. Vaccine should be administered early in the autumn before influenza outbreaks occur and should then be given annually to maintain immunity against the most current influenza virus strains.

Although antiviral drugs provide chemoprophylaxis against influenza, their use for that purpose has been limited because of concern about current and future development of resistance. Chemoprophylaxis with oseltamivir or zanamivir has been 84–89% efficacious against influenza A and B (Table 224-3). Chemoprophylaxis with amantadine or rimantadine is no longer recommended because of widespread resistance to these drugs. In earlier studies with sensitive viruses, prophylaxis with amantadine or rimantadine was 70–100% effective against illness associated with influenza A virus.

Chemoprophylaxis for healthy persons after community exposure generally is not recommended but may be considered for individuals at high risk of complications who have had close contact with an acutely ill person with influenza. During an outbreak, antiviral chemoprophylaxis can be administered simultaneously with inactivated vaccine because the drugs do not interfere with an immune response to the vaccine. However, concurrent administration of chemoprophylaxis and live attenuated vaccine may interfere with the immune response to the latter. Antiviral drugs should not be administered until at least 2 weeks after administration of live vaccine, and administration of live vaccine should not begin until at least 48 h after antiviral drug administration has been stopped. Chemoprophylaxis may also be considered to control nosocomial outbreaks of influenza. For that purpose, prophylaxis should be instituted promptly when influenza activity is detected and must be continued daily for the duration of the outbreak.

SECTION 14 INFECTIONS DUE TO HUMAN IMMUNODEFICIENCY VIRUS AND OTHER HUMAN RETROVIRUSES

225e The Human Retroviruses

Dan L. Longo, Anthony S. Fauci

This is a digital-only chapter. It is available on the DVD that accompanies this book, as well as on Access Medicine/Harrison's Online, and the eBook and "app" editions of HPIM 19e.

The retroviruses, which make up a large family (Retroviridae), infect mainly vertebrates. These viruses have a unique replication cycle whereby their genetic information is encoded by RNA rather than DNA. Retroviruses contain an RNA-dependent DNA polymerase (a reverse transcriptase) that directs the synthesis of a DNA form of the viral genome after infection of a host cell. The designation *retrovirus* denotes that information in the form of RNA is transcribed into DNA in the host cell—a sequence that overturned a central dogma of molecular biology: that information passes unidirectionally from DNA to RNA to protein. The observation that RNA was the source of genetic information in the causative agents of certain animal tumors led to a number of paradigm-shifting biologic insights regarding not only the direction of genetic information passage but also the viral etiology of certain cancers and the concept of oncogenes as normal host genes scavenged and altered by a viral vector.

226 Human Immunodeficiency Virus Disease: AIDS and Related Disorders

Anthony S. Fauci, H. Clifford Lane

AIDS was first recognized in the United States in the summer of 1981, when the U.S. Centers for Disease Control and Prevention (CDC) reported the unexplained occurrence of *Pneumocystis jiroveci* (formerly *P. carinii*) pneumonia in five previously healthy homosexual men in Los Angeles and of Kaposi's sarcoma (KS) with or without *P. jiroveci* pneumonia and other opportunistic infections in 26 previously healthy homosexual men in New York, San Francisco, and Los Angeles. The disease was soon recognized in male and female injection drug users; in hemophiliacs and blood transfusion recipients; among female sexual partners of men with AIDS; and among infants born to mothers with AIDS. In 1983, human immunodeficiency virus (HIV) was isolated from a patient with lymphadenopathy, and by 1984 it was demonstrated clearly to be the causative agent of AIDS. In 1985, a sensitive enzyme-linked immunosorbent assay (ELISA) was developed; this led to an appreciation of the scope and evolution of the HIV epidemic at first in the United States and other developed nations and ultimately among developing nations throughout the world (see "HIV Infection and AIDS Worldwide," below). The staggering worldwide evolution of the HIV pandemic has been matched by an explosion of information in the areas of HIV virology, pathogenesis (both immunologic and virologic), treatment of HIV disease, treatment and prophylaxis of the opportunistic diseases associated with HIV infection, and prevention of HIV infection. The information flow related to HIV disease is enormous and continues to expand, and it has become almost impossible for the health care generalist to stay abreast of the literature.

The purpose of this chapter is to present the most current information available on the scope of the epidemic; on its pathogenesis, treatment, and prevention; and on prospects for vaccine development. Above all, the aim is to provide a solid scientific basis and practical clinical guidelines for a state-of-the-art approach to the HIV-infected patient.

DEFINITION

The current U.S. CDC classification system for HIV infection and AIDS categorizes people on the basis of clinical conditions associated with HIV infection and CD4+ T lymphocyte measurement. A confirmed HIV case can be classified in one of five HIV infection stages (0, 1, 2, 3, or unknown). If there was a negative HIV test within 6 months of the first HIV infection diagnosis, the stage is 0, and remains 0 until 6 months after diagnosis. Advanced HIV disease (AIDS) is classified as stage 3 if one or more specific opportunistic illness has been diagnosed (Table 226-1). Otherwise, the stage is determined by CD4 test results and immunologic criteria (Table 226-2). If none of these criteria apply (e.g., because of missing information on CD4 test results), the stage is U (unknown).

The definition and staging criteria of AIDS are complex and comprehensive and were established for surveillance purposes rather than for the practical care of patients. Thus, the clinician should not focus

TABLE 226-1 CDC STAGE 3 (AIDS)-DEFINING OPPORTUNISTIC ILLNESSES IN HIV INFECTION

Bacterial infections, multiple or recurrent[a]
Candidiasis of bronchi, trachea, or lungs
Candidiasis of esophagus
Cervical cancer, invasive[b]
Coccidioidomycosis, disseminated or extrapulmonary
Cryptococcosis, extrapulmonary
Cryptosporidiosis, chronic intestinal (>1 month's duration)
Cytomegalovirus disease (other than liver, spleen, or nodes), onset at age >1 month
Cytomegalovirus retinitis (with loss of vision)
Encephalopathy attributed to HIV
Herpes simplex: chronic ulcers (>1 month's duration) or bronchitis, pneumonitis, or esophagitis (onset at age >1 month)
Histoplasmosis, disseminated or extrapulmonary
Isosporiasis, chronic intestinal (>1 month's duration)
Kaposi's sarcoma
Lymphoma, Burkitt's (or equivalent term)
Lymphoma, immunoblastic (or equivalent term)
Lymphoma, primary, of brain
Mycobacterium avium complex or *Mycobacterium kansasii*, disseminated or extrapulmonary
Mycobacterium tuberculosis of any site, pulmonary,[b] disseminated, or extrapulmonary
Mycobacterium, other species or unidentified species, disseminated or extrapulmonary
Pneumocystis jirovecii (previously known as *Pneumocystis carinii*) pneumonia
Pneumonia, recurrent[b]
Progressive multifocal leukoencephalopathy
Salmonella septicemia, recurrent
Toxoplasmosis of brain, onset at age >1 month
Wasting syndrome attributed to HIV

[a]Only among children age <6 years. [b]Only among adults, adolescents, and children age ≥6 years.

Source: MMWR 63(No. RR-03), April 11, 2014.

TABLE 226-2 CDC HIV INFECTION STAGES 1–3 BASED ON AGE-SPECIFIC CD4+ T LYMPHOCYTE COUNT OR CD4+ T LYMPHOCYTE PERCENTAGE OF TOTAL LYMPHOCYTES[a]

	Age on Date of CD4 T+ Lymphocyte Test					
	<1 Year		1–5 Years		6 Years through Adult	
Stage[a]	Cells/μL	%	Cells/μL	%	Cells/μL	%
1	≥1,500	≥34	≥1,000	≥30	≥500	≥26
2	750–1,499	26–33	500–999	22–29	200–499	14–25
3	<750	<26	<500	<22	<200	<14

[a]The stage is based primarily on the CD4+ T-lymphocyte count; the CD4+ T-lymphocyte count takes precedence over the CD4 T-lymphocyte percentage, and the percentage is considered only if the count is missing.

Source: MMWR 63(No. RR-03), April 11, 2014.

on whether the patient fulfills the strict definition of AIDS, but should view HIV disease as a spectrum ranging from primary infection, with or without the acute syndrome, to the asymptomatic stage, to advanced stages associated with opportunistic diseases (see "Pathophysiology and Pathogenesis," below).

ETIOLOGIC AGENT

HIV is the etiologic agent of AIDS; it belongs to the family of human retroviruses (Retroviridae) and the subfamily of lentiviruses (Chap. 225e). Nononcogenic lentiviruses cause disease in other animal species, including sheep, horses, goats, cattle, cats, and monkeys. The four retroviruses known to cause human disease belong to two distinct groups: the human T lymphotropic viruses (HTLV)-1 and HTLV-2, which are transforming retroviruses; and the human immunodeficiency viruses, HIV-1 and HIV-2, which cause cytopathic effects either directly or indirectly (Chap. 225e). The most common cause of HIV disease throughout the world, and certainly in the United States, is HIV-1, which comprises several subtypes with different geographic distributions (see "Molecular Heterogeneity of HIV-1," below). HIV-2 was first identified in 1986 in West African patients and was originally confined to West Africa. However, a number of cases that generally can be traced to West Africa or to sexual contacts with West Africans have been identified throughout the world. The currently defined groups of HIV-1 (M, N, O, P) and the HIV-2 groups A through H each are likely derived from a separate transfer to humans from a nonhuman primate reservoir. HIV-1 viruses likely came from chimpanzees and/or gorillas, and HIV-2 from sooty mangabeys. The AIDS pandemic is primarily caused by the HIV-1 M group viruses. Although HIV-1 group O and HIV-2 viruses have been found in numerous countries, including those in the developed world, they have caused much more localized epidemics. The taxonomic relationship between primate lentiviruses is shown in Fig. 226-1.

MORPHOLOGY OF HIV

Electron microscopy shows that the HIV virion is an icosahedral structure (Fig. 226-2) containing numerous external spikes formed by the two major envelope proteins, the external gp120 and the transmembrane gp41. The HIV envelope exists as a trimeric heterodimer. The virion buds from the surface of the infected cell and incorporates a variety of host proteins into its lipid bilayer. The structure of HIV-1 is schematically diagrammed in Fig. 226-2B.

REPLICATION CYCLE OF HIV

HIV is an RNA virus whose hallmark is the reverse transcription of its genomic RNA to DNA by the enzyme *reverse transcriptase*. The replication cycle of HIV begins with the high-affinity binding of the gp120 protein via a portion of its V1 region near the N terminus to its receptor on the host cell surface, the CD4 molecule (Fig. 226-3). The CD4 molecule is a 55-kDa protein found predominantly on a subset of T lymphocytes that are responsible for helper function in the immune system (Chap. 372e). It is also expressed on the surface of monocytes/macrophages and dendritic/Langerhans cells. Once it binds to CD4, the gp120 protein undergoes a conformational change that facilitates binding to one of two major co-receptors. The two major co-receptors for HIV-1 are CCR5 and CXCR4. Both receptors belong to the family of seven-transmembrane-domain G protein–coupled cellular receptors, and the use of one or the other or both receptors by the virus for entry into the cell is an important determinant of the cellular tropism of the virus. Certain dendritic cells (DCs) express a diversity of C-type lectin receptors on their surface—one of which is called *DC-SIGN*—that also bind with high affinity to the HIV gp120 envelope protein, allowing DCs to facilitate virus spread to CD4+ T cells. Following binding of the envelope protein to the CD4 molecule associated with the above-mentioned conformational change in the viral envelope gp120, fusion with the host cell membrane occurs via the newly exposed gp41 molecule penetrating the plasma membrane of the target cell and then coiling upon itself to bring the virion and target cell together (Fig. 226-4). Following fusion, uncoating of the capsid protein shell is initiated—a step that facilitates reverse transcription and leads to formation of the preintegration complex, composed of viral RNA, enzymes, and accessory proteins and surrounded by capsid and matrix proteins (Fig. 226-3). As the preintegration complex traverses

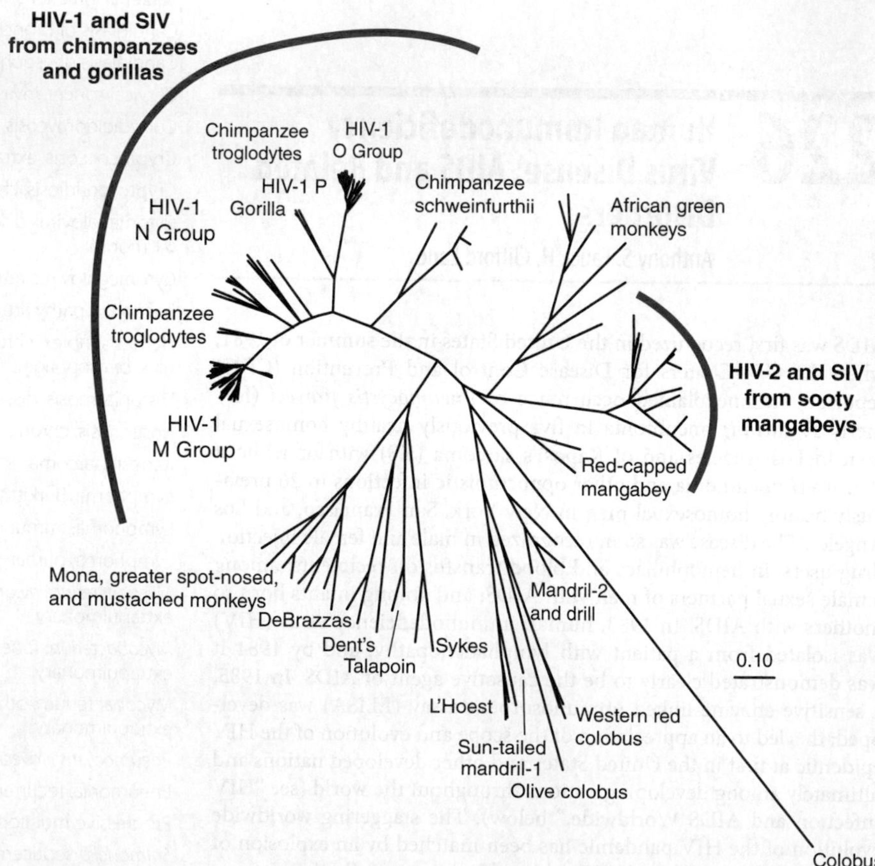

FIGURE 226-1 A phylogenetic tree based on the complete genomes of primate immunodeficiency viruses. The scale (0.10) indicates a 10% difference at the nucleotide level. *(Prepared by Brian Foley, PhD, of the HIV Sequence Database, Theoretical Biology and Biophysics Group, Los Alamos National Laboratory; additional information at www.hiv.lanl.gov/content/sequence/HelpDocs/subtypes.html.)*

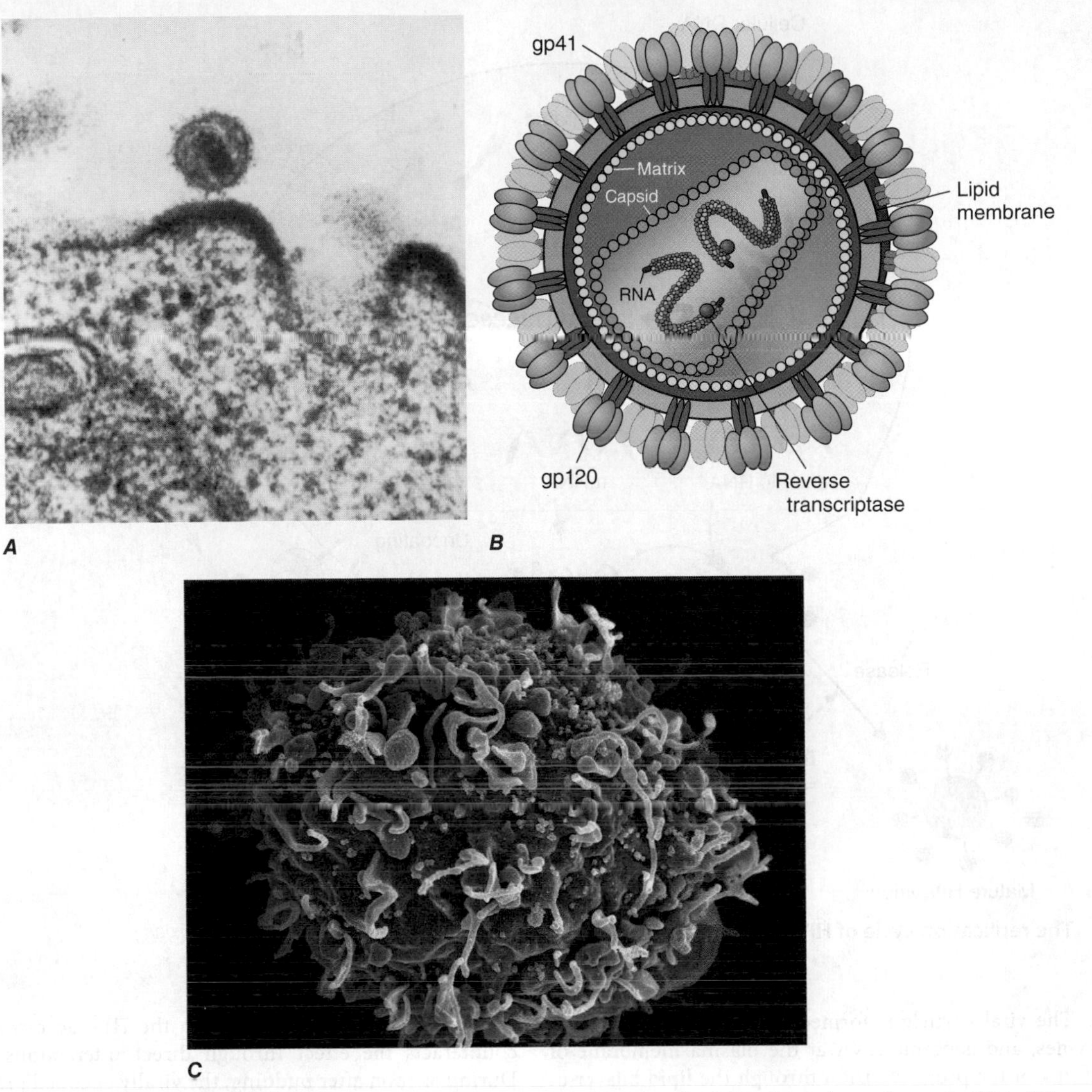

FIGURE 226-2 ***A.*** Electron micrograph of HIV. Figure illustrates a typical virion following budding from the surface of a CD4+ T lymphocyte, together with two additional incomplete virions in the process of budding from the cell membrane. ***B.*** Structure of HIV-1, including the gp120 envelope, gp41 transmembrane components of the envelope, genomic RNA, enzyme reverse transcriptase, p18(17) inner membrane (matrix), and p24 core protein (capsid). *(Copyright by George V. Kelvin.) (Adapted from RC Gallo: Sci Am 256:46, 1987.)* ***C.*** Scanning electron micrograph of HIV-1 virions infecting a human CD4+ T lymphocyte. The original photograph was imaged at 8000× magnification. *(Courtesy of Elizabeth R. Fischer, Rocky Mountain Laboratories, National Institute of Allergy and Infectious Diseases; with permission.)*

the cytoplasm to reach the nucleus, the viral reverse transcriptase enzyme catalyzes the reverse transcription of the genomic RNA into DNA, resulting in the formation of double-stranded proviral HIV-DNA. At the preintegration steps of the replication cycle, the viral genome is vulnerable to cellular factors that can block the progression of infection. In particular, the cytoplasmic tripartite motif-containing protein 5-α (TRIM5-α) is a host restriction factor that interacts with retroviral capsids (Fig. 226-3). Although the exact mechanisms of action of TRIM5-α remain unclear, the HIV-1 capsid is not recognized by the human form of TRIM5-α. Thus this host factor is not effective in restricting HIV-1 replication in human cells. The apolipoprotein B mRNA editing enzyme (catalytic polypeptide-like 3 [APOBEC3]) family of cellular proteins also inhibits progression of virus infection after virus has entered the cell and prior to entering the nucleus (Fig. 226-3). APOBEC3 proteins, which are incorporated into virions and released into the cytoplasm of a newly infected cell, bind to the single minus-strand DNA intermediate and deaminate viral cytidine, causing hypermutation of retroviral genomes. HIV has evolved a powerful strategy to protect itself from APOBEC. The viral protein Vif targets APOBEC3 for proteasomal degradation.

With activation of the cell, the viral DNA accesses the nuclear pore and is exported from the cytoplasm to the nucleus, where it is integrated into the host cell chromosomes through the action of another virally encoded enzyme, *integrase* (Fig. 226-3). HIV provirus (DNA) integrates into the nuclear DNA preferentially within introns of active genes and regional hotspots. This provirus may remain transcriptionally inactive (latent) or it may manifest varying levels of gene expression, up to active production of virus.

Cellular activation plays an important role in the replication cycle of HIV and is critical to the pathogenesis of HIV disease (see "Pathogenesis and Pathophysiology," below). Following initial binding, fusion, and internalization of the nucleic acid contents of virions into the target cell, incompletely reverse-transcribed DNA intermediates are labile in quiescent cells and do not integrate efficiently into the host cell genome unless cellular activation occurs shortly after infection. Furthermore, some degree of activation of the host cell is required for the initiation of transcription of the integrated proviral DNA into either genomic RNA or mRNA. This latter process may not necessarily be associated with the detectable expression of the classic cell-surface markers of activation. In this regard, activation of HIV expression from the latent state depends on the interaction of a number of cellular and viral factors. Following transcription, HIV mRNA is translated into proteins that undergo modification through glycosylation, myristoylation, phosphorylation,

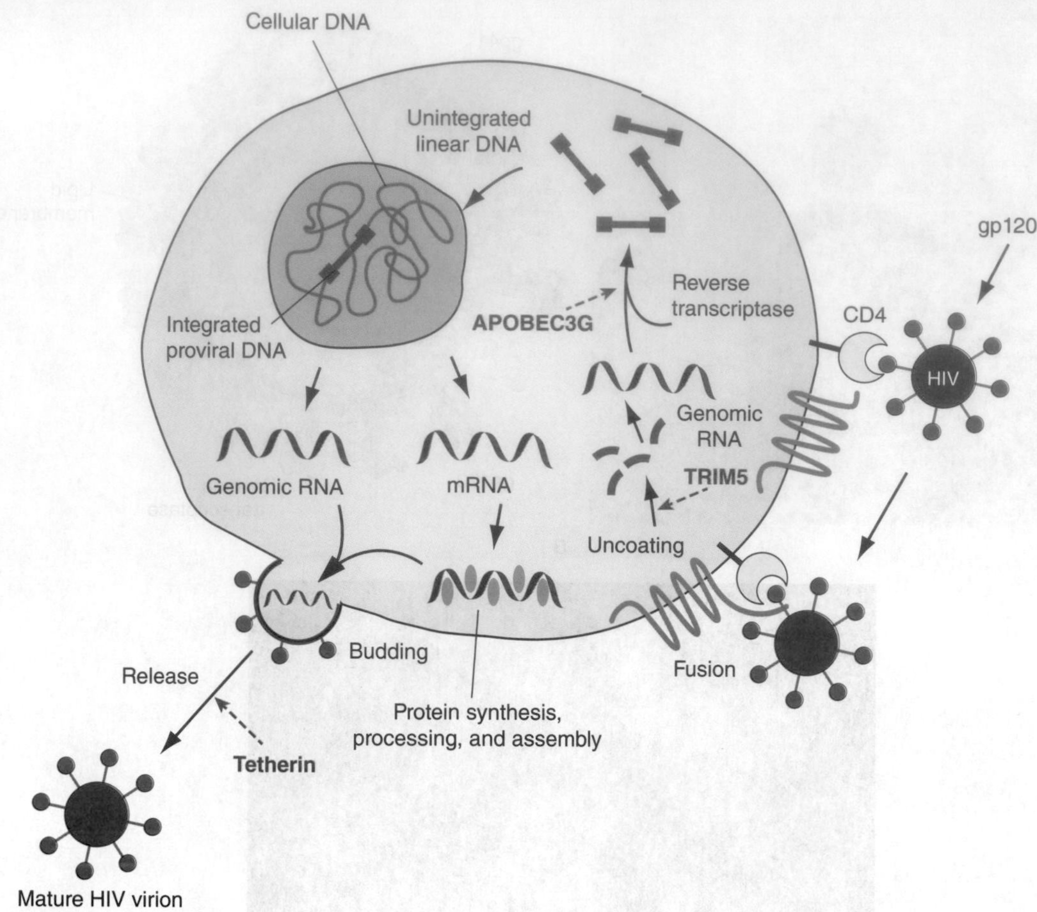

FIGURE 226-3 **The replication cycle of HIV.** See text for description. *(Adapted from AS Fauci: Nature 384:529, 1996.)*

and cleavage. The viral particle is formed by the assembly of HIV proteins, enzymes, and genomic RNA at the plasma membrane of the cells. Budding of the progeny virion through the lipid bilayer of the host cell membrane is the point at which the core acquires its external envelope and where the host restriction factor tetherin can inhibit the release of budding particles (Fig. 226-3). Tetherin is an interferon (IFN)-induced type II transmembrane protein that interferes with virion detachment, although the HIV accessory protein Vpu counteracts the effect through direct interactions with tetherin. During or soon after budding, the virally encoded protease catalyzes the cleavage of the gag-pol precursor to yield the mature virion. Progression through the virus replication cycle is profoundly influenced by a variety of viral regulatory gene products. Likewise, each point in the replication cycle of HIV is a real or potential target for therapeutic intervention. Thus far, the reverse transcriptase, protease, and integrase enzymes as well as the process of virus–target cell binding and fusion have proved clinically to be susceptible to pharmacologic disruption.

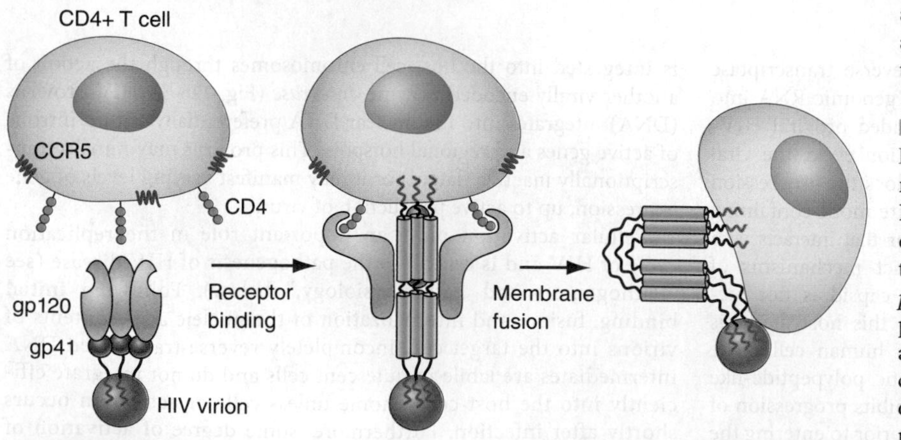

FIGURE 226-4 **Binding and fusion of HIV-1 with its target cell.** HIV-1 binds to its target cell via the CD4 molecule, leading to a conformational change in the gp120 molecule that allows it to bind to the co-receptor CCR5 (for R5-using viruses). The virus then firmly attaches to the host cell membrane in a coiled-spring fashion via the newly exposed gp41 molecule. Virus-cell fusion occurs as the transitional intermediate of gp41 undergoes further changes to form a hairpin structure that draws the two membranes into close proximity (see text for details). *(Adapted from D Montefiori, JP Moore: Science 283:336, 1999; with permission.)*

HIV GENOME

Figure 226-5 illustrates schematically the arrangement of the HIV genome. Like other retroviruses, HIV-1 has genes that encode the structural proteins of the virus: *gag* encodes the proteins that form the core of the virion (including p24 antigen); *pol* encodes the enzymes responsible for protease processing of viral proteins, reverse transcription, and integration; and *env* encodes the envelope glycoproteins. However, HIV-1 is more complex than other retroviruses, particularly those of the nonprimate group, in that it also contains at least six other genes (*tat, rev, nef, vif, vpr,* and *vpu*), which code for proteins involved in the modification of the host cell to enhance virus growth and the regulation of viral gene expression. Several of these proteins are thought to play a role in the pathogenesis of HIV disease; their various functions are listed in Fig. 226-5. Flanking these genes are the long terminal repeats (LTRs), which contain regulatory elements

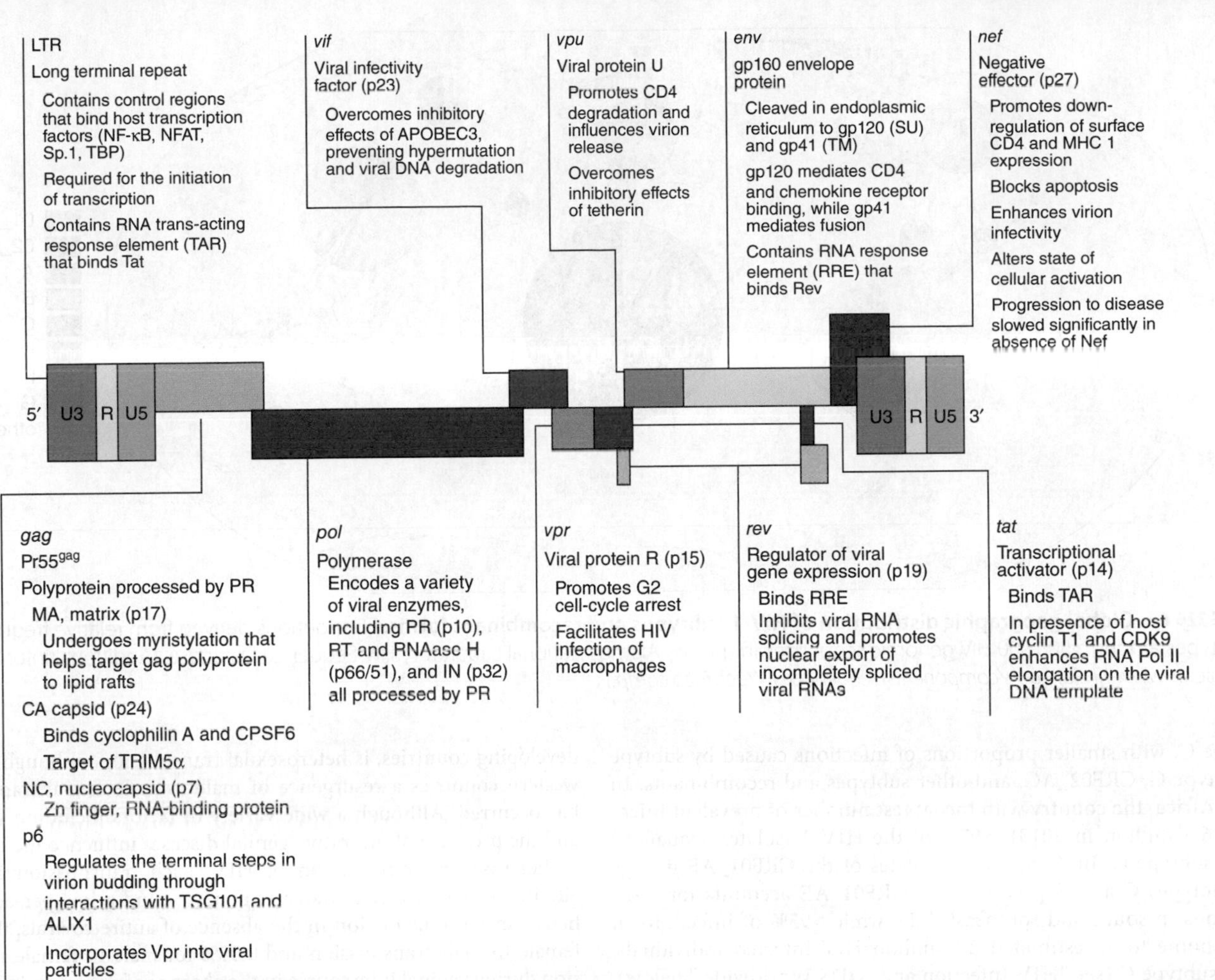

LTR
Long terminal repeat
Contains control regions that bind host transcription factors (NF-κB, NFAT, Sp.1, TBP)
Required for the initiation of transcription
Contains RNA trans-acting response element (TAR) that binds Tat
vif
Viral infectivity factor (p23)
Overcomes inhibitory effects of APOBEC3, preventing hypermutation and viral DNA degradation
vpu
Viral protein U
Promotes CD4 degradation and influences virion release
Overcomes inhibitory effects of tetherin
env
gp160 envelope protein
Cleaved in endoplasmic reticulum to gp120 (SU) and gp41 (TM)
gp120 mediates CD4 and chemokine receptor binding, while gp41 mediates fusion
Contains RNA response element (RRE) that binds Rev
nef
Negative effector (p27)
Promotes down-regulation of surface CD4 and MHC 1 expression
Blocks apoptosis
Enhances virion infectivity
Alters state of cellular activation
Progression to disease slowed significantly in absence of Nef
5′ U3 R U5
U3 R U5 3′
gag
Pr55gag
Polyprotein processed by PR
MA, matrix (p17)
Undergoes myristylation that helps target gag polyprotein to lipid rafts
CA capsid (p24)
Binds cyclophilin A and CPSF6
Target of TRIM5α
NC, nucleocapsid (p7)
Zn finger, RNA-binding protein
p6
Regulates the terminal steps in virion budding through interactions with TSG101 and ALIX1
Incorporates Vpr into viral particles
pol
Polymerase
Encodes a variety of viral enzymes, including PR (p10), RT and RNAase H (p66/51), and IN (p32) all processed by PR
vpr
Viral protein R (p15)
Promotes G2 cell-cycle arrest
Facilitates HIV infection of macrophages
rev
Regulator of viral gene expression (p19)
Binds RRE
Inhibits viral RNA splicing and promotes nuclear export of incompletely spliced viral RNAs
tat
Transcriptional activator (p14)
Binds TAR
In presence of host cyclin T1 and CDK9 enhances RNA Pol II elongation on the viral DNA template

FIGURE 226-5 **Organization of the genome of the HIV provirus** together with a summary description of its 9 genes encoding 15 proteins. *(Adapted from WC Greene, BM Peterlin: Nat Med 8:673, 2002.)*

involved in gene expression (Fig. 226-5). The major difference between the genomes of HIV-1 and HIV-2 is the fact that HIV-2 lacks the *vpu* gene and has a *vpx* gene not contained in HIV-1.

MOLECULAR HETEROGENEITY OF HIV-1

Molecular analyses of HIV isolates reveal varying levels of sequence diversity over all regions of the viral genome. For example, the degree of difference in the coding sequences of the viral envelope protein ranges from a few percent (very close, among isolates from the same infected individual) to more than 50% (extreme diversity, between isolates from the different groups of HIV-1, M, N, O, and P). The changes tend to cluster in hypervariable regions. HIV can evolve by several means, including simple base substitution, insertions and deletions, recombination, and gain and loss of glycosylation sites. HIV sequence diversity arises directly from the limited fidelity of the reverse transcriptase. The balance of immune pressure and functional constraints on proteins influences the regional level of variation within proteins. For example, Envelope, which is exposed on the surface of the virion and is under immune selective pressure from both antibodies and cytolytic T lymphocytes, is extremely variable, with clusters of mutations in hypervariable domains. In contrast, reverse transcriptase, with important enzymatic functions, is relatively conserved, particularly around the active site. The extraordinary variability of HIV-1 contrasts markedly with the relative stability of HTLV-1 and -2.

The four groups (M, N, O and P) of HIV-1 are the result of four separate chimpanzee-to-human (or possibly gorilla-to-human for groups O and P) transfers. Group M (major), which is responsible for most of the infections in the world, has diversified into subtypes and intersubtype recombinant forms, due to "sub-epidemics" within humans after one of those transfers.

Among primate lentiviruses, HIV-1 is most closely related to viruses isolated from chimpanzees and gorillas (Fig. 226-1). The chimpanzee subspecies *Pan troglodytes troglodytes* has been established to be the natural reservoir of the HIV-1 M and N groups. The rare viruses of the HIV-1 O and P groups are most closely related to viruses found in Cameroonian gorillas. The M group comprises nine subtypes, or *clades*, designated A, B, C, D, F, G, H, J, and K, as well as more than 60 known circulating recombinant forms (CRFs) and numerous unique recombinant forms. Intersubtype recombinants are generated by infection of an individual with two subtypes that then recombine and create a virus with a selective advantage. These CRFs range from highly prevalent forms such as CRF01_AE, common in southeast Asia, and CRF02_AG from west and central Africa, to a large number of CRFs that are relatively rare, either because they are of a more recent origin (newly recombined) or because they have not broken out into a major population. The subtypes and CRFs create the major lineages of the M group of HIV-1. HIV-1 M group subtype C dominates the global pandemic, and there is much speculation that it is more transmissible than other subtypes, but solid data on transmissibility variations between subtypes are rare. Human population densities, access to prevention and treatment, prevalence of genital ulcers, iatrogenic transmissions, and other confounding host factors are all possible reasons why one subtype has spread more than another.

Figure 226-6 schematically diagrams the worldwide distribution of HIV-1 subtypes by region. Seven strains account for the vast majority of HIV infections globally: HIV-1 subtypes A, B, C, D, G and two of the CRFs, CRF01_AE and CRF02_AG. Subtype C viruses (of the M group) are by far the most common form worldwide, likely accounting for ~50% of prevalent infections worldwide. In sub-Saharan Africa, home to approximately two-thirds of all individuals living with HIV/AIDS, the majority of infections are caused by

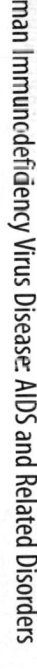

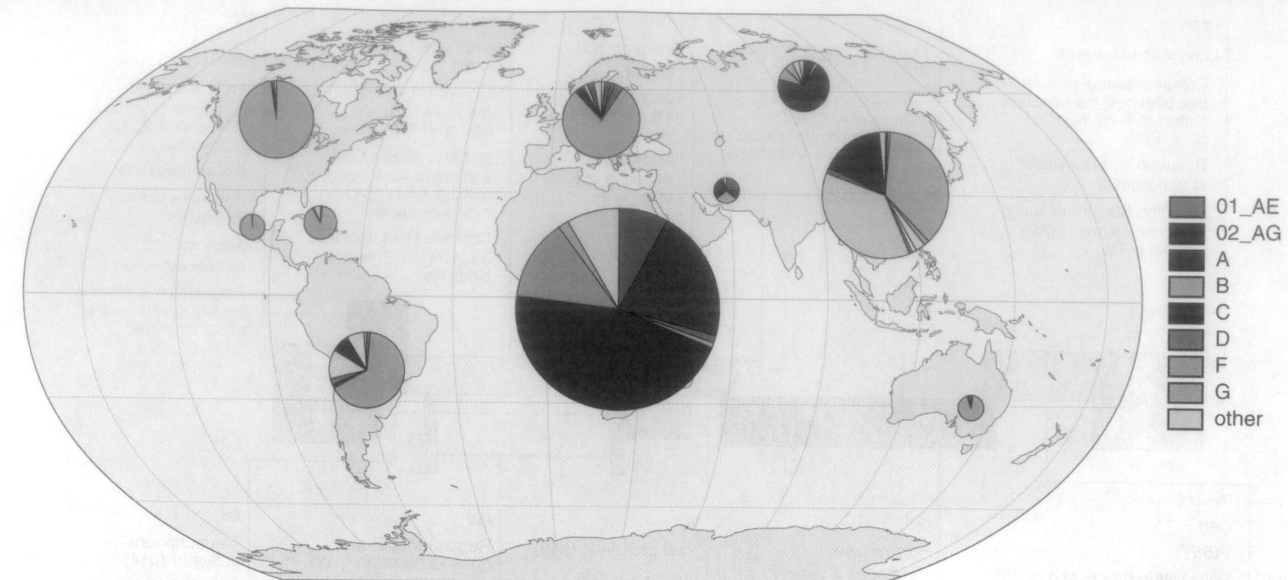

FIGURE 226-6 Global geographic distribution of HIV-1 subtypes and recombinant forms. Distributions derived from relative frequency of subtypes among >500,000 HIV genomic sequences in the Los Alamos National Laboratory HIV Sequence Database. (Additional information available at *www.hiv.lanl.gov/components/sequence/HIV/geo/geo.comp.*)

subtype C, with smaller proportions of infections caused by subtype A, subtype G, CRF02_AG, and other subtypes and recombinants. In South Africa, the country with the largest number of prevalent infections (6.3 million in 2013), >97% of the HIV-1 isolates sequenced are of subtype C. In Asia, HIV-1 isolates of the CRF01_AE lineage and subtypes C and B predominate. CRF01_AE accounts for most infections in south and southeast Asia, while >95% of infections in India, home to an estimated 2.1 million HIV-infected individuals, are of subtype C (see "HIV Infection and AIDS Worldwide," below). Subtype B viruses are the overwhelmingly predominant viruses seen in the United States, Canada, certain countries in South America, western Europe, and Australia. It is thought that, purely by chance, subtype B was seeded into the United States and Europe in the late 1970s, thereby establishing an overwhelming founder effect. Many countries have co-circulating viral subtypes that are giving rise to new CRFs. Sequence analyses of HIV-1 isolates from infected individuals indicate that recombination among viruses of different clades likely occurs as a result of infection of an individual with viruses of more than one subtype, particularly in geographic areas where subtypes overlap, and more often in sub-epidemics driven by IV drug use than in those driven by sexual transmission.

The extraordinary diversity of HIV, reflected by the presence of multiple subtypes, circulating recombinant forms, and continuous viral evolution, has implications for possible differential rates of transmission, rates of disease progression, responses to therapy, and the development of resistance to antiretroviral drugs. This diversity is also a formidable obstacle to HIV vaccine development, as a broadly useful vaccine would need to induce protective responses against a wide range of viral strains.

TRANSMISSION

HIV is transmitted primarily by sexual contact (both heterosexual and male to male); by blood and blood products; and by infected mothers to infants intrapartum, perinatally, or via breast milk. After more than 30 years of experience and observations regarding other potential modalities of transmission, there is no evidence that HIV is transmitted by casual contact or that the virus can be spread by insects, such as by a mosquito bite. Table 226-3 lists the estimated risk of HIV transmission for various types of exposures.

SEXUAL TRANSMISSION

HIV infection is predominantly a sexually transmitted infection (STI) worldwide. By far the most common mode of infection, particularly in developing countries, is heterosexual transmission, although in many western countries a resurgence of male-to-male sexual transmission has occurred. Although a wide variety of factors including viral load and the presence of ulcerative genital diseases influence the efficiency of heterosexual transmission of HIV, such transmission is generally inefficient. A recent systemic review found a low per-act risk of heterosexual transmission in the absence of antiretrovirals: 0.04% for female-to-male transmission and 0.08% for male-to-female transmission during vaginal intercourse in the absence of antiretroviral therapy or condom use (Table 226-3).

HIV has been demonstrated in seminal fluid both within infected mononuclear cells and in cell-free material. The virus appears to concentrate in the seminal fluid, particularly in situations where there are increased numbers of lymphocytes and monocytes in the fluid,

TABLE 226-3 ESTIMATED PER-ACT PROBABILITY OF ACQUIRING HIV FROM AN INFECTED SOURCE, BY EXPOSURE ACT

Type of Exposure	Risk per 10,000 Exposures
Parenteral	
Blood transfusion	9250
Needle-sharing during injection drug use	63
Percutaneous (needle-stick)	23
Sexual	
Receptive anal intercourse	138
Insertive anal intercourse	11
Receptive penile-vaginal intercourse	8
Insertive penile-vaginal intercourse	4
Receptive oral intercourse	Low
Insertive oral intercourse	Low
Other[a]	
Biting	Negligible
Spitting	Negligible
Throwing body fluids (including semen or saliva)	Negligible
Sharing sex toys	Negligible

[a]HIV transmission through these exposure routes is technically possible but unlikely and not well documented.

Sources: CDC, *www.cdc.gov/hiv/policies/law/risk.html*; P Patel: AIDS 28:1509, 2014.

as in genital inflammatory states such as urethritis and epididymitis, conditions closely associated with other STIs. The virus has also been demonstrated in cervical smears and vaginal fluid. There is an elevated risk of HIV transmission associated with unprotected receptive anal intercourse (URAI) among both men and women compared to the risk associated with receptive vaginal intercourse. Although data are limited, the per-act risk for HIV transmission via URAI has been estimated to be ~1.4% (Table 226-3). The risk of HIV acquisition associated with URAI is probably higher than that seen in penile-vaginal intercourse because only a thin, fragile rectal mucosal membrane separates the deposited semen from potentially susceptible cells in and beneath the mucosa, and micro-trauma of the mucosal membrane may be associated with anal intercourse. Anal douching and sexual practices that traumatize the rectal mucosa also increase the likelihood of infection. It is likely that anal intercourse provides at least two modalities of infection: (1) direct inoculation into blood in cases of traumatic tears in the mucosa; and (2) infection of susceptible target cells, such as Langerhans cells, in the mucosal layer in the absence of trauma. Insertive anal intercourse also confers an increased risk of HIV acquisition compared to insertive vaginal intercourse. Although the vaginal mucosa is several layers thicker than the rectal mucosa and less likely to be traumatized during intercourse, the virus can be transmitted to either partner through vaginal intercourse. As noted in Table 226-3, male-to-female HIV transmission is usually more efficient than female-to-male transmission. The differences in reported transmission rates between men and women may be due in part to the prolonged exposure to infected seminal fluid of the vaginal and cervical mucosa, as well as the endometrium (when semen enters through the cervical os). By comparison, the penis and urethral orifice are exposed relatively briefly to infected vaginal fluid. Among various cofactors examined in studies of heterosexual HIV transmission, the presence of other STIs has been strongly associated with HIV transmission. In this regard, there is a close association between genital ulcerations and transmission, owing to both susceptibility to infection and infectivity. Infections with microorganisms such as *Treponema pallidum* (Chap. 206), *Haemophilus ducreyi* (Chap. 182), and herpes simplex virus (HSV; Chap. 216) are important causes of genital ulcerations linked to transmission of HIV. In addition, pathogens responsible for non-ulcerative inflammatory STIs such as those caused by *Chlamydia trachomatis* (Chap. 213), *Neisseria gonorrhoeae* (Chap. 181), and *Trichomonas vaginalis* (Chap. 254) also are associated with an increased risk of transmission of HIV infection. Bacterial vaginosis, an infection related to sexual behavior, but not strictly an STI, also may be linked to an increased risk of transmission of HIV infection. Several studies suggest that treating other STIs and genital tract syndromes may help prevent transmission of HIV. This effect is most prominent in populations in which the prevalence of HIV infection is relatively low. It is noteworthy that this principle may not apply to the treatment of HSV infections since it has been shown that even following anti-HSV therapy with resulting healing of HSV-related genital ulcers, HIV acquisition is not reduced. Biopsy studies revealed the likely explanation is that HIV receptor–positive inflammatory cells persisted in the genital tissue despite the healing of ulcers, and so HIV-susceptible targets remained at the site.

The quantity of HIV-1 in plasma is a primary determinant of the risk of HIV-1 transmission. In a cohort of heterosexual couples in Uganda discordant for HIV infection and not receiving antiretroviral therapy, the mean serum HIV RNA level was significantly higher among HIV-infected subjects whose partners seroconverted than among those whose partners did not seroconvert. In fact, transmission was rare when the infected partner had a plasma level of <1700 copies of HIV RNA per milliliter, even when genital ulcer disease was present (Fig. 226-7). The rate of HIV transmission per coital act was highest during the early stage of HIV infection when plasma HIV RNA levels were high and in advanced disease as the viral set point increased.

Antiretroviral therapy dramatically reduces plasma viremia in most HIV-infected individuals (see "Treatment," below) and is associated with a reduction in risk of transmission. In a large study of serodiscordant couples, earlier treatment of the HIV-infected partner with

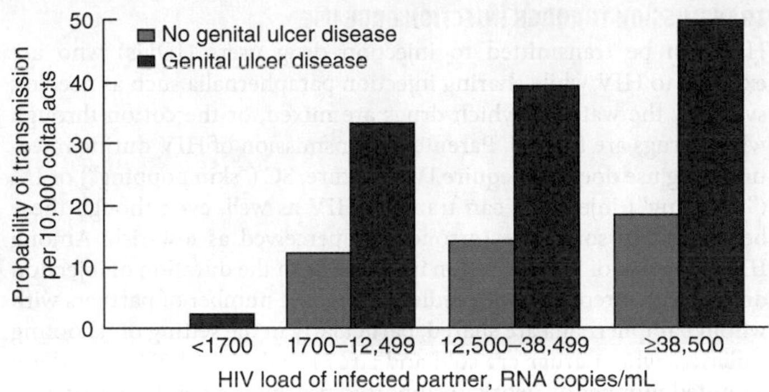

FIGURE 226-7 Probability of HIV transmission per coital act among monogamous, heterosexual, HIV-serodiscordant couples in Uganda. *(From RH Gray et al: Lancet 357:1149, 2001.)*

antiretroviral therapy rather than treatment delayed until the CD4+ T cells count fell below 250 cells per μL was associated with a 96% reduction in HIV transmission to the uninfected partner. This approach has been widely referred to as *treatment as prevention* or TasP. Several studies also have suggested a beneficial effect of antiretroviral treatment at the community level.

A number of studies including large, randomized, controlled trials clearly have indicated that male *circumcision* is associated with a lower risk of acquisition of HIV infection for heterosexual men. Studies are conflicting as to whether circumcision protects against HIV acquisition among men who have sex with men, but data suggest that circumcision is protective in those men who have sex with men who are insertive only. The benefit of circumcision may be due to increased susceptibility of uncircumcised men to ulcerative STIs, as well as to other factors such as microtrauma to the foreskin and glans penis. In addition, the highly vascularized inner foreskin tissue contains a high density of Langerhans cells as well as increased numbers of CD4+ T cells, macrophages, and other cellular targets for HIV. Finally, the moist environment under the foreskin may promote the presence or persistence of microbial flora that, via inflammatory changes, may lead to even higher concentrations of target cells for HIV in the foreskin. In addition, randomized trials have demonstrated that male circumcision also reduces hepatitis C virus (HCV) type 2, human papillomavirus virus (HPV), and genital ulcer disease in men as well as HPV, genital ulcer disease, bacterial vaginosis, and *Trichomonas vaginalis* infections among female partners of circumcised men. Thus, there may be an added benefit of diminution of risk for HIV acquisition to the female sexual partners of circumcised men.

In some studies the use of oral contraceptives was associated with an increase in incidence of HIV infection over and above that which might be expected by not using a condom for birth control. This phenomenon may be due to drug-induced changes in the cervical mucosa, rendering it more vulnerable to penetration by the virus. Adolescent girls might also be more susceptible to infection upon exposure due to the properties of an immature genital tract with increased cervical ectopy or exposed columnar epithelium.

Oral sex is a much less efficient mode of transmission of HIV than is anal intercourse or vaginal intercourse (Table 226-3). A number of studies have reported that the incidence of transmission of infection by oral sex among couples discordant for HIV was extremely low. However, there have been well-documented reports of HIV transmission that likely resulted from fellatio or cunnilingus. Therefore, the assumption that oral sex is completely safe is not warranted.

The association of alcohol consumption and illicit drug use with unsafe sexual behavior, both homosexual and heterosexual, leads to an increased risk of sexual transmission of HIV. Methamphetamine and other so-called club drugs (e.g., ecstasy, ketamine, and gamma hydroxybutyrate), sometimes taken in conjunction with PDE-5 inhibitors such as sildenafil (Viagra), tadalafil (Cialis), or vardenafil (Levitra), have been associated with risky sexual practices and increased risk of HIV infection, particularly among men who have sex with men.

TRANSMISSION THROUGH INJECTION DRUG USE

HIV can be transmitted to injection drug users (IDUs) who are exposed to HIV while sharing injection paraphernalia such as needles, syringes, the water in which drugs are mixed, or the cotton through which drugs are filtered. Parenteral transmission of HIV during injection drug use does not require IV puncture; SC ("skin popping") or IM ("muscling") injections can transmit HIV as well, even though these behaviors are sometimes erroneously perceived as low-risk. Among IDUs, the risk of HIV infection increases with the duration of injection drug use; the frequency of needle sharing; the number of partners with whom paraphernalia are shared, particularly in the setting of "shooting galleries" where drugs are sold and large numbers of IDUs may share a limited number of "works"; comorbid psychiatric conditions such as antisocial personality disorder; the use of cocaine in injectable form or smoked as "crack"; and the use of injection drugs in a geographic location with a high prevalence of HIV infection, such as certain inner-city areas in the United States. As noted in Table 226-3, the per-act risk of transmission from injection drug use with a contaminated needle has been estimated to be approximately 0.6%.

TRANSMISSION BY TRANSFUSED BLOOD AND BLOOD PRODUCTS

HIV can be transmitted to individuals who receive HIV-tainted blood transfusions, blood products, or transplanted tissue. The first cases of AIDS among transfusion recipients and individuals with hemophilia or other clotting disorders were reported in 1982. The vast majority of HIV infections acquired via contaminated blood transfusions, blood components, or transplanted tissue in resource-rich countries occurred prior to the spring of 1985, when mandatory testing of donated blood for HIV-1 was initiated. It is estimated that >90% of individuals exposed to HIV-contaminated blood products become infected (Table 226-3). Although blood screening for HIV is becoming more universal even in the developing world, unfortunately, in some resource-poor countries, HIV continues to be transmitted by blood, blood products, and tissues due to inadequate screening. Transfusions of whole blood, packed red blood cells, platelets, leukocytes, and plasma are all capable of transmitting HIV infection. In contrast, hyperimmune gamma globulin, hepatitis B immune globulin, plasma-derived hepatitis B vaccine, and Rh_0 immune globulin have not been associated with transmission of HIV infection. The procedures involved in processing these products either inactivate or remove the virus.

Currently, in the United States and in most developed countries, the following measures have made the risk of transmission of HIV infection by transfused blood or blood products extremely small: the screening of blood donations for antibodies to HIV-1 and HIV-2 and determination of the presence of HIV nucleic acid usually in minipools of several specimens; the careful selection of potential blood donors with health history questionnaires to exclude individuals with risk behavior; and opportunities for self-deferral and the screening out of HIV-negative individuals with serologic testing for infections that have shared risk factors with HIV, such as hepatitis B and C and syphilis. The chance of infection of a hemophiliac via clotting factor concentrates has essentially been eliminated because of the added layer of safety resulting from heat treatment of the concentrates. It is currently estimated that the risk of infection with HIV in the United States via transfused screened blood is approximately 1 in 2 million units. Therefore, since ~16 million donations are collected in the United States each year, despite the best efforts of science, one cannot completely eliminate the risk of transfusion-related transmission of HIV. In this regard, a case of transfusion-related transmission of HIV was reported in the United States in 2010, which was tracked to a blood donation in 2008; this was the first such reported case since 2002. Transmission of HIV (both HIV-1 and HIV-2) by blood or blood products is still an ongoing threat in certain developing countries, particularly in sub-Saharan Africa, where routine screening of blood is not universally practiced. In other countries, there have been reports of sporadic breakdowns in routinely available screening procedures in which contaminated blood was allowed to be transfused, resulting in small clusters of patients becoming infected. For example, in China in the 1990s, a disturbingly large number of persons became infected by selling blood in situations where the collectors reused needles that were contaminated and, in some instances, mixed blood products from a number of individuals, separated the plasma, and reinfused mixed red blood cells back into the individual donors.

OCCUPATIONAL TRANSMISSION OF HIV: HEALTH CARE WORKERS, LABORATORY WORKERS, AND THE HEALTH CARE SETTING

There is a small but definite occupational risk of HIV transmission to health care workers and laboratory personnel and potentially others who work with HIV-containing materials, particularly when sharp objects are used. An estimated 600,000 to 800,000 health care workers are stuck with needles or other sharp medical instruments in the United States each year. The global number of HIV infections among health care workers attributable to sharps injuries has been estimated to be 1000 cases (range, 200–5000) per year. As of 2010, there had been 57 documented cases of occupational HIV transmission to health care workers in the United States and 143 possible transmissions. There have been no confirmed cases reported since 1999.

Exposures that place a health care worker at potential risk of HIV infection are percutaneous injuries (e.g., a needle stick or cut with a sharp object) or contact of mucous membrane or nonintact skin (e.g., exposed skin that is chapped, abraded, or afflicted with dermatitis) with blood, tissue, or other potentially infectious body fluids. Large, multi-institutional studies have indicated that the risk of HIV transmission following skin puncture from a needle or a sharp object that was contaminated with blood from a person with documented HIV infection is ~0.3% and after a mucous membrane exposure it is 0.09% (see "HIV and the Health Care Worker," below) if the injured and/or exposed person is not treated within 24 h with antiretroviral drugs. The risk of hepatitis B virus (HBV) infection following a similar type of exposure is ~6–30% in nonimmune individuals; if a susceptible worker is exposed to HBV, postexposure prophylaxis with hepatitis B immune globulin and initiation of HBV vaccine is >90% effective in preventing HBV infection. The risk of HCV infection following percutaneous injury is ~1.8% (Chap. 360).

Rare HIV transmission after nonintact skin exposure has been documented, but the average risk for transmission by this route has not been precisely determined; however, it is estimated to be less than the risk for mucous membrane exposure. Transmission of HIV through intact skin has not been documented. Currently in developed countries, virtually all puncture wounds and mucous membrane exposures in health care workers involving blood from a patient with documented HIV infection are treated prophylactically with combination antiretroviral therapy (cART). This practice, referred to as *postexposure prophylaxis* or PEP, has dramatically reduced the occurrence of puncture-related transmissions of HIV to health care workers.

In addition to blood and visibly bloody body fluids, semen and vaginal secretions also are considered potentially infectious; however, they have not been implicated in occupational transmission from patients to health care workers. The following fluids also are considered potentially infectious: cerebrospinal fluid, synovial fluid, pleural fluid, peritoneal fluid, pericardial fluid, and amniotic fluid. The risk for transmission after exposure to fluids or tissues other than HIV-infected blood also has not been quantified, but it is probably considerably lower than the risk after blood exposures. Feces, nasal secretions, saliva, sputum, sweat, tears, urine, and vomitus are not considered potentially infectious for HIV unless they are visibly bloody. Rare cases of HIV transmission via human bites have been reported, but not in the setting of occupational exposure.

An increased risk for HIV infection following percutaneous exposures to HIV-infected blood is associated with exposures involving a relatively large quantity of blood, as in the case of a device visibly contaminated with the patient's blood, a procedure that involves a hollow-bore needle placed directly in a vein or artery, or a deep injury. Factors that might be associated with mucocutaneous transmission of HIV include exposure to an unusually large volume of blood and prolonged contact. In addition, the risk increases for exposures to blood from untreated patients with advanced-stage disease or those patients in the acute stage of HIV infection, owing to the higher levels of HIV in the blood under those circumstances. Since the beginning of the HIV epidemic, there have been rare instances where transmission of infection from a health care worker to patients seemed highly probable. Despite these small number of documented cases, the risk of HIV transmission involving health care workers (infected or not) to patients is extremely low in developed countries—in fact, too low to be measured accurately. In this regard, several epidemiologic studies have been performed tracing thousands of patients of HIV-infected dentists, physicians, surgeons, obstetricians, and gynecologists, and no other cases of HIV transmission that could be linked to the health care providers were identified.

Breaches in infection control and the reuse of contaminated syringes, failure to properly sterilize surgical instruments, and/or hemodialysis equipment have also resulted rarely in the transmission of HIV from patient to patient in hospitals, nursing homes, and outpatient settings. Finally, these very rare occurrences of transmission of HIV as well as HBV and HCV to and from health care workers in the workplace underscore the importance of the use of universal precautions when caring for all patients (see below and Chap. 168).

MOTHER-TO-CHILD TRANSMISSION OF HIV

HIV infection can be transmitted from an infected mother to her fetus during pregnancy, during delivery, or by breast-feeding. This remains an important form of transmission of HIV infection in certain developing countries, where the proportion of infected women to infected men is ~1:1. Virologic analyses of aborted fetuses indicate that HIV can be transmitted to the fetus during the first or second trimesters of pregnancy. However, maternal transmission to the fetus occurs most commonly in the perinatal period. Two studies performed in Rwanda and the Democratic Republic of Congo (then called Zaire) indicated that among all mother-to-child transmissions of HIV, the relative proportions were 23–30% before birth, 50–65% during birth, and 12–20% via breast-feeding.

In the absence of prophylactic antiretroviral therapy to the mother during pregnancy, labor, and delivery, and to the fetus following birth, the probability of transmission of HIV from mother to infant/fetus ranges from 15% to 25% in industrialized countries and from 25% to 35% in developing countries. These differences may relate to the adequacy of prenatal care as well as to the stage of HIV disease and the general health of the mother during pregnancy. Higher rates of transmission have been reported to be associated with many factors—the best documented of which is the presence of high maternal levels of plasma viremia, with the risk increasing linearly with the level of maternal plasma viremia. It is very unlikely that mother-to-child transmission will occur if the mother's level of plasma viremia is <1000 copies of HIV RNA/mL of blood and extremely unlikely if the level is undetectable (i.e., <50 copies/mL). However, there may not be a lower "threshold" below which transmission never occurs, since certain studies have reported rare transmission by women with viral RNA levels <50 copies/mL. Increased mother-to-child transmission is also correlated with closer human leukocyte antigen (HLA) match between mother and child. A prolonged interval between membrane rupture and delivery is another well-documented risk factor for transmission. Other conditions that are potential risk factors, but that have not been consistently demonstrated, are the presence of chorioamnionitis at delivery; STIs during pregnancy; illicit drug use during pregnancy; cigarette smoking; preterm delivery; and obstetric procedures such as amniocentesis, amnioscopy, fetal scalp electrodes, and episiotomy. In a seminal study conducted in the United States and France in the 1990s, zidovudine treatment of HIV-infected pregnant women from the beginning of the second trimester through delivery and of the infant for 6 weeks following birth dramatically decreased the rate of intrapartum and perinatal transmission of HIV infection from 22.6% in the untreated group to <5%. Today, the rate of mother-to-child transmission has fallen to 1% or less in pregnant women who are receiving combination antiretroviral therapy (cART) for their HIV infection. Such treatment, combined with cesarean section delivery, has rendered mother-to-child transmission of HIV an unusual event in the United States and other developed nations. In this regard, both the United States Public Health Service and the World Health Organization guidelines recommend that all pregnant HIV-infected women should receive cART for the health of the mother and to prevent perinatal transmission regardless of plasma HIV RNA copy number or CD4+ T cell counts.

Breast-feeding is an important modality of transmission of HIV infection in developing countries, particularly where mothers continue to breast-feed for prolonged periods. The risk factors for mother-to-child transmission of HIV via breast-feeding are not fully understood; factors that increase the likelihood of transmission include detectable levels of HIV in breast milk, the presence of mastitis, low maternal CD4+ T cell counts, and maternal vitamin A deficiency. The risk of HIV infection via breast-feeding is highest in the early months of breast-feeding. In addition, exclusive breast-feeding has been reported to carry a lower risk of HIV transmission than mixed feeding. In developed countries, breast feeding of babies by an HIV-infected mother is contraindicated since alternative forms of adequate nutrition, i.e., formulas, are readily available. In developing countries, where breast-feeding may be essential for the overall health of the infant, the continuation of cART in the infected mother during the period of breastfeeding markedly diminishes the risk of transmission of HIV to the infant. In fact, once cART has been initiated in a pregnant woman, many experts recommend that therapy be continued for life.

TRANSMISSION OF HIV BY OTHER BODY FLUIDS

Although HIV can be isolated typically in low titers from saliva of a small proportion of infected individuals, there is no convincing evidence that saliva can transmit HIV infection, either through kissing or through other exposures, such as occupationally to health care workers. Saliva contains endogenous antiviral factors; among these factors, HIV-specific immunoglobulins of IgA, IgG, and IgM isotypes are detected readily in salivary secretions of infected individuals. It has been suggested that large glycoproteins such as mucins and thrombospondin 1 sequester HIV into aggregates for clearance by the host. In addition, a number of soluble salivary factors inhibit HIV to various degrees in vitro, probably by targeting host cell receptors rather than the virus itself. Perhaps the best studied of these, secretory leukocyte protease inhibitor (SLPI), blocks HIV infection in several cell culture systems, and it is found in saliva at levels that approximate those required for inhibition of HIV in vitro. In this regard, higher salivary levels of SLPI in breast-fed infants were associated with a decreased risk of HIV transmission through breast milk. It has also been suggested that submandibular saliva reduces HIV infectivity by stripping gp120 from the surface of virions, and that saliva-mediated disruption and lysis of HIV-infected cells occurs because of the hypotonicity of oral secretions. There have been outlier cases of suspected transmission by saliva, but these have probably been blood-to-blood transmissions. Transmission of HIV by a human bite can occur but is a rare event. Although virus can be identified, if not isolated, from virtually any body fluid, there is no evidence that HIV transmission can occur as a result of exposure to tears, sweat, or urine. However, there have been isolated cases of transmission of HIV infection by body fluids that may or may not have been contaminated with blood. Most of these situations occurred in the setting of a close relative providing intensive nursing care for an HIV-infected person without observing universal precautions, underscoring the importance of adhering to such precautions in the handling of body fluids and wastes from HIV-infected individuals.

EPIDEMIOLOGY

HIV INFECTION AND AIDS WORLDWIDE

HIV infection/AIDS is a global pandemic, with cases reported from virtually every country. At the end of 2013, an estimated 35.0 million individuals were living with HIV infection, according to the Joint United Nations Programme on HIV/AIDS (UNAIDS). An estimated 95% of people living with HIV/AIDS reside in low- and middle-income countries; ~50% are female, and 3.2 million are children <15 years. The distribution of these cases is illustrated in Fig. 226-8. The estimated number of people living with HIV—i.e.,

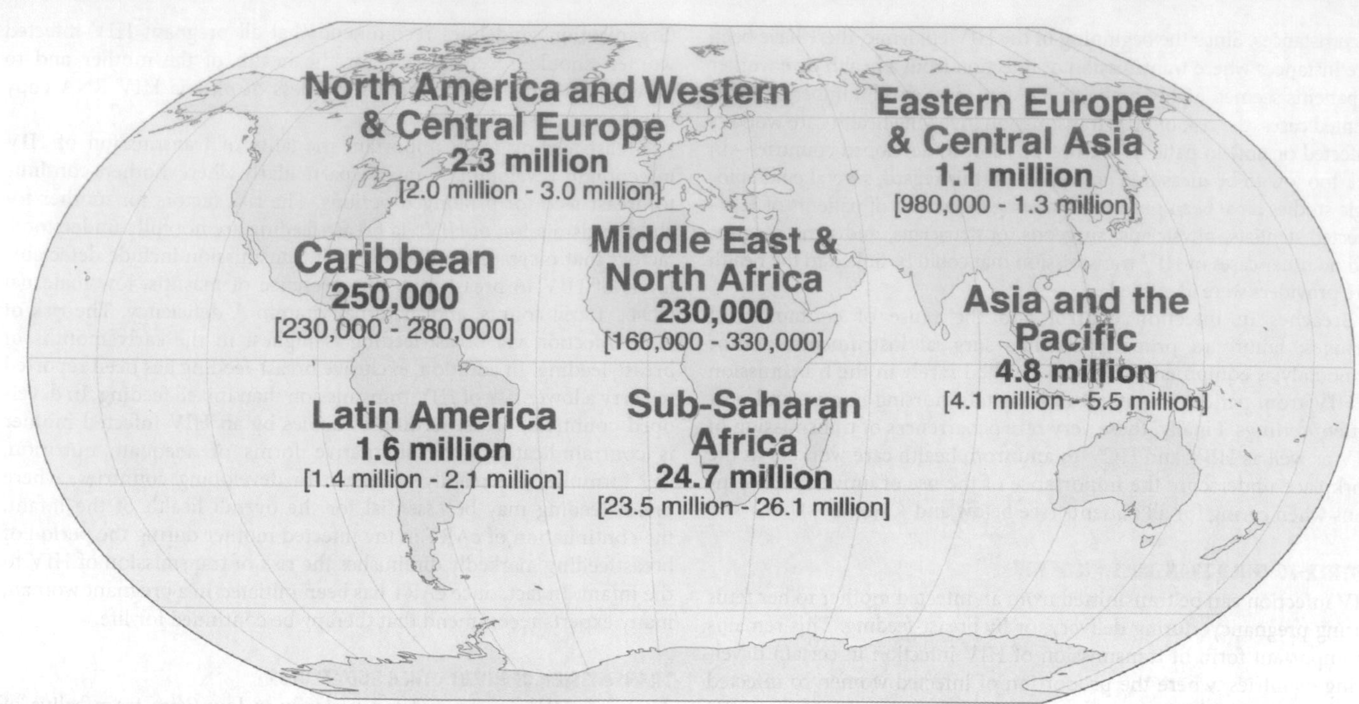

FIGURE 226-8 Estimated number of adults and children living with HIV infection as of December, 2013. Total: 35.0 (33.2 million–37.2 million). *(From Joint United Nations Programme on HIV/AIDS [UNAIDS].)*

the global prevalence—has increased more than fourfold since 1990, reflecting the combined effects of continued high rates of new HIV infections and the life-prolonging impact of antiretroviral therapy (Fig. 226-9). In 2013, the global prevalence rate among persons age 15–49 years was 0.8%, with rates varying widely by country and region as illustrated in Fig. 226-10.

In 2013, an estimated 2.1 million new cases of HIV infection occurred worldwide, including 240,000 among children <15 years; about 40% of new infections were among persons under age 25. Between 2001 and 2013, the estimated number of new HIV infections globally fell by 38% (Fig. 226-9). Recent reductions in global HIV incidence likely reflect progress with HIV prevention efforts and the increased provision to HIV-infected people of antiretroviral therapy, which makes them much less likely to transmit the virus to sexual partners. In 2013, global AIDS deaths totaled 1.5 million (including 190,000 children <15 years), a 35% decrease since 2005 that coincides with a rapid expansion of access to antiretroviral therapy (Fig. 226-9). Since the beginning of the pandemic, an estimated 39 million people have died of an AIDS-related illness.

The HIV epidemic has occurred in "waves" in different regions of the world, each wave having somewhat different characteristics depending on the demographics of the country and region in question and the timing of the introduction of HIV into the population. Although the AIDS epidemic was first recognized in the United States and shortly thereafter in Western Europe, it very likely began in sub-Saharan Africa (see above), which has been particularly devastated by the epidemic. More than 70% of all people with HIV infection (~25 million), and nearly 90% of all HIV-infected children live in that region, even though sub-Saharan Africa is home to just 12% of the world's population (Fig. 226-8). Within the region, southern Africa is worst-affected. In nine southern African countries, seroprevalence data indicate that >10% of the adult population age 15–49 is HIV-infected (Fig. 226-10). In addition, among high-risk individuals (e.g., commercial sex workers, patients attending STI clinics) who live in urban areas of sub-Saharan Africa, seroprevalence is now >50% in some places. Recent data offer promising signs of declining HIV incidence and prevalence in many countries in the region, although frequently at levels that remain high. Heterosexual exposure is

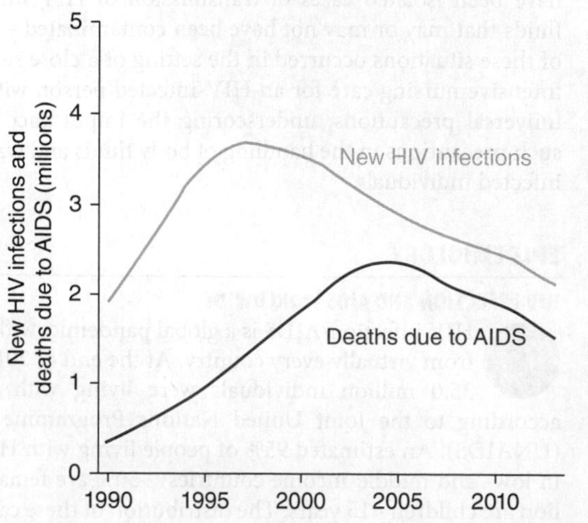

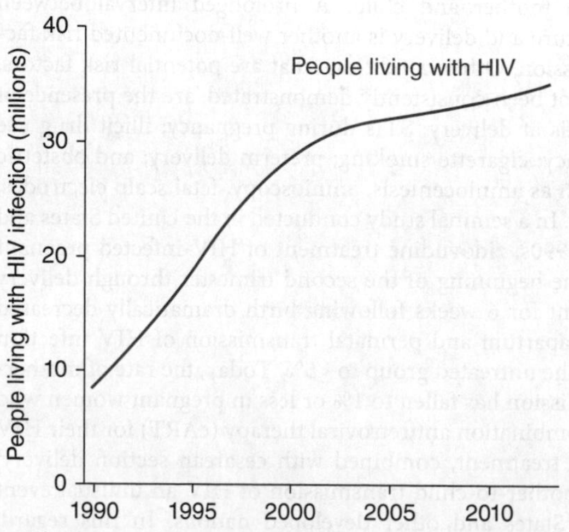

FIGURE 226-9 Global estimates of HIV incidence and AIDS deaths (*left*) and, HIV prevalence (*right*), 1990–2013. *(From UNAIDS.)*

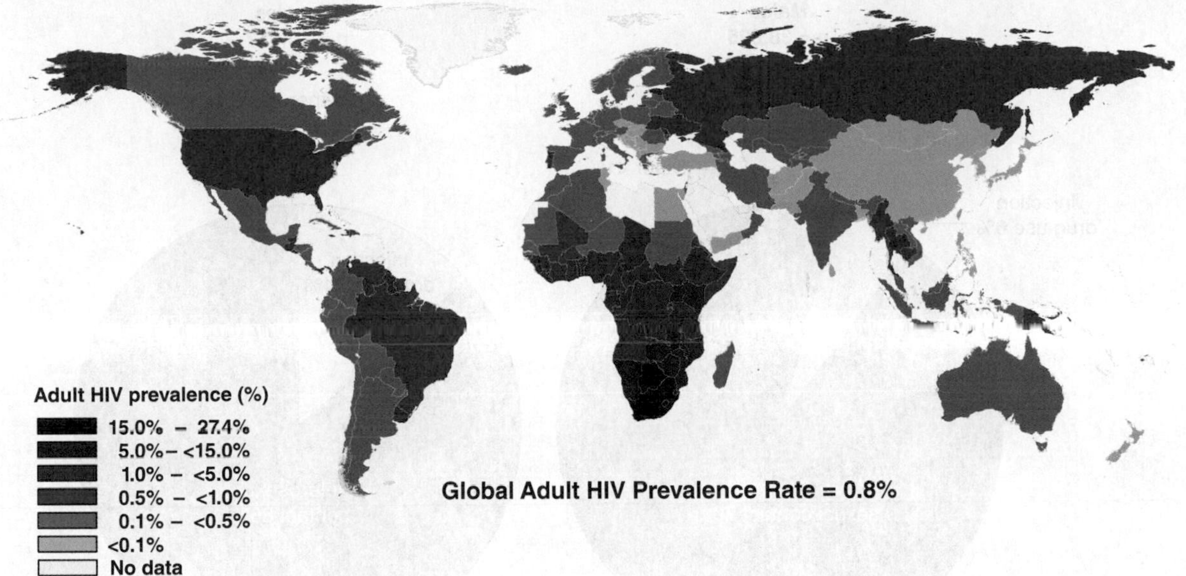

FIGURE 226-10 Global adult HIV prevalence rate, 2013. Data are estimates for adults aged 15-49 years. *(From UNAIDS.)*

the primary mode of HIV transmission in sub-Saharan Africa, with women and girls disproportionately affected, accounting for ~60 percent of all HIV infections in that region. In 2013, an estimated 230,000 people were living with HIV in the Middle East/North Africa region. Cases are largely concentrated among IDUs, men who have sex with men, and sex workers and their clients.

In Asia and the Pacific, an estimated 4.8 million people were living with HIV at the end of 2013. In this region of the world, HIV prevalence is highest in southeast Asian countries, with wide variation in trends between different countries. Among countries in Asia, only Thailand has an adult seroprevalence rate of >1%. However, the populations of many Asian nations are so large (especially India and China) that even low infection and seroprevalence rates result in large numbers of people living with HIV. Although Asia's epidemic has been concentrated for some time among specific populations—sex workers and their clients, men who have sex with men, and IDUs—it is expanding to the heterosexual partners of those most at risk.

The epidemic is expanding in Eastern Europe and Central Asia, where ~1.1 million people were living with HIV at the end of 2013. The Russian Federation and Ukraine account for the majority of HIV cases in the region. Driven initially by injection drug use and increasingly by heterosexual transmission, the number of new infections in this region has increased dramatically over the past decade.

Approximately 1.9 million people are living with HIV/AIDS in Central and South America and the Caribbean. Brazil is home to the largest number of HIV-infected people in the region. However, the epidemic has been slowed in that country due to successful treatment and prevention efforts. Men who have sex with men account for the largest proportion of HIV infections in Central and South America. The Caribbean region has the highest regional adult seroprevalence rate after Africa. Heterosexual transmission, often tied to sex work, is the main driver of transmission in the region.

Approximately 2.3 million people are living with HIV/AIDS in North America and western and central Europe. The number of new infections among men who have sex with men has increased over the past decade in these mostly high-income areas, while rates of new infections among heterosexuals have stabilized and infections among women and IDUs have fallen.

HIV INFECTION AND AIDS IN THE UNITED STATES

About 1.7 million people have been infected with HIV in the United States since the beginning of the epidemic, of whom >630,000 have died. Approximately 1.1 million individuals in the United States are living with HIV infection, ~16–18% of whom are unaware of their infection, according to recent estimates. As illustrated in Fig. 226-11, only a fraction of HIV-infected people are able to negotiate the steps in the HIV "care continuum," from diagnosis, to entering into and staying in care, to receiving antiretroviral therapy, and ultimately to achieving a suppressed viral load (see "Treatment," below).

More than 60% of those living with HIV/AIDS are Black/African-American or Hispanic/Latino, and more than half are men who have sex with men. The estimated HIV seroprevalence rate among all individuals age 13 years or older in the United States is ~0.5%. Approximately 2% of Black/African-American adults are HIV-infected in the United States, higher than any other group.

The number of new HIV infections in the United States, *HIV incidence*, peaked at about 130,000 per year in the late 1980s, followed by declines. For more than a decade, HIV incidence has remained stable at approximately 50,000 per year, with the proportion of new infections increasing in recent years among men who have sex with men and falling among women and IDUs. Among adults and adolescents newly diagnosed with HIV infection in 2011 (regardless of stage of infection), ~79% were males and ~21% were women. Of new HIV diagnoses among men, ~79% were attributed to male-to-male sexual contact, ~12% to heterosexual contact, ~6% to injection drug use, and ~4% to a combination of male-to-male sexual contact and injection drug use. Of new HIV diagnoses among women, ~86% were due to heterosexual contact and ~14% to injection drug use

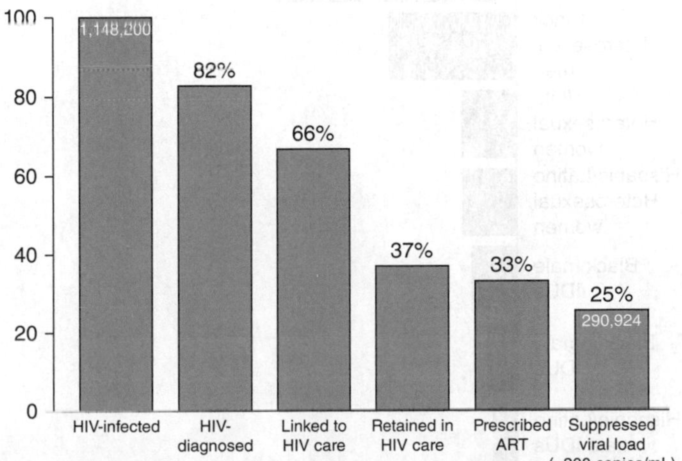

FIGURE 226-11 Estimated percentage of HIV-infected people engaged in selected stages of the continuum of HIV care in the United States. *(Adapted from HI Hall et al: JAMA Intern Med 173:1337, 2013.)*

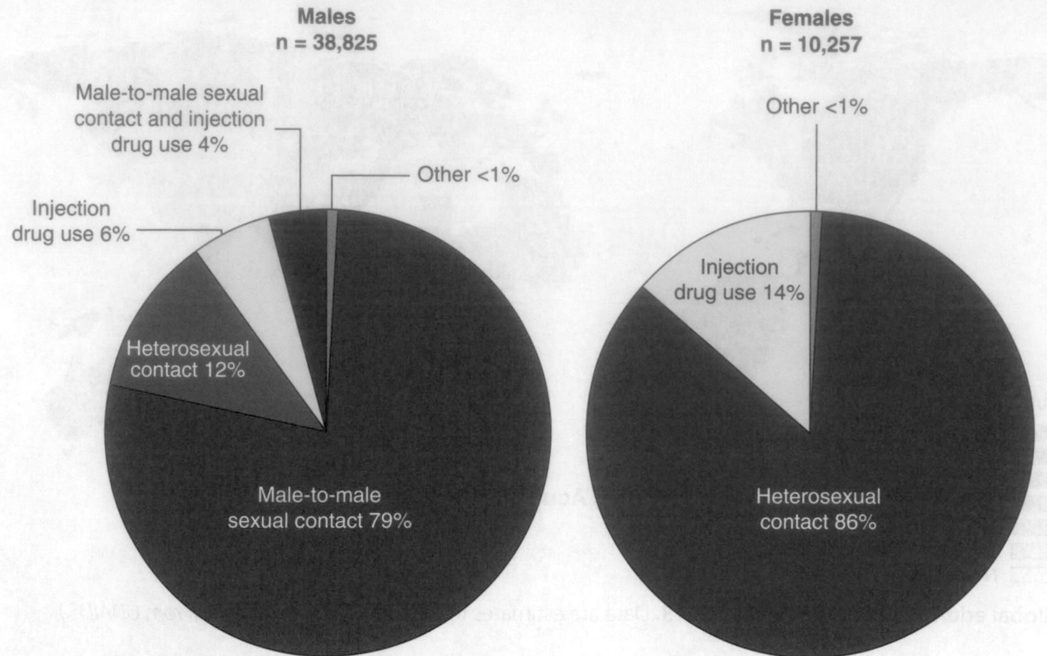

FIGURE 226-12 Transmission categories of adults and adolescents diagnosed with HIV infection (regardless of stage) in 2011, United States. *(From CDC.)*

(Fig. 226-12). The estimated numbers of new HIV infections in 2011 in the United States for the 10 most affected subpopulations are shown in Fig. 226-13.

Perinatal HIV transmission, from an HIV-infected mother to her baby, has declined significantly in the United States, largely due to the implementation of guidelines for the universal counseling and voluntary HIV testing of pregnant women and the use of antiretroviral therapy for pregnant women and newborn infants to prevent infection (Fig. 226-14). In 2011, fewer than 200 children were diagnosed with HIV infection in the United States.

HIV infection and AIDS have disproportionately affected minority populations in the United States. Among those diagnosed with HIV (regardless of stage of infection) in 2011, 47% percent were Blacks/African Americans, a group that constitutes only 12% of the U.S. population (Fig. 226-15A). The estimated rate of new HIV diagnoses in 2011 by race/ethnicity per 100,000 population in the United States is shown in Fig. 226-15B.

The number of individuals diagnosed with AIDS and deaths among persons with AIDS in the United States rose steadily through the 1980s; AIDS cases peaked in 1993 and deaths in 1995 (Fig. 226-16). Since then, the annual numbers of AIDS-related deaths in the United States have fallen ~70%. This trend is due to several factors, including improved prophylaxis and treatment of opportunistic infections, growing experience among the health professions in caring for HIV-infected individuals, improved access to health care, and a decrease in new infections due to saturational effects and prevention efforts.

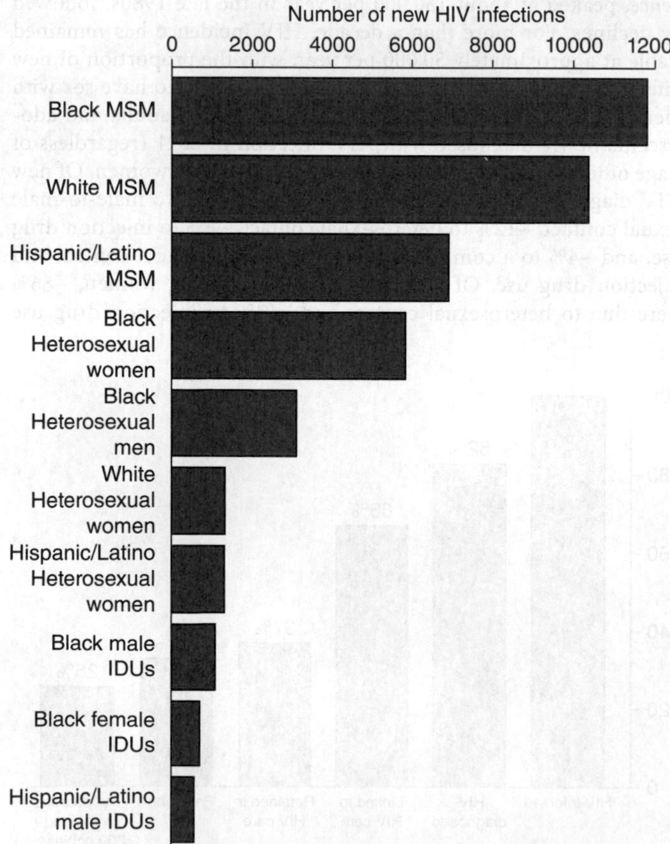

FIGURE 226-13 Estimated number of new HIV infections in the United States, 2011, for the most affected subpopulations. *(From CDC.)*

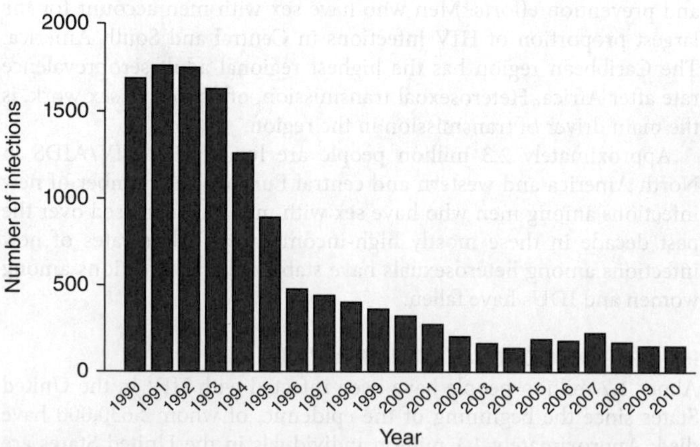

FIGURE 226-14 Estimated number of HIV-infected infants, United States, 1990–2010. *(From CDC.)*

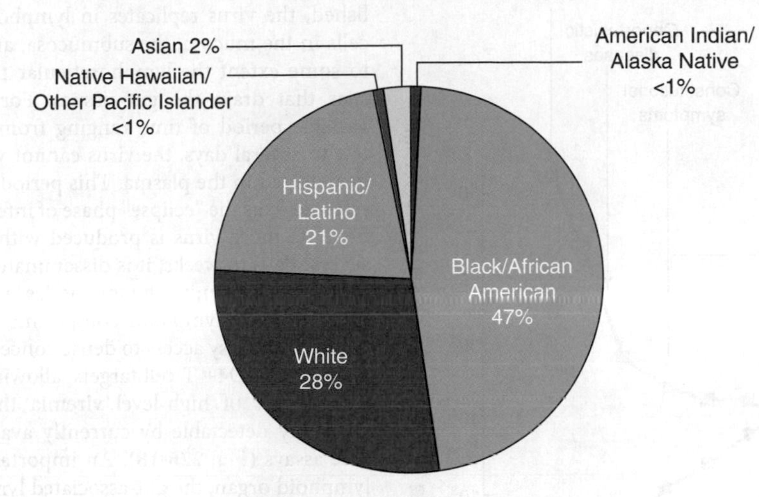

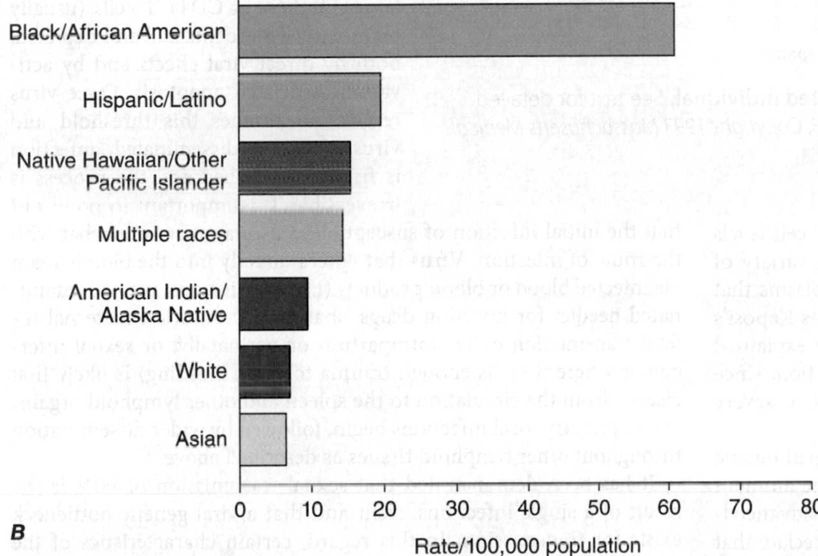

FIGURE 226-15 Race/ethnicity of persons (including children) diagnosed with HIV infection (regardless of stage) during 2011 in the United States. ***A.*** Estimated proportion of new infections by race/ethnicity. ***B.*** Estimated rate of new infections by race/ethnicity (per 100,000 population). *(From CDC.)*

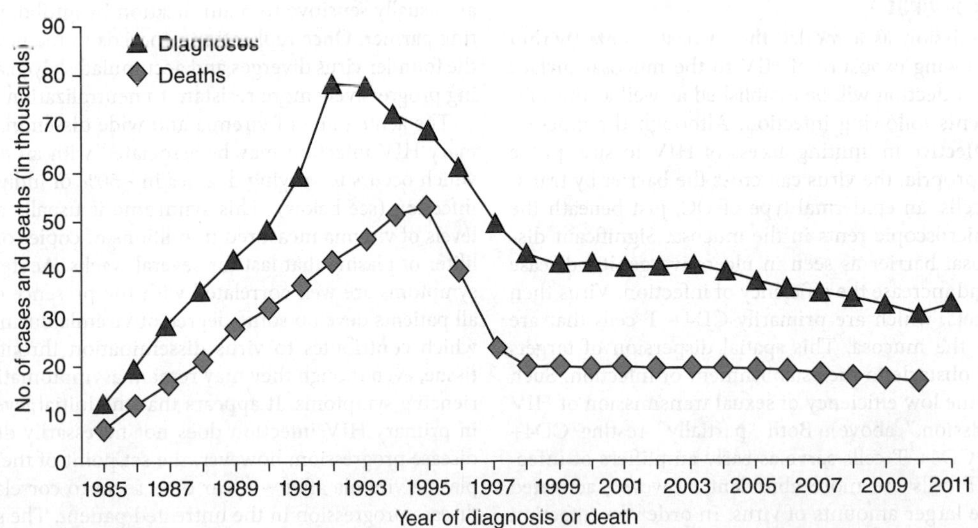

FIGURE 226-16 Estimated number of AIDS cases and AIDS deaths, United States, 1985–2011. *(From CDC.)*

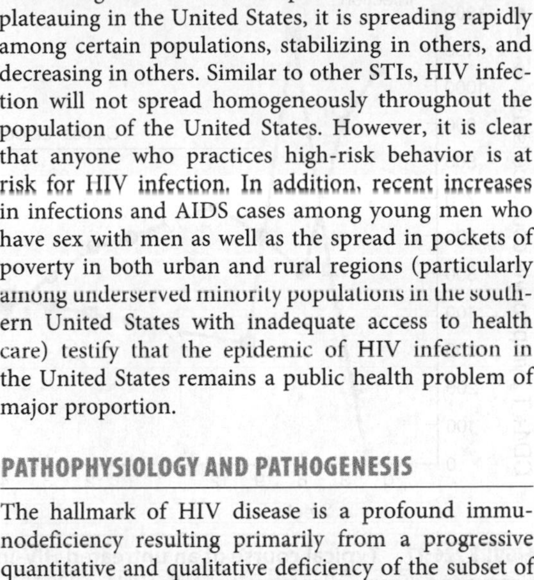

However, the most influential factor clearly has been the increased use of potent antiretroviral drugs, generally administered in a combination of three or four agents.

Although the HIV/AIDS epidemic on the whole is plateauing in the United States, it is spreading rapidly among certain populations, stabilizing in others, and decreasing in others. Similar to other STIs, HIV infection will not spread homogeneously throughout the population of the United States. However, it is clear that anyone who practices high-risk behavior is at risk for HIV infection. In addition, recent increases in infections and AIDS cases among young men who have sex with men as well as the spread in pockets of poverty in both urban and rural regions (particularly among underserved minority populations in the southern United States with inadequate access to health care) testify that the epidemic of HIV infection in the United States remains a public health problem of major proportion.

PATHOPHYSIOLOGY AND PATHOGENESIS

The hallmark of HIV disease is a profound immunodeficiency resulting primarily from a progressive quantitative and qualitative deficiency of the subset of T lymphocytes referred to as *helper T cells* occurring in a setting of polyclonal immune activation. The *helper* subset of T cells is defined phenotypically by the presence on its surface of the CD4 molecule (Chap. 372e), which serves as the primary cellular receptor for HIV. A co-receptor must also be present together with CD4 for efficient binding, fusion, and entry of HIV-1 into its target cells (Figs. 226-3 and 226-4). HIV uses two major co-receptors, CCR5 and CXCR4, for fusion and entry; these co-receptors are also the primary receptors for certain chemoattractive cytokines termed *chemokines* and belong to the seven-transmembrane-domain G protein–coupled family of receptors. A number of mechanisms responsible for cellular depletion and/or immune dysfunction of CD4+ T cells have been demonstrated in vitro; these include direct infection and destruction of these cells by HIV, as well as indirect effects such as immune clearance of infected cells, cell death associated with aberrant immune activation, and immune exhaustion due to aberrant cellular activation

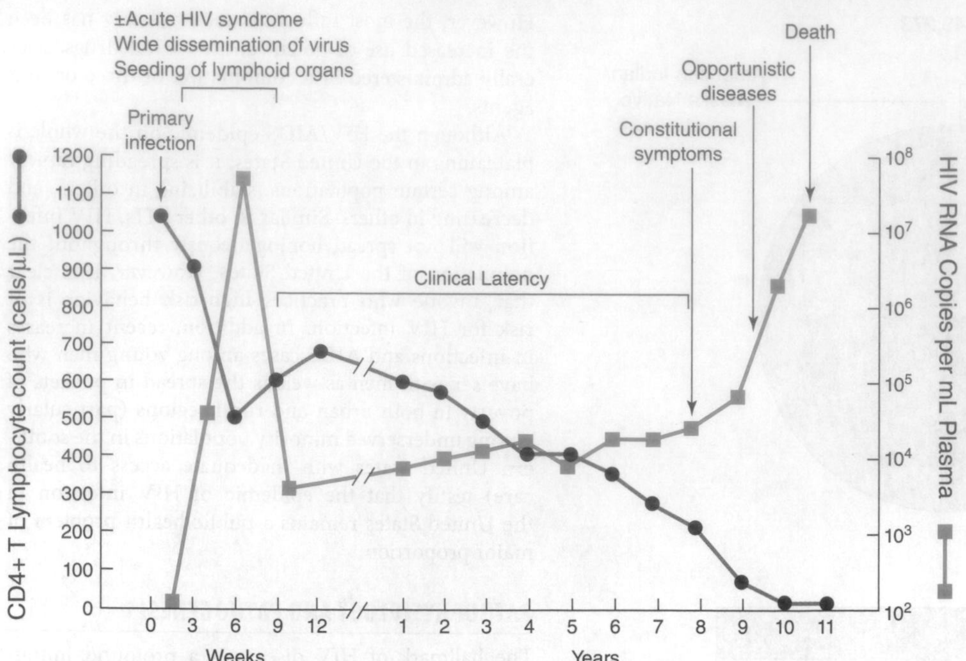

FIGURE 226-17 Typical course of an untreated HIV-infected individual. See text for detailed description. *(From G Pantaleo et al: N Engl J Med 328:327, 1993. Copyright 1993 Massachusetts Medical Society. All rights reserved.)*

with resulting cellular dysfunction. Patients with CD4+ T cell levels below certain thresholds are at high risk of developing a variety of opportunistic diseases, particularly the infections and neoplasms that are AIDS-defining illnesses. Some features of AIDS, such as Kaposi's sarcoma and certain neurologic abnormalities, cannot be explained completely by the immunodeficiency caused by HIV infection, since these complications may occur prior to the development of severe immunologic impairment.

The combination of viral pathogenic and immunopathogenic events that occurs during the course of HIV disease from the moment of initial (primary) infection through the development of advanced-stage disease is complex and varied. It is important to appreciate that the pathogenic mechanisms of HIV disease are multifactorial and multiphasic and are different at different stages of the disease. Therefore, it is essential to consider the typical clinical course of an untreated HIV-infected individual in order to more fully appreciate these pathogenic events (Fig. 226-17).

EARLY EVENTS IN HIV INFECTION: PRIMARY INFECTION AND INITIAL DISSEMINATION OF VIRUS

Using mucosal transmission as a model, the earliest events (within hours) that occur following exposure of HIV to the mucosal surface determine whether an infection will be established as well as the subsequent course of events following infection. Although the mucosal barrier is relatively effective in limiting access of HIV to susceptible targets in the lamina propria, the virus can cross the barrier by transport on Langerhans cells, an epidermal type of DC, just beneath the surface or through microscopic rents in the mucosa. Significant disruptions in the mucosal barrier as seen in ulcerative genital disease facilitate viral entry and increase the efficiency of infection. Virus then seeks susceptible targets, which are primarily CD4+ T cells that are spatially dispersed in the mucosa. This spatial dispersion of targets provides a significant obstacle to the establishment of infection. Such obstacles account for the low efficiency of sexual transmission of HIV (see "Sexual Transmission," above). Both "partially" resting CD4+ T cells and activated CD4+ T cells serve as early amplifiers of infection. Resting CD4+ T cells are more abundant; however, activated CD4+ T cells produce larger amounts of virus. In order for infection to become established, the basic reproductive rate (R_0) must become equal to or greater than 1, i.e., each infected cell would infect at least one other cell. Once infection is established, the virus replicates in lymphoid cells in the mucosa, the submucosa, and to some extent the lymphoreticular tissues that drain the gut tissues. For a variable period of time ranging from a few to several days, the virus cannot yet be detected in the plasma. This period is referred to as the "eclipse" phase of infection. As more virus is produced within several days to weeks, it is disseminated, first to the draining lymph nodes and then to other lymphoid compartments where it has easy access to dense concentrations of CD4+ T cell targets, allowing for a burst of high-level viremia that is readily detectable by currently available assays (Fig. 226-18). An important lymphoid organ, the gut-associated lymphoid tissue (GALT), is a major target of HIV infection and the location where large numbers of CD4+ T cells (usually memory cells) are infected and depleted, both by direct viral effects and by activation-associated apoptosis. Once virus replication reaches this threshold and virus is widely disseminated, infection is firmly established and the process is irreversible. It is important to point out that the initial infection of susceptible cells may vary somewhat with the route of infection. Virus that enters directly into the bloodstream via infected blood or blood products (i.e., transfusions, use of contaminated needles for injection drugs, sharp-object injuries, maternal-to-fetal transmission either intrapartum or perinatally, or sexual intercourse where there is enough trauma to cause bleeding) is likely first cleared from the circulation to the spleen and other lymphoid organs, where primary focal infections begin, followed by wider dissemination throughout other lymphoid tissues as described above.

It has been demonstrated that sexual transmission of HIV is the result of a single infectious event and that a viral genetic bottleneck exists for transmission. In this regard, certain characteristics of the HIV envelope glycoprotein have a major influence on transmission, at least in subtype A and C viruses. Transmitting viruses, often referred to as "founder viruses," are usually underrepresented in the circulating viremia of the transmitting partner and are less-diverged viruses with signature sequences including shorter V1–V2 loop sequences and fewer predicted N-linked glycosylation sites relative to the major circulating variants. These viruses are almost exclusively R5 strains and are usually sensitive to neutralization by antibody from the transmitting partner. Once replication proceeds in the newly infected partner, the founder virus diverges and accumulates glycosylation sites, becoming progressively more resistant to neutralization (Fig. 226-19).

The acute burst of viremia and wide dissemination of virus in primary HIV infection may be associated with an *acute HIV syndrome,* which occurs to varying degrees in ~50% of individuals with primary infection (see below). This syndrome is usually associated with high levels of viremia measured in millions of copies of HIV RNA per milliliter of plasma that last for several weeks. Acute mononucleosis-like symptoms are well correlated with the presence of viremia. Virtually all patients develop some degree of viremia during primary infection, which contributes to virus dissemination throughout the lymphoid tissue, even though they may remain asymptomatic or not recall experiencing symptoms. It appears that the initial level of plasma viremia in primary HIV infection does not necessarily determine the rate of disease progression; however, the set point of the level of steady-state plasma viremia after ~1 year does seem to correlate with the slope of disease progression in the untreated patient. The strikingly high levels of viremia observed in many patients with acute HIV infection is felt to be associated with a higher likelihood of transmission of the virus

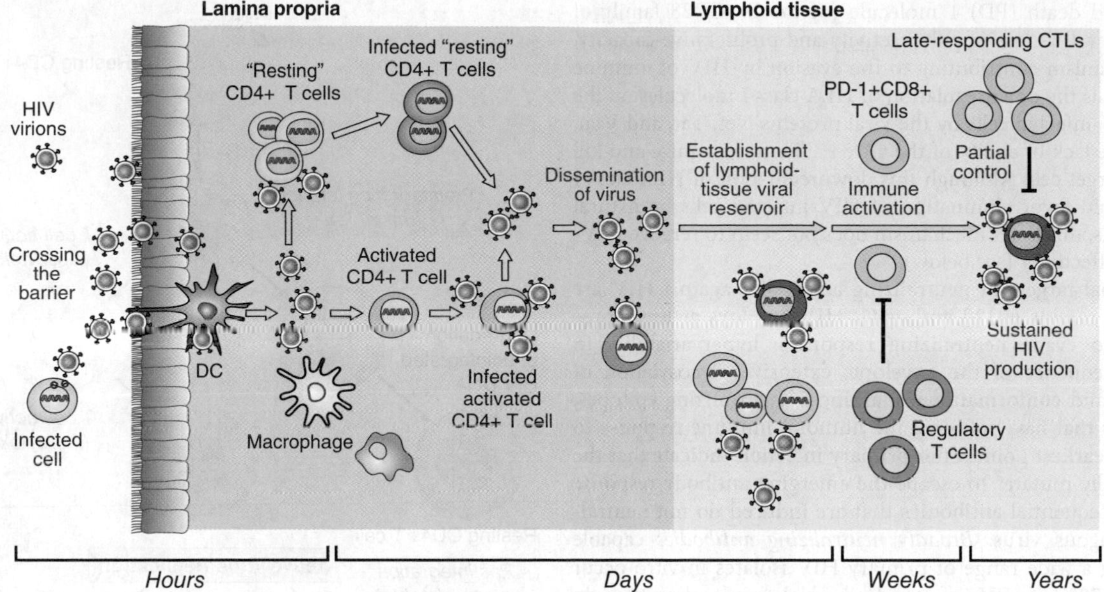

FIGURE 226-18 Summary of early events in HIV infection. See text for detailed description. CTLs, cytolytic T lymphocytes; HIV, human immunodeficiency virus. *(Adapted from AT Haase: Nat Rev Immunol 5:783, 2005.)*

to others by a variety of routes including sexual transmission, shared needles and syringes, and mother-to-child transmission intrapartum, perinatally, or via breast milk.

ESTABLISHMENT OF CHRONIC AND PERSISTENT INFECTION

Persistence of Virus Replication HIV infection is unique among human viral infections. Despite the robust cellular and humoral immune responses that are mounted following primary infection (see "Immune Response to HIV," below), once infection has been established the virus succeeds in escaping complete immune-mediated clearance, paradoxically seems to thrive on immune activation, and is never eliminated completely from the body. Rather, a chronic infection develops and persists with varying degrees of continual virus replication in the untreated patient for a median of ~10 years before the patient becomes clinically ill (see "Advanced HIV Disease," below). It is this establishment of a chronic, persistent infection that is the hallmark of HIV disease. Throughout the often protracted course of chronic infection, virus replication can invariably be detected in untreated patients by widely available assays that measure copies of HIV RNA per milliliter of plasma. Levels of virus vary greatly in most untreated patients, ranging from several thousand to a few million copies of HIV RNA per milliliter of plasma. Studies using highly sensitive molecular techniques have demonstrated that even in certain patients in whom plasma viremia is suppressed to below detection (lower limit, 20–50 copies of HIV RNA/mL depending on manufacturer) by cART, there is a continual low level of virus replication. In other human viral infections, with very few exceptions, if the host survives, the virus is completely cleared from the body and a state of immunity against subsequent infection develops. HIV infection very rarely kills the host during primary infection. Certain viruses, such as HSV (Chap. 216), are not completely cleared from the body after infection, but instead enter a latent state; in these cases, clinical latency is accompanied by microbiologic latency. This is not the case with HIV infection as described above. Chronicity associated with persistent virus replication can also be seen in certain cases of HBV and HCV infections (Chap. 362); however, in these infections the immune system is not a target of the virus.

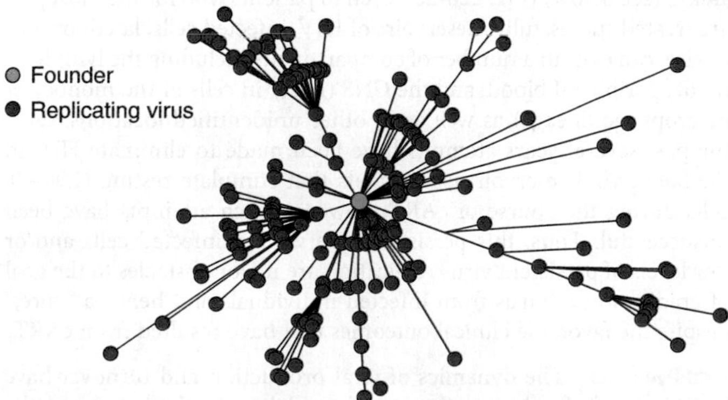

FIGURE 226-19 As HIV diverges from founder to chronically replicating virus, it accumulates N-linked glycosylation sites. See text for detailed description. *(Adapted from CA Derdeyn et al: Science 303:2019, 2004; B Chohan et al: J Virol 79:6528, 2005; and BF Keele et al: Proc Natl Acad Sci USA 105:7552, 2008.)*

Escape of HIV from Effective Immune System Control Inherent to the establishment of chronicity of HIV infection is the ability of the virus to evade adequate control and elimination by both the cellular and humoral limbs of the immune system. There are a number of mechanisms whereby the virus accomplishes this evasion. Paramount among these is the establishment of a sustained level of replication associated with the generation of viral diversity via mutation and recombination. The selection of mutants that escape control by CD8+ cytolytic T lymphocytes (CTLs) is critical to the propagation and progression of HIV infection. The high rate of virus replication associated with inevitable mutations also contributes to the inability of antibody to neutralize the autologous virus and thus to contain the virus quasispecies present in an individual at any given time. Extensive analyses of sequential HIV isolates and host responses have demonstrated that viral escape from B cell and CD8+ T cell epitopes occurs early after infection and allows the virus to stay one step ahead of effective immune responses. Virus-specific CD8+ CTLs expand greatly during primary HIV infection, and likely represent the high-affinity responses that would be expected to be most efficient in eliminating virus-infected cells; however, the restriction is generally incomplete as viral replication persists at relatively high levels in the majority of individuals. In addition to viral escape from CTLs through high rates of mutation, it is thought that the initially strong response becomes qualitatively dysfunctional owing to the overwhelming immune activation resulting from persistent viral replication, similar to the exhaustion of CD8+ CTLs that has been reported in the murine model of lymphocytic choriomeningitis virus (LCMV) infection. Several studies have indicated that exhaustion of HIV-specific CD8+ T cells during prolonged immune activation is associated with expression of inhibitory receptors, such as programmed death (PD) 1 molecule (of the B7-CD28 family of molecules), as well as loss of polyreactivity and proliferative capacity. Another mechanism contributing to the evasion by HIV of immune system control is the downregulation of HLA class I molecules on the surface of HIV-infected cells by the viral proteins Nef, Tat, and Vpu, resulting in the lack of ability of the CD8+ CTL to recognize and kill the infected target cell. Although this downregulation of HLA class I molecules would favor elimination of HIV-infected cells by natural killer (NK) cells, this latter mechanism does not seem to remove HIV-infected cells effectively (see below).

The principal targets of neutralizing antibodies against HIV are the envelope proteins gp120 and gp41. HIV employs at least three mechanisms to evade neutralizing responses: hypervariability in the primary sequence of the envelope, extensive glycosylation of the envelope, and conformational masking of neutralizing epitopes. Several studies that have followed the humoral immune response to HIV from the earliest points after primary infection indicate that the virus continually mutates to escape the emerging antibody response such that the sequential antibodies that are induced do not neutralize the autologous virus. *Broadly neutralizing antibodies* capable of neutralizing a wide range of primary HIV isolates in vitro occur in only about 20% of HIV-infected individuals, and, when they do occur, it generally requires 2 to 3 years of infection with continual virus replication to drive the affinity maturation of the antibodies. Unfortunately, by the time these broadly neutralizing antibodies are formed, they are ineffective in containing the virus replication in the patient. Persistent viremia also results in exhaustion of B cells similar to the exhaustion reported for CD4+ T cells, adding to the defects in the humoral response to HIV.

CD4+ T cell help is essential for the integrity of antigen-specific immune responses, both humoral and cell-mediated. HIV preferentially infects activated CD4+ T cells including HIV-specific CD4+ T cells, and so this loss of viral-specific helper T cell responses has profound negative consequences for the immunologic control of HIV replication. Furthermore, this loss occurs early in the course of infection, and animal studies indicate that 40–70% of all memory CD4+ T cells in the GALT are eliminated during acute infection. Another potential means of escape of HIV-infected cells from elimination by CD8+ CTLs is the sequestration of infected cells in immunologically privileged sites such as the central nervous system (CNS).

Finally, the escape of HIV from immune-mediated elimination during primary infection allows the formation of a pool of latently infected cells that may not be recognized or completely eliminated by virus-specific CTLs or by ART (see below). Thus, despite a potent immune response and the marked downregulation of virus replication following primary HIV infection, HIV succeeds in establishing a state of chronic infection with a variable degree of persistent virus replication. During this period most patients make the clinical transition from acute primary infection to variable periods of clinical latency or smoldering disease activity (see below).

The HIV Reservoir: Obstacles to the Eradication of Virus A pool of latently infected, resting CD4+ T cells that serves as at least one component of the persistent reservoir of virus exists in virtually all HIV-infected individuals, including those who are receiving cART. Such cells carry an integrated form of HIV DNA in the genome of the host and can remain in this state until an activation signal drives the expression of HIV transcripts and ultimately replication-competent virus. This form of latency is to be distinguished from preintegration latency, in which HIV enters a resting CD4+ T cell and, in the absence of an activation signal, reverse transcription of the HIV genome occurs to a certain extent but the resulting proviral DNA fails to integrate into the host genome. This period of preintegration latency may last hours to days, and if no activation signal is delivered to the cell, the proviral DNA loses its capacity to initiate a productive infection. If these cells do become activated prior to decay of the preintegration complex, reverse transcription proceeds to completion and the virus continues along its replication cycle (see above and Fig. 226-20). The pool of cells that are in the postintegration state of latency is established early during the course of primary HIV infection. Despite the suppression of plasma viremia to <50 copies of HIV RNA per milliliter by potent regimens of cART administered over several years, this pool of latently infected cells persists and can give rise to replication-competent virus upon cellular activation. Modeling studies built on projections of decay curves have estimated that in such a setting of prolonged suppression, it would require a few to several years for the pool of latently infected cells to be completely eliminated. This has not been documented to occur spontaneously in any patients very likely because the latent viral reservoir is continually replenished by the low levels of persistent virus replication that may remain below the limits of detection of current assays (see below) (Fig. 226-20), even in patients who for the most part are treated successfully. Reservoirs of HIV-infected cells, latent or otherwise, can exist in a number of compartments including the lymphoid tissue, peripheral blood, and the CNS (likely in cells of the monocyte/macrophage lineage) as well as in other unidentified locations. Over the past several years attempts have been made to eliminate HIV in the latent viral reservoir using agents that stimulate resting CD4+ T cells during the course of cART; however, such attempts have been unsuccessful. Thus, this persistent reservoir of infected cells and/or low levels of persistent virus replication are major obstacles to the goal of eradication of virus from infected individuals and hence a "cure," despite the favorable clinical outcomes that have resulted from cART.

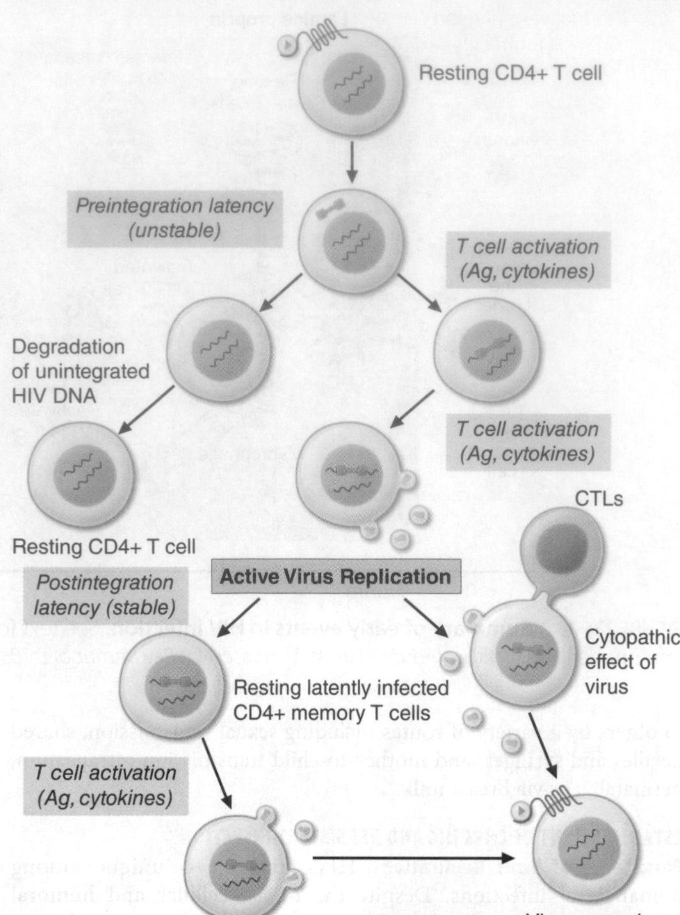

FIGURE 226-20 Generation of latently infected, resting CD4+ T cells in HIV-infected individuals. See text for details. Ag, antigen; CTLs, cytolytic T lymphocytes. *(Courtesy of TW Chun; with permission.)*

Viral Dynamics The dynamics of viral production and turnover have been quantified using mathematical modeling in the setting of the administration of reverse transcriptase and protease inhibitors to HIV-infected individuals in clinical studies. Treatment with these drugs resulted in a precipitous decline in the level of plasma viremia, which typically fell by well over 90% within 2 weeks. The number of CD4+ T cells in the blood increased concurrently, which suggested that the

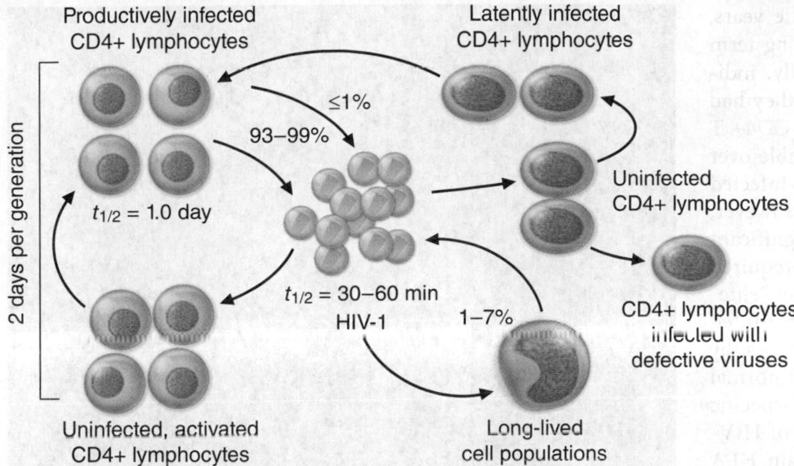

FIGURE 226-21 Dynamics of HIV infection in vivo. See text for detailed description. *(From AS Perelson et al: Science 271:1582, 1996.)*

killing of CD4+ T cells was linked directly to the levels of replicating virus. However, a significant component of the early rise in CD4+ T cell numbers following the initiation of therapy may be due to the redistribution of cells into the peripheral blood from other tissue compartments throughout the body as a consequence of therapy-related diminution in viremia-associated immune system activation. It was determined on the basis of modeling the kinetics of viral decline and the emergence of resistant mutants during therapy that 93–99% of the circulating virus originated from recently infected, rapidly turning over CD4+ T cells and that ~1–7% of circulating virus originated from longer-lived cells, likely monocytes/macrophages. A negligible amount of circulating virus originated from the pool of latently infected cells (Fig. 226-21). It was also determined that the half-life of a circulating virion was ~30–60 min and that of productively infected cells was 1 day. Given the relatively steady level of plasma viremia and of infected cells, it appears that extremely large amounts of virus (~10^{10}–10^{11} virions) are produced and cleared from the circulation each day. In addition, data suggest that the minimal duration of the HIV-1 replication cycle in vivo is ~2 days. Other studies have demonstrated that the decrease in plasma viremia that results from cART correlates closely with a decrease in virus replication in lymph nodes, further confirming that lymphoid tissue is the main site of HIV replication and the main source of plasma viremia.

The level of steady-state viremia, called the viral *set point*, at ~1 year following acquisition of HIV infection has important prognostic implications for the progression of HIV disease in the untreated patient. It has been demonstrated that as a group untreated HIV-infected individuals who have a low set point at 6 months to 1 year following infection progress to AIDS much more slowly than individuals whose set point is very high at that time (Fig. 226-22).

Clinical Latency versus Microbiologic Latency With the exception of long-term nonprogressors (see "Long-Term Survivors and Long-Term Nonprogressors," below), the level of CD4+ T cells in the blood decreases progressively in HIV-infected individuals in the absence of cART. The decline in CD4+ T cells may be gradual or abrupt, the latter usually reflecting a significant spike in the level of plasma viremia. Most patients are relatively asymptomatic while this progressive decline is taking place (see below) and are often described as being in a state of *clinical latency*. However, this term is misleading; it does not mean disease latency, since progression, although slow in many cases, is generally relentless during this period. Furthermore, clinical latency should not be confused with microbiologic latency, since varying levels of virus replication inevitably occur during this period of clinical latency. Even in those rare patients who have <50 copies of HIV RNA per milliliter in the absence of therapy, there is virtually always some degree of ongoing virus replication.

ADVANCED HIV DISEASE

In untreated patients or in patients in whom therapy has not adequately controlled virus replication, after a variable period, usually measured in years, the CD4+ T cell count falls below a critical level (<200/μL) and the patient becomes highly susceptible to opportunistic disease (Fig. 226-17). For this reason, the CDC case definition of AIDS includes all HIV-infected individuals over 5 years of age with CD4+ T cell counts below this level (Table 226-2). Patients may experience constitutional signs and symptoms or may develop an opportunistic disease abruptly without any prior symptoms, although the latter scenario is unusual. The depletion of CD4+ T cells continues to be progressive and unrelenting in this phase. It is not uncommon for CD4+ T cell counts in the untreated patient to drop to as low as 10/μL or even to zero. In countries where cART and prophylaxis and treatment for opportunistic infections are readily accessible to such patients, survival is increased dramatically even in those patients with advanced HIV disease. In contrast, untreated patients who progress to this severest form of immunodeficiency usually succumb to opportunistic infections or neoplasms (see below).

LONG-TERM SURVIVORS AND LONG-TERM NONPROGRESSORS

It is important to distinguish between the terms *long-term survivor* and *long-term nonprogressor*. Long-term nonprogressors are by definition long-term survivors; however, the reverse is not always true. Predictions from one study that antedated the availability of effective cART estimated that ~13% of homosexual/bisexual men who were infected at an early age may remain free of clinical AIDS for >20 years. Many of these individuals may have progressed in their degree of immune deficiency; however, they certainly survived for a considerable period of time. With the advent of effective cART, the survival of HIV-infected individuals has dramatically increased. Early in the AIDS epidemic, prior to the availability of therapy, if a patient presented with a life-threatening opportunistic infection, the median survival was 26 weeks from the time of presentation. Currently, an HIV-infected 20-year-old individual in a high-income country who is appropriately treated with cART can expect to live at least 50 years according to mathematical model projections. In the face of cART, long-term survival is becoming commonplace. Definitions of

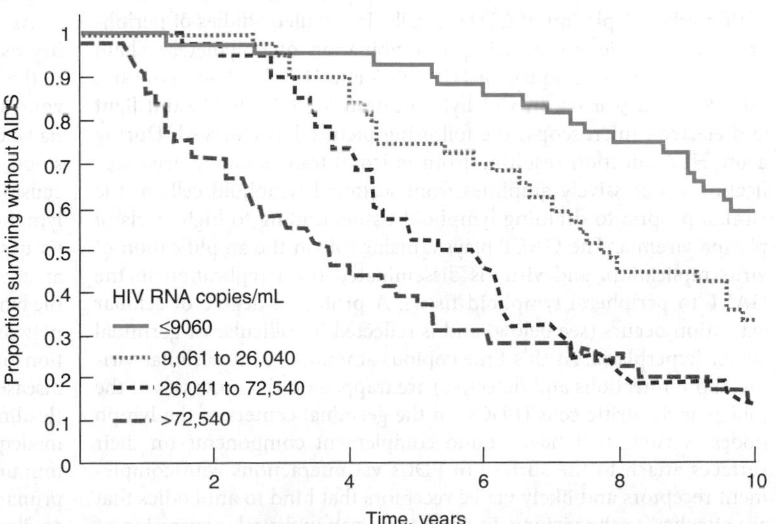

FIGURE 226-22 Relationship between levels of virus and rates of disease progression. Kaplan-Meier curves for AIDS-free survival stratified by baseline HIV-1 RNA categories (copies per milliliter). *(From JW Mellors et al: Science 272:1167, 1996.)*

long-term nonprogressors have varied considerably over the years, and so such individuals constitute a heterogeneous group. Long-term nonprogressors were first described in the 1990s. Originally, individuals were considered to be long-term nonprogressors if they had been infected with HIV for a long period (≥10 years), their CD4+ T cell counts were in the normal range, and they remained stable over years without receiving cART. Approximately 5–15% of HIV-infected individuals fell into this broader nonprogressor category. However, this group was rather heterogenous and over time a significant proportion of these individuals progressed and ultimately required therapy. From this broader group, a much smaller subgroup of "elite" controllers or nonprogressors was identified, and they constituted less than 1% of HIV-infected individuals. These elite controllers, by definition, have extremely low levels of plasma viremia and normal CD4+ T cell counts. It is noteworthy that certain of their HIV-specific immune responses are robust and clearly superior to those of HIV-infected progressors. In this group of elite controllers certain HLA class I haplotypes are overrepresented, particularly HLA-B57-01 and HLA-B27-05. Outside of the subgroup of elite controllers, a number of other genetic factors have been shown to be involved to a greater or lesser degree in the control of virus replication and thus in the rate of HIV disease progression (see "Genetic Factors in HIV-1 and AIDS Pathogenesis," below).

LYMPHOID ORGANS AND HIV PATHOGENESIS

Regardless of the portal of entry of HIV, lymphoid tissues are the major anatomic sites for the establishment and propagation of HIV infection. Despite the use of measurements of plasma viremia to determine the level of disease activity, virus replication occurs mainly in lymphoid tissue and not in blood; indeed, the level of plasma viremia directly reflects virus production in lymphoid tissue.

Some patients experience progressive generalized lymphadenopathy early in the course of the infection; others experience varying degrees of transient lymphadenopathy. Lymphadenopathy reflects the cellular activation and immune response to the virus in the lymphoid tissue, which is generally characterized by follicular or germinal center hyperplasia. Lymphoid tissue involvement is a common denominator of virtually all patients with HIV infection, even those without easily detectable lymphadenopathy.

Simultaneous examinations of lymph tissue and peripheral blood in patients and monkeys during various stages of HIV and SIV infection, respectively, have led to substantial insight into the pathogenesis of HIV disease. In most of the original human studies, peripheral lymph nodes have been used predominantly as the source of lymphoid tissue. More recent studies in monkeys and humans have also focused on the GALT, where the earliest burst of virus replication occurs associated with marked depletion of CD4+ T cells. In detailed studies of peripheral lymph node tissue, using a combination of polymerase chain reaction (PCR) techniques for HIV DNA and HIV RNA in tissue and HIV RNA in plasma, in situ hybridization for HIV RNA, and light and electron microscopy, the following picture has emerged. During acute HIV infection resulting from mucosal transmission, virus replication progressively amplifies from scattered lymphoid cells in the lamina propria to draining lymphoid tissue, leading to high levels of plasma viremia. The GALT plays a major role in the amplification of virus replication, and virus is disseminated from replication in the GALT to peripheral lymphoid tissue. A profound degree of cellular activation occurs (see below) and is reflected in follicular or germinal center hyperplasia. At this time copious amounts of extracellular virions (both infectious and defective) are trapped on the processes of the follicular dendritic cells (FDCs) in the germinal centers of the lymph nodes. Virions that have bound complement components on their surfaces attach to the surface of FDCs via interactions with complement receptors and likely via Fc receptors that bind to antibodies that are attached to the virions. In situ hybridization reveals expression of virus in individual cells of the paracortical area and, to a lesser extent, the germinal center (Fig. 226-23). The persistence of trapped virus after the transition from acute to chronic infection likely reflects a steady state whereby trapped virus turns over and is replaced by fresh virions that are continually produced. The trapped virus, either as whole virion or shed envelope, serves as a continual activator of CD4+ T cells, thus driving further virus replication.

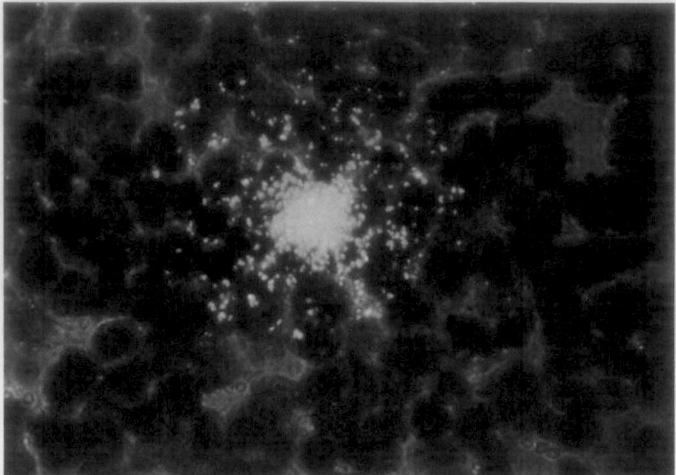

FIGURE 226-23 HIV in the lymph node of an HIV-infected individual. An individual cell infected with HIV shown expressing HIV RNA by in situ hybridization using a radiolabeled molecular probe. Original ×500. *(Adapted from G Pantaleo, AS Fauci et al: Nature 362:355, 1993.)*

During early and chronic/asymptomatic stages of HIV disease, the architecture of lymphoid tissues is generally preserved and may even be hyperplastic owing to an increased presence of B cells and specialized CD4+ T cells called follicular helper CD4+ T cells (TF_H) in prominent germinal centers. Extracellular virions can be seen by electron microscopy attached to FDC processes. The trapping of antigen is a physiologically normal function for the FDCs, which present antigen to B cells and, along with the action of TF_H cells, contribute to the generation of B cell memory. However, in the case of HIV, persistent cellular activation, resulting in the secretion of proinflammatory cytokines such as interleukin (IL) 1β, tumor necrosis factor (TNF) α, IFN-γ, and IL-6, which can induce viral replication (see below) and diminish the effectiveness of the immune response against the virus. In addition, the CD4+ TF_H cells that are recruited into the germinal center to provide help to B cells in the generation of an HIV-specific immune response are highly susceptible to infection by virus either trapped on FDC or propagated locally. Thus, in HIV infection, a normal physiologic function of the immune system that contributes to the clearance of virus, as well as to the generation of a specific immune response, can also have deleterious consequences.

As the disease progresses, the architecture of lymphoid tissues begins to show disruption. Confocal microscopy reveals destruction of the fibroblastic reticular cell (FRC) and FDC networks in the T cell zone and B cell follicles, respectively, and an incapacity to replenish naïve cells. The mechanisms of destruction are not completely understood, but they are thought to be associated with collagen deposition causing fibrosis and loss of production of cytokines such as IL-7 and lymphotoxin-α, which are critical to the maintenance of lymphoid tissues and their lymphocyte constituents. As the disease progresses to an advanced stage, there is complete disruption of the architecture of the lymphoid tissues, accompanied by dissolution of the FRC and FDC networks. At this point, the lymph nodes are "burnt out." This destruction of lymphoid tissue compounds the immunodeficiency of HIV disease and contributes both to the inability to control HIV replication (leading usually to high levels of plasma viremia in the untreated or inadequately treated patient) and to the inability to mount adequate immune responses against opportunistic pathogens. The events from primary infection to the ultimate destruction of the immune system are illustrated in Fig. 226-24. Recently, nonhuman primate studies and some human studies have examined GALT at various stages of HIV disease. Within the GALT, the basal level of activation combined with virus-mediated cellular activation results in the infection and elimination of an estimated 50–90% of CD4+ T cells in the gut. The extent of

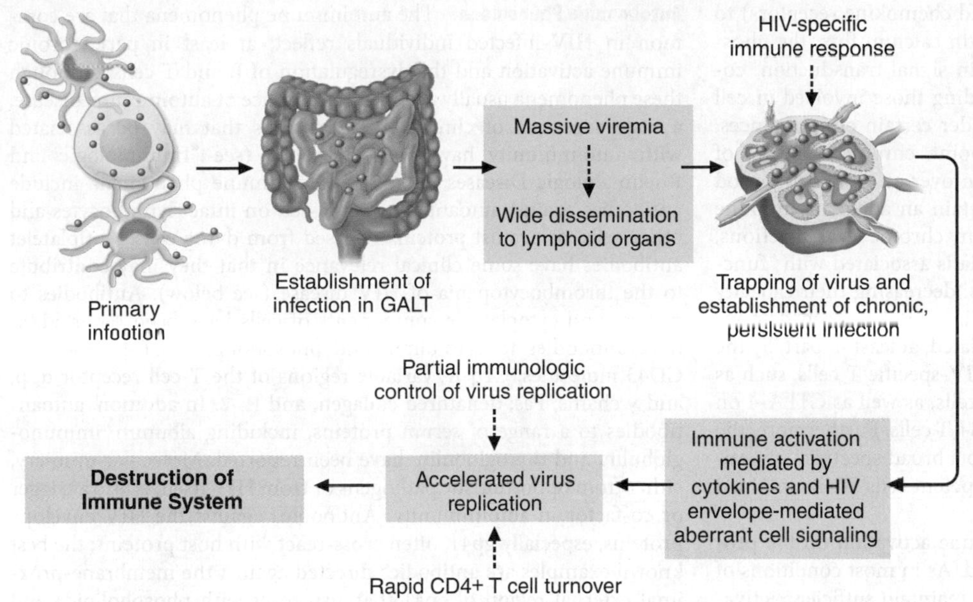

FIGURE 226-24 Events that transpire from primary HIV infection through the establishment of chronic persistent infection to the ultimate destruction of the immune system. See text for details. CTLs, cytolytic T lymphocytes; GALT, gut-associated lymphoid tissue.

this early damage to GALT, which constitutes a major component of lymphoid tissue in the body, may play a role in determining the potential for immunologic recovery of the memory cell subset.

IMMUNE ACTIVATION, INFLAMMATION, AND HIV PATHOGENESIS

Activation of the immune system and variable degrees of inflammation are essential components of any appropriate immune response to a foreign antigen. However, immune activation and inflammation, which can be considered aberrant in HIV-infected individuals, play a critical role in the pathogenesis of HIV disease and other chronic conditions associated with HIV disease. Immune activation and inflammation in the HIV-infected individual contribute substantially to (1) the replication of HIV, (2) the induction of immune dysfunction, and (3) the increased incidence of chronic conditions associated with persistent immune activation and inflammation (Table 226-4).

INDUCTION OF HIV REPLICATION BY ABERRANT IMMUNE ACTIVATION The immune system is normally in a state of homeostasis, awaiting perturbation by foreign antigenic stimuli. Once the immune response deals with and clears the antigen, the system returns to relative quiescence (Chap. 372e). This is generally not the case in HIV infection where, in the untreated patient, virus replication is invariably persistent with very few exceptions and immune activation is persistent. HIV replicates most efficiently in activated CD4+ T cells; in HIV infection, chronic activation provides the cell substrates necessary for persistent virus replication throughout the course of HIV disease, particularly in the untreated patient and to variable degrees even in certain patients receiving cART whose levels of plasma viremia are suppressed to below the level of detection by standard assays. From a virologic standpoint, although quiescent CD4+ T cells can be infected with HIV, reverse transcription, integration, and virus spread are much more efficient in activated cells. Furthermore, cellular activation induces expression of virus in cells latently infected with HIV. In essence, immune activation and inflammation provide the engine that drives HIV replication. In addition to endogenous factors such as cytokines, a number of exogenous factors such as other microbes that are associated with heightened cellular activation can enhance HIV replication and thus may have important effects on HIV pathogenesis. Co-infection in vivo or in vitro with a range of viruses, such as HSV types 1 and 2, cytomegalovirus (CMV), human herpesvirus (HHV) 6, Epstein-Barr virus (EBV), HBV, adenovirus, and HTLV-1 have been shown to upregulate HIV expression. In addition, infestation with nematodes has been shown to be associated with a heightened state of immune activation that facilitates HIV replication; in certain studies deworming of the infected host has resulted in a decrease in plasma viremia. Two diseases of extraordinary global health significance, malaria and tuberculosis (TB), have been shown to increase HIV viral load in dually infected individuals. Globally, *Mycobacterium tuberculosis* is the most common opportunistic infection in HIV-infected individuals (Chap. 202). In addition to the fact that HIV-infected individuals are more likely to develop active TB after exposure, it has been demonstrated that active TB can accelerate the course of HIV infection. It has also been shown that levels of plasma viremia are greatly elevated in HIV-infected individuals with active TB who are not on cART, compared with pre-TB levels and levels of viremia after successful treatment of the active TB. The situation is similar in the interaction between HIV and malaria parasites (Chap. 248). Acute infection of HIV-infected individuals with *Plasmodium falciparum* increases HIV viral load, and the increased viral load is reversed by effective malaria treatment.

MICROBIAL TRANSLOCATION AND PERSISTENT IMMUNE ACTIVATION One proposed mechanism of persistent immune activation involves the disruption of the mucosal barrier in the gut due to HIV replication in and disruption of submucosal lymphoid tissue. As a result of this disruption, there is an increase in the products, particularly lipopolysaccharide (LPS), of bacteria that translocate from the bowel lumen through the damaged mucosa to the circulation, leading to persistent systemic immune activation and inflammation. This effect can persist even after the HIV viral load is brought to <50 copies/mL by cART. Depletion in the GALT of IL-17–producing T cells, which are responsible for defense against extracellular bacteria and fungi, also is thought to contribute to HIV pathogenesis.

PERSISTENT IMMUNE ACTIVATION AND INFLAMMATION INDUCE IMMUNE DYSFUNCTION The activated state in HIV infection is reflected by hyperactivation of B cells leading to hypergammaglobulinemia; increased lymphocyte turnover; activation of monocytes; expression of activation markers on CD4+ and CD8+ T cells; increased activation-associated cellular apoptosis; lymph node hyperplasia, particularly early in the course of disease; increased secretion of proinflammatory cytokines, particularly IL-6; elevated levels of high-sensitivity C-reactive protein, fibrinogen, D-dimer, neopterin, β_2-microglobulin, acid-labile interferon, soluble (s) IL-2 receptors (R), sTNFR, sCD27, and sCD40L; and autoimmune phenomena (see "Autoimmune Phenomena," below). Even in the absence of direct infection of a target cell, HIV envelope proteins can interact

TABLE 226-4 CONDITIONS ASSOCIATED WITH PERSISTENT IMMUNE ACTIVATION AND INFLAMMATION IN PATIENTS WITH HIV INFECTION

- Accelerated aging syndrome
- Bone fragility
- Cancers
- Cardiovascular disease
- Diabetes
- Kidney disease
- Liver disease
- Neurocognitive dysfunction

with cellular receptors (CD4 molecules and chemokine receptors) to deliver potent activation signals resulting in calcium flux, the phosphorylation of certain proteins involved in signal transduction, colocalization of cytoplasmic proteins including those involved in cell trafficking, immune dysfunction, and, under certain circumstances, apoptosis. From an immunologic standpoint, chronic exposure of the immune system to a particular antigen over an extended period may ultimately lead to an inability to sustain an adequate immune response to the antigen in question. In many chronic viral infections, including HIV infection, persistent viremia is associated with "functional exhaustion" of virus-specific T cells, decreasing their capacity to proliferate and perform effector functions. It has been demonstrated that this phenomenon may be mediated, at least in part, by the upregulation of inhibitory receptors on HIV-specific T cells, such as PD-1 shared by both CD4+ and CD8+ T cells, as well as CTLA-4 on CD4+ and Tim-3, 2B4, and CD106 on CD8+ T cells. Furthermore, the ability of the immune system to respond to a broad spectrum of antigens may be compromised if immunocompetent cells are maintained in a state of chronic activation.

The deleterious effects of chronic immune activation on the progression of HIV disease are well established. As in most conditions of persistent antigen exposure, the host must maintain sufficient activation of antigen (HIV)-specific responses but must also prevent excessive activation and potential immune-mediated damage to tissues. Certain studies suggest that normal immunosuppressive mechanisms that act to keep hyperimmune activation in check, particularly CD4+, FoxP3+, CD25+ regulatory T cells (T-regs), may be dysfunctional or depleted in the context of advanced HIV disease.

MEDICAL CONDITIONS ASSOCIATED WITH PERSISTENT IMMUNE ACTIVATION AND INFLAMMATION IN HIV DISEASE It has become clear, as the survival of HIV-infected individuals has increased, that a number of previously unrecognized medical complications are associated with HIV disease—and that these complications relate to chronic immune activation and inflammation (Table 226-4). These complications can appear even after patients have experienced years of adequate control of viral replication (plasma viremia below detectable levels) for several years. Of particular note are endothelial cell dysfunction and its relationship to cardiovascular disease. Other chronic conditions that have been reported include bone fragility, certain cancers, persistent immune dysfunction, diabetes, kidney and liver disease, and neurocognitive dysfunction, thus presenting an overall picture of accelerated aging.

Apoptosis *Apoptosis* is a form of programmed cell death that is a normal mechanism for the elimination of effete cells in organogenesis as well as in the cellular proliferation that occurs during a normal immune response (Chap. 372e). Apoptosis is largely dependent on cellular activation, and the aberrant cellular activation associated with HIV disease is correlated with a heightened state of apoptosis. HIV can trigger both Fas-dependent and Fas-independent pathways of apoptosis, the former of which is generally referred to as activation-induced cell death through an extrinsic pathway and involves the upregulation of the death receptor Fas and Fas ligand. Fas-independent pathways can be either extrinsic with different death receptors or intrinsic due to the downregulation of the antiapoptotic proteins such as Bcl-2. More recently, the phenomenon of *pyroptosis*, an inflammatory form of cell death involving the upregulation of the proinflammatory enzyme caspase-1 and release of the proinflammatory cytokine IL-1 β, has been linked to a bystander effect of HIV replication on CD4+ T cells. Certain viral gene products have been associated with enhanced susceptibility to apoptosis; these include Env, Tat, and Vpr. In contrast, Nef has been shown to possess antiapoptotic properties. A number of studies, including those examining lymphoid tissue, have demonstrated that the rate of apoptosis is elevated in HIV infection and that apoptosis is seen in "bystander" cells such as CD8+ T cells and B cells as well as in uninfected CD4+ T cells. The intensity of apoptosis correlates with the general state of activation of the immune system and not with the stage of disease or with viral burden. It is likely that nonspecific apoptosis of immunocompetent cells related to immune activation contributes to the immune abnormalities in HIV disease.

Autoimmune Phenomena The autoimmune phenomena that are common in HIV-infected individuals reflect, at least in part, chronic immune activation and the dysregulation of B and T cells. Although these phenomena usually occur in the absence of autoimmune disease, a wide spectrum of clinical manifestations that may be associated with autoimmunity have been described (see "Immunologic and Rheumatologic Diseases," below). Autoimmune phenomena include antibodies against autoantigens expressed on intact lymphocytes and other cells, or against proteins released from dying cells. Antiplatelet antibodies have some clinical relevance in that they may contribute to the thrombocytopenia of HIV disease (see below). Antibodies to nuclear and cytoplasmic components of cells have been reported, as have antibodies to cardiolipin and phospholipids; CD4 molecules; CD43 molecules; C1q-A; variable regions of the T cell receptor α, β, and γ chains; Fas; denatured collagen; and IL-2. In addition, autoantibodies to a range of serum proteins, including albumin, immunoglobulin, and thyroglobulin, have been reported. Molecular mimicry, either from opportunistic pathogens or from HIV itself, is also a trigger or co-factor in autoimmunity. Antibodies against the HIV envelope proteins, especially gp41, often cross-react with host proteins; the best known examples are antibodies directed against the membrane-proximal external region of gp41 that also react with phospholipids and cardiolipin. The phenomenon of polyreactive HIV-specific antibodies may be beneficial to the host (see "Immune Response to HIV," below).

The increased occurrence and/or exacerbation of certain autoimmune diseases have been reported in HIV infection; these diseases include psoriasis, idiopathic thrombocytopenic purpura, Graves' disease, antiphospholipid syndrome, and primary biliary cirrhosis. The majority of these manifestations were described prior to the advent of cART and have decreased in frequency since its widespread use. However, with increasing availability of cART, an *immune reconstitution inflammatory syndrome* (IRIS) has become increasingly common in infected individuals, particularly those with low CD4+ T cell counts. IRIS is an autoimmune-like phenomenon characterized by a paradoxical deterioration of clinical condition, which is usually compartmentalized to a particular organ system, in individuals in whom cART has recently been initiated. It is associated with a decrease in viral load and at least partial recovery of immune competence, which is usually associated with increases in CD4+ T cell counts. The immunopathogenesis is felt to be related to an increase in immune response against the presence of residual antigens that are usually microbial and is commonly seen with underlying *Mycobacterium tuberculosis* and cryptococcosis. This syndrome is discussed in more detail below.

CYTOKINES AND OTHER SOLUBLE FACTORS IN HIV PATHOGENESIS

The immune system is homeostatically regulated by a complex network of immunoregulatory cytokines, which are pleiotropic and redundant and operate in an autocrine and paracrine manner. They are expressed continuously, even during periods of apparent quiescence of the immune system. On perturbation of the immune system by antigenic challenge, the expression of cytokines increases to varying degrees (Chap. 372e). Cytokines that are important components of this immunoregulatory network are thought to play major roles in HIV disease, during both the early and chronic phases of infection. A potent pro-inflammatory "cytokine storm" is induced during the acute phase of HIV infection, likely a response by inflammatory cells recruited to mucosal tissues where the virus initially replicates at very high levels. Cytokines that are induced during this early phase include IFN-α, IL-15, and the CXC chemokine IP-10 (CXCL10), followed by IL-6, IL-12, and TNF-α, and a delayed peak of the anti-inflammatory cytokine IL-10. Soluble factors of innate immunity are also induced shortly after infection, including neopterin and β-microglobulin. Several of these early-expressed cytokines and factors are not downregulated following the early phase of HIV infection, as seen in self-resolving viral infections, and persist during the chronic phase of infection and contribute to maintaining high levels of immune activation. Among the cytokines and factors associated with early innate immune responses, they are intended to contain viral replication, although most are potent inducers of HIV expression/replication because of their ability to induce immune activation that leads to enhanced viral production and an increase in readily available target cells for HIV (activated CD4+ T cells). The induction of IFN-α, one of the first cytokines induced during primary HIV infection, is thought to play a particularly important role in HIV pathogenesis by inducing a large number of IFN-associated genes that activate the immune system and alter the homeostasis of CD4+ T cells. Other cytokines that are elevated during the chronic phase of HIV infection and linked to immune activation include IFN-γ, the *CC-chemokine* RANTES (CCL5), macrophage inflammatory protein (MIP)-1β (CCL4), and IL-18.

Several specific cytokines and soluble factors have been associated with HIV pathogenesis at various stages of disease, in various tissues or organs, and in the regulation of HIV replication. Plasma levels of IP-10 are predictive of disease progression, whereas the proinflammatory cytokine IL-6, soluble CD14 (sCD14), and coagulation marker D-dimer are associated with increased risk of all-cause mortality in HIV-infected individuals. In particular, IL-6, sCD14, and D-dimer are associated with increased risk of cardiovascular disease and other causes of death, even in individuals receiving cART. IL-18 has also been shown to play a role in the development of the HIV-associated lipodystrophy syndrome, whereas increased levels of transforming growth factor (TGF)-β are associated with the induction of collagen deposition in lymph nodes (see above). Elevated levels of TNF-α and IL-6 have been demonstrated in plasma and cerebrospinal fluid (CSF), and increased expression of TNF-α, IL-1β, IFN-γ, and IL-6 has been demonstrated in the lymph nodes of HIV-infected individuals. RANTES, MIP-1α (CCL3), and MIP-1β (CCL4) (Chap. 372e) inhibit infection by and spread of R5 HIV-1 strains, while *stromal cell–derived factor* (SDF) 1 inhibits infection by and spread of X4 strains. The mechanisms whereby the CC-chemokines RANTES (CCL5), MIP-1α (CCL3), and MIP-1β (CCL4) inhibit infection of R5 strains of HIV, or SDF-1 blocks X4 strains of HIV, involve blocking of the binding of the virus to its co-receptors, the CC-chemokine receptor CCR5 and the CXC-chemokine receptor CXCR4, respectively. Other soluble factors that have not yet been fully characterized have also been shown to suppress HIV replication, independent of co-receptor usage.

LYMPHOCYTE TURNOVER IN HIV INFECTION

The immune systems of patients with HIV infection are characterized by a profound increase in lymphocyte turnover that is immediately reduced with effective cART. Studies utilizing in vivo or in vitro labeling of lymphocytes in the S-phase of the cell cycle have demonstrated a tight correlation between the degree of lymphocyte turnover and plasma levels of HIV RNA. This increase in turnover is seen in CD4+ and CD8+ T lymphocytes as well as B lymphocytes and can be observed in peripheral blood and lymphoid tissue. Mathematical models derived from these data suggest that one can view the lymphoid pool as consisting of dynamically distinct subpopulations of cells that are differentially affected by HIV infection. A major consequence of HIV infection appears to be a shift in cells from a more quiescent pool to a pool with a higher turnover rate. It is likely that a consequence of a higher rate of turnover is a higher rate of cell death. The role of the thymus in adult human T cell homeostasis and HIV pathogenesis is an area of controversy. While some data point to an important role for the thymus in maintaining T cell numbers and suggest that impairment of thymic function may be responsible for the declines in CD4+ T cells seen in the setting of HIV infection, other studies have concluded that the thymus plays a minor role in HIV pathogenesis. More recently, it has been suggested that the more rapid decline in CD4+ compared to CD8+ T cells may be linked to alterations in inflammatory and homeostatic cytokines that caused increased activation-induced death of CD4+ but not CD8+ T cells (see Table 226-5 for additional mechanisms of depletion).

TABLE 226-5 PROPOSED MECHANISMS OF CD4+ T CELL DYSFUNCTION AND DEPLETION

Direct Mechanisms	Indirect Mechanisms
Loss of plasma membrane integrity due to viral budding	Aberrant intracellular signaling events
Accumulation of unintegrated viral DNA	Autoimmunity
Activation of DNA-dependent protein kinase during viral integration into host genome	
Interference with cellular RNA processing	Innocent bystander killing of viral antigen–coated cells
Intracellular gp120-CD4 autofusion events	Apoptosis, pyroptosis (caspase-1 associated inflammation), autophagy
Syncytia formation	Inhibition of lymphopoiesis from reduced survival cytokines and lymphoid tissue integrity
	Activation-induced cell death
	Elimination of HIV-infected cells by virus-specific immune responses

THE ROLE OF VIRAL RECEPTORS AND CO-RECEPTORS IN HIV PATHOGENESIS

As mentioned above, HIV-1 utilizes two major co-receptors along with CD4 to bind to, fuse with, and enter target cells; these co-receptors are CCR5 and CXCR4, which are also receptors for certain endogenous chemokines. Strains of HIV that utilize CCR5 as a co-receptor are referred to as *R5 viruses*. Strains of HIV that utilize CXCR4 are referred to as *X4 viruses*. Many virus strains are *dual tropic* in that they utilize both CCR5 and CXCR4; these are referred to as *R5X4 viruses*.

The natural chemokine ligands for the major HIV co-receptors can readily block entry of HIV. For example, the CC-chemokines RANTES (CCL5), MIP-1α (CCL3), and MIP-1β (CCL4), which are the natural ligands for CCR5, block entry of R5 viruses, whereas SDF-1, the natural ligand for CXCR4, blocks entry of X4 viruses. The mechanism of inhibition of viral entry is a steric inhibition of binding that is not dependent on signal transduction (Fig. 226-25).

The transmitting virus is almost invariably an R5 virus that predominates during the early stages of HIV disease. In ~40% of HIV-infected individuals, there is a transition to a predominantly X4 virus that is associated with a relatively rapid progression of disease. However, at least 60% of infected individuals progress in their disease while maintaining predominance of an R5 virus. It should be pointed out that clade C viruses, unlike other subgroups, almost never switch from CCR5 tropism to CXCR4 tropism; the reason for this difference is unclear.

The basis for the tropism of different envelope glycoproteins for either CCR5 or CXCR4 relates to the ability of the HIV envelope, including the third variable region (V3 loop) of gp120, to interact with these co-receptors. In this regard, binding of gp120 to CD4 induces a conformational change in gp120 that increases its affinity for CCR5 (see above). Finally, R5 viruses are more efficient in infecting monocytes/macrophages and microglial cells of the brain (see "Neuropathogenesis in HIV Disease," below).

THE INTEGRIN α4β7 AND MUCOSAL TRANSMISSION OF HIV Several "accessory receptors" for HIV have been reported over the years, although only a few have withstood the test of time. These receptors are not necessary for virus binding and fusion to its target CD4+ T cell or for virus replication. However, the integrin *α4β7* is an accessory receptor for HIV and it likely plays an important role in the transmission of HIV at mucosal surfaces such as the genital tract and gut. The integrin α4β7, which is the gut homing receptor for peripheral T cells, binds in its activated form to a specific tripeptide in the V2 loop of gp120, resulting in rapid activation of leukocyte function–associated antigen 1 (LFA-1), the central integrin in the establishment of virologic synapses, which facilitate efficient cell-to-cell spread of HIV. It has been demonstrated that $α4β7^{high}$ CD4+ T cells are more susceptible to productive infection than are $α4β7^{low-neg}$ CD4+ T cells because this cellular subset is enriched with metabolically active CD4+ T cells that are $CCR5^{high}$. These cells are present at the gut and genital tract mucosal surfaces. Importantly, it has been demonstrated that the virus that is transmitted during sexual exposure binds much more efficiently to α4β7 than does the virus that diversifies from the transmitting virus over time by mutation,

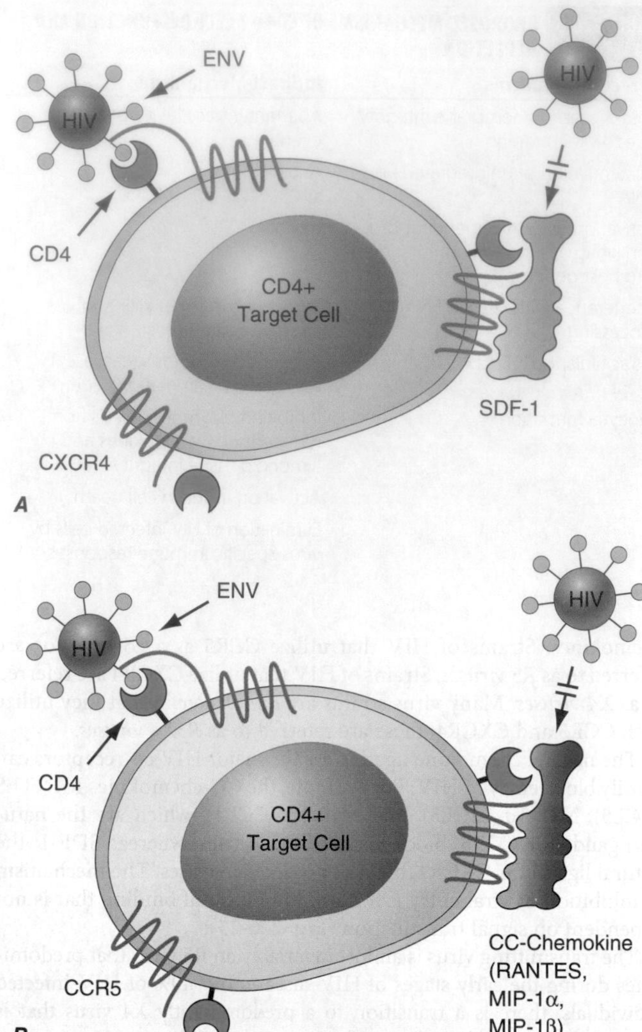

FIGURE 226-25 Model for the role of co-receptors CXCR4 and CCR5 in the efficient binding and entry of X4 (***A***) and R5 (***B***) strains of HIV-1, respectively, into CD4+ target cells. Blocking of this initial event in the virus life cycle can be accomplished by inhibition of binding to the co-receptor by the normal ligand for the receptor in question. The ligand for CXCR4 is stromal cell–derived factor (SDF-1); the ligands for CCR5 are RANTES, MIP-1α, and MIP-1β.

particularly involving the accumulation of glycosylation sites (see "Early Events in HIV Infection: Primary Infection and Initial Dissemination of Virus," above).

CELLULAR TARGETS OF HIV

Although the CD4+ T lymphocytes and to a lesser extent CD4+ cells of monocyte lineage are the principal targets of HIV, virtually any cell that expresses the CD4 molecule together with co-receptor molecules (see above and below) can potentially be infected with HIV. Circulating DCs have been reported to express low levels of CD4, and, depending on their stage of maturation, these cells can be infected with HIV. Epidermal Langerhans cells express CD4 and have been infected by HIV in vivo, although, as has been shown in vivo for DCs, FDCs, and B cells, these cells are more likely to bind and transfer virus to activated CD4+ T cells than to be productively infected themselves.

In vitro, HIV has been reported also to infect a wide range of cells and cell lines that express low levels of CD4, no detectable CD4, or only CD4 mRNA. However, since the only cells that have been shown unequivocally to be infected with HIV and to support replication of the virus are CD4+ T lymphocytes and cells of monocyte/macrophage lineage, the physiologic relevance of the in vitro infection of these other cell types is unclear.

Of potentially important clinical relevance is the demonstration that thymic precursor cells, which were assumed to be negative for CD3, CD4, and CD8 molecules, actually do express low levels of CD4 and can be infected with HIV in vitro. In addition, human thymic epithelial cells transplanted into an immunodeficient mouse can be infected with HIV by direct inoculation of virus into the thymus. Since these cells may play a role in the normal regeneration of CD4+ T cells, it is possible that their infection and depletion contribute, at least in part, to the impaired ability of the CD4+ T cell pool to completely reconstitute itself in certain infected individuals in whom cART has suppressed viral replication to <50 copies of HIV RNA per milliliter (see below). In addition, CD34+ monocyte precursor cells have been shown to be infected in vivo in patients with advanced HIV disease. It is likely that these cells express low levels of CD4, and therefore it is not essential to invoke CD4-independent mechanisms to explain the infection.

ABNORMALITIES OF MONONUCLEAR CELLS

CD4+ T Cells The primary immunopathogenic lesion in HIV infection involves CD4+ T cells, and the range of CD4+ T cell abnormalities in advanced HIV infection is broad. The defects are both quantitative and qualitative and ultimately impact virtually every limb of the immune system, indicating the critical dependence of the integrity of the immune system on the inducer/helper function of CD4+ T cells. In advanced HIV disease, most of the observed immune defects can ultimately be explained by the quantitative depletion of CD4+ T cells. However, T cell dysfunction can be demonstrated in patients early in the course of infection, even when the CD4+ T cell count is in the low-normal range. The degree and spectrum of dysfunctions increase as the disease progresses, reflecting the range of CD4+ T cell functional heterogeneity, especially in lymphoid tissues. One of the first sites of intense HIV replication is in the GALT where CD4+ T_H17 cells reside; they are important for host defense against extracellular pathogens in the intestinal mucosa and help maintain the integrity of the gut epithelium. In HIV infection, they are depleted by direct and indirect effects of viral replication and cause loss of gut homeostasis and integrity, as well as a shift to a more T_H1 phenotype. Studies have shown that even after many years of cART, normalization of the CD4+ T cells in the GALT remains incomplete. In lymph nodes, HIV perturbs another important subset of the CD4+ helper T lineage, namely TF_H cells (see "Lymphoid Organs and HIV Pathogenesis," above). TF_H cells, which are either derived directly from naïve CD4+ T cells or other T_H precursors, migrate into B follicles during germinal center reactions and provide help to antigen-specific B cells through cell–cell interactions and secretion of cytokines to which B cells respond, the most important of which is IL-21. As with T_H17 cells, TF_H cells are highly susceptible to HIV infection. However, in contrast to T_H17 and most other CD4+ T cell subsets, the number of TF_H cells is increased in lymph nodes of HIV-infected individuals, especially those who are viremic. It is unclear whether this increase is helpful to responding B cells, although the likely outcome is that the increase in numbers is detrimental to the quality of the humoral immune response against HIV (see "Immune Response to HIV," below). In addition, defects of central memory cells are a critical component of HIV immunopathogenesis. The progressive loss of antigen-specific CD4+ T cells has important implications for the control of HIV infection. In this regard, there is a correlation between the maintenance of HIV-specific CD4+ T cell proliferative responses and improved control of infection. Essentially every T cell function has been reported to be abnormal at some stage of HIV infection. Loss of polyfunctional HIV-specific CD4+ T cells, especially those that produce IL-2, occurs early in disease, whereas IFN-producing CD4+ T cells are maintained longer and do not correlate with control of HIV viremia. Other abnormalities include impaired expression of IL-2 receptors, defective IL-2 production, reduced expression of the IL-7 receptor (CD127), and a decreased proportion of CD4+ T cells that express CD28, a major co-stimulatory molecule necessary for the normal activation of T cells, which is also depleted as a result of aging. Cells lacking expression of CD28 do not respond normally to activation signals and may express markers of terminal activation including HLA-DR, CD38, and CD45RO. As mentioned above ("Immune Activation, Inflammation, and HIV Pathogenesis"), a subset of CD4+ T cells referred to as *T regulatory cells*, or T-regs, may be involved in damping aberrant immune activation that propagates HIV replication. The presence of these T-reg cells correlates with lower viral loads and higher CD4+/CD8+ T cell ratios. A loss of this T-reg capability with advanced disease may be detrimental to the control of virus replication.

It is difficult to explain completely the profound immunodeficiency noted in HIV-infected individuals solely on the basis of direct infection and quantitative depletion of CD4+ T cells. This is particularly apparent during the early stages of HIV disease, when CD4+ T cell numbers may be only marginally decreased. In this regard, it is likely that CD4+ T cell dysfunction results from a combination of depletion of cells due to direct infection of the cell and a number of virus-related but indirect effects on the cell (Table 226-5). Several of these effects have been demonstrated ex vivo and/or by the analysis of cells isolated from the peripheral blood. However, as explained above, many of the defects are related to specialized CD4+ T cells that reside in lymphoid tissues. Furthermore, since the main targets of HIV infection are immunocompetent cells, these responses may contribute to immune cell depletion and immunologic dysfunction by eliminating both infected cells and "innocent bystander" cells. Soluble viral proteins, particularly gp120, can bind with high affinity to the CD4 molecules on uninfected T cells and monocytes; in addition, virus and/or viral proteins can bind to DCs or FDCs. HIV-specific antibody can recognize these bound molecules and potentially collaborate in the elimination of the cells by ADCC. HIV envelope glycoproteins gp120 and gp160 manifest high-affinity binding to the CD4 molecule as well as to various chemokine receptors. Intracellular signals transduced by gp120 through both CD4 and CCR5/CXCR4 have been associated with a number of immunopathogenic processes including anergy, apoptosis, and abnormalities of cell trafficking. The molecular mechanisms responsible for these abnormalities include dysregulation of the T cell receptor–phosphoinositide pathway, p56lck activation, phosphorylation of focal adhesion kinase, activation of the MAP kinase and ras signaling pathways, and downregulation of the co-stimulatory molecules CD40 ligand and CD80.

The inexorable decline in CD4+ T cell counts that occurs in most HIV-infected individuals may result in part from the inability of the immune system to regenerate over an extended period of time the rapidly turning over CD4+ T cell pool efficiently enough to compensate for both HIV-mediated and naturally occurring attrition of cells. In this regard, the degree and duration of decline of CD4+ T cells at the time of initiation of therapy is an important predictor of the restoration of these cells. A person who maintains a very low CD4+ T cell count for a considerable period of time before the initiation of cART almost invariably has an incomplete reconstitution of such cells. At least two major mechanisms may contribute to the failure of the CD4+ T cell pool to reconstitute itself adequately over the course of HIV infection. The first is the destruction of lymphoid precursor cells, including thymic and bone marrow progenitor cells; the other is the gradual disruption of the lymphoid tissue microenvironment, which is essential for efficient regeneration of immunocompetent cells. Finally, during the advanced stages of CD4+ T lymphopenia, there are increased serum levels of the homeostatic cytokine IL-7. It was initially felt that this elevation was a homeostatic response to the lymphopenia; however, recent findings suggest that the increase in serum IL-7 was a result of reduced utilization of the cytokine related to the loss of cells expressing the IL-7 receptor, CD127, which serves as a normal physiologic regulator of IL-7 production.

CD8+ T Cells A relative CD8+ T lymphocytosis is generally associated with high levels of HIV plasma viremia and likely reflects an immune response to the virus as well as dysregulated homeostasis associated with generalized immune activation. During the late stages of HIV infection, there may be a significant reduction in the numbers of CD8+ T cells despite the presence of high levels of viremia. HIV-specific CD8+ CTLs have been demonstrated in HIV-infected individuals early in the course of disease, and their emergence often coincides with a decrease in plasma viremia—an observation that is a factor in the proposal that virus-specific CTLs can control HIV disease for a finite period of time in a certain percentage of infected individuals. However, emergence of HIV escape mutants that ultimately evade these HIV-specific CD8+ T cells has been described in the majority of HIV-infected individuals who are not receiving cART. In addition, as the disease progresses, the functional capability of these cells gradually decreases, at least in part due to the persistent nature of HIV infection that causes functional exhaustion via the upregulation of inhibitory receptors such as PD-1 on HIV-specific CD8+ T cells (see "Immune Activation, Inflammation, and HIV Pathogenesis," above). As chronic immune activation persists, there are also systemic effects on CD8+ T cells, such that as a population they assume an abnormal phenotype characterized by expression of activation markers such as HLA-DR and CD38 with an absence of expression of the IL-2 receptor (CD25) and a reduced expression of the IL-7 receptor (CD127). In addition, CD8+ T cells lacking CD28 expression are increased in HIV disease, reflecting a skewed expansion of a less differentiated CD8+ T cell subset. This skewing of subsets is also associated with diminished polyfunctionality, a qualitative difference that distinguishes nonprogressors from progressors. It has been reported that nonprogressors can also be distinguished from progressors by the maintenance in the former of a high proliferative capacity of their HIV-specific CD8+ T cells coupled to increases in perforin expression, characteristics that are markedly diminished in advanced HIV disease. It has been reported that the phenotype of CD8+ T cells in HIV-infected individuals may be of prognostic significance. Those individuals whose CD8+ T cells developed a phenotype of HLA-DR+/CD38– following seroconversion had stabilization of their CD4+ T cell counts, whereas those whose CD8+ T cells developed a phenotype of HLA-DR+/CD38+ had a more aggressive course and a poorer prognosis. In addition to the defects in HIV-specific CD8+ CTLs, functional defects in other MHC restricted CTLs, such as those directed against influenza and CMV, have been demonstrated. CD8+ T cells secrete a variety of soluble factors that inhibit HIV replication, including the CC-chemokines RANTES (CCL5), MIP-1α (CCL3), and MIP-1β (CCL4) as well as potentially a number of unidentified factors. The presence of high levels of HIV viremia in vivo as well as exposure of CD8+ T cells in vitro to HIV envelope, both of which are associated with aberrant immune activation, have been shown to be associated with a variety of cellular functional abnormalities. Furthermore, since the integrity of CD8+ T cell function depends in part on adequate inductive signals from CD4+ T cells, the defect in CD8+ CTLs is likely compounded by the quantitative loss and qualitative dysfunction of CD4+ T cells.

B Cells The predominant defect in B cells from HIV-infected individuals is one of aberrant cellular activation, which is reflected by increased propensity to terminal differentiation and immunoglobulin secretion and increased expression of markers of activation and exhaustion. As a result of activation and differentiation in vivo, B cells from HIV viremic patients manifest a decreased capacity to mount a proliferative response to ligation of the B cell antigen receptor and other B cell stimuli in vitro. B cells from HIV-infected individuals manifest enhanced spontaneous secretion of immunoglobulins in vitro, a process that reflects their highly differentiated state in vivo. There is also an increased incidence of EBV-related B cell lymphomas in HIV-infected individuals that are likely due to combined effects of defective T cell immune surveillance and increased turnover that increases the risk of oncogenesis. Untransformed B cells cannot be infected with HIV, although HIV or its products can activate B cells directly. B cells from patients with high levels of viremia bind virions to their surface via the CD21 complement receptor. It is likely that in vivo activation of B cells by replication-competent or defective virus as well as viral products during the viremic state accounts at least in part for their activated phenotype. B cell subpopulations from HIV-infected individuals undergo a number of changes over the course of HIV disease, including the attrition of resting memory B cells and replacement with several aberrant memory and differentiated B cell subpopulations that collectively express reduced levels of CD21 and either increased expression of activation markers or inhibitory receptors associated with functional exhaustion. The more activated and differentiated B cells are also responsible for increased secretion of immunoglobulins and increased susceptibility to Fas-mediated apoptosis. In more advanced disease, there is also the appearance of immature B cells associated with CD4+ T cell lymphopenia. Cognate B cell–CD4+ T cell interactions are abnormal in viremic HIV-infected individuals in that B cells respond poorly to CD4+ T cell help and CD4+ T cells receive inadequate co-stimulatory signals from activated B cells. In vivo, the aberrant activated state of B cells manifests itself by hypergammaglobulinemia and by the presence of circulating immune complexes and autoantibodies. HIV-infected individuals respond poorly to primary and secondary immunizations with protein and polysaccharide antigens. Using immunization with influenza vaccine, it has been demonstrated that there is a memory B cell defect in HIV-infected individuals, particularly those with high levels of HIV viremia. There is also evidence that responses to HIV and non-HIV antigens in infected individuals, especially those who remain viremic, are enriched in abnormal subsets of B cells that either are highly prone to apoptosis or show signs of functional exhaustion. Taken together, these B cell defects are likely responsible in part for the inadequate response to HIV as well as to decreased response to vaccinations and the increase in certain bacterial infections seen in advanced HIV disease in adults, as well as for the important role of bacterial infections in the morbidity and mortality rates of HIV-infected children, who cannot mount an adequate humoral response to common bacterial pathogens. The absolute number of circulating B cells may be depressed in HIV infection; this phenomenon likely reflects increased activation-induced apoptosis as well as a redistribution of cells out of the circulation and into the lymphoid tissue—phenomena that are associated with ongoing viral replication.

Monocytes/Macrophages Circulating monocytes are generally normal in number in HIV-infected individuals; however, there is evidence of increased activation within this lineage. The increased level of sCD14 and other biomarkers (see above) reported in HIV-infected individuals is an indirect marker of monocyte activation in vivo. A number of other abnormalities of circulating monocytes have been reported in HIV-infected individuals, many of which may be related directly or indirectly to aberrant in vivo immune activation. In this regard, increased levels of lipopolysaccharide (LPS) are found in the sera of HIV-infected individuals due, at least in part, to translocation across the gut mucosal barrier (see above). LPS is a highly inflammatory bacterial product that preferentially binds to macrophages through CD14 and Toll-like receptors, resulting in cellular activation. Functional abnormalities of monocyte/macrophages in HIV disease include decreased secretion of IL-1 and IL-12; increased secretion of IL-10 and IL-18; defects in antigen presentation and induction of T cell responses due to decreased MHC class II expression; and abnormalities of Fc receptor function, C3 receptor–mediated clearance, oxidative burst responses, and certain cytotoxic functions such as ADCC, possibly related to low levels of expression of Fc and complement receptors. Monocytes express the CD4 molecule and several co-receptors for HIV on their surface, including CCR5, CXCR4, and CCR3, and thus are potential targets of HIV infection. The degree of cytopathicity of HIV for cells of the monocyte lineage is low, and HIV can replicate in cells of the monocyte lineage with relatively little cytopathic effect. Hence, monocyte-lineage cells may play a role in the dissemination of HIV in the body and can serve as reservoirs of HIV infection, thus representing an obstacle to the eradication of HIV by antiretroviral drugs. In vivo infection of circulating monocytes is difficult to demonstrate; however, infection of tissue macrophages and macrophage-lineage cells in the brain (infiltrating macrophages or resident microglial cells) and lung (pulmonary alveolar macrophages) can be demonstrated easily. Tissue macrophages are an important source of HIV during the inflammatory response associated with opportunistic infections. Infection of monocyte precursors in the bone marrow may directly or indirectly be responsible for certain of the hematologic abnormalities in HIV-infected individuals. However, as with DCs, monocytes and macrophages express high levels of host restriction factors that likely help explain the low contribution of myeloid cells to the overall viral burden in HIV-infected individuals.

Dendritic and Langerhans Cells DCs and Langerhans cells are thought to play an important role in the initiation of HIV infection by virtue of the ability of HIV to bind to cell-surface C-type lectin receptors, particularly DC-SIGN (see above) and Langerin. This allows efficient presentation of virus to CD4+ T cell targets that become infected; complexes of infected CD4+ T cells and DCs provide an optimal microenvironment for virus replication. There was once considerable disagreement regarding the HIV infectibility and hence the depletion as well as the dysfunction of DCs themselves. However, since the recognition of myeloid (mDC) and plasmacytoid (pDC) subsets, there has been a better appreciation of specific DC dysfunction in HIV disease. pDCs are an important component of the innate immune system and secrete large amounts of IFN-α in response to viral infections. The numbers of circulating pDCs are decreased in HIV infection through mechanisms that remain unclear, and there are conflicting reports regarding the frequency of pDCs in lymphoid tissues, with some studies suggesting that their increased tissue presence and secretion of inflammatory cytokines such as IFN-α contributes to lymphoid hyperplasia. The mDCs or conventional DCs are involved in the initiation of adaptive immunity in draining lymph nodes by presenting antigen to T cells and B cells, as well as by secreting cytokines such as IL-12, IL-15, and IL-18 that activate other immune cells. There are also indications that the relatively low infectibility of DCs may be associated with the expression of host restriction factors, including APOBEC3G (see above).

Natural Killer Cells The role of NK cells is to provide immunosurveillance against virus-infected cells, certain tumor cells, and allogeneic cells (Chap. 372e). There are no convincing data that HIV productively infects NK cells in vivo; however, functional abnormalities in NK cells have been observed throughout the course of HIV disease, and the severity of these abnormalities increases as disease progresses. NK cells are part of the innate immune system and act by direct killing of infected cells and secretion of antiviral cytokines. In early HIV infection there is an increase in the activation of NK cells, and the capacity to secrete IFN-γ is maintained, although they manifest reduced cytotoxic function. During chronic HIV infection, both NK cell cytotoxicity and cytokine secretion become impaired. Given that HIV infection of target cells downregulates HLA-A and -B, but not HLA-C and -D molecules, this may explain in part the relative inability of NK cells to kill HIV-infected target cells. However, the NK cell impairments, especially in patients with high levels of virus replication, are associated with an expansion of an "anergic" CD56–/CD16+ NK cell subset. This abnormal subset of NK cells manifests an increased expression of inhibitory NK cell receptors (iNKRs) and a substantial decrease in expression of natural cytotoxicity receptors (NCRs) and shows a markedly impaired lytic activity. The overrepresentation of this abnormal subset of NK cells may explain in part the observed defects in NK cell function in HIV-infected individuals and likely begins to occur during primary infection. NK cells also serve as important sources of HIV-inhibitory CC-chemokines. NK cells isolated from HIV-infected individuals constitutively produce high levels of MIP-1α (CCL3), MIP-1β (CCL4), and RANTES (CCL5), although the impact of these chemokines on HIV replication in vivo is unclear. Finally, NK cell–DC interactions are important for normal immune function. NK cells and DCs reciprocally modulate each other's activation and maturation. These interactions are markedly impaired in HIV-infected individuals with high levels of plasma viremia.

GENETIC FACTORS IN HIV-1 AND AIDS PATHOGENESIS

PHENOTYPES OF SUSCEPTIBILITY AND RESPONSE TO HIV INFECTION It is well known that individuals vary in their susceptibility to acquiring HIV infection and that there is wide variation in both the steady-state level of HIV that is established soon after infection (virologic setpoint) as well as the rate at which HIV-infected patients progress to AIDS. Some striking examples include sex workers who remain uninfected despite repeated exposure to HIV; HIV-infected individuals who spontaneously control viral replication in the absence of cART (HIV controllers); patients who resist disease progression for at least 8–10 years, despite viremia; and those progressing to AIDS within 3 years. Investigators have hypothesized that genetic differences may partly explain this interindividual variation in risk of acquiring HIV infection and disease progression rates. In addition to these phenotypes, it has been hypothesized that genetic variation may partly underpin the risk of developing specific AIDS-defining illnesses (e.g., renal and neurologic diseases) and non-AIDS comorbidities (e.g., cardiovascular disease), as well as the variable recovery in CD4+ T cell counts observed while receiving cART.

Candidate gene approaches and genome-wide association studies (GWAS) have demonstrated associations between gene variations and the above-mentioned phenotypes. A list of some of these associations is shown in Table 226-6. While in vitro genome-wide functional scanning using RNA interference has identified hundreds of host factors that may be involved in the HIV life cycle, the association of these genes with HIV susceptibility and/or disease progression remains largely undefined. Below is a discussion of a few key genes with strong associations and their implications for improving clinical care.

ASSOCIATIONS WITH CCR5 AND TRANSLATION OF GENETIC FINDINGS TO THE CLINIC Possibly, the most dramatic example of the importance of genetic studies for identifying host factors that influence HIV-AIDS pathogenesis is from studies related to the gene that encodes for CC chemokine receptor 5 (CCR5). While in vitro studies established that CCR5 is the major HIV co-receptor for the cell entry of HIV-1 into the host, it was genetic studies that established the seminal in vivo role of this receptor for the initial entry of HIV and AIDS pathogenesis.

Genetic analysis revealed that the in vitro resistance to CCR5-using R5 strains of HIV is in some instances due to carriage of two defective *CCR5* alleles. This defect is a 32-bp deletion in the coding sequence (designated as the *Δ32* allele). The *CCR5 Δ32* allele encodes a truncated protein that is not expressed on the cell surface.

Approximately 1% of individuals of European ancestry are homozygous for the *CCR5 Δ32* allele. Depending on the geographic region in Europe, up to 20% of individuals are heterozygous for the *CCR5 Δ32* allele. The *CCR5 Δ32* allele is either absent or extremely rare in other populations. The evolutionary pressure that resulted in the emergence of the *CCR5 Δ32* allele in the European population remains unknown and has been speculated to be secondary to an ancestral pandemic such as the plague.

Individuals homozygous for the *CCR5 Δ32* allele (*Δ32/Δ32*) lack CCR5 surface expression and are highly resistant to acquiring HIV infection. Heterozygosity for the *CCR5 Δ32* allele is also associated with a reduced risk of acquiring HIV. Consequently, the frequency of the *CCR5 Δ32* allele is enriched in individuals of European descent who remain uninfected despite exposure to the virus. Although the *CCR5 Δ32/Δ32* genotype is associated with profound resistance to acquiring HIV, a few individuals with this genotype have become infected with the X4 HIV strain and, in some instances, experienced an accelerated disease course. In general, *CCR5 Δ32* heterozygosity is associated with a slower HIV disease course.

Subsequent studies identified single nucleotide polymorphisms (SNPs) in the promoter (regulatory region) of CCR5 that influence its expression levels. Alleles bearing specific cassettes of linked polymorphisms (haplotypes) were identified and designated as human haplogroups A to G*2 (HHA to HHG*2). The *CCR5 Δ32* is found on the HHG*2 haplotype. The *CCR5* HHE haplotype was associated with higher CCR5 expression, and genetic association studies have shown that homozygosity for the CCR5 HHE haplotype is associated with an increased risk of acquiring HIV, progressing rapidly to AIDS, and reduced immune recovery on cART. The *CCR2*-64I-bearing HHF*2 haplotype is associated with a slower HIV disease course. The *CCR5* HHA haplotype is the ancestral CCR5 haplotype and is associated with a lower CCR5 expression. The HHA haplotype was associated with slower disease progression in African populations and has been speculated to be a basis for why SIV-infected chimpanzees (who all carry the ancestral *CCR5* HHA haplotype) may resist disease progression. The *CCR5* haplotypes also influence cell-mediated immunity and immune recovery on cART.

The association of variations in the *CCR5* gene with HIV-AIDS phenotypes is also an example of how discoveries made in the laboratory (bench) have been translated to improve health outcomes (bedside). The discovery that the *CCR5 Δ32/Δ32* genotype is associated with strong resistance to HIV infection, and that uninfected Caucasians bearing this genotype did not appear to have impaired immunity, led to the development of two kinds of therapies. First, it spurred the development of a new class of FDA-approved therapies, entry inhibitors (e.g., maraviroc), that block the interaction of CCR5 with the HIV envelope. Second, it led to the development of novel experimental cellular therapies. An HIV-infected patient with acute myelogenous leukemia was given an allogeneic stem-cell transplantation from an HLA-compatible person whose cells lacked expression of CCR5 due to the *Δ32/Δ32* genotype. There has been no evidence of HIV-1 infection in the transplanted patient thus far (6 years). This observation spurred the hope of an HIV cure and led to the development of additional novel cellular therapies involving autologous transplantation of CD4+ T-cells in which the *CCR5* gene is inactivated ex vivo using new gene editing procedures.

DISCOVERY OF HLA CLASS I ALLELES THAT ASSOCIATE WITH VIROLOGIC CONTROL OF HIV INFECTION There is a strong association between variations within the *HLA-B* gene with protective (e.g., HLA-B*57 and -B*27 alleles) or detrimental (e.g., HLA-B*35 allele) outcomes during HIV infection. Carriage of the HLA-B*57 and/or HLA-B*27 alleles is associated with slower disease progression. The beneficial effects of these alleles may relate in part to their consistent associations with a lower virologic setpoint as well as to higher cell-mediated immunity. The protective effect of the HLA-B*57 and -B*27 alleles on HIV disease course is underscored by the finding that the prevalence of these alleles is higher among long-term nonprogressors and HIV elite controllers (see above). On the other hand, the HLA-B*35 allele has been associated with faster progression to AIDS and higher viral load. The prevalence of the *HLA-B* alleles differs between populations. HLA-B*57:01 in Europeans and HLA-B*57:03 in African Americans are the protective alleles. In some populations (e.g., Japanese) where the HLA-B*57/-B*27 alleles are absent, HLA-B*51 is associated with a protective phenotype.

Possession of the protective *HLA-B* alleles is associated with broader and stronger CD8+ T cell responses to HIV epitopes. The mechanisms underlying the differential effects of the *HLA-B* alleles on HIV disease course may relate to differences in the ability of antigen-presenting cells to present immunodominant HIV epitopes to T helper or cytotoxic T lymphocytes in the context of MHC-encoded molecules. This may result in differential immune responses that influence viral replication. In this regard, the *HLA-B* alleles that impact HIV disease course differ in their amino acid residues in the HLA-B peptide-binding groove—and this may play a critical role in virologic control.

Investigators have also examined the influence of extended *HLA* haplotypes (linked alleles) on HIV disease course. The extended *HLA* ancestral haplotype (AH) 8.1 is defined by the presence of HLA-A1, HLA-B8, and HLA-DR3 alleles. AH 8.1 is the most common ancestral haplotype in Caucasians (present in 10%) and is associated with multiple autoimmune diseases in HIV-uninfected persons. These associations of AH 8.1 are thought to be due to a genetically determined hyperresponsiveness characterized by high TNF-α production and lack of complement C4A. Strong epidemiologic data indicate that carriage of AH 8.1 in HIV-infected persons is associated with a rapid decline in CD4+ T cells and faster progression to AIDS development. Gene–gene interactions between HLA alleles and other genes (e.g., killer cell immunoglobulin-like receptors) also may influence HIV disease progression rates.

POLYMORPHISMS IDENTIFIED BY GWAS THAT ASSOCIATE WITH VIROLOGIC CONTROL Large scale GWASs have been conducted for the phenotype of viral load, including in a large group of HIV controllers. GWAS in HIV-infected persons of European ancestry identified four SNPs in genes in the HLA class I loci that associated with virologic control.

TABLE 226-6 HOST GENETIC FACTORS THAT INFLUENCE RISK OF HIV-1 ACQUISITION AND RATES OF HIV-1 DISEASE PROGRESSION

Gene[a]	Genetic Variation	Mechanisms[b]	Genetic Effect on HIV-AIDS[c]
Genes in MHC Locus			
HLA-B	B*27 and B*57	Presentation of specific HIV antigens	Slower progression to AIDS; lower viral load
	B*35	Restriction of specific HIV peptide presentation	Faster progression to AIDS; higher viral load
	HLA-Bw4	Providing ligands for activating KIR	Slower progression to AIDS
HLA class I allele	Homozygosity of *HLA*-class I alleles	Reduced repertoire for epitope recognition	Faster progression to AIDS; increased risk of mother-to-child transmission
	Shared donor-recipient *HLA* alleles	Preadaptation of HIV strains	Faster disease progression
	Rare *HLA* alleles	Limited adaptation of HIV strains; less frequent escape mutants	Protection against HIV infection
HLA class II allele	*HLA-DRB1* alleles	Influences protein specificity of CD4+ T cell responses to HIV Gag and Nef proteins	HLA-DRB1*15:02—lower viral load; HLA-DRB1*03:01—higher viral load
HLA extended haplotype	A1-B8-DR3-DQ2 (AH 8.1)	Increased proinflammatory responses; higher TNF-α production	Faster progression to AIDS
HLA-C	35 kb upstream, rs9264942-C	Increased expression of HLA-C	Decreased viral load set point
HCP5	rs2395029-G	Linkage disequilibrium with HLA-B*57:01	Lower viral load
MICA	Noncoding SNP near *MICA*, rs4418214-T	May affect HLA class I peptide presentation—linkage with protective *HLA-B* alleles	Enriched in HIV-1 controllers
PSORS1C3	rs3131018-A	May affect HLA class I peptide presentation	Enriched in HIV-1 controllers
ZNRD1	rs9261174-C	Possible interference in processing of HIV transcripts; influences ZNRD1 expression; linkage disequilibrium with *HLA-A10*	AIDS disease retardation
Chemokine Receptors			
CCR5	32-bp deletion in the ORF (Δ32), rs333	Truncated CCR5 protein	Δ32/Δ32: resistance to acquiring HIV infection Δ32/wild type: delays AIDS onset; improves immune reconstitution during ART
	Promoter SNPs, haplotypes (HHA to HHG*2)	Altered CCR5 expression, e.g., HHE allele correlates with high CCR5 expression	HHE/HHE: increased HIV/AIDS susceptibility
CCR2	SNP in ORF (64 V→I), rs1799864	Possibly due to linkage with polymorphism in *CCR5* promoter	64I: delayed AIDS onset
CXCR6	rs2234358 G→T in the 3′UTR	Trafficking of effector T cells and activation of NK T cells Minor HIV co-receptor	Prevalence of rs2234358-T was lower in long-term nonprogressors
CX3CR1	SNPs in ORF (249 V→I; and 280 T→M, rs3732378)	280M reduces receptor expression and binding of fractalkine, the CX3CR1 ligand	249I and 280M are associated with faster AIDS onset in some Caucasian cohorts; inconsistent effects were detected in other cohorts
DARC	African-specific promoter SNP (–46T→C), rs2814778	–46C/C associates with low neutrophil counts; influences circulating chemokine levels; alters HIV binding to RBCs and transinfection of HIV-1	–46C/C: increased risk of acquiring HIV but slower HIV disease progression; Duffy-null-associated low neutrophil trait associated with increased HIV risk in Africans
Chemokines			
CCL3L, *CCL4L*	Gene copy number of *CCL3L* and *CCL4L*	High numbers of *CCL3L* and *CCL4L* gene-containing segmental duplications correlate with high CCL3L and CCL4L levels	Gene copy number lower than population median associates with increased HIV/AIDS susceptibility and reduced immune reconstitution during ART
CCL5	Promoter SNPs	Altered gene expression	Altered HIV-AIDS susceptibility
CCL2	Promoter SNP (–2578 T→G), rs1024611	–2578G allele: increased CCL2 expression and monocyte recruitment	–2578G/G associates with increased risk of developing HIV-1-associated dementia and a rapid AIDS onset
Cytokines			
IL-6	Promoter SNP (–174 G→C), rs1800795	–174G/G associates with increased IL-6 and CRP levels	–174G/G associates with high risk of KS development and variable recovery of CD4 cells during ART
IL-10	Promoter SNP (–592 C→A), rs1800872	–592A results in decreased IL-10 levels	–592A associates with increased HIV-AIDS susceptibility
Innate Immunity Genes			
MBL	Coding alleles (O)	Low plasma concentration and structural variation of MBL protein	Slow progression to AIDS in heterozygous subjects (A/O)
	X allele (promoter SNP –221)	Decreased levels of MBL protein	Faster progression to AIDS in homozygous X/X subjects
Apobec-3G	ORF SNP (186 H→R), rs8177832	Reduced anti-HIV-1 activity	186R associates with rapid AIDS onset in African Americans
TLR7	ORF SNP (Gln11Leu), rs179008	Decreased expression of TLR7 leading to lack of recognition of HIV-infected cells	The Leu-containing protein associated with higher viral load and faster progression to AIDS

(Continued)

TABLE 226-6 HOST GENETIC FACTORS THAT INFLUENCE RISK OF HIV-1 ACQUISITION AND RATES OF HIV-1 DISEASE PROGRESSION (*CONTINUED*)

Gene[a]	Genetic Variation	Mechanisms[b]	Genetic Effect on HIV-AIDS[c]
PARD3B	rs11884476 (C→G), near exon 20	Direct interaction with HIV, signaling through SMAD family of proteins	rs11884476-G associated with slower progression to AIDS
Others			
ApoE	E4 allele	E4 enhances HIV cell entry in vitro	ApoE4/E4 associates with rapid AIDS onset and dementia
ApoL1/MYH9	Several risk haplotypes including G1	Unknown	Increased risk for HIV-associated nephropathy
RYR3	ORF SNP (A→G), rs2229116	Unknown, potential impact on calcium signaling and homeostasis	rs2229116-G associated with subclinical atherosclerosis
PROX1	rs17762192-G, 36kb upstream of *PROX1*	Unknown, presumably due to its impact on PROX1 expression, which is a negative regulator of IFN-γ	rs17762192-G: reduced rate of disease progression
Gene–Gene Interaction			
KIR+HLA	KIR3DS1 + HLA Bw4 80Ile	Altered NK cell activity required to eliminate HIV-infected cells	KIR3DS1 with HLA Bw4-80I +: delayed AIDS onset
	HLA-C1 + KIR2DL3,	Reduction of inhibitory KIR likely results in increased immune activation; impaired killing of latently infected cells; and a higher proviral burden	HLA-C1+/KIR2DL3+: better immune recovery after viral load suppression on ART
LILRB2+HLA	LILRB2 + HLA class I	Regulation of dendritic cells by LILRB2-HLA engagement	Control of HIV-1
CCL3L1+CCR5	Low *CCL3L1* gene copies + detrimental *CCR5* genotypes	Low CCL3L1 and high CCR5 expression	Increased HIV/AIDS susceptibility and reduced immune reconstitution during ART

[a]Representative genes and polymorphisms and [b]possible mechanisms are listed. [c]Some of the associations are population specific and may display cohort-specific effects.

Note: Apobec, apolipoprotein B mRNA editing enzyme, catalytic polypeptide-like; ApoE, apolipoprotein E; ART, antiretroviral therapy; CCL, CC ligand; CCL3L, CCL3-like; CCR5, CC chemokine receptor 5; CRP, C-reactive protein; CXCR6, chemokine (C-X-C motif) receptor 6; DARC, Duffy antigen receptor for chemokines; HCP5, HLA class I histocompatibility antigen protein P5, HHE, human haplogroup E; HLA, human leukocyte antigen; IFN, interferon; IL, interleukin; LILRB2, leukocyte immunoglobulin-like receptor B2; KIR, killer cell immunoglobulin-like receptors; KS, Kaposi's sarcoma; MBL, mannose-binding lectin; MHC, major histocompatibility complex; MICA: MHC class I polypeptide-related sequence A; ORF, open reading frame; PARD3B, par-3 family cell polarity regulator beta; PROX1, prospero homeobox 1; PSORS1C3, psoriasis susceptibility 1 candidate 3; SNP, single nucleotide polymorphism; rs#, SNP identification number in SNP database from NCBI; UTR, untranslated region; ZNRD1, zinc ribbon domain containing 1; +, present, –, absent.

Sources: Sunil K Ahuja, MD, Weijing He, MD, and Gabriel Catano, MD. Reviews for additional information: P An et al: Trends Genet 26:119, 2010; J Fellay: Antivir Ther 14:731, 2009; RA Kaslow et al: J Infect Dis 191:S68, 2005; D van Manen et al: Retrovirology 9:70, 2012; MP Martin et al: Immunol Rev 254:245, 2013; S Limou et al. Front Immunol 4:118, 2013.

These SNPs are within or in the vicinity of *HCP5*, *HLA-C*, *MICA*, and *PSORS1C3* genes. The protective effects of the SNPs in *HCP5* and *MICA* may relate to their linkage with known protective *HLA-B* alleles. The protective *HCP5* allele is in linkage disequilibrium with the HLA B*57:01, and the protective *MICA* allele tags with the HLA-B*57:01 and B*27:05 alleles. The protective *HLA-C* SNP is associated with higher HLA-C expression, and this effect is thought to be due to the altered binding of a microRNA to the *HLA-C* mRNA. Higher HLA-C expression has been associated with beneficial HIV phenotypes. The mechanism associated with the SNP in *PSORS1C3* is unknown. GWAS in African Americans identified a SNP that tags the HLA-B*57:03 allele that is known to associate with lower virologic setpoint and slower disease course. Together these GWAS data underscore the importance of variations in HLA class I loci in control of viral replication.

GENETIC ASSOCIATIONS WITH SPECIFIC AIDS AND NON-AIDS CONDITIONS • Carotid artery disease Many of the non-AIDS events in HIV-infected individuals resemble those related to immune senescence and those found in the HIV-uninfected aging population. A functional SNP in the ryanodine receptor 3 (*RYR3*) gene was found to be associated with an increased risk of common carotid intima–media thickness (cIMT), which is a surrogate for subclinical atherosclerosis. Functional studies on RYR3 and its isoforms demonstrate a major role of these receptors in modulating endothelial function and atherogenesis via calcium signaling pathways, providing a biologically plausible mechanism by which the SNP in *RYR3* may associate with increased cIMT risk.

Renal disease HIV-1-associated nephropathy (HIVAN) is a form of focal sclerosing glomerulonephritis caused by direct infection of kidney epithelial cells with HIV. HIVAN is more common in persons of African descent. There is evidence that polymorphisms in the *MYH9* gene and in the neighboring *APOL1* gene are a strong determinant of susceptibility to HIVAN in African Americans. The effect of carrying two *APOL1* risk alleles explains nearly 35% of HIVAN. The mechanisms by which *MYH9*/*APOL1* variants predispose to HIVAN are currently unknown.

HIV-associated neurocognitive disorder HIV-associated neurocognitive disorder (HAND) comprises a spectrum of neurocognitive deficits due to HIV infection. Variations in the apolipoprotein E (ApoE) gene have strong associations with Alzheimer's disease in the HIV-uninfected population. In HIV-infected persons, possession of the *ApoE4* allele has been associated with several cognitive outcomes including dementia, peripheral neuropathy, and impairment in cognition and immediate and delayed verbal memory. Macrophage recruitment and activation plays a central role in the development of many of the HAND syndromes. Variations in chemokines that play an influential role in macrophage activation and recruitment, namely *CCL2* (MCP-1) and *CCL3* (MIP-1α), have been shown to alter the risk of developing HAND. Variations in mitochondrial genes also have been associated with risk of AIDS and HAND.

ASSOCIATIONS WITH ART-RELATED ADVERSE EVENTS Abacavir, an effective antiretroviral agent, is associated with significant risk of hypersensitivity reactions (2–9% of cases). Interestingly, while the *HLA-B*57:01* allele is associated with a slower HIV disease course, possession of this allele is associated with a higher risk of abacavir-associated hypersensitivity. Pharmacogenetic screening for the HLA-B*57:01 allele is recommended before initiation of abacavir treatment.

NEUROPATHOGENESIS IN HIV DISEASE

While there has been a remarkable decrease in the incidence in the severe forms of HIV encephalopathy among those with access to treatment in the era of effective cART, HIV-infected individuals can still experience milder forms of neurocognitive impairment despite adequate cART. A variety of factors may contribute to the neurocognitive decline, which includes lack of complete control of HIV replication in the brain, production of HIV proteins that may be neurotoxic, low CD4+ T cell nadir, chronic immune activation, comorbidities such as drug abuse, and the potential for neurotoxicity of certain of the antiretroviral drugs. HIV has been demonstrated in the brain and CSF of infected individuals with and without neuropsychiatric abnormalities. As opposed to lymphoid tissues, there are no resident lymphocytes in the brain. The main cell types that are infected in the brain in vivo are the perivascular macrophages and the microglial cells; low-level viral replication is also seen in perivascular astrocytes. Monocytes that have already been infected in the blood can migrate into the brain, where they then reside as macrophages, or macrophages can be directly infected within the brain. The precise mechanisms whereby HIV enters the brain are unclear; however, they are thought to relate, at least in part, to the ability of virus-infected and immune-activated macrophages to induce adhesion molecules such as E-selectin and vascular cell adhesion molecule 1 (VCAM-1) on brain endothelium. Other studies have demonstrated that HIV gp120 enhances the expression of intercellular adhesion molecule 1 (ICAM-1) in glial cells; this effect may facilitate entry of HIV-infected cells into the CNS. Virus isolates from the brain are preferentially R5 strains as opposed to X4 strains; in this regard, HIV-infected individuals who are heterozygous for *CCR5-Δ32* appear to be relatively protected against the development of HIV encephalopathy. Once HIV enters the brain due to pressures of the local environment, it evolves to develop distinct sequences in the env, tat, and LTR genes. These unique sequences have been associated with neurocognitive dysfunction; however, it is unclear if they are causal (see below).

HIV-infected individuals may manifest white matter lesions as well as neuronal loss. The white matter lesions are due to axonal injury and a disruption of the blood-brain barrier and not due to demyelination. Given the absence of evidence of HIV infection of neurons either in vivo or in vitro, it is highly unlikely that direct infection of these cells accounts for their loss. Rather, the HIV-mediated effects on neurons are thought to involve indirect pathways whereby viral proteins, particularly gp120 and Tat, trigger the release of endogenous neurotoxins from macrophages and to a lesser extent from astrocytes. In addition, it has been demonstrated that both HIV-1 Nef and Tat can induce chemotaxis of leukocytes, including monocytes, into the CNS. Neurotoxins can be released from monocytes as a consequence of infection and/or immune activation. Monocyte-derived neurotoxic factors have been reported to kill neurons via the *N*-methyl-D-aspartate (NMDA) receptor. In addition, HIV gp120 shed by virus-infected monocytes could cause neurotoxicity by antagonizing the function of vasoactive intestinal peptide (VIP), by elevating intracellular calcium levels, and by decreasing nerve growth factor levels in the cerebral cortex. A variety of monocyte-derived cytokines can contribute directly or indirectly to the neurotoxic effects in HIV infection; these include TNF-α, IL-1, IL-6, TGF-β, IFN-γ, platelet-activating factor, and endothelin. Furthermore, among the CC-chemokines, elevated levels of monocyte chemotactic protein-1 (MCP-1 or CCL-2) in the brain and CSF have been shown to correlate best with the presence and degree of HIV encephalopathy. In addition, infection and/or activation of monocyte-lineage cells can result in increased production of eicosanoids, quinolinic acid, nitric oxide, excitatory amino acids such as L-cysteine and glutamate, arachidonic acid, platelet activating factor, free radicals, TNF-α, and TGF-β, which may contribute to neurotoxicity. Astrocytes may play diverse roles in HIV neuropathogenesis. Reactive gliosis or astrocytosis has been demonstrated in the brains of HIV-infected individuals, and TNF-α and IL-6 have been shown to induce astrocyte proliferation. In addition, astrocyte-derived IL-6 can induce HIV expression in infected cells in vitro. Furthermore, it has been suggested that astrocytes may downregulate macrophage-produced neurotoxins. Treatment with cART leads to improvement in neuropsychiatric manifestations and a decrease in these cytokine levels in CSF, suggesting that they are driven by the virus or by its products. However, even in patients on long-term cART, there may be evidence of persistently activated lymphocytes in the CSF. It is unclear if these lymphocytes may contribute to neuronal injury in the brain or are critical for controlling the CNS viral reservoir. The contribution of host genetic factors to development of neuropsychiatric manifestations of HIV infection has not been well studied. However, evidence supports the role of the E4 allele for apoE in an increased risk of HIV-associated neurocognitive disorders and peripheral neuropathy.

It has also been suggested that the CNS may serve as a relatively sequestered site for a reservoir of latently infected cells that might be a barrier for the eradication of virus by cART (see "Reservoirs of HIV-Infected Cells: Obstacles to the Eradication of Virus," above).

PATHOGENESIS OF KAPOSI'S SARCOMA

There are at least four distinct epidemiologic forms of KS: (1) the classic form that occurs in older men of predominantly Mediterranean or eastern European Jewish backgrounds with no recognized contributing factors; (2) the equatorial African form that occurs in all ages, also without any recognized precipitating factors; (3) the form associated with organ transplantation and its attendant iatrogenic immunosuppressed state; and (4) the form associated with HIV-1 infection. In the latter two forms, KS is an opportunistic disease; in HIV-infected individuals, unlike typical opportunistic infections, its occurrence is not strictly related to the level of depression of CD4+ T cell counts. The pathogenesis of KS is complex; fundamentally, it is an angioproliferative disease that is not a true neoplastic sarcoma, at least not in its early stages. It is a manifestation of excessive proliferation of spindle cells that are believed to be of vascular origin and have features in common with endothelial and smooth-muscle cells. In HIV disease the development of KS is dependent on the interplay of a variety of factors including HIV-1 itself, human herpes virus 8 (HHV-8), immune activation, and cytokine secretion. A number of epidemiologic and virologic studies have clearly linked HHV-8, which is also referred to as *Kaposi's sarcoma–associated herpesvirus* (KSHV), to KS not only in HIV-infected individuals but also in individuals with the other forms of KS. HHV-8 is a γ-herpesvirus related to EBV and *herpesvirus saimiri*. It encodes a homologue to human IL-6 and, in addition to KS, has been implicated in the pathogenesis of body cavity lymphoma, multiple myeloma, and monoclonal gammopathy of undetermined significance. Sequences of HHV-8 are found universally in the lesions of KS, and patients with KS are virtually all seropositive for HHV-8. HHV-8 DNA sequences can be found in the B cells of 30–50% of patients with KS and 7% of patients with AIDS without clinically apparent KS.

Between 1 and 2% of eligible blood donors are positive for antibodies to HHV-8, while the prevalence of HHV-8 seropositivity in HIV-infected men is 30–35%. The prevalence of HHV-8 seropositivity in HIV-infected women is ~4%. This finding is reflective of the lower incidence of KS in women. It has been debated whether HHV-8 is actually the transforming agent in KS; the bulk of the cells in the tumor lesions of KS are not neoplastic cells. However, it has been demonstrated that endothelial cells can be transformed in vitro by HHV-8. In this regard, HHV-8 possesses a number of genes, including homologues of the IL-8 receptor, Bcl-2, and cyclin D, that can potentially transform the host cell. Despite the complexity of the pathogenic events associated with the development of KS in HIV-infected individuals, HHV-8 is the etiologic agent of this disease. The initiation and/or propagation of KS requires an activated state and is mediated, at least in part, by cytokines. A number of factors, including TNF-α, IL-1β, IL-6, granulocyte-macrophage colony-stimulating factor (GM-CSF), basic fibroblast growth factor, and oncostatin M, function in an autocrine and paracrine manner to sustain the growth and chemotaxis of the KS spindle cells. In this regard, KSHV-derived IL-6 has been demonstrated to induce proliferation of lymphoma cells and to inhibit the cytostatic effects of IFN-α on KSHV-infected lymphoma cells.

IMMUNE RESPONSE TO HIV

As detailed above and below, following the initial burst of viremia during primary infection, HIV-infected individuals mount robust immune responses that in most cases substantially curtail the levels of plasma viremia and likely contribute to delaying the ultimate development of clinically apparent disease for a median of 10 years in untreated individuals. This immune response contains elements of both humoral and cell-mediated immunity involving both innate and adaptive immune responses (Table 226-7; Fig. 226-26). It is directed against multiple antigenic determinants of the HIV virion as

TABLE 226-7 ELEMENTS OF THE IMMUNE RESPONSE TO HIV

Humoral immunity
- Binding antibodies
- Neutralizing antibodies
  - Type specific
  - Group specific
  - Broadly neutralizing
- Antibodies participating in antibody-dependent cellular cytotoxicity (ADCC)
  - Protective
  - Pathogenic (bystander killing)
- Enhancing antibodies
- Complement

Cell-mediated immunity
- Helper CD4+ T lymphocytes
- Class I MHC–restricted cytotoxic CD8+ T lymphocytes
- CD8+ T cell–mediated inhibition (noncytolytic)
- ADCC
- Natural killer cells

Abbreviation: MHC, major histocompatibility complex.

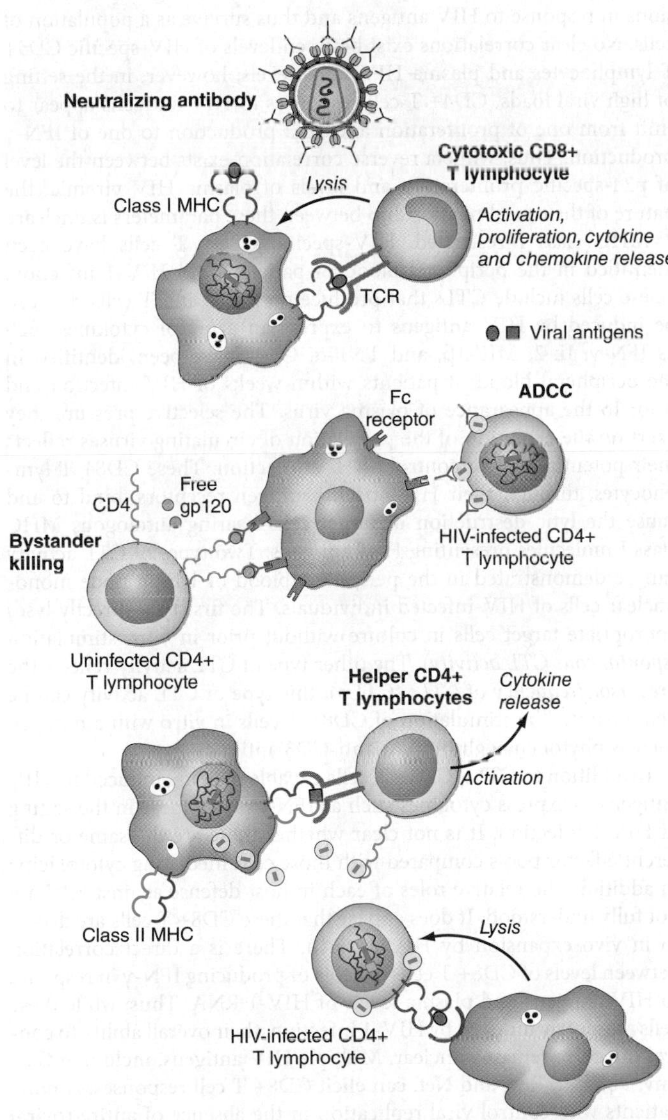

FIGURE 226-26 Schematic representation of the different immunologic effector mechanisms thought to be active in the setting of HIV infection. Detailed descriptions are given in the text. ADCC, antibody-dependent cellular cytotoxicity; MHC, major histocompatibility complex; TCR, T cell receptor.

well as against viral proteins expressed on the surface of infected cells. Ironically, those CD4+ T cells with T cell receptors specific for HIV are theoretically those CD4+ T cells most likely to be activated—and thus to serve as early targets for productive HIV infection and the cell death or dysfunction associated with infection. Thus, an early consequence of HIV infection is interference with and decrease of the helper T cell population needed to generate an effective immune response.

Although a great deal of investigation has been directed toward delineating and better understanding the components of this immune response, it remains unclear which immunologic effector mechanisms are most important in delaying progression of infection and which, if any, play a role in the pathogenesis of HIV disease. This lack of knowledge has also hampered the ability to develop an effective vaccine for HIV disease.

HUMORAL IMMUNE RESPONSE

Antibodies to HIV usually appear within 3–6 weeks and almost invariably within 12 weeks of primary infection (Fig. 226-27); rare exceptions are in individuals who have defects in the ability to produce HIV-specific antibodies. Detection of these antibodies forms the basis of most diagnostic screening tests for HIV infection. The appearance of HIV-binding antibodies detected by ELISA and Western blot assays occurs prior to the appearance of neutralizing antibodies; the latter generally appear following the initial decreases in plasma viremia and are more closely related to the appearance of HIV-specific CD8+ T lymphocytes. The first antibodies detected are those directed against the immunodominant region of the envelope gp41, followed by the appearance of antibodies to the structural or gag protein p24 and the gag precursor p55. Antibodies to p24 gag are followed by the appearance of antibodies to the outer envelope glycoprotein (gp120), the gag protein p17, and the products of the *pol* gene (p31 and p66). In addition, one may see antibodies to the low-molecular-weight regulatory proteins encoded by the HIV genes *vpr, vpu, vif, rev, tat,* and *nef.* On rare occasion, levels of HIV-specific antibodies may decline during treatment of acute HIV infection.

While antibodies to multiple antigens of HIV are produced, the precise functional significance of these different antibodies is unclear. The only viral proteins that elicit neutralizing antibodies are the envelope proteins gp120 and gp41. Antibodies directed toward the envelope proteins of HIV have been characterized both as being protective and as possibly contributing to the pathogenesis of HIV disease. Among the protective antibodies are those that function to neutralize HIV directly and prevent the spread of infection to additional cells, as well as those that participate in ADCC. The first neutralizing antibodies are directed against the autologous infecting

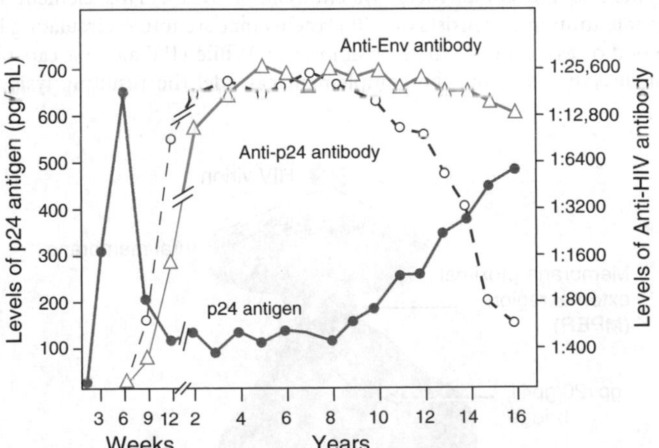

FIGURE 226-27 Relationship between antigenemia and the development of antibodies to HIV. Levels of plasma HIV parallel those of p24 antigen. Antibodies to HIV proteins are generally seen 6–12 weeks following infection and 3–6 weeks after the development of plasma viremia. Late in the course of illness, antibody levels to p24 decline, generally in association with a rising titer of p24 antigen.

virus and appear after approximately 12 weeks of infection. Due to its high rate of mutation the virus is usually able to quickly escape these (and subsequent) neutralizing antibodies. One important mechanism of immune escape is the addition of N-linked glycosylation sites, forming a glycan shield that interferes with envelope recognition by these initial antibodies.

A number of broad and potent HIV-neutralizing envelope-specific antibodies have been isolated from HIV-infected individuals in studies designed to better understand the host response to HIV infection. Approximately 20% of patients develop antibodies capable of neutralizing highly diverse strains. These studies have revealed at least five major sites within the HIV envelope that are able to elicit broadly-neutralizing antibodies. These sites include antibodies directed toward the CD4 binding site (CD4bs) of gp120, those binding glycan-dependent epitopes in the V1/V2 region of gp120, those near the base of the V3 region of gp120, those binding to the gp120/gp41 bridge, and those binding to the membrane-proximal region of gp41 (Fig. 226-28). Several of these antibodies contain unique features including high levels of somatic hypermutation, selective germline gene usage (especially for CD4bs antibodies) and long heavy chain complementary determining regions (especially CDRH3). Of note, while these antibodies are broadly neutralizing in vitro, their precise in vivo significance is unclear and the patients from whom they were derived demonstrate evidence of ongoing viral replication unless treated with cART.

The other major class of protective antibodies are those that participate in ADCC, a form of cell-mediated immunity (Chap. 372e) in which NK cells that bear Fc receptors are armed with specific anti-HIV antibodies that bind to the NK cells via their Fc portion. These armed NK cells then bind to and destroy cells expressing HIV antigens. The levels of anti-envelope antibodies capable of mediating ADCC are highest in the earlier stages of HIV infection. Antibodies to both gp120 and gp41 have been shown to participate in ADCC-mediated killing of HIV-infected cells. In vitro, IL-2 can augment ADCC-mediated killing.

In addition to playing a role in host defense, HIV-specific antibodies have also been implicated in disease pathogenesis. Antibodies directed to gp41, when present in low titer, have been shown in vitro to be capable of facilitating infection of cells through an Fc receptor–mediated mechanism known as *antibody enhancement*. Thus, the same regions of the envelope protein of HIV that give rise to antibodies capable of mediating ADCC can also elicit the production of antibodies that can facilitate infection of cells in vitro. In addition, it has been postulated that anti-gp120 antibodies that participate in the ADCC killing of HIV-infected cells might also kill uninfected CD4+ T cells if the uninfected cells had bound free gp120, a phenomenon referred to as *bystander killing*.

One of the most primitive components of the humoral immune system is the complement system (Chap. 372e). This element of innate immunity consists of ~30 proteins that are found circulating in blood or associated with cell membranes. While HIV alone is capable of directly activating the complement cascade, the resulting lysis is

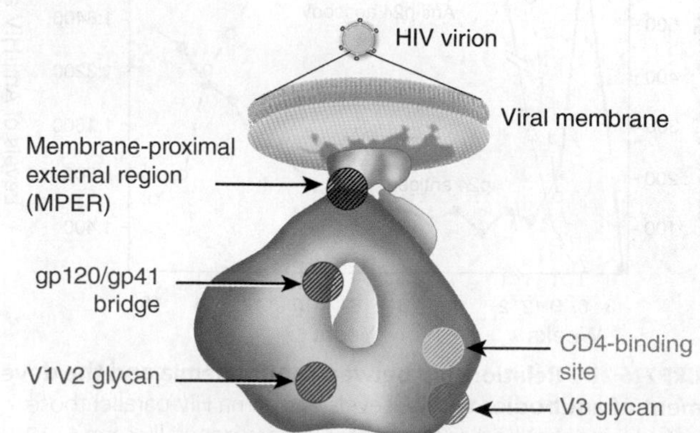

FIGURE 226-28 Known targets of broadly neutralizing antibodies against HIV-1. *(Adapted from PD Kwong, JR Mascola: Immunity 37:412, 2012.)*

weak due to the presence of host cell regulatory proteins captured in the virion envelope during budding. It is possible that complement-opsonized HIV virions have increased infectivity in a manner analogous to antibody-mediated enhancement.

CELLULAR IMMUNE RESPONSE

Given that T cell–mediated immunity is known to play a major role in host defense against most viral infections (Chap. 372e), it is generally thought to be an important component of the host immune response to HIV. T cell immunity can be divided into two major categories: that mediated by *helper/inducer CD4+ T cells* and that mediated by *cytotoxic/immunoregulatory CD8+ T cells*.

HIV-specific CD4+ T cells can be detected in the majority of HIV-infected patients through the use of flow cytometry to measure intracellular cytokine production in response to MHC class II tetramers pulsed with HIV peptides or through lymphocyte proliferation assays utilizing HIV antigens such as p24. These cells likely play a critical role in the orchestration of the immune response to HIV by providing help to HIV-specific B cells and CD8+ T cells. They may also be capable of directly killing HIV-infected cells. HIV-specific CD4+ T cells may be preferential targets of HIV infection by HIV-infected antigen-presenting cells during the generation of an immune response to HIV (Fig. 226-26). However, they also are likely to undergo clonal expansions in response to HIV antigens and thus survive as a population of cells. No clear correlations exist between levels of HIV-specific CD4+ T lymphocytes and plasma HIV RNA levels; however, in the setting of high viral loads, CD4+ T cell responses to HIV antigens appear to shift from one of proliferation and IL-2 production to one of IFN-γ production. Thus, while a reverse correlation exists between the level of p24-specific proliferation and levels of plasma HIV viremia, the nature of the causal relationship between these parameters is unclear.

MHC class I–restricted, HIV-specific CD8+ T cells have been identified in the peripheral blood of patients with HIV-1 infection. These cells include CTLs that produce perforins and T cells that can be induced by HIV antigens to express an array of cytokines such as IFN-γ, IL-2, MIP-1β, and TNF-α. CTLs have been identified in the peripheral blood of patients within weeks of HIV infection and prior to the appearance of plasma virus. The selective pressure they exert on the evolution of the population of circulating viruses reflects their potential role in control of HIV infection. These CD8+ T lymphocytes, through their HIV-specific antigen receptors, bind to and cause the lytic destruction of target cells bearing autologous MHC class I molecules presenting HIV antigens. Two types of CTL activity can be demonstrated in the peripheral blood or lymph node mononuclear cells of HIV-infected individuals. The first type directly lyses appropriate target cells in culture without prior in vitro stimulation (*spontaneous CTL activity*). The other type of CTL activity reflects the *precursor frequency of CTLs* (CTLp); this type of CTL activity can be demonstrated by stimulation of CD8+ T cells in vitro with a mitogen such as phytohemagglutinin or anti-CD3 antibody.

In addition to CTLs, CD8+ T cells capable of being induced by HIV antigens to express cytokines such as IFN-γ also appear in the setting of HIV-1 infection. It is not clear whether these are the same or different effector pools compared with those cells mediating cytotoxicity; in addition, the relative roles of each in host defense against HIV are not fully understood. It does appear that these CD8+ T cells are driven to in vivo expansion by HIV antigen. There is a direct correlation between levels of CD8+ T cells capable of producing IFN-γ in response to HIV antigens and plasma levels of HIV-1 RNA. Thus, while these cells are clearly induced by HIV-1 infection, their overall ability to control infection remains unclear. Multiple HIV antigens, including Gag, Env, Pol, Tat, Rev, and Nef, can elicit CD8+ T cell responses. Among patients who control viral replication in the absence of antiretroviral drugs are a subset of patients referred to as elite nonprogressors (see "Long-Term Survivors and Long-Term Nonprogressors," above) whose peripheral blood contains a population of CD8+ T cells that undergo substantial proliferation and perforin expression in response to HIV antigens. It is possible that these cells play an important role in HIV-specific host defense.

At least three other forms of cell-mediated immunity to HIV have been described: non-cytolytic CD8+ T cell–mediated suppression of HIV replication, ADCC, and NK cell activity. *Non-cytolytic CD8+ T cell–mediated suppression of HIV replication* refers to the ability of CD8+ T cells from an HIV-infected patient to inhibit the replication of HIV in tissue culture without killing infected targets. There is no requirement for HLA compatibility between the CD8+ T cells and the HIV-infected cells. This effector mechanism is thus nonspecific and appears to be mediated by soluble factor(s) including the CC-chemokines RANTES (CCL5), MIP-1α (CCL3), and MIP-1β (CCL4). These CC-chemokines are potent suppressors of HIV replication and operate at least in part via blockade of the HIV co-receptor (*CCR5*) for R5 (macrophage-tropic) strains of HIV-1 (see above). *ADCC*, as described above in relation to humoral immunity, involves the killing of HIV-expressing cells by NK cells armed with specific antibodies directed against HIV antigens. Finally, *NK cells* alone have been shown to be capable of killing HIV-infected target cells in tissue culture. This primitive cytotoxic mechanism of host defense is directed toward nonspecific surveillance for neoplastic transformation and viral infection through recognition of altered class I MHC molecules.

DIAGNOSIS AND LABORATORY MONITORING OF HIV INFECTION

The establishment of HIV as the causative agent of AIDS and related syndromes early in 1984 was followed by the rapid development of sensitive screening tests for HIV infection. By March 1985, blood donors in the United States were routinely screened for antibodies to HIV. In 1996, blood banks in the United States added the p24 antigen capture assay to the screening process to help identify the rare infected individuals who were donating blood in the time (up to 3 months) between infection and the development of antibodies. In 2002, the ability to detect early infection with HIV was further enhanced by the licensure of nucleic acid testing (NAT) as a routine part of blood donor screening. These refinements decreased the interval between infection and detection (window period) from 22 days for antibody testing to 16 days with p24 antigen testing and subsequently to 12 days with NAT. The development of sensitive assays for monitoring levels of plasma viremia ushered in a new era of being able to monitor the progression of HIV disease more closely. Utilization of these tests, coupled with the measurement of levels of CD4+ T lymphocytes in peripheral blood, is essential in the management of patients with HIV infection.

DIAGNOSIS OF HIV INFECTION

The CDC has recommended that screening for HIV infection be performed as a matter of routine health care. The diagnosis of HIV infection depends on the demonstration of antibodies to HIV and/or the direct detection of HIV or one of its components. As noted above, antibodies to HIV generally appear in the circulation 3–12 weeks following infection.

The standard blood screening tests for HIV infection are based on the detection of antibodies to HIV. A common platform is the ELISA, also referred to as an *enzyme immunoassay* (EIA). This solid-phase assay is an extremely good screening test with a sensitivity of >99.5%. Most diagnostic laboratories use commercial kits that contain antigens from both HIV-1 and HIV-2 and thus are able to detect antibodies to either. These kits use both natural and recombinant antigens and are continuously updated to increase their sensitivity to newly discovered species, such as group O viruses (Fig. 226-1). The fourth-generation EIA tests combine detection of antibodies to HIV with detection of the p24 antigen of HIV. EIA tests are generally scored as positive (highly reactive), negative (nonreactive), or indeterminate (partially reactive). While the EIA is an extremely sensitive test, it is not optimal with regard to specificity. This is particularly true in studies of low-risk individuals, such as volunteer blood donors. In this latter population, only 10% of EIA-positive individuals are subsequently confirmed to have HIV infection. Among the factors associated with false-positive EIA tests are antibodies to class II antigens (such as may be seen following pregnancy, blood transfusion, or transplantation), autoantibodies, hepatic disease, recent influenza vaccination, and acute viral infections. For these reasons, anyone suspected of having HIV infection based on a positive or inconclusive EIA result should ideally have the result confirmed with a more specific assay such as the Western blot. One can estimate whether an individual has a recent infection with HIV-1 by comparing the results on a standard EIA test that will score positive for all infected individuals with the results on an assay modified to be less sensitive ("detuned assay") that will score positive for individuals with established HIV infection and negative for individuals with recent infection. In rare instances, an HIV-infected individual treated early in the course of infection may revert to a negative EIA. This does *not* indicate clearing of infection; rather, it signifies levels of ongoing exposure to virus or viral proteins insufficient to maintain a measurable antibody response. When these individuals have discontinued therapy, viruses and antibodies have reappeared.

The most commonly used confirmatory test is the Western blot (Fig. 226-29). This assay takes advantage of the fact that multiple HIV antigens of different, well-characterized molecular weights elicit the production of specific antibodies. These antigens can be separated on the basis of molecular weight, and antibodies to each component can be detected as discrete bands on the Western blot. A negative Western blot is one in which no bands are present at molecular weights corresponding to HIV gene products. In a patient with a positive or indeterminate EIA and a negative Western blot, one can conclude with certainty that the EIA reactivity was a false positive. On the other hand, a Western blot demonstrating antibodies to products of all three of the major genes of HIV (*gag*, *pol*, and *env*) is conclusive evidence of infection with HIV. Criteria established by the U.S. Food and Drug Administration (FDA) in 1993 for a positive Western blot state that a result is considered positive if antibodies exist to two of the three HIV proteins: p24, gp41, and gp120/160. Using these criteria, ~10% of all blood donors deemed positive for HIV-1 infection lacked an antibody band to the *pol* gene product p31. Some 50% of these blood donors were subsequently found to be false positives. Thus, the absence of the p31 band should increase the suspicion that one may be dealing with a false-positive test result. In this setting it is prudent to obtain additional confirmation with an RNA-based test for HIV-1 and/or a follow-up Western blot. By definition, Western blot patterns of reactivity that do not fall into the positive or negative categories are considered "indeterminate." There are two possible explanations for an indeterminate Western blot result. The most likely explanation in a low-risk individual is that the patient being tested has antibodies that cross-react with one of the proteins of HIV. The most common patterns of cross-reactivity are antibodies that react with p24 and/or p55. The least likely explanation in this setting is that the individual is infected with HIV and is in the process of mounting a classic antibody response. In either instance, the Western blot should be repeated in 1 month to determine whether the indeterminate pattern is a pattern in evolution. In addition, one may attempt to confirm a diagnosis of HIV infection with the p24 antigen capture assay or one of the tests for HIV RNA (discussed below). While the Western blot is an excellent confirmatory test for HIV infection in patients with a positive or indeterminate EIA, it is a poor screening test. Among individuals with a negative EIA and PCR for HIV, 20–30% may show one or more bands on Western blot. While these bands are usually faint and represent cross-reactivity, their presence creates a situation in which other diagnostic modalities (such as DNA PCR, RT-PCR, or p24 antigen capture) must be employed to ensure that the bands do not indicate early HIV infection.

A guideline for the use of these serologic tests in attempting to make a diagnosis of HIV infection is depicted in Fig. 226-30. In patients in whom HIV infection is suspected, the appropriate initial test is the EIA. If the result is negative, unless there is strong reason to suspect early HIV infection (as in a patient exposed within the previous 3 months), the diagnosis is ruled out and retesting should be performed only as clinically indicated. If the EIA is indeterminate or positive, the test should be repeated. If the repeat is negative on two occasions, one can assume that the initial positive reading was due to a technical error in the performance of the assay and that the patient is negative. If the repeat is indeterminate or positive, one should proceed to the HIV-1 Western blot. If the Western blot is positive, the diagnosis is HIV-1

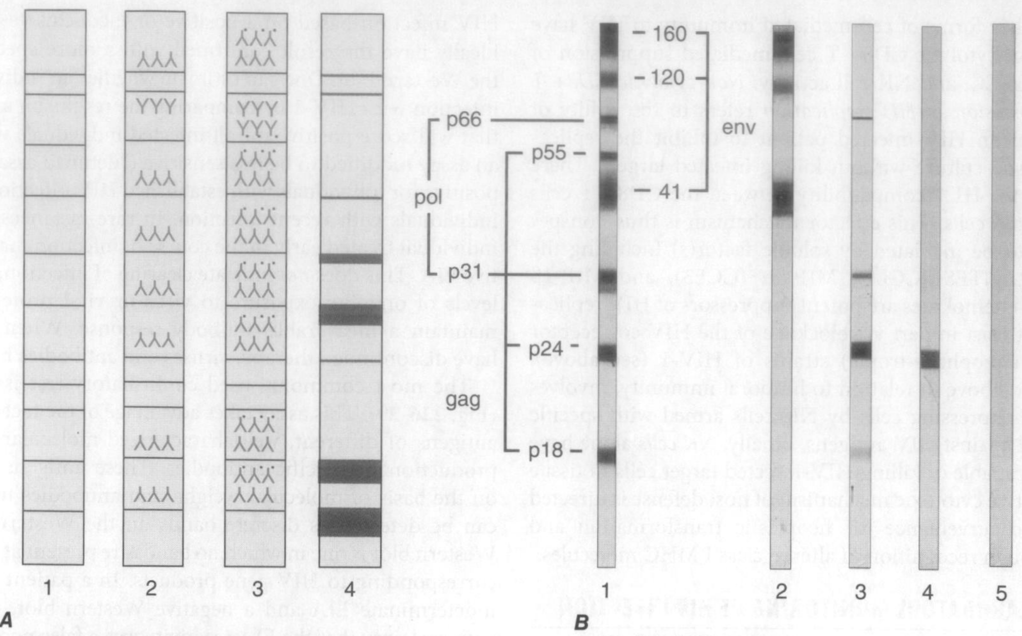

A
1. Virus digested: digest separated into components by molecular weight
2. Proteins transferred to filter paper: reaction with test serum
3. Enzyme-conjugated antihuman antibody added
4. Substrate added and color noted

B
1. Positive HIV-1 infection
2. gp 160 immunization
3. Indeterminate (HIV-2 infection)
4. Indeterminate (cross-reacting antibody to p24)
5. Negative

FIGURE 226-29 Western blot assay for detection of antibodies to HIV. ***A.*** Schematic representation of how a Western blot is performed. ***B.*** Examples of patterns of Western blot reactivity. In each instance the Western blot strip contains antigens to HIV-1. The serum from the patient immunized to the HIV-1 envelope gp160 contains only antibodies to the HIV-1 envelope proteins. The serum from the patient with HIV-2 infection cross-reacts with both *reverse transcriptase* and *gag* gene products of HIV-1.

infection. If the Western blot is negative, the EIA can be assumed to have been a false positive for HIV-1 and the diagnosis of HIV-1 infection is ruled out. It would also be prudent at this point to perform specific serologic testing for HIV-2 following the same type of algorithm. If the Western blot for HIV-1 is indeterminate, it should be repeated in 4–6 weeks; in addition, one may proceed to a p24 antigen capture assay, HIV-1 RNA assay, or HIV-1 DNA PCR and specific serologic testing for HIV-2. If the p24 and HIV RNA assays are negative and

SEROLOGIC TESTS IN THE DIAGNOSIS OF HIV-1 OR HIV-2 INFECTION

Screening HIV-1/HIV-2 EIA
(+) → Repeat HIV-1/HIV-2 EIA
(–) → Retest in 3–6 months if clinically indicated
Repeat HIV-1/HIV-2 EIA (+) → HIV-1 Western blot
Repeat HIV-1/HIV-2 EIA (–) → HIV-2 EIA
HIV-1 Western blot (+) → Diagnosis of HIV-1 infection
HIV-1 Western blot (–) → HIV-2 EIA
HIV-1 Western blot Indeterminate → Repeat in 4–6 weeks*
Repeat in 4–6 weeks* Indeterminate → HIV-2 Western blot
HIV-2 EIA (–) → Retest in 3–6 months if clinically indicated
HIV-2 EIA (+) → HIV-2 Western blot
HIV-2 Western blot (+) → Diagnosis of HIV-2 infection
HIV-2 Western blot (–) → Retest in 3–6 months if clinically indicated

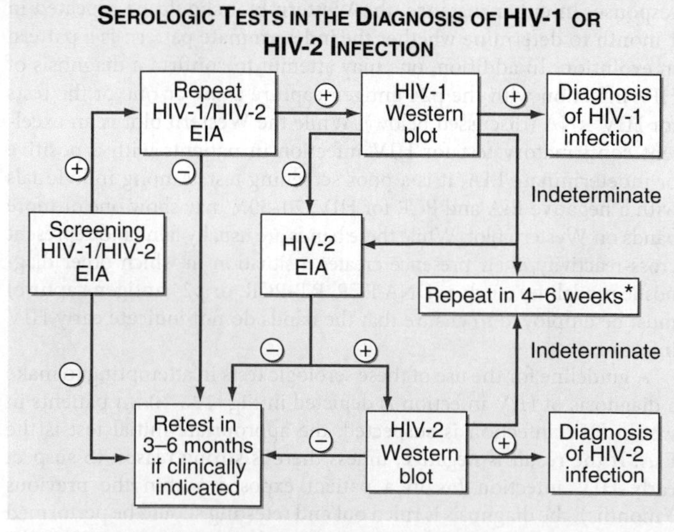

FIGURE 226-30 Algorithm for the use of serologic tests in the diagnosis of HIV-1 or HIV-2 infection. *Stable indeterminate Western blot 4–6 weeks later makes HIV infection unlikely. However, it should be repeated twice at 3-month intervals to rule out HIV infection. Alternatively, one may test for HIV-1 p24 antigen or HIV RNA. EIA, enzyme immunoassay.

there is no progression in the Western blot, a diagnosis of HIV-1 is ruled out. If either the p24 or HIV-1 RNA assay is positive and/or the HIV-1 Western blot shows progression, a tentative diagnosis of HIV-1 infection can be made and later confirmed with a follow-up Western blot demonstrating a positive pattern. In addition to these standard laboratory-based assays for detecting antibodies to HIV, an series of point-of-care tests can provide results in 1–60 min. Among the most popular of these is the OraQuick Rapid HIV-1 antibody test that can be run on blood, plasma, or saliva. The sensitivity and specificity of this test is ~99% when run on whole blood. Specificity remains the same but sensitivity drops to 98% when the test is run on saliva. While negative results from this test are adequate to rule out a diagnosis of HIV infection, a positive finding should be considered preliminary and confirmed with standard serologic testing, as described above. Two rapid test kits are licensed for home use. They are the OraQuick In-Home HIV test and the Home Access HIV-1 test system.

A variety of laboratory tests are available for the direct detection of HIV or its components (Table 226-8). These tests may be of considerable help in making a diagnosis of HIV infection when the Western blot results are indeterminate. In addition, the tests detecting levels of HIV RNA can be used to determine prognosis and to assess the response to antiretroviral therapies. The simplest of the direct detection tests is the *p24 antigen capture assay*. This is an EIA-type assay in which the solid phase consists of antibodies to the p24 antigen of HIV. It detects the viral protein p24 in the blood of HIV-infected individuals where it exists either as free antigen or complexed to anti-p24 antibodies. Overall, ~30% of individuals with untreated HIV infection have detectable levels of free p24 antigen. This increases to ~50% when samples are treated with a weak acid to dissociate antigen-antibody complexes. Throughout the course of HIV infection, an equilibrium exists between p24 antigen and anti-p24 antibodies. During the first few weeks of infection, before an immune response develops, there is a brisk rise in p24 antigen levels (Fig. 226-27). After the development of anti-p24 antibodies, these levels decline. Late in the course of infection, when circulating levels of virus are high, p24 antigen levels

TABLE 226-8 CHARACTERISTICS OF TESTS FOR DIRECT DETECTION OF HIV

Test	Technique	Sensitivity[a]	Cost/Test[b]
Immune complex–dissociated p24 antigen capture assay	Measurement of levels of HIV-1 core protein in an EIA-based format following dissociation of antigen-antibody complexes by weak acid treatment	Positive in 50% of patients; detects down to 15 pg/mL of p24 protein	$1–2
HIV RNA by PCR	Target amplification of HIV-1 RNA via reverse transcription followed by PCR	Reliable to 40 copies/mL of HIV RNA	$75–150
HIV RNA by bDNA	Measurement of levels of particle-associated HIV RNA in a nucleic acid capture assay employing signal amplification	Reliable to 50 copies/mL of HIV RNA	$75–150
HIV RNA by TMA	Target amplification of HIV-1 RNA via reverse transcription followed by T7 RNA polymerase	Reliable to 100 copies/mL of HIV RNA	$225
HIV RNA by NASBA	Isothermal nucleic acid amplification with internal controls	Reliable to 80 copies/mL of HIV RNA	$75–150

[a]Sensitivity figures refer to those approved by the U.S. Food and Drug Administration. [b]Prices may be lower in large-volume settings.

Abbreviations: bDNA, branched DNA; cDNA, complementary DNA; EIA, enzyme immunoassay; TMA, transcription-mediated amplification; NASBA, nucleic acid sequence–based amplification; PCR, polymerase chain reaction.

also increase, particularly when detected by techniques involving dissociation of antigen-antibody complexes. The p24 antigen capture assay has its greatest use as a screening test for HIV infection in patients suspected of having the acute HIV syndrome, as high levels of p24 antigen are present prior to the development of antibodies. Its use as a stand-alone test for routine blood donor screening for HIV infection has been replaced by use of NAT or "fourth-generation" assays that combine antigen and antibody testing. The ability to measure and monitor levels of HIV RNA in the plasma of patients with HIV infection has been of extraordinary value in furthering our understanding of the pathogenesis of HIV infection, in monitoring the response to cART, and in providing a diagnostic tool in settings where measurements of anti-HIV antibodies may be misleading, such as in acute infection and neonatal infection. Four assays are predominantly used for this purpose. They are reverse transcriptase PCR (*RT-PCR*; Amplicor); branched DNA (*bDNA*; VERSANT); transcription-mediated amplification (*TMA*; APTIMA); and nucleic acid sequence based amplification (*NASBA*; NucliSENS). These tests are of value in making a diagnosis of HIV infection, in establishing initial prognosis, and in monitoring the effects of therapy. In addition to these four commercially available tests, the *DNA PCR* also is employed by research laboratories for making a diagnosis of HIV infection by amplifying HIV proviral DNA from peripheral blood mononuclear cells. The commercially available RNA detection tests have a sensitivity of 40–8100 copies of HIV RNA per milliliter of plasma. Research laboratory–based RNA assays can detect as few as one HIV RNA copy per milliliter, while the DNA PCR tests can detect proviral DNA at a frequency of one copy per 10,000–100,000 cells. Thus, these tests are extremely sensitive. One frequent consequence of a high degree of sensitivity is some loss of specificity, and false-positive results have been reported with each of these techniques. For this reason, a positive EIA with a confirmatory Western blot remains the "gold standard" for a diagnosis of HIV infection, and the interpretation of other test results must be done with this in mind.

In the RT-PCR technique, following DNAse treatment, a cDNA copy is made of all RNA species present in plasma. Because HIV is an RNA virus, this will result in the production of DNA copies of the HIV genome in amounts proportional to the amount of HIV RNA present in plasma. This cDNA is then amplified and characterized using standard PCR techniques, employing primer pairs that can distinguish genomic cDNA from messenger cDNA. The bDNA assay involves the use of a solid-phase nucleic acid capture system and signal amplification through successive nucleic acid hybridizations to detect small quantities of HIV RNA. Both tests can achieve a tenfold increase in sensitivity to 40–50 copies of HIV RNA per milliliter with a preconcentration step in which plasma undergoes ultracentrifugation to pellet the viral particles. In the TMA assay, a cDNA copy of viral RNA is made using primers that contain a promoter sequence for T7 RNA polymerase. T7 polymerase is then added to produce multiple copies of RNA amplicon from the DNA template. It is qualified at 100 copies/mL. The NASBA technique involves the isothermal amplification of a sequence within the gag region of HIV in the presence of internal standards and employs the production of multiple RNA copies through the action of T7-RNA polymerase. The resulting RNA species are quantitated through hybridization with a molecular beacon DNA probe that is quenched in the absence of hybridization. The lower limit of detection for the NucliSENS assay is 80 copies/mL.

In addition to being a diagnostic and prognostic tool, RT-PCR and DNA-PCR are also useful for amplifying defined areas of the HIV genome for sequence analysis and have become an important technique for studies of sequence diversity and microbial resistance to antiretroviral agents. In patients with a positive or indeterminate EIA test and an indeterminate Western blot, and in patients in whom serologic testing may be unreliable (such as patients with hypogammaglobulinemia or advanced HIV disease), these tests for quantitating HIV RNA in plasma or detecting proviral DNA in peripheral blood mononuclear cells are valuable tools for making a diagnosis of HIV infection; however, they should be used for diagnosis only when standard serologic testing has failed to provide a definitive result.

LABORATORY MONITORING OF PATIENTS WITH HIV INFECTION

The epidemic of HIV infection and AIDS has provided the clinician with new challenges for integrating clinical and laboratory data to effect optimal patient management. The close relationship between clinical manifestations of HIV infection and CD4+ T cell count has made measurement of CD4+ T cell numbers a routine part of the evaluation of HIV-infected individuals. The discovery of HIV as the cause of AIDS led to the development of sensitive tests that allow one to monitor the levels of HIV in the blood. Determinations of peripheral blood CD4+ T cell counts and measurements of the plasma levels of HIV RNA provide a powerful set of tools for determining prognosis and monitoring response to therapy.

CD4+ T Cell Counts The CD4+ T cell count is the laboratory test generally accepted as the best indicator of the immediate state of immunologic competence of the patient with HIV infection. This measurement, which can be made directly or calculated as the product of the percentage of CD4+ T cells (determined by flow cytometry) and the total lymphocyte count (determined by the white blood cell count [WBC] multiplied by the lymphocyte differential percentage), has been shown to correlate very well with the level of immunologic competence. Patients with CD4+ T cell counts <200/μL are at high risk of disease from *P. jiroveci*, while patients with CD4+ T cell counts <50/μL are at high risk of disease from CMV, mycobacteria of the *M. avium* complex (MAC), and/or *T. gondii* (Fig. 226-31). Once the CD4+ T cell count is <200/μL, patients should be placed on a regimen for *P. jiroveci* prophylaxis, and once the count is <50/μL, primary prophylaxis for MAC infection is indicated. As with any laboratory measurement, one may wish to obtain two determinations prior to any significant changes in patient management based on CD4+ T cell count alone. Patients with HIV infection should have CD4+ T cell measurements performed at the time of diagnosis and every 3–6 months thereafter. More frequent measurements should be made if a declining trend is noted. For patients who have been on cART for at least 2 years

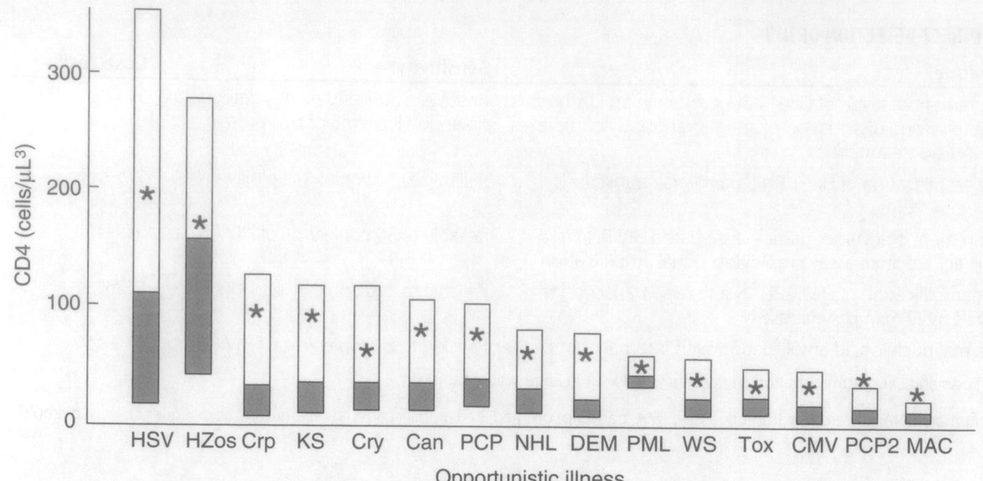

FIGURE 226-31 Relationship between CD4+ T cell counts and the development of opportunistic diseases. Boxplot of the median (line inside the box), first quartile (bottom of the box), third quartile (top of the box), and mean (asterisk) CD4+ lymphocyte count at the time of the development of opportunistic disease. Can, candidal esophagitis; CMV, cytomegalovirus infection; Crp, cryptosporidiosis; Cry, cryptococcal meningitis; DEM, AIDS dementia complex; HSV, herpes simplex virus infection; HZos, herpes zoster; KS, Kaposi's sarcoma; MAC, *Mycobacterium avium* complex bacteremia; NHL, non-Hodgkin's lymphoma; PCP, primary *Pneumocystis jiroveci* pneumonia; PCP2, secondary *P. jiroveci* pneumonia; PML, progressive multifocal leukoencephalopathy; Tox, *Toxoplasma gondii* encephalitis; WS, wasting syndrome. *(From RD Moore, RE Chaisson: Ann Intern Med 124:633, 1996.)*

with HIV RNA levels persistently <50 copies/mL, the monitoring of the CD4 count is felt by many to be optional. There are a handful of clinical situations in which the CD4+ T cell count may be misleading. Patients with HTLV-1/HIV co-infection may have elevated CD4+ T cell counts that do not accurately reflect their degree of immune competence. In patients with hypersplenism or those who have undergone splenectomy, and in patients receiving medications that suppress the bone marrow such as IFN-α, the CD4+ T cell percentage may be a more reliable indication of immune function than the CD4+ T cell count. A CD4+ T cell percentage of 15 is comparable to a CD4+ T cell count of 200/µL.

HIV RNA Determinations Facilitated by highly sensitive techniques for the precise quantitation of small amounts of nucleic acids, the measurement of serum or plasma levels of HIV RNA has become an essential component in the monitoring of patients with HIV infection. As discussed in "Diagnosis of HIV Infection," above, the most commonly used technique is the RT-PCR assay. This assay generates data in the form of number of copies of HIV RNA per milliliter of serum or plasma and can reliably detect as few as 40 copies of HIV RNA per milliliter of plasma. Research-based assays can detect down to one copy per milliliter. While it is common practice to describe levels of HIV RNA below these cut-offs as "undetectable," this is a term that should be avoided as it is imprecise and leaves the false impression that the level of virus is 0. By utilizing more sensitive, nested PCR techniques and by studying tissue levels of virus as well as plasma levels, HIV RNA can be detected in virtually every patient with HIV infection. The one notable exception to this is a patient who underwent cytoreductive therapy followed by a bone marrow transplant from a CCR5Δ32 homozygous donor.

Measurements of changes in HIV RNA levels over time have been of great value in delineating the relationship between levels of virus and rates of disease progression (Fig. 226-22), the rates of viral turnover, the relationship between immune system activation and viral replication, and the time to development of drug resistance. HIV RNA measurements are greatly influenced by the state of activation of the immune system and may fluctuate greatly in the setting of secondary infections or immunization. For these reasons, decisions based on HIV RNA levels should never be made on a single determination. Measurements of plasma HIV RNA levels should be made at the time of HIV diagnosis and every 3–6 months thereafter in the untreated patient. Following the initiation of therapy or any change in therapy, plasma HIV RNA levels should be monitored approximately every 4 weeks until the effectiveness of the therapeutic regimen is determined by the development of a new steady-state level of HIV RNA. In most instances of effective antiretroviral therapy the plasma level of HIV RNA will drop to <50 copies/mL within 6 months of the initiation of treatment. During therapy, levels of HIV RNA should be monitored every 3–6 months to evaluate the continuing effectiveness of therapy.

HIV Resistance Testing The availability of multiple antiretroviral drugs as treatment options has generated a great deal of interest in the potential for measuring the sensitivity of an individual's HIV virus(es) to different antiretroviral agents. HIV resistance testing can be done through either genotypic or phenotypic measurements. In the genotypic assays, sequence analyses of the HIV genomes obtained from patients are compared with sequences of viruses with known antiretroviral resistance profiles. In the phenotypic assays, the in vivo growth of viral isolates obtained from the patient is compared to the growth of reference strains of the virus in the presence or absence of different antiretroviral drugs. A modification of this phenotypic approach utilizes a comparison of the enzymatic activities of the reverse transcriptase, protease, or integrase genes obtained by molecular cloning of patients' isolates to the enzymatic activities of genes obtained from reference strains of HIV in the presence or absence of different drugs targeted to these genes. These tests are quite good in identifying those antiretroviral agents that have been utilized in the past and suggesting agents that may be of future value in a given patient. Resistance testing is recommended at the time of initial diagnosis and, if therapy is not initiated at that time, at the time of initiation of cART. Drug resistance testing is also indicated in the setting of virologic failure and should be performed while the patient is still on the failing regimen because of the propensity for the pool of HIV quasispecies to rapidly revert to wild-type in the absence of the selective pressures of cART. In the hands of experts, resistance testing enhances the short-term ability to decrease viral load by ~0.5 log compared with changing drugs merely on the basis of drug history. In addition to the use of resistance testing to help in the selection of new drugs in patients with virologic failure, it may also be of value in selecting an initial regimen for treatment of therapy-naïve individuals. This is particularly true in geographic areas with a high level of background resistance. The patient needs to have an HIV-1 RNA level above 500–1000 copies/mL for an accurate resistance determination. Resistance assays lose their consistency at lower levels of plasma viremia.

Co-Receptor Tropism Assays Following the licensure of maraviroc as the first CCR5 antagonist for the treatment of HIV infection (see below), it became necessary to be able to determine whether a patient's virus was likely to respond to this treatment. Patients tend to have CCR5-tropic virus early in the course of infection, with a trend toward CXCR4 viruses later in disease. The antiretroviral agent maraviroc is effective only against CCR5-tropic viruses. Because the genotypic determinants of cellular tropism are poorly defined, a phenotypic assay is necessary to determine this property of HIV. Two commercial assays, the Trofile assay (Monogram Biosciences) and the Phenoscript assay (VIRalliance), are available to make this determination. These assays clone the envelope regions of the patient's virus into an indicator virus that is then used to infect target cells expressing either CCR5 or CXCR4 as their

TABLE 226-9 ASSOCIATION BETWEEN HIGH-SENSITIVITY CRP, IL-6, AND D-DIMER WITH ALL-CAUSE MORTALITY IN PATIENTS WITH HIV INFECTION

	Unadjusted		Adjusted	
Marker	**Odds Ratio (Fourth/First)**	***p***	**Odds Ratio (Fourth/First)**	***p***
Hs-CRP	2.0	.05	2.8	.03
IL-6	8.3	<.0001	11.8	<.0001
D-dimer	12.4	<.0001	26.5	<.0001

Abbreviations: Hs-CRP, high-sensitivity C-reactive protein; IL-6, interleukin 6.

Source: From LH Kuller et al: PLoS Med 5:e203, 2008.

co-receptor. These assays take weeks to perform and are expensive. Another, less costly option is to obtain a genotypic assay of the V3 region of HIV-1 and then employ a computer algorithm to predict viral tropism from the sequence. While this approach is less expensive than the classic phenotypic assay, there are fewer data to validate its predictive value.

Other Tests A variety of other laboratory tests have been studied as potential markers of HIV disease activity. Among these are quantitative culture of replication-competent HIV from plasma, peripheral blood mononuclear cells, or resting CD4+ T cells; circulating levels of β_2-microglobulin, soluble IL-2 receptor, IgA, acid-labile endogenous IFN, or TNF-α; and the presence or absence of activation markers such as CD38, HLA-DR, and PD-1 on CD4+ or CD8+ T cells. Nonspecific serologic markers of inflammation and/or coagulation such as IL-6, D-dimer, and sCD14 have been shown to have a high correlation with all cause mortality (Table 226-9). While these measurements have value as markers of disease activity and help to increase our understanding of the pathogenesis of HIV disease, they do not currently play a major role in the monitoring of patients with HIV infection.

CLINICAL MANIFESTATIONS

The clinical consequences of HIV infection encompass a spectrum ranging from an acute syndrome associated with primary infection to a prolonged asymptomatic state to advanced disease. It is best to regard HIV disease as beginning at the time of primary infection and progressing through various stages. As mentioned above, active virus replication and progressive immunologic impairment occur throughout the course of HIV infection in most patients. With the exception of the rare, true, "elite" virus controllers or long-term nonprogressors (see "Long-Term Survivors and Long-Term Nonprogressors," above), HIV disease in untreated patients inexorably progresses even during the clinically latent stage. Since the mid-1990s, cART has had a major impact on preventing and reversing the progression of disease over extended periods of time in a substantial proportion of adequately treated patients.

ACUTE HIV INFECTION

It is estimated that 50–70% of individuals with HIV infection experience an acute clinical syndrome ~3–6 weeks after primary infection (Fig. 226-32). Varying degrees of clinical severity have been reported, and although it has been suggested that symptomatic seroconversion leading to the seeking of medical attention indicates an increased risk for an accelerated course of disease, there does not appear to be a correlation between the level of the initial burst of viremia in acute HIV infection and the subsequent course of disease. The typical clinical findings in the acute HIV syndrome are listed in Table 226-10; they occur along with a burst of plasma viremia. It has been reported that several symptoms of the acute HIV syndrome (fever, skin rash, pharyngitis, and myalgia) occur less frequently in those infected by injection drug use compared with those infected by sexual contact. The syndrome is typical of an acute viral syndrome and has been likened to acute infectious mononucleosis. Symptoms usually persist for one to several weeks and gradually subside as an immune response to HIV develops and the levels of plasma viremia decrease. Opportunistic infections have been reported during this stage of infection, reflecting the immunodeficiency that results from reduced numbers of CD4+ T cells and likely also from the dysfunction of CD4+ T cells owing to viral protein and endogenous cytokine-induced perturbations of cells (Table 226-5) associated with the extremely high levels of plasma viremia. A number of immunologic abnormalities accompany the acute HIV syndrome, including multiphasic perturbations of the numbers of circulating lymphocyte subsets. The number of total lymphocytes and T cell subsets (CD4+ and CD8+) are initially reduced. An inversion of the CD4+/CD8+ T cell ratio occurs later because of a rise in the number of CD8+ T cells. In fact, there may be a selective and transient expansion of CD8+ T cell subsets, as determined by T cell receptor analysis (see above). The total circulating CD8+ T cell count may remain elevated or return to normal; however, CD4+ T cell levels usually remain somewhat depressed, although there may be a slight rebound toward normal. Lymphadenopathy occurs in ~70% of individuals with primary HIV infection. Most patients recover spontaneously from this syndrome and many are left with only a mildly depressed CD4+ T cell count that remains stable for a variable period before beginning its progressive decline; in some individuals, the CD4+ T cell count returns to the normal range. Approximately 10% of patients manifest a fulminant course of immunologic and clinical deterioration after primary infection, even after the disappearance of initial symptoms. In most patients, primary infection with or without the acute syndrome is followed by a prolonged period of clinical latency or smoldering low disease activity.

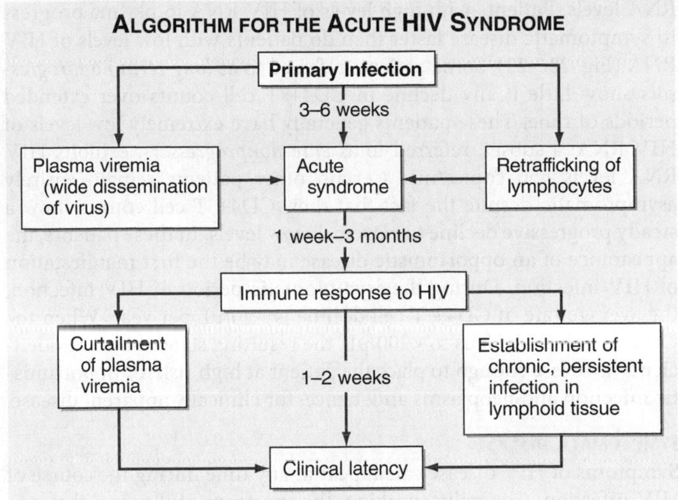

FIGURE 226-32 The acute HIV syndrome. See text for detailed description. *(Adapted from G Pantaleo et al: N Engl J Med 328:327, 1993. Copyright 1993 Massachusetts Medical Society. All rights reserved.)*

THE ASYMPTOMATIC STAGE—CLINICAL LATENCY

Although the length of time from initial infection to the development of clinical disease varies greatly, the median time for untreated patients is ~10 years. As emphasized above, HIV disease with active virus replication is ongoing and progressive during this asymptomatic period. The rate of disease progression is directly correlated with HIV

TABLE 226-10 CLINICAL FINDINGS IN THE ACUTE HIV SYNDROME

General	Neurologic
Fever	Meningitis
Pharyngitis	Encephalitis
Lymphadenopathy	Peripheral neuropathy
Headache/retroorbital pain	Myelopathy
Arthralgias/myalgias	**Dermatologic**
Lethargy/malaise	Erythematous maculopapular rash
Anorexia/weight loss	Mucocutaneous ulceration
Nausea/vomiting/diarrhea	

Source: From B Tindall, DA Cooper: AIDS 5:1, 1991.

RNA levels. Patients with high levels of HIV RNA in plasma progress to symptomatic disease faster than do patients with low levels of HIV RNA (Fig. 226-22). Some patients referred to as *long-term nonprogressors* show little if any decline in CD4+ T cell counts over extended periods of time. These patients generally have extremely low levels of HIV RNA; a subset, referred to as *elite nonprogressors*, exhibits HIV RNA levels <50 copies/mL. Certain other patients remain entirely asymptomatic despite the fact that their CD4+ T cell counts show a steady progressive decline to extremely low levels. In these patients, the appearance of an opportunistic disease may be the first manifestation of HIV infection. During the asymptomatic period of HIV infection, the average rate of CD4+ T cell decline is ~50/μL per year. When the CD4+ T cell count falls to <200/μL, the resulting state of immunodeficiency is severe enough to place the patient at high risk for opportunistic infection and neoplasms and, hence, for clinically apparent disease.

SYMPTOMATIC DISEASE

Symptoms of HIV disease can appear at any time during the course of HIV infection. Generally speaking, the spectrum of illnesses that one observes changes as the CD4+ T cell count declines. The more severe and life-threatening complications of HIV infection occur in patients with CD4+ T cell counts <200/μL. A diagnosis of AIDS is made in individuals age 6 years and older with HIV infection and a CD4+ T cell count <200/μL (Stage 3, Table 226-2) and in anyone with HIV infection who develops one of the HIV-associated diseases considered to be indicative of a severe defect in cell-mediated immunity (Table 226-1). While the causative agents of the secondary infections are characteristically opportunistic organisms such as *P. jiroveci*, atypical mycobacteria, CMV, and other organisms that do not ordinarily cause disease in the absence of a compromised immune system, they also include common bacterial and mycobacterial pathogens. Following the widespread use of cART and implementation of guidelines for the prevention of opportunistic infections (Table 226-11), the incidence of these secondary infections has decreased dramatically (Fig. 226-33). Overall, the clinical spectrum of HIV disease is constantly changing as patients live longer and new and better approaches to treatment and prophylaxis are developed. In addition to the classic AIDS-defining illnesses, patients with HIV infection also have an increase in serious non-AIDS illnesses, including non-AIDS related cancers and cardiovascular, renal, and hepatic disease. Non-AIDS events dominate the disease burden for patients with HIV infection receiving cART (Table 226-4). While AIDS-related illnesses are the leading cause of death in patients with HIV infection, they account for fewer than 50% of deaths. Non-AIDS-defining malignancies, liver disease, and cardiovascular disease each account for 10–15% of deaths in patients with HIV infection. The physician providing care to a patient with HIV infection must be well versed in general internal medicine as well as HIV-related opportunistic diseases. In general, it should be stressed that a key element of treatment of symptomatic complications of HIV disease, whether they are primary or secondary, is achieving good control of HIV replication through the use of cART and instituting primary and secondary prophylaxis for opportunistic infections as indicated.

Diseases of the Respiratory System Acute bronchitis and sinusitis are prevalent during all stages of HIV infection. The most severe cases tend to occur in patients with lower CD4+ T cell counts. Sinusitis presents as fever, nasal congestion, and headache. The diagnosis is made by CT or MRI. The maxillary sinuses are most commonly involved; however, disease is also frequently seen in the ethmoid, sphenoid, and frontal sinuses. While some patients may improve without antibiotic therapy, radiographic improvement is quicker and more pronounced in patients who have received antimicrobial therapy. It is postulated that this high incidence of sinusitis results from an increased frequency of infection with encapsulated organisms such as *H. influenzae* and *Streptococcus pneumoniae*. In patients with low CD4+ T cell counts one may see mucormycosis infections of the sinuses. In contrast to the course of this infection in other patient populations, mucormycosis of the sinuses in patients with HIV infection may progress more slowly. In this setting aggressive, frequent local debridement in addition to local and systemic amphotericin B may result in effective treatment.

Pulmonary disease is one of the most frequent complications of HIV infection. The most common manifestation of pulmonary disease is pneumonia. Three of the 10 most common AIDS-defining illnesses are recurrent bacterial pneumonia, tuberculosis, and pneumonia due to the unicellular fungus *P. jiroveci*. Other major causes of pulmonary infiltrates include other mycobacterial infections, other fungal infections, nonspecific interstitial pneumonitis, KS, and lymphoma.

Bacterial pneumonia is seen with an increased frequency in patients with HIV infection, with 0.8–2.0 cases per 100 person-years. Patients with HIV infection are particularly prone to infections with encapsulated organisms. *S. pneumoniae* (Chap. 171) and *H. influenzae* (Chap. 182) are responsible for most cases of bacterial pneumonia in patients with AIDS. This may be a consequence of altered B cell function and/or defects in neutrophil function that may be secondary to HIV disease (see above). Pneumonias due to *S. aureus* (Chap. 172) and *P. aeruginosa* (Chap. 189) also are reported to occur with an increased frequency in patients with HIV infection. *S. pneumoniae* (pneumococcal) infection may be the earliest serious infection to occur in patients with HIV disease. This can present as pneumonia, sinusitis, and/or bacteremia. Patients with untreated HIV infection have a sixfold increase in the incidence of pneumococcal pneumonia and a 100-fold increase in the incidence of pneumococcal bacteremia. Pneumococcal disease may be seen in patients with relatively intact immune systems. In one study, the baseline CD4+ T cell count at the time of a first episode of pneumococcal pneumonia was ~300/μL. Of interest is the fact that the inflammatory response to pneumococcal infection appears proportional to the CD4+ T cell count. Due to this high risk of pneumococcal disease, immunization with the conjugated pneumococcal vaccine followed by booster immunization with the 23-valent pneumococcal polysaccharide vaccine is one of the generally recommended prophylactic measures for patients with HIV infection. This is likely most effective if given while the CD4+ T cell count is >200/μL and, if given to patients with lower CD4+ T cell counts, should be repeated once the count has been above 200 for 6 months. Although clear guidelines do not exist, it also makes sense to repeat immunization every 5 years. The incidence of bacterial pneumonia is cut in half when patients quit smoking.

Pneumocystis pneumonia (PCP), once the hallmark of AIDS, has dramatically declined in incidence following the development of effective prophylactic regimens and the widespread use of cART. It is, however, still the single most common cause of pneumonia in patients with HIV infection in the United States and can be identified as a likely etiologic agent in 25% of cases of pneumonia in patients with HIV infection, with an incidence in the range of 2–3 cases per 100 person-years. Approximately 50% of cases of HIV-associated PCP occur in patients who are unaware of their HIV status. The risk of PCP is greatest among those who have experienced a previous bout of PCP and those who have CD4+ T cell counts of <200/μL. Overall, 79% of patients with PCP have CD4+ T cell counts <100/μL and 95% of patients have CD4+ T cell counts <200/μL. Recurrent fever, night sweats, thrush, and unexplained weight loss also are associated with an increased incidence of PCP. For these reasons, it is strongly recommended that all patients with CD4+ T cell counts <200/μL (or a CD4 percentage <15) receive some form of PCP prophylaxis. The incidence of PCP is approaching zero in patients with known HIV infection receiving appropriate cART and prophylaxis. In the United States, primary PCP is now occurring at a median CD4+ T cell count of 36/μL, while secondary PCP is occurring at a median CD4+ T cell count of 10/μL. Patients with PCP generally present with fever and a cough that is usually nonproductive or productive of only scant amounts of white sputum. They may complain of a characteristic retrosternal chest pain that is worse on inspiration and is described as sharp or burning. HIV-associated PCP may have an indolent course characterized by weeks of vague symptoms and should be included in the differential diagnosis of fever, pulmonary complaints, or unexplained weight loss in any patient with HIV infection and <200 CD4+ T cells/μL. The most

TABLE 226-11 NIH/CDC/IDSA 2013 GUIDELINES FOR THE PREVENTION OF OPPORTUNISTIC INFECTIONS IN PERSONS INFECTED WITH HIV

Pathogen	Indications	First Choice(s)	Alternatives
Recommended as Standard of Care for Primary and Secondary Prophylaxis			
Pneumocystis jiroveci	CD4+ T cell count <200/μL *or* Oropharyngeal candidiasis *or* Prior bout of PCP May stop prophylaxis if CD4+ T cell count >200/μL for ≥3 months	Trimethoprim/sulfamethoxazole (TMP/SMX), 1 DS tablet qd PO *or* TMP/SMX, 1 SS tablet qd PO	Dapsone 50 mg bid PO or 100 mg/d PO *or* Dapsone 50 mg/d PO + Pyrimethamine 50 mg/week PO + Leucovorin 25 mg/week PO *or* (Dapsone 200 mg PO + Pyrimethamine 75 mg PO + Leucovorin 25 mg) weekly PO *or* Aerosolized pentamidine, 300 mg via Respirgard II nebulizer every month *or* Atovaquone 1500 mg/d PO *or* TMP/SMX 1 DS tablet 3×/week PO
Mycobacterium tuberculosis			
Isoniazid sensitive	Skin test >5 mm *or* Positive IFN-γ release assay *or* Prior positive test without treatment *or* Close contact with case of active pulmonary TB	(Isoniazid 300 mg PO + Pyridoxine 25 mg PO) qd × 9 months *or* Isoniazid 900 mg PO twice weekly + Pyridoxine 25 mg PO daily × 9 months	Rifabutin (dose adjusted based on cART regimen) or rifampin 600 mg PO qd × 4 months
Drug resistant	Same with high probability of exposure to drug-resistant TB	Consult local public health authorities	
Mycobacterium-avium complex	CD4+ T cell count <50/μL	Azithromycin 1200 mg weekly PO or 600 mg twice weekly PO *or* Clarithromycin 500 mg bid PO	Rifabutin (dose adjusted based upon cART regimen)
	Prior documented disseminated disease May stop prophylaxis if CD4+ T cell count >100/μL for ≥6 months	Clarithromycin 500 mg bid PO + Ethambutol 15 (mg/kg)/d PO	Azithromycin 500–600 mg/d PO + Ethambutol 15 (mg/kg)/d PO
Toxoplasma gondii	TOXO IgG antibody positive and CD4+ T cell count <100/μL	TMP/SMX 1 DS tablet PO qd	TMP/SMX 1 DS 3× weekly PO *or* TMP/SMX, 1 SS PO daily *or* Dapsone 50 mg/d PO + Pyrimethamine 50 mg weekly PO + Leucovorin 25 mg weekly PO *or* (Dapsone 200 mg PO + Pyrimethamine 75 mg PO + Leucovorin 25 mg PO) weekly *or* Atovaquone 1500 mg PO daily ± (Pyrimethamine 25 mg PO + Leucovorin 10 mg PO) daily
	Prior toxoplasmic encephalitis and CD4+ T cell count <200/μL	Sulfadiazine 2000–4000 mg in 2–4 divided doses daily PO + Pyrimethamine 25–50 mg/d PO + Leucovorin 10–25 mg/d PO	Clindamycin 600 mg q8h PO + Pyrimethamine 25–50 mg/d PO + Leucovorin 10–25 mg/d PO *or*

(*Continued*)

TABLE 226-11 NIH/CDC/IDSA 2013 GUIDELINES FOR THE PREVENTION OF OPPORTUNISTIC INFECTIONS IN PERSONS INFECTED WITH HIV (*CONTINUED*)

Pathogen	Indications	First Choice(s)	Alternatives
Toxoplasma gondii	May stop prophylaxis if CD4+ T cell count >200/μL for ≥3 months		TMP/SMX 1 DS tablet bid *or* Atovaquone 750–1500 mg PO bid ± (Pyrimethamine 25 mg/d PO + Leucovorin 10 mg/d PO) or Sulfadiazine 2000–4000 mg/d (in 2–4 divided doses) PO
Varicella zoster virus	Significant exposure to chickenpox or shingles in a patient with no history of immunization or prior exposure to either	Varicella zoster immune globulin, IM, within 10 d of exposure (1-800-843-7477)	Acyclovir 800 mg PO 5 × day for 5–7 days *or* Valacyclovir 1 g PO tid for 5–7 days
Cryptococcus neoformans	Prior documented disease May stop prophylaxis if CD4+ T cell count >100/μL, no evidence of active fungal infection, and HIV RNA levels <500 copies/mL for >3 months	Fluconazole 200 mg/d PO	Itraconazole 200 mg/d PO
Histoplasma capsulatum	Prior documented disease or CD4+ T cell count <150μL and high risk (endemic area or occupational exposure) May stop prophylaxis after 1 year if CD4+ T cell count >150/μL and patient on cART for ≥6 months	Itraconazole 200 mg bid PO	Fluconazole 400 mg/d PO
Coccidioides immitis	Prior documented disease *or* positive serology and CD4+ T cell count <250/μL if from a disease endemic area. (For this indication prophylaxis can be stopped if CD4+ T cell count ≥250 for 6 months.)	Fluconazole 400 mg/d PO	
Penicillium marneffei	Prior documented disease Patients with CD4+T cell counts <100 who live or stay in northern Thailand, Southern China, or Vietnam May stop secondary prophylaxis in patients on ARV therapy with CD4+ T cell count >100/μL for ≥6 months	Itraconazole 200 mg/d PO	Fluconazole 400 mg PO once weekly
Salmonella species	Prior recurrent bacteremia	Ciprofloxacin 500 mg bid PO for ≥6 months	
Bartonella	Prior infection May stop if CD4+ T cell count >200/μL for >3 months	Doxycycline 200 mg/d PO *or* Azithromycin 1200 mg weekly PO *or* Clarithromycin 500 mg bid PO	
Cytomegalovirus	Prior end-organ disease May stop prophylaxis if CD4+ T cell count >100/μL for 6 months and no evidence of active CMV disease Restart if prior retinitis and CD4+ T cells <100/μL	Valganciclovir 900 mg bid PO	Cidofovir 5 mg/kg every other week IV + Probenecid *or* Foscarnet 90–120 (mg/kg)/d IV
Immunizations Generally Recommended			
Hepatitis B virus	All susceptible (anti-HBc- and anti-HBs-negative) patients	Hepatitis B vaccine: 3 doses	
Hepatitis A virus	All susceptible (anti-HAV-negative) patients	Hepatitis A vaccine: 2 doses	
Influenza virus	All patients annually	Inactivated trivalent influenza virus vaccine 1 dose yearly	Oseltamivir 75 mg PO qd *or* Rimantadine or amantadine 100 mg PO bid (influenza A only)
Streptococcus pneumoniae	All patients, preferably before CD4+ T cell count ≤200/μL	Pneumococcal conjugated vaccine (13) 0.5 mL IM × 1 followed in 8 weeks or more by pneumococcal polysaccharide vaccine (23) if CD4+ T cell count >200/μL	

(*Continued*)

TABLE 226-11 NIH/CDC/IDSA 2013 GUIDELINES FOR THE PREVENTION OF OPPORTUNISTIC INFECTIONS IN PERSONS INFECTED WITH HIV (*CONTINUED*)

Pathogen	Indications	First Choice(s)	Alternatives
Streptococcus pneumoniae		Reimmunize patients initially immunized at a CD4+ T cell count <100/μL whose CD4+ T cell count then increases to >200/μL	
Human papillomavirus	All patients 13–26 years of age	HPV vaccine; 3 doses	
Recommended for Prevention of Severe or Frequent Recurrences			
Herpes simplex	Frequent/severe recurrences	Valacyclovir 500 mg bid PO *or* Acyclovir 400 mg bid PO *or* Famciclovir 500 mg bid PO	
Candida	Frequent/severe recurrences	Fluconazole 100–200 mg/d PO	Posaconazole 400 mg bid PO

Abbreviations: ARV, antiretroviral; bid, twice daily; DS, double-strength; PCP, *Pneumocystis jiroveci* pneumonia; PO, by mouth; SS, single-strength; TB, tuberculosis.

common finding on chest x-ray is either a normal film, if the disease is suspected early, or a faint bilateral interstitial infiltrate. The classic finding of a dense perihilar infiltrate is unusual in patients with AIDS. In patients with PCP who have been receiving aerosolized pentamidine for prophylaxis, one may see an x-ray picture of upper lobe cavitary disease, reminiscent of TB. Other less common findings on chest x-ray include lobar infiltrates and pleural effusions. Thin-section CT

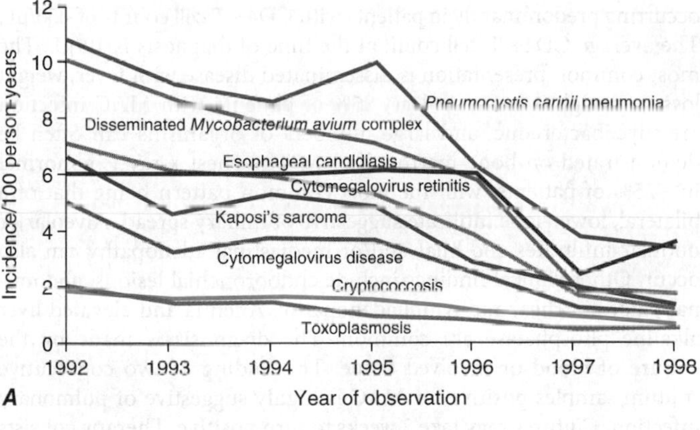

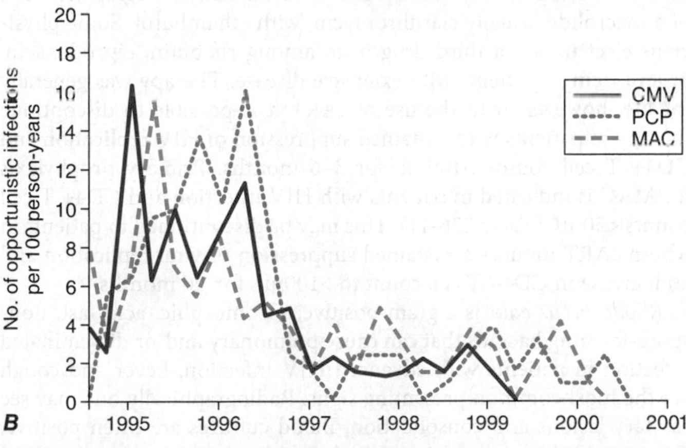

FIGURE 226-33 **A.** Decrease in the incidence of opportunistic infections and Kaposi's sarcoma in HIV-infected individuals with CD4+ T cell counts <100/μL from 1992 through 1998. *(Adapted and updated from FJ Palella et al: N Engl J Med 338:853, 1998, and JE Kaplan et al: Clin Infect Dis 30[S1]:S5, 2000, with permission.)* **B.** Quarterly incidence rates of cytomegalovirus (CMV), *Pneumocystis jiroveci* pneumonia (PCP), and *Mycobacterium avium* complex (MAC) from 1995 to 2001. *(From FJ Palella et al: AIDS 16:1617, 2002.)*

may demonstrate a patchy ground-glass appearance. Routine laboratory evaluation is usually of little help in the differential diagnosis of PCP. A mild leukocytosis is common, although this may not be obvious in patients with prior neutropenia. Elevation of lactate dehydrogenase is common. Arterial blood-gases may indicate hypoxemia with a decline in Pa_{O_2} and an increase in the arterial-alveolar (a–A) gradient. Arterial blood-gas measurements not only aid in making the diagnosis of PCP but also provide important information for staging the severity of the disease and directing treatment (see below). A definitive diagnosis of PCP requires demonstration of the organism in samples obtained from induced sputum, bronchoalveolar lavage, transbronchial biopsy, or open-lung biopsy. PCR has been used to detect specific DNA sequences for *P. jiroveci* in clinical specimens where histologic examinations have failed to make a diagnosis.

In addition to pneumonia, a number of other clinical problems have been reported in HIV-infected patients as a result of infection with *P. jiroveci*. Otic involvement may be seen as a primary infection, presenting as a polypoid mass involving the external auditory canal. In patients receiving aerosolized pentamidine for prophylaxis against PCP, one may see a variety of extrapulmonary manifestations of *P. jiroveci*. These include ophthalmic lesions of the choroid, a necrotizing vasculitis that resembles Burger's disease, bone marrow hypoplasia, and intestinal obstruction. Other organs that have been involved include lymph nodes, spleen, liver, kidney, pancreas, pericardium, heart, thyroid, and adrenals. Organ infection may be associated with cystic lesions that may appear calcified on CT or ultrasound.

The standard treatment for PCP or disseminated pneumocystosis is trimethoprim/sulfamethoxazole (TMP/SMX). A high (20–85%) incidence of side effects, particularly skin rash and bone marrow suppression, is seen with TMP/SMX in patients with HIV infection. Alternative treatments for mild to moderate PCP include dapsone/trimethoprim, clindamycin/primaquine, and atovaquone. IV pentamidine is the treatment of choice for severe disease in the patient unable to tolerate TMP/SMX. For patients with a Pa_{O_2} <70 mmHg or with an a–A gradient >35 mmHg, adjunct glucocorticoid therapy should be used in addition to specific antimicrobials. Overall, treatment should be continued for 21 days and followed by secondary prophylaxis. Prophylaxis for PCP is indicated for any HIV-infected individual who has experienced a prior bout of PCP, any patient with a CD4+ T cell count of <200/μL or a CD4 percentage <15, any patient with unexplained fever for >2 weeks, and any patient with a recent history of oropharyngeal candidiasis. The preferred regimen for prophylaxis is TMP/SMX, one double-strength tablet daily. This regimen also provides protection against toxoplasmosis and some bacterial respiratory pathogens. For patients who cannot tolerate TMP/SMX, alternatives for prophylaxis include dapsone plus pyrimethamine plus leucovorin, aerosolized pentamidine administered by the Respirgard II nebulizer, and atovaquone. Primary or secondary prophylaxis for PCP can be discontinued in those patients treated with cART who maintain good suppression of HIV (<50 copies/mL) and CD4+ T cell counts >200/μL for at least 3 months.

M. tuberculosis, once thought to be on its way to extinction in the United States, experienced a resurgence associated with the HIV epidemic (Chap. 202). Worldwide, approximately one-third of all AIDS-related deaths are associated with TB, and TB is the primary cause of death for 10–15% of patients with HIV infection. In the United States ~5% of AIDS patients have active TB. Patients with HIV infection are more likely to have active TB by a factor of 100 when compared with an HIV-negative population. For an asymptomatic HIV-negative person with a positive purified protein derivative (PPD) skin test, the risk of reactivation TB is around 1% per year. For the patient with untreated HIV infection, a positive PPD skin test, and no signs or symptoms of TB, the rate of reactivation TB is 7–10% per year. Untreated TB can accelerate the course of HIV infection. Levels of plasma HIV RNA increase in the setting of active TB and decline in the setting of successful TB treatment. Active TB is most common in patients 25–44 years of age, in African Americans and Hispanics, in patients in New York City and Miami, and in patients in developing countries. In these demographic groups, 20–70% of the new cases of active TB are in patients with HIV infection. The epidemic of TB embedded in the epidemic of HIV infection probably represents the greatest health risk to the general public and the health care profession associated with the HIV epidemic. In contrast to infection with atypical mycobacteria such as MAC, active TB often develops relatively early in the course of HIV infection and may be an early clinical sign of HIV disease. In one study, the median CD4+ T cell count at presentation of TB was 326/μL. The clinical manifestations of TB in HIV-infected patients are quite varied and generally show different patterns as a function of the CD4+ T cell count. In patients with relatively high CD4+ T cell counts, the typical pattern of pulmonary reactivation occurs: patients present with fever, cough, dyspnea on exertion, weight loss, night sweats, and a chest x-ray revealing cavitary apical disease of the upper lobes. In patients with lower CD4+ T cell counts, disseminated disease is more common. In these patients the chest x-ray may reveal diffuse or lower-lobe bilateral reticulonodular infiltrates consistent with miliary spread, pleural effusions, and hilar and/or mediastinal adenopathy. Infection may be present in bone, brain, meninges, GI tract, lymph nodes (particularly cervical lymph nodes), and viscera. Some patients with advanced HIV infection and active TB may have no symptoms of illness, and thus screening for TB should be part of the initial evaluation of every patient with HIV infection. Approximately 60–80% of HIV-infected patients with TB have pulmonary disease, and 30–40% have extrapulmonary disease. Respiratory isolation and a negative-pressure room should be used for patients in whom a diagnosis of pulmonary TB is being considered. This approach is critical to limit nosocomial and community spread of infection. Culture of the organism from an involved site provides a definitive diagnosis. Blood cultures are positive in 15% of patients. This figure is higher in patients with lower CD4 +T cell counts. In the setting of fulminant disease one cannot rely on the accuracy of a negative PPD skin test to rule out a diagnosis of TB. In addition, IFN-γ release assays may be difficult to interpret due to high backgrounds as a consequence of HIV-associated immune activation. TB is one of the conditions associated with HIV infection for which cure is possible with appropriate therapy. Therapy for TB is generally the same in the HIV-infected patient as in the HIV-negative patient (Chap. 202). Due to the possibility of multidrug-resistant or extensively drug-resistant TB, drug susceptibility testing should be performed to guide therapy. Due to pharmacokinetic interactions, adjusted doses of rifabutin should be substituted for rifampin in patients receiving the HIV protease inhibitors or nonnucleoside reverse transcriptase inhibitors. Treatment is most effective in programs that involve directly observed therapy. Initiation of cART and/or anti-TB therapy may be associated with clinical deterioration due to immune reconstitution inflammatory syndrome (IRIS) reactions. These are most common in patients initiating both treatments at the same time, may occur as early as 1 week after initiation of cART therapy, and are seen more frequently in patients with advanced HIV disease. For these reasons it is recommended that initiation of cART be delayed in antiretroviral-naïve patients with CD4 counts >50 cells/μL until 2–4 weeks following the initiation of treatment for TB. For patients with lower CD4 counts the benefits of more immediate cART outweigh the risks of IRIS, and cART should be started as soon as possible in those patients. Effective prevention of active TB can be a reality if the health care professional is aggressive in looking for evidence of latent or active TB by making sure that all patients with HIV infection receive a PPD skin test or evaluation with an IFN-γ release assay. Anergy testing is not of value in this setting. Since these tests rely on the host mounting an immune response to *M. tuberculosis*, patients with CD4+ T cell counts <200 cells/μL should be retested if their CD4+ T cell counts rise to persistently above 200. Patients at risk of continued exposure to TB should be tested annually. HIV-infected individuals with a skin-test reaction of >5 mm, those with a positive IFN-γ release assay, or those who are close household contacts of persons with active TB should receive treatment with 9 months of isoniazid and pyridoxine.

Atypical mycobacterial infections are also seen with an increased frequency in patients with HIV infection. Infections with at least 12 different mycobacteria have been reported, including *M. bovis* and representatives of all four Runyon groups. The most common atypical mycobacterial infection is with *M. avium* or *M. intracellulare* species—the *Mycobacterium avium* complex (MAC). Infections with MAC are seen mainly in patients in the United States and are rare in Africa. It has been suggested that prior infection with *M. tuberculosis* decreases the risk of MAC infection. MAC infections probably arise from organisms that are ubiquitous in the environment, including both soil and water. There is little evidence for person-to-person transmission of MAC infection. The presumed portals of entry are the respiratory and GI tracts. MAC infection is a late complication of HIV infection, occurring predominantly in patients with CD4+ T cell counts of <50/μL. The average CD4+ T cell count at the time of diagnosis is 10/μL. The most common presentation is disseminated disease with fever, weight loss, and night sweats. At least 85% of patients with MAC infection are mycobacteremic, and large numbers of organisms can often be demonstrated on bone marrow biopsy. The chest x-ray is abnormal in ~25% of patients, with the most common pattern being that of a bilateral, lower-lobe infiltrate suggestive of miliary spread. Alveolar or nodular infiltrates and hilar and/or mediastinal adenopathy can also occur. Other clinical findings include endobronchial lesions, abdominal pain, diarrhea, and lymphadenopathy. Anemia and elevated liver alkaline phosphatase are common. The diagnosis is made by the culture of blood or involved tissue. The finding of two consecutive sputum samples positive for MAC is highly suggestive of pulmonary infection. Cultures may take 2 weeks to turn positive. Therapy consists of a macrolide, usually clarithromycin, with ethambutol. Some physicians elect to add a third drug from among rifabutin, ciprofloxacin, or amikacin in patients with extensive disease. Therapy was generally for life; however, with the use of cART it is possible to discontinue therapy in patients with sustained suppression of HIV replication and CD4+ T cell counts >100/μL for 3–6 months. Primary prophylaxis for MAC is indicated in patients with HIV infection and CD4+ T cell counts <50/μL (Table 226-11). This may be discontinued in patients in whom cART induces a sustained suppression of viral replication and an increase in CD4+ T cell count to >100/μL for ≥6 months.

Rhodococcus equi is a gram-positive, pleomorphic, acid-fast, non-spore-forming bacillus that can cause pulmonary and/or disseminated infection in patients with advanced HIV infection. Fever and cough are the most common presenting signs. Radiographically one may see cavitary lesions and consolidation. Blood cultures are often positive. Treatment is based on antimicrobial sensitivity testing.

Fungal infections of the lung, in addition to PCP, can be seen in patients with AIDS. Patients with pulmonary cryptococcal disease present with fever, cough, dyspnea, and, in some cases, hemoptysis. A focal or diffuse interstitial infiltrate is seen on chest x-ray in >90% of patients. In addition, one may see lobar disease, cavitary disease, pleural effusions, and hilar or mediastinal adenopathy. More than half of patients are fungemic, and 90% of patients have concomitant CNS infection. *Coccidioides immitis* is a mold that is endemic in the southwest United States. It can cause a reactivation pulmonary syndrome in patients with HIV infection. Most patients with this condition will have CD4+ T cell counts <250/μL. Patients present with fever, weight loss, cough, and extensive, diffuse reticulonodular infiltrates on chest x-ray. One may also see nodules, cavities, pleural effusions, and hilar adenopathy. While serologic testing is of value in the immunocompetent host, serologies are negative in 25% of HIV-infected patients with coccidioidal infection. Invasive aspergillosis is not an AIDS-defining illness and is generally not seen in patients with AIDS in the absence of neutropenia or administration of glucocorticoids. When it does occur, *Aspergillus* infection may have an unusual presentation in the respiratory tract of patients with AIDS, where it gives the appearance of a pseudomembranous tracheobronchitis. Primary pulmonary infection of the lung may be seen with *histoplasmosis*. The most common pulmonary manifestation of histoplasmosis, however, is in the setting of disseminated disease, presumably due to reactivation. In this setting respiratory symptoms are usually minimal, with cough and dyspnea occurring in 10–30% of patients. The chest x-ray is abnormal in ~50% of patients, showing either a diffuse interstitial infiltrate or diffuse small nodules, and the urine will often be positive for *Histoplasma* antigen.

Two forms of *idiopathic interstitial pneumonia* have been identified in patients with HIV infection: lymphoid interstitial pneumonitis (LIP) and nonspecific interstitial pneumonitis (NIP). LIP, a common finding in children, is seen in about 1% of adult patients with untreated HIV infection. This disorder is characterized by a benign infiltrate of the lung and is thought to be part of the polyclonal activation of lymphocytes seen in the context of HIV and EBV infections. Transbronchial biopsy is diagnostic in 50% of the cases, with an open-lung biopsy required for diagnosis in the remainder of cases. This condition is generally self-limited and no specific treatment is necessary. Severe cases have been managed with brief courses of glucocorticoids. Although rarely a clinical problem since the use of cART, evidence of NIP may be seen in up to half of all patients with untreated HIV infection. Histologically, interstitial infiltrates of lymphocytes and plasma cells in a perivascular and peribronchial distribution are present. When symptomatic, patients present with fever and nonproductive cough occasionally accompanied by mild chest discomfort. Chest x-ray is usually normal or may reveal a faint interstitial pattern. Similar to LIP, NIP is a self-limited process for which no therapy is indicated other than appropriate management of the underlying HIV infection. HIV-related pulmonary arterial hypertension (HIV-PAH) is seen in ~0.5% of HIV-infected individuals. Patients may present with an array of symptoms including shortness of breath, fatigue, syncope, chest pain, and signs of right-sided heart failure. Chest x-ray reveals dilated pulmonary vessels and right-sided cardiomegaly with right ventricular hypertrophy seen on electrocardiogram. cART does not appear to be of clear benefit, and the prognosis is quite poor with a median survival in the range of 2 years.

Neoplastic diseases of the lung including KS and lymphoma are discussed below in the section on neoplastic diseases.

Diseases of the Cardiovascular System Heart disease is a relatively common postmortem finding in HIV-infected patients (25–75% in autopsy series). The most common form of heart disease is coronary heart disease. In one large series the overall rate of myocardial infarction (MI) was 3.5/1000 patient-years, 28% of these events were fatal, and MI was responsible for 7% of all deaths in the cohort. In patients with HIV infection, cardiovascular disease may be associated with classic risk factors such as smoking, a direct consequence of HIV infection, or a complication of cART. Patients with HIV infection have higher levels of triglycerides, lower levels of high-density lipoprotein cholesterol, and a higher prevalence of smoking than cohorts of individuals without HIV infection. The finding that the rate of cardiovascular disease events was lower in patients on antiretroviral therapy than in those randomized to undergo a treatment interruption identified a clear association between HIV replication and risk of cardiovascular disease. In one study, a baseline CD4+ T cell count of <500/μL was found to be an independent risk factor for cardiovascular disease comparable in magnitude to that attributable to smoking. While the precise pathogenesis of this association remains unclear, it is likely related to the immune activation and increased propensity for coagulation seen as a consequence of HIV replication. Exposure to HIV protease inhibitors and certain reverse transcriptase inhibitors has been associated with increases in total cholesterol and/or risk of MI. Any increases in the risk of death from MI resulting from the use of certain antiretrovirals must be balanced against the marked increases in overall survival brought about by these drugs.

Another form of heart disease associated with HIV infection is a dilated cardiomyopathy associated with congestive heart failure (CHF) referred to as *HIV-associated cardiomyopathy*. This generally occurs as a late complication of HIV infection and, histologically, displays elements of myocarditis. For this reason some have advocated treatment with IV immunoglobulin (IVIg). HIV can be directly demonstrated in cardiac tissue in this setting, and there is debate over whether it plays a direct role in this condition. Patients present with typical findings of CHF including edema and shortness of breath. Patients with HIV infection may also develop cardiomyopathy as side effects of IFN-α or nucleoside analogue therapy. These are reversible once therapy is stopped. KS, cryptococcosis, Chagas' disease, and toxoplasmosis can involve the myocardium, leading to cardiomyopathy. In one series, most patients with HIV infection and a treatable myocarditis were found to have myocarditis associated with toxoplasmosis. Most of these patients also had evidence of CNS toxoplasmosis. Thus, MRI or double-dose contrast CT scan of the brain should be included in the workup of any patient with advanced HIV infection and cardiomyopathy.

A variety of other cardiovascular problems are found in patients with HIV infection. Pericardial effusions may be seen in the setting of advanced HIV infection. Predisposing factors include TB, CHF, mycobacterial infection, cryptococcal infection, pulmonary infection, lymphoma, and KS. While pericarditis is quite rare, in one series 5% of patients with HIV disease had pericardial effusions that were considered to be moderate or severe. Tamponade and death have occurred in association with pericardial KS, presumably owing to acute hemorrhage. Nonbacterial thrombotic endocarditis has been reported and should be considered in patients with unexplained embolic phenomena. IV pentamidine, when given rapidly, can result in hypotension as a consequence of cardiovascular collapse.

Diseases of the Oropharynx and Gastrointestinal System Oropharyngeal and GI diseases are common features of HIV infection. They are most frequently due to secondary infections. In addition, oral and GI lesions may occur with KS and lymphoma.

Oral lesions, including *thrush, hairy leukoplakia*, and *aphthous ulcers* (Fig. 226-34), are particularly common in patients with untreated HIV infection. Thrush, due to *Candida* infection, and oral hairy leukoplakia, presumed due to EBV, are usually indicative of fairly advanced immunologic decline; they generally occur in patients with CD4+ T cell counts of <300/μL. In one study, 59% of patients with oral candidiasis went on to develop AIDS in the next year. Thrush appears as a white, cheesy exudate, often on an erythematous mucosa in the posterior oropharynx. While most commonly seen on the soft palate, early lesions are often found along the gingival border. The diagnosis is made by direct examination of a scraping for pseudohyphal elements. Culturing is of no diagnostic value, as patients with HIV infection may have a positive throat culture for *Candida* in the absence of thrush. Oral hairy leukoplakia presents as white, frondlike lesions, generally along the lateral borders of the tongue and sometimes on the adjacent buccal mucosa (Fig. 226-34). Despite its name, oral hairy leukoplakia is not considered a premalignant condition. Lesions are associated with florid replication of EBV. While usually more disconcerting as a sign of HIV-associated immunodeficiency than a clinical problem in need of treatment, severe cases have been reported to respond to topical podophyllin or systemic therapy with anti-herpesvirus agents. Aphthous ulcers of the posterior oropharynx also are seen with regularity in patients with untreated HIV infection

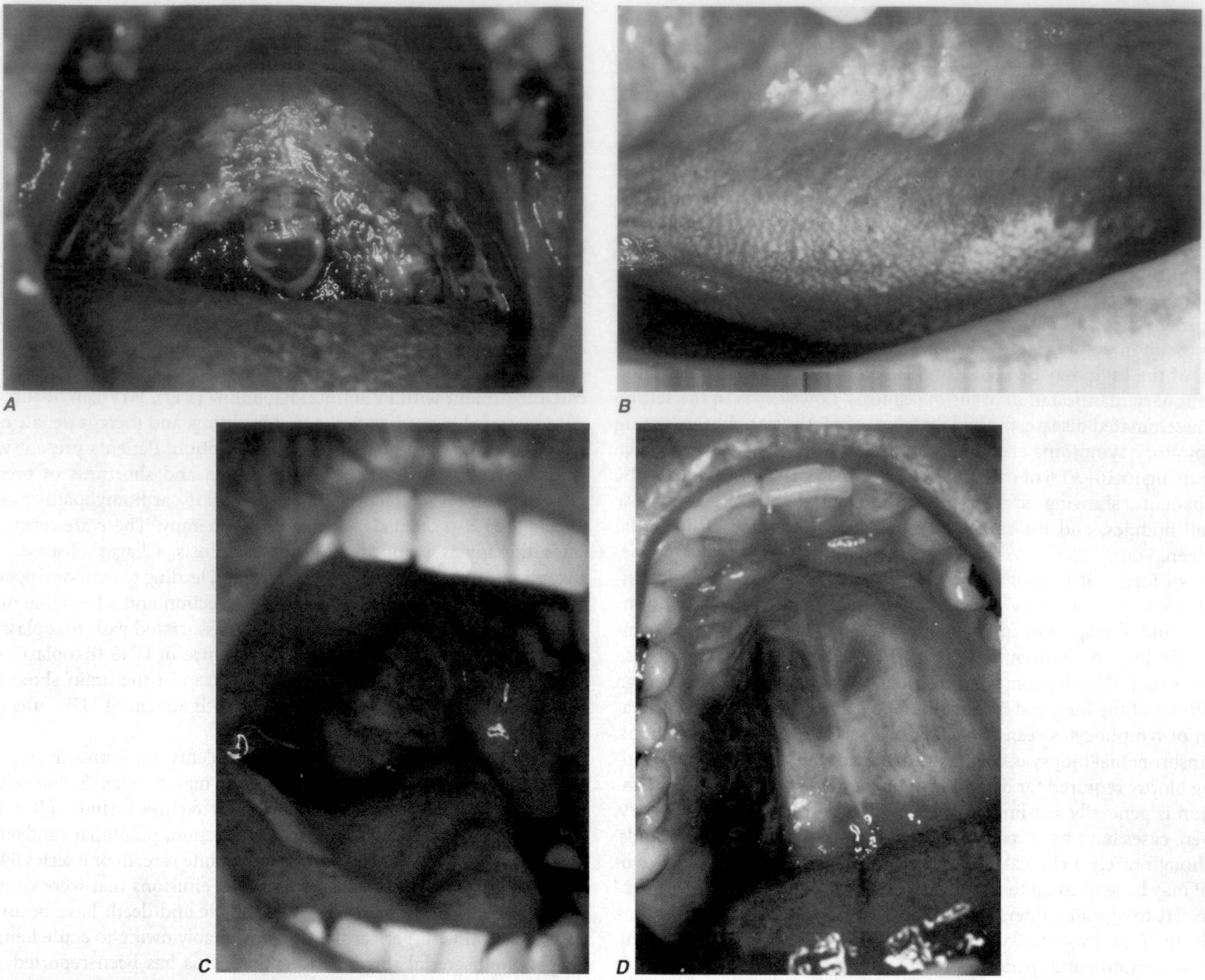

A B C D

FIGURE 226-34 Various oral lesions in HIV-infected individuals. *A.* Thrush. ***B.*** Hairy leukoplakia. ***C.*** Aphthous ulcer. ***D.*** Kaposi's sarcoma.

(Fig. 226-34). These lesions are of unknown etiology and can be quite painful and interfere with swallowing. Topical anesthetics provide immediate symptomatic relief of short duration. The fact that thalidomide is an effective treatment for this condition suggests that the pathogenesis may involve the action of tissue-destructive cytokines. Palatal, glossal, or gingival ulcers may also result from cryptococcal disease or histoplasmosis.

Esophagitis (Fig. 226-35) may present with odynophagia and retrosternal pain. Upper endoscopy is generally required to make an accurate diagnosis. Esophagitis may be due to *Candida*, CMV, or HSV. While CMV tends to be associated with a single large ulcer, HSV infection is more often associated with multiple small ulcers. The esophagus may also be the site of KS and lymphoma. Like the oral mucosa, the esophageal mucosa may have large, painful ulcers of unclear etiology that may respond to thalidomide. While achlorhydria is a common problem in patients with HIV infection, other gastric problems are generally rare. Among the neoplastic conditions involving the stomach are KS and lymphoma.

Infections of the small and large intestine leading to diarrhea, abdominal pain, and occasionally fever are among the most significant GI problems in HIV-infected patients. They include infections with bacteria, protozoa, and viruses.

Bacteria may be responsible for secondary infections of the GI tract. Infections with enteric pathogens such as *Salmonella, Shigella*, and *Campylobacter* are more common in men who have sex with men and are often more severe and more apt to relapse in patients with HIV infection. Patients with untreated HIV have approximately a 20-fold increased risk of infection with *S. typhimurium*.

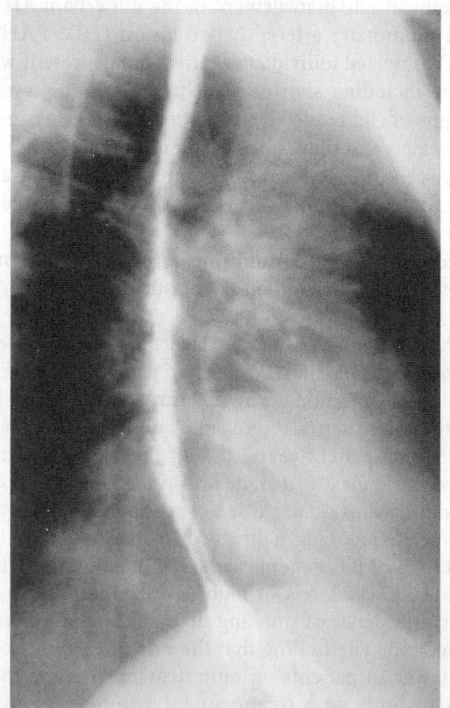

FIGURE 226-35 Barium swallow of a patient with *Candida* esophagitis. The flow of barium along the mucosal surface is grossly irregular.

They may present with a variety of nonspecific symptoms including fever, anorexia, fatigue, and malaise of several weeks' duration. Diarrhea is common but may be absent. Diagnosis is made by culture of blood and stool. Long-term therapy with ciprofloxacin is the recommended treatment. HIV-infected patients also have an increased incidence of *S. typhi* infection in areas of the world where typhoid is a problem. *Shigella* spp., particularly *S. flexneri*, can cause severe intestinal disease in HIV-infected individuals. Up to 50% of patients will develop bacteremia. *Campylobacter* infections occur with an increased frequency in patients with HIV infection. While *C. jejuni* is the strain most frequently isolated, infections with many other strains have been reported. Patients usually present with crampy abdominal pain, fever, and bloody diarrhea. Infection may also present as proctitis. Stool examination reveals the presence of fecal leukocytes. Systemic infection can occur, with up to 10% of infected patients exhibiting bacteremia. Most strains are sensitive to erythromycin. Abdominal pain and diarrhea may be seen with MAC infection.

Fungal infections may also be a cause of diarrhea in patients with HIV infection. Histoplasmosis, coccidioidomycosis, and penicilliosis have all been identified as a cause of fever and diarrhea in patients with HIV infection. Peritonitis has been seen with *C. immitis*.

Cryptosporidia, microsporidia, and *Isospora belli* (Chap. 254) are the most common opportunistic protozoa that infect the GI tract and cause diarrhea in HIV-infected patients. Cryptosporidial infection may present in a variety of ways, ranging from a self-limited or intermittent diarrheal illness in patients in the early stages of HIV infection to a severe, life-threatening diarrhea in severely immunodeficient individuals. In patients with untreated HIV infection and CD4+ T cell counts of <300/μL, the incidence of cryptosporidiosis is ~1% per year. In 75% of cases the diarrhea is accompanied by crampy abdominal pain, and 25% of patients have nausea and/or vomiting. Cryptosporidia may also cause biliary tract disease in the HIV-infected patient, leading to cholecystitis with or without accompanying cholangitis and pancreatitis secondary to papillary stenosis. The diagnosis of cryptosporidial diarrhea is made by stool examination or biopsy of the small intestine. The diarrhea is noninflammatory, and the characteristic finding is the presence of oocysts that stain with acid-fast dyes. Therapy is predominantly supportive, and marked improvements have been reported in the setting of effective cART. Treatment with up to 2000 mg/d of nitazoxanide (NTZ) is associated with improvement in symptoms or a decrease in shedding of organisms in about half of patients. Its overall role in the management of this condition remains unclear. Patients can minimize their risk of developing cryptosporidiosis by avoiding contact with human and animal feces, by not drinking untreated water from lakes or rivers, and by not eating raw shellfish.

Microsporidia are small, unicellular, obligate intracellular parasites that reside in the cytoplasm of enteric cells (Chap. 254). The main species causing disease in humans is *Enterocytozoon bieneusi*. The clinical manifestations are similar to those described for cryptosporidia and include abdominal pain, malabsorption, diarrhea, and cholangitis. The small size of the organism may make it difficult to detect; however, with the use of chromotrope-based stains, organisms can be identified in stool samples by light microscopy. Definitive diagnosis generally depends on electron-microscopic examination of a stool specimen, intestinal aspirate, or intestinal biopsy specimen. In contrast to cryptosporidia, microsporidia have been noted in a variety of extraintestinal locations, including the eye, brain, sinuses, muscle, and liver, and they have been associated with conjunctivitis and hepatitis. The most effective way to deal with microsporidia in a patient with HIV infection is to restore the immune system by treating the HIV infection with cART. Albendazole, 400 mg bid, has been reported to be of benefit in some patients.

I. belli is a coccidian parasite (Chap. 254) most commonly found as a cause of diarrhea in patients from tropical and subtropical regions. Its cysts appear in the stool as large, acid-fast structures that can be differentiated from those of cryptosporidia on the basis of size, shape, and number of sporocysts. The clinical syndromes of *Isospora* infection are identical to those caused by cryptosporidia. The important distinction is that infection with *Isospora* is generally relatively easy to treat with TMP/SMX. While relapses are common, a thrice-weekly regimen of TMP/SMX appears adequate to prevent recurrence.

CMV colitis was once seen as a consequence of advanced immunodeficiency in 5–10% of patients with AIDS. It is much less common with the advent of cART. CMV colitis presents as diarrhea, abdominal pain, weight loss, and anorexia. The diarrhea is usually nonbloody, and the diagnosis is achieved through endoscopy and biopsy. Multiple mucosal ulcerations are seen at endoscopy, and biopsies reveal characteristic intranuclear and cytoplasmic inclusion bodies. Secondary bacteremias may result as a consequence of thinning of the bowel wall. Treatment is with either ganciclovir or foscarnet for 3–6 weeks. Relapses are common, and maintenance therapy is typically necessary in patients whose HIV infection is poorly controlled. Patients with CMV disease of the GI tract should be carefully monitored for evidence of CMV retinitis.

In addition to disease caused by specific secondary infections, patients with HIV infection may also experience a chronic diarrheal syndrome for which no etiologic agent other than HIV can be identified. This entity is referred to as *AIDS enteropathy* or *HIV enteropathy*. It is most likely a direct result of HIV infection in the GI tract. Histologic examination of the small bowel in these patients reveals low-grade mucosal atrophy with a decrease in mitotic figures, suggesting a hyporegenerative state. Patients often have decreased or absent small-bowel lactase and malabsorption with accompanying weight loss.

The initial evaluation of a patient with HIV infection and diarrhea should include a set of stool examinations, including culture, examination for ova and parasites, and examination for *Clostridium difficile* toxin. Approximately 50% of the time this workup will demonstrate infection with pathogenic bacteria, mycobacteria, or protozoa. If the initial stool examinations are negative, additional evaluation, including upper and/or lower endoscopy with biopsy, will yield a diagnosis of microsporidial or mycobacterial infection of the small intestine ~30% of the time. In patients for whom this diagnostic evaluation is nonrevealing, a presumptive diagnosis of HIV enteropathy can be made if the diarrhea has persisted for >1 month. An algorithm for the evaluation of diarrhea in patients with HIV infection is given in Fig. 226-36.

Rectal lesions are common in HIV-infected patients, particularly the perirectal ulcers and erosions due to the reactivation of HSV

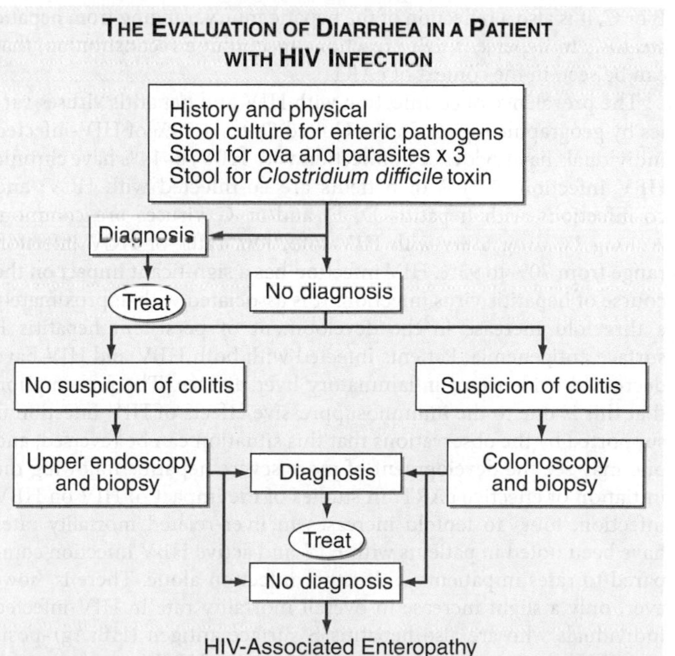

FIGURE 226-36 Algorithm for the evaluation of diarrhea in a patient with HIV infection. HIV-associated enteropathy is a diagnosis of exclusion and can be made only after other, generally treatable, forms of diarrheal illness have been ruled out.

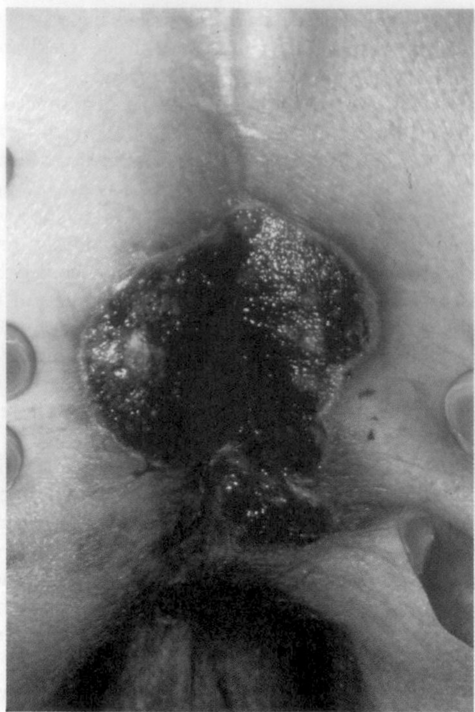

FIGURE 226-37 Severe, erosive perirectal herpes simplex in a patient with AIDS.

(Fig. 226-37). These lesions may appear quite atypical, as denuded skin without vesicles. They typically respond well to treatment with acyclovir, famciclovir, or foscarnet. Other rectal lesions encountered in patients with HIV infection include condylomata acuminata, KS, and intraepithelial neoplasia (see below).

Hepatobiliary Diseases Diseases of the hepatobiliary system are a major problem in patients with HIV infection. It has been estimated that approximately 15% of the deaths of patients with HIV infection are related to liver disease. While this is predominantly a reflection of the problems encountered in the setting of co-infection with hepatitis B or C, it is also a reflection of the hepatic injury, ranging from hepatic steatosis to hypersensitivity reactions to immune reconstitution, that can be seen in the context of cART.

The prevalence of co-infection with HIV and hepatitis viruses varies by geographic region. In the United States, ~90% of HIV-infected individuals have evidence of infection with HBV; 6–14% have chronic HBV infection; 5–50% of patients are co-infected with HCV; and co-infections with hepatitis D, E, and/or G viruses are common. Among IV drug users with HIV infection, rates of HCV infection range from 70% to 95%. HIV infection has a significant impact on the course of hepatitis virus infection. It is associated with approximately a threefold increase in the development of persistent hepatitis B surface antigenemia. Patients infected with both HBV and HIV have decreased evidence of inflammatory liver disease. The presumption that this is due to the immunosuppressive effects of HIV infection is supported by the observations that this situation can be reversed, and one may see the development of more severe hepatitis following the initiation of effective cART. In studies of the impact of HIV on HBV infection, four- to tenfold increases in liver-related mortality rates have been noted in patients with HIV and active HBV infection compared to rates in patients with either infection alone. There is, however, only a slight increase in overall mortality rate in HIV-infected individuals who are also hepatitis B surface antigen (HBsAg)–positive. IFN-α is less successful as treatment for HBV in patients with HIV co-infection. Lamivudine, emtricitabine, adefovir/tenofovir/entecavir, and telbivudine alone or in combination are useful in the treatment of hepatitis B in patients with HIV infection. It is important to remember that all the above-mentioned drugs also have activity against HIV and should not be used alone in patients with HIV infection, in order to avoid the emergence of quasispecies of HIV resistant to these drugs. For this reason, the need to treat hepatitis B infection in a patient with HIV infection is an indication to treat HIV infection in that same patient, regardless of CD4+ T cell count. HCV infection is more severe in the patient with HIV infection; it does not appear to affect overall mortality rates in HIV-infected individuals when other variables such as age, baseline CD4+ T cell count, and use of cART are taken into account. In the setting of HIV and HCV co-infection, levels of HCV are approximately tenfold higher than in the HIV-negative patient with HCV infection. There is a 50% higher overall mortality rate with a five-fold increased risk of death due to liver disease in patients chronically infected with both HCV and HIV. Use of directly acting agents for the treatment for HCV leads to cure rates approaching 100%, even in patients with HIV co-infection. Successful treatment of HCV in HIV-infected patients decreases mortality. Hepatitis A virus infection is not seen with an increased frequency in patients with HIV infection. It is recommended that all patients with HIV infection who have not experienced natural infection be immunized with hepatitis A and/or hepatitis B vaccines. Infection with hepatitis G virus, also known as GB virus C, is seen in ~50% of patients with HIV infection. For reasons that are currently unclear, there are data to suggest that patients with HIV infection co-infected with this virus have a decreased rate of progression to AIDS.

A variety of other infections also may involve the liver. Granulomatous hepatitis may be seen as a consequence of mycobacterial or fungal infections, particularly MAC infection. Hepatic masses may be seen in the context of TB, peliosis hepatis, or fungal infection. Among the fungal opportunistic infections, *C. immitis* and *Histoplasma capsulatum* are those most likely to involve the liver. Biliary tract disease in the form of papillary stenosis or sclerosing cholangitis has been reported in the context of cryptosporidiosis, CMV infection, and KS. When no diagnosis can be made, the term AIDS cholangiopathy is used. Hemophagocytic lymphohistiocytosis of the liver has been seen in the setting of Hodgkin's disease.

Many of the drugs used to treat HIV infection are metabolized by the liver and can cause liver injury. Fatal hepatic reactions have been reported with a wide array of antiretrovirals including nucleoside analogues, nonnucleoside analogues, and protease inhibitors. Nucleoside analogues work by inhibiting DNA synthesis. This can result in toxicity to mitochondria, which can lead to disturbances in oxidative metabolism. This may manifest as hepatic steatosis and, in severe cases, lactic acidosis and fulminant liver failure. It is important to be aware of this condition and to watch for it in patients with HIV infection receiving nucleoside analogues. It is reversible if diagnosed early and the offending agent(s) discontinued. Nevirapine has been associated with at times fatal fulminant and cholestatic hepatitis, hepatic necrosis, and hepatic failure. Indinavir may cause mild to moderate elevations in serum bilirubin in 10–15% of patients in a syndrome similar to Gilbert's syndrome. A similar pattern of hepatic injury may be seen with atazanavir. In the patient receiving cART with an unexplained increase in hepatic transaminases, strong consideration should be given to drug toxicity.

Pancreatic injury is most commonly a consequence of drug toxicity, notably that secondary to pentamidine or dideoxynucleosides. While up to half of patients in some series have biochemical evidence of pancreatic injury, <5% of patients show any clinical evidence of pancreatitis that is not linked to a drug toxicity.

Diseases of the Kidney and Genitourinary Tract Diseases of the kidney or genitourinary tract may be a direct consequence of HIV infection, due to an opportunistic infection or neoplasm, or related to drug toxicity. Overall, microalbuminuria is seen in ~20% of untreated HIV-infected patients; significant proteinuria is seen in closer to 2%. The presence of microalbuminuria has been associated with an increase in all-cause mortality rate. *HIV-associated nephropathy* (HIVAN) was first described in IDUs and was initially thought to be IDU nephropathy in patients with HIV infection; it is now recognized as a true direct complication of HIV infection. Although the majority of patients with this condition have CD4+ T cell counts <200/μL,

HIV-associated nephropathy can be an early manifestation of HIV infection and is also seen in children. Over 90% of reported cases have been in African-American or Hispanic individuals; the disease is not only more prevalent in these populations but also more severe and is the third leading cause of end-stage renal failure among African Americans age 20–64 in the United States. Proteinuria is the hallmark of this disorder. Edema and hypertension are rare. Ultrasound examination reveals enlarged, hyperechogenic kidneys. A definitive diagnosis is obtained through renal biopsy. Histologically, focal segmental glomerulosclerosis is present in 80%, and mesangial proliferation in 10–15% of cases. Prior to effective antiretroviral therapy, this disease was characterized by relatively rapid progression to end-stage renal disease. Patients with HIV-associated nephropathy should be treated for their HIV infection regardless of CD4+ T cell count. Treatment with angiotensin-converting enzyme (ACE) inhibitors and/or prednisone, 60 mg/d, also has been reported to be of benefit in some cases. The incidence of this disease in patients receiving adequate cART has not been well defined; however, the impression is that it has decreased in frequency and severity. It is the leading cause of end-stage renal disease in patients with HIV infection.

Among the drugs commonly associated with renal damage in patients with HIV disease are pentamidine, amphotericin, adefovir, cidofovir, tenofovir, and foscarnet. TMP/SMX may compete for tubular secretion with creatinine and cause an increase in the serum creatinine level. Sulfadiazine may crystallize in the kidney and result in an easily reversible form of renal shutdown, while indinavir or atazanavir may form renal calculi. Adequate hydration is the mainstay of treatment and prevention for these latter two conditions.

Genitourinary tract infections are seen with a high frequency in patients with HIV infection; they present with skin lesions, dysuria, hematuria, and/or pyuria and are managed in the same fashion as in patients without HIV infection. Infections with HSV are covered below ("Dermatologic Diseases"). Infections with *T. pallidum*, the etiologic agent of *syphilis*, play an important role in the HIV epidemic. In HIV-negative individuals, genital syphilitic ulcers as well as the ulcers of chancroid are major predisposing factors for heterosexual transmission of HIV infection. While most HIV-infected individuals with syphilis have a typical presentation, a variety of formerly rare clinical problems may be encountered in the setting of dual infection. Among them are *lues maligna*, an ulcerating lesion of the skin due to a necrotizing vasculitis; unexplained fever; nephrotic syndrome; and neurosyphilis. The most common presentation of syphilis in the HIV-infected patient is that of *condylomata lata*, a form of secondary syphilis. Neurosyphilis may be asymptomatic or may present as acute meningitis, neuroretinitis, deafness, or stroke. The rate of neurosyphilis may be as high as 1% in patients with HIV infection, and one should consider a lumbar puncture to look for neurosyphilis in all patients with HIV infection and secondary syphilis. As a consequence of the immunologic abnormalities seen in the setting of HIV infection, diagnosis of syphilis through standard serologic testing may be challenging. On the one hand, a significant number of patients have false-positive Venereal Disease Research Laboratory (VDRL) tests due to polyclonal B cell activation. On the other hand, the development of a new positive VDRL may be delayed in patients with new infections, and the anti–fluorescent treponemal antibody (anti-FTA) test may be negative due to immunodeficiency. Thus, dark-field examination of appropriate specimens should be performed in any patient in whom syphilis is suspected, even if the patient has a negative VDRL. Similarly, any patient with a positive serum VDRL test, neurologic findings, and an abnormal spinal fluid examination should be considered to have neurosyphilis and treated accordingly, regardless of the CSF VDRL result. In any setting, patients treated for syphilis need to be carefully monitored to ensure adequate therapy. Approximately one-third of patients with HIV infection will experience a Jarisch-Herxheimer reaction upon initiation of therapy for syphilis.

Vulvovaginal candidiasis is a common problem in women with HIV infection. Symptoms include pruritus, discomfort, dyspareunia, and dysuria. Vulvar infection may present as a morbilliform rash that may extend to the thighs. Vaginal infection is usually associated with a white discharge, and plaques may be seen along an erythematous vaginal wall. Diagnosis is made by microscopic examination of the discharge for pseudohyphal elements in a 10% potassium hydroxide solution. Mild disease can be treated with topical therapy. More serious disease can be treated with fluconazole. Other causes of vaginitis include *Trichomonas* and mixed bacteria.

Diseases of the Endocrine System and Metabolic Disorders A variety of endocrine and metabolic disorders are seen in the context of HIV infection. These may be a direct consequence of HIV infection, secondary to opportunistic infections or neoplasms, or related to medication side effects. Between 33% and 75% of patients with HIV infection receiving thymidine analogues or protease inhibitors as a component of cART develop a syndrome often referred to as *lipodystrophy*, consisting of elevations in plasma triglycerides, total cholesterol, and apolipoprotein B, as well as hyperinsulinemia and hyperglycemia. Many of the patients have been noted to have a characteristic set of body habitus changes associated with fat redistribution, consisting of truncal obesity coupled with peripheral wasting (Fig. 226-38). Truncal obesity is apparent as an increase in abdominal girth related to increases in mesenteric fat, a dorsocervical fat pad ("buffalo hump") reminiscent of patients with Cushing's syndrome, and enlargement of the breasts. The peripheral wasting, or lipoatrophy, is particularly noticeable in the face and buttocks and by the prominence of the veins in the legs. These changes may develop at any time ranging from ~6 weeks to several years following the initiation of cART. Approximately 20% of the patients with HIV-associated lipodystrophy meet the criteria for the *metabolic syndrome* as defined by The International Diabetes Federation or The U.S. National Cholesterol Education Program Adult Treatment Panel III. The lipodystrophy syndrome has been reported in association with regimens containing a variety of different drugs, and while initially reported in the setting of protease inhibitor therapy, it appears that similar changes can also be induced by protease-sparing regimens. It has been suggested that the lipoatrophy changes are particularly severe in patients receiving the thymidine analogues stavudine and zidovudine. National Cholesterol Education Program (NCEP) guidelines should be followed in the management of these lipid abnormalities (Chap. 291e), and consideration should be given to changing the components of cART with avoidance of thymidine analogues (azidothymidine and stavudine) and protease inhibitors. Due to concerns regarding drug interactions, the most commonly utilized lipid-lowering agents in this setting are gemfibrozil and atorvastatin. In addition, lactic acidosis is associated with cART. This is most commonly seen with nucleoside analogue reverse transcriptase inhibitors and can be fatal (see below).

Patients with advanced HIV disease may develop hyponatremia due to the syndrome of inappropriate antidiuretic hormone (vasopressin) secretion (SIADH) as a consequence of increased free-water intake and decreased free-water excretion. SIADH is usually seen in conjunction with pulmonary or CNS disease. Low serum sodium may also be due to adrenal insufficiency; a concomitant high serum potassium should alert one to this possibility. Hyperkalemia may be secondary to adrenal insufficiency; HIV nephropathy; or medications, particularly trimethoprim and pentamidine. Hypokalemia may be seen in the setting of tenofovir or amphotericin therapy. Adrenal gland disease may be due to mycobacterial infections, CMV disease, cryptococcal disease, histoplasmosis, or ketoconazole toxicity. Iatrogenic Cushing's syndrome with suppression of the hypothalamic-pituitary-adrenal axis may be seen with the use of local glucocorticoids (injected or inhaled) in patients receiving ritonavir. This is due to inhibition of the hepatic enzyme CYP3A4 by ritonavir leading to prolongation of the glucocorticoid half-life.

Thyroid function may be altered in 10–15% of patients with HIV infection. Both hypo- and hyperthyroidism may be seen. The predominant abnormality is subclinical hypothyroidism. In the setting of cART, up to 10% of patients have been noted to have elevated thyroid-stimulating hormone levels, suggesting that this may be

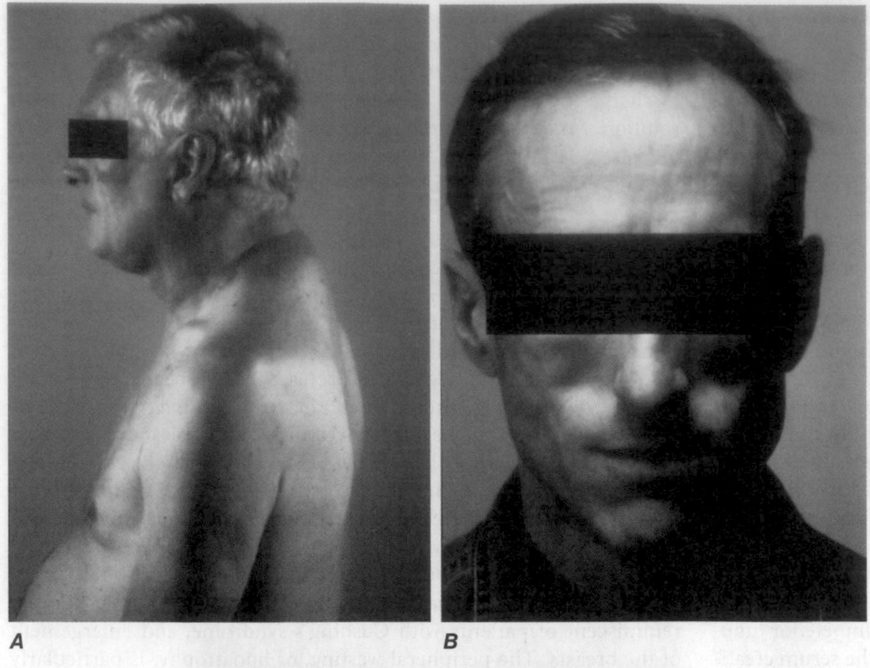

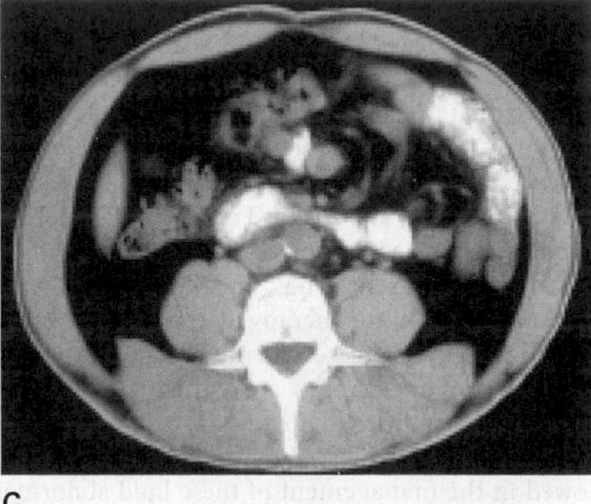

FIGURE 226-38 Characteristics of lipodystrophy. ***A.*** Truncal obesity and buffalo hump. ***B.*** Facial wasting. ***C.*** Accumulation of intraabdominal fat on CT scan.

a manifestation of immune reconstitution. Immune-reconstitution Graves' disease may occur as a late (9–48 months) complication of cART. In advanced HIV disease, infection of the thyroid gland may occur with opportunistic pathogens, including *P. jiroveci*, CMV, mycobacteria, *Toxoplasma gondii*, and *Cryptococcus neoformans*. These infections are generally associated with a nontender, diffuse enlargement of the thyroid gland. Thyroid function is usually normal. Diagnosis is made by fine-needle aspirate or open biopsy.

Depending on the severity of disease, HIV infection is associated with *hypogonadism* in 20–50% of men. While this is generally a complication of underlying illness, testicular dysfunction may also be a side effect of ganciclovir therapy. In some surveys, up to two-thirds of patients report decreased libido and one-third complain of erectile dysfunction. Androgen-replacement therapy should be considered in patients with symptomatic hypogonadism. HIV infection does not seem to have a significant effect on the menstrual cycle outside the setting of advanced disease.

Immunologic and Rheumatologic Diseases Immunologic and rheumatologic disorders are common in patients with HIV infection and range from excessive immediate-type hypersensitivity reactions (Chap. 376) to an increase in the incidence of reactive arthritis (Chap. 384) to conditions characterized by a diffuse infiltrative lymphocytosis. The occurrence of these phenomena is an apparent paradox in the setting of the profound immunodeficiency and immunosuppression that characterizes HIV infection and reflects the complex nature of the immune system and its regulatory mechanisms.

Drug allergies are the most significant allergic reactions occurring in HIV-infected patients and appear to become more common as the disease progresses. They occur in up to 65% of patients who receive therapy with TMP/SMX for PCP. In general, these drug reactions are characterized by erythematous, morbilliform eruptions that are pruritic, tend to coalesce, and are often associated with fever. Nonetheless, ~33% of patients can be maintained on the offending therapy, and thus these reactions are not an immediate indication to stop the drug. Anaphylaxis is extremely rare in patients with HIV infection, and patients who have a cutaneous reaction during a single course of therapy can still be considered candidates for future treatment or prophylaxis with the same agent. The one exception to this is the nucleoside analogue abacavir, where fatal hypersensitivity reactions have been reported with rechallenge. This hypersensitivity is strongly associated with the HLA-B5701 haplotype, and a hypersensitivity reaction to abacavir is an absolute contraindication to future therapy. For other agents, including TMP/SMX, desensitization regimens are moderately successful. While the mechanisms underlying these allergic-type reactions remain unknown, patients with HIV infection have been noted to have elevated IgE levels that increase as the CD4+ T cell count declines. The numerous examples of patients with multiple drug reactions suggest that a common pathway is involved.

HIV infection shares many similarities with a variety of autoimmune diseases, including a substantial polyclonal B cell activation that is associated with a high incidence of antiphospholipid antibodies, such as anticardiolipin antibodies, VDRL antibodies, and lupus-like anticoagulants. In addition, HIV-infected individuals have an increased incidence of antinuclear antibodies. Despite these serologic findings, there is no evidence that HIV-infected individuals have an increase in two of the more common autoimmune diseases, i.e., systemic lupus erythematosus and rheumatoid arthritis. In fact, it has been observed that these diseases may be somewhat ameliorated by the concomitant presence of HIV infection, suggesting that an intact CD4+ T cell limb of the immune response plays an integral role in the pathogenesis of these conditions. Similarly, there are anecdotal reports of patients with common variable immunodeficiency (Chap. 374), characterized by hypogammaglobulinemia, who have had a normalization of Ig levels following the development of HIV infection, suggesting a possible role for overactive CD4+ T cell immunity in certain forms of that syndrome. The one autoimmune disease that may occur with an increased frequency in patients with HIV infection is a variant of primary Sjögren's syndrome (Chap. 383). Patients with HIV infection may develop a syndrome consisting of parotid gland enlargement, dry eyes, and dry mouth that is associated with lymphocytic infiltrates of the salivary gland and lung. One also can see peripheral neuropathy, polymyositis, renal tubular acidosis, and hepatitis. In contrast to Sjögren's syndrome, in which the lymphocytic infiltrates are composed predominantly of CD4+ T cells, in patients with HIV infection the infiltrates are composed predominantly of CD8+ T cells. In addition, while patients with Sjögren's syndrome are mainly women who have autoantibodies to Ro and La and who frequently have HLA-DR3 or -B8 MHC haplotypes, HIV-infected individuals with this syndrome are usually African-American men who do not have anti-Ro or anti-La and who most often are HLA-DR5. This syndrome appears to be less common with the increased use of effective cART. The term *diffuse infiltrative lymphocytosis syndrome* (DILS) is used to describe this entity and to distinguish it from Sjögren's syndrome.

Approximately one-third of HIV-infected individuals experience arthralgias; furthermore, 5–10% are diagnosed as having some form of reactive arthritis, such as Reiter's syndrome or psoriatic arthritis as well as undifferentiated spondyloarthropathy (Chap. 384). These syndromes occur with increasing frequency as the competency of the immune system declines. This association may be related to an increase in the number of infections with organisms that may trigger a reactive arthritis with progressive immunodeficiency or to a loss of important regulatory T cells. Reactive arthritides in HIV-infected individuals generally respond well to standard treatment; however, therapy with methotrexate has been associated with an increase in the incidence of opportunistic infections and should be used with caution and only in severe cases.

HIV-infected individuals also experience a variety of joint problems without obvious cause that are referred to generically as *HIV-* or *AIDS-associated arthropathy*. This syndrome is characterized by subacute oligoarticular arthritis developing over a period of 1–6 weeks and lasting 6 weeks to 6 months. It generally involves the large joints, predominantly the knees and ankles, and is nonerosive with only a mild inflammatory response. X-rays are nonrevealing. Nonsteroidal anti-inflammatory drugs are only marginally helpful; however, relief has been noted with the use of intraarticular glucocorticoids. A second form of arthritis also thought to be secondary to HIV infection is called *painful articular syndrome*. This condition, reported as occurring in as many as 10% of AIDS patients, presents as an acute, severe, sharp pain in the affected joint. It affects primarily the knees, elbows, and shoulders; lasts 2–24 h; and may be severe enough to require narcotic analgesics. The cause of this arthropathy is unclear; however, it is thought to result from a direct effect of HIV on the joint. This condition is reminiscent of the fact that other lentiviruses, in particular the caprine arthritis-encephalitis virus, are capable of directly causing arthritis.

A variety of other immunologic or rheumatologic diseases have been reported in HIV-infected individuals, either de novo or in association with opportunistic infections or drugs. Using the criteria of widespread musculoskeletal pain of at least 3 months' duration and the presence of at least 11 of 18 possible tender points by digital palpation, 11% of an HIV-infected cohort containing 55% IDUs were diagnosed as having *fibromyalgia* (Chap. 396). While the incidence of frank arthritis was less in this population than in other studied populations that consisted predominantly of men who have sex with men, these data support the concept that there are musculoskeletal problems that occur as a direct result of HIV infection. In addition there have been reports of leukocytoclastic vasculitis in the setting of zidovudine therapy. CNS angiitis and polymyositis also have been reported in HIV-infected individuals. Septic arthritis is surprisingly rare, especially given the increased incidence of staphylococcal bacteremias seen in this population. When septic arthritis has been reported, it has usually been due to *Staphylococcus aureus*, systemic fungal infection with *C. neoformans, Sporothrix schenckii*, or *H. capsulatum* or to systemic mycobacterial infection with *M. tuberculosis, M. haemophilum, M. avium*, or *M. kansasii*.

Patients with HIV infection treated with cART have been found to have an increased incidence of osteonecrosis or avascular necrosis of the hip and shoulders. In a study of asymptomatic patients, 4.4% were found to have evidence of osteonecrosis on MRI. While precise cause-and-effect relationships have been difficult to establish, this complication has been associated with the use of lipid-lowering agents, systemic glucocorticoids, and testosterone; bodybuilding exercise; alcohol consumption; and the presence of anticardiolipin antibodies. Osteoporosis has been reported in 7% of women with HIV infection, with 41% of women demonstrating some degree of osteopenia. Several studies have documented decreases in bone mineral density of 2–6% in the first 2 years following the initiation of cART. This may be particularly apparent with tenofovir-containing regimens.

TABLE 226-12 CHARACTERISTICS OF IMMUNE RECONSTITUTION INFLAMMATORY SYNDROME (IRIS)

- Paradoxical worsening of an existing clinical condition or abrupt appearance of a new clinical finding (unmasking) is seen following the initiation of antiretroviral therapy
- Occurs weeks to months following the initiation of antiretroviral therapy
- Is most common in patients starting therapy with a CD4+ T cell count <50/μL who experience a precipitous drop in viral load
- Is frequently seen in the setting of tuberculosis; particularly when cART is starting soon after initiation of anti-TB therapy
- Can be fatal

Immune Reconstitution Inflammatory Syndrome (IRIS)

Following the initiation of effective cART, a paradoxical worsening of preexisting, untreated, or partially treated opportunistic infections may be noted. One may also see exacerbations of pre-existing or the development of new autoimmune conditions following the initiation of antiretrovirals (Table 226-12). IRIS related to a known pre-existing infection or neoplasm is referred to as *paradoxical IRIS*, while IRIS associated with a previously undiagnosed condition is referred to as *unmasking IRIS*. The term *immune reconstitution disease (IRD)* is sometimes used to distinguish IRIS manifestations related to opportunistic diseases from IRIS manifestations related to autoimmune diseases. IRD is particularly common in patients with underlying untreated mycobacterial or fungal infections. IRIS is seen in 10–30% of patients, depending on the clinical setting, and is most common in patients starting therapy with CD4+ T cell counts <50 cells/μL who have a precipitous drop in HIV RNA levels following the initiation of cART. Signs and symptoms may appear anywhere from 2 weeks to 2 years after the initiation of cART and can include localized lymphadenitis, prolonged fever, pulmonary infiltrates, hepatitis, increased intracranial pressure, uveitis, sarcoidosis, and Graves' disease. The clinical course can be protracted, and severe cases can be fatal. The underlying mechanism appears to be related to a phenomenon similar to type IV hypersensitivity reactions and reflects the immediate improvements in immune function that occur as levels of HIV RNA drop and the immunosuppressive effects of HIV infection are controlled. In severe cases, the use of immunosuppressive drugs such as glucocorticoids may be required to blunt the inflammatory component of these reactions while specific antimicrobial therapy takes effect.

Diseases of the Hematopoietic System Disorders of the hematopoietic system including lymphadenopathy, anemia, leukopenia, and/or thrombocytopenia are common throughout the course of HIV infection and may be the direct result of HIV, manifestations of secondary infections and neoplasms, or side effects of therapy (Table 226-13). Direct histologic examination and culture of lymph node or bone marrow tissue are often diagnostic. A significant percentage of bone marrow aspirates from patients with HIV infection have been reported to contain lymphoid aggregates, the precise significance of which is unknown. Initiation of cART will lead to reversal of most hematologic complications that are the direct result of HIV infection.

TABLE 226-13 CAUSES OF BONE MARROW SUPPRESSION IN PATIENTS WITH HIV INFECTION

HIV infection	Medications
Mycobacterial infections	Zidovudine
Fungal infections	Dapsone
B19 parvovirus infection	Trimethoprim/sulfamethoxazole
Lymphoma	Pyrimethamine
	5-Flucytosine
	Ganciclovir
	Interferon α
	Trimetrexate
	Foscarnet

Some patients, otherwise asymptomatic, may develop *persistent generalized lymphadenopathy* as an early clinical manifestation of HIV infection. This condition is defined as the presence of enlarged lymph nodes (>1 cm) in two or more extrainguinal sites for >3 months without an obvious cause. The lymphadenopathy is due to marked follicular hyperplasia in the node in response to HIV infection. The nodes are generally discrete and freely movable. This feature of HIV disease may be seen at any point in the spectrum of immune dysfunction and is not associated with an increased likelihood of developing AIDS. Paradoxically, a loss in lymphadenopathy or a decrease in lymph node size outside the setting of cART may be a prognostic marker of disease progression. In patients with CD4+ T cell counts >200/µL, the differential diagnosis of lymphadenopathy includes KS, TB, Castleman's disease, and lymphoma. In patients with more advanced disease, lymphadenopathy may also be due to atypical mycobacterial infection, toxoplasmosis, systemic fungal infection, or bacillary angiomatosis. While indicated in patients with CD4+ T cell counts <200/µL, lymph node biopsy is not indicated in patients with early-stage disease unless there are signs and symptoms of systemic illness, such as fever and weight loss, or unless the nodes begin to enlarge, become fixed, or coalesce. Monoclonal gammopathy of unknown significance (MGUS) (Chap. 136), defined as the presence of a serum monoclonal IgG, IgA, or IgM in the absence of a clear cause, has been reported in 3% of patients with HIV infection. The overall clinical significance of this finding in patients with HIV infection is unclear, although it has been associated with other viral infections, non-Hodgkin's lymphoma, and plasma cell malignancy.

Anemia is the most common hematologic abnormality in HIV-infected patients and, in the absence of a specific treatable cause, is independently associated with a poor prognosis. While generally mild, anemia can be quite severe and require chronic blood transfusions. Among the specific reversible causes of anemia in the setting of HIV infection are drug toxicity, systemic fungal and mycobacterial infections, nutritional deficiencies, and parvovirus B19 infections. Zidovudine may block erythroid maturation prior to its effects on other marrow elements. A characteristic feature of zidovudine therapy is an elevated mean corpuscular volume (MCV). Another drug used in patients with HIV infection that has a selective effect on the erythroid series is dapsone. This drug can cause a serious hemolytic anemia in patients who are deficient in glucose-6-phosphate dehydrogenase and can create a functional anemia in others through induction of methemoglobinemia. Folate levels are usually normal in HIV-infected individuals; however, vitamin B_{12} levels may be depressed as a consequence of achlorhydria or malabsorption. True autoimmune hemolytic anemia is rare, although ~20% of patients with HIV infection may have a positive direct antiglobulin test as a consequence of polyclonal B cell activation. Infection with parvovirus B19 may also cause anemia. It is important to recognize this possibility given the fact that it responds well to treatment with IVIg. Erythropoietin levels in patients with HIV infection and anemia are generally lower than expected given the degree of anemia. Treatment with erythropoietin may result in an increase in hemoglobin levels. An exception to this is a subset of patients with zidovudine-associated anemia in whom erythropoietin levels may be quite high.

During the course of HIV infection, neutropenia may be seen in approximately half of patients. In most instances it is mild; however, it can be severe and can put patients at risk of spontaneous bacterial infections. This is most frequently seen in patients with severely advanced HIV disease and in patients receiving any of a number of potentially myelosuppressive therapies. In the setting of neutropenia, diseases that are not commonly seen in HIV-infected patients, such as aspergillosis or mucormycosis, may occur. Both granulocyte colony-stimulating factor (G-CSF) and GM-CSF increase neutrophil counts in patients with HIV infection regardless of the cause of the neutropenia. Earlier concerns about the potential of these agents to also increase levels of HIV were not confirmed in controlled clinical trials.

Thrombocytopenia may be an early consequence of HIV infection. Approximately 3% of patients with untreated HIV infection and CD4+ T cell counts ≥400/µL have platelet counts <150,000/µL. For untreated patients with CD4+ T cell counts <400/µL, this incidence increases to 10%. In patients receiving antiretrovirals, thrombocytopenia is associated with hepatitis C, cirrhosis, and ongoing high-level HIV replication. Thrombocytopenia is rarely a serious clinical problem in patients with HIV infection and generally responds well to successful cART. Clinically, it resembles the thrombocytopenia seen in patients with idiopathic thrombocytopenic purpura (Chap. 140). Immune complexes containing anti-gp120 antibodies and anti-anti-gp120 antibodies have been noted in the circulation and on the surface of platelets in patients with HIV infection. Patients with HIV infection have also been noted to have a platelet-specific antibody directed toward a 25-kDa component of the surface of the platelet. Other data suggest that the thrombocytopenia in patients with HIV infection may be due to a direct effect of HIV on megakaryocytes. Whatever the cause, it is very clear that the most effective medical approach to this problem has been the use of cART. For patients with platelet counts <20,000/µL, a more aggressive approach combining IVIg or anti-Rh Ig for an immediate response and cART for a more lasting response is appropriate. Rituximab has been used with some success in otherwise refractory cases. Splenectomy is a rarely needed option and is reserved for patients refractory to medical management. Because of the risk of serious infection with encapsulated organisms, all patients with HIV infection about to undergo splenectomy should be immunized with pneumococcal polysaccharide. It should be noted that, in addition to causing an increase in the platelet count, removal of the spleen will result in an increase in the peripheral blood lymphocyte count, making CD4+ T cell counts unreliable markers of immunocompetence. In this setting, the clinician should rely on the CD4+ T cell percentage for making diagnostic decisions with respect to the likelihood of opportunistic infections. A CD4+ T cell percentage of 15 is approximately equivalent to a CD4+ T cell count of 200/µL. In patients with early HIV infection, thrombocytopenia has also been reported as a consequence of classic thrombotic thrombocytopenic purpura (Chap. 140). This clinical syndrome, consisting of fever, thrombocytopenia, hemolytic anemia, and neurologic and renal dysfunction, is a rare complication of early HIV infection. As in other settings, the appropriate management is the use of salicylates and plasma exchange. Other causes of thrombocytopenia include lymphoma, mycobacterial infections, and fungal infections.

The incidence of venous thromboembolic disease such as deep-vein thrombosis or pulmonary embolus is approximately 1% per year in patients with HIV infection. This is approximately 10 times higher than that seen in an age-matched population. Factors associated with an increased risk of clinical thrombosis include age over 45, history of an opportunistic infection, lower CD4 count, and estrogen use. Abnormalities of the coagulation cascade including decreased protein S activity, increases in factor VIII, anticardiolipin antibodies, or lupus-like anticoagulant have been reported in more than 50% of patients with HIV infection. The clinical significance of this increased propensity toward thromboembolic disease is likely reflected in the observation that elevations in D-dimer are strongly associated with all-cause mortality in patients with HIV infection (Table 226-9).

Dermatologic Diseases Dermatologic problems occur in >90% of patients with HIV infection. From the macular, roseola-like rash seen with the acute seroconversion syndrome to extensive end-stage KS, cutaneous manifestations of HIV disease can be seen throughout the course of HIV infection. Among the more common nonneoplastic problems are seborrheic dermatitis, folliculitis, and opportunistic infections. Extrapulmonary pneumocystosis may cause a necrotizing vasculitis. Neoplastic conditions are covered below.

Seborrheic dermatitis occurs in 3% of the general population and in up to 50% of patients with HIV infection. Seborrheic dermatitis increases in prevalence and severity as the CD4+ T cell count declines. In HIV-infected patients, seborrheic dermatitis may be aggravated by concomitant infection with *Pityrosporum*, a yeastlike fungus; use of topical antifungal agents has been recommended in cases refractory to standard topical treatment.

Folliculitis is among the most prevalent dermatologic disorders in patients with HIV infection and is seen in ~20% of patients. It is more common in patients with CD4+ T cell counts <200 cells/μL. Pruritic papular eruption is one of the most common pruritic rashes in patients with HIV infection. It appears as multiple papules on the face, trunk, and extensor surfaces and may improve with cART. *Eosinophilic pustular folliculitis* is a rare form of folliculitis that is seen with increased frequency in patients with HIV infection. It presents as multiple, urticarial perifollicular papules that may coalesce into plaquelike lesions. Skin biopsy reveals an eosinophilic infiltrate of the hair follicle, which in certain cases has been associated with the presence of a mite. Patients typically have an elevated serum IgE level and may respond to treatment with topical anthelmintics. Pruritus is a common symptom in patients with HIV infection and can lead to prurigo nodularis. Patients with HIV infection have also been reported to develop a severe form of *Norwegian scabies* with hyperkeratotic psoriasiform lesions.

Both *psoriasis* and *ichthyosis*, although they are not reported to be increased in frequency, may be particularly severe when they occur in patients with HIV infection. Preexisting psoriasis may become guttate in appearance and more refractory to treatment in the setting of HIV infection.

Reactivation herpes zoster (*shingles*) is seen in 10–20% of patients with HIV infection. This reactivation syndrome of varicella-zoster virus indicates a modest decline in immune function and may be the first indication of clinical immunodeficiency. In one series, patients who developed shingles did so an average of 5 years after HIV infection. In a cohort of patients with HIV infection and localized zoster, the subsequent rate of the development of AIDS was 1% per month. In that study, AIDS was more likely to develop if the outbreak of zoster was associated with severe pain, extensive skin involvement, or involvement of cranial or cervical dermatomes. The clinical manifestations of reactivation zoster in HIV-infected patients, although indicative of immunologic compromise, are not as severe as those seen in other immunodeficient conditions. Thus, while lesions may extend over several dermatomes, involve the spinal cord, and/or be associated with frank cutaneous dissemination, visceral involvement has not been reported. In contrast to patients without a known underlying immunodeficiency state, patients with HIV infection tend to have recurrences of zoster with a relapse rate of ~20%. Valacyclovir, acyclovir, or famciclovir is the treatment of choice. Foscarnet may be of value in patients with acyclovir-resistant virus.

Infection with *herpes simplex virus* in HIV-infected individuals is associated with recurrent orolabial, genital, and perianal lesions as part of recurrent reactivation syndromes (Chap. 216). As HIV disease progresses and the CD4+ T cell count declines, these infections become more frequent and severe. Lesions often appear as beefy red, are exquisitely painful, and have a tendency to occur high in the gluteal cleft (Fig. 226-37). Perirectal HSV may be associated with proctitis and anal fissures. HSV should be high in the differential diagnosis of any HIV-infected patient with a poorly healing, painful perirectal lesion. In addition to recurrent mucosal ulcers, recurrent HSV infection in the form of *herpetic whitlow* can be a problem in patients with HIV infection, presenting with painful vesicles or extensive cutaneous erosion. Valacyclovir, acyclovir or famciclovir is the treatment of choice in these settings. It is noteworthy that even subclinical reactivation of herpes simplex may be associated with increases in plasma HIV RNA levels.

Diffuse skin eruptions due to *Molluscum contagiosum* may be seen in patients with advanced HIV infection. These flesh-colored, umbilicated lesions may be treated with local therapy. They tend to regress with effective cART. Similarly, *condyloma acuminatum* lesions may be more severe and more widely distributed in patients with low CD4+ T cell counts. Imiquimod cream may be helpful in some cases. Atypical mycobacterial infections may present as erythematous cutaneous nodules, as may fungal infections, *Bartonella, Acanthamoeba*, and KS. Cutaneous infections with *Aspergillus* have been noted at the site of IV catheter placement.

The skin of patients with HIV infection is often a target organ for drug reactions (Chap. 74). Although most skin reactions are mild and not necessarily an indication to discontinue therapy, patients may have particularly severe cutaneous reactions, including erythroderma, *Stevens-Johnson syndrome*, and toxic epidermal necrolysis, as a reaction to drugs—particularly sulfa drugs, nonnucleoside reverse transcriptase inhibitors, abacavir, amprenavir, darunavir, fosamprenavir, and tipranavir. Similarly, patients with HIV infection are often quite photosensitive and burn easily following exposure to sunlight or as a side effect of radiation therapy (Chap. 75).

HIV infection and its treatment may be accompanied by cosmetic changes of the skin that are not of great clinical importance but may be troubling to patients. Yellowing of the nails and straightening of the hair, particularly in African-American patients, have been reported as a consequence of HIV infection. Zidovudine therapy has been associated with elongation of the eyelashes and the development of a bluish discoloration to the nails, again more common in African-American patients. Therapy with clofazimine may cause a yellow-orange discoloration of the skin and urine.

Neurologic Diseases Clinical disease of the nervous system accounts for a significant degree of morbidity in a high percentage of patients with HIV infection (Table 226-14). The neurologic problems that occur in HIV-infected individuals may be either primary to the pathogenic processes of HIV infection or secondary to opportunistic infections or neoplasms. Among the more frequent opportunistic diseases that involve the CNS are toxoplasmosis, cryptococcosis, progressive multifocal leukoencephalopathy, and primary CNS lymphoma. Other less common problems include mycobacterial infections; syphilis; and infection with CMV, HTLV-1, *Trypanosoma cruzi*, or *Acanthamoeba*. Overall, secondary diseases of the CNS have been reported to occur in approximately one-third of patients with AIDS. These data antedate the widespread use of cART, and this frequency is considerably lower in patients receiving effective antiretroviral drugs. Primary processes related to HIV infection of the nervous system are reminiscent of those seen with other lentiviruses, such as the Visna-Maedi virus of sheep.

Neurologic problems directly attributable to HIV occur throughout the course of infection and may be inflammatory, demyelinating, or degenerative in nature. The term *HIV-associated neurocognitive disorders* (HAND) is used to describe a spectrum of disorders that range from asymptomatic neurocognitive impairment (ANI) to minor neurocognitive disorder (MND) to clinically severe dementia. The most severe form, *HIV-associated dementia* (HAD), also referred to as the *AIDS dementia complex*, or *HIV encephalopathy*, is considered an AIDS-defining illness. Most HIV-infected patients have some neurologic problem during the course of their disease. Even in the setting of suppressive cART, approximately 50% of HIV-infected individuals can be shown to have mild to moderate neurocognitive impairment using sensitive neuropsychiatric testing. As noted in the section on

TABLE 226-14 NEUROLOGIC DISEASES IN PATIENTS WITH HIV INFECTION

Opportunistic infections	HIV-1 infection
Toxoplasmosis	Aseptic meningitis
Cryptococcosis	HIV-associated neurocognitive disorders (HAND), including HIV encephalopathy/AIDS dementia complex
Progressive multifocal leukoencephalopathy	Myelopathy
Cytomegalovirus	Vacuolar myelopathy
Syphilis	Pure sensory ataxia
Mycobacterium tuberculosis	Paresthesia/dysesthesia
HTLV-1 infection	Peripheral neuropathy
Amebiasis	Acute inflammatory demyelinating polyneuropathy (Guillain-Barré syndrome)
Neoplasms	Chronic inflammatory demyelinating polyneuropathy (CIDP)
Primary CNS lymphoma	Mononeuritis multiplex
Kaposi's sarcoma	Distal symmetric polyneuropathy
	Myopathy

pathogenesis, damage to the CNS may be a direct result of viral infection of the CNS macrophages or glial cells or may be secondary to the release of neurotoxins and potentially toxic cytokines such as IL-1β, TNF-α, IL-6, and TGF-β. It has been reported that HIV-infected individuals with the E4 allele for apoE are at increased risk for AIDS encephalopathy and peripheral neuropathy. Virtually all patients with HIV infection have some degree of nervous system involvement with the virus. This is evidenced by the fact that CSF findings are abnormal in ~90% of patients, even during the asymptomatic phase of HIV infection. CSF abnormalities include pleocytosis (50–65% of patients), detection of viral RNA (~75%), elevated CSF protein (35%), and evidence of intrathecal synthesis of anti-HIV antibodies (90%). It is important to point out that evidence of infection of the CNS with HIV does not imply impairment of cognitive function. The neurologic function of an HIV-infected individual should be considered normal unless clinical signs and symptoms suggest otherwise.

Aseptic meningitis may be seen in any but the very late stages of HIV infection. In the setting of acute primary infection, patients may experience a syndrome of headache, photophobia, and meningismus. Rarely, an acute encephalopathy due to encephalitis may occur. Cranial nerve involvement may be seen, predominantly cranial nerve VII but occasionally V and/or VIII. CSF findings include a lymphocytic pleocytosis, elevated protein level, and normal glucose level. This syndrome, which cannot be clinically differentiated from other viral meningitides (Chap. 165), usually resolves spontaneously within 2–4 weeks; however, in some patients, signs and symptoms may become chronic. Aseptic meningitis may occur any time in the course of HIV infection; however, it is rare following the development of AIDS. This suggests that clinical aseptic meningitis in the context of HIV infection is an immune-mediated disease.

Cryptococcus is the leading infectious cause of meningitis in patients with AIDS (Chap. 239). While the vast majority of these are due to *C. neoformans*, up to 12% may be due to *C. gattii*. Cryptococcal meningitis is the initial AIDS-defining illness in ~2% of patients and generally occurs in patients with CD4+ T cell counts <100/μL. Cryptococcal meningitis is particularly common in untreated patients with AIDS in Africa, occurring in ~5% of patients. Most patients present with a picture of subacute meningoencephalitis with fever, nausea, vomiting, altered mental status, headache, and meningeal signs. The incidence of seizures and focal neurologic deficits is low. The CSF profile may be normal or may show only modest elevations in WBC or protein levels and decreases in glucose. The opening pressure in the CSF is usually elevated. In addition to meningitis, patients may develop cryptococcomas and cranial nerve involvement. Approximately one-third of patients also have pulmonary disease. Uncommon manifestations of cryptococcal infection include skin lesions that resemble *molluscum contagiosum*, lymphadenopathy, palatal and glossal ulcers, arthritis, gastroenteritis, myocarditis, and prostatitis. The prostate gland may serve as a reservoir for smoldering cryptococcal infection. The diagnosis of cryptococcal meningitis is made by identification of organisms in spinal fluid with india ink examination or by the detection of cryptococcal antigen. Blood cultures for fungus are often positive. A biopsy may be needed to make a diagnosis of CNS cryptococcoma. Treatment is with IV amphotericin B 0.7 mg/kg daily, or liposomal amphotericin 4–6 mg/kg daily, with flucytosine 25 mg/kg qid for at least 2 weeks if possible, continuing with amphotericin alone ideally until the CSF culture turns negative. Decreases in renal function in association with amphotericin can lead to increases in flucytosine levels and subsequent bone marrow suppression. Amphotericin is followed by fluconazole 400 mg/d PO for 8 weeks, and then fluconazole 200 mg/d until the CD4+ T cell count has increased to >200 cells/μL for 6 months in response to cART. Repeated lumbar puncture may be required to manage increased intracranial pressure. Symptoms may recur with initiation of cART as an immune reconstitution syndrome (see above). Other fungi that may cause meningitis in patients with HIV infection are *C. immitis* and *H. capsulatum*. Meningoencephalitis has also been reported due to *Acanthamoeba* or *Naegleria*.

HIV-associated dementia consists of a constellation of signs and symptoms of CNS disease. While this is generally a late complication of HIV infection that progresses slowly over months, it can be seen in patients with CD4+ T cell counts >350 cells/μL. A major feature of this entity is the development of dementia, defined as a decline in cognitive ability from a previous level. It may present as impaired ability to concentrate, increased forgetfulness, difficulty reading, or increased difficulty performing complex tasks. Initially these symptoms may be indistinguishable from findings of situational depression or fatigue. In contrast to "cortical" dementia (such as Alzheimer's disease), aphasia, apraxia, and agnosia are uncommon, leading some investigators to classify HIV encephalopathy as a "subcortical dementia" characterized by defects in short-term memory and executive function (see below). In addition to dementia, patients with HIV encephalopathy may also have motor and behavioral abnormalities. Among the motor problems are unsteady gait, poor balance, tremor, and difficulty with rapid alternating movements. Increased tone and deep tendon reflexes may be found in patients with spinal cord involvement. Late stages may be complicated by bowel and/or bladder incontinence. Behavioral problems include apathy, irritability, and lack of initiative, with progression to a vegetative state in some instances. Some patients develop a state of agitation or mild mania. These changes usually occur without significant changes in level of alertness. This is in contrast to the finding of somnolence in patients with dementia due to toxic/metabolic encephalopathies.

HIV-associated dementia is the initial AIDS-defining illness in ~3% of patients with HIV infection and thus only rarely precedes clinical evidence of immunodeficiency. Clinically significant encephalopathy eventually develops in ~25% of untreated patients with AIDS. As immunologic function declines, the risk and severity of HIV-associated dementia increases. Autopsy series suggest that 80–90% of patients with HIV infection have histologic evidence of CNS involvement. Several classification schemes have been developed for grading HIV encephalopathy; a commonly used clinical staging system is outlined in Table 226-15.

The precise cause of HIV-associated dementia remains unclear, although the condition is thought to be a result of a combination of direct effects of HIV on the CNS and associated immune activation. HIV has been found in the brains of patients with HIV encephalopathy by Southern blot, in situ hybridization, PCR, and electron microscopy. Multinucleated giant cells, macrophages, and microglial cells appear to be the main cell types harboring virus in the CNS. Histologically, the major changes are seen in the subcortical areas of the brain and include pallor and gliosis, multinucleated giant cell encephalitis, and vacuolar myelopathy. Less commonly, diffuse or focal spongiform changes occur in the white matter. Areas of the brain involved in motor function, language, and judgment are most severely affected.

There are no specific criteria for a diagnosis of HIV-associated dementia, and this syndrome must be differentiated from a number of other diseases that affect the CNS of HIV-infected patients (Table 226-14). The diagnosis of dementia depends on demonstrating a decline in

TABLE 226-15 CLINICAL STAGING OF HAND ACCORDING TO FRASCATI CRITERIA

Stage	Neurocognitive Status[a]	Functional Status[b]
Asymptomatic	1 SD below mean in 2 cognitive domains	No impairments in activities of daily living
Mild neurocognitive disorder	1 SD below mean in 2 cognitive domains	Impairments in activities of daily living
HIV-associated dementia	2 SD below mean in 2 cognitive domains	Notable impairments in activities of daily living

[a]Neurocognitive testing should include assessment of at least 5 domains, including attention-information processing, language, abstraction-executive, complex perceptual motor skills, memory (including learning and recall), simple motor skills, or sensory perceptual skills. Appropriate norms must be available to establish the number of domains in which performance is below 1 SD. [b]Functional status is typically assessed by self-reporting but might be corroborated by a collateral source. No agreed measures exist for HIV-associated neurocognitive disorder criteria. Note that, for diagnosis of HIV-associated neurocognitive disorder, other causes of dementia must be ruled out and potential confounding effects of substance use or psychiatric illness should be considered.

Source: Adapted from A Antinori et al: Neurology 69:1789, 2007.

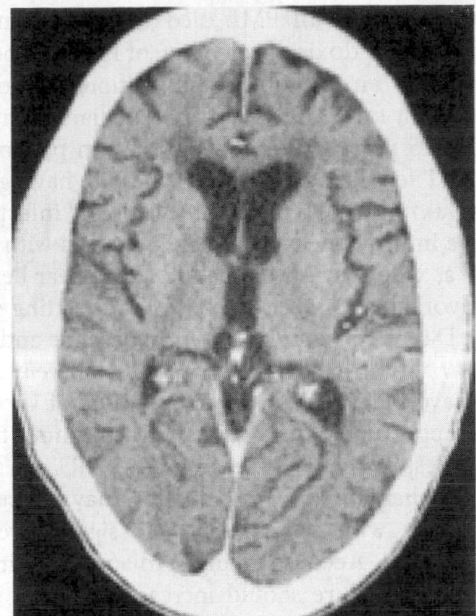

FIGURE 226-39 AIDS dementia complex. Postcontrast CT scan through the lateral ventricles of a 47-year-old man with AIDS, altered mental status, and dementia. The lateral and third ventricles and the cerebral sulci are abnormally prominent. Mild white matter hypodensity is seen adjacent to the frontal horns of the lateral ventricles.

cognitive function. This can be accomplished objectively with the use of a Mini-Mental Status Examination (MMSE) in patients for whom prior scores are available. For this reason, it is advisable for all patients with a diagnosis of HIV infection to have a baseline MMSE. However, changes in MMSE scores may be absent in patients with mild HIV encephalopathy. Imaging studies of the CNS, by either MRI or CT, often demonstrate evidence of cerebral atrophy (Fig. 226-39). MRI may also reveal small areas of increased density on T2-weighted images. Lumbar puncture is an important element of the evaluation of patients with HIV infection and neurologic abnormalities. It is generally most helpful in ruling out or making a diagnosis of opportunistic infections. In HIV encephalopathy, patients may have the nonspecific findings of an increase in CSF cells and protein level. While HIV RNA can often be detected in the spinal fluid and HIV can be cultured from the CSF, this finding is not specific for HIV encephalopathy. There appears to be no correlation between the presence of HIV in the CSF and the presence of HIV encephalopathy. Elevated levels of macrophage chemoattractant protein (MCP-1), β_2-microglobulin, neopterin, and quinolinic acid (a metabolite of tryptophan reported to cause CNS injury) have been noted in the CSF of patients with HIV encephalopathy. These findings suggest that these factors as well as inflammatory cytokines may be involved in the pathogenesis of this syndrome.

Combination antiretroviral therapy is of benefit in patients with HIV-associated dementia. Improvement in neuropsychiatric test scores has been noted for both adult and pediatric patients treated with antiretrovirals. The rapid improvement in cognitive function noted with the initiation of cART suggests that at least some component of this problem is quickly reversible, again supporting at least a partial role of soluble mediators in the pathogenesis. It should also be noted that these patients have an increased sensitivity to the side effects of neuroleptic drugs. The use of these drugs for symptomatic treatment is associated with an increased risk of extrapyramidal side effects; therefore, patients with HIV encephalopathy who receive these agents must be monitored carefully. It is felt by many physicians that the decrease in the prevalence of severe cases of HAND brought about by cART has resulted in an increase in the prevalence of milder forms of this disorder.

Seizures may be a consequence of opportunistic infections, neoplasms, or HIV encephalopathy (Table 226-16). The seizure threshold is often lower than normal in patients with advanced HIV infection due in part to the frequent presence of electrolyte abnormalities. Seizures are seen in 15–40% of patients with cerebral toxoplasmosis,

TABLE 226-16 CAUSES OF SEIZURES IN PATIENTS WITH HIV INFECTION

Disease	Overall Contribution to First Seizure, %	Fraction of Patients Who Have Seizures, %
HIV encephalopathy	24–47	7–50
Cerebral toxoplasmosis	28	15–40
Cryptococcal meningitis	13	8
Primary central nervous system lymphoma	4	15–30
Progressive multifocal leukoencephalopathy	1	20

Source: From DM Holtzman et al: Am J Med 87:173, 1989.

15–35% of patients with primary CNS lymphoma, 8% of patients with cryptococcal meningitis, and 7–50% of patients with HIV encephalopathy. Seizures may also be seen in patients with CNS tuberculosis, aseptic meningitis, and progressive multifocal leukoencephalopathy. Seizures may be the presenting clinical symptom of HIV disease. In one study of 100 patients with HIV infection presenting with a first seizure, cerebral mass lesions were the most common cause, responsible for 32 of the 100 new-onset seizures. Of these 32 cases, 28 were due to toxoplasmosis and 4 to lymphoma. HIV encephalopathy accounted for an additional 24 new-onset seizures. Cryptococcal meningitis was the third most common diagnosis, responsible for 13 of the 100 seizures. In 23 cases, no cause could be found, and it is possible that these cases represent a subcategory of HIV encephalopathy. Of these 23 cases, 16 (70%) had 2 or more seizures, suggesting that anticonvulsant therapy is indicated in all patients with HIV infection and seizures unless a rapidly correctable cause is found. While phenytoin remains the initial treatment of choice, hypersensitivity reactions to this drug have been reported in >10% of patients with AIDS, and therefore the use of phenobarbital or valproic acid should be considered as alternatives. Due to a variety of drug-drug interactions between antiseizure medications and antiretrovirals, drug levels need to be monitored carefully.

Patients with HIV infection may present with *focal neurologic deficits* from a variety of causes. The most common causes are toxoplasmosis, progressive multifocal leukoencephalopathy, and CNS lymphoma. Other causes include cryptococcal infections (discussed above; also Chap. 239), stroke, and reactivation of Chagas' disease.

Toxoplasmosis has been one of the most common causes of secondary CNS infections in patients with AIDS, but its incidence is decreasing in the era of cART. It is most common in patients from the Caribbean and from France, where the seroprevalence of *T. gondii* is around 50%. This figure is closer to 15% in the United States. Toxoplasmosis is generally a late complication of HIV infection and usually occurs in patients with CD4+ T cell counts <200/μL. Cerebral toxoplasmosis is thought to represent a reactivation of latent tissue cysts. It is 10 times more common in patients with antibodies to the organism than in patients who are seronegative. Patients diagnosed with HIV infection should be screened for IgG antibodies to *T. gondii* during the time of their initial workup. Those who are seronegative should be counseled about ways to minimize the risk of primary infection including avoiding the consumption of undercooked meat and careful hand washing after contact with soil or changing the cat litter box. The most common clinical presentation of cerebral toxoplasmosis in patients with HIV infection is fever, headache, and focal neurologic deficits. Patients may present with seizure, hemiparesis, or aphasia as a manifestation of these focal deficits or with a picture more influenced by the accompanying cerebral edema and characterized by confusion, dementia, and lethargy, which can progress to coma. The diagnosis is usually suspected on the basis of MRI findings of multiple lesions in multiple locations, although in some cases only a single lesion is seen. Pathologically, these lesions generally exhibit inflammation and central necrosis and, as a result, demonstrate ring enhancement on contrast MRI (Fig. 226-40) or, if MRI is unavailable or contraindicated, on double-dose contrast CT. There is usually evidence of surrounding edema. In addition to toxoplasmosis, the differential diagnosis of single or multiple enhancing mass lesions in

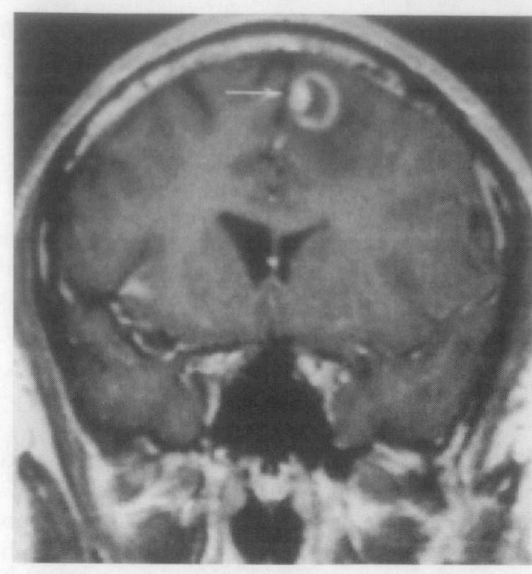

FIGURE 226-40 Central nervous system toxoplasmosis. A coronal postcontrast T1-weighted MRI scan demonstrates a peripheral enhancing lesion in the left frontal lobe, associated with an eccentric nodular area of enhancement (*arrow*); this so-called eccentric target sign is typical of toxoplasmosis.

the HIV-infected patient includes primary CNS lymphoma and, less commonly, TB or fungal or bacterial abscesses. The definitive diagnostic procedure is brain biopsy. However, given the morbidity rate that can accompany this procedure, it is usually reserved for the patient who has failed 2–4 weeks of empiric therapy for toxoplasmosis. If the patient is seronegative for *T. gondii*, the likelihood that a mass lesion is due to toxoplasmosis is <10%. In that setting, one may choose to be more aggressive and perform a brain biopsy sooner. Standard treatment is sulfadiazine and pyrimethamine with leucovorin as needed for a minimum of 4–6 weeks. Alternative therapeutic regimens include clindamycin in combination with pyrimethamine; atovaquone plus pyrimethamine; and azithromycin plus pyrimethamine plus rifabutin. Relapses are common, and it is recommended that patients with a history of prior toxoplasmic encephalitis receive maintenance therapy with sulfadiazine, pyrimethamine, and leucovorin as long as their CD4+ T cell counts remain <200 cells/μL. Patients with CD4+ T cell counts <100/μL and IgG antibody to *Toxoplasma* should receive primary prophylaxis for toxoplasmosis. Fortunately, the same daily regimen of a single double-strength tablet of TMP/SMX used for *P. jiroveci* prophylaxis provides adequate primary protection against toxoplasmosis. Secondary prophylaxis/maintenance therapy for toxoplasmosis may be discontinued in the setting of effective cART and increases in CD4+ T cell counts to >200/μL for 6 months.

JC virus, a human polyomavirus that is the etiologic agent of *progressive multifocal leukoencephalopathy* (PML), is an important opportunistic pathogen in patients with AIDS **(Chap. 164)**. While ~80% of the general adult population has antibodies to JC virus, indicative of prior infection, <10% of healthy adults show any evidence of ongoing viral replication. PML is the only known clinical manifestation of JC virus infection. It is a late manifestation of AIDS and is seen in ~1–4% of patients with AIDS. The lesions of PML begin as small foci of demyelination in subcortical white matter that eventually coalesce. The cerebral hemispheres, cerebellum, and brainstem may all be involved. Patients typically have a protracted course with multifocal neurologic deficits, with or without changes in mental status. Approximately 20% of patients experience seizures. Ataxia, hemiparesis, visual field defects, aphasia, and sensory defects may occur. Headache, fever, nausea, and vomiting are rarely seen. Their presence should suggest another diagnosis. MRI typically reveals multiple, nonenhancing white matter lesions that may coalesce and have a predilection for the occipital and parietal lobes. The lesions show signal hyperintensity on T2-weighted images and diminished signal on T1-weighted images. The measurement of JC virus DNA levels in CSF has a diagnostic sensitivity of 76% and a specificity of close to 100%. Prior to the availability of cART, the majority of patients with PML died within 3–6 months of the onset of symptoms. Paradoxical worsening of PML has been seen with initiation of cART as an immune reconstitution syndrome. There is no specific treatment for PML; however, a median survival of 2 years and survival of >15 years have been reported in patients with PML treated with cART for their HIV disease. Despite having a significant impact on survival, only ~50% of patients with HIV infection and PML show neurologic improvement with cART. Studies with other antiviral agents such as cidofovir have failed to show clear benefit. Factors influencing a favorable prognosis for PML in the setting of HIV infection include a CD4+ T cell count >100/μL at baseline and the ability to maintain an HIV viral load of <500 copies/mL. Baseline HIV-1 viral load does not have independent predictive value of survival. PML is one of the few opportunistic infections that continues to occur with some frequency despite the widespread use of cART.

Reactivation American trypanosomiasis may present as acute meningoencephalitis with focal neurologic signs, fever, headache, vomiting, and seizures. Accompanying cardiac disease in the form of arrhythmias or heart failure should increase the index of suspicion. The presence of antibodies to *T. cruzi* supports the diagnosis. In South America, reactivation of *Chagas' disease* is considered to be an AIDS-defining condition and may be the initial AIDS-defining condition. The majority of cases occur in patients with CD4+ T cell counts <200 cells/μL. Lesions appear radiographically as single or multiple hypodense areas, typically with ring enhancement and edema. They are found predominantly in the subcortical areas, a feature that differentiates them from the deeper lesions of toxoplasmosis. *T. cruzi* amastigotes, or trypanosomes, can be identified from biopsy specimens or CSF. Other CSF findings include elevated protein and a mild (<100 cells/μL) lymphocytic pleocytosis. Organisms can also be identified by direct examination of the blood. Treatment consists of benzimidazole (2.5 mg/kg bid) or nifurtimox (2 mg/kg qid) for at least 60 days, followed by maintenance therapy for the duration of immunodeficiency with either drug at a dose of 5 mg/kg three times a week. As is the case with cerebral toxoplasmosis, successful therapy with antiretrovirals may allow discontinuation of therapy for Chagas' disease.

Stroke may occur in patients with HIV infection. In contrast to the other causes of focal neurologic deficits in patients with HIV infection, the symptoms of a stroke are sudden in onset. Patients with HIV infection have an increased prevalence of many classic risk factors associated with stroke, including smoking and diabetes. It has been reported that HIV infection itself can lead to an increase in carotid artery stiffness. The relative increase in risk for stroke as a consequence of HIV infection is more pronounced in women and in individuals between the ages of 18 and 29. Among the secondary infectious diseases in patients with HIV infection that may be associated with stroke are vasculitis due to cerebral varicella zoster or neurosyphilis and septic embolism in association with fungal infection. Other elements of the differential diagnosis of stroke in the patient with HIV infection include atherosclerotic cerebral vascular disease, thrombotic thrombocytopenic purpura, and cocaine or amphetamine use.

Primary CNS lymphoma is discussed below in the section on neoplastic diseases.

Spinal cord disease, or myelopathy, is present in ~20% of patients with AIDS, often as part of HIV-associated neurocognitive disorder. In fact, 90% of the patients with HIV-associated myelopathy have some evidence of dementia, suggesting that similar pathologic processes may be responsible for both conditions. Three main types of spinal cord disease are seen in patients with AIDS. The first of these is a vacuolar myelopathy, as mentioned above. This condition is pathologically similar to subacute combined degeneration of the cord, such as that occurring with pernicious anemia. Although vitamin B_{12} deficiency can be seen in patients with AIDS as a primary complication of HIV infection, it does not appear to be responsible for the myelopathy seen in the majority of patients. Vacuolar myelopathy is characterized by a subacute onset and often presents with gait disturbances, predominantly ataxia and spasticity; it may progress to include bladder and bowel dysfunction. Physical findings include evidence of increased deep tendon reflexes and extensor plantar responses. The second form of spinal cord disease involves the dorsal columns and presents as a pure sensory ataxia. The third form is also sensory in nature and presents with paresthesias and dysesthesias of the lower extremities. In contrast to the cognitive problems seen in patients with HIV encephalopathy, these spinal cord syndromes do not respond well to antiretroviral drugs, and therapy is mainly supportive.

One important disease of the spinal cord that also involves the peripheral nerves is a *myelopathy* and *polyradiculopathy* seen in association with CMV infection. This entity is generally seen late in the course of HIV infection and is fulminant in onset, with lower extremity and sacral paresthesias, difficulty in walking, areflexia, ascending sensory loss, and urinary retention. The clinical course is rapidly progressive over a period of weeks. CSF examination reveals a predominantly neutrophilic pleocytosis, and CMV DNA can be detected by CSF PCR. Therapy with ganciclovir or foscarnet can lead to rapid improvement, and prompt initiation of foscarnet or ganciclovir therapy is important in minimizing the degree of permanent neurologic damage. Combination therapy with both drugs should be considered in patients who have been previously treated for CMV disease. Other diseases involving the spinal cord in patients with HIV infection include HTLV-1-associated myelopathy (HAM) (Chap. 225e), neurosyphilis (Chap. 206), infection with herpes simplex (Chap. 216) or varicella-zoster (Chap. 217), TB (Chap. 202), and lymphoma (Chap. 134).

Peripheral neuropathies are common in patients with HIV infection. They occur at all stages of illness and take a variety of forms. Early in the course of HIV infection, an acute inflammatory demyelinating polyneuropathy resembling Guillain-Barré syndrome may occur (Chap. 460). In other patients, a progressive or relapsing remitting inflammatory neuropathy resembling chronic inflammatory demyelinating polyneuropathy (CIDP) has been noted. Patients commonly present with progressive weakness, areflexia, and minimal sensory changes. CSF examination often reveals a mononuclear pleocytosis, and peripheral nerve biopsy demonstrates a perivascular infiltrate suggesting an autoimmune etiology. Plasma exchange or IVIg has been tried with variable success. Because of the immunosuppressive effects of glucocorticoids, they should be reserved for severe cases of CIDP refractory to other measures. Another autoimmune peripheral neuropathy seen in patients with AIDS is mononeuritis multiplex (Chaps. 460 and 385) due to a necrotizing arteritis of peripheral nerves. The most common peripheral neuropathy in patients with HIV infection is a *distal sensory polyneuropathy* (DSPN) also referred to as painful sensory neuropathy (HIV-SN), predominantly sensory neuropathy, or distal symmetric peripheral neuropathy. This condition may be a direct consequence of HIV infection or a side effect of dideoxynucleoside therapy. It is more common in taller individuals, older individuals, and those with lower CD4 counts. Two-thirds of patients with AIDS may be shown by electrophysiologic studies to have some evidence of peripheral nerve disease. Presenting symptoms are usually painful burning sensations in the feet and lower extremities. Findings on examination include a stocking-type sensory loss to pinprick, temperature, and touch sensation and a loss of ankle reflexes. Motor changes are mild and are usually limited to weakness of the intrinsic foot muscles. Response of this condition to antiretrovirals has been variable, perhaps because antiretrovirals are responsible for the problem in some instances. When due to dideoxynucleoside therapy, patients with lower extremity peripheral neuropathy may complain of a sensation that they are walking on ice. Other entities in the differential diagnosis of peripheral neuropathy include diabetes mellitus, vitamin B_{12} deficiency, and side effects from metronidazole or dapsone. For distal symmetric polyneuropathy that fails to resolve following the discontinuation of dideoxynucleosides, therapy is symptomatic; gabapentin, carbamazepine, tricyclics, or analgesics may be effective for dysesthesias. Treatment-naïve patients may respond to cART.

Myopathy may complicate the course of HIV infection; causes include HIV infection itself, zidovudine, and the generalized wasting syndrome. HIV-associated myopathy may range in severity from an asymptomatic elevation in creatine kinase levels to a subacute syndrome characterized by proximal muscle weakness and myalgias. Quite pronounced elevations in creatine kinase may occur in asymptomatic patients, particularly after exercise. The clinical significance of this as an isolated laboratory finding is unclear. A variety of both inflammatory and noninflammatory pathologic processes have been noted in patients with more severe myopathy, including myofiber necrosis with inflammatory cells, nemaline rod bodies, cytoplasmic bodies, and mitochondrial abnormalities. Profound muscle wasting, often with muscle pain, may be seen after prolonged zidovudine therapy. This toxic side effect of the drug is dose-dependent and is related to its ability to interfere with the function of mitochondrial polymerases. It is reversible following discontinuation of the drug. Red ragged fibers are a histologic hallmark of zidovudine-induced myopathy.

Ophthalmologic Diseases Ophthalmologic problems occur in ~50% of patients with advanced HIV infection. The most common abnormal findings on funduscopic examination are cotton-wool spots. These are hard white spots that appear on the surface of the retina and often have an irregular edge. They represent areas of retinal ischemia secondary to microvascular disease. At times they are associated with small areas of hemorrhage and thus can be difficult to distinguish from CMV retinitis. In contrast to CMV retinitis, however, these lesions are not associated with visual loss and tend to remain stable or improve over time.

One of the most devastating consequences of HIV infection is CMV retinitis. Patients at high risk of CMV retinitis (CD4+ T cell count <100/μL) should undergo an ophthalmologic examination every 3–6 months. The majority of cases of CMV retinitis occur in patients with a CD4+ T cell count <50/μL. Prior to the availability of cART, this CMV reactivation syndrome was seen in 25–30% of patients with AIDS. In the cART era this has dropped to close to 2%. CMV retinitis usually presents as a painless, progressive loss of vision. Patients may also complain of blurred vision, "floaters," and scintillations. The disease is usually bilateral, although typically it affects one eye more than the other. The diagnosis is made on clinical grounds by an experienced ophthalmologist. The characteristic retinal appearance is that of perivascular hemorrhage and exudate. In situations where the diagnosis is in doubt due to an atypical presentation or an unexpected lack of response to therapy, vitreous or aqueous humor sampling with molecular diagnostic techniques may be of value. CMV infection of the retina results in a necrotic inflammatory process, and the visual loss that develops is irreversible. CMV retinitis may be complicated by rhegmatogenous retinal detachment as a consequence of retinal atrophy in areas of prior inflammation. Therapy for CMV retinitis consists of oral valganciclovir, IV ganciclovir, or IV foscarnet, with cidofovir as an alternative. Combination therapy with ganciclovir and foscarnet has been shown to be slightly more effective than either ganciclovir or foscarnet alone in the patient with relapsed CMV retinitis. A 3-week induction course is followed by maintenance therapy with oral valganciclovir. If CMV disease is limited to the eye, intravitreal injections of ganciclovir or foscarnet may be considered. Intravitreal injections of cidofovir are generally avoided due to the increased risk of uveitis and hypotony. Maintenance therapy is continued until the CD4+ T cell count remains >100 μL for >6 months. The majority of patients with HIV infection and CMV disease develop some degree of uveitis with the initiation of cART. The etiology of this is unknown; however, it has been suggested that this may be due to the generation of an enhanced immune response to CMV as an IRIS (see above). In some instances this has required the use of topical glucocorticoids.

Both HSV and varicella zoster virus can cause a rapidly progressing, bilateral necrotizing retinitis referred to as the *acute retinal necrosis syndrome*, or *progressive outer retinal necrosis* (PORN). This syndrome, in contrast to CMV retinitis, is associated with pain, keratitis, and iritis. It is often associated with orolabial HSV or trigeminal zoster. Ophthalmologic examination reveals widespread pale gray peripheral lesions. This condition is often complicated by retinal detachment. It is important to recognize and treat this condition with IV acyclovir as quickly as possible to minimize the loss of vision.

Several other secondary infections may cause ocular problems in HIV-infected patients. *P. jiroveci* can cause a lesion of the choroid that may be detected as an incidental finding on ophthalmologic examination. These lesions are typically bilateral, are from half to twice the disc diameter in size, and appear as slightly elevated yellow-white plaques. They are usually asymptomatic and may be confused with cotton-wool spots. Chorioretinitis due to toxoplasmosis can be seen alone or, more commonly, in association with CNS toxoplasmosis. KS may involve the eyelid or conjunctiva, while lymphoma may involve the retina. Syphilis may lead to a uveitis that is highly associated with the presence of neurosyphilis.

Additional Disseminated Infections and Wasting Syndrome Infections with species of the small, gram-negative, *Rickettsia*-like organism *Bartonella* (Chap. 197) are seen with increased frequency in patients with HIV infection. While it is not considered an AIDS-defining illness by the CDC, many experts view infection with *Bartonella* as indicative of a severe defect in cell-mediated immunity. It is usually seen in patients with CD4+ T cell counts <100/μL and is a significant cause of unexplained fever in patients with advanced HIV infection. Among the clinical manifestations of *Bartonella* infection are bacillary angiomatosis, cat-scratch disease, and trench fever. *Bacillary angiomatosis* is usually due to infection with *B. henselae* and is linked to exposure to flea-infested cats. It is characterized by a vascular proliferation that leads to a variety of skin lesions that have been confused with the skin lesions of KS. In contrast to the lesions of KS, the lesions of bacillary angiomatosis generally blanch, are painful, and typically occur in the setting of systemic symptoms. Infection can extend to the lymph nodes, liver (peliosis hepatis), spleen, bone, heart, CNS, respiratory tract, and GI tract. *Cat-scratch disease* also is due to *B. henselae* and generally begins with a papule at the site of inoculation. This is followed several weeks later by the development of regional adenopathy and malaise. Infection with *B. quintana* is transmitted by lice and has been associated with case reports of trench fever, endocarditis, adenopathy, and bacillary angiomatosis. The organism is quite difficult to culture, and diagnosis often relies on identifying the organism in biopsy specimens using the Warthin-Starry or similar stains. Treatment is with either doxycycline or erythromycin for at least 3 months.

Histoplasmosis is an opportunistic infection that is seen most frequently in patients in the Mississippi and Ohio River valleys, Puerto Rico, the Dominican Republic, and South America. These are all areas in which infection with *H. capsulatum* is endemic (Chap. 236). Because of this limited geographic distribution, the percentage of AIDS cases in the United States with histoplasmosis is only ~0.5. Histoplasmosis is generally a late manifestation of HIV infection; however, it may be the initial AIDS-defining condition. In one study, the median CD4+ T cell count for patients with histoplasmosis and AIDS was 33/μL. While disease due to *H. capsulatum* may present as a primary infection of the lung, disseminated disease, presumably due to reactivation, is the most common presentation in HIV-infected patients. Patients usually present with a 4- to 8-week history of fever and weight loss. Hepatosplenomegaly and lymphadenopathy are each seen in about 25% of patients. CNS disease, either meningitis or a mass lesion, is seen in 15% of patients. Bone marrow involvement is common, with thrombocytopenia, neutropenia, and anemia occurring in 33% of patients. Approximately 7% of patients have mucocutaneous lesions consisting of a maculopapular rash and skin or oral ulcers. Respiratory symptoms are usually mild, with chest x-ray showing a diffuse infiltrate or diffuse small nodules in ~50% of cases. The gastrointestinal tract may be involved. Diagnosis is made by silver staining of tissue, by culturing the organisms from blood, bone marrow, or tissue, or by detecting antigen in blood or urine. Treatment is typically with liposomal amphotericin B followed by maintenance therapy with oral itraconazole until the serum histoplasma antigen is <2 units, the patient has been on antiretrovirals for at least 6 months, and the CD4 count is >150 cells/μL. In the setting of mild infection, it may be appropriate to initiate therapy with itraconazole alone.

Following the spread of HIV infection to southeast Asia, disseminated infection with the fungus *Penicillium marneffei* was recognized as a complication of HIV infection and is considered an AIDS-defining condition in those parts of the world where it occurs. *P. marneffei* is the third most common AIDS-defining illness in Thailand, following TB and cryptococcosis. It is more frequently diagnosed in the rainy than the dry season. Clinical features include fever, generalized lymphadenopathy, hepatosplenomegaly, anemia, thrombocytopenia, and papular skin lesions with central umbilication. Treatment is with amphotericin B followed by itraconazole until the CD4+ T cell count is >100 cells/μL for at least 6 months.

Visceral leishmaniasis (Chap. 251) is recognized with increasing frequency in patients with HIV infection who live in or travel to areas endemic for this protozoal infection transmitted by sandflies. The clinical presentation is one of hepatosplenomegaly, fever, and hematologic abnormalities. Lymphadenopathy and other constitutional symptoms may be present. A chronic, relapsing course is seen in two-thirds of co-infected patients. Organisms can be isolated from cultures of bone marrow aspirates. Histologic stains may be negative, and antibody titers are of little help. Patients with HIV infection usually respond well initially to standard therapy with amphotericin B or pentavalent antimony compounds. Eradication of the organism is difficult, however, and relapses are common.

Patients with HIV infection are at a slightly increased risk of clinical malaria. This is particularly true for patients from nonendemic areas with presumed primary infection and in patients with lower CD4+ T cell counts. HIV-positive individuals with CD4+ T cell counts <300 cells/μL have a poorer response to malaria treatment than others. Co-infection with malaria is associated with a modest increase in HIV viral load. The risk of malaria may be decreased with TMP/SMX prophylaxis.

Generalized wasting is an AIDS-defining condition; it is defined as involuntary weight loss of >10% associated with intermittent or constant fever and chronic diarrhea or fatigue lasting >30 days in the absence of a defined cause other than HIV infection. Prior to the widespread use of cART it was the initial AIDS-defining condition in ~10% of patients with AIDS in the United States and is an indication for initiation of cART. Generalized wasting is rarely seen today with the earlier initiation of antiretrovirals. A constant feature of this syndrome is severe muscle wasting with scattered myofiber degeneration and occasional evidence of myositis. Glucocorticoids may be of some benefit; however, this approach must be carefully weighed against the risk of compounding the immunodeficiency of HIV infection. Androgenic steroids, growth hormone, and total parenteral nutrition have been used as therapeutic interventions with variable success.

Neoplastic Diseases The neoplastic diseases considered to be AIDS-defining conditions are Kaposi's sarcoma, non-Hodgkin's lymphoma, and invasive cervical carcinoma. In addition, there is also an increase in the incidence of a variety of non-AIDS-defining malignancies including Hodgkin's disease; multiple myeloma; leukemia; melanoma; and cervical, brain, testicular, oral, lung, gastric, liver, renal, and anal cancers. Since the introduction of potent cART, there has been a marked reduction in the incidence of KS (Fig. 226-33) and CNS lymphoma, such that the non-AIDS-defining malignancies now account for more morbidity and mortality in patients with HIV infection than the AIDS-defining malignancies. Rates of non-Hodgkin's lymphoma have declined as well; however, this decline has not been as dramatic as the decline in rates of KS. In contrast, cART has had little effect on human papillomavirus (HPV)-associated malignancies. As patients with HIV infection live longer, a wider array of cancers is seen in this population. While some may only reflect known risk factors (e.g., smoking, alcohol consumption, co-infection with other viruses such as hepatitis B) that are increased in patients with HIV infection, some may be a direct consequence of HIV and are clearly increased in patients with lower CD4+ T cell counts.

Kaposi's sarcoma is a multicentric neoplasm consisting of multiple vascular nodules appearing in the skin, mucous membranes, and viscera. The course ranges from indolent, with only minor skin or lymph node involvement, to fulminant, with extensive cutaneous and visceral involvement. In the initial period of the AIDS epidemic, KS was a prominent clinical feature of the first cases of AIDS, occurring in 79% of the patients diagnosed in 1981. By 1989 it was seen in only 25% of cases, by 1992 the number had decreased to 9%, and by 1997 the number was <1%. HHV-8 (KSHV) has been strongly implicated as a viral cofactor in the pathogenesis of KS.

Clinically, KS has varied presentations and may be seen at any stage of HIV infection, even in the presence of a normal CD4+ T cell

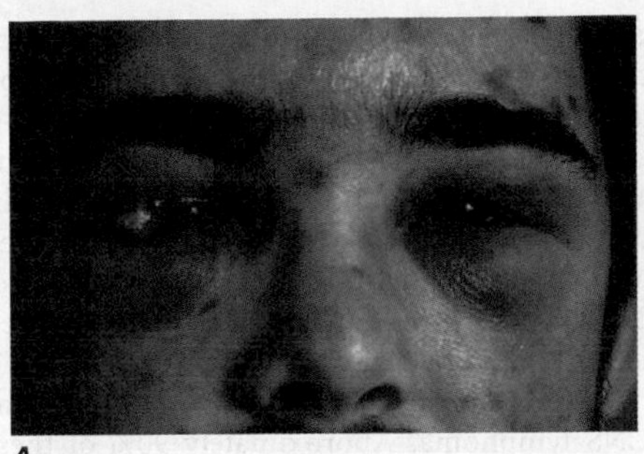
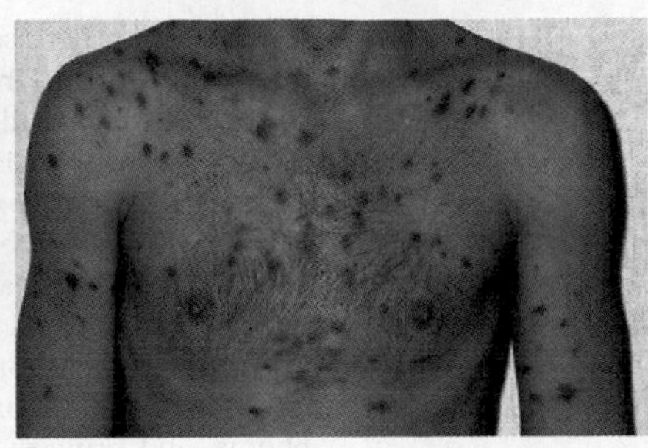
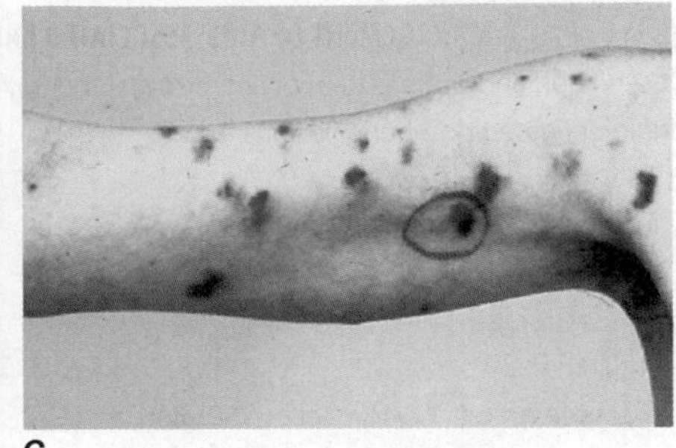

FIGURE 226-41 Kaposi's sarcoma in three patients with AIDS demonstrating (***A***) periorbital edema and bruising; (***B***) classic truncal distribution of lesions; and (***C***) upper extremity lesions.

count. The initial lesion may be a small, raised reddish-purple nodule on the skin (Fig. 226-41), a discoloration on the oral mucosa (Fig. 226-34*D*), or a swollen lymph node. Lesions often appear in sun-exposed areas, particularly the tip of the nose, and have a propensity to occur in areas of trauma (Koebner phenomenon). Because of the vascular nature of the tumors and the presence of extravasated red blood cells in the lesions, their colors range from reddish to purple to brown and often take the appearance of a bruise, with yellowish discoloration and tattooing. Lesions range in size from a few millimeters to several centimeters in diameter and may be either discrete or confluent. KS lesions most commonly appear as raised macules; however, they can also be papular, particularly in patients with higher CD4+ T cell counts. Confluent lesions may give rise to surrounding lymphedema and may be disfiguring when they involve the face and disabling when they involve the lower extremities or the surfaces of joints. Apart from skin, the lymph nodes, GI tract, and lung are the organ systems most commonly affected by KS. Lesions have been reported in virtually every organ, including the heart and the CNS. In contrast to most malignancies, in which lymph node involvement implies metastatic spread and a poor prognosis, lymph node involvement may be seen very early in KS and is of no special clinical significance. In fact, some patients may present with disease limited to the lymph nodes. These are generally patients with relatively intact immune function and thus the patients with the best prognosis. Pulmonary involvement with KS generally presents with shortness of breath. Some 80% of patients with pulmonary KS also have cutaneous lesions. The chest x-ray characteristically shows bilateral lower lobe infiltrates that obscure the margins of the mediastinum and diaphragm (Fig. 226-42). Pleural effusions are seen in 70% of cases of pulmonary KS, a fact that is often helpful in the differential diagnosis. GI involvement is seen in 50% of patients with KS and usually takes one of two forms: (1) mucosal involvement, which may lead to bleeding that can be severe; these patients sometimes also develop symptoms of GI obstruction if lesions become large; and (2) biliary tract involvement. KS lesions may infiltrate the gallbladder and biliary tree, leading to a clinical picture of obstructive jaundice similar to that seen with sclerosing cholangitis. Several staging systems have been proposed for KS. One in common use was developed by the National Institute of Allergy and Infectious Diseases AIDS Clinical Trials Group; it distinguishes patients on the basis of tumor extent, immunologic function, and presence or absence of systemic disease (Table 226-17).

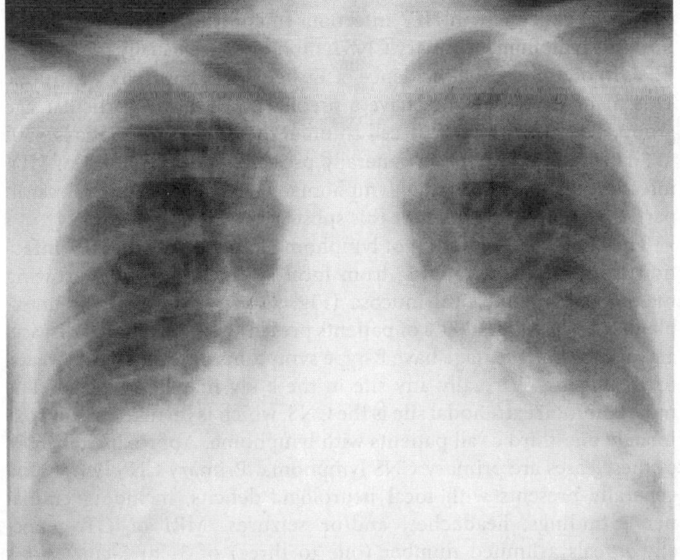

FIGURE 226-42 Chest x-ray of a patient with AIDS and pulmonary Kaposi's sarcoma. The characteristic findings include dense bilateral lower lobe infiltrates obscuring the heart borders and pleural effusions.

A diagnosis of KS is based on biopsy of a suspicious lesion. Histologically one sees a proliferation of spindle cells and endothelial cells, extravasation of red blood cells, hemosiderin-laden macrophages, and, in early cases, an inflammatory cell infiltrate. Included in the differential diagnosis are lymphoma (particularly for oral lesions), bacillary angiomatosis, and cutaneous mycobacterial infections.

Management of KS (Table 226-18) should be carried out in consultation with an expert since definitive treatment guidelines do not exist. In the majority of cases, effective cART will go a long way in achieving control. Antiretroviral therapy has been associated with the spontaneous regression of KS lesions. Paradoxically, it has also been associated with the initial appearance of KS as a form of IRIS. For patients in whom tumor persists or is compromising vital functions or in whom control of HIV replication is not possible, a variety of options exist. In some cases, lesions remain quite indolent, and many of these patients can be managed with no specific treatment. Fewer than 10% of AIDS patients with KS die as a consequence of their malignancy,

TABLE 226-17 NATIONAL INSTITUTE OF ALLERGY AND INFECTIOUS DISEASES AIDS CLINICAL TRIALS GROUP TIS STAGING SYSTEM FOR KAPOSI'S SARCOMA

Parameter	Good Risk (Stage 0): All of the Following	Poor Risk (Stage 1): Any of the Following
Tumor (T)	Confined to skin and/or lymph nodes and/or minimal oral disease	Tumor-associated edema or ulceration
		Extensive oral lesions
		GI lesions
		Nonnodal visceral lesions
Immune system (I)	CD4+ T cell count ≥200/μL	CD4+ T cell count <200/μL
Systemic illness (S)	No B symptoms[a]	B symptoms[a] present
	Karnofsky performance status ≥70	Karnofsky performance status <70
	No history of opportunistic infection, neurologic disease, lymphoma, or thrush	History of opportunistic infection, neurologic disease, lymphoma, or thrush

[a]Defined as unexplained fever, night sweats, >10% involuntary weight loss, or diarrhea persisting for more than 2 weeks.

TABLE 226-18 MANAGEMENT OF AIDS-ASSOCIATED KAPOSI'S SARCOMA

Observation and optimization of antiretroviral therapy
Single or limited number of lesions
  Radiation
  Intralesional vinblastine
  Cryotherapy
Extensive disease
  Initial therapy
    Interferon α (if CD4+ T cells >150/μL)
    Liposomal daunorubicin
  Subsequent therapy
    Liposomal doxorubicin
    Paclitaxel
Combination chemotherapy with low-dose doxorubicin, bleomycin, and vinblastine (ABV)
Targeted radiation

and death from secondary infections is considerably more common. Thus, whenever possible one should avoid treatment regimens that may further suppress the immune system and increase susceptibility to opportunistic infections. Treatment is indicated under two main circumstances. The first is when a single lesion or a limited number of lesions are causing significant discomfort or cosmetic problems, such as with prominent facial lesions, lesions overlying a joint, or lesions in the oropharynx that interfere with swallowing or breathing. Under these circumstances, treatment with localized radiation, intralesional vinblastine, topical 9-*cis*-retinoic acid, or cryotherapy may be helpful. It should be noted that patients with HIV infection are particularly sensitive to the side effects of radiation therapy. This is especially true with respect to the development of radiation-induced mucositis; doses of radiation directed at mucosal surfaces, particularly in the head and neck region, should be adjusted accordingly. The use of systemic therapy, either IFN-α or chemotherapy, should be considered in patients with a large number of lesions or in patients with visceral involvement. The single most important determinant of response appears to be the CD4+ T cell count. This relationship between response rate and baseline CD4+ T cell count is particularly true for IFN-α. The response rate to IFN-α for patients with CD4+ T cell counts >600/μL is ~80%, while the response rate for patients with counts <150/μL is <10%. In contrast to the other systemic therapies, IFN-α provides an added advantage of having antiretroviral activity; thus, it may be the appropriate first choice for single-agent systemic therapy for early patients with disseminated disease. A variety of chemotherapeutic agents also have been shown to have activity against KS. Four of them—liposomal daunorubicin, liposomal doxorubicin, vinblastine, and paclitaxel—have been approved by the FDA for this indication. Liposomal daunorubicin is approved as first-line therapy for patients with advanced KS. It has fewer side effects than conventional chemotherapy. In contrast, liposomal doxorubicin and paclitaxel are approved only for KS patients who have failed standard chemotherapy. Response rates vary from 23 to 88%, appear to be comparable to what had been achieved earlier with combination chemotherapy regimens, and are greatly influenced by CD4+ T cell count.

Lymphomas occur with an increased frequency in patients with congenital or acquired T cell immunodeficiencies (Chap. 374). AIDS is no exception; at least 6% of all patients with AIDS develop lymphoma at some time during the course of their illness. This is a 120-fold increase in incidence compared with the general population. In contrast to the situation with KS, primary CNS lymphoma, and most opportunistic infections, the incidence of AIDS-associated systemic lymphomas has not experienced a dramatic decrease as a consequence of the widespread use of effective cART. Lymphoma occurs in all risk groups, with the highest incidence in patients with hemophilia and the lowest incidence in patients from the Caribbean or Africa with heterosexually acquired infection. Lymphoma is a late manifestation of HIV infection, generally occurring in patients with CD4+ T cell counts <200/μL. As HIV disease progresses, the risk of lymphoma increases. The attack rate for lymphoma increases exponentially with increasing duration of HIV infection and decreasing level of immunologic function. At 3 years following a diagnosis of HIV infection, the risk of lymphoma is 0.8% per year; by 8 years after infection, it is 2.6% per year. As individuals with HIV infection live longer as a consequence of improved cART and better treatment and prophylaxis of opportunistic infections, it is anticipated that the incidence of lymphomas may increase.

Three main categories of lymphoma are seen in patients with HIV infection: grade III or IV immunoblastic lymphoma, Burkitt's lymphoma, and primary CNS lymphoma. Approximately 90% of these lymphomas are B cell in phenotype; more than half contain EBV DNA. Some are associated with KSHV. These tumors may be either monoclonal or oligoclonal in nature and are probably in some way related to the pronounced polyclonal B cell activation seen in patients with AIDS.

Immunoblastic lymphomas account for ~60% of the cases of lymphoma in patients with AIDS. The majority of these are diffuse large B cell lymphomas (DLBCL). They are generally high grade and would have been classified as diffuse histiocytic lymphomas in earlier classification schemes. This tumor is more common in older patients, increasing in incidence from 0% in HIV-infected individuals <1 year old to >3% in those >50 years of age. Two variants of immunoblastic lymphoma that are seen primarily in HIV-infected patients are primary effusion lymphoma (PEL) and its solid variant, plasmacytic lymphoma of the oral cavity. PEL, also referred to as body cavity lymphoma, presents with lymphomatous pleural, pericardial, and/or peritoneal effusions in the absence of discrete nodal or extranodal masses. The tumor cells do not express surface markers for B cells or T cells and are felt to represent a preplasmacytic stage of differentiation. While both HHV-8 and EBV DNA sequences have been found in the genomes of the malignant cells from patients with body cavity lymphoma, KSHV is felt to be the driving force behind the oncogenesis (see above).

Small noncleaved cell lymphoma (*Burkitt's lymphoma*) accounts for ~20% of the cases of lymphoma in patients with AIDS. It is most frequent in patients 10–19 years old and usually demonstrates characteristic c-*myc* translocations from chromosome 8 to chromosomes 14 or 22. Burkitt's lymphoma is not commonly seen in the setting of immunodeficiency other than HIV-associated immunodeficiency, and the incidence of this particular tumor is more than 1000-fold higher in the setting of HIV infection than in the general population. In contrast to African Burkitt's lymphoma, where 97% of the cases contain EBV genome, only 50% of HIV-associated Burkitt's lymphomas are EBV-positive.

Primary CNS lymphoma accounts for ~20% of the cases of lymphoma in patients with HIV infection. In contrast to HIV-associated Burkitt's lymphoma, primary CNS lymphomas are usually positive for EBV. In one study, the incidence of Epstein-Barr positivity was 100%. This malignancy does not have a predilection for any particular age group. The median CD4+ T cell count at the time of diagnosis is ~50/μL. Thus, CNS lymphoma generally presents at a later stage of HIV infection than does systemic lymphoma. This may explain, at least in part, the poorer prognosis for this subset of patients.

The clinical presentation of lymphoma in patients with HIV infection is quite varied, ranging from focal seizures to rapidly growing mass lesions in the oral mucosa (Fig. 226-43) to persistent unexplained fever. At least 80% of patients present with extranodal disease, and a similar percentage have B-type symptoms of fever, night sweats, or weight loss. Virtually any site in the body may be involved. The most common extranodal site is the CNS, which is involved in approximately one-third of all patients with lymphoma. Approximately 60% of these cases are primary CNS lymphoma. Primary CNS lymphoma generally presents with focal neurologic deficits, including cranial nerve findings, headaches, and/or seizures. MRI or CT generally reveals a limited number (one to three) of 3- to 5-cm lesions (Fig. 226-44). The lesions often show ring enhancement on contrast administration and may occur in any location. Contrast enhancement is usually less pronounced than that seen with toxoplasmosis.

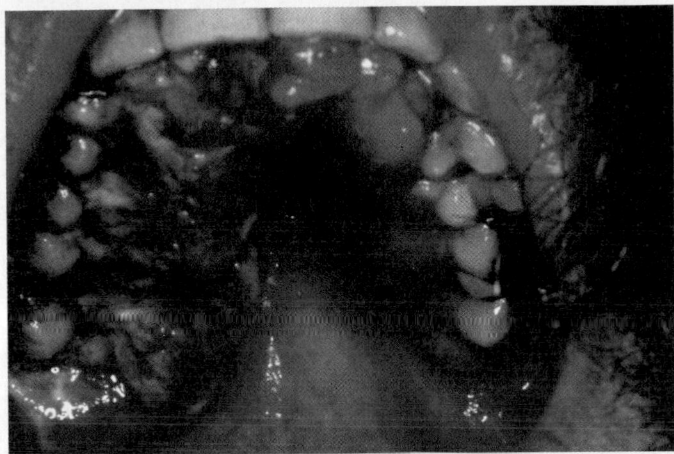

FIGURE 226-43 Immunoblastic lymphoma involving the hard palate of a patient with AIDS.

Locations that are most commonly involved with CNS lymphoma are deep in the white matter. The main diseases in the differential diagnosis are cerebral toxoplasmosis and cerebral Chagas' disease. In addition to the 20% of lymphomas in HIV-infected individuals that are primary CNS lymphomas, CNS disease is also seen in HIV-infected patients with systemic lymphoma. Approximately 20% of patients with systemic lymphoma have CNS disease in the form of leptomeningeal involvement. This fact underscores the importance of lumbar puncture in the staging evaluation of patients with systemic lymphoma.

Systemic lymphoma is seen at earlier stages of HIV infection than primary CNS lymphoma. In one series the mean CD4+ T cell count was 226/μL. In addition to lymph node involvement, systemic lymphoma may commonly involve the GI tract, bone marrow, liver, and lung. GI tract involvement is seen in ~25% of patients. Any site in the GI tract may be involved, and patients may complain of difficulty swallowing or abdominal pain. The diagnosis is usually suspected on the basis of CT or MRI of the abdomen. Bone marrow involvement is seen in ~20% of patients and may lead to pancytopenia. Liver and lung involvement are each seen in ~10% of patients. Pulmonary disease may present as a mass lesion, multiple nodules, or an interstitial infiltrate.

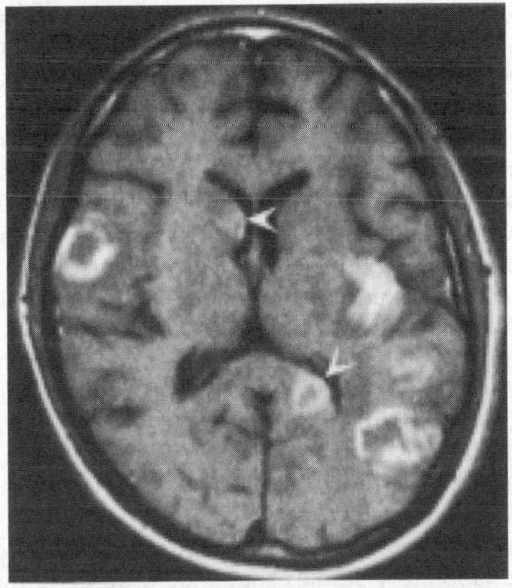

FIGURE 226-44 Central nervous system lymphoma. Postcontrast T1-weighted MRI scan in a patient with AIDS, an altered mental status, and hemiparesis. Multiple enhancing lesions, some ring-enhancing, are present. The left sylvian lesion shows gyral and subcortical enhancement, and the lesions in the caudate and splenium (*arrowheads*) show enhancement of adjacent ependymal surfaces.

Both conventional and unconventional approaches have been employed in an attempt to treat HIV-related lymphomas. Systemic lymphoma is generally treated by the oncologist with combination chemotherapy. Earlier disappointing figures are being replaced with more optimistic results for the treatment of systemic lymphoma following the availability of more effective cART and the use of rituximab in CD20+ tumors. While there is some controversy regarding the use of antiretrovirals during chemotherapy, there is no question that their use overall in patients with HIV lymphoma has improved survival. Concerns regarding synergistic bone marrow toxicities with chemotherapy and cART are mitigated with the use of cART regimens that avoid bone marrow–toxic antiretrovirals. As in most situations in patients with HIV disease, those with higher CD4+ T cell counts tend to fare better. Response rates as high as 72% with a median survival of 33 months and disease-free intervals up to 9 years have been reported. Treatment of primary CNS lymphoma remains a significant challenge. Treatment is complicated by the fact that this illness usually occurs in patients with advanced HIV disease. Palliative measures such as radiation therapy provide some relief. The prognosis remains poor in this group, with a 2-year survival of 29%.

Multicentric Castleman's disease is a KSHV-associated lymphoproliferative disorder that is seen with an increased frequency in patients with HIV infection. While not a true malignancy, it shares many features with lymphoma including generalized lymphadenopathy, hepatosplenomegaly, and systemic symptoms of fever, fatigue, and weight loss. Pulmonary symptoms may be seen in ~50% of patients. KS is present in 75–82% of cases. Lymph node biopsies reveal a predominance of interfollicular plasma cells and/or germinal centers with vascularization and an "onionskin" (hyaline vascular) appearance. Prior to the availability of cART, HIV-infected patients with multicentric Castleman's disease had a 15-fold increased risk of developing non-Hodgkin's lymphoma compared with HIV-infected patients in general. Treatment typically involves chemotherapy. Anecdotal reports of success with rituximab suggest that more specific treatment may be successful, although, in one series treatment with rituximab was associated with worsening of coexisting KS. The median survival of patients with treated multicentric Castleman's disease pre-cART was initially reported as 14 months. This has increased to a 2-year survival of more than 90% in the era of cART.

Evidence of infection with *human papillomavirus* (HPV), associated with *intraepithelial dysplasia of the cervix* or *anus*, is approximately twice as common in HIV-infected individuals as in the general population and can lead to intraepithelial neoplasia and eventually invasive cancer. In a series of studies, HIV-infected men were examined for evidence of anal dysplasia, and Papanicolaou (Pap) smears were found to be abnormal in 20–80%. These changes tend to persist and are generally not affected by cART, raising the possibility of a subsequent transition to a more malignant condition. While the incidence of an abnormal Pap smear of the cervix is ~5% in otherwise healthy women, the incidence of abnormal cervical smears in women with HIV infection is 30–60%, and *invasive cervical cancer* is included as an AIDS-defining condition. While only small increases in the absolute numbers of cervical or anal cancers have been seen as a consequence of HIV infection, the relative risk of these conditions when one compares HIV-infected to -noninfected men and women is on the order of 10- to 100-fold. Given the high rates of dysplasia and relative risks for cervical and anal cancer, a comprehensive gynecologic and rectal examination, including Pap smear, is indicated at the initial evaluation and 6 months later for all patients with HIV infection. If these examinations are negative at both time points, the patient should be followed with yearly evaluations. If an initial or repeat Pap smear shows evidence of severe inflammation with reactive squamous changes, the next Pap smear should be performed at 3 months. If, at any time, a Pap smear shows evidence of squamous intraepithelial lesions, colposcopic examination with biopsies as indicated should be performed. The 2-year survival rate for HIV-infected patients with invasive cervical cancer is 64% compared with 79% in non-HIV-infected patients. In addition to rectal and cervical lesions, HPV can also lead to head and neck cancers. In one study of men who have sex with men, 25% were found to have oral HPV; high-risk HPV genotypes were three times more common in the HIV-infected men. The most common HPV genotypes in the general population and the genotypes upon which current HPV vaccines are based are 6, 11, 16, and 18. This is not the case in the HIV-infected population, where other genotypes such as 58 and 53 also are prominent. This raises concerns about the level of effectiveness of the current HPV vaccines for HIV-infected patients. Despite this, it is recommended that patients with HIV infection be vaccinated against HPV.

IDIOPATHIC CD4+ T LYMPHOCYTOPENIA

A syndrome was recognized in 1992 characterized by an absolute CD4+ T cell count of <300/μL or <20% of total T cells on a minimum of two occasions at least 6 weeks apart; no evidence of HIV-1, HIV-2, HTLV-1, or HTLV-2 on testing; and the absence of any defined immunodeficiency or therapy associated with decreased levels of CD4+ T cells. By mid-1993, ~100 patients had been described. After extensive multicenter investigations, a series of reports were published in early 1993, which together allowed a number of conclusions. Idiopathic CD4+ lymphocytopenia (ICL) is a very rare syndrome, as determined by studies of blood donors and cohorts of HIV-seronegative men who have sex with men. Cases were clearly identified as early as 1983 and were remarkably similar to the clinical features of ICL that had been identified decades earlier. The definition of ICL based on CD4+ T cell counts coincided with the ready availability of testing for CD4+ T cells in patients suspected of being immunodeficient. Although, as a result of immune deficiency, certain patients with ICL develop some of the opportunistic diseases (particularly cryptococcosis, nontuberculous mycobacterial infections, and cervical dysplasia) seen in HIV-infected patients, the syndrome is demographically, clinically, and immunologically unlike HIV infection and AIDS. Fewer than half of the reported ICL patients had risk factors for HIV infection, and there were wide geographic and age distributions. The fact that a significant proportion of patients did have risk factors probably reflects a selection bias, in that physicians who take care of HIV-infected patients are more likely to monitor CD4+ T cells. Approximately half of the patients are women, compared with approximately one-third among HIV-infected individuals in the United States. Many patients with ICL remained clinically stable, and their condition did not deteriorate progressively as is common with seriously immunodeficient HIV-infected patients. Approximately 15% of patients with ICL experience spontaneous reversal of the CD4+ T lymphocytopenia. Immunologic abnormalities in ICL are somewhat different from those of HIV infection. ICL patients often have increases in CD4+ T cell activation with decreases in CD8+ T cells and B cells. Furthermore, immunoglobulin levels are either normal or, more commonly, decreased in patients with ICL, compared with the usual hypergammaglobulinemia of HIV-infected individuals. Virologic studies of these patients have revealed no evidence of HIV-1, HIV-2, HTLV-1, or HTLV-2 or of any other mononuclear cell–tropic virus. Furthermore, there has been no epidemiologic evidence to suggest that a transmissible microbe was involved. The cases of ICL have been widely dispersed, with no clustering. Close contacts and sexual partners who were studied were clinically well and were serologically, immunologically, and virologically negative for HIV. ICL is a heterogeneous syndrome, and it is highly likely that there is no common cause; however, there may be common causes among subgroups of patients that are currently unrecognized.

Patients who present with laboratory data consistent with ICL should be worked up for underlying diseases that could be responsible for the immune deficiency. If no underlying cause is detected, no specific therapy should be initiated. However, if opportunistic diseases occur, they should be treated appropriately (see above). Depending on the level of the CD4+ T cell count, patients should receive prophylaxis for the commonly encountered opportunistic infections.

TREATMENT AIDS AND RELATED DISORDERS

GENERAL PRINCIPLES OF PATIENT MANAGEMENT

The CDC guidelines call for the testing for HIV infection to be a part of routine medical care. It is recommended that the patient be informed of the intention to test, as is the case with other routine laboratory determinations, and be given the opportunity to "opt out." Such an approach is critical to the goal of identifying as many infected individuals as possible since 16–18% of the >1.1 million individuals in the United States who are HIV-infected are not aware of their status. Under these circumstances of routine testing, although it is desirable, pretest counseling may not always be built into the testing process. However, no matter how well prepared a patient is for adversity, the discovery of a diagnosis of HIV infection is a devastating event. Thus, physicians should be sensitive to this fact and, where possible, execute some degree of pretest counseling to at least partially prepare the patient should the results demonstrate the presence of HIV infection. Following a diagnosis of HIV infection, the health care provider should be prepared to immediately activate support systems for the newly diagnosed patient. These should include an experienced social worker or nurse who can spend time talking to the person and ensuring that he or she is emotionally stable. Most communities have HIV support centers that can be of great help in these difficult situations.

The treatment of patients with HIV infection requires not only a comprehensive knowledge of the possible disease processes that may occur and up-to-date knowledge of and experience with cART, but also the ability to deal with the problems of a chronic, potentially life-threatening illness. A comprehensive knowledge of internal medicine is required to deal with the changing spectrum of illnesses associated with HIV infection, many of which are similar to a state of accelerated aging. Great advances have been made in the treatment of patients with HIV infection. The appropriate use of potent cART and other treatment and prophylactic interventions are of critical importance in providing each patient with the best opportunity to live a long and healthy life despite the presence of HIV infection. In contrast to the earlier days of this epidemic, a diagnosis of HIV infection need no longer be equated with having an inevitably fatal disease. In addition to medical interventions, the health care provider has a responsibility to provide each patient with appropriate counseling and education concerning their disease as part of a comprehensive care plan. Patients must be educated about the potential transmissibility of their infection and about the fact that while health care providers may refer to levels of the virus as "undetectable," this is more a reflection of the sensitivity of the assay being used to measure the virus than a comment on the presence or absence of the virus. It is important for patients to be aware that the virus is still present and capable of being transmitted at all stages of HIV disease. Thus, there must be frank discussions concerning sexual practices and the sharing of syringes and other paraphernalia used in illicit drug use. The treating physician not only must be aware of the latest medications available for patients with HIV infection but also must educate patients concerning the natural history of their illness and listen and be sensitive to their fears and concerns. As with other diseases, therapeutic decisions should be made in consultation with the patient, when possible, and with the patient's proxy if the patient is incapable of making decisions. In this regard, it is recommended that all patients with HIV infection, and in particular those with CD4+ T cell counts <200/μL, designate a trusted individual with durable power of attorney to make medical decisions on their behalf, if necessary.

Following a diagnosis of HIV infection, there are several examinations and laboratory studies that should be performed to help determine the extent of disease and provide baseline standards for future reference (**Table 226-19**). In addition to routine chemistry, fasting lipid profile, aspartate aminotransferase, alanine aminotransferase, total and direct bilirubin, fasting glucose and hematology screening panels, Pap smear, urinalysis, and chest x-ray, one should also obtain a CD4+ T cell count, two separate plasma HIV

TABLE 226-19 INITIAL EVALUATION OF THE PATIENT WITH HIV INFECTION

History and physical examination
Routine chemistry and hematology
AST, ALT, direct and indirect bilirubin
Lipid profile and fasting glucose
CD4+ T lymphocyte count
Two plasma HIV RNA levels
HIV resistance testing
HLA-B5701 screening
RPR or VDRL test
Anti-*Toxoplasma* antibody titer
PPD skin test or IFN-γ release assay
Mini-Mental Status Examination
Serologies for hepatitis A, hepatitis B, and hepatitis C
Immunization with pneumococcal polysaccharide; influenza as indicated
Immunization with hepatitis A and hepatitis B if seronegative
Counseling regarding natural history and transmission
Help contacting others who might be infected

Abbreviations: ALT, alanine aminotransferase; AST, aspartate aminotransferase; PPD, purified protein derivative; RPR, rapid plasma reagin; VDRL, Venereal Disease Research Laboratory.

RNA levels, an HIV resistance test, a rapid plasma reagin or VDRL test, an anti-*Toxoplasma* antibody titer, and serologies for hepatitis A, B, and C. A PPD test or IFN-γ release assay should be done and an MMSE performed and recorded. A pregnancy test should be done in women in whom the drug efavirenz is being considered, and HLA-B5701 testing should be done in all patients in whom the drug abacavir is being considered. Patients should be immunized with pneumococcal polysaccharide, with annual influenza shots, and, if seronegative for these viruses, with HPV, hepatitis A, and hepatitis B vaccines. The status of hepatitis C infection should be determined. In addition, patients should be counseled with regard to sexual practices and needle sharing, and counseling should be offered to those whom the patient knows or suspects may also be infected. Once these baseline activities are performed, short- and long-term medical management strategies should be developed based on the most recent information available and modified as new information becomes available. The field of HIV medicine is changing rapidly, and it is difficult to remain fully up to date. Fortunately there are a series of excellent sites on the Internet that are frequently updated, and they provide the most recent information on a variety of topics, including consensus panel reports on treatment (**Table 226-20**).

ANTIRETROVIRAL THERAPY

Combination antiretroviral therapy (cART), also referred to as highly active antiretroviral therapy (HAART), is the cornerstone of management of patients with HIV infection. Following the initiation of widespread use of cART in the United States in 1995–1996, marked declines were noted in the incidence of most AIDS-defining conditions (Fig. 226-33). Suppression of HIV replication is an important component in prolonging life as well as in improving the quality of life in patients with HIV infection. Adequate suppression requires strict adherence to prescribed regimens of antiretroviral drugs. This has been facilitated by the coformulations of antiretrovirals and the development of once-daily regimens. Unfortunately, many of the most important questions related to the treatment of HIV disease currently lack definitive answers. Among them are the questions of when therapy should be started, what the best initial regimen is, when a given regimen should be changed, and what it should be changed to when a change is made. Notwithstanding these uncertainties, the physician and patient must come to a mutually agreeable plan based on the best available data. In an effort to facilitate this process, the U.S. Department of Health and Human Services makes available on the Internet (*www.aidsinfo.nih.gov*) a series of periodically updated guidelines, including *"Guidelines for the Use of Antiretroviral Agents in HIV-Infected Adults and Adolescents"* and *"Guidelines for the Prevention of Opportunistic Infections in Persons Infected with Human Immunodeficiency Virus."* At present, an extensive clinical trials network, involving both clinical investigators and patient advocates, is in place attempting to develop improved approaches to therapy. Consortia comprising representatives of academia, industry, independent foundations, and the federal government are involved in the process of drug development, including a wide-ranging series of clinical trials. As a result, new therapies and new therapeutic strategies are continually emerging. New drugs are often available through expanded-access programs prior to official licensure. Given the complexity of this field, decisions regarding cART are best made in consultation with experts.

TABLE 226-20 RESOURCES AVAILABLE ON THE WORLD WIDE WEB ON HIV DISEASE

www.aidsinfo.nih.gov	AIDSinfo, a service of the U.S. Department of Health and Human Services, posts federally approved treatment guidelines for HIV and AIDS; provides information on federally funded and privately funded clinical trials and CDC publications and data
www.cdcnpin.org	Updates on epidemiologic data and prevention information from the CDC

Abbreviation: CDC, Centers for Disease Control and Prevention.

Currently available drugs for the treatment of HIV infection as part of a combination regimen fall into four categories: those that inhibit the viral reverse transcriptase enzyme (nucleoside and nucleotide reverse transcriptase inhibitors; nonnucleoside reverse transcriptase inhibitors), those that inhibit the viral protease enzyme (protease inhibitors), those that inhibit the viral integrase enzyme (integrase inhibitors), and those that interfere with viral entry (fusion inhibitors; CCR5 antagonists) (**Table 226-21; Fig. 226-45**).

The FDA-approved reverse transcriptase inhibitors include the *nucleoside analogues* zidovudine, didanosine, zalcitabine, stavudine, lamivudine, abacavir, and emtricitabine; the *nucleotide analogue* tenofovir; and the *nonnucleoside reverse transcriptase inhibitors* nevirapine, delavirdine, efavirenz, and etravirine (Table 226-21; Fig. 226-45). These represent the first class of drugs licensed for the treatment of HIV infection. They are indicated for this use as part of combination regimens. It should be stressed that none of these drugs should be used as monotherapy for HIV infection due to the relative ease with which drug resistance may develop under such circumstances. Thus, when lamivudine, emtricitabine, or tenofovir is used to treat hepatitis B infection in the setting of HIV infection, one should ensure that the patient is also on additional antiretroviral medication. The reverse transcriptase inhibitors block the HIV replication cycle at the point of RNA-dependent DNA synthesis, the reverse transcription step. While the nonnucleoside reverse transcriptase inhibitors are quite selective for the HIV-1 reverse transcriptase, the nucleoside and nucleotide analogues inhibit a variety of DNA polymerases in addition to those of the HIV-1 reverse transcriptase. For this reason, serious side effects are more varied with the nucleoside analogues and include mitochondrial damage that can lead to hepatic steatosis and lactic acidosis as well as peripheral neuropathy and pancreatitis. The use of either of the thymidine analogues zidovudine and stavudine has been associated with a syndrome of hyperlipidemia, glucose intolerance/insulin resistance, and fat redistribution often referred to as *lipodystrophy syndrome* (discussed in "Diseases of the Endocrine System and Metabolic Disorders," above). The reverse transcriptase inhibitors preferred for use according to the DHHS Panel on the use of antiretroviral drugs are lamivudine, emtricitabine, abacavir, tenofovir, and rilpivirine.

Lamivudine (3TC; 2′,3′-dideoxy-3′-thiacytidine) is the fifth of the nucleoside analogues to be licensed in the United States. It is the negative enantiomer of a dideoxy analogue of cytidine. In actual practice, lamivudine or the closely related drug emtricitabine (see

TABLE 226-21 ANTIRETROVIRAL DRUGS USED IN THE TREATMENT OF HIV INFECTION

Drug	Status	Indication	Dose in Combination	Supporting Data	Toxicity
Nucleoside or Nucleotide Reverse Transcriptase Inhibitors					
Zidovudine (AZT, azidothymidine, Retrovir, 3′azido-3′-deoxythymidine)	Licensed	Treatment of HIV infection in combination with other antiretroviral agents	200 mg q8h or 300 mg bid	19 vs 1 death in original placebo-controlled trial in 281 patients with AIDS or ARC	Anemia, granulocytopenia, myopathy, lactic acidosis, hepatomegaly with steatosis, headache, nausea, nail pigmentation, lipid abnormalities, lipoatrophy, hyperglycemia
		Prevention of maternal-fetal HIV transmission		In pregnant women with CD4+ T cell count ≥200/μL, AZT PO beginning at weeks 14–34 of gestation plus IV drug during labor and delivery plus PO AZT to infant for 6 weeks decreased transmission of HIV by 67.5% (from 25.5% to 8.3%), n = 363	
Lamivudine (Epivir, 2′3′-dideoxy-3′-thiacytidine, 3TC)	Licensed	In combination with other antiretroviral agents for the treatment of HIV infection	150 mg bid 300 mg qd	In combination with AZT superior to AZT alone with respect to changes in CD4+ T cell counts in 495 patients who were zidovudine-naïve and 477 patients who were zidovudine-experienced; overall CD4+ T cell counts for the zidovudine group were at baseline by 24 weeks, while in the group treated with zidovudine plus lamivudine, they were 10–50 cells/μL above baseline; 54% decrease in progression to AIDS/death compared with AZT alone	Flare of hepatitis in HBV-co-infected patients who discontinue drug
Emtricitabine (FTC, Emtriva)	Licensed	In combination with other antiretroviral agents for the treatment of HIV infection	200 mg qd	Comparable to stavudine in combination with didanosine and efavirenz in 571 treatment-naïve patients; similar to 3TC in combination with AZT or stavudine + NNRTI or PI in 440 patients doing well for ≥12 weeks on a 3TC regimen	Hepatotoxicity in HBV-co-infected patients who discontinue drug, skin discoloration
Abacavir (Ziagen)	Licensed	For treatment of HIV infection in combination with other antiretroviral agents	300 mg bid	Abacavir + AZT + 3TC equivalent to indinavir + AZT + 3TC with regard to viral load suppression (~60% in each group with <400 HIV RNA copies/mL plasma) and CD4+ T cell increase (~100/μL in each group) at 24 weeks	Hypersensitivity reaction In HLA-B5701+ individuals (can be fatal); fever, rash, nausea, vomiting, malaise or fatigue, and loss of appetite
Tenofovir (Viread)	Licensed	For use in combination with other antiretroviral agents when treatment is indicated	300 mg qd	Reduction of ~0.6 log in HIV-1 RNA levels when added to background regimen in treatment-experienced patients	Renal, osteomalacia, flare of hepatitis in HBV-co-infected patients who discontinue drug
Non-Nucleoside Reverse Transcriptase Inhibitors					
Nevirapine (Viramune)	Licensed	In combination with other antiretroviral agents for treatment of progressive HIV infection	200 mg/d × 14 days then 200 mg bid *or* 400 mg extended release qd	Increase in CD4+ T cell count, decrease in HIV RNA when used in combination with nucleosides	Skin rash, hepatotoxicity
Efavirenz (Sustiva)	Licensed	For treatment of HIV infection in combination with other antiretroviral agents	600 mg qhs	Efavirenz + AZT + 3TC comparable to indinavir + AZT + 3TC with regard to viral load suppression (a higher percentage of the efavirenz group achieved viral load <50 copies/mL, but the discontinuation rate in the indinavir group was unexpectedly high, accounting for most treatment "failures"); CD4 cell increase (~140/μL in each group) at 24 weeks	Rash, dysphoria, elevated liver function tests, drowsiness, abnormal dreams, depression, lipid abnormalities, potentially teratogenic
Etravirine (Intelence)	Licensed	In combination with other antiretroviral agents in treatment-experienced patients whose HIV is resistant to nonnucleoside reverse transcriptase inhibitors and other antiretroviral medications	200 mg bid	Higher rates of HIV RNA suppression to <50 copies/mL (56% vs 39%); greater increases in CD4+ T cell count (89 vs 64 cells) compared to placebo when given in combination with an optimized background regimen	Rash, nausea, hypersensitivity reactions

(Continued)

TABLE 226-21 ANTIRETROVIRAL DRUGS USED IN THE TREATMENT OF HIV INFECTION (*CONTINUED*)

Drug	Status	Indication	Dose in Combination	Supporting Data	Toxicity
Rilpivirine (Edurant)	Licensed	In combination with other drugs in previously untreated patients when treatment is indicated.	25 mg qd	Noninferior to efavirenz with respect to suppression at week 48 in 1368 treatment-naive individuals except in patients with pretherapy HIV RNA levels >100,000 where it was inferior	Nausea, dizziness, somnolence, vertigo, less CNS toxicity and rash than Efavirenz
Protease Inhibitors					
Ritonavir (Norvir)	Licensed	In combination with other antiretroviral agents for treatment of HIV infection when treatment is warranted	600 mg bid (also used in lower doses as pharmacokinetic booster)	Reduction in the cumulative incidence of clinical progression or death from 34% to 17% in patients with CD4+ T cell count <100/μL treated for a median of 6 months	Nausea, abdominal pain, hyperglycemia, fat redistribution, lipid abnormalities, may alter levels of many other drugs, paresthesias, hepatitis
Atazanavir (Reyataz)	Licensed	For treatment of HIV infection in combination with other antiretroviral agents	400 mg qd or 300 mg qd + ritonavir 100 mg qd when given with efavirenz	Comparable to efavirenz when given in combination with AZT + 3TC in a study of 810 treatment-naïve patients; comparable to nelfinavir when given in combination with stavudine + 3TC in a study of 467 treatment-naïve patients	Hyperbilirubinemia, PR prolongation, nausea, vomiting, hyperglycemia, fat maldistribution, rash transaminase elevations, renal stones
Darunavir (Prezista)	Licensed	In combination with 100 mg ritonavir for combination therapy in treatment-experienced adults	600 mg + 100 mg ritonavir twice daily with food	At 24 weeks, patients with prior extensive exposure to antiretrovirals treated with a new combination including darunavir showed a −1.89-log change in HIV RNA levels and a 92-cell increase in CD4+ T cells compared with −0.48 log and 17 cells in the control arm	Diarrhea, nausea, headache, skin rash, hepatotoxicity, hyperlipidemia, hyperglycemia
Entry Inhibitors					
Enfuvirtide (Fuzeon)	Licensed	In combination with other agents in treatment-experienced patients with evidence of HIV-1 replication despite ongoing antiretroviral therapy	90 mg SC bid	In treatment of experienced patients, superior to placebo when added to new optimized background (37% vs 16% with <400 HIV RNA copies/mL at 24 weeks; + 71 vs + 35 CD4+ T cells at 24 weeks)	Local injection reactions, hypersensitivity reactions, increased rate of bacterial pneumonia
Maraviroc (Selzentry)	Licensed	In combination with other antiretroviral agents in adults infected with only CCR5-tropic HIV-1	150–600 mg bid depending on concomitant medications (see text)	At 24 weeks, among 635 patients with CCR5 tropic virus and HIV-1 RNA >5000 copies/mL despite at least 6 months of prior therapy with at least 1 agent from 3 of the 4 antiretroviral drug classes, 61% of patients randomized to maraviroc achieved HIV RNA levels <400 copies/mL compared with 28% of patients randomized to placebo	Hepatotoxicity, nasopharyngitis, fever, cough, rash, abdominal pain, dizziness, musculoskeletal symptoms
Integrase Inhibitor					
Raltegravir (Isentress)	Licensed	In combination with other antiretroviral agents	400 mg bid	At 24 weeks, among 436 patients with 3-class drug resistance, 76% of patients randomized to receive raltegravir achieved HIV RNA levels <400 copies/mL compared with 41% of patients randomized to receive placebo	Nausea, headache, diarrhea, CPK elevation, muscle weakness, rhabdomyolysis
Elvitegravir (Available only in combination with cobicistat, tenofovir, and emtricitabine [Stribild])	Licensed	Fixed-dose combination	1 tablet daily	Noninferior to raltegravir or atazanavir/ritonavir in treatment-experienced patients.	Diarrhea, nausea, upper respiratory infections, headache
Dolutegravir (Tivicay)	Licensed	In combination with other antiretroviral agents	50 mg daily for treatment-naïve patients 50 mg twice daily for treatment-experienced patients or those also receiving efavirenz or rifampin	Noninferior to raltegravir, superior to efavirenz or darunavir/ritonavir	Insomnia, headache, hypersensitivity reactions, hepatotoxicity

Abbreviations: ARC, AIDS-related complex; NRTIs, nonnucleoside reverse transcriptase inhibitors.

 below) is a frequent element of many different combination regimens currently in use. These two drugs and the nucleotide reverse transcriptase inhibitor tenofovir (see below) also have activity against hepatitis B virus. For this reason flares of hepatitis may be seen in co-infected patients starting and/or or stopping any of these three agents due to the confounding issues of direct effects on hepatitis B, direct effects on HIV, and immune reconstitution (see above). To prevent the development of resistant strains of HIV, these drugs should never be used on their own for the treatment of hepatitis B in the patient with HIV infection. Lamivudine is available either alone or in coformulations including zidovudine and/or abacavir (Table 226-22). One reason behind the excellent synergy

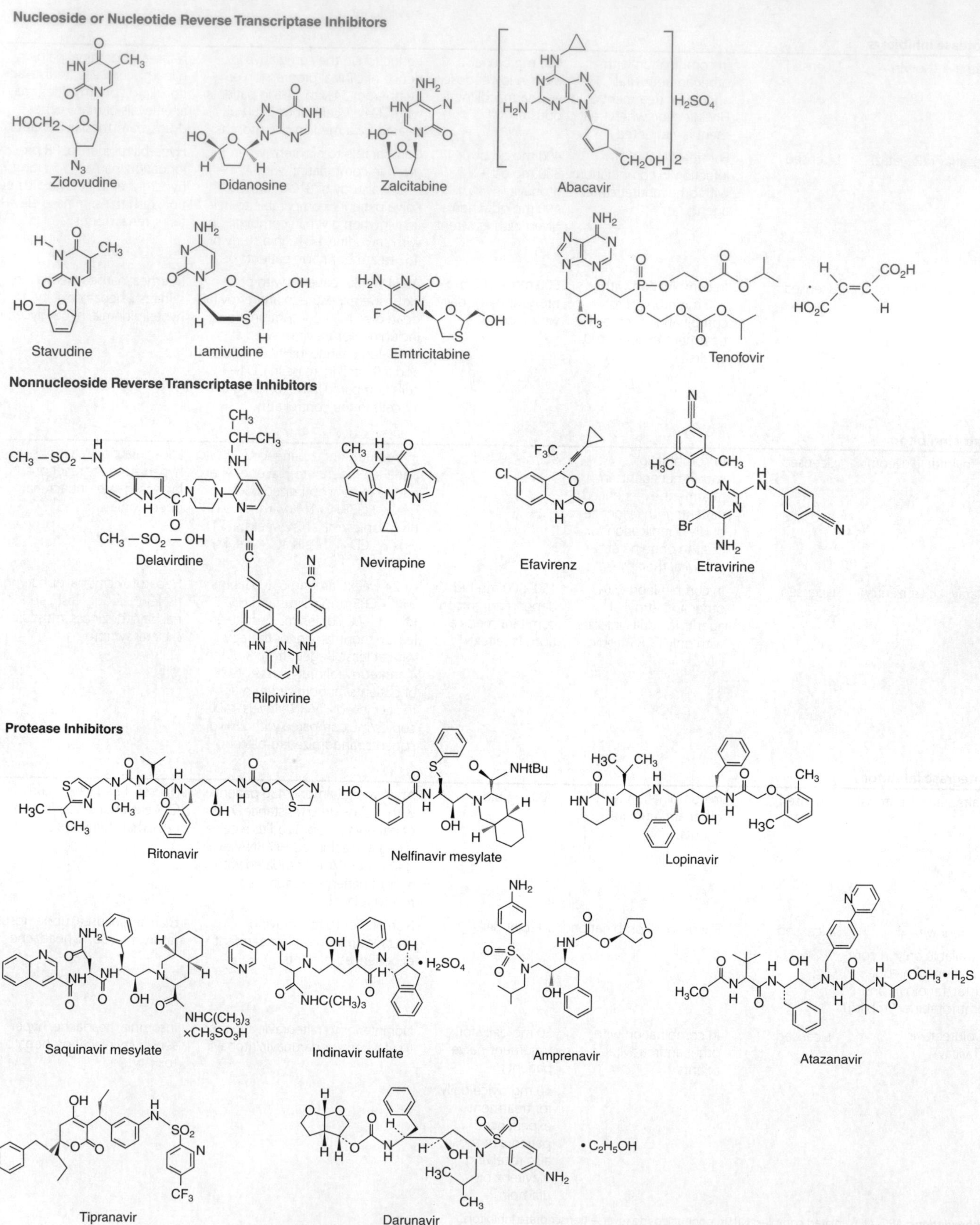

FIGURE 226-45 Molecular structures of antiretroviral agents.

Entry Inhibitors

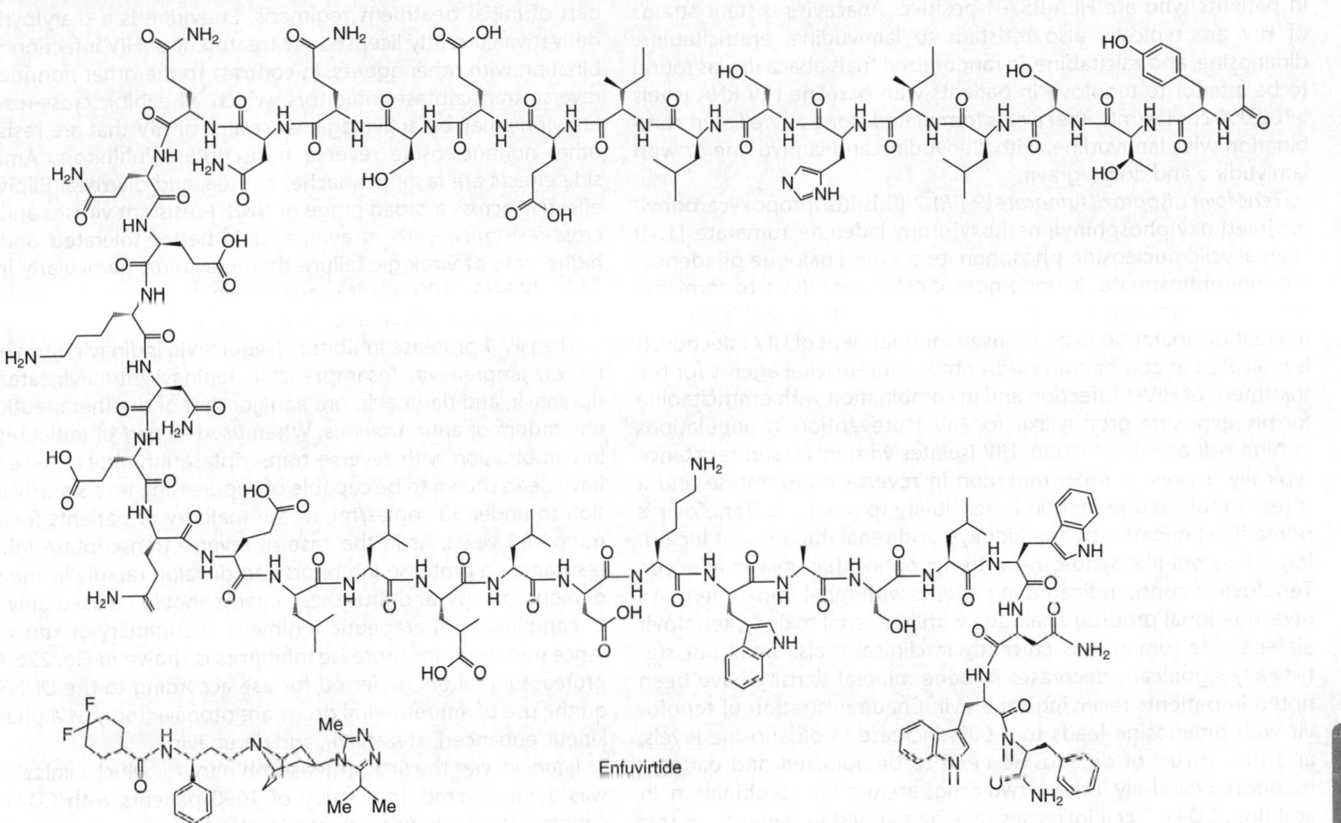

Enfuvirtide

Maraviroc

Integrase Inhibitors

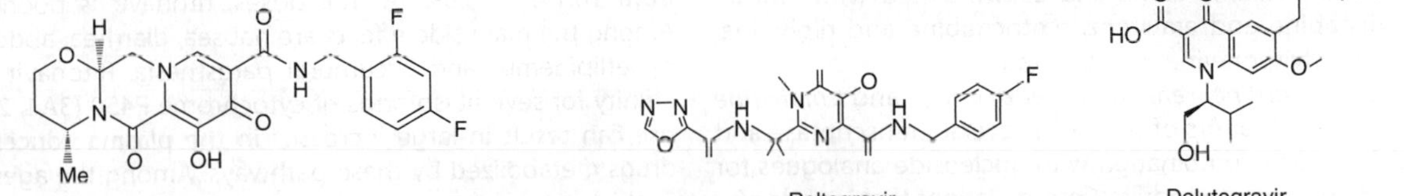

Elvitegravir

Raltegravir

Dolutegravir

FIGURE 226-45 *(Continued)*

seen between lamivudine and the other nucleoside analogues may be that strains of HIV resistant to lamivudine (M184V substitution) appear to have enhanced sensitivity to other nucleosides, and thus development of dual resistance is more difficult. In addition, there is a suggestion that 3TC-resistant strains of HIV may be less virulent and are less able to generate new mutants than are strains of HIV that are 3TC-sensitive. Lamivudine is among the best tolerated and least toxic of the nucleoside analogues.

TABLE 226-22 COMBINATION FORMULATIONS OF ANTIRETROVIRAL DRUGS

Name	Combination
Combivir	Zidovudine + lamivudine
Complera	Tenofovir + emtricitabine + rilpivirine
Epzicom	Abacavir + lamivudine
Stribild	Tenofovir + emtricitabine + elvitegravir + cobicistat
Triumeq	Abacavir + lamivudine + dolutegravir
Trizivir	Zidovudine + lamivudine + abacavir
Truvada	Tenofovir + emtricitabine
Atripla	Tenofovir + emtricitabine + efavirenz
Triomune[a]	Stavudine + lamivudine + nevirapine

[a]Not licensed in the United States.

Emtricitabine (FTC; 5-fluoro-1-(2R,5S)-[2-(hydroxymethyl)-1,3-oxathiolan-5-yl]cytosine) is the negative enantiomer of a thio analogue of cytidine with a fluorine in the 5 position. It is licensed for use in combination with other antiretroviral agents for treatment of HIV-1 infection in adults. Compared with lamivudine, it is similar in activity and has a longer half-life. It is available either alone or coformulated with tenofovir or tenofovir and efavirenz (Table 226-22). As with lamivudine, resistance to emtricitabine is associated with the M184V mutation in reverse transcriptase. Viruses showing the K65R mutation in reverse transcriptase may have reduced susceptibility to emtricitabine.

Abacavir {(1*S*,*cis*)-4-[2-amino-6-(cyclopropylamino)-9H-purin-9-yl]-2-cyclopentene-1-methanol sulfate (salt)(2:1)} is a synthetic carbocyclic analogue of the nucleoside guanosine. It is licensed to be used in combination with other antiretroviral agents for the treatment of HIV-1 infection. Hypersensitivity reactions that may occur with initial therapy or rechallenge have been reported in ~4% of patients treated with this drug, and patients developing signs or symptoms of hypersensitivity such as fever, skin rash, fatigue, and GI symptoms should discontinue the drug and not restart it. Fatal hypersensitivity reactions have been reported with rechallenge. Abacavir hypersensitivity occurs with a higher frequency in patients who are HLA-B5701-positive. It is recommended that patients be screened for HLA-B5701 prior to initiation of abacavir and that abacavir only be used as a last resort and with close monitoring in patients who are HLA-B5701-positive. Abacavir-resistant strains of HIV are typically also resistant to lamivudine, emtricitabine, didanosine, and zalcitabine. In randomized trials abacavir was found to be inferior to tenofovir in patients with baseline HIV RNA levels >100,000 copies/mL. Abacavir is formulated alone as well as in combination with lamivudine, with zidovudine and lamivudine or with lamivudine and dolutegravir.

Tenofovir disoproxil fumarate (9-[(*R*)-2-[[bis[[(isopropoxycarbonyl)oxy]methoxy]phosphinyl]methoxy]propyl]adenine fumarate [1:1]) is an acyclic nucleoside phosphonate diester analogue of adenosine monophosphate. It undergoes diester hydrolysis to form the nucleoside monophosphate (nucleotide) tenofovir and is the first nucleotide analogue to be licensed for treatment of HIV infection. It is indicated in combination with other antiretroviral agents for the treatment of HIV-1 infection and in combination with emtricitabine for pre-exposure prophylaxis for HIV-1 prevention in populations at high risk of HIV infection. HIV isolates with increased resistance typically express a K65R mutation in reverse transcriptase and a three- to fourfold reduction in sensitivity to tenofovir. Tenofovir is primarily eliminated by the kidneys, and renal impairment including a Fanconi-like syndrome with hypophosphatemia may occur. Tenofovir is contraindicated in patients with renal impairment. An investigational prodrug analogue with less renal toxicity, tenofovir alafenamide fumarate is currently in clinical trials. Small but statistically significant decreases in bone mineral density have been noted in patients receiving tenofovir. Coadministration of tenofovir with didanosine leads to a 60% increase in didanosine levels, and thus doses of didanosine need to be adjusted and patients monitored carefully if these two drugs are used in combination. In addition, CD4+ T cell increases may be blunted in patients on this combination. Coadministration of tenofovir with atazanavir leads to a decrease in atazanavir levels, and thus low-dose ritonavir (see below) needs to be added when these drugs are used in combination. Tenofovir is available alone and coformulated with emtricitabine, emtricitabine and efavirenz, emtricitabine and rilpivirine, or emtricitabine, elvitegravir and cobicistat.

Nevirapine, delavirdine, efavirenz, etravirine, and *rilpivirine* are nonnucleoside inhibitors of the HIV-1 reverse transcriptase and are licensed for use in combination with nucleoside analogues for the treatment of HIV-infected adults. Coformulations that include efavirenz or nevirapine are available (Table 226-22). These agents inhibit reverse transcriptase by binding to regions of the enzyme outside the active site and causing conformational changes in the enzyme that render it inactive. Although these agents are active in the nanomolar range, they are also very selective for the reverse transcriptase of HIV-1, have no activity against HIV-2, and, when used as monotherapy, are associated with the rapid emergence of drug-resistant mutants (Table 226-21; **Fig. 226-46**). Efavirenz and rilpivirine are administered once a day, nevirapine and etravirine twice a day, and delavirdine three times a day. All are associated with the development of a maculopapular rash, generally seen within the first few weeks of therapy. While it is possible to treat through this rash, it is important to be sure that one is not dealing with a more severe eruption such as Stevens-Johnson syndrome by looking carefully for signs of mucosal involvement, significant fever, or painful lesions with desquamation. Severe, life-threatening, and in some cases fatal hepatotoxicity, including fulminant and cholestatic hepatitis, hepatic necrosis, and hepatic failure, have been reported in patients treated with nevirapine. There is a suggestion that this is more common in women with higher CD4+ T cell counts. Many patients treated with efavirenz note a feeling of light-headedness, dizziness, or out of sorts following the initiation of therapy. Some complain of vivid dreams. These symptoms tend to disappear after several weeks of therapy. Aside from difficulties with dreams, taking efavirenz at bedtime may minimize the side effects. Efavirenz may cause fetal harm when administered during the first trimester to a pregnant woman. Women of childbearing potential should undergo pregnancy testing prior to initiation of efavirenz. Efavirenz is commonly used in combination with two nucleoside analogues as part of initial treatment regimens. Etravirine is a diarylpyrimidine derivative currently licensed for treatment of HIV infection in combination with other agents. In contrast to the other nonnucleoside reverse transcriptase inhibitors, which all exhibit cross-resistance, etravirine may be active against strains of HIV that are resistant to other nonnucleoside reverse transcriptase inhibitors. Among its side effects are rash, headache, nausea, and diarrhea. Rilpivirine is effective across a broad range of NNRTI-resistant viruses and shares cross-resistance with etravirine. It is better tolerated and a has higher rate of virologic failure than efavirenz, particularly in those with HIV RNA >100,000. It is only available as part of a combination regimen with tenofovir and emtricitabine.

The HIV-1 protease inhibitors (saquinavir, indinavir, ritonavir, nelfinavir, amprenavir, fosamprenavir, lopinavir/ritonavir, atazanavir, tipranavir, and darunavir) are a major part of the therapeutic armamentarium of antiretrovirals. When used as part of initial regimens in combination with reverse transcriptase inhibitors, these agents have been shown to be capable of suppressing levels of HIV replication to under 50 copies/mL in the majority of patients for a minimum of 5 years. As in the case of reverse transcriptase inhibitors, resistance to protease inhibitors can develop rapidly in the setting of monotherapy, and thus these agents should be used only as part of combination therapeutic regimens. A summary of known resistance mutations for protease inhibitors is shown in Fig. 226-46. The protease inhibitors preferred for use according to the DHHS Panel on the use of antiretroviral drugs are ritonavir (only as a pharmacokinetic enhancer), atazanavir, and darunavir.

Ritonavir was the first protease inhibitor for which clinical efficacy was demonstrated. In a study of 1090 patients with CD4+ T cell counts <100/μL who were randomized to receive either placebo or ritonavir in addition to any other licensed medications, patients receiving ritonavir had a reduction in the cumulative incidence of clinical progression or death from 34% to 17%. Mortality decreased from 10.1% to 5.8%. At full doses, ritonavir is poorly tolerated. Among the main side effects are nausea, diarrhea, abdominal pain, hyperlipidemia, and circumoral paresthesia. Ritonavir has a high affinity for several isoforms of cytochrome P450 (3A4, 2D6), and its use can result in large increases in the plasma concentrations of drugs metabolized by these pathways. Among the agents affected in this manner are most other protease inhibitors, macrolide antibiotics, *R*-warfarin, ondansetron, rifabutin, most calcium channel blockers, glucocorticoids, and some of the chemotherapeutic agents used to treat KS and/or lymphomas. In addition, ritonavir may increase the activity of glucuronyltransferases, thus decreasing the levels of drugs metabolized by this pathway. Overall, great care must be taken when prescribing additional drugs to patients taking protease inhibitors in general and ritonavir in particular. As mentioned above, the pharmacodynamic boosting property of ritonavir, seen with doses as low as 100–200 mg once or twice a day, is often used in the setting of cART for HIV infection to derive more convenient regimens. For example, when given with low-dose ritonavir, saquinavir and indinavir can be given on twice-a-day schedules and taken with food.

Atazanavir is an azapeptide inhibitor of the HIV-1 protease that was licensed in 2003. An advantage of atazanavir is that total cholesterol and triglyceride levels do not increase as much with atazanavir as with other protease inhibitors. This coupled with the fact that it can be given on a once-daily schedule made atazanavir a popular component of initial treatment regimens following its licensure. Atazanavir is associated with increases in serum bilirubin, renal stones, and prolongations of the ECG PR interval. Atazanavir-resistant isolates emerging in previously treatment-naïve individuals frequently harbor an I50L substitution. This mutation in some instances is associated with increased sensitivity to other protease inhibitors. Atazanavir requires an acidic gastric pH for absorption, and its use in combination with a proton pump inhibitor is contraindicated due to concerns about absorption. Atazanavir is an inhibitor of cytochrome P3A, and its use may be associated with

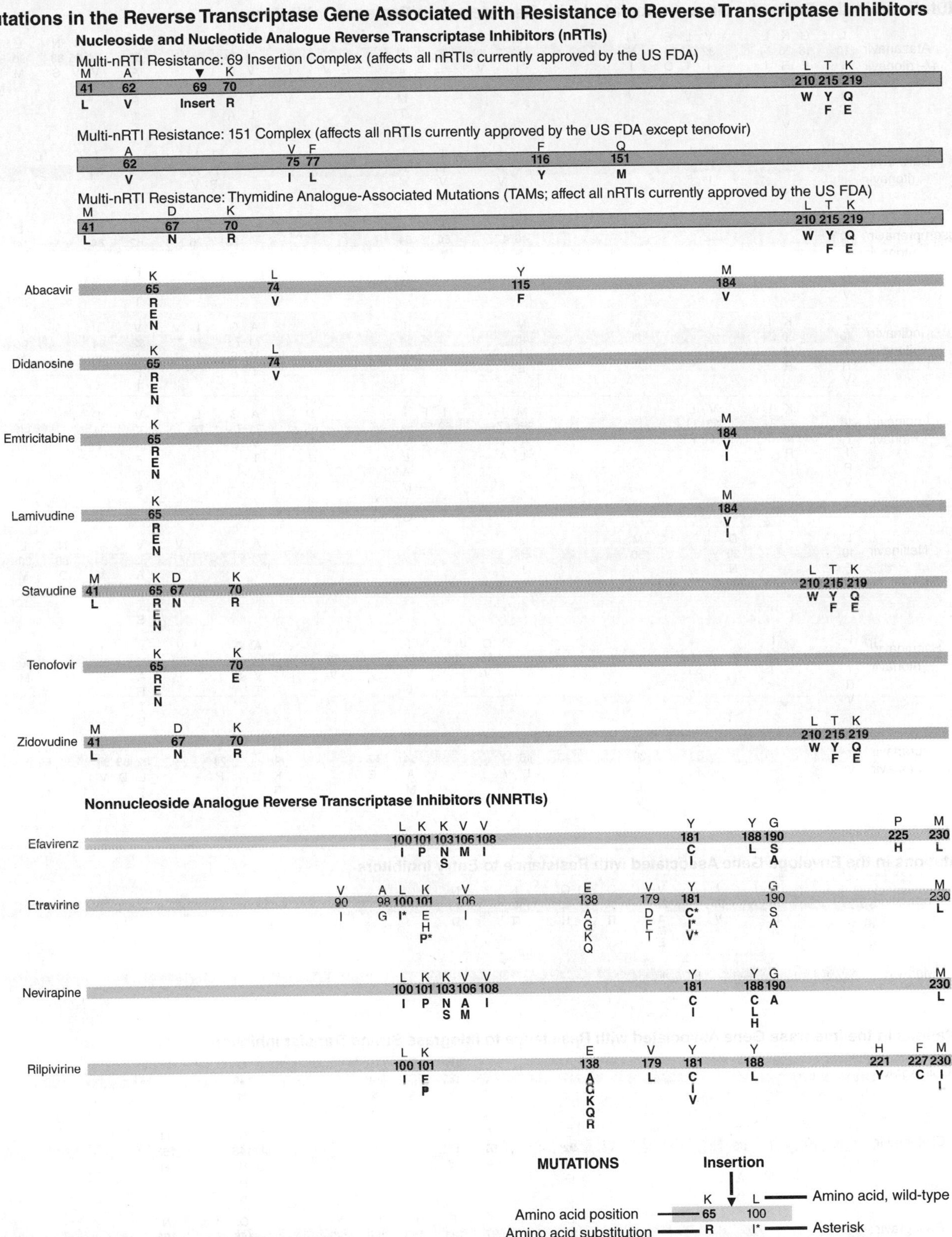

FIGURE 226-46 Amino acid substitutions conferring resistance to antiretroviral drugs. For each amino acid residue, the letter above the bar indicates the amino acid associated with wild-type virus and the letter(s) below indicate the substitution(s) that confer viral resistance. The number shows the position of the mutation in the protein. Mutations selected by protease inhibitors in Gag cleavage sites are not listed. HR1 indicates first heptad repeat; NAMs indicates nRTI-associated mutations; nRTI indicates nucleoside reverse transcriptase inhibitor; NNRTI indicates nonnucleoside reverse transcriptase inhibitor; PI indicates protease inhibitor. Amino acid abbreviations: A, alanine; C, cysteine; D, aspartate; E, glutamic acid; F, phenylalanine; G, glycine; H, histidine; I, isoleucine; K, lysine; L, leucine; M, methionine; N, asparagine; P, proline; Q, glutamine; R, arginine; S, serine; T, threonine; V, valine; W, tryptophan; Y, tyrosine. *(Reprinted with permission from the International Antiviral Society—USA. AM Wensing, V Calvez, HR Günthard et al: 2014 Update of the Drug Resistance Mutations in HIV-1. Top Antivir Med. 2014; 22(3):642–650. Updated information [and thorough explanatory notes] is available at www.iasusa.org.)*

Mutations in the Protease Gene Associated with Resistance to Protease Inhibitors

Atazanavir +/– ritonavir

Wild type	L	G	K	L	V	L	E	M	M	G	I	F	I	D	I	I	A	G	V	I	I	N	L	I
Position	10	16	20	24	32	33	34	36	46	48	**50**	53	54	60	62	64	71	73	82	**84**	85	**88**	90	93
Mutations	I, F, V, C	E	R, M, I, T, V	I	I	I, F, V	Q	I, L, V	I, L	V	L	L, Y	L, V, M, T, A	E	V	L, M, V	V, I, T, L	C, S, T, A	A, T, F, I	V	V	S	M	L, M

Darunavir/ritonavir

Wild type	V	V	L	I	I	I	T	L	I	L
Position	11	32	33	**47**	**50**	**54**	74	**76**	**84**	89
Mutations	I	I	F	V	V	M, L	P	V	V	V

Fosamprenavir/ritonavir

Wild type	L	V	M	I	I	I	G	L	V	I	L
Position	10	32	46	47	**50**	**54**	73	76	82	**84**	90
Mutations	F, I, R, V	I	I, L	V	V	L, V, M	S	V	A, F, S, T	V	M

Indinavir/ritonavir

Wild type	L	K	L	V	M	M	I	A	G	L	V	V	I	L
Position	10	20	24	32	36	**46**	54	71	73	76	77	**82**	**84**	90
Mutations	I, R, V	M, R	I	I	I	I, L	V	V, T	S, A	V	I	A, F, T	V	M

Lopinavir/ritonavir

Wild type	L	K	L	V	L	M	I	I	F	I	L	A	G	L	V	I	L
Position	10	20	24	**32**	33	46	**47**	50	53	54	63	71	73	**76**	**82**	84	90
Mutations	F, I, R, V	M, R	I	I	F	I, L	V, A	V	L	V, L, A, M, T, S	P	V, T	S	V	A, F, T, S	V	M

Nelfinavir

Wild type	L	D	M	M	A	V	V	I	N	L
Position	10	**30**	36	46	71	77	82	84	88	**90**
Mutations	F, I	N	I	I, L	V, T	I	A, F, T, S	V	D, S	M

Saquinavir/ritonavir

Wild type	L	L	G	I	I	A	G	V	V	I	L
Position	10	24	**48**	54	62	71	73	77	82	84	**90**
Mutations	I, R, V	I	V	V, L	V	V, T	S	I	A, F, T, S	V	M

Tipranavir ritonavir

Wild type	L	L	M	K	M	I	I	Q	H	T	V	N	I	L
Position	10	33	36	43	46	**47**	54	**58**	69	**74**	**82**	**83**	**84**	89
Mutations	V	F	I, L, V	T	L	V	A, M, V	E	K, R	P	L, T	D	V	I, M, V

Mutations in the Envelope Gene Associated with Resistance to Entry Inhibitors

Enfuvirtide

Wild type	G	I	V	Q	Q	N	N
Position	**36**	**37**	**38**	**39**	**40**	**42**	**43**
Mutations	**D, S**	**V**	**A, M, E**	**R**	**H**	**T**	**D**

Maraviroc: Activity limited to patients with R5 viruses

Mutations in the Integrase Gene Associated with Resistance to Integrase Strand Transfer Inhibitors

Dolutegravir

Wild type	F	E	G	Q
Position	**121**	**138**	**140**	**148**
Mutations	Y	A, K	**S**, A	**H**

Elvitegravir

Wild type	T	E	T	F	S	Q	N
Position	**66**	**92**	**97**	**121**	**147**	**148**	**155**
Mutations	**I**, A, K	**Q**, G	A	**Y**	**G**	**H**, H, K	**H**

Raltegravir

Wild type	L	E	T	F	E	G	Y	Q	N
Position	**74**	**92**	**97**	**121**	**138**	**140**	**143**	**148**	**155**
Mutations	M	Q	A	**Y**	A, K	A, S	**R, H, C**	**H, K, R**	**H**

FIGURE 226-46 *(Continued)*

increased levels of calcium channel blockers, macrolide antibiotics, HMG-CoA reductase inhibitors, and sildenafil. Levels of atazanavir are lower in the presence of tenofovir or efavirenz. In these settings, levels of atazanavir should be boosted with the use of low-dose ritonavir. In a head-to-head comparison, more patients discontinued atazanavir than either darunavir or raltegravir. The main reasons for discontinuation were bilirubin elevations and gastrointestinal side effects.

Darunavir is a nonpeptidic HIV protease inhibitor initially licensed in 2006. It is indicated for coadministration with 100 mg of ritonavir and other antiretroviral agents for the treatment of HIV infection. In initial studies in treatment-experienced subjects, 46% of patients achieved a reduction in HIV RNA viral loads to <50 copies/mL. Studies in treatment-naïve patients demonstrated efficacy superior to lopinavir/ritonavir-containing regimens but inferior to dolutegravir. Skin rash, which may be severe, is seen in 7% of patients and may be related to the sulfonamide moiety contained in the molecule. GI intolerance and headache are the other most frequent side effects.

Entry inhibitors act by interfering with the binding of HIV to its receptor or co-receptor or by interfering with the process of fusion (see above). The first drug in this class to be licensed was the fusion inhibitor *enfuvirtide*, or T-20, followed by the CCR5 antagonist *maraviroc*. A variety of additional small molecules that bind to HIV-1 co-receptors are currently in clinical trials.

Enfuvirtide is a linear 36-amino-acid synthetic peptide with the *N* terminus acetylated and the *C* terminus a carboxamide. It is composed of naturally occurring L-amino acid residues and interferes with the fusion of the viral and cellular membranes by binding to the HR1 region in the gp41 subunit of the HIV-1 envelope. This binding interferes with the coil-coil interaction required to approximate the viral envelope and the host cell membrane during the process of viral fusion. Enfuvirtide was licensed in 2003 for treatment of HIV-1 infection in combination with other antiretroviral agents in treatment-experienced patients with ongoing viral replication despite antiretroviral therapy. Enfuvirtide is not active against HIV-2. Enfuvirtide-resistant isolates of HIV exhibit amino acid changes in positions 36–45 of gp41. In two independent studies, patients who had persistent viremia despite prior treatment with agents from all three available classes of drugs were randomized to receive an individualized regimen (based on prior treatment history and resistance profile) with or without enfuvirtide. The change in plasma HIV-1 RNA from baseline was ~1 log greater (–1.53 vs –0.68) in patients randomized to receive enfuvirtide. Among the drawbacks of this agent are the requirement for twice-a-day injection, the occurrence of injection-site reactions in close to 100% of patients, and an increase in bacterial pneumonia in the enfuvirtide-treated patients compared with the control patients (4.68 vs 0.61 events per 100 patient-years) in the phase III studies.

Maraviroc is a CCR5 antagonist that interferes with HIV binding at the stage of co-receptor engagement. It was licensed in 2007 for treatment of HIV infection in combination with other agents in treatment-experienced patients infected with only CCR5-tropic (R5) virus resistant to multiple agents. The license was extended in 2009 to include treatment naïve patients with R5 virus. A co-receptor tropism assay should be performed if one is considering the use of maraviroc to ensure that the potential patient is only harboring R5 viruses. In phase III trials of treatment-experienced patients randomized to receive optimal therapy plus maraviroc or placebo, 61% of patients randomized to maraviroc achieved HIV RNA levels <400 copies/mL compared with 28% of patients randomized to placebo. An allergic reaction–associated hepatotoxicity has been reported with maraviroc. Among the most common side effects of maraviroc are dizziness due to postural hypotension, cough, fever, colds, rash, muscle and joint pain, and stomach pain. Maraviroc is a substrate of CYP3A and Pgp, and the recommend dose varies depending on concomitant medications. In combination with nucleoside analogues, tipranavir/ritonavir, enfuvirtide, and/or nevirapine, the dose is 300 mg twice daily. In the presence of CYP3A inhibitors, such as most protease inhibitors, the dose is 150 mg twice daily. In the presence of CYP3A inducers such as efavirenz, the dose is 600 mg twice daily.

Integrase inhibitors act by blocking the action of the HIV integrase enzyme and thus preventing integration of the HIV provirus into the host cell genome. They are among the most potent and safest of the antiretroviral drugs and frequently part of initial combination regimens. The three licensed integrase inhibitors are raltegravir, elvitegravir and dolutegravir.

Raltegravir is an inhibitor of the viral enzyme integrase and the first of this class to be approved. It acts by interfering with the binding of the preintegration complex to host DNA and as such is referred to as an integrase strand transfer inhibitor (INSTI). Raltegravir was approved in 2007 for treatment of HIV infection in combination with other agents in treatment-experienced patients, and the approval was extended in 2009 to include treatment-naïve patients. Raltegravir exhibits a wide range of activity against HIV-1 and HIV-2, including viruses with multiple resistance mutations to other classes of drugs. As with several other compounds, resistance to raltegravir comes at the expense of replicative fitness. In two phase III studies in which 436 patients with 3-class antiretroviral drug resistance were randomized to an optimized background regimen with raltegravir or placebo, 76% of patients receiving raltegravir achieved HIV RNA levels <400 copies/mL compared with 41% of patients randomized to the placebo arm. In contrast to many other antiretroviral drugs the side-effect profile of raltegravir is minimal, with similar side-effect profiles noted for the raltegravir and placebo groups.

Elvitegravir is an integrase inhibitor that was approved in 2012 as part of a fixed-dose combination tablet also containing tenofovir, emtricitabine, and cobicistat (Stribild). The cobicistat acts much in the same way as low-dose ritonavir to boost the concentrations of elvitegravir by inhibiting CYP3A such that once-a-day dosing of Stribild is sufficient. Elvitegravir demonstrates cross-resistance with raltegravir. In two randomized, controlled trials, elvitegravir was found to be noninferior to efavirenz in one study and noninferior to atazanavir/ritonavir in the other. The most common side effects experienced with elvitegravir are diarrhea, nausea, upper respiratory infection, and headache. The cobicistat component of the fixed-dose tablet inhibits tubular secretion of creatinine, resulting in increases in serum creatinine, and is not recommended for patients with estimated creatinine clearances <70 mL/min.

Dolutegravir was approved in 2013 for use as part of a combination regimen in either treatment-naïve or -experienced patients. It comes as a 50-mg tablet and is given once daily in treatment-naïve patients and twice daily in treatment-experienced patients. Isolates of HIV that have developed resistance to raltegravir or elvitegravir may still be sensitive to dolutegravir. Its main side effects are insomnia and headache. In two randomized, controlled trials it has been shown to be superior to either efavirenz (n = 833) or darunavir/ritonavir (n = 484) in combination with nucleos(t)ide analogues due to lower rates of discontinuation. In a third trial of 822 patients it was shown to be noninferior to raltegravir.

PRINCIPLES OF THERAPY

The principles of therapy for HIV infection have been articulated by a panel sponsored by the U.S. Department of Health and Human Services as a working group of the NIH Office of AIDS Research Advisory Council. These principles are summarized in **Table 226-23**. As noted in these guidelines, cART of HIV infection does not lead to eradication or cure of HIV. The single possible exception to this is an individual with HIV infection who received an allogeneic stem cell transplant for treatment of acute myelogenous leukemia. His conditioning regimen included cytotoxic chemotherapy, total-body irradiation, and antithymocyte immunoglobulin. The donor cells were homozygous for the CCR5Δ32 mutation (see above) and thus resistant to HIV infection. Despite cART being stopped the day of the transplant, the patient has exhibited no signs of active HIV infection for more than 8 years.

Treatment decisions must take into account the fact that one is dealing with a chronic infection that requires daily therapy. While early therapy is generally the rule in infectious diseases, immediate treatment of every HIV-infected individual upon diagnosis may not be prudent, and therapeutic decisions must take into account the balance between risks and benefits. Patients initiating antiretroviral therapy must be willing to commit to life-long treatment and understand the importance of adherence to their prescribed regimen. The importance of adherence is illustrated by the observation that treatment interruption is associated with rapid increases in HIV RNA levels, rapid declines in CD4+ T cell counts, and an increased risk of clinical progression. While it seems reasonable to assume that the complications associated with cART could be minimized by

TABLE 226-23 PRINCIPLES OF THERAPY OF HIV INFECTION

1. Ongoing HIV replication leads to immune system damage, progression to AIDS, and systemic immune activation.
2. Plasma HIV RNA levels indicate the magnitude of HIV replication and the rate of CD4+ T cell destruction. CD4+ T cell counts indicate the current level of competence of the immune system.
3. Maximal suppression of viral replication is a goal of therapy; the greater the suppression the less likely the appearance of drug-resistant quasispecies.
4. The most effective therapeutic strategies involve the simultaneous initiation of combinations of effective anti-HIV drugs with which the patient has not been previously treated and that are not cross-resistant with antiretroviral agents that the patient has already received.
5. The antiretroviral drugs used in combination regimens should be used according to optimum schedules and dosages.
6. The number of available drugs is limited. Any decisions on antiretroviral therapy have a long-term impact on future options for the patient.
7. Women should receive optimal antiretroviral therapy regardless of pregnancy status.
8. The same principles apply to children and adults. The treatment of HIV-infected children involves unique pharmacologic, virologic, and immunologic considerations.
9. Compliance is an important part of ensuring maximal effect from a given regimen. The simpler the regimen, the easier it is for the patient to be compliant.

Source: Modified from *Principles of Therapy of HIV Infection*, USPHS, and the Henry J. Kaiser Family Foundation.

TABLE 226-24 INITIAL COMBINATION REGIMENS FOR ANY TREATMENT-NAÏVE PATIENT REGARDLESS OF HIV RNA LEVEL OR CD4 COUNT

I. Non-Nucleoside Reverse Transcriptase Inhibitor Based:
   - Efavirenz + tenofovir + emtricitabine

II. Protease Inhibitor Based:
   - Atazanavir/ritonavir + tenofovir + emtricitabine
   - Darunavir/ritonavir + tenofovir + emtricitabine

III. Integrase Inhibitor Based:
   - Dolutegravir + tenofovir + emtricitabine
   - Raltegravir + tenofovir + emtricitabine

Source: *Guidelines for the Use of Antiretroviral Agents in HIV-Infected Adults and Adolescents*, USPHS.

intermittent treatment regimens designed to minimize exposure to the drugs in question, all efforts to do so have paradoxically been associated with an increase in serious adverse events in the patients randomized to intermittent therapy, suggesting that some "non-AIDS-associated" serious adverse events such as heart attack and stroke may be linked to HIV replication. Thus, unless contraindicated for reasons of toxicity, patients started on cART should remain on cART.

At present, the U.S. Department of Health and Human Services Guidelines panel recommends that everyone with HIV infection be treated with cART. The evidence for this is strongest for patients with CD4+ T cell counts <350/μL. Clinical trials are underway to more carefully determine the benefit of initiating therapy in patients with CD4+ T cell counts ≥350/μL. In addition, one may wish to administer a 6-week course of therapy to uninfected individuals immediately following a high-risk exposure to HIV. The combination of tenofovir and emtricitabine is also indicated for pre-exposure prophylaxis in individuals at high risk of HIV infection. For patients diagnosed with an opportunistic infection and HIV infection at the same time, one may consider a 2- to 4-week delay in the initiation of antiretroviral therapy during which time treatment is focused on the opportunistic infection. This delay may decrease the severity of any subsequent immune reconstitution inflammatory syndrome by lowering the antigenic burden of the opportunistic infection. For patients with advanced HIV infection (CD4+ <50 cells/μL), however, cART should be initiated as soon as possible.

Once the decision has been made to initiate therapy, the health care provider must decide which drugs to use as the first regimen. The decision regarding choice of drugs not only will affect the immediate response to therapy but also will have implications regarding options for future therapeutic regimens. The initial regimen is usually the most effective insofar as the virus has yet to develop significant resistance. HIV is capable of rapidly developing resistance to any single agent, and therapy must be given as a multidrug combination. Given that patients can be infected with viruses that harbor drug resistance mutations, it is recommended that a viral genotype be done prior to the initiation of therapy to optimize the selection of antiretroviral agents. The combination regimens currently recommended for initial therapy in any treatment-naïve patient are listed in **Table 226-24**. Other regimens containing abacavir and rilpivirine may be appropriate for patients with HIV RNA levels <100,000 copies/mL. It is currently unclear whether treatment-naïve individuals with <50 copies/mL of HIV RNA benefit from cART. Following the initiation of therapy one should expect a rapid, at least 1-log (tenfold) reduction in plasma HIV RNA levels within 1–2 months and then a slower decline in plasma HIV RNA levels to <50 copies/mL within 6 months. During this same time there should be a rise in the CD4+ T cell count of 100–150/μL that is also particularly brisk during the first month of therapy. Subsequently, one should anticipate a CD4+ T cell count increase of 50–100 cells/year until numbers approach normal. Many clinicians feel that failure to achieve these endpoints is an indication for a change in therapy. Other reasons for a change in therapy include a persistently declining CD4+ T cell count, a consistent increase in HIV RNA levels to >200 copies/mL, clinical deterioration, or drug toxicity (**Table 226-25**). As in the case of initiating therapy, changing therapy may have a lasting impact on future therapeutic options. When changing therapy because of treatment failure (clinical progression or worsening laboratory parameters), it is important to attempt to provide a regimen with at least two new active drugs. This decision can be guided by resistance testing (see below). In the patient in whom a change is made for reasons of drug toxicity, a simple replacement of one drug is reasonable. It should be stressed that in attempting to sort out a drug toxicity it may be advisable to hold all therapy for a period of time to distinguish between drug toxicity and disease progression. Drug toxicity will usually begin to show signs of reversal within 1–2 weeks. Prior to changing a treatment regimen because of drug failure, it is important to ensure that the patient has been adherent to the prescribed regimen. As in the case of initial therapy, the simpler the new therapeutic regimen, the easier it is for the patient to be compliant. Plasma HIV RNA levels should be monitored every 3–6 months during therapy and more frequently if one is contemplating a change in regimen due to an increase in viral load or immediately following a change in regimen.

In order to determine an optimal therapeutic regimen for initial therapy or for a patient on a failing regimen, one may attempt to measure antiretroviral drug susceptibility through genotyping or phenotyping of HIV quasispecies and to determine adequacy of dosing through measurement of drug levels. Genotyping may be done through cDNA sequencing. Phenotypic assays typically measure the

TABLE 226-25 INDICATIONS FOR CHANGING ANTIRETROVIRAL THERAPY IN PATIENTS WITH HIV INFECTION[a]

- Less than a 1-log drop in plasma HIV RNA by 4 weeks following the initiation of therapy
- A reproducible significant increase (defined as threefold or greater) from the nadir of plasma HIV RNA level not attributable to intercurrent infection, vaccination, or test methodology
- Persistently declining CD4+ T cell numbers
- Clinical deterioration
- Side effects

[a]Generally speaking, a change should involve the initiation of at least two drugs felt to be effective in the given patient. The exception to this is when change is being made to manage toxicity, in which case a single substitution is reasonable.

Source: *Guidelines for the Use of Antiretroviral Agents in HIV-Infected Adults and Adolescents*, USPHS.

enzymatic activity of viral enzymes in the presence or absence of different concentrations of different drugs and have also been used to determine co-receptor tropism. These assays will generally detect quasispecies present at a frequency of ≥10%. NextGen sequencing may allow detection of quasispecies at frequencies down to 1%. It is generally recommended that resistance testing be used in selecting initial therapy in settings where the risk of transmission of resistant virus is high (such as the United States and Europe) and in determining new regimens for patients experiencing virologic failure while on therapy. Resistance testing may be of particular value in distinguishing drug-resistant virus from poor patient compliance. Due to the rapid rate at which drug-resistant viruses revert to wild-type, it is recommended that resistance testing performed in the setting of drug failure be carried out while the patient is still on the failing regimen. Measurement of plasma drug levels can also be used to tailor an individual treatment. The inhibitory quotient, defined as the trough blood level/IC_{50} of the patient's virus, is used by some to determine the adequacy of dosing of a given treatment regimen. Despite the best of efforts there will still be patients with ongoing high levels of HIV replication while receiving the best available therapy. These patients will receive benefit from remaining on antiretroviral therapy even though it is not fully suppressive.

In addition to the licensed medications discussed above, a large number of experimental agents are being evaluated as possible therapies for HIV infection. Therapeutic strategies are being developed to interfere with virtually every step of the replication cycle of the virus (Fig. 226-3). In addition, as more is discovered about the role of the immune system in controlling viral replication, additional strategies, generically referred to as "immune based therapies," are being developed as a complement to antiviral therapy. Among the antiviral agents in early clinical trials are additional nucleoside and nucleotide analogues, protease inhibitors, fusion inhibitors, receptor and co-receptor antagonists, and integrase inhibitors as well as new antiviral strategies including antisense nucleic acids and maturation inhibitors. Among the immune-based therapies being evaluated are IFN-α, bone marrow transplantation, adoptive transfer of lymphocytes genetically modified to resist infection or enhance HIV-specific immunity, active immunotherapy with inactivated HIV or its components, IL-7, and IL-15.

HIV AND THE HEALTH CARE WORKER

Health care workers, especially those who deal with large numbers of HIV-infected patients, have a small but definite risk of becoming infected with HIV as a result of professional activities (see "Occupational Transmission of HIV: Health Care Workers, Laboratory Workers, and the Health Care Setting," above). The first case of HIV transmission from a patient to health care worker was reported in 1984. Occupational transmission of HIV has been reported in most countries; as noted above, the global number of HIV infections among health care workers attributable to punctures/cuts has been estimated to be 1000 cases (range, 200–5000) per year.

In the United States 57 health care workers for whom case investigations were completed as of 2010 had documented seroconversions to HIV following occupational exposures. The routes of exposure resulting in infection were as follows: 48 percutaneous (puncture/cut injury); 5 mucocutaneous (mucous membrane and/or skin); 2 both percutaneous and mucocutaneous; and 2 of unknown route. Of the 57 health care personnel, 49 were exposed to HIV-infected blood; 3 to concentrated virus in a laboratory; 1 to visibly bloody fluid; and 4 to an unspecified fluid. The individuals with documented seroconversions included 19 laboratory workers (16 of whom were clinical laboratory workers), 24 nurses, 6 physicians, 2 surgical technicians, 1 dialysis technician, 1 respiratory therapist, 1 health aide, 1 embalmer/morgue technician, and 2 housekeeper/maintenance workers. In addition, more than 140 possible cases of occupationally acquired HIV infection have been reported among health care personnel in the United States. The number of these workers who actually acquired their infection through occupational exposures is not known. Taken together, data from several large studies suggest that the risk of HIV infection following a percutaneous exposure to HIV-contaminated blood is ~0.3%, and after a mucous membrane exposure, ~0.09%. Although episodes of HIV transmission after nonintact skin exposure have been documented, the average risk for transmission by this route has not been precisely quantified but is estimated to be less than the risk for mucous membrane exposures. The risk for transmission after exposure to fluids or tissues other than HIV-infected blood also has not been quantified but is probably considerably lower than for blood exposures. A seroprevalence survey of 3420 orthopedic surgeons, 75% of whom practiced in an area with a relatively high prevalence of HIV infection and 39% of whom reported percutaneous exposure to patient blood, usually through an accident involving a suture needle, failed to reveal any cases of possible occupational infection, suggesting that the risk of infection with a suture needle may be considerably less than that with a blood-drawing (hollow-bore) needle.

Most cases of health care worker seroconversion occur as a result of needle-stick injuries. When one considers the circumstances that result in needle-stick injuries, it is immediately obvious that adhering to the standard guidelines for dealing with sharp objects would result in a significant decrease in this type of accident. In one study, 27% of needle-stick injuries resulted from improper disposal of the needle (over half of these were due to recapping the needle), 23% occurred during attempts to start an IV line, 22% occurred during blood drawing, 16% were associated with an IM or SC injection, and 12% were associated with giving an IV infusion.

Clinicians should consider potential occupational exposures to HIV as urgent medical concerns to ensure timely postexposure management and possible administration of postexposure antiretroviral prophylaxis (PEP). Recommendations regarding PEP must take into account that a variety of circumstances determine the risk of transmission of HIV following occupational exposure. In this regard, several factors have been associated with an increased risk for occupational transmission of HIV infection, including deep injury, the presence of visible blood on the instrument causing the exposure, injury with a device that had been placed in the vein or artery of the source patient, terminal illness in the source patient, and lack of postexposure cART in the exposed health care worker. Other important considerations when considering PEP in the health care worker include known or suspected pregnancy or breast-feeding, the possibility of exposure to drug-resistant virus, and toxicities of PEP regimens. Regardless of the decision to use PEP, the wound should be cleansed immediately and antiseptic applied. If a decision is made to offer PEP, U.S. Public Health Service guidelines recommend (1) a combination of two nucleoside analogue reverse transcriptase inhibitors given for 4 weeks for less severe exposures, or (2) a combination of two nucleoside analogue reverse transcriptase inhibitors plus a third drug given for 4 weeks for more severe exposures. Most clinicians administer the latter regimen in all cases in which a decision is made to treat. Detailed guidelines are available from the *Updated U.S. Public Health Service Guidelines for the Management of Occupational Exposures to HIV and Recommendations for Postexposure Prophylaxis* (CDC, 2005). The report emphasizes the importance of adherence to PEP when it is indicated, follow-up of exposed workers to improve PEP adherences, monitoring for adverse events (including seroconversion), and expert consultation in the management of exposures.

For consultation on the treatment of occupational exposures to HIV and other bloodborne pathogens, the clinician managing the exposed patient can call the National Clinicians' Post-Exposure Prophylaxis Hotline (PEPline) at 888-448-4911. This service is available 24 hours a day at no charge. (Additional information on the Internet is available at *www.nccc.ucsf.edu*.) PEPline support may be especially useful in challenging situations, such as when drug-resistant HIV strains are suspected or the health care worker is pregnant.

Health care workers can minimize their risk of occupational HIV infection by following the CDC guidelines of July 1991, which include adherence to universal precautions, refraining from direct patient care if one has exudative lesions or weeping dermatitis, and disinfecting and sterilizing reusable devices employed in invasive procedures.

The premise of universal precautions is that every specimen should be handled as if it came from someone infected with a bloodborne pathogen. All samples should be double-bagged, gloves should be worn when drawing blood, and spills should be immediately disinfected with bleach.

In attempting to put this small but definite risk to the health care worker in perspective, it is important to point out that ~200 health care workers die each year as a result of occupationally acquired hepatitis B infection. The tragedy in this instance is that these infections and deaths due to HBV could be greatly decreased by more extended use of the HBV vaccine. The risk of HBV infection following a needle-stick injury from a hepatitis antigen–positive patient is much higher than the risk of HIV infection (see "Transmission," above). There are multiple examples of needle-stick injuries where the patient was positive for both HBV and HIV and the health care worker became infected only with HBV. For these reasons, it is advisable, given the high prevalence of HBV infection in HIV-infected individuals, that all health care workers dealing with HIV-infected patients be immunized with the HBV vaccine.

TB is another infection common to HIV-infected patients that can be transmitted to the health care worker. For this reason, all health care workers should know their PPD status, have it checked yearly, and receive 6 months of isoniazid treatment if their skin test converts to positive. In addition, all patients in whom a diagnosis of TB is being entertained should be placed immediately in respiratory isolation, pending results of the diagnostic evaluation. The emergence of drug-resistant organisms, including the extensively drug-resistant TB strains that have been identified in Africa, has made TB an increasing problem for health care workers. This is particularly true for the health care worker with preexisting HIV infection.

One of the most charged issues ever to come between health care workers and patients is that of transmission of infection from HIV-infected health care workers to their patients. This is discussed in "Occupational Transmission of HIV: Health Care Workers, Laboratory Workers, and the Health Care Setting," above. Theoretically, the same universal precautions that are used to protect the health care worker from the HIV-infected patient will also protect the patient from the HIV-infected health care worker.

A PREVENTIVE VACCINE AGAINST HIV INFECTION

Given that human behavior, especially human sexual behavior, is extremely difficult to change, a critical modality for preventing the spread of HIV infection is the development of a safe and effective vaccine. Historically, vaccines have provided a safe, cost-effective, and efficient means of preventing illness, disability, and death from infectious diseases. Successful vaccines for the most part are predicated on the assumptions that the body can mount an adequate immune response to the microbe or virus in question during natural infection and that the vaccine will mimic the natural response to infection. Even with serious diseases, such as smallpox, poliomyelitis, measles, and influenza among others, the body in the vast majority of cases clears the infectious agent and provides protection, which is usually life-long against future exposure. Unfortunately, this is not the case with HIV infection since the natural immune response to HIV infection is unable to clear the virus from the body and cases of superinfection are not uncommon. Some of the factors that contribute to the problematic nature of development of a preventive HIV vaccine are the high mutability of the virus, the fact that the infection can be transmitted by cell-free or cell-associated virus, the fact that the HIV provirus integrates itself into the genome of the target cell and may remain in a latent form unexposed to the immune system, the likely need for the development of effective mucosal immunity, and the fact that it has been difficult to establish the precise correlates of protective immunity to HIV infection. A fraction of a percent of HIV-infected individuals are "elite controllers" in that they maintain extremely low and even undetectable levels of viremia in the absence of cART, and a number of individuals have been exposed to HIV multiple times but remain uninfected; these facts suggest that there are elements of host defense or an HIV-specific immune response that have the potential to be protective. Early attempts to develop a vaccine with the envelope protein gp120 aimed at inducing neutralizing antibodies in humans were unsuccessful in that the elicited antisera failed to neutralize primary isolates of HIV cultured and tested in fresh peripheral blood mononuclear cells. In this regard, two phase 3 trials were undertaken in the United States and Thailand using soluble gp120, and the vaccines failed to protect human volunteers from HIV infection. In addition, two separate vaccine trials aimed at eliciting CD8+ T cell responses to prevent infection and, if unsuccessful in preventing infection to control postinfection viremia, also failed at both goals. Recently, a vaccine using a poxvirus vector prime expressing various viral proteins followed by an envelope protein boost was tested in a 16,000-person clinical trial (RV144) conducted in Thailand among predominantly low-prevalence heterosexuals. The vaccine provided the first positive, albeit very modest, signal ever reported in an HIV vaccine trial, showing 31% protection against acquisition of infection. Such a result is certainly not sufficient justification for clinical use of the vaccine, but it served as an important first step in the direction of the development of a safe and effective vaccine against HIV infection. Follow-up studies of RV144 indicate that nonneutralizing or weakly neutralizing antibody responses against certain constant epitopes in the otherwise highly variable V1-V2 region of the HIV envelope may be associated with the modest degree of protection observed in that clinical trial. Additional studies are planned in attempts to improve on the results of RV144 by a variety of approaches, including increasing the number of vaccine boosts with envelope protein.

An area of HIV vaccine research that is currently being actively pursued is the attempt to induce broadly neutralizing antibodies by developing as immunogens for vaccination certain epitopes on the HIV envelope that are the targets of naturally occurring broadly neutralizing antibodies during HIV infection. It is curious that only about 20% of HIV-infected individuals develop broadly neutralizing antibodies in response to natural infection and they do so only after 2 to 3 years of ongoing infection. By the time these antibodies appear, they can neutralize a broad range of primary HIV isolates, but they appear to be ineffective against the autologous virus in the infected subject. Upon close examination, these broadly neutralizing antibodies manifest a high degree of somatic mutations that were accumulated over time and are responsible for their affinity maturation and broadly neutralizing capacity. The goal of current efforts is to develop the conformationally correct HIV envelope epitopes that, when used as immunogens, would direct the immune response of an uninfected individual to the production of broadly neutralizing antibodies over a reasonable time frame by sequential immunizations. It remains to be seen whether this approach will be feasible.

PREVENTION

Education, counseling, and behavior modification are the cornerstones of any HIV prevention strategy. A major problem in the United States and elsewhere is that many infections are passed on by those who do not know that they are infected. Of the ~1.1 million persons in the United States who are HIV-infected, it is estimated that ~16–18% do not know their HIV status and approximately 49% of all new infections are transmitted by those people who are not aware that they are infected. In this regard, the CDC has recommended that HIV testing become part of routine medical care and that all individuals between the ages of 13 and 64 years be tested at least one time. These individuals should be informed of the testing and be tested without the need for written informed consent. Each individual could "opt out" of testing, but testing would otherwise be routinely administered. Individuals who are practicing high-risk behavior should be tested more often. In addition to identifying individuals who might benefit from cART, information gathered from such an approach should serve as the basis for behavior-modification programs, both for infected individuals who may be unaware of their HIV status and who could infect others and for uninfected individuals practicing high-risk behavior. The practice of "safer sex" is the most effective way for sexually active uninfected individuals to avoid contracting HIV infection and for infected individuals to avoid spreading infection. Abstinence from sexual relations is the only absolute way to prevent sexual transmission of HIV infection. However, for many individuals this may not be feasible, and there are a number of relatively safe practices that can markedly decrease the chances of transmission of HIV infection. Partners engaged in monogamous sexual relationships who wish to be assured of safety should both be tested for HIV antibody. If both are negative, it must be understood that any divergence from monogamy puts both partners at risk; open discussion of the importance of honesty in such relationships should be encouraged. When the HIV status of either partner is not known, or when one partner is positive, there are a number of options. Use of condoms can markedly decrease the chance of HIV transmission. It should be remembered that condoms are not 100% effective in preventing transmission of HIV infection, and there is a ~10% failure rate of condoms used for contraceptive purposes. Most condom failures result from breakage or improper usage, such as not wearing the condom for the entire period of intercourse. Latex condoms are preferable, since virus has been shown to leak through natural skin condoms. Petroleum-based gels should never be used for lubrication of the condom, since they increase the likelihood of condom rupture. Some men who have sex with men practice fellatio as a "minimal risk" activity compared with anal intercourse. It should be emphasized that receptive fellatio is definitely not safe sex, and although the incidence of transmission via fellatio is considerably less than that of rectal or vaginal intercourse, there has been documentation of transmission of HIV where receptive fellatio was the only sexual act performed (see "Transmission," above). Topical microbicides composed of gels containing antiretroviral drugs have been shown to be efficacious in preventing acquisition of HIV infection in women engaging in vaginal intercourse. However, there has been a considerable degree of variability in efficacy related to the variable adherence of participants to the use of the intervention. In general, it is felt that microbicides can be quite efficacious; however, adherence is a major stumbling block to their broad effectiveness. Pre-exposure prophylaxis (PreP) using oral antiretroviral drugs on a daily basis in uninfected men who have sex with men and transgender women has been shown to be efficacious in preventing acquisition of HIV infection. The degree of efficacy can be very high (>90%) if subjects adhere strictly to the regimen. However, adherence has proven to be a problem in maximizing the overall effectiveness of this approach.

Adult male circumcision has been shown to result in a 50% to 65% reduction in HIV acquisition in the circumcised subject. Clearly, this approach has considerable potential as a preventive strategy for HIV infection and is currently being pursued, particularly in developing nations, as a component of HIV prevention. The most effective way to prevent transmission of HIV infection among IDUs is to stop the use of injectable drugs. Unfortunately, that is extremely difficult to accomplish unless the individual enters a treatment program. For those who will not or cannot participate in a drug treatment program and who will continue to inject drugs, the avoidance of sharing of needles and other paraphernalia ("works") is the next best way to avoid transmission of infection. However, the cultural and social factors that contribute to the sharing of paraphernalia are complex and difficult to overcome. In addition, needles and syringes may be in short supply. Under these circumstances, paraphernalia should be cleaned after each usage with a virucidal solution, such as undiluted sodium hypochlorite (household bleach). Programs that provide sterile needles to addicts in exchange for used needles have resulted in a marked decrease in HIV transmission without increasing the use of injection drugs. It is important for IDUs to be tested for HIV infection and counseled to avoid transmission to their sexual partners. Oral PreP also is effective in preventing acquisition of HIV infections among IDUs. Prevention of transmission through blood or blood products and prevention of mother-to-child transmission are discussed in "Transmission," above.

SECTION 15 INFECTIONS DUE TO RNA VIRUSES

227 Viral Gastroenteritis

Umesh D. Parashar, Roger I. Glass

Acute infectious gastroenteritis is a common illness that affects persons of all ages worldwide. It is a leading cause of mortality among children in developing countries, accounting for an estimated 0.7 million deaths each year, and is responsible for up to 10 12% of all hospitalizations among children in industrialized countries, including the United States. Elderly persons, especially those with debilitating health conditions, also are at risk of severe complications and death from acute gastroenteritis. Among healthy young adults, acute gastroenteritis is rarely fatal but incurs substantial medical and social costs, including those of time lost from work.

Several enteric viruses have been recognized as important etiologic agents of acute infectious gastroenteritis (Table 227-1, Fig. 227-1). Although most viral gastroenteritis is caused by RNA viruses, the DNA viruses that are occasionally involved (e.g., adenovirus types 40 and 41) are included in this chapter. Illness caused by these viruses is characterized by the acute onset of vomiting and/or diarrhea, which may be accompanied by fever, nausea, abdominal cramps, anorexia, and malaise. As shown in Table 227-2, several features can help distinguish gastroenteritis caused by viruses from that caused by bacterial agents. However, the distinction based on clinical and epidemiologic parameters alone is often difficult, and laboratory tests are required to confirm the diagnosis.

HUMAN CALICIVIRUSES

Etiologic Agent The Norwalk virus is the prototype strain of a group of small (27–40 nm), nonenveloped, round, icosahedral viruses with relatively amorphous surface features on visualization by electron microscopy. These viruses have been difficult to classify because they have not been adapted to growth in cell culture and no animal models are available. Molecular cloning and characterization have demonstrated that the viruses have a single, positive-strand RNA genome ~7.5 kb in length and possess a single virion-associated protein—similar to that of typical caliciviruses—with a molecular mass of 60 kDa. On the basis of these molecular characteristics, these viruses are presently classified in two genera belonging to the family Caliciviridae: the *noroviruses* and the *sapoviruses* (previously called Norwalk-like viruses and Sapporo-like viruses, respectively).

Epidemiology Infections with the Norwalk and related human caliciviruses are common worldwide, and most adults have antibodies to these viruses. Antibody is acquired at an earlier age in developing countries—a pattern consistent with the presumed fecal-oral mode of transmission. Infections occur year-round, although, in temperate climates, a distinct increase has been noted in cold-weather months. Noroviruses may be the most common infectious agents of mild gastroenteritis in the community and affect all age groups, whereas sapoviruses primarily cause gastroenteritis in children. Noroviruses also cause traveler's diarrhea, and outbreaks have occurred among military personnel deployed to various parts of the world. The limited data available indicate that norovirus may be the second most common viral agent (after rotavirus) among young

TABLE 227-1 VIRAL CAUSES OF GASTROENTERITIS AMONG HUMANS

Virus	Family	Genome	Primary Age Group at Risk	Clinical Severity	Detection Assays
Group A rotavirus	Reoviridae	Double-strand segmented RNA	Children <5 years	+ + +	EM, EIA (commercial), PAGE, RT-PCR
Norovirus	Caliciviridae	Positive-sense single-strand RNA	All ages	+ +	EM, RT-PCR
Sapovirus	Caliciviridae	Positive-sense single-strand RNA	Children <5 years	+	EM, RT-PCR
Astrovirus	Astroviridae	Positive-sense single-strand RNA	Children <5 years	+	EM, EIA, RT-PCR
Adenovirus (mainly types 40 and 41)	Adenoviridae	Double-strand DNA	Children <5 years	+/+ +	EM, EIA (commercial), PCR

Abbreviations: EIA, enzyme immunoassay; EM, electron microscopy; PAGE, polyacrylamide gel electrophoresis; PCR, polymerase chain reaction; RT-PCR, reverse-transcription PCR.

children and the most common agent among older children and adults. In the United States, with the decline in severe rotavirus disease following implementation of rotavirus vaccines, norovirus has become the leading cause of medically attended gastroenteritis in young children. Noroviruses are also recognized as the major cause of epidemics of gastroenteritis worldwide. In the United States, >90% of outbreaks of nonbacterial gastroenteritis are caused by noroviruses.

Virus is transmitted predominantly by the fecal-oral route but is also present in vomitus. Because an inoculum with very few viruses can be infectious, transmission can occur by aerosolization, by contact with contaminated fomites, and by person-to-person contact. Viral shedding and infectivity are greatest during the acute illness, but challenge studies with Norwalk virus in volunteers indicate that viral antigen may be shed by asymptomatically infected persons and also by symptomatic persons before the onset of symptoms and for several weeks after the resolution of illness. Viral shedding can be prolonged in immunocompromised individuals.

Pathogenesis The exact sites and cellular receptors for attachment of viral particles have not been determined. Data suggest that carbohydrates that are similar to human histo-blood group antigens and are present on the gastroduodenal epithelium of individuals with the secretor phenotype may serve as ligands for the attachment of Norwalk virus. Additional studies must more fully elucidate norovirus-carbohydrate interactions, including potential strain-specific variations. After the infection of volunteers, reversible lesions are noted in the upper jejunum, with broadening and blunting of the villi, shortening of the microvilli, vacuolization of the lining epithelium, crypt hyperplasia, and infiltration of the lamina propria by polymorphonuclear neutrophils and lymphocytes. The lesions persist for at least 4 days after the resolution of symptoms and are associated with malabsorption of carbohydrates and fats and a decreased level of brush-border enzymes.

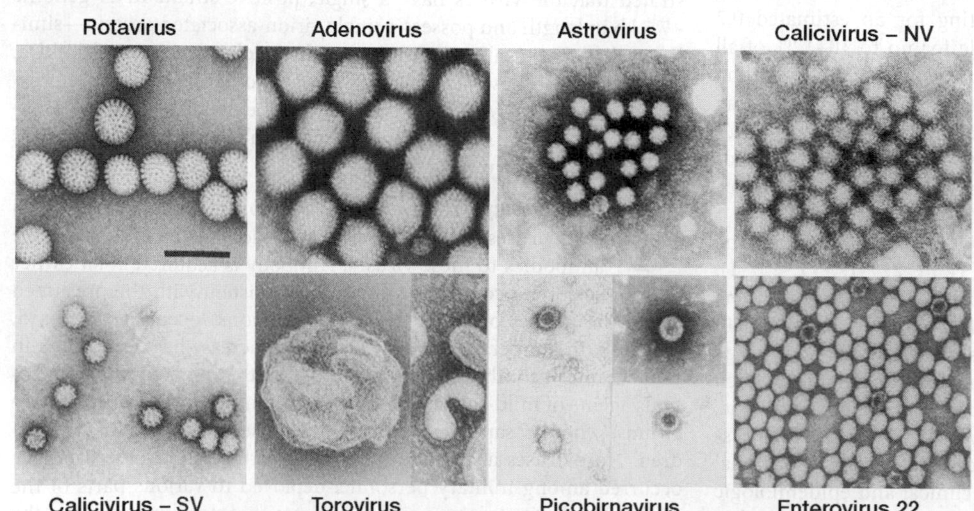

FIGURE 227-1 Viral agents of gastroenteritis. NV, norovirus; SV, sapovirus.

Adenylate cyclase activity is not altered. No histopathologic changes are seen in the stomach or colon, but gastric motor function is delayed, and this alteration is believed to contribute to the nausea and vomiting that are typical of this illness.

Clinical Manifestations Gastroenteritis caused by Norwalk and related human caliciviruses has a sudden onset following an average incubation period of 24 h (range, 12–72 h). The illness generally lasts 12–60 h and is characterized by one or more of the following symptoms: nausea, vomiting, abdominal cramps, and diarrhea. Vomiting is more prevalent among children, whereas a greater proportion of adults develop diarrhea. Constitutional symptoms are common, including headache, fever, chills, and myalgias. The stools are characteristically loose and watery, without blood, mucus, or leukocytes. White cell counts are generally normal; rarely, leukocytosis with relative lymphopenia may be observed. Death is a rare outcome and usually results from severe dehydration in vulnerable persons (e.g., elderly patients with debilitating health conditions).

Immunity Approximately 50% of persons challenged with Norwalk virus become ill and acquire short-term immunity against the infecting strain. Immunity to Norwalk virus appears to correlate inversely with level of antibody; i.e., persons with higher levels of preexisting antibody to Norwalk virus are more susceptible to illness. This observation suggests that some individuals have a genetic predisposition to illness. Specific ABO, Lewis, and secretor blood group phenotypes may influence susceptibility to norovirus infection.

Diagnosis Cloning and sequencing of the genomes of Norwalk and several other human caliciviruses have allowed the development of assays based on polymerase chain reaction (PCR) for detection of virus in stool and vomitus. Virus-like particles produced by expression of capsid proteins in a recombinant baculovirus vector have been used to develop enzyme immunoassays (EIAs) for detection of virus in stool or a serologic response to a specific viral antigen. These newer diagnostic techniques are considerably more sensitive than previous detection methods, such as electron microscopy, immune electron microscopy, and EIAs based on reagents derived from humans. However, no currently available single assay can detect all human caliciviruses because of their great genetic and antigenic diversity. In addition, the assays are still cumbersome and are available primarily in research laboratories, although they are increasingly being adopted by public health laboratories for routine screening of fecal specimens from patients affected by outbreaks of gastroenteritis. Commercial EIA kits have limited sensitivity and usefulness in clinical practice and are of greatest

TABLE 227-2 CHARACTERISTICS OF GASTROENTERITIS CAUSED BY VIRAL AND BACTERIAL AGENTS

Feature	Viral Gastroenteritis	Bacterial Gastroenteritis
Setting	Incidence similar in developing and developed countries	More common in settings with poor hygiene and sanitation
Infectious dose	Low (10–100 viral particles) for most agents	High (>10^5 bacteria) for *Escherichia coli, Salmonella, Vibrio;* medium (10^2–10^5 bacteria) for *Campylobacter jejuni;* low (10–100 bacteria) for *Shigella*
Seasonality	In temperate climates, winter seasonality for most agents; year-round occurrence in tropical areas	More common in summer or rainy months, particularly in developing countries with a high disease burden
Incubation period	1–3 days for most agents; can be shorter for norovirus	1–7 days for common agents (e.g., *Campylobacter, E. coli, Shigella, Salmonella);* a few hours for bacteria producing preformed toxins (e.g., *Staphylococcus aureus, Bacillus cereus)*
Reservoir	Primarily humans	Depending on species, human (e.g., *Shigella, Salmonella*), animal (e.g., *Campylobacter, Salmonella, E. coli*), and water (e.g., *Vibrio*) reservoirs exist
Fever	Common with rotavirus and norovirus; uncommon with other agents	Common with agents causing inflammatory diarrhea (e.g., *Salmonella, Shigella*)
Vomiting	Prominent and can be the only presenting feature, especially in children	Common with bacteria producing preformed toxins; less prominent in diarrhea due to other agents
Diarrhea	Common; nonbloody in almost all cases	Prominent and occasionally bloody with agents causing inflammatory diarrhea
Duration	1–3 days for norovirus and sapovirus; 2–8 days for other viruses	1–2 days for bacteria producing preformed toxins; 2–8 days for most other bacteria
Diagnosis	This is often a diagnosis of exclusion in clinical practice. Commercial enzyme immunoassays are available for detection of rotavirus and adenovirus, but identification of other agents is limited to research and public health laboratories.	Fecal examination for leukocytes and blood is helpful in differential diagnosis. Culture of stool specimens, sometimes on special media, can identify several pathogens. Molecular techniques are useful epidemiologic tools but are not routinely used in most laboratories.
Treatment	Supportive therapy to maintain adequate hydration and nutrition should be given. Antibiotics and antimotility agents are contraindicated.	Supportive hydration therapy is adequate for most patients. Antibiotics are recommended for patients with dysentery caused by *Shigella* or diarrhea caused by *Vibrio cholerae* and for some patients with *Clostridium difficile* colitis.

utility in outbreaks, in which many specimens are tested and only a few need be positive to identify norovirus as the cause.

TREATMENT INFECTIONS WITH NORWALK AND RELATED HUMAN CALICIVIRUSES

The disease is self-limited, and oral rehydration therapy is generally adequate. If severe dehydration develops, IV fluid therapy is indicated. No specific antiviral therapy is available.

Prevention Epidemic prevention relies on situation-specific measures, such as control of contamination of food and water, exclusion of ill food handlers, and reduction of person-to-person spread through good personal hygiene and disinfection of contaminated fomites. The role of immunoprophylaxis is not clear, given the lack of long-term immunity from natural disease, but efforts to develop norovirus vaccines are ongoing. In a clinical study, a candidate virus-like particle norovirus vaccine was shown to protect against homologous viral challenge.

ROTAVIRUS

Etiologic Agent Rotaviruses are members of the family Reoviridae. The viral genome consists of 11 segments of double-strand RNA that are enclosed in a triple-layered, nonenveloped, icosahedral capsid 75 nm in diameter. Viral protein 6 (VP6), the major structural protein, is the target of commercial immunoassays and determines the group specificity of rotaviruses. There are seven major groups of rotavirus (A through G); human illness is caused primarily by group A and, to a much lesser extent, by groups B and C. Two outer-capsid proteins, VP7 (G-protein) and VP4 (P-protein), determine serotype specificity, induce neutralizing antibodies, and form the basis for binary classification of rotaviruses (G and P types). The segmented genome of rotavirus allows genetic reassortment (i.e., exchange of genome segments between viruses) during co-infection—a property that may play a role in viral evolution and that has been utilized in the development of reassortant animal-human rotavirus–based vaccines.

Epidemiology Worldwide, nearly all children are infected with rotavirus by 3–5 years of age. Neonatal infections are common but are often asymptomatic or mild, presumably because of protection by maternal antibody or breast milk. Compared with rotavirus disease in industrialized countries, disease in developing countries occurs at a younger age, is less seasonal, and is more frequently caused by uncommon rotavirus strains. Moreover, because of suboptimal access to hydration therapy, rotavirus is a leading cause of diarrheal death among children in the developing world, with the highest mortality rates among children in sub-Saharan Africa and South Asia (Fig. 227-2).

First infections after 3 months of age are likely to be symptomatic, and the incidence of disease peaks among children 4–23 months of age. Reinfections are common, but the severity of disease decreases with each repeat infection. Therefore, severe rotavirus infections are less common among older children and adults than among younger individuals. Nevertheless, rotavirus can cause illness in parents and caretakers of children with rotavirus diarrhea, immunocompromised persons, travelers, and elderly individuals and should be considered in the differential diagnosis of gastroenteritis among adults.

In tropical settings, rotavirus disease occurs year-round, with less pronounced seasonal peaks than in temperate settings, where rotavirus disease occurs predominantly during the cooler fall and winter months. Before the introduction of rotavirus vaccine in the United States, the rotavirus season each year began in the Southwest during the autumn and early winter (October through December) and migrated across the continent, peaking in the Northeast during late winter and spring (March through May). The reasons for this characteristic pattern are not clear but may be correlated with state-specific differences in birth rates, which could influence the rate of accumulation of susceptible infants after each rotavirus season. After the implementation of routine vaccination of U.S. infants against rotavirus in 2006, the characteristic prevaccine geotemporal pattern of U.S. rotavirus was dramatically altered, and these changes were accompanied by substantial declines in rotavirus detections by a national network of sentinel laboratories (Fig. 227-3). During the latest two seasons with available data (spanning 2010–2012), the number of rotavirus detections declined by 74–90% from the prevaccine baseline, and the

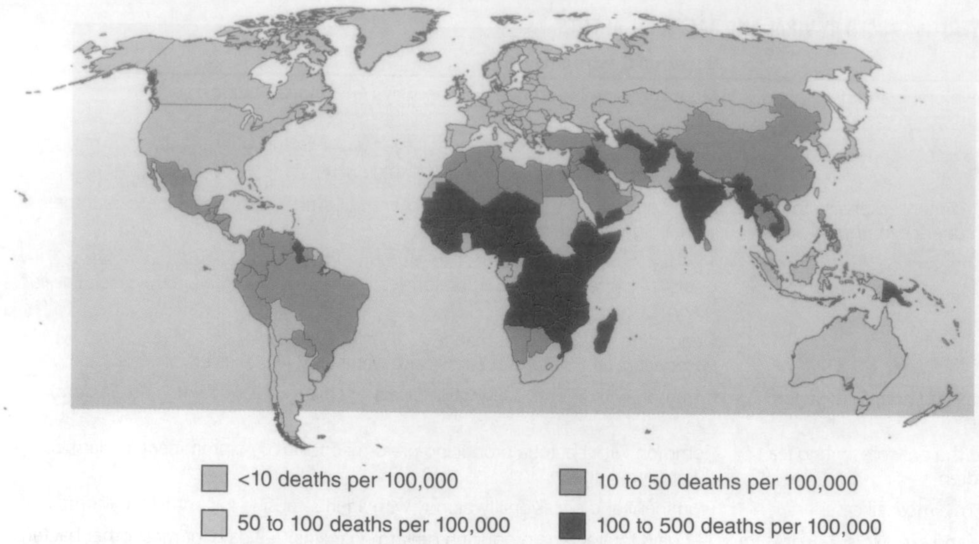

FIGURE 227-2 Rotavirus mortality rates by country, per 100,000 children <5 years of age. *(Reproduced with permission from UD Parashar et al: J Infect Dis 200:S9, 2009.)*

common. While human rotavirus strains that possess a high degree of genetic homology with animal strains have been identified, animal-to-human transmission appears to be uncommon.

Group B rotaviruses have been associated with several large epidemics of severe gastroenteritis among adults in China since 1982 and have also been identified in India. Group C rotaviruses have been associated with a small proportion of pediatric gastroenteritis cases in several countries worldwide.

annual proportion of rotavirus tests that were positive was below 10% in both seasons (compared with a prevaccine baseline median of 26%). A pattern of biennial increases in rotavirus activity has emerged during the five postvaccine seasons (2007–2012), but activity has remained substantially below prevaccine levels in each season.

During episodes of rotavirus-associated diarrhea, virus is shed in large quantities in stool (10^7–10^{12}/g). Viral shedding detectable by EIA usually subsides within 1 week but may persist for >30 days in immunocompromised individuals; it may be detected for longer periods by sensitive molecular assays, such as PCR. The virus is transmitted predominantly through the fecal-oral route. Spread through respiratory secretions, person-to-person contact, or contaminated environmental surfaces has been postulated to explain the rapid acquisition of antibody in the first 3 years of life, regardless of sanitary conditions.

At least 10 different G serotypes of group A rotavirus have been identified in humans, but only 5 types (G1 through G4 and G9) are

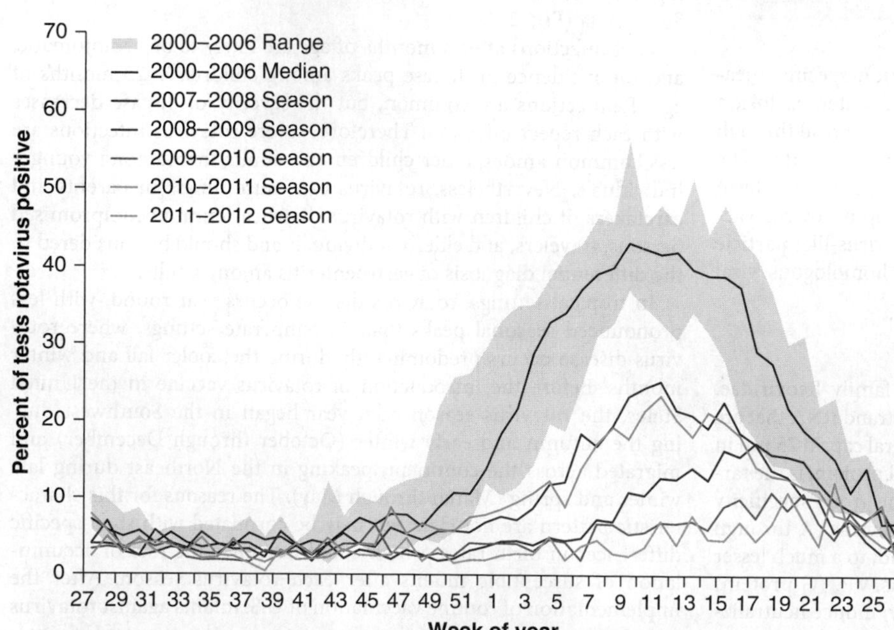

FIGURE 227-3 Percentage of rotavirus tests with positive results, by week of year, July–June, 2000–2012. The maximal or minimal percentage of rotavirus-positive tests for 2000–2006 may have occurred during any of the six baseline seasons. Data are from the National Respiratory and Enteric Virus Surveillance System. *(Adapted from Centers for Disease Control and Prevention, 2012.)*

Pathogenesis Rotaviruses infect and ultimately destroy mature enterocytes in the villous epithelium of the proximal small intestine. The loss of absorptive villous epithelium, coupled with the proliferation of secretory crypt cells, results in secretory diarrhea. Brush-border enzymes characteristic of differentiated cells are reduced, and this change leads to the accumulation of unmetabolized disaccharides and consequent osmotic diarrhea. Studies in mice indicate that a nonstructural rotavirus protein, NSP4, functions as an enterotoxin and contributes to secretory diarrhea by altering epithelial cell function and permeability. In addition, rotavirus may evoke fluid secretion through activation of the enteric nervous system in the intestinal wall. Data indicate that rotavirus antigenemia and viremia are common among children with acute rotavirus infection, although the antigen and RNA levels in serum are substantially lower than those in stool.

Clinical Manifestations The clinical spectrum of rotavirus infection ranges from subclinical infection to severe gastroenteritis leading to life-threatening dehydration. After an incubation period of 1–3 days, the illness has an abrupt onset, with vomiting frequently preceding the onset of diarrhea. Up to one-third of patients may have a temperature of >39°C. The stools are characteristically loose and watery and only infrequently contain red or white cells. Gastrointestinal symptoms generally resolve in 3–7 days.

Respiratory and neurologic features in children with rotavirus infection have been reported, but causal associations have not been proven. Moreover, rotavirus infection has been associated with a variety of other clinical conditions (e.g., sudden infant death syndrome, necrotizing enterocolitis, intussusception, Kawasaki's disease, and type 1 diabetes), but no causal relationship has been confirmed with any of these syndromes.

Rotavirus does not appear to be a major opportunistic pathogen in children with HIV infection. In severely immunodeficient children, rotavirus can cause protracted diarrhea with prolonged viral excretion and, in rare instances, can disseminate systemically. Persons who are immunosuppressed for bone marrow transplantation also are at risk for severe or even fatal rotavirus disease.

Immunity Protection against rotavirus disease is correlated with the presence of virus-specific secretory IgA antibodies in the intestine and, to some extent, the serum. Because virus-specific IgA production at the intestinal surface is short lived, complete protection against disease is only temporary. However, each infection and subsequent reinfection confers progressively greater immunity; thus severe disease is most common among young children with first or second infections. Immunologic memory is believed to be important in the attenuation of disease severity upon reinfection.

Diagnosis Illness caused by rotavirus is difficult to distinguish clinically from that caused by other enteric viruses. Because large quantities of virus are shed in feces, the diagnosis can usually be confirmed by a wide variety of commercially available EIAs or by techniques for detecting viral RNA, such as gel electrophoresis, probe hybridization, or PCR.

TREATMENT ROTAVIRUS INFECTIONS

Rotavirus gastroenteritis can lead to severe dehydration. Thus appropriate treatment should be instituted early. Standard oral rehydration therapy is successful for most children who can take fluids by mouth, but IV fluid replacement may be required for patients who are severely dehydrated or are unable to tolerate oral therapy because of frequent vomiting. The therapeutic roles of probiotics, bismuth subsalicylate, enkephalinase inhibitors, and nitazoxanide have been evaluated in clinical studies but are not clearly defined. Antibiotics and antimotility agents should be avoided. In immunocompromised children with chronic symptomatic rotavirus disease, orally administered immunoglobulins or colostrum may result in the resolution of symptoms, but the best choices regarding agents and their doses have not been well studied, and treatment decisions are often empirical.

Prevention Efforts to develop rotavirus vaccines were pursued because it was apparent—given the similar rates in less developed and industrialized nations—that improvements in hygiene and sanitation were unlikely to reduce disease incidence. The first rotavirus vaccine licensed in the United States in 1998 was withdrawn from the market within 1 year because it was linked with a low incidence of intussusception, a severe bowel obstruction.

In 2006, promising safety and efficacy results for two new rotavirus vaccines were reported from large clinical trials conducted in North America, Europe, and Latin America. Both vaccines are now recommended for routine immunization of all U.S. infants, and their use has rapidly led to a >70–80% decline in rotavirus hospitalizations and emergency department visits at hospitals across the United States. Indirect benefits from vaccination (i.e., herd immunity) have also been documented in many settings. In April 2009, the World Health Organization recommended the use of rotavirus vaccines in all countries worldwide. As of May 2013, a total of 42 countries, including 5 low-income countries in Africa and Asia, have incorporated rotavirus vaccine into their national childhood immunization programs. In Mexico and in Brazil, a decline in deaths from childhood diarrhea following introduction of rotavirus vaccines has been documented. Postmarketing surveillance has identified a low risk of intussusception in some countries; however, the benefits of vaccination exceed the risks, and no changes in vaccine administration policy have been implemented.

The different epidemiology of rotavirus disease and the greater prevalence of co-infection with other enteric pathogens, of comorbidities, and of malnutrition in developing countries may adversely affect the performance of oral rotavirus vaccines, as is the case with oral vaccines against poliomyelitis, cholera, and typhoid in these regions. Therefore, evaluation of the efficacy of rotavirus vaccines in resource-poor settings of Africa and Asia was specifically recommended, and these trials have now been completed. As anticipated, the efficacy of rotavirus vaccines was moderate (50–65%) in these settings when compared with that in industrialized countries. Nevertheless, even a moderately efficacious rotavirus vaccine would be likely to have substantial public health benefits in these areas with a high disease burden.

OTHER VIRAL AGENTS OF GASTROENTERITIS

Enteric *adenoviruses* of serotypes 40 and 41 belonging to subgroup F are 70- to 80-nm viruses with double-strand DNA that cause ~2–12% of all diarrhea episodes in young children. Unlike adenoviruses that cause respiratory illness, enteric adenoviruses are difficult to cultivate in cell lines, but they can be detected with commercially available EIAs. Adenovirus types 31 and 42–49 have been linked to diarrhea in HIV-infected and other immunocompromised persons.

Astroviruses are 28- to 30-nm viruses with a characteristic icosahedral structure and a positive-sense, single-strand RNA. At least seven serotypes have been identified, of which serotype 1 is most common. Astroviruses are primarily pediatric pathogens, causing ~2–10% of cases of mild to moderate gastroenteritis in children. The availability of simple immunoassays to detect virus in fecal specimens and of molecular methods to confirm and characterize strains will permit more comprehensive assessment of the etiologic role of these agents.

Toroviruses are 100- to 140-nm, enveloped, positive-strand RNA viruses that are recognized as causes of gastroenteritis in horses (Berne virus) and cattle (Breda virus). Their role as a cause of diarrhea in humans is still unclear, but studies from Canada have demonstrated associations between torovirus excretion and both nosocomial gastroenteritis and necrotizing enterocolitis in neonates. These associations require further evaluation.

Picobirnaviruses are small, bisegmented, double-strand RNA viruses that cause gastroenteritis in a variety of animals. Their role as primary causes of gastroenteritis in humans remains unclear, but several studies have found an association between picobirnaviruses and gastroenteritis in HIV-infected adults.

Several other viruses (e.g., enteroviruses, reoviruses, pestiviruses, and parvovirus B) have been identified in the feces of patients with diarrhea, but their etiologic role in gastroenteritis has not been proven. Diarrhea has also been noted as a manifestation of infection with recently recognized viruses that primarily cause severe respiratory illness: the severe acute respiratory syndrome–associated coronavirus (SARS-CoV), influenza A/H5N1 virus, and the current pandemic strain of influenza A/H1N1 virus.

228 Enterovirus, Parechovirus, and Reovirus Infections

Jeffrey I. Cohen

ENTEROVIRUSES

CLASSIFICATION AND CHARACTERIZATION

Enteroviruses, members of the family Picornaviridae, are so designated because of their ability to multiply in the gastrointestinal tract. Despite their name, these viruses are not a prominent cause of gastroenteritis. Enteroviruses encompass more than 100 human serotypes: 3 serotypes of poliovirus, 21 serotypes of coxsackievirus A, 6 serotypes of coxsackievirus B, 28 serotypes of echovirus, enteroviruses 68–71, and multiple new enteroviruses (beginning with enterovirus 73) that have been identified by molecular techniques. Human enteroviruses have been reclassified into four species designated A–D. Echoviruses 22 and 23 have been reclassified as parechoviruses 1 and 2 on the basis of low nucleotide homology and differences in viral proteins. Enterovirus surveillance conducted in the United States by the Centers for Disease Control and Prevention (CDC) in 2007–2008 showed that the most common enterovirus serotype, coxsackievirus B1, was followed in frequency by echoviruses 18, 9, and 6; together, these four viruses accounted for 52% of all isolates.

Human enteroviruses contain a single-stranded RNA genome surrounded by an icosahedral capsid comprising four viral proteins. These viruses have no lipid envelope and are stable in acidic environments, including the stomach. They are susceptible to chlorine-containing cleansers but resistant to inactivation by standard disinfectants (e.g., alcohol, detergents) and can persist for days at room temperature.

PATHOGENESIS AND IMMUNITY

Much of what is known about the pathogenesis of enteroviruses has been derived from studies of poliovirus infection. After ingestion, poliovirus is thought to infect epithelial cells in the mucosa of the gastrointestinal tract and then to spread to and replicate in the submucosal lymphoid tissue of the tonsils and Peyer's patches. The virus next spreads to the regional lymph nodes, a viremic phase ensues, and the virus replicates in organs of the reticuloendothelial system. In some cases, a second episode of viremia occurs and the virus replicates further in various tissues, sometimes causing symptomatic disease.

It is uncertain whether poliovirus reaches the central nervous system (CNS) during viremia or whether it also spreads via peripheral nerves. Since viremia precedes the onset of neurologic disease in humans, it has been assumed that the virus enters the CNS via the bloodstream. The poliovirus receptor is a member of the immunoglobulin superfamily. Poliovirus infection is limited to primates, largely because their cells express the viral receptor. Studies demonstrating the poliovirus receptor in the end-plate region of muscle at the neuromuscular junction suggest that, if the virus enters the muscle during viremia, it could travel across the neuromuscular junction up the axon to the anterior horn cells. Studies of monkeys and of transgenic mice expressing the poliovirus receptor show that, after IM injection, poliovirus does not reach the spinal cord if the sciatic nerve is cut. Taken together, these findings suggest that poliovirus can spread directly from muscle to the CNS by neural pathways.

Poliovirus can usually be cultured from the blood 3–5 days after infection, before the development of neutralizing antibodies. While viral replication at secondary sites begins to slow 1 week after infection, it continues in the gastrointestinal tract. Poliovirus is shed from the oropharynx for up to 3 weeks after infection and from the gastrointestinal tract for as long as 12 weeks; hypogammaglobulinemic patients can shed poliovirus for >20 years. During replication in the gastrointestinal tract, attenuated oral poliovirus can mutate, reverting to a more neurovirulent phenotype within a few days; however, additional mutations are probably required for full neurovirulence. One patient with hypogammaglobulinemia who had been infected 12 years earlier and was receiving IV immune globulin suddenly developed quadriplegia and respiratory muscle paralysis and died; analysis showed that the virus had reverted to a more wild-type sequence.

Humoral and secretory immunity in the gastrointestinal tract is important for the control of enterovirus infections. Enteroviruses induce specific IgM, which usually persists for <6 months, and specific IgG, which persists for life. Capsid protein VP1 is the predominant target of neutralizing antibody, which generally confers lifelong protection against subsequent disease caused by the same serotype but does not prevent infection or virus shedding. Enteroviruses also induce cellular immunity whose significance is uncertain. Patients with impaired cellular immunity are not known to develop unusually severe disease when infected with enteroviruses. In contrast, the severe infections in patients with agammaglobulinemia emphasize the importance of humoral immunity in controlling enterovirus infections. Disseminated enterovirus infections have occurred in hematopoietic cell transplant recipients. IgA antibodies are instrumental in reducing poliovirus replication in and shedding from the gastrointestinal tract. Breast milk contains IgA specific for enteroviruses and can protect humans from infection.

EPIDEMIOLOGY

Enteroviruses have a worldwide distribution. More than 50% of nonpoliovirus enterovirus infections and more than 90% of poliovirus infections are subclinical. When symptoms do develop, they are usually nonspecific and occur in conjunction with fever; only a minority of infections are associated with specific clinical syndromes. The incubation period for most enterovirus infections ranges from 2 to 14 days but usually is <1 week.

Enterovirus infection is more common in socioeconomically disadvantaged areas, especially in those where conditions are crowded and in tropical areas where hygiene is poor. Infection is most common among infants and young children; serious illness develops most often during the first few days of life and in older children and adults. In developing countries, where children are infected at an early age, poliovirus infection has less often been associated with paralysis; in countries with better hygiene, older children and adults are more likely to be seronegative, become infected, and develop paralysis. Passively acquired maternal antibody reduces the risk of symptomatic infection in neonates. Young children are the most frequent shedders of enteroviruses and are usually the index cases in family outbreaks. In temperate climates, enterovirus infections occur most often in the summer and fall; no seasonal pattern is apparent in the tropics.

Most enteroviruses are transmitted primarily by the fecal-oral or oral-oral route. Patients are most infectious shortly before and after the onset of symptomatic disease, when virus is present in the stool and throat. The ingestion of virus-contaminated food or water also can cause disease. Certain enteroviruses (such as enterovirus 70, which causes acute hemorrhagic conjunctivitis) can be transmitted by direct inoculation from the fingers to the eye. Airborne transmission is important for some viruses that cause respiratory tract disease, such as coxsackievirus A21. Enteroviruses can be transmitted across the placenta from mother to fetus, causing severe disease in the newborn. The transmission of enteroviruses through blood transfusions or insect bites has not been documented. Nosocomial spread of coxsackievirus and echovirus has taken place in hospital nurseries.

CLINICAL FEATURES

Poliovirus Infection Most infections with poliovirus are asymptomatic. After an incubation period of 3–6 days, ~5% of patients present with a minor illness (abortive poliomyelitis) manifested by fever, malaise, sore throat, anorexia, myalgias, and headache. This condition usually resolves in 3 days. About 1% of patients present with aseptic meningitis (nonparalytic poliomyelitis). Examination of cerebrospinal fluid (CSF) reveals lymphocytic pleocytosis, a normal glucose level, and a normal or slightly elevated protein level; CSF polymorphonuclear leukocytes may be present early. In some patients, especially children, malaise and fever precede the onset of aseptic meningitis.

PARALYTIC POLIOMYELITIS The least common presentation is that of paralytic disease. After one or several days, signs of aseptic meningitis are followed by severe back, neck, and muscle pain and by the rapid or gradual development of motor weakness. In some cases the disease appears to be biphasic, with aseptic meningitis followed first by apparent recovery but then (1–2 days later) by the return of fever and the development of paralysis; this form is more common among children than among adults. Weakness is generally asymmetric, is proximal more than distal, and may involve the legs (most commonly); the arms; or the abdominal, thoracic, or bulbar muscles. Paralysis develops during the febrile phase of the illness and usually does not progress after defervescence. Urinary retention may also occur. Examination reveals weakness, fasciculations, decreased muscle tone, and reduced or absent reflexes in affected areas. Transient hyperreflexia sometimes precedes the loss of reflexes. Patients frequently report sensory symptoms, but objective sensory testing usually yields normal results. Bulbar paralysis may lead to dysphagia, difficulty in handling secretions, or dysphonia. Respiratory insufficiency due to aspiration, involvement of the respiratory center in the medulla, or paralysis of the phrenic or intercostal nerves may develop, and severe medullary involvement may lead to circulatory collapse. Most patients with paralysis recover some function weeks to months after infection. About two-thirds of patients have residual neurologic sequelae.

Paralytic disease is more common among older individuals, pregnant women, and persons exercising strenuously or undergoing trauma at the time of CNS symptoms. Tonsillectomy predisposes to bulbar poliomyelitis, and IM injections increase the risk of paralysis in the involved limb(s).

VACCINE-ASSOCIATED POLIOMYELITIS The risk of developing poliomyelitis after oral vaccination is estimated at 1 case per 2.5 million doses. The risk is ~2000 times higher among immunodeficient persons, especially in persons with hypo- or agammaglobulinemia. Before 1997, an average of eight cases of vaccine-associated poliomyelitis occurred—in both vaccinees and their contacts—in the United States each year. With the change in recommendations first to a sequential regimen of inactivated poliovirus vaccine (IPV) and oral poliovirus vaccine (OPV) in 1997 and then to an all-IPV regimen in 2000, the number of cases of vaccine-associated polio declined. From 1997 to 1999, six such cases were reported in the United States; no cases have been reported since 1999.

POSTPOLIO SYNDROME The *postpolio syndrome* presents as a new onset of weakness, fatigue, fasciculations, and pain with additional atrophy of the muscle group involved during the initial paralytic disease 20–40 years earlier. The syndrome is more common among women and with increasing time after acute disease. The onset is usually insidious, and weakness occasionally extends to muscles that were not involved during the initial illness. The prognosis is generally good; progression to further weakness is usually slow, with plateau periods of 1–10 years. The postpolio syndrome is thought to be due to progressive dysfunction and loss of motor neurons that compensated for the neurons lost during the original infection and not to persistent or reactivated poliovirus infection.

Other Enteroviruses An estimated 5–10 million cases of symptomatic disease due to enteroviruses other than poliovirus occur in the United States each year. Among neonates, enteroviruses are the most common cause of aseptic meningitis and nonspecific febrile illnesses. Certain clinical syndromes are more likely to be caused by certain serotypes (Table 228-1).

NONSPECIFIC FEBRILE ILLNESS (SUMMER GRIPPE) The most common clinical manifestation of enterovirus infection is a nonspecific febrile illness. After an incubation period of 3–6 days, patients present with an acute onset of fever, malaise, and headache. Occasional cases are associated with upper respiratory symptoms, and some cases include nausea and vomiting. Symptoms often last for 3–4 days, and most cases resolve in a week. While infections with other respiratory viruses occur more often from late fall to early spring, febrile illness due to enteroviruses frequently occurs in the summer and early fall.

TABLE 228-1 MANIFESTATIONS COMMONLY ASSOCIATED WITH ENTEROVIRUS SEROTYPES

	Serotype(s) of Indicated Virus	
Manifestation	**Coxsackievirus**	**Echovirus (E) and Enterovirus (Ent)**
Acute hemorrhagic conjunctivitis	A24	E70
Aseptic meningitis	A2, 4, 7, 9, 10; B1–5	E4, 6, 7, 9, 11, 13, 16, 18, 19, 30, 33; Ent70, 71
Encephalitis	A9; B1–5	E3, 4, 6, 7, 9, 11, 18, 25, 30; Ent71
Exanthem	A4, 5, 9, 10, 16; B1, 3–5	E4–7, 9, 11, 16–19, 25, 30; Ent71
Generalized disease of the newborn	B1–5	E4–7, 9, 11, 14, 16, 18, 19
Hand-foot-and-mouth disease	A5–7, 9, 10, 16; B1, 2, 5	Ent71
Herpangina	A1–10, 16, 22; B1–5	E6, 9, 11, 16, 17, 25, 30; Ent71
Myocarditis, pericarditis	A4, 9, 16; B1–5	E6, 9, 11, 22
Paralysis	A4, 7, 9; B1–5	E2–4, 6, 7, 9, 11, 18, 30; Ent70, 71
Pleurodynia	A1, 2, 4, 6, 9, 10, 16; B1–6	E1–3, 6, 7, 9, 11, 12, 14, 16, 19, 24, 25, 30
Pneumonia	A9, 16; B1–5	E6, 7, 9, 11, 12, 19, 20, 30; Ent-D68, 71

GENERALIZED DISEASE OF THE NEWBORN Most serious enterovirus infections in infants develop during the first week of life, although severe disease can occur up to 3 months of age. Neonates often present with an illness resembling bacterial sepsis, with fever, irritability, and lethargy. Laboratory abnormalities include leukocytosis with a left shift, thrombocytopenia, elevated values in liver function tests, and CSF pleocytosis. The illness can be complicated by myocarditis and hypotension, fulminant hepatitis and disseminated intravascular coagulation, meningitis or meningoencephalitis, or pneumonia. It may be difficult to distinguish neonatal enterovirus infection from bacterial sepsis, although a history of a recent virus-like illness in the mother provides a clue.

ASEPTIC MENINGITIS AND ENCEPHALITIS In children and young adults, enteroviruses are the cause of up to 90% of cases of aseptic meningitis in which an etiologic agent can be identified. Patients with aseptic meningitis typically present with an acute onset of fever, chills, headache, photophobia, and pain on eye movement. Nausea and vomiting also are common. Examination reveals meningismus without localizing neurologic signs; drowsiness or irritability may also be apparent. In some cases, a febrile illness may be reported that remits but returns several days later in conjunction with signs of meningitis. Other systemic manifestations may provide clues to an enteroviral cause, including diarrhea, myalgias, rash, pleurodynia, myocarditis, and herpangina. Examination of the CSF invariably reveals pleocytosis; the CSF cell count shows a shift from neutrophil to lymphocyte predominance within 1 day of presentation, and the total cell count does not exceed 1000/μL. The CSF glucose level is usually normal (in contrast to the low CSF glucose level in mumps), with a normal or slightly elevated protein concentration. Partially treated bacterial meningitis may be particularly difficult to exclude in some instances. Enteroviral meningitis is more common in summer and fall in temperate climates, while viral meningitis of other etiologies is more common in winter and spring. Symptoms ordinarily resolve within a week, although CSF abnormalities can persist for several weeks. Enteroviral meningitis is often more severe in adults than in children. Neurologic sequelae are rare, and most patients have an excellent prognosis.

Enteroviral encephalitis is much less common than enteroviral aseptic meningitis. Occasional highly inflammatory cases of enteroviral meningitis may be complicated by a mild form of encephalitis that is recognized on the basis of progressive lethargy, disorientation, and sometimes seizures. Less commonly, severe primary encephalitis may develop. An estimated 10–35% of cases of viral encephalitis are due to enteroviruses. Immunocompetent patients generally have a good prognosis.

Patients with hypogammaglobulinemia, agammaglobulinemia, or severe combined immunodeficiency may develop chronic meningitis or encephalitis; about half of these patients have a dermatomyositis-like syndrome, with peripheral edema, rash, and myositis. They may also have chronic hepatitis. Patients may develop neurologic disease while receiving immunoglobulin replacement therapy. Echoviruses (especially echovirus 11) are the most common pathogens in this situation.

Paralytic disease due to enteroviruses other than poliovirus occurs sporadically and is usually less severe than poliomyelitis. Most cases are due to enterovirus 70 or 71 or to coxsackievirus A7 or A9. Guillain-Barré syndrome is also associated with enterovirus infection. While earlier studies suggested a link between enteroviruses and chronic fatigue syndrome, most recent studies have not demonstrated such an association.

PLEURODYNIA (BORNHOLM DISEASE) Patients with pleurodynia present with an acute onset of fever and spasms of pleuritic chest or upper abdominal pain. Chest pain is more common in adults, and abdominal pain is more common in children. Paroxysms of severe, knifelike pain usually last 15–30 min and are associated with diaphoresis and tachypnea. Fever peaks within an hour after the onset of paroxysms and subsides when pain resolves. The involved muscles are tender to palpation, and a pleural rub may be detected. The white blood cell count and chest x-ray results are usually normal. Most cases are due to coxsackievirus B and occur during epidemics. Symptoms resolve in a few days, and recurrences are rare. Treatment includes the administration of nonsteroidal anti-inflammatory agents or the application of heat to the affected muscles.

MYOCARDITIS AND PERICARDITIS Enteroviruses are estimated to cause up to one-third of cases of acute myocarditis. Coxsackievirus B and its RNA have been detected in pericardial fluid and myocardial tissue in some cases of acute myocarditis and pericarditis. Most cases of enteroviral myocarditis or pericarditis occur in newborns, adolescents, or young adults. More than two-thirds of patients are male. Patients often present with an upper respiratory tract infection that is followed by fever, chest pain, dyspnea, arrhythmias, and occasionally heart failure. A pericardial friction rub is documented in half of cases, and the electrocardiogram shows ST-segment elevations or ST- and T-wave abnormalities. Serum levels of myocardial enzymes are often elevated. Neonates commonly have severe disease, while most older children and adults recover completely. Up to 10% of cases progress to chronic dilated cardiomyopathy. Chronic constrictive pericarditis may also be a sequela.

EXANTHEMS Enterovirus infection is the leading cause of exanthems in children in the summer and fall. While exanthems are associated with many enteroviruses, certain types have been linked to specific syndromes. Echoviruses 9 and 16 have frequently been associated with exanthem and fever. Rashes may be discrete or confluent, beginning on the face and spreading to the trunk and extremities. Echovirus 9 is the most common cause of a rubelliform (discrete) rash. Unlike the rash of rubella, the enteroviral rash occurs in the summer and is not associated with lymphadenopathy. Roseola-like rashes develop after defervescence, with macules and papules on the face and trunk. The Boston exanthem, caused by echovirus 16, is a roseola-like rash. A variety of other rashes have been associated with enteroviruses, including erythema multiforme (see Fig. 25e-25) and vesicular, urticarial, petechial, or purpuric lesions. Enanthems also occur, including lesions that resemble the Koplik's spots seen with measles (see Fig. 25e-2).

HAND-FOOT-AND-MOUTH DISEASE (Fig. 228-1) After an incubation period of 4–6 days, patients with hand-foot-and-mouth disease present with fever, anorexia, and malaise; these manifestations are followed by the development of sore throat and vesicles (see Fig. 25e-23) on the buccal mucosa and often on the tongue and then by the appearance of tender vesicular lesions on the dorsum of the hands, sometimes with involvement of the palms. The vesicles may form bullae and quickly ulcerate. About one-third of patients also have lesions on the palate, uvula, or tonsillar pillars, and one-third have a rash on the feet (including the soles) or on the buttocks. The disease is highly infectious, with attack rates of close to 100% among young children. The lesions usually resolve in 1 week. Most cases are due to coxsackievirus A16 or enterovirus 71.

An epidemic of enterovirus 71 infection in Taiwan in 1998 resulted in thousands of cases of hand-foot-and-mouth disease or herpangina (see below). Severe complications included CNS disease, myocarditis, and pulmonary hemorrhage. About 90% of those who died were children ≤5 years old, and death was associated with pulmonary edema or pulmonary hemorrhage. CNS disease included aseptic meningitis, flaccid paralysis (similar to that seen in poliomyelitis), and rhombencephalitis with myoclonus and tremor or ataxia. The mean age of patients with CNS complications was 2.5 years, and MRI in cases with encephalitis usually showed brain-stem lesions. Follow-up of children at 6 months showed persistent dysphagia, cranial nerve palsies, hypoventilation, limb weakness, and atrophy; at 3 years, persistent neurologic sequelae were documented, with delayed development and impaired cognitive function.

Another epidemic of enterovirus 71 infection occurred in China in 2008–2010, with nearly 500,000 infections and 126 deaths. Infections were associated with fever, rash, brain-stem encephalitis with myoclonic jerks, and limb trembling; some cases progressed to seizures and coma. Lung findings included pulmonary edema and hemorrhage; while the level of creatine kinase MB was sometimes elevated, myocardial necrosis was generally not found.

Cyclic epidemics occur every 2–3 years in other Asian countries. However, the virus circulates at lower rates in the United States, Europe, and Africa. In the United States, hand-foot-and-mouth disease is most commonly associated with coxsackievirus A16. Between November 2011 and February 2012, outbreaks of hand-foot-and-mouth disease

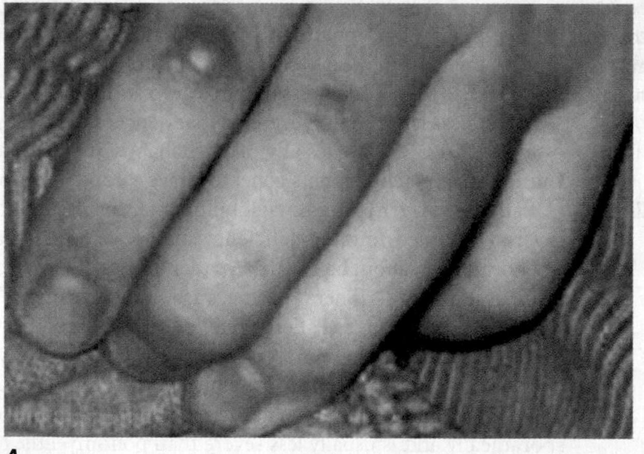
A

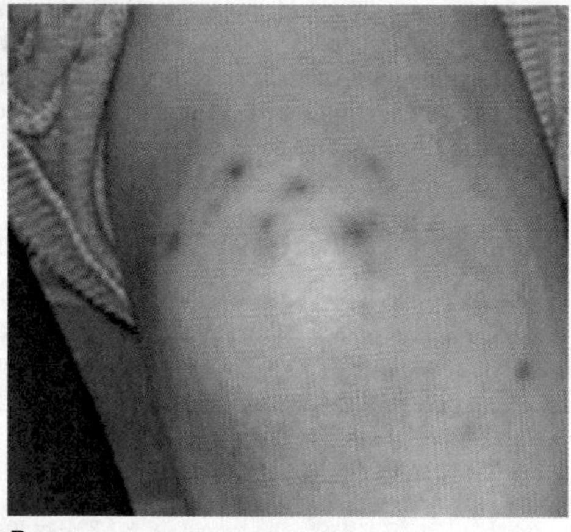
B

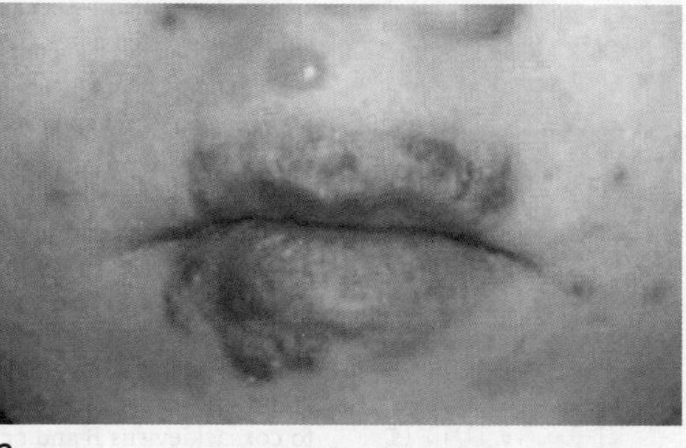
C

FIGURE 228-1 Vesicular eruptions of the hand (*A*), foot (*B*), and mouth (*C*) of a 6-year-old boy with coxsackievirus A6 infection. *(Images reprinted courtesy of Centers for Disease Control and Prevention/Emerging Infectious Diseases.)*

due to coxsackievirus A6 occurred in several U.S. states, and 19% of the affected persons were hospitalized.

HERPANGINA Herpangina is usually caused by coxsackievirus A and presents as acute-onset fever, sore throat, odynophagia, and grayish-white papulovesicular lesions on an erythematous base that ulcerate. The lesions can persist for weeks; are present on the soft palate, anterior pillars of the tonsils, and uvula; and are concentrated in the posterior portion of the mouth. In contrast to herpes stomatitis, enteroviral herpangina is not associated with gingivitis. Acute lymphonodular pharyngitis associated with coxsackievirus A10 presents as white or yellow nodules surrounded by erythema in the posterior oropharynx. The lesions do not ulcerate.

ACUTE HEMORRHAGIC CONJUNCTIVITIS Patients with acute hemorrhagic conjunctivitis present with an acute onset of severe eye pain, blurred vision, photophobia, and watery discharge from the eye. Examination reveals edema, chemosis, and subconjunctival hemorrhage and often shows punctate keratitis and conjunctival follicles as well (Fig. 228-2). Preauricular adenopathy is often found. Epidemics and nosocomial spread have been associated with enterovirus 70 and coxsackievirus A24. Systemic symptoms, including headache and fever, develop in 20% of cases, and recovery is usually complete in 10 days. The sudden onset and short duration of the illness help to distinguish acute hemorrhagic conjunctivitis from other ocular infections, such as those due to adenovirus and *Chlamydia trachomatis*. Paralysis has been associated with some cases of acute hemorrhagic conjunctivitis due to enterovirus 70 during epidemics.

OTHER MANIFESTATIONS Enteroviruses are an infrequent cause of childhood pneumonia and the common cold. In the fall of 2014, enterovirus D68 infection was confirmed in more than 500 persons with mild to severe respiratory illnesses in 43 U.S. states. Nearly all reported cases were in children, many of whom had asthma. Enterovirus D68 was detected in upper respiratory tract specimens from some patients with unexplained acute neurologic disease during outbreaks of infection with this virus; however, the virus was not detected in the CSF, and at present the link between the virus and neurologic disease is uncertain. Coxsackievirus B has been isolated at autopsy from the pancreas of a few children presenting with type 1 diabetes mellitus; however, most attempts to isolate the virus have been unsuccessful. Other diseases that have been associated with enterovirus infection include parotitis, bronchitis, bronchiolitis, croup, infectious lymphocytosis, polymyositis, acute arthritis, and acute nephritis.

DIAGNOSIS

Isolation of enterovirus in cell culture is the traditional diagnostic procedure. While cultures of stool, nasopharyngeal, or throat samples from patients with enterovirus diseases are often positive, isolation of the virus from these sites does not prove that it is directly associated with disease because these sites are frequently colonized for weeks in

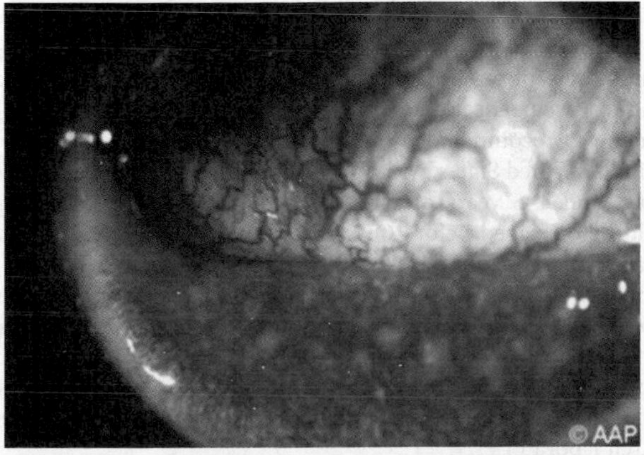

FIGURE 228-2 Acute hemorrhagic conjunctivitis due to enterovirus 70. *(Image reprinted with permission from Red Book 2012: Committee on Infectious Diseases, 29th ed. Used with permission of the American Academy of Pediatrics.)*

patients with subclinical infections. Isolation of virus from the throat is more likely to be associated with disease than is isolation from the stool since virus is shed for shorter periods from the throat. Cultures of CSF, serum, fluid from body cavities, or tissues are positive less frequently, but a positive result is indicative of disease caused by enterovirus. In some cases, the virus is isolated only from the blood or only from the CSF; therefore, it is important to culture multiple sites. Cultures are more likely to be positive earlier than later in the course of infection. Most human enteroviruses can be detected within a week after inoculation of cell cultures. Cultures may be negative because of the presence of neutralizing antibody, lack of susceptibility of the cells used, or inappropriate handling of the specimen. Coxsackievirus A may require inoculation into special cell-culture lines or into suckling mice.

Identification of the enterovirus serotype is useful primarily for epidemiologic studies and, with a few exceptions, has little clinical utility. It is important to identify serious infections with enterovirus during epidemics and to distinguish the vaccine strain of poliovirus from the other enteroviruses in the throat or in the feces. Stool and throat samples for culture as well as acute- and convalescent-phase serum specimens should be obtained from all patients with suspected poliomyelitis. In the absence of a positive CSF culture, a positive culture of stool obtained within the first 2 weeks after the onset of symptoms is most often used to confirm the diagnosis of poliomyelitis. If poliovirus infection is suspected, two or more fecal and throat swab samples should be obtained at least 1 day apart and cultured for enterovirus as soon as possible. If poliovirus is isolated, it should be sent to the CDC for identification as either wild-type or vaccine virus.

Reverse-transcriptase polymerase chain reaction (PCR) has been used to amplify viral nucleic acid from CSF, serum, urine, stool, conjunctiva, throat swabs, and tissues. A pan-enterovirus PCR assay can detect all human enteroviruses. With the proper controls, PCR of the CSF is highly sensitive (70–100%) and specific (>80%) and is more rapid than culture. PCR of the CSF is less likely to be positive when patients present ≥3 days after the onset of meningitis or with enterovirus 71 infection; in these cases, PCR of throat or rectal swabs—although less specific than PCR of CSF—should be considered.

PCR of serum is also highly sensitive and specific in the diagnosis of disseminated disease. PCR may be particularly helpful for the diagnosis and follow-up of enterovirus disease in immunodeficient patients receiving immunoglobulin therapy, whose viral cultures may be negative. Antigen detection is less sensitive than PCR.

Serologic diagnosis of enterovirus infection is limited by the large number of serotypes and the lack of a common antigen. Demonstration of seroconversion may be useful in rare cases for confirmation of culture results, but serologic testing is usually limited to epidemiologic studies. Serum should be collected and frozen soon after the onset of disease and again ~4 weeks later. Measurement of neutralizing titers is the most accurate method for antibody determination; measurement of complement-fixation titers is usually less sensitive. Titers of virus-specific IgM are elevated in both acute and chronic infection.

TREATMENT ENTEROVIRUS INFECTIONS

Most enterovirus infections are mild and resolve spontaneously; however, intensive supportive care may be needed for cardiac, hepatic, or CNS disease. IV, intrathecal, or intraventricular immunoglobulin has been used with apparent success in some cases for the treatment of chronic enterovirus meningoencephalitis and dermatomyositis in patients with hypogammaglobulinemia or agammaglobulinemia. The disease may stabilize or resolve during therapy; however, some patients decline inexorably despite therapy. IV immunoglobulin often prevents severe enterovirus disease in these patients. IV administration of immunoglobulin with high titers of antibody to the infecting virus has been used in some cases of life-threatening infection in neonates, who may not have maternally acquired antibody. In one trial involving neonates with enterovirus infections, immunoglobulin containing very high titers of antibody to the infecting virus reduced rates of viremia; however, the study was too small to show a substantial clinical benefit. The level of enteroviral antibodies varies with the immunoglobulin preparation. A phase 2 trial of pleconaril for severe neonatal enterovirus disease has been completed; however, as of this writing, the results have not been reported and the drug is not available on a compassionate-use basis. Glucocorticoids are contraindicated.

Good hand-washing practices and the use of gowns and gloves are important in limiting nosocomial transmission of enteroviruses during epidemics. Enteric precautions are indicated for 7 days after the onset of enterovirus infections. Enterovirus 71 vaccine candidates are under development.

PREVENTION AND ERADICATION OF POLIOVIRUS

(See also Chap. 148) After a peak of 57,879 cases of poliomyelitis in the United States in 1952, the introduction of IPV in 1955 and of OPV in 1961 ultimately eradicated disease due to wild-type poliovirus in the Western Hemisphere. Such disease has not been documented in the United States since 1979, when cases occurred among religious groups who had declined immunization. In the Western Hemisphere, paralysis due to wild-type poliovirus was last documented in 1991.

In 1988, the World Health Organization adopted a resolution to eradicate poliomyelitis by the year 2000. From 1988 to 2001, the number of cases worldwide decreased by >99%, with only 496 confirmed cases reported in 2001. Wild-type poliovirus type 2 has not been detected in the world since 1999. The Americas were certified free of indigenous wild-type poliovirus transmission in 1994, the Western Pacific Region in 2000, and the European Region in 2002. However, in 2002, there were 1922 cases of polio, with 1600 cases reported in India. In fact, after the nadir of 496 cases in 2001, 21 countries that had previously been free of polio reported cases imported from 6 polio-endemic countries in 2002–2005. By 2006, polio transmission had been reduced in most of these 21 countries. In 2012, 293 cases of polio were reported (the lowest number ever in a 1-year period); 85% were from Nigeria, Pakistan, and Afghanistan, the only countries where polio remains endemic (Table 228-2). As of November 2013, there had been 390 cases of polio in 2013 compared with 293 cases in 2012. The increase was associated with a marked rise in imported cases, including more than 180 cases in Somalia, more than 10 cases each in Kenya and Syria, and cases in Cameroon and Ethiopia. Also in 2013, wild-type poliovirus was detected in sewage in Israel, prompting a massive vaccination campaign with OPV. As of November 2013, India had not reported a case of polio since January 2011. Polio is a source of concern for unimmunized or partially immunized travelers. Importation of poliovirus accounted for ~50% of cases in 2013. Clearly, global eradication of polio is necessary to eliminate the risk of importation of wild-type virus. Outbreaks are thought to have been facilitated by suboptimal rates of vaccination, isolated pockets of unvaccinated children, poor sanitation and crowding, improper vaccine-storage conditions, and a reduced level of response to one of the serotypes in the vaccine.

TABLE 228-2 LABORATORY-CONFIRMED CASES OF POLIOMYELITIS IN 2012

Country	Type of Transmission	No. of Cases
Nigeria	Endemic	130[a]
Pakistan	Endemic	74[b]
Afghanistan	Endemic	46[c]
Chad	Imported	17[d]
Democratic Republic of the Congo	Vaccine-derived	17
Kenya	Vaccine-derived	3
Yemen	Vaccine-derived	2
China	Vaccine-derived	2
Niger	Imported	1
Somalia	Vaccine-derived	1
Total		**293**

[a]Of these cases, 8 were vaccine-derived. [b]Of these cases, 16 were vaccine-derived. [c]Of these cases, 9 were vaccine-derived. [d]Of these cases, 12 were vaccine-derived.

Source: World Health Organization.

While the global eradication campaign has markedly reduced the number of cases of endemic polio, doubts have been raised as to whether eradication is a realistic goal, given the large number of asymptomatic infections and the political instability in developing countries.

The occurrence of outbreaks of poliomyelitis due to circulating vaccine-derived poliovirus of all three types has been increasing, especially in areas with low vaccination rates. In Egypt, 32 cases of vaccine-derived polio occurred in 1983–1993; in the Dominican Republic and Haiti, 21 cases occurred in 2000–2001; in Indonesia, 46 cases were reported in 2005; in Nigeria, 385 cases occurred in 2005–2012; in the Democratic Republic of the Congo, 64 cases were reported in 2008–2012; in Pakistan, 16 cases occurred in 2012, and at least 30 cases occurred in 2013. These OPV-derived viruses reverted to a more neurovirulent phenotype after undetected circulation (probably for >2 years). The epidemic in Hispaniola was rapidly terminated after intensive vaccination with OPV. In 2005, a case of vaccine-derived polio occurred in an unvaccinated U.S. woman returning from a visit to Central and South America. In the same year, an unvaccinated immunocompromised infant in Minnesota was found to be shedding vaccine-derived poliovirus; further investigation identified 4 of 22 infants in the same community who were shedding the virus. All 5 infants were asymptomatic. These outbreaks emphasize the need for maintaining high levels of vaccine coverage and continued surveillance for circulating virus.

IPV is used in most industrialized countries and OPV in most developing countries, including those in which polio still is or recently was endemic. While IM injections of other vaccines (live or attenuated) can be given concurrently with OPV, unnecessary IM injections should be avoided during the first month after OPV vaccination because they increase the risk of vaccine-associated paralysis. Since 1988, an enhanced-potency inactivated poliovirus vaccine has been available in the United States.

After several doses of OPV alone, the seropositivity rate for individual poliovirus serotypes may still be suboptimal for children in developing countries; one or more supplemental doses of IPV can increase the rate of seropositivity for these serotypes. Against a given serotype, monovalent OPV containing only that serotype is more immunogenic than trivalent vaccine because of a lack of interference from other serotypes. With eradication of wild-type poliovirus type 2, bivalent OPV (types 1 and 3), which was shown to be superior to trivalent OPV, has been the vaccine of choice to eliminate polio and has markedly reduced rates of polio in Nigeria. As the frequency of wild-type polio declines and reports of polio associated with circulating vaccine-derived viruses increase, the World Health Organization is investigating whether IPV can be produced from OPV strains that require less biocontainment, ultimately replacing OPV.

OPV and IPV induce antibodies that persist for at least 5 years. Both vaccines induce IgG and IgA antibodies. Compared with recipients of IPV, recipients of OPV shed less virus and less frequently develop reinfection with wild-type virus after exposure to poliovirus. Although IPV is safe and efficacious, OPV offers the advantages of ease of administration, lower cost, and induction of intestinal immunity resulting in a reduction in the risk of community transmission of wild-type virus. Because of progress toward global eradication of polio and the continued occurrence of cases of vaccine-associated polio, an all-IPV regimen was recommended in 2000 for childhood poliovirus vaccination in the United States, with vaccine administration at 2, 4, and 6–18 months and 4–6 years of age. The risk of vaccine-associated polio should be discussed before OPV is administered. Recommendations for vaccination of adults are listed in Table 228-3.

There are concerns about discontinuing vaccination in the event that endemic spread of poliovirus is eliminated. Among the reasons for these concerns are that poliovirus is shed from some immunocompromised persons for >10 years, that vaccine-derived poliovirus can circulate and cause disease, and that wild-type poliovirus is present in research laboratories.

PARECHOVIRUSES

Human parechoviruses (HPeVs), like enteroviruses, are members of the family Picornaviridae. The 16 serotypes of HPeV commonly cause

TABLE 228-3 RECOMMENDATIONS FOR POLIOVIRUS VACCINATION OF ADULTS

1. Most adults in the United States have been vaccinated during childhood and are at little risk of exposure to wild-type virus in the United States. Immunization is recommended for those with a higher risk of exposure than the general population, including:
   a. travelers to areas where poliovirus is or may be epidemic or endemic;
   b. members of communities or population groups with disease caused by wild-type polioviruses;
   c. laboratory workers handling specimens that may contain wild-type polioviruses; and
   d. health care workers in close contact with patients who may be excreting wild-type polioviruses.
2. Three doses of IPV are recommended for adults who need to be immunized. The second dose should be given 1–2 months after the first dose; the third dose should be given 6–12 months after the second dose.
3. Adults who are at increased risk of exposure to wild-type poliovirus and who have previously completed primary immunization should receive a single dose of IPV. Adults who did not complete primary immunization should receive the remaining required doses of IPV.

Abbreviation: IPV, inactivated poliovirus vaccine.

Source: Modified from Pickering LK, ed. Red Book 2012: Committee on Infectious Diseases, 29th ed.

infections in early childhood. HPeV-1 infections occur throughout the year, while other parechovirus infections occur more commonly in summer and fall. Infections with HPeVs present similarly to those due to enteroviruses and may cause generalized disease of the newborn, aseptic meningitis, encephalitis, transient paralysis, exanthems, respiratory tract disease, and gastroenteritis. While HPeV-1 is the most common serotype and generally causes mild disease, deaths of infants in the United States have been associated with HPeV-1, HPeV-3, and HPeV-6. HPeVs can be isolated from the same sites as enteroviruses, including the nasopharynx, stool, and respiratory tract secretions. PCR using pan-enterovirus primers does not detect HPeVs, and while PCR assays are performed by the CDC and research laboratories, many commercial laboratories do not perform the test.

REOVIRUSES

Reoviruses are double-stranded RNA viruses encompassing three serotypes. Serologic studies indicate that most humans are infected with reoviruses during childhood. Most infections either are asymptomatic or cause mild upper respiratory tract symptoms. Reovirus is considered a rare cause of mild gastroenteritis or meningitis in infants and children. Speculation regarding an association of reovirus type 3 with idiopathic neonatal hepatitis and extrahepatic biliary atresia is based on an elevated prevalence of antibody to reovirus in some affected patients and the detection of viral RNA by PCR in hepatobiliary tissues in some studies. New orthoreoviruses have been associated with human disease—e.g., Melaka and Kampar viruses with fever and acute respiratory disease in Malaysia, and Nelson Bay virus with acute respiratory disease in a traveler from Bali.

229 Measles (Rubeola)

Kaitlin Rainwater-Lovett, William J. Moss

DEFINITION

Measles is a highly contagious viral disease that is characterized by a prodromal illness of fever, cough, coryza, and conjunctivitis followed by the appearance of a generalized maculopapular rash. Before the widespread use of measles vaccines, it was estimated that measles caused between 5 million and 8 million deaths worldwide each year.

GLOBAL CONSIDERATIONS

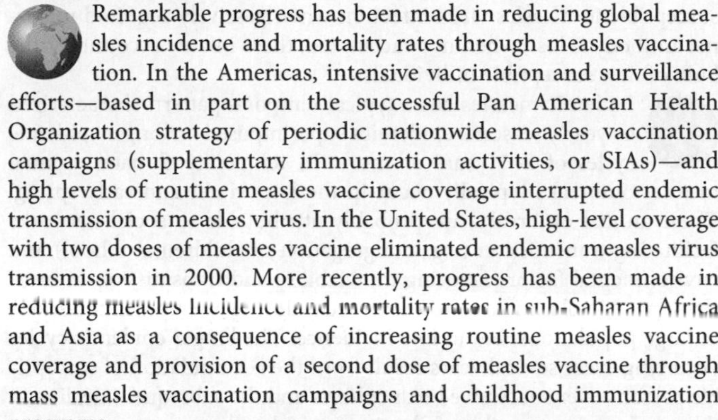

Remarkable progress has been made in reducing global measles incidence and mortality rates through measles vaccination. In the Americas, intensive vaccination and surveillance efforts—based in part on the successful Pan American Health Organization strategy of periodic nationwide measles vaccination campaigns (supplementary immunization activities, or SIAs)—and high levels of routine measles vaccine coverage interrupted endemic transmission of measles virus. In the United States, high-level coverage with two doses of measles vaccine eliminated endemic measles virus transmission in 2000. More recently, progress has been made in reducing measles incidence and mortality rates in sub-Saharan Africa and Asia as a consequence of increasing routine measles vaccine coverage and provision of a second dose of measles vaccine through mass measles vaccination campaigns and childhood immunization programs.

In 2003, the World Health Assembly endorsed a resolution urging member countries to reduce the number of deaths attributed to measles by 50% (compared with 1999 estimates) by the end of 2005. This target was met. Global measles mortality rates were further reduced in 2008; during that year, there were an estimated 164,000 deaths due to measles (uncertainty bounds: 115,000 and 222,000 deaths). These achievements attest to the enormous public-health significance of measles vaccination. However, recent large outbreaks of measles in Europe and Africa illustrate the challenges faced in sustaining measles control: in these outbreaks, measles was imported into countries that had eliminated indigenous transmission of measles virus.

The Measles and Rubella Initiative, a partnership led by the American Red Cross, the United Nations Foundation, UNICEF, the U.S. Centers for Disease Control and Prevention (CDC), and the World Health Organization (WHO), is playing an important role in reducing global measles incidence and mortality rates. Since its inception in 2001, the Initiative has provided governments and communities in more than 80 countries with technical and financial support for routine immunization activities, mass vaccination campaigns, and disease surveillance systems. Through its 2012–2020 Global Measles and Rubella Strategic Plan, the Initiative aims to reduce measles deaths by 95% (compared with year 2000 estimates) by 2015 and to eliminate measles from at least five of the six WHO regions by 2020. As regional goals for measles elimination are set, global measles eradication is likely to become a public health goal in the near future.

ETIOLOGY

Measles virus is a spherical, nonsegmented, single-stranded, negative-sense RNA virus and a member of the *Morbillivirus* genus in the family Paramyxoviridae. Measles was originally a zoonotic infection, arising from animal-to-human transmission of an ancestral morbillivirus ~10,000 years ago, when human populations had attained sufficient size to sustain virus transmission. Although RNA viruses typically have high mutation rates, measles virus is considered to be an antigenically monotypic virus; i.e., the surface proteins responsible for inducing protective immunity have retained their antigenic structure across time and distance. The public health significance of this stability is that measles vaccines developed decades ago from a single strain of measles virus remain protective worldwide. Measles virus is killed by ultraviolet light and heat, and attenuated measles vaccine viruses retain these characteristics, necessitating a cold chain for vaccine transport and storage.

EPIDEMIOLOGY

Measles virus is one of the most highly contagious directly transmitted pathogens. Outbreaks can occur in populations in which <10% of persons are susceptible. Chains of transmission are common among household contacts, school-age children, and health care workers. There are no latent or persistent measles virus infections that result in prolonged contagiousness, nor are there animal reservoirs for the virus. Thus, measles virus can be maintained in human populations only by an unbroken chain of acute infections, which requires a continuous supply of susceptible individuals. Newborns become susceptible to measles virus infection when passively acquired maternal antibody is lost; when not vaccinated, these infants account for the bulk of new susceptible individuals.

Endemic measles has a typical temporal pattern characterized by yearly seasonal epidemics superimposed on longer epidemic cycles of 2–5 years or more. In temperate climates, annual measles outbreaks typically occur in the late winter and early spring. These annual outbreaks are probably attributable to social networks facilitating transmission (e.g., congregation of children at school) and environmental factors favoring the viability and transmission of measles virus. Measles cases continue to occur during interepidemic periods in large populations, but at low incidence. The longer epidemic cycles occurring every several years result from the accumulation of susceptible persons over successive birth cohorts and the subsequent decline in the number of susceptibles following an outbreak.

Secondary attack rates among susceptible household and institutional contacts generally exceed 90%. The average age at which measles occurs depends on rates of contact with infected persons, protective maternal antibody decline, and vaccine coverage. In densely populated urban settings with low-level vaccination coverage, measles is a disease of infants and young children. The cumulative distribution can reach 50% by 1 year of age, with a significant proportion of children acquiring measles before 9 months—the age of routine vaccination in many countries, in line with the schedule recommended by the WHO's Expanded Programme on Immunization. As measles vaccine coverage increases or population density decreases, the age distribution shifts toward older children. In such situations, measles cases predominate in school-age children. Infants and young children, although susceptible if not protected by vaccination, are not exposed to measles virus at a rate sufficient to cause a large disease burden in this age group. As vaccination coverage increases further, the age distribution of cases may be shifted into adolescence and adulthood; this distribution is seen in measles outbreaks in the United States and necessitates targeted measles vaccination programs for these older age groups.

Persons with measles are infectious for several days before and after the onset of rash, when levels of measles virus in blood and body fluids are highest and when cough, coryza, and sneezing, which facilitate virus spread, are most severe. The contagiousness of measles before the onset of recognizable disease hinders the effectiveness of quarantine measures. Viral shedding by children with impaired cell-mediated immunity can be prolonged.

Medical settings are well-recognized sites of measles virus transmission. Children may present to health care facilities during the prodrome, when the diagnosis is not obvious although the child is infectious and is likely to infect susceptible contacts. Health care workers can acquire measles from infected children and transmit measles virus to others. Nosocomial transmission can be reduced by maintenance of a high index of clinical suspicion, use of appropriate isolation precautions when measles is suspected, administration of measles vaccine to susceptible children and health care workers, and documentation of health care workers' immunity to measles (i.e., proof of receipt of two doses of measles vaccine or detection of antibodies to measles virus).

As efforts at measles control are increasingly successful, public perceptions of the risk of measles as a disease diminish and are replaced by concerns about possible adverse events associated with measles vaccine. As a consequence, numerous measles outbreaks have occurred because of opposition to vaccination on religious or philosophical grounds or unfounded fears of serious adverse events (see "Active Immunization," below).

PATHOGENESIS

Measles virus is transmitted primarily by respiratory droplets over short distances and, less commonly, by small-particle aerosols that remain suspended in the air for long periods. Airborne transmission appears to be important in certain settings, including schools, physicians' offices, hospitals, and enclosed public places. The virus can be transmitted by direct contact with infected secretions but does not survive for long on fomites.

The incubation period for measles is ~10 days to fever onset and 14 days to rash onset. This period may be shorter in infants and longer (up to 3 weeks) in adults. Infection is initiated when measles virus is deposited on epithelial cells in the respiratory tract, oropharynx, or conjunctivae (Fig. 229-1*A*). During the first 2–4 days after infection, measles virus proliferates locally in the respiratory mucosa and spreads to draining lymph nodes. Virus then enters the bloodstream in infected leukocytes (primarily monocytes), producing the primary viremia that disseminates infection throughout the reticuloendothelial system. Further replication results in secondary viremia that begins 5–7 days after infection and disseminates measles virus throughout the body. Replication of measles virus in these target organs, together with the host's immune response, is responsible for the signs and symptoms of measles that occur 8–12 days after infection and mark the end of the incubation period (Fig. 229-1*B*).

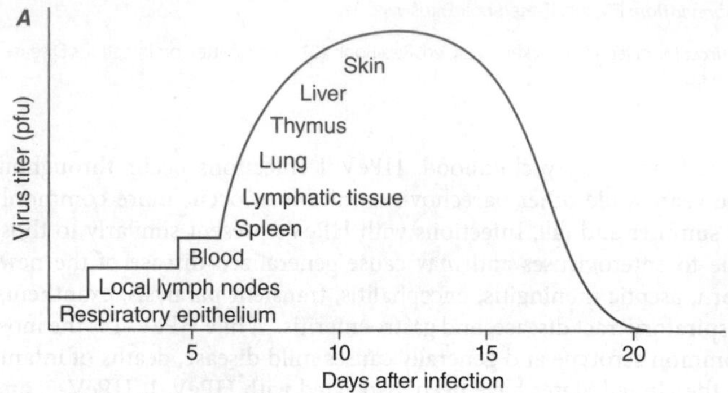

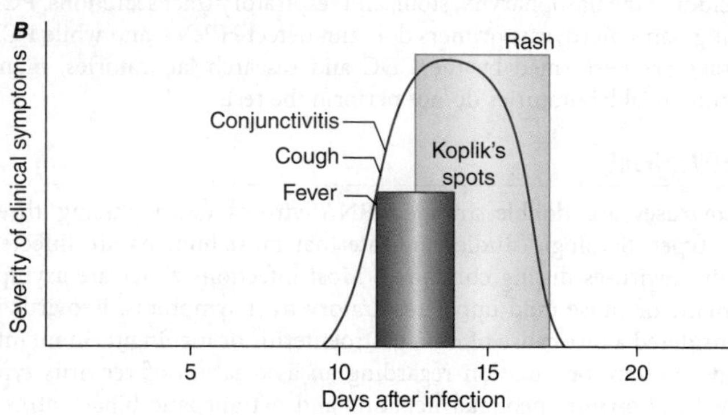

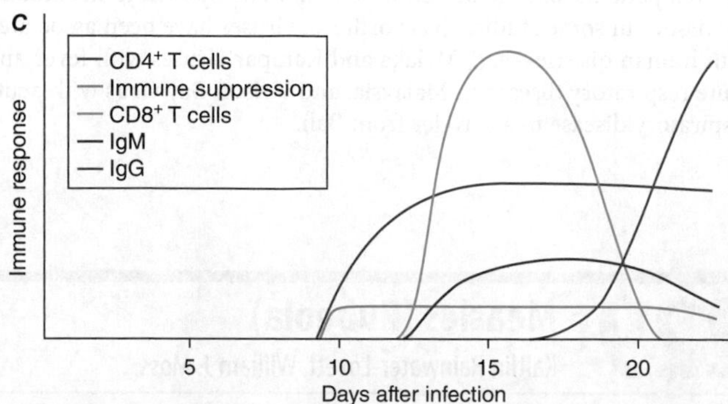

FIGURE 229-1 Measles virus infection: pathogenesis, clinical features, and immune responses. ***A.*** Spread of measles virus, from initial infection of the respiratory tract through dissemination to the skin. ***B.*** Appearance of clinical signs and symptoms, including Koplik's spots and rash. ***C.*** Antibody and T cell responses to measles virus. The signs and symptoms of measles arise coincident with the host immune response. *(Source: Modified from WJ Moss, DE Griffin: Nat Rev Microbiol 4:900, 2006.)*

IMMUNE RESPONSES

Host immune responses to measles virus are essential for viral clearance, clinical recovery, and the establishment of long-term immunity (Fig. 229-1C). Early nonspecific (innate) immune responses during the prodromal phase include activation of natural killer cells and increased production of antiviral proteins. The adaptive immune responses consist of measles virus–specific antibody and cellular responses. The protective efficacy of antibodies to measles virus is illustrated by the immunity conferred to infants from passively acquired maternal antibodies and the protection of exposed, susceptible individuals after administration of anti–measles virus immunoglobulin. The first measles virus–specific antibodies produced after infection are of the IgM subtype, with a subsequent switch to predominantly IgG1 and IgG4 isotypes. The IgM antibody response is typically absent following reexposure or revaccination and serves as a marker of primary infection.

The importance of cellular immunity to measles virus is demonstrated by the ability of children with agammaglobulinemia (congenital inability to produce antibodies) to recover fully from measles and the contrasting picture for children with severe defects in T lymphocyte function, who often develop severe or fatal disease (Chap. 374). The initial predominant T_H1 response (characterized by interferon γ) is essential for viral clearance, and the later T_H2 response (characterized by interleukin 4) promotes the development of measles virus–specific antibodies that are critical for protection against reinfection.

The duration of protective immunity following wild-type measles virus infection is generally thought to be lifelong. Immunologic memory to measles virus includes both continued production of measles virus–specific antibodies and circulation of measles virus–specific $CD4^+$ and $CD8^+$ T lymphocytes.

However, the intense immune responses induced by measles virus infection are paradoxically associated with depressed responses to unrelated (non–measles virus) antigens, which persist for several weeks to months beyond resolution of the acute illness. This state of immune suppression enhances susceptibility to secondary infections with bacteria and viruses that cause pneumonia and diarrhea and is responsible for a substantial proportion of measles-related morbidity and deaths. Delayed-type hypersensitivity responses to recall antigens, such as tuberculin, are suppressed, and cellular and humoral responses to new antigens are impaired. Reactivation of tuberculosis and remission of autoimmune diseases after measles have been described and are attributed to this period of immune suppression.

APPROACH TO THE PATIENT: Measles

Clinicians should consider measles in persons presenting with fever and generalized erythematous rash, particularly when measles virus is known to be circulating or the patient has a history of travel to endemic areas. Appropriate precautions must be taken to prevent nosocomial transmission. The diagnosis requires laboratory confirmation except during large outbreaks in which an epidemiologic link to a confirmed case can be established. Care is largely supportive and consists of the administration of vitamin A and antibiotics (see "Treatment," below). Complications of measles, including secondary bacterial infections and encephalitis, may occur after acute illness and require careful monitoring, particularly in immunocompromised persons.

CLINICAL MANIFESTATIONS

In most persons, the signs and symptoms of measles are highly characteristic (Fig. 229-1*B*). Fever and malaise beginning ~10 days after exposure are followed by cough, coryza, and conjunctivitis. These signs and symptoms increase in severity over 4 days. Koplik's spots (see Fig. 25e-2) develop on the buccal mucosa ~2 days before the rash appears. The characteristic rash of measles (see Fig. 25e-3) begins 2 weeks after infection, when the clinical manifestations are most severe, and signal the host's immune response to the replicating virus. Headache, abdominal pain, vomiting, diarrhea, and myalgia may be present.

Koplik's spots (see Fig. 25e-2) are pathognomonic of measles and consist of bluish white dots ~1 mm in diameter surrounded by erythema. The lesions appear first on the buccal mucosa opposite the lower molars but rapidly increase in number to involve the entire buccal mucosa. They fade with the onset of rash.

The rash of measles begins as erythematous macules behind the ears and on the neck and hairline. The rash progresses to involve the face, trunk, and arms (see Fig. 25e-3), with involvement of the legs and feet by the end of the second day. Areas of confluent rash appear on the trunk and extremities, and petechiae may be present. The rash fades slowly in the same order of progression as it appeared, usually beginning on the third or fourth day after onset. Resolution of the rash may be followed by desquamation, particularly in undernourished children.

Because the characteristic rash of measles is a consequence of the cellular immune response, it may not develop in persons with impaired cellular immunity (e.g., those with AIDS; Chap. 226). These persons have a high case-fatality rate and frequently develop giant-cell pneumonitis caused by measles virus. T lymphocyte defects due to causes other than HIV-1 infection (e.g., cancer chemotherapy) also are associated with increased severity of measles.

A severe atypical measles syndrome was observed in recipients of a formalin-inactivated measles vaccine (used in the United States from 1963 to 1967 and in Canada until 1970) who were subsequently exposed to wild-type measles virus. The atypical rash began on the palms and soles and spread centripetally to the proximal extremities and trunk, sparing the face. The rash was initially erythematous and maculopapular but frequently progressed to vesicular, petechial, or purpuric lesions (see Fig. 25e-22).

DIFFERENTIAL DIAGNOSIS

The differential diagnosis of measles includes other causes of fever, rash, and conjunctivitis, including rubella, Kawasaki disease, infectious mononucleosis, roseola, scarlet fever, Rocky Mountain spotted fever, enterovirus or adenovirus infection, and drug sensitivity. Rubella is a milder illness without cough and with distinctive lymphadenopathy. The rash of roseola (exanthem subitum) (see Fig. 25e-5) appears after fever has subsided. The atypical lymphocytosis in infectious mononucleosis contrasts with the leukopenia commonly observed in children with measles.

DIAGNOSIS

Measles is readily diagnosed on clinical grounds by clinicians familiar with the disease, particularly during outbreaks. Koplik's spots (see Fig. 25e-2) are especially helpful because they appear early and are pathognomonic. Clinical diagnosis is more difficult (1) during the prodromal illness; (2) when the rash is attenuated by passively acquired antibodies or prior immunization; (3) when the rash is absent or delayed in immunocompromised children or severely undernourished children with impaired cellular immunity; and (4) in regions where the incidence of measles is low and other pathogens are responsible for the majority of illnesses with fever and rash. The CDC case definition for measles requires (1) a generalized maculopapular rash of at least 3 days' duration; (2) fever of at least 38.3°C (101°F); and (3) cough, coryza, or conjunctivitis.

Serology is the most common method of laboratory diagnosis. The detection of measles virus–specific IgM in a single specimen of serum or oral fluid is considered diagnostic of acute infection, as is a fourfold or greater increase in measles virus–specific IgG antibody levels between acute- and convalescent-phase serum specimens. Primary infection in the immunocompetent host results in antibodies that are detectable within 1–3 days of rash onset and reach peak levels in 2–4 weeks. Measles virus–specific IgM antibodies may not be detectable until 4–5 days or more after rash onset and usually fall to undetectable levels within 4–8 weeks of rash onset.

Several methods for measurement of antibodies to measles virus are available. Neutralization tests are sensitive and specific, and the results are highly correlated with protective immunity; however, these tests require propagation of measles virus in cell culture and thus are expensive and laborious. Commercially available enzyme immunoassays are most frequently used. Measles can also be diagnosed by isolation of the virus in cell culture from respiratory secretions, nasopharyngeal or conjunctival swabs, blood, or urine. Direct detection of giant cells in respiratory secretions, urine, or tissue obtained by biopsy provides another method of diagnosis.

For detection of measles virus RNA by reverse-transcriptase polymerase chain reaction amplification of RNA extracted from clinical specimens, primers targeted to highly conserved regions of measles virus genes are used. Extremely sensitive and specific, this assay may also permit identification and characterization of measles virus genotypes for molecular epidemiologic studies and can distinguish wild-type from vaccine virus strains.

TREATMENT MEASLES

There is no specific antiviral therapy for measles. Treatment consists of general supportive measures, such as hydration and administration of antipyretic agents. Because secondary bacterial infections are a major cause of morbidity and death attributable to measles, effective case management involves prompt antibiotic treatment for patients who have clinical evidence of bacterial infection, including pneumonia and otitis media. *Streptococcus pneumoniae* and *Haemophilus influenzae* type b are common causes of bacterial pneumonia following measles; vaccines against these pathogens probably lower the incidence of secondary bacterial infections following measles.

Vitamin A is effective for the treatment of measles and can markedly reduce rates of morbidity and mortality. The WHO recommends administration of once-daily doses of 200,000 IU of vitamin A for 2 consecutive days to all children with measles who are ≥12 months of age. Lower doses are recommended for younger children: 100,000 IU per day for children 6–12 months of age and 50,000 IU per day for children <6 months old. A third dose is recommended 2–4 weeks later for children with evidence of vitamin A deficiency. While such deficiency is not a widely recognized problem in the United States, many American children with measles do, in fact, have low serum levels of vitamin A, and these children experience increased measles-associated morbidity. The Committee on Infectious Diseases of the American Academy of Pediatrics recommends that the administration of two consecutive daily doses of vitamin A be considered for children who are hospitalized with measles and its complications as well as for children with measles who are immunodeficient; who have ophthalmologic evidence of vitamin A deficiency, impaired intestinal absorption, or moderate to severe malnutrition; or who have recently immigrated from areas with high measles mortality rates. Parenteral and oral formulations of vitamin A are available.

Anecdotal reports have described the recovery of previously healthy pregnant and immunocompromised patients with measles pneumonia and of immunocompromised patients with measles encephalitis after treatment with aerosolized and IV ribavirin. However, the clinical benefits of ribavirin in measles have not been conclusively demonstrated in clinical trials.

COMPLICATIONS

Most complications of measles involve the respiratory tract and include the effects of measles virus replication itself and secondary bacterial infections. Acute laryngotracheobronchitis (croup) can occur during measles and may result in airway obstruction, particularly in young children. Giant-cell pneumonitis due to replication of measles virus in the lungs can develop in immunocompromised children, including those with HIV-1 infection. Many children with measles develop diarrhea, which contributes to undernutrition.

Most complications of measles result from secondary bacterial infections of the respiratory tract that are attributable to a state of immune suppression lasting for several weeks to months after acute measles. Otitis media and bronchopneumonia are most common and may be caused by *S. pneumoniae*, *H. influenzae* type b, or staphylococci. Recurrence of fever or failure of fever to subside with the rash suggests secondary bacterial infection.

Rare but serious complications of measles involve the central nervous system (CNS). Postmeasles encephalomyelitis complicates ~1 in 1000 cases, affecting mainly older children and adults. Encephalomyelitis occurs within 2 weeks of rash onset and is characterized by fever, seizures, and a variety of neurologic abnormalities. The finding of periventricular demyelination, the induction of immune responses to myelin basic protein, and the absence of measles virus in the brain suggest that postmeasles encephalomyelitis is an autoimmune disorder triggered by measles virus infection. Other CNS complications that occur months to years after acute infection are measles inclusion body encephalitis (MIBE) and subacute sclerosing panencephalitis (SSPE). In contrast to postmeasles encephalomyelitis, MIBE and SSPE are caused by persistent measles virus infection. MIBE is a rare but fatal complication that affects individuals with defective cellular immunity and typically occurs months after infection. SSPE is a slowly progressive disease characterized by seizures and progressive deterioration of cognitive and motor functions, with death occurring 5–15 years after measles virus infection. SSPE most often develops in persons infected with measles virus at <2 years of age.

PROGNOSIS

Most persons with measles recover and develop long-term protective immunity to reinfection. Measles case-fatality proportions vary with the average age of infection, the nutritional and immunologic status of the population, measles vaccine coverage, and access to health care. Among previously vaccinated persons who do become infected, disease is less severe and mortality rates are significantly lower. In developed countries, <1 in 1000 children with measles die. In endemic areas of sub-Saharan Africa, the measles case-fatality proportion may be 5–10% or even higher. Measles is a major cause of childhood deaths in refugee camps and in internally displaced populations, where case-fatality proportions have been as high as 20–30%.

PREVENTION

Passive Immunization Human immunoglobulin given shortly after exposure can attenuate the clinical course of measles. In immunocompetent persons, administration of immunoglobulin within 72 h of exposure usually prevents measles virus infection and almost always prevents clinical measles. Administered up to 6 days after exposure, immunoglobulin will still prevent or modify the disease. Prophylaxis with immunoglobulin is recommended for susceptible household and nosocomial contacts who are at risk of developing severe measles, particularly children <1 year of age, immunocompromised persons (including HIV-infected persons previously immunized with live attenuated measles vaccine), and pregnant women. Except for premature infants, children <6 months of age usually will be partially or completely protected by passively acquired maternal antibody. If measles is diagnosed in a household member, all unimmunized children in the household should receive immunoglobulin. The recommended dose is 0.25 mL/kg given intramuscularly. Immunocompromised persons should receive 0.5 mL/kg. The maximum total dose is 15 mL. IV immunoglobulin contains antibodies to measles virus; the usual dose of 100–400 mg/kg generally provides adequate prophylaxis for measles exposures occurring as long as 3 weeks or more after IV immunoglobulin administration.

Active Immunization The first live attenuated measles vaccine was developed by passage of the Edmonston strain in chick embryo fibroblasts to produce the Edmonston B virus, which was licensed in 1963 in the United States. Further passage of Edmonston B virus produced the more attenuated Schwarz vaccine that currently serves as the standard in much of the world. The Moraten ("more attenuated Enders") strain, which was licensed in 1968 and is used in the United States, is genetically closely related to the Schwarz strain.

Lyophilized measles vaccines are relatively stable, but reconstituted vaccine rapidly loses potency. Live attenuated measles vaccines are inactivated by light and heat and lose about half their potency at 20°C and almost all their potency at 37°C within 1 h after reconstitution. Therefore, a cold chain must be maintained before and after reconstitution. Antibodies first appear 12–15 days after vaccination, and titers peak at 1–3 months. Measles vaccines are often combined with other live attenuated virus vaccines, such as those for mumps and rubella (MMR) and for mumps, rubella, and varicella (MMR-V).

The recommended age of first vaccination varies from 6 to 15 months and represents a balance between the optimal age for seroconversion and the probability of acquiring measles before that age. The proportions of children who develop protective levels of antibody after measles vaccination approximate 85% at 9 months of age and 95% at 12 months. Common childhood illnesses concomitant with vaccination may reduce the level of immune response, but such illness is not a valid reason to withhold vaccination. Measles vaccines have been well tolerated and immunogenic in HIV-1-infected children and adults, although antibody levels may wane. Because of the potential severity of wild-type measles virus infection in HIV-1-infected children, routine measles vaccination is recommended except for those who are severely immunocompromised. Measles vaccination is contraindicated in individuals with other severe deficiencies of cellular immunity because of the possibility of disease due to progressive pulmonary or CNS infection with the vaccine virus.

The duration of vaccine-induced immunity is at least several decades if not longer. Rates of secondary vaccine failure 10–15 years after immunization have been estimated at ~5% but are probably lower when vaccination takes place after 12 months of age. Decreasing antibody concentrations do not necessarily imply a complete loss of protective immunity: a secondary immune response usually develops after reexposure to measles virus, with a rapid rise in antibody titers in the absence of overt clinical disease.

Standard doses of currently licensed measles vaccines are safe for immunocompetent children and adults. Fever to 39.4°C (103°F) occurs in ~5% of seronegative vaccine recipients, and 2% of vaccine recipients develop a transient rash. Mild transient thrombocytopenia has been reported, with an incidence of ~1 case per 40,000 doses of MMR vaccine.

Since the publication of a report in 1998 hypothesizing that MMR vaccine may cause a syndrome of autism and intestinal inflammation, much public attention has focused on this purported association. The events that followed publication of this report led to diminished vaccine coverage in the United Kingdom and provide important lessons in the misinterpretation of epidemiologic evidence and the communication of scientific results to the public. The publication that incited the concern was a case series describing 12 children with a regressive developmental disorder and chronic enterocolitis; 9 of these children had autism. In 8 of the 12 cases, the parents associated onset of the developmental delay with MMR vaccination. This simple temporal association was misinterpreted and misrepresented as a possible causal relationship, first by the lead author of the study and then by elements of the media and the public. Subsequently, several comprehensive reviews and additional epidemiologic studies refuted evidence of a causal relationship between MMR vaccination and autism.

PROSPECTS FOR MEASLES ERADICATION

Progress in global measles control has renewed discussion of measles eradication. In contrast to poliovirus eradication, the eradication of measles virus will not entail challenges posed by prolonged shedding of potentially virulent vaccine viruses and environmental viral reservoirs. However, in comparison with smallpox eradication, higher levels of population immunity will be necessary to interrupt measles virus transmission, more highly skilled health care workers will be required to administer measles vaccines, and containment through case detection and ring vaccination will be more difficult for measles virus because of infectivity before rash onset. New tools, such as aerosol administration of measles vaccines, will facilitate mass vaccination campaigns. Despite enormous progress, measles remains a leading vaccine-preventable cause of childhood mortality worldwide and continues to cause outbreaks in communities with low vaccination coverage rates in industrialized nations.

230e Rubella (German Measles)

Laura A. Zimmerman, Susan E. Reef

This is a digital-only chapter. It is available on the DVD that accompanies this book, as well as on Access Medicine/Harrison's Online, and the eBook and "app" editions of HPIM 19e.

Rubella was historically viewed as a variant of measles or scarlet fever. Not until 1962 was a separate viral agent for rubella isolated. After an epidemic of rubella in Australia in the early 1940s, the ophthalmologist Norman Gregg noticed the occurrence of congenital cataracts among infants whose mothers had reported rubella infection during early pregnancy, and congenital rubella syndrome (CRS) was first described.

231e Mumps

Steven A. Rubin, Kathryn M. Carbone

This is a digital-only chapter. It is available on the DVD that accompanies this book, as well as on Access Medicine/Harrison's Online, and the eBook and "app" editions of HPIM 19e.

DEFINITION

Mumps is an illness characterized by acute-onset unilateral or bilateral tender, self-limited swelling of the parotid or other salivary gland(s) that lasts at least 2 days and has no other apparent cause.

232 Rabies and Other Rhabdovirus Infections

Alan C. Jackson

RABIES

Rabies is a rapidly progressive, acute infectious disease of the central nervous system (CNS) in humans and animals that is caused by infection with rabies virus. The infection is normally transmitted from animal vectors. Rabies has encephalitic and paralytic forms that progress to death.

ETIOLOGIC AGENT

Rabies virus is a member of the family Rhabdoviridae. Two genera in this family, *Lyssavirus* and *Vesiculovirus*, contain species that cause human disease. Rabies virus is a lyssavirus that infects a broad range of animals and causes serious neurologic disease when transmitted to humans. This single-strand RNA virus has a nonsegmented, negative-sense (antisense) genome that consists of 11,932 nucleotides and encodes 5 proteins: nucleocapsid protein, phosphoprotein, matrix protein, glycoprotein, and a large polymerase protein. Rabies virus variants, which can be characterized by distinctive nucleotide sequences, are associated with specific animal reservoirs. Six other non–rabies virus species in the *Lyssavirus* genus have been reported to cause a clinical picture similar to rabies. Vesicular stomatitis virus, a vesiculovirus, causes vesiculation and ulceration in cattle, horses, and other animals and causes a self-limited, mild, systemic illness in humans (see "Other Rhabdoviruses," below).

Rabies is a zoonotic infection that occurs in a variety of mammals throughout the world except in Antarctica and on some islands. Rabies virus is usually transmitted to humans by the bite of an infected animal. Worldwide, endemic canine rabies is estimated to cause 55,000 human deaths annually. Most of these deaths occur in Asia and Africa, with rural populations and children most frequently affected. Thus, in many resource-poor and resource-limited countries, canine rabies continues to be a threat to humans. However, in Latin America, rabies control efforts in dogs have been quite successful in recent years. Endemic canine rabies has been eliminated from the United States and most other resource-rich countries. Rabies is endemic in wildlife species, and a variety of animal reservoirs have been identified in different countries. Surveillance data from 2012 identified 6162 confirmed animal cases of rabies in the United States (including Puerto Rico). Only 8% of these cases were in domestic animals, including 257 cases in cats, 84 in dogs, and 115 in cattle. In North American wildlife reservoirs, including bats, raccoons, skunks, and foxes, the infection is endemic, with involvement of one or more rabies virus variants in each reservoir species (Fig. 232-1). "Spillover" of rabies to other wildlife species and to domestic animals occurs. Bat rabies virus variants are present in every state except Hawaii and are responsible for most indigenously acquired human rabies cases in the United States. Raccoon rabies is endemic along the entire eastern coast of the United States. Skunk rabies is present in the midwestern states, with another focus in California. Rabies in foxes occurs in Texas, New Mexico, Arizona, and Alaska.

In Canada and Europe, epizootics of rabies in red foxes have been well controlled with the use of baits containing rabies vaccine. A similar approach is used in Canada to control raccoon rabies.

Rabies virus variants isolated from humans or other mammalian species can be identified by reverse-transcription polymerase chain reaction (RT-PCR) amplification and sequencing or by characterization with monoclonal antibodies. These techniques are helpful in human cases with no known history of exposure. Worldwide, most human rabies is transmitted from dogs in countries with endemic canine rabies and dog-to-dog transmission, and human cases can be imported by travelers returning from these regions. In North America, human disease is usually associated with transmission from bats; there may be no known history of bat bite or other bat exposure in these cases. Most human cases are due to a bat rabies virus variant associated with silver-haired and tricolored bats. These are small bats whose bite may not be recognized, and the virus has adapted for replication at skin temperature and in cell types that are present in the skin.

Transmission from nonbite exposures is relatively uncommon. Aerosols generated in the laboratory or in caves containing millions of Brazilian free-tail bats have rarely caused human rabies. Transmission has resulted from corneal transplantation and also from solid organ transplantation and a vascular conduit (for a liver transplant) from undiagnosed donors with rabies in Texas, Florida, and Germany. Human-to-human transmission is extremely rare, although hypothetical concern about transmission to health care workers has prompted the implementation of barrier techniques to prevent exposures.

PATHOGENESIS

The incubation period of rabies (defined as the interval between exposure and the onset of clinical disease) is usually 20–90 days but in rare cases is as short as a few days or >1 year. During most of the incubation period, rabies virus is thought to be present at or close to the site of inoculation (Fig. 232-2). In muscles, the virus is known to bind to nicotinic acetylcholine receptors on postsynaptic membranes at neuromuscular junctions, but the exact details of viral entry into the skin and SC tissues have not yet been clarified. Rabies virus spreads centripetally along peripheral nerves toward the CNS at a rate of up to ~250 mm/d via retrograde fast axonal transport to the spinal cord or brainstem. Once the virus enters the CNS, it rapidly disseminates to other regions of the CNS via fast axonal transport along neuroanatomic connections. Neurons are prominently infected in rabies; infection of astrocytes is unusual. After CNS infection becomes established, there is centrifugal spread along sensory and autonomic nerves to other tissues, including the salivary glands, heart, adrenal glands, and skin. Rabies virus replicates in acinar cells of the salivary glands and is secreted in the saliva of rabid animals that serve as vectors of

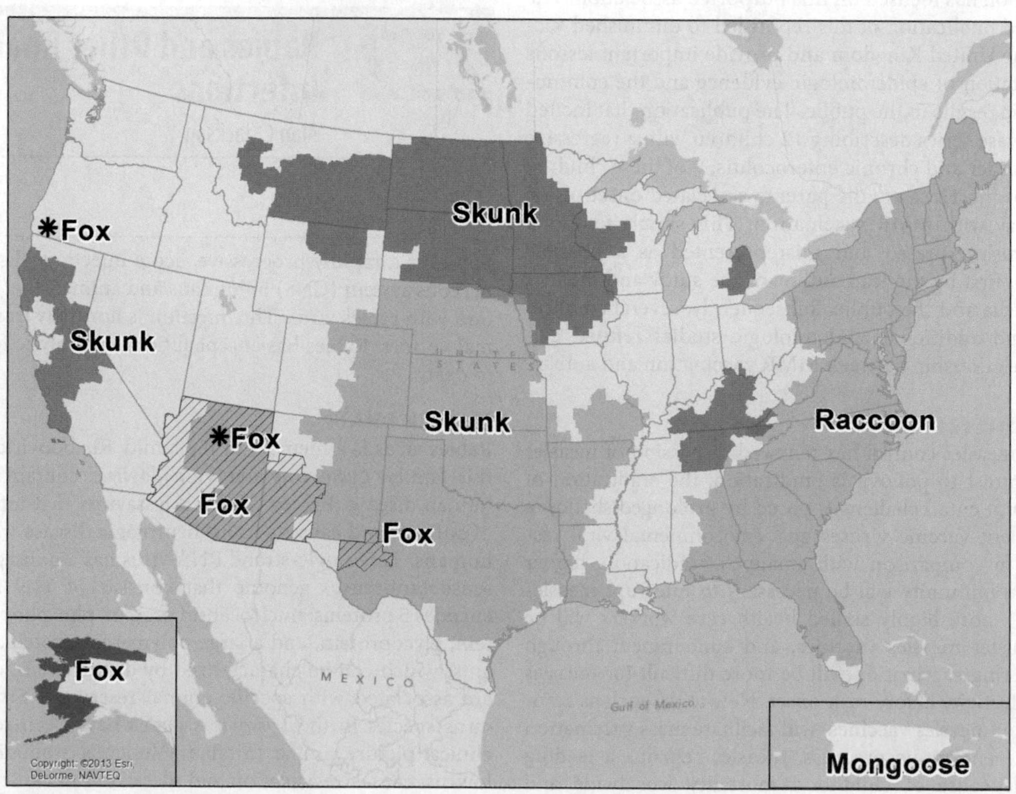

FIGURE 232-1 Distribution of the major rabies virus variants among wild terrestrial reservoirs in the United States and Puerto Rico, 2008–2012. *Potential host-shift event. *(From JL Dyer et al: J Am Vet Med Assoc 243:805, 2013.)*

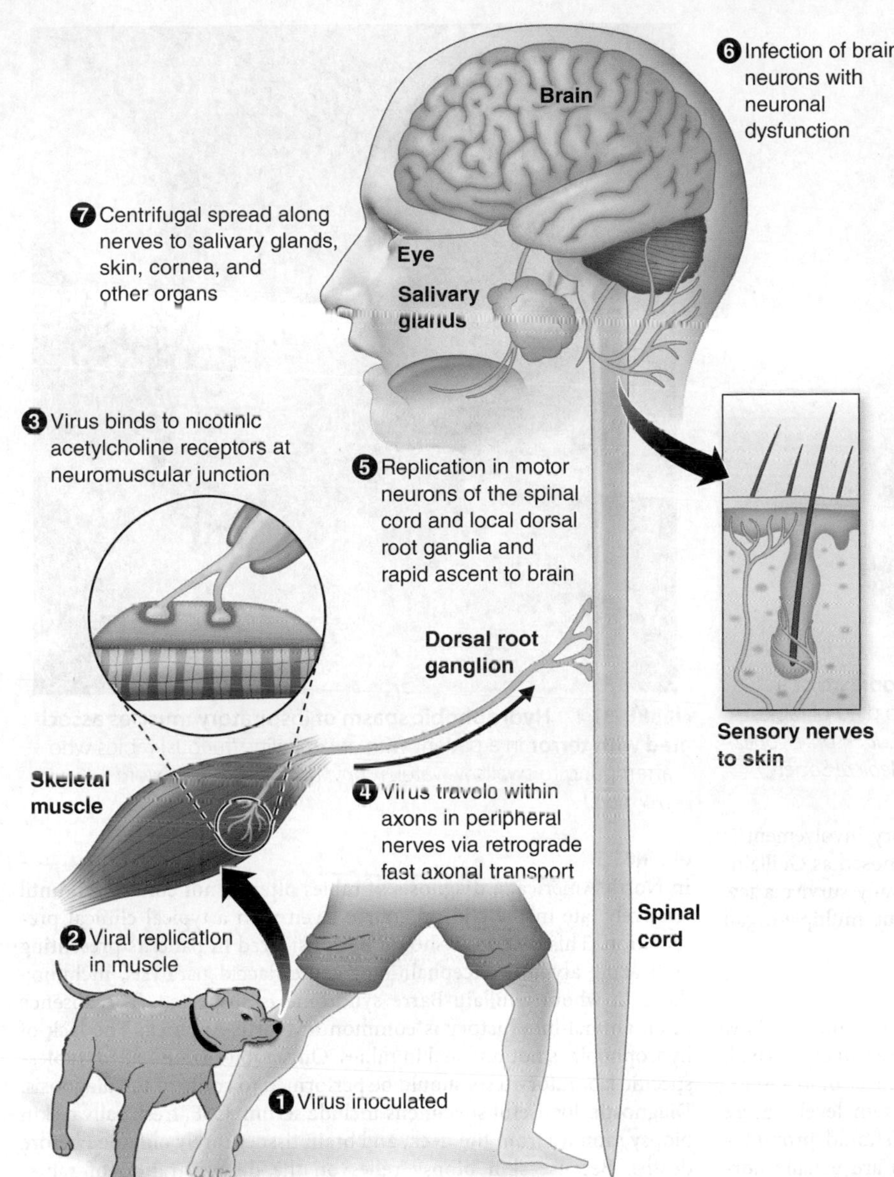

6 Infection of brain neurons with neuronal dysfunction
Brain
7 Centrifugal spread along nerves to salivary glands, skin, cornea, and other organs
Eye
Salivary glands
3 Virus binds to nicotinic acetylcholine receptors at neuromuscular junction
5 Replication in motor neurons of the spinal cord and local dorsal root ganglia and rapid ascent to brain
Dorsal root ganglion
Sensory nerves to skin
Skeletal muscle
4 Virus travels within axons in peripheral nerves via retrograde fast axonal transport
Spinal cord
2 Viral replication in muscle
1 Virus inoculated

FIGURE 232-2 Schematic representation of the pathogenetic events following peripheral inoculation of rabies virus by an animal bite. *(Adapted from Jackson AC: Human disease, in Rabies: scientific basis of the disease and its management, 3rd ed., AC Jackson [ed], Oxford, UK, Elsevier Academic Press, 2013, pp 269–298; with permission.)*

the disease. There is no well-documented evidence for hematogenous spread of rabies virus.

Pathologic studies show mild inflammatory changes in the CNS in rabies, with mononuclear inflammatory infiltration in the leptomeninges, perivascular regions, and parenchyma, including microglial nodules called *Babes nodules*. Degenerative neuronal changes usually are not prominent, and there is little evidence of neuronal death; neuronophagia is observed occasionally. The pathologic changes are surprisingly mild in light of the clinical severity and fatal outcome of the disease. The most characteristic pathologic finding in rabies is the *Negri body* (Fig. 232-3). Negri bodies are eosinophilic cytoplasmic inclusions in brain neurons that are composed of rabies virus proteins and viral RNA. These inclusions occur in a minority of infected neurons, are commonly observed in Purkinje cells of the cerebellum and in pyramidal neurons of the hippocampus, and are less frequently seen in cortical and brainstem neurons. Negri bodies are not observed in all cases of rabies. The lack of prominent degenerative neuronal changes has led to the concept that neuronal dysfunction—rather than neuronal death—is responsible for clinical disease in rabies. The basis for behavioral changes, including the aggressive behavior of rabid animals, is not well understood.

CLINICAL MANIFESTATIONS

In rabies, the emphasis must be on postexposure prophylaxis (PEP) initiated before any symptoms or signs develop. Rabies should usually be suspected on the basis of the clinical presentation. The disease usually presents as atypical encephalitis with relative preservation of consciousness. Rabies may be difficult to recognize late in the clinical course when progression to coma has occurred. A minority of patients present with acute flaccid paralysis. There are prodromal, acute neurologic, and comatose phases that usually progress to death despite aggressive therapy (Table 232-1).

Prodromal Features The clinical features of rabies begin with nonspecific prodromal manifestations, including fever, malaise, headache, nausea, and vomiting. Anxiety or agitation may also occur. The earliest specific neurologic symptoms of rabies include paresthesias, pain, or pruritus near the site of the exposure, one or more of which occur in 50–80% of patients and strongly suggest rabies. The wound has usually healed by this point, and these symptoms probably reflect infection with associated inflammatory changes in local dorsal root or cranial sensory ganglia.

Encephalitic Rabies Two acute neurologic forms of rabies are seen in humans: encephalitic (furious) in 80% and paralytic in 20%. Some of the manifestations of encephalitic rabies, including fever, confusion, hallucinations, combativeness, and seizures, may be seen in other viral encephalitides as well. Autonomic dysfunction is common and may result in hypersalivation, gooseflesh, cardiac arrhythmia, and priapism. In encephalitic rabies, episodes of hyperexcitability are typically followed by periods of complete lucidity that become shorter as the disease progresses. Rabies encephalitis is distinguished by early brainstem involvement, which results in the classic features of *hydrophobia* (involuntary, painful contraction of the diaphragm and accessory respiratory, laryngeal, and pharyngeal muscles in response to swallowing liquids) and *aerophobia* (the same features caused by stimulation from a draft of air). These symptoms are probably due to dysfunction of infected brainstem neurons that normally inhibit inspiratory neurons near the nucleus ambiguus, resulting in exaggerated defense reflexes that protect the respiratory tract. The combination of hypersalivation and pharyngeal dysfunction is also responsible for the classic appearance of "foaming at the mouth" (Fig. 232-4). Brainstem dysfunction progresses rapidly, and coma—followed within days by death—is the rule unless the course is prolonged by supportive measures. With such measures, late complications can include cardiac and/or respiratory failure, disturbances of water balance (syndrome of inappropriate antidiuretic hormone secretion or diabetes insipidus), noncardiogenic pulmonary edema, and gastrointestinal hemorrhage. Cardiac arrhythmias may be due to dysfunction affecting vital centers in the brainstem or to myocarditis. Multiple-organ failure is common in patients treated aggressively in critical care units.

Paralytic Rabies About 20% of patients have paralytic rabies in which muscle weakness predominates and cardinal features of encephalitic rabies (hyperexcitability, hydrophobia, and aerophobia) are lacking. There is early and prominent flaccid muscle weakness, often beginning in the bitten extremity and spreading to produce quadriparesis and facial

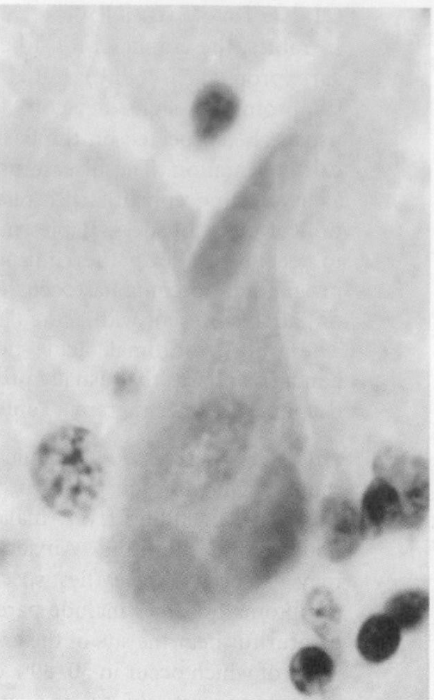

FIGURE 232-3 Three large Negri bodies in the cytoplasm of a cerebellar Purkinje cell from an 8-year-old boy who died of rabies after being bitten by a rabid dog in Mexico. *(From AC Jackson, E Lopez-Corella: N Engl J Med 335:568, 1996. © Massachusetts Medical Society.)*

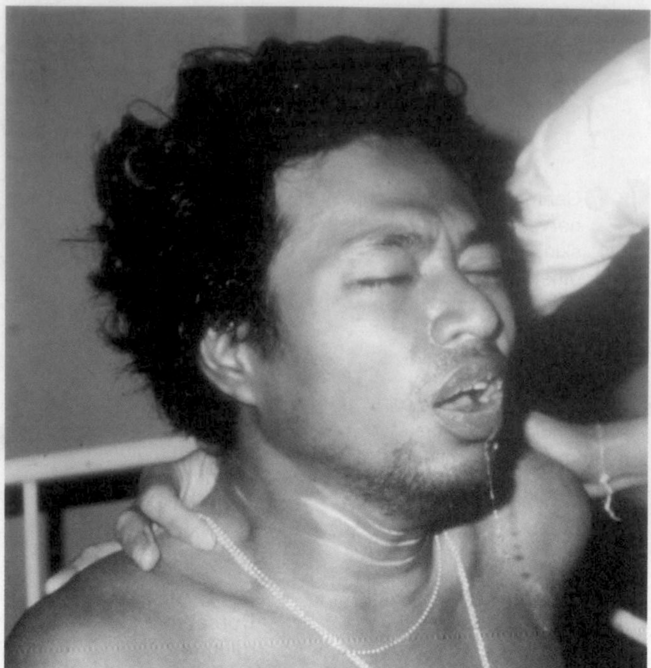

FIGURE 232-4 Hydrophobic spasm of inspiratory muscles associated with terror in a patient with encephalitic (furious) rabies who is attempting to swallow water. *(Copyright DA Warrell, Oxford, UK; with permission.)*

weakness. Sphincter involvement is common, sensory involvement is usually mild, and these cases are commonly misdiagnosed as Guillain-Barré syndrome. Patients with paralytic rabies generally survive a few days longer than those with encephalitic rabies, but multiple-organ failure nevertheless ensues.

LABORATORY INVESTIGATIONS

Most routine laboratory tests in rabies yield normal results or show nonspecific abnormalities. Complete blood counts are usually normal. Examination of cerebrospinal fluid (CSF) often reveals mild mononuclear cell pleocytosis with a mildly elevated protein level. Severe pleocytosis (>1000 white cells/μL) is unusual and should prompt a search for an alternative diagnosis. CT head scans are usually normal in rabies. MRI brain scans may show signal abnormalities in the brainstem or other gray-matter areas, but these findings are variable and nonspecific. Electroencephalograms show only nonspecific abnormalities. Of course, important tests in suspected cases of rabies include those that may identify an alternative, potentially treatable diagnosis (see "Differential Diagnosis," below).

TABLE 232-1 CLINICAL STAGES OF RABIES

Phase	Typical Duration	Symptoms and Signs
Incubation period	20–90 days	None
Prodrome	2–10 days	Fever, malaise, anorexia, nausea, vomiting; paresthesias, pain, or pruritus at the wound site
Acute neurologic disease		
Encephalitic (80%)	2–7 days	Anxiety, agitation, hyperactivity, bizarre behavior, hallucinations, autonomic dysfunction, hydrophobia
Paralytic (20%)	2–10 days	Flaccid paralysis in limb(s) progressing to quadriparesis with facial paralysis
Coma, death[a]	0–14 days	

[a]Recovery is rare.

Source: MAW Hattwick: Rabies virus, in *Principles and Practice of Infectious Diseases*, GL Mandell et al (eds). New York, Wiley, 1979, pp 1217–1228. Adapted with permission from Elsevier.

DIAGNOSIS

In North America, a diagnosis of rabies often is not considered until relatively late in the clinical course, even with a typical clinical presentation. This diagnosis should be considered in patients presenting with acute atypical encephalitis or acute flaccid paralysis, including those in whom Guillain-Barré syndrome is suspected. The absence of an animal-bite history is common in North America. The lack of hydrophobia is not unusual in rabies. Once rabies is suspected, rabies-specific laboratory tests should be performed to confirm the diagnosis. Diagnostically useful specimens include serum, CSF, fresh saliva, skin biopsy samples from the neck, and brain tissue (rarely obtained before death). Because skin biopsy relies on the demonstration of rabies virus antigen in cutaneous nerves at the base of hair follicles, samples are usually taken from hairy skin at the nape of the neck. Corneal impression smears are of low diagnostic yield and are generally not performed. Negative antemortem rabies-specific laboratory tests never exclude a diagnosis of rabies, and tests may need to be repeated after an interval for diagnostic confirmation.

Rabies Virus–Specific Antibodies In a previously unimmunized patient, serum neutralizing antibodies to rabies virus are diagnostic. However, because rabies virus infects immunologically privileged neuronal tissues, serum antibodies may not develop until late in the disease. Antibodies may be detected within a few days after the onset of symptoms, but some patients die without detectable antibodies. The presence of rabies virus–specific antibodies in the CSF suggests rabies encephalitis, regardless of immunization status. A diagnosis of rabies is questionable in patients who recover from rabies without developing serum neutralizing antibodies to rabies virus.

RT-PCR Amplification Detection of rabies virus RNA by RT-PCR is highly sensitive and specific. This technique can detect virus in fresh saliva samples, skin, CSF, and brain tissues. In addition, RT-PCR with genetic sequencing can distinguish among rabies virus variants, permitting identification of the probable source of an infection.

Direct Fluorescent Antibody Testing Direct fluorescent antibody (DFA) testing with rabies virus antibodies conjugated to fluorescent dyes is highly sensitive and specific and can be performed quickly and applied to skin biopsies and brain tissue. In skin biopsies, rabies virus antigen may be detected in cutaneous nerves at the base of hair follicles.

DIFFERENTIAL DIAGNOSIS

The diagnosis of rabies may be difficult without a history of animal exposure, and no exposure to an animal (e.g., a bat) may be recalled. The presentation of rabies is usually quite different from that of acute viral encephalitis due to most other causes, including herpes simplex encephalitis and arboviral (e.g., West Nile) encephalitis. Early neurologic symptoms may occur at the site of the bite, and there may be early features of brainstem involvement with preservation of consciousness. Anti-*N*-methyl-D-aspartate receptor (anti-NMDA) encephalitis occurs in young patients (especially females) and is characterized by behavioral changes, autonomic instability, hypoventilation, and seizures. Postinfectious (immune-mediated) encephalomyelitis may follow influenza, measles, mumps, and other infections; it may also occur as a sequela of immunization with rabies vaccine derived from neural tissues, which are used only in resource-limited and resource-poor countries. Rabies may present with unusual neuropsychiatric symptoms and may be misdiagnosed as a psychiatric disorder. Rabies hysteria may occur as a psychological response to the fear of rabies and is often characterized by a shorter incubation period than rabies, aggressive behavior, inability to communicate, and a long course with recovery.

As previously mentioned, paralytic rabies may mimic Guillain-Barré syndrome. In these cases, fever, bladder dysfunction, a normal sensory examination, and CSF pleocytosis favor a diagnosis of rabies. Conversely, Guillain-Barré syndrome may occur as a complication of rabies vaccination with a neural tissue–derived product (e.g., suckling mouse brain vaccine) and may be mistaken for paralytic rabies (i.e., vaccine failure).

TREATMENT RABIES

There is no established treatment for rabies. There have been many recent treatment failures with the combination of antiviral drugs, ketamine, and therapeutic (induced) coma—measures that were used in a healthy survivor in whom antibodies to rabies virus were detected at presentation. Expert opinion should be sought before a course of experimental therapy is embarked upon. A palliative approach may be appropriate for some patients.

PROGNOSIS

Rabies is an almost uniformly fatal disease but is nearly always preventable with appropriate postexposure therapy during the early incubation period (see below). There are seven well-documented cases of survival from rabies. All but one of these patients had received rabies vaccine before disease onset. The single survivor who had not received vaccine had neutralizing antibodies to rabies virus in serum and CSF at clinical presentation. Most patients with rabies die within several days of the onset of illness, despite aggressive care in a critical care unit.

PREVENTION

Postexposure Prophylaxis Since there is no effective therapy for rabies, it is extremely important to prevent the disease after an animal exposure. Figure 232-5 shows the steps involved in making decisions about PEP. On the basis of the history of the exposure and local epidemiologic information, the physician must decide whether initiation of PEP is warranted. Healthy dogs, cats, or ferrets may be confined and observed for 10 days. PEP is not necessary if the animal remains healthy. If the animal develops signs of rabies during the observation period, it should be euthanized immediately; the head should be transported to the laboratory under refrigeration, rabies virus should be sought by DFA testing, and viral isolation should be attempted by cell culture and/or mouse inoculation. Any animal other than a dog, cat, or ferret should be euthanized immediately and the head submitted for laboratory examination. In high-risk exposures and in areas where canine rabies is endemic, rabies prophylaxis should be initiated without waiting for laboratory results. If the laboratory results prove to be negative, it may safely be concluded that the animal's saliva did not

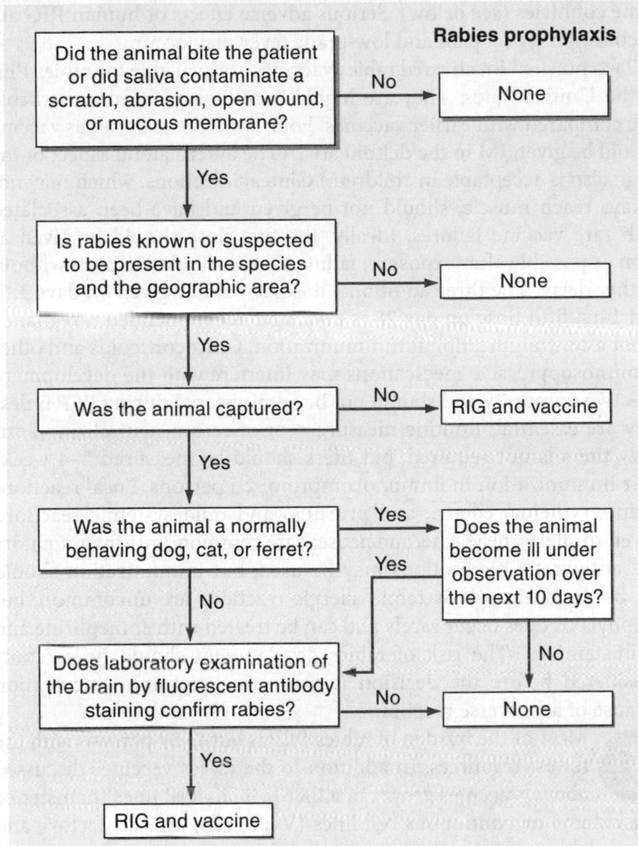

FIGURE 232-5 Algorithm for rabies postexposure prophylaxis. RIG, rabies immune globulin. (*From L Corey, in Harrison's Principles of Internal Medicine, 15th ed. E Braunwald et al [eds]: New York, McGraw-Hill, 2001; adapted with permission.*)

contain rabies virus, and immunization should be discontinued. If an animal escapes after an exposure, it must be considered rabid, and PEP must be initiated unless information from public health officials indicates otherwise (i.e., there is no endemic rabies in the area). Although controversial, the use of PEP may be warranted when a person (e.g., a small child or a sleeping adult) has been present in the same space as a bat and an unrecognized bite cannot be reliably excluded.

PEP includes local wound care and both active and passive immunization. Local wound care is essential and may greatly decrease the risk of rabies virus infection. Wound care should not be delayed, even if the initiation of immunization is postponed pending the results of the 10-day observation period. All bite wounds and scratches should be washed thoroughly with soap and water. Devitalized tissues should be debrided, tetanus prophylaxis given, and antibiotic treatment initiated whenever indicated.

All previously unvaccinated persons (but not those who have previously been immunized) should be passively immunized with rabies immune globulin (RIG). If RIG is not immediately available, it should be administered no later than 7 days after the first vaccine dose. After day 7, endogenous antibodies are being produced, and passive immunization may actually be counterproductive. If anatomically feasible, the entire dose of RIG (20 IU/kg) should be infiltrated at the site of the bite; otherwise, any RIG remaining after infiltration of the bite site should be administered IM at a distant site. With multiple or large wounds, the RIG preparation may need to be diluted in order to obtain a sufficient volume for adequate infiltration of all wound sites. If the exposure involves a mucous membrane, the entire dose should be administered IM. Rabies vaccine and RIG should never be administered at the same site or with the same syringe. Commercially available RIG in the United States is purified from the serum of hyperimmunized human donors. These human RIG preparations are much better tolerated than are the equine-derived preparations still in use in some countries (see below). Serious adverse effects of human RIG are uncommon. Local pain and low-grade fever may occur.

Two purified inactivated rabies vaccines are available for rabies PEP in the United States. They are highly immunogenic and remarkably safe compared with earlier vaccines. Four 1-mL doses of rabies vaccine should be given IM in the deltoid area. (The anterolateral aspect of the thigh also is acceptable in children.) Gluteal injections, which may not always reach muscle, should not be given and have been associated with rare vaccine failures. Ideally, the first dose should be given as soon as possible after exposure; failing that, it should be given without further delay. The three additional doses should be given on days 3, 7, and 14; a fifth dose on day 28 is no longer recommended. Pregnancy is not a contraindication for immunization. Glucocorticoids and other immunosuppressive medications may interfere with the development of active immunity and should not be administered during PEP unless they are essential. Routine measurement of serum neutralizing antibody titers is not required, but titers should be measured 2–4 weeks after immunization in immunocompromised persons. Local reactions (pain, erythema, edema, and pruritus) and mild systemic reactions (fever, myalgias, headache, and nausea) are common; anti-inflammatory and antipyretic medications may be used, but immunization should not be discontinued. Systemic allergic reactions are uncommon, but anaphylaxis does occur rarely and can be treated with epinephrine and antihistamines. The risk of rabies development should be carefully considered before the decision is made to discontinue vaccination because of an adverse reaction.

Most of the burden of rabies PEP is borne by persons with the fewest resources. In addition to the rabies vaccines discussed above, vaccines grown in either primary cell lines (hamster or dog kidney) or continuous cell lines (Vero cells) are satisfactory and are available in many countries outside the United States. Less expensive vaccines derived from neural tissues are still used in a diminishing number of developing countries; however, these vaccines are associated with serious neuroparalytic complications, including postinfectious encephalomyelitis and Guillain-Barré syndrome. The use of these vaccines should be discontinued as soon as possible, and progress has been made in this regard. Worldwide, >10 million individuals receive postexposure rabies vaccine each year.

If human RIG is unavailable, purified equine RIG can be used in the same manner at a dose of 40 IU/kg. Before the administration of equine RIG, hypersensitivity should be assessed by intradermal testing with a 1:10 dilution. The incidence of anaphylactic reactions and serum sickness has been low with recent equine RIG products.

Preexposure Rabies Vaccination Preexposure rabies prophylaxis should be considered for people with an occupational or recreational risk of rabies exposures, including certain travelers to rabies-endemic areas. The primary schedule consists of three doses of rabies vaccine given on days 0, 7, and 21 or 28. Serum neutralizing antibody tests help determine the need for subsequent booster doses. When a previously immunized individual is exposed to rabies, two booster doses of vaccine should be administered on days 0 and 3. Wound care remains essential. As stated above, RIG should not be administered to previously vaccinated persons.

OTHER RHABDOVIRUSES

OTHER LYSSAVIRUSES

A growing number of lyssaviruses other than rabies virus have been discovered to infect bat populations in Europe, Africa, Asia, and Australia. Six of these viruses have produced a very small number of cases of a human disease indistinguishable from rabies: European bat lyssaviruses 1 and 2, Australian bat lyssavirus, Irkut virus, and Duvenhage virus. Mokola virus, a lyssavirus that has been isolated from shrews with an unknown reservoir species in Africa, may also produce human disease indistinguishable from rabies.

VESICULAR STOMATITIS VIRUS

Vesicular stomatitis is a viral disease of cattle, horses, pigs, and some wild mammals. Vesicular stomatitis virus is a member of the genus *Vesiculovirus* in the family Rhabdoviridae. Outbreaks of vesicular stomatitis in horses and cattle occur sporadically in the southwestern United States. The animal infection is associated with severe vesiculation and ulceration of oral tissues, teats, and feet and may be clinically indistinguishable from the more dangerous foot-and-mouth disease. Epidemics are usually seasonal, typically beginning in the late spring, and are probably due to arthropod vectors. Direct animal-to-animal spread can also occur, although the virus cannot penetrate intact skin. Transmission to humans usually results from direct contact with infected animals (particularly cattle) and occasionally follows laboratory exposure. In human disease, early conjunctivitis is followed by an acute influenza-like illness with fever, chills, nausea, vomiting, headache, retrobulbar pain, myalgias, substernal pain, malaise, pharyngitis, and lymphadenitis. Small vesicular lesions may be present on the buccal mucosa or on the fingers. Encephalitis is very rare. The illness usually lasts 3–6 days, with complete recovery. Subclinical infections are common. A serologic diagnosis can be made on the basis of a rise in titer of complement-fixing or neutralizing antibodies. Therapy is symptom-based.

233 Arthropod-Borne and Rodent-Borne Virus Infections

Jens H. Kuhn, Clarence J. Peters

This chapter summarizes the major features of selected arthropod-borne and rodent-borne viruses. Numerous viruses of this category are transmitted in nature among animals without ever infecting humans. Other viruses incidentally infect humans, but only a proportion of these viruses induce human disease. In addition, certain viral agents are regularly introduced into human populations or spread among humans by certain arthropods (specifically, insects and ticks) or by chronically infected rodents. These zoonotic viruses are taxonomically diverse and therefore differ fundamentally from one another in terms of virion morphology, replication strategies, genomic organization, and genome sequence. While a virus's classification in a taxon is enlightening with regard to natural maintenance strategies, sensitivity to antiviral agents, and particular aspects of pathogenesis, the classification does not necessarily predict which clinical signs and symptoms (if any) the virus will cause in humans. Zoonotic viruses are evolving, and "new" zoonotic viruses are regularly discovered. The epizootiology and epidemiology of zoonotic viruses continue to change as a result of environmental alterations affecting vectors, reservoirs, wildlife, livestock, and humans. Zoonotic viruses are most numerous in the tropics but are also found in temperate and even frigid climates. The distribution and seasonal activity of a zoonotic virus may vary, and the rate at which it changes is likely to depend largely on ecologic conditions (e.g., rainfall and temperature), which can affect the density of virus vectors and reservoirs and the development of infection.

Arthropod-borne viruses (arboviruses) infect their vectors after ingestion of a blood meal from a viremic, usually nonhuman vertebrate; some arthropods may also become infected by saliva-activated transmission. The arthropod vectors then develop chronic, systemic infection as the viruses penetrate the gut and spread throughout the body to the salivary glands; such virus dissemination, referred to as *extrinsic incubation*, typically lasts 1–3 weeks in mosquitoes. At this point, if the salivary glands become involved, the arthropod vector is competent to continue the chain of transmission by infecting a vertebrate during a subsequent blood meal. An alternative mechanism for virus maintenance in its arthropod vector is *transovarial transmission*. The arthropod generally is unharmed by the infection, and the natural vertebrate partner usually has only transient viremia with no overt disease.

Rodent-borne viruses are maintained in nature by transmission between rodents, which become chronically infected. Usually a high degree of rodent–virus specificity is observed, and overt disease in the reservoir host is rare.

ETIOLOGY

Arthropod-borne and rodent-borne zoonotic viruses belong to at least seven families: Arenaviridae, Bunyaviridae, Flaviviridae, Orthomyxoviridae, Reoviridae, Rhabdoviridae, and Togaviridae (Table 233-1).

ARENAVIRIDAE

The members of the family Arenaviridae that infect humans are all assigned to the genus *Arenavirus*. The members of this genus are divided into two main phylogenetic branches: Old World viruses (the Lassa–lymphocytic choriomeningitis serocomplex) and New World viruses (the Tacaribe serocomplex). Human arenaviruses form spherical, oval, or pleomorphic enveloped and spiked virions (~50–300 nm in diameter) that bud from the infected cell's plasma membrane. The particles contain two genomic single-stranded RNAs (S, ~3.5 kb; and L, ~7.5 kb) encoding structural proteins in an ambisense orientation. Most arenaviruses persist in nature by chronically infecting rodents. The Old World viruses are maintained by murid rodents that often are persistently viremic and commonly transmit viruses vertically and horizontally. New World viruses are found in cricetid rodents; horizontal transmission is typical, vertical infection may occur, and persistent viremia may be observed. Strikingly, each arenavirus is predominantly adapted to one particular type of rodent. Humans usually become infected through inhalation of or direct contact with infected rodent excreta or secreta (e.g., aerosols of rodents in harvesting machines; aerosolized dried rodent urine or feces in barns or houses; direct contact with rodents in traps). Person-to-person transmission of arenaviruses is uncommon.

BUNYAVIRIDAE

The family Bunyaviridae includes four medically significant genera: *Hantavirus*, *Nairovirus*, *Orthobunyavirus*, and *Phlebovirus*. The members of all these genera form spherical to pleomorphic enveloped virions containing three genomic single-stranded RNAs (S, ~1–2 kb; M, 3.6–5.3 kb; and L, 6.4–12.3 kb) of negative (hantaviruses, nairoviruses, orthobunyaviruses) or ambisense (nairoviruses) polarity. Bunyaviruses mature into particles 80–120 nm in diameter in the Golgi complex of infected cells and exit these cells by exocytosis.

Hantaviruses are unique among the bunyaviruses in that they are not transmitted by arthropods but instead are maintained in nature by rodents that chronically shed virions. Old World hantaviruses are harbored by murid and cricetid rodents, and New World hantaviruses are maintained by cricetid rodents. As with arenaviruses, individual hantaviruses usually are specifically adapted to a particular type of rodent. However, hantaviruses do not cause chronic viremia in their rodent hosts and are transmitted only horizontally from rodent to rodent. Similar to arenaviruses, hantaviruses infect humans primarily through inhalation of or direct contact with rodent excreta or secreta, and person-to-person transmission is not a common event (with the notable exception of Andes virus). Although there is overlap, the human Old World hantaviruses usually are the etiologic agents of hemorrhagic fever with renal syndrome, whereas the New World viruses usually cause hantavirus pulmonary syndrome.

Nairoviruses are maintained by ixodid ticks, which vertically (transovarially and transstadially) transmit these viruses to progeny tick generations and horizontally spread them through viremic vertebrate hosts. Humans are usually infected via a tick bite or during handling of infected vertebrates.

Orthobunyaviruses are largely mosquito-borne and rarely midge-borne and have viremic vertebrate intermediate hosts. Many orthobunyaviruses are also transovarially transmitted in their mosquito host. Numerous orthobunyaviruses have been associated with human infection and disease. They have been considered to be members of ~19 serogroups based on antigenic cross-reactions, but this grouping is currently undergoing revision with the accumulation of new genomic data and phylogenetic analyses. Human viruses are found in at least nine serogroups.

Phleboviruses are transmitted vertically (transovarially) in their arthropod hosts and horizontally through viremic vertebrate hosts. Phleboviruses are divided into two groups: the phlebotomus group viruses are transmitted by sandflies and the Uukuniemi group viruses by ticks. Phleboviruses are assigned to at least 10 serocomplexes; human pathogens are found in at least four of these serocomplexes.

FLAVIVIRIDAE

The family Flaviviridae currently includes four genera, one of which (*Flavivirus*) comprises arthropod-borne human viruses. Flaviviruses sensu stricto have single-stranded positive-sense RNA genomes (~11 kb) and form spherical enveloped particles 40–60 nm in diameter. The flaviviruses discussed here belong to two phylogenetically and antigenically distinct groups and are transmitted among vertebrates by mosquitoes and ixodid ticks, respectively. Vectors are usually infected when they feed on viremic hosts; as in the case of most other viruses discussed here, humans are accidental hosts who usually are infected by arthropod bites. Arthropods maintain flavivirus infections horizontally, although transovarial transmission has been documented. Under certain circumstances, flaviviruses can also be transmitted by aerosols or via contaminated food products; in particular, raw milk can transmit tick-borne encephalitis virus.

ORTHOMYXOVIRIDAE

The family Orthomyxoviridae includes two genera of medically relevant arthropod-borne viruses: *Quaranjavirus* and *Thogotovirus*. Quaranjaviruses are transmitted among birds by ixodid ticks, whereas thogotoviruses have a predilection for mammalian host reservoirs and can be transmitted by both ixodid ticks and mosquitoes.

REOVIRIDAE

The family Reoviridae contains viruses with linear, multisegmented, double stranded RNA genomes (~16–29 kb in total). These viruses produce particles that have icosahedral symmetry and are 60–80 nm in diameter. In contrast to all other virions discussed here, reovirions are not enveloped and thus are insensitive to detergent inactivation. Fifteen genera of reoviruses are currently recognized. Human arthropod-borne viruses are found among the genera *Coltivirus* (subfamily Spinareovirinae), *Orbivirus*, and *Seadornavirus* (subfamily Sedoreovirinae). Arthropod-borne coltiviruses possess 12 genome segments. Coltiviruses are transmitted by numerous tick types transstadially but not transovarially. Overall maintenance of the transmission cycle, therefore, involves viremic mammalian hosts infected by tick bites. Arthropod-borne orbiviruses have 10 genome segments and are transmitted by mosquitoes or ixodid ticks, whereas relevant seadornaviruses have 12 genome segments and are transmitted exclusively by mosquitoes.

RHABDOVIRIDAE

The family Rhabdoviridae is included in the order *Mononegavirales*. Viruses of the nine rhabdovirus genera have linear, nonsegmented, single-stranded RNA genomes of negative polarity (~11–15 kb) and form bullet-shaped to pleomorphic enveloped particles (100–430 nm long and 45–100 nm wide). Only the genus *Vesiculovirus* includes human arthropod-borne viruses, all of which are transmitted by insects (biting midges, mosquitoes, and sandflies). The general properties of rhabdoviruses are discussed in more detail in Chap. 232.

TOGAVIRIDAE

The members of the family Togaviridae have linear, single- and positive-stranded RNA genomes (~9.7–11.8 kb) and form enveloped icosahedral virions (~60–70 nm in diameter) that bud from the plasma membrane of the infected cell. The togaviruses discussed here are all members of the genus *Alphavirus* and are transmitted among vertebrates by mosquitoes.

TABLE 233-1 ZOONOTIC ARTHROPOD- AND RODENT-BORNE VIRUSES THAT INFECT HUMANS

Virus Group	Virus (Abbreviation)	Principal Reservoir Host(s)	Vector(s)	Syndrome[a]
Alphaviruses (Barmah Forest serocomplex)	Barmah Forest virus (BFV)	Horses, marsupials	Biting midges (*Culicoides marksi*), mosquitoes (*Aedes camptorhynchus, A. normanensis, A. notoscriptus, A. vigilax, Culex annulirostris*)	A/R
Alphaviruses (Semliki Forest serocomplex)	Chikungunya virus (CHIKV)	Bats, nonhuman primates	Mosquitoes (*Aedes, Culex* spp.)	A/R[b]
	Mayaro virus (MAYV)	Nonhuman primates, possums, rodents	Mosquitoes (predominantly *Haemagogus* spp.)	A/R
	O'nyong-nyong virus (ONNV)	Unknown	Mosquitoes (in particular *Anopheles gambiae, A. funestus, Mansonia* spp.)	A/R
	Una virus (UNAV)	Birds, horses, rodents	Mosquitoes (*Aedes, Anopheles, Coquillettidia, Culex, Ochlerotatus, Psorophora* spp.)	F/M
	Ross River virus (RRV)	Macropods, rodents	Mosquitoes (*Aedes normanensis, A. vigilax, Culex annulirostris*)	A/R
	Semliki Forest virus (SFV)	Birds, rodents	Mosquitoes (*Aedes, Culex* spp.)	A/R
Alphaviruses (eastern equine encephalitis serocomplex)	Eastern equine encephalitis virus (EEEV)	Freshwater swamp birds	Mosquitoes (*Aedes, Coquillettidia, Culex* spp.; *Culiseta melanura, Mansonia perturbans, Psorophora* spp.)	E
Alphaviruses (Venezuelan equine encephalitis serocomplex)	Everglades virus (EVEV)	Hispid cotton rats (*Sigmodon hispidus*)	Mosquitoes (*Culex cedecei*)	F/M, E
	Mucambo virus (MUCV)	Nonhuman primates, rodents	Mosquitoes (*Culex, Ochlerotatus* spp.)	F/M, E
	Tonate virus (TONV)	Suriname crested oropendolas (*Psarocolius decumanus*)	Mosquitoes (*Culex portesi*)	F/M, E
	Venezuelan equine encephalitis virus (VEEV)	Horses, rodents	Mosquitoes (*Aedes, Culex* spp.; *Psorophora confinnis*)	F/M, E
Alphaviruses (western equine encephalitis serocomplex)	Sindbis virus (SINV)	Birds	Mosquitoes (*Culex, Culiseta* spp.)	A/R
	Western equine encephalitis virus (WEEV)	Lagomorphs, passerine birds	Mosquitoes (*Culex tarsalis*)	E
Arenaviruses (Old World)	Lassa virus (LASV)	Natal multimammate mice (*Mastomys natalensis*)	None	F/M, VHF
	Lujo virus (LUJV)	Unknown	None	VHF
	Lymphocytic choriomeningitis virus (LCMV)	House mice (*Mus musculus*)	None	E, F/M, (VHF)
Arenaviruses (New World)	Chapare virus (CHPV)	Unknown	None	VHF
	Guanarito virus (GTOV)	Short-tailed zygodonts (*Zygodontomys brevicauda*)	None	VHF
	Junín virus (JUNV)	Drylands lauchas (*Calomys musculinus*)	None	VHF
	Machupo virus (MACV)	Big lauchas (*Calomys callosus*)	None	VHF
	Sabiá virus (SABV)	Unknown	None	VHF
	Whitewater Arroyo virus (WWAV)[c]	White-throated woodrats (*Neotoma albigula*)	None	(E)
Bunyaviruses (genus undetermined)	Bangui virus (BGIV)	Unknown	Unknown	F/M
	Gan Gan virus (GGV)	Unknown	Mosquitoes (*Aedes, Culex* spp.)	A/R
	Tataguine virus (TATV)	Unknown	Mosquitoes (*Anopheles* spp.)	F/M
	Trubanaman virus (TRUV)	Unknown	Mosquitoes (*Anopheles, Culex* spp.)	(A/R)
Coltiviruses	Colorado tick fever virus (CTFV)	Bushy-tailed woodrats (*Neotoma cinerea*), Columbian ground squirrels (*Spermophilus columbianus*), deer mice (*Peromyscus maniculatus*), golden-mantled ground squirrels (*Spermophilus lateralis*), least chipmunks (*Tamias minimus*), North American porcupines (*Erethizon dorsata*), yellow pine chipmunks (*Tamias amoenus*)	Ixodid ticks (predominantly *Dermacentor andersoni*)	E, F/M
	Eyach virus (EYAV)	Lagomorphs, rodents	Ixodid ticks (*Ixodes ricinus, I. ventalloi*)	E, F/M
	Salmon River virus (SRV)	Unknown	Ixodid ticks (*Ixodes* spp.)	E, F/M
Flaviviruses (mosquito-borne)	Dengue viruses 1–4 (DENV 1–4)	Nonhuman primates	Mosquitoes (predominantly *Aedes aegypti, A. albopictus*)	F/M, VHF
	Japanese encephalitis virus (JEV)	Ardeid wading birds (in particular herons), horses, pigs	Mosquitoes (*Culex* spp., in particular *C. tritaeniorhynchus*)	E
	Kokobera virus (KOKV)	Macropods, horses	Mosquitoes (*Culex* spp.)	A/R
	Murray Valley encephalitis virus (MVEV)	Birds	Mosquitoes (predominantly *Culex annulirostris*)	E

(Continued)

TABLE 233-1 ZOONOTIC ARTHROPOD- AND RODENT-BORNE VIRUSES THAT INFECT HUMANS (*CONTINUED*)

Virus Group	Virus (Abbreviation)	Principal Reservoir Host(s)	Vector(s)	Syndrome[a]
	Rocio virus (ROCV)	Rufous-collared sparrows (*Zonotrichia capensis*)	Mosquitoes (*Aedes*, *Culex*, *Psorophora* spp.)	E
	St. Louis encephalitis virus (SLEV)	Columbiform and passeriform birds (finches, sparrows)	Mosquitoes (predominantly *Culex* spp., in particular *C. nigripalpus*, *C. pipiens*, *C. quinquefasciatus*, *C. tarsalis*)	E
	Usutu virus (USUV)	Passerine birds	Mosquitoes (*Culex* spp., in particular *C. pipiens*)	(E)
	West Nile virus (WNV)[d]	Passerine birds (blackbirds, crows, finches, sparrows), small mammals, horses	Mosquitoes (*Culex* spp., in particular *C. pipiens*, *C. quinquefasciatus*, *C. restuans*, *C. tarsalis*)	E
	Yellow fever virus (YFV)	Nonhuman primates (*Alouatta*, *Ateles*, *Cebus*, *Cercopithecus*, *Colobus* spp.)	Mosquitoes (*Aedes* spp., in particular *A. aegypti*)	VHF
	Zika virus (ZIKV)	Nonhuman primates (*Macaca*, *Pongo* spp.)	Mosquitoes (*Aedes* spp.)	A/R, F/M
Flaviviruses (tick-borne)	Kyasanur Forest disease virus (KFDV)[e]	Indomalayan vandeleurias (*Vandeleuria oleracea*), roof rats (*Rattus rattus*)	Ixodid ticks (predominantly *Haemaphysalis spinigera*); sand tampans (*Ornithodoros savignyi*)	VHF
	Omsk hemorrhagic fever virus (OHFV)	Migratory birds, rodents	Ixodid ticks (predominantly *Dermacentor* spp.)	VHF
	Powassan virus (POWV)	Red squirrels (*Tamiasciurus hudsonicus*), white-footed deer mice (*Peromyscus leucopus*), woodchucks (*Marmota monax*), other small mammals	Ixodid ticks (in particular *Ixodes cookei*, other *Ixodes* spp., *Dermacentor* spp.)	E
	Tick-borne encephalitis virus (TBEV)	Passerine birds, deer, eulipotyphla, goats, grouse, small mammals, rodents, sheep	Ixodid ticks (*Ixodes gibbosus*, *I. persulcatus*, *I. ricinus*; sporadically *Dermacentor*, *Haemaphysalis*, *Hyalomma* spp.)	E, F/M, (VHF)
Hantaviruses (Old World)	Amur/Soochong virus (ASV)	Korean field mice (*Apodemus peninsulae*)	None	VHF
	Dobrava-Belgrade virus (DOBV)	Caucasus field mice (*Apodemus ponticus*), striped field mice (*Apodemus agrarius*), yellow-necked field mice (*Apodemus flavicollis*)	None	VHF
	Gou virus (GOUV)	Brown rats (*Rattus norvegicus*), roof rats (*R. rattus*), Oriental house rats (*Rattus tanezumi*)	None	VHF
	Hantaan virus (HTNV)	Striped field mice (*A. agrarius*)	None	VHF
	Kurkino virus	Striped field mice (*A. agrarius*)	None	VHF
	Muju virus (MUJV)	Korean red-backed voles (*Myodes regulus*)	None	VHF
	Puumala virus (PUUV)	Bank voles (*Myodes glareolus*)	None	(P), VHF
	Saaremaa virus (SAAV)	Striped field mice (*A. agrarius*)	None	VHF
	Seoul virus (SEOV)	Brown rats (*R. norvegicus*), roof rats (*R. rattus*)	None	VHF
	Sochi virus	Caucasus field mice (*A. ponticus*)	None	VHF
	Tula virus (TULV)	Common voles (*Microtus arvalis*), East European voles (*Microtus levis*), field voles (*Microtus agrestis*)	None	(P), VHF
Hantaviruses (New World)	Anajatuba virus (ANJV)	Fornes' colilargos (*Oligoryzomys fornesi*)	None	P
	Andes virus (ANDV)	Long-tailed colilargos (*Oligoryzomys longicaudatus*)	None	P
	Araraquara virus (ARAV)	Hairy-tailed akodonts (*Necromys lasiurus*)	None	P
	Araucária virus (ARAUV)	Black-footed colilargos (*Oligoryzomys nigripes*)	None	P
	Bayou virus (BAYV)	Marsh rice rats (*Oryzomys palustris*)	None	P
	Bermejo virus (BMJV)	Chacoan colilargos (*Oligoryzomys chacoensis*)	None	P
	Black Creek Canal virus (BCCV)	Hispid cotton rats (*S. hispidus*)	None	P
	Blue River virus (BRV)	White-footed deer mice (*P. leucopus*)	None	P
	Castelo dos Sonhos virus (CASV)	Brazilian colilargos (*Oligoryzomys eliurus*)	None	P
	Choclo virus (CHOV)	Fulvous colilargos (*Oligoryzomys fulvescens*)	None	F/M

(*Continued*)

TABLE 233-1 ZOONOTIC ARTHROPOD- AND RODENT-BORNE VIRUSES THAT INFECT HUMANS (*CONTINUED*)

Virus Group	Virus (Abbreviation)	Principal Reservoir Host(s)	Vector(s)	Syndrome[a]
	El Moro Canyon virus (ELMCV)	Sumichrast's harvest mice (*Reithrodontomys sumichrasti*), western harvest mice (*Reithrodontomys megalotis*)	None	P
	Juquitiba virus (JUQV)	Black-footed colilargos (*O. nigripes*)	None	P
	Laguna Negra virus (LANV)	Little lauchas (*Calomys laucha*)	None	P
	Lechiguanas virus (LECV)	Flavescent colilargos (*Oligoryzomys flavescens*)	None	P
	Maciel virus (MCLV)	Dark-furred akodonts (*Necromys obscurus*)	None	P
	Maripa virus	Unknown	None	P
	Monongahela virus (MGLV)	North American deer mice (*P. maniculatus*)	None	P
	Muleshoe virus (MULV)	Hispid cotton rat (*S. hispidus*)	None	P
	New York virus (NYV)	White-footed deer mice (*P. leucopus*)	None	P
	Orán virus (ORNV)	Long-tailed colilargos (*O. longicaudatus*)	None	P
	Paranoá virus	Unknown	None	P
	Pergamino virus	Azara's akodonts (*Akodon azarae*)	None	P
	Río Mamoré virus (RIOMV)	Common bristly mice (*Neacomys spinosus*)	None	P
	Sin Nombre virus (SNV)	North American deer mice (*P. maniculatus*)	None	P
	Tunari virus (TUNV)	Unknown	None	P
Nairoviruses (Crimean-Congo hemorrhagic fever virus group)	Crimean-Congo hemorrhagic fever virus (CCHFV)	Cattle, dogs, goats, hares, hedgehogs, mice, ostriches, sheep	Predominantly ixodid ticks (*Hyalomma* spp.)	VHF
Nairoviruses (Dugbe virus group)	Dugbe virus (DUGV)	Northern giant pouched rats (*Cricetomys gambianus*), Zébu cattle (*Bos primigenius*)	Biting midges (*Culicoides* spp.), ixodid ticks (*Amblyomma, Hyalomma, Rhipicephalus* spp.)	F/M
	Nairobi sheep disease virus[f] (NSDV)	Sheep	Ixodid ticks (*Haemaphysalis, Rhipicephalus* spp.), mosquitoes (*Culex* spp.)	F/M
Nairoviruses (Sakhalin virus group)	Avalon virus (AVAV)	European herring gulls (*Larus argentatus*)	Ixodid ticks (*Ixodes uriae*)	(Polyradiculoneuritis?)
Nairoviruses (Thiafora virus group)	Erve virus (ERVEV)	Greater white-toothed shrews (*Crocidura russula*)	?	(Thunderclap headache?)
Orbiviruses	Kemerovo virus (KEMV)	Birds, rodents	Ixodid ticks (*Ixodes persulcatus*)	E, F/M
	Lebombo virus (LEBV)	Unknown	Mosquitoes (*Aedes, Mansonia* spp.)	F/M
	Orungo virus (ORUV)	Camels, cattle, goats, nonhuman primates, sheep	Mosquitoes (*Aedes, Anopheles, Culex* spp.)	E, F/M
	Tribeč virus (TRBV)[g]	Bank voles (*M. glareolus*), birds, common pine voles (*Microtus subterraneus*), goats, hares	Ixodid ticks (*Ixodes persulcatus, I. ricinus*)	F/M
Orthobunyaviruses (Anopheles A serogroup)	Tacaiuma virus (TCMV)	Nonhuman primates	Mosquitoes (*Anopheles, Haemagogus* spp.)	F/M
Orthobunyaviruses (Bunyamwera serogroup)	Batai virus (BATV)[h]	Birds, camels, cattle, goats, rodents, sheep	Mosquitoes (*Aedes abnormalis, A. curtipes, Anopheles barbirostris, Culex gelidus*, other spp.)	F/M
	Bunyamwera virus (BUNV)	Birds, cows, goats, horses, sheep	Mosquitoes (*Aedes* spp.)	F/M
	Cache Valley virus (CVV)	Cattle, deer, foxes, horses, nonhuman primates, raccoons	Mosquitoes (*Aedes, Anopheles, Culiseta* spp.)	F/M
	Fort Sherman virus (FSV)	Unknown	Mosquitoes?	F/M
	Germiston virus (GERV)	Rodents	Mosquitoes (*Culex* spp.)	F/M
	Guaroa virus (GROV)	Unknown	Mosquitoes (*Anopheles* spp.)	F/M
	Ilesha virus (ILEV)	Unknown	Mosquitoes (*Anopheles gambiae*)	F/M, (VHF)
	Ngari virus (NRIV)	Unknown	Mosquitoes (*Aedes, Anopheles* spp.)	F/M, VHF
	Shokwe virus (SHOV)	Rodents	Mosquitoes (*Aedes, Anopheles, Mansonia* spp.)	F/M
	Xingu virus (XINV)	Unknown	Unknown	F/M
Orthobunyaviruses (Bwamba serogroup)	Bwamba virus (BWAV)	Unknown	Mosquitoes (*Aedes, Anopheles, Mansonia* spp.)	F/M
	Pongola virus (PGAV)	Cattle, donkeys, goats, sheep	Mosquitoes (*Aedes, Anopheles, Mansonia* spp.)	F/M

(*Continued*)

TABLE 233-1 ZOONOTIC ARTHROPOD- AND RODENT-BORNE VIRUSES THAT INFECT HUMANS (*CONTINUED*)

Virus Group	Virus (Abbreviation)	Principal Reservoir Host(s)	Vector(s)	Syndrome[a]
Orthobunyaviruses (California serogroup)	California encephalitis virus (CEV)	Lagomorphs, rodents	Mosquitoes (*Aedes, Culex, Culiseta, Psorophora* spp.)	E, F/M
	Inkoo virus (INKV)	Cattle, foxes, hares, moose, rodents	Mosquitoes (*Aedes* spp.)	E, F/M
	Jamestown Canyon virus (JCV)	Bison, deer, elk, moose	Mosquitoes (*Aedes, Culiseta, Ochlerotatus* spp.)	E, F/M
	La Crosse virus (LACV)	Chipmunks, squirrels	Mosquitoes (*Ochlerotatus triseriatus*)	E, F/M
	Lumbo virus (LUMV)	Unknown	Mosquitoes (*Aedes pembaensis*)	E, F/M
	Snowshoe hare virus (SSHV)	Snowshoe hares, squirrels, other small mammals	Mosquitoes (*Aedes, Culiseta, Ochlerotatus* spp.)	E, F/M
	Tahyña virus (TAHV)	Cattle, dogs, eulipotyphla, foxes, hares, horses, pigs, rodents	Mosquitoes (*Aedes, Culex, Culiseta* spp.)	E, F/M
Orthobunyaviruses (group C serogroup)	Apeú virus (APEUV)	Bare-tailed woolly opossums (*Caluromys philander*) and other opossums; rodents; tufted capuchins (*Cebus apella*)	Mosquitoes (*Aedes, Culex* spp.)	F/M
	Caraparú virus (CARV)	Rodents, tufted capuchins (*C. apella*)	Mosquitoes (*Culex* spp.)	F/M
	Itaquí virus (ITQV)	Capuchins (*Cebus* spp.), opossums, rodents	Mosquitoes (*Culex* spp.)	F/M
	Madrid virus (MADV)	Capuchins (*Cebus* spp.), opossums, rodents	Mosquitoes (*Culex* spp.)	F/M
	Marituba virus (MTBV)	Capuchins (*Cebus* spp.), opossums, rodents	Mosquitoes (*Culex* spp.)	F/M
	Murutucú virus (MURV)	Capuchins (*Cebus* spp.), opossums, pale-throated sloths (*Bradypus tridactylus*), rodents	Mosquitoes (*Coquillettidia, Culex* spp.)	F/M
	Nepuyo virus (NEPV)	Bats (*Artibeus* spp.), rodents	Mosquitoes (*Culex* spp.)	F/M
	Oriboca virus (ORIV)	Capuchins (*Cebus* spp.), opossums, rodents	Mosquitoes (*Aedes, Culex, Mansonia, Psorophora* spp.)	F/M
	Ossa virus (OSSAV)	Rodents	Mosquitoes (*Culex* spp.)	F/M
	Restan virus (RESV)	Unknown	Mosquitoes (*Culex* spp.)	F/M
	Zungarococha virus (ZUNV)	Unknown	Unknown	F/M
Orthobunyaviruses (Guama serogroup)	Catu virus (CATUV)	Bats, capuchins (*Cebus* spp.), opossums, rodents	Mosquitoes (*Culex* spp.)	F/M
	Guama virus (GMAV)	Bats, capuchins (*Cebus* spp.), howlers (*Alouatta* spp.), marsupials, rodents	Mosquitoes (*Aedes, Culex, Limatus, Mansonia, Psorophora, Trichoprosopon* spp.)	F/M
Orthobunyaviruses (Nyando serogroup)	Nyando virus (NDV)	Unknown	Mosquitoes (*Aedes, Anopheles* spp.), sandflies (*Lutzomyia* spp.)	F/M
Orthobunyaviruses (Simbu serogroup)	Iquitos virus (IQTV)	Unknown	Unknown	F/M
	Oropouche virus (OROV)	Marmosets (*Callithrix* spp.), pale-throated sloth (*B. tridactylus*)	Biting midges (*Culicoides paraensis*), mosquitoes (*Coquillettidia venezuelensis, Culex quinquefasciatus, Mansonia* spp., *Ochlerotatus serratus*)	F/M
Orthobunyaviruses (Wyeomyia serogroup)	Wyeomyia virus (WYOV)	Unknown	Mosquitoes (*Wyeomyia* spp.)	F/M
Phleboviruses (Bhanja serocomplex)	Bhanja virus[i] (BHAV)	Cattle, four-toed hedgehog (*Atelerix albiventris*), goats, sheep, striped ground squirrels (*Xerus erythropus*)	Ixodid ticks (*Amblyomma, Dermacentor, Haemaphysalis, Hyalomma, Rhipicephalus* spp.)	E, F/M
	Heartland virus	Cattle, deer, elk, goats, sheep?	Ixodid ticks (*Amblyomma americanum*)	F/M
	"Severe fever with thrombocytopenia syndrome virus" ("SFTSV")	Cattle, chicken, dogs, goats, rodents, sheep?	Ixodid ticks (*Haemaphysalis longicornis, Rhipicephalus microplus*)	F/M, VHF
Phleboviruses (Candiru serocomplex)	Alenquer virus (ALEV)	Unknown	Unknown	F/M
	Candiru virus (CDUV)	Unknown	Unknown	F/M
	Escharate virus (ESCV)	Unknown	Unknown	F/M
	Maldonado virus (MLOV)	Unkown	Unknown	F/M
	Morumbi virus (MRBV)	Unknown	Unknown	F/M
	Serra Norte virus (SRNV)	Unknown	Unknown	F/M
Phleboviruses (Punta Toro serocomplex)	Punta Toro virus (PTV)	Unknown	Sandflies (*Lutzomyia* spp.)	F/M
Phleboviruses (sandfly fever serocomplex)	Chagres virus (CHGV)	Unknown	Sandflies (*Lutzomyia* spp.)	F/M
	Chios virus	Unknown	Unknown	E
	Rift Valley fever virus (RVFV)	Cattle, sheep	Mosquitoes (*Aedes, Anopheles, Coquillettidia, Culex, Eretmapodites, Mansonia* spp.)	E, F/M, VHF

(*Continued*)

TABLE 233-1 ZOONOTIC ARTHROPOD- AND RODENT-BORNE VIRUSES THAT INFECT HUMANS (CONTINUED)

Virus Group	Virus (Abbreviation)	Principal Reservoir Host(s)	Vector(s)	Syndrome[a]
	Sandfly fever Cyprus virus (SFCV)	Unknown	Unknown	F/M
	Sandfly fever Naples virus (SFNV)	Unknown	Sandflies (*Phlebotomus papatasi*, *P. perfiliewi*, *P. perniciosus*)	F/M
	Sandfly fever Sicilian virus (SFSV)	Eulipotyphla, least weasles (*Mustela nivalis*), rodents	Sandflies (particularly *Phlebotomus papatasi*)	F/M
	Sandfly fever Turkey virus (SFTV)	Unknown	Sandflies (*Phlebotomus* spp.)	F/M
	Toscana virus (TOSV)	Unknown	Sandflies (*Phlebotomus papatasi*, *P. perfiliewi*)	E, F/M
Phleboviruses (Uukuniemi serocomplex)	Uukuniemi virus (UUKV)	Birds, cattle, rodents	Ixodid ticks (*Ixodes* spp.)	F/M
Quaranjaviruses	Quaranfil virus (QRFV)	Birds	Ixodid ticks (*Argas arboreus*)	F/M
Seadornaviruses	Banna virus (BAV)	Cattle, pigs	Mosquitoes (*Aedes*, *Anopheles*, *Culiseta* spp.)	E
Thogotoviruses	Dhori virus (DHOV)[k]	Bats, camels, horses	Mosquitoes (*Aedes*, *Anopheles*, *Culex* spp.), ixodid ticks (*Dermacentor*, *Hyalomma*, *Ornithodoros* spp.)	E, F/M
	Thogoto virus (THOV)	Camels, cattle	Ixodid ticks (*Amblyomma*, *Hyalomma*, *Rhipicephalus* spp.)	E, F/M
Vesiculoviruses	Chandipura virus (CHPV)	Hedgehogs	Mosquitoes (*Aedes aegypti*), sandflies (*Phlebotomus*, *Sergentomyia* spp.)	E, F/M
	Isfahan virus (ISFV)	Great gerbils (*Rhombomys opimus*)	Sandflies (*Phlebotomus papatasi*)	F/M
	Piry virus (PIRYV)	Gray four-eyed opossums (*Philander opossum*)	Mosquitoes (*Aedes*, *Culex*, *Toxorhynchites* spp.)	F/M
	Vesicular stomatitis Indiana virus (VSIV)	Cattle, horses, pigs	Sandflies (*Lutzomyia* spp.)	F/M
	Vesicular stomatitis New Jersey virus (VSNJV)	Cattle, horses, pigs	Biting midges (*Culicoides* spp.), chloropid flies, mosquitoes (*Culex*, *Mansonia* spp.), muscoid flies (*Musca* spp.), simuliid flies	F/M

[a]Abbreviations refer to the syndrome most commonly associated with the virus: A/R, arthritis/rash; E, encephalitis; F/M, fever/myalgia; P, pulmonary; VHF, viral hemorrhagic fever. Abbreviations are placed in parentheses when cases are either extremely rare or controversial. [b]In the older literature, chikungunya virus often is also listed as a causative agent of VHF. However, later studies revealed that, in most cases, people with "chikungunya hemorrhagic fever" were co-infected with one or more dengue viruses, an observation suggesting that the VHF was actually severe dengue. [c]Whitewater Arroyo virus is often listed as a causative agent of VHF in the literature, but convincing data associating this virus with VHF have not been published. [d]Also includes Kunjin virus. [e]Includes the recently described Alkhurma/Alkhumra variant of Kyasanur Forest disease virus. [f]Also known as Ganjam virus. [g]Also known as Brezová virus, Cvilín virus, Kharagysh virus, Koliba virus, or Lipovník virus. [h]Also known as Čalovo virus or Chittoor virus. [i]Also known as Palma virus. [j]The final virus name has not yet been decided. Alternatives used in the literature are Huaiyangshan virus (HYSV) and Henan fever virus (HNFV). [k]Also known as Astra virus and Batken virus.

EPIDEMIOLOGY

The distributions of arthropod-borne and rodent-borne viruses are restricted by the areas inhabited by their reservoir hosts and/or vectors. Consequently, a patient's geographic origin or travel history can provide important clues in the differential diagnosis. Table 233-2 lists the approximate geographic distribution of most arthropod-borne and rodent-borne infections. Many of these diseases can be acquired in either rural or urban settings; these diseases include yellow fever, dengue (previously called dengue fever), severe dengue (previously called dengue hemorrhagic fever and dengue shock syndrome), chikungunya virus disease, hemorrhagic fever with renal syndrome caused by Seoul virus, sandfly fever caused by sandfly fever Naples and Sicilian viruses, and Oropouche virus disease.

DIAGNOSIS

In patients with suspected viral infection, a recognized history of mosquito bite has little diagnostic significance, but a history of tick bite is more diagnostically useful. Exposure to rodents is sometimes reported by persons infected with arenaviruses or hantaviruses. Laboratory diagnosis is required in all cases, although epidemics occasionally provide enough clinical and epidemiologic clues for a presumptive etiologic diagnosis. For most arthropod-borne and rodent-borne viruses, acute-phase serum samples (collected within 3 or 4 days of onset) have yielded isolates. Paired serum samples have been used to demonstrate rising antibody titers. Intensive efforts to develop rapid tests for viral hemorrhagic fevers have resulted in reliable antigen-detection enzyme-linked immunosorbent assays (ELISAs), IgM-capture ELISAs, and multiplex polymerase chain reaction (PCR) assays. These tests can provide a diagnosis based on a single serum sample within a few hours and are particularly useful in patients with severe disease. More sensitive reverse-transcription PCR (RT-PCR) assays may yield diagnoses based on samples without detectable antigen and may also provide useful genetic information about the etiologic agent.

Hantavirus infections differ from other viral infections discussed here in that severe acute disease is immunopathologic; patients present with serum IgM that serves as the basis for a sensitive and specific test. At diagnosis, patients with encephalitides generally are no longer viremic or antigenemic and usually do not have virions in cerebrospinal fluid (CSF). In this situation, the value of serologic methods for IgM determination and RT-PCR is high. IgM-capture ELISA is increasingly being used for the simultaneous testing of serum and CSF. IgG ELISA or classic serology is useful in the evaluation of past exposure to viruses, many of which circulate in areas with minimal medical infrastructures and sometimes cause only mild or subclinical infection.

SYNDROMES

The spectrum of possible human responses to infection with arthropod- or rodent-borne viruses is wide, and knowledge of the outcome of most of these infections is limited. People infected with these viruses may not develop signs of illness. If viral disease is recognized, it can usually be grouped into one of five broad categories: arthritis and rash, encephalitis, fever and myalgia, pulmonary disease, or viral hemorrhagic fever (VHF) (Table 233-3). These categories often overlap. For example, infections with West Nile and Venezuelan equine

TABLE 233-2 GEOGRAPHIC DISTRIBUTION (UNITED NATIONS GEOSCHEME) OF ZOONOTIC ARTHROPOD-BORNE OR RODENT-BORNE VIRAL DISEASES

Area	Type of Disease[a]						
	Arenaviral	Bunyaviral	Flaviviral	Orthomyxoviral	Reoviral	Rhabdoviral	Togaviral
Africa	Lassa fever; Lujo virus infection	Bangui, Batai, Bhanja, Bunyamwera, and Bwamba virus infections; Crimean-Congo hemorrhagic fever; Dugbe, Germiston, Ilesha virus infections; Nairobi sheep disease virus infection; Ngari, Nyando, and Pongola virus infections, Rift Valley fever, sandfly fever/Pappataci fever/phlebotomus fever; Shokwe, Tataguine virus infections	Dengue/severe dengue; (Usutu virus infection); West Nile virus infection; yellow fever; Zika virus infection	Dhori, Quaranfil, and Thogoto virus infections	Lebombo, Orungo, and Tribeč virus infections	—	Chikungunya virus disease; o'nyong-nyong fever; Semliki Forest and Sindbis virus infections
Central Asia	—	Bhanja virus infection; Crimean-Congo hemorrhagic fever	Tick-borne viral encephalitis	Dhori virus infection	—	Isfahan virus infection	—
Eastern Asia	—	Crimean-Congo hemorrhagic fever; hemorrhagic fever with renal syndrome; sandfly fever/Pappataci fever/phlebotomus fever; severe fever with thrombocytopenia syndrome	Dengue/severe dengue; Japanese encephalitis; Kyasanur Forest disease; tick-borne viral encephalitis	—	Banna virus infection	—	—
Southern Asia	—	Batai and Bhanja virus infections; Crimean-Congo hemorrhagic fever; hemorrhagic fever with renal syndrome; Nairobi sheep disease virus infection; sandfly fever/Pappataci fever/phlebotomus fever	Dengue/severe dengue; Japanese encephalitis; Kyasanur Forest disease; West Nile virus infection, Zika virus infection	Dhori, Quaranfil, and Thogoto virus infections	—	Chandipura and Isfahan virus infections	Chikungunya virus disease
South-Eastern Asia	—	Batai virus infection; hemorrhagic fever with renal syndrome	Dengue/severe dengue; Japanese encephalitis; West Nile virus infection; Zika virus infection	—	—	—	Chikungunya virus disease
Western Asia	—	Batai and Bhanja virus infections; Crimean-Congo hemorrhagic fever, hemorrhagic fever with renal syndrome; sandfly fever/Pappataci fever/phlebotomus fever	Dengue/severe dengue; Kyasanur Forest disease; tick-borne viral encephalitis; West Nile virus infection	Dhori and Quaranfil virus infections	—	—	Chikungunya virus disease
Latin America and the Caribbean	"Brazilian hemorrhagic fever"; Chapare virus infection; Junín/Argentinian hemorrhagic fever; lymphocytic choriomeningitis/meningoencephalitis; Machupo/Bolivian hemorrhagic fever; "Venezuelan hemorrhagic fever"	Alenquer, Apeú, Bunyamwera, Cache Valley, Candiru, Caraparú, Catu, Chagres, Escharate, Fort Sherman, Guama, and Guaroa virus infections; hantavirus pulmonary syndrome; Itaquí, Juquitiba, Madrid, Maldonado, Marituba, Mayaro, Morumbi, Murutucú, Nepuyo, and Oriboca virus infections; Oropouche virus disease; Ossa, Punta Toro, Restan, Serra Norte, Tacaiuma, Trinidad, Wyeomyia, Xingu, and Zungarococha virus infections	Dengue/severe dengue; Rocio virus disease; yellow fever	—		Piry virus disease; vesicular stomatitis virus disease/Indiana fever	Chikungunya virus disease; Mayaro virus infection; Mucambo, Tonate, and Una virus infections; Venezuelan equine fever
Northern America	Lymphocytic choriomeningitis/meningoencephalitis; (Whitewater Arroyo virus infection)	(Avalon) and Cache Valley virus infections; California (meningo)encephalitis; hantavirus pulmonary syndrome; Heartland virus and Nepuyo virus infections	Dengue/severe dengue; Powassan virus disease; St. Louis encephalitis; West Nile virus infection	—	Colorado tick fever; Salmon River virus infection	Vesicular stomatitis virus disease/Indiana fever	Eastern equine encephalitis; Everglades virus infection; western equine encephalitis

(Continued)

TABLE 233-2 GEOGRAPHIC DISTRIBUTION (UNITED NATIONS GEOSCHEME) OF ZOONOTIC ARTHROPOD-BORNE OR RODENT-BORNE VIRAL DISEASES (*CONTINUED*)

Area	Type of Disease[a]						
	Arenaviral	Bunyaviral	Flaviviral	Orthomyxoviral	Reoviral	Rhabdoviral	Togaviral
Europe	Lymphocytic choriomeningitis/ meningoen-cephalitis	(Avalon) and Bhanja virus infections; California (meningo)encephalitis; Crimean-Congo hemorrhagic fever; (Erve virus infection); hemorrhagic fever with renal syndrome; Inkoo virus infection; sandfly fever/Pappataci fever/phlebotomus fever; Uukuniemi virus infection	Dengue/severe dengue; tick-borne viral encephalitis; Omsk hemorrhagic fever; (Usutu virus infection); West Nile virus infection	Dhori and Thogoto virus infections	Eyach, Kemerovo, and Tribeč virus infections	—	Chikungunya virus disease; Sindbis virus infection
Oceania	—	Gan Gan and (Trubanaman virus) infections	Australian encephalitis; dengue/severe dengue; Japanese encephalitis; Kokobera virus infection; Murray Valley encephalitis; West Nile virus infection; Zika virus infection	—	—	—	Barmah Forest virus infection; Ross River disease; Sindbis virus infection

[a]Quotation marks indicate common usage in the absence of International Classification of Disease version 10 (ICD-10) recognition. Diseases not acknowledged by the ICD-10 are designated as "virus infection." Disease names are placed in parentheses when cases are either extremely rare or controversial.

TABLE 233-3 CLINICAL SYNDROMES CAUSED BY ZOONOTIC ARTHROPOD-BORNE OR RODENT-BORNE VIRUSES

Syndrome	Virus[a]
Arthritis and rash (A/R)	Bunyaviridae: Gan Gan and (Trubanaman) viruses
	Flaviviridae: Kokobera and Zika viruses
	Togaviridae: Barmah Forest, chikungunya, Mayaro, o'nyong-nyong, Ross River, Semliki Forest, and Sindbis viruses
Encephalitis (E)	Arenaviridae: lymphocytic choriomeningitis and (Whitewater Arroyo) viruses
	Bunyaviridae: Bhanja, California encephalitis, Chios, Inkoo, Jamestown Canyon, La Crosse, Lumbo, Rift Valley fever, snowshoe hare, Tahyňa, and Toscana viruses
	Flaviviridae: Japanese encephalitis, Murray Valley encephalitis, Powassan, Rocio, St. Louis encephalitis, tick-borne encephalitis, (Usutu), and West Nile viruses
	Orthomyxoviridae: Dhori and Thogoto viruses
	Reoviridae: Banna, Colorado tick fever, Eyach, Kemerovo, Orungo, and Salmon River viruses
	Rhabdoviridae: Chandipura virus
	Togaviridae: eastern equine encephalitis, Everglades, Mucambo, Tonate, Venezuelan equine encephalitis, and western equine encephalitis viruses
Fever and myalgia (F/M)	Arenaviridae: Lassa and lymphocytic choriomeningitis viruses
	Bunyaviridae: Alenquer, Apeú, Bangui, Batai, Bhanja, Bunyamwera, Bwamba, Cache Valley, California encephalitis, Candiru, Caraparú, Catu, Chagres, Choclo, Dugbe, Escharate, Fort Sherman, Germiston, Guama, Guaroa, Heartland, Ilesha, Inkoo, Iquitos, Itaquí, Jamestown Canyon, La Crosse, Lumbo, Madrid, Maldonado, Marituba, Morumbi, Nairobi sheep disease, Nepuyo, Ngari, Nyando, Oriboca, Oropouche, Ossa, Pongola, Punta Toro, Restan, Rift Valley fever, sandfly fever Cyprus, sandfly fever Naples, sandfly fever Sicilian, sandfly fever Turkey, Serra Norte, "severe fever with thrombocytopenia syndrome," Shokwe, snowshoe hare, Tacaiuma, Tahyňa, Tataguine, Thogoto, Toscana, Uukuniemi, Wyeomyia, Xingu, and Zungarococha viruses
	Flaviviridae: dengue 1–4, tick-borne encephalitis, and Zika viruses
	Orthomyxoviridae: Dhori and Quaranfil viruses
	Reoviridae: Colorado tick fever, Eyach, Kemerovo, Lebombo, Orungo, Salmon River, and Tribeč viruses
	Rhabdoviridae: Chandipura, Isfahan, Piry, vesicular stomatitis Indiana, and vesicular stomatitis New Jersey viruses
	Togaviridae: Everglades, Mucambo, Tonate, Una, and Venezuelan equine encephalitis viruses
Pulmonary disease (P)	Bunyaviridae: Anajatuba, Andes, Araucária, Bayou, Bermejo, Black Creek Canal, Blue River, Castelo dos Sonhos, El Moro Canyon, Juquitiba, Laguna Negra, Lechiguanas, Maciel, Monongahela, Muleshoe, New York, Orán, Paranoá, Pergamino, (Puumala), Río Mamoré, Sin Nombre, (Tula), and Tunari viruses
Viral hemorrhagic fever (VHF)	Arenaviridae: Chapare, Guanarito, Junín, Lassa, Lujo, (lymphocytic choriomeningitis), Machupo, and Sabiá viruses
	Bunyaviridae: Amur/Soochong, Crimean-Congo hemorrhagic fever, Dobrava-Belgrade, Gou, Hantaan, (Ilesha), Kurkino, Muju, Ngari, Puumala, Rift Valley fever, Saaremaa, Seoul, "severe fever with thrombocytopenia syndrome," Sochi, and Tula viruses
	Flaviviridae: dengue 1–4, Kyasanur Forest disease, Omsk hemorrhagic fever, (tick-borne encephalitis), and yellow fever viruses

[a]Virus names are placed in parentheses when human infections are either extremely rare or controversial.

encephalitis viruses are discussed here as encephalitides, but during epidemics many patients present with much milder febrile syndromes. Similarly, Rift Valley fever virus is best known as a cause of VHF, but the attack rates for febrile disease are far higher, and encephalitis and blindness occasionally occur as well. Lymphocytic choriomeningitis virus is classified here as a cause of fever and myalgia because this syndrome is the most common disease manifestation; even when central nervous system (CNS) disease evolves during infection with this virus, neural manifestations are usually mild and are preceded by fever and myalgia. Infection with any dengue virus type (1, 2, 3, or 4) is considered as a cause of fever and myalgia because this syndrome is by far the most common manifestation worldwide. However, severe dengue is a VHF with a complicated pathogenesis that is of tremendous importance in pediatric practice in certain areas of the world. Unfortunately, most of the known arthropod- or rodent-borne viral diseases have not been studied in detail with modern medical approaches; thus available data may be incomplete or biased. The reader must be aware that data on geographic distribution are often fuzzy: the literature frequently is not clear as to whether the data pertain to the distribution of a particular virus or the areas where human disease has been observed. In addition, the designations for viruses and viral diseases have changed multiple times over decades. Here, virus and taxon names are in line with the latest reports of the International Committee on Taxonomy of Viruses, and disease names are largely in accordance with the World Health Organization's International Classification of Disease version 10 (ICD-10) and more recent updates.

ARTHRITIS AND RASH

Arthritides are common accompaniments of several viral diseases, such as hepatitis B, parvovirus B19 infection, and rubella, and occasionally accompany infection due to adenoviruses, enteroviruses, herpesviruses, and mumps virus. Two ungrouped bunyaviruses, Gan Gan virus and Trubanaman virus, and the flavivirus Kokobera virus have been associated with single cases of polyarthritic disease. Arthropod-borne alphaviruses are also common causes of arthritides—usually acute febrile diseases accompanied by the development of a maculopapular rash. Rheumatic involvement includes arthralgia alone, periarticular swelling, and (less commonly) joint effusions. Most alphavirus infections are less severe and have fewer articular manifestations in children than in adults. In temperate climates, these ailments are summer diseases. No specific therapies or licensed vaccines exist. The most important alphavirus arthritides are Barmah Forest virus infection, chikungunya virus disease, Ross River disease, and Sindbis virus infection. A large (>2 million cases), albeit isolated, epidemic was caused by o'nyong nyong virus in 1959–1961 (o'nyong nyong fever). Mayaro, Semliki Forest, and Una viruses have caused isolated cases or limited and infrequent epidemics (30 to several hundred cases per year) in the past. Signs and symptoms of infections with these viruses often are similar to those observed with chikungunya virus disease.

Chikungunya Virus Disease Disease caused by chikungunya virus is endemic in rural areas of Africa. Intermittent epidemics take place in towns and cities of both Africa and Asia. *Aedes aegypti* mosquitoes are the usual vectors for the disease in urban areas. In 2004, a massive epidemic began in the Indian Ocean region (in particular on the islands of Réunion and Mauritius) and was most likely spread by travelers; *Aedes albopictus* was identified as the major vector of chikungunya virus during that epidemic. Between 2013 and 2014, several thousand chikungunya virus infections were reported (and several tens of thousands of cases were suspected) from Caribbean islands. The virus was imported to Italy, France, and the United States by travelers from the Caribbean. Chikungunya virus poses a threat to the continental United States as suitable vector mosquitoes are present in the southern states. The disease is most common among adults, in whom the clinical presentation may be dramatic. The abrupt onset of chikungunya virus disease follows an incubation period of 2–10 days. Fever (often severe) with a saddleback pattern and severe arthralgia are accompanied by chills and constitutional symptoms and signs, such as abdominal pain, anorexia, conjunctival injection, headache, nausea, and photophobia. Migratory polyarthritis mainly affects the small joints of the ankles, feet, hands, and wrists, but the larger joints are not necessarily spared. Rash may appear at the outset or several days into the illness; its development often coincides with defervescence, which occurs around day 2 or 3 of the disease. The rash is most intense on the trunk and limbs and may desquamate. Young children develop less prominent signs and are therefore less frequently hospitalized. Children also often develop a bullous rather than a maculopapular/petechial rash. Maternal–fetal transmission has been reported and in some cases has led to fetal death. Recovery may require weeks, and some elderly patients may continue to experience joint pain, recurrent effusions, or stiffness for several years. This persistence of signs and symptoms may be especially common in HLA-B27-positive patients. In addition to arthritis, petechiae are occasionally seen and epistaxis is not uncommon, but chikungunya virus should not be considered a VHF agent. A few patients develop leukopenia. Elevated concentrations of aspartate aminotransferase (AST) and C-reactive protein have been described, as have mildly decreased platelet counts. Treatment of chikungunya virus disease relies on nonsteroidal anti-inflammatory drugs and sometimes chloroquine for refractory arthritis.

Barmah Forest Virus Infection and Ross River Disease Barmah Forest virus and Ross River virus cause diseases that are indistinguishable on clinical grounds alone (hence the previously common disease designation *epidemic polyarthritis* for both infections). Ross River virus has caused epidemics in Australia, Papua New Guinea, and the South Pacific since the beginning of the twentieth century and continues to be responsible for ~4800 cases of disease in rural and suburban areas annually. In 1979–1980, the virus swept through the Pacific Islands, causing more than 500,000 infections. Ross River virus is predominantly transmitted by *Aedes normanensis*, *Aedes vigilax*, and *Culex annulirostris*. Wallabies and rodents are probably the main vertebrate hosts. Barmah Forest virus infections have been on the rise in recent years. In 2005–2006, roughly 2000 cases were recorded in Australia. Barmah Forest virus is transmitted by both *Aedes* and *Culex* mosquitoes and has been isolated from biting midges. The vertebrate hosts remain to be determined, but serologic studies implicate horses and possums.

Of the human Barmah Forest and Ross River virus infections surveyed, 55–75% were asymptomatic, however, these viral diseases can be debilitating. The incubation period is 7–9 days; the onset of illness is sudden, and disease is usually ushered in by disabling symmetrical joint pain. A nonitchy, diffuse, maculopapular rash (more common in Barmah Forest virus infection) generally develops coincidentally or follows shortly, but in some patients it can precede joint pains by several days. Constitutional symptoms such as low-grade fever, asthenia, headache, myalgia, and nausea are not prominent or are absent in many patients. Most patients are incapacitated for considerable periods (≥6 months) by joint involvement, which interferes with grasping, sleeping, and walking. Ankle, interphalangeal, knee, metacarpophalangeal, and wrist joints are most often involved, although elbows, shoulders, and toes may also be affected. Periarticular swelling and tenosynovitis are common, and one-third of patients have true arthritis (more common in Ross River disease). Myalgia and nuchal stiffness may accompany joint pains. Only half of all patients with arthritis can resume normal activities within 4 weeks, and 10% still must limit their activity after 3 months. Occasional patients are symptomatic for 1–3 years but without progressive arthropathy.

In the diagnosis of either infection, clinical laboratory values are normal or variable. Tests for rheumatoid factor and antinuclear antibodies are negative, and the erythrocyte sedimentation rate is acutely elevated. Joint fluid contains 1000–60,000 mononuclear cells/μL, and viral antigen can usually be detected in macrophages. IgM antibodies are valuable in the diagnosis of this infection, although such antibodies occasionally persist for years. Isolation of the virus from blood after mosquito inoculation or growth of the virus in cell culture is possible early in the illness. Because of the great economic impact of annual epidemics in Australia, an inactivated Ross River virus vaccine is under development. Nonsteroidal anti-inflammatory drugs such as naproxen or acetylsalicylic acid are effective for treatment.

Sindbis Virus Infection Sindbis virus is transmitted among birds by infected mosquitoes. Infections with northern European or southern African variants are particularly likely in rural environments. After an incubation period of <1 week, Sindbis virus infection begins with rash and arthralgia. Constitutional clinical signs are not marked, and fever is modest or lacking altogether. The rash, which lasts ~1 week, begins on the trunk, spreads to the extremities, and evolves from macules to papules that often vesiculate. The arthritis is multiarticular, migratory, and incapacitating, with resolution of the acute phase in a few days; the ankles, elbows, knees, phalangeal joints, wrists, and—to a much lesser extent—proximal and axial joints are involved. Persistence of joint pain and occasionally of arthritis is a major problem and may continue for months or even years despite lack of deformities.

Zika Virus Infection Zika virus is an emerging pathogen that is transmitted among nonhuman primates and humans by *Aedes* mosquitoes. Human infections are usually benign and are most likely misdiagnosed as dengue or influenza. Zika virus infection is characterized by influenza-like clinical signs, including fever, headaches, and malaise. A maculopapular rash, conjunctivitis, myalgia, and arthralgia usually accompany or follow those manifestations. Zika virus infection was first documented in Africa in 1947 and was later recognized in southeastern and southern Asia. In recent years, the number of Zika virus infections reported from Micronesia and Polynesia has increased steadily.

ENCEPHALITIS

The major encephalitis viruses are found in the families Bunyaviridae, Flaviviridae, Rhabdoviridae, and Togaviridae. However, individual agents of other families, including Dhori virus and thogotovirus (Orthomyxoviridae) as well as Banna virus (Reoviridae), have been known to cause isolated cases of encephalitis as well. Arboviral encephalitides are seasonal diseases, commonly occurring in the warmer months. Their incidence varies markedly with time and place, depending on ecologic factors. The causative viruses differ substantially in terms of case–infection ratio (i.e., the ratio of clinical to subclinical infections), lethality rate, and residual disease. Humans are not important amplifiers of these viruses.

All the viral encephalitides discussed in this section have a similar pathogenesis. An infected arthropod ingests blood from a human and thereby initiates infection. The initial viremia is thought to originate from the lymphoid system. Viremia leads to multifocal entry into the CNS, presumably through infection of olfactory neuroepithelium, with passage through the cribriform plate; "Trojan horse" entry with infected macrophages; or infection of brain capillaries. During the viremic phase, there may be little or no recognizable disease except in tick-borne flavivirus encephalitides, which may manifest with clearly delineated phases of fever and systemic illness.

CNS lesions arise partly from direct neuronal infection and subsequent damage and partly from edema, inflammation, and other indirect effects. The usual pathologic features of arboviral encephalitides are focal necroses of neurons, inflammatory glial nodules, and perivascular lymphoid cuffing. Involved areas display the "luxury perfusion" phenomenon, with normal or increased total blood flow and low oxygen extraction. The typical patient presents with a prodrome of nonspecific constitutional signs and symptoms, including fever, abdominal pain, sore throat, and respiratory signs. Headache, meningeal signs, photophobia, and vomiting follow quickly. The severity of human infection varies from an absence of signs/symptoms to febrile headache, aseptic meningitis, and full-blown encephalitis. The proportions and severity of these manifestations vary with the infecting virus. Involvement of deeper brain structures in less severe cases may be signaled by lethargy, somnolence, and intellectual deficit (as disclosed by the mental status examination). More severely affected patients are obviously disoriented and may become comatose. Tremors, loss of abdominal reflexes, cranial nerve palsies, hemiparesis, monoparesis, difficulty swallowing, limb-girdle syndrome, and frontal lobe signs are all common. Spinal and motor neuron diseases are documented after West Nile and Japanese encephalitis virus infections. Seizures and focal signs may be evident early or may appear during the course of the disease. Some patients present with an abrupt onset of fever, convulsions, and other signs of CNS involvement. The acute encephalitis usually lasts from a few days to as long as 2–3 weeks. The infections may be fatal, or recovery may be slow, with weeks or months required for the return of maximal recoupable function, or incomplete, with persisting long-term deficits. Difficulty concentrating, fatigability, tremors, and personality changes are common during recovery.

The diagnosis of arboviral encephalitides depends on the careful evaluation of a febrile patient with CNS disease and the performance of laboratory studies to determine etiology. Clinicians should (1) consider empirical acyclovir treatment for herpesvirus meningoencephalitis and antibiotic treatment for bacterial meningitis until test results are received; (2) exclude intoxination and metabolic or oncologic causes, including paraneoplastic syndromes, hyperammonemia, liver failure, and anti-NMDA receptor encephalitis; and (3) rule out a brain abscess or a stroke. Leptospirosis, neurosyphilis, Lyme disease, cat-scratch disease, and more recently described viral encephalitides (e.g., Nipah virus infection) should be considered if epidemiologically relevant. CSF examination usually shows a modest increase in leukocyte counts—in the tens or hundreds or perhaps a few thousand. Early in the process, a significant proportion of these leukocytes may be polymorphonuclear, but mononuclear cells are usually predominant later. CSF glucose concentrations are generally normal. There are exceptions to this pattern of findings: in eastern equine encephalitis, for example, polymorphonuclear leukocytes may predominate during the first 72 h of disease and hypoglycorrhachia may be detected. In lymphocytic choriomeningitis/meningoencephalitis, lymphocyte counts may be in the thousands, and the glucose concentration may be diminished. A humoral immune response is usually detectable at or near the onset of disease. Both serum (acute- or convalescent-phase) and CSF should be examined for IgM antibodies and viruses by plaque-reduction neutralization assay and/or (RT)-PCR. Virus generally cannot be isolated from blood or CSF, although Japanese encephalitis virus has been recovered from CSF of patients with severe disease. RT-PCR analysis of CSF may yield positive results. Viral antigen is present in brain tissue, although its distribution may be focal. Electroencephalography usually shows diffuse abnormalities and is not directly helpful.

Experience with medical imaging is still evolving. Both computed tomography (CT) and magnetic resonance imaging (MRI) scans may be normal except for evidence of preexisting conditions or occasional diffuse edema. Imaging is generally nonspecific in that most patients do not present with pathognomonic lesions, but it can be used to rule out other suspected causes of disease. It is important to remember that imaging may yield negative results if done early in the disease course but later may detect lesions. For example, eastern equine encephalitis (focal abnormalities) and severe Japanese encephalitis (hemorrhagic bilateral thalamic lesions) have caused lesions detectable by medical imaging.

Comatose patients may require management of intracranial pressure elevations, inappropriate secretion of antidiuretic hormone, respiratory failure, or seizures. Specific therapies for these viral encephalitides are not available. The only practical preventive measures are vector management and personal protection against the arthropod transmitting the virus. For Japanese encephalitis or tick-borne viral encephalitis, vaccination should be considered in certain circumstances (see relevant sections below).

Bunyaviruses: California (Meningo)encephalitis The isolation of California encephalitis virus established California serogroup orthobunyaviruses as causes of encephalitides. However, California encephalitis virus has been implicated in only a very few cases of encephalitis, whereas its close relative, La Crosse virus, is the major cause of encephalitis in this serogroup (~70 cases per year in the United States). California (meningo)encephalitis due to La Crosse virus infection is most commonly reported from the upper Midwest of the United States but is also found in other areas of the central and eastern parts of the country, most often in West Virginia, Tennessee, North Carolina, and Georgia. The serogroup includes 13 other viruses, some of which (e.g., Inkoo, Jamestown Canyon, Lumbo, snowshoe hare, and Tahyña viruses) also cause human disease. Transovarial transmission is a strong component of transmission of the California serogroup viruses in *Aedes* and *Ochlerotatus* mosquitoes. The mosquito vector of La Crosse virus is *Ochlerotatus triseriatus*. In addition to transovarial transmission, acquisition through feeding on viremic chipmunks and other mammals as well as venereal transmission can result in infection of this mosquito. *O. triseriatus* breeds in sites such as tree holes and abandoned tires and bites during daylight hours. The habits of this mosquito correlate with the risk factors for human cases: recreation in forested areas, residence at a forest's edge, and the presence of water-containing abandoned tires around the home. Intensive environmental modification based on these findings has reduced the incidence of disease in a highly endemic area in the U.S. Midwest.

Most humans are infected from July through September. The Asian tiger mosquito (*A. albopictus*) efficiently transmits La Crosse virus to mice and also transmits the agent transovarially in the laboratory; this aggressive anthropophilic mosquito has the capacity to urbanize, and its possible impact on transmission of virus to humans is of concern. The prevalence of antibody to La Crosse virus in humans is ≥20% in endemic areas, a figure indicating that infection is common but often asymptomatic. CNS disease has been recognized primarily in children <15 years of age.

The illness from La Crosse virus varies from aseptic meningitis accompanied by confusion to severe and occasionally fatal encephalitis (lethality rate, <0.5%). The incubation period is ~3–7 days. Although there may be prodromal symptoms/signs, the onset of CNS disease is sudden, with fever, headache, and lethargy often joined by nausea and vomiting, convulsions (in one-half of patients), and coma (in one-third of patients). Focal seizures, hemiparesis, tremor, aphasia, chorea, Babinski signs, and other evidence of significant neurologic dysfunction are common, but residual disease is not. Approximately 10% of patients have recurrent seizures in the succeeding months. Other serious sequelae of La Crosse virus infection are rare, although a decrease in scholastic standing in children has been reported and mild personality change has occasionally been suggested.

The blood leukocyte count is commonly elevated in patients with La Crosse virus infection, sometimes reaching 20,000/μL, and is usually accompanied by a left shift. CSF leukocyte counts are typically 30–500/μL with a mononuclear cell predominance (although 25–90% of cells are polymorphonuclear in some patients). The blood protein concentration is normal or slightly increased, and the glucose concentration is normal. Specific virologic diagnosis based on IgM-capture assays of serum and CSF is efficient. The only human anatomic site from which virus has been isolated is the brain.

Treatment is supportive over a 1- to 2-week acute phase during which status epilepticus, cerebral edema, and inappropriate secretion of antidiuretic hormone are important concerns. A phase 2B clinical trial of IV ribavirin in children with La Crosse virus infection was discontinued during dose escalation because of adverse effects.

Jamestown Canyon virus has been implicated in several cases of encephalitis in adults, usually with a significant respiratory illness at onset. Human infection with this virus has been documented in New York, Wisconsin, Ohio, Michigan, Ontario, and other areas of North America where the vector mosquito, *Aedes stimulans*, feeds on its main host, the white-tailed deer. Tahyña virus can be found in central Europe, Russia, China, and Africa. The virus is a prominent cause of febrile disease but can also cause pharyngitis, pulmonary syndromes, aseptic meningitis, or meningoencephalitis.

Flaviviruses The most important flavivirus encephalitides are Japanese encephalitis, St. Louis encephalitis, tick-borne encephalitis, and West Nile virus infection. Australian encephalitis (Murray Valley encephalitis) and Rocio virus infection resemble Japanese encephalitis but are documented only occasionally in Australia and Brazil, respectively. Powassan virus has caused ~50 cases of often-severe disease (lethality rate, ~10%), frequently occurring among children in eastern Canada and the United States. Usutu virus has caused only individual cases of human infection, but such infections may be underdiagnosed.

JAPANESE ENCEPHALITIS Japanese encephalitis is the most important viral encephalitis in Asia. Each year 35,000–50,000 cases and more than 15,000 deaths are reported. Japanese encephalitis virus is found throughout Asia, including far eastern Russia, Japan, China, India, Pakistan, and southeastern Asia, and causes occasional epidemics on western Pacific islands. The virus has been detected in the Torres Strait islands, and five human encephalitis cases have been identified on the nearby Australian mainland. The virus is particularly common in areas where irrigated rice fields attract the natural avian vertebrate hosts and provide abundant breeding sites for mosquitoes such as *Culex tritaeniorhynchus*, which transmit the virus to humans. Additional amplification by pigs, which suffer abortion, and horses, which develop encephalitis, may be significant as well. Vaccination of these additional amplifying hosts may reduce the transmission of the virus.

Clinical signs of Japanese encephalitis emerge after an incubation period of 5–15 days and range from an unspecific febrile presentation (nausea, vomiting, diarrhea, cough) to aseptic meningitis, meningoencephalitis, acute flaccid paralysis, and severe encephalitis. Common findings are cerebellar signs, cranial nerve palsies, and cognitive and speech impairments. A Parkinsonian presentation and seizures are typical in severe cases. Effective vaccines are available. Vaccination is indicated for summer travelers to rural Asia, where the risk of acquiring Japanese encephalitis is considered to be about 1 per 5000 to 1 per 20,000 travelers per week if travel duration exceeds 3 weeks. Usually two intramuscular doses of the vaccine are given 28 days apart, with the second dose administered at least 1 week prior to travel.

ST. LOUIS ENCEPHALITIS St. Louis encephalitis virus is transmitted between mosquitoes and birds. This virus causes a low-level endemic infection among rural residents of the western and central United States, where *Culex tarsalis* is the vector (see "Western Equine Encephalitis," below). The more urbanized mosquitoes *Culex pipiens* and *Culex quinquefasciatus* have been responsible for epidemics resulting in hundreds or even thousands of cases in cities of the central and eastern United States. Most cases occur in June through October. The urban mosquitoes breed in accumulations of stagnant water and sewage with high organic content and readily feed on humans in and around houses at dusk. The elimination of open sewers and trash-filled drainage systems is expensive and may not be possible, but screening of houses and implementation of personal protective measures may be an effective approach to the prevention of infection. The rural mosquito vector is most active at dusk and outdoors; its bites can be avoided by modification of activities and use of repellents.

Disease severity increases with age. St. Louis encephalitis virus infections that result in aseptic meningitis or mild encephalitis are concentrated among children and young adults, while severe and fatal cases primarily affect the elderly. Infection rates are similar in all age groups; thus the greater susceptibility of older persons to disease is a biologic consequence of aging. St. Louis encephalitis has an abrupt onset after an incubation period of 4–21 days, sometimes following a prodrome, and begins with fever, lethargy, confusion, and headache. In addition, nuchal rigidity, hypotonia, hyperreflexia, myoclonus, and tremors are common. Severe cases can include cranial nerve palsies, hemiparesis, and seizures. Patients often report dysuria and may have viral antigen in urine as well as pyuria. The overall rate of lethality is generally ~7% but may reach 20% among patients >60 years of age. Recovery is slow. Emotional lability, difficulties with concentration and memory, asthenia, and tremors are commonly prolonged in older convalescent patients. The CSF of patients with St. Louis encephalitis usually contains tens to hundreds of leukocytes, with a lymphocytic predominance and a left shift. The CSF glucose concentration is normal in these patients.

TICK-BORNE VIRAL ENCEPHALITIS Tick-borne encephalitis viruses are currently subdivided into four groups: the western/European subtype (previously called central European encephalitis virus), the (Ural-) Siberian subtype (previously called Russian spring-summer encephalitis virus), the Far Eastern subtype, and the louping ill subtype (previously called louping ill virus or, in Japan, Negishi virus). Small mammals and grouse, deer, and sheep are the vertebrate amplifiers for these viruses, which are transmitted by ticks. The risk of infection varies by geographic area and can be highly localized within a given area; human infections usually follow either outdoor activities resulting in tick bites or consumption of raw (unpasteurized) milk from infected goats or, less commonly, from other infected animals (cows, sheep). Milk seems to represent the main transmission route for louping ill viruses, which cause disease only very rarely. The western/European subtype viruses are transmitted mainly by *Ixodes ricinus* from Scandinavia to the Ural Mountains. (Ural-)Siberian viruses are transmitted predominantly by *Ixodes persulcatus* from Europe across the Ural Mountains to the Pacific Ocean; louping ill viruses seem to be confined primarily to Great Britain. Several thousand infections with tick-borne encephalitis virus are recorded each year among people of all ages. Human tick-borne viral encephalitis occurs between April and October, with a peak in June and July.

Western/European viruses classically caused bimodal disease. After an incubation period of 7–14 days, the illness begins with a *fever–myalgia phase* (arthralgia, fever, headaches, myalgia, nausea) that lasts for 2–4 days and is thought to correlate with viremia. A subsequent remission for several days is followed by the recurrence of fever and the onset of meningeal signs. The *CNS phase* (7–10 days before onset of improvement) varies from mild aseptic meningitis, which is more common among younger patients, to severe (meningo-)encephalitis with coma, seizures, tremors, and motor signs. Spinal and medullary involvement can lead to typical limb-girdle paralysis and respiratory paralysis. Most patients with western/European virus infections recover (lethality rate, 1%), and only a minority of patients have significant deficits. However, the lethality rate from (Ural-)Siberian virus infections reaches 7–8%.

Infections with Far Eastern viruses generally run a more abrupt course. The encephalitic syndrome caused by these viruses sometimes begins without a remission from the fever–myalgia phase and has more severe manifestations than the western/European syndrome. The lethality rate is high (20–40%), and major sequelae—most notably, lower motor neuron paralyses of the proximal muscles of the extremities, trunk, and neck—are common, developing in approximately one-half of patients. Thrombocytopenia sometimes develops during the initial febrile illness, resembling the early hemorrhagic phase of some other tick-borne flavivirus infections, such as Kyasanur Forest disease. In the early stage of the illness, virus may be isolated from the blood. In the CNS phase, IgM antibodies are detectable in serum and/or CSF.

Diagnosis of tick-borne viral encephalitis primarily relies on serology and detection of viral genomes by RT-PCR. There is no specific therapy for infection. However, effective alum-adjuvanted, formalin-inactivated virus vaccines are produced in Austria, Germany, and Russia in chicken embryo cells (FSME-Immun® and Encepur®). Two doses of the Austrian vaccine separated by an interval of 1–3 months appear to be effective in the field, and antibody responses are similar when vaccine is given on days 0 and 14. Because rare cases of postvaccination Guillain-Barré syndrome have been reported, vaccination should be reserved for persons likely to experience rural exposure in an endemic area during the season of transmission. Cross-neutralization for the western/European and Far Eastern variants has been established, but there are no published field studies on cross-protection among formalin-inactivated vaccines.

Because 0.2–4% of ticks in endemic areas may be infected, the use of immunoglobulin prophylaxis of tick-borne viral encephalitis has been raised. Prompt administration of high-titered specific antibody preparations should probably be undertaken, although no controlled data are available to prove the efficacy of this measure. Immunoglobulins should be considered because of the risk of antibody-mediated enhancement of infection or antigen–antibody complex deposition in tissues.

WEST NILE VIRUS INFECTION West Nile virus is now the primary cause of arboviral encephalitis in the United States. In 2012, 2873 cases of neuroinvasive disease (e.g., meningitis, encephalitis, acute flaccid paralysis), with 270 deaths, and 2801 cases of non-neuroinvasive infection were reported. West Nile virus was initially described as being transmitted among wild birds by *Culex* mosquitoes in Africa, Asia, and southern Europe. In addition, the virus has been implicated in severe and fatal hepatic necrosis in Africa. West Nile virus was introduced into New York City in 1999 and subsequently spread to other areas of the northeastern United States, causing die-offs among crows, exotic zoo birds, and other birds. The virus has continued to spread and is now found in almost all states as well as in Canada, Mexico, South America, and the Caribbean islands. *C. pipiens* remains the major vector in the northeastern United States, but several other *Culex* species and *A. albopictus* are also involved. Jays compete with crows and other corvids as amplifiers and lethal targets in other areas of the country.

West Nile virus is a common cause of febrile disease without CNS involvement (incubation period, 3–14 days), but it occasionally causes aseptic meningitis and severe encephalitis, particularly among the elderly. The fever–myalgia syndrome caused by West Nile virus differs from that caused by other viruses in terms of the frequent—rather than occasional—appearance of a maculopapular rash concentrated on the trunk (especially in children) and the development of lymphadenopathy. Back pain, fatigue, headache, myalgia, retroorbital pain, sore throat, nausea and vomiting, and arthralgia (but not arthritis) are common accompaniments that may persist for several weeks. Encephalitis, sequelae, and death are all more common among elderly, diabetic, and hypertensive patients and among patients with previous CNS insults. In addition to the more severe motor and cognitive sequelae, milder findings may include tremor, slight abnormalities in motor skills, and loss of executive functions. Intense clinical interest and the availability of laboratory diagnostic methods have made it possible to define a number of unusual clinical features. Such features include chorioretinitis, flaccid paralysis with histologic lesions resembling poliomyelitis, and initial presentation with fever and focal neurologic deficits in the absence of diffuse encephalitis. Immunosuppressed patients may have fulminant courses or develop persistent CNS infection. Virus transmission through both transplantation and blood transfusion has necessitated screening of blood and organ donors by nucleic acid–based tests. Occasionally, pregnant women infect their fetuses with West Nile virus.

Rhabdoviruses: Chandipura Virus Infection Chandipura virus seems to be an emerging and increasingly important human virus in India, where it is transmitted among hedgehogs by mosquitoes and sandflies. In humans, the disease begins as an influenza-like illness, with fever, headache, abdominal pain, nausea, and vomiting; these manifestations are followed by neurologic impairment and infection-related or autoimmune-mediated encephalitis. Chandipura virus infection is characterized by high lethality in children. Several hundred cases of infection are recorded in India every year. Infections with other arthropod-borne rhabdoviruses (Isfahan, Piry, vesicular stomatitis Indiana, vesicular stomatitis New Jersey) may imitate the early febrile stage of Chandipura virus infection.

Togaviruses • ***EASTERN EQUINE ENCEPHALITIS*** This disease is encountered primarily in swampy foci along the eastern coast of the United States, with a few inland foci as far removed as Michigan. Infected humans present for medical care from June through October. During this period, the bird–*Culiseta* mosquito cycle spills over into other mosquitoes such as *Aedes sollicitans* or *Aedes vexans*, which are more likely to feed on mammals. There is concern over the potential role of the introduced anthropophilic mosquito species *A. albopictus*, which has been found to be infected with eastern equine encephalitis virus and is an effective experimental vector in the laboratory. Horses are a common target for the virus. Contact with unvaccinated horses may be associated with human disease, but horses probably do not play a significant role in amplification of the virus.

Eastern equine encephalitis is one of the most destructive of the arboviral diseases, with a sudden onset after an incubation period of ~5–10 days, rapid progression, 50–75% lethality, and frequent sequelae in survivors. This severity is reflected in the extensive necrotic lesions and polymorphonuclear infiltrates found at postmortem examination of the brain. Acute polymorphonuclear CSF pleocytosis, often occurring during the first 1–3 days of disease, is another indication of severity. In addition, leukocytosis with a left shift is a common feature. A formalin-inactivated vaccine has been used to protect laboratory workers but is not generally available or applicable.

VENEZUELAN EQUINE ENCEPHALITIS Venezuelan equine encephalitis viruses are separated into epizootic viruses (subtypes IA/B and IC) and enzootic viruses (subtypes ID, IE, and IF). Closely related enzootic viruses are Everglades virus, Mucambo virus, and Tonate virus. Enzootic viruses are found primarily in humid tropical-forest habitats and are maintained between culicoid mosquitoes and rodents. These viruses cause human disease but are not pathogenic for horses and do not cause epizootics. Enzootic viruses are common causes of acute febrile disease. Everglades virus has caused encephalitis in humans in Florida. Extrapolation from the rate of genetic change suggests that Everglades virus may have been introduced into Florida <200 years ago. Everglades virus is most closely related to the ID subtype viruses that appear to have given evolutionary rise to the epizootic variants active in South America.

Epizootic viruses have an unknown natural cycle but periodically cause extensive epizootics/epidemics in equids and humans in the Americas. These epizootics/epidemics are the result of high-level viremia in horses and mules, which transmit the infection to several types of mosquitoes. Infected mosquitoes in turn infect humans and perpetuate virus transmission. Humans also have high-level viremia, but their role in virus transmission is unclear. Epizootics of Venezuelan equine fever occurred repeatedly in South America at intervals of ≤10 years from the 1930s until 1969, when a massive epizootic spread throughout Central America and Mexico, reaching southern Texas in 1971. Genetic sequencing suggested that the virus from that outbreak originated from residual "un-inactivated" IA/B subtype virus in veterinary vaccines. The outbreak was terminated in Texas with a live attenuated vaccine (TC-83) originally developed for human use by the U.S. Army; the epizootic virus was then used for further production of inactivated veterinary vaccines. No further epizootic disease was identified until 1995, when additional epizootics took place in Colombia, Venezuela, and Mexico. The viruses involved in these epizootics as well as previously epizootic IC viruses are close phylogenetic relatives of known enzootic ID viruses. This finding suggests that active evolution and selection of epizootic viruses are under way in South America.

During epizootics, extensive human infection is the rule, with clinical disease in 10–60% of infected individuals. Most infections result in notable acute febrile disease, while relatively few infections (5–15%) result in neurologic disease. A low rate of CNS invasion is supported by the absence of encephalitis among the many infections resulting from exposure to aerosols in the laboratory setting or from vaccination accidents. The most recent large epizootic of Venezuelan equine fever occurred in Colombia and Venezuela in 1995; of the more than 85,000 clinical cases, 4% (with a higher proportion among children than adults) included neurologic symptoms/signs, and 300 cases ended in death.

The prevention of epizootic Venezuelan equine fever depends on vaccination of horses with the attenuated TC-83 vaccine or with an inactivated vaccine prepared from that variant. Enzootic viruses are genetically and antigenically different from epizootic viruses, and protection against the former with vaccines prepared from the latter is relatively ineffective. Humans can be protected by immunization with similar vaccines prepared from Everglades virus, Mucambo virus, and Venezuelan equine encephalitis virus, but the use of the vaccines is restricted to laboratory personnel because of reactogenicity, possible fetal pathogenicity, and limited availability.

WESTERN EQUINE ENCEPHALITIS The primary maintenance cycle of western equine encephalitis virus in the United States is between *C. tarsalis* and birds, principally sparrows and finches. Equids and humans become infected, and both suffer encephalitis without amplifying the virus in nature. St. Louis encephalitis virus is transmitted in a similar cycle in the same regions harboring western equine encephalitis virus; disease caused by the former occurs about a month earlier than that caused by the latter (July through October). Large epidemics of western equine encephalitis occurred in the western and central United States and Canada during the 1930s through 1950s, but in recent years the disease has been uncommon. From 1964 through 2010, only 640 cases were reported in the United States. This decline in incidence may reflect in part the integrated approach to mosquito management that has been employed in irrigation projects and the increasing use of agricultural pesticides. The decreased incidence of western equine encephalitis almost certainly reflects the increased tendency for humans to be indoors behind closed windows at dusk—the peak biting period by the major vector.

After an incubation period of ~5–10 days, western equine encephalitis virus causes a typical diffuse viral encephalitis, with an increased attack rate and increased morbidity among the young, particularly children <2 years old. In addition, the lethality rate is high among the young and the very elderly (3–7% overall). One-third of individuals who have convulsions during the acute illness have subsequent seizure activity. Infants <1 year old—particularly those in the first months of life—are at serious risk of motor and intellectual damage. Twice as many males as females develop clinical encephalitis after 5–9 years of age. This difference in incidence may be related to greater outdoor exposure of boys to the vector but may also be due in part to biologic differences. A formalin-inactivated vaccine has been used to protect laboratory workers but is not generally available.

FEVER AND MYALGIA

The fever and myalgia syndrome is most commonly associated with zoonotic virus infection. Many of the numerous viruses listed in Table 233-1 probably cause at least a few cases of this syndrome, but only some of these viruses have prominent associations with the syndrome and are of biomedical importance. The fever and myalgia syndrome typically begins with the abrupt onset of fever, chills, intense myalgia, and malaise. Patients may also report joint or muscle pains, but true arthritis is not found. Anorexia is characteristic and may be accompanied by nausea or even vomiting. Headache is common and may be severe, with photophobia and retroorbital pain. Physical findings are minimal and are usually confined to conjunctival injection with pain on palpation of muscles or the epigastrium. The duration of symptoms/signs is quite variable (generally 2–5 days), with a biphasic course in some instances. The spectrum of disease varies from subclinical to temporarily incapacitating. Less constant findings include a nonpruritic maculopapular rash. Epistaxis may occur but does not necessarily indicate a bleeding diathesis. A minority of the patients may develop aseptic meningitis. This diagnosis is difficult to make in remote areas, given patients' photophobia and myalgia as well as the lack of opportunity to examine the CSF. Although pharyngitis or radiographic evidence of pulmonary infiltrates is found in some patients, the agents causing this syndrome are not primary respiratory pathogens.

The differential diagnosis includes anicteric leptospirosis, rickettsial diseases, and the early stages of other syndromes discussed in this chapter. The fever and myalgia syndrome is often described as "influenza-like," but the usual absence of cough and coryza makes influenza an unlikely confounder except at the earliest stages. Treatment is supportive, but acetylsalicylic acid is avoided because of the potential for exacerbated bleeding or Reye's syndrome. Complete recovery is the general outcome for people with this syndrome, although prolonged asthenia and nonspecific symptoms have been described in some patients, particularly after infection with lymphocytic choriomeningitis virus or dengue virus types 1–4.

Efforts at prevention of viral infection are best based on vector control, which, however, may be expensive or impossible. For mosquito control, destruction of breeding sites is generally the most economically and environmentally sound approach. Emerging containment technologies include the release of genetically modified mosquitoes and the spread of *Wolbachia* bacteria to limit mosquito multiplication rates. Depending on the vector and its habits, other possible approaches include the use of screens or other barriers (e.g., permethrin-impregnated bed nets) to prevent the vector from entering dwellings, judicious application of arthropod repellents such as *N,N*,-diethyltoluamide (DEET) to the skin, wearing of long-sleeved and ideally permethrin-impregnated clothing, and avoidance of the vectors' habitats and times of peak activity.

Arenaviruses Lymphocytic choriomeningitis/meningoencephalitis is the only human arenavirus infection resulting predominantly in fever and myalgia. Lymphocytic choriomeningitis virus is transmitted to humans from the common house mouse (*Mus musculus*) by aerosols of excreta and secreta. The virus is maintained in the mouse mainly by vertical transmission from infected dams. The vertically infected mouse remains viremic and sheds virus for life, with high concentrations of virus in all tissues. Infected colonies of pet hamsters also can serve as a link to humans. Infections among scientists and animal caretakers can occur because the virus is widely used in immunology laboratories as a model of T cell function and can silently infect cell cultures and passaged tumor lines. In addition, patients may have a history of residence in rodent-infested housing or other exposure to rodents. An antibody prevalence of ~5–10% has been reported among adults from Argentina, Germany, and the United States.

Lymphocytic choriomeningitis/meningoencephalitis differs from the general syndrome of fever and myalgia in that the onset is gradual. Conditions occasionally associated with the disease are orchitis, transient alopecia, arthritis, pharyngitis, cough, and maculopapular rash. An estimated one-fourth of patients (or fewer) experience a febrile phase of 3–6 days. After a brief remission, many develop renewed fever accompanied by severe headache, nausea and vomiting, and meningeal signs lasting for ~1 week (the CNS phase). These patients virtually always recover fully, as do the rare patients with clear-cut signs of encephalitis. Recovery may be delayed by transient hydrocephalus. During the initial febrile phase, leukopenia and thrombocytopenia are common, and virus can usually be isolated from blood. During the CNS phase, the virus may be found in the CSF, and antibodies are present in the blood. The pathogenesis of lymphocytic choriomeningitis/meningoencephalitis is thought to resemble that following direct intracranial inoculation of the virus into adult mice. The onset of the immune response leads to T cell–mediated immunopathologic meningitis. During the meningeal phase, CSF mononuclear-cell counts range from the hundreds to the low thousands per microliter, and hypoglycorrhachia is found in one-third of patients.

IgM-capture ELISA, immunochemistry, and RT-PCR are used in the diagnosis of lymphocytic choriomeningitis/meningoencephalitis. IgM-capture ELISA of serum and CSF usually yields positive results; RT-PCR assays have been developed for probing CSF. Because patients who have fulminant infections transmitted by recent organ transplantation do not mount an immune response, immunohistochemistry or RT-PCR is required for diagnosis. Infection should be suspected in acutely ill febrile patients with marked leukopenia and thrombocytopenia. In patients with aseptic meningitis, any of the following suggests lymphocytic choriomeningitis/meningoencephalitis: a well-marked febrile prodrome, adult age, occurrence in the autumn, low CSF glucose levels, or CSF mononuclear-cell counts of >1000/μL. In pregnant women, infection may lead to fetal invasion with consequent congenital hydrocephalus and chorioretinitis. Because the maternal infection may be mild, causing only a short febrile illness, antibodies to the virus should be sought in both the mother and the fetus under suspicious circumstances, particularly in TORCH (toxoplasmosis, rubella, cytomegalovirus, herpes simplex, and HIV)–negative neonatal hydrocephalus.

Bunyaviruses Numerous bunyaviruses cause fever and myalgia. Many of these viruses cause individual infections and usually do not result in epidemics—e.g., the viruses of the orthobunyavirus Anopheles A serogroup (e.g., Tacaiuma virus), Bwamba serogroup (Bwamba virus, Pongola virus), Guama serogroup (Catu virus, Guama virus), Nyando serogroup (Nyando virus), and Wyeomyia serogroup (Wyeomyia virus); the unclassified bunyavirus Tataguine virus; the phlebovirus Bhanja complex (Bhanja virus, Heartland virus) and Candiru complex (Alenquer, Candiru, Escharate, Maldonado, Morumbi, and Serra Norte viruses); the hantavirus Choclo virus; and the Dugbe and Nairobi sheep disease nairoviruses. In the relevant orthobunyaviral Bunyamwera serogroup (Bunyamwera, Batai, Cache Valley, Fort Sherman, Germiston, Guaroa, Ilesha, Ngari, Shokwe, and Xingu viruses), Ngari virus recently has been implicated in a large epidemic in Africa.

ORTHOBUNYAVIRUS GROUP C SEROGROUP Apeú, Caraparú, Itaquí, Madrid, Marituba, Murutucú, Nepuyo, Oriboca, Ossa, Restan, and Zungarococha viruses are among the most common causes of arboviral infection in humans entering South American jungles. These viruses cause acute febrile disease and are transmitted by mosquitoes in neotropical forests.

ORTHOBUNYAVIRUS SIMBU SEROGROUP Oropouche virus is transmitted in Central and South America by a biting midge, *Culicoides paraensis*, which often breeds to high density in cacao husks and other vegetable detritus found in towns and cities. Explosive epidemics involving thousands of patients have been reported from several towns in Brazil and Peru. Rash and aseptic meningitis have been detected in a number of patients. Iquitos virus, a recently discovered reassortant and close relative of Oropouche virus, causes disease that is easily mistaken for Oropouche virus disease; its overall epidemiologic significance remains to be determined.

PHLEBOVIRUS SANDFLY FEVER SEROGROUP A previous designation for sandfly fever, "3-day fever," instructively describes the brief debilitating course associated with this essentially benign infection. There is neither a rash nor CNS involvement, and complete recovery is the rule. Sandfly fever is caused by at least six distinct phleboviruses of the phlebovirus sandfly fever serocomplex (Chagres virus, sandfly fever Cyprus virus, sandfly fever Naples virus, sandfly fever Sicilian virus, sandfly fever Turkey virus, and Toscana virus). Sandfly fever Naples virus, sandfly fever Sicilian virus, and Toscana viruses are the most important human pathogens of this group. *Phlebotomus* sandflies transmit the viruses, probably among small mammals, and infect humans by bites. Female sandflies may be infected by the oral route as they take a blood meal and may transmit the virus to offspring when they lay their eggs after a second blood meal. This prominent transovarial transmission confounds virus control.

Sandfly fever is found in the circum-Mediterranean area, extending to the east through the Balkans into parts of China as well as into western Asia. Chagres virus is endemic in Panama. Sandflies are found in both rural and urban settings and are known for their short flight ranges and their small sizes; the latter enables them to penetrate standard mosquito screens and netting. Epidemics have been described in the wake of natural disasters and wars. After World War II, extensive spraying in parts of Europe to control malaria greatly reduced sandfly populations and sandfly fever Naples virus transmission; the incidence of sandfly fever continues to be low.

A common pattern of disease in endemic areas consists of high attack rates among travelers and military personnel and little or no disease in the local population, who are protected after childhood infection. Toscana virus infection is common during the summer among rural residents and vacationers, particularly in Italy, Spain, and Portugal; a number of cases have been identified in travelers returning to Germany and Scandinavia. The disease may manifest as an uncomplicated febrile illness but is often associated with aseptic meningitis, with virus isolated from the CSF.

Punta Toro virus is a phlebovirus that is not part of the sandfly fever serocomplex but that, like the members of this complex, is transmitted by sandflies. Punta Toro virus causes a sandfly fever–like disease in the Latin American tropical forest, where the vectors rest on tree buttresses. Epidemics have not been reported, but antibody prevalence among inhabitants of villages in endemic areas indicates a cumulative lifetime exposure rate of >50%.

Flaviviruses The most clinically important flaviviruses that cause the fever and myalgia syndrome are dengue viruses 1–4. In fact, dengue is probably the most important arthropod-borne viral disease worldwide, with 50–100 million infections occurring per year. Year-round transmission of dengue viruses 1–4 occurs between latitudes of 25°N and 25°S, but seasonal forays of the viruses into the United States and Europe have been documented. All four viruses have *A. aegypti* as their principal vector. Through increasing spread of mosquitoes throughout the tropics and subtropics and international travel of infected humans, large areas of the world have become vulnerable to the introduction of dengue viruses. Thus, dengue and severe dengue (see "Viral Hemorrhagic Fevers," below) are becoming increasingly common. For instance, conditions favorable to dengue virus 1–4 transmission via

A. aegypti exist in Hawaii and the southern United States. The range of a lesser dengue virus vector, *A. albopictus*, now extends from Asia to the United States, the Indian Ocean, parts of Europe, and Hawaii. *A. aegypti* typically breeds near human habitation, using relatively fresh water from sources such as water jars, vases, discarded containers, coconut husks, and old tires. The mosquito usually inhabits dwellings and bites during the day. Bursts of dengue cases are to be expected in the southern United States, particularly along the Mexican border, where containers of water may be infested with *A. aegypti*. Closed habitations with air-conditioning may inhibit transmission of many arboviruses, including dengue viruses 1–4.

Dengue begins after an incubation period averaging 4–7 days, when the typical patient experiences the sudden onset of fever, frontal headache, retroorbital pain, and back pain along with severe myalgias. These symptoms gave rise to the colloquial designation of dengue as "break-bone fever." Often a transient macular rash appears on the first day, as do adenopathy, palatal vesicles, and scleral injection. The illness may last a week, with additional symptoms and clinical signs usually including anorexia, nausea or vomiting, and marked cutaneous hypersensitivity. Near the time of defervescence on days 3–5, a maculopapular rash begins on the trunk and spreads to the extremities and the face. Epistaxis and scattered petechiae are often noted in uncomplicated dengue, and preexisting gastrointestinal lesions may bleed during the acute illness.

Laboratory findings of dengue include leukopenia, thrombocytopenia, and, in many cases, elevations of serum aminotransferase concentrations. The diagnosis is made by IgM ELISA or paired serology during recovery or by antigen-detection ELISA or RT-PCR during the acute phase. Virus is readily isolated from blood in the acute phase if mosquito inoculation or mosquito cell culture is used.

Reoviruses Several orbiviruses (Lebombo, Kemerovo, Orungo, and Tribeč viruses) and coltiviruses (Colorado tick fever, Eyach, and Salmon River viruses) can cause fever and myalgia in humans. With the exception of Lebombo and Orungo viruses, all of these viruses are transmitted by ticks. The most important reoviral arthropod-borne disease is Colorado tick fever. Several hundred patients with this disease are reported annually in the United States. The infection is acquired between March and November through the bite of an infected ixodid tick, the Rocky Mountain wood tick (*Dermacentor andersoni*), in mountainous western regions at altitudes of 1200–3000 m. Small mammals serve as amplifying hosts. The most common presentation is fever and myalgia; meningoencephalitis is not uncommon, and hemorrhagic disease, pericarditis, myocarditis, orchitis, and pulmonary presentations have also been reported. Rash develops in a minority of patients. Leukopenia and thrombocytopenia are also noted. The disease usually lasts 7–10 days and is often biphasic. The most important differential diagnostic considerations since the beginning of the twentieth century have been Rocky Mountain spotted fever (although Colorado tick fever is much more common in Colorado) and tularemia. Colorado tick fever virus replicates for several weeks in erythropoietic cells and can be found in erythrocytes. This feature, detected in erythroid smears stained by immunofluorescence, can be diagnostically helpful and is important during screening of blood donors.

PULMONARY DISEASE

Hantavirus pulmonary syndrome (HPS) was first described in 1993, but retrospective identification of cases by immunohistochemistry (1978) and serology (1959) support the idea that HPS is a recently discovered rather than a truly new disease. The causative agents are hantaviruses of a distinct phylogenetic lineage that is associated with the cricetid rodent subfamily Sigmodontinae. Sin Nombre virus, which chronically infects North American deer mice (*Peromyscus maniculatus*), is the most important agent of HPS in the United States. Several other related viruses (Anajatuba, Andes, Araraquara, Araucária, Bayou, Bermejo, Black Creek Canal, Blue River, Castelo dos Sonhos, El Moro Canyon, Juquitiba, Laguna Negra, Lechiguanas, Maciel, Monongahela, Muleshoe, New York, Orán, Paranoá, Pergamino, Río Mamoré, and Tunari) cause the disease in North and South America, but Andes virus is unusual in that it has been implicated in human-to-human transmission. HPS particularly affects rural residents living in dwellings permeable to rodent entry or working in occupations that pose a risk of rodent exposure. Each type of rodent has its own particular habits; in the case of deer mice, these behaviors include living in and around human habitation.

HPS begins with a prodrome of ~3–4 days (range, 1–11 days) comprising fever, malaise, myalgia, and—in many cases—gastrointestinal disturbances such as abdominal pain, nausea, and vomiting. Dizziness is common and vertigo occasional. Severe prodromal symptoms/signs may bring some patients to medical attention, but most cases are recognized as the pulmonary phase begins. Typical signs are slightly lowered blood pressure, tachycardia, tachypnea, mild hypoxemia, thrombocytopenia, and early radiographic signs of pulmonary edema. Physical findings in the chest are often surprisingly scant. The conjunctival and cutaneous signs of vascular involvement seen in hantavirus VHFs (see below) are uncommon. During the next few hours, decompensation may progress rapidly to severe hypoxemia and respiratory failure.

The HPS differential diagnosis includes abdominal surgical conditions and pyelonephritis as well as rickettsial disease, sepsis, meningococcemia, plague, tularemia, influenza, and relapsing fever. A specific diagnosis is best made by IgM antibody testing of acute-phase serum, which has yielded positive results even in the prodrome. Tests using a Sin Nombre virus antigen detect antibodies to the related HPS-causing hantaviruses. Occasionally, heterotypic viruses will react only in the IgG ELISA, but such a finding is highly suspicious given the very low seroprevalence of these viruses in normal populations. RT-PCR is usually positive when used to test blood clots obtained in the first 7–9 days of illness and when used to test tissues; this assay is useful in identifying the infecting virus in areas outside the home range of deer mice and in atypical cases.

During the prodrome, the differential diagnosis of HPS is difficult, but by the time of presentation or within 24 h thereafter, a number of diagnostically helpful clinical features become apparent. Cough usually is not present at the outset. Interstitial edema is evident on a chest x-ray. Later, bilateral alveolar edema with a central distribution develops in the setting of a normal-sized heart; occasionally, the edema is initially unilateral. Pleural effusions are often seen. Thrombocytopenia, circulating atypical lymphocytes, and a left shift (often with leukocytosis) are almost always evident; thrombocytopenia is a particularly important early clue. Hemoconcentration, hypoalbuminemia, and proteinuria should also be sought for diagnosis. Although thrombocytopenia virtually always develops and prolongation of the partial thromboplastin time is the rule, clinical evidence for coagulopathy or laboratory indications of disseminated intravascular coagulation (DIC) are found in only a minority of severely ill patients. Patients with severe illness also have acidosis and elevated serum lactate concentrations. Mildly increased values in renal function tests are common, but patients with severe HPS often have markedly elevated serum creatinine concentrations. Some New World hantaviruses other than Sin Nombre virus (e.g., Andes virus) have been associated with more kidney involvement, but few such cases have been studied.

Management of HPS during the first few hours after presentation is critical. The goal is to prevent severe hypoxemia by oxygen therapy, with intubation and intensive respiratory management if needed. During this period, hypotension and shock with increasing hematocrit invite aggressive fluid administration, but this intervention should be undertaken with great caution. Because of low cardiac output with myocardial depression and increased pulmonary vascular permeability, shock should be managed expectantly with pressors and modest infusion of fluid guided by pulmonary capillary wedge pressure. Mild cases can be managed by frequent monitoring and oxygen administration without intubation. Many patients require intubation to manage hypoxemia and developing shock. Extracorporeal membrane oxygenation is instituted in severe cases, ideally before the onset of shock. The procedure is indicated in patients who have a cardiac index of 2.3 L/min/m^2 or an arterial oxygen tension/fractional inspired oxygen (Pa_{O_2}/FI_{O_2}) ratio of

<50 and who are unresponsive to conventional support. Lethality rates remain at ~30–40% even with good management, but most patients surviving the first 48 h of hospitalization are extubated and discharged within a few days with no apparent long-term residua. The antiviral drug ribavirin inhibits hantaviruses in vitro but did not have a marked effect on patients treated in an open-label study.

VIRAL HEMORRHAGIC FEVER

VHF is a constellation of findings based on vascular instability and decreased vascular integrity. An assault, direct or indirect, on the microvasculature leads to increased permeability and (particularly when platelet function is decreased) to actual disruption and local hemorrhage (a positive tourniquet sign). Blood pressure is decreased, and in severe cases shock supervenes. Cutaneous flushing and conjunctival suffusion are examples of common, observable abnormalities in the control of local circulation. Hemorrhage occurs infrequently. In most patients, hemorrhage is an indication of widespread vascular damage rather than a life-threatening loss of blood volume. In some VHFs, specific organs may be particularly impaired. For instance, the kidneys are primary targets in hemorrhagic fever with renal syndrome (HFRS), and the liver is a primary target in yellow fever and filovirus diseases. However, in all of these diseases, generalized circulatory disturbance is critically important. The pathogenesis of VHF is poorly understood and varies among the viruses regularly implicated in the syndrome. In some viral infections, direct damage to the vascular system or even to parenchymal cells of target organs is an important factor; in other viral infections, soluble mediators are thought to play a major role in the development of hemorrhage or fluid redistribution.

The acute phase in most cases of VHF is associated with ongoing virus replication and viremia. VHFs begin with fever and myalgia, usually of abrupt onset. (Arenavirus infections are the exceptions as they often develop gradually.) Within a few days, the patient presents for medical attention because of increasing prostration that is often accompanied by abdominal or chest pain, anorexia, dizziness, severe headache, hyperesthesia, photophobia, and nausea or vomiting and other gastrointestinal disturbances. Initial examination often reveals only an acutely ill patient with conjunctival suffusion, tenderness to palpation of muscles or abdomen, and borderline hypotension or postural hypotension, perhaps with tachycardia. Petechiae (often best visualized in the axillae), flushing of the head and thorax, periorbital edema, and proteinuria are common. AST concentrations are usually elevated at presentation or within a day or two thereafter. Hemoconcentration from vascular leakage, which is usually evident, is most marked in HFRS and in severe dengue. The seriously ill patient progresses to more severe clinical signs and develops shock and other findings typical of the causative virus. Shock, multifocal bleeding, and CNS involvement (encephalopathy, coma, seizures) are all poor prognostic signs.

One of the major diagnostic clues to VHF is travel to an endemic area within the incubation period for a given syndrome. Except in infections with Seoul, dengue, and yellow fever viruses, which have urban hosts/vectors, travel to a rural setting is especially suggestive of a diagnosis of VHF. In addition, several diseases considered in the differential diagnosis—falciparum malaria, shigellosis, typhoid fever, leptospirosis, relapsing fever, and rickettsial diseases—are treatable and potentially lethal.

Early recognition of VHF is important because of the need for virus-specific therapy and supportive measures. Such measures include prompt, atraumatic hospitalization; judicious fluid therapy that takes into account the patient's increased capillary permeability; administration of cardiotonic drugs; use of pressors to maintain blood pressure at levels that will support renal perfusion; treatment of the relatively common secondary bacterial (and the more rare fungal) infections; replacement of clotting factors and platelets as indicated; and the usual precautionary measures used in the treatment of patients with hemorrhagic diatheses. DIC should be treated only if clear laboratory evidence of its existence is found and if laboratory monitoring of therapy is feasible; there is no proven benefit of such therapy. The available evidence suggests that VHF patients have decreased cardiac output and will respond poorly to fluid loading as it is often practiced in the treatment of shock associated with bacterial sepsis. Specific therapy is available for several of the VHFs. Strict barrier nursing and other precautions against infection of medical staff and visitors are indicated when VHFs are encountered except when the illness is due to dengue viruses, hantaviruses, Rift Valley fever virus, or yellow fever virus.

Novel VHF-causing agents are still being discovered. Besides the viruses listed below, the latest addition may be the unclassified rhabdovirus Bas-Congo virus, which has been associated with three cases of VHF in the Democratic Republic of the Congo. However, Koch's postulates have not yet been fulfilled to prove cause and effect.

Arenaviruses The most important arenaviruses causing VHF are Junín virus, Lassa virus, and Machupo virus. Chapare, Guanarito, Lujo, and Sabiá viruses have caused limited and/or infrequent outbreaks or individual cases.

JUNÍN/ARGENTINIAN AND MACHUPO/BOLIVIAN HEMORRHAGIC FEVERS These severe diseases (with fetal lethality rates reaching 15–30%) are caused by Junín virus and Machupo virus, respectively. Their clinical presentations are similar, but their epidemiology differs because of the distribution and behavior of the viruses' rodent reservoirs. Junín/Argentinian hemorrhagic fever has thus far been recorded only in rural areas of Argentina, whereas Machupo/Bolivian hemorrhagic fever seems to be confined to rural Bolivia. Infection with the causative agents almost always results in disease, and all ages and both sexes are affected. Person-to-person or nosocomial transmission is rare but has occurred. The transmission of Junín/Argentinian hemorrhagic fever from convalescing men to their wives suggests the need for counseling of patients with arenavirus hemorrhagic fever concerning the avoidance of intimate contacts for several weeks after recovery. Compared with the pattern in Lassa fever (see below), thrombocytopenia—often marked—is the rule, hemorrhage is common, and CNS dysfunction (e.g., marked confusion, tremors of the upper extremities and tongue, and cerebellar signs) is much more common in disease caused by Junín virus and Machupo virus. Some cases follow a predominantly neurologic course, with a poor prognosis.

The clinical laboratory is helpful in diagnosis since thrombocytopenia, leukopenia, and proteinuria are typical findings. Junín/Argentinian hemorrhagic fever is readily treated with convalescent-phase plasma given within the first 8 days of illness. In the absence of passive antibody therapy, IV ribavirin in the dose recommended for Lassa fever is likely to be effective in all the South American VHFs caused by arenaviruses. A safe, effective, live attenuated vaccine exists for Junín/Argentinian hemorrhagic fever. After vaccination of more than 250,000 high-risk persons in the endemic area, the incidence of this VHF decreased markedly. In experimental animals, this vaccine is cross-protective against Machupo/Bolivian hemorrhagic fever.

LASSA FEVER Lassa virus is known to cause endemic and epidemic disease in Nigeria, Sierra Leone, Guinea, and Liberia, although it is probably more widely distributed in western Africa. In countries where Lassa virus is endemic, Lassa fever can be a prominent cause of febrile disease. For example, in one hospital in Sierra Leone, laboratory-confirmed Lassa fever is consistently responsible for one-fifth of admissions to the medical wards. In western Africa alone, probably tens of thousands of Lassa virus infections occur annually. Lassa virus can be transmitted by close person-to-person contact. The virus is often present in urine during convalescence and is suspected to be present in seminal fluid early in recovery. Nosocomial spread has occurred but is uncommon if proper sterile parenteral techniques are used. All ages and both sexes are affected; the incidence of disease is highest in the dry season, but transmission takes place year-round.

Among the VHF agents, only arenaviruses are typically associated with a gradual onset of illness, which begins after an incubation period of 5–16 days. Hemorrhage is seen in only ~15–30% of Lassa fever patients; a maculopapular rash is often noted in light-skinned patients. Effusions are common, and male-dominant pericarditis may develop late. Maternal lethality is higher than the usual 15–30% and is especially increased during the last trimester. The fetal death rate reaches 90%. Excavation of the uterus may increase survival rates of pregnant women, but data on Lassa fever and pregnancy are still sparse. These figures suggest that interruption of the pregnancy of Lassa virus–infected women should be considered. White blood cell counts are normal or slightly elevated, and platelet counts are normal or somewhat low. Deafness coincides with clinical improvement in ~20% of patients and is permanent and bilateral in some patients. Reinfection may occur but has not been associated with severe disease.

High-level viremia or a high serum AST concentration statistically predicts a fatal outcome. Thus, patients with an AST concentration of >150 IU/mL should be treated with IV ribavirin. This antiviral nucleoside analogue appears to be effective in reducing case-fatality rates from those documented among retrospective controls. However, possible side effects, such as reversible anemia (which usually does not require transfusion), dependent hemolytic anemia, and bone marrow suppression, need to be kept in mind. Ribavirin should be given by slow IV infusion in a dose of 32 mg/kg; this dose should be followed by 16 mg/kg every 6 h for 4 days and then by 8 mg/kg every 8 h for 6 days. Inactivated Lassa virus vaccines failed in preclinical studies.

Bunyaviruses The most important VHF-causing bunyaviruses are Crimean-Congo hemorrhagic fever virus, hantaviruses, Rift Valley fever virus, and "severe fever with thrombocytopenia syndrome virus." Other bunyaviruses—e.g., the Garissa variant of Ngari virus and Ilesha virus—have caused sporadic VHF outbreaks in Africa.

CRIMEAN-CONGO HEMORRHAGIC FEVER (CCHF) This severe VHF has a wide geographic distribution, potentially emerging wherever virus-bearing ticks occur. Because of the propensity of CCHF virus–transmitting ticks to feed on domestic livestock and certain wild mammals, veterinary serosurveys are the most effective mechanism for the monitoring of virus circulation in a particular region. Human infections are acquired via tick bites or during the crushing of infected ticks. Domestic animals do not become ill but do develop viremia. Thus, there is risk of acquiring CCHF during sheep shearing, slaughter, and contact with infected hides or carcasses from recently slaughtered infected animals. Nosocomial epidemics are common and are usually related to extensive blood exposure or needlesticks.

Although generally similar to other VHFs, CCHF causes extensive liver damage, resulting in jaundice in some patients. Clinical laboratory values indicate DIC and show elevations in concentrations of AST, creatine phosphokinase, and bilirubin. Patients who do not survive generally have more distinct changes than survivors in the concentrations of these markers, even in the early days of illness, and also develop leukocytosis rather than leukopenia. In addition, thrombocytopenia is more marked and develops earlier in patients who do not survive than in survivors. The benefit of IV ribavirin for treatment remains hotly debated, but clinical experience and retrospective comparison of patients with ominous clinical laboratory values suggest that ribavirin may be efficacious. No human or veterinary vaccines are recommended.

HEMORRHAGIC FEVER WITH RENAL SYNDROME HFRS is the most important VHF today, with more than 100,000 cases of severe disease in Asia annually and milder infections numbering in the thousands in Europe. The disease is widely distributed in Eurasia. The major causative viruses are Puumala virus (Europe), Dobrava-Belgrade virus (the Balkans), and Hantaan virus (eastern Asia). Amur/Soochong, Gou, Kurkino, Muju, Saaremaa, Sochi, and Tula viruses also cause HFRS but much less frequently and in more geographically confined areas determined by the distribution of reservoir hosts. Seoul virus is exceptional in that it is associated with brown rats (*Rattus norvegicus*); therefore, the virus has a worldwide distribution because of the migration of these rodents on ships. Despite the wide distribution of Seoul virus, only mild or moderate HFRS occurs in Asia, and human disease has been difficult to identify in many areas of the world. Most cases of HFRS occur in rural residents or vacationers; the exception is Seoul virus infection, which may be acquired in an urban or rural setting or from contaminated laboratory-rat colonies. Classic Hantaan virus infection in Korea and in rural China is most common in the spring and fall and is related to rodent density and agricultural practices. Human infection is acquired primarily through aerosols of rodent urine, although virus is also present in rodent saliva and feces. Patients with HFRS are not infectious.

Severe cases of HFRS evolve in four identifiable stages. The *febrile stage* lasts 3 or 4 days and is identified by the abrupt onset of fever, headache, severe myalgia, thirst, anorexia, and often nausea and vomiting. Photophobia, retroorbital pain, and pain on ocular movement are common, and the vision may become blurred with ciliary body inflammation. Flushing over the face, the V area of the neck, and the back is characteristic, as are pharyngeal injection, periorbital edema, and conjunctival suffusion. Petechiae often develop in areas of pressure, the conjunctivae, and the axillae. Back pain and tenderness to percussion at the costovertebral angle reflect massive retroperitoneal edema. Laboratory evidence of mild to moderate DIC is present. Other laboratory findings of HFRS include proteinuria and active urinary sediment. The *hypotensive stage* lasts from a few hours to 48 h and begins with falling blood pressure and sometimes shock. The relative bradycardia typical of the febrile phase is replaced by tachycardia. Kinin activation is marked. The rising hematocrit reflects increasing vascular leakage. Leukocytosis with a left shift develops, and thrombocytopenia continues. Atypical lymphocytes—which in fact are activated CD8+ and, to a lesser extent, CD4+ T cells—circulate. Proteinuria is marked, and the urine's specific gravity falls to 1.010. Renal circulation is congested and compromised from local and systemic circulatory changes resulting in necrosis of tubules, particularly at the corticomedullary junction, and oliguria. During the *oliguric stage*, hemorrhagic tendencies continue, probably in large part because of uremic bleeding defects. Oliguria persists for 3–10 days before the return of renal function marks the onset of the *polyuric stage* (diuresis and hyposthenuria), which carries the danger of dehydration and electrolyte abnormalities.

Mild cases of HFRS may be much less stereotypical. The presentation may include only fever, gastrointestinal abnormalities, and transient oliguria followed by hyposthenuria. Infections with Puumala virus, the most common cause of HFRS in Europe (*nephropathia epidemica*), result in a much-attenuated picture but the same general presentation. Bleeding manifestations are found in only 10% of patients, hypotension rather than shock is usually documented, and oliguria is present in only about half of patients. The dominant features may be fever, abdominal pain, proteinuria, mild oliguria, and sometimes blurred vision or glaucoma followed by polyuria and hyposthenuria in recovery. The lethality rate is <1%.

HFRS should be suspected in patients with rural exposure in an endemic area. Prompt recognition of the disease permits rapid hospitalization and expectant management of shock and renal failure. Useful clinical laboratory parameters include leukocytosis, which may be leukemoid and is associated with a left shift; thrombocytopenia; and proteinuria. HFRS is readily diagnosed by an IgM capture ELISA that is positive at admission or within 24–48 h thereafter. The isolation of hantaviruses is difficult, but RT-PCR of a blood clot collected early in the clinical course or of tissues obtained postmortem should give positive results. Such testing is usually undertaken if definitive identification of the infecting virus is required.

Mainstays of therapy are management of shock, reliance on vasopressors, modest crystalloid infusion, IV human serum albumin administration, and treatment of renal failure with prompt dialysis to prevent overhydration that may result in pulmonary edema and to control hypertension that increases the possibility of intracranial hemorrhage. Use of IV ribavirin has reduced lethality and morbidity in severe cases, provided treatment is begun within the first 4 days of illness. Lethality may be as high as 15% but with proper therapy should be <5%. Sequelae have not been definitively established.

RIFT VALLEY FEVER The natural range of Rift Valley fever virus was previously confined to sub-Saharan Africa, with circulation of the virus markedly enhanced by substantial rainfall. The El Niño Southern Oscillation phenomenon of 1997 facilitated subsequent spread of Rift

Valley fever to the Arabian Peninsula, with epidemic disease in 2000. The virus has also been found in Madagascar and has been introduced into Egypt, where it caused major epidemics in 1977–1979, 1993, and thereafter. Rift Valley fever virus is maintained in nature by transovarial transmission in floodwater *Aedes* mosquitoes and presumably also has a vertebrate amplifier. Increased transmission during particularly heavy rains leads to epizootics characterized by high-level viremia in cattle, goats, or sheep. Numerous types of mosquitoes then feed on these animals and become infected, thereby increasing the possibility of human infections. Remote sensing via satellite can detect the ecologic changes associated with high rainfall that predict the likelihood of Rift Valley fever virus transmission. High-resolution satellites can also detect the special depressions in floodwaters from which the mosquitoes emerge. In addition, the virus can be transmitted by contact with blood or aerosols from domestic animals. Transmission risk is therefore high during birthing, and both abortuses and placentas need to be handled with caution. Slaughtered animals are not infectious because anaerobic glycolysis in postmortem tissues results in an acidic environment that rapidly inactivates bunyaviruses. Neither person-to-person nor nosocomial transmission of Rift Valley fever has been documented.

Rift Valley fever virus is unusual in that it causes several clinical syndromes. Most infections are manifested as the fever–myalgia syndrome. A small proportion of infections result in VHF with especially prominent liver involvement. Renal failure and DIC are also common features. Perhaps 10% of otherwise mild infections lead to retinal vasculitis, and some patients have permanently impaired vision. Funduscopic examination reveals edema, hemorrhages, and infarction of the retina as well as optic nerve degeneration. In a small proportion of patients (<1 in 200), retinal vasculitis is followed by viral encephalitis.

No proven therapy exists for Rift Valley fever. Both retinal disease and encephalitis occur after the acute febrile syndrome has resolved and serum neutralizing antibody has developed—events suggesting that only supportive care need be given. Epidemic disease is best prevented by vaccination of livestock. The ability of this virus to propagate after introduction into Egypt suggests that other potentially receptive areas, including the United States, should develop response plans. Rift Valley fever, like Venezuelan equine encephalitis, is likely to be controlled only with adequate stocks of an effective live attenuated vaccine, but such global stocks are unavailable. A formalin-inactivated vaccine confers immunity in humans, but quantities are limited and three injections are required; this vaccine is recommended for potentially exposed laboratory workers and for veterinarians working in sub-Saharan Africa. A new live attenuated vaccine, MP-12, is being tested in humans and may soon become available for general use. The vaccine is safe and licensed for use in sheep and cattle.

SEVERE FEVER WITH THROMBOCYTOPENIA SYNDROME This is a recently described tick-borne disease caused by a previously unknown and still-unclassified phlebovirus. Numerous human infections have been reported during the past few years from China, and several cases have also been detected in Japan and South Korea. The clinical presentation ranges from mild nonspecific fever to severe VHF with a high (>12%) lethality rate.

Flaviviruses The most important flaviviruses that cause VHF are the mosquito-borne dengue viruses 1–4 and yellow fever viruses. These viruses are widely distributed and cause tens to hundreds of thousands of infections each year. Kyasanur Forest disease virus and Omsk hemorrhagic fever virus are geographically very restricted but important tick-borne flaviviruses that cause VHF, sometimes with subsequent viral encephalitis. Tick-borne encephalitis virus has caused VHF in a few patients. There is currently no therapy for these VHFs, but an inactivated vaccine has been used in India to prevent Kyasanur Forest disease.

SEVERE DENGUE Several weeks after convalescence from infection with dengue virus 1, 2, 3, or 4, the transient protection conferred by that infection against reinfection with a heterotypic dengue virus usually wanes. Heterotypic reinfection may result in classic dengue or, less commonly, in severe dengue. In the past 20 years, *A. aegypti* has progressively reinvaded Latin America and other areas, and frequent travel by infected individuals has introduced multiple variants of dengue viruses 1–4 from many geographic areas. Thus the pattern of hyperendemic transmission of multiple dengue virus serotypes established in the Americas and the Caribbean has led to the emergence of severe dengue as a major problem. Among the millions of dengue virus 1–4 infections, ~500,000 cases of severe dengue occur annually, with a lethality rate of ~2.5%. The induction of vascular permeability and shock depends on multiple factors, such as the presence or absence of enhancing and nonneutralizing antibodies, age (susceptibility to severe dengue drops considerably after 12 years of age), sex (females are more often affected than males), race (whites are more often affected than blacks), nutritional status (malnutrition is protective), or sequence of infections (e.g., dengue virus 1 infection followed by dengue virus 2 infection seems to be more dangerous than dengue virus 4 infection followed by dengue virus 2 infection). In addition, considerable heterogeneity exists among each dengue virus population. For instance, Southeast Asian dengue virus 2 variants have more potential to cause severe dengue than do other variants.

Severe dengue is identified by the detection of bleeding tendencies (tourniquet test, petechiae) or overt bleeding in the absence of underlying causes, such as preexisting gastrointestinal lesions. Shock may result from increased vascular permeability. In milder cases of severe dengue, restlessness, lethargy, thrombocytopenia (<100,000/μL), and hemoconcentration are detected 2–5 days after the onset of typical dengue, usually at the time of defervescence. The maculopapular rash that often develops in dengue may also appear in severe dengue. In more severe cases, frank shock is apparent, with low pulse pressure, cyanosis, hepatomegaly, pleural effusions, and ascites; in some patients, severe ecchymoses and gastrointestinal bleeding develop. The period of shock lasts only 1 or 2 days.

A virologic diagnosis of severe dengue can be made by the usual means. However, multiple flavivirus infections result in broad immune responses to several members of the genus, and this situation may result in a lack of virus specificity of the IgM and IgG immune responses. A secondary antibody response can be sought with tests against several flavivirus antigens to demonstrate the characteristic wide spectrum of reactivity.

Most patients with shock respond promptly to close monitoring, oxygen administration, and infusion of crystalloid or—in severe cases—colloid. The case–fatality rates reported vary greatly with case ascertainment and quality of treatment; however, most patients with severe dengue respond well to supportive therapy, and the overall lethality rate at an experienced center in the tropics is probably as low as 1%.

The key to control of both dengue and severe dengue is the control of *A. aegypti*, which also reduces the risk of urban yellow fever and chikungunya virus circulation. Control efforts have been handicapped by the presence of nondegradable tires and long-lived plastic containers in trash repositories (perfect mosquito breeding grounds when filled with water during rainfall) and by insecticide resistance. Urban poverty and an inability of the public health community to mobilize the populace to respond to the need to eliminate mosquito breeding sites are also factors in lack of mosquito control. A tetravalent live attenuated dengue vaccine based on the attenuated yellow fever virus 17D platform is currently being evaluated in phase 3 clinical trials in Latin America, Asia, and Australia. At least two other live attenuated candidate vaccines based on modified recombinant dengue viruses have been evaluated in phase 1 clinical studies, but the results have not been promising.

YELLOW FEVER Yellow fever virus had caused major epidemics in Africa and Europe before its transmission by *A. aegypti* mosquitoes was discovered in 1900. Urban yellow fever became established in the New World as a result of colonization with *A. aegypti*, originally an African mosquito. Subsequently, different types of mosquitoes and nonhuman primates were found to maintain yellow fever virus in Africa and also in Central and South American jungles. Transmission to humans is incidental, occurring via bites from mosquitoes that have fed on viremic monkeys. After the identification of *A. aegypti* mosquitoes as vectors of yellow fever, containment strategies were aimed at increased mosquito control. Today, urban yellow fever transmission occurs only in some African cities, but the threat exists in the great cities of South America, where reinfestation by *A. aegypti* has taken place and dengue virus 1–4 transmission by the same mosquito is common. Despite the existence of a highly effective and safe vaccine, several hundred jungle yellow fever cases occur annually in South America, and thousands of jungle and urban cases occur each year in Africa (29,000–60,000 estimated for 2013).

Yellow fever is a typical VHF accompanied by prominent hepatic necrosis. A period of viremia, typically lasting 3 or 4 days, is followed by a period of "intoxication." During the latter phase in severe cases, characteristic jaundice, hemorrhages, black vomit, anuria, and terminal delirium occur, perhaps related in part to extensive hepatic involvement. Blood leukocyte counts may be normal or reduced and are often high in terminal stages. Albuminuria is usually noted and may be marked. As renal function fails in terminal or severe cases, the concentration of blood urea nitrogen rises proportionately. Abnormalities detected in liver function tests range from modest elevations of AST concentrations in mild cases to severe derangement.

Urban yellow fever can be prevented by the control of *A. aegypti*. The continuing sylvatic cycles require vaccination of all visitors to areas of potential transmission with live attenuated variant 17D vaccine virus, which cannot be transmitted by mosquitoes. With few exceptions, reactions to the vaccine are minimal; immunity is provided within 10 days and lasts for at least 25–35 years. An egg allergy mandates caution in vaccine administration. Although there are no documented harmful effects of the vaccine on fetuses, pregnant women should be immunized only if they are definitely at risk of exposure to yellow fever virus. Because vaccination has been associated with several cases of encephalitis in children <6 months of age, it is contraindicated in this age group, nor is it recommended for infants 6–8 months of age unless the risk of exposure is very high. Rare, serious, multisystemic adverse reactions (occasionally fatal) have been reported, particularly affecting the elderly, and risk-to-benefit should be weighed prior to vaccine administration to individuals ≥60 years of age. Nevertheless, the number of deaths of unvaccinated travelers with yellow fever exceeds the number of deaths from vaccination, and a liberal vaccination policy for travelers to involved areas should be pursued. Timely information on changes in yellow fever distribution and yellow fever vaccine requirements can be obtained from the U.S. Centers for Disease Control and Prevention (*http://www.cdc.gov/vaccines/vpd-vac/yf/default.htm*).

234 Ebolavirus and Marburgvirus Infections

Jens H. Kuhn

Several viruses of the family Filoviridae cause severe and frequently fatal viral hemorrhagic fevers in humans. Introduction of filoviruses into human populations is an extremely rare event that most likely occurs by direct or indirect contact with healthy mammalian filovirus hosts or by contact with infected, sick, or deceased nonhuman primates. Filoviruses are highly infectious but not very contagious. Natural human-to-human transmission takes place through direct person-to-person (usually skin-to-skin) contact or exposure to infected bodily fluids and tissues; there is no evidence of such transmission by aerosol or respiratory droplets. Infections progress rapidly from influenza-like to hemorrhagic manifestations and typically culminate in multiple-organ dysfunction syndrome and shock. Treatment of filovirus infections is of necessity entirely supportive because no specific efficacious antiviral agents or vaccines are yet available.

Filoviruses are categorized as World Health Organization (WHO) Risk Group 4 Pathogens. Consequently, all work with material suspected of containing filoviruses should be conducted only in maximal containment (biosafety level 4) laboratories. Experienced personnel handling these viruses must wear appropriate personal protective gear (see "Prevention," below) and follow rigorous standard operating procedures. The proper authorities and WHO reference laboratories should be contacted immediately when filovirus infections are suspected.

ETIOLOGY

The family Filoviridae includes three genera: *Cuevavirus*, *Ebolavirus*, and *Marburgvirus* (Table 234-1 and Fig. 234-1). The available data suggest that the only known cuevavirus, Lloviu virus (LLOV), and one ebolavirus, Reston virus (RESTV), are not pathogenic for humans. The remaining four ebolaviruses—Bundibugyo virus (BDBV), Ebola virus (EBOV), Sudan virus (SUDV), and Taï Forest virus (TAFV)—cause Ebola virus disease (EVD; International Classification of Disease, Tenth Revision [ICD-10], code A98.4). The two marburgviruses, Marburg virus (MARV) and Ravn virus (RAVV), are the etiologic agents of Marburg virus disease (MVD; ICD-10 code A98.3).

Filoviruses have linear, nonsegmented, single-stranded, negative-sense RNA genomes that are ~19 kb in length. These genomes contain six or seven genes that encode the following seven structural proteins: nucleoprotein, polymerase cofactor (VP35), matrix protein (VP40), glycoprotein ($GP_{1,2}$), transcriptional cofactor (VP30), secondary matrix protein (VP24), and RNA-dependent RNA polymerase (L protein). Cuevaviruses and ebolaviruses, but not marburgviruses, also encode three nonstructural proteins of unknown function (sGP, ssGP, and Δ-peptide). Filovirions are unique among human virus particles in that they are predominantly pleomorphic filaments but also assume torus- or 6-like shapes (width, ~80 nm; average length, ≥790 nm). These enveloped virions contain helical ribonucleocapsids and are covered with $GP_{1,2}$ spikes (Fig. 234-2).

TABLE 234-1 FILOVIRUS TAXONOMY

Current Taxonomy and Nomenclature	Previous Taxonomy and Nomenclature
Order Mononegavirales	Order Mononegavirales
Family Filoviridae	Family Filoviridae
Genus *Marburgvirus*	Genus *Marburgvirus*
Species *Marburg marburgvirus*	Species *Lake Victoria marburgvirus*
Virus 1: Marburg virus (MARV)	Virus: Lake Victoria marburgvirus (MARV)
Virus 2: Ravn virus (RAVV)	
Genus *Ebolavirus*	Genus *Ebolavirus*
Species *Taï Forest ebolavirus*	Species *Cote d'Ivoire ebolavirus* [sic[a]]
Virus: Taï Forest virus (TAFV)	Virus: Cote d'Ivoire ebolavirus [sic] (CIEBOV)
Species *Reston ebolavirus*	Species *Reston ebolavirus*
Virus: Reston virus (RESTV)	Virus: Reston ebolavirus (REBOV)
Species *Sudan ebolavirus*	Species *Sudan ebolavirus*
Virus: Sudan virus (SUDV)	Virus: Sudan ebolavirus (SEBOV)
Species *Zaire ebolavirus*	Species *Zaire ebolavirus*
Virus: Ebola virus (EBOV)	Virus: Zaire ebolavirus (ZEBOV)
Species *Bundibugyo ebolavirus*	
Virus: Bundibugyo virus (BDBV)	
Genus *Cuevavirus*	
Species *Lloviu cuevavirus*	
Virus: Lloviu virus (LLOV)	

[a]The correct spelling of the country for which this virus is named is Côte d'Ivoire. The lack of a circumflex in "Cote" in the virus designation produced a false country name. This fact is denoted by "[sic]."

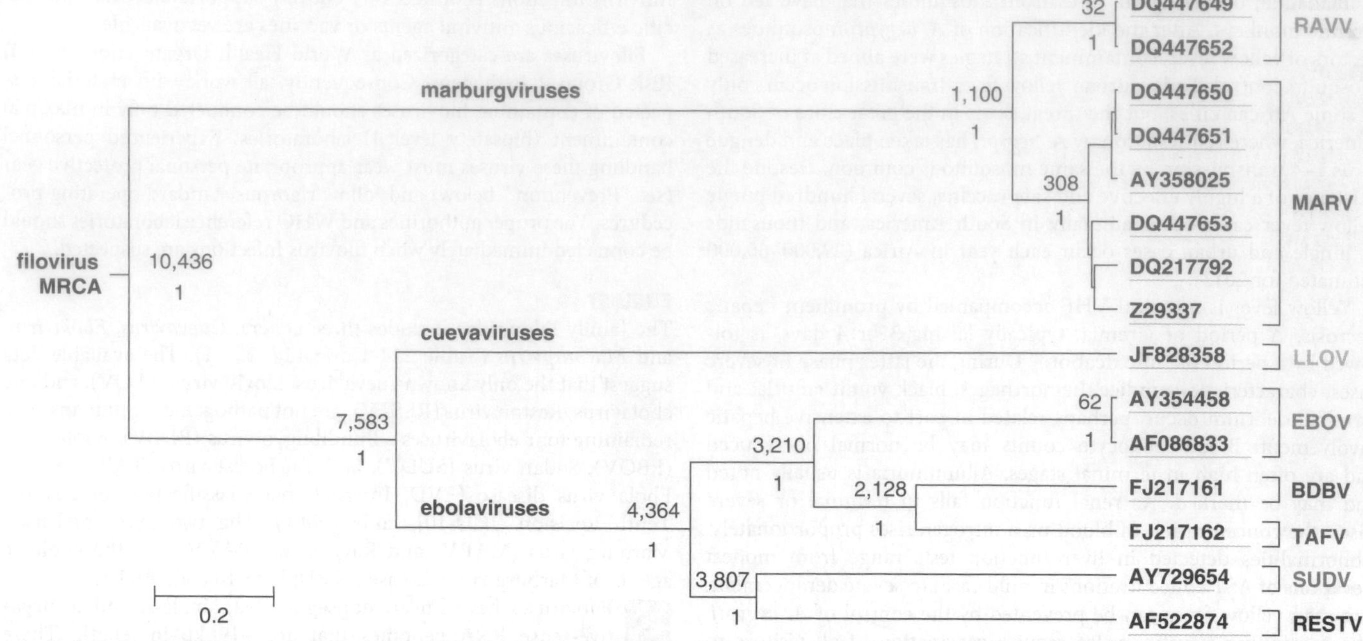

FIGURE 234-1 Filovirus phylogeny/evolution. Bayesian coalescent analysis of representative variants of all known filovirus clades (represented by underlined GenBank accession numbers). The maximal clade credibility tree is shown with the most recent common ancestor (MRCA) at each node. Posterior probability values are shown beneath MRCA estimates in years. Scale is in substitutions/site based on an analysis performed by Dr. Serena Carroll, Centers for Disease Control and Prevention. BDBV, Bundibugyo virus; EBOV, Ebola virus; LLOV, Lloviu virus; MARV, Marburg virus; RAVV, Ravn virus; RESTV, Reston virus; SUDV, Sudan virus; TAFV, Taï Forest virus.

EPIDEMIOLOGY

To date (i.e., as of December 3, 2014), a total of 20,012 human filovirus infections and 8058 fatalities have been recorded (Fig. 234-3). These numbers emphasize both the high degree of lethality (number of deaths per number of sick people; 40.3%) and the overall low mortality (impact on healthy population) of filovirus infections. At least for the moment, natural filovirus infections do not pose a global threat. Filoviruses pathogenic for humans appear to be exclusively endemic to Equatorial Africa, although this distribution may change if natural or artificial environmental alterations lead to filovirus host migration and increased contacts between nonhuman hosts and humans (Fig. 234-4). The majority of recorded EVD and MVD outbreaks can be traced back to single index cases who transmitted the infection to others. These chains of contacts suggest that only around 50 natural host-to-human spillover events have occurred since the discovery of filoviruses in 1967. Outbreak frequency, case numbers, and overall lethality probably depend on the particular etiologic agent, the geographic location and socioeconomic conditions of the affected country, and local customs. In particular, the availability of personal protective gear and reusable medical equipment, such as syringes and needles, has affected overall case numbers in the past, and outbreaks have been contained when local burial practices, such as ritual washing, have been either prevented or altered by the use of gloves. The incidence of EVD and MVD may have increased over the past two decades (Figs. 234-3 and 234-4), but researchers debate whether the observed change is due to increased filovirus activity, more frequent contact between filovirus hosts and humans, or continuous improvement in surveillance capabilities.

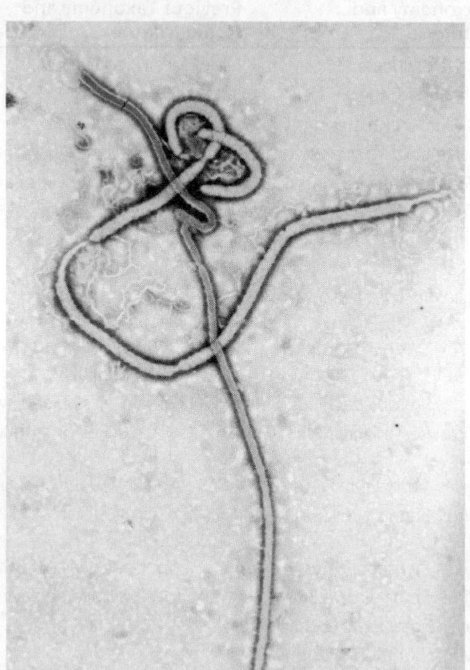

FIGURE 234-2 Ebola virus particle: the first transmission electron micrograph of an Ebola virion in a culture of Vero cells inoculated with a blood sample from a patient from the 1976 Zaire outbreak of Ebola virus disease. Shown is the typical and unique filamentous and pleomorphic structure of filovirions. *(PHIL ID#1833, taken by Dr. Fredrick A. Murphy, Centers for Disease Control and Prevention.)*

EVD and MVD outbreaks are associated with distinct meteorologic and geographic conditions and are probably associated with distinct hosts or reservoirs. The four ebolaviruses that cause disease in humans are endemic in humid rainforests. EVD outbreaks have often been linked to hunting or contact with bush meat (i.e., meat from apes, other nonhuman primates, duikers, or bush pigs) in forests. Ecologic studies indicate that EBOV may be the etiologic agent of extensive and frequently fatal epizootics among wild chimpanzee and gorilla populations. However, replicating isolates of ebolaviruses from wild nonhuman primates have thus far been obtained only in the case of TAFV, which was isolated from a succumbed western chimpanzee in Côte d'Ivoire in 1994. The marburgviruses MARV and RAVV, on the other hand, seem to infect hosts inhabiting arid woodlands. MVD outbreaks have almost always been epidemiologically linked to visits to or work in natural or artificial caves or mines. A pteropid (fruit) bat, the cave-dwelling Egyptian rousette (*Rousettus aegyptiacus*), serves as a natural and subclinically infected reservoir for both MARV and RAVV. Although bats are suspected to be the hosts for ebolaviruses as

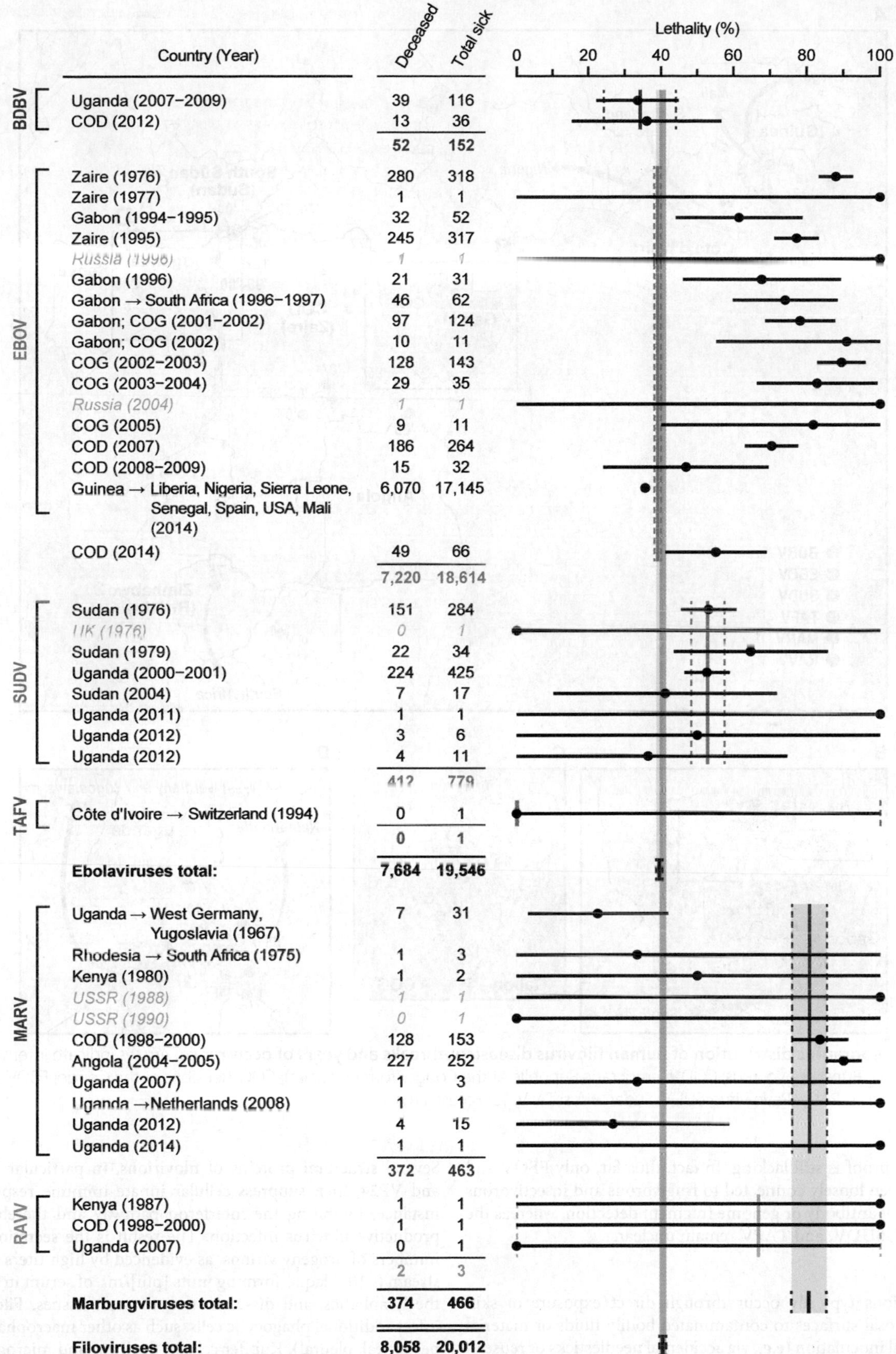

Country (Year)
Deceased
Total sick
Lethality (%)
0
20
40
60
80
100
BDBV
Uganda (2007–2009) 39 116
COD (2012) 13 36
52 152
EBOV
Zaire (1976) 280 318
Zaire (1977) 1 1
Gabon (1994–1995) 32 52
Zaire (1995) 245 317
Russia (1996) 1 1
Gabon (1996) 21 31
Gabon → South Africa (1996–1997) 46 62
Gabon; COG (2001–2002) 97 124
Gabon; COG (2002) 10 11
COG (2002–2003) 128 143
COG (2003–2004) 29 35
Russia (2004) 1 1
COG (2005) 9 11
COD (2007) 186 264
COD (2008–2009) 15 32
Guinea → Liberia, Nigeria, Sierra Leone, Senegal, Spain, USA, Mali (2014) 6,070 17,145
COD (2014) 49 66
7,220 18,614
SUDV
Sudan (1976) 151 284
UK (1976) 0 1
Sudan (1979) 22 34
Uganda (2000–2001) 224 425
Sudan (2004) 7 17
Uganda (2011) 1 1
Uganda (2012) 3 6
Uganda (2012) 4 11
412 779
TAFV
Côte d'Ivoire → Switzerland (1994) 0 1
0 1
Ebolaviruses total: 7,684 19,546
MARV
Uganda → West Germany, Yugoslavia (1967) 7 31
Rhodesia → South Africa (1975) 1 3
Kenya (1980) 1 2
USSR (1988) 1 1
USSR (1990) 0 1
COD (1998–2000) 128 153
Angola (2004–2005) 227 252
Uganda (2007) 1 3
Uganda →Netherlands (2008) 1 1
Uganda (2012) 4 15
Uganda (2014) 1 1
372 463
RAVV
Kenya (1987) 1 1
COD (1998–2000) 1 1
Uganda (2007) 0 1
2 3
Marburgviruses total: 374 466
Filoviruses total: 8,058 20,012

FIGURE 234-3 Characteristics of outbreaks of human filovirus disease. Six of eight known filoviruses have caused disease in humans in the past. Outbreaks are listed by virus in chronological order. Laboratory infections are shaded gray and italicized. *Arrows* indicate international case exportation. Total number of cases and total number of lethal cases are summarized in the middle column (2014 EBOV infections as of December 3). The lethality/case–fatality rate (*black dots*) for each outbreak is plotted on a 0–100% scale along with 99% confidence intervals (*black horizontal lines*). The overall case–fatality rate for disease caused by a particular virus is delineated by *vertical bold-colored lines*, with *vertical bold-colored dashed lines* indicating the corresponding 99% confidence intervals; the overall case–fatality rate for all ebolavirus infections, all marburgvirus infections, and all filovirus infections are shown by *vertical gray bars*. BDBV, Bundibugyo virus; COD, Democratic Republic of the Congo (formerly Zaire); COG, Republic of the Congo; EBOV, Ebola virus; MARV, Marburg virus; RAVV, Ravn virus; SUDV, Sudan virus; TAFV, Taï Forest virus; UK, United Kingdom; USSR, Union of Soviet Socialist Republics (today Russia).

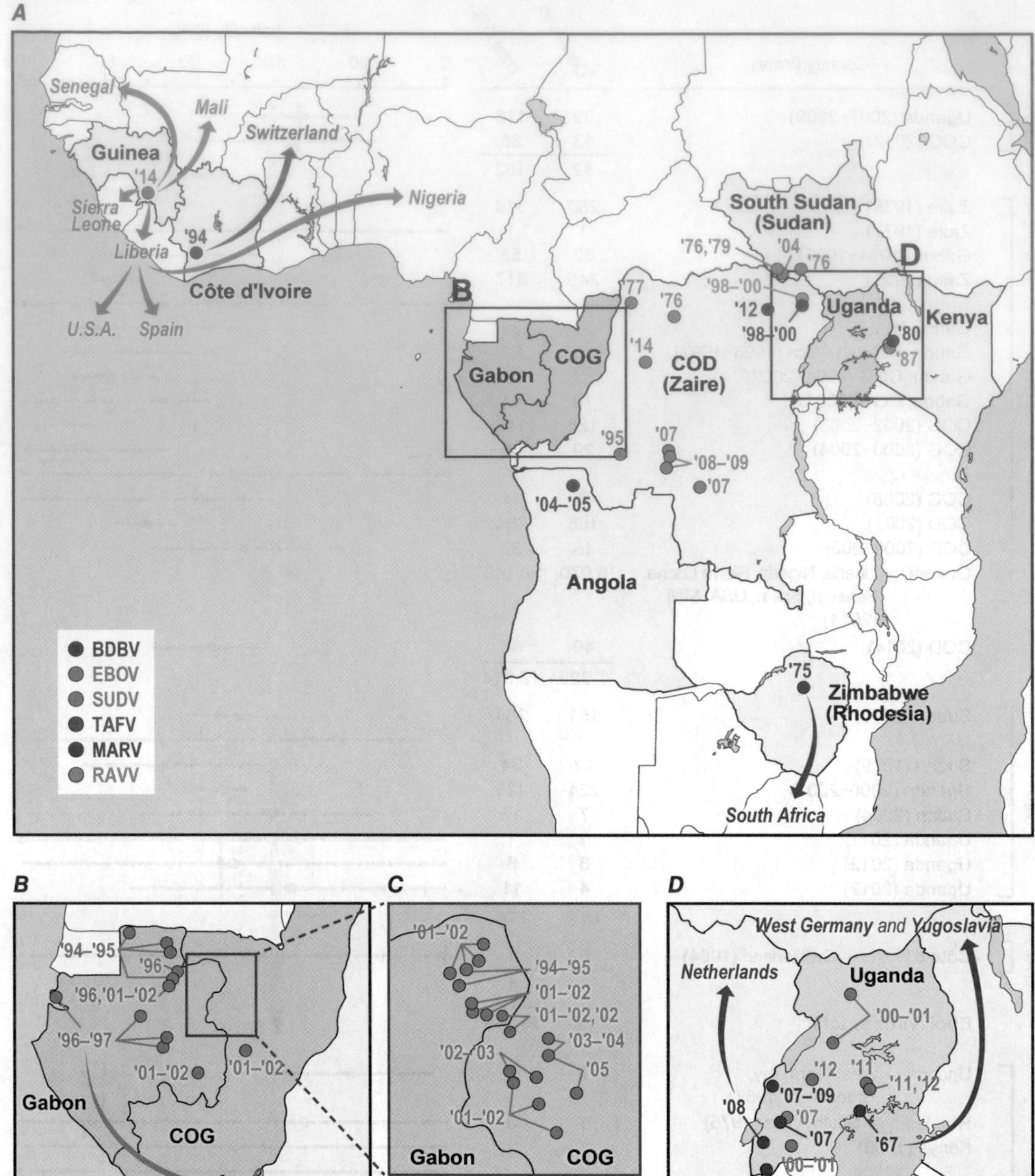

FIGURE 234-4 Geographic distribution of human filovirus disease outbreaks and years of occurrence. *Arrows* indicate international case exportation. BDBV, Bundibugyo virus; COD, Democratic Republic of the Congo (formerly Zaire); COG, Republic of the Congo; EBOV, Ebola virus; MARV, Marburg virus; RAVV, Ravn virus; SUDV, Sudan virus; TAFV, Taï Forest virus.

well, definitive proof is still lacking. In fact, thus far, only EBOV and RESTV have been loosely connected to frugivorous and insectivorous bats by means of antibody or genome fragment detection, whereas the hosts of BDBV, SUDV, and TAFV remain unclear.

PATHOGENESIS

Human infections typically occur through direct exposure of skin lesions or mucosal surfaces to contaminated bodily fluids or material or by parenteral inoculation (e.g., via accidental needlesticks or reuse of needles in poorly equipped hospitals). Numerous studies, both in vitro and in vivo (in several animal models of human disease), have shed light on key pathogenetic events that evolve subsequent to filovirion exposure. The $GP_{1,2}$ spikes on the surface of filovirions determine their cell and tissue tropism by engaging yet-unidentified cell-surface molecules and the intracellular receptor Niemann-Pick C1.

One of the pathogenetic hallmarks of filovirus infection is a pronounced suppression of the immune system. The first targets of filovirions are local macrophages, monocytes, and dendritic cells. Several structural proteins of filovirions, in particular VP35, VP40, and VP24, then suppress cellular innate immune responses by, for instance, inhibiting the interferon pathway and thereby enabling a productive filovirus infection. The result is the secretion of copious numbers of progeny virions, as evidenced by high titers in the bloodstream (>10^6 plaque-forming units [pfu]/mL of serum in humans) and the lymphatics, and dissemination to most tissues. Filovirions then infect additional phagocytic cells, such as other macrophages (alveolar, peritoneal, pleural), Kupffer cells in the liver, and microglia, as well as other targets, such as adrenal cortical cells, fibroblasts, hepatocytes, endothelial cells, and a variety of epithelial cells. Infection leads to the secretion of soluble signaling molecules (varying with the cell type) that most likely are crucial factors in immune response modulation and development of multiorgan dysfunction syndrome. For instance, infected macrophages react by secreting proinflammatory cytokines, a response that leads to further recruitment of macrophages to the site of infection. In contrast, infected dendritic cells are not activated to secrete cytokines, and expression of major histocompatibility class II antigens is partially suppressed. Immunosuppression occurs in part by massive lymphoid depletion in lymph nodes, spleen, and thymus in the absence of reactive inflammatory cellular responses. Results from animal studies suggest that depletion is a direct consequence of considerable bystander apoptosis of lymphocytes; this explanation would also account for the severe lymphopenia that develops in patients. The consequence of these events is not only florid filovirus dissemination but also a proclivity of the patient for secondary bacterial and fungal infections.

Other pathogenetic hallmarks of filovirus infections are a severe disturbance of the clotting system and the impairment of vascular integrity. Disseminated intravascular coagulation is the cause of the severe imbalance in the clotting system of filovirus-infected patients. Thrombocytopenia, increased concentrations of tissue factor, consumption of clotting factors, increased concentrations of fibrin degradation products (D-dimers), and declining concentrations of protein C are typical features of infection. Consequently, the occlusion of small vessels by widely distributed microthrombi leads to extensive necroses/hypoxic infarcts in target tissues (particularly the gonads, kidneys, liver, and spleen) in the absence of marked inflammatory responses. In addition, petechiae, ecchymoses, extensive visceral effusions, and other hemorrhagic signs are observed in internal organs, mucous membranes, and skin. Actual severe blood loss, however, is a rare event. Aberrance in cytokines or other factors such as nitric oxide and direct infection and activation of endothelial cells most likely are responsible for upregulated permeability of the endothelia of blood vessels. This upregulation leads to fluid redistribution (*third spacing*); interstitial and myocardial edema and hypovolemic shock are common developments. Clinical improvement is rare and is usually characterized by falling viral titers during the development of a virus-specific immune response.

CLINICAL MANIFESTATIONS

MVD and EVD cannot be differentiated by mere observation of clinical manifestations. The incidence of clinical signs does not differ significantly among infections caused by disparate filoviruses (Table 234-2). The incubation period ranges from 3 to 25 days, after which infected people develop a biphasic syndrome with a 1- to 2-day

TABLE 234-2 DISTRIBUTION OF CLINICAL SIGNS/SYMPTOMS OF FILOVIRUS-INFECTED PATIENTS IN THREE REPRESENTATIVE OUTBREAKS

	Frequency (%) Among Survivors			Frequency (%) Among Fatal Cases		
Sign/Symptom	**BDBV**	**EBOV**	**MARV**	**BDBV**	**EBOV**	**MARV**
Abdominal pain	88	68	59	93	62	57
Abortion	NR	5	NR	NR	2	NR
Anorexia	83	47	77	80	43	72
Anuria	NR	0	NR	NR	7	NR
Arthralgia or myalgia	83	79	55	86	50	55
Asthenia	NR	95	NR	NR	85	NR
Bleeding from puncture sites	NR	5	0	NR	8	7
Bleeding from the gums	NR	0	23	NR	15	36
Bleeding from any site	NR	NR	59	NR	NR	71
Bloody stools	NR	5	NR	NR	7	NR
Chest pain	NR	5	18	NR	10	4
Conjunctival injection	NR	47	14	NR	42	42
Convulsions	NR	0	NR	NR	2	NR
Cough	NR	26	9	NR	7	5
Diarrhea	92	84	59	87	86	56
Difficulty breathing	26	NR	36	57	NR	58
Dysesthesia	NR	5	NR	NR	0	NR
Epistaxis	NR	0	18	NR	2	34
Fever	100	95	100	100	93	92
Headaches	84	74	73	93	52	79
Hearing loss	NR	11	NR	NR	5	NR
Hematemesis	NR	0	68	NR	13	76
Hematoma	NR	0	0	NR	2	3
Hematuria	NR	16	NR	NR	7	NR
Hemoptysis	NR	11	9	NR	0	4
Hepatomegaly (without jaundice)	NR	5	NR	NR	2	NR
Hiccups	17	5	18	40	17	44
Lumbar pain	NR	26	5	NR	12	8
Maculopapular rash	35	16	NR	33	14	NR
Malaise or fatigue	96	NR	86	100	NR	83
Melena	NR	16	41	NR	8	58
Nausea and vomiting	92	68	77	87	73	76
Petechiae	NR	0	9	NR	8	7
Sore throat, odynophagia, or dysphagia	43	58	43	60	56	43
Splenomegaly	NR	5	NR	NR	2	NR
Tachypnea	NR	0	NR	NR	31	NR
Tinnitus	NR	11	NR	NR	1	NR

Abbreviations: BDBV, Bundibugyo virus; EBOV, Ebola virus; MARV, Marburg virus; NR, not reported.

relative remission separating the two phases. The first phase (disease onset until around day 5–7) resembles influenza and is characterized by sudden onset of fever and chills, severe headaches, cough, myalgia, pharyngitis, arthralgia of the larger joints, development of a maculopapular rash, and other signs/symptoms (Table 234-2). The second phase (approximately 5–7 days after disease onset and thereafter) involves the gastrointestinal tract (abdominal pain with vomiting and/or diarrhea), respiratory tract (chest pain, cough), vascular system (postural hypotension, edema), and central nervous system (confusion, coma, headache). Hemorrhagic manifestations such as subconjunctival injection, nosebleeds, hematemesis, hematuria, and melena are typical (Table 234-2).

Typical laboratory findings are leukopenia (with cell counts as low as 1000/μL) with a left shift prior to leukocytosis, thrombocytopenia (with counts as low as 50,000/μL), increased concentrations of liver and pancreatic enzymes (aspartate aminotransferase > alanine aminotransferase, γ-glutamyltransferase, serum amylase), hypokalemia, hypoproteinemia, increased creatinine and urea concentrations with proteinuria, and prolonged prothrombin and partial thromboplastin times.

Patients usually succumb to disease 4–14 days after infection. Patients who survive experience prolonged and sometimes incapacitating sequelae such as arthralgia, asthenia, iridocyclitis, hearing loss, myalgia, orchitis, parotitis, psychosis, recurrent hepatitis, transverse myelitis, or uveitis. Temporary hair loss and desquamation of skin areas previously affected by a typical maculopapular rash are visible consequences of the disease. Rarely, filoviruses can persist in the liver, eyes, or testicles of survivors and may cause recurrent disease months after convalescence.

DIAGNOSIS

Filovirus infections cannot be diagnosed on the basis of clinical presentation alone. Numerous diseases typical for Equatorial Africa need to be considered in the differential diagnosis of a febrile patient. Almost all of these diseases occur at a much higher incidence than filovirus infections and are therefore the more likely candidates during differential diagnostic deliberations. The most important of the infectious diseases that closely mimic EVD and MVD are falciparum malaria and typhoid fever; also important are enterohemorrhagic *Escherichia coli* enteritis, gram-negative septicemia (including shigellosis), meningococcal septicemia, rickettsial infections, fulminant viral hepatitis, leptospirosis, measles, and all other viral hemorrhagic fevers (in particular, yellow fever). Other ailments, such as venomous snakebites, warfarin intoxication, and the many transient or inherited platelet and vascular disorders, also must be considered. Visits to caves or mines and direct contact with bats, nonhuman primates (especially apes), or bush meat should raise suspicion of filovirus infection, as should admission to or treatment in rural hospitals or direct contact with severely ill local residents.

If EVD or MVD is suspected on the basis of epidemiologic history, exposure history, and/or clinical manifestations, infectious disease specialists and the proper public health authorities, including the WHO, should be notified immediately. Laboratory diagnosis of EVD and MVD is relatively straightforward but requires maximal containment (biosafety level 4), which usually is not available in filovirus-endemic countries, or the involvement of on-site personnel trained in the use of diagnostic assays adapted for field use. Consequently, diagnostic samples should be collected with great caution and with use of proper personal protective equipment and strict barrier nursing techniques. With adherence to established biosafety precautionary measures, samples should be sent in suitable transport media to national or international WHO reference laboratories. Acute-phase blood/serum is the preferred diagnostic specimen because it usually contains high titers of filovirions and filovirion-specific antibodies.

The current methods of choice for the diagnosis of filovirus infection are reverse-transcription polymerase chain reaction (detection limit, 1000–2000 virus genome copies per milliliter of serum) and antigen capture enzyme-linked immunosorbent assay (ELISA) for the detection of filovirus genomes and filovirion components, respectively. Direct IgM and IgG or IgM capture ELISA is used for the detection of filovirion-targeting antibodies from patients in later stages of disease—i.e., those who have been able to mount a detectable immune response, including survivors. All these assays can be conducted on samples treated with guanidinium isothiocyanate (for polymerase chain reaction) or cobalt-60 irradiation (for ELISA) or subjected to other effective measures that render filoviruses noninfectious. Virus isolation in cell culture and plaque assays for quantification or diagnostic confirmation is relatively easy but must be performed in maximal-containment laboratories. If available, electron microscopic examination of properly inactivated samples or cultures can confirm the diagnosis because filovirions have unique filamentous shapes (Fig. 234-2). Formalin-fixed skin biopsies can be useful for safe postmortem diagnoses.

TREATMENT FILOVIRUS INFECTIONS

Any treatment of patients with suspected or confirmed filovirus infection must be administered under increased safety precautions by experienced specialists using appropriate personal protective equipment (see "Prevention," below). Treatment of EVD and MVD is entirely supportive because no accepted/approved, efficacious, specific antiviral agents or vaccines are yet available. The one exception is hyperimmune equine immunoglobulin, which has been approved in Russia—in the absence of convincing efficacy data—for emergency treatment of laboratory infections. Given the extraordinarily high lethality of filoviruses, special protocols may be established by ad hoc expert groups to outline treatment of exposed individuals with one of several regimens that have shown promise in experimental nonhuman primates. Current options include postexposure vaccination with filovirus $GP_{1,2}$-expressing recombinant replicating vesicular stomatitis Indiana virus; administration of specific filovirus genome- or transcript-targeting small interfering RNAs or phosphorodiamidate morpholino oligomers; administration of filovirus-specific antibodies or antibody cocktails (convalescent sera have not yet been proven effective); and use of a synthetic adenosine analog (BCX4430) that acts as a non-obligate RNA chain terminator. In the absence of these candidate treatments, measures to stabilize patients include those generally recommended for severe septicemia/sepsis/shock. Countermeasures should address hypotension and hypoperfusion, vascular leakage in the systemic and pulmonary circulatory system, disseminated intravascular coagulation and overt hemorrhaging, acute kidney failure, and electrolyte (especially potassium) imbalances. Pain management and administration of antipyretics and antiemetics should always be considered.

COMPLICATIONS

Given the severe immunosuppression induced by filovirus infection, secondary infections should be kept in mind and appropriately treated as early as possible. Pregnancy and labor cause severe and frequently fatal complications in filovirus infections due to clotting factor consumption, fetal loss, and/or severe blood loss during birth.

PROGNOSIS

The prognosis of filovirus infections is generally poor, although outcome probably depends somewhat on which particular virus causes the infection (Fig. 234-3). Convalescence may take months, with skin peeling, alopecia, prostration, weight loss, orchitis, amnesia, confusion, and anxiety as typical sequelae. Rarely, filoviruses persist in apparently healthy survivors and are either reactivated by unknown means at a later point or transmitted sexually. Condom use or abstinence from sexual activity for at least 3 months after disappearance of clinical signs is therefore recommended for survivors.

CONTROL AND PREVENTION

Currently, filovirus vaccines are not available. Prevention of filovirus infection in nature is difficult because the ecology of the viruses is not completely understood. As stated above, frugivorous cave-dwelling pteropid bats (Egyptian rousettes) have been identified as healthy carriers of MARV and RAVV. Avoidance of direct or indirect contact with these bats is therefore useful advice to people entering or living in areas where the animals can be found. Prevention seems to be more difficult in the case of ebolaviruses, for which definite reservoirs have not yet been pinpointed. EVD outbreaks have been associated not with bats but rather with hunting or consumption of nonhuman primates. The mechanism of introduction of ebolaviruses into nonhuman primate populations is unclear. Therefore, the best advice to locals and travelers is to avoid contact with bush meat, nonhuman primates, and bats.

Relatively simple barrier nursing techniques, vigilant use of proper personal protective equipment, and quarantine measures usually suffice to terminate or at least contain filovirus disease outbreaks. Isolation of filovirus-infected people and avoidance of direct person-to-person contact without proper personal protective equipment usually suffice to prevent further spread as the pathogens are not transmitted through droplets or aerosols under natural conditions. Typical protective gear sufficient to prevent filovirus infections consists of disposable gloves, gowns, and shoe covers and a face shield and/or goggles. If available, N-95/N-100 respirators may be used to further limit infection risk. Positive air pressure respirators should be considered for high-risk medical procedures such as intubation or suctioning. Medical equipment used in the care of a filovirus-infected patient, such as gloves or syringes, should never be reused unless safety-tested sterilization or disinfection methods are properly applied. Because filovirions are enveloped, disinfection with detergents, such as 1% sodium deoxycholate, diethyl ether, or phenolic compounds, is relatively straightforward. Bleach solutions of 1:100 and 1:10 are recommended for surface disinfection and application to excreta/corpses, respectively. Whenever possible, potentially contaminated materials should be autoclaved, irradiated, or destroyed.

SECTION 16 FUNGAL INFECTIONS

235 Diagnosis and Treatment of Fungal Infections

John E. Edwards, Jr.

TERMINOLOGY AND MICROBIOLOGY

Traditionally, fungal infections have been classified into specific categories based on both anatomic location and epidemiology. The most common general anatomic categories are mucocutaneous and deep organ infection; the most common general epidemiologic categories are endemic and opportunistic infection. Although *mucocutaneous infections* can cause serious morbidity, they are rarely fatal. *Deep organ infections* also cause severe illness in many cases and, in contrast to mucocutaneous infections, are often fatal. The *endemic mycoses* (e.g., coccidioidomycosis) are caused by fungal organisms that are not part of the normal human microbiota but rather are acquired from environmental sources. In contrast, *opportunistic mycoses* are caused by organisms (e.g., *Candida* and *Aspergillus*) that commonly are components of the normal human microbiota and whose ubiquity in nature renders them easily acquired by the immunocompromised host (Table 235-1). Opportunistic fungi cause serious infections when the immunologic response of the host becomes ineffective, allowing the organisms to transition from harmless commensals to invasive pathogens. Frequently, the diminished effectiveness of the immune system is a result of advanced modern therapies that coincidentally either cause an imbalance in the host's microbiota or directly interfere with immunologic responses. Endemic mycoses cause more severe illness in immunocompromised patients than in immunocompetent individuals.

TABLE 235-1 ENDEMIC AND OPPORTUNISTIC MYCOSES

Endemic Mycoses[a]	Opportunistic Mycoses
Coccidioidomycosis	Candidiasis
Histoplasmosis	Aspergillosis
Blastomycosis	Cryptococcosis
Phaeohyphomycosis	Mucormycosis (zygomycosis)
Penicilliosis	Scedosporiosis
Sporotrichosis	Trichosporonosis
Paracoccidioidomycosis	Fusariosis
	Pneumocystosis

[a]The endemic mycoses can also occur as opportunistic infections.

Patients acquire deep organ infection with endemic fungi almost exclusively by inhalation. Cutaneous infections result either from hematogenous dissemination or, more often, from direct contact with soil—the natural reservoir for the vast majority of endemic mycoses. The dermatophytic fungi may be acquired by human-to-human transmission, but the majority of infections result from environmental contact. In contrast, the opportunistic fungus *Candida* invades the host from normal sites of colonization, usually the mucous membranes of the gastrointestinal tract. In general, innate immunity is the primary defense mechanism against fungi. Although antibodies are formed during many fungal infections (and even during commensalism), they generally do not constitute the primary mode of host defense. Nevertheless, in selected infections, as discussed below, measurement of antibody titers may be a useful diagnostic test.

Three other terms frequently used in clinical discussions of fungal infections are *yeast*, *mold*, and *dimorphic fungus*. *Yeasts* are seen as rounded single cells or as budding organisms. *Candida* and *Cryptococcus* are traditionally classified as yeasts. *Molds* grow as filamentous forms called *hyphae* both at room temperature and in invaded tissue. *Aspergillus*, *Rhizopus* (the genus that causes mucormycosis, also known as zygomycosis), and fungi commonly infecting the skin to cause ringworm and related cutaneous conditions are classified as molds. Variations occur within this classification of yeasts and molds. For instance, when *Candida* infects tissue, both yeasts and filamentous forms may be present (except with *C. glabrata*, which forms only yeasts in tissue); in contrast, *Cryptococcus* exists only in yeast form. *Dimorphic* is the term used to describe fungi that grow as yeasts or large spherical structures in tissue but as filamentous forms at room temperature in the environment. Classified in this group are the organisms causing blastomycosis, paracoccidioidomycosis, coccidioidomycosis, histoplasmosis, and sporotrichosis.

The incidence of nearly all fungal infections has risen substantially. Opportunistic infections have increased in frequency as a consequence of intentional immunosuppression in organ and stem cell transplantation and other disorders, the administration of cytotoxic chemotherapy for cancers, the liberal use of antibacterial agents, and, more recently, the increasing use of monoclonal antibodies.

Within a global context, the incidence of endemic mycoses has increased in geographic locations where there has been substantial population growth. When advances in medical care (e.g., more aggressive treatment of cancer or organ transplantation) are introduced into a given area, the opportunistic mycoses increase in incidence.

DIAGNOSIS

The definitive diagnosis of any fungal infection requires histopathologic identification of the fungus invading tissue and accompanying evidence of an inflammatory response. The identification of an inflammatory response has been especially important with regard to *Aspergillus* infection. *Aspergillus* is ubiquitous and can float in the air onto biopsy material. Therefore, in rare but important instances, this fungus is an ex vivo contaminant during processing of a specimen for microscopy, with a consequent incorrect diagnosis. The stains most commonly used to identify fungi are periodic acid–Schiff and Gomori methenamine silver. *Candida*, unlike other fungi, is visible on gram-stained tissue smears. Hematoxylin and eosin stain is not sufficient to identify *Candida* in tissue specimens. When positive, an india ink preparation of cerebrospinal fluid (CSF) is diagnostic for cryptococcosis. Most laboratories now use calcofluor white staining coupled with fluorescent microscopy to identify fungi in fluid specimens.

Extensive investigations of the diagnosis of deep organ fungal infections have yielded a variety of tests with different degrees of specificity and sensitivity. The most reliable tests are the detection of antibody to *Coccidioides immitis* in serum and CSF; of *Histoplasma capsulatum* antigen in urine, serum, and CSF; and of cryptococcal polysaccharide antigen in serum and CSF. These tests have a general sensitivity and specificity of 90%; however, because of variability among laboratories, testing on multiple occasions is advisable. The test for galactomannan has been used extensively in Europe and is now approved in the United States for diagnosis of aspergillosis. Sources of concern regarding galactomannan are the incidence of false-negative results and the need for multiple serial tests to reduce this incidence. The β-glucan test for *Candida* is also under evaluation but, like the galactomannan test, still requires additional validation; this test has a negative predictive value of ~90%. Both of these tests are being used with increasing frequency, especially for guiding the timing of initiation and duration of therapy. The galactomannan test is being evaluated in both serum and bronchoalveolar lavage fluid. Numerous polymerase chain reaction assays to detect antigens are in the developmental stages, as are nucleic acid hybridization techniques; currently, these tests are not widely available.

Of the fungal organisms, *Candida* is by far the most frequently recovered from blood. Although *Candida* species can be detected with any of the automated blood culture systems widely used at present, the lysis-centrifugation technique increases the sensitivity of blood cultures for *Candida* and for less common organisms (e.g., *H. capsulatum*). Lysis-centrifugation should be used when disseminated fungal infection is suspected.

Except in the cases of coccidioidomycosis, cryptococcosis, and histoplasmosis, there are no fully validated and widely used tests for serodiagnosis of disseminated fungal infection. Skin tests for the endemic mycoses are no longer available.

TREATMENT FUNGAL INFECTIONS

This discussion is intended as a brief overview of general strategies for the use of antifungal agents in the treatment of fungal infections. Regimens, schedules, and strategies are detailed in the chapters on specific mycoses that follow in this section. The doses cited here are standard doses for adults with invasive infection.

Since fungal organisms are eukaryotic cells that contain most of the same organelles (with many of the same physiologic functions) as human cells, the identification of drugs that selectively kill or inhibit fungi but are not toxic to human cells has been highly problematic. Far fewer antifungal than antibacterial agents have been introduced into clinical medicine.

AMPHOTERICIN B

The introduction of amphotericin B (AmB) in the late 1950s revolutionized the treatment of fungal infections in deep organs. Before AmB became available, cryptococcal meningitis and other disseminated fungal infections were nearly always fatal. For nearly a decade after AmB was introduced, it was the only effective agent for the treatment of life-threatening fungal infections. AmB remains the broadest-spectrum antifungal agent but carries several disadvantages, including significant nephrotoxicity, lack of an oral preparation, and unpleasant side effects (fever, chills, and nausea) during treatment. To circumvent nephrotoxicity and infusion side effects, lipid formulations of AmB were developed and have virtually replaced the original colloidal deoxycholate formulation in clinical use (although the older formulation is still available). The lipid formulations include liposomal AmB (L-AmB; 3–5 mg/kg per day) and AmB lipid complex (ABLC; 5 mg/kg per day). A third preparation, AmB colloidal dispersion (ABCD; 3–4 mg/kg per day), is rarely used because of the high incidence of side effects associated with infusion.

The lipid formulations of AmB have the disadvantage of being considerably more expensive than the deoxycholate formulation. Experience is still accumulating on the comparative efficacy, toxicity, and advantages of the different formulations for specific clinical fungal infections, including central nervous system (CNS) infection. Whether there is a clinically significant difference in these drugs with respect to CNS penetration or nephrotoxicity remains controversial. Despite these issues and despite the expense, the lipid formulations are now much more commonly used than AmB deoxycholate in developed countries. In developing countries, AmB deoxycholate is still preferred because of the expense of the lipid formulations.

AZOLES

This class of antifungal drugs offers important advantages over AmB: the azoles cause little or no nephrotoxicity and are available in oral formulations. Early azoles included ketoconazole and miconazole, which have been replaced by newer agents for the treatment of deep organ fungal infections. The azoles' mechanism of action is inhibition of ergosterol synthesis in the fungal cell wall. Unlike AmB, these drugs are considered fungistatic, not fungicidal.

Fluconazole Since its introduction, fluconazole has played an extremely important role in the treatment of a wide variety of serious fungal infections. Its major advantages are the availability of both oral and IV formulations, a long half-life, satisfactory penetration of most body fluids (including ocular fluid and CSF), and minimal toxicity (especially relative to that of AmB). Its disadvantages include (usually reversible) hepatotoxicity and—at high doses—alopecia, muscle weakness, and dry mouth with a metallic taste. Fluconazole is not effective for the treatment of aspergillosis, mucormycosis, or *Scedosporium apiospermum* infections. It is less effective than the newer azoles against *Candida glabrata* and *Candida krusei*.

Fluconazole has become the agent of choice for the treatment of coccidioidal meningitis, although relapses have followed therapy with this drug. In addition, fluconazole is useful as both consolidation and maintenance therapy for cryptococcal meningitis. This agent has been shown to be as efficacious as AmB in the treatment of candidemia. The effectiveness of fluconazole in candidemia and the drug's relatively minimal toxicity, in conjunction with the inadequacy of diagnostic tests for widespread hematogenously disseminated candidiasis, have led to a change in the paradigm for candidemia management. The standard of care is now to treat all candidemic patients with an antifungal agent and to change all their intravascular lines, if feasible, rather than merely removing a singular suspect intravascular line and then observing the patient. The usual fluconazole regimen for treatment of candidemia is 400 mg/d given until 2 weeks after the last positive blood culture.

Fluconazole is considered effective as fungal prophylaxis in bone marrow transplant recipients and high-risk liver transplant patients. Its general use for prophylaxis in patients with leukemia, in AIDS patients with low CD4+ T cell counts, and in patients on surgical intensive care units remains controversial. Because of concerns about the possibility of infection due to resistant *Candida* species and of infection with *Aspergillus* species, many clinicians are initiating therapy with an echinocandin, which is then replaced by fluconazole once a susceptible *Candida* species is recovered and concern about *Aspergillus* is diminished.

Voriconazole Voriconazole, which is available in both oral and IV formulations, has a broader spectrum than fluconazole against *Candida* species (including *C. glabrata* and *C. krusei*) and is active against *Aspergillus*, *Scedosporium*, and *Fusarium*. It is generally considered the first-line drug of choice for treatment of aspergillosis. A few case reports have shown voriconazole to be effective in individual patients with coccidioidomycosis, blastomycosis, and histoplasmosis, but because of limited data this agent is not recommended for primary treatment of the endemic mycoses. Among the disadvantages of voriconazole (compared with fluconazole) are its more numerous interactions with many of the drugs used in patients predisposed to fungal infections. Hepatotoxicity, skin rashes (including photosensitivity), and visual disturbances are relatively common. Skin cancer surveillance is now recommended for patients taking voriconazole. In addition, voriconazole is considerably more expensive than fluconazole. Moreover, it is advisable to monitor voriconazole levels in certain patients since (1) this drug is completely metabolized in the liver by CYP2C9, CYP3A4, and CYP2C19; and (2) human genetic variability in CYP2C19 activity exists. Dosages should be reduced accordingly in patients with liver failure. Dose adjustments for renal insufficiency are not necessary; however, because the IV formulation is prepared in cyclodextrin, it should not be given to patients with severe renal insufficiency.

Itraconazole Itraconazole is available in IV and oral (capsule and suspension) formulations. Varying blood levels among patients taking oral itraconazole reflect a disadvantage compared with the other azoles. Itraconazole is the drug of choice for mild to moderate histoplasmosis and blastomycosis and has often been used for chronic mucocutaneous candidiasis. It has been approved by the U.S. Food and Drug Administration (FDA) for use in febrile neutropenic patients. Itraconazole has also proved useful for the treatment of chronic coccidioidomycosis, sporotrichosis, and *S. apiospermum* infection. The mucocutaneous and cutaneous fungal infections that have been treated successfully with itraconazole include oropharyngeal candidiasis (especially in AIDS patients), tinea versicolor, tinea capitis, and onychomycosis. Disadvantages of itraconazole include its poor penetration into CSF, the use of cyclodextrin in both the oral suspension and the IV formulation, the variable absorption of the drug in capsule form, and the need for monitoring of blood levels in patients taking capsules for disseminated mycoses. Reported cases of severe congestive heart failure in patients taking itraconazole have been a source of concern. Like the other azoles, itraconazole can cause hepatic toxicity.

Posaconazole Posaconazole is approved by the FDA for prophylaxis of aspergillosis and candidiasis in patients at high risk for developing these infections because of severe immunocompromise. It has also been approved for the treatment of oropharyngeal candidiasis and has been evaluated as therapy for zygomycosis, fusariosis, aspergillosis, cryptococcosis, and various other forms of candidal infection. The relevant studies of posaconazole in zygomycosis, fusariosis, and aspergillosis have examined salvage therapy. A study of more than 90 patients whose zygomycosis was refractory to other therapy yielded encouraging results. No trials of posaconazole for the treatment of candidemia have yet been reported. Case reports have described the drug's efficacy in coccidioidomycosis and histoplasmosis. Controlled trials have shown its effectiveness as a prophylactic agent in patients with acute leukemia and in bone marrow transplant recipients. In addition, posaconazole has been found to be effective against fluconazole-resistant *Candida* species. The results of a large-scale study of the use of posaconazole as salvage therapy for aspergillosis indicated that it is an alternative to other agents for salvage therapy; however, that study predated the use of voriconazole and the echinocandins.

ECHINOCANDINS

The echinocandins, including the FDA-approved drugs caspofungin, anidulafungin, and micafungin, have added considerably to the antifungal armamentarium. All three of these agents inhibit β-1,3-glucan synthase, which is necessary for cell wall synthesis in fungi and is not a component of human cells. None of these agents is currently available in an oral formulation. The echinocandins are considered fungicidal for *Candida* and fungistatic for *Aspergillus*. Their greatest use to date is against candidal infections. They offer two advantages: broad-spectrum activity against all *Candida* species and relatively low toxicity. The minimal inhibitory concentrations (MICs) of all the echinocandins are highest against *Candida parapsilosis*; it is not clear whether these higher MIC values represent less clinical effectiveness against this species. The echinocandins are among the safest antifungal agents.

In controlled trials, *caspofungin* has been at least as efficacious as AmB for the treatment of candidemia and invasive candidiasis and as efficacious as fluconazole for the treatment of candidal esophagitis. In addition, caspofungin has been efficacious as salvage therapy for aspergillosis. *Anidulafungin* has been approved by the FDA as therapy for candidemia in nonneutropenic patients and for *Candida* esophagitis, intraabdominal infection, and peritonitis. In controlled trials, anidulafungin has been shown to be noninferior and possibly superior to fluconazole against candidemia and invasive candidiasis. It is as efficacious as fluconazole against candidal esophagitis. When anidulafungin is used with cyclosporine, tacrolimus, or voriconazole, no dosage adjustment is required for either drug in the combination. *Micafungin* has been approved for the treatment of esophageal candidiasis and candidemia and for prophylaxis in patients receiving stem cell transplants. In a head-to-head trial, micafungin was noninferior to caspofungin for the treatment of candidemia. Studies thus far have shown that coadministration of micafungin and cyclosporine does not require dose adjustments for either drug. When micafungin is given with sirolimus, the area under the plasma drug concentration–time curve rises for sirolimus, usually necessitating a reduction in its dose. In open-label trials, favorable results have been obtained with micafungin for the treatment of deep-seated *Aspergillus* and *Candida* infections.

FLUCYTOSINE (5-FLUOROCYTOSINE)

The use of flucytosine has diminished as newer antifungal drugs have been developed. This agent is now used most commonly in combination with AmB (deoxycholate or lipid formulations) for the initial treatment of cryptococcal meningitis. Flucytosine has a unique mechanism of action based on intrafungal conversion to 5-fluorouracil, which is toxic to the fungal cell. Development of resistance to the compound has limited its use as a single agent. Flucytosine is nearly always used in combination with AmB. Its good penetration into the CSF makes it attractive for use with AmB for treatment of cryptococcal meningitis. Flucytosine has also been recommended for the treatment of candidal meningitis in combination with AmB; comparative trials with AmB alone have not been done. Significant and frequent bone marrow depression is seen with flucytosine when this drug is used with AmB.

GRISEOFULVIN AND TERBINAFINE

Historically, griseofulvin has been useful primarily for ringworm infection. This agent is usually given for relatively long periods. Terbinafine has been used primarily for onychomycosis but also for ringworm. In comparative studies, terbinafine has been as effective as itraconazole and more effective than griseofulvin for both conditions.

TOPICAL ANTIFUNGAL AGENTS

A detailed discussion of the agents used for the treatment of cutaneous fungal infections and onychomycosis is beyond the scope of this chapter; the reader is referred to the dermatology literature. Many classes of compounds have been used to treat the common fungal infections of the skin. Among the azoles used are clotrimazole, econazole, miconazole, oxiconazole, sulconazole, ketoconazole, tioconazole, butoconazole, and terconazole. In general, topical treatment of vaginal candidiasis has been successful. Since little difference is thought to exist in the efficacy of the various vaginal preparations, the choice of agent is made by the physician and/or the patient on the basis of preference and availability. Fluconazole given orally at 150 mg has the advantage of not requiring repeated intravaginal application. Nystatin is a polyene that has been used for both oropharyngeal thrush and vaginal candidiasis. Useful agents in other classes include ciclopirox olamine, haloprogin, terbinafine, naftifine, tolnaftate, and undecylenic acid.

236 Histoplasmosis

Chadi A. Hage, L. Joseph Wheat

ETIOLOGY

Histoplasma capsulatum, a thermal dimorphic fungus, is the etiologic agent of histoplasmosis. In most endemic areas, *H. capsulatum* var. *capsulatum* is the causative agent. In Africa, *H. capsulatum* var. *duboisii* also is found; var. *duboisii* can be differentiated from var. *capsulatum* as the *duboisii* yeasts are larger. In Central and South America, histoplasmosis is common and is caused by clades of *H. capsulatum* var. *capsulatum* that differ genetically from those involved elsewhere.

Mycelia—the naturally infectious form of *Histoplasma*—have a characteristic appearance, with microconidial and macroconidial forms. Microconidia are oval and are small enough (2–4 μm) to reach the terminal bronchioles and alveoli. Shortly after infecting the host, mycelia transform into the yeasts that are found inside macrophages and other phagocytes. The yeast forms are characteristically small (2–5 μm), with occasional narrow budding. In the laboratory, mycelia are best grown at room temperature, whereas yeasts are grown at 37°C on enriched media.

EPIDEMIOLOGY

Histoplasmosis is the most prevalent endemic mycosis in North America. Although this fungal disease has been reported throughout the world, its endemicity is particularly notable in certain parts of North, Central, and South America; Africa; and Asia. In Europe, histoplasmosis is diagnosed fairly often, mostly in emigrants from or travelers to endemic areas on other continents. In the United States, the endemic areas spread over the Ohio and Mississippi river valleys. This pattern is related to the humid and acidic nature of the soil in these areas. Soil enriched with bird or bat droppings promotes the growth and sporulation of *Histoplasma*. Disruption of soil containing the organism leads to aerosolization of the microconidia and exposure of humans nearby. Activities associated with high-level exposure include spelunking, excavation, cleaning of chicken coops, demolition and remodeling of old buildings, and cutting of dead trees. Most cases seen outside of highly endemic areas represent imported disease—e.g., cases reported in Europe after travel to the Americas, Africa, or Asia.

PATHOGENESIS AND PATHOLOGY

Infection follows inhalation of microconidia (Fig. 236-1). Once they reach the alveolar spaces, microconidia are rapidly recognized and engulfed by alveolar macrophages. At this point, the microconidia transform into budding yeasts (Fig. 236-2), a process that is integral to the pathogenesis of histoplasmosis and is dependent on the availability of calcium and iron inside the phagocytes. The yeasts are capable of growing and multiplying inside resting macrophages. Neutrophils and then lymphocytes are attracted to the site of infection. Before the development of cellular immunity, yeasts use the phagosomes as a vehicle for translocation to local draining lymph nodes, whence they spread hematogenously throughout the reticuloendothelial system. Adequate cellular immunity develops ~2 weeks after infection. T cells produce interferon γ to assist the macrophages in killing the organism and controlling the progression of disease. Interleukin 12 and tumor necrosis factor α (TNF-α) play an essential role in cellular immunity to *H. capsulatum*. In the immunocompetent host, macrophages, lymphocytes, and epithelial cells eventually organize and form granulomas that contain the organisms. These granulomas typically fibrose and calcify; calcified mediastinal lymph nodes and hepatosplenic calcifications are frequently found in healthy individuals from endemic areas. In immunocompetent hosts, infection with *H. capsulatum* confers some immunity to reinfection. In patients with impaired cellular immunity, the infection is not contained and can disseminate. Progressive disseminated histoplasmosis (PDH) can involve multiple organs, most commonly the bone marrow, spleen, liver (Fig. 236-3), adrenal glands, and mucocutaneous membranes. Unlike latent tuberculosis, latent histoplasmosis rarely reactivates.

Structural lung disease (e.g., emphysema) impairs the clearance of pulmonary histoplasmosis, and chronic pulmonary disease can result. This chronic process is characterized by progressive inflammation, tissue necrosis, and fibrosis mimicking cavitary tuberculosis.

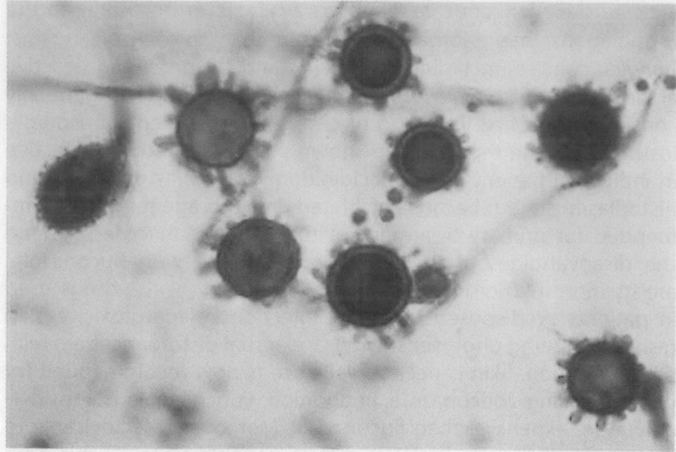

FIGURE 236-1 Spiked spherical conidia of *H. capsulatum* (lactophenol cotton blue stain).

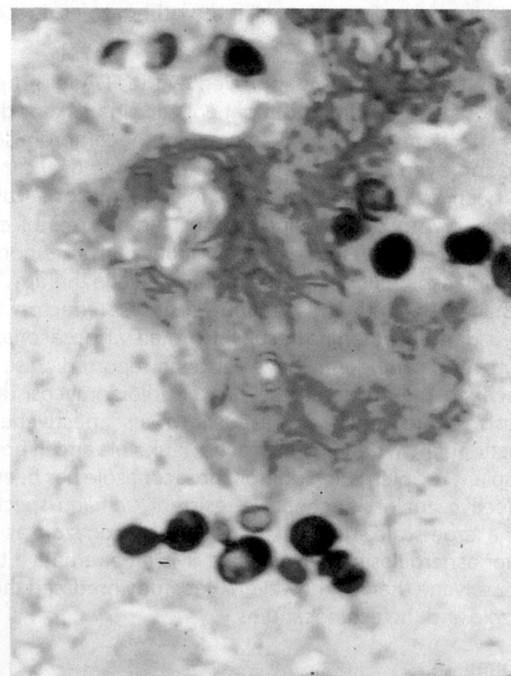

FIGURE 236-2 Small (2–5 μm) narrow budding yeasts of *H. capsulatum* from bronchoalveolar lavage fluid (Grocott's methenamine silver stain).

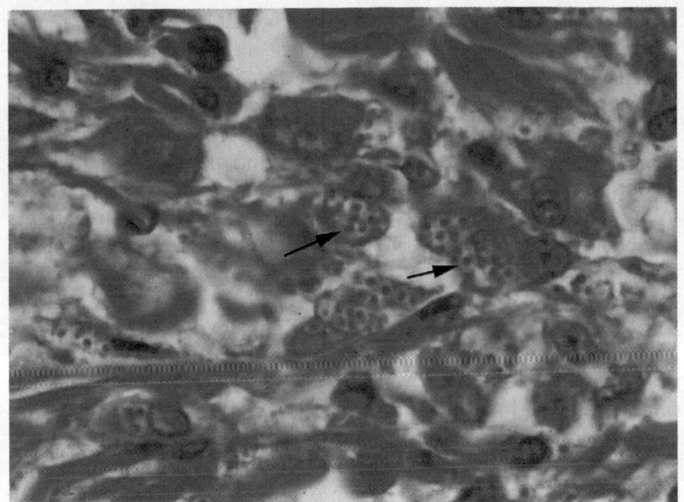

FIGURE 236-3 **Intracellular yeasts (*arrows*) of *H. capsulatum*** in a liver biopsy specimen (hematoxylin and eosin stain).

CLINICAL MANIFESTATIONS

The clinical spectrum of histoplasmosis ranges from asymptomatic infection to life-threatening illness. The attack rate and the extent and severity of the disease depend on the intensity of exposure, the immune status of the exposed individual, and the underlying lung architecture of the host.

In immunocompetent individuals with low-level exposure, most *Histoplasma* infections are either asymptomatic or mild and self-limited. Of adults residing in endemic areas, 50–80% have skin-test and/or radiographic evidence of previous infection without clinical manifestations. When symptoms do develop, they usually appear 1–4 weeks after exposure. Heavy exposure leads to a flulike illness with fever, chills, sweats, headache, myalgia, anorexia, cough, dyspnea, and chest pain. Chest radiographs usually show signs of pneumonitis with prominent hilar or mediastinal adenopathy. Pulmonary infiltrates may be focal with light exposure or diffuse with heavy exposure. Rheumatologic symptoms of arthralgia or arthritis, often associated with erythema nodosum, occur in 5–10% of patients with acute histoplasmosis. Pericarditis may also develop. These manifestations represent inflammatory responses to the acute infection rather than its direct effects. Hilar or mediastinal lymph nodes may undergo necrosis and coalesce to form large mediastinal masses that can cause compression of great vessels, proximal airways, and the esophagus. These necrotic lymph nodes may also rupture and create fistulas between mediastinal structures (e.g., bronchoesophageal fistulas).

PDH is typically seen in immunocompromised individuals, who account for ~70% of cases. Common risk factors include AIDS (CD4+ T cell count, <200/μL), extremes of age, immunosuppressive medications administered for prevention or treatment of rejection following transplantation (e.g., prednisone, mycophenolate, calcineurin inhibitors, and biologic response modifiers), and methotrexate, anti-TNF-α agents, or other biologic response modifiers given for inflammatory arthritis or Crohn's disease.

The spectrum of PDH ranges from an acute, rapidly fatal course—with diffuse interstitial or reticulonodular lung infiltrates causing respiratory failure, shock, coagulopathy, and multiorgan failure—to a more subacute course with a focal organ distribution. Common manifestations include fever and weight loss. Hepatosplenomegaly also is common. Other findings may include meningitis or focal brain lesions, ulcerations of the oral mucosa, gastrointestinal ulcerations, and adrenal insufficiency. Prompt recognition of this devastating illness is of paramount importance in patients with more severe manifestations or with underlying immunosuppression, especially AIDS (Chap. 226).

Chronic cavitary histoplasmosis is seen in smokers who have structural lung disease (e.g., bullous emphysema). This chronic illness is characterized by productive cough, dyspnea, low-grade fever, night sweats, and weight loss. Chest radiographs usually show upper-lobe infiltrates, cavitation, and pleural thickening—findings resembling those of tuberculosis. Without treatment, the course is slowly progressive.

Fibrosing mediastinitis is an uncommon and serious complication of histoplasmosis. In certain patients, acute infection is followed for unknown reasons by progressive fibrosis around the hilar and mediastinal lymph nodes. Involvement may be unilateral or bilateral; bilateral involvement carries a worse prognosis. Major manifestations include superior vena cava syndrome, obstruction of pulmonary vessels, and airway obstruction. Patients may experience recurrent pneumonia, hemoptysis, or respiratory failure. Fibrosing mediastinitis is fatal in up to one-third of cases.

In healed histoplasmosis, calcified mediastinal nodes or lung parenchyma may erode through the walls of the airways and cause hemoptysis. This condition is called *broncholithiasis*.

The clinical features and management of histoplasmosis caused by the genetically different clades in Central and South America are similar to those of the disease in North America. African histoplasmosis caused by var. *duboisii* is clinically distinct and is characterized by frequent skin and bone involvement.

DIAGNOSIS

Fungal culture remains the gold standard diagnostic test for histoplasmosis. However, culture results may not be known for up to 1 month, and cultures are often negative in less severe cases. Cultures are positive in ~75% of cases of PDH and chronic pulmonary histoplasmosis. Cultures of bronchoalveolar lavage (BAL) fluid are positive in about half of cases that include acute pulmonary histoplasmosis causing diffuse infiltrates with hypoxemia. In PDH, the culture yield is highest for BAL fluid, bone marrow aspirate, and blood. Cultures of sputum or bronchial washings are usually positive in chronic pulmonary histoplasmosis. Cultures are typically negative, however, in other forms of histoplasmosis.

Fungal stains of cytopathology or biopsy materials showing structures resembling *Histoplasma* yeasts are helpful in the diagnosis of PDH, yielding positive results in about half of cases. Yeasts can be seen in BAL fluid (Fig. 236-2) from patients with diffuse pulmonary infiltrates, in bone marrow biopsy samples, and in biopsy specimens of other involved organs (e.g., the adrenal glands). Occasionally, yeasts are seen in blood smears from patients with severe PDH. However, artifacts and other fungal elements sometimes stain positive and may be misidentified as *Histoplasma* yeasts.

The detection of *Histoplasma* antigen in body fluids is extremely useful in the diagnosis of PDH and acute diffuse pulmonary histoplasmosis. The sensitivity of this technique is >95% in patients with PDH and >80% in patients with acute pulmonary histoplasmosis if both urine and serum are tested. Antigen level correlates with severity of illness in PDH and can be used to follow disease progression as levels predictably decrease with effective therapy. An increase in antigen levels also predicts relapse. Antigen can be detected in cerebrospinal fluid from patients with meningitis and in BAL fluid from those with pneumonia. Cross-reactivity occurs with African histoplasmosis, blastomycosis, coccidioidomycosis, paracoccidioidomycosis, and *Penicillium marneffei* infection.

Serologic tests, including immunodiffusion and complement fixation, are useful for the diagnosis of histoplasmosis in immunocompetent patients. Serum antibody titers may rise fourfold in patients with acute histoplasmosis. Serologic tests are especially useful for the diagnosis of chronic pulmonary histoplasmosis. The limitations of serology, however, include insensitivity early in the course of infection (at least 1 month is required for the production of antibodies), insensitivity in immunosuppressed patients, and persistence of detectable antibody for several years after infection. Positive results from past infection may lead to a misdiagnosis of active histoplasmosis in a patient with another disease process.

TREATMENT HISTOPLASMOSIS

Treatment recommendations for histoplasmosis are summarized in Table 236-1. Treatment is indicated for all patients with PDH or chronic pulmonary histoplasmosis as well as for symptomatic

TABLE 236-1 RECOMMENDATIONS FOR THE TREATMENT OF HISTOPLASMOSIS

Type of Histoplasmosis	Treatment Recommendations	Comments
Acute pulmonary, moderate to severe illness with diffuse infiltrates and/or hypoxemia	Lipid AmB (3–5 mg/kg per day) ± glucocorticoids for 1–2 weeks; then itraconazole (200 mg bid) for 12 weeks. Monitor renal and hepatic function.	Patients with mild cases usually recover without therapy, but itraconazole should be considered if the patient's condition has not improved after 1 month.
Chronic/cavitary pulmonary	Itraconazole (200 mg qd or bid) for at least 12 months. Monitor hepatic function.	Continue treatment until radiographic findings show no further improvement. Monitor for relapse after treatment is stopped.
Progressive disseminated	Lipid AmB (3–5 mg/kg per day) for 1–2 weeks; then itraconazole (200 mg bid) for at least 12 months. Monitor renal and hepatic function.	Liposomal AmB is preferred, but the AmB lipid complex may be used because of cost. Chronic maintenance therapy may be necessary if the degree of immunosuppression cannot be reduced.
Central nervous system	Liposomal AmB (5 mg/kg per day) for 4–6 weeks; then itraconazole (200 mg bid or tid) for at least 12 months. Monitor renal and hepatic function.	A longer course of lipid AmB is recommended because of the high risk of relapse. Itraconazole should be continued until cerebrospinal fluid or CT abnormalities clear.

Abbreviation: AmB, amphotericin B.

patients with acute pulmonary histoplasmosis causing diffuse infiltrates, especially with hypoxemia. In most cases of pulmonary histoplasmosis, treatment is not recommended because the degree of exposure is not heavy; the infection is asymptomatic or symptoms are mild, subacute, and not progressive; and the illness resolves without therapy.

The preferred treatments for histoplasmosis include the lipid formulations of amphotericin B (AmB) in more severe cases and itraconazole in others. Liposomal AmB has been more effective than the deoxycholate formulation for treatment of PDH in patients with AIDS. The deoxycholate formulation is an alternative to lipid formulations for patients at low risk for nephrotoxicity. Posaconazole, voriconazole, and fluconazole are alternatives for patients who cannot take itraconazole.

In severe cases requiring hospitalization, a lipid formulation of AmB is followed by itraconazole. In patients with meningitis, a lipid formulation of AmB should be given for 4–6 weeks before the switch to itraconazole. In immunosuppressed patients, the degree of immunosuppression should be reduced if possible, although immune reconstitution inflammatory syndrome (IRIS) may ensue. Antiretroviral treatment improves the outcome of PDH in patients with AIDS and is recommended; however, whether antiretroviral treatment should be delayed to avoid IRIS is unknown.

Blood levels of itraconazole should be monitored to ensure adequate drug exposure, with target concentrations of the parent drug and its hydroxy metabolites of 1–5 μg/mL as measured by high-performance liquid chromatography and 2–10 μg/mL as measured by microbiologic assay. Drug interactions should be carefully assessed: itraconazole not only is cleared by cytochrome P450 metabolism but also inhibits cytochrome P450. This profile causes interactions with many other medications.

The duration of treatment for acute pulmonary histoplasmosis is 6–12 weeks, while that for PDH and chronic pulmonary histoplasmosis is ≥1 year. Antigen levels in urine and serum should be monitored during and for at least 1 year after therapy for PDH. Stable or rising antigen levels suggest treatment failure or relapse.

Previously, lifelong itraconazole maintenance therapy was recommended for patients with AIDS once histoplasmosis was diagnosed. Today, however, maintenance therapy is not required for patients who respond well to antiretroviral therapy, with CD4+ T cell counts of at least 150/μL (preferably >250/μL); who complete at least 1 year of itraconazole therapy; and who exhibit neither clinical evidence of active histoplasmosis nor an antigenuria level of >4 ng/mL. Maintenance therapy also appears to be unnecessary in patients receiving immunosuppressive treatment if the degree of immunosuppression can be reduced through an approach similar to that used for patients with AIDS.

Fibrosing mediastinitis, which represents a chronic fibrotic reaction to past mediastinal histoplasmosis rather than an active infection, does not respond to antifungal therapy. While treatment is often prescribed for patients with pulmonary histoplasmosis who have not recovered within 1 month and for those with persistent mediastinal lymphadenopathy, the effectiveness of antifungal therapy in these situations is unknown.

237 Coccidioidomycosis

Neil M. Ampel

DEFINITION AND ETIOLOGY

Coccidioidomycosis, commonly known as Valley fever (see "Epidemiology," below), is caused by dimorphic soil-dwelling fungi of the genus *Coccidioides*. Genetic analysis has demonstrated the existence of two species, *C. immitis* and *C. posadasii*. These species are indistinguishable with regard to the clinical disease they cause and their appearance on routine laboratory media. Thus, the organisms will be referred to simply as *Coccidioides* for the remainder of this chapter.

EPIDEMIOLOGY

Coccidioidomycosis is confined to the Western Hemisphere between the latitudes of 40°N and 40°S. In the United States, areas of high endemicity include the southern portion of the San Joaquin Valley of California and the south-central region of Arizona. However, infection may be acquired in other areas of the southwestern United States, including the southern coastal counties in California, southern Nevada, southwestern Utah, southern New Mexico, and western Texas, including the Rio Grande Valley. Outside the United States, coccidioidomycosis is endemic to northern Mexico as well as to localized regions of Central America. In South America, there are endemic foci in Colombia, Venezuela, northeastern Brazil, Paraguay, Bolivia, and north-central Argentina.

The risk of infection is increased by direct exposure to soil harboring *Coccidioides*. Because of difficulty in isolating *Coccidioides* from the soil, the precise characteristics of potentially infectious soil are not known. In the United States, several outbreaks of coccidioidomycosis have been associated with soil from archaeologic excavations of Amerindian sites both within and outside of the recognized endemic region. These cases often involved alluvial soils in regions of relative aridity with moderate temperature ranges. *Coccidioides* was isolated at depths of 2–20 cm below the surface. The recent identification of three cases of coccidioidomycosis in eastern Washington State may suggest that the endemic region is expanding.

In endemic areas, many cases of *Coccidioides* infection occur without obvious soil or dust exposure. Climatic factors appear to increase the infection rate in these regions. In particular, periods of aridity following rainy seasons have been associated with marked increases in the number of symptomatic cases. Overall, the incidence within the United States has increased substantially over the past decade, with nearly 43 cases per 100,000 residents of the endemic region in

2011. Most of that increase has occurred in south-central Arizona, where most of that state's population resides, and in the southern San Joaquin Valley of California, a much less populated region. The factors causing this increase have not been fully elucidated; however, an influx of older individuals without prior coccidioidal infection appears to be involved. Other variables, such as climate change, construction activity, and increased awareness and reporting, may also be factors. Health care providers should consider coccidioidomycosis when evaluating persons with pneumonia who live in or have traveled to endemic areas.

PATHOGENESIS, PATHOLOGY, AND IMMUNE RESPONSE

On agar media and in the soil, *Coccidioides* organisms exist as filamentous molds. Within this mycelial structure, individual filaments (*hyphae*) elongate and branch, some growing upward. Alternating cells within the hyphae degenerate, leaving barrel-shaped viable elements called *arthroconidia*. Measuring ~2 by 5 μm, arthroconidia may become airborne for extended periods. Their small size allows them to evade initial mechanical mucosal defenses and reach deep into the bronchial tree, where infection is initiated in the nonimmune host.

Once in a susceptible host, the arthroconidia enlarge, become rounded, and develop internal septations. The resulting structures, called *spherules* (Fig. 237-1), may attain sizes of 200 μm and are unique to *Coccidioides*. The septations encompass uninuclear elements called *endospores*. Spherules may rupture and release packets of endospores that can themselves develop into spherules, thus propagating infection locally. If returned to artificial media or the soil, the fungus reverts to its mycelial stage.

Clinical observations and data from studies of animals strongly support the critical role of a robust cellular immune response in the host's control of coccidioidomycosis. Necrotizing granulomas containing

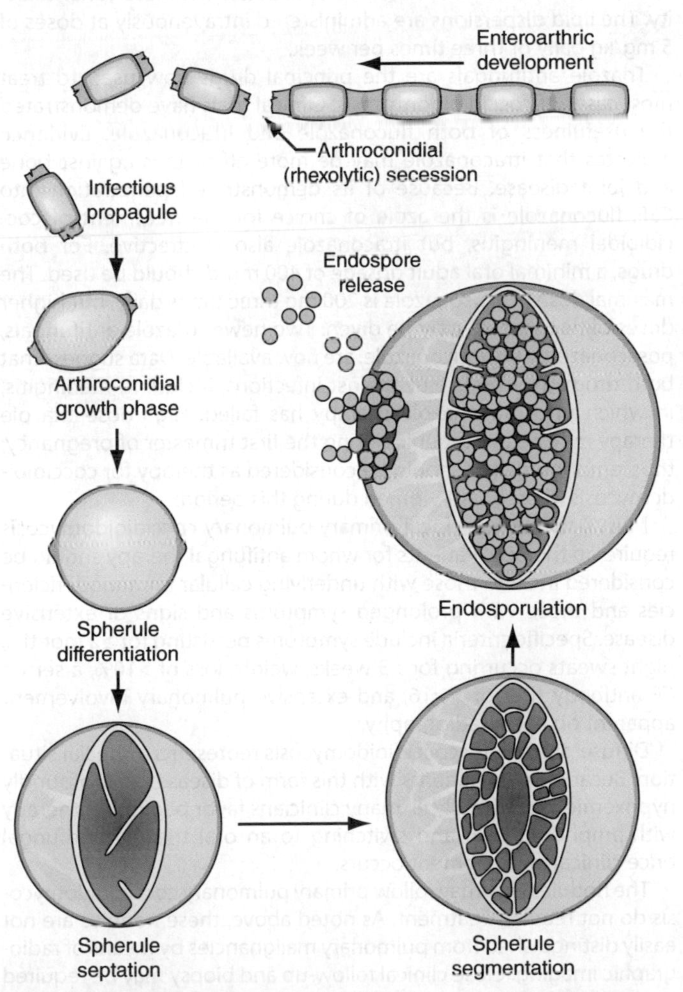

FIGURE 237-1 Life cycle of *Coccidioides*. *(From TN Kirkland, J Fierer: Emerg Infect Dis 2:192, 1996.)*

spherules are typically identified in patients with resolved pulmonary infection. In disseminated disease, granulomas are generally poorly formed or do not develop at all, and a polymorphonuclear leukocyte response occurs frequently. In patients who are asymptomatic or in whom the initial pulmonary infection resolves, delayed-type hypersensitivity to coccidioidal antigens has been routinely documented.

CLINICAL AND LABORATORY MANIFESTATIONS

Of infected individuals, 60% are completely asymptomatic, and the remaining 40% have symptoms that are related principally to pulmonary infection, including fever, cough, and pleuritic chest pain. The risk of symptomatic illness increases with age. Coccidioidomycosis is commonly misdiagnosed as community-acquired bacterial pneumonia.

There are several cutaneous manifestations of primary pulmonary coccidioidomycosis. Toxic erythema consisting of a maculopapular rash has been noted in some cases. Erythema nodosum (see Fig. 25e-40)—typically over the lower extremities—or erythema multiforme (see Fig. 25e-25)—usually in a necklace distribution—may occur; these manifestations are seen particularly often in women. Arthralgias and arthritis may develop. The diagnosis of primary pulmonary coccidioidomycosis is suggested by a history of night sweats or profound fatigue as well as by peripheral-blood eosinophilia and hilar or mediastinal lymphadenopathy on chest radiography. While pleuritic chest pain is common, pleural effusions occur in fewer than 10% of cases. Such effusions are invariably associated with a pulmonary infiltrate on the same side. The cellular content of these effusions is mononuclear in nature; *Coccidioides* is rarely grown from effusions.

In most patients, primary pulmonary coccidioidomycosis usually resolves without sequelae in weeks. However, several pneumonic complications may arise. Pulmonary nodules are residua of primary pneumonia. Generally single, frequently located in the upper lobes, and ≤4 cm in diameter, nodules are often discovered on a routine chest radiograph in an asymptomatic patient. Calcification is uncommon. Coccidioidal pulmonary nodules can be difficult to distinguish radiographically from pulmonary malignancies. Like malignancies, coccidioidal nodules often enhance on positron emission tomography. However, routine CT often demonstrates multiple nodules in coccidioidomycosis. Biopsy is often required to distinguish between these two conditions.

Pulmonary cavities occur when a nodule extrudes its contents into the bronchus, resulting in a thin-walled shell. These cavities can be associated with persistent cough, hemoptysis, and pleuritic chest pain. Rarely, a cavity may rupture into the pleural space, causing pyopneumothorax. In such cases, patients present with acute dyspnea, and the chest radiograph reveals a collapsed lung with a pleural air-fluid level. Chronic or persistent pulmonary coccidioidomycosis manifests with prolonged symptoms of fever, cough, and weight loss and is radiographically associated with pulmonary scarring, fibrosis, and cavities. It occurs most commonly in patients who already have chronic lung disease due to other etiologies.

In some cases, primary pneumonia presents as a diffuse reticulonodular pulmonary process (detected by plain chest radiography) in association with dyspnea and fever. Primary diffuse coccidioidal pneumonia may occur in settings of intense environmental exposure or profoundly suppressed cellular immunity (e.g., in patients with AIDS), with unrestrained fungal growth that is frequently associated with fungemia.

Clinical dissemination outside the thoracic cavity occurs in fewer than 1% of infected individuals. Dissemination is more likely to occur in male patients, particularly those of African-American or Filipino ancestry, and in persons with depressed cellular immunity, including patients with HIV infection and peripheral-blood CD4+ T cell counts of <250/μL; those receiving chronic glucocorticoid therapy; those with allogeneic solid-organ transplants; and those being treated with tumor necrosis factor α antagonists. Women who acquire infection during the second or third trimester of pregnancy also are at risk for disseminated disease. Common sites for dissemination include the skin, bone, joints, soft tissues, and meninges. Dissemination may follow symptomatic or asymptomatic pulmonary infection and may involve only one site or multiple anatomic foci. When it occurs, clinical dissemination is usually evident within the first few months after primary pulmonary infection.

Coccidioidal meningitis, if untreated, is uniformly fatal. Patients usually present with a persistent headache, which is sometimes accompanied by lethargy and confusion. Nuchal rigidity, if present, is not severe. Examination of cerebrospinal fluid (CSF) demonstrates lymphocytic pleocytosis with profound hypoglycorrhachia and elevated protein levels. CSF eosinophilia is occasionally documented. With or without appropriate therapy, patients may develop hydrocephalus, which presents clinically as a marked decline in mental status, often with gait disturbances.

DIAGNOSIS

As mentioned above, coccidioidomycosis is often misdiagnosed as community-acquired bacterial pneumonia. Clues that suggest a diagnosis of coccidioidomycosis include peripheral-blood eosinophilia, hilar or mediastinal adenopathy on radiographic imaging, marked fatigue, and failure to improve with antibiotic therapy.

Serology plays an important role in establishing a diagnosis of coccidioidomycosis. Several techniques are available, including the traditional tube-precipitin (TP) and complement-fixation (CF) assays, immunodiffusion (IDTP and IDCF), and enzyme immunoassay (EIA) to detect IgM and IgG antibodies. TP and IgM antibodies are found in serum soon after infection and persist for weeks. They are not useful for gauging disease progression and are not found in the CSF. The CF and IgG antibodies occur later in the course of the disease and persist longer than TP and IgM antibodies. Rising CF titers are associated with clinical progression, and the presence of CF antibody in CSF is indicative of coccidioidal meningitis. Antibodies disappear over time in persons whose clinical illness resolves.

Because of its commercial availability, the coccidioidal EIA is frequently used as a screening tool for coccidioidal serology. There has been concern that the IgM EIA is occasionally falsely positive, particularly in asymptomatic individuals. In addition, while the sensitivity and specificity of the IgG EIA appear to be higher than those of the CF and IDCF assays, the optical density obtained in the EIA does not correlate with the serologic titer of either of the latter tests.

Coccidioides grows within 3–7 days at 37°C on a variety of artificial media, including blood agar. Therefore, it is always useful to obtain samples of sputum or other respiratory fluids and tissues for culture in suspected cases of coccidioidomycosis. The clinical laboratory should be alerted to the possibility of this diagnosis, since *Coccidioides* poses a significant laboratory hazard if it is inadvertently inhaled. The organism can also be identified directly. While treatment of samples with potassium hydroxide is rarely fruitful in establishing the diagnosis, examination of sputum or other respiratory fluids after Papanicolaou or Gomori methenamine silver staining reveals spherules in a significant proportion of patients with pulmonary coccidioidomycosis. For fixed tissues (e.g., those obtained from biopsy specimens), spherules with surrounding inflammation can be demonstrated with hematoxylin-eosin or Gomori methenamine silver staining.

A commercially available test for coccidioidal antigenuria and antigenemia has been developed and appears to be particularly useful in immunosuppressed patients with severe or disseminated disease. False-positive results may occur in cases of histoplasmosis or blastomycosis. Some laboratories offer genomic detection by polymerase chain reaction.

TABLE 237-1 CLINICAL PRESENTATIONS OF COCCIDIOIDOMYCOSIS, THEIR FREQUENCY, AND RECOMMENDED INITIAL THERAPY FOR THE IMMUNOCOMPETENT HOST

Clinical Presentation	Frequency, %	Recommended Therapy
Asymptomatic infection	60	None
Primary pneumonia (focal)	40	In most cases, none[a]
Diffuse pneumonia	<1	Amphotericin B followed by prolonged oral triazole therapy
Pulmonary sequelae	5	
Nodule	—	None
Cavity	—	In most cases, none[b]
Chronic pneumonia	—	Prolonged triazole therapy
Disseminated disease	≤1	
Skin, bone, joint, soft tissue disease	—	Prolonged triazole therapy[c]
Meningitis	—	Lifelong triazole therapy[d]

[a]Treatment is indicated for hosts with depressed cellular immunity as well as for those with prolonged symptoms and signs of increased severity, including night sweats for >3 weeks, weight loss of >10%, a complement-fixation titer of >1:16, and extensive pulmonary involvement on chest radiography. [b]Treatment (usually with the oral triazoles fluconazole and itraconazole) is recommended for persistent symptoms. [c]In severe cases, some clinicians would use amphotericin B as initial therapy. [d]Intraventricular or intrathecal amphotericin B is recommended in cases of triazole failure. Hydrocephalus may occur, requiring a CSF shunt.

Note: See text for dosages and durations.

TREATMENT COCCIDIOIDOMYCOSIS

Currently, two main classes of antifungal agents are useful for the treatment of coccidioidomycosis (Table 237-1). While once prescribed routinely, amphotericin B in all its formulations is now reserved for only the most severe cases of dissemination and for intrathecal or intraventricular administration to patients with coccidioidal meningitis in whom triazole antifungal therapy has failed. The original formulation of amphotericin B, which is dispersed with deoxycholate, is usually administered intravenously in doses of 0.7–1.0 mg/kg either daily or three times per week. The newer lipid-based formulations—amphotericin B lipid complex (ABLC), amphotericin B colloidal dispersion (ABCD), and amphotericin B liposomal complex (L-AmB)—are associated with less renal toxicity. The lipid dispersions are administered intravenously at doses of 5 mg/kg daily or three times per week.

Triazole antifungals are the principal drugs now used to treat most cases of coccidioidomycosis. Clinical trials have demonstrated the usefulness of both fluconazole and itraconazole. Evidence indicates that itraconazole may be more efficacious against bone and joint disease. Because of its demonstrated penetration into CSF, fluconazole is the azole of choice for the treatment of coccidioidal meningitis, but itraconazole also is effective. For both drugs, a minimal oral adult dosage of 400 mg/d should be used. The maximal dose of itraconazole is 200 mg three times daily, but higher doses of fluconazole may be given. Two newer triazole antifungals, posaconazole and voriconazole, are now available. Data suggest that both drugs may be useful against infections, including meningitis, in which prior fluconazole therapy has failed. High-dose triazole therapy may be teratogenic during the first trimester of pregnancy; thus, amphotericin B should be considered as therapy for coccidioidomycosis in pregnant women during this period.

Most patients with focal primary pulmonary coccidioidomycosis require no therapy. Patients for whom antifungal therapy should be considered include those with underlying cellular immunodeficiencies and those with prolonged symptoms and signs of extensive disease. Specific criteria include symptoms persisting for ≥2 months, night sweats occurring for >3 weeks, weight loss of >10%, a serum CF antibody titer of >1:16, and extensive pulmonary involvement apparent on chest radiography.

Diffuse pulmonary coccidioidomycosis represents a special situation. Because most patients with this form of disease are profoundly hypoxemic and critically ill, many clinicians favor beginning therapy with amphotericin B and switching to an oral triazole antifungal once clinical improvement occurs.

The nodules that may follow primary pulmonary coccidioidomycosis do not require treatment. As noted above, these nodules are not easily distinguished from pulmonary malignancies by means of radiographic imaging. Close clinical follow-up and biopsy may be required to distinguish between these two entities. Most pulmonary cavities do not require therapy. Antifungal treatment should be considered in patients with persistent cough, pleuritic chest pain, and hemoptysis. Occasionally, pulmonary coccidioidal cavities become secondarily infected. This development is usually manifested by an air-fluid level within the cavity. Bacterial flora or *Aspergillus* species are commonly involved, and therapy directed at these organisms should be considered. Surgery is rarely required except in cases of persistent hemoptysis or pyopneumothorax. For chronic pulmonary coccidioidomycosis, prolonged antifungal therapy—lasting for at least 1 year—is usually required, with monitoring of symptoms, radiographic changes, sputum cultures, and serologic titers.

Most cases of disseminated coccidioidomycosis require prolonged antifungal therapy. Duration of treatment is based on resolution of the signs and symptoms of the lesions in conjunction with a significant decline in serum CF antibody titer. Such therapy routinely is continued for at least several years. Relapse occurs in 15–30% of individuals once therapy is discontinued.

Coccidioidal meningitis poses a special challenge. While most patients with this form of disease respond to treatment with oral triazoles, 80% experience relapse when therapy is stopped. Thus, lifelong therapy is recommended. In cases of triazole failure, intrathecal or intraventricular amphotericin B may be used. Installation requires considerable expertise and should be undertaken only by an experienced health care provider. Shunting of CSF in addition to appropriate antifungal therapy is required in cases of meningitis complicated by hydrocephalus. It is prudent to obtain expert consultation in all cases of coccidioidal meningitis.

PREVENTION

There are no proven methods to reduce the risk of acquiring coccidioidomycosis among residents of an endemic region, but avoidance of direct contact with uncultivated soil or with visible dust containing soil is reasonable. For individuals with suppressed cellular immunity, the risk of developing symptomatic coccidioidomycosis is greater than that in the general population. Among those about to undergo allogeneic solid-organ transplantation, antifungal therapy is appropriate when there is evidence of active or recent coccidioidomycosis. Several cases of donor-transmitted coccidioidomycosis have occurred during transplantation. If possible, donors from an endemic region should be screened for coccidioidomycosis before transplantation. Data on the use of antifungal agents for prophylaxis in other situations are limited. The administration of an antifungal drug to prevent symptomatic coccidioidomycosis is not recommended for HIV-1-infected patients who live in an endemic region. Most experts would administer a triazole to patients with a history of active coccidioidomycosis or a positive coccidioidal serology in whom therapy with tumor necrosis factor α antagonists is being initiated.

238 Blastomycosis

Donna C. Sullivan, Rathel L. Nolan, III

Blastomycosis is a systemic pyogranulomatous infection, involving primarily the lungs, that follows inhalation of the conidia of *Blastomyces dermatitidis*. Pulmonary blastomycosis varies from an asymptomatic infection to acute or chronic pneumonia. Hematogenous dissemination to skin, bones, and the genitourinary system is common; however, almost any organ can be involved.

ETIOLOGIC AGENT

B. dermatitidis is the asexual state of *Ajellomyces dermatitidis*. Two serotypes have been identified on the basis of the presence or absence of the A antigen. Distinct genotypic groups have been differentiated by rDNA polymerase chain reaction restriction fragment length polymorphisms and microsatellite markers. *B. dermatitidis* exhibits thermal dimorphism, growing as the mycelial phase at room temperature and as the yeast phase at 37°C. Primary isolation in the laboratory is most dependable for the mycelial phase incubated at 30°C. Definitive identification usually requires conversion to the yeast phase at 37°C or—now more commonly—the use of nucleic acid amplification techniques that detect mycelial-phase growth. Under the microscope, the yeast cells are usually 8–15 μm in diameter, have thick refractile cell walls, are multinucleate, and exhibit a single, large, broad-based bud (Fig. 238-1).

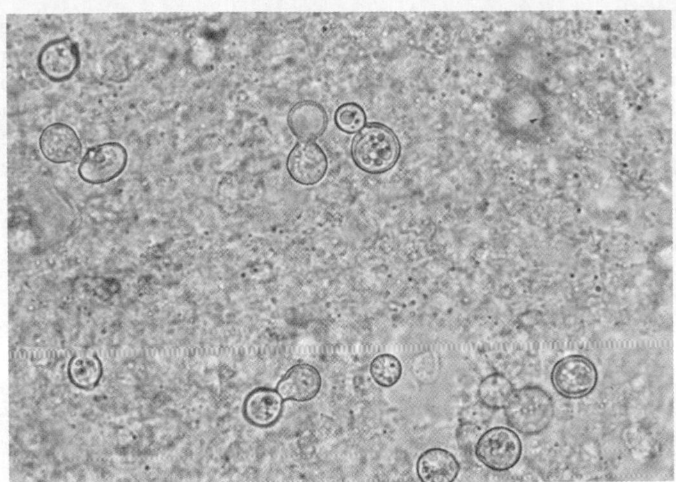

FIGURE 238-1 *Blastomyces dermatitidis* broad-based budding yeast in the aspirate of a chest wall abscess. Note the presence of multiple nuclei, the thickened cell wall, and the broad-based bud.

EPIDEMIOLOGY

Most cases of blastomycosis have been reported in North America. Endemic areas include the southeastern and south-central states bordering the Mississippi and Ohio river basins, the midwestern states, and the Canadian provinces bordering the Great Lakes. A small endemic area exists in New York and Canada along the St. Lawrence River. Acute blastomycosis is typically found only in North America, and the clinical presentation of blastomycosis in nonendemic areas is as a chronic disease.

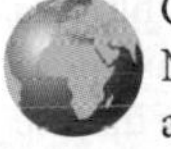

Outside North America, blastomycosis occurs sporadically in Nigeria, Zimbabwe, Tunisia, Saudi Arabia, Israel, Lebanon, and India. The disease has been reported most frequently in Africa.

Early studies indicated that middle-aged men with outdoor occupations were at greatest risk. Reported outbreaks, however, do not suggest a predilection according to sex, age, race, occupation, or season. The specific niche in nature in which the organism resides remains uncertain; *B. dermatitidis* probably grows as microfoci in the warm, moist soil of wooded areas rich in organic debris. Inhalation of conidia following exposure to soil, whether related to work or recreation, appears to be the common factor associated with infection. Outbreaks of human disease may be preceded by the occurrence of disease in simultaneously exposed dogs. Zoonotic transmission is rare but has been reported in association with dog bites, pet kinkajou bites, cat scratches, and animal necropsies.

PATHOGENESIS

Alveolar macrophages and polymorphonuclear leukocytes are critical for phagocytosis and killing of the inhaled conidia of *B. dermatitidis*. The interaction of these mediators of the innate immune response with local host factors, such as lung surfactant, plays a significant role in inhibiting conversion to the pathogenic yeast form. This inhibition prevents the establishment of symptomatic disease and may account for the high frequency of asymptomatic infections in outbreaks. Once conversion to the thick-walled yeast form has occurred, phagocytosis and killing are much more difficult, and the development of clinically apparent infection is much more likely. Ultimately, the T lymphocyte response—specifically, a T_H1 response—is the primary factor in limiting infection and dissemination. Moreover, yeast-phase conversion results in the expression of yeast phase–specific proteins such as the 120-kDa glycoprotein adhesin BAD-1 and the *Blastomyces* yeast phase–specific protein 1 (BYS1). BAD-1 has been well characterized as a virulence factor and is the major epitope for humoral and cellular immunity. The role of BYS1, putatively identified as a signal peptide, has not been determined.

APPROACH TO THE PATIENT: Blastomycosis

Blastomycosis most commonly presents as acute or chronic pneumonia that has been refractory to therapy with antibacterial drugs. Whether acute or chronic, blastomycosis may mimic many other disease processes. For example, acute pulmonary blastomycosis may present with signs and symptoms indistinguishable from those of bacterial pneumonia or influenza, and chronic pulmonary blastomycosis may mimic malignancy or tuberculosis. Skin lesions are often misdiagnosed as basal cell or squamous cell carcinoma, pyoderma gangrenosum, or keratoacanthoma. Laryngeal lesions are frequently mistaken for squamous cell carcinoma. Thus, the clinician must maintain a high index of suspicion and ensure that secretions or biopsy materials from patients who live in or have visited regions endemic for blastomycosis are subjected to careful histologic evaluation. This diligence is especially important in caring for individuals with pneumonia who fail to respond to treatment with antibacterial agents.

CLINICAL MANIFESTATIONS

Acute pulmonary infection is often diagnosed in association with point-source outbreaks. Typical symptoms include the abrupt onset of fever, chills, pleuritic chest pain, arthralgias, and myalgias. Cough is initially nonproductive but frequently becomes purulent as disease progresses. Chest radiographs usually reveal alveolar infiltrates with consolidation. Pleural effusions and hilar adenopathy are uncommon. Most patients diagnosed with pulmonary blastomycosis have chronic indolent pneumonia with signs and symptoms of fever, weight loss, productive cough, and hemoptysis. The most common radiologic findings are alveolar infiltrates with or without cavitation, mass lesions that mimic bronchogenic carcinoma, and fibronodular infiltrates. Hematogenous dissemination to the skin, bones, and genitourinary tract occurs most often in association with chronic pulmonary disease. Although blastomycosis is not considered an opportunistic infection, immunosuppression has been recognized as a risk factor for more serious pulmonary involvement, including respiratory failure (adult respiratory distress syndrome) associated with miliary disease or diffuse pulmonary infiltrates. In the late stages of AIDS, mortality rates of ≥50% have been documented. Most deaths occur within the first few days of therapy. Solid-organ transplant recipients with endemic fungal infections, including both histoplasmosis and blastomycosis, frequently have more severe pulmonary disease as well as dissemination. Blastomycosis has been associated with a mortality rate of 36% in these patients.

In Africa, pulmonary cases typically include bony involvement (frequently of the vertebrae), with subcutaneous abscesses of the chest wall or legs. All of the manifestations seen in African patients fall within the spectrum of blastomycosis observed in North America. The increased prevalence of chronic and disseminated bone disease in these patients may reflect a delay in diagnosis in regions where spinal disease is often treated empirically as tuberculosis.

Skin disease is the most common extrapulmonary manifestation of blastomycosis. Two types of skin lesions occur: verrucous (more common) and ulcerative. Osteomyelitis occurs in as many as one-fourth of *B. dermatitidis* infections. The vertebrae, pelvis, sacrum, skull, ribs, and long bones are most frequently involved. Patients with *B. dermatitidis* osteomyelitis often present with contiguous soft-tissue abscesses or chronic draining sinuses. In men, blastomycosis may involve the prostate and epididymis. Central nervous system (CNS) disease occurs in fewer than 5% of immunocompetent patients with blastomycosis. A recent multicenter review identified 22 patients with CNS disease, of whom 12 (54%) met at least one criterion for immunosuppression; although most cases of CNS blastomycosis are associated with infection at other sites, 22.7% of the reviewed cases had only CNS involvement. CNS disease, usually presenting as a brain abscess, has been reported in ~40% of cases in patients with AIDS. Less common forms of CNS disease are cranial or spinal epidural abscess and meningitis.

DIAGNOSIS

Definitive diagnosis of blastomycosis requires growth of the organism from sputum, bronchial washings, pus, or biopsy material. Specimens should be inoculated onto a fungal medium such as Sabouraud dextrose agar, with or without chloramphenicol. *B. dermatitidis* is generally visible in 5–10 days but may require incubation for up to 30 days if only a few organisms are present in the specimen. A presumptive diagnosis may be based on demonstration of the characteristic broad-based budding yeast by microscopic examination of wet preps of sputum in pneumonia or of skin-lesion scrapings. Serologic testing for antibodies to *B. dermatitidis* by complement fixation, immunodiffusion, or enzyme immunoassay is of little value for diagnosis because of limited sensitivity and specificity as well as cross-reactivity with other fungal antigens.

A *Blastomyces* antigen assay that detects antigen in urine and serum is commercially available and is reasonably sensitive and specific (MiraVista Diagnostics, Indianapolis, IN). Antigen detection appears to be more sensitive in urine than in serum. This antigen test may be useful for monitoring of patients during therapy or for early detection of relapse. Chemiluminescent DNA probes (AccuProbe; GenProbe Inc., San Diego, CA) are commonly used to confirm identification of *B. dermatitidis* once growth has been detected in culture. Repetitive sequence–based PCR is available (DiversiLab System; bioMérieux, Durham, NC). Molecular identification techniques are currently used only to supplement traditional diagnostic methods.

TREATMENT BLASTOMYCOSIS

The Infectious Diseases Society of America has published guidelines for the treatment of blastomycosis. Selection of an appropriate therapeutic regimen must be based on the clinical form and severity of the disease, the immune status of the patient, and the toxicity of the antifungal agent (Table 238-1). Although spontaneous cures of acute pulmonary infection are well documented, there are no criteria by which to distinguish patients whose disease will progress or resolve without treatment. Thus all patients with blastomycosis should be treated.

Itraconazole is the agent of choice for immunocompetent patients with mild to moderate pulmonary or non-CNS extrapulmonary disease. Therapy is continued for 6–12 months. Amphotericin B (AmB) is the preferred initial treatment for patients who are severely immunocompromised, who have life-threatening disease or CNS disease, or whose disease progresses during treatment with itraconazole. Although not rigorously studied, lipid formulations of AmB provide an alternative for patients who cannot tolerate AmB deoxycholate. Most patients with non-CNS disease whose clinical condition improves after an initial course of AmB (usually 2 weeks in duration) can be switched to itraconazole to complete 6–12 months of therapy. Fluconazole, because of its excellent penetration of the CNS, is useful in the treatment of patients with brain abscess or meningitis after an initial course of AmB.

Voriconazole has been used successfully to treat refractory blastomycosis, blastomycosis in immunosuppressed patients, and—given

TABLE 238-1 TREATMENT OF BLASTOMYCOSIS[a]

Disease	Primary Therapy	Alternative Therapy
Immunocompetent Patient/Life-Threatening Disease		
Pulmonary	Lipid AmB, 3–5 mg/kg qd, *or* AmB deoxycholate, 0.7–1.0 mg/kg qd (total dose: 1.5–2.5 g)	Itraconazole, 200–400 mg/d (once patient's condition has stabilized)
Disseminated		
CNS	Lipid AmB, 3–5 mg/kg qd, *or* AmB deoxycholate, 0.7–1.0 mg/kg qd (total dose: at least 2 g)	Fluconazole, 800 mg/d (if patient is intolerant to full course of AmB)
Non-CNS	Lipid AmB, 3–5 mg/kg qd, *or* AmB deoxycholate, 0.7–1.0 mg/kg qd (total dose: 1.5–2.5 g)	Itraconazole, 200–400 mg/d (once patient's condition has stabilized)
Immunocompetent Patient/Non-Life-Threatening Disease		
Pulmonary or disseminated (non-CNS)	Itraconazole, 200–400 mg/d, *or* Lipid AmB, 3–5 mg/kg qd, *or* AmB deoxycholate, 0.5–0.7 mg/kg qd (in patients intolerant to itraconazole or whose disease progresses despite therapy)	Fluconazole, 400–800 mg/d, *or* Ketoconazole, 400–800 mg/d
Immunocompromised Patient[b]		
All infections	Lipid AmB, 3–5 mg/kg qd, *or* AmB deoxycholate, 0.7–1.0 mg/kg qd (total dose: 1.5–2.5 g)	Itraconazole, 200–400 mg/d (non-CNS disease, once clinically improved)

[a]Therapy is generally given for 6–12 months. For bone and joint disease, a 12-month course is usually necessary. [b]Suppressive therapy with itraconazole may be considered for patients whose immunocompromised state continues. Fluconazole (800 mg/d) may be useful for patients who have CNS disease or cannot tolerate itraconazole.

Abbreviations: AmB, amphotericin B; CNS, central nervous system.

its good penetration of cerebrospinal fluid—CNS disease. Posaconazole has also been used for refractory pulmonary disease. The echinocandins have variable activity against *B. dermatitidis* and therefore are not used in the treatment of blastomycosis.

PROGNOSIS

Cure rates are 90–95% among compliant immunocompetent patients given itraconazole for mild to moderate pulmonary and extrapulmonary disease without CNS involvement. Bone and joint disease usually requires 12 months of therapy. The fewer than 5% of infections that relapse after an initial course of itraconazole usually respond well to a second treatment course.

ACKNOWLEDGMENT

The authors thank Dr. Stanley W. Chapman, Professor Emeritus, University of Mississippi, for his continued help and support and for his contributions to this chapter in an earlier edition.

239 Cryptococcosis

Arturo Casadevall

DEFINITION AND ETIOLOGY

Cryptococcus, a genus of yeast-like fungi, is the etiologic agent of cryptococcosis. Both species, *C. neoformans* and *C. gattii,* can cause cryptococcosis in humans. The two varieties of *C. neoformans—grubii* and *neoformans*—correlate with serotypes A and D, respectively. *C. gattii,* although not divided into varieties, also is antigenically diverse, encompassing serotypes B and C. Most clinical microbiology laboratories do not routinely distinguish between *C. neoformans* and *C. gattii,* or among varieties, but rather identify and report all isolates simply as *C. neoformans.*

EPIDEMIOLOGY

Cryptococcosis was first described in the 1890s but remained relatively rare until the mid-twentieth century, when advances in diagnosis and increases in the number of immunosuppressed individuals markedly raised its reported prevalence. Although serologic evidence of cryptococcal *infection* is common among immunocompetent individuals, cryptococcal *disease* (cryptococcosis) is relatively rare in the absence of impaired immunity. Individuals at high risk for disease due to *C. neoformans* include patients with hematologic malignancies, recipients of solid organ transplants who require ongoing immunosuppressive therapy, persons whose medical conditions necessitate glucocorticoid therapy, and patients with advanced HIV infection and CD4+ T lymphocyte counts of <200/μL. In contrast, *C. gattii*–related disease is not associated with specific immune deficits and often occurs in immunocompetent individuals.

Cryptococcal infection is acquired from the environment. *C. neoformans* and *C. gattii* inhabit different ecologic niches. *C. neoformans* is frequently found in soils contaminated with avian excreta and can easily be recovered from shaded and humid soils contaminated with pigeon droppings. In contrast, *C. gattii* is not found in bird feces. Instead, it inhabits a variety of arboreal species, including several types of eucalyptus tree. *C. neoformans* strains are found throughout the world; however, var. *grubii* (serotype A) strains are far more common than var. *neoformans* (serotype D) strains among both clinical and environmental isolates. The geographic distribution of *C. gattii* was thought to be largely limited to tropical regions until an outbreak of cryptococcosis caused by a new serotype B strain began in Vancouver in 1999. This outbreak has extended into the United States, and *C. gattii* infections are being encountered increasingly in several states in the Pacific Northwest.

The global burden of cryptococcosis was recently estimated at ~1 million cases, with >600,000 deaths annually. Thus cryptococci are important human pathogens. Since the onset of the HIV pandemic in the early 1980s, the overwhelming majority of cryptococcosis cases have occurred in patients with AIDS (Chap. 226). To comprehend the impact of HIV infection on the epidemiology of cryptococcosis, it is instructive to note that in the early 1990s there were >1000 cases of cryptococcal meningitis each year in New York City—a figure far exceeding that for all cases of bacterial meningitis. With the advent of effective antiretroviral therapy, the incidence of AIDS-related cryptococcosis has been sharply reduced among treated individuals. Thus most cases of cryptococcosis now occur in resource-limited regions of the world. The disease remains distressingly common in regions where antiretroviral therapy is not readily available (e.g., parts of Africa and Asia); in these regions, up to one-third of patients with AIDS have cryptococcosis. Among HIV-infected persons, those with a decreased percentage of memory B cells expressing IgM may be at greater risk for cryptococcosis.

PATHOGENESIS

Cryptococcal infection is acquired by inhalation of aerosolized infectious particles. The exact nature of these particles is not known; the two leading candidate forms are small desiccated yeast cells and basidiospores. Little is known about the pathogenesis of initial infection. Serologic studies have shown that cryptococcal infection is acquired in childhood, but it is not known whether the initial infection is symptomatic. Given that cryptococcal infection is common while disease is rare, the consensus is that pulmonary defense mechanisms in immunologically intact individuals are highly effective at containing this fungus. It is not clear whether initial infection leads to a state of immunity or whether most individuals are subject throughout life to frequent and recurrent infections that resolve without clinical disease. However, evidence indicates that some human cryptococcal infections lead to a state of latency in which viable organisms are harbored for prolonged periods, possibly in granulomas. Thus the inhalation of cryptococcal cells and/or spores can be followed by either clearance or establishment of the latent state. The consequences of prolonged harboring of cryptococcal cells in the lung are not known, but evidence from animal studies indicates that the organisms' prolonged presence could alter the immunologic milieu in the lung and predispose to allergic airway disease.

Cryptococcosis usually presents clinically as chronic meningoencephalitis. The mechanisms by which the fungus undergoes extrapulmonary dissemination and enters the central nervous system (CNS) remain poorly understood. The mechanism by which cryptococcal cells cross the blood–brain barrier is a subject of intensive study. Current evidence suggests that both direct fungal-cell migration across the endothelium and fungal-cell carriage inside macrophages as "Trojan horse" invaders can occur. *Cryptococcus* species have well-defined virulence factors that include the expression of the polysaccharide capsule, the ability to make melanin, and the elaboration of enzymes (e.g., phospholipase and urease) that enhance the survival of fungal cells in tissue. Among these virulence factors, the capsule and melanin production have been most extensively studied. The cryptococcal capsule is antiphagocytic, and the capsular polysaccharide has been associated with numerous deleterious effects on host immune function. Cryptococcal infections can elicit little or no tissue inflammatory response. The immune dysfunction seen in cryptococcosis has been attributed to the release of copious amounts of capsular polysaccharide into tissues, where it probably interferes with local immune responses (Fig. 239-1). In clinical practice, the capsular polysaccharide is the antigen that is measured as a diagnostic marker of cryptococcal infection.

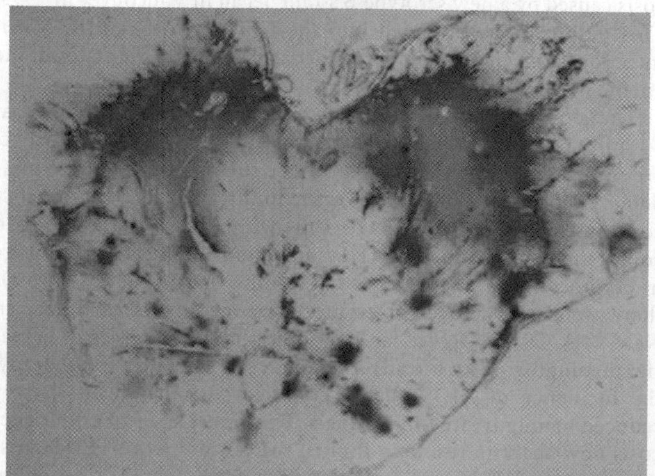

FIGURE 239-1 Cryptococcal antigen in human brain tissue, as revealed by immunohistochemical staining. Brown areas show polysaccharide deposits in the midbrain of a patient who died of cryptococcal meningitis. *(Reprinted with permission from SC Lee et al: Hum Pathol 27:839, 1996.)*

APPROACH TO THE PATIENT: Cryptococcosis

Cryptococcosis should be included in the differential diagnosis when any patient presents with findings suggestive of chronic meningitis. Concern about cryptococcosis is heightened by a history of headache and neurologic symptoms in a patient with an underlying immunosuppressive disorder or state that is associated with an increased incidence of cryptococcosis, such as advanced HIV infection or solid organ transplantation.

CLINICAL MANIFESTATIONS

The clinical manifestations of cryptococcosis reflect the site of fungal infection. The spectrum of disease caused by *Cryptococcus* species consists predominantly of meningoencephalitis and pneumonia, but skin and soft tissue infections also occur; in fact, cryptococcosis can affect any tissue or organ. CNS involvement usually presents as signs and symptoms of chronic meningitis, such as headache, fever, lethargy, sensory deficits, memory deficits, cranial nerve paresis, vision deficits, and meningismus. Cryptococcal meningitis differs from bacterial meningitis in that many *Cryptococcus*-infected patients present with symptoms of several weeks' duration. In addition, classic characteristics of meningeal irritation, such as meningismus, may be absent in cryptococcal meningitis. Indolent cases can present as subacute dementia. Meningeal cryptococcosis can lead to sudden catastrophic vision loss.

Pulmonary cryptococcosis usually presents as cough, increased sputum production, and chest pain. Patients infected with *C. gattii* can present with granulomatous pulmonary masses known as *cryptococcomas*. Fever develops in a minority of cases. Like CNS disease, pulmonary cryptococcosis can follow an indolent course, and the majority of cases probably do not come to clinical attention. In fact, many cases are discovered incidentally during the workup of an abnormal chest radiograph obtained for other diagnostic purposes. Pulmonary cryptococcosis can be associated with antecedent diseases such as malignancy, diabetes, and tuberculosis.

Skin lesions are common in patients with disseminated cryptococcosis and can be highly variable, including papules, plaques, purpura, vesicles, tumor-like lesions, and rashes. The spectrum of cryptococcosis in HIV-infected patients is so varied and has changed so much since the advent of antiretroviral therapy that a distinction between HIV-related and HIV-unrelated cryptococcosis is no longer pertinent. In patients with AIDS and solid organ transplant recipients, the lesions of cutaneous cryptococcosis often resemble those of molluscum contagiosum (Fig. 239-2; Chap. 220e).

DIAGNOSIS

A diagnosis of cryptococcosis requires the demonstration of yeast cells in normally sterile tissues. Visualization of the capsule of fungal cells in cerebrospinal fluid (CSF) mixed with India ink is a useful rapid diagnostic technique. Cryptococcal cells in India ink have a distinctive appearance because their capsules exclude ink particles. However, the CSF India ink examination may yield negative results in patients with a low fungal burden. This examination should be performed by a trained individual, since leukocytes and fat globules can sometimes be mistaken for fungal cells. Cultures of CSF and blood that are positive for cryptococcal cells are diagnostic for cryptococcosis. In cryptococcal meningitis, CSF examination usually reveals evidence of chronic meningitis with mononuclear cell pleocytosis and increased protein levels. A particularly useful test is cryptococcal antigen (CRAg) detection in CSF and blood. The assay is based on serologic detection of cryptococcal polysaccharide and is both sensitive and specific. A positive CRAg test provides strong presumptive evidence for cryptococcosis; however, because the result is often negative in pulmonary cryptococcosis, the test is less useful in the diagnosis of pulmonary disease and is of only limited usefulness in monitoring the response to therapy.

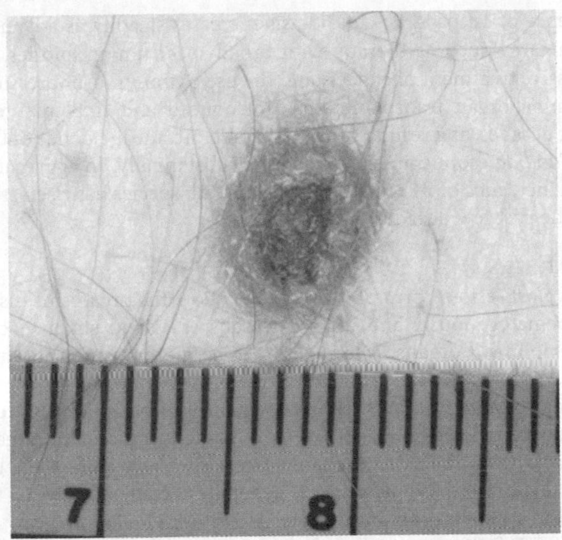

FIGURE 239-2 Disseminated fungal infection. A liver transplant recipient developed six cutaneous lesions similar to the one shown. Biopsy and serum antigen testing demonstrated *Cryptococcus*. Important features of the lesion include a benign-appearing fleshy papule with central umbilication resembling molluscum contagiosum. *(Photo courtesy of Dr. Lindsey Baden; with permission.)*

In areas of Africa where there is a high prevalence of HIV infection, routine screening of blood for CRAg in HIV-infected patients with low CD4+ T lymphocyte counts may identify individuals at high risk of cryptococcal disease who are candidates for antifungal therapy. Similarly, CRAg screening has shown that a significant proportion of HIV-infected patients hospitalized with pneumonia in Thailand harbor cryptococcal infection. Inexpensive point-of-care CRAg tests that are under development could be of great diagnostic benefit in resource-limited regions.

TREATMENT CRYPTOCOCCOSIS

Both the site of infection and the immune status of the host must be considered in the selection of therapy for cryptococcosis. The disease has two general patterns of manifestation: (1) pulmonary cryptococcosis, with no evidence of extrapulmonary dissemination; and (2) extrapulmonary (systemic) cryptococcosis, with or without meningoencephalitis. Pulmonary cryptococcosis in an immunocompetent host sometimes resolves without therapy. However, given the propensity of *Cryptococcus* species to disseminate from the lung, the inability to gauge the host's immune status precisely, and the availability of low-toxicity therapy in the form of fluconazole, the current recommendation is for pulmonary cryptococcosis in an immunocompetent individual to be treated with fluconazole (200 400 mg/d for 3–6 months). Extrapulmonary cryptococcosis without CNS involvement in an immunocompetent host can be treated with the same regimen, although amphotericin B (AmB; 0.5–1 mg/kg daily for 4–6 weeks) may be required for more severe cases. In general, extrapulmonary cryptococcosis without CNS involvement requires less intensive therapy, with the caveat that morbidity and death in cryptococcosis are associated with meningeal involvement. Thus the decision to categorize cryptococcosis as "extrapulmonary without CNS involvement" should be made only after careful evaluation of the CSF reveals no evidence of cryptococcal infection. For CNS involvement in a host without AIDS or obvious immune impairment, most authorities recommend initial therapy with AmB (0.5–1 mg/kg daily) during an induction phase, which is followed by prolonged therapy with fluconazole (400 mg/d) during a consolidation phase. For cryptococcal meningoencephalitis without a concomitant immunosuppressive condition, the recommended regimen is AmB (0.5–1 mg/kg) plus flucytosine (100 mg/kg) daily for 6–10 weeks. Alternatively, patients can be treated with AmB (0.5–1 mg/kg) plus flucytosine (100 mg/kg) daily for 2 weeks and then with fluconazole (400 mg/d) for at least 10 weeks. Patients with immunosuppression are treated with the same initial regimens except that consolidation therapy with fluconazole is given for a prolonged period to prevent relapse.

Cryptococcosis in patients with HIV infection always requires aggressive therapy and is considered incurable unless immune function improves. Consequently, therapy for cryptococcosis in the setting of AIDS has two phases: induction therapy (intended to reduce the fungal burden and alleviate symptoms) and lifelong maintenance therapy (to prevent a symptomatic clinical relapse). Pulmonary and extrapulmonary cryptococcosis without evidence of CNS involvement can be treated with fluconazole (200–400 mg/d). In patients who have more extensive disease, flucytosine (100 mg/kg per day) may be added to the fluconazole regimen for 10 weeks, with lifelong fluconazole maintenance therapy thereafter. For HIV-infected patients with evidence of CNS involvement, most authorities recommend induction therapy with AmB. An acceptable regimen is AmB (0.7–1 mg/kg) plus flucytosine (100 mg/kg) daily for 2 weeks followed by fluconazole (400 mg/d) for at least 10 weeks and then by lifelong maintenance therapy with fluconazole (200 mg/d). Fluconazole (400–800 mg/d) plus flucytosine (100 mg/kg per day) for 6–10 weeks followed by fluconazole (200 mg/d) as maintenance therapy is an alternative. Newer triazoles like voriconazole and posaconazole are highly active against cryptococcal strains and appear effective clinically, but clinical experience with these agents in the treatment of cryptococcosis is limited. Lipid formulations of AmB can be substituted for AmB deoxycholate in patients with renal impairment. Neither caspofungin nor micafungin is effective against *Cryptococcus* species; consequently, neither drug has a role in the treatment of cryptococcosis. Cryptococcal meningoencephalitis is often associated with increased intracranial pressure, which is believed to be responsible for damage to the brain and cranial nerves. Appropriate management of CNS cryptococcosis requires careful attention to the management of intracranial pressure, including the reduction of pressure by repeated therapeutic lumbar puncture and the placement of shunts. Recent studies suggest that the addition of a short course of interferon γ to antifungal therapy in patients with HIV infection increases clearance of cryptococci from the CSF.

In HIV-infected patients with previously treated cryptococcosis who are receiving fluconazole maintenance therapy, it may be possible to discontinue antifungal drug treatment if antiretroviral therapy results in immunologic improvement. However, certain recipients of maintenance therapy who have a history of successfully treated cryptococcosis can develop a troublesome immune reconstitution syndrome when antiretroviral therapy produces a rebound in immunologic function.

PROGNOSIS AND COMPLICATIONS

Even with antifungal therapy, cryptococcosis is associated with high rates of morbidity and death. For the majority of patients with cryptococcosis, the most important prognostic factors are the extent and the duration of the underlying immunologic deficits that predisposed them to develop the disease. Therefore, cryptococcosis is often curable with antifungal therapy in individuals with no apparent immunologic dysfunction, but, in patients with severe immunosuppression (e.g., those with AIDS), the best that can be hoped for is that antifungal therapy will induce remission, which can then be maintained with lifelong suppressive therapy. Before the advent of antiretroviral therapy, the median overall survival period for AIDS patients with cryptococcosis was <1 year. Cryptococcosis in patients with underlying neoplastic disease has a particularly poor prognosis. For CNS cryptococcosis, poor prognostic markers are a CSF assay positive for yeast cells on initial India ink examination (evidence of a heavy fungal burden), high CSF pressure, low CSF glucose levels, low CSF pleocytosis (<2/μL), recovery of yeast cells from extraneural sites, absence of antibody to capsular polysaccharide, a CSF or serum cryptococcal antigen level of ≥1:32, and concomitant glucocorticoid therapy or hematologic malignancy. A response to treatment does not guarantee cure since relapse of cryptococcosis is common even among patients with relatively intact immune systems. Complications of CNS cryptococcosis include cranial nerve deficits, vision loss, and cognitive impairment.

PREVENTION

No vaccine is available for cryptococcosis. In patients at high risk (e.g., those with advanced HIV infection and CD4+ T lymphocyte counts of <200/μL), primary prophylaxis with fluconazole (200 mg/d) is effective in reducing the prevalence of disease. Since antiretroviral therapy raises the CD4+ T lymphocyte count, it constitutes an immunologic form of prophylaxis. However, cryptococcosis in the setting of immune reconstitution has been reported in patients with HIV infection and in recipients of solid organ transplants.

240 Candidiasis

John E. Edwards, Jr.

The genus *Candida* encompasses more than 150 species, only a few of which cause disease in humans. With rare exceptions (although the exceptions are increasing in number), the human pathogens are *C. albicans, C. guilliermondii, C. krusei, C. parapsilosis, C. tropicalis, C. kefyr, C. lusitaniae, C. dubliniensis,* and *C. glabrata.* Ubiquitous in nature, they inhabit the gastrointestinal tract (including the mouth and oropharynx), the female genital tract, and the skin. Although cases of candidiasis have been described since antiquity in debilitated patients, the advent of *Candida* species as common human pathogens dates to the introduction of modern therapeutic approaches that suppress normal host defense mechanisms. Of these relatively recent advances, the most important is the use of antibacterial agents that alter the normal human microbiota and allow nonbacterial species to become more prevalent in the commensal flora. With the introduction of antifungal agents, the causes of *Candida* infections shifted from an almost complete dominance of *C. albicans* to the common involvement of *C. glabrata* and the other species listed above. The non-*albicans* species now account for approximately half of all cases of candidemia and hematogenously disseminated candidiasis. Recognition of this change is clinically important, since the various species differ in susceptibility to the newer antifungal agents. In developed countries, where medical therapeutics are commonly used, *Candida* species are now among the most common nosocomial pathogens.

Candida is a small, thin-walled, ovoid yeast that measures 4–6 μm in diameter and reproduces by budding. Organisms of this genus occur in three forms in tissue: blastospores, pseudohyphae, and hyphae. *Candida* grows readily on simple medium; lysis centrifugation enhances its recovery from blood. Species are identified by biochemical testing (currently with automated devices) or on special agar (e.g., CHROMagar).

EPIDEMIOLOGY

Candida organisms are ubiquitous in nature; worldwide, these fungi are present in humans as commensals, in animals, in foods, and on inanimate objects. In developed countries, where advanced medical therapeutics are commonly used (see "Treatment," below), *Candida* species are now among the most common health care–associated pathogens. In the United States, these species are the fourth most common isolates from the blood of hospitalized patients. In countries where advanced medical care is rarely available, mucocutaneous *Candida* infections, such as thrush, are more common than deep organ infections, which rarely occur; however, the incidence of deep organ candidiasis increases steadily as advances in health care—such as therapy with broad-spectrum antibiotics, more aggressive treatment of cancer, and the use of immunosuppression for sustaining organ transplants—are introduced and implemented. In recent decades, as a result of the HIV epidemic, the incidence of thrush and *Candida* esophagitis has increased substantially. In aggregate, the global incidence of infections due to *Candida* species has risen steadily over the past few decades.

PATHOGENESIS

In the most serious form of *Candida* infection, the organisms disseminate hematogenously and form microabscesses and small macroabscesses in major organs. Although the exact mechanism is not known, *Candida* probably enters the bloodstream from mucosal surfaces after growing to large numbers as a consequence of bacterial suppression by antibacterial drugs; alternatively, in some instances, the organism may enter from the skin. A change from the blastospore stage to the pseudohyphal and hyphal stages is generally considered integral to the organism's penetration into tissue. However, *C. glabrata* can cause extensive infection even though it does not transform into pseudohyphae or hyphae. Adherence to both epithelial and endothelial cells, thought to be the first step in invasion and infection, has been studied extensively, and several adhesins have been identified. Biofilm formation also is considered important in pathogenesis. Numerous reviews of cases of hematogenously disseminated candidiasis have identified the predisposing factors or conditions associated with disseminated disease (Table 240-1). Women who receive antibacterial agents may develop vaginal candidiasis.

Innate immunity is the most important defense mechanism against hematogenously disseminated candidiasis, and the neutrophil is the most important component of this defense. Macrophages also play an important defensive role. STAT1, Dectin-1, CARD9, and T_H1 and T_H17 lymphocytes contribute significantly to innate defense (see "Clinical Manifestations," below). Although many immunocompetent individuals have antibodies to *Candida*, the role of these antibodies in defense against the organism is not clear. Multiple genetic polymorphisms that predispose to disseminated candidiasis will most likely be identified in future studies.

CLINICAL MANIFESTATIONS

Mucocutaneous Candidiasis *Thrush* is characterized by white, adherent, painless, discrete or confluent patches in the mouth, on the tongue, or in the esophagus, occasionally with fissuring at the corners of the mouth. This form of disease caused by *Candida* can also occur at points of contact with dentures. Organisms are identifiable in gram-stained scrapings from lesions. The occurrence of thrush in a young, otherwise healthy-appearing person should prompt an investigation for underlying HIV infection. More commonly, thrush is seen as a nonspecific manifestation of severe debilitating illness. Vulvovaginal candidiasis is accompanied by pruritus, pain, and vaginal discharge which is usually thin but may contain whitish "curds" in severe cases. A subset of patients with recurrent vulvovaginitis have a deficiency in the surface expression of Dectin-1, a major recognition factor for β-glucan on *Candida*. This deficiency leads to suboptimal functioning of the CARD9 pathway, which ultimately increases the propensity for recurrent vaginal infections.

TABLE 240-1 WELL-RECOGNIZED FACTORS AND CONDITIONS PREDISPOSING TO HEMATOGENOUSLY DISSEMINATED CANDIDIASIS

Antibacterial agents	Abdominal and thoracic surgery
Indwelling intravenous catheters	Cytotoxic chemotherapy
Hyperalimentation fluids	Immunosuppressive agents for organ transplantation
Indwelling urinary catheters	Respirators
Parenteral glucocorticoids	Neutropenia
Severe burns	Low birth weight (neonates)
HIV-associated low CD4+ T cell counts	Diabetes

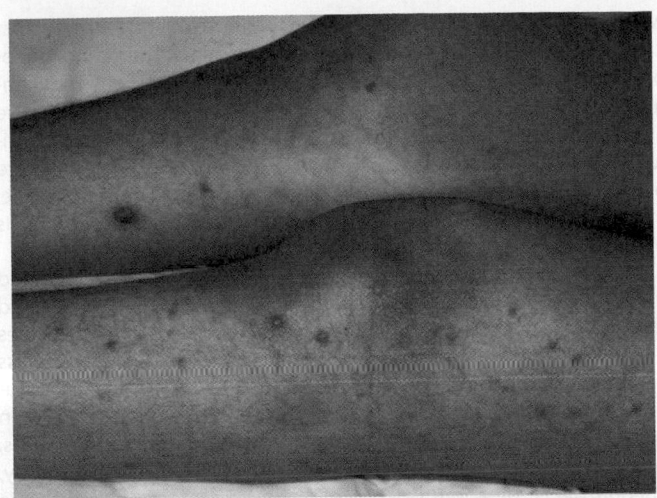

FIGURE 240-1 Macronodular skin lesions associated with hematogenously disseminated candidiasis. *Candida* organisms are usually but not always visible on histopathologic examination. The fungi grow when a portion of the biopsied specimen is cultured. Therefore, for optimal identification, both histopathology and culture should be performed. *(Image courtesy of Dr. Noah Craft and the Victor Newcomer collection at UCLA, archived by Logical Images, Inc.; with permission.)*

Other *Candida* skin infections include *paronychia*, a painful swelling at the nail-skin interface; *onychomycosis*, a fungal nail infection rarely caused by this genus; *intertrigo*, an erythematous irritation with redness and pustules in the skin folds; *balanitis*, an erythematous-pustular infection of the glans penis; *erosio interdigitalis blastomycetica*, an infection between the digits of the hands or toes; *folliculitis*, with pustules developing most frequently in the area of the beard; *perianal candidiasis*, a pruritic, erythematous, pustular infection surrounding the anus; and *diaper rash*, a common erythematous-pustular perineal infection in infants. *Generalized disseminated cutaneous candidiasis*, another form of infection that occurs primarily in infants, is characterized by widespread eruptions over the trunk, thorax, and extremities. The diagnostic macronodular lesions of hematogenously disseminated candidiasis (Fig. 240-1) indicate a high probability of dissemination to multiple organs as well as the skin. While the lesions are seen predominantly in immunocompromised patients treated with cytotoxic drugs, they may also develop in patients without neutropenia.

Chronic mucocutaneous candidiasis is a heterogeneous infection of the hair, nails, skin, and mucous membranes that persists despite intermittent therapy. The onset of disease usually comes in infancy or within the first two decades of life but in rare cases comes in later life. The condition may be mild and limited to a specific area of the skin or nails, or it may take a severely disfiguring form (*Candida* granuloma) characterized by exophytic outgrowths on the skin. Chronic mucocutaneous candidiasis is usually associated with specific immunologic dysfunction; most frequently reported is a failure of T lymphocytes to proliferate or to excrete cytokines in response to stimulation by *Candida* antigens in vitro. A subset of the affected patients have mutations in the STAT1 gene resulting in an insufficiency of interferon γ, interleukin 17, and interleukin 22.

Approximately half of patients with chronic mucocutaneous candidiasis have associated endocrine abnormalities that together are designated the *a*utoimmune *p*oly*e*ndocrinopathy–*c*andidiasis–*e*ctodermal *d*ystrophy (APECED) syndrome. This syndrome is due to mutations in the autoimmune regulator (*AIRE*) gene and is most prevalent among Finns, Iranian Jews, Sardinians, northern Italians, and Swedes. Conditions that usually follow the onset of the disease include hypoparathyroidism, adrenal insufficiency, autoimmune thyroiditis, Graves' disease, chronic active hepatitis, alopecia, juvenile-onset pernicious anemia, malabsorption, and primary hypogonadism. In addition, dental enamel dysplasia, vitiligo, pitted nail dystrophy, and calcification of the tympanic membranes may occur. Patients with chronic mucocutaneous candidiasis rarely develop hematogenously disseminated candidiasis, probably because their neutrophil function remains intact.

Deeply Invasive Candidiasis Deeply invasive *Candida* infections may or may not be due to hematogenous seeding. Deep esophageal infection may result from penetration by organisms from superficial esophageal erosions; joint or deep wound infection from contiguous spread of organisms from the skin; kidney infection from catheter-initiated spread of organisms through the urinary tract; infection of intraabdominal organs and the peritoneum from perforation of the gastrointestinal tract; and gallbladder infection from retrograde migration of organisms from the gastrointestinal tract into the biliary drainage system.

However, far more commonly, deeply invasive candidiasis results from hematogenous seeding of various organs as a complication of candidemia. Once the organism gains access to the intravascular compartment (either from the gastrointestinal tract or, less often, from the skin through the site of an indwelling intravascular catheter), it may spread hematogenously to a variety of deep organs. The brain, chorioretina (Fig. 240-2), heart, and kidneys are most commonly infected and the liver and spleen less commonly so (most often in neutropenic patients). In fact, nearly any organ can become involved, including the endocrine glands, pancreas, heart valves (native or prosthetic), skeletal muscle, joints (native or prosthetic), bone, and meninges. *Candida* organisms can also spread hematogenously to the skin and cause classic macronodular lesions (Fig. 240-1). Frequently, painful muscular involvement also is evident beneath the area of affected skin. Chorioretinal involvement and skin involvement are highly significant, since both findings are associated with a very high probability of abscess formation in multiple deep organs as a result of generalized hematogenous seeding. Ocular involvement (Fig. 240-2) may require specific treatment (e.g., partial vitrectomy or intraocular injection of antifungal agents) to prevent permanent blindness. An ocular examination is indicated for all patients with candidemia, whether or not they have ocular manifestations.

DIAGNOSIS

The diagnosis of *Candida* infection is established by visualization of pseudohyphae or hyphae on wet mount (saline and 10% KOH), tissue Gram's stain, periodic acid–Schiff stain, or methenamine silver stain in the presence of inflammation. Absence of organisms on hematoxylin-eosin staining does not reliably exclude *Candida* infection. The most

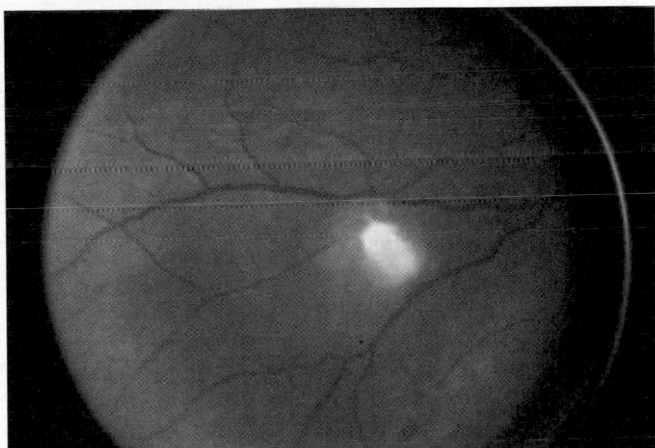

FIGURE 240-2 Hematogenous *Candida* endophthalmitis. A classic off-white lesion projecting from the chorioretina into the vitreous causes the surrounding haze. The lesion is composed primarily of inflammatory cells rather than organisms. Lesions of this type may progress to cause extensive vitreal inflammation and eventual loss of the eye. Partial vitrectomy, combined with IV and possibly intravitreal antifungal therapy, may be helpful in controlling the lesions. *(Image courtesy of Dr. Gary Holland; with permission.)*

TABLE 240-2 TREATMENT OF MUCOCUTANEOUS CANDIDAL INFECTIONS

Disease	Preferred Treatment	Alternatives
Cutaneous	Topical azole	Topical nystatin
Vulvovaginal	Oral fluconazole (150 mg) or azole cream or suppository	Nystatin suppository
Thrush	Clotrimazole troches	Nystatin, fluconazole
Esophageal	Fluconazole tablets (100–200 mg/d) or itraconazole solution (200 mg/d)	Caspofungin, micafungin, or amphotericin B

challenging aspect of diagnosis is determining which patients with *Candida* isolates have hematogenously disseminated candidiasis. For instance, recovery of *Candida* from sputum, urine, or peritoneal catheters may indicate mere colonization rather than deep-seated infection, and *Candida* isolation from the blood of patients with indwelling intravascular catheters may reflect inconsequential seeding of the blood from or growth of the organisms on the catheter. Despite extensive research into both antigen and antibody detection systems, there is currently no widely available and validated diagnostic test to distinguish patients with inconsequential seeding of the blood from those whose positive blood cultures represent hematogenous dissemination to multiple organs. Many studies are under way to establish the utility of the β-glucan test; at present, its greatest utility is its negative predictive value (~90%). Meanwhile, the presence of ocular or macronodular skin lesions is highly suggestive of widespread infection of multiple deep organs. Although extensive research is being conducted on other tests for infection, such as PCR, none of these tests is fully validated or widely available at present.

TREATMENT *CANDIDA* INFECTIONS

MUCOCUTANEOUS *CANDIDA* INFECTION

The treatment of mucocutaneous candidiasis is summarized in **Table 240-2**.

CANDIDEMIA AND SUSPECTED HEMATOGENOUSLY DISSEMINATED CANDIDIASIS

All patients with candidemia are treated with a systemic antifungal agent. A certain percentage of patients, including many of those who have candidemia associated with an indwelling intravascular catheter, probably have "benign" candidemia rather than deep-organ seeding. However, because there is no reliable way to distinguish benign candidemia from deep-organ infection, and because antifungal drugs less toxic than amphotericin B are available, antifungal treatment for candidemia—with or without clinical evidence of deep-organ involvement—has become the standard of practice. In addition, if an indwelling intravascular catheter is present, it is best to remove or replace the device whenever feasible.

The drugs used for the treatment of candidemia and suspected disseminated candidiasis are listed in **Table 240-3**. Various lipid formulations of amphotericin B, three echinocandins, and the azoles fluconazole and voriconazole are used; no agent within a given class has been clearly identified as superior to the others. Most institutions choose an agent from each class on the basis of their own specific microbial epidemiology, strategies to minimize toxicities, and cost considerations. Unless azole resistance is considered likely, fluconazole is the agent of choice for the treatment of candidemia and suspected disseminated candidiasis in nonneutropenic, hemodynamically stable patients. Initial treatment in the context of likely azole resistance depends, as mentioned above, on the epidemiology of the individual hospital. For example, certain hospitals have a high rate of recovery of *C. glabrata*, while others do not. At institutions where non-*albicans Candida* species are frequently recovered, therapy with an echinocandin is typically started while the results of sensitivity testing are awaited. For hemodynamically unstable or neutropenic patients, initial treatment with broader-spectrum agents is desirable; these drugs include polyenes, echinocandins, or later-generation azoles such as voriconazole. Once the clinical response has been assessed and the pathogen specifically identified, the regimen can be altered accordingly. At present, the vast majority of *C. albicans* isolates are sensitive to fluconazole. Isolates of *C. glabrata* and *C. krusei* are less sensitive to fluconazole and more sensitive to polyenes and echinocandins. *C. parapsilosis* is less sensitive to echinocandins in vitro; however, this lesser sensitivity is considered nonsignificant.

Some generalizations exist regarding the management of specific *Candida* infections. Recovery of *Candida* from sputum is almost never indicative of underlying pulmonary candidiasis and does not by itself warrant antifungal treatment. Similarly, *Candida* in the urine of a patient with an indwelling bladder catheter may represent colonization only rather than bladder or kidney infection; however, the threshold for systemic treatment is lower in severely ill patients in

TABLE 240-3 AGENTS FOR THE TREATMENT OF DISSEMINATED CANDIDIASIS

Agent	Route of Administration	Dose[a]	Comment
Amphotericin B deoxycholate	IV only	0.5–1.0 mg/kg daily	Being replaced by lipid formulations
Amphotericin B lipid formulations			Not FDA approved as primary therapy, but used commonly because less toxic than amphotericin B deoxycholate
Liposomal (AmBiSome, Abelcet)	IV only	3.0–5.0 mg/kg daily	
Lipid complex (ABLC)	IV only	3.0–5.0 mg/kg daily	
Colloidal dispersion (ABCD)	IV only	3.0–5.0 mg/kg daily	Associated with frequent infusion reactions
Azoles[b]			
Fluconazole	IV and oral	400 mg/d	Most commonly used
Voriconazole	IV and oral	400 mg/d	Multiple drug interactions Approved for candidemia in nonneutropenic patients
Echinocandins			Broad spectrum against *Candida* species; approved for disseminated candidiasis
Caspofungin	IV only	50 mg/d	
Anidulafungin	IV only	100 mg/d	
Micafungin	IV only	100 mg/d	

[a]For loading doses and adjustments in renal failure, see Pappas PG et al: Clinical practice guidelines for the management of candidiasis: 2009 update by the Infectious Diseases Society of America. Clin Infect Dis 48:503, 2009. The recommended duration of therapy is 2 weeks beyond the last positive blood culture and the resolution of signs and symptoms of infection. [b]Although ketoconazole is approved for the treatment of disseminated candidiasis, it has been replaced by the newer agents listed in this table. Posaconazole has been approved for prophylaxis in neutropenic patients and for oropharyngeal candidiasis. FDA, U.S. Food and Drug Administration.

this category since it is impossible to distinguish colonization from lower or upper urinary tract infection. If the isolate is *C. albicans*, most clinicians use oral fluconazole rather than a bladder washout with amphotericin B, which was more commonly used in the past. Caspofungin has been used with success; although echinocandins are poorly excreted into the urine, they may be an option, especially for non-*albicans* isolates. The doses and duration are the same as for disseminated candidiasis. The significance of the recovery of *Candida* from abdominal drains in postoperative patients is unclear, but again the threshold for treatment is generally low because most of the affected patients have been subjected to factors predisposing to disseminated candidiasis.

Removal of the infected valve and long-term antifungal therapy constitute appropriate treatment for *Candida* endocarditis. Although definitive studies are not available, patients usually are treated for weeks with a systemic antifungal agent (Table 240-2) and then given chronic suppressive therapy for months or years (sometimes indefinitely) with an oral azole (usually fluconazole at 400–800 mg/d).

Hematogenous *Candida* endophthalmitis is a special problem requiring ophthalmologic consultation. When lesions are expanding or are threatening the macula, an IV polyene combined with flucytosine (25 mg/kg four times daily) has been the regimen of choice, although comparative studies with other regimens have not yet been reported. As more data on the azoles and echinocandins become available, new strategies involving these agents are developing. Of paramount importance is the decision to perform a partial vitrectomy. This procedure debulks the infection and can preserve sight, which may otherwise be lost as a result of vitreal scarring. All patients with candidemia should undergo ophthalmologic examination because of the relatively high frequency of this ocular complication. Not only can this examination detect a developing eye lesion early in its course; in addition, identification of a lesion signifies a probability of ~90% of deep-organ abscesses and may prompt prolongation of therapy for candidemia beyond the recommended 2 weeks after the last positive blood culture. Although the basis for the consensus is a very small data set, the recommended treatment for *Candida* meningitis is a polyene (Table 240-3) plus flucytosine (25 mg/kg four times daily). Successful treatment of *Candida* infected prosthetic material (e.g., an artificial joint) nearly always requires removal of the infected material followed by long-term administration of an antifungal agent selected on the basis of the isolate's sensitivity and the logistics of administration.

PROPHYLAXIS

The use of antifungal agents to prevent *Candida* infections has been controversial, but some general principles have emerged. Most centers administer prophylactic fluconazole (400 mg/d) to recipients of allogeneic stem cell transplants. High-risk liver transplant recipients also are given fluconazole prophylaxis in most centers. The use of prophylaxis for neutropenic patients has varied considerably from center to center; many centers that elect to give prophylaxis to this population use either fluconazole (200–400 mg/d) or a lipid formulation of amphotericin B (AmBiSome, 1–2 mg/d). Caspofungin (50 mg/d) also has been recommended. Some centers have used itraconazole suspension (200 mg/d). Posaconazole (200 mg three times daily) also has been approved by the FDA for prophylaxis in neutropenic patients and is gaining in popularity.

Prophylaxis is sometimes given to surgical patients at very high risk. The widespread use of prophylaxis for nearly all patients in general surgical or medical intensive care units is not—and should not be—a common practice for three reasons: (1) the incidence of disseminated candidiasis is relatively low, (2) the cost-benefit ratio is suboptimal, and (3) increased resistance with widespread prophylaxis is a valid concern.

Prophylaxis for oropharyngeal or esophageal candidiasis in HIV-infected patients is not recommended unless there are frequent recurrences.

241 Aspergillosis

David W. Denning

Aspergillosis is the collective term used to describe all disease entities caused by any one of ~50 pathogenic and allergenic species of *Aspergillus*. Only those species that grow at 37°C can cause invasive infection, although some species without this ability can cause allergic syndromes. *A. fumigatus* is responsible for most cases of invasive aspergillosis, almost all cases of chronic aspergillosis, and most allergic syndromes. *A. flavus* is more prevalent in some hospitals and causes a higher proportion of cases of sinus infections, cutaneous infections, and keratitis than *A. fumigatus*. *A. niger* can cause invasive infection but more commonly colonizes the respiratory tract and causes external otitis. *A. terreus* causes only invasive disease, usually with a poor prognosis. *A. nidulans* occasionally causes invasive infection, primarily in patients with chronic granulomatous disease.

EPIDEMIOLOGY AND ECOLOGY

Aspergillus has a worldwide distribution, most commonly growing in decomposing plant materials (i.e., compost) and in bedding. This hyaline (nonpigmented), septate, branching mold produces vast numbers of conidia (spores) on stalks above the surface of mycelial growth. Aspergilli are found in indoor and outdoor air, on surfaces, and in water from surface reservoirs. Daily exposures vary from a few to many millions of conidia; the latter high numbers of conidia are encountered in hay barns and other very dusty environments. The required size of the infecting inoculum is uncertain; however, only intense exposures (e.g., during construction work, handling of moldy bark or hay, or composting) are sufficient to cause disease in healthy immunocompetent individuals. Allergic syndromes may be exacerbated by continuous antigenic exposure arising from sinus or airway colonization or from nail infection. High-efficiency particulate air (HEPA) filtration is often protective against infection; thus HEPA filters should be installed and monitored for efficiency in operating rooms and in areas of the hospital that house high-risk patients.

The incubation period of invasive aspergillosis after exposure is highly variable, extending in documented cases from 2 to 90 days. Thus community acquisition of an infecting strain frequently manifests as invasive infection during hospitalization, although nosocomial acquisition is also common. Outbreaks usually are directly related to a contaminated air source in the hospital.

Global aspergillosis incidence and prevalence have been estimated (Table 241-1). However, given the inadequate diagnostic capability in almost all low- and middle-income countries, the accuracy of these estimates is uncertain. The frequency of different manifestations of aspergillosis varies considerably with geographic location; most notably, chronic granulomatous sinusitis is rare outside the Middle East and India, and fungal keratitis is particularly common in Nepal, Myanmar, Bhutan, and India (800 and 113 cases/100,000 population, respectively). The potential effects of chronic pulmonary aspergillosis after pulmonary tuberculosis have only recently been appreciated and include life-threatening hemoptysis, misdiagnosis of smear-negative tuberculosis, and general exacerbation of posttuberculosis morbidity.

RISK FACTORS AND PATHOGENESIS

The primary risk factors for invasive aspergillosis are profound neutropenia and glucocorticoid use; risk increases with longer duration of these conditions. Higher doses of glucocorticoids increase the risk of both acquisition of invasive aspergillosis and death from the infection. Neutrophil and/or phagocyte dysfunction also is an important risk factor, as evidenced by aspergillosis in chronic granulomatous disease, advanced HIV infection, and relapsed leukemia. An increasing incidence of invasive aspergillosis in medical intensive care units suggests that, in patients who are not immunocompromised, temporary abrogation of protective responses as a result of glucocorticoid use or a general anti-inflammatory state is a significant risk factor. Many

TABLE 241-1 DISEASE FREQUENCY AND DIAGNOSTIC SENSITIVITY FOR DIFFERENT MANIFESTATIONS OF ASPERGILLOSIS

	Type of Disease		
Parameter	Invasive	Chronic	Allergic
Incidence/100,000[a]	8.6	10.4	?[b]
Prevalence/100,000[a]	—	32.8	286[c]
Global burden[d]	~200,000	~3,000,000	~10,000,000
Mortality rate without treatment	~100%	~50%	<1%
Respiratory Diagnostic Sensitivity[e]			
Culture	✓	✓	✓
Microscopy	✓	?	?
Antigen	✓✓✓	?	✓✓✓
Real-time PCR	✓✓✓	✓✓✓	✓✓✓
Blood Diagnostic Sensitivity[e]			
Culture	✗	✗	✗
Antigen	✓✓	✓	✗
β-D-glucan	✓✓	✓	?
Real-time PCR	✓✓	?	?
IgG antibody	✓	✓✓✓✓	✓✓
IgE antibody	✗	✓✓	✓✓✓✓

[a]Incidence and prevalence figures are for Europe. From *www.ecdc.europa.eu/en/publications/publications/risk-assessment-impact-environmental-usage-of-triazoles-on-aspergillus-spp-resistance-to-medical-triazoles.pdf.* [b]People are not born with allergic fungal disease; the annual frequency with which it occurs is not known. [c]Allergic bronchopulmonary aspergillosis and severe asthma with fungal sensitization. [d]GD Brown et al: Human fungal infections: the hidden killers. Sci Transl Med 2012:4:165rv13. [e]Key for sensitivity: 1 check = limited (as the text indicates, 10–30% for culture); 2 checks = higher; 3 checks = >80%; and 4 checks = ~95%.

Abbreviation: PCR, polymerase chain reaction.

patients have some evidence of prior pulmonary disease—typically, a history of pneumonia or chronic obstructive pulmonary disease. Therapy with infliximab, adalimumab, alemtuzumab, daclizumab, rituximab, and possibly bevacizumab therapy also carries an increased risk of invasive aspergillosis, as do severe liver disease and high levels of stored iron in bone marrow.

Patients with chronic pulmonary aspergillosis have a wide spectrum of underlying pulmonary disease, including tuberculosis, prior pneumothorax, or chronic obstructive pulmonary disease. These patients are immunocompetent except for some cytokine regulation defects, most of which are consistent with an inability to mount an inflammatory immune (T_H1-like) response or to control it adequately. Glucocorticoids accelerate disease progression.

Allergic bronchopulmonary aspergillosis (ABPA) is associated with polymorphisms of interleukin (IL) 4Ra, IL-10, and SPA2 genes (and others) and with heterozygosity of the cystic fibrosis transmembrane conductance regulator (*CFTR*) gene. These associations suggest a strong genetic basis for the development of a T_H2-like and "allergic" response to *A. fumigatus*.

CD4+CD25+ T (T_{reg}) cells also appear to be pivotal in determining disease phenotype. Remarkably, high-dose glucocorticoid treatment for exacerbations of ABPA almost never leads to invasive aspergillosis.

CLINICAL FEATURES AND APPROACH TO THE PATIENT
(Table 241-2)

Invasive Pulmonary Aspergillosis Both the frequency of invasive disease and the pace of its progression increase with greater degrees of immunocompromise. Invasive aspergillosis is arbitrarily classified as acute and subacute, with courses of ≤1 month and 1–3 months, respectively. More than 80% of cases of invasive aspergillosis involve the lungs. The most common clinical features are no symptoms at all, fever, cough (sometimes productive), nondescript chest discomfort, trivial hemoptysis, and shortness of breath. Although the fever often responds to glucocorticoids, the disease progresses. The keys to early diagnosis in at-risk patients are a high index of suspicion, screening for circulating antigen (in leukemia), and urgent CT of the thorax. Invasive aspergillosis is one of the most common diagnostic errors revealed at autopsy.

Invasive Sinusitis The sinuses are involved in 5–10% of cases of invasive aspergillosis, especially affecting patients with leukemia and recipients of hematopoietic stem cell transplants. In addition to fever, the most common features are nasal or facial discomfort, blocked nose, and nasal discharge (sometimes bloody). Endoscopic examination of the nose reveals pale, dusky or necrotic-looking tissue in any location. CT or MRI of the sinuses is essential but does not distinguish invasive *Aspergillus* sinusitis from preexisting allergic or bacterial sinusitis early in the disease process.

Tracheobronchitis Occasionally, only the airways are infected by *Aspergillus*. The resulting manifestations range from acute or chronic bronchitis to ulcerative or pseudomembranous tracheobronchitis. These entities are particularly common among lung transplant recipients. Obstruction with mucous plugs occurs in normal individuals; in persons with ABPA, cystic fibrosis, and/or bronchiectasis; and in immunocompromised patients.

Disseminated Aspergillosis In the most severely immunocompromised patients, *Aspergillus* disseminates from the lungs to multiple organs—most often to the brain but also to the skin, thyroid, bone, kidney, liver, gastrointestinal tract, eye (endophthalmitis), and heart valve. Aside from cutaneous lesions, the most common features are gradual clinical deterioration over 1–3 days, with low-grade fever and features of mild sepsis, and nonspecific abnormalities in laboratory tests. In most cases, at least one localization becomes apparent before death. Blood cultures are almost always negative.

Cerebral Aspergillosis Hematogenous dissemination to the brain is a devastating complication of invasive aspergillosis. Single or multiple lesions may develop. In acute disease, hemorrhagic infarction is most

TABLE 241-2 MAJOR MANIFESTATIONS OF ASPERGILLOSIS

	Type of Disease			
Organ	Invasive (Acute and Subacute)	Chronic	Saprophytic	Allergic
Lung	Angioinvasive (in neutropenia), non-angioinvasive, granulomatous	Chronic cavitary, chronic fibrosing	Aspergilloma (single), airway colonization	Allergic bronchopulmonary, severe asthma with fungal sensitization, extrinsic allergic alveolitis
Sinus	Acute invasive	Chronic invasive, chronic granulomatous	Maxillary fungal ball	Allergic fungal sinusitis, eosinophilic fungal rhinosinusitis
Brain	Abscess, hemorrhagic infarction, meningitis	Granulomatous, meningitis	None	None
Skin	Acute disseminated, locally invasive (trauma, burns, IV access)	External otitis, onychomycosis	None	None
Heart	Endocarditis (native or prosthetic), pericarditis	None	None	None
Eye	Keratitis, endophthalmitis	None	None	None described

typical, and cerebral abscess is common. Rarer manifestations include meningitis, mycotic aneurysm, and cerebral granuloma (mimicking a brain tumor). Local spread from cranial sinuses also occurs. Postoperative infection develops rarely and is exacerbated by glucocorticoids, often given after neurosurgery. The presentation can be either acute or subacute, with mood changes, focal signs, seizures, and decline in mental status. MRI is the most useful immediate investigation; unenhanced CT of the brain is usually nonspecific, and contrast is often contraindicated because of poor renal function.

Endocarditis Most cases of *Aspergillus* endocarditis are prosthetic valve infections resulting from contamination during surgery. Native valve disease is reported, especially as a feature of disseminated infection and in persons using illicit IV drugs. Culture-negative endocarditis with large vegetations is the most common presentation; embolectomy occasionally reveals the diagnosis.

Cutaneous Aspergillosis Dissemination of *Aspergillus* occasionally results in cutaneous features, usually an erythematous or purplish nontender area that progresses to a necrotic eschar. Direct invasion of the skin occurs in neutropenic patients at the site of IV catheter insertion and in burn patients; such invasion may also follow trauma. Wounds may become infected with *Aspergillus* (especially *A. flavus*) after surgery.

Chronic Pulmonary Aspergillosis The hallmark of chronic cavitary pulmonary aspergillosis (also called semi-invasive aspergillosis, chronic necrotizing aspergillosis, or complex aspergilloma) (Fig. 241-1) is one or more pulmonary cavities expanding over a period of months or years in association with pulmonary symptoms and systemic manifestations such as fatigue and weight loss. (Pulmonary aspergillosis developing over <3 months is better classified as subacute invasive aspergillosis.) Often mistaken initially for tuberculosis, almost all cases occur in patients with prior pulmonary disease (e.g., tuberculosis, atypical mycobacterial infection, sarcoidosis, rheumatoid lung disease, pneumothorax, bullae) or lung surgery. The onset is insidious, and systemic features may be more prominent than pulmonary symptoms. Cavities may have a fluid level or a well-formed fungal ball, but pericavitary infiltrates and multiple cavities—with or without pleural thickening—are typical. An irregular internal cavity surface and thickened cavity walls are indicative of disease activity.

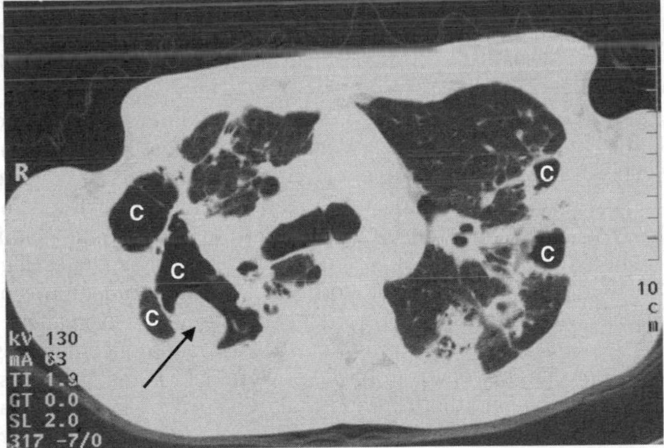

FIGURE 241-1 CT scan image of the chest in a patient with long-standing bilateral chronic cavitary pulmonary aspergillosis. This patient had a history of several bilateral pneumothoraces and had required bilateral pleurodesis in 1990. CT scan then demonstrated multiple bullae, and sputum cultures grew *A. fumigatus*. The patient had initially weakly and later strongly positive serum *Aspergillus* antibody tests (precipitins). This scan (2003) shows a mixture of thick- and thin-walled cavities in both lungs (each marked with *C*), with a probable fungal ball (*black arrow*) protruding into the large cavity on the patient's right side (*R*). There is also considerable pleural thickening bilaterally.

IgG antibodies (usually precipitating) to *Aspergillus* are almost always detectable in blood, and levels fall slowly with successful therapy. Some patients have concurrent infections—even without a fungal ball—with atypical mycobacteria and/or other bacterial pathogens. One or more *Aspergillus* nodules that resemble early lung carcinoma and may cavitate have been recognized. If untreated, chronic pulmonary aspergillosis typically progresses (sometimes relatively rapidly) to unilateral or upper-lobe fibrosis. This end-stage entity is termed *chronic fibrosing pulmonary aspergillosis*.

Aspergilloma Aspergilloma (fungal ball) occurs in up to 20% of residual pulmonary cavities ≥2.5 cm in diameter. Signs and symptoms associated with single (simple) aspergillomas are minor, including cough (sometimes productive), hemoptysis, wheezing, and mild fatigue. More significant signs and symptoms are associated with chronic cavitary pulmonary aspergillosis and should be treated as such. The vast majority of fungal balls are caused by *A. fumigatus*, but *A. niger* has been implicated, particularly in diabetic patients; aspergillomas due to *A. niger* can lead to oxalosis with renal dysfunction. The most significant complication of aspergilloma is life-threatening hemoptysis, which may be the presenting manifestation. Some fungal balls resolve spontaneously, but the cavity may still be infected.

Chronic *Aspergillus* Sinusitis Three entities are subsumed under this broad designation: fungal ball of the sinus, chronic invasive sinusitis, and chronic granulomatous sinusitis. *Fungal ball of the sinus* is limited to the maxillary sinus (except in rare cases involving the sphenoid sinus) and consists of a chronic saprophytic entity in which the sinus cavity is filled with a fungal ball. Maxillary disease is associated with prior upper-jaw root canal work and chronic (bacterial) sinusitis. About 90% of CT scans show focal hyperattenuation related to concretions; on MRI scans, the T2-weighted signal is decreased, whereas it is increased in bacterial sinusitis. Removal of the fungal ball is curative. No tissue invasion is demonstrable histologically or radiologically.

In contrast, *chronic invasive sinusitis* is a slowly destructive process that most commonly affects the ethmoid and sphenoid sinuses but can involve any sinus. Patients are usually but not always immunocompromised to some degree (e.g., as a result of diabetes or HIV infection). Imaging of the cranial sinuses shows opacification of one or more sinuses, local bone destruction, and invasion of local structures. The differential diagnosis is wide, including infections caused by numerous other fungi; sphenoid sinusitis is often caused by bacteria. Apart from a history of chronic nasal discharge and blockage, loss of the sense of smell, and persistent headache, the usual presenting features are related to local involvement of critical structures. The orbital apex syndrome (blindness and proptosis) is characteristic. Facial swelling, cavernous sinus thrombosis, carotid artery occlusion, pituitary fossa, and brain and skull base invasion have been described.

Chronic granulomatous sinusitis due to *Aspergillus* is most commonly seen in the Middle East and India and is often caused by *A. flavus*. It typically presents late, with facial swelling and unilateral proptosis. The prominent granulomatous reaction histologically distinguishes this disease from chronic invasive sinusitis, in which tissue necrosis with a low-grade mixed-cell infiltrate is typical. IgG antibodies to *A. flavus* are usually detectable.

Allergic Bronchopulmonary Aspergillosis In almost all cases, ABPA represents a hypersensitivity reaction to *A. fumigatus*; rare cases are due to other aspergilli and other fungi. ABPA occurs in ~2.5% of patients with asthma who are referred to secondary care and in up to 15% of adults with cystic fibrosis. Episodes of bronchial obstruction with mucous plugs leading to coughing fits, "pneumonia," consolidation, and breathlessness are typical. Many patients report coughing up thick sputum casts. Eosinophilia commonly develops before systemic glucocorticoids are given. The cardinal diagnostic tests include an elevated serum level of total IgE (usually >1000 IU/mL), a positive skin-prick test in response to *A. fumigatus* extract, or detection of *Aspergillus*-specific IgE and IgG antibodies. The presence of hyperattenuated mucus in airways is highly specific. Central bronchiectasis is characteristic, and some patients develop chronic cavitary pulmonary aspergillosis.

Severe Asthma with Fungal Sensitization Many adults with severe asthma do not fulfill the criteria for ABPA and yet are allergic to fungi. Although *A. fumigatus* is a common allergen, numerous other fungi (e.g., *Cladosporium* and *Alternaria* species) are implicated by skin-prick testing and/or specific IgE radioallergosorbent testing. Serum total IgE concentrations are <1000 IU/mL, and bronchiectasis is moderately common.

Allergic Sinusitis Like the lungs, the sinuses manifest allergic responses to *Aspergillus* and other fungi. The affected patients present with chronic (i.e., perennial) sinusitis that is relatively unresponsive to antibiotics. Many of these patients have nasal polyps, and all have congested nasal mucosae and sinuses full of mucoid material. The histologic hallmarks of allergic fungal sinusitis are local eosinophilia and Charcot-Leyden crystals. Removal of abnormal mucus and polyps, with local and occasionally systemic administration of glucocorticoids, usually leads to resolution. Persistent or recurrent signs and symptoms may require more extensive surgery (ethmoidectomy) and possibly local antifungal therapy. Recurrence is common, often after another bacterial or viral infection.

Superficial Aspergillosis *Aspergillus* can cause keratitis and otitis externa. The former may be difficult to diagnose early enough to save the patient's sight. Treatment requires local surgical debridement as well as intensive topical antifungal therapy. Otitis externa usually resolves with debridement and local application of antifungal agents.

DIAGNOSIS

Several techniques are required to establish the diagnosis of any form of aspergillosis with confidence (Table 241-1). Patients with acute invasive aspergillosis have a relatively heavy load of fungus in the affected organ; thus culture, molecular diagnosis, antigen detection, and histopathology usually confirm the diagnosis. However, the pace of progression leaves only a narrow window for making the diagnosis without losing the patient, and some invasive procedures are not possible because of coagulopathy, respiratory compromise, and other factors. Currently, ~40% of cases of invasive aspergillosis are missed clinically and are diagnosed only at autopsy. Histologic examination of affected tissue reveals either infarction, with invasion of blood vessels by many fungal hyphae, or acute necrosis, with limited inflammation and fewer hyphae. *Aspergillus* hyphae are hyaline, narrow, and septate, with branching at 45°; no yeast forms are present in infected tissue. Hyphae can be seen in cytology or microscopy preparations, which therefore provide a rapid means of presumptive diagnosis.

Culture is important in confirming the diagnosis, given that multiple other (rarer) fungi can mimic *Aspergillus* species histologically. Bacterial agar is less sensitive than fungal media for culture. Thus, if physicians do not request fungal culture, the diagnosis may be missed. Culture may be falsely positive (e.g., in patients whose airways are colonized by *Aspergillus*) or falsely negative. Only 10–30% of patients with invasive aspergillosis have a positive culture at any time. Both antigen detection and real-time polymerase chain reaction (PCR) are faster and much more sensitive than culture of respiratory samples and blood.

The *Aspergillus* antigen test relies on detection of galactomannan release from *Aspergillus* organisms during growth. Positive serum antigen results usually precede clinical or radiologic features by several days. The sensitivity of antigen detection is reduced by antifungal prophylaxis and empirical therapy.

Definitive confirmation of the diagnosis requires (1) a positive culture of a sample taken directly from an ordinarily sterile site (e.g., a brain abscess) or (2) positive results of both histologic testing and culture of a sample taken from an affected organ (e.g., sinuses or skin). Most diagnoses of invasive aspergillosis are inferred from fewer data, including the presence of the *halo sign* on a high-resolution thoracic CT scan, in which a localized ground-glass appearance representing hemorrhagic infarction surrounds a nodule. While a halo sign may be produced by other fungi, *Aspergillus* species are by far the most common cause. Halo signs are present for ~7 days early in the course of infection in neutropenic patients and are a good prognostic feature, reflecting an early diagnosis. Thick CT sections can give the false appearance of a halo sign, as can other technical factors. Other common radiologic features of invasive pulmonary aspergillosis include nodules and pleural-based infarction or cavitation, with pleural fluid apparent in 10% of patients.

For chronic invasive aspergillosis, *Aspergillus* antibody testing is invaluable although relatively imprecise. Biopsy of new nodules reveals hyphae surrounded by cells of chronic inflammation and sometimes granulomas. Antibody titers fall with successful therapy. Cultures are infrequently positive but are important in checking for azole resistance. Real-time PCR of sputum is often strongly positive. Some patients with chronic pulmonary aspergillosis also have elevated titers of total serum IgE and *Aspergillus*-specific IgE.

ABPA and severe asthma with fungal sensitization are diagnosed serologically with elevated total and specific serum IgE levels and with skin-prick tests. Allergic *Aspergillus* sinusitis is usually diagnosed histologically, although precipitating antibodies in blood also may be useful.

TREATMENT ASPERGILLOSIS

Antifungal drugs active against *Aspergillus* include voriconazole, itraconazole, posaconazole, caspofungin, micafungin, and amphotericin B (AmB). Drug interactions with azoles must be considered before these agents are prescribed. In addition, plasma azole concentrations vary substantially from one patient to another, and many authorities recommend monitoring to ensure that drug concentrations are adequate but not excessive. Initial IV administration is preferred for acute invasive aspergillosis and oral administration for all other disease that requires antifungal therapy. Current recommendations are shown in **Table 241-3**.

Voriconazole is the preferred agent for invasive aspergillosis; caspofungin, posaconazole, and lipid-associated AmB are second-line agents. AmB is not active against *A. terreus* or *A. nidulans*. An infectious disease consultation is advised for patients with invasive disease, given the complexity of management. Combination therapy (voriconazole plus an echinocandin) for acute invasive aspergillosis may be beneficial for non-neutropenic patients. Immune reconstitution can complicate recovery. The duration of therapy for invasive aspergillosis varies from ~3 months to several years, depending on the patient's immune status and response to therapy. Relapse occurs if the response is suboptimal and immune reconstitution is not complete.

Itraconazole is currently the preferred oral agent for chronic and allergic forms of aspergillosis. Voriconazole or posaconazole can be substituted when failure, emergence of resistance, or adverse events occur. An itraconazole dose of 200 mg twice daily is recommended, with monitoring of drug concentrations in the blood. Chronic cavitary pulmonary aspergillosis probably requires lifelong therapy, whereas the duration of treatment for other forms of chronic and allergic aspergillosis requires case-by-case evaluation.

Resistance to one or more azoles, although uncommon, is present in isolates from the environment in many regions, including northern Europe, India, China, and North America. Resistance may be derived from azole fungicide use for crops. In addition, resistance arising from multiple mechanisms may develop during long-term treatment, and a positive culture during antifungal therapy is an indication for susceptibility testing. Combined resistance to itraconazole and voriconazole is the most common type of cross-resistance. Glucocorticoids should be used in chronic cavitary pulmonary aspergillosis only if covered by adequate antifungal therapy.

Surgical treatment is important in several forms of aspergillosis, including fungal ball of the sinus and single aspergillomas, in which surgery is curative; invasive aspergillosis involving bone,

TABLE 241-3 TREATMENT OF ASPERGILLOSIS[a]

Indication	Primary Treatment	Evidence Level[b]	Precautions	Secondary Treatment	Comments
Invasive[c]	Voriconazole	AI	Drug interactions (especially with rifampin), renal failure (IV only)	AmB, caspofungin, posaconazole, micafungin	As primary therapy, voriconazole carries 20% more responses than AmB. Consider initial combination therapy with an echinocandin in non-neutropenic patients.
Prophylaxis	Posaconazole, itraconazole solution	AI	Diarrhea and vomiting with itraconazole, vincristine interaction	Micafungin, aerosolized AmB	Some centers monitor plasma levels of itraconazole and posaconazole.
Single aspergilloma	Surgery	BII	Multicavity disease: poor outcome of surgery, medical therapy preferable	Itraconazole, voriconazole, intracavity AmB	Single large cavities with an aspergilloma are best resected.
Chronic pulmonary[c]	Itraconazole, voriconazole	BII	Poor absorption of itraconazole capsules with proton pump inhibitors or H_2 blockers	Posaconazole, IV AmB, IV micafungin	Resistance may emerge during treatment, especially if plasma drug levels are subtherapeutic.
ABPA/SAFS	Itraconazole	AI	Some glucocorticoid interactions, including with inhaled formulations	Voriconazole, posaconazole	Long-term therapy is helpful in most cases. No evidence indicates whether therapy modifies progression to bronchiectasis/fibrosis.

[a]For information on duration of therapy, see text. [b]Evidence levels are those used in treatment guidelines (TJ Walsh et al: Treatment of aspergillosis: Clinical practice guidelines of the Infectious Diseases Society of America [IDSA]. Clin Infect Dis 46:327, 2008). [c]An infectious disease consultation is appropriate for these patients.

Note: The oral dose is usually 200 mg bid for voriconazole and itraconazole and 400 mg bid for posaconazole suspension. The IV dose of voriconazole for adults is 6 mg/kg twice at 12-h intervals (loading doses) followed by 4 mg/kg q12h; a larger dose is required for children and teenagers. Plasma monitoring is helpful in optimizing the dosage. Caspofungin is given as a single loading dose of 70 mg and then at 50 mg/d; some authorities use 70 mg/d for patients weighing >80 kg, and lower doses are required with hepatic dysfunction. Micafungin is given as 50 mg/d for prophylaxis and as at least 150 mg/d for treatment; this drug has not yet been approved by the U.S. Food and Drug Administration (FDA) for this indication. AmB deoxycholate is given at a daily dose of 1 mg/kg if tolerated. Several strategies are available for minimizing renal dysfunction. Lipid-associated AmB is given at 3 mg/kg (AmBisome) or 5 mg/kg (Abelcet). Different regimens are available for aerosolized AmB, but none is FDA approved. Other considerations that may alter dose selection or route include age; concomitant medications; renal, hepatic, or intestinal dysfunction; and drug tolerability.

Abbreviations: AmB, amphotericin B; ABPA, allergic bronchopulmonary aspergillosis; SAFS, severe asthma with fungal sensitization.

heart valve, sinuses, and proximal areas of the lung; brain abscess; keratitis; and endophthalmitis. In allergic fungal sinusitis, removal of abnormal mucus and polyps, with local and occasionally systemic glucocorticoid treatment, usually leads to resolution. Persistent or recurrent signs and symptoms may require more extensive surgery (ethmoidectomy) and possibly local antifungal therapy. Surgery is problematic in chronic pulmonary aspergillosis, usually resulting in serious complications. Bronchial artery embolization is preferred for problematic hemoptysis.

PROPHYLAXIS

In situations in which moderate or high risk is predicted (e.g., after induction therapy for acute myeloid leukemia), the need for antifungal prophylaxis for superficial and systemic candidiasis and for invasive aspergillosis is generally accepted. Fluconazole is commonly used in these situations but has no activity against *Aspergillus* species. Itraconazole capsules are ineffective, and itraconazole solution offers only modest efficacy. Posaconazole solution is more effective. Some data support the use of IV micafungin. No prophylactic regimen is completely successful.

OUTCOME

Invasive aspergillosis is curable if immune reconstitution occurs, whereas allergic and chronic forms are not. The mortality rate for invasive aspergillosis is ~50% if the infection is treated but is 100% if the diagnosis is missed. Infection with a voriconazole-resistant strain carries a mortality rate of 88%. Cerebral aspergillosis, *Aspergillus* endocarditis, and bilateral extensive invasive pulmonary aspergillosis have very poor outcomes, as does invasive infection in persons with late-stage AIDS or relapsed uncontrolled leukemia and in recipients of allogeneic hematopoietic stem cell transplants.

The mortality rate for chronic cavitary pulmonary aspergillosis is ~30% 6 months after presentation, falling to ~15% annually thereafter. After 12 months with no antifungal therapy, 70% of patients have deteriorated and 30% are stable (Fig. 241-2). Therapy fails in ~30% of recipients of antifungal therapy and still more often if azole resistance is present.

Both ABPA and SAFS patients respond to antifungal therapy; ~60% respond to itraconazole and ~80% to voriconazole and posaconazole (if tolerated). If the severity of asthma declines, the inhaled glucocorticoid dose can be reduced and oral glucocorticoids can be stopped.

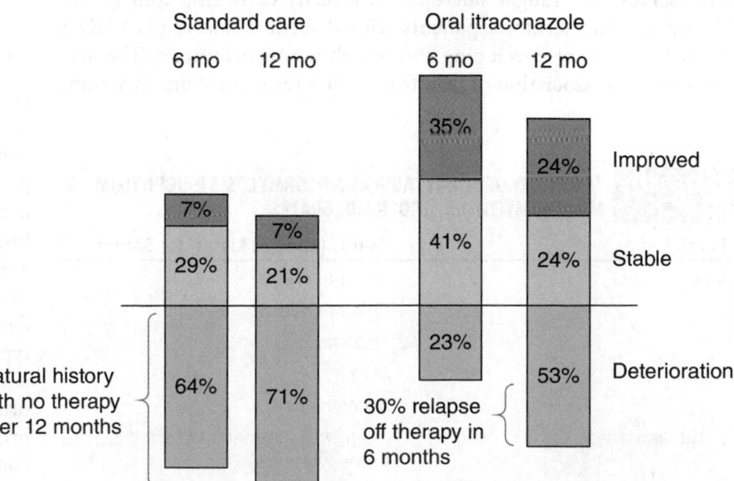

FIGURE 241-2 Comparison of the impact of itraconazole therapy (400 mg/d) and standard care on chronic cavitary pulmonary aspergillosis at 6 and 12 months. *(After R Agarwal et al: Itraconazole in chronic cavitary pulmonary aspergillosis: a randomised controlled trial and systematic review of literature. Mycoses 56:559, 2013.)*

242 Mucormycosis

Brad Spellberg, Ashraf S. Ibrahim

Mucormycosis represents a group of life-threatening infections caused by fungi of the order Mucorales of the subphylum Mucoromycotina (formerly known as the class Zygomycetes). Infection caused by the Mucorales is most accurately referred to as *mucormycosis*, although the term *zygomycosis* may still be used by some sources. Mucormycosis is highly invasive and relentlessly progressive, resulting in higher rates of morbidity and mortality than many other infections. However, recent studies have suggested that mortality rates from mucormycosis have declined with newer therapies. A high index of suspicion is critical for diagnosis, and early initiation of therapy—often before confirmation of the diagnosis—is necessary to optimize outcomes.

ETIOLOGY

Fungi of the order Mucorales belong to seven medically relevant families (Table 242-1), all of which can cause mucormycosis. Among the Mucorales, *Rhizopus oryzae* (in the family Mucoraceae) is by far the most common cause of infection in the Western Hemisphere. Less frequently isolated species of the Mucoraceae that cause a similar spectrum of infections include *Rhizopus microsporus*, *Rhizomucor pusillus*, *Lichtheimia corymbifera* (formerly *Absidia corymbifera*), *Apophysomyces elegans*, and *Mucor* species (which, despite its name, only rarely causes mucormycosis). Increasing numbers of cases of mucormycosis due to infection with *Cunninghamella* species (family Cunninghamellaceae) have also been reported, particularly in highly immunocompromised patients. Rare case reports have demonstrated the ability of fungi in the remaining families of the Mucorales to cause mucormycosis, although other Mucorales can be the major cause of disease in certain geographic areas (e.g., *A. elegans* in India and *Mucor irregularis* in China).

PATHOGENESIS

The Mucorales are ubiquitous environmental fungi to which humans are constantly exposed. These fungi cause infection primarily in patients with diabetes or defects in phagocytic function (e.g., those associated with neutropenia or glucocorticoid treatment). Patients with elevated levels of free iron, which supports fungal growth in serum and tissues, are likewise at increased risk for mucormycosis. In iron-overloaded patients with end-stage renal failure, treatment with deferoxamine predisposes to the development of rapidly fatal disseminated mucormycosis; this agent, an iron chelator for the human host, serves as a fungal siderophore, directly delivering iron to the Mucorales. Furthermore, patients with diabetic ketoacidosis (DKA) are at high risk of developing rhinocerebral mucormycosis. The acidosis causes dissociation of iron from sequestering proteins in serum, resulting in enhanced fungal survival and virulence. Nevertheless, the majority of diabetic patients who present with mucormycosis are not acidotic, and, even absent acidosis, hyperglycemia directly contributes to the risk of mucormycosis by at least three likely mechanisms: (1) hyperglycation of iron-sequestering proteins, disrupting normal iron sequestration; (2) upregulation of a mammalian cell receptor (GRP78) that binds to Mucorales, enabling tissue penetration (due to both a direct effect of hyperglycemia and increasing levels of free iron, which independently enhances GRP78 expression); and (3) induction of poorly characterized defects in phagocytic function.

TABLE 242-1 TAXONOMY OF FUNGI CAUSING MUCORMYCOSIS (SUBPHYLUM MUCOROMYCOTINA, ORDER MUCORALES)

Family	Genus (Species Listed for Some)
Mucoraceae	*Rhizopus oryzae*
	Rhizopus microsporus
	Rhizomucor
	Mucor
	Actinomucor
Lichtheimiaceae	*Lichtheimia* (formerly *Mycocladus*, formerly *Absidia*)
Cunninghamellaceae	*Cunninghamella*
Thamnidiaceae	*Cokeromyces*
Mortierellaceae	*Mortierella*
Saksenaceae	*Saksenaea*
	Apophysomyces
Syncephalastraceae	*Syncephalastrum*

EPIDEMIOLOGY

Mucormycosis typically occurs in patients with diabetes mellitus, solid organ or hematopoietic stem cell transplantation (HSCT), prolonged neutropenia, or malignancy. The majority of diabetic patients are not acidotic on presentation with mucormycosis. Furthermore, patients often have no previously recognized history of diabetes mellitus when they present with mucormycosis. In these instances, presentation for mucormycosis may result in the first clinical recognition of hyperglycemia, which may have been unmasked by recent glucocorticoid use. Thus a high index of suspicion of mucormycosis must be maintained, even in the absence of a known history of diabetes, if hyperglycemia is present. In patients undergoing HSCT, mucormycosis develops at least as commonly during nonneutropenic as during neutropenic periods, probably because of glucocorticoid treatment of graft-versus-host disease. Mucormycosis can occur as isolated cutaneous or subcutaneous infection in immunologically normal individuals after traumatic implantation of soil or vegetation (e.g., due to natural disasters or motor vehicle accidents) or in nosocomial settings via direct access through IV catheters, SC injections, or maceration of the skin by a moist dressing.

Patients receiving antifungal prophylaxis with either itraconazole or voriconazole may be at increased risk of mucormycosis. These patients typically present with disseminated mucormycosis, the most lethal form of disease. Breakthrough mucormycosis also has been described in patients receiving posaconazole or echinocandin prophylaxis.

CLINICAL MANIFESTATIONS

Mucormycosis can be divided into at least six clinical categories based on clinical presentation and the involvement of a particular anatomic site: rhino-orbital-cerebral, pulmonary, cutaneous, gastrointestinal, disseminated, and miscellaneous. These categories of invasive mucormycosis tend to affect patients with specific defects in host defense. For example, patients with DKA typically develop the rhino-orbital-cerebral form and much more rarely develop pulmonary or disseminated disease. In contrast, pulmonary mucormycosis occurs most commonly in leukemic patients who are receiving chemotherapy and in patients undergoing HSCT.

Rhino-Orbital-Cerebral Disease Rhino-orbital-cerebral mucormycosis continues to be the most common form of the disease. Most cases occur in patients with diabetes, although such cases (probably due to glucocorticoid use) are increasingly being described in the transplantation setting, often along with glucocorticoid-induced diabetes mellitus. The initial symptoms of rhino-orbital-cerebral mucormycosis are nonspecific and include eye or facial pain and facial numbness followed by the onset of conjunctival suffusion and blurry vision. Fever may be absent in up to half of cases. White blood cell counts are typically elevated as long as the patient has functioning bone marrow. If untreated, infection usually spreads from the ethmoid sinus to the orbit, resulting in compromise of extraocular muscle function and proptosis, typically with chemosis. Onset of signs and symptoms in the contralateral eye, with resulting bilateral proptosis, chemosis, vision loss, and ophthalmoplegia, is ominous, suggesting the development of cavernous sinus thrombosis.

Upon visual inspection, infected tissue may appear to be normal during the earliest stages of fungal spread, then progressing through an erythematous phase, with or without edema, before the onset of a violaceous appearance and finally the development of a black necrotic eschar. Infection can sometimes extend from the sinuses into the mouth and produce painful necrotic ulcerations of the hard palate, but this is a late finding that suggests extensive, well-established infection.

Pulmonary Disease Pulmonary mucormycosis is the second most common manifestation. Symptoms include dyspnea, cough, and chest pain; fever is often but not invariably present. Angioinvasion results in necrosis, cavitation, and/or hemoptysis. Lobar consolidation, isolated masses, nodular disease, cavities, or wedge-shaped infarcts may be seen on chest radiography. High-resolution chest CT is the best method for determining the extent of pulmonary mucormycosis and may demonstrate evidence of infection before it is seen on chest x-ray. In the setting of cancer, where mucormycosis may be difficult to differentiate from aspergillosis, the presence of ≥10 pulmonary nodules, pleural effusion, or concomitant sinusitis makes mucormycosis more likely. It is critical to distinguish mucormycosis from aspergillosis as rapidly as possible because treatments for these infections differ. Indeed, voriconazole—the first-line treatment for aspergillosis—exacerbates mucormycosis in mouse and fly models of infection.

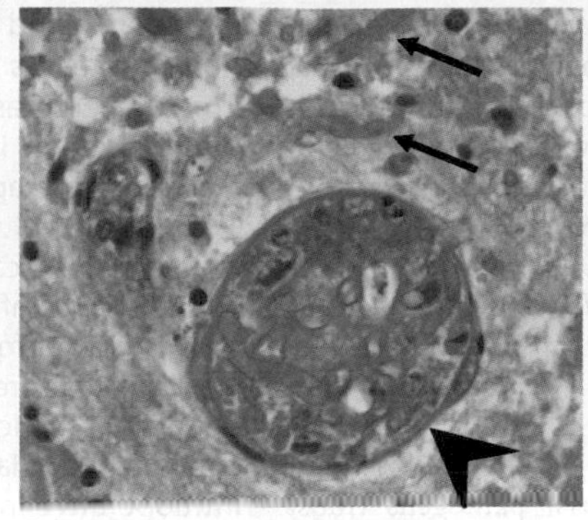

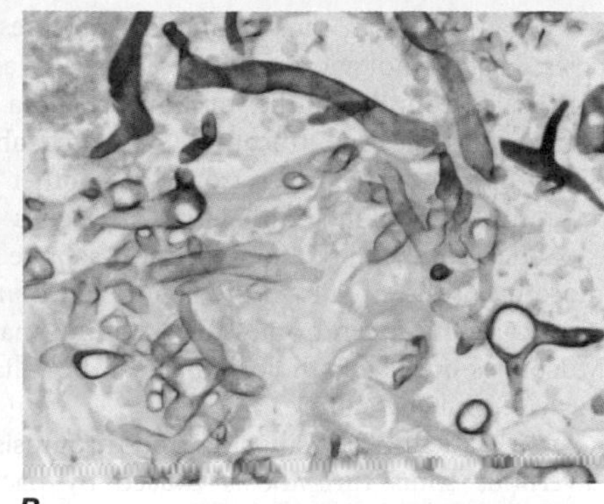

FIGURE 242-1 Histopathology sections of *Rhizopus oryzae* in infected brain. ***A.*** Broad, ribbon-like, nonseptate hyphae in the parenchyma (*arrows*) and a thrombosed blood vessel with extensive intravascular hyphae (*arrowhead*) (hematoxylin and eosin). ***B.*** Extensive, broad, ribbon-like hyphae invading the parenchyma (Gomori methenamine silver).

Cutaneous Disease Cutaneous mucormycosis may result from external implantation of the fungus or conversely from hematogenous dissemination. External implantation–related infection has been described in the setting of soil exposure from trauma (e.g., in a motor vehicle accident or natural disaster), penetrating injury with plant material (e.g., a thorn), injections of medications (e.g., insulin), catheter insertion, contamination of surgical dressings, and use of tape to secure endotracheal tubes. Cutaneous disease can be highly invasive, penetrating into muscle, fascia, and even bone. In mucormycosis, necrotizing fasciitis carries a mortality rate approaching 80%. Necrotic cutaneous lesions in the setting of hematogenous dissemination also are associated with an extremely high mortality rate. However, with prompt, aggressive surgical debridement, isolated cutaneous mucormycosis has a favorable prognosis and a low mortality rate.

Gastrointestinal Disease In the past, gastrointestinal mucormycosis occurred primarily in premature neonates in association with disseminated disease and necrotizing enterocolitis. However, there has been a marked increase in case reports describing adults with neutropenia or other immunocompromising conditions. In addition, gastrointestinal disease has been reported as a nosocomial process following administration of medications mixed with contaminated wooden applicator sticks. Nonspecific abdominal pain and distention associated with nausea and vomiting are the most common symptoms. Gastrointestinal bleeding is common, and fungating masses may be seen in the stomach at endoscopy. The disease may progress to visceral perforation, with extremely high mortality rates.

Disseminated and Miscellaneous Forms of Disease Hematogenously disseminated mucormycosis may originate from any primary site of infection. The most common site of dissemination is the brain, but metastatic lesions may also be found in any other organ. The mortality rate associated with dissemination to the brain approaches 100%. Even without central nervous system (CNS) involvement, mortality rates for disseminated mucormycosis exceed 90%. Miscellaneous forms of mucormycosis may affect any body site, including bones, mediastinum, trachea, kidneys, and (in association with dialysis) peritoneum.

DIAGNOSIS

A high index of suspicion is required for diagnosis of mucormycosis. Unfortunately, autopsy series have shown that up to half of cases are diagnosed only post-mortem. Because the Mucorales are environmental isolates, definitive diagnosis requires a positive culture from a sterile site (e.g., a needle aspirate, a tissue biopsy specimen, or pleural fluid) or histopathologic evidence of invasive mucormycosis. A probable diagnosis of mucormycosis can be established by culture from a nonsterile site (e.g., sputum or bronchoalveolar lavage) when a patient has appropriate risk factors as well as clinical and radiographic evidence of disease. However, given the urgency of administering therapy early, the patient should be treated while confirmation of the diagnosis is awaited.

Biopsy with histopathologic examination remains the most sensitive and specific modality for definitive diagnosis (Fig. 242-1). Biopsy reveals characteristic wide (≥6- to 30-μm), thick-walled, ribbon-like, aseptate hyphal elements that branch at right angles. Other fungi, including *Aspergillus*, *Fusarium*, and *Scedosporium* species, have septa, are thinner, and branch at acute angles. Because artificial septa may result from folding of tissue during processing (which may also alter the appearance of the angle of branching), the width and the ribbon-like form of the fungus are the most reliable features distinguishing mucormycosis. The Mucorales are visualized most effectively with periodic acid–Schiff or methenamine silver stain or, if the organism burden is high, with hematoxylin and eosin. While histopathology can identify the Mucorales, specific species can be identified only by culture. Polymerase chain reaction (PCR) is being investigated as a diagnostic tool for mucormycosis but is not yet approved by the U.S. Food and Drug Administration (FDA) for this purpose and is not generally available.

Unfortunately, cultures are positive in fewer than half of cases of mucormycosis. Nevertheless, the Mucorales are not fastidious organisms and tend to grow quickly (i.e., within 48 h) on culture media. The likely explanation for the low sensitivity of culture is that the Mucorales form long filamentous structures that are killed by tissue homogenization—the standard method for preparing tissue cultures in the clinical microbiology laboratory. Thus the laboratory should be advised when a diagnosis of mucormycosis is suspected, and the tissue should be cut into sections and placed in the center of culture dishes rather than homogenized. There is also substantial variability among isolates in optimal growth temperature, so growth at both room temperature and 37°C is advisable.

Imaging techniques often yield subtle findings that underestimate the extent of disease. For example, the most common finding on CT or MRI of the head or sinuses of a patient with rhino-orbital mucormycosis is sinusitis that is indistinguishable from bacterial sinusitis. It is also common to detect no abnormalities in sinus bones despite clinical evidence of progressive disease. MRI is more sensitive (~80%) for detecting orbital and CNS disease than is CT. High-risk patients should always undergo endoscopy and/or surgical exploration, with biopsy of the areas of suspected infection. If mucormycosis is suspected, initial empirical therapy with a polyene antifungal agent should be initiated while the diagnosis is being confirmed.

DIFFERENTIAL DIAGNOSIS

Other mold infections, including aspergillosis, scedosporiosis, fusariosis, and infections caused by the dematiaceous fungi (brown-pigmented soil organisms), can cause clinical syndromes identical to mucormycosis. Histopathologic examination usually allows distinction of the Mucorales from these other organisms, and a positive culture permits definitive species identification. As stated above, it is important to distinguish the Mucorales from these other fungi, as the preferred antifungal treatments differ (i.e., polyenes for the Mucorales vs. expanded-spectrum triazoles for most septate molds). The entomophthoromycoses caused by *Basidiobolus* and *Conidiobolus* also can cause identical clinical syndromes. These fungi may appear similar to the Mucorales on histopathology and can be reliably distinguished from the latter only by culture.

In a patient with sinusitis and proptosis, orbital cellulitis and cavernous sinus thrombosis caused by bacterial pathogens (most commonly *Staphylococcus aureus*, but also streptococcal and gram-negative species) must be excluded. *Klebsiella rhinoscleromatis* is a rare cause of an indolent facial rhinoscleroma syndrome that may appear similar to mucormycosis. Finally, the Tolosa-Hunt syndrome causes painful ophthalmoplegia, ptosis, headache, and cavernous sinus inflammation; biopsies and clinical follow-up may be needed to distinguish the Tolosa-Hunt syndrome from mucormycosis by the lack of progression of the former entity.

TREATMENT MUCORMYCOSIS

GENERAL PRINCIPLES

The successful treatment of mucormycosis requires four steps: (1) early diagnosis; (2) reversal of underlying predisposing risk factors, if possible; (3) surgical debridement; and (4) prompt antifungal therapy. Early diagnosis of mucormycosis is critical, since early initiation of therapy is associated with improved survival rates. It is also crucial to reverse (or prevent) underlying defects in host defense during treatment (e.g., by stopping or reducing the dosage of immunosuppressive medications or by rapidly restoring euglycemia and normal acid-base status). Finally, iron administration to patients with active mucormycosis should be avoided, as iron exacerbates infection in animal models. Blood transfusion typically results in some liberation of free iron due to hemolysis, so a conservative approach to red blood cell transfusions is advisable.

Blood vessel thrombosis and resulting tissue necrosis during mucormycosis can result in poor penetration of antifungal agents to the site of infection. Therefore, debridement of all necrotic tissues is critical for eradication of disease. Surgery has been found (by logistic regression and in multiple case series) to be an independent variable for favorable outcome in patients with mucormycosis. Limited data from a retrospective study support the use of intraoperative frozen sections to delineate the margins of infected tissues, with sparing of tissues lacking evidence of infection. A multidisciplinary team, including an internist, an infectious disease specialist, and surgical specialists whose expertise is relevant to the sites of infection, is typically required for the management of mucormycosis.

ANTIFUNGAL THERAPY

Primary therapy for mucormycosis should be based on a polyene antifungal agent (Table 242-2), except perhaps for mild localized infection (e.g., isolated suprafascial cutaneous infection) that has been eradicated surgically in an immunocompetent patient. Amphotericin B (AmB) deoxycholate remains the only licensed antifungal agent for the treatment of mucormycosis. However, lipid formulations of AmB are significantly less nephrotoxic, can be administered at higher doses, and are probably more effective than AmB deoxycholate for this purpose. Liposomal amphotericin B (LAmB) is preferred to amphotericin B lipid complex (ABLC) for management of CNS infection on the basis of retrospective survival data and superior brain penetration; there is no clear advantage of either agent for non-CNS infections.

TABLE 242-2 FIRST-LINE ANTIFUNGAL OPTIONS FOR THE TREATMENT OF MUCORMYCOSIS[a]

Drug	Recommended Dosage	Advantages and Supporting Studies	Disadvantages
Primary Antifungal Therapy			
AmB deoxycholate	1.0–1.5 mg/kg qd	• >5 decades of clinical experience • Inexpensive • Only licensed agent for treatment of mucormycosis	• Highly toxic • Poor CNS penetration
LAmB	5–10 mg/kg qd	• Less nephrotoxic than AmB deoxycholate • Better CNS penetration than AmB deoxycholate or ABLC • Better outcomes than with AmB deoxycholate in murine models and a retrospective clinical review	• Expensive
ABLC	5 mg/kg qd	• Less nephrotoxic than AmB deoxycholate • Murine and retrospective clinical data suggest benefit of combination therapy with echinocandins	• Expensive • Possibly less efficacious than LAmB for CNS infection
Primary Combination Therapy[b]			
Caspofungin plus lipid polyene	70-mg IV loading dose, then 50 mg/d for ≥2 weeks 50 mg/m² IV in children	• Favorable toxicity profile • Synergistic in murine disseminated mucormycosis • Retrospective clinical data suggest superior outcomes for rhino-orbital-cerebral mucormycosis.	• Very limited clinical data on combination therapy
Micafungin or anidulafungin plus lipid polyene	100 mg/d for ≥2 weeks Micafungin: 4 mg/kg qd in children Micafungin: 10 mg/kg qd in low-birth-weight infants Anidulafungin: 1.5 mg/kg qd in children	• Favorable toxicity profile • Synergistic with LAmB in murine model of disseminated mucormycosis	• No clinical data

[a]Primary therapy should generally include a polyene. Non-polyene-based regimens may be appropriate for patients who refuse or are intolerant of polyene therapy or for relatively immunocompetent patients with mild disease (e.g., isolated suprafascial cutaneous infection) that can be surgically eradicated. [b]Prospective randomized trials are necessary to confirm the suggested benefit (from animal and small retrospective human studies) of combination therapy for mucormycosis. Dose escalation of any echinocandin is not recommended because of a paradoxical loss of benefit of combination therapy at echinocandin doses of ≥3 mg/kg qd.

Abbreviations: ABLC, AmB lipid complex; AmB, amphotericin B; CNS, central nervous system; LAmB, liposomal AmB.

Source: Modified from B Spellberg et al: Clin Infect Dis 48:1743, 2009.

The optimal dosages for antifungal treatment of mucormycosis are not known. Starting dosages of 1 mg/kg per day for AmB deoxycholate and 5 mg/kg per day for LAmB and ABLC are commonly given to adults and children. Dose escalation of LAmB to 7.5 or 10 mg/kg per day for CNS mucormycosis may be considered in light of the limited penetration of polyenes into the brain. Because of auto-induction of metabolism, which results in paradoxically lower drug levels, there is no advantage to escalating the LAmB dose above 10 mg/kg per day, and doses of 5 mg/kg per day are probably adequate for non-CNS infections. ABLC dose escalation above 5 mg/kg per day is not advisable given the lack of relevant data and the drug's potential toxicity.

Echinocandin lipid polyene combinations improved survival rates among mice with disseminated mucormycosis (including CNS disease) and were associated with significantly better outcomes than polyene monotherapy in a small retrospective clinical study involving patients with rhino-orbital-cerebral mucormycosis. Although combination therapy may be considered on the basis of these limited data sets, definitive clinical trials are needed to establish whether it offers any real advantage over monotherapy for mucormycosis. Echinocandins should be administered at standard, FDA-approved doses, since dose escalation has resulted in paradoxical loss of efficacy in preclinical models.

In contrast to deferoxamine, the iron chelator deferasirox is fungicidal against clinical isolates of the Mucorales. In mice with DKA and disseminated mucormycosis, combination deferasirox-LAmB therapy resulted in synergistic improvement of survival rates and reduced the fungal burden in brain. Unfortunately, a randomized, double-blind, phase 2 safety clinical trial of adjunctive therapy with deferasirox (plus LAmB) documented excess mortality in the patients treated with deferasirox. It is noteworthy that the study population included primarily patients with active malignancy, and few patients in the study had diabetes mellitus as their only risk factor. Deferasirox is therefore contraindicated as therapy in patients with active malignancy, but its role in patients who have diabetes mellitus without malignancy (the setting in which its preclinical efficacy was optimal) remains uncertain.

Posaconazole is the only FDA-approved azole with in vitro activity against the Mucorales. However, pharmacokinetic/pharmacodynamic data raise concerns about the reliability with which adequate in vivo levels of orally administered posaconazole are attained. Furthermore, posaconazole is inferior in efficacy to AmB for the treatment of murine mucormycosis and is not superior to placebo for treatment of murine infection with *R. oryzae*. Moreover, posaconazole-polyene combination therapy is not superior to polyene monotherapy for mucormycosis in mice, and no comparative data are available for combination therapy in humans.

The roles of recombinant cytokines and neutrophil transfusions in the primary treatment of mucormycosis are not clear, although it is intuitive that earlier recovery of neutrophil counts should improve survival rates. Limited data indicate that hyperbaric oxygen may be useful in centers with the appropriate technical expertise and facilities.

In general, antifungal therapy for mucormycosis should be continued until resolution of clinical signs and symptoms of infection and resolution of underlying immunosuppression. For patients with mucormycosis who are receiving immunosuppressive medications, secondary antifungal prophylaxis is typically continued for as long as the immunosuppressive regimen is administered.

The role of radiographic follow-up in determining prognosis and therapeutic duration is being studied. Analysis of data from the phase 2 DEFEAT Mucor study indicated that early radiographic progression (within the first 2 weeks) did not predict long-term mortality risk, nor did early radiographic stability/regression predict long-term survival. Therefore, caution should be used in reacting to short-term, serial radiographic results, and greater emphasis should be placed on clinical response, particularly within the first 2–4 weeks after initiation of therapy.

243 Superficial Mycoses and Less Common Systemic Mycoses

Carol A. Kauffman

ENDEMIC MYCOSES (DIMORPHIC FUNGI)

Dimorphic fungi exist in discrete environmental niches as molds that produce conidia, which are their infectious form. In tissues and at temperatures of >35°C, the mold converts to the yeast form. Other endemic mycoses—histoplasmosis, coccidioidomycosis, and blastomycosis—are discussed in Chaps. 236, 237, and 238, respectively.

SPOROTRICHOSIS

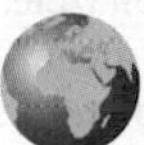

Etiologic Agent *Sporothrix schenckii* is a thermally dimorphic fungus that is found worldwide in sphagnum moss, decaying vegetation, and soil.

Epidemiology and Pathogenesis Sporotrichosis most commonly infects persons who participate in outdoor activities such as landscaping, gardening, and tree farming. Infected animals can transmit *S. schenckii* to humans. An outbreak of sporotrichosis in Rio de Janeiro that began in 1998 and that has involved >2000 people has been traced to cats, which are highly susceptible to this infection. Sporotrichosis is primarily a localized infection of skin and subcutaneous tissues that follows traumatic inoculation of conidia. Osteoarticular sporotrichosis is uncommon, occurring most often in middle aged men who abuse alcohol, and pulmonary sporotrichosis occurs almost exclusively in persons with chronic obstructive pulmonary disease who have inhaled the organism from the environment. Dissemination occurs rarely, almost always in markedly immunocompromised patients, especially those with AIDS.

Clinical Manifestations Days or weeks after inoculation, a papule develops at the site and then usually ulcerates but is not very painful. Similar lesions develop sequentially along the lymphatic channels proximal to the original lesion (Fig. 243-1). Some patients develop a fixed cutaneous lesion that can be verrucous or ulcerative and that remains localized without lymphatic extension. The differential diagnosis of lymphocutaneous sporotrichosis includes nocardiosis, tularemia, nontuberculous mycobacterial infection (especially that due to *Mycobacterium marinum*), and leishmaniasis. Osteoarticular sporotrichosis can present as chronic synovitis or septic arthritis. Pulmonary sporotrichosis must be differentiated from tuberculosis and from other fungal pneumonias.

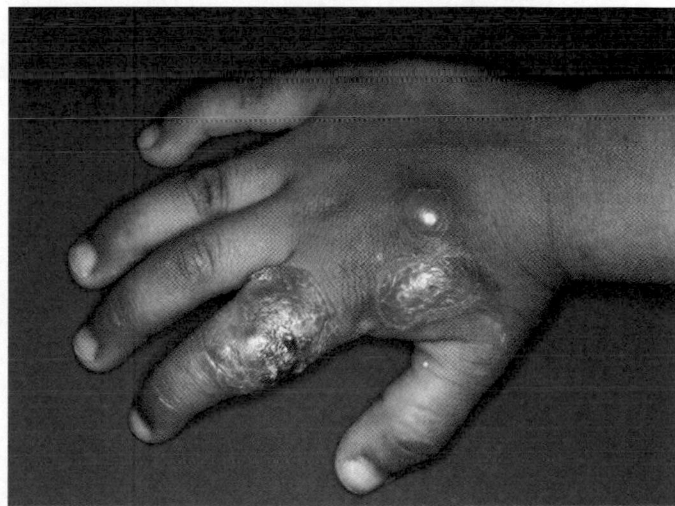

FIGURE 243-1 **Several nodular lesions** that developed after a young boy pricked his index finger with a thorn. A culture yielded *S. schenckii*. *(Courtesy of Dr. Angela Restrepo.)*

Numerous ulcerated skin lesions, with or without spread to visceral organs (including the central nervous system [CNS]), are characteristic of disseminated sporotrichosis.

Diagnosis *S. schenckii* usually grows readily as a mold when material from a cutaneous lesion is incubated at room temperature. Histopathologic examination of biopsy material shows a mixed granulomatous and pyogenic reaction, and tiny oval or cigar-shaped yeasts are sometimes visualized with special stains. Serologic testing is not useful.

Treatment and Prognosis Guidelines for the management of the various forms of sporotrichosis have been published by the Infectious Diseases Society of America (Table 243-1). Itraconazole is the drug of choice for lymphocutaneous sporotrichosis. Fluconazole is less effective; voriconazole and posaconazole have not been used for sporotrichosis. Saturated solution of potassium iodide (SSKI) also is effective for lymphocutaneous infection and costs much less than itraconazole. However, SSKI is poorly tolerated because of adverse reactions, including metallic taste, salivary gland swelling, rash, and fever. Terbinafine appears to be effective but has been used in few patients. Treatment for lymphocutaneous sporotrichosis is continued for 2–4 weeks after all lesions have resolved, usually for a total of 3–6 months. Pulmonary and osteoarticular forms of sporotrichosis are treated with itraconazole for at least 1 year. Severe pulmonary infection and disseminated sporotrichosis, including that involving the CNS, are treated initially with amphotericin B (AmB), which is followed by itraconazole after improvement has been noted. Lifelong suppressive therapy with itraconazole is required for AIDS patients. The success rate for treatment of lymphocutaneous sporotrichosis is 90–100%, but other forms of the disease respond poorly to antifungal therapy.

TABLE 243-1 SUGGESTED TREATMENT FOR ENDEMIC MYCOSES

Disease	First-Line Therapy	Alternatives/Comments
Sporotrichosis		
Cutaneous, lymphocutaneous	Itraconazole, 200 mg/d until 2–4 weeks after lesions resolve	SSKI, increasing doses[a] Terbinafine, 500 mg bid
Pulmonary, osteoarticular	Itraconazole, 200 mg bid for 12 months	Lipid AmB[b] for severe pulmonary disease until stable; then itraconazole
Disseminated, central nervous system	Lipid AmB[b] for 4–6 weeks	Itraconazole, 200 mg bid after AmB for 12 months Itraconazole maintenance for AIDS patients: 200 mg/d until CD4+ T cell count has been >200/μL for 12 months
Paracoccidioidomycosis		
Chronic (adult form)	Itraconazole, 100–200 mg/d for 6–12 months	TMP-SMX, 160/800 mg bid for 12–36 months
Acute (juvenile form)	AmB[c] until improvement	Itraconazole, 200 mg bid after AmB for 12 months
Penicilliosis		
Mild or moderate	Itraconazole, 200 mg bid for 12 weeks	Itraconazole maintenance for AIDS patients: 200 mg/d until CD4+ T cell count has been >100/μL for 6 months
Severe	AmB[c] until improvement	Itraconazole, 200 mg bid after AmB for 12 weeks Itraconazole maintenance: as for mild or moderate disease

[a]The starting dosage is 5–10 drops tid in water or juice. The dosage is increased weekly by 10 drops per dose, as tolerated, up to 40–50 drops tid. [b]The dosage of lipid AmB is 3–5 mg/kg daily; the higher dosage should be used when the central nervous system is involved. [c]The dosage of AmB deoxycholate is 0.6–1.0 mg/kg daily.

Abbreviations: AmB, amphotericin B; SSKI, saturated solution of potassium iodide; TMP-SMX, trimethoprim-sulfamethoxazole.

PARACOCCIDIOIDOMYCOSIS

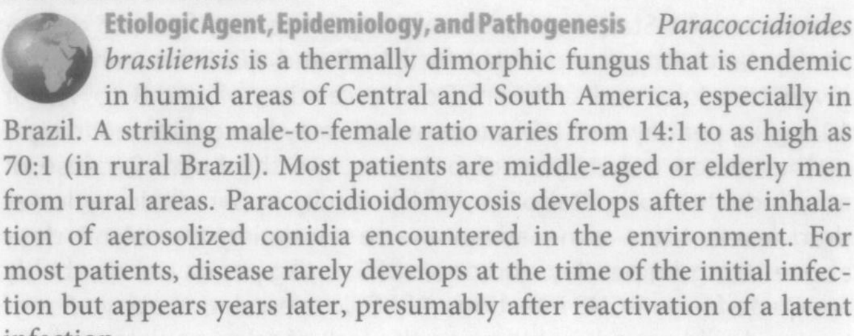

Etiologic Agent, Epidemiology, and Pathogenesis *Paracoccidioides brasiliensis* is a thermally dimorphic fungus that is endemic in humid areas of Central and South America, especially in Brazil. A striking male-to-female ratio varies from 14:1 to as high as 70:1 (in rural Brazil). Most patients are middle-aged or elderly men from rural areas. Paracoccidioidomycosis develops after the inhalation of aerosolized conidia encountered in the environment. For most patients, disease rarely develops at the time of the initial infection but appears years later, presumably after reactivation of a latent infection.

Clinical Manifestations Two major syndromes are associated with paracoccidioidomycosis: the acute or juvenile form and the chronic or adult form. The acute form is uncommon, occurs mostly in persons <30 years old, and manifests as disseminated infection of the reticuloendothelial system. Immunocompromised individuals also manifest this type of rapidly progressive disease. The chronic form of paracoccidioidomycosis accounts for ~90% of cases and predominantly affects older men. The primary manifestation is progressive pulmonary disease, primarily in the lower lobes, with fibrosis. Ulcerative and nodular mucocutaneous lesions in the nares and mouth—another common manifestation of chronic paracoccidioidomycosis—must be differentiated from leishmaniasis (Chap. 251) and squamous cell carcinoma (Chap. 105).

Diagnosis The diagnosis is established by growth of the organism in culture. A presumptive diagnosis can be made by detection of the distinctive thick-walled yeast, with multiple narrow-necked buds attached circumferentially, in purulent material or tissue biopsies.

Treatment and Prognosis Itraconazole is the treatment of choice for paracoccidioidomycosis (Table 243-1). Ketoconazole is also effective but more toxic; voriconazole and posaconazole have been used with success in a few cases. Sulfonamides also are effective and are the least costly agents, but the response is slower and the relapse rate higher. Seriously ill patients should be treated with AmB initially. Patients with paracoccidioidomycosis have an excellent response to therapy, but pulmonary fibrosis is often progressive in those with chronic disease.

PENICILLIOSIS

Etiologic Agent, Epidemiology, and Pathogenesis *Penicillium marneffei* is a thermally dimorphic fungus that is endemic in the soil in certain areas of Vietnam, Thailand, and several other southeastern Asian countries. The epidemiology of penicilliosis is linked to bamboo rats, which are infected with the fungus but rarely manifest disease. The disease occurs most often among persons living in rural areas in which the rats are found, but there is no evidence for transmission of the infection directly from rats to humans. Infection is rare in immunocompetent hosts, and most cases are reported in persons who have advanced AIDS. Infection results from the inhalation of conidia from the environment. The organism converts to the yeast phase in the lungs and then spreads hematogenously to the reticuloendothelial system.

Clinical Manifestations The clinical manifestations of penicilliosis mimic those of disseminated histoplasmosis and include fever, fatigue, weight loss, dyspnea, diarrhea (in some cases), lymphadenopathy, hepatosplenomegaly, and skin lesions, which appear as papules that often umbilicate and resemble molluscum contagiosum (Chap. 220e).

Diagnosis Penicilliosis is diagnosed by culture of *P. marneffei* from blood or from biopsy samples of skin, bone marrow, or lymph node. The organism usually grows within 1 week as a mold that produces a distinctive red pigment. Histopathologic examination of tissues and smears of blood or material from skin lesions shows oval or elliptical yeast-like organisms with central septation and can quickly establish a presumptive diagnosis.

Treatment and Prognosis Patients who have severe disease should be treated initially with AmB until their condition improves; therapy can then be changed to itraconazole (Table 243-1). Patients who have mild symptoms can be treated from the start with itraconazole. For patients with AIDS, suppressive therapy with itraconazole is recommended until immune reconstitution (related to successful therapy for HIV infection with antiretroviral drugs) is evident. Disseminated penicilliosis is usually fatal if not treated. With treatment, the mortality rate is ~10%.

PHAEOHYPHOMYCOSES

In these common soil organisms (also called *dematiaceous* fungi), melanin causes the hyphae and/or conidia to be darkly pigmented. The term *phaeohyphomycosis* is used to describe any infection with a pigmented mold. This definition encompasses two specific syndromes—eumycetoma and chromoblastomycosis—as well as all other types of infections caused by these organisms. It is important to note that eumycetomas can be caused by hyaline molds as well as brown-black molds and that only about half of all mycetomas are due to fungi. Actinomycetes cause the remainder (Chap. 199). Most of the involved fungi cause localized subcutaneous infections after direct inoculation, but disseminated infection and serious focal visceral infections also occur, especially in immunocompromised patients.

Etiologic Agents A large number of pigmented molds can cause human infection. All are found in the soil or on plants, and some cause economically important plant diseases. The most common cause of eumycetoma is *Madurella* species. *Fonsecaea* and *Cladophialophora* species are responsible for most cases of chromoblastomycosis. Disseminated infection and focal visceral infections are caused by a variety of dematiaceous fungi; *Alternaria, Exophiala, Curvularia,* and *Wangiella* species are among the more common molds reported to cause human infection. Recently, *Exserohilum* species have caused a large outbreak of severe, sometimes fatal CNS and osteoarticular infections following the injection of methylprednisolone contaminated with this fungus.

Epidemiology and Pathogenesis Eumycetoma and chromoblastomycosis are acquired by inoculation through the skin. These two syndromes are seen almost entirely in tropical and subtropical areas and occur mostly in rural laborers who are frequently exposed to the organisms. Other infections with dematiaceous molds are acquired by inhalation, by traumatic inoculation into the eye or through the skin, or by injection of contaminated medication. Melanin is a virulence factor for all the pigmented molds. Several organisms, specifically *Cladophialophora bantiana* and *Rhinocladiella mackenziei,* are neurotropic and likely to cause CNS infection. In an immunocompromised patient or when a pigmented mold is injected directly into a deep structure, these organisms become opportunists, invading blood vessels and mimicking better-known opportunistic infections, such as aspergillosis.

Clinical Manifestations Eumycetoma is a chronic subcutaneous and cutaneous infection that usually occurs on the lower extremities and that is characterized by swelling, development of sinus tracts, and the appearance of grains that are actually colonies of fungi discharged from the sinus tract. As the infection progresses, adjacent fascia and bony structures become involved. The disease is indolent and disfiguring, progressing slowly over years. Complications include fractures of infected bone and bacterial superinfection.

Chromoblastomycosis is an indolent subcutaneous infection characterized by nodular, verrucous, or plaque-like painless lesions that occur predominantly on the lower extremities and grow slowly over months to years. There is hardly ever extension to adjacent structures, as is seen with eumycetoma. Long-term consequences include bacterial superinfection, chronic lymphedema, and (rarely) the development of squamous cell carcinoma.

Dematiaceous molds are the most common cause of allergic fungal sinusitis and a less common cause of invasive fungal sinusitis. Keratitis occurs with traumatic corneal inoculation. Even in many immunocompromised patients, inoculation through the skin generally produces localized cyst-like, nodular lesions at the entry site. However, other immunocompromised patients develop pneumonia, brain abscess, or disseminated infection. Epidural injection of *Exserohilum*-contaminated steroids has led to meningitis, basilar stroke, epidural abscess or phlegmon, vertebral osteomyelitis, and arachnoiditis.

Diagnosis The specific diagnosis of infection with a pigmented mold is established by growth of the organism in culture. However, in eumycetoma, a tentative clinical diagnosis can be made when a patient presents with a lesion characterized by swelling, sinus tracts, and grains. Histopathologic examination and culture are necessary to confirm that the etiologic agent is a mold and not an actinomycete. In chromoblastomycosis, the diagnosis rests on the histologic demonstration of sclerotic bodies (dark brown, thick-walled, septate fungal forms that resemble large yeasts) in the tissues; culture establishes which pigmented mold is causing the infection. For other infections, growth of the organism is essential to differentiate infection with a hyaline mold (e.g., *Aspergillus* or *Fusarium*) from that due to a pigmented mold. No serologic assays for pigmented molds are available. Polymerase chain reaction (PCR) assays are increasingly used in the diagnosis of infection due to pigmented molds but are available only through fungal reference laboratories.

Treatment and Prognosis Treatment of eumycetoma and chromoblastomycosis involves both surgical extirpation of the lesion and use of antifungal agents. Surgical removal of the lesions of both eumycetoma and chromoblastomycosis is most effective if performed before extensive spread has occurred. In chromoblastomycosis, cryosurgery and laser therapy have been used with variable success. The antifungal agents of choice are itraconazole, voriconazole, and posaconazole. The most experience has accrued with itraconazole; less experience has been gained with the newer azoles, which are active in vitro and have been reported to be effective in a few patients. Flucytosine and terbinafine also have been used to treat chromoblastomycosis. Chromoblastomycosis and eumycetoma are chronic indolent infections that are difficult to cure but are not life-threatening.

Disseminated and focal visceral infections are treated with the appropriate antifungal agent; the choice of agent is based on the location and extent of the infection, in vitro testing, and clinical experience with the specific infecting organism. AmB is not effective against many of these organisms but has been used successfully against others. The most experience has accrued with itraconazole in the treatment of localized infections. Voriconazole is increasingly used when infections are disseminated or involve the CNS because this drug reaches adequate concentrations within the CNS and because both IV and well-absorbed oral formulations are available. The role of posaconazole has not been established but will likely expand. Disseminated and focal visceral infections, especially those involving the CNS, are associated with high mortality rates.

OPPORTUNISTIC FUNGAL INFECTIONS

Two genera of hyaline (nonpigmented) molds, *Fusarium* and *Scedosporium*, and one yeast-like genus, *Trichosporon*, have become prominent pathogens among immunocompromised patients. Infections caused by *Fusarium* and *Scedosporium* species overlap with invasive aspergillosis in their clinical manifestations, and, when seen in tissues, these organisms appear similar to *Aspergillus*. In the immunocompetent host, these fungi cause localized infections of skin, skin structures, and subcutaneous tissues, but their role as causes of infection in immunocompromised patients will be emphasized in this section.

FUSARIOSIS

Etiologic Agent, Epidemiology, and Pathogenesis *Fusarium* species, which are found worldwide in soil and on plants, have emerged as major opportunists in markedly immunocompromised patients. Most human infections follow inhalation of conidia, but ingestion and direct inoculation also can lead to disease. An outbreak of severe *Fusarium* keratitis among soft contact lens wearers was traced back to a particular brand of contact lens solution and individual contact lens cases that had been contaminated. Disseminated infection is reported most often in patients who have a hematologic malignancy, are neutropenic, have received a stem cell or solid organ transplant, or have a severe burn.

Clinical Manifestations In immunocompetent persons, *Fusarium* species cause localized infections of various organs. These organisms commonly cause fungal keratitis, which can extend into the anterior chamber of the eye; cause loss of vision; and require corneal transplantation. Onychomycosis due to *Fusarium* species, while basically an annoyance in immunocompetent patients, is a source of subsequent hematogenous dissemination and should be aggressively sought and treated in neutropenic patients. In profoundly immunocompromised patients, fusariosis is angioinvasive, and clinical manifestations mimic those of aspergillosis. Pulmonary infection is characterized by multiple nodular lesions. Sinus infection is likely to lead to invasion of adjacent structures. Disseminated fusariosis occurs primarily in neutropenic patients with hematologic malignancies and in allogeneic stem cell transplant recipients, especially those with graft-versus-host disease. Disseminated fusariosis differs from disseminated aspergillosis in that skin lesions are extremely common with fusariosis; the lesions are nodular or necrotic, are usually painful, and appear over time in different locations (Fig. 243-2).

Diagnosis The diagnostic approach usually includes both documentation of the growth of *Fusarium* species from involved tissue and demonstration of invasion by histopathologic techniques that show septate hyphae in tissues. The organism is difficult to differentiate from *Aspergillus* species in tissues; thus, identification with culture is imperative. An extremely helpful diagnostic clue is growth in blood cultures, which are positive in as many as 50% of patients with disseminated fusariosis. There are no serologic assays for *Fusarium*. PCR techniques have proved useful but are available only through fungal reference laboratories.

Treatment and Prognosis *Fusarium* species are resistant to many antifungal agents. A lipid formulation of AmB (at least 5 mg/kg daily), voriconazole (200–400 mg twice daily), or posaconazole (300 mg daily) is recommended. Many physicians use both a lipid formulation of AmB and either voriconazole or posaconazole because susceptibility information is not available when therapy must be initiated. Serum drug levels should be monitored with either azole to ensure that absorption is adequate and with voriconazole to avoid toxicity. Mortality rates for disseminated fusariosis have been as high as 85%. With the improved antifungal therapy now available, mortality rates have fallen to ~50%. However, if neutropenia persists, the mortality rate approaches 100%.

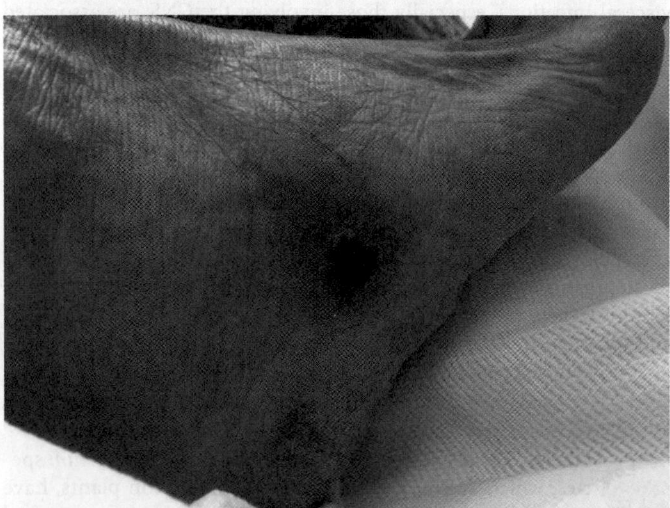

FIGURE 243-2 Painful necrotic foot lesion that developed over a week in a woman who had acute leukemia and who had been neutropenic for 2 months. *Fusarium* species were grown from a punch biopsy. *(Courtesy of Dr. Nessrine Ktaich.)*

SCEDOSPORIOSIS

Etiologic Agent The genus *Scedosporium* includes several pathogens. The major causes of human infections are *Scedosporium apiospermum*, which in its sexual state is termed *Pseudallescheria boydii*, and *S. prolificans*. The *S. apiospermum* complex encompasses several species but will be referred to here simply as *S. apiospermum*.

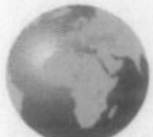

Epidemiology and Pathogenesis *S. apiospermum* is found worldwide in temperate climates in tidal flats, swamps, ponds, manure, and soil. This organism is known as a cause of pneumonia, disseminated infection, and brain abscess in near-drowning victims. *S. prolificans* is also found in soil but is more geographically restricted. Infection occurs predominantly through inhalation of conidia, but direct inoculation through the skin or into the eye also can occur.

Clinical Manifestations Among immunocompetent persons, *Scedosporium* species are a prominent cause of eumycetoma. Keratitis as a result of accidental corneal inoculation is a sight-threatening infection. In patients who have hematologic malignancies (especially acute leukemia with neutropenia), recipients of solid organ or stem cell transplants, and patients receiving glucocorticoids, *Scedosporium* species are angioinvasive, causing pneumonia and widespread dissemination with abscesses. Pulmonary infection mimics aspergillosis; nodules, cavities, and lobar infiltrates are common. Disseminated infection involves the skin, heart, brain, and many other organs. Skin lesions are not as common or as painful as those of fusariosis.

Diagnosis Diagnosis depends on the growth of *Scedosporium* species from involved tissue and the demonstration of invasion by histopathologic techniques that show septate hyphae in tissues. Culture evidence is essential because *Scedosporium* species are difficult to differentiate from *Aspergillus* in tissues. Demonstration of tissue invasion is essential because these ubiquitous environmental molds can be mere contaminants or colonizers. *S. prolificans* can grow in blood cultures, but *S. apiospermum* usually does not. There are no serologic assays for *Scedosporium*. PCR techniques have proved useful but are available only through fungal reference laboratories.

Treatment and Prognosis *Scedosporium* species are resistant to AmB, echinocandins, and some azoles. Voriconazole is the agent of choice for *S. apiospermum*, and posaconazole also has been used for this infection. *S. prolificans* is resistant in vitro to almost every available antifungal agent; the addition of agents such as terbinafine to a voriconazole regimen has been attempted because in vitro data suggest possible synergy against some strains of *S. prolificans*. Mortality rates for invasive *S. apiospermum* infection are ~50%, but those for invasive *S. prolificans* infection remain as high as 85–100%.

TRICHOSPORONOSIS

Etiologic Agent The genus *Trichosporon* contains many species, some of which cause localized infection of hair and nails. The major pathogen responsible for invasive infection is *Trichosporon asahii*. *Trichosporon* species grow as yeast-like colonies in vitro; in vivo, however, hyphae, pseudohyphae, and arthroconidia can also be seen.

Epidemiology and Pathogenesis These yeasts are commonly found in soil, sewage, and water and in rare instances can colonize human skin and the human gastrointestinal tract. Most infections follow fungal inhalation or entry via central venous catheters. Systemic infection occurs almost exclusively in immunocompromised hosts, including those who have hematologic malignancies, are neutropenic, have received a solid organ transplant, or are receiving glucocorticoids.

Clinical Manifestations Disseminated trichosporonosis resembles invasive candidiasis, and fungemia is often the initial manifestation of infection. Pneumonia, skin lesions, and sepsis syndrome are common. The skin lesions begin as papules or nodules surrounded by erythema and progress to central necrosis. A chronic form of infection mimics hepatosplenic candidiasis (chronic disseminated candidiasis).

Diagnosis The diagnosis of systemic *Trichosporon* infection is established by growth of the organism from involved tissues or from blood. Histopathologic examination of a skin lesion showing a mixture of yeast forms, arthroconidia, and hyphae can lead to an early presumptive diagnosis of trichosporonosis. The serum cryptococcal antigen latex agglutination test may be positive in patients with disseminated trichosporonosis because *T. asahii* and *Cryptococcus neoformans* share polysaccharide antigens.

Treatment and Prognosis Rates of response to AmB have been disappointing, and many *Trichosporon* isolates are resistant in vitro. Voriconazole appears to be the antifungal agent of choice and is used at a dosage of 200–400 mg twice daily. The mortality rates for disseminated *Trichosporon* infection have been as high as 70% but are decreasing with the use of newer azoles, such as voriconazole; however, patients who remain neutropenic are likely to succumb to this infection.

SUPERFICIAL CUTANEOUS INFECTIONS

Fungal infections of the skin and skin structures are caused by molds and yeasts that do not invade deeper tissues but rather cause disease merely by inhabiting the superficial layers of skin, hair follicles, and nails. These agents are the most common cause of fungal infections of humans but only rarely cause serious infections.

YEAST INFECTIONS

Etiologic Agents The lipophilic yeast *Malassezia* is dimorphic in that it lives on the skin in the yeast phase but transforms to the mold phase as it causes disease. Most species require exogenous lipids for growth.

Epidemiology and Pathogenesis *Malassezia* species are part of the indigenous human flora found in the stratum corneum of the back, chest, scalp, and face—areas rich in sebaceous glands. Disease is more common in humid areas. The organisms do not invade below the stratum corneum and generally elicit little if any inflammatory response.

Clinical Manifestations *Malassezia* species cause tinea versicolor (also called *pityriasis versicolor*), folliculitis, and seborrheic dermatitis. Tinea versicolor presents as flat round scaly patches of hypo- or hyperpigmented skin on the neck, chest, or upper arms. The lesions are usually asymptomatic but can be pruritic. They can be mistaken for vitiligo, but the latter is not scaly. Folliculitis occurs over the back and chest and mimics bacterial folliculitis. Seborrheic dermatitis manifests as erythematous pruritic scaly lesions in the eyebrows, moustache, nasolabial folds, and scalp. The scalp lesions are termed *cradle cap* in babies and *dandruff* in adults. Seborrheic dermatitis can be severe in patients with advanced AIDS. Fungemia and disseminated infection occur rarely with *Malassezia* species—almost always in premature neonates receiving parenteral lipid preparations through a central venous catheter.

Diagnosis *Malassezia* infections are diagnosed clinically in most cases. If scrapings are collected on a microscope slide on which a drop of potassium hydroxide has been placed, a mixture of budding yeasts and short septate hyphae is seen. In order to culture *M. furfur* from those patients in whom disseminated infection is suspected, sterile olive oil must be added to the medium.

Treatment and Prognosis Topical creams and lotions, including selenium sulfide shampoo, ketoconazole shampoo or cream, terbinafine cream, and ciclopirox cream, are effective in treating *Malassezia* infections and are usually given for 2 weeks. Mild topical steroid creams are sometimes used to treat seborrheic dermatitis. For extensive disease, itraconazole (200 mg/d) or fluconazole (200 mg/d) can be used for 5–7 days. The rare cases of fungemia caused by *Malassezia* species are treated with AmB or fluconazole, prompt removal of the catheter, and discontinuance of parenteral lipid infusions. *Malassezia* skin infections are benign and self-limited, although recurrences are the rule. The outcome of systemic infection depends on the host's underlying conditions, but most infected infants do well.

DERMATOPHYTE (MOLD) INFECTIONS

Etiologic Agents The molds that cause skin infections in humans include the genera *Trichophyton*, *Microsporum*, and *Epidermophyton*. These organisms, which are not components of the normal skin flora, can live within the keratinized structures of the skin—hence the term *dermatophytes*.

Epidemiology and Pathogenesis Dermatophytes occur worldwide, and infections with these organisms are extremely common. Some organisms cause disease only in humans and can be transmitted by person-to-person contact and by fomites, such as hairbrushes or wet floors, that have been contaminated by infected individuals. Several species cause infections in cats and dogs and can readily be transmitted from these animals to humans. Finally, some dermatophytes are spread from contact with soil. The characteristic ring shape of cutaneous lesions is the result of the organisms' outward growth in a centrifugal pattern in the stratum corneum. Fungal invasion of the nail usually occurs through the lateral or superficial nail plates and then spreads throughout the nail; when hair shafts are invaded, the organisms can be found either within the shaft or surrounding it. Symptoms are caused by the inflammatory reaction elicited by fungal antigens and not by tissue invasion. Dermatophyte infections occur more commonly in male than in female patients, and progesterone has been shown to inhibit dermatophyte growth.

Clinical Manifestations Dermatophyte infection of the skin is often called *ringworm*. This term is confusing because worms are not involved. *Tinea*, the Latin word for *worm*, describes the serpentine nature of the skin lesions and is a less confusing designation that is used in conjunction with the name of the body part affected—e.g., tinea capitis (head), tinea pedis (feet), tinea corporis (body), tinea cruris (crotch), and tinea unguium (nails, although infection at this site is more often termed *onychomycosis*).

Tinea capitis occurs most commonly in children 3–7 years old. Children with tinea capitis usually present with well-demarcated scaly patches in which hair shafts are broken off right above the skin; alopecia can result. Tinea corporis is manifested by well-demarcated, annular, pruritic, scaly lesions that undergo central clearing. Usually one or several small lesions are present. In some cases, tinea corporis can involve much of the trunk or manifest as folliculitis with pustule formation. The rash should be differentiated from contact dermatitis, eczema, and psoriasis. Tinea cruris is seen almost exclusively in men. The perineal rash is erythematous and pustular, has a discrete scaly border, is without satellite lesions, and is usually pruritic. The rash must be differentiated from intertriginous candidiasis, erythrasma, and psoriasis.

Tinea pedis also is more common among men than among women. It usually starts in the web spaces of the toes; peeling, maceration, and pruritus are followed by development of a scaly pruritic rash along the lateral and plantar surfaces of the feet. Hyperkeratosis of the soles of the feet often ensues. Tinea pedis has been implicated in lower-extremity cellulitis, as streptococci and staphylococci can gain entrance to the tissues through fissures between the toes. Onychomycosis affects toenails more often than fingernails and is most common among persons who have tinea pedis. The nail becomes thickened and discolored and may crumble; onycholysis almost always occurs. Onychomycosis is more common in older adults and in persons with vascular disease, diabetes mellitus, and trauma to the nails. Fungal infection must be differentiated from psoriasis, which can mimic onychomycosis but usually has associated skin lesions.

Diagnosis Many dermatophyte infections are diagnosed by their clinical appearance. If the diagnosis is in doubt, as is often the case in children with tinea capitis, scrapings should be taken from the edge of a lesion with a scalpel blade, transferred to a slide to which a drop of potassium hydroxide is added, and examined under a microscope for the presence of hyphae. Cultures are indicated if an outbreak is suspected or the patient does not respond to therapy. Culture of the nail is especially useful as an aid to decisions about both diagnosis and treatment.

Treatment and Prognosis Dermatophyte infections usually respond to topical therapy. Lotions or sprays are easier than creams to apply to large or hairy areas. Particularly for tinea cruris, the affected

TABLE 243-2 SUGGESTED ORAL TREATMENT FOR EXTENSIVE TINEA INFECTIONS AND ONYCHOMYCOSIS

Antifungal Agent	Suggested Dosage	Comments
Extensive Tinea Skin Infection		
Terbinafine	250 mg/d for 1–2 weeks	Adverse reactions minimal with short treatment period
Itraconazole[a]	200 mg/d for 1–2 weeks	Adverse reactions minimal with short treatment period except for drug interactions
Onychomycosis		
Terbinafine	250 mg/d for 3 months	Slightly superior to itraconazole; monitor for hepatotoxicity
Itraconazole[a]	200 mg/d for 3 months or 200 mg bid for 1 week each month for 3 months	Drug interactions frequent; monitor for hepatotoxicity; rarely causes hypokalemia, hypertension, edema; use with caution in patients with congestive heart failure

[a]Itraconazole capsules require food and gastric acid for absorption, whereas itraconazole solution is taken on an empty stomach.

area should be kept as dry as possible. When patients have extensive skin lesions, oral itraconazole or terbinafine can hasten resolution (Table 243-2). Terbinafine interacts with fewer drugs than itraconazole and is generally the first-line agent. Onychomycosis does not respond to topical therapy, although ciclopirox nail lacquer applied daily for a year is occasionally beneficial. Itraconazole and terbinafine both accumulate in the nail plate and can be used to treat onychomycosis (Table 243-2). These agents are more effective and better tolerated than griseofulvin and ketoconazole. The major decision to be made with regard to therapy is whether the extent of nail involvement justifies the use of systemic antifungal agents that have adverse effects, may interact with other drugs, and are costly. Treating for cosmetic reasons alone is discouraged. Relapses of tinea cruris and tinea pedis are common and should be treated early with topical creams to avoid development of more extensive disease. Relapses of onychomycosis follow treatment in 25–30% of cases.

244 *Pneumocystis* Infections

Henry Masur, Alison Morris

DEFINITION AND DESCRIPTION

Pneumocystis is an opportunistic pathogen that is an important cause of pneumonia in immunocompromised hosts, particularly those with HIV infection (Chap. 226), and in individuals with organ transplants, those with hematologic malignancies, and those receiving immunosuppressive therapy. The organism was discovered in rodents in 1906 and was initially believed to be a protozoan. Because *Pneumocystis* cannot be cultured, our understanding of its biology has been limited, but molecular techniques have demonstrated that the organism is actually a fungus. Formerly known as *Pneumocystis carinii*, the species infecting humans has been renamed *Pneumocystis jirovecii*.

EPIDEMIOLOGY

P. jirovecii pneumonia (PCP) came to medical attention when cases were reported in malnourished orphans in Europe during World War II. The disease was later recognized in other immunosuppressed populations but was rare in the era before HIV/AIDS and before intensive immunosuppressive therapy for organ transplantation and autoimmune disorders. In 1981, PCP was first reported in men who had sex with men and in IV drug users who had no obvious cause of immunosuppression. These cases were subsequently recognized as the first cases of what came to be known as the acquired immunodeficiency syndrome (AIDS) (Chap. 226). The incidence of PCP increased dramatically as the AIDS epidemic grew: without chemoprophylaxis or antiretroviral therapy (ART), 80–90% of patients with HIV/AIDS in North America and Western Europe ultimately develop one or more episodes of PCP. While its incidence declined with the introduction of anti-*Pneumocystis* prophylaxis and combination ART, PCP has continued to be a leading cause of AIDS-associated morbidity in the United States and Western Europe, particularly in individuals who do not know they are infected with HIV until they are profoundly immunosuppressed and in HIV-infected patients who are not receiving ART or PCP prophylaxis.

PCP also develops in HIV-uninfected patients who are immunocompromised secondary to hematologic or malignant neoplasms, stem cell or solid organ transplantation, and immunosuppressive medications. The incidence of PCP depends on the degree of immunosuppression. PCP is increasingly reported among individuals receiving tumor necrosis factor α inhibitors and antilymphocyte monoclonal antibodies for rheumatologic or other diseases. While clinical PCP in immunocompetent hosts has not been clearly documented, studies have shown that *Pneumocystis* organisms can colonize the airways of children and adults who are not overtly immunocompromised. The relevance of these organisms to acute or chronic syndromes, such as chronic obstructive pulmonary disease (COPD), in immunocompetent patients is being investigated.

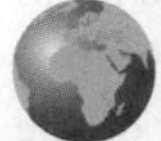

In some developing countries, the incidence of PCP among HIV-infected individuals has been found to be lower than that in industrialized countries. This lower incidence may be due to competing mortality from infectious diseases such as tuberculosis and bacterial pneumonia, which typically occur before patients become immunosuppressed enough to develop PCP. Geographic variations in *Pneumocystis* exposure and underdiagnosis also may explain the apparent lower frequency of PCP in some countries.

PATHOGENESIS AND PATHOLOGY

Life Cycle and Transmission The life cycle of *Pneumocystis* involves both sexual and asexual reproduction, and the organism exists as a trophic form, a cyst, and a precyst at various points. Serologic and molecular studies have demonstrated that most humans are exposed to *Pneumocystis* early in life. It was historically thought that *Pneumocystis* developed from reactivation of latent infection, but *de novo* infections from environmental sources and person-to-person transmission occur as well. Outbreaks of PCP suggest that nosocomial transmission can take place, and studies with rodents show that immunocompetent animals can serve as reservoirs for transmission of *P. carinii* (the infecting species in rodents) to immunocompetent and immunosuppressed animals. However, *Pneumocystis* organisms are species specific, and thus humans are infected only by other humans who transmit *P. jirovecii*; humans cannot be infected with animal species of *Pneumocystis* such as *P. murina* (mice) or *P. oryctolagi* (rabbits). The utility of respiratory isolation in preventing transmission from patients with PCP to other immunosuppressed individuals has been debated; no clear evidence exists, although it seems prudent to isolate patients with active PCP from other immunosuppressed patients.

Role of Immunity Defects in cellular and/or humoral immunity predispose to development of PCP. CD4+ T cells are critical in host defense against *Pneumocystis*. For HIV-infected patients, the incidence is inversely related to the CD4+ T cell count: at least 80% of cases occur at counts of <200 cells/μL, and most of these cases develop at counts of <100 cells/μL. CD4+ T cell counts are less specific and thus less useful in predicting the risk of PCP in HIV-uninfected, immunosuppressed patients.

Lung Pathology *Pneumocystis* has a unique tropism for the lung. It is presumably inhaled into the alveolar space. Clinically apparent pneumonia occurs only if an individual is immunocompromised. *Pneumocystis* proliferates in the lung, provoking a mononuclear cell

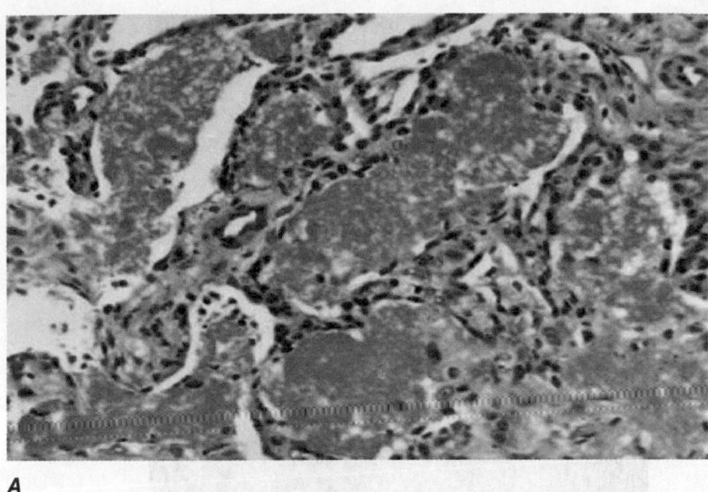

A

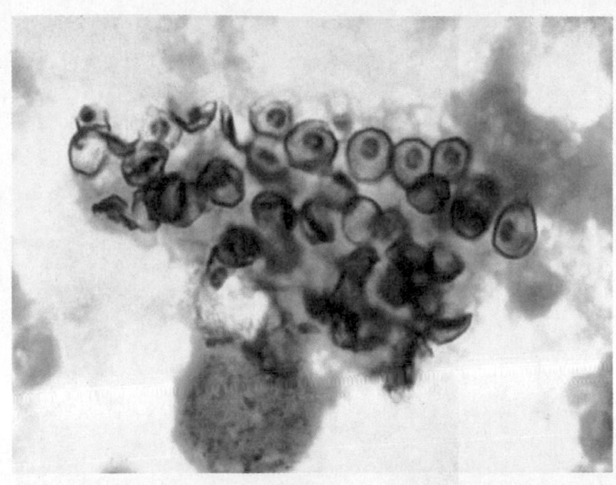

B

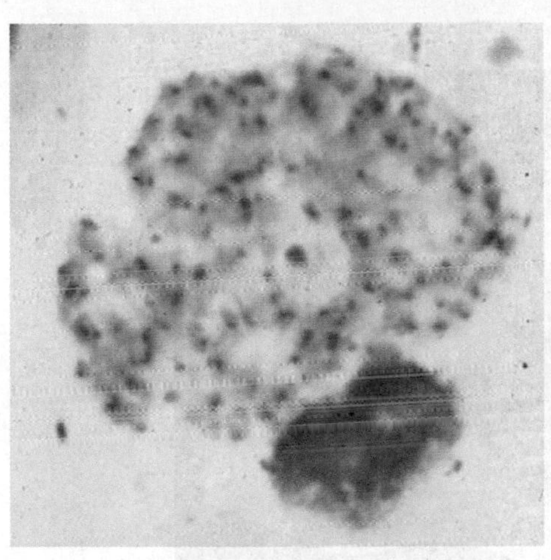

C

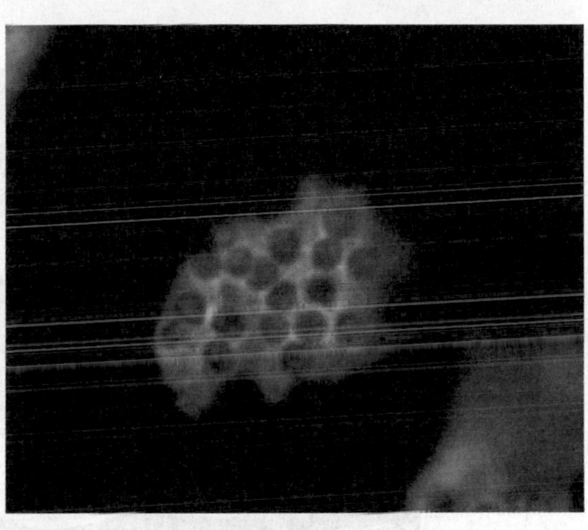

D

FIGURE 244-1 Direct microscopy of *Pneumocystis* pneumonia. ***A.*** Transbronchial lung biopsy stained with hematoxylin and eosin shows eosinophilic alveolar filling. ***B.*** Methenamine silver–stained bronchoalveolar lavage (BAL) fluid. ***C.*** Giemsa-stained BAL fluid. ***D.*** Immunofluorescent stain of BAL fluid.

response. The alveoli become filled with proteinaceous material, and alveolar damage results in increased alveolar-capillary injury and surfactant abnormalities. Stained lung sections typically show foamy, vacuolated alveolar exudates composed largely of viable and nonviable organisms (Fig. 244-1*A*). Interstitial edema and fibrosis may develop, and organisms can be seen in the alveolar space with silver or other stains. Moreover, the organisms can be seen when tissue is subjected to colorimetric or immunofluorescent staining (Fig. 244-1*B–D*).

CLINICAL FEATURES

Clinical Presentation PCP presents as acute or subacute pneumonia that may initially be characterized by a vague sense of dyspnea alone but that subsequently manifests as fever and nonproductive cough with progressive shortness of breath ultimately resulting in respiratory failure and death. Extrapulmonary manifestations of PCP are rare but can include involvement of almost any organ, most notably lymph nodes, spleen, and liver.

Physical Examination The physical examination findings in PCP are nonspecific. Patients have decreased oxygen saturation—at rest or with exertion—that, without treatment, progresses to severe hypoxemia. Patients may initially have a normal chest examination and no adventitious sounds but later, without treatment, develop diffuse rales and signs of consolidation. Oral thrush in a patient with HIV infection indicates an increased risk for PCP.

Laboratory Findings The results of routine laboratory tests are nonspecific in PCP. Serum levels of lactate dehydrogenase (LDH) are often elevated due to pulmonary damage; however, a normal LDH level does not rule out PCP, nor is an elevated LDH value specific for PCP. The peripheral white blood cell count may be elevated, but the increase is usually modest. Hepatic and renal function are typically normal.

Radiographic Findings Although the initial chest radiograph may be normal when patients have mild symptoms, the classic radiographic appearance of PCP consists of diffuse bilateral interstitial infiltrates that are perihilar and symmetric (Fig. 244-2*A*)—yet another finding that is not specific for PCP. The interstitial infiltrates can progress to alveolar filling (Fig. 244-2*B*). High-resolution chest CT shows diffuse ground-glass opacities in virtually all patients with PCP (Fig. 244-2*C*). A normal chest CT essentially rules out the diagnosis of PCP. Cysts and pneumothoraces are common chest radiographic findings (Fig. 244-2*D*). A wide variety of atypical radiographic findings have been described, including asymmetric patterns, upper lobe infiltrates, mediastinal adenopathy, nodules, cavities, and effusions.

DIAGNOSIS

The optimal sample for diagnostic examination depends on how ill the patient is and what resources are available. Before the 1990s, diagnoses of PCP were usually established by open lung biopsy; later, transbronchial lung biopsy was employed. Hematoxylin and eosin staining of pulmonary

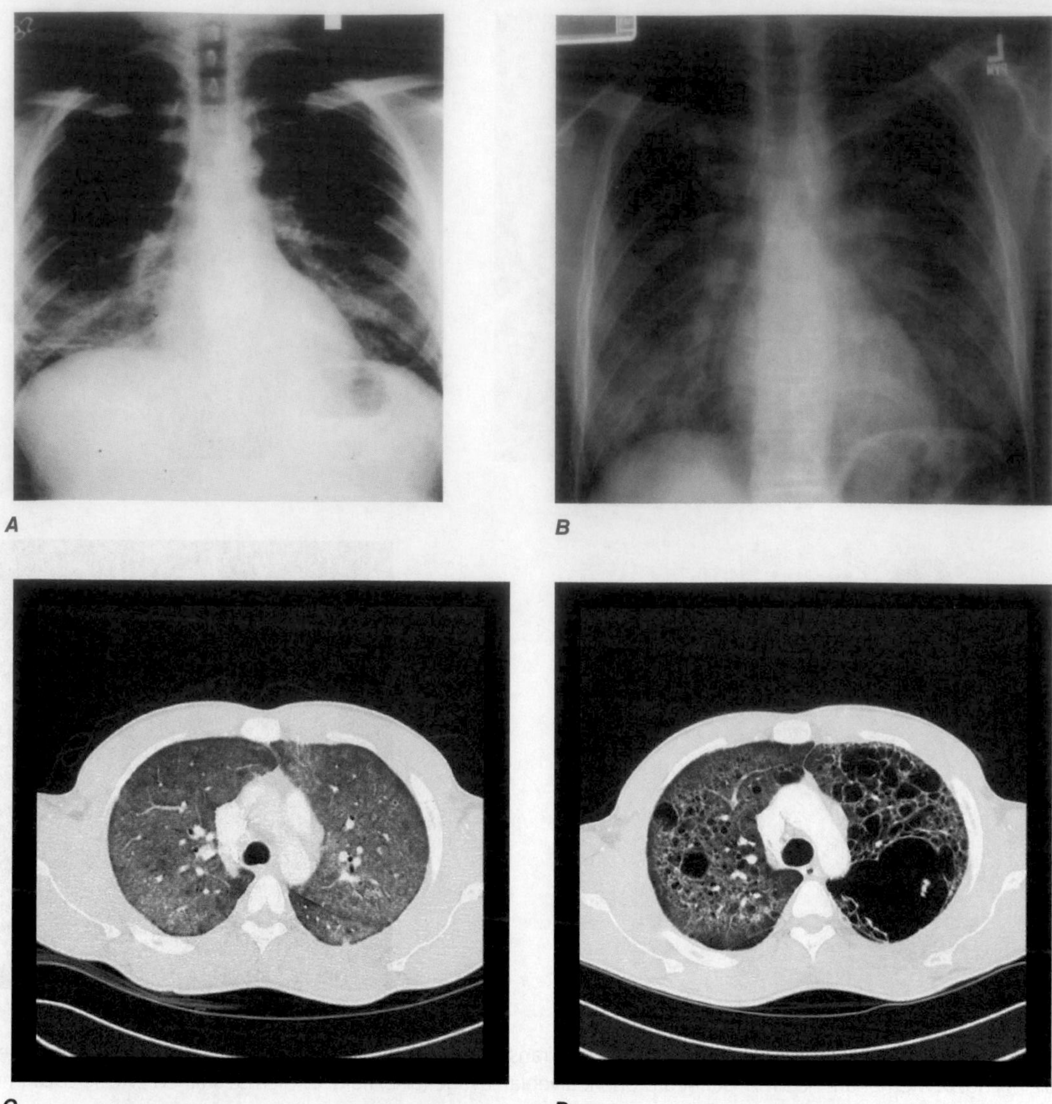

FIGURE 244-2 Radiographs in *Pneumocystis* pneumonia. ***A.*** Posterior-anterior chest radiograph showing symmetric interstitial infiltrates. ***B.*** Posterior-anterior chest radiograph showing symmetric alveolar infiltrates (courtesy of Alison Morris). ***C.*** CT image demonstrating symmetric interstitial infiltrates and ground-glass opacities. ***D.*** CT image showing symmetric interstitial infiltrates, ground-glass opacities, and pneumatoceles.

tissue demonstrates a foamy alveolar infiltrate and a mononuclear interstitial infiltrate (Fig. 244-2*A*). This appearance is pathognomonic for PCP even though the organisms cannot be specifically identified with this stain. The diagnosis is typically established in lung tissue or pulmonary secretions by highly specific staining of the cyst—e.g., with methenamine silver (Fig. 244-2*B*), toluidine blue O, or Giemsa (Fig. 244-2*C*)—or by staining with a specific immunofluorescent antibody (Fig. 244-2*D*).

The demonstration of organisms in bronchoalveolar lavage fluid is almost 100% sensitive and specific for PCP in patients with either HIV infection or immunosuppression of other etiologies. The organisms are identified with the specific stains indicated above for lung biopsy. While expectorated sputum or throat swabs have very low sensitivity, an induced sputum sample obtained and interpreted by an experienced provider can be highly sensitive and specific. The reported sensitivity of induced sputum for PCP is widely variable (55–90%), however, and is dependent on both the characteristics of the patient and the experience of the center conducting the test.

Recently, many laboratories have offered polymerase chain reaction (PCR) testing of respiratory specimens for *Pneumocystis*. However, these PCR tests are so sensitive that it is difficult to distinguish patients with colonization (i.e., those whose acute lung disease is due to some other process but who have low levels of *Pneumocystis* DNA in the lungs) from those with acute pneumonia due to *Pneumocystis*. Such PCR tests on appropriate samples may be more useful for ruling out a diagnosis of PCP if they are negative than for definitively attributing the disease to *Pneumocystis*.

There has been considerable interest in serologic tests such as assays for (1→3)-β-D-glucan, levels of which are frequently elevated in patients with PCP. However, no serologic assays developed to date offer substantial sensitivity or specificity.

COURSE AND PROGNOSIS

Untreated, PCP is invariably fatal. Patients with HIV infection often have an indolent course that presents as mild exercise intolerance or chest tightness without fever or cough and a normal or nearly normal posterior-anterior chest radiograph, with progression over days, weeks, or even a few months to fever, cough, diffuse alveolar infiltrates, and profound hypoxemia. Some patients with HIV infection and most patients with other types of immunosuppression have more acute disease that progresses over a few days to respiratory failure. Rare patients also develop distributive shock. A few unusual patients present with extrapulmonary manifestations in the skin or soft tissue, retina, brain, liver, kidney, or spleen that are nonspecific in presentation and can be diagnosed only by histology.

Factors that influence mortality risk include the patient's age and degree of immunosuppression as well as the presence of preexisting lung disease, a low serum albumin level, the need for mechanical ventilation, and the development of pneumothorax. With advances in supportive critical care, the prognosis for patients with PCP who require intubation and respiratory support has improved and now depends to a large extent on comorbidities and the prognosis of the underlying disease. Since patients typically do not respond to therapy for 4–8 days, supportive care for a minimum of 10 days is a reasonable consideration if such support is compatible with the patient's wishes and the prognosis of comorbidities. Patients whose condition continues to deteriorate after 3 or 4 days or has not improved after 7–10 days should be reevaluated to determine whether other infectious processes are present (either having been missed on initial evaluation or having developed during treatment) or whether noninfectious processes (e.g., congestive heart failure, pulmonary emboli, pulmonary hypertension, drug toxicity, or a neoplastic process) are causing pulmonary dysfunction.

TREATMENT *P. JIROVECII* PNEUMONIA

The treatment of choice for PCP is trimethoprim-sulfamethoxazole (TMP-SMX), given either IV or PO for 14–21 days (Table 244-1). TMP-SMX, which interferes with the organism's folate metabolism, is at least as effective as alternative agents and is better tolerated. However, TMP-SMX can cause leukopenia, hepatitis, rash, and fever as well as anaphylactic and anaphylactoid reactions, and patients with HIV infection have an unusually high incidence of hypersensitivity to TMP-SMX. Monitoring of serum drug levels is useful if renal function or toxicities are issues. Maintenance of a 2-h post-dose sulfamethoxazole level of 100–150 μg/mL has been associated with a successful outcome. Resistance to TMP-SMX cannot be measured by organism growth inhibition in the laboratory because *Pneumocystis* cannot be cultured. However, mutations in the target gene for sulfamethoxazole that confer in vitro sulfa resistance to other organisms have been found in *Pneumocystis*. The clinical relevance of these mutations for the response to therapy is unknown. Sulfadiazine plus pyrimethamine, an oral regimen more often used for treatment of toxoplasmosis, also is highly effective. Dapsone plus pyrimethamine or dapsone plus trimethoprim also can be used.

Intravenous pentamidine or the combination of clindamycin plus primaquine is an option for patients who cannot tolerate TMP-SMX and for patients in whose treatment TMP-SMX appears to be failing. Pentamidine must be given IV over at least 60 min to avoid potentially lethal hypotension. Adverse effects can be severe and irreversible and include renal dysfunction, dysglycemia (life-threatening hypoglycemia that can occur days or weeks after initial infusion and be followed by hyperglycemia), neutropenia, and torsades des pointes. Clindamycin plus primaquine is effective, but primaquine can be given only by the oral route—a disadvantage for patients who cannot ingest or absorb oral drugs.

A major advance in therapy for PCP was the recognition that glucocorticoids could improve survival rates among HIV-infected patients with moderate to severe disease (room air PO_2, <70 mmHg; or alveolar-arterial oxygen gradient, ≥35 mmHg). Glucocorticoids appear to reduce the pulmonary inflammation that occurs after specific therapy is started and organisms begin to die, eliciting inflammation. Therapy with glucocorticoids should be the standard of care for patients with HIV infection and probably is also effective for patients with other immunodeficiencies. This treatment should be started for moderate or severe disease when therapy for PCP is initiated, even if the diagnosis has not yet been confirmed. If HIV-infected or HIV-uninfected patients are receiving high-dose glucocorticoids when they develop PCP, there are theoretical advantages to increasing or decreasing the steroid dose, but there is no convincing evidence on which to base any specific strategy.

No definitive trials have defined the best therapeutic algorithm for patients in whom TMP-SMX treatment for PCP is failing. If no other treatable infectious or noninfectious processes are detected and pulmonary dysfunction appears to be due to PCP alone, many authorities would switch from TMP-SMX to either IV pentamidine or IV clindamycin plus oral primaquine. Some authorities would add the second drug or drug combination to TMP-SMX rather than switching regimens. If patients are not already receiving them, glucocorticoids should be added to the regimen; the dosage and regimen, which are usually chosen empirically, depend on what glucocorticoid regimen (if any) the patient was receiving when PCP therapy was begun.

For patients with HIV infection who present with PCP before the initiation of ART, ART should be started within the first 2 weeks of therapy for PCP in most cases. Immune reconstitution inflammatory syndrome (IRIS) can occur, however, and the decision to initiate ART thus requires considerable expertise in terms of optimal timing relative to PCP recovery as well as in the other factors that are relevant when ART is initiated in any patient.

TABLE 244-1 TREATMENT OF PNEUMOCYSTOSIS (14–21 DAYS)

Drug(s)	Dose, Route	Adverse Effects
First-Choice Agent		
TMP-SMX	TMP (5 mg/kg) plus SMX (25 mg/kg) q6–8h PO or IV (2 double-strength tablets tid or qid)	Fever, rash, cytopenias, hepatitis, hyperkalemia
Alternative Agents		
TMP ***plus*** Dapsone	5 mg/kg q6–8h PO 100 mg qd PO	Hemolysis (G6PD deficiency), methemoglobinemia, rash, fever, gastrointestinal disturbances
Atovaquone	750 mg bid PO	Rash, fever, hepatitis
Clindamycin ***plus*** Primaquine	300–450 mg q6h PO or 600 mg q6–8h IV 15–30 mg qd PO	Hemolysis (G6PD deficiency), methemoglobinemia, neutropenia, rash
Pentamidine	3–4 mg/kg qd IV	Hypotension, azotemia, cardiac arrhythmias (torsades des pointes), pancreatitis, dysglycemias, hypocalcemia, neutropenia, hepatitis
Adjunctive Agent		
Prednisone or methylprednisolone	40 mg bid × 5 d, 40 mg qd × 5 d, 20 mg qd × 11 d; PO or IV	Peptic ulcer disease, hyperglycemia, mood alteration, hypertension

Abbreviations: G6PD, glucose-6-phosphate dehydrogenase; TMP-SMX, trimethoprim-sulfamethoxazole.

PREVENTION

The most effective method for preventing PCP is to eliminate the cause of immunosuppression by withdrawing immunosuppressive therapy or treating the underlying cause, e.g., HIV infection. Patients who are susceptible to PCP benefit from chemoprophylaxis during the period of susceptibility. For patients with HIV infection, CD4+ T cell counts are a reliable marker of susceptibility, and counts below 200 cells/μL are an indication to start prophylaxis (Table 244-2). For patients with HIV infection who are not receiving ART, oral candidiasis or prior PCP also is an indication for chemoprophylaxis, regardless of CD4+ T cell count. For such patients not receiving ART, any prior episode of an AIDS-defining illness or pneumonia should encourage the use of chemoprophylaxis. However, patients who are not adherent to ART are not likely to take PCP chemoprophylaxis.

For patients without HIV infection, there is no laboratory parameter, including the CD4+ T cell count, that predicts susceptibility to PCP with adequate positive and negative accuracy. The period of susceptibility is usually estimated on the basis of experience with the

TABLE 244-2 PROPHYLAXIS OF PNEUMOCYSTOSIS

Drug(s)	Dose, Route	Comments
First-Choice Agent		
TMP-SMX	1 tablet (double- or single-strength) qd PO	Incidence of hypersensitivity is high. Rechallenge for non-life-threatening hypersensitivity; consider dose-escalation protocol.
Alternative Agents		
Dapsone	50 mg bid or 100 mg qd PO	Hemolysis is associated with G6PD deficiency.
Dapsone *plus*	50 mg qd PO	Leucovorin ameliorates cytopenias due to pyrimethamine.
Pyrimethamine *plus*	50 mg weekly PO	
Leucovorin	25 mg weekly PO	
Dapsone *plus*	200 mg weekly PO	Leucovorin ameliorates cytopenias due to pyrimethamine.
Pyrimethamine *plus*	75 mg weekly PO	
Leucovorin	25 mg weekly PO	
Pentamidine	300 mg monthly via Respirgard II nebulizer	Aerosol may cause bronchospasm. Pentamidine is probably less effective than TMP-SMX or dapsone regimens.
Atovaquone	1500 mg qd PO	Requires fatty meal for optimal absorption.

Abbreviations: G6PD, glucose-6-phosphate dehydrogenase; TMP-SMX, trimethoprim-sulfamethoxazole.

underlying disease and immunosuppressive regimen. Patients receiving a prolonged course of high-dose glucocorticoids appear to be particularly susceptible to PCP. The glucocorticoid exposure threshold that warrants chemoprophylaxis is controversial, but such preventive therapy should be strongly considered for any patient receiving more than the equivalent of 20 mg of prednisone daily for 30 days.

TMP-SMX is the most effective prophylactic drug: few patients experience a PCP breakthrough when they are reliably taking a recommended TMP-SMX chemoprophylactic regimen. Several TMP-SMX regimens have been used successfully. One double-strength tablet daily is the regimen with which there is the most experience, but either one single-strength tablet daily or one double-strength tablet two or three times weekly also has been recommended for various populations of patients.

For patients who cannot tolerate TMP-SMX (usually because of hypersensitivity or bone marrow suppression), alternative drugs include daily dapsone, weekly dapsone-pyrimethamine, and monthly aerosol pentamidine. Patients who develop hypersensitivity to TMP-SMX can sometimes tolerate the drug if a gradual dose-escalation protocol is used. Dapsone cross-reacts with sulfonamides in a substantial fraction of patients and therefore is rarely useful in patients with a history of life-threatening reactions to TMP-SMX. Aerosolized pentamidine is highly effective, but it is not as effective as TMP-SMX and may not provide protection in areas of the lung that are not well ventilated. Atovaquone is also effective and well tolerated; however, this drug is available only as an oral preparation, and gastrointestinal absorption is unpredictable in patients with abnormal gastrointestinal motility or function.

SECTION 17 PROTOZOAL AND HELMINTHIC INFECTIONS: GENERAL CONSIDERATIONS

245e Laboratory Diagnosis of Parasitic Infections

Sharon L. Reed, Charles E. Davis

This is a digital-only chapter. It is available on the DVD that accompanies this book, as well as on Access Medicine/Harrison's Online, and the eBook and "app" editions of HPIM 19e.

The cornerstone for the diagnosis of parasitic infections is a thorough history of the patient's illness. Epidemiologic aspects of the illness are especially important because the risks of acquiring many parasites are closely related to occupation, recreation, or travel to areas of high endemicity. Without a basic knowledge of the epidemiology and life cycles of the major parasites, it is difficult to approach the diagnosis of parasitic infections systematically. Accordingly, the medical classification of important human parasites in this chapter emphasizes their geographic distribution, their transmission, and the anatomic location and stages of their life cycle in humans. The text and tables are intended to serve as a guide to the correct diagnostic procedures for the major parasitic infections; in addition, the reader is referred to other chapters that contain more comprehensive information about each infection (Chaps. 247–260). This chapter summarizes the geographic distributions, the anatomic locations, and the methods employed for the diagnosis of flatworm, roundworm, and protozoal infections, respectively.

In addition to selecting the correct diagnostic procedures, physicians must counsel their patients to ensure that specimens are collected properly and arrive at the laboratory promptly. For example, the diagnosis of bancroftian filariasis is unlikely to be confirmed by the laboratory unless blood is drawn near midnight, when the nocturnal microfilariae are active. Laboratory personnel and surgical pathologists should be notified in advance when a parasitic infection is suspected. Continuing interaction with the laboratory staff and the surgical pathologists increases the likelihood that parasites in body fluids or biopsy specimens will be examined carefully by the most capable individuals.

246e Agents Used to Treat Parasitic Infections

Thomas A. Moore

This is a digital-only chapter. It is available on the DVD that accompanies this book, as well as on Access Medicine/Harrison's Online, and the eBook and "app" editions of HPIM 19e.

This chapter deals exclusively with the agents used to treat infections due to parasites. Specific treatment recommendations for the parasitic diseases of humans are listed in chapters on individual pathogens.

Parasitic infections afflict more than half of the world's population and impose a substantial health burden, particularly in underdeveloped nations, where they are most prevalent. The reach of some parasitic diseases, including malaria, has expanded over the past few decades as a result of factors such as deforestation, population shifts, global warming, and other climatic events. Despite major efforts at vaccine development and vector control, chemotherapy remains the single most effective means of controlling parasitic infections. Efforts to combat the spread of some diseases are hindered by the development and spread of drug resistance, the limited introduction of new antiparasitic agents, and the proliferation of counterfeit medications. However, there are good reasons to be optimistic. Ambitious global initiatives aimed at controlling or eliminating threats such as AIDS, tuberculosis, and malaria have demonstrated some early successes. Recognition of the substantial burden imposed by the "neglected" tropical diseases has generated multinational partnerships to develop and deploy effective antiparasitic agents. Vaccines against several tropical diseases are being developed, and clinical trials for vaccines against parasites continue.

SECTION 18 PROTOZOAL INFECTIONS

247 Amebiasis and Infection with Free-Living Amebas

Rosa M. Andrade, Sharon L. Reed

AMEBIASIS

DEFINITION

Amebiasis is an infection with the intestinal protozoan *Entamoeba histolytica*. About 90% of infections are asymptomatic, and the remaining 10% produce a spectrum of clinical syndromes ranging from dysentery to abscesses of the liver or other organs.

LIFE CYCLE AND TRANSMISSION

E. histolytica is acquired by ingestion of viable cysts from fecally contaminated water, food, or hands. Food-borne exposure is most prevalent and is particularly likely when food handlers are shedding cysts or food is being grown with feces-contaminated soil, fertilizer, or water. Besides the drinking of contaminated water, less common means of transmission include oral and anal sexual practices and—in rare instances—direct rectal inoculation through colonic irrigation devices. Motile trophozoites are released from cysts in the small intestine and, in most patients, remain as harmless commensals in the large bowel. After encystation, infectious cysts are shed in the stool and can survive for several weeks in a moist environment. In some patients, the trophozoites invade either the bowel mucosa, causing symptomatic colitis, or the bloodstream, causing distant abscesses of the liver, lungs, or brain. The trophozoites may not encyst in patients with active dysentery, and motile hematophagous trophozoites are frequently present in fresh stools. Trophozoites are rapidly killed by exposure to air or stomach acid, however, and therefore cannot transmit infection.

EPIDEMIOLOGY

About 10% of the world's population is infected with *Entamoeba*, the majority with noninvasive *Entamoeba dispar*. Amebiasis results from infection with *E. histolytica* and is the third most common cause of death from parasitic disease (after schistosomiasis and malaria). Invasive colitis and liver abscesses are sevenfold more common among men than among women; this difference has been attributed to a disparity in complement-mediated killing. The wide spectrum of clinical disease caused by *Entamoeba* is due in part to the differences between these two infecting species. *E. histolytica* has unique isoenzymes, surface antigens, DNA markers, and virulence properties that distinguish it from other genetically related and morphologically identical species, such as *E. dispar* and *E. moshkovskii*.

Most asymptomatic carriers, including men who have sex with men (MSM) and patients with AIDS, harbor *E. dispar* and have self-limited infections. In this respect, *E. dispar* is dissimilar to other enteric pathogens such as *Cryptosporidium* and *Cystoisospora belli*, which can cause self-limited illnesses in immunocompetent hosts but devastating diarrhea in patients with AIDS. These observations indicate that *E. dispar* is incapable of causing invasive disease. Unlike *E. dispar*, *E. histolytica* can cause invasive disease, as demonstrated in recent reports from Korea, China, and India that suggest higher prevalences of amebic seroconversion, invasive amebiasis, and amebic liver abscesses among HIV positive than HIV-negative patients. In another study, 10% of asymptomatic patients who were colonized with *E. histolytica* went on to develop amebic colitis, while the rest remained asymptomatic and cleared the infection within 1 year.

The potential of *E. moshkovskii* to cause diarrhea, weight loss, and colitis was recently demonstrated in a mouse model of cecal infection. However, the pathogenic potential of this species is not clear. A prospective evaluation of children from the Mirpur community of Dhaka, Bangladesh, found that most children who had diarrheal diseases associated with *E. moshkovskii* were simultaneously infected with at least one other enteric pathogen.

Areas of highest incidence of *Entamoeba* infection (due to inadequate sanitation and crowding) include most developing countries in the tropics, particularly Mexico, India, and nations of Central and South America, tropical Asia, and Africa. In a 4-year follow-up study of preschool children in a highly endemic area of Bangladesh, 80% of children had at least one episode of *E. histolytica* infection and 53% had more than one episode. Naturally acquired immunity did develop but was usually short-lived and correlated with the presence in the stool of secretory IgA antibody to the major adherence lectin galactose *N*-acetylgalactosamine (Gal/GalNAc). The main groups at risk for amebiasis in developed countries are returned travelers, recent immigrants, MSM, military personnel, and inmates of institutions. Data from the GeoSentinel Surveillance Network, which come from tropical medicine clinics on six continents, showed that, among long-term travelers (trip duration, >6 months), diarrhea due to *E. histolytica* was among the most common diagnoses.

Both trophozoites (Fig. 247-1) and cysts (Fig. 247-2) are found in the intestinal lumen, but only trophozoites of *E. histolytica* invade tissue. The trophozoite is 20–60 μm in diameter and contains vacuoles and a nucleus with a characteristic central nucleolus. In animals, depletion of intestinal mucus, diffuse inflammation, and disruption of the epithelial barrier precede trophozoite contact with the colonic mucosa. Trophozoites attach to colonic mucus and epithelial cells by their Gal/GalNAc lectin. The earliest intestinal lesions are microulcerations of the mucosa of the cecum, sigmoid colon, or rectum that release erythrocytes, inflammatory cells, and epithelial cells. Proctoscopy reveals small ulcers with heaped-up margins and normal intervening mucosa (Fig. 247-3*A*). Submucosal extension of ulcerations under viable-appearing surface mucosa causes the classic "flask-shaped" ulcer containing trophozoites at the margins of dead and viable tissues. Although neutrophilic infiltrates may accompany the early lesions in animals, human intestinal infection is marked by a paucity of inflammatory cells, probably in part because of the killing of neutrophils by trophozoites (Fig. 247-3*B*). Treated ulcers characteristically heal with little or no scarring. Occasionally, however, full-thickness necrosis and perforation occur.

Rarely, intestinal infection results in the formation of a mass lesion, or *ameboma*, in the bowel lumen. The overlying mucosa is usually thin and ulcerated, while other layers of the wall are thickened, edematous, and hemorrhagic; this condition results in exuberant formation of granulation tissue with little fibrous-tissue response.

A number of virulence factors have been linked to the ability of *E. histolytica* to invade through the interglandular epithelium. One factor consists of the extracellular cysteine proteinases that degrade collagen, elastin, IgA, IgG, and the anaphylatoxins C3a and C5a. Other enzymes may disrupt glycoprotein bonds between mucosal epithelial cells in the gut. Amebas can lyse neutrophils, monocytes, lymphocytes, and cells of colonic and hepatic lines. The cytolytic effect of amebas appears to require direct contact with target cells and may be linked to the release of phospholipase A and pore-forming peptides. *E. histolytica* trophozoites also cause apoptosis of human cells. Phagocytosis is a virulence factor that leads to defective parasite proliferation if inhibited. This process is potentially modulated by calmodulin-like calcium-binding protein 3, which pairs with actin and myosin during initiation and formation of phagosomes. Another virulence factor is the ability to resist reactive oxygen species, reactive nitrogen species such as nitric oxide, or S-nitrosothiols such as S-nitrosoglutathione (GSNO) and S-nitrosocysteine (CySNO). *E. histolytica* trophozoites are constantly exposed to reactive oxygen and nitrogen species from their own metabolism and host defenses during tissue invasion. Overexpression of hydrogen peroxide regulatory motif–binding protein appears to increase *E. histolytica* cytotoxicity. Since *E. histolytica* lacks glutathione and glutathione reductase, it relies on its thioredoxin/thioredoxin reductase system to prevent, regulate, and repair the damage caused by oxidative stress. This antioxidant system is versatile in that it can reduce

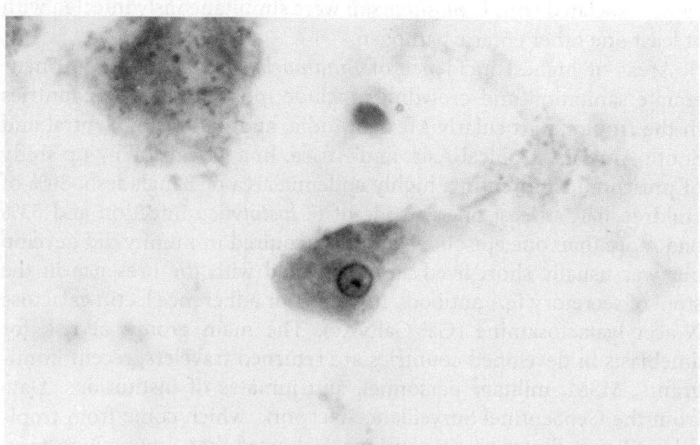

FIGURE 247-1 Trophozoite of *E. histolytica*. A single nucleus with a central, dot-like nucleolus is seen (trichrome stain).

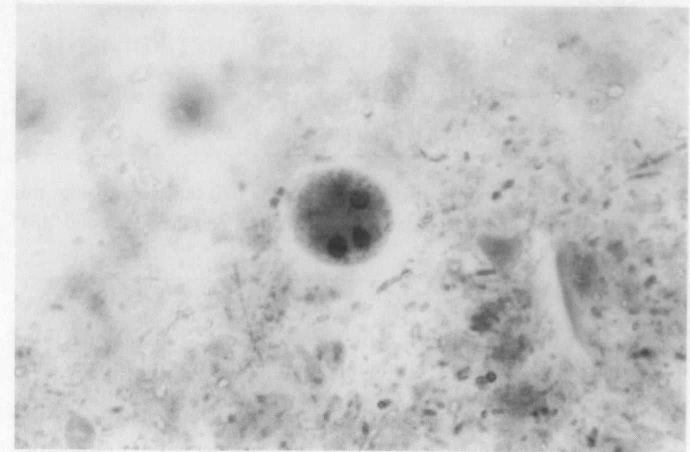

FIGURE 247-2 Cyst of *E. histolytica*. Three of the four nuclei are visible (trichrome stain).

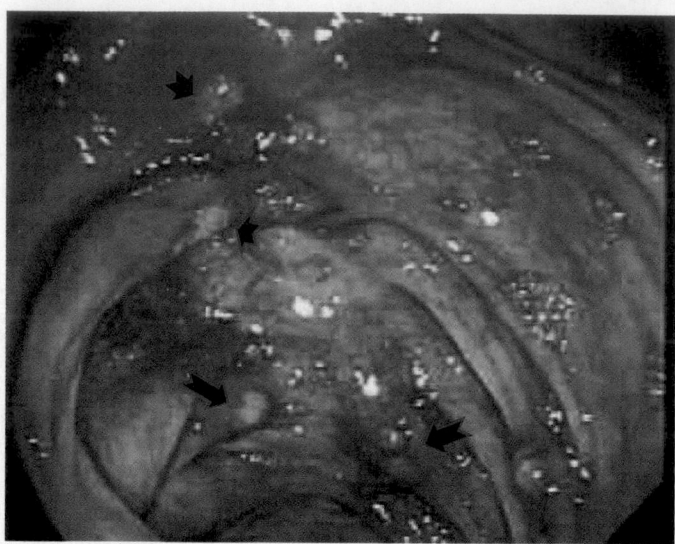

A

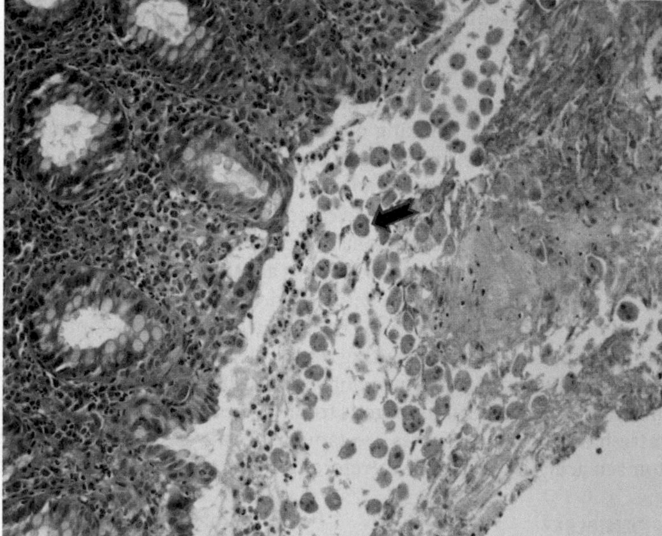

B

FIGURE 247-3 Endoscopic and histopathologic features of intestinal amebiasis. *A.* Appearance of ulcers on colonoscopy (*arrows*). ***B.*** Inflammatory infiltrate and *E. histolytica* trophozoites (*arrow*) in invasive amebic colitis (hematoxylin and eosin). *(Courtesy of the Department of Pathology and Gastroenterology, VA San Diego Medical Center.)*

reactive nitrogen species and use an alternative electron donor such as the reduced form of nicotinamide adenine dinucleotide. Metronidazole, the current standard of therapy for amebiasis, seems to exert its antiparasitic effect through the inhibition of this antioxidant system. Newer therapeutic candidates targeting this system, such as auranofin, also have demonstrated in vitro and in vivo efficacy against this parasite.

Liver abscesses are always preceded by intestinal colonization, which may be asymptomatic. Blood vessels may be compromised early by wall lysis and thrombus formation. Trophozoites invade veins to reach the liver through the portal venous system. *E. histolytica* is resistant to complement-mediated lysis—a property critical to survival in the bloodstream. In contrast, *E. dispar* is rapidly lysed by complement and is thus restricted to the bowel lumen. Inoculation of amebas into the portal system of hamsters results in an acute cellular infiltrate consisting predominantly of neutrophils. Later, the neutrophils are lysed by contact with amebas, and the release of neutrophil toxins may contribute to necrosis of hepatocytes. The liver parenchyma is replaced by necrotic material that is surrounded by a thin rim of congested liver tissue. The necrotic contents of a liver abscess are classically described as "anchovy paste," although the fluid is variable in color and is composed of bacteriologically sterile granular debris with few or no cells. Amebas, if seen, tend to be found near the capsule of the abscess.

Host innate and adaptive immunity are important factors that determine susceptibility to invasive disease and its clinical outcome. While neutrophils were thought to contribute to tissue damage in intestinal and liver amebiasis due to their cytotoxic effects on host epithelial cells, a recent report suggests that they may exert a protective effect in susceptible mice. Neutropenia, induced with an antibody to Gr-1 (i.e., to peripheral neutrophils), led to death in C3H/HeJ mice and to severe disease in CBA mice (both of which are relatively susceptible to *E. histolytica* infection), while it had no effect on C57BL/6 mice, which are known for their intrinsic resistance to infection with this parasite.

Antimicrobial peptides, such as cathelicidins, are an important part of innate immunity and are induced by *E. histolytica* upon intestinal invasion in a mouse model. In this model, cecal cathelicidin-related antimicrobial peptide (CRAMP) mRNA increased more than fourfold by 3 days and more than 100-fold at 7 days. However, *E. histolytica* remained resistant to cathelicidin-mediated killing, probably because the antimicrobial peptide was digested by amebic cysteine proteinases.

IgA plays a critical role in acquired immunity to *E. histolytica*. A study in Bangladeshi schoolchildren revealed that an intestinal IgA response to Gal/GalNAc reduced the risk of new *E. histolytica* infection by 64%. Serum IgG antibody is not protective; titers correlate with the duration of illness rather than with the severity of disease. Indeed, Bangladeshi children with a serum IgG response were more likely than those without such a response to develop new *E. histolytica* infection. In infants from this same Bangladeshi community, passive immunity conferred by maternal parasite-specific IgA via breastfeeding resulted in a 39% reduction in risk of infection and a 64% reduction in risk of diarrheal disease from *E. histolytica* during the first year of life.

A link between nutrition and immunity is demonstrated by the elevated rate of infections due to protozoan parasites, including *E. histolytica*, among undernourished children in developing countries. Resistance to amebiasis is associated with a polymorphism in the receptor for the adipocytokine leptin. Children in a Bangladeshi cohort with a mutant R223 leptin receptor allele were nearly four times more likely to be infected with *E. histolytica* than those carrying the ancestral Q223 allele. This mutant allele is overrepresented in many geographic areas with a high prevalence of amebiasis, such as Bangladesh and India.

CLINICAL SYNDROMES

Intestinal Amebiasis The most common type of amebic infection is asymptomatic cyst passage. Even in highly endemic areas, most patients harbor *E. dispar*.

Symptomatic amebic colitis develops 2–6 weeks after the ingestion of infectious *E. histolytica* cysts. A gradual onset of lower abdominal pain and mild diarrhea is followed by malaise, weight loss, and diffuse lower abdominal or back pain. Cecal involvement may mimic acute appendicitis. Patients with full-blown dysentery may pass 10–12 stools per day. The stools contain little fecal material and consist mainly of blood and mucus. In contrast to those with bacterial diarrhea, fewer than 40% of patients with amebic dysentery are febrile. Virtually all patients have heme-positive stools.

More fulminant intestinal infection, with severe abdominal pain, high fever, and profuse diarrhea, is rare and occurs predominantly in children. Patients may develop toxic megacolon, in which there is severe bowel dilation with intramural air. Patients receiving glucocorticoids are at risk for severe amebiasis. Uncommonly, patients develop a chronic form of amebic colitis, which can be confused with inflammatory bowel disease. The association between severe amebiasis complications and glucocorticoid therapy emphasizes the importance of excluding amebiasis when inflammatory bowel disease is suspected. An occasional patient presents with only an asymptomatic or tender abdominal mass caused by an ameboma, which is easily confused with cancer on barium studies. A positive serologic test or biopsy can prevent unnecessary surgery in this setting. The syndrome of post–amebic colitis—i.e., persistent diarrhea following documented cure of amebic colitis—is controversial; no evidence of recurrent amebic infection can be found, and re-treatment usually has no effect.

Amebic Liver Abscess Extraintestinal infection by *E. histolytica* most often involves the liver. Of travelers who develop an amebic liver abscess after leaving an endemic area, 95% do so within 5 months. Young patients with an amebic liver abscess are more likely than older patients to present in the acute phase with prominent symptoms of <10 days' duration. Most patients are febrile and have right-upper-quadrant pain, which may be dull or pleuritic in nature and may radiate to the shoulder. Point tenderness over the liver and right-sided pleural effusion are common. Jaundice is rare. Although the initial site of infection is the colon, fewer than one-third of patients with an amebic abscess have active diarrhea. Older patients from endemic areas are more likely to have a subacute course lasting 6 months, with weight loss and hepatomegaly. About one-third of patients with chronic presentations are febrile. Thus, the clinical diagnosis of an amebic liver abscess may be difficult to establish because the symptoms and signs are often nonspecific. Since 10–15% of patients present only with fever, amebic liver abscess must be considered in the differential diagnosis of fever of unknown origin (Chap. 26).

Complications of Amebic Liver Abscess Pleuropulmonary involvement, which is reported in 20–30% of patients, is the most frequent complication of amebic liver abscess. Manifestations include sterile effusions, contiguous spread from the liver, and rupture into the pleural space. Sterile effusions and contiguous spread usually resolve with medical therapy, but frank rupture into the pleural space requires drainage. A hepatobronchial fistula may cause cough productive of large amounts of necrotic material that may contain amebas. This dramatic complication carries a good prognosis. Abscesses that rupture into the peritoneum may present as an indolent leak or an acute abdomen and require both percutaneous catheter drainage and medical therapy. Rupture into the pericardium, usually from abscesses of the left lobe of the liver, carries the gravest prognosis; it can occur during medical therapy and requires surgical drainage.

Other Extraintestinal Sites The genitourinary tract may become involved by direct extension of amebiasis from the colon or by hematogenous spread of the infection. Painful genital ulcers, characterized by a punched-out appearance and profuse discharge, may develop secondary to extension from either the intestine or the liver. Both of these conditions respond well to medical therapy. Cerebral involvement has been reported in fewer than 0.1% of patients in large clinical series. Symptoms and prognosis depend on the size and location of the lesion.

DIAGNOSTIC TESTS

Laboratory Diagnosis Stool examinations, serologic tests, and noninvasive imaging of the liver are the most important procedures in the diagnosis of amebiasis. Fecal findings suggestive of amebic colitis include a positive test for heme, a paucity of neutrophils, and amebic cysts or trophozoites. The definitive diagnosis of amebic colitis is made by the demonstration of hematophagous trophozoites of *E. histolytica* (Fig. 247-1). Because trophozoites are killed rapidly by water, drying, or barium, it is important to examine at least three fresh stool specimens. Examination of a combination of wet mounts, iodine-stained concentrates, and trichrome-stained preparations of fresh stool and concentrates for cysts (Fig. 247-2) or trophozoites (Fig. 247-1) confirms the diagnosis in 75–95% of cases. Culture of amebas is more sensitive, but this diagnostic method is not routinely available. If stool examinations are negative, sigmoidoscopy with biopsy of the edge of ulcers may increase the yield, but this procedure is dangerous during fulminant colitis because of the risk of perforation. Trophozoites in a biopsy specimen from a colonic mass confirm the diagnosis of ameboma, but trophozoites are rare in liver aspirates because they are found in the abscess capsule and not in the readily aspirated necrotic center. Accurate diagnosis requires experience, since the trophozoites may be confused with neutrophils and the cysts must be differentiated morphologically from those of *Entamoeba hartmanni*, *Entamoeba coli*, and *Endolimax nana*, which do not cause clinical disease and do not warrant therapy. Unfortunately, the cysts of *E. histolytica* cannot be distinguished microscopically from those of *E. dispar* or *E. moshkovskii*. Therefore, the microscopic diagnosis of *E. histolytica* can be made only by the detection of *Entamoeba* trophozoites that have ingested erythrocytes. In terms of sensitivity, stool diagnostic tests based on the detection of the Gal/GalNAc lectin of *E. histolytica* compare favorably with the polymerase chain reaction and with isolation in culture followed by isoenzyme analysis.

Serology is an important addition to the methods used for parasitologic diagnosis of invasive amebiasis. Enzyme-linked immunosorbent assays and agar gel diffusion assays are positive in more than 90% of patients with colitis, amebomas, or liver abscess. Positive results in conjunction with the appropriate clinical syndrome suggest active disease because serologic findings usually revert to negative within 6–12 months. Even in highly endemic areas such as South Africa, fewer than 10% of asymptomatic individuals have a positive amebic serology. The interpretation of the indirect hemagglutination test is more difficult because titers may remain positive for as long as 10 years.

Up to 10% of patients with acute amebic liver abscess may have negative serologic findings; in suspected cases with an initially negative result, testing should be repeated in 1 week. In contrast to carriers of *E. dispar*, most asymptomatic carriers of *E. histolytica* develop antibodies. Thus, serologic tests are helpful in assessing the risk of invasive amebiasis in asymptomatic, cyst-passing individuals in nonendemic areas. Serologic tests also should be performed in patients with ulcerative colitis before the institution of glucocorticoid therapy to prevent the development of severe colitis or toxic megacolon owing to unsuspected amebiasis.

Routine hematology and chemistry tests usually are not very helpful in the diagnosis of invasive amebiasis. About three-fourths of patients with an amebic liver abscess have leukocytosis (>10,000 cells/μL); this condition is particularly likely if symptoms are acute or complications have developed. Invasive amebiasis does not elicit eosinophilia. Anemia, if present, is usually multifactorial. Even with large liver abscesses, liver enzyme levels are normal or minimally elevated. The alkaline phosphatase level is most often elevated and may remain so for months. Aminotransferase elevations suggest acute disease or a complication.

Radiographic Studies Radiographic barium studies are potentially dangerous in acute amebic colitis. Amebomas are usually identified first by a barium enema, but biopsy is necessary for differentiation from carcinoma.

Radiographic techniques such as ultrasonography, CT, and MRI are all useful for detection of the round or oval hypoechoic cyst of an amebic liver abscess. More than 80% of patients who have had symptoms for >10 days have a single abscess of the right lobe of the liver (Fig. 247-4). Approximately 50% of patients who have had symptoms for <10 days have multiple abscesses. Findings associated

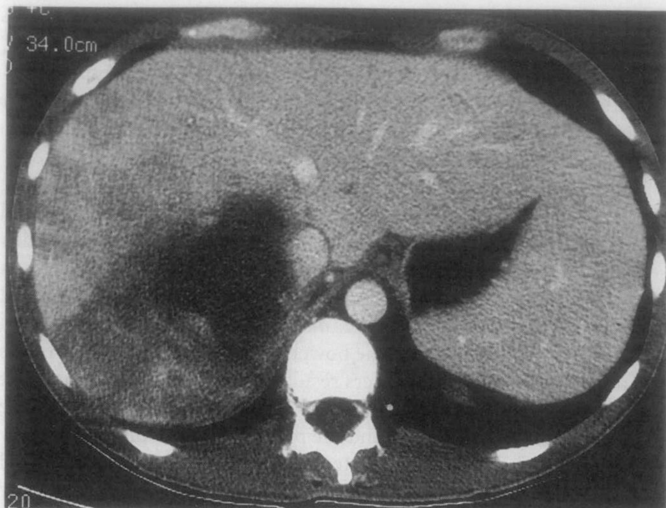

FIGURE 247-4 Abdominal CT scan of a large amebic abscess of the right lobe of the liver. *(Courtesy of the Department of Radiology, UCSD Medical Center, San Diego; with permission.)*

with complications include large abscesses (>10 cm) in the superior part of the right lobe, which may rupture into the pleural space; multiple lesions, which must be differentiated from pyogenic abscesses; and lesions of the left lobe, which may rupture into the pericardium. Because abscesses resolve slowly and may increase in size in patients who are responding clinically to therapy, frequent follow-up ultrasonography may prove confusing. Complete resolution of a liver abscess within 6 months can be anticipated in two-thirds of patients, but 10% may have persistent abnormalities for a year.

Differential Diagnosis The differential diagnosis of intestinal amebiasis includes bacterial diarrheas (Chap. 160) caused by *Campylobacter* (Chap. 192); enteroinvasive *Escherichia coli* (Chap. 186); and species of *Shigella* (Chap. 191), *Salmonella* (Chap. 190), and *Vibrio* (Chap. 193). Although the typical patient with amebic colitis has less prominent fever than in these other conditions as well as heme-positive stools with few neutrophils, correct diagnosis requires bacterial cultures, microscopic examination of stools, and amebic serologic testing. As has already been mentioned, amebiasis must be ruled out in any patient thought to have inflammatory bowel disease.

Because of the variety of presenting signs and symptoms, amebic liver abscess can easily be confused with pulmonary or gallbladder disease or with any febrile illness with few localizing signs, such as malaria (Chap. 248) or typhoid fever (Chap. 190). The diagnosis should be considered in members of high-risk groups who have recently traveled outside the United States (Chap. 149) and in inmates of institutions. Once radiographic studies have identified an abscess in the liver, the most important differential diagnosis is between amebic and pyogenic abscess. Patients with pyogenic abscess typically are older and have a history of underlying bowel disease or recent surgery. Amebic serology is helpful, but aspiration of the abscess, with Gram's staining and culture of the material, may be required for differentiation of the two diseases.

TREATMENT AMEBIASIS

INTESTINAL DISEASE

The drugs used to treat amebiasis can be classified according to their primary site of action (Table 247-1). *Luminal* amebicides are poorly absorbed; they reach high concentrations in the bowel, but their activity is limited to cysts and trophozoites close to the mucosa. Only two luminal drugs are available in the United States: iodoquinol and paromomycin. Indications for the use of luminal agents include eradication of cysts in patients with colitis or a liver abscess and treatment of asymptomatic carriers. The majority of

TABLE 247-1 DRUG THERAPY FOR AMEBIASIS

Indication	Therapy
Asymptomatic carriage	Luminal agent: iodoquinol (650-mg tablets), 650 mg tid for 20 days; *or* paromomycin (250-mg tablets), 500 mg tid for 10 days
Acute colitis	Metronidazole (250- or 500-mg tablets), 750 mg PO or IV tid for 5–10 days; *or* tinidazole, 2 g/d PO for 3 days *plus* Luminal agent as above
Amebic liver abscess	Metronidazole, 750 mg PO or IV for 5–10 days; *or* tinidazole, 2 g PO once; *or* ornidazole,[a] 2 g PO once *plus* Luminal agent as above

[a]Not available in the United States.

asymptomatic individuals who pass cysts are colonized with *E. dispar*, which does not warrant specific therapy. However, it is prudent to treat asymptomatic individuals who pass cysts unless *E. dispar* colonization can be definitively demonstrated by specific antigen-detection tests.

Tissue amebicides reach high concentrations in the blood and tissue after oral or parenteral administration. The development of nitroimidazole compounds, especially metronidazole, was a major advance in the treatment of invasive amebiasis. Patients with amebic colitis should be treated with IV or oral metronidazole. Side effects include nausea, vomiting, abdominal discomfort, and a disulfiram like reaction. Another longer-acting imidazole compound, tinidazole, is also effective and available in the United States. All patients should also receive a full course of therapy with a luminal agent, since metronidazole does not eradicate cysts. Resistance to metronidazole has been selected in the laboratory but has not been found in clinical isolates. Relapses are not uncommon and probably represent reinfection or failure to eradicate amebas from the bowel because of an inadequate dosage or duration of therapy.

AMEBIC LIVER ABSCESS

Metronidazole is the drug of choice for amebic liver abscess. Longer-acting nitroimidazoles (tinidazole and ornidazole) have been effective as single-dose therapy in developing countries. With early diagnosis and therapy, mortality rates from uncomplicated amebic liver abscess are <1%. There is no evidence that combined therapy with two drugs is more effective than the single-drug regimen. Studies of South Africans with liver abscesses demonstrated that 72% of patients without intestinal symptoms had bowel infection with *E. histolytica*; thus, all treatment regimens should include a luminal agent to eradicate cysts and prevent further transmission. Amebic liver abscess recurs rarely.

More than 90% of patients respond dramatically to metronidazole therapy with decreases in both pain and fever within 72 h. Indications for aspiration of liver abscesses are (1) the need to rule out a pyogenic abscess, particularly in patients with multiple lesions; (2) the lack of a clinical response in 3–5 days; (3) the threat of imminent rupture; and (4) the need to prevent rupture of left-lobe abscesses into the pericardium. There is no evidence that aspiration, even of large abscesses (up to 10 cm), accelerates healing. Percutaneous drainage may be successful even if the liver abscess has already ruptured. Surgery should be reserved for instances of bowel perforation and rupture into the pericardium.

PREVENTION

Amebic infection is spread by ingestion of food or water contaminated with cysts. Since an asymptomatic carrier may excrete up to 15 million cysts per day, prevention of infection requires adequate sanitation and eradication of cyst carriage. In high-risk areas, infection can be minimized by the avoidance of unpeeled fruits and vegetables and the use of bottled water. Because cysts are resistant to readily attainable levels of chlorine, disinfection by iodination (tetraglycine hydroperiodide) is recommended. There is no effective prophylaxis.

INFECTION WITH FREE-LIVING AMEBAS

EPIDEMIOLOGY

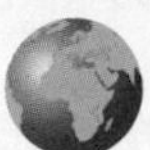

Free-living amebas of the genera *Acanthamoeba* and *Naegleria* are distributed throughout the world and have been isolated from a wide variety of fresh and brackish water, including that from lakes, taps, hot springs, swimming pools, and heating and air-conditioning units, and even from the nasal passages of healthy children. Encystation may protect the protozoa from desiccation and food deprivation. The persistence of *Legionella pneumophila* in water supplies may be attributable in part to chronic infection of free-living amebas, particularly *Naegleria*. Free-living amebas of the genus *Balamuthia* have been isolated from soil samples, including a sample from a flowerpot linked to a fatal infection in a child.

NAEGLERIA INFECTIONS

Primary amebic meningoencephalitis caused by *Naegleria fowleri* follows the aspiration of water contaminated with trophozoites or cysts or the inhalation of contaminated dust, leading to invasion of the olfactory neuroepithelium. Infection is most common among otherwise healthy children or young adults, who often report recent swimming in lakes or heated swimming pools. Rarely, some cases occur when contaminated water is used for nasal irrigation. After an incubation period of 2–15 days, severe headache, high fever, nausea, vomiting, and meningismus develop. Photophobia and palsies of the third, fourth, and sixth cranial nerves are common. Rapid progression to seizures and coma may follow. The prognosis is uniformly poor: most patients die within a week. Recently, two surviving children were treated with miltefosine, an investigational drug that is available through the Centers for Disease Control and Prevention (CDC) for the treatment of *Naegleria* infections.

The diagnosis of *Naegleria* infection should be considered in any patient who has purulent meningitis without evidence of bacteria on Gram's staining, antigen detection assay, and culture. Other laboratory findings resemble those for fulminant bacterial meningitis, with elevated intracranial pressure, high white blood cell counts (up to 20,000/μL), and elevated protein concentrations and low glucose levels in cerebrospinal fluid (CSF). Diagnosis depends on the detection of motile trophozoites in wet mounts of fresh spinal fluid. Antibodies to *Naegleria* species have been detected in healthy adults; serologic testing is not useful in the diagnosis of acute infection.

ACANTHAMOEBA INFECTIONS

Granulomatous Amebic Encephalitis Infection with *Acanthamoeba* species follows a more indolent course and typically occurs in chronically ill or debilitated patients. Risk factors include lymphoproliferative disorders, chemotherapy, glucocorticoid therapy, lupus erythematosus, and AIDS. Infection usually reaches the central nervous system hematogenously from a primary focus in the sinuses, skin, or lungs. In the central nervous system, the onset is insidious, and the syndrome often mimics a space-occupying lesion. Altered mental status, headache, and stiff neck may be accompanied by focal findings such as cranial nerve palsies, ataxia, and hemiparesis. Cutaneous ulcers or hard nodules containing amebas are frequently detected in AIDS patients with disseminated *Acanthamoeba* infection and can be an important diagnostic site.

Examination of the CSF for trophozoites may be diagnostically helpful, but lumbar puncture may be contraindicated because of increased intracerebral pressure. CT frequently reveals cortical and subcortical lesions of decreased density consistent with embolic infarcts. In other patients, multiple enhancing lesions with edema may mimic the computed tomographic appearance of toxoplasmosis (Chap. 253). Demonstration of the trophozoites and cysts of *Acanthamoeba* on wet mounts or in biopsy specimens establishes the diagnosis. Culture on nonnutrient agar plates seeded with *Escherichia coli* also may be helpful. Fluorescein-labeled antiserum is available

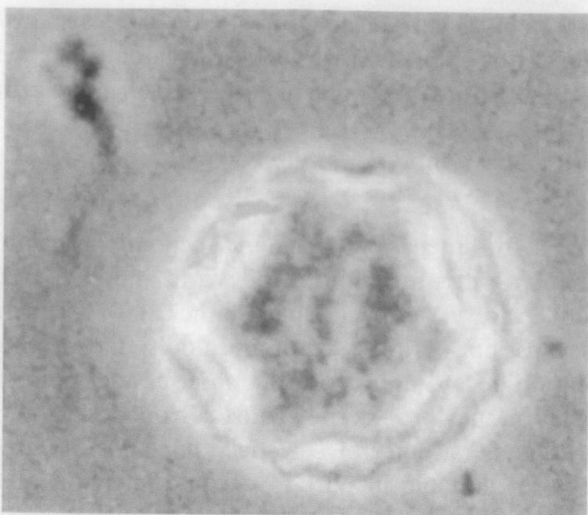

FIGURE 247-5 Double-walled cyst of *Acanthamoeba castellanii*, as seen by phase-contrast microscopy. *(From DJ Krogstad et al, in A Balows et al [eds]: Manual of Clinical Microbiology, 5th ed. Washington, DC, American Society for Microbiology, 1991.)*

from the CDC for the detection of protozoa in biopsy specimens. Granulomatous amebic encephalitis in patients with AIDS may have an accelerated course (with survival for only 3–40 days) because of poor granuloma formation in these individuals. Various antimicrobial agents have been used to treat *Acanthamoeba* infection, but the infection is almost uniformly fatal. The CDC has now made miltefosine available because of improved survival rates when the drug is included in treatment regimens.

Keratitis The incidence of keratitis caused by *Acanthamoeba* has increased in the past 30 years, in part as a result of improved diagnosis. Earlier infections were associated with trauma to the eye and exposure to contaminated water. At present, most infections are linked to extended-wear contact lenses, and rare cases are associated with laser-assisted in situ keratomileusis (LASIK). Risk factors include the use of homemade saline, the wearing of lenses while swimming, and inadequate disinfection. Since contact lenses presumably cause microscopic trauma, the early corneal findings may be nonspecific. The first symptoms usually include tearing and the painful sensation of a foreign body. Once infection is established, progression is rapid; the characteristic clinical sign is an annular, paracentral corneal ring representing a corneal abscess. Deeper corneal invasion and loss of vision may follow.

The differential diagnosis includes bacterial, mycobacterial, and herpetic infection. The irregular polygonal cysts of *Acanthamoeba* (Fig. 247-5) may be identified in corneal scrapings or biopsy material, and trophozoites can be grown on special media. Cysts are resistant to available drugs, and the results of medical therapy have been disappointing. Some reports have suggested partial responses to propamidine isethionate eyedrops. Severe infections usually require keratoplasty.

BALAMUTHIA INFECTIONS

Balamuthia mandrillaris, a free-living ameba previously referred to as a leptomyxid ameba, is an important etiologic agent of amebic meningoencephalitis in immunocompetent hosts. The course is typically subacute, with focal neurologic signs, fever, seizures, and headaches leading to death within 1 week to several months after onset. Examination of CSF reveals mononuclear or neutrophilic pleocytosis, elevated protein levels, and normal to low glucose concentrations. Multiple hypodense lesions are usually detected with imaging studies (Fig. 247-6). This mixed picture of space-occupying lesions with CSF pleocytosis is suggestive of *Balamuthia*. Fluorescent antibody is available from the CDC for brain biopsy specimens. The variety of drugs used to treat the few surviving patients (i.e., fewer than five reported in the United States) includes pentamidine, flucytosine, sulfadiazine, and macrolides. The CDC recommends that miltefosine now be included, as for the other free-living amebas. The differential diagnosis includes tuberculomas (Chap. 202) and neurocysticercosis (Chap. 260).

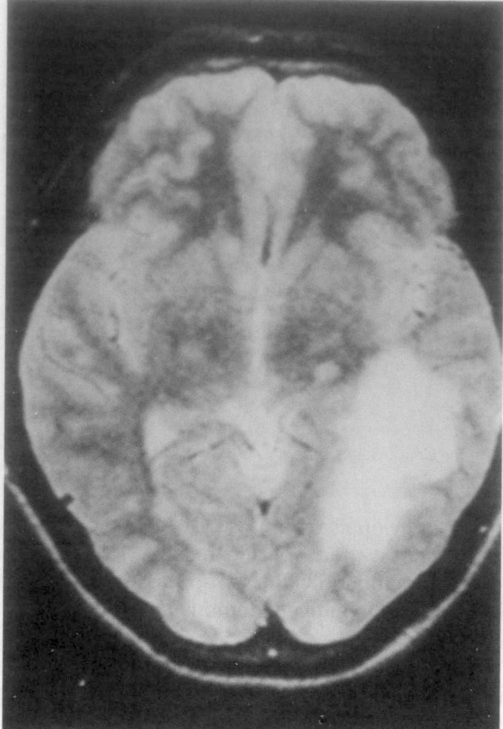

FIGURE 247-6 Brain MRI of amebic meningoencephalitis due to *Balamuthia mandrillaris*. A large lesion in the parieto-occipital lobe and other smaller lesions are seen. *(Courtesy of the Department of Radiology, UCSD Medical Center, San Diego.)*

248 Malaria

Nicholas J. White, Joel G. Breman

Humanity has but three great enemies: Fever, famine, and war; of these by far the greatest, by far the most terrible, is fever.

—William Osler

Malaria is a protozoan disease transmitted by the bite of infected *Anopheles* mosquitoes. The most important of the parasitic diseases of humans, it is transmitted in 106 countries containing 3 billion people and causes approximately 2000 deaths each day; mortality rates are decreasing as a result of highly effective control programs in several countries. Malaria has been eliminated from the United States, Canada, Europe, and Russia; in the late twentieth and early twenty-first centuries, however, its prevalence rose in many parts of the tropics. Increases in the drug resistance of the parasite, the insecticide resistance of its vectors, and human travel and migration have contributed to this resurgence. Occasional local transmission after importation of malaria has occurred in several southern and eastern areas of the United States and in Europe, indicating the continual danger to nonmalarious countries. Although there are many successful new control initiatives as well as promising research initiatives, malaria remains today, as it has been for centuries, a heavy burden on tropical communities, a threat to nonendemic countries, and a danger to travelers.

ETIOLOGY AND PATHOGENESIS

Six species of the genus *Plasmodium* cause nearly all malarial infections in humans. These are *P. falciparum*, *P. vivax*, two morphologically identical sympatric species of *P. ovale* (as suggested by recent evidence), *P. malariae*, and—in Southeast Asia—the monkey malaria parasite *P. knowlesi* (Table 248-1). While almost all deaths are caused

TABLE 248-1 CHARACTERISTICS OF *PLASMODIUM* SPECIES INFECTING HUMANS

	Finding for Indicated Species[a]			
Characteristic	*P. falciparum*	*P. vivax*	*P. ovale*	*P. malariae*
Duration of intrahepatic phase (days)	5.5	8	9	15
Number of merozoites released per infected hepatocyte	30,000	10,000	15,000	15,000
Duration of erythrocytic cycle (hours)	48	48	50	72
Red cell preference	Younger cells (but can invade cells of all ages)	Reticulocytes and cells up to 2 weeks old	Reticulocytes	Older cells
Morphology	Usually only ring forms[b]; banana-shaped gametocytes	Irregularly shaped large rings and trophozoites; enlarged erythrocytes; Schüffner's dots	Infected erythrocytes, enlarged and oval with tufted ends; Schüffner's dots	Band or rectangular forms of trophozoites common
Pigment color	Black	Yellow-brown	Dark brown	Brown-black
Ability to cause relapses	No	Yes	Yes	No

[a]In Southeast Asia, the monkey malaria parasite *P. knowlesi* also causes disease in humans. Young ring forms resemble those of *P. falciparum*, while older trophozoites resemble those of *P. malariae*. Reliable identification requires molecular genotyping. [b]Parasitemias of >2% are suggestive of *P. falciparum* infection.

by falciparum malaria, *P. knowlesi* and occasionally *P. vivax* also can cause severe illness. Human infection begins when a female anopheline mosquito inoculates plasmodial *sporozoites* from its salivary gland during a blood meal (Fig. 248-1). These microscopic motile forms of the malaria parasite are carried rapidly via the bloodstream to the liver, where they invade hepatic parenchymal cells and begin a period of asexual reproduction. By this amplification process (known as *intrahepatic* or *preerythrocytic schizogony* or *merogony*), a single sporozoite eventually may produce from 10,000 to >30,000 daughter merozoites. The swollen infected liver cells eventually burst, discharging motile *merozoites* into the bloodstream. These merozoites then invade the red blood cells (RBCs) and multiply six- to twentyfold every 48 h (*P. knowlesi*, 24 h; *P. malariae*, 72 h). When the parasites reach densities of ~50/μL of blood (~100 million parasites in the blood of an adult), the symptomatic stage of the infection begins. In *P. vivax* and *P. ovale* infections, a proportion of the intrahepatic forms do not divide immediately but remain inert for a period ranging from 3 weeks to ≥1 year before reproduction begins. These dormant forms, or *hypnozoites*, are the cause of the relapses that characterize infection with these two species.

After entry into the bloodstream, merozoites rapidly invade erythrocytes and become *trophozoites*. Attachment is mediated via a specific erythrocyte surface receptor. For *P. falciparum*, the reticulocyte-binding protein homologue 5 (PfRh5) is indispensable for erythrocyte invasion. Basigin (CD147, EMMPRIN) is the erythrocyte receptor of PfRh5. In the case of *P. vivax*, this receptor is related to the Duffy blood-group antigen Fy^a or Fy^b. Most West Africans and people with origins in that region carry the Duffy-negative FyFy phenotype and are therefore resistant to *P. vivax* malaria. During the early stage of intraerythrocytic development, the small "ring forms" of the different parasitic species appear similar under light microscopy. As the trophozoites enlarge, species-specific characteristics become evident, pigment becomes visible, and the parasite assumes an irregular or ameboid shape. By the end of the intraerythrocytic life cycle, the parasite has consumed two-thirds of the RBC's hemoglobin and has grown to occupy most of the cell. It is now called a *schizont*. Multiple nuclear divisions have taken place (*schizogony* or *merogony*). The RBC then ruptures to release 6–30 daughter merozoites, each potentially capable of invading a new RBC and repeating the cycle. The disease in human beings is caused by the direct effects of the asexual parasite—RBC invasion and destruction—and by the host's reaction. After release from the liver (*P. vivax, P. ovale, P. malariae, P. knowlesi*), some of the blood-stage parasites develop into morphologically distinct,

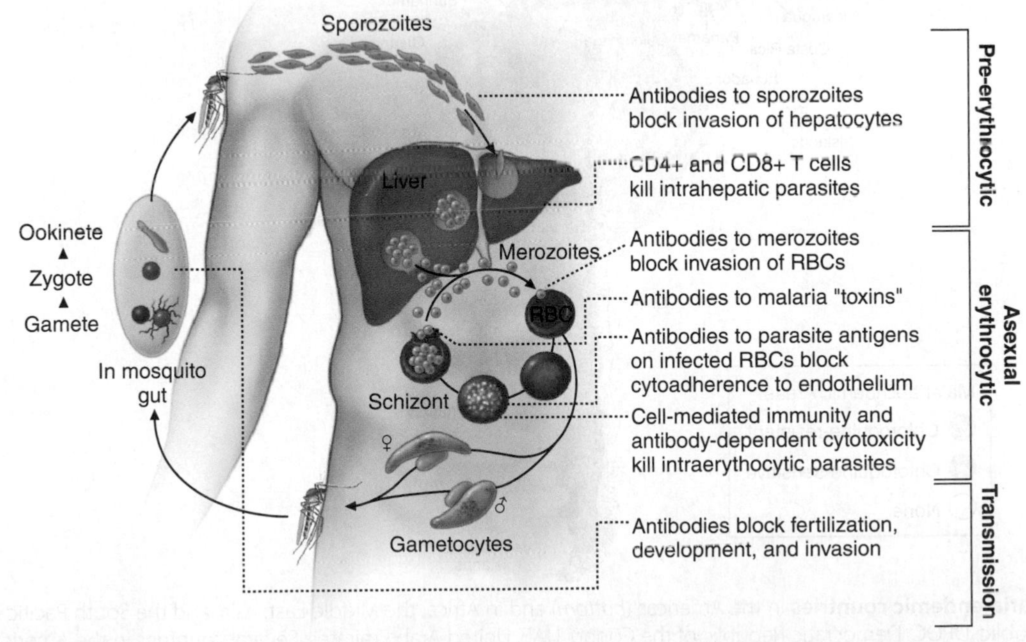

FIGURE 248-1 The malaria transmission cycle from mosquito to human and targets of immunity. RBC, red blood cell.

longer-lived sexual forms (*gametocytes*) that can transmit malaria. In falciparum malaria, a delay of several asexual cycles precedes this switch to gametocytogenesis.

After being ingested in the blood meal of a biting female anopheline mosquito, the male and female gametocytes form a zygote in the insect's midgut. This zygote matures into an ookinete, which penetrates and encysts in the mosquito's gut wall. The resulting oocyst expands by asexual division until it bursts to liberate myriad motile sporozoites, which then migrate in the hemolymph to the salivary gland of the mosquito to await inoculation into another human at the next feeding.

EPIDEMIOLOGY

Malaria occurs throughout most of the tropical regions of the world (Fig. 248-2). *P. falciparum* predominates in Africa, New Guinea, and Hispaniola (i.e., the Dominican Republic and Haiti); *P. vivax* is more common in Central America. The prevalence of these two species is approximately equal in South America, the Indian subcontinent, eastern Asia, and Oceania. *P. malariae* is found in most endemic areas, especially throughout sub-Saharan Africa, but is much less common. *P. ovale* is relatively unusual outside of Africa and, where it is found, comprises <1% of isolates. Patients infected with *P. knowlesi* have been

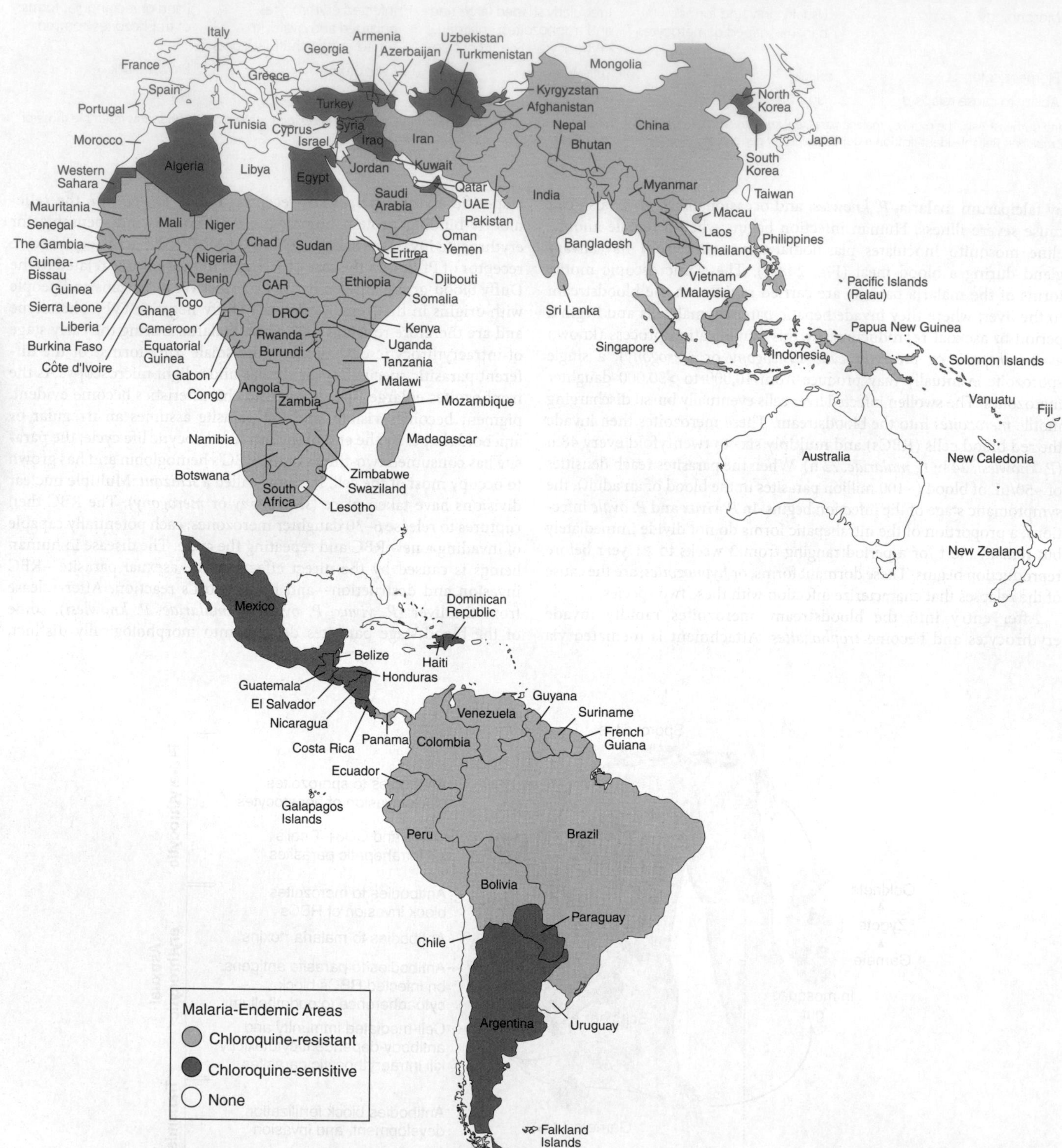

FIGURE 248-2 Malaria-endemic countries in the Americas (*bottom*) and in Africa, the Middle East, Asia, and the South Pacific (*top*), 2007. CAR, Central African Republic; DROC, Democratic Republic of the Congo; UAE, United Arab Emirates. Several countries in the Americas, the Middle East, and North Africa are close to eliminating malaria.

identified on the island of Borneo and, to a lesser extent, elsewhere in Southeast Asia, where the main hosts, long-tailed and pig-tailed macaques, are found.

The epidemiology of malaria is complex and may vary considerably even within relatively small geographic areas. Endemicity traditionally has been defined in terms of parasitemia rates or palpable-spleen rates in children 2–9 years of age and classified as hypoendemic (<10%), mesoendemic (11–50%), hyperendemic (51–75%), and holoendemic (>75%). Until recently, it was uncommon to use these indices for planning control programs; however, many countries are now conducting national surveys to assess program progress. In holo- and hyperendemic areas (e.g., certain regions of tropical Africa or coastal New Guinea) where there is intense *P. falciparum* transmission, people may sustain more than one infectious mosquito bite per day and are infected repeatedly throughout their lives. In such settings, rates of morbidity and mortality due to malaria are considerable during early childhood. Immunity against disease is hard won in these areas, and the burden of disease in young children is high; by adulthood, however, most malarial infections are asymptomatic. As control measures progress and urbanization expands, environmental conditions become less conducive to transmission, and all age groups may lose protective immunity and become susceptible to illness. Constant, frequent, year-round infection is termed *stable transmission*. In areas where transmission is low, erratic, or focal, full protective immunity is not acquired, and symptomatic disease may occur at all ages. This situation usually exists in hypoendemic areas and is termed *unstable transmission*. Even in stable-transmission areas, there is often an increased incidence of symptomatic malaria coinciding with increased mosquito breeding and transmission during the rainy season. Malaria can behave like an epidemic disease in some areas, particularly those with unstable malaria, such as northern India (the Punjab region), the horn of Africa, Rwanda, Burundi, southern Africa, and Madagascar. An epidemic can develop when there are changes in environmental, economic, or social conditions, such as heavy rains following drought or migrations (usually of refugees or workers) from a nonmalarious region to an area of high transmission, along with failure to invest in national programs; a breakdown in malaria control and prevention services caused by war or civil disorder can intensify epidemic conditions. This situation usually results in considerable mortality among all age groups.

The principal determinants of the epidemiology of malaria are the number (density), the human-biting habits, and the longevity of the anopheline mosquito vectors. More than 100 of the >400 anopheline species can transmit malaria, but the ~40 species that do so commonly vary considerably in their efficiency as malaria vectors. More specifically, the transmission of malaria is directly proportional to the density of the vector, the square of the number of human bites per day per mosquito, and the tenth power of the probability of the mosquito's surviving for 1 day. Mosquito longevity is particularly important because the portion of the parasite's life cycle that takes place within the mosquito—from gametocyte ingestion to subsequent inoculation (*sporogony*)—lasts 8–30 days, depending on ambient temperature; thus, to transmit malaria, the mosquito must survive for >7 days. Sporogony is not completed at cooler temperatures—i.e., <16°C (60.8°F) for *P. vivax* and <21°C (69.8°F) for *P. falciparum*; thus transmission does not occur below these temperatures or at high altitudes, although malaria outbreaks and transmission have occurred in the highlands (>1500 m) of eastern Africa, which were previously free of vectors. The most effective mosquito vectors of malaria are those, such as *Anopheles gambiae* in Africa, that are long-lived, occur in high densities in tropical climates, breed readily, and bite humans in preference to other animals. The entomologic inoculation rate (i.e., the number of sporozoite-positive mosquito bites per person per year) is the most common measure of malaria transmission and varies from <1 in some parts of Latin America and Southeast Asia to >300 in parts of tropical Africa.

ERYTHROCYTE CHANGES IN MALARIA

After invading an erythrocyte, the growing malarial parasite progressively consumes and degrades intracellular proteins, principally hemoglobin. The potentially toxic heme is detoxified by lipid-mediated crystallization to biologically inert hemozoin (malaria pigment). The parasite also alters the RBC membrane by changing its transport properties, exposing cryptic surface antigens, and inserting new parasite-derived proteins. The RBC becomes more irregular in shape, more antigenic, and less deformable.

In *P. falciparum* infections, membrane protuberances appear on the erythrocyte's surface 12–15 h after the cell's invasion. These "knobs" extrude a high-molecular-weight, antigenically variant, strain-specific erythrocyte membrane adhesive protein (PfEMP1) that mediates attachment to receptors on venular and capillary endothelium—an event termed *cytoadherence*. Several vascular receptors have been identified, of which intercellular adhesion molecule 1 is probably the most important in the brain, chondroitin sulfate B in the placenta, and CD36 in most other organs. Thus, the infected erythrocytes stick inside and eventually block capillaries and venules. At the same stage, these *P. falciparum*–infected RBCs may also adhere to uninfected RBCs (to form rosettes) and to other parasitized erythrocytes (agglutination). The processes of cytoadherence, rosetting, and agglutination are central to the pathogenesis of falciparum malaria. They result in the sequestration of RBCs containing mature forms of the parasite in vital organs (particularly the brain), where they interfere with microcirculatory flow and metabolism. Sequestered parasites continue to develop out of reach of the principal host defense mechanism: splenic processing and filtration. As a consequence, only the younger ring forms of the asexual parasites are seen circulating in the peripheral blood in falciparum malaria, and the level of peripheral parasitemia underestimates the true number of parasites within the body. Severe malaria is also associated with reduced deformability of the uninfected erythrocytes, which compromises their passage through the partially obstructed capillaries and venules and shortens RBC survival.

In the other human malarias, sequestration does not occur, and all stages of the parasite's development are evident on peripheral-blood smears. Whereas *P. vivax*, *P. ovale*, and *P. malariae* show a marked predilection for either young RBCs (*P. vivax*, *P. ovale*) or old cells (*P. malariae*) and produce a level of parasitemia that is seldom >2%, *P. falciparum* can invade erythrocytes of all ages and may be associated with very high levels of parasitemia.

HOST RESPONSE

Initially, the host responds to plasmodial infection by activating nonspecific defense mechanisms. Splenic immunologic and filtrative clearance functions are augmented in malaria, and the removal of both parasitized and uninfected erythrocytes is accelerated. The spleen is able to remove damaged ring-form parasites and return the once-infected erythrocytes to the circulation, where their survival period is shortened. The parasitized cells escaping splenic removal are destroyed when the schizont ruptures. The material released induces the activation of macrophages and the release of proinflammatory cytokines, which cause fever and exert other pathologic effects. Temperatures of >40°C (104°F) damage mature parasites; in untreated infections, the effect of such temperatures is to further synchronize the parasitic cycle, with eventual production of the regular fever spikes and rigors that originally served to characterize the different malarias. These regular fever patterns (quotidian, daily; tertian, every 2 days; quartan, every 3 days) are seldom seen today in patients who receive prompt and effective antimalarial treatment.

The geographic distributions of sickle cell disease, hemoglobins C and E, hereditary ovalocytosis, the thalassemias, and glucose-6-phosphate dehydrogenase (G6PD) deficiency closely resemble that of falciparum malaria before the introduction of control measures. This similarity suggests that these genetic disorders confer protection against death from falciparum malaria. For example, HbA/S heterozygotes (sickle cell trait) have a sixfold reduction in the risk of dying from severe falciparum malaria. Hemoglobin S–containing RBCs impair parasite growth at low oxygen tensions, and *P. falciparum*–infected RBCs containing hemoglobins S and C exhibit reduced cytoadherence because of reduced surface presentation of the adhesin PfEMP1. Parasite multiplication in HbA/E heterozygotes is reduced at high parasite densities. In Melanesia, children with α-thalassemia appear to have more frequent malaria (both vivax and falciparum) in the early years of life, and this pattern of infection appears to protect them against severe disease. In Melanesian ovalocytosis, rigid erythrocytes resist merozoite invasion, and the intraerythrocytic milieu is hostile.

Nonspecific host defense mechanisms stop the infection's expansion, and the subsequent strain-specific immune response then controls the infection. Eventually, exposure to sufficient strains confers protection from high-level parasitemia and disease but not from infection. As a result of this state of infection without illness (*premunition*), asymptomatic parasitemia is common among adults and older children living in regions with stable and intense transmission (i.e., holo- or hyperendemic areas) and also in parts of low-transmission areas. Immunity is mainly specific for both the species and the strain of infecting malarial parasite. Both humoral immunity and cellular immunity are necessary for protection, but the mechanisms of each are incompletely understood (Fig. 248-1). Immune individuals have a polyclonal increase in serum levels of IgM, IgG, and IgA, although much of this antibody is unrelated to protection. Antibodies to a variety of parasitic antigens presumably act in concert to limit in vivo replication of the parasite. In the case of falciparum malaria, the most important of these antigens is the surface adhesin—the variant protein PfEMP1. Passively transferred IgG from immune adults has been shown to reduce levels of parasitemia in children. Passive transfer of maternal antibody contributes to the relative (but not complete) protection of infants from severe malaria in the first months of life. This complex immunity to disease declines when a person lives outside an endemic area for several months or longer.

Several factors retard the development of cellular immunity to malaria. These factors include the absence of major histocompatibility antigens on the surface of infected RBCs, which precludes direct T cell recognition; malaria antigen–specific immune unresponsiveness; and the enormous strain diversity of malarial parasites, along with the ability of the parasites to express variant immunodominant antigens on the erythrocyte surface that change during the course of infection. Parasites may persist in the blood for months or years (or, in the case of *P. malariae*, for decades) if treatment is not given. The complexity of the immune response in malaria, the sophistication of the parasites' evasion mechanisms, and the lack of a good in vitro correlate with clinical immunity have all slowed progress toward an effective vaccine.

CLINICAL FEATURES

Malaria is a very common cause of fever in tropical countries. The first symptoms of malaria are nonspecific; the lack of a sense of well-being, headache, fatigue, abdominal discomfort, and muscle aches followed by fever are all similar to the symptoms of a minor viral illness. In some instances, a prominence of headache, chest pain, abdominal pain, cough, arthralgia, myalgia, or diarrhea may suggest another diagnosis. Although headache may be severe in malaria, the neck stiffness and photophobia seen in meningitis do not occur. While myalgia may be prominent, it is not usually as severe as in dengue fever, and the muscles are not tender as in leptospirosis or typhus. Nausea, vomiting, and orthostatic hypotension are common. The classic malarial paroxysms, in which fever spikes, chills, and rigors occur at regular intervals, are relatively unusual and suggest infection with *P. vivax* or *P. ovale*. The fever is usually irregular at first (that of falciparum malaria may never become regular); the temperature of nonimmune individuals and children often rises above 40°C (104°F) in conjunction with tachycardia and sometimes delirium. Although childhood febrile convulsions may occur with any of the malarias, generalized seizures are specifically associated with falciparum malaria and may herald the development of encephalopathy (cerebral malaria). Many clinical abnormalities have been described in acute malaria, but most patients with uncomplicated infections have few abnormal physical findings other than fever, malaise, mild anemia, and (in some cases) a palpable spleen. Anemia is common among young children living in areas with stable transmission, particularly where resistance has compromised the efficacy of antimalarial drugs. In nonimmune individuals with acute malaria, the spleen takes several days to become palpable, but splenic enlargement is found in a high proportion of otherwise healthy individuals in malaria-endemic areas and reflects repeated infections. Slight enlargement of the liver is also common, particularly among young children. Mild jaundice is common among adults; it may develop in patients with otherwise uncomplicated malaria and usually resolves over 1–3 weeks. Malaria is not associated with a rash like those seen in meningococcal septicemia, typhus, enteric fever, viral exanthems, and drug reactions. Petechial hemorrhages in the skin or mucous membranes—features of viral hemorrhagic fevers and leptospirosis—develop only very rarely in severe falciparum malaria.

SEVERE FALCIPARUM MALARIA

Appropriately and promptly treated, uncomplicated falciparum malaria (i.e., the patient can swallow medicines and food) carries a mortality rate of <0.1%. However, once vital-organ dysfunction occurs or the total proportion of erythrocytes infected increases to >2% (a level corresponding to >10^{12} parasites in an adult), mortality risk rises steeply. The major manifestations of severe falciparum malaria are shown in Table 248-2, and features indicating a poor prognosis are listed in Table 248-3.

TABLE 248-2 MANIFESTATIONS OF SEVERE FALCIPARUM MALARIA

Signs	Manifestations
Major	
Unarousable coma/cerebral malaria	Failure to localize or respond appropriately to noxious stimuli; coma persisting for >30 min after generalized convulsion
Acidemia/acidosis	Arterial pH of <7.25 or plasma bicarbonate level of <15 mmol/L; venous lactate level of >5 mmol/L; manifests as labored deep breathing, often termed "respiratory distress"
Severe normochromic, normocytic anemia	Hematocrit of <15% or hemoglobin level of <50 g/L (<5 g/dL) with parasitemia <10,000/μL
Renal failure	Serum or plasma creatinine level of >265 μmol/L (>3 mg/dL); urine output (24 h) of <400 mL in adults or <12 mL/kg in children; no improvement with rehydration
Pulmonary edema/adult respiratory distress syndrome	Noncardiogenic pulmonary edema, often aggravated by overhydration
Hypoglycemia	Plasma glucose level of <2.2 mmol/L (<40 mg/dL)
Hypotension/shock	Systolic blood pressure of <50 mmHg in children 1–5 years or <80 mmHg in adults; core/skin temperature difference of >10°C; capillary refill >2 s
Bleeding/disseminated intravascular coagulation	Significant bleeding and hemorrhage from the gums, nose, and gastrointestinal tract and/or evidence of disseminated intravascular coagulation
Convulsions	More than two generalized seizures in 24 h; signs of continued seizure activity, sometimes subtle (e.g., tonic-clonic eye movements without limb or face movement)
Other	
Hemoglobinuria[a]	Macroscopic black, brown, or red urine; not associated with effects of oxidant drugs and red blood cell enzyme defects (such as G6PD deficiency)
Extreme weakness	Prostration; inability to sit unaided[b]
Hyperparasitemia	Parasitemia level of >5% in nonimmune patients (>10% in any patient)
Jaundice	Serum bilirubin level of >50 mmol/L (>3 mg/dL) if combined with a parasite density of 100,000/μL or other evidence of vital-organ dysfunction

[a]Hemoglobinuria may also occur in uncomplicated malaria and in patients with G6PD deficiency who take primaquine. [b]In children who are normally able to sit.

Abbreviation: G6PD, glucose-6-phosphate dehydrogenase.

TABLE 248-3 FEATURES INDICATING A POOR PROGNOSIS IN SEVERE FALCIPARUM MALARIA

Clinical
Marked agitation
Hyperventilation (respiratory distress)
Hypothermia (<36.5°C; <97.7°F)
Bleeding
Deep coma
Repeated convulsions
Anuria
Shock
Laboratory
Biochemistry
Hypoglycemia (<2.2 mmol/L)
Hyperlactatemia (>5 mmol/L)
Acidosis (arterial pH <7.3, serum HCO_3 <15 mmol/L)
Elevated serum creatinine (>265 μmol/L)
Elevated total bilirubin (>50 μmol/L)
Elevated liver enzymes (AST/ALT 3 times upper limit of normal)
Elevated muscle enzymes (CPK ↑, myoglobin ↑)
Elevated urate (>600 μmol/L)
Hematology
Leukocytosis (>12,000/μL)
Severe anemia (PCV <15%)
Coagulopathy
Decreased platelet count (<50,000/μL)
Prolonged prothrombin time (>3 s)
Prolonged partial thromboplastin time
Decreased fibrinogen (<200 mg/dL)
Parasitology
Hyperparasitemia
Increased mortality at >100,000/μL
High mortality at >500,000/μL
>20% of parasites identified as pigment-containing trophozoites and schizonts
>5% of neutrophils with visible pigment

Abbreviations: ALT, alanine aminotransferase; AST, aspartate aminotransferase; CPK, creatine phosphokinase; PCV, packed cell volume.

Cerebral Malaria Coma is a characteristic and ominous feature of falciparum malaria and, despite treatment, is associated with death rates of ~20% among adults and 15% among children. Any obtundation, delirium, or abnormal behavior should be taken very seriously. The onset may be gradual or sudden following a convulsion.

Cerebral malaria manifests as diffuse symmetric encephalopathy; focal neurologic signs are unusual. Although some passive resistance to head flexion may be detected, signs of meningeal irritation are absent. The eyes may be divergent and a pout reflex is common, but other primitive reflexes are usually absent. The corneal reflexes are preserved, except in deep coma. Muscle tone may be either increased or decreased. The tendon reflexes are variable, and the plantar reflexes may be flexor or extensor; the abdominal and cremasteric reflexes are absent. Flexor or extensor posturing may be seen. On routine funduscopy, ~15% of patients have retinal hemorrhages; with pupillary dilation and indirect ophthalmoscopy, this figure increases to 30–40%. Other funduscopic abnormalities (Fig. 248-3) include discrete spots of retinal opacification (30–60%), papilledema (8% among children, rare among adults), cotton wool spots (<5%), and decolorization of a retinal vessel or segment of vessel (occasional cases). Convulsions, usually generalized and often repeated, occur in ~10% of adults and up to 50% of children with cerebral malaria. More covert seizure activity also is common, particularly among children, and may manifest as repetitive tonic-clonic eye movements or even hypersalivation. Whereas adults

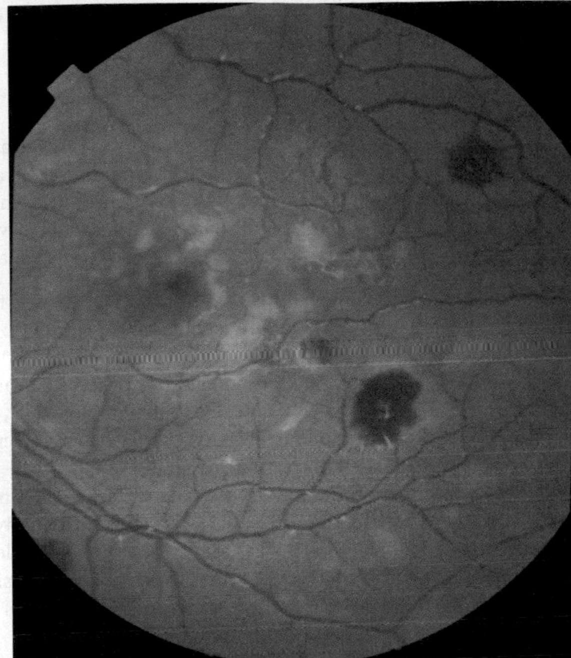

FIGURE 248-3 The eye in cerebral malaria: perimacular whitening and pale-centered retinal hemorrhages. *(Courtesy of N. Beare, T. Taylor, S. Harding, S. Lewallen, and M. Molyneux; with permission.)*

rarely (i.e., in <3% of cases) suffer neurologic sequelae, ~10% of children surviving cerebral malaria—especially those with hypoglycemia, severe anemia, repeated seizures, and deep coma—have residual neurologic deficits when they regain consciousness; hemiplegia, cerebral palsy, cortical blindness, deafness, and impaired cognition have been reported. The majority of these deficits improve markedly or resolve completely within 6 months. However, the prevalence of some other deficits increases over time; ~10% of children surviving cerebral malaria have a persistent language deficit. There may also be deficits in learning, planning and executive functions, attention, memory, and nonverbal functioning. The incidence of epilepsy is increased and life expectancy decreased among these children.

Hypoglycemia Hypoglycemia, an important and common complication of severe malaria, is associated with a poor prognosis and is particularly problematic in children and pregnant women. Hypoglycemia in malaria results from a failure of hepatic gluconeogenesis and an increase in the consumption of glucose by both the host and, to a much lesser extent, the malaria parasites. To compound the situation, quinine, which is still widely used for the treatment of both severe and uncomplicated falciparum malaria, is a powerful stimulant of pancreatic insulin secretion. Hyperinsulinemic hypoglycemia is especially troublesome in pregnant women receiving quinine treatment. In severe disease, the clinical diagnosis of hypoglycemia is difficult: the usual physical signs (sweating, gooseflesh, tachycardia) are absent, and the neurologic impairment caused by hypoglycemia cannot be distinguished from that caused by malaria.

Acidosis Acidosis, an important cause of death from severe malaria, results from accumulation of organic acids. Hyperlactatemia commonly coexists with hypoglycemia. In adults, coexisting renal impairment often compounds the acidosis; in children, ketoacidosis also may contribute. Other, still-unidentified organic acids are major contributors to acidosis. Acidotic breathing, sometimes called "respiratory distress," is a sign of poor prognosis. It is followed often by circulatory failure refractory to volume expansion or inotropic drug treatment and ultimately by respiratory arrest. The plasma concentrations of bicarbonate or lactate are the best biochemical prognosticators in severe malaria. Hypovolemia is not a major contributor to acidosis. Lactic acidosis is caused by the combination of anaerobic glycolysis in tissues where sequestered parasites interfere with microcirculatory flow, lactate production by the parasites, and a failure of hepatic and renal lactate clearance. The prognosis of severe acidosis is poor.

Noncardiogenic Pulmonary Edema Adults with severe falciparum malaria may develop noncardiogenic pulmonary edema even after several days of antimalarial therapy. The pathogenesis of this variant of the adult respiratory distress syndrome is unclear. The mortality rate is >80%. This condition can be aggravated by overly vigorous administration of IV fluid. Noncardiogenic pulmonary edema can also develop in otherwise uncomplicated vivax malaria, where recovery is usual.

Renal Impairment Acute kidney injury is common in severe falciparum malaria, but oliguric renal failure is rare among children. The pathogenesis of renal failure is unclear but may be related to erythrocyte sequestration and agglutination interfering with renal microcirculatory flow and metabolism. Clinically and pathologically, this syndrome manifests as acute tubular necrosis. Renal cortical necrosis never develops. Acute renal failure may occur simultaneously with other vital-organ dysfunction (in which case the mortality risk is high) or may progress as other disease manifestations resolve. In survivors, urine flow resumes in a median of 4 days, and serum creatinine levels return to normal in a mean of 17 days (Chap. 334). Early dialysis or hemofiltration considerably enhances the likelihood of a patient's survival, particularly in acute hypercatabolic renal failure.

Hematologic Abnormalities Anemia results from accelerated RBC removal by the spleen, obligatory RBC destruction at parasite schizogony, and ineffective erythropoiesis. In severe malaria, both infected and uninfected RBCs show reduced deformability, which correlates with prognosis and development of anemia. Splenic clearance of all RBCs is increased. In nonimmune individuals and in areas with unstable transmission, anemia can develop rapidly and transfusion is often required. As a consequence of repeated malarial infections, children in many areas of Africa and on the island of New Guinea may develop severe anemia resulting from both shortened survival of uninfected RBCs and marked dyserythropoiesis. Anemia is a common consequence of antimalarial drug resistance, which results in repeated or continued infection.

Slight coagulation abnormalities are common in falciparum malaria, and mild thrombocytopenia is usual (a normal platelet count should raise questions about the diagnosis of malaria). Of patients with severe malaria, <5% have significant bleeding with evidence of disseminated intravascular coagulation. Hematemesis from stress ulceration or acute gastric erosions also may occur rarely.

Liver Dysfunction Mild hemolytic jaundice is common in malaria. Severe jaundice is associated with *P. falciparum* infections; is more common among adults than among children; and results from hemolysis, hepatocyte injury, and cholestasis. When accompanied by other vital-organ dysfunction (often renal impairment), liver dysfunction carries a poor prognosis. Hepatic dysfunction contributes to hypoglycemia, lactic acidosis, and impaired drug metabolism. Occasional patients with falciparum malaria may develop deep jaundice (with hemolytic, hepatic, and cholestatic components) without evidence of other vital-organ dysfunction, in which case the prognosis is good.

Other Complications HIV/AIDS and malnutrition predispose to more severe malaria in nonimmune individuals; malaria anemia is worsened by concurrent infections with intestinal helminths, hookworm in particular. Septicemia may complicate severe malaria, particularly in children. Differentiating severe malaria from sepsis with incidental parasitemia in childhood is very difficult. In endemic areas, *Salmonella* bacteremia has been associated specifically with *P. falciparum* infections. Chest infections and catheter-induced urinary tract infections are common among patients who are unconscious for >3 days. Aspiration pneumonia may follow generalized convulsions. The frequencies of complications of severe falciparum malaria are summarized in Table 248-4.

TABLE 248-4 RELATIVE INCIDENCE OF SEVERE COMPLICATIONS OF FALCIPARUM MALARIA

Complication	Nonpregnant Adults	Pregnant Women	Children
Anemia	+	++	+++
Convulsions	+	+	+++
Hypoglycemia	+	+++	+++
Jaundice	+++	+++	+
Renal failure	+++	+++	–
Pulmonary edema	++	+++	+

Note: –, rare; +, infrequent; ++, frequent; +++, very frequent.

MALARIA IN PREGNANCY

Malaria in early pregnancy causes abortion. In areas of high malaria transmission, falciparum malaria in primi- and secundigravid women is associated with low birth weight (average reduction, ~170 g) and consequently increased infant mortality rates. In general, infected mothers in areas of stable transmission remain asymptomatic despite intense accumulation of parasitized erythrocytes in the placental microcirculation. Maternal HIV infection predisposes pregnant women to more frequent and higher-density malaria infections, predisposes their newborns to congenital malarial infection, and exacerbates the reduction in birth weight associated with malaria.

In areas with unstable transmission of malaria, pregnant women are prone to severe infections and are particularly vulnerable to high parasitemias with anemia, hypoglycemia, and acute pulmonary edema. Fetal distress, premature labor, and stillbirth or low birth weight are common results. Fetal death is usual in severe malaria. Congenital malaria occurs in <5% of newborns whose mothers are infected; its frequency and the level of parasitemia are related directly to the parasite density in maternal blood and in the placenta. *P. vivax* malaria in pregnancy is also associated with a reduction in birth weight (average, 110 g), but, in contrast to the situation in falciparum malaria, this effect is more pronounced in multigravid than in primigravid women. About 350,000 women die in childbirth yearly, with most deaths occurring in low-income countries; maternal death from hemorrhage at childbirth is correlated with malaria-induced anemia.

MALARIA IN CHILDREN

Most of the 660,000 persons who die of falciparum malaria each year are young African children. Convulsions, coma, hypoglycemia, metabolic acidosis, and severe anemia are relatively common among children with severe malaria, whereas deep jaundice, oliguric acute kidney injury, and acute pulmonary edema are unusual. Severely anemic children may present with labored deep breathing, which in the past has been attributed incorrectly to "anemic congestive cardiac failure" but in fact is usually caused by metabolic acidosis, often compounded by hypovolemia. In general, children tolerate antimalarial drugs well and respond rapidly to treatment.

TRANSFUSION MALARIA

Malaria can be transmitted by blood transfusion, needle-stick injury, sharing of needles by infected injection drug users, or organ transplantation. The incubation period in these settings is often short because there is no preerythrocytic stage of development. The clinical features and management of these cases are the same as for naturally acquired infections. Radical chemotherapy with primaquine is unnecessary for transfusion-transmitted *P. vivax* and *P. ovale* infections.

CHRONIC COMPLICATIONS OF MALARIA

TROPICAL SPLENOMEGALY (HYPERREACTIVE MALARIAL SPLENOMEGALY)

Chronic or repeated malarial infections produce hypergammaglobulinemia; normochromic, normocytic anemia; and, in certain situations, splenomegaly. Some residents of malaria-endemic areas in tropical Africa and Asia exhibit an abnormal immunologic response to repeated infections that is characterized by massive splenomegaly, hepatomegaly, marked elevations in serum titers of IgM and malarial antibody, hepatic sinusoidal lymphocytosis, and (in Africa) peripheral B cell lymphocytosis. This syndrome has been associated with the production of cytotoxic IgM antibodies to CD8+ T lymphocytes, antibodies to CD5+ T lymphocytes, and an increase in the ratio of CD4+ to CD8+ T cells. These events may lead to uninhibited B cell production of IgM and the formation of cryoglobulins (IgM aggregates and immune complexes). This immunologic process stimulates reticuloendothelial hyperplasia and clearance activity and eventually produces splenomegaly. Patients with hyperreactive malarial splenomegaly present with an abdominal mass or a dragging sensation in the abdomen and occasional sharp abdominal pains suggesting perisplenitis. Anemia and some degree of pancytopenia are usually evident, and in some cases malarial parasites cannot be found in peripheral-blood smears. Vulnerability to respiratory and skin infections is increased; many patients die of overwhelming sepsis. Persons with hyperreactive malarial splenomegaly who are living in endemic areas should receive antimalarial chemoprophylaxis; the results are usually good. In nonendemic areas, antimalarial treatment is advised. In some cases refractory to therapy, clonal lymphoproliferation may develop and can then evolve into a malignant lymphoproliferative disorder.

QUARTAN MALARIAL NEPHROPATHY

Chronic or repeated infections with *P. malariae* (and possibly with other malarial species) may cause soluble immune complex injury to the renal glomeruli, resulting in the nephrotic syndrome. Other unidentified factors must contribute to this process since only a very small proportion of infected patients develop renal disease. The histologic appearance is that of focal or segmental glomerulonephritis with splitting of the capillary basement membrane. Subendothelial dense deposits are seen on electron microscopy, and immunofluorescence reveals deposits of complement and immunoglobulins; in samples of renal tissue from children, *P. malariae* antigens are often visible. A coarse-granular pattern of basement membrane immunofluorescent deposits (predominantly IgG3) with selective proteinuria carries a better prognosis than a fine-granular, predominantly IgG2 pattern with nonselective proteinuria. Quartan nephropathy usually responds poorly to treatment with either antimalarial agents or glucocorticoids and cytotoxic drugs.

BURKITT'S LYMPHOMA AND EPSTEIN-BARR VIRUS INFECTION

It is possible that malaria-related immune dysregulation provokes infection with lymphoma viruses. Burkitt's lymphoma is strongly associated with Epstein-Barr virus. The prevalence of this childhood tumor is high in malarious areas of Africa.

DIAGNOSIS

DEMONSTRATION OF THE PARASITE

The diagnosis of malaria rests on the demonstration of asexual forms of the parasite in stained peripheral-blood smears. After a negative blood smear, repeat smears should be made if there is a high degree of suspicion. Of the Romanowsky stains, Giemsa at pH 7.2 is preferred; Field's, Wright's, or Leishman's stain can also be used. Both thin (Figs. 248-4 and 248-5; see also Figs. 250e-3 and 250e-4) and thick (Figs. 248-6, 248-7, 248-8, and 248-9) blood smears should be examined. The thin blood smear should be rapidly air-dried, fixed in anhydrous methanol, and stained; the RBCs in the tail of the film should then be examined under oil immersion (×1000 magnification). The level of parasitemia is expressed as the number of parasitized erythrocytes per 1000 RBCs. The thick blood film should be of uneven thickness. The smear should be dried thoroughly and stained without fixing. As many layers of erythrocytes overlie one another and are lysed during the staining procedure, the thick film has the advantage of concentrating the parasites (by 40- to 100-fold compared with a thin blood film) and thus increasing diagnostic sensitivity. Both parasites and white blood cells (WBCs) are counted, and the number of parasites per unit volume is calculated from the total leukocyte count. Alternatively, a WBC count of 8000/μL is assumed. This figure is converted to the number of parasitized erythrocytes per microliter. A minimum of 200 WBCs should be counted under oil immersion. Interpretation of blood smear films requires some experience because artifacts are common. Before a thick smear is judged to be negative, 100–200 fields should be examined under oil immersion. In high-transmission areas, the presence of up to 10,000 parasites/μL of blood may be tolerated without symptoms or signs in partially immune individuals. Thus in these areas the detection of malaria parasites is sensitive but has low specificity in identifying

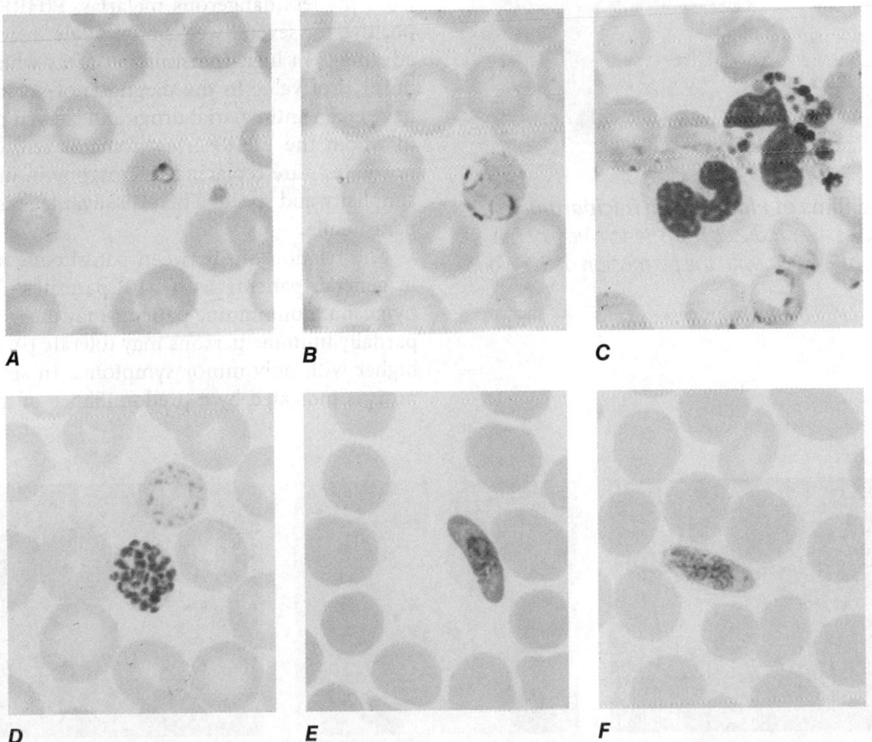

FIGURE 248-4 Thin blood films of *Plasmodium falciparum*. ***A.*** Young trophozoites. ***B.*** Old trophozoites. ***C.*** Pigment in polymorphonuclear cells and trophozoites. ***D.*** Mature schizonts. ***E.*** Female gametocytes. ***F.*** Male gametocytes. *(Reproduced from Bench Aids for the Diagnosis of Malaria Infections, 2nd ed, with the permission of the World Health Organization.)*

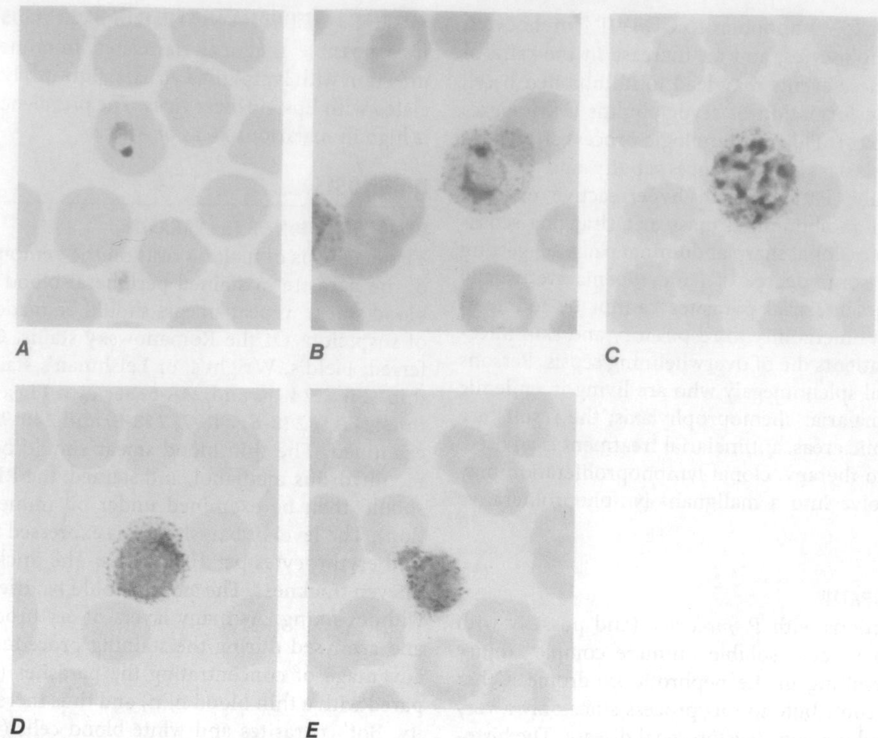

FIGURE 248-5 Thin blood films of *Plasmodium vivax*. ***A.*** Young trophozoites. ***B.*** Old trophozoites. ***C.*** Mature schizonts. ***D.*** Female gametocytes. ***E.*** Male gametocytes. *(Reproduced from Bench Aids for the Diagnosis of Malaria Infections, 2nd ed, with the permission of the World Health Organization.)*

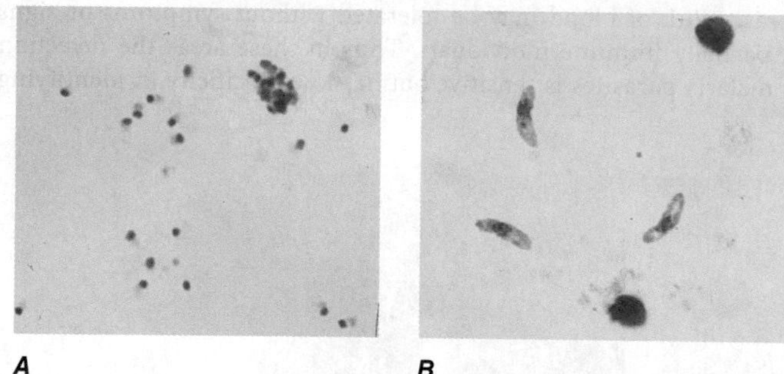

FIGURE 248-6 Thick blood films of *Plasmodium falciparum*. ***A.*** Trophozoites. ***B.*** Gametocytes. *(Reproduced from Bench Aids for the Diagnosis of Malaria Infections, 2nd ed, with the permission of the World Health Organization.)*

malaria as the cause of illness. Low-density parasitemia is common in other conditions causing fever.

Rapid, simple, sensitive, and specific antibody-based diagnostic stick or card tests that detect *P. falciparum*–specific, histidine-rich protein 2 (PfHRP2), lactate dehydrogenase, or aldolase antigens in finger-prick blood samples are now being used widely in control programs (Table 248-5). Some of these rapid diagnostic tests carry a second antibody, which allows falciparum malaria to be distinguished from the less dangerous malarias. PfHRP2-based tests may remain positive for several weeks after acute infection. This feature is a disadvantage in high-transmission areas where infections are frequent, but it is of value in the diagnosis of severe malaria in patients who have taken antimalarial drugs and cleared peripheral parasitemia (but in whom the PfHRP2 test remains strongly positive). Rapid diagnostic tests are replacing microscopy in many areas because of their simplicity and speed. Their disadvantage is that they do not quantify parasitemia.

The relationship between parasitemia and prognosis is complex; in general, patients with $>10^5$ parasites/μL are at increased risk of dying, but nonimmune patients may die with much lower counts, and partially immune persons may tolerate parasitemia levels many times higher with only minor symptoms. In severe malaria, a poor prognosis is indicated by a predominance of more mature *P. falciparum*

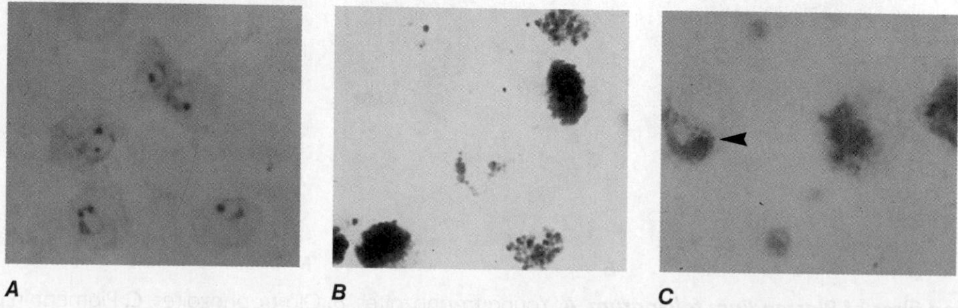

FIGURE 248-7 Thick blood films of *Plasmodium vivax*. ***A.*** Trophozoites. ***B.*** Schizonts. ***C.*** Gametocytes. *(Reproduced from Bench Aids for the Diagnosis of Malaria Infections, 2nd ed, with the permission of the World Health Organization.)*

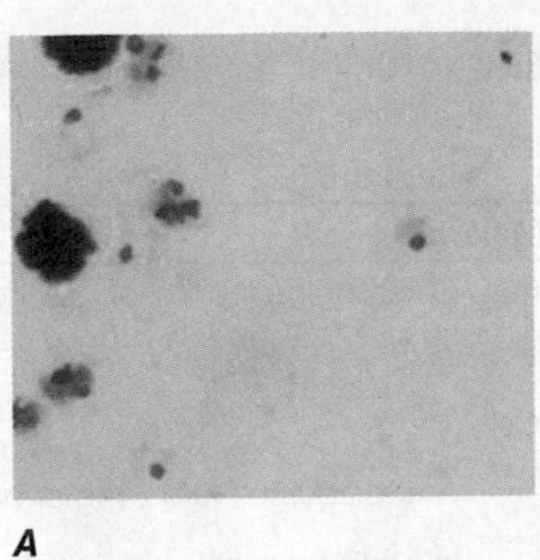
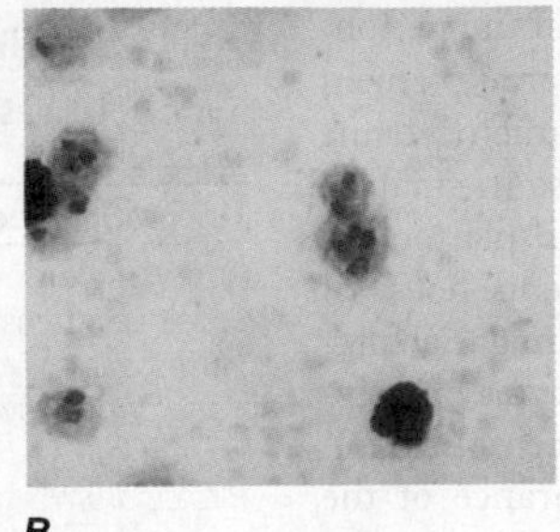
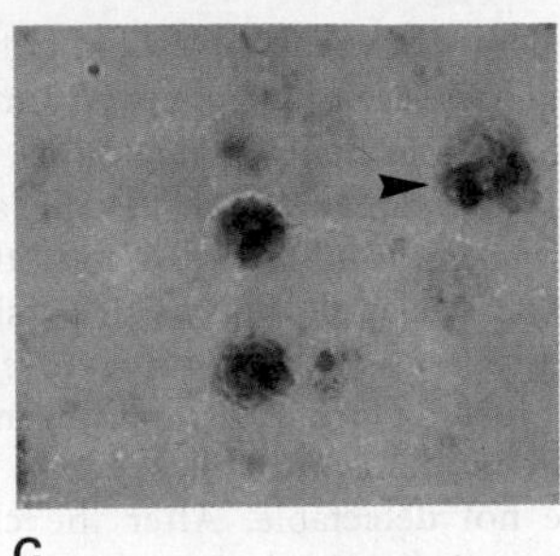

FIGURE 248-8 **Thick blood films of *Plasmodium ovale*. *A.*** Trophozoites. ***B.*** Schizonts. ***C.*** Gametocytes. *(Reproduced from Bench Aids for the Diagnosis of Malaria Infections, 2nd ed, with the permission of the World Health Organization.)*

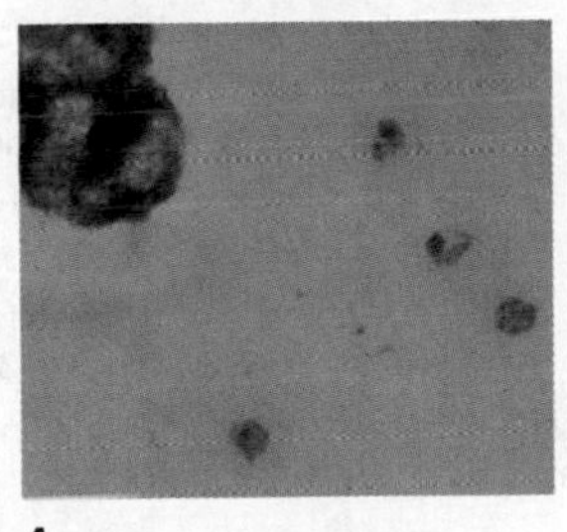
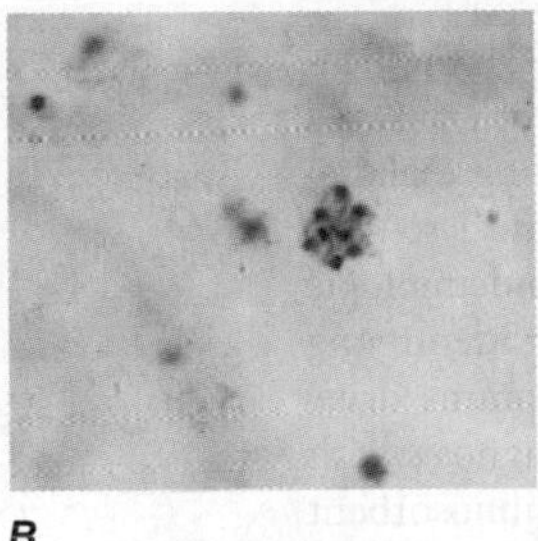
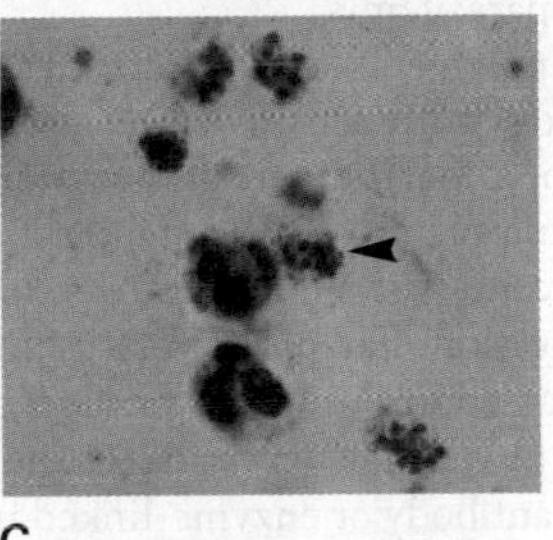

FIGURE 248-9 **Thick blood films of *Plasmodium malariae*. *A.*** Trophozoites. ***B.*** Schizonts. ***C.*** Gametocytes. *(Reproduced from Bench Aids for the Diagnosis of Malaria Infections, 2nd ed, with the permission of the World Health Organization.)*

TABLE 248-5 STANDARD METHODS FOR THE DIAGNOSIS OF MALARIA[a]

Method	Procedure	Advantages	Disadvantages
Thick blood film[b]	Blood should be uneven in thickness but thin enough that the hands of a watch can be read through part of the spot. Stain dried, unfixed blood spot with Giemsa, Field's, or another Romanowsky stain. Count number of asexual parasites per 200 WBCs (or per 500 at low densities). Count gametocytes separately.[c]	Sensitive (0.001% parasitemia); species specific; inexpensive	Requires experience (artifacts may be misinterpreted as low-level parasitemia); underestimates true count
Thin blood film[d]	Stain fixed smear with Giemsa, Field's, or another Romanowsky stain. Count number of RBCs containing asexual parasites per 1000 RBCs. In severe malaria, assess stage of parasite development and count neutrophils containing malaria pigment.[e] Count gametocytes separately.[c]	Rapid; species specific; inexpensive; in severe malaria, provides prognostic information[e]	Insensitive (<0.05% parasitemia); uneven distribution of *P. vivax*, as enlarged infected red cells concentrate at leading edge
PfHRP2 dipstick or card test	A drop of blood is placed on the stick or card, which is then immersed in washing solutions. Monoclonal antibody capture of parasitic antigens reads out as a colored band.	Robust and relatively inexpensive; rapid; sensitivity similar to or slightly lower than that of thick films (~0.001% parasitemia)	Detects only *Plasmodium falciparum*; remains positive for weeks after infection[f]; does not quantitate *P. falciparum* parasitemia
Plasmodium LDH dipstick or card test	A drop of blood is placed on the stick or card, which is then immersed in washing solutions. Monoclonal antibody capture of parasitic antigens reads out as two colored bands. One band is genus specific (all malarias), and the other is specific for *P. falciparum*.	Rapid; sensitivity similar to or slightly lower than that of thick films for *P. falciparum* (~0.001% parasitemia)	Slightly more difficult preparation than PfHRP2 tests; may miss low-level parasitemia with *P. vivax*, *P. ovale*, and *P. malariae* and may not speciate these organisms; does not quantitate *P. falciparum* parasitemia
Microtube concentration methods with acridine orange staining	Blood is collected in a specialized tube containing acridine orange, anticoagulant, and a float. After centrifugation, which concentrates the parasitized cells around the float, fluorescence microscopy is performed.	Sensitivity similar or superior to that of thick films (~0.001% parasitemia); ideal for processing large numbers of samples rapidly	Does not speciate or quantitate; requires fluorescence microscopy

[a]Malaria cannot be diagnosed clinically with accuracy, but treatment should be started on clinical grounds if laboratory confirmation is likely to be delayed. In areas of the world where malaria is endemic and transmission is high, low-level asymptomatic parasitemia is common in otherwise healthy people. Thus malaria may not be the cause of a fever, although in this context the presence of >10,000 parasites/μL (~0.2% parasitemia) does indicate that malaria is the cause. Antibody and polymerase chain reaction tests have no role in the diagnosis of malaria except that PCR is increasingly used for genotyping and speciation in mixed infections and for detection of low-level parasitemias in asymptomatic residents of endemic areas. [b]Asexual parasites/200 WBCs × 40 = parasite count/μL (assumes a WBC count of 8000/μL). See Figs. 248-6 through 248-9. [c]*P. falciparum* gametocytemia may persist for days or weeks after clearance of asexual parasites. Gametocytemia without asexual parasitemia does not indicate active infection. [d]Parasitized RBCs (%) × hematocrit × 1256 = parasite count/μL. See Figs. 248-4 and 248-5. [e]The presence of >100,000 parasites/μL (~2% parasitemia) is associated with an increased risk of severe malaria, but some patients have severe malaria with lower counts. At any level of parasitemia, the finding that >50% of parasites are tiny rings (cytoplasm thickness less than half of nucleus width) carries a relatively good prognosis. The presence of visible pigment in >20% of parasites or of phagocytosed pigment in >5% of polymorphonuclear leukocytes (indicating massive recent schizogony) carries a worse prognosis. [f]Persistence of PfHRP2 is a disadvantage in high-transmission settings, where many asymptomatic people have positive tests, but can be used to diagnostic advantage in low-transmission settings when a sick patient has previously received unknown treatment (which, in endemic areas, often consists of antimalarial drugs). A positive PfHRP2 test indicates that the illness is falciparum malaria, even if the blood smear is negative.

Abbreviations: LDH, lactate dehydrogenase; PfHRP2, *P. falciparum* histidine-rich protein 2; RBCs, red blood cells; WBCs, white blood cells.

parasites (i.e., >20% of parasites with visible pigment) in the peripheral-blood film or by the presence of phagocytosed malarial pigment in >5% of neutrophils. In *P. falciparum* infections, gametocytemia peaks 1 week after the peak of asexual parasites. Because the mature gametocytes of *P. falciparum* (unlike those of other plasmodia) are not affected by most antimalarial drugs, their persistence does not constitute evidence of drug resistance. Phagocytosed malarial pigment is sometimes seen inside peripheral-blood monocytes or polymorphonuclear leukocytes and may provide a clue to recent infection if malaria parasites are not detectable. After the clearance of the parasites, this intraphagocytic malarial pigment is often evident for several days in the peripheral blood films or for longer in bone marrow aspirates or smears of fluid expressed after intradermal puncture. Staining of parasites with the fluorescent dye acridine orange allows more rapid diagnosis of malaria (but not speciation of the infection) in patients with low-level parasitemia.

Molecular diagnosis by polymerase chain reaction (PCR) amplification of parasite nucleic acid is more sensitive than microscopy or rapid diagnostic tests for detecting malaria parasites and defining malarial species. While currently impractical in the standard clinical setting, PCR is used in reference centers in endemic areas. In epidemiologic surveys, sensitive PCR detection may prove very useful in identifying asymptomatic infections as control and eradication programs drive parasite prevalence down to very low levels. Serologic diagnosis with either indirect fluorescent antibody or enzyme-linked immunosorbent assays may prove useful as measures of transmission intensity in future epidemiologic studies. Serology has no place in the diagnosis of acute illness.

LABORATORY FINDINGS

Normochromic, normocytic anemia is usual. The leukocyte count is generally normal, although it may be raised in very severe infections. There is slight monocytosis, lymphopenia, and eosinopenia, with reactive lymphocytosis and eosinophilia in the weeks after the acute infection. The erythrocyte sedimentation rate, plasma viscosity, and levels of C-reactive protein and other acute-phase proteins are high. The platelet count is usually reduced to ~10^5/μL. Severe infections may be accompanied by prolonged prothrombin and partial thromboplastin times and by more severe thrombocytopenia. Levels of antithrombin III are reduced even in mild infection. In uncomplicated malaria, plasma concentrations of electrolytes, blood urea nitrogen (BUN), and creatinine are usually normal. Findings in severe malaria may include metabolic acidosis, with low plasma concentrations of glucose, sodium, bicarbonate, calcium, phosphate, and albumin together with elevations in lactate, BUN, creatinine, urate, muscle and liver enzymes, and conjugated and unconjugated bilirubin. Hypergammaglobulinemia is usual in immune and semi-immune subjects. Urinalysis generally gives normal results. In adults and children with cerebral malaria, the mean cerebrospinal fluid (CSF) opening pressure at lumbar puncture is ~160 mm; usually the CSF content is normal or there is a slight elevation of total protein level (<1.0 g/L [<100 mg/dL]) and cell count (<20/μL).

TREATMENT MALARIA

(Table 248-6) When a patient in or from a malarious area presents with fever, thick and thin blood smears should be prepared and *examined immediately* to confirm the diagnosis and identify the species of infecting parasite (Figs. 248-4 through 248-9). Repeat blood smears should be performed at least every 12–24 h for 2 days if the first smears are negative and malaria is strongly suspected. Alternatively, a rapid antigen detection card or stick test should be performed. Patients with severe malaria or those unable to take oral drugs should receive parenteral antimalarial therapy. If there is any doubt about the resistance status of the infecting organism, it should be considered resistant. Antimalarial drug susceptibility testing can be performed but is rarely available, has poor predictive value in an individual case, and yields results too slowly to influence the choice of treatment. Several drugs are available for oral treatment. The choice of drug depends on the likely sensitivity of

TABLE 248-6 REGIMENS FOR THE TREATMENT OF MALARIA[a]

Type of Disease or Treatment	Regimen(s)
Uncomplicated Malaria	
Known chloroquine-sensitive strains of *Plasmodium vivax, P. malariae, P. ovale, P. knowlesi, P. falciparum*[b]	Chloroquine (10 mg of base/kg stat followed by 5 mg/kg at 12, 24, and 36 h or by 10 mg/kg at 24 h and 5 mg/kg at 48 h)
	or
	Amodiaquine (10–12 mg of base/kg qd for 3 days)
Radical treatment for *P. vivax* or *P. ovale* infection	In addition to chloroquine or amodiaquine as detailed above, primaquine (0.5 mg of base/kg qd in tropical regions and 0.25 mg/kg for temperate-origin *P. vivax*) should be given for 14 days to prevent relapse. In mild G6PD deficiency, 0.75 mg of base/kg should be given once weekly for 8 weeks. Primaquine should not be given in severe G6PD deficiency.
Sensitive *P. falciparum* malaria[c]	Artesunate[d] (4 mg/kg qd for 3 days) *plus* sulfadoxine (25 mg/kg)/pyrimethamine (1.25 mg/kg) as a single dose
	or
	Artesunate[d] (4 mg/kg qd for 3 days) *plus* amodiaquine (10 mg of base/kg qd for 3 days)[e]
Multidrug-resistant *P. falciparum* malaria	Either artemether-lumefantrine[d] (1.5/9 mg/kg bid for 3 days with food)
	or
	Artesunate[d] (4 mg/kg qd for 3 days) *plus* mefloquine (24–25 mg of base/kg—either 8 mg/kg qd for 3 days or 15 mg/kg on day 2 and then 10 mg/kg on day 3)[e]
	or
	Dihydroartemisinin-piperaquine[d] (2.5/20 mg/kg qd for 3 days)
Second-line treatment/treatment of imported malaria	Either artesunate[d] (2 mg/kg qd for 7 days) or quinine (10 mg of salt/kg tid for 7 days) *plus 1 of the following 3:*
	1. Tetracycline[f] (4 mg/kg qid for 7 days)
	2. Doxycycline[f] (3 mg/kg qd for 7 days)
	3. Clindamycin (10 mg/kg bid for 7 days)
	or
	Atovaquone-proguanil (20/8 mg/kg qd for 3 days with food)
Severe Falciparum Malaria[g]	
	Artesunate[d] (2.4 mg/kg stat IV followed by 2.4 mg/kg at 12 and 24 h and then daily if necessary)[h]
	or, if unavailable,
	Artemether[d] (3.2 mg/kg stat IM followed by 1.6 mg/kg qd)
	or, if unavailable,
	Quinine dihydrochloride (20 mg of salt/kg[i] infused over 4 h, followed by 10 mg of salt/kg infused over 2–8 h q8h[j])
	or, if unavailable,
	Quinidine (10 mg of base/kg[i] infused over 1–2 h, followed by 1.2 mg of base/kg per hour[j] with electrocardiographic monitoring)

[a]In endemic areas, except in pregnant women and infants, a single dose of primaquine (0.25 mg of base/kg) should be added as a gametocytocide to all falciparum malaria treatments to prevent transmission. This addition is considered safe even in G6PD deficiency. [b]Very few areas now have chloroquine-sensitive *P. falciparum* malaria (Fig. 248-2). [c]In areas where the partner drug to artesunate is known to be effective. [d]Artemisinin derivatives are not readily available in some temperate countries. [e]Fixed-dose coformulated combinations are available. The World Health Organization now recommends artemisinin combination regimens as first-line therapy for falciparum malaria in all tropical countries and advocates use of fixed-dose combinations. [f]Tetracycline and doxycycline should not be given to pregnant women or to children <8 years of age. [g]Oral treatment should be substituted as soon as the patient recovers sufficiently to take fluids by mouth. [h]Artesunate is the drug of choice when available. The doses in children weighing <20 kg should be 3 mg/kg. The data from large studies in Southeast Asia showed a 35% lower mortality rate than with quinine, and very large studies in Africa showed a 22.5% reduction in mortality rate compared with quinine. [i]A loading dose should not be given if therapeutic doses of quinine or quinidine have definitely been administered in the previous 24 h. Some authorities recommend a lower dose of quinidine. [j]Infusions can be given in 0.9% saline and 5–10% dextrose in water. Infusion rates for quinine and quinidine should be carefully controlled.

Abbreviation: G6PD, glucose-6-phosphate dehydrogenase.

the infecting parasites. Despite increasing evidence of chloroquine resistance in *P. vivax* (from parts of Indonesia, Oceania, eastern and southern Asia, and Central and South America), chloroquine remains a first-line treatment for the non-falciparum malarias (*P. vivax*, *P. ovale*, *P. malariae*, *P. knowlesi*) except in Indonesia and Papua New Guinea, where high levels of resistance in *P. vivax* are prevalent.

The treatment of falciparum malaria has changed radically in recent years. In all endemic areas, the World Health Organization (WHO) now recommends artemisinin-based combinations (ACTs) as first-line treatment for uncomplicated falciparum malaria. These combinations are also highly effective for the other malarias. These rapidly and reliably effective drugs are sometimes unavailable in temperate countries, where treatment recommendations are limited by the registered available drugs. Fake or substandard antimalarials are commonly sold in many Asian and African countries. Thus, careful attention is required at the time of purchase and later, especially if the patient fails to respond as expected. Characteristics of antimalarial drugs are shown in **Table 248-7**.

SEVERE MALARIA

In large studies, parenteral artesunate, a water-soluble artemisinin derivative, has reduced mortality rates in severe falciparum malaria among Asian adults and children by 35% and among African children by 22.5% compared with mortality rates with quinine treatment. Artesunate has therefore become the drug of choice for all patients with severe malaria everywhere. Artesunate is given by IV injection but can also be given by IM injection. Artemether and the closely related drug artemotil (arteether) are oil-based formulations given by IM injection; they are erratically absorbed and do not confer the same survival benefit as artesunate. A rectal formulation of artesunate has been developed as a community-based pre-referral treatment for patients in the rural tropics who cannot take oral medications. Pre-referral administration of rectal artesunate has been shown to decrease mortality risk among severely ill children in communities without access to immediate parenteral treatment. Although the artemisinin compounds are safer than quinine and considerably safer than quinidine, only one formulation is available in the United States. IV artesunate has been approved by the U.S. Food and Drug Administration for emergency use against severe malaria and can be obtained through the Centers for Disease Control and Prevention (CDC) Drug Service (see end of chapter for contact information). The antiarrhythmic quinidine gluconate is as effective as quinine and, as it was more readily available, replaced quinine for the treatment of malaria in the United States. The administration of quinidine must be closely monitored if dysrhythmias and hypotension are to be avoided. If total plasma levels exceed 8 μg/mL or the QT_c interval exceeds 0.6 s or the QRS complex widens by more than 25% of baseline, then infusion rates should be slowed or infusion stopped temporarily. If arrhythmia or saline-unresponsive hypotension develops, treatment with this drug should be discontinued. Quinine is safer than quinidine; cardiovascular monitoring is not required except when the recipient has cardiac disease.

Severe falciparum malaria constitutes a medical emergency requiring intensive nursing care and careful management. The patient should be weighed and, if comatose, placed on his or her side. Frequent evaluation of the patient's condition is essential. Adjunctive treatments such as high-dose glucocorticoids, urea, heparin, dextran, desferrioxamine, antibody to tumor necrosis factor α, high-dose phenobarbital (20 mg/kg), mannitol, or large-volume fluid or albumin boluses have proved either ineffective or harmful in clinical trials and should not be used. In acute renal failure or severe metabolic acidosis, hemofiltration or hemodialysis should be started as early as possible.

In severe malaria, parenteral antimalarial treatment should be started immediately. Artesunate, given by either IV or IM injection, is the agent of choice; it is simple to administer, safe, and rapidly effective. It does not require dose adjustments in liver dysfunction or renal failure, and it should be used in pregnant women with severe malaria. If artesunate is unavailable and artemether, quinine, or quinidine is used, an initial loading dose must be given so that therapeutic concentrations are reached as soon as possible. Both quinine and quinidine will cause dangerous hypotension if injected rapidly; when given IV, they must be administered carefully by rate-controlled infusion only. If this approach is not possible, quinine may be given by deep IM injections into the anterior thigh. The optimal therapeutic range for quinine and quinidine in severe malaria is not known with certainty, but total plasma concentrations of 8–15 mg/L for quinine and 3.5–8.0 mg/L for quinidine are effective and do not cause serious toxicity. The systemic clearance and apparent volume of distribution of these alkaloids are markedly reduced and plasma protein binding is increased in severe malaria, so that the blood concentrations attained with a given dose are higher. If the patient remains seriously ill or in acute renal failure for >2 days, maintenance doses of quinine or quinidine should be reduced by 30–50% to prevent toxic accumulation of the drug. The initial doses should never be reduced. If safe and feasible, exchange transfusion may be considered for patients with severe malaria, although the precise indications for this procedure have not been agreed upon and there is no clear evidence that this measure is beneficial, particularly with artesunate treatment. Convulsions should be treated promptly with IV (or rectal) benzodiazepines. The role of prophylactic anticonvulsants in children is uncertain. If respiratory support is not available, then a full loading dose of phenobarbital (20 mg/kg) to prevent convulsions should not be given as it may cause respiratory arrest.

When the patient is unconscious, the blood glucose level should be measured every 4–6 h. All patients should receive a continuous infusion of dextrose, and blood concentrations ideally should be maintained above 4 mmol/L. Hypoglycemia (<2.2 mmol/L or 40 mg/dL) should be treated immediately with bolus glucose. The parasite count and hematocrit level should be measured every 6–12 h. Anemia develops rapidly; if the hematocrit falls to <20%, then whole blood (preferably fresh) or packed cells should be transfused slowly, with careful attention to circulatory status. Renal function should be checked daily. Children presenting with severe anemia and acidotic breathing require immediate blood transfusion. Accurate assessment is vital. Management of fluid balance is difficult in severe malaria, particularly in adults, because of the thin dividing line between overhydration (leading to pulmonary edema) and underhydration (contributing to renal impairment). As soon as the patient can take fluids, oral therapy should be substituted for parenteral treatment.

UNCOMPLICATED MALARIA

Infections due to sensitive strains of *P. vivax*, *P. knowlesi*, *P. malariae*, and *P. ovale* should be treated with oral chloroquine (total dose, 25 mg of base/kg) or with an ATC known to be efficacious. In much of the tropics, drug-resistant *P. falciparum* has been increasing in distribution, frequency, and intensity. It is now accepted that, to prevent resistance, falciparum malaria should be treated with drug combinations and not with single drugs in endemic areas; the same rationale has been applied successfully to the treatment of tuberculosis, HIV/AIDS, and cancers. This combination strategy is based on simultaneous use of two or more drugs with different modes of action. ACT regimens are now recommended as first-line treatment for falciparum malaria throughout the malaria-affected world. These regimens are safe and effective in adults, children, and after the first trimester of pregnancy (uncertainty regarding safety currently precludes their use in the first trimester). The rapidly eliminated artemisinin component is usually an artemisinin derivative (artesunate, artemether, or dihydroartemisinin) given for 3 days, and the partner drug is usually a more slowly eliminated antimalarial to which *P. falciparum* is sensitive. Five ACT regimens are currently recommended by the WHO. In areas with multidrug-resistant falciparum malaria (parts of Asia and South America, including those with mefloquine-resistant parasites; **Fig. 248-10**), artemether-lumefantrine, artesunate-mefloquine, or dihydroartemisinin-piperaquine should be used; these regimens provide cure rates of >90%. In areas with sensitive parasites, the aforementioned combinations, artesunate-sulfadoxine-pyrimethamine, or artesunate-amodiaquine also may be

TABLE 248-7 PROPERTIES OF ANTIMALARIAL DRUGS

Drug(s)	Pharmacokinetic Properties	Antimalarial Activity	Minor Toxicity	Major Toxicity
Quinine, quinidine	Good oral and IM absorption (quinine); *Cl* and V_d reduced, but plasma protein binding (principally to ∝1 acid glycoprotein) increased (90%) in malaria; quinine $t_{1/2}$: 16 h in malaria, 11 h in healthy persons; quinidine $t_{1/2}$: 13 h in malaria, 8 h in healthy persons	Acts mainly on trophozoite blood stage; kills gametocytes of *P. vivax, P. ovale,* and *P. malariae* (but not *P. falciparum*); no action on liver stages	*Common:* "Cinchonism": tinnitus, high-tone hearing loss, nausea, vomiting, dysphoria, postural hypotension; ECG QT_c interval prolongation (quinine usually by <10% but quinidine by up to 25%) *Rare:* Diarrhea, visual disturbance, rashes *Note:* Very bitter taste	*Common:* Hypoglycemia *Rare:* Hypotension, blindness, deafness, cardiac arrhythmias, thrombocytopenia, hemolysis, hemolytic-uremic syndrome, vasculitis, cholestatic hepatitis, neuromuscular paralysis *Note:* Quinidine more cardiotoxic
Chloroquine	Good oral absorption, very rapid IM and SC absorption; complex pharmacokinetics; enormous *Cl* and V_d (unaffected by malaria); blood concentration profile determined by distribution processes in malaria; $t_{1/2}$: 1–2 months	As for quinine but acts slightly earlier in asexual cycle	*Common:* Nausea, dysphoria, pruritus in dark-skinned patients, postural hypotension, slight ECG QTC prolongation *Rare:* Accommodation difficulties, keratopathy, rash *Note:* Bitter taste, well tolerated	*Acute:* Hypotensive shock (parenteral), cardiac arrhythmias, neuropsychiatric reactions *Chronic:* Retinopathy (cumulative dose, >100 g), skeletal and cardiac myopathy
Piperaquine	Adequate oral absorption, may be enhanced by fats; similar pharmacokinetics to chloroquine; $t_{1/2}$: 21–28 days	As for chloroquine, but retains activity against multidrug-resistant *P. falciparum*	Epigastric pain, diarrhea, slight ECG QT_c prolongation	None identified
Amodiaquine	Good oral absorption; largely converted to active metabolite desethylamodiaquine	As for chloroquine	Nausea (tastes better than chloroquine)	Agranulocytosis; hepatitis, mainly with prophylactic use; should not be used with efavirenz
Primaquine	Complete oral absorption; active metabolite not known; $t_{1/2}$: 5–7 h	Radical cure; eradicates hepatic forms of *P. vivax* and *P. ovale;* kills all stages of gametocyte development of *P. falciparum*	Nausea, vomiting, diarrhea, abdominal pain, hemolysis, methemoglobinemia	Massive hemolysis in subjects with severe G6PD deficiency
Mefloquine	Adequate oral absorption; no parenteral preparation; $t_{1/2}$: 14–20 days (shorter in malaria)	As for quinine	Nausea, giddiness, dysphoria, fuzzy thinking, sleeplessness, nightmares, sense of dissociation	Neuropsychiatric reactions, convulsions, encephalopathy
Halofantrine[a]	Highly variable absorption related to fat intake; $t_{1/2}$: 1–3 days (active desbutyl metabolite $t_{1/2}$: 3–7 days)	As for quinine	Diarrhea	Cardiac conduction disturbances; atrioventricular block; marked ECG QT_c interval prolongation; potentially lethal ventricular tachyarrhythmias
Lumefantrine	Highly variable absorption related to fat intake; $t_{1/2}$: 3–4 days	As for quinine	None identified	None identified
Artemisinin and derivatives (artemether, artesunate)	Good oral absorption, slow and variable absorption of IM artemether; artesunate and artemether biotransformed to active metabolite dihydroartemisinin; all drugs eliminated very rapidly; $t_{1/2}$: <1 h	Broader stage specificity and more rapid than other drugs; no action on liver stages; kills all but fully mature gametocytes of *P. falciparum*	Reduction in reticulocyte count (but not anemia); neutropenia at high doses; in some cases, delayed anemia after treatment of severe malaria with hyperparasitemia	Anaphylaxis, urticaria, fever
Pyrimethamine	Good oral absorption, variable IM absorption; $t_{1/2}$: 4 days	For blood stages, acts mainly on mature forms; causal prophylactic	Well tolerated	Megaloblastic anemia, pancytopenia, pulmonary infiltration
Proguanil (chloroguanide)	Good oral absorption; biotransformed to active metabolite cycloguanil; $t_{1/2}$: 16 h; biotransformation reduced by oral contraceptive use and in pregnancy	Causal prophylactic; not used alone for treatment	Well tolerated; mouth ulcers and rare alopecia	Megaloblastic anemia in renal failure
Atovaquone	Highly variable absorption related to fat intake; $t_{1/2}$: 30–70 h	Acts mainly on trophozoite blood stage	None identified	None identified
Tetracycline, doxycycline[b]	Excellent absorption; $t_{1/2}$: 8 h for tetracycline, 18 h for doxycycline	Weak antimalarial activity; should not be used alone for treatment	Gastrointestinal intolerance, deposition in growing bones and teeth, photosensitivity, moniliasis, benign intracranial hypertension	Renal failure in patients with impaired renal function (tetracycline)

[a]Halofantrine should not be used by patients with long ECG QT_c intervals or known conduction disturbances or by those taking drugs that may affect ventricular repolarization—e.g., quinidine, quinine, mefloquine, chloroquine, neuroleptics, antiarrhythmics, tricyclic antidepressants, and some antihistamines. [b]Tetracycline and doxycycline should not be given to pregnant women or to children <8 years of age.

Abbreviations: *Cl*, systemic clearance; ECG, electrocardiogram; G6PD, glucose-6-phosphate dehydrogenase; V_d, total apparent volume of distribution.

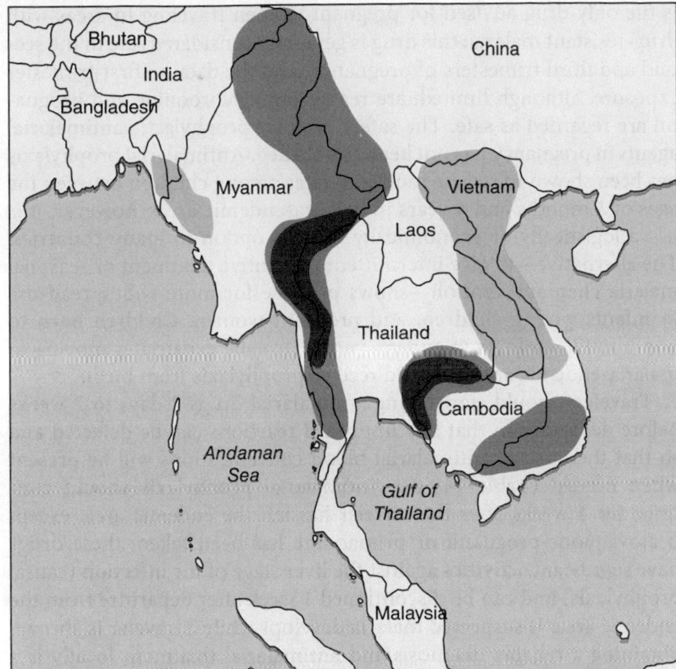

FIGURE 248-10 Mefloquine and artemisinin resistance in *Plasmodium falciparum* in Southeast Asia: high-level mefloquine resistance (*dark red*), low-level mefloquine resistance (*pink*), and mefloquine sensitivity (failure rate, <20%; *green*). There is insufficient information for other areas. Artemisinin resistance is now prevalent in areas where mefloquine resistance has been reported (*pink areas*).

used. Pyronaridine-artesunate is still under evaluation. Atovaquone-proguanil is highly effective everywhere, although it is seldom used in endemic areas because of its high cost and the propensity for rapid emergence of resistance. Of great concern is the emergence of artemisinin-resistant *P. falciparum* in western Cambodia and eastern Myanmar. Infections with these parasites are cleared slowly from the blood, with clearance times typically exceeding 3 days, and cure rates with ACTs are reduced.

The 3-day ACT regimens are all well tolerated, although mefloquine is associated with increased rates of vomiting and dizziness. As second-line treatments for recrudescence following first-line therapy, a different ACT regimen may be given; another alternative is a 7-day course of either artesunate or quinine plus tetracycline, doxycycline, or clindamycin. Tetracycline and doxycycline cannot be given to pregnant women or to children <8 years of age. Oral quinine is extremely bitter and regularly produces cinchonism comprising tinnitus, high-tone deafness, nausea, vomiting, and dysphoria. Adherence is poor with the required 7-day regimens of quinine.

Patients should be monitored for vomiting for 1 h after the administration of any oral antimalarial drug. If there is vomiting, the dose should be repeated. Symptom-based treatment, with tepid sponging and acetaminophen administration, lowers fever and thereby reduces the patient's propensity to vomit these drugs. Minor central nervous system reactions (nausea, dizziness, sleep disturbances) are common. The incidence of serious adverse neuropsychiatric reactions to mefloquine treatment is ~1 in 1000 in Asia but may be as high as 1 in 200 among Africans and Caucasians. All the antimalarial quinolines (chloroquine, mefloquine, and quinine) exacerbate the orthostatic hypotension associated with malaria, and all are tolerated better by children than by adults. Pregnant women, young children, patients unable to tolerate oral therapy, and nonimmune individuals (e.g., travelers) with suspected malaria should be evaluated carefully and hospitalization considered. If there is any doubt as to the identity of the infecting malarial species, treatment for falciparum malaria should be given. A negative blood smear makes malaria unlikely but does not rule it out completely; thick blood films should be checked again 1 and 2 days later to exclude the diagnosis. Nonimmune patients receiving treatment for malaria should have daily parasite counts performed until the thick films are negative. If the level of parasitemia does not fall below 25% of the admission value in 48 h or if parasitemia has not cleared by 7 days (and adherence is assured), drug resistance is likely and the regimen should be changed.

To eradicate persistent liver stages and prevent relapse (radical treatment), primaquine (0.5 mg of base/kg or, in infections acquired in temperate areas, 0.25 mg/kg) should be given daily for 14 days to patients with *P. vivax* or *P. ovale* infections after laboratory tests for G6PD deficiency have proved negative. If the patient has a mild variant of G6PD deficiency, primaquine can be given in a dose of 0.75 mg of base/kg (45 mg maximum) once weekly for 8 weeks. Pregnant women with vivax or ovale malaria should not be given primaquine but should receive suppressive prophylaxis with chloroquine (5 mg of base/kg per week) until delivery, after which radical treatment can be given.

COMPLICATIONS

Acute Renal Failure If the plasma level of BUN or creatinine rises despite adequate rehydration, fluid administration should be restricted to prevent volume overload. As in other forms of hypercatabolic acute renal failure, renal replacement therapy is best performed early (Chap. 334). Hemofiltration and hemodialysis are more effective than peritoneal dialysis and are associated with lower mortality risk. Some patients with renal impairment pass small volumes of urine sufficient to allow control of fluid balance; these cases can be managed conservatively if other indications for dialysis do not arise. Renal function usually improves within days, but full recovery may take weeks.

Acute Pulmonary Edema (Acute Respiratory Distress Syndrome) Patients should be positioned with the head of the bed at a 45° elevation and given oxygen and IV diuretics. Pulmonary artery occlusion pressures may be normal, indicating increased pulmonary capillary permeability. Positive-pressure ventilation should be started early if the immediate measures fail (Chap. 326).

Hypoglycemia An initial slow injection of 50% dextrose (0.5 g/kg) should be followed by an infusion of 10% dextrose (0.10 g/kg per hour). The blood glucose level should be checked regularly thereafter as recurrent hypoglycemia is common, particularly among patients receiving quinine or quinidine. In severely ill patients, hypoglycemia commonly occurs together with metabolic (lactic) acidosis and carries a poor prognosis.

Other Complications Patients who develop spontaneous bleeding should be given fresh blood and IV vitamin K. Convulsions should be treated with IV or rectal benzodiazepines and, if necessary, respiratory support. Aspiration pneumonia should be suspected in any unconscious patient with convulsions, particularly with persistent hyperventilation; IV antimicrobial agents and oxygen should be administered, and pulmonary toilet should be undertaken. Hypoglycemia or gram-negative septicemia should be suspected when the condition of any patient suddenly deteriorates for no obvious reason during antimalarial treatment. In malaria-endemic areas where a high proportion of children are parasitemic, it is usually impossible to distinguish severe malaria from bacterial sepsis with confidence. These children should be treated with both antimalarials and broad-spectrum antibiotics from the outset. Because nontyphoidal *Salmonella* infections are particularly common, empirical antibiotics should be selected to cover these organisms. Antibiotics should be considered for severely ill patients of any age who are not responding to antimalarial treatment.

PREVENTION

In recent years, considerable progress has been made in malaria prevention, control, and research. Distribution of insecticide-treated bed-nets (ITNs) has been shown to reduce all-cause mortality in African children by 20%. New drugs have been discovered and developed, and one vaccine candidate (the RTS,S vaccine) will soon be considered for registration. Highly effective drugs, long-lasting ITNs, and insecticides for spraying dwellings are being purchased for endemic countries by the Global Fund to Fight AIDS, Tuberculosis, and Malaria; the President's Malaria Initiative (funded by the U.S. Agency for International Development and managed by the CDC in partnership with endemic countries); UNICEF; and other organizations. Malaria research and control are being strongly supported by the National Institute of Allergy and Infectious Diseases, the CDC, the Wellcome Trust, the Bill & Melinda Gates Foundation, the Multilateral Initiative on Malaria, the Roll Back Malaria Partnership, and the WHO among others. While a laudable goal, the global eradication of malaria is not feasible in the immediate future because of the widespread distribution of *Anopheles* breeding sites; the great number of infected persons; the continued use of ineffective antimalarial drugs; and inadequacies in human and material resources, infrastructure, and control programs. The call for and commitment to ultimate eradication of malaria by the Gates Foundation in 2007—seconded by Margaret Chan, Director General of the WHO—added great impetus to all malaria initiatives, especially those aimed at discovery and implementation of new interventions. Malaria may be contained by judicious use of insecticides to kill the mosquito vector, rapid diagnosis, patient management, and—where effective and feasible—administration of intermittent preventive treatment, seasonal malaria chemoprevention, or chemoprophylaxis to high-risk groups such as pregnant women, young children, and travelers from nonendemic regions. Malaria researchers are intensifying their efforts to gain a better understanding of parasite-human-mosquito interactions and to develop more effective control and prevention interventions. Despite the enormous investment in efforts to develop a malaria vaccine and the 30–60% efficacy in African children of a recombinant protein sporozoite-targeted adjuvanted vaccine (RTS,S) in field trials, no safe, highly effective, long-lasting vaccine is likely to be available for general use in the near future (Chap. 148). Indeed, protection from RTS,S in the very youngest recipients dropped to 16% only 4 years after vaccination. While there is great promise for one or several malaria vaccines on the more distant horizon, prevention and control measures continue to rely on antivector and drug-use strategies. Furthermore, recent gains are threatened by increasing insecticide resistance and behavioral changes (to avoid ITN contact) in anopheline mosquito vectors and by spreading artemisinin resistance in *P. falciparum*.

PERSONAL PROTECTION AGAINST MALARIA

Simple measures to reduce the frequency of infected-mosquito bites in malarious areas are very important. These measures include the avoidance of exposure to mosquitoes at their peak feeding times (usually dusk to dawn) and the use of insect repellents containing 10–35% DEET (or, if DEET is unacceptable, 7% picaridin), suitable clothing, and ITNs or other insecticide-impregnated materials. Widespread use of bed nets treated with residual pyrethroids reduces the incidence of malaria in areas where vectors bite indoors at night.

CHEMOPROPHYLAXIS

(Table 248-8; *wwwnc.cdc.gov/travel/yellowbook/2014/chapter-3-infectious-diseases-related-to-travel/malaria*) Recommendations for prophylaxis depend on knowledge of local patterns of *Plasmodium* species drug sensitivity and the likelihood of acquiring malarial infection. When there is uncertainty, drugs effective against resistant *P. falciparum* should be used (atovaquone-proguanil [Malarone], doxycycline, or mefloquine). Chemoprophylaxis is never entirely reliable, and malaria should always be considered in the differential diagnosis of fever in patients who have traveled to endemic areas, even if they are taking prophylactic antimalarial drugs.

Pregnant women traveling to malarious areas should be warned about the potential risks. All pregnant women at risk in endemic areas should be encouraged to attend regular antenatal clinics. Mefloquine is the only drug advised for pregnant women traveling to areas with drug-resistant malaria; this drug is generally considered safe in the second and third trimesters of pregnancy, and the data on first-trimester exposure, although limited, are reassuring. Chloroquine and proguanil are regarded as safe. The safety of other prophylactic antimalarial agents in pregnancy has not been established. Antimalarial prophylaxis has been shown to reduce mortality rates among children between the ages of 3 months and 4 years in malaria-endemic areas; however, it is not a logistically or economically feasible option in many countries. The alternative—to give intermittent preventive treatment or seasonal malaria chemoprevention—shows promise for more widespread use in infants, young children, and pregnant women. Children born to nonimmune mothers in endemic areas (usually expatriates moving to malaria-endemic areas) should receive prophylaxis from birth.

Travelers should start taking antimalarial drugs 2 days to 2 weeks before departure so that any untoward reactions can be detected and so that therapeutic antimalarial blood concentrations will be present when needed (Table 248-8). Antimalarial prophylaxis should continue for 4 weeks after the traveler has left the endemic area, except if atovaquone-proguanil or primaquine has been taken; these drugs have significant activities against the liver stage of the infection (causal prophylaxis) and can be discontinued 1 week after departure from the endemic area. If suspected malaria develops while a traveler is abroad, obtaining a reliable diagnosis and antimalarial treatment locally is a top priority. Presumptive self-treatment for malaria with atovaquone-proguanil (for 3 consecutive days) or another drug can be considered under special circumstances; medical advice on self-treatment should be sought before departure for malarious areas and as soon as possible after illness begins. Every effort should be made to confirm the diagnosis by parasitologic studies.

Atovaquone-proguanil (Malarone; 3.75/1.5 mg/kg or 250/100 mg, daily adult dose) is a fixed-combination, once-daily prophylactic agent that is very well tolerated by adults and children, with fewer adverse gastrointestinal effects than chloroquine-proguanil and fewer adverse central nervous system effects than mefloquine. It is proguanil itself, rather than the antifolate metabolite cycloguanil, that acts synergistically with atovaquone. This combination is effective against all types of malaria, including multidrug-resistant falciparum malaria. Atovaquone-proguanil is best taken with food or a milky drink to optimize absorption. There are insufficient data on the safety of this regimen in pregnancy.

Mefloquine (250 mg of salt weekly, adult dose) has been widely used for malarial prophylaxis because it is usually effective against multidrug-resistant falciparum malaria and is reasonably well tolerated. The drug has been associated with rare episodes of psychosis and seizures at prophylactic doses; these reactions are more frequent at the higher doses used for treatment. More common side effects with prophylactic doses of mefloquine include mild nausea, dizziness, fuzzy thinking, disturbed sleep patterns, vivid dreams, and malaise. The drug is contraindicated for use by travelers with known hypersensitivity to mefloquine or related compounds (e.g., quinine, quinidine) and by persons with active or recent depression, anxiety disorder, psychosis, schizophrenia, another major psychiatric disorder, or seizures; mefloquine is not recommended for persons with cardiac conduction abnormalities although the evidence that it is cardiotoxic is very weak. Confidence is increasing with regard to the safety of mefloquine prophylaxis during pregnancy; in studies in Africa, mefloquine prophylaxis was found to be effective and safe during pregnancy. However, in one study from Thailand, treatment of malaria with mefloquine was associated with an increased risk of stillbirth; this effect was not seen subsequently.

Daily administration of doxycycline (100 mg daily, adult dose) is an effective alternative to atovaquone-proguanil or mefloquine. Doxycycline is generally well tolerated but may cause vulvovaginal thrush, diarrhea, and photosensitivity and cannot be used by children <8 years old or by pregnant women.

Chloroquine can no longer be relied upon to prevent *P. falciparum* infections in most areas but is used to prevent and treat malaria due to the other human *Plasmodium* species and for *P. falciparum* malaria in Central American countries west and north of the Panama

TABLE 248-8 DRUGS USED IN THE PROPHYLAXIS OF MALARIA

Drug	Usage	Adult Dose	Pediatric Dose	Comments
Atovaquone-proguanil (Malarone)	Prophylaxis in areas with chloroquine- or mefloquine-resistant *Plasmodium falciparum*	1 adult tablet PO[a]	5–8 kg: ½ pediatric tablet[b] daily ≥8–10 kg: ¾ pediatric tablet daily ≥10–20 kg: 1 pediatric tablet daily ≥20–30 kg: 2 pediatric tablets daily ≥30–40 kg: 3 pediatric tablets daily ≥40 kg: 1 adult tablet daily	Begin 1–2 days before travel to malarious areas. Take daily at the same time each day while in the malarious areas and for 7 days after leaving such areas. Atovaquone-proguanil is contraindicated in persons with severe renal impairment (creatinine clearance rate <30 mL/min). In the absence of data, it is not recommended for children weighing <5 kg, pregnant women, or women breast-feeding infants weighing <5 kg. Atovaquone-proguanil should be taken with food or a milky drink.
Chloroquine phosphate (Aralen and generic)	Prophylaxis only in areas with chloroquine-sensitive *P. falciparum*[c] or areas with *P. vivax* only	300 mg of base (500 mg of salt) PO once weekly	5 mg/kg of base (8.3 mg of salt/kg) PO once weekly, up to maximum adult dose of 300 mg of base	Begin 1–2 weeks before travel to malarious areas. Take weekly on the same day of the week while in the malarious areas and for 4 weeks after leaving such areas. Chloroquine phosphate may exacerbate psoriasis.
Doxycycline (many brand names and generic)	Prophylaxis in areas with chloroquine- or mefloquine-resistant *P. falciparum*	100 mg PO qd (except in pregnant women; see Comments)	≥8 years of age: 2 mg/kg, up to adult dose	Begin 1–2 days before travel to malarious areas. Take daily at the same time each day while in the malarious areas and for 4 weeks after leaving such areas. Doxycycline is contraindicated in children <8 years of age and in pregnant women.
Hydroxychloroquine sulfate (Plaquenil)	An alternative to chloroquine for primary prophylaxis only in areas with chloroquine-sensitive *P. falciparum*[c] or areas with *P. vivax* only	310 mg of base (400 mg of salt) PO once weekly	5 mg of base/kg (6.5 mg of salt/kg) PO once weekly, up to maximum adult dose of 310 mg of base	Begin 1–2 weeks before travel to malarious areas. Take weekly on the same day of the week while in the malarious areas and for 4 weeks after leaving such areas. Hydroxychloroquine may exacerbate psoriasis.
Mefloquine (Lariam and generic)	Prophylaxis in areas with chloroquine-resistant *P. falciparum*[c]	228 mg of base (250 mg of salt) PO once weekly	≤9 kg: 4.6 mg of base/kg (5 mg of salt/kg) PO once weekly 10–19 kg: ¼ tablet once weekly 20–30 kg: ½ tablet once weekly 31–45 kg: ¾ tablet once weekly ≥46 kg: 1 tablet once weekly	Begin 1–2 weeks before travel to malarious areas. Take weekly on the same day of the week while in the malarious areas and for 4 weeks after leaving such areas. Mefloquine is contraindicated in persons allergic to this drug or related compounds (e.g., quinine and quinidine) and in persons with active or recent depression, generalized anxiety disorder, psychosis, schizophrenia, other major psychiatric disorders, or seizures. Use with caution in persons with psychiatric disturbances or a history of depression. Mefloquine is not recommended for persons with cardiac conduction abnormalities.
Primaquine	For prevention of malaria in areas with mainly *P. vivax*	30 mg of base (52.6 mg of salt) PO qd	0.5 mg of base/kg (0.8 mg of salt/kg) PO qd, up to adult dose; should be taken with food	Begin 1–2 days before travel to malarious areas. Take daily at the same time each day while in the malarious areas and for 7 days after leaving such areas. Primaquine is contraindicated in persons with G6PD deficiency. It is also contraindicated during pregnancy and in lactation unless the infant being breast-fed has a documented normal G6PD level.
Primaquine	Used for presumptive antirelapse therapy (terminal prophylaxis) to decrease risk of relapses of *P. vivax* and *P. ovale*	30 mg of base (52.6 mg of salt) PO qd for 14 days after departure from the malarious area	0.5 mg of base/kg (0.8 mg of salt/kg), up to adult dose, PO qd for 14 days after departure from the malarious area	This therapy is indicated for persons who have had prolonged exposure to *P. vivax* and/or *P. ovale*. It is contraindicated in persons with G6PD deficiency as well as during pregnancy and in lactation unless the infant being breast-fed has a documented normal G6PD level.

[a]An adult tablet contains 250 mg of atovaquone and 100 mg of proguanil hydrochloride. [b]A pediatric tablet contains 62.5 mg of atovaquone and 25 mg of proguanil hydrochloride. [c]Very few areas now have chloroquine-sensitive malaria (Fig. 248-2).

Source: CDC: *www.cdc.gov/malaria/travelers/drugs.html.*

Canal, Caribbean countries, and some countries in the Middle East. Chloroquine-resistant *P. vivax* has been reported from parts of eastern Asia, Oceania, and Central and South America. This drug is generally well tolerated, although some patients cannot take it because of malaise, headache, visual symptoms (due to reversible keratopathy), gastrointestinal intolerance, or pruritus. Chloroquine is considered safe in pregnancy. With chronic administration for >5 years, a characteristic dose-related retinopathy may develop, but this condition is rare at the doses used for antimalarial prophylaxis. Idiosyncratic or allergic reactions are also rare. Skeletal and/or cardiac myopathy is a potential problem with protracted prophylactic use; such myopathy is more likely to occur at the high doses used in the treatment of rheumatoid arthritis. Neuropsychiatric reactions and skin rashes are unusual. When used continuously, amodiaquine, a related aminoquinoline, is associated with a high risk of agranulocytosis (~1 person in 2000) and hepatotoxicity (~1 person in 16,000); thus this agent should not be used for prophylaxis.

Primaquine (daily adult dose, 0.5 mg of base/kg or 30 mg taken with food), an 8-aminoquinoline compound, has proved safe and effective in the prevention of drug-resistant falciparum and vivax malaria in adults. This drug can be considered for persons who are traveling to areas with or without drug-resistant *P. falciparum* and who are intolerant to other recommended drugs. Abdominal pain and oxidant hemolysis—the principal adverse effects—are not common as long as the drug is taken with food and is not given to G6PD-deficient persons, in whom it can cause serious hemolysis. Travelers must be tested for G6PD deficiency and be shown to have a level in the normal range before receiving primaquine. Primaquine should not be given to pregnant women or neonates. Primaquine, given in a single dose of 0.25 mg/kg as a gametocytocide, together with an ACT is recommended in falciparum malaria treatment regimens in malaria elimination programs.

In the past, the dihydrofolate reductase inhibitors pyrimethamine and proguanil (chloroguanide) were administered widely, but the rapid selection of resistance in both *P. falciparum* and *P. vivax* has limited their use. Whereas antimalarial quinolines such as chloroquine (a 4-aminoquinoline) act on the erythrocyte stage of parasitic development, the dihydrofolate reductase inhibitors also inhibit preerythrocytic growth in the liver (causal prophylaxis) and development in the mosquito (sporontocidal activity). Proguanil is safe and well tolerated, although mouth ulceration occurs in ~8% of persons using this drug; it is considered safe for antimalarial prophylaxis in pregnancy. The prophylactic use of the combination of pyrimethamine and sulfadoxine is not recommended because of an unacceptable incidence of severe toxicity, principally exfoliative dermatitis and other skin rashes, agranulocytosis, hepatitis, and pulmonary eosinophilia (incidence, 1:7000; fatal reactions, 1:18,000). The combination of pyrimethamine with dapsone (0.2/1.5 mg/kg weekly; 12.5/100 mg, adult dose) has been used in some countries. Dapsone may cause methemoglobinemia and allergic reactions and (at higher doses) may pose a significant risk of agranulocytosis. Proguanil and the pyrimethamine-dapsone combination are not available in the United States.

Because of the increasing spread and intensity of antimalarial drug resistance (Figs. 248-2 and 248-10), the CDC recommends that travelers and their providers consider their destination, type of travel, and current medications and health risks when choosing antimalarial chemoprophylaxis. There is an increasingly appreciated problem of counterfeit and substandard antimalarial drugs (and other medicines) on the shelves of pharmacies in Southeast Asia and sub-Saharan Africa; hence, travelers should purchase their preventive drugs from a reputable source before going to a malarious country. Consultation for the evaluation of prophylaxis failures or treatment of malaria can be obtained from state and local health departments and the CDC Malaria Hotline (770-488-7788) or the CDC Emergency Operations Center (770-488-7100).

249 Babesiosis

Edouard G. Vannier, Peter J. Krause

Babesiosis is an emerging tick-borne infectious disease caused by protozoan parasites of the genus *Babesia* that invade and eventually lyse red blood cells (RBCs). Most cases are due to *Babesia microti* and occur in the United States, particularly in the Northeast and upper Midwest. The infection typically is mild in young and otherwise healthy individuals but can be severe and sometimes fatal in persons >50 years of age and in immunocompromised patients. Sporadic cases have been reported in Europe and the rest of the world.

ETIOLOGY AND EPIDEMIOLOGY

Geographic Distribution More than 100 *Babesia* species are found in wild and domestic animals; a few of these species cause infection in humans (Fig. 249-1). *B. microti*, a parasite of small rodents, is the most common etiologic agent of human babesiosis and is endemic in the northeastern and upper midwestern United States. Seven states in these two regions (Connecticut, Massachusetts, Minnesota, New Jersey, New York, Rhode Island, and Wisconsin) account for >95% of the reported cases. Other etiologic agents include *Babesia duncani* and *B. duncani*–type organisms on the West Coast and *Babesia divergens*–like organisms in Kentucky, Missouri, and Washington State.

The primary causative agent of human babesiosis in Europe is *B. divergens*, but *Babesia venatorum* and *B. microti* also have been reported. In Asia, cases due to *B. microti*–like organisms have been documented in Japan, Taiwan, and the People's Republic of China. A case caused by *B. venatorum* also has been reported from the People's Republic of China. A case of *B. microti* infection was described in Australia. Sporadic cases due to uncharacterized species have been reported in Colombia, Egypt, India, Mozambique, and South Africa.

Incidence More than 1100 cases were reported in the United States in 2011, the year the disease became nationally notifiable. This figure represents a fivefold increase in incidence over the past decade. The incidence of babesiosis is markedly underestimated because symptoms are nonspecific and because young healthy individuals typically experience a mild or asymptomatic infection and may not seek medical attention. Fewer than 50 cases of *B. divergens*, *B. divergens*–like, and *B. venatorum* infections have been reported. Babesiosis caused by *B. duncani* and *B. duncani*–type organisms has also been sporadic, with fewer than 10 reported cases.

Modes of Transmission In the United States, *B. microti* is transmitted to humans primarily by the nymphal stage of the deer tick (*Ixodes scapularis*), the same tick that transmits the causative agents of Lyme disease (Chap. 210) and human granulocytotropic anaplasmosis (Chap. 211). Transmission generally occurs from May through October, with three-fourths of cases presenting in July and August. The vectors for transmission of *B. duncani* and *B. divergens*–like organisms are thought to be *Ixodes pacificus* and *Ixodes dentatus*, respectively. In Europe, *Ixodes ricinus* is the vector for *B. divergens* and *B. venatorum*. In Japan, *B. microti*–like organisms have been found in *Ixodes ovatus* ticks.

Babesiosis occasionally is acquired through transfusion of blood or blood products. *B. microti* is the most common transfusion-transmitted pathogen reported to the U.S. Food and Drug Administration, and more than 170 such cases have been identified. Three transfusion-transmitted cases caused by *B. duncani* have been documented. Transfusion-transmitted cases occur year-round, although most cases occur from June through November. More than 80% of cases occur in endemic areas. Transfusion-transmitted babesiosis occurs in nonendemic areas when unrecognized *Babesia*-contaminated blood products are imported from endemic areas: asymptomatically infected residents of endemic areas donate blood in nonendemic areas, or residents of nonendemic areas travel to endemic areas, become infected, and donate blood after they return home. Approximately three-quarters of the transfusion-transmitted babesiosis cases reported between 1979 and 2009 occurred in the last decade of this period, and about one-fifth of patients died.

Seven cases of probable or confirmed congenital *B. microti* infection have been described. Other cases of neonatal babesiosis have been acquired by transfusion or tick bite.

CLINICAL MANIFESTATIONS

Asymptomatic *B. microti* Infection At least 20% of adults and 40% of children do not experience symptoms following *B. microti* infection. Asymptomatic infection, whether treated or not, may persist for >1 year after acute babesial illness. There is no evidence of long-term complications following asymptomatic infection; however, people who are asymptomatically infected may transmit the infection when they donate blood.

Mild to Moderate *B. microti* Illness Symptoms typically develop following an incubation period of 1–4 weeks after tick bite and 1–9 weeks (but as long as 6 months) after transfusion of blood products. Patients experience a gradual onset of malaise, fatigue, and weakness. Fever

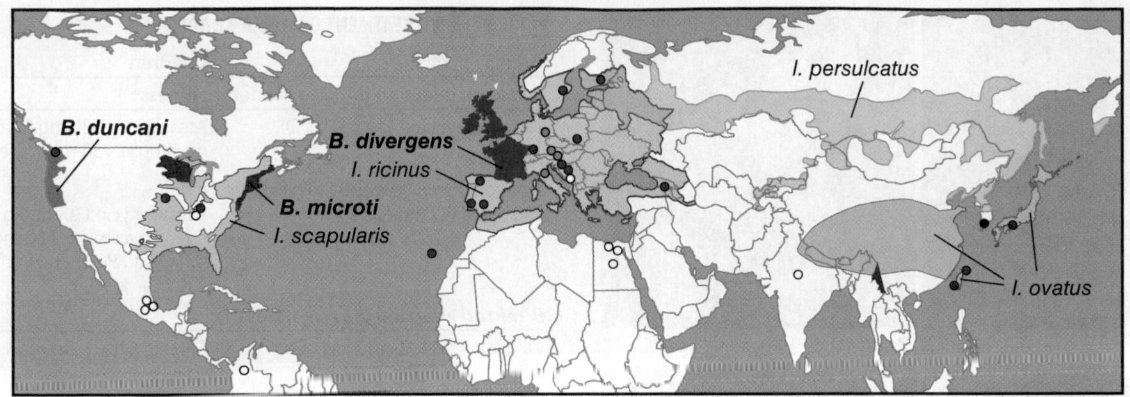

FIGURE 249-1 Worldwide distribution of human babesiosis. *Dark colors* designate areas where human babesiosis is either endemic or sporadic (as defined by more than three tick-borne cases reported in a country or state). Isolated cases of babesiosis are denoted by *circles*. Colors designate causative *Babesia* species: *Babesia microti* and *B. microti*–like organisms in *red*, *Babesia duncani* and *B. duncani*–type organisms in *orange*, *Babesia divergens* and *B. divergens*–like organisms in *blue*, *Babesia venatorum* in *purple*, KO1 in *black*, and unspeciated *Babesia* organisms in *white*. Due to space constraints, the 10 cases reported from Montenegro are denoted by a single *white circle*, and those from Australia, Mozambique, and South Africa are not shown. *Light colors* denote areas that are enzootic for *Ixodes* tick species known to transmit one or several *Babesia* species but where human babesiosis has yet to be documented. *(Adapted from E Vannier, PJ Krause: N Engl J Med 366:2397, 2012.)*

can reach 40.9°C (105.6°F) and is accompanied by one or more of the following: chills, sweats, headache, myalgia, arthralgia, nausea, anorexia, and dry cough. Less common symptoms include sore throat, photophobia, abdominal pain, vomiting, weight loss, shortness of breath, and depression. On physical examination, fever is the salient feature. Ecchymoses and petechiae have been reported. An erythema migrans rash signifies concurrent Lyme disease (Chap. 210). Splenomegaly and hepatomegaly occasionally are noted. Lymphadenopathy is absent. Jaundice, slight pharyngeal erythema, and retinopathy with splinter hemorrhages and retinal infarcts rarely occur. Symptoms typically last 1–2 weeks, but fatigue may persist for several months.

Severe *B. microti* Illness Severe babesiosis requires hospital admission and typically occurs in patients with one or more of the following: age of >50 years, neonatal prematurity, male gender, asplenia, HIV/AIDS, malignancy, hemoglobinopathy, and immunosuppressive therapy. More than one-third of hospitalized patients develop complications, including acute respiratory distress syndrome, disseminated intravascular coagulation, congestive heart failure, renal failure, splenic infarcts, and splenic rupture. Patients who develop complications tend to have severe anemia (hemoglobin, ≤10 g/L). Laboratory prognostic factors for severe outcome—defined by hospitalization for >14 days, an intensive care unit stay of >2 days, or death—include an elevated alkaline phosphatase level (>125 U/L) and parasitemia of >4%. The fatality rate is 5–9% among hospitalized patients but is ~20% among immunocompromised patients and patients with transfusion-transmitted babesiosis.

Other *Babesia* Infections Cases of *B. duncani* infection range in severity from asymptomatic to fatal. Clinical manifestations are similar to those reported for *B. microti* infection. All three patients infected with *B. divergens*–like organisms in the United States required hospitalization; one died. Most cases of *B. divergens* infection in Europe have occurred in people lacking a spleen. The incubation period is 1–3 weeks. Symptoms appear suddenly and consist of fever (>41°C or 105.8°F), shaking chills, drenching sweats, headache, myalgia, and lumbar and abdominal pain. Hemoglobinuria and jaundice are commonly noted, and mild hepatomegaly may occur. If the infection is not treated, patients often develop pulmonary edema and renal failure. All four patients infected with *B. venatorum* in Europe had been splenectomized; their illness ranged from mild to severe, and none died. A child in China who developed *B. venatorum* illness had an intact spleen and survived the infection.

PATHOGENESIS

Anemia is a key feature of the pathogenesis of babesiosis. Hemolytic anemia caused by rupture of infected RBCs generates cell debris that may accumulate in the kidney and cause renal failure. Anemia also results from the clearance of intact RBCs as they pass through the splenic red pulp and encounter resident macrophages. *Babesia* antigens expressed at the RBC membrane promote opsonization and facilitate uptake by splenic macrophages. In addition, RBCs are poorly deformable as a result of oxidation generated by the parasite and the host immune response and are filtered out as they attempt to squeeze across the venous vasculature. Bone marrow suppression due to cytokine production may also contribute to anemia.

An appropriate immune response is necessary for the control and clearance of *Babesia*. However, several lines of evidence suggest that an excessive response contributes to pathogenesis. Studies using laboratory mice have clearly established that CD4+ T cells are critical for resistance to and resolution of *B. microti* infection. CD4+ T cells are a major source of interferon γ (IFN-γ), and lack of this cytokine causes resistant mice to become highly susceptible to *B. microti*. IFN-γ is central to host resistance in *B. duncani* infection, but natural killer cells are its main source. *B. duncani* infection is more severe than *B. microti* infection in rodents and is characterized by pulmonary inflammation. Tumor necrosis factor α is expressed around alveolar septa, whereas IFN-γ is detected around pulmonary vessels. Blockade of either cytokine promotes the survival of mice infected with *B. duncani*.

DIAGNOSIS

A diagnosis of babesiosis should be considered for any patient who lives or travels in a *Babesia*-endemic area and presents with a febrile illness in the late spring, summer, or early autumn or within 6 months after a blood transfusion. Co-infection with *Babesia* should be considered in cases of Lyme disease or human granulocytotropic anaplasmosis when symptoms are more severe or prolonged than usual.

Screening laboratory tests can help support the diagnosis of babesiosis. A complete blood count often shows anemia and thrombocytopenia. Low hematocrit, hemoglobin, and haptoglobin levels and elevated reticulocyte counts and lactate dehydrogenase levels are consistent with hemolytic anemia. Liver enzyme tests often reveal elevated levels of alkaline phosphatase, aspartate and alanine aminotransferases, and bilirubin. Urinalysis may show hemoglobinuria, excess urobilinogen, and proteinuria. Elevated levels of blood urea nitrogen and serum creatinine indicate renal compromise.

A specific diagnosis usually is established by microscopic examination of Giemsa-stained thin blood smears (Fig. 249-2). *Babesia* trophozoites appear round, pear-shaped, or ameboid. The ring form is most common and lacks the central brownish deposit (hemozoin) typical of *Plasmodium falciparum* trophozoites (see Fig. 250e-1C). Other distinguishing features are the absence of schizonts and gametocytes and the occasional presence of tetrads ("Maltese cross").

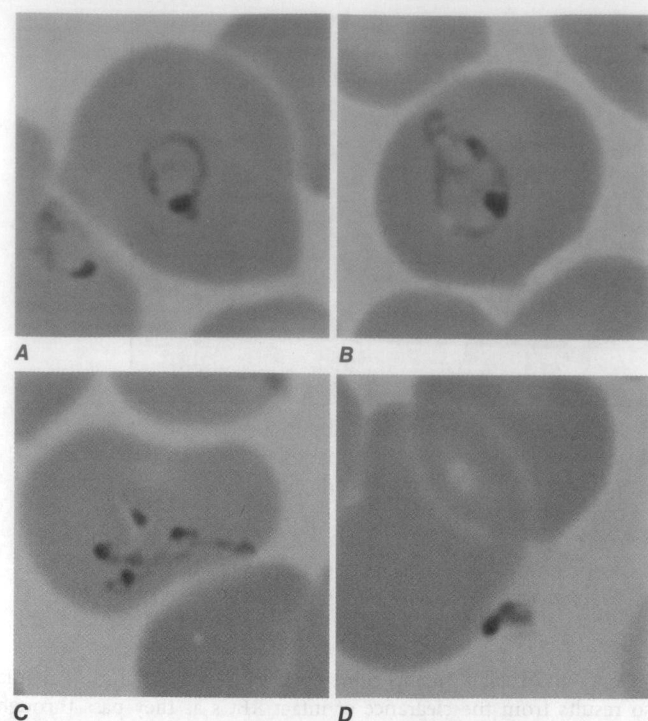

FIGURE 249-2 Giemsa-stained thin blood films showing *Babesia microti* parasites. *B. microti* are obligate parasites of erythrocytes. Trophozoites may appear as ring forms (***A***) or as ameboid forms (***B***). Merozoites can be arranged in tetrads and are pathognomonic (***C***). Extracellular parasites can be noted, particularly when parasitemia is high (***D***). *(Adapted from E Vannier, PJ Krause: N Engl J Med 366:2397, 2012.)*

Tetrads are characteristic of *B. microti*, *B. duncani*, and *B. divergens*–like organisms in human erythrocytes. Because the number of parasitized RBCs may be low, particularly at the onset of symptoms, identification of the parasite may require multiple blood smears over several days. Parasitemia levels can range from 1% to 20% in immunocompetent hosts and can be as high as 85% in immunocompromised patients. If parasites cannot be identified by microscopy and the disease is still suspected, amplification of the babesial 18S rRNA gene by polymerase chain reaction (PCR) is recommended. Quantitative PCR has greatly lowered the threshold for detection of *B. microti* DNA.

Serology can suggest or confirm the diagnosis of babesiosis. An indirect immunofluorescent antibody test for *B. microti* is most commonly used. IgM titers of ≥1:64 and IgG titers of ≥1:1024 suggest active or recent infection. Titers typically decline over 6–12 months. Antibodies to *B. microti* do not cross-react with *B. duncani* or *B. divergens* antigen. In *B. divergens* infection, serology is of limited use because symptoms often appear before antibodies can be detected. Sera from patients infected with *B. divergens*–like organisms or *B. venatorum* are reactive against *B. divergens* antigen.

TREATMENT BABESIOSIS

ASYMPTOMATIC *B. MICROTI* INFECTION

People who experience asymptomatic *B. microti* infection often are not diagnosed and treated. Current guidelines recommend antibiotic therapy for asymptomatic carriers only if parasitemia persists for >3 months. Laboratory-based tests are being developed for the purpose of screening the blood supply and will result in the identification of a greater number of asymptomatic *B. microti* carriers, raising the question of whether they should be treated.

MILD TO MODERATE *B. MICROTI* ILLNESS

Atovaquone plus azithromycin, given orally for 7–10 days, is the recommended antibiotic treatment combination for mild to moderate babesiosis (**Table 249-1**). Clindamycin plus quinine is a second choice. Symptoms usually begin to resolve within 48 h of therapy initiation, but complete resolution may take weeks to months. An atypical or poor response to therapy should raise concern about the possibility of concurrent Lyme disease (**Chap. 210**) or human granulocytotropic anaplasmosis (**Chap. 211**). In the first prospective trial of antibabesial therapy, the combination of atovaquone plus azithromycin was compared with clindamycin plus quinine in adults. These two drug combinations were equally effective in resolving symptoms and clearing parasitemia. Adverse effects were reported in 15% of trial participants who received atovaquone plus azithromycin but in 72% of those who received clindamycin plus quinine. Adverse reactions were so severe that treatment had to be stopped in about one-third of participants taking clindamycin plus quinine but in only 2% of those taking atovaquone plus azithromycin.

TABLE 249-1 TREATMENT OF HUMAN BABESIOSIS

Adults	Children
***B. microti* Infection (Mild to Moderate Illness[a,b])**	
Atovaquone (750 mg q12h PO) ***plus*** Azithromycin (500 mg/d PO on day 1, 250 mg/d PO thereafter)	Atovaquone (20 mg/kg q12h PO; maximum, 750 mg/dose) ***plus*** Azithromycin (10 mg/kg qd PO on day 1 [maximum, 500 mg/dose], 5 mg/kg qd PO thereafter [maximum, 250 mg/dose])
***B. microti* Infection (Severe Illness[c,d])**	
Clindamycin (300–600 mg q6h IV or 600 mg q8h PO) ***plus*** Quinine (650 mg q6–8h PO) ***plus*** Consider exchange transfusion	Clindamycin (7–10 mg/kg q6–8h IV or 7–10 mg/kg q6–8h PO; maximum, 600 mg/dose) ***plus*** Quinine (8 mg/kg q8h PO; maximum, 650 mg/dose) ***plus*** Consider exchange transfusion
***B. divergens* Infection**	
Immediate complete exchange transfusion ***plus*** Clindamycin (600 mg q6–8h IV) ***plus*** Quinine (650 mg q8h PO)	Immediate complete exchange transfusion ***plus*** Clindamycin (7–10 mg/kg q6–8h IV; maximum, 600 mg/dose) ***plus*** Quinine (8 mg/kg q8h PO; maximum, 650 mg/dose)

[a]Treatment duration, 7–10 days. [b]A high dose of azithromycin (600–1000 mg) combined with atovaquone has been recommended for immunocompromised hosts. [c]Treatment typically is given for 7–10 days, but its duration may vary. In severely immunocompromised patients, therapy should be continued for at least 6 weeks, including 2 weeks after parasites are no longer detected on blood smear. [d]Several alternative regimens have been used in a limited number of cases of *B. microti* infection, and their efficacy is uncertain. These regimens include atovaquone, azithromycin, and clindamycin; atovaquone, azithromycin, and doxycycline; atovaquone, clindamycin, and doxycycline; atovaquone, doxycycline, and artemisinin; atovaquone-proguanil; azithromycin and quinine; and azithromycin, clindamycin, and doxycycline.

Sources: (1) ME Falagas, MS Klempner: Clin Infect Dis 22:809, 1996. (2) PJ Krause et al: N Engl J Med 343:1454, 2000. (3) PJ Krause et al: Clin Infect Dis 46:370, 2008. (4) CM Shih, CC Wang: Am J Trop Med Hyg 59:509, 1998. (5) CP Stowell et al: N Engl J Med 356:2313, 2007. (6) JM Vyas et al: Clin Infect Dis 45:1588, 2007. (7) GP Wormser et al: Clin Infect Dis 50:381, 2010.

SEVERE *B. MICROTI* ILLNESS

Clindamycin given intravenously plus quinine given orally for 7–10 days constitute the recommended treatment for severe babesiosis. Intravenous quinidine may be used instead of oral quinine but requires cardiac monitoring because of the risk of QT prolongation and polymorphic ventricular tachycardia.

Standard antimicrobial therapy is sometimes insufficient to resolve symptoms and clear parasitemia, especially in patients with marked immunosuppression due to splenectomy, HIV/AIDS, malignancy, and/or immunosuppressive therapy (including rituximab for B cell lymphomas). In such patients, antimicrobial therapy should be administered for at least 6 weeks, including 2 weeks after parasites are no longer observed on blood smear. High-dose azithromycin (600–1000 mg/d) plus atovaquone have been successfully used in immunocompromised patients. Resistance to atovaquone plus azithromycin has occurred in a few cases. In patients who are unresponsive to atovaquone plus azithromycin or who do not tolerate clindamycin plus quinine, alternative regimens have been used (Table 249-1).

Partial or complete RBC exchange transfusion is recommended in patients with high-grade parasitemia (≥10%), severe anemia (hemoglobin <10 g/dL), or pulmonary, hepatic, or renal compromise. Parasitemia and hematocrit should be monitored daily until symptoms recede and the parasitemia level is <5%.

OTHER *BABESIA* INFECTIONS

The regimen for *B. duncani* infections typically consists of intravenous clindamycin (600 mg tid/qid or 1200 mg bid) plus oral quinine (600–650 mg tid) for 7–10 days. A regimen often used for *B. divergens*–like infections is intravenous clindamycin (600 mg tid/qid, 900 mg tid, or 1200 mg bid) plus oral quinine or quinidine (650 mg tid).

In Europe, *B. divergens* infection is considered a medical emergency. The recommended treatment is immediate complete blood exchange transfusion and therapy with intravenous clindamycin plus either oral quinine or intravenous quinidine. Some cases have been cured with exchange transfusion and clindamycin monotherapy. Anemia may persist for >1 month and require additional transfusion.

PREVENTION

No vaccine is available for human use. There is no role for antibiotic prophylaxis. Individuals who reside in endemic areas, especially those at risk for severe babesiosis, should wear clothing that covers the lower part of the body, apply tick repellents (such as DEET) to clothing, and limit outdoor activities where ticks may abound from May through October. The skin should be thoroughly examined after outdoor activities, and ticks should be removed with tweezers. Individuals with a history of symptomatic babesiosis or with positive *Babesia* serology are indefinitely deferred from donating blood.

250e Atlas of Blood Smears of Malaria and Babesiosis

Nicholas J. White, Joel G. Breman

This is a digital-only chapter. It is available on the DVD that accompanies this book, as well as on Access Medicine/Harrison's Online, and the eBook and "app" editions of HPIM 19e.

Six species of blood protozoan parasites cause human malaria (Chap. 248): the potentially lethal and often drug-resistant *Plasmodium falciparum;* the relapsing parasites *Plasmodium vivax* and *Plasmodium ovale* (with what appear to be two morphologically identical sympatric species of *P. ovale*); *Plasmodium malariae*, which can persist at low densities for years; and, in infections in individuals living in or close to tropical forests in Southeast Asia, *Plasmodium knowlesi*, a monkey parasite that microscopically resembles *P. falciparum* (young forms) and *P. malariae* (older forms) but is identified definitively by molecular methods.

251 Leishmaniasis

Shyam Sundar

DEFINITION

Encompassing a complex group of disorders, leishmaniasis is caused by unicellular eukaryotic obligatory intracellular protozoa of the genus *Leishmania* and primarily affects the host's reticuloendothelial system. *Leishmania* species produce widely varying clinical syndromes ranging from self-healing cutaneous ulcers to fatal visceral disease. These syndromes fall into three broad categories: visceral leishmaniasis (VL), cutaneous leishmaniasis (CL), and mucosal leishmaniasis (ML).

ETIOLOGY AND LIFE CYCLE

Leishmaniasis is caused by ~20 species of the genus *Leishmania* in the order Kinetoplastida and the family Trypanosomatidae (Table 251-1). Several clinically important species are of the subspecies *Viannia*. The organisms are transmitted by phlebotomine sandflies of the genus *Phlebotomus* in the "Old World" (Asia, Africa, and Europe) and the genus *Lutzomyia* in the "New World" (the Americas). Transmission may be anthroponotic (i.e., the vector transmits the infection from infected humans to healthy humans) or zoonotic (i.e., the vector transmits the infection from an animal reservoir to humans). Human-to-human transmission via shared infected needles has been documented in IV drug users in the Mediterranean region. In utero transmission to the fetus occurs rarely.

Leishmania organisms occur in two forms: extracellular, flagellate promastigotes (length, 10–20 μm) in the sandfly vector and intracellular, nonflagellate amastigotes (length, 2–4 μm; Fig. 251-1) in vertebrate hosts, including humans. Promastigotes are introduced through the proboscis of the female sandfly into the skin of the vertebrate host. Neutrophils predominate among the host cells that first encounter and take up promastigotes at the site of parasite delivery. The infected neutrophils may undergo apoptosis and release viable parasites that are taken up by macrophages, or the apoptotic cells may themselves be taken up by macrophages and dendritic cells. The parasites multiply as amastigotes inside macrophages, causing cell rupture with subsequent invasion of other macrophages. While feeding on infected hosts, sandflies pick up amastigotes, which transform into the flagellate form in the flies' posterior midgut and multiply by binary fission; the promastigotes then migrate to the anterior midgut and can infect a new host when flies take another blood meal.

EPIDEMIOLOGY

Leishmaniasis occurs in 98 countries—most of them developing—in tropical and temperate regions (Fig. 251-2). More than 1.5 million cases occur annually, of which 0.7–1.2 million are CL (and its variations) and 200,000–400,000 are VL. More than 350 million people are at risk, with an overall prevalence of 12 million. Although the distribution of *Leishmania* is limited by the distribution of sandfly vectors, human leishmaniasis is on the increase worldwide.

VISCERAL LEISHMANIASIS

VL (also known as *kala-azar*, a Hindi term meaning "black fever") is caused by the *Leishmania donovani* complex, which includes *L. donovani* and *Leishmania infantum* (the latter designated *Leishmania chagasi* in the New World); these species are responsible for anthroponotic and zoonotic transmission, respectively. India and neighboring Bangladesh, Sudan, South Sudan, Ethiopia, and Brazil are the four largest foci of VL and account for 90% of the world's VL burden, with India being the worst affected. Zoonotic VL is reported from all countries in the Middle East, Pakistan, and other countries from western Asia to China. Endemic foci also exist in the independent states of the former Soviet Union, mainly Georgia and Azerbaijan. In the Horn of Africa, Sudan, South Sudan, Ethiopia, Kenya, Uganda, and Somalia report VL. In Sudan and South Sudan, large outbreaks are thought to be anthroponotic, although zoonotic transmission also occurs. VL is rare in West and sub-Saharan Africa.

TABLE 251-1 GEOGRAPHIC DISTRIBUTION AND CHARACTERISTIC EPIDEMIOLOGY OF LEISHMANIASES

Organism, Endemic Region	Clinical Syndrome	Species	Vector	Reservoir	Transmission	Setting
***Leishmania donovani* Complex**						
South Asia	VL, PKDL	*L. donovani*	*Phlebotomus argentipes*	Humans	Anthroponotic	Rural, domestic
Sudan, South Sudan, Somalia, Ethiopia, Kenya, Uganda	VL, PKDL	*L. donovani*	*P. orientalis, P. martini*	Humans, rodents in Sudan, canines	Anthroponotic, occasionally zoonotic	Majority peridomestic, occasionally sylvatic
Mediterranean basin, Middle East, central Asia, China	VL, CL	*L. infantum*	*P. perniciosus, P. ariasi*	Dogs, foxes, jackals	Zoonotic	Domestic, peridomestic
Middle East, Saudi Arabia, Yemen	VL	*L. donovani*	*P. perniciosus, P. ariasi*	Dogs, foxes, jackals	Zoonotic	Domestic, peridomestic
Central and South America	VL, CL	*L. infantum*[a]	*Lutzomyia longipalpis*	Foxes, dogs, opossums	Zoonotic	Domestic, peridomestic, periurban
Azerbaijan, Armenia, Georgia, Kazakhstan, Kyrgyzstan, Tajikistan, Turkmenistan, Uzbekistan	VL	*L. infantum*	*P. turanicus*	Humans, dogs, foxes	Anthroponotic, zoonotic	Domestic
L. tropica						
Western India to Turkey, parts of North and East Africa	CL, leishmaniasis recidivans	*L. tropica*	*P. sergenti*	Humans	Anthroponotic	Urban domestic, peridomestic
L. major						
Western and Central Asia, North and sub-Saharan Africa	CL	*L. major*	*P. papatasi, P. duboscqi*	Nile rats, rodents	Zoonotic	Sylvatic, peridomestic
Kazakhstan, Turkmenistan, Uzbekistan	CL	*L. major*	*P. papatasi, P. duboscqi*	Gerbils	Zoonotic	Rural
L. aethiopica						
Ethiopia, Uganda, Kenya	CL, DCL	*L. aethiopica*	*P. longipes, P. pedifer*	Hyraxes	Zoonotic	Sylvatic, peridomestic
Subspecies *Viannia*						
Peru, Ecuador	CL, ML	*L. (V.) peruviana*	*Lutzomyia verrucarum, L. peruensis*	Wild rodents	Zoonotic	Andean Valleys
Guyana, Surinam, French Guyana, Ecuador, Brazil, Colombia, Bolivia	CL, ML	*L. (V.) guyanensis*	*L. umbratilis*	Sloths, arboreal anteaters, opossums	Zoonotic	Tropical forest
Central America, Ecuador, Colombia	CL, ML	*L. (V.) panamensis*	*L. trapidoi*	Sloths	Zoonotic	Tropical forest and deforested areas
South and Central America	CL, ML	*L. (V.) braziliensis*	*Lutzomyia* spp., *L. umbratilis, Psychodopygus wellcomei*	Forest rodents, peridomestic animals	Zoonotic	Tropical forest and deforested areas
***L. mexicana* Complex**						
Central America and northern parts of South America	CL, ML, DCL	*L. amazonensis*	*L. flaviscutellata*	Forest rodents	Zoonotic	Tropical forest and deforested areas
	CL, ML, DCL	*L. mexicana*	*L. olmeca*	Variety of forest rodents and marsupials	Zoonotic	Tropical forest and deforested areas
	CL, DCL	*L. pifanoi*	*L. olmeca*	Variety of forest rodents and marsupials	Zoonotic	Tropical forest and deforested areas

[a]*L. infantum* is designated *L. chagasi* in the New World.

Abbreviations: CL, cutaneous leishmaniasis; DCL, diffuse cutaneous leishmaniasis; ML, mucosal leishmaniasis; PKDL, post–kala-azar dermal leishmaniasis; VL, visceral leishmaniasis.

Mediterranean VL, long an established endemic disease due to *L. infantum*, has a large canine reservoir and was seen primarily in infants before the advent of HIV infection. In Mediterranean Europe, 70% of adult VL cases are associated with HIV co-infection. The combination is deadly because of the impact of the two infections together on the immune system. IV drug users are at particular risk. Other forms of immunosuppression (e.g., that associated with organ transplantation) also predispose to VL. In the Americas, disease caused by *L. infantum* is endemic from Mexico to Argentina, but 90% of cases in the New World are reported from northeastern Brazil.

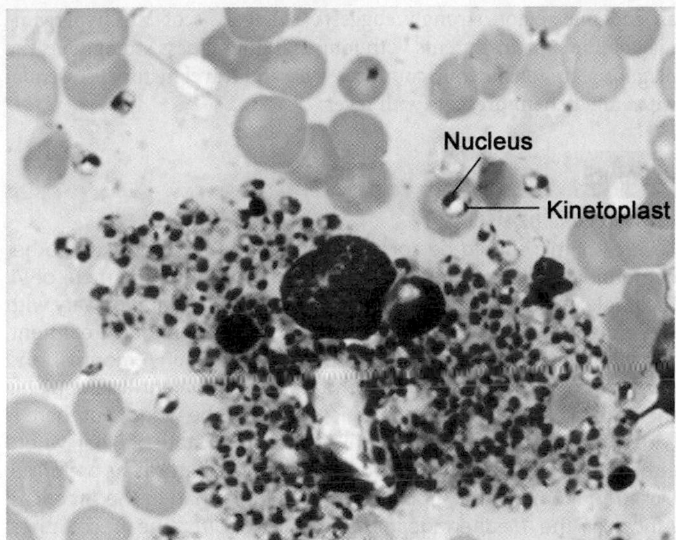

FIGURE 251-1 A macrophage with numerous intracellular amastigotes (2–4 μm) in a Giemsa-stained splenic smear from a patient with visceral leishmaniasis. Each amastigote contains a nucleus and a characteristic kinetoplast consisting of multiple copies of mitochondrial DNA. A few extracellular parasites are also visible.

Immunopathogenesis The majority of individuals infected by *L. donovani* or *L. infantum* mount a successful immune response and control the infection, never developing symptomatic disease. Forty-eight hours after intradermal injection of killed promastigotes, these individuals exhibit delayed-type hypersensitivity (DTH) to leishmanial antigens in the leishmanin skin test (also called the Montenegro skin test). Results in mouse models indicate that the development of acquired resistance to leishmanial infection is controlled by the production of interleukin (IL) 12 by antigen-presenting cells and the subsequent secretion of interferon (IFN) γ, tumor necrosis factor (TNF) α, and other proinflammatory cytokines by the T helper 1 (T_H1) subset of T lymphocytes. The immune response in patients developing active VL is complex; in addition to increased production of multiple proinflammatory cytokines and chemokines, patients with active disease have markedly elevated levels of IL-10 in serum as well as enhanced IL-10 mRNA expression in lesional tissues. The main disease-promoting activity of IL-10 in VL may be to condition host macrophages for enhanced survival and growth of the parasite. IL-10 can render macrophages unresponsive to activation signals and inhibit killing of amastigotes by downregulating the production of TNF-α and nitric oxide. Multiple antigen-presentation functions of dendritic cells and macrophages are also suppressed by IL-10. Patients with such suppression do not have positive leishmanin skin tests, nor do their peripheral-blood mononuclear cells respond to leishmanial antigens in vitro. Organs of the reticuloendothelial system are predominantly affected, with remarkable enlargement of the spleen, liver, and lymph nodes in some regions. The tonsils and intestinal submucosa are also heavily infiltrated with parasites. Bone marrow dysfunction results in pancytopenia.

Clinical Features On the Indian subcontinent and in the Horn of Africa, persons of all ages are affected by VL. In endemic areas of the Americas and the Mediterranean basin, immunocompetent infants and small children as well as immunodeficient adults are affected especially often. The most common presentation of VL is an abrupt onset of moderate- to high-grade fever associated with rigor and chills. Fever may continue for several weeks with decreasing intensity, and the patient may become afebrile for a short period before experiencing another bout of fever. The spleen may be palpable by the second week of illness and, depending on the duration of illness, may become hugely enlarged (Fig. 251-3). Hepatomegaly (usually moderate in degree) soon follows. Lymphadenopathy is common in most endemic regions of the world except the Indian subcontinent, where it is rare. Patients lose weight and feel weak, and the skin gradually develops dark discoloration due to hyperpigmentation that is most easily seen in brown-skinned individuals. In advanced illness, hypoalbuminemia may manifest as pedal edema and ascites. Anemia appears early and may become severe enough to cause congestive heart failure. Epistaxis, retinal hemorrhages, and gastrointestinal bleeding are associated with thrombocytopenia. Secondary infections such as measles, pneumonia, tuberculosis, bacillary or amebic dysentery, and gastroenteritis are common. Herpes zoster, chickenpox, boils in the skin, and scabies may also occur. Untreated, the disease is fatal in most patients, including 100% of those with HIV co-infection.

Leukopenia and anemia occur early and are followed by thrombocytopenia. There is a marked polyclonal increase in serum immunoglobulins. Serum levels of hepatic aminotransferases are raised in a significant proportion of patients, and serum bilirubin levels are elevated occasionally. Renal dysfunction is uncommon.

Laboratory Diagnosis Demonstration of amastigotes in smears of tissue aspirates is the gold standard for the diagnosis of VL (Fig. 251-1). The

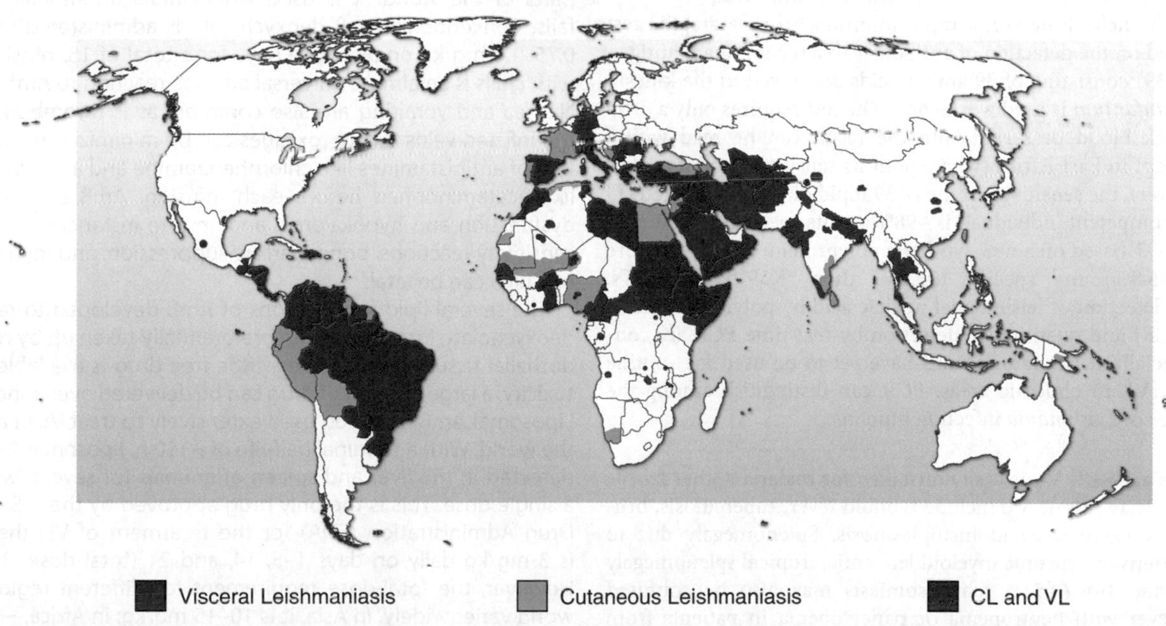

FIGURE 251-2 Worldwide distribution of human leishmaniasis. CL, cutaneous leishmaniasis; VL, visceral leishmaniasis.

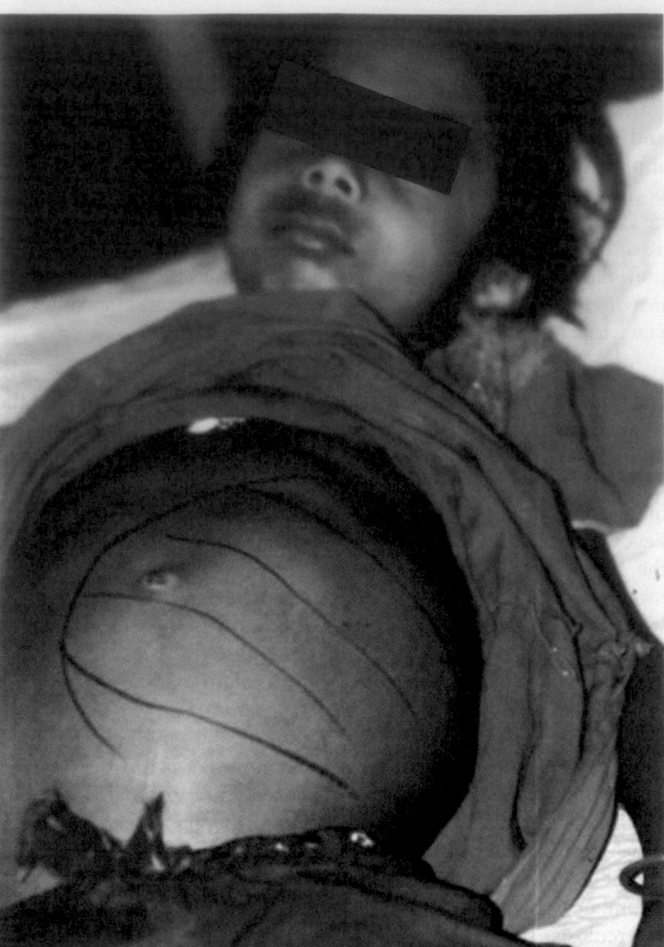

FIGURE 251-3 A patient with visceral leishmaniasis has a hugely enlarged spleen visible through the surface of the abdomen. Splenomegaly is the most important feature of visceral leishmaniasis.

sensitivity of splenic smears is >95%, whereas smears of bone marrow (60–85%) and lymph node aspirates (50%) are less sensitive. Culture of tissue aspirates increases sensitivity. Splenic aspiration is invasive and may be dangerous in untrained hands. Several serologic techniques are currently used to detect antibodies to *Leishmania*. An enzyme-linked immunosorbent assay (ELISA) and the indirect immunofluorescent antibody test (IFAT) are used in sophisticated laboratories.

In the field, however, a rapid immunochromatographic test based on the detection of antibodies to a recombinant antigen (rK39) consisting of 39 amino acids conserved in the kinesin region of *L. infantum* is used worldwide. The test requires only a drop of fingerprick blood or serum, and the result can be read within 15 min. Except in East Africa (where both its sensitivity and its specificity are lower), the sensitivity of the rK39 rapid diagnostic test (RDT) in immunocompetent individuals is ~98% and its specificity is 90%. In Sudan, an RDT based on a new synthetic polyprotein, rK28, was more sensitive (96.8%) and specific (96.2%) than rK39-based RDTs. Qualitative detection of leishmanial nucleic acid by polymerase chain reaction (PCR) and quantitative detection by real-time PCR are confined to specialized laboratories and have yet to be used for routine diagnosis of VL in endemic areas. PCR can distinguish among the major species of *Leishmania* infecting humans.

Differential Diagnosis VL is easily mistaken for malaria. Other febrile illnesses that may mimic VL include typhoid fever, tuberculosis, brucellosis, schistosomiasis, and histoplasmosis. Splenomegaly due to portal hypertension, chronic myeloid leukemia, tropical splenomegaly syndrome, and (in Africa) schistosomiasis may also be confused with VL. Fever with neutropenia or pancytopenia in patients from an endemic region strongly suggests a diagnosis of VL; hypergammaglobulinemia in patients with long-standing illness strengthens the diagnosis. In nonendemic countries, a careful travel history is essential when any patient presents with fever.

TREATMENT VISCERAL LEISHMANIASIS

GENERAL CONSIDERATIONS

Severe anemia should be corrected by blood transfusion, and other comorbid conditions should be managed promptly. Treatment of VL is complex because the optimal drug, dosage, and duration vary with the endemic region. Despite completing recommended treatment, some patients experience relapse (most often within 6 months), and prolonged follow-up is recommended. A pentavalent antimonial is the drug of choice in most endemic regions of the world, but there is widespread resistance to antimony in the Indian state of Bihar, where either amphotericin B (AmB) deoxycholate or miltefosine is preferred. Dose requirements for AmB are lower in India than in the Americas, Africa, or the Mediterranean region. In Mediterranean countries, where cost is seldom an issue, liposomal AmB is the drug of choice. In immunocompetent patients, relapses are uncommon with AmB in its deoxycholate and lipid formulations. Antileishmanial therapy has recently evolved as new drugs and delivery systems have become available and resistance to antimonial compounds has emerged.

Except for AmB (deoxycholate and lipid formulations), antileishmanial drugs are available in the United States only from the Centers for Disease Control and Prevention.

PENTAVALENT ANTIMONIAL COMPOUNDS

Two pentavalent antimonial (Sb^V) preparations are available: sodium stibogluconate (100 mg of Sb^V/mL) and meglumine antimoniate (85 mg of Sb^V/mL). The daily dose is 20 mg/kg by IV infusion or IM injection, and therapy continues for 28–30 days. Cure rates exceed 90% in Africa, the Americas, and most of the Old World but are <50% in Bihar, India, as a result of resistance. Adverse reactions to Sb^V treatment are common and include arthralgia, myalgia, and elevated serum levels of aminotransferases. Electrocardiographic changes are common. Concave ST-segment elevation is not significant, but prolongation of QT_c to >0.5 s may herald ventricular arrhythmia and sudden death. Chemical pancreatitis is common but usually does not require discontinuation of treatment; severe clinical pancreatitis occurs in immunosuppressed patients.

AMPHOTERICIN B

AmB is currently used as a first-line drug in Bihar, India. In other parts of the world, it is used when initial antimonial treatment fails. Conventional AmB deoxycholate is administered in doses of 0.75–1.0 mg/kg on alternate days for a total of 15 infusions. Fever with chills is an almost universal adverse reaction to AmB infusions. Nausea and vomiting are also common, as is thrombophlebitis in the infused veins. Acute toxicities can be minimized by administration of antihistamines like chlorpheniramine and antipyretic agents like acetaminophen before each infusion. AmB can cause renal dysfunction and hypokalemia and, in rare instances, elicits hypersensitivity reactions, bone marrow suppression, and myocarditis, all of which can be fatal.

The several lipid formulations of AmB developed to replace the deoxycholate formulation are preferentially taken up by reticuloendothelial tissues. Because very little free drug is available to cause toxicity, a large amount of drug can be delivered over a short period. Liposomal AmB has been used extensively to treat VL in all parts of the world. With a terminal half-life of ~150 h, liposomal AmB can be detected in the liver and spleen of animals for several weeks after a single dose. This is the only drug approved by the U.S. Food and Drug Administration (FDA) for the treatment of VL; the regimen is 3 mg/kg daily on days 1–5, 14, and 21 (total dose, 21 mg/kg). However, the total-dose requirement for different regions of the world varies widely. In Asia, it is 10–15 mg/kg; in Africa, ~18 mg/kg;

and in Mediterranean/American regions, ≥20 mg/kg. The daily dose is flexible (1–10 mg/kg). In a study in India, a single dose of 10 mg/kg cured infection in 96% of patients. Adverse effects of liposomal AmB are usually mild and include infusion reactions, backache, and occasional reversible nephrotoxicity.

PAROMOMYCIN

Paromomycin (aminosidine) is an aminocyclitol-aminoglycoside antibiotic with antileishmanial activity. Its mechanism of action against *Leishmania* has yet to be established. Paromomycin is approved in India for the treatment of VL at an IM dose of 11 mg of base/kg daily for 21 days; this regimen produces a cure rate of 95%. However, the optimal dose has not been established in other endemic regions. Paromomycin is a relatively safe drug, but some patients develop hepatotoxicity, reversible ototoxicity, and (in rare instances) nephrotoxicity and tetany.

MILTEFOSINE

Miltefosine, an alkylphosphocholine, is the first oral compound approved for the treatment of leishmaniasis. This drug has a long half-life (150–200 h); its mechanism of action is not clearly understood. The recommended therapeutic regimens for patients on the Indian subcontinent are a daily dose of 50 mg for 28 days for patients weighing <25 kg, a twice-daily dose of 50 mg for 28 days for patients weighing ≥25 kg, and 2.5 mg/kg for 28 days for children 2–11 years of age. These regimens have resulted in a cure rate of 94% in India. However, recent studies from the Indian subcontinent indicate a decline in the cure rate. Doses in other regions remain to be established. Because of its long half-life, miltefosine is prone to induce resistance in *Leishmania*. Its adverse effects include mild to moderate vomiting and diarrhea in 40% and 20% of patients, respectively; these reactions usually clear spontaneously after a few days. Rare cases of severe allergic dermatitis, hepatotoxicity, and nephrotoxicity have been reported. Because miltefosine is expensive and is associated with significant adverse events, it is best administered as directly observed therapy to ensure completion of treatment and to minimize the risk of resistance induction. Because miltefosine is teratogenic in rats, its use is contraindicated during pregnancy and (unless contraceptive measures are strictly adhered to for at least 3 months after treatment) in women of childbearing age.

MULTIDRUG THERAPY

Multidrug therapy for leishmaniasis is likely to be preferred in the future. Its potential advantages in VL include (1) better compliance and lower costs associated with shorter treatment courses and decreased hospitalization, (2) less toxicity due to lower drug doses and/or shorter duration of treatment, and (3) a reduced likelihood that resistance to either agent will develop. In a study from India, one dose of liposomal AmB (5 mg/kg) followed by miltefosine for 7 days, paromomycin for 10 days, or both miltefosine and paromomycin simultaneously for 10 days (in their usual daily doses) produced a cure rate of >97% (all three combinations). In Africa, a combination of Sb^V and paromomycin given for 17 days was as effective and safe as Sb^V given for 30 days.

PROGNOSIS OF TREATED VL PATIENTS

Recovery from VL is quick. Within a week after the start of treatment, defervescence, regression of splenomegaly, weight gain, and recovery of hematologic parameters are evident. With effective treatment, no parasites are recovered from tissue aspirates at the posttreatment evaluation. Continued clinical improvement over 6–12 months is suggestive of cure. A small percentage of patients (with the exact figure depending on the regimen used) relapse but respond well to treatment with AmB deoxycholate or lipid formulations.

VL IN THE IMMUNOCOMPROMISED HOST

HIV/VL co-infection has been reported from 35 countries. Where both infections are endemic, VL behaves as an opportunistic infection in HIV-1-infected patients. HIV infection can increase the risk of developing VL by severalfold in endemic areas. Co-infected patients usually show the classic signs of VL, but they may present with atypical features due to loss of immunity and involvement of unusual anatomic locations, with, for example, infiltration of the skin, oral mucosa, gastrointestinal tract, lungs, and other organs. Serodiagnostic tests are commonly negative. Parasites can be recovered from unusual sites such as bronchoalveolar lavage fluid and buffy coat. Liposomal AmB is the drug of choice for HIV/VL co-infection—both for primary treatment and for treatment of relapses. A total dose of 40 mg/kg, administered as 4 mg/kg on days 1–5, 10, 17, 24, 31, and 38, is considered optimal and is approved by the FDA, but most patients experience a relapse within 1 year. Pentavalent antimonials and AmB deoxycholate can also be used where liposomal AmB is not accessible. Reconstitution of patients' immunity by antiretroviral therapy has led to a dramatic decline in the incidence of co-infection in the Mediterranean basin. In contrast, HIV/VL co-infection is on the rise in African and Asian countries. Ethiopia is worst affected: up to 30% of VL patients are also infected with HIV. Because restoration of the CD4+ T cell count to >200/μL does decrease the frequency of relapse, antiretroviral therapy (in addition to antileishmanial therapy) is a cornerstone for the management of HIV/VL co-infection. Secondary prophylaxis with liposomal AmB has been shown to delay relapses, but no regimen has been established as optimal.

POST–KALA-AZAR DERMAL LEISHMANIASIS

On the Indian subcontinent and in Sudan and other East African countries, 2–50% of patients develop skin lesions concurrent with or after the cure of VL. Most common are hypopigmented macules, papules, and/or nodules or diffuse infiltration of the skin and sometimes of the oral mucosa. The African and Indian diseases differ in several respects; important features of post–kala-azar dermal leishmaniasis (PKDL) in these two regions are listed in Table 251-2, and disease in an Indian patient is depicted in Fig. 251-4.

In PKDL, parasites are scanty in hypopigmented macules but may be seen and cultured more easily from nodular lesions. Cellular infiltrates are heavier in nodules than in macules. Lymphocytes are the dominant cells; next most common are histiocytes and plasma

TABLE 251-2 CLINICAL, EPIDEMIOLOGIC, AND THERAPEUTIC FEATURES OF POST–KALA-AZAR DERMAL LEISHMANIASIS: EAST AFRICA AND THE INDIAN SUBCONTINENT

Feature	East Africa	Indian Subcontinent
Most affected country	Sudan and South Sudan	Bangladesh
Incidence among patients with VL	~50%	~2–17%
Interval between VL and PKDL	During VL to 6 months	6 months to 3 years
Age distribution	Mainly children	Any age
History of prior VL	Yes	Not necessarily
Rashes of PKDL in presence of active VL	Yes	No
Treatment with sodium stibogluconate	2–3 months	2–4 months
Natural course	Spontaneous cure in majority of patients	Spontaneous cure in minority of patients

Abbreviations: PKDL, post–kala-azar dermal leishmaniasis; VL, visceral leishmaniasis.

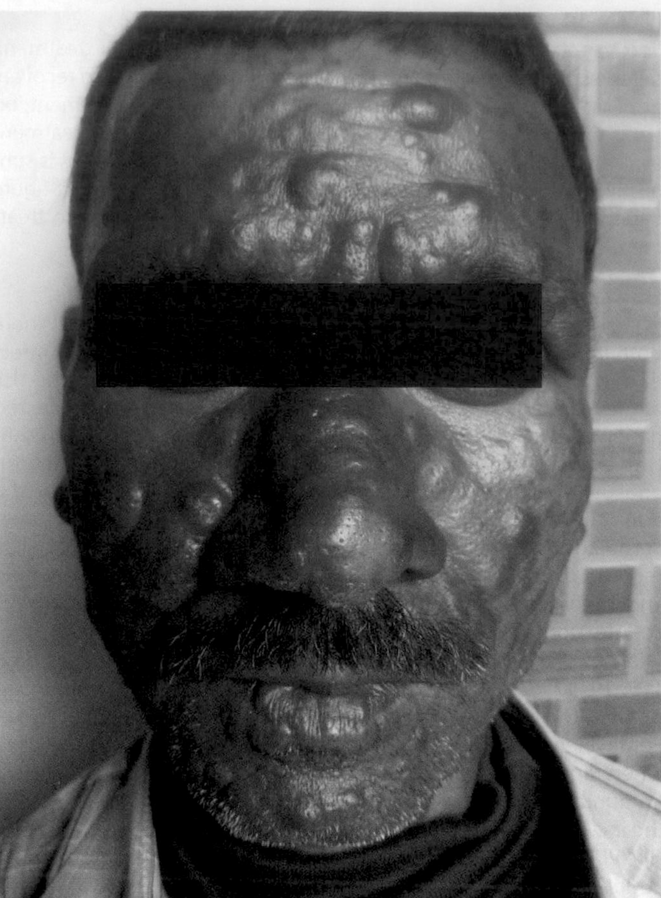

FIGURE 251-4 Post–kala-azar dermal leishmaniasis in an Indian patient. Note nodules of varying size involving the entire face. The face is erythematous, and the surface of some of the large nodules is discolored.

cells. In about half of cases, epithelioid cells—scattered individually or forming compact granulomas—are seen. The diagnosis is based on history and clinical findings, but rK39 and other serologic tests are positive in most cases. Indian PKDL is treated with pentavalent antimonials for 60–120 days. This prolonged course frequently leads to noncompliance. The alternative—several courses of AmB spread over several months—is expensive and unacceptable for most patients. Oral miltefosine for 12 weeks, in the usual daily doses, cures most patients with Indian PKDL. In East Africa, a majority of patients experience spontaneous healing. In those with persistent lesions, the response to 60 days of treatment with a pentavalent antimonial is good.

CUTANEOUS LEISHMANIASIS

CL can be broadly divided into Old World and New World forms. Old World CL caused by *Leishmania tropica* is anthroponotic and is confined to urban or suburban areas throughout its range. Zoonotic CL is most commonly due to *Leishmania major*, which naturally parasitizes several species of desert rodents that act as reservoirs over wide areas of the Middle East, Africa, and central Asia. Local outbreaks of human disease are common. Major outbreaks currently affect Afghanistan and Pakistan in association with refugees and population movement. CL is increasingly seen in tourists and military personnel on mission in CL-endemic regions of countries like Afghanistan and as a co-infection in HIV-infected patients. *Leishmania aethiopica* is restricted to the highlands of Ethiopia, Kenya, and Uganda, where it is a natural parasite of hyraxes. New World CL is mainly zoonotic and is most often caused by *Leishmania mexicana*, *Leishmania (Viannia) panamensis*, and *Leishmania amazonensis*. A wide range of forest animals act as reservoirs, and human infections with these species are predominantly rural. As a result of extensive urbanization and deforestation, *Leishmania (Viannia) braziliensis* has adapted to peridomestic and urban animals, and CL due to this organism is increasingly becoming an urban disease. In the United States, a few cases of CL have been acquired indigenously in Texas.

Immunopathogenesis As in VL, the proinflammatory (T_H1) response in CL may result in either asymptomatic or subclinical infection. However, in some individuals, the immune response causes ulcerative skin lesions, the majority of which heal spontaneously, leaving a scar. Healing is usually followed by immunity to reinfection with that species of parasite.

Clinical Features A few days or weeks after the bite of a sandfly, a papule develops and grows into a nodule that ulcerates over some weeks or months. The base of the ulcer, which is usually painless, consists of necrotic tissue and crusted serum, but secondary bacterial infection sometimes occurs. The margins of the ulcer are raised and indurated. Lesions may be single or multiple and vary in size from 0.5 to >3 cm (Fig. 251-5). Lymphatic spread and lymph gland involvement may be palpable and may precede the appearance of the skin lesion. There may be satellite lesions, especially in *L. major* and *L. tropica* infections. The lesions usually heal spontaneously after 2–15 months. Lesions due to *L. major* and *L. mexicana* tend to heal rapidly, whereas those due to *L. tropica* and parasites of subspecies *Viannia* heal more slowly. In CL caused by *L. tropica*, new lesions—usually scaly, erythematous papules and nodules—develop in the center or periphery of a healed sore, a condition known as *leishmaniasis recidivans*. Lesions of *L. mexicana* and *Leishmania (Viannia) peruviana* closely resemble those seen in the Old World; however, lesions on the pinna of the ear are common, chronic, and destructive in the former infections. *L. mexicana* is responsible for chiclero's ulcer, the so-called self-healing sore of Mexico. CL lesions on exposed body parts (e.g., the face and hands), permanent scar formation, and social stigmatization may cause anxiety and depression and may affect the quality of life of CL patients.

Differential Diagnosis A typical history (an insect bite followed by the events leading to ulceration) in a resident of or a traveler to an endemic focus strongly suggests CL. Cutaneous tuberculosis, fungal infections, leprosy, sarcoidosis, and malignant ulcers are sometimes mistaken for CL.

Laboratory Diagnosis Demonstration of amastigotes in material obtained from a lesion remains the diagnostic gold standard. Microscopic examination of slit skin smears, aspirates, or biopsies of the lesion is used for detection of parasites. Culture of smear or biopsy material may yield *Leishmania*. PCR is more sensitive than microscopy and culture and allows identification of *Leishmania* to the species level. This information is important in decisions about therapy because responses to treatment can vary with the species. Isoenzyme profiling is used to determine species for research purposes.

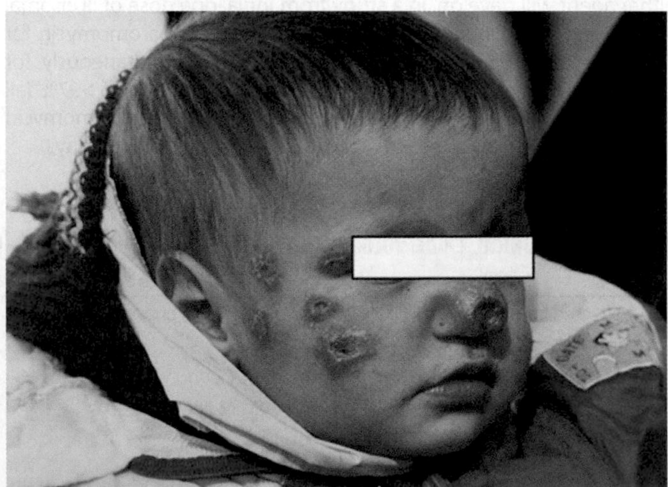

FIGURE 251-5 Cutaneous leishmaniasis in a Bolivian child. There are multiple ulcers resulting from several sandfly bites. The edges of the ulcers are raised. *(Courtesy of P. Desjeux, Retired Medical Officer, World Health Organization, Geneva, Switzerland.)*

TREATMENT CUTANEOUS LEISHMANIASIS

Although lesions heal spontaneously in the majority of cases, their spread or persistence indicates that treatment may be needed. One or a few small lesions due to "self-healing species" can be treated with topical agents. Systemic treatment is required for lesions over the face, hands, or joints; multiple lesions; large ulcers; lymphatic spread; New World CL with the potential for development of ML; and CL in HIV co-infected patients.

A pentavalent antimonial is the first-line drug for all forms of CL and is used in a dose of 20 mg/kg for 20 days, as for VL. The exceptions to this rule are CL caused by *Leishmania (Viannia) guyanensis*, for which pentamidine isethionate is the drug of choice (two injections of 4 mg of salt/kg separated by a 48-h interval), and CL due to *L. aethiopica*, which responds to paromomycin (16 mg/kg daily) but not to antimonials. Relapses usually respond to a second course of treatment. In Peru, topical imiquimod (5–7.5%) plus parenteral antimonials have been shown to cure CL more rapidly than antimonials alone. Azoles and triazoles have been used with mixed responses in both Old and New World CL but have not been adequately assessed for this indication in clinical trials. In *L. major* infection, oral fluconazole (200 mg/d for 6 weeks) resulted in a higher rate of cure than placebo (79% vs 34%) and also cured infection faster. Adverse effects include gastrointestinal symptoms and hepatotoxicity. Ketoconazole (600 mg/d for 28 days) is 76–90% effective in CL due to *L. (V.) panamensis* and *L. mexicana* in Panama and Guatemala. Miltefosine has been used in CL in doses of 2.5 mg/kg for 28 days. This agent is effective against *L. major* infections. In Colombia, where CL is due to *L. (V.) panamensis*, miltefosine was also effective, with a cure rate of 91%. For *L. (V.) braziliensis* infections, however, the results with miltefosine are less consistent. In Brazil, miltefosine cured 71% of patients with *L. (V.) guyanensis* infection. Other drugs, such as dapsone, allopurinol, rifampin, azithromycin, and pentoxifylline, have been used either alone or in combinations, but most of the relevant studies have had design limitations that preclude meaningful conclusions.

Small lesions (≤3 cm in diameter) may conveniently be treated weekly until cure with an intralesional injection of a pentavalent antimonial at a dose adequate to blanch the lesion (0.2–2.0 mL). An ointment containing 15% paromomycin sulfate, either alone or with 0.5% gentamicin or 12% methylbenzonium chloride, cured 70–82% of lesions due to *L. major* in 20 days and may be suitable for lesions caused by other species. Heat therapy with an FDA-approved radiofrequency generator and cryotherapy with liquid nitrogen have also been used successfully.

Diffuse Cutaneous Leishmaniasis (DCL) DCL is a rare form of leishmaniasis caused by *L. amazonensis* and *L. mexicana* in South and Central America and by *L. aethiopica* in Ethiopia and Kenya. DCL is characterized by the lack of a cell-mediated immune response to the parasite, the uncontrolled multiplication of which thus continues unabated. The DTH response does not develop, and lymphocytes do not respond to leishmanial antigens in vitro. DCL patients have a polarized immune response with high levels of immunosuppressive cytokines, including IL-10, transforming growth factor (TGF) β, and IL-4, and low concentrations of IFN-γ. Profound immunosuppression leads to widespread cutaneous disease. Lesions may initially be confined to the face or a limb but spread over months or years to other areas of the skin. They may be symmetrically or asymmetrically distributed and include papules, nodules, plaques, and areas of diffuse infiltration. These lesions do not ulcerate. The overlying skin is usually erythematous in pale-skinned patients. The lesions are teeming with parasites, which are therefore easy to recover. DCL does not heal spontaneously and is difficult to treat. If relapse and drug resistance are to be prevented, treatment should be continued for some time after lesions have healed and parasites can no longer be isolated. In the New World, repeated 20-day courses of pentavalent antimonials are given, with an intervening drug-free period of 10 days. Miltefosine has been used for several months with a good initial response. Combinations should be tried. In Ethiopia, a combination of paromomycin (14 mg/kg per day) and sodium stibogluconate (10 mg/kg per day) is effective.

MUCOSAL LEISHMANIASIS

The subgenus *Viannia* is widespread from the Amazon basin to Paraguay and Costa Rica and is responsible for deep sores and for ML (Table 251-1). In *L. (V.) braziliensis* infections, cutaneous lesions may be simultaneously accompanied by mucosal spread of the disease or followed by spread years later. ML is typically caused by *L. (V.) braziliensis* and rarely by *L. amazonensis*, *L. (V.) guyanensis*, and *L. (V.) panamensis*. Young men with chronic lesions of CL are at particular risk. Overall, ~3% of infected persons develop ML. Not every patient with ML has a history of prior CL. ML is almost entirely confined to the Americas. In rare cases, ML may also be caused by Old World species like *L. major*, *L. infantum* (*L. chagasi*), or *L. donovani*.

Immunopathogenesis and Clinical Features The immune response is polarized toward a T_H1 response, with marked increases of IFN-γ and TNF-α and varying levels of T_H2 cytokines (IL-10 and TGF-β). Patients have a stronger DTH response with ML than with CL, and their peripheral-blood mononuclear cells respond strongly to leishmanial antigens. The parasite spreads via the lymphatics or the bloodstream to mucosal tissues of the upper respiratory tract. Intense inflammation leads to destruction, and severe disability ensues. Lesions in or around the nose or mouth (espundia; Fig. 251-6) are the typical presentation of ML. Patients usually provide a history of self-healed CL preceding ML by 1–5 years. Typically, ML presents as nasal stuffiness and bleeding followed by destruction of nasal cartilage, perforation of the nasal septum, and collapse of the nasal bridge. Subsequent involvement of the pharynx and larynx leads to difficulty in swallowing and phonation.

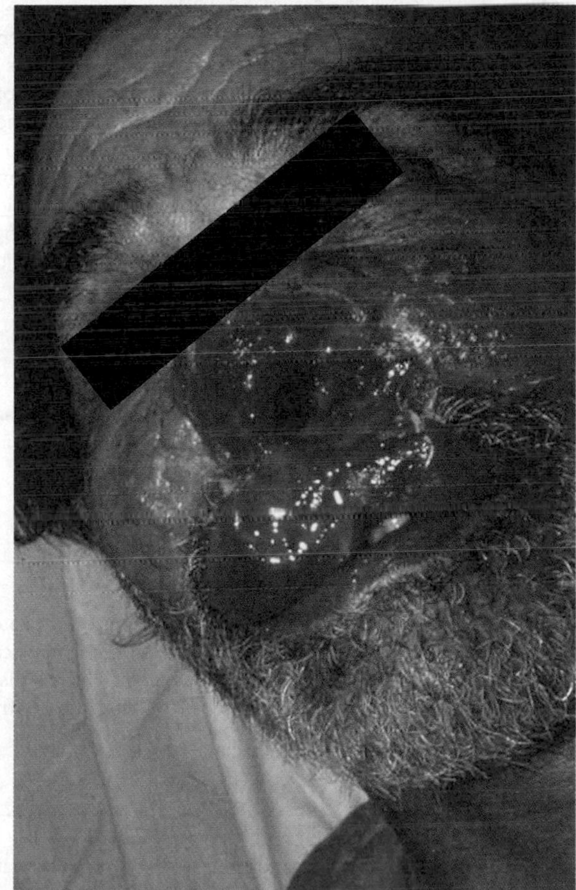

FIGURE 251-6 Mucosal leishmaniasis in a Brazilian patient. There is extensive inflammation around the nose and mouth, destruction of the nasal mucosa, ulceration of the upper lip and nose, and destruction of the nasal septum. *(Courtesy of R. Dietz, Universidade Federal do Espírito Santo, Vitória, Brazil.)*

The lips, cheeks, and soft palate may also be affected. Secondary bacterial infection is common, and aspiration pneumonia may be fatal. Despite the high degree of T_H1 immunity and the strong DTH response, ML does not heal spontaneously.

Laboratory Diagnosis Tissue biopsy is essential for identification of parasites, but the rate of detection is poor unless PCR techniques are used. The strongly positive DTH response fails to distinguish between past and present infection.

TREATMENT MUCOSAL LEISHMANIASIS

The regimen of choice is a pentavalent antimonial agent administered at a dose of 20 mg of Sb^V/kg for 30 days. Patients with ML require long-term follow-up with repeated oropharyngeal and nasal examination. With failure of therapy or relapse, patients may receive another course of an antimonial but then become unresponsive, presumably because of resistance in the parasite. In this situation, AmB should be used. An AmB deoxycholate dose totaling 25–45 mg/kg is appropriate. There are no controlled trials of liposomal AmB, but administration of 2–3 mg/kg for 20 days is considered adequate. Miltefosine (2.5 mg/kg for 28 days) cured 71% of ML patients in Bolivia. The more extensive the disease, the worse the prognosis; thus prompt, effective treatment and regular follow-up are essential.

PREVENTION OF LEISHMANIASIS

No vaccine is available for any form of leishmaniasis. Inoculation with live *L. major* ("leishmanization") is practiced in Iran. Anthroponotic leishmaniasis is controlled by case finding, treatment, and vector control with insecticide-impregnated bed nets and curtains and residual insecticide spraying. Control of zoonotic leishmaniasis is more difficult. Use of insecticide-impregnated collars for dogs, treatment of infected domestic dogs, and culling of street dogs are measures that have been used with uncertain efficacy to prevent transmission of *L. infantum*. In Brazil, a canine vaccine has been found to promote a decrease in the human and canine incidence of zoonotic VL. Two vaccines, Leishmune® and Leish-Tec®, are licensed in Brazil; Leishmune provides significant protection to vaccinated dogs. CaniLeish® is the first licensed canine vaccine developed in Europe. Personal prophylaxis with bed nets and repellants may reduce the risk of CL infections in the New World.

252 Chagas Disease and African Trypanosomiasis

Louis V. Kirchhoff, Anis Rassi Jr.

Although the genus *Trypanosoma* contains many species of protozoans, only *T. cruzi*, *T. brucei gambiense*, and *T. brucei rhodesiense* cause disease in humans. *T. cruzi* is the etiologic agent of Chagas disease in the Americas; *T. b. gambiense* and *T. b. rhodesiense* cause African trypanosomiasis.

CHAGAS DISEASE (AMERICAN TRYPANOSOMIASIS)

DEFINITION

Chagas disease, or American trypanosomiasis, is a zoonosis caused by the protozoan parasite *T. cruzi*. Acute Chagas disease is usually a mild febrile illness that results from initial infection with the organism. After spontaneous resolution of the acute illness, most infected persons remain for life in the indeterminate phase of chronic Chagas disease, which is characterized by subpatent parasitemia, easily detectable IgG antibodies to *T. cruzi*, and an absence of associated signs and symptoms. In 10–30% of chronically infected patients, cardiac and/or gastrointestinal symptoms develop that can lead to serious morbidity and even death.

LIFE CYCLE AND TRANSMISSION

T. cruzi is transmitted among its mammalian hosts by hematophagous triatomine insects, often called reduviid bugs. The insects become infected by sucking blood from animals or humans with circulating parasites. Ingested organisms multiply in the gut of the triatomines, and infective forms are discharged with the feces at the time of subsequent blood meals. Transmission to a second vertebrate host occurs when breaks in the skin, mucous membranes, or conjunctivae become contaminated with bug feces that contain infective parasites. *T. cruzi* can also be transmitted by transfusion of blood donated by infected persons, by organ transplantation, from mother to unborn child, by ingestion of contaminated food or drink, and in laboratory accidents.

PATHOLOGY

Initial infection at the site of parasite entry is characterized by local histologic changes that include the presence of parasites within leukocytes and cells of subcutaneous tissues and the development of interstitial edema, lymphocytic infiltration, and reactive hyperplasia of adjacent lymph nodes. After dissemination of the organisms through the lymphatics and the bloodstream, primarily muscles (including the myocardium) (Fig. 252-1) and ganglion cells may become heavily parasitized. The characteristic pseudocysts present in sections of infected tissues are intracellular aggregates of multiplying parasites.

In persons with chronic *T. cruzi* infections who develop related clinical manifestations, the heart is the organ most commonly affected. Changes include thinning of the ventricular walls, biventricular enlargement, apical aneurysms, and mural thrombi. Widespread lymphocytic infiltration, diffuse interstitial fibrosis, and atrophy of myocardial cells are often apparent. Although parasites are difficult to find in myocardial tissue by conventional histologic methods, more sensitive techniques of parasite detection, such as immunohistochemistry and polymerase chain reaction (PCR), have more frequently demonstrated *T. cruzi* antigens and parasite DNA in chronic lesions. Conduction-system abnormalities often affect the right branch and the left anterior branch of the bundle of His. In chronic Chagas disease of the gastrointestinal tract (*megadisease*), the esophagus and colon may exhibit varying degrees of dilation. On microscopic examination, focal inflammatory lesions with lymphocytic infiltration are seen, and the number of neurons in the myenteric plexus may be markedly reduced. Accumulating evidence implicates the persistence of parasites and the accompanying chronic inflammation—rather than autoimmune mechanisms—as the basis for the pathology in patients with chronic *T. cruzi* infection.

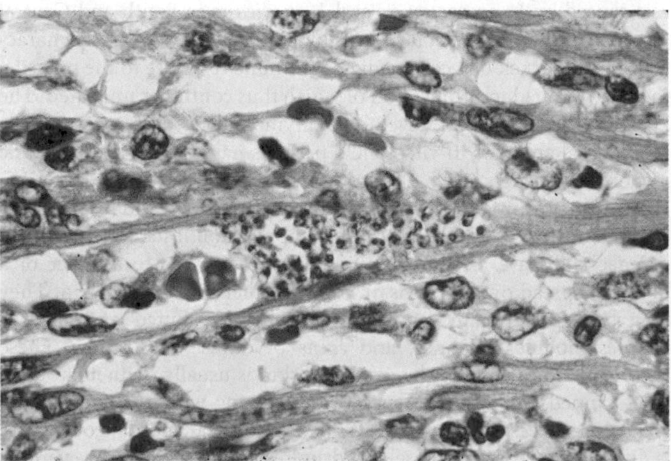

FIGURE 252-1 ***Trypanosoma cruzi* in the heart muscle of a child** who died of acute Chagas myocarditis. An infected myocyte containing several dozen *T. cruzi* amastigotes is in the center of the field (hematoxylin and eosin, 900 ×).

EPIDEMIOLOGY

T. cruzi is found only in the Americas. Wild and domestic mammals harboring *T. cruzi* and infected triatomines are found in spotty distributions from the southern United States to southern Argentina. Humans become involved in the cycle of transmission when infected vectors take up residence in the primitive wood, adobe, and stone houses common in much of Latin America. Thus human *T. cruzi* infection is a health problem primarily among the poor in rural areas of Mexico and Central and South America. Most new *T. cruzi* infections in rural settings occur in children, but the incidence is unknown because most cases go undiagnosed. Historically, transfusion-associated transmission of *T. cruzi* was a serious public health problem in many endemic countries. Transmission by this route has been largely eliminated, however, as effective programs for serologic screening of donated blood have been implemented. Several dozen patients with HIV and chronic *T. cruzi* infections who underwent acute recrudescence of the latter have been described. These patients generally presented with *T. cruzi* brain abscesses, a manifestation of the illness that does not occur in immunocompetent persons. Currently, it is estimated that 8 million people are chronically infected with *T. cruzi* and that 14,000 deaths due to the illness occur each year. The resulting morbidity and mortality make Chagas disease the most important parasitic disease burden in Latin America.

In recent years, the rate of *T. cruzi* transmission has decreased markedly in several endemic countries as a result of successful programs involving vector control, screening of donated blood, and education of at-risk populations. A major program, which began in 1991 in the "southern cone" nations of South America (Uruguay, Paraguay, Bolivia, Brazil, Chile, and Argentina), has provided the framework for much of this progress. Uruguay and Chile were certified free of transmission by the main domiciliary vector species (*Triatoma infestans*) in the late 1990s, and Brazil was declared transmission-free in 2006. Transmission has been reduced markedly in Argentina as well. Similar control programs have been initiated in the countries of northern South America and in the Central American nations.

Acute Chagas disease is rare in the United States, where 22 cases of autochthonous transmission and seven instances of transmission by blood transfusion have been reported. Moreover, *T. cruzi* was transmitted to five recipients of organs from three *T. cruzi*–infected donors, two of whom became infected through cardiac transplants. Acute Chagas disease has been reported in only one tourist returning to the United States from Latin America, although three such instances have been reported in Europe as well as one in Canada. In contrast, the prevalence of chronic *T. cruzi* infections in the United States has increased considerably in recent years. An estimated 23 million immigrants from Chagas-endemic countries currently live in the United States, ~17 million of whom are Mexicans. The total number of *T. cruzi*–infected persons living in the United States is estimated to be 300,000. Screening of the U.S. blood supply for *T. cruzi* infection began in January 2007. The overall prevalence of *T. cruzi* infection among donors is ~1 in 13,300, and to date nearly 2000 infected donors have been identified and deferred permanently (see "Diagnosis," below).

CLINICAL COURSE

The first signs of acute Chagas disease develop at least 1 week after invasion by the parasites. When the organisms enter through a break in the skin, an indurated area of erythema and swelling (the *chagoma*), accompanied by local lymphadenopathy, may appear. *Romaña sign*—the classic finding in acute Chagas disease, which consists of unilateral painless edema of the palpebrae and periocular tissues—can result when the conjunctiva is the portal of entry. These initial local signs may be followed by malaise, fever, anorexia, and edema of the face and lower extremities. Generalized lymphadenopathy and hepatosplenomegaly may develop. Severe myocarditis develops rarely; most deaths in acute Chagas disease are due to heart failure. Neurologic signs are not common, but meningoencephalitis occurs occasionally, especially in children <2 years old. Usually within 4–8 weeks, acute signs and symptoms resolve spontaneously in virtually all patients, with commencement of the asymptomatic or indeterminate form of chronic *T. cruzi* infection.

Symptomatic chronic Chagas disease becomes apparent years or even decades after the initial infection. The heart is commonly involved, and symptoms are caused by rhythm disturbances, segmental or dilated cardiomyopathy, and thromboembolism. Right bundle branch block is a common electrocardiographic abnormality, but other types of intraventricular and atrioventricular blocks, premature ventricular contractions, and tachy- and bradyarrhythmias occur frequently. Cardiomyopathy often results in biventricular heart failure, with a predominance of right-sided failure at advanced stages. Embolization of mural thrombi to the brain or other areas may take place. Sudden death is the main cause of death in Chagas heart disease; congestive heart failure and stroke are next most common. Patients with megaesophagus suffer from dysphagia, odynophagia, chest pain, and regurgitation. Aspiration can occur (especially during sleep) in patients with severe esophageal dysfunction, and repeated episodes of aspiration pneumonitis are common. Weight loss, cachexia, and pulmonary infection can result in death. Patients with megacolon are plagued by abdominal pain and chronic constipation, which predisposes to fecaloma formation. Advanced megacolon can cause obstruction, volvulus, septicemia, and death.

DIAGNOSIS

The diagnosis of acute Chagas disease requires the detection of parasites. Microscopic examination of fresh anticoagulated blood or the buffy coat is the simplest way to see the motile organisms. Parasites also can be seen in Giemsa-stained thin and thick blood smears. Microhematocrit tubes containing acridine orange as a stain can be used for the same purpose. When used repeatedly by experienced personnel, all of these methods yield positive results in a high proportion of cases of acute Chagas disease. Serologic testing does not play a major role in diagnosing acute Chagas disease. PCR assays often give positive results in infected patients in whom traditional parasitologic tests are negative, including infants with congenital Chagas disease.

Chronic Chagas disease is diagnosed by the detection of specific IgG antibodies that bind to *T. cruzi* antigens. Demonstration of the parasite is not of primary importance. In Latin America, ~30 assays are commercially available, including several based on recombinant antigens. Although these tests usually show good sensitivity and reasonable specificity, false-positive reactions may occur—typically with samples from patients who have other infectious and parasitic diseases or autoimmune disorders. In addition, confirmatory testing has presented a persistent challenge. For these reasons, the World Health Organization recommends that specimens be tested in at least two assays and that well-characterized positive and negative comparison samples be included in each run. The Chagas radioimmune precipitation assay (RIPA), a highly sensitive and specific confirmatory method for detecting antibodies to *T. cruzi*, is approved under the Clinical Laboratory Improvement Amendment and available in the laboratory of one of the authors (L.V.K.). In 2006, the U.S. Food and Drug Administration (FDA) approved a test to screen blood and organ donors for *T. cruzi* infection (Ortho *T. cruzi* ELISA Test System; Ortho-Clinical Diagnostics, Raritan, NJ). Since January 2007, the vast majority of U.S. blood donors have been screened, and positive units have undergone confirmatory testing with the Chagas RIPA. A second test for donor screening was approved by the FDA in 2010 (Abbott PRISM® Chagas Assay; Abbott Laboratories, Abbott Park, IL), as was an enzyme strip assay (Abbott ESA Chagas) in 2011. The use of PCR assays to detect *T. cruzi* DNA in chronically infected persons has been studied extensively; unfortunately, the sensitivity of this approach has not been shown to be reliably greater than that of serology.

TREATMENT CHAGAS DISEASE

Therapy for Chagas disease is still unsatisfactory. For many years now, only two drugs—nifurtimox and benznidazole—have been available for this purpose. Regrettably, both drugs lack efficacy and may cause bothersome side effects.

In acute Chagas disease, nifurtimox markedly reduces the duration of symptoms and parasitemia and decreases the mortality rate.

Nevertheless, limited studies have shown that only ~70% of acute infections are cured by a full course of treatment. Common adverse effects of nifurtimox include anorexia, nausea, vomiting, weight loss, and abdominal pain. Neurologic reactions to the drug may include restlessness, disorientation, insomnia, twitching, paresthesia, polyneuritis, and seizures. These symptoms usually disappear when the dosage is reduced or treatment is discontinued. The recommended daily dosage is 8–10 mg/kg for adults, 12.5–15 mg/kg for adolescents, and 15–20 mg/kg for children 1–10 years of age. The drug should be given orally in four divided doses each day, and therapy should be continued for 90–120 days. Nifurtimox is available from the Drug Service of the Centers for Disease Control and Prevention (CDC) in Atlanta (telephone number, 404-639-3670).

The efficacy of benznidazole is similar or even superior to that of nifurtimox. A cure rate of >90% among congenitally infected infants treated before their first birthday has been reported. Adverse effects include rash, peripheral neuropathy, and rare instances of granulocytopenia. The recommended oral dosage is 5 mg/kg per day for 60 days for adults and 5–10 mg/kg per day for 60 days for children, with administration of two or three divided doses. Benznidazole is generally considered the drug of choice in Latin America.

The question of whether adults in the indeterminate or chronic symptomatic phase of Chagas disease should be treated with nifurtimox or benznidazole has been debated for years. The fact that cure rates in persons with long-established chronic infection are notably inferior to those in patients with acute or recent chronic infection is central to this controversy. No convincing evidence from randomized controlled trials indicates that nifurtimox or benznidazole treatment of adults in the indeterminate or chronic symptomatic phase reduces either the appearance or progression of symptoms or mortality rates. On the basis of results of some observational studies, a panel of experts convened by the CDC in 2006 recommended that adults <50 years old with presumably long-standing indeterminate *T. cruzi* infections—or even with mild to moderate disease—be offered treatment. A large randomized clinical trial (the BENEFIT multicenter trial) designed to assess the parasitologic and clinical efficacy of benznidazole in 2856 adults (18–75 years old) with chronic Chagas heart disease (without advanced lesions) is being performed in Brazil, Argentina, Colombia, Bolivia, and El Salvador, but results will not be available until 2015. In contrast, randomized studies have shown that treatment of children is useful, and the current consensus of Latin American authorities and the CDC panel of experts is that all *T. cruzi*–infected persons up to 18 years old and all adults known to have become infected recently should be given benznidazole or nifurtimox.

The usefulness of antifungal azoles for the treatment of Chagas disease has been studied in laboratory animals and to a lesser extent in humans. To date, none of these drugs has exhibited a level of anti–*T. cruzi* activity that would justify its use in humans. Several newer drugs in this class have shown promise in animal studies and are currently being evaluated in phase 2 clinical trials.

Patients who develop cardiac and/or gastrointestinal disease in association with *T. cruzi* infection should be referred to appropriate subspecialists for further evaluation and treatment. Pacemakers can be useful in patients with ominous arrhythmias. The usefulness of implantable cardioverter defibrillators in persons with Chagas heart disease has not been established and currently is being studied in a prospective randomized trial. Cardiac transplantation is an option for patients with end-stage chagasic cardiomyopathy; more than 150 such transplantations have been done in Brazil and the United States. The survival rate among Chagas disease cardiac transplant recipients seems to be higher than that among persons receiving cardiac transplants for other reasons. This better outcome may be due to the fact that lesions are limited to the heart in most patients with symptomatic chronic Chagas disease.

PREVENTION

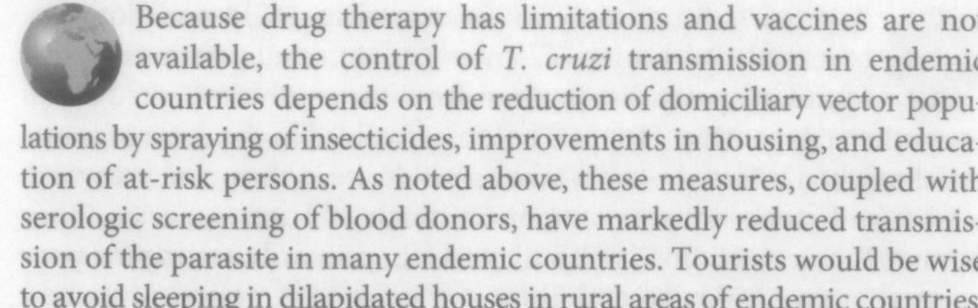

Because drug therapy has limitations and vaccines are not available, the control of *T. cruzi* transmission in endemic countries depends on the reduction of domiciliary vector populations by spraying of insecticides, improvements in housing, and education of at-risk persons. As noted above, these measures, coupled with serologic screening of blood donors, have markedly reduced transmission of the parasite in many endemic countries. Tourists would be wise to avoid sleeping in dilapidated houses in rural areas of endemic countries. Mosquito nets and insect repellent can provide additional protection.

In view of the possibly serious consequences of chronic *T. cruzi* infection, it would be prudent for all immigrants from endemic regions who are living in the United States to be tested for evidence of infection. Identification of persons harboring the parasite would permit periodic electrocardiographic monitoring, which is important to detect incipient heart disease and guide further diagnostic studies and treatment. The possibility of congenital transmission is yet another justification for screening. *T. cruzi* is classified as a Risk Group 2 agent in the United States and a Risk Group 3 agent in some European countries. Laboratory staff should work with the parasite or infected vectors and mammals at containment levels consistent with the risk group designation in their areas.

SLEEPING SICKNESS (AFRICAN TRYPANOSOMIASIS)

DEFINITION

Sleeping sickness, or human African trypanosomiasis (HAT), is caused by flagellated protozoan parasites that belong to the *T. brucei* complex and are transmitted to humans by tsetse flies. In untreated patients, the trypanosomes first cause a febrile illness that is followed months or years later by progressive neurologic impairment and death.

THE PARASITES AND THEIR TRANSMISSION

The East African (*rhodesiense*) and the West African (*gambiense*) forms of sleeping sickness are caused, respectively, by two trypanosome subspecies: *T. b. rhodesiense* and *T. b. gambiense*. These subspecies are morphologically indistinguishable but cause illnesses that are epidemiologically and clinically distinct (Table 252-1). The parasites are transmitted by blood-sucking tsetse flies of the genus *Glossina*. The insects acquire the infection when they ingest blood from infected mammalian hosts. After many cycles of multiplication in the midgut of the vector, the parasites migrate to the salivary glands. Their transmission takes place when they are inoculated into a mammalian host during a subsequent blood meal. The injected trypanosomes multiply in the blood (Fig. 252-2) and other extracellular spaces and evade immune destruction for long periods by undergoing antigenic variation, a process driven by gene switching in which the antigenic structure of the organisms' surface coat of glycoproteins changes periodically.

TABLE 252-1 COMPARISON OF WEST AFRICAN AND EAST AFRICAN TRYPANOSOMIASES

Point of Comparison	West African (*gambiense*)	East African (*rhodesiense*)
Organism	*T. b. gambiense*	*T. b. rhodesiense*
Vectors	Tsetse flies (palpalis group)	Tsetse flies (morsitans group)
Primary reservoir	Humans	Antelope and cattle
Human illness	Chronic (late CNS disease)	Acute (early CNS disease)
Duration of illness	Months to years	<9 months
Lymphadenopathy	Prominent	Minimal
Parasitemia	Low	High
Epidemiology	Rural populations	Workers in wild areas, rural populations, tourists in game parks

Abbreviation: CNS, central nervous system.

Source: Reprinted with permission from LV Kirchhoff, in GL Mandell et al (eds): *Principles and Practice of Infectious Diseases*, 7th ed. Philadelphia, Elsevier Churchill Livingstone, 2010.

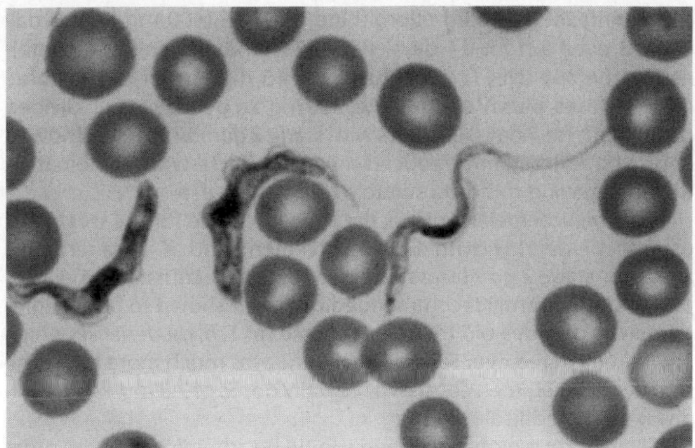

FIGURE 252-2 ***Trypanosoma brucei rhodesiense*** **parasites in rat blood.** The slender parasite is thought to be the form that multiplies in mammalian hosts, whereas the stumpy forms are nondividing and are capable of infecting insect vectors (Giemsa, 1200 ×). *(Courtesy of Dr. G. A. Cook, Madison, WI; with permission.)*

PATHOGENESIS AND PATHOLOGY

A self-limited inflammatory lesion (*trypanosomal chancre*) may appear a week or so after the bite of an infected tsetse fly. A systemic febrile illness then evolves as the parasites are disseminated through the lymphatics and bloodstream. Systemic HAT without central nervous system (CNS) involvement is generally referred to as *stage 1 disease*. In this stage, widespread lymphadenopathy and splenomegaly reflect marked lymphocytic and histiocytic proliferation and invasion of morular cells, which are plasmacytes that may be involved in the production of IgM. Endarteritis, with perivascular infiltration of both parasites and lymphocytes, may develop in lymph nodes and the spleen. Myocarditis develops frequently in patients with stage 1 disease and is especially common in *T. b. rhodesiense* infections.

Hematologic manifestations that accompany stage 1 HAT include moderate leukocytosis, thrombocytopenia, and anemia. High levels of immunoglobulins, consisting primarily of polyclonal IgM, are a constant feature, and heterophile antibodies, antibodies to DNA, and rheumatoid factor are often detected. High levels of antigen–antibody complexes may play a role in the tissue damage and increased vascular permeability that facilitate dissemination of the parasites.

Stage 2 disease involves invasion of the CNS. The presence of trypanosomes in perivascular areas is accompanied by intense infiltration of mononuclear cells. Abnormalities in cerebrospinal fluid (CSF) include increased pressure, elevated total protein concentration, and pleocytosis. In addition, trypanosomes are frequently found in CSF.

EPIDEMIOLOGY

The trypanosomes that cause sleeping sickness are found only in sub-Saharan Africa. After its near-eradication in the mid-1960s, sleeping sickness underwent a resurgence in the 1990s, primarily in Uganda, Sudan, the Central African Republic, the Democratic Republic of the Congo, and Angola. A subsequent increase in control activities reduced the incidence in many endemic areas, however, and in 2009 fewer than 10,000 cases were reported to the World Health Organization. Although underreporting is a persistent problem, the level of control achieved to date was the basis for convening a panel of experts in 2009 to develop a vision for eradication of HAT.

Humans are the only reservoir of *T. b. gambiense*, which occurs in widely distributed foci in tropical rain forests of Central and West Africa. *Gambiense* trypanosomiasis is primarily a problem in rural populations; tourists rarely become infected. Trypanotolerant antelope species in savanna and woodland areas of Central and East Africa are the principal reservoir of *T. b. rhodesiense*. Cattle can also be infected with this and other trypanosome species but generally succumb to the infection. Because risk results from contact with tsetse flies that feed on wild animals, humans acquire *T. b. rhodesiense* infection only incidentally, usually while visiting or working in areas where infected game and vectors are present. Roughly one or two imported cases of HAT acquired in East African parks are reported to the CDC each year.

CLINICAL COURSE

A painful trypanosomal chancre appears in some patients at the site of inoculation of the parasite. Hematogenous and lymphatic dissemination (stage 1 disease) is marked by the onset of fever. Typically, bouts of high temperatures lasting several days are separated by afebrile periods. Lymphadenopathy is prominent in *T. b. gambiense* trypanosomiasis. The nodes are discrete, movable, rubbery, and nontender. Cervical nodes are often visible, and enlargement of the nodes of the posterior cervical triangle, or *Winterbottom's sign*, is a classic finding. Pruritus and maculopapular rashes are common. Inconstant findings include malaise, headache, arthralgias, weight loss, edema, hepatosplenomegaly, and tachycardia. The differential diagnosis of stage 1 HAT includes many diseases that are common in the tropics and are associated with fevers. HIV infection, malaria, and typhoid fever are common in populations at risk for HAT and need to be considered.

CNS invasion (stage 2 disease) is characterized by the insidious development of protean neurologic manifestations that are accompanied by progressive abnormalities in the CSF. A picture of progressive indifference and daytime somnolence develops (hence the designation "sleeping sickness"), sometimes alternating with restlessness and insomnia at night. A listless gaze accompanies a loss of spontaneity, and speech may become halting and indistinct. Extrapyramidal signs may include choreiform movements, tremors, and fasciculations. Ataxia is frequent, and the patient may appear to have Parkinson's disease, with a shuffling gait, hypertonia, and tremors. In the final phase, progressive neurologic impairment ends in coma and death.

The most striking difference between the *gambiense* and *rhodesiense* forms of HAT is that the latter illness tends to follow a more acute course. Typically, in tourists with *T. b. rhodesiense* disease, systemic signs of infection, such as fever, malaise, and headache, appear before the end of the trip or shortly after the return home. Persistent tachycardia unrelated to fever is common early in the course of *T. b. rhodesiense* trypanosomiasis, and death may result from arrhythmias and congestive heart failure before CNS disease develops. In general, untreated *T. b. rhodesiense* trypanosomiasis leads to death in a matter of weeks to months, often without a clear distinction between the hemolymphatic and CNS stages. In contrast, *T. b. gambiense* disease can smolder for many months or even for years.

DIAGNOSIS

A definitive diagnosis of HAT requires detection of the parasite. If a chancre is present, fluid should be expressed and examined directly by light microscopy for the highly motile trypanosomes. The fluid also should be fixed and stained with Giemsa. Material obtained by needle aspiration of lymph nodes early in the illness should be examined similarly. Examination of wet preparations and Giemsa-stained thin and thick films of serial blood samples is also useful. If parasites are not seen initially in blood, efforts should be made to concentrate the organisms, which can be done in microhematocrit tubes containing acridine orange. Alternatively, the buffy coat from 10–15 mL of anticoagulated blood can be examined directly under a microscope. The likelihood of finding parasites in blood is higher in stage 1 than in stage 2 disease and in patients infected with *T. b. rhodesiense* rather than *T. b. gambiense*. Trypanosomes may also be seen in material aspirated from the bone marrow; the aspirate can be inoculated into liquid culture medium, as can blood, buffy coat, lymph node aspirates, and CSF. It is essential to examine CSF from all patients in whom HAT is suspected. Abnormalities in the CSF that may be associated with stage 2 disease include an increase in the CSF cell count as well as increases in opening pressure and in levels of total protein and IgM. Trypanosomes may be seen in the sediment of centrifuged CSF. Any CSF abnormality in a patient in whom trypanosomes have been found at other sites must be viewed as pathognomonic for CNS involvement and thus must prompt specific treatment for CNS disease. In patients with CSF pleocytosis in whom parasites are not found, tuberculous meningitis and HIV-associated CNS infections such as cryptococcosis should be considered in the differential diagnosis.

A number of serologic assays, such as the card agglutination test for trypanosomes (CATT) for *T. b. gambiense*, are available to aid in the diagnosis of HAT. Their ease of use makes them valuable for epidemiologic surveys, but their variable sensitivity and specificity mandate that decisions about treatment be based on demonstration of the parasite. Accurate PCR assays for detecting African trypanosomes in humans have been developed, but the lack of the necessary technical and human resources in most endemic areas stands in the way of their widespread use.

TREATMENT SLEEPING SICKNESS

The drugs used for treatment of HAT are suramin, pentamidine, eflornithine, and the organic arsenical melarsoprol. In the United States, these drugs can be obtained from the CDC. Therapy for HAT must be individualized on the basis of the infecting subspecies, the presence or absence of CNS disease, adverse reactions, and occasionally drug resistance. The choices of drugs for the treatment of HAT are summarized in **Table 252-2**.

Suramin is highly effective against stage 1 *rhodesiense* HAT. However, it can cause serious adverse effects and must be administered under the close supervision of a physician. A 100- to 200-mg IV test dose should be given to detect hypersensitivity. The dosage for adults is 20 mg/kg on days 1, 5, 12, 18, and 26. The drug is given by slow IV infusion of a freshly prepared 10% aqueous solution. Approximately 1 patient in 20,000 has an immediate, severe, and potentially fatal reaction to the drug, developing nausea, vomiting, shock, and seizures. Less severe reactions include fever, photophobia, pruritus, arthralgias, and skin eruptions. Renal damage is the most common important adverse effect of suramin. Transient proteinuria often appears during treatment. A urinalysis should be done before each dose, and treatment should be discontinued if proteinuria increases or if casts and red cells appear in the sediment. Suramin should not be given to patients with renal insufficiency.

Pentamidine is the first-line drug for treatment of stage 1 *gambiense* HAT. The dose for both adults and children is 4 mg/kg per day, given IM or IV for 7–10 days. Frequent, immediate adverse reactions include nausea, vomiting, tachycardia, and hypotension. These reactions are usually transient and do not warrant cessation of therapy. Other adverse reactions include nephrotoxicity, abnormal liver function tests, neutropenia, rashes, hypoglycemia, and sterile abscesses. Suramin is an alternative agent for stage 1 *T. b. gambiense* disease.

Eflornithine is highly effective for treatment of both stages of *gambiense* sleeping sickness. In the trials on which the FDA based its approval, this agent cured >90% of 600 patients with stage 2 disease. The recommended treatment schedule is 400 mg/kg per day, given IV in four divided doses, for 2 weeks. Adverse reactions include diarrhea, anemia, thrombocytopenia, seizures, and hearing loss. The high dosage and duration of therapy required are disadvantages that make widespread use of eflornithine difficult. A randomized trial comparing the standard eflornithine regimen (400 mg/kg per day infused over 6 h for 14 days) with nifurtimox-eflornithine combination therapy (NECT; oral nifurtimox, 15 mg/kg per day in three divided doses, plus IV eflornithine, 200 mg/kg per day in two divided doses, both for 7 days) in adults with stage 2 *gambiense* HAT showed improved efficacy and reduced adverse effects with combination therapy, making this drug suitable for first-line use.

The arsenical melarsoprol is the drug of choice for the treatment of *rhodesiense* HAT with CNS involvement and is an alternative agent for stage 2 *gambiense* disease. The "short course" of melarsoprol that is currently recommended has been shown to be noninferior to the decades-old treatment course for *T. b. rhodesiense*, which was administered over several weeks and was much more toxic. The short-course regimen consists of 10 daily doses of 2.2 mg/kg IV, each given with prednisolone (1 mg/kg).

Melarsoprol is highly toxic and should be administered with great care. As noted, all patients receiving melarsoprol should be given prednisolone to reduce the likelihood of drug-induced encephalopathy. Without prednisolone prophylaxis, the incidence of reactive encephalopathy has been as high as 18% in some series. Clinical manifestations of reactive encephalopathy include high fever, headache, tremor, impaired speech, seizures, and even coma and death. Treatment with melarsoprol should be discontinued at the first sign of encephalopathy but may be restarted cautiously at lower doses a few days after signs have resolved. Extravasation of the drug results in intense local reactions. Vomiting, abdominal pain, nephrotoxicity, and myocardial damage can occur.

TABLE 252-2 TREATMENT OF HUMAN AFRICAN TRYPANOSOMIASIS[a]

	Clinical Stage	
Causative Organism	**1 (Normal CSF)**	**2 (Abnormal CSF)**
T. b. gambiense	Pentamidine	Eflornithine
(West African)	Alternative: Suramin	Alternatives:
		NECT
		Melarsoprol[b]
T. b. rhodesiense	Suramin	Melarsoprol[b]
(East African)	Alternative: Pentamidine	

[a]For doses and duration, see text. [b]Short course.

Abbreviations: CSF, cerebrospinal fluid; NECT, nifurtimox-eflornithine combination therapy.

PREVENTION

HAT poses complex public-health and epizootic problems in Africa. Considerable progress has been made in many areas through control programs that focus on eradication of vectors and drug treatment of infected humans. People can reduce their risk of acquiring trypanosomiasis by avoiding areas known to harbor infected insects, by wearing protective clothing, and by using insect repellent. Chemoprophylaxis is not recommended, and no vaccine is available to prevent transmission of the parasites.

253 *Toxoplasma* Infections

Kami Kim, Lloyd H. Kasper

DEFINITION

Toxoplasmosis is caused by infection with the obligate intracellular parasite *Toxoplasma gondii*. Acute infection acquired after birth may be asymptomatic but is thought to result in the lifelong chronic persistence of cysts in the host's tissues. In both acute and chronic toxoplasmosis, the parasite is responsible for clinically evident disease, including lymphadenopathy, encephalitis, myocarditis, and pneumonitis. *Congenital* toxoplasmosis is an infection of newborns that results from the transplacental passage of parasites from an infected mother to the fetus. These infants may be asymptomatic at birth, but most later manifest a wide range of signs and symptoms, including chorioretinitis, strabismus, epilepsy, and psychomotor retardation. In immunocompetent individuals, toxoplasmosis can also present as acute disease (typically chorioretinitis) associated with food- or waterborne sources.

ETIOLOGY

T. gondii is an intracellular coccidian that infects both birds and mammals. There are two distinct stages in the life cycle of *T. gondii* that yield transmissible forms of the parasite (Fig. 253-1). In the *asexual* stages, tissue cysts that contain bradyzoites or sporulated oocysts that contain sporozoites are ingested by an intermediate host (e.g., a human, mouse, sheep, pig, or bird). The cyst is rapidly digested by the

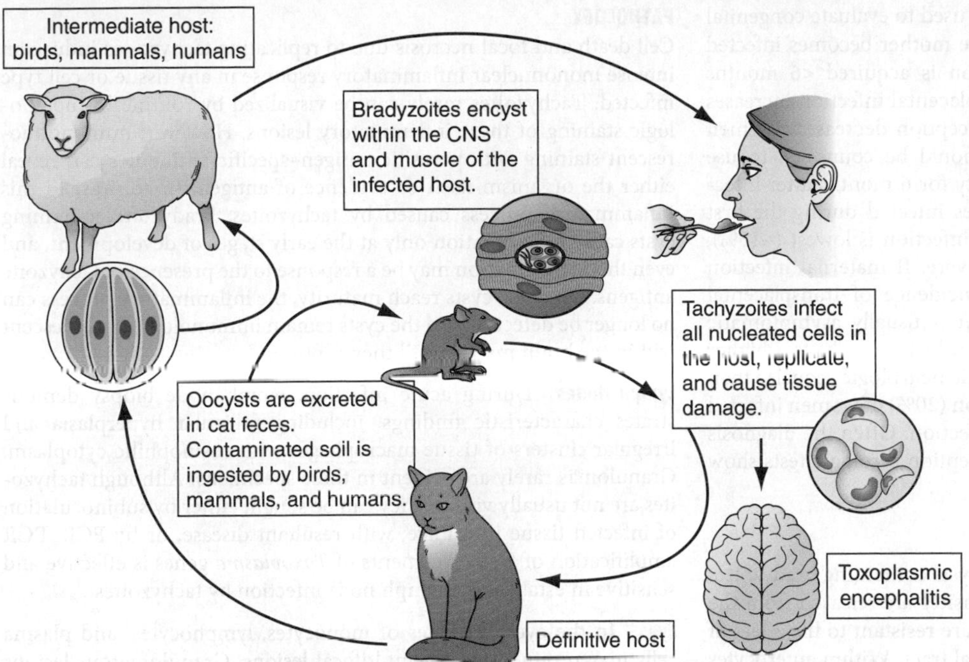
Intermediate host:
birds, mammals, humans
Bradyzoites encyst
within the CNS
and muscle of the
infected host.
Tachyzoites infect
all nucleated cells in
the host, replicate,
and cause tissue
damage.
Oocysts are excreted
in cat feces.
Contaminated soil is
ingested by birds,
mammals, and humans.
Toxoplasmic
encephalitis
Definitive host

FIGURE 253-1 Life cycle of *Toxoplasma gondii*. The cat is the definitive host in which the sexual phase of the cycle is completed. Oocysts shed in cat feces can infect a wide range of animals, including birds, rodents, grazing domestic animals, and humans. The bradyzoites found in the muscle of food animals may infect humans who eat insufficiently cooked meat products, particularly lamb and pork. Although human disease can take many forms, congenital infection and encephalitis from reactivation of latent infection in the brains of immunosuppressed persons are the most important manifestations. CNS, central nervous system. *(Courtesy of Dominique Buzoni-Gatel, Institut Pasteur, Paris; with permission.)*

acidic-pH gastric secretions. Bradyzoites or sporozoites are released, enter the small-intestinal epithelium, and transform into rapidly dividing tachyzoites. The tachyzoites can infect and replicate in all mammalian cells except red blood cells. The parasite actively penetrates the cell and forms a parasitophorous vacuole. Parasite replication continues within the vacuole. After the parasites reach a critical mass, intracellular signaling within the host and the parasite, including calcium fluxes, result in parasite egress from the vacuole. The host cell is destroyed, and the released tachyzoites infect adjoining cells. The tachyzoite replication cycle within an infected organ causes cytopathology. Most tachyzoites are eliminated by the host's humoral and cell-mediated immune responses. Tissue cysts containing many bradyzoites develop 7–10 days after systemic tachyzoite infection. These tissue cysts occur in various host organs but persist principally within the central nervous system (CNS) and muscle. The development of this chronic stage completes the asexual portion of the life cycle. Active infection in the immunocompromised host is most likely to be due to the spontaneous release of encysted parasites that undergo rapid transformation into tachyzoites within the CNS and are not contained by the immune system.

The *sexual* stage in the life cycle takes place in the cat (the definitive host). The parasite's sexual phase is defined by the formation of oocysts within the feline host. This enteroepithelial cycle begins with the ingestion of the bradyzoite tissue cysts and, after several intermediate stages, culminates in the production of gametes. Gamete fusion produces a zygote, which envelops itself in a rigid wall and is secreted in the feces as an unsporulated oocyst. After 2–3 days of exposure to air at ambient temperature, the noninfectious oocyst sporulates to produce eight sporozoite progeny. The sporulated oocyst can be ingested by an intermediate host, such as a person emptying a cat's litter box or a pig rummaging in a barnyard. It is in the intermediate host that *T. gondii* completes its life cycle.

Sporulated oocysts are environmentally hardy and very infectious; they are thought to be sources of waterborne outbreaks such as those reported in Victoria (British Columbia, Canada) and in South America.

EPIDEMIOLOGY

T. gondii infects a wide range of mammals and birds. Its seroprevalence depends on the locale and the age of the population. Generally, hot arid climatic conditions are associated with a low prevalence of infection. In the United States and most European countries, the seroprevalence increases with age and exposure. For example, in the United States, 5–30% of individuals 10–19 years old and 10–67% of those >50 years old have serologic evidence of exposure. In Central America, France, Turkey, and Brazil, the seroprevalence is higher. Because of increased awareness of foodborne infections, the prevalence of seropositivity has decreased worldwide.

TRANSMISSION

Oral Transmission Most cases of human *Toxoplasma* infection are thought to be acquired by the oral route. Transmission can be attributable to ingestion of sporulated oocysts from contaminated soil, food, or water. During acute feline infection, a cat may excrete as many as 100 million parasites per day. These very stable sporozoite-containing oocysts are highly infectious and may remain viable for many years in soil or water. Humans infected during an oocyst-transmitted infection develop stage-specific antibodies to the oocyst/sporozoite.

Children and adults also can acquire infection from tissue cysts containing bradyzoites. The ingestion of a single cyst is all that is required for human infection. Undercooking or insufficient freezing of meat is an important source of infection in the developed world. In the United States, lamb products and pork products may yield evidence of cysts that contain bradyzoites, but the overall prevalence of *T. gondii* has been gradually decreasing. The incidence in beef is much lower—perhaps as low as 1%. Direct ingestion of bradyzoite cysts in these various meat products leads to acute infection.

Transmission via Blood or Organs In addition to being transmitted orally, *T. gondii* can be transmitted directly from a seropositive donor to a seronegative recipient in a transplanted heart, heart-lung, kidney, liver, or pancreas. Viable parasites can be cultured from refrigerated anticoagulated blood, which may be a source of infection in individuals receiving blood transfusions. *T. gondii* reactivation has been reported in bone marrow, hematopoietic stem cell, and liver transplant recipients as well as in individuals with AIDS. Although antibody titers generally are not useful in monitoring *T. gondii* infection, individuals with higher antibody titers may be at relatively high risk for reactivation after hematopoietic stem cell transplantation; thus routine polymerase chain reaction (PCR) screening of blood from these patients may be in order. Finally, laboratory personnel can be infected after contact with contaminated needles or glassware or with infected tissue.

Transplacental Transmission On average, about one-third of all women who acquire infection with *T. gondii* during pregnancy transmit the parasite to the fetus; the remainder give birth to normal, uninfected babies. Of the various factors that influence fetal outcome, gestational age at the time of infection is the most critical (see below). Few data support a role for recrudescent maternal infection as the source of congenital disease, although rare cases of transmission by immunocompromised women (e.g., those infected with HIV or those receiving high-dose glucocorticoids) have been reported. Thus, women who are seropositive before pregnancy usually are protected against acute infection and do not give birth to congenitally infected neonates.

The following general guidelines can be used to evaluate congenital infection. There is essentially no risk if the mother becomes infected ≥6 months before conception. If infection is acquired <6 months before conception, the likelihood of transplacental infection increases as the interval between infection and conception decreases. Women with documented acute toxoplasmosis should be counseled to use appropriate measures to prevent pregnancy for 6 months after infection. In pregnancy, if the mother becomes infected during the first trimester, the incidence of transplacental infection is lowest (~15%), but the disease in the neonate is most severe. If maternal infection occurs during the third trimester, the incidence of transplacental infection is greatest (65%), but the infant is usually asymptomatic at birth. Infected infants who are normal at birth may have a higher incidence of learning disabilities and chronic neurologic sequelae than uninfected children. Only a small proportion (20%) of women infected with *T. gondii* develop clinical signs of infection. Often the diagnosis is first appreciated when routine postconception serologic tests show evidence of specific antibody.

PATHOGENESIS

Upon the host's ingestion of either tissue cysts containing bradyzoites or oocysts containing sporozoites, the parasites are released from the cysts by the digestive process. Bradyzoites are resistant to the effect of pepsin and invade the host's gastrointestinal tract. Within enterocytes (or other gut-associated cells), the parasites undergo morphologic transformation, giving rise to invasive tachyzoites. These tachyzoites induce a parasite-specific secretory IgA response. From the gastrointestinal tract, parasites disseminate to a variety of organs, particularly lymphatic tissue, skeletal muscle, myocardium, retina, placenta, and the CNS. At these sites, the parasite infects host cells, replicates, and invades the adjoining cells. In this fashion, the hallmarks of the infection develop: cell death and focal necrosis surrounded by an acute inflammatory response.

In the immunocompetent host, both the humoral and the cellular immune responses control infection; parasite virulence and tissue tropism may be strain specific. Tachyzoites are sequestered by a variety of immune mechanisms, including induction of parasiticidal antibody, activation of macrophages with radical intermediates, production of interferon γ (IFN-γ), and stimulation of CD8+ cytotoxic T lymphocytes. These antigen-specific lymphocytes are capable of killing both extracellular parasites and target cells infected with parasites. As tachyzoites are cleared from the acutely infected host, tissue cysts containing bradyzoites begin to appear, usually within the CNS and the retina. Studies indicate that *Toxoplasma* secretes signaling molecules into infected host cells and that these molecules modulate host gene expression, host metabolism, and host immune response. While it was initially thought that cysts with bradyzoites are not eliminated by the immune system, recent studies in the murine model indicate that both CD8+ T cells and alternatively activated macrophages are able to kill cysts in vivo; some cysts persist, however, and the ability to eliminate cysts may depend on the genetic background of the infected host.

In the immunocompromised or fetal host, the immune factors necessary to control the spread of tachyzoite infection are lacking. This altered immune state allows the persistence of tachyzoites and gives rise to progressive focal destruction that results in organ failure (i.e., necrotizing encephalitis, pneumonia, and myocarditis).

It is thought that all infected individuals have persistent infection with cysts containing bradyzoites, but this lifelong infection usually remains subclinical. Although bradyzoites are in a slow metabolic phase, cysts do degenerate and rupture within the CNS. This degenerative process, with the development of new bradyzoite-containing cysts, is the most probable source of recrudescent infection in immunocompromised individuals and the most likely stimulus for the persistence of antibody titers in the immunocompetent host. Although the concept is controversial, the persistence of toxoplasmosis has been hypothesized to be a contributing factor to a variety of neuropsychiatric conditions, including schizophrenia and bipolar disease. In rodents, infection clearly has significant effects on behavior, increasing predation.

PATHOLOGY

Cell death and focal necrosis due to replicating tachyzoites induce an intense mononuclear inflammatory response in any tissue or cell type infected. Tachyzoites rarely can be visualized by routine histopathologic staining of these inflammatory lesions. However, immunofluorescent staining with parasitic antigen–specific antibodies can reveal either the organism itself or evidence of antigen. In contrast to this inflammatory process caused by tachyzoites, bradyzoite-containing cysts cause inflammation only at the early stages of development, and even this inflammation may be a response to the presence of tachyzoite antigens. Once the cysts reach maturity, the inflammatory process can no longer be detected, and the cysts remain immunologically quiescent within the brain matrix until they rupture.

Lymph Nodes During acute infection, lymph node biopsy demonstrates characteristic findings, including follicular hyperplasia and irregular clusters of tissue macrophages with eosinophilic cytoplasm. Granulomas rarely are evident in these specimens. Although tachyzoites are not usually visible, they can be sought either by subinoculation of infected tissue into mice, with resultant disease, or by PCR. PCR amplification of DNA fragments of *Toxoplasma* genes is effective and sensitive in establishing lymph node infection by tachyzoites.

Eyes In the eye, infiltrates of monocytes, lymphocytes, and plasma cells may produce uni- or multifocal lesions. Granulomatous lesions and chorioretinitis can be observed in the posterior chamber after acute necrotizing retinitis. Other ocular complications include iridocyclitis, cataracts, and glaucoma.

Central Nervous System During CNS involvement, both focal and diffuse meningoencephalitis can be documented, with evidence of necrosis and microglial nodules. Necrotizing encephalitis in patients without AIDS is characterized by small diffuse lesions with perivascular cuffing in contiguous areas. In the AIDS population, polymorphonuclear leukocytes may be present in addition to monocytes, lymphocytes, and plasma cells. Cysts containing bradyzoites frequently are found contiguous with the necrotic tissue border. As a consequence of combined antiretroviral therapy (cART) for AIDS, the incidence of toxoplasmosis has decreased in the developed world. Its incidence in under-resourced settings is not known.

Lungs and Heart Among patients with AIDS who die of toxoplasmosis, 40–70% have involvement of the lungs and heart. Interstitial pneumonitis can develop in neonates and immunocompromised patients. Thickened and edematous alveolar septa infiltrated with mononuclear and plasma cells are apparent. This inflammation may extend to the endothelial walls. Tachyzoites and bradyzoite-containing cysts have been observed within the alveolar membrane. Superimposed bronchopneumonia can be caused by other microbial agents. Cysts and aggregates of parasites in cardiac muscle tissue are evident in patients with AIDS who die of toxoplasmosis. Focal necrosis surrounded by inflammatory cells is associated with hyaline necrosis and disrupted myocardial cells. Pericarditis is associated with toxoplasmosis in some patients.

Gastrointestinal Tract Rare cases of human gastrointestinal tract infection with *T. gondii* have presented as ulcerations in the mucosa. Acute infection in certain strains of inbred mice (C57BL/6) results in lethal ileitis within 7–9 days. This inflammatory bowel disease has been recognized in several other mammalian species, including pigs and nonhuman primates. Although the association between human inflammatory bowel disease and either acute or recurrent *Toxoplasma* infection has not been established, studies have demonstrated recognition of the infection by human intestinal epithelial cells, as evidenced by mitogen-activated protein kinase phosphorylation, nuclear factor κB translocation, and interleukin (IL) 8 secretion.

Other Sites Pathologic changes during disseminated infection are similar to those described for the lymph nodes, eyes, and CNS. In patients with AIDS, the skeletal muscle, pancreas, stomach, and kidneys can be involved, with necrosis, invasion by inflammatory cells, and (rarely) tachyzoites detectable by routine staining. Large necrotic lesions may cause direct tissue destruction. In addition, secondary effects from acute infection of these various organs, including pancreatitis, myositis, and glomerulonephritis, have been reported.

HOST IMMUNE RESPONSE

Acute *Toxoplasma* infection evokes a cascade of protective immune responses in the immunocompetent host. *Toxoplasma* enters the host at the gut mucosal level and evokes a mucosal immune response that includes the production of antigen-specific secretory IgA. Titers of serum IgA antibody directed at p30 (SAG1) are a useful marker for congenital and acute toxoplasmosis. Milk-whey IgA from acutely infected mothers contains a high titer of antibody to *T. gondii* and can block infection of enterocytes in vitro. In mice, IgA intestinal secretions directed at the parasite are abundant and are associated with the induction of mucosal T cells.

Within the host, *T. gondii* rapidly induces detectable levels of both IgM and IgG serum antibodies. Monoclonal gammopathy of the IgG class can occur in congenitally infected infants. IgM levels may be increased in newborns with congenital infection. The polyclonal IgG antibodies evoked by infection are parasiticidal in vitro in the presence of serum complement and are the basis for the Sabin-Feldman dye test. However, cell-mediated immunity is the major protective response evoked by the parasite during host infection. Macrophages are activated after phagocytosis of antibody-opsonized parasites. This activation can lead to death of the parasite by either an oxygen-dependent or an oxygen-independent process. If the parasite is not phagocytosed and enters the macrophage by active penetration, it continues to replicate, and this replication may represent the mechanism for transport and dissemination to distant organs. *Toxoplasma* stimulates a robust IL-12 response by human dendritic cells. The requirement for costimulation via CD40/154 has been established. The CD4+ and CD8+ T cell responses are antigen-specific and further stimulate the production of a variety of important lymphokines that expand the T cell and natural killer cell repertoire. *T. gondii* is a potent inducer of a T_H1 phenotype, with IL-12 and IFN-γ playing an essential role in the control of the parasites' growth in the host. Regulation of the inflammatory response is at least partially under the control of a T_H2 response that includes the production of IL-4 and IL-10 in seropositive individuals. Both asymptomatic patients and those with active infection may have a depressed CD4+-to-CD8+ ratio. This shift may be correlated with a disease syndrome but is not necessarily correlated with disease outcome. Human T cell clones of both the CD4+ and the CD8+ phenotypes are cytolytic against parasite-infected macrophages. These T cell clones produce cytokines that are "microbistatic." IL-18, IL-7, and IL-15 upregulate the production of IFN-γ and may be important during acute and chronic infection. The effect of IFN-γ may be paradoxical, with stimulation of a host down-regulatory response as well.

Although *T. gondii* infection is believed to be recrudescent in patients with AIDS or other immunocompromised states, antibody titers are not useful in establishing reactivation or in following the activity of infection. An absence of positive serologies suggests an alternative diagnosis, although AIDS patients may have borderline positive or low serologies. T cells from AIDS patients with reactivation of toxoplasmosis fail to secrete both IFN-γ and IL-2. This alteration in the production of these critical immune cytokines contributes to the persistence of infection. *Toxoplasma* infection frequently develops late in the course of AIDS, when the loss of T cell–dependent protective mechanisms, particularly CD8+ T cells, becomes most pronounced.

CLINICAL MANIFESTATIONS

In persons whose immune systems are intact, acute toxoplasmosis is usually asymptomatic and self-limited. This condition can go unrecognized in 80–90% of adults and children with acquired infection. The asymptomatic nature of this infection makes diagnosis difficult in mothers infected during pregnancy. In contrast, the wide range of clinical manifestations in congenitally infected children includes severe neurologic complications such as hydrocephalus, microcephaly, mental retardation, and chorioretinitis. If prenatal infection is severe, multiorgan failure and subsequent intrauterine fetal death can occur. In children and adults, chronic infection can persist throughout life, with little consequence to the immunocompetent host.

Toxoplasmosis in Immunocompetent Patients The most common manifestation of acute toxoplasmosis is cervical lymphadenopathy. The nodes may be single or multiple, are usually nontender, are discrete, and vary in firmness. Lymphadenopathy also may be found in suboccipital, supraclavicular, inguinal, and mediastinal areas. Generalized lymphadenopathy occurs in 20–30% of symptomatic patients. Between 20% and 40% of patients with lymphadenopathy also have headache, malaise, fatigue, and fever (usually with a temperature of <40°C [<104°F]). A smaller proportion of symptomatic individuals have myalgia, sore throat, abdominal pain, maculopapular rash, meningoencephalitis, and confusion. Rare complications associated with infection in the normal immune host include pneumonia, myocarditis, encephalopathy, pericarditis, and polymyositis. Signs and symptoms associated with acute infection usually resolve within several weeks, although the lymphadenopathy may persist for some months. In one epidemic, toxoplasmosis was diagnosed correctly in only 3 of the 25 patients who consulted physicians. If toxoplasmosis is considered in the differential diagnosis, routine laboratory and serologic screening should precede node biopsy.

It is now appreciated that genotypes of *T. gondii* prevalent in South America may be more virulent than those typically seen in North America or Europe. These genotypes may be associated with acute or recurrent ocular disease in immunocompetent individuals and have also been associated with pneumonitis and a fulminant sepsis picture in immunologically normal individuals. Thus a detailed history is critical for establishing a diagnosis.

The results of routine laboratory studies are usually unremarkable except for minimal lymphocytosis, an elevated erythrocyte sedimentation rate, and a nominal increase in serum aminotransferase levels. Evaluation of cerebrospinal fluid (CSF) in cases with evidence of encephalopathy or meningoencephalitis shows an elevation of intracranial pressure, mononuclear pleocytosis (10–50 cells/mL), a slight increase in protein concentration, and (occasionally) an increase in the gamma globulin level. PCR amplification of the *Toxoplasma* DNA target sequence in CSF may be beneficial. The CSF of chronically infected individuals is normal.

Infection of Immunocompromised Patients Patients with AIDS and those receiving immunosuppressive therapy for lymphoproliferative disorders are at greatest risk for developing acute toxoplasmosis. Toxoplasmosis has also been reported after treatment with antibodies to tumor necrosis factor. The infection may be due either to reactivation of latent infection or to acquisition of parasites from exogenous sources such as blood or transplanted organs. In individuals with AIDS, >95% of cases of *Toxoplasma* encephalitis (TE) are believed to be due to recrudescent infection. In most of these cases, encephalitis develops when the CD4+ T cell count falls below 100/μL. In immunocompromised hosts, the disease may be rapidly fatal if untreated. Thus, accurate diagnosis and initiation of appropriate therapy are necessary to prevent fulminant infection.

Toxoplasmosis is a principal opportunistic infection of the CNS in persons with AIDS. Although geographic origin may be related to frequency of infection, it has no correlation with the severity of disease in immunocompromised hosts. Individuals with AIDS who are seropositive for *T. gondii* are at high risk for encephalitis. Before the advent of current cART, about one-third of the 15–40% of adult AIDS patients in the United States who were latently infected with *T. gondii* developed TE. TE may still be a presenting infection in individuals who are unaware of their positive HIV status.

The signs and symptoms of acute toxoplasmosis in immunocompromised patients principally involve the CNS (Fig. 253-2). More than 50% of patients with clinical manifestations have intracerebral involvement. Clinical findings at presentation range from nonfocal to focal dysfunction. CNS findings include encephalopathy, meningoencephalitis, and mass lesions. Patients may present with altered mental status (75%), fever (10–72%), seizures (33%), headaches (56%), and focal neurologic findings (60%), including motor deficits, cranial nerve

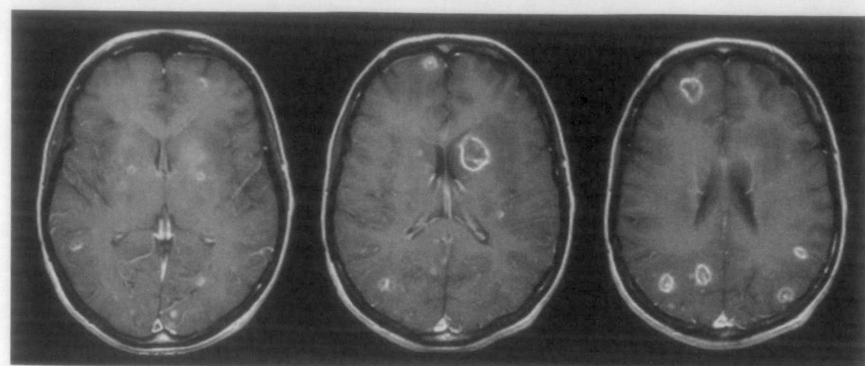

FIGURE 253-2 Toxoplasmic encephalitis in a 36-year-old patient with AIDS. The multiple lesions are demonstrated by MRI scanning (T1-weighted with gadolinium enhancement). *(Courtesy of Clifford Eskey, Dartmouth Hitchcock Medical Center, Hanover, NH; with permission.)*

palsies, movement disorders, dysmetria, visual-field loss, and aphasia. Patients who present with evidence of diffuse cortical dysfunction develop evidence of focal neurologic disease as infection progresses. This altered condition is due not only to the necrotizing encephalitis caused by direct invasion by the parasite but also to secondary effects, including vasculitis, edema, and hemorrhage. The onset of infection can range from an insidious process over several weeks to an acute presentation with fulminant focal deficits, including hemiparesis, hemiplegia, visual-field defects, localized headache, and focal seizures.

Although lesions can occur anywhere in the CNS, the areas most often involved appear to be the brainstem, basal ganglia, pituitary gland, and corticomedullary junction. Brainstem involvement gives rise to a variety of neurologic dysfunctions, including cranial nerve palsy, dysmetria, and ataxia. With basal ganglionic infection, patients may develop hydrocephalus, choreiform movements, and choreoathetosis. *Toxoplasma* usually causes encephalitis, and meningeal involvement is uncommon. CSF findings may be unremarkable or may include a modest increase in cell count and in protein—but not glucose—concentration. Nonetheless, the parasite may be detected by PCR in CSF from many patients with TE.

Cerebral toxoplasmosis must be differentiated from other opportunistic infections or tumors in the CNS of AIDS patients. The differential diagnosis includes herpes simplex encephalitis, cryptococcal meningitis, progressive multifocal leukoencephalopathy, and primary CNS lymphoma. Involvement of the pituitary gland can give rise to panhypopituitarism and hyponatremia from inappropriate secretion of vasopressin (antidiuretic hormone). HIV-associated neurocognitive disorder (HAND) may present as cognitive impairment, attention loss, and altered memory. Brain biopsy in patients who have been treated for TE but who continue to exhibit neurologic dysfunction often fails to identify organisms.

Autopsies of *Toxoplasma*-infected patients have demonstrated the involvement of multiple organs, including the lungs, gastrointestinal tract, pancreas, skin, eyes, heart, and liver. *Toxoplasma* pneumonia can be confused with *Pneumocystis* pneumonia (PcP). Respiratory involvement usually presents as dyspnea, fever, and a nonproductive cough and may rapidly progress to acute respiratory failure with hemoptysis, metabolic acidosis, hypotension, and (occasionally) disseminated intravascular coagulation. Histopathologic studies demonstrate necrosis and a mixed cellular infiltrate. The presence of organisms is a helpful diagnostic indicator, but organisms can also be found in healthy tissue. Infection of the heart is usually asymptomatic but can be associated with cardiac tamponade or biventricular failure. Infections of the gastrointestinal tract and the liver have been documented.

Congenital Toxoplasmosis Between 400 and 4000 infants born each year in the United States are affected by congenital toxoplasmosis. Acute infection in mothers acquiring *T. gondii* during pregnancy is usually asymptomatic; most such women are diagnosed via prenatal serologic screening. Infection of the placenta leads to hematogenous infection of the fetus. As gestation proceeds, the proportion of fetuses that become infected increases, but the clinical severity of the infection declines. Although infected children may initially be asymptomatic, the persistence of *T. gondii* can result in reactivation and clinical disease—most frequently chorioretinitis—decades later. Factors associated with relatively severe disabilities include delays in diagnosis and in initiation of therapy, neonatal hypoxia and hypoglycemia, profound visual impairment (see "Ocular Infection," below), uncorrected hydrocephalus, and increased intracranial pressure. If treated appropriately, upwards of 70% of children have normal developmental, neurologic, and ophthalmologic findings at follow-up evaluations. Treatment for 1 year with pyrimethamine, a sulfonamide, and folinic acid is tolerated with minimal toxicity (see "Treatment," below).

Ocular Infection Infection with *T. gondii* is estimated to cause 35% of all cases of chorioretinitis in the United States and Europe. It was formerly thought that the majority of cases of ocular disease were due to congenital infection. New ocular toxoplasmosis in immunocompetent individuals occurs more commonly than was previously appreciated and has been associated with outbreaks in Victoria (British Columbia) and in South America. A variety of ocular manifestations are documented, including blurred vision, scotoma, photophobia, and eye pain. Macular involvement occurs, with loss of central vision, and nystagmus is secondary to poor fixation. Involvement of the extraocular muscles may lead to disorders of convergence and to strabismus. Ophthalmologic examination should be undertaken in newborns with suspected congenital infection. As the inflammation resolves, vision improves, but episodic flare-ups of chorioretinitis, which progressively destroy retinal tissue and lead to glaucoma, are common. The ophthalmologic examination reveals yellow-white, cotton-like patches with indistinct margins of hyperemia. As the lesions age, white plaques with distinct borders and black spots within the retinal pigment become more apparent. Lesions usually are located near the posterior pole of the retina; they may be single but are more commonly multiple. Congenital lesions may be unilateral or bilateral and show evidence of massive chorioretinal degeneration with extensive fibrosis. Surrounding these areas of involvement are a normal retina and vasculature. In patients with AIDS, retinal lesions are often large, with diffuse retinal necrosis, and include both free tachyzoites and cysts containing bradyzoites. Toxoplasmic chorioretinitis may be a prodrome to the development of encephalitis.

DIAGNOSIS

Tissue and Body Fluids The differential diagnosis of acute toxoplasmosis can be made by appropriate culture, serologic testing, and PCR (Table 253-1). Although available only at specialized laboratories, the isolation of *T. gondii* from blood or other body fluids can be accomplished after subinoculation of the sample into the peritoneal cavity of mice. If no parasites are found in the mouse's peritoneal fluid 6–10 days after inoculation, its anti-*Toxoplasma* serum titer can be evaluated 4–6 weeks after inoculation. Isolation of *T. gondii* from the patient's body fluids reflects acute infection, whereas isolation from biopsied tissue is an indication only of the presence of tissue cysts and should not be misinterpreted as evidence of acute toxoplasmosis. Persistent parasitemia in patients with latent, asymptomatic infection is rare. Histologic examination of lymph nodes may suggest the characteristic changes described above. Demonstration of tachyzoites in lymph nodes establishes the diagnosis of acute toxoplasmosis. Like subinoculation into mice, histologic demonstration of cysts containing bradyzoites confirms prior infection with *T. gondii* but is nondiagnostic for acute infection.

Serology The procedures mentioned above have great diagnostic value but are limited by difficulties encountered either in the growth

TABLE 253-1 DIFFERENTIAL LABORATORY DIAGNOSIS OF TOXOPLASMOSIS

Clinical Setting	Alternative Diagnosis	Distinguishing Characteristics
Mononucleosis syndrome	Epstein-Barr virus infection	Serology
	Cytomegalovirus infection	Serology/PCR or culture
	HIV infection	Serology/viral load
	Bartonella infection (cat-scratch disease)	Biopsy (PCR or culture)/serology
	Lymphoma	Biopsy
Congenital infection	Cytomegalovirus infection	Viral culture/PCR
	Herpes simplex virus infection	Viral culture/PCR
	Rubella virus infection	Viral culture/serology
	Syphilis	Serology
	Listeriosis	Bacterial culture
Chorioretinitis in immunocompetent individual	Tuberculosis	Bacterial culture
	Syphilis	Serology
	Histoplasmosis	Serology/culture
Chorioretinitis in AIDS patient	Cytomegalovirus infection	Viral culture/PCR
	Syphilis	Serology
	Herpes simplex virus infection	Viral culture/PCR
	Varicella-zoster virus infection	Viral culture/PCR
	Fungal infection	Culture
CNS lesions in AIDS patient	Lymphoma or metastatic tumor	Tissue biopsy
	Brain abscess	Biopsy and culture
	Progressive multifocal leukoencephalopathy	PCR for JC virus
	Fungal infection	Biopsy and culture
	Mycobacterial infection	Biopsy and culture

Abbreviations: CNS, central nervous system; PCR, polymerase chain reaction.

Source: Adapted from JD Schwartzman: Toxoplasmosis, *in Principles and Practice of Clinical Parasitology*. Hoboken, Wiley, 2001.

of parasites in vivo or in the identification of tachyzoites by histochemical methods. Serologic testing has become the routine method of diagnosis.

Diagnosis of acute infection with *T. gondii* can be established by detection of the simultaneous presence of IgG and IgM antibodies to *Toxoplasma* in serum. The presence of circulating IgA favors the diagnosis of an acute infection. The Sabin-Feldman dye test, the indirect fluorescent antibody test, and the enzyme-linked immunosorbent assay (ELISA) all satisfactorily measure circulating IgG antibody to *Toxoplasma*. Positive IgG titers (>1:10) can be detected as early as 2–3 weeks after infection. These titers usually peak at 6–8 weeks and decline slowly to a new baseline level that persists for life. Antibody avidity increases with time and can be useful in difficult cases during pregnancy for establishing when infection may have occurred. The serum IgM titer should be measured in concert with the IgG titer to better establish the time of infection; either the double-sandwich IgM-ELISA or the IgM-immunosorbent assay (IgM-ISAGA) should be used. Both assays are specific and sensitive, with fewer false-positive results than other commercial tests. The double-sandwich IgA-ELISA is more sensitive than the IgM-ELISA for detecting congenital infection in the fetus and newborn. Although a negative IgM result with a positive IgG titer indicates distant infection, IgM can persist for >1 year and should not necessarily be considered a reflection of acute disease. If acute toxoplasmosis is suspected, a more extensive panel of serologic tests can be performed. In the United States, testing is available at the *Toxoplasma* Serology Laboratory at Palo Alto Medical Foundation (*http://www.pamf.org/serology/clinicianguide.html*).

Molecular Diagnostics Molecular approaches can directly detect *T. gondii* in biologic samples independent of the serologic response. Results obtained with PCR have suggested high sensitivity, specificity, and clinical utility in the diagnosis of TE, and PCR technology may be becoming more readily available in resource-poor settings. Real-time PCR is a promising technique that can provide quantitative results. Isolates can be genotyped and polymorphic sequences can be obtained, with consequent identification of the precise strain. Molecular epidemiologic studies with polymorphic markers have been useful in correlating clinical signs and symptoms of disease with different *T. gondii* genotypes.

The Immunocompetent Adult or Child For the patient who presents with lymphadenopathy only, a positive IgM titer is an indication of acute infection—and an indication for therapy, if clinically warranted (see "Treatment," below). The serum IgM titer should be determined again in 3 weeks. An elevation in the IgG titer without an increase in the IgM titer suggests that infection is present but is not acute. If there is a borderline increase in either IgG or IgM, the titers should be reassessed in 3–4 weeks.

The Immunocompromised Host A presumptive clinical diagnosis of TE in patients with AIDS is based on clinical presentation, history of exposure (as evidenced by positive serology), and radiologic evaluation. To detect latent infection with *T. gondii*, HIV-infected persons should be tested for IgG antibody to *Toxoplasma* soon after HIV infection is diagnosed. When these criteria are used, the predictive value is as high as 80%. More than 97% of patients with AIDS and toxoplasmosis have IgG antibody to *T. gondii* in serum. IgM serum antibody usually is not detectable. Although IgG titers do not correlate with active infection, serologic evidence of infection virtually always precedes the development of TE. It is therefore important to determine the *Toxoplasma* antibody status of all patients infected with HIV. Antibody titers may range from negative to 1:1024 in patients with AIDS and TE. Fewer than 3% of patients have no demonstrable antibody to *Toxoplasma* at diagnosis of TE.

Patients with TE have focal or multifocal abnormalities demonstrable by CT or MRI. Neuroradiologic evaluation should include double-dose contrast CT of the head. By this test, single and frequently multiple contrast-enhancing lesions (<2 cm) may be identified. MRI usually demonstrates multiple lesions located in both hemispheres, with the basal ganglia and corticomedullary junction most commonly involved; MRI provides a more sensitive evaluation of the efficacy of therapy than does CT (Fig. 253-2). These findings are not pathognomonic of *Toxoplasma* infection, because 40% of CNS lymphomas are multifocal and 50% are ring-enhancing. For both MRI and CT scans, the rate of false-negative results is ~10%. The finding of a single lesion on an MRI scan increases the likelihood of primary CNS lymphoma (in which solitary lesions are four times more likely than in TE) and strengthens the argument for the performance of a brain biopsy. A therapeutic trial of anti-*Toxoplasma* medications is frequently used to assess the diagnosis. Treatment of presumptive TE with pyrimethamine plus sulfadiazine or clindamycin results in quantifiable clinical improvement in >50% of patients by day 3. Leucovorin is administered to prevent bone marrow toxicity. By day 7, >90% of treated patients show evidence of improvement. In contrast, if patients fail to respond or have lymphoma, clinical signs and symptoms worsen by day 7. Patients in this category require brain biopsy with or without a change in therapy. This procedure can now be performed by a stereotactic CT-guided method that reduces the potential for complications. Brain biopsy for *T. gondii* identifies organisms in 50–75% of cases. PCR amplification of CSF may also confirm toxoplasmosis or suggest alternative diagnoses (Table 253-1), such as progressive multifocal leukoencephalopathy (JC virus positive) or primary CNS lymphoma (Epstein-Barr virus positive).

CT and MRI with contrast are currently the standard diagnostic imaging tests for TE. As in other conditions, the radiologic response may lag behind the clinical response. Resolution of lesions may take from 3 weeks to 6 months. Some patients show clinical improvement despite worsening radiographic findings.

Congenital Infection The issue of concern when a pregnant woman has evidence of recent *T. gondii* infection is whether the fetus is infected. PCR analysis of the amniotic fluid for the B1 gene of *T. gondii* has replaced fetal blood sampling. Serologic diagnosis is based on the persistence of IgG antibody or a positive IgM titer after the first week of life (a time frame that excludes placental leak). The IgG determination should be repeated every 2 months. An increase in IgM beyond the first week of life is indicative of acute infection. Up to 25% of infected newborns may be seronegative and have normal routine physical examinations. Thus assessment of the eye and the brain, with ophthalmologic testing, CSF evaluation, and radiologic studies, is important in establishing the diagnosis.

Ocular Toxoplasmosis The serum antibody titer may not correlate with the presence of active lesions in the fundus, particularly in cases of congenital toxoplasmosis. In general, a positive IgG titer (measured in undiluted serum if necessary) in conjunction with typical lesions establishes the diagnosis. Antibody production in ocular fluids, expressed in terms of the Goldmann-Witmer coefficient, has been described for diagnosis of ocular disease but does not always correlate with PCR results. If lesions are atypical and the serum antibody titer is in the low-positive range, the diagnosis is presumptive. The parasitic antigen–specific polyclonal IgG assay as well as parasite-specific PCR may facilitate the diagnosis. Accordingly, the clinical diagnosis of ocular toxoplasmosis can be supported in 60–90% of cases by laboratory tests, depending on the time of anterior chamber puncture and the panel of antibody analyses used. In the remaining cases, the possibility of a falsely negative laboratory diagnosis or of an incorrect clinical diagnosis cannot be clarified further.

TREATMENT TOXOPLASMOSIS

CONGENITAL INFECTION

Congenitally infected neonates are treated with daily oral pyrimethamine (1 mg/kg) and sulfadiazine (100 mg/kg) with folinic acid for 1 year. Depending on the signs and symptoms, prednisone (1 mg/kg per day) may be used for congenital infection. Some U.S. states and some countries routinely screen pregnant women (France, Austria) and/or newborns (Denmark, Massachusetts). Management and treatment regimens vary with the country and the treatment center. Most experts use spiramycin to treat pregnant women who have acute toxoplasmosis early in pregnancy and use pyrimethamine/sulfadiazine/folinic acid to treat women who seroconvert after 18 weeks of pregnancy or in cases of documented fetal infection. This treatment is somewhat controversial: clinical studies, which have included few untreated women, have not proven the efficacy of such therapy in preventing congenital toxoplasmosis. However, studies do suggest that treatment during pregnancy decreases the severity of infection. Many women who are infected in the first trimester elect termination of pregnancy. Those who do not terminate pregnancy are offered prenatal antibiotic therapy to reduce the frequency and severity of *Toxoplasma* infection in the infant. The optimal duration of treatment for a child with asymptomatic congenital toxoplasmosis is not clear, although most clinicians in the United States would treat the child for 1 year in light of cohort investigations conducted by the National Collaborative Chicago-Based, Congenital Toxoplasmosis Study.

INFECTION IN IMMUNOCOMPETENT PATIENTS

Immunologically competent adults and older children who have only lymphadenopathy do not require specific therapy unless they have persistent, severe symptoms. Patients with ocular toxoplasmosis are usually treated for 1 month with pyrimethamine plus either sulfadiazine or clindamycin and sometimes with prednisone. Treatment should be supervised by an ophthalmologist familiar with *Toxoplasma* disease. Ocular disease can be self-limited without treatment, but therapy is typically considered for lesions that are severe or close to the fovea or optic disc.

INFECTION IN IMMUNOCOMPROMISED PATIENTS

Primary Prophylaxis Patients with AIDS should be treated for acute toxoplasmosis; in immunocompromised patients, toxoplasmosis is rapidly fatal if untreated. Before the introduction of cART, the median survival time was >1 year for patients who could tolerate treatment for TE. Despite their toxicity, the drugs used to treat TE were required for survival prior to cART. The incidence of TE has declined as the survival of patients with HIV infection has increased through the use of cART.

In Africa, many patients are diagnosed with HIV infection only after developing opportunistic infections. Hence, the optimal management of these opportunistic infections is important if the benefits of subsequent cART are to be realized. The incidence of TE in under-resourced settings is not clear because of a lack of facilities for serologic testing and imaging. AIDS patients who are seropositive for *T. gondii* and who have a CD4+ T lymphocyte count of <100/μL should receive prophylaxis against TE.

Of the currently available agents, trimethoprim-sulfamethoxazole (TMP-SMX) appears to be an effective alternative for treatment of TE in resource-poor settings where the preferred combination of pyrimethamine plus sulfadiazine is not available. The daily dose of TMP-SMX (one double-strength tablet) that is recommended as the preferred regimen for prophylaxis of PcP is effective against TE. If patients cannot tolerate TMP-SMX, the recommended alternative is dapsone-pyrimethamine, which likewise is effective against PcP. Atovaquone with or without pyrimethamine also can be considered. Prophylactic monotherapy with dapsone, pyrimethamine, azithromycin, clarithromycin, or aerosolized pentamidine is probably insufficient. AIDS patients who are seronegative for *Toxoplasma* and are not receiving prophylaxis for PcP should be retested for IgG antibody to *Toxoplasma* if their CD4+ T cell count drops to <100/μL. If seroconversion has taken place, then the patient should be given prophylaxis as described above.

Discontinuing Primary Prophylaxis Current studies indicate that prophylaxis against TE can be discontinued in patients who have responded to cART and whose CD4+ T lymphocyte count has been >200/μL for 3 months. Although patients with CD4+ T lymphocyte counts of <100/μL are at greatest risk for developing TE, the risk that this condition will develop when the count has increased to 100–200/μL has not been established. Thus, prophylaxis should be discontinued when the count has increased to >200/μL. Discontinuation of therapy reduces the pill burden; the potential for drug toxicity, drug interaction, or selection of drug-resistant pathogens; and cost. Prophylaxis should be recommenced if the CD4+ T lymphocyte count again decreases to <100–200/μL.

Individuals who have completed initial therapy for TE should receive treatment indefinitely unless immune reconstitution, with a CD4+ T cell count of >200/μL, occurs as a consequence of cART. Combination therapy with pyrimethamine plus sulfadiazine plus leucovorin is effective for this purpose. An alternative to sulfadiazine in this regimen is clindamycin.

Discontinuing Secondary Prophylaxis (Long-Term Maintenance Therapy) Patients receiving secondary prophylaxis for TE are at low risk for recurrence when they have completed initial therapy for TE, remain asymptomatic, and have evidence of restored immune function. Individuals with HIV infection should have a CD4+ T lymphocyte count of >200/μL for at least 6 months after cART. This recommendation is consistent with more extensive data indicating the safety of discontinuing secondary prophylaxis for other opportunistic infections during advanced HIV disease. A repeat MRI brain scan is recommended. Secondary prophylaxis should be reintroduced if the CD4+ T lymphocyte count decreases to <200/μL.

PREVENTION

All HIV-infected persons should be counseled regarding sources of *Toxoplasma* infection. The chances of primary infection with *Toxoplasma* can be reduced by not eating undercooked meat and by avoiding oocyst-contaminated material (i.e., a cat's litter box). Specifically, lamb, beef, and pork should be cooked to an internal temperature of 165°–170°F; from a more practical perspective, meat cooked until it is no longer pink inside usually satisfies this requirement. Hands should be washed thoroughly after work in the garden, and all fruits and vegetables should be washed. Ingestion of raw shellfish is a risk factor for toxoplasmosis, given that the filter-feeding mechanism of clams and mussels concentrates oocysts.

If the patient owns a cat, the litter box should be cleaned or changed daily, preferably by an HIV-negative, nonpregnant person; alternatively, patients should wash their hands thoroughly after changing the litter box. Litter boxes should be changed daily if possible, as freshly excreted oocysts will not have sporulated and will not be infectious. Patients should be encouraged to keep their cats inside and not to adopt or handle stray cats. Cats should be fed only canned or dried commercial food or well-cooked table food, not raw or undercooked meats. Patients need not be advised to part with their cats or to have their cats tested for toxoplasmosis. Blood intended for transfusion into *Toxoplasma*-seronegative immunocompromised individuals should be screened for antibody to *T. gondii*. Although such serologic screening is not routinely performed, seronegative women should be screened for evidence of infection several times during pregnancy if they are exposed to environmental conditions that put them at risk for infection with *T. gondii*. HIV-positive individuals should adhere closely to these preventive measures.

254 Protozoal Intestinal Infections and Trichomoniasis

Peter F. Weller

PROTOZOAL INFECTIONS

GIARDIASIS

Giardia intestinalis (also known as *G. lamblia* or *G. duodenalis*) is a cosmopolitan protozoal parasite that inhabits the small intestines of humans and other mammals. Giardiasis is one of the most common parasitic diseases in both developed and developing countries worldwide, causing both endemic and epidemic intestinal disease and diarrhea.

Life Cycle and Epidemiology (Fig. 254-1) Infection follows the ingestion of environmentally hardy cysts, which excyst in the small intestine, releasing flagellated trophozoites (Fig. 254-2) that multiply by binary fission. *Giardia* remains a pathogen of the proximal small bowel and does not disseminate hematogenously. Trophozoites remain free in the lumen or attach to the mucosal epithelium by means of a ventral sucking disk. As a trophozoite encounters altered conditions, it forms a morphologically distinct cyst, which is the stage of the parasite usually found in the feces. Trophozoites may be present and even predominate in loose or watery stools, but it is the resistant cyst that survives outside the body and is responsible for transmission. Cysts do not tolerate heating or desiccation, but they do remain viable for months in cold fresh water. The number of cysts excreted varies widely but can approach 10^7 per gram of stool.

Ingestion of as few as 10 cysts is sufficient to cause infection in humans. Because cysts are infectious when excreted, person-to-person transmission occurs where fecal hygiene is poor. Giardiasis is especially prevalent in day-care centers; person-to-person spread also takes place in other institutional settings with poor fecal hygiene and during anal-oral contact. If food is contaminated with *Giardia* cysts after cooking or preparation, food-borne transmission can occur. Waterborne transmission accounts for episodic infections (e.g., in campers and travelers) and for major epidemics in metropolitan areas.

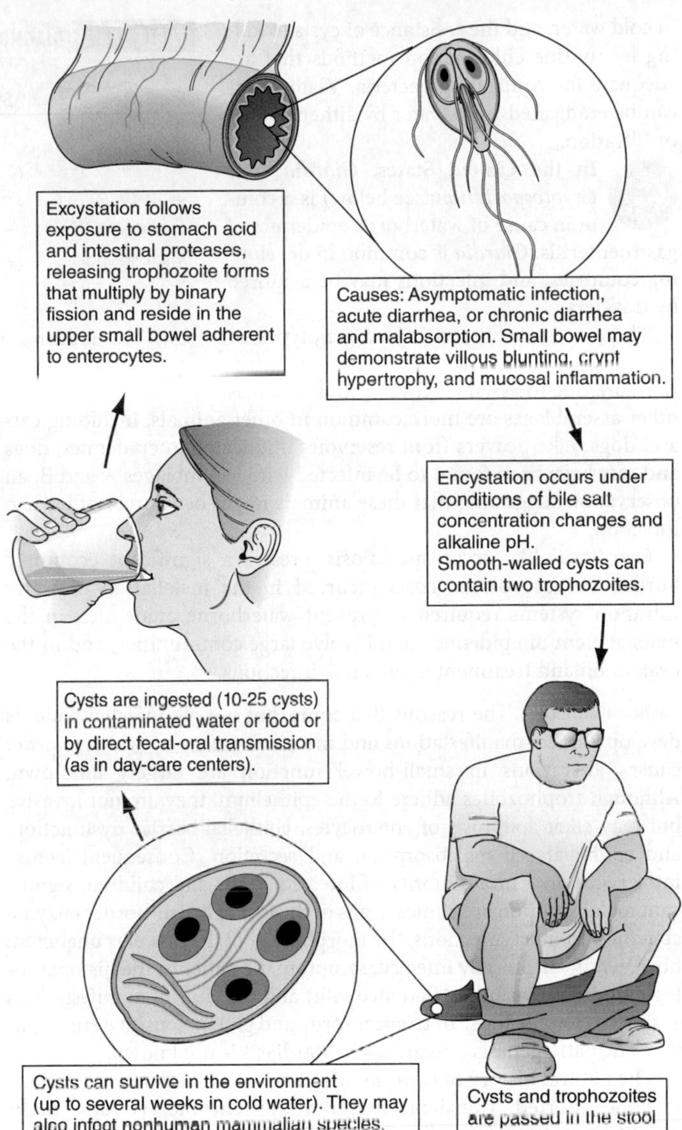

Excystation follows exposure to stomach acid and intestinal proteases, releasing trophozoite forms that multiply by binary fission and reside in the upper small bowel adherent to enterocytes.
Causes: Asymptomatic infection, acute diarrhea, or chronic diarrhea and malabsorption. Small bowel may demonstrate villous blunting, crypt hypertrophy, and mucosal inflammation.
Encystation occurs under conditions of bile salt concentration changes and alkaline pH. Smooth-walled cysts can contain two trophozoites.
Cysts are ingested (10-25 cysts) in contaminated water or food or by direct fecal-oral transmission (as in day-care centers).
Cysts can survive in the environment (up to several weeks in cold water). They may also infect nonhuman mammalian species.
Cysts and trophozoites are passed in the stool into the environment.

FIGURE 254-1 Life cycle of *Giardia*. *(Reprinted with permission from RL Guerrant et al [eds]: Tropical Infectious Diseases: Principles, Pathogens and Practice, 2nd ed, p 987. © 2006, with permission from Elsevier Science.)*

Surface water, ranging from mountain streams to large municipal reservoirs, can become contaminated with fecally derived *Giardia* cysts. The efficacy of water as a means of transmission is enhanced by the small infectious inoculum of *Giardia*, the prolonged survival of cysts

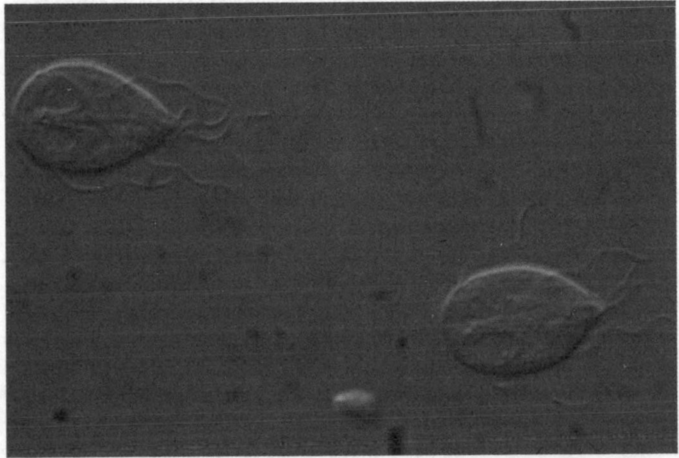

FIGURE 254-2 Flagellated, binucleate *Giardia* trophozoites.

in cold water, and the resistance of cysts to killing by routine chlorination methods that are adequate for controlling bacteria. Viable cysts can be eradicated from water by either boiling or filtration.

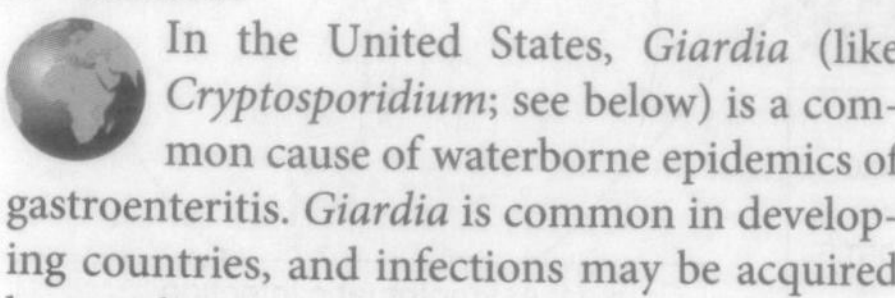

In the United States, *Giardia* (like *Cryptosporidium*; see below) is a common cause of waterborne epidemics of gastroenteritis. *Giardia* is common in developing countries, and infections may be acquired by travelers.

There are several recognized genotypes or assemblages of *G. intestinalis*. Human infections are due to assemblages A and B, whereas other assemblages are more common in other animals, including cats and dogs. Like beavers from reservoirs implicated in epidemics, dogs and cats have been found to be infected with assemblages A and B, an observation suggesting that these animals might be sources of human infection.

TABLE 254-1 DIAGNOSIS OF INTESTINAL PROTOZOAL INFECTIONS

Parasite	Stool O+P[a]	Fecal Acid-Fast Stain	Fecal Antigen Immunoassays	Fecal NAATs[b]	Other
Giardia	+		+	+	
Cryptosporidium	–	+	+	+	
Isospora	–	+		+	
Cyclospora	–	+		+	
Microsporidia	–			+	Special fecal stains, tissue biopsies

[a]O+P, ova and parasites. [b]Nucleic acid amplification tests.

Giardiasis, like cryptosporidiosis, creates a significant economic burden because of the costs incurred in the installation of water filtration systems required to prevent waterborne epidemics, in the management of epidemics that involve large communities, and in the evaluation and treatment of endemic infections.

Pathophysiology The reasons that some, but not all, infected patients develop clinical manifestations and the mechanisms by which *Giardia* causes alterations in small-bowel function are largely unknown. Although trophozoites adhere to the epithelium, they are not invasive but may elicit apoptosis of enterocytes, epithelial barrier dysfunction, and epithelial cell malabsorption and secretion. Consequent lactose intolerance and, in a minority of infected adults and children, significant malabsorption are clinical signs of the loss of brush-border enzyme activities. In most infections, the morphology of the bowel is unaltered; however, in chronically infected, symptomatic patients, the histopathologic findings (including flattened villi) and the clinical manifestations at times resemble those of tropical sprue and gluten-sensitive enteropathy. The pathogenesis of diarrhea in giardiasis is not known.

The natural history of *Giardia* infection varies markedly. Infections may be aborted, transient, recurrent, or chronic. *G. intestinalis* parasites vary genotypically, and such variations might contribute to different courses of infection. Parasite as well as host factors may be important in determining the course of infection and disease. Both cellular and humoral responses develop in human infections, but their precise roles in disease pathogenesis and/or control of infection are unknown. Because patients with hypogammaglobulinemia suffer from prolonged, severe infections that are poorly responsive to treatment, humoral immune responses appear to be important. The greater susceptibilities of the young than of the old and of newly exposed persons than of chronically exposed populations suggest that at least partial protective immunity may develop.

Clinical Manifestations Disease manifestations of giardiasis range from asymptomatic carriage to fulminant diarrhea and malabsorption. Most infected persons are asymptomatic, but in epidemics the proportion of symptomatic cases may be higher. Symptoms may develop suddenly or gradually. In persons with acute giardiasis, symptoms develop after an incubation period that lasts at least 5–6 days and usually 1–3 weeks. Prominent early symptoms include diarrhea, abdominal pain, bloating, belching, flatus, nausea, and vomiting. Although diarrhea is common, upper intestinal manifestations such as nausea, vomiting, bloating, and abdominal pain may predominate. The duration of acute giardiasis is usually >1 week, although diarrhea often subsides. Individuals with chronic giardiasis may present with or without having experienced an antecedent acute symptomatic episode. Diarrhea is not necessarily prominent, but increased flatus, loose stools, sulfurous belching, and (in some instances) weight loss occur. Symptoms may be continual or episodic and may persist for years. Some persons who have relatively mild symptoms for long periods recognize the extent of their discomfort only in retrospect. Fever, the presence of blood and/or mucus in the stools, and other signs and symptoms of colitis are uncommon and suggest a different diagnosis or a concomitant illness. Symptoms tend to be intermittent yet recurring and gradually debilitating, in contrast with the acute disabling symptoms associated with many enteric bacterial infections. Because of the less severe illness and the propensity for chronic infections, patients may seek medical advice late in the course of the illness; however, disease can be severe, resulting in malabsorption, weight loss, growth retardation, and dehydration. A number of extraintestinal manifestations have been described, such as urticaria, anterior uveitis, and arthritis; whether these are caused by giardiasis or concomitant processes is unclear.

Giardiasis can be severe in patients with hypogammaglobulinemia and can complicate other preexisting intestinal diseases, such as that occurring in cystic fibrosis. In patients with AIDS, *Giardia* can cause enteric illness that is refractory to treatment.

Diagnosis (Table 254-1) Giardiasis is diagnosed by detection of parasite antigens in the feces, by identification of cysts in the feces or of trophozoites in the feces or small intestines, or by nucleic acid amplification tests (NAATs). Cysts are oval, measure 8–12 μm × 7–10 μm, and characteristically contain four nuclei. Trophozoites are pear-shaped, dorsally convex, flattened parasites with two nuclei and four pairs of flagella (Fig. 254-2). The diagnosis is sometimes difficult to establish. Direct examination of fresh or properly preserved stools as well as concentration methods should be used. Because cyst excretion is variable and may be undetectable at times, repeated examination of stool, sampling of duodenal fluid, and biopsy of the small intestine may be required to detect the parasite. Tests for parasitic antigens in stool are at least as sensitive and specific as good microscopic examinations and are easier to perform. Newer NAATs are highly sensitive but are not always available for clinical use at present.

TREATMENT GIARDIASIS

Cure rates with metronidazole (250 mg thrice daily for 5 days) are usually >90%. Tinidazole (2 g once by mouth) may be more effective than metronidazole. Albendazole (400 mg daily for 5–10 days) is as effective as metronidazole and is associated with fewer side effects. Nitazoxanide (500 mg twice daily for 3 days) is an alternative agent for treatment of giardiasis. Paromomycin, an oral aminoglycoside that is not well absorbed, can be given to symptomatic pregnant patients, although information is limited on how effectively this agent eradicates infection.

Almost all patients respond to therapy and are cured, although some with chronic giardiasis experience delayed resolution of symptoms after eradication of *Giardia*. For many of the latter patients, residual symptoms probably reflect delayed regeneration of intestinal brush-border enzymes. Continued infection should be documented by stool examinations before treatment is repeated. Patients who remain infected after repeated treatments should be evaluated for reinfection through family members, close personal contacts, and environmental sources as well as for hypogammaglobulinemia. In cases refractory to multiple treatment courses, prolonged therapy with metronidazole (750 mg thrice daily for 21 days) or therapy with varied combinations of multiple agents has been successful.

Prevention Giardiasis can be prevented by consumption of uncontaminated food and water and by personal hygiene during the provision of care for infected children. Boiling or filtering potentially contaminated water prevents infection.

CRYPTOSPORIDIOSIS

The coccidian parasite *Cryptosporidium* causes diarrheal disease that is self-limited in immunocompetent human hosts but can be severe in persons with AIDS or other forms of immunodeficiency. Two species of *Cryptosporidium*, *C. hominis* (especially in the United States, sub-Saharan Africa, and Asia) and *C. parvum* (in Europe), cause most human infections.

Life Cycle and Epidemiology *Cryptosporidium* species are widely distributed in the world. Cryptosporidiosis is acquired by the consumption of oocysts (50% infectious dose: ~132 *C. parvum* oocysts in nonimmune individuals), which excyst to liberate sporozoites that in turn enter and infect intestinal epithelial cells. The parasite's further development involves both asexual and sexual cycles, which produce forms capable of infecting other epithelial cells and of generating oocysts that are passed in the feces. *Cryptosporidium* species infect a number of animals, and *C. parvum* can spread from infected animals to humans. Since oocysts are immediately infectious when passed in feces, person-to-person transmission takes place in day-care centers and among household contacts and medical providers. Waterborne transmission (especially that of *C. hominis*) accounts for infections in travelers and for common-source epidemics. Oocysts are quite hardy and resist killing by routine chlorination. Both drinking water and recreational water (e.g., pools, waterslides) have been increasingly recognized as sources of infection.

Pathophysiology Although intestinal epithelial cells harbor cryptosporidia in an intracellular vacuole, the means by which secretory diarrhea is elicited remain uncertain. No characteristic pathologic changes are found by biopsy. The distribution of infection can be spotty within the principal site of infection, the small bowel. Cryptosporidia are found in the pharynx, stomach, and large bowel of some patients and at times in the respiratory tract. Especially in patients with AIDS, involvement of the biliary tract can cause papillary stenosis, sclerosing cholangitis, or cholecystitis.

Clinical Manifestations Asymptomatic infections can occur in both immunocompetent and immunocompromised hosts. In immunocompetent persons, symptoms develop after an incubation period of ~1 week and consist principally of watery nonbloody diarrhea, sometimes in conjunction with abdominal pain, nausea, anorexia, fever, and/or weight loss. In these hosts, the illness usually subsides after 1–2 weeks. In contrast, in immunocompromised hosts (especially those with AIDS and CD4+ T cell counts <100/μL), diarrhea can be chronic, persistent, and remarkably profuse, causing clinically significant fluid and electrolyte depletion. Stool volumes may range from 1 to 25 L/d. Weight loss, wasting, and abdominal pain may be severe. Biliary tract involvement can manifest as mid-epigastric or right upper quadrant pain.

Diagnosis (Table 254-1) Evaluation starts with fecal examination for small oocysts, which are smaller (4–5 μm in diameter) than the fecal stages of most other parasites. Because conventional stool examination for ova and parasites (O+P) does not detect *Cryptosporidium*, specific testing must be requested. Detection is enhanced by evaluation of stools (obtained on multiple days) by several techniques, including modified acid-fast and direct immunofluorescent stains and enzyme immunoassays. Newer NAATs are being employed. Cryptosporidia can also be identified by light and electron microscopy at the apical surfaces of intestinal epithelium from biopsy specimens of the small bowel and, less frequently, the large bowel.

TREATMENT CRYPTOSPORIDIOSIS

Nitazoxanide, approved by the U.S. Food and Drug Administration (FDA) for the treatment of cryptosporidiosis, is available in tablet form for adults (500 mg twice daily for 3 days) and as an elixir for children. To date, however, this agent has not been effective for the treatment of HIV-infected patients, in whom improved immune status due to antiretroviral therapy can lead to amelioration of cryptosporidiosis. Otherwise, treatment includes supportive care with replacement of fluids and electrolytes and administration of antidiarrheal agents. Biliary tract obstruction may require papillotomy or T-tube placement. Prevention requires minimizing exposure to infectious oocysts in human or animal feces. Use of submicron water filters may minimize acquisition of infection from drinking water.

CYSTOISOSPORIASIS

The coccidian parasite *Cystoisospora belli* causes human intestinal disease. Infection is acquired by the consumption of oocysts, after which the parasite invades intestinal epithelial cells and undergoes both sexual and asexual cycles of development. Oocysts excreted in stool are not immediately infectious but must undergo further maturation.

Although *C. belli* infects many animals, little is known about the epidemiology or prevalence of this parasite in humans. It is most common in tropical and subtropical countries. Acute infections can begin abruptly with fever, abdominal pain, and watery nonbloody diarrhea and can last for weeks or months. In patients who have AIDS or are immunocompromised for other reasons, infections often are not self-limited but rather resemble cryptosporidiosis, with chronic, profuse watery diarrhea. Eosinophilia, which is not found in other enteric protozoan infections, may be detectable. The diagnosis (Table 254-1) is usually made by detection of the large (~25-μm) oocysts in stool by modified acid-fast staining. Oocyst excretion may be low-level and intermittent; if repeated stool examinations are unrevealing, sampling of duodenal contents by aspiration or small-bowel biopsy (often with electron microscopic examination) may be necessary. NAATs are promising newer diagnostic tools.

TREATMENT CYSTOISOSPORIASIS

Trimethoprim-sulfamethoxazole (TMP-SMX, 160/800 mg four times daily for 10 days, and for HIV-infected patients, then continuing three times daily for 3 weeks) is effective. For patients intolerant of sulfonamides, pyrimethamine (50–75 mg/d) can be used. Relapses can occur in persons with AIDS and necessitate maintenance therapy with TMP-SMX (160/800 mg three times per week).

CYCLOSPORIASIS

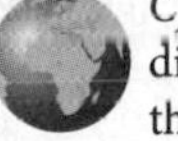

Cyclospora cayetanensis, a cause of diarrheal illness, is globally distributed: illness due to *C. cayetanensis* has been reported in the United States, Asia, Africa, Latin America, and Europe. The epidemiology of this parasite has not yet been fully defined, but waterborne transmission and food-borne transmission (e.g., by basil, sweet peas, and imported raspberries) have been recognized. The full spectrum of illness attributable to *Cyclospora* has not been delineated. Some infected patients may be without symptoms, but many have diarrhea, flulike symptoms, and flatulence and belching. The illness can be self-limited, can wax and wane, or, in many cases, can involve prolonged diarrhea, anorexia, and upper gastrointestinal symptoms, with sustained fatigue and weight loss in some instances. Diarrheal illness may persist for >1 month. *Cyclospora* can cause enteric illness in patients infected with HIV.

The parasite is detectable in epithelial cells of small-bowel biopsy samples and elicits secretory diarrhea by unknown means. The absence of fecal blood and leukocytes indicates that disease due to *Cyclospora* is not caused by destruction of the small-bowel mucosa. The diagnosis (Table 254-1) can be made by detection of spherical 8- to 10-μm oocysts in the stool, although routine stool O+P examinations are not sufficient. Specific fecal examinations must be requested to detect the oocysts, which are variably acid-fast and are fluorescent when viewed with ultraviolet light microscopy. Newer NAATs are proving to be sensitive. Cyclosporiasis should be considered in the differential diagnosis of prolonged diarrhea, with or without a history of travel by the patient to other countries.

TREATMENT CYCLOSPORIASIS

Cyclosporiasis is treated with TMP-SMX (160/800 mg twice daily for 7–10 days). HIV-infected patients may experience relapses after such treatment and thus may require longer-term suppressive maintenance therapy.

MICROSPORIDIOSIS

Microsporidia are obligate intracellular spore-forming protozoa that infect many animals and cause disease in humans, especially as opportunistic pathogens in AIDS. Microsporidia are members of a distinct phylum, Microspora, which contains dozens of genera and hundreds of species. The various microsporidia are differentiated by their developmental life cycles, ultrastructural features, and molecular taxonomy based on ribosomal RNA. The complex life cycles of the organisms result in the production of infectious spores (Fig. 254-3). Currently, eight genera of microsporidia—*Encephalitozoon, Pleistophora, Nosema, Vittaforma, Trachipleistophora, Anncalia, Microsporidium,* and *Enterocytozoon*—are recognized as causes of human disease. Although some microsporidia are probably prevalent causes of self-limited or asymptomatic infections in immunocompetent patients, little is known about how microsporidiosis is acquired.

Microsporidiosis is most common among patients with AIDS, less common among patients with other types of immunocompromise, and rare among immunocompetent hosts. In patients with AIDS, intestinal infections with *Enterocytozoon bieneusi* and *Encephalitozoon* (formerly *Septata*) *intestinalis* are recognized to contribute to chronic diarrhea and wasting; these infections had been found in 10–40% of patients with chronic diarrhea. Both organisms have been found in the biliary tracts of patients with cholecystitis. *E. intestinalis* may also disseminate to cause fever, diarrhea, sinusitis, cholangitis, and bronchiolitis. In patients with AIDS, *Encephalitozoon hellem* has caused superficial keratoconjunctivitis as well as sinusitis, respiratory tract disease, and disseminated infection. Myositis due to *Pleistophora* has been documented. *Nosema, Vittaforma,* and *Microsporidium* have caused stromal keratitis associated with trauma in immunocompetent patients.

Microsporidia are small gram-positive organisms with mature spores measuring 0.5–2 μm × 1–4 μm. Diagnosis of microsporidial infections in tissue often requires electron microscopy, although intracellular spores can be visualized by light microscopy with hematoxylin and eosin, Giemsa, or tissue Gram's stain. For the diagnosis of intestinal microsporidiosis, modified trichrome or chromotrope 2R-based staining and Uvitex 2B or calcofluor fluorescent staining reveal spores in smears of feces or duodenal aspirates. Definitive therapies for microsporidial infections remain to be established. For superficial keratoconjunctivitis due to *E. hellem*, topical therapy with fumagillin suspension has shown promise (Chap. 246e). For enteric infections with *E. bieneusi* and *E. intestinalis* in HIV-infected patients, therapy with albendazole may be efficacious (Chap. 246e).

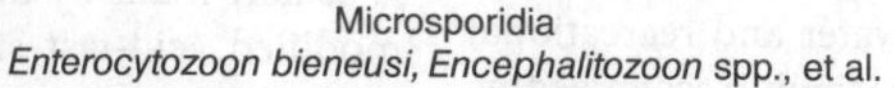

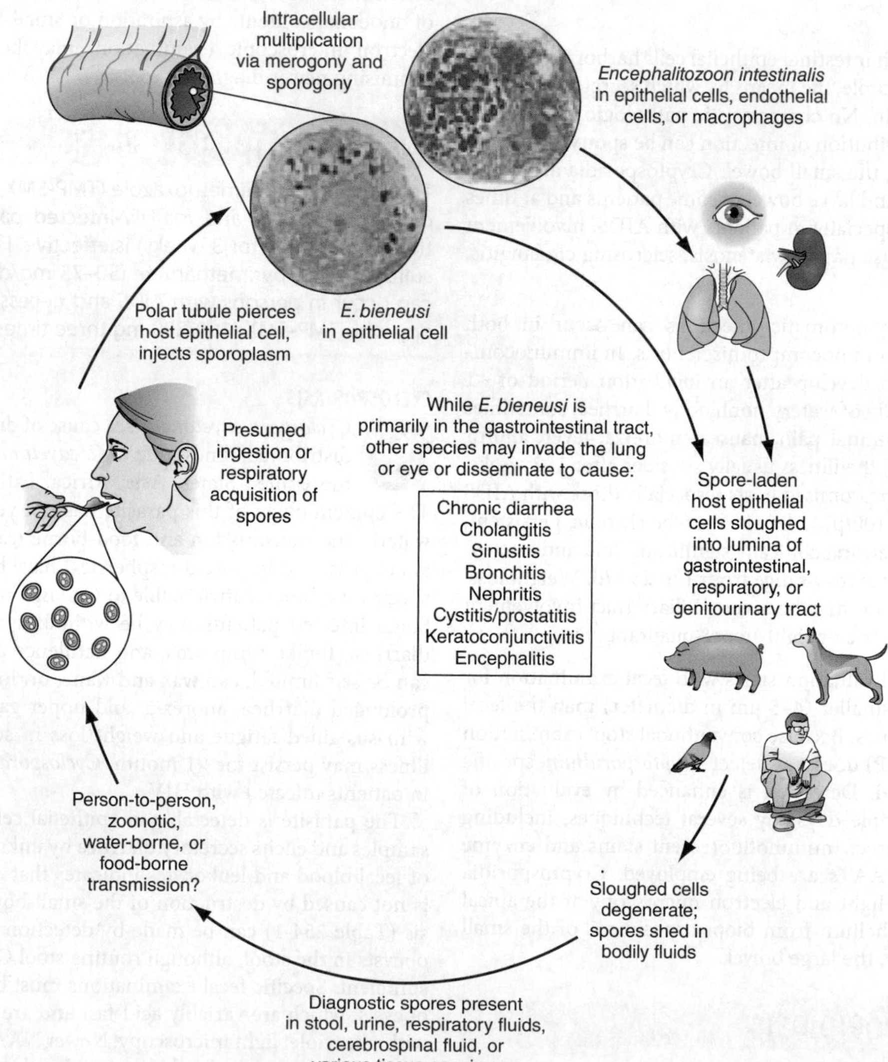

FIGURE 254-3 Life cycle of microsporidia. *(Reprinted with permission from RL Guerrant et al [eds]: Tropical Infectious Diseases: Principles, Pathogens and Practice, 2nd ed, p 1128. © 2006, with permission from Elsevier Science.)*

OTHER INTESTINAL PROTOZOA

Balantidiasis *Balantidium coli* is a large ciliated protozoal parasite that can produce a spectrum of large-intestinal disease analogous to amebiasis. The parasite is widely distributed in the world. Since it infects pigs, cases in humans are more common where pigs are raised. Infective cysts can be transmitted from person to person and through water, but many cases are due to the ingestion of cysts derived from porcine feces in association with slaughtering, with use of pig feces for fertilizer, or with contamination of water supplies by pig feces.

Ingested cysts liberate trophozoites, which reside and replicate in the large bowel. Many patients remain asymptomatic, but some have persisting intermittent diarrhea, and a few develop more fulminant dysentery. In symptomatic individuals, the pathology in the bowel—both gross and microscopic—is similar to that seen in amebiasis, with varying degrees of mucosal invasion, focal necrosis, and ulceration. Balantidiasis, unlike amebiasis, only rarely spreads hematogenously to other organs. The diagnosis is made by detection of the trophozoite stage in stool or sampled colonic tissue. Tetracycline (500 mg four times daily for 10 days) is an effective therapeutic agent.

Blastocystosis *Blastocystis hominis* remains an organism of uncertain pathogenicity. Some patients who pass *B. hominis* in their stools are asymptomatic, whereas others have diarrhea and associated intestinal symptoms. Diligent evaluation reveals other potential bacterial, viral, or protozoal causes of diarrhea in some but not all patients with symptoms. Because the pathogenicity of *B. hominis* is uncertain and because therapy for *Blastocystis* infection is neither specific nor uniformly effective, patients with prominent intestinal symptoms should be fully evaluated for other infectious causes of diarrhea. If diarrheal symptoms associated with *Blastocystis* are prominent, either metronidazole (750 mg thrice daily for 10 days) or TMP-SMX (160 mg/800 mg twice daily for 7 days) can be used.

Dientamoebiasis *Dientamoeba fragilis* is unique among intestinal protozoa in that it has a trophozoite stage but not a cyst stage. How trophozoites survive to transmit infection is not known. When symptoms develop in patients with *D. fragilis* infection, they are generally mild and include intermittent diarrhea, abdominal pain, and anorexia. The diagnosis is made by the detection of trophozoites in stool; the lability of these forms accounts for the greater yield when fecal samples are preserved immediately after collection. Since fecal excretion rates vary, examination of several samples obtained on alternate days increases the rate of detection. Iodoquinol (650 mg three times daily for 20 days) or paromomycin (25–35 mg/kg per day in three doses for 7 days) is appropriate for treatment.

TRICHOMONIASIS

Various species of trichomonads can be found in the mouth (in association with periodontitis) and occasionally in the gastrointestinal tract. *Trichomonas vaginalis*—one of the most prevalent protozoal parasites in the United States—is a pathogen of the genitourinary tract and a major cause of symptomatic vaginitis (Chap. 163).

Life Cycle and Epidemiology *T. vaginalis* is a pear-shaped, actively motile organism that measures about 10 × 7 μm, replicates by binary fission, and inhabits the lower genital tract of females and the urethra and prostate of males. In the United States, it accounts for ~3 million infections per year in women. While the organism can survive for a few hours in moist environments and could be acquired by direct contact, person-to-person venereal transmission accounts for virtually all cases of trichomoniasis. Its prevalence is greatest among persons with multiple sexual partners and among those with other sexually transmitted diseases (Chap. 163).

Clinical Manifestations Many men infected with *T. vaginalis* are asymptomatic, although some develop urethritis and a few have epididymitis or prostatitis. In contrast, infection in women, which has an incubation period of 5–28 days, is usually symptomatic and manifests with malodorous vaginal discharge (often yellow), vulvar erythema and itching, dysuria or urinary frequency (in 30–50% of patients), and dyspareunia. These manifestations, however, do not clearly distinguish trichomoniasis from other types of infectious vaginitis.

Diagnosis Detection of motile trichomonads by microscopic examination of wet mounts of vaginal or prostatic secretions has been the conventional means of diagnosis. Although this approach provides an immediate diagnosis, its sensitivity for the detection of *T. vaginalis* is only ~50–60% in routine evaluations of vaginal secretions. Direct immunofluorescent antibody staining is more sensitive (70–90%) than wet-mount examinations. *T. vaginalis* can be recovered from the urethra of both males and females and is detectable in males after prostatic massage. A new NAAT, APTIMA, is FDA approved and is highly sensitive and specific for urine and for endocervical and vaginal swabs from women.

TREATMENT TRICHOMONIASIS

Metronidazole (either a single 2-g dose or 500-mg doses twice daily for 7 days) or tinidazole (a single 2-g dose) is effective. All sexual partners must be treated concurrently to prevent reinfection, especially from asymptomatic males. In males with persistent symptomatic urethritis after therapy for nongonococcal urethritis, metronidazole therapy should be considered for possible trichomoniasis. Alternatives to metronidazole for treatment during pregnancy are not readily available. Reinfection often accounts for apparent treatment failures, but strains of *T. vaginalis* exhibiting high-level resistance to metronidazole have been encountered. Treatment of these resistant infections with higher oral doses, parenteral doses, or concurrent oral and vaginal doses of metronidazole or with tinidazole has been successful.

SECTION 19 HELMINTHIC INFECTIONS

255e Introduction to Helminthic Infections

Peter F. Weller

This is a digital-only chapter. It is available on the DVD that accompanies this book, as well as on Access Medicine/Harrison's Online, and the eBook and "app" editions of HPIM 19e.

The word *helminth* is derived from the Greek *helmins* ("parasitic worm"). Helminthic worms are highly prevalent and, depending on the species, may exist as free-living organisms or as parasites of plant or animal hosts. The parasitic helminths have co-evolved with specific mammalian and other host species. Accordingly, most helminthic infections are restricted to nonhuman hosts, and only rarely do these zoonotic helminths accidentally cause human infections.

256 Trichinellosis and Other Tissue Nematode Infections

Peter F. Weller

Nematodes are elongated, symmetric roundworms. Parasitic nematodes of medical significance may be broadly classified as either predominantly intestinal or tissue nematodes. This chapter covers the tissue nematodes that cause trichinellosis, visceral and ocular larva migrans, cutaneous larva migrans, cerebral angiostrongyliasis, and gnathostomiasis. All of these zoonotic infections result from incidental exposure to infectious nematodes. The clinical symptoms of these infections are due largely to invasive larval stages that (except in the case of *Trichinella*) do not reach maturity in humans.

TRICHINELLOSIS

Trichinellosis develops after the ingestion of meat containing cysts of *Trichinella* (e.g., pork or other meat from a carnivore). Although most infections are mild and asymptomatic, heavy infections can cause severe enteritis, periorbital edema, myositis, and (infrequently) death.

Life Cycle and Epidemiology Eight species of *Trichinella* are recognized as causes of infection in humans. Two species are distributed worldwide: *T. spiralis*, which is found in a great variety of carnivorous and omnivorous animals, and *T. pseudospiralis*, which is found in mammals and birds. *T. nativa* is present in Arctic regions and infects bears; *T. nelsoni* is found in equatorial eastern Africa, where it is common among felid predators and scavengers such as hyenas and bush pigs; and *T. britovi* is found in Europe, western Africa, and western Asia among carnivores but not among domestic swine. *T. murrelli* is present in North American game animals.

After human consumption of trichinous meat, encysted larvae are liberated by digestive acid and proteases (Fig. 256-1). The larvae invade the small-bowel mucosa and mature into adult worms. After ~1 week, female worms release newborn larvae that migrate via the circulation to striated muscle. The larvae of all species except *T. pseudospiralis*, *T. papuae*, and *T. zimbabwensis* then encyst by inducing a radical transformation in the muscle cell architecture. Although host immune responses may help to expel intestinal adult worms, they have few deleterious effects on muscle-dwelling larvae.

Human trichinellosis is often caused by the ingestion of infected pork products and thus can occur in almost any location where the meat of domestic or wild swine is eaten. Human trichinellosis may also be acquired from the meat of other animals, including dogs (in parts of Asia and Africa), horses (in Italy and France), and bears and walruses (in northern regions). Although cattle (being herbivores) are not natural hosts of *Trichinella*, beef has been implicated in outbreaks when contaminated or adulterated with trichinous pork. Laws that prohibit the feeding of uncooked garbage to pigs have greatly reduced the transmission of trichinellosis in the United States. About 12 cases of trichinellosis are reported annually in this country, but most mild cases probably remain undiagnosed. Recent U.S. and Canadian outbreaks have been attributable to consumption of wild game (especially bear meat) and, less frequently, of pork.

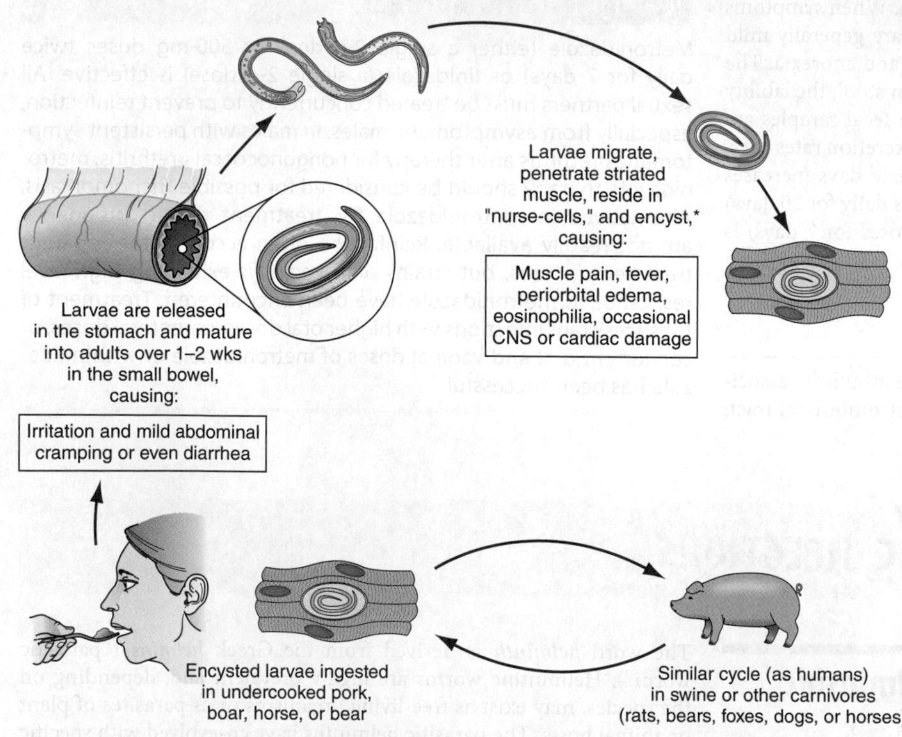

Larvae migrate, penetrate striated muscle, reside in "nurse-cells," and encyst,* causing:
Muscle pain, fever, periorbital edema, eosinophilia, occasional CNS or cardiac damage
Larvae are released in the stomach and mature into adults over 1–2 wks in the small bowel, causing:
Irritation and mild abdominal cramping or even diarrhea
Encysted larvae ingested in undercooked pork, boar, horse, or bear
Similar cycle (as humans) in swine or other carnivores (rats, bears, foxes, dogs, or horses)
*T. papuae, T. zimbabwensis, and T. pseudospiralis do not encyst.

FIGURE 256-1 Life cycle of *Trichinella* *spiralis* (cosmopolitan); *nelsoni* (equatorial Africa); *britovi* (Europe, western Africa, western Asia); *nativa* (Arctic); *murrelli* (North America); *papuae* (Papua New Guinea); *zimbabwensis* (Tanzania); and *pseudospiralis* (cosmopolitan). CNS, central nervous system. *(Reprinted from RL Guerrant et al [eds]: Tropical Infectious Diseases: Principles, Pathogens and Practice, 2nd ed, p 1218. © 2006, with permission from Elsevier Science.)*

Pathogenesis and Clinical Features Clinical symptoms of trichinellosis arise from the successive phases of parasite enteric invasion, larval migration, and muscle encystment (Fig. 256-1). Most light infections (those with <10 larvae per gram of muscle) are asymptomatic, whereas heavy infections (which can involve >50 larvae per gram of muscle) can be life-threatening. Invasion of the gut by large numbers of parasites occasionally provokes diarrhea during the first week after infection. Abdominal pain, constipation, nausea, or vomiting also may be prominent.

Symptoms due to larval migration and muscle invasion begin to appear in the second week after infection. The migrating *Trichinella* larvae provoke a marked local and systemic hypersensitivity reaction, with fever and hypereosinophilia. Periorbital and facial edema is common, as are hemorrhages in the subconjunctivae, retina, and nail beds ("splinter" hemorrhages). A maculopapular rash, headache, cough, dyspnea, or dysphagia sometimes develops. Myocarditis with tachyarrhythmias or heart failure—and, less commonly, encephalitis or pneumonitis—may develop and accounts for most deaths of patients with trichinellosis.

Upon onset of larval encystment in muscle 2–3 weeks after infection, symptoms of myositis with myalgias, muscle edema, and weakness develop, usually overlapping with the inflammatory reactions to migrating larvae. The most commonly involved muscle groups include the extraocular muscles; the biceps; and the muscles of the jaw, neck, lower back, and diaphragm. Peaking ~3 weeks after infection, symptoms subside only gradually during a prolonged convalescence. Uncommon infections with *T. pseudospiralis*, whose larvae do not encapsulate in muscles, elicit prolonged polymyositis-like illness.

Laboratory Findings and Diagnosis Blood eosinophilia develops in >90% of patients with symptomatic trichinellosis and may peak at a level of >50% 2–4 weeks after infection. Serum levels of muscle enzymes, including creatine phosphokinase, are elevated in most symptomatic patients. Patients should be questioned thoroughly about their consumption of pork or wild animal meat and about illness in other individuals who ate the same meat. A presumptive clinical diagnosis can be based on fevers, eosinophilia, periorbital edema, and myalgias after a suspect meal. A rise in the titer of parasite-specific antibody, which usually does not occur until after the third week

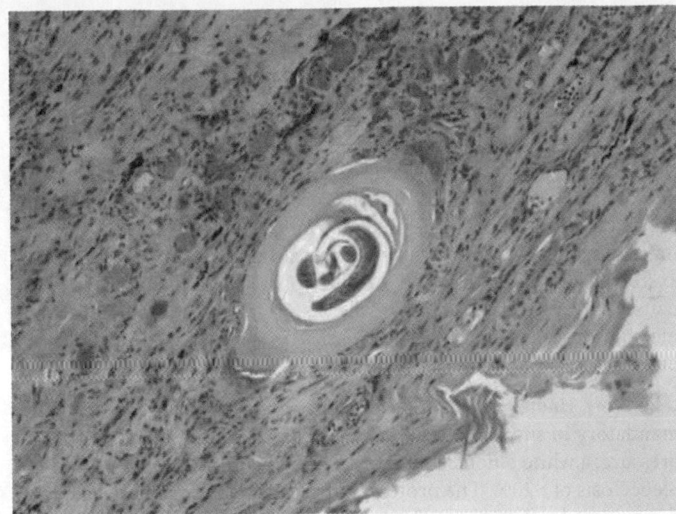

FIGURE 256-2 ***Trichinella* larva** encysted in a characteristic hyalinized capsule in striated muscle tissue. *(Photo/Wadsworth Center, New York State Department of Health. Reprinted from MMWR 53:606, 2004; public domain.)*

of infection, confirms the diagnosis. Alternatively, a definitive diagnosis requires surgical biopsy of at least 1 g of involved muscle; the yields are highest near tendon insertions. The fresh muscle tissue should be compressed between glass slides and examined microscopically (Fig. 256-2), because larvae may be missed by examination of routine histopathologic sections alone.

TREATMENT TRICHINELLOSIS

Most lightly infected patients recover uneventfully with bed rest, antipyretics, and analgesics. Glucocorticoids like prednisone (Table 256-1) are beneficial for severe myositis and myocarditis. Mebendazole and albendazole are active against enteric stages of the parasite, but their efficacy against encysted larvae has not been conclusively demonstrated.

Prevention Larvae may be killed by cooking pork until it is no longer pink or by freezing it at −15°C for 3 weeks. However, Arctic *T. nativa* larvae in walrus or bear meat are relatively resistant and may remain viable despite freezing.

TABLE 256-1 THERAPY FOR TISSUE NEMATODE INFECTIONS

Infection	Severity	Treatment
Trichinellosis	Mild	Supportive
	Moderate	Albendazole (400 mg bid × 8–14 days) or Mebendazole (200–400 mg tid × 3 days, then 400 mg tid × 8–14 days)
	Severe	Add glucocorticoids (e.g., prednisone, 1 mg/kg qd × 5 days)
Visceral larva migrans	Mild to moderate	Supportive
	Severe	Glucocorticoids (as above)
	Ocular	Not fully defined; albendazole (800 mg bid for adults, 400 mg bid for children) with glucocorticoids × 5–20 days has been effective
Cutaneous larva migrans		Ivermectin (single dose, 200 µg/kg) or Albendazole (200 mg bid × 3 days)
Angiostrongyliasis	Mild to moderate	Supportive
	Severe	Glucocorticoids (as above)
Gnathostomiasis		Ivermectin (200 µg/kg per day × 2 days) or Albendazole (400 mg bid × 21 days)

VISCERAL AND OCULAR LARVA MIGRANS

Visceral larva migrans is a syndrome caused by nematodes that are normally parasitic for nonhuman host species. In humans, these nematode larvae do not develop into adult worms but instead migrate through host tissues and elicit eosinophilic inflammation. The most common form of visceral larva migrans is toxocariasis due to larvae of the canine ascarid *Toxocara canis*; the syndrome is due less commonly to the feline ascarid *T. cati* and even less commonly to the pig ascarid *Ascaris suum*. Rare cases with eosinophilic meningoencephalitis have been caused by the raccoon ascarid *Baylisascaris procyonis*.

Life Cycle and Epidemiology The canine roundworm *T. canis* is distributed among dogs worldwide. Ingestion of infective eggs by dogs is followed by liberation of *Toxocara* larvae, which penetrate the gut wall and migrate intravascularly into canine tissues, where most remain in a developmentally arrested state. During pregnancy, some larvae resume migration in bitches and infect puppies prenatally (through transplacental transmission) or after birth (through suckling). Thus, in lactating bitches and puppies, larvae return to the intestinal tract and develop into adult worms, which produce eggs that are released in the feces. Eggs must undergo embryonation over several weeks to become infectious. Humans acquire toxocariasis mainly by eating soil contaminated by puppy feces that contains infective *T. canis* eggs. Visceral larva migrans is most common among children who habitually eat dirt.

Pathogenesis and Clinical Features Clinical disease most commonly afflicts preschool children. After humans ingest *Toxocara* eggs, the larvae hatch and penetrate the intestinal mucosa, from which they are carried by the circulation to a wide variety of organs and tissues. The larvae invade the liver, lungs, central nervous system (CNS), and other sites, provoking intense local eosinophilic granulomatous responses. The degree of clinical illness depends on larval number and tissue distribution, reinfection, and host immune responses. Most light infections are asymptomatic and may be manifest only by blood eosinophilia. Characteristic symptoms of visceral larva migrans include fever, malaise, anorexia and weight loss, cough, wheezing, and rashes. Hepatosplenomegaly is common. These features may be accompanied by extraordinary peripheral eosinophilia, which may approach 90%. Uncommonly, seizures or behavioral disorders develop. Rare deaths are due to severe neurologic, pneumonic, or myocardial involvement.

The ocular form of the larva migrans syndrome occurs when *Toxocara* larvae invade the eye. An eosinophilic granulomatous mass, most commonly in the posterior pole of the retina, develops around the entrapped larva. The retinal lesion can mimic retinoblastoma in appearance, and mistaken diagnosis of the latter condition can lead to unnecessary enucleation. The spectrum of eye involvement also includes endophthalmitis, uveitis, and chorioretinitis. Unilateral visual disturbances, strabismus, and eye pain are the most common presenting symptoms. In contrast to visceral larva migrans, ocular toxocariasis usually develops in older children or young adults with no history of pica; these patients seldom have eosinophilia or visceral manifestations.

Diagnosis In addition to eosinophilia, leukocytosis and hypergammaglobulinemia may be evident. Transient pulmonary infiltrates are apparent on chest x-rays of about one-half of patients with symptoms of pneumonitis. The clinical diagnosis can be confirmed by an enzyme-linked immunosorbent assay for toxocaral antibodies. Stool examination for parasite eggs is worthless in toxocariasis, since the larvae do not develop into egg-producing adults in humans.

TREATMENT VISCERAL AND OCULAR LARVA MIGRANS

The vast majority of *Toxocara* infections are self-limited and resolve without specific therapy. In patients with severe myocardial, CNS, or pulmonary involvement, glucocorticoids may be employed to reduce inflammatory complications. Available anthelmintic drugs, including mebendazole and albendazole, have not been shown conclusively to alter the course of larva migrans. Control measures include prohibiting dog excreta in public parks and playgrounds, deworming dogs, and preventing pica in children. Treatment of ocular disease is not fully defined, but the administration of albendazole in conjunction with glucocorticoids has been effective (Table 256-1).

CUTANEOUS LARVA MIGRANS

Cutaneous larva migrans ("creeping eruption") is a serpiginous skin eruption caused by burrowing larvae of animal hookworms, usually the dog and cat hookworm *Ancylostoma braziliense*. The larvae hatch from eggs passed in dog and cat feces and mature in the soil. Humans become infected after skin contact with soil in areas frequented by dogs and cats, such as areas underneath house porches. Cutaneous larva migrans is prevalent among children and travelers in regions with warm humid climates, including the southeastern United States.

After larvae penetrate the skin, erythematous lesions form along the tortuous tracks of their migration through the dermal-epidermal junction; the larvae advance several centimeters in a day. The intensely pruritic lesions may occur anywhere on the body and can be numerous if the patient has lain on the ground. Vesicles and bullae may form later. The animal hookworm larvae do not mature in humans and, without treatment, will die after an interval ranging from weeks to a couple of months, with resolution of skin lesions. The diagnosis is made on clinical grounds. Skin biopsies only rarely detect diagnostic larvae. Symptoms can be alleviated by ivermectin or albendazole (Table 256-1).

ANGIOSTRONGYLIASIS

Angiostrongylus cantonensis, the rat lungworm, is the most common cause of human eosinophilic meningitis (Fig. 256-3).

Life Cycle and Epidemiology This infection occurs principally in Southeast Asia and the Pacific Basin but has spread to other areas of the world, including the Caribbean islands, countries in Central and South America, and the southern United States. *A. cantonensis* larvae produced by adult worms in the rat lung migrate to the gastrointestinal tract and are expelled with the feces. They develop into infective larvae in land snails and slugs. Humans acquire the infection by ingesting raw infected mollusks; vegetables contaminated by mollusk slime; or crabs, freshwater shrimp, and certain marine fish that have themselves eaten infected mollusks. The larvae then migrate to the brain.

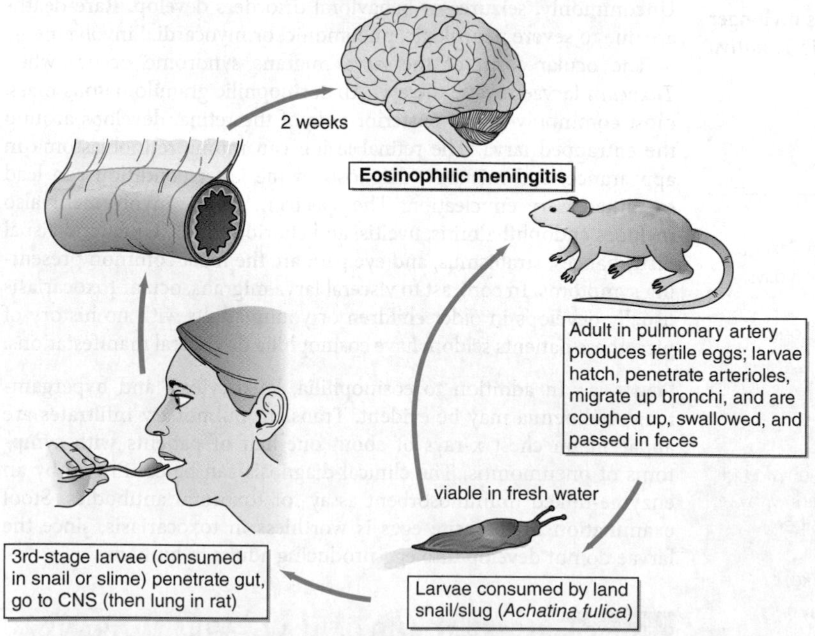

Pathogenesis and Clinical Features The parasites eventually die in the CNS, but not before initiating pathologic consequences that, in heavy infections, can result in permanent neurologic sequelae or death. Migrating larvae cause marked local eosinophilic inflammation and hemorrhage, with subsequent necrosis and granuloma formation around dying worms. Clinical symptoms develop 2–35 days after the ingestion of larvae. Patients usually present with an insidious or abrupt excruciating frontal, occipital, or bitemporal headache. Neck stiffness, nausea and vomiting, and paresthesias are also common. Fever, cranial and extraocular nerve palsies, seizures, paralysis, and lethargy are uncommon.

Laboratory Findings Examination of cerebrospinal fluid (CSF) is mandatory in suspected cases and usually reveals an elevated opening pressure, a white blood cell count of 150–2000/μL, and an eosinophilic pleocytosis of >20%. The protein concentration is usually elevated and the glucose level normal. The larvae of *A. cantonensis* are only rarely seen in CSF. Peripheral-blood eosinophilia may be mild. The diagnosis is generally based on the clinical presentation of eosinophilic meningitis together with a compatible epidemiologic history.

TREATMENT ANGIOSTRONGYLIASIS

Specific chemotherapy is not of benefit in angiostrongyliasis; larvicidal agents may exacerbate inflammatory brain lesions. Management consists of supportive measures, including the administration of analgesics, sedatives, and—in severe cases—glucocorticoids (Table 256-1). Repeated lumbar punctures with removal of CSF can relieve symptoms. In most patients, cerebral angiostrongyliasis has a self-limited course, and recovery is complete. The infection may be prevented by adequately cooking snails, crabs, and prawns and inspecting vegetables for mollusk infestation. Other parasitic or fungal causes of eosinophilic meningitis in endemic areas may include gnathostomiasis (see below), paragonimiasis (Chap. 259), schistosomiasis (Chap. 259), neurocysticercosis (Chap. 260), and coccidioidomycosis (Chap. 237).

FIGURE 256-3 Life cycle of *Angiostrongylus cantonensis* (rat lung worm), found in Southeast Asia, Pacific Islands, Cuba, Australia, Japan, China, Mauritius, and U.S. ports. CNS, central nervous system. *(Reprinted from RL Guerrant et al [eds]: Tropical Infectious Diseases: Principles, Pathogens and Practice, 2nd ed, p 1225. © 2006, with permission from Elsevier Science.)*

GNATHOSTOMIASIS

Infection of human tissues with larvae of *Gnathostoma spinigerum* can cause eosinophilic meningoencephalitis, migratory cutaneous swellings, or invasive masses of the eye and visceral organs.

Life Cycle and Epidemiology Human gnathostomiasis occurs in many countries and is notably endemic in Southeast Asia and parts of China and Japan. In nature, the mature adult worms parasitize the gastrointestinal tract of dogs and cats. First-stage larvae hatch from eggs passed into water and are ingested by *Cyclops* species (water fleas). Infective third-stage larvae develop in the flesh of many animal species (including fish, frogs, eels, snakes, chickens, and ducks) that have eaten either infected *Cyclops* or another infected second intermediate host. Humans typically acquire the infection by eating raw or undercooked fish or poultry. Raw fish dishes, such as *som fak* in Thailand and *sashimi* in Japan, account for many cases of human gnathostomiasis. Some cases in Thailand result from the local practice of applying frog or snake flesh as a poultice.

Pathogenesis and Clinical Features Clinical symptoms are due to the aberrant migration of a single larva into cutaneous, visceral, neural, or ocular tissues. After invasion, larval migration may cause local inflammation, with pain, cough, or hematuria accompanied by fever and eosinophilia. Painful, itchy, migratory swellings may develop in the skin, particularly in the distal extremities or periorbital area. Cutaneous swellings usually last ~1 week but often recur intermittently over many years. Larval invasion of the eye can provoke a sight-threatening inflammatory response. Invasion of the CNS results in eosinophilic meningitis with myeloencephalitis, a serious complication due to ascending larval migration along a large nerve track. Patients characteristically present with agonizing radicular pain and paresthesias in the trunk or a limb, which are followed shortly by paraplegia. Cerebral involvement, with focal hemorrhages and tissue destruction, is often fatal.

Diagnosis and Treatment Cutaneous migratory swellings with marked peripheral eosinophilia, supported by an appropriate geographic and dietary history, generally constitute an adequate basis for a clinical diagnosis of gnathostomiasis. However, patients may present with ocular or cerebrospinal involvement without antecedent cutaneous swellings. In the latter case, eosinophilic pleocytosis is demonstrable (usually along with hemorrhagic or xanthochromic CSF), but worms are almost never recovered from CSF. Surgical removal of the parasite from subcutaneous or ocular tissue, though rarely feasible, is both diagnostic and therapeutic. Albendazole or ivermectin may be helpful (Table 256-1). At present, cerebrospinal involvement is managed with supportive measures and generally with a course of glucocorticoids. Gnathostomiasis can be prevented by adequate cooking of fish and poultry in endemic areas.

257 Intestinal Nematode Infections

Peter F. Weller, Thomas B. Nutman

More than a billion persons worldwide are infected with one or more species of intestinal nematodes. Table 257-1 summarizes biologic and clinical features of infections due to the major intestinal parasitic nematodes. These parasites are most common in regions with poor fecal sanitation, particularly in resource-poor countries in the tropics and subtropics, but they have also been seen with increasing frequency among immigrants and refugees to resource-rich countries. Although nematode infections are not usually fatal, they contribute to malnutrition and diminished work capacity. It is interesting that these helminth infections may protect some individuals from allergic disease. Humans may on occasion be infected with nematode parasites that ordinarily infect animals; these zoonotic infections produce diseases such as trichostrongyliasis, anisakiasis, capillariasis, and abdominal angiostrongyliasis.

Intestinal nematodes are roundworms; they range in length from 1 mm to many centimeters when mature (Table 257-1). Their life cycles are complex and highly varied; some species, including *Strongyloides stercoralis* and *Enterobius vermicularis*, can be transmitted directly from person to person, while others, such as *Ascaris lumbricoides*, *Necator americanus*, and *Ancylostoma duodenale*, require a soil phase for development. Because most helminth parasites do not self-replicate, the acquisition of a heavy burden of adult worms requires repeated exposure to the parasite in its infectious stage, whether larva or egg. Hence, clinical disease, as opposed to asymptomatic infection, generally develops only with prolonged residence in an endemic area and is typically related to infection intensity. In persons with marginal nutrition, intestinal helminth infections may impair growth and development. Eosinophilia and elevated serum IgE levels are features of many helminth infections and, when unexplained, should always prompt a search for intestinal helminths. Significant protective immunity to intestinal nematodes appears not to develop in humans, although mechanisms of parasite immune evasion and host immune responses to these infections have not been elucidated in detail.

ASCARIASIS

A. lumbricoides is the largest intestinal nematode parasite of humans, reaching up to 40 cm in length. Most infected individuals have low worm burdens and are asymptomatic. Clinical disease arises from larval migration in the lungs or effects of the adult worms in the intestines.

Life Cycle Adult worms live in the lumen of the small intestine. Mature female *Ascaris* worms are extraordinarily fecund, each producing up to 240,000 eggs a day, which pass with the feces. Ascarid eggs, which are remarkably resistant to environmental stresses, become infective after several weeks of maturation in the soil and can remain infective for years. After infective eggs are swallowed, larvae hatched in the intestine invade the mucosa, migrate through the circulation to the lungs, break into the alveoli, ascend the bronchial tree, and return—through swallowing—to the small intestine, where they develop into adult worms. Between 2 and 3 months elapse between initial infection and egg production. Adult worms live for 1–2 years.

Epidemiology *Ascaris* is widely distributed in tropical and subtropical regions as well as in other humid areas, including the rural southeastern United States. Transmission typically occurs through fecally contaminated soil and is due either to a lack of sanitary facilities or to the use of human feces as fertilizer. With their propensity for hand-to-mouth fecal carriage, younger children are most affected. Infection outside endemic areas, though uncommon, can occur when eggs on transported vegetables are ingested.

Clinical Features During the lung phase of larval migration, ~9–12 days after egg ingestion, patients may develop an irritating nonproductive cough and burning substernal discomfort that is aggravated by coughing or deep inspiration. Dyspnea and blood-tinged sputum are less common. Fever is usually reported. Eosinophilia develops during this symptomatic phase and subsides slowly over weeks. Chest x-rays may reveal evidence of eosinophilic pneumonitis (Löffler's syndrome), with rounded infiltrates a few millimeters to several centimeters in size. These infiltrates may be transient and intermittent, clearing after several weeks. Where there is seasonal transmission of the parasite, seasonal pneumonitis with eosinophilia may develop in previously infected and sensitized hosts.

In established infections, adult worms in the small intestine usually cause no symptoms. In heavy infections, particularly in children, a large bolus of entangled worms can cause pain and small-bowel obstruction, sometimes complicated by perforation, intussusception, or volvulus. Single worms may cause disease when they migrate into aberrant sites. A large worm can enter and occlude the biliary tree, causing biliary colic, cholecystitis, cholangitis, pancreatitis, or (rarely) intrahepatic abscesses. Migration of an adult worm up the esophagus can provoke coughing and oral expulsion of the worm. In highly endemic areas, intestinal and biliary ascariasis can rival acute appendicitis and gallstones as causes of surgical acute abdomen.

Laboratory Findings Most cases of ascariasis can be diagnosed by microscopic detection of characteristic *Ascaris* eggs (65 by 45 μm) in fecal samples. Occasionally, patients present after passing an adult worm—identifiable by its large size and smooth cream-colored surface—in the stool or, much less commonly, through the mouth or nose. During the early transpulmonary migratory phase, when eosinophilic pneumonitis occurs, larvae can be found in sputum or gastric aspirates before diagnostic eggs appear in the stool. The eosinophilia that is prominent during this early stage usually decreases to minimal levels in established infection. Adult worms may be visualized, occasionally serendipitously, on contrast studies of the gastrointestinal tract. A plain abdominal film may reveal masses of worms in gas-filled loops of bowel in patients with intestinal obstruction. Pancreaticobiliary worms can be detected by ultrasound and endoscopic retrograde cholangiopancreatography; the latter method also has been used to extract biliary *Ascaris* worms.

TREATMENT ASCARIASIS

Ascariasis should always be treated to prevent potentially serious complications. Albendazole (400 mg once), mebendazole (100 g twice daily for 3 days or 500 mg once), or ivermectin (150–200 μg/kg

TABLE 257-1 MAJOR HUMAN INTESTINAL PARASITIC NEMATODES

	Parasitic Nematode				
Feature	*Ascaris lumbricoides* (Roundworm)	*Necator americanus, Ancylostoma duodenale* (Hookworm)	*Strongyloides stercoralis*	*Trichuris trichiura* (Whipworm)	*Enterobius vermicularis* (Pinworm)
Global prevalence in humans (millions)	807	576	100	604	209
Endemic areas	Worldwide	Hot, humid regions	Hot, humid regions	Worldwide	Worldwide
Infective stage	Egg	Filariform larva	Filariform larva	Egg	Egg
Route of infection	Oral	Percutaneous	Percutaneous or autoinfection	Oral	Oral
Gastrointestinal location of worms	Jejunal lumen	Jejunal mucosa	Small-bowel mucosa	Cecum, colonic mucosa	Cecum, appendix
Adult worm size	15–40 cm	7–12 mm	2 mm	30–50 mm	8–13 mm (female)
Pulmonary passage of larvae	Yes	Yes	Yes	No	No
Incubation period[a] (days)	60–75	40–100	17–28	70–90	35–45
Longevity	1 year	*N. americanus*: 2–5 years *A. duodenale*: 6–8 years	Decades (owing to autoinfection)	5 years	2 months
Fecundity (eggs/day/worm)	240,000	*N. americanus*: 4000–10,000 *A. duodenale*: 10,000–25,000	5000–10,000	3000–7000	2000
Principal symptoms	Rarely, biliary obstruction or, in heavy infections, gastrointestinal obstruction	Iron-deficiency anemia in heavy infection	Gastrointestinal symptoms; malabsorption or sepsis in hyperinfection	Gastrointestinal symptoms or anemia in heavy infection	Perianal pruritus
Diagnostic stage	Eggs in stool	Eggs in fresh stool, larvae in old stool	Larvae in stool or duodenal aspirate; sputum in hyperinfection	Eggs in stool	Eggs from perianal skin on cellulose acetate tape
Treatment	Mebendazole Albendazole Ivermectin	Mebendazole Albendazole	Ivermectin Albendazole	Mebendazole Albendazole Ivermectin	Mebendazole Albendazole

[a]Time from infection to egg production by mature female worm.

once) is effective. These medications are contraindicated in pregnancy, however. Mild diarrhea and abdominal pain are uncommon side effects of these agents. Partial intestinal obstruction should be managed with nasogastric suction, IV fluid administration, and instillation of piperazine through the nasogastric tube, but complete obstruction and its severe complications require immediate surgical intervention.

HOOKWORM

Two hookworm species (*A. duodenale* and *N. americanus*) are responsible for human infections. Most infected individuals are asymptomatic. Hookworm disease develops from a combination of factors—a heavy worm burden, a prolonged duration of infection, and an inadequate iron intake—and results in iron-deficiency anemia and, on occasion, hypoproteinemia.

Life Cycle Adult hookworms, which are ~1 cm long, use buccal teeth (*Ancylostoma*) or cutting plates (*Necator*) to attach to the small-bowel mucosa and suck blood (0.2 mL/d per *Ancylostoma* adult) and interstitial fluid. The adult hookworms produce thousands of eggs daily. The eggs are deposited with feces in soil, where rhabditiform larvae hatch and develop over a 1-week period into infectious filariform larvae. Infective larvae penetrate the skin and reach the lungs by way of the bloodstream. There they invade alveoli and ascend the airways before being swallowed and reaching the small intestine. The prepatent period from skin invasion to appearance of eggs in the feces is ~6–8 weeks, but it may be longer with *A. duodenale*. Larvae of *A. duodenale*, if swallowed, can survive and develop directly in the intestinal mucosa. Adult hookworms may survive over a decade but usually live ~6–8 years for *A. duodenale* and 2–5 years for *N. americanus*.

Epidemiology *A. duodenale* is prevalent in southern Europe, North Africa, and northern Asia, and *N. americanus* is the predominant species in the Western Hemisphere and equatorial Africa. The two species overlap in many tropical regions, particularly Southeast Asia. In most areas, older children have the highest incidence and greatest intensity of hookworm infection. In rural areas where fields are fertilized with human feces, older working adults also may be heavily infected.

Clinical Features Most hookworm infections are asymptomatic. Infective larvae may provoke pruritic maculopapular dermatitis ("ground itch") at the site of skin penetration as well as serpiginous tracks of subcutaneous migration (similar to those of cutaneous larva migrans; Chap. 256) in previously sensitized hosts. Larvae migrating through the lungs occasionally cause mild transient pneumonitis, but this condition develops less frequently in hookworm infection than in ascariasis. In the early intestinal phase, infected persons may develop epigastric pain (often with postprandial accentuation), inflammatory diarrhea, or other abdominal symptoms accompanied by eosinophilia. The major consequence of chronic hookworm infection is iron deficiency. Symptoms are minimal if iron intake is adequate, but marginally nourished individuals develop symptoms of progressive iron-deficiency anemia and hypoproteinemia, including weakness and shortness of breath.

Laboratory Findings The diagnosis is established by the finding of characteristic 40- by 60-μm oval hookworm eggs in the feces. Stool-concentration procedures may be required to detect light infections. Eggs of the two species are indistinguishable by light microscopy. In a stool sample that is not fresh, the eggs may have hatched to release rhabditiform larvae, which need to be differentiated from those of *S. stercoralis*. Hypochromic microcytic anemia, occasionally with eosinophilia or hypoalbuminemia, is characteristic of hookworm disease.

TREATMENT HOOKWORM INFECTION

Hookworm infection can be eradicated with several safe and highly effective anthelmintic drugs, including albendazole (400 mg once) and mebendazole (500 mg once). Mild iron-deficiency anemia can often be treated with oral iron alone. Severe hookworm disease with protein loss and malabsorption necessitates nutritional support and oral iron replacement along with deworming. There is some concern that the benzimidazoles (mebendazole and albendazole) are becoming less effective against human hookworms.

Ancylostoma caninum* and *Ancylostoma braziliense *A. caninum*, the canine hookworm, has been identified as a cause of human eosinophilic enteritis, especially in northeastern Australia. In this zoonotic infection, adult hookworms attach to the small intestine (where they may be visualized by endoscopy) and elicit abdominal pain and intense local eosinophilia. Treatment with mebendazole (100 mg twice daily for 3 days) or albendazole (400 mg once) or endoscopic removal is effective. Both of these animal hookworm species can cause cutaneous larva migrans ("creeping eruption"; Chap. 256).

STRONGYLOIDIASIS

S. stercoralis is distinguished by its ability—unique among helminths (except for *Capillaria*; see below)—to replicate in the human host. This capacity permits ongoing cycles of autoinfection as infective larvae are internally produced. Strongyloidiasis can thus persist for decades without further exposure of the host to exogenous infective larvae. In immunocompromised hosts, large numbers of invasive *Strongyloides* larvae can disseminate widely and can be fatal.

Life Cycle In addition to a parasitic cycle of development, *Strongyloides* can undergo a free-living cycle of development in the soil (Fig. 257-1). This adaptability facilitates the parasite's survival in the absence of mammalian hosts. Rhabditiform larvae passed in feces can transform into infectious filariform larvae either directly or after a free-living phase of development. Humans acquire strongyloidiasis when filariform larvae in fecally contaminated soil penetrate the skin or mucous membranes. The larvae then travel through the bloodstream to the lungs, where they break into the alveolar spaces, ascend the bronchial tree, are swallowed, and thereby reach the small intestine. There the larvae mature into adult worms that penetrate the mucosa of the proximal small bowel. The minute (2-mm-long) parasitic adult female worms reproduce by parthenogenesis; adult males do not exist. Eggs hatch in the intestinal mucosa, releasing rhabditiform larvae that migrate to the lumen and pass with the feces into soil. Alternatively, rhabditiform larvae in the bowel can develop directly into filariform larvae that penetrate the colonic wall or perianal skin and enter the circulation to repeat the migration that establishes ongoing internal reinfection. This autoinfection cycle allows strongyloidiasis to persist for decades.

Epidemiology *S. stercoralis* is spottily distributed in tropical areas and other hot, humid regions and is particularly common in Southeast Asia, sub-Saharan Africa, and Brazil. In the United States, the parasite is endemic in parts of the Southeast and is found in immigrants, refugees, travelers, and military personnel who have lived in endemic areas.

Clinical Features In uncomplicated strongyloidiasis, many patients are asymptomatic or have mild cutaneous and/or abdominal symptoms. Recurrent urticaria, often involving the buttocks and wrists, is the most common cutaneous manifestation. Migrating larvae can elicit a pathognomonic serpiginous eruption, *larva currens* ("running larva"). This pruritic, raised, erythematous lesion advances as rapidly as 10 cm/h along the course of larval migration. Adult parasites burrow into the duodenojejunal mucosa and can cause abdominal (usually midepigastric) pain, which resembles peptic ulcer pain except that it is aggravated by food ingestion. Nausea, diarrhea, gastrointestinal bleeding, mild chronic colitis, and weight loss can occur. Small-bowel obstruction may develop with early, heavy infection. Pulmonary symptoms are rare in uncomplicated strongyloidiasis. Eosinophilia is common, with levels fluctuating over time.

The ongoing autoinfection cycle of strongyloidiasis is normally constrained by unknown factors of the host's immune system. Abrogation of host immunity, especially with glucocorticoid therapy and much less commonly with other immunosuppressive medications, leads to hyperinfection, with the generation of large numbers of filariform larvae. Colitis, enteritis, or malabsorption may develop. In disseminated strongyloidiasis, larvae may invade not only gastrointestinal tissues and the lungs but also the central nervous system, peritoneum, liver, and kidneys. Moreover, bacteremia may develop because of the passage of enteric flora through disrupted mucosal barriers. Gram-negative sepsis, pneumonia, or meningitis may complicate or dominate the clinical course. Eosinophilia is often absent in severely infected patients. Disseminated strongyloidiasis, particularly in patients with unsuspected infection who are given glucocorticoids, can be fatal. Strongyloidiasis is a frequent complication of infection with human T cell lymphotropic virus type 1, but disseminated strongyloidiasis is not common among patients infected with HIV-1.

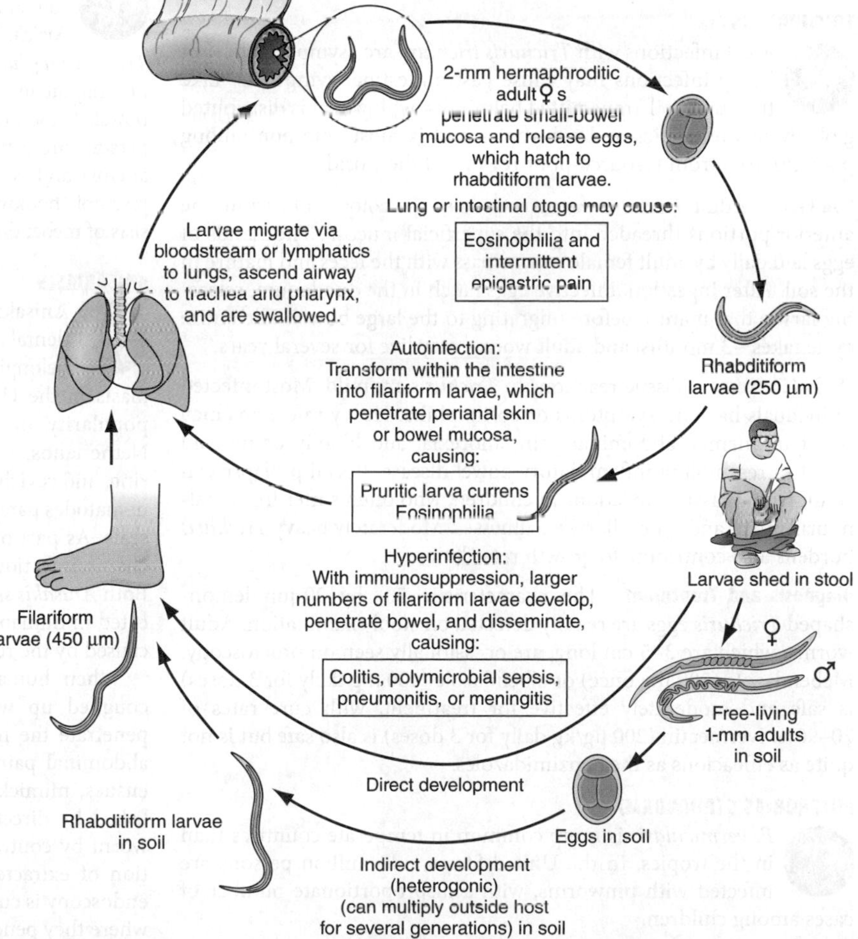

FIGURE 257-1 Life cycle of *Strongyloides stercoralis*. *(Adapted from Guerrant RL et al [eds]: Tropical Infectious Diseases: Principles, Pathogens and Practice, 2nd ed, p 1276. © 2006, with permission from Elsevier Science.)*

Diagnosis In uncomplicated strongyloidiasis, the finding of rhabditiform larvae in feces is diagnostic. Rhabditiform larvae are ~250 μm long, with a short buccal cavity that distinguishes them from hookworm larvae. In uncomplicated infections, few larvae are passed and single stool examinations detect only about one-third of cases. Serial examinations and the use of the agar plate detection method improve the sensitivity of stool diagnosis. In uncomplicated strongyloidiasis (but not in hyperinfection), stool examinations may be repeatedly negative. *Strongyloides* larvae may also be found by sampling of the duodenojejunal contents by aspiration or biopsy. An enzyme-linked immunosorbent assay for serum antibodies to antigens of *Strongyloides* is a sensitive method for diagnosing uncomplicated infections. Such serologic testing should be performed for patients whose geographic histories indicate potential exposure, especially those who exhibit eosinophilia and/or are candidates for glucocorticoid treatment of other conditions. In disseminated strongyloidiasis, filariform larvae should be sought in stool as well as in samples obtained from sites of potential larval migration, including sputum, bronchoalveolar lavage fluid, or surgical drainage fluid.

TREATMENT STRONGYLOIDIASIS

Even in the asymptomatic state, strongyloidiasis must be treated because of the potential for subsequent dissemination and fatal hyperinfection. Ivermectin (200 μg/kg daily for 2 days) is consistently more effective than albendazole (400 mg daily for 3 days). For disseminated strongyloidiasis, treatment with ivermectin should be extended for at least 5–7 days or until the parasites have been eradicated. In immunocompromised hosts, the course of ivermectin should be repeated 2 weeks after initial treatment.

TRICHURIASIS

Most infections with *Trichuris trichiura* are asymptomatic, but heavy infections may cause gastrointestinal symptoms. Like the other soil-transmitted helminths, whipworm is distributed globally in the tropics and subtropics and is most common among poor children from resource-poor regions of the world.

Life Cycle Adult *Trichuris* worms reside in the colon and cecum, the anterior portions threaded into the superficial mucosa. Thousands of eggs laid daily by adult female worms pass with the feces and mature in the soil. After ingestion, infective eggs hatch in the duodenum, releasing larvae that mature before migrating to the large bowel. The entire cycle takes ~3 months, and adult worms may live for several years.

Clinical Features Tissue reactions to *Trichuris* are mild. Most infected individuals have no symptoms or eosinophilia. Heavy infections may result in anemia, abdominal pain, anorexia, and bloody or mucoid diarrhea resembling inflammatory bowel disease. Rectal prolapse can result from massive infections in children, who often suffer from malnourishment and other diarrheal illnesses. Moderately heavy *Trichuris* burdens also contribute to growth retardation.

Diagnosis and Treatment The characteristic 50- by 20-μm lemon-shaped *Trichuris* eggs are readily detected on stool examination. Adult worms, which are 3–5 cm long, are occasionally seen on proctoscopy. Mebendazole (500 mg once) or albendazole (400 mg daily for 3 doses) is safe and moderately effective for treatment, with cure rates of 70–90%. Ivermectin (200 μg/kg daily for 3 doses) is also safe but is not quite as efficacious as the benzimidazoles.

ENTEROBIASIS (PINWORM)

E. vermicularis is more common in temperate countries than in the tropics. In the United States, ~40 million persons are infected with pinworms, with a disproportionate number of cases among children.

Life Cycle and Epidemiology *Enterobius* adult worms are ~1 cm long and dwell in the cecum. Gravid female worms migrate nocturnally into the perianal region and release up to 2000 immature eggs each. The eggs become infective within hours and are transmitted by hand-to-mouth passage. From ingested eggs, larvae hatch and mature into adults. This life cycle takes ~1 month, and adult worms survive for ~2 months. Self-infection results from perianal scratching and transport of infective eggs on the hands or under the nails to the mouth. Because of the ease of person-to-person spread, pinworm infections are common among family members.

Clinical Features Most pinworm infections are asymptomatic. Perianal pruritus is the cardinal symptom. The itching, which is often worse at night as a result of the nocturnal migration of the female worms, may lead to excoriation and bacterial superinfection. Heavy infections have been alleged to cause abdominal pain and weight loss. On rare occasions, pinworms invade the female genital tract, causing vulvovaginitis and pelvic or peritoneal granulomas. Eosinophilia is uncommon.

Diagnosis Since pinworm eggs are not released in feces, the diagnosis cannot be made by conventional fecal ova and parasite tests. Instead, eggs are detected by the application of clear cellulose acetate tape to the perianal region in the morning. After the tape is transferred to a slide, microscopic examination will detect pinworm eggs, which are oval, measure 55 by 25 μm, and are flattened along one side.

TREATMENT ENTEROBIASIS

Infected children and adults should be treated with mebendazole (100 mg once) or albendazole (400 mg once), with the same treatment repeated after 2 weeks. Treatment of household members is advocated to eliminate asymptomatic reservoirs of potential reinfection.

TRICHOSTRONGYLIASIS

Trichostrongylus species, which are normally parasites of herbivorous animals, occasionally infect humans, particularly in Asia and Africa. Humans acquire the infection by accidentally ingesting *Trichostrongylus* larvae on contaminated leafy vegetables. The larvae do not migrate in humans but mature directly into adult worms in the small bowel. These worms ingest far less blood than hookworms; most infected persons are asymptomatic, but heavy infections may give rise to mild anemia and eosinophilia. In stool examinations, *Trichostrongylus* eggs resemble hookworm eggs but are larger (85 by 115 μm). Treatment consists of mebendazole or albendazole (Chap. 246e).

ANISAKIASIS

Anisakiasis is a gastrointestinal infection caused by the accidental ingestion in uncooked saltwater fish of nematode larvae belonging to the family Anisakidae. The incidence of anisakiasis in the United States has increased as a result of the growing popularity of raw fish dishes. Most cases occur in Japan, the Netherlands, and Chile, where raw fish—sashimi, pickled green herring, and ceviche, respectively—are national culinary staples. Anisakid nematodes parasitize large sea mammals such as whales, dolphins, and seals. As part of a complex parasitic life cycle involving marine food chains, infectious larvae migrate to the musculature of a variety of fish. Both *Anisakis simplex* and *Pseudoterranova decipiens* have been implicated in human anisakiasis, but an identical gastric syndrome may be caused by the red larvae of eustrongylid parasites of fish-eating birds.

When humans consume infected raw fish, live larvae may be coughed up within 48 h. Alternatively, larvae may immediately penetrate the mucosa of the stomach. Within hours, violent upper abdominal pain accompanied by nausea and occasionally vomiting ensues, mimicking an acute abdomen. The diagnosis can be established by direct visualization on upper endoscopy, outlining of the worm by contrast radiographic studies, or histopathologic examination of extracted tissue. Extraction of the burrowing larvae during endoscopy is curative. In addition, larvae may pass to the small bowel, where they penetrate the mucosa and provoke a vigorous eosinophilic granulomatous response. Symptoms may appear 1–2 weeks after the infective meal, with intermittent abdominal pain, diarrhea, nausea, and fever resembling the manifestations of Crohn's disease. The diagnosis may be suggested by barium studies and confirmed by curative surgical resection of a granuloma in which the worm is embedded. Anisakid eggs are not found in the stool, since the larvae do not mature in humans. Serologic tests have been developed but are not widely available.

Anisakid larvae in saltwater fish are killed by cooking to 60°C, freezing at -20°C for 3 days, or commercial blast freezing, but usually not by salting, marinating, or cold smoking. No medical treatment is available; surgical or endoscopic removal should be undertaken.

CAPILLARIASIS

Intestinal capillariasis is caused by ingestion of raw fish infected with *Capillaria philippinensis*. Subsequent autoinfection can lead to a severe wasting syndrome. The disease occurs in the Philippines and Thailand and, on occasion, elsewhere in Asia. The natural cycle of *C. philippinensis* involves fish from fresh and brackish water. When humans eat infected raw fish, the larvae mature in the intestine into adult worms, which produce invasive larvae that cause intestinal inflammation and villus loss. Capillariasis has an insidious onset with nonspecific abdominal pain and watery diarrhea. If untreated, progressive autoinfection can lead to protein-losing enteropathy, severe malabsorption, and ultimately death from cachexia, cardiac failure, or superinfection. The diagnosis is established by identification of the characteristic peanut-shaped (20- by 40-μm) eggs on stool examination. Severely ill patients require hospitalization and supportive therapy in addition to prolonged anthelmintic treatment with albendazole (200 mg twice daily for 10 days; Chap. 246e).

ABDOMINAL ANGIOSTRONGYLIASIS

Abdominal angiostrongyliasis is found in Latin America and Africa. The zoonotic parasite *Angiostrongylus costaricensis* causes eosinophilic ileocolitis after the ingestion of contaminated vegetation. *A. costaricensis* normally parasitizes the cotton rat and other rodents, with slugs and snails serving as intermediate hosts. Humans become infected by accidentally ingesting infective larvae in mollusk slime deposited on fruits and vegetables; children are at highest risk. The larvae penetrate the gut wall and migrate to the mesenteric artery, where they develop into adult worms. Eggs deposited in the gut wall provoke an intense eosinophilic granulomatous reaction, and adult worms may cause mesenteric arteritis, thrombosis, or frank bowel infarction. Symptoms may mimic those of appendicitis, including abdominal pain and tenderness, fever, vomiting, and a palpable mass in the right iliac fossa. Leukocytosis and eosinophilia are prominent. CT with contrast medium typically shows inflamed bowel, often with concomitant obstruction, but a definitive diagnosis is usually made surgically with partial bowel resection. Pathologic study reveals a thickened bowel wall with eosinophilic granulomas surrounding the *Angiostrongylus* eggs. In nonsurgical cases, the diagnosis rests solely on clinical grounds because larvae and eggs cannot be detected in the stool. Medical therapy for abdominal angiostrongyliasis is of uncertain efficacy. Careful observation and surgical resection for severe symptoms are the mainstays of treatment.

258 Filarial and Related Infections

Thomas B. Nutman, Peter F. Weller

Filarial worms are nematodes that dwell in the subcutaneous tissues and the lymphatics. Eight filarial species infect humans (Table 258-1); of these, four—*Wuchereria bancrofti, Brugia malayi, Onchocerca volvulus*, and *Loa loa*—are responsible for most serious filarial infections. Filarial parasites, which infect an estimated 170 million persons worldwide, are transmitted by specific species of mosquitoes or other arthropods and have a complex life cycle, including infective larval stages carried by insects and adult worms that reside in either lymphatic or subcutaneous tissues of humans. The offspring of adults are microfilariae, which, depending on their species, are 200–250 μm long and 5–7 μm wide, may or may not be enveloped in a loose sheath, and either circulate in the blood or migrate through the skin (Table 258-1). To complete the life cycle, microfilariae are ingested by the arthropod vector and develop over 1–2 weeks into new infective larvae. Adult worms live for many years, whereas microfilariae survive for 3–36 months. The bacterial endosymbiont *Wolbachia* has been found intracellularly in all stages of *Brugia, Wuchereria, Mansonella*, and *Onchocerca* species and has become a target for antifilarial chemotherapy.

Usually, infection is established only with repeated, prolonged exposures to infective larvae. Since the clinical manifestations of filarial diseases develop relatively slowly, these infections should be considered to induce chronic infections with possible long-term debilitating effects. In terms of the nature, severity, and timing of clinical manifestations, patients with filarial infections who are native to endemic areas and have lifelong exposure may differ significantly from those who are travelers or who have recently moved to these areas. Characteristically, filarial disease is more acute and intense in newly exposed individuals than in natives of endemic areas.

LYMPHATIC FILARIASIS

Lymphatic filariasis is caused by *W. bancrofti, B. malayi*, or *B. timori*. The threadlike adult parasites reside in lymphatic channels or lymph nodes, where they may remain viable for more than two decades.

EPIDEMIOLOGY

W. bancrofti, the most widely distributed filarial parasite of humans, affects an estimated 110 million people and is found throughout the tropics and subtropics, including Asia and the Pacific Islands, Africa, areas of South America, and the Caribbean basin. Humans are the only definitive host for the parasite. Generally, the subperiodic form is found only in the Pacific Islands; elsewhere, *W. bancrofti* is nocturnally periodic. Nocturnally periodic forms of microfilariae are scarce in peripheral blood by day and increase at night, whereas subperiodic forms are present in peripheral blood at all times and reach maximal levels in the afternoon. Natural vectors for *W. bancrofti* are *Culex fatigans* mosquitoes in urban settings and *Anopheles* or *Aedes* mosquitoes in rural areas.

Brugian filariasis due to *B. malayi* occurs primarily in eastern India, Indonesia, Malaysia, and the Philippines. *B. malayi* also has two forms distinguished by the periodicity of microfilaremia. The more common nocturnal form is transmitted in areas of coastal rice fields, while the subperiodic form is found in forests. *B. malayi* naturally infects cats as well as humans. The distribution of *B. timori* is limited to the islands of southeastern Indonesia.

PATHOLOGY

The principal pathologic changes result from inflammatory damage to the lymphatics, which is typically caused by adult worms and not by microfilariae. Adult worms live in afferent lymphatics or sinuses of lymph nodes and cause lymphatic dilation and thickening of the vessel walls. The infiltration of plasma cells, eosinophils, and macrophages in and around the infected vessels, along with endothelial and connective tissue proliferation, leads to tortuosity of the lymphatics and damaged or incompetent lymph valves. Lymphedema and chronic stasis changes with hard or brawny edema develop in the overlying skin. These consequences of filarial infection are due both to the direct effects of the worms and to the host's inflammatory response to the parasite. Inflammatory responses are believed to cause the granulomatous and proliferative processes that precede total lymphatic obstruction. It is thought that the lymphatic vessel remains patent as long as the worm remains viable and that the death of the worm leads to enhanced granulomatous reactions and fibrosis. Lymphatic obstruction results, and, despite collateralization, lymphatic function is compromised.

CLINICAL FEATURES

The most common presentations of the lymphatic filariases are asymptomatic (or subclinical) microfilaremia, hydrocele (Fig. 258-1), acute

TABLE 258-1 CHARACTERISTICS OF THE FILARIAE

Organism	Periodicity	Distribution	Vector	Location of Adult	Microfilarial Location	Sheath
Wuchereria bancrofti	Nocturnal	Cosmopolitan areas worldwide, including South America, Africa, southern Asia, Papua New Guinea, China, Indonesia	*Culex, Anopheles* (mosquitoes)	Lymphatic tissue	Blood	+
	Subperiodic	Eastern Pacific	*Aedes* (mosquitoes)	Lymphatic tissue	Blood	+
Brugia malayi	Nocturnal	Southeast Asia, Indonesia, India	*Mansonia, Anopheles* (mosquitoes)	Lymphatic tissue	Blood	+
	Subperiodic	Indonesia, Southeast Asia	*Coquillettidia, Mansonia* (mosquitoes)	Lymphatic tissue	Blood	+
B. timori	Nocturnal	Indonesia	*Anopheles* (mosquitoes)	Lymphatic tissue	Blood	+
Loa loa	Diurnal	West and Central Africa	*Chrysops* (deerflies)	Subcutaneous tissue	Blood	+
Onchocerca volvulus	None	South and Central America, Africa	*Simulium* (blackflies)	Subcutaneous tissue	Skin, eye	–
Mansonella ozzardi	None	South and Central America	*Culicoides* (midges)	Undetermined site	Blood	–
		Caribbean	*Simulium* (blackflies)			
M. perstans	None	South and Central America, Africa	*Culicoides* (midges)	Body cavities, mesentery, perirenal tissue	Blood	–
M. streptocerca	None	West and Central Africa	*Culicoides* (midges)	Subcutaneous tissue	Skin	–

adenolymphangitis (ADL), and chronic lymphatic disease. In areas where *W. bancrofti* or *B. malayi* is endemic, the overwhelming majority of infected individuals have few overt clinical manifestations of filarial infection despite large numbers of circulating microfilariae in the peripheral blood. Although they may be clinically asymptomatic, virtually all persons with *W. bancrofti* or *B. malayi* microfilaremia have some degree of subclinical disease that includes microscopic hematuria and/or proteinuria, dilated (and tortuous) lymphatics (visualized by imaging), and—in men with *W. bancrofti* infection—scrotal lymphangiectasia (detectable by ultrasound). Despite these findings, the majority of individuals appear to remain clinically asymptomatic for years; in relatively few does the infection progress to either acute or chronic disease.

ADL is characterized by high fever, lymphatic inflammation (lymphangitis and lymphadenitis), and transient local edema. The lymphangitis is retrograde, extending peripherally from the lymph node

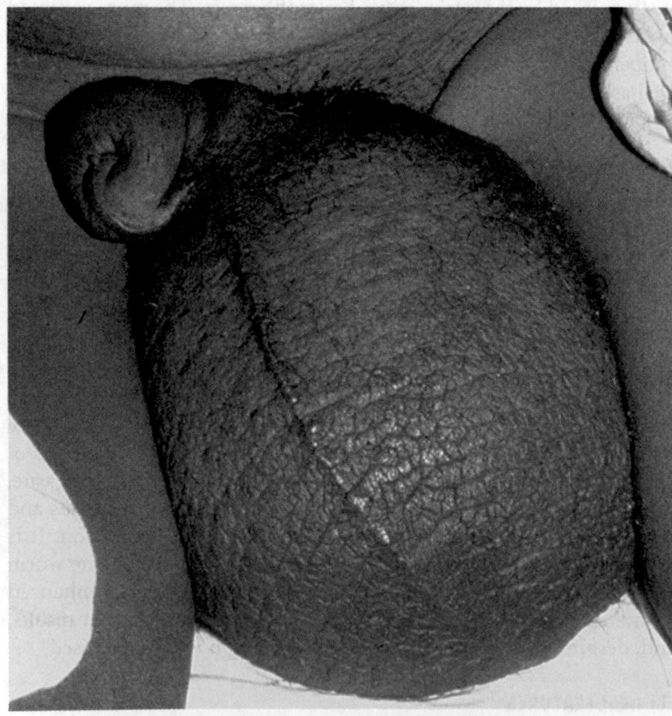

FIGURE 258-1 Hydrocele associated with *Wuchereria bancrofti* infection.

draining the area where the adult parasites reside. Regional lymph nodes are often enlarged, and the entire lymphatic channel can become indurated and inflamed. Concomitant local thrombophlebitis can occur as well. In brugian filariasis, a single local abscess may form along the involved lymphatic tract and subsequently rupture to the surface. The lymphadenitis and lymphangitis can involve both the upper and lower extremities in both bancroftian and brugian filariasis, but involvement of the genital lymphatics occurs almost exclusively with *W. bancrofti* infection. This genital involvement can be manifested by funiculitis, epididymitis, and scrotal pain and tenderness. In endemic areas, another type of acute disease—dermatolymphangioadenitis (DLA)—is recognized as a syndrome that includes high fever, chills, myalgias, and headache. Edematous inflammatory plaques clearly demarcated from normal skin are seen. Vesicles, ulcers, and hyperpigmentation may also be noted. There is often a history of trauma, burns, irradiation, insect bites, punctiform lesions, or chemical injury. Entry lesions, especially in the interdigital area, are common. DLA is often diagnosed as cellulitis.

If lymphatic damage progresses, transient lymphedema can develop into lymphatic obstruction and the permanent changes associated with elephantiasis (Fig. 258-2). Brawny edema follows early pitting edema, the subcutaneous tissues thicken, and hyperkeratosis occurs. Fissuring of the skin develops, as do hyperplastic changes. Superinfection of these poorly vascularized tissues becomes a problem. In bancroftian filariasis, in which genital involvement is common, hydroceles may develop (Fig. 258-1); in advanced stages, this condition may evolve into scrotal lymphedema and scrotal elephantiasis. Furthermore, if there is obstruction of the retroperitoneal lymphatics, increased renal lymphatic pressure leads to rupture of the renal lymphatics and the development of chyluria, which is usually intermittent and most prominent in the morning.

The clinical manifestations of filarial infections in travelers or transmigrants who have recently entered an endemic region are distinctive. Given a sufficient number of bites by infected vectors, usually over a 3- to 6-month period, recently exposed patients can develop acute lymphatic or scrotal inflammation with or without urticaria and localized angioedema. Lymphadenitis of epitrochlear, axillary, femoral, or inguinal lymph nodes is often followed by retrogradely evolving lymphangitis. Acute attacks are short-lived and are not usually accompanied by fever. With prolonged exposure to infected mosquitoes, these attacks, if untreated, become more severe and lead to permanent lymphatic inflammation and obstruction.

DIAGNOSIS

A definitive diagnosis can be made only by detection of the parasites and hence can be difficult. Adult worms localized in lymphatic

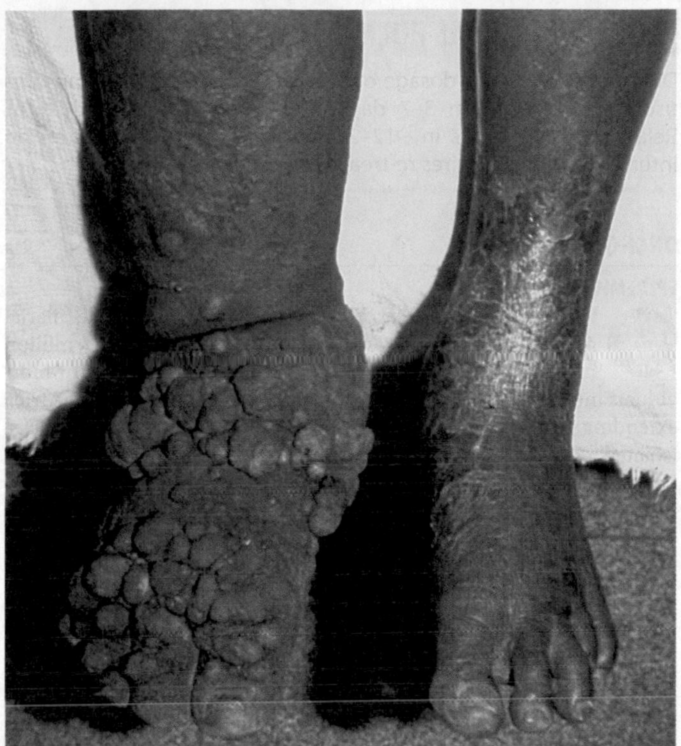

FIGURE 258-2 Elephantiasis of the lower extremity associated with *Wuchereria bancrofti* infection.

vessels or nodes are largely inaccessible. Microfilariae can be found in blood, in hydrocele fluid, or (occasionally) in other body fluids. Such fluids can be examined microscopically, either directly or—for greater sensitivity—after concentration of the parasites by the passage of fluid through a polycarbonate cylindrical-pore filter (pore size, 3 μm) or by the centrifugation of fluid fixed in 2% formalin (Knott's concentration technique). The timing of blood collection is critical and should be based on the periodicity of the microfilariae in the endemic region involved. Many infected individuals do not have microfilaremia, and definitive diagnosis in such cases can be difficult. Assays for circulating antigens of *W. bancrofti* permit the diagnosis of microfilaremic and cryptic (amicrofilaremic) infection. Two tests are commercially available: an enzyme-linked immunosorbent assay (ELISA) and a rapid-format immunochromatographic card test. Both assays have sensitivities of 93–100% and specificities approaching 100%. There are currently no tests for circulating antigens in brugian filariasis.

Polymerase chain reaction (PCR)–based assays for DNA of *W. bancrofti* and *B. malayi* in blood have been developed. A number of studies indicate that the sensitivity of this diagnostic method is equivalent to or greater than that of parasitologic methods.

In cases of suspected lymphatic filariasis, examination of the scrotum, the lymph nodes, or (in female patients) the breast by means of high-frequency ultrasound in conjunction with Doppler techniques may result in the identification of motile adult worms within dilated lymphatics. Worms may be visualized in the lymphatics of the spermatic cord in up to 80% of men infected with *W. bancrofti*. Live adult worms have a distinctive pattern of movement within the lymphatic vessels (termed the *filarial dance sign*). Radionuclide lymphoscintigraphic imaging of the limbs reliably demonstrates widespread lymphatic abnormalities in both subclinical microfilaremic persons and those with clinical manifestations of lymphatic pathology. Although of potential utility in the delineation of anatomic changes associated with infection, lymphoscintigraphy is unlikely to assume primacy in the diagnostic evaluation of individuals with suspected infection; it is principally a research tool, although it has been used more widely for assessment of lymphedema of any cause. Eosinophilia and elevated serum concentrations of IgE and antifilarial antibody support the diagnosis of lymphatic filariasis. There is, however, extensive cross-reactivity between filarial antigens and antigens of other helminths, including the common intestinal roundworms; thus, interpretations of serologic findings can be difficult. In addition, residents of endemic areas can become sensitized to filarial antigens (and thus be serologically positive) through exposure to infected mosquitoes without having patent filarial infections.

The ADL associated with lymphatic filariasis must be distinguished from thrombophlebitis, infection, and trauma. Retrograde evolution is a characteristic feature that helps distinguish filarial lymphangitis from ascending bacterial lymphangitis. Chronic filarial lymphedema must also be distinguished from the lymphedema of malignancy, postoperative scarring, trauma, chronic edematous states, and congenital lymphatic system abnormalities.

TREATMENT LYMPHATIC FILARIASIS

With newer definitions of clinical syndromes in lymphatic filariasis and new tools to assess clinical status (e.g., ultrasound, lymphoscintigraphy, circulating filarial antigen assays, PCR), approaches to treatment based on infection status can be considered.

Orally administered diethylcarbamazine (DEC; 6 mg/kg daily for 12 days), which has both macro- and microfilaricidal properties, remains the drug of choice for the treatment of active lymphatic filariasis (defined by microfilaremia, antigen positivity, or adult worms on ultrasound), although albendazole (400 mg twice daily by mouth for 21 days) has also demonstrated macrofilaricidal efficacy. A 4- to 6-week course of oral doxycycline (targeting the intracellular *Wolbachia*) also has significant macrofilaricidal activity, as does DEC/albendazole used daily for 7 days. The addition of DEC to a 3-week course of doxycycline is efficacious in lymphatic filariasis.

Regimens that combine single doses of albendazole (400 mg) with either DEC (6 mg/kg) or ivermectin (200 μg/kg) all have a sustained microfilaricidal effect and are the mainstay of programs for the eradication of lymphatic filariasis in Africa (albendazole/ivermectin) and elsewhere (albendazole/DEC) (see "Prevention and Control," below).

As has already been mentioned, a growing body of evidence indicates that, although they may be asymptomatic, virtually all persons with *W. bancrofti* or *B. malayi* microfilaremia have some degree of subclinical disease (hematuria, proteinuria, abnormalities on lymphoscintigraphy). Thus, early treatment of asymptomatic persons who have microfilaremia is recommended to prevent further lymphatic damage. For ADL, supportive treatment (including the administration of antipyretics and analgesics) is recommended, as is antibiotic therapy if secondary bacterial infection is likely. Similarly, because lymphatic disease is associated with the presence of adult worms, treatment with DEC is recommended for microfilaria-negative carriers of adult worms.

In persons with chronic manifestations of lymphatic filariasis, treatment regimens that emphasize hygiene, prevention of secondary bacterial infections, and physiotherapy have gained wide acceptance for morbidity control. These regimens are similar to those recommended for lymphedema of most nonfilarial causes and are known by a variety of names, including *complex decongestive physiotherapy* and *complex lymphedema therapy*. Hydroceles (Fig. 258-1) can be managed surgically. With chronic manifestations of lymphatic filariasis, drug treatment should be reserved for individuals who have evidence of active infection; however, a 6-week course of doxycycline has been shown to provide improvement in filarial lymphedema irrespective of disease activity.

Side effects of DEC treatment include fever, chills, arthralgias, headaches, nausea, and vomiting. Both the development and the severity of these reactions are directly related to the number of microfilariae circulating in the bloodstream. The adverse reactions may represent either an acute hypersensitivity reaction to the antigens being released by dead and dying parasites or an inflammatory reaction induced by the intracellular *Wolbachia* endosymbionts freed from their intracellular niche.

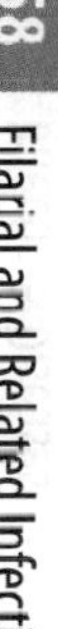

Ivermectin has a side effect profile similar to that of DEC when used in lymphatic filariasis. In patients infected with *L. loa* who have high levels of microfilaremia, DEC—like ivermectin (see "Loiasis," below)—can elicit severe encephalopathic complications. When used in single-dose regimens for the treatment of lymphatic filariasis, albendazole is associated with relatively few side effects.

PREVENTION AND CONTROL

To protect themselves against filarial infection, individuals must avoid contact with infected mosquitoes by using personal protective measures, including bed nets, particularly those impregnated with insecticides such as permethrin. Community-based intervention is the current approach to elimination of lymphatic filariasis as a public health problem. The underlying tenet of this approach is that mass annual distribution of antimicrofilarial chemotherapy—albendazole with either DEC (for all areas except those where onchocerciasis is coendemic; see section on onchocerciasis treatment, below) or ivermectin—will profoundly suppress microfilaremia. If the suppression is sustained, then transmission can be interrupted.

Created by the World Health Organization in 1997, the Global Programme to Eliminate Lymphatic Filariasis is based on mass administration of single annual doses of DEC plus albendazole in non-African regions and of albendazole plus ivermectin in Africa. Available information from late 2013 indicated that more than 792 million persons in 53 countries had thus far participated. Not only has lymphatic filariasis been eliminated in some defined areas, but collateral benefits—avoidance of disability and treatment of intestinal helminths and other conditions (e.g., scabies and louse infestation)—have also been noted. The strategy of the global program is being refined, and attempts are being made to integrate this effort with other mass-treatment strategies (e.g., deworming programs, malaria control, and trachoma control) in an integrated control strategy.

TROPICAL PULMONARY EOSINOPHILIA

Tropical pulmonary eosinophilia (TPE) is a distinct syndrome that develops in some individuals infected with the lymphatic-dwelling filarial species. This syndrome affects males and females in a ratio of 4:1, often during the third decade of life. The majority of cases have been reported from India, Pakistan, Sri Lanka, Brazil, Guyana, and Southeast Asia.

Clinical Features The main features include a history of residence in filarial-endemic regions, paroxysmal cough and wheezing (usually nocturnal and probably related to the nocturnal periodicity of microfilariae), weight loss, low-grade fever, lymphadenopathy, and pronounced blood eosinophilia (>3000 eosinophils/μL). Chest x-rays or CT scans may be normal but generally show increased bronchovascular markings. Diffuse miliary lesions or mottled opacities may be present in the middle and lower lung fields. Tests of pulmonary function show restrictive abnormalities in most cases and obstructive defects in half. Characteristically, total serum IgE levels (4–40 KIU/mL) and antifilarial antibody titers are markedly elevated.

Pathology In TPE, microfilariae and parasite antigens are rapidly cleared from the bloodstream by the lungs. The clinical symptoms result from allergic and inflammatory reactions elicited by the cleared parasites. In some patients, trapping of microfilariae in other reticuloendothelial organs can cause hepatomegaly, splenomegaly, or lymphadenopathy. A prominent, eosinophil-enriched, intraalveolar infiltrate is often reported, and with it comes the release of cytotoxic proinflammatory eosinophil granule proteins that may mediate some of the pathology seen in TPE. In the absence of successful treatment, interstitial fibrosis can lead to progressive pulmonary damage.

Differential Diagnosis TPE must be distinguished from asthma, Löffler's syndrome, allergic bronchopulmonary aspergillosis, allergic granulomatosis with angiitis (Churg-Strauss syndrome), the systemic vasculitides (most notably, periarteritis nodosa and granulomatosis with polyangiitis), chronic eosinophilic pneumonia, and the idiopathic hypereosinophilic syndrome.

TREATMENT TROPICAL PULMONARY EOSINOPHILIA

DEC is used at a daily dosage of 4–6 mg/kg for 14 days. Symptoms usually resolve within 3–7 days after the initiation of therapy. Relapse, which occurs in ~12–25% of cases (sometimes after an interval of years), requires re-treatment.

ONCHOCERCIASIS

EPIDEMIOLOGY

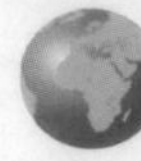

Onchocerciasis ("river blindness") is caused by the filarial nematode *O. volvulus*, which infects an estimated 37 million individuals in 35 countries worldwide. The majority of individuals infected with *O. volvulus* live in the equatorial region of Africa extending from the Atlantic coast to the Red Sea. In the Americas, isolated foci were identified in Mexico, Guatemala, Colombia, Ecuador, Venezuela, and Brazil. The infection is also found in Yemen.

ETIOLOGY

Infection in humans begins with the deposition of infective larvae on the skin by the bite of an infected blackfly. The larvae develop into adults, which are typically found in subcutaneous nodules. About 7 months to 3 years after infection, the gravid female releases microfilariae that migrate out of the nodule and throughout the tissues, concentrating in the dermis. Infection is transmitted to other persons when a female fly ingests microfilariae from the host's skin and these microfilariae then develop into infective larvae. Adult *O. volvulus* females and males are ~40–60 cm and ~3–6 cm in length, respectively. The life span of adults can be as long as 18 years, with an average of ~9 years. Because the blackfly vector breeds along free-flowing rivers and streams (particularly in rapids) and generally restricts its flight to an area within several kilometers of these breeding sites, both biting and disease transmission are most intense in these locations.

PATHOLOGY

Onchocerciasis primarily affects the skin, eyes, and lymph nodes. In contrast to the pathology in lymphatic filariasis, the damage in onchocerciasis is elicited by microfilariae and not by adult parasites. In the skin, there are mild but chronic inflammatory changes that can result in loss of elastic fibers, atrophy, and fibrosis. The subcutaneous nodules (*onchocercomata*) consist primarily of fibrous tissues surrounding the adult worm, often with a peripheral ring of inflammatory cells (characterized as lymphatic in origin) surrounded by an endothelial layer. In the eye, neovascularization and corneal scarring lead to corneal opacities and blindness. Inflammation in the anterior and posterior chambers frequently results in anterior uveitis, chorioretinitis, and optic atrophy. Although punctate opacities are due to an inflammatory reaction surrounding dead or dying microfilariae, the pathogenesis of most manifestations of onchocerciasis is still unclear.

CLINICAL FEATURES

Skin Pruritus and rash are the most common manifestations of onchocerciasis. The pruritus can be incapacitating; the rash is typically a papular eruption (Fig. 258-3) that is generalized rather than localized to a particular region of the body. Long-term infection results in exaggerated and premature wrinkling of the skin, loss of elastic fibers, and epidermal atrophy that can lead to loose, redundant skin and hypo- or hyperpigmentation. Localized eczematoid dermatitis can cause hyperkeratosis, scaling, and pigmentary changes. In an immunologically hyperreactive form of onchodermatitis (commonly termed *sowdah* or *localized onchodermatitis*), the affected skin darkens as a consequence of the profound inflammation that occurs as microfilariae in the skin are cleared.

Onchocercomata These subcutaneous nodules, which can be palpable and/or visible, contain the adult worm. In African patients, they are common over the coccyx and sacrum, the trochanter of the femur, the lateral anterior crest, and other bony prominences; in patients from South and Central America, nodules

FIGURE 258-3 Papular eruption as a consequence of onchocerciasis.

tend to develop preferentially in the upper part of the body, particularly on the head, neck, and shoulders. Nodules vary in size and characteristically are firm and not tender. It has been estimated that, for every palpable nodule, there are four deeper nonpalpable ones.

Ocular Tissue Visual impairment is the most serious complication of onchocerciasis and usually affects only those persons with moderate or heavy infections. Lesions may develop in all parts of the eye. The most common early finding is conjunctivitis with photophobia. Punctate keratitis—acute inflammatory reactions surrounding dying microfilariae and manifested as "snowflake" opacities—is common among younger patients and resolves without apparent complications.

Sclerosing keratitis occurs in 1–5% of infected persons and is the leading cause of onchocercal blindness in Africa. Anterior uveitis and iridocyclitis develop in ~5% of infected persons in Africa. In Latin America, complications of the anterior uveal tract (pupillary deformity) may cause secondary glaucoma. Characteristic chorioretinal lesions develop as a result of atrophy and hyperpigmentation of the retinal pigment epithelium. Constriction of the visual fields and overt optic atrophy may occur.

Lymph Nodes Mild to moderate lymphadenopathy is common, particularly in the inguinal and femoral areas, where the enlarged nodes may hang down in response to gravity ("hanging groin"), sometimes predisposing to inguinal and femoral hernias.

Systemic Manifestations Some heavily infected individuals develop cachexia with loss of adipose tissue and muscle mass. Among adults who become blind, there is a three- to fourfold increase in the mortality rate.

DIAGNOSIS

Definitive diagnosis depends on the detection of an adult worm in an excised nodule or, more commonly, of microfilariae in a skin snip. Skin snips are obtained with a corneal-scleral punch, which collects a blood-free skin biopsy sample extending to just below the epidermis, or by lifting of the skin with the tip of a needle and excision of a small (1- to 3-mm) piece with a sterile scalpel blade. The biopsy tissue is incubated in tissue culture medium or in saline on a glass slide or flat-bottomed microtiter plate. After incubation for 2–4 h (or occasionally overnight in light infections), microfilariae emergent from the skin can be seen by low-power microscopy.

Eosinophilia and elevated serum IgE levels are common but, because they occur in many parasitic infections, are not diagnostic in themselves. Assays to detect specific antibodies to *Onchocerca* and PCR to detect onchocercal DNA in skin snips are used in specialized laboratories and are highly sensitive and specific.

TREATMENT ONCHOCERCIASIS

The main goals of therapy are to prevent the development of irreversible lesions and to alleviate symptoms. Surgical excision is recommended when nodules are located on the head (because of the proximity of microfilaria-producing adult worms to the eye), but chemotherapy is the mainstay of management. Ivermectin, a semisynthetic macrocyclic lactone active against microfilariae, is the first-line agent for the treatment of onchocerciasis. It is given orally in a single dose of 150 μg/kg, either yearly or semiannually. More frequent ivermectin administration (every 3 months) has been suggested to ameliorate pruritus and skin disease

After treatment, most individuals have few or no reactions. Pruritus, cutaneous edema, and/or maculopapular rash occurs in ~1–10% of treated individuals. In areas of Africa coendemic for *O. volvulus* and *L. loa*, however, ivermectin is contraindicated (as it is for pregnant or breast-feeding women) because of severe posttreatment encephalopathy, especially in patients who are heavily microfilaremic for *L. loa* (>8000 microfilariae/mL). Although ivermectin treatment results in a marked drop in microfilarial density, its effect can be short-lived (<3 months in some cases). Thus, it is occasionally necessary to give ivermectin more frequently for persistent symptoms.

A 6-week course of doxycycline is macrofilaristatic, rendering female adult worms sterile for long periods.

PREVENTION

Vector control has been beneficial in highly endemic areas in which breeding sites are vulnerable to insecticide spraying, but most areas endemic for onchocerciasis are not suited to this type of control. Community-based administration of ivermectin every 6–12 months is being used to interrupt transmission in endemic areas. This measure, in conjunction with vector control, has already helped eliminate the infection in most of Latin America and has reduced the prevalence of disease in many endemic foci in Africa. No drug has proved useful for prophylaxis of *O. volvulus* infection.

LOIASIS

ETIOLOGY AND EPIDEMIOLOGY

Loiasis is caused by *L. loa* (the African eye worm), which is present in the rainforests of West and Central Africa. Adult parasites (females, 50–70 mm long and 0.5 mm wide; males, 25–35 mm long and 0.25 mm wide) live in subcutaneous tissues. Microfilariae circulate in the blood with a diurnal periodicity that peaks between 12:00 noon and 2:00 P.M.

CLINICAL FEATURES

Manifestations of loiasis in natives of endemic areas may differ from those in temporary residents or visitors. Among the indigenous population, loiasis is often an asymptomatic infection with microfilaremia. Infection may be recognized only after subconjunctival migration of an adult worm (Fig. 258-4) or may be manifested by episodic *Calabar swellings*—evanescent localized areas of angioedema and erythema developing on the extremities and less frequently at other sites. Nephropathy, encephalopathy, and cardiomyopathy can occur but are rare. In patients who are not residents of endemic areas, allergic symptoms predominate, episodes of Calabar swelling tend to be more frequent and debilitating, microfilaremia is less common, and eosinophilia and increased levels of antifilarial antibodies are characteristic.

PATHOLOGY

The pathogenesis of the manifestations of loiasis is poorly understood. Calabar swellings are thought to result from a hypersensitivity reaction to adult worm antigens.

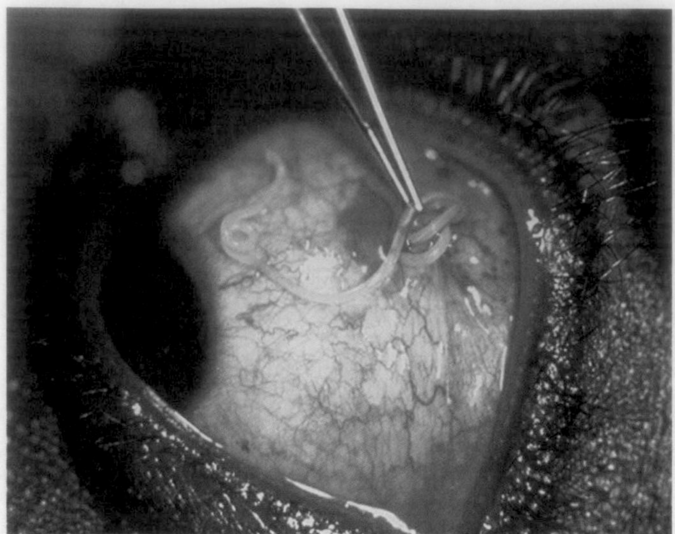

FIGURE 258-4 **Adult *Loa loa* worm** being surgically removed after its subconjunctival migration.

DIAGNOSIS

Definitive diagnosis of loiasis requires the detection of microfilariae in the peripheral blood or the isolation of the adult worm from the eye (Fig. 258-4) or from a subcutaneous biopsy specimen collected from a site of swelling developing after treatment. PCR-based assays for the detection of *L. loa* DNA in blood are available in specialized laboratories and are highly sensitive and specific, as are some newer recombinant antigen–based serologic techniques. In practice, the diagnosis must often be based on a characteristic history and clinical presentation, blood eosinophilia, and elevated levels of antifilarial antibodies, particularly in travelers to an endemic region, who are usually amicrofilaremic. Other clinical findings in travelers include hypergammaglobulinemia, elevated levels of serum IgE, and elevated leukocyte and eosinophil counts.

TREATMENT LOIASIS

DEC (8–10 mg/kg per day administered orally for 21 days) is effective against both the adult and the microfilarial forms of *L. loa*, but multiple courses are frequently necessary before loiasis resolves completely. In cases of heavy microfilaremia, allergic or other inflammatory reactions can take place during treatment, including central nervous system involvement with coma and encephalitis. Heavy infections can be treated initially with apheresis to remove the microfilariae and with glucocorticoids (40–60 mg of prednisone per day) followed by doses of DEC (0.5 mg/kg per day). If antifilarial treatment has no adverse effects, the prednisone dose can be rapidly tapered and the dose of DEC gradually increased to 8–10 mg/kg per day.

Albendazole or ivermectin is effective in reducing microfilarial loads, although neither is approved for this purpose by the U.S. Food and Drug Administration. Moreover, ivermectin is contraindicated in patients with >8000 microfilariae/mL because this drug has been associated with severe adverse events (including encephalopathy and death) in heavily infected patients with loiasis in West and Central Africa. DEC (300 mg weekly) is an effective prophylactic regimen for loiasis.

STREPTOCERCIASIS

Mansonella streptocerca, found mainly in the tropical forest belt of Africa from Ghana to the Democratic Republic of the Congo, is transmitted by biting midges. The major clinical manifestations involve the skin and include pruritus, papular rashes, and pigmentation changes. Many infected individuals have inguinal adenopathy, although most are asymptomatic. The diagnosis is made by detection of the characteristic microfilariae in skin snips. Ivermectin at a single dose of 150 μg/kg leads to sustained suppression of microfilariae in the skin and is probably the treatment of choice for streptocerciasis.

MANSONELLA PERSTANS INFECTION

M. perstans, distributed across the center of Africa and in northeastern South America, is transmitted by midges. Adult worms reside in serous cavities—pericardial, pleural, and peritoneal—as well as in the mesentery and the perirenal and retroperitoneal tissues. Microfilariae circulate in the blood without periodicity. The clinical and pathologic features of the infection are poorly defined. Most patients appear to be asymptomatic, but manifestations may include transient angioedema and pruritus of the arms, face, or other parts of the body (analogous to the Calabar swellings of loiasis); fever; headache; arthralgias; and right-upper-quadrant pain. Occasionally, pericarditis and hepatitis occur. The diagnosis is based on the demonstration of microfilariae in blood or serosal effusions. Perstans filariasis is often associated with peripheral-blood eosinophilia and antifilarial antibody elevations.

With the identification of a *Wolbachia* endosymbiont in *M. perstans*, doxycycline (200 mg twice a day) for 6 weeks has been established as the first effective treatment for this infection.

MANSONELLA OZZARDI INFECTION

The distribution of *M. ozzardi* is restricted to Central and South America and certain Caribbean islands. Adult worms are rarely recovered from humans. Microfilariae circulate in the blood without periodicity. Although this organism has often been considered nonpathogenic, headache, articular pain, fever, pulmonary symptoms, adenopathy, hepatomegaly, pruritus, and eosinophilia have been ascribed to *M. ozzardi* infection. The diagnosis is made by detection of microfilariae in peripheral blood. Ivermectin is effective in treating this infection.

DRACUNCULIASIS (GUINEA WORM INFECTION)

ETIOLOGY AND EPIDEMIOLOGY

The incidence of dracunculiasis, caused by *Dracunculus medinensis*, has declined dramatically because of global eradication efforts. In 2012, only 542 cases worldwide had been identified. The infection is currently endemic only in Chad, Ethiopia, Mali, and South Sudan.

Humans acquire *D. medinensis* when they ingest water containing infective larvae derived from *Cyclops*, a crustacean that is the intermediate host. Larvae penetrate the stomach or intestinal wall, mate, and mature. The adult male probably dies; the female worm develops over a year and migrates to subcutaneous tissues, usually in the lower extremity. As the thin female worm, ranging in length from 30 cm to 1 m, approaches the skin, a blister forms that, over days, breaks down and forms an ulcer. When the blister opens, large numbers of motile, rhabditiform larvae can be released into stagnant water; ingestion by *Cyclops* completes the life cycle.

CLINICAL FEATURES

Few or no clinical manifestations of dracunculiasis are evident until just before the blister forms, when there is an onset of fever and generalized allergic symptoms, including periorbital edema, wheezing, and urticaria. The emergence of the worm is associated with local pain and swelling. When the blister ruptures (usually as a result of immersion in water) and the adult worm releases larva-rich fluid, symptoms are relieved. The shallow ulcer surrounding the emerging adult worm heals over weeks to months. Such ulcers, however, can become secondarily infected, the result being cellulitis, local inflammation, abscess formation, or (uncommonly) tetanus. Occasionally, the adult worm does not emerge but becomes encapsulated and calcified.

DIAGNOSIS

The diagnosis is based on the findings developing with the emergence of the adult worm, as described above.

TREATMENT DRACUNCULIASIS

Gradual extraction of the worm by winding of a few centimeters on a stick each day remains the common and effective practice. Worms may be excised surgically. No drug is effective in treating dracunculiasis.

PREVENTION

Prevention, which remains the only real control measure, depends on the provision of safe drinking water.

ZOONOTIC FILARIAL INFECTIONS

Dirofilariae that affect primarily dogs, cats, and raccoons occasionally infect humans incidentally, as do *Brugia* and *Onchocerca* parasites that affect small mammals. Because humans are an abnormal host, the parasites never develop fully. Pulmonary dirofilarial infection caused by the canine heartworm *Dirofilaria immitis* generally presents in humans as a solitary pulmonary nodule. Chest pain, hemoptysis, and cough are uncommon. Infections with *D. repens* (from dogs) or *D. tenuis* (from raccoons) can cause local subcutaneous nodules in humans. Zoonotic *Brugia* infection can produce isolated lymph node enlargement, whereas zoonotic *Onchocerca* can cause subconjunctival masses. Eosinophilia levels and antifilarial antibody titers are not commonly elevated. Excisional biopsy is both diagnostic and curative. These infections usually do not respond to chemotherapy.

259 Schistosomiasis and Other Trematode Infections

Charles H. King, Adel A. F. Mahmoud

Trematodes, or flatworms, are a group of morphologically and biologically heterogeneous organisms that belong to the phylum Platyhelminthes. Human infection with trematodes occurs in many geographic areas and can cause considerable morbidity and mortality. The dependence on one drug—praziquantel—for treatment of most infections caused by trematodes raises the specter of developing resistance in these worms; several instances of reduced drug efficacy have already been reported. The widespread use of oxamniquine in the 1970s to reduce the impact of schistosomiasis resulted in the development of significant resistance. Recently, a single quantitative trait locus on schistosomal chromosome 6 was identified as the genetic basis for resistance.

ETIOLOGIC AGENTS AND THEIR LIFE CYCLES

For clinical purposes, significant trematode infections of humans may be divided according to the tissues invaded by the adult stage of the fluke, whether bloodstream, biliary tree, intestines, or lungs (Table 259-1). Trematodes share some common morphologic features, including macroscopic size (from one to several centimeters); dorsoventral, flattened, bilaterally symmetric bodies (adult worms); and the prominence of two suckers. Except for schistosomes, all human parasitic trematodes are hermaphroditic. Their life cycles involve a definitive host (mammalian/human), in which adult worms initiate sexual reproduction, and an intermediate host (snail), in which asexual multiplication of larvae occurs. More than one intermediate host may be necessary for some species of trematodes. Human infection is initiated either by direct penetration of intact skin or by ingestion. Upon maturation within humans, adult flukes initiate sexual reproduction and egg production. Helminth ova leave the definitive host in excreta or sputum and, upon reaching suitable environmental conditions, they hatch, releasing free-living miracidia that seek specific snail intermediate hosts. After asexual reproduction, cercariae are released from infected snails. In certain species, these organisms infect humans; in others, they find a second intermediate host to allow encystment into metacercariae—the infective stage for humans.

TABLE 259-1 MAJOR HUMAN TREMATODE INFECTIONS

Trematode	Transmission	Endemic Area(s)
Blood Flukes		
Schistosoma mansoni	Skin penetration by cercariae released from snails	Africa, South America, Middle East
S. japonicum	Skin penetration by cercariae released from snails	China, Philippines, Indonesia
S. intercalatum	Skin penetration by cercariae released from snails	West Africa
S. mekongi	Skin penetration by cercariae released from snails	Southeast Asia
S. haematobium	Skin penetration by cercariae released from snails	Africa, Middle East
Biliary (Hepatic) Flukes		
Clonorchis sinensis	Ingestion of metacercariae in freshwater fish	Eastern Asia
Opisthorchis viverrini	Ingestion of metacercariae in freshwater fish	Eastern Asia, Thailand
O. felineus	Ingestion of metacercariae in freshwater fish	Eastern Asia, Europe
Fasciola hepatica	Ingestion of metacercariae on aquatic plants or in water	Worldwide
F. gigantica	Ingestion of metacercariae on aquatic plants or in water	Sporadic, Africa
Intestinal Flukes		
Fasciolopsis buski	Ingestion of metacercariae on aquatic plants	Southeast Asia
Heterophyes heterophyes	Ingestion of metacercariae in freshwater or brackish-water fish	Eastern Asia, North Africa
Lung Flukes		
Paragonimus westermani and related species	Ingestion of metacercariae in crayfish or crabs	Global except North America and Europe

The host-parasite relationship in trematode infections is a product of certain biologic features of these organisms: they are multicellular, undergo several developmental changes within the host, and usually result in chronic infections. In general, the distribution of worm infections in human populations is *overdispersed*; i.e., it follows a negative binomial statistical distribution in which most infected individuals harbor low worm burdens while a small percentage are heavily infected. It is the heavily infected minority who are particularly prone to disease sequelae and who constitute an epidemiologically significant reservoir of infection in endemic areas. Recent evidence indicates that the prevalence of morbidity in infected populations is greater than was previously thought. Morbidity and death due to trematode infections reflect a multifactorial process that results from the tipping of a delicate balance between intensity of infection and host reactions, which initiate and modulate immunologic and pathologic outcome. Furthermore, the genetics of the parasite and of the human host contribute to the outcome of infection and disease. Infections with trematodes that migrate through or reside in host tissues are associated with a moderate to high degree of peripheral-blood eosinophilia; this association is of significance in protective and immunopathologic sequelae and is a useful clinical indicator of infection.

APPROACH TO THE PATIENT: Trematode Infection

The approach to individuals with suspected trematode infection begins with a question: Where have you been? Details of geographic history, exposure to freshwater bodies, and indulgence in local eating habits (without ensuring safety of food and drink) are all essential elements in eliciting the history of the present illness. The workup plan must include a detailed physical examination and tests appropriate for suspected infection. Diagnosis is based either on detection of the relevant stage of the parasite in excreta, sputum, or (rarely) tissue samples or on sensitive and specific serologic tests. Consultation with physicians familiar with these infections or with the U.S. Centers for Disease Control and Prevention (CDC) is helpful in guiding diagnosis and selecting therapy.

GLOBAL CONSIDERATIONS: EPIDEMIOLOGY OF TREMATODE INFECTIONS

Except among international travelers, trematode infections are quite rare in high-income countries because good sanitation and hygiene block trematode transmission and because transmission is tied to the distribution of the specific snail species that serve as intermediate hosts during the parasites' life cycle. In contrast, parasitic fluke infections are quite common in underdeveloped areas of Africa, Asia, and South America, with an estimated 440 million people affected by past or present *Schistosoma* infection and another 60 million people affected by the other foodborne trematodes. These infections are not benign; they result in multiyear chronic inflammatory disorders that significantly affect performance status and health-related quality of life. Global disease burden estimates indicate that at least 5 million years of healthy life are lost each year in the more than 90 endemic countries around the world.

BLOOD FLUKES: SCHISTOSOMIASIS

Human schistosomiasis is caused by five species of the parasitic trematode genus *Schistosoma*: *S. mansoni*, *S. japonicum*, *S. mekongi*, and *S. intercalatum* cause intestinal and hepatic schistosomiasis, and *S. haematobium* causes urogenital schistosomiasis. Infection may cause considerable morbidity in the intestines, liver, or urinary tract, and a small proportion of affected individuals die. Other schistosomes (e.g., avian species) may invade human skin but then die in subcutaneous tissue, producing only self-limiting cutaneous manifestations.

ETIOLOGY

Human infection is initiated by penetration of intact skin with infective cercariae. These organisms, which are released from infected snails in freshwater bodies, measure ~2 mm in length and possess an anterior and a ventral sucker that attach to the skin and facilitate penetration. Once in subcutaneous tissue, cercariae transform into schistosomula, with morphologic, membrane, and immunologic changes. The cercarial outer membrane changes from a trilaminar to a heptalaminar structure that is then maintained throughout the organism's life span in humans. This transformation is thought to be the schistosome's main adaptive mechanism for survival in humans. Schistosomula begin their migration within 2–4 days via venous or lymphatic vessels, reaching the lungs and finally the liver parenchyma. Sexually mature worms descend into the venous system at specific anatomic locations: intestinal veins (*S. mansoni*, *S. japonicum*, *S. mekongi*, and *S. intercalatum*) and vesical and other pelvic veins (*S. haematobium*). After mating, adult gravid females travel against venous blood flow to small tributaries, where they deposit their ova intravascularly. Schistosome ova (Fig. 259-1) have specific morphologic features that vary with the species. Aided by enzymatic secretions through minipores in eggshells, ova move through the venous wall, traversing host tissues to reach the lumen of the intestinal or urinary tract, and are voided with stools or urine. Approximately 50% of ova are retained in host tissues locally (intestines or urinary tract) or are carried by venous blood flow to the liver and other organs. Schistosome ova that reach freshwater bodies hatch, releasing free-living miracidia that seek the snail intermediate host and undergo several cycles of asexual multiplication. Finally, infective cercariae are shed from snails to complete the transmission cycle.

Adult schistosomes are ~1–2 cm long. Males are slightly shorter than females, with flattened bodies and anteriorly curved edges forming the gynecophoral canal, in which mature adult females are usually held. Females are longer, slender, and rounded in cross-section. The precise nature of biochemical and reproductive exchanges between the two sexes is unknown, as are the regulatory mechanisms for pairing. Adult schistosomes parasitize specific sites in the host venous system. What guides adult intestinal schistosomes to branches of the superior or inferior mesenteric veins or adult *S. haematobium* worms to the vesical plexus is unknown. In addition, adult worms inhibit the coagulation cascade and evade the effector arms of the host immune responses by still-undetermined mechanisms. The genome of schistosomes is relatively large (~270 Mb) and is arrayed on seven pairs of autosomes and one pair of sex chromosomes. Sequencing of the *S. japonicum*, *S. mansoni*, and *S. haematobium* genomes has provided insight into the worms' genomic and proteomic features, offering an opportunity to

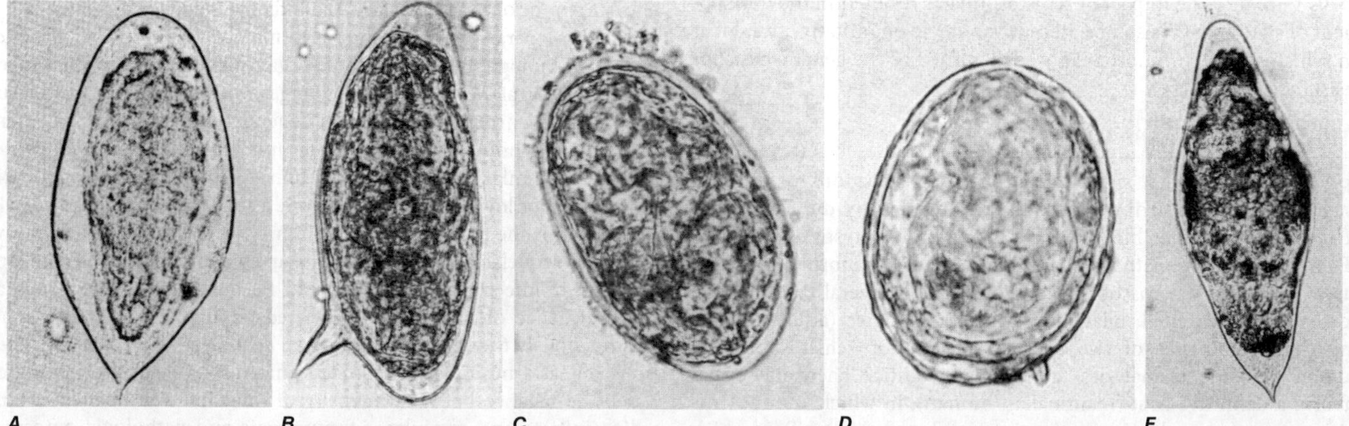

FIGURE 259-1 Morphology of schistosome eggs, the diagnostic stage of the parasite's life cycle. ***A.*** *Schistosoma haematobium* egg (in a urine sample) is large (~140 mm long), with a terminal spine. ***B.*** *S. mansoni* egg (in a fecal sample) is large (~150 mm long), with a thin shell and lateral spine. ***C.*** *S. japonicum* egg (fecal) is smaller than that of *S. mansoni* (~90 mm long), with a small spine or hooklike structure. ***D.*** *S. mekongi* egg (fecal) is similar to that of *S. japonicum* but smaller (~65 mm long). ***E.*** *S. intercalatum* egg (fecal) is larger than that of *S. haematobium* (~190 mm long), with a longer, sharply pointed spine. *(From LR Ash, TC Orihel: Atlas of Human Parasitology, 3rd ed. Chicago, ASCP Press, 1990; with permission.)*

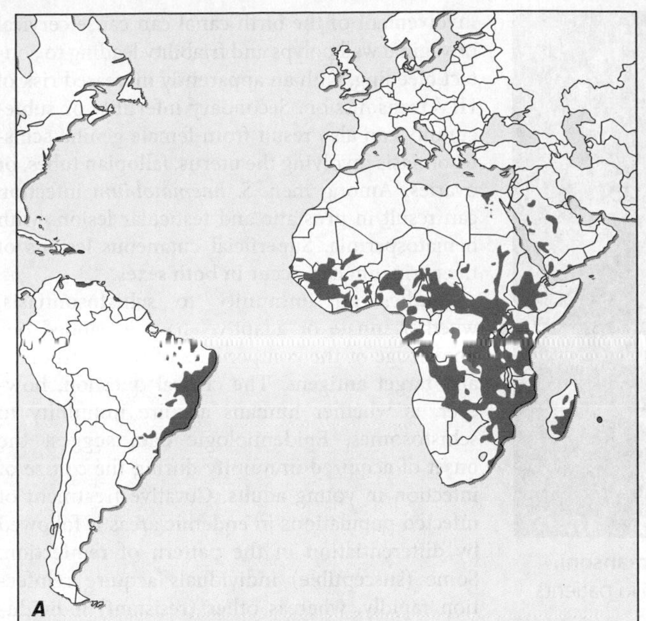

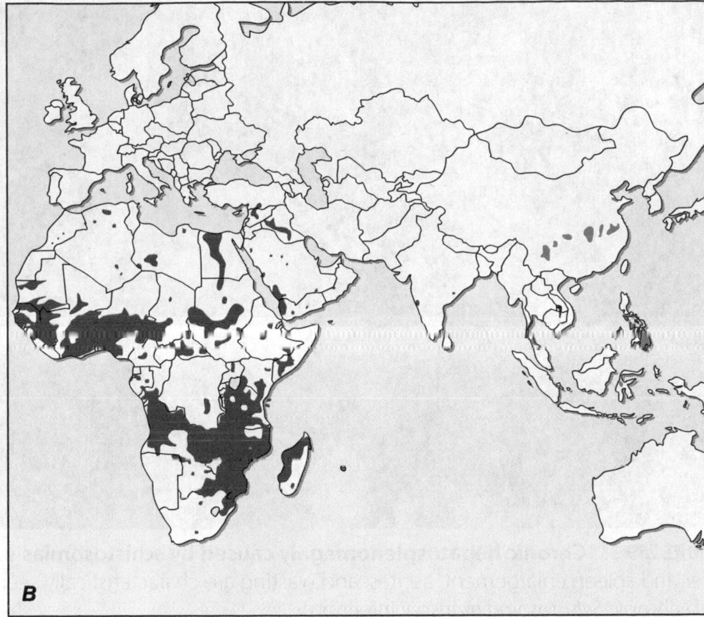

FIGURE 259-2 Global distribution of schistosomiasis. *A.* *Schistosoma mansoni* infection (*dark blue*) is endemic in Africa, the Middle East, South America, and a few Caribbean countries. *S. intercalatum* infection (*green*) is endemic in sporadic foci in West and Central Africa. ***B.*** *S. haematobium* infection (*purple*) is endemic in Africa and the Middle East. The major endemic countries for *S. japonicum* infection (*green*) are China, the Philippines, and Indonesia. *S. mekongi* infection (*red*) is endemic in sporadic foci in Southeast Asia.

discover new drug targets and to understand the molecular basis of pathogenesis.

EPIDEMIOLOGY

The global distribution of schistosome infection in human populations (Fig. 259-2) is dependent on both parasite and host factors. Information on prevalence and global distribution is inexact. At present, the five *Schistosoma* species are estimated to infect 200–300 million individuals (mostly children and young adults) in South America, the Caribbean, Africa, the Middle East, and Southeast Asia. Notably, parasite-related disease persists after active infection resolves, leaving a substantial health burden among adult populations. Thus, the overall number of humans likely to be affected by *Schistosoma*-related disease is now ~440 million. The total population living under conditions favoring transmission risk numbers ~700 million—a fact reflecting the global public health significance of schistosomiasis.

In endemic areas, the rate of yearly onset of new infection (incidence) is generally low. Prevalence, on the other hand, starts to be appreciable by the age of 3–4 years and builds to a maximum that varies by endemic region (up to 100%) in the 12- to 20-year age group. Prevalence then stabilizes or decreases slightly in older age groups (>40 years). Intensity of infection (as measured by fecal or urinary egg counts, which correlate with adult worm burdens in most circumstances) follows the increase in prevalence up to the age of 12–20 years and then declines markedly in older age groups. This decline may reflect acquisition of resistance or may be due to changes in water contact patterns, since older people have less exposure. Infection with schistosomes in human populations has a peculiar pattern. Most infected individuals harbor low worm burdens, and only a small proportion suffer from high-intensity infection. This pattern may be due to differences in worm infectivity or to a spectrum of genetic susceptibilities in human populations.

Disease due to schistosome infection is the consequence of parasitologic, host, and associated viral infections and of nutritional and environmental factors. Most disease syndromes relate to the presence of one or more of the parasite stages in humans. Disease manifestations in the populations of endemic areas correlate, in general, with intensity and duration of infection as well as with age and genetic susceptibility of the host. Overall, severe *Schistosoma*-specific disease manifestations are relatively rare among persons infected with any of the intestinal schistosomes. In contrast, symptoms of urogenital schistosomiasis manifest clinically in most *S. haematobium*-infected individuals. In addition, all forms of *Schistosoma* infection are associated with subclinical systemic morbidities that can significantly affect physical and cognitive performance, causing, for example, growth stunting, undernutrition, and anemia of chronic inflammation. New estimates of total morbidity due to chronic schistosomiasis indicate a significantly greater burden than was previously appreciated.

Schistosomiasis appears to be a cofactor in the spread and progression of HIV/AIDS in areas where both diseases are endemic. Increased emphasis should be placed on the treatment of schistosome infections in persons at risk of HIV/AIDS.

PATHOGENESIS AND IMMUNITY

Cercarial invasion is associated with dermatitis arising from dermal and subdermal inflammatory responses, both humoral and cell-mediated. As the parasites approach sexual maturity in the liver of infected individuals and as oviposition commences, acute schistosomiasis or Katayama syndrome (a serum sickness–like illness; see "Clinical Features," below) may occur. The associated antigen excess results in formation of soluble immune complexes, which may be deposited in several tissues, initiating multiple pathologic events. In chronic schistosomiasis, most disease manifestations are due to eggs retained in host tissues. The granulomatous response around these ova is cell-mediated and is regulated both positively and negatively by a cascade of cytokine, cellular, and humoral responses. Granuloma formation begins with recruitment of a host of inflammatory cells in response to antigens secreted by the living organism within the ova. Cells recruited initially include phagocytes, antigen-specific T cells, and eosinophils. Fibroblasts, giant cells, and B lymphocytes predominate later. Over time, these cumulative lesions reach a size many times that of parasite eggs, thus inducing organomegaly and obstruction. Immunomodulation or downregulation of host responses to schistosome eggs plays a significant role in limiting the extent of the granulomatous lesions—and consequently disease—in chronically infected experimental animals or humans. The underlying mechanisms involve another cascade of regulatory cytokines and idiotypic antibodies. Subsequent to the granulomatous response, fibrosis sets in, resulting in more permanent disease sequelae. Because schistosomiasis is also a

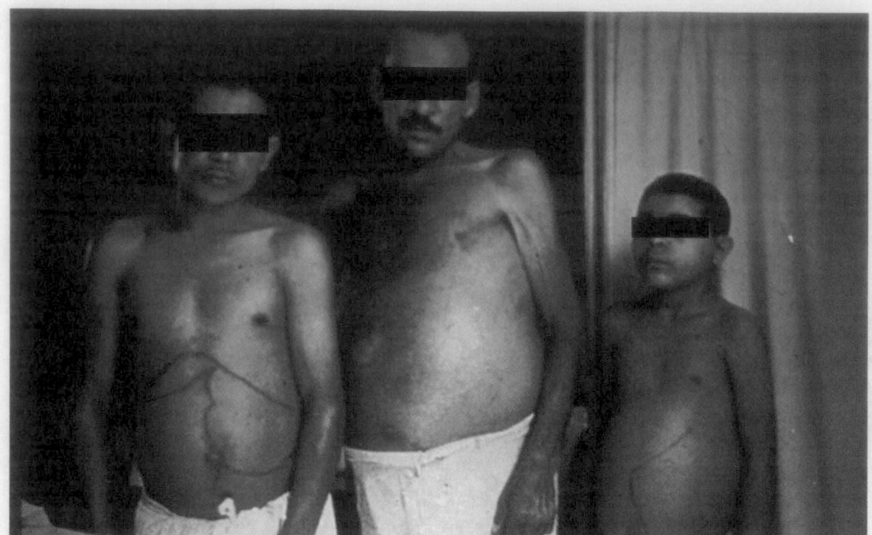

FIGURE 259-3 Chronic hepatosplenomegaly caused by schistosomiasis mansoni. Liver and spleen enlargement, ascites, and wasting are characteristically seen in patients with chronic *Schistosoma mansoni* infection.

chronic infection, the accumulation of antigen–antibody complexes results in deposits in renal glomeruli and may cause significant kidney disease.

The better-studied pathologic sequelae in schistosomiasis are those observed in liver disease. Ova that are carried by portal blood embolize to the liver. Because of their size (~150 × 60 μm in the case of *S. mansoni*), they lodge at presinusoidal sites, where granulomas are formed. These granulomas contribute to the hepatomegaly observed in infected individuals (Fig. 259-3). Schistosomal liver enlargement is also associated with certain class I and class II human leukocyte antigen (HLA) haplotypes and markers; its genetic basis appears to be polygenic. Presinusoidal portal blockage causes several hemodynamic changes, including portal hypertension and associated development of portosystemic collaterals at the esophagogastric junction and other sites. Esophageal varices are most likely to break and cause repeated episodes of hematemesis. Because changes in hepatic portal blood flow occur slowly, compensatory arterialization of the blood flow through the liver is established. Although this compensatory mechanism may be associated with certain metabolic side effects, retention of hepatocyte perfusion permits maintenance of normal liver function for several years.

The second most significant pathologic change in the liver relates to fibrosis. It is characteristically periportal (Symmers' clay pipe–stem fibrosis) but may be diffuse. Fibrosis, when diffuse, may be seen in areas of egg deposition and granuloma formation but is also seen in distant locations such as portal tracts. Schistosomiasis results in pure fibrotic lesions in the liver; cirrhosis occurs only when other toxic factors or infectious agents (e.g., hepatitis B or C virus) are involved. Deposition of fibrotic tissue in the extracellular matrix results from the interaction of T lymphocytes with cells of the fibroblast series; several cytokines, such as interleukin (IL) 2, IL-4, IL-1, and transforming growth factor β, are known to stimulate fibrogenesis. The process may be dependent on the genetic constitution of the host. Furthermore, regulatory cytokines that can suppress T cell responses and fibrogenesis, such as IL-10, interferon γ, or IL-12, may play a role in modulating the response.

Although the above description focuses on granuloma formation and fibrosis of the liver, similar processes occur in urogenital schistosomiasis. Granuloma formation at the lower end of the ureters obstructs urinary flow, with subsequent development of hydroureter and hydronephrosis. Similar lesions in the urinary bladder cause the protrusion of papillomatous structures into its cavity; these may ulcerate and/or bleed. The chronic stage of infection is associated with scarring and deposition of calcium in the bladder wall. Among women, involvement of the birth canal can cause cervical or vaginal wall polyps and friability leading to contact bleeding, with an apparently increased risk of HIV transmission. Secondary infertility or subfecundity can also result from female genital schistosomiasis involving the uterus, fallopian tubes, or ovaries. Among men, *S. haematobium* infection can result in prostatic and testicular lesions with hematospermia. Superficial cutaneous lesions of the perineum can occur in both sexes.

Studies on immunity to schistosomiasis, whether innate or adaptive, have expanded our knowledge of the components of these responses and target antigens. The critical question, however, is whether humans acquire immunity to schistosomes. Epidemiologic data suggest the onset of acquired immunity during the course of infection in young adults. Curative treatment of infected populations in endemic areas is followed by differentiation in the pattern of reinfection. Some (susceptible) individuals acquire reinfection rapidly, whereas other (resistant) individuals are reinfected slowly. This difference may be explained by differences in transmission, immunologic response, or genetic susceptibility. The mechanism of acquired immunity involves antibodies, complement, and several effector cells, particularly eosinophils. Furthermore, the intensity of schistosome infection has been correlated with a region in chromosome 5. In several studies, a few protective schistosome antigens have been identified as vaccine candidates, but none has been fully evaluated in human populations to date.

CLINICAL FEATURES

In general, disease manifestations of schistosomiasis occur in three stages, which vary not only by species but also by intensity of infection and other host factors, such as age and genetics of the human host. During the phase of cercarial invasion, a form of dermatitis may be observed. This so-called swimmers' itch occurs most often with *S. mansoni* and *S. japonicum* infections, manifesting 2 or 3 days after invasion as an itchy maculopapular rash on the affected areas of the skin. The condition is particularly severe when humans are exposed to avian schistosomes. This form of cercarial dermatitis is also seen around freshwater lakes in the northern United States, particularly in the spring and summer months. Cercarial dermatitis is a self-limiting clinical entity. During worm maturation and at the beginning of oviposition (i.e., 4–8 weeks after skin invasion), acute schistosomiasis or Katayama syndrome—a serum sickness–like illness with fever, generalized lymphadenopathy, and hepatosplenomegaly—may develop. Individuals with acute schistosomiasis have a high degree of peripheral-blood eosinophilia. Parasite-specific antibodies may be detected before schistosome eggs are identified in excreta.

Acute schistosomiasis has become an important clinical entity worldwide because of increased travel to endemic areas. Travelers are exposed to parasites while swimming or wading in freshwater bodies and upon their return present with acute manifestations. The course of acute schistosomiasis is generally benign, but central nervous system (CNS) schistosomiasis and even deaths are occasionally reported in association with heavy exposure to schistosomes among travelers and migrants.

The main clinical manifestations of chronic schistosomiasis are species-dependent. Intestinal species (*S. mansoni*, *S. japonicum*, *S. mekongi*, and *S. intercalatum*) cause intestinal and hepatosplenic disease as well as several manifestations associated with portal hypertension. During the intestinal phase, which may begin a few months after infection and may last for years, symptomatic patients characteristically have colicky abdominal pain, bloody diarrhea, and anemia. Patients may also report fatigue and an inability to perform daily routine functions and may show evidence of growth retardation and anemia. This more subtle form of schistosomiasis morbidity is generally underappreciated. The severity of intestinal schistosomiasis is often related to the intensity of the worm burden. The disease runs a chronic course and may result in colonic polyposis, which has been reported from some endemic areas, such as Egypt and Uganda.

The hepatosplenic phase of disease manifests early (during the first year of infection, particularly in children) with liver enlargement due to parasite-induced granulomatous lesions. Hepatomegaly is seen in ~15–20% of infected individuals; it correlates roughly with intensity of infection, occurs more often in children, and may be related to specific HLA haplotypes. In subsequent phases of infection, presinusoidal blockage of blood flow leads to portal hypertension and splenomegaly (Fig. 259-3). Moreover, portal hypertension may lead to varices at the lower end of the esophagus and at other sites. Patients with schistosomal liver disease may have right-upper-quadrant "dragging" pain during the hepatomegaly phase, and this pain may move to the left upper quadrant as splenomegaly progresses. Bleeding from esophageal varices may, however, be the first clinical manifestation of this phase. Patients may experience repeated bleeding but seem to tolerate its impact, because an adequate total hepatic blood flow permits normal liver function for a considerable period. In late-stage disease, typical fibrotic changes occur along with liver function deterioration and the onset of ascites, hypoalbuminemia, and defects in coagulation. Intercurrent viral infections of the liver (especially hepatitis B and C), toxic insults (excessive ethanol ingestion or exposure to organic poisons or aflatoxin), or nutritional deficiencies may well accelerate or exacerbate the deterioration of hepatic function.

The extent and severity of intestinal and hepatic disease in schistosomiasis mansoni and japonica have been well described. Although it was originally thought that *S. japonicum* might induce more severe disease manifestations because the adult worms can produce 10 times more eggs than *S. mansoni*, subsequent field studies have not supported this claim. Clinical observations of individuals infected with *S. mekongi* or *S. intercalatum* have been less detailed, partly because of the limited geographic distribution of these organisms.

The clinical manifestations of *S. haematobium* infection occur relatively early and involve a high percentage of infected individuals. Up to 80% of children infected with *S. haematobium* have dysuria, frequency, and hematuria. Hematuria may sometimes occur only at the end of voiding. Urine examination reveals blood and albumin as well as an unusually high frequency of bacterial urinary tract infections and urinary sediment cellular metaplasia. These manifestations correlate with the intensity of infection, the presence of urinary bladder granulomas, and subsequent ulceration. Along with local effects of granuloma formation in the urinary bladder, obstruction of the lower end of the ureters results in hydroureter and hydronephrosis, which may be seen in 25–50% of infected children. As infection progresses, bladder granulomas undergo fibrosis, which results in typical sandy patches visible on cystoscopy. In many endemic areas, an association between squamous cell carcinoma of the bladder and *S. haematobium* infection has been observed. Such malignancy is detected in a younger age group than is transitional cell carcinoma. In fact, *S. haematobium* has now been classified as a human carcinogen. Genital schistosomiasis (described in the previous section) is a common presenting symptom among adults of both sexes.

Significant disease may occur in other organs during chronic schistosomiasis. Lung and CNS disease have been documented; other sites, such as the skin and the genital organs, are less frequently affected. In pulmonary schistosomiasis, embolized eggs lodge in small arterioles, producing acute necrotizing arteriolitis and granuloma formation. During *S. mansoni* and *S. japonicum* infection, schistosome eggs reach the lungs after the development of portosystemic collateral circulation; in *S. haematobium* infection, ova may reach the lungs directly via connections between the vesical and systemic circulation. Subsequent fibrous tissue deposition leads to endarteritis obliterans, pulmonary hypertension, and cor pulmonale. The most common symptoms are cough, fever, and dyspnea. Cor pulmonale may be diagnosed radiologically on the basis of prominence of the right side of the heart and dilation of the pulmonary artery. Frank evidence of right-sided heart failure may be seen in late cases.

Although less common than pulmonary manifestations, CNS schistosomiasis is important, characteristically occurring in association with *S. japonicum* infection. Migratory worms deposit eggs in the brain and induce a granulomatous response. The frequency of this manifestation among infected individuals in some endemic areas (e.g., the Philippines) is calculated at 2–4%. Jacksonian epilepsy due to *S. japonicum* infection is the second most common cause of epilepsy in these areas. *S. mansoni* and *S. haematobium* infections have been associated with transverse myelitis. This syndrome is thought to be due to eggs traveling to the venous plexus around the spinal cord. In schistosomiasis mansoni, transverse myelitis is usually seen in the chronic stage after the development of portal hypertension and portosystemic shunts, which allow ova to travel to the spinal cord veins. This proposed sequence of events has been challenged because of a few reports of transverse myelitis occurring early in the course of *S. mansoni* infection. More information is needed to confirm these observations. During schistosomiasis caused by *Schistosoma haematobium*, ova may travel through communication between vesical and systemic veins, resulting in spinal cord disease that may be detected at any stage of infection. Pathologic study of lesions in schistosomal transverse myelitis may reveal eggs along with necrotic or granulomatous lesions. Patients usually present with acute or rapidly progressing lower-leg weakness accompanied by sphincter dysfunction.

DIAGNOSIS

Physicians in areas not endemic for schistosomiasis face considerable diagnostic challenges. In the most common clinical presentation, a traveler returns with symptoms and signs of acute syndromes of schistosomiasis—namely, cercarial dermatitis or Katayama syndrome. Central to a correct diagnosis is a thorough inquiry into the patient's history of travel and exposure to freshwater bodies—whether slow- or fast-running—in an endemic area. Differential diagnosis of fever in returned travelers includes a spectrum of infections whose etiologies are viral (e.g., dengue fever), bacterial (e.g., enteric fever, leptospirosis), rickettsial, or protozoal (e.g., malaria). In cases of Katayama syndrome, prompt diagnosis is essential and is based on clinical presentation, high-level peripheral-blood eosinophilia, and a positive serologic assay for schistosomal antibodies. Two tests are available at the CDC: the Falcon assay screening test/enzyme-linked immunosorbent assay (FAST-ELISA) and the confirmatory enzyme-linked immunoelectrotransfer blot (EITB). Both tests are highly sensitive and ~96% specific. In some instances, examination of stool or urine for ova may yield positive results.

Individuals with established infection are diagnosed by a combination of geographic history, characteristic clinical presentation, and presence of schistosome ova in excreta. The diagnosis may also be established with the serologic assays mentioned above or with those that detect circulating schistosome antigens. These assays can be applied to blood, urine, or other body fluids (e.g., cerebrospinal fluid). For suspected schistosome infection, stool examination by the Kato thick smear or any other concentration method generally identifies most patients with heavy infection but does not identify all lightly infected individuals. For the latter patients, a point-of-care test to detect parasite circulating cathodic antigen in urine may prove very useful in establishing the presence of active *S. mansoni* infection and in monitoring the clearance of infection after treatment. For *S. haematobium*, urine may be examined by microscopy of sediment or by filtration of a known volume through Nuclepore filters. Sensitivity can be further improved by testing for parasite DNA in urine sediment. The Kato thick smear and Nuclepore filtration provide quantitative data on the intensity of infection, which is of value in assessing the degree of tissue damage and in monitoring the effect of chemotherapy. Schistosome infection may also be diagnosed by examination of tissue specimens, typically rectal biopsy samples; except in rare circumstances, other biopsy procedures (e.g., liver biopsy) are not needed.

The differential diagnosis of schistosomal hepatomegaly must include viral hepatitis of all etiologies, miliary tuberculosis, malaria, visceral leishmaniasis, ethanol abuse, and causes of hepatic and portal vein obstruction. The differential diagnosis of hematuria in *S. haematobium* infection includes bacterial cystitis, tuberculosis, urinary stones, and malignancy.

TREATMENT SCHISTOSOMIASIS

Treatment of schistosomiasis depends on the stage of infection and the clinical presentation. Other than topical dermatologic applications for relief of itching, no specific treatment is indicated for cercarial dermatitis caused by avian schistosomes. Therapy for acute schistosomiasis or Katayama syndrome needs to be adjusted appropriately for each case. Although antischistosomal chemotherapy may be used, it does not have a significant impact on maturing worms. In severe acute schistosomiasis, management in an acute-care setting is necessary, with supportive measures and consideration of glucocorticoid treatment to reduce inflammation. Once the acute critical phase is over, specific chemotherapy is indicated for parasite elimination. For all individuals with established infection, treatment to eradicate the parasite should be administered. The drug of choice is praziquantel, which—depending on the infecting species (Table 259-2)—is administered PO as a total of 40 or 60 mg/kg in two or three doses over a single day. Praziquantel treatment results in parasitologic cure in ~85% of cases and reduces egg counts by >90%. Efficacy rates among children <5 years old have been reported to be lower. These children are more likely to need re-treatment to effect a cure. Few side effects have been encountered, and those that do develop usually do not interfere with completion of treatment. Dependence on a single chemotherapeutic agent has raised the possibility of development of resistance in schistosomes; to date, such resistance does not seem to be clinically significant. The effect of antischistosomal treatment on disease manifestations varies by stage. Early hepatomegaly and bladder lesions are known to resolve after chemotherapy, but the late established manifestations, such as fibrosis, do not recede. Additional management modalities are needed for individuals with other manifestations, such as hepatocellular failure or recurrent hematemesis. The use of these interventions is guided by general medical and surgical principles.

PREVENTION AND CONTROL

Transmission of schistosomiasis is dependent on human behavior. Because the geographic distribution of infections in endemic regions of the world is not clearly demarcated, it is prudent for travelers to endemic areas to avoid contact with *all* freshwater bodies, irrespective of the speed of water flow or unsubstantiated claims of safety. Some topical agents, when applied to the skin, may inhibit cercarial penetration, but none is currently available. If exposure occurs, a follow-up visit with a health care provider is strongly recommended. Prevention of infection in inhabitants of endemic areas is a significant challenge. Residents of these regions use freshwater bodies for sanitary, domestic, recreational, and agricultural purposes. Several control measures have been used, including application of molluscicides, provision of sanitary water and sewage disposal, chemotherapy, and health education to effect behavioral change in terms of water-contact activities. Current recommendations to countries endemic for schistosomiasis emphasize the use of multiple approaches. With the advent of an oral, safe, and effective broad-spectrum antischistosomal agent (praziquantel), chemotherapy has been most successful in reducing the intensity of infection and reversing disease. The duration of this positive impact depends on the transmission dynamics of the parasite in any specific endemic region. The ultimate goal of research on prevention and control is the development of a vaccine. Although there are a few promising leads, this goal probably is not within reach during the next decade.

TABLE 259-2 DRUG THERAPY FOR HUMAN TREMATODE INFECTIONS

Infection	Drug of Choice	Adult Dose and Duration
Blood Flukes		
S. mansoni, S. intercalatum, S. haematobium	Praziquantel	20 mg/kg, 2 doses in 1 day
S. japonicum, S. mekongi	Praziquantel	20 mg/kg, 3 doses in 1 day
Biliary (Hepatic) Flukes		
Clonorchis sinensis, Opisthorchis viverrini, O. felineus	Praziquantel	25 mg/kg, 3 doses in 1 day
Fasciola hepatica, F. gigantica	Triclabendazole	10 mg/kg once
Intestinal Flukes		
Fasciolopsis buski, Heterophyes heterophyes	Praziquantel[a]	25 mg/kg, 3 doses in 1 day
Lung Flukes		
Paragonimus westermani	Praziquantel[a]	25 mg/kg, 3 doses per day for 2 days

[a]Not approved by the U.S. Food and Drug Administration for this indication.

LIVER (BILIARY) FLUKES

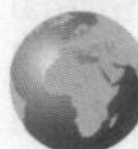

Several species of biliary fluke infecting humans are particularly common in Southeast Asia and Russia. Other species are transmitted in Europe, Africa, and the Americas. On the basis of their migratory pathway in humans, these infections may be divided into the *Clonorchis* and *Fasciola* groups (Table 259-1).

CLONORCHIASIS AND OPISTHORCHIASIS

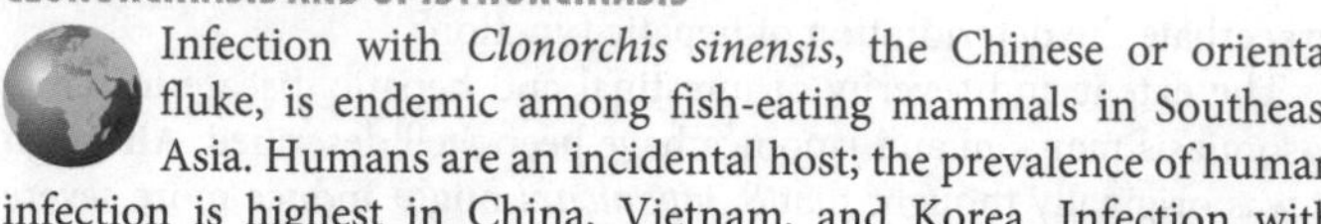

Infection with *Clonorchis sinensis*, the Chinese or oriental fluke, is endemic among fish-eating mammals in Southeast Asia. Humans are an incidental host; the prevalence of human infection is highest in China, Vietnam, and Korea. Infection with *Opisthorchis viverrini* and *O. felineus* is zoonotic in cats and dogs. Transmission to humans occurs occasionally, particularly in Thailand (*O. viverrini*) and in Southeast Asia and eastern Europe (*O. felineus*). Data on the exact geographic distribution of these infectious agents in human populations are rudimentary.

Infection with any of these three species is established by ingestion of raw or inadequately cooked freshwater fish harboring metacercariae. These organisms excyst in the duodenum, releasing larvae that travel through the ampulla of Vater and mature into adult worms in bile canaliculi. Mature flukes are flat and elongated, measuring 1–2 cm in length. The hermaphroditic worms reproduce by releasing small operculated eggs, which pass with bile into the intestines and are voided with stools. The life cycle is completed in the environment in specific freshwater snails (the first intermediate host) along with later encystment of snail-derived cercariae as infectious metacercariae in freshwater fish.

Except for late sequelae, the exact clinical syndromes caused by clonorchiasis and opisthorchiasis are not well defined. Because most infected individuals harbor a low worm burden, many are minimally symptomatic. Moderate to heavy infection may be associated with vague right-upper-quadrant pain. In contrast, chronic or repeated infection is associated with manifestations such as cholangitis, cholangiohepatitis, and biliary obstruction. Cholangiocarcinoma is epidemiologically related to *C. sinensis* infection in China and to *O. viverrini* infection in northeastern Thailand. This association has resulted in classification of these infectious agents as human carcinogens.

FASCIOLIASIS

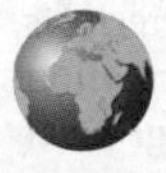

Infections with *Fasciola hepatica* and *F. gigantica* are worldwide zoonoses that are particularly endemic in sheep-raising countries. Human cases have been reported in South America, Europe, Africa, and Australia. Recent estimates indicate a worldwide prevalence of 17 million cases. High endemicity has been reported in certain areas of Peru and Bolivia. In most endemic areas the predominant species is *F. hepatica*, but in Asia and Africa a varying degree of overlap with *F. gigantica* has been observed.

Humans acquire fascioliasis by ingestion of metacercariae attached to certain aquatic plants, such as watercress, water caltrop, and water chestnuts. Infection may also be acquired by consumption of contaminated water or ingestion of food items washed with such water. Acquisition of human infection through consumption of freshly prepared raw liver containing immature flukes has been reported. Infection is initiated when metacercariae excyst, penetrate the gut wall, and travel through the peritoneal cavity to invade the liver capsule. Adult worms migrate through the liver parenchyma and finally reach bile ducts, where they produce large operculated eggs that are voided in bile through the gastrointestinal tract to the outside environment. The flukes' life cycle is completed in specific snails (the first intermediate host) followed by encystment on aquatic plants.

Clinical features of fascioliasis relate to the stage and intensity of infection. Acute disease develops during parasite migration (1–2 weeks after infection) and includes fever, right upper quadrant pain, hepatomegaly, and eosinophilia. Computed tomography (CT) of the liver may show multiple parenchymal holes/or migratory tracks. Symptoms and signs usually subside as the parasites reach their final habitat. In individuals with chronic infection, bile duct obstruction and biliary cirrhosis are infrequently demonstrated. No relation to hepatic malignancy has been ascribed to fascioliasis.

DIAGNOSIS

Diagnosis of infection with any of the biliary flukes depends on a high degree of suspicion, elicitation of an appropriate geographic history, and stool examination for characteristically shaped parasite ova. Additional evidence may be obtained by documenting peripheral-blood eosinophilia or imaging the liver. Serologic testing is helpful, particularly in lightly infected individuals.

TREATMENT BILIARY FLUKES

Drug therapy (praziquantel or triclabendazole) is summarized in Table 259-2. Patients with anatomic lesions in the biliary tract or malignancy are managed according to general medical guidelines.

INTESTINAL FLUKES

Two species of intestinal flukes cause human infection in defined geographic areas worldwide (Table 259-1). The large *Fasciolopsis buski* (adults measure 2 × 7 cm) is endemic in Southeast Asia, whereas the smaller *Heterophyes heterophyes* is found in the Nile Delta of Egypt. Infection is initiated by ingestion of metacercariae attached to aquatic plants (*F. buski*) or encysted in freshwater or brackish-water fish (*H. heterophyes*). Flukes mature in human intestines, and eggs are passed with stools. Most individuals infected with intestinal flukes are asymptomatic. In heavy *F. buski* infection, diarrhea, abdominal pain, and malabsorption may be encountered. Heavy infection with *H. heterophyes* may be associated with abdominal pain and mucous diarrhea. The diagnosis is established by detection of characteristically shaped ova in stool samples. The drug of choice for treatment is praziquantel (Table 259-2).

LUNG FLUKES

Infection with the lung fluke *Paragonimus westermani* (Table 259-1) and related species (e.g., *P. africanus*) is endemic in many parts of the world, excluding North America and Europe. Endemicity is particularly noticeable in West Africa, Central and South America, and Asia. In nature, the reservoir hosts of *P. westermani* are wild and domestic felines. In Africa, *P. africanus* has been found in other species, such as dogs. Adult lung flukes, which are 7–12 mm in length, are found encapsulated in the lungs of infected persons. In rare circumstances, flukes are found encysted in the CNS (cerebral paragonimiasis) or the abdominal cavity. Humans acquire lung fluke infection by ingesting infective metacercariae encysted in the muscles and viscera of crayfish and freshwater crabs. In endemic areas, these crustaceans are consumed raw, marinated, or pickled. Once the organisms reach the duodenum, they excyst, penetrate the gut wall, and travel through the peritoneal cavity, diaphragm, and pleural space to reach the lungs. Mature flukes are found in the bronchioles surrounded by cystic lesions. Parasite eggs are either expectorated with sputum or swallowed and passed to the outside environment with feces. The life cycle is completed in snails and freshwater crustaceans.

When maturing flukes lodge in lung tissues, they cause hemorrhage and necrosis, resulting in cyst formation. The adjacent lung parenchyma shows evidence of inflammatory infiltration, predominantly by eosinophils. Cysts usually measure 1–2 cm in diameter and may contain one or two worms each. With the onset of oviposition, cysts usually rupture in adjacent bronchioles—an event allowing ova to exit the human host. Older cysts develop thickened walls, which may undergo calcification. During the active phase of paragonimiasis, lung tissues surrounding parasite cysts may show evidence of pneumonia, bronchitis, bronchiectasis, and fibrosis.

Pulmonary paragonimiasis is particularly symptomatic in persons with moderate to heavy infection. Productive cough with brownish sputum or frank hemoptysis associated with peripheral-blood eosinophilia is usually the presenting feature. Chest examination may reveal signs of pleurisy. In chronic cases, bronchitis or bronchiectasis may predominate, but these conditions rarely proceed to lung abscess. Imaging of the lungs demonstrates characteristic features, including patchy densities, cavities, pleural effusion, and ring shadows. Cerebral paragonimiasis presents as either space-occupying lesions or epilepsy.

DIAGNOSIS

Pulmonary paragonimiasis is diagnosed by detection of parasite ova in sputum and/or stools. Serology is of considerable help in egg-negative cases and in cerebral paragonimiasis. The differential diagnosis includes active tuberculosis, bacterial lung abscess, and lung carcinoma.

TREATMENT LUNG FLUKES

The drug of choice for treatment is praziquantel (Table 259-2). Other medical or surgical management may be needed for pulmonary or cerebral lesions.

CONTROL AND PREVENTION OF TISSUE FLUKES

For residents of nonendemic areas who are visiting an endemic region, the only effective preventive measure is to avoid ingestion of local plants, fish, or crustaceans; if their ingestion is necessary, these items should be washed and cooked thoroughly. Instruction on water and food preparation and consumption should be included in physicians' advice to travelers (Chap. 149). Interruption of transmission among residents of endemic areas depends on avoiding ingestion of infective stages and disposing of feces and sputum appropriately to prevent hatching of eggs in the environment. These two approaches rely greatly on socioeconomic development, health education, and significant behavioral change. In countries where economic progress has resulted in financial and social improvements, transmission has decreased. The third approach to control in endemic communities entails selective use of chemotherapy for individuals posing the highest risk of transmission (i.e., those with heavy infections). The availability of praziquantel—a broad-spectrum, safe, and effective anthelmintic agent—provides a means for reducing the reservoirs of infection in human populations. However, the existence of most of these helminthic infections as zoonoses in several animal species complicates control efforts.

260 Cestode Infections

A. Clinton White, Jr., Peter F. Weller

Cestodes, or tapeworms, are segmented worms. The adults reside in the gastrointestinal tract, but the larvae can be found in almost any organ. Human tapeworm infections can be divided into two major clinical groups. In one group, humans are the definitive hosts, with the adult tapeworms living in the gastrointestinal tract (*Taenia saginata, Diphyllobothrium, Hymenolepis,* and *Dipylidium caninum*). In the other, humans are intermediate hosts, with larval-stage parasites present in the tissues; diseases in this category include echinococcosis, sparganosis, and coenurosis. Humans may be either the definitive or the intermediate hosts for *Taenia solium*. Both stages of *Hymenolepis nana* are found simultaneously in the human intestines.

The ribbon-shaped tapeworm attaches to the intestinal mucosa by means of sucking cups or hooks located on the scolex. Behind the scolex is a short, narrow neck from which proglottids (segments) form. As each proglottid matures, it is displaced further back from the neck by the formation of new, less mature segments. The progressively elongating chain of attached proglottids, called the *strobila*, constitutes the bulk of the tapeworm. The length varies among species. In some, the tapeworm may consist of more than 1000 proglottids and may be several meters long. The mature proglottids are hermaphroditic and produce eggs, which are subsequently released. Because eggs of the different *Taenia* species are morphologically identical, differences in the morphology of the scolex or proglottids provide the basis for diagnostic identification to the species level.

Most human tapeworms require at least one intermediate host for complete larval development. After ingestion of the eggs or proglottids by an intermediate host, the larval oncospheres are activated, escape the egg, and penetrate the intestinal mucosa. The oncosphere migrates to tissues and develops into an encysted form known as a *cysticercus* (single scolex), a *coenurus* (multiple scolices), or a *hydatid* (cyst with daughter cysts, each containing several protoscolices). The definitive host's ingestion of tissues containing a cyst enables a scolex to develop into a tapeworm.

TAENIASIS SAGINATA AND TAENIASIS ASIATICA

The beef tapeworm *T. saginata* occurs in all countries where raw or undercooked beef is eaten. It is most prevalent in sub-Saharan African and Middle Eastern countries. *T. asiatica* is closely related to *T. saginata* and is found in Asia, with pigs as intermediate hosts. The clinical manifestations and morphology of these two species are very similar and are therefore discussed together.

Etiology and Pathogenesis Humans are the only definitive host for the adult stage of *T. saginata* and *T. asiatica*. The tapeworms, which can reach 8 m in length with 1000–2000 proglottids, inhabit the upper jejunum. The scolex of *T. saginata* has four prominent suckers, whereas *T. asiatica* has an unarmed rostellum. Each gravid segment has 15–30 uterine branches (in contrast to 8–12 for *T. solium*). The eggs are indistinguishable from those of *T. solium*; they measure 30–40 μm, contain the oncosphere, and have a thick brown striated shell. Eggs deposited on vegetation can live for months or years until they are ingested by cattle or other herbivores (*T. saginata*) or pigs (*T. asiatica*). The embryo released after ingestion invades the intestinal wall and is carried to striated muscle or viscera, where it transforms into the cysticercus. When ingested in raw or undercooked meat, this form can infect humans. After the cysticercus is ingested, it takes ~2 months for the mature adult worm to develop.

Clinical Manifestations Patients become aware of the infection most commonly by noting passage of proglottids in their feces. The proglottids are often motile, and patients may experience perianal discomfort when proglottids are discharged. Mild abdominal pain or discomfort, nausea, change in appetite, weakness, and weight loss can occur.

Diagnosis The diagnosis is made by the detection of eggs or proglottids in the stool. Eggs may also be present in the perianal area; thus, if proglottids or eggs are not found in the stool, the perianal region should be examined with use of a cellophane-tape swab (as in pinworm infection; Chap. 257). Distinguishing *T. saginata* or *T. asiatica* from *T. solium* requires examination of mature proglottids. All three species can be distinguished by examining the scolex. Available serologic tests are not helpful diagnostically. Eosinophilia and elevated levels of serum IgE may be detected.

TREATMENT TAENIASIS SAGINATA AND TAENIASIS ASIATICA

A single dose of praziquantel (10 mg/kg) is highly effective.

Prevention The major method of preventing infection is the adequate cooking of beef or pork viscera; exposure to temperatures as low as 56°C for 5 min will destroy cysticerci. Refrigeration or salting for long periods or freezing at −10°C for 9 days also kills cysticerci in beef. General preventive measures include inspection of beef and proper disposal of human feces.

TAENIASIS SOLIUM AND CYSTICERCOSIS

The pork tapeworm *T. solium* can cause two distinct forms of infection in humans: adult tapeworms in the intestine or larval forms in the tissues (cysticercosis). Humans are the only definitive hosts for *T. solium*; pigs are the usual intermediate hosts, although other animals may harbor the larval forms.

T. solium is found worldwide in areas where pigs are raised and have access to human feces. However, it is most prevalent in Latin America, sub-Saharan Africa, China, India, and Southeast Asia. Cysticercosis occurs in industrialized nations largely as a result of the immigration of infected persons from endemic areas.

Etiology and Pathogenesis The adult tapeworm generally resides in the upper jejunum. The scolex attaches by both sucking disks and two rows of hooklets. The adult worm usually lives for a few years. The tapeworm, usually ~3 m in length, may have as many as 1000 proglottids, each of which produces up to 50,000 eggs. Proglottids are released and excreted into the feces, and the eggs in these proglottids are infective for both humans and animals. The eggs may survive in the environment for several months. After ingestion of eggs by the pig intermediate host, the larvae are activated, escape the egg, penetrate the intestinal wall, and are carried to many tissues; they are most frequently identified in striated muscle of the neck, tongue, and trunk. Within 60–90 days, the encysted larval stage develops. These cysticerci can survive for months to years. By ingesting undercooked pork containing cysticerci, humans acquire infections that lead to intestinal tapeworms. Infections that cause human cysticercosis follow the ingestion of *T. solium* eggs, usually from close contact with a tapeworm carrier. Autoinfection may occur if an individual with an egg-producing tapeworm ingests eggs derived from his or her own feces.

Clinical Manifestations Intestinal infections with *T. solium* may be asymptomatic. Fecal passage of proglottids may be noted by patients. Other symptoms are infrequent.

In cysticercosis, the clinical manifestations are variable. Cysticerci can be found anywhere in the body but are most commonly detected in the brain, cerebrospinal fluid (CSF), skeletal muscle, subcutaneous tissue, or eye. The clinical presentation of cysticercosis depends on the number and location of cysticerci as well as on the extent of associated inflammatory responses or scarring. Neurologic manifestations are the most common (Fig. 260-1). Seizures are associated with inflammation surrounding cysticerci in the brain parenchyma. These seizures may be generalized, focal, or Jacksonian. Hydrocephalus results from CSF flow obstruction by cysticerci and accompanying inflammation or by CSF outflow obstruction from arachnoiditis. Symptoms of increased intracranial pressure, including headache, nausea, vomiting, changes in

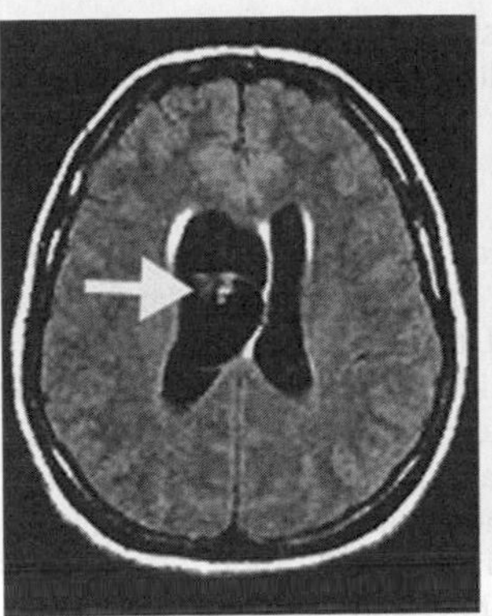

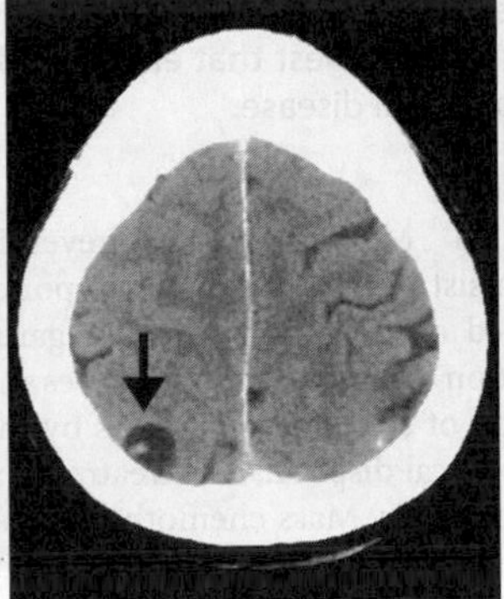

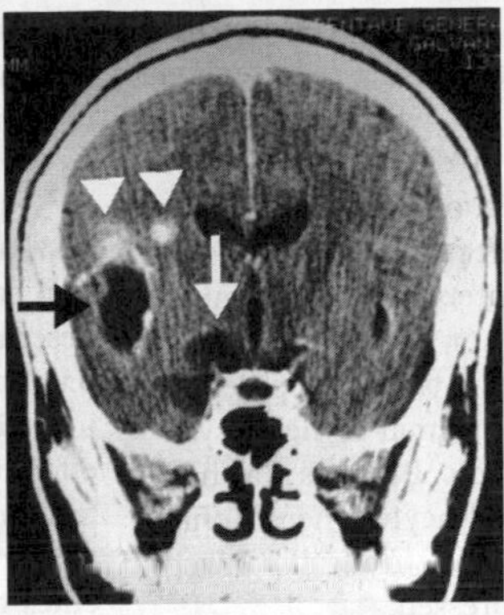

FIGURE 260-1 Neurocysticercosis is caused by *Taenia solium*. Neurologic infection can be classified on the basis of the location and viability of the parasites. When the parasites are in the ventricles, they often cause obstructive hydrocephalus. ***Left:*** Magnetic resonance imaging showing a cysticercus in the lateral ventricle, with resultant hydrocephalus. The *arrow* points to the scolex within the cystic parasite. ***Center:*** CT showing a parenchymal cysticercus, with enhancement of the cyst wall and an internal scolex (*arrow*). ***Right:*** Multiple cysticerci, including calcified lesions from prior infection (*arrowheads*), viable cysticerci in the basilar cisterns (*white arrow*), and a large degenerating cysticercus in the Sylvian fissure (*black arrow*). *(Modified with permission from JC Bandres et al: Clin Infect Dis 15:799, 1992. © The University of Chicago Press.)*

vision, dizziness, ataxia, or confusion, are often evident. Patients with hydrocephalus may develop papilledema or display altered mental status. When cysticerci develop at the base of the brain or in the subarachnoid space, they may cause chronic meningitis or arachnoiditis, communicating hydrocephalus, hemorrhages, or strokes.

Diagnosis The diagnosis of intestinal *T. solium* infection is made by the detection of eggs or proglottids, as described for *T. saginata*. More sensitive methods, including antigen-capture enzyme-linked immunosorbent assay (ELISA), polymerase chain reaction (PCR), and serology for tapeworm stage-specific antigens, are currently available only as research techniques. In cysticercosis, diagnosis can be difficult. A consensus conference has delineated absolute, major, minor, and epidemiologic criteria for diagnosis (Table 260-1). Diagnostic certainty is possible only with definite demonstration of the parasite (absolute criteria). This task can be accomplished by histologic observation of the parasite in excised tissue, by funduscopic visualization of the parasite in the eye (in the anterior chamber, vitreous, or subretinal spaces), or by neuroimaging studies demonstrating cystic lesions containing a characteristic scolex (Fig. 260-1). With improving resolution of neuroimaging studies, the scolex can now be identified in many cases. In other instances, a clinical diagnosis is based on a combination of clinical presentation, radiographic studies, serologic tests, and exposure history.

Neuroimaging findings suggestive of neurocysticercosis constitute the primary major diagnostic criterion (Fig. 260-1). These findings include cystic lesions with or without enhancement (e.g., ring enhancement), one or more nodular calcifications (which may also have associated enhancement), or focal enhancing lesions. Cysticerci in the brain parenchyma are usually 5–20 mm in diameter and rounded. Cystic lesions in the subarachnoid space or fissures may enlarge up to 6 cm in diameter and may be lobulated. For cysticerci within the subarachnoid space or ventricles, the walls may be very thin and the cyst fluid is often isodense with CSF. Thus, obstructive hydrocephalus or enhancement of the basilar meninges may be the only finding on CT in extraparenchymal neurocysticercosis. Cysticerci in the ventricles or subarachnoid space are usually visible to an experienced neuroradiologist on MRI or on CT with intraventricular contrast injection. CT is more sensitive than MRI in identifying calcified lesions, whereas MRI is better for identifying cystic lesions, scolices, and enhancement.

The second major diagnostic criterion is detection of specific antibodies to cysticerci. Although most tests using unfractionated antigen have high rates of false-positive and false-negative results, this problem can be overcome by using the more specific immunoblot assay. An immunoblot assay using lentil lectin purified glycoproteins is >99% specific and highly sensitive. However, patients with single intracranial lesions or with calcifications may be seronegative. With this assay, serum samples provide greater diagnostic sensitivity than CSF. All of the diagnostic antigens have been cloned, and assays using recombinant antigens are being developed. Antigen detection assays using monoclonal antibodies to detect parasite antigen in the blood or CSF may also facilitate diagnosis and patient follow-up. These assays are only now becoming available for patient care.

Studies have demonstrated that clinical criteria can aid in diagnosis in selected cases. In patients from endemic areas who had single enhancing lesions presenting with seizures, a normal physical examination, and no evidence of systemic disease (e.g., no fever, adenopathy, or chest radiographic abnormalities), the constellation of rounded CT lesions 5–20 mm in diameter with no midline shift was almost always caused by neurocysticercosis. Finally, spontaneous resolution or resolution after therapy with albendazole alone is consistent with neurocysticercosis.

Minor diagnostic criteria include neuroimaging findings consistent with but less characteristic of cysticercosis, clinical manifestations suggestive of neurocysticercosis (e.g., seizures, hydrocephalus, or altered mental status), evidence of cysticercosis outside the central nervous system (CNS) (e.g., cigar-shaped soft-tissue calcifications), or detection of antibody in CSF by ELISA. Epidemiologic criteria include

TABLE 260-1 DIAGNOSTIC CRITERIA FOR HUMAN CYSTICERCOSIS[a]

1. Absolute criteria
   a. Demonstration of cysticerci by histologic or microscopic examination of biopsy material
   b. Visualization of the parasite in the eye by funduscopy
   c. Neuroradiologic demonstration of cystic lesions containing a characteristic scolex
2. Major criteria
   a. Neuroradiologic lesions suggestive of neurocysticercosis
   b. Demonstration of antibodies to cysticerci in serum by enzyme-linked immunoelectrotransfer blot
   c. Resolution of intracranial cystic lesions spontaneously or after therapy with albendazole or praziquantel alone
3. Minor criteria
   a. Lesions compatible with neurocysticercosis detected by neuroimaging studies
   b. Clinical manifestations suggestive of neurocysticercosis
   c. Demonstration of antibodies to cysticerci or cysticercal antigen in cerebrospinal fluid by enzyme-linked immunosorbent assay
   d. Evidence of cysticercosis outside the central nervous system (e.g., cigar-shaped soft-tissue calcifications)
4. Epidemiologic criteria
   a. Residence in a cysticercosis-endemic area
   b. Frequent travel to a cysticercosis-endemic area
   c. Household contact with an individual infected with *Taenia solium*

[a]Diagnosis is confirmed by either one absolute criterion or a combination of two major criteria, one minor criterion, and one epidemiologic criterion. A probable diagnosis is supported by the fulfillment of (1) one major criterion plus two minor criteria; (2) one major criterion plus one minor criterion and one epidemiologic criterion; or (3) three minor criteria plus one epidemiologic criterion.

Source: Modified from OH Del Brutto et al: Neurology 57:177, 2001.

exposure to a tapeworm carrier or household member infected with *T. solium*, current or prior residence in an endemic area, and frequent travel to an endemic area.

The diagnosis is confirmed in patients with either one absolute criterion or a combination of two major criteria, one minor criterion, and one epidemiologic criterion (Table 260-1). A probable diagnosis is supported by the fulfillment of (1) one major criterion plus two minor criteria; (2) one major criterion plus one minor criterion and one epidemiologic criterion; or (3) three minor criteria plus one epidemiologic criterion. Although the CSF is usually abnormal in neurocysticercosis, CSF abnormalities are not pathognomonic. Patients may have CSF pleocytosis with a predominance of lymphocytes, neutrophils, or eosinophils. The protein level in CSF may be elevated; the glucose concentration is usually normal but may be depressed.

TREATMENT TAENIASIS SOLIUM AND CYSTICERCOSIS

Intestinal *T. solium* infection is treated with a single dose of praziquantel (10 mg/kg). However, praziquantel occasionally evokes an inflammatory response in the CNS if concomitant cryptic cysticercosis is present. Niclosamide (2 g) is also effective but is not widely available.

The initial management of neurocysticercosis should focus on symptom-based treatment of seizures or hydrocephalus. Seizures can usually be controlled with antiepileptic treatment. If parenchymal lesions resolve without development of calcifications and patients remain free of seizures, antiepileptic therapy can usually be discontinued after 1–2 years. Placebo-controlled trials are clarifying the clinical advantage of antiparasitic drugs for parenchymal neurocysticercosis. Trends toward faster resolution of neuroradiologic abnormalities have been observed in most studies. The clinical benefits are less dramatic and consist mainly of shortening the period during which recurrent seizures occur and decreasing the number of patients who have many recurrent seizures. For the treatment of patients with brain parenchymal cysticerci, most authorities favor antiparasitic drugs, including albendazole (15 mg/kg per day for 8–28 days) or praziquantel (50–100 mg/kg daily in three divided doses for 15–30 days). A combination of albendazole and praziquantel (50 mg/kg per day) may be more effective in patients with multiple lesions. A longer course or combination therapy is often needed in patients with multiple subarachnoid cysticerci. Both agents may exacerbate the inflammatory response around the dying parasite, thereby exacerbating seizures or hydrocephalus as well. Thus, patients receiving these drugs should be carefully monitored. High-dose glucocorticoids should be used during treatment. Because glucocorticoids induce first-pass metabolism of praziquantel and may decrease its antiparasitic effect, cimetidine should be co-administered to inhibit praziquantel metabolism.

For patients with hydrocephalus, the emergent reduction of intracranial pressure is the mainstay of therapy. In the case of obstructive hydrocephalus, the preferred approach is removal of the cysticercus via endoscopic surgery. However, this intervention is not always possible. An alternative approach is initially to perform a diverting procedure, such as ventriculoperitoneal shunting. Historically, shunts have usually failed, but low failure rates have been attained with administration of antiparasitic drugs and glucocorticoids. Open craniotomy to remove cysticerci is now required only infrequently but is an alternative for fourth-ventricular cysticerci. For patients with subarachnoid cysts or giant cysticerci, anti-inflammatory medications such as glucocorticoids are needed to reduce arachnoiditis and accompanying vasculitis. Most authorities recommend prolonged courses of antiparasitic drugs as well as shunting when hydrocephalus is present. Methotrexate should be used as a steroid-sparing agent in patients requiring prolonged therapy. In patients with diffuse cerebral edema and elevated intracranial pressure due to multiple inflamed lesions, glucocorticoids are the mainstay of therapy, and antiparasitic drugs should be avoided. For ocular and spinal medullary lesions, drug-induced inflammation may cause irreversible damage. Ocular disease should be managed surgically. Recent data suggest that either medical or surgical therapy can be used for spinal disease.

Prevention Measures for the prevention of intestinal *T. solium* infection consist of the application to pork of precautions similar to those described above for beef with regard to *T. saginata* infection. The prevention of cysticercosis involves minimizing the opportunities for ingestion of fecally derived eggs by means of good personal hygiene, effective fecal disposal, and treatment and prevention of human intestinal infections. Mass chemotherapy has been administered to human and porcine populations in efforts at disease eradication. Finally, vaccines to prevent porcine cysticercosis have shown promise in studies and are under development.

ECHINOCOCCOSIS

Echinococcosis is an infection caused in humans by the larval stage of the *Echinococcus granulosus* complex, *E. multilocularis*, or *E. vogeli*. *E. granulosus* complex parasites produce cystic hydatid disease, with unilocular cystic lesions. These infections are prevalent in most areas where livestock is raised in association with dogs. Molecular evidence suggests that *E. granulosus* strains may actually belong to more than one species; specifically, strains from sheep, cattle, pigs, horses, and camels probably represent separate species. These parasites are found on all continents, with areas of high prevalence in China, central Asia, the Middle East, the Mediterranean region, eastern Africa, and parts of South America. *E. multilocularis*, which causes multilocular alveolar lesions that are locally invasive, is found in Alpine, sub-Arctic, or Arctic regions, including Canada, the United States, and central and northern Europe; China; and central Asia. *E. vogeli* causes polycystic hydatid disease and is found only in Central and South America.

Like other cestodes, echinococcal species have both intermediate and definitive hosts. The definitive hosts are canines that pass eggs in their feces. After the ingestion of eggs, cysts develop in the intermediate hosts—sheep, cattle, humans, goats, camels, and horses for the *E. granulosus* complex and mice and other rodents for *E. multilocularis*. When a dog (*E. granulosus*) or fox (*E. multilocularis*) ingests infected meat containing cysts, the life cycle is completed.

Etiology The small (5-mm-long) adult *E. granulosus* complex worms, which live for 5–20 months in the jejunum of dogs, have only three proglottids: one immature, one mature, and one gravid. The gravid segment splits to release eggs that are morphologically similar to *Taenia* eggs and are extremely hardy. After humans ingest the eggs, embryos escape from the eggs, penetrate the intestinal mucosa, enter the portal circulation, and are carried to various organs, most commonly the liver and lungs. Larvae develop into fluid-filled unilocular hydatid cysts that consist of an external membrane and an inner germinal layer. Daughter cysts develop from the inner aspect of the germinal layer, as do germinating cystic structures called *brood capsules*. New larvae, called *protoscolices*, develop in large numbers within the brood capsule. The cysts expand slowly over a period of years.

The life cycle of *E. multilocularis* is similar except that wild canines, such as foxes, serve as the definitive hosts and small rodents serve as the intermediate hosts. The larval form of *E. multilocularis*, however, is quite different in that it remains in the proliferative phase, the parasite is always multilocular, and vesicles without brood capsule or protoscolices progressively invade the host tissue by peripheral extension of processes from the germinal layer.

Clinical Manifestations Slowly enlarging echinococcal cysts generally remain asymptomatic until their expanding size or their space-occupying effect in an involved organ elicits symptoms. The liver and the lungs are the most common sites of these cysts. The liver is involved in about two-thirds of *E. granulosus* infections and in nearly all *E. multilocularis* infections. Because a period of years elapses before cysts enlarge sufficiently to cause symptoms, they may be discovered incidentally on a routine x-ray or ultrasound study.

Patients with hepatic echinococcosis who are symptomatic most often present with abdominal pain or a palpable mass in the right upper quadrant. Compression of a bile duct or leakage of cyst fluid into the biliary tree may mimic recurrent cholelithiasis, and biliary obstruction can result in jaundice. Rupture of or episodic leakage from a hydatid cyst may produce fever, pruritus, urticaria, eosinophilia, or anaphylaxis. Pulmonary hydatid cysts may rupture into the bronchial tree or pleural cavity and produce cough, salty phlegm, dyspnea, chest pain, or hemoptysis. Rupture of hydatid cysts, which can occur spontaneously or at surgery, may lead to multifocal dissemination of protoscolices, which can form additional cysts. Other presentations are due to the involvement of bone (invasion of the medullary cavity with slow bone erosion producing pathologic fractures), the CNS (space-occupying lesions), the heart (conduction defects, pericarditis), and the pelvis (pelvic mass).

The larval forms of *E. multilocularis* characteristically present as a slowly growing hepatic tumor, with progressive destruction of the liver and extension into vital structures. Patients commonly report upper-quadrant and epigastric pain. Liver enlargement and obstructive jaundice may be apparent. The lesions may infiltrate adjoining organs (e.g., diaphragm, kidneys, or lungs) or may metastasize to the spleen, lungs, or brain.

Diagnosis Radiographic and related imaging studies are important in detecting and evaluating echinococcal cysts. Plain x-rays will define pulmonary cysts of *E. granulosus*—usually as rounded masses of uniform density—but may miss cysts in other organs unless there is cyst wall calcification (as occurs in the liver). MRI, CT, and ultrasound reveal well-defined cysts with thick or thin walls. When older cysts contain a layer of hydatid sand that is rich in accumulated protoscolices, these imaging methods may detect this fluid layer of different density. However, the most pathognomonic finding, if demonstrable, is that of daughter cysts within the larger cyst. This finding, like eggshell or mural calcification on CT, is indicative of *E. granulosus* infection and helps to distinguish the cyst from carcinomas, bacterial or amebic liver abscesses, or hemangiomas. In contrast, ultrasound or CT of alveolar hydatid cysts reveals indistinct solid masses with central necrosis and plaquelike calcifications.

A specific diagnosis of *E. granulosus* infection can be made by the examination of aspirated fluids for protoscolices or hooklets, but diagnostic aspiration is not usually recommended because of the risk of fluid leakage resulting in either dissemination of infection or anaphylactic reactions. Serodiagnostic assays can be useful, although a negative test does not exclude the diagnosis of echinococcosis. Cysts in the liver elicit positive antibody responses in ~90% of cases, whereas up to 50% of individuals with cysts in the lungs are seronegative. Detection of antibody to specific echinococcal antigens by immunoblotting has the highest degree of specificity.

TREATMENT ECHINOCOCCOSIS

Therapy for cystic echinococcosis is based on considerations of the size, location, and manifestations of cysts and the overall health of the patient. Surgery has traditionally been the principal definitive method of treatment. Currently, ultrasound staging is recommended for *E. granulosus* infections (Fig. 260-2). Small CL, CE1, and CE3 lesions may respond to chemotherapy with albendazole. For CE1 lesions and uncomplicated CE3 lesions, PAIR (*p*ercutaneous *a*spiration, *i*nfusion of scolicidal agents, and *r*easpiration) is now recommended instead of surgery. PAIR is contraindicated for superficially located cysts (because of the risk of rupture), for cysts with multiple thick internal septal divisions (honeycombing pattern), and for cysts communicating with the biliary tree. For prophylaxis of secondary peritoneal echinococcosis due to inadvertent spillage of fluid during PAIR, the administration of albendazole (15 mg/kg daily in two divided doses) should be initiated at least 2 days before the procedure and continued for at least 4 weeks afterward. Ultrasound- or CT-guided aspiration allows confirmation of the diagnosis by demonstration of protoscolices in the aspirate. After aspiration, contrast material should be injected to detect occult communications with the biliary tract. Alternatively, the fluid should be checked for bile staining visually and by dipstick. If no bile is found and no communication is visualized, the contrast material is reaspirated, with subsequent infusion of scolicidal agents (usually 95% ethanol; alternatively, hypertonic saline). This approach, when implemented by a skilled practitioner, yields rates of cure and relapse equivalent to those following surgery, with less perioperative morbidity and shorter hospitalization. In experienced hands, some CE2 lesions can be treated by aspiration with a trocar. Daughter cysts within the primary cyst may need to be punctured separately, and catheter drainage may be required.

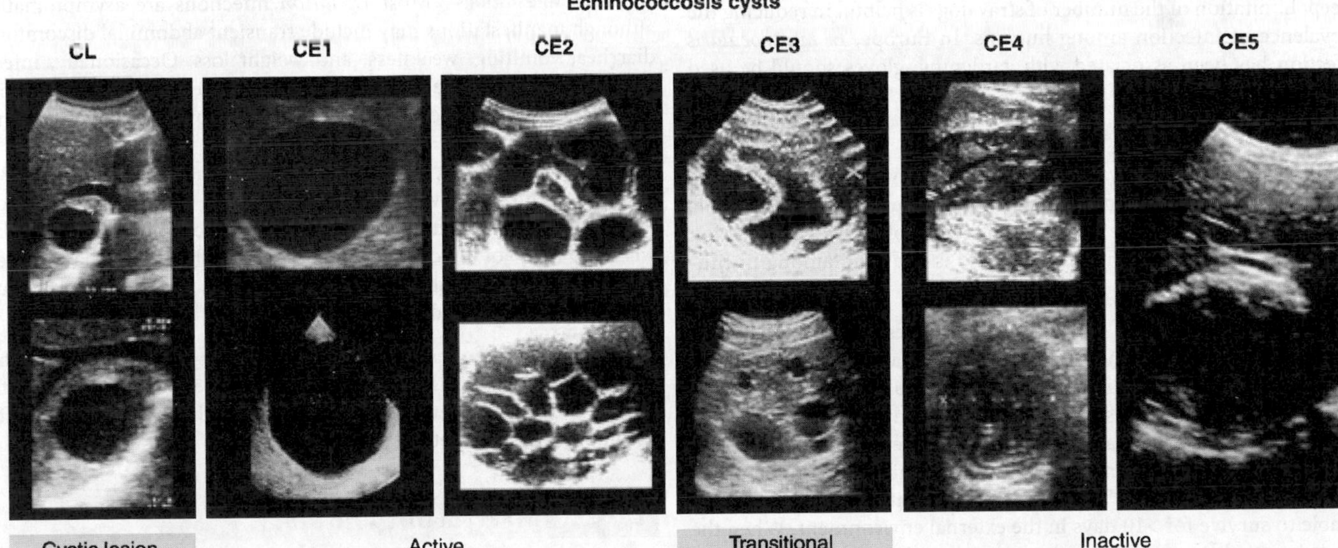

FIGURE 260-2 Management of cystic hydatid disease caused by *Echinococcus granulosus* should be based on viability of the parasite, which can be estimated from radiographic appearance. The ultrasound appearance includes lesions classified as active, transitional, and inactive. *Active* cysts include types CL (with a cystic lesion and no visible cyst wall), CE1 (with a visible cyst wall and internal echoes [*snowflake sign*]), and CE2 (with a visible cyst wall and internal septation). *Transitional* cysts (CE3) may have detached laminar membranes or may be partially collapsed. *Inactive cysts* include types CE4 (a nonhomogeneous mass) and CE5 (a cyst with a thick calcified wall). *(Adapted from RL Guerrant et al [eds]: Tropical Infectious Diseases: Principles, Pathogens and Practice, 2nd ed, p 1312. © 2005, with permission from Elsevier Science.)*

Surgery remains the treatment of choice for complicated *E. granulosus* cysts (e.g., those communicating with the biliary tract), for most thoracic and intracranial cysts, and for areas where PAIR is not possible. For *E. granulosus* of the liver, the preferred surgical approach is pericystectomy, in which the entire cyst and the surrounding fibrous tissue are removed. The risks posed by leakage of fluid during surgery or PAIR include anaphylaxis and dissemination of infectious protoscolices. The latter complication has been minimized by careful attention to the prevention of spillage of the cyst and by soaking of the drapes with hypertonic saline. Infusion of scolicidal agents is no longer recommended because of problems with hypernatremia, intoxication, or sclerosing cholangitis. Albendazole, which is active against *Echinococcus*, should be administered adjunctively, beginning several days before resection of the liver and continuing for several weeks for *E. granulosus*. Praziquantel (50 mg/kg daily for 2 weeks) may hasten the death of the protoscolices. Medical therapy with albendazole alone for 12 weeks to 6 months results in cure in ~30% of cases and in improvement in another 50%. In many instances of treatment failure, *E. granulosus* infections are subsequently treated successfully with PAIR or additional courses of medical therapy. Response to treatment is best assessed by serial imaging studies, with attention to cyst size and consistency. Some cysts may not demonstrate complete radiologic resolution even though no viable protoscolices are present. Some of these cysts with partial radiologic resolution (e.g., CE4 or CE5) can be managed with observation only.

Surgical resection remains the treatment of choice for *E. multilocularis* infection. Complete removal of the parasite continues to offer the best chance for cure. Ongoing therapy with albendazole for at least 2 years after presumptively curative surgery is recommended. Positron emission tomography can be used to follow disease activity. Most cases are diagnosed at a stage at which complete resection is not possible; in these cases, albendazole treatment should be continued indefinitely, with careful monitoring. In some cases, liver transplantation has been used because of the size of the necessary liver resection. However, continuous immunosuppression favors the proliferation of *E. multilocularis* larvae and reinfection of the transplant. Thus, indefinite treatment with albendazole is required.

Prevention In endemic areas, echinococcosis can be prevented by administering praziquantel to infected dogs, by denying dogs access to infected animals, or by vaccinating sheep. Limitation of the number of stray dogs is helpful in reducing the prevalence of infection among humans. In Europe, *E. multilocularis* infection has been associated with gardening; gloves should be used when working with soil.

HYMENOLEPIASIS NANA

Infection with *Hymenolepis nana*, the dwarf tapeworm, is the most common of all the cestode infections. *H. nana* is endemic in both temperate and tropical regions of the world. Infection is spread by fecal/oral contamination and is common among institutionalized children.

Etiology and Pathogenesis *H. nana* is the only cestode of humans that does not require an intermediate host. Both the larval and adult phases of the life cycle take place in the human. The adult—the smallest tapeworm parasitizing humans—is ~2 cm long and dwells in the proximal ileum. Proglottids, which are small and rarely seen in the stool, release spherical eggs 30–44 μm in diameter, each of which contains an oncosphere with six hooklets. The eggs are immediately infective and are unable to survive for >10 days in the external environment. When the egg is ingested by a new host, the oncosphere is freed and penetrates the intestinal villi, becoming a cysticercoid larva. Larvae migrate back into the intestinal lumen, attach to the mucosa, and mature into adult worms over 10–12 days. Eggs may also hatch before passing into the stool, causing internal autoinfection with increasing numbers of intestinal worms. Although the life span of adult *H. nana* worms is only ~4–10 weeks, the autoinfection cycle perpetuates the infection.

Clinical Manifestations *H. nana* infection, even with many intestinal worms, is usually asymptomatic. When infection is intense, anorexia, abdominal pain, and diarrhea develop.

Diagnosis Infection is diagnosed by the finding of eggs in the stool.

TREATMENT HYMENOLEPIASIS NANA

Praziquantel (25 mg/kg once) is the treatment of choice, because it acts against both the adult worms and the cysticercoids in the intestinal villi. Nitazoxanide (500 mg bid for 3 days) may be used as an alternative.

Prevention Good personal hygiene and improved sanitation can eradicate the disease. Epidemics have been controlled by mass chemotherapy coupled with improved hygiene.

HYMENOLEPIASIS DIMINUTA

Hymenolepis diminuta, a cestode of rodents, occasionally infects small children, who ingest the larvae in uncooked cereal foods contaminated by fleas and other insects in which larvae develop. Infection is usually asymptomatic and is diagnosed by the detection of eggs in the stool. Treatment with praziquantel results in cure in most cases.

DIPHYLLOBOTHRIASIS

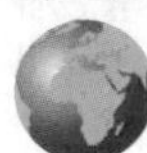

Diphyllobothrium latum and other *Diphyllobothrium* species are found in the lakes, rivers, and deltas of the Northern Hemisphere, central Africa, and South America.

Etiology and Pathogenesis The adult worm—the longest tapeworm (up to 25 m)—attaches to the ileal and occasionally to the jejunal mucosa by its suckers, which are located on its elongated scolex. The adult worm has 3000–4000 proglottids, which release ~1 million eggs daily into the feces. If an egg reaches water, it hatches and releases a free-swimming embryo that can be eaten by small freshwater crustaceans (*Cyclops* or *Diaptomus* species). After an infected crustacean containing a developed procercoid is swallowed by a fish, the larva migrates into the fish's flesh and grows into a plerocercoid, or sparganum larva. Humans acquire the infection by ingesting infected raw or smoked fish. Within 3–5 weeks, the tapeworm matures into an adult in the human intestine.

Clinical Manifestations Most *D. latum* infections are asymptomatic, although manifestations may include transient abdominal discomfort, diarrhea, vomiting, weakness, and weight loss. Occasionally, infection can cause acute abdominal pain and intestinal obstruction; in rare cases, cholangitis or cholecystitis may be produced by migrating proglottids.

Because the tapeworm absorbs large quantities of vitamin B_{12} and interferes with ileal B_{12} absorption, vitamin B_{12} deficiency can develop, but this effect has been noted only in Scandinavia, where up to 2% of infected patients, especially the elderly, have megaloblastic anemia resembling pernicious anemia and may exhibit neurologic sequelae of B_{12} deficiency.

Diagnosis The diagnosis is made readily by the detection of the characteristic eggs in the stool. The eggs possess a single shell with an operculum at one end and a knob at the other. Mild to moderate eosinophilia may be detected.

TREATMENT DIPHYLLOBOTHRIASIS

Praziquantel (5–10 mg/kg once) is highly effective. Parenteral vitamin B_{12} should be given if B_{12} deficiency is manifest.

Prevention Infection can be prevented by heating fish to 54°C for 5 min or by freezing it at −18°C for 24 h. Placing fish in brine with a high salt concentration for long periods kills the eggs.

DIPYLIDIASIS

Dipylidium caninum, a common tapeworm of dogs and cats, may accidentally infect humans. Dogs, cats, and occasionally humans become infected by ingesting fleas harboring cysticercoids. Children are more likely to become infected than adults. Most infections are asymptomatic, but abdominal pain, diarrhea, anal pruritus, urticaria, eosinophilia, or passage of segments in the stool may occur. The diagnosis is made by the detection of proglottids or ova in the stool. As in *D. latum* infection, therapy consists of praziquantel. Prevention requires anthelmintic treatment and flea control for pet dogs or cats.

SPARGANOSIS

Humans can be infected by the sparganum, or plerocercoid larva, of a diphyllobothrid tapeworm of the genus *Spirometra*. Infection can be acquired by the consumption of water containing infected *Cyclops*; by the ingestion of infected snakes, birds, or mammals; or by the application of infected flesh as poultices. The worm migrates slowly in tissues, and infection commonly presents as a subcutaneous swelling. Periorbital tissues can be involved, and ocular sparganosis may destroy the eye. Surgical excision is used to treat localized sparganosis.

COENUROSIS

This rare infection of humans by the larval stage (coenurus) of the dog tapeworm *Taenia multiceps* or *T. serialis* results in a space-occupying cystic lesion. As in cysticercosis, involvement of the CNS and subcutaneous tissue is most common. Both definitive diagnosis and treatment require surgical excision of the lesion. Chemotherapeutic agents generally are not effective.

261e Microbial Bioterrorism

H. Clifford Lane, Anthony S. Fauci

This is a digital-only chapter. It is available on the DVD that accompanies this book, as well as on Access Medicine/Harrison's Online, and the eBook and "app" editions of HPIM 19e.

Descriptions of the use of microbial pathogens as potential weapons of war or terrorism date from ancient times. Among the most frequently cited of such episodes are the poisoning of water supplies in the sixth century B.C. with the fungus *Claviceps purpurea* (rye ergot) by the Assyrians, the hurling of the dead bodies of plague victims over the walls of the city of Kaffa by the Tartar army in 1346, and the efforts by the British to spread smallpox to the Native American population loyal to the French via contaminated blankets in 1763. The tragic attacks on the World Trade Center and the Pentagon on September 11, 2001, followed closely by the mailing of letters containing anthrax spores to media and congressional offices through the U.S. Postal Service, dramatically changed the mindset of the American public regarding both our vulnerability to microbial bioterrorist attacks and the seriousness and intent of the federal government to protect its citizens against future attacks. Modern science has revealed methods of deliberately spreading or enhancing disease in ways not appreciated by our ancestors. The combination of basic research, good medical practice, and constant vigilance will be needed to defend against such attacks.

262e Chemical Terrorism

Charles G. Hurst, Jonathan Newmark, James A. Romano, Jr.

This is a digital-only chapter. It is available on the DVD that accompanies this book, as well as on Access Medicine/Harrison's Online, and the eBook and "app" editions of HPIM 19e.

The use of chemical warfare agents (CWAs) in modern warfare dates back to World War I (WWI). Sulfur mustard and nerve agents were used by Iraq against the Iranian military and Kurdish civilians. Most recently the nerve agent Sarin, GB, was used by the Syrian military against their civilian population. Since the Japanese sarin attacks in 1994–1995 and the terrorist strikes of September 11, 2001, the all-too-real possibility of chemical or biological terrorism against civilian populations anywhere in the world has attracted increased attention.

Military planners consider the WWI blistering agent sulfur mustard and the organophosphorus nerve agents as the most likely agents to be used on the battlefield. In a civilian or terrorist scenario, the choice widens considerably. For example, many of the CWAs of WWI, including chlorine, phosgene, and cyanide, are used today in large amounts in industry. They are produced in chemical plants, are stockpiled in large tanks, and travel up and down highways and railways in large tanker cars. The rupture of any of these stores by accident or on purpose could cause many injuries and deaths. In three attacks in February 2007, for example, insurgents in Iraq used chlorine gas released from tankers after explosions as a crude form of chemical weaponry; these attacks killed 12 people and intoxicated more than 140 others. Countless hazardous materials (HAZMATs) that are not used on the battlefield can be used as terrorist weapons. Some of them, including insecticides and ammonia, could wreak as much damage and injury as the weaponized chemical agents.

263e Radiation Terrorism

Christine E. Hill-Kayser, Eli Glatstein, Zelig A. Tochner

This is a digital-only chapter. It is available on the DVD that accompanies this book, as well as on Access Medicine/Harrison's Online, and the eBook and "app" editions of HPIM 19e.

The threat of a terror attack employing nuclear or radiation-related devices is unequivocal in the twenty-first century. Such an attack would certainly have the potential to cause unique and devastating medical and psychological effects that would require prompt action by members of the medical community. This chapter outlines the most probable scenarios for an attack involving radiation as well as the medical principles for handling such threats.

PART 10: Disorders of the Cardiovascular System

SECTION 1 INTRODUCTION TO CARDIOVASCULAR DISORDERS

264 Approach to the Patient with Possible Cardiovascular Disease

Joseph Loscalzo

THE MAGNITUDE OF THE PROBLEM

Cardiovascular diseases comprise the most prevalent serious disorders in industrialized nations and are a rapidly growing problem in developing nations (Chap. 266e). Age-adjusted death rates for coronary heart disease have declined by two-thirds in the last four decades in the United States, reflecting the identification and reduction of risk factors as well as improved treatments and interventions for the management of coronary artery disease, arrhythmias, and heart failure. Nonetheless, cardiovascular diseases remain the most common causes of death, responsible for 35% of all deaths, almost 1 million deaths each year. Approximately one-fourth of these deaths are sudden. In addition, cardiovascular diseases are highly prevalent, diagnosed in 80 million adults, or ~35% of the adult population. The growing prevalence of obesity (Chap. 416), type 2 diabetes mellitus (Chap. 417), and metabolic syndrome (Chap. 422), which are important risk factors for atherosclerosis, now threatens to reverse the progress that has been made in the age-adjusted reduction in the mortality rate of coronary heart disease.

For many years cardiovascular disease was considered to be more common in men than in women. In fact, the percentage of all deaths secondary to cardiovascular disease is higher among women (43%) than among men (37%) (Chap. 6e). In addition, although the absolute number of deaths secondary to cardiovascular disease has declined over the past decades in men, this number has actually risen in women. Inflammation, obesity, type 2 diabetes mellitus, and the metabolic syndrome appear to play more prominent roles in the development of coronary atherosclerosis in women than in men. Coronary artery disease (CAD) is more frequently associated with dysfunction of the coronary microcirculation in women than in men. Exercise electrocardiography has a lower diagnostic accuracy in the prediction of epicardial obstruction in women than in men.

NATURAL HISTORY

Cardiovascular disorders often present acutely, as in a previously asymptomatic person who develops an acute myocardial infarction (Chap. 295), or a previously asymptomatic patient with hypertrophic cardiomyopathy (Chap. 287), or with a prolonged QT interval (Chap. 277) whose first clinical manifestation is syncope or even sudden death. However, the alert physician may recognize the patient at risk for these complications long before they occur and often can take measures to prevent their occurrence. For example, a patient with acute myocardial infarction will often have had risk factors for atherosclerosis for many years. Had these risk factors been recognized, their elimination or reduction might have delayed or even prevented the infarction. Similarly, a patient with hypertrophic cardiomyopathy may have had a heart murmur for years and a family history of this disorder. These findings could have led to an echocardiographic examination, recognition of the condition, and appropriate therapy long before the occurrence of a serious acute manifestation.

Patients with valvular heart disease or idiopathic dilated cardiomyopathy, by contrast, may have a prolonged course of gradually increasing dyspnea and other manifestations of chronic heart failure that is punctuated by episodes of acute deterioration only late in the course of the disease. Understanding the natural history of various cardiac disorders is essential for applying appropriate diagnostic and therapeutic measures to each stage of the condition, as well as for providing the patient and family with the likely prognosis.

CARDIAC SYMPTOMS

The symptoms caused by heart disease result most commonly from myocardial ischemia, disturbance of the contraction and/or relaxation of the myocardium, obstruction to blood flow, or an abnormal cardiac rhythm or rate. Ischemia, which is caused by an imbalance between the heart's oxygen supply and demand, is manifest most frequently as chest discomfort (Chap. 19), whereas reduction of the pumping ability of the heart commonly leads to fatigue and elevated intravascular pressure upstream of the failing ventricle. The latter results in abnormal fluid accumulation, with peripheral edema (Chap. 50) or pulmonary congestion and dyspnea (Chap. 47e). Obstruction to blood flow, as occurs in valvular stenosis, can cause symptoms resembling those of myocardial failure (Chap. 279). Cardiac arrhythmias often develop suddenly, and the resulting symptoms and signs—palpitations (Chap. 52), dyspnea, hypotension, and syncope (Chap. 27)—generally occur abruptly and may disappear as rapidly as they develop.

Although dyspnea, chest discomfort, edema, and syncope are cardinal manifestations of cardiac disease, they occur in other conditions as well. Thus, dyspnea is observed in disorders as diverse as pulmonary disease, marked obesity, and anxiety (Chap. 47e). Similarly, chest discomfort may result from a variety of noncardiac and cardiac causes other than myocardial ischemia (Chap. 19). Edema, an important finding in untreated or inadequately treated heart failure, also may occur with primary renal disease and in hepatic cirrhosis (Chap. 50). Syncope occurs not only with serious cardiac arrhythmias but in a number of neurologic conditions as well (Chap. 27). Whether heart disease is responsible for these symptoms frequently can be determined by carrying out a careful clinical examination (Chap. 267), supplemented by noninvasive testing using electrocardiography at rest and during exercise (Chap. 268), echocardiography, roentgenography, and other forms of myocardial imaging (Chap. 270e).

Myocardial or coronary function that may be adequate at rest may be insufficient during exertion. Thus, dyspnea and/or chest discomfort that appear during activity are characteristic of patients with heart disease, whereas the opposite pattern, i.e., the appearance of these symptoms at rest and their remission during exertion, is rarely observed in such patients. It is important, therefore, to question the patient carefully about the relation of symptoms to exertion.

Many patients with cardiovascular disease may be asymptomatic both at rest and during exertion but may present with an abnormal physical finding such as a heart murmur, elevated arterial pressure, or an abnormality of the electrocardiogram (ECG) or imaging test. It is important to assess the global risk of CAD in asymptomatic individuals, using a combination of clinical assessment and measurement of cholesterol and its fractions, as well as other biomarkers, such as C-reactive protein, in some patients (Chap. 291e). Since the first clinical manifestation of CAD may be catastrophic—sudden cardiac death, acute myocardial infarction, or stroke in previous asymptomatic persons—it is mandatory to identify those at high risk of such events and institute further testing and preventive measures.

DIAGNOSIS

As outlined by the New York Heart Association (NYHA), the elements of a complete cardiac diagnosis include the systematic consideration of the following:

1. *The underlying etiology.* Is the disease congenital, hypertensive, ischemic, or inflammatory in origin?

TABLE 264-1 NEW YORK HEART ASSOCIATION FUNCTIONAL CLASSIFICATION

Class I	Class III
No limitation of physical activity	Marked limitation of physical activity
No symptoms with ordinary exertion	Less than ordinary activity causes symptoms
Class II	Asymptomatic at rest
Slight limitation of physical activity	**Class IV**
Ordinary activity causes symptoms	Inability to carry out any physical activity without discomfort
	Symptoms at rest

Source: Modified from The Criteria Committee of the New York Heart Association.

2. *The anatomic abnormalities.* Which chambers are involved? Are they hypertrophied, dilated, or both? Which valves are affected? Are they regurgitant and/or stenotic? Is there pericardial involvement? Has there been a myocardial infarction?
3. *The physiologic disturbances.* Is an arrhythmia present? Is there evidence of congestive heart failure or myocardial ischemia?
4. *Functional disability.* How strenuous is the physical activity required to elicit symptoms? The classification provided by the NYHA has been found to be useful in describing functional disability (Table 264-1).

One example may serve to illustrate the importance of establishing a complete diagnosis. In a patient who presents with exertional chest discomfort, the identification of myocardial ischemia as the etiology is of great clinical importance. However, the simple recognition of ischemia is insufficient to formulate a therapeutic strategy or prognosis until the underlying anatomic abnormalities responsible for the myocardial ischemia, e.g., coronary atherosclerosis or aortic stenosis, are identified and a judgment is made about whether other physiologic disturbances that cause an imbalance between myocardial oxygen supply and demand, such as severe anemia, thyrotoxicosis, or supraventricular tachycardia, play contributory roles. Finally, the severity of the disability should govern the extent and tempo of the workup and strongly influence the therapeutic strategy that is selected.

The establishment of a correct and complete cardiac diagnosis usually commences with the history and physical examination (Chap. 267). Indeed, the clinical examination remains the basis for the diagnosis of a wide variety of disorders. The clinical examination may then be supplemented by five types of laboratory tests: (1) ECG (Chap. 268), (2) noninvasive imaging examinations (chest roentgenogram, echocardiogram, radionuclide imaging, computed tomographic imaging, positron emission tomography, and magnetic resonance imaging) (Chap. 270e), (3) blood tests to assess risk (e.g., lipid determinations, C-reactive protein [Chap. 291e]) or cardiac function (e.g., brain natriuretic peptide [BNP] [Chap. 279]), (4) occasionally specialized invasive examinations (i.e., cardiac catheterization and coronary arteriography [Chap. 272]), and (5) genetic tests to identify monogenic cardiac diseases (e.g., hypertrophic cardiomyopathy [Chap. 287], Marfan's syndrome [Chap. 427], and abnormalities of cardiac ion channels that lead to prolongation of the QT interval and an increase in the risk of sudden death [Chap. 276]). These tests are becoming more widely available.

FAMILY HISTORY

In eliciting the history of a patient with known or suspected cardiovascular disease, particular attention should be directed to the family history. Familial clustering is common in many forms of heart disease. Mendelian transmission of single-gene defects may occur, as in hypertrophic cardiomyopathy (Chap. 287), Marfan's syndrome (Chap. 427), and sudden death associated with a prolonged QT syndrome (Chap. 277). Premature coronary disease and essential hypertension, type 2 diabetes mellitus, and hyperlipidemia (the most important risk factors for CAD) are usually polygenic disorders. Although familial transmission may be less obvious than in the monogenic disorders, it is helpful in assessing risk and prognosis in polygenic disorders, as well. Familial clustering of cardiovascular diseases not only may occur on a genetic basis but also may be related to familial dietary or behavior patterns, such as excessive ingestion of salt or calories and cigarette smoking.

ASSESSMENT OF FUNCTIONAL IMPAIRMENT

When an attempt is made to determine the severity of functional impairment in a patient with heart disease, it is helpful to ascertain the level of activity and the rate at which it is performed before symptoms develop. Thus, it is not sufficient to state that the patient complains of dyspnea. The breathlessness that occurs after running up two long flights of stairs denotes far less functional impairment than do similar symptoms that occur after taking a few steps on level ground. Also, the degree of customary physical activity at work and during recreation should be considered. The development of two-flight dyspnea in a well-conditioned marathon runner may be far more significant than the development of one-flight dyspnea in a previously sedentary person. The history should include a detailed consideration of the patient's therapeutic regimen. For example, the persistence or development of edema, breathlessness, and other manifestations of heart failure in a patient who is receiving optimal doses of diuretics and other therapies for heart failure (Chap. 279) is far graver than are similar manifestations in the absence of treatment. Similarly, the presence of angina pectoris despite treatment with optimal doses of multiple antianginal drugs (Chap. 293) is more serious than it is in a patient on no therapy. In an effort to determine the progression of symptoms, and thus the severity of the underlying illness, it may be useful to ascertain what, if any, specific tasks the patient could have carried out 6 months or 1 year earlier that he or she cannot carry out at present.

ELECTROCARDIOGRAM

(See also Chap. 268) Although an ECG usually should be recorded in patients with known or suspected heart disease, with the exception of the identification of arrhythmias, conduction abnormalities, ventricular hypertrophy, and acute myocardial infarction, it generally does not establish a specific diagnosis. The range of normal electrocardiographic findings is wide, and the tracing can be affected significantly by many noncardiac factors, such as age, body habitus, and serum electrolyte concentrations. In general, electrocardiographic changes should be interpreted in the context of other abnormal cardiovascular findings.

ASSESSMENT OF THE PATIENT WITH A HEART MURMUR

(Fig. 264-1) The cause of a heart murmur can often be readily elucidated from a systematic evaluation of its major attributes: timing, duration, intensity, quality, frequency, configuration, location, and radiation when considered in the light of the history, general physical examination, and other features of the cardiac examination, as described in Chap. 267.

The majority of heart murmurs are midsystolic and soft (grades I–II/VI). When such a murmur occurs in an asymptomatic child or young adult *without* other evidence of heart disease on clinical examination, it is usually benign and echocardiography generally is not required. By contrast, two-dimensional and Doppler echocardiography (Chap. 270e) are indicated in patients with loud systolic murmurs (grades ≥III/VI), especially those that are holosystolic or late systolic, and in most patients with diastolic or continuous murmurs.

PITFALLS IN CARDIOVASCULAR MEDICINE

Increasing subspecialization in internal medicine and the perfection of advanced diagnostic techniques in cardiology can lead to several undesirable consequences. Examples include the following:

1. Failure by the *noncardiologist* to recognize important cardiac manifestations of systemic illnesses. For example, the presence of mitral stenosis, patent foramen ovale, and/or transient atrial arrhythmia should be considered in a patient with stroke, or the presence of pulmonary hypertension and cor pulmonale should be considered in a patient with scleroderma or Raynaud's syndrome. A cardiovascular examination should be carried out to identify and estimate

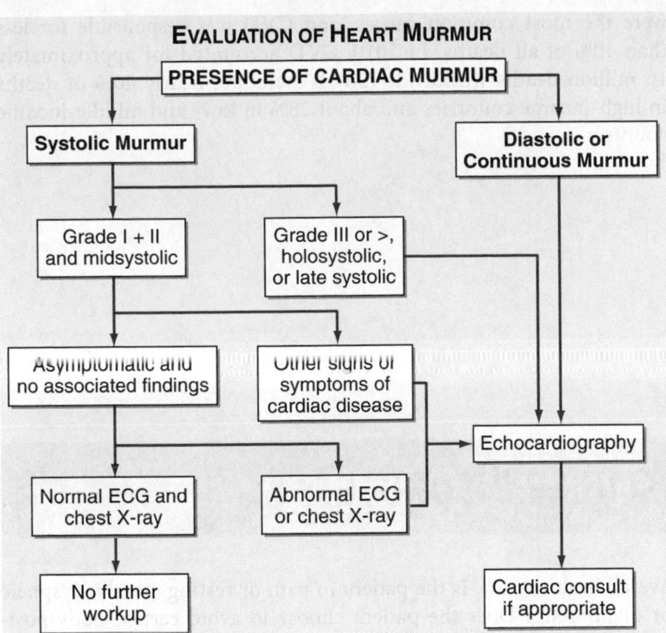

FIGURE 264-1 Approach to the evaluation of a heart murmur. ECG, electrocardiogram. *(From RA O'Rourke, in Primary Cardiology, 2nd ed, E Braunwald, L Goldman [eds]. Philadelphia, Saunders, 2003.)*

the severity of the cardiovascular involvement that accompanies many noncardiac disorders.

2. Failure by the *cardiologist* to recognize underlying systemic disorders in patients with heart disease. For example, hyperthyroidism should be considered in an elderly patient with atrial fibrillation and unexplained heart failure, and Lyme disease should be considered in a patient with unexplained fluctuating atrioventricular block. A cardiovascular abnormality may provide the clue critical to the recognition of some systemic disorders. For example, an unexplained pericardial effusion may provide an early clue to the diagnosis of tuberculosis or a neoplasm.
3. Overreliance on and overutilization of laboratory tests, particularly invasive techniques, for the evaluation of the cardiovascular system. Cardiac catheterization and coronary arteriography (Chap. 272) provide precise diagnostic information that may be crucial in developing a therapeutic plan in patients with known or suspected CAD. Although a great deal of attention has been directed to these examinations, it is important to recognize that they serve to *supplement*, not *supplant*, a careful examination carried out with clinical and noninvasive techniques. A coronary arteriogram should not be performed in lieu of a careful history in patients with chest pain suspected of having ischemic heart disease. Although coronary arteriography may establish whether the coronary arteries are obstructed and to what extent, the results of the procedure by themselves often do not provide a definitive answer to the question of whether a patient's complaint of chest discomfort is attributable to coronary atherosclerosis and whether or not revascularization is indicated.

Despite the value of invasive tests in certain circumstances, they entail some small risk to the patient, involve discomfort and substantial cost, and place a strain on medical facilities. Therefore, they should be carried out only if the results can be expected to modify the patient's management.

DISEASE PREVENTION AND MANAGEMENT

The prevention of heart disease, especially of CAD, is one of the most important tasks of primary care health givers as well as cardiologists. Prevention begins with risk assessment, followed by attention to lifestyle, such as achieving optimal weight, physical activity, and smoking cessation, and then aggressive treatment of all abnormal risk factors, such as hypertension, hyperlipidemia, and diabetes mellitus (Chap. 417).

After a complete diagnosis has been established in patients with known heart disease, a number of management options are usually available. Several examples may be used to demonstrate some of the principles of cardiovascular therapeutics:

1. In the absence of evidence of heart disease, the patient should be clearly informed of this assessment and *not* be asked to return at intervals for repeated examinations. If there is no evidence of disease, such continued attention may lead to the patient's developing inappropriate concern about the possibility of heart disease.
2. If there is no evidence of cardiovascular disease but the patient has one or more risk factors for the development of ischemic heart disease (Chap. 293), a plan for their reduction should be developed and the patient should be retested at intervals to assess compliance and efficacy in risk reduction.
3. Asymptomatic or mildly symptomatic patients with valvular heart disease that is anatomically severe should be evaluated periodically, every 6 to 12 months, by clinical and noninvasive examinations. Early signs of deterioration of ventricular function may signify the need for surgical treatment before the development of disabling symptoms, irreversible myocardial damage, and excessive risk of surgical treatment (Chap. 283).
4. In patients with CAD (Chap. 293), available practice guidelines should be considered in the decision on the form of treatment (medical, percutaneous coronary intervention, or surgical revascularization). Mechanical revascularization may be employed too frequently in the United States and too infrequently in Eastern Europe and developing nations. The mere presence of angina pectoris and/or the demonstration of critical coronary arterial narrowing at angiography should not reflexively evoke a decision to treat the patient by revascularization. Instead, these interventions should be limited to patients with CAD whose angina has not responded adequately to medical treatment or in whom revascularization has been shown to improve the natural history (e.g., acute coronary syndrome or multivessel CAD with left ventricular dysfunction).

265e Basic Biology of the Cardiovascular System

Joseph Loscalzo, Peter Libby, Jonathan A. Epstein

This is a digital-only chapter. It is available on the DVD that accompanies this book, as well as on Access Medicine/Harrison's Online, and the eBook and "app" editions of HPIM 19e.

THE BLOOD VESSEL

VASCULAR ULTRASTRUCTURE

Blood vessels participate in homeostasis on a moment-to-moment basis and contribute to the pathophysiology of diseases of virtually every organ system. Hence, an understanding of the fundamentals of vascular biology furnishes a foundation for understanding the normal function of all organ systems and many diseases. The smallest blood vessels—capillaries—consist of a monolayer of endothelial cells apposed to a basement membrane, adjacent to occasional smooth-muscle-like cells known as *pericytes*. Unlike larger vessels, pericytes do not invest the entire microvessel to form a continuous sheath. Arteries typically have a trilaminar structure. The *intima* consists of a monolayer of endothelial cells continuous with those of the capillaries. The middle layer, or *tunica media*, consists of layers of smooth-muscle cells; in veins, the media can contain just a few layers of smooth-muscle cells. The outer layer, the *adventitia*, consists of looser extracellular matrix with occasional fibroblasts, mast cells, and nerve terminals. Larger arteries have their own vasculature, the *vasa vasorum*, which nourishes the outer aspects of the tunica media. The adventitia of many veins surpasses the intima in thickness.

266e Epidemiology of Cardiovascular Disease

Thomas A. Gaziano, J. Michael Gaziano

This is a digital-only chapter. It is available on the DVD that accompanies this book, as well as on Access Medicine/Harrison's Online, and the eBook and "app" editions of HPIM 19e.

Cardiovascular disease (CVD) is now the most common cause of death worldwide. Before 1900, infectious diseases and malnutrition were the most common causes, and CVD was responsible for less than 10% of all deaths. In 2010, CVD accounted for approximately 16 million deaths worldwide (30%), including nearly 40% of deaths in high-income countries and about 28% in low- and middle-income countries.

SECTION 2 DIAGNOSIS OF CARDIOVASCULAR DISORDERS

267 Physical Examination of the Cardiovascular System

Patrick T. O'Gara, Joseph Loscalzo

The approach to a patient with known or suspected cardiovascular disease begins with the time-honored traditions of a directed history and a targeted physical examination. The scope of these activities depends on the clinical context at the time of presentation, ranging from an elective ambulatory follow-up visit to a more focused emergency department encounter. There has been a gradual decline in physical examination skills over the last two decades at every level, from student to faculty specialist, a development of great concern to both clinicians and medical educators. Classic cardiac findings are recognized by only a minority of internal medicine and family practice residents. Despite popular perceptions, clinical performance does not improve predictably as a function of experience; instead, the acquisition of new examination skills may become more difficult for a busy individual practitioner. Less time is now devoted to mentored cardiovascular examinations during the training of students and residents. One widely recognized outcome of these trends is the progressive overutilization of noninvasive imaging studies to establish the presence and severity of cardiovascular disease even when the examination findings imply a low pretest probability of significant pathology. Educational techniques to improve bedside skills include repetition, patient-centered teaching conferences, and visual display feedback of auscultatory events with Doppler echocardiographic imaging.

The evidence base that links the findings from the history and physical examination to the presence, severity, and prognosis of cardiovascular disease has been established most rigorously for coronary artery disease, heart failure, and valvular heart disease. For example, observations regarding heart rate, blood pressure, signs of pulmonary congestion, and the presence of mitral regurgitation (MR) contribute importantly to bedside risk assessment in patients with acute coronary syndromes. Observations from the physical examination in this setting can inform clinical decision making before the results of cardiac biomarkers testing are known. The prognosis of patients with systolic heart failure can be predicted on the basis of the jugular venous pressure (JVP) and the presence or absence of a third heart sound (S_3). Accurate characterization of cardiac murmurs provides important insight into the natural history of many valvular and congenital heart lesions. Finally, the important role played by the physical examination in enhancing the clinician-patient relationship cannot be overestimated.

THE GENERAL PHYSICAL EXAMINATION

Any examination begins with an assessment of the general appearance of the patient, with notation of age, posture, demeanor, and overall health status. Is the patient in pain or resting quietly, dyspneic or diaphoretic? Does the patient choose to avoid certain body positions to reduce or eliminate pain, as might be the case with suspected acute pericarditis? Are there clues indicating that dyspnea may have a pulmonary cause, such as a barrel chest deformity with an increased anterior-posterior diameter, tachypnea, and pursed-lip breathing? Skin pallor, cyanosis, and jaundice can be appreciated readily and provide additional clues. A chronically ill-appearing emaciated patient may suggest the presence of long-standing heart failure or another systemic disorder, such as a malignancy. Various genetic syndromes, often with cardiovascular involvement, can also be recognized easily, such as trisomy 21, Marfan's syndrome, and Holt-Oram syndrome. Height and weight should be measured routinely, and both body mass index and body surface area should be calculated. Knowledge of the waist circumference and the waist-to-hip ratio can be used to predict long-term cardiovascular risk. Mental status, level of alertness, and mood should be assessed continuously during the interview and examination.

Skin Central cyanosis occurs with significant right-to-left shunting at the level of the heart or lungs, allowing deoxygenated blood to reach the systemic circulation. Peripheral cyanosis or acrocyanosis, in contrast, is usually related to reduced extremity blood flow due to small vessel constriction, as seen in patients with severe heart failure, shock, or peripheral vascular disease; it can be aggravated by the use of β-adrenergic blockers with unopposed α-mediated constriction. Differential cyanosis refers to isolated cyanosis affecting the lower but not the upper extremities in a patient with a large patent ductus arteriosus (PDA) and secondary pulmonary hypertension with right-to-left to shunting at the great vessel level. Hereditary telangiectasias on the lips, tongue, and mucous membranes, as part of the Osler-Weber-Rendu syndrome (hereditary hemorrhagic telangiectasia), resemble spider nevi and can be a source of right-to-left shunting when also present in the lung. Malar telangiectasias also are seen in patients with advanced mitral stenosis and scleroderma. An unusually tan or bronze discoloration of the skin may suggest hemochromatosis as the cause of the associated systolic heart failure. Jaundice, which may be visible first in the sclerae, has a broad differential diagnosis but, in the appropriate setting, can be consistent with advanced right heart failure and congestive hepatomegaly or late-term "cardiac cirrhosis." Cutaneous ecchymoses are seen frequently among patients taking vitamin K antagonists or antiplatelet agents such as aspirin and thienopyridines. Various lipid disorders sometimes are associated with subcutaneous xanthomas, particularly along the tendon sheaths or over the extensor surfaces of the extremities. Severe hypertriglyceridemia can be associated with eruptive xanthomatosis and lipemia retinalis. Palmar crease xanthomas are specific for type III hyperlipoproteinemia. Pseudoxanthoma elasticum, a disease associated with premature atherosclerosis, is manifested by a leathery, cobblestoned appearance of the skin in the axilla and neck creases and by angioid streaks on funduscopic examination. Extensive lentiginoses have been described in a variety of development delay–cardiovascular syndromes, including Carney's syndrome, which includes multiple atrial myxomas. Cutaneous manifestations of sarcoidosis such as lupus pernio and erythema nodosum may suggest this disease as a cause of an associated dilated cardiomyopathy, especially with heart block, intraventricular conduction delay, or ventricular tachycardia.

Head and Neck Dentition and oral hygiene should be assessed in every patient both as a source of potential infection and as an index of general health. A high-arched palate is a feature of Marfan's syndrome and other connective tissue disease syndromes. Bifid uvula has been described in patients with Loeys-Dietz syndrome, and orange tonsils are characteristic of Tangier disease. The ocular manifestations of hyperthyroidism have been well described. Many patients with congenital heart disease have associated hypertelorism, low-set ears, or micrognathia. Blue sclerae are a feature of osteogenesis imperfecta. An arcus senilis pattern lacks specificity as an index of coronary heart disease risk. The funduscopic examination is an often underused method by which to assess the microvasculature, especially among patients with established atherosclerosis, hypertension, or diabetes mellitus. A mydriatic agent may be necessary for optimal visualization. A funduscopic examination should be performed routinely in the assessment of patients with suspected endocarditis and those with a history of acute visual change. Branch retinal artery occlusion or visualization of a Hollenhorst plaque can narrow the differential diagnosis rapidly in the appropriate setting. Relapsing polychondritis may manifest as an inflamed pinna or, in its later stages, as a saddle-nose deformity because of destruction of nasal cartilage; granulomatosis with polyangiitis (Wegener's) can also lead to a saddle-nose deformity.

Chest Midline sternotomy, left posterolateral thoracotomy, or infraclavicular scars at the site of pacemaker/defibrillator generator implantation should not be overlooked and may provide the first clue regarding an underlying cardiovascular disorder in patients unable to provide a relevant history. A prominent venous collateral pattern may suggest subclavian or vena caval obstruction. If the head and neck appear dusky and slightly cyanotic and the venous pressure is grossly elevated without visible pulsations, a diagnosis of superior vena cava syndrome should be entertained. Thoracic cage abnormalities have been well described among patients with connective tissue disease syndromes. They include pectus carinatum ("pigeon chest") and pectus excavatum ("funnel chest"). Obstructive lung disease is suggested by a barrel chest deformity, especially with tachypnea, pursed-lip breathing, and use of accessory muscles. The characteristically severe kyphosis and compensatory lumbar, pelvic, and knee flexion of ankylosing spondylitis should prompt careful auscultation for a murmur of aortic regurgitation (AR). Straight back syndrome refers to the loss of the normal kyphosis of the thoracic spine and has been described in patients with mitral valve prolapse (MVP) and its variants. In some patients with cyanotic congenital heart disease, the chest wall appears to be asymmetric, with anterior displacement of the left hemithorax. The respiratory rate and pattern should be noted during spontaneous breathing, with additional attention to depth, audible wheezing, and stridor. Lung examination can reveal adventitious sounds indicative of pulmonary edema, pneumonia, or pleuritis.

Abdomen In some patients with advanced obstructive lung disease, the point of maximal cardiac impulse may be in the epigastrium. The liver is frequently enlarged and tender in patients with chronic heart failure. Systolic pulsations over the liver signify severe tricuspid regurgitation (TR). Splenomegaly may be a feature of infective endocarditis, particularly when symptoms have persisted for weeks or months. Ascites is a nonspecific finding but may be present with advanced chronic right heart failure, constrictive pericarditis, hepatic cirrhosis, or an intraperitoneal malignancy. The finding of an elevated JVP implies a cardiovascular etiology. In nonobese patients, the aorta typically is palpated between the epigastrium and the umbilicus. The sensitivity of palpation for the detection of an abdominal aortic aneurysm (pulsatile and expansile mass) decreases as a function of body size. Because palpation alone is not sufficiently accurate to establish this diagnosis, a screening ultrasound examination is advised. The presence of an arterial bruit over the abdomen suggests high-grade atherosclerotic disease, although precise localization is difficult.

Extremities The temperature and color of the extremities, the presence of clubbing, arachnodactyly, and pertinent nail findings can be surmised quickly during the examination. Clubbing implies the presence of central right-to-left shunting, although it has also been described in patients with endocarditis. Its appearance can range from cyanosis and softening of the root of the nail bed, to the classic loss of the normal angle between the base of the nail and the skin, to the skeletal and periosteal bony changes of hypertrophic osteoarthropathy, which is seen rarely in patients with advanced lung or liver disease. Patients with the Holt-Oram syndrome have an unopposable, "fingerized" thumb, whereas patients with Marfan's syndrome may have arachnodactyly and a positive "wrist" (overlapping of the thumb and fifth finger around the wrist) or "thumb" (protrusion of the thumb beyond the ulnar aspect of the hand when the fingers are clenched over the thumb in a fist) sign. The Janeway lesions of endocarditis are nontender, slightly raised hemorrhages on the palms and soles, whereas Osler's nodes are tender, raised nodules on the pads of the fingers or toes. Splinter hemorrhages are classically identified as linear petechiae in the midposition of the nail bed and should be distinguished from the more common traumatic petechiae, which are seen closer to the distal edge.

Lower extremity or presacral edema in the setting of an elevated JVP defines volume overload and may be a feature of chronic heart failure or constrictive pericarditis. Lower extremity edema in the absence of jugular venous hypertension may be due to lymphatic or venous obstruction or, more commonly, to venous insufficiency, as further suggested by the appearance of varicosities, venous ulcers (typically medial in location), and brownish cutaneous discoloration from hemosiderin deposition (eburnation). Pitting edema can also be seen in patients who use dihydropyridine calcium channel blockers. A Homan's sign (posterior calf pain on active dorsiflexion of the foot against resistance) is neither specific nor sensitive for deep venous thrombosis. Muscular atrophy or the absence of hair along an extremity is consistent with severe arterial insufficiency or a primary neuromuscular disorder.

CARDIOVASCULAR EXAMINATION

Jugular Venous Pressure and Waveform JVP is the single most important bedside measurement from which to estimate the volume status. The internal jugular vein is preferred because the external jugular vein is valved and not directly in line with the superior vena cava and right atrium. Nevertheless, the external jugular vein has been used to discriminate between high and low central venous pressure (CVP) when tested among medical students, residents, and attending physicians. Precise estimation of the central venous or right atrial pressure from bedside assessment of the jugular venous waveform has proved difficult. Venous pressure traditionally has been measured as the vertical distance between the top of the jugular venous pulsation and the sternal inflection point (angle of Louis). A distance >4.5 cm at 30° elevation is considered abnormal. However, the actual distance between the mid-right atrium and the angle of Louis varies considerably as a function of both body size and the patient angle at which the assessment is made (30°, 45°, or 60°). The use of the sternal angle as a reference point leads to systematic underestimation of CVP, and this method should be used less for semiquantification than to distinguish a normal from an abnormally elevated CVP. The use of the clavicle may provide an easier reference for standardization. Venous pulsations above this level in the sitting position are clearly abnormal, as the distance between the clavicle and the right atrium is at least 10 cm. The patient should always be placed in the sitting position, with the legs dangling below the bedside, when an elevated pressure is suspected in the semisupine position. It should also be noted that bedside estimates of CVP are made in centimeters of water but must be converted to millimeters of mercury to provide correlation with accepted hemodynamic norms (1.36 cmH_2O = 1.0 mmHg).

The venous waveform sometimes can be difficult to distinguish from the carotid pulse, especially during casual inspection. Nevertheless, the venous waveform has several characteristic features, and its individual components can be appreciated in most patients (Fig. 267-1). The arterial pulsation is not easily obliterated with palpation; the venous waveform in patients with sinus rhythm is usually biphasic, while the carotid pulse is monophasic; and the jugular venous pulsation should change with changes in posture or inspiration (unless the venous pressure is quite elevated).

The venous waveform is divided into several distinct peaks. The *a* wave reflects right atrial presystolic contraction and occurs just after the electrocardiographic P wave, preceding the first heart sound (S_1). A prominent *a* wave is seen in patients with reduced right ventricular compliance; a cannon *a* wave occurs with atrioventricular (AV) dissociation and right atrial contraction against a closed tricuspid valve. In a patient with a wide complex tachycardia, the appreciation of cannon *a* waves in the jugular venous waveform identifies the rhythm as ventricular in origin. The *a* wave is not present with atrial fibrillation. The *x* descent defines the fall in right atrial pressure after inscription of the *a* wave. The *c* wave interrupts this *x* descent and is followed by a further descent. The *v* wave represents atrial filling (atrial diastole) and occurs during ventricular systole. The height of the *v* wave is determined by right atrial compliance as well as the volume of blood returning to the right atrium either antegrade from the cavae or retrograde through an incompetent tricuspid valve. In patients with TR, the *v* wave is accentuated and the subsequent fall in pressure (*y* descent) is rapid. With progressive degrees of TR, the *v* wave merges with the *c* wave, and the right atrial and jugular vein waveforms become "ventricularized." The *y* descent, which follows the peak of the *v* wave, can become prolonged or blunted with obstruction to right ventricular inflow, as may occur with tricuspid stenosis or pericardial tamponade. Normally, the venous pressure should fall by at least 3 mmHg with inspiration. Kussmaul's sign is defined by either a rise or a lack of fall of the JVP with inspiration and is classically associated with constrictive pericarditis, although it has been reported in patients with restrictive cardiomyopathy, massive pulmonary embolism, right ventricular infarction, and advanced left ventricular systolic heart failure. It is also a common, isolated finding in patients after cardiac surgery without other hemodynamic abnormalities.

Venous hypertension sometimes can be elicited by performance of the abdominojugular reflex or with passive leg elevation. When these signs are positive, a volume-overloaded state with limited compliance of an overly distended or constricted venous system is present. The abdominojugular reflex is elicited with firm and consistent pressure over the upper portion of the abdomen, preferably over the right upper quadrant, for at least 10 s. A positive response is defined by a sustained rise of more than 3 cm in JVP for at least 15 s after release of the hand. Patients must be coached to refrain from breath holding or a Valsalva-like maneuver during the procedure. The abdominojugular reflex is useful in predicting a pulmonary artery wedge pressure in excess of 15 mmHg in patients with heart failure.

Although the JVP estimates right ventricular filling pressure, it has a predictable relationship with the pulmonary artery wedge pressure. In a large study of patients with advanced heart failure, the presence of a right atrial pressure >10 mmHg (as predicted on bedside examination) had a positive value of 88% for the prediction of a pulmonary artery wedge pressure of >22 mmHg. In addition, an elevated JVP has prognostic significance in patients with both symptomatic heart failure and asymptomatic left ventricular systolic dysfunction. The presence of an elevated JVP is associated with a higher risk of subsequent hospitalization for heart failure, death from heart failure, or both.

Assessment of Blood Pressure Measurement of blood pressure usually is delegated to a medical assistant but should be repeated by the clinician. Accurate measurement depends on body position, arm size, time of measurement, place of measurement, device, device size, technique, and examiner. In general, physician-recorded blood pressures are higher than both nurse-recorded pressures and self-recorded pressures at home. Blood pressure is best measured in the seated position with

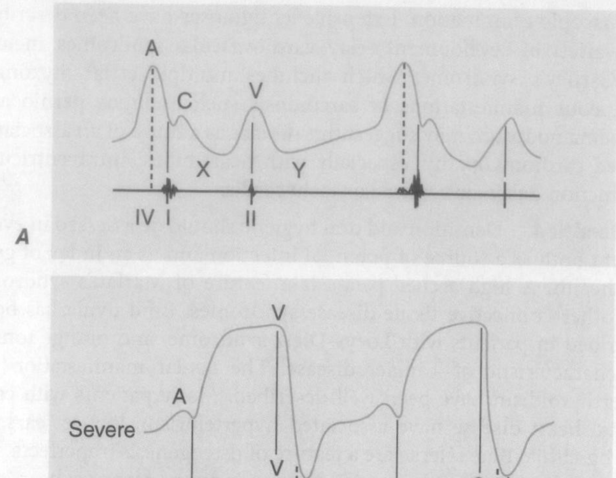

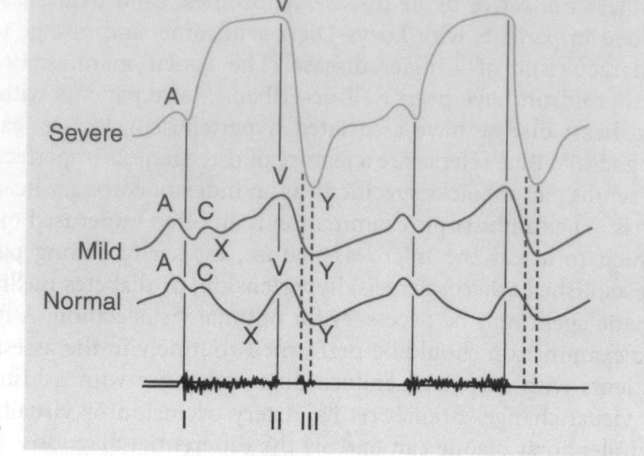

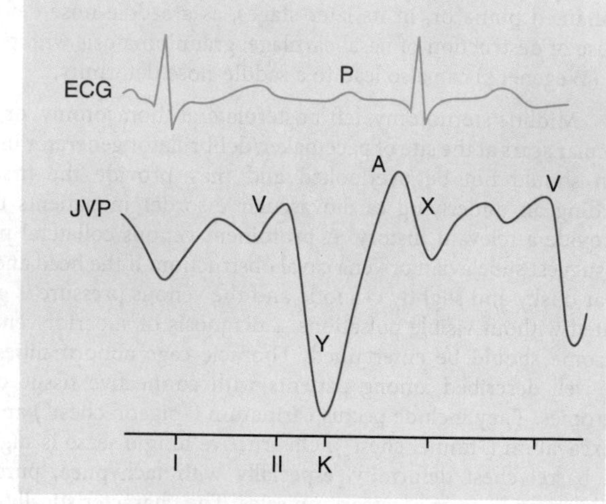

FIGURE 267-1 ***A.*** Jugular venous pulse wave tracing (*top*) with heart sounds (*bottom*). The A wave represents right atrial presystolic contraction and occurs just after the electrocardiographic P wave and just before the first heart sound (I). In this example, the A wave is accentuated and larger than normal due to decreased right ventricular compliance, as also suggested by the right-sided S_4 (IV). The C wave may reflect the carotid pulsation in the neck and/or an early systolic increase in right atrial pressure as the right ventricle pushes the closed tricuspid valve into the right atrium. The *x* descent follows the A wave just as atrial pressure continues to fall. The V wave represents atrial filling during ventricular systole and peaks at the second heart sound (II). The *y* descent corresponds to the fall in right atrial pressure after tricuspid valve opening. ***B.*** Jugular venous wave forms in mild (*middle*) and severe (*top*) tricuspid regurgitation, compared with normal, with phonocardiographic representation of the corresponding heart sounds below. With increasing degrees of tricuspid regurgitation, the waveform becomes "ventricularized." ***C.*** Electrocardiogram (ECG) (*top*), jugular venous waveform (JVP) (*middle*), and heart sounds (*bottom*) in pericardial constriction. Note the prominent and rapid *y* descent, corresponding in timing to the pericardial knock (K). *(From J Abrams: Synopsis of Cardiac Physical Diagnosis, 2nd ed. Boston, Butterworth Heinemann, 2001, pp 25–35.)*

the arm at the level of the heart, using an appropriately sized cuff, after 5–10 min of relaxation. When it is measured in the supine position, the arm should be raised to bring it to the level of the mid-right atrium. The length and width of the blood pressure cuff bladder should be 80% and 40% of the arm's circumference, respectively. A common source of error in practice is to use an inappropriately small cuff, resulting in marked overestimation of true blood pressure, or an inappropriately large cuff, resulting in underestimation of true blood pressure. The cuff should be inflated to 30 mmHg above the expected systolic pressure and the pressure released at a rate of 2–3 mmHg/s. Systolic and diastolic pressures are defined by the first and fifth Korotkoff sounds, respectively. Very low (even 0 mmHg) diastolic blood pressures may be recorded in patients with chronic, severe AR or a large arteriovenous fistula because of enhanced diastolic "run-off." In these instances, both the phase IV and phase V Korotkoff sounds should be recorded. Blood pressure is best assessed at the brachial artery level, though it can be measured at the radial, popliteal, or pedal pulse level. In general, systolic pressure increases and diastolic pressure decreases when measured in more distal arteries. Blood pressure should be measured in both arms, and the difference should be less than 10 mmHg. A blood pressure differential that exceeds this threshold may be associated with atherosclerotic or inflammatory subclavian artery disease, supravalvular aortic stenosis, aortic coarctation, or aortic dissection. Systolic leg pressures are usually as much as 20 mmHg higher than systolic arm pressures. Greater leg–arm pressure differences are seen in patients with chronic severe AR as well as patients with extensive and calcified lower extremity peripheral arterial disease. The ankle-brachial index (lower pressure in the dorsalis pedis or posterior tibial artery divided by the higher of the two brachial artery pressures) is a powerful predictor of long-term cardiovascular mortality.

The blood pressure measured in an office or hospital setting may not accurately reflect the pressure in other venues. "White coat hypertension" is defined by at least three separate clinic-based measurements >140/90 mmHg and at least two non-clinic-based measurements <140/90 mmHg in the absence of any evidence of target organ damage. Individuals with white coat hypertension may not benefit from drug therapy, although they may be more likely to develop sustained hypertension over time. Masked hypertension should be suspected when normal or even low blood pressures are recorded in patients with advanced atherosclerotic disease, especially when evidence of target organ damage is present or bruits are audible.

Orthostatic hypotension is defined by a fall in systolic pressure >20 mmHg or in diastolic pressure >10 mmHg in response to assumption of the upright posture from a supine position within 3 min. There may also be a lack of a compensatory tachycardia, an abnormal response that suggests autonomic insufficiency, as may be seen in patients with diabetes or Parkinson's disease. Orthostatic hypotension is a common cause of postural lightheadedness/syncope and should be assessed routinely in patients for whom this diagnosis might pertain. It can be exacerbated by advanced age, dehydration, certain medications, food, deconditioning, and ambient temperature.

Arterial Pulse The carotid artery pulse occurs just after the ascending aortic pulse. The aortic pulse is best appreciated in the epigastrium, just above the level of the umbilicus. Peripheral arterial pulses that should be assessed routinely include the subclavian, brachial, radial, ulnar, femoral, popliteal, dorsalis pedis, and posterior tibial. In patients in whom the diagnosis of either temporal arteritis or polymyalgia rheumatica is suspected, the temporal arteries also should be examined. Although one of the two pedal pulses may not be palpable in up to 10% of normal subjects, the pair should be symmetric. The integrity of the arcuate system of the hand is assessed by Allen's test, which is performed routinely before instrumentation of the radial artery. The pulses should be examined for their symmetry, volume, timing, contour, amplitude, and duration. If necessary, simultaneous auscultation of the heart can help identify a delay in the arrival of an arterial pulse. Simultaneous palpation of the radial and femoral pulses may reveal a femoral delay in a patient with hypertension and suspected aortic coarctation. The carotid upstrokes should never be examined simultaneously or before listening for a bruit. Light pressure should always be used to avoid precipitation of carotid hypersensitivity syndrome and syncope in a susceptible elderly individual. The arterial pulse usually becomes more rapid and spiking as a function of its distance from the heart, a phenomenon that reflects the muscular status of the more peripheral arteries and the summation of the incident and reflected waves. In general, the character and contour of the arterial pulse depend on the stroke volume, ejection velocity, vascular compliance, and systemic vascular resistance. The pulse examination can be misleading in patients with reduced cardiac output and in those with stiffened arteries from aging, chronic hypertension, or peripheral arterial disease.

The character of the pulse is best appreciated at the carotid level (Fig. 267-2). A weak and delayed pulse (*pulsus parvus et tardus*) defines severe aortic stenosis (AS). Some patients with AS may also have a slow, notched, or interrupted upstroke (anacrotic pulse) with a thrill or shudder. With chronic severe AR, by contrast, the carotid upstroke has a sharp rise and rapid fall-off (Corrigan's or water-hammer pulse). Some patients with advanced AR may have a bifid or bisferiens pulse, in which two systolic peaks can be appreciated. A bifid pulse is also described in patients with hypertrophic obstructive cardiomyopathy (HOCM), with inscription of percussion and tidal waves. A bifid pulse is easily appreciated in patients on intraaortic balloon counterpulsation (IABP), in whom the second pulse is diastolic in timing.

Pulsus paradoxus refers to a fall in systolic pressure >10 mmHg with inspiration that is seen in patients with pericardial tamponade but also is described in those with massive pulmonary embolism, hemorrhagic shock, severe obstructive lung disease, and tension pneumothorax.

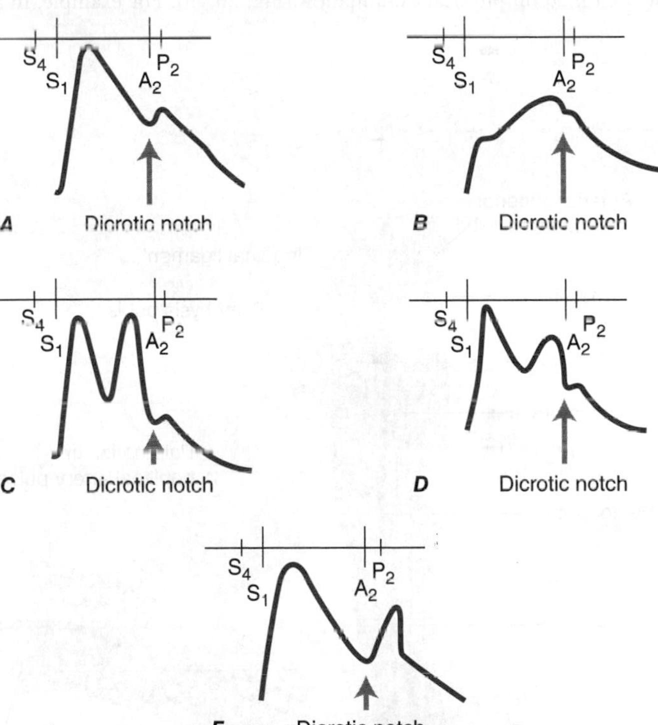

FIGURE 267-2 Schematic diagrams of the configurational changes in carotid pulse and their differential diagnoses. Heart sounds are also illustrated. ***A.*** Normal. S_4, fourth heart sound; S_1, first heart sound; A_2 aortic component of second heart sound; P_2 pulmonic component of second heart sound. ***B.*** Aortic stenosis. Anacrotic pulse with slow upstroke to a reduced peak. ***C.*** Bisferiens pulse with two peaks in systole. This pulse is rarely appreciated in patients with severe aortic regurgitation. ***D.*** Bisferiens pulse in hypertrophic obstructive cardiomyopathy. There is a rapid upstroke to the first peak (percussion wave) and a slower rise to the second peak (tidal wave). ***E.*** Dicrotic pulse with peaks in systole and diastole. This waveform may be seen in patients with sepsis or during intraaortic balloon counterpulsation with inflation just after the dicrotic notch. *(From K Chatterjee, W Parmley [eds]: Cardiology: An Illustrated Text/Reference. Philadelphia, Gower Medical Publishers, 1991.)*

 Pulsus paradoxus is measured by noting the difference between the systolic pressure at which the Korotkoff sounds are first heard (during expiration) and the systolic pressure at which the Korotkoff sounds are heard with each heartbeat, independent of the respiratory phase. Between these two pressures, the Korotkoff sounds are heard only intermittently and during expiration. The cuff pressure must be decreased slowly to appreciate the finding. It can be difficult to measure pulsus paradoxus in patients with tachycardia, atrial fibrillation, or tachypnea. A pulsus paradoxus may be palpable at the brachial artery or femoral artery level when the pressure difference exceeds 15 mmHg. This inspiratory fall in systolic pressure is an exaggerated consequence of interventricular dependence.

Pulsus alternans, in contrast, is defined by beat-to-beat variability of pulse amplitude. It is present only when every other phase I Korotkoff sound is audible as the cuff pressure is lowered slowly, typically in a patient with a regular heart rhythm and independent of the respiratory cycle. Pulsus alternans is seen in patients with severe left ventricular systolic dysfunction and is thought to be due to cyclic changes in intracellular calcium and action potential duration. When pulsus alternans is associated with electrocardiographic T-wave alternans, the risk for an arrhythmic event appears to be increased.

Ascending aortic aneurysms can rarely be appreciated as a pulsatile mass in the right parasternal area. Appreciation of a prominent abdominal aortic pulse should prompt noninvasive imaging for better characterization. Femoral and/or popliteal artery aneurysms should be sought in patients with abdominal aortic aneurysm disease.

The level of a claudication-producing arterial obstruction can often be identified on physical examination (Fig. 267-3). For example, in a patient with calf claudication, a decrease in pulse amplitude between the common femoral and popliteal arteries will localize the obstruction to the level of the superficial femoral artery, although inflow obstruction above the level of the common femoral artery may coexist. Auscultation for carotid, subclavian, abdominal aortic, and femoral artery bruits should be routine. However, the correlation between the presence of a bruit and the degree of vascular obstruction is poor. A cervical bruit is a weak indicator of the degree of carotid artery stenosis; the absence of a bruit does not exclude the presence of significant luminal obstruction. If a bruit extends into diastole or if a thrill is present, the obstruction is usually severe. Another cause of an arterial bruit is an arteriovenous fistula with enhanced flow.

The likelihood of significant lower extremity peripheral arterial disease increases with typical symptoms of claudication, cool skin, abnormalities on pulse examination, or the presence of a vascular bruit. Abnormal pulse oximetry (a >2% difference between finger and toe oxygen saturation) can be used to detect lower extremity peripheral arterial disease and is comparable in its performance characteristics to the ankle-brachial index.

Inspection and Palpation of the Heart The left ventricular apex beat may be visible in the midclavicular line at the fifth intercostal space in thin-chested adults. Visible pulsations anywhere other than this expected location are abnormal. The left anterior chest wall may heave in patients with an enlarged or hyperdynamic left or right ventricle. As noted previously, a visible right upper parasternal pulsation may be suggestive of ascending aortic aneurysm disease. In thin, tall patients and patients with advanced obstructive lung disease and flattened

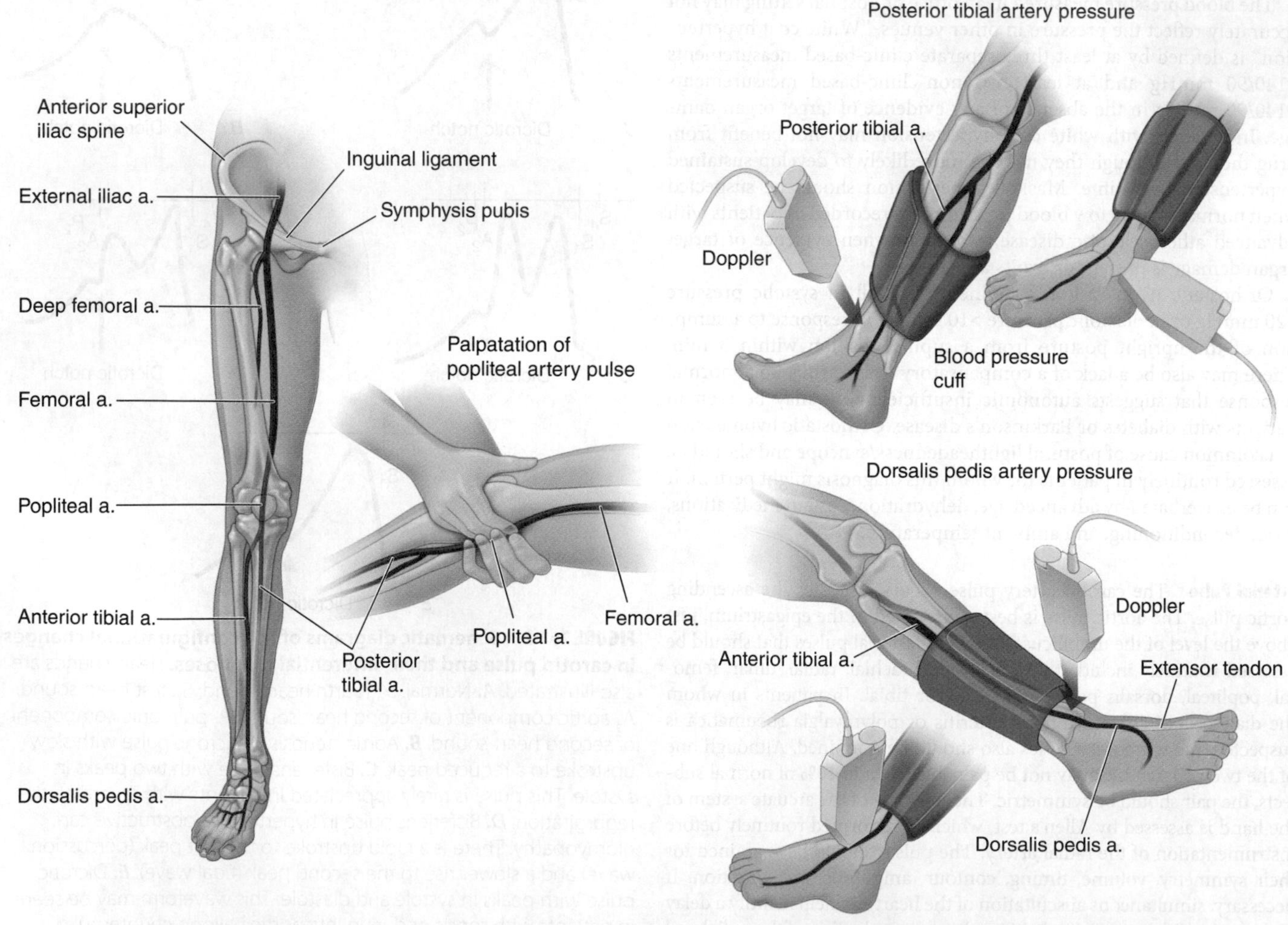

FIGURE 267-3 ***A.*** Anatomy of the major arteries of the leg. ***B.*** Measurement of the ankle systolic pressure. *(From NA Khan et al: JAMA 295:536, 2006.)*

diaphragms, the cardiac impulse may be visible in the epigastrium and should be distinguished from a pulsatile liver edge.

Palpation of the heart begins with the patient in the supine position at 30° and can be enhanced by placing the patient in the left lateral decubitus position. The normal left ventricular impulse is less than 2 cm in diameter and moves quickly away from the fingers; it is better appreciated at end expiration, with the heart closer to the anterior chest wall. Characteristics such as size, amplitude, and rate of force development should be noted.

Enlargement of the left ventricular cavity is manifested by a leftward and downward displacement of an enlarged apex beat. A sustained apex beat is a sign of pressure overload, such as that which may be present in patients with AS or chronic hypertension. A palpable presystolic impulse corresponds to the fourth heart sound (S_4) and is indicative of reduced left ventricular compliance and the forceful contribution of atrial contraction to ventricular filling. A palpable third sound (S_3), which is indicative of a rapid early filling wave in patients with heart failure, may be present even when the gallop itself is not audible. A large left ventricular aneurysm may sometimes be palpable as an ectopic impulse, discrete from the apex beat. HOCM may very rarely cause a triple cadence beat at the apex with contributions from a palpable S_4 and the two components of the bisferiens systolic pulse.

Right ventricular pressure or volume overload may create a sternal lift. Signs of either TR (*cv* waves in the jugular venous pulse) and/or pulmonary arterial hypertension (a loud single or palpable P_2) would be confirmatory. The right ventricle can enlarge to the extent that left-sided events cannot be appreciated. A zone of retraction between the right and left ventricular impulses sometimes can be appreciated in patients with right ventricle pressure or volume overload when they are placed in the left lateral decubitus position. Systolic and diastolic thrills signify turbulent and high-velocity blood flow. Their locations help identify the origin of heart murmurs.

CARDIAC AUSCULTATION

Heart Sounds Ventricular systole is defined by the interval between the first (S_1) and second (S_2) heart sounds (Fig. 267-4). The first heart sound (S_1) includes mitral and tricuspid valve closure. Normal splitting can be appreciated in young patients and those with right bundle branch block, in whom tricuspid valve closure is relatively delayed. The intensity of S_1 is determined by the distance over which the anterior leaflet of the mitral valve must travel to return to its annular plane, leaflet mobility, left ventricular contractility, and the PR interval. S_1 is classically loud in the early phases of rheumatic mitral stenosis (MS) and in patients with hyperkinetic circulatory states or short PR intervals. S_1 becomes softer in the later stages of MS when the leaflets are rigid and calcified, after exposure to β-adrenergic receptor blockers, with long PR intervals, and with left ventricular contractile dysfunction. The intensity of heart sounds, however, can be reduced by any process that increases the distance between the stethoscope and the responsible cardiac event, including mechanical ventilation, obstructive lung disease, obesity, pneumothorax, and a pericardial effusion.

Aortic and pulmonic valve closure constitutes the second heart sound (S_2). With normal or physiologic splitting, the A_2–P_2 interval increases with inspiration and narrows during expiration. This physiologic interval will widen with right bundle branch block because of the further delay in pulmonic valve closure and in patients with severe MR because of the premature closure of the aortic valve. An unusually narrowly split or even a singular S_2 is a feature of pulmonary arterial hypertension. Fixed splitting of S_2, in which the A_2–P_2 interval is wide and does not change during the respiratory cycle, occurs in patients with a secundum atrial septal defect. Reversed or paradoxical splitting refers to a pathologic delay in aortic valve closure, such as that which occurs in patients with left bundle branch block, right ventricular pacing, severe AS, HOCM, and acute myocardial ischemia. With reversed or paradoxical splitting, the individual components of S_2 are audible at end expiration, and their interval narrows with inspiration, the opposite of what would be expected under normal physiologic conditions. P_2 is considered loud when its intensity exceeds that of A_2 at the base, when it can be palpated in the area of the proximal main pulmonary

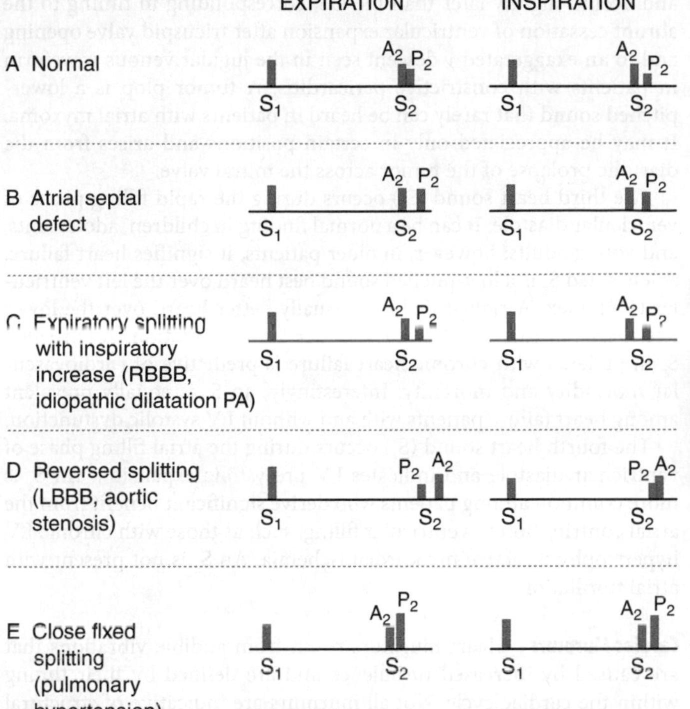

FIGURE 267-4 Heart sounds. ***A.*** Normal. S_1, first heart sound; S_2, second heart sound; A_2, aortic component of the second heart sound; P_2, pulmonic component of the second heart sound. ***B.*** Atrial septal defect with fixed splitting of S_2. ***C.*** Physiologic but wide splitting of S_2 with right bundle branch block (RBBB). PA, pulmonary artery. ***D.*** Reversed or paradoxical splitting of S_2 with left bundle branch block (LBBB). ***E.*** Narrow splitting of S_2 with pulmonary hypertension. *(From NO Fowler: Diagnosis of Heart Disease. New York, Springer-Verlag, 1991, p 31.)*

artery (second left interspace), or when both components of S_2 can be appreciated at the lower left sternal border or apex. The intensity of A_2 and P_2 decreases with aortic and pulmonic stenosis, respectively. In these conditions, a single S_2 may result.

Systolic Sounds An ejection sound is a high-pitched early systolic sound that corresponds in timing to the upstroke of the carotid pulse. It usually is associated with congenital bicuspid aortic or pulmonic valve disease; however, ejection sounds are also sometimes audible in patients with isolated aortic or pulmonary root dilation and normal semilunar valves. The ejection sound that accompanies bicuspid aortic valve disease becomes softer and then inaudible as the valve calcifies and becomes more rigid. The ejection sound that accompanies pulmonic stenosis (PS) moves closer to the first heart sound as the severity of the stenosis increases. In addition, the pulmonic ejection sound is the only right-sided acoustic event that decreases in intensity with inspiration. Ejection sounds are often heard more easily at the lower left sternal border than they are at the base. Nonejection sounds (clicks), which occur after the onset of the carotid upstroke, are related to MVP and may be single or multiple. The nonejection click may introduce a murmur. This click-murmur complex will move away from the first heart sound with maneuvers that increase ventricular preload, such as squatting. On standing, the click and murmur move closer to S_1.

Diastolic Sounds The high-pitched opening snap (OS) of MS occurs after a very short interval after the second heart sound. The A_2–OS interval is inversely proportional to the height of the left atrial–left ventricular diastolic pressure gradient. The intensity of both S_1 and the OS of MS decreases with progressive calcification and rigidity of the anterior mitral leaflets. The pericardial knock (PK) is also high-pitched and occurs slightly later than the OS, corresponding in timing to the abrupt cessation of ventricular expansion after tricuspid valve opening and to an exaggerated *y* descent seen in the jugular venous waveform in patients with constrictive pericarditis. A tumor plop is a lower-pitched sound that rarely can be heard in patients with atrial myxoma. It may be appreciated only in certain positions and arises from the diastolic prolapse of the tumor across the mitral valve.

The third heart sound (S_3) occurs during the rapid filling phase of ventricular diastole. It can be a normal finding in children, adolescents, and young adults; however, in older patients, it signifies heart failure. A left-sided S_3 is a low-pitched sound best heard over the left ventricular (LV) apex. A right-sided S_3 is usually better heard over the lower left sternal border and becomes louder with inspiration. A left-sided S_3 in patients with chronic heart failure is predictive of cardiovascular morbidity and mortality. Interestingly, an S_3 is equally prevalent among heart failure patients with and without LV systolic dysfunction.

The fourth heart sound (S_4) occurs during the atrial filling phase of ventricular diastole and indicates LV presystolic expansion. An S_4 is more common among patients who derive significant benefit from the atrial contribution to ventricular filling, such as those with chronic LV hypertrophy or active myocardial ischemia. An S_4 is not present with atrial fibrillation.

Cardiac Murmurs Heart murmurs result from audible vibrations that are caused by increased turbulence and are defined by their timing within the cardiac cycle. Not all murmurs are indicative of structural heart disease, and the accurate identification of a benign or functional systolic murmur often can obviate the need for additional testing in healthy subjects. The duration, frequency, configuration, and intensity of a heart murmur are dictated by the magnitude, variability, and duration of the responsible pressure difference between two cardiac chambers, the two ventricles, or the ventricles and their respective great arteries. The intensity of a heart murmur is graded on a scale of 1 to 6; a thrill is present with murmurs of grade 4 or greater intensity. Other attributes of the murmur that aid in its accurate identification include its location, radiation, and response to bedside maneuvers. Although clinicians can detect and correctly identify heart murmurs with only fair reliability, a careful and complete bedside examination usually can identify individuals with valvular heart disease for whom transthoracic echocardiography and clinical follow-up are indicated and exclude subjects for whom no further evaluation is necessary.

Systolic murmurs can be early, mid, late, or holosystolic in timing (Fig. 267-5). Acute severe MR results in a decrescendo early systolic murmur, the characteristics of which are related to the progressive attenuation of the left ventricular to left atrial pressure gradient during systole because of the steep and rapid rise in left atrial pressure in this context. Severe MR associated with posterior leaflet prolapse or flail radiates anteriorly and to the base, where it can be confused with the murmur of AS. MR that is due to anterior leaflet involvement radiates posteriorly and to the axilla. With acute TR in patients with normal pulmonary artery pressures, an early systolic murmur that may increase in intensity with inspiration may be heard at the left lower sternal border, with regurgitant *cv* waves visible in the jugular venous pulse.

A midsystolic murmur begins after S_1 and ends before S_2; it is typically crescendo-decrescendo in configuration. AS is the most common cause of a midsystolic murmur in an adult. It is often difficult to estimate the severity of the valve lesion on the basis of the physical examination findings, especially in older hypertensive patients with stiffened carotid arteries or patients with low cardiac output in whom the intensity of the systolic heart murmur is misleadingly soft. Examination findings consistent with severe AS would include *parvus et tardus* carotid upstrokes, a late-peaking grade 3 or greater midsystolic murmur, a soft A_2, a sustained LV apical impulse, and an S_4. It is sometimes difficult to distinguish aortic sclerosis from more advanced degrees of valve stenosis. The former is defined by focal thickening and calcification of the aortic valve leaflets that is not severe enough to result in obstruction. These valve changes are associated with a Doppler jet velocity across the aortic valve of 2.5 m/s or less. Patients

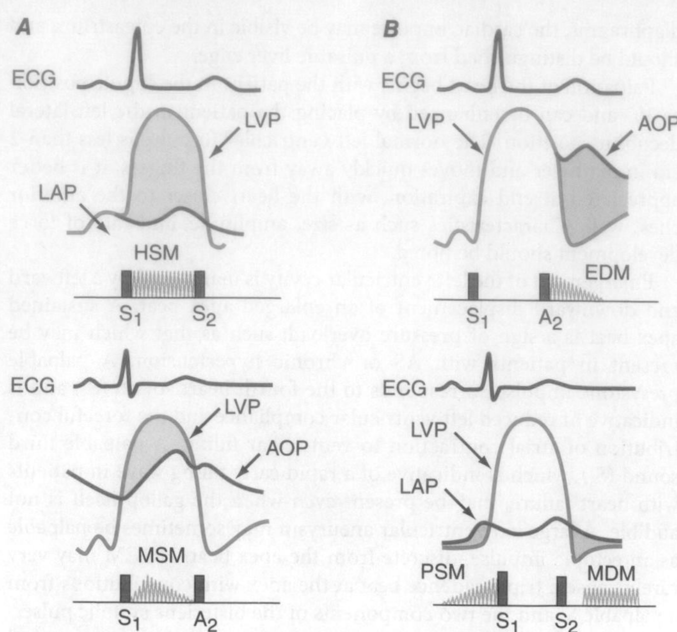

FIGURE 267-5 ***A. Top.*** Graphic representation of the systolic pressure difference (green shaded area) between left ventricle and left atrium with phonocardiographic recording of a holosystolic murmur (HSM) indicative of mitral regurgitation. ECG, electrocardiogram; LAP, left atrial pressure; LVP, left ventricular pressure; S_1, first heart sound; S_2 second heart sound. ***Bottom.*** Graphic representation of the systolic pressure gradient (green shaded area) between left ventricle and aorta in patient with aortic stenosis. A midsystolic murmur (MSM) with a crescendo-decrescendo configuration is recorded. AOP, aortic pressure. ***B. Top.*** Graphic representation of the diastolic pressure difference between the aorta and left ventricle (blue shaded area) in a patient with aortic regurgitation, resulting in a decrescendo, early diastolic murmur (EDM) beginning with A_2. ***Bottom.*** Graphic representation of the diastolic left atrial–left ventricular gradient (blue areas) in a patient with mitral stenosis with a mid-diastolic murmur (MDM) and late presystolic murmurs (PSM).

with aortic sclerosis can have grade 2 or 3 midsystolic murmurs identical in their acoustic characteristics to the murmurs heard in patients with more advanced degrees of AS. Other causes of a midsystolic heart murmur include pulmonic valve stenosis (with or without an ejection sound), HOCM, increased pulmonary blood flow in patients with a large atrial septal defect and left-to-right shunting, and several states associated with accelerated blood flow in the absence of structural heart disease, such as fever, thyrotoxicosis, pregnancy, anemia, and normal childhood/adolescence.

The murmur of HOCM has features of both obstruction to LV outflow and MR, as would be expected from knowledge of the pathophysiology of this condition. The systolic murmur of HOCM usually can be distinguished from other causes on the basis of its response to bedside maneuvers, including Valsalva, passive leg raising, and standing/squatting. In general, maneuvers that decrease LV preload (or increase LV contractility) will cause the murmur to intensify, whereas maneuvers that increase LV preload or afterload will cause a decrease in the intensity of the murmur. Accordingly, the systolic murmur of HOCM becomes louder during the strain phase of the Valsalva maneuver and after standing quickly from a squatting position. The murmur becomes softer with passive leg raising and when squatting. The murmur of AS is typically loudest in the second right interspace with radiation into the carotids, whereas the murmur of HOCM is best heard between the lower left sternal border and the apex. The murmur of PS is best heard in the second left interspace. The midsystolic murmur associated with enhanced pulmonic blood flow in the setting of a large atrial septal defect (ASD) is usually loudest at the mid-left sternal border.

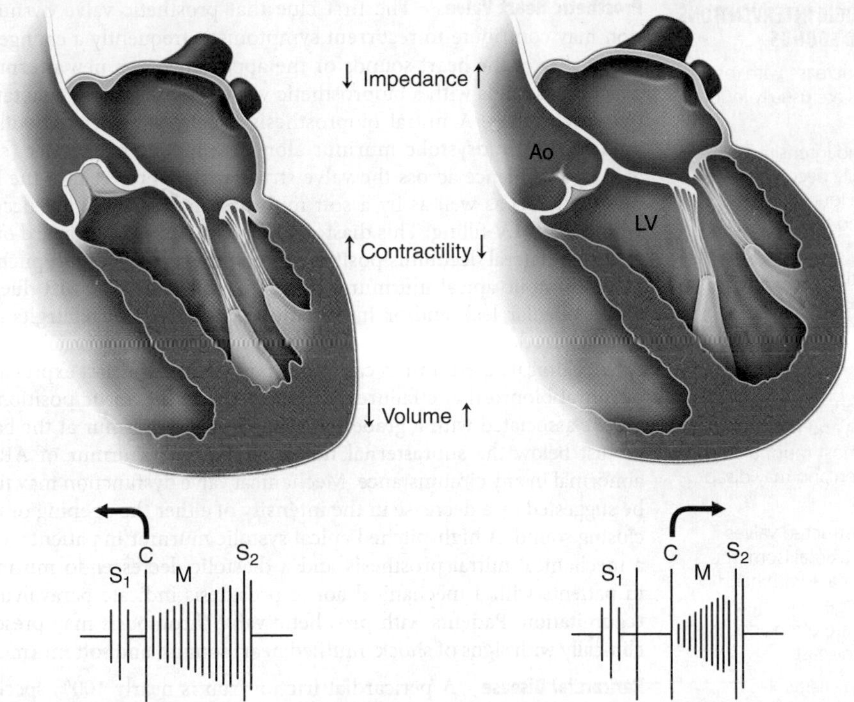

FIGURE 267-6 Behavior of the click (C) and murmur (M) of mitral valve prolapse with changes in loading (volume, impedance) and contractility. S_1, first heart sound; S_2, second heart sound. With standing (left side of figure), volume and impedance decrease, as a result of which the click and murmur move closer to S_1. With squatting (right), the click and murmur move away from S_1 due to the increases in left ventricular volume and impedance (afterload). Ao, aorta; LV, left ventricle. *(Adapted from RA O'Rourke, MH Crawford: Curr Prob Cardiol 1:9, 1976.)*

A late systolic murmur, heard best at the apex, indicates MVP. As previously noted, the murmur may or may not be introduced by a nonejection click. Differential radiation of the murmur, as previously described, may help identify the specific leaflet involved by the myxomatous process. The click-murmur complex behaves in a manner directionally similar to that demonstrated by the murmur of HOCM during the Valsalva and stand/squat maneuvers (Fig. 267-6). The murmur of MVP can be identified by the accompanying nonejection click.

Holosystolic murmurs are plateau in configuration and reflect a continuous and wide pressure gradient between the left ventricle and left atrium with chronic MR, the left ventricle and right ventricle with a ventricular septal defect (VSD), and the right ventricle and right atrium with TR. In contrast to acute MR, in chronic MR the left atrium is enlarged and its compliance is normal or increased to the extent that there is little if any further increase in left atrial pressure from any increase in regurgitant volume. The murmur of MR is best heard over the cardiac apex. The intensity of the murmur increases with maneuvers that increase LV afterload, such as sustained hand grip. The murmur of a VSD (without significant pulmonary hypertension) is holosystolic and loudest at the mid-left sternal border, where a thrill is usually present. The murmur of TR is loudest at the lower left sternal border, increases in intensity with inspiration (Carvallo's sign), and is accompanied by visible *cv* waves in the jugular venous wave form and, on occasion, by pulsatile hepatomegaly.

Diastolic Murmurs In contrast to some systolic murmurs, diastolic heart murmurs always signify structural heart disease (Fig. 267-5). The murmur associated with acute, severe AR is relatively soft and of short duration because of the rapid rise in LV diastolic pressure and the progressive diminution of the aortic-LV diastolic pressure gradient. In contrast, the murmur of chronic severe AR is classically heard as a decrescendo, blowing diastolic murmur along the left sternal border in patients with primary valve pathology and sometimes along the right sternal border in patients with primary aortic root pathology. With chronic AR, the pulse pressure is wide and the arterial pulses are bounding in character. These signs of significant diastolic run-off are absent in the acute phase. The murmur of pulmonic regurgitation is also heard along the left sternal border. It is most commonly due to pulmonary hypertension and enlargement of the annulus of the pulmonic valve. S_2 is single and loud and may be palpable. There is a right ventricular/parasternal lift that is indicative of chronic right ventricular pressure overload. A less impressive murmur of PR is present after repair of tetralogy of Fallot or pulmonic valve atresia. In this postoperative setting, the murmur is softer and lower-pitched, and the severity of the accompanying pulmonic regurgitation can be underestimated significantly.

MS is the classic cause of a mid- to late diastolic murmur, which is best heard over the apex in the left lateral decubitus position, is low-pitched or rumbling, and is introduced by an OS in the early stages of the rheumatic disease process. Presystolic accentuation refers to an increase in the intensity of the murmur just before the first heart sound and occurs in patients with sinus rhythm. It is absent in patients with atrial fibrillation. The auscultatory findings in patients with rheumatic tricuspid stenosis typically are obscured by left-sided events, although they are similar in nature to those described in patients with MS. "Functional" mitral or tricuspid stenosis refers to the generation of mid-diastolic murmurs that are created by increased and accelerated transvalvular diastolic flow, even in the absence of valvular obstruction, in the setting of severe MR, severe TR, or a large ASD with left-to-right shunting. The Austin Flint murmur of chronic severe AR is a low-pitched mid- to late apical diastolic murmur that sometimes can be confused with MS. The Austin Flint murmur typically decreases in intensity after exposure to vasodilators, whereas the murmur of MS may be accompanied by an opening snap and also may increase in intensity after vasodilators because of the associated increase in cardiac output. Unusual causes of a mid-diastolic murmur include atrial myxoma, complete heart block, and acute rheumatic mitral valvulitis.

Continuous Murmur A continuous murmur is predicated on a pressure gradient that persists between two cardiac chambers or blood vessels across systole and diastole. The murmurs typically begin in systole, envelop the second heart sound (S_2), and continue through some portion of diastole. They can often be difficult to distinguish from individual systolic and diastolic murmurs in patients with mixed valvular heart disease. The classic example of a continuous murmur is that associated with a PDA, which usually is heard in the second or third interspace at a slight distance from the sternal border. Other causes of a continuous murmur include a ruptured sinus of Valsalva aneurysm with creation of an aortic–right atrial or right ventricular fistula, a coronary or great vessel arteriovenous fistula, and an arteriovenous fistula constructed to provide dialysis access. There are two types of benign continuous murmurs. The cervical venous hum is heard in children or adolescents in the supraclavicular fossa. It can be obliterated with firm pressure applied to the diaphragm of the stethoscope, especially when the subject turns his or her head toward the examiner. The mammary soufflé of pregnancy relates to enhanced arterial blood flow through engorged breasts. The diastolic component of the murmur can be obliterated with firm pressure over the stethoscope.

Dynamic Auscultation Diagnostic accuracy can be enhanced by the performance of simple bedside maneuvers to identify heart murmurs and characterize their significance (Table 267-1). Except for the pulmonic

TABLE 267-1 EFFECTS OF PHYSIOLOGIC AND PHARMACOLOGIC INTERVENTIONS ON THE INTENSITY OF HEART MURMURS AND SOUNDS

Respiration Right-sided murmurs and sounds generally increase with inspiration, except for the PES. Left-sided murmurs and sounds are usually louder during expiration.

Valsalva maneuver Most murmurs decrease in length and intensity. Two exceptions are the systolic murmur of HOCM, which usually becomes much louder, and that of MVP, which becomes longer and often louder. After release of the Valsalva maneuver, right-sided murmurs tend to return to control intensity earlier than do left-sided murmurs.

After VPB or AF Murmurs originating at normal or stenotic semilunar valves increase in the cardiac cycle after a VPB or in the cycle after a long cycle length in AF. By contrast, systolic murmurs due to AV valve regurgitation do not change, diminish (papillary muscle dysfunction), or become shorter (MVP).

Positional changes With *standing*, most murmurs diminish, with two exceptions being the murmur of HOCM, which becomes louder, and that of MVP, which lengthens and often is intensified. With *squatting*, most murmurs become louder, but those of HOCM and MVP usually soften and may disappear. Passive leg raising usually produces the same results.

Exercise Murmurs due to blood flow across normal or obstructed valves (e.g., PS, MS) become louder with both isotonic and submaximal isometric (hand grip) exercise. Murmurs of MR, VSD, and AR also increase with hand grip exercise. However, the murmur of HOCM often decreases with nearly maximum hand grip exercise. Left-sided S_4 and S_3 sounds are often accentuated by exercise, particularly when due to ischemic heart disease.

Abbreviations: AF, atrial fibrillation; AR, aortic regurgitation; HOCM, hypertrophic obstructive cardiomyopathy; MR, mitral regurgitation; MS, mitral stenosis; MVP, mitral valve prolapse; PES, pulmonic ejection sound; PR, pulmonic regurgitation; PS, pulmonic stenosis; TR, tricuspid regurgitation; TS, tricuspid stenosis; VPB, ventricular premature beat; VSD, ventricular septal defect.

ejection sound, right-sided events increase in intensity with inspiration and decrease with expiration; left-sided events behave oppositely (100% sensitivity, 88% specificity). As previously noted, the intensity of the murmurs associated with MR, VSD, and AR will increase in response to maneuvers that increase LV afterload, such as hand grip and vasopressors. The intensity of these murmurs will decrease after exposure to vasodilating agents. Squatting is associated with an abrupt increase in LV preload and afterload, whereas rapid standing results in a sudden decrease in preload. In patients with MVP, the click and murmur move away from the first heart sound with squatting because of the delay in onset of leaflet prolapse at higher ventricular volumes. With rapid standing, however, the click and murmur move closer to the first heart sound as prolapse occurs earlier in systole at a smaller chamber dimension. The murmur of HOCM behaves similarly, becoming softer and shorter with squatting (95% sensitivity, 85% specificity) and longer and louder on rapid standing (95% sensitivity, 84% specificity). A change in the intensity of a systolic murmur in the first beat after a premature beat or in the beat after a long cycle length in patients with atrial fibrillation suggests valvular AS rather than MR, particularly in an older patient in whom the murmur of the AS may be well transmitted to the apex (Gallavardin effect). Of note, however, the systolic murmur of HOCM also increases in intensity in the beat after a premature beat. This increase in intensity of any LV outflow murmur in the beat after a premature beat relates to the combined effects of enhanced LV filling (from the longer diastolic period) and postextrasystolic potentiation of LV contractile function. In either instance, forward flow will accelerate, causing an increase in the gradient across the LV outflow tract (dynamic or fixed) and a louder systolic murmur. In contrast, the intensity of the murmur of MR does not change in a postpremature beat, because there is relatively little change in the nearly constant LV to left atrial pressure gradient or further alteration in mitral valve flow. Bedside exercise can sometimes be performed to increase cardiac output and, secondarily, the intensity of both systolic and diastolic heart murmurs. Most left-sided heart murmurs decrease in intensity and duration during the strain phase of the Valsalva maneuver. The murmurs associated with MVP and HOCM are the two notable exceptions. The Valsalva maneuver also can be used to assess the integrity of the heart and vasculature in the setting of advanced heart failure.

Prosthetic Heart Valves The first clue that prosthetic valve dysfunction may contribute to recurrent symptoms is frequently a change in the quality of the heart sounds or the appearance of a new murmur. The heart sounds with a bioprosthetic valve resemble those generated by native valves. A mitral bioprosthesis usually is associated with a grade 2 or 3 midsystolic murmur along the left sternal border (created by turbulence across the valve struts as they project into the LV outflow tract) as well as by a soft mid-diastolic murmur that occurs with normal LV filling. This diastolic murmur often can be heard only in the left lateral decubitus position and after exercise. A high pitched or holosystolic apical murmur is indicative of pathologic MR due to a paravalvular leak and/or intra-annular bioprosthetic regurgitation from leaflet degeneration, for which additional imaging is usually indicated. Clinical deterioration can occur rapidly after the first expression of mitral bioprosthetic failure. A tissue valve in the aortic position is always associated with a grade 2 to 3 midsystolic murmur at the base or just below the suprasternal notch. A diastolic murmur of AR is abnormal in any circumstance. Mechanical valve dysfunction may first be suggested by a decrease in the intensity of either the opening or the closing sound. A high-pitched apical systolic murmur in patients with a mechanical mitral prosthesis and a diastolic decrescendo murmur in patients with a mechanical aortic prosthesis indicate paravalvular regurgitation. Patients with prosthetic valve thrombosis may present clinically with signs of shock, muffled heart sounds, and soft murmurs.

Pericardial Disease A pericardial friction rub is nearly 100% specific for the diagnosis of acute pericarditis, although the sensitivity of this finding is not nearly as high, because the rub may come and go over the course of an acute illness or be very difficult to elicit. The rub is heard as a leathery or scratchy three-component or two-component sound, although it may be monophasic. Classically, the three components are ventricular systole, rapid early diastolic filling, and late presystolic filling after atrial contraction in patients in sinus rhythm. It is necessary to listen to the heart in several positions. Additional clues may be present from the history and 12-lead electrocardiogram. The rub typically disappears as the volume of any pericardial effusion increases. Pericardial tamponade can be diagnosed with a sensitivity of 98%, a specificity of 83%, and a positive likelihood ratio of 5.9 (95% confidence interval 2.4–14) by a pulsus paradoxus that exceeds 12 mmHg in a patient with a large pericardial effusion.

The findings on physical examination are integrated with the symptoms previously elicited with a careful history to construct an appropriate differential diagnosis and proceed with indicated imaging and laboratory assessment. The physical examination is an irreplaceable component of the diagnostic algorithm and in selected patients can inform prognosis. Educational efforts to improve clinician competence eventually may result in cost saving, particularly if the indications for imaging can be influenced by the examination findings.

268 Electrocardiography

Ary L. Goldberger

An electrocardiogram (ECG or EKG) is a graphic recording of electric potentials generated by the heart. The signals are detected by means of metal electrodes attached to the extremities and chest wall and then are amplified and recorded by the electrocardiograph. ECG *leads* actually display the instantaneous *differences* in potential between the electrodes.

The clinical utility of the ECG derives from its immediate availability as a noninvasive, inexpensive, and highly versatile test. In addition to its use in detecting arrhythmias, conduction disturbances, and myocardial ischemia, electrocardiography may reveal findings related to life-threatening metabolic disturbances (e.g., hyperkalemia) or increased susceptibility to sudden cardiac death (e.g., QT prolongation syndromes).

ELECTROPHYSIOLOGY

(See also Chaps. 274 and 276) Depolarization of the heart is the initiating event for cardiac contraction. The electric currents that spread through the heart are produced by three components: cardiac pacemaker cells, specialized conduction tissue, and the heart muscle itself. The ECG, however, records only the depolarization (stimulation) and repolarization (recovery) potentials generated by the "working" atrial and ventricular myocardium.

The depolarization stimulus for the normal heartbeat originates in the *sinoatrial* (SA) *node* (Fig. 268-1), or *sinus node*, a collection of *pacemaker cells*. These cells fire spontaneously; that is, they exhibit *automaticity*. The first phase of cardiac electrical activation is the spread of the depolarization wave through the right and left atria, followed by atrial contraction. Next, the impulse stimulates pacemaker and specialized conduction tissues in the atrioventricular (AV) nodal and His bundle areas; together, these two regions constitute the AV junction. The bundle of His bifurcates into two main branches, the right and left bundles, which rapidly transmit depolarization wavefronts to the right and left ventricular myocardium by way of Purkinje fibers. The main left bundle bifurcates into two primary subdivisions: a left anterior fascicle and a left posterior fascicle. The depolarization wavefronts then spread through the ventricular wall, from endocardium to epicardium, triggering ventricular contraction.

Since the cardiac depolarization and repolarization waves have direction and magnitude, they can be represented by vectors. Vector analysis illustrates a central concept of electrocardiography: The ECG records the complex spatial and temporal summation of electrical potentials from multiple myocardial fibers conducted to the surface of the body. This principle accounts for inherent limitations in both ECG *sensitivity* (activity from certain cardiac regions may be canceled out or may be too weak to be recorded) and *specificity* (the same vectorial sum can result from either a selective gain or a loss of forces in opposite directions).

ECG WAVEFORMS AND INTERVALS

The ECG waveforms are labeled alphabetically, beginning with the P wave, which represents atrial depolarization (Fig. 268-2). The QRS complex represents ventricular depolarization, and the ST-T-U complex (ST segment, T wave, and U wave) represents ventricular repolarization. The J point is the junction between the end of the QRS complex and the beginning of the ST segment. Atrial repolarization (ST_a and T_a) is usually too low in amplitude to be detected, but it may become apparent in conditions such as acute pericarditis and atrial infarction.

The QRS-T waveforms of the surface ECG correspond in a general way with the different phases of simultaneously obtained ventricular *action potentials*, the intracellular recordings from single myocardial fibers (Chap. 274). The rapid upstroke (phase 0) of the action potential corresponds to the onset of QRS. The plateau (phase 2) corresponds to the isoelectric ST segment, and active repolarization (phase 3) corresponds to the inscription of the T wave. Factors that decrease the slope of phase 0 by impairing the influx of Na^+ (e.g., hyperkalemia and drugs such as flecainide) tend to increase QRS duration. Conditions that prolong phase 2 (amiodarone, hypocalcemia) increase the QT interval. In contrast, shortening of ventricular repolarization (phase 2), such as by digitalis administration or hypercalcemia, abbreviates the ST segment.

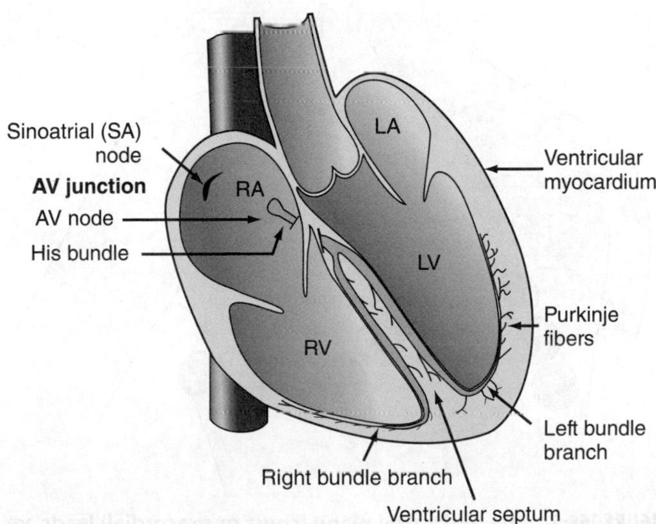

FIGURE 268-1 Schematic of the cardiac conduction system.

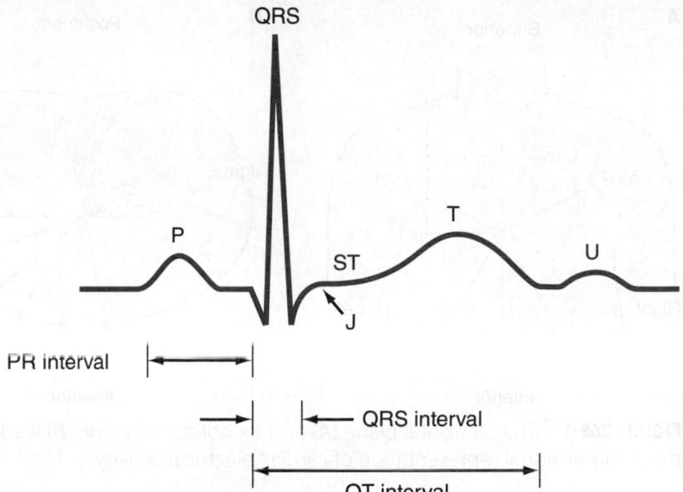

FIGURE 268-2 Basic ECG waveforms and intervals. Not shown is the RR interval, the time between consecutive QRS complexes.

The ECG ordinarily is recorded on special graph paper that is divided into 1-mm^2 gridlike boxes. Since the usual ECG paper speed is 25 mm/s, the smallest (1 mm) horizontal divisions correspond to 0.04 (40 ms), with heavier lines at intervals of 0.20 s (200 ms). Vertically, the ECG graph measures the amplitude of a specific wave or deflection (1 mV = 10 mm with standard calibration; the voltage criteria for hypertrophy mentioned below are given in millimeters). There are four major ECG intervals: RR, PR, QRS, and QT (Fig. 268-2). The heart rate (beats per minute) can be computed readily from the interbeat (RR) interval by dividing the number of large (0.20 s) time units between consecutive R waves into 300 or the number of small (0.04 s) units into 1500. The PR interval measures the time (normally 120–200 ms) between atrial and ventricular depolarization, which includes the physiologic delay imposed by stimulation of cells in the AV junction area. The QRS interval (normally 100–110 ms or less) reflects the duration of ventricular depolarization. The QT interval includes both ventricular depolarization and repolarization times and varies inversely with the heart rate. A rate-related ("corrected") QT interval, QT_c, can be calculated as $QT/\sqrt{RR}$ and normally is ≤0.44 s. (Some references give QT_c upper normal limits as 0.43 s in men and 0.45 s in women. Also, a number of different formulas have been proposed, without consensus, for calculating the QT_c.)

The QRS complex is subdivided into specific deflections or waves. If the initial QRS deflection in a particular lead is negative, it is termed a *Q wave*; the first positive deflection is termed an *R wave*. A negative deflection after an R wave is an *S wave*. Subsequent positive or negative waves are labeled R′ and S′, respectively. Lowercase letters (qrs) are used for waves of relatively small amplitude. An entirely negative QRS complex is termed a *QS wave*.

ECG LEADS

The 12 conventional ECG leads record the difference in potential between electrodes placed on the surface of the body. These leads are divided into two groups: six limb (extremity) leads and six chest (precordial) leads. The limb leads record potentials transmitted onto the *frontal plane* (Fig. 268-3A), and the chest leads record potentials transmitted onto the *horizontal plane* (Fig. 268-3B).

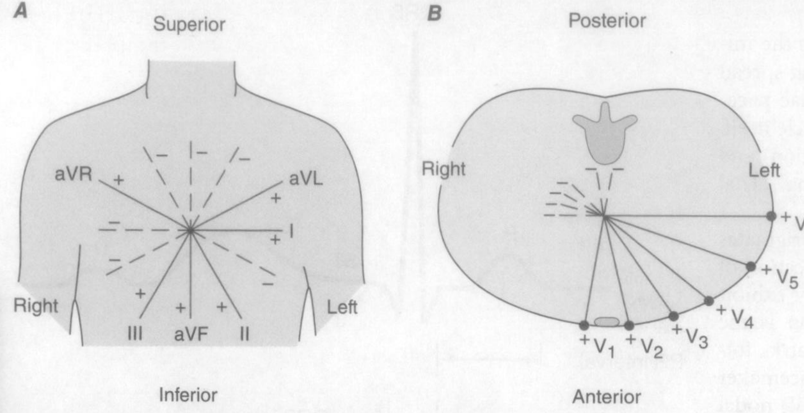

FIGURE 268-3 The six frontal plane (*A*) and six horizontal plane (*B*) leads provide a three-dimensional representation of cardiac electrical activity.

The spatial orientation and polarity of the six frontal plane leads is represented on the hexaxial diagram (Fig. 268-4). The six chest leads (Fig. 268-5) are unipolar recordings obtained by electrodes in the following positions: lead V_1, fourth intercostal space, just to the right of the sternum; lead V_2, fourth intercostal space, just to the left of the sternum; lead V_3, midway between V_2 and V_4; lead V_4, midclavicular line, fifth intercostal space; lead V_5, anterior axillary line, same level as V_4; and lead V_6, midaxillary line, same level as V_4 and V_5. Additional posterior leads are sometimes placed on the same horizontal plane as V_4 to facilitate detection of acute posterolateral infarction (V_7, midaxillary line; V_8 posterior axillary line; and V_9, posterior scapular line).

Together, the frontal and horizontal plane electrodes provide a three-dimensional representation of cardiac electrical activity. Each lead can be likened to a different video camera angle "looking" at the same events—atrial and ventricular depolarization and repolarization—from different spatial orientations. The conventional 12-lead ECG can be supplemented with additional leads in special circumstances. For example, right precordial leads V_3R, V_4R, etc., are useful in detecting evidence of acute right ventricular ischemia. Bedside monitors and ambulatory ECG (Holter) recordings usually employ only one or two modified leads. Intracardiac electrocardiography and electrophysiologic testing are discussed in Chaps. 274 and 276.

The ECG leads are configured so that a positive (upright) deflection is recorded in a lead if a wave of depolarization spreads toward the positive pole of that lead, and a negative deflection is recorded if the wave spreads toward the negative pole. If the *mean* orientation of the depolarization vector is at right angles to a particular lead axis, a biphasic (equally positive and negative) deflection will be recorded.

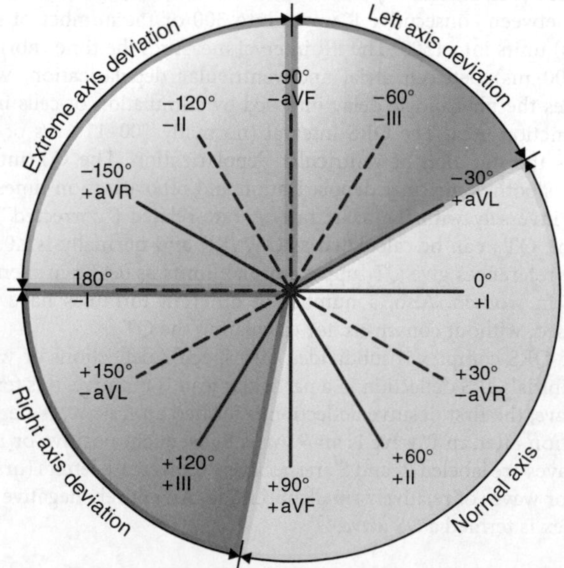

FIGURE 268-4 The frontal plane (limb or extremity) leads are represented on a hexaxial diagram. Each ECG lead has a specific spatial orientation and polarity. The positive pole of each lead axis (*solid line*) and the negative pole (*hatched line*) are designated by their angular position relative to the positive pole of lead I (0°). The mean electrical axis of the QRS complex is measured with respect to this display.

GENESIS OF THE NORMAL ECG

P WAVE

The normal atrial depolarization vector is oriented downward and toward the subject's left, reflecting the spread of depolarization from the sinus node to the right and then the left atrial myocardium. Since this vector points toward the positive pole of lead II and toward the negative pole of lead aVR, the normal P wave will be positive in lead II and negative in lead aVR. By contrast, activation of the atria from an ectopic pacemaker in the lower part of either atrium or in the AV junction region may produce retrograde P waves (negative in lead II, positive in lead aVR). The normal P wave in lead V_1 may be biphasic with a positive component reflecting right atrial depolarization, followed by a small (<1 mm^2) negative component reflecting left atrial depolarization.

QRS COMPLEX

Normal ventricular depolarization proceeds as a rapid, continuous spread of activation wave fronts. This complex process can be divided into two major sequential phases, and each phase can be represented by a mean vector (Fig. 268-6). The first phase is depolarization of the interventricular septum from the left to the right and anteriorly (vector 1). The second results from the simultaneous depolarization of the right and left ventricles; it normally is dominated by the more massive left ventricle, so that vector 2 points leftward and posteriorly. Therefore, a right precordial lead (V_1) will record this biphasic depolarization process with a small positive deflection (septal r wave) followed by a larger negative deflection (S wave). A left precordial lead, e.g., V_6, will record the same sequence with a small negative deflection (septal q wave) followed by a relatively tall positive deflection (R wave). Intermediate leads show a relative increase in R-wave amplitude (normal R-wave progression) and a decrease in S-wave amplitude progressing across the chest from right to left. The precordial lead where

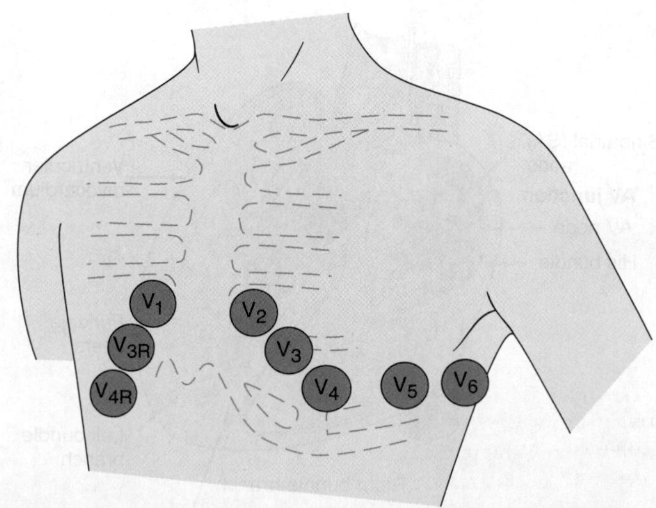

FIGURE 268-5 The horizontal plane (chest or precordial) leads are obtained with electrodes in the locations shown.

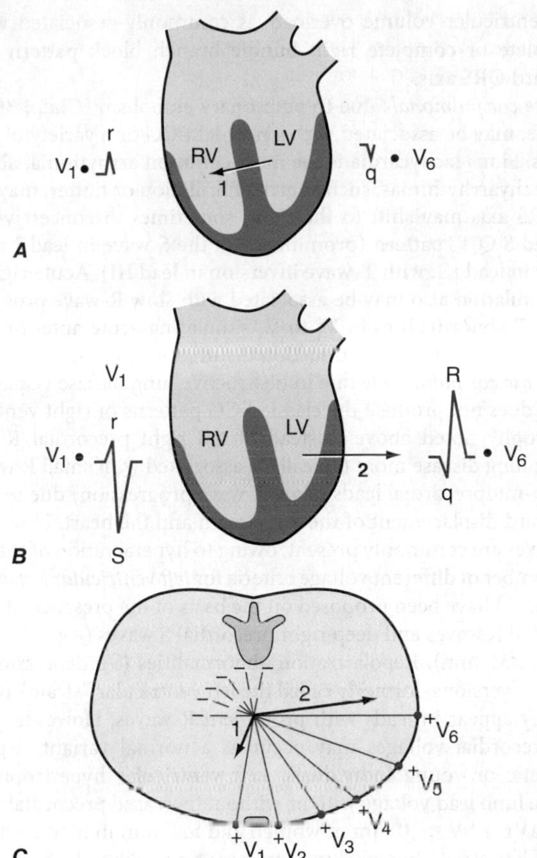

FIGURE 268-6 Ventricular depolarization can be divided into two major phases, each represented by a vector. ***A.*** The first phase (*arrow 1*) denotes depolarization of the ventricular septum, beginning on the left side and spreading to the right. This process is represented by a small "septal" r wave in lead V_1 and a small septal q wave in lead V_6. ***B.*** Simultaneous depolarization of the left and right ventricles (LV and RV) constitutes the second phase. Vector 2 is oriented to the left and posteriorly, reflecting the electrical predominance of the LV. ***C.*** Vectors (*arrows*) representing these two phases are shown in reference to the horizontal plane leads. *(After AL Goldberger et al: Goldberger's Clinical Electrocardiography: A Simplified Approach, 8th ed. Philadelphia, Elsevier/Saunders, 2013.)*

the R and S waves are of approximately equal amplitude is referred to as the *transition zone* (usually V_3 or V_4) (Fig. 268-7).

The QRS pattern in the extremity leads may vary considerably from one normal subject to another depending on the *electrical axis* of the QRS, which describes the mean orientation of the QRS vector with reference to the six frontal plane leads. Normally, the QRS axis ranges from −30° to +100° (Fig. 268-4). An axis more negative than −30° is referred to as *left axis deviation*, and an axis more positive than +100° is referred to as *right axis deviation.* Left axis deviation may occur as a normal variant but is more commonly associated with left ventricular hypertrophy, a block in the anterior fascicle of the left bundle system (left anterior fascicular block or hemiblock), or inferior myocardial infarction. Right axis deviation also may occur as a normal variant (particularly in children and young adults), as a spurious finding due to reversal of the left and right arm electrodes, or in conditions such as right ventricular overload (acute or chronic), infarction of the lateral wall of the left ventricle, dextrocardia, left pneumothorax, and left posterior fascicular block.

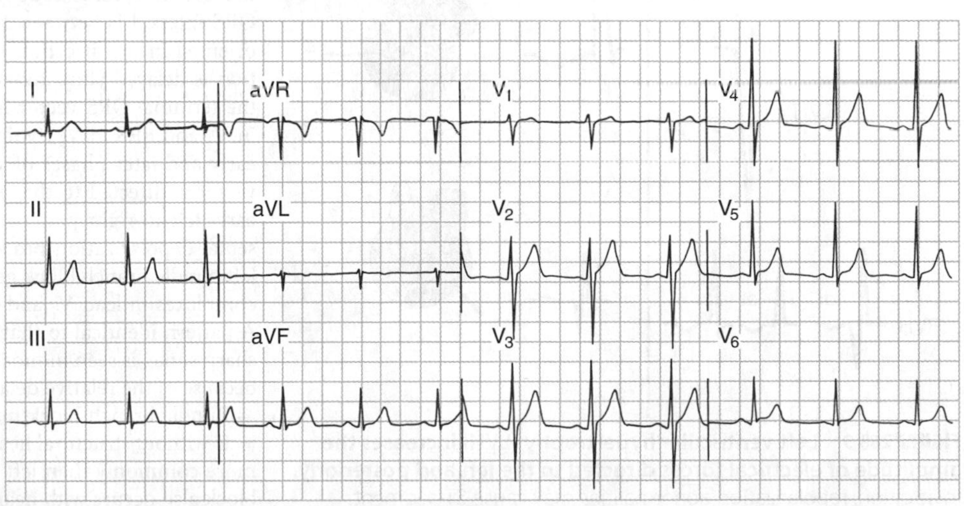

FIGURE 268-7 Normal electrocardiogram from a healthy subject. Sinus rhythm is present with a heart rate of 75 beats per minute. PR interval is 0.16 s; QRS interval (duration) is 0.08 s; QT interval is 0.36 s; QT_c is 0.40 s; the mean QRS axis is about +70°. The precordial leads show normal R-wave progression with the transition zone (R wave = S wave) in lead V_3.

T WAVE AND U WAVE

Normally, the mean T-wave vector is oriented roughly concordant with the mean QRS vector (within about 45° in the frontal plane). Since depolarization and repolarization are electrically opposite processes, this normal QRS–T-wave vector concordance indicates that repolarization normally must proceed in the reverse direction from depolarization (i.e., from ventricular epicardium to endocardium). The normal U wave is a small, rounded deflection (≤1 mm) that follows the T wave and usually has the same polarity as the T wave. An abnormal increase in U-wave amplitude is most commonly due to drugs (e.g., dofetilide, amiodarone, sotalol, quinidine) or to hypokalemia. Very prominent U waves are a marker of increased susceptibility to the *torsades de pointes* type of ventricular tachycardia (Chap. 276). Inversion of the U wave in the precordial leads is abnormal and may be a subtle sign of ischemia.

MAJOR ECG ABNORMALITIES

CARDIAC ENLARGEMENT AND HYPERTROPHY

Right atrial overload (acute or chronic) may lead to an increase in P-wave amplitude (≥2.5 mm) (Fig. 268-8), sometimes referred to as "P-pulmonale." Left atrial overload typically produces a biphasic P wave in V_1 with a broad negative component or a broad (≥120 ms), often notched P wave in one or more limb leads (Fig. 268-8). This pattern, previously referred to as "P-mitrale," may also occur with left atrial conduction delays in the absence of actual atrial enlargement, leading to the more general designation of *left atrial abnormality.*

Right ventricular hypertrophy due to a sustained, severe pressure load (e.g., due to tight pulmonic valve stenosis or certain pulmonary artery hypertension syndromes) is characterized by a relatively tall R wave in lead V_1 (R ≥ S wave), usually with right axis deviation (Fig. 268-9); alternatively, there may be a qR pattern in V_1 or V_3R. ST depression and T-wave inversion in the right-to-midprecordial leads are also often present. This pattern, formerly called right ventricular "strain," is attributed to repolarization abnormalities in acutely or chronically overloaded muscle. Prominent S waves may occur in the left lateral precordial leads. Right ventricular hypertrophy due to ostium secundum–type atrial septal defects, with the accompanying

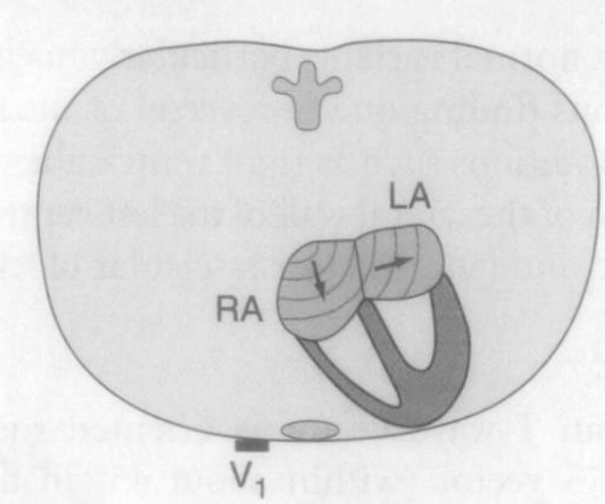

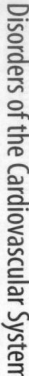

FIGURE 268-8 Right atrial (RA) overload may cause tall, peaked P waves in the limb or precordial leads. Left atrial (LA) abnormality may cause broad, often notched P waves in the limb leads and a biphasic P wave in lead V_1 with a prominent negative component representing delayed depolarization of the LA. *(After MK Park, WG Guntheroth: How to Read Pediatric ECGs, 4th ed. St. Louis, Mosby/Elsevier, 2006.)*

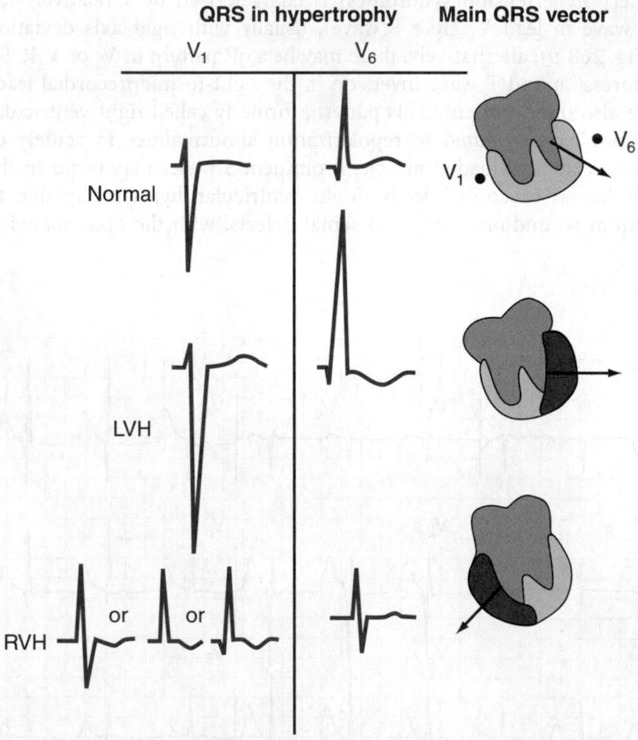

FIGURE 268-9 Left ventricular hypertrophy (LVH) increases the amplitude of electrical forces directed to the left and posteriorly. In addition, repolarization abnormalities may cause ST-segment depression and T-wave inversion in leads with a prominent R wave. Right ventricular hypertrophy (RVH) may shift the QRS vector to the right; this effect usually is associated with an R, RS, or qR complex in lead V_1. T-wave inversions may be present in right precordial leads.

right ventricular volume overload, is commonly associated with an incomplete or complete right bundle branch block pattern with a rightward QRS axis.

Acute cor pulmonale due to pulmonary embolism (Chap. 300), for example, may be associated with a normal ECG or a variety of abnormalities. Sinus tachycardia is the most common arrhythmia, although other tachyarrhythmias, such as atrial fibrillation or flutter, may occur. The QRS axis may shift to the right, sometimes in concert with the so-called $S_1Q_3T_3$ pattern (prominence of the S wave in lead I and the Q wave in lead III, with T-wave inversion in lead III). Acute right ventricular dilation also may be associated with slow R-wave progression and ST-T abnormalities in V_1 to V_4 simulating acute anterior infarction. A right ventricular conduction disturbance may appear.

Chronic cor pulmonale due to obstructive lung disease (Chap. 279) usually does not produce the classic ECG patterns of right ventricular hypertrophy noted above. Instead of tall right precordial R waves, chronic lung disease more typically is associated with small R waves in right-to-midprecordial leads (slow R-wave progression) due in part to downward displacement of the diaphragm and the heart. Low-voltage complexes are commonly present, owing to hyperaeration of the lungs.

A number of different voltage criteria for *left ventricular hypertrophy* (Fig. 268-9) have been proposed on the basis of the presence of tall left precordial R waves and deep right precordial S waves (e.g., SV_1 + [RV_5 or RV_6] >35 mm). Repolarization abnormalities (ST depression with T-wave inversions, formerly called the left ventricular "strain" pattern) also may appear in leads with prominent R waves. However, prominent precordial voltages may occur as a normal variant, especially in athletic or young individuals. Left ventricular hypertrophy may increase limb lead voltage with or without increased precordial voltage (e.g., RaVL + SV_3 >20 mm in women and >28 mm in men). The presence of left atrial abnormality increases the likelihood of underlying left ventricular hypertrophy in cases with borderline voltage criteria. Left ventricular hypertrophy often progresses to incomplete or complete left bundle branch block. The sensitivity of conventional voltage criteria for left ventricular hypertrophy is decreased in obese persons and smokers. ECG evidence for left ventricular hypertrophy is a major noninvasive marker of increased risk of cardiovascular morbidity and mortality rates, including sudden cardiac death. However, because of false-positive and false-negative diagnoses, the ECG is of limited utility in diagnosing atrial or ventricular enlargement. More definitive information is provided by echocardiography (Chap. 270e).

BUNDLE BRANCH BLOCKS AND RELATED PATTERNS

Intrinsic impairment of conduction in either the right or the left bundle system (intraventricular conduction disturbances) leads to prolongation of the QRS interval. With complete bundle branch blocks, the QRS interval is ≥120 ms in duration; with incomplete blocks, the QRS interval is between 100 and 120 ms. The QRS vector usually is oriented in the direction of the myocardial region where depolarization is delayed (Fig. 268-10). Thus, with right bundle branch block, the terminal QRS vector is oriented to the right and anteriorly (rSR′ in V_1 and qRS in V_6, typically). Left bundle branch block alters both early and later phases of ventricular depolarization. The major QRS vector is directed to the left and posteriorly. In addition, the normal early left-to-right pattern of septal activation is disrupted such that septal depolarization proceeds from right to left as well. As a result, left bundle branch block generates wide, predominantly negative (QS) complexes in lead V_1 and entirely positive (R) complexes in lead V_6. A pattern identical to that of left bundle branch block, preceded by a sharp spike, is seen in most cases of electronic right ventricular pacing because of the relative delay in left ventricular activation.

Bundle branch block may occur in a variety of conditions. In subjects without structural heart disease, right bundle branch block is seen more commonly than left bundle branch block. Right bundle branch block also occurs with heart disease, both congenital (e.g., atrial septal defect) and acquired (e.g., valvular, ischemic). Left bundle branch block is often a marker of one of four underlying conditions associated with increased risk of cardiovascular morbidity and mortality rates: coronary heart disease (frequently with impaired left ventricular

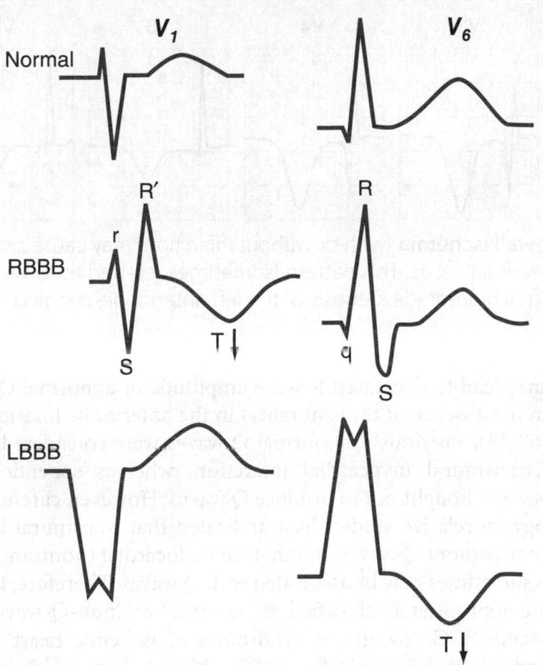

FIGURE 268-10 Comparison of typical QRS-T patterns in right bundle branch block (RBBB) and left bundle branch block (LBBB) with the normal pattern in leads V_1 and V_6. Note the secondary T-wave inversions (*arrows*) in leads with an rSR′ complex with RBBB and in leads with a wide R wave with LBBB.

function), hypertensive heart disease, aortic valve disease, and cardiomyopathy. Bundle branch blocks may be chronic or intermittent. A bundle branch block may be rate-related; for example, it often occurs when the heart rate exceeds some critical value.

Bundle branch blocks and depolarization abnormalities secondary to artificial pacemakers not only affect ventricular depolarization (QRS) but also are characteristically associated with *secondary repolarization* (ST-T) abnormalities. With bundle branch blocks, the T wave is typically opposite in polarity to the last deflection of the QRS (Fig. 268-10). This discordance of the QRS–T-wave vectors is caused by the altered sequence of repolarization that occurs secondary to altered depolarization. In contrast, *primary repolarization* abnormalities are independent of QRS changes and are related instead to actual alterations in the electrical properties of the myocardial fibers themselves (e.g., in the resting membrane potential or action potential duration), not just to changes in the sequence of repolarization. Ischemia, electrolyte imbalance, and drugs such as digitalis all cause such primary ST–T-wave changes. Primary and secondary T-wave changes may coexist. For example, T-wave inversions in the right precordial leads with left bundle branch block or in the left precordial leads with right bundle branch block may be important markers of underlying ischemia or other abnormalities.

A distinctive abnormality simulating right bundle branch block with ST-segment elevations in the right chest leads is seen with the Brugada pattern (Chap. 276).

Partial blocks (fascicular or "hemiblocks") in the left bundle system (left anterior or posterior fascicular blocks) generally do not prolong the QRS duration substantially but instead are associated with shifts in the frontal plane QRS axis (leftward or rightward, respectively). Left anterior fascicular block (QRS axis more negative than −45°) is probably the most common cause of marked left axis deviation in adults. In contrast, left posterior fascicular block (QRS axis more rightward than +110–120°) is extremely rare as an isolated finding and requires exclusion of other factors causing right axis deviation mentioned earlier.

More complex combinations of fascicular and bundle branch blocks may occur that involve the left and right bundle system. Examples of *bifascicular block* include right bundle branch block and left posterior fascicular block, right bundle branch block with left anterior fascicular block, and complete left bundle branch block. Chronic bifascicular block in an asymptomatic individual is associated with a relatively low risk of progression to high-degree AV heart block. In contrast, new bifascicular block with acute anterior myocardial infarction carries a much greater risk of complete heart block. Alternation of right and left bundle branch block is a sign of *trifascicular disease. However, the presence of a prolonged PR interval and bifascicular block does not necessarily indicate trifascicular involvement, since this combination may arise with AV node disease and bifascicular block.* Intraventricular conduction delays also can be caused by extrinsic (toxic) factors that slow ventricular conduction, particularly hyperkalemia or drugs (e.g., class 1 antiarrhythmic agents, tricyclic antidepressants, phenothiazines).

Prolongation of QRS duration does not necessarily indicate a conduction delay but may be due to *preexcitation* of the ventricles via a bypass tract, as in Wolff-Parkinson-White (WPW) patterns (Chap. 276) and related variants. The diagnostic triad of WPW consists of a wide QRS complex associated with a relatively short PR interval and slurring of the initial part of the QRS (delta wave), with the latter effect being due to aberrant activation of ventricular myocardium. The presence of a bypass tract predisposes to reentrant supraventricular tachyarrhythmias.

MYOCARDIAL ISCHEMIA AND INFARCTION

(See also Chap. 295) The ECG is a cornerstone in the diagnosis of acute and chronic ischemic heart disease. The findings depend on several key factors: the nature of the process (reversible [i.e., ischemia] versus irreversible [i.e., infarction]), the duration (acute versus chronic), the extent (transmural versus subendocardial), and localization (anterior versus inferoposterior), as well as the presence of other underlying abnormalities (ventricular hypertrophy, conduction defects).

Ischemia exerts complex time-dependent effects on the electrical properties of myocardial cells. Severe, acute ischemia lowers the resting membrane potential and shortens the duration of the action potential. Such changes cause a voltage gradient between normal and ischemic zones. As a consequence, current flows between those regions. These currents of injury are represented on the surface ECG by deviation of the ST segment (Fig. 268-11). When the acute ischemia is *transmural*, the ST vector usually is shifted in the direction of the outer (epicardial) layers, producing ST elevations and sometimes, in the earliest stages of ischemia, tall, positive so-called hyperacute T waves over the ischemic zone. With ischemia confined primarily to the *subendocardium*, the ST vector typically shifts toward the subendocardium and ventricular cavity, so that overlying (e.g., anterior precordial) leads show ST-segment depression (with ST elevation in lead aVR). Multiple factors affect the amplitude of acute ischemic ST deviations. Profound ST elevation or depression in multiple leads usually indicates very severe ischemia.

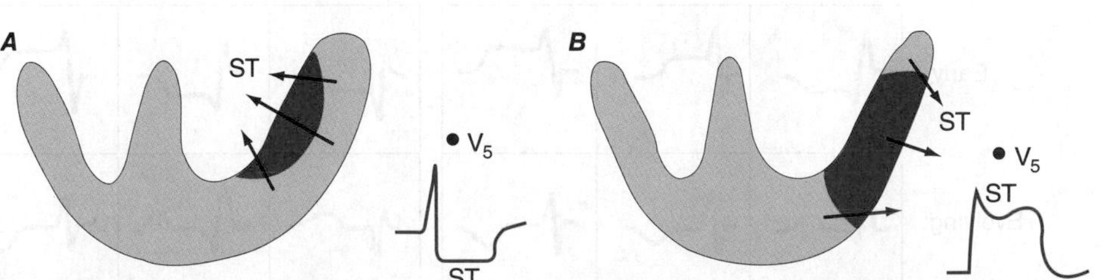

FIGURE 268-11 Acute ischemia causes a current of injury. With predominant subendocardial ischemia (***A***), the resultant ST vector will be directed toward the inner layer of the affected ventricle and the ventricular cavity. Overlying leads therefore will record ST depression. With ischemia involving the outer ventricular layer (***B***) (transmural or epicardial injury), the ST vector will be directed outward. Overlying leads will record ST elevation.

From a clinical viewpoint, the division of acute myocardial infarction into ST-segment elevation and non-ST elevation types is useful since the efficacy of acute reperfusion therapy is limited to the former group.

The ECG leads are usually more helpful in localizing regions of ST elevation than non-ST elevation ischemia. For example, acute transmural anterior (including apical and lateral) wall ischemia is reflected by ST elevations or increased T-wave positivity in one or more of the precordial leads (V_1–V_6) and leads I and aVL. Inferior wall ischemia produces changes in leads II, III, and aVF. "Posterior" wall ischemia (usually associated with lateral or inferior involvement) may be indirectly recognized by *reciprocal* ST depressions in leads V_1 to V_3 (thus constituting an ST elevation "equivalent" acute coronary syndrome). Right ventricular ischemia usually produces ST elevations in right-sided chest leads (Fig. 268-5). When ischemic ST elevations occur as the earliest sign of acute infarction, they typically are followed within a period ranging from hours to days by evolving T-wave inversions and often by Q waves occurring in the same lead distribution. Reversible transmural ischemia, for example, due to coronary vasospasm (Prinzmetal's variant angina and possibly the Tako-tsubo "stress" cardiomyopathy syndrome), may cause transient ST-segment elevations without development of Q waves, as may very early reperfusion in acute coronary syndromes. Depending on the severity and duration of ischemia, the ST elevations may resolve completely in minutes or be followed by T-wave inversions that persist for hours or even days. Patients with ischemic chest pain who present with deep T-wave inversions in multiple precordial leads (e.g., V_1–V_4, I, and aVL) with or without cardiac enzyme elevations typically have severe obstruction in the left anterior descending coronary artery system (Fig. 268-12). In contrast, patients whose baseline ECG already shows abnormal T-wave inversions may develop T-wave normalization (*pseudonormalization*) during episodes of acute transmural ischemia.

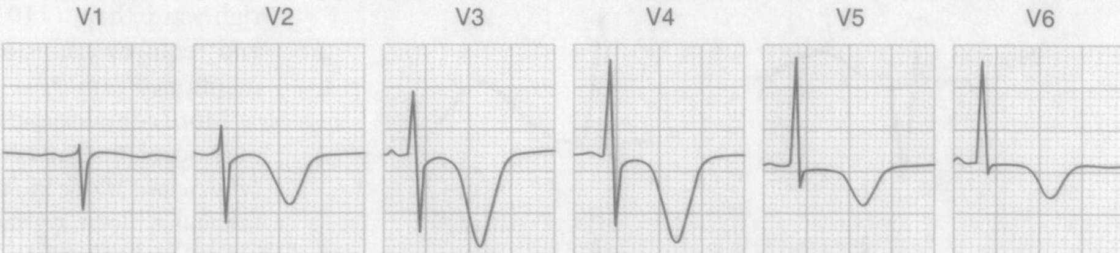

FIGURE 268-12 Severe anterior wall ischemia (with or without infarction) may cause prominent T-wave inversions in the precordial leads. This pattern (sometimes referred to as Wellens T waves) is usually associated with a high-grade stenosis of the left anterior descending coronary artery.

With infarction, depolarization (QRS) changes often accompany repolarization (ST-T) abnormalities. Necrosis of sufficient myocardial tissue may lead to decreased R-wave amplitude or abnormal Q waves (even in the absence of transmurality) in the anterior or inferior leads (Fig. 268-13). Previously, abnormal Q waves were considered markers of transmural myocardial infarction, whereas subendocardial infarcts were thought not to produce Q waves. However, careful ECG-pathology correlative studies have indicated that transmural infarcts may occur without Q waves and that subendocardial (nontransmural) infarcts sometimes may be associated with Q waves. Therefore, infarcts are more appropriately classified as "Q-wave" or "non-Q-wave." The major acute ECG changes in syndromes of ischemic heart disease are summarized schematically in Fig. 268-14. Loss of depolarization forces due to posterior or lateral infarction may cause reciprocal increases in R-wave amplitude in leads V_1 and V_2 without diagnostic Q waves in any of the conventional leads. Atrial infarction may be associated with PR-segment deviations due to an atrial current of injury, changes in P-wave morphology, or atrial arrhythmias. In the weeks and months after infarction, these ECG changes may persist or begin to resolve. Complete normalization of the ECG after Q-wave infarction is uncommon but may occur, particularly with smaller infarcts. In contrast, ST-segment elevations that persist for several weeks or more after a Q-wave infarct usually correlate with a severe underlying wall motion disorder (akinetic or dyskinetic zone), although not necessarily a frank ventricular aneurysm. ECG changes due to ischemia may occur spontaneously or may be provoked by various exercise protocols (stress electrocardiography; Chap. 293).

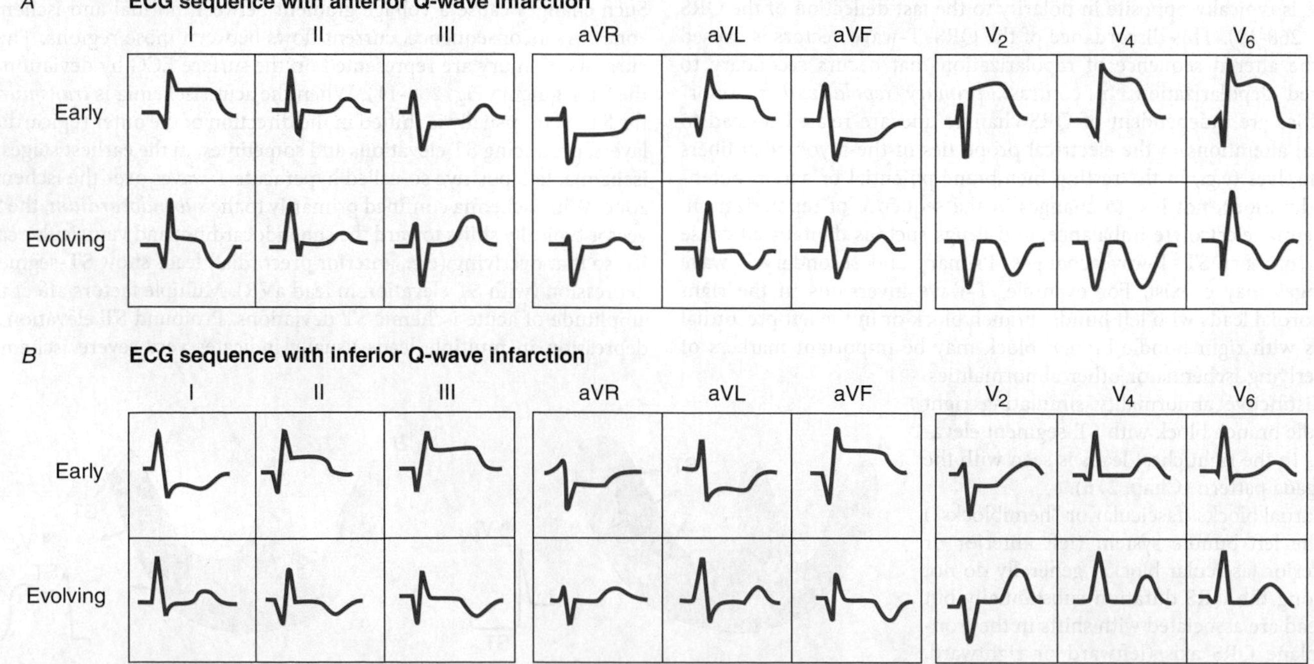

FIGURE 268-13 Sequence of depolarization and repolarization changes with (*A*) acute anterior and (*B*) acute inferior wall Q-wave infarctions. With anterior infarcts, ST elevation in leads I and aVL and the precordial leads may be accompanied by reciprocal ST depressions in leads II, III, and aVF. Conversely, acute inferior (or posterolateral) infarcts may be associated with reciprocal ST depressions in leads V_1 to V_3. *(After AL Goldberger et al: Goldberger's Clinical Electrocardiography: A Simplified Approach, 8th ed. Philadelphia, Elsevier/Saunders, 2013.)*

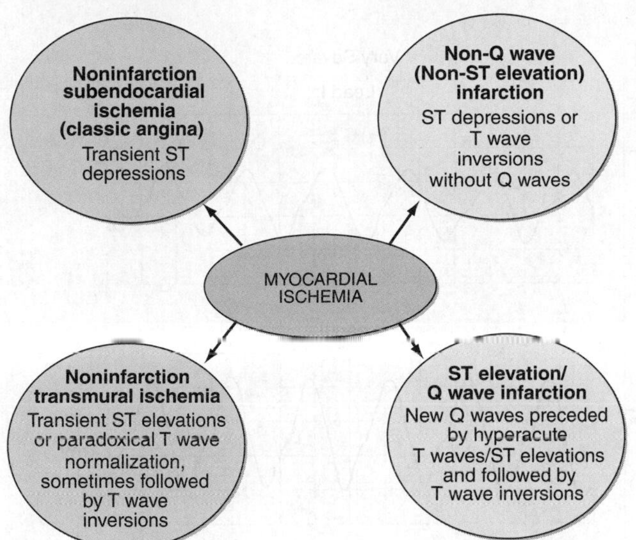

FIGURE 268-14 Variability of ECG patterns with acute myocardial ischemia. The ECG also may be normal or nonspecifically abnormal. Furthermore, these categorizations are not mutually exclusive. *(After AL Goldberger et al: Goldberger's Clinical Electrocardiography: A Simplified Approach, 8th ed. Philadelphia, Elsevier/Saunders, 2013.)*

The ECG has important limitations in both sensitivity and specificity in the diagnosis of ischemic heart disease. Although a single normal ECG does not exclude ischemia or even acute infarction, a normal ECG *throughout* the course of an acute infarct is distinctly uncommon. Prolonged chest pain without diagnostic ECG changes therefore should always prompt a careful search for other noncoronary causes of chest pain (Chap. 19). Furthermore, the diagnostic changes of acute or evolving ischemia are often masked by the presence of left bundle branch block, electronic ventricular pacemaker patterns, and Wolff-Parkinson-White preexcitation. However, clinicians continue to overdiagnose ischemia or infarction based on the presence of ST-segment elevations or depressions; T-wave inversions; tall, positive T waves; or Q waves *not* related to ischemic heart disease (pseudoinfarct patterns). For example, ST-segment elevations simulating ischemia may occur with acute pericarditis or myocarditis, as a normal variant (including the typical "early repolarization" pattern), or in a variety of other conditions (Table 268-1). Similarly, tall, positive T waves do not invariably represent hyperacute ischemic changes but may also be caused by normal variants, hyperkalemia, cerebrovascular injury, and left ventricular volume overload due to mitral or aortic regurgitation, among other causes.

ST-segment elevations and tall, positive T waves are common findings in leads V_1 and V_2 in left bundle branch block or left ventricular hypertrophy in the absence of ischemia. The differential diagnosis of Q waves includes physiologic or positional variants, ventricular hypertrophy, acute or chronic noncoronary myocardial injury, hypertrophic cardiomyopathy, and ventricular conduction disorders. Digoxin, ventricular hypertrophy, hypokalemia, and a variety of other factors may cause ST-segment depression mimicking subendocardial ischemia. Prominent T-wave inversion may occur with ventricular hypertrophy, cardiomyopathies, myocarditis, and cerebrovascular injury (particularly intracranial bleeds), among many other conditions.

METABOLIC FACTORS AND DRUG EFFECTS

A variety of metabolic and pharmacologic agents alter the ECG and, in particular, cause changes in repolarization (ST-T-U) and sometimes QRS prolongation. Certain life-threatening electrolyte disturbances may be diagnosed initially and monitored from the ECG. *Hyperkalemia* produces a sequence of changes (Fig. 268-15), usually beginning with narrowing and peaking (tenting) of the T waves. Further elevation of extracellular K^+ leads to AV conduction disturbances, diminution in P-wave amplitude, and widening of the QRS interval. Severe hyperkalemia eventually causes cardiac arrest with a slow sinusoidal type of mechanism ("sine-wave" pattern) followed by asystole. *Hypokalemia* (Fig. 268-16) prolongs ventricular repolarization, often with prominent U waves. Prolongation of the QT interval is also seen with drugs that increase the duration of the ventricular action potential: class 1A antiarrhythmic agents and related drugs (e.g., quinidine, disopyramide, procainamide, tricyclic antidepressants, phenothiazines) and class III agents (e.g., amiodarone [Fig. 268-16], dofetilide, dronedarone, sotalol, ibutilide). Marked QT prolongation, sometimes with deep, wide T-wave inversions, may occur with intracranial bleeds, particularly subarachnoid hemorrhage ("CVA T-wave" pattern) (Fig. 268-16). Systemic *hypothermia* also prolongs repolarization, usually with a distinctive convex elevation of the J point (Osborn wave). *Hypocalcemia* typically prolongs the QT interval (ST portion), whereas *hypercalcemia* shortens it (Fig. 268-17). Digitalis glycosides also shorten the QT interval, often with a characteristic "scooping" of the ST–T-wave complex (*digitalis effect*).

Many other factors are associated with ECG changes, particularly alterations in ventricular repolarization. T-wave flattening, minimal T-wave inversions, or slight ST-segment depression ("nonspecific ST–T-wave changes") may occur with a variety of electrolyte and acid-base disturbances, a number of infectious processes, central nervous system disorders, endocrine abnormalities, many drugs, ischemia, hypoxia, and virtually any type of cardiopulmonary abnormality. Although subtle ST–T-wave changes may be markers of ischemia, transient nonspecific repolarization changes may also occur after a meal or with postural (orthostatic) change, hyperventilation, or exercise in healthy individuals.

TABLE 268-1 DIFFERENTIAL DIAGNOSIS OF ST-SEGMENT ELEVATIONS

Ischemia/myocardial infarction
Noninfarction, transmural ischemia (Prinzmetal's angina, and probably Tako-tsubo syndrome, which may also exactly simulate classical acute infarction)
Acute myocardial infarction
Postmyocardial infarction (ventricular aneurysm pattern)
Acute pericarditis
Normal variants (including benign "early repolarization" patterns)
Left ventricular hypertrophy/left bundle branch block[a]
Other (rarer)
Acute pulmonary embolism[a]
Brugada patterns (right bundle branch block–like pattern with ST elevations in right precordial leads)[a]
Class 1C antiarrhythmic drugs[a]
DC cardioversion
Hypercalcemia[a]
Hyperkalemia[a]
Hypothermia (J [Osborn] waves)
Nonischemic myocardial injury
Myocarditis
Tumor invading left ventricle
Trauma to ventricles

[a]Usually localized to V_1–V_2 or V_3.

Source: Modified from AL Goldberger et al: *Goldberger's Clinical Electrocardiography: A Simplified Approach*, 8th ed. Philadelphia, Elsevier/Saunders, 2013.

LOW QRS VOLTAGE

Low QRS voltage is arbitrarily defined as peak-to-trough QRS amplitudes of ≤5 mm in the six limb leads and/or ≤10 mm in the chest leads. Multiple factors may be responsible. Among the most serious include pericardial (Fig. 268-18) or pleural effusions, chronic obstructive pulmonary disease, infiltrative cardiomyopathies, and anasarca.

ELECTRICAL ALTERNANS

Electrical alternans—a beat-to-beat alternation in one or more components of the ECG signal—is a common type of nonlinear cardiovascular response to a variety of hemodynamic and electrophysiologic

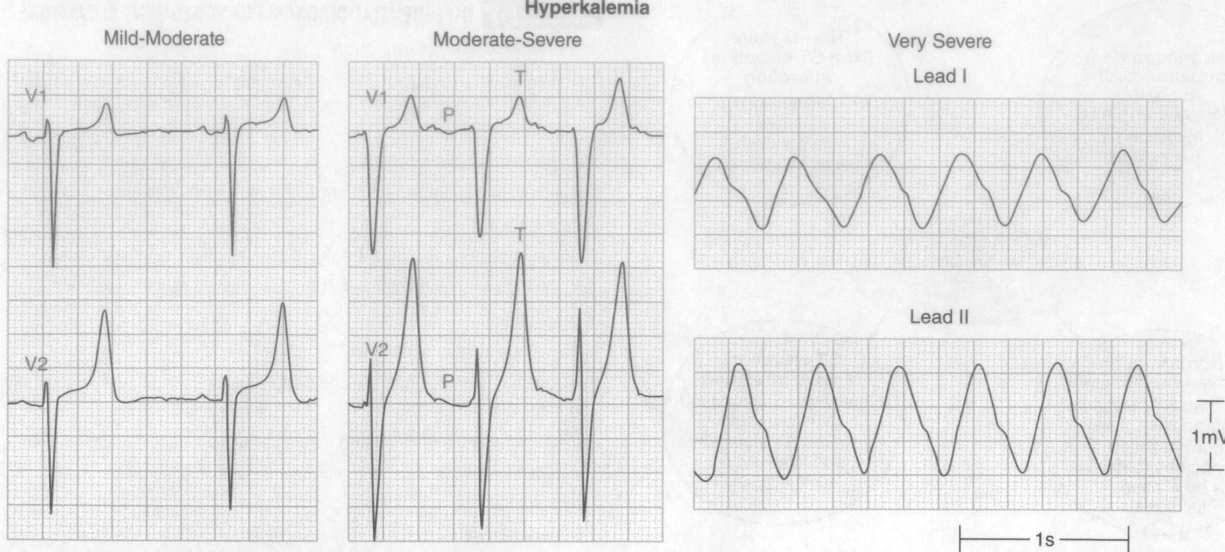

FIGURE 268-15 The earliest ECG change with hyperkalemia is usually peaking ("tenting") of the T waves. With further increases in the serum potassium concentration, the QRS complexes widen, the P waves decrease in amplitude and may disappear, and finally a sine-wave pattern leads to asystole unless emergency therapy is given. *(After AL Goldberger et al: Goldberger's Clinical Electrocardiography: A Simplified Approach, 8th ed. Philadelphia, Elsevier/Saunders, 2013.)*

perturbations. Total electrical alternans (P-QRS-T) with sinus tachycardia is a relatively specific sign of pericardial effusion, usually with cardiac tamponade **(Fig. 268-18)**. The mechanism relates to a periodic swinging motion of the heart in the effusion at a frequency exactly one-half the heart rate. In contrast, pure repolarization (ST-T or U wave) alternans is a sign of electrical instability and may precede ventricular tachyarrhythmias.

CLINICAL INTERPRETATION OF THE ECG

Accurate analysis of ECGs requires thoroughness and care. The patient's age, gender, and clinical status should always be taken into account. Many mistakes in ECG interpretation are errors of omission. Therefore, a systematic approach is essential. The following 14 points should be analyzed carefully in every ECG: (1) standardization (calibration) and technical features (including lead placement and artifacts), (2) rhythm, (3) heart rate, (4) PR interval/AV conduction, (5) QRS interval, (6) QT/QT$_c$ intervals, (7) mean QRS electrical axis, (8) P waves, (9) QRS voltages, (10) precordial R-wave progression,

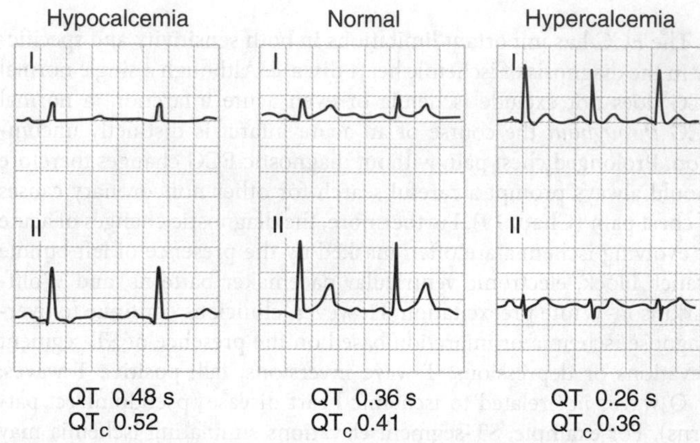

FIGURE 268-17 Prolongation of the Q-T interval (ST-segment portion) is typical of hypocalcemia. Hypercalcemia may cause abbreviation of the ST segment and shortening of the QT interval.

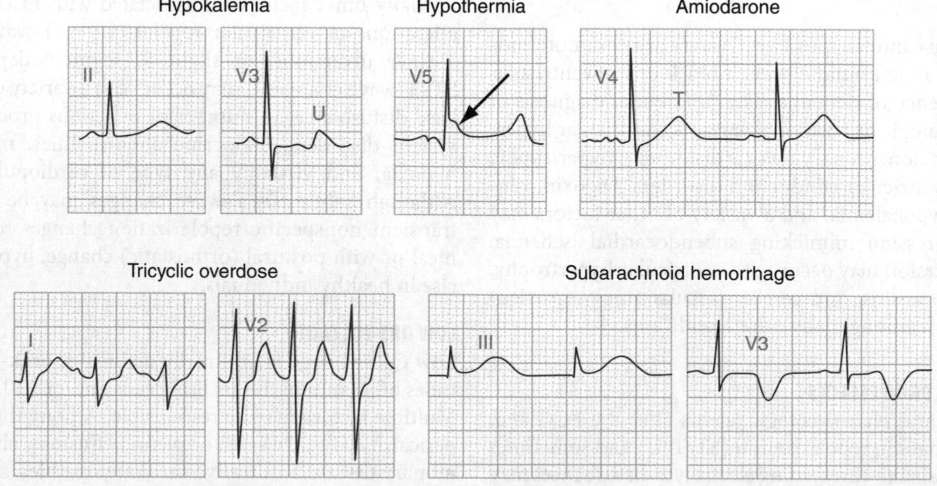

FIGURE 268-16 A variety of metabolic derangements, drug effects, and other factors may prolong ventricular repolarization with QT prolongation or prominent U waves. Prominent repolarization prolongation, particularly if due to hypokalemia, inherited "channelopathies," or certain pharmacologic agents, indicates increased susceptibility to *torsades des pointes*–type ventricular tachycardia **(Chap. 277)**. Marked systemic hypothermia is associated with a distinctive convex "hump" at the J point (Osborn wave, *arrow*) due to altered ventricular action potential characteristics. Note QRS and QT prolongation along with sinus tachycardia in the case of tricyclic antidepressant overdose.

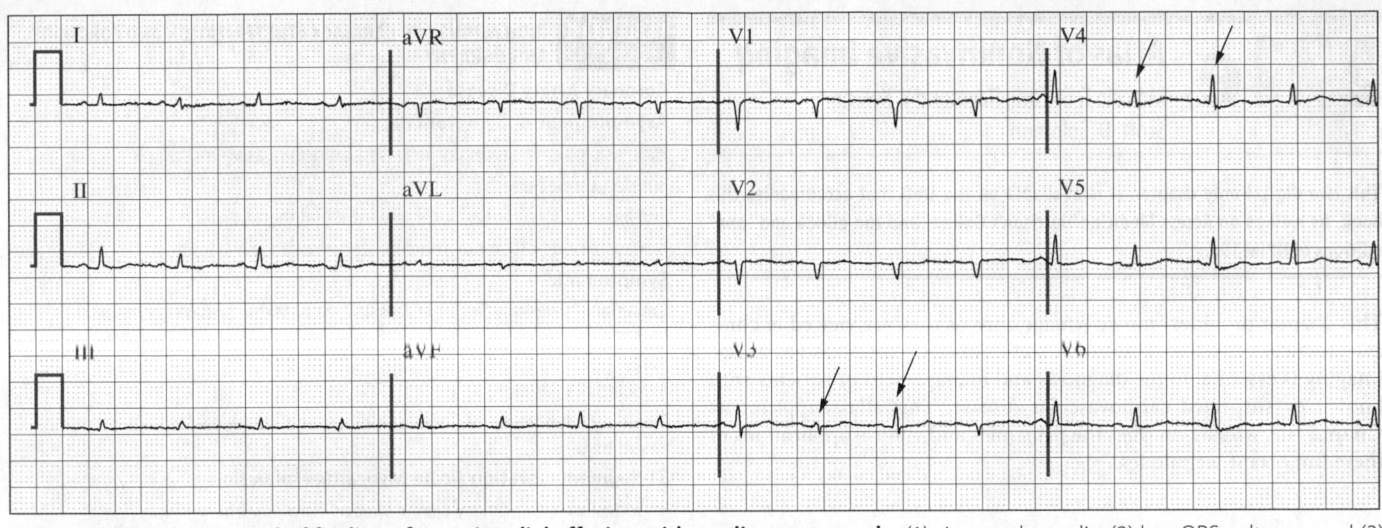

FIGURE 268-18 Classic triad of findings for pericardial effusion with cardiac tamponade: (1) sinus tachycardia; (2) low QRS voltages; and (3) electrical alternans (best seen in leads V_3 and V_4 in this case; *arrows*). This triad is highly specific for pericardial effusion, usually with tamponade physiology, but of limited sensitivity. *(Adapted from LA Nathanson et al: ECG Wave-Maven. http://ecg.bidmc.harvard.edu.)*

(11) abnormal Q waves, (12) ST segments, (13) T waves, and (14) U waves. Comparison with any previous ECGs is invaluable. The diagnosis and management of specific cardiac arrhythmias and conduction disturbances are discussed in Chaps. 274 and 276.

COMPUTERIZED ELECTROCARDIOGRAPHY

Computerized ECG systems are widely used for immediate retrieval of thousands of ECG records. Computer interpretation of ECGs still has major limitations. Incomplete or inaccurate readings are most likely with arrhythmias and complex abnormalities. Therefore, computerized interpretation (including measurements of basic ECG intervals) should not be accepted without careful clinician review.

269e Atlas of Electrocardiography

Ary L. Goldberger

This is a digital-only chapter. It is available on the DVD that accompanies this book, as well as on Access Medicine/Harrison's Online, and the eBook and "app" editions of HPIM 19e.

The electrocardiograms (ECGs) in this atlas supplement those illustrated in Chap. 268. The interpretations emphasize findings of specific teaching value.

270e Noninvasive Cardiac Imaging: Echocardiography, Nuclear Cardiology, and Magnetic Resonance/Computed Tomography Imaging

Marcelo F. Di Carli, Raymond Y. Kwong, Scott D. Solomon

This is a digital-only chapter. It is available on the DVD that accompanies this book, as well as on Access Medicine/Harrison's Online, and the eBook and "app" editions of HPIM 19e.

The ability to image the heart and blood vessels noninvasively has been one of the greatest advances in cardiovascular medicine since the development of the electrocardiogram. Cardiac imaging complements history taking and physical examination, blood and laboratory testing, and exercise testing in the diagnosis and management of most diseases of the cardiovascular system. Modern cardiovascular imaging consists of echocardiography (cardiac ultrasound), nuclear scintigraphy including positron emission tomography (PET) imaging, magnetic resonance imaging (MRI), and computed tomography (CT). These studies, often used in conjunction with exercise testing, can be used independently or in concert depending on the specific diagnostic needs. In this chapter, we review the principles of each of these modalities and the utility and relative benefits of each for the most common cardiovascular diseases.

271e Atlas of Noninvasive Imaging

Marcelo F. Di Carli, Raymond Y. Kwong, Scott D. Solomon

This is a digital-only chapter. It is available on the DVD that accompanies this book, as well as on Access Medicine/Harrison's Online, and the eBook and "app" editions of HPIM 19e.

This chapter provides "movie" image clips as they are viewed in clinical practice, as well as additional static images. Noninvasive cardiac imaging is essential to the diagnosis and management of patients with known or suspected cardiovascular disease. This atlas supplements Chap. 270e, which describes the principles and clinical applications of these important techniques.

272 Diagnostic Cardiac Catheterization and Coronary Angiography

Jane A. Leopold, David P. Faxon

Diagnostic cardiac catheterization and coronary angiography are considered the gold standard in the assessment of the anatomy and physiology of the heart and its associated vasculature. In 1929, Forssmann demonstrated the feasibility of cardiac catheterization in humans when he passed a urological catheter from a vein in his arm to his right atrium and documented the catheter's position in the heart by x-ray. In the 1940s, Cournand and Richards applied this technique to patients with cardiovascular disease to evaluate cardiac function. These three physicians were awarded the Nobel Prize in 1956. In 1958, Sones inadvertently performed the first selective coronary angiography when a catheter in the left ventricle slipped back across the aortic valve, engaged the right coronary artery, and power-injected 40 mL of contrast down the vessel. The resulting angiogram provided superb anatomic detail of the artery, and the patient suffered no adverse effects. Sones went on to develop selective coronary catheters, which were modified further by Judkins, who developed preformed catheters and allowed coronary artery angiography to gain widespread use as a diagnostic tool. In the United States, cardiac catheterization is the second most common operative procedure, with more than one million procedures performed annually.

CARDIAC CATHETERIZATION

INDICATIONS, RISKS, AND PREPROCEDURE MANAGEMENT

Cardiac catheterization and coronary angiography are indicated to evaluate the extent and severity of cardiac disease in symptomatic patients and to determine if medical, surgical, or catheter-based interventions are warranted (Table 272-1). They are also used to exclude severe disease in symptomatic patients with equivocal findings on noninvasive studies and in patients with chest-pain syndromes of unclear etiology for whom a definitive diagnosis is necessary for management. Cardiac catheterization is not mandatory prior to cardiac surgery in some younger patients who have congenital or valvular heart disease that is well defined by noninvasive imaging and who do not have symptoms or risk factors that suggest concomitant coronary artery disease.

The risks associated with elective cardiac catheterization are relatively low, with a reported risk of 0.05% for myocardial infarction, 0.07% for stroke, and 0.08–0.14% for death. These risks increase substantially if the catheterization is performed emergently, during acute myocardial infarction or in hemodynamically unstable patients.

TABLE 272-1 INDICATIONS FOR CARDIAC CATHETERIZATION AND CORONARY ANGIOGRAPHY

Coronary Artery Disease
Asymptomatic or Symptomatic
High risk for adverse outcome based on noninvasive testing
Sudden cardiac death
Sustained (>30 s) monomorphic ventricular tachycardia
Nonsustained (<30 s) polymorphic ventricular tachycardia
Symptomatic
Canadian Cardiology Society Class II, III, or IV stable angina on medical therapy
Acute coronary syndrome (unstable angina and non-ST-segment elevation myocardial infarction)
Chest-pain syndrome of unclear etiology and equivocal findings on noninvasive tests
ST-Segment Elevation Acute Myocardial Infarction
Reperfusion with primary percutaneous coronary intervention
Persistent or recurrent ischemia
Pulmonary edema and/or reduced ejection fraction
Cardiogenic shock or hemodynamic instability
Risk stratification or positive stress test after acute myocardial infarction
Mechanical complications—mitral regurgitation, ventricular septal defect
Valvular Heart Disease
Suspected severe valve disease in symptomatic patients—dyspnea, angina, heart failure, syncope
Infective endocarditis with need for cardiac surgery
Asymptomatic patients with aortic regurgitation and cardiac enlargement or ↓ ejection fraction
Prior to cardiac surgery in patients with suspected coronary artery disease
Congestive Heart Failure
New onset with angina or suspected undiagnosed coronary artery disease
New-onset cardiomyopathy of uncertain cause or suspected to be due to coronary artery disease
Congenital Heart Disease
Prior to surgical correction, when symptoms or noninvasive testing suggests coronary disease
Suspicion for congenital coronary anomalies
Pericardial Disease
Symptomatic patients with suspected cardiac tamponade or constrictive pericarditis
Cardiac Transplantation
Preoperative and postsurgical evaluation
Other Conditions
Hypertrophic cardiomyopathy with angina
Diseases of the aorta when knowledge of coronary artery involvement is necessary for management

Additional risks of the procedure include tachy- or bradyarrhythmias that require countershock or pharmacologic therapy, acute renal failure leading to transient or permanent dialysis, vascular complications that necessitate surgical repair, and significant access-site bleeding. Of these risks, vascular access-site bleeding is the most common complication, occurring in 1.5–2.0% of patients, with major bleeding events associated with a worse short- and long-term outcome.

In patients who understand and accept the risks associated with cardiac catheterization, there are no absolute contraindications when the procedure is performed in anticipation of a life-saving intervention. Relative contraindications do, however, exist; these include decompensated congestive heart failure; acute renal failure; severe chronic renal insufficiency, unless dialysis is planned; bacteremia; acute stroke; active gastrointestinal bleeding; severe, uncorrected electrolyte abnormalities; a history of an anaphylactic/anaphylactoid reaction to iodinated contrast agents; and a history of allergy/bronchospasm to aspirin in patients for whom progression to a percutaneous coronary intervention is likely and aspirin desensitization has not been performed.

Contrast allergy and contrast-induced acute kidney injury merit further consideration, because these adverse events may occur in otherwise healthy individuals and prophylactic measures exist to reduce risk. Allergic reactions to contrast agents occur in <5% of cases, with severe anaphylactoid (clinically indistinguishable from anaphylaxis, but not mediated by an IgE mechanism) reactions occurring in 0.1%–0.2% of patients. Mild reactions manifest as nausea, vomiting, and urticaria, while severe anaphylactoid reactions lead to hypotensive shock, pulmonary edema, and cardiorespiratory arrest. Patients with a history of significant contrast allergy should be premedicated with corticosteroids and antihistamines (H_1- and H_2-blockers) and studies performed with nonionic, low-osmolar contrast agents that have a lower reported rate of allergic reactions.

Contrast-induced acute kidney injury, defined as an increase in creatinine >0.5 mg/dL or 25% above baseline that occurs 48–72 hours after contrast administration, occurs in ~2–7% of patients with rates of 20–30% reported in high-risk patients, including those with diabetes mellitus, congestive heart failure, chronic kidney disease, anemia, and older age. Dialysis is required in 0.3–0.7% of patients and is associated with a fivefold increase in in-hospital mortality. For all patients, adequate intravascular volume expansion with intravenous 0.9% saline (1.0–1.5 mL/kg per hour) for 3–12 hours before and continued 6–24 hours after the procedure limits the risk of contrast-induced acute kidney injury. Pretreatment with *N*-acetylcysteine (Mucomyst) has not reduced the risk of contrast-induced acute kidney injury consistently and, therefore, is no longer recommended routinely. Diabetic patients treated with metformin should stop the drug 48 hours prior to the procedure to limit the associated risk of lactic acidosis. Other strategies to decrease risk include the administration of sodium bicarbonate (3 mL/kg per hour) 1 hour before and 6 hours after the procedure; use of low- or iso-osmolar contrast agents; and limiting the volume of contrast to <100 mL per procedure.

Cardiac catheterization is performed after the patient has fasted for 6 hours and has received intravenous conscious sedation to remain awake but sedated during the procedure. All patients with suspected coronary artery disease are pretreated with 325 mg aspirin. In patients in whom the procedure is likely to progress to a percutaneous coronary intervention, an additional antiplatelet agent should be started: clopidogrel (600-mg loading dose and 75 mg daily) or prasugrel (60-mg loading dose and 10 mg daily), or ticagrelor (180-mg loading and 90 mg twice daily). Prasugrel should not be selected for individuals with prior stroke or transient ischemic attack. Warfarin is held starting 2–3 days prior to the catheterization to allow the international normalized ratio (INR) to fall to <1.7 and limit access site bleeding complications. Cardiac catheterization is a sterile procedure, so antibiotic prophylaxis is not required.

TECHNIQUE

Cardiac catheterization and coronary angiography provide a detailed hemodynamic and anatomic assessment of the heart and coronary arteries. The selection of procedures is dependent on the patient's symptoms and clinical condition, with some direction provided by noninvasive studies.

Vascular Access Cardiac catheterization procedures are performed using a percutaneous technique to enter the femoral artery and vein as the preferred access sites for left and right heart catheterization, respectively. A flexible sheath is inserted into the vessel over a guidewire, allowing diagnostic catheters to be introduced into the vessel and advanced toward the heart using fluoroscopic guidance. The radial artery (or brachial artery) may also be used as an arterial access site in patients, particularly those with peripheral arterial disease that involves the abdominal aorta, iliac, or femoral vessels; severe iliac artery tortuosity; morbid obesity; or preference for early postprocedure ambulation. Use of radial-artery access is gaining popularity due to a lower rate of access-site bleeding complications. A normal Allen's test confirming dual blood supply to the hand from the radial and ulnar arteries is recommended prior to access at this site. The internal jugular or antecubital veins serve as alternate access sites to the right heart when the patient has an inferior vena cava filter in place or requires prolonged hemodynamic monitoring.

Right Heart Catheterization This procedure measures pressures in the right heart. Right heart catheterization is no longer a routine part of diagnostic cardiac catheterization, but it is reasonable in patients with unexplained dyspnea, valvular heart disease, pericardial disease, right and/or left ventricular dysfunction, congenital heart disease, and suspected intracardiac shunts. Right heart catheterization uses a balloon-tipped flotation catheter that is advanced sequentially to the right atrium, right ventricle, pulmonary artery, and pulmonary wedge position (as a surrogate for left atrial pressure) using fluoroscopic guidance; in each cardiac chamber, pressure is measured and blood samples are obtained for oxygen saturation analysis to screen for intracardiac shunts.

Left Heart Catheterization This procedure measures pressures in the left heart as a determinant of left ventricular performance. With the aid of fluoroscopy, a catheter is guided to the ascending aorta and across the aortic valve into the left ventricle to provide a direct measure of left ventricular pressure. In patients with a tilting-disc prosthetic aortic valve, crossing the valve with a catheter is contraindicated, and the left heart may be accessed via a transseptal technique from the right atrium using a needle-tipped catheter to puncture the atrial septum at the fossa ovalis. Once the catheter crosses from the right to the left atrium, it can be advanced across the mitral valve to the left ventricle. This technique is also used for mitral valvuloplasty. Heparin is given for prolonged procedures to limit the risk of stroke from embolism of clots that may form on the catheter. For patients with heparin-induced thrombocytopenia, the direct thrombin inhibitors bivalirudin (0.75 mg/kg bolus, 1.75 mg/kg per hour for the duration of the procedure) or argatroban (350 μg/kg bolus, 15 μg/kg per minute for the duration of the procedure) may be used.

HEMODYNAMICS

A comprehensive hemodynamic assessment involves obtaining pressure measurements in the right and left heart and peripheral arterial system and determining the cardiac output (Table 272-2). The shape

TABLE 272-2 NORMAL VALUES FOR HEMODYNAMIC MEASUREMENTS

Pressures (mmHg)	
Right atrium	
Mean	0–5
a wave	1–7
v wave	1–7
Right ventricle	
Peak systolic/end diastolic	17–32/1–7
Pulmonary artery	
Peak systolic/end diastolic	17–32/1–7
Mean	9–19
Pulmonary capillary wedge (mean)	4–12
Left atrium	
Mean	4–12
a wave	4–15
v wave	4–15
Left ventricle	
Peak systolic/end diastolic	90–130/5–12
Aorta	
Peak systolic/end diastolic	90–130/60–85
Mean	70–100
(Resistances [dyn-s]/cm⁵)	
Systemic vascular resistance	900–1400
Pulmonary vascular resistance	40–120
Oxygen Consumption Index ([L-min]/m²)	115–140
Arteriovenous oxygen difference (vol %)	3.5–4.8
Cardiac index ([L-min]/m²)	2.8–4.2

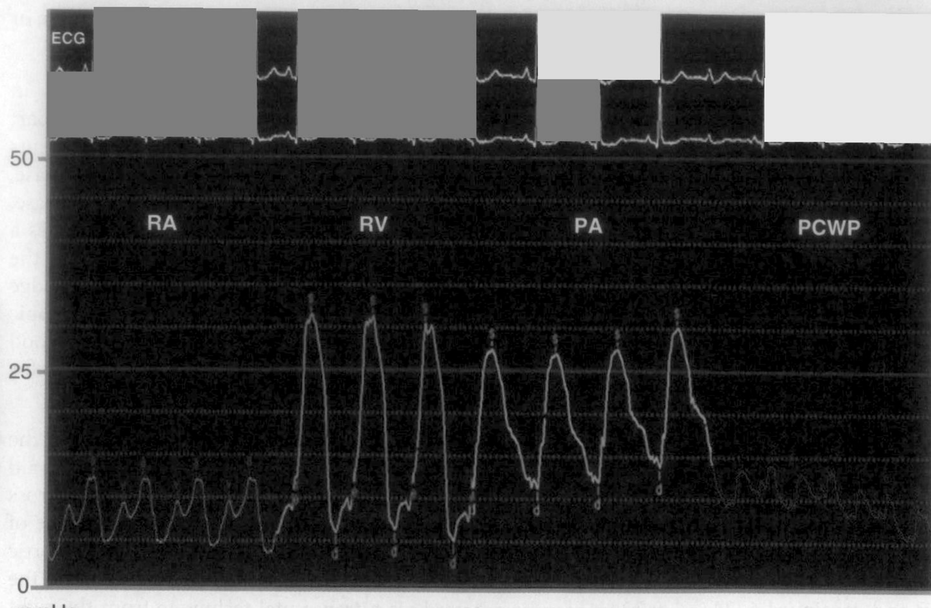

FIGURE 272-1 Normal hemodynamic waveforms recorded during right heart catheterization. Atrial pressure tracings have a characteristic "*a*" wave that reflects atrial contraction and a "*v*" wave that reflects pressure changes in the atrium during ventricular systole. Ventricular pressure tracings have a low-pressure diastolic filling period and a sharp rise in pressure that occurs during ventricular systole. d, diastole; PA, pulmonary artery; PCWP, pulmonary capillary wedge pressure; RA, right atrium; RV, right ventricle; s, systole.

and magnitude of the pressure waveforms provide important diagnostic information; an example of normal pressure tracings is shown in Fig. 272-1. In the absence of valvular heart disease, the atria and ventricles are "one chamber" during diastole when the tricuspid and mitral valves are open while in systole, when the pulmonary and aortic valves are open, the ventricles and their respective outflow tracts are considered "one chamber." These concepts form the basis by which hemodynamic measurements are used to assess valvular stenosis. When aortic stenosis is present, there is a systolic pressure gradient between the left ventricle and the aorta; when mitral stenosis is present, there is a diastolic pressure gradient between the pulmonary capillary wedge (left atrial) pressure and the left ventricle (Fig. 272-2). Hemodynamic measurements also discriminate between aortic stenosis and hypertrophic obstructive cardiomyopathy where the asymmetrically hypertrophied septum creates a dynamic intraventricular pressure gradient during ventricular systole. The magnitude of this obstruction is measured using an end-hole catheter positioned at the left ventricular apex that is pulled back while recording pressure; once the catheter has passed the septal obstruction and is positioned in the apex of the left ventricle, a gradient can be measured between the left ventricular apex and the aorta. Hypertrophic obstructive cardiomyopathy is confirmed by the Brockenbrough-Braunwald sign: following a premature ventricular contraction, there is an increase in the left ventricular–aorta pressure gradient with a simultaneous decrease in the aortic pulse pressure. These findings are absent in aortic stenosis.

Regurgitant valvular lesions increase volume (and pressure) in the "receiving" cardiac chamber. In severe mitral and tricuspid regurgitation, the increase in blood flow to the atria takes place during ventricular systole, leading to an increase in the *v* wave (two times greater than the mean pressure). Severe aortic regurgitation leads to a decrease in aortic diastolic pressure with a concomitant rise in left ventricular end-diastolic pressure, resulting in equalization of pressures between the two chambers at end-diastole.

Hemodynamic measurements are also used to differentiate between cardiac tamponade, constrictive pericarditis, and restrictive cardiomyopathy (Table 272-3). In cardiac tamponade, right atrial pressure is increased with a decreased or absent "y" descent, indicative of impaired right atrial emptying in diastole, and there is diastolic equalization of pressures in all cardiac chambers. In constrictive pericarditis, right atrial pressure is elevated with a prominent "y" descent, indicating rapid filling of the right ventricle during early diastole. A diastolic dip and plateau or "square root sign," in the ventricular waveforms due to an abrupt halt in ventricular filling during diastole; right ventricular and pulmonary artery pressures are elevated; and discordant pressure changes in the right and left ventricles with inspiration (right ventricular systolic pressure increases while left ventricular systolic pressure decreases) are observed. The latter hemodynamic phenomenon is the most specific for constriction. Restrictive cardiomyopathy may be distinguished from constrictive pericarditis by a marked increase in right ventricular and pulmonary artery systolic pressures (usually >60 mmHg), a separation of the left and right ventricular diastolic pressures by >5 mmHg (at baseline or with acute volume loading), and concordant changes in left and right ventricular diastolic filling pressures with inspiration (both increase).

Cardiac Output Cardiac output is measured by the Fick method or the thermodilution technique. Typically, the Fick method and thermodilution technique are both performed during cardiac catheterization, although the Fick method is considered more reliable in the presence of tricuspid regurgitation and in low-output states. The Fick method

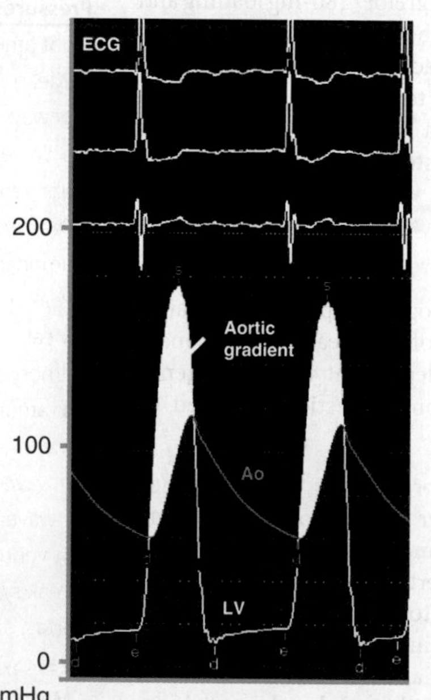

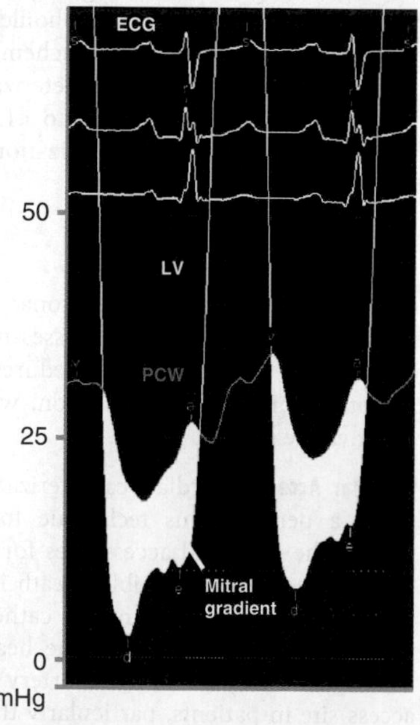

FIGURE 272-2 Severe aortic and mitral stenosis. Simultaneous recording of left ventricular (LV) and aortic (Ao) pressure tracings demonstrates a 62-mmHg mean systolic gradient (*shaded area*) that corresponds to an aortic valve area of 0.6 cm^2 (*left*). Simultaneous recording of LV and pulmonary capillary wedge (PCW) pressure tracings reveals a 14-mmHg mean diastolic gradient (*shaded area*) that is consistent with critical mitral stenosis (mitral valve area = 0.5 cm^2). d, diastole; e, end diastole; s, systole.

TABLE 272-3 HEMODYNAMIC FINDINGS IN TAMPONADE, CONSTRICTIVE PERICARDITIS, AND RESTRICTIVE CARDIOMYOPATHY

	Cardiac Tamponade	Constrictive Pericarditis	Effusive-Constrictive Pericarditis	Restrictive Cardiomyopathy
Pericardial pressure	↑	↑	↑	Normal
Right atrium pressure	↑	↑	↑ (Fails to decrease by 50% or to <10 mmHg after pericardiocentesis)	↑
Right atrium pressure waveform	Prominent "x" descent	Prominent "x" descent	Prominent "x" descent	Prominent "y" descent
	Diminished or absent "y" descent	Prominent "y" descent	"y" descent less prominent than expected	
Right ventricle systolic pressure	<50 mmHg	<50 mmHg	<50 mmHg	>60 mmHg
Right ventricle end-diastolic pressure		>1/3 right ventricular systolic pressure	>1/3 right ventricular systolic pressure	<1/3 right ventricular systolic pressure
	Equals left ventricular end-diastolic pressure within 5 mmHg	Equals left ventricular end-diastolic pressure within 5 mmHg	Equals left ventricular end-diastolic pressure within 5 mmHg	Less than left ventricular end-diastolic pressure by ≥5 mmHg
Right ventricle pressure waveform		Dip and plateau or "square root" sign	Dip and plateau or "square root" sign	Dip and plateau or "square root" sign
Right ventricle–left ventricle systolic pressure relationship with inspiration	Discordant	Discordant	Discordant	Concordant

uses oxygen as the indicator substance and is based on the principle that the amount of a substance taken up or released by an organ (oxygen consumption) is equal to the product of its blood flow (cardiac output) and the difference in the concentration of the substance in the arterial and venous circulation (arterial-venous oxygen difference). Thus, the formula for calculating the Fick cardiac output is:

Cardiac output (L/min) = (oxygen consumption [mL/min])/(arterial-venous oxygen difference [mL/L])

Oxygen consumption is estimated as 125 mL oxygen/minute × body surface area, and the arterial venous oxygen difference is determined by first calculating the oxygen carrying capacity of blood (hemoglobin [g/100 mL] × 1.36 [mL oxygen/g hemoglobin] × 10) and multiplying this product by the fractional oxygen saturation. The thermodilution method measures a substance that is injected into and adequately mixes with blood. In contemporary practice, thermodilution cardiac outputs are measured using temperature as the indicator. Measurements are made with a thermistor-tipped catheter that detects temperature deviations in the pulmonary artery after the injection of 10 mL of room-temperature normal saline into the right atrium.

Vascular Resistance Resistance across the systemic and pulmonary circulations is calculated by extrapolating from Ohm's law of electrical resistance and is equal to the mean pressure gradient divided by the mean flow (cardiac output). Therefore, systemic vascular resistance is ([mean aortic pressure – mean right atrial pressure]/cardiac output) multiplied by 80 to convert the resistance from Wood units to dyn-s-cm^{-5}. Similarly, the pulmonary vascular resistance is ([mean pulmonary artery – mean pulmonary capillary wedge pressure]/cardiac output) × 80. Pulmonary vascular resistance is lowered by oxygen, nitroprusside, calcium channel blockers, prostacyclin infusions, and inhaled nitric oxide; these therapies may be administered during catheterization to determine if increased pulmonary vascular resistance is fixed or reversible.

Valve Area Hemodynamic data may also be used to calculate the valve area using the Gorlin formula that equates the area to the flow across the valve divided by the pressure gradient between the cardiac chambers surrounding the valve. The formula for the assessment of valve area is: Area = (cardiac output [cm^3/min]/[systolic ejection period or diastolic filling period][heart rate])/44.3 C × square root of the pressure gradient, where C = 1 for aortic valve and 0.85 for the mitral valve. A valve area of <1.0 cm^2 and a mean gradient of greater than 40 mmHg indicate severe aortic stenosis, while a valve area of <1.5 cm^2 and a mean gradient >5–10 mmHg is consistent with moderate-to-severe mitral stenosis; in symptomatic patients with a mitral valve area >1.5 cm^2, a mean gradient >15 mmHg, pulmonary artery pressure >60 mmHg, or a pulmonary artery wedge pressure >25 mmHg after exercise is also considered significant and may warrant intervention. The modified Hakki formula has also been used to estimate aortic valve area. This formula calculates the valve area as the cardiac output (L/min) divided by the square root of the pressure gradient. Aortic valve area calculations based on the Gorlin formula are flow-dependent and, therefore, for patients with low cardiac outputs, it is imperative to determine if a decreased valve area actually reflects a fixed stenosis or is overestimated by a low cardiac output and stroke volume that is insufficient to open the valve leaflets fully. In these instances, cautious hemodynamic manipulation using dobutamine to increase the cardiac output and recalculation of the aortic valve area may be necessary.

Intracardiac Shunts In patients with congenital heart disease, detection, localization, and quantification of the intracardiac shunt should be evaluated. A shunt should be suspected when there is unexplained arterial desaturation or increased oxygen saturation of venous blood. A "step up" or increase in oxygen content indicates the presence of a left-to-right shunt while a "step down" indicates a right-to-left shunt. The shunt is localized by detecting a difference in oxygen saturation levels of 5–7% between adjacent cardiac chambers. The severity of the shunt is determined by the ratio of pulmonary blood flow (Q_p) to the systemic blood flow (Q_s), or Q_p/Q_s = ([systemic arterial oxygen content – mixed venous oxygen content]/pulmonary vein oxygen content – pulmonary artery oxygen content). For an atrial septal defect, a shunt ratio of 1.5 is considered significant and factored with other clinical variables to determine the need for intervention. When a congenital ventricular septal defect is present, a shunt ratio of ≥2.0 with evidence of left ventricular volume overload is a strong indication for surgical correction.

VENTRICULOGRAPHY AND AORTOGRAPHY

Ventriculography to assess left ventricular function may be performed during cardiac catheterization. A pigtail catheter is advanced retrograde across the aortic valve into the left ventricle and 30–45 mL of contrast is power-injected to visualize the left ventricular chamber during the cardiac cycle. The ventriculogram is usually performed in the right anterior oblique projection to examine wall motion and mitral valve function. Normal wall motion is observed as symmetric contraction of all segments; hypokinetic segments have decreased contraction, akinetic segments do not contract, and dyskinetic segments appear to bulge paradoxically during systole (Fig. 272-3). Ventriculography may also reveal a left ventricular aneurysm, pseudoaneurysm, or diverticulum and can be used to assess mitral valve prolapse and the severity of mitral regurgitation. The degree of mitral regurgitation is estimated

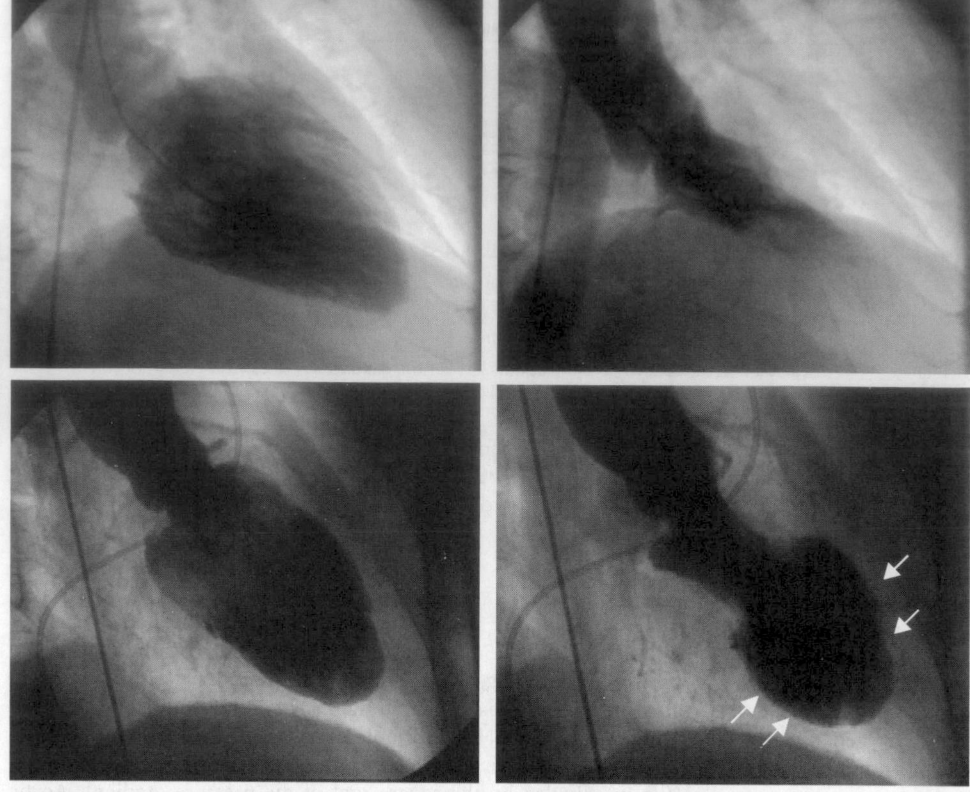

FIGURE 272-3 Left ventriculogram at end diastole (*left*) and end systole (*right*). In patients with normal left ventricular function, the ventriculogram reveals symmetric contraction of all walls (*top*). Patients with coronary artery disease may have wall motion abnormalities on ventriculography as seen in this 60-year-old male following a large anterior myocardial infarction. In systole, the anterior, apical, and inferior walls are akinetic (*white arrows*) (*bottom*).

lumina. Aortography can also be used to identify patent saphenous vein grafts that elude selective cannulation, identify shunts that involve the aorta such as a patent ductus arteriosus, and provide a qualitative assessment of aortic regurgitation using a 1+–4+ scale similar to that used for mitral regurgitation.

CORONARY ANGIOGRAPHY

Selective coronary angiography is almost always performed during cardiac catheterization and is used to define the coronary anatomy and determine the extent of epicardial coronary artery and coronary artery bypass graft disease. Specially shaped coronary catheters are used to engage the left and right coronary ostia. Hand injection of radiopaque contrast agents creates a coronary "luminogram" that is recorded as radiographic images (cine angiography). Because the coronary arteries are three-dimensional objects that are in motion with the cardiac cycle, angiograms of the vessels using several different orthogonal projections are taken to best visualize the vessels without overlap or foreshortening.

The normal coronary anatomy is highly variable between individuals, but, in general, there are two coronary ostia and three major coronary vessels—the left anterior descending, the left circumflex, and the right coronary arteries with the left anterior descending and left circumflex arteries arising from the left main coronary artery (Fig. 272-4). When the right coronary artery is the origin of the atrioventricular nodal branch, the posterior descending artery, and the posterior lateral vessels, the circulation is defined as right dominant; this is found in ~85% of individuals. When these branches arise from the left circumflex artery as occurs in ~5% of individuals, the circulation is defined as left dominant. The remaining ~10% of patients have a codominant circulation with vessels arising from both the right and left coronary circulation. In some patients, a ramus intermedius branch arises directly from the left main coronary artery; this finding is a normal variant. Coronary artery anomalies occur in 1–2% of patients, with separate ostia for the left anterior descending and left circumflex arteries being the most common (0.41%).

by comparing the density of contrast opacification of the left atrium with that of the left ventricle. Minimal contrast reflux into the left atrium is considered 1+ mitral regurgitation, while contrast density in the left atrium that is greater than that in the left ventricle with reflux of contrast into the pulmonary veins within three beats defines 4+ mitral regurgitation. Ventriculography performed in the left anterior oblique projection can be used to identify a ventricular septal defect. Calculation of the ventricular volumes in systole and diastole allows calculation of stroke volume and cardiac output.

Aortography in the cardiac catheterization laboratory visualizes abnormalities of the ascending aorta, including aneurysmal dilation and involvement of the great vessels, as well as dissection with compression of the true lumen by an intimal flap that separates the true and false

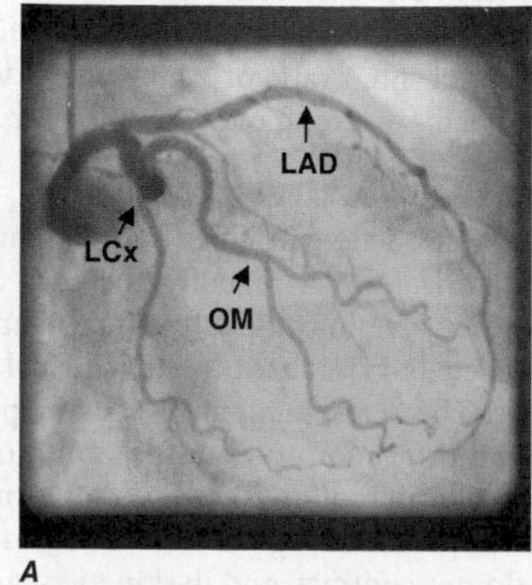

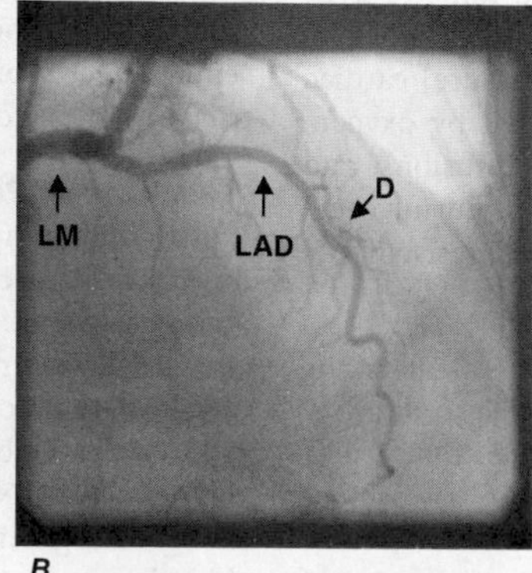

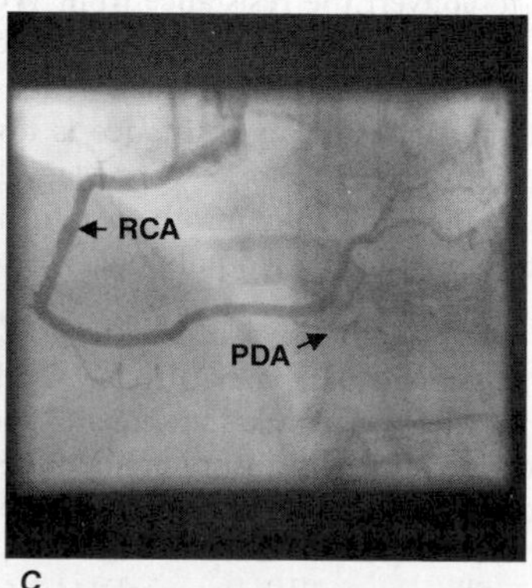

FIGURE 272-4 Normal coronary artery anatomy. ***A.*** Coronary angiogram showing the left circumflex (LCx) artery and its obtuse marginal (OM) branches. The left anterior descending artery (LAD) is also seen but may be foreshortened in this view. ***B.*** The LAD and its diagonal (D) branches are best seen in cranial views. In this angiogram, the left main (LM) coronary artery is also seen. ***C.*** The right coronary artery (RCA) gives off the posterior descending artery (PDA), so this is a right dominant circulation.

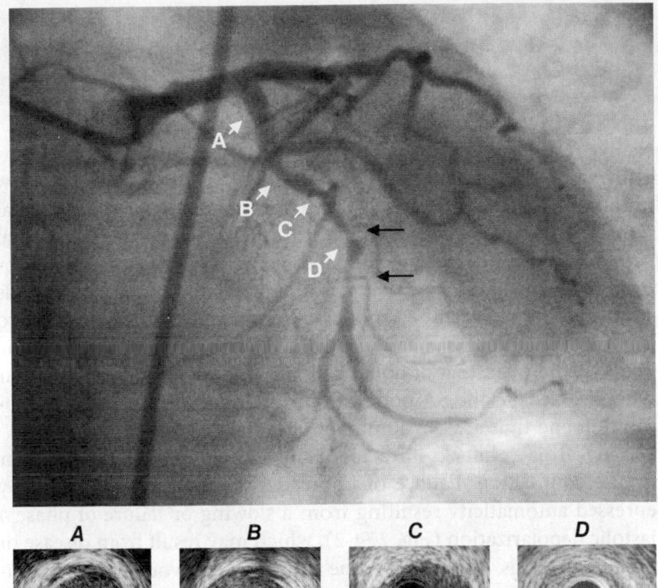

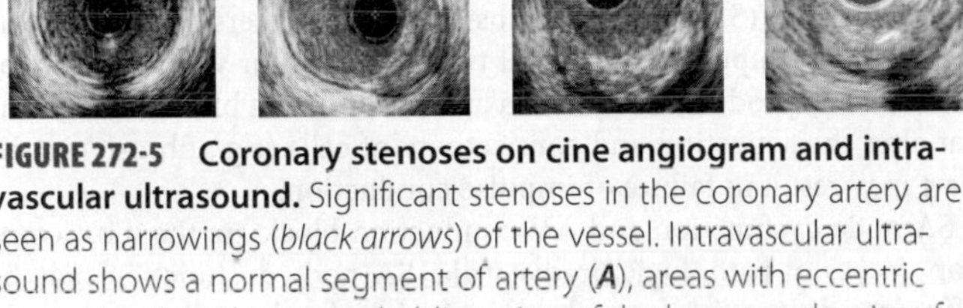

FIGURE 272-5 Coronary stenoses on cine angiogram and intravascular ultrasound. Significant stenoses in the coronary artery are seen as narrowings (*black arrows*) of the vessel. Intravascular ultrasound shows a normal segment of artery (*A*), areas with eccentric plaque (*B, C*), and near total obliteration of the lumen at the site of the significant stenosis (*D*). Note that the intravascular ultrasound catheter is present in the images as a black circle.

Coronary angiography visualizes coronary artery stenoses as luminal narrowings on the cine angiogram. The degree of narrowing is referred to as the percent stenosis and is determined visually by comparing the most severely diseased segment with a proximal or distal "normal segment"; a stenosis >50% is considered significant (Fig. 272-5). Online quantitative coronary angiography can provide a more accurate assessment of the percent stenosis and lessen the tendency to overestimate lesion severity visually. The presence of a myocardial bridge, which most commonly involves the left anterior descending artery, may be mistaken for a significant stenosis; this occurs when a portion of the vessel dips below the epicardial surface into the myocardium and is subject to compressive forces during ventricular systole. The key to differentiating a myocardial bridge from a fixed stenosis is that the "stenosed" part of the vessel returns to normal during diastole. Coronary calcification is also seen during angiography prior to the injection of contrast agents. Collateral blood vessels may be seen traversing from one vessel to the distal vasculature of a severely stenosed or totally occluded vessel. Thrombolysis in myocardial infarction (TIMI) flow grade, a measure of the relative duration of time that it takes for contrast to opacify the coronary artery fully, may provide an additional clue to the degree of lesion severity, and the presence of TIMI grade 1 (minimal filling) or 2 (delayed filling) suggests that a significant coronary artery stenosis is present.

INTRAVASCULAR ULTRASOUND, OPTICAL COHERENCE TOMOGRAPHY, AND FRACTIONAL FLOW RESERVE

During coronary angiography, intermediate stenoses (40–70%), indeterminate findings, or anatomic findings that are incongruous with the patient's symptoms may require further interrogation. In these cases, intravascular ultrasound provides a more accurate anatomic assessment of the coronary artery and the degree of coronary atherosclerosis (Fig. 272-5). Intravascular ultrasound (IVUS) is performed using a small flexible catheter with a 40-mHz transducer at its tip that is advanced into the coronary artery over a guidewire. Data from intravascular ultrasound studies may be used to image atherosclerotic plaque precisely, determine luminal cross-sectional area, and measure vessel size; it is also used during or following percutaneous coronary intervention to assess the stenosis and determine the adequacy of stent placement. Optical coherence tomography (OCT) is a catheter-based imaging technique that uses near-infrared light to generate images with better spatial resolution than IVUS; however, the depth of field is smaller. The advantage of OCT imaging over IVUS lies in its ability to image characteristics of the atherosclerotic plaque (lipid, fibrous cap) with high definition and to assess coronary stent placement, apposition, and patency (Fig. 272-6).

Measurement of the fractional flow reserve provides a functional assessment of the stenosis and is more accurate in predicting long-term clinical outcome than imaging techniques. The fractional flow reserve is the ratio of the pressure in the coronary artery distal to the stenosis divided by the pressure in the artery proximal to the stenosis at maximal vasodilation. Fractional flow reserve is measured using a coronary pressure–sensor guidewire at rest and at maximal hyperemia following the injection of adenosine. A fractional flow reserve of <0.80 indicates a hemodynamically significant stenosis that would benefit from intervention.

POSTPROCEDURE CARE

Once the procedure is completed, vascular access sheaths are removed. If the femoral approach is used, direct manual compression or vascular closure devices that immediately close the arteriotomy site with a staple/clip, collagen plug, or sutures are used to achieve hemostasis. These devices decrease the length of supine bed rest (from 6 hours to 2–4 hours) and improve patient satisfaction but have not been shown definitively to be superior to manual compression with respect to access-site complications. With radial-artery access, bed rest is needed for only 2 hours. When cardiac catheterization is performed as an elective outpatient procedure, the patient completes postprocedure bed rest in a monitored setting and is discharged home with instructions to liberalize fluids because contrast agents promote an osmotic diuresis, to avoid strenuous activity, and to observe the vascular access site for signs of complications. Overnight hospitalization may be required for high-risk patients with significant comorbidities, patients with complications occurring during the catheterization, or patients who have undergone a percutaneous coronary intervention. Hypotension early after the procedure may be due to inadequate fluid replacement or retroperitoneal bleeding from the access site. Patients who received >2 Gy of radiation during the procedure should be examined for signs of erythema. For patients who received higher doses (>5 Gy), clinical follow-up within 1 month to assess for skin injury is recommended.

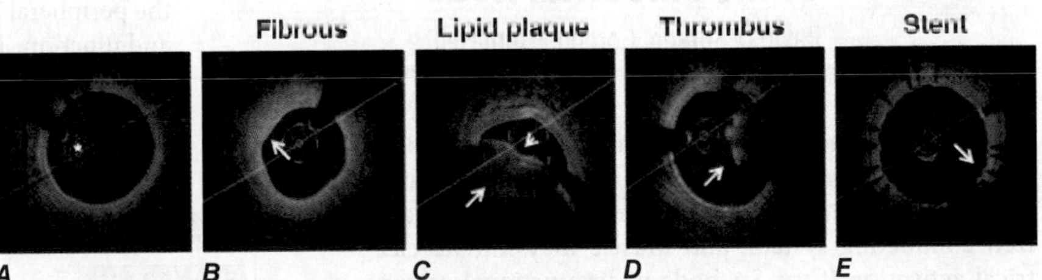

FIGURE 272-6 Optical coherence tomography imaging. ***A.*** The optical coherence tomography (OCT) catheter (*) in the lumen of a coronary artery with limited neointima formation. The intima is seen with high definition, but unlike intravascular ultrasound imaging, the vessel media and adventitia are not well visualized. ***B.*** A fibrous plaque (*arrow*) is characterized by a bright signal. ***C.*** A large, eccentric, lipid-rich plaque obscures part of the vessel lumen. Because lipid in the plaque absorbs light, the lipid-rich plaque appears as a dark area with irregular borders (*arrow*). The plaque is covered by a thin fibrous cap (*arrowhead*) typical of a vulnerable plaque. ***D.*** A thrombus (*arrow*) adherent to a ruptured plaque that is protruding into the vessel lumen. ***E.*** A coronary stent is that is well opposed to the vessel wall. The stent struts appear as short bright lines with dropout behind the struts (*arrow*).

273e Principles of Electrophysiology

David D. Spragg, Gordon F. Tomaselli

This is a digital-only chapter. It is available on the DVD that accompanies this book, as well as on Access Medicine/Harrison's Online, and the eBook and "app" editions of HPIM 19e.

HISTORY AND INTRODUCTION

The field of cardiac electrophysiology was ushered in with the development of the electrocardiogram (ECG) by Einthoven at the turn of the twentieth century. Subsequent recording of cellular membrane currents demonstrated that the body surface ECG is the timed sum of the cellular action potentials in the atria and ventricles. In the late 1960s, the development of intracavitary recording, in particular His bundle electrograms, marked the beginning of contemporary clinical electrophysiology. Adoption of radiofrequency technology to ablate cardiac tissue in the early 1990s heralded the birth of interventional cardiac electrophysiology.

The clinical problem of sudden death caused by ventricular arrhythmias, most commonly in the setting of coronary artery obstruction, was recognized as early as the late nineteenth century. The problem was vexing and led to the development of pharmacologic and nonpharmacologic therapies, including transthoracic defibrillators, cardiac massage, and, most recently, implantable defibrillators. Over time the limitations of antiarrhythmic drug therapy have been highlighted repeatedly in clinical trials, and now ablation and devices are first-line therapy for a number of cardiac arrhythmias.

In the last two decades, the genetic basis of a number of heritable arrhythmias has been elucidated, revealing important insights into the mechanisms not only of these rare arrhythmias but also of similar rhythm disturbances observed in more common forms of heart disease.

274 The Bradyarrhythmias: Disorders of the Sinoatrial Node

David D. Spragg, Gordon F. Tomaselli

Electrical activation of the heart normally originates in the sinoatrial (SA) node, the predominant pacemaker. Other subsidiary pacemakers in the atrioventricular (AV) node, specialized conducting system, and muscle may initiate electrical activation if the SA node is dysfunctional or suppressed. Typically, subsidiary pacemakers discharge at a slower rate and, in the absence of an appropriate increase in stroke volume, may result in tissue hypoperfusion.

Spontaneous activation and contraction of the heart are a consequence of the specialized pacemaking tissue in these anatomic locales. As described in Chap. 273e, action potentials in the heart are regionally heterogeneous. The action potentials in cells isolated from nodal tissue are distinct from those recorded from atrial and ventricular myocytes (Fig. 274-1). The complement of ionic currents present in nodal cells results in a less negative resting membrane potential compared with atrial or ventricular myocytes. Electrical diastole in nodal cells is characterized by slow diastolic depolarization (phase 4), which generates an action potential as the membrane voltage reaches threshold. The action potential upstrokes (phase 0) are slow compared with atrial or ventricular myocytes, being mediated by calcium rather than sodium current. Cells with properties of SA and AV nodal tissue are electrically connected to the remainder of the myocardium by cells with an electrophysiologic phenotype between that of nodal cells and that of atrial or ventricular myocytes. Cells in the SA node exhibit the most rapid phase 4 depolarization and thus are the dominant pacemakers in a normal heart.

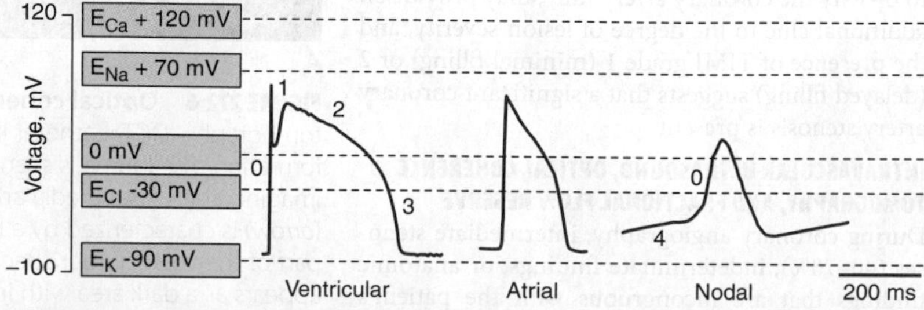

FIGURE 274-1 Action potential profiles recorded in cells isolated from sinoatrial or atrioventricular nodal tissue compared with those of cells from atrial or ventricular myocardium. Nodal cell action potentials exhibit more depolarized resting membrane potentials, slower phase 0 upstrokes, and phase 4 diastolic depolarization.

Bradycardia results from a failure of either impulse initiation or impulse conduction. Failure of impulse initiation may be caused by depressed automaticity resulting from a slowing or failure of phase 4 diastolic depolarization (Fig. 274-2), which may result from disease or exposure to drugs. Prominently, the autonomic nervous system modulates the rate of phase 4 diastolic depolarization and thus the firing rate of both primary (SA node) and subsidiary pacemakers. Failure of conduction of an impulse from nodal tissue to atrial or ventricular myocardium may produce bradycardia as a result of exit block. Conditions that alter the activation and connectivity of cells (e.g., fibrosis) in the heart may result in failure of impulse conduction.

SA node dysfunction and AV conduction block are the most common causes of pathologic bradycardia. SA node dysfunction may be difficult to distinguish from physiologic sinus bradycardia, particularly in the young. SA node dysfunction increases in frequency between the fifth and sixth decades of life and should be considered in patients with fatigue, exercise intolerance, or syncope and sinus bradycardia.

Permanent pacemaking is the only reliable therapy for symptomatic bradycardia in the absence of extrinsic and reversible etiologies such as increased vagal tone, hypoxia, hypothermia, and drugs (Table 274-1). Approximately 50% of the 150,000 permanent pacemakers implanted in the United States and 20–30% of the 150,000 of those in Europe were implanted for SA node disease.

STRUCTURE AND PHYSIOLOGY OF THE SA NODE

The SA node is composed of a cluster of small fusiform cells in the sulcus terminalis on the epicardial surface of the heart at the right atrial–superior vena caval junction, where they envelop the SA nodal artery. The SA node is structurally heterogeneous, but the central prototypic nodal cells have fewer distinct myofibrils than does the surrounding atrial myocardium, no intercalated disks visible on light microscopy, a poorly developed sarcoplasmic reticulum, and no T-tubules. Cells in the peripheral regions of the SA node are transitional in both structure and function. The SA nodal artery arises from the right coronary artery in 55–60% and the left circumflex artery in 40–45% of persons. The SA node is richly innervated by sympathetic and parasympathetic nerves and ganglia.

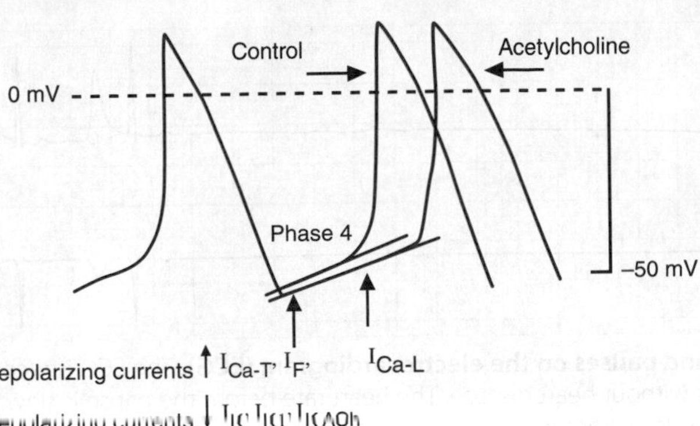

FIGURE 274-2 Schematics of nodal action potentials and the currents that contribute to phase 4 depolarization. Relative increases in depolarizing L- (I_{Ca-L}) and T- (I_{Ca-T}) type calcium and pacemaker currents (I_f) along with a reduction in repolarizing inward rectifier (I_{K1}) and delayed rectifier (I_K) potassium currents result in depolarization. Activation of ACh-gated (I_{KACh}) potassium current and beta blockade slow the rate of phase 4 and decrease the pacing rate. *(Modified from J Jalife et al: Basic Cardiac Electrophysiology for the Clinician, Blackwell Publishing, 1999.)*

Irregular and slow propagation of impulses from the SA node can be explained by the electrophysiology of nodal cells and the structure of the SA node itself. The action potentials of SA nodal cells are characterized by a relatively depolarized membrane potential (Fig. 274-1) of –40 to –60 mV, slow phase 0 upstroke, and relatively rapid phase 4 diastolic depolarization compared with the action potentials recorded in cardiac muscle cells. The relative absence of inward rectifier potassium current (I_{K1}) accounts for the depolarized membrane potential; the slow upstroke of phase 0 results from the absence of available fast sodium current (I_{Na}) and is mediated by L-type calcium current (I_{Ca-L}); and phase 4 depolarization is a result of the aggregate activity of a number of ionic currents. Prominently, both L- and T-type (I_{Ca-T}) calcium currents, the pacemaker current (so-called funny current, or I_f) formed by hyperpolarization-activated cyclic nucleotide-gated channels, and the electrogenic sodium-calcium exchanger provide depolarizing current that is antagonized by delayed rectifier (I_{Kr}) and acetylcholine-gated (I_{KACh}) potassium currents. I_{Ca-L}, I_{Ca-T}, and I_f are modulated by β-adrenergic stimulation and I_{KACh} by vagal stimulation, explaining the exquisite sensitivity of diastolic depolarization to autonomic nervous system activity. The slow conduction within the SA node is explained by the absence of I_{Na} and poor electrical coupling of cells in the node, resulting from sizable amounts of interstitial tissue and a low abundance of gap junctions. The poor coupling allows for graded electrophysiologic properties within the node, with the peripheral transitional cells being silenced by electrotonic coupling to atrial myocardium.

TABLE 274-1 ETIOLOGIES OF SA NODE DYSFUNCTION

Extrinsic	Intrinsic
Autonomic	Sick-sinus syndrome (SSS)
Carotid sinus hypersensitivity	Coronary artery disease (chronic and acute MI)
Vasovagal (cardioinhibitory) stimulation	Inflammatory
Drugs	Pericarditis
Beta blockers	Myocarditis (including viral)
Calcium channel blockers	Rheumatic heart disease
Digoxin	Collagen vascular diseases
Ivabradine	Lyme disease
Antiarrhythmics (class I and III)	Senile amyloidosis
Adenosine	Congenital heart disease
Clonidine (other sympatholytics)	TGA/Mustard and Fontan repairs
Lithium carbonate	Iatrogenic
Cimetidine	Radiation therapy
Amitriptyline	Postsurgical
Phenothiazines	Chest trauma
Narcotics (methadone)	Familial
Pentamidine	SSS2, AD, OMIM #163800 (15q24-25)
Hypothyroidism	SSS1, AR OMIM #608567 (3p21)
Sleep apnea	SSS3, AD, OMIM #614090 (14q11.2)
Hypoxia	SA node disease with myopia, OMIM #182190
Endotracheal suctioning (vagal maneuvers)	Kearns-Sayre syndrome, OMIM #530000
Hypothermia	Myotonic dystrophy
Increased intracranial pressure	Type 1, OMIM #160900 (19q13.2-13.3)
	Type 2, OMIM #602668 (3q13.3-q24)
	Friedreich's ataxia, OMIM #229300 (9q13, 9p23-p11)

Abbreviations: AD, autosomal dominant; AR, autosomal recessive; MI, myocardial infarction; OMIM, Online Mendelian Inheritance in Man (database); TGA, transposition of the great arteries.

ETIOLOGY OF SA NODAL DISEASE

SA nodal dysfunction has been classified as intrinsic or extrinsic. The distinction is important because extrinsic dysfunction is often reversible and generally should be corrected before pacemaker therapy is considered (Table 274-1). The most common causes of extrinsic SA node dysfunction are drugs and autonomic nervous system influences that suppress automaticity and/or compromise conduction. Other extrinsic causes include hypothyroidism, sleep apnea, and conditions likely to occur in critically ill patients such as hypothermia, hypoxia, increased intracranial pressure (Cushing's response), and endotracheal suctioning via activation of the vagus nerve.

Intrinsic sinus node dysfunction is degenerative and often is characterized pathologically by fibrous replacement of the SA node or its connections to the atrium. Acute and chronic coronary artery disease (CAD) may be associated with SA node dysfunction, although in the setting of acute myocardial infarction (MI; typically inferior), the abnormalities are transient. Inflammatory processes may alter SA node function, ultimately producing replacement fibrosis. Pericarditis, myocarditis, and rheumatic heart disease have been associated with SA nodal disease with sinus bradycardia, sinus arrest, and exit block. Carditis associated with systemic lupus erythematosus (SLE), rheumatoid arthritis (RA), and mixed connective tissue disorders (MCTDs) may also affect SA node structure and function. Senile amyloidosis is an infiltrative disorder in patients typically in the ninth decade of life; deposition of amyloid protein in the atrial myocardium can impair SA node function. Some SA node disease is iatrogenic and results from direct injury to the SA node during cardiothoracic surgery.

Rare heritable forms of sinus node disease have been described, and several have been characterized genetically. Autosomal dominant sinus node dysfunction in conjunction with supraventricular tachycardia (i.e., tachycardia-bradycardia variant of sick-sinus syndrome [SSS2]) has been linked to mutations in the pacemaker current (I_f) subunit gene *HCN4* on chromosome 15. An autosomal recessive form of SSS1 with the prominent feature of atrial inexcitability and absence of P waves on the electrocardiogram (ECG) is caused by mutations in the cardiac sodium channel gene, *SCN5A*, on chromosome 3. Variants in myosin heavy chain 6 (*MYH6*) increase the susceptibility to SSS (SSS3). SA node dysfunction associated with myopia has been described but not genetically characterized. There are several neuromuscular diseases, including Kearns-Sayre syndrome (ophthalmoplegia, pigmentary degeneration of the retina, and cardiomyopathy) and myotonic dystrophy, that have a predilection for the conducting system and SA node.

SSS in both the young and the elderly is associated with an increase in fibrous tissue in the SA node. The onset of SSS may be hastened by coexisting disease, such as CAD, diabetes mellitus, hypertension, and valvular diseases and cardiomyopathies.

CLINICAL FEATURES OF SA NODE DISEASE

SA node dysfunction may be completely asymptomatic and manifest as an ECG anomaly such as sinus bradycardia; sinus arrest and exit block; or alternating supraventricular tachycardia, usually atrial fibrillation, and bradycardia. Symptoms associated with SA node dysfunction, in particular tachycardia-bradycardia syndrome, may be related to both slow and fast heart rates. For example, tachycardia may be associated with palpitations, angina pectoris, and heart failure, and bradycardia may be associated with hypotension, syncope, presyncope, fatigue, and weakness. In the setting of SSS, overdrive suppression of the SA node may result in prolonged pauses and syncope upon termination of the tachycardia. In many cases, symptoms associated with SA node dysfunction result from concomitant cardiovascular disease. A significant minority of patients with SSS develop signs and symptoms of heart failure that may be related to slow or fast heart rates.

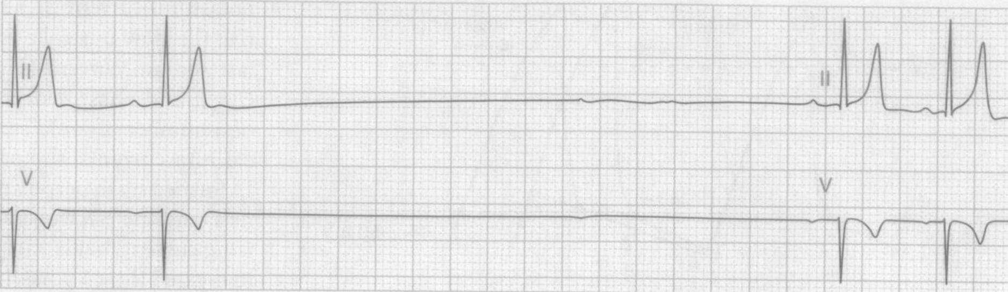

FIGURE 274-3 Sinus slowing and pauses on the electrocardiogram (ECG). The ECG is recorded during sleep in a young patient without heart disease. The heart rate before the pause is slow, and the PR interval is prolonged, consistent with an increase in vagal tone. The P waves have a morphology consistent with sinus rhythm. The recording is from a two-lead telemetry system in which the tracing labeled II mimics frontal lead II and V represents Modified Central Lead 1, which mimics lead V_1 of the standard 12-lead ECG.

One-third to one-half of patients with SA node dysfunction develop supraventricular tachycardia, usually atrial fibrillation or atrial flutter. The incidence of persistent atrial fibrillation in patients with SA node dysfunction increases with advanced age, hypertension, diabetes mellitus, left ventricular dilation, valvular heart disease, and ventricular pacing. Remarkably, some symptomatic patients may experience an improvement in symptoms with the development of atrial fibrillation, presumably from an increase in their average heart rate. Patients with the tachycardia-bradycardia variant of SSS, similar to patients with atrial fibrillation, are at risk for thromboembolism, and *those at greatest risk*, including patients ≥65 years and patients with a prior history of stroke, valvular heart disease, left ventricular dysfunction, or atrial enlargement, should be treated with anticoagulants. Up to one-quarter of patients with SA node disease will have concurrent AV conduction disease, although only a minority will require specific therapy for high-grade AV block.

The natural history of SA node dysfunction is one of varying intensity of symptoms even in patients who present with syncope. Symptoms related to SA node dysfunction may be significant, but overall mortality usually is not compromised in the absence of other significant comorbid conditions. These features of the natural history need to be taken into account in considering therapy for these patients.

ELECTROCARDIOGRAPHY OF SA NODE DISEASE

The electrocardiographic manifestations of SA node dysfunction include sinus bradycardia, sinus pauses, sinus arrest, sinus exit block, tachycardia (in SSS), and chronotropic incompetence. It is often difficult to distinguish pathologic from physiologic sinus bradycardia. By definition, sinus bradycardia is a rhythm driven by the SA node with a rate of <60 beats/min; sinus bradycardia is very common and typically benign. Resting heart rates <60 beats/min are very common in young healthy individuals and physically conditioned subjects. A sinus rate of <40 beats/min in the awake state in the absence of physical conditioning generally is considered abnormal. Sinus pauses and sinus arrest result from failure of the SA node to discharge, producing a pause without P waves visible on the ECG (Fig. 274-3). Sinus pauses of up to 3 s are common in awake athletes, and pauses of this duration or longer may be observed in asymptomatic elderly subjects. Intermittent failure of conduction from the SA node produces sinus exit block. The severity of sinus exit block may vary in a manner similar to that of AV block (Chap. 275). Prolongation of conduction from the sinus node will not be apparent on the ECG; second-degree SA block will produce intermittent conduction from the SA node and a regularly irregular atrial rhythm.

Type I second-degree SA block results from progressive prolongation of SA node conduction with intermittent failure of the impulses originating in the sinus node to conduct to the surrounding atrial tissue. Second-degree SA block appears on the ECG as an intermittent absence of P waves (Fig. 274-4). In type II second-degree SA block, there is no change in SA node conduction before the pause. Complete or third-degree SA block results in no P waves on the ECG. Tachycardia-bradycardia syndrome is manifest as alternating sinus bradycardia and atrial tachyarrhythmias. Although atrial tachycardia, atrial flutter, and atrial fibrillation may be observed, the latter is the most common tachycardia. Chronotropic incompetence is the inability to increase the heart rate in response to exercise or other stress appropriately and is defined in greater detail below.

DIAGNOSTIC TESTING

SA node dysfunction is most commonly a clinical or electrocardiographic diagnosis. Sinus bradycardia or pauses on the resting ECG are rarely sufficient to diagnose SA node disease, and longer-term recording and symptom correlation generally are required. Symptoms in the absence of sinus bradyarrhythmias may be sufficient to exclude a diagnosis of SA node dysfunction.

Electrocardiographic recording plays a central role in the diagnosis and management of SA node dysfunction. Despite the limitations of the resting ECG, longer-term recording employing Holter or event monitors may permit correlation of symptoms with the cardiac rhythm. Many contemporary event monitors may be automatically triggered to record the ECG when certain programmed heart rate criteria are met. Implantable ECG monitors permit long-term recording (12–18 months) in particularly challenging patients.

Failure to increase the heart rate with exercise is referred to as *chronotropic incompetence*. This is alternatively defined as failure to reach 85% of predicted maximal heart rate at peak exercise or failure to achieve a heart rate >100 beats/min with exercise or a maximal heart rate with exercise less than two standard deviations below that of an age-matched control population. Exercise testing may be useful in dis-

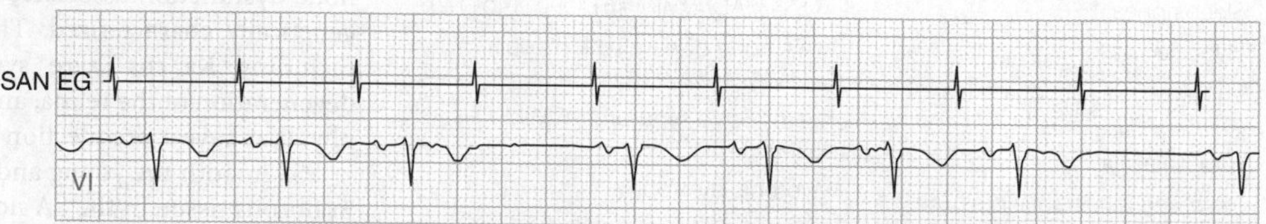

FIGURE 274-4 Mobitz type I SA nodal exit block. A theoretical SA node electrogram (SAN EG) is shown. Note that there is grouped beating producing a regularly irregular heart rhythm. The SA node EG rate is constant with progressive delay in exit from the node and activation of the atria, inscribing the P wave. This produces subtly decreasing P-P intervals before the pause, and the pause is less than twice the cycle length of the last sinus interval.

criminating chronotropic incompetence from resting bradycardia and may aid in the identification of the mechanism of exercise intolerance.

Autonomic nervous system testing is useful in diagnosing carotid sinus hypersensitivity; pauses >3 s are consistent with the diagnosis but may be present in asymptomatic elderly subjects. Determining the intrinsic heart rate (IHR) may distinguish SA node dysfunction from slow heart rates that result from high vagal tone. The normal IHR after administration of 0.2 mg/kg propranolol and 0.04 mg/kg atropine is 117.2 – (0.53 × age) in beats/min; a low IHR is indicative of SA disease.

Electrophysiologic testing may play a role in the assessment of patients with presumed SA node dysfunction and in the evaluation of syncope, particularly in the setting of structural heart disease. In this circumstance, electrophysiologic testing is used to rule out more malignant etiologies of syncope, such as ventricular tachyarrhythmias and AV conduction block. There are several ways to assess SA node function invasively. They include the sinus node recovery time (SNRT), defined as the longest pause after cessation of overdrive pacing of the right atrium near the SA node (normal: <1500 ms or, corrected for sinus cycle length, <550 ms), and the sinoatrial conduction time (SACT), defined as one-half the difference between the intrinsic sinus cycle length and a noncompensatory pause after a premature atrial stimulus (normal <125 ms). The combination of an abnormal SNRT, an abnormal SACT, and a low IHR is a sensitive and specific indicator of intrinsic SA node disease.

TREATMENT SINOATRIAL NODE DYSFUNCTION

Since SA node dysfunction is not associated with increased mortality rates, the aim of therapy is alleviation of symptoms. Exclusion of extrinsic causes of SA node dysfunction and correlation of the cardiac rhythm with symptoms is an essential part of patient management. Pacemaker implantation is the primary therapeutic intervention in patients with symptomatic SA node dysfunction. Pharmacologic considerations are important in the evaluation and management of patients with SA nodal disease. A number of drugs modulate SA node function and are extrinsic causes of dysfunction (Table 274-1). Beta blockers and calcium channel blockers increase SNRT in patients with SA node dysfunction, and antiarrhythmic drugs with class I and III action may promote SA node exit block. In general, such agents should be discontinued before decisions regarding the need for permanent pacing in patients with SA node disease are made. Chronic pharmacologic therapy for sinus bradyarrhythmias is limited. Some pharmacologic agents may improve SA node function; digitalis, for example, has been shown to shorten SNRT in patients with SA node dysfunction. Isoproterenol or atropine administered IV may increase the sinus rate acutely. Theophylline has been used both acutely and chronically to increase heart rate but has liabilities when used in patients with tachycardia-bradycardia syndrome, increasing the frequency of supraventricular tachyarrhythmias, and in patients with structural heart disease, increasing the risk of potentially serious ventricular arrhythmias. Currently, there is only a single randomized study of therapy for SA node dysfunction. In patients with resting heart rates <50 and >30 beats/min on a Holter monitor, patients who received dual-chamber pacemakers experienced significantly fewer syncopal episodes and had symptomatic improvement compared with patients randomized to theophylline or no treatment.

In certain circumstances, sinus bradycardia requires no specific treatment or only temporary rate support. Sinus bradycardia is common in patients with acute inferior or posterior MI and can be exacerbated by vagal activation induced by pain or the use of drugs such as morphine. Ischemia of the SA nodal artery probably occurs in acute coronary syndromes more typically with involvement with the right coronary artery, and even with infarction, the effect on SA node function most often is transient.

Sinus bradycardia is a prominent feature of carotid sinus hypersensitivity and neurally mediated hypotension associated with vasovagal syncope that responds to pacemaker therapy. Carotid hypersensitivity with recurrent syncope or presyncope associated with a predominant cardioinhibitory component responds to pacemaker implantation. Several randomized trials have investigated the efficacy of permanent pacing in patients with drug-refractory vasovagal syncope, with mixed results. Although initial trials suggested that patients undergoing pacemaker implantation have fewer recurrences and a longer time to recurrence of symptoms, at least one follow-up study did not confirm these results.

PERMANENT PACEMAKERS

Nomenclature and Complications The main therapeutic intervention in SA node dysfunction is permanent pacing. Since the first implementation of permanent pacing in the 1950s, many advances in technology have resulted in miniaturization, increased longevity of pulse generators, improvement in leads, and increased functionality. To better understand pacemaker therapy for bradycardias, it is important to be familiar with the fundamentals of pacemaking. Pacemaker modes and function are named using a five-letter code. The first letter indicates the chamber(s) that is paced (O, none; A, atrium; V, ventricle; D, dual; S, single), the second is the chamber(s) in which sensing occurs (O, none; A, atrium; V, ventricle; D, dual; S, single), the third is the response to a sensed event (O, none; I, inhibition; T, triggered; D, inhibition + triggered), the fourth refers to the programmability or rate response (R, rate responsive), and the fifth refers to the existence of antitachycardia functions if present (O, none; P, antitachycardia pacing; S, shock; D, pace + shock). Almost all modern pacemakers are multiprogrammable and have the capability for rate responsiveness using one of several rate sensors: activity or motion, minute ventilation, or QT interval. The most commonly programmed modes of implanted single- and dual-chamber pacemakers are VVIR and DDDR, respectively, although multiple modes can be programmed in modern pacemakers.

Although pacemakers are highly reliable, they are subject to a number of complications related to implantation and electronic function. In adults, permanent pacemakers are most commonly implanted with access to the heart by way of the subclavian–superior vena cava venous system. Rare, but possible, acute complications of transvenous pacemaker implantation include infection, hematoma, pneumothorax, cardiac perforation, diaphragmatic/phrenic nerve stimulation, and lead dislodgment. Limitations of chronic pacemaker therapy include infection, erosion, lead failure, and abnormalities resulting from inappropriate programming or interaction with the patient's native electrical cardiac function. Rotation of the pacemaker pulse generator in its subcutaneous pocket, either intentionally or inadvertently, often referred to as "twiddler's syndrome," can wrap the leads around the generator and produce dislodgment with failure to sense or pace the heart. The small size and light weight of contemporary pacemakers make this a rare complication.

Complications stemming from chronic cardiac pacing also result from disturbances in atrioventricular synchrony and/or left ventricular mechanical synchrony. Pacing modes that interrupt or fail to restore atrioventricular synchrony may lead to a constellation of signs and symptoms, collectively referred to as pacemaker syndrome, that include neck pulsation, fatigue, palpitations, cough, confusion, exertional dyspnea, dizziness, syncope, elevation in jugular venous pressure, canon A waves, and stigmata of congestive heart failure, including edema, rales, and a third heart sound. Right ventricular apical pacing can induce dyssynchronous activation of the left ventricle, leading to compromised left ventricular systolic function, mitral valve regurgitation, and the previously mentioned stigmata of congestive heart failure. Maintenance of AV synchrony can minimize the sequelae of pacemaker syndrome. Selection of pacing modes that minimize unnecessary ventricular pacing or implantation of a device capable of right and left ventricular pacing (biventricular pacing) can help minimize the deleterious consequences of pacing-induced mechanical dyssynchrony at the ventricular level.

Pacemaker Therapy in SA Node Dysfunction Pacing in SA nodal disease is indicated to alleviate symptoms of bradycardia. Consensus guidelines published by the American Heart Association (AHA)/American College of Cardiology/Heart Rhythm Society (ACC/HRS) outline the indications for the use of pacemakers and categorize them by class based on levels of evidence. Class I conditions are those for which there is evidence or consensus of opinion that therapy is useful and effective. In class II conditions, there is conflicting evidence or a divergence of opinion about the efficacy of a procedure or treatment; in class IIa conditions, the weight of evidence or opinion favors treatment; and in class IIb conditions, efficacy is less well established by the evidence or opinion of experts. In class III conditions, the evidence or weight of opinion indicates that the therapy is not efficacious or useful and may be harmful.

Class I indications for pacing in SA node dysfunction include documented symptomatic bradycardia, sinus node dysfunction–associated long-term drug therapy for which there is no alternative, and symptomatic chronotropic incompetence. Class IIa indications include those outlined previously in which sinus node dysfunction is suspected but not documented and for syncope of unexplained origin in the presence of major abnormalities of SA node dysfunction. Mildly symptomatic individuals with heart rates consistently <40 beats/min constitute a class IIb indication for pacing. Pacing is not indicated in patients with SA node dysfunction who do not have symptoms and in those in whom bradycardia is associated with the use of nonessential drugs (Table 274-2).

There is some controversy about the mode of pacing that should be employed in SA node disease. A number of randomized, single-blind trials of pacing mode have been performed. There are no trials that demonstrate an improvement in mortality rate with AV synchronous pacing compared with single-chamber pacing in SA node disease. In some of these studies, the incidence of atrial fibrillation and thromboembolic events was reduced with AV synchronous pacing. In trials of patients with dual-chamber pacemakers designed to compare single-chamber with dual-chamber pacing by crossover design, the need for AV synchronous pacing due to pacemaker syndrome was common. Pacing modes that preserve AV synchrony appear to be associated with a reduction in the incidence of atrial fibrillation and improved quality of life. Because of the low but finite incidence of AV conduction disease, patients with SA node dysfunction usually undergo dual-chamber pacemaker implantation.

TABLE 274-2 SUMMARY OF GUIDELINES FOR PACEMAKER IMPLANTATION IN SA NODE DYSFUNCTION

Class I

1. SA node dysfunction with symptomatic bradycardia or sinus pause
2. Symptomatic SA node dysfunction as a result of essential long-term drug therapy with no acceptable alternatives
3. Symptomatic chronotropic incompetence
4. Atrial fibrillation with bradycardia and pauses >5 s

Class IIa

1. SA node dysfunction with heart rates <40 beats/min without a clear and consistent relationship between bradycardia and symptoms
2. SA node dysfunction with heart rates <40 beats/min on an essential long-term drug therapy with no acceptable alternatives, without a clear and consistent relationship between bradycardia and symptoms
3. Syncope of unknown origin when major abnormalities of SA node dysfunction are discovered or provoked by electrophysiologic testing

Class IIb

1. Mildly symptomatic patients with waking chronic heart rates <40 beats/min

Class III

1. SA node dysfunction in asymptomatic patients, even those with heart rates <40 beats/min
2. SA node dysfunction in which symptoms suggestive of bradycardia are not associated with a slow heart rate
3. SA node dysfunction with symptomatic bradycardia due to nonessential drug therapy

Source: Modified from AE Epstein et al: J Am Coll Cardiol 51:e1, 2008 and CM Tracy et al: J Am Coll Cardiol 61:e6, 2013.

Pacemaker Therapy in Carotid Sinus Hypersensitivity and Vasovagal Syncope Carotid sinus hypersensitivity, if accompanied by a significant cardioinhibitory component, responds well to pacing. In this circumstance, pacing is required only intermittently and single-chamber ventricular pacing is often sufficient. The mechanism of vasovagal syncope is incompletely understood but appears to involve activation of cardiac mechanoreceptors with consequent activation of neural centers that mediate vagal activation and withdrawal of sympathetic nervous system tone. Several randomized clinical trials have been performed in patients with drug-refractory vasovagal syncope, with some studies suggesting reduction in the frequency and the time to recurrent syncope in patients who were paced compared with those who were not. A recent follow-up study to one of those initial trials, however, found less convincing results, casting some doubt on the utility of pacing for vagally mediated syncope.

275 The Bradyarrhythmias: Disorders of the Atrioventricular Node

David D. Spragg, Gordon F. Tomaselli

Impulses generated in the sinoatrial (SA) node or in ectopic atrial loci are conducted to the ventricles through the electrically and anatomically complex atrioventricular (AV) node. As described in Chap. 274, the electrophysiologic properties of nodal tissue are distinct from atrial and ventricular myocardium. Cells located in the AV node sit at a relatively higher resting membrane potential than surrounding atrial and ventricular myocytes, exhibit spontaneous depolarization during phase 4 of the action potential, and have slower phase 0 depolarization (mediated by calcium influx in nodal tissue) than that seen in ventricular tissue (mediated by sodium influx).

Bradycardia may occur when conduction across the AV node is compromised, resulting in ineffective ventricular rates, with the possibility of attendant symptoms, including fatigue, syncope, and (if subsidiary pacemaker activity is insufficient) even death. It is important to recognize that in the setting of disturbed AV conduction, SA activation and atrial systole may occur at normal or even accelerated rates, while ventricular activation is either slowed or nonexistent. Transient AV conduction block is common in the young and is most likely the result of high vagal tone found in up to 10% of young adults. Acquired and persistent failure of AV conduction is decidedly rare in healthy adult populations, with an estimated incidence of 200 per million population per year. In the setting of myocardial ischemia, aging and fibrosis, or cardiac infiltrative diseases, however, persistent AV block is much more common.

As with symptomatic bradycardia arising from SA node dysfunction, permanent pacing is the only reliable therapy for symptoms arising from AV conduction block. Approximately 50% of the 150,000 permanent pacemakers implanted in the United States and 70–80% of those in Europe are implanted for disorders of AV conduction.

STRUCTURE AND PHYSIOLOGY OF THE AV NODE

The AV conduction axis is structurally complex, involving the atria and ventricles as well as the AV node. Unlike the SA node, the AV node is a subendocardial structure originating in the transitional zone, which is composed of aggregates of cells in the posterior-inferior right atrium. Superior, medial, and posterior transitional atrionodal bundles converge on the compact AV node. The compact AV node (~1 × 3 × 5 mm) is situated at the apex of the triangle of Koch, which is defined by the coronary sinus ostium posteriorly, the septal tricuspid valve annulus anteriorly, and the tendon of Todaro superiorly. The compact AV node continues as the penetrating AV bundle where it immediately traverses the central fibrous body and is in close proximity to the aortic, mitral, and tricuspid valve annuli; thus, it is subject to injury in the setting of valvular heart disease or its surgical treatment. The penetrating AV bundle continues through the annulus fibrosis and emerges along the ventricular septum adjacent to the membranous septum as the bundle of His. The right bundle branch (RBB) emerges from the distal AV bundle in a band that traverses the right ventricle (moderator band). In contrast, the left bundle branch (LBB) is a broad subendocardial sheet of tissue on the septal left ventricle. The Purkinje fiber network emerges from the RBB and LBB and extensively ramifies on the endocardial surfaces of the right and left ventricles, respectively.

The blood supply to the penetrating AV bundle is from the AV nodal artery and first septal perforator of the left anterior descending coronary artery. The bundle branches also have a dual blood supply from the septal perforators of the left anterior descending coronary artery and branches of the posterior descending coronary artery. The AV node is highly innervated with postganglionic sympathetic and parasympathetic nerves. The bundle of His and distal conducting system are minimally influenced by autonomic tone.

The cells that constitute the AV node complex are heterogeneous with a range of action potential profiles. In the transitional zones, the cells have an electrical phenotype between those of atrial myocytes and cells of the compact node (see Fig. 274-1). Atrionodal transitional connections may exhibit *decremental conduction*, defined as slowing of conduction with increasingly rapid rates of stimulation. Fast and slow AV nodal pathways have been described, but it is controversial whether these two types of pathway are anatomically distinct or represent functional heterogeneities in different regions of the AV nodal complex. Myocytes that constitute the compact node are depolarized (resting membrane potential ~ 60 mV) and exhibit action potentials with low amplitudes, slow upstrokes of phase 0 (<10 V/s), and phase 4 diastolic depolarization; high-input resistance; and relative insensitivity to external [K+]. The action potential phenotype is explained by the complement of ionic currents expressed. AV nodal cells lack a robust inward rectifier potassium current (I_{K1}) and fast sodium current (I_{Na}); L-type calcium current (I_{Ca-L}) is responsible for phase 0; and phase 4 depolarization reflects the composite activity of the depolarizing currents—funny current (I_f), I_{Ca-L}, T-type calcium current (I_{Ca-T}), and sodium calcium exchanger current (I_{NCX})—and the repolarizing currents—delayed rectifier (I_{Kr}) and acetylcholine-gated (I_{KACh}) potassium currents. Electrical coupling between cells in the AV node is tenuous due to the relatively sparse expression of gap junction channels (predominantly connexin 40) and increased extracellular volume.

The His bundle and the bundle branches are insulated from ventricular myocardium. The most rapid conduction in the heart is observed in these tissues. The action potentials exhibit very rapid upstrokes (phase 0), prolonged plateaus (phase 2), and modest automaticity (phase 4 depolarization). Gap junctions, composed largely of connexin-40, are abundant, but bundles are poorly connected transversely to ventricular myocardium.

TABLE 275-1 ETIOLOGIES OF ATRIOVENTRICULAR BLOCK

Autonomic	
Carotid sinus hypersensitivity	Vasovagal
Metabolic/Endocrine	
Hyperkalemia	Hypothyroidism
Hypermagnesemia	Adrenal insufficiency
Drug-Related	
Beta blockers	Adenosine
Calcium channel blockers	Antiarrhythmics (class I and III)
Digitalis	Lithium
Infectious	
Endocarditis	Tuberculosis
Lyme disease	Diphtheria
Chagas' disease	Toxoplasmosis
Syphilis	
Heritable/Congenital	
Congenital heart disease	Facioscapulohumeral MD, OMIM #158900 (4q35)
Maternal SLE	Emery-Dreifuss MD, OMIM #310300 (Xq28)
Kearns-Sayre syndrome, OMIM #530000	Progressive familial heart block, type IA OMIM #113900 (3p21)
Myotonic dystrophy Type 1, OMIM #160900 (19q13.2-13.3) Type 2, OMIM #602668 (3q13.3 q24)	Progressive familial heart block, type IB, OMIM #604559 (19q13.32) Progressive familial heart block, type II, OMIM %140400
Inflammatory	
SLE	MCTD
Rheumatoid arthritis	Scleroderma
Infiltrative	
Amyloidosis	Hemochromatosis
Sarcoidosis	
Neoplastic/Traumatic	
Lymphoma	Radiation
Mesothelioma	Catheter ablation
Melanoma	
Degenerative	
Lev's disease	Lenègre's disease
Coronary Artery Disease	
Acute MI	

Abbreviations: MCTD, mixed connective tissue disease; MI, myocardial infarction; OMIM, Online Mendelian Inheritance in Man (database; designations: #, phenotypic description, molecular basis known; %, phenotypic description); SLE, systemic lupus erythematosus.

ETIOLOGY OF AV CONDUCTION DISEASE

Conduction block from the atrium to the ventricle can occur for a variety of reasons in a number of clinical situations, and AV conduction block may be classified in a number of ways. The etiologies may be functional or structural, in part analogous to extrinsic and intrinsic causes of SA nodal dysfunction. The block may be classified by its severity from first to third degree or complete AV block or by the location of block within the AV conduction system. Table 275-1 summarizes the etiologies of AV conduction block. Those that are functional (autonomic, metabolic/endocrine, and drug-related) tend to be reversible. Most other etiologies produce structural changes, typically fibrosis, in segments of the AV conduction axis that are generally permanent. Heightened vagal tone during sleep or in well-conditioned individuals can be associated with all grades of AV block. Carotid sinus hypersensitivity, vasovagal syncope, and cough and micturition syncope may be associated with SA node slowing and AV conduction block. Transient metabolic and endocrinologic disturbances as well as a number of pharmacologic agents also may produce reversible AV conduction block.

Several infectious diseases have a predilection for the conducting system. Lyme disease may involve the heart in up to 50% of cases; 10% of patients with Lyme carditis develop AV conduction block, which is generally reversible but may require temporary pacing support. Chagas' disease, which is common in Latin America, and syphilis may produce more persistent AV conduction disturbances. Some autoimmune and infiltrative diseases may produce AV conduction block, including systemic lupus erythematosus (SLE), rheumatoid arthritis, mixed connective tissue disease, scleroderma, amyloidosis (primary and secondary), sarcoidosis, and hemochromatosis; rare malignancies also may impair AV conduction.

Idiopathic progressive fibrosis of the conduction system is one of the more common and degenerative causes of AV conduction block. Aging is associated with degenerative changes in the summit of the ventricular septum, central fibrous body, and aortic and mitral annuli and has been described as "sclerosis of the left cardiac skeleton." The process typically begins in the fourth decade of life and may be accelerated by atherosclerosis, hypertension, and diabetes mellitus. Accelerated forms

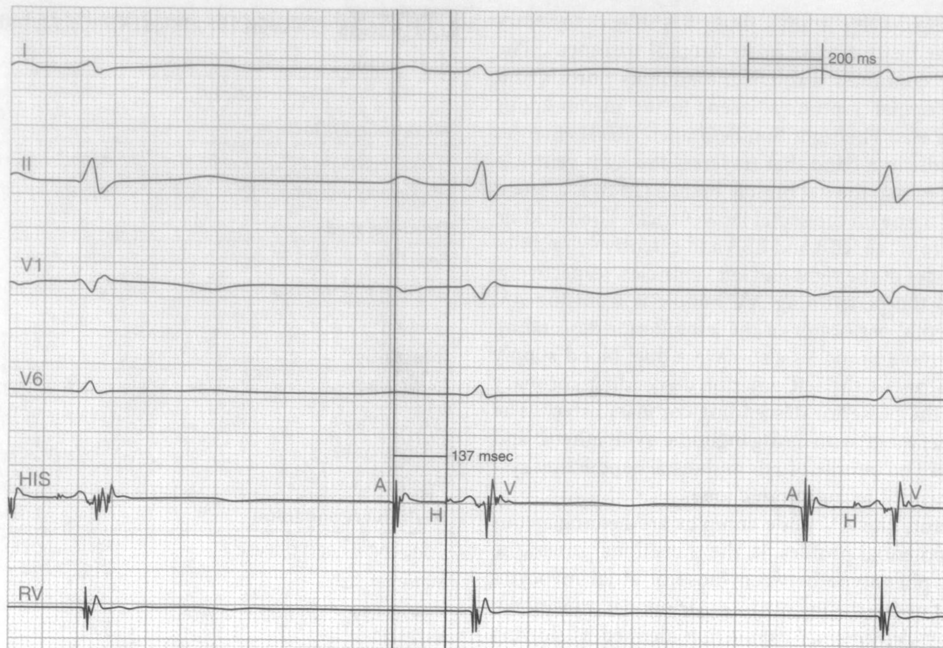

FIGURE 275-1 First-degree AV block with slowing of conduction in the AV node as indicated by the prolonged atrial-to-His bundle electrogram (AH) interval, in this case 157 ms. The His bundle-to-earliest ventricular activation on the surface ECG (HV) interval is normal. The normal HV interval suggests normal conduction below the AV node to the ventricle. I and V_1 are surface ECG leads, and HIS is the recording of the endocavitary electrogram at the His bundle position. A, H, and V are labels for the atrial, His bundle, and right ventricular electrograms, respectively.

of progressive familial heart block have been identified in families with mutations in the cardiac sodium channel gene (*SCN5A*) and other loci that have been mapped to chromosomes 1 and 19.

AV conduction block has been associated with heritable neuromuscular diseases, including the nucleotide repeat disease myotonic dystrophy, the mitochondrial myopathy Kearns-Sayre syndrome (Chap. 462e), and several of the monogenic muscular dystrophies. Congenital AV block may be observed in complex congenital cardiac anomalies (Chap. 282), such as transposition of the great arteries, ostium primum atrial septal defects (ASDs), ventricular septal defects (VSDs), endocardial cushion defects, and some single-ventricle defects. Congenital AV block in the setting of a structurally normal heart has been seen in children born to mothers with SLE. Iatrogenic AV block may occur during mitral or aortic valve surgery, rarely in the setting of thoracic radiation, and as a consequence of catheter ablation. AV block is a decidedly rare complication of the surgical repair of VSDs or ASDs but may complicate repairs of transposition of the great arteries.

Coronary artery disease may produce transient or persistent AV block. In the setting of coronary spasm, ischemia, particularly in the right coronary artery distribution, may produce transient AV block. In acute myocardial infarction (MI), AV block transiently develops in 10–25% of patients; most commonly, this is first-or second-degree AV block, but complete heart block (CHB) may also occur. Second-degree and higher-grade AV block tends to occur more often in inferior than in anterior acute MI; however, the level of block in inferior MI tends to be in the AV node with more stable, narrow escape rhythms. In contrast, acute anterior MI is associated with block in the distal AV nodal complex, His bundle, or bundle branches and results in wide complex, unstable escape rhythms and a worse prognosis with high mortality rates.

ELECTROCARDIOGRAPHY AND ELECTROPHYSIOLOGY OF AV CONDUCTION BLOCK

AV conduction block typically is diagnosed electrocardiographically, which characterizes the severity of the conduction disturbance and allows one to draw inferences about the location of the block. AV conduction block manifests as slow conduction in its mildest forms and failure to conduct, either intermittent or persistently, in more severe varieties. First-degree AV block (PR interval >200 ms) is a slowing of conduction through the AV junction (Fig. 275-1). The site of delay is typically in the AV node but may be in the atria, bundle of His, or His-Purkinje system. A wide QRS is suggestive of delay in the distal conduction system, whereas a narrow QRS suggests delay in the AV node proper or, less commonly, in the bundle of His. In second-degree AV block there is an intermittent failure of electrical impulse conduction from atrium to ventricle. Second-degree AV block is subclassified as Mobitz type I (Wenckebach) or Mobitz type II. The periodic failure of conduction in Mobitz type I block is characterized by a progressively lengthening PR interval, shortening of the RR interval, and a pause that is less than two times the immediately preceding RR interval on the electrocardiogram (ECG). The ECG complex after the pause exhibits a shorter PR interval than that immediately preceding the pause (Fig. 275-2). This ECG pattern most often arises because of decremental conduction of electrical impulses in the AV node.

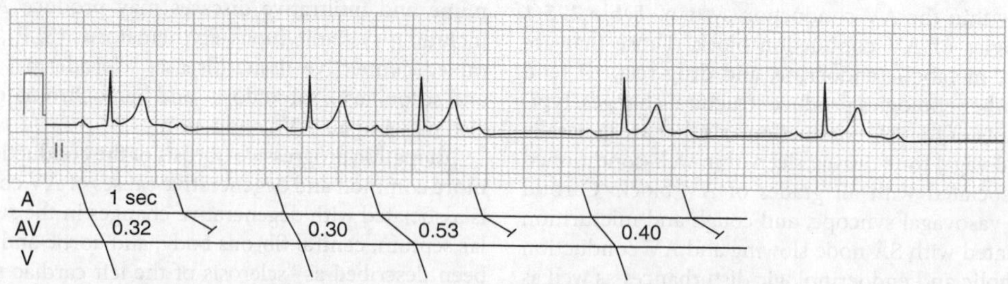

FIGURE 275-2 Mobitz type I second-degree AV block. The PR interval prolongs before the pause, as shown in the ladder diagram. The ECG pattern results from slowing of conduction in the AV node.

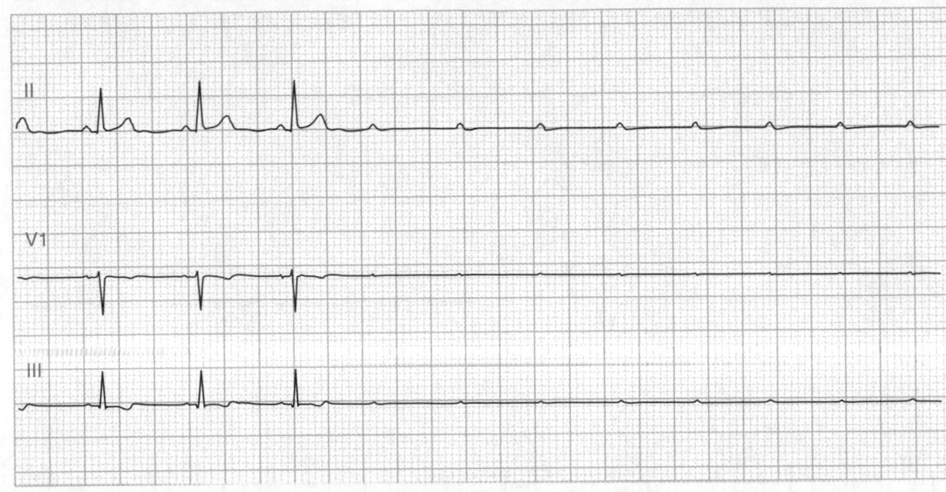

FIGURE 275-3 Paroxysmal AV block. Multiple nonconducted P waves after a period of sinus bradycardia with a normal PR interval. This implies significant conduction system disease, requiring permanent pacemaker implantation.

It is important to distinguish type I from type II second-degree AV nodal block because the latter has more serious prognostic implications. Type II second-degree AV block is characterized by intermittent failure of conduction of the P wave without changes in the preceding PR or RR intervals. When AV block is 2:1, it may be difficult to distinguish type I from type II block. Type II second-degree AV block typically occurs in the distal or infra-His conduction system, is often associated with intraventricular conduction delays (e.g., bundle branch block), and is more likely to proceed to higher grades of AV block than is type I second-degree AV block. Second-degree AV block (particularly type II) may be associated with a series of nonconducted P waves, referred to as *paroxysmal AV block* (Fig. 275-3), and implies significant conduction system disease and is an indication for permanent pacing. Complete failure of conduction from atrium to ventricle is referred to as complete or third-degree AV block. AV block that is intermediate between second degree and third degree is referred to as high-grade AV block and, as with CHB, implies advanced AV conduction system disease. In both cases, the block is most often distal to the AV node, and the duration of the QRS complex can be helpful in determining the level of the block. In the absence of a preexisting bundle branch block, a wide QRS escape rhythm (Fig. 275-4*B*) implies a block in the distal His or bundle branches; in contrast, a narrow QRS rhythm implies a block in the AV node or proximal His and an escape rhythm originating in the AV junction (Fig. 275-4*A*). Narrow QRS escape rhythms are typically faster and more stable than wide QRS escape rhythms and originate more proximally in the AV conduction system.

DIAGNOSTIC TESTING

Diagnostic testing in the evaluation of AV block is aimed at determining the level of conduction block, particularly in asymptomatic patients, since the prognosis and therapy depend on whether the block is in or below the AV node. Vagal maneuvers, carotid sinus massage, exercise, and administration of drugs such as atropine and isoproterenol may be diagnostically informative. Owing to the differences in the innervation of the AV node and infranodal conduction system, vagal stimulation and carotid sinus massage slow conduction in the AV node but have less of an effect on infranodal tissue and may even improve conduction due to a reduced rate of activation of distal tissues. Conversely, atropine, isoproterenol, and exercise improve conduction through the AV node and impair infranodal conduction. In patients with congenital CHB and a narrow QRS complex, exercise typically increases heart rate; by contrast, those with acquired CHB, particularly with wide QRS, do not respond to exercise with an increase in heart rate.

Additional diagnostic evaluation, including electrophysiologic testing, may be indicated in patients with syncope and suspected high-grade AV block. This is particularly relevant if noninvasive testing does not reveal the cause of syncope or if the patient has structural heart disease with ventricular tachyarrhythmias as a cause of symptoms. Electrophysiologic testing provides more precise information regarding the location of AV conduction block and permits studies of AV conduction under conditions of pharmacologic stress and exercise. Recording of the His bundle electrogram by a catheter positioned at the superior margin of the tricuspid valve annulus provides information about conduction at all levels of the AV conduction axis. A properly recorded His bundle electrogram reveals local atrial activity, the His electrogram, and local ventricular activation; when it is monitored simultaneously with recorded body surface electrocardiographic traces, intraatrial, AV nodal, and infranodal conduction times can be assessed (Fig. 275-1). The time from the most rapid deflection of the

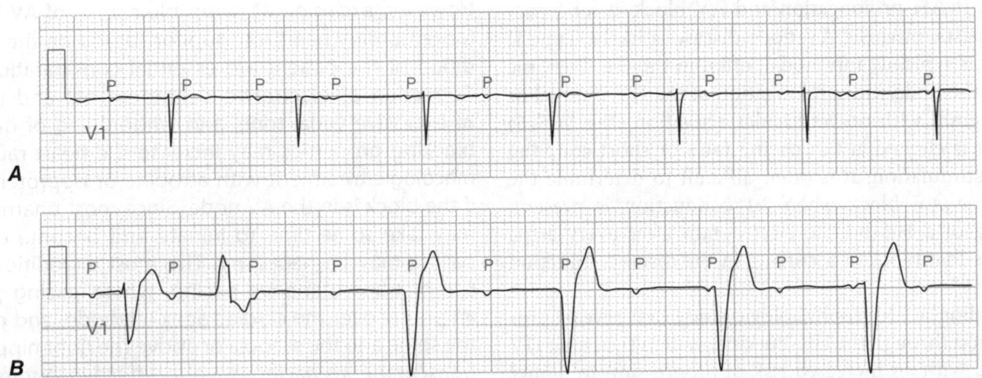

FIGURE 275-4 High-grade AV block. ***A.*** Multiple nonconducted P waves with a regular narrow complex QRS escape rhythm probably emanating from the AV junction. ***B.*** A wide complex QRS escape and a single premature ventricular contraction. In both cases, there is no consistent temporal relationship between the P waves and QRS complexes.

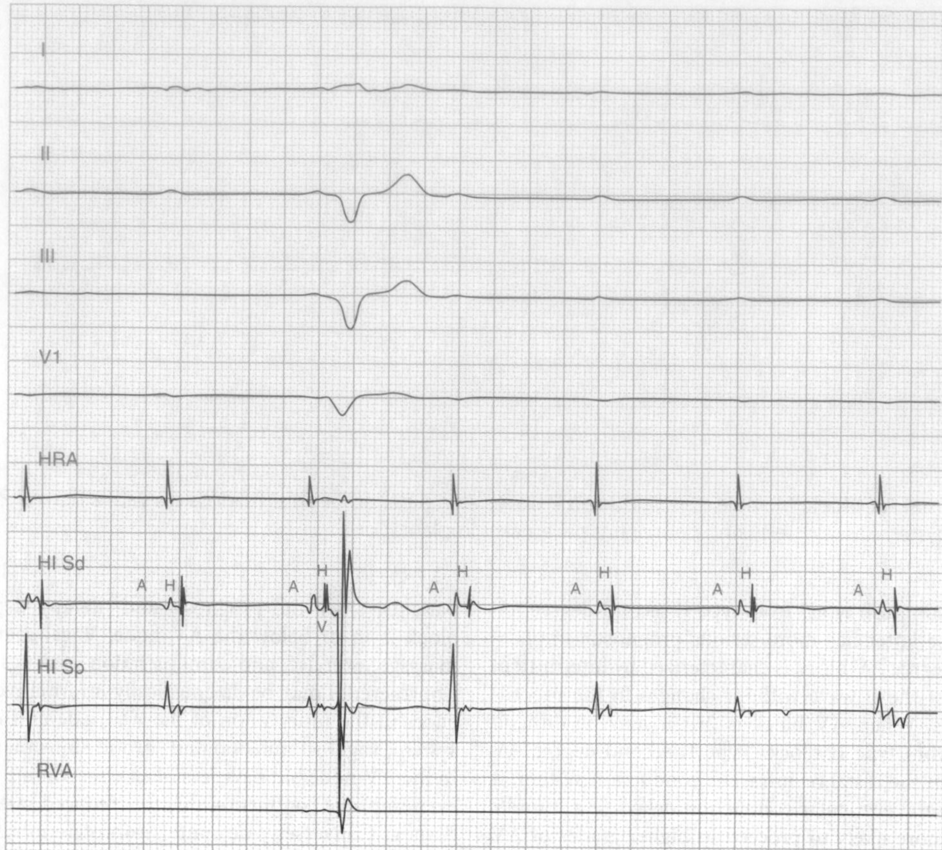

FIGURE 275-5 High-grade AV block below the His. The AH interval is normal and is not changing before the block. Atrial and His bundle electrograms are recorded consistent with block below the distal AV junction. I, II, III, and V_1 are surface ECG leads. HISp, HISd, and RVA are the proximal HIS, distal HIS, and right ventricular apical electrical recordings, respectively. A, H, and V represent the atrial, His, and ventricular electrograms on the His bundle recording, respectively. *(Tracing courtesy of Dr. Joseph Marine; with permission.)*

atrial electrogram in the His bundle recording to the His electrogram (*AH interval*) represents conduction through the AV node and is normally <130 ms. The time from the His electrogram to the earliest onset of the QRS on the surface ECG (*HV interval*) represents the conduction time through the His-Purkinje system and is normally ≤55 ms.

Rate stress produced by pacing can unveil abnormal AV conduction. Mobitz I second-degree AV block at short atrial paced cycle lengths is a normal response. However, when it occurs at atrial cycle lengths >500 ms (<120 beats/min) in the absence of high vagal tone, it is abnormal. Typically, type I second-degree AV block is associated with prolongation of the AH interval, representing conduction slowing and block in the AV node. AH prolongation occasionally is due to the effect of drugs (beta blockers, calcium channel blockers, digitalis) or increased vagal tone. Atropine can be used to reverse high vagal tone; however, if AH prolongation and AV block at long pacing cycle lengths persists, intrinsic AV node disease is likely. Type II second-degree block is typically infranodal, often in the His-Purkinje system. Block below the node with prolongation of the HV interval or a His bundle electrogram with no ventricular activation (Fig. 275-5) is abnormal unless it is elicited at fast pacing rates or short coupling intervals with extra stimulation. It is often difficult to determine the type of second-degree AV block when 2:1 conduction is present; however, the finding of a His bundle electrogram after every atrial electrogram indicates that block is occurring in the distal conduction system.

Intracardiac recording at electrophysiologic study that reveals prolongation of conduction through the His-Purkinje system (i.e., long HV interval) is associated with an increased risk of progression to higher grades of block and is generally an indication for pacing. In the setting of bundle branch block, the HV interval may reveal the condition of the unblocked bundle and the prognosis for developing more advanced AV conduction block. Prolongation of the HV interval in patients with asymptomatic bundle branch block is associated with an increased risk of developing higher-grade AV block. The risk increases with greater prolongation of the HV interval such that in patients with an HV interval >100 ms, the annual incidence of complete AV block approaches 10%, indicating a need for pacing. In patients with acquired CHB, even if intermittent, there is little role for electrophysiologic testing, and pacemaker implantation is almost always indicated.

TREATMENT MANAGEMENT OF AV CONDUCTION BLOCK

Temporary or permanent artificial pacing is the most reliable treatment for patients with symptomatic AV conduction system disease. However, exclusion of reversible causes of AV block and the need for temporary heart rate support based on the hemodynamic condition of the patient are essential considerations in each patient. Correction of electrolyte derangements and ischemia, inhibition of excessive vagal tone, and withholding of drugs with AV nodal blocking properties may increase the heart rate. Adjunctive pharmacologic treatment with atropine or isoproterenol may be useful if the block is in the AV node. Since most pharmacologic treatment may take some time to initiate and become effective, temporary pacing may be necessary. The most expeditious technique is the use of transcutaneous pacing, where pacing patches are placed anteriorly over the cardiac apex (cathode) and posteriorly between the spine and the scapula or above the right nipple (anode). Acutely, transcutaneous pacing is highly effective, but its duration is limited by patient discomfort and longer-term failure to capture the ventricle owing to changes in lead impedance. If a patient requires more

TABLE 275-2 GUIDELINE SUMMARY FOR PACEMAKER IMPLANTATION IN ACQUIRED AV BLOCK

Class I

1. Third-degree or high-grade AV block at any anatomic level associated with:
   a. Symptomatic bradycardia
   b. Essential drug therapy that produces symptomatic bradycardia
   c. Periods of asystole >3 s or any escape rate <40 beats/min while awake, or an escape rhythm originating below the AV node
   d. Postoperative AV block not expected to resolve
   e. Catheter ablation of the AV junction
   f. Neuromuscular diseases such as myotonic dystrophy, Kearns-Sayre syndrome, Erb dystrophy, and peroneal muscular atrophy, regardless of the presence of symptoms
2. Second degree AV block with symptomatic bradycardia
3. Type II second-degree AV block with a wide QRS complex with or without symptoms
4. Exercise-induced second-or third-degree AV block in the absence of ischemia
5. Atrial fibrillation with bradycardia and pauses >5 s

Class IIa

1. Asymptomatic third-degree AV block regardless of level
2. Asymptomatic type II second-degree AV block with a narrow QRS complex
3. Asymptomatic type II second-degree AV block with block within or below the His at electrophysiologic study
4. First- or second-degree AV block with symptoms similar to pacemaker syndrome

Class IIb

1. AV block in the setting of drug use/toxicity, when the block is expected to recur even with drug discontinuation
2. Neuromuscular diseases such as myotonic dystrophy, Kearns-Sayre syndrome, Erb dystrophy, and peroneal muscular atrophy with any degree of AV block regardless of the presence of symptoms

Class III

1. Asymptomatic first-degree AV block
2. Asymptomatic type I second-degree AV block at the AV node level
3. AV block that is expected to resolve or is unlikely to recur (Lyme disease, drug toxicity)

Source: Modified from AE Epstein et al: J Am Coll Cardiol 51:e1, 2008.

than a few minutes of pacemaker support, transvenous temporary pacing should be instituted. Temporary pacing leads can be placed from the jugular or subclavian venous system and advanced to the right ventricle, permitting stable temporary pacing for many days, if necessary. In most circumstances, in the absence of prompt resolution, conduction block distal to the AV node requires permanent pacemaking.

PACEMAKERS IN AV CONDUCTION DISEASE

There are no randomized trials that evaluate the efficacy of pacing in patients with AV block, as there are no reliable therapeutic alternatives for AV block and untreated high-grade AV block is potentially lethal. The consensus guidelines for pacing in acquired AV conduction block in adults provide a general outline for situations in which pacing is indicated (Table 275-2). Pacemaker implantation should be performed in any patient with symptomatic bradycardia and irreversible second-or third-degree AV block, regardless of the cause or level of block in the conducting system. Symptoms may include those directly related to bradycardia and low cardiac output or to worsening heart failure, angina, or intolerance to an essential medication. Pacing in patients with asymptomatic AV block should be individualized; situations in which pacing should be considered are patients with acquired CHB, particularly in the setting of cardiac enlargement; left ventricular dysfunction; and waking heart rates ≤40 beats/min. Patients who have asymptomatic second-degree AV block of either type should be considered for pacing if the block is demonstrated to be intra- or infra-His or is associated with a wide QRS complex. Pacing may be indicated in asymptomatic patients in special circumstances, in patients with profound first-degree AV block and left ventricular dysfunction in whom a shorter AV interval produces hemodynamic improvement, and in the setting of milder forms of AV conduction delay (first-degree AV block, intraventricular conduction delay) in patients with neuromuscular diseases that have a predilection for the conduction system, such as myotonic dystrophy and other muscular dystrophies, and Kearns-Sayre syndrome.

PACEMAKER THERAPY IN MYOCARDIAL INFARCTION

AV block in acute MI is often transient, particularly in inferior infarction. The circumstances in which pacing is indicated in acute MI are persistent second or third degree AV block, particularly if symptomatic, and transient second-or third-degree AV block associated with bundle branch block (Table 275-3). Pacing is generally not indicated in the setting of transient AV block in the absence of intraventricular conduction delays or in the presence of fascicular block

TABLE 275-3 GUIDELINE SUMMARY FOR PACEMAKER IMPLANTATION IN AV CONDUCTION BLOCK IN ACUTE MYOCARDIAL INFARCTION (AMI)

Class I

1. Persistent second-degree AV block in the His-Purkinje system with bilateral bundle branch block or third-degree block within or below the His after AMI
2. Transient advanced (second-or third-degree) infranodal AV block and associated bundle branch block. If the site of block is uncertain, an electrophysiologic study may be necessary
3. Persistent and symptomatic second-or third-degree AV block

Class IIb

1. Persistent second- or third-degree AV block at the AV node level

Class III

1. Transient AV block in the absence of intraventricular conduction defects
2. Transient AV block in the presence of isolated left anterior fascicular block
3. Acquired left anterior fascicular block in the absence of AV block
4. Persistent first-degree AV block in the presence of bundle branch block that is old or age-indeterminate

Source: Modified from AE Epstein et al: J Am Coll Cardiol 51:e1, 2008.

TABLE 275-4 INDICATIONS FOR PACEMAKER IMPLANTATION IN CHRONIC BIFASCICULAR AND TRIFASCICULAR BLOCK

Class I
1. Intermittent third-degree AV block
2. Type II second-degree AV block
3. Alternating bundle branch block
Class IIa
1. Syncope not demonstrated to be due to AV block when other likely causes (e.g., ventricular tachycardia) have been excluded
2. Incidental finding at electrophysiologic study of a markedly prolonged HV interval (>100 ms) in asymptomatic patients
3. Incidental finding at electrophysiologic study of pacing-induced infra-His block that is not physiologic
Class IIb
1. Neuromuscular diseases such as myotonic dystrophy, Kearns-Sayre syndrome, Erb dystrophy, and peroneal muscular atrophy with any degree of fascicular block regardless of the presence of symptoms, because there may be unpredictable progression of AV conduction disease
Class III
1. Fascicular block without AV block or symptoms
2. Fascicular block with first-degree AV block without symptoms

Source: Modified from AE Epstein et al: J Am Coll Cardiol 51:e1, 2008.

or first-degree AV block that develops in the setting of preexisting bundle branch block. Fascicular blocks that develop in acute MI in the absence of other forms of AV block also do not require pacing (Table 275-3 and Table 275-4).

PACEMAKER THERAPY IN BIFASCICULAR AND TRIFASCICULAR BLOCK

Distal forms of AV conduction block may require pacemaker implantation in certain clinical settings. Patients with bifascicular or trifascicular block and symptoms, particularly syncope that is not attributable to other causes, should undergo pacemaker implantation. Pacemaking is indicated in asymptomatic patients with bifascicular or trifascicular block who experience intermittent third-degree, type II second-degree AV block or alternating bundle branch block. In patients with fascicular block who are undergoing electrophysiologic study, a markedly prolonged HV interval or block below the His at long cycle lengths also may constitute an indication for permanent pacing. Patients with fascicular block and the neuromuscular diseases previously described should also undergo pacemaker implantation (Table 275-4).

SELECTION OF PACING MODE

In general, a pacing mode that maintains AV synchrony reduces complications of pacing such as pacemaker syndrome and pacemaker-mediated tachycardia. This is particularly true in younger patients; the importance of dual-chamber pacing in the elderly, however, is not well established. Several studies have failed to demonstrate a difference in mortality rate in older patients with AV block treated with a single-(VVI) compared with a dual-(DDD) chamber pacing mode. In some of the studies that randomized pacing mode, the risk of chronic atrial fibrillation and stroke risk decreased with physiologic pacing. In patients with sinus rhythm and AV block, the very modest increase in risk with dual-chamber pacemaker implantation appears to be justified to avoid the possible complications of single-chamber pacing.

276 Supraventricular Tachyarrhythmias

Gregory F. Michaud, William G. Stevenson

Supraventricular tachyarrhythmias originate from or are dependent on conduction through the atrium or atrioventricular (AV) node to the ventricles. Most produce narrow QRS-complex tachycardia (QRS duration <120 ms) characteristic of ventricular activation over the Purkinje system. Conduction block in the left or right bundle branch or activation of the ventricles from an accessory pathway produces a wide QRS complex during supraventricular tachycardia that must be distinguished from ventricular tachycardia (Chap. 277). Supraventricular tachyarrhythmia may be divided into physiologic sinus tachycardia and pathologic tachycardia (Table 276-1). The prognosis and treatment vary considerably depending on the mechanism and underlying heart disease.

Supraventricular tachycardia can be of brief duration, termed *nonsustained*, or can be sustained such that an intervention, such as cardioversion or drug administration, is required for termination. Episodes that occur with sudden onset and termination are referred to as paroxysmal. *Paroxysmal supraventricular tachycardia* (PSVT) refers to a family of tachycardias including AV node reentry, AV reentry using an accessory pathway, and atrial tachycardia.

CLINICAL PRESENTATION

Symptoms of supraventricular arrhythmia vary depending on the rate, duration, associated heart disease, and comorbidities and include palpitations, chest pain, dyspnea, diminished exertional capacity, and occasionally syncope. Rarely, a supraventricular arrhythmia precipitates cardiac arrest in patients with the Wolff-Parkinson-White syndrome or severe heart disease, such as hypertrophic cardiomyopathy.

Diagnosis requires obtaining an electrocardiogram (ECG) at the time of symptoms. For transient arrhythmia, ambulatory ECG recording is warranted (see Table 277-1). Exercise testing is useful for assessing exercise-related symptoms. Occasionally an invasive electrophysiology study is warranted to provoke the arrhythmia with pacing, confirm the mechanism, and often, perform catheter ablation.

Physiologic Sinus Tachycardia The sinus node is comprised of a group of cells dispersed within the superior aspect of the thick ridge of muscle known as the crista terminalis where the posterior smooth atrial wall derived from the sinus venosus meets the trabeculated anterior portion of the right atrium (Fig. 276-1). Sinus p waves are characterized by a frontal plane axis directed inferiorly and leftward, with positive p waves in leads II, III, and aVF; a negative p wave in aVR; and an initially positive biphasic p wave in V1. Normal sinus rhythm has a rate of 60–100 beats/min. Sinus tachycardia (>100 beats/min) typically occurs in response to sympathetic stimulation and vagal withdrawal, whereby the rate of spontaneous depolarization of the sinus node increases and the focus of earliest activation within the node typically shifts more leftward and closer to the superior septal aspect of the crista terminalis, thus producing taller p waves in the inferior limb leads when compared to normal sinus rhythm.

Sinus tachycardia is considered physiologic when it is an appropriate response to exercise, stress, or illness. Sinus tachycardia can be difficult to distinguish from focal atrial tachycardia (see below) that originates from a focus near the sinus node. A causative factor (such as exertion) and a gradual increase and decrease in rate favors sinus tachycardia, whereas an abrupt onset and offset favor atrial tachycardia. The distinction can be difficult and occasionally requires extended ECG monitoring or even invasive electrophysiology study. Treatment for physiologic sinus tachycardia is aimed at the underlying condition (Table 276-2).

Nonphysiologic Sinus Tachycardia *Inappropriate sinus tachycardia* is an uncommon condition in which the sinus rate increases spontaneously at rest or out of proportion to physiologic stress or exertion.

TABLE 276-1 SUPRAVENTRICULAR TACHYCARDIA

I. Physiologic sinus tachycardia

Defining feature: normal sinus mechanism precipitated by exertion, stress, concurrent illness (Table 276-2)

II. Pathologic supraventricular tachycardia

A. Tachycardia originating from the atrium

Defining feature: tachycardia may continue despite beats that fail to conduct to the ventricles, indicating that the AV node is not participating in the tachycardia circuit

1. Inappropriate sinus tachycardia

Defining feature: tachycardia from the normal sinus node area that occurs without an identifiable precipitating factor as a result of dysfunctional autonomic regulation

2. Focal atrial tachycardia

***Defining feature*: Regular atrial tachycardia with defined p wave; may be sustained, nonsustained, paroxysmal, or incessant.** Frequent sites of origin occur along the valve annuli of left or right atrium, pulmonary veins, coronary sinus musculature, superior vena cava

3. Atrial flutter – macroreentrant atrial tachycardia

Defining feature: organized reentry creates organized atrial activity, commonly seen as sawtooth flutter waves at rates typically faster than 200 beats/min

a. Common atrial flutter

i. Right atrial reentry parallel to the tricuspid annulus and dependent on conduction through the isthmus between the inferior vena cava and tricuspid annulus

1. Counterclockwise (as viewed from the ventricular aspect)

2. Clockwise

b. Atypical atrial flutter

i. Usually due to reentry in left or right atrium associated with scars usually from prior surgery or catheter ablation for atrial fibrillation, but may be idiopathic

4. Atrial fibrillation

Defining feature: chaotic rapid atrial electrical activity with variable ventricular rate; the most common sustained cardiac arrhythmia in older adults

5. Multifocal atrial tachycardia

Defining feature: multiple discrete p waves often seen in patients with pulmonary disease during acute exacerbations of pulmonary insufficiency

B. AV nodal reentry tachycardia

Defining feature: paroxysmal regular tachycardia with P waves visible at the end of the QRS complex or not visible at all; the most common paroxysmal sustained tachycardia in healthy young adults; more common in women

C. Tachycardias associated with accessory atrioventricular pathways

a. Orthodromic AV reentry tachycardia

Defining feature: paroxysmal sustained tachycardia similar to AV nodal reentry; during sinus rhythm, evidence of ventricular preexcitation may be present (Wolff-Parkinson-White syndrome) or absent (concealed accessory pathway)

b. Preexcited tachycardia

Defining feature: wide QRS tachycardia with QRS morphology similar to VT

1. Antidromic AV reentry – regular paroxysmal tachycardia

2. Atrial fibrillation with preexcitation – irregular wide complex, or intermittently wide complex tachycardia, some with dangerously rapid rates faster than 250/min

3. Atrial tachycardia or flutter with preexcitation

Abbreviations: AV, atrioventricular; VT, ventricular tachycardia.

Affected individuals are often women in the third or fourth decade of life. Fatigue, dizziness, and even syncope may accompany palpitations, which can be disabling. Additional symptoms of chest pain, headaches, and gastrointestinal upset are common. It must be distinguished from appropriate sinus tachycardia and from focal atrial tachycardia, as discussed above. Misdiagnosis of physiologic sinus tachycardia with an anxiety disorder is common. Therapy is often ineffective or poorly tolerated. Careful titration of beta blockers and/or calcium channel blockers may reduce symptoms. Clonidine and serotonin reuptake inhibitors have also been used. Ivabradine, a drug that blocks the I_f current causing sinus node depolarization, is promising but is not approved for use in the United States. Catheter ablation of the sinus node has been used, but long-term control of symptoms is usually poor, and it often leaves young individuals with a permanent pacemaker.

When symptomatic sinus tachycardia occurs with postural hypotension, the syndrome is called *postural orthostatic tachycardia syndrome* (POTS). Symptoms are often similar to those in patients with inappropriate sinus tachycardia. POTS is sometimes due to autonomic dysfunction following a viral illness and may resolve spontaneously over 3–12 months. Volume expansion with salt supplementation, oral fludrocortisone, compression stockings, and the α-agonist midodrine, often in combination, can be helpful. Exercise training has also been purported to improve symptoms.

Focal Atrial Tachycardia Focal atrial tachycardia (AT) can be due to abnormal automaticity, triggered automaticity, or a small reentry circuit confined to the atrium or atrial tissue extending into a pulmonary vein, the coronary sinus, or vena cava. It can be sustained, nonsustained, paroxysmal, or incessant. Focal AT accounts for approximately 10% of PSVT referred for catheter ablation. Nonsustained AT is commonly observed on 24-h ambulatory ECG recordings, and the prevalence increases with age. Tachycardia can occur in the absence of structural heart disease or can be associated with any form of heart disease that affects the atrium. Sympathetic stimulation is a promoting factor such that AT can be a sign of underlying illness. AT with AV block can occur in digitalis toxicity. Symptoms are similar to other supraventricular tachycardias (SVTs). Incessant AT can cause tachycardia-induced cardiomyopathy.

AT typically presents as an SVT either with 1:1 AV conduction or with AV block that can be Wenckebach type conduction or fixed (e.g., 2:1 or 3:1) block. Because it is not dependent on AV nodal conduction, AT will not terminate with AV block, and the atrial rate will not be affected, which distinguishes AT from most AV nodal–dependent SVTs, such as AV nodal reentry and AV reentry using an accessory pathway (see below). An accelerated warm-up phase after initiation or cool-down phase prior to termination also favors AT rather than AV nodal–dependent SVT. P waves are often discrete, with an intervening isoelectric segment, in contrast to atrial flutter and macroreentrant AT (see below). When 1:1 conduction to the ventricles is present, the arrhythmia can resemble sinus tachycardia typically with a P-R interval shorter than the R-P interval (Fig. 276-2). It can be distinguished from sinus tachycardia by the p-wave morphology, which usually differs from sinus p waves depending on the location of the focus. Focal AT tends to originate in areas of complex atrial anatomy, such as the crista terminalis, valve annuli, atrial septum, and atrial muscle extending along cardiac thoracic veins (superior vena cava, coronary sinus, and pulmonary veins) (Fig. 276-3), and the location can often be estimated by the P-wave morphology. AT from the right atrium has a positive P-wave morphology in lead I and biphasic P-wave morphology in lead V_1. AT from the atrial septum will frequently have a narrower P-wave duration than sinus rhythm. AT from the left atrium will usually have a monophasic, positive P wave in lead V_1. AT that originates from superior atrial locations, such as the superior vena cava or superior pulmonary veins, will be positive in the inferior limb leads II, III, and aVF, whereas AT from a more inferior location, such as the ostium of the coronary sinus, will inscribe negative P waves in these same leads. When the focus is in the superior aspect of the crista terminalis, close to the sinus node, however, the p wave will resemble that of sinus tachycardia. Abrupt onset and offset then favor AT rather than sinus tachycardia. Depending on the atrial rate, the P wave may fall on top of the t wave or, during 2:1 conduction, may fall coincident with the QRS. Maneuvers that increase AV block, such as carotid sinus massage, Valsalva maneuver, or administration of AV nodal–blocking agents, such as adenosine, are useful to create AV block that will expose the p wave (Fig. 276-4).

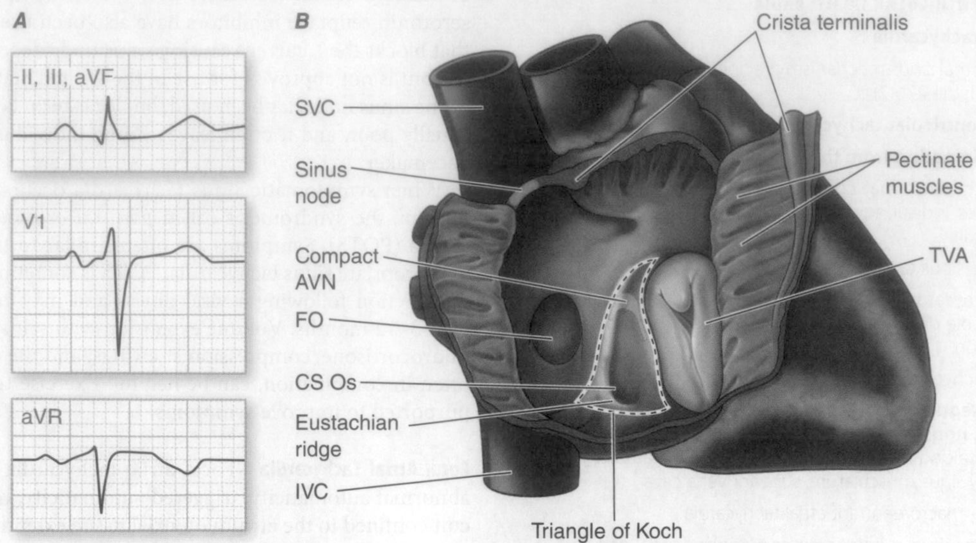

FIGURE 276-1 Right atrial anatomy pertinent to normal sinus rhythm and supraventricular tachycardia. ***A.*** Typical P-wave morphology during normal sinus rhythm based on standard 12-lead electrocardiogram. There is a positive P wave in leads II, III, and aVF; biphasic, initially positive P wave in V_1; and negative P wave in aVR. ***B.*** Right atrial anatomy seen from a right lateral perspective with the lateral wall opened to view the septum. AVN, atrioventricular node; CS Os, coronary sinus ostium; FO, fossa ovalis; IVC, inferior vena cava; SVC, superior vena cava; TVA, tricuspid valve annulus.

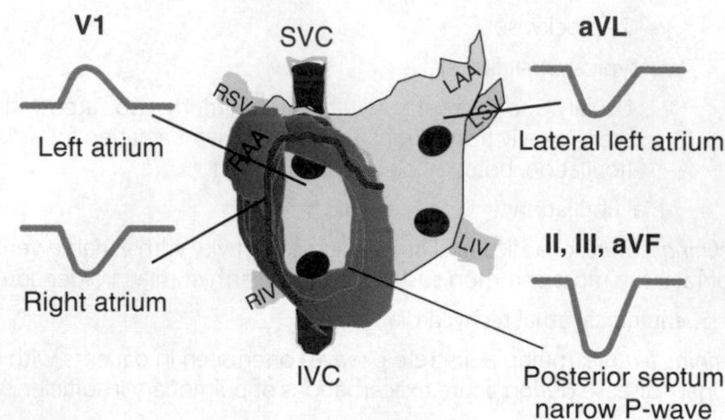

FIGURE 276-3 Location of focal atrial tachycardia focus estimated by P-wave morphology. LAA, left atrial appendage; LIV, left inferior pulmonary vein; LSV, left superior pulmonary vein; RAA, right atrial appendage; RIV, right inferior pulmonary vein; RSV, right superior pulmonary vein; SVC, superior vena cava.

TABLE 276-2 COMMON CAUSES OF PHYSIOLOGIC SINUS TACHYCARDIA

1. Exercise
2. Acute illness with fever, infection, pain
3. Hypovolemia, anemia
4. Hyperthyroidism
5. Pulmonary insufficiency
6. Drugs that have sympathomimetic, vagolytic, or vasodilator properties, e.g., albuterol, theophylline, tricyclic antidepressants, nifedipine, hydralazine
7. Pheochromocytoma

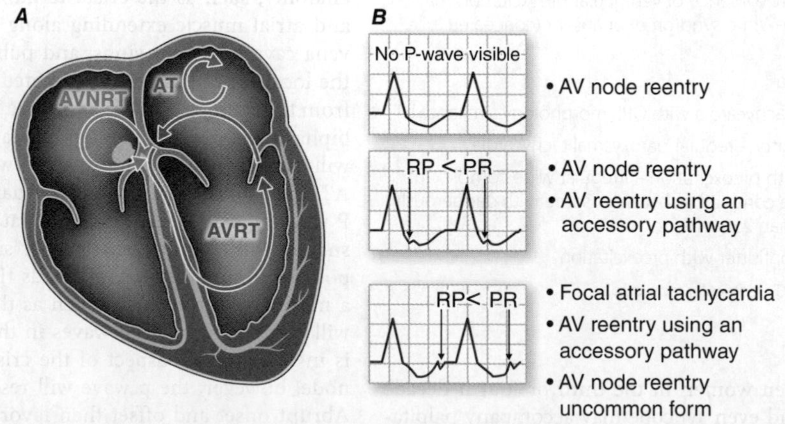

FIGURE 276-2 Common mechanisms underlying paroxysmal supraventricular tachycardia along with typical R-P relationships. ***A.*** Schematic showing a four-chamber view of the heart with atrioventricular node in *green* and an accessory pathway between the left atrium and left ventricle in *yellow*. Atrial tachycardia (AT; *red circuit*) is confined completely to atrial tissue. Atrioventricular nodal reentry tachycardia (AVNRT; *blue circuit*) uses atrioventricular (AV) nodal and perinodal atrial tissue. Atrioventricular reentry tachycardia (AVRT; *black circuit*) uses atrial and ventricular tissue, accessory pathway, AV node, and specialized conduction fibers (His-Purkinje) as part of the reentry circuit. ***B.*** Typical relation of the p wave to QRS, commonly described as the R-P to P-R relationships for the different tachycardia mechanisms.

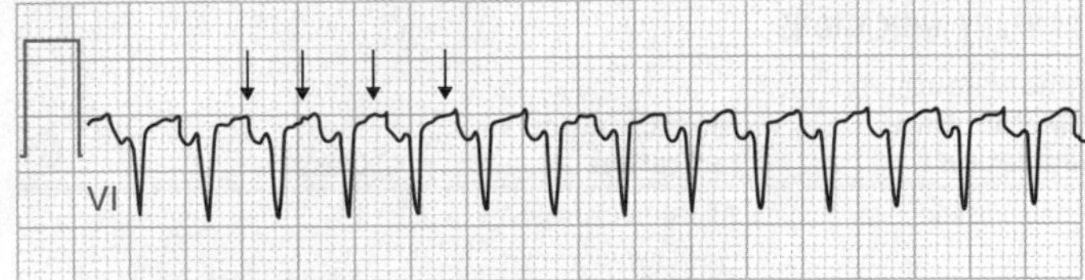

A

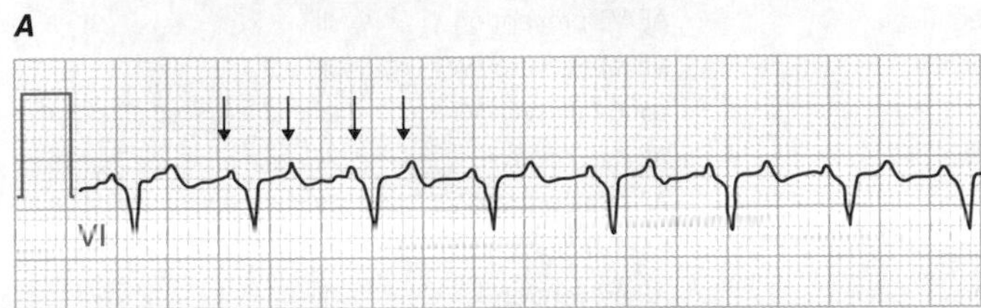

B

FIGURE 276-4 Atrial tachycardia (AT) with 1:1 and 2:1 atrioventricular (AV) conduction. *Arrows* indicate p waves. ***A.*** AT with 1:1 AV relationship and R-P > P-R. ***B.*** Same AT with 2:1 AV relationship after AV nodal–blocking agent administered. *(Adapted from F Marchlinski: The tachyarrhythmias. In Longo DL et al [eds]: Harrison's Principles of Internal Medicine, 18th ed. New York, McGraw-Hill, 2012, pp 1878–1900.)*

Acute management of sudden-onset, sustained AT is the same as for PSVT (see below), but the response to pharmacologic therapy is variable, likely depending on the mechanism. For AT due to reentry, administration of adenosine or vagal maneuvers may transiently increase AV block without terminating tachycardia. Some ATs terminate with a sufficient dose of adenosine, consistent with triggered activity as the mechanism. Cardioversion can be effective in some, but fails in others, suggesting automaticity as the mechanism. Beta blockers and calcium channel blockers may slow the ventricular rate by increasing AV block, which can improve tolerance of the arrhythmias. Potential precipitating factors and intercurrent illness should be sought and corrected. Underlying heart disease should be considered and excluded.

For patients with recurrent episodes, beta blockers, the calcium channel blockers diltiazem or verapamil, and the antiarrhythmic drugs flecainide, propafenone, disopyramide, sotalol, and amiodarone can be effective, but potential toxicities and adverse effects often warrant avoiding these agents (Tables 276-3, 276-4, and 276-5). Catheter ablation targeting the AT focus is effective in more than 80% of patients and is recommended for recurrent symptomatic AT when drugs fail or are not desired or for incessant AT causing tachycardia-induced cardiomyopathy.

Atrioventricular Nodal Reentry Tachycardia AV nodal reentry tachycardia (AVNRT) is the most common form of PSVT, representing approximately 60% of cases referred for catheter ablation. It most commonly manifests in the second to fourth decades of life, often in women. It is often well tolerated, but rapid tachycardia, particularly in the elderly, may cause angina, pulmonary edema, hypotension, or syncope. It is not usually associated with structural heart disease.

The mechanism is reentry involving the AV node and likely the perinodal atrium, made possible by the existence of multiple pathways for conduction from the atrium into the AV node (Fig. 276-5). In the most common form, a slowly conducting AV nodal pathway extends from the compact AV node near the bundle of His, inferiorly along the tricuspid annulus, adjacent to the coronary sinus os. The reentry wavefront propagates up this slow pathway to the compact AV node and then exits from the fast pathway at the top of the AV node. The path back to the slow pathway to complete the circuit is not defined. The conduction time from the compact AV node region to the atrium is similar to that from the compact node to the His bundle and ventricles, such that atrial activation occurs at about the same time as ventricular activation. The p wave is therefore inscribed during, slightly before, or slightly after the QRS and can be difficult to discern. Often the P wave is seen at the end of the QRS complex as a pseudo-r′ in lead V_1 and pseudo-S waves in leads II, III, and aVF (Fig. 276-5*A*). The rate can vary with sympathetic tone. Simultaneous atrial and ventricular contraction results in atrial contraction against a closed tricuspid valve that produces cannon a waves visible in the jugular venous pulse and that the patient often perceives as a fluttering sensation in the neck. Elevated venous pressures may also lead to release of natriuretic peptides that cause posttachycardia diuresis. Less frequently, the AV nodal reentry circuit revolves in the opposite direction and gives rise to a tachycardia with an R-P interval longer than the P-R interval, similar to AT. The p wave will have the morphology noted above, and in contrast to ATs, maneuvers or medications that produce AV block terminate the arrhythmia.

Acute treatment is the same as for PSVT (discussed below). Whether ongoing therapy is warranted depends on the severity of symptoms and frequency of episodes. Reassurance and instruction as to performance of the Valsalva maneuver to terminate episodes are sufficient for many patients. Administration of an oral beta blocker, verapamil, or diltiazem at the onset of an episode has been used to

TABLE 276-3 COMMONLY USED ANTIARRHYTHMIC AGENTS—INTRAVENOUS DOSE RANGE/PRIMARY INDICATION

Drug	Loading	Maintenance	Primary Indication	Class[a]
Adenosine	6–18 mg (rapid bolus)	N/A	Terminate reentrant SVT involving AV node	—
Amiodarone	15 mg/min for 10 min, 1 mg/min for 6 h	0.5–1 mg/min	AF, AFL, SVT, VT/VF	III
Digoxin	0.25 mg q2h until 1 mg total	0.125–0.25 mg/d	AF/AFL rate control	—
Diltiazem	0.25 mg/kg over 3–5 min (max 20 mg)	5–15 mg/h	SVT, AF/AFL rate control	IV
Esmolol	500 μg/kg over 1 min	50 μg/kg per min	AF/AFL rate control	II
Ibutilide	1 mg over 10 min if over 60 kg	N/A	Terminate AF/AFL	III
Lidocaine	1–3 mg/kg at 20–50 mg/min	1–4 mg/min	VT	IB
Metoprolol	5 mg over 3–5 min × 3 doses	1.25–5 mg q6h	SVT, AF rate control; exercise-induced VT; long QT	II
Procainamide	15 mg/kg over 60 min	1–4 mg/min	Convert/prevent AF/VT	IA
Quinidine	6–10 mg/kg at 0.3–0.5 mg/kg per min	N/A	Convert/prevent AF/VT	IA
Verapamil	5–10 mg over 3–5 min	2.5–10 mg/h	SVT, AF rate control	IV

[a]Classification of antiarrhythmic drugs: class I—agents that primarily block inward sodium current; class IA agents also prolong action potential duration; class II—antisympathetic agents; class III—agents that primarily prolong action potential duration; class IV—calcium channel–blocking agents.

Abbreviations: AF, atrial fibrillation; AFL, atrial flutter; AV, atrioventricular; SVT, supraventricular tachycardia; VF, ventricular fibrillation; VT, ventricular tachycardia.

TABLE 276-4 COMMONLY USED ANTIARRHYTHMIC AGENTS: CHRONIC ORAL DOSING/PRIMARY INDICATIONS

Drug	Dosing Oral, mg, Maintenance	Half-Life, h	Primary Route(s) of Metabolism/ Elimination	Most Common Indication	Class[a]
Acebutolol	200–400 q12h	6–7	Renal/hepatic	AF rate control/SVT Long QT/RVOT VT	II
Amiodarone	100–400 qd	40–55 d	Hepatic	AF/VT prevention	III[b]
Atenolol	25–100 per d	6–9	Renal	AF rate control/SVT Long QT/RVOT VT	II
Digoxin	0.125–0.25 qd	38–48	Renal	AF rate control	—
Diltiazem	30–60 q6h	3–4.5	Hepatic	AF rate control/SVT	IV
Disopyramide	100–300 q6–8h	4–10	Renal 50%/hepatic	AF/SVT prevention	Ia
Dofetilide	0.125–0.5 q12h	10	Renal	AF prevention	III
Dronedarone	400 q12h	13–19	Hepatic	AF prevention	IIIb
Flecainide	50–200 q12h	7–22	Hepatic 75%/renal	AF/SVT/VT prevention	Ic
Metoprolol	25–100 q6h	3–8	Hepatic	AF rate control/SVT Long QT/RVOT VT	II
Mexiletine	150–300 q8–12h	10–14	Hepatic	VT prevention	Ib
Nadolol	40–240 per d	10–24	Renal	Same as metoprolol	II
Propafenone	150–300 q8h	2–8	Hepatic	AF/SVT/VT prevention	Ic
Quinidine	300–600 q6h	6–8	Hepatic 75%/renal	AF/SVT/VT prevention	Ia
Sotalol	80–160 q12h	12	Renal	AF/VT prevention	III
Verapamil	80–120 q6–8h	4.5–12	Hepatic/renal	AF rate control/RVOT VT Idiopathic LV VT	IV

[a]Classification of antiarrhythmic drugs: class I—agents that primarily block inward sodium current; class II—antisympathetic agents; class III—agents that primarily prolong action potential duration; class IV—calcium channel-blocking agents. [b]Amiodarone and dronedarone both are grouped in class III, but both also have class I, II, and IV properties.

Abbreviations: AF, atrial fibrillation; LV, left ventricular; RVOT, right ventricular outflow tract; SVT, supraventricular tachycardia; VT, ventricular tachycardia.

facilitate termination. Chronic therapy with these medications or flecainide is an option if prophylactic therapy is needed. Catheter ablation of the slow AV nodal pathway is recommended for patients with recurrent or severe episodes or when drug therapy is ineffective, not tolerated, or not desired by the patient. Catheter ablation is curative in over 95% of patients. The major risk is heart block requiring permanent pacemaker implantation, which occurs in less than 1% of patients.

Junctional Tachycardia Junctional ectopic tachycardia (JET) is due to automaticity within the AV node. It is rare in adults and more frequently encountered as an incessant tachycardia in children, often in the perioperative period of surgery for congenital heart disease. It presents as a narrow QRS tachycardia, often with ventriculoatrial (VA) block, such that AV dissociation is present. JET can occur as a manifestation of increased adrenergic tone and may be seen after administration of isoproterenol. It may also occur for a short period of time after ablation for AVNRT.

Accelerated junctional rhythm is a junctional automatic rhythm between 50 and 100 beats/min. Initiation may occur with gradual acceleration in rate, suggesting an automatic focus, or after a premature

TABLE 276-5 COMMON AND PROARRHYTHMIC TOXICITIES OF ANTIARRHYTHMIC AGENTS

Drug	Potential Proarrhythmic Toxicities	Common Toxicities
Amiodarone	Sinus bradycardia, AV block, increase in defibrillation threshold. Rare: long QT and torsades des pointes, incessant slow VT in heart disease	Tremor, peripheral neuropathy, pulmonary fibrosis or inflammation, hypo- and hyperthyroidism, hepatitis, photosensitivity
Adenosine	Transient profound pauses, atrial fibrillation	Cough, flushing, chest pain, anxiety
Digoxin	AV block, fascicular tachycardia, accelerated junctional rhythm, atrial tachycardia with AV block	Anorexia, nausea, vomiting, visual changes
Disopyramide	Long QT and torsades des pointes, 1:1 ventricular response to atrial flutter	Anticholinergic effects, acute urinary retention (males), negative inotropy
Dofetilide	Long QT and torsades des pointes	Nausea
Dronedarone	Bradyarrhythmias and AV block, long QT and torsades des pointes (rare)	Gastrointestinal intolerance, exacerbation of heart failure
Flecainide	1:1 Ventricular response to atrial flutter; increased risk of ventricular tachycardias in patients with structural heart disease; sinus bradycardia	Dizziness, nausea, headache, decreased myocardial contractility
Ibutilide	Long QT and torsades des pointes	Nausea
Lidocaine	Slow VT in some patients with structural heart disease	Dizziness, confusion, delirium, seizures, coma
Mexiletine	Slow VT in patients with structural heart disease	Ataxia, tremor, gait disturbances, rash, nausea
Procainamide	Long QT and torsades des pointes, accelerated ventricular rate in AF or flutter	Lupus erythematosus–like syndrome (more common in slow acetylators), anorexia, nausea, neutropenia
Propafenone	1:1 Ventricular response to atrial flutter; increased risk ventricular tachycardias in patients with structural heart disease; sinus bradycardia	Taste disturbance, dyspepsia, nausea, vomiting
Quinidine	Long QT and torsades des pointes, accelerated ventricular rate in AF or flutter	Diarrhea, nausea, vomiting, cinchonism, thrombocytopenia
Sotalol	Long QT and torsades des pointes	Hypotension, bronchospasm from β-blocking effect

Abbreviations: AF, atrial fibrillation; AV, atrioventricular; VT, ventricular tachycardia.

A

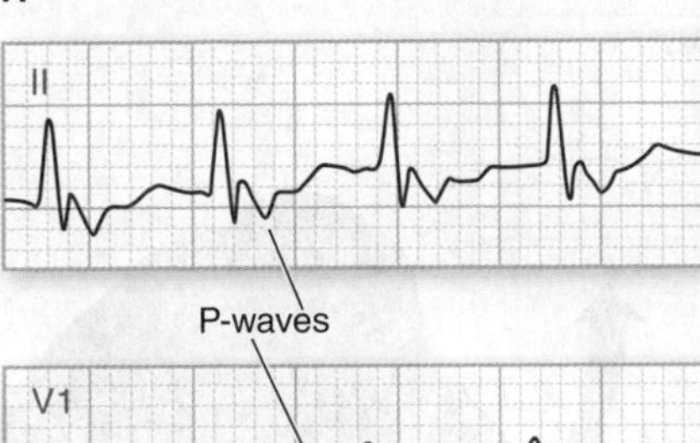

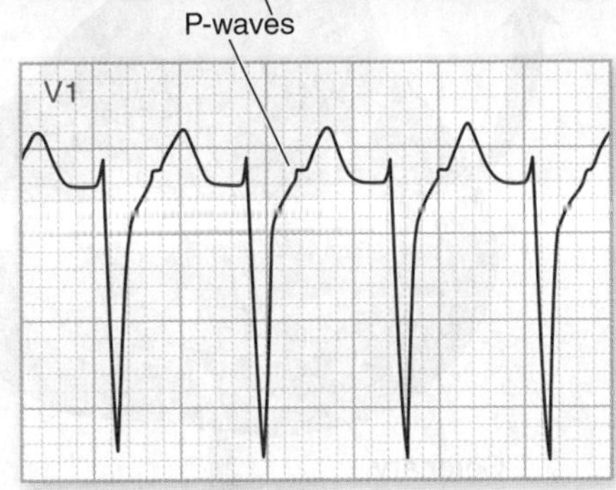

B

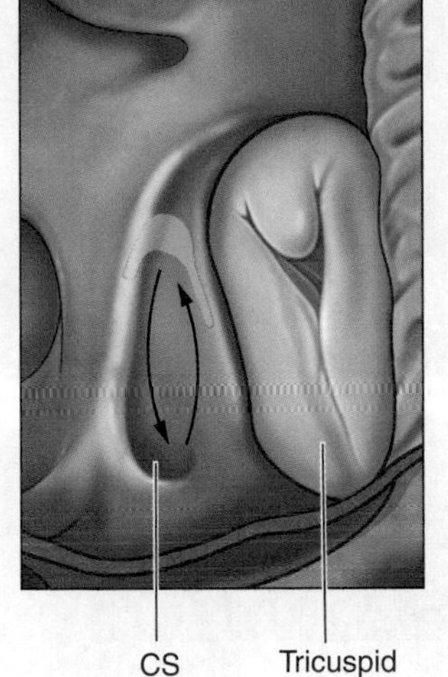

FIGURE 276-5 Atrioventricular (AV) node reentry. ***A.*** Leads II and V_1 are shown. P waves are visible at the end of the QRS complex and are negative in lead II, and may give the impression of S waves in the inferior limb leads II, III, and aVF and an R′ in lead V_1. ***B.*** Stylized version of the AV nodal reentry circuit within the triangle of Koch (Fig. 276-1) that involves AV node and its extensions along with perinodal atrial tissue.

ventricular contraction, suggesting a focus of triggered automaticity. VA conduction is usually present, with p-wave morphology and timing such that it resembles slow AVNRT.

ACCESSORY PATHWAYS AND THE WOLFF-PARKINSON-WHITE SYNDROME

Accessory pathways (APs) occur in 1 in 1500–2000 people and are associated with a variety of arrhythmias including narrow-complex PSVT, wide-complex tachycardias, and, rarely, sudden death. Most patients have structurally normal hearts, but APs are associated with Ebstein's anomaly of the tricuspid valve and forms of hypertrophic cardiomyopathy including *PRKAG2* mutations, Danon's disease, and Fabry's disease.

APs are abnormal connections that allow conduction between the atrium and ventricles across the AV ring (Fig. 276-6). They are present from birth and are due to failure of complete partitioning of atrium and ventricle by the fibrous AV rings. They occur across either an AV valve annulus or the septum, most frequently between the left atrium and free wall of the left ventricle, followed by posteroseptal, right free wall, and anteroseptal locations. If the AP conducts from atrium to ventricle (antegrade) with a shorter conduction time than the AV node and His bundle, then the ventricles are preexcited during sinus rhythm, and the ECG shows a short P-R interval (<0.12 s), slurred initial portion of the QRS (delta wave), and prolonged QRS duration produced by slow conduction through direct activation of ventricular myocardium over the AP (Fig. 276-6*A*). The morphology of the QRS and delta wave is determined by the AP location (Fig. 276-7) and the degree of fusion between the excitation wavefronts from conduction over the AV node and conduction over the AP. Right-sided pathways preexcite the right ventricle, producing a left bundle branch block–like configuration in lead V_1, and often show marked preexcitation because of relatively close proximity of the AP to the sinus node (Fig. 276-7). Left-sided pathways preexcite the left ventricle and may produce a right bundle branch–like configuration in lead V_1 and a negative delta wave in aVL, indicating initial depolarization of the lateral portion of the left ventricle that can mimic q waves of lateral wall infarction (Fig. 276-7). Preexcitation due to an AP at the diaphragmatic surface of the heart, typically in the paraseptal region, produces delta waves that are negative in leads III and aVF, mimicking the q waves of inferior wall infarction (Fig. 276-7). Preexcitation can be intermittent and disappear during exercise as conduction over the AV node accelerates and takes over ventricular activation completely.

Wolff-Parkinson-White (WPW) syndrome is defined as a preexcited QRS during sinus rhythm and episodes of PSVT. There are a number of variations of APs, which may not cause preexcitation and/or arrhythmias. Concealed APs allow only retrograde conduction, from ventricle to atrium, so no preexcitation is present during sinus rhythm, but SVT can occur. Fasciculoventricular connections between the His bundle and ventricular septum produce preexcitation but do not cause arrhythmia, nor do fibers such as atrio-Hisian connections, probably because the circuit is too short to promote reentry. Atriofascicular pathways, also known as Mahaim fibers, probably represent a duplicate AV node and His-Purkinje system that connect the right atrium to fascicles of the right bundle branch and conduct slowly only in the anterograde direction.

AV Reentry Tachycardia The most common tachycardia caused by an AP is the PSVT designated *orthodromic AV reentry.* The circulating reentry wavefront propagates from the atrium anterogradely over the AV node and His-Purkinje system to the ventricles and then reenters the atria via retrograde conduction over the AP (Fig. 276-6*B*). The QRS is narrow or may have typical right or left bundle branch block, but without preexcitation during tachycardia. Because excitation through the normal AV conduction system and AP are necessary, AV or VA block results in tachycardia termination. During sinus rhythm, preexcitation is seen if the pathway also allows anterograde conduction (Fig. 276-6*A*). Most commonly, during tachycardia the R-P interval is shorter than the P-R interval and can resemble AVNRT (Fig. 276-1). Unlike typical AVNRT, P-wave timing is never simultaneous with a narrow QRS complex because the ventricles must be activated before the reentry wavefront reaches the AP and conducts back to the atrium. The morphology of the P wave is determined by the pathway location, but can be difficult to assess because it is usually inscribed during the ST segment. The p wave in posteroseptal APs is negative in leads II, III, and aVF, similar to that of AV nodal reentry, but P-wave morphology differs from AV nodal reentry for pathways in other locations (Fig. 276-7).

Occasionally, an AP conducts extremely slowly in the retrograde direction, which results in tachycardia with a long R-P interval, similar to most ATs. These pathways are usually located in the septal region and have negative p waves in leads II, III, and aVF. Slow conduction facilitates reentry, often leading to nearly incessant tachycardia, known as *paroxysmal junctional reciprocating tachycardia* (PJRT). Tachycardia-induced cardiomyopathy can occur. Without an invasive electrophysiology study, it may be difficult to distinguish this form of orthodromic AV reentry from atypical AV nodal reentry or AT.

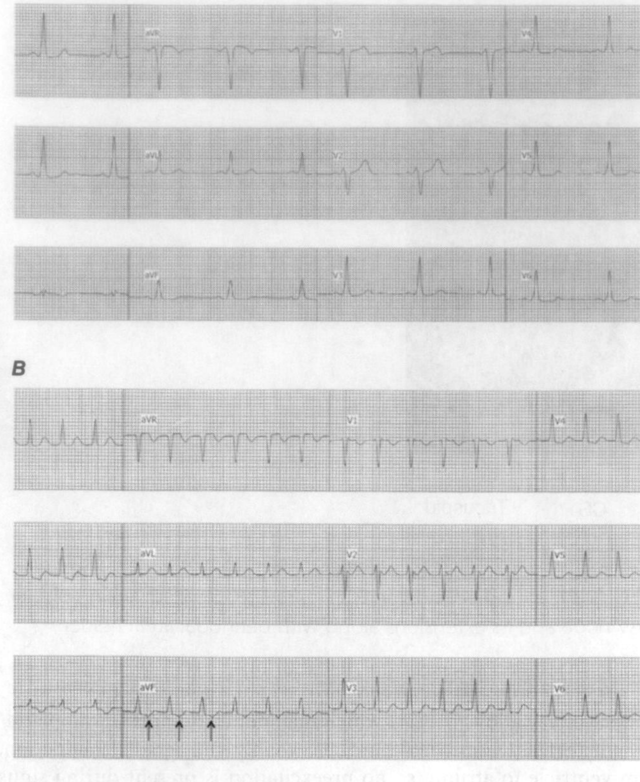

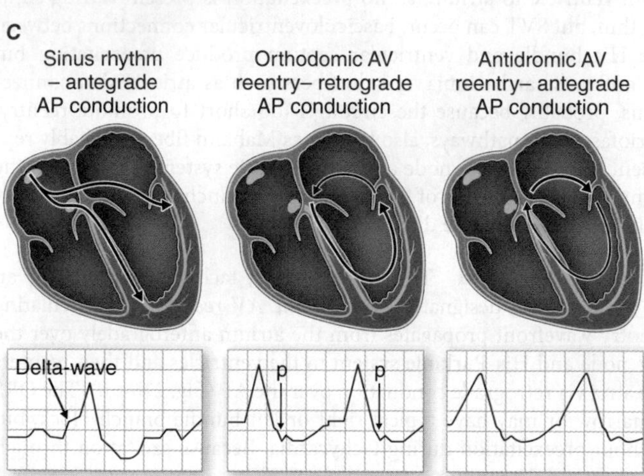

FIGURE 276-6 Wolff-Parkinson-White (WPW) syndrome. ***A.*** A 12-lead electrocardiogram in sinus rhythm (SR) of a patient with WPW demonstrating short P-R interval, delta waves, and widened QRS complex. This patient had an anteroseptal location of the AP. ***B.*** Orthodromic AV reentry in a patient with WPW syndrome using a posteroseptal AP. Note the P waves in the ST segment (*arrows*) seen in lead III and normal appearance of QRS complex. ***C.*** Three most common rhythms associated with WPW syndrome: sinus rhythm demonstrating antegrade conduction over the AP and AV node; orthodromic AVRT using retrograde conduction over the AP and antegrade conduction over the AV node; and antidromic AVRT using retrograde conduction over the AV node and antegrade conduction over the AP. AP, accessory pathway; AV, atrioventricular; AVRT, atrioventricular reentry tachycardia; WPW, Wolff-Parkinson-White.

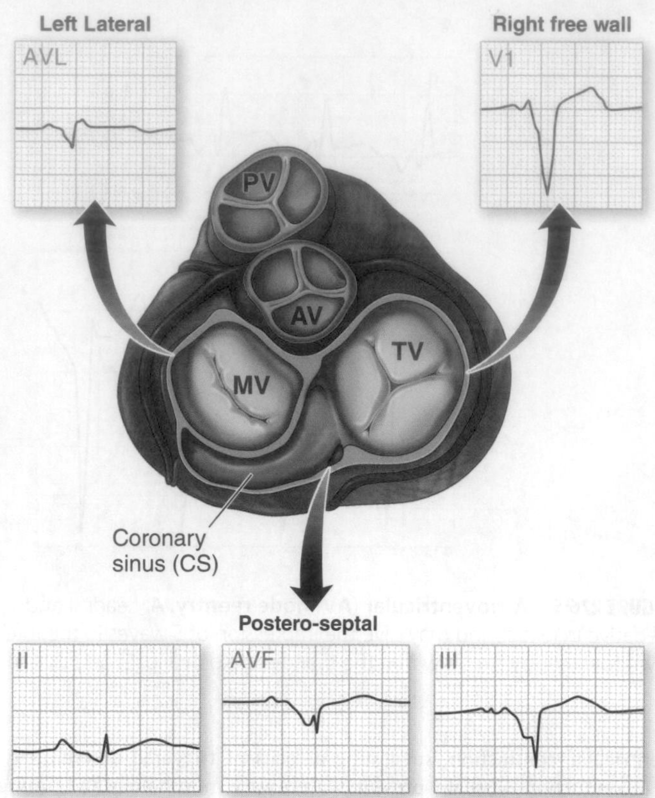

FIGURE 276-7 Potential locations for accessory pathways in patients with Wolff-Parkinson-White Syndrome and typical QRS appearance of delta waves that can mimic underlying structural heart disease such as myocardial infraction of bundle branch block. AV, aortic valve; MV, mitral valve; PV, pulmonary valve; TV, tricuspid valve.

Preexcited Tachycardias Preexcitated tachycardia occurs when the ventricles are activated by antegrade conduction over the AP (Fig. 276-6C). The most common is *antidromic AV reentry* in which activation propagates from atrium to ventricle via the AP and then conducts retrogradely to the atria via the His-Purkinje system and the AV node (or rarely a second AP). The wide QRS complex is produced entirely via ventricular excitation over the AP because there is no contribution of ventricular activation over more rapidly conducting specialized His-Purkinje fibers. This tachycardia is often indistinguishable from monomorphic ventricular tachycardia. The presence of preexcitation in sinus rhythm suggests the diagnosis.

Preexcitated tachycardia also occurs if an AP allows antegrade conduction to the ventricles during AT, atrial flutter, atrial fibrillation (Fig. 276-8), or AV nodal reentry. Atrial fibrillation and atrial flutter are potentially life threatening if the AP allows very rapid repetitive conduction. Approximately 25% of APs causing preexcitation allow minimum R-to-R intervals of less than 250 ms during atrial fibrillation are therefore associated with a risk of inducing ventricular fibrillation and sudden death. Preexcited atrial fibrillation presents as a wide-complex, very irregular rhythm. During atrial fibrillation, the ventricular rate is determined by the conduction properties of the AP and AV node. The QRS complex can appear quite bizarre and change on a beat-to-beat basis due to the variability in the degree of fusion from activation over the AV node and AP, or all beats may be due to conduction over the AP (Fig. 276-8). Ventricular activation from the Purkinje system may depolarize the ventricular end of the AP and prevent 1:1 atrial wavefront conduction over the AP. Slowing AV nodal conduction can thereby facilitate AP conduction and dangerously accelerate the ventricular rate. Administration of AV nodal–blocking agents including oral or intravenous verapamil, diltiazem, beta blockers, intravenous adenosine, and intravenous amiodarone are contraindicated. Preexcited tachycardias should be treated with electrical cardioversion or intravenous procainamide or ibutilide, which may terminate or slow the ventricular rate.

Management of Patients with Accessory Pathways Acute management of orthodromic AV reentry is discussed below for PSVT. Patients

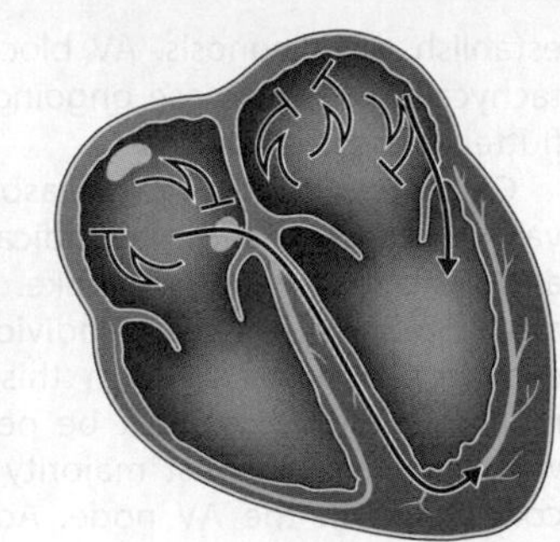

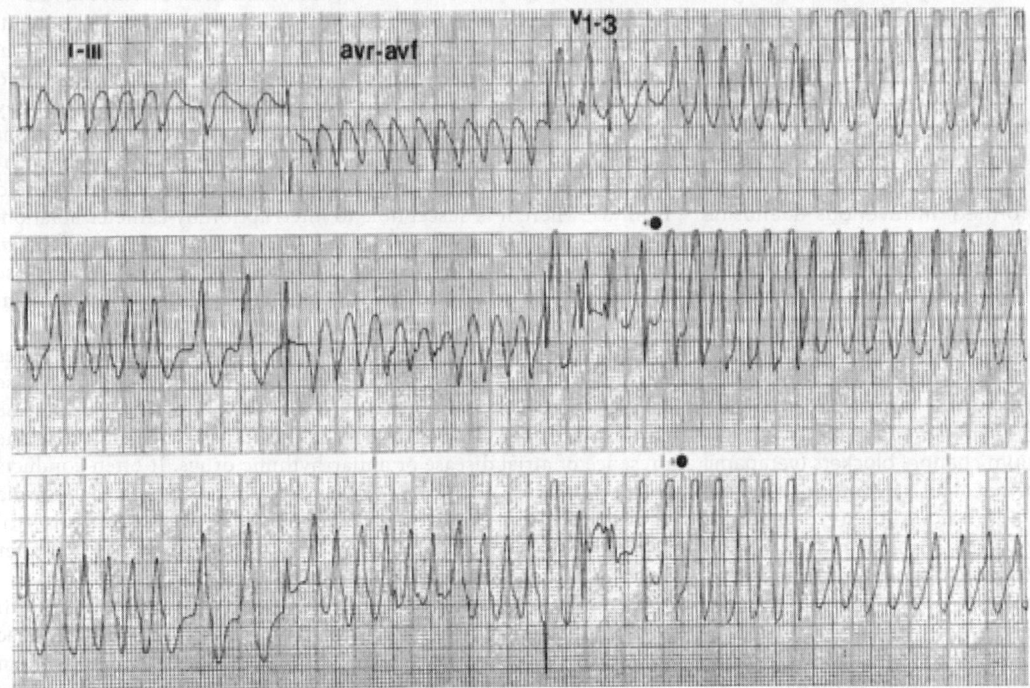

FIGURE 276-8 Preexcited atrial fibrillation (AF) due to conduction over a left free wall accessory pathway (AP). The electrocardiogram shows rapid irregular QRS complexes that represent fusion between conduction over the atrioventricular node and left free wall AP. Shortest R-R intervals between preexcited QRS complexes of less than 250 ms, as in this case, indicate a risk of sudden death with this arrhythmia.

with WPW syndrome may have wide-complex tachycardia due to antidromic AV reentry, orthodromic AV with bundle branch block, or a preexcited tachycardia, and treatment depends on the underlying rhythm.

Initial patient evaluation should include assessment for aggravating factors, including intercurrent illness and factors that increase sympathetic tone. Examination should focus on excluding underlying heart disease. An echocardiogram is reasonable to exclude Ebstein's anomaly and hypertrophic cardiomyopathy.

Patients with preexcitation who have symptoms of arrhythmia are at risk for developing atrial fibrillation and sudden death if they have an AP with high-risk properties. The risk of cardiac arrest is in the range of 2 per 1000 patients in adults but is likely greater in children. An invasive electrophysiology study is warranted to determine if the AP is high enough risk to warrant potentially curative catheter ablation. For patients with concealed APs or known low-risk APs causing orthodromic AV reentry, chronic therapy is guided by symptoms and frequency of events. Vagal maneuvers may terminate episodes, as may a dose of beta blocker, verapamil, or diltiazem taken at the onset of an episode. Chronic therapy with these agents or flecainide can reduce the frequency of episodes in some patients. Catheter ablation is warranted for recurrent arrhythmias when drugs are ineffective, not tolerated, or not desired by the patient or if the AP is considered high risk (Fig. 276-8). Efficacy is in the range of 95% depending on the location of the AP. Serious complications occur in fewer than 3% of patients, but can include AV block, cardiac tamponade, thromboemboli, coronary artery injury, and vascular access complications. Mortality occurs in less than 1 in 1000 patients.

Adults who have preexcitation but no arrhythmia symptoms have a risk of sudden death estimated to be 1 per 1000 patient-years. Electrophysiology study is usually advised for people in occupations for which an arrhythmia occurrence would place them or others at risk, such as police, military, and pilots, or for individuals who desire evaluation for risk. Routine follow-up without therapy is reasonable in others. Children are at greater risk of sudden death, approximately 2 per 1000 patient-years.

TREATMENT PAROXYSMAL SUPRAVENTRICULAR TACHYCARDIA

Acute management of narrow QRS PSVT is guided by the clinical presentation. Continuous ECG monitoring should be implemented and a 12-lead ECG should always be obtained when possible. In the presence of hypotension with unconsciousness or respiratory distress, QRS-synchronous direct current cardioversion is warranted, but this is rarely needed, because intravenous adenosine works promptly in most situations (see below). For stable individuals, initial therapy takes advantage of the fact that most PSVTs are dependent on AV nodal conduction (AV nodal reentry or orthodromic AV reentry) and therefore likely to respond to sympatholytic and vagotonic maneuvers and drugs (Fig. 276-9). As these are administered, the ECG should be continuously recorded, because the response can

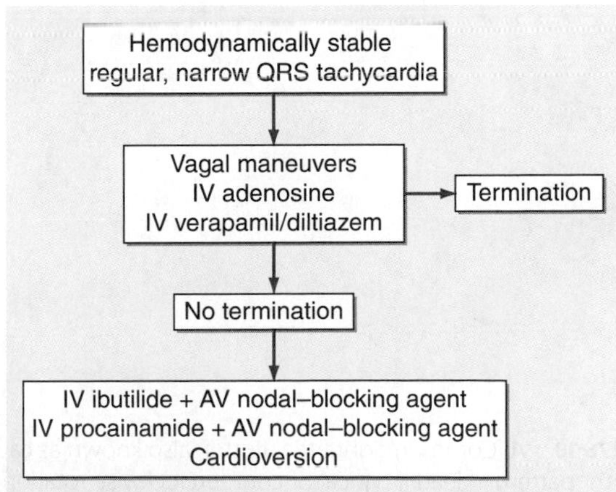

FIGURE 276-9 Treatment algorithm for patients presenting with hemodynamically stable paroxysmal supraventricular tachycardia. AV, atrioventricular.

establish the diagnosis. AV block with only transient slowing of tachycardia may expose ongoing p waves, indicating AT or atrial flutter as the mechanism.

Carotid sinus massage is reasonable provided the risk of carotid vascular disease is low, as indicated by absence of carotid bruits and no prior history of stroke. A Valsalva maneuver should be attempted in cooperative individuals, and if effective, the patient can be taught to perform this maneuver as needed. If vagal maneuvers fail or cannot be performed, intravenous adenosine will terminate the vast majority of PSVT by transiently blocking conduction in the AV node. Adenosine may produce transient chest pain, dyspnea, and anxiety. It is contraindicated in patients with prior cardiac transplantation due to potential hypersensitivity. It can theoretically aggravate bronchospasm. Adenosine precipitates atrial fibrillation, which is usually brief, in up to 15% of patients, so it should be used cautiously in patients with WPW syndrome in whom AF may produce hemodynamic instability. Intravenous beta blockers and calcium channel blockers (verapamil or diltiazem) are also effective but may cause hypotension before and after arrhythmia termination and have a longer duration of action. These agents can also be given orally and can be taken by the patient on an as-needed basis to slow ventricular rate and facilitate termination by Valsalva maneuver.

The differential diagnosis of wide-complex tachycardia includes ventricular tachycardia (Chap. 277), PSVT with bundle branch block aberrancy, and preexcited tachycardia (see above). In general, these should be managed as ventricular tachycardia until proven otherwise. If the tachycardia is regular and the patient is stable, a trial of intravenous adenosine is reasonable. Very irregular wide-complex tachycardia should be managed with cardioversion, intravenous procainamide, or ibutilide, which presumes preexcited atrial fibrillation or flutter (see above). If the diagnosis of PSVT with aberrancy is unequivocal, as may be the case in patients with prior episodes, treatment for PSVT is reasonable. In all cases, continuous ECG monitoring should be implemented, and emergency cardioversion and defibrillation should be available.

COMMON ATRIAL FLUTTER AND MACROREENTRANT ATRIAL TACHYCARDIAS

Macrorrentrant atrial tachycardia is due to a large reentry circuit, often associated with areas of scar in the atria. *Common or typical right atrial flutter* is due to a circuit that revolves around the tricuspid valve annulus, bounded anteriorly by the annulus and posteriorly by functional conduction block in the crista terminalis. The wavefront passes through an isthmus between the inferior vena cava and the tricuspid valve annulus, known as the sub-Eustachian or cavotricuspid isthmus, where it is susceptible to interruption by catheter ablation. Thus, common atrial flutter is *cavotricuspid isthmus-dependent atrial flutter*. This circuit most commonly revolves in a counterclockwise direction (as viewed looking toward the tricuspid annulus from the ventricular aspect), which produces the characteristic negative sawtooth flutter waves in leads II, III, and aVF and positive P waves in lead V_1 (Fig. 276-10). When the direction is reversed, clockwise rotation produces the opposite P-wave vector in those leads. The atrial rate is typically 240–300 beats/min but may be slower in the presence of atrial disease or antiarrhythmic drugs. It often conducts to the ventricles with 2:1 AV block, creating a regular tachycardia at 150 beats/min, with p waves that may be difficult to discern. Maneuvers that increase AV nodal block will typically expose flutter waves, allowing diagnosis.

Common right atrial flutter often occurs in association with atrial fibrillation and with atrial scar from senescence or prior cardiac surgery. Some patients with atrial fibrillation that is treated with an antiarrhythmic drug, particularly flecainide, propafenone, or amiodarone, will present with atrial flutter rather than fibrillation.

Macroreentrant ATs that are not dependent on conduction through the cavotricuspid isthmus are referred to as *atypical atrial flutters*. They can occur in either atrium and are usually associated with areas of scar. Left atrial flutter and perimitral left atrial flutter are commonly seen after extensive left atrial ablation for atrial fibrillation or atrial surgery. The clinical presentation is similar to common atrial flutter, but with different P-wave morphologies. They can be difficult to distinguish from focal AT, and in most cases, the mechanism can only be confirmed by an electrophysiology study.

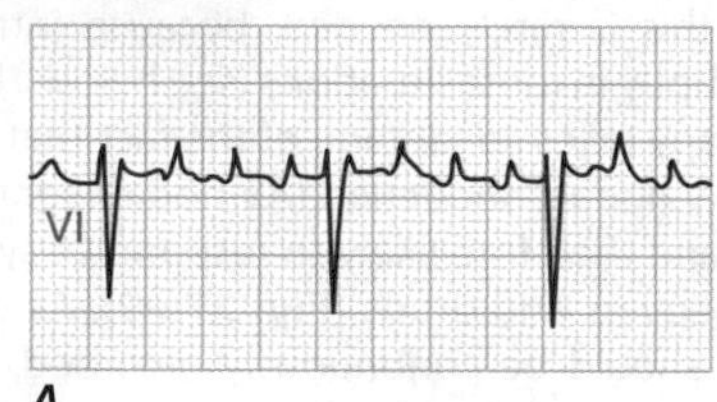

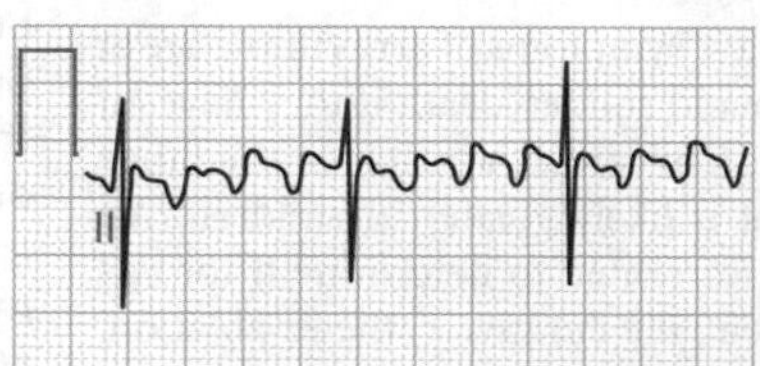

A

Counterclockwise flutter

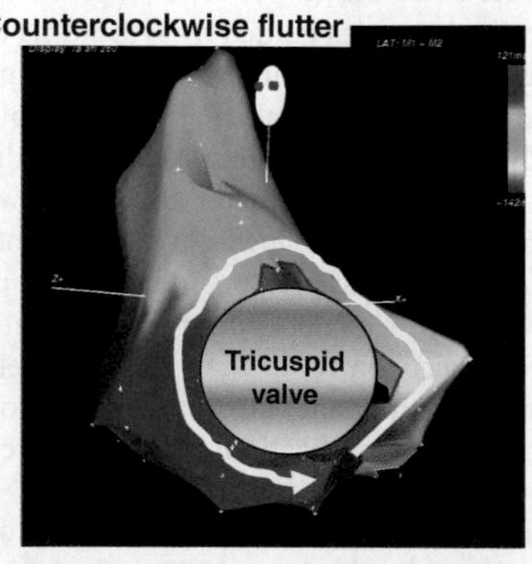

B

FIGURE 276-10 ***A.*** Common right atrial flutter, also known as cavotricuspid isthmus flutter, showing positive P waves in lead V_1 and negative "sawtooth" pattern in lead II typical of counterclockwise rotation relative to the tricuspid valve annulus. *(Adapted from F Marchlinski: The tachyarrhythmias. In Longo DL et al [eds]: Harrison's Principles of Internal Medicine, 18th ed. New York, McGraw-Hill, 2012, pp 1878–1900.)* ***B.*** A right atrial map of common counterclockwise flutter is shown. Colors indicate activation time, progressing from red to yellow to green, blue, and purple. The reentry path parallels the tricuspid annulus.

TREATMENT ATRIAL FLUTTER AND MACROREENTRANT ATRIAL TACHYCARDIAS

Initial management of atrial flutter is similar to that for atrial fibrillation, discussed in more detail below. Electrical cardioversion is warranted for hemodynamic instability or severe symptoms. Otherwise, rate control can be achieved with administration of AV nodal–blocking agents, but this is often more difficult than for atrial fibrillation. The risk of thromboembolic events is felt to be similar to that associated with atrial fibrillation. Anticoagulation is warranted prior to conversion for episodes more than 48 h in duration and chronically for patients at increased risk of thromboembolic stroke based on the CHA_2DS_2-VASc scoring system (Table 276-6).

For a first episode of atrial flutter, conversion to sinus rhythm with no antiarrhythmic drug therapy is reasonable. For recurrent episodes, antiarrhythmic drug therapy with sotalol, dofetilide, disopyramide, and amiodarone may be considered, but more than 70% of patients experience recurrences. For recurrent episodes of common atrial flutter, catheter ablation of the cavotricuspid isthmus abolishes the arrhythmia in over 90% of patients with a low risk of complications that are largely related to vascular access and infrequent heart block. Approximately 50% of patients presenting with atrial flutter develop atrial fibrillation within the next 5 years.

MULTIFOCAL ATRIAL TACHYCARDIA

Multifocal AT (MAT) is characterized by at least three distinct P-wave morphologies with rates typically between 100 and 150 beats/min. Unlike atrial fibrillation, there are clear isoelectric intervals between P waves (Fig. 276-11). The mechanism is likely triggered automaticity from multiple atrial foci. It is usually encountered in patients with chronic pulmonary disease and acute illness.

TREATMENT MULTIFOCAL ATRIAL TACHYCARDIA

Therapy for MAT is directed at treating the underlying disease and correcting any metabolic abnormalities. Electrical cardioversion has no effect. The calcium channel blockers verapamil or diltiazem may slow the atrial and ventricular rate. Patients with severe pulmonary disease often do not tolerate beta blocker therapy. MAT may respond to amiodarone, but long-term therapy with this agent is usually avoided due to its toxicities, particularly pulmonary fibrosis.

ATRIAL FIBRILLATION

Atrial fibrillation (AF) is characterized by disorganized, rapid, and irregular atrial activation with loss of atrial contraction and with an irregular ventricular rate that is determined by AV nodal conduction (Fig. 276-12). In an untreated patient, the ventricular rate also tends

TABLE 276-6 CHA_2DS_2-VASc RISK ASSESSMENT AND ORAL ANTICOAGULANTS

Risk Factors	Points	CHA_2DS_2-VASc Score	Estimated Annual Stroke Rate[a]
C – congestive heart failure	1	0	0
H – hypertension	1	1	1.3%
A – age ≥75 y	2	2	2.2%
D – diabetes mellitus	1	3	3.2%
S – stroke or TIA, embolus	2	4	4.0%
V – vascular disease	1	5	6.7%
A – age 65–75 y	1	6–9	>9%
Sex – female	1		

Anticoagulants	Mechanism	Excretion	Dosing Considerations	Risk/Benefit
Warfarin	Vitamin K antagonist	Liver	Adjusted to INR 2–3	Major hemorrhage: 1% per year
			Days to therapeutic effect	Intracranial hemorrhage: 0.1–0.6% per year
			Multiple drug/food interactions (e.g., amiodarone)	Risk of bleeding increases with INR >3.5
				Inexpensive
Dabigatran[b]	Thrombin inhibitor	Kidney		
		CCr >30 mL/min	150 mg bid	Onset of action within hours
		CCr 15–30 mL/min	75 mg bid	No reversal agent for bleeding
			P-glycoprotein substrate (inducers – rifampin, reduce concentration)	
			(inhibitors – amiodarone, verapamil, dronedarone, quinidine),	
			Proton pump inhibitors may reduce absorption	
Rivaroxaban	Xa inhibitor	Kidney	P-glycoprotein substrate	No reversal agent for bleeding
		CCr ≥50 mL/min	20 mg daily	
		CCr 15–50 mL/min	15 mg daily	
Apixaban	Xa inhibitor	Kidney and liver	P-glycoprotein substrate	No reversal agent for bleeding
		Cr >1.5 mg/dL	2.5 mg bid	

[a]Modified from GY Lip et al: Lancet 379:648, 2012. [b]U.S. Food and Drug Administration recommended dosing; other regimens are available outside the United States.

Abbreviations: CCr, creatinine clearance; Cr, creatinine; INR, international normalized ratio; TIA, transient ischemic attack.

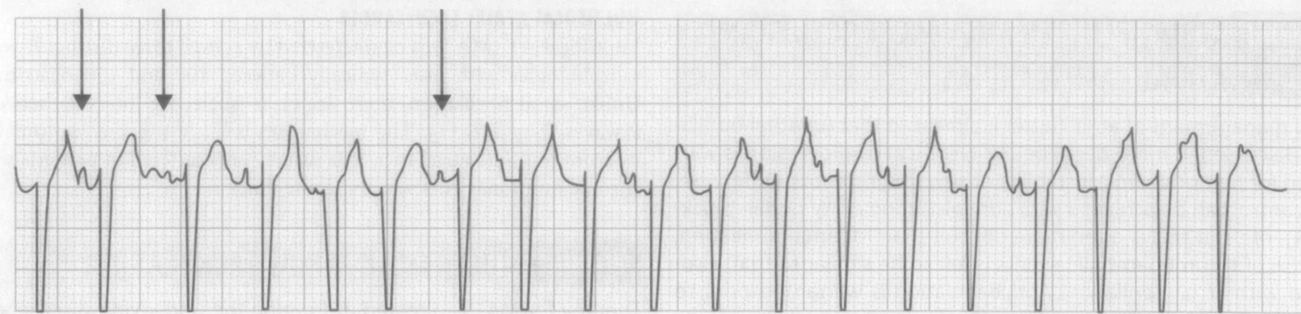

FIGURE 276-11 Multifocal atrial tachycardia. Rhythm strip obtained from a patient with severe pulmonary disease during an acute illness. *Arrows* note three distinct P-wave morphologies.

to be rapid and variable, between 120 and 160 beats/min, but in some patients, it may exceed 200 beats/min. Patients with high vagal tone or AV nodal conduction disease may have slow rates.

AF is the most common sustained arrhythmia and is a major public health problem. Prevalence increases with age, and more than 95% of AF patients are older than 60 years of age. The prevalence by age 80 is approximately 10%. The lifetime risk of developing AF for individuals 40 years old is approximately 25%. AF is slightly more common in men than women and more common in whites than blacks. Risk factors for developing AF in addition to age include hypertension, diabetes mellitus, cardiac disease, and sleep apnea. AF is a marker for heart disease, the severity of heart disease, and age, and it is therefore difficult to determine the extent to which AF itself contributes to associated increased mortality and morbidity. AF is associated with increased risk of developing heart failure. AF increases the risk of stroke by fivefold and is estimated to be the cause of 25% of strokes. It also increases the risk of dementia.

AF is occasionally associated with an acute precipitating factor such as hyperthyroidism, acute alcohol intoxication, or an acute illness including myocardial infarction or pulmonary embolism. AF occurs in up to 30% of patients recovering from cardiac surgery, associated with inflammatory pericarditis.

The clinical type of AF suggests the underlying pathophysiology (Fig. 276-12). Paroxysmal AF is defined as episodes that start and stop spontaneously. It is often initiated by small reentrant or rapidly firing foci in sleeves of atrial muscle along the pulmonary veins. Catheter ablation that isolates these foci usually abolishes the AF. Persistent AF has a longer duration, exceeding 7 days, and, in many cases, will continue unless cardioversion is performed. Cardioversion can be followed by prolonged periods of sinus rhythm. Episodes may be initiated by rapidly firing foci, but persistence of the arrhythmia is likely due to single or multiple areas of reentry facilitated by structural and electrophysiologic atrial abnormalities. In patients with long-standing persistent AF (>1 year), significant structural changes are present in the atrium that support reentry and automaticity, making it difficult to restore and maintain sinus rhythm. Some patients progress over years from paroxysmal to persistent AF. Fibrosis that develops with

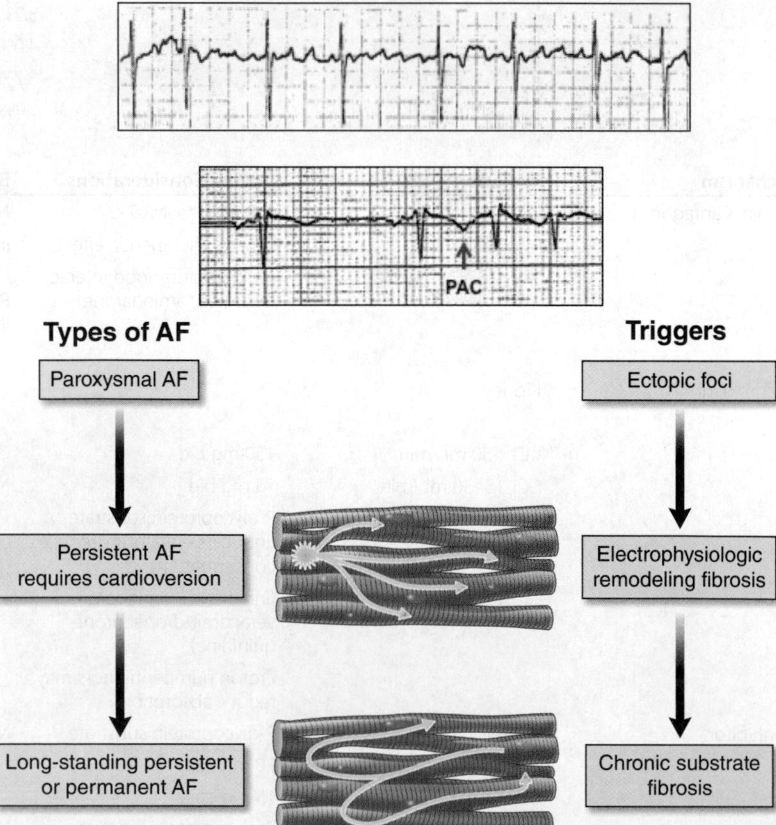

FIGURE 276-12 A rhythm strip of atrial fibrillation (AF) showing no distinct P-wave morphology and irregular ventricular response. Diagram depicts atrial fibrillation types. Paroxysmal AF is initiated by premature beats, as shown in the rhythm strip (*arrow*) after two sinus beats. Triggering foci are often an important cause of this arrhythmia. Persistent AF is associated with atrial structural and electrophysiologic remodeling, as well as with triggering foci in many patients. Long-standing persistent AF is associated with greater structural remodeling with atrial fibrosis and electrophysiologic remodeling.

aging and atrial hypertrophy in response to hypertension and other cardiac disease may be an important promoting factor, although electrophysiologic changes to conduction and refractoriness occur as well in response to chronic tachycardia in the atrium.

Clinical consequences are related to rapid ventricular rates, loss of atrial contribution to ventricular filling, and predisposition to thrombus formation in the left atrial appendage with potential embolization. Presentations vary with the ventricular rate and underlying heart disease and comorbidities. Many patients are asymptomatic. Rapid rates may cause hemodynamic collapse or heart failure exacerbations particularly in patients with impaired cardiac function, hypertrophic cardiomyopathy, and heart failure with preserved systolic function. Exercise intolerance and easy fatigability are common. Occasionally, dizziness or syncope occurs due to pauses when AF terminates to sinus rhythm (Fig. 276-13).

TREATMENT ATRIAL FIBRILLATION

Treatment for AF is primarily guided by patients' symptoms, the hemodynamic effect of AF, the duration of AF if there are persistent risk factors for stroke, and underlying heart disease. Oral anticoagulation in high-risk patients with AF includes vitamin K antagonists or the newer anticoagulants such as thrombin inhibitors (dabigatran) or factor Xa inhibitors (rivaroxaban, apixaban), but not antiplatelet agents (aspirin and clopidogrel), which have substantially less effect.

New-onset AF that produces severe hypotension, pulmonary edema, or angina should be electrically cardioverted starting with a QRS synchronous shock of 200 J, ideally after sedation or anesthesia is achieved. Greater shock energy and different electrode placements may be tried if the shock fails to terminate AF. If AF terminates and reinitiates, administration of an antiarrhythmic drug, such as ibutilide, and repeat cardioversion may be considered. If the patient is stable, immediate management involves rate control to alleviate or prevent symptoms, anticoagulation if appropriate, and cardioversion to restore sinus rhythm if AF is persistent. Anticoagulation strategies for new-onset AF are debated. In the absence of contraindications, it is usually appropriate to initiate systemic anticoagulation with heparin immediately, while evaluation and other therapies are implemented.

CARDIOVERSION AND ANTICOAGULATION

Cardioversion *within 48 h of the onset of AF* is common practice in patients who have not been anticoagulated, provided that they are not at high risk for stroke due to a prior history of embolic events, rheumatic mitral stenosis, or hypertrophic cardiomyopathy with marked left atrial enlargement. These patients are usually at risk of recurrence, such that initiation of anticoagulation is considered based on the patient's individual risk for stroke, commonly assessed from the CHA_2DS_2-VASc score.

If the duration of AF exceeds 48 h or is unknown, there is greater concern for thromboembolism with cardioversion, even in patients considered low risk for stroke. There are two approaches to mitigate the risk related to cardioversion. One option is to anticoagulate continuously for 3 weeks before and a minimum of 4 weeks after cardioversion. A second approach is to start anticoagulation and perform a transesophageal echocardiogram to determine if thrombus is present in the left atrial appendage. If thrombus is absent, cardioversion can be performed and anticoagulation continued for a minimum of 4 weeks because recovery of atrial mechanical function after electrical or pharmacologic cardioversion may be delayed and thrombus can form and embolize days after cardioversion. Some patients may merit ongoing anticoagulation after cardioversion, depending on stroke risk profile.

RATE CONTROL

Acute rate control can be achieved with beta blockers and/or the calcium channel blockers verapamil and diltiazem administered either intravenously or orally, as warranted by the urgency of the clinical situation. Digoxin may be added, particularly in heart failure

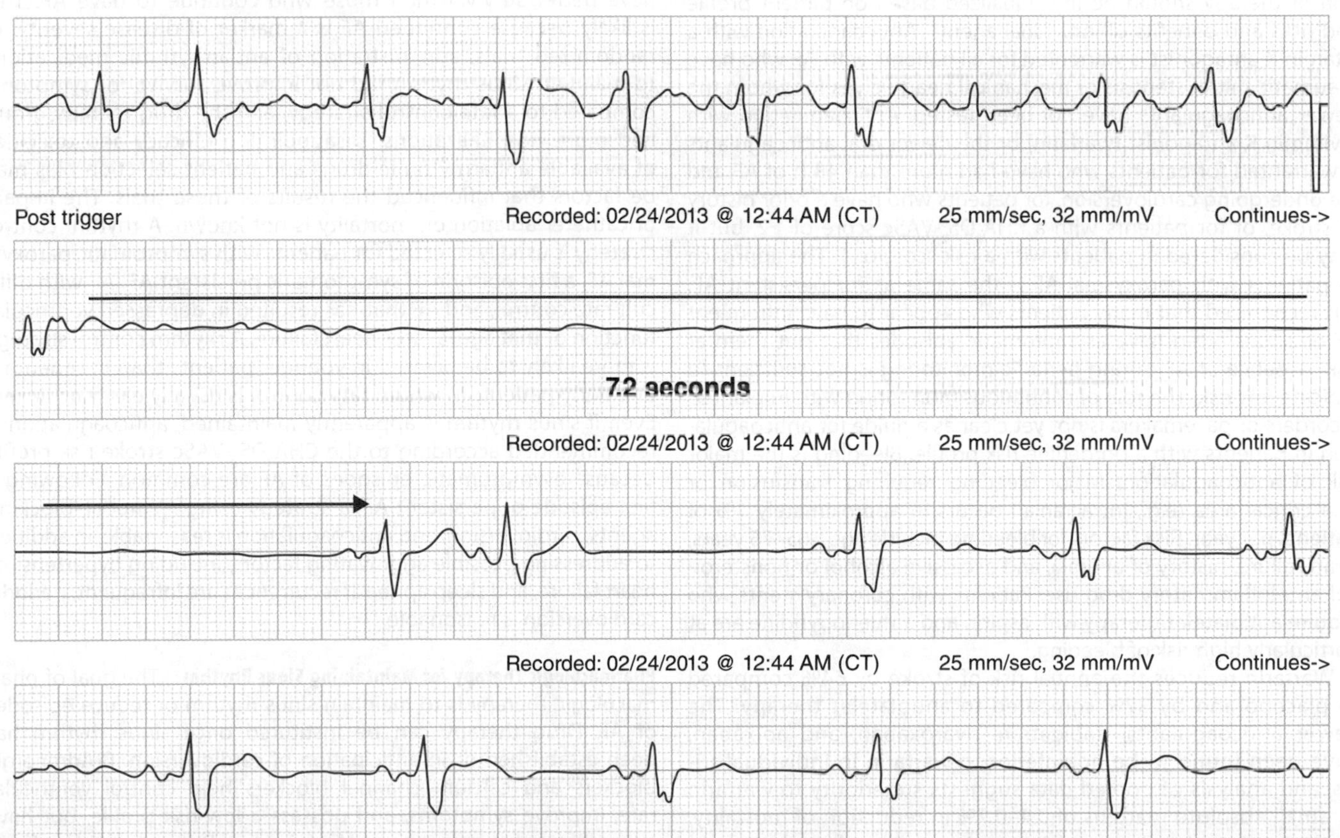

FIGURE 276-13 A continuous rhythm strip is shown. Atrial fibrillation is present at the top and abruptly terminates in the second tracing, with atrial and ventricular standstill for 7.2 s until resumption of sinus rhythm. The patient experienced syncope.

patients, because it does not have negative inotropic effects, particularly if use of AV nodal–blocking agents is limited by poor tolerance or is contraindicated. Its effect is modest but synergistic with the other AV nodal–blocking agents, but it is particularly limited when sympathetic tone is elevated. Typically, the goal of acute rate control is to reduce the ventricular rate to less than 100/min, but the goal must be guided by the clinical situation.

CHRONIC RATE CONTROL

For patients who remain in AF chronically, the goal of rate control is to alleviate and prevent symptoms and prevent deterioration of ventricular function from excessive rates. β-Adrenergic blockers, calcium channel blockers, and digoxin are used, sometimes in combination. Rate should be assessed with exertion and medications adjusted accordingly. Exertion-related symptoms are often an indication of inadequate rate control. The initial goal is a resting heart rate of less than 80 beats/min that increases to less than 100 beats/min with light exertion, such as walking. If it is difficult to slow the ventricular rate to that degree, allowing a resting rate of up to 110 beats/min is acceptable provided it does not cause symptoms and ventricular function remains normal. Periodic assessment of ventricular function is warranted because some patients develop tachycardia-induced cardiomyopathy.

If adequate rate control in AF is difficult to achieve, further consideration should be given to restoring sinus rhythm. Catheter ablation of the AV junction to create heart block and implantation of a permanent pacemaker reliably achieve rate control without the need for AV nodal agents, but implement life-long permanent pacing. Right ventricular apical pacing induces dyssynchronous ventricular activation that can be symptomatic or depress ventricular function in some patients. Biventricular pacing may be used to minimize the degree of ventricular dyssynchrony.

STROKE PREVENTION IN ATRIAL FIBRILLATION

The majority of patients warrant chronic anticoagulation, but selection of therapy should be individualized based on patient profile and risks and benefits of individual agents. Anticoagulation with a vitamin K antagonist is warranted for all patients with AF who have rheumatic mitral stenosis or mechanical heart valves for whom the newer anticoagulants have not been tested. Anticoagulation with a vitamin K antagonist (warfarin) or the newer oral anticoagulants is warranted for patients who have had more than 48 h of AF and are undergoing cardioversion, for patients who have a prior history of stroke, or for patients with a CHA_2DS_2-VASc score of ≥2, but it may be considered in patients with a risk score of 1. The approach to patients with paroxysmal AF is the same as for persistent AF. It is recognized that many patients who appear to have infrequent AF episodes often have asymptomatic episodes that put them at risk. Absence of AF during periodic monitoring is not sufficient to indicate low risk. The role of continuous monitoring with implanted recorders or pacemakers is not yet clear as a guide for anticoagulation in patients with a borderline risk profile. Bleeding is the major risk of anticoagulation. Major bleeding requiring transfusion or in a critical area (e.g., intracranial) occurs in approximately 1% of patients per year. Risk factors for bleeding include age >65–75 years, heart failure, history of anemia, and excessive alcohol or nonsteroidal anti-inflammatory drug use. Patients with coronary stents who require antiplatelet therapy with aspirin and a thienopyridine are at particularly high risk of bleeding.

Warfarin reduces the annual risk of stroke by 64% compared to placebo and by 37% compared to antiplatelet therapy. The newer anticoagulants, dabigatran, rivaroxaban, and apixaban, have been found to be noninferior to warfarin in individual trials, and analysis of pooled data suggests superiority to warfarin by small absolute margins of 0.4–0.7% in reduction of mortality, stroke, major bleeding, and intracranial hemorrhage. Warfarin is an inconvenient agent that requires several days to achieve a therapeutic effect (prothrombin time [PT]/international normalized ratio [INR] >2), requires monitoring of PT/INR to adjust dose, and has many drug and food interactions, thus limiting patient compliance. The newer agents are easier to use and achieve reliable anticoagulation promptly without requiring dosage adjustment based on blood tests. Dabigatran, rivaroxaban, and apixaban have renal excretion, cannot be used with severe renal insufficiency, and require dose adjustment for modest renal impairment, which is of particular concern in the elderly, who are at increased bleeding risk. Excretion can also be influenced by P-glycoprotein inducers and inhibitors. Warfarin anticoagulation can be reversed by administration of fresh frozen plasma and vitamin K. Reversing agents for the newer anticoagulants are lacking (but in development), and bleeding must be managed with supportive care, with the expectation that clotting will improve over 12 h as the anticoagulant is excreted.

The antiplatelet agents aspirin and clopidogrel are inferior to warfarin for stroke prevention in AF and do not reduce the risk of bleeding. Clopidogrel combined with aspirin is better than aspirin alone but inferior to warfarin and has greater bleeding risk than aspirin alone.

Chronic anticoagulation is contraindicated in some patients due to bleeding risks. Because most atrial thrombi are felt to originate in the left atrial appendage, surgical removal of the appendage, combined with atrial maze surgery, may be considered for patients undergoing surgery, although removal of the appendage has not been unequivocally shown to reduce the risk of thromboembolism. Percutaneous devices that occlude or ligate the left atrial appendage are being studied for safety and efficacy.

RHYTHM CONTROL

The decision to administer antiarrhythmic drugs or perform catheter ablation to attempt maintenance of sinus rhythm (commonly referred to as the "rhythm control strategy") is mainly guided by patient symptoms and preferences regarding the benefits and risks of therapies. In general, patients who maintain sinus rhythm have better survival than those who continue to have AF. This is likely because continued AF is a marker of disease severity. In randomized trials, administration of antiarrhythmic medications to maintain sinus rhythm did not improve survival or symptoms compared to a rate control strategy, and the drug therapy group had more hospitalizations. Disappointing efficacy and toxicities of available antiarrhythmic drugs and patient selection bias may be factors that influenced the results of these trials. The impact of catheter ablation on mortality is not known. A rhythm control strategy is usually selected for patients with symptomatic paroxysmal AF, a first episode of symptomatic persistent AF, AF with difficult rate control, and AF that has resulted in depressed ventricular function or that aggravates heart failure. A rhythm control strategy is more likely to be favored in younger patients than in sedentary or elderly patients in whom rate control is usually easily achieved. Even if sinus rhythm is apparently maintained, anticoagulation is recommended according to the CHA_2DS_2-VASc stroke risk profile because asymptomatic episodes of AF are common. Following a first episode of persistent AF, a strategy using AV nodal–blocking agents, cardioversion, and anticoagulation is reasonable, in addition to addressing possible aggravating factors, including hypertension, heart failure, and sleep apnea. If recurrences are infrequent, periodic cardioversion is reasonable.

Pharmacologic Therapy for Maintaining Sinus Rhythm The goal of pharmacologic therapy is to maintain sinus rhythm or reduce episodes of AF. Drug therapy can be instituted once sinus rhythm has been established or in anticipation of cardioversion. β-Adrenergic blockers and calcium channel blockers help control ventricular rate, improve symptoms, and possess a low-risk profile, but have low efficacy for preventing AF episodes. Risks and side effects of antiarrhythmic drugs are a major consideration in selecting therapy. Class I sodium channel–blocking agents (e.g., flecainide, propafenone, disopyramide) are options for subjects without significant structural heart disease, but they have negative inotropic and proarrhythmic effects that warrant avoidance in patients with coronary artery disease or heart failure. The class III agents sotalol and dofetilide can be administered to patients with coronary artery disease or structural heart disease but have approximately a 3% risk of inducing excessive QT prolongation and torsades des pointes. Dofetilide should be initiated only in a hospital with ECG monitoring, and many physicians take this approach with sotalol as well. Dronedarone increases mortality in patients with heart failure. All of these agents have modest efficacy in patients with paroxysmal AF, of whom approximately 30–50% will benefit. Amiodarone is more effective, maintaining sinus rhythm in approximately two-thirds of patients. It can be administered to patients with heart failure and coronary artery disease. Over 20% of patients experience toxicities during long-term therapy.

CATHETER AND SURGICAL ABLATION FOR ATRIAL FIBRILLATION

Catheter ablation avoids antiarrhythmic drug toxicities but has procedural risks and requires an experienced center. For patients with previously untreated but recurrent paroxysmal AF, catheter ablation has similar efficacy to antiarrhythmic drug therapy and is superior to antiarrhythmic drugs for patients who have recurrent AF despite drug treatment. The procedure involves cardiac catheterization, transatrial septal puncture, and radiofrequency ablation or cryoablation to electrically isolate the regions around the pulmonary veins, abolishing the effect of triggering foci to interact with the left atrial AF substrate. Extensive areas of ablation are required, and gaps in healed ablation areas necessitate a repeat procedure in 20–50% of patients. Sinus rhythm is maintained for more than 1 year after one procedure in approximately 60% of patients and in 70–80% of patients after multiple procedures. Some patients become more responsive to antiarrhythmic drugs.

There is a 2–7% risk of major complications, including stroke (0.5–1%), cardiac tamponade (1%), phrenic nerve paralysis, bleeding from femoral access sites, and fluid overload with heart failure, that can emerge 1–3 days after the procedure. It is important to recognize the potential for delayed presentation of some complications. Ablation within the pulmonary veins can lead to pulmonary vein stenosis, presenting weeks to months after the procedure with dyspnea or hemoptysis. Esophageal ulcers can form immediately after the procedure and may rarely lead to a fistula between the left atrium and esophagus (estimated incidence of 0.1%) that presents as endocarditis and stroke 10 days to 3 weeks after the procedure.

Catheter ablation is less effective for persistent AF. More extensive ablation is often required, including areas that likely support reentry in regions outside the pulmonary venous antra, but individual strategies are debated. More than one ablation procedure is often required to maintain sinus rhythm.

Surgical ablation of AF is typically performed concomitant with cardiac valve or coronary artery surgery and less commonly as a stand-alone procedure; however, for patients with persistent AF, surgical or hybrid procedures may have higher single-procedure efficacy. Risks include sinus node injury requiring pacemaker implantation. Surgical removal of the left atrial appendage may reduce stroke risk, although thrombus can form in the remnant of the appendage or if the appendage is not completely ligated.

ACKNOWLEDGMENT

Portions of this chapter were retained from the work of the previous author, Francis Marchlinski.

277 Ventricular Arrhythmias

Roy M. John, William G. Stevenson

Arrhythmias that originate in the ventricular myocardium or His-Purkinje system include premature ventricular beats, ventricular tachycardias that can be sustained or nonsustained, and ventricular fibrillation. Arrhythmia may emerge from a focus of myocardial or Purkinje cells capable of automaticity, or triggered automaticity, or from reentry through areas of scar or a diseased Purkinje system. Ventricular arrhythmias are often associated with structural heart disease and are an important cause of sudden death (Chap. 327). They also occur in some structurally normal hearts, in which case they are usually benign. Evaluation and management are guided by the risk of arrhythmic death, which is assessed based on symptoms, type of arrhythmia, and associated underlying heart disease.

DEFINITIONS

Ventricular arrhythmias are characterized by their electrocardiographic appearance and duration. Conduction away from the ventricular focus through the ventricular myocardium is slower than activation of the ventricles over the Purkinje system. Hence, the QRS complex during ventricular arrhythmias will be wide, typically >0.12 s.

Premature ventricular beats (also referred to as *premature ventricular contractions* [PVCs]) are single ventricular beats that fall earlier than the next anticipated supraventricular beat (Fig. 277-1). PVCs that originate from the same focus will have the same QRS morphology and are referred to as unifocal (Fig. 277-1*A*). PVCs that originate from different ventricular sites have different QRS morphologies and are referred to as multifocal (Fig. 277-1*B*). Two consecutive ventricular beats are *ventricular couplets*.

Ventricular tachycardia (VT) is three or more consecutive beats at a rate faster than 100 beats/min. Three or more consecutive beats at slower rates are designated an *idioventricular rhythm* (Fig. 277-1*C*). VT that terminates spontaneously within 30 s is designated *nonsustained* (Fig. 277-2), whereas *sustained VT* persists longer than 30 s or is terminated by an active intervention, such as administration of an intravenous medication, external cardioversion, or pacing or a shock from an implanted cardioverter-defibrillator.

Monomorphic VT has the same QRS complex from beat to beat, indicating that the activation sequence is the same from beat to beat and that each beat likely originates from the same source (Fig. 277-3*A*). The initial site of ventricular activation largely determines the sequence of ventricular activation. Therefore, the QRS morphology of PVCs and monomorphic VT provides an indication of the site of origin within the ventricles (Fig. 277-4). The likely origin often suggests whether an arrhythmia is idiopathic or associated with structural disease. Arrhythmias that originate from the right ventricle or septum result in late activation of much of the left ventricle, thereby producing a prominent S wave in V_1 referred to as a left bundle branch block–like configuration. Arrhythmias that originate from the free wall of the left ventricle have a prominent positive deflection in V_1, thereby producing a right bundle branch block–like morphology in V_1. The frontal plane axis of the QRS is also useful. An axis that is directed inferiorly, as indicated by dominant R waves in leads II, III, and AVF, suggests initial activation of the cranial portion of the ventricle, whereas a frontal plane axis that is directed superiorly (dominant S waves in II, III, and AVF) suggests initial activation at the inferior wall.

Very rapid monomorphic VT has a sinusoidal appearance, also called *ventricular flutter*, because it is not possible to distinguish the QRS complex from the T wave (Fig. 277-3*B*). Relatively slow *sinusoidal* VTs have a wide QRS indicative of slowed ventricular conduction (Fig. 277-3*C*). Hyperkalemia, toxicity from excessive effects of drugs that blocks sodium channels (e.g., flecainide, propafenone, or

A

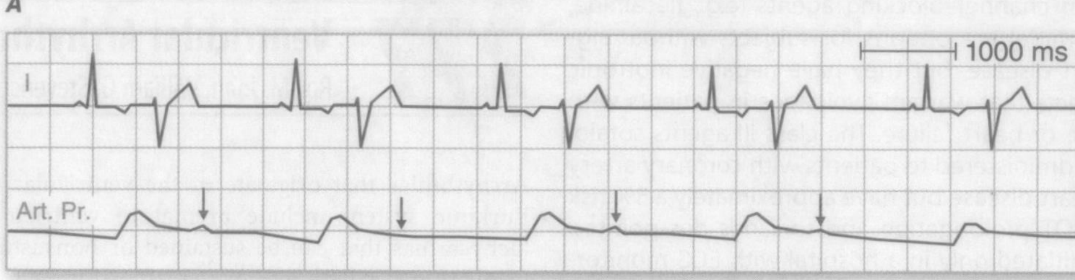

B

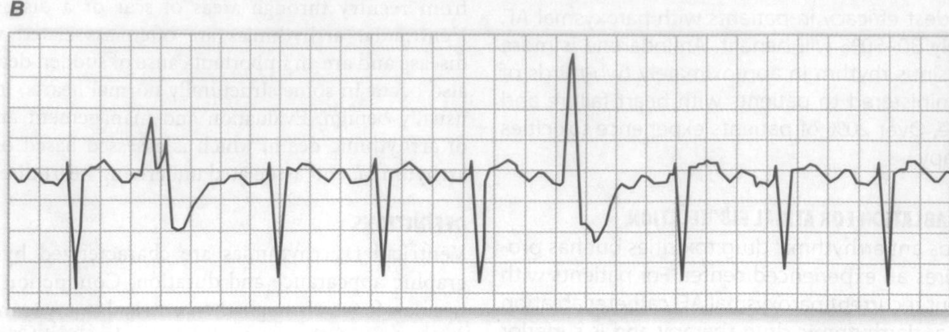

C

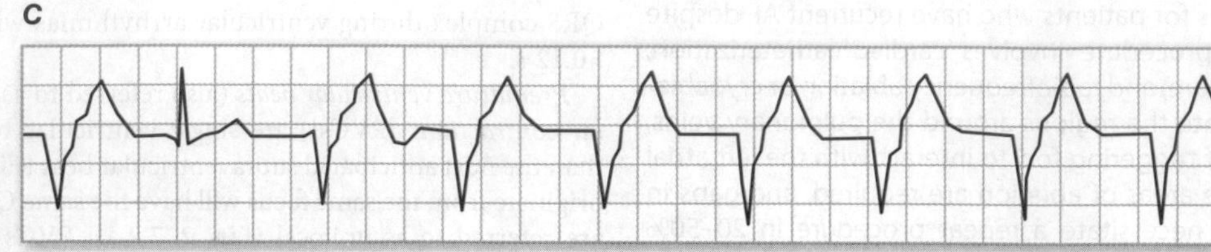

FIGURE 277-1 Examples of types of premature ventricular contractions (PVCs). ***A.*** Unifocal PVCs follow every sinus beat in a bigeminal frequency. Trace shows electrocardiogram lead 1 and arterial pressure (Art. Pr.). Sinus rhythm beats are followed by normal arterial waveform. The arterial pressure following premature beats is attenuated (*arrows*) and imperceptible to palpation. The pulse in this patient is registered at half the heart rate. ***B.*** Multifocal PVCs. The two PVCs shown have different morphologies. ***C.*** Example of accelerated idioventricular rhythm. The second QRS is a normally conducted beat. All other QRS complexes on this rhythm strip are ventricular due to accelerated idioventricular rhythm.

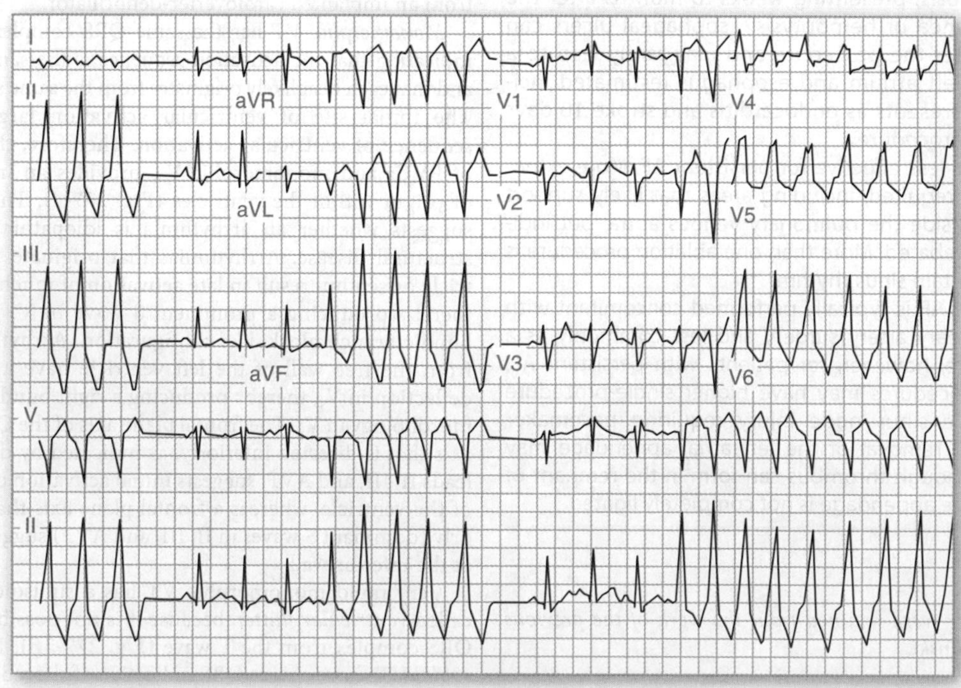

FIGURE 277-2 Repetitive monomorphic nonsustained ventricular tachycardia (VT) of right ventricular outflow tract origin. The VT has a left bundle branch block pattern with inferior axis with tall QRS complexes in the inferior leads.

tricyclic antidepressants), and severe global myocardial ischemia are causes.

Polymorphic VT has a continually changing QRS morphology indicating a changing ventricular activation sequence. Polymorphic VT that occurs in the context of congenital or acquired prolongation of the QT interval often has a waxing and waning QRS amplitude creating a "twisting about the points" appearance referred to as *Torsade de Pointes* (Fig. 277-3D).

Ventricular fibrillation (VF) has continuous irregular activation with no discrete QRS complexes (Fig. 277-3E). Monomorphic or polymorphic VT may transition to VF in susceptible patients.

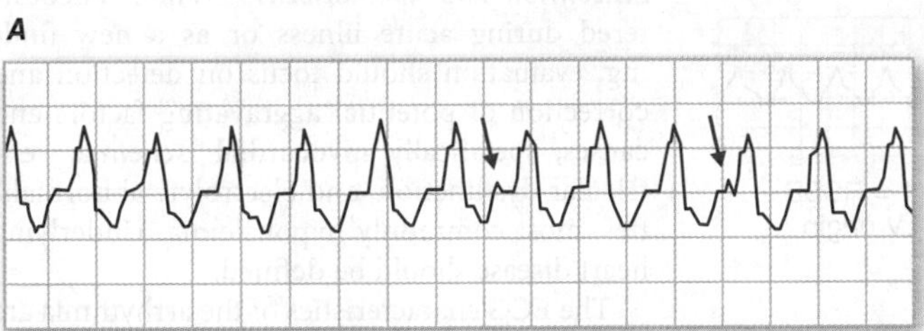

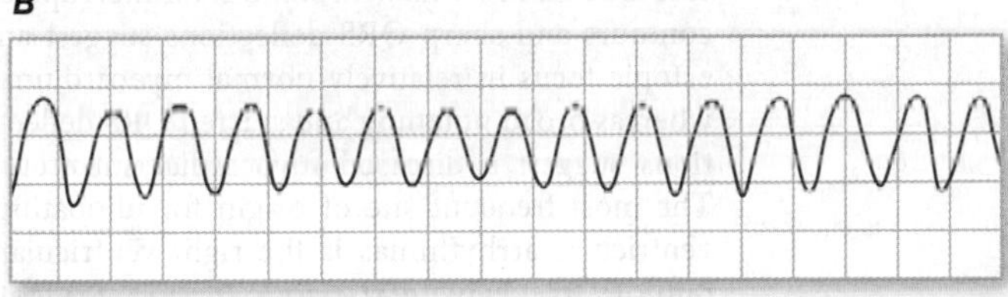

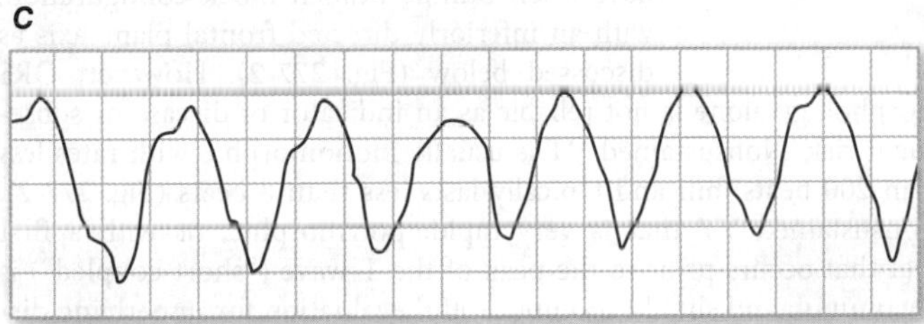

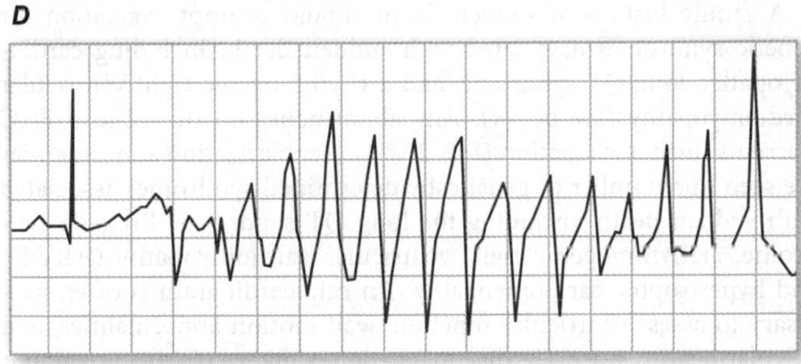

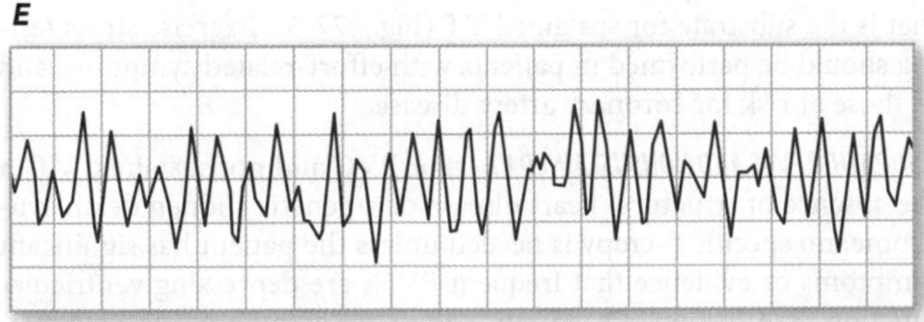

FIGURE 277-3 Examples of types of ventricular tachycardia (VT). ***A.*** Monomorphic VT with dissociated P waves (*short arrows*). ***B.*** Ventricular flutter. ***C.*** Sinusoidal VT due to electrolyte disturbance or drug effects. ***D.*** Polymorphic VT resulting from prolongation of QT interval (torsade de pointes VT). ***E.*** Ventricular fibrillation.

CLINICAL MANIFESTATIONS AND DIAGNOSIS

Common symptoms of ventricular arrhythmias include palpitations, dizziness, exercise intolerance, episodes of lightheadedness, syncope, or sudden death. These arrhythmias can be asymptomatic and encountered unexpectedly as an irregular pulse or heart sounds on examination, or seen on a routine electrocardiogram (ECG), exercise test, or cardiac ECG monitoring.

Syncope is a concerning symptom that can be due to an episode of VT with hypotension. Syncope due to a ventricular arrhythmia often indicates that there is a significant risk for subsequent cardiac arrest and sudden death with arrhythmia recurrence. Although benign causes of syncope, such as reflex-mediated neurocardiogenic (vasovagal) syncope and orthostatic hypotension, are generally more common, it is important to consider the possibility of heart disease or a genetic syndrome causing VT. When these are suspected, hospitalization for further evaluation and monitoring is often appropriate.

Sustained VT may present with cardiac arrest, often with degeneration of the VT to VF. Occasionally a sustained VT will be hemodynamically tolerated and present with diminished exercise capacity or exacerbation of heart failure. Many patients who are at risk for VT have known heart disease and may have an implantable cardioverter-defibrillator (ICD). In patients with an ICD, spontaneous episodes of VT may elicit an episode of transient lightheadedness, palpitations, or syncope that may be followed by a shock from the ICD (see below).

The diagnosis of ventricular arrhythmias is established by recording of the arrhythmia on an ECG or, in some cases, initiation of the arrhythmia during an electrophysiologic study (Table 277-1). A 12-lead ECG of the arrhythmia should be obtained when possible and often provides clues to the potential site of origin and possible presence of underlying heart disease (see above). When the arrhythmia is intermittent with days to weeks between symptoms, prolonged ambulatory monitoring to capture the ECG at the time of symptoms is required to make the diagnosis. Continuous ambulatory monitoring or looping event recording monitors are options. Exercise testing should be considered in patients with exercise-induced symptoms.

APPROACH TO THE PATIENT: Documented or Suspected Ventricular Arrhythmias

Initial assessment focuses on hemodynamic stability and evaluation for underlying heart disease. A family history of sudden death or cardiomyopathy suggests the possibility of a genetic basis for the arrhythmia and greater risk. The electrocardiogram can provide important clues. Patients with benign idiopathic arrhythmias usually have a completely normal ECG during sinus rhythm.

Cardiac imaging is warranted to assess ventricular function and look for evidence of depressed ventricular function indicative of a cardiomyopathy or ventricular hypertrophy that may indicate hypertrophic cardiomyopathy. Cardiac magnetic resonance imaging (MRI) with late gadolinium enhancement can detect areas of ventricular scar, which are usually present in patients who are at risk for sustained monomorphic VT (Fig. 277-5). Evaluation to exclude atherosclerotic coronary artery disease should be performed in patients at risk, guided by age and other risk factors.

SPECIFIC ARRHYTHMIAS

PVCs and Nonsustained VT Ventricular extrasystoles (Fig. 277-1*A*) can be due to automaticity or reentry (Chap. 278e). PVCs can be a sign of increased sympathetic tone; myocardial ischemia; hypoxia; electrolyte abnormalities, particularly hypokalemia; or underlying heart disease. During myocardial ischemia or in association with other heart disease, PVCs can be a harbinger of sustained VT or

VF. In patients with heart disease, a higher frequency of ectopy and complexity (couplets and nonsustained VT) are associated with more severe disease and, in those with heart failure, with increased mortality. However, suppression of these arrhythmias with antiarrhythmic drugs does not improve survival. In the absence of cardiac disease, PVCs and nonsustained VT generally have a benign prognosis. PVCs that occur at a bigeminal frequency may not generate sufficient cardiac output for a radial pulse and hence may register at rates half that of the heart rate (Fig. 277-1*A*). Very frequent PVCs can depress ventricular function (see below).

EVALUATION AND MANAGEMENT When encountered during acute illness or as a new finding, evaluation should focus on detection and correction of potential aggravating factors and causes, specifically myocardial ischemia, ventricular dysfunction, and electrolyte abnormalities, most commonly hypokalemia. Underlying heart disease should be defined.

The ECG characteristics of the arrhythmia are often suggestive of whether structural heart disease is present. PVCs with smooth uninterrupted contours and sharp QRS deflections suggest an ectopic focus in relatively normal myocardium, whereas broad notching and slurred QRS deflections suggest a diseased myocardial substrate. The most frequent site of origin for idiopathic ventricular arrhythmias is the right ventricular outflow tract, giving rise to PVCs or VT that have a left bundle branch block configuration, with an inferiorly directed frontal plane axis as discussed below (Fig. 277-2). However, QRS morphology alone is not reliable as an indicator of disease or subsequent risk. Nonsustained VT is usually monomorphic with rates less than 200 beats/min and typically lasts less than 8 beats (Fig. 277-2). Nonsustained VT that is very rapid, polymorphic, or with a first beat that occurs prior to the peak of the T wave ("short-coupled") is uncommon and should prompt careful evaluation for underlying disease or genetic syndromes associated with sudden death.

A family history of sudden death should prompt evaluation for genetic syndromes associated with sudden death, including cardiomyopathy, long QT syndrome, and arrhythmogenic right ventricular cardiomyopathy (see below). Any abnormality on the 12-lead ECG warrants further evaluation (Fig. 277-6). Repolarization abnormalities are seen in a number of genetically determined syndromes associated with sudden death, including the long QT syndrome, Brugada syndrome, arrhythmogenic right ventricular cardiomyopathy (ARVC), and hypertrophic cardiomyopathy. An echocardiogram is often necessary to assess ventricular function, wall motion abnormalities, and valvular heart disease. Cardiac magnetic resonance (CMR) imaging is also useful for this purpose and for the detection of ventricular scarring that is the substrate for sustained VT (Fig. 277-5). Exercise stress testing should be performed in patients with effort-related symptoms and in those at risk for coronary artery disease.

IDIOPATHIC PVCS AND NONSUSTAINED VT For PVC and nonsustained VT in the absence of structural heart disease or a genetic sudden death syndrome, no specific therapy is needed unless the patient has significant symptoms or evidence that frequent PVCs are depressing ventricular function (see below). Reassurance that the arrhythmia is benign is often sufficient to allow the patient to cope with the symptoms, which will often wax and wane in frequency over years. Avoiding stimulants, such as caffeine, is helpful in some patients. If symptoms require treatment, β-adrenergic blockers and nondihydropyridine calcium channel blockers (verapamil and diltiazem) are sometimes helpful (see Table 276-3). If these fail, more potent antiarrhythmic drugs or catheter

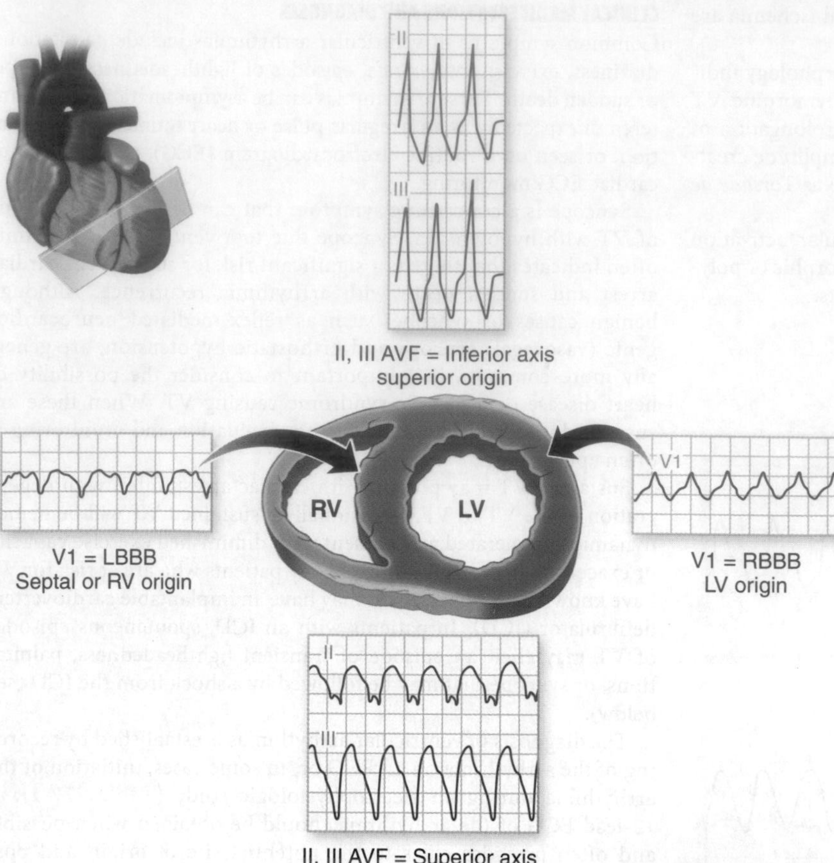

FIGURE 277-4 Site of VT origin based on QRS morphology. LBBB, left bundle branch block; LV, left ventricle; RBBB, right bundle branch block; RV, right ventricle.

TABLE 277-1 DIAGNOSTIC TESTS FOR VENTRICULAR ARRHYTHMIAS

I. 12-Lead ECG
   A. Should be obtained for PVCs, nonsustained VT, and monomorphic VT when possible
   B. QRS morphology suggests ventricular region of origin
      V1 – dominant S = septum or RV
      V1 – dominant R = LV
      Superior axis = inferior wall origin
      Inferior axis = outflow region or anterior wall
II. Ambulatory monitoring
   A. 24- to 48-h continuous Holter monitor
      Useful for evaluation of daily symptoms to quantitate PVCs
   B. Event recorder: can be used for weeks at a time
      Useful for evaluation of infrequent symptoms
      Some require patient activation and will miss asymptomatic arrhythmias
III. Exercise testing
   A. Useful for evaluating exercise-induced arrhythmias and symptoms
   B. QT interval response to exercise may be abnormal in long QT syndrome
IV. Invasive electrophysiology study
   A. Can establish definitive diagnosis of VT versus supraventricular tachycardia with aberrancy or ventricular preexcitation
   B. Can provoke some arrhythmias that are otherwise infrequent
   C. Allows potential catheter ablation
   D. Procedural risks determined by vascular access, whether ablation is performed, and the location of the arrhythmia substrate

Abbreviation: RV, right ventricle. See text for other abbreviations.

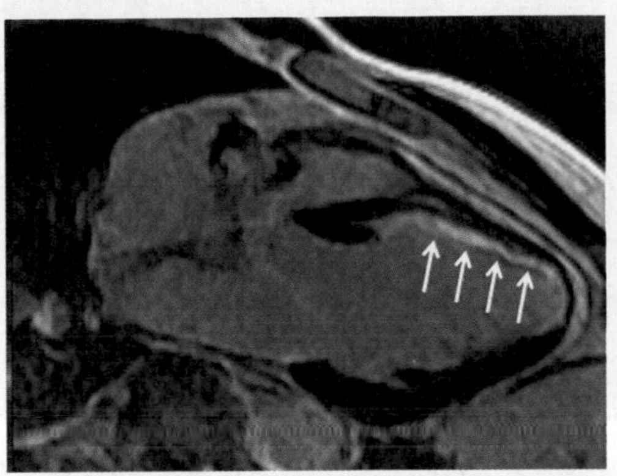

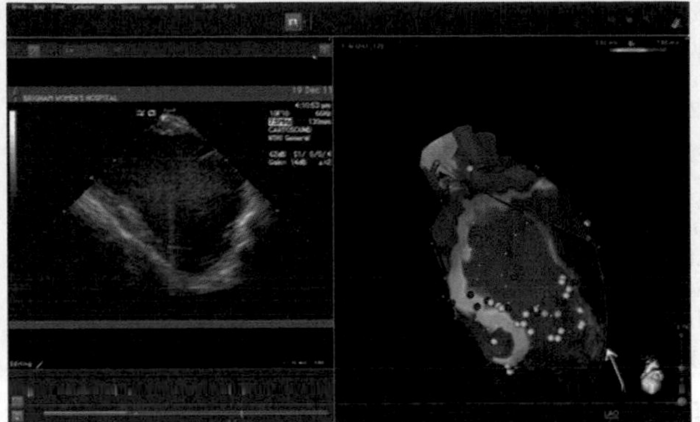

FIGURE 277-5 Imaging studies of the left ventricle (LV) used to assist ablation for ventricle tachycardia (VT). *Left panel* is a magnetic resonance image of a longitudinal section demonstrating thinning of the anterior wall and late gadolinium enhancement in a subendocardial scar (*white arrows*). The *middle panel* shows a two-dimensional image of the LV in long axis corresponding to the sector through the mid LV (*arrow, right panel*) obtained by an intracardiac echo probe positioned in the right ventricle. An electroanatomic three-dimensional map of the LV in the left anterior oblique projection is displayed in the right panel. The purple color depicts areas of normal voltage (>1.5 mV). Blue, green, and yellow represent progressively lower voltages with the red areas indicating scar (<0.5 mV). Channels of viable myocardium with slow conduction within the scar are identified with the light blue dots. Areas of ablation delivered to regions involved in reentrant VT are indicated by maroon dots.

ablation can be considered. The antiarrhythmic agents flecainide, propafenone, mexiletine, and amiodarone can be effective, but the potential for side effects warrants careful consideration. Catheter ablation can be effective if the arrhythmia occurs with sufficient frequency or is readily provoked such that its origin can be identified for ablation in a similar manner to that for idiopathic monomorphic VT as discussed below. Benefit must be carefully weighed against the procedure-related risks (see below).

PVCS AND NONSUSTAINED VT ASSOCIATED WITH ACUTE CORONARY SYNDROMES During and early after acute myocardial infarction (MI), PVCs and nonsustained VT are common and can be an early manifestation of ischemia and a harbinger of subsequent VF. Treatment with β-adrenergic blockers and correction of hypokalemia and hypomagnesemia reduce the risk of VF. Routine administration of the antiarrhythmic drugs such as lidocaine has not been shown to reduce mortality and is not indicated for suppression of PVCs or asymptomatic nonsustained VT.

Following recovery from acute MI, frequent PVCs (typically >10 PVCs per hour), repetitive PVCs with couplets, and nonsustained VT are markers for depressed ventricular function and increased mortality, but routine antiarrhythmic drug therapy to suppress these arrhythmias is not warranted. Treatment with the sodium channel blocker flecainide increased mortality. Amiodarone therapy reduces sudden death, but does not improve total mortality. Therefore, amiodarone is an option for treatment of symptomatic arrhythmias in this population when the potential benefit outweighs its potential toxicities. β-Adrenergic blockers reduce sudden death but have limited effect on spontaneous arrhythmias.

For survivors of an acute MI, an ICD reduces mortality in certain high-risk groups: patients who have survived >40 days after the acute MI and have a left ventricular (LV) ejection fraction of ≤0.30 or who have an ejection fraction <0.35 and have symptomatic heart failure (functional class II or III); and patients >5 days after MI who have a reduced LV ejection fraction, nonsustained VT, and inducible sustained VT or VF on electrophysiologic testing. ICDs do not reduce mortality when routinely implanted soon after MI or in patients after recent coronary artery revascularization surgery.

PVCS AND NONSUSTAINED VT ASSOCIATED WITH DEPRESSED VENTRICULAR FUNCTION AND HEART FAILURE PVCs and nonsustained VT are common in patients with depressed ventricular function and heart failure and are markers for disease severity and increased mortality, but antiarrhythmic drug therapy to suppress these arrhythmias has not been shown to improve survival. Antiarrhythmic drugs whose major action is blockade of the cardiac sodium channel (flecainide, propafenone, mexiletine, quinidine, and disopyramide) are avoided in patients with structural heart disease because of a risk of proarrhythmia, negative inotropic effects, and increased mortality. Therapy with the potassium channel blockers, e.g., dofetilide, does not reduce mortality. Amiodarone suppresses ventricular ectopy and reduces sudden death but does not improve overall survival. ICDs are the major

FIGURE 277-6 Precordial chest leads V_1–V_3 showing typical abnormalities of arrhythmogenic right ventricular cardiomyopathy (ARVC) (*A*) and Brugada syndrome (*B*). In ARVC, there is T inversion and delayed ventricular activation manifest as epsilon waves (*arrows*). Panel B shows ST elevation in V_1 and V_2 typical of the Brugada syndrome. *(Figures reproduced from F Marchlinski: The tachyarrhythmias. In Longo DL et al [eds]: Harrison's Principles of Internal Medicine, 18th edition. New York, McGraw-Hill, 2012, pp 1878–1900.)*

therapy to protect against sudden death in patients at high risk and are recommended for those with LV ejection fraction <0.35 and New York Heart Association class II and III heart failure, in whom they reduce mortality by 20%, from 36% to 29%, over 5 years.

OTHER CARDIAC DISEASES Ventricular ectopy is associated with increased mortality in patients with *hypertrophic cardiomyopathy* (Chap. 287) or with *congenital heart disease* (Chap. 282) associated with right ventricular or LV dysfunction. In these patients, management is similar to that for patients with ventricular dysfunction. Pharmacologic suppression of the arrhythmia has not been shown to improve mortality. ICDs are indicated for patients considered at high risk for sudden cardiac death.

PVC-INDUCED VENTRICULAR DYSFUNCTION Very frequent ventricular ectopy and repetitive nonsustained VT (Fig. 277-2) can depress ventricular function, possibly through an effect similar to chronic tachycardia or by inducing ventricular dyssynchrony. Depression of ventricular function rarely occurs unless PVCs account for more than 10–20% of total beats over a 24-h period. Often the PVCs are idiopathic and unifocal, most commonly originating from the LV papillary muscles or outflow tract regions where they can be targeted for ablation. The distinction between PVC-induced ventricular dysfunction as compared to a cardiomyopathic process causing ventricular dysfunction and arrhythmia is difficult and in some cases can be made only retrospectively by observing an improvement in ventricular function after the arrhythmia is suppressed with an antiarrhythmic drug, such as amiodarone, or by catheter ablation.

Idioventricular Rhythms Three or more ventricular beats at a rate slower than 100 beats/min are termed *idioventricular rhythm* (Fig. 277-1C). Automaticity is the likely mechanism. Idioventricular rhythms are common during acute MI (Chap. 295) and may emerge during sinus bradycardia. Atropine may be administered to increase the sinus rates if the loss of atrioventricular synchrony leads to hemodynamic compromise. This rhythm is also common in patients with cardiomyopathies or sleep apnea. It can also be idiopathic, often emerging when the sinus rate slows during sleep. Therapy should target any underlying cause and correction of bradycardia. Specific therapy for asymptomatic idioventricular rhythm is not necessary.

Sustained Monomorphic VT Sustained monomorphic VT presents as a wide QRS tachycardia that has the same QRS configuration from beat to beat, indicating an identical sequence of ventricular depolarization for each beat (Fig. 277-3A). VT originates from a stable focus or reentry circuit. In structural heart disease, the substrate is often an area of patchy replacement fibrosis due to infarction, inflammation, or prior cardiac surgery that creates anatomical or functional reentry pathways (Fig. 277-5). Less commonly, VT is related to reentry or automaticity in a diseased Purkinje system. In the absence of structural heart disease, idiopathic VT can present as sustained monomorphic VTs that are due to focal automaticity or reentry involving a portion of the Purkinje system.

The clinical presentation can vary depending on the rate of the arrhythmia, underlying cardiac function, and autonomic adaptation in response to the arrhythmia. Whereas patients with normal cardiac function might tolerate rapid VTs, those with severe LV dysfunction often experience symptoms of hypotension, even if VT is not particularly fast. Monomorphic VT may deteriorate to VF, which may be the initial cardiac rhythm recorded at the time of resuscitation.

DIAGNOSIS Sustained monomorphic VT has to be distinguished from other causes of uniform wide QRS tachycardia. These include supraventricular tachycardia with left or right bundle branch block aberrant conduction, supraventricular tachycardias conducted to the ventricles over an accessory pathway (Chap. 276), and rapid cardiac pacing in a patient with a pacemaker or defibrillator. In the presence of known heart disease, VT is the most likely diagnosis of a wide QRS tachycardia. Hemodynamic stability during the arrhythmia does not exclude VT. A number of ECG criteria have been evaluated. The presence of AV dissociation is usually a reliable marker for VT (Fig. 277-7), but P waves can be difficult to define. A P wave following each QRS does not exclude VT because 1:1 conduction from ventricle to atrium can occur. A monophasic R wave or Rs complex in AVR or concordance from V_1 to V_6 of monophasic R or S waves is also relatively specific for VT (Fig. 277-7). Other QRS morphology criteria have also been described, but all have limitations and are not very reliable in patients with severe heart disease. In patients with known bundle branch block, the same QRS morphology during tachycardia as during sinus rhythm suggests supraventricular tachycardia rather than VT, but is not absolutely reliable. An electrophysiologic study is sometimes required for definitive diagnosis. Rarely, noise and movement artifacts on telemetry recordings can simulate VT; prompt recognition can avoid unnecessary tests and interventions.

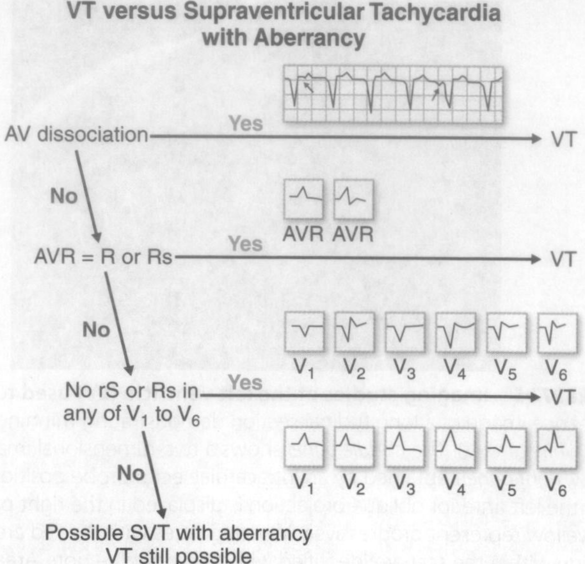

FIGURE 277-7 Algorithm for differentiation of ventricular tachycardia (VT) from supraventricular tachycardia (SVT) with aberration. AV, atrioventricular.

When LV function is depressed or there is evidence of structural myocardial disease, scar-related reentry is the most likely diagnosis. Scars are suggested by pathologic Q waves on the ECG, segmental left or right ventricular wall motion abnormalities on echocardiogram or nuclear imaging, and areas of delayed gadolinium enhancement during MRI (Fig. 277-5).

TREATMENT AND PROGNOSIS Initial management follows Advanced Cardiac Life Support (ACLS) guidelines. If hypotension, impaired consciousness, or pulmonary edema is present, QRS synchronous electrical cardioversion should be performed, ideally after sedation if the patient is conscious. For stable tachycardia, a trial of adenosine is reasonable, as this may clarify a supraventricular tachycardia with aberrancy (Chap. 276). Intravenous amiodarone is the drug of choice if heart disease is present. Following restoration of sinus rhythm, hospitalization and evaluation to define underlying heart disease are required. Assessment of cardiac biomarkers for evidence of MI is appropriate, but acute MI is rarely a cause of sustained monomorphic VT, and elevations in troponin or creatine kinase (CK)-MB are more likely to indicate myocardial damage that is secondary to hypotension and ischemia from the VT. Subsequent management is determined by the underlying heart disease and frequency of VT. If VT recurs frequently or is incessant, administration of antiarrhythmic medications or catheter ablation may be required to restore stability. More commonly, sustained monomorphic VT occurs as an isolated episode, but with a risk of recurrence. ICDs are usually considered for VT associated with structural heart disease.

Sustained Monomorphic VT in Specific Diseases • ***CORONARY ARTERY DISEASE*** Patients who present with sustained VT associated with coronary artery disease typically have a history of prior large MI and present years after the acute infarct with a remodeled ventricle and markedly depressed LV function. Even when there is biomarker evidence of acute MI, a preexisting scar from previous MI should be suspected as the cause of the VT. Infarct scars provide a durable substrate for sustained VT, and up to 70% of patients have a recurrence of the arrhythmia within 2 years. Scar-related reentry is not dependent on recurrent acute myocardial ischemia, so coronary revascularization cannot be anticipated to prevent recurrent VT, even when it may be appropriate for other indications. Depressed ventricular function, which is a risk factor for sudden death, is usually present. Implantation of an ICD is warranted for most patients provided that there is a reasonable expectation of survival with acceptable functional status for the next year after recovery from the VT episode. ICDs reduce annual mortality from 12.3% to 8.8% and lower arrhythmic deaths by 50% in patients with hemodynamically significant sustained VT or a history of cardiac arrest compared with pharmacologic therapy. Chronic amiodarone therapy may be considered for patients who are not candidates for or who decline ICD placement.

Following ICD implantation, patients remain at risk for heart failure, recurrent ischemic events, and recurrent VT, with a 5-year mortality that exceeds 30%. Attention to therapies with survival benefit, including β-adrenergic blocking agents, angiotensin-converting enzyme inhibitors, and statins, is important. Patients with frequent symptomatic recurrences of VT require antiarrhythmic drug therapy or catheter ablation.

NONISCHEMIC DILATED CARDIOMYOPATHY Sustained monomorphic VT associated with nonischemic cardiomyopathy is usually due to scar-related reentry. The etiology of scar is often unclear, but progressive replacement fibrosis is the likely cause. On cardiac MRI, scars are detectable as areas of delayed gadolinium enhancement and are more often intramural or subepicardial in location as compared with patients with prior MI. Scars that cause VT are often located adjacent to a valve annulus and can occur in either ventricle. Any cardiomyopathic process can cause scars and VT, but cardiac sarcoidosis (Chap. 390) and Chagas' disease (Chap. 252) are particularly associated with monomorphic VT (Table 277-2). An ICD is usually indicated with additional drugs or ablation for control of recurrent VT.

MONOMORPHIC VT IN ARVC ARVC (Chap. 287) is a rare genetic disorder most commonly due to mutations in genes encoding for cardiac desmosomal proteins. Approximately 50% have a familial transmission with autosomal dominant inheritance. A less common, autosomal recessive form is associated with cardiocutaneous syndromes that include Naxos disease and Carvajal syndrome. Patients typically present between the second and fifth decade with palpitations, syncope, or cardiac arrest owing to sustained monomorphic VT, although polymorphic VT can also occur. Fibrosis and fibro-fatty replacement most commonly involve the right ventricular myocardium and provide the substrate for reentrant VT that usually has a left bundle branch block–like configuration, consistent with the right ventricular origin. The sinus rhythm ECG suggests the disease in more than 85% of patients, most often showing T-wave inversions in V_1–V_3 (Fig. 277-6). Delayed activation of the right ventricle may cause a widened QRS (≥110 ms) in the right precordial leads and a prolonged S-wave upstroke in those leads, and occasionally a deflection at the end of the QRS known as an *epsilon wave* (Fig. 277-6). Cardiac imaging may show right ventricular enlargement or areas of abnormal motion or reveal areas of scar on CMR imaging with gadolinium. The monomorphic VT of early ARVC can sometimes be difficult to differentiate from idiopathic right ventricular outflow tract VT.

LV involvement can occur and occasionally precede manifest right ventricular disease. Heart failure is rare except in late stages, and survival to advanced age can be anticipated provided that VT can be controlled. An ICD is recommended. When VT is exercise-induced, it may respond to β-adrenergic blockers and limiting exercise. Sotalol, amiodarone, and catheter ablation have been used to reduce recurrences. Ablation targets are often located in the subepicardium of the RV.

TETRALOGY OF FALLOT VT occurs in 3–14% of patients late after repair of tetralogy of Fallot (Chap. 282) and contributes to a 2% per decade risk of

TABLE 277-2 VENTRICULAR ARRHYTHMIAS ASSOCIATED WITH DIFFERENT FORMS OF HEART DISEASE

I. Idiopathic VT without structural heart disease
  - A. Outflow tract origin
    1. RV outflow tract: left bundle branch block pattern with inferior axis (tall QRS in inferior leads) and late transition in the precordial leads
    2. LV outflow tract: prominent R in V_1 with inferior axis
  - B. Left posterior fascicular VT
    1. Right bundle branch block pattern with left axis deviation (most common)

II. Ischemic cardiomyopathy
  - A. Monomorphic VT is common with prior large myocardial infarction
  - B. Polymorphic VT and VF should prompt ischemia evaluation

III. Nonischemic cardiomyopathy
  - A. Polymorphic VT and VF more common but fibrotic scars can cause monomorphic VT especially with sarcoidosis and Chagas' disease

IV. Arrhythmogenic right ventricular cardiomyopathy
  - A. Monomorphic VT usually of right ventricular origin (left bundle branch morphology)
  - B. Polymorphic VT and VF can occur independently or through degeneration of monomorphic VT

V. Repaired tetralogy of Fallot
  - A. Monomorphic VT of right ventricular origin (usually left bundle branch morphology)

VI. Hypertrophic cardiomyopathy
  - A. Polymorphic VT or ventricular fibrillation
  - B. Less commonly, monomorphic VT associated with myocardial scars

VIII. Genetic arrhythmia syndromes
  - A. Long QT syndrome: torsade de pointes VT
  - B. Brugada syndrome: VF
  - C. Catecholaminergic polymorphic VT: polymorphic VT or bidirectional VT
  - D. Short QT syndrome: ventricular fibrillation
  - E. Early repolarization syndrome: polymorphic VT or VF

Abbreviation: RV, right ventricle. See text for other abbreviations.

sudden death. Monomorphic VT is due to reentry around areas of surgically created scar in the RV (Table 277-2). Factors associated with VT risk include age >5 years at the time of repair, high-grade ventricular ectopy, inducible VT on an electrophysiologic study, abnormal right ventricular hemodynamics, and sinus rhythm QRS duration >180 ms. An ICD is usually warranted for patients who have a spontaneous episode of VT, but criteria for a prophylactic ICD in other patients have not been established. Catheter ablation is used to control recurrent episodes.

BUNDLE BRANCH REENTRY VT Reentry through the Purkinje system occurs in approximately 5% of patients with monomorphic VT in the presence of structural heart disease. The reentry circuit typically revolves retrograde via the left bundle and anterograde down the right bundle, thereby producing VT that has a left bundle branch block configuration. Catheter ablation of the right bundle branch abolishes this VT. Bundle branch reentry is usually associated with severe underlying heart disease. Other scar-related VTs are often present and often require additional therapy or ICD implantation.

IDIOPATHIC MONOMORPHIC VT Idiopathic VT in patients without structural heart disease usually presents with palpitations, lightheadedness, and occasionally syncope, often provoked by sympathetic stimulation during exercise or emotional upset. The QRS morphology of the arrhythmia suggests the diagnosis (see below). The sinus rhythm ECG is normal. Cardiac imaging shows normal ventricular function and no evidence of ventricular scar. Occasionally a patient with structural heart disease is found to have concomitant idiopathic VT, unrelated to the structural disease. Sudden death is rare.

Outflow tract VTs originate from a focus, usually with features consistent with triggered automaticity. The arrhythmia may present with

TABLE 277-3 CAUSES OF QT PROLONGATION AND TORSADE DE POINTES VENTRICULAR TACHYCARDIA

1. Congenital long QT syndromes (see text for details)
   - Long QT syndrome type 1: Reduced repolarizing current I_{Ks} due to mutation in *KCNQ1* gene
   - Long QT syndrome type 2: Reduced repolarizing current I_{Kr} due to mutation in *KCNH2* gene
   - Long QT syndrome type 3: Delayed inactivation of the I_{Na} due to mutations in *SCN5A* gene
   - Others: Several other types of long QT syndromes have been described; long QT types 1, 2, and 3 account for 80–90% of cases
2. Acquired prolongation of QT interval
   - Electrolyte abnormalities
     - Hypokalemia
     - Hypomagnesemia
     - Hypocalcemia
   - Drugs
     - Antiarrhythmic drugs
       - Class IA: Quinidine, disopyramide, procainamide
       - Class III: Sotalol, amiodarone (QT prolongation common but torsade ventricular tachycardia is rare), ibutilide, dofetilide, almokalant
     - Antibiotics
       - Macrolides: Erythromycin, clarithromycin, azithromycin
       - Fluoroquinolones: Levofloxacin, moxifloxacin, gatifloxacin
       - Trimethoprim-sulfamethoxazole
       - Clindamycin
       - Pentamidine
       - Chloroquine
       - Antifungals: Ketoconazole, itraconazole
       - Antivirals: Amantadine
     - Antipsychotics
       - Haloperidol, phenothiazines, thioridazine, trifluoperazine, sertindole, zimelidine, ziprasidone
       - Tricyclic and tetracyclic antidepressants
     - Antihistamines (histamine 1-receptor antagonists)
       - Terfenadine, astemizole, diphenhydramine, hydroxyzine
     - Cholinergic antagonists: Cisapride, organophosphates
     - Citrate (massive blood transfusions)
     - Cocaine
     - Methadone
     - Fluoxetine (in conjunction with other drugs that prolong QT)
   - Cardiac conditions
     - Myocardial ischemia and infarction
     - Myocarditis
     - Marked bradycardia
     - Stress cardiomyopathy
   - Endocrine disorders
     - Hypothyroidism
     - Hyperparathyroidism
     - Pheochromocytoma
     - Hyperaldosteronism
   - Intracranial disorders
     - Subarachnoid hemorrhage
     - Thalamic hematoma
     - Cerebrovascular accident
     - Encephalitis
     - Head injury
   - Nutritional disorders
     - Anorexia nervosa
     - Starvation
     - Liquid protein diets
     - Gastroplasty and ileojejunal bypass
     - Celiac disease

sustained VT, nonsustained VT, or PVCs often provoked by exercise or emotional upset. Repeated bursts of nonsustained VTs, which may occur incessantly, are known as repetitive monomorphic VTs and can cause tachycardia-induced cardiomyopathy with depressed ventricular function that recovers after suppression of the arrhythmia (Fig. 277-2). Most originate in the right ventricular outflow tract, which gives rise to VT that has a left bundle branch block configuration in V_1 and an axis that is directed inferiorly, with tall R waves in leads II, III, and AVF (Fig. 277-2). Idiopathic VT can also arise in the LV outflow tract or in sleeves of myocardium that extend along the aortic root. LV origin is suspected when lead V_1 or V_2 has prominent R waves. Although this typical outflow tract QRS morphology favors idiopathic VT, some cardiomyopathies, notably ARVC, can cause PVCs or VT from this region. Excluding these diseases is an initial focus of evaluation.

LV intrafascicular VT presents with sustained VT that has a right bundle branch block–like configuration. It is often exercise-induced and occurs more often in men than women. The mechanism is reentry in or near the septal ramifications of the LV Purkinje system. This VT can be terminated by intravenous administration of verapamil.

MANAGEMENT OF IDIOPATHIC VT Treatment is required for symptoms or when frequent or incessant arrhythmias depress ventricular function. β-Adrenergic blockers are first-line therapy. Nondihydropyridine calcium channel blockers (diltiazem and verapamil) are sometimes effective. Catheter ablation is warranted for severe symptoms or when beta blockers or calcium channel blockers are not effective or not desired. Efficacy and risks of catheter ablation vary with the specific site of origin of the VT, being most favorable for arrhythmias originating in the right ventricular outflow tract.

LV fascicular VT can be terminated by intravenous administration of verapamil, although chronic therapy with oral verapamil is not always effective. Catheter ablation is recommended if β-adrenergic blockers or calcium channel blockers are ineffective or not desired.

Polymorphic VT Sustained polymorphic VT can be seen with any form of structural heart disease (Table 277-2). However, unlike sustained monomorphic VT, polymorphic VT does not always indicate a structural abnormality or focus of automaticity. Reentry with continually changing reentrant paths, spiral wave reentry, and multiple automatic foci are potential mechanisms (Chap. 278e). Sustained polymorphic VT usually degenerates into VF. Polymorphic VT is typically seen in association with acute MI or myocardial ischemia, ventricular hypertrophy, and a number of genetic mutations that affect cardiac ion channels (Table 277-3).

POLYMORPHIC VT ASSOCIATED WITH ACUTE MI/MYOCARDIAL ISCHEMIA Acute MI or ischemia is a common cause of polymorphic VT and should be the initial consideration in management. Approximately 10% of patients with acute MI develop VT that degenerates to VF, related to reentry through the infarct border zone. The risk is greatest in the first hour of acute MI. Following resuscitation as per the ACLS guidelines, management is as for acute MI (Chap. 295). β-Adrenergic blockers, correction of electrolyte abnormalities, and prompt myocardial reperfusion are required. Repeated episodes of polymorphic VT suggest ongoing myocardial ischemia and warrant assessment of adequacy of myocardial reperfusion. Polymorphic VT and VF that occur within the first 48 h of acute MI are associated with greater in-hospital mortality, but those who survive past hospital discharge are not at increased risk for arrhythmic sudden death. Long-term therapy for postinfarct ventricular arrhythmia is determined by residual LV function, with an ICD being indicated for persistent severe LV dysfunction (LV ejection fraction <0.35).

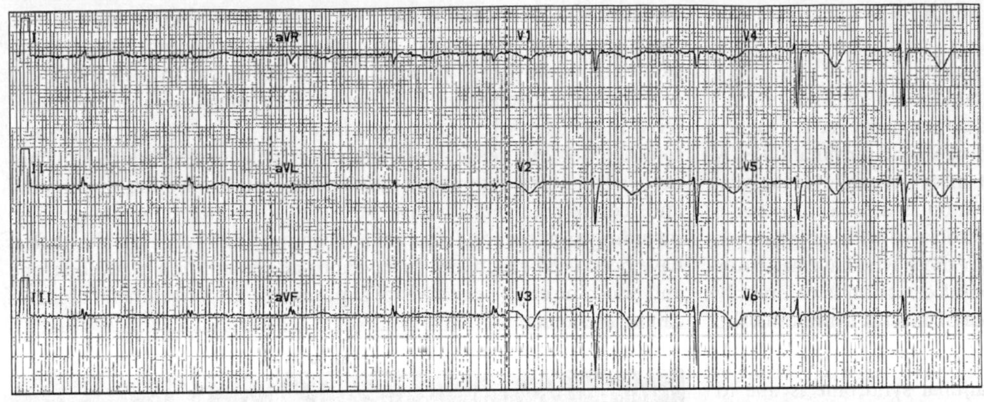

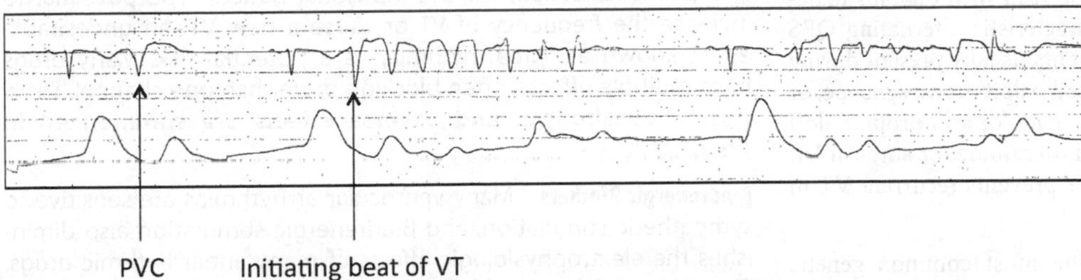

FIGURE 277-8 Electrocardiogram (ECG) of a patient with prolonged QT and episodes of torsade de pointes ventricular tachycardia (VT). ***A.*** Twelve-lead ECG showing a heart rate of 54, anterior wall T inversion, and QT interval of 600 ms. The corrected QT interval (QTc) is 585 ms. ***B.*** Telemetry ECG tracing with digital pulse waveform demonstrating bursts of torsade de pointes VT. The initiating sequence of the VT is characteristic, with a PVC inducing a pause followed by a sinus beat that had a longer QT and interruption of the T wave by a PVC that is the first beat of VT. The VT is self-terminating in this case.

REPOLARIZATION ABNORMALITIES AND GENETIC ARRHYTHMIA SYNDROMES • Acquired long QT Abnormal prolongation of the QT interval is associated with the polymorphic VT Torsade de Pointes (Fig. 277-8). The VT often has a characteristic initiation sequence of a premature ventricular beat that induces a pause, followed by a sinus beat that has a longer QT interval and interruption of the T wave by the PVC that is the first beat of the polymorphic VT. This characteristic initiation is termed "pause-dependent" (Fig. 277-8). Causes of QT prolongation include electrolyte abnormalities, bradycardia, and a number of medications that block repolarizing potassium currents, notably the antiarrhythmic drugs sotalol, dofetilide, and ibutilide, but also a number of other medications used for noncardiac diseases, including erythromycin, pentamidine, haloperidol, phenothiazines, and methadone (Table 277-3). Individual susceptibility may be related to genetic polymorphisms or mutations that influence repolarization.

Patients typically present with near-syncope, syncope, or cardiac arrest. Sustained episodes degenerate to VF requiring defibrillation. PVCs and nonsustained VT often precede episodes of sustained VT. Intravenous administration of 1–2 g of magnesium sulphate usually suppresses recurrent episodes. If magnesium alone is ineffective, increasing heart rate with isoproterenol infusion or pacing, to a rate of 100–120 beats/min as required to suppress PVCs, usually suppresses VT recurrences. These maneuvers allow time for correction of associated electrolyte disturbance (hypokalemia and hypocalcemia) and bradycardia and removal of any causative drugs (Table 277-3). Drug interactions that elevate levels of the offending agent are often a precipitating factor. Patients who experience a polymorphic VT induced by QT prolongation should be considered to have a susceptibility to the arrhythmia and should avoid all future exposure to medications known to prolong the QT interval.

Congenital long QT syndrome The congenital long QT syndrome (LQTS) is caused by mutations in genes coding for cardiac ion channels responsible for ventricular repolarization. The corrected QT (QTc) is typically prolonged to greater than 440 ms in men and 460 ms in women. Symptoms are due to Torsade de Pointes VT (Fig. 277-8). Several forms of congenital LQTS have been identified, but three groups of mutations that lead to LQTS type 1 (LQTS-1), LQTS type 2 (LQTS-2), or LQTS type 3 (LQTS-3) account for 90% of cases. The most frequently encountered mutations, *LQTS1* and *LQTS2*, are due to abnormalities of potassium channels, but mutations affecting the sodium channel (*LQTS3*) and calcium channels have also been described (Table 277-3).

Patients often present with syncope or cardiac arrest, usually during childhood. In LQTS-1, episodes tend to occur during exertion, particularly swimming. In LQTS-2, sudden auditory stimuli or emotional upset predispose to events. In LQTS-3, sudden death during sleep is a notable feature. Asymptomatic patients may be discovered in the course of family screening or on a routine ECG. Genotyping can be helpful for family screening and to provide reassurance regarding the diagnosis. Correlations of genotype with risk and response to therapy are beginning to emerge. In most patients with LQTS-1 or LQTS-2, adequate doses of beta blocker therapy (the nonselective agents nadolol or propranolol) are sufficient protection from arrhythmia episodes. Markers of increased risk include QTc interval exceeding 0.5 s, female gender, and a history of syncope or cardiac arrest. Recurrent syncope despite beta blocker therapy or a high-risk profile merits consideration of an ICD. Avoidance of QT-prolonging drugs is critical for all patients with LQTS, including those who are genotype positive but have normal QT intervals.

Short QT syndrome Short QT syndrome is very rare compared to LQTS. The QTc is shorter than 0.36 s, and usually less than 0.3 s. The genetic abnormality causes a gain of function of the potassium channel (I_{Kr}) or reduced inward depolarizing currents. The abnormality is associated with atrial fibrillation, polymorphic VT, and sudden death.

Brugada syndrome Brugada syndrome is a rare syndrome characterized by >0.2 mV of ST-segment elevation with a coved ST segment and negative T wave in more than one anterior precordial lead (V_1–V_3) (Fig. 277-6) and episodes of syncope or cardiac arrest due to polymorphic VT in the absence of structural heart disease. Cardiac arrest may occur during sleep or be provoked by febrile illness. Males are more commonly affected than females. Mutations involving cardiac sodium channels are identified in approximately 25% of cases. Distinction from patients with similar ST elevation owing to LV hypertrophy, pericarditis, myocardial ischemia or MI hyperkalemia, hypothermia, right bundle branch block, and ARVC is often difficult. Furthermore, the characteristic ST-segment elevation can wax and wane over time and may become pronounced during acute illness and fever. Administration of the sodium channel blocking drug flecainide, ajmaline, or procainamide can augment or unmask ST elevation in affected individuals. An ICD is indicated for individuals who have had unexplained syncope or been resuscitated from cardiac arrest.

Quinidine has been used successfully to suppress frequent episodes of VT.

Early repolarization syndrome Patients resuscitated from VF who have no structural heart disease or other identified abnormality have a higher prevalence of J-point elevation with notching in the terminal QRS. A family history of sudden death is present in some patients, suggesting a potential genetic basis. J-point elevation is also seen in some patients with the Brugada syndrome and associated with a higher risk of arrhythmias. An ICD is recommended for those who have had prior cardiac arrest. It should be noted that J-point elevation is commonly seen as a normal variant, and in the absence of specific symptoms, the clinical relevance is not known.

Catecholaminergic polymorphic VT This rare familial syndrome is due to mutations in the cardiac ryanodine receptor and, less commonly, the sarcoplasmic calcium binding protein, calsequestin 2. These mutations result in abnormal sarcoplasmic calcium handling and polymorphic ventricular arrhythmias that resemble those seen with digitalis toxicity. The VT is polymorphic or has a characteristic alternating QRS morphology termed bidirectional VT. Patients usually present during childhood with exercise- or emotion-induced palpitations, syncope, or cardiac arrest. β-Adrenergic blockers (e.g., nadolol and propranolol) and an ICD are recommended. Verapamil, flecainide, or surgical left cardiac sympathetic denervation reduces or prevents recurrent VT in some patients.

Hypertrophic cardiomyopathy (HCM) HCM is the most common genetic cardiovascular disorder, occurring in 1 in 500 individuals, and is a prominent cause of sudden death before the age of 35 years (Chap. 287). Sudden death can be due to polymorphic VT/VF. Rarely, sustained monomorphic VT occurs related to areas of ventricular scar. Risk factors include young age, nonsustained VT, failure of blood pressure to increase during exercise, recent (within 6 months) syncope, ventricular wall thickness >3 cm, and possibly the severity of LV outflow obstruction. An ICD is generally indicated for high-risk patients, but the specific risk profile warranting an ICD continues to be debated. Surgical myectomy, performed to relieve outflow obstruction, has been associated with a sudden death rate of less than 1% per year. The reported annual rate of sustained VT or sudden death after transcoronary ethanol septal ablation done to relieve outflow obstruction has been reported to range between 1 and 5%.

Genetic dilated cardiomyopathies Genetic dilated cardiomyopathies account for 30–40% of cases of nonischemic dilated cardiomyopathies. Some are associated with muscular dystrophy. Autosomal dominant, recessive, X-linked, and mitochondrial inheritance patterns are recognized. Mutations in genes coding for structural proteins of the nuclear lamina (lamin A and C) and the *SCN5A* gene are particularly associated with conduction system disease and ventricular arrhythmias. Patients can experience polymorphic VT and cardiac arrest or develop areas of scar causing sustained monomorphic VT. ICDs are recommended for those who have had a sustained VT or are at high risk due to significantly depressed ventricular function (LV ejection fraction of ≤0.35 and associated with heart failure) or a malignant family history of sudden death.

Ventricular Fibrillation VF is characterized by disordered electrical ventricular activation without identifiable QRS complexes (Fig. 277-3*E*). Spiral wave reentry and multiple circulating reentry wavefronts are possible mechanisms. Sustained polymorphic or monomorphic VT that degenerates to VF is a common cause of out-of-hospital cardiac arrest. Treatment follows ACLS guidelines with defibrillation to restore sinus rhythm. If resuscitation is successful, further evaluation is performed to identify and treat underlying heart disease and potential causes of the arrhythmia, including the possibility that monomorphic or polymorphic VT could have initiated VF. If a transient reversible cause such as acute MI is not identified, therapy to reduce the risk of sudden death with an ICD is often warranted. Chronic amiodarone therapy may be considered for individuals who are not ICD candidates.

Incessant VT and Electrical Storm VT is incessant when it continues to recur shortly after electrical, pharmacologic, or spontaneous conversion to sinus rhythm. "VT storm" or "electrical storm" refers to three or more separate episodes of VT within 24 h, most commonly encountered in patients with ICDs. Slow incessant VT is sometimes asymptomatic, but can cause heart failure or tachycardia-induced cardiomyopathy. More commonly, these presentations are life-threatening and require emergent therapy. Measures to reduce sympathetic tone, including β-adrenergic blockade, sedation, and general anesthesia, have been used effectively. Intravenous administration of amiodarone and lidocaine can be effective for suppression. Urgent catheter ablation can be lifesaving.

TREATMENT VENTRICULAR ARRHYTHMIAS

ANTIARRHYTHMIC DRUGS

Use of antiarrhythmic drugs is based on consideration of the risks and potential benefit for the individual patient. The potential to increase the frequency of VT or cause a new VT, an undesirable effect known as "proarrhythmia," is a potential risk. Many drugs have multiple effects, often blocking more than one channel. **Drug doses, metabolism, and adverse effects are summarized in Chap. 277.**

β-Adrenergic Blockers Many ventricular arrhythmias are sensitive to sympathetic stimulation, and β-adrenergic stimulation also diminishes the electrophysiologic effects of many antiarrhythmic drugs. The safety of β-blocking agents makes them the first choice of therapy for most ventricular arrhythmias. They are particularly useful for exercise-induced arrhythmias and idiopathic arrhythmias, but have limited efficacy for most arrhythmias associated with heart disease. Bradyarrhythmias are the major cardiac toxicity.

Calcium Channel Blockers The nondihydropyridine calcium channel blockers diltiazem and verapamil can be effective for some idiopathic VTs. The risk of proarrhythmia is low, but they have negative inotropic and vasodilatory effects that can aggravate hypotension.

Sodium Channel-Blocking Agents Drugs whose major effect is mediated through sodium channel blockade include mexiletine, quinidine, disopyramide, flecainide, and propafenone, which are available for chronic oral therapy (Table 277-3). Lidocaine, quinidine, and procainamide are available as intravenous formulations. Quinidine, disopyramide, and procainamide also have potassium channel-blocking effects that prolong the QT interval. These agents have potential proarrhythmic effects and, with the possible exception of quinidine, also have negative inotropic effects that may contribute to increased mortality observed in patients with prior MI. Long-term therapy is generally avoided in patients with structural heart disease but may be used to reduce symptomatic arrhythmias in patients with ICDs.

Potassium Channel-Blocking Agents Sotalol and dofetilide block the delayed rectifier potassium channel I_{Kr} thereby prolonging the QT interval. Sotalol also has nonselective β-adrenergic blocking activity. It has a modest effect on reducing ICD shocks due to ventricular and atrial arrhythmias. Proarrhythmia with Torsade de Pointes due to QT prolongation occurs in 3–5% of patients. Both sotalol and dofetilide are excreted via the kidneys, necessitating dose adjustment or avoidance in renal insufficiency. These drugs must be avoided in patients with other risk factors for Torsade de Pointes, including QT prolongation, hypokalemia, and significant bradycardia.

Amiodarone and Dronedarone Amiodarone, which blocks multiple cardiac ionic currents and has sympatholytic activity, suppresses a variety of ventricular arrhythmias. It is administered intravenously for life-threatening arrhythmias. During chronic oral therapy, electrophysiologic effects develop over several days. It is more effective than sotalol in reducing ICD shocks and is the preferred drug for ventricular arrhythmias in patients with heart disease who are not candidates for an ICD. Bradyarrhythmias are the major cardiac adverse effect. Ventricular proarrhythmia can occur, but Torsade de Pointes VT is rare. Noncardiac toxicities are a major problem and contribute to drug discontinuation in approximately a third of patients during long-term therapy. Pneumonitis or pulmonary fibrosis occurs in approximately 1% of patients. Photosensitivity is common, and neuropathy and ocular toxicity can occur. Systematic monitoring is recommended during chronic therapy, including assessment for thyroid and liver toxicity every 6 months and lung toxicity with a chest radiograph and/or determination of lung diffusing capacity annually. Dronedarone has structural similarities to amiodarone but without the iodine moiety. Efficacy for ventricular arrhythmias is poor, and it increases mortality in patients with heart failure.

IMPLANTABLE CARDIOVERTER-DEFIBRILLATORS

ICDs are highly effective for termination of VT and VF and also provide bradycardia pacing. ICDs decrease mortality in patients at risk for sudden death due to structural heart diseases. In all cases, ICDs are recommended only if there is also expectation for survival of at least a year with acceptable functional capacity. The exception is in cases of patients with end-stage heart disease who are awaiting cardiac transplantation outside the hospital, or who have left bundle branch block QRS prolongation such that they are likely to have improvement in ventricular function with cardiac resynchronization therapy from a biventricular ICD.

ICDs can often terminate monomorphic VT by a burst of rapid pacing faster than the VT, known as antitachycardia pacing (ATP) (**Fig. 277-9A**). If ATP fails or is not a programmed treatment, as is often the case for rapid VT or VF, a shock is delivered (**Fig. 277-9B**). Shocks are painful if the patient is conscious. The most common ICD complication is the delivery of unnecessary therapy (either ATP or shocks) in response to a rapid supraventricular tachycardia or electrical noise as a result of an ICD lead fracture. Interrogation of the ICD, which can be performed remotely and communicated via Internet, is critical after an ICD shock to determine the arrhythmia diagnosis and exclude an unnecessary therapy. Device infection occurs in approximately 1% of patients.

Despite prompt termination of VT or VF by an ICD, the occurrence of these arrhythmias predicts subsequent increased mortality and risk of heart failure. Occurrence of VT or VF should therefore prompt assessment for potential causes including worsening heart failure, electrolyte abnormalities, and ischemia. Repeated shocks, even if appropriate, often induce posttraumatic stress disorder. Antiarrhythmic drugs mostly in the form of amiodarone or catheter ablation are often required for suppression of recurrent arrhythmias. Antiarrhythmic drug therapy can alter the VT rate and the energy required for defibrillation, thereby necessitating programming changes in the ICD's algorithms for detection and therapy.

CATHETER ABLATION FOR VT

Catheter ablation is performed by guiding an electrode catheter to the arrhythmia origin and producing a thermal injury with radiofrequency current. The size and location of the arrhythmia substrate determine the ease and likely effectiveness of the procedure, as well as potential complications. The most common complications, which occur in <5% of patients, are related to vascular access, including bleeding, femoral hematomas, arteriovenous fistulae, and pseudoaneurysms.

Catheter ablation is a reasonable first-line therapy for many patients with symptomatic idiopathic VTs. Success rates for those originating from a focus in the right ventricular outflow tract are in the range of 80–90% but lower for idiopathic VTs arising in less common locations such as from the LV outflow tract or aortic root, along the atrioventricular valve annuli, and from the papillary muscles. Failure of ablation is often due to inability to induce the

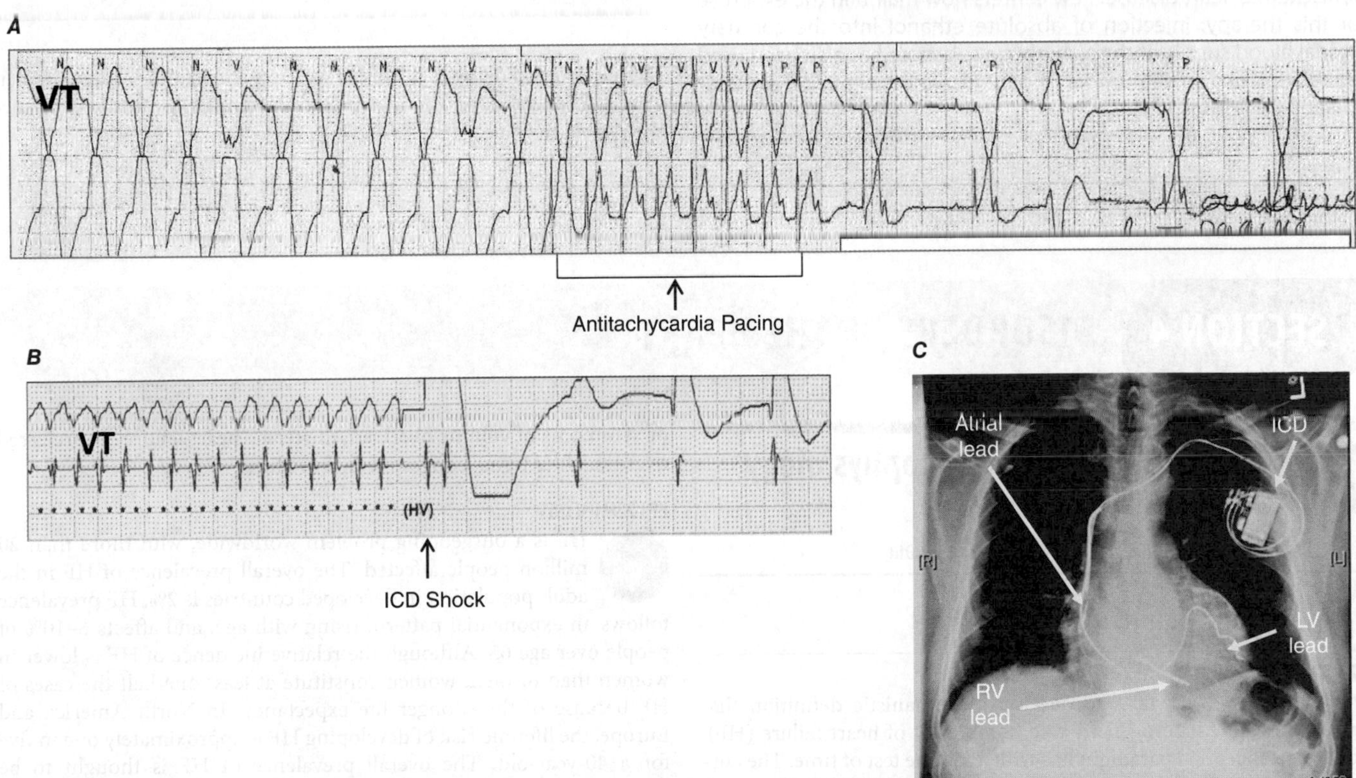

FIGURE 277-9 Implantable cardioverter-defibrillator (ICD) and therapies for ventricular arrhythmias. ***A.*** A monomorphic ventricular tachycardia (VT) is terminated by a burst of pacing impulses at a rate faster than VT (antitachycardia pacing). ***B.*** A rapid VT is converted with a high-voltage shock (*arrow*). The chest x-ray in panel ***C*** shows the components of an ICD capable of biventricular pacing. ICD generator in the subcutaneous tissue of the left upper chest, pacing leads in the right atrium and the left ventricular (LV) branch of the coronary sinus (LV lead), and a pacing/defibrillating lead in the right ventricle (RV lead) are shown.

arrhythmia for precise localization or because the origin of the VT is from a site that is inaccessible or in close proximity to a coronary artery. Complications are infrequent but can include perforation with cardiac tamponade, atrioventricular block due to injury to the conduction system, and coronary artery injury for foci in proximity to a coronary vessel.

In patients with scar-related VT due to prior infarction or cardiomyopathy, ablation targets abnormal regions in the scar. Because these scars often contain multiple reentry circuits over relatively large regions, extensive areas of ablation are required, and these areas are often identified as regions of low voltage displayed on anatomic reconstructions of the ventricle (Fig. 277-5). If the circuits are not confined to the subendocardial scar, epicardial mapping and ablation can be performed via a subxiphoid pericardial puncture, similar to a pericardiocentesis. Epicardial mapping and ablation are often required for VTs due to nonischemic cardiomyopathy, but also have potentially greater risks of bleeding, coronary injury, and post-procedure pericarditis, which is usually transient. For drug-refractory VT due to prior MI, ablation abolishes VT in approximately half of patients and reduces the frequency of VT in an additional 20%. More than one procedure is necessary in up to 30% of patients. Ablation can be lifesaving for patients with very frequent or incessant VT. Procedure-related mortality is in the range of 3%, with most mortality due to continued uncontrollable VT when the procedure fails. In nonischemic heart disease, the arrhythmia substrate locations are more variable and outcomes are less well defined.

Catheter ablation can also be lifesaving for rare patients with recurrent polymorphic VT and VF that is repeatedly initiated by a uniform PVC. The initiating ectopic beat often originates from the Purkinje system or the right ventricular outflow tract and can be targeted for ablation.

When antiarrhythmic drug therapy and catheter ablation fail or are not options, surgical cryoablation, often combined with aneurysmectomy, can be effective therapy for recurrent VT due to prior MI and has also been used successfully in a few patients with nonischemic heart disease. Few centers now maintain the expertise for this therapy. Injection of absolute ethanol into the coronary arterial blood supply of the arrhythmia substrate has also been used for ablation in a small number of patients who have failed catheter ablation and drugs.

SUMMARY

Patients with ventricular arrhythmias fall into three general groups. The first are those who have associated structural heart disease that must be detected. The risk of life-threatening arrhythmias causing sudden death is indicated by the nature of the arrhythmia—sustained (or causing cardiac arrest) or nonsustained, in which case the risk of life-threatening arrhythmias is assessed from the severity of the heart disease, usually the severity of ventricular dysfunction. ICDs provide the most protection from sudden arrhythmic death. The second group comprises those who do not have recognizable structural heart disease, but have a genetic syndrome associated with increased risk of sudden death. A family history of sudden death and abnormal electrocardiogram most frequently suggest the diagnosis. The third group includes individuals with benign idiopathic arrhythmias who may require therapy to control symptoms, but who are not at significant risk for life-threatening arrhythmias. The appropriate recognition of these patients is facilitated by thoughtful application of ECG and cardiac imaging. High-risk individuals benefit from specialized care for consideration of ICDs, catheter ablation, and antiarrhythmic drug therapy.

278e Atlas of Cardiac Arrhythmias

Ary L. Goldberger

This is a digital-only chapter. It is available on the DVD that accompanies this book, as well as on Access Medicine/Harrison's Online, and the eBook and "app" editions of HPIM 19e.

The electrocardiograms in this atlas supplement those illustrated in Chaps. 274 and 276. The interpretations emphasize findings of specific teaching value.

SECTION 4 DISORDERS OF THE HEART

279 Heart Failure: Pathophysiology and Diagnosis

Douglas L. Mann, Murali Chakinala

HEART FAILURE

DEFINITION

Despite repeated attempts to develop a mechanistic definition that encompasses the heterogeneity and complexity of heart failure (HF), no single conceptual paradigm has withstood the test of time. The current American College of Cardiology Foundation (ACCF)/American Heart Association (AHA) guidelines define HF as a complex clinical syndrome that results from structural or functional impairment of ventricular filling or ejection of blood, which in turn leads to the cardinal clinical symptoms of dyspnea and fatigue and signs of HF, namely edema and rales. Because many patients present without signs or symptoms of volume overload, the term "heart failure" is preferred over the older term "congestive heart failure."

EPIDEMIOLOGY

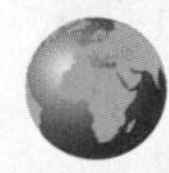

HF is a burgeoning problem worldwide, with more than 20 million people affected. The overall prevalence of HF in the adult population in developed countries is 2%. HF prevalence follows an exponential pattern, rising with age, and affects 6–10% of people over age 65. Although the relative incidence of HF is lower in women than in men, women constitute at least one-half the cases of HF because of their longer life expectancy. In North America and Europe, the lifetime risk of developing HF is approximately one in five for a 40-year-old. The overall prevalence of HF is thought to be increasing, in part because current therapies for cardiac disorders, such as myocardial infarction (MI), valvular heart disease, and arrhythmias, are allowing patients to survive longer. Very little is known about the prevalence or risk of developing HF in emerging nations because of the lack of population-based studies in those countries. HF was once thought to arise primarily in the setting of a depressed left ventricular (LV) ejection fraction (EF); however, epidemiologic studies have shown that approximately one-half of patients who develop HF have a normal or preserved EF (EF ≥50%). Accordingly, the historical terms "systolic" and "diastolic" HF have been abandoned, and HF patients are now broadly categorized into HF with a reduced EF (HFrEF; formerly *systolic failure*) or HF with a preserved EF (HRpEF; formerly *diastolic failure*).

ETIOLOGY

As shown in Table 279-1, any condition that leads to an alteration in LV structure or function can predispose a patient to developing HF. Although the etiology of HF in patients with a preserved EF differs from that of patients with depressed EF, there is considerable overlap between the etiologies of these two conditions. In industrialized countries, coronary artery disease (CAD) has become the predominant cause in men and women and is responsible for 60–75% of cases of HF. Hypertension contributes to the development of HF in 75% of patients, including most patients with CAD. Both CAD and hypertension interact to augment the risk of HF, as does diabetes mellitus.

In 20–30% of the cases of HF with a depressed EF, the exact etiologic basis is not known. These patients are referred to as having nonischemic, dilated, or idiopathic cardiomyopathy if the cause is unknown (Chap. 287). Prior viral infection or toxin exposure (e.g., alcoholic or chemotherapeutic) also may lead to a dilated cardiomyopathy. Moreover, it is becoming increasingly clear that a large number of cases of dilated cardiomyopathy are secondary to specific genetic defects, most notably those in the cytoskeleton. Most forms of familial dilated cardiomyopathy are inherited in an autosomal dominant fashion. Mutations of genes that encode cytoskeletal proteins (desmin, cardiac myosin, vinculin) and nuclear membrane proteins (laminin) have been identified thus far. Dilated cardiomyopathy also is associated with Duchenne's, Becker's, and limb-girdle muscular dystrophies. Conditions that lead to a high cardiac output (e.g., arteriovenous fistula, anemia) are seldom responsible for the development of HF in a normal heart; however, in the presence of underlying structural heart disease, these conditions can lead to overt HF.

TABLE 279-1 ETIOLOGIES OF HEART FAILURE

Depressed Ejection Fraction (<40%)	
Coronary artery disease	Nonischemic dilated cardiomyopathy
Myocardial infarction[a]	Familial/genetic disorders
Myocardial ischemia[a]	Infiltrative disorders[a]
Chronic pressure overload	Toxic/drug-induced damage
Hypertension[a]	Metabolic disorder[a]
Obstructive valvular disease[a]	Viral
Chronic volume overload	Chagas' disease
Regurgitant valvular disease	Disorders of rate and rhythm
Intracardiac (left-to-right) shunting	Chronic bradyarrhythmias
Extracardiac shunting	Chronic tachyarrhythmias
Chronic lung disease	
Cor pulmonale	
Pulmonary vascular disorders	
Preserved Ejection Fraction (>40–50%)	
Pathologic hypertrophy	Restrictive cardiomyopathy
Primary (hypertrophic cardiomyopathies)	Infiltrative disorders (amyloidosis, sarcoidosis)
Secondary (hypertension)	Storage diseases (hemochromatosis)
Aging	Fibrosis
	Endomyocardial disorders
High-Output States	
Metabolic disorders	Excessive blood flow requirements
Thyrotoxicosis	Systemic arteriovenous shunting
Nutritional disorders (beriberi)	Chronic anemia

[a]Indicates conditions that can also lead to heart failure with a preserved ejection fraction.

TABLE 279-2 NEW YORK HEART ASSOCIATION CLASSIFICATION

Functional Capacity	Objective Assessment
Class I	Patients with cardiac disease but without resulting limitation of physical activity. Ordinary physical activity does not cause undue fatigue, palpitations, dyspnea, or anginal pain.
Class II	Patients with cardiac disease resulting in slight limitation of physical activity. They are comfortable at rest. Ordinary physical activity results in fatigue, palpitation, dyspnea, or anginal pain.
Class III	Patients with cardiac disease resulting in marked limitation of physical activity. They are comfortable at rest. Less than ordinary activity causes fatigue, palpitation, dyspnea, or anginal pain.
Class IV	Patients with cardiac disease resulting in inability to carry on any physical activity without discomfort. Symptoms of heart failure or the anginal syndrome may be present even at rest. If any physical activity is undertaken, discomfort is increased.

Source: Adapted from New York Heart Association, Inc., *Diseases of the Heart and Blood Vessels: Nomenclature and Criteria for Diagnosis*, 6th ed. Boston, Little Brown, 1964, p. 114.

GLOBAL CONSIDERATIONS

Rheumatic heart disease remains a major cause of HF in Africa and Asia, especially in the young. Hypertension is an important cause of HF in the African and African-American populations. Chagas' disease is still a major cause of HF in South America. Not surprisingly, anemia is a frequent concomitant factor in HF in many developing nations. As developing nations undergo socioeconomic development, the epidemiology of HF is becoming similar to that of Western Europe and North America, with CAD emerging as the single most common cause of HF. Although the contribution of diabetes mellitus to HF is not well understood, diabetes accelerates atherosclerosis and often is associated with hypertension.

PROGNOSIS

Despite many recent advances in the evaluation and management of HF, the development of symptomatic HF still carries a poor prognosis. Community-based studies indicate that 30–40% of patients die within 1 year of diagnosis and 60–70% die within 5 years, mainly from worsening HF or as a sudden event (probably because of a ventricular arrhythmia). Although it is difficult to predict prognosis in an individual, patients with symptoms at rest (New York Heart Association [NYHA] class IV) have a 30–70% annual mortality rate, whereas patients with symptoms with moderate activity (NYHA class II) have an annual mortality rate of 5–10%. Thus, functional status is an important predictor of patient outcome (Table 279-2).

PATHOGENESIS

Figure 279-1 provides a general conceptual framework for considering the development and progression of HFrEF. As shown, HF may be viewed as a progressive disorder that is initiated after an *index event* either damages the heart muscle, with a resultant loss of functioning cardiac myocytes, or, alternatively, disrupts the ability of the myocardium to generate force, thereby preventing the heart from contracting normally. This index event may have an abrupt onset, as in the case of an MI; it may have a gradual or insidious onset, as in the case of hemodynamic pressure or volume overloading; or it may be hereditary, as in the case of many of the genetic cardiomyopathies. Regardless of the nature of the inciting event, the feature that is common to each of these index events is that they all in some manner produce a decline in the pumping capacity of the heart. In most instances, patients remain asymptomatic or minimally symptomatic after the initial decline in pumping capacity of the heart or develop symptoms only after the dysfunction has been present for some time.

Although the precise reasons why patients with LV dysfunction may remain asymptomatic is not certain, one potential explanation is that a number of compensatory mechanisms become activated in the presence of cardiac injury and/or LV dysfunction allowing patients

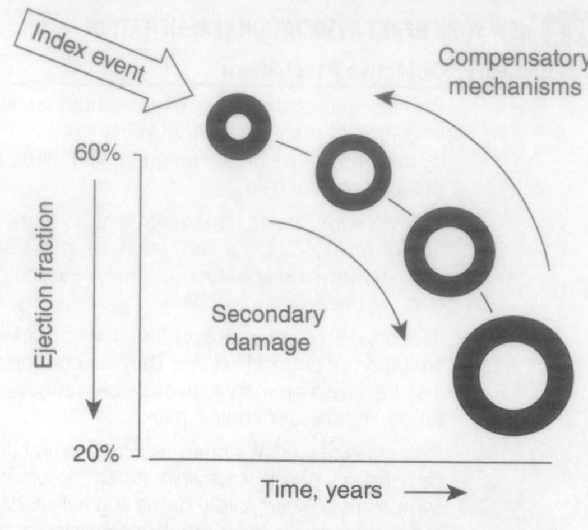

FIGURE 279-1 Pathogenesis of heart failure with a depressed ejection fraction. Heart failure begins after an index event produces an initial decline in the heart's pumping capacity. After this initial decline in pumping capacity, a variety of compensatory mechanisms are activated, including the adrenergic nervous system, the renin-angiotensin-aldosterone system, and the cytokine system. In the short term, these systems are able to restore cardiovascular function to a normal homeostatic range with the result that the patient remains asymptomatic. However, with time, the sustained activation of these systems can lead to secondary end-organ damage within the ventricle, with worsening left ventricular remodeling and subsequent cardiac decompensation. *(From D Mann: Circulation 100:999, 1999.)*

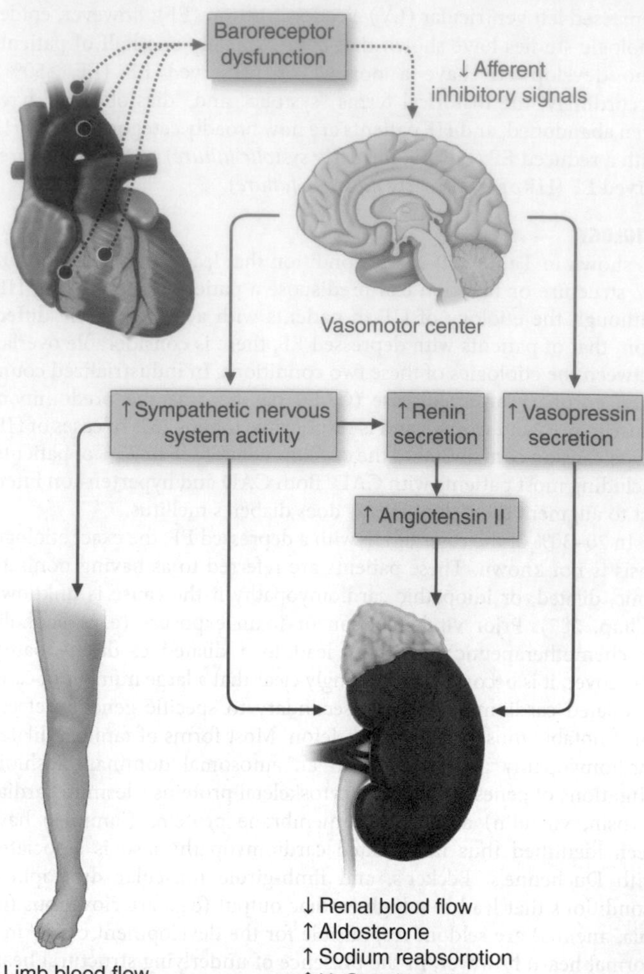

FIGURE 279-2 Activation of neurohormonal systems in heart failure. The decreased cardiac output in heart failure (HF) patients results in an "unloading" of high-pressure baroreceptors (*circles*) in the left ventricle, carotid sinus, and aortic arch. This unloading of the peripheral baroreceptors leads to a loss of inhibitory parasympathetic tone to the central nervous system (CNS), with a resultant generalized increase in efferent sympathetic tone, and nonosmotic release of arginine vasopressin (AVP) from the pituitary. AVP (or antidiuretic hormone [ADH]) is a powerful vasoconstrictor that increases the permeability of the renal collecting ducts, leading to the reabsorption of free water. These afferent signals to the CNS also activate efferent sympathetic nervous system pathways that innervate the heart, kidney, peripheral vasculature, and skeletal muscles.

Sympathetic stimulation of the kidney leads to the release of renin, with a resultant increase in the circulating levels of angiotensin II and aldosterone. The activation of the renin-angiotensin-aldosterone system promotes salt and water retention and leads to vasoconstriction of the peripheral vasculature, myocyte hypertrophy, myocyte cell death, and myocardial fibrosis. Although these neurohormonal mechanisms facilitate short-term adaptation by maintaining blood pressure, and hence perfusion to vital organs, the same neurohormonal mechanisms are believed to contribute to end-organ changes in the heart and the circulation and to the excessive salt and water retention in advanced HF. *(Modified from A Nohria et al: Neurohormonal, renal and vascular adjustments, in Atlas of Heart Failure: Cardiac Function and Dysfunction, 4th ed, WS Colucci [ed]. Philadelphia, Current Medicine Group 2002, p. 104.)*

to sustain and modulate LV function for a period of months to years. The compensatory mechanisms that have been described thus far include (1) activation of the renin-angiotensin-aldosterone (RAA) and adrenergic nervous systems, which are responsible, respectively, for maintaining cardiac output through increased retention of salt and water (Fig. 279-2), and (2) increased myocardial contractility. In addition, there is activation of a family of countervailing vasodilatory molecules, including the atrial and brain natriuretic peptides (ANP and BNP), prostaglandins (PGE_2 and PGI_2), and nitric oxide (NO), that offsets the excessive peripheral vascular vasoconstriction. Genetic background, sex, age, or environment may influence these compensatory mechanisms, which are able to modulate LV function within a physiologic/homeostatic range so that the functional capacity of the patient is preserved or is depressed only minimally. Thus, patients may remain asymptomatic or minimally symptomatic for a period of years; however, at some point patients become overtly symptomatic, with a resultant striking increase in morbidity and mortality rates. Although the exact mechanisms that are responsible for this transition are not known, as will be discussed below, the transition to symptomatic HF is accompanied by increasing activation of neurohormonal, adrenergic, and cytokine systems that lead to a series of adaptive changes within the myocardium collectively referred to as *LV remodeling*.

In contrast to our understanding of the pathogenesis of HF with a depressed EF, our understanding of the mechanisms that contribute to the development of HF with a preserved EF is still evolving. That is, although diastolic dysfunction (see below) was thought to be the only mechanism responsible for the development of HF with a preserved EF, community-based studies suggest that additional extracardiac mechanisms may be important, such as increased vascular stiffness and impaired renal function.

BASIC MECHANISMS OF HEART FAILURE

Heart Failure with a Reduced Ejection Fraction LV remodeling develops in response to a series of complex events that occur at the cellular and molecular levels (Table 279-3). These changes include (1) myocyte hypertrophy; (2) alterations in the contractile properties of the myocyte; (3) progressive loss of myocytes through necrosis, apoptosis, and autophagic cell death; (4) β-adrenergic desensitization; (5) abnormal myocardial energetics and metabolism; and (6) reorganization of the extracellular matrix with dissolution of the organized structural collagen weave surrounding myocytes and subsequent replacement by an interstitial collagen matrix that does not

TABLE 279-3 OVERVIEW OF LEFT VENTRICULAR REMODELING

Alterations in Myocyte Biology
Excitation-contraction coupling
Myosin heavy chain (fetal) gene expression
β-Adrenergic desensitization
Hypertrophy
Myocytolysis
Cytoskeletal proteins
Myocardial Changes
Myocyte loss
Necrosis
Apoptosis
Autophagy
Alterations in extracellular matrix
Matrix degradation
Myocardial fibrosis
Alterations in Left Ventricular Chamber Geometry
Left ventricular (LV) dilation
Increased LV sphericity
LV wall thinning
Mitral valve incompetence

Source: Adapted from D. Mann: Pathophysiology of heart failure, in *Braunwald's Heart Disease*, 8th ed, PL Libby et al (eds). Philadelphia, Elsevier, 2008, p. 550.

provide structural support to the myocytes. The biologic stimuli for these profound changes include mechanical stretch of the myocyte, circulating neurohormones (e.g., norepinephrine, angiotensin II), inflammatory cytokines (e.g., tumor necrosis factor [TNF]), other peptides and growth factors (e.g., endothelin), and reactive oxygen species (e.g., superoxide). The sustained overexpression of these biologically active molecules is believed to contribute to the progression of HF by virtue of the deleterious effects they exert on the heart and the circulation. Indeed, this insight forms the clinical rationale for using pharmacologic agents that antagonize these systems (e.g., angiotensin-converting enzyme [ACE] inhibitors and beta blockers) in treating patients with HF (Chap. 280).

To understand how the changes that occur in the failing cardiac myocyte contribute to depressed LV systolic function in HF, it is instructive first to review the biology of the cardiac muscle cell (Chap. 265e). Sustained neurohormonal activation and mechanical overload result in transcriptional and posttranscriptional changes in the genes and proteins that regulate excitation-contraction coupling and cross-bridge interaction (see Figs. 265e-6 and 265e-7). The changes that regulate excitation-contraction include decreased function of sarcoplasmic reticulum Ca^{2+} adenosine triphosphatase (SERCA2A), resulting in decreased calcium uptake into the sarcoplasmic reticulum (SR), and hyperphosphorylation of the ryanodine receptor, leading to calcium leakage from the SR. The changes that occur in the cross-bridges include decreased expression of α-myosin heavy chain and increased expression of β-myosin heavy chain, myocytolysis, and disruption of the cytoskeletal links between the sarcomeres and the extracellular matrix. Collectively, these changes impair the ability of the myocyte to contract and therefore contribute to the depressed LV systolic function observed in patients with HF.

Myocardial relaxation is an adenosine triphosphate (ATP)-dependent process that is regulated by uptake of cytoplasmic calcium into the SR by SERCA2A and extrusion of calcium by sarcolemmal pumps (see Fig. 265e-7). Accordingly, reductions in ATP concentration, as occurs in ischemia, may interfere with these processes and lead to slowed myocardial relaxation. Alternatively, if LV filling is delayed because LV compliance is reduced (e.g., from hypertrophy or fibrosis), LV filling pressures will similarly remain elevated at end diastole (see Fig. 265e-11). An increase in heart rate disproportionately shortens the time for diastolic filling, which may lead to elevated LV filling pressures, particularly in noncompliant ventricles. Elevated LV end-diastolic filling pressures result in increases in pulmonary capillary pressures, which can contribute to the dyspnea experienced by patients with diastolic dysfunction. In addition to impaired myocardial relaxation, increased myocardial stiffness secondary to cardiac hypertrophy and increased myocardial collagen content may contribute to diastolic failure. Importantly, diastolic dysfunction can occur alone or in combination with systolic dysfunction in patients with HF.

Left Ventricular Remodeling *Ventricular remodeling* refers to the changes in LV mass, volume, and shape and the composition of the heart that occur after cardiac injury and/or abnormal hemodynamic loading conditions. LV remodeling may contribute independently to the progression of HF by virtue of the mechanical burdens that are engendered by the changes in the geometry of the remodeled LV. In addition to the increase in LV end-diastolic volume, LV wall thinning occurs as the left ventricle begins to dilate. The increase in wall thinning, along with the increase in afterload created by LV dilation, leads to a functional *afterload mismatch* that may contribute further to a decrease in stroke volume. Moreover, the high end-diastolic wall stress might be expected to lead to (1) hypoperfusion of the subendocardium, with resultant worsening of LV function; (2) increased oxidative stress, with the resultant activation of families of genes that are sensitive to free radical generation (e.g., TNF and interleukin 1β); and (3) sustained expression of stretch-activated genes (angiotensin II, endothelin, and TNF) and/or stretch activation of hypertrophic signaling pathways. Increasing LV dilation also results in tethering of the papillary muscles with resulting incompetence of the mitral valve apparatus and functional mitral regurgitation, which in turn leads to further hemodynamic overloading of the ventricle. Taken together, the mechanical burdens that are engendered by LV remodeling contribute to the progression of HF. Recent studies have shown that LV remodeling can be reversed following medical and device therapy and that reverse LV remodeling is associated with improved clinical outcomes in patients with HFrEF. Indeed, one of the goals of therapy for HF is to prevent and/or reverse LV remodeling.

CLINICAL MANIFESTATIONS

Symptoms The cardinal symptoms of HF are fatigue and shortness of breath. Although fatigue traditionally has been ascribed to the low cardiac output in HF, it is likely that skeletal-muscle abnormalities and other noncardiac comorbidities (e.g., anemia) also contribute to this symptom. In the early stages of HF, dyspnea is observed only during exertion; however, as the disease progresses, dyspnea occurs with less strenuous activity, and it ultimately may occur even at rest. The origin of dyspnea in HF is probably multifactorial (Chap. 47e). The most important mechanism is pulmonary congestion with accumulation of interstitial or intra-alveolar fluid, which activates juxtacapillary J receptors, which in turn stimulate the rapid, shallow breathing characteristic of cardiac dyspnea. Other factors that contribute to dyspnea on exertion include reductions in pulmonary compliance, increased airway resistance, respiratory muscle and/or diaphragm fatigue, and anemia. Dyspnea may become less frequent with the onset of right ventricular (RV) failure and tricuspid regurgitation.

ORTHOPNEA Orthopnea, which is defined as dyspnea occurring in the recumbent position, is usually a later manifestation of HF than is exertional dyspnea. It results from redistribution of fluid from the splanchnic circulation and lower extremities into the central circulation during recumbency, with a resultant increase in pulmonary capillary pressure. Nocturnal cough is a common manifestation of this process and a frequently overlooked symptom of HF. Orthopnea generally is relieved by sitting upright or sleeping with additional pillows. Although orthopnea is a relatively specific symptom of HF, it may occur in patients with abdominal obesity or ascites and patients with pulmonary disease whose lung mechanics favor an upright posture.

PAROXYSMAL NOCTURNAL DYSPNEA (PND) This term refers to acute episodes of severe shortness of breath and coughing that generally occur at night and awaken the patient from sleep, usually 1–3 h after the patient retires. PND may manifest as coughing or wheezing, possibly because of increased pressure in the bronchial arteries leading to airway compression, along with interstitial pulmonary edema that leads to increased airway resistance. Whereas orthopnea may be relieved by sitting upright at the side of the bed with the legs in a dependent position, patients with PND often have persistent coughing and wheezing even after they have assumed the upright position. *Cardiac asthma* is closely related to PND, is characterized by wheezing secondary to bronchospasm, and must be differentiated from primary asthma and pulmonary causes of wheezing.

CHEYNE-STOKES RESPIRATION Also referred to as periodic respiration or cyclic respiration, Cheyne-Stokes respiration is present in 40% of patients with advanced HF and usually is associated with low cardiac output. Cheyne-Stokes respiration is caused by an increased sensitivity of the respiratory center to arterial PCO_2. There is an apneic phase, during which arterial PO_2 falls and arterial PCO_2 rises. These changes in the arterial blood gas content stimulate the respiratory center, resulting in hyperventilation and hypocapnia, followed by recurrence of apnea. Cheyne-Stokes respirations may be perceived by the patient or the patient's family as severe dyspnea or as a transient cessation of breathing.

ACUTE PULMONARY EDEMA See Chap. 326

Other Symptoms Patients with HF also may present with gastrointestinal symptoms. Anorexia, nausea, and early satiety associated with abdominal pain and fullness are common complaints and may be related to edema of the bowel wall and/or a congested liver. Congestion of the liver and stretching of its capsule may lead to right upper-quadrant pain. Cerebral symptoms such as confusion, disorientation, and sleep and mood disturbances may be observed in patients with severe HF, particularly elderly patients with cerebral arteriosclerosis and reduced cerebral perfusion. Nocturia is common in HF and may contribute to insomnia.

PHYSICAL EXAMINATION

A careful physical examination is always warranted in the evaluation of patients with HF. The purpose of the examination is to help determine the cause of HF as well as to assess the severity of the syndrome. Obtaining additional information about the hemodynamic profile and the response to therapy and determining the prognosis are important additional goals of the physical examination.

General Appearance and Vital Signs In mild or moderately severe HF, the patient appears to be in no distress at rest except for feeling uncomfortable when lying flat for more than a few minutes. In more severe HF, the patient must sit upright, may have labored breathing, and may not be able to finish a sentence because of shortness of breath. Systolic blood pressure may be normal or high in early HF, but it generally is reduced in advanced HF because of severe LV dysfunction. The pulse pressure may be diminished, reflecting a reduction in stroke volume. Sinus tachycardia is a nonspecific sign caused by increased adrenergic activity. Peripheral vasoconstriction leading to cool peripheral extremities and cyanosis of the lips and nail beds is also caused by excessive adrenergic activity.

Jugular Veins (See also Chap. 267) Examination of the jugular veins provides an estimation of right atrial pressure. The jugular venous pressure is best appreciated with the patient lying recumbent, with the head tilted at 45°. The jugular venous pressure should be quantified in centimeters of water (normal ≤8 cm) by estimating the height of the venous column of blood above the sternal angle in centimeters and then adding 5 cm. In the early stages of HF, the venous pressure may be normal at rest but may become abnormally elevated with sustained (~15 seconds) pressure on the abdomen (positive abdominojugular reflux). Giant *v* waves indicate the presence of tricuspid regurgitation.

Pulmonary Examination Pulmonary crackles (rales or crepitations) result from the transudation of fluid from the intravascular space into the alveoli. In patients with pulmonary edema, rales may be heard widely over both lung fields and may be accompanied by expiratory wheezing (cardiac asthma). When present in patients without concomitant lung disease, rales are specific for HF. Importantly, rales are frequently absent in patients with chronic HF, even when LV filling pressures are elevated, because of increased lymphatic drainage of alveolar fluid. Pleural effusions result from the elevation of pleural capillary pressure and the resulting transudation of fluid into the pleural cavities. Since the pleural veins drain into both the systemic and the pulmonary veins, pleural effusions occur most commonly with biventricular failure. Although pleural effusions are often bilateral in HF, when they are unilateral, they occur more frequently in the right pleural space.

Cardiac Examination Examination of the heart, although essential, frequently does not provide useful information about the severity of HF. If cardiomegaly is present, the point of maximal impulse (PMI) usually is displaced below the fifth intercostal space and/or lateral to the midclavicular line, and the impulse is palpable over two interspaces. Severe LV hypertrophy leads to a sustained PMI. In some patients, a third heart sound (S_3) is audible and palpable at the apex. Patients with enlarged or hypertrophied right ventricles may have a sustained and prolonged left parasternal impulse extending throughout systole. An S_3 (or *protodiastolic gallop*) is most commonly present in patients with volume overload who have tachycardia and tachypnea, and it often signifies severe hemodynamic compromise. A fourth heart sound (S_4) is not a specific indicator of HF but is usually present in patients with diastolic dysfunction. The murmurs of mitral and tricuspid regurgitation are frequently present in patients with advanced HF.

Abdomen and Extremities Hepatomegaly is an important sign in patients with HF. When it is present, the enlarged liver is frequently tender and may pulsate during systole if tricuspid regurgitation is present. Ascites, a late sign, occurs as a consequence of increased pressure in the hepatic veins and the veins draining the peritoneum. Jaundice, also a late finding in HF, results from impairment of hepatic function secondary to hepatic congestion and hepatocellular hypoxemia and is associated with elevations of both direct and indirect bilirubin.

Peripheral edema is a cardinal manifestation of HF, but it is nonspecific and usually is absent in patients who have been treated adequately with diuretics. Peripheral edema is usually symmetric and dependent in HF and occurs predominantly in the ankles and the pretibial region in ambulatory patients. In bedridden patients, edema may be found in the sacral area (*presacral edema*) and the scrotum. Long-standing edema may be associated with indurated and pigmented skin.

Cardiac Cachexia With severe chronic HF, there may be marked weight loss and cachexia. Although the mechanism of cachexia is not entirely understood, it is probably multifactorial and includes elevation of the resting metabolic rate; anorexia, nausea, and vomiting due to congestive hepatomegaly and abdominal fullness; elevation of circulating concentrations of cytokines such as TNF; and impairment of intestinal absorption due to congestion of the intestinal veins. When present, cachexia augurs a poor overall prognosis.

DIAGNOSIS

The diagnosis of HF is relatively straightforward when the patient presents with classic signs and symptoms of HF; however, the signs and symptoms of HF are neither specific nor sensitive. Accordingly, the key to making the diagnosis is to have a high index of suspicion, particularly for high-risk patients. When these patients present with signs or symptoms of HF, additional laboratory testing should be performed.

Routine Laboratory Testing Patients with new-onset HF and those with chronic HF and acute decompensation should have a complete blood count, a panel of electrolytes, blood urea nitrogen, serum creatinine, hepatic enzymes, and a urinalysis. Selected patients should have assessment for diabetes mellitus (fasting serum glucose or oral glucose tolerance test), dyslipidemia (fasting lipid panel), and thyroid abnormalities (thyroid-stimulating hormone level).

Electrocardiogram (ECG) A routine 12-lead ECG is recommended. The major importance of the ECG is to assess cardiac rhythm and determine the presence of LV hypertrophy or a prior MI (presence or absence of Q waves) as well as to determine QRS width to ascertain whether the patient may benefit from resynchronization therapy (see below). A normal ECG virtually excludes LV systolic dysfunction.

Chest X-Ray A chest x-ray provides useful information about cardiac size and shape, as well as the state of the pulmonary vasculature, and may identify noncardiac causes of the patient's symptoms. Although patients with acute HF have evidence of pulmonary hypertension, interstitial edema, and/or pulmonary edema, the majority of patients with chronic HF do not. The absence of these findings in patients with chronic HF reflects the increased capacity of the lymphatics to remove interstitial and/or pulmonary fluid.

Assessment of LV Function Noninvasive cardiac imaging (Chap. 270e) is essential for the diagnosis, evaluation, and management of HF. The most useful test is the two-dimensional (2-D) echocardiogram/Doppler, which can provide a semiquantitative assessment of LV size and function as well as the presence or absence of valvular and/or regional wall motion abnormalities (indicative of a prior MI). The presence of left atrial dilation and LV hypertrophy, together with abnormalities of LV diastolic filling provided by pulse-wave and tissue Doppler, is useful for the assessment of HF with a preserved EF. The 2-D echocardiogram/Doppler is also invaluable in assessing RV size and pulmonary pressures, which are critical in the evaluation and management of cor pulmonale (see below). Magnetic resonance imaging (MRI) also provides a comprehensive analysis of cardiac anatomy and function and is now the gold standard for assessing LV mass and volumes. MRI also is emerging as a useful and accurate imaging modality for evaluating patients with HF, both in terms of assessing LV structure and for determining the cause of HF (e.g., amyloidosis, ischemic cardiomyopathy, hemochromatosis).

The most useful index of LV function is the EF (stroke volume divided by end-diastolic volume). Because the EF is easy to measure by noninvasive testing and easy to conceptualize, it has gained wide acceptance among clinicians. Unfortunately, the EF has a number of limitations as a true measure of contractility, since it is influenced by alterations in afterload and/or preload. Nonetheless, with the exceptions indicated above, when the EF is normal (≥50%), systolic function is usually adequate, and when the EF is significantly depressed (<30–40%), contractility is usually depressed.

Biomarkers Circulating levels of natriuretic peptides are useful and important adjunctive tools in the diagnosis of patients with HF. Both B-type natriuretic peptide (BNP) and N-terminal pro-BNP (NT-proBNP), which are released from the failing heart, are relatively sensitive markers for the presence of HF with depressed EF; they also are elevated in HF patients with a preserved EF, albeit to a lesser degree. In ambulatory patients with dyspnea, the measurement of BNP or NT-proBNP is useful to support clinical decision making regarding the diagnosis of HF, especially in the setting of clinical uncertainty. Moreover, the measurement of BNP or NT-proBNP is useful for establishing prognosis or disease severity in chronic HF and can be useful to achieve optimal dosing of medical therapy in select clinically euvolemic patients. However, it is important to recognize that natriuretic peptide levels increase with age and renal impairment, are more elevated in women, and can be elevated in right HF from any cause. Levels can be falsely low in obese patients. Other biomarkers, such as soluble ST-2 and galectin-3, are newer biomarkers that can be used for determining the prognosis of HF patients.

Exercise Testing Treadmill or bicycle exercise testing is not routinely advocated for patients with HF, but either is useful for assessing the need for cardiac transplantation in patients with advanced HF (Chap. 281). A peak oxygen uptake (vo_2) <14 mL/kg per min is associated with a relatively poor prognosis. Patients with a vo_2 <14 mL/kg per min have been shown, in general, to have better survival when transplanted than when treated medically.

DIFFERENTIAL DIAGNOSIS

HF resembles but should be distinguished from (1) conditions in which there is circulatory congestion secondary to abnormal salt and water retention but in which there is no disturbance of cardiac structure or function (e.g., renal failure), and (2) noncardiac causes of pulmonary edema (e.g., acute respiratory distress syndrome). In most patients who present with classic signs and symptoms of HF, the diagnosis is relatively straightforward. However, even experienced clinicians have difficulty differentiating the dyspnea that arises from cardiac and pulmonary causes (Chap. 47e). In this regard, noninvasive cardiac imaging, biomarkers, pulmonary function testing, and chest x-ray may be useful. A very low BNP or NT-proBNP may be helpful in excluding a cardiac cause of dyspnea in this setting. Ankle edema may arise secondary to varicose veins, obesity, renal disease, or gravitational effects. When HF develops in patients with a preserved EF, it may be difficult to determine the relative contribution of HF to the dyspnea that occurs in chronic lung disease and/or obesity.

COR PULMONALE

DEFINITION

Cor pulmonale, often referred to as *pulmonary heart disease*, can be defined as altered RV structure and/or function in the context of chronic lung disease and is triggered by the onset of pulmonary hypertension. Although RV dysfunction is also an important sequela of HFpEF and HFrEF, this is not considered as cor pulmonale.

ETIOLOGY AND EPIDEMIOLOGY

Cor pulmonale develops in response to acute or chronic changes in the pulmonary vasculature and/or the lung parenchyma that are sufficient to cause pulmonary hypertension. The true prevalence of cor pulmonale is difficult to ascertain. First, not all patients with chronic lung disease will develop cor pulmonale, which may be subclinical in compensated individuals. Second, our ability to diagnose pulmonary hypertension and cor pulmonale by routine physical examination and laboratory testing is relatively insensitive. However, advances in 2-D echo/Doppler imaging and biomarkers (BNP) can make it easier to identify cor pulmonale.

Once patients with chronic pulmonary or pulmonary vascular disease develop cor pulmonale, the prognosis worsens. Although chronic obstructive pulmonary disease (COPD) and chronic bronchitis are responsible for approximately 50% of the cases of cor pulmonale in North America (Chap. 314), any disease that affects the pulmonary vasculature (Chap. 304) or parenchyma can lead to cor pulmonale (Table 279-4). Primary pulmonary vascular disorders are relatively rare causes of cor pulmonale, but cor pulmonale is extremely common with these conditions, given the magnitude of pulmonary hypertension present.

PATHOPHYSIOLOGY AND BASIC MECHANISMS

Although many conditions can lead to cor pulmonale, the common pathophysiologic mechanism is pulmonary hypertension that is sufficient to alter RV structure (i.e., dilation with or without hypertrophy) and function. Normally, pulmonary artery pressures are only ~15 mmHg and do not increase even with multiples of resting cardiac output, because of vasodilation and blood vessel recruitment of the pulmonary circulatory bed. But, in the setting of parenchymal lung diseases, primary pulmonary vascular disorders, or chronic (alveolar) hypoxia, the circulatory bed undergoes varying degrees of vascular remodeling, vasoconstriction, and destruction. As a result, pulmonary artery pressures and RV afterload increase, setting the stage for cor pulmonale (Table 279-4). The systemic consequences of cor pulmonale relate to alterations in cardiac output as well as salt and

TABLE 279-4 ETIOLOGY OF CHRONIC COR PULMONALE

Diseases of the Lung Parenchyma
Chronic obstructive pulmonary disease
Emphysema
Chronic bronchitis
Cystic fibrosis
Idiopathic interstitial pneumonitis
Idiopathic pulmonary fibrosis
Nonspecific interstitial pneumonitis
Sarcoidosis
Bronchiectasis
Pulmonary Langerhans cell histiocytosis
Lymphangioleiomyomatosis
Disorders of Chronic (Alveolar) Hypoxia
Alveolar hypoventilation syndromes
Obesity hypoventilation syndrome
Central hypoventilation syndrome
Neuromuscular respiratory failure
Chest wall disorders
Kyphoscoliosis
Living at high altitude
Diseases of the Pulmonary Vasculature
Pulmonary arterial hypertension (PAH)
Idiopathic PAH
Heritable PAH
Associated PAH
Venoocclusive disease
Chronic thromboembolic pulmonary hypertension
Pulmonary tumor thrombotic microangiopathy

water homeostasis. Anatomically, the RV is a thin-walled, compliant chamber that is better suited to handle volume overload than pressure overload. Thus, the sustained pressure overload imposed by pulmonary hypertension and increased pulmonary vascular resistance eventually causes the RV to fail.

The response of the RV to pulmonary hypertension depends on the acuteness and severity of the pressure overload. Acute cor pulmonale occurs after a sudden and severe stimulus (e.g., massive pulmonary embolus), with RV dilatation and failure but no RV hypertrophy (Chap. 300). Chronic cor pulmonale, however, is associated with a more slowly evolving and progressive pulmonary hypertension that leads to initial modest RV hypertrophy and subsequent RV dilation. Acute decompensation of previously compensated chronic cor pulmonale is a common clinical occurrence. Triggers include worsening hypoxia from any cause (e.g., pneumonia), acidemia (e.g., exacerbation of COPD), acute pulmonary embolus, atrial tachyarrhythmia, hypervolemia, and mechanical ventilation that leads to compressive forces on alveolar blood vessels.

CLINICAL MANIFESTATIONS

Symptoms The symptoms of chronic cor pulmonale generally are related to the underlying pulmonary disorder. Dyspnea, the most common symptom, is usually the result of the increased work of breathing secondary to changes in elastic recoil of the lung (fibrosing lung diseases), altered respiratory mechanics (e.g., overinflation with COPD), or inefficient ventilation (e.g., primary pulmonary vascular disease). Orthopnea and PND are rarely symptoms of isolated right HF and usually point toward concurrent left heart dysfunction. Rarely, these symptoms reflect increased work of breathing in the supine position resulting from compromised diaphragmatic excursion. Abdominal pain and ascites that occur with cor pulmonale are similar to the right HF that ensues in chronic HF. Lower-extremity edema may occur secondary to neurohormonal activation, elevated RV filling pressures, or increased levels of carbon dioxide and hypoxemia, which can lead to peripheral vasodilation and edema formation.

Signs Many of the signs encountered in cor pulmonale are also present in HF patients with a depressed EF, including tachypnea, elevated jugular venous pressures, hepatomegaly, and lower-extremity edema. Patients may have prominent *v* waves in the jugular venous pulse as a result of tricuspid regurgitation. Other cardiovascular signs include an RV heave palpable along the left sternal border or in the epigastrium. The increase in intensity of the holosystolic murmur of tricuspid regurgitation with inspiration ("Carvallo's sign") may be lost eventually as RV failure worsens. Cyanosis is a late finding in cor pulmonale and is secondary to a low cardiac output with systemic vasoconstriction and ventilation-perfusion mismatches in the lung.

DIAGNOSIS

The most common cause of right HF is not pulmonary parenchymal or vascular disease but left HF. Therefore, it is important to evaluate the patient for LV systolic and diastolic dysfunction. The ECG in severe pulmonary hypertension shows P pulmonale, right axis deviation, and RV hypertrophy. Radiographic examination of the chest may show enlargement of the main central pulmonary arteries and hilar vessels. Spirometry and lung volumes can identify obstructive and/or restrictive defects indicative of parenchymal lung diseases; arterial blood gases can demonstrate hypoxemia and/or hypercapnia. Spiral computed tomography (CT) scans of the chest are useful in diagnosing acute thromboembolic disease; however, ventilation-perfusion lung scanning remains best suited for diagnosing *chronic thromboembolic disease* (Chap. 300). A high-resolution CT scan of the chest can identify interstitial lung disease.

Two-dimensional echocardiography is useful for measuring RV thickness and chamber dimensions. Location of the RV behind the sternum and its crescent shape challenge assessment of RV function by echocardiography, especially when parenchymal lung disease is present. Calculated measures of RV function (e.g., tricuspid annular plane systolic excursion [TAPSE] or the Tei Index) supplement more subjective assessments of RV function. The interventricular septum may move paradoxically during systole in the presence of pulmonary hypertension. As noted, Doppler echocardiography can be used to assess pulmonary artery pressures. MRI is also useful for assessing RV structure and function, particularly in patients who are difficult to image with 2-D echocardiography because of severe lung disease. Right-heart catheterization is useful for confirming the diagnosis of pulmonary hypertension and for excluding elevated left-heart pressures (measured as the pulmonary capillary wedge pressure) as a cause for right HF. BNP and N-terminal BNP levels are elevated in patients with cor pulmonale secondary to RV myocardial stretch and may be dramatically elevated in acute pulmonary embolism.

280 Heart Failure: Management

Mandeep R. Mehra

Distinctive phenotypes of presentation with diverse management targets exemplify the vast syndrome of heart failure. These range from chronic heart failure with reduced ejection fraction (HFrEF) or heart failure with preserved ejection fraction (HFpEF), acute decompensated heart failure (ADHF), and advanced heart failure. Early management evolved from symptom control to disease-modifying therapy in HFrEF with the advent of renin-angiotensin-aldosterone system (RAAS)–directed therapy, beta receptor antagonists, mineralocorticoid receptor antagonists, cardiac resynchronization therapy, and implantable cardio-defibrillators. However, similar advances have been elusive in the syndromes of HFpEF and ADHF, which have remained devoid of convincing therapeutic advances to alter their natural history. In advanced heart failure, a stage of disease typically encountered in HFrEF, the patient remains markedly symptomatic with demonstrated refractoriness or inability to tolerate full-dose neurohormonal antagonism, often requires escalating doses of diuretics, and exhibits persistent hyponatremia and renal insufficiency with frequent episodes of heart failure decompensation requiring recurrent hospitalizations. Such individuals are at the highest risk of sudden or progressive pump failure–related deaths (Chap. 281). In contrast, early-stage asymptomatic left ventricular dysfunction is amenable to preventive care, and its natural history is modifiable by neurohormonal antagonism (not further discussed).

HEART FAILURE WITH PRESERVED EJECTION FRACTION

GENERAL PRINCIPLES

Therapeutic targets in HFpEF include control of congestion, stabilization of heart rate and blood pressure, and efforts at improving exercise tolerance. Addressing surrogate targets, such as regression of ventricular hypertrophy in hypertensive heart disease, and use of lusitropic agents, such as calcium channel blockers and beta receptor antagonists, have been disappointing. Experience has demonstrated that lowering blood pressure alleviates symptoms more effectively than targeted therapy with specific agents.

CLINICAL TRIALS IN HFpEF

The Candesartan in Heart Failure—Assessment of Mortality and Morbidity (CHARM) Preserved study showed a statistically significant reduction in hospitalizations but no difference in all-cause mortality in patients with HFpEF who were treated with the angiotensin receptor blocker (ARB), candesartan. Similarly, the Irbesartan in Heart Failure with Preserved Systolic Function (I-PRESERVE) trial demonstrated no differences in meaningful endpoints in such patients treated with irbesartan. An earlier analysis of a subset of the Digitalis Investigation Group (DIG) trial found no role for digoxin in the treatment of HFpEF. In the Study of the Effects of Nebivolol Intervention on Outcomes and Rehospitalization in Seniors with Heart Failure (SENIORS) trial of nebivolol, a vasodilating beta blocker, the subgroup of elderly patients with prior hospitalization and HFpEF did not appear to benefit in terms of all-cause or cardiovascular mortality. Much smaller mechanistic studies in the elderly with the angiotensin-converting enzyme inhibitor (ACEI) enalapril showed no effect on peak exercise oxygen consumption, 6-minute walk distance, aortic distensibility, left ventricular mass, or peripheral neurohormone expression.

NOVEL TARGETS

A small trial demonstrated that the phosphodiesterase-5 inhibitor *sildenafil* improved filling pressures and right ventricular function in a cohort of HFpEF patients with pulmonary venous hypertension. This finding led to the phase II trial, Phosphodiesterase-5 Inhibition to Improve Clinical Status and Exercise Capacity in Diastolic Heart Failure (RELAX), in HFpEF patients (left ventricular ejection fraction [LVEF] >50%) with New York Heart Association (NYHA) functional class II or III symptoms, who received sildenafil at 20 mg three times daily for 3 months, followed by 60 mg three times daily for another 3 months, compared with a placebo. There was no improvement in functional capacity, quality of life, or other clinical and surrogate parameters. Conceptually targeting myocardial fibrosis in HFpEF, the large-scale Aldosterone Antagonist Therapy in Adults with Preserved Ejection Fraction Congestive Heart Failure (TOPCAT) trial has been completed. This trial demonstrated no improvement in the primary composite end-point, but did show a secondary signal of benefit on HF hospitalizations, counterbalanced, however, by an increase in adverse effects, particularly hyperkalemia. However, pessimism has been generated by the negative outcome of the Aldosterone Receptor Blockade in Diastolic Heart Failure (ALDO-DHF) study wherein *spironolactone* improved echocardiographic indices of diastolic dysfunction but failed to improve exercise capacity, symptoms, or quality-of-life measures. A unique molecule that hybridizes an *ARB with an endopeptidase inhibitor*, LCZ696, increases the generation of myocardial cyclic guanosine 3′,5′-monophosphate, enhances myocardial relaxation, and reduces ventricular hypertrophy. This dual blocker has been shown to reduce circulating natriuretic peptides and reduce left atrial size to a significantly greater extent than valsartan alone in patients with HFpEF.

CLINICAL PEARLS

Even as efforts to control hypertension in HFpEF are critical, evaluation for and correction of underlying ischemia may be beneficial. Appropriate identification and treatment of sleep-disordered breathing should be strongly considered. Excessive decrease in preload with vasodilators may lead to underfilling the ventricle and subsequent hypotension and syncope. Some investigators have suggested that the exercise intolerance in HFpEF is a manifestation of chronotropic insufficiency and that such aberrations could be corrected with use of rate responsive pacemakers, but this remains an inadequately investigated contention (Fig. 280-1).

ACUTE DECOMPENSATED HEART FAILURE

GENERAL PRINCIPLES

ADHF is a heterogeneous clinical syndrome most often resulting in need for hospitalization due to confluence of interrelated abnormalities of decreased cardiac performance, renal dysfunction, and alterations in vascular compliance. Admission with a diagnosis of ADHF is associated with excessive morbidity and mortality, with nearly half of these patients readmitted for management within 6 months, and a high short-term (5–8% in-hospital) and long-term mortality (20% at 1 year). Importantly, long-term aggregate outcomes remain poor, with a combined incidence of cardiovascular deaths, heart failure hospitalizations, myocardial infarction, strokes, or sudden death reaching 50% at 12 months after hospitalization. The management of these patients has remained difficult and principally revolves around volume control and decrease of vascular impedance while maintaining attention to end-organ perfusion (coronary and renal).

The first principle of management of these patients is to identify and tackle known precipitants of decompensation. Identification and management of medication nonadherence and use of prescribed medicines such as nonsteroidal anti-inflammatory drugs, cold and flu preparations with cardiac stimulants, and herbal preparations, including licorice, ginseng, and ma huang (an herbal form of ephedrine now banned in most places), are required. Active infection and overt or covert pulmonary thromboembolism should be sought, identified, and treated when clinical clues suggest such direction. When possible, arrhythmias should be corrected by controlling heart rate or restoring sinus rhythm in patients with poorly tolerated rapid atrial fibrillation and by correcting ongoing ischemia with coronary revascularization or by correcting offenders such as ongoing bleeding in demand-related ischemia. A parallel step in management involves stabilization of hemodynamics in those with instability. The routine use of a pulmonary artery catheter is not recommended and should be restricted to those who respond poorly to diuresis or experience hypotension or signs and symptoms suggestive of a low cardiac output where therapeutic targets are unclear. Analysis of in-hospital registries has identified several

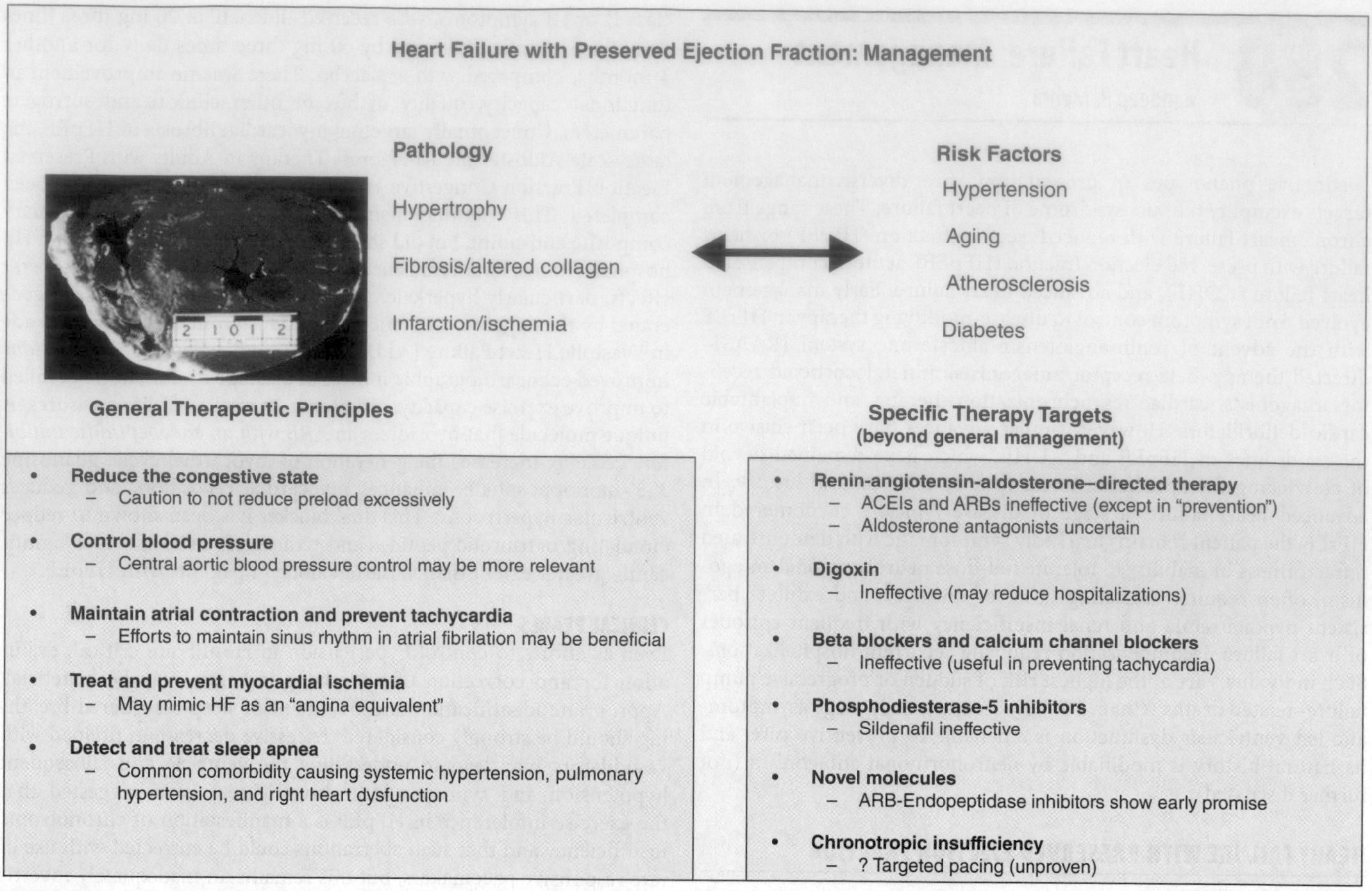

Heart Failure with Preserved Ejection Fraction: Management

General Therapeutic Principles

- **Reduce the congestive state**
  - Caution to not reduce preload excessively
- **Control blood pressure**
  - Central aortic blood pressure control may be more relevant
- **Maintain atrial contraction and prevent tachycardia**
  - Efforts to maintain sinus rhythm in atrial fibrillation may be beneficial
- **Treat and prevent myocardial ischemia**
  - May mimic HF as an "angina equivalent"
- **Detect and treat sleep apnea**
  - Common comorbidity causing systemic hypertension, pulmonary hypertension, and right heart dysfunction

Specific Therapy Targets (beyond general management)

- **Renin-angiotensin-aldosterone–directed therapy**
  - ACEIs and ARBs ineffective (except in "prevention")
  - Aldosterone antagonists uncertain
- **Digoxin**
  - Ineffective (may reduce hospitalizations)
- **Beta blockers and calcium channel blockers**
  - Ineffective (useful in preventing tachycardia)
- **Phosphodiesterase-5 inhibitors**
  - Sildenafil ineffective
- **Novel molecules**
  - ARB-Endopeptidase inhibitors show early promise
- **Chronotropic insufficiency**
  - ? Targeted pacing (unproven)

FIGURE 280-1 Pathophysiologic correlations, general therapeutic principles, and results of specific "directed" therapy in heart failure (HF) with preserved ejection fraction. ACEI, angiotensin-converting enzyme inhibitor; ARB, angiotensin receptor blocker.

parameters associated with worse outcomes: a blood urea nitrogen level greater than 43 mg/dL (to convert to mmol/L, multiply by 0.357), systolic blood pressure less than 115 mmHg, a serum creatinine level greater than 2.75 mg/dL (to convert to μmol/L, multiply by 88.4), and an elevated troponin I level. A useful clinical schema to identify treatment targets for the various phenotypic presentations and management goals in ADHF is depicted in Fig. 280-2.

VOLUME MANAGEMENT

Intravenous Diuretic Agents Intravenous diuretic agents rapidly and effectively relieve symptoms of congestion and are essential when oral drug absorption is impaired. When high doses of diuretic agents are required or when the effect is suboptimal, a continuous infusion may be needed to reduce toxicity and maintain stable serum drug levels. Randomized clinical trials of high-versus low-dose or bolus versus continuous infusion diuresis have not provided clear justification for the best diuretic strategy in ADHF, and as such, the use of diuretic regimens remains an art rather than science. Addition of a thiazide diuretic agent such as metolazone in combination provides a synergistic effect and is often required in patients receiving long-term therapy with loop diuretic agents. Change in weight is often used as a surrogate for adequate diuresis, but this objective measure of volume status may be surprisingly difficult to interpret, and weight loss during hospitalization does not necessarily correlate closely with outcomes. It is generally advisable to continue diuresis until euvolemia has been achieved. Physical examination findings, specifically the jugular venous pressure coupled with biomarker trends, are useful in timing discharge planning.

The Cardiorenal Syndrome The cardiorenal syndrome is being recognized increasingly as a complication of ADHF. Multiple definitions have been proposed for the cardiorenal syndrome, but at its simplest, it can be thought to reflect the interplay between abnormalities of heart and kidney function, with deteriorating function of one organ while therapy is administered to preserve the other. Approximately 30% of patients hospitalized with ADHF exhibit abnormal renal function at baseline, and this is associated with longer hospitalizations and increased mortality. However, mechanistic studies have been largely unable to find correlation between deterioration in renal function, cardiac output, left-sided filling pressures, and reduced renal perfusion; most patients with cardiorenal syndrome demonstrate a preserved cardiac output. It is hypothesized that in patients with established heart failure, this syndrome represents a complex interplay of neurohormonal factors, potentially exacerbated by "backward failure" resulting from increased intra-abdominal pressure and impairment in return of renal venous blood flow. Continued use of diuretic therapy may be associated with a reduction in glomerular filtration rate and a worsening of the cardiorenal syndrome when right-sided filling pressures remain elevated. In patients in the late stages of disease characterized by profound low cardiac output state, inotropic therapy or mechanical circulatory support has been shown to preserve or improve renal function in selected individuals in the short term until more definitive therapy such as assisted circulation or cardiac transplantation is implemented.

Ultrafiltration Ultrafiltration (UF) is an invasive fluid removal technique that may supplement the need for diuretic therapy. Proposed benefits of UF include controlled rates of fluid removal, neutral effects on serum electrolytes, and decreased neurohormonal activity. This technique has also been referred to as aquapheresis in recognition of its electrolyte depletion–sparing effects. Current UF systems function with two large-bore, peripherally inserted venous lines. In a pivotal study evaluating UF versus conventional therapy, fluid removal was improved and subsequent heart failure hospitalizations and urgent clinic visits were reduced with UF; however, no improvement in renal function and no subjective differences in dyspnea scores or adverse outcomes were noted. More recently, in the Cardiorenal Rescue Study in Acute Decompensated Heart Failure (CARRESS-HF) trial,

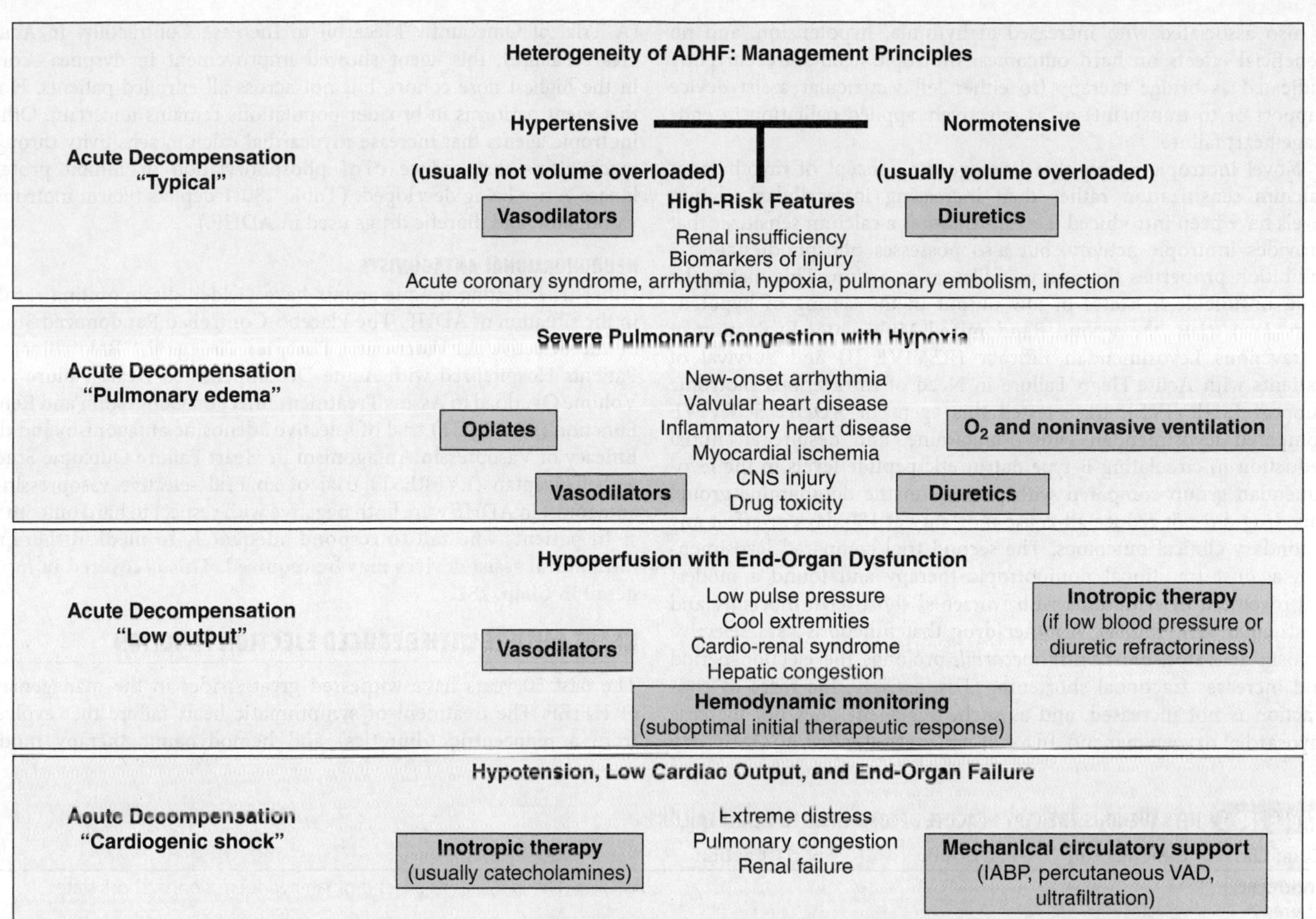

FIGURE 280-2 The distinctive phenotypes of acute decompensated heart failure (ADHF), their presentations, and suggested therapeutic routes. (Unique causes of ADHF, such as isolated right heart failure and pericardial disease, and rare causes, such as aortic and coronary dissection or ruptured valve structures or sinuses of Valsalva, are not delineated and are covered elsewhere.) IABP, intraaortic balloon pump; VAD, ventricular assist device.

188 patients with ADHF and worsening renal failure were randomized to stepped pharmacologic care or UF. The primary endpoint was a change in serum creatinine and change in weight (reflecting fluid removal) at 96 hours. Although similar weight loss occurred in both groups (approximately 5.5 kg), there was worsening in creatinine in the UF group. Deaths and hospitalizations for heart failure were no different between groups, but there were more severe adverse events in the UF group, mainly due to kidney failure, bleeding complications, and intravenous catheter-related complications. This investigation argues against using UF as a primary strategy in patients with ADHF who are nonetheless responsive to diuretics. Whether UF is useful in states of diuretic unresponsiveness remains an open question, and this strategy continues to be employed judiciously in such situations.

VASCULAR THERAPY

Vasodilators including *intravenous nitrates, nitroprusside,* and *nesiritide* (a recombinant brain-type natriuretic peptide) have been advocated for upstream therapy in an effort to stabilize ADHF. The latter agent was introduced in a fixed dose for therapy after a comparison with intravenous nitrates suggested more rapid and greater reduction in pulmonary capillary wedge pressure. Enthusiasm for nesiritide waned due to concerns within the pivotal trials for development of renal insufficiency and an increase in mortality. To address these concerns, a large-scale morbidity and mortality trial, the Acute Study of Clinical Effectiveness of Nesiritide in Decompensated Heart Failure (ASCEND-HF) study was completed in 2011 and randomly enrolled 7141 patients with ADHF to nesiritide or placebo for 24 to 168 hours in addition to standard care. Nesiritide was not associated with an increase or a decrease in the rates of death and rehospitalization and had a clinically insignificant benefit on dyspnea. Renal function did not worsen, but increased rates of hypotension were noted. Although this trial established the safety for this drug, the routine use cannot be advocated due to lack of significant efficacy. *Recombinant human relaxin-2*, or serelaxin, is a peptide upregulated in pregnancy and examined in ADHF patients with a normal or elevated blood pressure. In the Relaxin in Acute Heart Failure (RELAX-AHF) trial, serelaxin or placebo was added to a regimen of standard therapy in 1161 patients hospitalized with ADHF, evidence of congestion, and systolic pressure >125 mmHg. Serelaxin improved dyspnea, reduced signs and symptoms of congestion, and was associated with less early worsening of HF. Exploratory endpoints of hard outcomes at 6 months suggested positive signals in favor of mortality reduction. This agent is being tested in a large, more confirmatory trial setting.

INOTROPIC THERAPY

Impairment of myocardial contractility often accompanies ADHF, and pharmacologic agents that increase intracellular concentration of cyclic adenosine monophosphate via direct or indirect pathways, such as sympathomimetic amines (dobutamine) and phosphodiesterase-3 inhibitors (milrinone), respectively, serve as positive inotropic agents. Their activity leads to an increase in cytoplasmic calcium. Inotropic therapy in those with a low-output state augments cardiac output, improves perfusion, and relieves congestion acutely. Although milrinone and dobutamine have similar hemodynamic profiles, milrinone is slower acting and is renally excreted and thus requires dose adjustments in the setting of kidney dysfunction. Since milrinone acts downstream from the β_1-adrenergic receptor, it may provide an advantage in patients receiving beta blockers when admitted to the hospital. Studies are in universal agreement that long-term inotropic therapy increases mortality. However, the short-term use of inotropic agents in ADHF is also associated with increased arrhythmia, hypotension, and no beneficial effects on hard outcomes. Inotropic agents are currently indicated as bridge therapy (to either left ventricular assist device support or to transplant) or as selectively applied palliation in end-stage heart failure.

Novel inotropic agents that leverage the concept of myofilament calcium sensitization rather than increasing intracellular calcium levels have been introduced. *Levosimendan* is a calcium sensitizer that provides inotropic activity, but also possesses phosphodiesterase-3 inhibition properties that are vasodilators in action. This makes the drug unsuitable in states of low output in the setting of hypotension. Two trials, the second Randomized Multicenter Evaluation of Intravenous Levosimendan Efficacy (REVIVE II) and Survival of Patients with Acute Heart Failure in Need of Intravenous Inotropic Support (SURVIVE), have tested this agent in ADHF. SURVIVE compared levosimendan with dobutamine, and despite an initial reduction in circulating B-type natriuretic peptide levels in the levosimendan group compared with patients in the dobutamine group, this drug did not reduce all-cause mortality at 180 days or affect any secondary clinical outcomes. The second trial compared levosimendan against traditional noninotropic therapy and found a modest improvement in symptoms with worsened short-term mortality and ventricular arrhythmias. Another drug that functions as a selective myosin activator, *omecamtiv mecarbil*, prolongs the ejection period and increases fractional shortening. Distinctively, the force of contraction is not increased, and as such, this agent does not increase myocardial oxygen demand. In a 600-patient trial called ATOMIC-HF (A Trial of Omecamtiv Mecarbil to Increase Contractility in Acute Heart Failure), this agent showed improvement in dyspnea scores in the highest dose cohort, but not across all enrolled patients. How this agent performs in broader populations remains uncertain. Other inotropic agents that increase myocardial calcium sensitivity through mechanisms that reduce cTnI phosphorylation or inhibit protein kinase A are being developed. (Table 280-1 depicts typical inotropic, vasodilator, and diuretic drugs used in ADHF.)

NEUROHORMONAL ANTAGONISTS

Other trials testing unique agents have yielded disappointing results in the situation of ADHF. The Placebo-Controlled Randomized Study of the Selective A1 Adenosine Receptor Antagonist Rolofylline for Patients Hospitalized with Acute Decompensated Heart Failure and Volume Overload to Assess Treatment Effect on Congestion and Renal Function (PROTECT) trial of selective adenosine antagonism and the Efficacy of Vasopressin Antagonism in Heart Failure Outcome Study with Tolvaptan (EVEREST) trial of an oral selective vasopressin-2 antagonist in ADHF were both negative with respect to hard outcomes.

In patients who fail to respond adequately to medical therapy, mechanical assist devices may be required. This is covered in more detail in Chap. 281.

HEART FAILURE WITH REDUCED EJECTION FRACTION

The past 50 years have witnessed great strides in the management of HFrEF. The treatment of symptomatic heart failure that evolved from a renocentric (diuretics) and hemodynamic therapy model

TABLE 280-1 INTRAVENOUS THERAPY IN ACUTE DECOMPENSATED HEART FAILURE

Drug Class	Generic Drug	Usual Dosing	Special Caution	Comments
Inotropic therapy				Use in hypotension, end-organ hypoperfusion, or shock states
	Dobutamine	2–20 μg/kg per min	Increased myocardial oxygen demand, arrhythmia	Short acting, an advantage; variable efficacy in presence of beta blockers (requires higher doses); clinical tolerance to prolonged infusions; concerns with hypersensitivity carditis (rare)
	Milrinone	0.375–0.75 μg/kg per min	Hypotension, arrhythmia	Decrease dose in renal insufficiency; avoid initial bolus; effectiveness retained in presence of beta blockers
	Levosimendan	0.1 μg/kg per min, range, 0.05–0.2 μg/kg per min	Hypotension, arrhythmia	Long acting; should not be used in presence of low blood pressure; similar effectiveness as dobutamine but effectiveness retained in presence of beta blockers
	Omecamtiv Mecarbil	N/A	*In trials	Increases contractility without increasing myocardial oxygen demand; in confirmatory trials
Vasodilators				Use in presence of pulmonary congestion for rapid relief of dyspnea, in presence of a preserved blood pressure
	Nitroglycerine	10–20 μg/min, increase up to 200 μg/min	Headache, flushing, tolerance	Most common vasodilator but often underdosed; effective in higher doses
	Nesiritide	Bolus 2 μg/kg and infusion at 0.01 μg/kg per min	Hypotension	Decrease in blood pressure may reduce renal perfusion pressure; bolus may be avoided since it increases hypotension predilection
	Nitroprusside	0.3 μg/kg per min titrated to 5 μg/kg per min	Thiocyanate toxicity in renal insufficiency (>72 hours)	Requires arterial line placement for titration for precise blood pressure management and prevention of hypotension
	Serelaxin	N/A (tested at 30 μg/kg per d)	Baseline blood pressure should be >125 mmHg	Not widely commercially available; undergoing confirmatory trials
Diuretics				First line of therapy in volume overload with congestion; may use bolus or continuous dosing; initial low dose (1× home dose) or high dose (2.5 × home dose) equally effective with higher risk of renal worsening with higher dose
	Furosemide	20–240 mg daily	Monitor for electrolyte loss	In severe congestion, use intravenously and consider continuous infusion (not trial supported)
	Torsemide	10–100 mg daily	Monitor for electrolyte loss	High bioavailability, can be given orally; anecdotally more effective in advanced heart failure states if furosemide less bioavailable (due to gut congestion)
	Bumetanide	0.5–5 mg daily	Monitor for electrolyte loss	Can be used orally; intermediate bioavailability
	Adjuvant diuretics for augmentation	n/a	Metolazone, chlorthalidone, spironolactone, acetazolamide	Acetazolamide is useful in presence of alkalosis; metolazone given in 2.5- to 10-mg doses; causes severe electrolyte imbalance; spironolactone is useful in presence of severe hypokalemia and normal renal function

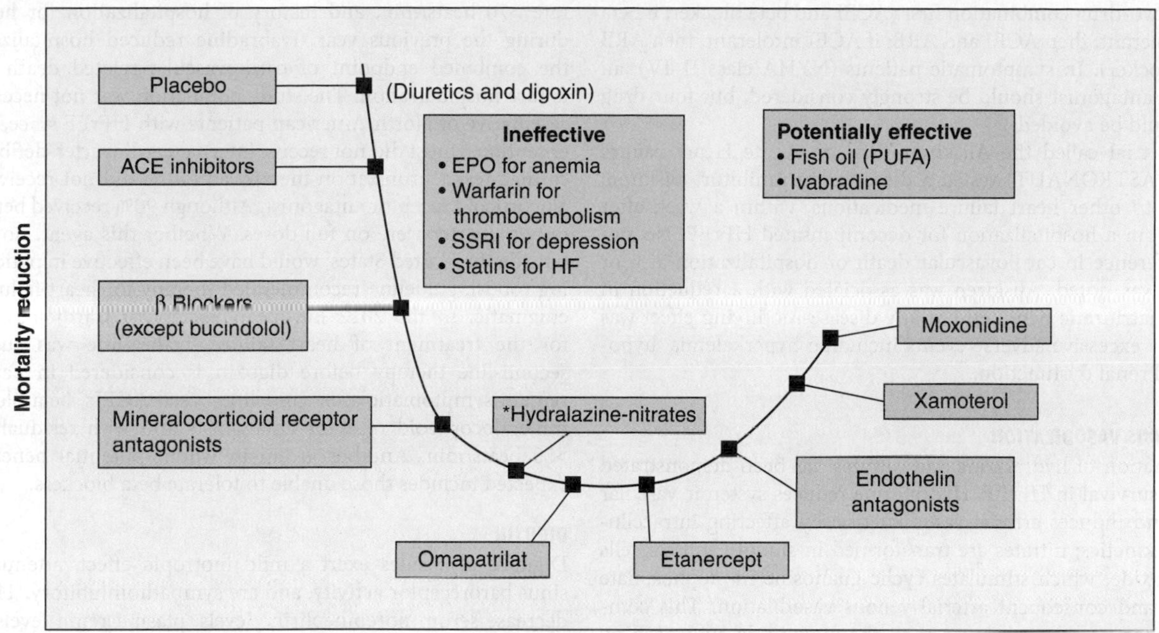

FIGURE 280-3 Progressive decline in mortality with angiotensin-converting enzyme (ACE) inhibitors or angiotensin receptor blockers (ARBs), beta blockers, mineralocorticoid receptor antagonists, and balanced vasodilators (*selected populations such as African Americans); further stack on neurohormonal therapy is ineffective or results in worse outcome; management of comorbidity is of unclear efficacy. EPO, erythropoietin; HF, heart failure; HFrEF, heart failure with reduced ejection fraction; PUFA, polyunsaturated fatty acid; SSRI, selective serotonin reuptake inhibitor.

(digoxin, inotropic therapy) ushered in the era of disease-modifying therapy with neurohormonal antagonism. In this regard, ACEIs and beta blockers form the cornerstone of pharmacotherapy and lead to attenuation of decline and improvement in cardiac structure and function with consequent reduction in symptoms, improvement in quality of life, decreased burden of hospitalizations, and a decline in mortality from both pump failure and arrhythmic deaths (Fig. 280-3).

NEUROHORMONAL ANTAGONISM

Meta-analyses suggest a 23% reduction in mortality and a 35% reduction in the combination endpoint of mortality and hospitalizations for heart failure in patients treated with ACEIs. Patients treated with beta blockers provide a further 35% reduction in mortality on top of the benefit provided by ACEIs alone. Increased experience with both agents in a broad range of patients with HFrEF has demonstrated the safety of ACEIs in treating patients with mild renal insufficiency and the tolerability of beta blockers in patients with moderately controlled diabetes, asthma, and obstructive lung disease. The benefits of ACEIs and beta blockers extend to advanced symptoms of disease (NYHA class IIIb–IV). However, a substantial number of patients with advanced heart failure may not be able to achieve optimal doses of neurohormonal inhibitors and require cautious reduction in dose exposure to maintain clinical stability. Such individuals with lower exposure to ACEIs and beta blockers represent a high-risk cohort with poor prognosis.

Class Effect and Sequence of Administration ACEIs exert their beneficial effects in HFrEF as a class; however, the beneficial effects of beta blockers are thought to be limited to specific drugs. Beta blockers with intrinsic sympathomimetic activity (xamoterol) and other agents, including bucindolol, have not demonstrated a survival benefit. On the basis of investigations, beta blocker use in HFrEF should be restricted to carvedilol, bisoprolol, and metoprolol succinate—agents tested and proven to improve survival in clinical trials. Whether beta blockers or ACEIs should be started first was answered by the Cardiac Insufficiency Bisoprolol Study (CIBIS) III, in which outcomes did not vary when either agent was initiated first. Thus, it matters little which agent is initiated first; what does matter is that optimally titrated doses of both ACEIs and beta blockers be established in a timely manner.

Dose and Outcome A trial has indicated that higher tolerated doses of ACEIs achieve greater reduction in hospitalizations without materially improving survival. Beta blockers demonstrate a dose-dependent improvement in cardiac function and reductions in mortality and hospitalizations. Clinical experience suggests that, in the absence of symptoms to suggest hypotension (fatigue and dizziness), pharmacotherapy may be up-titrated every 2 weeks in hemodynamically stable and euvolemic ambulatory patients as tolerated.

MINERALOCORTICOID ANTAGONISTS

Aldosterone antagonism is associated with a reduction in mortality in all stages of symptomatic NYHA class II to IV HFrEF. Elevated aldosterone levels in HFrEF promote sodium retention, electrolyte imbalance, and endothelial dysfunction and may directly contribute to myocardial fibrosis. The selective agent eplerenone (tested in NYHA class II and post–myocardial infarction heart failure) and the nonselective antagonist spironolactone (tested in NYHA class III and IV heart failure) reduce mortality and hospitalizations, with significant reductions in sudden cardiac death (SCD). Hyperkalemia and worsening renal function are concerns, especially in patients with underlying chronic kidney disease, and renal function and serum potassium levels must be closely monitored.

RAAS THERAPY AND NEUROHORMONAL "ESCAPE"

Neurohormonal "escape" has been witnessed in patients with HFrEF by the finding that circulating levels of angiotensin II return to pretreatment levels with long-term ACEI therapy. ARBs blunt this phenomenon by binding competitively to the AT_1 receptor. A large meta-analysis of 24 randomized trials showed the superiority of ARBs to placebo in patients with intolerable adverse effects with ACEIs and their noninferiority in all-cause mortality or hospitalizations when compared with ACEIs. The Valsartan Heart Failure Trial (Val-HeFT) suggested that addition of valsartan in patients already receiving treatment with ACEIs and beta blockers was associated with a trend toward worse outcomes. Similarly, adding valsartan to captopril in patients with heart failure after myocardial infarction who were receiving background beta blocker therapy was associated with an increase in adverse events without any added benefit compared with monotherapy for either group. Thus, the initial clinical strategy should be to use a two-drug combination first (ACEI and beta blocker; if beta blocker intolerant, then ACEI and ARB; if ACEI intolerant, then ARB and beta blocker). In symptomatic patients (NYHA class II–IV), an aldosterone antagonist should be strongly considered, but four-drug therapy should be avoided.

A recent trial called the Aliskiren Trial on Acute Heart Failure Outcomes (ASTRONAUT) tested a direct renin inhibitor, aliskiren, in addition to other heart failure medications, within a week after discharge from a hospitalization for decompensated HFrEF. No significant difference in cardiovascular death or hospitalization at 6 or 12 months was noted. Aliskiren was associated with a reduction in circulating natriuretic peptides, but any disease-modifying effect was overcome by excessive adverse events including hyperkalemia, hypotension, and renal dysfunction.

ARTERIOVENOUS VASODILATION

The combination of hydralazine and nitrates has been demonstrated to improve survival in HFrEF. Hydralazine reduces systemic vascular resistance and induces arterial vasodilatation by affecting intracellular calcium kinetics; nitrates are transformed in smooth muscle cells into nitric oxide, which stimulates cyclic guanosine monophosphate production and consequent arterial-venous vasodilation. This combination improves survival, but not to the magnitude evidenced by ACEIs or ARBs. However, in individuals with HFrEF unable to tolerate renin-angiotensin-aldosterone–based therapy for reasons such as renal insufficiency or hyperkalemia, this combination is preferred as a disease-modifying approach. A trial conducted in self-identified African Americans, the African-American Heart Failure Trial (A-Heft), studied a fixed dose of isosorbide dinitrate with hydralazine in patients with advanced symptoms of HFrEF who were receiving standard background therapy. The study demonstrated benefit in survival and hospitalization recidivism in the treatment group. Adherence to this regimen is limited by the thrice-daily dosing schedule. Table 280-2 lists the common neurohormonal and vasodilator regimens for HFrEF.

HEART RATE MODIFICATION

Ivabradine, an inhibitor of the I_f current in the sinoatrial node, slows the heart rate without a negative inotropic effect. The Systolic Heart Failure Treatment with Ivabradine Compared with Placebo Trial (SHIFT) was conducted in patients with class II or III HFrEF, a heart rate >70 beats/min, and history of hospitalization for heart failure during the previous year. Ivabradine reduced hospitalizations and the combined endpoint of cardiovascular-related death and heart failure hospitalization. The study population was not necessarily representative of North American patients with HFrEF since, with a few exceptions, most did not receive internal cardioverter-defibrillation or cardiac resynchronization therapy and 40% did not receive a mineralocorticoid receptor antagonist. Although 90% received beta blockers, only a quarter were on full doses. Whether this agent, now available outside the United States, would have been effective in patients receiving robust, guideline-recommended therapy for heart failure remains enigmatic. In the 2012 European Society of Cardiology guidelines for the treatment of heart failure, ivabradine was suggested as second-line therapy before digoxin is considered in patients who remain symptomatic after guideline-based ACEIs, beta blockers, and mineralocorticoid receptor antagonists and with residual heart rate >70 beats/min. Another group in whom potential benefit may be expected includes those unable to tolerate beta blockers.

DIGOXIN

Digitalis glycosides exert a mild inotropic effect, attenuate carotid sinus baroreceptor activity, and are sympathoinhibitory. These effects decrease serum norepinephrine levels, plasma renin levels, and possibly aldosterone levels. The DIG trial demonstrated a reduction in heart failure hospitalizations in the treatment group but no reduction in mortality or improvement in quality of life. Importantly, treatment with digoxin resulted in a higher mortality rate in women than men. Furthermore, the effects of digoxin in reducing hospitalizations were lower in women than in men. It should be noted that low doses of digoxin are sufficient to achieve any potentially beneficial outcomes, and higher doses breach the therapeutic safety index. Although digoxin levels should be checked to minimize toxicity and although dose reductions are indicated for higher levels, no adjustment is made for low levels. Generally, digoxin is now relegated as therapy for patients who remain profoundly symptomatic despite optimal neurohormonal blockade and adequate volume control.

ORAL DIURETICS

Neurohormonal activation results in avid salt and water retention. Loop diuretic agents are often required because of their increased potency,

TABLE 280-2 PHARMACOLOGIC THERAPY AND TARGET DOSES IN HEART FAILURE WITH REDUCED EJECTION FRACTION

Drug Class	Generic Drug	Mean Daily Dose in Clinical Trials (mg)	Initiation (mg)	Target Dose (mg)
Angiotensin-Converting Enzyme Inhibitors				
	Lisinopril	4.5–33	2.5–5 qd	20–35 qd
	Enalapril	17	2.5 bid	10–20 bid
	Captopril	123	6.25 tid	50 tid
	Trandolapril	N/A	0.5–1 qd	4 qd
Angiotensin Receptor Blockers				
	Losartan	129	50 qd	150 qd
	Valsartan	254	40 bid	160 bid
	Candesartan	24	4–8 qd	32 qd
Aldosterone Antagonists				
	Eplerenone	42.6	25 qd	50 qd
	Spironolactone	26	12.5–25 qd	25–50 qd
Beta Blockers				
	Metoprolol succinate CR/XL	159	12.5–25 qd	200 qd
	Carvedilol	37	3.125 bid	25–50 bid
	Bisoprolol	8.6	1.25 qd	10 qd
Arteriovenous Vasodilators				
	Hydralazine isosorbide dinitrate	270/136	37.5/20 tid	75/40 tid
	Fixed-dose hydralazine/isosorbide dinitrate	143/76	37.5/20 qid	75/40 qid

and frequent dose adjustments may be necessary because of variable oral absorption and fluctuations in renal function. Importantly, clinical trial data confirming efficacy are limited, and no data suggest that these agents improve survival. Thus, diuretic agents should ideally be used in tailored dosing schedules to avoid excessive exposure. Indeed, diuretics are essential at the outset to achieve volume control before neurohormonal therapy is likely to be well tolerated or titrated.

CALCIUM CHANNEL ANTAGONISTS

Amlodipine and felodipine, second-generation calcium channel-blocking agents, safely and effectively reduce blood pressure in HFrEF but do not affect morbidity, mortality, or quality of life. The first-generation agents, including verapamil and diltiazem, may exert negative inotropic effects and destabilize previously asymptomatic patients. Their use should be discouraged.

NOVEL NEUROHORMONAL ANTAGONISM

Despite an abundance of animal and clinical data demonstrating deleterious effects of activated neurohormonal pathways beyond the RAAS and sympathetic nervous system, targeting such pathways with incremental blockade has been largely unsuccessful. As an example, the endothelin antagonist bosentan is associated with worsening heart failure in HFrEF despite demonstrating benefits in right sided heart failure due to pulmonary arterial hypertension. Similarly, the centrally acting sympatholytic agent moxonidine worsens outcomes in left heart failure. The combined drug omapatrilat hybridizes an ACEI with a neutral endopeptidase inhibitor, and this agent was tested in the Omapatrilat Versus Enalapril Randomized Trial of Utility in Reducing Events (OVERTURE) trial. This drug did not favorably influence the primary outcome measure of the combined risk of death or hospitalization for heart failure requiring intravenous treatment. The risk of angioedema was notably higher with omapatrilat than ACEIs alone. LCZ696 and ARB with an endopeptidase inhibitor have shown benefit in a large trial versus ARB alone.

INFLAMMATION

Targeting inflammatory cytokines such as tumor necrosis factor α (TNF-α) by using anticytokine agents such as infliximab and etanercept has been unsuccessful and associated with worsening heart failure. Nonspecific immunomodulation has been tested in the large Advanced Chronic Heart Failure Clinical Assessment of Immune Modulation Therapy (ACCLAIM-HF) trial of 2426 HFrEF patients with NYHA functional class II to IV symptoms. Ex vivo exposure of a blood sample to controlled oxidative stress initiates apoptosis of leukocytes soon after intramuscular gluteal injection of the treated sample. The physiologic response to apoptotic cells results in a reduction in inflammatory cytokine production and upregulation of anti-inflammatory cytokines. This promising hypothesis was not proven, although certain subgroups (those with no history of previous myocardial infarction and those with mild heart failure) showed signals in favor of immunomodulation. Use of intravenous immunoglobulin therapy in nonischemic etiology of heart failure has not been shown to result in beneficial outcomes.

STATINS

Potent lipid-altering and pleiotropic effects of statins reduce major cardiovascular events and improve survival in non–heart failure populations. Once heart failure is well established, this therapy may not be as beneficial and theoretically could even be detrimental by depleting ubiquinone in the electron transport chain. Two trials, Controlled Rosuvastatin Multinational Trial in Heart Failure (CORONA) and Gruppo Italiano per lo Studio della Sopravvivenza nell'Insufficienza Cardiac (GISSI-HF), have tested low-dose rosuvastatin in patients with HFrEF and demonstrated no improvement in aggregate clinical outcomes. If statins are required to treat progressive coronary artery disease in the background setting of heart failure, then they should be employed. However, no rationale appears to exist for routine statin therapy in nonischemic heart failure.

ANTICOAGULATION AND ANTIPLATELET THERAPY

HFrEF is accompanied by a hypercoagulable state and therefore a high risk of thromboembolic events, including stroke, pulmonary embolism, and peripheral arterial embolism. Although long-term oral anticoagulation is established in certain groups, including patients with atrial fibrillation, the data are insufficient to support the use of warfarin in patients in normal sinus rhythm without a history of thromboembolic events or echocardiographic evidence of left ventricular thrombus. In the large Warfarin versus Aspirin in Reduced Cardiac Ejection Fraction (WARCEF) trial, 2305 patients with HFrEF were randomly allocated to either full-dose aspirin or international normalized ratio–controlled warfarin with follow-up for 6 years. Among patients with reduced LVEF who were in sinus rhythm, there was no significant overall difference in the primary outcome between treatment with warfarin and treatment with aspirin. A reduced risk of ischemic stroke with warfarin was offset by an increased risk of major hemorrhage. Aspirin blunts ACEI-mediated prostaglandin synthesis, but the clinical importance of this finding remains unclear. Current guidelines support the use of aspirin in patients with ischemic cardiomyopathy.

FISH OIL

Treatment with long-chain omega-3 polyunsaturated fatty acids (ω-3 PUFAs) has been shown to be associated with modestly improved clinical outcomes in patients with HFrEF. This observation from the GISSI-HF trial was extended to measurements of ω-3 PUFAs in plasma phospholipids at baseline and after 3 months. Three-month treatment with ω-3 PUFAs enriched circulating eicosapentaenoic acid (EPA) and docosahexaenoic acid (DHA). Low EPA levels are inversely related to total mortality in patients with HFrEF.

MICRONUTRIENTS

A growing body of evidence suggests an association between heart failure and micronutrient status. Reversible heart failure has been described as a consequence of severe thiamine and selenium deficiency. Thiamine deficiency has received attention in heart failure due to the fact that malnutrition and diuretics are prime risk factors for thiamine loss. Small exploratory randomized studies have suggested a benefit of supplementation of thiamine in HFrEF with evidence of improved cardiac function. This finding is restricted to chronic heart failure states and does not appear to be beneficial in the ADHF phenotype. Due to the preliminary nature of the evidence, no recommendations for routine supplementation or testing for thiamine deficiency can be made.

ENHANCED EXTERNAL COUNTERPULSATION (EECP)

Peripheral lower extremity therapy using graded external pneumatic compression at high pressure is administered in 1-hour sessions for 35 treatments (7 weeks) and has been proposed to reduce angina symptoms and extend time to exercise-induced ischemia in patients with coronary artery disease. The Prospective Evaluation of Enhanced External Counterpulsation in Congestive Heart Failure (PEECH) study assessed the benefits of enhanced external counterpulsation in the treatment of patients with mild-to-moderate heart failure. This randomized trial improved exercise tolerance, quality of life, and NYHA functional classification but without an accompanying increase in peak oxygen consumption. A placebo effect due to the nature of the intervention simply cannot be excluded.

EXERCISE

The Heart Failure: A Controlled Trial Investigating Outcomes of Exercise Training (HF-ACTION) study investigated short-term (3-month) and long-term (12-month) effects of a supervised exercise training program in patients with moderate HFrEF. Exercise was safe, improved patients' sense of well-being, and correlated with a trend toward mortality reduction. Maximal changes in 6-minute walk distance were evident at 3 months with significant improvements in cardiopulmonary exercise time and peak oxygen consumption persisting at 12 months. Therefore, exercise training is recommended as an adjunctive treatment in patients with heart failure.

Sleep-disordered breathing is common in HF and particularly in HFrEF. A range of presentations exemplified by obstructive sleep apnea, central sleep apnea, and its extreme form of Cheyne-Stokes breathing are noted. Frequent periods of hypoxia and repeated micro- and macro-arousals trigger adrenergic surges, which can worsen hypertension and impair systolic and diastolic function. A high index of suspicion is required, especially in patients with difficult-to-control hypertension or with predominant symptoms of fatigue despite reverse remodeling in response to optimal medical therapy. Worsening of right heart function with improvement of left ventricular function noted on medical therapy should immediately trigger a search for underlying sleep-disordered breathing or pulmonary complications such as occult embolism or pulmonary hypertension. Treatment with nocturnal positive airway pressure improves oxygenation, LVEF, and 6-minute walk distance. However, no conclusive data exist to support this therapy as a disease-modifying approach with reduction in mortality.

Anemia is common in heart failure patients, reduces functional status and quality of life, and is associated with increased proclivity for hospital admissions and mortality. Anemia in heart failure is more common in the elderly, in those with advanced stages of HFrEF, in the presence of renal insufficiency, and in women and African Americans. The mechanisms include iron deficiency, dysregulation of iron metabolism, and occult gastrointestinal bleeding. Intravenous iron using either iron sucrose or carboxymaltose (Ferric Carboxymaltose Assessment in Patients with Iron Deficiency and Chronic Heart Failure [FAIR-HF] trial) has been shown to correct anemia and improve functional capacity. Erythropoiesis-regulating agents such as erythropoietin analogues have been studied with disappointing results. The Reduction of Events by Darbepoetin Alfa in Heart Failure (RED-HF) trial evaluated 2278 mild-to-moderate anemia patients with HFrEF and demonstrated that treatment with darbepoetin alfa did not improve clinical outcomes in patients with systolic heart failure.

Depression is common in HFrEF, with a reported prevalence of one in five patients, and is associated with a poor quality of life, limited functional status, and increased risk of morbidity and mortality in this population. Antidepressants may improve depression, promote vascular health, and decrease systemic inflammation in HFrEF. However, the largest randomized study of depression in HFrEF, the Sertraline Against Depression and Heart Disease in Chronic Heart Failure (SADHART-CHF) trial, showed that sertraline was safe, but did not provide greater reduction in depression or improve cardiovascular status among patients with heart failure and depression compared with nurse-driven multidisciplinary management.

Atrial arrhythmias, especially atrial fibrillation, are common and serve as a harbinger of worse prognosis in patients with heart failure. When rate control is inadequate or symptoms persist, pursuing a rhythm control strategy is reasonable. Rhythm control may be achieved via pharmacotherapy or by percutaneous or surgical techniques, and referral to practitioners or centers experienced in these modalities is recommended. Antiarrhythmic drug therapy should be restricted to amiodarone and dofetilide, both of which have been shown to be safe and effective but do not alter the natural history of the underlying disease. The Antiarrhythmic Trial with Dronedarone in Moderate-to-Severe Congestive Heart Failure Evaluating Morbidity Decrease (ANDROMEDA) studied the effects of the novel antiarrhythmic agent dronedarone and found an increased mortality due to worsening heart failure. Catheter ablation and pulmonary vein isolation appear to be safe and effective in this high-risk cohort and compare favorably with the more established practice of atrioventricular node ablation and biventricular pacing.

CARDIAC RESYNCHRONIZATION THERAPY

Nonsynchronous contraction between the walls of the left ventricle (intraventricular) or between the ventricular chambers (interventricular) impairs systolic function, decreases mechanical efficiency of contraction, and adversely affects ventricular filling. Mechanical dyssynchrony results in an increase in wall stress and worsens functional mitral regurgitation. The single most important association of extent of dyssynchrony is a widened QRS interval on the surface electrocardiogram, particularly in the presence of a left bundle branch block pattern. With placement of a pacing lead via the coronary sinus to the lateral wall of the ventricle, cardiac resynchronization therapy (CRT) enables a more synchronous ventricular contraction by aligning the timing of activation of the opposing walls. Early studies showed improved exercise capacity, reduction in symptoms, and evidence of reverse remodeling. The Cardiac Resynchronization in Heart Failure Study (CARE-HF) trial was the first study to demonstrate a reduction in all-cause mortality with CRT placement in patients with HFrEF on optimal therapy with continued moderate-to-severe residual symptoms of NYHA class III or IV heart failure. More recent clinical trials have demonstrated disease-modifying properties of CRT in even minimally symptomatic patients with HFrEF, including the Resynchronization–Defibrillation for Ambulatory Heart Failure Trial (RAFT) and Multicenter Automatic Defibrillator Implantation Trial with Cardiac Resynchronization Therapy (MADIT-CRT), both of which sought to use CRT in combination with an implantable defibrillator. Most benefit in mildly symptomatic HFrEF patients accrues from applying this therapy in those with a QRS width of >149 ms and a left bundle branch block pattern. Attempts to further optimize risk stratification and expand indications for CRT using modalities other than electrocardiography have proven disappointing. In particular, echocardiographically derived measures of dyssynchrony vary tremendously, and narrow QRS dyssynchrony has not proven to be a good target for treatment. Uncertainty surrounds the benefits of CRT in those with ADHF, a predominant right bundle branch block pattern, atrial fibrillation, and evidence of scar in the lateral wall, which is the precise location where the CRT lead is positioned.

SUDDEN CARDIAC DEATH PREVENTION IN HEART FAILURE

SCD due to ventricular arrhythmias is the mode of death in approximately half of patients with heart failure and is particularly proportionally prevalent in HFrEF patients with early stages of the disease. Patients who survive an episode of SCD are considered to be at very high risk and qualify for placement of an implantable cardioverter-defibrillator (ICD). Although primary prevention is challenging, the degree of residual left ventricular dysfunction despite optimal medical therapy (≤35%) to allow for adequate remodeling and the underlying etiology (post–myocardial infarction or ischemic cardiomyopathy) are the two single most important risk markers for stratification of need and benefit. Currently, patients with NYHA class II or III symptoms of heart failure and an LVEF <35%, irrespective of etiology of heart failure, are appropriate candidates for ICD prophylactic therapy. In patients with a myocardial infarction and optimal medical therapy with residual LVEF ≤30% (even when asymptomatic), placement of an ICD is appropriate. In patients with a terminal illness and a predicted life span of less than 6 months or in those with NYHA class IV symptoms who are refractory to medications and who are not candidates for transplant, the risks of multiple ICD shocks must be carefully weighed against the survival benefits. If a patient meets the QRS criteria for CRT, combined CRT with ICD is often employed (Table 280-3).

SURGICAL THERAPY IN HEART FAILURE

Coronary artery bypass grafting (CABG) is considered in patients with ischemic cardiomyopathy with multivessel coronary artery disease. The recognition that hibernating myocardium, defined as myocardial tissue with abnormal function but maintained cellular function, could recover after revascularization led to the notion that revascularization with CABG would be useful in those with living myocardium. Revascularization is most robustly supported in individuals with ongoing angina and left ventricular failure. Revascularizing those with left ventricular failure in the absence of angina remains controversial. The Surgical Treatment for Ischemic Heart Failure (STICH) trial enrolled 1212 patients with an ejection fraction of 35% or less and coronary artery disease amenable to CABG and randomly assigned them to

TABLE 280-3 PRINCIPLES OF ICD IMPLANTATION FOR PRIMARY PREVENTION OF SUDDEN DEATH

Principle	Comment
Arrhythmia–sudden death mismatch	Sudden death in heart failure patients is generally due to progressive LVD, not a focal arrhythmia substrate (except in patients with post-MI HF)
Diminishing returns with advanced disease	Intervention at early stages of HF most successful since sudden death diminishes as cause of death with advanced HF
Timing of benefits	LVEF should be evaluated on optimal medical therapy or after revascularization before ICD therapy is employed; no benefit to ICD implant within 40 days of an MI (unless for secondary prevention)
Estimation of benefits and prognosis	Patients and clinicians often overestimate benefits of ICDs; an ICD discharge is not equivalent to an episode of sudden death (some ventricular arrhythmias terminate spontaneously); appropriate ICD discharges are associated with a worse near-term prognosis

Abbreviations: HF, heart failure; ICD, implantable cardioverter-defibrillator; LVD, left ventricular disease; LVEF, left ventricular ejection fraction; MI, myocardial infarction.

medical therapy alone or medical therapy plus CABG. There was no significant difference between groups with respect to the primary endpoint of death from any cause. Patients assigned to CABG had lower rates of death from cardiovascular causes and of death from any cause or hospitalization for cardiovascular causes. An ancillary study of this trial also determined that the detection of hibernation pre-revascularization did not materially influence the efficacy of this approach, nor did it help to define a population unlikely to benefit if hibernation was not detected.

Surgical ventricular restoration (SVR), a technique characterized by infarct exclusion to remodel the left ventricle by reshaping it surgically in patients with ischemic cardiomyopathy and dominant anterior left ventricular dysfunction, has been proposed. However, in a 1000-patient trial in patients with HFrEF who underwent CABG alone or CABG plus SVR, the addition of SVR to CABG had no disease-modifying effect. Cardiac symptoms and exercise tolerance improved from baseline to a similar degree in both study groups. SVR resulted in lower left ventricular volumes at 4 months after operation. However, left ventricular aneurysm surgery is still advocated in those with refractory heart failure, ventricular arrhythmias, or thromboembolism arising from an akinetic aneurysmal segment of the ventricle. Other remodeling procedures, such as use of an external mesh-like net attached around the heart to limit further enlargement, have not been shown to provide hard clinical benefits, although favorable cardiac remodeling was noted.

Mitral regurgitation (MR) occurs with varying degrees in patients with HFrEF and dilated ventricles. Annular dilatation and leaflet noncoaptation in the setting of anatomically normal papillary muscles, chordal structures, and valve leaflets characterize functional MR. In patients who are not candidates for surgical coronary revascularization, mitral valve repair remains controversial. Ischemic MR (or infarct-related MR) is typically associated with leaflet tethering and displacement related to abnormal left ventricular wall motion and geometry. No evidence to support the use of surgical or percutaneous valve correction for functional MR exists as disease-modifying therapy even though MR can be corrected.

CELLULAR AND GENE-BASED THERAPY

The cardiomyocyte is no longer considered a terminally differentiated cell and possesses regenerative capacity. Such renewal is accelerated under conditions of stress and injury, such as an ischemic event or heart failure. Investigations that use either bone marrow–derived precursor cells or autologous cardiac-derived cells have gained traction. A number of small- and moderate-scale trials of such therapy have focused on post–myocardial infarction patients and have used autologous bone marrow–derived progenitor or stem cells. These trials have had variable results, with most demonstrating modest improvements in parameters of cardiac structure and remodeling. More promising, however, are cardiac-derived stem cells. Two preliminary pilot trials delivering cells via an intracoronary approach have been reported. In one, autologous c-kit–positive cells isolated from the atria obtained from patients undergoing CABG were cultured and reinfused. In another, cardiosphere-derived cells grown from endomyocardial biopsy specimens were used. These small trials demonstrated improvements in left ventricular function but require far more work to usher in a clinical therapeutic success. The appropriate route of administration, the quantity of cells to achieve a minimal therapeutic threshold, the constitution of these cells (single source or mixed), the mechanism by which benefit accrues, and short- and long-term safety remain to be elucidated.

Targeting molecular aberrations using gene transfer therapy, mostly with an adenoviral vector, is emerging in HFrEF. Several methods of gene delivery have been developed, including direct intramyocardial injection, coronary artery or venous infusion, and injection into the pericardial space. Cellular targets under consideration include β_2-adrenergic receptors and calcium cycling proteins such as inhibitors of phospholamban. SERCA2a is deficient in patients with HFrEF and is primarily responsible for reincorporating calcium into the sarcoplasmic reticulum during diastole. A phase II randomized, double-blind, placebo-controlled trial called CUPID (Efficacy and Safety Study of Genetically Targeted Enzyme Replacement Therapy for Advanced Heart Failure) was completed. This study used coronary arterial infusion of adeno-associated virus type 1 carrying the gene for SERCA2a and demonstrated that natriuretic peptides were decreased, reverse remodeling was noted, and symptomatic improvements were forthcoming. Stromal derived factor 1 enhances myocardial repair and facilitates "homing" of stem cells to the site of tissue injury. Strategies using intramyocardial injections to deploy this gene at sites of injury are being studied.

More advanced therapies for late-stage heart failure such as left ventricular assist devices and cardiac transplantation are covered in detail in Chap. 281.

DISEASE MANAGEMENT AND SUPPORTIVE CARE

Despite stellar outcomes with medical therapy, admission rates following heart failure hospitalization remain high, with nearly half of all patients readmitted to hospital within 6 months of discharge. Recurrent heart failure and related cardiovascular conditions account for only half of readmissions in patients with heart failure, whereas other comorbidity-related conditions account for the rest. The key to achieving enhanced outcomes must begin with the attention to transitional care at the index hospitalization with facilitated discharge through comprehensive discharge planning, patient and caregiver education, appropriate use of visiting nurses, and planned follow-up. Early postdischarge follow-up, whether by telephone or clinic-based, may be critical to ensuring stability because most heart failure–related readmissions tend to occur within the first 2 weeks after discharge. Although routinely advocated, intensive surveillance of weight and vital signs with use of telemonitoring has not decreased hospitalizations. Intrathoracic impedance measurements have been advocated for the identification of early rise in filling pressure and worsened hemodynamics so that preemptive management may be employed. However, this has not been successful and may worsen outcomes in the short term. Implantable pressure monitoring systems do tend to provide signals for early decompensation, and in patients with moderately advanced symptoms, such systems have been shown to provide information that can allow implementation of therapy to avoid hospitalizations by as much as 39% (in the CardioMEMS Heart Sensor Allows Monitoring of Pressure to Improve Outcomes in NYHA Class III Heart

Failure Patients [CHAMPION] trial). Once heart failure becomes advanced, regularly scheduled review of the disease course and options with the patient and family is recommended including discussions surrounding end-of-life preferences when patients are comfortable in an outpatient setting. As the disease state advances further, integrating care with social workers, pharmacists, and community-based nursing may be critical in improving patient satisfaction with the therapy, enhancing quality of life, and avoiding heart failure hospitalizations. Equally important is attention to seasonal influenza vaccinations and periodic pneumococcal vaccines that may obviate non–heart failure hospitalizations in these ill patients. When nearing end of life, facilitating a shift in priorities to outpatient and hospice palliation is key, as are discussions around advanced therapeutics and continued use of ICD prophylaxis, which may worsen quality of life and prolong death.

GLOBAL CONSIDERATIONS

Substantial differences exist in the practice of heart failure therapeutics and outcomes by geographic location. International guidelines produced by the American College of Cardiology/American Heart Association, European Society of Cardiology, and National Institute for Health and Clinical Excellence (United Kingdom) differ in their approach to evaluation of evidence and prioritization of therapy. The penetrance of CRT and ICD is higher in the United States than in Europe. Conversely, therapy unavailable in the United States, such as ivabradine and levosimendan, is designated as useful in Europe. Although ACEIs appear to be similarly effective across populations, variation in the benefits of beta blockers based on world region remains an area of controversy. In oral pharmacologic therapy trials of HFrEF, patients from southwest Europe have a lower incidence of ischemic cardiomyopathy and those in North America tend to have more diabetes and prior coronary revascularization. There is also regional variation in medication use even after accounting for indication. In trials of ADHF, patients in Eastern Europe tend to be younger, with higher ejection fractions and lower natriuretic peptide levels. Patients from South America tend to have the lowest rates of comorbidities, revascularization, and device use. In contrast, patients from North America have the highest comorbidity burden with high revascularization and device use rates. Given geographic differences in baseline characteristics and clinical outcomes, the generalizability of therapeutic outcomes in patients in the United States and Western Europe may require verification.

281 Cardiac Transplantation and Prolonged Assisted Circulation

Sharon A. Hunt, Hari R. Mallidi

Advanced or end-stage heart failure is an increasingly frequent sequela of many types of heart disease, as progressively more effective palliation for the earlier stages of heart disease and prevention of sudden death associated with heart disease become more widely recognized and employed (Chap. 279). When patients with end-stage or refractory heart failure are identified, the physician is faced with the decision of advising compassionate end-of-life care or choosing to recommend extraordinary life-extending measures. For the occasional patient who is relatively young and without serious comorbidities, the latter may represent a reasonable option. Current therapeutic options are limited to cardiac transplantation (with the option of mechanical cardiac assistance as a "bridge" to transplantation) or permanent mechanical assistance of the circulation. In the future, it is possible that genetic modulation of ventricular function or cell-based cardiac repair will be options for such patients. Currently, both of the latter approaches are considered to be experimental.

CARDIAC TRANSPLANTATION

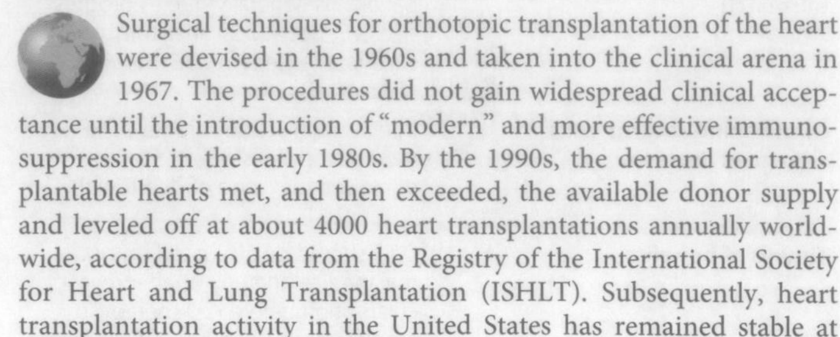

Surgical techniques for orthotopic transplantation of the heart were devised in the 1960s and taken into the clinical arena in 1967. The procedures did not gain widespread clinical acceptance until the introduction of "modern" and more effective immunosuppression in the early 1980s. By the 1990s, the demand for transplantable hearts met, and then exceeded, the available donor supply and leveled off at about 4000 heart transplantations annually worldwide, according to data from the Registry of the International Society for Heart and Lung Transplantation (ISHLT). Subsequently, heart transplantation activity in the United States has remained stable at ~2200 per year, but worldwide activity reported to this registry has decreased somewhat. This apparent decline in numbers may be a result of the fact that reporting is legally mandated in the United States but not elsewhere, and several countries have started their own databases.

SURGICAL TECHNIQUE

Donor and recipient hearts are excised in virtually identical operations with incisions made across the atria and atrial septum at the mid-atrial level (with the posterior walls of the atria left in place) and across the great vessels just above the semilunar valves. The donor heart is generally "harvested" by a separate surgical team, transported from the donor hospital in a bag of iced saline solution, and reanastomosed into the waiting recipient in the orthotopic or normal anatomic position. The only change in surgical technique since this method was first described has been a movement in recent years to move the right atrial anastomosis back to the level of the superior and inferior venae cavae to better preserve right atrial geometry and prevent atrial arrhythmias. Both methods of implantation leave the recipient with a surgically denervated heart that does not respond to any direct sympathetic or parasympathetic stimuli but does respond to circulating catecholamines. The physiologic responses of the denervated heart to the demands of exercise are atypical but quite adequate for continuation of normal physical activity.

DONOR ALLOCATION SYSTEM

In the United States, the allocation of donor organs is accomplished under the supervision of the United Network for Organ Sharing, a private organization under contract to the federal government. The United States is divided geographically into eleven regions for donor heart allocation. Allocation of donor hearts within a region is decided according to a system of priority that takes into account (1) the severity of illness, (2) the geographic distance from the donor, and (3) the patient's time on the waiting list. A physiologic limit of ~3 h of "ischemic" (out-of-body) time for hearts precludes a national sharing of hearts. This allocation system design is reissued annually and is responsive to input from a variety of constituencies, including both donor families and transplantation professionals.

At the current time, the highest priority according to severity of illness is assigned to patients requiring hospitalization at the transplantation center for IV inotropic support, with a pulmonary artery catheter in place for hemodynamic monitoring, or to patients requiring mechanical circulatory support—i.e., use of an intra-aortic balloon pump or a right or left ventricular assist device (RVAD, LVAD), extracorporeal membrane oxygenation, or mechanical ventilation. The second highest priority is given to patients requiring ongoing inotropic support, but without a pulmonary artery catheter in place. All other patients are assigned a priority according to time accrued on the waiting list, and matching generally is based only on compatibility in terms of ABO blood group and gross body size.

While HLA matching of donor and recipient would be ideal, the relatively small numbers of patients as well as the time constraints involved make such matching impractical. However, some patients who are "presensitized" and have preexisting antibodies to human leukocyte antigens (HLAs) undergo prospective cross-matching with the

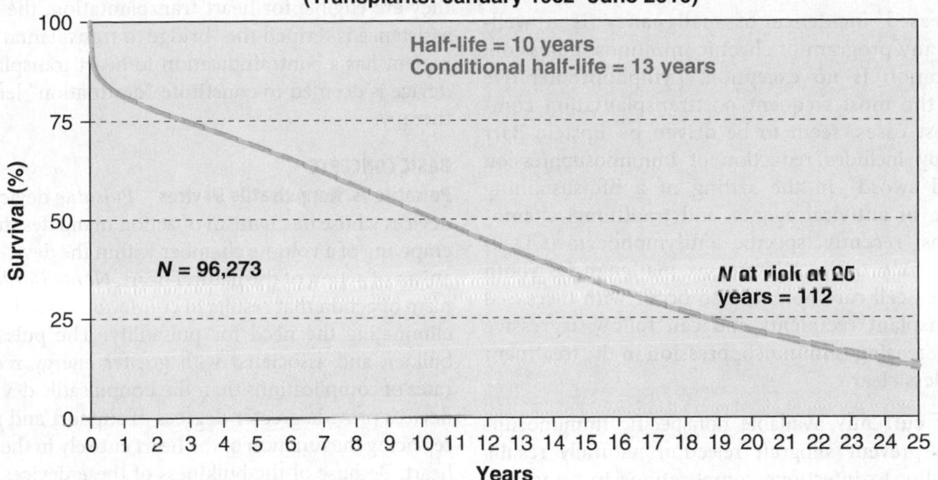

FIGURE 281-1 Global survival rates after heart transplantation since 1982. Rates were calculated by the Kaplan-Meier method, which incorporates information from all transplant recipients for whom any follow-up has been provided. Because many patients are still alive and some patients have been lost to follow-up, the survival rates are estimates rather than exact figures because the time of death is not known for all patients. Therefore, 95% confidence limits are provided. *(From J Stehlik et al: J Heart Lung Transplant 31:1052, 2012.)*

donor; these patients are commonly multiparous women or patients who have received multiple transfusions.

INDICATIONS/CONTRAINDICATIONS

Heart failure is an increasingly common cause of death, particularly in the elderly. Most patients who reach what has recently been categorized as stage D, or refractory end-stage heart failure, are appropriately treated with compassionate end-of-life care. A subset of such patients who are younger and without significant comorbidities can be considered as candidates for heart transplantation. Exact criteria vary in different centers but generally take into consideration the patient's physiologic age and the existence of comorbidities such as peripheral or cerebrovascular disease, obesity, diabetes, cancer, or chronic infection.

RESULTS

A registry organized by the ISHLT has tracked worldwide and U.S. survival rates after heart transplantation since 1982. The most recent update reveals survival rates of 83% and 76% 1 and 3 years after transplantation, respectively, or a posttransplantation "half-life" of 10.00 years (Fig. 281-1). The quality of life of survivors is generally excellent, with well over 90% of patients in the registry returning to normal and unrestricted function after transplantation.

IMMUNOSUPPRESSION

Medical regimens employed to suppress the normal immune response to a solid organ allograft vary from center to center and are in a constant state of evolution, as more effective agents with improved side-effect profiles and less toxicity are introduced. All currently used regimens are nonspecific, providing general hyporeactivity to foreign antigens rather than donor-specific hyporeactivity and also causing the attendant, and unwanted, susceptibility to infections and malignancy. Most cardiac transplantation programs currently use a three-drug regimen that includes a calcineurin inhibitor (cyclosporine or tacrolimus), an inhibitor of T cell proliferation or differentiation (azathioprine, mycophenolate mofetil, or sirolimus), and at least a short initial course of glucocorticoids. Many programs also include an initial "induction" course of polyclonal or monoclonal antibodies to T cells in the perioperative period to decrease the frequency or severity of early posttransplantation rejection. Most recently introduced have been monoclonal antibodies (daclizumab and basiliximab) that block the interleukin 2 receptor and may prevent allograft rejection without additional global immunosuppression.

Cardiac allograft rejection is usually diagnosed by endomyocardial biopsy conducted either on a surveillance basis or in response to clinical deterioration. Biopsy surveillance is performed on a regular basis in most programs for the first year postoperatively (or the first 5 years in many programs). Therapy consists of augmentation of immunosuppression, the intensity and duration of which are dictated by the severity of rejection.

LATE POSTTRANSPLANTATION MANAGEMENT ISSUES

Increasing numbers of heart transplant recipients are surviving for years following transplantation and constitute a population of patients with a number of long-term management issues.

Allograft Coronary Artery Disease Despite usually having young donor hearts, cardiac allograft recipients are prone to develop coronary artery disease (CAD). This CAD is generally a diffuse, concentric, and longitudinal process that is quite different from "ordinary" atherosclerotic CAD, which is more focal and often eccentric. The underlying etiology most likely is primarily immunologic injury of the vascular endothelium, but a variety of risk factors influence the existence and progression of CAD, including nonimmunologic factors such as dyslipidemia, diabetes mellitus, and cytomegalovirus (CMV) infection. It is hoped that newer and improved immunosuppressive modalities will reduce the incidence and impact of these devastating complications, which currently account for the majority of late posttransplantation deaths. Thus far, the immunosuppressive agents mycophenolate mofetil and the mammalian target of the rapamycin (mTOR) inhibitors sirolimus and everolimus have been shown to be associated with short-term lower incidence and extent of coronary intimal thickening; in anecdotal reports, institution of sirolimus was associated with some reversal of CAD. The use of statins also is associated with a reduced incidence of this vasculopathy, and these drugs are now used almost universally in transplant recipients unless contraindicated. Palliation of CAD with percutaneous interventions is probably safe and effective in the short term, although the disease often advances relentlessly. Because of the denervated status of the organ, patients rarely experience angina pectoris, even in advanced stages of disease.

Retransplantation is the only definitive form of therapy for advanced allograft CAD. However, the scarcity of donor hearts makes the decision to pursue retransplantation in an individual patient difficult and ethically complex.

Malignancy An increased incidence of malignancy is a well-recognized sequela of any program of chronic immunosuppression, and organ transplantation is no exception. Lymphoproliferative disorders are among the most frequent posttransplantation complications and, in most cases, seem to be driven by Epstein-Barr virus. Effective therapy includes reduction of immunosuppression (a clear "double-edged sword" in the setting of a life-sustaining organ), administration of antiviral agents, and traditional chemo- and radiotherapy. Most recently, specific antilymphocyte (CD20) therapy has shown great promise. Cutaneous malignancies (both basal cell and squamous cell carcinomas) also occur with increased frequency among transplant recipients and can follow aggressive courses. The role of decreasing immunosuppression in the treatment of these cancers is far less clear.

Infections The use of currently available nonspecific immunosuppressive modalities to prevent allograft rejection naturally results in increased susceptibility to infectious complications in transplant recipients. Although the incidence has decreased since the introduction of cyclosporine, infections with unusual and opportunistic organisms are still the major cause of death during the first postoperative year and remain a threat to the chronically immunosuppressed patient throughout life. Effective therapy depends on careful surveillance for early signs and symptoms of opportunistic infection, an extremely aggressive approach to obtaining a specific diagnosis, and expertise in recognizing the more common clinical presentations of infections caused by CMV, *Aspergillus*, and other opportunistic agents.

PROLONGED ASSISTED CIRCULATION

The modern era of mechanical circulatory support can be traced back to 1953, when cardiopulmonary bypass was first used in a clinical setting and ushered in the possibility of brief periods of circulatory support to permit open-heart surgery. Subsequently, a variety of extracorporeal pumps to provide circulatory support for brief periods have been developed. The use of a mechanical device to support the circulation for more than a few hours initially progressed slowly, with the implantation of a total artificial heart in 1969 in Texas by Cooley. This patient survived for 60 h until a donor organ became available, at which point he underwent transplantation. Unfortunately, the patient died of pulmonary complications after transplantation. The entire field of mechanical replacement of the heart then took a decade-long hiatus until the 1980s, when total artificial hearts were reintroduced with much publicity; however, they failed to produce the hoped-for treatment of end-stage heart disease. Starting in the 1970s, in parallel with the development of the total artificial heart, intense research had addressed the development of ventricular assist devices, which provide mechanical assistance for (rather than replacing) the failing ventricle.

Although conceived of initially as alternatives to biologic replacement of the heart, LVADs were introduced—and are still employed primarily—as temporary "bridges" to heart transplantation in candidates in whom medical therapy begins to fail before a donor heart becomes available. Several devices are approved by the U.S. Food and Drug Administration (FDA) and are in widespread use (see later). Those that are implantable within the body are compatible with hospital discharge and offer the patient a chance for life at home during a wait for a donor heart. However successful such "bridging" is for the individual patient, it does nothing to alleviate the scarcity of donor hearts; the ultimate goal in the field remains that of providing a reasonable alternative to biologic replacement of the heart—one that is widely and easily available and cost-effective.

CURRENT INDICATIONS AND APPLICATIONS OF VENTRICULAR ASSIST DEVICES

Currently, there are two major indications for ventricular assistance. First, patients at risk of imminent death from cardiogenic shock are eligible for mechanical support. These patients are generally managed with temporary cardiac assist devices. Second, if patients have a left ventricular ejection fraction <25% or a peak VO_2 <14 mL/kg per min or are dependent on inotropic therapy or support with intra-aortic balloon counterpulsation, they may be eligible for mechanical support. If they are eligible for heart transplantation, the mechanical circulatory assistance is termed the "bridge to transplantation." By contrast, if the patient has a contraindication to heart transplantation, the use of the device is deemed to constitute "destination" left ventricular assistance therapy.

BASIC CONCEPTS

Pulsatile vs. Nonpulsatile Devices *Pulsatile* devices are ventricular assist devices whose mechanism of action mandates the alternating filling and emptying of a volume chamber within the device that mimics the mechanism of action of the natural heart. *Nonpulsatile* devices have a mechanism of action that results in continuous blood flow through the device, eliminating the need for pulsatility. The pulsatile devices are larger, bulkier, and associated with greater energy requirements and higher rates of complications than the nonpulsatile devices. However, pulsatile devices provide greater degrees of support and may even be capable of replacing the function of the heart entirely in the form of a total artificial heart. Because of the bulkiness of these devices, many patients are too small to be supported with intracorporeal pulsatile pumps. However, paracorporeal versions are available. These devices are versatile and can be used for right, left, or biventricular assistance/replacement.

Continuous-flow (nonpulsatile) devices are further categorized on the basis of impeller design and mechanism. The older designs have tended to be axial-flow pumps, which operate on the Archimedes screw principle. These devices have an impeller that is in line with the direction of blood flow, and the inlet direction of blood is the same as the outlet direction. Continuous-flow devices have been dependent on the presence of blood-washed bearings within the pump housing and may be associated with an increased risk of blood and platelet activation. The newer devices are centrifugal in design; the blood flow takes a 90° turn between the inlet section of the pump and the outlet section. Another major difference in the newer devices is the absence of blood-washed bearings (with most devices having magnetically levitated impellers). This design allows the construction of smaller pumps with less blood-element activation than the axial-flow designs.

Available Devices In the United States, there are currently four FDA-approved devices that are used as bridges to transplantation in adults. Of these four devices, one is also approved for use as destination therapy or as long-term mechanical support of the heart. A number of other devices are approved only for short-term support in post–cardiac surgery shock or in cardiogenic shock secondary to acute myocardial infarction or fulminant myocarditis; these will not be considered here. So far, no long-term device is totally implantable, and, because of the need for transcutaneous connections, all share a common problem with infectious complications. Likewise, all share some tendency to thromboembolic complications and are subject to the possibility of mechanical failure common to any machine.

The total artificial heart (TAH) (Syncardia, Tucson, AZ) is a pneumatic, biventricular, orthotopically implanted ventricular assist device with an externalized driveline connecting it to its console. The TAH is currently the only FDA-approved device for use in patients who have severe biventricular failure.

The Thoratec LVAD (Thoratec Corp., Pleasanton, CA) is an extracorporeal pump that takes blood from a large cannula placed in the left ventricular apex and propels it forward through an outflow cannula inserted into the ascending aorta. The extracorporeal nature of this pump allows its use in small adults for whom intracorporeal pumps would be too large. This device provides not only left but also right ventricular assistance and can be utilized for biventricular support within the same patient (BiVentricular Assist Device).

The HeartMate II LVAD (Thoratec) similarly uses a drainage cannula in the left ventricular apex to drain blood into a small chamber, where the blood is driven by an electrically powered motor that spins a rotor, accelerating blood outflow into the ascending aorta (Fig. 281-2). This device is currently the only FDA-approved axial-flow pump that can be used both as a bridge to transplantation and as destination therapy.

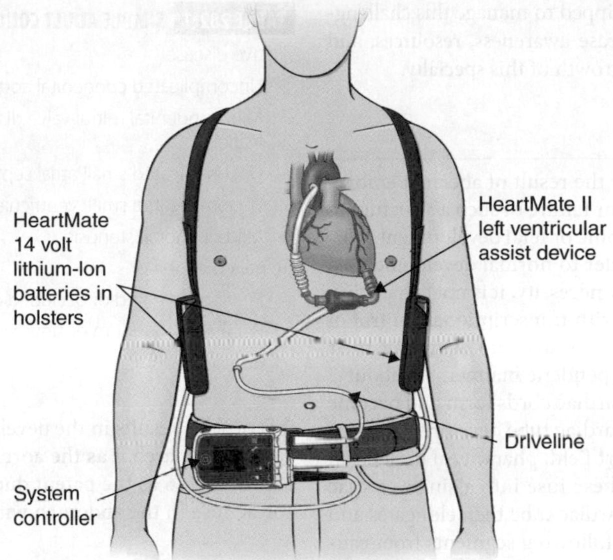

FIGURE 281-2 Diagram of HeartMate II left ventricular assist device (LVAD). *(Reprinted with permission from Thoratec Corp., Pleasanton, CA.)*

The HeartWare Ventricular Assist System with the HVAD pump (HeartWare Inc., Framingham, MA) is the first third-generation device to be granted FDA approval for use in patients as a bridge to transplantation. The device is a centrifugal pump that is housed completely within the patient's pericardial cavity and provides adequate support for many patients.

RESULTS

The use of these devices in the United States is limited mainly to patients with post–cardiac surgery shock and to those who are bridged to transplantation. The results of bridging to transplantation with the available devices are quite good, with nearly 75% of younger patients receiving a transplant by 1 year and having excellent posttransplantation survival rates.

Publication of the REMATCH (Randomized Evaluation of Mechanical Assistance in the Treatment of Heart Failure) trial in 2001 documented a somewhat improved survival rate in patients who had end-stage heart disease, were not candidates for transplantation, and were randomized to a pulsatile LVAD (albeit with a high rate of complications, especially neurologic issues) as opposed to continued medical therapy. This result led to renewed interest in use of the devices for nonbiologic permanent replacement of heart function as well. Subsequently, this device was supplanted by the HeartMate II axial-flow device, which has dramatically improved the survival of patients with severe end-stage heart disease in whom medical therapy has failed. The patients who had this device implanted had a 2-year survival rate of 58%, whereas the survival rate for patients in the medically treated arm of the original REMATCH trial was only 8%. More recent experience has shown that the mean survival period of patients with a continuous-flow LVAD for destination therapy is approaching 5 years.

Several studies have evaluated the benefit of LVAD therapy as a bridge to transplantation. The most recent data come from a series of 140 patients who underwent implantation of a HeartWare HVAD. Of these patients, 94% achieved the principal outcome (defined as survival to transplantation, recovery of heart function, or ongoing device support) at 180 days. With increased experience and improved outcomes using LVADs as a bridge to transplantation, the ability to maintain end-organ function and limit the progression of pulmonary hypertension—or even to decrease pulmonary vascular resistance—makes mechanical unloading a more attractive option than continued inotropic support. The early bridge-to-transplantation experience demonstrated reduced posttransplantation survival compared with medical management; however, more recent experience has shown equivalent outcomes following transplantation. This result is likely secondary to a trend toward earlier device implantation—i.e., prior to the onset of irreversible end-organ damage.

282 Congenital Heart Disease in the Adult

Jamil A. Aboulhosn, John S. Child

Over a hundred years ago, Sir William Osler, in his classic textbook *The Principles and Practice of Medicine* (New York, Appleton & Co, 1892, pp 659–663), devoted only five pages to "Congenital Affections of the Heart," with the first sentence declaring that "[t]hese [disorders] have only limited clinical interest, as in a large proportion of cases the anomaly is not compatible with life, and in others nothing can be done to remedy the defect or even to relieve symptoms." Fortunately, in the intervening century, considerable progress has been made in understanding the basis for these disorders and their effective treatment.

The most common birth defects are cardiovascular in origin. These malformations are due to complex multifactorial genetic and environmental causes. Recognized chromosomal aberrations and mutations of single genes account for <10% of all cardiac malformations. Congenital heart disease (CHD) complicates ~1% of all live births in the general population—about 40,000 births/year—but occurs more frequently in the offspring (about 4–10%, depending on maternal CHD type) of women with CHD. Owing to the remarkable surgical advances over the last 60 years, >90% of afflicted neonates and children now reach adulthood; women with CHD may now frequently successfully bear children after competent repairs. As such, the population with CHD is steadily increasing. Women with CHD are at increased risk for peri- and postpartum complications, but maternal CHD is generally not considered an absolute contraindication to pregnancy unless the mother has certain high-risk features (e.g., cyanosis, pulmonary hypertension, decompensated heart failure, arrhythmias, aortic aneurysm, among others). Consultation with an adult CHD expert is warranted for all females with CHD who desire to become pregnant.

Nearly one and a half million adults with operated or unoperated CHD live in the United States today; there are now more adults than children with CHD in the United States. Because true surgical cures are rare, and all repairs—be they palliative or corrective—may leave residua, sequelae, or complications, most require some degree of lifetime expert surveillance. The anatomic and physiologic changes in the heart and circulation due to any specific CHD lesion are not static but, rather, progress from prenatal life to adulthood. Malformations that are benign or escape detection in childhood may become clinically significant in the adult. Unfortunately, the growing number of adults with CHD has not been paralleled by an adequate increase in the number of specialists and specialty centers that are trained and equipped to manage this challenging population. Ongoing efforts to increase awareness, resources, and advocacy are essential for the necessary growth of this specialty.

CARDIAC DEVELOPMENT

(See also Chap. 265e) CHD is generally the result of aberrant embryonic development of a normal structure or failure of such a structure to progress beyond an early stage of embryonic or fetal development. This brief section serves to introduce the reader to normal development so that defects may be better understood; by necessity, it is not exhaustive. Cardiogenesis is a finely tuned process with transcriptional control of a complex group of regulatory proteins that activate or inhibit their gene targets in a location- and time-dependent manner. At about 3 weeks of embryonic development, two cardiac cords form and become canalized; at that point, the primordial cardiac tube develops from two sources (cardiac crescent or the first heart field, pharyngeal mesoderm or the second heart field); by 21 days, these fuse into a single cardiac tube beginning at the cranial end. The cardiac tube then elongates and develops discrete constrictions with the following segments from caudal to cranial location: sinus venosus receives the umbilical, vitelline, and common cardinal veins: atrium, ventricle, bulbus cordis, truncus arteriosus, aortic sac, and the aortic arches. The cardiac tube is fixed at the sinus venosus and arterial ends.

Subsequently, in the next few weeks, differential growth of cells causes the tube to elongate and loop as an "S" with the bulboventricular portion moving rightward and the atrium and sinus venosus moving posterior to the ventricle. The primitive atrium and ventricle communicate via the atrioventricular canal from which the endocardial cushion develops into two parts (ventrally and dorsally). The cushions fuse and divide the atrioventricular canal into two atrioventricular inlets and also migrate to help form the ventricular septum. The primitive atrium is divided first by a septum primum membrane, which grows down from the superior wall to the cushions; as this fusion occurs, the mid-portion resorbs in the center forming the ostium secundum. Rightward of the septum primum, a second septum secundum membrane grows down from the ventral-cranial wall toward—but not reaching—the cushions, and covering most, but not all, of the ostium secundum, resulting in a flap of the foramen ovale. The primitive ventricle is partitioned by a finely tuned set of events. The interventricular septum grows up toward the cushions, and the cushions form an upper inlet septum; between the two portions is a hole called the interventricular foramen. The left and right ventricles begin to develop side by side, and the atria and their respective inlet valves align over their ventricles. Finally, these two parts of the septum fuse with the bulboventricular ridges, which, once having septated the truncus arteriosus, extend into the ventricle. The bulbocordis divides into a subaortic portion as the muscular conus resorbs, whereas the subpulmonary section has elongation of its muscular conus. Spiral division of the common truncus arteriosus rotates and aligns the pulmonary artery and aortic portions over their respective outflow tracts, the aortic valve moving posterior over the left ventricle (LV) outflow tract and the pulmonary valve moving anterior over the right ventricle (RV) outflow tract, with a wraparound relationship of the two great arteries.

Early on, the venous systems are bilateral and symmetric and enter two horns of the sinus venosus. Ultimately, except for the coronary sinus, most of the left-sided portions and the left sinus–venosus horn regress, and the systemic venous system empties into the right horn via the inferior and superior vena cavae. The pulmonary venous system, initially connecting to the systemic venous system, develops as buds from the developing lungs, which fuse together in the pulmonary venous confluence, at which point the connection to the systemic system regresses. Simultaneously, a projection from the back wall of the left atrium (the common pulmonary vein) grows posteriorly to merge with the confluence, which then becomes a part of the posterior left atrial wall.

The truncus arteriosus and aortic sac initially develop six paired symmetric arches, which curve posteriorly and become the paired dorsal aortae. The detailed description of the selective regression of some of the arches is not presented in this chapter. In brief summary, this process results in the development of arch 3 as the internal carotid arteries, left arch 4 as the aortic arch and right subclavian artery, and part of arch 6 as the patent ductus arteriosus. The two dorsal thoracic aortae fuse in the abdomen with persistence of the left dorsal aorta.

TABLE 282-1 SIMPLE ADULT CONGENITAL HEART DISEASE

Native disease
Uncomplicated congenital aortic valve disease
Mild congenital mitral valve disease (e.g., except parachute valve, cleft leaflet)
Uncomplicated small atrial septal defect
Uncomplicated small ventricular septal defect
Mild pulmonic stenosis
Repaired conditions
Previously ligated or occluded ductus arteriosus
Repaired secundum or sinus venosus atrial septal defect without residua
Repaired ventricular septal defect without residua

SPECIFIC CARDIAC DEFECTS

Tables 282-1, 282-2, and 282-3 list CHD malformations as simple, intermediate, or complex. Simple defects generally are single lesions with a shunt or a valvular malformation. Intermediate defects may have two or more simple defects. Complex defects generally have components of an intermediate defect plus more complex cardiac and vascular anatomy, often with cyanosis, and frequently with transposition complexes. The goal of these tables is to suggest when cardiology consultation or advanced CHD specialty care is needed. Patients with complex CHD (which includes most "named" surgeries that usually involve complex CHD) should virtually always be managed in conjunction with an experienced specialty adult CHD center. Patients with intermediate lesions should have an initial consultation and subsequent occasional intermittent follow-up with an adult CHD specialist. Patients with simple lesions often may be managed by a well-informed internist or general cardiologist, although consultation with a specifically trained adult congenital cardiologist is occasionally advisable.

ATRIAL SEPTAL DEFECT

Atrial septal defect (ASD) is a common cardiac anomaly that may be first encountered in the adult and occurs more frequently in females. Sinus venosus ASD occurs high in the atrial septum near the entry of the superior vena cava into the right atrium and is associated frequently with anomalous pulmonary venous connection from the right lung to the superior vena cava or right atrium (Fig. 282-1). Ostium primum ASDs lie adjacent to the atrioventricular valves, either of which may be deformed and regurgitant. Ostium primum ASDs are common in Down's syndrome, often as part of complex atrioventricular septal defects with a common atrioventricular valve and a posterior defect of the basal portion of the interventricular septum. The most common ostium secundum ASD involves the fossa ovalis and is midseptal in location; this should not be confused with a patent foramen

TABLE 282-2 INTERMEDIATE COMPLEXITY CONGENITAL HEART DISEASE

Ostium primum or sinus venosus atrial septal defect
Anomalous pulmonary venous drainage, partial or total
Atrioventricular canal defects (partial or complete)
Ventricular septal defect, complicated (e.g., absent or abnormal valves or with associated obstructive lesions, aortic regurgitation)
Coarctation of the aorta
Pulmonic valve stenosis (moderate to severe)
Infundibular right ventricular outflow obstruction of significance
Pulmonary valve regurgitation (moderate to severe)
Patent ductus arteriosus (nonclosed)—moderate to large
Sinus of Valsalva fistula/aneurysm
Subvalvular or supravalvular aortic stenosis

TABLE 282-3 COMPLEX ADULT CONGENITAL HEART DISEASE

Cyanotic congenital heart diseases (all forms)
Eisenmenger's syndrome
Ebstein's anomaly
Tetralogy of Fallot or pulmonary atresia (all forms)
Transposition of the great arteries
Single ventricle; tricuspid or mitral atresia
Double-outlet ventricle
Truncus arteriosus
Fontan or Rastelli procedures

ovale. Anatomic obliteration of the foramen ovale ordinarily follows its functional closure soon after birth, but residual "probe patency" is a common normal variant; ASD denotes a true deficiency of the atrial septum and implies functional and anatomic patency. The magnitude of the left-to-right shunt depends on the ASD size, ventricular diastolic properties, and the relative impedance in the pulmonary and systemic circulations. The left-to-right shunt causes diastolic overloading of the RV and increased pulmonary blood flow. Patients with ASD are usually asymptomatic in early life, although there may be some physical underdevelopment and an increased tendency for respiratory infections; cardiorespiratory symptoms occur in many older patients. Beyond the fourth decade, a significant number of patients develop atrial arrhythmias, pulmonary arterial hypertension, and right heart failure. Patients exposed to the chronic environmental hypoxemia of high altitude tend to develop pulmonary hypertension at younger ages. In older patients, left-to-right shunting across the ASD increases as progressive systemic hypertension and/or coronary artery disease (CAD) result in reduced compliance of the LV.

Physical Examination Examination usually reveals a prominent RV impulse and palpable pulmonary artery pulsation. The first heart sound is normal or split, with accentuation of the tricuspid valve closure sound. Increased flow across the pulmonic valve is responsible for a midsystolic pulmonary outflow murmur. The second heart sound is widely split and is fixed in relation to respiration. A mid-diastolic rumbling murmur, loudest at the fourth intercostal space and along the left sternal border, reflects increased flow across the tricuspid valve. In ostium primum ASD, an apical holosystolic murmur indicates associated mitral or tricuspid regurgitation or a ventricular septal defect (VSD).

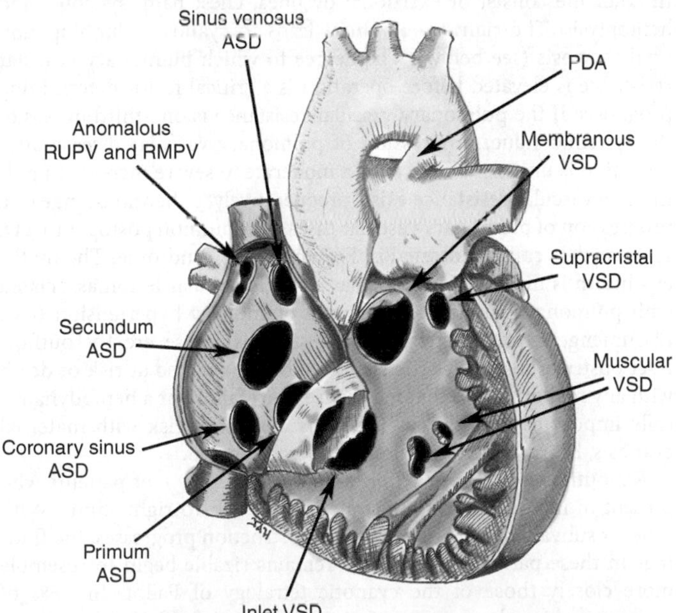

FIGURE 282-1 Types and locations of congenital cardiac defects. ASD, atrial septal defect; PDA, patent ductus arteriosus; RMPV, right middle pulmonary vein; RUPV, right upper pulmonary vein; VSD, ventricular septal defect.

These findings are altered when increased pulmonary vascular resistance causes diminution of the left-to-right shunt. Both the pulmonary outflow and tricuspid inflow murmurs decrease in intensity, the pulmonic component of the second heart sound and a systolic ejection sound are accentuated, the two components of the second heart sound may fuse, and a diastolic murmur of pulmonic regurgitation appears. Cyanosis and clubbing accompany the development of a right-to-left shunt (see "Ventricular Septal Defect" later in this chapter). In adults with an ASD and atrial fibrillation, the physical findings may be confused with mitral stenosis with pulmonary hypertension because the tricuspid diastolic flow murmur and widely split second heart sound may be mistakenly thought to represent the diastolic murmur of mitral stenosis and the mitral "opening snap," respectively.

Electrocardiogram In ostium secundum ASD, electrocardiogram (ECG) usually shows right-axis deviation and an rSr′ pattern in the right precordial leads representing enlargement of the RV outflow tract. An ectopic atrial pacemaker or first-degree heart block may occur with the sinus venous ASD. In ostium primum ASD, the RV conduction defect is accompanied by left superior axis deviation and counterclockwise rotation of the frontal plane QRS loop. Varying degrees of RV and right atrial (RA) enlargement or hypertrophy may occur with each type of defect, depending on the presence and degree of pulmonary hypertension. Chest x-ray shows an enlarged RA and RV, and pulmonary artery and its branches; increased pulmonary vascular markings of left-to-right shunt vascularity will diminish if pulmonary vascular disease develops.

Echocardiogram Echocardiography reveals pulmonary arterial and RV and RA dilatation with abnormal (paradoxical) ventricular septal motion in the presence of a significant right heart volume overload. The ASD may be visualized directly by two-dimensional imaging, color-flow imaging, or echocontrast. Echocardiography and Doppler examination have supplanted cardiac catheterization. Transesophageal echocardiography is indicated if the transthoracic echocardiogram is ambiguous, which is often the case with sinus venosus defects, or for guiding catheter device closure (Fig. 282-2). Cardiac catheterization is performed if inconsistencies exist in the clinical data, if significant pulmonary hypertension or associated malformations are suspected, if CAD is a possibility, or when attempting transcatheter closure of the ASD.

TREATMENT ATRIAL SEPTAL DEFECT

Operative repair, usually with a patch of pericardium or of prosthetic material or percutaneous transcatheter device closure, if the ASD is of an appropriate size and shape, should be advised for all patients with uncomplicated secundum ASD with significant left-to-right shunting, i.e., pulmonary-to-systemic flow ratios ≥1.5:1. Excellent results may be anticipated, at low risk, even in patients >40 years, in the absence of severe pulmonary hypertension. In ostium primum ASD, cleft mitral valves may require repair in addition to patch closure of the ASD. Closure is not usually carried out in patients with small defects and trivial left-to-right shunts or in those with severe pulmonary vascular disease without a significant left-to-right shunt. However, the use of pulmonary vasodilators with resultant reduction in pulmonary artery pressure and resistance may allow closure of ASD in patients with pulmonary vascular disease.

Patients with sinus venosus or ostium secundum ASDs rarely die before the fifth decade. During the fifth and sixth decades, the incidence of progressive symptoms, often leading to severe disability, increases substantially. Medical management should include prompt treatment of respiratory tract infections; antiarrhythmic medications for atrial fibrillation or supraventricular tachycardia; and the usual measures for hypertension, coronary disease, or heart failure (Chap. 279), if these complications occur. The risk of infective endocarditis is low, and antibiotic prophylaxis is not recommended (Chap. 155).

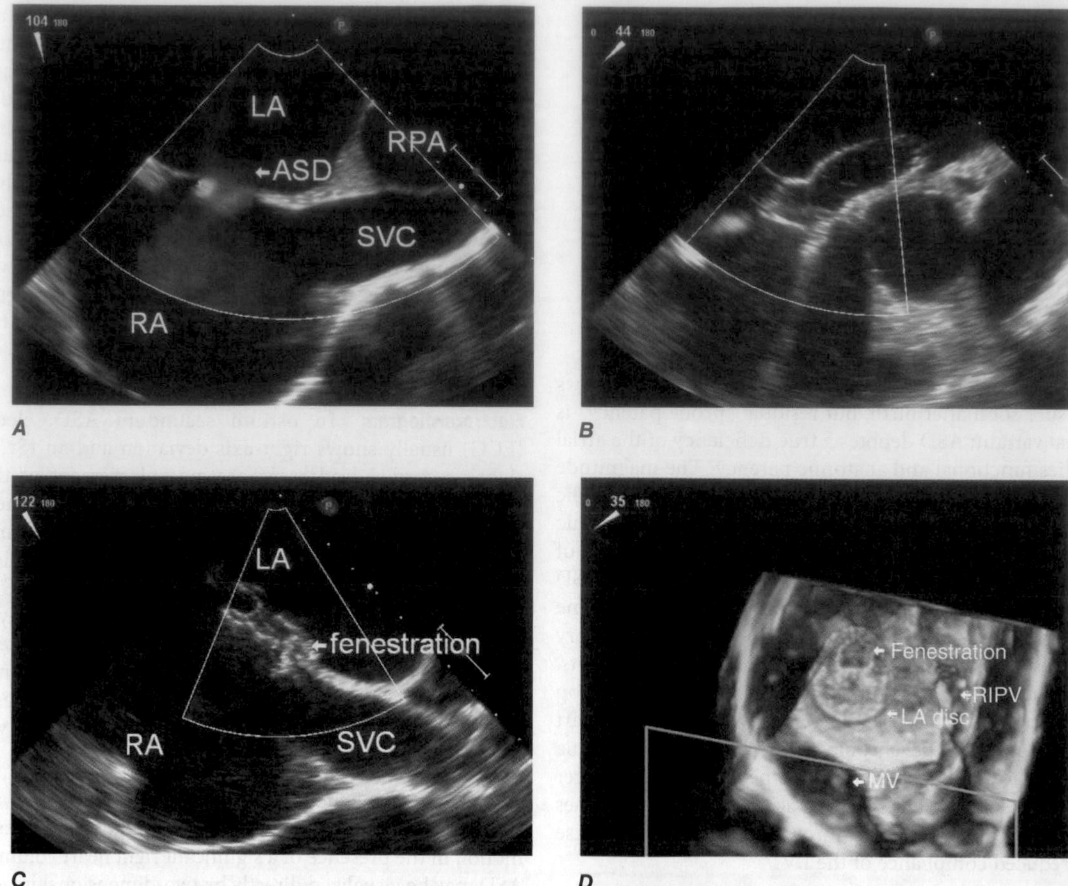

FIGURE 282-2 ***A.*** Transesophageal echocardiogram demonstrating a secundum-type atrial septal defect (ASD) with shunting from the left atrium (LA) to the right atrium (RA). The right pulmonary artery (RPA) and superior vena cava (SVC) are labeled. ***B.*** Transcatheter balloon sizing of the ASD. ***C.*** Atrial septal occluder placement with a small manually created "fenestration" within the device that continues to allow a small amount of flow from the LA to the RA; this is used as a means of preventing left atrial hypertension after ASD closure. Left atrial hypertension may occur in older patients with decreased left ventricular compliance. ***D.*** Three-dimensional image of the septal occluder en-face; note the fenestration in the LA disc. The mitral valve (MV) and right inferior pulmonary vein (RIPV) are labeled.

VENTRICULAR SEPTAL DEFECT

VSD is one of the most common of all cardiac birth defects, either as an isolated defect or as a component of a combination of anomalies (Fig. 282-1). The VSD is usually single and situated in the membranous or midmuscular portion of the septum. The functional disturbance depends on its size and on the status of the pulmonary vascular bed. Only small- or moderate-size VSDs are seen initially in adulthood, as most patients with an isolated large VSD come to medical or surgical attention early in life.

A wide spectrum exists in the natural history of VSD, ranging from spontaneous closure to congestive cardiac failure and death in infancy. Included within this spectrum is the possible development of pulmonary vascular obstruction, RV outflow tract obstruction, aortic regurgitation, or infective endocarditis. Spontaneous closure is more common in patients born with a small VSD, which occurs in early childhood in most. The pulmonary vascular bed is often a principal determinant of the clinical manifestations and course of a given VSD and feasibility of surgical repair. Increased pulmonary arterial pressure results from increased pulmonary blood flow and/or resistance, the latter usually the result of obstructive, obliterative structural changes within the pulmonary vascular bed. It is important to quantitate and compare pulmonary-to-systemic flows and resistances in patients with severe pulmonary hypertension. The term Eisenmenger's syndrome is applied to patients with a large communication between the two circulations at the aortopulmonary, ventricular, or atrial levels and bidirectional or predominantly right-to-left shunts because of high resistance and obstructive pulmonary hypertension.

Patients with large VSDs and pulmonary hypertension are at greatest risk for developing pulmonary vascular disease. Large VSDs should be corrected early in life when pulmonary vascular disease is not severely elevated. In patients with Eisenmenger's syndrome, symptoms in adult life consist of exertional dyspnea, chest pain, syncope, and hemoptysis. The right-to-left shunt leads to cyanosis, clubbing, and erythrocytosis (see below). The degree to which pulmonary vascular resistance is elevated before operation is a critical factor determining prognosis. If the pulmonary vascular resistance is one-third or less of the systemic value, progression of pulmonary vascular disease after operation is unusual; however, if a moderate to severe increase in pulmonary vascular resistance exists preoperatively, either no change or a progression of pulmonary vascular disease is common postoperatively. Pregnancy is contraindicated in Eisenmenger's syndrome. The mother's health is most at risk if she has a cardiovascular lesion associated with pulmonary vascular disease and pulmonary hypertension (e.g., Eisenmenger's physiology or mitral stenosis) or severe LV outflow tract obstruction (e.g., aortic stenosis), but she is also at risk of death with any malformation that may cause heart failure or a hemodynamically important arrhythmia. The fetus is most at risk with maternal cyanosis, heart failure, or pulmonary hypertension.

RV outflow tract obstruction develops in ~5–10% of patients who present in infancy with a moderate to large left-to-right shunt. With time, as subvalvular RV outflow tract obstruction progresses, the findings in these patients whose VSD remains sizable begin to resemble more closely those of the cyanotic tetralogy of Fallot. In ~5% of patients, aortic valve regurgitation results from insufficient cusp tissue or prolapse of the cusp through the interventricular defect; the aortic regurgitation then complicates and dominates the clinical course. Echocardiography with spectral and color Doppler examination defines the number and location of defects in the ventricular septum and associated anomalies and the hemodynamic physiology of the defect(s). Hemodynamic and angiographic study may be occasionally required to assess the status of the pulmonary vascular bed and clarify details of the altered anatomy. Cross-sectional imaging modalities such as computed tomography (CT) or magnetic resonance imaging (MRI) are useful in delineating complex anatomy and assessing extra-cardiac structures.

TREATMENT VENTRICULAR SEPTAL DEFECT

Closure is not recommended for patients with normal pulmonary arterial pressures with small shunts (pulmonary-to-systemic flow ratios of <1.5:1). Operative correction or transcatheter closure is indicated when there is a moderate to large left-to-right shunt with a pulmonary-to-systemic flow ratio >1.5:1, in the absence of prohibitively high levels of pulmonary vascular resistance (pulmonary arterial resistance is less than two-thirds of systemic arterial resistance).

In patients with Eisenmenger's VSD, pulmonary arterial vasodilators and both single- or double-lung transplantation with intracardiac defect repair or heart/lung transplantation show promise for improvement in symptoms (Chaps. 281 and 320e). Chronic hypoxemia in cyanotic CHD results in secondary erythrocytosis due to increased erythropoietin production (Chap. 49). The term polycythemia is a misnomer; white cell counts are normal, and platelet counts are normal to decreased. Compensated erythrocytosis with iron-replete equilibrium hematocrits rarely results in symptoms of hyperviscosity at hematocrits <65% and occasionally not even with hematocrits ≥70%. For this reason, therapeutic phlebotomy is rarely required in compensated erythrocytosis. In contrast, patients with decompensated erythrocytosis fail to establish equilibrium with unstable, rising hematocrits and recurrent hyperviscosity symptoms. Therapeutic phlebotomy, a two-edged sword, allows temporary relief of symptoms but limits oxygen delivery, begets instability of the hematocrit, and compounds the problem by iron depletion. Iron-deficiency symptoms are usually indistinguishable from those of hyperviscosity; progressive symptoms after recurrent phlebotomy are usually due to iron depletion with hypochromic microcytosis. Iron depletion results in a larger number of smaller (microcytic) hypochromic red cells that are less capable of carrying oxygen and less deformable in the microcirculation; with more of them relative to plasma volume, viscosity is greater than for an equivalent hematocrit with fewer, larger, iron-replete, deformable cells. As such, iron-depleted erythrocytosis results in increasing symptoms due to decreased oxygen delivery to the tissues.

Hemostasis is abnormal in cyanotic CHD, due, in part, to the increased blood volume and engorged capillaries, abnormalities in platelet function, and sensitivity to aspirin or nonsteroidal anti-inflammatory agents, as well as abnormalities of the extrinsic and intrinsic coagulation system. Oral contraceptives are often contraindicated for cyanotic women because of the enhanced risk of vascular thrombosis. Symptoms of hyperviscosity can be produced in any cyanotic patient with erythrocytosis if dehydration reduces plasma volume. Phlebotomy for symptoms of hyperviscosity not due to dehydration or iron deficiency is a simple outpatient removal of 500 mL of blood over 45 min with isovolumetric replacement with isotonic saline. Acute phlebotomy without volume replacement is contraindicated. Iron repletion in decompensated iron-depleted erythrocytosis reduces iron-deficiency symptoms, but must be done gradually to avoid an excessive rise in hematocrit and resulting hyperviscosity.

PATENT DUCTUS ARTERIOSUS

The ductus arteriosus is a vessel leading from the bifurcation of the pulmonary artery to the aorta just distal to the left subclavian artery (Fig. 282-1). Normally, the vascular channel is open in the fetus but closes immediately after birth. The flow across the ductus is determined by the pressure and resistance relationships between the systemic and pulmonary circulations and by the cross-sectional area and length of the ductus. In most adults with this anomaly, pulmonary pressures are normal, and a gradient and shunt from aorta to pulmonary artery persist throughout the cardiac cycle, resulting in a characteristic thrill and a continuous "machinery" murmur with late systolic accentuation at the upper left sternal edge. In adults who were born with a large left-to-right shunt through the ductus arteriosus, pulmonary vascular obstruction (Eisenmenger's syndrome) with pulmonary hypertension, right-to-left shunting, and cyanosis have usually developed. Severe pulmonary vascular disease results in reversal of flow through the ductus; unoxygenated blood is shunted to the descending aorta; and the toes—but not the fingers—become cyanotic and clubbed, a finding termed differential cyanosis (Fig. 282-3). The leading causes of death in adults with patent ductus arteriosus are cardiac failure and infective endocarditis; occasionally, severe pulmonary vascular obstruction may cause aneurysmal dilatation, calcification, and rupture of the ductus.

TREATMENT PATENT DUCTUS ARTERIOSUS

In the absence of severe pulmonary vascular disease and predominant left-to-right shunting of blood, the patent ductus should be surgically ligated or divided. Transcatheter closure has become common for appropriately shaped defects. Operation should be deferred for several months in patients treated successfully for infective endocarditis because the ductus may remain somewhat edematous and friable.

AORTIC ROOT–TO–RIGHT-HEART SHUNTS

The three most common causes of aortic root to right-heart shunts are congenital aneurysm of an aortic sinus of Valsalva with fistula, coronary arteriovenous fistula, and anomalous origin of the left coronary artery from the pulmonary trunk. Aneurysm of an aortic sinus of Valsalva consists of a separation or lack of fusion between the media of the aorta and the annulus of the aortic valve. Rupture usually occurs in the third or fourth decade of life; most often, the aorticocardiac fistula is between the right coronary cusp and the RV; but occasionally, when the noncoronary cusp is involved, the fistula drains into the RA. Abrupt rupture causes chest pain, bounding pulses, a continuous murmur accentuated in diastole, and volume overload of the heart. Diagnosis is confirmed by two-dimensional and Doppler echocardiographic studies; cardiac catheterization quantitates the left-to-right shunt, and thoracic aortography visualizes the fistula. Medical management is directed at cardiac failure, arrhythmias, or endocarditis. At operation, the aneurysm is closed and amputated, and the aortic wall is reunited with the heart, either by direct suture or with a patch or prosthesis. Transcatheter device closure is a less invasive and effective alternative to surgery.

Coronary arteriovenous fistula, an unusual anomaly, consists of a communication between a coronary artery and another cardiac chamber, usually the coronary sinus, RA, or RV. The shunt is usually of small magnitude, and myocardial blood flow is not usually compromised; if the shunt is large, there may be a coronary "steal" syndrome with myocardial ischemia and possible angina or ventricular arrhythmias. Potential complications include infective endocarditis; thrombus formation with occlusion or distal embolization with myocardial infarction; rupture of an aneurysmal fistula; and, rarely, pulmonary hypertension and congestive failure. A loud, superficial, continuous murmur at the lower or midsternal border usually prompts a further evaluation of asymptomatic patients. Doppler echocardiography demonstrates the site of drainage; if the site of origin is proximal, it may be detectable by two-dimensional echocardiography. Angiography (classic catheterization, CT, or magnetic resonance angiography) permits identification of the size and anatomic features of the fistulous tract, which may be closed by suture or transcatheter obliteration.

The third anomaly causing a shunt from the aortic root to the right heart is anomalous origin of the left coronary artery from the pulmonary artery. In this condition, oxygenated blood from the aortic root flows via a dilated right coronary artery and collaterals to the left coronary artery and retrograde to the lower pressure pulmonary artery circulation via the anomalous left main coronary artery (which emerges from the pulmonary artery). Myocardial infarction and

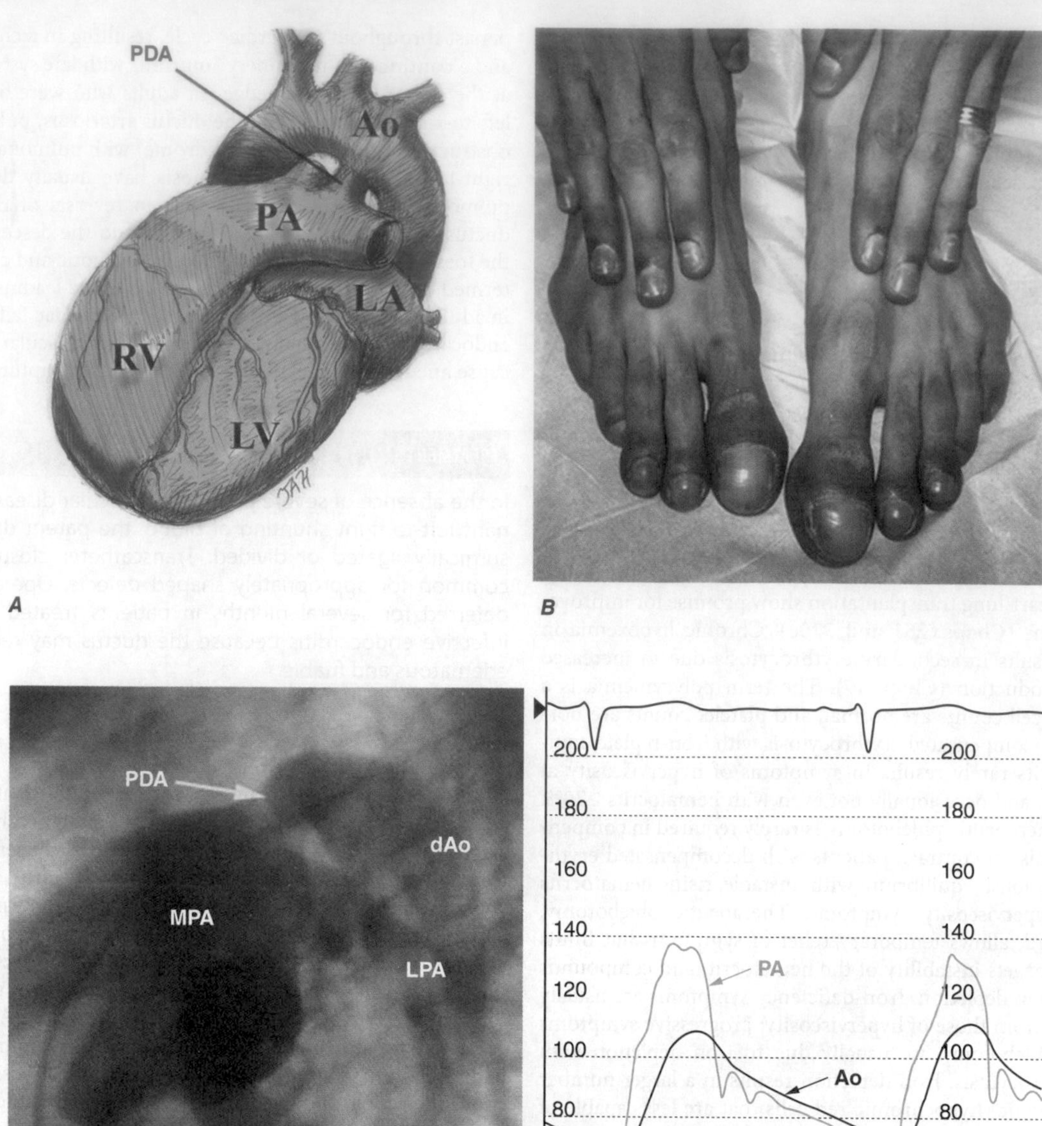

FIGURE 282-3 *A.* Patent ductus arteriosus (PDA) in a patient with severe pulmonary hypertension (Eisenmenger's syndrome). Due to the suprasystemic pulmonary arterial resistance, deoxygenated (cyanotic) blood from the right ventricle (RV) and pulmonary artery (PA) is shunted across the PDA to the aorta (Ao). The left atrium (LA) and left ventricle (LV) are labeled. *B.* Differential clubbing and cyanosis of the toes due to lower extremity perfusion by the deoxygenated blood crossing the PDA. *C.* Angiogram in a dilated main pulmonary artery (MPA) with shunting noted across the PDA to the descending aorta (dAo). The left pulmonary artery (LPA) is labeled. *D.* Direct pressure recordings in the Ao and PA demonstrating suprasystemic PA systolic pressure.

fibrosis commonly lead to death within the first year, although up to 20% of patients survive to adolescence and beyond without surgical correction. The diagnosis is supported by the ECG findings of an anterolateral myocardial infarction and left ventricular hypertrophy (LVH). Operative management of adults consists of coronary artery reimplantation, coronary artery bypass with an internal mammary artery graft, or saphenous vein–coronary artery graft.

CONGENITAL AORTIC STENOSIS

Malformations that cause obstruction to LV outflow include congenital valvular aortic stenosis, discrete subaortic stenosis, or supravalvular aortic stenosis. Bicuspid aortic valves are more common in males than in females. The congenital bicuspid aortic valve, which may initially be functionally normal, is one of the most common congenital malformations of the heart and may go undetected in early life. Because bicuspid valves may develop stenosis or regurgitation with time or be the site of infective endocarditis, the lesion may be difficult to distinguish in older adults from acquired rheumatic or degenerative calcific aortic valve disease. The dynamics of blood flow associated with a congenitally deformed, rigid aortic valve commonly lead to thickening of the cusps and, in later life, to calcification. Hemodynamically significant obstruction causes concentric hypertrophy of the LV wall. The ascending aorta is often dilated, misnamed "poststenotic" dilatation; this is due to histologic abnormalities of the aortic media and may result in aortic dissection. Diagnosis is made by echocardiography, which reveals the morphology of the aortic valve and aortic root and quantitates severity of stenosis or regurgitation. **The clinical manifestations and hemodynamic abnormalities are discussed in Chap. 283.**

TREATMENT VALVULAR AORTIC STENOSIS

In patients with diminished cardiac reserve, medical management includes the administration of digoxin and diuretics and sodium restriction while awaiting operation. A dilated aortic root may require beta blockers, angiotensin receptor blockers, or angiotensin-converting enzyme inhibitors. Aortic valve replacement is indicated in adults with critical obstruction, i.e., with an aortic valve area <0.45 cm²/m², with symptoms secondary to LV dysfunction or myocardial ischemia, or with hemodynamic evidence of LV dysfunction. In asymptomatic children or adolescents or young adults with critical aortic stenosis without valvular calcification or these features, aortic balloon valvuloplasty is often useful (Chap. 296e). If surgery is contraindicated in older patients because of a complicating medical problem such as malignancy or renal or hepatic failure, balloon valvuloplasty may provide short-term improvement. This procedure may serve as a bridge to aortic valve replacement in patients with severe heart failure. Transcatheter aortic valve replacement is a potential alternative to surgery.

SUBAORTIC STENOSIS The discrete form of subaortic stenosis consists of a membranous diaphragm or fibromuscular ring encircling the LV outflow tract just beneath the base of the aortic valve. The jet impact from the subaortic stenotic jet on the underside of the aortic valve often begets progressive aortic valve fibrosis and valvular regurgitation. Echocardiography demonstrates the anatomy of the subaortic obstruction; Doppler studies show turbulence proximal to the aortic valve and can quantitate the pressure gradient and severity of aortic regurgitation. Treatment consists of complete excision of the membrane or fibromuscular ring.

SUPRAVALVULAR AORTIC STENOSIS This is a localized or diffuse narrowing of the ascending aorta originating just above the level of the coronary arteries at the superior margin of the sinuses of Valsalva. In contrast to other forms of aortic stenosis, the coronary arteries are subjected to elevated systolic pressures from the LV, are often dilated and tortuous, and are susceptible to premature atherosclerosis. The coronary ostia may also become obstructed by the aortic valve leaflets. In most patients, a genetic defect for the anomaly is located in the same chromosomal region as elastin on chromosome 7. Supravalvular aortic stenosis is the most commonly associated cardiac defect in Williams-Beuren syndrome, typically comprising the following: "elfin" facies, low nasal bridge, cheerful demeanor, mental retardation with retained language skills and love of music, supravalvular aortic stenosis, and transient hypercalcemia.

COARCTATION OF THE AORTA

Narrowing or constriction of the lumen of the aorta may occur anywhere along its length but is most common distal to the origin of the left subclavian artery near the insertion of the ligamentum arteriosum. Coarctation occurs in ~7% of patients with CHD, is more common in males than females, and is particularly frequent in patients with gonadal dysgenesis (e.g., Turner's syndrome). Clinical manifestations depend on the site and extent of obstruction and the presence of associated cardiac anomalies, most commonly a bicuspid aortic valve. Circle of Willis aneurysms may occur in up to 10%.

Most children and young adults with isolated, discrete coarctation are asymptomatic. Headache, epistaxis, chest pressure, and claudication with exercise may occur, and attention is usually directed to the cardiovascular system when a heart murmur or hypertension in the upper extremities and absence, marked diminution, or delayed pulsations in the femoral arteries are detected on physical examination. Enlarged and pulsatile collateral vessels may be palpated in the intercostal spaces anteriorly, in the axillae, or posteriorly in the interscapular area. The upper extremities and thorax may be more developed than the lower extremities. A midsystolic murmur over the left interscapular space may become continuous if the lumen is narrowed sufficiently to result in a high-velocity jet across the lesion throughout the cardiac cycle. Additional systolic and continuous murmurs over the lateral thoracic wall may reflect increased flow through dilated and tortuous collateral vessels. The ECG usually reveals LV hypertrophy. Chest x-ray may show a dilated left subclavian artery high on the left mediastinal border and a dilated ascending aorta. Indentation of the aorta at the site of coarctation and pre- and poststenotic dilatation (the "3" sign) along the left paramediastinal shadow are essentially pathognomonic. Notching of the third to ninth ribs, an important radiographic sign, is due to inferior rib erosion by dilated collateral vessels. Two-dimensional echocardiography from suprasternal windows identifies the site of coarctation; Doppler quantitates the pressure gradient. Transesophageal echocardiography and MRI or CT allow visualization of the length and severity of the obstruction and associated collateral arteries. In adults, cardiac catheterization is indicated primarily to evaluate the coronary arteries or to perform catheter-based intervention (angioplasty and stent of the coarctation).

The chief hazards of proximal aortic severe hypertension include cerebral aneurysms and hemorrhage, aortic dissection and rupture, premature coronary arteriosclerosis, aortic valve failure, and LV failure; infective endarteritis may occur on the coarctation site or endocarditis may settle on an associated bicuspid aortic valve, which is estimated to be present in 50% of patients.

TREATMENT COARCTATION OF THE AORTA

Treatment is surgical or involves percutaneous catheter balloon dilatation with stent placement; the details of selection of therapy are beyond this review; however, the use of transcatheter treatment techniques has increased dramatically, and many previously "surgical" cases are treated via percutaneous or hybrid techniques. Late postoperative systemic hypertension in the absence of residual coarctation is related partly to the duration of preoperative hypertension. Follow-up of rest and exercise blood pressures is important; many have systolic hypertension only during exercise, in part due to a diffuse vasculopathy and to noncompliance of the stented or surgically reconstructed region. All operated or stented coarctation patients deserve a high-quality MRI or CT procedure in follow-up.

PULMONARY STENOSIS WITH INTACT VENTRICULAR SEPTUM

Obstruction to RV outflow may be localized to the supravalvular, valvular, or subvalvular levels or occur at a combination of these sites. Multiple sites of narrowing of the peripheral pulmonary arteries are a feature of rubella embryopathy and may occur with both the familial and sporadic forms of supravalvular aortic stenosis. Valvular pulmonic stenosis (PS) is the most common form of isolated RV obstruction.

The severity of the obstructing lesion, rather than the site of narrowing, is the most important determinant of the clinical course. In the presence of a normal cardiac output, a peak systolic pressure gradient <30 mmHg indicates mild PS and >50 mmHg indicates severe PS; pressures between these limits are considered to indicate moderate stenosis. Patients with mild PS are generally asymptomatic and demonstrate little or no progression in the severity of obstruction with age. In patients with more significant stenosis, the severity may increase with time. Symptoms vary with the degree of obstruction. Fatigue, dyspnea, RV failure, and syncope may limit the activity of older patients, in whom moderate or severe obstruction may prevent an augmentation of cardiac output with exercise. In patients with severe obstruction, the systolic pressure in the RV may exceed that in the LV, because the ventricular septum is intact. RV ejection is prolonged with moderate or severe stenosis, and the sound of pulmonary valve closure is delayed and soft. RV hypertrophy reduces the compliance of that chamber, and a forceful RA contraction is necessary to augment RV filling. A fourth heart sound; prominent a waves in the jugular venous pulse; and, occasionally, presystolic pulsations of the liver reflect vigorous atrial contraction. The clinical diagnosis is supported by a left parasternal lift and harsh systolic crescendo-decrescendo murmur and thrill at the upper left sternal border, typically preceded by a systolic ejection sound if the obstruction is due to a mobile nondysplastic pulmonary valve. The holosystolic murmur of tricuspid regurgitation may accompany severe PS, especially in the presence of congestive heart failure. Cyanosis usually reflects right-to-left shunting through a patent foramen ovale or ASD. In patients with supravalvular or peripheral pulmonary arterial stenosis, the murmur is systolic or continuous and is best heard over the area of narrowing, with radiation to the peripheral lung fields.

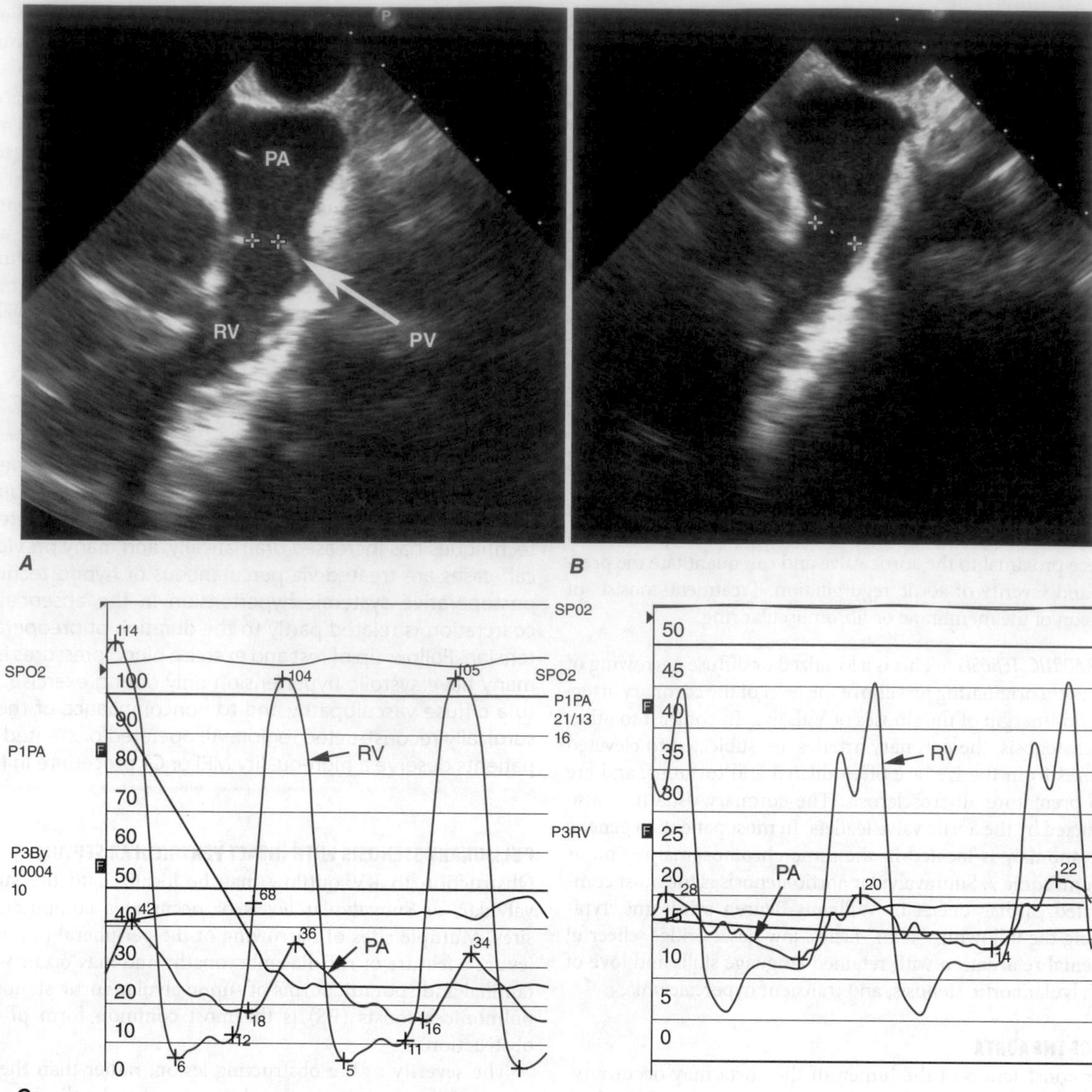

FIGURE 282-4 ***A.*** Transesophageal echocardiogram of a patient with severe pulmonary stenosis due to a mobile and doming pulmonary valve (PV). The pulmonary artery (PA) and the right ventricle (RV) are labeled. ***B.*** Following balloon valvuloplasty, the pulmonary valve orifice is larger. ***C.*** Simultaneous RV and PA pressure tracings before balloon valvuloplasty; the peak-to-peak gradient across the pulmonary valve is ~70 mmHg. ***D.*** After balloon valvuloplasty, the peak-to-peak gradient is reduced to ~25 mmHg.

In mild cases, the ECG is normal, whereas moderate and severe stenoses are associated with RV hypertrophy. The chest x-ray with mild or moderate PS shows a heart of normal size with normal lung vascularity. In pulmonary valvular stenosis, dilatation of the main and left pulmonary arteries occurs in part due to the direction of the PS jet and in part due to intrinsic tissue weakness. With severe obstruction, RV hypertrophy is generally evident. The pulmonary vascularity may be reduced with severe stenosis, RV failure, and/or a right-to-left shunt at the atrial level. Two- and three-dimensional echocardiography visualizes pulmonary valve morphology; the outflow tract pressure gradient is quantitated by Doppler echocardiography (Fig. 282-4).

TREATMENT PULMONARY STENOSIS

The cardiac catheter technique of balloon valvuloplasty (Chap. 272) is usually effective, and the surgery is rarely necessary. Multiple stenoses of the peripheral pulmonary arteries are effectively treated with transcatheter angioplasty or stenting.

TETRALOGY OF FALLOT

The four components of the tetralogy of Fallot are malaligned VSD, obstruction to RV outflow, aortic override of the VSD, and RV hypertrophy due to the RV's response to aortic pressure via the large VSD.

The severity of RV outflow obstruction determines the clinical presentation. The severity of hypoplasia of the RV outflow tract varies from mild to complete (pulmonary atresia). Pulmonary valve stenosis and supravalvular and peripheral pulmonary arterial obstruction may coexist; rarely, there is unilateral absence of a pulmonary artery (usually the left). A right-sided aortic arch and descending thoracic aorta occur in ~25%.

The relationship between the resistance of blood flow from the ventricles into the aorta and into the pulmonary artery plays a major role in determining the hemodynamic and clinical picture. When the RV outflow obstruction is severe, pulmonary blood flow is reduced markedly, and a large volume of desaturated systemic venous blood shunts right-to-left across the VSD. Severe cyanosis and erythrocytosis occur, and symptoms of systemic hypoxemia are prominent. In many infants and children, the obstruction is mild but progressive.

The ECG shows RV hypertrophy. Chest x-ray shows a normal-sized, boot-shaped heart (*coeur en sabot*) with a prominent RV and a concavity in the region of the pulmonary conus. Pulmonary vascular markings are typically diminished, and the aortic arch and knob may be on the right side. Echocardiography demonstrates the malaligned VSD with the overriding aorta and the site and severity of PS, which may be subpulmonic (fixed or dynamic), at the pulmonary valve or in the main or branch pulmonary arteries. Classic contrast angiography may provide details regarding the RV outflow tract, pulmonary valve and annulus, and caliber of the main branches of the pulmonary artery, as well as about possible associated aortopulmonary collaterals. Coronary arteriography identifies the anatomy and course of the coronary arteries, which may be anomalous. Cardiac MRI and CT complement echocardiography and provide much of the information gathered by angiography as well as additional functional information. MRI is considered the clinical gold standard for quantification of RV volume and function as well as quantification of the pulmonary regurgitation severity.

TREATMENT TETRALOGY OF FALLOT

For a variety of reasons, only a few adults with tetralogy of Fallot have not had some form of previous surgical intervention. Reoperation in adults is most commonly for severe pulmonary regurgitation or pulmonary stenosis. Long-term concerns about ventricular function persist. Ventricular and atrial arrhythmias occur, respectively, in 15% and 25% of adults and may require medical treatment, electrophysiologic study and ablation, defibrillator placement, or transcatheter or surgical intervention, usually including pulmonary valve replacement. Transcatheter pulmonary valve replacement is widely used in patients meeting anatomic criteria. The aortic root has a medial tissue defect; it is commonly enlarged and associated with aortic regurgitation. Endocarditis remains a risk despite surgical repair.

COMPLETE TRANSPOSITION OF THE GREAT ARTERIES

This condition is commonly called *dextro-* or D-*transposition of the great arteries*. The aorta arises rightward anteriorly from the RV, and the pulmonary artery emerges leftward and posteriorly from the LV, which results in two separate parallel circulations; some communication between them must exist after birth to sustain life. Most patients have an interatrial communication, two-thirds have a patent ductus arteriosus, and about one-third have an associated VSD. Transposition is more common in males and accounts for ~10% of cyanotic heart disease. The course is determined by the degree of tissue hypoxemia, the ability of each ventricle to sustain an increased workload in the presence of reduced coronary arterial oxygenation, the nature of the associated cardiovascular anomalies, and the status of the pulmonary vascular bed. Patients who do not undergo surgical palliation generally do not survive to reach adulthood. The long-term outcomes in those that have undergone surgery are in large part determined by the type of surgery performed. By the third decade of life, ~30% of patients with "atrial switch" operations will have developed decreased RV function and progressive tricuspid regurgitation, which may lead to congestive heart failure. Pulmonary vascular obstruction develops by 1–2 years of age in patients with an associated large VSD or large patent ductus arteriosus in the absence of obstruction to LV outflow.

TREATMENT TRANSPOSITION OF THE GREAT ARTERIES

The balloon or blade catheter or surgical creation or enlargement of an interatrial communication in the neonate is the simplest procedure for providing increased intracardiac mixing of systemic and pulmonary venous blood. Systemic pulmonary artery anastomosis may be indicated in the patient with severe obstruction to LV outflow and diminished pulmonary blood flow. Intracardiac repair may be accomplished by rearranging the venous returns (intraatrial switch, i.e., Mustard or Senning operation) so that the systemic venous blood is directed to the mitral valve and, thence, to the LV and pulmonary artery, while the pulmonary venous blood is diverted through the tricuspid valve and RV to the aorta. The late survival after these repairs is good, but arrhythmias (e.g., atrial flutter) or conduction defects (e.g., sick sinus syndrome) occur in ~50% of such patients by 30 years after the intraatrial switch surgery. Progressive dysfunction of the systemic subaortic RV, tricuspid regurgitation, ventricular arrhythmias, cardiac arrest, and late sudden death are worrisome features. Preferably, this malformation is corrected in infancy by transposing both coronary arteries to the posterior artery and transecting, contraposing, and anastomosing the aorta and pulmonary arteries (arterial-switch operation). For patients with a VSD in whom it is necessary to bypass a severely obstructed LV outflow tract, corrective operation employs an intracardiac ventricular baffle and extracardiac prosthetic conduit to replace the pulmonary artery (Rastelli procedure).

SINGLE VENTRICLE

This is a family of complex lesions with both atrioventricular valves or a common atrioventricular valve opening to a single ventricular chamber. Associated anomalies include abnormal great artery positional relationships, pulmonic valvular or subvalvular stenosis, and subaortic stenosis. Survival to adulthood depends on a relatively normal pulmonary blood flow, yet normal pulmonary resistance and good ventricular function. Modifications of the Fontan approach are generally applied to carefully selected patients with creation of a pathway(s) from the systemic veins to the pulmonary arteries.

TRICUSPID ATRESIA

This malformation is characterized by atresia of the tricuspid valve; an interatrial communication; and, frequently, hypoplasia of the RV and pulmonary artery. The clinical picture is usually dominated by severe cyanosis due to obligatory admixture of systemic and pulmonary venous blood in the LV. The ECG characteristically shows RA enlargement, left-axis deviation, and LV hypertrophy.

Atrial septostomy and palliative operations to increase pulmonary blood flow, often by anastomosis of a systemic artery or vein to a pulmonary artery, may allow survival to the second or third decade. A Fontan atriopulmonary or total cavopulmonary connection may then allow functional correction in patients with normal or low pulmonary arterial resistance pressure and good LV function. There are a number of important long-term considerations with the Fontan circulation, including the development of arrhythmias, progressive liver dysfunction, thromboembolic complications, and potential long-term need for heart or heart and liver transplantation.

EBSTEIN'S ANOMALY

Characterized by a downward displacement of the tricuspid valve into the RV, due to anomalous attachment of the tricuspid leaflets, the Ebstein tricuspid valve tissue is dysplastic and results in tricuspid regurgitation. The abnormally situated tricuspid orifice produces an "atrialized" portion of the RV lying between the atrioventricular ring and the origin of the valve, which is continuous with the RA chamber. Often, the RV is hypoplastic. Although the clinical manifestations are variable, some patients come to initial attention because of either (1) progressive cyanosis from right-to-left atrial shunting, (2) symptoms due to tricuspid regurgitation and RV dysfunction, or (3) paroxysmal atrial tachyarrhythmias with or without atrioventricular bypass tracts (Wolff-Parkinson-White [WPW] syndrome). Diagnostic findings by two-dimensional echocardiography include the abnormal positional relation between the tricuspid and mitral valves with abnormally increased apical displacement of the septal tricuspid leaflet. Tricuspid regurgitation is quantitated by Doppler examination. Surgical approaches include prosthetic replacement of the tricuspid valve when the leaflets are tethered or repair of the native valve.

The two fundamental anatomic abnormalities in this malformation are transposition of the ascending aorta and pulmonary trunk and inversion of the ventricles. This arrangement results in desaturated systemic venous blood passing from the RA through the mitral valve to the LV and into the pulmonary trunk, whereas oxygenated pulmonary venous blood flows from the left atrium through the tricuspid valve to the RV and into the aorta. Thus, the circulation is corrected functionally. The clinical presentation, course, and prognosis of patients with congenitally corrected transposition vary depending on the nature and severity of any complicating intracardiac anomalies and of development of dysfunction of the systemic subaortic RV. Progressive RV dysfunction and tricuspid regurgitation may also develop in one-third of patients by age 30; Ebstein-type anomalies of the left-side tricuspid atrioventricular valve are common. VSD or PS due to obstruction to outflow from the right-sided subpulmonary (anatomic left) ventricle may coexist. Complete heart block occurs at a rate of 2–10% per decade. The diagnosis of the malformation and associated lesions can be established by comprehensive two-dimensional echocardiography and Doppler examination.

MALPOSITIONS OF THE HEART

Positional anomalies refer to conditions in which the cardiac apex is in the right side of the chest (*dextrocardia*) or at the midline (*mesocardia*), or in which there is a normal location of the heart in the left side of the chest but abnormal position of the viscera (*isolated levocardia*). Knowledge of the position of the abdominal organs and of the branching pattern of the main stem bronchi is important in categorizing these malpositions. When dextrocardia occurs without situs inversus, when the visceral situs is indeterminate, or if isolated levocardia is present, associated, often complex, multiple cardiac anomalies are usually present. In contrast, mirror-image dextrocardia is usually observed with complete situs inversus, which occurs most frequently in individuals whose hearts are otherwise normal.

SURGICALLY MODIFIED CONGENITAL HEART DISEASE

Owing to the enormous strides in cardiovascular surgical techniques that have occurred in the past 70 years, a large number of long-term survivors of palliative or corrective operations in infancy and childhood have reached adulthood. These patients are often challenging because of the diversity of anatomic, hemodynamic, and electrophysiologic residua and sequelae of cardiac operations.

The proper care of the survivor of an operation for CHD requires that the clinician understand the details of the malformation before operation; pay meticulous attention to the details of the operative procedure; and recognize the postoperative residua (conditions left totally or partially uncorrected), the sequelae (conditions caused by surgery), and the complications that may have resulted from the operation. Except for ligation of an uncomplicated patent ductus arteriosus, almost every other surgical repair leaves behind or causes some abnormality of the heart and circulation that may range from trivial to serious. Thus, even with results that are considered clinically to be good to excellent, continued long-term postoperative follow-up is advisable.

Cardiac operations involving the atria, such as closure of ASD, repair of total or partial anomalous pulmonary venous return, or venous switch corrections of complete transposition of the great arteries (the Mustard or Senning operations), may be followed years later by sinus node or atrioventricular node dysfunction and/or by atrial arrhythmias (especially atrial flutter). Intraventricular surgery may also result in electrophysiologic consequences, including complete heart block necessitating pacemaker insertion to avoid sudden death. Valvular problems may arise late after initial cardiac operation. An example is the progressive stenosis of an initially nonobstructive bicuspid aortic valve in the patient who underwent aortic coarctation repair. Such aortic valves may also be the site of infective endocarditis. After repair of the ostium primum ASD, the cleft mitral valve may become progressively regurgitant. Tricuspid regurgitation may also be progressive in the postoperative patient with tetralogy of Fallot if RV outflow tract obstruction was not relieved adequately at initial surgery. In many patients with surgically modified CHD, inadequate relief of an obstructive lesion, a residual regurgitant lesion, or a residual shunt will cause or hasten the onset of clinical signs and symptoms of myocardial dysfunction. Despite a good hemodynamic repair, many patients with a subaortic RV develop RV decompensation and signs of left heart failure. In many patients, particularly those who were cyanotic for many years before operation, a preexisting compromise in ventricular performance is due to the original underlying malformation.

A final category of postoperative problems involves the use of prosthetic valves, patches, or conduits in the operative repair. The special risks include infective endocarditis, thrombus formation, and premature degeneration and calcification of the prosthetic materials. There are many patients in whom extracardiac conduits are required to correct the circulation functionally and often to carry blood to the lungs from the RA or RV. These conduits may develop intraluminal obstruction, and if they include a prosthetic valve, it may show progressive calcification and thickening. Many such patients face reintervention (interventional cardiac catheterization or surgical reoperation) one or more times in their lives. Such care should be directed to centers specializing in adults with complex congenital cardiovascular malformations. The effect of pregnancy in postoperative patients depends on the outcome of the repair, including the presence and severity of residua, sequelae, or complications. Contraception is an important topic with such patients. Tubal ligation should be considered in those in whom pregnancy is strictly contraindicated.

Endocarditis Prophylaxis Two major predisposing causes of infective endocarditis are a susceptible cardiovascular substrate and a source of bacteremia. The clinical and bacteriologic profile of infective endocarditis in patients with CHD has changed with the advent of intracardiac surgery and of prosthetic devices. Prophylaxis includes both antimicrobial and hygienic measures. Meticulous dental and skin care are required. Routine antimicrobial prophylaxis is recommended for bacteremic dental procedures or instrumentation through an infected site in most patients with operated CHD, particularly if foreign material, such as a prosthetic valve, conduit, or surgically constructed shunt, is in place. In the case of patches, in the absence of a high-pressure patch leak, or transcatheter devices, prophylaxis is usually recommended for 6 months until there is endothelialization. Individuals with unrepaired cyanotic heart disease are also generally recommended to receive prophylaxis (Chap. 155).

283 Aortic Valve Disease

Patrick T. O'Gara, Joseph Loscalzo

GLOBAL BURDEN OF VALVULAR HEART DISEASE

Primary valvular heart disease ranks well below coronary heart disease, stroke, hypertension, obesity, and diabetes as a major threat to the public health. Nevertheless, it is the source of significant morbidity and mortality rates. Rheumatic fever (Chap. 381) is the dominant cause of valvular heart disease in developing and low-income countries. Its prevalence has been estimated to range from as low as 1 per 100,000 school-age children in Costa Rica to as high as 150 per 100,000 in China. Rheumatic heart disease accounts for 12–65% of hospital admissions related to cardiovascular disease and 2–10% of hospital discharges in some developing countries. Prevalence and mortality rates vary among communities even within the same country as a function of overcrowding and the availability of medical resources and population-wide programs for detection and treatment of group A streptococcal pharyngitis. In economically deprived areas, tropical and subtropical climates (particularly on the Indian subcontinent), Central

America, and the Middle East, rheumatic valvular disease progresses more rapidly than in more-developed nations and frequently causes serious symptoms in patients younger than 20 years of age. This accelerated natural history may be due to repeated infections with more virulent strains of rheumatogenic streptococci. Approximately 15 million to 20 million people live with rheumatic heart disease worldwide, an estimated prevalence characterized by 300,000 new cases and 233,000 case fatalities per year, with the highest mortality rates reported from Southeast Asia (~7.6 per 100,000).

Although there have been recent reports of isolated outbreaks of streptococcal infection in North America, valve disease in high-income countries is dominated by degenerative or inflammatory processes that lead to valve thickening, calcification, and dysfunction. The prevalence of valvular heart disease increases with age for both men and women. Important left-sided valve disease may affect as many as 12–13% of adults older than the age of 75. In the United States, there were 85,000 hospital discharges with valvular heart disease in 2010, and the vast majority of these were related to surgical procedures for heart valve disease (mostly involving the aortic and mitral valves).

The incidence of infective endocarditis (Chap. 155) has increased with the aging of the population, the more widespread prevalence of vascular grafts and intracardiac devices, the emergence of more virulent multidrug-resistant microorganisms, and the growing epidemic of diabetes. The more restricted use of antibiotic prophylaxis since 2007 has thus far not been associated with an increase in incidence rates. Infective endocarditis has become a relatively more frequent cause of acute valvular regurgitation.

Bicuspid aortic valve disease affects as many as 0.5–1.4% of the general population, with an associated incidence of aortopathy involving root or ascending aortic aneurysm disease or coarctation. An increasing number of childhood survivors of congenital heart disease present later in life with valvular dysfunction. The global burden of valvular heart disease is expected to progress.

As is true for many other chronic health conditions, disparities in access to and quality of care for patients with valvular heart disease have been well documented. Management decisions and outcome differences based on age, gender, race, and geography require educational efforts across all levels of providers.

The role of the physical examination in the evaluation of patients with valvular heart disease is also considered in Chaps. 51e and 267; of electrocardiography (ECG) in Chap. 268; of echocardiography and other noninvasive imaging techniques in Chap. 270e; and of cardiac catheterization and angiography in Chap. 272.

AORTIC STENOSIS

Aortic stenosis (AS) occurs in about one-fourth of all patients with chronic valvular heart disease; approximately 80% of adult patients with symptomatic, valvular AS are male.

ETIOLOGY AND PATHOGENESIS

(Table 283-1) AS in adults is due to degenerative calcification of the aortic cusps and occurs most commonly on a substrate of congenital disease (bicuspid aortic valve), chronic (trileaflet) deterioration, or previous rheumatic inflammation. A pathologic study of specimens removed at the time of aortic valve replacement for AS showed that 53% were bicuspid and 4% unicuspid. The process of aortic valve deterioration and calcification is not a passive one, but rather one that shares many features with vascular atherosclerosis, including endothelial dysfunction, lipid accumulation, inflammatory cell activation, cytokine release, and upregulation of several signaling pathways (Fig. 283-1). Eventually, valvular myofibroblasts differentiate phenotypically into osteoblasts and actively produce bone matrix proteins that allow for the deposition of calcium hydroxyapatite crystals. Genetic polymorphisms involving the vitamin D receptor, the estrogen receptor in postmenopausal women, interleukin 10, and apolipoprotein E4 have been linked to the development of calcific AS, and a strong familial clustering of cases has been reported from western France. Several traditional atherosclerotic risk factors have also been associated with the development and progression of calcific AS, including low-density lipoprotein (LDL) cholesterol, lipoprotein a (Lp[a]), diabetes mellitus, smoking, chronic kidney disease, and the metabolic syndrome. The presence of aortic valve sclerosis (focal thickening and calcification of the leaflets not severe enough to cause obstruction) is associated with an excess risk of cardiovascular death and myocardial infarction (MI) among persons older than age 65. Approximately 30% of persons older than 65 years exhibit aortic valve sclerosis, whereas 2% exhibit frank stenosis.

Rheumatic disease of the aortic leaflets produces commissural fusion, sometimes resulting in a bicuspid-appearing valve. This condition, in turn, makes the leaflets more susceptible to trauma and ultimately leads to fibrosis, calcification, and further narrowing. By the time the obstruction to left ventricular (LV) outflow causes serious clinical disability, the valve is usually a rigid calcified mass, and careful examination may make it difficult or even impossible to determine the etiology of the underlying process. Rheumatic AS is almost always associated with involvement of the mitral valve and with aortic regurgitation. Mediastinal radiation can also result in late scarring, fibrosis, and calcification of the leaflets with AS.

TABLE 283-1 MAJOR CAUSES OF AORTIC VALVE DISEASE

Valve Lesion	Etiologies
Aortic stenosis	Congenital (bicuspid, unicuspid)
	Degenerative calcific
	Rheumatic fever
	Radiation
Aortic regurgitation	Valvular
	Congenital (bicuspid)
	Endocarditis
	Rheumatic fever
	Myxomatous (prolapse)
	Traumatic
	Syphilis
	Ankylosing spondylitis
	Root disease
	Aortic dissection
	Cystic medial degeneration
	Marfan's syndrome
	Bicuspid aortic valve
	Nonsyndromic familial aneurysm
	Aortitis
	Hypertension

BICUSPID AORTIC VALVE DISEASE

A bicuspid aortic valve (BAV) is the most common congenital heart valve defect and occurs in 0.5–1.4% of the population with a 2–4:1 male-to-female predominance. The inheritance pattern appears to be autosomal dominant with incomplete penetrance, although some have questioned an X-linked component as suggested by the prevalence of BAV disease among patients with Turner's syndrome. The prevalence of BAV disease among first-degree relatives of an affected individual is approximately 10%. A single gene defect to explain the majority of cases has not been identified, although a mutation in the *NOTCH1* gene has been described in some families. Abnormalities in endothelial nitric oxide synthase and NKX2.5 have been implicated as well. Medial degeneration with ascending aortic aneurysm formation occurs commonly among patients with BAV disease; aortic coarctation is less frequently encountered. Patients with BAV disease have larger aortas than patients with comparable tricuspid aortic valve disease. The aortopathy develops independent of the hemodynamic severity of the valve lesion and is a risk factor for aneurysm formation and/or dissection. A BAV can be a component of more complex congenital heart disease with or without other left heart obstructing lesions, as seen in Shone's complex.

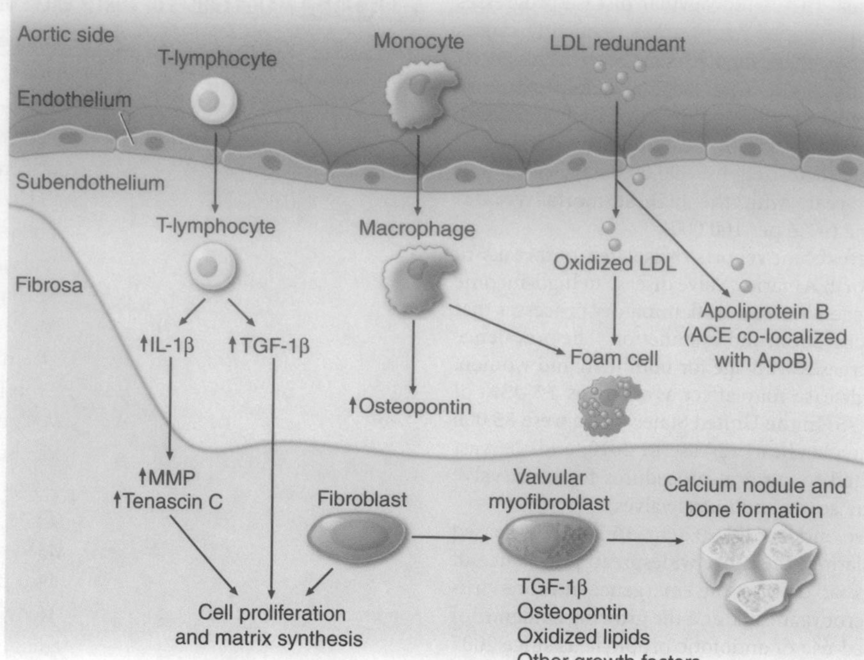

FIGURE 283-1 Pathogenesis of calcific aortic stenosis. Inflammatory cells infiltrate across the endothelial barrier and release cytokines that act on fibroblasts to promote cellular proliferation and matrix remodeling. LDL is oxidatively modified and taken up by macrophage scavengers to become foam cells. Angiotensin-converting enzyme colocalizes with ApoB. A subset of myofibroblasts differentiates into an osteoblast phenotype capable of promoting bone formation. ACE, angiotensin-converting enzyme; ApoB, apolipoprotein B; LDL, low-density lipoprotein; IL, interleukin; MMP, matrix metalloproteinase; TGF, transforming growth factor. *(From RV Freeman, CM Otto: Circulation 111:3316, 2005; with permission.)*

OTHER FORMS OF OBSTRUCTION TO LEFT VENTRICULAR OUTFLOW

In addition to valvular AS, three other lesions may be responsible for obstruction to LV outflow: *hypertrophic obstructive cardiomyopathy* (Chap. 287), *discrete fibromuscular/membranous subaortic stenosis*, and *supravalvular AS* (Chap. 282). The causes of LV outflow obstruction can be differentiated on the basis of the cardiac examination and Doppler echocardiographic findings.

PATHOPHYSIOLOGY

The obstruction to LV outflow produces a systolic pressure gradient between the LV and aorta. When severe obstruction is suddenly produced experimentally, the LV responds by dilation and reduction of stroke volume. However, in some patients, the obstruction may be present at birth and/or increase gradually over the course of many years, and LV contractile performance is maintained by the presence of concentric LV hypertrophy. Initially, this serves as an adaptive mechanism because it reduces toward normal the systolic stress developed by the myocardium, as predicted by the Laplace relation ($S = Pr/h$, where S = systolic wall stress, P = pressure, r = radius, and h = wall thickness). A large transaortic valve pressure gradient may exist for many years without a reduction in cardiac output (CO) or LV dilation; ultimately, however, excessive hypertrophy becomes maladaptive, LV systolic function declines because of afterload mismatch, abnormalities of diastolic function progress, and irreversible myocardial fibrosis develops.

A mean systolic pressure gradient >40 mmHg with a normal CO or an effective aortic orifice area of approximately <1 cm^2 (or approximately <0.6 cm^2/m^2 body surface area in a normal-sized adult)—i.e., less than approximately one-third of the normal orifice area—is generally considered to represent severe obstruction to LV outflow. The elevated LV end-diastolic pressure observed in many patients with severe AS and preserved ejection fraction (EF) signifies the presence of diminished compliance of the hypertrophied LV. Although the CO at rest is within normal limits in most patients with severe AS, it usually fails to rise normally during exercise. Loss of an appropriately timed, vigorous atrial contraction, as occurs in atrial fibrillation (AF) or atrioventricular dissociation, may cause rapid progression of symptoms. Late in the course, contractile function deteriorates because of afterload excess, the CO and LV–aortic pressure gradient decline, and the mean left atrial (LA), pulmonary artery (PA), and right ventricular (RV) pressures rise. LV performance can be further compromised by superimposed coronary artery disease (CAD). Stroke volume (and thus CO) can also be reduced in patients with significant hypertrophy and a small LV cavity despite a normal EF. Low-flow, low-gradient AS (with either reduced or normal LV systolic function) is both a diagnostic and therapeutic challenge.

The hypertrophied LV causes an increase in myocardial oxygen requirements. In addition, even in the absence of obstructive CAD, coronary blood flow is impaired to the extent that ischemia can be precipitated under conditions of excess demand. Capillary density is reduced relative to wall thickness, compressive forces are increased, and the elevated LV end-diastolic pressure reduces the coronary driving pressure. The subendocardium is especially vulnerable to ischemia by this mechanism.

SYMPTOMS

AS is rarely of clinical importance until the valve orifice has narrowed to approximately 1 cm^2. Even severe AS may exist for many years without producing any symptoms because of the ability of the hypertrophied LV to generate the elevated intraventricular pressures required to maintain a normal stroke volume. Once symptoms occur, valve replacement is indicated.

Most patients with pure or predominant AS have gradually increasing obstruction over years but do not become symptomatic until the sixth to eighth decades. Adult patients with BAV disease, however, develop significant valve dysfunction and symptoms one to two decades sooner. Exertional dyspnea, angina pectoris, and syncope are the three cardinal symptoms. Often, there is a history of insidious progression of fatigue and dyspnea associated with gradual curtailment of activities and reduced effort tolerance. *Dyspnea* results primarily from elevation of the pulmonary capillary pressure caused by elevations of LV diastolic pressures secondary to impaired relaxation and reduced LV compliance. *Angina pectoris* usually develops somewhat later and reflects an imbalance between the augmented myocardial oxygen requirements and reduced oxygen availability. CAD may or may not be present, although its coexistence is common among AS patients older than age 65. *Exertional syncope* may result from a decline in arterial pressure caused by vasodilation in the exercising muscles and inadequate vasoconstriction in nonexercising muscles in the face of a fixed CO, or from a sudden fall in CO produced by an arrhythmia.

Because the CO at rest is usually well maintained until late in the course, marked fatigability, weakness, peripheral cyanosis, cachexia, and other clinical manifestations of a low CO are usually not prominent until this stage is reached. Orthopnea, paroxysmal nocturnal dyspnea, and pulmonary edema, i.e., symptoms of LV failure, also occur only in the advanced stages of the disease. Severe pulmonary hypertension leading to RV failure and systemic venous hypertension, hepatomegaly, AF, and tricuspid regurgitation (TR) are usually late findings in patients with isolated severe AS.

When AS and mitral stenosis (MS) coexist, the reduction in flow (CO) induced by MS lowers the pressure gradient across the aortic valve and, thereby, masks many of the clinical findings produced by AS. The transaortic pressure gradient can be increased in patients with concomitant aortic regurgitation (AR) due to higher aortic valve flow rates.

PHYSICAL FINDINGS

The rhythm is generally regular until late in the course; at other times, AF should suggest the possibility of associated mitral valve disease. The systemic arterial pressure is usually within normal limits. In the late stages, however, when stroke volume declines, the systolic pressure may fall and the pulse pressure narrow. The carotid arterial pulse rises slowly to a delayed peak (*pulsus parvus et tardus*). A thrill or anacrotic "shudder" may be palpable over the carotid arteries, more commonly the left. In the elderly, the stiffening of the arterial wall may mask this important physical sign. In many patients, the *a* wave in the jugular venous pulse is accentuated. This results from the diminished distensibility of the RV cavity caused by the bulging, hypertrophied interventricular septum.

The LV impulse is sometimes displaced laterally in the later stages of the disease. A double apical impulse (with a palpable S_4) may be recognized, particularly with the patient in the left lateral recumbent position. A systolic thrill may be present at the base of the heart to the right of the sternum when leaning forward or in the suprasternal notch.

Auscultation An early systolic ejection sound is frequently audible in children, adolescents, and young adults with congenital BAV disease. This sound usually disappears when the valve becomes calcified and rigid. As AS increases in severity, LV systole may become prolonged so that the aortic valve closure sound no longer precedes the pulmonic valve closure sound, and the two components may become synchronous, or aortic valve closure may even follow pulmonic valve closure, causing paradoxical splitting of S_2 (Chap. 267). The sound of aortic valve closure can be heard most frequently in patients with AS who have pliable valves, and calcification diminishes the intensity of this sound. Frequently, an S_4 is audible at the apex and reflects the presence of LV hypertrophy and an elevated LV end-diastolic pressure; an S_3 generally occurs late in the course, when the LV dilates and its systolic function becomes severely compromised.

The murmur of AS is characteristically an ejection (mid) systolic murmur that commences shortly after the S_1, increases in intensity to reach a peak toward the middle of ejection, and ends just before aortic valve closure. It is characteristically low-pitched, rough and rasping in character, and loudest at the base of the heart, most commonly in the second right intercostal space. It is transmitted upward along the carotid arteries. Occasionally it is transmitted downward and to the apex, where it may be confused with the systolic murmur of mitral regurgitation (MR) (Gallavardin effect). In almost all patients with severe obstruction and preserved CO, the murmur is at least grade III/VI. In patients with mild degrees of obstruction or in those with severe stenosis with heart failure and low CO in whom the stroke volume and, therefore, the transvalvular flow rate are reduced, the murmur may be relatively soft and brief.

LABORATORY EXAMINATION

ECG In most patients with severe AS, there is LV hypertrophy. In advanced cases, ST-segment depression and T-wave inversion (LV "strain") in standard leads I and aVL and in the left precordial leads are evident. However, there is no close correlation between the ECG and the hemodynamic severity of obstruction, and the absence of ECG signs of LV hypertrophy does not exclude severe obstruction. Many patients with AS have systemic hypertension, which can also contribute to the development of hypertrophy.

Echocardiogram The key findings on TTE are thickening, calcification, and reduced systolic opening of the valve leaflets and LV hypertrophy. Eccentric closure of the aortic valve cusps is characteristic of congenitally bicuspid valves. TEE imaging can display the obstructed orifice extremely well, but it is not routinely required for accurate characterization of AS. The valve gradient and aortic valve area can be estimated by Doppler measurement of the transaortic velocity. Severe AS is defined by a valve area <1 cm², whereas moderate AS is defined by a valve area of 1–1.5 cm² and mild AS by a valve area of 1.5–2 cm². Aortic valve sclerosis, conversely, is accompanied by a jet velocity of less than 2.5 meters/s (peak gradient <25 mmHg). LV dilation and reduced systolic shortening reflect impairment of LV function. There is increasing experience with the use of longitudinal strain and strain rate to characterize earlier changes in LV systolic function, well before a decline in EF can be appreciated. Doppler indices of impaired diastolic function are frequently seen.

Echocardiography is useful for identifying coexisting valvular abnormalities; for differentiating valvular AS from other forms of LV outflow obstruction; and for measurement of the aortic root and proximal ascending aortic dimensions. These aortic measurements are particularly important for patients with BAV disease. Dobutamine stress echocardiography is useful for the evaluation of patients with AS and severe LV systolic dysfunction (low-flow, low-gradient, severe AS with reduced EF), in whom the severity of the AS can often be difficult to judge. Patients with severe AS (i.e., valve area <1 cm²) with a relatively low mean gradient (<40 mmHg) despite a normal EF (low-flow, low-gradient, severe AS with normal EF) are often hypertensive, and efforts to control their systemic blood pressure should be optimized before Doppler echocardiography is repeated. The use of dobutamine stress echocardiography in this setting is under investigation. When there is continued uncertainty regarding the severity of AS in patients with reduced CO, quantitative analysis of the amount of aortic valve calcium with chest computed tomography (CT) may be helpful.

Chest X-Ray The chest x-ray may show no or little overall cardiac enlargement for many years. Hypertrophy without dilation may produce some rounding of the cardiac apex in the frontal projection and slight backward displacement in the lateral view. A dilated proximal ascending aorta may be seen along the upper right heart border in the frontal view. Aortic valve calcification may be discernible in the lateral view, but is usually readily apparent on fluoroscopic examination or by echocardiography; the absence of valvular calcification on fluoroscopy in an adult suggests that severe valvular AS is *not* present. In later stages of the disease, as the LV dilates, there is increasing roentgenographic evidence of LV enlargement, pulmonary congestion, and enlargement of the LA, PA, and right heart chambers.

Catheterization Right and left heart catheterization for invasive assessment of AS is performed infrequently but can be useful when there is a discrepancy between the clinical and noninvasive findings. Concern has been raised that attempts to cross the aortic valve for measurement of LV pressures are associated with a risk of cerebral embolization. Catheterization is also useful in three distinct categories of patients: (1) *patients with multivalvular disease*, in whom the role played by each valvular deformity should be defined to aid in the planning of operative treatment; (2) *young, asymptomatic patients with noncalcific congenital AS*, to define the severity of obstruction to LV outflow, because operation or percutaneous aortic balloon valvuloplasty (PABV) may be indicated in these patients if severe AS is present, even in the absence of symptoms; and (3) *patients in whom it is suspected that the obstruction to LV outflow may not be at the level of the aortic valve* but rather at the sub- or supravalvular level.

Coronary angiography is indicated to screen for CAD in appropriate patients with severe AS who are being considered for surgery. The incidence of significant CAD for which bypass grafting is indicated at the time of aortic valve replacement (AVR) exceeds 50% among adult patients.

NATURAL HISTORY

Death in patients with severe AS occurs most commonly in the seventh and eighth decades. Based on data obtained at postmortem examination in patients before surgical treatment became widely available, the average time to death after the onset of various symptoms was as follows: angina pectoris, 3 years; syncope, 3 years; dyspnea, 2 years; congestive heart failure, 1.5–2 years. Moreover, in >80% of patients who died with AS, symptoms had existed for <4 years. Among adults dying with valvular AS, sudden death, which presumably resulted from an arrhythmia, occurred in 10–20%; however, most sudden deaths occurred in patients who had previously been symptomatic. Sudden death as the first manifestation of severe AS is very uncommon (<1% per year) in asymptomatic adult patients. Calcific AS is a progressive disease, with an annual reduction in valve area averaging 0.1 cm^2 and annual increases in the peak jet velocity and mean valve gradient averaging 0.3 meters/s and 7 mmHg, respectively (Table 283-2).

TREATMENT AORTIC STENOSIS (FIG. 283-2)

MEDICAL TREATMENT

In patients with severe AS (valve area <1 cm^2), strenuous physical activity and competitive sports should be avoided, even in the asymptomatic stage. Care must be taken to avoid dehydration and hypovolemia to protect against a significant reduction in CO. Medications used for the treatment of hypertension or CAD, including beta blockers and angiotensin-converting enzyme (ACE) inhibitors, are generally safe for asymptomatic patients with preserved LV systolic function. Nitroglycerin is helpful in relieving angina pectoris in patients with CAD. Retrospective studies have shown that patients with degenerative calcific AS who receive HMG-CoA reductase inhibitors ("statins") exhibit slower progression of leaflet calcification and aortic valve area reduction than those who do not. However, randomized prospective studies with either high-dose atorvastatin or combination simvastatin/ezetimibe have failed to show a measurable effect on valve-related outcomes. The use of statin medications should continue to be driven by considerations regarding primary and secondary prevention of atherosclerotic cardiovascular disease (ASCVD) events. ACE inhibitors have not been studied prospectively for AS-related outcomes. The need for endocarditis prophylaxis is restricted to AS patients with a prior history of endocarditis.

SURGICAL TREATMENT

Asymptomatic patients with calcific AS and severe obstruction should be followed carefully for the development of symptoms and by serial echocardiograms for evidence of deteriorating LV function. Operation is indicated in patients with severe AS (valve area <1 cm^2 or 0.6 cm^2/m^2 body surface area) who are symptomatic, those who exhibit LV systolic dysfunction (EF <50%), and those with BAV disease and an aneurysmal root or ascending aorta (maximal dimension >5.5 cm). Operation for aneurysm disease is recommended at smaller aortic diameters (4.5–5.0 cm) for patients with a family history of an aortic catastrophe and for patients who exhibit rapid aneurysm growth (>0.5 cm/year). Patients with asymptomatic moderate or severe AS who are referred for coronary artery bypass grafting surgery should also have AVR. In patients without heart failure, the operative risk of AVR (including patients with AS or AR) is approximately 2% (Table 283-2) but increases as a function of age and the need for concomitant aortic surgery or coronary revascularization with bypass grafting. The indications for AVR in the asymptomatic patient have been the subject of intense debate over the past 5 years, as surgical outcomes in selected patients have continued to improve. Relative indications for which surgery can be considered include an abnormal response to treadmill exercise; rapid progression of AS, especially when urgent access to medical care might be compromised; very severe AS, defined by an aortic valve jet velocity >5 meters/s or mean gradient >60 mmHg and low operative risk; and excessive LV hypertrophy in the absence of systemic hypertension. Exercise testing can be safely performed in the asymptomatic patient, as many as one-third of whom will show signs of functional impairment.

Operation should be carried out promptly after symptom onset. In patients with low-flow, low-gradient severe AS with reduced LVEF, the perioperative mortality risk is high (15–20%), and evidence of myocardial disease may persist even when the operation is technically successful. Long-term postoperative survival correlates with preoperative LV function. Nonetheless, in view of the even worse prognosis of such patients when they are treated medically, there is usually little choice but to advise valve replacement, especially in patients in whom contractile reserve can be demonstrated by dobutamine stress echocardiography (defined by a ≥20% increase in stroke volume after dobutamine challenge). Patients in this high surgical risk group may benefit from transcatheter aortic valve replacement (TAVR, see below). The treatment of patients with low-flow, low-gradient severe AS with normal LVEF is also difficult. Outcomes appear to be better with surgery compared with conservative medical care for symptomatic patients with this type of "paradoxical" low-flow AS, but more research is needed to guide therapeutic decision-making. In patients in whom severe AS and CAD coexist, relief of the AS and revascularization may sometimes result in striking clinical and hemodynamic improvement (Table 283-2).

Because many patients with calcific AS are elderly, particular attention must be directed to the adequacy of hepatic, renal, and pulmonary function before AVR is recommended. Age alone is not a contraindication to AVR for AS. The perioperative mortality rate depends to a substantial extent on the patient's preoperative clinical and hemodynamic state. Treatment decisions for AS patients who are not at low operative risk should be made by a multidisciplinary heart team with representation from general cardiology, interventional cardiology, imaging, cardiac surgery, and other allied specialties as needed, including geriatrics. The 10-year survival rate of older adult patients with AVR is approximately 60%. Approximately 30% of bioprosthetic valves evidence primary valve failure in 10 years, requiring re-replacement, and an approximately equal percentage of patients with mechanical prostheses develop significant hemorrhagic complications as a consequence of treatment with vitamin K antagonists. Homograft AVR is usually reserved for patients with aortic valve endocarditis.

The Ross procedure involves replacement of the diseased aortic valve with the autologous pulmonic valve and implantation of a homograft in the native pulmonic position. Its use has declined considerably in the United States because of the technical complexity of the procedure and the incidence of late postoperative aortic root dilation and autograft failure with AR. There is also a low incidence of pulmonary homograft stenosis.

TABLE 283-2 MORTALITY RATES AFTER AORTIC VALVE SURGERY[a]

Operation	Number	Unadjusted Operative Mortality (%)
AVR (isolated)	14,795	2.3
AVR + CAB	9158	4.2
AVR + MVR	876	8.8

[a]Data are for the first two quarters of calendar year 2013, during which 1004 sites reported a total of 135,666 procedures. Data are available from the Society of Thoracic Surgeons at *http://www.sts.org/sites/default/files/documents/2013_3rdHarvestExecutiveSummary.pdf.*

Abbreviations: AVR, aortic valve replacement; CAB, coronary artery bypass; MVR, mitral valve replacement.

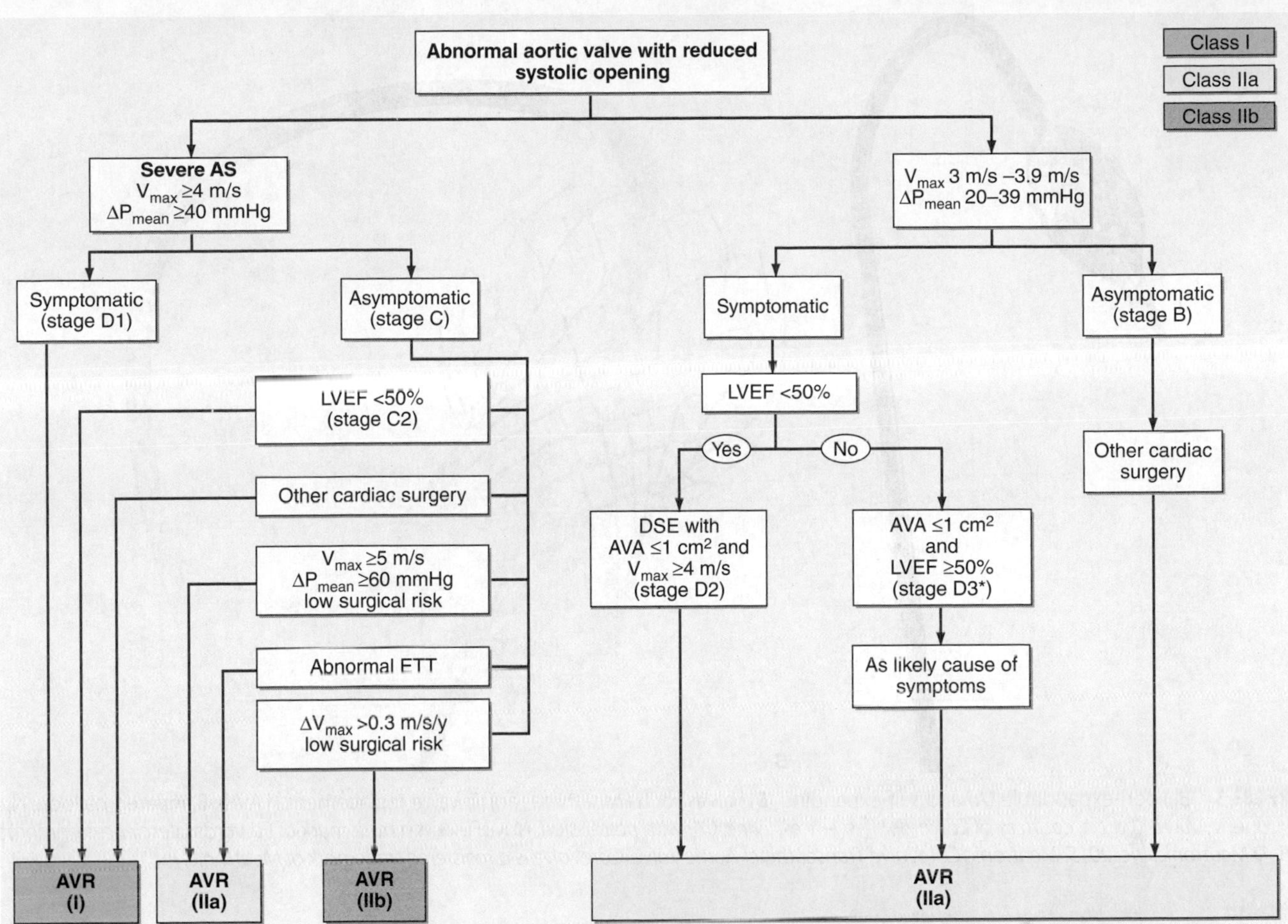

FIGURE 283-2 Management strategy for patients with aortic stenosis. Preoperative coronary angiography should be performed routinely as determined by age, symptoms, and coronary risk factors. Cardiac catheterization and angiography may also be helpful when there is a discrepancy between clinical and noninvasive findings. Patients who do not meet criteria for intervention should be monitored periodically with clinical and echocardiographic follow-up. The class designations refer to the American College of Cardiology/American Heart Association methodology for treatment recommendations. Class I recommendations should be performed or are indicated; Class IIa recommendations are considered reasonable to perform; Class IIb recommendations may be considered. The stages refer to the stages of progression of the disease. At disease stage A, risk factors are present for the development of valve dysfunction; stage B refers to progressive, mild-moderate, asymptomatic valve disease; stage C disease is severe in nature but clinically asymptomatic; stage C1 characterizes asymptomatic patients with severe valve disease but compensated ventricular function; stage C2 refers to asymptomatic, severe disease with ventricular decompensation; stage D refers to severe, symptomatic valve disease. With aortic stenosis, stage D1 refers to symptomatic patients with severe aortic stenosis and a high valve gradient (>40 mmHg mean gradient); stage D2 comprises patients with symptomatic, severe, low-flow, low-gradient aortic stenosis and low left ventricular ejection fraction; and stage D3 characterizes patients with symptomatic, severe, low-flow, low-gradient aortic stenosis and preserved left ventricular ejection fraction (paradoxical, low-flow, low-gradient severe aortic stenosis). AS, aortic stenosis; AVA; aortic valve area; AVR, aortic valve replacement by either surgical or transcatheter approach; BP, blood pressure; DSE, dobutamine stress echocardiography; ETT, exercise treadmill test; LVEF, left ventricular ejection fraction; ΔP_{mean}, mean pressure gradient; and V_{max}, maximum velocity. *(Adapted from RA Nishimura et al: 2014 AHA/ACC Guideline for the Management of Patients with Valvular Heart Disease. J Am Coll Cardiol doi: 10.1016/j.jacc.2014.02.536, 2014, with permission.)*

PERCUTANEOUS AORTIC BALLOON VALVULOPLASTY (PABV)

This procedure is preferable to operation in many children and young adults with congenital, noncalcific AS (Chap. 282). It is not commonly used as definitive therapy in adults with severe calcific AS because of a very high restenosis rate (80% within 1 year) and the risk of procedural complications, but on occasion, it has been used successfully as a "bridge to operation" in patients with severe LV dysfunction and shock who are too ill to tolerate surgery. It is performed routinely as part of the TAVR procedure (see below).

TRANSCATHETER AORTIC VALVE REPLACEMENT

TAVR for treatment of AS has been performed in more than 50,000 prohibitive- or high-surgical-risk adult patients worldwide using one of two available systems, a balloon-expandable valve and a self-expanding valve, both of which incorporate a pericardial prosthesis (Fig. 283-3). More than 250 U.S. centers now offer this procedure. TAVR is most frequently performed via the transfemoral route, although trans-LV apical, subclavian, carotid, and ascending aortic routes have been used. Aortic balloon valvuloplasty under rapid RV pacing is performed as a first step to create an orifice of sufficient size for the prosthesis. Procedural success rates exceed 90%. Among elderly patients with severe AS who are considered inoperable (i.e., prohibitive surgical risk), 1- and 2-year survival rates are significantly higher with TAVR compared with medical therapy (including PABV) (Fig. 283-4). One- and 2-year survival rates are essentially equal for high-surgical-risk patients treated with TAVR or surgical AVR (SAVR) (Fig. 283-5). TAVR is associated with an early hazard for stroke and a higher incidence of postprocedural, paravalvular AR, a risk factor for mortality over the next 2 years. Postprocedural heart block requiring permanent pacemaker therapy is observed significantly more frequently with the self-expanding valve. Valve performance characteristics are excellent. Overall outcomes with this

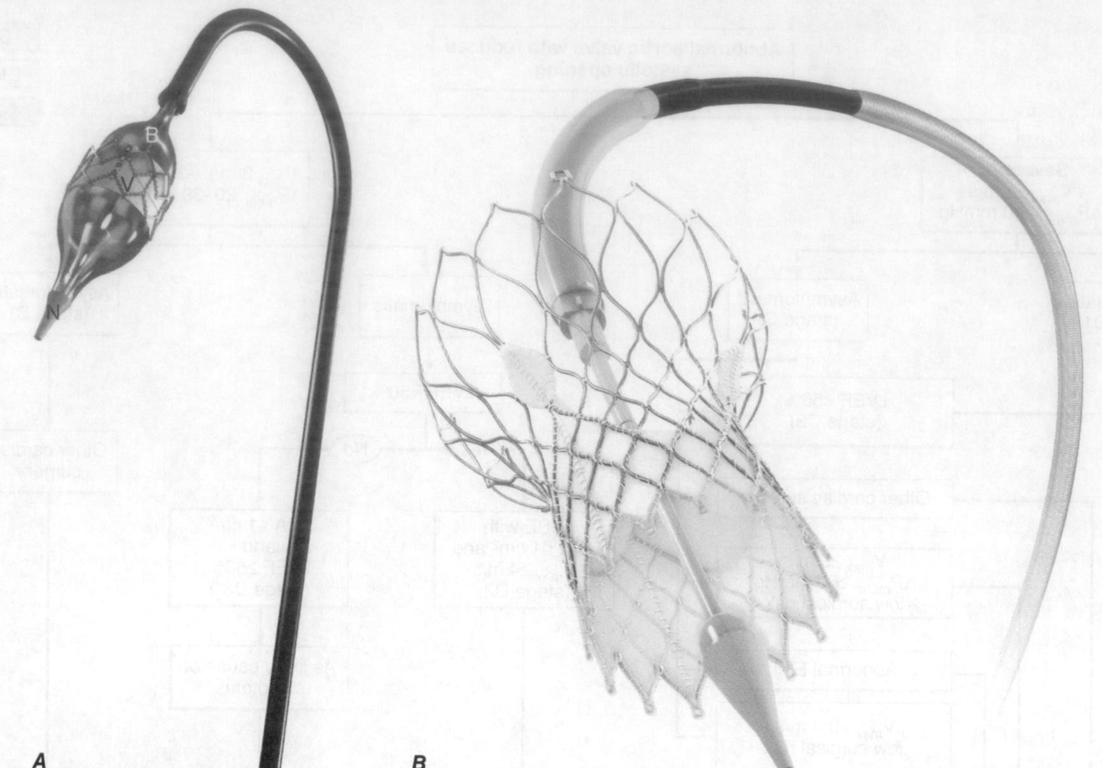

FIGURE 283-3 Balloon-expandable (*A*) and self-expanding (*B*) valves for transcatheter aortic valve replacement (TAVR). B, inflated balloon; N, nose cone; V, valve. *(Part A, courtesy of Edwards Lifesciences, Irvine, CA; with permission. NovaFlex+ is a trademark of Edwards Lifesciences Corporation. Part B, © Medtronic, Inc. 2015. Medtronic CoreValve Transcatheter Aortic Valve. CoreValve is a registered trademark of Medtronic, Inc.)*

transformative technology have been very favorable and have allowed the extension of AVR to groups of patients previously considered at high or prohibitive risk for conventional surgery. Nevertheless, some patients are not candidates for this procedure because their comorbidity profile, including an assessment of frailty, would make its undertaking inappropriate. The heart team is specifically charged with making challenging decisions of this nature. The use of these devices for the treatment of patients at intermediate operative risk and for those with structural deterioration of bioprosthetic aortic and mitral valves ("valve-in-valve"), as an alternative to reoperative valve replacement, is under active study.

Hazard ratio, 0.56 (95% CI, 0.43–0.73)
P<0.001
Standard therapy 68.0
TAVR 43.3
Death from any cause (%)
Months since randomization

No. at Risk

	0	6	12	18	24
TAVR	179	138	124	110	83
Standard therapy	179	121	85	62	42

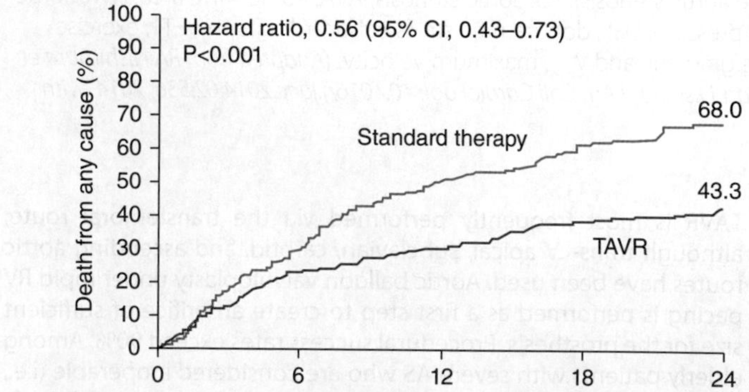

FIGURE 283-4 Twenty-four-month outcomes following transcatheter aortic valve replacement (TAVR) for inoperable patients in the PARTNER I trial (cohort B). CI, confidence interval. *(Adapted from RR Makkar et al: N Engl J Med 366:1696, 2012; with permission.)*

AORTIC REGURGITATION

ETIOLOGY

(Table 283-1) AR may be caused by primary valve disease or by primary aortic root disease.

Primary Valve Disease Rheumatic disease results in thickening, deformity, and shortening of the individual aortic valve cusps, changes that prevent their proper opening during systole and closure during diastole. A rheumatic origin is much less common in patients with isolated AR who do not have associated rheumatic mitral valve disease. Patients with congenital BAV disease may develop predominant AR,

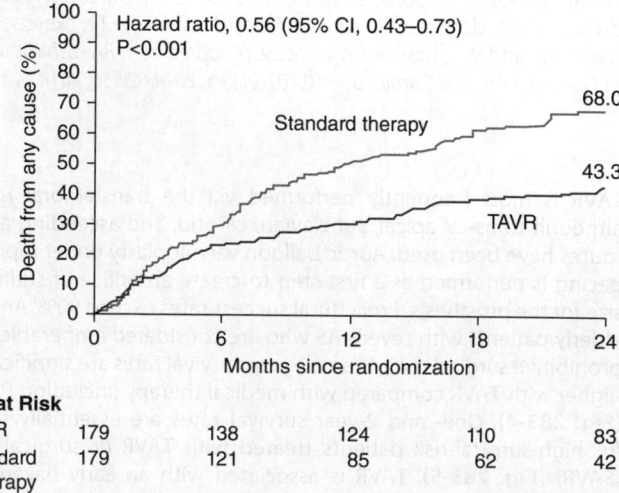

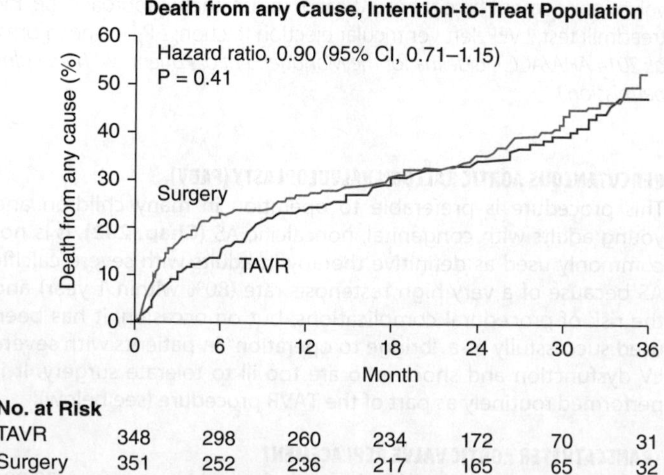

FIGURE 283-5 Thirty-six-month outcomes following transcatheter aortic valve replacement (TAVR) for high-surgical-risk patients (cohort A) in the PARTNER I trial. CI, confidence interval. *(Adapted from SK Kodali et al: New Engl J Med 366:1686, 2012.)*

and approximately 20% of patients will require aortic valve surgery between 10 and 40 years of age. Congenital fenestrations of the aortic valve occasionally produce mild AR. Membranous subaortic stenosis often leads to thickening and scarring of the aortic valve leaflets with secondary AR. Prolapse of an aortic cusp, resulting in progressive chronic AR, occurs in approximately 15% of patients with ventricular septal defect (Chap. 282) but may also occur as an isolated phenomenon or as a consequence of myxomatous degeneration sometimes associated with mitral and/or tricuspid valve involvement.

AR may result from infective endocarditis, which can develop on a valve previously affected by rheumatic disease, a congenitally deformed valve, or on a normal aortic valve, and may lead to perforation or erosion of one or more leaflets. The aortic valve leaflets may become scarred and retracted during the course of syphilis or ankylosing spondylitis and contribute further to the AR that derives primarily from the associated root disease. Although traumatic rupture or avulsion of an aortic cusp is an uncommon cause of acute AR, it represents the most frequent serious lesion in patients surviving nonpenetrating cardiac injuries. The coexistence of hemodynamically significant AS with AR usually excludes all the rarer forms of AR because it occurs almost exclusively in patients with rheumatic or congenital AR. In patients with AR due to primary valvular disease, dilation of the aortic annulus may occur secondarily and lead to worsening regurgitation.

Primary Aortic Root Disease AR also may be due entirely to marked aortic annular dilation, i.e., aortic root disease, without primary involvement of the valve leaflets; widening of the aortic annulus and separation of the aortic leaflets are responsible for the AR (Chap. 301). Medial degeneration of the ascending aorta, which may or may not be associated with other manifestations of Marfan's syndrome, idiopathic dilation of the aorta; annuloaortic ectasia; osteogenesis imperfecta; and severe, chronic hypertension may all widen the aortic annulus and lead to progressive AR. Occasionally AR is caused by retrograde dissection of the aorta involving the aortic annulus. Syphilis and ankylosing spondylitis, both of which may affect the aortic leaflets, may also be associated with cellular infiltration and scarring of the media of the thoracic aorta, leading to aortic dilation, aneurysm formation, and severe regurgitation. In syphilis of the aorta (Chap. 206), now a very rare condition, the involvement of the intima may narrow the coronary ostia, which in turn may be responsible for myocardial ischemia.

PATHOPHYSIOLOGY

The total stroke volume ejected by the LV (i.e., the sum of the effective forward stroke volume and the volume of blood that regurgitates back into the LV) is increased in patients with AR. In patients with severe AR, the volume of regurgitant flow may equal the effective forward stroke volume. In contrast to MR, in which a portion of the LV stroke volume is delivered into the low-pressure LA, in AR the entire LV stroke volume is ejected into a high-pressure zone, the aorta. An increase in the LV end-diastolic volume (increased preload) constitutes the major hemodynamic compensation for AR. The dilation and eccentric hypertrophy of the LV allow this chamber to eject a larger stroke volume without requiring any increase in the relative shortening of each myofibril. Therefore, severe AR may occur with a normal effective forward stroke volume and a normal LVEF (total [forward plus regurgitant] stroke volume/end-diastolic volume), together with an elevated LV end-diastolic pressure and volume. However, through the operation of Laplace's law, LV dilation increases the LV systolic tension required to develop any given level of systolic pressure. Chronic AR is, thus, a state in which LV preload and afterload are both increased. Ultimately, these adaptive measures fail. As LV function deteriorates, the end-diastolic volume rises further and the forward stroke volume and EF decline. Deterioration of LV function often precedes the development of symptoms. Considerable thickening of the LV wall also occurs with chronic AR, and at autopsy, the hearts of these patients may be among the largest encountered, sometimes weighing >1000 g.

The reverse pressure gradient from aorta to LV, which drives the AR flow, falls progressively during diastole, accounting for the decrescendo nature of the diastolic murmur. Equilibration between aortic and LV pressures may occur toward the end of diastole in patients with chronic severe AR, particularly when the heart rate is slow. In patients with acute severe AR, the LV is unprepared for the regurgitant volume load. LV compliance is normal or reduced, and LV diastolic pressures rise rapidly, occasionally to levels >40 mmHg. The LV pressure may exceed the LA pressure toward the end of diastole, and this reversed pressure gradient closes the mitral valve prematurely.

In patients with chronic severe AR, the effective forward CO usually is normal or only slightly reduced at rest, but often it fails to rise normally during exertion. An early sign of LV dysfunction is a reduction in the EF. In advanced stages, there may be considerable elevation of the LA, PA wedge, PA, and RV pressures and lowering of the forward CO at rest.

Myocardial ischemia may occur in patients with AR because myocardial oxygen requirements are elevated by LV dilation, hypertrophy, and elevated LV systolic tension, and coronary blood flow may be compromised. A large fraction of coronary blood flow occurs during diastole, when arterial pressure is low, thereby reducing coronary perfusion or driving pressure. This combination of increased oxygen demand and reduced supply may cause myocardial ischemia, particularly of the subendocardium, even in the absence of epicardial CAD.

HISTORY

Approximately three-fourths of patients with pure or predominant valvular AR are men; women predominate among patients with primary valvular AR who have associated rheumatic mitral valve disease. A history compatible with infective endocarditis may sometimes be elicited from patients with rheumatic or congenital involvement of the aortic valve, and the infection often precipitates or seriously aggravates preexisting symptoms.

In patients with *acute severe AR*, as may occur in infective endocarditis, aortic dissection, or trauma, the LV cannot dilate sufficiently to maintain stroke volume, and LV diastolic pressure rises rapidly with associated marked elevations of LA and PA wedge pressures. Pulmonary edema and/or cardiogenic shock may develop rapidly.

Chronic severe AR may have a long latent period, and patients may remain relatively asymptomatic for as long as 10–15 years. However, uncomfortable awareness of the heartbeat, especially on lying down, may be an early complaint. Sinus tachycardia, during exertion or with emotion, or premature ventricular contractions may produce particularly uncomfortable palpitations as well as head pounding. These complaints may persist for many years before the development of exertional dyspnea, usually the first symptom of diminished cardiac reserve. The dyspnea is followed by orthopnea, paroxysmal nocturnal dyspnea, and excessive diaphoresis. Anginal chest pain even in the absence of CAD may occur in patients with severe AR, even in younger patients. Anginal pain may develop at rest as well as during exertion. Nocturnal angina may be a particularly troublesome symptom, and it may be accompanied by marked diaphoresis. The anginal episodes can be prolonged and often do not respond satisfactorily to sublingual nitroglycerin. Systemic fluid accumulation, including congestive hepatomegaly and ankle edema, may develop late in the course of the disease.

PHYSICAL FINDINGS

In chronic severe AR, the jarring of the entire body and the bobbing motion of the head with each systole can be appreciated, and the abrupt distention and collapse of the larger arteries are easily visible. The examination should be directed toward the detection of conditions predisposing to AR, such as bicuspid valve, endocarditis, Marfan's syndrome, and ankylosing spondylitis.

Arterial Pulse A rapidly rising "water-hammer" pulse, which collapses suddenly as arterial pressure falls rapidly during late systole and diastole (Corrigan's pulse), and capillary pulsations, an alternate flushing and paling of the skin at the root of the nail while pressure is applied to the tip of the nail (Quincke's pulse), are characteristic of chronic severe AR. A booming "pistol-shot" sound can be heard over the femoral arteries (Traube's sign), and a to-and-fro murmur (Duroziez's sign) is audible if the femoral artery is lightly compressed with a stethoscope.

The arterial pulse pressure is widened as a result of both systolic hypertension and a lowering of the diastolic pressure. The measurement of arterial diastolic pressure with a sphygmomanometer may be complicated by the fact that systolic sounds are frequently heard with the cuff completely deflated. However, the level of cuff pressure at the time of muffling of the Korotkoff sounds (phase IV) generally corresponds fairly closely to the true intraarterial diastolic pressure. As the disease progresses and the LV end-diastolic pressure rises, the arterial diastolic pressure may actually rise as well, because the aortic diastolic pressure cannot fall below the LV end-diastolic pressure. For the same reason, acute severe AR may also be accompanied by only a slight widening of the pulse pressure. Such patients are invariably tachycardic as the heart rate increases in an attempt to preserve the CO.

Palpation In patients with chronic severe AR, the LV impulse is heaving and displaced laterally and inferiorly. The systolic expansion and diastolic retraction of the apex are prominent. A diastolic thrill may be palpable along the left sternal border in thin-chested individuals, and a prominent systolic thrill may be palpable in the suprasternal notch and transmitted upward along the carotid arteries. This systolic thrill and the accompanying murmur do not necessarily signify the coexistence of AS. In some patients with AR or with combined AS and AR, the carotid arterial pulse may be bisferiens, i.e., with two systolic waves separated by a trough (see Fig. 267-2*D*).

Auscultation In patients with severe AR, the aortic valve closure sound (A_2) is usually absent. A systolic ejection sound is audible in patients with BAV disease, and occasionally an S_4 also may be heard. The murmur of chronic AR is typically a high-pitched, blowing, decrescendo diastolic murmur, heard best in the third intercostal space along the left sternal border (see Fig. 267-5*B*). In patients with mild AR, this murmur is brief, but as the severity increases, it generally becomes louder and longer, indeed holodiastolic. When the murmur is soft, it can be heard best with the diaphragm of the stethoscope and with the patient sitting up, leaning forward, and with the breath held in forced expiration. In patients in whom the AR is caused by primary valvular disease, the diastolic murmur is usually louder along the left than the right sternal border. However, when the murmur is heard best along the right sternal border, it suggests that the AR is caused by aneurysmal dilation of the aortic root. "Cooing" or musical diastolic murmurs suggest eversion of an aortic cusp vibrating in the regurgitant stream.

A mid-systolic ejection murmur is frequently audible in isolated AR. It is generally heard best at the base of the heart and is transmitted along the carotid arteries. This murmur may be quite loud without signifying aortic obstruction. A third murmur sometimes heard in patients with severe AR is the *Austin Flint murmur*, a soft, low-pitched, rumbling mid-to-late diastolic murmur. It is probably produced by the diastolic displacement of the anterior leaflet of the mitral valve by the AR stream and is not associated with hemodynamically significant mitral obstruction. The auscultatory features of AR are intensified by strenuous and sustained handgrip, which augments systemic vascular resistance.

In acute severe AR, the elevation of LV end-diastolic pressure may lead to early closure of the mitral valve, a soft S_1, a pulse pressure that is not particularly wide, and a soft, short, early diastolic murmur of AR.

LABORATORY EXAMINATION

ECG In patients with chronic severe AR, the ECG signs of LV hypertrophy become manifest (Chap. 268). In addition, these patients frequently exhibit ST-segment depression and T-wave inversion in leads I, aVL, V_5, and V_6 ("LV strain"). Left-axis deviation and/or QRS prolongation denote diffuse myocardial disease, generally associated with patchy fibrosis, and usually signify a poor prognosis.

Echocardiogram LV size is increased in chronic AR and systolic function is normal or even supernormal until myocardial contractility declines, as signaled by a decrease in EF or increase in the end-systolic dimension. A rapid, high-frequency diastolic fluttering of the anterior mitral leaflet produced by the impact of the regurgitant jet is a characteristic finding. The echocardiogram is also useful in determining the cause of AR, by detecting dilation of the aortic annulus and root, aortic dissection (see Fig. 270e-5), or primary leaflet pathology. With severe AR, the central jet width assessed by color flow Doppler imaging exceeds 65% of the LV outflow tract, the regurgitant volume is ≥60 mL/beat, the regurgitant fraction is ≥50%, and there is diastolic flow reversal in the proximal descending thoracic aorta. The continuous-wave Doppler profile of the AR jet shows a rapid deceleration time in patients with acute severe AR, due to the rapid increase in LV diastolic pressure. Surveillance transthoracic echocardiography forms the cornerstone of longitudinal follow-up and allows for the early detection of changes in LV size and/or function. For patients in whom transthoracic echocardiography (TTE) is limited by poor acoustical windows or inadequate semiquantitative assessment of LV function or the severity of the regurgitation, cardiac magnetic resonance imaging (MRI) can be performed. This modality also allows for accurate assessment of aortic size and contour. Transesophageal echocardiography (TEE) can also provide detailed anatomic assessment of the valve, root, and portions of the aorta.

Chest X-Ray In chronic severe AR, the apex is displaced downward and to the left in the frontal projection. In the left anterior oblique and lateral projections, the LV is displaced posteriorly and encroaches on the spine. When AR is caused by primary disease of the aortic root, aneurysmal dilation of the aorta may be noted, and the aorta may fill the retrosternal space in the lateral view. Echocardiography, cardiac MRI, and chest CT angiography are more sensitive than the chest x-ray for the detection of root and ascending aortic enlargement.

Cardiac Catheterization and Angiography When needed, right and left heart catheterization with contrast aortography can provide confirmation of the magnitude of regurgitation and the status of LV function. Coronary angiography is performed routinely in appropriate patients prior to surgery.

TREATMENT AORTIC REGURGITATION

ACUTE AORTIC REGURGITATION (FIG. 283-6)

Patients with acute severe AR may respond to intravenous diuretics and vasodilators (such as sodium nitroprusside), but stabilization is usually short-lived and operation is indicated urgently. Intraaortic balloon counterpulsation is contraindicated. Beta blockers are also best avoided so as not to reduce the CO further or slow the heart rate, thus allowing more time for diastolic filling of the LV. Surgery is the treatment of choice and is usually necessary within 24 h of diagnosis.

CHRONIC AORTIC REGURGITATION

Early symptoms of dyspnea and effort intolerance respond to treatment with diuretics; vasodilators (ACE inhibitors, dihydropyridine calcium channel blockers, or hydralazine) may be useful as well. Surgery can then be performed in a more controlled setting. The use of vasodilators to extend the compensated phase of chronic severe AR before the onset of symptoms or the development of LV dysfunction is more controversial and less well established. Systolic blood pressure should be controlled (goal <140 mmHg) in patients with chronic AR, and vasodilators are an excellent first choice as antihypertensive agents. It is often difficult to achieve adequate control because of the increased stroke volume that accompanies severe AR. Cardiac arrhythmias and systemic infections are poorly tolerated in patients with severe AR and must be treated promptly and vigorously. Although nitroglycerin and long-acting nitrates are not as helpful in relieving anginal pain as they are in patients with ischemic heart disease, they are worth a trial. Patients with

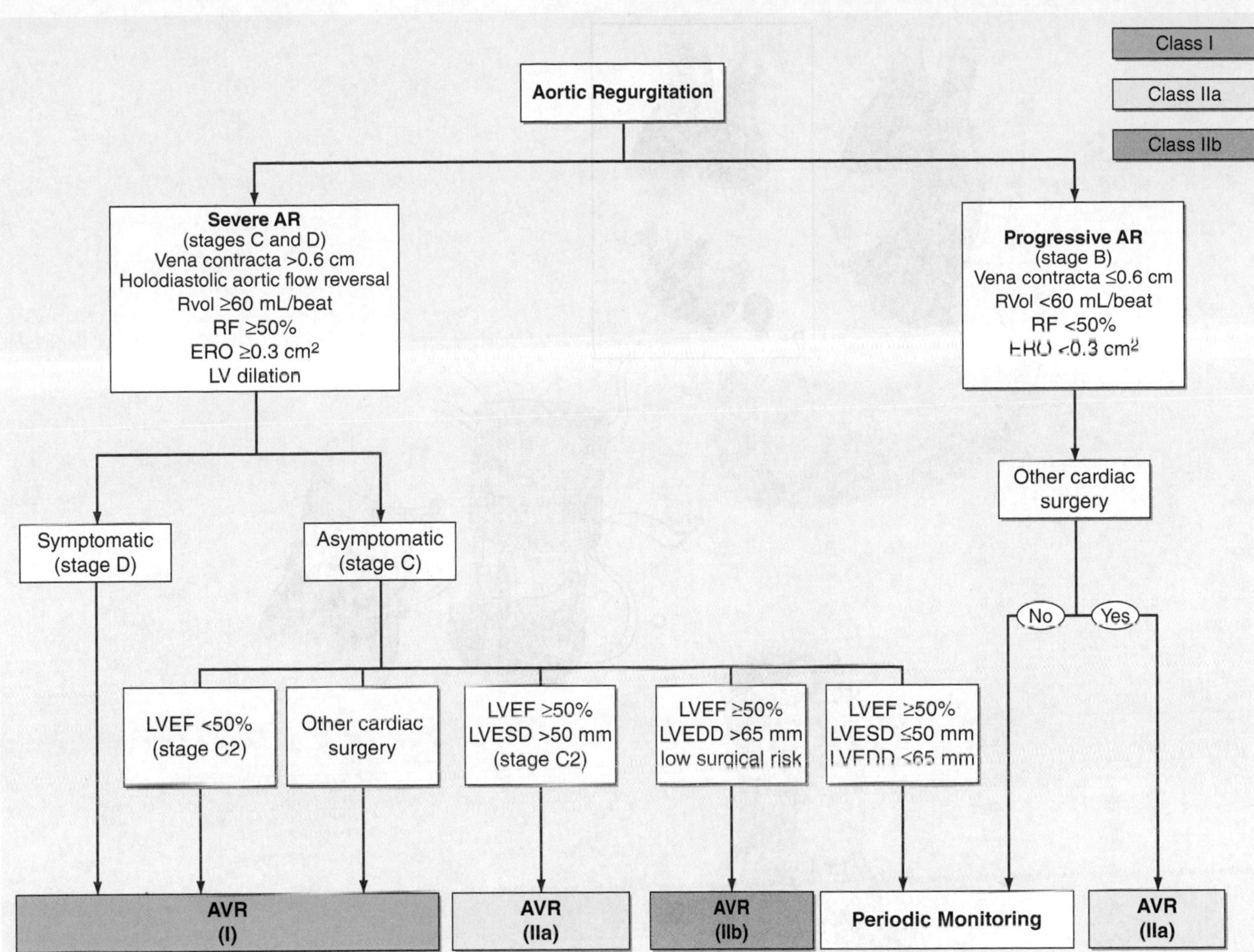

FIGURE 283-6 Management of patients with aortic regurgitation. See legend for Fig. 283-2 for explanation of treatment recommendations (Class I, IIa, and IIb) and disease stages (B, C1, C2, D). Preoperative coronary angiography should be performed routinely as determined by age, symptoms, and coronary risk factors. Cardiac catheterization and angiography may also be helpful when there is a discrepancy between clinical and noninvasive findings. Patients who do not meet criteria for intervention should be monitored periodically with clinical and echocardiographic follow-up. AR, aortic regurgitation; AVR, aortic valve replacement (valve repair may be appropriate in selected patients); ERO, effective regurgitant orifice; LV, left ventricular; LVEDD, left ventricular end-diastolic dimension; LVEF, left ventricular ejection fraction; LVESD, left ventricular end-systolic dimension; RF, regurgitant fraction; RVol, regurgitant volume. *(Adapted from RA Nishimura et al: 2014 AHA/ACC Guideline for the Management of Patients with Valvular Heart Disease. J Am Coll Cardiol doi: 10.1016/j.jacc.2014.02.536, 2014, with permission.)*

syphilitic aortitis should receive a full course of penicillin therapy (Chap. 206). Beta blockers and the angiotensin receptor blocker losartan may be useful to retard the rate of aortic root enlargement in young patients with Marfan's syndrome and aortic root dilation. Early reports of the efficacy of losartan in patients with Marfan's syndrome have led to its use in other populations of patients including those with BAV disease and aortopathy. The use of beta blockers in patients with valvular AR was previously felt to be relatively contraindicated due to concerns that the resulting slowing of the heart rate would allow more time for diastolic regurgitation. More recent observational reports, however, suggest that beta blockers may provide functional benefit in patients with chronic AR. Beta blockers can sometimes provide incremental blood pressure lowering in patients with chronic AR and hypertension. Patients with severe AR, particularly those with an associated aortopathy, should avoid isometric exercises.

SURGICAL TREATMENT

In deciding on the advisability and proper timing of surgical treatment, two points should be kept in mind: (1) patients with chronic severe AR usually do not become symptomatic until *after* the development of myocardial dysfunction; and (2) when delayed too long (defined as >1 year from onset of symptoms or LV dysfunction), surgical treatment often does not restore normal LV function. Therefore, in patients with chronic severe AR, careful clinical follow-up and noninvasive testing with echocardiography at approximately 6- to 12-month intervals are necessary if operation is to be undertaken at the optimal time, i.e., *after* the onset of LV dysfunction but *prior to* the development of severe symptoms. Exercise testing may be helpful to assess effort tolerance more objectively. Operation can be deferred as long as the patient both remains asymptomatic and retains normal LV function without severe chamber dilation.

AVR is indicated for the treatment of severe AR in symptomatic patients irrespective of LV function. In general, the operation should be carried out in asymptomatic patients with severe AR and progressive LV dysfunction defined by an LVEF <50%, an LV end-systolic dimension >50 mm, or an LV diastolic dimension >65 mm. Smaller dimensions may be appropriate thresholds in individuals of smaller stature. Patients with severe AR without indications for operation should be followed by clinical and echocardiographic examination every 6–12 months.

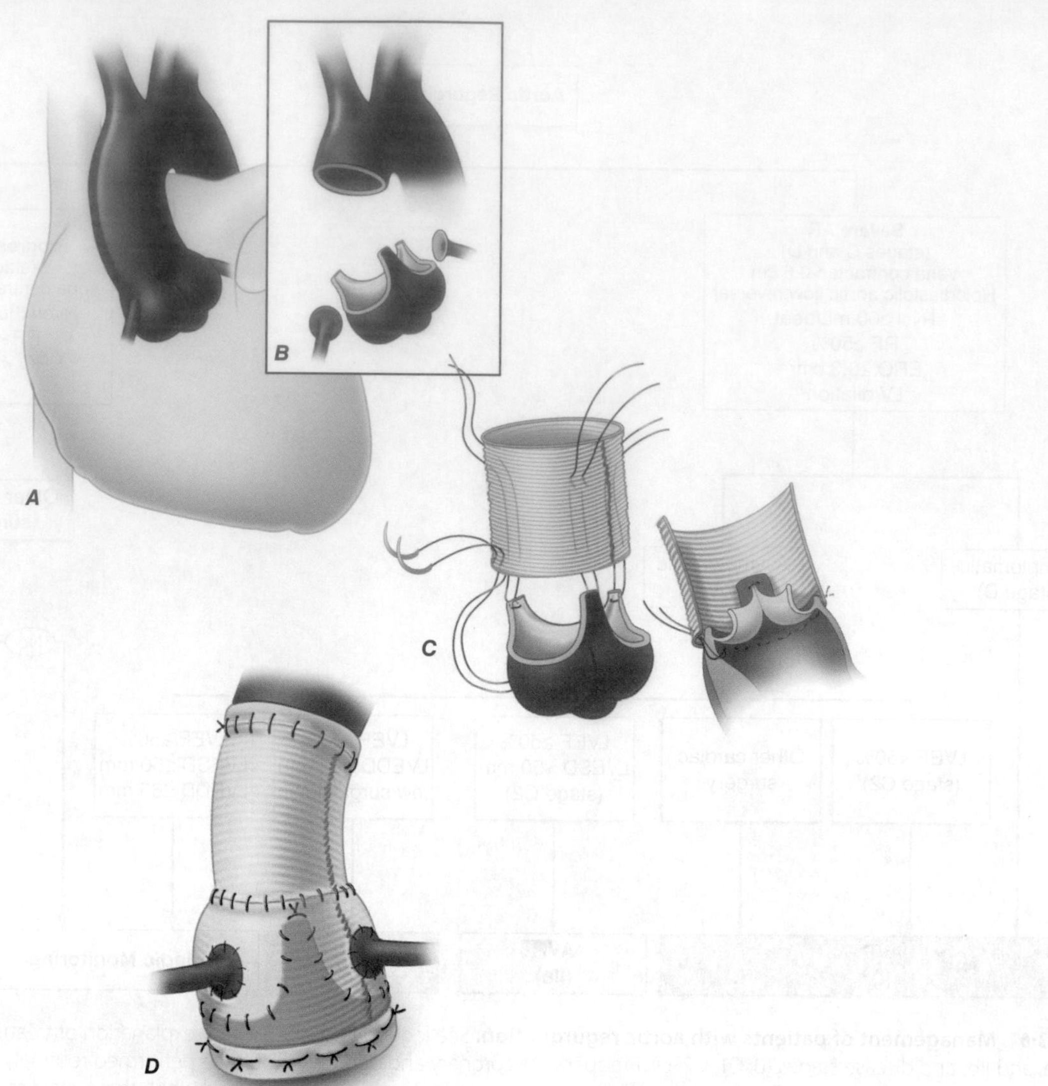

FIGURE 283-7 Valve-sparing aortic root reconstruction (David procedure). *(From P Steltzer et al [eds]: Valvular Heart Disease: A Companion to Braunwald's Heart Disease, 3rd ed, Fig 12-27, p. 200.)*

Surgical options for management of aortic valve and root disease have expanded considerably over the past decade. AVR with a suitable mechanical or tissue prosthesis is generally necessary in patients with rheumatic AR and in many patients with other forms of regurgitation. Rarely, when a leaflet has been perforated during infective endocarditis or torn from its attachments to the aortic annulus by thoracic trauma, primary surgical repair may be possible. When AR is due to aneurysmal dilation of the root or proximal ascending aorta rather than to primary valve involvement, it may be possible to reduce or eliminate the regurgitation by narrowing the annulus or by excising a portion of the aortic root without replacing the valve. Elective, valve-sparing aortic root reconstruction generally involves reimplantation of the valve in a contoured graft with reattachment of the coronary artery buttons into the side of the graft and is best undertaken in specialized surgical centers (Fig. 283-7). Resuspension of the native aortic valve leaflets is possible in approximately 50% of patients with acute AR in the setting of type A aortic dissection. In other conditions, however, regurgitation can be effectively eliminated only by replacing the aortic valve, the dilated or aneurysmal ascending aorta responsible for the regurgitation, and implanting a composite valve-graft conduit. This formidable procedure entails a higher risk than isolated AVR.

As in patients with other valvular abnormalities, both the operative risk and the late mortality rate are largely dependent on the stage of the disease and myocardial function at the time of operation. The overall operative mortality rate for isolated AVR (performed for either or both AS or AR) is approximately 2% (Table 283-2). However, patients with AR, marked cardiac enlargement, and prolonged LV dysfunction experience an operative mortality rate of approximately 10% and a late mortality rate of approximately 5% per year due to LV failure despite a technically satisfactory operation. Nonetheless, because of the very poor prognosis with medical management, even patients with LV systolic failure should be considered for operation.

Patients with acute severe AR require prompt surgical treatment, which may be lifesaving.

284 Mitral Valve Disease

Patrick T. O'Gara, Joseph Loscalzo

The role of the physical examination in the evaluation of patients with valvular heart disease is also considered in Chaps. 51e and 267; of electrocardiography (ECG) in Chap. 268; of echocardiography and other noninvasive imaging techniques in Chap. 270e; and of cardiac catheterization and angiography in Chap. 272.

MITRAL STENOSIS

ETIOLOGY AND PATHOLOGY

Rheumatic fever is the leading cause of mitral stenosis (MS) (Table 284-1). Other less common etiologies of obstruction to left ventricular inflow include congenital mitral valve stenosis, cor triatriatum, mitral annular calcification with extension onto the leaflets, systemic lupus erythematosus, rheumatoid arthritis, left atrial myxoma, and infective endocarditis with large vegetations. Pure or predominant MS occurs in approximately 40% of all patients with rheumatic heart disease and a history of rheumatic fever (Chap. 381). In other patients with rheumatic heart disease, lesser degrees of MS may accompany mitral regurgitation (MR) and aortic valve disease. With reductions in the incidence of acute rheumatic fever, particularly in temperate climates and developed countries, the incidence of MS has declined considerably over the past several decades. However, it remains a major problem in developing nations, especially in tropical and semitropical climates.

In rheumatic MS, chronic inflammation leads to diffuse thickening of the valve leaflets with formation of fibrous tissue and/or calcific deposits. The mitral commissures fuse, the chordae tendineae fuse and shorten, the valvular cusps become rigid, and these changes, in turn, lead to narrowing at the apex of the funnel-shaped ("fish-mouth") valve. Although the initial insult to the mitral valve is rheumatic, later changes may be exacerbated by a nonspecific process resulting from trauma to the valve due to altered flow patterns. Calcification of the stenotic mitral valve immobilizes the leaflets and narrows the orifice further. Thrombus formation and arterial embolization may arise from the calcific valve itself, but in patients with atrial fibrillation (AF), thrombi arise more frequently from the dilated left atrium (LA), particularly from within the LA appendage.

TABLE 284-1 MAJOR CAUSES OF MITRAL VALVE DISEASE

Valve Lesion	Etiologies
Mitral stenosis	Rheumatic fever
	Congenital
	Severe mitral annular calcification
	SLE, RA
Mitral regurgitation	Acute
	Endocarditis
	Papillary muscle rupture (post-MI)
	Trauma
	Chordal rupture/leaflet flail (MVP, IE)
	Chronic
	Myxomatous (MVP)
	Rheumatic fever
	Endocarditis (healed)
	Mitral annular calcification
	Congenital (cleft, AV canal)
	HOCM with SAM
	Ischemic (LV remodeling)
	Dilated cardiomyopathy
	Radiation

Abbreviations: AV, atrioventricular; IE, infective endocarditis; HOCM, hypertrophic obstructive cardiomyopathy; LV, left ventricular; MI, myocardial infarction; MVP, mitral valve prolapse; RA, rheumatoid arthritis; SAM, systolic anterior motion; SLE, systemic lupus erythematosus.

PATHOPHYSIOLOGY

In normal adults, the area of the mitral valve orifice is 4–6 cm². In the presence of significant obstruction, i.e., when the orifice area is reduced to < ~2 cm², blood can flow from the LA to the left ventricle (LV) only if propelled by an abnormally elevated left atrioventricular pressure gradient, the hemodynamic hallmark of MS. When the mitral valve opening is reduced to ≤1.5 cm², referred to as "severe" MS, an LA pressure of ~25 mmHg is required to maintain a normal cardiac output (CO). The elevated pulmonary venous and pulmonary arterial (PA) wedge pressures reduce pulmonary compliance, contributing to exertional dyspnea. The first bouts of dyspnea are usually precipitated by clinical events that increase the rate of blood flow across the mitral orifice, resulting in further elevation of the LA pressure (see below).

To assess the severity of obstruction hemodynamically, both the transvalvular pressure gradient and the flow rate must be measured (Chap. 272). The latter depends not only on the CO but on the heart rate, as well. An increase in heart rate shortens diastole proportionately more than systole and diminishes the time available for flow across the mitral valve. Therefore, at any given level of CO, tachycardia, including that associated with rapid AF, augments the transvalvular pressure gradient and elevates further the LA pressure. Similar considerations apply to the pathophysiology of tricuspid stenosis.

The LV diastolic pressure and ejection fraction (EF) are normal in isolated MS. In MS and sinus rhythm, the elevated LA and PA wedge pressures exhibit a prominent atrial contraction pattern (*a* wave) and a gradual pressure decline after the *v* wave and mitral valve opening (*y* descent). In severe MS and whenever pulmonary vascular resistance is significantly increased, the PA pressure (PAP) is elevated at rest and rises further during exercise, often causing secondary elevations of right ventricular (RV) end-diastolic pressure and volume.

Cardiac Output In patients with severe MS (mitral valve orifice 1–1.5 cm²), the CO is normal or almost so at rest, but rises subnormally during exertion. In patients with very severe MS (valve area <1 cm²), particularly those in whom pulmonary vascular resistance is markedly elevated, the CO is subnormal at rest and may fail to rise or may even decline during activity.

Pulmonary Hypertension The clinical and hemodynamic features of MS are influenced importantly by the level of the PAP. Pulmonary hypertension results from: (1) passive backward transmission of the elevated LA pressure; (2) pulmonary arteriolar constriction (the so-called "second stenosis"), which presumably is triggered by LA and pulmonary venous hypertension (reactive pulmonary hypertension); (3) interstitial edema in the walls of the small pulmonary vessels; and (4) at end stage, organic obliterative changes in the pulmonary vascular bed. Severe pulmonary hypertension results in RV enlargement, secondary tricuspid regurgitation (TR), and pulmonic regurgitation (PR), as well as right-sided heart failure.

SYMPTOMS

In temperate climates, the latent period between the initial attack of rheumatic carditis (in the increasingly rare circumstances in which a history of one can be elicited) and the development of symptoms due to MS is generally about two decades; most patients begin to experience disability in the fourth decade of life. Studies carried out before the development of mitral valvotomy revealed that once a patient with MS became seriously symptomatic, the disease progressed inexorably to death within 2–5 years.

In patients whose mitral orifices are large enough to accommodate a normal blood flow with only mild elevations of LA pressure, marked elevations of this pressure leading to dyspnea and cough may be precipitated by sudden changes in the heart rate, volume status, or CO, as, for example, with severe exertion, excitement, fever, severe anemia, paroxysmal AF and other tachycardias, sexual intercourse, pregnancy, and thyrotoxicosis. As MS progresses, lesser degrees of stress precipitate dyspnea, the patient becomes limited in daily activities, and orthopnea and paroxysmal nocturnal dyspnea develop. The development of persistent AF often marks a turning point in the patient's course and is generally associated with acceleration of the rate at which symptoms progress. *Hemoptysis* (Chap. 48) results from rupture of pulmonary-bronchial venous connections secondary to pulmonary venous hypertension. It occurs most frequently in patients who have elevated LA pressures without markedly elevated pulmonary vascular resistances and is rarely fatal. *Recurrent pulmonary emboli* (Chap. 300), sometimes with infarction, are an important cause of morbidity and mortality late in the course of MS. *Pulmonary infections*, i.e., bronchitis, bronchopneumonia, and lobar pneumonia, commonly complicate untreated MS, especially during the winter months.

Pulmonary Changes In addition to the aforementioned changes in the pulmonary vascular bed, fibrous thickening of the walls of the alveoli and pulmonary capillaries occurs commonly in MS. The vital capacity, total lung capacity, maximal breathing capacity, and oxygen uptake per unit of ventilation are reduced (Chap. 306e). Pulmonary compliance falls further as pulmonary capillary pressure rises during exercise.

Thrombi and Emboli *Thrombi* may form in the left atria, particularly within the enlarged atrial appendages of patients with MS. Systemic embolization, the incidence of which is 10–20%, occurs more frequently in patients with AF, in patients >65 years of age, and in those with a reduced CO. However, systemic embolization may be the presenting feature in otherwise asymptomatic patients with only mild MS.

PHYSICAL FINDINGS

(See also Chaps. 51e and 267)

Inspection and Palpation In patients with severe MS, there may be a malar flush with pinched and blue facies. In patients with sinus rhythm and severe pulmonary hypertension or associated tricuspid stenosis (TS), the jugular venous pulse reveals prominent *a* waves due to vigorous right atrial systole. The systemic arterial pressure is usually normal or slightly low. An RV tap along the left sternal border signifies an enlarged RV. A diastolic thrill may rarely be present at the cardiac apex, with the patient in the left lateral recumbent position.

Auscultation The first heart sound (S_1) is usually accentuated in the early stages of the disease and slightly delayed. The pulmonic component of the second heart sound (P_2) also is often accentuated with elevated PA pressures, and the two components of the second heart sound (S_2) are closely split. The opening snap (OS) of the mitral valve is most readily audible in expiration at, or just medial to, the cardiac apex. This sound generally follows the sound of aortic valve closure (A_2) by 0.05–0.12 s. The time interval between A_2 and OS varies inversely with the severity of the MS. The OS is followed by a low-pitched, rumbling, diastolic murmur, heard best at the apex with the patient in the left lateral recumbent position (see Fig. 267-5); it is accentuated by mild exercise (e.g., a few rapid sit-ups) carried out just before auscultation. In general, the duration of this murmur correlates with the severity of the stenosis in patients with preserved CO. In patients with sinus rhythm, the murmur often reappears or becomes louder during atrial systole (presystolic accentuation). Soft, grade I or II/VI systolic murmurs are commonly heard at the apex or along the left sternal border in patients with pure MS and do not necessarily signify the presence of MR. Hepatomegaly, ankle edema, ascites, and pleural effusion, particularly in the right pleural cavity, may occur in patients with MS and RV failure.

Associated Lesions With severe pulmonary hypertension, a pansystolic murmur produced by functional TR may be audible along the left sternal border. This murmur is usually louder during inspiration and diminishes during forced expiration (Carvallo's sign). When the CO is markedly reduced in MS, the typical auscultatory findings, including the diastolic rumbling murmur, may not be detectable (silent MS), but they may reappear as compensation is restored. The *Graham Steell murmur* of PR, a high-pitched, diastolic, decrescendo blowing murmur along the left sternal border, results from dilation of the pulmonary valve ring and occurs in patients with mitral valve disease and severe pulmonary hypertension. This murmur may be indistinguishable from the more common murmur produced by aortic regurgitation (AR), although it may increase in intensity with inspiration and is accompanied by a loud and often palpable P_2.

LABORATORY EXAMINATION

ECG In MS and sinus rhythm, the P wave usually suggests LA enlargement (see Fig. 268-8). It may become tall and peaked in lead II and upright in lead V_1 when severe pulmonary hypertension or TS complicates MS and right atrial (RA) enlargement occurs. The QRS complex is usually normal. However, with severe pulmonary hypertension, right axis deviation and RV hypertrophy are often present.

Echocardiogram (See also Chap. 270e) Transthoracic echocardiography (TTE) with color flow and spectral Doppler imaging provides critical information, including measurements of mitral inflow velocity during early (E wave) and late (A wave in patients in sinus rhythm) diastolic filling, estimates of the transvalvular peak and mean gradients and of the mitral orifice area, the presence and severity of any associated MR, the extent of leaflet calcification and restriction, the degree of distortion of the subvalvular apparatus, and the anatomic suitability for percutaneous mitral balloon valvotomy (percutaneous mitral balloon valvuloplasty [PMBV]; see below). In addition, TTE provides an assessment of LV and RV function, chamber sizes, an estimation of the PAP based on the tricuspid regurgitant jet velocity, and an indication of the presence and severity of any associated valvular lesions, such as aortic stenosis and/or regurgitation. Transesophageal echocardiography (TEE) provides superior images and should be used when TTE is inadequate for guiding management decisions. TEE is especially indicated to exclude the presence of LA thrombus prior to PMBV. The performance of TTE with exercise to evaluate the mean mitral diastolic gradient and PA pressures can be very helpful in the evaluation of patients with MS when there is a discrepancy between the clinical findings and the resting hemodynamics.

Chest X-Ray The earliest changes are straightening of the upper left border of the cardiac silhouette, prominence of the main PAs, dilation of the upper lobe pulmonary veins, and posterior displacement of the esophagus by an enlarged LA. Kerley B lines are fine, dense, opaque, horizontal lines that are most prominent in the lower and mid-lung fields and that result from distention of interlobular septae and lymphatics with edema when the resting mean LA pressure exceeds approximately 20 mmHg.

DIFFERENTIAL DIAGNOSIS

Like MS, significant MR may also be associated with a prominent diastolic murmur at the apex due to increased antegrade transmitral flow, but in patients with isolated MR, this diastolic murmur commences slightly later than in patients with MS, and there is often clear-cut evidence of LV enlargement. An OS and increased P_2 are absent, and S_1 is soft or absent. An apical pansystolic murmur of at least grade III/VI intensity as well as an S_3 suggest significant MR. Similarly, the apical mid-diastolic murmur associated with severe AR (*Austin Flint murmur*) may be mistaken for MS but can be differentiated from it because it is not intensified in presystole and becomes softer with administration of amyl nitrite or other arterial vasodilators. TS, which occurs rarely in the absence of MS, may mask many of the clinical features of MS or be clinically silent; when present, the diastolic murmur of TS increases with inspiration and the *y* descent in the jugular venous pulse is delayed.

Atrial septal defect (Chap. 282) may be mistaken for MS; in both conditions, there is often clinical, ECG, and chest x-ray evidence of RV enlargement and accentuation of pulmonary vascularity. However, the absence of LA enlargement and of Kerley B lines and the demonstration of fixed splitting of S_2 with a grade II or III mid-systolic murmur at the mid to upper left sternal border all favor atrial septal defect over MS. Atrial septal defects with large left-to-right shunts may result in functional TS because of the enhanced diastolic flow.

Left atrial myxoma (Chap. 289e) may obstruct LA emptying, causing dyspnea, a diastolic murmur, and hemodynamic changes resembling those of MS. However, patients with an LA myxoma often have features suggestive of a systemic disease, such as weight loss, fever, anemia, systemic emboli, and elevated serum IgG and interleukin 6 (IL-6) concentrations. The auscultatory findings may change markedly with body position. The diagnosis can be established by the demonstration of a characteristic echo-producing mass in the LA with TTE.

CARDIAC CATHETERIZATION

Left and right heart catheterization can be useful when there is a discrepancy between the clinical and noninvasive findings, including those from TEE and exercise echocardiographic testing as appropriate. Catheterization is helpful in assessing associated lesions, such as aortic stenosis (AS) and AR. Catheterization and coronary angiography are not usually necessary to aid in decision-making about surgery in patients younger than 65 years of age with typical findings of severe mitral obstruction on physical examination and TTE. In men older than 40 years of age, women older than 45 years of age, and younger patients with coronary risk factors, especially those with positive noninvasive stress tests for myocardial ischemia, coronary angiography is advisable preoperatively to identify patients with critical coronary obstructions that should be bypassed at the time of operation. Computed tomographic coronary angiography (CTCA) (Chap. 270e) is now often used to screen preoperatively for the presence of coronary artery disease (CAD) in patients with valvular heart disease and low pretest likelihood of CAD. Catheterization and left ventriculography may be useful in patients who have undergone PMBV or previous mitral valve surgery for MS, and who have redeveloped limiting symptoms, especially if questions regarding the severity of the valve lesion(s) remain after noninvasive study.

TREATMENT MITRAL STENOSIS

(Fig. 284-1) Penicillin prophylaxis of group A β-hemolytic streptococcal infections (Chap. 381) for secondary prevention of rheumatic fever is important for at-risk patients with rheumatic MS. Recommendations for infective endocarditis prophylaxis are similar to those for other valve lesions and are restricted to patients at high risk for complications from infection, including patients with a history of endocarditis. In symptomatic patients, some improvement usually occurs with restriction of sodium intake and small doses of oral diuretics. Beta blockers, nondihydropyridine calcium channel blockers (e.g., verapamil or diltiazem), and digitalis glycosides are useful in slowing the ventricular rate of patients with AF. Warfarin therapy targeted to an international normalized ratio (INR) of 2–3 should be administered indefinitely to patients with MS who have AF or a history of thromboembolism. The routine use of warfarin in patients in sinus rhythm with LA enlargement (maximal dimension

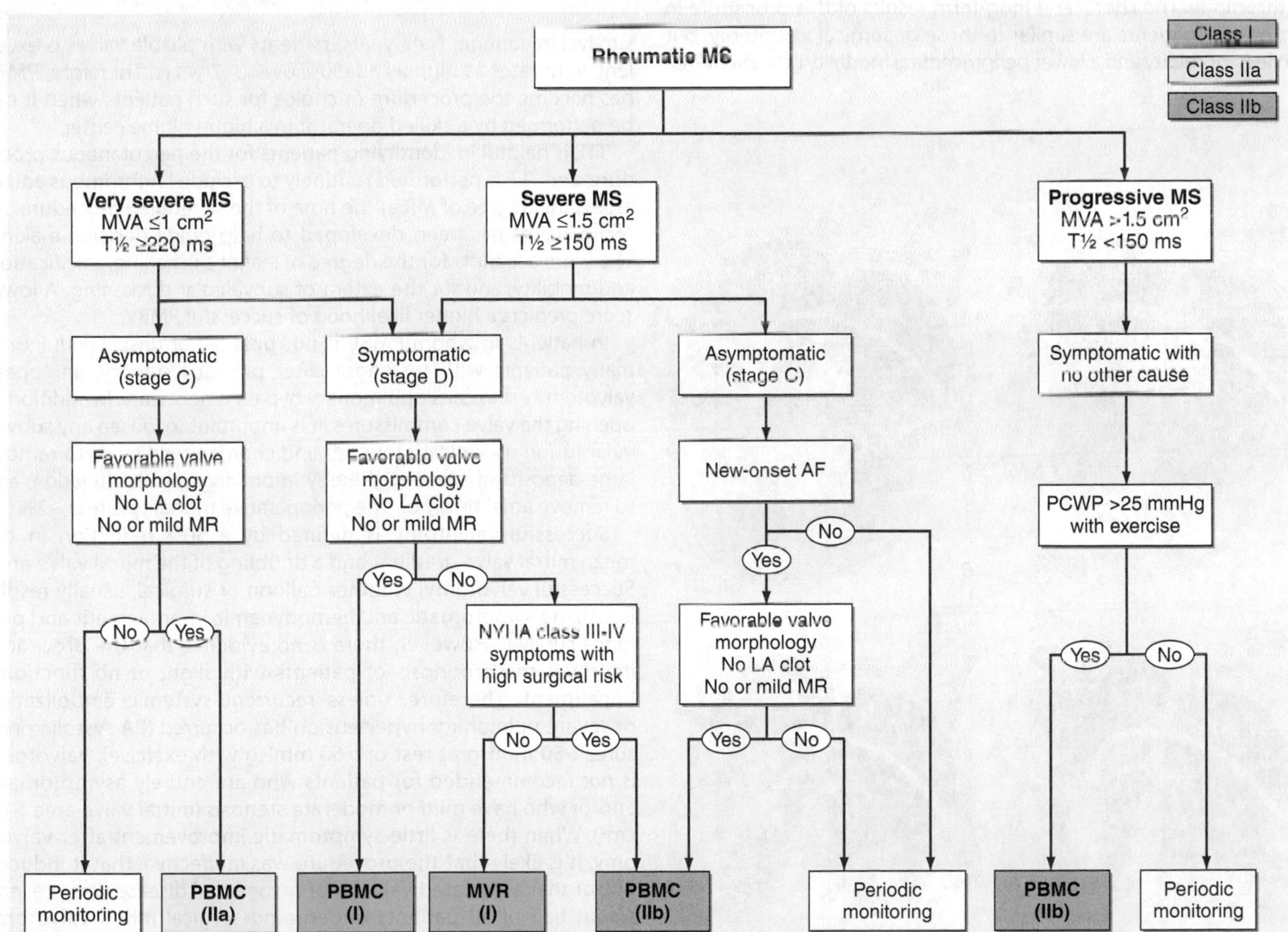

FIGURE 284-1 Management of rheumatic mitral stenosis. See legend for Fig. 283-2 for explanation of treatment recommendations (class I, IIa, IIb) and disease stages (C, D). Preoperative coronary angiography should be performed routinely as determined by age, symptoms, and coronary risk factors. Cardiac catheterization and angiography may also be helpful when there is a discrepancy between clinical and noninvasive findings. AF, atrial fibrillation; LA, left atrial; MR, mitral regurgitation; MS, mitral stenosis; MVA, mitral valve area; MVR, mitral valve surgery (repair or replacement); NYHA, New York Heart Association; PCWP, pulmonary capillary wedge pressure; PMBC, percutaneous mitral balloon commissurotomy; and T ½, pressure half-time. *(Adapted from RA Nishimura et al: 2014 AHA/ACC Guideline for the Management of Patients with Valvular Heart Disease. J Am Coll Cardiol doi: 10.1016/j.jacc.2014.02.536, 2014, with permission.)*

>5.5 cm) with or without spontaneous echo contrast is more controversial. The novel oral anticoagulants are not approved for use in patients with significant valvular heart disease.

If AF is of relatively recent onset in a patient whose MS is not severe enough to warrant PMBV or surgical commissurotomy, reversion to sinus rhythm pharmacologically or by means of electrical countershock is indicated. Usually, cardioversion should be undertaken after the patient has had at least 3 consecutive weeks of anticoagulant treatment to a therapeutic INR. If cardioversion is indicated more urgently, then intravenous heparin should be provided and TEE performed to exclude the presence of LA thrombus before the procedure. Conversion to sinus rhythm is rarely successful or sustained in patients with severe MS, particularly those in whom the LA is especially enlarged or in whom AF has been present for more than 1 year.

MITRAL VALVOTOMY

Unless there is a contraindication, mitral valvotomy is indicated in symptomatic (New York Heart Association [NYHA] Functional Class II–IV) patients with isolated severe MS, whose effective orifice (valve area) is < ~1 cm^2/m^2 body surface area, or <1.5 cm^2 in normal-sized adults. Mitral valvotomy can be carried out by two techniques: PMBV and surgical valvotomy. In PMBV **(Figs. 284-2 and 284-3)**, a catheter is directed into the LA after transseptal puncture, and a single balloon is directed across the valve and inflated in the valvular orifice. Ideal patients have relatively pliable leaflets with little or no commissural calcium. In addition, the subvalvular structures should not be significantly scarred or thickened, and there should be no LA thrombus. The short- and long-term results of this procedure in appropriate patients are similar to those of surgical valvotomy, but with less morbidity and a lower periprocedural mortality rate. Event-free survival in younger (<45 years) patients with pliable valves is excellent, with rates as high as 80–90% over 3–7 years. Therefore, PMBV has become the procedure of choice for such patients when it can be performed by a skilled operator in a high-volume center.

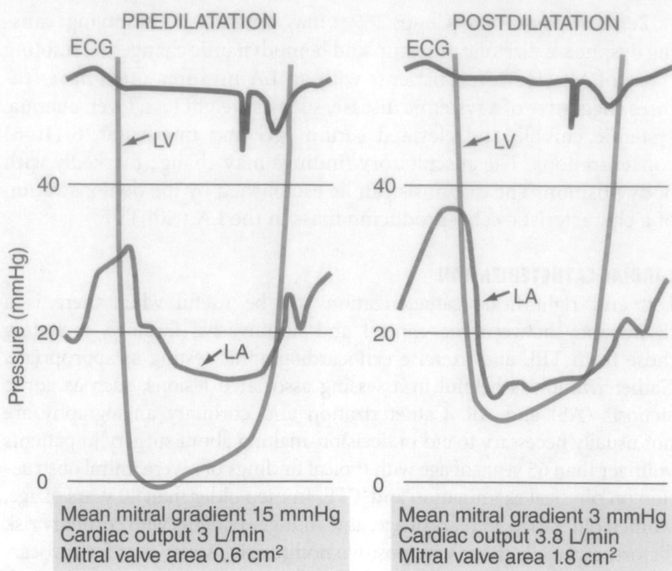

FIGURE 284-3 Simultaneous left atrial (LA) and left ventricular (LV) pressure before and after percutaneous mitral balloon valvuloplasty (PMBV) in a patient with severe mitral stenosis. ECG, electrocardiogram. *(Courtesy of Raymond G. McKay, MD; with permission.)*

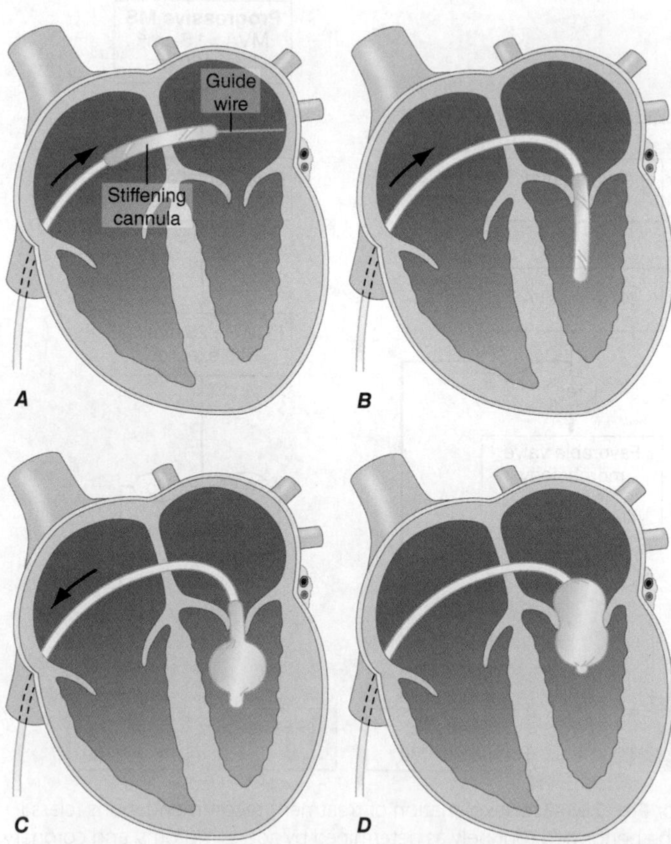

FIGURE 284-2 Inoue balloon technique for percutaneous mitral balloon valvotomy. *A.* After transseptal puncture, the deflated balloon catheter is advanced across the interatrial septum, then across the mitral valve and into the left ventricle. ***B–D.*** The balloon is inflated stepwise within the mitral orifice.

TTE is helpful in identifying patients for the percutaneous procedure, and TEE is performed routinely to exclude LA thrombus and to assess the degree of MR at the time of the scheduled procedure. An "echo score" has been developed to help guide decision-making. The score accounts for the degree of leaflet thickening, calcification, and mobility, and for the extent of subvalvular thickening. A lower score predicts a higher likelihood of successful PMBV.

In patients in whom PMBV is not possible or unsuccessful, or in many patients with restenosis after previous surgery, an "open" valvotomy using cardiopulmonary bypass is necessary. In addition to opening the valve commissures, it is important to loosen any subvalvular fusion of papillary muscles and chordae tendineae; to remove large deposits of calcium, thereby improving valvular function; and to remove atrial thrombi. The perioperative mortality rate is ~2%.

Successful valvotomy is defined by a 50% reduction in the mean mitral valve gradient and a doubling of the mitral valve area. Successful valvotomy, whether balloon or surgical, usually results in striking symptomatic and hemodynamic improvement and prolongs survival. However, there is no evidence that the procedure improves the prognosis of patients with slight or no functional impairment. Therefore, unless recurrent systemic embolization or severe pulmonary hypertension has occurred (PA systolic pressures >50 mmHg at rest or >60 mmHg with exercise), valvotomy is *not* recommended for patients who are entirely asymptomatic and/or who have mild or moderate stenosis (mitral valve area >1.5 cm^2). When there is little symptomatic improvement after valvotomy, it is likely that the procedure was ineffective, that it induced MR, or that associated valvular or myocardial disease was present. About half of all patients undergoing surgical mitral valvotomy require reoperation by 10 years. In the pregnant patient with MS, valvotomy should be carried out if pulmonary congestion occurs despite intensive medical treatment. PMBV is the preferred strategy in this setting and is performed with TEE and no or minimal x-ray exposure.

Mitral valve replacement (MVR) is necessary in patients with MS and significant associated MR, those in whom the valve has been severely distorted by previous transcatheter or operative

Operation	Number	Unadjusted Operative Mortality (%)
MVR (isolated)	3154	5.2
MVR + CAB	1184	10.0
MVRp	4215	1.0
MVRp + CAB	2330	4.8

TABLE 284-2 MORTALITY RATES AFTER MITRAL VALVE SURGERY[a]

[a]Data are for the first two quarters of calendar year 2013, during which 1004 sites reported a total of 135,666 procedures. Data are available from the Society of Thoracic Surgeons at *http://www.sts.org/sites/default/files/documents/2013_3rdHarvestExecutiveSummary.pdf.*

Abbreviations: CAB, coronary artery bypass; MVR, mitral valve replacement; MVRp, mitral valve repair.

manipulation, or those in whom the surgeon does not find it possible to improve valve function significantly with valvotomy. MVR is now routinely performed with preservation of the chordal attachments to optimize LV functional recovery. Perioperative mortality rates with MVR vary with age, LV function, the presence of CAD, and associated comorbidities. They average 5% overall but are lower in young patients and may be twice as high in patients >65 years of age with significant comorbidities (Table 284-2). Because there are also long-term complications of valve replacement, patients in whom preoperative evaluation suggests the possibility that MVR may be required should be operated on only if they have severe MS—i.e., an orifice area ≤1.5 cm²—and are in NYHA Class III, i.e., symptomatic with ordinary activity despite optimal medical therapy. The overall 10-year survival of surgical survivors is ~70%. Long-term prognosis is worse in patients >65 years of age and those with marked disability and marked depression of the CO preoperatively. Pulmonary hypertension and RV dysfunction are additional risk factors for poor outcome.

MITRAL REGURGITATION

ETIOLOGY

MR may result from an abnormality or disease process that affects any one or more of the five functional components of the mitral valve apparatus (leaflets, annulus, chordae tendineae, papillary muscles, and subjacent myocardium) (Table 284-1). Acute MR can occur in the setting of acute myocardial infarction (MI) with papillary muscle rupture (Chap. 295), following blunt chest wall trauma, or during the course of infective endocarditis. With acute MI, the posteromedial papillary muscle is involved much more frequently than the anterolateral papillary muscle because of its singular blood supply. Transient, acute MR can occur during periods of active ischemia and bouts of angina pectoris. Rupture of chordae tendineae can result in "acute-on-chronic MR" in patients with myxomatous degeneration of the valve apparatus.

Chronic MR can result from rheumatic disease, mitral valve prolapse (MVP), extensive mitral annular calcification, congenital valve defects, hypertrophic obstructive cardiomyopathy (HOCM), and dilated cardiomyopathy (Chap. 287). Distinction also should be drawn between primary (degenerative, organic) MR, in which the leaflets and/or chordae tendineae are primarily responsible for abnormal valve function, and functional (secondary) MR, in which the leaflets and chordae tendineae are structurally normal but the regurgitation is caused by annular enlargement, papillary muscle displacement, leaflet tethering, or their combination. The rheumatic process produces rigidity, deformity, and retraction of the valve cusps and commissural fusion, as well as shortening, contraction, and fusion of the chordae tendineae. The MR associated with both MVP and HOCM is usually dynamic in nature. MR in HOCM occurs as a consequence of anterior papillary muscle displacement and systolic anterior motion of the anterior mitral valve leaflet into the narrowed LV outflow tract. Annular calcification is especially prevalent among patients with advanced renal disease and is commonly observed in women >65 years of age with hypertension and diabetes. MR may occur as a congenital anomaly (Chap. 282), most commonly as a defect of the endocardial cushions (atrioventricular cushion defects). A cleft anterior mitral valve leaflet accompanies primum atrial septal defect. Chronic MR is frequently secondary to ischemia and may occur as a consequence of ventricular remodeling, papillary muscle displacement, and leaflet tethering, or with fibrosis of a papillary muscle, in patients with healed MI(s) and ischemic cardiomyopathy. Similar mechanisms of annular dilation and ventricular remodeling contribute to the MR that occurs among patients with nonischemic forms of dilated cardiomyopathy once the LV end-diastolic dimension reaches 6 cm.

Irrespective of cause, chronic severe MR is often progressive, because enlargement of the LA places tension on the posterior mitral leaflet, pulling it away from the mitral orifice and thereby aggravating the valvular dysfunction. Similarly, LV dilation increases the regurgitation, which, in turn, enlarges the LA and LV further, resulting in a vicious circle; hence the aphorism, "mitral regurgitation begets mitral regurgitation."

PATHOPHYSIOLOGY

The resistance to LV emptying (LV afterload) is reduced in patients with MR. As a consequence, the LV is decompressed into the LA during ejection, and with the reduction in LV size during systole, there is a rapid decline in LV tension. The initial compensation to MR is more complete LV emptying. However, LV volume increases progressively with time as the severity of the regurgitation increases and as LV contractile function deteriorates. This increase in LV volume is often accompanied by a reduced forward CO. LV compliance is often increased, and thus, LV diastolic pressure does not increase until late in the course. The regurgitant volume varies directly with the LV systolic pressure and the size of the regurgitant orifice; the latter, in turn, is influenced by the extent of LV and mitral annular dilation. Because EF rises in severe MR in the presence of normal LV function, even a modest reduction in this parameter (<60%) reflects significant dysfunction.

During early diastole, as the distended LA empties, there is a particularly rapid *y* descent in the absence of accompanying MS. A brief, early diastolic LA-LV pressure gradient (often generating a rapid filling sound [S_3] and mid-diastolic murmur masquerading as MS) may occur in patients with pure, severe MR as a result of the very rapid flow of blood across a normal-sized mitral orifice.

Semiquantitative estimates of LV ejection fraction (LVEF), CO, PA systolic pressure, regurgitant volume, regurgitant fraction (RF), and the effective regurgitant orifice area can be obtained during a careful Doppler echocardiographic examination. These measurements can also be obtained accurately with cardiac magnetic resonance (CMR) imaging, although this technology is not widely available. Left and right heart catheterization with contrast ventriculography is used less frequently. Severe, nonischemic MR is defined by a regurgitant volume ≥60 mL/beat, RF ≥50%, and effective regurgitant orifice area ≥0.40 cm². Severe ischemic MR, however, is usually associated with an effective regurgitant orifice area of >0.2 cm². In the latter instance, lesser degrees of MR carry relatively greater prognostic weight.

LA Compliance In acute severe MR, the regurgitant volume is delivered into a normal-sized LA having normal or reduced compliance. As a result, LA pressures rise markedly for any increase in LA volume. The *v* wave in the LA pressure pulse is usually prominent, LA and pulmonary venous pressures are markedly elevated, and pulmonary edema is common. Because of the rapid rise in LA pressures during ventricular systole, the murmur of acute MR is early in timing and decrescendo in configuration ending well before S_2, as a reflection of the progressive diminution in the LV-LA pressure gradient. LV systolic function in acute MR may be normal, hyperdynamic, or reduced, depending on the clinical context.

Patients with chronic severe MR, on the other hand, develop marked LA enlargement and *increased* LA compliance with little if any increase in LA and pulmonary venous pressures for any increase in LA volume. The LA *v* wave is relatively less prominent. The murmur of chronic MR is classically holosystolic in timing and plateau in configuration, as a reflection of the near-constant LV-LA pressure gradient. These patients usually complain of severe fatigue and exhaustion secondary to a low forward CO, whereas symptoms resulting from pulmonary congestion are less prominent initially; AF is almost invariably present once the LA dilates significantly.

SYMPTOMS

Patients with chronic mild-to-moderate, isolated MR are usually asymptomatic. This form of LV volume overload is well tolerated. Fatigue, exertional dyspnea, and orthopnea are the most prominent complaints in patients with chronic severe MR. Palpitations are common and may signify the onset of AF. Right-sided heart failure, with painful hepatic congestion, ankle edema, distended neck veins, ascites, and secondary TR, occurs in patients with MR who have associated pulmonary vascular disease and pulmonary hypertension. Acute pulmonary edema is common in patients with acute severe MR.

PHYSICAL FINDINGS

In patients with chronic severe MR, the arterial pressure is usually normal, although the carotid arterial pulse may show a sharp, low-volume upstroke owing to the reduced forward CO. A systolic thrill is often palpable at the cardiac apex, the LV is hyperdynamic with a brisk systolic impulse and a palpable rapid-filling wave (S_3), and the apex beat is often displaced laterally.

In patients with acute severe MR, the arterial pressure may be reduced with a narrow pulse pressure, the jugular venous pressure and wave forms may be normal or increased and exaggerated, the apical impulse is not displaced, and signs of pulmonary congestion are prominent.

Auscultation S_1 is generally absent, soft, or buried in the holosystolic murmur of chronic, severe MR. In patients with severe MR, the aortic valve may close prematurely, resulting in wide but physiologic splitting of S_2. A low-pitched S_3 occurring 0.12–0.17 s after the aortic valve closure sound, i.e., at the completion of the rapid-filling phase of the LV, is believed to be caused by the sudden tensing of the papillary muscles, chordae tendineae, and valve leaflets. It may be followed by a short, rumbling, mid-diastolic murmur, even in the absence of structural MS. A fourth heart sound is often audible in patients with *acute* severe MR who are in sinus rhythm. A presystolic murmur is not ordinarily heard with isolated MR.

A systolic murmur of at least grade III/VI intensity is the most characteristic auscultatory finding in chronic severe MR. It is usually holosystolic (see Fig. 267-5A), but as previously noted, it is decrescendo and ceases in mid to late systole in patients with acute severe MR. The systolic murmur of chronic MR is usually most prominent at the apex and radiates to the axilla. However, in patients with ruptured chordae tendineae or primary involvement of the posterior mitral leaflet with prolapse or flail, the regurgitant jet is eccentric, directed anteriorly, and strikes the LA wall adjacent to the aortic root. In this situation, the systolic murmur is transmitted to the base of the heart and, therefore, may be confused with the murmur of AS. In patients with ruptured chordae tendineae, the systolic murmur may have a cooing or "seagull" quality, whereas a flail leaflet may produce a murmur with a musical quality. The systolic murmur of chronic MR not due to MVP is intensified by isometric exercise (handgrip) but is reduced during the strain phase of the Valsalva maneuver because of the associated decrease in LV preload.

LABORATORY EXAMINATION

ECG In patients with sinus rhythm, there is evidence of LA enlargement, but RA enlargement also may be present when pulmonary hypertension is significant and affects RV function. Chronic severe MR is frequently associated with AF. In many patients, there is no clear-cut ECG evidence of enlargement of either ventricle. In others, the signs of eccentric LV hypertrophy are present.

Echocardiogram TTE is indicated to assess the mechanism of the MR and its hemodynamic severity. LV function can be assessed from LV end-diastolic and end-systolic volumes and EF. Observations can be made regarding leaflet structure and function, chordal integrity, LA and LV size, annular calcification, and regional and global LV systolic function. Doppler imaging should demonstrate the width or area of the color flow MR jet within the LA, the duration and intensity of the continuous wave Doppler signal, the pulmonary venous flow contour, the early peak mitral inflow velocity, and quantitative measures of regurgitant volume, RF, and effective regurgitant orifice area. In addition, the PAPs can be estimated from the TR jet velocity. TTE is also indicated to follow the course of patients with chronic MR and to provide rapid assessment for any clinical change. The echocardiogram in patients with MVP is described in the next section. TEE provides greater anatomic detail than TTE (see Fig. 270e-5). Exercise testing with TTE can be useful to assess exercise capacity as well as any dynamic change in MR severity, PA systolic pressures, and biventricular function, for patients in whom there is a discrepancy between clinical findings and the results of functional testing performed at rest.

Chest X-Ray The LA and LV are the dominant chambers in chronic MR. Late in the course of the disease, the LA may be massively enlarged and forms the right border of the cardiac silhouette. Pulmonary venous congestion, interstitial edema, and Kerley B lines are sometimes noted. Marked calcification of the mitral leaflets occurs commonly in patients with long-standing, combined rheumatic MR and MS. Calcification of the mitral annulus may be visualized, particularly on the lateral view of the chest. Patients with acute severe MR may have asymmetric pulmonary edema if the regurgitant jet is directed predominantly to the orifice of an upper lobe pulmonary vein.

TREATMENT MITRAL REGURGITATION

MEDICAL TREATMENT (FIG. 284-4)

The management of chronic severe MR depends to some degree on its cause. Warfarin should be provided once AF intervenes with a target INR of 2–3. Novel oral anticoagulants are not approved for this indication. Cardioversion should be considered depending on the clinical context and LA size. In contrast to the acute setting, there are no large, long-term prospective studies to substantiate the use of vasodilators for the treatment of chronic, isolated severe MR with preserved LV systolic function *in the absence of systemic hypertension*. The severity of MR in the setting of an ischemic or nonischemic dilated cardiomyopathy may diminish with aggressive guideline-directed treatment of heart failure including the use of diuretics, beta blockers, angiotensin-converting enzyme (ACE) inhibitors, digitalis, and biventricular pacing (cardiac resynchronization therapy [CRT]) when otherwise indicated. Asymptomatic patients with severe MR in sinus rhythm with normal LV size and systolic function should avoid isometric forms of exercise.

Patients with acute severe MR require urgent stabilization and preparation for surgery. Diuretics, intravenous vasodilators (particularly sodium nitroprusside), and even intraaortic balloon counterpulsation may be needed for patients with post-MI papillary muscle rupture or other forms of acute severe MR.

SURGICAL TREATMENT

In the selection of patients with chronic, nonischemic, primary or organic, severe MR for surgical treatment, the often slowly progressive nature of the condition must be balanced against the immediate and long-term risks associated with operation. These risks are significantly lower for primary valve repair than for valve replacement (**Table 287-2**). Repair usually consists of valve reconstruction using a variety of valvuloplasty techniques and insertion of an annuloplasty ring. Repair spares the patient the long-term adverse consequences of valve replacement, including thromboembolic and hemorrhagic complications in the case of mechanical prostheses and late valve failure necessitating repeat valve replacement in the case of bioprostheses. In addition, by preserving the integrity of the papillary muscles, subvalvular apparatus, and chordae tendineae, mitral repair and valvuloplasty maintain LV function to a relatively greater degree.

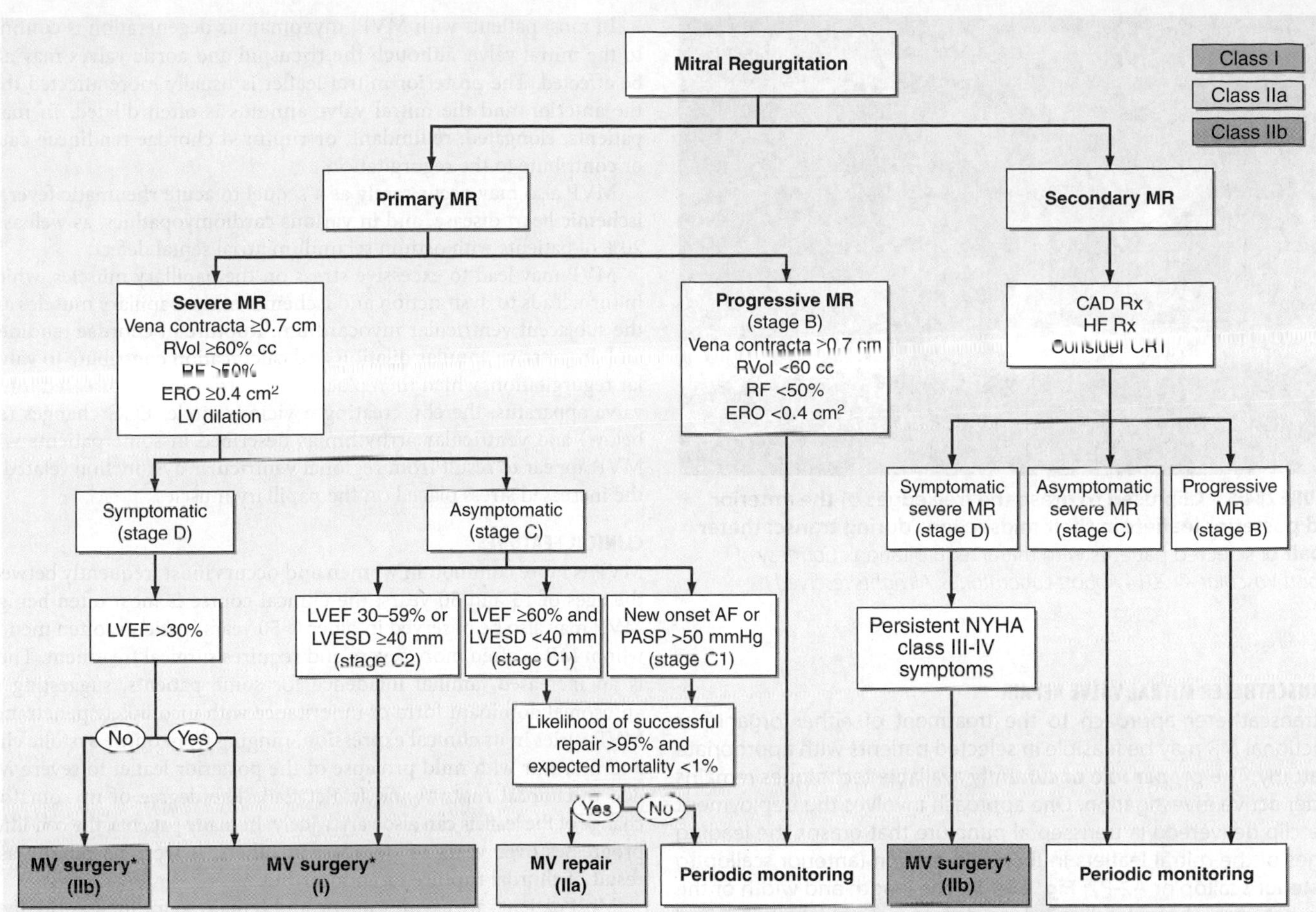

FIGURE 284-4 Management of mitral regurgitation. See legend for **Fig. 283-2** for explanation of treatment recommendations (class I, IIa, IIb) and disease stages (B, C1, C2, D). Preoperative coronary angiography should be performed routinely as determined by age, symptoms, and coronary risk factors. Cardiac catheterization and angiography may also be helpful when there is a discrepancy between clinical and noninvasive findings. AF, atrial fibrillation; CAD, coronary artery disease; CRT, cardiac resynchronization therapy; ERO, effective regurgitant orifice; HF, heart failure; LV, left ventricular; LVEF, left ventricular ejection fraction; LVESD, left ventricular end-systolic dimension; MR, mitral regurgitation, MV, mitral valve; MVR, mitral valve replacement; NYHA, New York Heart Association; PASP, pulmonary artery systolic pressure; RF, regurgitant fraction; RVol, regurgitant volume; and Rx, therapy. *Mitral valve repair preferred over MVR when possible. *(Adapted from RA Nishimura et al: 2014 AHA/ACC Guideline for the Management of Patients with Valvular Heart Disease. J Am Coll Cardiol doi: 10.1016/j.jacc.2014.02.536, 2014, with permission.)*

Surgery for chronic nonischemic severe MR is indicated once symptoms occur, especially if valve repair is feasible (Fig. 284-4). Other indications for early consideration of mitral valve repair include recent-onset AF and pulmonary hypertension defined as a systolic PA pressure ≥50 mmHg at rest or ≥60 mmHg with exercise. Surgical treatment of chronic nonischemic severe MR is indicated for asymptomatic patients when LV dysfunction is progressive with the LVEF falling below 60% and/or end-systolic dimension increasing beyond 40 mm. These aggressive recommendations for surgery are predicated on the outstanding results achieved with mitral valve repair particularly when applied to patients with myxomatous disease such as that associated with prolapse or flail leaflet. Indeed primary valvuloplasty repair of patients younger than 75 years with normal LV systolic function and no CAD can now be performed by experienced surgeons with <1% perioperative mortality risk. The risk of stroke, however, is also approximately 1%. Repair is feasible in up to 95% of patients with myxomatous disease operated on by a high-volume surgeon in a referral center of excellence. Long-term durability is excellent; the incidence of reoperative surgery for failed primary repair is ~1% per year for the first 10 years after surgery. For patients with AF, left or biatrial maze surgery, or radiofrequency, isolation of the pulmonary veins is often performed to reduce the risk of recurrent postoperative AF.

The surgical management of patients with functional, ischemic MR is more complicated and most often involves simultaneous coronary artery revascularization. Current surgical practice includes annuloplasty repair with an undersized, rigid ring or chord-sparing valve replacement for patients with moderate or greater degrees of MR. Valve repair for ischemic MR is associated with lower perioperative mortality rates but higher rates of recurrent MR over time. In patients with ischemic MR and significantly impaired LV systolic function (EF <30%), the risk of surgery is higher, recovery of LV performance is incomplete, and long-term survival is reduced. Referral for surgery must be individualized and made only after aggressive attempts with guideline-directed medical therapy and CRT, when indicated. The routine performance of valve repair in patients with significant MR in the setting of severe, functional, nonischemic dilated cardiomyopathy has not been shown to improve long-term survival compared with optimal medical therapy. Patients with acute severe MR can often be stabilized temporarily with appropriate medical therapy, but surgical correction will be necessary emergently in the case of papillary muscle rupture and within days to weeks in most other settings.

When surgical treatment is contemplated, left and right heart catheterization and left ventriculography *may* be helpful in confirming the presence of severe MR in patients in whom there is a discrepancy between the clinical and TTE findings that cannot be resolved with TEE or CMR. Coronary angiography identifies patients who require concomitant coronary revascularization.

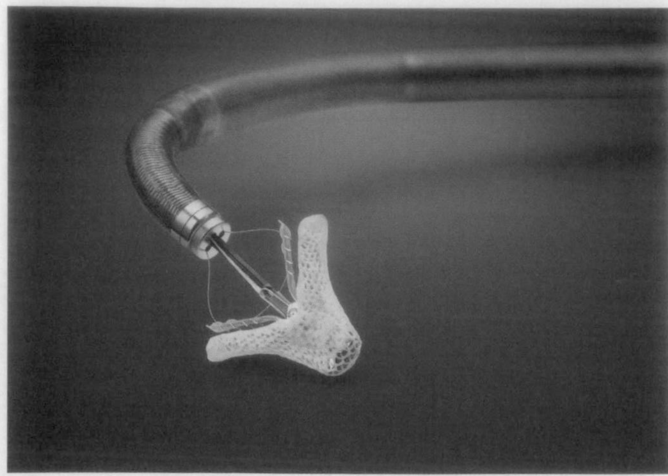

FIGURE 284-5 Clip used to grasp the free edges of the anterior and posterior leaflets in their midsections during transcatheter repair of selected patients with mitral regurgitation. *(Courtesy of Abbott Vascular. © 2014 Abbott Laboratories. All rights reserved.)*

TRANSCATHETER MITRAL VALVE REPAIR

A transcatheter approach to the treatment of either organic or functional MR may be feasible in selected patients with appropriate anatomy. The proper role of currently available techniques remains under active investigation. One approach involves the deployment of a clip delivered via transseptal puncture that grasps the leading edges of the mitral leaflets in their mid-portion (anterior scallop to posterior scallop or A2-P2; Fig. 284-5). The length and width of the gap between these leading edges dictate patient eligibility. The device is commercially available for the treatment of prohibitive surgical risk patients with severe, degenerative (organic) MR and is undergoing study in the United States for treatment of patients with symptomatic heart failure, reduced LVEF, and severe, functional MR despite guideline-directed medical therapy. A second approach involves the deployment of a device within the coronary sinus that can be adjusted to reduce its circumference, thus secondarily decreasing the circumference of the mitral annulus and the effective orifice area of the valve much like a surgically implanted ring. Variations in the anatomic relationship of the coronary sinus to the mitral annulus and circumflex coronary artery have limited the applicability of this technique. Attempts to reduce the septal-lateral dimension of a dilated annulus using adjustable cords placed across the LV in a subvalvular location have also been investigated.

MITRAL VALVE PROLAPSE

MVP, also variously termed the *systolic click-murmur syndrome, Barlow's syndrome, floppy-valve syndrome*, and *billowing mitral leaflet syndrome*, is a relatively common but highly variable clinical syndrome resulting from diverse pathologic mechanisms of the mitral valve apparatus. Among these are excessive or redundant mitral leaflet tissue, which is commonly associated with myxomatous degeneration and greatly increased concentrations of certain glycosaminoglycans.

In most patients with MVP, the cause is unknown, but in some, it appears to be genetically determined. A reduction in the production of type III collagen has been incriminated, and electron microscopy has revealed fragmentation of collagen fibrils.

MVP is a frequent finding in patients with heritable disorders of connective tissue, including Marfan's syndrome (Chap. 427), osteogenesis imperfecta, and Ehlers-Danlos syndrome. MVP may be associated with thoracic skeletal deformities similar to but not as severe as those in Marfan's syndrome, such as a high-arched palate and alterations of the chest and thoracic spine, including the so-called straight back syndrome.

In most patients with MVP, myxomatous degeneration is confined to the mitral valve, although the tricuspid and aortic valves may also be affected. The posterior mitral leaflet is usually more affected than the anterior, and the mitral valve annulus is often dilated. In many patients, elongated, redundant, or ruptured chordae tendineae cause or contribute to the regurgitation.

MVP also may occur rarely as a sequel to acute rheumatic fever, in ischemic heart disease, and in various cardiomyopathies, as well as in 20% of patients with ostium secundum atrial septal defect.

MVP may lead to excessive stress on the papillary muscles, which, in turn, leads to dysfunction and ischemia of the papillary muscles and the subjacent ventricular myocardium. Rupture of chordae tendineae and progressive annular dilation and calcification contribute to valvular regurgitation, which then places more stress on the diseased mitral valve apparatus, thereby creating a vicious circle. ECG changes (see below) and ventricular arrhythmias described in some patients with MVP appear to result from regional ventricular dysfunction related to the increased stress placed on the papillary muscles.

CLINICAL FEATURES

MVP is more common in women and occurs most frequently between the ages of 15 and 30 years; the clinical course is most often benign. MVP may also be observed in older (>50 years) patients, often men, in whom MR is often more severe and requires surgical treatment. There is an increased familial incidence for some patients, suggesting an autosomal dominant form of inheritance with incomplete penetrance. MVP varies in its clinical expression, ranging from only a systolic click and murmur with mild prolapse of the posterior leaflet to severe MR due to chordal rupture and leaflet flail. The degree of myxomatous change of the leaflets can also vary widely. In many patients, the condition progresses over years or decades; in others, it worsens rapidly as a result of chordal rupture or endocarditis.

Most patients are asymptomatic and remain so for their entire lives. However, in North America, MVP is now the most common cause of isolated severe MR requiring surgical treatment. Arrhythmias, most commonly ventricular premature contractions and paroxysmal supraventricular and ventricular tachycardia, as well as AF, have been reported and may cause palpitations, light-headedness, and syncope. Sudden death is a very rare complication and occurs most often in patients with severe MR and depressed LV systolic function. There may be an excess risk of sudden death among patients with a flail leaflet. Many patients have chest pain that is difficult to evaluate; it is often substernal, prolonged, and not related to exertion, but may rarely resemble angina pectoris. Transient cerebral ischemic attacks secondary to emboli from the mitral valve due to endothelial disruption have been reported. Infective endocarditis may occur in patients with MR and/or leaflet thickening.

Auscultation A frequent finding is the mid or late (nonejection) systolic click, which occurs 0.14 s or more after S_1 and is thought to be generated by the sudden tensing of slack, elongated chordae tendineae or by the prolapsing mitral leaflet when it reaches its maximal excursion. Systolic clicks may be multiple and may be followed by a high-pitched, mid-late systolic crescendo-decrescendo murmur, which occasionally is "whooping" or "honking" and is heard best at the apex. The click and murmur occur earlier with standing, during the strain phase of the Valsalva maneuver, and with any intervention that decreases LV volume, exaggerating the propensity of mitral leaflet prolapse. Conversely, squatting and isometric exercises, which increase LV volume, diminish MVP; the click-murmur complex is delayed, moves away from S_1, and may even disappear. Some patients have a mid-systolic click without a murmur; others have a murmur without a click. Still others have both sounds at different times.

LABORATORY EXAMINATION

The ECG most commonly is normal but may show biphasic or inverted T waves in leads II, III, and aVF, and occasionally supraventricular or ventricular premature beats. TTE is particularly effective in identifying the abnormal position and prolapse of the mitral valve leaflets. A useful echocardiographic definition of MVP is systolic displacement (in the parasternal long axis view) of the mitral valve leaflets by at least 2 mm into the LA superior to the plane of the mitral annulus. Color flow and continuous wave Doppler imaging is helpful to evaluate the associated MR and provide semiquantitative estimates of severity. The jet lesion of MR due to MVP is most often eccentric, and assessment of RF and effective regurgitant orifice area can be difficult. TEE is indicated when more accurate information is required and is performed routinely for intraoperative guidance for valve repair. Invasive left ventriculography is rarely necessary but can also show prolapse of the posterior and sometimes of both mitral valve leaflets.

TREATMENT MITRAL VALVE PROLAPSE

Infective endocarditis prophylaxis is indicated only for patients with a prior history of endocarditis. Beta blockers sometimes relieve chest pain and control palpitations. If the patient is symptomatic from severe MR, mitral valve repair (or rarely, chord-sparing replacement) is indicated (Fig. 284-4). Antiplatelet agents, such as aspirin, should be given to patients with transient ischemic attacks, and if these are not effective, warfarin should be considered. Warfarin is also indicated once AF intervenes.

285 Tricuspid and Pulmonic Valve Disease

Patrick T. O'Gara, Joseph Loscalzo

TRICUSPID STENOSIS

Tricuspid stenosis (TS), which is much less prevalent than mitral stenosis (MS) in North America and Western Europe, is generally rheumatic in origin, and is more common in women than men (Table 285-1). It does not occur as an isolated lesion and is usually associated with MS. Hemodynamically significant TS occurs in 5–10% of patients with severe MS; rheumatic TS is commonly associated with some degree of tricuspid regurgitation (TR). Nonrheumatic causes of TS are rare.

PATHOPHYSIOLOGY

A diastolic pressure gradient between the right atrium (RA) and right ventricle (RV) defines TS. It is augmented when the transvalvular blood flow increases during inspiration and declines during expiration. A mean diastolic pressure gradient of 4 mmHg is usually sufficient to elevate the mean RA pressure to levels that result in systemic venous congestion. Unless sodium intake has been restricted and diuretics administered, this venous congestion is associated with hepatomegaly, ascites, and edema, sometimes severe. In patients with sinus rhythm, the RA *a* wave may be extremely tall and may even approach the level of the RV systolic pressure. The *y* descent is prolonged. The cardiac output (CO) at rest is usually depressed, and it fails to rise during exercise. The low CO is responsible for the normal or only slightly elevated left atrial (LA), pulmonary artery (PA), and RV systolic pressures despite the presence of MS. Thus, the presence of TS can mask the hemodynamic and clinical features of any associated MS.

SYMPTOMS

Because the development of MS generally precedes that of TS, many patients initially have symptoms of pulmonary congestion and fatigue. Characteristically, patients with severe TS complain of relatively little dyspnea for the degree of hepatomegaly, ascites, and edema that they have. However, fatigue secondary to a low CO and discomfort due to refractory edema, ascites, and marked hepatomegaly are common in patients with advanced TS and/or TR. In some patients, TS may be suspected for the first time when symptoms of right-sided failure persist after an adequate mitral valvotomy.

TABLE 285-1 CAUSES OF TRICUSPID AND PULMONIC VALVE DISEASES

Valve Lesion	Etiologies
Tricuspid stenosis	Rheumatic
	Congenital
Tricuspid regurgitation	Primary (organic)
	Rheumatic
	Endocarditis
	Myxomatous (TVP)
	Carcinoid
	Radiation
	Congenital (Ebstein's)
	Trauma
	Papillary muscle injury (post-MI)
	Secondary (functional)
	RV and tricuspid annular dilatation due to multiple causes of RV enlargement (e.g., long-standing pulmonary HTN, remodeling post-RV MI)
	Chronic RV apical pacing
Pulmonic stenosis	Congenital
	Carcinoid
	Tumor
	Endocarditis
Pulmonic regurgitation	Primary valve disease
	Congenital
	Postvalvotomy
	Endocarditis
	Carcinoid
	Annular enlargement
	Pulmonary hypertension
	Idiopathic dilation
	Marfan's syndrome

Abbreviations: HTN, hypertension; MI, myocardial infarction; RV, right ventricular; TVP, tricuspid valve prolapse.

PHYSICAL FINDINGS

Because TS usually occurs in the presence of other obvious valvular disease, the diagnosis may be missed unless it is considered. Severe TS is associated with marked hepatic congestion, often resulting in cirrhosis, jaundice, serious malnutrition, anasarca, and ascites. Congestive hepatomegaly and, in cases of severe tricuspid valve disease, splenomegaly are present. The jugular veins are distended, and in patients with sinus rhythm, there may be giant *a* waves. The *v* waves are less conspicuous, and because tricuspid obstruction impedes RA emptying during diastole, there is a slow *y* descent. In patients with sinus rhythm, there may be prominent presystolic pulsations of the enlarged liver as well.

On auscultation, an opening snap (OS) of the tricuspid valve may rarely be heard approximately 0.06 s after pulmonic valve closure. The diastolic murmur of TS has many of the qualities of the diastolic murmur of MS, and because TS almost always occurs in the presence of MS, it may be missed. However, the tricuspid murmur is generally heard best along the left lower sternal border and over the xiphoid process, and is most prominent during presystole in patients with sinus rhythm. The murmur of TS is augmented during inspiration, and it is reduced during expiration and particularly during the strain phase of the Valsalva maneuver, when tricuspid transvalvular flow is reduced.

LABORATORY EXAMINATION

The electrocardiogram (ECG) features of RA enlargement (see Fig. 268-8) include tall, peaked P waves in lead II, as well as prominent, upright P waves in lead V_1. The *absence* of ECG evidence of RV hypertrophy (RVH) in a patient with right-sided heart failure who is believed to have MS should suggest associated tricuspid valve disease. The chest x-ray in patients with combined TS and MS shows particular prominence of the RA and superior vena cava without much enlargement of the PA and with less evidence of pulmonary vascular congestion than occurs in patients with isolated MS. On echocardiographic examination, the tricuspid valve is usually thickened and domes in diastole; the transvalvular gradient can be estimated by continuous wave Doppler echocardiography. Severe TS is characterized by a valve area ≤1 cm² or pressure half-time of ≥190 ms. The RA and inferior vena cava (IVC) are enlarged. Transthoracic echocardiography (TTE) provides additional information regarding the severity of any associated TR, mitral valve structure and function, left ventricle (LV) and RV size and function, and PA pressure. Cardiac catheterization is not routinely necessary for assessment of TS.

TREATMENT TRICUSPID STENOSIS

Patients with TS generally exhibit marked systemic venous congestion; salt restriction, bed rest, and diuretic therapy are required during the preoperative period. Such a preparatory period may diminish hepatic congestion and thereby improve hepatic function sufficiently so that the risks of operation, particularly bleeding, are diminished. Surgical relief of the TS should be carried out, preferably at the time of surgical mitral valvotomy or mitral valve replacement (MVR) for mitral valve disease, in patients with moderate or severe TS who have mean diastolic pressure gradients exceeding ~4 mmHg and tricuspid orifice areas <1.5–2 cm². TS is almost always accompanied by significant TR. Operative repair may permit substantial improvement of tricuspid valve function. If repair cannot be accomplished, the tricuspid valve may have to be replaced. Meta-analysis has shown no difference in overall survival between mechanical and tissue valve replacement. Mechanical valves in the tricuspid position are more prone to thromboembolic complications than in other positions. Percutaneous tricuspid balloon valvuloplasty for isolated severe TS without significant TR is very rarely performed.

TRICUSPID REGURGITATION

In at least 80% of cases, TR is secondary to marked dilation of the tricuspid annulus from RV enlargement due to PA hypertension (Table 285-1). Functional TR may complicate RV enlargement of any cause, however, including an inferior myocardial infarction (MI) that involves the RV. It is commonly seen in the late stages of heart failure due to rheumatic or congenital heart disease with severe PA hypertension (PA systolic pressure >55 mmHg), as well as in ischemic and idiopathic dilated cardiomyopathies. It is reversible in part if PA hypertension can be relieved. Functional TR can also develop from chronic RV apical pacing. Rheumatic fever may produce primary (organic) TR, often associated with TS. Infarction of RV papillary muscles, tricuspid valve prolapse, carcinoid heart disease, endomyocardial fibrosis, radiation, infective endocarditis, and leaflet trauma all may produce TR. Less commonly, TR results from congenitally deformed tricuspid valves, and it occurs with defects of the atrioventricular canal, as well as with Ebstein's malformation of the tricuspid valve (Chap. 282).

PATHOPHYSIOLOGY

The incompetent tricuspid valve allows blood to flow backward from the RV into the RA, the volume of which is dependent on the driving pressure (i.e., RV systolic pressure) and the size of the regurgitant orifice. The severity and physical signs of TR can vary as a function of PA systolic pressure (in the absence of RV outflow tract stenosis), the dimension of the tricuspid valve annulus, the respiratory cycle–dependent changes in RV preload, and RA compliance. RV filling is increased during inspiration. Forward CO is reduced and does not augment with exercise. Significant degrees of TR will lead to RA enlargement and elevation of the RA and jugular venous pressures with prominent *c-v* waves in the pulse tracings. Progressively severe TR can lead to "ventricularization" of the RA wave form (see Fig. 267-1*B*). Severe TR is also characterized by RV dilation (RV volume overload) and eventual systolic dysfunction, the rate of which can be accelerated by a concomitant pressure load from PA hypertension or by myocardial fibrosis from previous injury.

SYMPTOMS

Mild or moderate degrees of TR are usually well tolerated in the absence of other hemodynamic disturbances. Because TR most often coexists with left-sided valve lesions, LV dysfunction, and/or PA hypertension, symptoms related to these lesions may dominate the clinical picture. Fatigue and exertional dyspnea owing to reduced forward CO are early symptoms of isolated, severe TR. As the disease progresses and RV function declines, patients may report cervical pulsations, abdominal fullness/bloating, diminished appetite, and muscle wasting, although with progressive weight gain and painful swelling of the lower extremities.

PHYSICAL FINDINGS

The neck veins in patients with severe TR are distended with prominent *c-v* waves and rapid *y* descents (in the absence of TS). TR is more often diagnosed by examination of the neck veins than by auscultation of the heart sounds. Other findings may include marked hepatomegaly with systolic pulsations, ascites, pleural effusions, edema, and a positive hepatojugular reflex. A prominent RV pulsation along the left parasternal region and a blowing holosystolic murmur along the lower left sternal margin, which may be intensified during inspiration (Carvallo's sign) and reduced during expiration or the strain phase of the Valsalva maneuver, are characteristic findings. The murmur of TR may sometimes be confused with that of MR unless attention is paid to its variation during the respiratory cycle and the extent of RV enlargement is appreciated. Atrial fibrillation (AF) is usually present in the chronic phase of the disease.

LABORATORY EXAMINATION

The ECG may show changes characteristic of the lesion responsible for the TR, e.g., an inferior Q-wave MI suggestive of a prior RV MI, RVH, or a bizarre right bundle branch block type pattern with preexcitation in patients with Ebstein's anomaly. ECG signs of RA enlargement may be present in patients with sinus rhythm; AF is frequently noted. The chest x-ray may show RA and RV enlargement, depending on the chronicity and severity of TR. TTE is usually definitive with demonstration of RA dilation and RV volume overload and prolapsing, flail, scarred, or displaced/tethered tricuspid leaflets; the diagnosis and assessment of TR can be made by color flow Doppler imaging (see Fig. 270e-8). Severe TR is accompanied by hepatic vein systolic flow reversal. Continuous wave Doppler of the TR velocity profile is useful in estimating PA systolic pressure. Accurate assessment of TR severity, PA pressures, and RV size and systolic function with TTE can be quite challenging in many patients. Real-time three-dimensional echocardiography and cardiac magnetic resonance (CMR) imaging provide alternative imaging modalities, although they are not widely available. In patients with severe TR, the CO is usually markedly reduced, and the RA pressure pulse may exhibit no *x* descent during early systole but a prominent *c-v* wave with a rapid *y* descent. The mean RA and RV end-diastolic pressures are often elevated. Exercise testing can be used to assess functional capacity in patients with asymptomatic severe TR. The prognostic significance of exercise-induced changes in TR severity and RV function has not been well studied.

TREATMENT TRICUSPID REGURGITATION (FIG. 285-1)

Diuretics can be useful for patients with severe TR and signs of right heart failure. An aldosterone antagonist may be particularly helpful because many patients have secondary hyperaldosteronism from marked hepatic congestion. Therapies to reduce elevated PA pressures and/or pulmonary vascular resistance, including those targeted at left-sided heart disease, can also be considered for patients with PA hypertension and severe functional TR. Tricuspid valve surgery is recommended for patients with severe TR who are undergoing

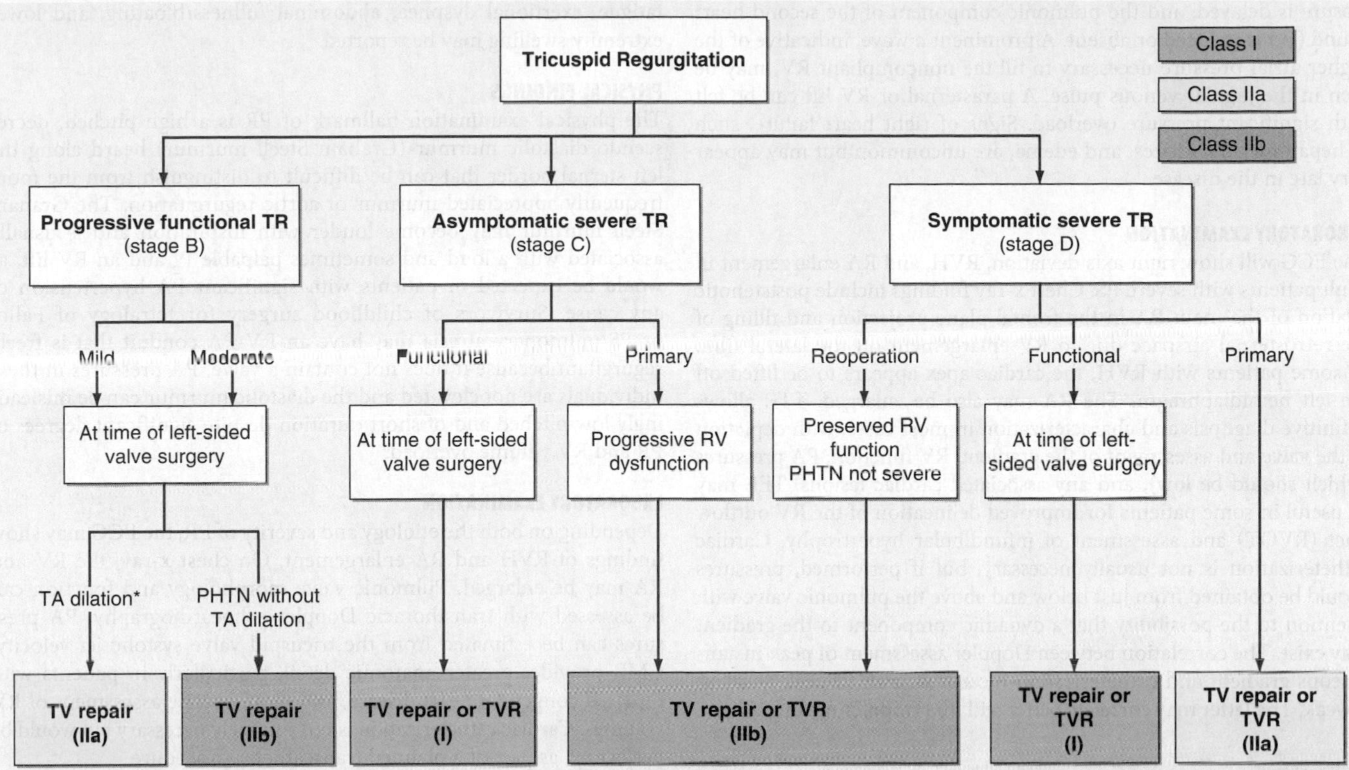

FIGURE 285-1 Management of tricuspid regurgitation. See legend for Fig. 283-2 for explanation of treatment recommendations (Class I, IIa, IIb) and disease stages (B, C, D). Preoperative coronary angiography should be performed routinely as determined by age, symptoms, and coronary risk factors. Cardiac catheterization and angiography may also be helpful when there is a discrepancy between clinical and noninvasive findings. PHTN, pulmonary hypertension; RV, right ventricular; TA, tricuspid annular; TTE, transthoracic echocardiogram; TR, tricuspid regurgitation; TV, tricuspid valve; TVR, tricuspid valve replacement. *TA dilation is defined by >40 mm on TTE (>21 mm/m2) or >70 mm on direct intraoperative measurement. *(Adapted from RA Nishimura et al: 2014 AHA/ACC Guideline for the Management of Patients with Valvular Heart Disease. J Am Coll Cardiol doi: 10.1016/j.jacc.2014.02.536, 2014, with permission.)*

left-sided valve surgery and is also undertaken frequently for treatment of even moderate TR in patients undergoing left-sided valve surgery who have tricuspid annular dilation (>40 mm), a history of right heart failure, or PA hypertension. Operation most often comprises repair rather than replacement in these settings and has become routine in most major surgical centers. Surgery may also infrequently be required for treatment of severe, primary TR with right heart failure not responsive to standard medical therapy or because of progressively declining RV systolic function. Reported perioperative mortality rates for isolated tricuspid valve surgery (repair and replacement) are high (~8-9%) and likely are influenced by the hazards encountered during reoperation on patients who have undergone previous left-sided valve surgery and have reduced RV function. Indwelling pacemaker or defibrillator leads can also pose technical challenges.

PULMONIC STENOSIS

Pulmonic valve stenosis (PS) is essentially a congenital disorder (Table 285-1). With isolated PS, the valve is typically domed. Dysplastic pulmonic valves are seen as part of the Noonan's syndrome (Chap. 302), which maps to chromosome 12. Much less common etiologies include carcinoid and obstructing tumors or bulky vegetations. The pulmonic valve is only very rarely affected by the rheumatic process.

PATHOPHYSIOLOGY

PS is defined hemodynamically by a systolic pressure gradient between the RV and main PA. RV hypertrophy develops as a consequence of sustained obstruction to RV outflow, and systolic ejection is prolonged. Compared with the ability of the LV to compensate for the pressure overload imposed by aortic stenosis (AS), RV dysfunction from afterload mismatch occurs earlier in the course of PS and at lower peak systolic pressures, because the RV adapts less well to this type of hemodynamic burden. With normal systolic function and CO, severe PS is defined by a peak systolic gradient across the pulmonic valve of >50 mmHg; moderate PS correlates with a peak gradient of 30–50 mmHg. PS rarely progresses in patients with peak gradients less than 30 mmHg, but may worsen in those with moderate disease due to valve thickening and calcification with age. The RA *a* wave elevates in relation to the higher pressures needed to fill a noncompliant, hypertrophied RV. A prominent RA *v* wave signifies functional TR from RV and annular dilation. The CO is maintained until late in the course of the disease.

SYMPTOMS

Patients with mild or even moderate PS are usually asymptomatic and first come to medical attention because of a heart murmur that leads to echocardiography. With severe PS, patients may report exertional dyspnea or early onset fatigue. Anginal chest pain from RV oxygen supply-demand mismatch and syncope may occur with very severe forms of obstruction, particularly in the presence of a destabilizing trigger such as atrial fibrillation, fever, infection, or anemia.

PHYSICAL FINDINGS

The murmur of mild or moderate PS is mid-systolic in timing, crescendo-decrescendo in configuration, heard best in the left second interspace, and usually introduced by an ejection sound (click) in younger adults whose valves are still pliable. The ejection sound is the only right-sided acoustic event that decreases in intensity with inspiration. This phenomenon reflects premature opening of the pulmonic valve by the elevated RV end-diastolic (postatrial *a* wave) pressure. The systolic murmur increases in intensity during inspiration. With progressively severe PS, the ejection sound moves closer to the first heart sound and eventually becomes inaudible. A right-sided fourth heart sound may emerge. The systolic murmur peaks later and may persist through the aortic component of the second heart sound (A_2). Pulmonic valve closure is delayed, and the pulmonic component of the second heart sound (P_2) is reduced or absent. A prominent *a* wave, indicative of the higher atrial pressure necessary to fill the noncompliant RV, may be seen in the jugular venous pulse. A parasternal or RV lift can be felt with significant pressure overload. Signs of right heart failure, such as hepatomegaly, ascites, and edema, are uncommon but may appear very late in the disease.

LABORATORY EXAMINATION

The ECG will show right axis deviation, RVH, and RA enlargement in adult patients with severe PS. Chest x-ray findings include poststenotic dilation of the main PA in the frontal plane projection and filling of the retrosternal airspace due to RV enlargement on the lateral film. In some patients with RVH, the cardiac apex appears to be lifted off the left hemidiaphragm. The RA may also be enlarged. TTE allows definitive diagnosis and characterization in most cases, with depiction of the valve and assessment of the gradient, RV function, PA pressures (which should be low), and any associated cardiac lesions. TEE may be useful in some patients for improved delineation of the RV outflow tract (RVOT) and assessment of infundibular hypertrophy. Cardiac catheterization is not usually necessary, but if performed, pressures should be obtained from just below and above the pulmonic valve with attention to the possibility that a dynamic component to the gradient may exist. The correlation between Doppler assessment of peak instantaneous gradient and catheterization-measured peak-to-peak gradient is weak. The latter may correlate better with the Doppler mean gradient.

TREATMENT PULMONIC STENOSIS

Diuretics can be used to treat symptoms and signs of right heart failure. Provided there is less than moderate pulmonic regurgitation, pulmonic balloon valvotomy is recommended for symptomatic patients with a domed valve and a peak gradient >50 mmHg (or mean gradient >30 mmHg) and for asymptomatic patients with a peak gradient >60 mmHg (or mean gradient >40 mmHg). Surgery may be required when the valve is dysplastic (as seen in patients with Noonan's syndrome and other disorders). A multidisciplinary heart team is best positioned to make treatment decisions of this nature.

PULMONIC REGURGITATION

Pulmonic regurgitation (PR) may develop as a consequence of primary valve pathology, annular enlargement, or their combination; after surgical treatment of RVOT obstruction in children with such disorders as tetralogy of Fallot; or after pulmonic balloon valvotomy (Table 285-1). Carcinoid usually causes mixed pulmonic valve disease with PR and PS. Long-standing severe PA hypertension from any cause can result in dilation of the pulmonic valve ring and PR.

PATHOPHYSIOLOGY

Severe PR results in RV chamber enlargement and eccentric hypertrophy. As is the case for aortic regurgitation (AR), PR is a state of increased preload and afterload. The reverse pressure gradient from the PA to the RV, which drives the PR, progressively decreases throughout diastole and accounts for the decrescendo nature of the diastolic murmur. As RV diastolic pressure increases, the murmur becomes shorter in duration. The forward CO is preserved during the early stages of the disease, but may not increase normally with exercise and declines over time. A reduction in RV ejection fraction may be an early indicator of hemodynamic compromise. In advanced stages, there is significant enlargement of the RV and RA with marked elevation of the jugular venous pressure.

SYMPTOMS

Mild or moderate degrees of PR do not, by themselves, result in symptoms. Other problems, such as PA hypertension, may dominant the clinical picture. With progressively severe PR and RV dysfunction, fatigue, exertional dyspnea, abdominal fullness/bloating, and lower extremity swelling may be reported.

PHYSICAL FINDINGS

The physical examination hallmark of PR is a high-pitched, decrescendo diastolic murmur (Graham Steell murmur) heard along the left sternal border that can be difficult to distinguish from the more frequently appreciated murmur of aortic regurgitation. The Graham Steell murmur may become louder with inspiration and is usually associated with a loud and sometimes palpable P_2 and an RV lift, as would be expected in patients with significant PA hypertension of any cause. Survivors of childhood surgery for tetralogy of Fallot or PS/pulmonary atresia may have an RV-PA conduit that is freely regurgitant because it does not contain a valve. PA pressures in these individuals are not elevated and the diastolic murmur can be misleadingly low pitched and of short duration despite significant degrees of PR and RV volume overload.

LABORATORY EXAMINATION

Depending on both the etiology and severity of PR, the ECG may show findings of RVH and RA enlargement. On chest x-ray, the RV and RA may be enlarged. Pulmonic valve morphology and function can be assessed with transthoracic Doppler echocardiography. PA pressures can be estimated from the tricuspid valve systolic jet velocity. CMR provides greater anatomic detail, particularly in patients with repaired congenital heart disease, and more precise assessment of RV volumes. Cardiac catheterization is not routinely necessary but would be performed as part of a planned transcatheter procedure.

TREATMENT PULMONIC REGURGITATION

In patients with functional PR due to PA hypertension and annular dilation, efforts to reduce PA vascular resistance and pressure should be optimized. Such efforts may include pharmacologic/vasodilator and/or surgical/interventional strategies, depending on the cause of the PA hypertension. Diuretics can be used to treat the manifestations of right heart failure. Surgical valve replacement for primary, severe, pulmonic valve disease, such as carcinoid or endocarditis, is rarely undertaken. Transcatheter pulmonic valve replacement has been successfully performed in many patients with severe PR after childhood repair of tetralogy of Fallot or pulmonic valve stenosis or atresia. This procedure was introduced clinically prior to transcatheter aortic valve replacement.

286 Multiple and Mixed Valvular Heart Disease

Patrick T. O'Gara, Joseph Loscalzo

Many acquired and congenital cardiac lesions may result in stenosis and/or regurgitation of one or more heart valves. For example, rheumatic heart disease can involve the mitral (mitral stenosis [MS], mitral regurgitation [MR], or MS and MR), aortic (aortic stenosis [AS], aortic regurgitation [AR], or AS and AR), and/or tricuspid (tricuspid stenosis [TS], tricuspid regurgitation [TR], or TS and TR) valve, alone or in combination. The common association of functional TR with significant mitral valve disease is discussed in Chap. 285. Severe mitral annular calcification can result in regurgitation (due to decreased annular shortening during systole) and mild stenosis (caused by extension of the calcification onto the leaflets resulting in restricted valve opening). Patients with severe AS may develop functional MR that may not improve after isolated aortic valve replacement (AVR). Chordal rupture has been described infrequently in patients with severe AS. Aortic valve infective endocarditis may secondarily involve the mitral apparatus either by abscess formation and contiguous spread via the intervalvular fibrosa or by "drop metastases" from the aortic leaflets onto the anterior leaflet of the mitral valve. Mediastinal radiation may result in aortic, mitral, and even tricuspid valve disease, most often with mixed stenosis and regurgitation. Carcinoid heart disease may cause mixed lesions of either or both the tricuspid and pulmonic valves. Ergotamines, and the previously used combination of fenfluramine and phentermine, can rarely result in mixed lesions of the aortic and/or mitral valve. Patients with Marfan's syndrome may have both AR from aortic root dilation and MR due to mitral valve prolapse (MVP). Myxomatous degeneration causing prolapse of multiple valves (mitral, aortic, tricuspid) can also occur in the absence of an identifiable connective tissue disorder. Bicuspid aortic or pulmonic valve disease can result in mixed stenosis and regurgitation.

PATHOPHYSIOLOGY

In patients with multivalvular heart disease, the pathophysiologic derangements associated with the more proximal valve disease can mask the full expression of the attributes of the more distal valve lesion. For example, in patients with rheumatic mitral and aortic valve disease, the reduction in cardiac output (CO) imposed by the mitral valve disease will decrease the magnitude of the hemodynamic derangements related to the severity of the aortic valve lesion (stenotic, regurgitant, or both). Alternatively, the development of atrial fibrillation (AF) during the course of MS can lead to sudden worsening in a patient whose aortic valve disease was not previously felt to be significant. The development of reactive pulmonary vascular disease, sometimes referred to as a "secondary obstructive lesion in series," can impose an additional challenge in these settings. As CO falls with progressive tricuspid valve disease, the severity of any associated mitral or aortic disease can be underestimated.

One of the most common examples of multivalve disease is that of functional TR in the setting of significant mitral valve disease. Functional TR occurs as a consequence of right ventricular and annular dilation; pulmonary artery (PA) hypertension is often present. The tricuspid leaflets are morphologically normal. Progressive degrees of TR lead to right ventricular volume overload and continued chamber and annular dilation. The TR is usually central in origin; reflux into the right atrium (RA) is expressed as large, systolic *c-v* waves in the RA pressure pulse. The height of the *c-v* wave is dependent on RA compliance and the volume of regurgitant flow. The RA wave form may become "ventricularized" in advanced stages of chronic, severe TR with PA hypertension. CO falls and the severity of the associated mitral valve disease may become more difficult to appreciate. Primary rheumatic tricuspid valve disease may occur with rheumatic mitral disease and cause hemodynamic changes reflective of TR, TS, or their combination. With TS, the *y* descent in the RA pressure pulse is prolonged.

Another example of rheumatic, multivalve disease involves the combination of mitral and aortic valve pathology, frequently characterized by MS and AR. In isolated MS, left ventricular (LV) preload and diastolic pressure are reduced as a function of the severity of inflow obstruction. With concomitant AR, however, LV filling is enhanced and diastolic pressure may rise depending on the compliance characteristics of the chamber. Because the CO falls with progressive degrees of MS, transaortic valve flows will decline, masking the potential severity of the aortic valve lesion (AR, AS, or its combination). As noted above, onset of AF in such patients can be especially deleterious.

Functional MR may complicate the course of some patients with severe AS. The mitral valve leaflets and chordae tendineae are usually normal. Incompetence is related to changes in LV geometry (remodeling) and abnormal systolic tethering of the leaflets in the context of markedly elevated LV systolic pressures. Relief of the excess afterload with surgical or transcatheter AVR often, but not always, results in reduction or elimination of the MR. Persistence of significant MR following AVR is associated with impaired functional outcomes and reduced survival. Identification of patients who would benefit from concomitant treatment of their functional MR at time of AVR is quite challenging. Most surgeons advocate for repair of moderate-to-severe or severe functional MR at time of surgical AVR.

In patients with mixed AS and AR, assessment of valve stenosis can be influenced by the magnitude of the regurgitant valve flow. Because transvalvular systolic flow velocities are augmented in patients with AR and preserved LV systolic function, the LV-aortic Doppler-derived pressure gradient and the intensity of the systolic murmur will be elevated to values higher than expected for the true systolic valve orifice size as delineated by planimetry. Uncorrected, the Gorlin formula, which relies on forward CO (systolic transvalvular flow) and the mean pressure gradient for calculation of valve area, is not accurate in the setting of mixed aortic valve disease. Similar considerations apply to patients with mixed mitral valve disease. The peak mitral valve Doppler E wave velocity (v_0) is increased in the setting of severe MR because of enhanced early diastolic flow and may not accurately reflect the contribution to left atrial (LA) hypertension from any associated MS. When either AR or MR is the dominant lesion in patients with mixed aortic or mitral valve disease, respectively, the LV is dilated. When AS or MS predominates, LV chamber size will be normal or small. It can sometimes be difficult to ascertain whether stenosis or regurgitation is the dominant lesion in patients with mixed valve disease, although an integrated clinical and noninvasive assessment can usually provide clarification for purposes of patient management and follow-up.

Patients with significant AS, a nondilated LV chamber, and concentric hypertrophy will poorly tolerate the abrupt development of aortic regurgitation, as may occur, for example, with infective endocarditis or after surgical or transcatheter AVR complicated by paravalvular leakage. The noncompliant LV is not prepared to accommodate the sudden volume load, and as a result, LV diastolic pressure rises rapidly and severe heart failure develops. Indeed, paravalvular regurgitation is a significant risk factor for short- to intermediate-term death following transcatheter AVR. Conditions in which the LV may not be able to dilate in response to chronic AR (or MR) include radiation heart disease and, in some patients, the cardiomyopathy associated with obesity and diabetes. Noncompliant ventricles of small chamber size predispose to earlier onset diastolic dysfunction and heart failure in response to any further perturbation in valve function.

SYMPTOMS

Compared with patients with isolated, single-lesion valve disease, patients with multiple or mixed valve disease may develop symptoms at a relatively earlier stage in the natural history of their disease. Symptoms such as exertional dyspnea and fatigue are usually related to elevated filling pressures, reduced CO, or their combination. Palpitations may signify AF and identify mitral valve disease as an important component of the clinical presentation, even when not previously suspected. Chest pain compatible with angina could reflect left or right ventricular oxygen supply/demand mismatch on a substrate of hypertrophy and pressure/volume overload with or without superimposed coronary artery disease. Symptoms related to right heart failure (abdominal fullness/bloating, edema) are late manifestations of advanced disease.

PHYSICAL FINDINGS

Mixed disease of a single valve is most often manifested by systolic and diastolic murmurs, each with the attributes expected for the valve in question. Thus, patients with AS and AR will have characteristic mid-systolic, crescendo-decrescendo and blowing, decrescendo diastolic murmurs at the base of the heart in the second right interspace and along the left sternal edge, respectively. Many patients with significant AR have mid-systolic outflow murmurs even in the absence of valve sclerosis/stenosis, and other findings of AS must be sought. The separate murmurs of AS and AR can occasionally be difficult to distinguish from the continuous murmurs associated with either a patent ductus arteriosus (PDA) or ruptured sinus of Valsalva aneurysm. With mixed aortic valve disease, the systolic murmur should end before, and not envelope or extend through, the second heart sound (S_2). The murmur associated with a PDA is heard best to the left of the upper sternum. The continuous murmur heard with a ruptured sinus of Valsalva aneurysm is often first appreciated after an episode of acute chest pain. An early ejection click, which usually defines bicuspid aortic valve disease in young adults, is often not present in patients with congenital, mixed AS and AR. As noted above, both the intensity and duration of these separate murmurs can be influenced by a reduction in CO and transvalvular flow due to coexistent mitral valve disease. In patients with isolated MS and MR, expected findings would include a blowing, holosystolic murmur and a mid-diastolic rumble (with or without an opening snap) best heard at the cardiac apex. An irregularly irregular heart rhythm in such patients would likely signify AF. Findings with TS and TR would mimic those of left-sided MS and MR, save for the expected changes in the murmurs with respiration. The murmurs of pulmonic stenosis and regurgitation behave in a fashion directionally similar to AS and AR; dynamic changes during respiration should be noted. Specific attributes of these cardiac murmurs are reviewed in Chap. 285.

LABORATORY EXAMINATION

The electrocardiogram (ECG) may show evidence of ventricular hypertrophy and/or atrial enlargement. ECG signs indicative of right-sided cardiac abnormalities in patients with left-sided valve lesions should prompt additional assessment for PA hypertension and/or right-sided valve disease. The presence of AF in patients with aortic valve disease may be a clue to the presence of previously unsuspected mitral valve disease in the appropriate context. The chest x-ray can be reviewed for evidence of cardiac chamber enlargement, valve and/or annular calcification, and any abnormalities in the appearance of the pulmonary vasculature. The latter could include enlargement of the main and proximal pulmonary arteries with PA hypertension and pulmonary venous redistribution/engorgement or Kerley B lines with increasing degrees of LA hypertension. An enlarged azygos vein in the frontal projection indicates RA hypertension. Roentgenographic findings not expected based on a single or mixed valve lesion may reflect other valve disease.

Transthoracic echocardiography (TTE) is the most commonly used imaging modality for the diagnosis and characterization of multiple and/or mixed valvular heart disease and may often demonstrate findings not clinically suspected. Transesophageal echocardiography (TEE) may sometimes be required for more accurate assessment of valve anatomy (specifically, the mitral valve) and when infective endocarditis (IE) is considered responsible for the clinical presentation. TTE findings of particular interest include those related to valve morphology and function, calcification, chamber size, ventricular wall thickness, estimated PA systolic pressure, and the dimensions of the great vessels, including the root and ascending aorta, PA, and inferior vena cava. Exercise testing (with or without echocardiography) can be useful when the degree of functional limitation reported by the patient is not adequately explained by the findings on TTE performed at rest. An integrated assessment of the clinical and TTE findings is needed to help determine the dominant valve lesion(s) and establish an appropriate plan for treatment and follow-up. Natural history is usually influenced to a relatively greater degree by the dominant lesion. Exercise testing (with or without echocardiography) can

Cardiac magnetic resonance (CMR) can be used to provide additional anatomic and physiologic information when echocardiography proves suboptimal, but is less well suited to the evaluation of valve morphology. Cardiac computed tomography (CT) has been used to assess intracardiac structures in patients with complicated IE. Coronary CT angiography provides a noninvasive alternative for the assessment of coronary artery anatomy prior to surgery.

Invasive hemodynamic evaluation with right and left heart catheterization may be required to characterize more completely the individual contributions of each lesion in patients with either multiple or mixed valvular heart disease. Measurement of PA pressures and calculation of pulmonary vascular resistance (PVR) can help inform clinical decision-making in certain patient subsets, such as those with advanced mitral and tricuspid valve disease. Attention to the accurate assessment of CO is essential. Coronary angiography (if indicated) can be performed as part of the procedure. Contrast ventriculography and great vessel angiography are performed infrequently.

TREATMENT MULTIPLE AND MIXED VALVE DISEASE

Management of patients with multiple or mixed valve disease can be challenging. As noted above, it is helpful to determine the dominant valve lesion and proceed according to the treatment and follow-up recommendations for it (Chaps. 283 to 285), being mindful of deviations from the expected course because of problems related to another valve disorder. For example, AF that emerges in the course of moderate mitral valve disease may precipitate heart failure in patients with concomitant, severe aortic valve disease.

Medical therapies are limited and include diuretics when indicated for relief of congestion and vitamin K antagonists for anticoagulation to prevent stroke and thromboembolism in patients with AF. The novel oral anticoagulants are not approved for use in the setting of significant valvular heart disease. Blood pressure–lowering medications may be needed to treat systemic hypertension, which may aggravate left-sided regurgitant valve lesions, but should be initiated and titrated carefully. Pulmonary vasodilators to lower PVR are not generally effective in this context.

There is a paucity of evidence to inform practice guidelines for surgical and/or transcatheter valve intervention in patients with multiple or mixed valve disease. When there is a clear, dominant lesion, as for example in a patient with severe AS and mild AR, indications for intervention are straightforward and follow those recommended for patients with AS (Chap. 283). In other patients, however, there is less clarity, and decisions regarding intervention should be based on several considerations, including those related to lesion severity, ventricular remodeling, functional capacity, and PA pressures. In this regard, it is important to realize that patients with multiple and/or mixed valve disease may develop limiting symptoms or signs of physiologic impairment even with moderate valve lesions.

Concomitant aortic and mitral valve replacement surgery is associated with a significantly higher perioperative mortality risk than replacement of either valve alone (see Tables 283-2 and 284-2), and operation should be carefully considered. Double valve replacement surgery is usually performed for treatment of severe (unrepairable) valve disease at both locations and for the combination of severe disease at one location with moderate disease at the other, so as to avoid the hazards of reoperation in the intermediate to late term for progressive disease of the unoperated valve. In addition, the presence of a prosthesis in the aortic position significantly restricts surgical exposure of the native mitral valve. The need for double valve replacement may also impact the decision regarding the type of prosthesis (i.e., mechanical vs tissue).

Tricuspid valve repair for moderate or severe functional TR at the time of left-sided valve surgery is now commonplace, particularly if there is dilation of the tricuspid annulus (>40 mm). The addition of tricuspid valve repair, consisting usually of insertion of an annuloplasty ring, adds little time or complexity to the procedure and is well tolerated. Reoperation for repair (or replacement) of progressive TR years after initial surgery for left-sided valve disease, on the other hand, is associated with a relatively high perioperative mortality risk. Repair of moderate or severe functional MR at time of AVR for AS can usually be undertaken with acceptable risk for perioperative death or major complication.

The presence of moderate or severe MR in patients with rheumatic MS is a contraindication to percutaneous mitral balloon valvotomy (PMBV). Likewise, the presence of significant AR in patients with AS disqualifies them from percutaneous aortic balloon valvotomy (PABV). The presence of severe, coexistent AR was an exclusion criterion for enrollment in the initial PARTNER trials of transcatheter AVR (TAVR) in prohibitive- and high-surgical-risk patients with severe, calcific AS. Transcatheter management of both severe AS (with TAVR) and functional MR (with deployment of a MitralClip) has been reported. Further advances in transcatheter treatments for multiple and mixed valve disease are anticipated.

287 Cardiomyopathy and Myocarditis

Neal K. Lakdawala, Lynne Warner Stevenson, Joseph Loscalzo

DEFINITION AND CLASSIFICATION

Cardiomyopathy is disease of the heart muscle. It is estimated that cardiomyopathy accounts for 5–10% of the heart failure in the 5–6 million patients carrying that diagnosis in the United States. This term is intended to exclude cardiac dysfunction that results from other structural heart disease, such as coronary artery disease, primary valve disease, or severe hypertension; however, in general usage, the phrase *ischemic cardiomyopathy* is sometimes applied to describe diffuse dysfunction attributed to multivessel coronary artery disease, and *nonischemic cardiomyopathy* to describe cardiomyopathy from other causes. As of 2006, cardiomyopathies are defined as "a heterogeneous group of diseases of the myocardium associated with mechanical and/or electrical dysfunction that usually (but not invariably) exhibit inappropriate ventricular hypertrophy or dilatation and are due to a variety of causes that frequently are genetic."[1]

The traditional classification of cardiomyopathies into a triad of dilated, restrictive, and hypertrophic was based initially on autopsy specimens and later on echocardiographic findings. Dilated and hypertrophic cardiomyopathies can be distinguished on the basis of left ventricular wall thickness and cavity dimension; however, restrictive cardiomyopathy can have variably increased wall thickness and chamber dimensions that range from reduced to slightly increased, with prominent atrial enlargement. Restrictive cardiomyopathy is now defined more on the basis of abnormal diastolic function, which is also present but initially less prominent in dilated and hypertrophic cardiomyopathy. Restrictive cardiomyopathy can overlap in presentation, gross morphology, and etiology with both hypertrophic and dilated cardiomyopathies (Table 287-1).

Expanding information renders this classification triad based on phenotype increasingly inadequate to define disease or therapy. Identification of more genetic determinants of cardiomyopathy has suggested a four-way classification scheme of etiology as primary (affecting primarily the heart) and secondary to other systemic disease. The primary causes are then divided into genetic, mixed genetic and acquired, and acquired; however, genetic information is often unavailable at the time of initial presentation, the phenotypic expression of a given mutation varies widely, and genetic predisposition influences the clinical phenotype of acquired cardiomyopathies, as well. Although the proposed genetic classification does not yet guide many current clinical strategies, it will likely become increasingly relevant as classification of disease moves beyond individual organ pathology to more integrated systems approaches.

GENERAL PRESENTATION

For all cardiomyopathies, the early symptoms often relate to exertional intolerance with breathlessness or fatigue, usually from inadequate cardiac reserve during exercise. These symptoms may initially go unnoticed or be attributed to other causes, commonly lung disease or age-dependent exercise limitation. As fluid retention leads to elevation of resting filling pressures, shortness of breath may occur during routine daily activity such as dressing and may manifest as dyspnea or cough when lying down at night. Although often considered the hallmark of congestion, peripheral edema may be absent despite severe fluid retention, particularly in younger patients in whom ascites and abdominal discomfort may dominate. The nonspecific term *congestive heart failure* describes only the resulting syndrome of fluid retention, which is common to all three types of cardiomyopathy and also to cardiac structural diseases associated with elevated filling pressures. All three types of cardiomyopathy can be associated with atrioventricular valve regurgitation, typical and atypical chest pain, atrial and ventricular tachyarrhythmias, and embolic events (Table 287-1). Initial evaluation begins with a detailed clinical history and examination, looking for clues to cardiac, extracardiac, and familial disease (Table 287-2).

GENETIC ETIOLOGIES OF CARDIOMYOPATHY

Estimates for the prevalence of genetic etiology for cardiomyopathy continue to rise, with increasing attention paid to the family history and the availability of genetic testing. Well-recognized in hypertrophic cardiomyopathy, heritability is also present in at least 30% of dilated cardiomyopathy without other clear etiology. Careful family history should elicit not only known cardiomyopathy and heart failure, but also family members who have had sudden death, often incorrectly attributed to "a massive heart attack," who have had atrial fibrillation or pacemaker implantation by middle age, or who have muscular dystrophy.

Most familial cardiomyopathies are inherited in an autosomal dominant pattern, with occasional autosomal recessive and X-linked inheritance (Table 287-3). Missense mutations with amino acid substitutions are the most common in cardiomyopathy. Expressed mutant proteins may interfere with function of the normal allele through a dominant negative mechanism. Mutations introducing a premature stop codon (nonsense) or shift in the reading frame (frameshift) may create a truncated or unstable protein the lack of which causes cardiomyopathy (haploinsufficiency). Deletions or duplications of an entire exon or gene are uncommon causes of cardiomyopathy, except for the dystrophinopathies.

Many different genes have been implicated in human cardiomyopathy (locus heterogeneity), and many mutations within those genes have been associated with disease (allelic heterogeneity). Although most identified mutations are "private" to individual families, several specific mutations are found repeatedly, either due to a founder effect or recurrent mutations at a common residue.

Genetic cardiomyopathy is characterized by age dependence and incomplete penetrance. The defining phenotype of cardiomyopathy is rarely present at birth and, in some individuals, may never manifest. Related individuals who carry the *same* mutation may differ in the severity of cardiomyopathy and associated consequences of rhythm disorders and need for transplantation, indicating the important role of other genetic, epigenetic, and environmental modifiers in disease expression. Sex appears to play a role, as penetrance and clinical severity may be greater in men for most cardiomyopathies. Clinical disease expression is generally more severe in the 3–5% of individuals who harbor two or more mutations linked to cardiomyopathy. However, the clinical course of a patient usually cannot be predicted based on which mutation is present; thus, current therapy is based on the phenotype rather than the genetic defect. Currently, the greatest utility of genetic testing for cardiomyopathy is to inform family evaluations. However, genetic testing occasionally enables the detection of a disease for which specific therapy is indicated, such as the replacements for defective metabolic enzymes in Fabry's disease and Gaucher disease.

GENES AND PATHWAYS IN CARDIOMYOPATHY

Mutations in sarcomeric genes, encoding the thick and thin myofilament proteins, are the best characterized. While the majority are associated with hypertrophic cardiomyopathy, an increasing number of sarcomeric mutations have now been implicated in dilated cardiomyopathy, and some in left ventricular noncompaction. Few mutations have been identified in excitation-contraction coupling proteins, perhaps because they are too crucial for survival to allow variation. The most commonly recognized genetic causes of dilated cardiomyopathy are structural mutations of the giant protein titin, encoded *TTN*, which maintains sarcomere structure and acts as a key signaling molecule.

As cytoskeletal proteins play crucial roles in the structure, connection, and stability of the myocyte, multiple defects in these proteins can lead to cardiomyopathy, usually with a dilated phenotype (Fig. 287-1). For example, desmin forms intermediate filaments that connect the nuclear and plasma membranes, Z-lines,

[1]From BJ Maron et al: Circulation 113:1807, 2006.

TABLE 287-1 PRESENTATION WITH SYMPTOMATIC CARDIOMYOPATHY

	Dilated	Restrictive	Hypertrophic
Ejection fraction (normal >55%)	Usually <30% when symptoms severe	25–50%	>60%
Left ventricular diastolic dimension (normal <55 mm)	≥60 mm	<60 mm (may be decreased)	Often decreased
Left ventricular wall thickness	Normal or decreased	Normal or increased	Markedly increased
Atrial size	Increased, may also be primarily affected	Increased; may be massive	Increased; related to elevated filling pressures
Valvular regurgitation	Related to annular dilation; mitral appears earlier during decompensation; tricuspid regurgitation with right ventricular dysfunction	Related to endocardial involvement; frequent mitral and tricuspid regurgitation, rarely severe	Related to valve-septum interaction; mitral regurgitation
Common first symptoms	Exertional intolerance	Exertional intolerance, fluid retention early, may have dominant right-sided symptoms	Exertional intolerance; may have chest pain
Congestive symptoms[a]	Left before right, except right prominent in young adults	Right often dominates	Left-sided congestion at rest may develop late
Arrhythmias	Ventricular tachyarrhythmia; conduction block in Chagas' disease, and some families. Atrial fibrillation.	Ventricular uncommon except in sarcoidosis, conduction block in sarcoidosis and amyloidosis. Atrial fibrillation.	Ventricular tachyarrhythmias; atrial fibrillation

[a]Left-sided symptoms of pulmonary congestion: dyspnea on exertion, orthopnea, paroxysmal nocturnal dyspnea. Right-sided symptoms of systemic venous congestion: hepatic and abdominal distention, discomfort on bending, peripheral edema.

TABLE 287-2 INITIAL EVALUATION OF CARDIOMYOPATHY

Clinical Evaluation
Thorough history and physical examination to identify cardiac and noncardiac disorders[a]
Detailed family history of heart failure, cardiomyopathy, skeletal myopathy, conduction disorders, tachyarrhythmias, and sudden death
History of alcohol, illicit drugs, chemotherapy or radiation therapy[a]
Assessment of ability to perform routine and desired activities[a]
Assessment of volume status, orthostatic blood pressure, body mass index[a]
Laboratory Evaluation
Electrocardiogram[a]
Chest radiograph[a]
Two-dimensional and Doppler echocardiogram[a]
Magnetic resonance imaging for evidence of myocardial inflammation and fibrosis
Chemistry:
Serum sodium,[a] potassium,[a] calcium,[a] magnesium[a]
Fasting glucose (glycohemoglobin in diabetes mellitus)
Creatinine,[a] blood urea nitrogen[a]
Albumin,[a] total protein,[a] liver function tests[a]
Lipid profile
Thyroid-stimulating hormone[a]
Serum iron, transferrin saturation
Urinalysis
Creatine kinase isoforms
Cardiac troponin levels
Hematology:
Hemoglobin/hematocrit[a]
White blood cell count with differential,[a] including eosinophils
Erythrocyte sedimentation rate
Initial Evaluation When Specific Diagnoses Are Suspected
Titers for infection in the setting of clinical suspicion:
Acute viral (coxsackie, echovirus, influenza)
Human immunodeficiency virus
Chagas' (*Trypanosoma cruzi*), Lyme (*Borrelia burgdorferi*), toxoplasmosis
Catheterization with coronary angiography in patients with angina who are candidates for intervention[a]
Serologies for active rheumatologic disease
Endomyocardial biopsy including sample for electron microscopy when suspecting specific diagnosis with therapeutic implications
Screening for sleep-disordered breathing

[a]Level I recommendations from ACC/AHA Practice Guidelines for Chronic Heart Failure in the Adult.

and the intercalated disks between muscle cells. Desmin mutations impair the transmission of force and signaling for both cardiac and skeletal muscle and may cause combined cardiac and skeletal myopathy.

Sarcolemmal membrane protein defects are associated with dilated cardiomyopathy. The best known is dystrophin, encoded by the X chromosome gene *DMD*, abnormalities of which cause Duchenne's and Becker's muscle dystrophy. (Interestingly, abnormal dystrophin can be acquired when the coxsackie virus cleaves dystrophin during viral myocarditis.) This protein provides a network that supports the sarcolemma and also connects to the sarcomere. The progressive functional defect in both cardiac and skeletal muscle reflects vulnerability to mechanical stress. Dystrophin is associated at the membrane with a complex of other proteins, such as metavinculin, abnormalities of which also cause dilated cardiomyopathy. Defects in the sarcolemmal channel proteins (*channelopathies*) are generally associated with primary arrhythmias, but mutations in *SCN5A*, distinct from those that cause the Brugada or long-QT syndromes, have been implicated in dilated cardiomyopathy with conduction disease.

Nuclear membrane protein defects in cardiac and skeletal muscle occur in either autosomal (lamin A/C) or X-linked (emerin) patterns. These defects are associated with a high prevalence of atrial arrhythmias and conduction system disease, which can occur in some family members without or before detectable cardiomyopathy.

Intercalated disks contribute to intracellular connections, allowing mechanical and electrical coupling between cells and also connections to desmin filaments within the cell. Mutations in proteins of the desmosomal complex compromise attachment of the myocytes, which can become disconnected and die, to be replaced by fat and fibrous tissue. These areas are highly arrhythmogenic and may dilate to form aneurysms. Although more often noted in the right ventricle (arrhythmogenic right ventricular dysplasia), this condition can affect both ventricles and has also been termed "arrhythmogenic cardiomyopathy."

Owing to the conservation of signaling pathways in multiple systems, we may expect to discover more extracardiac manifestations of genetic abnormalities initially considered to manifest exclusively in the heart. In contrast, the monogenic disorders of metabolism that affect the heart are already clearly recognized to affect multiple organ systems. Currently, it is most important to diagnose defective enzymes for which specific enzyme replacement therapy can now ameliorate the course of disease, such as with alpha-galactosidase A deficiency (Fabry's disease). Abnormalities of mitochondrial DNA (maternally transmitted) impair energy production with multiple clinical manifestations, including impaired cognitive function and skeletal myopathy. The phenotypic expression is highly variable depending on the

TABLE 287-3 SELECTED GENETIC DEFECTS ASSOCIATED WITH CARDIOMYOPATHY

	Gene Product	Inheritance	Cardiac Phenotype	Isolated Cardiac Phenotype	Extracardiac Manifestations
Sarcomere	*MYH7* (β myosin heavy chain)	AD	HCM, DCM, LVNC	Yes	Skeletal myopathy
	MYBPC3 (myosin binding protein C)	AD	HCM	Yes	
	TNNT2 (cardiac troponin T)	AD	HCM, DCM, LVNC	Yes	
	TNNI3 (cardiac troponin I)	AD, AR	HCM, DCM, RCM	Yes	
	TTN (Titin)	AD	DCM	Yes	
	TPM1 (α-tropomyosin)	AD	HCM, DCM	Yes	
	TNNC1 (cardiac troponin C)	AD	DCM	Yes	
	ACTC (α-actin)	AD	HCM, DCM, (LVNC)	Yes	
	MYL2 (myosin regulatory light chain)	AD	HCM	Yes	Skeletal myopathy
	MYL3 (myosin essential light chain)	AD	HCM	Yes	
Z-disk and Cytoskeleton	*DES* (Desmin)	AD	DCM, RCM	Yes	Skeletal myopathy
	LDB3 (Cypher-ZASP)	AD	DCM, LVNC	Yes	Skeletal myopathy
	MYOZ2 (Myozenin)	AD	HCM	Yes	
	TCAP (Telethonin)	AD	DCM, HCM	Yes	
	ANKRD1 (CARP)	AD	HCM, (DCM)	Yes	
	CSRP3 (MLP)	AD	DCM, (HCM)	Yes	
	ACTN2 (α-actinin-2)	AD	DCM	Yes	
	CRYAB (αB-crystallin)	AD	DCM	Yes	
Nuclear Membrane	*LMNA* (Lamin A/C)	AD, AR	CDDC	Yes	Skeletal myopathy
	EMD (Emerin)	X-linked	CDDC	No	Skeletal myopathy, contractures
Excitation-Contraction Coupling	*PLN* (Phospholamban)	AD	DCM	Yes	
	SCN5A (NAV 1.5)	AD	CDDC	Yes	Note other mutations associated with Brugada syndrome
	RYR2 (cardiac ryanodine receptor)	AD	ARVC	Yes	
	CASQ2 (calsequestrin 2)	AR	ARVC	Yes	
Cellular Metabolism	*PRKAG2* (γ-subunit of AMP kinase)	AD	HCM+	Yes	
	LAMP2 (lysosomal associated membrane protein)	X-linked	HCM+	No[a]	Danon's disease: skeletal myopathy, cognitive impairment
	TAZ (Tafazzin)	X-linked	DCM, LVNC	No	Barth's syndrome: skeletal myopathy, cognitive impairment, neutropenia
	FXN (Frataxin)	AR	HCM	No	Friedreich's ataxia: ataxia, diabetes mellitus type 2
	TMEM43 (transmembrane protein 43)	AD	ARVC	Yes	
	GLA (α-galactosidase-A)	X-linked	HCM+	Yes	Fabry's disease: renal failure, angiokeratomas and painful neuropathy
Mitochondria	Mitochondrial DNA	Maternal transmission	DCM, HCM	No	MELAS, MERRF, Kearns-Sayre syndrome, ocular myopathy
Sarcolemmal Membrane	*DMD* (Dystrophin)	X-linked	DCM	No[a]	Duchenne's and Becker's muscular dystrophy
	DMPK (dystrophica myotonica protein kinase)	AD	DCM	No	Myotonic dystrophy type 1
	SGCD (δ-sarcoglycan)	AD	DCM	Yes	
Desmosome	*DSP* (Desmoplakin) *JUP* (Plakoglobin)	AD, AR	ARVC	Yes	Carvajal syndrome (AR), Naxos syndrome (AR), "woolly hair" and hyperkeratosis of palms and soles
	DSG2 (Desmoglein 2) *DSC2* (Desmocollin 2) *PKP2* (Plakophilin 2)	AD	ARVC	Yes	
Other Examples	*RBM20* (RNA binding motif 20)	AD	DCM	Yes	
	PSEN1 (Presenilin-1,2)	AD	DCM	Yes	Dementia
	BAG3 (BCL2-associated athanogene 3)	AD	DCM	Yes	

[a]Indicates that isolated cardiac phenotype can occur in women with the X-linked defects.

Abbreviations: AD, autosomal dominant; AR, autosomal recessive; ARVC, arrhythmogenic right ventricular cardiomyopathy; CDDC, conduction disease with dilated cardiomyopathy; DCM, dilated cardiomyopathy; HCM, hypertrophic cardiomyopathy; HCM+, HCM with preexcitation; HCMc, HCM with conduction disease; LVNC, left ventricular noncompaction; MELAS, (mitochondrial) myopathy, encephalopathy, lactic acidosis, and strokelike episodes syndrome; MERRF, myoclonic epilepsy with ragged red fibers; RCM, restrictive cardiomyopathy.

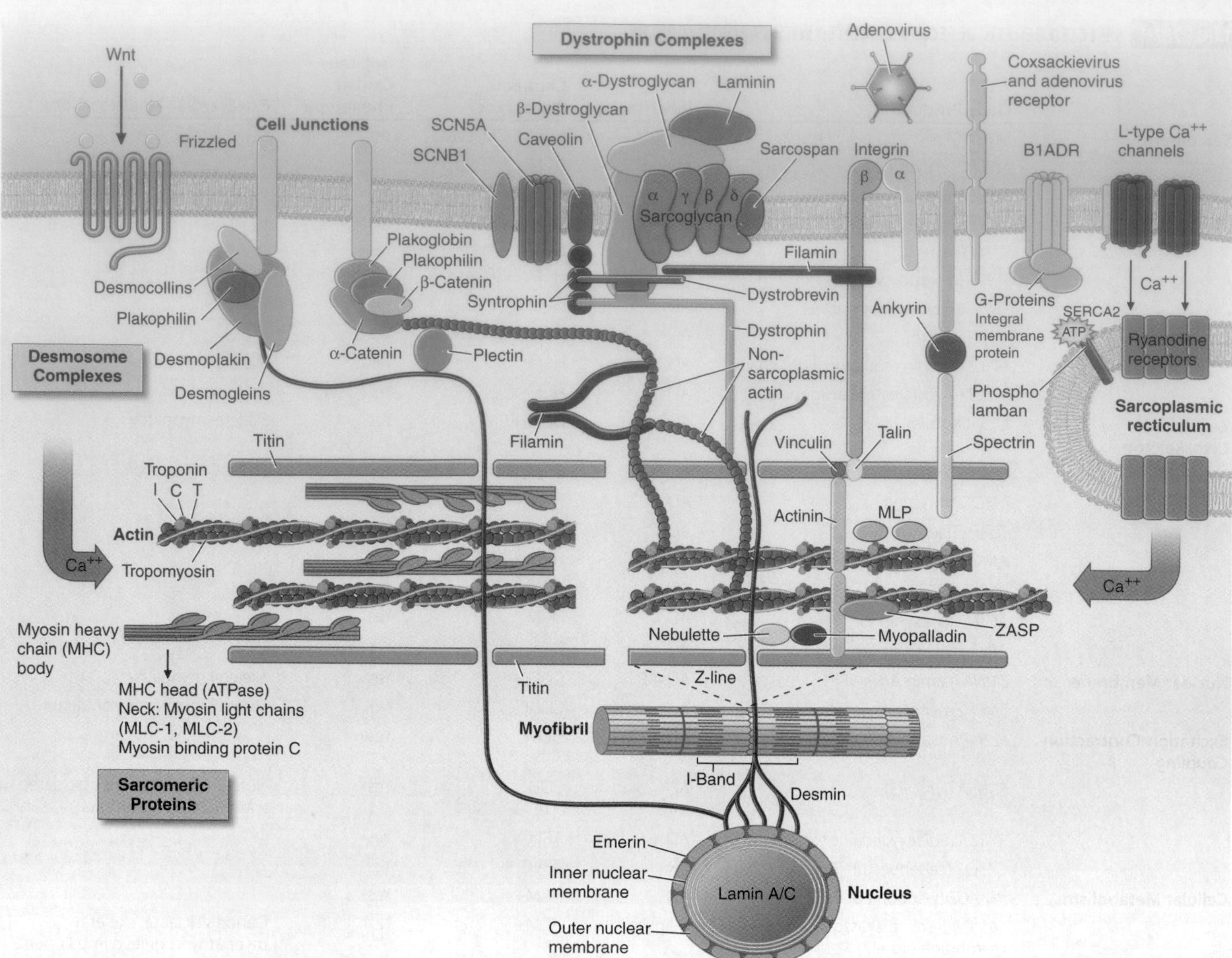

FIGURE 287-1 Drawing of myocyte indicating multiple sites of abnormal gene products associated with cardiomyopathy. Major functional groups include the sarcomeric proteins (actin, myosin, tropomyosin, and the associated regulatory proteins), the dystrophin complex stabilizing and connecting the cell membrane to intracellular structures, the desmosome complexes associated with cell-cell connections and stability, and multiple cytoskeletal proteins that integrate and stabilize the myocyte. ATP, adenosine triphosphate. *(Figure adapted from Jeffrey A. Towbin, MD, University of Cincinnati, with permission.)*

distribution of the maternal mitochondria during embryonic development. Heritable systemic diseases, such as familial amyloidosis and hemochromatosis, can affect the heart without mutation of genes expressed in the heart.

For any patient with suspected or proven genetic disease, family members should be considered and evaluated in a longitudinal fashion. Screening includes an echocardiogram and electrocardiogram (ECG). The indications and implications for confirmatory specific genetic testing vary depending on the specific mutation. The profound questions raised by families about diseases shared and passed down merit serious and sensitive discussion, ideally provided by a trained genetic counselor.

DILATED CARDIOMYOPATHY

An enlarged left ventricle with decreased systolic function as measured by left ventricular ejection fraction characterizes dilated cardiomyopathy (Figs. 287-2, 287-3, and 287-4). *Systolic failure* is more marked than diastolic dysfunction. Although the syndrome of dilated cardiomyopathy has multiple etiologies (Table 287-4), there appear to be common pathways of secondary response and disease progression. When myocardial injury is acquired, some myocytes may die initially, whereas others survive only to have later programmed cell death (apoptosis), and remaining myocytes hypertrophy in response to increased wall stress. Local and circulating factors stimulate deleterious secondary responses that contribute to progression of disease. Dynamic remodeling of the interstitial scaffolding affects diastolic function and the amount of ventricular dilation. Mitral regurgitation commonly develops as the valvular apparatus is distorted and is usually substantial by the time heart failure is severe. Many cases that present "acutely" have progressed silently through these stages over months to years. Dilation and decreased function of the right ventricle may result from the initial injury and occasionally dominate, but more commonly appear later in relation to mechanical interactions with the failing left ventricle and the elevated afterload presented by secondary pulmonary hypertension.

Regardless of the nature and degree of direct cell injury, the resulting functional impairment often includes some contribution from secondary responses that may be modifiable or reversible. Almost half of all patients with new-onset cardiomyopathy demonstrate substantial spontaneous recovery. Even with long-standing disease, some patients have dramatic improvement to near-normal ejection fractions during pharmacologic therapy, particularly notable with the β-adrenergic antagonists coupled with renin-angiotensin system inhibition. For patients in whom left bundle branch block precedes clinical heart failure by many years, cardiac resynchronization pacing may be particularly likely to improve ejection fraction and decrease ventricular size. Interest in the potential for recovery of cardiomyopathy has been

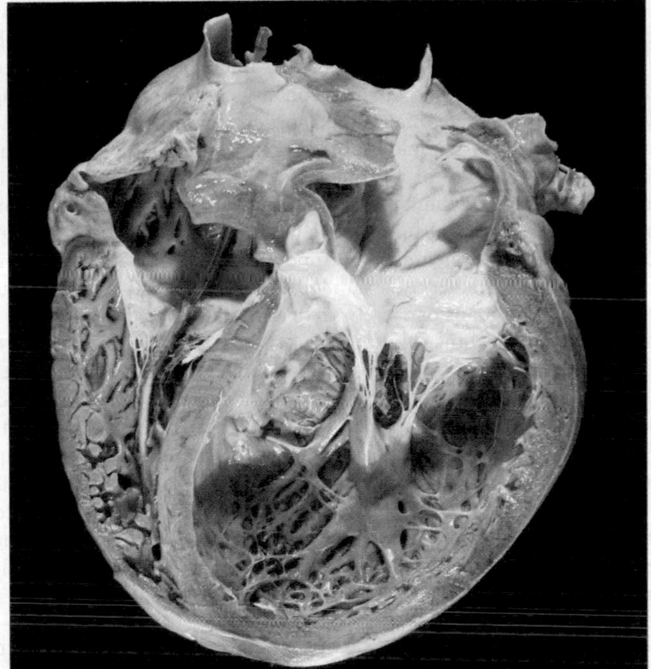

FIGURE 287-2 Dilated cardiomyopathy. This gross specimen of a heart removed at the time of transplantation shows massive left ventricular dilation and moderate right ventricular dilation. Although the left ventricular wall in particular appears thinned, there is significant hypertrophy of this heart, which weighs more than 800 g (upper limit of normal = 360 g). A defibrillator lead is seen traversing the tricuspid valve into the right ventricular apex. *(Image courtesy of Robert Padera, MD, PhD, Department of Pathology, Brigham and Women's Hospital, Boston.)*

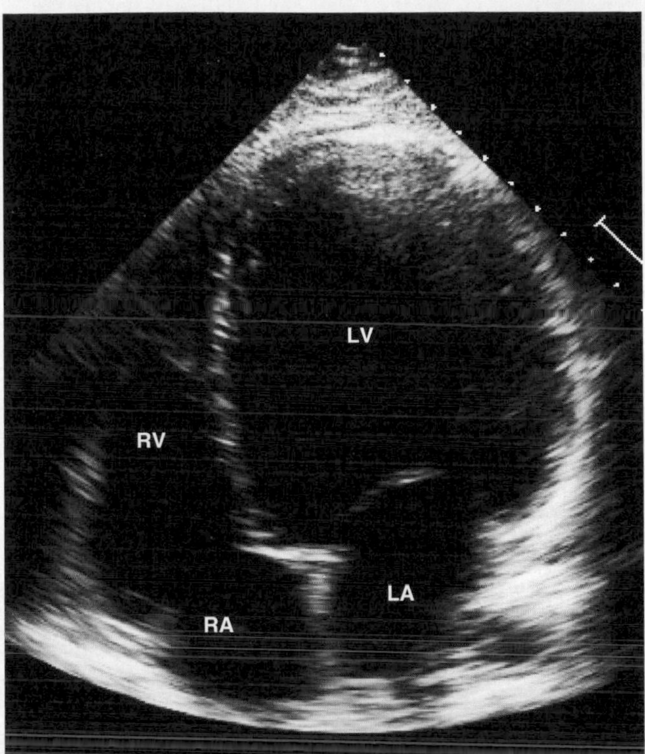

FIGURE 287-3 Dilated cardiomyopathy. This echocardiogram of a young man with dilated cardiomyopathy shows massive global dilation and thinning of the walls of the left ventricle (LV). The left atrium (LA) is also enlarged compared to normal. Note that the echocardiographic and pathologic images are vertically opposite, such that the LV is by convention on the top right in the echocardiographic image and bottom right in the pathologic images. RA, right atrium; RV, right ventricle. *(Image courtesy of Justina Wu, MD, Brigham and Women's Hospital, Boston.)*

further stimulated by occasional "recovery" of left ventricular function after prolonged mechanical circulatory support. The diagnosis and therapy for dilated cardiomyopathy are generally dictated by the stage of heart failure (Chap. 279), with specific aspects discussed for relevant etiologies below.

MYOCARDITIS

Myocarditis (inflammation of the heart) can result from multiple causes but is most commonly attributed to infective agents that can injure the myocardium through direct invasion, production of cardiotoxic substances, or chronic inflammation with or without persistent infection. Myocarditis cannot be assumed from a presentation of decreased systolic function in the setting of an acute infection, as any severe infection causing systemic cytokine release can depress cardiac function transiently. Infectious myocarditis has been reported with almost all types of infective agents but is most commonly associated with viruses and the protozoan *Trypanosoma cruzi.*

INFECTIVE MYOCARDITIS

The pathogenesis of viral myocarditis has been extensively studied in murine models. After viruses gain entry through the respiratory or gastrointestinal tract, they can infect organs possessing specific receptors, such as the coxsackie-adenovirus receptor on the heart. Viral infection and replication can cause myocardial injury and lysis. For example, the enteroviral protease 2A facilitates viral replication and infection through degradation of the myocyte protein dystrophin, which is crucial for myocyte stability. Activation of viral receptor proteins can also activate host tyrosine kinases, which modify the cytoskeleton to facilitate further viral entry.

The first host response to infection is the nonspecific innate immune response, heavily dependent on Toll-like receptors that recognize common antigenic patterns. Cytokine release is rapid, followed by triggered activation and expansion of specific T- and B-cell populations. This initial response appears to be crucial, as early immunosuppression in animal models can increase viral replication and worsen cardiac injury. However, successful recovery from viral infection depends not only on the efficacy of the immune response to limit viral infection, but also on timely downregulation to prevent overreaction and autoimmune injury to the host.

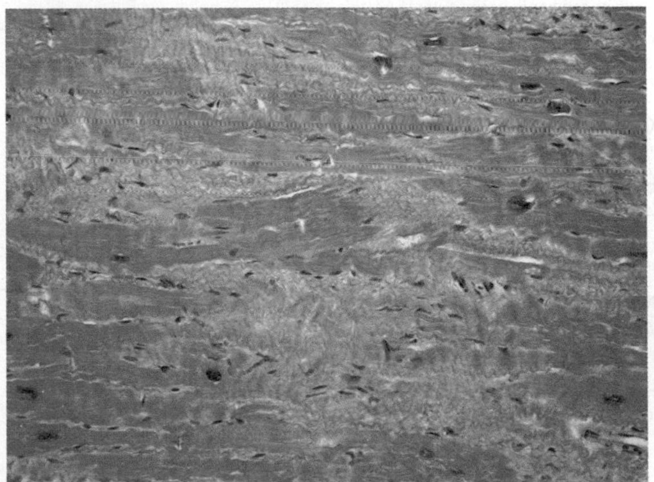

FIGURE 287-4 Dilated cardiomyopathy. Microscopic specimen of a dilated cardiomyopathy showing the nonspecific changes of interstitial fibrosis and myocyte hypertrophy characterized by increased myocyte size and enlarged, irregular nuclei. Hematoxylin and eosin–stained section, 100× original magnification. *(Image courtesy of Robert Padera, MD, PhD, Department of Pathology, Brigham and Women's Hospital, Boston.)*

TABLE 287-4 MAJOR CAUSES OF DILATED CARDIOMYOPATHY (WITH COMMON EXAMPLES)

Inflammatory Myocarditis
Infective
Viral (coxsackie,[a] adenovirus,[a] HIV, hepatitis C)
Parasitic (*T. cruzi*—Chagas' disease, trypanosomiasis, toxoplasmosis)
Bacterial (diphtheria)
Spirochetal (*Borrelia burgdorferi*—Lyme disease)
Rickettsial (Q fever)
Fungal (with systemic infection)
Noninfective
Granulomatous inflammatory disease
Sarcoidosis
Giant cell myocarditis
Eosinophilic myocarditis
Polymyositis, dermatomyositis
Collagen vascular disease
Peripartum cardiomyopathy
Transplant rejection
Toxic
Alcohol
Catecholamines: amphetamines, cocaine
Chemotherapeutic agents (anthracyclines, trastuzumab)
Interferon
Other therapeutic agents (hydroxychloroquine, chloroquine)
Drugs of misuse (emetine, anabolic steroids)
Heavy metals: lead, mercury
Occupational exposure: hydrocarbons, arsenicals
Metabolic[a]
Nutritional deficiencies: thiamine, selenium, carnitine
Electrolyte deficiencies: calcium, phosphate, magnesium
Endocrinopathy
Thyroid disease
Pheochromocytoma
Diabetes
Obesity
Hemochromatosis
Inherited Metabolic Pathway Defects[a]
Familial[a] (See Table 287-3)
Skeletal and cardiac myopathy
Dystrophin-related dystrophy (Duchenne's, Becker's)
Mitochondrial myopathies (e.g., Kearns-Sayre syndrome)
Arrhythmogenic ventricular dysplasia
Hemochromatosis
Associated with other systemic diseases
Susceptibility to immune-mediated myocarditis
Overlap with Nondilated Cardiomyopathy
"Minimally dilated cardiomyopathy"
Hemochromatosis[a]
Amyloidosis[a]
Hypertrophic cardiomyopathy[a] ("burned-out")
"Idiopathic"[a]
Miscellaneous (Shared Elements of Above Etiologies)
Arrhythmogenic right ventricular dysplasia (may also affect left ventricle)[a]
Left ventricular noncompaction[a]
Peripartum cardiomyopathy
Tachycardia-related cardiomyopathy
Supraventricular arrhythmias with uncontrolled rate
Very frequent nonsustained ventricular tachycardia or high premature ventricular complex burden
Left bundle branch block (LBBB) has been implicated as a cause of dilated cardiomyopathy appearing late after idiopathic LBBB and responding with near-normal left ventricle size and function after cardiac resynchronization therapy.

[a]Some specific cases can be linked now to specific genetic mutation in a familial cardiomyopathy; others with similar phenotypes that appear to be acquired or idiopathic may represent genetic factors not yet identified.

The secondary acquired immune response is more specifically addressed against the viral proteins and can include both T-cell infiltration and antibodies to viral proteins. If unchecked, the acquired immune response can perpetuate secondary cardiac damage. Ongoing cytokine release activates matrix metalloproteinases that can disrupt the collagen and elastin scaffolding of the heart, potentiating ventricular dilation. Stimulation of profibrotic factors leads to pathologic interstitial fibrosis. Some of the antibodies triggered through co-stimulation or molecular mimicry also recognize targets within the host myocyte, such as the β-adrenergic receptor, troponin, and Na^+/K^+ ATPase, but it remains unclear whether these antibodies contribute actively to cardiac dysfunction in humans or merely serve as markers of cardiac injury.

It is not known how long the viruses persist in the human heart, whether late persistence of the viral genome continues to be deleterious, or how often a dormant virus can again become pathogenic. Genomes of common viruses have frequently been detected in patients with clinical diagnoses of myocarditis or dilated cardiomyopathy, but there is little information on how often these are present in patients without cardiac disease (see below). Further information is needed to understand the relative timing and contribution of infection, immune responses, and secondary adaptations in the progression of heart failure after viral myocarditis (Fig 287-5).

Clinical Presentation of Viral Myocarditis *Acute viral myocarditis* often presents with symptoms and signs of heart failure. Some patients present with chest pain suggestive of pericarditis or acute myocardial infarction. Occasionally, the presentation is dominated by atrial or ventricular tachyarrhythmias, or by pulmonary or systemic emboli from intracardiac thrombi. Electrocardiographic or echocardiographic abnormalities may also be detected incidentally during evaluation for other diagnoses. The typical patient with presumed viral myocarditis is a young to middle-aged adult who develops progressive dyspnea and weakness within a few days to weeks after a viral syndrome that was accompanied by fever and myalgias.

A small number of patients present with fulminant myocarditis, with rapid progression from a severe febrile respiratory syndrome to cardiogenic shock that may involve multiple organ systems, leading to renal failure, hepatic failure, and coagulopathy. These patients are typically young adults who have recently been dismissed from urgent care settings with antibiotics for bronchitis or oseltamivir for viral syndromes, only to return within a few days in rapidly progressive cardiogenic shock. Prompt triage is vital to provide aggressive support with high-dose intravenous catecholamine therapy and sometimes with temporary mechanical circulatory support. Recognition of patients with this fulminant presentation is potentially life-saving as more than half can survive, with marked improvement demonstrable within the first few weeks. The ejection fraction function of these patients often recovers to near-normal, although residual diastolic dysfunction may limit vigorous exercise for some survivors.

Chronic viral myocarditis is often invoked, but rarely proven, as a diagnosis when no other cause of dilated cardiomyopathy can be identified. However, some cases of otherwise unexplained cardiomyopathy will later be recognized to have a genetic basis, or ultimately found to have resulted from excess alcohol consumption or illicit drugs. There are likely many other causes that cannot yet be identified. The prevalence of previous or persistent viral infection as the cause for chronic dilated cardiomyopathy remains highly controversial.

Laboratory evaluation for myocarditis The initial evaluation for suspected myocarditis includes an ECG, an echocardiogram, and serum levels of troponin and creatine phosphokinase fractions. Magnetic resonance imaging is increasingly used for the diagnosis of myocarditis, which is supported by evidence of increased tissue edema and gadolinium enhancement (Fig. 287-6), particularly in the mid-wall (as distinct from usual coronary artery territories).

Endomyocardial biopsy is not often indicated for the initial evaluation of suspected viral myocarditis unless ventricular tachyarrhythmias suggest possible etiologies of sarcoidosis or giant cell myocarditis. The indications and benefit of endomyocardial biopsy for evaluation of myocarditis or new-onset cardiomyopathy remain controversial.

FIGURE 287-5 Schematic diagram demonstrating the possible progression from infection through direct, secondary, and autoimmune responses to dilated cardiomyopathy. Most of the supporting evidence for this sequence is derived from animal models. It is not known to what degree persistent infection and/or ongoing immune responses contribute to ongoing myocardial injury in the chronic phase.

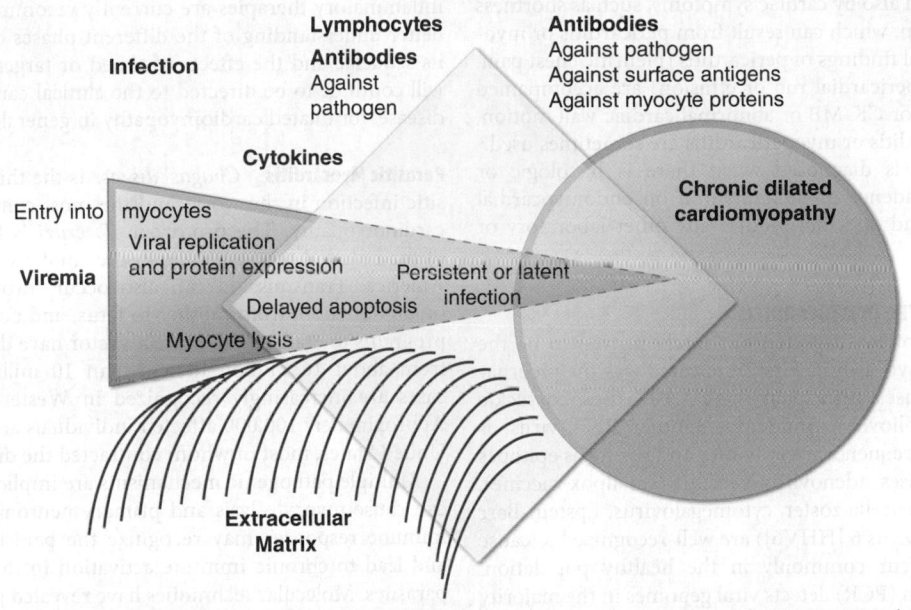

The Dallas Criteria for myocarditis on endomyocardial biopsy include lymphocytic infiltrate with evidence of myocyte necrosis (Fig. 287-7) and are negative in 80–90% of patients with clinical myocarditis. Negative Dallas Criteria can reflect sampling error or early resolution of lymphocytic infiltrates, but also the insensitivity of the test when inflammation results from cytokines and antibody-mediated injury. Routine histologic examination of endomyocardial biopsy rarely reveals a specific infective etiology, such as toxoplasmosis or *Cytomegalovirus*. Immunohistochemistry of myocardial biopsy samples is commonly used to identify active lymphocyte subtypes and may also detect upregulation of HLA antigens and the presence of complement components attributed to inflammation, but the specificity and significance of these findings are uncertain.

An increase in circulating viral titers between acute and convalescent blood samples supports a diagnosis of acute viral myocarditis with potential spontaneous improvement. There is no established role for measuring circulating anti-heart antibodies, which may be the result, rather than a cause, of myocardial injury and have been found also in patients with coronary artery disease and genetic cardiomyopathy.

FIGURE 287-6 Magnetic resonance image of myocarditis showing the typical mid-wall location (*arrow*) for late gadolinium enhancement from cardiac inflammation and scarring. *(Image courtesy of Ron Blankstein, MD, and Marcelo Di Carli, MD, Division of Nuclear Medicine, Brigham and Women's Hospital, Boston.)*

Patients with recent or ongoing viral syndromes can be classified into three levels of diagnosis:

1. Possible subclinical acute myocarditis is diagnosed when a patient has a typical viral syndrome but *no* cardiac symptoms, with one or more of the following:
   - Elevated biomarkers of cardiac injury (troponin or CK-MB)
   - ECG findings suggestive of acute injury
   - Reduced left ventricular ejection fraction or regional wall motion
   - Abnormality on cardiac imaging, usually echocardiography

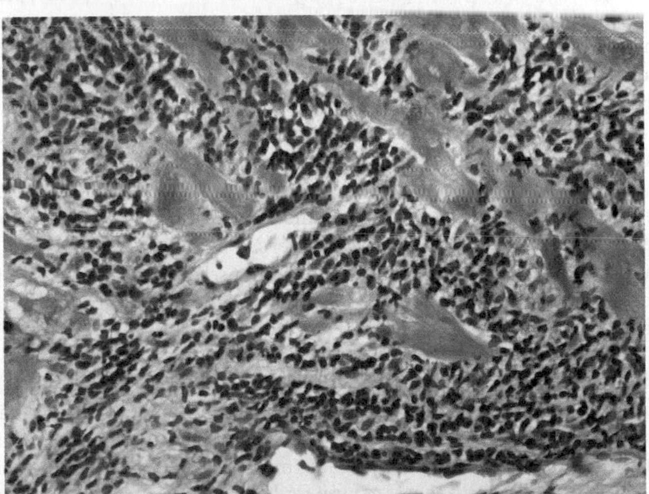

FIGURE 287-7 Acute myocarditis. Microscopic image of an endomyocardial biopsy showing massive infiltration with mononuclear cells and occasional eosinophils associated with clear myocyte damage. The myocyte nuclei are enlarged and reactive. Such extensive involvement of the myocardium would lead to extensive replacement fibrosis even if the inflammatory response could be suppressed. Hematoxylin and eosin–stained section, 200× original magnification. *(Image courtesy of Robert Padera, MD, PhD, Department of Pathology, Brigham and Women's Hospital, Boston.)*

2. Probable acute myocarditis is diagnosed when the above criteria are met and accompanied also by cardiac symptoms, such as shortness of breath or chest pain, which can result from pericarditis or myocarditis. When clinical findings of pericarditis (pleuritic chest pain, ECG abnormalities, pericardial rub or effusion) are accompanied by elevated troponin or CK-MB or abnormal cardiac wall motion, the terms perimyocarditis or myopericarditis are sometimes used.
3. Definite myocarditis is diagnosed when there is histologic or immunohistologic evidence of inflammation on endomyocardial biopsy (see below) and does *not* require any other laboratory or clinical criteria.

SPECIFIC VIRUSES IMPLICATED IN MYOCARDITIS

In humans, viruses are often suspected but rarely proven to be the direct cause of clinical myocarditis. First implicated was the picornavirus family of RNA viruses, principally the enteroviruses, coxsackie virus, echovirus, and poliovirus. Influenza, another RNA virus, is implicated with varying frequency every winter and spring as epitopes change. Of the DNA viruses, adenovirus, vaccinia (smallpox vaccine), and the herpesviruses (varicella zoster, cytomegalovirus, Epstein-Barr virus, and human herpesvirus 6 [HHV6]) are well-recognized to cause myocarditis but also occur commonly in the healthy population. Polymerase chain reaction (PCR) detects viral genomes in the majority of patients with dilated cardiomyopathy, but also in normal "control" hearts. Most often detected are parvovirus B19 and HHV6, which may affect the cardiovascular system, in part, through infection of vascular endothelial cells. However, their contribution to chronic cardiomyopathy is uncertain, as serologic evidence of exposure is present in many children and most adults.

Human immunodeficiency virus (HIV) was associated with an incidence of dilated cardiomyopathy of 1–2%; however, with the advent of highly active antiretroviral therapy (HAART), HIV has been associated with a significantly lower incidence of cardiac disease. Cardiomyopathy in HIV may result from cardiac involvement with other associated viruses, such as cytomegalovirus and hepatitis C, as well as by HIV directly. Antiviral drugs to treat chronic HIV can cause cardiomyopathy, both directly and through drug hypersensitivity. The clinical picture may be complicated by pericardial effusions and pulmonary hypertension. There is a high frequency of lymphocytic myocarditis found at autopsy, and viral particles have been demonstrated in the myocardium in some cases, consistent with direct causation.

Hepatitis C has been repeatedly implicated in cardiomyopathy, particularly in Germany and Asia. Cardiac dysfunction may improve after interferon therapy. As this cytokine itself often depresses cardiac function transiently, careful coordination of administration and ongoing clinical evaluation are critical. Involvement of the heart with hepatitis B is uncommon, but can be seen when associated with systemic vasculitis (polyarteritis nodosa).

Additional viruses implicated specifically in myocarditis include *mumps, respiratory syncytial virus,* the *arboviruses (dengue fever and yellow fever),* and *arenaviruses (Lassa fever).* However, for any serious infection, the systemic inflammatory response can cause nonspecific depression of cardiac function, which is generally reversible if the patient survives.

THERAPY

There is currently no specific therapy recommended during any stage of viral myocarditis. During acute infection, therapy with anti-inflammatory or immunosuppressive medications is avoided, as their use has been shown to increase viral replication and myocardial injury in animal models. Therapy with specific antiviral agents (such as oseltamivir) has not been studied in relation to cardiac involvement. There is ongoing investigation into the impact of antiviral therapy to treat chronic viral persistence identified from endomyocardial biopsy. Large trials of immunosuppressive therapy for Dallas Criteria–positive myocarditis have been negative. There are some initial encouraging results and ongoing investigations with immunosuppressive therapy for immune-mediated myocarditis defined by immunohistologic criteria on biopsy or circulating anti-heart antibodies in the absence of myocardial viral genomes. However, neither antiviral nor anti-inflammatory therapies are currently recommended. Until we have a better understanding of the different phases of viral myocarditis and its sequelae and the effects of timed or targeted therapies, treatment will continue to be directed to the clinical cardiovascular stage of the disease, for dilated cardiomyopathy in general.

Parasitic Myocarditis *Chagas' disease* is the third most common parasitic infection in the world and the most common infective cause of cardiomyopathy. The protozoan *T. cruzi* is transmitted by the bite of the reduviid bug, endemic in the rural areas of South and Central America. Transmission can also occur through blood transfusion, organ donation, from mother to fetus, and occasionally orally. While programs to eradicate the insect vector have decreased the prevalence from about 16 million to less than 10 million in South America, cases are increasingly recognized in Western developed countries. Approximately 100,000 affected individuals are currently living in the United States, most of whom contracted the disease in endemic areas.

Multiple pathogenic mechanisms are implicated. The parasite itself can cause myocyte lysis and primary neuronal damage, and specific immune responses may recognize the parasites or related antigens and lead to chronic immune activation in the absence of detectable parasites. Molecular techniques have revealed persistent parasite DNA fragments in infected individuals. Further evidence for persistent infection is the eruption of parasitic skin lesions during immunosuppression after cardiac transplantation. As with viral myocarditis, the relative roles of persistent infection and of secondary autoimmune injury have not been resolved (Fig. 287-5). An additional factor in the progression of Chagas' disease is the autonomic dysfunction and microvascular damage that may contribute to cardiac and gastrointestinal disease.

The acute phase of Chagas' disease with parasitemia is usually unrecognized, but in fewer than 5% of cases, it presents clinically within a few weeks of infection, with nonspecific symptoms or occasionally with acute myocarditis and meningoencephalitis. In the absence of antiparasitic therapy, the silent stage progresses slowly over 10–30 years in almost half of patients to manifest in the cardiac and gastrointestinal systems in the chronic stages. Features typical of Chagas' disease are conduction system abnormalities, particularly sinus node and atrioventricular (AV) node dysfunction and right bundle branch block. Atrial fibrillation and ventricular tachyarrhythmias also occur. Small ventricular aneurysms are common, particularly at the ventricular apex. These dilated ventricles are particularly thrombogenic, giving rise to pulmonary and systemic emboli. Xenodiagnosis, detection of the parasite itself, is rarely performed. The serologic tests for specific IgG antibodies against the trypanosome lack sufficient specificity and sensitivity, thereby requiring two separate positive tests required to make a diagnosis.

Treatment of the advanced stages focuses on clinical manifestations of the disease and includes heart failure medications, pacemaker-defibrillators, and anticoagulation. Increasing attention is directed to antiparasitic therapy even in chronic disease without obvious active infection. The most common effective antiparasitic therapies are benznidazole and nifurtimox, both associated with multiple severe reactions, including dermatitis, gastrointestinal distress, and neuropathy. Survival is less than 30% at 5 years after the onset of overt clinical heart failure. Patients without major extracardiac disease have occasionally undergone transplantation, after which they may require lifelong therapy to suppress reactivation of infection.

African trypanosomiasis infection results from the tsetse fly bite and can occur in travelers exposed during trips to Africa. The West African form is caused by *Trypanosoma brucei gambiense* and progresses silently over years. The East African form caused by *T. brucei rhodesiense* can progress rapidly through perivascular infiltration to myocarditis and heart failure, with frequent arrhythmias. The diagnosis is made by identification of trypanosomes in blood, lymph nodes, or other affected sites. Antiparasitic therapy has limited efficacy and is determined by the specific type and the stage of infection (hemolymphatic or neurologic).

Toxoplasmosis is contracted through undercooked infected beef or pork, transmission from feline feces, organ transplantation, transfusion, or maternal-fetal transmission. Immunocompromised hosts are most likely to experience reactivation of latent infection from cysts. The cysts have been found in up to 40% of autopsies of patients dying from HIV infection. Toxoplasmosis may present with encephalitis or chorioretinitis and, in the heart, can cause myocarditis, pericardial effusion, constrictive pericarditis, and heart failure. The diagnosis in an immunocompetent patient is made when the IgM is positive and the IgG becomes positive later. Active toxoplasmosis may be suspected in an immunocompromised patient with myocarditis and a positive IgG titer for toxoplasmosis, particularly when avidity testing identifies high specificity of the antibody. Fortuitous sampling occasionally reveals the cysts in the myocardium. Combination therapy can include pyrimethamine and sulfadiazine or clindamycin.

Trichinellosis is caused by *Trichinella spiralis* larva ingested with undercooked meat. Larvae migrating into skeletal muscles cause myalgias, weakness, and fever. Periorbital and facial edema and conjunctival and retinal hemorrhage may also be seen. Although the larva may occasionally invade the myocardium, clinical heart failure is rare and, when observed, attributed to the eosinophilic inflammatory response. The diagnosis is made from the specific serum antibody and is further supported by the presence of eosinophilia. Treatment includes antihelminthic drugs (albendazole, mebendazole) and glucocorticoids if inflammation is severe.

Cardiac involvement with *Echinococcus* is rare, but cysts can form and rupture in the myocardium and pericardium.

Bacterial Infections Most bacterial infections can involve the heart occasionally through direct invasion and abscess formation, but do so rarely. More commonly, systemic inflammatory responses depress contractility in severe infection and sepsis. *Diphtheria* specifically affects the heart in almost one-half of cases, and cardiac involvement is the most common cause of death in patients with this infection. The prevalence of vaccines has shifted the incidence of diphtheria from children worldwide to countries without routine immunization and to older populations who have lost their immunity. The bacillus releases a toxin that impairs protein synthesis and may particularly affect the conduction system. The specific antitoxin should be administered as soon as possible, with higher priority than antibiotic therapy. Other systemic bacterial infections that can involve the heart include *brucellosis, chlamydophila, legionella, meningococcus, mycoplasma, psittacosis,* and *salmonellosis,* for which specific treatment is directed at the systemic infection.

Clostridial infections cause myocardial damage from the released toxin. Gas bubbles can be detected in the myocardium, and occasionally abscesses can form in the myocardium and pericardium. *Streptococcal infection* with β-hemolytic streptococci is most commonly associated with acute rheumatic fever and is characterized by inflammation and fibrosis of cardiac valves and systemic connective tissue, but it can also lead to a myocarditis with focal or diffuse infiltrates of mononuclear cells.

Tuberculosis can involve the myocardium directly as well as through tuberculous pericarditis, but rarely does so when the disease is treated with antibiotics. *Whipple's disease* is caused by *Tropheryma whipplei.* The usual manifestations are in the gastrointestinal tract, but pericarditis, coronary arteritis, valvular lesions, and occasionally clinical heart failure may also occur. Multidrug antituberculous regimens are effective, but the disease tends to relapse even with appropriate treatment.

Other Infections **Spirochetal myocarditis** has been diagnosed from myocardial biopsies containing *Borrelia burgdorferi* that causes *Lyme disease.* Lyme carditis most often presents with arthritis and conduction system disease that resolves within 1–2 weeks of antibiotic treatment, only rarely implicated in chronic heart failure.

Fungal myocarditis can occur due to hematogenous or direct spread of infection from other sites, as has been described for aspergillosis, actinomycosis, blastomycosis, candidiasis, coccidioidomycosis, cryptococcosis, histoplasmosis, and mucormycosis. However, cardiac involvement is rarely the dominant clinical feature of these infections.

The **rickettsial infections,** *Q fever, Rocky Mountain spotted fever, and scrub typhus* are frequently accompanied by ECG changes, but most clinical manifestations relate to systemic vascular involvement.

NONINFECTIVE MYOCARDITIS

Myocardial inflammation can occur without apparent preceding infection. The paradigm of noninfective inflammatory myocarditis is cardiac transplant rejection, from which we have learned that myocardial depression can develop and reverse quickly, that noncellular mediators such as antibodies and cytokines play a major role in addition to lymphocytes, and that myocardial antigens are exposed by prior physical injury and viral infection.

The most commonly diagnosed noninfective inflammation is granulomatous myocarditis, including both sarcoidosis and giant cell myocarditis. Sarcoidosis, as discussed in Chap. 390, is a multisystem disease most commonly affecting the lungs. Although classically presenting with higher prevalence in young African-American men, the epidemiology appears to be changing, with increasing recognition of sarcoidosis in Caucasian patients in nonurban areas. Patients with pulmonary sarcoid are at high risk for cardiac involvement, but cardiac sarcoidosis also occurs without clinical lung disease. Regional clustering of the disease supports the suspicion that the granulomatous reaction is triggered by an infectious or environmental allergen not yet identified.

The sites and density of cardiac granulomata, the time course, and the degree of extracardiac involvement are remarkably variable. Patients may present with rapid-onset heart failure and ventricular tachyarrhythmias, conduction block, chest pain syndromes, or minor cardiac findings in the setting of ocular involvement, an infiltrative skin rash, or a nonspecific febrile illness. They may also present less acutely after months to years of fluctuating cardiac symptoms. When ventricular tachycardia or conduction block dominates the initial presentation of heart failure without coronary artery disease, suspicion should be high for these granulomatous myocarditides.

Depending on the time course, the ventricles may appear restrictive or dilated. There is often right ventricular predominance of both dilation and ventricular arrhythmias, sometimes initially attributed to arrhythmogenic right ventricular dysplasia. Small ventricular aneurysms are common. Computed tomography of the chest often reveals pulmonary lymphadenopathy even in the absence of clinical lung disease. Metabolic imaging (positron emission tomography (PET]) of the whole chest can highlight active sarcoid lesions that are avid for glucose. Magnetic resonance imaging (MRI) of the heart can identify areas likely to be inflammatory. To rule out chronic infections, such as tuberculosis or histoplasmosis as the cause of adenopathy, the diagnosis usually requires pathologic confirmation. Biopsy of enlarged mediastinal nodes may provide the highest yield. The scattered granulomata of sarcoidosis can easily be missed on cardiac biopsy (Fig. 287-8).

Immunosuppressive treatment for sarcoidosis is initiated with high-dose glucocorticoids, which are often more effective for arrhythmias than for the heart failure. Patients with sarcoid lesions that persist or recur during tapering of corticosteroids are considered candidates for other immunosuppressive therapies, frequently with agents also used for cardiac transplantation. Pacemakers and implantable defibrillators are generally indicated to prevent life-threatening heart block or ventricular tachycardia, respectively. Because the inflammation often resolves into extensive fibrosis that impairs cardiac function and provides pathways for reentrant arrhythmias, the prognosis for improvement is best when the granulomata are not extensive and the ejection fraction is not severely reduced.

Giant cell myocarditis is less common than sarcoidosis, but accounts for 10–20% of biopsy-positive cases of myocarditis. Giant cell myocarditis typically presents with rapidly progressive heart failure and tachyarrhythmias. Diffuse granulomatous lesions are surrounded by extensive inflammatory infiltrate unlikely to be missed on endomyocardial biopsy, often with extensive eosinophilic infiltration. Associated conditions are thymomas, thyroiditis, pernicious anemia, other autoimmune diseases, and occasionally recent infections. Glucocorticoid therapy is less effective than for sarcoidosis and is

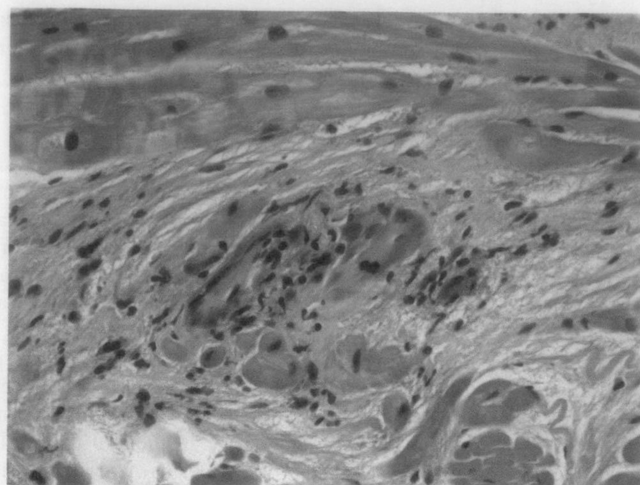

FIGURE 287-8 Sarcoidosis. Microscopic image of an endomyocardial biopsy showing a noncaseating granuloma and associated interstitial fibrosis typical of sarcoidosis. No microorganisms were present on special stains, and no foreign material was identified. Hematoxylin and eosin–stained section, 200× original magnification. *(Image courtesy of Robert Padera, MD, PhD, Department of Pathology, Brigham and Women's Hospital, Boston.)*

sometimes combined with other immunosuppressive agents. The course is generally of rapid deterioration requiring urgent transplantation. Although the severity of presentation and myocardial histology are more fulminant than with sarcoidosis, the occasional finding of giant cell myocarditis after sarcoidosis suggests that they may in some cases represent different stages of the same disease spectrum.

Eosinophilic myocarditis can be an important manifestation of the hypereosinophilic syndrome, which in Western countries is often idiopathic, although in Mediterranean and African countries, it is likely a consequence of antecedent infection. It may also be seen with systemic eosinophilic syndromes such as Churg-Strauss syndrome or malignancies. *Hypersensitivity myocarditis* is often an unexpected diagnosis, made when the biopsy reveals infiltration with lymphocytes and mononuclear cells with a high proportion of eosinophils. Most commonly, the reaction is attributed to antibiotics, particularly those taken chronically, but thiazides, anticonvulsants, indomethacin, and methyldopa have also been implicated. Occasional associations with the smallpox vaccine have been reported. Although the circulating eosinophil count may be slightly elevated in hypersensitivity myocarditis, it does not reach the high levels of the hypereosinophilic syndrome. High-dose glucocorticoids and discontinuation of the trigger agent can be curative for hypersensitivity myocarditis.

Myocarditis is often associated with systemic inflammatory diseases, such as polymyositis and *dermatomyositis,* which affect skeletal and cardiac muscle. Although noninfective inflammatory myocarditis is sometimes included in the differential diagnosis of cardiac findings in patients with connective tissue disease such as systemic lupus erythematosus, pericarditis, vasculitis, pulmonary hypertension, and accelerated coronary artery disease are more common cardiac manifestations of connective tissue disease.

Peripartum cardiomyopathy (PPCM) develops during the last trimester or within the first 6 months after pregnancy, with a frequency between 1:2000 and 1:15,000 deliveries. Risk factors are increased maternal age, increased parity, twin pregnancy, malnutrition, use of tocolytic therapy for premature labor, and preeclampsia or toxemia of pregnancy. Heart failure early after delivery was previously common in Nigeria, when the custom for new mothers included salt ingestion while reclining on a warm bed, which likely impaired mobilization of the excess circulating volume after delivery. In the Western world, lymphocytic myocarditis has sometimes been found on myocardial biopsy. This inflammation has been hypothesized to reflect increased susceptibility to viral myocarditis or an autoimmune myocarditis due to cross-reactivity of anti-uterine antibodies against cardiac muscle. Another proposed mechanism invokes an abnormal prolactin cleavage fragment, which is induced by oxidative stress and may trigger myocardial apoptosis; this observation has led to preliminary investigation of bromocriptine as possible therapy.

Very recently, PPCM has been found to be associated with increased antiangiogenic signaling, a process that is exacerbated by preeclampsia. In animal models of this disease, proangiogenic therapies have proven curative.

As the increased circulatory demand of pregnancy can aggravate other cardiac disease that was clinically unrecognized, it is crucial to the diagnosis of PPCM that there be no evidence for a preexisting cardiac disorder. By contrast, heart failure presenting earlier in pregnancy has been termed pregnancy-associated cardiomyopathy (PACM). Both PPCM and PACM have been found in some families with other presentations of dilated cardiomyopathy, in some cases with known sarcomeric protein mutations. Pregnancy may, thus, represent an environmental trigger for accelerated phenotypic expression of genetic cardiomyopathy.

TOXIC CARDIOMYOPATHY

Cardiotoxicity has been reported with multiple environmental and pharmacologic agents. Often these associations are seen only with very high levels of exposure or acute overdoses, in which acute electrocardiographic and hemodynamic abnormalities may reflect both direct drug effect and systemic toxicity.

Alcohol is the most common toxin implicated in chronic dilated cardiomyopathy. Excess consumption may contribute to more than 10% of cases of heart failure, including exacerbation of cases with other primary etiologies such as valvular disease or previous infarction. Toxicity is attributed both to alcohol and to its primary metabolite, acetaldehyde. Polymorphisms of the genes encoding alcohol dehydrogenase and the angiotensin-converting enzyme increase the likelihood of alcoholic cardiomyopathy in an individual with excess consumption. Superimposed vitamin deficiencies and toxic alcohol additives are rarely implicated. The alcohol consumption necessary to produce cardiomyopathy in an otherwise normal heart has been estimated to be five to six drinks (about 4 ounces of pure ethanol) daily for 5–10 years, but frequent binge drinking may also be sufficient. Many patients with alcoholic cardiomyopathy are fully functional in their daily lives without apparent stigmata of alcoholism. The cardiac impairment in severe alcoholic cardiomyopathy is the sum of both permanent damage and a substantial component that is reversible after cessation of alcohol consumption. Atrial fibrillation occurs commonly both early in the disease ("holiday heart") and in advanced stages. Medical therapy includes neurohormonal antagonists and diuretics as needed for fluid management. Withdrawal should be supervised to avoid exacerbations of heart failure or arrhythmias, and ongoing support arranged. Even with severe disease, marked improvement can occur within 3–6 months of abstinence. Implantable defibrillators are generally deferred until an adequate period of abstinence, after which they may not be necessary if the ejection fraction has improved. With continued consumption, the prognosis is grim.

Cocaine, amphetamines, and related catecholaminergic stimulants can produce chronic cardiomyopathy as well as acute ischemia and tachyarrhythmias. Pathology reveals microinfarcts consistent with small vessel ischemia, similar to those seen with pheochromocytoma.

Chemotherapy agents are the most common drugs implicated in toxic cardiomyopathy. Judicious use of these drugs requires balancing the risks of the malignancy and the risks of cardiotoxicity, as many cancers have a chronic course with better prognosis than heart failure.

Anthracyclines cause characteristic histologic changes of vacuolar degeneration and myofibrillar loss. Generation of reactive oxygen species involving heme compounds is currently the favored explanation for myocyte injury and fibrosis. Disruption of the large titin protein may contribute to loss of sarcomere organization. Risk for cardiotoxicity increases with higher doses, preexisting cardiac disease, and concomitant chest irradiation. There are three different presentations of anthracycline-induced cardiomyopathy. (1) Heart failure can develop acutely during administration of a single dose, but may clinically resolve in a few weeks. (2) Early-onset doxorubicin cardiotoxicity develops in about 3% of patients during or shortly after a chronic course, relating closely to total dose. It may be rapidly progressive, but may also resolve to good, but not normal, ventricular function. (3) The chronic presentation differs according to whether therapy was given before or after puberty. Patients who received doxorubicin while still growing may have impaired development of the heart, which leads to clinical heart failure by the time the patient reaches the early twenties. Late after adult exposure, patients may develop the gradual onset of symptoms or an acute onset precipitated by a reversible second insult, such as influenza or atrial fibrillation. Doxorubicin cardiotoxicity leads to a relatively nondilated ventricle, perhaps due to the accompanying fibrosis. Thus, the stroke volume may be severely reduced with an ejection fraction of 30–40%, which would be well tolerated in a patient with a larger ventricle typical of other cardiomyopathies with systolic dysfunction. Therapy includes angiotensin-converting enzyme inhibitors and β-adrenergic blocking agents used for other causes of heart failure, with careful suppression of "inappropriate" sinus tachycardia, and attention to postural hypotension that can occur in these patients. Once thought to have an inexorable downward course, some patients with doxorubicin cardiotoxicity improve under careful management to near-normal clinical function for many years.

Trastuzumab (Herceptin) is a monoclonal antibody that interferes with cell surface receptors crucial for some tumor growth and for cardiac adaptation. The incidence of cardiotoxicity is lower than for anthracyclines but enhanced by coadministration with them. Although considered to be more often reversible, trastuzumab cardiotoxicity does not always resolve, and some patients progress to clinical heart failure and death. As with anthracycline cardiotoxicity, therapy is as usual for heart failure, but it is not clear whether the spontaneous rate of improvement is enhanced by neurohormonal antagonists.

Cardiotoxicity with *cyclophosphamide and ifosfamide* generally occurs acutely and with very high doses. 5-Fluorouracil, cisplatin, and some other alkylating agents can cause recurrent coronary spasm that occasionally leads to depressed contractility. Acute administration of *interferon-α* can cause hypotension and arrhythmias. Clinical heart failure occurring during repeated chronic administration usually resolves after discontinuation.

Many small-molecule *tyrosine kinase inhibitors* are under development for different malignancies. Although these agents are "targeted" at specific tumor receptors or pathways, the biologic conservation of signaling pathways can cause these inhibitors to have "off target" effects that include the heart and vasculature. Recognition of cardiotoxicity during therapy with these agents is complicated because they occasionally cause peripheral fluid accumulation (ankle edema, periorbital swelling, pleural effusions) due to local factors rather than elevated central venous pressures. Therapeutic approaches include withdrawal of the tyrosine kinase inhibitor (when possible) and substitution with a congener (when available), as well as conventional treatment for heart failure. Prophylactic treatment with beta blockers and angiotensin-converting enzyme inhibitors prior to and during chemotherapy is a topic of ongoing investigation.

Other therapeutic drugs that can cause cardiotoxicity during chronic use include hydroxychloroquine, chloroquine, emetine, and antiretroviral therapies.

Toxic exposures can cause arrhythmias or respiratory injury acutely during accidents. Chronic exposures implicated in cardiotoxicity include hydrocarbons, fluorocarbons, arsenicals, lead, and mercury.

METABOLIC CAUSES OF CARDIOMYOPATHY

Endocrine disorders affect multiple organ systems, including the heart. *Hyperthyroidism and hypothyroidism* do not often cause clinical heart failure in an otherwise normal heart, but commonly exacerbate heart failure. Clinical signs of thyroid disease may be masked, so tests of thyroid function are part of the routine evaluation of cardiomyopathy. Hyperthyroidism should always be considered with new-onset atrial fibrillation or ventricular tachycardia or atrial fibrillation in which the rapid ventricular response is difficult to control. The most common current reason for thyroid abnormalities in the cardiac population is the treatment of tachyarrhythmias with amiodarone, a drug with substantial iodine content. Hypothyroidism should be treated with very slow escalation of thyroid supplements to avoid exacerbating tachyarrhythmias and heart failure. Hyperthyroidism and heart failure are a dangerous combination that merits very close supervision, often hospitalization, during titration of antithyroid medications, during which decompensation of heart failure may occur precipitously and fatally.

Pheochromocytoma is rare, but should be considered when a patient has heart failure and very labile blood pressure and heart rate, sometimes with episodic palpitations (Chap. 407). Patients with pheochromocytoma often have postural hypotension. In addition to α-adrenergic receptor antagonists, definitive therapy requires surgical extirpation. Very high renin states, such as those caused by renal artery stenosis, can lead to modest depression in ejection fraction with little or no ventricular dilation and markedly labile symptoms with flash pulmonary edema, related to sudden shifts in vascular tone and intravascular volume.

Controversies remain regarding whether *diabetes* and *obesity* are sufficient to cause cardiomyopathy. Most heart failure in diabetes results from epicardial coronary disease, with further increase in coronary artery risk due to accompanying hypertension and renal dysfunction. Cardiomyopathy may result in part from insulin resistance and increased advanced-glycosylation end products, which impair both systolic and diastolic function. However, much of the dysfunction can be attributed to scattered focal ischemia resulting from distal coronary artery tapering and limited microvascular perfusion even without proximal focal stenoses. Diabetes is a typical factor in heart failure with "preserved" ejection fraction, along with hypertension, advanced age, and female gender.

The existence of a cardiomyopathy due to *obesity* is generally accepted. In addition to cardiac involvement from associated diabetes, hypertension, and vascular inflammation of the metabolic syndrome, obesity alone is associated with impaired excretion of excess volume load, which, over time, can lead to increased wall stress and secondary adaptive neurohumoral responses. Fluid retention may be aggravated by large fluid intake and the rapid clearance of natriuretic peptides by adipose tissue. In the absence of another obvious cause of cardiomyopathy in an obese patient with systolic dysfunction without marked ventricular dilation, effective weight reduction is often associated with major improvement in ejection fraction and clinical function. Improvement in cardiac function has been described after successful bariatric surgery, although all major surgical therapy poses increased risk for patients with heart failure. Postoperative malabsorption and nutritional deficiencies, such as calcium and phosphate deficiencies, may be particularly deleterious for patients with cardiomyopathy.

Nutritional deficiencies can occasionally cause dilated cardiomyopathy but are not commonly implicated in developed Western countries. *Beri-beri heart disease* due to thiamine deficiency can result from poor nutrition in undernourished populations and in patients deriving most of their calories from alcohol, and has been reported in teenagers subsisting only on highly processed foods. This disease is initially a vasodilated state with very high output heart failure that can later progress to a low output state; thiamine repletion can lead to prompt recovery of cardiovascular function. Abnormalities in *carnitine* metabolism can cause dilated or restrictive cardiomyopathies, usually in children. Deficiency of trace elements such as *selenium* can cause cardiomyopathy (Keshan's disease).

Calcium is essential for excitation-contraction coupling. Chronic deficiencies of calcium, such as can occur with hypoparathyroidism (particularly postsurgical) or intestinal dysfunction (from diarrheal syndromes and following extensive resection), can cause severe chronic heart failure that responds over days or weeks to vigorous calcium repletion. *Phosphate* is a component of high-energy compounds needed for efficient energy transfer and multiple signaling pathways. *Hypophosphatemia* can develop during starvation and early refeeding following a prolonged fast, and occasionally during hyperalimentation. *Magnesium* is a cofactor for thiamine-dependent reactions and for the sodium-potassium adenosine triphosphatase (ATPase), but

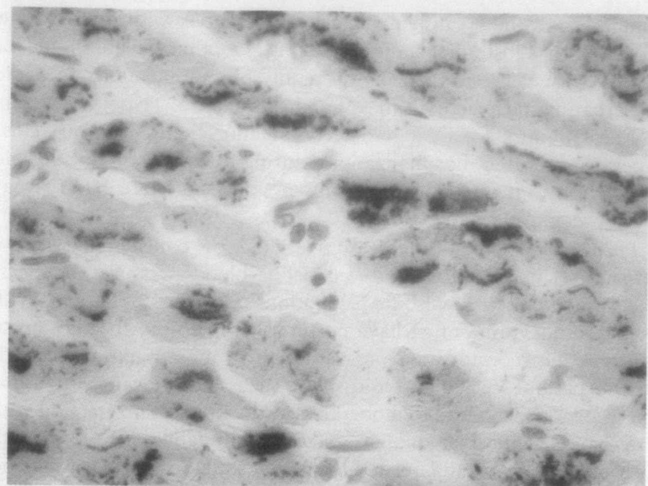

FIGURE 287-9 Hemochromatosis. Microscopic image of an endomyocardial biopsy showing extensive iron deposition within the cardiac myocytes with the Prussian blue stain (400× original magnification). *(Image courtesy of Robert Padera, MD, PhD, Department of Pathology, Brigham and Women's Hospital, Boston.)*

hypomagnesemia rarely becomes sufficiently profound to cause clinical cardiomyopathy.

Hemochromatosis is variably classified as a metabolic or storage disease (Chap. 428). It is included among the causes of restrictive cardiomyopathy, but the clinical presentation is often that of a dilated cardiomyopathy. The autosomal recessive form is related to the *HFE* gene. With up to 10% of the population heterozygous for one mutation, the clinical prevalence might be as high as 1 in 500. The lower observed rates highlight the limited penetrance of the disease, suggesting the role of additional genetic and environmental factors for clinical expression. Hemochromatosis can also be acquired from iron overload due to hemolytic anemia and transfusions. Excess iron is deposited in the perinuclear compartment of cardiomyocytes, with resulting disruption of intracellular architecture and mitochondrial function. Diagnosis is easily made from measurement of serum iron and transferrin saturation, with a threshold of >60% for men and >45–50% for women. MRI can help to quantitate iron stores in the liver and heart, and endomyocardial biopsy tissue can be stained for iron (Fig. 287-9), which is particularly important if the patient has another cause for cardiomyopathy. If diagnosed early, hemochromatosis can often be managed by repeated phlebotomy to remove iron. For more severe iron overload, iron chelation therapy with desferrioxamine (deferoxamine) or deferasirox can help to improve cardiac function if myocyte loss and replacement fibrosis are not too severe.

Inborn disorders of metabolism occasionally present with dilated cardiomyopathy, although they are most often associated with restrictive cardiomyopathy (Table 287-4).

FAMILIAL DILATED CARDIOMYOPATHY

The genetic basis for cardiomyopathy is discussed in the section, "Genetic Etiologies of Cardiomyopathy." The recognized frequency of familial involvement in dilated cardiomyopathy has increased to over 30%. Mutations in *TTN*, encoding the giant sarcomeric protein titin, are the most common cause of dilated cardiomyopathy, accounting for up to 25% of familial disease. On average, men with *TTN* mutations develop cardiomyopathy a decade before women, without distinctive clinical features. Mutations in thick and thin filament genes account for ~8% of dilated cardiomyopathy and may manifest in early childhood.

The most recognizable familial cardiomyopathy syndromes with extracardiac manifestations are the *muscular dystrophies.* Both Duchenne's and the milder Becker's dystrophy result from abnormalities in the X-linked dystrophin gene of the sarcolemmal membrane. Skeletal myopathy is present in multiple other genetic cardiomyopathies (Table 287-3), some of which are associated with creatine kinase elevations.

Families with a history of atrial arrhythmias, conduction system disease, and cardiomyopathy may have abnormalities of the nuclear membrane lamin proteins. While all dilated cardiomyopathies carry a risk of sudden death, a family history of cardiomyopathy with sudden death raises suspicion for a particularly arrhythmogenic mutation; affected family members may be considered for implantable defibrillators even before meeting the reduced ejection fraction threshold for primary prevention of sudden death.

A prominent family history of sudden death or ventricular tachycardia before clinical cardiomyopathy suggests genetic defects in the desmosomal proteins (Fig. 287-10). Originally described as affecting the right ventricle (arrhythmogenic right ventricular dysplasia [ARVD]), this disorder (arrhythmogenic ventricular dysplasia) can affect either or both ventricles. Patients often present first with ventricular tachycardia. Genetic defects in proteins of the desmosomal complex disrupt myocyte junctions and adhesions, leading to replacement of myocardium by deposits of fat. Thin ventricular walls may be recognized on echocardiography but are better visualized on MRI. Because desmosomes are also important for elasticity of hair and skin, some of the defective desmosomal proteins are associated with striking "woolly hair" and thickened skin on the palms and soles. Implantable defibrillators are usually indicated to prevent sudden death. There is variable progression to right, left, or biventricular failure.

Left ventricular noncompaction is a condition of unknown prevalence that is increasingly revealed with the refinement of imaging techniques. The diagnostic criteria include the presence of multiple trabeculations in the left ventricle distal to the papillary muscles, creating a "spongy" appearance of the apex. Noncompaction has been associated with multiple genetic variants in the sarcomeric and other genes, such as *TAZ* (encoding tafazzin). The diagnosis may be made incidentally or in patients previously diagnosed with cardiomyopathy, in whom the criteria for noncompaction may appear and resolve with changing left ventricular size and function. The three cardinal clinical features are ventricular arrhythmias, embolic events, and heart failure. Treatment generally includes anticoagulation and early consideration for an implantable defibrillator, in addition to neurohormonal antagonists as indicated by stage of disease.

Some families inherit a susceptibility to viral-induced myocarditis. This propensity may relate to abnormalities in cell surface receptors, such as the coxsackie-adenovirus receptor, that bind viral proteins.

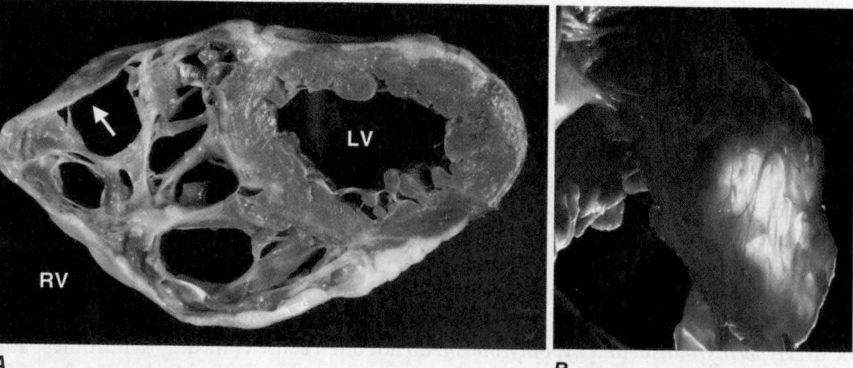

FIGURE 287-10 Arrhythmogenic right ventricular dysplasia. *A.* Cross-sectional slice of a pathology specimen removed at transplantation, showing severe dysplasia of the right ventricle (RV) with extensive fatty replacement of right ventricular myocardium. ***B.*** The remarkably thin right ventricular free wall is revealed by transillumination. LV, left ventricle. *(Images courtesy of Gayle Winters, MD, and Richard Mitchell, MD, PhD, Division of Pathology, Brigham and Women's Hospital, Boston.)*

Some may have partial homology with viral proteins such that an autoimmune response is triggered against the myocardium.

Prognosis and therapy of familial dilated cardiomyopathy are dictated primarily by the stage of clinical disease and the risk for sudden death. In some cases, the familial etiology facilitates prognostic decisions, particularly regarding the likelihood of recovery after a new diagnosis, which is unlikely for familial disease. The rate of progression of disease, once manifest, is, to some extent, heritable, although marked variation can be seen. However, there have been cases of remarkable clinical remission after acute presentation, likely after a reversible additional insult, such as prolonged tachycardia or infective myocarditis.

TAKOTSUBO CARDIOMYOPATHY

The apical ballooning syndrome, or stress-induced cardiomyopathy, occurs typically in older women after sudden intense emotional or physical stress. The ventricle shows global ventricular dilation with basal contraction, forming the shape of the narrow-necked jar (*takotsubo*) used in Japan to trap octopi. Originally described in Japan, it is increasingly recognized elsewhere during emergency cardiac catheterization and intensive care unit admissions for noncardiac conditions. Presentations include pulmonary edema, hypotension, and chest pain with ECG changes mimicking an acute infarction. The left ventricular dysfunction extends beyond a specific coronary artery distribution and generally resolves within days to weeks. Animal models and ventricular biopsies suggest that this acute cardiomyopathy may result from intense sympathetic activation with heterogeneity of myocardial autonomic innervation, diffuse microvascular spasm, and/or direct catecholamine toxicity. Coronary angiography may be required to rule out acute coronary occlusion. No therapies have been proven beneficial, but reasonable strategies include nitrates for pulmonary edema, intraaortic balloon pump if needed for low output, combined alpha and beta blockers rather than selective beta blockade if hemodynamically stable, and magnesium for arrhythmias related to QT prolongation. Anticoagulation is generally withheld due to the occasional occurrence of ventricular rupture. While the prognosis is generally good, recurrences have been described in up to 10% of patients.

IDIOPATHIC DILATED CARDIOMYOPATHY

Idiopathic dilated cardiomyopathy is a diagnosis of exclusion, when all other known factors have been excluded. Approximately two-thirds of dilated cardiomyopathies are still labeled as idiopathic; however, a substantial proportion of these may reflect unrecognized genetic disease. Continued reconsideration of etiology during chronic heart failure management often reveals specific causes later in a patient's course.

OVERLAPPING TYPES OF CARDIOMYOPATHY

The limitations of our phenotypic classification are revealed through the multiple overlaps between the etiologies and presentations of the three types. Cardiomyopathy with reduced systolic function but without severe dilation can represent early dilated cardiomyopathy, "minimally dilated cardiomyopathy," or restrictive diseases without marked increases in ventricular wall thickness. For example, sarcoidosis and hemochromatosis can present as dilated or restrictive disease. Early stages of amyloidosis are often mistaken for hypertrophic cardiomyopathy. Progression of hypertrophic cardiomyopathy into a "burned-out" phase occurs occasionally, with decreased contractility and modest ventricular dilation. Overlaps are particularly common with the inherited metabolic disorders, which can present as any of the three major phenotypes (Fig. 287-4).

DISORDERS OF METABOLIC PATHWAYS

Multiple genetic disorders of metabolic pathways can cause myocardial disease, due to infiltration of abnormal products or cells containing them between the myocytes, and storage disease, due to their accumulation within cells (see HPIM 18e, Table 238-4, and 287-5). The restrictive phenotype is most common, but mildly dilated cardiomyopathy may occur. Hypertrophic cardiomyopathy may be mimicked by the myocardium thickened with these abnormal products causing "pseudohypertrophy." Most of these diseases are diagnosed during childhood.

TABLE 287-5 CAUSES OF RESTRICTIVE CARDIOMYOPATHIES

Infiltrative (Between Myocytes)
Amyloidosis
Primary (light chain amyloid)
Familial (abnormal transthyretin)[a]
Senile (normal transthyretin or atrial peptides)
Inherited metabolic defects[a]
Storage (Within Myocytes)
Hemochromatosis (iron)[a]
Inherited metabolic defects[a]
Fabry's disease
Glycogen storage disease (II, III)
Fibrotic
Radiation
Scleroderma
Endomyocardial
Possibly related fibrotic diseases
Tropical endomyocardial fibrosis
Hypereosinophilic syndrome (Löffler's endocarditis)
Carcinoid syndrome
Radiation
Drugs: e.g., serotonin, ergotamine
Overlap with Other Cardiomyopathies
Hypertrophic cardiomyopathy/"pseudohypertrophic"[a]
"Minimally dilated" cardiomyopathy
Early-stage dilated cardiomyopathy
Partial recovery from dilated cardiomyopathy
Sarcoidosis
Idiopathic[a]

[a]Can be familial.

Fabry's disease results from a deficiency of the lysosomal enzyme alpha galactosidase A caused by one of more than 160 mutations. This disorder of glycosphingolipid metabolism is an X-linked recessive disorder that may also cause clinical disease in female carriers. Glycolipid accumulation may be limited to the cardiac tissues or may also involve the skin and kidney. Electron microscopy of endomyocardial biopsy tissue shows diagnostic vesicles containing concentric lamellar figures (Fig. 287-11). Diagnosis is crucial because enzyme replacement can reduce abnormal deposits and improve cardiac and clinical function. The magnitude of clinical impact has not been well-established for this therapy, which requires frequent infusions of the enzyme at a cost of over $100,000 a year. Enzyme replacement can also improve the course of Gaucher's disease, in which cerebroside-rich cells accumulate in multiple organs due to a deficiency of beta-glucosidase. Cerebroside-rich cells infiltrate the heart, which can also lead to a hemorrhagic pericardial effusion and valvular disease.

Glycogen storage diseases lead to accumulation of lysosomal storage products and intracellular glycogen accumulation, particularly with *glycogen storage disease type III,* due to a defective debranching enzyme. There are more than 10 types of *mucopolysaccharidoses,* in which autosomal dominant or X-linked deficiencies of lysosomal enzymes lead to the accumulation of glycosaminoglycans in the skeleton, nervous system, and occasionally the heart. With characteristic facies, short stature, and frequent cognitive impairment, most individuals are diagnosed early in childhood and die before adulthood.

Carnitine is an essential cofactor in long-chain fatty acid metabolism. Multiple defects have been described that lead to carnitine deficiency, causing intracellular lipid inclusions and restrictive or dilated cardiomyopathy, often presenting in children. Fatty acid oxidation requires many metabolic steps with specific enzymes that can be deficient, with complex interactions with carnitine. Depending on the defect, cardiac and skeletal myopathy can be ameliorated with replacement of fatty acid intermediates and carnitine.

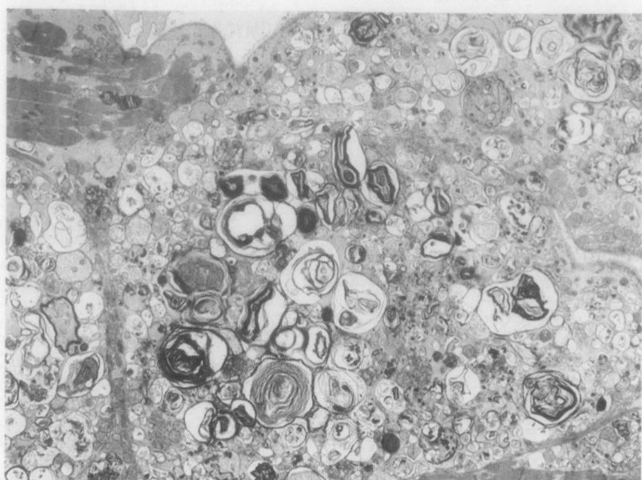

FIGURE 287-11 Fabry's disease. Transmission electron micrograph of a right ventricular endomyocardial biopsy specimen at high magnification showing the characteristic concentric lamellar inclusions of glycosphingolipids accumulating as a result of deficiency of the lysosomal enzyme alpha-galactosidase A. Image taken at 15,000× original magnification. *(Image courtesy of Robert Padera, MD, PhD, Department of Pathology, Brigham and Women's Hospital, Boston.)*

Two monogenic metabolic cardiomyopathies have recently been described as causes of increased ventricular wall thickness without an increase of muscle subunits or an increase in contractility. Mutations in the gamma-2 regulatory subunit of the adenosine monophosphate (AMP)-activated protein kinase important for glucose metabolism (*PRKAG2*) have been associated with a high prevalence of conduction abnormalities, such as AV block and ventricular preexcitation (Wolff-Parkinson-White syndrome). Several defects have been reported in an X-linked lysosome-associated membrane protein (*LAMP2*). This defect can be maternally transmitted or sporadic and has occasionally been isolated to the heart, although it often leads to a syndrome of skeletal myopathy, mental retardation, and hepatic dysfunction referred to as *Danon's disease.* Extreme left ventricular hypertrophy appears early, often in childhood, and can progress rapidly to end-stage heart failure with low ejection fraction. Electron microscopy of these metabolic disorders shows that the myocytes are enlarged by multiple intracellular vacuoles of metabolic by-products.

RESTRICTIVE CARDIOMYOPATHY

The least common of the physiologic triad of cardiomyopathies is restrictive cardiomyopathy, which is dominated by abnormal diastolic function, often with mildly decreased contractility and ejection fraction (usually >30–50%). Both atria are enlarged, sometimes massively. Modest left ventricular dilation can be present, usually with an end-diastolic dimension <6 cm. End-diastolic pressures are elevated in both ventricles, with preservation of cardiac output until late in the disease. Subtle exercise intolerance is usually the first symptom but is often not recognized until after clinical presentation with congestive symptoms. The restrictive diseases often present with relatively more right-sided symptoms, such as edema, abdominal discomfort, and ascites, although filling pressures are elevated in both ventricles. The cardiac impulse is less displaced than in dilated cardiomyopathy and less dynamic than in hypertrophic cardiomyopathy. A fourth heart sound is more common than a third heart sound in sinus rhythm, but atrial fibrillation is common. Jugular venous pressures often show rapid Y descents and may increase during inspiration (positive Kussmaul's sign). Most restrictive cardiomyopathies are due to infiltration of abnormal substances between myocytes, storage of abnormal metabolic products within myocytes, or fibrotic injury (Table 287-5). The differential diagnosis should include constrictive pericardial disease, which may also be dominated by right-sided heart failure.

INFILTRATIVE DISEASE

Amyloidosis is the major cause of restrictive cardiomyopathy (Figs. 287-12, 287-13, and 287-14). Several proteins can self-assemble to form the beta-sheets of amyloid proteins, which deposit with different consequences depending on the type of protein. The systemic amyloidoses are discussed in Chap. 137. In addition to cardiac infiltration, neurologic involvement occurs commonly with primary amyloidosis (immunoglobulin light chains) and with familial amyloidosis (genetic abnormalities of transthyretin). There are over 100 identified mutations in transthyretin on chromosome 13, among which the V122I transthyretin mutation has been identified in about 4% of African Americans and in 10% of African Americans with heart failure and may contribute importantly to heart failure in general in the elderly African-American population. Organ dysfunction was previously attributed solely to physical disruption from the infiltrating amyloid fibrils, but newer information suggests additional direct toxicity from the immunoglobulin light chain and abnormal transthyretin protein aggregates themselves. In senile amyloidosis, there is abnormal accumulation of normal transthyretin or natriuretic peptide folding, detected in 10% of people over 80 years and half of those over 90 years but often without apparent clinical disease. Men show a greater burden of amyloid deposition and 20-fold greater likelihood of clinical disease with senile amyloidosis. The aging of the population will soon render senile amyloidosis the most common of the amyloidoses.

Cardiac amyloid is classically suspected from thickened ventricular walls with an ECG that shows low voltage. However, low voltage is not always present and is less common in familial or senile amyloidosis than in primary AL amyloidosis. A characteristic refractile brightness in the septum on echocardiography is suggestive of the diagnosis, but neither sensitive nor specific. Both atria are dilated, often dramatically, and diastolic dysfunction may be more obvious than in left ventricular hypertrophy from other causes. Amyloid infiltration can also be detected with gadolinium enhancement in MRI.

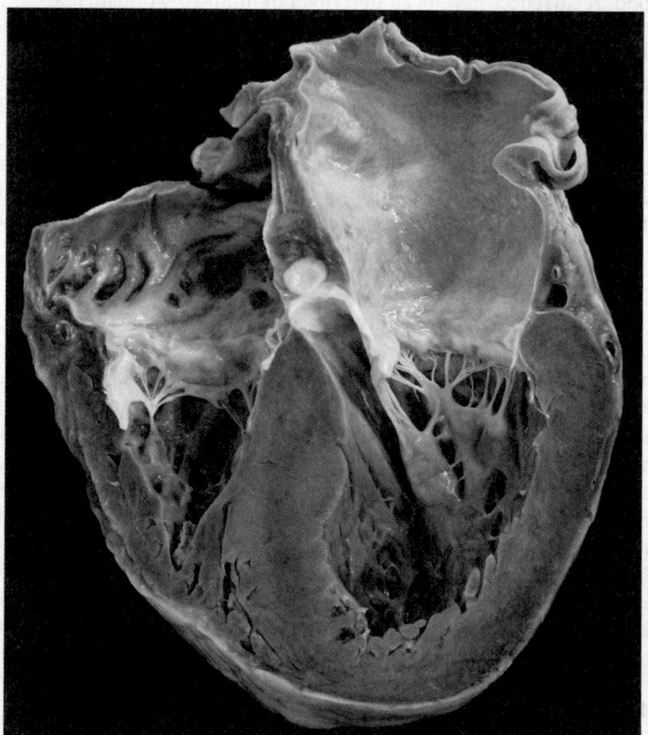

FIGURE 287-12 Restrictive cardiomyopathy—amyloidosis. Gross specimen of a heart with amyloidosis. The heart is firm and rubbery with a waxy cut surface. The atria are markedly dilated, and the left atrial endocardium, normally smooth, has yellow-brown amyloid deposits that give texture to the surface. *(Image courtesy of Robert Padera, MD, PhD, Department of Pathology, Brigham and Women's Hospital, Boston.)*

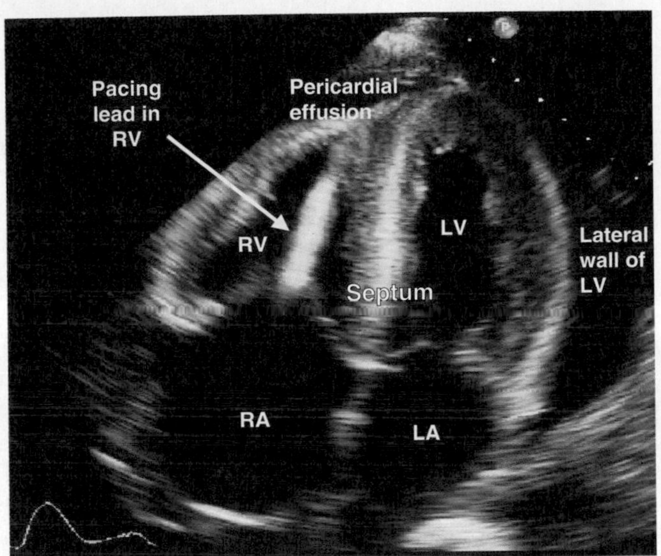

FIGURE 287-13 Restrictive cardiomyopathy—amyloidosis. Echocardiogram showing thickened walls of both ventricles without major chamber dilation. The atria are markedly dilated, consistent with chronically elevated ventricular filling pressures. In this example, there is a characteristic hyperrefractile "glittering" of the myocardium typical of amyloid infiltration, which is often absent (especially with more recent echocardiographic systems of better resolution). The mitral and tricuspid valves are thickened. A pacing lead is visible in the right ventricle (RV), and a pericardial effusion is evident. Note that the echocardiographic and pathologic images are vertically opposite, such that the left ventricle (LV) is by convention on the top right in the echocardiographic image and bottom right in the pathologic images. LA, left atrium; RA, right atrium. *(Image courtesy of Justina Wu, MD, Brigham and Women's Hospital, Boston.)*

The diagnosis of primary or familial amyloidosis can sometimes be made from biopsies of an abdominal fat pad or the rectum, but cardiac amyloidosis is most reliably identified from a biopsy of the heart, in which amyloid fibrils infiltrate the myocardium diffusely, particularly around the conduction system and coronary vessels (Fig. 287-14). Diagnosis of the type of amyloid protein requires immunohistochemistry of biopsied tissue rather than serum or urine electrophoresis, which can lead to incorrect classification.

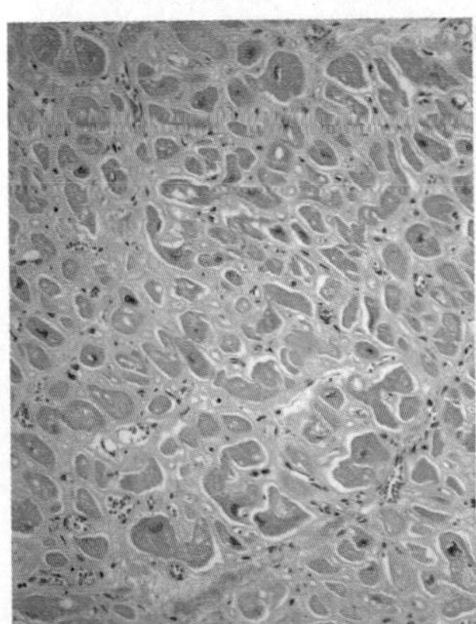

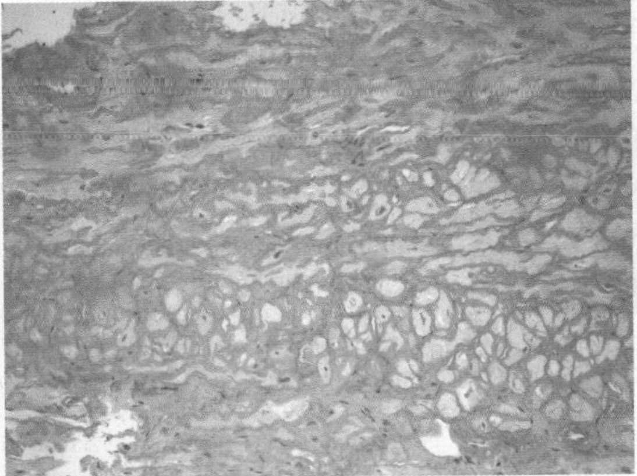

FIGURE 287-14 Amyloidosis—microscopic images of amyloid involving the myocardium. The left panel (hematoxylin and eosin stain) shows glassy, grey-pink amorphous material infiltrating between cardiomyocytes, which stain a darker pink. The right panel shows a sulfated blue stain that highlights the amyloid green and stains the cardiac myocytes yellow. (The Congo red stain can also be used to highlight amyloid; under polarized light, amyloid will have an apple-green birefringence when stained with Congo red.) Images at 100× original magnification. *(Image courtesy of Robert Padera, MD, PhD, Department of Pathology, Brigham and Women's Hospital, Boston.)*

Therapy for all types of amyloid is predominantly for symptoms of fluid retention, which often requires high doses of loop diuretics. Digoxin bound to the amyloid fibrils can reach toxic levels, and should therefore be used only in very low doses, if at all. There is no evidence regarding use of neurohormonal antagonists in amyloid heart disease, where the possible theoretical benefit has to be balanced against the possibility of aggravating postural hypotension and diminishing the crucial heart rate reserve. The risk of intracardiac thrombi may warrant chronic anticoagulation.

The prognosis is worst for primary amyloid, with a median survival of 6–12 months after symptoms of heart failure. If present, multiple myeloma is treated with chemotherapy, the extent of which is often limited by the potential of worsening cardiac dysfunction. Immunoglobulin-associated amyloid has occasionally been treated with sequential heart transplantation and delayed bone marrow transplant, with frequent recurrence of amyloid in the transplanted heart. Abnormal transthyretin-associated cardiac amyloid has a somewhat better prognosis and can be treated in selected patients with heart and liver transplantation. Senile cardiac amyloid has the slowest progression and best overall prognosis.

FIBROTIC RESTRICTIVE CARDIOMYOPATHY

Progressive fibrosis can cause restrictive myocardial disease without ventricular dilation. Thoracic radiation, common for breast and lung cancer or mediastinal lymphoma, can produce early or late restrictive cardiomyopathy. Patients with *radiation cardiomyopathy* may present with a possible diagnosis of constrictive pericarditis, as the two conditions often coexist. Careful hemodynamic evaluation and, often, endomyocardial biopsy should be performed if considering pericardial stripping surgery, which is unlikely to be successful in the presence of underlying restrictive cardiomyopathy.

Scleroderma causes small vessel spasm and ischemia that can lead to a small, stiff heart with reduced ejection fraction without dilation. The pulmonary hypertension associated with scleroderma may lead to more clinical right heart failure because of concomitant fibrotic disease of the right ventricle. Doxorubicin causes direct myocyte injury usually leading to dilated cardiomyopathy, but the limited degree of dilation may result from increased fibrosis, which restricts remodeling.

ENDOMYOCARDIAL DISEASE

The physiologic picture of elevated filling pressures with atrial enlargement and preserved ventricular contractility with normal or reduced ventricular volumes can result from extensive fibrosis of the endocardium, without transmural myocardial disease. For patients who have not lived in the equatorial regions, this picture is rare, and when seen is often associated with a history of chronic hypereosinophilic syndrome (*Löffler's endocarditis*), which is more common in men than women. In this disease, persistent hypereosinophilia of >1500 eos/mm^3 for at least 6 months can cause an acute phase of eosinophilic injury in the endocardium (see earlier discussion of eosinophilic myocarditis), with systemic illness and injury to other organs. There is usually no obvious cause, but the hypereosinophilia can occasionally be explained by allergic, parasitic, or malignant disease. It is postulated to be followed by a period in which cardiac inflammation is replaced by evidence of fibrosis with superimposed thrombosis. In severe disease, the dense fibrotic layer can obliterate the ventricular apices and extend to thicken and tether the AV valve leaflets. The clinical disease may present with heart failure, embolic events, and atrial arrhythmias. While plausible, the sequence of transition from eosinophilic myocarditis or Löffler's endocarditis to endomyocardial fibrosis has not been clearly demonstrated.

In tropical countries, up to one-quarter of heart failure may be due to *endomyocardial fibrosis*, affecting either or both ventricles. This condition shares with the previous condition the partial obliteration of the ventricular apex with fibrosis extending into the valvular inflow tract and leaflets; however, it is not clear that the etiologies are the same for all cases. Pericardial effusions frequently accompany endomyocardial fibrosis but are not common in Löffler's endocarditis. For endomyocardial fibrosis, there is no gender difference, but a higher prevalence in African-American populations. While tropical endomyocardial fibrosis could represent the end-stage of previous hypereosinophilic disease triggered by endemic parasites, neither prior parasitic infection nor hypereosinophilia is usually documented. Geographic nutritional deficiencies have also been proposed as an etiology.

Medical treatment focuses on glucocorticoids and chemotherapy to suppress hypereosinophilia when present. Fluid retention may become increasingly resistant to diuretic therapy. Anticoagulation is recommended. Atrial fibrillation is associated with worse symptoms and prognosis, but may be difficult to suppress. Surgical resection of the apices and replacement of the fibrotic valves can improve symptoms, but surgical morbidity and mortality and later recurrence rates are high.

The serotonin secreted by *carcinoid* tumors can produce fibrous plaques in the endocardium and right-sided cardiac valves, occasionally affecting left-sided valves, as well. Valvular lesions may be stenotic or regurgitant. Systemic symptoms include flushing and diarrhea. Liver disease from hepatic metastases may play a role by limiting hepatic function and thereby allowing more serotonin to reach the venous circulation.

HYPERTROPHIC CARDIOMYOPATHY

Hypertrophic cardiomyopathy is defined as left ventricular hypertrophy that develops in the absence of causative hemodynamic factors, such as hypertension, aortic valve disease, or systemic infiltrative or storage diseases (Figs. 287-15 and 287-16). It has previously been termed *hypertrophic obstructive cardiomyopathy* (HOCM), *asymmetric septal hypertrophy* (ASH), and *idiopathic hypertrophic subaortic stenosis* (IHSS). However, the accepted terminology is now hypertrophic cardiomyopathy with or without obstruction. Prevalence in North America, Japan, and China is about 1:500. It is the leading cause of sudden death in the young and is an important cause of heart failure. Although pediatric presentation is associated with increased early morbidity and mortality, the prognosis for patients diagnosed as adults is generally favorable.

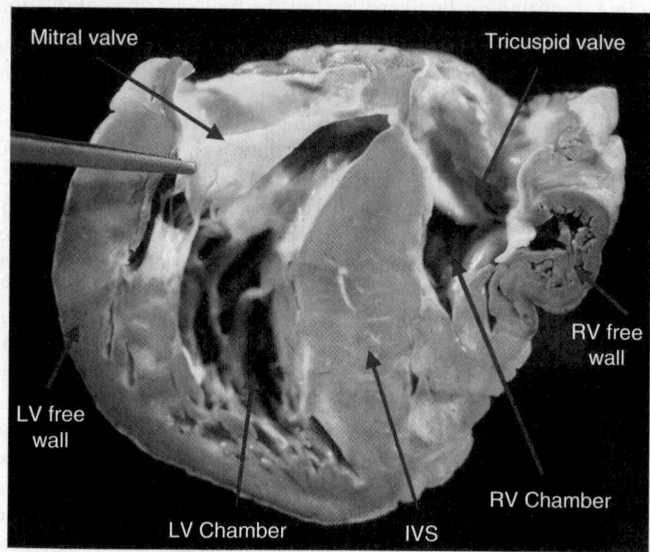

FIGURE 287-15 Hypertrophic cardiomyopathy. Gross specimen of a heart with hypertrophic cardiomyopathy removed at the time of transplantation, showing asymmetric septal hypertrophy (septum much thicker than left ventricular free wall) with the septum bulging into the left ventricular outflow tract causing obstruction. The forceps are retracting the anterior leaflet of the mitral valve, demonstrating the characteristic plaque of systolic anterior motion, manifest as endocardial fibrosis on the interventricular septum in a mirror-image pattern to the valve leaflet. There is patchy replacement fibrosis, and small thick-walled arterioles can be appreciated grossly, especially in the interventricular septum. IVS, interventricular septum; LV, left ventricle; RV, right ventricle. *(Image courtesy of Robert Padera, MD, PhD, Department of Pathology, Brigham and Women's Hospital, Boston.)*

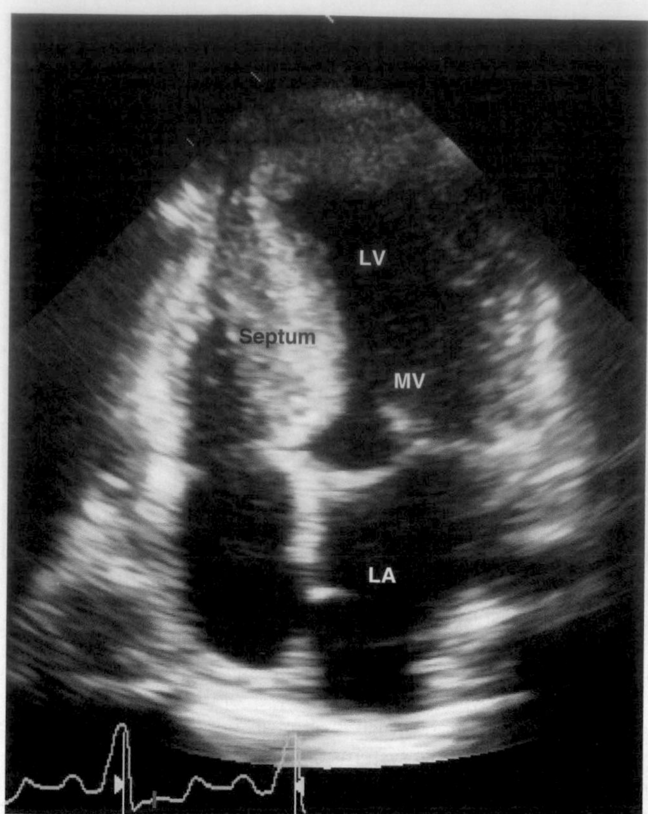

FIGURE 287-16 Hypertrophic cardiomyopathy. This echocardiogram of hypertrophic cardiomyopathy shows asymmetric hypertrophy of the septum compared to the lateral wall of the left ventricle (LV). The mitral valve (MV) is moving anteriorly toward the hypertrophied septum in systole. The left atrium (LA) is enlarged. Note that the echocardiographic and pathologic images are vertically opposite, such that the LV is by convention on the top right in the echocardiographic image and bottom right in the pathologic images. *(Image courtesy of Justina Wu, MD, Brigham and Women's Hospital, Boston.)*

The clustering of hypertrophic cardiomyopathy within families has been appreciated since recognition of the disease approximately 55 years ago. Echocardiographic screening of families revealed an autosomal dominant pattern of inheritance. Initial genetic studies using linkage analysis in large families identified disease-causing mutations in sarcomeric genes. A sarcomere mutation is present in ~60% of patients with hypertrophic cardiomyopathy and is more common in those with familial disease and characteristic asymmetric septal hypertrophy. More than nine different sarcomere genes with over 1400 mutations have been implicated, although ~80% of patients have a mutation in either *MYH7* or *MYBPC3* (Table 287-3), most of which are unique to individual families ("private" mutations).

Hypertrophic cardiomyopathy is characterized by age-dependent and incomplete penetrance. The defining phenotype of left ventricular hypertrophy is rarely present at birth and usually develops later in life. Accordingly, screening of family members should begin in adolescence and extend through adulthood. In *MYBPC3* mutation carriers, the average age of disease development is 40 years, while 30% remain free from hypertrophy after 70 years. Related individuals who carry the *same* mutation may have a different extent and pattern of hypertrophy (e.g., asymmetric versus concentric), occurrence of outflow tract obstruction, and associated clinical outcomes (e.g., sudden death, atrial fibrillation).

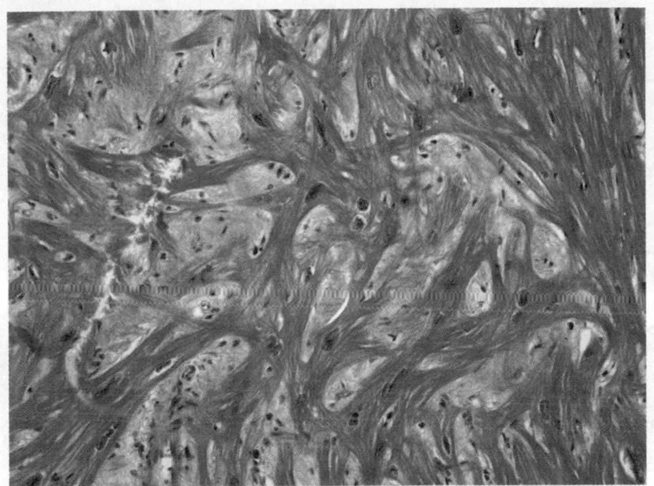

FIGURE 287-17 Hypertrophic cardiomyopathy. Microscopic image of hypertrophic cardiomyopathy showing the characteristic disordered myocyte architecture with swirling and branching rather than the usual parallel arrangement of myocyte fibers. Myocyte nuclei vary markedly in size and interstitial fibrosis is present. *(Image courtesy of Robert Padera, MD, PhD, Department of Pathology, Brigham and Women's Hospital, Boston.)*

At the level of the sarcomere, hypertrophic cardiomyopathy mutations lead to enhanced calcium sensitivity, maximal force generation, and ATPase activity. Calcium handling is affected through modification of regulatory proteins. Sarcomere mutations lead to abnormal energetics and impaired relaxation, both directly and as a result of hypertrophy. Hypertrophic cardiomyopathy is characterized by misalignment and disarray of the enlarged myofibrils and myocytes (Fig. 287-17), which can also occur to a lesser extent in other cardiac diseases. Although hypertrophy is the defining feature of hypertrophic cardiomyopathy, fibrosis and microvascular disease are also present. Interstitial fibrosis is detectable before overt hypertrophy develops and likely results from early activation of profibrotic pathways. In the majority of patients with overt cardiomyopathy, focal areas of replacement fibrosis can be readily detected with MRI. These areas of "scar" may represent substrate for the development of ventricular arrhythmias. Increased thickness and decreased luminal area of the intramural vessels in hypertrophied myocardium contribute to microvascular ischemia and angina. Microinfarction of hypertrophied myocardium is a hypothesized mechanism for replacement scar formation.

Macroscopically, hypertrophy is typically manifest as nonuniform ventricular thickening (Fig. 287-15). The interventricular septum is the typical location of maximal hypertrophy, although other patterns of hypertrophic remodeling include concentric and midventricular. Hypertrophy confined to the ventricular apex (apical hypertrophic cardiomyopathy) is less often familial and has a different genetic substrate, with sarcomere mutations present in only ~15%. Left ventricular outflow tract obstruction represents the most common focus of diagnosis and intervention, although diastolic dysfunction, myocardial fibrosis, and microvascular ischemia also contribute to contractile dysfunction and elevated intracardiac pressures. Obstruction is present in ~30% of patients at rest and can be provoked by exercise in another ~30%. Systolic obstruction is initiated by drag forces, which push an anteriorly displaced and enlarged anterior mitral leaflet into contact with the hypertrophied ventricular septum. Mitral leaflet coaptation may ensue, leading to posteriorly directed mitral regurgitation. In order to maintain stroke volume across outflow tract obstruction, the ventricle generates higher pressures, leading to higher wall stress and myocardial oxygen demand. Smaller chamber size and increased contractility exacerbate the severity of obstruction. Conditions of low preload, such as dehydration, and low afterload, such as arterial vasodilation, may lead to transient hypotension and near-syncope. The systolic ejection murmur of left ventricular outflow tract obstruction is harsh and late peaking and can be enhanced by bedside maneuvers that diminish ventricular volume and transiently worsen obstruction, such as standing from a squatting position or the Valsalva maneuver.

DIAGNOSIS

The substantial variability of hypertrophic cardiomyopathy pathology is reflected in the diversity of clinical presentations. Patients may be diagnosed after undergoing evaluations triggered by the abnormal physical findings (murmur) or symptoms of exertional dyspnea, angina, or syncope. Alternatively, diagnosis may follow evaluations prompted by the detection of disease in family members. Cardiac imaging (Fig. 287-16) is central to diagnosis due to the insensitivity of examination and ECG and the need to exclude other causes for hypertrophy. The identification of a disease-causing mutation in a proband can focus family evaluations on mutation carriers, but this strategy requires a high degree of certainty that the mutation is truly pathogenic and not a benign DNA variant. Biopsy is not needed to diagnose hypertrophic cardiomyopathy but can be used to exclude infiltrative and metabolic diseases. Rigorous athletic training (athlete's heart) may cause intermediate degrees of physiologic hypertrophy difficult to differentiate from mild hypertrophic cardiomyopathy. Unlike hypertrophic cardiomyopathy, hypertrophy in the athlete's heart regresses with cessation of training, and is accompanied by supernormal exercise capacity (VO_{2max} >50 mL/kg/min), mild ventricular dilation, and normal diastolic function.

TREATMENT HYPERTROPHIC CARDIOMYOPATHY

Management focuses on treatment of symptoms and prevention of sudden death and stroke (Fig. 287-18). Left ventricular outflow tract obstruction can be controlled medically in the majority of patients. β-Adrenergic blocking agents and L-type calcium channel blockers (e.g., verapamil) are first-line agents that reduce the severity of obstruction by slowing heart rate, enhancing diastolic filling, and decreasing contractility. Persistent symptoms of exertional dyspnea or chest pain can sometimes be controlled with the addition of disopyramide, an antiarrhythmic agent with potent negative inotropic properties. Patients with or without obstruction may develop heart failure symptoms due to fluid retention and require diuretic therapies for venous congestion. Severe medically refractory symptoms develop in ~5% of patients, for whom surgical myectomy or alcohol septal ablation may be effective. Developed over 50 years ago, surgical myectomy effectively relieves outflow tract obstruction by excising part of the septal myocardium involved in the dynamic obstruction. In selected patients, perioperative mortality is extremely low with excellent long-term survival free from recurrent obstruction and symptoms. Mitral valve repair or replacement is usually unnecessary as associated eccentric mitral regurgitation resolves with myectomy alone. Alcohol septal ablation in patients with suitable coronary anatomy can relieve outflow tract obstruction via a controlled infarction of the proximal septum, which produces similar periprocedural outcomes and gradient reduction as surgical myomectomy. Until long-term outcomes are demonstrated for this procedure, it is relegated primarily to patients who wish to avoid surgery or who have limiting comorbidities. Neither procedure has been shown to improve outcomes other than symptoms. With both procedures, the most common complication is the development of complete heart block necessitating permanent pacing. However, ventricular pacing as a primary therapy for outflow tract obstruction is ineffective and not generally advised.

Patients with hypertrophic cardiomyopathy have an increased risk of sudden cardiac death from ventricular tachyarrhythmias. Vigorous physical activity and competitive sport are prohibited. Factors that increase the risk of sudden death from a baseline of 0.5% per year are presented in Table 287-6. As sudden death has not been reduced by medical or procedural interventions, an implantable cardioverter-defibrillator is advised for patients with two or more risk factors and is advised on a selected basis for patient with one risk factor. Nevertheless, the positive predictive value of most risk factors is low, and many patients receiving a defibrillator

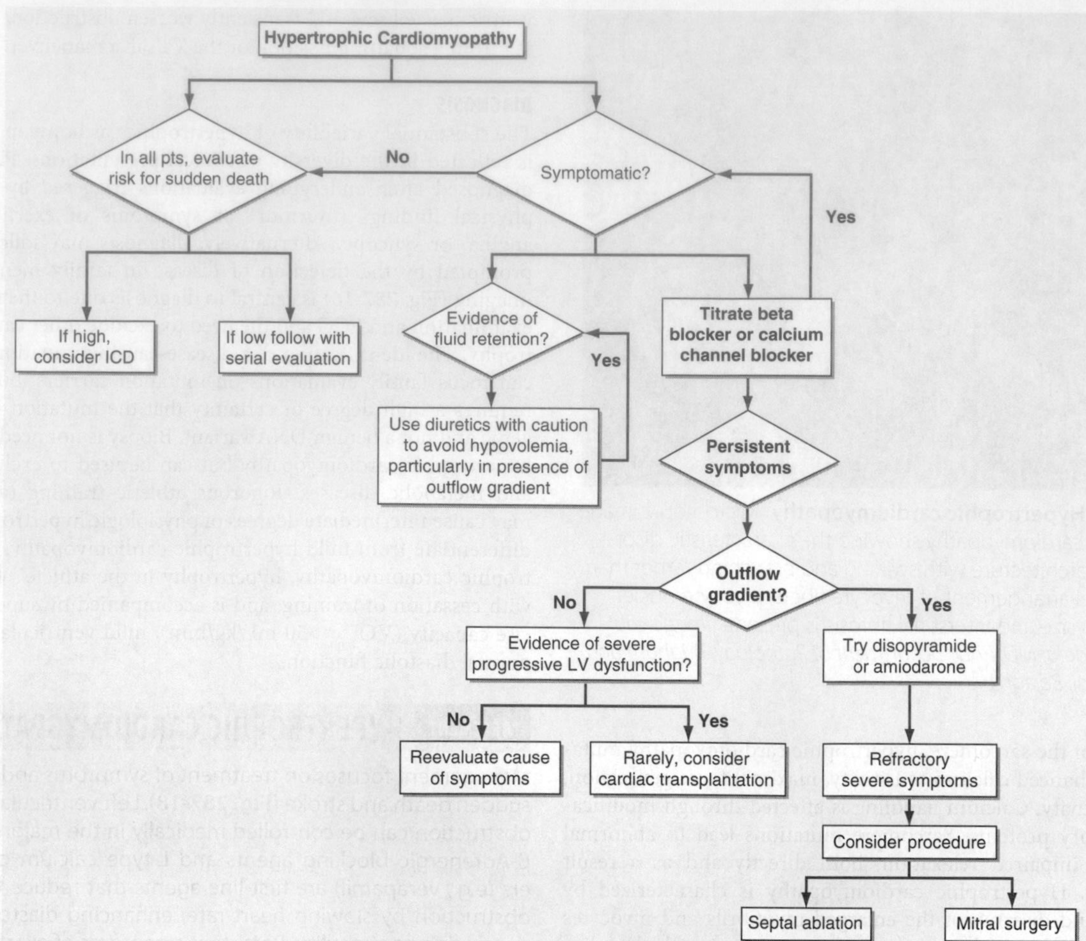

FIGURE 287-18 Treatment algorithm for hypertrophic cardiomyopathy depending on the presence and severity of symptoms and the presence of an intraventricular gradient with obstruction to outflow. Note that all patients with hypertrophic cardiomyopathy should be evaluated for atrial fibrillation and risk of sudden death, whether or not they require treatment for symptoms. ICD, implantable cardioverter-defibrillator; LV, left ventricular.

never receive an appropriate therapy. Long-term use of a defibrillator may be associated with serious device-related complications, particularly in young active patients. Refinement of sudden death risk through the application of contemporary technologies such as cardiac MRI is ongoing.

TABLE 287-6 RISK FACTORS FOR SUDDEN DEATH IN HYPERTROPHIC CARDIOMYOPATHY

Major Risk Factor		Screening Technique
History of cardiac arrest or spontaneous sustained ventricular tachycardia[a]		History
Syncope	Nonvagal, often with or after exertion	History
Family history of sudden cardiac death		Family history
Spontaneous nonsustained ventricular tachycardia[b]	>3 beats at rate >120	Exercise or 24- to 48-hour ambulatory recording
LV thickness >30 mm	Present in <10% of patients	Echocardiography
Abnormal blood pressure response to exercise[b]	Systolic blood pressure fall or failure to increase at peak exercise	Maximal upright exercise testing

[a]Implantable cardioverter-defibrillator advised for patients with prior arrest or sustained ventricular tachycardia regardless of other risk factors. [b] Prognostic value most applicable to patients less than 40 years old.

Abbreviation: LV, left ventricle.

Atrial fibrillation is common in patients with hypertrophic cardiomyopathy and may lead to hemodynamic deterioration and embolic stroke. Rapid ventricular response is poorly tolerated and may worsen outflow tract obstruction. β-Adrenergic blocking agents and L-type calcium channel blockers slow AV nodal conduction and improve symptoms; cardiac glycosides should be avoided, as they may increase contractility and worsen obstruction. Symptoms exacerbated by atrial fibrillation may persist despite adequate rate control due to loss of AV synchrony and may require restoration of sinus rhythm. Disopyramide and amiodarone are the preferred antiarrhythmic agents, with radiofrequency ablation considered for medically refractory cases. Anticoagulation to prevent embolic stroke in atrial fibrillation is recommended.

PROGNOSIS The general prognosis for hypertrophic cardiomyopathy is good, better than in early studies of referral populations. For patients diagnosed as adults, survival is comparable to an age-matched population without cardiomyopathy. The sudden death risk is less than 1% per year; however, up to 1 in 20 patients will progress to overt systolic dysfunction with a reduced ejection fraction with or without dilated remodeling ("burned out" or end-stage hypertrophic cardiomyopathy). These patients suffer from low cardiac output and have a high risk of death from progressive heart failure and sudden death unless they undergo cardiac transplantation.

288 Pericardial Disease

Eugene Braunwald

NORMAL FUNCTIONS OF THE PERICARDIUM

The normal pericardium is a double-layered sac; the visceral pericardium is a serous membrane that is separated by a small quantity (15–50 mL) of fluid, an ultrafiltrate of plasma, from the fibrous parietal pericardium. The normal pericardium, by exerting a restraining force, prevents sudden dilation of the cardiac chambers, especially the right atrium and ventricle, during exercise and with hypervolemia. It also restricts the anatomic position of the heart, and probably retards the spread of infections from the lungs and pleural cavities to the heart. Nevertheless, *total* absence of the pericardium, either congenital or after surgery, does not produce obvious clinical disease. In *partial* left pericardial defects, the main pulmonary artery and left atrium may bulge through the defect; very rarely, herniation and subsequent strangulation of the left atrium may cause sudden death.

ACUTE PERICARDITIS

Acute pericarditis, by far the most common pathologic process involving the pericardium (Table 288-1), has four principal diagnostic features:

1. *Chest pain* is usually present in acute infectious pericarditis and in many of the forms presumed to be related to hypersensitivity or autoimmunity. The pain of acute pericarditis is often severe, retrosternal, and left precordial, and referred to the neck, arms, or left shoulder. Frequently the pain is pleuritic, consequent to accompanying pleural inflammation (i.e., sharp and aggravated by inspiration and coughing), but sometimes it is steady, constricting, radiates into either arm or both arms, and resembles that of myocardial ischemia; therefore, confusion with acute myocardial infarction (AMI) is common. Characteristically, however, pericardial pain may be relieved by sitting up and leaning forward and is intensified by lying supine (Chap. 19). Pain is often absent in slowly developing tuberculous, postirradiation, and neoplastic, uremic, and constrictive pericarditis.

   The differentiation of AMI from acute pericarditis may become perplexing when, with acute pericarditis, serum biomarkers of myocardial damage such as troponin and creatine kinase-MB rise, presumably because of concomitant involvement of the epicardium in the inflammatory process (an epi-myocarditis) with resulting myocyte necrosis. However, these elevations, if they occur, are quite modest given the extensive electrocardiographic ST-segment elevation in pericarditis. This dissociation is useful in differentiating between these conditions.
2. A *pericardial friction rub* is audible at some point in about 85% of patients with acute pericarditis, may have up to three components per cardiac cycle, is high-pitched, and is described as rasping, scratching, or grating (Chap. 267). It is heard most frequently at end expiration with the patient upright and leaning forward.
3. The *electrocardiogram* (ECG) in acute pericarditis without massive effusion usually displays changes secondary to acute subepicardial inflammation (Fig. 288-1). It typically evolves through four stages. In stage 1, there is widespread elevation of the ST segments, often with upward concavity, involving two or three standard limb leads and V_2 to V_6, with reciprocal depressions only in aVR and sometimes V_1. Also, there is depression of the PR segment below the TP segment, reflecting atrial involvement. Usually there are no significant changes in QRS complexes. After several days, the ST segments return to normal (stage 2), and only then, or even later, do the T waves become inverted (stage 3). Weeks or months after the onset of acute pericarditis, the ECG returns to normal (stage 4). In contrast, in AMI, ST elevations are convex, and reciprocal depression is usually more prominent; these changes may return to normal within a day or two. Q waves may develop, with loss of R-wave amplitude, and T-wave inversions are usually seen within hours *before* the ST segments have become isoelectric (Chaps. 294 and 295).
4. *Pericardial effusion* is usually associated with pain and/or the ECG changes mentioned above, as well as electrical alternans.

TABLE 288-1 CLASSIFICATION OF PERICARDITIS

Clinical Classification
I. Acute pericarditis (<6 weeks)
A. Fibrinous
B. Effusive (serous or sanguineous)
II. Subacute pericarditis (6 weeks to 6 months)
A. Effusive-constrictive
B. Constrictive
III. Chronic pericarditis (>6 months)
A. Constrictive
B. Effusive
C. Adhesive (nonconstrictive)
Etiologic Classification
I. Infectious pericarditis
A. Viral (coxsackievirus A and B, echovirus, mumps, adenovirus, hepatitis, HIV)
B. Pyogenic (pneumococcus, *Streptococcus, Staphylococcus, Neisseria, Legionella*)
C. Tuberculous
D. Fungal (histoplasmosis, coccidioidomycosis, *Candida*, blastomycosis)
E. Other infections (syphilitic, protozoal, parasitic)
II. Noninfectious pericarditis
A. Acute myocardial infarction
B. Uremia
C. Neoplasia
1. Primary tumors (benign or malignant, mesothelioma)
2. Tumors metastatic to pericardium (lung and breast cancer, lymphoma, leukemia)
D. Myxedema
E. Cholesterol
F. Chylopericardium
G. Trauma
1. Penetrating chest wall
2. Nonpenetrating
H. Aortic dissection (with leakage into pericardial sac)
I. Postirradiation
J. Familial Mediterranean fever
K. Familial pericarditis
1. Mulibrey nanism[a]
L. Acute idiopathic
M. Whipple's disease
N. Sarcoidosis
III. Pericarditis presumably related to hypersensitivity or autoimmunity
A. Rheumatic fever
B. Collagen vascular disease (systemic lupus erythematosus, rheumatoid arthritis, ankylosing spondylitis, scleroderma, acute rheumatic fever, granulomatosis with polyangiitis [Wegener's])
C. Drug-induced (e.g., procainamide, hydralazine, phenytoin, isoniazid, minoxidil, anticoagulants, methysergide)
D. Postcardiac injury
1. Postmyocardial infarction (Dressler's syndrome)
2. Postpericardiotomy
3. Posttraumatic

[a]An autosomal recessive syndrome characterized by growth failure, muscle hypotonia, hepatomegaly, ocular changes, enlarged cerebral ventricles, mental retardation, ventricular hypertrophy, and chronic constrictive pericarditis

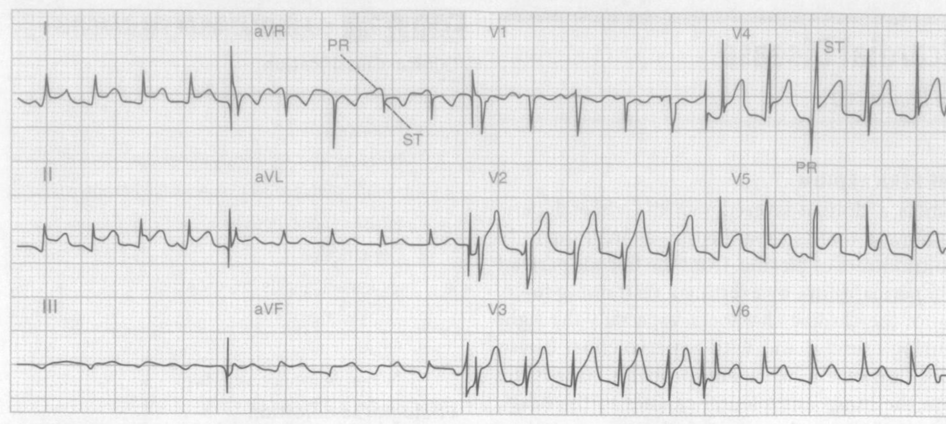

FIGURE 288-1 Acute pericarditis. There are diffuse ST-segment elevations (in this case in leads I, II, aVF, and V_2 to V_6) due to a ventricular current of injury. There is PR-segment deviation (opposite in polarity to the ST segment) due to a concomitant atrial injury current.

Pericardial effusion is especially important clinically when it develops within a relatively short time because it may lead to cardiac tamponade (see below). Differentiation from cardiac enlargement may be difficult on physical examination, but heart sounds may be fainter with pericardial effusion. The friction rub and the apex impulse may disappear. The base of the left lung may be compressed by pericardial fluid, producing *Ewart's sign*, a patch of dullness and increased fremitus (and egophony) beneath the angle of the left scapula. The chest roentgenogram may show enlargement of the cardiac silhouette, with a "water bottle" configuration, but may be normal.

Diagnosis *Echocardiography* (Chap. 270e) is the most widely used imaging technique. It is sensitive, specific, simple, noninvasive, may be performed at the bedside, and can identify accompanying cardiac tamponade (see below) (Fig. 288-2). The presence of pericardial fluid is recorded by two-dimensional transthoracic echocardiography as a relatively echo-free space between the posterior pericardium and left ventricular epicardium in patients with small effusions and as a space between the anterior right ventricle and the parietal pericardium just beneath the anterior chest wall. In patients with large effusions, the heart may swing freely within the pericardial sac. When severe, the extent of this motion alternates and may be associated with electrical alternans (Fig. 288-3). Echocardiography allows localization and identification of the quantity of pericardial fluid.

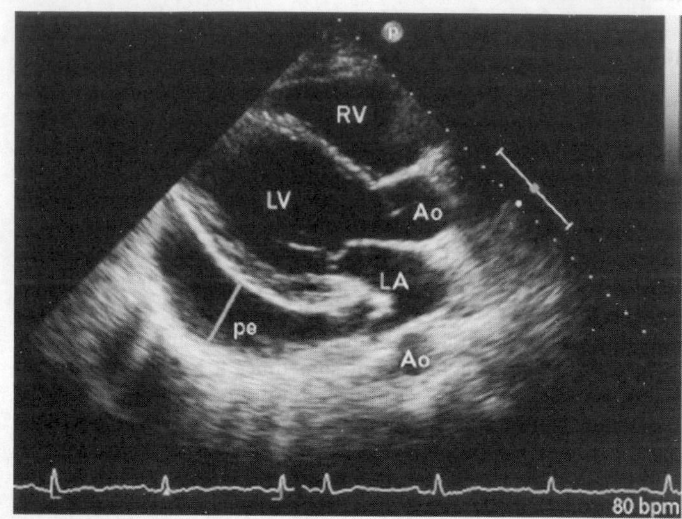

FIGURE 288-2 Two-dimensional echocardiogram in lateral view in a patient with a large pericardial effusion. Ao, aorta; LV, left ventricle; pe, pericardial effusion; RV, right ventricle. *(From M Imazio: Curr Opin Cardiol 27:308, 2012.)*

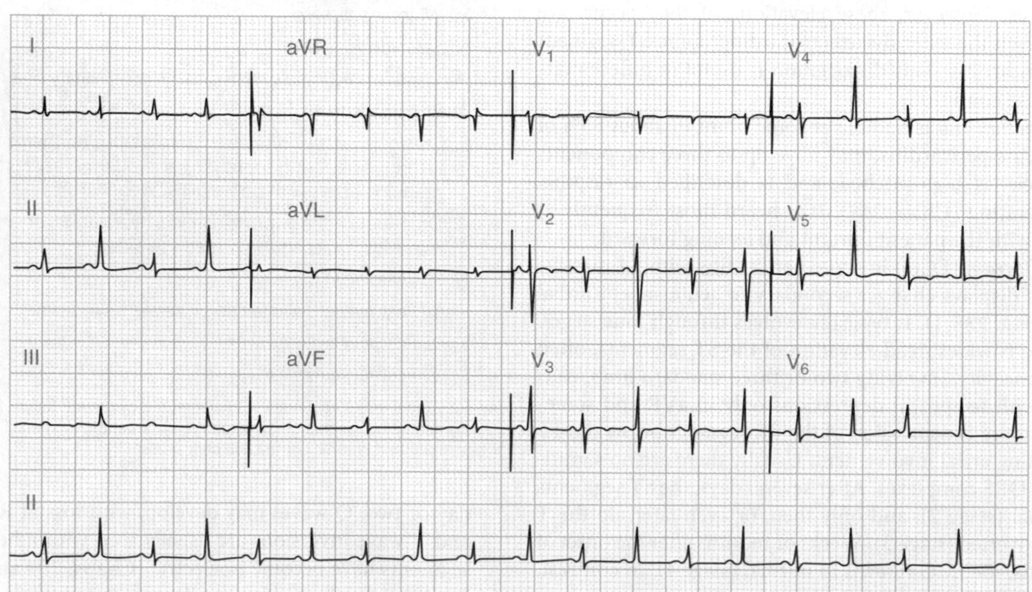

FIGURE 288-3 Electrical alternans. This tracing was obtained from a patient with a large pericardial effusion with tamponade. *(Reproduced from DM Mirvis, AL Goldberger: Electrocardiography, in RO Bonow et al [eds]: Braunwald's Heart Disease, 9th ed. Philadelphia: Elsevier, 2012.)*

The diagnosis of pericardial fluid or thickening may be confirmed by computed tomography (CT) or magnetic resonance imaging (MRI). These techniques may be superior to echocardiography in detecting loculated pericardial effusions, pericardial thickening, and the identification of pericardial masses.

TREATMENT ACUTE PERICARDITIS

There is no specific therapy for acute idiopathic pericarditis, but bed rest and anti-inflammatory treatment with aspirin (2–4 g/d), with gastric protection (e.g., omeprazole 20 mg/d), may be given. If this is ineffective, one of the nonsteroidal anti-inflammatory drugs (NSAIDs), such as ibuprofen (400–600 mg tid) or indomethacin (25–50 mg tid), should be tried. In responsive patients, these doses should be continued for 1–2 weeks and then tapered over several weeks. In patients who are unresponsive, colchicine (0.5 mg bid, given for 4–8 weeks) has been found to be effective, not only in acute pericarditis, but also in reducing the risk of recurrent pericarditis. Colchicine is concentrated in and interferes with the migration of neutrophils, is contraindicated in patients with hepatic or renal dysfunction, and may cause diarrhea and other gastrointestinal side effects. Glucocorticoids (e.g., prednisone 1 mg/kg per day) usually suppress the clinical manifestations of acute pericarditis in patients who have failed therapy with the anti-inflammatory therapies described above, but appear to increase the risk of subsequent recurrence. Therefore, full-dose corticosteroids should be given for only 2–4 days and then tapered. Anticoagulants should be avoided because their use could cause bleeding into the pericardial cavity and tamponade.

In patients with recurrences that are multiple, frequent, disabling, continue for more than 2 years, and are not prevented by colchicine and other NSAIDs and are not controlled by glucocorticoids, pericardial stripping may be necessary to terminate the illness, and usually does so.

CARDIAC TAMPONADE

The accumulation of fluid in the pericardial space in a quantity sufficient to cause serious obstruction of the inflow of blood into the ventricles results in cardiac tamponade. This complication may be fatal if it is not recognized and treated promptly. The most common causes of tamponade are idiopathic pericarditis and pericarditis secondary to neoplastic disease. Tamponade may also result from bleeding into the pericardial space after leakage from an aortic dissection, cardiac operations, trauma, and treatment of patients with acute pericarditis with anticoagulants.

The three principal features of tamponade (*Beck's triad*) are hypotension, soft or absent heart sounds, and jugular venous distention with a prominent *x* descent but an absent *y* descent. The limitations of ventricular filling are responsible for a reduction of cardiac output. The quantity of fluid necessary to produce cardiac tamponade may be as small as 200 mL when the fluid develops rapidly to as much as >2000 mL in slowly developing effusions when the pericardium has had the opportunity to stretch and adapt to an increasing volume. Tamponade may also develop more slowly, and in these circumstances, the clinical manifestations can resemble those of heart failure, including dyspnea, orthopnea, and hepatic engorgement.

A high index of suspicion for cardiac tamponade is required because in many instances no obvious cause for pericardial disease is apparent, and this diagnosis should be considered in any patient with otherwise unexplained enlargement of the cardiac silhouette, hypotension, and elevation of jugular venous pressure. There may be reduction in amplitude of the QRS complexes, and *electrical alternans* of the P, QRS, or T waves should raise the suspicion of cardiac tamponade (Fig. 288-3). Table 288-2 lists the features that distinguish acute cardiac tamponade from constrictive pericarditis.

TABLE 288-2 FEATURES THAT DISTINGUISH CARDIAC TAMPONADE FROM CONSTRICTIVE PERICARDITIS AND SIMILAR CLINICAL DISORDERS

Characteristic	Tamponade	Constrictive Pericarditis	Restrictive Cardiomyopathy	RVMI	Effusive Constrictive Pericarditis
Clinical					
Pulsus paradoxus	+++	+	+	+	+++
Jugular veins					
Prominent *y* descent	−	++	+	+	−
Prominent *x* descent	+++	++	+++	+	+++
Kussmaul's sign	−	+++	+	+++	++
Third heart sound	−	−	+	+	+
Pericardial knock	−	++	−	−	−
Electrocardiogram					
Low ECG voltage	++	++	++	−	++
Electrical alternans	++	−	−	−	+
Echocardiogram					
Thickened pericardium	−	+++	−	−	++
Pericardial calcification	−	++	−	−	
Pericardial effusion	+++	−	−	++	
RV size	Usually small	Usually normal	Usually normal	Enlarged	
RA and RV	+++		−	−	
Exaggerated respiratory variation in flow velocity	+++	+++	−	+++	
CT/MRI					
Thickened pericardium	−	+++	−	++	
Cardiac catheterization					
Equalization of diastolic pressures	+++	+++	−	++	

Abbreviations: +++, always present; ++, usually present; +, rare;–, absent; DC, diastolic collapse; ECG, electrocardiograph; RA, right atrium; RV, right ventricle; RVMI, right ventricular myocardial infarction.

Source: Adapted from GM Brockington et al: Cardiol Clin 8:645, 1990, with permission.

Paradoxical Pulse This important clue to the presence of cardiac tamponade consists of a greater than normal (10 mmHg) inspiratory decline in systolic arterial pressure. When severe, it may be detected by palpating weakness or disappearance of the arterial pulse during inspiration, but usually sphygmomanometric measurement of systolic pressure during slow respiration is required.

Because both ventricles share a tight incompressible covering, i.e., the pericardial sac, the inspiratory enlargement of the right ventricle in cardiac tamponade compresses and reduces left ventricular volume; leftward bulging of the interventricular septum reduces further the left ventricular cavity as the right ventricle enlarges during inspiration. Thus, in cardiac tamponade, the normal inspiratory augmentation of right ventricular volume causes an exaggerated reduction of left ventricular volume, stroke volume, and systolic pressure. Paradoxical pulse also occurs in approximately one-third of patients with constrictive pericarditis (see below), and in some cases of hypovolemic shock, acute and chronic obstructive airway disease, and pulmonary embolus. Right ventricular infarction (Chap. 295) may resemble cardiac tamponade with hypotension, elevated jugular venous pressure, an absent *y* descent in the jugular venous pulse, and, occasionally, a paradoxical pulse (Table 288-2).

Low-pressure tamponade refers to mild tamponade in which the intrapericardial pressure is increased from its slightly subatmospheric levels to +5 to +10 mmHg; in some instances, hypovolemia coexists. As a consequence, the central venous pressure is normal or only slightly elevated, whereas arterial pressure is unaffected and there is no paradoxical pulse. These patients are asymptomatic or complain of mild weakness and dyspnea. The diagnosis is aided by echocardiography, and both hemodynamic and clinical manifestations improve after pericardiocentesis.

Diagnosis Because immediate treatment of cardiac tamponade may be lifesaving, prompt measures to establish the diagnosis by echocardiography should be undertaken. When pericardial effusion causes tamponade, Doppler ultrasound shows that tricuspid and pulmonic valve flow velocities increase markedly during inspiration, whereas pulmonic vein, mitral, and aortic flow velocities diminish (as in constrictive pericarditis, see below) (Fig. 288-4). In tamponade, there is late diastolic inward motion (collapse) of the right ventricular free wall and the right atrium. Transesophageal echocardiography, CT, or cardiac MRI may be necessary to diagnose a loculated effusion responsible for cardiac tamponade.

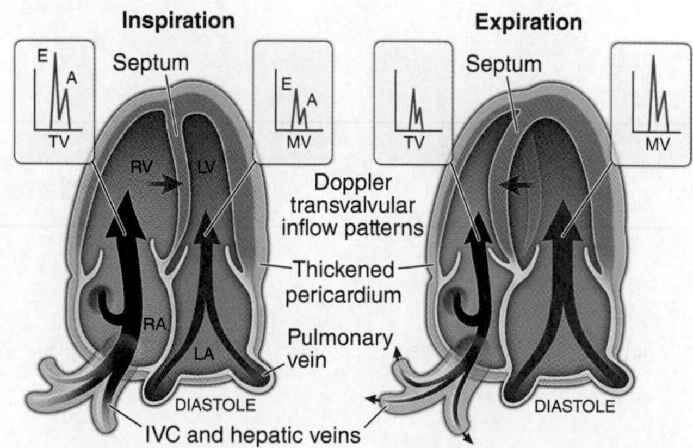

FIGURE 288-4 Constrictive pericarditis. Doppler schema of respirophasic changes in mitral and tricuspid inflow. Reciprocal patterns of ventricular filling are assessed on pulsed Doppler examination of mitral valve (MV) and tricuspid valve (TV) inflow. IVC, inferior vena cava; LA, left atrium; LV, left ventricle; RA, right atrium; RV, right ventricle. *(Courtesy of Bernard E. Bulwer, MD; with permission.)*

TREATMENT CARDIAC TAMPONADE

Patients with acute pericarditis should be observed frequently for the development of an effusion; if a large effusion is present, pericardiocentesis should be carried out or the patient watched closely for signs of tamponade. Arterial and venous pressures should be monitored and serial echocardiograms obtained.

PERICARDIOCENTESIS

If manifestations of tamponade appear, echocardiographically guided pericardiocentesis using an apical, parasternal, or, most commonly, subxiphoid approach must be carried out at once because reduction of the elevated intrapericardial pressure may be lifesaving. Intravenous saline may be administered as the patient is being readied for the procedure, but the pericardiocentesis must not be delayed. If possible, intrapericardial pressure should be measured before fluid is withdrawn, and the pericardial cavity should be drained as completely as possible. A small, multiholed catheter advanced over the needle inserted into the pericardial cavity may be left in place to allow draining of the pericardial space if fluid reaccumulates. Surgical drainage through a limited (subxiphoid) thoracotomy may be required in recurrent tamponade, when it is necessary to remove loculated effusions, and/or when it is necessary to obtain tissue for diagnosis.

Pericardial fluid obtained from an effusion often has the physical characteristics of an exudate. Bloody fluid is most commonly due to neoplasm, renal failure, or dialysis in the United States and tuberculosis in developing nations but may also be found in the effusion of acute rheumatic fever, after cardiac injury, and after myocardial infarction. Transudative pericardial effusions may occur in heart failure.

The pericardial fluid should be analyzed for red and white blood cells and cytologic studies, and cultures should be obtained. The presence of DNA of *Mycobacterium tuberculosis* determined by the polymerase chain reaction strongly supports the diagnosis of tuberculous pericarditis (Chap. 202).

VIRAL OR IDIOPATHIC ACUTE PERICARDITIS

In many instances, acute pericarditis occurs in association with illnesses of known or presumed viral origin and probably is caused by the same agent. Commonly, there is an antecedent infection of the respiratory tract, and viral isolation and serologic studies are negative. In some cases, coxsackievirus A or B or the virus of influenza, echovirus, mumps, herpes simplex, chickenpox, adenovirus, or cytomegalovirus has been isolated from pericardial fluid and/or appropriate elevations in viral antibody titers have been noted. Pericardial effusion is a common cardiac manifestation of HIV; it is usually secondary to infection (often mycobacterial) or neoplasm, most often lymphoma. Frequently, a viral cause cannot be established, and the term *idiopathic acute pericarditis* is then appropriate.

Viral or idiopathic acute pericarditis occurs at all ages but is more common in young adults and is often associated with pleural effusions and pneumonitis. The almost simultaneous development of fever and precordial pain, often 10–12 days after a presumed viral illness, constitutes an important feature in the differentiation of acute pericarditis from AMI, in which chest pain precedes fever. The constitutional symptoms are usually mild to moderate, and a pericardial friction rub is often audible. The disease ordinarily runs its course in a few days to 4 weeks. The ST-segment alterations in the ECG usually disappear after 1 or more weeks, but the abnormal T waves may persist for several years and be a source of confusion in persons without a clear history of pericarditis. Pleuritis and pneumonitis frequently accompany viral or idiopathic acute pericarditis. Accumulation of some pericardial fluid is common, and both tamponade and constrictive pericarditis are possible, but infrequent, complications.

The most frequent complication is recurrent (relapsing) pericarditis, which occurs in about one-fourth of patients with acute idiopathic pericarditis. In a smaller number, there are multiple recurrences. For treatment, see earlier section on treatment of acute pericarditis.

Postcardiac Injury Syndrome Acute pericarditis may appear in a variety of circumstances that have one common feature—previous injury to the myocardium with blood in the pericardial cavity. The syndrome may develop after a cardiac operation (postpericardiotomy syndrome), after blunt or penetrating cardiac trauma (Chap. 289e), or after perforation of the heart with a catheter. Rarely, it follows AMI.

The clinical picture mimics acute viral or idiopathic pericarditis. The principal symptom is the pain of acute pericarditis, which usually develops 1–4 weeks after the cardiac injury but earlier (1–3 days) after AMI. Recurrences are common and may occur up to 2 years or more following the injury. Fever, pleuritis, and pneumonitis are the outstanding features, and the bout of illness usually subsides in 1 or 2 weeks. The pericarditis may be of the fibrinous variety, or it may be a pericardial effusion, which is often serosanguineous but rarely causes tamponade. ECG changes typical of acute pericarditis may also occur. This syndrome is probably the result of a hypersensitivity reaction to antigen(s) that originate from injured myocardial tissue and/or pericardium.

Often no treatment is necessary aside from aspirin and analgesics. When the illness is severe or followed by a series of disabling recurrences, therapy with an NSAID, colchicine, or a glucocorticoid, such as described for treatment of acute pericarditis, is usually effective.

DIFFERENTIAL DIAGNOSIS

Because there is no specific test for *acute idiopathic pericarditis*, the diagnosis is one of exclusion. Consequently, all other disorders that may be associated with acute fibrinous pericarditis must be considered. A common diagnostic error is mistaking acute viral or idiopathic pericarditis for AMI and vice versa. When acute fibrinous pericarditis is associated with AMI (Chap. 295), it is characterized by fever, pain, and a friction rub in the first 4 days after the development of the infarct. ECG abnormalities (such as the appearance of Q waves, brief ST-segment elevations with reciprocal changes, and earlier T-wave changes in AMI) and the extent of the elevations of markers of myocardial necrosis (higher in AMI) are helpful in differentiating pericarditis from AMI.

Pericarditis secondary to postcardiac injury is differentiated from acute idiopathic pericarditis chiefly by timing. If it occurs within a few days or weeks of an AMI, a chest blow, a cardiac perforation, or a cardiac operation, it may be justified to conclude that the two are probably related.

It is important to distinguish *pericarditis due to collagen vascular disease* from acute idiopathic pericarditis. Most important in the differential diagnosis is the pericarditis due to systemic lupus erythematosus (SLE; Chap. 378) or drug-induced (procainamide or hydralazine) lupus. When pericarditis occurs in the absence of any obvious underlying disorder, the diagnosis of SLE may be suggested by a rise in the titer of antinuclear antibodies. Acute pericarditis is an occasional complication of *rheumatoid arthritis*, *scleroderma*, and *polyarteritis nodosa*, and other evidence of these diseases is usually obvious.

Pyogenic (purulent) pericarditis is usually secondary to cardiothoracic operations, by extension of infection from the lungs or pleural cavities, from rupture of the esophagus into the pericardial sac, or from rupture of a ring abscess in a patient with infective endocarditis. It may also complicate the viral, pyogenic, mycobacterial, and fungal infections that occur with HIV infection. It is generally accompanied by fever, chills, septicemia, and evidence of infection elsewhere and generally has a poor prognosis. The diagnosis is made by examination of the pericardial fluid. It requires drainage as well as vigorous antibiotic treatment.

Pericarditis of renal failure occurs in up to one-third of patients with chronic uremia (*uremic pericarditis*), and is also seen in patients undergoing chronic dialysis who have normal levels of blood urea and creatinine (*dialysis-associated pericarditis*). These two forms of pericarditis may be fibrinous and are generally associated with serosanguineous effusions. A pericardial friction rub is common, but pain is usually absent or mild. Treatment with an NSAID and intensification of dialysis are usually adequate. Occasionally, tamponade occurs and pericardiocentesis is required. When the pericarditis of renal failure is recurrent or persistent, a pericardial window should be created or pericardiectomy may be necessary.

Pericarditis due to *neoplastic diseases* results from extension or invasion of metastatic tumors (most commonly carcinoma of the lung and breast, malignant melanoma, lymphoma, and leukemia) to the pericardium; pain, atrial arrhythmias, and tamponade are complications that occur occasionally. Diagnosis is made by pericardial fluid cytology or pericardial biopsy. *Mediastinal irradiation* for neoplasm may cause acute pericarditis and/or chronic constrictive pericarditis. Unusual causes of acute pericarditis include syphilis, fungal infection (histoplasmosis, blastomycosis, aspergillosis, and candidiasis), and parasitic infestation (amebiasis, toxoplasmosis, echinococcosis, and trichinosis).

CHRONIC PERICARDIAL EFFUSIONS

Chronic pericardial effusions are sometimes encountered in patients without an antecedent history of acute pericarditis. They may cause few symptoms per se, and their presence may be detected by finding an enlarged cardiac silhouette on a chest roentgenogram. Tuberculosis is a common cause. *Myxedema* may be responsible for chronic pericardial effusion that is sometimes massive but rarely, if ever, causes cardiac tamponade. The cardiac silhouette may be markedly enlarged, and an echocardiogram distinguishes cardiomegaly from pericardial effusion. The diagnosis of myxedema can be confirmed by tests of thyroid function (Chap. 405). Myxedematous pericardial effusion responds to thyroid hormone replacement. Neoplasms, SLE, rheumatoid arthritis, mycotic infections, radiation therapy to the chest, pyogenic infections, and chylopericardium may also cause chronic pericardial effusion and should be considered and specifically sought in such patients.

Aspiration and analysis of the pericardial fluid are often helpful in diagnosis. Pericardial fluid should be analyzed as described in pericardiocentesis. Grossly sanguineous pericardial fluid results most commonly from a neoplasm, tuberculosis, renal failure, or slow leakage from an aortic dissection. Pericardiocentesis may resolve large effusions, but pericardiectomy may be required in patients with recurrence. Intrapericardial instillation of sclerosing agents may be used to prevent reaccumulation of fluid.

CHRONIC CONSTRICTIVE PERICARDITIS

This disorder results when the healing of an acute fibrinous or serofibrinous pericarditis or the resorption of a chronic pericardial effusion is followed by obliteration of the pericardial cavity with the formation of granulation tissue. The latter gradually contracts and forms a firm scar encasing the heart, which may be calcified. In developing nations where the condition is prevalent, a high percentage of cases are of tuberculous origin, but this is now an uncommon cause in North America. Chronic constrictive pericarditis may follow acute or relapsing viral or idiopathic pericarditis, trauma with organized blood clot, or cardiac surgery of any type or result from mediastinal irradiation, purulent infection, histoplasmosis, neoplastic disease (especially breast cancer, lung cancer, and lymphoma), rheumatoid arthritis, SLE, or chronic renal failure treated by chronic dialysis. In many patients, the cause of the pericardial disease is undetermined, and in these patients, an asymptomatic or forgotten bout of viral pericarditis, acute or idiopathic, may have been the inciting event.

The basic physiologic abnormality in patients with chronic constrictive pericarditis is the inability of the ventricles to fill because of the limitations imposed by the rigid, thickened pericardium. Ventricular filling is unimpeded during early diastole but is reduced abruptly when the elastic limit of the pericardium is reached, whereas in cardiac tamponade, ventricular filling is impeded throughout diastole. In both conditions, ventricular end-diastolic and stroke volumes are reduced and the end-diastolic pressures in both ventricles and the mean pressures in the atria, pulmonary veins, and systemic veins are all elevated to similar levels (i.e., within 5 mmHg of one another). Despite these hemodynamic changes, systolic function may be normal or only slightly impaired. However, in advanced cases, the fibrotic process may extend into the myocardium and cause myocardial scarring and atrophy, and venous congestion may then be due to the combined effects of the pericardial and myocardial lesions.

In constrictive pericarditis, the right and left atrial pressure pulses display an M-shaped contour, with prominent *x* and *y* descents. The *y* descent, which is absent or diminished in cardiac tamponade, is the most prominent deflection in constrictive pericarditis; it reflects rapid early filling of the ventricles. The *y* descent is interrupted by a rapid rise in atrial pressure during early diastole, when ventricular filling is impeded by the constricting pericardium. These characteristic changes are transmitted to the jugular veins, where they may be recognized by inspection. In constrictive pericarditis, the ventricular pressure pulses in both ventricles exhibit characteristic "square root" signs during diastole. These hemodynamic changes, although characteristic, are not pathognomonic of constrictive pericarditis and may also be observed in restrictive cardiomyopathies (Chap. 287, Table 287-2).

CLINICAL AND LABORATORY FINDINGS

Weakness, fatigue, weight gain, increased abdominal girth, abdominal discomfort, and edema are common. The patient often appears chronically ill, and in advanced cases, anasarca, skeletal muscle wasting, and cachexia may be present. Exertional dyspnea is common, and orthopnea may occur, although it is usually not severe. Acute left ventricular failure (acute pulmonary edema) is very uncommon. The cervical veins are distended and may remain so even after intensive diuretic treatment, and venous pressure may fail to decline during inspiration (*Kussmaul's sign*). The latter is common in chronic pericarditis but may also occur in tricuspid stenosis, right ventricular infarction, and restrictive cardiomyopathy.

The pulse pressure is normal or reduced. A paradoxical pulse can be detected in about one-third of cases. Congestive hepatomegaly is pronounced and may impair hepatic function and cause jaundice; ascites is common and is usually more prominent than dependent edema. The apical pulse is reduced and may retract in systole (*Broadbent's sign*). The heart sounds may be distant; an early third heart sound (i.e., a pericardial knock, occurring at the cardiac apex 0.09–0.12 s after aortic valve closure) with the abrupt cessation of ventricular filling is often conspicuous.

The *ECG* frequently displays low voltage of the QRS complexes and diffuse flattening or inversion of the T waves. Atrial fibrillation is present in about one-third of patients. The *chest roentgenogram* shows a normal or slightly enlarged heart. Pericardial calcification is most common in tuberculous pericarditis. Pericardial calcification may, however, occur in the absence of constriction, and constriction may occur without calcification.

Inasmuch as the usual physical signs of cardiac disease (murmurs, cardiac enlargement) may be inconspicuous or absent in chronic constrictive pericarditis, hepatic enlargement and dysfunction associated with jaundice and intractable ascites may lead to a mistaken diagnosis of hepatic cirrhosis. This error can be avoided if the neck veins are inspected and found to be distended.

The transthoracic *echocardiogram* typically shows pericardial thickening, dilation of the inferior vena cava and hepatic veins, and a sharp halt in ventricular filling in early diastole, with normal ventricular systolic function and flattening of the left ventricular posterior wall. There is a distinctive pattern of transvalvular flow velocity on Doppler echocardiography. During inspiration, there is an exaggerated reduction in blood flow velocity in the pulmonary veins and across the mitral valve and a leftward shift of the ventricular septum; the opposite occurs during expiration. Diastolic flow velocity in the inferior vena cava into the right atrium and across the tricuspid valve increases in an exaggerated manner during inspiration and declines during expiration (Fig. 288-4). However, echocardiography cannot definitively exclude the diagnosis of constrictive pericarditis. CT and MRI scanning (Fig. 288-5) are more accurate than echocardiography in establishing or excluding the presence of a thickened pericardium.

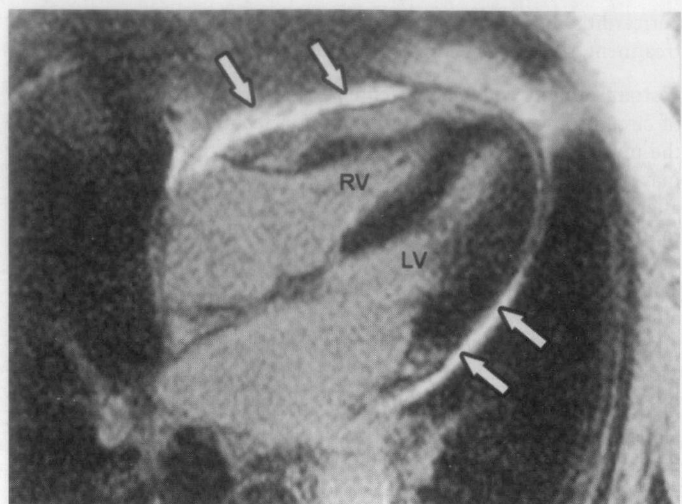

FIGURE 288-5 Magnetic resonance imaging in chronic constrictive pericarditis. The *arrows* point to a thickened pericardium, which shows late enhancement after gadolinium, characteristic of intense inflammation. LV, left ventricle; RV, right ventricle. *(From RY Kwong: Cardiovascular magnetic resonance imaging, in RO Bonow et al [eds]: Braunwald's Heart Disease, 9th ed. Philadelphia: Elsevier, 2012.)*

DIFFERENTIAL DIAGNOSIS

Like chronic constrictive pericarditis, cor pulmonale (Chap. 279) may be associated with severe systemic venous hypertension but little pulmonary congestion; the heart is usually not enlarged, and a paradoxical pulse may be present. However, in cor pulmonale, advanced parenchymal pulmonary disease is usually apparent and venous pressure *falls* during inspiration (i.e., Kussmaul's sign is negative). *Tricuspid stenosis* (Chap. 283) may also simulate chronic constrictive pericarditis; congestive hepatomegaly, splenomegaly, ascites, and venous distention may be equally prominent. However, in tricuspid stenosis, a characteristic murmur and the murmur of accompanying mitral stenosis are usually present.

Because constrictive pericarditis can be corrected surgically, it is important to distinguish chronic constrictive pericarditis from restrictive cardiomyopathy (Chap. 287), which has a similar physiologic abnormality (i.e., restriction of ventricular filling). The differentiating features are summarized in Table 288-2. When a patient has progressive, disabling, and unresponsive congestive heart failure and displays any of the features of constrictive heart disease, Doppler echocardiography to record respiratory effects on transvalvular flow and an MRI or CT scan should be obtained to detect or exclude constrictive pericarditis, because the latter is usually correctable.

TREATMENT CONSTRICTIVE PERICARDITIS

Pericardial resection is the only definitive treatment of constrictive pericarditis and should be as complete as possible. Dietary sodium restriction and diuretics are useful during preoperative preparation. Coronary arteriography should be carried out preoperatively in patients older than 50 years to exclude unsuspected accompanying coronary artery disease. The benefits derived from cardiac decortication are usually progressive over a period of months. The risk of this operation depends on the extent of penetration of the myocardium by the fibrotic and calcific process, the severity of myocardial atrophy, the extent of secondary impairment of hepatic and/or renal function, and the patient's general condition. Operative mortality is in the range of 5 to 10% even in experienced centers; the patients with the most severe disease are at highest risk. Therefore, surgical treatment should, if possible, be carried out as early as possible in the course.

Subacute Effusive-Constrictive Pericarditis This form of pericardial disease is characterized by the combination of a tense effusion in the pericardial space and constriction of the heart by thickened pericardium. It shares a number of features with both chronic pericardial effusion producing cardiac compression and with pericardial constriction. It may be caused by tuberculosis (see below), multiple attacks of acute idiopathic pericarditis, radiation, traumatic pericarditis, renal failure, scleroderma, and neoplasms. The heart is generally enlarged, and a paradoxical pulse and a prominent *x* descent (without a prominent *y* descent) are present in the atrial and jugular venous pressure pulses. After pericardiocentesis, the physiologic findings may change from those of cardiac tamponade to those of pericardial constriction. Furthermore, the intrapericardial pressure and the central venous pressure may decline, but not to normal. The diagnosis can be established by pericardiocentesis followed by pericardial biopsy. Wide excision of both the visceral and parietal pericardium is usually effective therapy.

Tuberculous Pericardial Disease This chronic infection is a common cause of chronic pericardial effusion, although less so in North America than in the developing world where active tuberculosis is endemic. The clinical picture is that of a chronic, systemic illness in a patient with pericardial effusion. It is important to consider this diagnosis in a patient with known tuberculosis, with HIV, and with fever, chest pain, weight loss, and enlargement of the cardiac silhouette of undetermined origin. If the etiology of chronic pericardial effusion remains obscure despite detailed analysis of the pericardial fluid (see above), a pericardial biopsy, preferably by a limited thoracotomy, should be performed. If definitive evidence is still lacking but the specimen shows granulomas with caseation, antituberculous chemotherapy (Chap. 202) is indicated.

If the biopsy specimen shows a thickened pericardium after 2–4 weeks of antituberculin therapy, pericardiectomy should be carried out to prevent the development of constriction. Tubercular cardiac constriction should be treated surgically while the patient is receiving antituberculous chemotherapy.

OTHER DISORDERS OF THE PERICARDIUM

Pericardial cysts appear as rounded or lobulated deformities of the cardiac silhouette, most commonly at the right cardiophrenic angle. They usually do not cause symptoms, and their major clinical significance lies in the possibility of confusion with a tumor, ventricular aneurysm, or massive cardiomegaly. *Tumors* involving the pericardium are most commonly secondary to malignant neoplasms originating in or invading the mediastinum, including carcinoma of the bronchus and breast, lymphoma, and melanoma. Mesothelioma is the most common *primary* malignant tumor. The usual clinical picture of malignant pericardial tumor is an insidiously developing, often bloody pericardial effusion. Surgical exploration is required to establish a definitive diagnosis and to carry out definitive or, more commonly, palliative treatment.

289e Tumors and Trauma of the Heart

Eric H. Awtry, Wilson S. Colucci

This is a digital-only chapter. It is available on the DVD that accompanies this book, as well as on Access Medicine/Harrison's Online, and the eBook and "app" editions of HPIM 19e.

TUMORS OF THE HEART

PRIMARY TUMORS

Primary tumors of the heart are rare. Approximately three-quarters are histologically benign, and the majority of these tumors are myxomas. Malignant tumors, almost all of which are sarcomas, account for 25% of primary cardiac tumors. All cardiac tumors, regardless of pathologic type, have the potential to cause life-threatening complications. Many tumors are now surgically curable; thus, early diagnosis is imperative.

Clinical Presentation Cardiac tumors may present with a wide array of cardiac and noncardiac manifestations. These manifestations depend in large part on the location and size of the tumor and are often nonspecific features of more common forms of heart disease, such as chest pain, syncope, heart failure, murmurs, arrhythmias, conduction disturbances, and pericardial effusion with or without tamponade. Additionally, embolic phenomena and constitutional symptoms may occur.

290e Cardiac Manifestations of Systemic Disease

Eric H. Awtry, Wilson S. Colucci

This is a digital-only chapter. It is available on the DVD that accompanies this book, as well as on Access Medicine/Harrison's Online, and the eBook and "app" editions of HPIM 19e.

The common systemic disorders that have associated cardiac manifestations are summarized in this chapter.

DIABETES MELLITUS

(See also Chap. 417) Diabetes mellitus, both insulin- and non-insulin-dependent, is an independent risk factor for coronary artery disease (CAD; Chap. 291e) and accounts for 14–50% of new cases of cardiovascular disease. Furthermore, CAD is the most common cause of death in adults with diabetes mellitus. In the diabetic population, the incidence of CAD relates to the duration of diabetes and the level of glycemic control, and its pathogenesis involves endothelial dysfunction, increased lipoprotein peroxidation, increased inflammation, a prothrombotic state, and associated metabolic abnormalities.

291e The Pathogenesis, Prevention, and Treatment of Atherosclerosis

Peter Libby

This is a digital-only chapter. It is available on the DVD that accompanies this book, as well as on Access Medicine/Harrison's Online, and the eBook and "app" editions of HPIM 19e.

PATHOGENESIS

Atherosclerosis remains the major cause of death and premature disability in developed societies. Moreover, current predictions estimate that by the year 2020 cardiovascular diseases, notably atherosclerosis, will become the leading global cause of total disease burden. Although many generalized or systemic risk factors predispose to its development, atherosclerosis affects various regions of the circulation preferentially and has distinct clinical manifestations that depend on the particular circulatory bed affected. Atherosclerosis of the coronary arteries commonly causes myocardial infarction (MI) (Chap. 295) and angina pectoris (Chap. 293). Atherosclerosis of the arteries supplying the central nervous system frequently provokes strokes and transient cerebral ischemia (Chap. 446). In the peripheral circulation, atherosclerosis causes intermittent claudication and gangrene and can jeopardize limb viability. Involvement of the splanchnic circulation can cause mesenteric ischemia. Atherosclerosis can affect the kidneys either directly (e.g., renal artery stenosis) or as a common site of atheroembolic disease (Chap. 301).

292e Atlas of Atherosclerosis

Peter Libby

This is a digital-only chapter. It is available on the DVD that accompanies this book, as well as on Access Medicine/Harrison's Online, and the eBook and "app" editions of HPIM 19e.

Knowledge about the biology of human atherosclerosis and the risk factors for the disease has expanded considerably. The application of vascular biology to human atherosclerosis has revealed many new insights into the mechanisms that promote clinical events. The series of animated video presentations presented here illustrates some of the evolving information about risk factors for atherosclerosis and the pathophysiology of clinical events.

The importance of blood pressure as a risk factor for atherosclerosis and cardiovascular events has long been recognized. More recent clinical information has highlighted the importance of pulse pressure—the difference between the systolic pressure and minimum diastolic arterial pressure—as a prognostic indicator of cardiovascular risk. The video clip on pulse pressure explains the pathophysiology of this readily measured clinical variable.

293 Ischemic Heart Disease

Elliott M. Antman, Joseph Loscalzo

Ischemic heart disease (IHD) is a condition in which there is an inadequate supply of blood and oxygen to a portion of the myocardium; it typically occurs when there is an imbalance between myocardial oxygen supply and demand. The most common cause of myocardial ischemia is atherosclerotic disease of an epicardial coronary artery (or arteries) sufficient to cause a regional reduction in myocardial blood flow and inadequate perfusion of the myocardium supplied by the involved coronary artery. Chapter 291e deals with the development and treatment of atherosclerosis. This chapter focuses on the chronic manifestations and treatment of IHD. The subsequent chapters address the acute phases of IHD.

EPIDEMIOLOGY AND GLOBAL TRENDS

IHD causes more deaths and disability and incurs greater economic costs than any other illness in the developed world. IHD is the most common, serious, chronic, life-threatening illness in the United States, where 13 million persons have IHD, >6 million have angina pectoris, and >7 million have sustained a myocardial infarction. Genetic factors, a high-fat and energy-rich diet, smoking, and a sedentary lifestyle are associated with the emergence of IHD (Chap. 291e). In the United States and Western Europe, IHD is growing among low-income groups, but primary prevention has delayed the disease to later in life in all socioeconomic groups. Despite these sobering statistics, it is worth noting that epidemiologic data show a decline in the rate of deaths due to IHD, about half of which is attributable to treatments and half to prevention by risk factor modification.

Obesity, insulin resistance, and type 2 diabetes mellitus are increasing and are powerful risk factors for IHD. These trends are occurring in the general context of population growth and as a result of the increase in the average age of the world's population. With urbanization in countries with emerging economies and a growing middle class, elements of the energy-rich Western diet are being adopted. As a result, the prevalence of risk factors for IHD and the prevalence of IHD itself are both increasing rapidly, so that in analyses of the global burden of disease, there is a shift from communicable to noncommunicable diseases. Population subgroups that appear to be particularly affected are men in South Asian countries, especially India and the Middle East. In light of the projection of large increases in IHD throughout the world, IHD is likely to become the most common cause of death worldwide by 2020.

PATHOPHYSIOLOGY

Central to an understanding of the pathophysiology of myocardial ischemia is the concept of myocardial supply and demand. In normal conditions, for any given level of a demand for oxygen, the myocardium will control the supply of oxygen-rich blood to prevent underperfusion of myocytes and the subsequent development of ischemia and infarction. The major determinants of myocardial oxygen demand (MVO_2) are heart rate, myocardial contractility, and myocardial wall tension (stress). An adequate supply of oxygen to the myocardium requires a satisfactory level of oxygen-carrying capacity of the blood (determined by the inspired level of oxygen, pulmonary function, and hemoglobin concentration and function) and an adequate level of coronary blood flow. Blood flows through the coronary arteries in a phasic fashion, with the majority occurring during diastole. About 75% of the total coronary resistance to flow occurs across three sets of arteries: (1) large epicardial arteries (Resistance 1 = R_1), (2) prearteriolar vessels (R_2), and (3) arteriolar and intramyocardial capillary vessels (R_3). In the absence of significant flow-limiting atherosclerotic obstructions, R_1 is trivial; the major determinant of coronary resistance is found in R_2 and R_3.

The normal coronary circulation is dominated and controlled by the heart's requirements for oxygen. This need is met by the ability of the coronary vascular bed to vary its resistance (and, therefore, blood flow) considerably while the myocardium extracts a high and relatively fixed percentage of oxygen. Normally, intramyocardial resistance vessels demonstrate a great capacity for dilation (R_2 and R_3 decrease). For example, the changing oxygen needs of the heart with exercise and emotional stress affect coronary vascular resistance and in this manner regulate the supply of oxygen and substrate to the myocardium (*metabolic regulation*). The coronary resistance vessels also adapt to physiologic alterations in blood pressure to maintain coronary blood flow at levels appropriate to myocardial needs (*autoregulation*).

By reducing the lumen of the coronary arteries, atherosclerosis limits appropriate increases in perfusion when the demand for flow is augmented, as occurs during exertion or excitement. When the luminal reduction is severe, myocardial perfusion in the basal state is reduced. Coronary blood flow also can be limited by spasm (see Prinzmetal's angina in Chap. 294), arterial thrombi, and, rarely, coronary emboli as well as by ostial narrowing due to aortitis. Congenital abnormalities such as the origin of the left anterior descending coronary artery from the pulmonary artery may cause myocardial ischemia and infarction in infancy, but this cause is very rare in adults.

Myocardial ischemia also can occur if myocardial oxygen demands are markedly increased and particularly when coronary blood flow may be limited, as occurs in severe left ventricular hypertrophy due to aortic stenosis. The latter can present with angina that is indistinguishable from that caused by coronary atherosclerosis largely owing to subendocardial ischemia (Chap. 283). A reduction in the oxygen-carrying capacity of the blood, as in extremely severe anemia or in the presence of carboxyhemoglobin, rarely causes myocardial ischemia by itself but may lower the threshold for ischemia in patients with moderate coronary obstruction.

Not infrequently, two or more causes of ischemia coexist in a patient, such as an increase in oxygen demand due to left ventricular hypertrophy secondary to hypertension and a reduction in oxygen supply secondary to coronary atherosclerosis and anemia. Abnormal constriction or failure of normal dilation of the coronary resistance vessels also can cause ischemia. When it causes angina, this condition is referred to as *microvascular angina*.

CORONARY ATHEROSCLEROSIS

Epicardial coronary arteries are the major site of atherosclerotic disease. The major risk factors for atherosclerosis (high levels of plasma low-density lipoprotein [LDL], low plasma high-density lipoprotein [HDL], cigarette smoking, hypertension, and diabetes mellitus [Chap. 291e]) disturb the normal functions of the vascular endothelium. These functions include local control of vascular tone, maintenance of an antithrombotic surface, and control of inflammatory cell adhesion and diapedesis. The loss of these defenses leads to inappropriate constriction, luminal thrombus formation, and abnormal interactions between blood cells, especially monocytes and platelets, and the activated vascular endothelium. Functional changes in the vascular milieu ultimately result in the subintimal collections of fat, smooth muscle cells, fibroblasts, and intercellular matrix that define the atherosclerotic plaque. Rather than viewing atherosclerosis strictly as a vascular problem, it is useful to consider it in the context of alterations in the nature of the circulating blood (hyperglycemia; increased concentrations of LDL cholesterol, tissue factor, fibrinogen, von Willebrand factor, coagulation factor VII, and platelet microparticles). The combination of a "vulnerable vessel" in a patient with "vulnerable blood" promotes a state of hypercoagulability and hypofibrinolysis. This is especially true in patients with diabetes mellitus.

Atherosclerosis develops at irregular rates in different segments of the epicardial coronary tree and leads eventually to segmental reductions in cross-sectional area, i.e., plaque formation. There is also a predilection for atherosclerotic plaques to develop at sites of increased turbulence in coronary flow, such as at branch points in the epicardial arteries. When a stenosis reduces the diameter of an epicardial artery by 50%, there is a limitation of the ability to increase flow to meet increased myocardial demand. When the diameter is reduced by ~80%, blood flow at rest may be reduced, and further minor decreases in the stenotic orifice area can reduce coronary flow dramatically to cause myocardial ischemia at rest or with minimal stress.

Segmental atherosclerotic narrowing of epicardial coronary arteries is caused most commonly by the formation of a plaque, which is subject to rupture or erosion of the cap separating the plaque from the bloodstream. Upon exposure of the plaque contents to blood, two important and interrelated processes are set in motion: (1) platelets are activated and aggregate, and (2) the coagulation cascade is activated, leading to deposition of fibrin strands. A thrombus composed of platelet aggregates and fibrin strands traps red blood cells and can reduce coronary blood flow, leading to the clinical manifestations of myocardial ischemia.

The location of the obstruction influences the quantity of myocardium rendered ischemic and determines the severity of the clinical manifestations. Thus, critical obstructions in vessels, such as the left main coronary artery and the proximal left anterior descending coronary artery, are particularly hazardous. Chronic severe coronary narrowing and myocardial ischemia frequently are accompanied by the development of collateral vessels, especially when the narrowing develops gradually. When well developed, such vessels can by themselves provide sufficient blood flow to sustain the viability of the myocardium at rest but not during conditions of increased demand.

With progressive worsening of a stenosis in a proximal epicardial artery, the distal resistance vessels (when they function normally) dilate to reduce vascular resistance and maintain coronary blood flow. A pressure gradient develops across the proximal stenosis, and poststenotic pressure falls. When the resistance vessels are maximally dilated, myocardial blood flow becomes dependent on the pressure in the coronary artery distal to the obstruction. In these circumstances, ischemia, manifest clinically by angina or electrocardiographically by ST-segment deviation, can be precipitated by increases in myocardial oxygen demand caused by physical activity, emotional stress, and/or tachycardia. Changes in the caliber of the stenosed coronary artery due to physiologic vasomotion, loss of endothelial control of dilation (as occurs in atherosclerosis), pathologic spasm (Prinzmetal's angina), or small platelet-rich plugs also can upset the critical balance between oxygen supply and demand and thereby precipitate myocardial ischemia.

EFFECTS OF ISCHEMIA

During episodes of inadequate perfusion caused by coronary atherosclerosis, myocardial tissue oxygen tension falls and may cause transient disturbances of the mechanical, biochemical, and electrical functions of the myocardium (Fig. 293-1). Coronary atherosclerosis is a focal process that usually causes nonuniform ischemia. During ischemia, regional disturbances of ventricular contractility cause segmental hypokinesia, akinesia, or, in severe cases, bulging (dyskinesia), which can reduce myocardial pump function.

The abrupt development of severe ischemia, as occurs with total or subtotal coronary occlusion, is associated with almost instantaneous failure of normal muscle relaxation and then contraction. The relatively poor perfusion of the subendocardium causes more intense ischemia of this portion of the wall (compared with the subepicardial region). Ischemia of large portions of the ventricle causes transient left ventricular failure, and if the papillary muscle apparatus is involved, mitral regurgitation can occur. When ischemia is transient, it may be associated with angina pectoris; when it is prolonged, it can lead to myocardial necrosis and scarring with or without the clinical picture of acute myocardial infarction (Chap. 295).

A wide range of abnormalities in cell metabolism, function, and structure underlie these mechanical disturbances during ischemia. The normal myocardium metabolizes fatty acids and glucose to carbon

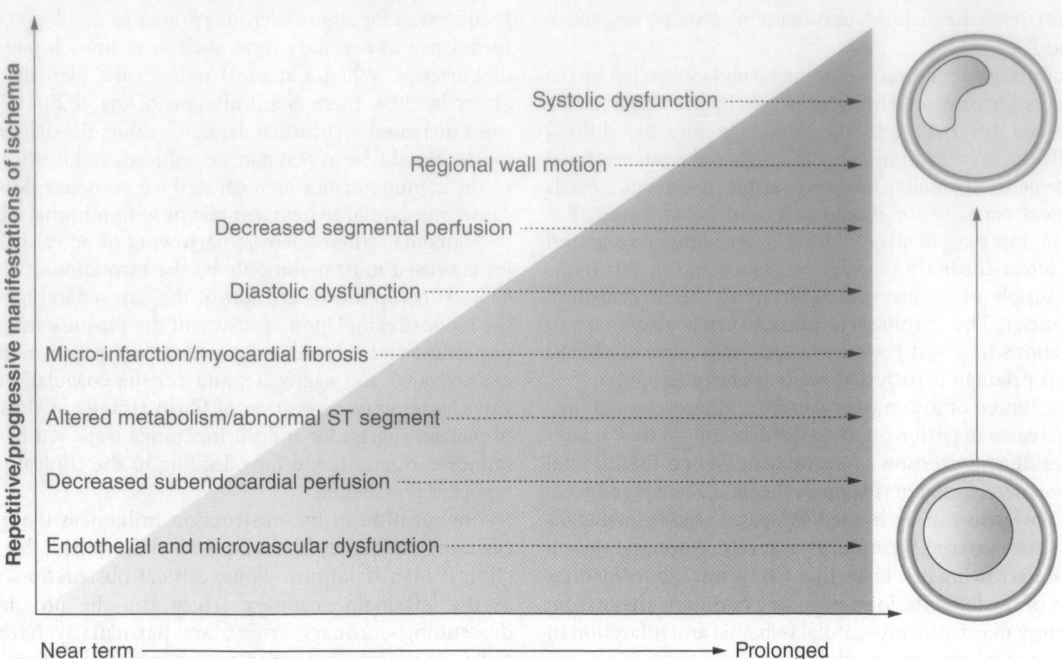

FIGURE 293-1 Cascade of mechanisms and manifestations of ischemia. *(Modified from LJ Shaw et al: J Am Coll Cardiol 54:1561, 2009. Original figure illustration by Rob Flewell.)*

dioxide and water. With severe oxygen deprivation, fatty acids cannot be oxidized, and glucose is converted to lactate; intracellular pH is reduced, as are the myocardial stores of high-energy phosphates, i.e., ATP and creatine phosphate. Impaired cell membrane function leads to the leakage of potassium and the uptake of sodium by myocytes as well as an increase in cytosolic calcium. The severity and duration of the imbalance between myocardial oxygen supply and demand determine whether the damage is reversible (≤20 min for total occlusion in the absence of collaterals) or permanent, with subsequent myocardial necrosis (>20 min).

Ischemia also causes characteristic changes in the electrocardiogram (ECG) such as repolarization abnormalities, as evidenced by inversion of T waves and, when more severe, displacement of ST segments (Chap. 268). Transient T-wave inversion probably reflects nontransmural, intramyocardial ischemia; transient ST-segment depression often reflects patchy subendocardial ischemia; and ST-segment elevation is thought to be caused by more severe transmural ischemia. Another important consequence of myocardial ischemia is electrical instability, which may lead to isolated ventricular premature beats or even ventricular tachycardia or ventricular fibrillation (Chap. 277). Most patients who die suddenly from IHD do so as a result of ischemia-induced ventricular tachyarrhythmias (Chap. 327).

ASYMPTOMATIC VERSUS SYMPTOMATIC IHD

Although the prevalence is decreasing, postmortem studies of accident victims and military casualties in Western countries still show that coronary atherosclerosis can begin before age 20 and is present even among adults who were asymptomatic during life. Exercise stress tests in asymptomatic persons may show evidence of silent myocardial ischemia, i.e., exercise-induced ECG changes not accompanied by angina pectoris; coronary angiographic studies of such persons may reveal coronary artery plaques and previously unrecognized obstructions (Chap. 272). Postmortem examination of patients with such obstructions without a history of clinical manifestations of myocardial ischemia often shows macroscopic scars secondary to myocardial infarction in regions supplied by diseased coronary arteries, with or without collateral circulation. According to population studies, ~25% of patients who survive acute myocardial infarction may not come to medical attention, and these patients have the same adverse prognosis as do those who present with the classic clinical picture of acute myocardial infarction (Chap. 295). Sudden death may be unheralded and is a common presenting manifestation of IHD (Chap. 327).

Patients with IHD also can present with cardiomegaly and heart failure secondary to ischemic damage of the left ventricular myocardium that may have caused no symptoms before the development of heart failure; this condition is referred to as *ischemic cardiomyopathy*. In contrast to the asymptomatic phase of IHD, the symptomatic phase is characterized by chest discomfort due to either angina pectoris or acute myocardial infarction (Chap. 295). Having entered the symptomatic phase, the patient may exhibit a stable or progressive course, revert to the asymptomatic stage, or die suddenly.

STABLE ANGINA PECTORIS

This episodic clinical syndrome is due to transient myocardial ischemia. Various diseases that cause myocardial ischemia and the numerous forms of discomfort with which it may be confused are discussed in Chap. 19. Males constitute ~70% of all patients with angina pectoris and an even greater proportion of those less than 50 years of age. It is, however, important to note that angina pectoris in women is often atypical in presentation (see below).

HISTORY

The typical patient with angina is a man >50 years or a woman >60 years of age who complains of episodes of chest discomfort, usually described as heaviness, pressure, squeezing, smothering, or choking and only rarely as frank pain. When the patient is asked to localize the sensation, he or she typically places a hand over the sternum, sometimes with a clenched fist, to indicate a squeezing, central, substernal discomfort (Levine's sign). Angina is usually crescendo-decrescendo in nature, typically lasts 2 to 5 min, and can radiate to either shoulder and to both arms (especially the ulnar surfaces of the forearm and hand). It also can arise in or radiate to the back, interscapular region, root of the neck, jaw, teeth, and epigastrium. Angina is rarely localized below the umbilicus or above the mandible. A useful finding in assessing a patient with chest discomfort is the fact that myocardial ischemic discomfort does not radiate to the trapezius muscles; that radiation pattern is more typical of pericarditis.

Although episodes of angina typically are caused by exertion (e.g., exercise, hurrying, or sexual activity) or emotion (e.g., stress, anger, fright, or frustration) and are relieved by rest, they also may occur at rest (Chap. 294) and while the patient is recumbent (angina decubitus). The patient may be awakened at night by typical chest discomfort and dyspnea. Nocturnal angina may be due to episodic tachycardia, diminished oxygenation as the respiratory pattern changes during sleep, or expansion of the intrathoracic blood volume that occurs with recumbency; the latter causes an increase in cardiac size (end-diastolic volume), wall tension, and myocardial oxygen demand that can lead to ischemia and transient left ventricular failure.

The threshold for the development of angina pectoris may vary by time of day and emotional state. Many patients report a fixed threshold for angina, which occurs predictably at a certain level of activity, such as climbing two flights of stairs at a normal pace. In these patients, coronary stenosis and myocardial oxygen supply are fixed, and ischemia is precipitated by an increase in myocardial oxygen demand; they are said to have stable exertional angina. In other patients, the threshold for angina may vary considerably within any particular day and from day to day. In such patients, variations in myocardial oxygen supply, most likely due to changes in coronary vasomotor tone, may play an important role in defining the pattern of angina. A patient may report symptoms upon minor exertion in the morning (a short walk or shaving) yet by midday be capable of much greater effort without symptoms. Angina may also be precipitated by unfamiliar tasks, a heavy meal, exposure to cold, or a combination of these factors.

Exertional angina typically is relieved in 1–5 min by slowing or ceasing activities and even more rapidly by rest and sublingual nitroglycerin (see below). Indeed, the diagnosis of angina should be suspect if it does not respond to the combination of these measures. The severity of angina can be conveniently summarized by the Canadian Cardiac Society functional classification (Table 293-1). Its impact on the patient's functional capacity can be described by using the New York Heart Association functional classification (Table 293-1).

TABLE 293-1 CARDIOVASCULAR DISEASE CLASSIFICATION CHART

Class	New York Heart Association Functional Classification	Canadian Cardiovascular Society Functional Classification
I	Patients have cardiac disease but *without* the resulting *limitations* of physical activity. Ordinary physical activity does not cause undue fatigue, palpitation, dyspnea, or anginal pain.	Ordinary physical activity, such as walking and climbing stairs, *does not cause angina*. Angina present with strenuous or rapid or prolonged exertion at work or recreation.
II	Patients have cardiac disease resulting in *slight limitation* of physical activity. They are comfortable at rest. Ordinary physical activity results in fatigue, palpitation, dyspnea, or anginal pain.	*Slight limitation* of ordinary activity. Walking or climbing stairs rapidly, walking uphill, walking or stair climbing after meals, in cold, or when under emotional stress or only during the few hours after awakening. Walking more than two blocks on the level and climbing more than one flight of stairs at a normal pace and in normal conditions.
III	Patients have cardiac disease resulting in *marked limitation* of physical activity. They are comfortable at rest. Less than ordinary physical activity causes fatigue, palpitation, dyspnea, or anginal pain.	*Marked limitation* of ordinary physical activity. Walking one to two blocks on the level and climbing more than one flight of stairs in normal conditions.
IV	Patients have cardiac disease resulting in *inability* to carry on any physical activity without discomfort. Symptoms of cardiac insufficiency or of the anginal syndrome may be present even at rest. If any physical activity is undertaken, discomfort is increased.	*Inability* to carry on any physical activity without discomfort—anginal syndrome *may* be present at rest.

Source: Modified from L Goldman et al: Circulation 64:1227, 1981.

Sharp, fleeting chest pain or a prolonged, dull ache localized to the left submammary area is rarely due to myocardial ischemia. However, especially in women and diabetic patients, angina pectoris may be atypical in location and not strictly related to provoking factors. In addition, this symptom may exacerbate and remit over days, weeks, or months. Its occurrence can be seasonal, occurring more frequently in the winter in temperate climates. Anginal "equivalents" are symptoms of myocardial ischemia other than angina. They include dyspnea, nausea, fatigue, and faintness and are more common in the elderly and in diabetic patients.

Systematic questioning of a patient with suspected IHD is important to uncover the features of an unstable syndrome associated with increased risk, such as angina occurring with less exertion than in the past, occurring at rest, or awakening the patient from sleep. Since coronary atherosclerosis often is accompanied by similar lesions in other arteries, a patient with angina should be questioned and examined for peripheral arterial disease (intermittent claudication [Chap. 302]), stroke, or transient ischemic attacks (Chap. 446). It is also important to uncover a family history of premature IHD (<55 years in first-degree male relatives and <65 in female relatives) and the presence of diabetes mellitus, hyperlipidemia, hypertension, cigarette smoking, and other risk factors for coronary atherosclerosis (Chap. 291e).

The history of typical angina pectoris establishes the diagnosis of IHD until proven otherwise. The coexistence of advanced age, male sex, the postmenopausal state, and risk factors for atherosclerosis increase the likelihood of hemodynamically significant coronary disease. A particularly challenging problem is the evaluation and management of patients with persistent ischemic-type chest discomfort but no flow-limiting obstructions in their epicardial coronary arteries. This situation arises more often in women than in men. Potential etiologies include microvascular coronary disease (detectable on coronary reactivity testing in response to vasoactive agents such as intracoronary adenosine, acetylcholine, and nitroglycerin) and abnormal cardiac nociception. Treatment of microvascular coronary disease should focus on efforts to improve endothelial function, including nitrates, beta blockers, calcium antagonists, statins, and angiotensin-converting enzyme (ACE) inhibitors. Abnormal cardiac nociception is more difficult to manage and may be ameliorated in some cases by imipramine.

PHYSICAL EXAMINATION

The physical examination is often normal in patients with stable angina when they are asymptomatic. However, because of the increased likelihood of IHD in patients with diabetes and/or peripheral arterial disease, clinicians should search for evidence of atherosclerotic disease at other sites, such as an abdominal aortic aneurysm, carotid arterial bruits, and diminished arterial pulses in the lower extremities. The physical examination also should include a search for evidence of risk factors for atherosclerosis such as xanthelasmas and xanthomas (Chap. 291e). Evidence for peripheral arterial disease should be sought by evaluating the pulse contour at multiple locations and comparing the blood pressure between the arms and between the arms and the legs (ankle-brachial index). Examination of the fundi may reveal an increased light reflex and arteriovenous nicking as evidence of hypertension. There also may be signs of anemia, thyroid disease, and nicotine stains on the fingertips from cigarette smoking.

Palpation may reveal cardiac enlargement and abnormal contraction of the cardiac impulse (left ventricular dyskinesia). Auscultation can uncover arterial bruits, a third and/or fourth heart sound, and, if acute ischemia or previous infarction has impaired papillary muscle function, an apical systolic murmur due to mitral regurgitation. These auscultatory signs are best appreciated with the patient in the left lateral decubitus position. Aortic stenosis, aortic regurgitation (Chap. 283), pulmonary hypertension (Chap. 304), and hypertrophic cardiomyopathy (Chap. 287) must be excluded, since these disorders may cause angina in the absence of coronary atherosclerosis. Examination during an anginal attack is useful, since ischemia can cause transient left ventricular failure with the appearance of a third and/or fourth heart sound, a dyskinetic cardiac apex, mitral regurgitation, and even pulmonary edema. Tenderness of the chest wall, localization of the discomfort with a single fingertip on the chest, or reproduction of the pain with palpation of the chest makes it unlikely that the pain is caused by myocardial ischemia. A protuberant abdomen may indicate that the patient has the metabolic syndrome and is at increased risk for atherosclerosis.

LABORATORY EXAMINATION

Although the diagnosis of IHD can be made with a high degree of confidence from the history and physical examination, a number of simple laboratory tests can be helpful. The urine should be examined for evidence of diabetes mellitus and renal disease (including microalbuminuria) since these conditions accelerate atherosclerosis. Similarly, examination of the blood should include measurements of lipids (cholesterol—total, LDL, HDL—and triglycerides), glucose (hemoglobin A_{1C}), creatinine, hematocrit, and, if indicated based on the physical examination, thyroid function. A chest x-ray is important as it may show the consequences of IHD, i.e., cardiac enlargement, ventricular aneurysm, or signs of heart failure. These signs can support the diagnosis of IHD and are important in assessing the degree of cardiac damage. Evidence exists that an elevated level of high-sensitivity C-reactive protein (CRP) (specifically, between 0 and 3 mg/dL) is an independent risk factor for IHD and may be useful in therapeutic decision making about the initiation of hypolipidemic treatment. The major benefit of high-sensitivity CRP is in reclassifying the risk of IHD in patients in the "intermediate" risk category on the basis of traditional risk factors.

ELECTROCARDIOGRAM

A 12-lead ECG recorded at rest may be normal in patients with typical angina pectoris, but there may also be signs of an old myocardial infarction (Chap. 268). Although repolarization abnormalities, i.e., ST-segment and T-wave changes, as well as left ventricular hypertrophy and disturbances of cardiac rhythm or intraventricular conduction are suggestive of IHD, they are nonspecific, since they also can occur in pericardial, myocardial, and valvular heart disease or, in the case of the former, transiently with anxiety, changes in posture, drugs, or esophageal disease. The presence of left ventricular hypertrophy (LVH) is a significant indication of increased risk of adverse outcomes from IHD. Of note, even though LVH and cardiac rhythm disturbances are nonspecific indicators of the development of IHD, they may be contributing factors to episodes of angina in patients in whom IHD has developed as a consequence of conventional risk factors. Dynamic ST-segment and T-wave changes that accompany episodes of angina pectoris and disappear thereafter are more specific.

STRESS TESTING

Electrocardiographic The most widely used test for both the diagnosis of IHD and the estimation of risk and prognosis involves recording the 12-lead ECG before, during, and after exercise, usually on a treadmill (Fig. 293-2). The test consists of a standardized incremental increase in external workload (Table 293-2) while symptoms, the ECG, and arm blood pressure are monitored. Exercise duration is usually symptom-limited, and the test is discontinued upon evidence of chest discomfort, severe shortness of breath, dizziness, severe fatigue, ST-segment depression >0.2 mV (2 mm), a fall in systolic blood pressure >10 mmHg, or the development of a ventricular tachyarrhythmia. This test is used to discover any limitation in exercise performance, detect typical ECG signs of myocardial ischemia, and establish their relationship to chest discomfort. The ischemic ST-segment response generally is defined as flat or downsloping depression of the ST segment >0.1 mV below baseline (i.e., the PR segment) and lasting longer than 0.08 s (Fig. 293-1). Upsloping or junctional ST-segment changes are not considered characteristic of ischemia and do not constitute a positive test. Although T-wave abnormalities, conduction disturbances, and ventricular arrhythmias that develop during exercise should be noted, they are also not diagnostic. Negative exercise tests in which the target heart rate (85% of maximal predicted heart rate for age and sex) is not achieved are considered nondiagnostic.

In interpreting ECG stress tests, the probability that coronary artery disease (CAD) exists in the patient or population under study (i.e., pretest probability) should be considered. Overall, false-positive or false-negative results occur in one-third of cases. However, a positive result on exercise indicates that the likelihood of CAD is 98% in males who are >50 years with a history of typical angina pectoris and who develop chest discomfort during the test. The likelihood decreases if the patient has atypical or no chest pain by history and/or during the test.

The incidence of false-positive tests is significantly increased in patients with low probabilities of IHD, such as asymptomatic men age <40 or premenopausal women with no risk factors for premature atherosclerosis. It is also increased in patients taking cardioactive drugs, such as digitalis and antiarrhythmic agents, and in those with intraventricular conduction disturbances, resting ST-segment and T-wave abnormalities, ventricular hypertrophy, or abnormal serum potassium levels. Obstructive disease limited to the circumflex coronary artery may result in a false-negative stress test since the lateral portion of the heart that this vessel supplies is not well represented on the surface 12-lead ECG. Since the overall sensitivity of exercise stress electrocardiography is only ~75%, a negative result does not exclude CAD, although it makes the likelihood of three-vessel or left main CAD extremely unlikely.

A medical professional should be present throughout the exercise test. It is important to measure total duration of exercise, the times to the onset of ischemic ST-segment change and chest discomfort, the external work performed (generally expressed as the stage of exercise), and the internal cardiac work performed, i.e., by the heart rate–blood pressure product. The depth of the ST-segment depression and the time needed for recovery of these ECG changes are also important. Because the risks of exercise testing are small but real—estimated at one fatality and two nonfatal complications per 10,000 tests—equipment for resuscitation should be available. Modified (heart rate–limited rather than symptom-limited) exercise tests can be performed safely in patients as early as 6 days after uncomplicated myocardial infarction (Table 293-2). Contraindications to exercise stress testing include rest angina within 48 h, unstable rhythm, severe aortic stenosis, acute myocarditis, uncontrolled heart failure, severe pulmonary hypertension, and active infective endocarditis.

The normal response to graded exercise includes progressive increases in heart rate and blood pressure. Failure of the blood pressure to increase or an actual decrease with signs of ischemia during the test is an important adverse prognostic sign, since it may reflect ischemia-induced global left ventricular dysfunction. The development of angina and/or severe (>0.2 mV) ST-segment depression at a low workload, i.e., before completion of stage II of the Bruce protocol, and/or ST-segment depression that persists >5 min after the termination of exercise increases the specificity of the test and suggests severe IHD and a high risk of future adverse events.

Cardiac Imaging (See also Chap. 270e) When the resting ECG is abnormal (e.g., preexcitation syndrome, >1 mm of resting ST-segment depression, left bundle branch block, paced ventricular rhythm), information gained from an exercise test can be enhanced by stress myocardial radionuclide perfusion imaging after the intravenous administration of thallium-201 or 99m-technetium sestamibi during exercise (or with pharmacologic) stress. Contemporary data also suggest positron emission tomography (PET) imaging (with exercise or pharmacologic stress) using N-13 ammonia or rubidium-82 nuclide as another technique for assessing perfusion. Images obtained immediately after cessation of exercise to detect regional ischemia are compared with those obtained at rest to confirm reversible ischemia and regions of persistently absent uptake that signify infarction.

A sizable fraction of patients who need noninvasive stress testing to identify myocardial ischemia and increased risk of coronary events cannot exercise because of peripheral vascular or musculoskeletal disease, exertional dyspnea, or deconditioning. In these circumstances, an intravenous pharmacologic challenge is used in place of exercise. For example, dipyridamole or adenosine can be given to create a coronary "steal" by temporarily increasing flow in nondiseased

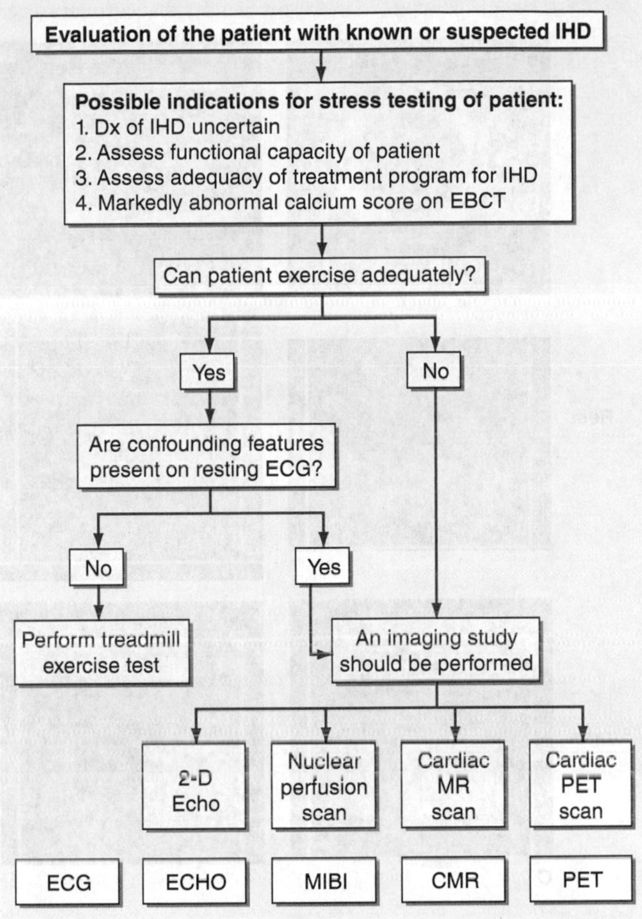

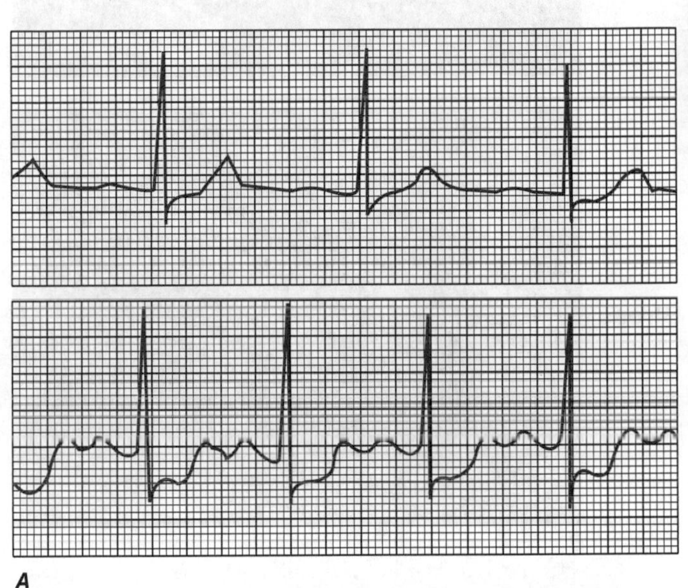

FIGURE 293-2 Evaluation of the patient with known or suspected ischemic heart disease. On the left of the figure is an algorithm for identifying patients who should be referred for stress testing and the decision pathway for determining whether a standard treadmill exercise with electrocardiogram (ECG) monitoring alone is adequate. A specialized imaging study is necessary if the patient cannot exercise adequately (pharmacologic challenge is given) or if there are confounding features on the resting ECG (symptom-limited treadmill exercise may be used to stress the coronary circulation). Panels B–E, continued on the next page, are examples of the data obtained with ECG monitoring and specialized imaging procedures. CMR, cardiac magnetic resonance; EBCT, electron beam computed tomography; ECHO, echocardiography; IHD, ischemic heart disease; MIBI, methoxyisobutyl isonitrite; MR, magnetic resonance; PET, positron emission tomography. ***A.*** Lead V_4 at rest (*top panel*) and after 4.5 min of exercise (*bottom panel*). There is 3 mm (0.3 mV) of horizontal ST-segment depression, indicating a positive test for ischemia. *(Modified from BR Chaitman, in E Braunwald et al [eds]: Heart Disease, 8th ed, Philadelphia, Saunders, 2008.)* ***B.*** A 45-year-old avid jogger who began experiencing classic substernal chest pressure underwent an exercise echo study. With exercise the patient's heart rate increased from 52 to 153 beats/min. The left ventricular chamber dilated with exercise, and the septal and apical portions became akinetic to dyskinetic (*red arrow*). These findings are strongly suggestive of a significant flow-limiting stenosis in the proximal left anterior descending artery, which was confirmed at coronary angiography. *(Modified from SD Solomon, in E. Braunwald et al [eds]: Primary Cardiology, 2nd ed, Philadelphia, Saunders, 2003.)* ***C.*** Stress and rest myocardial perfusion single-photon emission computed tomography images obtained with 99m-technetium sestamibi in a patient with chest pain and dyspnea on exertion. The images demonstrate a medium-size and severe stress perfusion defect involving the inferolateral and basal inferior walls, showing nearly complete reversibility, consistent with moderate ischemia in the right coronary artery territory (*red arrows*). *(Images provided by Dr. Marcello Di Carli, Nuclear Medicine Division, Brigham and Women's Hospital, Boston, MA.)* ***D.*** A patient with a prior myocardial infarction presented with recurrent chest discomfort. On cardiac magnetic resonance (CMR) cine imaging, a large area of anterior akinesia was noted (marked by the *arrows* in the top left and right images, systolic frame only). This area of akinesia was matched by a larger extent of late gadolinium-DTPA enhancements consistent with a large transmural myocardial infarction (marked by *arrows* in the middle left and right images). Resting (*bottom left*) and adenosine vasodilating stress (*bottom right*) first-pass perfusion images revealed reversible perfusion abnormality that extended to the inferior septum. This patient was found to have an occluded proximal left anterior descending coronary artery with extensive collateral formation. This case illustrates the utility of different modalities in a CMR examination in characterizing ischemic and infarcted myocardium. DTPA, diethylenetriamine penta-acetic acid. *(Images provided by Dr. Raymond Kwong, Cardiovascular Division, Brigham and Women's Hospital, Boston, MA.)* ***E.*** Stress and rest myocardial perfusion PET images obtained with rubidium-82 in a patient with chest pain on exertion. The images demonstrate a large and severe stress perfusion defect involving the mid and apical anterior, anterolateral, and anteroseptal walls and the left ventricular apex, showing complete reversibility, consistent with extensive and severe ischemia in the mid-left anterior descending coronary artery territory (*red arrows*). *(Images provided by Dr. Marcello Di Carli, Nuclear Medicine Division, Brigham and Women's Hospital, Boston, MA.)*

Rest

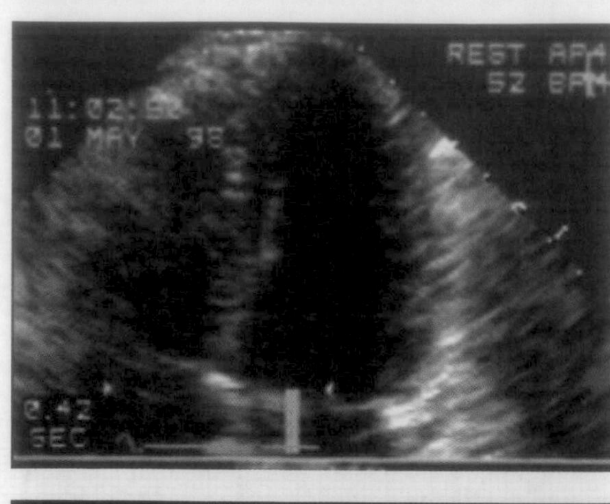

Stress

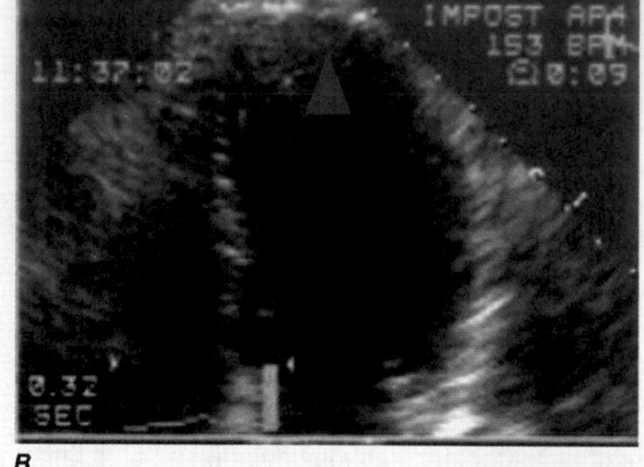

B

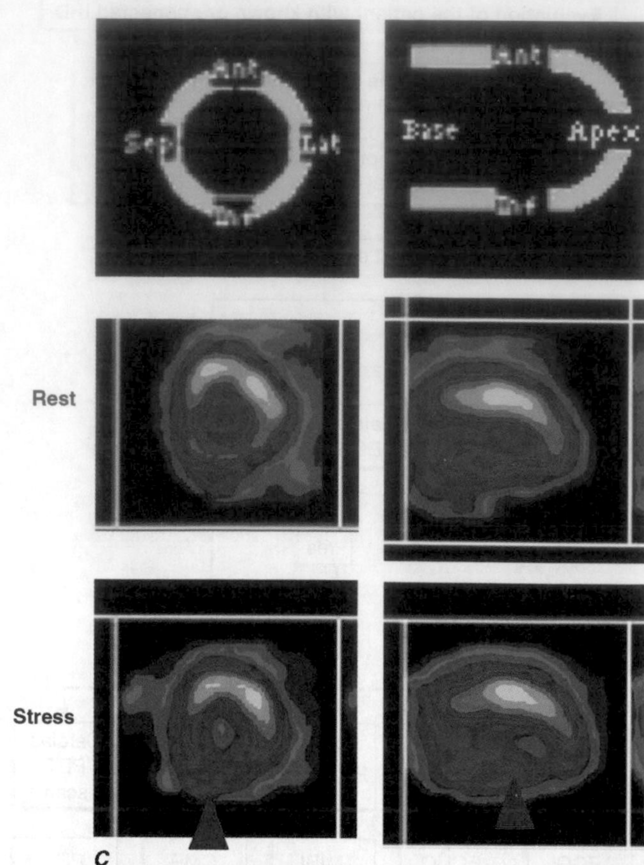

C

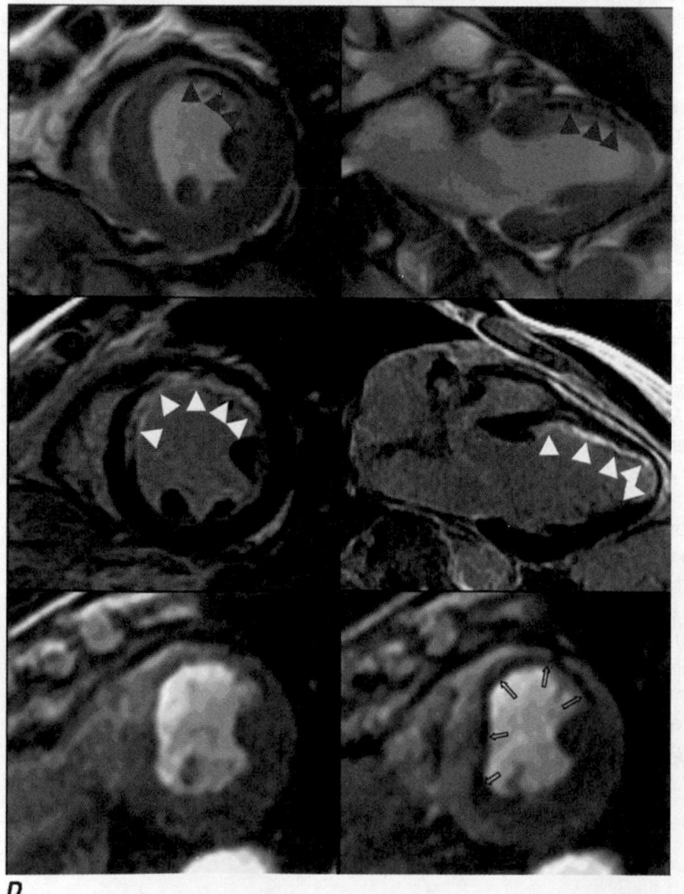
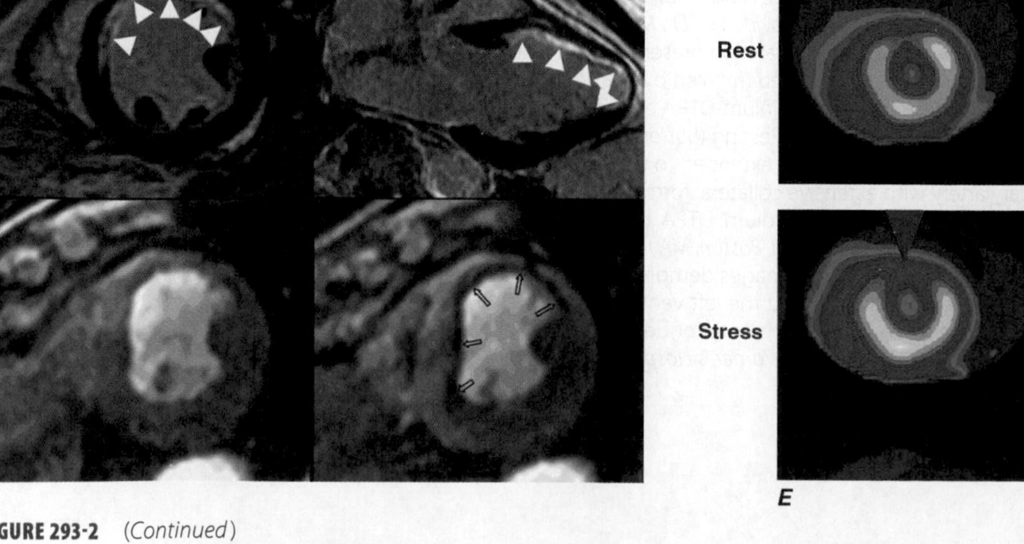

D

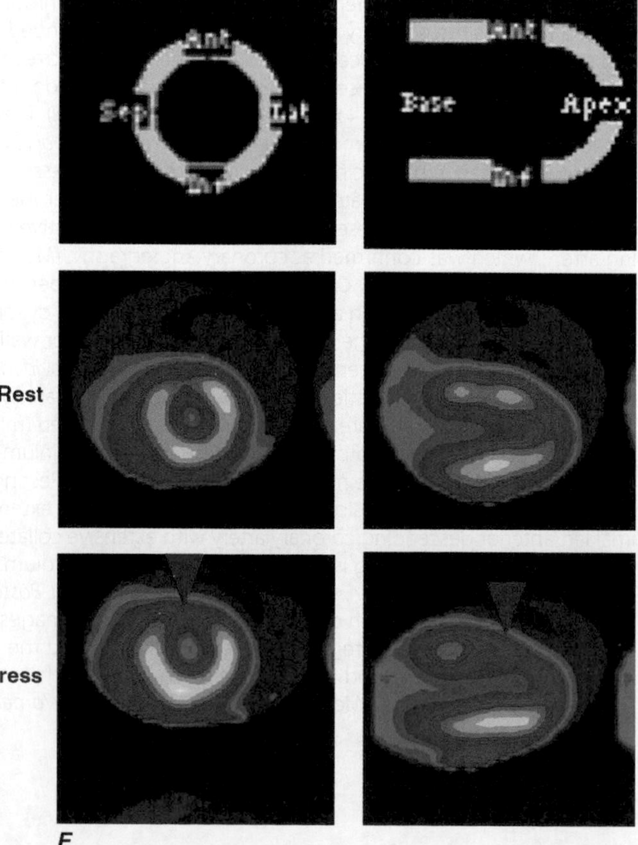

E

FIGURE 293-2 *(Continued)*

TABLE 293-2 RELATION OF METABOLIC EQUIVALENT TASKS (METs) TO STAGES IN VARIOUS TESTING PROTOCOLS

<table>
<tr><th rowspan="3">Functional Class</th><th rowspan="3" colspan="4">Clinical Status</th><th rowspan="3">O_2 Cost mL/kg/min</th><th rowspan="3">METs</th><th colspan="4">Treadmill Protocols</th></tr>
<tr><th colspan="2">BRUCE Modified 3 min Stages</th><th colspan="2">BRUCE 3 min Stages</th></tr>
<tr><th>MPH</th><th>%GR</th><th>MPH</th><th>%GR</th></tr>
<tr><td rowspan="13">NORMAL AND I</td><td rowspan="19">HEALTHY, DEPENDENT ON AGE, ACTIVITY</td><td rowspan="9"></td><td rowspan="12"></td><td rowspan="14"></td><td></td><td></td><td>6.0</td><td>22</td><td>6.0</td><td>22</td></tr>
<tr><td></td><td></td><td>5.5</td><td>20</td><td>5.2</td><td>20</td></tr>
<tr><td></td><td></td><td>5.0</td><td>18</td><td>5.0</td><td>18</td></tr>
<tr><td>56.0</td><td>16</td><td></td><td></td><td></td><td></td></tr>
<tr><td>52.5</td><td>15</td><td></td><td></td><td></td><td></td></tr>
<tr><td>49.0</td><td>14</td><td></td><td></td><td></td><td></td></tr>
<tr><td>45.5</td><td>13</td><td>4.2</td><td>16</td><td>4.2</td><td>16</td></tr>
<tr><td>42.0</td><td>12</td><td></td><td></td><td></td><td></td></tr>
<tr><td>38.5</td><td>11</td><td>3.4</td><td>14</td><td>3.4</td><td>14</td></tr>
<tr><td rowspan="7">SEDENTARY HEALTHY</td><td>35.0</td><td>10</td><td></td><td></td><td></td><td></td></tr>
<tr><td>31.5</td><td>9</td><td></td><td></td><td></td><td></td></tr>
<tr><td>28.0</td><td>8</td><td></td><td></td><td></td><td></td></tr>
<tr><td rowspan="6">LIMITED</td><td>24.5</td><td>7</td><td>2.5</td><td>12</td><td>2.5</td><td>12</td></tr>
<tr><td rowspan="2">II</td><td>21.0</td><td>6</td><td></td><td></td><td></td><td></td></tr>
<tr><td rowspan="5">SYMPTOMATIC</td><td>17.5</td><td>5</td><td>1.7</td><td>10</td><td>1.7</td><td>10</td></tr>
<tr><td rowspan="3">III</td><td>14.0</td><td>4</td><td></td><td></td><td></td><td></td></tr>
<tr><td rowspan="3"></td><td>10.5</td><td>3</td><td>1.7</td><td>5</td><td></td><td></td></tr>
<tr><td>7.0</td><td>2</td><td>1.7</td><td>0</td><td></td><td></td></tr>
<tr><td>IV</td><td></td><td>3.5</td><td>1</td><td></td><td></td><td></td><td></td></tr>
</table>

Abbreviations: GR, grade; MPH, miles per hour.

Source: Modified from GF Fletcher et al: Circulation 104:1694, 2001.

segments of the coronary vasculature at the expense of diseased segments. Alternatively, a graded incremental infusion of dobutamine may be administered to increase MVO_2. A variety of imaging options are available to accompany these pharmacologic stressors (Fig. 293-2). The development of a transient perfusion defect with a tracer such as thallium-201 or 99m-technetium sestamibi is used to detect myocardial ischemia.

Echocardiography is used to assess left ventricular function in patients with chronic stable angina and patients with a history of a prior myocardial infarction, pathologic Q waves, or clinical evidence of heart failure. Two-dimensional echocardiography can assess both global and regional wall motion abnormalities of the left ventricle that are transient when due to ischemia. Stress (exercise or dobutamine) echocardiography may cause the emergence of regions of akinesis or dyskinesis that are not present at rest. Stress echocardiography, like stress myocardial perfusion imaging, is more sensitive than exercise electrocardiography in the diagnosis of IHD. Cardiac magnetic resonance (CMR) stress testing is also evolving as an alternative to radionuclide, PET, or echocardiographic stress imaging. CMR stress testing performed with dobutamine infusion can be used to assess wall motion abnormalities accompanying ischemia, as well as myocardial perfusion. CMR can be used to provide more complete ventricular evaluation using multislice magnetic resonance imaging (MRI) studies.

Atherosclerotic plaques become progressively calcified over time, and coronary calcification in general increases with age. For this reason, methods for detecting coronary calcium have been developed as a measure of the presence of coronary atherosclerosis. These methods involve computed tomography (CT) applications that achieve rapid acquisition of images (electron beam [EBCT] and multidetector [MDCT] detection). Coronary calcium detected by these imaging techniques most commonly is quantified by using the Agatston score, which is based on the area and density of calcification. Although the diagnostic accuracy of this imaging method is high (sensitivity, 90–94%; specificity, 95–97%; negative predictive value, 93–99%), its prognostic utility has not been defined. Thus, its role in CT, EBCT, and MDCT scans for the detection and management of patients with IHD has not been clarified.

CORONARY ARTERIOGRAPHY

(See also Chap. 272) This diagnostic method outlines the lumina of the coronary arteries and can be used to detect or exclude serious coronary obstruction. However, coronary arteriography provides no information about the arterial wall, and severe atherosclerosis that does not encroach on the lumen may go undetected. Of note, atherosclerotic plaques characteristically are scattered throughout the coronary tree, tend to occur more frequently at branch points, and grow progressively in the intima and media of an epicardial coronary artery at first without encroaching on the lumen, causing an outward bulging of the artery—a process referred to as remodeling (Chap. 291e). Later in the course of the disease, further growth causes luminal narrowing.

Indications Coronary arteriography is indicated in (1) patients with chronic stable angina pectoris who are severely symptomatic despite medical therapy and are being considered for revascularization, i.e., a percutaneous coronary intervention (PCI) or coronary artery bypass grafting (CABG); (2) patients with troublesome symptoms that present diagnostic difficulties in whom there is a need to confirm or rule out the diagnosis of IHD; (3) patients with known or possible angina pectoris who have survived cardiac arrest; (4) patients with angina or evidence of ischemia on noninvasive testing with clinical or laboratory evidence of ventricular dysfunction; and (5) patients judged to be at high risk of sustaining coronary events based on signs of severe ischemia on noninvasive testing, regardless of the presence or severity of symptoms (see below).

Examples of other indications for coronary arteriography include the following:

1. Patients with chest discomfort suggestive of angina pectoris but a negative or nondiagnostic stress test who require a definitive diagnosis for guiding medical management, alleviating psychological stress, career or family planning, or insurance purposes.
2. Patients who have been admitted repeatedly to the hospital for a suspected acute coronary syndrome (Chaps. 294 and 295), but in whom this diagnosis has not been established and in whom the presence or absence of CAD should be determined.

3. Patients with careers that involve the safety of others (e.g., pilots, firefighters, police) who have questionable symptoms or suspicious or positive noninvasive tests and in whom there are reasonable doubts about the state of the coronary arteries.
4. Patients with aortic stenosis or hypertrophic cardiomyopathy and angina in whom the chest pain could be due to IHD.
5. Male patients >45 years and females >55 years who are to undergo a cardiac operation such as valve replacement or repair and who may or may not have clinical evidence of myocardial ischemia.
6. Patients after myocardial infarction, especially those who are at high risk after myocardial infarction because of the recurrence of angina or the presence of heart failure, frequent ventricular premature contractions, or signs of ischemia on the stress test.
7. Patients with angina pectoris, regardless of severity, in whom noninvasive testing indicates a high risk of coronary events (poor exercise performance or severe ischemia).
8. Patients in whom coronary spasm or another nonatherosclerotic cause of myocardial ischemia (e.g., coronary artery anomaly, Kawasaki disease) is suspected.

Noninvasive alternatives to diagnostic coronary arteriography include CT angiography and CMR angiography (Chap. 270e). Although these new imaging techniques can provide information about obstructive lesions in the epicardial coronary arteries, their exact role in clinical practice has not been rigorously defined. Important aspects of their use that should be noted include the substantially higher radiation exposure with CT angiography compared to conventional diagnostic arteriography and the limitations on CMR imposed by cardiac movement during the cardiac cycle, especially at high heart rates.

PROGNOSIS

The principal prognostic indicators in patients known to have IHD are age, the functional state of the left ventricle, the location(s) and severity of coronary artery narrowing, and the severity or activity of myocardial ischemia. Angina pectoris of recent onset, unstable angina (Chap. 294), early postmyocardial infarction angina, angina that is unresponsive or poorly responsive to medical therapy, and angina accompanied by symptoms of congestive heart failure all indicate an increased risk for adverse coronary events. The same is true for the physical signs of heart failure, episodes of pulmonary edema, transient third heart sounds, and mitral regurgitation and for echocardiographic or radioisotopic (or roentgenographic) evidence of cardiac enlargement and reduced (<0.40) ejection fraction.

Most important, any of the following signs during noninvasive testing indicates a high risk for coronary events: inability to exercise for 6 min, i.e., stage II (Bruce protocol) of the exercise test; a strongly positive exercise test showing onset of myocardial ischemia at low workloads (≥0.1 mV ST-segment depression before completion of stage II, ≥0.2 mV ST-segment depression at any stage, ST-segment depression for >5 min after the cessation of exercise, a decline in systolic pressure >10 mmHg during exercise, or the development of ventricular tachyarrhythmias during exercise); the development of large or multiple perfusion defects or increased lung uptake during stress radioisotope perfusion imaging; and a decrease in left ventricular ejection fraction during exercise on radionuclide ventriculography or during stress echocardiography. Conversely, patients who can complete stage III of the Bruce exercise protocol and have a normal stress perfusion scan or negative stress echocardiographic evaluation are at very low risk for future coronary events. The finding of frequent episodes of ST-segment deviation on ambulatory ECG monitoring (even in the absence of symptoms) is also an adverse prognostic finding.

On cardiac catheterization, elevations of left ventricular end-diastolic pressure and ventricular volume and reduced ejection fraction are the most important signs of left ventricular dysfunction and are associated with a poor prognosis. Patients with chest discomfort but normal left ventricular function and normal coronary arteries have an excellent prognosis. Obstructive lesions of the left main (>50% luminal diameter) or left anterior descending coronary artery proximal to the origin of the first septal artery are associated with a greater risk than are lesions of the right or left circumflex coronary artery because of the greater quantity of myocardium at risk. Atherosclerotic plaques in epicardial arteries with fissuring or filling defects indicate increased risk. These lesions go through phases of inflammatory cellular activity, degeneration, endothelial dysfunction, abnormal vasomotion, platelet aggregation, and fissuring or hemorrhage. These factors can temporarily worsen the stenosis and cause thrombosis and/or abnormal reactivity of the vessel wall, thus exacerbating the manifestations of ischemia. The recent onset of symptoms, the development of severe ischemia during stress testing (see above), and unstable angina pectoris (Chap. 294) all reflect episodes of rapid progression in coronary lesions.

With any degree of obstructive CAD, mortality is greatly increased when left ventricular function is impaired; conversely, at any level of left ventricular function, the prognosis is influenced importantly by the quantity of myocardium perfused by critically obstructed vessels. Therefore, it is essential to collect all the evidence substantiating past myocardial damage (evidence of myocardial infarction on ECG, echocardiography, radioisotope imaging, or left ventriculography), residual left ventricular function (ejection fraction and wall motion), and risk of future damage from coronary events (extent of coronary disease and severity of ischemia defined by noninvasive stress testing). The larger the quantity of established myocardial necrosis is, the less the heart is able to withstand additional damage and the poorer the prognosis is. Risk estimation must include age, presenting symptoms, all risk factors, signs of arterial disease, existing cardiac damage, and signs of impending damage (i.e., ischemia).

The greater the number and severity of risk factors for coronary atherosclerosis (advanced age [>75 years], hypertension, dyslipidemia, diabetes, morbid obesity, accompanying peripheral and/or cerebrovascular disease, previous myocardial infarction), the worse the prognosis of an angina patient. Evidence exists that elevated levels of CRP in the plasma, extensive coronary calcification on electron beam CT (see above), and increased carotid intimal thickening on ultrasound examination also indicate an increased risk of coronary events.

TREATMENT STABLE ANGINA PECTORIS

Once the diagnosis of IHD has been made, each patient must be evaluated individually with respect to his or her level of understanding, expectations and goals, control of symptoms, and prevention of adverse clinical outcomes such as myocardial infarction and premature death. The degree of disability and the physical and emotional stress that precipitates angina must be recorded carefully to set treatment goals. The management plan should include the following components: (1) explanation of the problem and reassurance about the ability to formulate a treatment plan, (2) identification and treatment of aggravating conditions, (3) recommendations for adaptation of activity as needed, (4) treatment of risk factors that will decrease the occurrence of adverse coronary outcomes, (5) drug therapy for angina, and (6) consideration of revascularization.

EXPLANATION AND REASSURANCE

Patients with IHD need to understand their condition and realize that a long and productive life is possible even though they have angina pectoris or have experienced and recovered from an acute myocardial infarction. Offering results of clinical trials showing improved outcomes can be of great value in encouraging patients to resume or maintain activity and return to work. A planned program of rehabilitation can encourage patients to lose weight, improve exercise tolerance, and control risk factors with more confidence.

IDENTIFICATION AND TREATMENT OF AGGRAVATING CONDITIONS

A number of conditions may increase oxygen demand or decrease oxygen supply to the myocardium and may precipitate or exacerbate angina in patients with IHD. Left ventricular hypertrophy, aortic valve disease, and hypertrophic cardiomyopathy may cause or contribute to angina and should be excluded or treated. Obesity, hypertension, and hyperthyroidism should be treated aggressively to reduce the frequency and severity of anginal episodes. Decreased myocardial oxygen supply may be due to reduced oxygenation of the arterial blood (e.g., in pulmonary disease or, when carboxyhemoglobin is present, due to cigarette or cigar smoking) or decreased oxygen-carrying capacity (e.g., in anemia). Correction of these abnormalities, if present, may reduce or even eliminate angina pectoris.

ADAPTATION OF ACTIVITY

Myocardial ischemia is caused by a discrepancy between the demand of the heart muscle for oxygen and the ability of the coronary circulation to meet that demand. Most patients can be helped to understand this concept and utilize it in the rational programming of activity. Many tasks that ordinarily evoke angina may be accomplished without symptoms simply by reducing the speed at which they are performed. Patients must appreciate the diurnal variation in their tolerance of certain activities and should reduce their energy requirements in the morning, immediately after meals, and in cold or inclement weather. On occasion, it may be necessary to recommend a change in employment or residence to avoid physical stress.

Physical conditioning usually improves the exercise tolerance of patients with angina and has substantial psychological benefits. A regular program of isotonic exercise that is within the limits of the individual patient's threshold for the development of angina pectoris and that does not exceed 80% of the heart rate associated with ischemia on exercise testing should be strongly encouraged. Based on the results of an exercise test, the number of metabolic equivalent tasks (METs) performed at the onset of ischemia can be estimated (Table 293-2) and a practical exercise prescription can be formulated to permit daily activities that will fall below the ischemic threshold (Table 293-3).

TREATMENT OF RISK FACTORS

A *family history* of premature IHD is an important indicator of increased risk and should trigger a search for treatable risk factors such as hyperlipidemia, hypertension, and diabetes mellitus. *Obesity* impairs the treatment of other risk factors and increases the risk of adverse coronary events. In addition, obesity often is accompanied by three other risk factors: diabetes mellitus, hypertension, and hyperlipidemia. The treatment of obesity and these accompanying risk factors is an important component of any management plan. A diet low in saturated and *trans*-unsaturated fatty acids and a reduced caloric intake to achieve optimal body weight are a cornerstone in the management of chronic IHD. It is especially important to emphasize weight loss and regular exercise in patients with the metabolic syndrome or overt diabetes mellitus.

Cigarette smoking accelerates coronary atherosclerosis in both sexes and at all ages and increases the risk of thrombosis, plaque instability, myocardial infarction, and death (Chap. 291e). In addition, by increasing myocardial oxygen needs and reducing oxygen supply, it aggravates angina. Smoking cessation studies have demonstrated important benefits with a significant decline in the occurrence of these adverse outcomes. The physician's message must be clear and strong and supported by programs that achieve and monitor abstinence (Chap. 470). *Hypertension* (Chap. 298) is associated with an increased risk of adverse clinical events from coronary atherosclerosis as well as stroke. In addition, the left ventricular hypertrophy that results from sustained hypertension aggravates ischemia. There is evidence that long-term effective treatment of hypertension can decrease the occurrence of adverse coronary events.

Diabetes mellitus (Chap. 417) accelerates coronary and peripheral atherosclerosis and is frequently associated with dyslipidemias and increases in the risk of angina, myocardial infarction, and sudden coronary death. Aggressive control of the dyslipidemia (target LDL cholesterol <70 mg/dL) and hypertension (target blood pressure 120/80 mmHg) that are frequently found in diabetic patients is highly effective and therefore essential, as described below.

TABLE 293-3 ENERGY REQUIREMENTS FOR SOME COMMON ACTIVITIES

Less Than 3 METs	3–5 METs	5–7 METs	7–9 METs	More Than 9 METs
Self-Care				
Washing/shaving	Cleaning windows	Easy digging in garden	Heavy shovelling	Carrying loads up stairs (objects more than 90 lb)
Dressing	Raking	Level hand lawn mowing	Carrying objects (60–90 lb)	Climbing stairs (quickly)
Light housekeeping	Power lawn mowing	Carrying objects (30–60 lb)		Shoveling heavy snow
Desk work	Bed making/stripping			
Driving auto	Carrying objects (15–30 lb)			
Occupational				
Sitting (clerical/assembly)	Stocking shelves (light objects)	Carpentry (exterior)	Digging ditches (pick and shovel)	Heavy labor
Desk work	Light welding/carpentry	Shoveling dirt		
Standing (store clerk)		Sawing wood		
Recreational				
Golf (cart)	Dancing (social)	Tennis (singles)	Canoeing	Squash
Knitting	Golf (walking)	Snow skiing (downhill)	Mountain climbing	Ski touring
	Sailing	Light backpacking		Vigorous basketball
	Tennis (doubles)	Basketball		
		Stream fishing		
Physical Conditioning				
Walking (2 mph)	Level walking (3–4 mph)	Level walking (4.5–5.0 mph)	Level jogging (5 mph)	Running more than 6 mph
Stationary bike	Level biking (6–8 mph)	Bicycling (9–10 mph)	Swimming (crawl stroke)	Bicycling (more than 13 mph)
Very light calisthenics	Light calisthenics	Swimming, breast stroke	Rowing machine	Rope jumping
			Heavy calisthenics	Walking uphill (5 mph)
			Bicycling (12 mph)	

Abbreviation: METs, metabolic equivalent tasks.

Source: Modified from WL Haskell: Rehabilitation of the coronary patient, in NK Wenger, HK Hellerstein (eds): *Design and Implementation of Cardiac Conditioning Program*. New York, Churchill Livingstone, 1978.

DYSLIPIDEMIA

The treatment of dyslipidemia is central in aiming for long-term relief from angina, reduced need for revascularization, and reduction in myocardial infarction and death. The control of lipids can be achieved by the combination of a diet low in saturated and *trans*-unsaturated fatty acids, exercise, and weight loss. Nearly always, HMG-CoA reductase inhibitors (statins) are required and can lower LDL cholesterol (25–50%), raise HDL cholesterol (5–9%), and lower triglycerides (5–30%). A powerful treatment effect of statins on atherosclerosis, IHD, and outcomes is seen regardless of the pretreatment LDL cholesterol level. Fibrates or niacin can be used to raise HDL cholesterol and lower triglycerides (Chaps. 291e and 421). Controlled trials with lipid-regulating regimens have shown equal proportional benefit for men, women, the elderly, diabetic patients, and smokers.

Compliance with the health-promoting behaviors listed above is generally very poor, and a conscientious physician must not underestimate the major effort required to meet this challenge. Many patients who are discharged from the hospital with proven coronary disease do not receive adequate treatment for dyslipidemia. In light of the proof that treating dyslipidemia brings major benefits, physicians need to establish treatment pathways, monitor compliance, and follow up regularly.

RISK REDUCTION IN WOMEN WITH IHD

The incidence of clinical IHD in premenopausal women is very low; however, after menopause, the atherogenic risk factors increase (e.g., increased LDL, reduced HDL) and the rate of clinical coronary events accelerates to the levels observed in men. Women have not given up cigarette smoking as effectively as have men. Diabetes mellitus, which is more common in women, greatly increases the occurrence of clinical IHD and amplifies the deleterious effects of hypertension, hyperlipidemia, and smoking. Cardiac catheterization and coronary revascularization are underused in women and are performed at a later and more severe stage of the disease than in men. When cholesterol lowering, beta blockers after myocardial infarction, and coronary artery bypass grafting are applied in the appropriate patient groups, women benefit to the same degree as men.

DRUG THERAPY

The commonly used drugs for the treatment of angina pectoris are summarized in Tables 293-4 through 293-6. Pharmacotherapy for IHD is designed to reduce the frequency of anginal episodes, myocardial infarction, and coronary death. There is a wealth of trial data to emphasize how important this medical management is when added to the health-promoting behaviors discussed above. To achieve maximum benefit from medical therapy for IHD, it is frequently necessary to combine agents from different classes and titrate the doses as guided by the individual profile of risk factors, symptoms, hemodynamic responses, and side effects.

TABLE 293-4 NITRATE THERAPY IN PATIENTS WITH ISCHEMIC HEART DISEASE

Preparation of Agent	Dose	Schedule
Nitroglycerin[a]		
Ointment	0.5–2 inches	Two or three times daily
Transdermal patch	0.2–0.8 mg/h	Every 24 h; remove at bedtime for 12–14 h
Sublingual tablet	0.3–0.6 mg	As needed, up to three doses 5 min apart
Spray	One or two sprays	As needed, up to three doses 5 min apart
Isosorbide dinitrate[a]		
Oral	10–40 mg	Two or three times daily
Oral sustained release	80–120 mg	Once or twice daily (eccentric schedules)
Isosorbide 5-mononitrate		
Oral	20 mg	Twice daily (given 7–8 h apart)
Oral sustained release	30–240 mg	Once daily

[a]A 10- to 12-h nitrate-free interval is recommended.

Source: Modified from DA Morrow, WE Boden: Stable ischemic heart disease. In RO Bonow et al (eds): *Braunwald's Heart Disease: A Textbook of Cardiovascular Medicine*. 9th edition. Philadelphia, Saunders, 2012, p. 1224.

NITRATES

The organic nitrates are a valuable class of drugs in the management of angina pectoris (Table 293-4). Their major mechanisms of action include systemic venodilation with concomitant reduction in left ventricular end-diastolic volume and pressure, thereby reducing myocardial wall tension and oxygen requirements; dilation of epicardial coronary vessels; and increased blood flow in collateral vessels. When metabolized, organic nitrates release nitric oxide (NO) that binds to guanylyl cyclase in vascular smooth muscle cells, leading to an increase in cyclic guanosine monophosphate, which causes relaxation of vascular smooth muscle. Nitrates also exert antithrombotic activity by NO-dependent activation of platelet guanylyl cyclase, impairment of intraplatelet calcium flux, and platelet activation.

The absorption of these agents is most rapid and complete through the mucous membranes. For this reason, nitroglycerin is most commonly administered sublingually in tablets of 0.4 or 0.6 mg. Patients with angina should be instructed to take the medication both to relieve angina and also approximately 5 min before stress that is likely to induce an episode. The value of this prophylactic use of the drug cannot be overemphasized.

Nitrates improve exercise tolerance in patients with chronic angina and relieve ischemia in patients with unstable angina as well as patients with Prinzmetal's variant angina (Chap. 294). A diary of angina and nitroglycerin use may be valuable for detecting changes in the frequency, severity, or threshold for discomfort that may signify the development of unstable angina pectoris and/or herald an impending myocardial infarction.

Long-Acting Nitrates None of the long-acting nitrates are as effective as sublingual nitroglycerin for the acute relief of angina. These organic nitrate preparations can be swallowed, chewed, or administered as a patch or paste by the transdermal route (Table 293-4). They can provide effective plasma levels for up to 24 h, but the therapeutic response is highly variable. Different preparations and/or administration during the daytime should be tried only to prevent discomfort while avoiding side effects such as headache and dizziness. Individual dose titration is important to prevent side effects. To minimize the effects of tolerance, the minimum effective dose should be used and a minimum of 8 h each day kept free of the drug to restore any useful response(s).

β-Adrenergic Blockers These drugs represent an important component of the pharmacologic treatment of angina pectoris (Table 293-5). They reduce myocardial oxygen demand by inhibiting the increases in heart rate, arterial pressure, and myocardial contractility caused by adrenergic activation. Beta blockade reduces these variables most strikingly during exercise but causes only small reductions at rest. Long-acting beta-blocking drugs or sustained-release formulations offer the advantage of once-daily dosing (Table 293-5). The therapeutic aims include relief of angina and ischemia. These drugs also can reduce mortality and reinfarction rates in patients after myocardial infarction and are moderately effective antihypertensive agents.

Relative contraindications include asthma and reversible airway obstruction in patients with chronic lung disease, atrioventricular conduction disturbances, severe bradycardia, Raynaud's phenomenon, and a history of mental depression. Side effects include fatigue, reduced exercise tolerance, nightmares, impotence, cold extremities, intermittent claudication, bradycardia (sometimes severe), impaired atrioventricular conduction, left ventricular failure, bronchial asthma, worsening claudication, and intensification of the hypoglycemia produced by oral hypoglycemic agents and insulin.

TABLE 293-5 PROPERTIES OF BETA BLOCKERS IN CLINICAL USE FOR ISCHEMIC HEART DISEASE

Drugs	Selectivity	Partial Agonist Activity	Usual Dose for Angina
Acebutolol	β_1	Yes	200–600 mg twice daily
Atenolol	β_1	No	50–200 mg/d
Betaxolol	β_1	No	10–20 mg/d
Bisoprolol	β_1	No	10 mg/d
Esmolol (intravenous)[a]	β_1	No	50–300 μg/kg/min
Labetalol[b]	None	Yes	200–600 mg twice daily
Metoprolol	β_1	No	50–200 mg twice daily
Nadolol	None	No	40–80 mg/d
Nebivolol	β_1 (at low doses)	No	5–40 mg/d
Pindolol	None	Yes	2.5–7.5 mg 3 times daily
Propranolol	None	No	80–120 mg twice daily
Timolol	None	No	10 mg twice daily

[a]Esmolol is an ultra-short-acting beta blocker that is administered as a continuous intravenous infusion. Its rapid offset of action makes esmolol an attractive agent to use in patients with relative contraindications to beta blockade. [b]Labetolol is a combined alpha and beta blocker.

Note: This list of beta blockers that may be used to treat patients with angina pectoris is arranged alphabetically. The agents for which there is the greatest clinical experience include atenolol, metoprolol, and propranolol. It is preferable to use a sustained-release formulation that may be taken once daily to improve the patient's compliance with the regimen.

Source: Modified from RJ Gibbons et al: J Am Coll Cardiol 41:159, 2003.

Reducing the dose or even discontinuation may be necessary if these side effects develop and persist. Since sudden discontinuation can intensify ischemia, the doses should be tapered over 2 weeks. Beta blockers with relative β_1-receptor specificity such as metoprolol and atenolol may be preferable in patients with mild bronchial obstruction and insulin-requiring diabetes mellitus.

Calcium Channel Blockers Calcium channel blockers (Table 293-6) are coronary vasodilators that produce variable and dose-dependent reductions in myocardial oxygen demand, contractility, and arterial pressure. These combined pharmacologic effects are advantageous and make these agents as effective as beta blockers in the treatment of angina pectoris. They are indicated when beta blockers are contraindicated, poorly tolerated, or ineffective. Because of differences in the dose-response relationship on cardiac electrical activity between the dihydropyridine and nondihydropyridine calcium channel blockers, verapamil and diltiazem may produce symptomatic disturbances in cardiac conduction and bradyarrhythmias. They also exert negative inotropic actions and are more likely to aggravate left ventricular failure, particularly when used in patients with left ventricular dysfunction, especially if the patients are also receiving beta blockers. Although useful effects usually are achieved when calcium channel blockers are combined with beta blockers and nitrates, individual titration of the doses is essential with these combinations. Variant (Prinzmetal's) angina responds particularly well to calcium channel blockers (especially members of the dihydropyridine class), supplemented when necessary by nitrates (Chap. 294).

Verapamil ordinarily should not be combined with beta blockers because of the combined adverse effects on heart rate and contractility. Diltiazem can be combined with beta blockers in patients with normal ventricular function and no conduction disturbances. Amlodipine and beta blockers have complementary actions on coronary blood supply and myocardial oxygen demands. Whereas the former decreases blood pressure and dilates coronary arteries, the latter slows heart rate and decreases contractility. Amlodipine and the other second-generation dihydropyridine calcium antagonists (nicardipine, isradipine, long-acting nifedipine, and felodipine) are

TABLE 293-6 CALCIUM CHANNEL BLOCKERS IN CLINICAL USE FOR ISCHEMIC HEART DISEASE

Drugs	Usual Dose	Duration of Action	Side Effects
Dihydropyridines			
Amlodipine	5–10 mg qd	Long	Headache, edema
Felodipine	5–10 mg qd	Long	Headache, edema
Isradipine	2.5–10 mg bid	Medium	Headache, fatigue
Nicardipine	20–40 mg tid	Short	Headache, dizziness, flushing, edema
Nifedipine	Immediate release:[a] 30–90 mg daily orally	Short	Hypotension, dizziness, flushing, nausea, constipation, edema
	Slow release: 30–180 mg orally		
Nisoldipine	20–40 mg qd	Short	Similar to nifedipine
Nondihydropyridines			
Diltiazem	Immediate release: 30–80 mg 4 times daily	Short	Hypotension, dizziness, flushing, bradycardia, edema
	Slow release: 120–320 mg qd	Long	
Verapamil	Immediate release: 80–160 mg tid	Short	Hypotension, myocardial depression, heart failure, edema, bradycardia
	Slow release: 120–480 mg qd	Long	

[a]May be associated with increased risk of mortality if administered during acute myocardial infarction.

Note: This list of calcium channel blockers that may be used to treat patients with angina pectoris is divided into two broad classes, dihydropyridines and nondihydropyridines, and arranged alphabetically within each class. Among the dihydropyridines, the greatest clinical experience has been obtained with amlodipine and nifedipine. After the initial period of dose titration with a short-acting formulation, it is preferable to switch to a sustained-release formulation that may be taken once daily to improve patient compliance with the regimen.

Source: Modified from RJ Gibbons et al: J Am Coll Cardiol 41:159, 2003.

potent vasodilators and are useful in the simultaneous treatment of angina and hypertension. Short-acting dihydropyridines should be avoided because of the risk of precipitating infarction, particularly in the absence of concomitant beta blocker therapy.

Choice Between Beta Blockers and Calcium Channel Blockers for Initial Therapy Since beta blockers have been shown to improve life expectancy after acute myocardial infarction (Chaps. 294 and 295) and calcium channel blockers have not, the former may also be preferable in patients with angina and a damaged left ventricle. However, calcium channel blockers are indicated in patients with the following: (1) inadequate responsiveness to the combination of beta blockers and nitrates; many of these patients do well with a combination of a beta blocker and a dihydropyridine calcium channel blocker; (2) adverse reactions to beta blockers such as depression, sexual disturbances, and fatigue; (3) angina and a history of asthma or chronic obstructive pulmonary disease; (4) sick-sinus syndrome or significant atrioventricular conduction disturbances; (5) Prinzmetal's angina; or (6) symptomatic peripheral arterial disease.

Antiplatelet Drugs Aspirin is an irreversible inhibitor of platelet cyclooxygenase and thereby interferes with platelet activation. Chronic administration of 75–325 mg orally per day has been shown to reduce coronary events in asymptomatic adult men over age 50, patients with chronic stable angina, and patients who have or have survived unstable angina and myocardial infarction. There is a dose-dependent increase in bleeding when aspirin is used chronically. It is preferable to use an enteric-coated formulation in the range of 81–162 mg/d. Administration of this drug should be considered in all patients with IHD in the absence of gastrointestinal bleeding, allergy, or dyspepsia. Clopidogrel (300–600 mg loading and 75 mg/d) is an oral agent that blocks P2Y12 ADP receptor–mediated platelet aggregation. It provides benefits similar to those of aspirin in patients with stable chronic IHD and may be substituted for aspirin if aspirin causes the side effects listed above. Clopidogrel combined with aspirin reduces death and coronary ischemic events in patients with an acute coronary syndrome (Chap. 294) and also reduces the risk of thrombus formation in patients undergoing implantation of a stent in a coronary artery (Chap. 296e). Alternative antiplatelet agents that block the P2Y12 platelet receptor such as prasugrel and ticagrelor have been shown to be more effective than clopidogrel for prevention of ischemic events after placement of a stent for an acute coronary syndrome but are associated with an increased risk of bleeding. Although combined treatment with clopidogrel and aspirin for at least a year is recommended in patients with an acute coronary syndrome treated with implantation of a drug-eluting stent, studies have not shown any benefit from the routine addition of clopidogrel to aspirin in patients with chronic stable IHD.

OTHER THERAPIES

The angiotensin-converting enzyme (ACE) inhibitors are widely used in the treatment of survivors of myocardial infarction, patients with hypertension or chronic IHD including angina pectoris, and those at high risk of vascular diseases such as diabetes. The benefits of ACE inhibitors are most evident in IHD patients at increased risk, especially if diabetes mellitus or left ventricle dysfunction is present, and those who have not achieved adequate control of blood pressure and LDL cholesterol on beta blockers and statins. However, the routine administration of ACE inhibitors to IHD patients who have normal left ventricular function and have achieved blood pressure and LDL goals on other therapies does not reduce the incidence of events and therefore is not cost-effective.

Despite treatment with nitrates, beta blockers, or calcium channel blockers, some patients with IHD continue to experience angina, and additional medical therapy is now available to alleviate their symptoms. Ranolazine, a piperazine derivative, may be useful for patients with chronic angina despite standard medical therapy. Its antianginal action is believed to occur via inhibition of the late inward sodium current (I_{Na}). The benefits of I_{Na} inhibition include limitation of the Na overload of ischemic myocytes and prevention of Ca^{2+} overload via the Na^+–Ca^{2+} exchanger. A dose of 500–1000 mg orally twice daily is usually well tolerated. Ranolazine is contraindicated in patients with hepatic impairment or with conditions or drugs associated with QT_c prolongation and when drugs that inhibit the CYP3A metabolic system (e.g., ketoconazole, diltiazem, verapamil, macrolide antibiotics, HIV protease inhibitors, and large quantities of grapefruit juice) are being used.

Nonsteroidal anti-inflammatory drug (NSAID) use in patients with IHD may be associated with a small but finite increased risk of myocardial infarction and mortality. For this reason, they generally should be avoided in IHD patients. If they are required for symptom relief, it is advisable to coadminister aspirin and strive to use an NSAID associated with the lowest risk of cardiovascular events, in the lowest dose required, and for the shortest period of time.

Another class of agents opens ATP-sensitive potassium channels in myocytes, leading to a reduction of free intracellular calcium ions. The major drug in this class is nicorandil, which typically is administered orally in a dose of 20 mg twice daily for prevention of angina. (Nicorandil is not available for use in the United States but is used in several other countries.)

Angina and Heart Failure Transient left ventricular failure with angina can be controlled by the use of nitrates. For patients with established congestive heart failure, the increased left ventricular wall tension raises myocardial oxygen demand. Treatment of congestive heart failure with an ACE inhibitor, a diuretic, and digoxin (Chap. 279) reduces heart size, wall tension, and myocardial oxygen demand, which helps control angina and ischemia. If the symptoms and signs of heart failure are controlled, an effort should be made to use beta blockers not only for angina but because trials in heart failure have shown significant improvement in survival. A trial of the intravenous ultra-short-acting beta blocker esmolol may be useful to establish the safety of beta blockade in selected patients. Nocturnal angina often can be relieved by the treatment of heart failure.

The combination of congestive heart failure and angina in patients with IHD usually indicates a poor prognosis and warrants serious consideration of cardiac catheterization and coronary revascularization.

CORONARY REVASCULARIZATION

Clinical trials have confirmed that with the initial diagnosis of stable IHD, it is first appropriate to initiate a thorough medical regimen as described above. Revascularization should be considered in the presence of unstable phases of the disease, intractable symptoms, severe ischemia or high-risk coronary anatomy, diabetes, and impaired left ventricular (LV) function. *Revascularization should be employed in conjunction with but not replace the continuing need to modify risk factors and assess medical therapy.* An algorithm for integrating medical therapy and revascularization options in patients with IHD is shown in Fig. 293-3.

PERCUTANEOUS CORONARY INTERVENTION

(See also Chap. 296e) Percutaneous coronary intervention (PCI) involving balloon dilatation usually accompanied by coronary stenting is widely used to achieve revascularization of the myocardium in patients with symptomatic IHD and suitable stenoses of epicardial coronary arteries. Whereas patients with stenosis of the left main coronary artery and those with three-vessel IHD (especially with diabetes and/or impaired LV function) who require revascularization are best treated with CABG, PCI is widely employed in patients with symptoms and evidence of ischemia due to stenoses of one or two vessels and even in selected patients with three-vessel disease (and, perhaps, in some patients with left main disease) and may offer many advantages over surgery.

Indications and Patient Selection The most common clinical indication for PCI is symptom-limiting angina pectoris, despite medical therapy, accompanied by evidence of ischemia during a stress test. PCI is more effective than medical therapy for the relief of angina. PCI improves

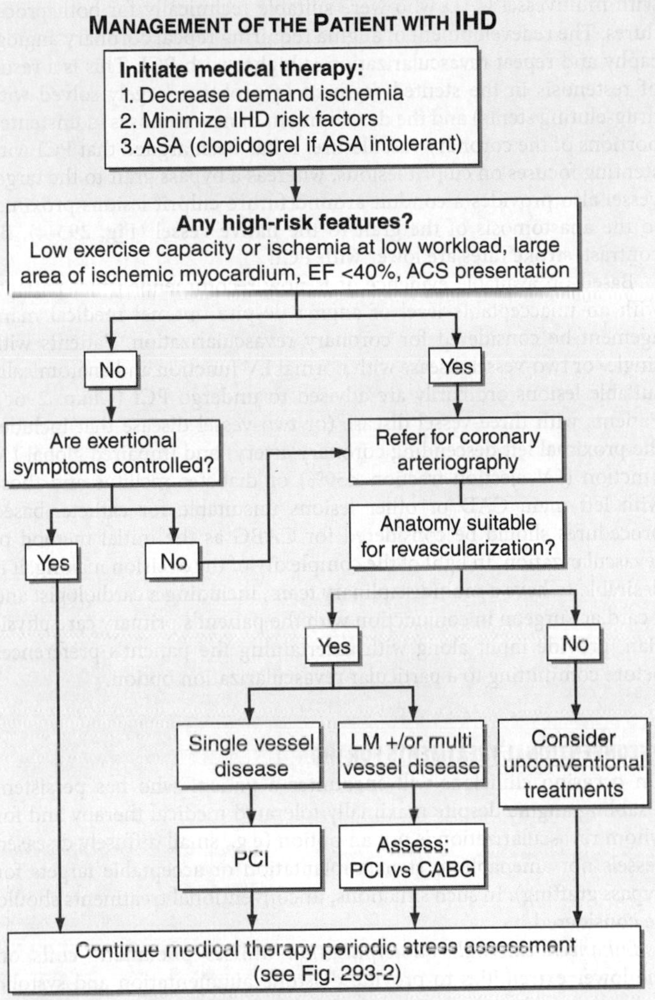

Management of the Patient with IHD

Initiate medical therapy:
1. Decrease demand ischemia
2. Minimize IHD risk factors
3. ASA (clopidogrel if ASA intolerant)

Any high-risk features?
Low exercise capacity or ischemia at low workload, large area of ischemic myocardium, EF <40%, ACS presentation

No → Are exertional symptoms controlled? → Yes / No

Yes → Refer for coronary arteriography → Anatomy suitable for revascularization? → Yes / No

Single vessel disease → PCI

LM +/or multi vessel disease → Assess: PCI vs CABG

Consider unconventional treatments

Continue medical therapy periodic stress assessment (see Fig. 293-2)

FIGURE 293-3 Algorithm for management of a patient with ischemic heart disease. All patients should receive the core elements of medical therapy as shown at the top of the algorithm. If high-risk features are present, as established by the clinical history, exercise test data, and imaging studies, the patient should be referred for coronary arteriography. Based on the number and location of the diseased vessels and their suitability for revascularization, the patient is treated with a percutaneous coronary intervention (PCI) or coronary artery bypass graft (CABG) surgery or should be considered for unconventional treatments. See text for further discussion. ACS, acute coronary syndrome; ASA, aspirin; EF, ejection fraction; IHD, ischemic heart disease; LM, left main.

outcomes in patients with unstable angina or when used early in the course of myocardial infarction with and without cardiogenic shock. However, in patients with stable exertional angina, clinical trials have confirmed that PCI does not reduce the occurrence of death or myocardial infarction compared to optimum medical therapy. PCI can be used to treat stenoses in native coronary arteries as well as in bypass grafts in patients who have recurrent angina after CABG.

Risks When coronary stenoses are discrete and symmetric, two and even three vessels can be treated in sequence. However, case selection is essential to avoid a prohibitive risk of complications, which are usually due to dissection or thrombosis with vessel occlusion, uncontrolled ischemia, and ventricular failure (Chap. 296e). Oral aspirin, a P2Y12 antagonist, and an antithrombin agent are given to reduce coronary thrombus formation. Left main coronary artery stenosis generally is regarded as a contraindication to PCI; such patients should be treated with CABG. In selected cases such as patients with prohibitive surgical risks, PCI of an unprotected left main can be considered, but such a procedure should be performed only by a highly skilled operator; importantly, there are regional differences in the use of this approach internationally.

Efficacy Primary success, i.e., adequate dilation (an increase in luminal diameter >20% to a residual diameter obstruction <50%) with relief of angina, is achieved in >95% of cases. Recurrent stenosis of the dilated vessels occurs in ~20% of cases within 6 months of PCI with bare metal stents, and angina will recur within 6 months in 10% of cases. Restenosis is more common in patients with diabetes mellitus, arteries with small caliber, incomplete dilation of the stenosis, long stents, occluded vessels, obstructed vein grafts, dilation of the left anterior descending coronary artery, and stenoses containing thrombi. In diseased vein grafts, procedural success has been improved by the use of capture devices or filters that prevent embolization, ischemia, and infarction.

It is usual clinical practice to administer aspirin indefinitely and a P2Y12 antagonist for 1–3 months after the implantation of a bare metal stent. Although aspirin in combination with a thienopyridine may help prevent coronary thrombosis during and shortly after PCI with stenting, there is no evidence that these medications reduce the incidence of restenosis.

The use of drug-eluting stents that locally deliver antiproliferative drugs can reduce restenosis to less than 10%. Advances in PCI, especially the availability of drug-eluting stents, have vastly extended the use of this revascularization option in patients with IHD. Of note, however, the delayed endothelial healing in the region of a drug-eluting stent also extends the period during which the patient is at risk for subacute stent thrombosis. Current recommendations are to administer aspirin indefinitely and a P2Y12 antagonist daily for at least 1 year after implantation of a drug-eluting stent. When a situation arises in which temporary discontinuation of antiplatelet therapy is necessary, the clinical circumstances should be reviewed with the operator who performed the PCI and a coordinated plan should be established for minimizing the risk of late stent thrombus; central to this plan is the discontinuation of antiplatelet therapy for the shortest acceptable period. The risk of stent thrombosis is dependent on stent size and length, complexity of the lesions, age, diabetes, and technique. However, compliance with dual antiplatelet therapy and individual responsiveness to platelet inhibition are very important factors as well.

Successful PCI produces effective relief of angina in >95% of cases. The majority of patients with symptomatic IHD who require revascularization can be treated initially by PCI. Successful PCI is less invasive and expensive than CABG and permits savings in the *initial* cost of care. Successful PCI avoids the risk of stroke associated with CABG surgery, allows earlier return to work, and allows the resumption of an active life. However, the early health-related and economic benefit of PCI is reduced over time because of the greater need for follow-up and the increased need for repeat procedures. When directly compared in patients with diabetes or three-vessel or left main CAD, CABG was superior to PCI in preventing major adverse cardiac or cerebrovascular events over a 12-month follow-up.

CORONARY ARTERY BYPASS GRAFTING

Anastomosis of one or both of the internal mammary arteries or a radial artery to the coronary artery distal to the obstructive lesion is the preferred procedure. For additional obstructions that cannot be bypassed by an artery, a section of a vein (usually the saphenous) is used to form a connection between the aorta and the coronary artery distal to the obstructive lesion.

Although some indications for CABG are controversial, certain areas of agreement exist:

1. The operation is relatively safe, with mortality rates <1% in patients without serious comorbid disease and normal LV function and when the procedure is performed by an experienced surgical team.
2. Intraoperative and postoperative mortality rates increase with the severity of ventricular dysfunction, comorbidities, age >80 years, and lack of surgical experience. The effectiveness and risk of CABG vary widely depending on case selection and the skill and experience of the surgical team.

3. Occlusion of *venous* grafts is observed in 10–20% of patients during the first postoperative year and in approximately 2% per year during 5- to 7-year follow-up and 4% per year thereafter. Long-term patency rates are considerably higher for internal mammary and radial artery implantations than for saphenous vein grafts. In patients with left anterior descending coronary artery obstruction, survival is better when coronary bypass involves the internal mammary artery rather than a saphenous vein. Graft patency and outcomes are improved by meticulous treatment of risk factors, particularly dyslipidemia.
4. Angina is abolished or greatly reduced in ~90% of patients after complete revascularization. Although this usually is associated with graft patency and restoration of blood flow, the pain may also have been alleviated as a result of infarction of the ischemic segment or a placebo effect. Within 3 years, angina recurs in about one-fourth of patients but is rarely severe.
5. Survival may be improved by operation in patients with stenosis of the left main coronary artery as well as in patients with three- or two-vessel disease with significant obstruction of the proximal left anterior descending coronary artery. The survival benefit is greater in patients with abnormal LV function (ejection fraction <50%). Survival *may* also be improved in the following patients: (a) patients with obstructive CAD who have survived sudden cardiac death or sustained ventricular tachycardia; (b) patients who have undergone previous CABG and have multiple saphenous vein graft stenoses, especially of a graft supplying the left anterior descending coronary artery; and (c) patients with recurrent stenosis after PCI and high-risk criteria on noninvasive testing.
6. Minimally invasive CABG through a small thoracotomy and/or off-pump surgery can reduce morbidity and shorten convalescence in suitable patients but does not appear to reduce significantly the risk of neurocognitive dysfunction postoperatively.
7. Among patients with type 2 diabetes mellitus and multivessel coronary disease, CABG surgery plus optimal medical therapy is superior to optimal medical therapy alone in preventing major cardiovascular events, a benefit mediated largely by a significant reduction in nonfatal myocardial infarction. The benefits of CABG are especially evident in diabetic patients treated with an insulin-sensitizing strategy as opposed to an insulin-providing strategy. CABG has also been shown to be superior to PCI (including the use of drug-eluting stents) in preventing death, myocardial infarction, and repeat revascularization in patients with diabetes mellitus and multivessel IHD.

Indications for CABG usually are based on the severity of symptoms, coronary anatomy, and ventricular function. The ideal candidate is male, <80 years of age, has no other complicating disease, and has troublesome or disabling angina that is not adequately controlled by medical therapy or does not tolerate medical therapy. The patient wishes to lead a more active life and has severe stenoses of two or three epicardial coronary arteries with objective evidence of myocardial ischemia as a cause of the chest discomfort. Great symptomatic benefit can be anticipated in such patients. Congestive heart failure and/or LV dysfunction, advanced age (>80 years), reoperation, urgent need for surgery, and the presence of diabetes mellitus are all associated with a higher perioperative mortality rate.

LV dysfunction can be due to noncontractile or hypocontractile segments that are viable but are chronically ischemic (hibernating myocardium). As a consequence of chronic reduction in myocardial blood flow, these segments downregulate their contractile function. They can be detected by using radionuclide scans of myocardial perfusion and metabolism, PET, cardiac MRI, or delayed scanning with thallium-201 or by improvement of regional functional impairment provoked by low-dose dobutamine. In such patients, revascularization improves myocardial blood flow, can return function, and can improve survival.

The Choice Between PCI and CABG All the clinical characteristics of each individual patient must be used to decide on the method of revascularization (e.g., LV function, diabetes, lesion complexity). A number of randomized clinical trials have compared PCI and CABG in patients with multivessel CAD who were suitable technically for both procedures. The redevelopment of angina requiring repeat coronary angiography and repeat revascularization is higher with PCI. This is a result of restenosis in the stented segment (a problem largely solved with drug-eluting stents) and the development of new stenoses in unstented portions of the coronary vasculature. It has been argued that PCI with stenting focuses on culprit lesions, whereas a bypass graft to the target vessel also provides a conduit around future culprit lesions proximal to the anastomosis of the graft to the native vessel (Fig. 293-4). By contrast, stroke rates are lower with PCI.

Based on available evidence, it is now recommended that patients with an unacceptable level of angina despite optimal medical management be considered for coronary revascularization. Patients with single- or two-vessel disease with normal LV function and anatomically suitable lesions ordinarily are advised to undergo PCI (Chap. 296e). Patients with three-vessel disease (or two-vessel disease that includes the proximal left descending coronary artery) and impaired global LV function (LV ejection fraction <50%) or diabetes mellitus and those with left main CAD or other lesions unsuitable for catheter-based procedures should be considered for CABG as the initial method of revascularization. In light of the complexity of the decision making, it is desirable to have a multidisciplinary team, including a cardiologist and a cardiac surgeon in conjunction with the patient's primary care physician, provide input along with ascertaining the patient's preferences before committing to a particular revascularization option.

UNCONVENTIONAL TREATMENTS FOR IHD

On occasion clinicians will encounter a patient who has persistent disabling angina despite maximally tolerated medical therapy and for whom revascularization is not an option (e.g., small diffusely diseased vessels not amenable to stent implantation or acceptable targets for bypass grafting). In such situations, unconventional treatments should be considered.

Enhanced external counterpulsation utilizes pneumatic cuffs on the lower extremities to provide diastolic augmentation and systolic unloading of blood pressure to decrease cardiac work and oxygen consumption while enhancing coronary blood flow. Clinical trials have shown that regular application improves angina, exercise capacity, and regional myocardial perfusion. Experimental approaches such as gene and stem cell therapies are also under active study.

ASYMPTOMATIC (SILENT) ISCHEMIA

Obstructive CAD, acute myocardial infarction, and transient myocardial ischemia are frequently asymptomatic. During continuous ambulatory ECG monitoring, the majority of ambulatory patients with typical chronic stable angina are found to have objective evidence of myocardial ischemia (ST-segment depression) during episodes of chest discomfort while they are active outside the hospital. In addition, many of these patients also have more frequent episodes of asymptomatic ischemia. Frequent episodes of ischemia (symptomatic and asymptomatic) during daily life appear to be associated with an increased likelihood of adverse coronary events (death and myocardial infarction). In addition, patients with asymptomatic ischemia after a myocardial infarction are at greater risk for a second coronary event. The widespread use of exercise ECG during routine examinations has also identified some of these previously unrecognized patients with asymptomatic CAD. Longitudinal studies have demonstrated an increased incidence of coronary events in asymptomatic patients with positive exercise tests.

TREATMENT ASYMPTOMATIC ISCHEMIA

The management of patients with asymptomatic ischemia must be individualized. When coronary disease has been confirmed, the aggressive treatment of hypertension and dyslipidemia is essential and will decrease the risk of infarction and death. In addition, the

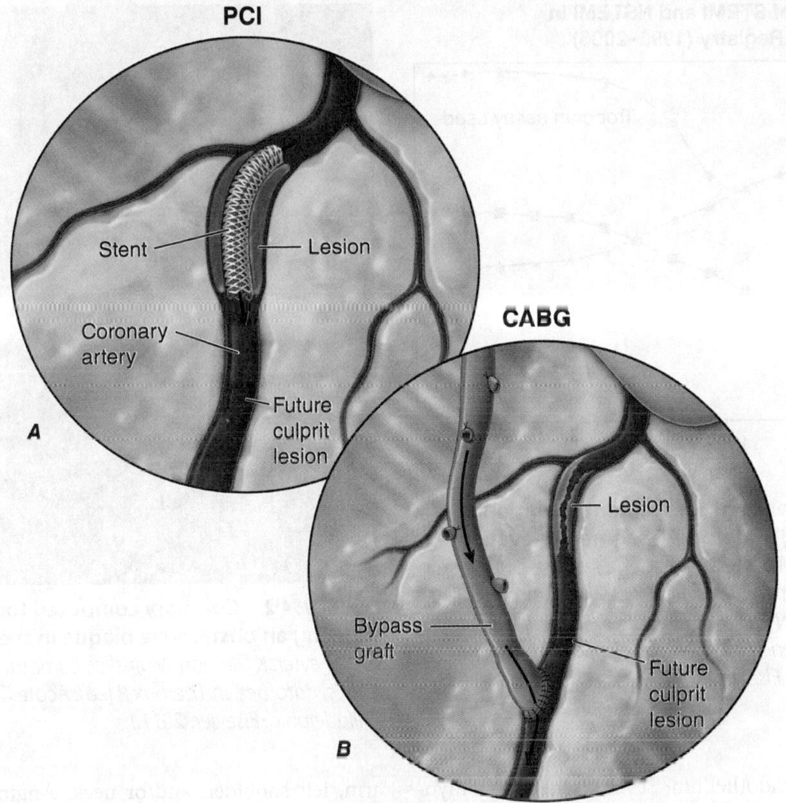

FIGURE 293-4 Difference in the approach to the lesion with percutaneous coronary intervention (PCI) and coronary artery bypass grafting (CABG). PCI is targeted at the "culprit" lesion or lesions, whereas CABG is directed at the epicardial vessel, including the culprit lesion or lesions and future culprits, proximal to the insertion of the vein graft, a difference that may account for the superiority of CABG, at least in the intermediate term, in patients with multivessel disease. *(Reproduced from BJ Gersh, RL Frye: N Engl J Med 352:2235, 2005.)*

physician should consider the following: (1) the degree of positivity of the stress test, particularly the stage of exercise at which ECG signs of ischemia appear; the magnitude and number of the ischemic zones of myocardium on imaging; and the change in LV ejection fraction that occurs on radionuclide ventriculography or echocardiography during ischemia and/or during exercise; (2) the ECG leads showing a positive response, with changes in the anterior precordial leads indicating a less favorable prognosis than changes in the inferior leads; and (3) the patient's age, occupation, and general medical condition.

Most would agree that an asymptomatic 45-year-old commercial airline pilot with significant (0.4-mV) ST-segment depression in leads V_1 to V_4 during mild exercise should undergo coronary arteriography, whereas an asymptomatic, sedentary 85-year-old retiree with 0.1-mV ST-segment depression in leads II and III during maximal activity need not. However, there is no consensus about the most appropriate approach in the large majority of patients for whom the situation is less extreme. Asymptomatic patients with silent ischemia, three-vessel CAD, and impaired LV function may be considered appropriate candidates for CABG.

The treatment of risk factors, particularly lipid lowering and blood pressure control as described above, and the use of aspirin, statins, and beta blockers after infarction have been shown to reduce events and improve outcomes in asymptomatic as well as symptomatic patients with ischemia and proven CAD. Although the incidence of asymptomatic ischemia can be reduced by treatment with beta blockers, calcium channel blockers, and long-acting nitrates, it is not clear whether this is necessary or desirable in patients who have not had a myocardial infarction.

294 Non-ST-Segment Elevation Acute Coronary Syndrome (Non-ST-Segment Elevation Myocardial Infarction and Unstable Angina)

Christopher P. Cannon, Eugene Braunwald

Patients with ischemic heart disease fall into two large groups: patients with chronic coronary artery disease (CAD) who most commonly present with stable angina (Chap. 293) and patients with acute coronary syndromes (ACSs). These include patients with acute myocardial infarction with ST-segment elevation (STEMI) on their presenting electrocardiogram (Chap. 295) and those with non-ST-segment elevation acute coronary syndrome (NSTE-ACS). The latter include patients with non-ST-segment elevation myocardial infarction (NSTEMI), who, by definition, have evidence of myocyte necrosis, and those with unstable angina (UA), who do not. The relative incidence of NSTEMI compared to STEMI appears to be increasing (Fig. 294-1). Every year in the United States, approximately 1.1 million patients are admitted to hospitals with NSTE-ACS as compared with ~300,000 patients with acute STEMI. Women comprise more than one-third of patients with NSTE-ACS, but less than one-fourth of patients with STEMI.

PATHOPHYSIOLOGY

NSTE-ACS is most commonly caused by an imbalance between oxygen supply and oxygen demand resulting from a partially occluding thrombus forming on a disrupted atherothrombotic coronary plaque

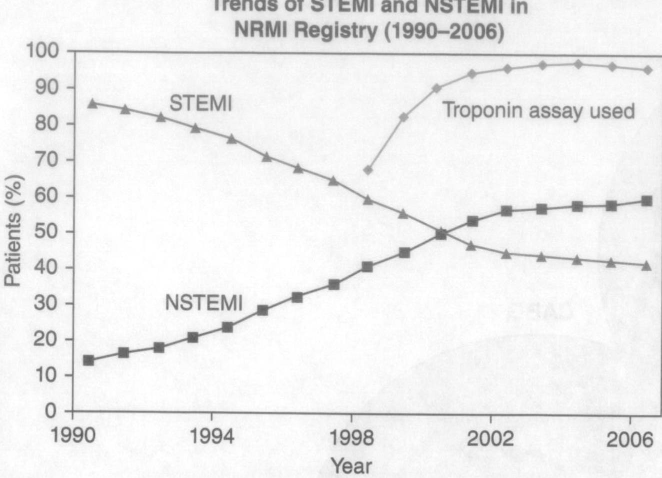

FIGURE 294-1 Trends of incidence of ST-segment elevation myocardial infarction (STEMI) and non-ST-segment elevation myocardial infarction (NSTEMI) and of frequency of use of troponin assay to diagnose acute myocardial infarction. NRMI, National Registry of Myocardial Infarction. *(From N Arora, RG Brindis, CP Cannon: Acute coronary syndrome in North America, in Theroux P [ed]: Acute Coronary Syndromes, 2nd ed. Philadelphia: Elsevier, 2011.)*

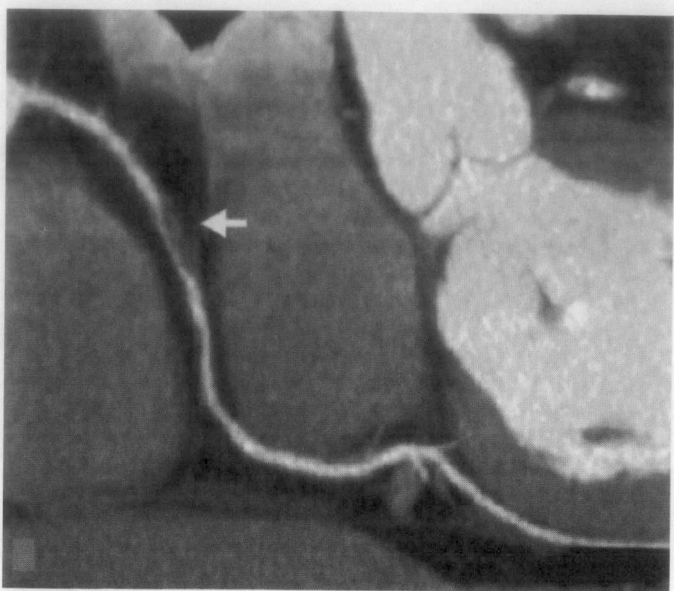

FIGURE 294-2 Coronary computed tomographic angiogram showing an obstructive plaque in the right coronary artery. *(From PJ de Feyter, K Nieman. Multislice computed tomography in acute coronary syndromes, in Theroux P [ed]: Acute Coronary Syndromes, 2nd ed. Philadelphia: Elsevier, 2011.)*

or on eroded coronary artery endothelium. Severe ischemia or myocardial necrosis may occur consequent to the reduction of coronary blood flow caused by the thrombus and by downstream embolization of platelet aggregates and/or atherosclerotic debris. Other causes of NSTE-ACS include: (1) dynamic obstruction (e.g., coronary spasm, as in Prinzmetal's variant angina [see "Prinzmetal's Variant Angina" later]); (2) severe mechanical obstruction due to progressive coronary atherosclerosis; and (3) increased myocardial oxygen demand produced by conditions such as fever, tachycardia, and thyrotoxicosis in the presence of fixed epicardial coronary obstruction. More than one of these processes may be involved.

Among patients with NSTE-ACS studied at angiography, approximately 10% have stenosis of the left main coronary artery, 35% have three-vessel CAD, 20% have two-vessel disease, 20% have single-vessel disease, and 15% have no apparent critical epicardial coronary artery stenosis; some of the latter may have obstruction of the coronary microcirculation and/or spasm. The "culprit lesion" responsible for ischemia may show an eccentric stenosis with scalloped or overhanging edges and a narrow neck on coronary angiography. Optical coherence tomography (an invasive technique) and contrast-enhanced coronary computed tomographic angiography (CCTA), a noninvasive technique (Fig. 294-2), have shown that culprit lesions are composed of a lipid-rich core with a thin fibrous cap. Patients with NSTE-ACS frequently have multiple such plaques that are at risk of disruption (vulnerable plaques).

CLINICAL PRESENTATION

Diagnosis The diagnosis of NSTE-ACS is based largely on the clinical presentation. Typically, chest discomfort is severe and has at least one of three features: (1) it occurs at rest (or with minimal exertion), lasting >10 minutes; (2) it is of relatively recent onset (i.e., within the prior 2 weeks); and/or (3) it occurs with a crescendo pattern (i.e., distinctly more severe, prolonged, or frequent than previous episodes). The diagnosis of NSTEMI is established if a patient with these clinical features develops evidence of myocardial necrosis, as reflected in abnormally elevated levels of biomarkers of cardiac necrosis (see below).

History and Physical Examination The chest discomfort, often severe enough to be described as frank pain, is typically located in the substernal region or sometimes in the epigastrium, and radiates to the left arm, left shoulder, and/or neck. Anginal "equivalents" such as dyspnea, epigastric discomfort, nausea, or weakness may occur instead of chest pain and appear to be more frequent in women, the elderly, and patients with diabetes mellitus. The physical examination resembles that in patients with stable angina (Chap. 293) and may be unremarkable. If the patient has a large area of myocardial ischemia or a large NSTEMI, the physical findings can include diaphoresis; pale, cool skin; sinus tachycardia; a third and/or fourth heart sound; basilar rales; and, sometimes, hypotension.

Electrocardiogram ST-segment depression occurs in 20 to 25% of patients; it may be transient in patients without biomarker evidence of myocardial necrosis, but may be persistent for several days in NSTEMI. T-wave changes are common but are less specific signs of ischemia, unless they are new and deep T-wave inversions (≥0.3 mV).

Cardiac Biomarkers Patients with NSTEMI have elevated biomarkers of necrosis, such as cardiac troponin I or T, which are specific, sensitive, and the preferred markers of myocardial necrosis. The MB isoform of creatine kinase (CK-MB) is a less sensitive alternative. Elevated levels of these markers distinguish patients with NSTEMI from those with UA. There is a characteristic temporal rise and fall of the plasma concentration of these markers and a direct relationship between the degree of elevation and mortality (see Fig. 294-4*B*). However, in patients *without* a clear clinical history of myocardial ischemia, minor cardiac troponin (cTn) elevations have been reported and can be caused by congestive heart failure, myocarditis, or pulmonary embolism, or using high-sensitivity assays, they may occur in ostensibly normal subjects. Thus, in patients with an *unclear* history, small elevations of cTn, especially if they are persistent, may not be diagnostic of an ACS.

With more widespread measurement of troponin, especially using high-sensitivity assays, an increasing fraction of patients with NSTE-ACS are found to have NSTEMI, whereas the fraction of patients with UA is dwindling.

DIAGNOSTIC EVALUATION

In addition to the clinical examination, three major noninvasive tools are used in the evaluation of NSTEMI-ACS: the electrocardiogram (ECG), cardiac biomarkers, and stress testing. CCTA is an additional emerging option (Fig. 294-2). The goals are to: (1) recognize or exclude myocardial infarction (MI) using cardiac biomarkers, preferably cTn;

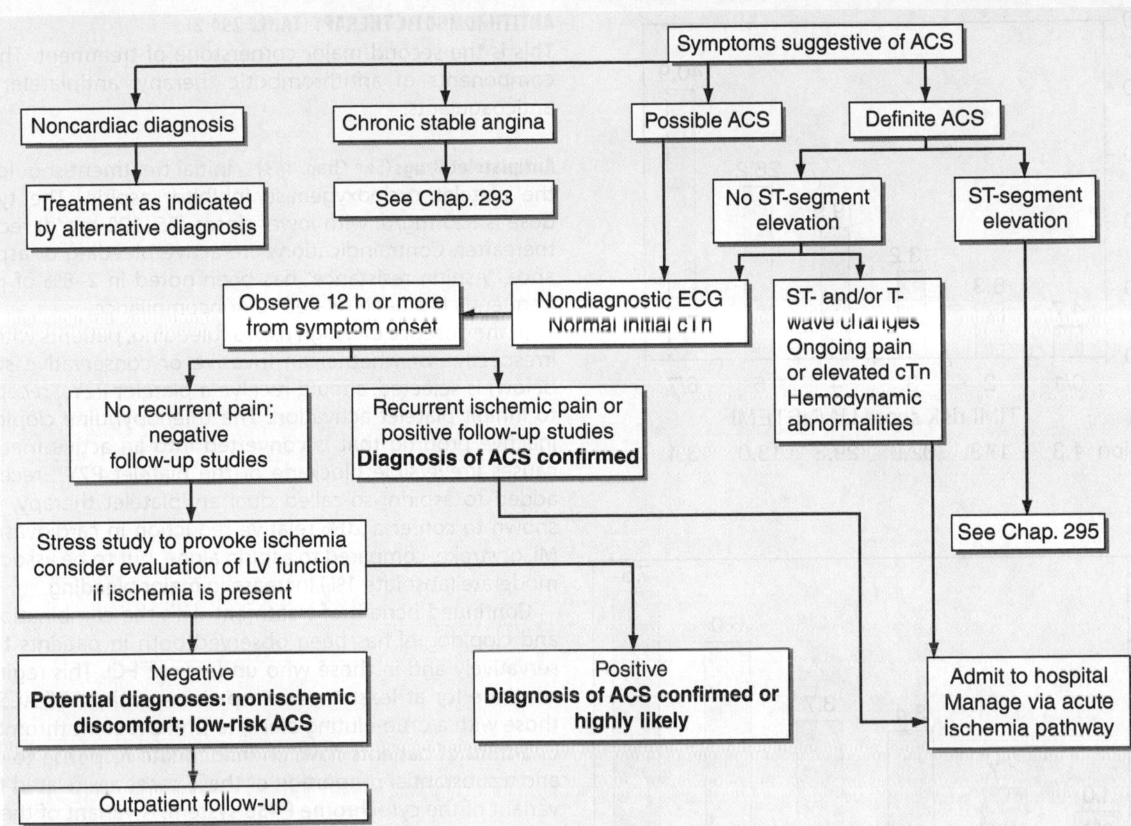

FIGURE 294-3 Algorithm for evaluation and management of patients with suspected acute coronary syndrome (ACS). Follow-up studies refer to ST deviations and elevation of troponin levels. cTn, cardiac troponin; ECG, electrocardiogram; LV, left ventricular. *(Modified from JL Anderson et al: J Am Coll Cardiol 61:e179, 2013.)*

(2) detect rest ischemia (using serial or continuous ECGs); and (3) detect significant coronary obstruction at rest with CCTA and myocardial ischemia using stress testing (Chap 270e).

Patients with a low likelihood of ischemia are usually managed with an emergency department–based critical pathway (which, in some institutions, is carried out in a "chest pain unit") (Fig. 294-3). Evaluation of such patients includes clinical monitoring for recurrent ischemic discomfort and continuous monitoring of ECGs and cardiac markers, typically obtained at baseline and at 4–6 h and 12 h after presentation. If new elevations in cardiac markers or ST-T-wave changes on the ECG are noted, the patient should be admitted to the hospital. Patients who remain pain free with negative markers may proceed to stress testing to determine the presence of ischemia or CCTA to detect coronary luminal obstruction (Fig. 294-2).

RISK STRATIFICATION

Patients with documented NSTE-ACS exhibit a wide spectrum of early (30 days) risk of death, ranging from 1 to 10%, and a recurrent ACS rate of 5 to 15% during the first year. Assessment of risk can be accomplished by clinical risk scoring systems such as that developed from the Thrombolysis in Myocardial Infarction (TIMI) Trials, which includes seven independent risk factors (Fig. 294-4*A*). The presence of an abnormally elevated cTn is especially important, as is its peak level, which correlates with the extent of myocardial damage (Fig. 294-4*B*). Other risk factors include diabetes mellitus, left ventricular dysfunction, renal dysfunction, and elevated levels of B-type natriuretic peptides and C-reactive protein. Multimarker strategies are now gaining favor, both to define more fully the pathophysiologic mechanisms underlying a given patient's presentation and to stratify the patient's risk further. Patients with ACS without elevated levels of cTn (infrequently encountered with the new sensitive troponin assays) are considered to have UA and have a more favorable prognosis than those with cTn elevations (NSTEMI).

Early risk assessment is useful both in predicting the risk of recurrent cardiac events and in identifying patients who would derive the greatest benefit from an early invasive strategy. For example, in the TACTICS-TIMI 18 Trial, an early invasive strategy conferred a 40% reduction in recurrent cardiac events in patients with an elevated cTn level, whereas no benefit was observed in those without detectable troponin.

TREATMENT NON-ST-SEGMENT ELEVATION ACUTE CORONARY SYNDROME (NON-ST-SEGMENT ELEVATION MYOCARDIAL INFARCTION AND UNSTABLE ANGINA)

MEDICAL TREATMENT

Patients should be placed at bed rest with continuous ECG monitoring for ST-segment deviation and cardiac arrhythmias. Ambulation is permitted if the patient shows no recurrence of ischemia (symptoms or ECG changes) and does not develop an elevation of a biomarker of necrosis for 12–24 h. Medical therapy involves simultaneous anti-ischemic and antithrombotic treatments and consideration of coronary revascularization.

ANTI-ISCHEMIC TREATMENT (TABLE 294-1)

To provide relief and prevention of recurrence of chest pain, initial treatment should include bed rest, nitrates, beta adrenergic blockers, and inhaled oxygen in the presence of hypoxemia.

Nitrates These should first be given sublingually or by buccal spray (0.3–0.6 mg) if the patient is experiencing ischemic pain. If pain persists after three doses given 5 min apart, intravenous nitroglycerin (5–10 μg/min using nonabsorbing tubing) is recommended. The rate of the infusion may be increased by 10 μg/min every 3–5 min until symptoms are relieved, systolic arterial pressure falls to

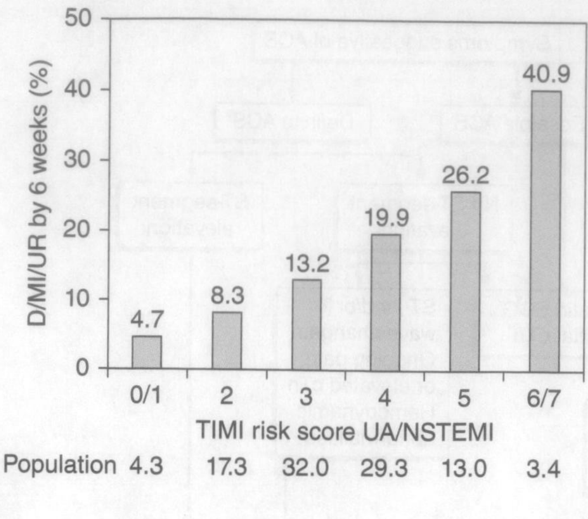

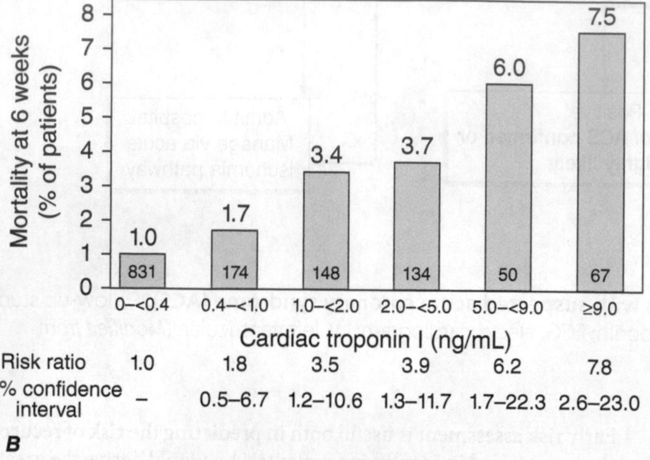

FIGURE 294-4 ***A.*** Death (D), myocardial infarction (MI), or need for urgent revascularization (UR) through 6 weeks by Thrombolysis in Myocardial Infarction (TIMI) Risk Score in the unfractionated heparin arm of the TIMI 11B trial. *(From EM Antman et al: JAMA 284:835, 2000.)* ***B.*** Mortality rate at 42 days by baseline cardiac troponin I levels in the TIMI 3B trial. *(From EM Antman et al: N Engl J Med 335:1342, 1996.)*

<100 mmHg, or the dose reaches 200 μg/min. Topical or oral nitrates **(Chap. 293)** can be used when the pain has resolved, or they may replace intravenous nitroglycerin when the patient has been pain-free for 12–24 h. The only absolute contraindications to the use of nitrates are hypotension or the use of sildenafil or other phosphodiesterase-5 inhibitors within the previous 24–48 h.

Beta Adrenergic Blockers and Other Agents Beta blockers are the other mainstay of anti-ischemic treatment. They may be started by the intravenous route in patients with severe ischemia, but this is contraindicated in the presence of heart failure. Ordinarily, oral beta blockade targeted to a heart rate of 50–60 beats/min is recommended. Heart rate–slowing calcium channel blockers, e.g., verapamil or diltiazem, are recommended for patients who have persistent symptoms or ECG signs of ischemia after treatment with full-dose nitrates and beta blockers and in patients with contraindications to either class of these agents. Additional medical therapy includes angiotensin-converting enzyme (ACE) inhibitors or, if these are not tolerated, angiotensin receptor blockers. Early administration of intensive HMG-CoA reductase inhibitors (statins), such as atorvastatin 80 mg/d, prior to percutaneous coronary intervention (PCI), and continued thereafter, has been shown to reduce complications of the procedure and recurrences of ACS.

ANTITHROMBOTIC THERAPY (TABLE 294-2)

This is the second major cornerstone of treatment. There are two components of antithrombotic therapy: antiplatelet drugs and anticoagulants.

Antiplatelet Drugs (See Chap. 143) Initial treatment should begin with the platelet cyclooxygenase inhibitor aspirin. The typical initial dose is 325 mg/d, with lower doses (75–100 mg/d) recommended thereafter. Contraindications are active bleeding or aspirin intolerance. "Aspirin resistance" has been noted in 2–8% of patients but frequently has been related to noncompliance.

In the absence of a high risk for bleeding, patients with NSTE-ACS, irrespective of whether an invasive or conservative strategy (see below) is selected, should receive a platelet $P2Y_{12}$ receptor blocker to inhibit platelet activation. The thienopyridine clopidogrel is an inactive prodrug that is converted into an active metabolite that causes irreversible blockade of the platelet $P2Y_{12}$ receptor. When added to aspirin, so-called dual antiplatelet therapy, it has been shown to confer a 20% relative reduction in cardiovascular death, MI, or stroke, compared to aspirin alone, but to be associated with a moderate (absolute 1%) increase in major bleeding.

Continued benefit of treatment with the combination of aspirin and clopidogrel has been observed both in patients treated conservatively and in those who underwent PCI. This regimen should continue for at least 1 year in patients with NSTE-ACS, especially those with a drug-eluting stent, to prevent stent thrombosis. Up to one-third of patients have an inadequate response to clopidogrel, and a substantial proportion of these cases are related to a genetic variant of the cytochrome P450 system. A variant of the 2C19 gene leads to reduced conversion of clopidogrel into its active metabolite, which, in turn, reduces platelet inhibition and is associated with increases in the incidence of adverse cardiovascular events. Alternate $P2Y_{12}$ blockers, such as prasugrel or ticagrelor (see below) used with aspirin, should be considered in patients with NSTE-ACS who develop a coronary event while receiving clopidogrel and aspirin or who are hyporesponsive to clopidogrel as identified by platelet and/or genetic testing, although such testing is not yet widespread.

A second $P2Y_{12}$ blocker, prasugrel, also a thienopyridine, achieves a more rapid onset and higher level of platelet inhibition than clopidogrel. It has been approved for ACS patients following angiography in whom PCI is planned. It should be administered at a loading dose of 60 mg followed by 10 mg/d for up to 15 months. The TRITON-TIMI 38 trial showed that relative to clopidogrel, prasugrel reduced the risk of cardiovascular death, MI, or stroke significantly, albeit with an increase in major bleeding. Stent thrombosis was reduced by half. This agent is contraindicated in patients with prior stroke or transient ischemic attack or at high risk for bleeding. It has not been found to be effective in patients treated by a conservative strategy (see below).

Ticagrelor is a novel, potent, *reversible* platelet $P2Y_{12}$ inhibitor. It has been shown in the PLATO trial to reduce the risk of cardiovascular death, MI, or stroke compared with clopidogrel in ACS patients who are treated by either an invasive or a conservative strategy. This agent reduced mortality but increased the risk of bleeding not associated with coronary artery bypass grafting. After a loading dose of 180 mg, 90 mg bid is administered as maintenance.

Prior to the development of the oral $P2Y_{12}$ receptor blockers, many trials had shown the benefit of intravenous glycoprotein IIb/IIIa inhibitors. Their benefit, however, has been small (i.e., only a 10% reduction in death or MI, with a significant increase in major bleeding). Two recent studies failed to show a benefit of routine early initiation of a drug in this class compared with their use only in patients who undergo PCI. The addition of these agents to aspirin and a $P2Y_{12}$ inhibitor (i.e., triple antiplatelet therapy) should be reserved for unstable patients with recurrent rest pain, elevated cTn, and ECG changes, as well as those who have a coronary thrombus evident on angiography when they undergo PCI.

TABLE 294-1 DRUGS COMMONLY USED IN INTENSIVE MEDICAL MANAGEMENT OF PATIENTS WITH UNSTABLE ANGINA AND NON-ST-SEGMENT ELEVATION MYOCARDIAL INFARCTION

Drug Category	Clinical Condition	When to Avoid[a]	Dosage
Nitrates	Administer sublingually, and, if symptoms persist, intravenously	Hypotension	Topical, oral, or buccal nitrates are acceptable alternatives for patients without ongoing or refractory symptoms
		Patient receiving sildenafil or other PDE-5 inhibitor	5–10 μg/min by continuous infusion titrated up to 75–100 μg/min until relief of symptoms or limiting side effects (headache or hypotension with a systolic blood pressure <90 mmHg or more than 30% below starting mean arterial pressure levels if significant hypertension is present)
Beta blockers[b]	Unstable angina	PR interval (ECG) <0.24 s	Metoprolol 25–50 mg by mouth every 6 h
		2° or 3° atrioventricular block	If needed, and no heart failure, 5-mg increments by slow (over 1–2 min) IV administration
		Heart rate <60 beats/min	
		Systolic pressure <90 mmHg	
		Shock	
		Left ventricular failure	
		Severe reactive airway disease	
Calcium channel blockers	Patients whose symptoms are not relieved by adequate doses of nitrates and beta blockers, or in patients unable to tolerate adequate doses of one or both of these agents, or in patients with variant angina	Pulmonary edema	Dependent on specific agent
		Evidence of left ventricular dysfunction (for diltiazem or verapamil)	
Morphine sulfate	Patients whose symptoms are not relieved after three serial sublingual nitroglycerin tablets or whose symptoms recur with adequate anti-ischemic therapy	Hypotension	2–5 mg IV dose
		Respiratory depression	May be repeated every 5–30 min as needed to relieve symptoms and maintain patient comfort
		Confusion	
		Obtundation	

[a]Allergy or prior intolerance is a contraindication for all categories of drugs listed in this chart. [b]Choice of the specific agent is not as important as ensuring that appropriate candidates receive this therapy. If there are concerns about patient intolerance due to existing pulmonary disease, especially asthma, left ventricular dysfunction, risk of hypotension, or severe bradycardia, initial selection should favor a short-acting agent, such as propranolol or metoprolol or the ultra-short-acting agent esmolol. Mild wheezing or a history of chronic obstructive pulmonary disease should prompt a trial of a short-acting agent at a reduced dose (e.g., 2.5 mg IV metoprolol, 12.5 mg oral metoprolol, or 25 μg/kg per min esmolol as initial doses) rather than complete avoidance of beta blocker therapy.

Note: Some of the recommendations in this guide suggest the use of agents for purposes or in doses other than those specified by the U.S. Food and Drug Administration. Such recommendations are made after consideration of concerns regarding nonapproved indications. Where made, such recommendations are based on more recent clinical trials or expert consensus. 2°, second-degree; 3°, third-degree; ECG, electrocardiogram; IV, intravenous.

Source: Modified from J Anderson et al: J Am Coll Cardiol 61:e179, 2013.

Anticoagulants **(See Chap. 143)** Four options are available for anticoagulant therapy to be added to antiplatelet agents: (1) unfractionated heparin (UFH), long the mainstay of therapy; (2) the low-molecular-weight heparin (LMWH), enoxaparin, which has been shown to be superior to UFH in reducing recurrent cardiac events, especially in patients managed by a conservative strategy but with some increase in bleeding; (3) bivalirudin, a direct thrombin inhibitor that is similar in efficacy to either UFH or LMWH but causes less bleeding and is used just prior to and/or during PCI; and (4) the indirect factor Xa inhibitor, fondaparinux, which is equivalent in efficacy to enoxaparin but appears to have a lower risk of major bleeding.

Excessive bleeding is the most important adverse effect of all antithrombotic agents, including both antiplatelet agents and anticoagulants. Therefore, attention must be directed to the doses of antithrombotic agents, accounting for body weight, creatinine clearance, and a previous history of excessive bleeding, as a means of reducing the risk of bleeding. Patients who have experienced a stroke are at higher risk of intracranial bleeding with potent antiplatelet agents and combinations of antithrombotic drugs.

INVASIVE VERSUS CONSERVATIVE STRATEGY

Multiple clinical trials have demonstrated the benefit of an early invasive strategy in high-risk patients (i.e., patients with multiple clinical risk factors, ST-segment deviation, and/or positive biomarkers) (Table 294-3). In this strategy, following treatment with anti-ischemic and antithrombotic agents, coronary arteriography is carried out within ~48 h of presentation, followed by coronary revascularization (PCI or coronary artery bypass grafting), depending on the coronary anatomy. In low-risk patients, the outcomes from an invasive strategy are similar to those obtained from a conservative strategy. The latter consists of anti-ischemic and antithrombotic therapy followed by "watchful waiting," in which the patient is closely observed and coronary arteriography is carried out only if rest pain or ST-segment changes recur, a biomarker of necrosis becomes positive, or there is evidence of severe ischemia on a stress test.

LONG-TERM MANAGEMENT

The time of hospital discharge is a "teachable moment" for the patient with NSTE-ACS, when the physician can review and optimize the medical regimen. Risk-factor modification is key, and the caregiver should discuss with the patient the importance of smoking cessation, achieving optimal weight, daily exercise, blood-pressure control, following an appropriate diet, control of hyperglycemia (in diabetic patients), and lipid management as recommended for patients with chronic stable angina (Chap. 293).

TABLE 294-2 CLINICAL USE OF ANTITHROMBOTIC THERAPY

Oral Antiplatelet Therapy	
Aspirin	Initial dose of 325 mg nonenteric formulation followed by 75–100 mg/d of an enteric or a nonenteric formulation
Clopidogrel	Loading dose of 300–600 mg followed by 75 mg/d
Prasugrel	Pre-PCI: Loading dose 60 mg followed by 10 mg/d
Ticagrelor	Loading dose of 180 mg followed by 90 mg twice daily
Intravenous Antiplatelet Therapy	
Abciximab	0.25 mg/kg bolus followed by infusion of 0.125 μg/kg per min (maximum 10 μg/min) for 12–24 h
Eptifibatide	180 μg/kg bolus followed 10 min later by second bolus of 180 μg with infusion of 2.0 μg/kg per min for 72–96 h following first bolus
Tirofiban	25 μg/kg per min followed by infusion of 0.15 μg/kg per min for 48–96 h
Heparins[a]	
Unfractionated heparin (UFH)	[b]Bolus 70–100 U/kg (maximum 5000 U) IV followed by infusion of 12–15 U/kg per h (initial maximum 1000 U/h) titrated to ACT 250–300 s
Enoxaparin	1 mg/kg SC every 12 h; the first dose may be preceded by a 30-mg IV bolus; renal adjustment to 1 mg/kg once daily if creatine clearance <30 cc/min
Fondaparinux	2.5 mg SC qd
Bivalirudin	Initial IV bolus of 0.75 mg/kg and an infusion of 1.75 mg/kg per h.

[a]Other low-molecular-weight heparins exist beyond those listed. [b]If no glycoprotein IIb/IIIa inhibitor planned.

Abbreviations: ACT, activated clotting time for HemoTec; IV, intravenous; SC, subcutaneously.

Source: Modified from J Anderson et al: J Am Coll Cardiol 61:e179, 2013.

There is evidence of benefit with long-term therapy with five classes of drugs that are directed at different components of the atherothrombotic process. Beta blockers, statins (at a high dose, e.g., atorvastatin 80 mg/d), and ACE inhibitors or angiotensin receptor blockers are recommended for long-term plaque stabilization. Antiplatelet therapy, now recommended to be the combination of low-dose (75–100 mg/d) aspirin and a $P2Y_{12}$ inhibitor (clopidogrel, prasugrel, or ticagrelor) for 1 year, with aspirin continued thereafter, prevents or reduces the severity of any thrombosis that would occur if a plaque were to rupture.

Registries have shown that women and racial minorities, as well as patients with NSTE-ACS at high risk, including the elderly and patients with diabetes or chronic kidney disease, are less likely to receive evidence-based pharmacologic and interventional therapies with resultant poorer clinical outcomes and quality of life. Special attention should be directed to these groups.

TABLE 294-3 CLASS I RECOMMENDATIONS FOR USE OF AN EARLY INVASIVE STRATEGY IN PATIENTS WITH NON-ST-SEGMENT ELEVATION ACUTE CORONARY SYNDROME[a]

Class I (Level of Evidence: A) Indications
Recurrent angina at rest/low-level activity despite treatment
Elevated TnT or TnI
New ST-segment depression
CHF symptoms, rales, MR
EF <0.40
Sustained VT
PCI <6 months, prior CABG
High-risk findings from noninvasive testing
Hemodynamic instability
Mild-to-moderate renal dysfunction
Diabetes mellitus
High TIMI Risk Score (>3)[b]

[a]Any one of the high-risk indicators. [b]See Antman (JAMA 284:835, 2000).

Abbreviations: CABG, coronary artery bypass grafting; CHF, congestive heart failure; EF, ejection fraction; MR, mitral regurgitation; PCI, percutaneous coronary intervention; TIMI, Thrombolysis in Myocardial Infarction; TnI, troponin I; TnT, troponin T; VT, ventricular tachycardia.

Source: Modified from J Anderson et al: J Am Coll Cardiol 61:e179, 2013.

PRINZMETAL'S VARIANT ANGINA

In 1959 Prinzmetal et al. described a syndrome of severe ischemic pain that usually occurs at rest and is associated with transient ST-segment elevation. Prinzmetal's variant angina (PVA) is caused by focal spasm of an epicardial coronary artery, leading to severe transient myocardial ischemia and occasionally infarction. The cause of the spasm is not well defined, but it may be related to hypercontractility of vascular smooth muscle due to adrenergic vasoconstrictors, leukotrienes, or serotonin. For reasons that are not clear, the prevalence of PVA has decreased substantially during the past few decades.

Clinical and Angiographic Manifestations Patients with PVA are generally younger and have fewer coronary risk factors (with the exception of cigarette smoking) than do patients with NSTE-ACS. Cardiac examination is usually unremarkable in the absence of ischemia. The clinical diagnosis of PVA is made by the detection of transient ST-segment *elevation* with rest pain. Many patients also exhibit multiple episodes of asymptomatic ST-segment elevation (*silent ischemia*). Small elevations of troponin may occur in patients with prolonged attacks.

Coronary angiography demonstrates transient coronary spasm as the diagnostic hallmark of PVA. Atherosclerotic plaques in at least one proximal coronary artery occur in about half of patients, and in these patients, spasm usually occurs within 1 cm of the plaque. Focal spasm is most common in the right coronary artery, and it may occur at one or more sites in one artery or in multiple arteries simultaneously. Hyperventilation or intracoronary acetylcholine has been used to provoke focal coronary stenosis on angiography or to provoke rest angina with ST-segment elevation to establish the diagnosis.

TREATMENT PRINZMETAL'S VARIANT ANGINA

Nitrates and calcium channel blockers are the main therapeutic agents. Aspirin may actually increase the severity of ischemic episodes, possibly as a result of the sensitivity of coronary tone to modest changes in the synthesis of prostacyclin. The response to beta blockers is variable. Coronary revascularization may be helpful in patients who also have discrete, flow-limiting, proximal fixed obstructive lesions.

Prognosis Many patients with PVA pass through an acute, active phase, with frequent episodes of angina and cardiac events during the first 6 months after presentation. Survival at 5 years is excellent (~90–95%). Patients with no or mild fixed coronary obstruction tend to experience a more benign course than do patients with associated severe obstructive lesions. Nonfatal MI occurs in up to 20% of patients by 5 years. Patients with PVA who develop serious arrhythmias during spontaneous episodes of pain are at a higher risk for sudden cardiac death. In most patients who survive an infarction or the initial 3- to 6-month period of frequent episodes, there is a tendency for symptoms and cardiac events to diminish over time.

295 ST-Segment Elevation Myocardial Infarction

Elliott M. Antman, Joseph Loscalzo

Acute myocardial infarction (AMI) is one of the most common diagnoses in hospitalized patients in industrialized countries. In the United States, approximately 525,000 patients experience a new AMI, and 190,000 experience a recurrent AMI each year. More than half of AMI-related deaths occur before the stricken individual reaches the hospital. The in-hospital mortality rate after admission for AMI has declined from 10% to about 6% over the past decade. The 1-year mortality rate after AMI is about 15%. Mortality is approximately fourfold higher in elderly patients (over age 75) as compared with younger patients.

When patients with prolonged ischemic discomfort at rest are first seen, the working clinical diagnosis is that they are suffering from an acute coronary syndrome (Fig. 295-1). The 12-lead electrocardiogram (ECG) is a pivotal diagnostic and triage tool because it is at the center of the decision pathway for management; it permits distinction of those patients presenting with ST-segment elevation from those presenting without ST-segment elevation. Serum cardiac biomarkers are obtained to distinguish unstable angina (UA) from non-ST-segment elevation myocardial infarction (NSTEMI) and to assess the magnitude of an ST-segment elevation myocardial infarction (STEMI). This chapter focuses on the evaluation and management of patients with STEMI, while Chap. 294 discusses UA/NSTEMI.

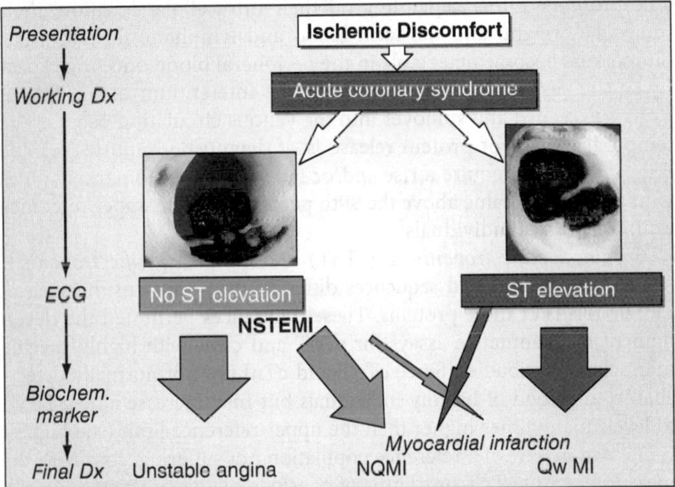

FIGURE 295-1 Acute coronary syndromes. Following disruption of a vulnerable plaque, patients experience ischemic discomfort resulting from a reduction of flow through the affected epicardial coronary artery. The flow reduction may be caused by a completely occlusive thrombus (*right*) or subtotally occlusive thrombus (*left*). Patients with ischemic discomfort may present with or without ST-segment elevation. Of patients with ST-segment elevation, the majority (*wide red arrow*) ultimately develop a Q wave on the ECG (Qw MI), while a minority (*thin red arrow*) do not develop Q wave and, in older literature, were said to have sustained a non-Q-wave MI (NQMI). Patients who present without ST-segment elevation are suffering from either unstable angina or a non-ST-segment elevation MI (NSTEMI) (*wide green arrows*), a distinction that is ultimately made based on the presence or absence of a serum cardiac marker such as CK-MB or a cardiac troponin detected in the blood. The majority of patients presenting with NSTEMI do not develop a Q wave on the ECG; a minority develop a Qw MI (*thin green arrow*). Dx, diagnosis; ECG, electrocardiogram; MI, myocardial infarction. *(Adapted from CW Hamm et al: Lancet 358:1533, 2001, and MJ Davies: Heart 83:361, 2000; with permission from the BMJ Publishing Group.)*

PATHOPHYSIOLOGY: ROLE OF ACUTE PLAQUE RUPTURE

STEMI usually occurs when coronary blood flow decreases abruptly after a thrombotic occlusion of a coronary artery previously affected by atherosclerosis. Slowly developing, high-grade coronary artery stenoses do not typically precipitate STEMI because of the development of a rich collateral network over time. Instead, STEMI occurs when a coronary artery thrombus develops rapidly at a site of vascular injury. This injury is produced or facilitated by factors such as cigarette smoking, hypertension, and lipid accumulation. In most cases, STEMI occurs when the surface of an atherosclerotic plaque becomes disrupted (exposing its contents to the blood) and conditions (local or systemic) favor thrombogenesis. A mural thrombus forms at the site of plaque disruption, and the involved coronary artery becomes occluded. Histologic studies indicate that the coronary plaques prone to disruption are those with a rich lipid core and a thin fibrous cap (Chap. 291e). After an initial platelet monolayer forms at the site of the disrupted plaque, various agonists (collagen, ADP, epinephrine, serotonin) promote platelet activation. After agonist stimulation of platelets, thromboxane A_2 (a potent local vasoconstrictor) is released, further platelet activation occurs, and potential resistance to fibrinolysis develops.

In addition to the generation of thromboxane A_2, activation of platelets by agonists promotes a conformational change in the glycoprotein IIb/IIIa receptor (Chap. 140). Once converted to its functional state, this receptor develops a high affinity for soluble adhesive proteins (i.e., integrins) such as fibrinogen. Since fibrinogen is a multivalent molecule, it can bind to two different platelets simultaneously, resulting in platelet cross-linking and aggregation.

The coagulation cascade is activated on exposure of tissue factor in damaged endothelial cells at the site of the disrupted plaque. Factors VII and X are activated, ultimately leading to the conversion of prothrombin to thrombin, which then converts fibrinogen to fibrin (Chap. 141). Fluid-phase and clot-bound thrombin participates in an autoamplification reaction leading to further activation of the coagulation cascade. The culprit coronary artery eventually becomes occluded by a thrombus containing platelet aggregates and fibrin strands.

In rare cases, STEMI may be due to coronary artery occlusion caused by coronary emboli, congenital abnormalities, coronary spasm, and a wide variety of systemic—particularly inflammatory—diseases. The amount of myocardial damage caused by coronary occlusion depends on (1) the territory supplied by the affected vessel, (2) whether or not the vessel becomes totally occluded, (3) the duration of coronary occlusion, (4) the quantity of blood supplied by collateral vessels to the affected tissue, (5) the demand for oxygen of the myocardium whose blood supply has been suddenly limited, (6) endogenous factors that can produce early spontaneous lysis of the occlusive thrombus, and (7) the adequacy of myocardial perfusion in the infarct zone when flow is restored in the occluded epicardial coronary artery.

Patients at increased risk for developing STEMI include those with multiple coronary risk factors (Chap. 291e) and those with UA (Chap. 294). Less common underlying medical conditions predisposing patients to STEMI include hypercoagulability, collagen vascular disease, cocaine abuse, and intracardiac thrombi or masses that can produce coronary emboli.

There have been major advances in the management of STEMI with recognition that the "chain of survival" involves a highly integrated system starting with prehospital care and extending to early hospital management so as to provide expeditious implementation of a reperfusion strategy.

CLINICAL PRESENTATION

In up to one-half of cases, a precipitating factor appears to be present before STEMI, such as vigorous physical exercise, emotional stress, or a medical or surgical illness. Although STEMI may commence at any time of the day or night, circadian variations have been reported such that clusters are seen in the morning within a few hours of awakening.

Pain is the most common presenting complaint in patients with STEMI. The pain is deep and visceral; adjectives commonly used to describe it are *heavy*, *squeezing*, and *crushing*, although, occasionally, it is described as stabbing or burning (Chap. 19). It is similar in character to the discomfort of angina pectoris (Chap. 293) but commonly occurs at rest, is usually more severe, and lasts longer. Typically, the pain involves the central portion of the chest and/or the epigastrium, and, on occasion, it radiates to the arms. Less common sites of radiation include the abdomen, back, lower jaw, and neck. The frequent location of the pain beneath the xiphoid and epigastrium and the patients' denial that they may be suffering a heart attack are chiefly responsible for the common mistaken impression of indigestion. The pain of STEMI may radiate as high as the occipital area but not below the umbilicus. It is often accompanied by weakness, sweating, nausea, vomiting, anxiety, and a sense of impending doom. The pain may commence when the patient is at rest, but when it begins during a period of exertion, it does not usually subside with cessation of activity, in contrast to angina pectoris.

The pain of STEMI can simulate pain from acute pericarditis (Chap. 288), pulmonary embolism (Chap. 300), acute aortic dissection (Chap. 301), costochondritis, and gastrointestinal disorders. These conditions should therefore be considered in the differential diagnosis. Radiation of discomfort to the trapezius is not seen in patients with STEMI and may be a useful distinguishing feature that suggests pericarditis is the correct diagnosis. However, *pain is not uniformly present in patients with STEMI*. The proportion of painless STEMIs is greater in patients with diabetes mellitus, and it increases with age. In the elderly, STEMI may present as sudden-onset breathlessness, which may progress to pulmonary edema. Other less common presentations, with or without pain, include sudden loss of consciousness, a confusional state, a sensation of profound weakness, the appearance of an arrhythmia, evidence of peripheral embolism, or merely an unexplained drop in arterial pressure.

PHYSICAL FINDINGS

Most patients are anxious and restless, attempting unsuccessfully to relieve the pain by moving about in bed, altering their position, and stretching. Pallor associated with perspiration and coolness of the extremities occurs commonly. The combination of substernal chest pain persisting for >30 min and diaphoresis strongly suggests STEMI. Although many patients have a normal pulse rate and blood pressure within the first hour of STEMI, about one-fourth of patients with anterior infarction have manifestations of sympathetic nervous system hyperactivity (tachycardia and/or hypertension), and up to one-half with inferior infarction show evidence of parasympathetic hyperactivity (bradycardia and/or hypotension).

The precordium is usually quiet, and the apical impulse may be difficult to palpate. In patients with anterior wall infarction, an abnormal systolic pulsation caused by dyskinetic bulging of infarcted myocardium may develop in the periapical area within the first days of the illness and then may resolve. Other physical signs of ventricular dysfunction include fourth and third heart sounds, decreased intensity of the first heart sound, and paradoxical splitting of the second heart sound (Chap. 267). A transient midsystolic or late systolic apical systolic murmur due to dysfunction of the mitral valve apparatus may be present. A pericardial friction rub may be heard in patients with transmural STEMI at some time in the course of the disease, if they are examined frequently. The carotid pulse is often decreased in volume, reflecting reduced stroke volume. Temperature elevations up to 38°C may be observed during the first week after STEMI. The arterial pressure is variable; in most patients with transmural infarction, systolic pressure declines by approximately 10–15 mmHg from the preinfarction state.

LABORATORY FINDINGS

STEMI progresses through the following temporal stages: (1) acute (first few hours–7 days), (2) healing (7–28 days), and (3) healed (≥29 days). When evaluating the results of diagnostic tests for STEMI, the temporal phase of the infarction must be considered. The laboratory tests of value in confirming the diagnosis may be divided into four groups: (1) ECG, (2) serum cardiac biomarkers, (3) cardiac imaging, and (4) nonspecific indices of tissue necrosis and inflammation.

ELECTROCARDIOGRAM

The electrocardiographic manifestations of STEMI are described in Chap. 268. During the initial stage, total occlusion of an epicardial coronary artery produces ST-segment elevation. Most patients initially presenting with ST-segment elevation ultimately evolve Q waves on the ECG. However, Q waves in the leads overlying the infarct zone may vary in magnitude and even appear only transiently, depending on the reperfusion status of the ischemic myocardium and restoration of transmembrane potentials over time. A small proportion of patients initially presenting with ST-segment elevation will not develop Q waves when the obstructing thrombus is not totally occlusive, obstruction is transient, or if a rich collateral network is present. Among patients presenting with ischemic discomfort but *without* ST-segment elevation, if a serum cardiac biomarker of necrosis (see below) is detected, the diagnosis of NSTEMI is ultimately made (Fig. 295-1). A minority of patients who present initially without ST-segment elevation may develop a Q-wave MI. Previously, it was believed that transmural myocardial infarction (MI) is present if the ECG demonstrates Q waves or loss of R waves, and nontransmural MI may be present if the ECG shows only transient ST-segment and T-wave changes. However, electrocardiographic-pathologic correlations are far from perfect and terms such as *Q-wave MI*, *non-Q-wave MI*, *transmural MI*, and *nontransmural MI*, have been replaced by STEMI and NSTEMI (Fig. 295-1). Contemporary studies using magnetic resonance imaging (MRI) suggest that the development of a Q wave on the ECG is more dependent on the volume of infarcted tissue rather than the transmurality of infarction.

SERUM CARDIAC BIOMARKERS

Certain proteins, called serum cardiac biomarkers, are released from necrotic heart muscle after STEMI. The rate of liberation of specific proteins differs depending on their intracellular location, their molecular weight, and the local blood and lymphatic flow. Cardiac biomarkers become detectable in the peripheral blood once the capacity of the cardiac lymphatics to clear the interstitium of the infarct zone is exceeded and spillover into the venous circulation occurs. The temporal pattern of protein release is of diagnostic importance. The criteria for AMI require a rise and/or fall in cardiac biomarker values with at least one value above the 99th percentile of the upper reference limit for normal individuals

Cardiac-specific troponin T (cTnT) and *cardiac-specific troponin I* (cTnI) have amino-acid sequences different from those of the skeletal muscle forms of these proteins. These differences permitted the development of quantitative assays for cTnT and cTnI with highly specific monoclonal antibodies. Since cTnT and cTnI are not normally detectable in the blood of healthy individuals but may increase after STEMI to levels many times higher than the upper reference limit (the highest value seen in 99% of a reference population not suffering from MI), the measurement of cTnT or cTnI is of considerable diagnostic usefulness, and they are now the preferred biochemical markers for MI (Fig. 295-2). With improvements in the assays for the cardiac-specific troponins, it is now possible to detect concentrations <1 ng/L in patients without ischemic-type chest discomfort. The cardiac troponins are particularly valuable when there is clinical suspicion of either skeletal muscle injury or a small MI that may be below the detection limit for creatine phosphokinase (CK) and its MB isoenzyme (CK-MB) measurements, and they are, therefore, of particular value in distinguishing UA from NSTEMI. In practical terms, the high-sensitivity troponin assays are of less immediate value in patients with STEMI. Contemporary urgent reperfusion strategies necessitate making a decision (based largely on a combination of clinical and ECG findings) before the results of blood tests have returned from the laboratory. Levels of cTnI and cTnT may remain elevated for 7–10 days after STEMI.

CK rises within 4–8 h and generally returns to normal by 48–72 h (Fig. 295-2). An important drawback of total CK measurement is its lack of specificity for STEMI, as CK may be elevated with skeletal muscle disease or trauma, including intramuscular injection. The MB isoenzyme of CK has the advantage over total CK that it is not present in significant concentrations in extracardiac tissue and, therefore,

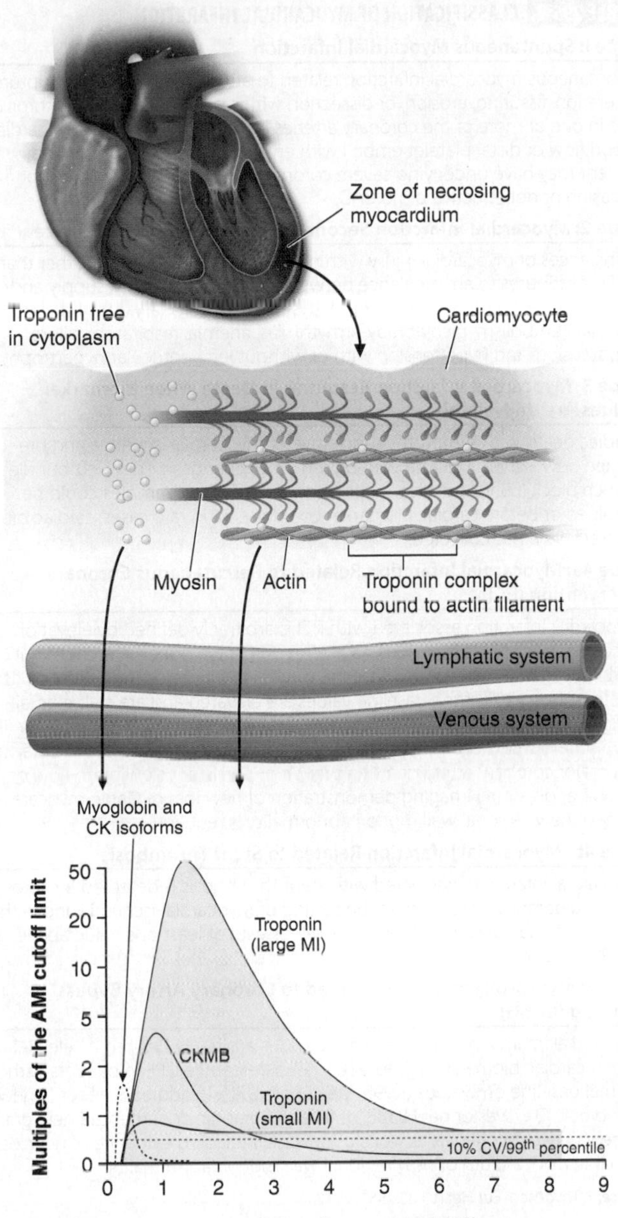

FIGURE 295-2 The zone of necrosing myocardium is shown at the top of the figure, followed in the middle portion of the figure by a diagram of a cardiomyocyte that is in the process of releasing biomarkers. The biomarkers that are released into the interstitium are first cleared by lymphatics followed subsequently by spillover into the venous system. After disruption of the sarcolemmal membrane of the cardiomyocyte, the cytoplasmic pool of biomarkers is released first (*left-most arrow in bottom portion of figure*). Markers such as myoglobin and CK isoforms are rapidly released, and blood levels rise quickly above the cutoff limit; this is then followed by a more protracted release of biomarkers from the disintegrating myofilaments that may continue for several days. Cardiac troponin levels rise to about 20 to 50 times the upper reference limit (the 99th percentile of values in a reference control group) in patients who have a "classic" acute myocardial infarction (MI) and sustain sufficient myocardial necrosis to result in abnormally elevated levels of the MB fraction of creatine kinase (CK-MB). Clinicians can now diagnose episodes of microinfarction by sensitive assays that detect cardiac troponin elevations above the upper reference limit, even though CK-MB levels may still be in the normal reference range (not shown). CV, coefficient of variation. *(Modified from EM Antman: Decision making with cardiac troponin tests. N Engl J Med 346:2079, 2002 and AS Jaffe, L Babiun, FS Apple: Biomarkers in acute cardiac disease: The present and the future. J Am Coll Cardiol 48:1, 2006.)*

is considerably more specific. However, cardiac surgery, myocarditis, and electrical cardioversion often result in elevated serum levels of the MB isoenzyme. A ratio (relative index) of CK-MB mass to CK activity ≥2.5 suggests but is not diagnostic of a myocardial rather than a skeletal muscle source for the CK-MB elevation.

Many hospitals are using cTnT or cTnI rather than CK-MB as the routine serum cardiac marker for diagnosis of STEMI, although any of these analytes remain clinically acceptable. It is *not* cost-effective to measure both a cardiac-specific troponin and CK-MB at all time points in every patient.

While it has long been recognized that the total quantity of protein released correlates with the size of the infarct, the peak protein concentration correlates only weakly with infarct size. Recanalization of a coronary artery occlusion (either spontaneously or by mechanical or pharmacologic means) in the early hours of STEMI causes earlier peaking of biomarker measurements (Fig. 295-2) because of a rapid washout from the interstitium of the infarct zone, quickly overwhelming lymphatic clearance of the proteins.

The *nonspecific reaction* to myocardial injury is associated with polymorphonuclear leukocytosis, which appears within a few hours after the onset of pain and persists for 3–7 days; the white blood cell count often reaches levels of 12,000–15,000/μL. The erythrocyte sedimentation rate rises more slowly than the white blood cell count, peaking during the first week and sometimes remaining elevated for 1 or 2 weeks.

CARDIAC IMAGING

Abnormalities of wall motion on *two-dimensional echocardiography* (Chap. 270e) are almost universally present. Although acute STEMI cannot be distinguished from an old myocardial scar or from acute severe ischemia by echocardiography, the ease and safety of the procedure make its use appealing as a screening tool in the Emergency Department setting. When the ECG is not diagnostic of STEMI, early detection of the presence or absence of wall motion abnormalities by echocardiography can aid in management decisions, such as whether the patient should receive reperfusion therapy (e.g., fibrinolysis or a percutaneous coronary intervention [PCI]). Echocardiographic estimation of left ventricular (LV) function is useful prognostically; detection of reduced function serves as an indication for therapy with an inhibitor of the renin-angiotensin-aldosterone system. Echocardiography may also identify the presence of right ventricular (RV) infarction, ventricular aneurysm, pericardial effusion, and LV thrombus. In addition, Doppler echocardiography is useful in the detection and quantitation of a ventricular septal defect and mitral regurgitation, two serious complications of STEMI.

Several *radionuclide imaging techniques* (Chap. 270e) are available for evaluating patients with suspected STEMI. However, these imaging modalities are used less often than echocardiography because they are more cumbersome and lack sensitivity and specificity in many clinical circumstances. Myocardial perfusion imaging with [^{201}Tl] or [^{99m}Tc]-sestamibi, which are distributed in proportion to myocardial blood flow and concentrated by viable myocardium (Chap. 293), reveals a defect ("cold spot") in most patients during the first few hours after development of a transmural infarct. Although perfusion scanning is extremely sensitive, it cannot distinguish acute infarcts from chronic scars and, thus, is not specific for the diagnosis of *acute* MI. Radionuclide ventriculography, carried out with [^{99m}Tc]-labeled red blood cells, frequently demonstrates wall motion disorders and reduction in the ventricular ejection fraction in patients with STEMI. While of value in assessing the hemodynamic consequences of infarction and in aiding in the diagnosis of RV infarction when the RV ejection fraction is depressed, this technique is nonspecific, as many cardiac abnormalities other than MI alter the radionuclide ventriculogram.

MI can be detected accurately with high-resolution cardiac MRI (Chap. 270e) using a technique referred to as late enhancement. A standard imaging agent (gadolinium) is administered and images are obtained after a 10-min delay. Since little gadolinium enters normal myocardium, where there are tightly packed myocytes, but does percolate into the expanded intercellular region of the infarct zone, there

TABLE 295-1 DEFINITION OF MYOCARDIAL INFARCTION

Criteria for Acute Myocardial Infarction
The term acute myocardial infarction (MI) should be used when there is evidence of myocardial necrosis in a clinical setting consistent with acute myocardial ischemia. Under these conditions, any one of the following criteria meets the diagnosis for MI:
• Detection of a rise and/or fall of cardiac biomarker values (preferably cardiac troponin [cTn]) with at least one value above the 99th percentile upper reference limit (URL) and with at least one of the following: ◦ Symptoms of ischemia ◦ New or presumed new significant ST-segment T-wave (ST-T) changes or new left bundle branch block (LBBB) ◦ Development of pathologic Q waves in the electrocardiogram (ECG) ◦ Imaging evidence of new loss of viable myocardium or new regional wall motion abnormality ◦ Identification of an intracoronary thrombus by angiography or autopsy
• Cardiac death with symptoms suggestive of myocardial ischemia and presumed new ischemic ECG changes of new LBBB, but death occurred before cardiac biomarkers were obtained or before cardiac biomarker values would be increased.
• Percutaneous coronary intervention (PCI)–related MI is arbitrarily defined by elevation of cTn values (>5 × 99th percentile URL) in patients with normal baseline values (≤99th percentile URL) or a rise of cTn values >20% if the baseline values are elevated and are stable or falling. In addition, either (i) symptoms suggestive of myocardial ischemia, or (ii) new ischemic ECG changes, or (iii) angiographic findings consistent with a procedural complication, or (iv) imaging demonstration of new loss of viable myocardium or new regional wall motion abnormality are required.
• Stent thrombosis associated with MI when detected by coronary angiography or autopsy in the setting of myocardial ischemia and with a rise and/or fall of cardiac biomarker values with at least one value above the 99th percentile URL.
• Coronary artery bypass grafting (CABG)–related MI is arbitrarily defined by elevation of cardiac biomarker values (>10 × 99th percentile URL) in patients with normal baseline cTn values (≤99th percentile URL). In addition, either (i) new pathologic Q waves or new LBBB, or (ii) angiographic documented new graft or new native coronary artery occlusion, or (iii) imaging evidence of new loss of viable myocardium or new regional wall motion abnormality.
Criteria for Prior Myocardial Infarction
Any one of the following criteria meets the diagnosis for prior MI:
• Pathologic Q waves with or without symptoms in the absence of nonischemic causes.
• Imaging evidence of a region of loss of viable myocardium that is thinned and fails to contract, in the absence of a nonischemic cause.
• Pathologic findings of a prior MI.

Source: K Thygesen: Eur Heart J 33:2551, 2012.

TABLE 295-2 CLASSIFICATION OF MYOCARDIAL INFARCTION

Type 1: Spontaneous Myocardial Infarction
Spontaneous myocardial infarction related to atherosclerotic plaque rupture, ulceration, fissuring, erosion, or dissection with resulting intraluminal thrombus in one or more of the coronary arteries leading to decreased myocardial blood flow or distal platelet emboli with ensuing myocyte necrosis. The patient may have underlying severe coronary artery disease (CAD) but on occasion nonobstructive or no CAD.
Type 2: Myocardial Infarction Secondary to an Ischemic Imbalance
In instances of myocardial injury with necrosis where a condition other than CAD contributes to an imbalance between myocardial oxygen supply and/or demand, e.g., coronary endothelial dysfunction, coronary artery spasm, coronary embolism, tachy-brady-arrhythmias, anemia, respiratory failure, hypotension, and hypertension with or without left ventricular hypertrophy.
Type 3: Myocardial Infarction Resulting in Death When Biomarker Values Are Unavailable
Cardiac death with symptoms suggestive of myocardial ischemia and presumed new ischemic electrocardiogram (ECG) changes or new left bundle branch block (LBBB), but death occurring before blood samples could be obtained or before cardiac biomarker could rise, or in rare cases, cardiac biomarkers were not collected.
Type 4a: Myocardial Infarction Related to Percutaneous Coronary Intervention (PCI)
Myocardial infarction associated with PCI is arbitrarily defined by elevation of cardiac troponin (cTn) values >5 × 99th percentile upper reference limit (URL) in patients with normal baseline values (≤99th percentile URL) or a rise of cTn values >20% if the baseline values are elevated and are stable or falling. In addition, either (i) symptoms suggestive of myocardial ischemia, or (ii) new ischemic ECG changes or new LBBB, or (iii) angiographic loss of patency of a major coronary artery or a side branch or persistent slow or no flow or embolization, or (iv) imaging demonstration of new loss of viable myocardium or new regional wall motion abnormality is required.
Type 4b: Myocardial Infarction Related to Stent Thrombosis
Myocardial infarction associated with stent thrombosis is detected by coronary angiography or autopsy in the setting of myocardial ischemia and with a rise and/or fall of cardiac biomarker values with at least one value above the 99th percentile URL.
Type 5: Myocardial Infarction Related to Coronary Artery Bypass Grafting (CABG)
Myocardial infarction associated with CABG is arbitrarily defined by elevation of cardiac biomarker values >10 × 99th percentile URL in patients with normal baseline cTn values (≤99th percentile URL). In addition, either (i) new pathologic Q waves or new LBBB, or (ii) angiographic documented new graft or new native coronary artery occlusion, or (iii) imaging evidence of new loss of viable myocardium or new regional wall motion abnormality.

Source: K Thygesen: Eur Heart J 33:2551, 2012.

is a bright signal in areas of infarction that appears in stark contrast to the dark areas of normal myocardium.

An Expert Consensus Task Force for the Universal Definition of Myocardial Infarction has provided a comprehensive set of criteria for the definition of MI that integrates the clinical and laboratory findings discussed earlier (Table 295-1) as well as a classification of MI into five types that reflect the clinical circumstances in which it may occur (Table 295-2).

INITIAL MANAGEMENT

PREHOSPITAL CARE

The prognosis in STEMI is largely related to the occurrence of two general classes of complications: (1) electrical complications (arrhythmias) and (2) mechanical complications ("pump failure"). Most out-of-hospital deaths from STEMI are due to the sudden development of ventricular fibrillation. The vast majority of deaths due to ventricular fibrillation occur within the first 24 h of the onset of symptoms, and of these, over half occur in the first hour. Therefore, the major elements of prehospital care of patients with suspected STEMI include (1) recognition of symptoms by the patient and prompt seeking of medical attention; (2) rapid deployment of an emergency medical team capable of performing resuscitative maneuvers, including defibrillation; (3) expeditious transportation of the patient to a hospital facility that is continuously staffed by physicians and nurses skilled in managing arrhythmias and providing advanced cardiac life support; and (4) expeditious implementation of reperfusion therapy (Fig. 295-3). The greatest delay usually occurs not during transportation to the hospital but, rather, between the onset of pain and the patient's decision to call for help. This delay can best be reduced by health care professionals educating the public concerning the significance of chest discomfort and the importance of seeking early medical attention. Regular office visits with patients having a history of or who are at risk for ischemic heart disease are important "teachable moments" for clinicians to review the symptoms of STEMI and the appropriate action plan.

Increasingly, monitoring and treatment are carried out by trained personnel in the ambulance, further shortening the time between the onset of the infarction and appropriate treatment. General guidelines for initiation of fibrinolysis in the prehospital setting include the ability to transmit 12-lead ECGs to confirm the diagnosis, the presence of paramedics in the ambulance, training of paramedics in the interpretation of ECGs and management of STEMI, and online medical command and control that can authorize the initiation of treatment in the field.

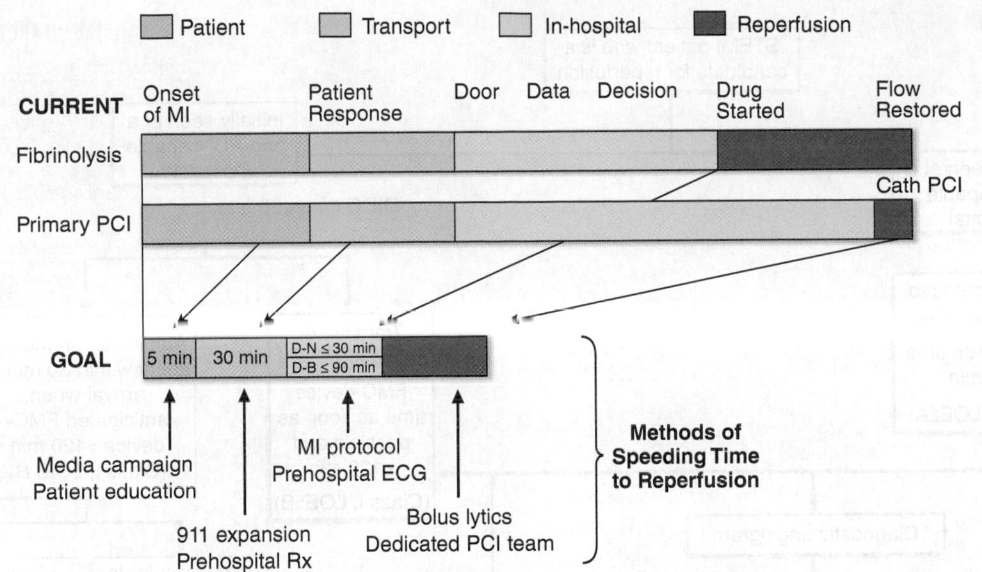

FIGURE 295-3 Major components of time delay between onset of symptoms from ST-segment elevation myocardial infarction and restoration of flow in the infarct-related artery. Plotted sequentially from left to right are the times for patients to recognize symptoms and seek medical attention, transportation to the hospital, in-hospital decision making, implementation of reperfusion strategy, and restoration of flow once the reperfusion strategy has been initiated. The time to initiate fibrinolytic therapy is the "door-to-needle" (D-N) time; this is followed by the period of time required for pharmacologic restoration of flow. More time is required to move the patient to the catheterization laboratory for a percutaneous coronary interventional (PCI) procedure, referred to as the "door-to-balloon" (D-B) time, but restoration of flow in the epicardial infarct-related artery occurs promptly after PCI. At the bottom is a variety of methods for speeding the time to reperfusion along with the goals for the time intervals for the various components of the time delay. *(Adapted from CP Cannon et al: J Thromb Thrombol 1:27, 1994.)*

MANAGEMENT IN THE EMERGENCY DEPARTMENT

In the Emergency Department, the goals for the management of patients with suspected STEMI include control of cardiac discomfort, rapid identification of patients who are candidates for urgent reperfusion therapy, triage of lower-risk patients to the appropriate location in the hospital, and avoidance of inappropriate discharge of patients with STEMI. Many aspects of the treatment of STEMI are initiated in the Emergency Department and then continued during the in-hospital phase of management (Fig. 295-4). The overarching goal is to minimize the time from first medical contact to initiation of reperfusion therapy. This may involve transfer from a non-PCI hospital to one that is PCI capable, with a goal of initiating PCI within 120 min of first medical contact (Fig. 295-4).

Aspirin is essential in the management of patients with suspected STEMI and is effective across the entire spectrum of acute coronary syndromes (Fig. 295-1). Rapid inhibition of cyclooxygenase-1 in platelets followed by a reduction of thromboxane A_2 levels is achieved by buccal absorption of a chewed 160–325-mg tablet in the Emergency Department. This measure should be followed by daily oral administration of aspirin in a dose of 75–162 mg.

In patients whose arterial O_2 saturation is normal, supplemental O_2 is of limited if any clinical benefit and therefore is not cost-effective. However, when hypoxemia is present, O_2 should be administered by nasal prongs or face mask (2–4 L/min) for the first 6–12 h after infarction; the patient should then be reassessed to determine if there is a continued need for such treatment.

CONTROL OF DISCOMFORT

Sublingual *nitroglycerin* can be given safely to most patients with STEMI. Up to three doses of 0.4 mg should be administered at about 5-min intervals. In addition to diminishing or abolishing chest discomfort, nitroglycerin may be capable of both decreasing myocardial oxygen demand (by lowering preload) and increasing myocardial oxygen supply (by dilating infarct-related coronary vessels or collateral vessels). In patients whose initially favorable response to sublingual nitroglycerin is followed by the return of chest discomfort, particularly if accompanied by other evidence of ongoing ischemia such as further ST-segment or T-wave shifts, the use of intravenous nitroglycerin should be considered. Therapy with nitrates should be avoided in patients who present with low systolic arterial pressure (<90 mmHg) or in whom there is clinical suspicion of RV infarction (inferior infarction on ECG, elevated jugular venous pressure, clear lungs, and hypotension). Nitrates should not be administered to patients who have taken a phosphodiesterase-5 inhibitor for erectile dysfunction within the preceding 24 h, because it may potentiate the hypotensive effects of nitrates. An idiosyncratic reaction to nitrates, consisting of sudden marked hypotension, sometimes occurs but can usually be reversed promptly by the rapid administration of intravenous atropine.

Morphine is a very effective analgesic for the pain associated with STEMI. However, it may reduce sympathetically mediated arteriolar and venous constriction, and the resulting venous pooling may reduce cardiac output and arterial pressure. These hemodynamic disturbances usually respond promptly to elevation of the legs, but in some patients, volume expansion with intravenous saline is required. The patient may experience diaphoresis and nausea, but these events usually pass and are replaced by a feeling of well-being associated with the relief of pain. Morphine also has a vagotonic effect and may cause bradycardia or advanced degrees of heart block, particularly in patients with inferior infarction. These side effects usually respond to atropine (0.5 mg intravenously). Morphine is routinely administered by repetitive (every 5 min) intravenous injection of small doses (2–4 mg), rather than by the subcutaneous administration of a larger quantity, because absorption may be unpredictable by the latter route.

Intravenous *beta blockers* are also useful in the control of the pain of STEMI. These drugs control pain effectively in some patients, presumably by diminishing myocardial O_2 demand and hence ischemia. More important, there is evidence that intravenous beta blockers reduce the risks of reinfarction and ventricular fibrillation (see "Beta-Adrenoceptor Blockers" below). However, patient selection is important when considering beta blockers for STEMI. Oral beta blocker therapy should be initiated in the first 24 h for patients who do not have any of the following: (1) signs of heart failure, (2) evidence of a low-output state, (3) increased risk for cardiogenic shock, or (4) other

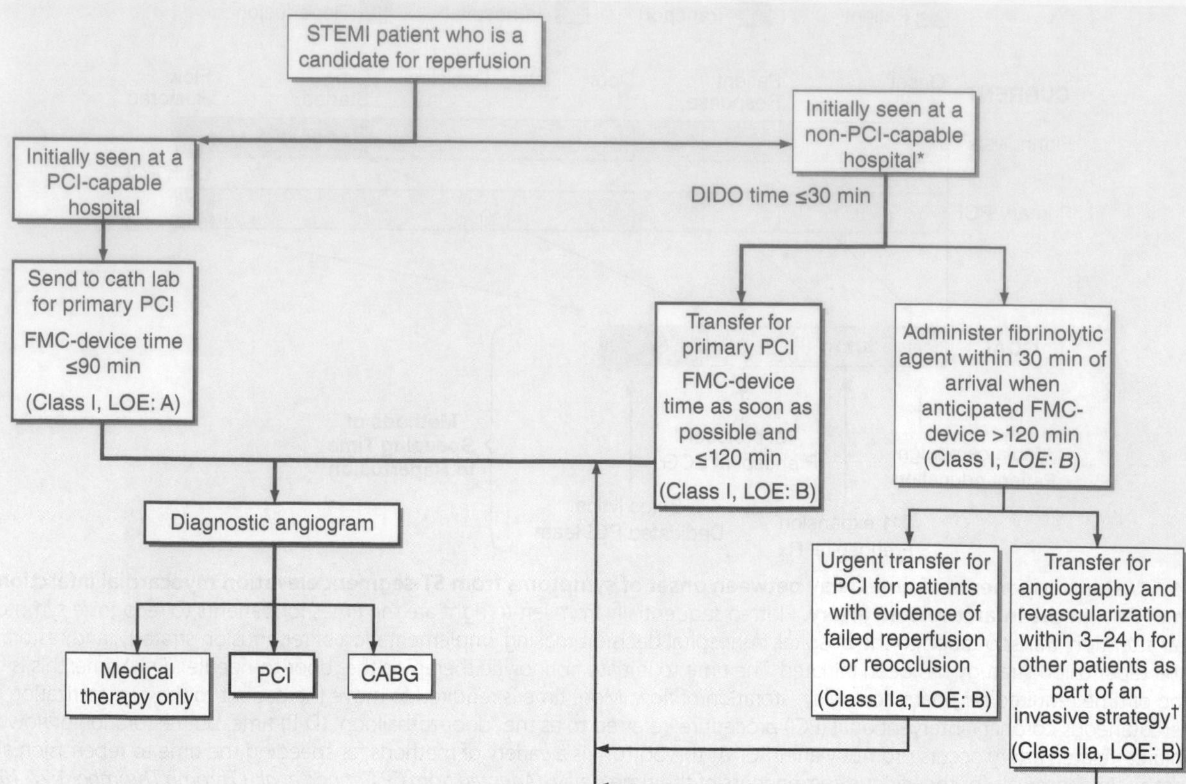

FIGURE 295-4 Reperfusion therapy for patients with ST-segment elevation myocardial infarction (STEMI). The *bold arrows* and *boxes* are the preferred strategies. Performance of percutaneous coronary intervention (PCI) is dictated by an anatomically appropriate culprit stenosis. *Patients with cardiogenic shock or severe heart failure initially seen at a non–PCI-capable hospital should be transferred for cardiac catheterization and revascularization as soon as possible, irrespective of time delay from myocardial infarction (MI) onset (Class I, LOE: B). †Angiography and revascularization should not be performed within the first 2 to 3 hours after administration of fibrinolytic therapy. CABG, coronary artery bypass graft; DIDO, door-in–door-out; FMC, first medical contact; LOE, level of evidence; STEMI, ST-elevation myocardial infarction. *(Adapted with permission from P O'Gara et al: Circulation 127:e362, 2013.)*

relative contraindications to beta blockade (PR interval greater than 0.24 seconds, second- or third-degree heart block, active asthma, or reactive airway disease). A commonly employed regimen is metoprolol, 5 mg every 2–5 min for a total of three doses, provided the patient has a heart rate >60 beats/min, systolic pressure >100 mmHg, a PR interval <0.24 s, and rales that are no higher than 10 cm up from the diaphragm. Fifteen minutes after the last intravenous dose, an oral regimen is initiated of 50 mg every 6 h for 48 h, followed by 100 mg every 12 h.

Unlike beta blockers, calcium antagonists are of little value in the acute setting, and there is evidence that short-acting dihydropyridines may be associated with an increased mortality risk.

MANAGEMENT STRATEGIES

The primary tool for screening patients and making triage decisions is the initial 12-lead ECG. When ST-segment elevation of at least 2 mm in two contiguous precordial leads and 1 mm in two adjacent limb leads is present, a patient should be considered a candidate for *reperfusion therapy* (Fig. 295-4). The process of selecting patients for fibrinolysis versus primary PCI (angioplasty or stenting; Chap. 296e) is discussed below. In the absence of ST-segment elevation, fibrinolysis is not helpful, and evidence exists suggesting that it may be harmful.

LIMITATION OF INFARCT SIZE

The quantity of myocardium that becomes necrotic as a consequence of a coronary artery occlusion is determined by factors other than just the site of occlusion. While the central zone of the infarct contains necrotic tissue that is irretrievably lost, the fate of the surrounding ischemic myocardium (ischemic penumbra) may be improved by timely restoration of coronary perfusion, reduction of myocardial O_2 demands, prevention of the accumulation of noxious metabolites, and blunting of the impact of mediators of reperfusion injury (e.g., calcium overload and oxygen-derived free radicals). Up to one-third of patients with STEMI may achieve *spontaneous* reperfusion of the infarct-related coronary artery within 24 h and experience improved healing of infarcted tissue. Reperfusion, either pharmacologically (by fibrinolysis) or by PCI, accelerates the opening of infarct-related arteries in those patients in whom spontaneous fibrinolysis ultimately would have occurred and also greatly increases the number of patients in whom restoration of flow in the infarct-related artery is accomplished. Timely restoration of flow in the epicardial infarct–related artery combined with improved perfusion of the downstream zone of infarcted myocardium results in a limitation of infarct size. Protection of the ischemic myocardium by the maintenance of an optimal balance between myocardial O_2 supply and demand through pain control, treatment of congestive heart failure (CHF), and minimization of tachycardia and hypertension extends the "window" of time for the salvage of myocardium by reperfusion strategies.

Glucocorticoids and nonsteroidal anti-inflammatory agents, with the exception of aspirin, should be avoided in patients with STEMI. They can impair infarct healing and increase the risk of myocardial rupture, and their use may result in a larger infarct scar. In addition, they can increase coronary vascular resistance, thereby potentially reducing flow to ischemic myocardium.

PRIMARY PERCUTANEOUS CORONARY INTERVENTION

(See also Chap. 296e) PCI, usually angioplasty and/or stenting without preceding fibrinolysis, referred to as *primary PCI*, is effective in restoring perfusion in STEMI when carried out on an emergency basis in the first few hours of MI. It has the advantage of being applicable to patients who have contraindications to fibrinolytic therapy (see below) but otherwise are considered appropriate candidates for reperfusion. It appears to be more effective than fibrinolysis in opening occluded coronary arteries and, *when performed by experienced operators in dedicated medical centers*, is associated with better short-term and long-term clinical outcomes. Compared with fibrinolysis, primary PCI is generally preferred when the diagnosis is in doubt, cardiogenic shock is present, bleeding risk is increased, or symptoms have been present for at least 2–3 h when the clot is more mature and less easily lysed by fibrinolytic drugs. However, PCI is expensive in terms of personnel and facilities, and its applicability is limited by its availability, around the clock, in only a minority of hospitals (Fig. 295-4).

FIBRINOLYSIS

If no contraindications are present (see below), fibrinolytic therapy should ideally be initiated within 30 min of presentation (i.e., door-to-needle time ≤30 min). The principal goal of fibrinolysis is prompt restoration of full coronary arterial patency. The fibrinolytic agents tissue plasminogen activator (tPA), streptokinase, tenecteplase (TNK), and reteplase (rPA) have been approved by the U.S. Food and Drug Administration for intravenous use in patients with STEMI. These drugs all act by promoting the conversion of plasminogen to plasmin, which subsequently lyses fibrin thrombi. Although considerable emphasis was first placed on a distinction between more fibrin-specific agents, such as tPA, and non-fibrin-specific agents, such as streptokinase, it is now recognized that these differences are only relative, as some degree of systemic fibrinolysis occurs with the former agents. TNK and rPA are referred to as *bolus fibrinolytics* since their administration does not require a prolonged intravenous infusion.

When assessed angiographically, flow in the culprit coronary artery is described by a simple qualitative scale called the *Thrombolysis in Myocardial Infarction (TIMI) grading system*: grade 0 indicates complete occlusion of the infarct-related artery; grade 1 indicates some penetration of the contrast material beyond the point of obstruction but without perfusion of the distal coronary bed; grade 2 indicates perfusion of the entire infarct vessel into the distal bed, but with flow that is delayed compared with that of a normal artery; and grade 3 indicates full perfusion of the infarct vessel with normal flow. The latter is the goal of reperfusion therapy, because full perfusion of the infarct-related coronary artery yields far better results in terms of limiting infarct size, maintenance of LV function, and reduction of both short- and long-term mortality rates. Additional methods of angiographic assessment of the efficacy of fibrinolysis include counting the number of frames on the cine film required for dye to flow from the origin of the infarct-related artery to a landmark in the distal vascular bed (*TIMI frame count*) and determining the rate of entry and exit of contrast dye from the microvasculature in the myocardial infarct zone (*TIMI myocardial perfusion grade*). These methods have an even tighter correlation with outcomes after STEMI than the more commonly employed TIMI flow grade.

tPA and the other relatively fibrin-specific plasminogen activators, rPA and TNK, are more effective than streptokinase at restoring full perfusion—i.e., TIMI grade 3 coronary flow—and have a small edge in improving survival as well. The current recommended regimen of tPA consists of a 15-mg bolus followed by 50 mg intravenously over the first 30 min, followed by 35 mg over the next 60 min. Streptokinase is administered as 1.5 million units (MU) intravenously over 1 h. rPA is administered in a double-bolus regimen consisting of a 10-MU bolus given over 2–3 min, followed by a second 10-MU bolus 30 min later. TNK is given as a single weight-based intravenous bolus of 0.53 mg/kg over 10 s. In addition to the fibrinolytic agents discussed earlier, pharmacologic reperfusion typically involves adjunctive antiplatelet and antithrombotic drugs, as discussed subsequently.

Clear contraindications to the use of fibrinolytic agents include a history of cerebrovascular hemorrhage at any time, a nonhemorrhagic stroke or other cerebrovascular event within the past year, marked hypertension (a reliably determined systolic arterial pressure >180 mmHg and/or a diastolic pressure >110 mmHg) at any time during the acute presentation, suspicion of aortic dissection, and active internal bleeding (excluding menses). While advanced age is associated with an increase in hemorrhagic complications, the benefit of fibrinolytic therapy in the elderly appears to justify its use if no other contraindications are present and the amount of myocardium in jeopardy appears to be substantial.

Relative contraindications to fibrinolytic therapy, which require assessment of the risk-to-benefit ratio, include current use of anticoagulants (international normalized ratio ≥2), a recent (<2 weeks) invasive or surgical procedure or prolonged (>10 min) cardiopulmonary resuscitation, known bleeding diathesis, pregnancy, a hemorrhagic ophthalmic condition (e.g., hemorrhagic diabetic retinopathy), active peptic ulcer disease, and a history of severe hypertension that is currently adequately controlled. Because of the risk of an allergic reaction, patients should not receive streptokinase if that agent had been received within the preceding 5 days to 2 years.

Allergic reactions to streptokinase occur in ~2% of patients who receive it. While a minor degree of hypotension occurs in 4–10% of patients given this agent, marked hypotension occurs, although rarely, in association with severe allergic reactions.

Hemorrhage is the most frequent and potentially the most serious complication. Because bleeding episodes that require transfusion are more common when patients require invasive procedures, unnecessary venous or arterial interventions should be avoided in patients receiving fibrinolytic agents. Hemorrhagic stroke is the most serious complication and occurs in ~0.5–0.9% of patients being treated with these agents. This rate increases with advancing age, with patients >70 years experiencing roughly twice the rate of intracranial hemorrhage as those <65 years. Large-scale trials have suggested that the rate of intracranial hemorrhage with tPA or rPA is slightly higher than with streptokinase.

INTEGRATED REPERFUSION STRATEGY

Evidence has emerged that suggests PCI plays an increasingly important role in the management of STEMI. Prior approaches that segregated the pharmacologic and catheter-based approaches to reperfusion have now been replaced with an integrated approach to triage and transfer of STEMI patients to receive PCI (Fig. 295-4). To achieve the degree of integration required to care for a patient with STEMI, all communities should create and maintain a regional system of STEMI care that includes assessment and continuous quality improvement of emergency medical services and hospital-based activities.

Cardiac catheterization and coronary angiography should be carried out after fibrinolytic therapy if there is evidence of either (1) failure of reperfusion (persistent chest pain and ST-segment elevation >90 min), in which case a *rescue PCI* should be considered; or (2) coronary artery reocclusion (re-elevation of ST segments and/or recurrent chest pain) or the development of recurrent ischemia (such as recurrent angina in the early hospital course or a positive exercise stress test before discharge), in which case an *urgent PCI* should be considered. Routine angiography and *elective PCI* even in asymptomatic patients following administration of fibrinolytic therapy are used with less frequency, given the numerous technologic advances that have occurred in the catheterization laboratory and the increasing number of skilled interventionalists. Coronary artery bypass surgery should be reserved for patients whose coronary anatomy is unsuited to PCI but in whom revascularization appears to be advisable because of extensive jeopardized myocardium or recurrent ischemia.

HOSPITAL PHASE MANAGEMENT

CORONARY CARE UNITS

These units are routinely equipped with a system that permits continuous monitoring of the cardiac rhythm of each patient and hemodynamic monitoring in selected patients. Defibrillators, respirators, noninvasive transthoracic pacemakers, and facilities for introducing pacing catheters and flow-directed balloon-tipped catheters are also usually available. Equally important is the organization of a highly trained team of nurses who can recognize arrhythmias; adjust the dosage of antiarrhythmic, vasoactive, and anticoagulant drugs; and perform cardiac resuscitation, including electroshock, when necessary.

Patients should be admitted to a coronary care unit early in their illness when it is expected that they will derive benefit from the sophisticated and expensive care provided. The availability of electrocardiographic monitoring and trained personnel outside the coronary care unit has made it possible to admit lower-risk patients (e.g., those not hemodynamically compromised and without active arrhythmias) to "intermediate care units."

The duration of stay in the coronary care unit is dictated by the ongoing need for intensive care. If symptoms are controlled with oral therapy, patients may be transferred out of the coronary care unit. Also, patients who have a confirmed STEMI but who are considered to be at low risk (no prior infarction and no persistent chest discomfort, CHF, hypotension, or cardiac arrhythmias) may be safely transferred out of the coronary care unit within 24 h.

Activity Factors that increase the work of the heart during the initial hours of infarction may increase the size of the infarct. Therefore, patients with STEMI should be kept at bed rest for the first 6–12 h. However, in the absence of complications, patients should be encouraged, under supervision, to resume an upright posture by dangling their feet over the side of the bed and sitting in a chair within the first 24 h. This practice is psychologically beneficial and usually results in a reduction in the pulmonary capillary wedge pressure. In the absence of hypotension and other complications, by the second or third day, patients typically are ambulating in their room with increasing duration and frequency, and they may shower or stand at the sink to bathe. By day 3 after infarction, patients should be increasing their ambulation progressively to a goal of 185 m (600 ft) at least three times a day.

Diet Because of the risk of emesis and aspiration soon after STEMI, patients should receive either nothing or only clear liquids by mouth for the first 4–12 h. The typical coronary care unit diet should provide ≤30% of total calories as fat and have a cholesterol content of ≤300 mg/d. Complex carbohydrates should make up 50–55% of total calories. Portions should not be unusually large, and the menu should be enriched with foods that are high in potassium, magnesium, and fiber, but low in sodium. Diabetes mellitus and hypertriglyceridemia are managed by restriction of concentrated sweets in the diet.

Bowel Management Bed rest and the effect of the narcotics used for the relief of pain often lead to constipation. A bedside commode rather than a bedpan, a diet rich in bulk, and the routine use of a stool softener such as dioctyl sodium sulfosuccinate (200 mg/d) are recommended. If the patient remains constipated despite these measures, a laxative can be prescribed. Contrary to prior belief, it is safe to perform a gentle rectal examination on patients with STEMI.

Sedation Many patients require sedation during hospitalization to withstand the period of enforced inactivity with tranquility. Diazepam (5 mg), oxazepam (15–30 mg), or lorazepam (0.5–2 mg), given three to four times daily, is usually effective. An additional dose of any of the above medications may be given at night to ensure adequate sleep. Attention to this problem is especially important during the first few days in the coronary care unit, where the atmosphere of 24-h vigilance may interfere with the patient's sleep. However, sedation is no substitute for reassuring, quiet surroundings. Many drugs used in the coronary care unit, such as atropine, H_2 blockers, and narcotics, can produce delirium, particularly in the elderly. This effect should not be confused with agitation, and it is wise to conduct a thorough review of the patient's medications before arbitrarily prescribing additional doses of anxiolytics.

PHARMACOTHERAPY

ANTITHROMBOTIC AGENTS

The use of antiplatelet and anticoagulant therapy during the initial phase of STEMI is based on extensive laboratory and clinical evidence that thrombosis plays an important role in the pathogenesis of this condition. The primary goal of treatment with antiplatelet and anticoagulant agents is to maintain patency of the infarct-related artery, in conjunction with reperfusion strategies. A secondary goal is to reduce the patient's tendency to thrombosis and, thus, the likelihood of mural thrombus formation or deep venous thrombosis, either of which could result in pulmonary embolization. The degree to which antiplatelet and anticoagulant therapy achieves these goals partly determines how effectively it reduces the risk of mortality from STEMI.

As noted previously (see "Management in the Emergency Department" earlier), aspirin is the standard antiplatelet agent for patients with STEMI. The most compelling evidence for the benefits of antiplatelet therapy (mainly with aspirin) in STEMI is found in the comprehensive overview by the Antiplatelet Trialists' Collaboration. Data from nearly 20,000 patients with MI enrolled in 15 randomized trials were pooled and revealed a relative reduction of 27% in the mortality rate, from 14.2% in control patients to 10.4% in patients receiving antiplatelet agents.

Inhibitors of the $P2Y_{12}$ ADP receptor prevent activation and aggregation of platelets. The addition of the $P2Y_{12}$ inhibitor clopidogrel to background treatment with aspirin to STEMI patients reduces the risk of clinical events (death, reinfarction, stroke) and, in patients receiving fibrinolytic therapy, has been shown to prevent reocclusion of a successfully reperfused infarct artery. New $P2Y_{12}$ ADP receptor antagonists, such as prasugrel and ticagrelor, are more effective than clopidogrel in preventing ischemic complications in STEMI patients undergoing PCI, but are associated with an increased risk of bleeding. Glycoprotein IIb/IIIa receptor inhibitors appear useful for preventing thrombotic complications in patients with STEMI undergoing PCI.

The standard anticoagulant agent used in clinical practice is unfractionated heparin (UFH). The available data suggest that when UFH is added to a regimen of aspirin and a non-fibrin-specific thrombolytic agent such as streptokinase, additional mortality benefit occurs (about 5 lives saved per 1000 patients treated). It appears that the immediate administration of intravenous UFH, in addition to a regimen of aspirin and relatively fibrin-specific fibrinolytic agents (tPA, rPA, or TNK), helps to maintain patency of the infarct-related artery. This effect is achieved at the cost of a small increased risk of bleeding. The recommended dose of UFH is an initial bolus of 60 U/kg (maximum 4000 U) followed by an initial infusion of 12 U/kg per hour (maximum 1000 U/h). The activated partial thromboplastin time during maintenance therapy should be 1.5–2 times the control value.

Alternatives to UFH for anticoagulation of patients with STEMI are the low-molecular-weight heparin (LMWH) preparations, a synthetic version of the critical pentasaccharide sequence (fondaparinux), and the direct antithrombin bivalirudin. Advantages of LMWHs include high bioavailability permitting administration subcutaneously, reliable anticoagulation without monitoring, and greater antiXa:IIa activity. Enoxaparin has been shown to reduce significantly the composite endpoints of death/nonfatal reinfarction and death/nonfatal reinfarction/urgent revascularization compared with UFH in STEMI patients who receive fibrinolysis. Treatment with enoxaparin is associated with higher rates of serious bleeding, but net clinical benefit—a composite endpoint that combines efficacy and safety—still favors enoxaparin over UFH. Interpretation of the data on fondaparinux is difficult because of the complex nature of the pivotal clinical trial evaluating it in STEMI (OASIS-6). Fondaparinux appears superior to placebo in STEMI patients not receiving reperfusion therapy, but its relative efficacy and safety compared with UFH is less certain. Due to the risk of catheter thrombosis, fondaparinux should not be used alone at the time of coronary angiography and PCI but should be combined with another anticoagulant with antithrombin activity such as UFH or bivalirudin. Contemporary trials of bivalirudin used an open-label design to evaluate its efficacy and safety compared with UFH plus a glycoprotein IIb/IIIa inhibitor. Bivalirudin was associated with a lower rate of bleeding, largely driven by reductions in vascular access site hematomas ≥5 cm or the administration of blood transfusions.

Patients with an anterior location of the infarction, severe LV dysfunction, heart failure, a history of embolism, two-dimensional echocardiographic evidence of mural thrombus, or atrial fibrillation are at increased risk of systemic or pulmonary thromboembolism. Such individuals should receive full therapeutic levels of anticoagulant therapy (LMWH or UFH) while hospitalized, followed by at least 3 months of warfarin therapy.

BETA-ADRENOCEPTOR BLOCKERS

The benefits of beta blockers in patients with STEMI can be divided into those that occur immediately when the drug is given acutely and those that accrue over the long term when the drug is given for secondary prevention after an infarction. Acute intravenous beta blockade improves the myocardial O_2 supply-demand relationship, decreases pain, reduces infarct size, and decreases the incidence of serious ventricular arrhythmias. In patients who undergo fibrinolysis soon after the onset of chest pain, no incremental reduction in mortality rate is seen with beta blockers, but recurrent ischemia and reinfarction are reduced.

Thus, beta-blocker therapy after STEMI is useful for most patients (including those treated with an angiotensin-converting enzyme [ACE] inhibitor) except those in whom it is specifically contraindicated (patients with heart failure or severely compromised LV function, heart block, orthostatic hypotension, or a history of asthma) and perhaps those whose excellent long-term prognosis (defined as an expected mortality rate of <1% per year, patients <55 years, no previous MI, with normal ventricular function, no complex ventricular ectopy, and no angina) markedly diminishes any potential benefit.

INHIBITION OF THE RENIN-ANGIOTENSIN-ALDOSTERONE SYSTEM

ACE inhibitors reduce the mortality rate after STEMI, and the mortality benefits are additive to those achieved with aspirin and beta blockers. The maximum benefit is seen in high-risk patients (those who are elderly or who have an anterior infarction, a prior infarction, and/or globally depressed LV function), but evidence suggests that a short-term benefit occurs when ACE inhibitors are prescribed unselectively to all hemodynamically stable patients with STEMI (i.e., those with a systolic pressure >100 mmHg). The mechanism involves a reduction in ventricular remodeling after infarction (see "Ventricular Dysfunction" later) with a subsequent reduction in the risk of CHF. The rate of recurrent infarction may also be lower in patients treated chronically with ACE inhibitors after infarction.

Before hospital discharge, LV function should be assessed with an imaging study. ACE inhibitors should be continued indefinitely in patients who have clinically evident CHF, in patients in whom an imaging study shows a reduction in global LV function or a large regional wall motion abnormality, or in those who are hypertensive.

Angiotensin receptor blockers (ARBs) should be administered to STEMI patients who are intolerant of ACE inhibitors and who have either clinical or radiologic signs of heart failure. Long-term aldosterone blockade should be prescribed for STEMI patients without significant renal dysfunction (creatinine ≥2.5 mg/dL in men and ≥2.0 mg/dL in women) or hyperkalemia (potassium ≥5.0 mEq/L) who are already receiving therapeutic doses of an ACE inhibitor, have an LV ejection fraction ≤40%, and have either symptomatic heart failure or diabetes mellitus. A multidrug regimen for inhibiting the renin-angiotensin-aldosterone system has been shown to reduce both heart failure–related and sudden cardiac death–related cardiovascular mortality after STEMI, but has not been as thoroughly explored as ACE inhibitors in STEMI patients.

OTHER AGENTS

Favorable effects on the ischemic process and ventricular remodeling (see below) previously led many physicians to routinely use *intravenous nitroglycerin* (5–10 μg/min initial dose and up to 200 μg/min as long as hemodynamic stability is maintained) for the first 24–48 h after the onset of infarction. However, the benefits of routine use of intravenous nitroglycerin are less in the contemporary era where beta-adrenoceptor blockers and ACE inhibitors are routinely prescribed for patients with STEMI.

Results of multiple trials of different calcium antagonists have failed to establish a role for these agents in the treatment of most patients with STEMI. Therefore, the routine use of calcium antagonists cannot be recommended. Strict control of blood glucose in diabetic patients with STEMI has been shown to reduce the mortality rate. Serum magnesium should be measured in all patients on admission, and any demonstrated deficits should be corrected to minimize the risk of arrhythmias.

COMPLICATIONS AND THEIR MANAGEMENT

VENTRICULAR DYSFUNCTION

After STEMI, the left ventricle undergoes a series of changes in shape, size, and thickness in both the infarcted and noninfarcted segments. This process is referred to as *ventricular remodeling* and generally precedes the development of clinically evident CHF in the months to years after infarction. Soon after STEMI, the left ventricle begins to dilate. Acutely, this results from expansion of the infarct, i.e., slippage of muscle bundles, disruption of normal myocardial cells, and tissue loss within the necrotic zone, resulting in disproportionate thinning and elongation of the infarct zone. Later, lengthening of the noninfarcted segments occurs as well. The overall chamber enlargement that occurs is related to the size and location of the infarct, with greater dilation following infarction of the anterior wall and apex of the left ventricle and causing more marked hemodynamic impairment, more frequent heart failure, and a poorer prognosis. Progressive dilation and its clinical consequences may be ameliorated by therapy with ACE inhibitors and other vasodilators (e.g., nitrates). In patients with an ejection fraction <40%, regardless of whether or not heart failure is present, ACE inhibitors or ARBs should be prescribed (see "Inhibition of the Renin-Angiotensin-Aldosterone System" earlier).

HEMODYNAMIC ASSESSMENT

Pump failure is now the primary cause of in-hospital death from STEMI. The extent of infarction correlates well with the degree of pump failure and with mortality, both early (within 10 days of infarction) and later. The most common clinical signs are pulmonary rales and S_3 and S_4 gallop sounds. Pulmonary congestion is also frequently seen on the chest roentgenogram. Elevated LV filling pressure and elevated pulmonary artery pressure are the characteristic hemodynamic findings, but these findings may result from a reduction of ventricular compliance (diastolic failure) and/or a reduction of stroke volume with secondary cardiac dilation (systolic failure) (Chap. 279).

A classification originally proposed by Killip divides patients into four groups: class I, no signs of pulmonary or venous congestion; class II, moderate heart failure as evidenced by rales at the lung bases, S_3 gallop, tachypnea, or signs of failure of the right side of the heart, including venous and hepatic congestion; class III, severe heart failure, pulmonary edema; and class IV, shock with systolic pressure <90 mmHg and evidence of peripheral vasoconstriction, peripheral cyanosis, mental confusion, and oliguria. When this classification was established in 1967, the expected hospital mortality rate of patients in these classes was as follows: class I, 0–5%; class II, 10–20%; class III, 35–45%; and class IV, 85–95%. With advances in management, the mortality rate in each class has fallen, perhaps by as much as one-third to one-half.

Hemodynamic evidence of abnormal global LV function appears when contraction is seriously impaired in 20–25% of the left ventricle. Infarction of ≥40% of the left ventricle usually results in cardiogenic shock (Chap. 326). Positioning of a balloon flotation (Swan-Ganz) catheter in the pulmonary artery permits monitoring of LV filling pressure; this technique is useful in patients who exhibit hypotension and/or clinical evidence of CHF. Cardiac output can also be determined with a pulmonary artery catheter. With the addition of intra-arterial pressure monitoring, systemic vascular resistance can be calculated as a guide to adjusting vasopressor and vasodilator therapy. Some patients with STEMI have markedly elevated LV filling pressures (>22 mmHg) and normal cardiac indices (2.6–3.6 L/[min/m^2]), while others have relatively low LV filling pressures (<15 mmHg) and reduced cardiac indices. The former patients usually benefit from diuresis, while the latter may respond to volume expansion.

HYPOVOLEMIA

This is an easily corrected condition that may contribute to the hypotension and vascular collapse associated with STEMI in some patients. It may be secondary to previous diuretic use, to reduced fluid intake during the early stages of the illness, and/or to vomiting associated with pain or medications. Consequently, hypovolemia should be identified and corrected in patients with STEMI and hypotension before more vigorous forms of therapy are begun. Central venous pressure reflects RV rather than LV filling pressure and is an inadequate guide for adjustment of blood volume, because LV function is almost always affected much more adversely than RV function in patients with STEMI. The optimal LV filling or pulmonary artery wedge pressure may vary considerably among patients. Each patient's ideal level (generally ~20 mmHg) is reached by cautious fluid administration during careful monitoring of oxygenation and cardiac output. Eventually, the cardiac output level plateaus, and further increases in LV filling pressure only increase congestive symptoms and decrease systemic oxygenation without raising arterial pressure.

TREATMENT CONGESTIVE HEART FAILURE

The management of CHF in association with STEMI is similar to that of acute heart failure secondary to other forms of heart disease (avoidance of hypoxemia, diuresis, afterload reduction, inotropic support) (Chap. 279), except that the benefits of digitalis administration to patients with STEMI are unimpressive. By contrast, diuretic agents are extremely effective, as they diminish pulmonary congestion in the presence of systolic and/or diastolic heart failure. LV filling pressure falls and orthopnea and dyspnea improve after the intravenous administration of furosemide or other loop diuretics. These drugs should be used with caution, however, as they can result in a massive diuresis with associated decreases in plasma volume, cardiac output, systemic blood pressure, and, hence, coronary perfusion. Nitrates in various forms may be used to decrease preload and congestive symptoms. Oral isosorbide dinitrate, topical nitroglycerin ointment, and intravenous nitroglycerin all have the advantage over a diuretic of lowering preload through venodilation without decreasing the total plasma volume. In addition, nitrates may improve ventricular compliance if ischemia is present, as ischemia causes an elevation of LV filling pressure. Vasodilators must be used with caution to prevent serious hypotension. As noted earlier, ACE inhibitors are an ideal class of drugs for management of ventricular dysfunction after STEMI, especially for the long term. (See "Inhibition of the Renin-Angiotensin-Aldosterone System" earlier.)

CARDIOGENIC SHOCK

Prompt reperfusion, efforts to reduce infarct size and treatment of ongoing ischemia and other complications of MI appear to have reduced the incidence of cardiogenic shock from 20% to about 7%. Only 10% of patients with this condition present with it on admission, while 90% develop it during hospitalization. Typically, patients who develop cardiogenic shock have severe multivessel coronary artery disease with evidence of "piecemeal" necrosis extending outward from the original infarct zone. The evaluation and management of cardiogenic shock and severe power failure after STEMI are discussed in detail in Chap. 326.

RIGHT VENTRICULAR INFARCTION

Approximately one-third of patients with inferior infarction demonstrate at least a minor degree of RV necrosis. An occasional patient with inferoposterior LV infarction also has extensive RV infarction, and rare patients present with infarction limited primarily to the RV. Clinically significant RV infarction causes signs of severe RV failure (jugular venous distention, Kussmaul's sign, hepatomegaly [Chap. 267]) with or without hypotension. ST-segment elevations of right-sided precordial ECG leads, particularly lead V_4R, are frequently present in the first 24 h in patients with RV infarction. Two-dimensional echocardiography is helpful in determining the degree of RV dysfunction. Catheterization of the right side of the heart often reveals a distinctive hemodynamic pattern resembling constrictive pericarditis (steep right atrial "y" descent and an early diastolic dip and plateau in RV waveforms) (Chap. 288). Therapy consists of volume expansion to maintain adequate RV preload and efforts to improve LV performance with attendant reduction in pulmonary capillary wedge and pulmonary arterial pressures.

ARRHYTHMIAS

(See also Chaps. 274 and 276) The incidence of arrhythmias after STEMI is higher in patients seen early after the onset of symptoms. The mechanisms responsible for infarction-related arrhythmias include autonomic nervous system imbalance, electrolyte disturbances, ischemia, and slowed conduction in zones of ischemic myocardium. An arrhythmia can usually be managed successfully if trained personnel and appropriate equipment are available when it develops. Since most deaths from arrhythmia occur during the first few hours after infarction, the effectiveness of treatment relates directly to the speed with which patients come under medical observation. The prompt management of arrhythmias constitutes a significant advance in the treatment of STEMI.

Ventricular Premature Beats Infrequent, sporadic ventricular premature depolarizations occur in almost all patients with STEMI and do not require therapy. Whereas in the past, frequent, multifocal, or early diastolic ventricular extrasystoles (so-called warning arrhythmias) were routinely treated with antiarrhythmic drugs to reduce the risk of development of ventricular tachycardia and ventricular fibrillation, pharmacologic therapy is now reserved for patients with sustained ventricular arrhythmias. Prophylactic antiarrhythmic therapy (either intravenous lidocaine early or oral agents later) is contraindicated for ventricular premature beats in the absence of clinically important ventricular tachyarrhythmias, because such therapy may actually increase the mortality rate. Beta-adrenoceptor blocking agents are effective in abolishing ventricular ectopic activity in patients with STEMI and in the prevention of ventricular fibrillation. As described earlier (see "Beta-Adrenoceptor Blockers"), they should be used routinely in patients without contraindications. In addition, hypokalemia and hypomagnesemia are risk factors for ventricular fibrillation in patients with STEMI; to reduce the risk, the serum potassium concentration should be adjusted to approximately 4.5 mmol/L and magnesium to about 2.0 mmol/L.

Ventricular Tachycardia and Fibrillation Within the first 24 h of STEMI, ventricular tachycardia and fibrillation can occur without prior warning arrhythmias. The occurrence of ventricular fibrillation can be reduced by prophylactic administration of intravenous lidocaine. However, prophylactic use of lidocaine has not been shown to reduce overall mortality from STEMI. In fact, in addition to causing possible noncardiac complications, lidocaine may predispose to an excess risk of bradycardia and asystole. For these reasons, and with earlier treatment of active ischemia, more frequent use of beta-blocking agents, and the nearly universal success of electrical cardioversion or defibrillation, routine prophylactic antiarrhythmic drug therapy *is no longer recommended.*

Sustained ventricular tachycardia that is well tolerated hemodynamically should be treated with an intravenous regimen of amiodarone (bolus of 150 mg over 10 min, followed by infusion of 1.0 mg/min for 6 h and then 0.5 mg/min) or procainamide (bolus of 15 mg/kg over 20–30 min; infusion of 1–4 mg/min); if it does not stop promptly, electroversion should be used (Chap. 276). An unsynchronized discharge of 200–300 J (monophasic waveform; approximately 50% of these energies with biphasic waveforms) is used immediately in patients with ventricular fibrillation or when ventricular tachycardia causes hemodynamic deterioration. Ventricular tachycardia or fibrillation that is refractory to electroshock may be more responsive after the patient is treated with epinephrine (1 mg intravenously or 10 mL of a 1:10,000 solution via the intracardiac route) or amiodarone (a 75–150-mg bolus).

Ventricular arrhythmias, including the unusual form of ventricular tachycardia known as torsades des pointes (Chaps. 276 and 277), may occur in patients with STEMI as a consequence of other concurrent problems (such as hypoxia, hypokalemia, or other electrolyte disturbances) or of the toxic effects of an agent being administered to the patient (such as digoxin or quinidine). A search for such secondary causes should always be undertaken.

Although the in-hospital mortality rate is increased, the long-term survival is excellent in patients who survive to hospital discharge after *primary* ventricular fibrillation; i.e., ventricular fibrillation that is a primary response to acute ischemia that occurs during the first 48 h and is not associated with predisposing factors such as CHF, shock, bundle branch block, or ventricular aneurysm. This result is in sharp contrast to the poor prognosis for patients who develop ventricular fibrillation *secondary* to severe pump failure. For patients who develop ventricular tachycardia or ventricular fibrillation late in their hospital course (i.e., after the first 48 h), the mortality rate is increased both in-hospital and during long-term follow-up. Such patients should be considered for electrophysiologic study and implantation of a cardioverter-defibrillator (ICD) (Chap. 276). A more challenging issue is the prevention of sudden cardiac death from ventricular fibrillation late after STEMI in patients who have not exhibited sustained ventricular tachyarrhythmias during their index hospitalization. An algorithm for selection of patients who warrant prophylactic implantation of an ICD is shown in Fig. 295-5.

Accelerated Idioventricular Rhythm Accelerated idioventricular rhythm (AIVR, "slow ventricular tachycardia"), a ventricular rhythm with a rate of 60–100 beats/min, often occurs transiently during fibrinolytic therapy at the time of reperfusion. For the most part, AIVR, whether it occurs in association with fibrinolytic therapy or spontaneously, is benign and does not presage the development of classic ventricular tachycardia. Most episodes of AIVR do not require treatment if the patient is monitored carefully, as degeneration into a more serious arrhythmia is rare.

Supraventricular Arrhythmias Sinus tachycardia is the most common supraventricular arrhythmia. If it occurs secondary to another cause

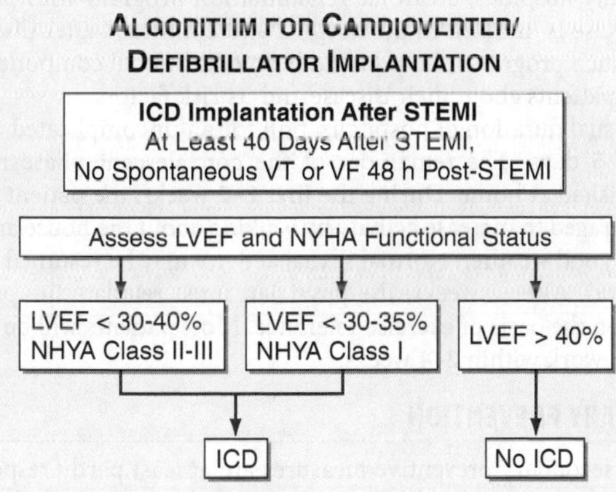

FIGURE 295-5 Algorithm for assessment of need for implantation of a cardioverter-defibrillator. The appropriate management is selected based on measurement of left ventricular ejection fraction and assessment of the New York Heart Association (NYHA) functional class. Patients with depressed left ventricular function at least 40 days after ST-segment elevation myocardial infarction (STEMI) are referred for insertion of an implantable cardioverter-defibrillator (ICD) if the left ventricular ejection fraction (LVEF) is <30–40% and they are in NYHA class II–III or if the LVEF is <30–35% and they are in NYHA class I functional status. Patients with preserved left ventricular function (LVEF >40%) do not receive an ICD regardless of NYHA functional class. All patients are treated with medical therapy after STEMI. VF, ventricular fibrillation; VT, ventricular tachycardia. *(Adapted from data contained in DP Zipes et al: ACC/AHA/ESC 2006 guidelines for management of patients with ventricular arrhythmias and the prevention of sudden cardiac death; a report of the American College of Cardiology/American Heart Association Task Force and the European Society of Cardiology Committee for Practice Guidelines [Writing Committee to Develop Guidelines for Management of Patients with Ventricular Arrhythmias and the Prevention of Sudden Cardiac Death]. J Am Coll Cardiol 48:1064, 2006.)*

(such as anemia, fever, heart failure, or a metabolic derangement), the primary problem should be treated first. However, if it appears to be due to sympathetic overstimulation (e.g., as part of a hyperdynamic state), then treatment with a beta blocker is indicated. Other common arrhythmias in this group are atrial flutter and atrial fibrillation, which are often secondary to LV failure. Digoxin is usually the treatment of choice for supraventricular arrhythmias if heart failure is present. If heart failure is absent, beta blockers, verapamil, or diltiazem are suitable alternatives for controlling the ventricular rate, as they may also help to control ischemia. If the abnormal rhythm persists for >2 h with a ventricular rate >120 beats/min, or if tachycardia induces heart failure, shock, or ischemia (as manifested by recurrent pain or ECG changes), a synchronized electroshock (100–200 J monophasic waveform) should be used.

Accelerated junctional rhythms have diverse causes but may occur in patients with inferoposterior infarction. Digitalis excess must be ruled out. In some patients with severely compromised LV function, the loss of appropriately timed atrial systole results in a marked reduction of cardiac output. Right atrial or coronary sinus pacing is indicated in such instances.

Sinus Bradycardia Treatment of sinus bradycardia is indicated if hemodynamic compromise results from the slow heart rate. Atropine is the most useful drug for increasing heart rate and should be given intravenously in doses of 0.5 mg initially. If the rate remains <50–60 beats/min, additional doses of 0.2 mg, up to a total of 2.0 mg, may be given. Persistent bradycardia (<40 beats/min) despite atropine may be treated with electrical pacing. Isoproterenol should be avoided.

Atrioventricular and Intraventricular Conduction Disturbances (See also Chap. 274) Both the in-hospital mortality rate and the postdischarge mortality rate of patients who have complete atrioventricular (AV) block in association with anterior infarction are markedly higher than those of patients who develop AV block with inferior infarction. This difference is related to the fact that heart block in inferior infarction is commonly a result of increased vagal tone and/or the release of adenosine and therefore is transient. In anterior wall infarction, however, heart block is usually related to ischemic malfunction of the conduction system, which is commonly associated with extensive myocardial necrosis.

Temporary electrical pacing provides an effective means of increasing the heart rate of patients with bradycardia due to AV block. However, acceleration of the heart rate may have only a limited impact on prognosis in patients with anterior wall infarction and complete heart block in whom the large size of the infarct is the major factor determining outcome. It should be carried out if it improves hemodynamics. Pacing does appear to be beneficial in patients with inferoposterior infarction who have complete heart block associated with heart failure, hypotension, marked bradycardia, or significant ventricular ectopic activity. A subgroup of these patients, those with RV infarction, often respond poorly to ventricular pacing because of the loss of the atrial contribution to ventricular filling. In such patients, dual-chamber AV sequential pacing may be required.

External noninvasive pacing electrodes should be positioned in a "demand" mode for patients with sinus bradycardia (rate <50 beats/min) that is unresponsive to drug therapy, Mobitz II second-degree AV block, third-degree heart block, or bilateral bundle branch block (e.g., right bundle branch block plus left anterior fascicular block). Retrospective studies suggest that permanent pacing may reduce the long-term risk of sudden death due to bradyarrhythmias in the rare patient who develops combined persistent bifascicular and transient third-degree heart block during the acute phase of MI.

OTHER COMPLICATIONS

Recurrent Chest Discomfort Because recurrent or persistent ischemia often heralds extension of the original infarct or reinfarction in a new myocardial zone and is associated with a near tripling of mortality after STEMI, patients with these symptoms should be referred for prompt coronary arteriography and mechanical revascularization.

Administration of a fibrinolytic agent is an alternative to early mechanical revascularization.

Pericarditis (See also Chap. 288) Pericardial friction rubs and/or pericardial pain are frequently encountered in patients with STEMI involving the epicardium. This complication can usually be managed with aspirin (650 mg four times daily). It is important to diagnose the chest pain of pericarditis accurately, because failure to recognize it may lead to the erroneous diagnosis of recurrent ischemic pain and/or infarct extension, with resulting inappropriate use of anticoagulants, nitrates, beta blockers, or coronary arteriography. When it occurs, complaints of pain radiating to either trapezius muscle is helpful, because such a pattern of discomfort is typical of pericarditis but rarely occurs with ischemic discomfort. Anticoagulants potentially could cause tamponade in the presence of acute pericarditis (as manifested by either pain or persistent rub) and therefore should not be used unless there is a compelling indication.

Thromboembolism Clinically apparent thromboembolism complicates STEMI in ~10% of cases, but embolic lesions are found in 20% of patients in necropsy series, suggesting that thromboembolism is often clinically silent. Thromboembolism is considered to be an important contributing cause of death in 25% of patients with STEMI who die after admission to the hospital. Arterial emboli originate from LV mural thrombi, while most pulmonary emboli arise in the leg veins.

Thromboembolism typically occurs in association with large infarcts (especially anterior), CHF, and an LV thrombus detected by echocardiography. The incidence of arterial embolism from a clot originating in the ventricle at the site of an infarction is small but real. Two-dimensional echocardiography reveals LV thrombi in about one-third of patients with anterior wall infarction but in few patients with inferior or posterior infarction. Arterial embolism often presents as a major complication, such as hemiparesis when the cerebral circulation is involved or hypertension if the renal circulation is compromised. When a thrombus has been clearly demonstrated by echocardiographic or other techniques or when a large area of regional wall motion abnormality is seen even in the absence of a detectable mural thrombus, systemic anticoagulation should be undertaken (in the absence of contraindications), as the incidence of embolic complications appears to be markedly lowered by such therapy. The appropriate duration of therapy is unknown, but 3–6 months is probably prudent.

Left Ventricular Aneurysm The term *ventricular aneurysm* is usually used to describe *dyskinesis* or local expansile paradoxical wall motion. Normally functioning myocardial fibers must shorten more if stroke volume and cardiac output are to be maintained in patients with ventricular aneurysm; if they cannot, overall ventricular function is impaired. True aneurysms are composed of scar tissue and neither predispose to nor are associated with cardiac rupture.

The complications of LV aneurysm do not usually occur for weeks to months after STEMI; they include CHF, arterial embolism, and ventricular arrhythmias. Apical aneurysms are the most common and the most easily detected by clinical examination. The physical finding of greatest value is a double, diffuse, or displaced apical impulse. Ventricular aneurysms are readily detected by two-dimensional echocardiography, which may also reveal a mural thrombus in an aneurysm.

Rarely, myocardial rupture may be contained by a local area of pericardium, along with organizing thrombus and hematoma. Over time, this *pseudoaneurysm* enlarges, maintaining communication with the LV cavity through a narrow neck. Because a pseudoaneurysm often ruptures spontaneously, it should be surgically repaired if recognized.

POSTINFARCTION RISK STRATIFICATION AND MANAGEMENT

Many clinical and laboratory factors have been identified that are associated with an increase in cardiovascular risk after initial recovery from STEMI. Some of the most important factors include persistent ischemia (spontaneous or provoked), depressed LV ejection fraction (<40%), rales above the lung bases on physical examination or congestion on chest radiograph, and symptomatic ventricular arrhythmias. Other features associated with increased risk include a history of previous MI, age >75, diabetes mellitus, prolonged sinus tachycardia, hypotension, ST-segment changes at rest without angina ("silent ischemia"), an abnormal signal-averaged ECG, nonpatency of the infarct-related coronary artery (if angiography is undertaken), and persistent advanced heart block or a new intraventricular conduction abnormality on the ECG. Therapy must be individualized on the basis of the relative importance of the risk(s) present.

The goal of preventing reinfarction and death after recovery from STEMI has led to strategies to evaluate risk after infarction. In stable patients, submaximal exercise stress testing may be carried out before hospital discharge to detect residual ischemia and ventricular ectopy and to provide the patient with a guideline for exercise in the early recovery period. Alternatively, or in addition, a maximal (symptom-limited) exercise stress test may be carried out 4–6 weeks after infarction. Evaluation of LV function is usually warranted as well. Recognition of a depressed LV ejection fraction by echocardiography or radionuclide ventriculography identifies patients who should receive medications to inhibit the renin-angiotensin-aldosterone system. Patients in whom angina is induced at relatively low workloads, those who have a large reversible defect on perfusion imaging or a depressed ejection fraction, those with demonstrable ischemia, and those in whom exercise provokes symptomatic ventricular arrhythmias should be considered at high risk for recurrent MI or death from arrhythmia (Fig. 295-5). Cardiac catheterization with coronary angiography and/or invasive electrophysiologic evaluation is advised.

Exercise tests also aid in formulating an individualized exercise prescription, which can be much more vigorous in patients who tolerate exercise without any of the previously mentioned adverse signs. In addition, predischarge stress testing may provide an important psychological benefit, building the patient's confidence by demonstrating a reasonable exercise tolerance.

In many hospitals, a cardiac rehabilitation program with progressive exercise is initiated in the hospital and continued after discharge. Ideally, such programs should include an educational component that informs patients about their disease and its risk factors.

The usual duration of hospitalization for an uncomplicated STEMI is about 5 days. The remainder of the convalescent phase may be accomplished at home. During the first 1–2 weeks, the patient should be encouraged to increase activity by walking about the house and outdoors in good weather. Normal sexual activity may be resumed during this period. After 2 weeks, the physician must regulate the patient's activity on the basis of exercise tolerance. Most patients will be able to return to work within 2–4 weeks.

SECONDARY PREVENTION

Various secondary preventive measures are at least partly responsible for the improvement in the long-term mortality and morbidity rates after STEMI. Long-term treatment with an antiplatelet agent (usually aspirin) after STEMI is associated with a 25% reduction in the risk of recurrent infarction, stroke, or cardiovascular mortality (36 fewer events for every 1000 patients treated). An alternative antiplatelet agent that may be used for secondary prevention in patients intolerant of aspirin is clopidogrel (75 mg orally daily). ACE inhibitors or ARBs and, in appropriate patients, aldosterone antagonists should be used indefinitely by patients with clinically evident heart failure, a moderate decrease in global ejection fraction, or a large regional wall motion abnormality to prevent late ventricular remodeling and recurrent ischemic events.

The chronic routine use of oral beta-adrenoceptor blockers for at least 2 years after STEMI is supported by well-conducted, placebo-controlled trials.

Evidence suggests that warfarin lowers the risk of late mortality and the incidence of reinfarction after STEMI. Most physicians prescribe aspirin routinely for all patients without contraindications and add warfarin for patients at increased risk of embolism (see "Thromboembolism" earlier). Several studies suggest that in patients

<75 years old a low dose of aspirin (75–81 mg/d) in combination with warfarin administered to achieve an international normalized ratio >2.0 is more effective than aspirin alone for preventing recurrent MI and embolic cerebrovascular accident. However, there is an increased risk of bleeding and a high rate of discontinuation of warfarin that has limited clinical acceptance of combination antithrombotic therapy. There is increased risk of bleeding when warfarin is added to dual antiplatelet therapy (aspirin and clopidogrel). However, patients who have had a stent implanted and have an indication for anticoagulation should receive dual antiplatelet therapies in combination with warfarin. Such patients should also receive a proton pump inhibitor to minimize the risk of gastrointestinal bleeding and should have regular monitoring of their hemoglobin levels and stool hematest while on combination antithrombotic therapy.

Finally, risk factors for *atherosclerosis* (Chap. 265e) should be discussed with the patient and, when possible, favorably modified.

296e Percutaneous Coronary Interventions and Other Interventional Procedures

David P. Faxon, Deepak L. Bhatt

This is a digital-only chapter. It is available on the DVD that accompanies this book, as well as on Access Medicine/Harrison's Online, and the eBook and "app" editions of HPIM 19e.

Percutaneous transluminal coronary angioplasty (PTCA) was first introduced by Andreas Gruentzig in 1977 as an alternative to coronary bypass surgery. The concept was initially demonstrated by Charles Dotter in 1964 in peripheral vessels. The development of a small inelastic balloon catheter by Gruentzig allowed expansion of the technique into smaller peripheral and coronary vessels. Initial coronary experience was limited to single-vessel coronary disease and discrete proximal lesions due to the technical limitations of the equipment. Advances in technology and greater operator experience allowed the procedure to grow rapidly with expanded use in patients with more complex lesions and multivessel disease. The introduction of coronary stents in 1994 was one of the major advances in the field. These devices reduced acute complications and reduced by half the significant problem of restenosis (or recurrence of the stenosis). Further reductions in restenosis were achieved by the introduction of drug-eluting stents in 2003. These stents slowly release antiproliferative drugs directly into the plaque over a few months. Percutaneous coronary intervention (PCI) is the most common revascularization procedure in the United States and is performed more than twice as often as coronary artery bypass surgery: nearly 600,000 patients a year.

Interventional cardiology is a separate discipline in cardiology that requires a dedicated 1-year interventional cardiology fellowship following a 3-year general cardiology fellowship in order to obtain a separate board certification. The discipline has also expanded to include interventions for structural heart disease including treatment of congenital heart disease and valvular heart disease; it also includes interventions to treat peripheral vascular disease, including atherosclerotic and nonatherosclerotic lesions in the carotid, renal, aortic, and peripheral circulations.

297e Atlas of Percutaneous Revascularization

Jane A. Leopold, Deepak L. Bhatt, David P. Faxon

This is a digital-only chapter. It is available on the DVD that accompanies this book, as well as on Access Medicine/Harrison's Online, and the eBook and "app" editions of HPIM 19e.

Percutaneous coronary intervention (PCI) is the most widely employed coronary revascularization procedure worldwide (Chap. 296e). It is now applied to patients with stable angina; patients with acute coronary syndromes, including unstable angina and non-ST-segment elevation myocardial infarction (NSTEMI); and as a primary treatment strategy in patients with ST-segment elevation myocardial infarction (STEMI). PCI is also applicable to patients with either single-vessel or multivessel disease.

In this chapter, the use of PCI will be illustrated in a variety of commonly encountered clinical and anatomic situations, such as chronic total occlusion of a coronary artery, bifurcation disease, acute STEMI, saphenous vein graft disease, left main coronary artery disease, multivessel disease, and stent thrombosis. In addition, the use of interventional techniques to treat structural heart disease will be shown, including closure of an atrial septal defect (ASD) and transcatheter aortic valve replacement (TAVR).

298 Hypertensive Vascular Disease

Theodore A. Kotchen

Hypertension is one of the leading causes of the global burden of disease. Approximately 7.6 million deaths (13–15% of the total) and 92 million disability-adjusted life years worldwide were attributable to high blood pressure in 2001. Hypertension doubles the risk of cardiovascular diseases, including coronary heart disease (CHD), congestive heart failure (CHF), ischemic and hemorrhagic stroke, renal failure, and peripheral arterial disease. It often is associated with additional cardiovascular disease risk factors, and the risk of cardiovascular disease increases with the total burden of risk factors. Although antihypertensive therapy reduces the risks of cardiovascular and renal disease, large segments of the hypertensive population are either untreated or inadequately treated.

EPIDEMIOLOGY

Blood pressure levels, the rate of age-related increases in blood pressure, and the prevalence of hypertension vary among countries and among subpopulations within a country. Hypertension is present in all populations except for a small number of individuals living in developing countries. In industrialized societies, blood pressure increases steadily during the first two decades of life. In children and adolescents, blood pressure is associated with growth and maturation. Blood pressure "tracks" over time in children and between adolescence and young adulthood. In the United States, average systolic blood pressure is higher for men than for women during early adulthood, although among older individuals the age-related rate of rise is steeper for women. Consequently, among individuals age 60 and older, systolic blood pressures of women are higher than those of men. Among adults, diastolic blood pressure also increases progressively with age until ~55 years, after which it tends to decrease. The consequence is a widening of pulse pressure (the difference between systolic and diastolic blood pressure) beyond age 60.

In the United States, based on results of the National Health and Nutrition Examination Survey (NHANES), approximately 30% (age-adjusted prevalence) of adults, or at least 65 million individuals, have hypertension (defined as any one of the following: systolic blood pressure ≥140 mmHg, diastolic blood pressure ≥90 mmHg, taking antihypertensive medications). Hypertension prevalence is 33.5% in non-Hispanic blacks, 28.9% in non-Hispanic whites, and 20.7% in Mexican Americans. The likelihood of hypertension increases with age, and among individuals age ≥60, the prevalence is 65.4%. Recent evidence suggests that the prevalence of hypertension in the United States may be increasing, possibly as a consequence of increasing obesity. The prevalence of hypertension and stroke mortality rates are higher in the southeastern United States than in other regions. In African Americans, hypertension appears earlier, is generally more severe, and results in higher rates of morbidity and mortality from stroke, left ventricular hypertrophy, CHF, and end-stage renal disease (ESRD) than in white Americans.

Both environmental and genetic factors may contribute to regional and racial variations in hypertension prevalence. Studies of societies undergoing "acculturation" and studies of migrants from a less to a more urbanized setting indicate a profound environmental contribution to blood pressure. Obesity and weight gain are strong, independent risk factors for hypertension. It has been estimated that 60% of hypertensives are >20% overweight. Among populations, hypertension prevalence is related to dietary NaCl intake, and the age-related increase in blood pressure may be augmented by a high NaCl intake. Low dietary intakes of calcium and potassium also may contribute to the risk of hypertension. The urine sodium-to-potassium ratio (an index of both sodium and potassium intakes) is a stronger correlate of blood pressure than is either sodium or potassium alone. Alcohol consumption, psychosocial stress, and low levels of physical activity also may contribute to hypertension.

Adoption, twin, and family studies document a significant heritable component to blood pressure levels and hypertension. Family studies controlling for a common environment indicate that blood pressure heritabilities are in the range 15–35%. In twin studies, heritability estimates of blood pressure are ~60% for males and 30–40% for females. High blood pressure before age 55 occurs 3.8 times more frequently among persons with a positive family history of hypertension. However, to date, only a fraction of high heritability estimates are accounted for by specific genetic determinants.

GENETIC CONSIDERATIONS

Although specific genetic variants have been identified in rare Mendelian forms of hypertension (Table 298–5), these variants are not applicable to the vast majority (>98%) of patients with hypertension. For most individuals, it is likely that hypertension represents a polygenic disorder in which a combination of genes acts in concert with environmental exposures to make only a modest contribution to blood pressure. Further, different subsets of genes may lead to different phenotypes associated with hypertension, e.g., obesity, dyslipidemia, insulin resistance.

Several strategies are being used in the search for specific hypertension-related genes. Animal models (including selectively bred rats and congenic rat strains) provide a powerful approach for evaluating genetic loci and genes associated with hypertension. Comparative mapping strategies allow for the identification of syntenic genomic regions between the rat and human genomes that may be involved in blood pressure regulation. In association studies, different alleles (or combinations of alleles at different loci) of specific candidate genes or chromosomal regions are compared in hypertensive patients and normotensive control subjects. Current evidence suggests that genes that encode components of the renin-angiotensin-aldosterone system, along with angiotensinogen and angiotensin-converting enzyme (ACE) polymorphisms, may be related to hypertension and to blood pressure sensitivity to dietary NaCl. The alpha-adducin gene is thought to be associated with increased renal tubular absorption of sodium, and variants of this gene may be associated with hypertension and salt sensitivity of blood pressure. Other genes possibly related to hypertension include genes encoding the AT_1 receptor, aldosterone synthase, atrial natriuretic peptide, and the β_2 adrenoreceptor. Genomewide association studies involve rapidly scanning markers across the entire genome to identify loci (not specific genes) associated with an observable trait (e.g., blood pressure) or a particular disease. This strategy has been facilitated by the availability of dense genotyping chips and the International HapMap. Results of candidate gene studies often have not been replicated, and in contrast to several other polygenic disorders, genomewide association studies have had limited success in identifying genetic determinants of hypertension.

Preliminary evidence suggests that there may also be genetic determinants of target organ damage attributed to hypertension. Family studies indicate significant heritability of left ventricular mass, and there is considerable individual variation in the responses of the heart to hypertension. Family studies and variations in candidate genes associated with renal damage suggest that genetic factors also may contribute to hypertensive nephropathy. Specific genetic variants have been linked to CHD and stroke.

In the future, it is possible that DNA analysis will predict individual risk for hypertension and target organ damage and will identify responders to specific classes of antihypertensive agents. However, with the exception of the rare, monogenic hypertensive diseases, the genetic variants associated with hypertension remain to be confirmed, and the intermediate steps by which these variants affect blood pressure remain to be determined.

MECHANISMS OF HYPERTENSION

To provide a framework for understanding the pathogenesis of and treatment options for hypertensive disorders, it is useful to understand factors involved in the regulation of both normal and elevated arterial pressure. Cardiac output and peripheral resistance are the two determinants of arterial pressure (Fig. 298-1). Cardiac output is determined by stroke volume and heart rate; stroke volume is related to myocardial contractility and to the size of the vascular compartment. Peripheral resistance is determined by functional and anatomic changes in small arteries (lumen diameter 100–400 μm) and arterioles.

INTRAVASCULAR VOLUME

Sodium is predominantly an extracellular ion and is a primary determinant of the extracellular fluid volume. When NaCl intake exceeds the capacity of the kidney to excrete sodium, vascular volume may initially expand and cardiac output may increase. However, many vascular beds have the capacity to autoregulate blood flow, and if constant blood flow is to be maintained in the face of increased arterial pressure, resistance within that bed must increase, since

$$\text{Blood flow} = \frac{\text{pressure across the vascular bed}}{\text{vascular resistance}}$$

The initial elevation of blood pressure in response to vascular volume expansion may be related to an increase of cardiac output; however, over time, peripheral resistance increases and cardiac output reverts toward normal. Whether this hypothesized sequence of events occurs in the pathogenesis of hypertension is not clear. What is clear is that salt can activate a number of neural, endocrine/paracrine, and vascular mechanisms, all of which have the potential to increase arterial pressure. The effect of sodium on blood pressure is related to the provision of sodium with chloride; nonchloride salts of sodium have

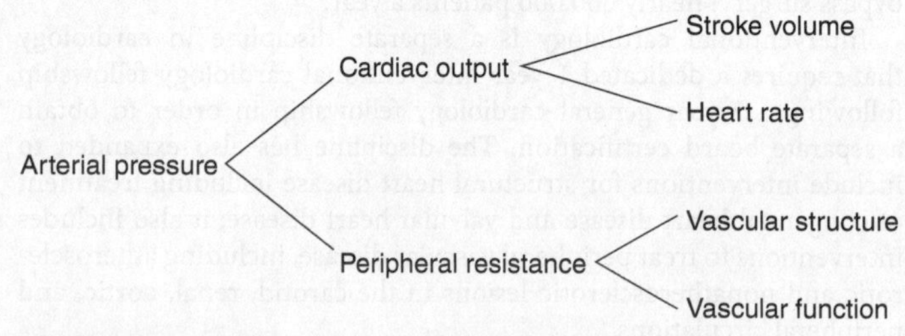

FIGURE 298-1 Determinants of arterial pressure.

little or no effect on blood pressure. As arterial pressure increases in response to a high NaCl intake, urinary sodium excretion increases and sodium balance is maintained at the expense of an increase in arterial pressure. The mechanism for this "pressure-natriuresis" phenomenon may involve a subtle increase in the glomerular filtration rate, decreased absorbing capacity of the renal tubules, and possibly hormonal factors such as atrial natriuretic factor. In individuals with an impaired capacity to excrete sodium, greater increases in arterial pressure are required to achieve natriuresis and sodium balance.

NaCl-dependent hypertension may be a consequence of a decreased capacity of the kidney to excrete sodium, due either to intrinsic renal disease or to increased production of a salt-retaining hormone (mineralocorticoid) resulting in increased renal tubular reabsorption of sodium. Renal tubular sodium reabsorption also may be augmented by increased neural activity to the kidney. In each of these situations, a higher arterial pressure may be required to achieve sodium balance. Conversely, salt-wasting disorders are associated with low blood pressure levels. ESRD is an extreme example of volume-dependent hypertension. In ~80% of these patients, vascular volume and hypertension can be controlled with adequate dialysis; in the other 20%, the mechanism of hypertension is related to increased activity of the renin-angiotensin system and is likely to be responsive to pharmacologic blockade of renin-angiotensin.

AUTONOMIC NERVOUS SYSTEM

Adrenergic reflexes modulate blood pressure over the short term, and adrenergic function, in concert with hormonal and volume-related factors, contributes to the long-term regulation of arterial pressure. Norepinephrine, epinephrine, and dopamine all play important roles in tonic and phasic cardiovascular regulation.

The activities of the adrenergic receptors are mediated by guanosine nucleotide-binding regulatory proteins (G proteins) and by intracellular concentrations of downstream second messengers. In addition to receptor affinity and density, physiologic responsiveness to catecholamines may be altered by the efficiency of receptor-effector coupling at a site "distal" to receptor binding. The receptor sites are relatively specific both for the transmitter substance and for the response that occupancy of the receptor site elicits. Based on their physiology and pharmacology, adrenergic receptors have been divided into two principal types: α and β. These types have been differentiated further into α_1, α_2, β_1, and β_2 receptors. Recent molecular cloning studies have identified several additional subtypes. α Receptors are occupied and activated more avidly by norepinephrine than by epinephrine, and the reverse is true for β receptors. α_1 Receptors are located on postsynaptic cells in smooth muscle and elicit vasoconstriction. α_2 Receptors are localized on presynaptic membranes of postganglionic nerve terminals that synthesize norepinephrine. When activated by catecholamines, α_2 receptors act as negative feedback controllers, inhibiting further norepinephrine release. In the kidney, activation of α_1 adrenergic receptors increases renal tubular reabsorption of sodium. Different classes of antihypertensive agents either inhibit α_1 receptors or act as agonists of α_2 receptors and reduce systemic sympathetic outflow. Activation of myocardial β_1 receptors stimulates the rate and strength of cardiac contraction and consequently increases cardiac output. β_1 Receptor activation also stimulates renin release from the kidney. Another class of antihypertensive agents acts by inhibiting β_1 receptors. Activation of β_2 receptors by epinephrine relaxes vascular smooth muscle and results in vasodilation.

Circulating catecholamine concentrations may affect the number of adrenoreceptors in various tissues. Downregulation of receptors may be a consequence of sustained high levels of catecholamines and provides an explanation for decreasing responsiveness, or tachyphylaxis, to catecholamines. For example, orthostatic hypotension frequently is observed in patients with pheochromocytoma, possibly due to the lack of norepinephrine-induced vasoconstriction with assumption of the upright posture. Conversely, with chronic reduction of neurotransmitter substances, adrenoreceptors may increase in number or be upregulated, resulting in increased responsiveness to the neurotransmitter. Chronic administration of agents that block adrenergic receptors may result in upregulation, and abrupt withdrawal of those agents may produce a condition of temporary hypersensitivity to sympathetic stimuli. For example, clonidine is an antihypertensive agent that is a centrally acting α_2 agonist that inhibits sympathetic outflow. Rebound hypertension may occur with the abrupt cessation of clonidine therapy, probably as a consequence of upregulation of α_1 receptors.

Several reflexes modulate blood pressure on a minute-to-minute basis. One arterial baroreflex is mediated by stretch-sensitive sensory nerve endings in the carotid sinuses and the aortic arch. The rate of firing of these baroreceptors increases with arterial pressure, and the net effect is a decrease in sympathetic outflow, resulting in decreases in arterial pressure and heart rate. This is a primary mechanism for rapid buffering of acute fluctuations of arterial pressure that may occur during postural changes, behavioral or physiologic stress, and changes in blood volume. However, the activity of the baroreflex declines or adapts to sustained increases in arterial pressure such that the baroreceptors are reset to higher pressures. Patients with autonomic neuropathy and impaired baroreflex function may have extremely labile blood pressures with difficult-to-control episodic blood pressure spikes associated with tachycardia.

In both normal-weight and obese individuals, hypertension often is associated with increased sympathetic outflow. Based on recordings of postganglionic muscle nerve activity (detected by a microelectrode inserted in a peroneal nerve in the leg), sympathetic outflow tends to be higher in hypertensive than in normotensive individuals. Sympathetic outflow is increased in obesity-related hypertension and in hypertension associated with obstructive sleep apnea. Baroreceptor activation via electrical stimulation of carotid sinus afferent nerves lowers blood pressure in patients with "resistant" hypertension. Drugs that block the sympathetic nervous system are potent antihypertensive agents, indicating that the sympathetic nervous system plays a permissive, although not necessarily a causative, role in the maintenance of increased arterial pressure.

Pheochromocytoma is the most blatant example of hypertension related to increased catecholamine production, in this instance by a tumor. Blood pressure can be reduced by surgical excision of the tumor or by pharmacologic treatment with an α_1 receptor antagonist or with an inhibitor of tyrosine hydroxylase, the rate-limiting step in catecholamine biosynthesis.

RENIN-ANGIOTENSIN-ALDOSTERONE

The renin-angiotensin-aldosterone system contributes to the regulation of arterial pressure primarily via the vasoconstrictor properties of angiotensin II and the sodium-retaining properties of aldosterone. Renin is an aspartyl protease that is synthesized as an enzymatically inactive precursor, prorenin. Most renin in the circulation is synthesized in the renal afferent renal arteriole. Prorenin may be secreted directly into the circulation or may be activated within secretory cells and released as active renin. Although human plasma contains two to five times more prorenin than renin, there is no evidence that prorenin contributes to the physiologic activity of this system. There are three primary stimuli for renin secretion: (1) decreased NaCl transport in the distal portion of the thick ascending limb of the loop of Henle that abuts the corresponding afferent arteriole (macula densa), (2) decreased pressure or stretch within the renal afferent arteriole (baroreceptor mechanism), and (3) sympathetic nervous system stimulation of renin-secreting cells via β_1 adrenoreceptors. Conversely, renin secretion is inhibited by increased NaCl transport in the thick ascending limb of the loop of Henle, by increased stretch within the renal afferent arteriole, and by β_1 receptor blockade. In addition, angiotensin II directly inhibits renin secretion due to angiotensin II type 1 receptors on juxtaglomerular cells, and renin secretion increases in response to pharmacologic blockade of either ACE or angiotensin II receptors.

Once released into the circulation, active renin cleaves a substrate, angiotensinogen, to form an inactive decapeptide, angiotensin I (Fig. 298-2). A converting enzyme, located primarily but not exclusively in the pulmonary circulation, converts angiotensin I to the active octapeptide, angiotensin II, by releasing the C-terminal histidylleucine dipeptide. The same converting enzyme cleaves a number

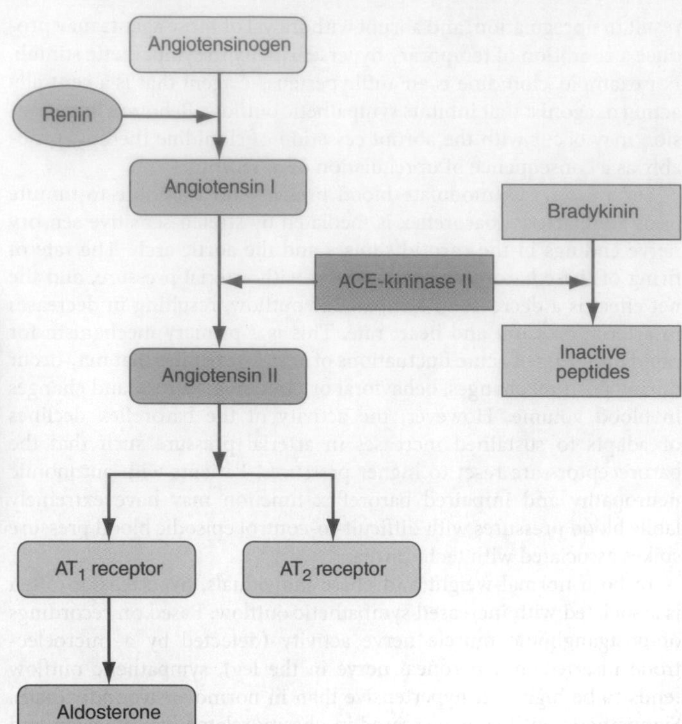

FIGURE 298-2 Renin-angiotensin-aldosterone axis. ACE, angiotensin-converting enzyme.

of other peptides, including and thereby inactivating the vasodilator bradykinin. Acting primarily through angiotensin II type 1 (AT_1) receptors on cell membranes, angiotensin II is a potent pressor substance, the primary tropic factor for the secretion of aldosterone by the adrenal zona glomerulosa, and a potent mitogen that stimulates vascular smooth muscle cell and myocyte growth. Independent of its hemodynamic effects, angiotensin II may play a role in the pathogenesis of atherosclerosis through a direct cellular action on the vessel wall. The angiotensin II type 2 (AT_2) receptor has the opposite functional effects of the AT_1 receptor. The AT_2 receptor induces vasodilation, sodium excretion, and inhibition of cell growth and matrix formation. Experimental evidence suggests that the AT_2 receptor improves vascular remodeling by stimulating smooth muscle cell apoptosis and contributes to the regulation of glomerular filtration rate. AT_1 receptor blockade induces an increase in AT_2 receptor activity.

Renin-secreting tumors are clear examples of renin-dependent hypertension. In the kidney, these tumors include benign hemangiopericytomas of the juxtaglomerular apparatus and, infrequently, renal carcinomas, including Wilms' tumors. Renin-producing carcinomas also have been described in lung, liver, pancreas, colon, and adrenals. In these instances, in addition to excision and/or ablation of the tumor, treatment of hypertension includes pharmacologic therapies targeted to inhibit angiotensin II production or action. Renovascular hypertension is another renin-mediated form of hypertension. Obstruction of the renal artery leads to decreased renal perfusion pressure, thereby stimulating renin secretion. Over time, possibly as a consequence of secondary renal damage, this form of hypertension may become less renin dependent.

Angiotensinogen, renin, and angiotensin II are also synthesized locally in many tissues, including the brain, pituitary, aorta, arteries, heart, adrenal glands, kidneys, adipocytes, leukocytes, ovaries, testes, uterus, spleen, and skin. Angiotensin II in tissues may be formed by the enzymatic activity of renin or by other proteases, e.g., tonin, chymase, and cathepsins. In addition to regulating local blood flow, tissue angiotensin II is a mitogen that stimulates growth and contributes to modeling and repair. Excess tissue angiotensin II may contribute to atherosclerosis, cardiac hypertrophy, and renal failure and consequently may be a target for pharmacologic therapy to prevent target organ damage.

Angiotensin II is the primary tropic factor regulating the synthesis and secretion of aldosterone by the zona glomerulosa of the adrenal cortex. Aldosterone synthesis is also dependent on potassium, and aldosterone secretion may be decreased in potassium-depleted individuals. Although acute elevations of adrenocorticotropic hormone (ACTH) levels also increase aldosterone secretion, ACTH is not an important tropic factor for the chronic regulation of aldosterone.

Aldosterone is a potent mineralocorticoid that increases sodium reabsorption by amiloride-sensitive epithelial sodium channels (ENaC) on the apical surface of the principal cells of the renal cortical collecting duct (Chap. 332e). Electric neutrality is maintained by exchanging sodium for potassium and hydrogen ions. Consequently, increased aldosterone secretion may result in hypokalemia and alkalosis.

Cortisol also binds to the mineralocorticoid receptor but normally functions as a less potent mineralocorticoid than aldosterone because cortisol is converted to cortisone by the enzyme 11 β-hydroxysteroid dehydrogenase type 2. Cortisone has no affinity for the mineralocorticoid receptor. Primary aldosteronism is a compelling example of mineralocorticoid-mediated hypertension. In this disorder, adrenal aldosterone synthesis and release are independent of renin-angiotensin, and renin release is suppressed by the resulting volume expansion.

Mineralocorticoid receptors are expressed in a number of tissues in addition to the kidney, and mineralocorticoid receptor activation induces structural and functional alterations in the heart, kidney, and blood vessels, leading to myocardial fibrosis, nephrosclerosis, and vascular inflammation and remodeling, perhaps as a consequence of oxidative stress. These effects are amplified by a high salt intake. In animal models, high circulating aldosterone levels stimulate cardiac fibrosis and left ventricular hypertrophy, and spironolactone (an aldosterone antagonist) prevents aldosterone-induced myocardial fibrosis. Pathologic patterns of left ventricular geometry also have been associated with elevations of plasma aldosterone concentration in hypertensive patients. In patients with CHF, low-dose spironolactone reduces the risk of progressive heart failure and sudden death from cardiac causes by 30%. Due to a renal hemodynamic effect, in patients with primary aldosteronism, high circulating levels of aldosterone also may cause glomerular hyperfiltration and albuminuria. These renal effects are reversible after removal of the effects of excess aldosterone by adrenalectomy or spironolactone.

Increased activity of the renin-angiotensin-aldosterone axis is not invariably associated with hypertension. In response to a low-NaCl diet or to volume contraction, arterial pressure and volume homeostasis may be maintained by increased activity of the renin-angiotensin-aldosterone axis. Secondary aldosteronism (i.e., increased aldosterone secondary to increased renin-angiotensin), but not hypertension, also is observed in edematous states such as CHF and liver disease.

VASCULAR MECHANISMS

Vascular radius and compliance of resistance arteries are important determinants of arterial pressure. Resistance to flow varies inversely with the fourth power of the radius, and consequently, small decreases in lumen size significantly increase resistance. In hypertensive patients, structural, mechanical, or functional changes may reduce the lumen diameter of small arteries and arterioles. Remodeling refers to geometric alterations in the vessel wall without a change in vessel volume. Hypertrophic (increased cell size, and increased deposition of intercellular matrix) or eutrophic vascular remodeling results in decreased lumen size and, hence, increased peripheral resistance. Apoptosis, low-grade inflammation, and vascular fibrosis also contribute to remodeling. Lumen diameter also is related to elasticity of the vessel. Vessels with a high degree of elasticity can accommodate an increase of volume with relatively little change in pressure, whereas in a semirigid vascular system, a small increment in volume induces a relatively large increment of pressure.

Hypertensive patients may have stiffer arteries due to arteriosclerosis, and high systolic blood pressures and wide pulse pressures are a consequence of decreased vascular compliance. Due to arterial stiffness, central blood pressures (aortic, carotid) may not correspond to brachial artery pressures. Ejection of blood into the aorta elicits a pressure wave that is propagated at a given velocity. The forward travelling wave generates a reflected wave that travels backward toward the ascending aorta. Although mean arterial pressure is determined by cardiac output and peripheral resistance, pulse pressure is related to the functional properties of large arteries and the amplitude and timing of the incident and reflected waves. Increased arterial stiffness results in increased pulse wave velocity of both incident and reflected waves. Due to the timing of these waves, the consequence is augmentation of aortic systolic pressure and a reduction of aortic diastolic pressure, i.e., an increase in pulse pressure. The aortic augmentation index, an index of arterial stiffening, is calculated as the ratio of central arterial pressure-to-pulse pressure. Central blood pressure may be measured directly by placing a sensor in the aorta or noninvasively by radial tonometry using commercially available devices. Central blood pressure and the aortic augmentation index are strong, independent predictors of cardiovascular disease and all-cause mortality.

Ion transport by vascular smooth muscle cells may contribute to hypertension-associated abnormalities of vascular tone and vascular growth, both of which are modulated by intracellular pH (pH_i). Three ion transport mechanisms participate in the regulation of pH_i: (1) Na^+-H^+ exchange, (2) Na^+-dependent HCO_3^--Cl^- exchange, and (3) cation-independent HCO_3^--Cl^- exchange. Based on measurements in cell types that are more accessible than vascular smooth muscle (e.g., leukocytes, erythrocytes, platelets, skeletal muscle), activity of the Na^+-H^+ exchanger is increased in hypertension, and this may result in increased vascular tone by two mechanisms. First, increased sodium entry may lead to increased vascular tone by activating Na^+-Ca^{2+} exchange and thereby increasing intracellular calcium. Second, increased pH_i enhances calcium sensitivity of the contractile apparatus, leading to an increase in contractility for a given intracellular calcium concentration. Additionally, increased Na^+-H^+ exchange may stimulate growth of vascular smooth muscle cells by enhancing sensitivity to mitogens.

Vascular endothelial function also modulates vascular tone. The vascular endothelium synthesizes and releases several vasoactive substances, including nitric oxide, a potent vasodilator. Endothelium-dependent vasodilation is impaired in hypertensive patients. This impairment often is assessed with high-resolution ultrasonography before and after the hyperemic phase of reperfusion that follows 5 minutes of forearm ischemia. Alternatively, endothelium-dependent vasodilation may be assessed in response to an intra-arterially infused endothelium-dependent vasodilator, e.g., acetylcholine. Endothelin is a vasoconstrictor peptide produced by the endothelium, and orally active endothelin antagonists may lower blood pressure in patients with resistant hypertension.

Currently, it is not known if the hypertension-related vascular abnormalities of ion transport and endothelial function are primary alterations or secondary consequences of elevated arterial pressure. Limited evidence suggests that vascular compliance and endothelium-dependent vasodilation may be improved by aerobic exercise, weight loss, and antihypertensive agents. It remains to be determined whether these interventions affect arterial structure and stiffness via a blood pressure–independent mechanism and whether different classes of antihypertensive agents preferentially affect vascular structure and function.

PATHOLOGIC CONSEQUENCES OF HYPERTENSION

Hypertension is an independent predisposing factor for heart failure, coronary artery disease, stroke, renal disease, and peripheral arterial disease (PAD).

HEART

Heart disease is the most common cause of death in hypertensive patients. Hypertensive heart disease is the result of structural and functional adaptations leading to left ventricular hypertrophy, CHF, abnormalities of blood flow due to atherosclerotic coronary artery disease and microvascular disease, and cardiac arrhythmias.

Individuals with left ventricular hypertrophy are at increased risk for CHD, stroke, CHF, and sudden death. Aggressive control of hypertension can regress or reverse left ventricular hypertrophy and reduce the risk of cardiovascular disease. It is not clear whether different classes of antihypertensive agents have an added impact on reducing left ventricular mass, independent of their blood pressure–lowering effect.

CHF may be related to systolic dysfunction, diastolic dysfunction, or a combination of the two. Abnormalities of diastolic function that range from asymptomatic heart disease to overt heart failure are common in hypertensive patients. Approximately one-third of patients with CHF have normal systolic function but abnormal diastolic function. Diastolic dysfunction is an early consequence of hypertension-related heart disease and is exacerbated by left ventricular hypertrophy and ischemia. Cardiac catheterization provides the most accurate assessment of diastolic function. Alternatively, diastolic function can be evaluated by several noninvasive methods, including echocardiography and radionuclide angiography.

BRAIN

Stroke is the second most frequent cause of death in the world; it accounts for 5 million deaths each year, with an additional 15 million persons having nonfatal strokes. Elevated blood pressure is the strongest risk factor for stroke. Approximately 85% of strokes are due to infarction, and the remainder are due to either intracerebral or subarachnoid hemorrhage. The incidence of stroke rises progressively with increasing blood pressure levels, particularly systolic blood pressure in individuals >65 years. Treatment of hypertension decreases the incidence of both ischemic and hemorrhagic strokes.

Hypertension also is associated with impaired cognition in an aging population, and longitudinal studies support an association between midlife hypertension and late-life cognitive decline. Hypertension-related cognitive impairment and dementia may be a consequence of a single infarct due to occlusion of a "strategic" larger vessel or multiple lacunar infarcts due to occlusive small vessel disease resulting in subcortical white matter ischemia. Several clinical trials suggest that antihypertensive therapy has a beneficial effect on cognitive function, although this remains an active area of investigation.

Cerebral blood flow remains unchanged over a wide range of arterial pressures (mean arterial pressure of 50–150 mmHg) through a process termed *autoregulation* of blood flow. In patients with the clinical syndrome of malignant hypertension, encephalopathy is related to failure of autoregulation of cerebral blood flow at the upper pressure limit, resulting in vasodilation and hyperperfusion. Signs and symptoms of hypertensive encephalopathy may include severe headache, nausea and vomiting (often of a projectile nature), focal neurologic signs, and alterations in mental status. Untreated, hypertensive encephalopathy may progress to stupor, coma, seizures, and death within hours. It is important to distinguish hypertensive encephalopathy from other neurologic syndromes that may be associated with hypertension, e.g., cerebral ischemia, hemorrhagic or thrombotic stroke, seizure disorder, mass lesions, pseudotumor cerebri, delirium tremens, meningitis, acute intermittent porphyria, traumatic or chemical injury to the brain, and uremic encephalopathy.

KIDNEY

The kidney is both a target and a cause of hypertension. Primary renal disease is the most common etiology of secondary hypertension. Mechanisms of kidney-related hypertension include a diminished capacity to excrete sodium, excessive renin secretion in relation to volume status, and sympathetic nervous system overactivity. Conversely, hypertension is a risk factor for renal injury and ESRD. The increased risk associated with high blood pressure is graded, continuous, and present throughout the distribution of blood pressure above optimal pressure. Renal risk appears to be more closely related to systolic than to diastolic blood pressure, and black men are at greater risk than white men for developing ESRD at every level of blood pressure.

Atherosclerotic, hypertension-related vascular lesions in the kidney primarily affect preglomerular arterioles, resulting in ischemic changes in the glomeruli and postglomerular structures. Glomerular injury also may be a consequence of direct damage to the glomerular capillaries due to glomerular hyperperfusion. Studies of hypertension-related renal damage, primarily in experimental animals, suggest that loss of autoregulation of renal blood flow at the afferent arteriole results in transmission of elevated pressures to an unprotected glomerulus with ensuing hyperfiltration, hypertrophy, and eventual focal segmental glomerular sclerosis. With progressive renal injury there is a loss of autoregulation of renal blood flow and glomerular filtration rate, resulting in a lower blood pressure threshold for renal damage and a steeper slope between blood pressure and renal damage. The result may be a vicious cycle of renal damage and nephron loss leading to more severe hypertension, glomerular hyperfiltration, and further renal damage. Glomerular pathology progresses to glomerulosclerosis, and eventually the renal tubules may also become ischemic and gradually atrophic. The renal lesion associated with malignant hypertension consists of fibrinoid necrosis of the afferent arterioles, sometimes extending into the glomerulus, and may result in focal necrosis of the glomerular tuft.

Clinically, macroalbuminuria (a random urine albumin/creatinine ratio >300 mg/g) or microalbuminuria (a random urine albumin/creatinine ratio 30–300 mg/g) are early markers of renal injury. These are also risk factors for renal disease progression and cardiovascular disease.

PERIPHERAL ARTERIES

In addition to contributing to the pathogenesis of hypertension, blood vessels are a target organ for atherosclerotic disease secondary to long-standing elevated blood pressure. In hypertensive patients, vascular disease is a major contributor to stroke, heart disease, and renal failure. Further, hypertensive patients with arterial disease of the lower extremities are at increased risk for future cardiovascular disease. Although patients with stenotic lesions of the lower extremities may be asymptomatic, intermittent claudication is the classic symptom of PAD. The ankle-brachial index is a useful approach for evaluating PAD and is defined as the ratio of noninvasively assessed ankle to brachial (arm) systolic blood pressure. An ankle-brachial index <0.90 is considered diagnostic of PAD and is associated with >50% stenosis in at least one major lower limb vessel. An ankle-brachial index <0.80 is associated with elevated blood pressure, particularly systolic blood pressure.

DEFINING HYPERTENSION

From an epidemiologic perspective, there is no obvious level of blood pressure that defines hypertension. In adults, there is a continuous, incremental risk of cardiovascular disease, stroke, and renal disease across levels of both systolic and diastolic blood pressure. The Multiple Risk Factor Intervention Trial (MRFIT), which included >350,000 male participants, demonstrated a continuous and graded influence of both systolic and diastolic blood pressure on CHD mortality, extending down to systolic blood pressures of 120 mmHg. Similarly, results of a meta-analysis involving almost 1 million participants indicate that ischemic heart disease mortality, stroke mortality, and mortality from other vascular causes are directly related to the height of the blood pressure, beginning at 115/75 mmHg, without evidence of a threshold. Cardiovascular disease risk doubles for every 20-mmHg increase in systolic and 10-mmHg increase in diastolic pressure. Among older individuals, systolic blood pressure and pulse pressure are more powerful predictors of cardiovascular disease than is diastolic blood pressure.

Clinically, hypertension may be defined as that level of blood pressure at which the institution of therapy reduces blood pressure–related morbidity and mortality. Current clinical criteria for defining hypertension generally are based on the average of two or more seated blood pressure readings during each of two or more outpatient visits. A recent classification recommends blood pressure criteria for defining normal blood pressure, prehypertension, hypertension (stages I and II), and isolated systolic hypertension, which is frequent among the elderly (Table 298-1). In children and adolescents, hypertension generally is defined as systolic and/or diastolic blood pressure consistently >95th percentile for age, sex, and height. Blood pressures between the 90th and 95th percentiles are considered prehypertensive and are an indication for lifestyle interventions.

TABLE 298-1 BLOOD PRESSURE CLASSIFICATION

Blood Pressure Classification	Systolic, mmHg	Diastolic, mmHg
Normal	<120	*and* <80
Prehypertension	120–139	*or* 80–89
Stage 1 hypertension	140–159	*or* 90–99
Stage 2 hypertension	≥160	*or* ≥100
Isolated systolic hypertension	≥140	*and* <90

Source: Adapted from AV Chobanian et al: JAMA 289:2560, 2003.

Home blood pressure and average 24-h ambulatory blood pressure measurements are generally lower than clinic blood pressures. Because ambulatory blood pressure recordings yield multiple readings throughout the day and night, they provide a more comprehensive assessment of the vascular burden of hypertension than do a limited number of office readings. Increasing evidence suggests that home blood pressures, including 24-h blood pressure recordings, more reliably predict target organ damage than do office blood pressures. Blood pressure tends to be higher in the early morning hours, soon after waking, than at other times of day. Myocardial infarction and stroke are more common in the early morning hours. Nighttime blood pressures are generally 10–20% lower than daytime blood pressures, and an attenuated nighttime blood pressure "dip" may be associated with increased cardiovascular disease risk. Recommended criteria for a diagnosis of hypertension, based on 24-h blood pressure monitoring, are average awake blood pressure ≥135/85 mmHg and asleep blood pressure ≥120/75 mmHg. These levels approximate a clinic blood pressure of 140/90 mmHg.

Approximately 15–20% of patients with stage 1 hypertension (as defined in Table 298-1) based on office blood pressures have average ambulatory readings <135/85 mmHg. This phenomenon, so-called white coat hypertension, also may be associated with an increased risk of target organ damage, although to a lesser extent than in individuals with elevated office and ambulatory readings. Individuals with white coat hypertension are also at increased risk for developing sustained hypertension.

CLINICAL DISORDERS OF HYPERTENSION

Depending on methods of patient ascertainment, ~80–95% of hypertensive patients are diagnosed as having primary, or "essential," hypertension. In the remaining 5–20% of hypertensive patients, a specific underlying disorder causing the elevation of blood pressure can be identified (Tables 298-2 and 298-3). In individuals with "secondary" hypertension, a specific mechanism for the blood pressure elevation is often more apparent.

PRIMARY HYPERTENSION

Primary hypertension tends to be familial and is likely to be the consequence of an interaction between environmental and genetic factors. The prevalence of primary hypertension increases with age, and individuals with relatively high blood pressures at younger ages are at increased risk for the subsequent development of hypertension. It is

TABLE 298-2 SYSTOLIC HYPERTENSION WITH WIDE PULSE PRESSURE

1. Decreased vascular compliance (arteriosclerosis)
2. Increased cardiac output
    a. Aortic regurgitation
    b. Thyrotoxicosis
    c. Hyperkinetic heart syndrome
    d. Fever
    e. Arteriovenous fistula
    f. Patent ductus arteriosus

TABLE 298-3 SECONDARY CAUSES OF SYSTOLIC AND DIASTOLIC HYPERTENSION

Renal	Parenchymal diseases, renal cysts (including polycystic kidney disease), renal tumors (including renin-secreting tumors), obstructive uropathy
Renovascular	Arteriosclerotic, fibromuscular dysplasia
Adrenal	Primary aldosteronism, Cushing's syndrome, 17α-hydroxylase deficiency, 11β-hydroxylase deficiency, 11-hydroxysteroid dehydrogenase deficiency (licorice), pheochromocytoma
Aortic coarctation	
Obstructive sleep apnea	
Preeclampsia/eclampsia	
Neurogenic	Psychogenic, diencephalic syndrome, familial dysautonomia, polyneuritis (acute porphyria, lead poisoning), acute increased intracranial pressure, acute spinal cord section
Miscellaneous endocrine	Hypothyroidism, hyperthyroidism, hypercalcemia, acromegaly
Medications	High-dose estrogens, adrenal steroids, decongestants, appetite suppressants, cyclosporine, tricyclic antidepressants, monoamine oxidase inhibitors, erythropoietin, nonsteroidal anti-inflammatory agents, cocaine
Mendelian forms of hypertension	See Table 298-4

likely that primary hypertension represents a spectrum of disorders with different underlying pathophysiologies. In the majority of patients with established hypertension, peripheral resistance is increased and cardiac output is normal or decreased; however, in younger patients with mild or labile hypertension, cardiac output may be increased and peripheral resistance may be normal.

When plasma renin activity (PRA) is plotted against 24-h sodium excretion, ~10–15% of hypertensive patients have high PRA and 25% have low PRA. High-renin patients may have a vasoconstrictor form of hypertension, whereas low-renin patients may have volume-dependent hypertension. Inconsistent associations between plasma aldosterone and blood pressure have been described in patients with primary hypertension. The association between aldosterone and blood pressure is more striking in African Americans, and PRA tends to be low in hypertensive African Americans. This raises the possibility that subtle increases in aldosterone may contribute to hypertension in at least some groups of patients who do not have overt primary aldosteronism. Furthermore, spironolactone, an aldosterone antagonist, may be a particularly effective antihypertensive agent for some patients with primary hypertension, including some patients with "drug-resistant" hypertension.

OBESITY AND THE METABOLIC SYNDROME

(See also Chap. 422) There is a well-documented association between obesity (body mass index >30 kg/m^2) and hypertension. Further, cross-sectional studies indicate a direct linear correlation between body weight (or body mass index) and blood pressure. Centrally located body fat is a more important determinant of blood pressure elevation than is peripheral body fat. In longitudinal studies, a direct correlation exists between change in weight and change in blood pressure over time. Sixty percent of hypertensive adults are more than 20% overweight. It has been established that 60–70% of hypertension in adults may be directly attributable to adiposity.

Hypertension and dyslipidemia frequently occur together and in association with resistance to insulin-stimulated glucose uptake. This clustering of risk factors is often, but not invariably, associated with obesity, particularly abdominal obesity. Insulin resistance also is associated with an unfavorable imbalance in the endothelial production of mediators that regulate platelet aggregation, coagulation, fibrinolysis, and vessel tone. When these risk factors cluster, the risks for CHD, stroke, diabetes, and cardiovascular disease mortality are increased further.

Depending on the populations studied and the methodologies for defining insulin resistance, ~25–50% of nonobese, nondiabetic hypertensive persons are insulin resistant. The constellation of insulin resistance, abdominal obesity, hypertension, and dyslipidemia has been designated as the *metabolic syndrome*. As a group, first-degree relatives of patients with primary hypertension are also insulin resistant, and hyperinsulinemia (a surrogate marker of insulin resistance) may predict the eventual development of hypertension and cardiovascular disease. Although the metabolic syndrome may in part be heritable as a polygenic condition, the expression of the syndrome is modified by environmental factors, such as degree of physical activity and diet. Insulin sensitivity increases and blood pressure decreases in response to weight loss. The recognition that cardiovascular disease risk factors tend to cluster within individuals has important implications for the evaluation and treatment of hypertension. Evaluation of both hypertensive patients and individuals at risk for developing hypertension should include assessment of overall cardiovascular disease risk. Similarly, introduction of lifestyle modification strategies and drug therapies should address overall risk and not focus exclusively on hypertension.

RENAL PARENCHYMAL DISEASES

Virtually all disorders of the kidney may cause hypertension (Table 298-3), and renal disease is the most common cause of secondary hypertension. Hypertension is present in >80% of patients with chronic renal failure. In general, hypertension is more severe in glomerular diseases than in interstitial diseases such as chronic pyelonephritis. Conversely, hypertension may cause nephrosclerosis, and in some instances it may be difficult to determine whether hypertension or renal disease was the initial disorder. Proteinuria >1000 mg/d and an active urine sediment are indicative of primary renal disease. In either instance, the goals are to control blood pressure and retard the rate of progression of renal dysfunction.

RENOVASCULAR HYPERTENSION

Hypertension due to an occlusive lesion of a renal artery, renovascular hypertension, is a potentially curable form of hypertension. In the initial stages, the mechanism of hypertension generally is related to activation of the renin-angiotensin system. However, renin activity and other components of the renin-angiotensin system may be elevated only transiently; over time, recruitment of other pressure mechanisms may contribute to elevated arterial pressure. Two groups of patients are at risk for this disorder: older arteriosclerotic patients who have a plaque obstructing the renal artery, frequently at its origin, and patients with fibromuscular dysplasia. Atherosclerosis accounts for the large majority of patients with renovascular hypertension. Although fibromuscular dysplasia may occur at any age, it has a strong predilection for young white women. The prevalence in females is eightfold that in males. There are several histologic variants of fibromuscular dysplasia, including medial fibroplasia, perimedial fibroplasia, medial hyperplasia, and intimal fibroplasia. Medial fibroplasia is the most common variant and accounts for approximately two-thirds of patients. The lesions of fibromuscular dysplasia are frequently bilateral and, in contrast to atherosclerotic renovascular disease, tend to affect more distal portions of the renal artery.

Several clues from the history and physical examination may suggest renovascular hypertension. The diagnosis should be considered in patients with other evidence of atherosclerotic vascular disease. Although response to antihypertensive therapy does not exclude the diagnosis, severe or refractory hypertension, recent loss of hypertension control or recent onset of moderately severe hypertension, and unexplained deterioration of renal function or deterioration of renal function associated with an ACE inhibitor should raise the possibility of renovascular hypertension. Approximately 50% of patients with renovascular hypertension have an abdominal or flank bruit, and the bruit is more likely to be hemodynamically significant if it lateralizes or extends throughout systole into diastole.

If blood pressure is adequately controlled with a simple antihypertensive regimen and renal function remains stable, there may be little impetus to pursue an evaluation for renal artery stenosis, particularly in an older patient with atherosclerotic disease and comorbid conditions. Patients with long-standing hypertension, advanced renal insufficiency, or diabetes mellitus are less likely to benefit from renal vascular repair. The most effective medical therapies include an ACE inhibitor or an angiotensin II receptor blocker; however, these agents decrease glomerular filtration rate in a stenotic kidney owing to efferent renal arteriolar dilation. In the presence of bilateral renal artery stenosis or renal artery stenosis to a solitary kidney, progressive renal insufficiency may result from the use of these agents. Importantly, the renal insufficiency is generally reversible after discontinuation of the offending drug.

If renal artery stenosis is suspected and if the clinical condition warrants an intervention such as percutaneous transluminal renal angioplasty (PTRA), placement of a vascular endoprosthesis (stent), or surgical renal revascularization, imaging studies should be the next step in the evaluation. As a screening test, renal blood flow may be evaluated with a radionuclide [^{131}I]-orthoiodohippurate (OIH) scan, or glomerular filtration rate may be evaluated with a [^{99}mTc]-diethylenetriamine pentaacetic acid (DTPA) scan before and after a single dose of captopril (or another ACE inhibitor). The following are consistent with a positive study: (1) decreased relative uptake by the involved kidney, which contributes <40% of total renal function, (2) delayed uptake on the affected side, and (3) delayed washout on the affected side. In patients with normal, or nearly normal, renal function, a normal captopril renogram essentially excludes functionally significant renal artery stenosis; however, its usefulness is limited in patients with renal insufficiency (creatinine clearance <20 mL/min) or bilateral renal artery stenosis. Additional imaging studies are indicated if the scan is positive. Doppler ultrasound of the renal arteries produces reliable estimates of renal blood flow velocity and offers the opportunity to track a lesion over time. Positive studies usually are confirmed at angiography, whereas false-negative results occur frequently, particularly in obese patients. Gadolinium-contrast magnetic resonance angiography offers clear images of the proximal renal artery but may miss distal lesions. An advantage is the opportunity to image the renal arteries with an agent that is not nephrotoxic. Contrast arteriography remains the "gold standard" for evaluation and identification of renal artery lesions. Potential risks include nephrotoxicity, particularly in patients with diabetes mellitus or preexisting renal insufficiency.

Some degree of renal artery obstruction may be observed in almost 50% of patients with atherosclerotic disease, and there are several approaches for evaluating the functional significance of such a lesion to predict the effect of vascular repair on blood pressure control and renal function. Each approach has varying degrees of sensitivity and specificity, and no single test is sufficiently reliable to determine a causal relationship between a renal artery lesion and hypertension. Functionally significant lesions generally occlude more than 70% of the lumen of the affected renal artery. On angiography, the presence of collateral vessels to the ischemic kidney suggests a functionally significant lesion. A lateralizing renal vein renin ratio (ratio >1.5 of affected side/contralateral side) has a 90% predictive value for a lesion that would respond to vascular repair; however, the false-negative rate for blood pressure control is 50–60%. Measurement of the pressure gradient across a renal artery lesion does not reliably predict the response to vascular repair.

In the final analysis, a decision concerning vascular repair vs. medical therapy and the type of repair procedure should be individualized. Patients with fibromuscular disease have more favorable outcomes than do patients with atherosclerotic lesions, presumably owing to their younger age, shorter duration of hypertension, and less systemic disease. Because of its low risk-versus-benefit ratio and high success rate (improvement or cure of hypertension in 90% of patients and restenosis rate of 10%), PTRA is the initial treatment of choice for these patients. Surgical revascularization may be undertaken if PTRA is unsuccessful or if a branch lesion is present. In atherosclerotic patients, vascular repair should be considered if blood pressure cannot be controlled adequately despite optimal medical therapy or if renal function deteriorates. Surgery may be the preferred initial approach for younger atherosclerotic patients without comorbid conditions; however, for most atherosclerotic patients, depending on the location of the lesion, the initial approach may be PTRA and/or stenting. Surgical revascularization may be indicated if these approaches are unsuccessful, the vascular lesion is not amenable to PTRA or stenting, or concomitant aortic surgery is required, e.g., to repair an aneurysm. A National Institutes of Health–sponsored prospective, randomized clinical trial is in progress comparing medical therapy alone with medical therapy plus renal artery stenting regarding Cardiovascular Outcomes for Renal Atherosclerotic Lesions (CORAL).

PRIMARY ALDOSTERONISM

Excess aldosterone production due to primary aldosteronism is a potentially curable form of hypertension. In patients with primary aldosteronism, increased aldosterone production is independent of the renin-angiotensin system, and the consequences are sodium retention, hypertension, hypokalemia, and low PRA. The reported prevalence of this disorder varies from <2% to ~15% of hypertensive individuals. In part, this variation is related to the intensity of screening and the criteria for establishing the diagnosis.

History and physical examination provide little information about the diagnosis. The age at the time of diagnosis is generally the third through fifth decade. Hypertension is usually mild to moderate but occasionally may be severe; primary aldosteronism should be considered in all patients with refractory hypertension. Hypertension in these patients may be associated with glucose intolerance. Most patients are asymptomatic; however, infrequently, polyuria, polydipsia, paresthesias, or muscle weakness may be present as a consequence of hypokalemic alkalosis. Although aldosterone is a salt-retaining hormone, patients with primary aldosteronism rarely have edema. Renal dysfunction and cardiovascular disease are strikingly increased in patients with primary aldosteronism compared to those with primary hypertension.

In a hypertensive patient with unprovoked hypokalemia (i.e., unrelated to diuretics, vomiting, or diarrhea), the prevalence of primary aldosteronism approaches 40–50%. In patients on diuretics, serum potassium <3.1 mmol/L (<3.1 meq/L) also raises the possibility of primary aldosteronism; however, serum potassium is an insensitive and nonspecific screening test. Serum potassium is normal in ~25% of patients subsequently found to have an aldosterone-producing adenoma, and higher percentages of patients with other etiologies of primary aldosteronism are not hypokalemic. Additionally, hypokalemic hypertension may be a consequence of secondary aldosteronism, other mineralocorticoid- and glucocorticoid-induced hypertensive disorders, and pheochromocytoma.

The ratio of plasma aldosterone to plasma renin activity (PA/PRA) is a useful screening test. These measurements preferably are obtained in ambulatory patients in the morning. A ratio >30:1 in conjunction with a plasma aldosterone concentration >555 pmol/L (>20 ng/dL) reportedly has a sensitivity of 90% and a specificity of 91% for an aldosterone-producing adenoma. In a Mayo Clinic series, an aldosterone-producing adenoma subsequently was confirmed surgically in >90% of hypertensive patients with a PA/PRA ratio ≥20 and a plasma aldosterone concentration ≥415 pmol/L (≥15 ng/dL). There are, however, several caveats to interpreting the ratio. The cutoff for a "high" ratio is laboratory- and assay-dependent. Some antihypertensive agents may affect the ratio (e.g., aldosterone antagonists, angiotensin receptor antagonists, and ACE inhibitors may increase renin; aldosterone antagonists may increase aldosterone). Current recommendations are to withdraw aldosterone antagonists for at least 4–6 weeks before obtaining these measurements. Because aldosterone biosynthesis is potassium-dependent, hypokalemia should be corrected with oral potassium supplements prior to screening. With these caveats, the ratio has been reported to be useful as a screening test in measurements obtained with patients taking their usual antihypertensive medications. A high ratio in the absence of an elevated plasma aldosterone level is considerably less specific for primary aldosteronism since many patients with primary hypertension have low renin levels in this setting, particularly African Americans and elderly patients.

In patients with renal insufficiency, the ratio may also be elevated because of decreased aldosterone clearance. In patients with an elevated PA/PRA ratio, the diagnosis of primary aldosteronism can be confirmed by demonstrating failure to suppress plasma aldosterone to <277 pmol/L (<10 ng/dL) after IV infusion of 2 L of isotonic saline over 4 h; post-saline infusion plasma aldosterone values between 138 and 277 pmol/L (5–10 ng/dL) are not determinant. Alternative confirmatory tests include failure to suppress aldosterone (based on test specific criteria) in response to an oral NaCl load, fludrocortisone, or captopril.

Several sporadic and familial adrenal abnormalities may culminate in the syndrome of primary aldosteronism, and appropriate therapy depends on the specific etiology. The two most common causes of sporadic primary aldosteronism are an aldosterone-producing adenoma and bilateral adrenal hyperplasia. Together, they account for >90% of all patients with primary aldosteronism. The tumor is almost always unilateral, and most often measures <3 cm in diameter. Most of the remainder of these patients have bilateral adrenocortical hyperplasia (idiopathic hyperaldosteronism). Rarely, primary aldosteronism may be caused by an adrenal carcinoma or an ectopic malignancy, e.g., ovarian arrhenoblastoma. Most aldosterone-producing carcinomas, in contrast to adrenal adenomas and hyperplasia, produce excessive amounts of other adrenal steroids in addition to aldosterone. Functional differences in hormone secretion may assist in the diagnosis of adenoma vs. hyperplasia. Aldosterone biosynthesis is more responsive to ACTH in patients with adenoma and more responsive to angiotensin in patients with hyperplasia. Consequently, patients with adenoma tend to have higher plasma aldosterone in the early morning that decreases during the day, reflecting the diurnal rhythm of ACTH, whereas plasma aldosterone tends to increase with upright posture in patients with hyperplasia, reflecting the normal postural response of the renin-angiotensin-aldosterone axis. However, there is overlap in the ability of these measurements to discriminate between adenoma and hyperplasia. Rare familial forms of primary aldosteronism include glucocorticoid-remediable primary aldosteronism and familial aldosteronism types II and III. Genetic testing may assist in the diagnosis of these familial disorders.

Adrenal computed tomography (CT) should be carried out in all patients diagnosed with primary aldosteronism. High-resolution CT may identify tumors as small as 0.3 cm and is positive for an adrenal tumor 90% of the time. If the CT is not diagnostic, an adenoma may be detected by adrenal scintigraphy with 6 β [I^{131}] iodomethyl-19-norcholesterol after dexamethasone suppression (0.5 mg every 6 h for 7 days); however, this technique has decreased sensitivity for adenomas <1.5 cm.

When carried out by an experienced radiologist, bilateral adrenal venous sampling for measurement of plasma aldosterone is the most accurate means of differentiating unilateral from bilateral forms of primary aldosteronism. The sensitivity and specificity of adrenal venous sampling (95% and 100%, respectively) for detecting unilateral aldosterone hypersecretion are superior to those of adrenal CT; success rates are 90–96%, and complication rates are <2.5%. One frequently used protocol involves sampling for aldosterone and cortisol levels in response to ACTH stimulation. An ipsilateral/contralateral aldosterone ratio >4, with symmetric ACTH-stimulated cortisol levels, is indicative of unilateral aldosterone production.

Hypertension generally is responsive to surgery in patients with adenoma but not in patients with bilateral adrenal hyperplasia. Unilateral adrenalectomy, often done via a laparoscopic approach, is curative in 40–70% of patients with an adenoma. Transient hypoaldosteronism may occur up to 3 months postoperatively, resulting in hyperkalemia. Potassium should be monitored during this time, and hyperkalemia should be treated with potassium-wasting diuretics and with fludrocortisone, if needed. Patients with bilateral hyperplasia should be treated medically. The drug regimen for these patients, as well as for patients with an adenoma who are poor surgical candidates, should include an aldosterone antagonist and, if necessary, other potassium-sparing diuretics.

Glucocorticoid-remediable hyperaldosteronism is a rare, monogenic autosomal dominant disorder characterized by moderate to severe hypertension, often occurring at an early age. These patients may have a family history of hemorrhagic stroke at a young age. Hypokalemia is usually mild or absent. Normally, angiotensin II stimulates aldosterone production by the adrenal zona glomerulosa, whereas ACTH stimulates cortisol production in the zona fasciculata. Owing to a chimeric gene on chromosome 8, ACTH also regulates aldosterone secretion by the zona fasciculata in patients with glucocorticoid-remediable hyperaldosteronism. The consequence is overproduction in the zona fasciculata of both aldosterone and hybrid steroids (18-hydroxycortisol and 18-oxocortisol) due to oxidation of cortisol. The diagnosis may be established by urine excretion rates of these hybrid steroids that are 20 to 30 times normal or by direct genetic testing. Therapeutically, suppression of ACTH with low-dose glucocorticoids corrects the hyperaldosteronism, hypertension, and hypokalemia. Aldosterone antagonists are also therapeutic options. Patients with familial aldosteronism types II and III are treated with aldosterone antagonists or adrenalectomy.

CUSHING'S SYNDROME

(See also Chap. 406) Cushing's syndrome is related to excess cortisol production due either to excess ACTH secretion (from a pituitary tumor or an ectopic tumor) or to ACTH-independent adrenal production of cortisol. Hypertension occurs in 75–80% of patients with Cushing's syndrome. The mechanism of hypertension may be related to stimulation of mineralocorticoid receptors by cortisol and increased secretion of other adrenal steroids. If clinically suspected based on phenotypic characteristics, in patients not taking exogenous glucocorticoids, laboratory screening may be carried out with measurement of 24-h excretion rates of urine free cortisol or an overnight dexamethasone-suppression test. Late night salivary cortisol is also a sensitive and convenient screening test. Further evaluation is required to confirm the diagnosis and identify the specific etiology of Cushing's syndrome. Appropriate therapy depends on the etiology.

PHEOCHROMOCYTOMA

(See also Chap. 407) Catecholamine-secreting tumors are located in the adrenal medulla (pheochromocytoma) or in extra-adrenal paraganglion tissue (paraganglioma) and account for hypertension in ~0.05% of patients. If unrecognized, pheochromocytoma may result in lethal cardiovascular consequences. Clinical manifestations, including hypertension, are primarily related to increased circulating catecholamines, although some of these tumors may secrete a number of other vasoactive substances. In a small percentage of patients, epinephrine is the predominant catecholamine secreted by the tumor, and these patients may present with hypotension rather than hypertension. The initial suspicion of the diagnosis is based on symptoms and/or the association of pheochromocytoma with other disorders (Table 298-4). Approximately 20% of pheochromocytomas are familial with autosomal dominant inheritance. Inherited pheochromocytomas may be associated with multiple endocrine neoplasia (MEN) type 2A and type 2B, von Hippel-Lindau disease, and neurofibromatosis (Table 298-4). Each of these syndromes is related to specific, identifiable germ-line mutations. Additionally, mutations of succinate dehydrogenase genes are associated with paraganglioma syndromes, generally characterized by head and neck paragangliomas. Laboratory testing consists of measuring catecholamines in either urine or plasma, e.g., 24-h urine metanephrine excretion or fractionated plasma free metanephrines. The urine measurement is less sensitive but more specific. Genetic screening is available for evaluating patients and relatives suspected of harboring a pheochromocytoma associated with a familial syndrome. Surgical excision is the definitive treatment of pheochromocytoma and results in cure in ~90% of patients.

MISCELLANEOUS CAUSES OF HYPERTENSION

Independent of obesity, hypertension occurs in >50% of individuals with *obstructive sleep apnea*. The severity of hypertension correlates with the severity of sleep apnea. Approximately 70% of patients with obstructive sleep apnea are obese. Hypertension related to obstructive sleep apnea also should be considered in patients with drug-resistant

TABLE 298-4 RARE MENDELIAN FORMS OF HYPERTENSION

Disease	Phenotype	Genetic Cause
Glucocorticoid-remediable hyperaldosteronism	Autosomal dominant Absent or mild hypokalemia	Chimeric 11β-hydroxylase/aldosterone gene on chromosome 8
17α-hydroxylase deficiency	Autosomal recessive Males: pseudohermaphroditism Females: primary amenorrhea, absent secondary sexual characteristics	Random mutations of the *CYP17* gene on chromosome 10
11β-hydroxylase deficiency	Autosomal recessive Masculinization	Mutations of the *CYP11B1* gene on chromosome 8q21-q22
11β-hydroxysteroid dehydrogenase deficiency (apparent mineralocorticoid excess syndrome)	Autosomal recessive Hypokalemia, low renin, low aldosterone	Mutations in the 11β-hydroxysteroid dehydrogenase gene
Liddle's syndrome	Autosomal dominant Hypokalemia, low renin, low aldosterone	Mutation subunits of the epithelial sodium channel *SCNN1B* and *SCNN1C* genes
Pseudohypoaldosteronism type II (Gordon's syndrome)	Autosomal dominant Hyperkalemia, normal glomerular filtration rate	Linkage to chromosomes 1q31-q42 and 17p11-q21
Hypertension exacerbated in pregnancy	Autosomal dominant Severe hypertension in early pregnancy	Missense mutation with substitution of leucine for serine at codon 810 (MR_{L810})
Polycystic kidney disease	Autosomal dominant Large cystic kidneys, renal failure, liver cysts, cerebral aneurysms, valvular heart disease	Mutations in the *PKD1* gene on chromosome 16 and *PKD2* gene on chromosome 4
Pheochromocytoma	Autosomal dominant	
	(a) Multiple endocrine neoplasia, type 2A Medullary thyroid carcinoma, hyperparathyroidism	(a) Mutations in the *RET* protooncogene
	(b) Multiple endocrine neoplasia, type 2B Medullary thyroid carcinoma, mucosal neuromas, thickened corneal nerves, alimentary ganglioneuromatoses, marfanoid habitus	(b) Mutations in the *RET* protooncogene
	(c) von Hippel-Lindau disease Retinal angiomas, hemangioblastomas of the cerebellum and spinal cord, renal cell carcinoma	(c) Mutations in the *VHL* tumor-suppressor gene
	(d) Neurofibromatosis type 1 Multiple neurofibromas, café-au-lait spots	(d) Mutations in the *NF1* tumor-suppressor gene

hypertension and patients with a history of snoring. The diagnosis can be confirmed by polysomnography. In obese patients, weight loss may alleviate or cure sleep apnea and related hypertension. Continuous positive airway pressure (CPAP) or bilevel positive airway pressure (BiPAP) administered during sleep is an effective therapy for obstructive sleep apnea. With CPAP or BiPAP, patients with apparently drug-resistant hypertension may be more responsive to antihypertensive agents.

Coarctation of the aorta is the most common congenital cardiovascular cause of hypertension (Chap. 282). The incidence is 1–8 per 1000 live births. It is usually sporadic but occurs in 35% of children with Turner's syndrome. Even when the anatomic lesion is surgically corrected in infancy, up to 30% of patients develop subsequent hypertension and are at risk of accelerated coronary artery disease and cerebrovascular events. Patients with less severe lesions may not be diagnosed until young adulthood. Physical findings include diminished and delayed femoral pulses and a systolic pressure gradient between the right arm and the legs and, depending on the location of the coarctation, between the right and left arms. A blowing systolic murmur may be heard in the posterior left interscapular areas. The diagnosis may be confirmed by chest x-ray and transesophageal echocardiography. Therapeutic options include surgical repair and balloon angioplasty, with or without placement of an intravascular stent. Subsequently, many patients do not have a normal life expectancy but may have persistent hypertension, with death due to ischemic heart disease, cerebral hemorrhage, or aortic aneurysm.

Several additional endocrine disorders, including *thyroid diseases* and *acromegaly*, cause hypertension. Mild diastolic hypertension may be a consequence of hypothyroidism, whereas hyperthyroidism may result in systolic hypertension. *Hypercalcemia* of any etiology, the most common being primary hyperparathyroidism, may result in hypertension. Hypertension also may be related to a number of prescribed or over-the-counter *medications*.

MONOGENIC HYPERTENSION

In addition to glucocorticoid-remediable primary aldosteronism, a number of rare forms of monogenic hypertension have been identified (Table 298-4). These disorders may be recognized by their characteristic phenotypes, and in many instances the diagnosis may be confirmed by genetic analysis. Several inherited defects in adrenal steroid biosynthesis and metabolism result in mineralocorticoid-induced hypertension and hypokalemia. In patients with a 17α-hydroxylase deficiency, synthesis of sex hormones and cortisol is decreased (Fig. 298-3). Consequently, these individuals do not mature sexually; males may present with pseudohermaphroditism and females with primary amenorrhea and absent secondary sexual characteristics. Because cortisol-induced negative feedback on pituitary ACTH production is diminished, ACTH-stimulated adrenal steroid synthesis proximal to the enzymatic block is increased. Hypertension and hypokalemia are consequences of increased synthesis of mineralocorticoids proximal to the enzymatic block, particularly desoxycorticosterone. Increased steroid production and, hence, hypertension may be treated with low-dose glucocorticoids. An 11β-hydroxylase deficiency results in a salt-retaining adrenogenital syndrome that occurs in 1 in 100,000 live births. This enzymatic defect results in decreased cortisol synthesis, increased synthesis of mineralocorticoids (e.g., desoxycorticosterone), and shunting of steroid biosynthesis into the androgen pathway. In the severe form, the syndrome may present early in life, including the

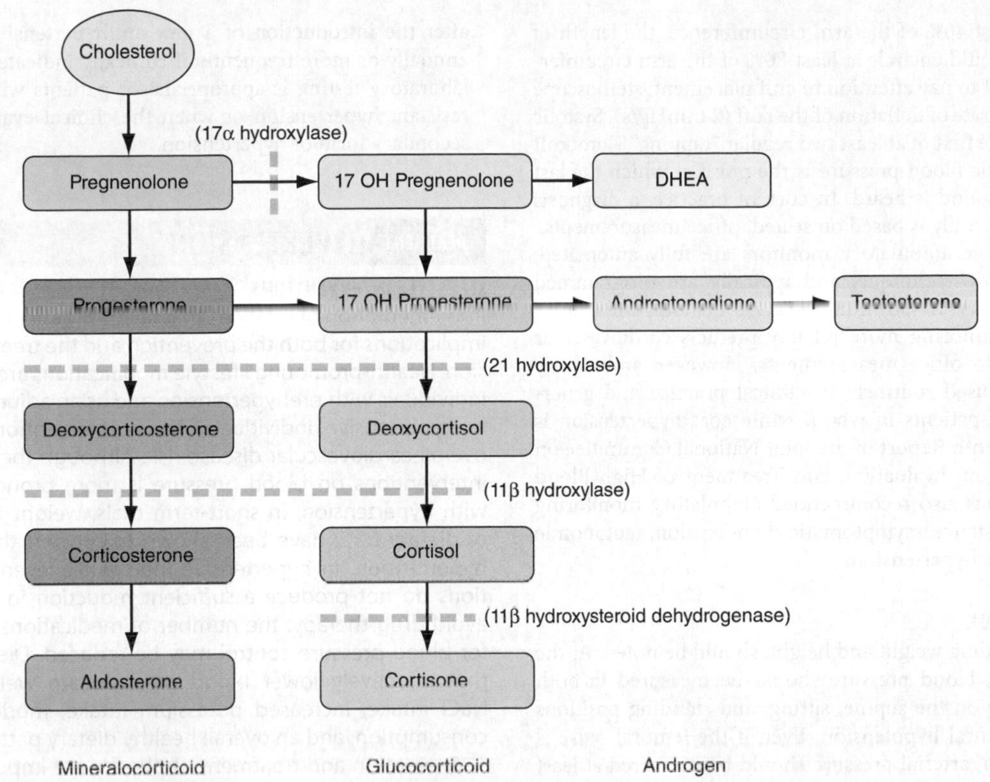

FIGURE 298-3 Adrenal enzymatic defects. DHEA, dehydroepiandrosterone.

newborn period, with virilization and ambiguous genitalia in females and penile enlargement in males, or in older children as precocious puberty and short stature. Acne, hirsutism, and menstrual irregularities may be the presenting features when the disorder is first recognized in adolescence or early adulthood. Hypertension is less common in the late-onset forms. Patients with an 11β-hydroxysteroid dehydrogenase deficiency have an impaired capacity to metabolize cortisol to its inactive metabolite, cortisone, and hypertension is related to activation of mineralocorticoid receptors by cortisol. This defect may be inherited or acquired, due to licorice-containing glycyrrhizin acid. The same substance is present in the paste of several brands of chewing tobacco. The defect in Liddle's syndrome **(Chaps. 63 and 406)** results from constitutive activation of amiloride-sensitive epithelial sodium channels on the distal renal tubule, resulting in excess sodium reabsorption; the syndrome is ameliorated by amiloride. Hypertension exacerbated in pregnancy **(Chap. 8)** may be due to activation of the mineralocorticoid receptor by progesterone.

APPROACH TO THE PATIENT: Hypertension

HISTORY

The initial assessment of a hypertensive patient should include a complete history and physical examination to confirm a diagnosis of hypertension, screen for other cardiovascular disease risk factors, screen for secondary causes of hypertension, identify cardiovascular consequences of hypertension and other comorbidities, assess blood pressure–related lifestyles, and determine the potential for intervention.

Most patients with hypertension have no specific symptoms referable to their blood pressure elevation. Although popularly considered a symptom of elevated arterial pressure, headache generally occurs only in patients with severe hypertension. Characteristically, a "hypertensive headache" occurs in the morning and is localized to the occipital region. Other nonspecific symptoms that may be related to elevated blood pressure include dizziness, palpitations, easy fatigability, and impotence. When symptoms are present, they are generally related to hypertensive cardiovascular disease or to manifestations of secondary hypertension. Table 298-5 lists salient features that should be addressed in obtaining a history from a hypertensive patient.

MEASUREMENT OF BLOOD PRESSURE

Reliable measurements of blood pressure depend on attention to the details of the technique and conditions of the measurement. Proper training of observers, positioning of the patient, and selection of cuff size are essential. Owing to recent regulations preventing the use of mercury because of concerns about its potential toxicity, most office measurements are made with aneroid sphygmomanometers or with oscillometric devices. These instruments should be calibrated periodically, and their accuracy confirmed. Before the blood pressure measurement is taken, the individual should be seated quietly in a chair (not the exam table) with feet on the floor for 5 min in a private, quiet setting with a comfortable room temperature. At least two measurements should be made. The center of the cuff should be at heart level, and the width of the bladder cuff

TABLE 298-5 PATIENT'S RELEVANT HISTORY

Duration of hypertension
Previous therapies: responses and side effects
Family history of hypertension and cardiovascular disease
Dietary and psychosocial history
Other risk factors: weight change, dyslipidemia, smoking, diabetes, physical inactivity
Evidence of secondary hypertension: history of renal disease; change in appearance; muscle weakness; spells of sweating, palpitations, tremor; erratic sleep, snoring, daytime somnolence; symptoms of hypo-or hyperthyroidism; use of agents that may increase blood pressure
Evidence of target organ damage: history of TIA, stroke, transient blindness; angina, myocardial infarction, congestive heart failure; sexual function
Other comorbidities

Abbreviation: TIA, transient ischemic attack.

should equal at least 40% of the arm circumference; the length of the cuff bladder should encircle at least 80% of the arm circumference. It is important to pay attention to cuff placement, stethoscope placement, and the rate of deflation of the cuff (2 mmHg/s). Systolic blood pressure is the first of at least two regular "tapping" Korotkoff sounds, and diastolic blood pressure is the point at which the last regular Korotkoff sound is heard. In current practice, a diagnosis of hypertension generally is based on seated, office measurements.

Currently available ambulatory monitors are fully automated, use the oscillometric technique, and typically are programmed to take readings every 15–30 min. Twenty-four-hour ambulatory blood pressure monitoring more reliably predicts cardiovascular disease risk than do office measurements. However, ambulatory monitoring is not used routinely in clinical practice and generally is reserved for patients in whom white coat hypertension is suspected. The Seventh Report of the Joint National Committee on Prevention, Detection, Evaluation, and Treatment of High Blood Pressure (JNC 7) has also recommended ambulatory monitoring for treatment resistance, symptomatic hypotension, autonomic failure, and episodic hypertension.

PHYSICAL EXAMINATION

Body habitus, including weight and height, should be noted. At the initial examination, blood pressure should be measured in both arms and preferably in the supine, sitting, and standing positions to evaluate for postural hypotension. Even if the femoral pulse is normal to palpation, arterial pressure should be measured at least once in the lower extremity in patients in whom hypertension is discovered before age 30. Heart rate also should be recorded. Hypertensive individuals have an increased prevalence of atrial fibrillation. The neck should be palpated for an enlarged thyroid gland, and patients should be assessed for signs of hypo- and hyperthyroidism. Examination of blood vessels may provide clues about underlying vascular disease and should include funduscopic examination, auscultation for bruits over the carotid and femoral arteries, and palpation of femoral and pedal pulses. The retina is the only tissue in which arteries and arterioles can be examined directly. With increasing severity of hypertension and atherosclerotic disease, progressive funduscopic changes include increased arteriolar light reflex, arteriovenous crossing defects, hemorrhages and exudates, and, in patients with malignant hypertension, papilledema. Examination of the heart may reveal a loud second heart sound due to closure of the aortic valve and an S_4 gallop attributed to atrial contraction against a noncompliant left ventricle. Left ventricular hypertrophy may be detected by an enlarged, sustained, and laterally displaced apical impulse. An abdominal bruit, particularly a bruit that lateralizes and extends throughout systole into diastole, raises the possibility of renovascular hypertension. Kidneys of patients with polycystic kidney disease may be palpable in the abdomen. The physical examination also should include evaluation for signs of CHF and a neurologic examination.

LABORATORY TESTING

Table 298-6 lists recommended laboratory tests in the initial evaluation of hypertensive patients. Repeat measurements of renal function, serum electrolytes, fasting glucose, and lipids may be obtained after the introduction of a new antihypertensive agent and then annually or more frequently if clinically indicated. More extensive laboratory testing is appropriate for patients with apparent drug-resistant hypertension or when the clinical evaluation suggests a secondary form of hypertension.

TREATMENT HYPERTENSION

LIFESTYLE INTERVENTIONS

Implementation of lifestyles that favorably affect blood pressure has implications for both the prevention and the treatment of hypertension. Health-promoting lifestyle modifications are recommended for individuals with prehypertension and as an adjunct to drug therapy in hypertensive individuals. These interventions should address overall cardiovascular disease risk. Although the impact of lifestyle interventions on blood pressure is more pronounced in persons with hypertension, in short-term trials, weight loss and reduction of dietary NaCl have been shown to prevent the development of hypertension. In hypertensive individuals, even if these interventions do not produce a sufficient reduction in blood pressure to avoid drug therapy, the number of medications or doses required for blood pressure control may be reduced. Dietary modifications that effectively lower blood pressure are weight loss, reduced NaCl intake, increased potassium intake, moderation of alcohol consumption, and an overall healthy dietary pattern (Table 298-7).

Prevention and treatment of obesity are important for reducing blood pressure and cardiovascular disease risk. In short-term trials, even modest weight loss can lead to a reduction of blood pressure and an increase in insulin sensitivity. Average blood pressure reductions of 6.3/3.1 mmHg have been observed with a reduction in mean body weight of 9.2 kg. Regular physical activity facilitates weight loss, decreases blood pressure, and reduces the overall risk of cardiovascular disease. Blood pressure may be lowered by 30 min of moderately intense physical activity, such as brisk walking, 6–7 days a week, or by more intense, less frequent workouts.

There is individual variability in the sensitivity of blood pressure to NaCl, and this variability may have a genetic basis. Based on results of meta-analyses, lowering of blood pressure by limiting daily NaCl intake to 4.4–7.4 g (75–125 meq) results in blood pressure reductions of 3.7–4.9/0.9–2.9 mmHg in hypertensive individuals and lesser reductions in normotensive individuals. Several long-term, prospective, randomized clinical trials have reported that a reduced salt intake results in a decreased incidence of cardiovascular events. Although reduced salt intakes are generally recommended for both the prevention and treatment of hypertension, overly rigorous salt restriction may have adverse cardiovascular outcomes in diabetic patients and in patients with CHF aggressively treated with diuretics. Potassium and calcium supplementation have inconsistent, modest antihypertensive effects, and, independent of blood pressure, potassium supplementation may be associated with reduced stroke mortality. Consuming three or more alcoholic drinks per day (a standard drink contains ~14 g ethanol) is associated with higher blood pressures, and a reduction of alcohol consumption is associated with a

TABLE 298-6 BASIC LABORATORY TESTS FOR INITIAL EVALUATION

System	Test
Renal	Microscopic urinalysis, albumin excretion, serum BUN and/or creatinine
Endocrine	Serum sodium, potassium, calcium, ?TSH
Metabolic	Fasting blood glucose, total cholesterol, HDL and LDL (often computed) cholesterol, triglycerides
Other	Hematocrit, electrocardiogram

Abbreviations: BUN, blood urea nitrogen; HDL, high-density lipoprotein; LDL, low-density lipoprotein; TSH, thyroid-stimulating hormone.

TABLE 298-7 LIFESTYLE MODIFICATIONS TO MANAGE HYPERTENSION

Weight reduction	Attain and maintain BMI <25 kg/m^2
Dietary salt reduction	<6 g NaCl/d
Adapt DASH-type dietary plan	Diet rich in fruits, vegetables, and low-fat dairy products with reduced content of saturated and total fat
Moderation of alcohol consumption	For those who drink alcohol, consume ≤2 drinks/day in men and ≤1 drink/day in women
Physical activity	Regular aerobic activity, e.g., brisk walking for 30 min/d

Abbreviations: BMI, body mass index; DASH, Dietary Approaches to Stop Hypertension (trial).

reduction of blood pressure. In patients with advanced renal disease, dietary protein restriction may have a modest effect in mitigating renal damage by reducing the intrarenal transmission of systemic arterial pressure.

The DASH (Dietary Approaches to Stop Hypertension) trial convincingly demonstrated that over an 8-week period a diet high in fruits, vegetables, and low-fat dairy products lowers blood pressure in individuals with high-normal blood pressures or mild hypertension. Reduction of daily NaCl intake to <6 g (100 meq) augmented the effect of this diet on blood pressure. Fruits and vegetables are enriched sources of potassium, magnesium, and fiber, and dairy products are an important source of calcium.

PHARMACOLOGIC THERAPY

Drug therapy is recommended for individuals with blood pressures ≥140/90 mmHg. The degree of benefit derived from antihypertensive agents is related to the magnitude of the blood pressure reduction. Lowering systolic blood pressure by 10–12 mmHg and diastolic blood pressure by 5–6 mmHg confers relative risk reductions of 35–40% for stroke and 12–16% for CHD within 5 years of the initiation of treatment. Risk of heart failure is reduced by >50%. Hypertension control is the single most effective intervention for slowing the rate of progression of hypertension-related kidney disease.

There is considerable variation in individual responses to different classes of antihypertensive agents, and the magnitude of response to any single agent may be limited by activation of counter-regulatory mechanisms. Most available agents reduce systolic blood pressure by 7–13 mmHg and diastolic blood pressure by 4–8 mmHg when corrected for placebo effect. More often than not, combinations of agents, with complementary antihypertensive mechanisms, are required to achieve goal blood pressure reductions. Selection of antihypertensive agents and combinations of agents should be individualized, taking into account age, severity of hypertension, other cardiovascular disease risk factors, comorbid conditions, and practical considerations related to cost, side effects, and frequency of dosing (Table 298-8).

Diuretics Low-dose thiazide diuretics may be used alone or in combination with other antihypertensive drugs. Thiazides inhibit the Na^+/Cl^- pump in the distal convoluted tubule and hence increase sodium excretion. In the long term, they also may act as vasodilators. Thiazides are safe, efficacious, inexpensive, and reduce clinical events. They provide additive blood pressure–lowering effects when combined with beta blockers, angiotensin-converting enzyme inhibitors (ACEIs), or angiotensin receptor blockers (ARBs). In contrast, addition of a diuretic to a calcium channel blocker is less effective. Usual doses of hydrochlorothiazide range from 6.25–50 mg/d. Owing to an increased incidence of metabolic side effects (hypokalemia, insulin resistance, increased cholesterol), higher doses generally are not recommended. Chlorthalidone is a diuretic structurally similar to hydrochlorothiazide, and like hydrochlorothiazide, it blocks sodium-chloride cotransport in the early distal tubule. However, chlorthalidone has a longer half-life (40–60 h vs. 9–15 h) and an antihypertensive potency ~1.5–2.0 times that of hydrochlorothiazide. Potassium loss is also greater with chlorthalidone. Two potassium-sparing diuretics, amiloride and triamterene, act by inhibiting epithelial sodium channels in the distal nephron. These agents are weak antihypertensive agents but may be used in combination with a thiazide to protect against hypokalemia. The main pharmacologic target for loop diuretics is the Na^+-K^+-$2Cl^-$ cotransporter in the thick ascending limb of the loop of Henle. Loop diuretics generally are reserved for hypertensive patients with reduced glomerular filtration rates (reflected in serum creatinine >220 μmol/L [>2.5 mg/dL]), CHF, or sodium retention and edema for some other reason, such as treatment with a potent vasodilator, e.g., minoxidil.

Blockers of the Renin–Angiotensin System ACEIs decrease the production of angiotensin II, increase bradykinin levels, and reduce sympathetic nervous system activity. ARBs provide selective blockade of AT_1 receptors, and the effect of angiotensin II on unblocked AT_2 receptors may augment their hypotensive effect. Both classes of agents are effective antihypertensive agents that may be used as monotherapy or in combination with diuretics, calcium antagonists, and alpha blocking agents. ACEIs and ARBs improve insulin action and ameliorate the adverse effects of diuretics on glucose metabolism. Although the overall impact on the incidence of diabetes is modest, compared with amlodipine (a calcium antagonist), valsartan (an ARB) has been shown to reduce the risk of developing diabetes in high-risk hypertensive patients. ACEI/ARB combinations are less effective in lowering blood pressure than is the case when either class of these agents is used in combination with other classes of agents. In patients with vascular disease or a high risk of diabetes, combination ACEI/ARB therapy has been associated with more adverse events (e.g., cardiovascular death, myocardial infarction, stroke, and hospitalization for heart failure) without increases in benefit.

Side effects of ACEIs and ARBs include functional renal insufficiency due to efferent renal arteriolar dilation in a kidney with a stenotic lesion of the renal artery. Additional predisposing conditions to renal insufficiency induced by these agents include dehydration, CHF, and use of nonsteroidal anti-inflammatory drugs. Dry cough occurs in ~15% of patients, and angioedema occurs in <1% of patients taking ACEIs. Angioedema occurs most commonly in individuals of Asian origin and more commonly in African Americans than in whites. Hyperkalemia due to hypoaldosteronism is an occasional side effect of both ACEIs and ARBs.

An alternative approach to blocking the renin-angiotensin system has recently been introduced into clinical practice for the treatment of hypertension: direct renin inhibitors. Blockade of the renin-angiotensin system is more complete with renin inhibitors than with ACEIs or ARBs. Aliskiren is the first of a class of oral, nonpeptide competitive inhibitors of the enzymatic activity of renin. Monotherapy with aliskiren seems to be as effective as an ACEI or ARB for lowering blood pressure, but not more effective. Further blood reductions may be achieved when aliskiren is used in combination with a thiazide diuretic or a calcium antagonist. Currently, aliskiren is not considered a first-line antihypertensive agent.

Aldosterone Antagonists Spironolactone is a nonselective aldosterone antagonist that may be used alone or in combination with a thiazide diuretic. It may be a particularly effective agent in patients with low-renin primary hypertension, resistant hypertension, and primary aldosteronism. In patients with CHF, low-dose spironolactone reduces mortality and hospitalizations for heart failure when given in addition to conventional therapy with ACEIs, digoxin, and loop diuretics. Because spironolactone binds to progesterone and androgen receptors, side effects may include gynecomastia, impotence, and menstrual abnormalities. These side effects are circumvented by a newer agent, eplerenone, which is a selective aldosterone antagonist.

Beta Blockers β-Adrenergic receptor blockers lower blood pressure by decreasing cardiac output, due to a reduction of heart rate and contractility. Other proposed mechanisms by which beta blockers lower blood pressure include a central nervous system effect and inhibition of renin release. Beta blockers are particularly effective in hypertensive patients with tachycardia, and their hypotensive potency is enhanced by coadministration with a diuretic. In lower doses, some beta blockers selectively inhibit cardiac β_1 receptors and have less influence on β_2 receptors on bronchial and vascular smooth muscle cells; however, there seems to be no difference in the antihypertensive potencies of cardioselective and nonselective beta blockers. Some beta blockers have intrinsic sympathomimetic activity, although it is uncertain whether this constitutes an overall advantage or disadvantage in cardiac therapy. Beta blockers without intrinsic sympathomimetic activity decrease the rate of sudden death, overall mortality, and recurrent myocardial infarction. In patients with CHF, beta blockers have been shown to reduce the risks of hospitalization and mortality. Overall, beta blockers

TABLE 298-8 EXAMPLES OF ORAL DRUGS USED IN TREATMENT OF HYPERTENSION

Drug Class	Examples	Usual Total Daily Dose[a] (Dosing Frequency/Day)	Other Indications	Contraindications/Cautions
Diuretics				
Thiazides	Hydrochlorothiazide	6.25–50 mg (1–2)		Diabetes, dyslipidemia, hyperuricemia, gout, hypokalemia
	Chlorthalidone	25–50 mg (1)		
Loop diuretics	Furosemide	40–80 mg (2–3)	CHF due to systolic dysfunction, renal failure	Diabetes, dyslipidemia, hyperuricemia, gout, hypokalemia
	Ethacrynic acid	50–100 mg (2–3)		
Aldosterone antagonists	Spironolactone	25–100 mg (1–2)	CHF due to systolic dysfunction, primary aldosteronism	Renal failure, hyperkalemia
	Eplerenone	50–100 mg (1–2)		
K+ retaining	Amiloride	5–10 mg (1–2)		Renal failure, hyperkalemia
	Triamterene	50–100 mg (1–2)		
Beta blockers				
Cardioselective	Atenolol	25–100 mg (1)	Angina, CHF due to systolic dysfunction, post-MI, sinus tachycardia, ventricular tachyarrhythmias	Asthma, COPD, 2nd- or 3rd-degree heart block, sick-sinus syndrome
	Metoprolol	25–100 mg (1–2)		
Nonselective	Propranolol	40–160 mg (2)		
	Propranolol LA	60–180 (1)		
Combined alpha/beta	Labetalol	200–800 mg (2)	?Post-MI, CHF	
	Carvedilol	12.5–50 mg (2)		
Alpha antagonists				
Selective	Prazosin	2–20 mg (2–3)	Prostatism	
	Doxazosin	1–16 mg (1)		
	Terazosin	1–10 mg (1–2)		
Nonselective	Phenoxybenzamine	20–120 mg (2–3)	Pheochromocytoma	
Sympatholytics				
Central	Clonidine	0.1–0.6 mg (2)		
	Clonidine patch	0.1–0.3 mg (1/week)		
	Methyldopa	250–1000 mg (2)		
	Reserpine	0.05–0.25 mg (1)		
	Guanfacine	0.5–2 mg (1)		
ACE inhibitors	Captopril	25–200 mg (2)	Post-MI, coronary syndromes, CHF with low ejection fraction, nephropathy	Acute renal failure, bilateral renal artery stenosis, pregnancy, hyperkalemia
	Lisinopril	10–40 mg (1)		
	Ramipril	2.5–20 mg (1–2)		
Angiotensin II antagonists	Losartan	25–100 mg (1–2)	CHF with low ejection fraction, nephropathy, ACE inhibitor cough	Renal failure, bilateral renal artery stenosis, pregnancy, hyperkalemia
	Valsartan	80–320 mg (1)		
	Candesartan	2–32 mg (1–2)		
Renin inhibitors	Aliskiren	150–300 mg (1)	Diabetic nephropathy	Pregnancy
Calcium antagonists				
Dihydropyridines	Nifedipine (long-acting)	30–60 mg (1)		
Nondihydropyridines	Verapamil (long-acting)	120–360 mg (1–2)	Post-MI, supraventricular tachycardias, angina	2nd- or 3rd-degree heart block
	Diltiazem (long-acting)	180-420 mg (1)		
Direct vasodilators	Hydralazine	25–100 mg (2)		Severe coronary artery disease
	Minoxidil	2.5–80 mg (1–2)		

[a]At the initiation of therapy, lower doses may be preferable for elderly patients and for select combinations of antihypertensive agents.

Abbreviations: ACE, angiotensin-converting enzyme; CHF, congestive heart failure; COPD, chronic obstructive pulmonary disease; MI, myocardial infarction.

may be less protective against cardiovascular and cerebrovascular endpoints, and some beta blockers may have less effect on central aortic pressure than other classes of antihypertensive agents. However, beta blockers remain appropriate therapy for hypertensive patients with concomitant heart disease and related comorbidities. Carvedilol and labetalol block both β receptors and peripheral α-adrenergic receptors. The potential advantages of combined β- and α-adrenergic blockade in treating hypertension remain to be determined. Nebivolol represents another class of cardioselective beta blockers that has additional vasodilator actions related to enhancement of nitric oxide activity. Whether this confers greater clinical effectiveness remains to be determined.

α-Adrenergic Blockers Postsynaptic, selective α-adrenoreceptor antagonists lower blood pressure by decreasing peripheral vascular resistance. They are effective antihypertensive agents used either as monotherapy or in combination with other agents. However, in clinical trials of hypertensive patients, alpha blockade has not been shown to reduce cardiovascular morbidity and mortality or to provide as much protection against CHF as other classes of antihypertensive agents. These agents are also effective in treating lower urinary tract symptoms in men with prostatic hypertrophy. Nonselective α-adrenoreceptor antagonists bind to postsynaptic and presynaptic receptors and are used primarily for the management of patients with pheochromocytoma.

Sympatholytic Agents Centrally acting α_2 sympathetic agonists decrease peripheral resistance by inhibiting sympathetic outflow. They may be particularly useful in patients with autonomic neuropathy who have wide variations in blood pressure due to baroreceptor denervation. Drawbacks include somnolence, dry mouth, and rebound hypertension on withdrawal. Peripheral sympatholytics decrease peripheral resistance and venous constriction by depleting nerve terminal norepinephrine. Although they are potentially effective antihypertensive agents, their usefulness is limited by orthostatic hypotension, sexual dysfunction, and numerous drug-drug interactions. Rebound hypertension is another concern with abrupt cessation of drugs with a short half-life.

Calcium Channel Blockers Calcium antagonists reduce vascular resistance through L-channel blockade, which reduces intracellular calcium and blunts vasoconstriction. This is a heterogeneous group of agents that includes drugs in the following three classes: phenylalkylamines (verapamil), benzothiazepines (diltiazem), and 1,4-dihydropyridines (nifedipine-like). Used alone and in combination with other agents (ACEIs, beta blockers, α_1-adrenergic blockers), calcium antagonists effectively lower blood pressure; however, it is unclear if adding a diuretic to a calcium blocker results in a further lowering of blood pressure. Side effects of flushing, headache, and edema with dihydropyridine use are related to their potencies as arteriolar dilators; edema is due to an increase in transcapillary pressure gradients, not to net salt and water retention.

Direct Vasodilators Direct vasodilators decrease peripheral resistance and concomitantly activate mechanisms that defend arterial pressure, notably the sympathetic nervous system, the renin-angiotensin-aldosterone system, and sodium retention. Usually, they are not considered first-line agents but are most effective when added to a combination that includes a diuretic and a beta blocker. Hydralazine is a potent direct vasodilator that has antioxidant and nitric oxide–enhancing actions, and minoxidil is a particularly potent agent and is used most frequently in patients with renal insufficiency who are refractory to all other drugs. Hydralazine may induce a lupus-like syndrome, and side effects of minoxidil include hypertrichosis and pericardial effusion. Intravenous nitroprusside can be used to treat malignant hypertension and life-threatening left ventricular heart failure associated with elevated arterial pressure.

COMPARISONS OF ANTIHYPERTENSIVES

Based on pooling results from clinical trials, meta-analyses of the efficacy of different classes of antihypertensive agents suggest essentially equivalent blood pressure–lowering effects of the following six major classes of antihypertensive agents when used as monotherapy: thiazide diuretics, beta blockers, ACEIs, ARBs, calcium antagonists, and α_1 blockers. On average, standard doses of most antihypertensive agents reduce blood pressure by 8–10/4–7 mmHg; however, there may be subgroup differences in responsiveness. Younger patients may be more responsive to beta blockers and ACEIs, whereas patients over age 50 may be more responsive to diuretics and calcium antagonists. There is a limited relationship between plasma renin and blood pressure response. Patients with high-renin hypertension may be more responsive to ACEIs and ARBs than to other classes of agents, whereas patients with low-renin hypertension are more responsive to diuretics and calcium antagonists. Hypertensive African Americans tend to have low renin and may require higher doses of ACEIs and ARBs than whites for optimal blood pressure control, although this difference is abolished when these agents are combined with a diuretic. Beta blockers also appear to be less effective than thiazide diuretics in African Americans than in non-African Americans. Early pharmacogenetic studies, utilizing either a candidate gene approach or genome-wide scans, have shown associations of gene polymorphisms with blood pressure responsiveness to specific antihypertensive drugs. However, the reported effects have generally been too small to affect clinical decisions, and associated polymorphisms remain to be confirmed. Currently, in practical terms, the presence of comorbidities often influences the selection of antihypertensive agents.

A meta-analysis of more than 30 randomized trials of blood pressure–lowering therapy indicates that for a given reduction in blood pressure, the major drug classes seem to produce similar overall net effects on total cardiovascular events. In both nondiabetic and diabetic hypertensive patients, most trials have failed to show significant differences in cardiovascular outcomes with different drug regimens as long as equivalent decreases in blood pressure were achieved. For example, the Antihypertensive and Lipid-Lowering Treatment to Prevent Heart Attack Trial (ALLHAT) demonstrated that the occurrence of CHD and nonfatal myocardial infarction, as well as overall mortality, was virtually identical in hypertensive patients treated with either an ACEI (lisinopril), a diuretic (chlorthalidone), or a calcium antagonist (amlodipine).

However, in specific patient groups, ACEIs may have particular advantages, beyond that of blood pressure control, in reducing cardiovascular and renal outcomes. ACEIs and ARBs decrease intraglomerular pressure and proteinuria and may retard the rate of progression of renal insufficiency, not totally accounted for by their hypotensive effects, in both diabetic and nondiabetic renal diseases. In patients with type 2 diabetes, treatment with an ACEI, an ARB, or aliskiren decreases proteinuria and delays the progression of renal disease. In experimental models of hypertension and diabetes, renal protection with aliskiren is comparable to that with ACEIs and ARBs. However, in patients with type 2 diabetes, addition of aliskiren to an ACEI provides no additional protection against cardiovascular or renal disease and may be associated with more adverse outcomes. Among African Americans with hypertension-related renal disease, ACEIs appear to be more effective than beta blockers or dihydropyridine calcium channel blockers in slowing, although not preventing, the decline of glomerular filtration rate. The renoprotective effect of these renin-angiotensin blockers, compared with other antihypertensive drugs, is less obvious at lower blood pressures. In most patients with hypertension and heart failure due to systolic and/or diastolic dysfunction, the use of diuretics, ACEIs or ARBs, and beta blockers is recommended to improve survival. Independent of blood pressure, in both hypertensive and normotensive individuals, ACEIs attenuate the development of left ventricular hypertrophy, improve symptomatology and risk of death from CHF, and reduce morbidity and mortality rates in post-myocardial infarction patients. Similar benefits in cardiovascular morbidity and mortality rates in patients with CHF have been observed with the use of ARBs. ACEIs provide better coronary protection than do calcium channel blockers, whereas calcium channel blockers provide more stroke protection than do either ACEIs or beta blockers. Results of a large, double-blind, prospective clinical trial (Avoiding Cardiovascular Events through Combination Therapy in Patients Living with Systolic Hypertension [ACCOMPLISH Trial]) indicated that combination treatment with an ACEI (benazepril) plus a calcium antagonist (amlodipine) was superior to treatment with the ACEI plus a diuretic (hydrochlorothiazide) in reducing the risk of cardiovascular events and death among high-risk patients with hypertension. However, the combination of an ACEI and a diuretic has recently been shown to produce major reductions in morbidity and mortality in the very elderly.

After a stroke, combination therapy with an ACEI and a diuretic, but not with an ARB, has been reported to reduce the rate of recurrent stroke. Some of these apparent differences may reflect differences in trial design and/or patient groups.

There is a recent resurgence of interest in two nonpharmacologic, antihypertensive therapies that interrupt sympathetic outflow: (1) device-based carotid baroreflex activation by electrical stimulation of the carotid sinus; and (2) endovascular radiofrequency ablation of the renal sympathetic nerves. Whereas renal denervation is a minimally invasive procedure, carotid baroreceptor stimulation is a surgical procedure, usually performed under general anesthesia, that currently involves implanting electrodes on both the right and left carotid arteries. Both interventions inhibit sympathetic drive and decrease blood pressure by increasing the capacity of the kidney to excrete sodium and by decreasing renin release. Sustained activation of the baroreflex most likely lowers blood pressure by other mechanisms as well. Clinical experience with these interventions is limited. In the short term, blood pressure is lowered in 75–80% of patients, and the magnitude of the blood pressure reduction is similar for both procedures. To date, the most impressive results have been observed in patients with "resistant" hypertension and patients with obesity-related hypertension. Awaiting the results of long-term, multicenter clinical trials to evaluate their efficacy and safety, it remains to be seen whether these interventions will be adopted into clinical practice.

BLOOD PRESSURE GOALS OF ANTIHYPERTENSIVE THERAPY

Based on clinical trial data, the maximum protection against combined cardiovascular endpoints is achieved with pressures <135–140 mmHg for systolic blood pressure and <80–85 mmHg for diastolic blood pressure; however, treatment has not reduced cardiovascular disease risk to the level in nonhypertensive individuals. In diabetic patients, effective blood pressure control reduces the risk of cardiovascular events and death as well as the risk for microvascular disease (nephropathy, retinopathy). Although guidelines for hypertension control have recommended more aggressive blood pressure targets (e.g., office or clinic blood pressure <130/80 mmHg) for patients with diabetes, CHD, chronic kidney disease, or additional cardiovascular disease risk factors, recent evidence suggests that overly aggressive targets for blood pressure control may not be advantageous, particularly in high-risk patients. For example, among hypertensive patients with diabetes and coronary heart disease, "tight control" of systolic blood pressure (<130 mmHg) is not associated with improved cardiovascular outcomes. The concept of a "J-curve" suggests that the risk of cardiovascular events increases at blood pressures that are either too high or too low. Theoretically blood pressures that are too low may exceed the autoregulatory capacity of cerebral, coronary, and renal blood flows. There is some suggestive evidence from recent randomized clinical trials for a J-shaped relationship between blood pressure and cardiovascular outcomes (including all-cause mortality) in high-risk patients. Consequently, caution should be exercised in lowering blood pressure <130/80 mmHg in patients with diabetes, CHD, and other high-risk patients. In patients with chronic renal insufficiency, a small, nonprogressive increase in the serum creatinine concentration may occur. This generally reflects a hemodynamic response, not structural renal injury, indicating that intraglomerular pressure has been reduced. Blood pressure control should not be allowed to deteriorate in order to prevent the modest creatinine rise. Among older patients with isolated systolic hypertension, further lowering of diastolic blood pressure does not result in harm. However, relatively little information is available concerning the risk-versus-benefit ratio of antihypertensive therapy in individuals >80 years of age, and in this population, gradual blood pressure reduction to a less aggressive target level of control may be appropriate.

To achieve recommended blood pressure goals, the majority of individuals with hypertension will require treatment with more than one drug. Three or more drugs frequently are needed in patients with diabetes and renal insufficiency. For most agents, reduction of blood pressure at half-standard doses is only ~20% less than at standard doses. Appropriate combinations of agents at these lower doses may have additive or almost additive effects on blood pressure with a lower incidence of side effects.

The term *resistant hypertension* refers to patients with blood pressures persistently >140/90 mmHg despite taking three or more antihypertensive agents, including a diuretic. Resistant or difficult-to-control hypertension is more common in patients >60 years than in younger patients. Resistant hypertension may be related to "pseudoresistance" (high office blood pressures and lower home blood pressures), nonadherence to therapy, identifiable causes of hypertension (including obesity and excessive alcohol intake), and the use of any of a number of nonprescription and prescription drugs (Table 298-3). Rarely, in older patients, pseudohypertension may be related to the inability to measure blood pressure accurately in severely sclerotic arteries. This condition is suggested if the radial pulse remains palpable despite occlusion of the brachial artery by the cuff (Osler maneuver). The actual blood pressure can be determined by direct intra-arterial measurement. Evaluation of patients with resistant hypertension might include home blood pressure monitoring to determine if office blood pressures are representative of the usual blood pressure. A more extensive evaluation for a secondary form of hypertension should be undertaken if no other explanation for hypertension resistance becomes apparent.

HYPERTENSIVE EMERGENCIES

Probably due to the widespread availability of antihypertensive therapy, in the United States there has been a decline in the numbers of patients presenting with "crisis levels" of blood pressure. Most patients who present with severe hypertension are chronically hypertensive, and in the absence of acute end organ damage, precipitous lowering of blood pressure may result in significant morbidity and should be avoided. The key to successful management of severe hypertension is to differentiate hypertensive crises from hypertensive urgencies. The degree of target organ damage, rather than the level of blood pressure alone, determines the rapidity with which blood pressure should be lowered. **Tables 298-9 and 298-10** list a number of hypertension-related emergencies and recommended therapies.

Malignant hypertension is a syndrome associated with an abrupt increase of blood pressure in a patient with underlying hypertension or related to the sudden onset of hypertension in a previously normotensive individual. The absolute level of blood pressure is not as important as its rate of rise. Pathologically, the syndrome is associated with diffuse necrotizing vasculitis, arteriolar thrombi, and fibrin deposition in arteriolar walls. Fibrinoid necrosis has been observed in arterioles of kidney, brain, retina, and other organs. Clinically, the syndrome is recognized by progressive retinopathy (arteriolar spasm, hemorrhages, exudates, and papilledema), deteriorating renal function with proteinuria, microangiopathic hemolytic anemia, and encephalopathy. Historic inquiry should include questions about the use of monoamine oxidase inhibitors and recreational drugs (e.g., cocaine, amphetamines).

Although blood pressure should be lowered rapidly in patients with hypertensive encephalopathy, there are inherent risks of overly aggressive therapy. In hypertensive individuals, the upper and lower limits of autoregulation of cerebral blood flow are shifted to higher levels of arterial pressure, and rapid lowering of blood pressure to below the lower limit of autoregulation may precipitate cerebral ischemia or infarction as a consequence of decreased cerebral blood flow. Renal and coronary blood flows also may decrease with overly aggressive acute therapy. The initial goal of therapy is to reduce

TABLE 298-9 PREFERRED PARENTERAL DRUGS FOR SELECTED HYPERTENSIVE EMERGENCIES

Hypertensive encephalopathy	Nitroprusside, nicardipine, labetalol
Malignant hypertension (when IV therapy is indicated)	Labetalol, nicardipine, nitroprusside, enalaprilat
Stroke	Nicardipine, labetalol, nitroprusside
Myocardial infarction/unstable angina	Nitroglycerin, nicardipine, labetalol, esmolol
Acute left ventricular failure	Nitroglycerin, enalaprilat, loop diuretics
Aortic dissection	Nitroprusside, esmolol, labetalol
Adrenergic crisis	Phentolamine, nitroprusside
Postoperative hypertension	Nitroglycerin, nitroprusside, labetalol, nicardipine
Preeclampsia/eclampsia of pregnancy	Hydralazine, labetalol, nicardipine

Source: Adapted from DG Vidt, in S Oparil, MA Weber (eds): *Hypertension*, 2nd ed. Philadelphia, Elsevier Saunders, 2005.

TABLE 298-10 USUAL INTRAVENOUS DOSES OF ANTIHYPERTENSIVE AGENTS USED IN HYPERTENSIVE EMERGENCIES[a]

Antihypertensive Agent	Intravenous Dose
Nitroprusside	Initial 0.3 (μg/kg)/min; usual 2–4 (μg/kg)/min; maximum 10 (μg/kg)/min for 10 min
Nicardipine	Initial 5 mg/h; titrate by 2.5 mg/h at 5–15 min intervals; max 15 mg/h
Labetalol	2 mg/min up to 300 mg *or* 20 mg over 2 min, then 40–80 mg at 10-min intervals up to 300 mg total
Enalaprilat	Usual 0.625–1.25 mg over 5 min every 6–8 h; maximum 5 mg/dose
Esmolol	Initial 80–500 μg/kg over 1 min, then 50–300 (μg/kg)/min
Phentolamine	5–15 mg bolus
Nitroglycerin	Initial 5 μg/min, then titrate by 5 μg/min at 3–5-min intervals; if no response is seen at 20 μg/min, incremental increases of 10–20 μg/min may be used
Hydralazine	10–50 mg at 30-min intervals

[a]Constant blood pressure monitoring is required. Start with the lowest dose. Subsequent doses and intervals of administration should be adjusted according to the blood pressure response and duration of action of the specific agent.

mean arterial blood pressure by no more than 25% within minutes to 2 h or to a blood pressure in the range of 160/100–110 mmHg. This may be accomplished with IV nitroprusside, a short-acting vasodilator with a rapid onset of action that allows for minute-to-minute control of blood pressure. Parenteral labetalol and nicardipine are also effective agents for the treatment of hypertensive encephalopathy.

In patients with malignant hypertension without encephalopathy or another catastrophic event, it is preferable to reduce blood pressure over hours or longer rather than minutes. This goal may effectively be achieved initially with frequent dosing of short-acting oral agents such as captopril, clonidine, and labetalol.

Acute, transient blood pressure elevations that last days to weeks frequently occur after thrombotic and hemorrhagic strokes. Autoregulation of cerebral blood flow is impaired in ischemic cerebral tissue, and higher arterial pressures may be required to maintain cerebral blood flow. Although specific blood pressure targets have not been defined for patients with acute cerebrovascular events, aggressive reductions of blood pressure are to be avoided. With the increasing availability of improved methods for measuring cerebral blood flow (using CT technology), studies are in progress to evaluate the effects of different classes of antihypertensive agents on both blood pressure and cerebral blood flow after an acute stroke. Currently, in the absence of other indications for acute therapy, for patients with cerebral infarction who are not candidates for thrombolytic therapy, one recommended guideline is to institute antihypertensive therapy only for patients with a systolic blood pressure >220 mmHg or a diastolic blood pressure >130 mmHg. If thrombolytic therapy is to be used, the recommended goal blood pressure is <185 mmHg systolic pressure and <110 mmHg diastolic pressure. In patients with hemorrhagic stroke, suggested guidelines for initiating antihypertensive therapy are systolic >180 mmHg or diastolic pressure >130 mmHg. The management of hypertension after subarachnoid hemorrhage is controversial. Cautious reduction of blood pressure is indicated if mean arterial pressure is >130 mmHg.

In addition to pheochromocytoma, an adrenergic crisis due to catecholamine excess may be related to cocaine or amphetamine overdose, clonidine withdrawal, acute spinal cord injuries, and an interaction of tyramine-containing compounds with monoamine oxidase inhibitors. These patients may be treated with phentolamine or nitroprusside.

Treatment of hypertension in patients with acute aortic dissection is discussed in Chap. 301, and treatment of hypertension in pregnancy is discussed in Chap. 8.

299 Renovascular Disease

Stephen C. Textor

The renal vasculature is unusually complex with rich arteriolar flow to the cortex in excess of metabolic requirements, consistent with its primary function as a filtering organ. After delivering blood to cortical glomeruli, the postglomerular circulation supplies deeper medullary segments that support energy-dependent solute transport at multiple levels of the renal tubule. These postglomerular vessels carry less blood, and high oxygen consumption leaves the deeper medullary regions at the margin of hypoxemia. Vascular disorders that commonly threaten the blood supply of the kidney include large-vessel atherosclerosis, fibromuscular diseases, and embolic disorders. **Microvascular injury, including inflammatory and primary hematologic disorders, is described in Chap. 341.**

The glomerular capillary endothelium shares susceptibility to oxidative stress, pressure injury, and inflammation with other vascular territories. Rates of urinary albumin excretion (UAE) are predictive of systemic atherosclerotic disease events. Increased UAE may develop years before cardiovascular events. UAE and the risk of cardiovascular events are both reduced with pharmacologic therapy such as statins. Experimental studies demonstrate functional changes and rarefaction of renal microvessels under conditions of accelerated atherosclerosis and/or compromise of proximal perfusion pressures with large-vessel disease (Fig. 299-1).

MACROVASCULAR DISEASE

Large-vessel renal artery occlusive disease can result from extrinsic compression of the vessel, fibromuscular dysplasia, or, most commonly, atherosclerotic disease. Any disorder that reduces perfusion pressure to the kidney can activate mechanisms that tend to restore renal pressures at the expense of developing systemic hypertension. Because restoration of perfusion pressures can reverse these pathways, renal artery stenosis is considered a specifically treatable "secondary" cause of hypertension.

Renal artery stenosis is common and often has only minor hemodynamic effects. Fibromuscular dysplasia (FMD) is reported in 3–5% of normal subjects presenting as potential kidney donors without hypertension. It may present clinically with hypertension in younger individuals (between age 15 and 50), most often women. FMD does not often threaten kidney function, but sometimes produces total occlusion and can be associated with renal artery aneurysms. Atherosclerotic renal artery stenosis (ARAS) is common in the general population (6.8% of a community-based sample above age 65), and the prevalence increases with age and for patients with other vascular conditions such as coronary artery disease (18–23%) and/or peripheral aortic or lower extremity disease (>30%). If untreated, ARAS progresses in nearly 50% of cases over a 5 year period, sometimes to total occlusion. Intensive treatment of arterial blood pressure and statin therapy appear to slow these rates and improve clinical outcomes.

Critical levels of stenosis lead to a reduction in perfusion pressure that activates the renin-angiotensin system, reduces sodium excretion, and activates sympathetic adrenergic pathways. These events lead to systemic hypertension characterized by angiotensin dependence in the early stages, widely varying pressures, loss of circadian blood pressure (BP) rhythms, and accelerated target organ injury, including left ventricular hypertrophy and renal fibrosis. Renovascular hypertension can be treated with agents that block the renin-angiotensin system and other drugs that modify these pressor pathways. It can also be treated with restoration of renal blood flow by either endovascular or surgical revascularization. Most patients require continued antihypertensive drug therapy because revascularization alone rarely lowers BP to normal.

ARAS and systemic hypertension tend to affect both the post-stenotic and contralateral kidneys, reducing overall glomerular filtration rate (GFR) in ARAS. When kidney function is threatened by

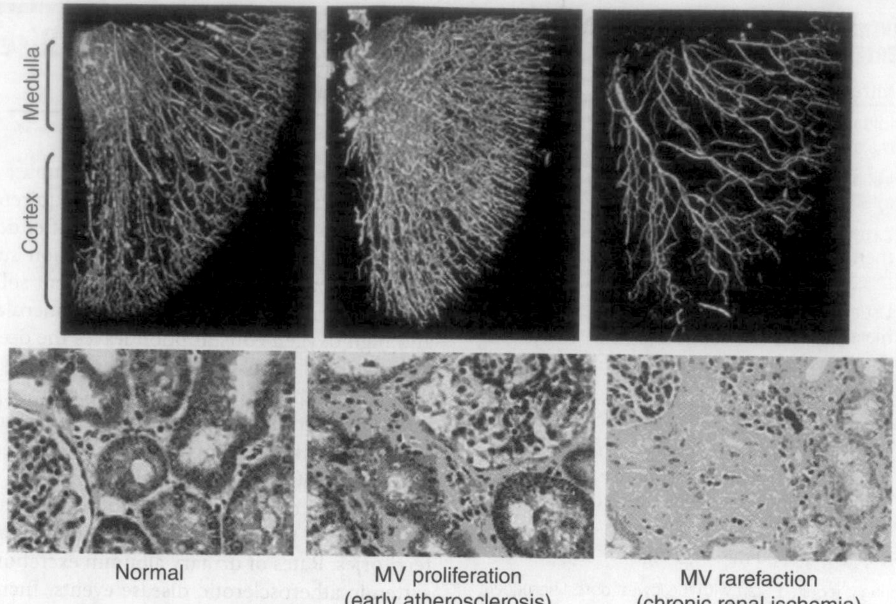

FIGURE 299-1 Examples of micro-CT images from vessels defined by radiopaque casts injected into the renal vasculature. These illustrate the complex, dense cortical capillary network supplying the kidney cortex that can either proliferate or succumb to rarefaction under the influence of atherosclerosis and/or occlusive disease. Changes in blood supply are followed by tubulointerstitial fibrosis and loss of kidney function. MV, microvascular. *(From LO Lerman, AR Chade: Curr Opin Nephrol Hyper 18:160, 2009, with permission.)*

large-vessel disease primarily, it has been labeled ischemic nephropathy. Moderately reduced blood flow that develops gradually is associated with reduced GFR and limited oxygen consumption with preserved tissue oxygenation. Hence, kidney function can remain stable during medical therapy, sometimes for years. With more advanced disease, reductions in cortical perfusion and frank tissue hypoxia develop. Unlike FMD, ARAS develops in patients with other risk factors for atherosclerosis and is commonly superimposed upon preexisting small-vessel disease in the kidney resulting from hypertension, aging, and diabetes. Nearly 85% of patients considered for renal revascularization have stage 3–5 chronic kidney disease (CKD) with GFR below 60 mL/min per 1.73 m^2. The presence of ARAS is a strong predictor of morbidity- and mortality-related cardiovascular events, independent of whether renal revascularization is undertaken.

Diagnostic approaches to renal artery stenosis depend partly on the specific issues to be addressed. Noninvasive characterization of the renal vasculature may be achieved by several techniques, summarized in Table 299-1. Although activation of the renin-angiotensin system is a key step in developing renovascular hypertension, it is transient. Levels of renin activity are therefore subject to timing, the effects of drugs, and sodium intake, and do not reliably predict the response to vascular therapy. Renal artery velocities by Doppler ultrasound above 200 cm/s generally predict hemodynamically important lesions (above 60% vessel lumen occlusion), although treatment trials require velocity above 300 cm/s to avoid false positives. The renal resistive index has predictive value regarding the viability of the kidney. It remains operator- and institution-dependent, however. Captopril-enhanced renography has a strong negative predictive value when entirely normal. Magnetic resonance angiography (MRA) is now less often used, as gadolinium contrast has been associated with nephrogenic systemic fibrosis. Contrast-enhanced computed tomography (CT) with vascular reconstruction provides excellent vascular images and functional assessment, but carries a small risk of contrast toxicity.

TREATMENT RENAL ARTERY STENOSIS

While restoring renal blood flow and perfusion seems intuitively beneficial for high-grade occlusive lesions, revascularization procedures also pose hazards and expense. Patients with FMD are commonly younger females with otherwise normal vessels and a

TABLE 299-1 SUMMARY OF IMAGING MODALITIES FOR EVALUATING THE KIDNEY VASCULATURE

Perfusion Studies to Assess Differential Renal Blood Flow			
Captopril renography with technetium ^{99m}Tc mertiatide (^{99m}Tc MAG3)	Captopril-mediated fall in filtration pressure amplifies differences in renal perfusion	Normal study excludes renovascular hypertension	Multiple limitations in patients with advanced atherosclerosis or creatinine >2.0 mg/dL (177 μmol/L)
Vascular Studies to Evaluate the Renal Arteries			
Duplex ultrasonography	Shows the renal arteries and measures flow velocity as a means of assessing the severity of stenosis	Inexpensive; widely available	Heavily dependent on operator's experience; less useful than invasive angiography for the diagnosis of fibromuscular dysplasia and abnormalities in accessory renal arteries
Magnetic resonance angiography	Shows the renal arteries and perirenal aorta	Not nephrotoxic, but concerns for gadolinium toxicity exclude use in GFR <30 mL/min/1.73 m^2; provides excellent images	Expensive; gadolinium excluded in renal failure, unable to visualize stented vessels
Computed tomographic angiography	Shows the renal arteries and perirenal aorta	Provides excellent images; stents do not cause artifacts	Expensive, moderate volume of contrast required, potentially nephrotoxic
Intraarterial angiography	Shows location and severity of vascular lesion	Considered "gold standard" for diagnosis of large-vessel disease, usually performed simultaneous with planned intervention	Expensive, associated hazard of atheroemboli, contrast toxicity, procedure-related complications, e.g., dissection

Abbreviation: GFR, glomerular filtration rate.

long life expectancy. These patients often respond well to percutaneous renal artery angioplasty. If BP can be controlled to goal levels and kidney function remains stable in patients with ARAS, it may be argued that medical therapy with follow-up for disease progression is equally effective. Prospective trials up to now have failed to identify compelling benefits for interventional procedures regarding short-term results of BP and renal function, and long-term studies regarding cardiovascular outcomes, such as stroke, congestive heart failure, myocardial infarction, and end-stage renal failure, are not yet complete. Medical therapy should include blockade of the renin-angiotensin system, attainment of goal BPs, cessation of tobacco, statins, and aspirin. Renal revascularization is now often reserved for patients failing medical therapy or developing additional complications.

Techniques of renal revascularization are improving. With experienced operators, major complications occur in about 9% of cases, including renal artery dissection, capsular perforation, hemorrhage, and occasional atheroembolic disease. Although not common, atheroembolic disease can be catastrophic and accelerate both hypertension and kidney failure, precisely the events that revascularization is intended to prevent. Although renal blood flow usually can be restored by endovascular stenting, recovery of renal function is limited to about 25% of cases, with no change in 50% and some deterioration evident in others. Patients with rapid loss of kidney function, sometimes associated with antihypertensive drug therapy, or with vascular disease affecting the entire functioning kidney mass are more likely to recover function after restoring blood flow. When hypertension is refractory to effective therapy, revascularization offers real benefits. Table 299-2 summarizes currently accepted guidelines for considering renal revascularization.

ATHEROEMBOLIC RENAL DISEASE

Emboli to the kidneys arise most frequently as a result of cholesterol crystals breaking free of atherosclerotic vascular plaque and lodging in downstream microvessels. Most clinical atheroembolic events follow angiographic procedures, often of the coronary vessels. It has been argued that nearly all vascular interventional procedures lead to plaque fracture and release of microemboli, but clinical manifestations develop only in a fraction of these. The incidence of clinical atheroemboli has been increasing with more vascular procedures and

TABLE 299-2 CLINICAL FACTORS FAVORING MEDICAL THERAPY AND REVASCULARIZATION OR SURVEILLANCE FOR RENAL ARTERY STENOSIS

Factors Favoring Medical Therapy and Revascularization for Renal Artery Stenosis

- Progressive decline in GFR during treatment of systemic hypertension
- Failure to achieve adequate blood pressure control with optimal medical therapy (medical failure)
- Rapid or recurrent decline in the GFR in association with a reduction in systemic pressure
- Decline in the GFR during therapy with ACE inhibitors or ARBs
- Recurrent congestive heart failure in a patient in whom the adequacy of left ventricular function does not explain a cause

Factors Favoring Medical Therapy and Surveillance of Renal Artery Disease

- Controlled blood pressure with stable renal function (e.g., stable renal insufficiency)
- Stable renal artery stenosis without progression on surveillance studies (e.g., serial duplex ultrasound)
- Very advanced age and/or limited life expectancy
- Extensive comorbidity that make revascularization too risky
- High risk for or previous experience with atheroembolic disease
- Other concomitant renal parenchymal diseases that cause progressive renal dysfunction (e.g., interstitial nephritis, diabetic nephropathy)

Abbreviations: ACE, angiotensin-converting enzyme; ARBs, angiotensin receptor blockers; GFR, glomerular filtration rate.

longer life spans. Atheroembolic renal disease is suspected in more than 3% of elderly subjects with end-stage renal disease (ESRD) and is likely underdiagnosed. It is more frequent in males with a history of diabetes, hypertension, and ischemic cardiac disease. Atheroemboli in the kidney are strongly associated with aortic aneurysmal disease and renal artery stenosis. Most clinical cases can be linked to precipitating events, such as angiography, vascular surgery, anticoagulation with heparin, thrombolytic therapy, or trauma. Clinical manifestations of this syndrome commonly develop between 1 and 14 days after an inciting event and may continue to develop for weeks thereafter. Systemic embolic disease manifestations, such as fever, abdominal pain, and weight loss, are present in less than half of patients, although cutaneous manifestations including livedo reticularis and localized toe gangrene may be more common. Worsening hypertension and deteriorating kidney function are common, sometimes reaching a malignant phase. Progressive renal failure can occur and require dialytic support. These cases often develop after a stuttering onset over many weeks and have an ominous prognosis. Mortality rate after 1 year reaches 38%, and although some may eventually recover sufficiently to no longer require dialysis, many do not.

Beyond the clinical manifestations above, laboratory findings include rising creatinine, transient eosinophilia (60–80%), elevated sedimentation rate, and hypocomplementemia (15%). Establishing this diagnosis can be difficult and is often by exclusion. Definitive diagnosis depends on kidney biopsy demonstrating microvessel occlusion with cholesterol crystals that leave a "cleft" in the vessel. Biopsies obtained from patients undergoing surgical revascularization of the kidney indicate that silent cholesterol emboli are frequently present before any further manipulation is performed.

No effective therapy is available for atheroembolic disease once it has developed. Withdrawal of anticoagulation is recommended. Late recovery of kidney function after supportive measures sometimes occurs, and statin therapy may improve outcome. The role of embolic protection devices in the renal circulation is unclear, but a few prospective trials have failed to demonstrate major benefits. These devices are limited to distal protection during the endovascular procedure and offer no protection from embolic debris after removal.

THROMBOEMBOLIC RENAL DISEASE

Thrombotic occlusion of renal vessels or branch arteries can lead to declining renal function and hypertension. It is difficult to diagnose and is often overlooked, especially in elderly patients. Thrombosis can develop as a result of local vessel abnormalities, such as local dissection, trauma, or inflammatory vasculitis. Local microdissections sometimes lead to patchy, transient areas of infarctions labeled "segmental arteriolar mediolysis." Although hypercoagulability conditions sometimes present as renal artery thrombosis, this is rare. It can also derive from distant embolic events, e.g., the left atrium in patients with atrial fibrillation or from fat emboli originating from traumatized tissue, most commonly large bone fractures. Cardiac sources include vegetations from subacute bacterial endocarditis. Systemic emboli to the kidneys may also arise from the venous circulation if right-to-left shunting occurs, e.g., through a patent foramen ovale.

Clinical manifestations vary depending on the rapidity of onset and extent of occlusion. Acute arterial thrombosis may produce flank pain, fever, leukocytosis, nausea, and vomiting. If kidney infarction results, enzymes such as lactate dehydrogenase (LDH) rise to extreme levels. If both kidneys are affected, renal function will decline precipitously with a drop in urine output. If a single kidney is involved, renal functional changes may be minor. Hypertension related to sudden release of renin from ischemic tissue can develop rapidly, as long as some viable tissue in the "peri-infarct" border zone remains. If the infarct zone demarcates precisely, the rise in BP and renin activity may resolve. Diagnosis of renal infarction may be established by vascular imaging with MRI, CT angiography, or arteriography (Fig. 299-2).

MANAGEMENT OF ARTERIAL THROMBOSIS OF THE KIDNEY

Options for interventions of newly detected arterial occlusion include surgical reconstruction, anticoagulation, thrombolytic therapy,

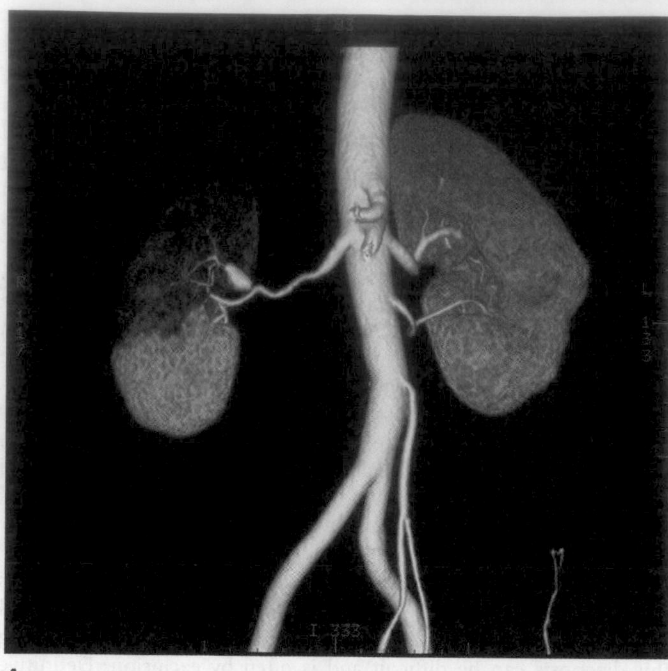

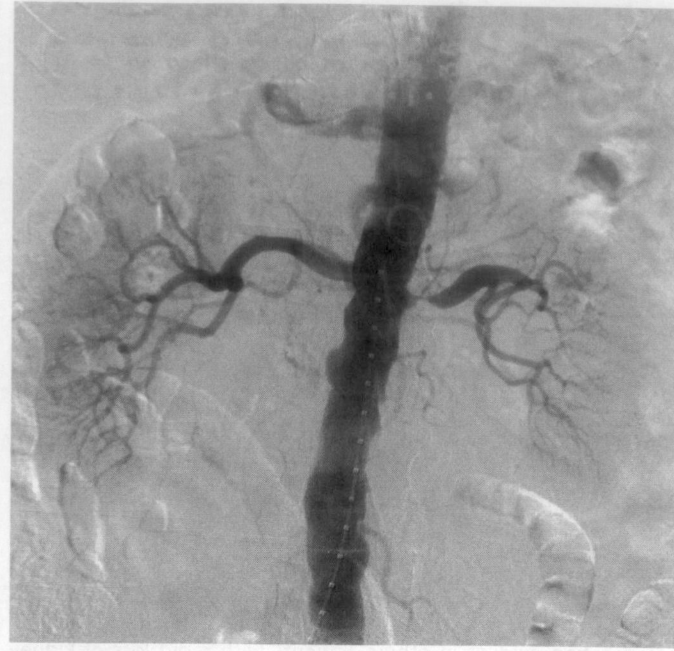

A B

FIGURE 299-2 ***A.*** CT angiogram illustrating loss of circulation to the upper pole of the right kidney in a patient with fibromuscular disease and a renal artery aneurysm. Activation of the renin-angiotensin system produced rapidly developing hypertension. ***B.*** Angiogram illustrating high-grade renal artery stenosis affecting the left kidney. This lesion is often part of widespread atherosclerosis and sometimes is an extension of aortic plaque. This lesion develops in older individuals with preexisting atherosclerotic risk factors.

endovascular procedures, and supportive care, particularly antihypertensive drug therapy. Application of these methods depends on the patient's overall condition, the precipitating factors (e.g., local trauma or systemic illness), the magnitude of renal tissue and function at risk, and the likelihood of recurrent events in the future. For unilateral disease, e.g., arterial dissection with thrombosis, supportive care with anticoagulation may suffice. Acute, bilateral occlusion is potentially catastrophic, producing anuric renal failure. Depending on the precipitating event, surgical or thrombolytic therapies can sometimes restore kidney viability.

MICROVASCULAR INJURY ASSOCIATED WITH HYPERTENSION

ARTERIOLONEPHROSCLEROSIS

"Malignant" Hypertension Although BP rises with age, it has long been recognized that some individuals develop rapidly progressive BP elevations with target organ injury including retinal hemorrhages, encephalopathy, and declining kidney function. Placebo arms during the controlled trials of hypertension therapy identified progression to severe levels in 20% of subjects over 5 years. If untreated, patients with target organ injury including papilledema and declining kidney function suffered mortality rates in excess of 50% over 6–12 months, hence the designation "malignant." Postmortem studies of such patients identified vascular lesions, designated "fibrinoid necrosis," with breakdown of the vessel wall, deposition of eosinophilic material including fibrin, and a perivascular cellular infiltrate. A separate lesion was identified in the larger interlobular arteries in many patients with hyperplastic proliferation of the vascular wall cellular elements, deposition of collagen, and separation of layers, designated the "onionskin" lesion. For many of these patients, fibrinoid necrosis led to obliteration of glomeruli and loss of tubular structures. Progressive kidney failure ensued and, without dialysis support, led to early mortality in untreated malignant-phase hypertension. These vascular changes could develop with pressure-related injury from a variety of hypertensive pathways, including but not limited to activation of the renin-angiotensin system and severe vasospasm associated with catecholamine release. Occasionally, endothelial injury is sufficient to induce microangiopathic hemolysis, as discussed below.

Antihypertensive therapy is the mainstay of therapy for malignant hypertension. With effective BP reduction, manifestations of vascular injury including microangiopathic hemolysis and renal dysfunction can improve over time. Whereas series reported before the era of drug therapy suggested that 1-year mortality rates exceeded 90%, current survival over 5 years exceeds 50%.

Malignant hypertension is less common in Western countries, although it persists in parts of the world where medical care and antihypertensive drug therapy are less available. It most commonly develops in patients with treated hypertension who neglect to take medications or who may use vasospastic drugs, such as cocaine. Renal abnormalities typically include rising serum creatinine and occasionally hematuria and proteinuria. Biochemical findings may include evidence of hemolysis (anemia, schistocytes, and reticulocytosis) and changes associated with kidney failure. African-American males are more likely to develop rapidly progressive hypertension and kidney failure than are whites in the United States. Genetic polymorphisms (first identified as *MYH9*, but now thought to be *APOL1*) that are common in the African-American population predispose to subtle focal sclerosing glomerular disease, with severe hypertension developing at younger ages secondary to renal disease in this instance.

"Hypertensive Nephrosclerosis" Based on experience with malignant hypertension and epidemiologic evidence linking BP with long-term risks of kidney failure, it has long been assumed that lesser degrees of hypertension induce less severe, but prevalent, changes in kidney vessels and loss of kidney function. As a result, a large portion of patients reaching ESRD without a specific etiologic diagnosis are assigned the designation "hypertensive nephrosclerosis." Pathologic examination commonly identifies afferent arteriolar thickening with deposition of homogeneous eosinophilic material (hyaline arteriolosclerosis) associated with narrowing of vascular lumina. Clinical manifestations include retinal vessel changes associated with hypertension (arteriolar narrowing, crossing changes), left ventricular hypertrophy, and elevated BP. The role of these vascular changes in kidney function is unclear. Postmortem and biopsy samples from normotensive kidney donors demonstrate similar vessel changes associated with aging, dyslipidemia, and glucose intolerance. Although BP reduction does slow progression of proteinuric kidney diseases and is warranted to reduce the excessive cardiovascular risks associated with CKD, antihypertensive therapy does not alter the course of kidney dysfunction identified specifically as hypertensive nephrosclerosis.

300 Deep Venous Thrombosis and Pulmonary Thromboembolism

Samuel Z. Goldhaber

EPIDEMIOLOGY

Venous thromboembolism (VTE) encompasses deep venous thrombosis (DVT) and pulmonary embolism (PE) and causes cardiovascular death and disability. In the United States, the Surgeon General estimates there are 100,000 to 180,000 deaths annually from PE and has declared that PE is the most common preventable cause of death among hospitalized patients. Survivors may succumb to the disabilities of chronic thromboembolic pulmonary hypertension or postthrombotic syndrome. Chronic thromboembolic pulmonary hypertension causes breathlessness, especially with exertion. Postthrombotic syndrome (also known as *chronic venous insufficiency*) damages the venous valves of the leg and causes ankle or calf swelling and leg aching, especially after prolonged standing. In its most severe form, postthrombotic syndrome causes skin ulceration (Fig. 300-1).

PATHOPHYSIOLOGY

Inflammation and Platelet Activation Virchow's triad of inflammation, hypercoagulability, and endothelial injury leads to recruitment of activated platelets, which release microparticles. These microparticles contain proinflammatory mediators that bind neutrophils, stimulating them to release their nuclear material and form web-like extracellular networks called neutrophil extracellular traps. These prothrombotic networks contain histones that stimulate platelet aggregation and promote platelet-dependent thrombin generation. Venous thrombi form and flourish in an environment of stasis, low oxygen tension, and upregulation of proinflammatory genes.

Prothrombotic States The two most common autosomal dominant genetic mutations are factor V Leiden, which causes resistance to the

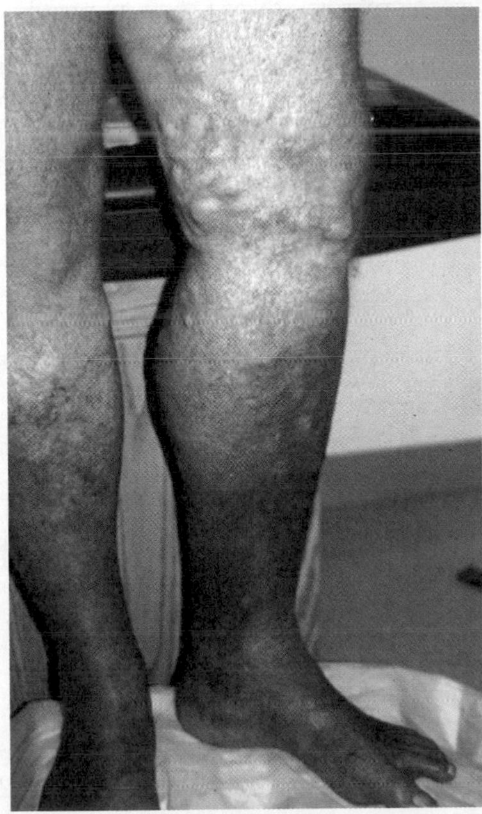

FIGURE 300-1 Skin ulceration in the lateral malleolus from postthrombotic syndrome of the leg.

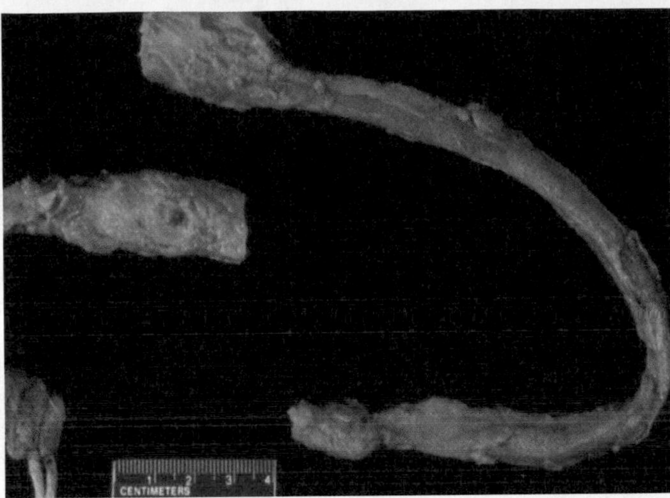

FIGURE 300-2 Deep venous thrombosis at autopsy.

endogenous anticoagulant, activated protein C (which inactivates clotting factors V and VIII), and the prothrombin gene mutation, which increases the plasma prothrombin concentration (Chaps. 78 and 142). Antithrombin, protein C, and protein S are naturally occurring coagulation inhibitors. Deficiencies of these inhibitors are associated with VTE but are rare. Antiphospholipid antibody syndrome is the most common acquired cause of thrombophilia and is associated with venous or arterial thrombosis. Other common predisposing factors include cancer, obesity, cigarette smoking, systemic arterial hypertension, chronic obstructive pulmonary disease, chronic kidney disease, blood transfusion, long-haul air travel, air pollution, oral contraceptives, pregnancy, postmenopausal hormone replacement, surgery, and trauma.

Embolization When deep venous thrombi (Fig. 300-2) detach from their site of formation, they embolize to the vena cava, right atrium, and right ventricle, and lodge in the pulmonary arterial circulation, thereby causing acute PE. Paradoxically, these thrombi occasionally embolize to the arterial circulation through a patent foramen ovale or atrial septal defect. Many patients with PE have no evidence of DVT because the clot has already embolized to the lungs.

Physiology The most common gas exchange abnormalities are arterial hypoxemia and an increased alveolar-arterial O_2 tension gradient, which represents the inefficiency of O_2 transfer across the lungs. Anatomic dead space increases because breathed gas does not enter gas exchange units of the lung. Physiologic dead space increases because ventilation to gas exchange units exceeds venous blood flow through the pulmonary capillaries.

Other pathophysiologic abnormalities include:

1. *Increased pulmonary vascular resistance* due to vascular obstruction or platelet secretion of vasoconstricting neurohumoral agents such as serotonin. Release of vasoactive mediators can produce ventilation-perfusion mismatching at sites remote from the embolus, thereby accounting for discordance between a small PE and a large alveolar-arterial O_2 gradient.
2. *Impaired gas exchange* due to increased alveolar dead space from vascular obstruction, hypoxemia from alveolar hypoventilation relative to perfusion in the nonobstructed lung, right-to-left shunting, or impaired carbon monoxide transfer due to loss of gas exchange surface.
3. *Alveolar hyperventilation* due to reflex stimulation of irritant receptors.
4. *Increased airway resistance* due to constriction of airways distal to the bronchi.
5. *Decreased pulmonary compliance* due to lung edema, lung hemorrhage, or loss of surfactant.

Pulmonary Hypertension, Right Ventricular (RV) Dysfunction, and RV Microinfarction Pulmonary artery obstruction causes a rise in pulmonary artery pressure and in pulmonary vascular resistance. When RV wall tension rises, RV dilation and dysfunction ensue, with release of the cardiac biomarker, brain natriuretic peptide. The interventricular septum bulges into and compresses an intrinsically normal left ventricle (LV). Diastolic LV dysfunction reduces LV distensibility and impairs LV filling. Increased RV wall tension also compresses the right coronary artery, limits myocardial oxygen supply, and precipitates right coronary artery ischemia and RV microinfarction, with release of cardiac biomarkers such as troponin. Underfilling of the LV may lead to a fall in LV cardiac output and systemic arterial pressure, with consequent circulatory collapse and death.

CLASSIFICATION OF PULMONARY EMBOLISM AND DEEP VENOUS THROMBOSIS

Pulmonary Embolism **Massive PE** accounts for 5–10% of cases, and is characterized by extensive thrombosis affecting at least half of the pulmonary vasculature. Dyspnea, syncope, hypotension, and cyanosis are hallmarks of massive PE. Patients with massive PE may present in cardiogenic shock and can die from multisystem organ failure. **Submassive PE** accounts for 20–25% of patients, and is characterized by RV dysfunction despite normal systemic arterial pressure. The combination of right heart failure and release of cardiac biomarkers indicates an increased likelihood of clinical deterioration. **Low-risk PE** constitutes about 70–75% of cases. These patients have an excellent prognosis.

Deep Venous Thrombosis **Lower extremity DVT** usually begins in the calf and propagates proximally to the popliteal vein, femoral vein, and iliac veins. Leg DVT is about 10 times more common than **upper extremity DVT,** which is often precipitated by placement of pacemakers, internal cardiac defibrillators, or indwelling central venous catheters. The likelihood of upper extremity DVT increases as the catheter diameter and number of lumens increase. **Superficial venous thrombosis** usually presents with erythema, tenderness, and a "palpable cord." Patients are at risk for extension of the thrombosis to the deep venous system.

DIAGNOSIS

Clinical Evaluation PE is known as "the Great Masquerader." Diagnosis is difficult because symptoms and signs are nonspecific. The most common symptom is unexplained breathlessness. When occult PE occurs concomitantly with overt congestive heart failure or pneumonia, clinical improvement often fails to occur despite standard medical treatment of the concomitant illness. This scenario presents a clinical clue to the possible coexistence of PE.

With DVT, the most common symptom is a cramp or "charley horse" in the lower calf that persists and intensifies over several days. Point score criteria help estimate the clinical likelihood of DVT and PE (Table 300-1). Patients with a low-to-moderate likelihood of DVT or PE should undergo initial diagnostic evaluation with D-dimer testing alone (see "Blood Tests") without obligatory imaging tests (Fig. 300-3). However, patients with a high clinical likelihood of VTE should skip D-dimer testing and undergo imaging as the next step in the diagnostic algorithm.

Clinical Pearls Not all leg pain is due to DVT, and not all dyspnea is due to PE (Table 300-2). Sudden, severe calf discomfort suggests a ruptured Baker's cyst. Fever and chills usually herald cellulitis rather than DVT. Physical findings, if present, may consist only of mild palpation discomfort in the lower calf. However, massive DVT often presents with marked thigh swelling, tenderness, and erythema. If the leg is diffusely edematous, DVT is unlikely. More probable is an acute exacerbation of venous insufficiency due to postthrombotic syndrome. Upper extremity venous thrombosis may present with asymmetry in the supraclavicular fossa or in the circumference of the upper arms.

Pulmonary infarction usually indicates a small PE. This condition is exquisitely painful because the thrombus lodges peripherally, near the innervation of pleural nerves. *Nonthrombotic PE* etiologies include fat embolism after pelvic or long bone fracture, tumor embolism, bone marrow, and air embolism. Cement embolism and bony fragment embolism

TABLE 300-1 CLINICAL DECISION RULES

Low Clinical Likelihood of DVT if Point Score Is Zero or Less; Moderate Likelihood if Score Is 1 to 2; High Likelihood if Score Is 3 or Greater	
Clinical Variable	**DVT Score**
Active cancer	1
Paralysis, paresis, or recent cast	1
Bedridden for >3 days; major surgery <12 weeks	1
Tenderness along distribution of deep veins	1
Entire leg swelling	1
Unilateral calf swelling >3 cm	1
Pitting edema	1
Collateral superficial nonvaricose veins	1
Alternative diagnosis at least as likely as DVT	−2
High Clinical Likelihood of PE if Point Score Exceeds 4	
Clinical Variable	**PE Score**
Signs and symptoms of DVT	3.0
Alternative diagnosis less likely than PE	3.0
Heart rate >100/min	1.5
Immobilization >3 days; surgery within 4 weeks	1.5
Prior PE or DVT	1.5
Hemoptysis	1.0
Cancer	1.0

can occur after total hip or knee replacement. Intravenous drug users may inject themselves with a wide array of substances that can embolize such as hair, talc, and cotton. *Amniotic fluid embolism* occurs when fetal membranes leak or tear at the placental margin.

Nonimaging Diagnostic Modalities • *BLOOD TESTS* The quantitative *plasma D-dimer enzyme-linked immunosorbent assay (ELISA)* rises in the presence of DVT or PE because of the breakdown of fibrin by plasmin. Elevation of D-dimer indicates endogenous although often clinically ineffective thrombolysis. The sensitivity of the D-dimer is >80% for DVT (including isolated calf DVT) and >95% for PE. The D-dimer is less sensitive for DVT than for PE because the DVT thrombus size is smaller. A normal D-dimer is a useful "rule out" test. However, the D-dimer assay is not specific. Levels increase in patients with myocardial infarction, pneumonia, sepsis, cancer, and the postoperative state and those in the second or third trimester of pregnancy. Therefore, D-dimer rarely has a useful role among hospitalized patients, because levels are frequently elevated due to systemic illness.

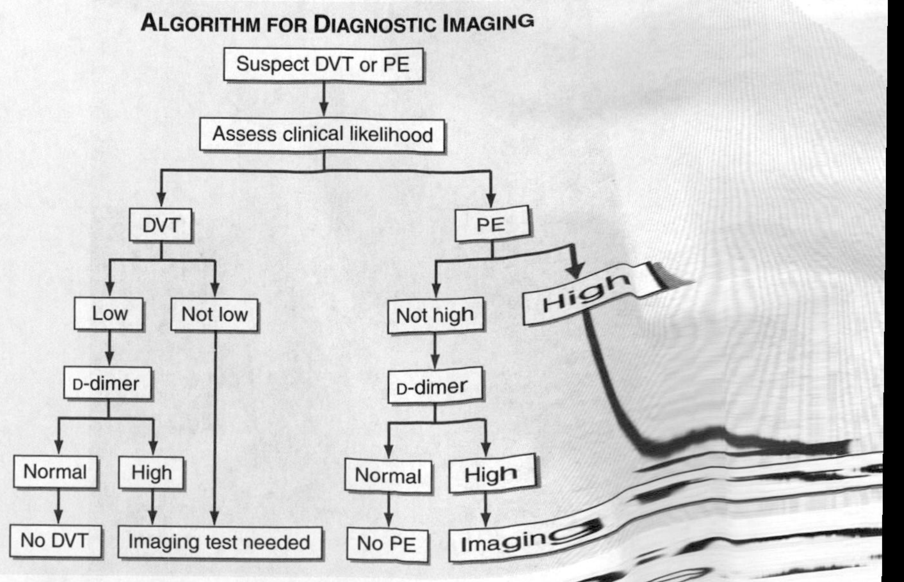

ALGORITHM FOR DIAGNOSTIC IMAGING
Suspect DVT or PE
Assess clinical likelihood
DVT
PE
Low
Not low
Not high
High
D-dimer
D-dimer
Normal
High
Normal
High
No DVT
Imaging test needed
No PE
Imaging

FIGURE 300-3 **How to decide whether diagnostic im... needed.** For assessment of clinical likelihood, see Tabl...

TABLE 300-2 DIFFERENTIAL DIAGNOSIS

DVT
Ruptured Baker's cyst
Cellulitis
Postphlebitic syndrome/venous insufficiency
PE
Pneumonia, asthma, chronic obstructive pulmonary disease
Congestive heart failure
Pericarditis
Pleurisy: "viral syndrome," costochondritis, musculoskeletal discomfort
Rib fracture, pneumothorax
Acute coronary syndrome
Anxiety

ELEVATED CARDIAC BIOMARKERS Serum troponin and plasma heart-type fatty acid–binding protein levels increase because of RV microinfarction. Myocardial stretch causes release of brain natriuretic peptide or NT-pro-brain natriuretic peptide.

ELECTROCARDIOGRAM The most frequently cited abnormality, in addition to sinus tachycardia, is the S1Q3T3 sign: an S wave in lead I, a Q wave in lead III, and an inverted T wave in lead III (Chap. 268). This finding is relatively specific but insensitive. RV strain and ischemia cause the most common abnormality, T-wave inversion in leads V_1 to V_4.

Noninvasive Imaging Modalities • ***VENOUS ULTRASONOGRAPHY*** Ultrasonography of the deep venous system relies on loss of vein compressibility as the primary criterion for DVT. When a normal vein is imaged in cross-section, it readily collapses with gentle manual pressure from the ultrasound transducer. This creates the illusion of a "wink." With acute DVT, the vein loses its compressibility because of passive distention by acute thrombus. The diagnosis of acute DVT is even more secure when thrombus is directly visualized. It appears homogeneous and has low echogenicity (Fig. 300-4). The vein itself often appears mildly dilated, and collateral channels may be absent.

Venous flow dynamics can be examined with Doppler imaging. Normally, manual calf compression causes augmentation of the Doppler flow pattern. Loss of normal respiratory variation is caused by an obstructing DVT or by any obstructive process within the pelvis. For patients with a technically poor or nondiagnostic venous ultrasound, one should consider alternative imaging modalities for DVT, such as computed tomography (CT) and magnetic resonance imaging.

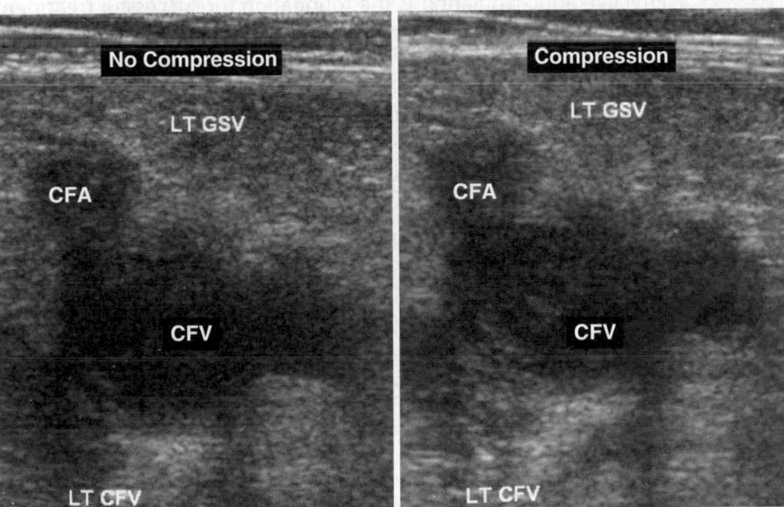

FIGURE 300-4 Venous ultrasound, with and without compression of the leg veins. CFA, common femoral artery; CFV, common femoral vein; GSV, great saphenous vein; LT, left.

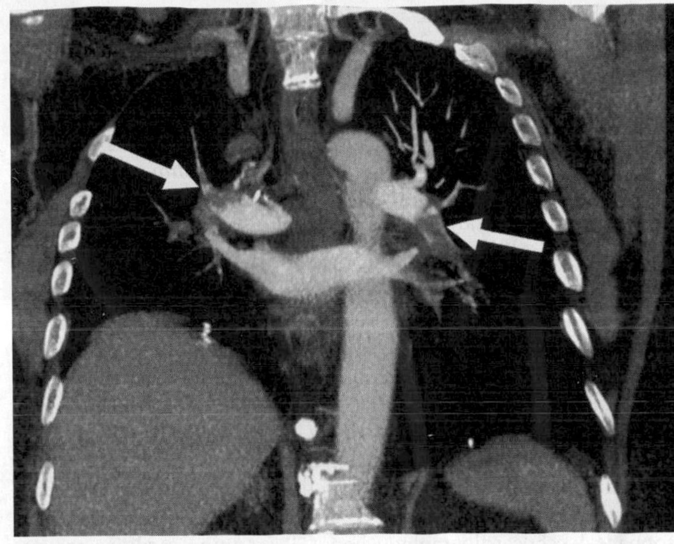

FIGURE 300-5 Large bilateral proximal PE on a coronal chest CT image in a 54-year-old man with lung cancer and brain metastases. He had developed sudden onset of chest heaviness and shortness of breath while at home. There are filling defects in the main and segmental pulmonary arteries bilaterally (*white arrows*). Only the left upper lobe segmental artery is free of thrombus.

CHEST ROENTGENOGRAPHY A normal or nearly normal chest x-ray often occurs in PE. Well-established abnormalities include focal oligemia (Westermark's sign), a peripheral wedged-shaped density above the diaphragm (Hampton's hump), and an enlarged right descending pulmonary artery (Palla's sign).

CHEST CT CT of the chest with intravenous contrast is the principal imaging test for the diagnosis of PE (Fig. 300-5). Multidetector-row spiral CT acquires all chest images with ≤1 mm of resolution during a short breath hold. Sixth-order branches can be visualized with resolution superior to that of conventional invasive contrast pulmonary angiography. The CT scan also provides an excellent four-chamber view of the heart. RV enlargement on chest CT indicates an increased likelihood of death within the next 30 days compared with PE patients who have normal RV size. When imaging is continued below the chest to the knee, pelvic and proximal leg DVT also can be diagnosed by CT scanning. In patients without PE, the lung parenchymal images may establish alternative diagnoses not apparent on chest x-ray that explain the presenting symptoms and signs such as pneumonia, emphysema, pulmonary fibrosis, pulmonary mass, and aortic pathology. Sometimes asymptomatic early-stage lung cancer is diagnosed incidentally.

LUNG SCANNING Lung scanning has become a second-line diagnostic test for PE, used mostly for patients who cannot tolerate intravenous contrast. Small particulate aggregates of albumin labeled with a gamma-emitting radionuclide are injected intravenously and are trapped in the pulmonary capillary bed. The perfusion scan defect indicates absent or decreased blood flow, possibly due to PE. Ventilation scans, obtained with a radiolabeled inhaled gas such as xenon or krypton, improve the specificity of the perfusion scan. Abnormal ventilation scans indicate abnormal nonventilated lung, thereby providing possible explanations for perfusion defects other than acute PE, such as asthma and chronic obstructive pulmonary disease. A high-probability scan for PE is defined as two or more segmental perfusion defects in the presence of normal ventilation.

The diagnosis of PE is very unlikely in patients with normal and nearly normal scans and is about 90% certain in patients with high-probability scans. Unfortunately, most patients have nondiagnostic scans, and fewer than one-half of patients with angiographically confirmed PE have a high probability scan. As many as 40% of patients with high clinical suspicion for PE but "low-probability" scans do, in fact, have PE at angiography.

MAGNETIC RESONANCE (MR) (CONTRAST-ENHANCED) IMAGING When ultrasound is equivocal, MR venography with gadolinium contrast is an excellent imaging modality to diagnose DVT. MR pulmonary angiography may detect large proximal PE but is not reliable for smaller segmental and subsegmental PE.

ECHOCARDIOGRAPHY Echocardiography is *not* a reliable diagnostic imaging tool for acute PE because most patients with PE have normal echocardiograms. However, echocardiography is a very useful diagnostic tool for detecting conditions that may mimic PE, such as acute myocardial infarction, pericardial tamponade, and aortic dissection. Transthoracic echocardiography rarely images thrombus directly. The best-known indirect sign of PE on transthoracic echocardiography is McConnell's sign: hypokinesis of the RV free wall with normal or hyperkinetic motion of the RV apex. One should consider transesophageal echocardiography when CT scanning facilities are not available or when a patient has renal failure or severe contrast allergy that precludes administration of contrast despite premedication with high-dose steroids. This imaging modality can identify saddle, right main, or left main PE.

Invasive Diagnostic Modalities • *PULMONARY ANGIOGRAPHY* Chest CT with contrast (see above) has virtually replaced invasive pulmonary angiography as a diagnostic test. Invasive catheter-based diagnostic testing is reserved for patients with technically unsatisfactory chest CTs and for those in whom an interventional procedure such as catheter-directed thrombolysis is planned. A definitive diagnosis of PE depends on visualization of an intraluminal filling defect in more than one projection. Secondary signs of PE include abrupt occlusion ("cut-off") of vessels, segmental oligemia or avascularity, a prolonged arterial phase with slow filling, and tortuous, tapering peripheral vessels.

CONTRAST PHLEBOGRAPHY Venous ultrasonography has virtually replaced contrast phlebography as the diagnostic test for suspected DVT.

Integrated Diagnostic Approach An integrated diagnostic approach (Fig. 300-3) streamlines the workup of suspected DVT and PE (Fig. 300-6).

TREATMENT DEEP VENOUS THROMBOSIS

PRIMARY THERAPY

Primary therapy consists of clot dissolution with pharmacomechanical therapy that usually includes low-dose catheter-directed thrombolysis. This approach is reserved for patients with extensive femoral, iliofemoral, or upper extremity DVT. The open vein hypothesis postulates that patients who receive primary therapy will sustain less long-term damage to venous valves, with consequent lower rates of postthrombotic syndrome. A National Heart, Lung, and Blood Institute–sponsored randomized controlled trial called ATTRACT (NCT00790335) is testing this hypothesis.

SECONDARY PREVENTION

Anticoagulation or placement of an inferior vena caval filter constitutes *secondary prevention* of VTE. To lessen the severity of postthrombotic syndrome of the legs, below-knee graduated compression stockings may be prescribed, 30–40 mmHg, for 2 years after the DVT episode. They should be replaced every 3 months because they lose their elasticity.

TREATMENT PULMONARY EMBOLISM

RISK STRATIFICATION

Hemodynamic instability, RV dysfunction on echocardiography, RV enlargement on chest CT, or elevation of the troponin level due to RV microinfarction portend a high risk of an adverse clinical outcome. When RV function remains normal in a hemodynamically stable patient, a good clinical outcome is highly likely with anticoagulation alone (Fig. 300-7).

ANTICOAGULATION

Effective anticoagulation is the foundation for successful treatment of DVT and PE. There are three options: (1) the conventional strategy

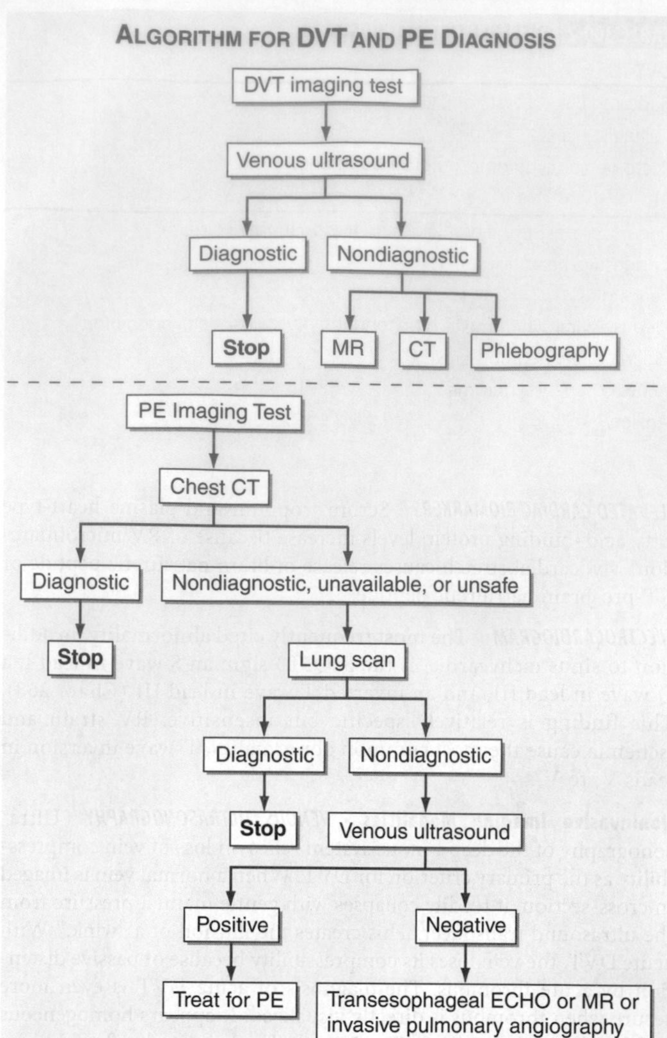

FIGURE 300-6 Imaging tests to diagnose DVT and PE. ECHO, echocardiography.

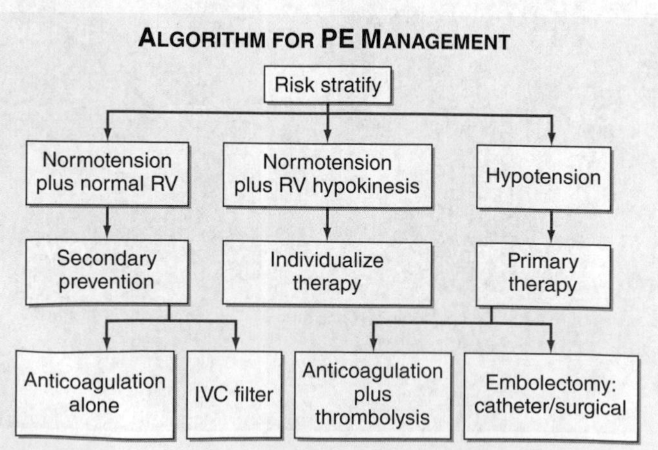

FIGURE 300-7 Acute management of pulmonary thromboembolism. RV, right ventricular; IVC, inferior vena cava.

TABLE 300-3 ANTICOAGULATION OF VTE

Immediate Anticoagulation
Unfractionated heparin, bolus and continuous infusion, to achieve aPTT 2–3 times the upper limit of the laboratory normal, *or*
Enoxaparin 1 mg/kg twice daily with normal renal function, *or*
Dalteparin 200 U/kg once daily or 100 U/kg twice daily, with normal renal function, *or*
Tinzaparin 175 U/kg once daily with normal renal function, *or*
Fondaparinux weight-based once daily; adjust for impaired renal function
Direct thrombin inhibitors: argatroban or bivalirudin
Rivaroxaban 15 mg twice daily for 3 weeks, followed by 20 mg once daily with the dinner meal thereafter
Apixaban (not yet licensed)
Warfarin Anticoagulation
Requires 5–10 days of administration to achieve effectiveness as monotherapy
(Unfractionated heparin, low-molecular-weight heparin, and fondaparinux are the usual immediately effective "bridging agents" used when initiating warfarin)
Usual start dose is 5 mg
Titrate to INR, target 2.0–3.0
Continue parenteral anticoagulation for a minimum of 5 days and until two sequential INR values, at least 1 day apart, achieve the target INR range
Novel Oral Anticoagulants for Extended-Duration Anticoagulation following Initial Parenteral Anticoagulation
Edoxaban (not yet licensed)
Dabigatran (not yet licensed)

of parenteral therapy "bridged" to warfarin, (2) parenteral therapy "bridged" to a novel oral anticoagulant such as dabigatran (a direct thrombin inhibitor) or edoxaban (an anti-Xa agent), or (3) oral anticoagulation with rivaroxaban or apixaban (both are anti-Xa agents) with a loading dose followed by a maintenance dose as monotherapy without parenteral anticoagulation.

The three heparin-based parenteral anticoagulants are (1) unfractionated heparin (UFH), (2) low-molecular-weight heparin (LMWH), and (3) fondaparinux. For patients with suspected or proven heparin-induced thrombocytopenia, there are two parenteral direct thrombin inhibitors: argatroban and bivalirudin (Table 300-3).

Unfractionated Heparin UFH anticoagulates by binding to and accelerating the activity of antithrombin, thus preventing additional thrombus formation. UFH is dosed to achieve a target activated partial thromboplastin time (aPTT) of 60–80 s. The most popular nomogram uses an initial bolus of 80 U/kg, followed by an initial infusion rate of 18 U/kg per h.

The major advantage of UFH is its short half-life, which is especially useful in patients in whom hour-to-hour control of the intensity of anticoagulation is desired.

Low-Molecular-Weight Heparins These fragments of UFH exhibit less binding to plasma proteins and endothelial cells and consequently have greater bioavailability, a more predictable dose response, and a longer half-life than does UFH. No monitoring or dose adjustment is needed unless the patient is markedly obese or has chronic kidney disease.

Fondaparinux Fondaparinux, an anti-Xa pentasaccharide, is administered as a weight-based once-daily subcutaneous injection in a prefilled syringe. No laboratory monitoring is required. Fondaparinux is synthesized in a laboratory and, unlike LMWH or UFH, is not derived from animal products. It does not cause heparin-induced thrombocytopenia. The dose must be adjusted downward for patients with renal dysfunction.

Warfarin This vitamin K antagonist prevents carboxylation activation of coagulation factors II, VII, IX, and X. The full effect of warfarin requires at least 5 days, even if the prothrombin time, used for monitoring, becomes elevated more rapidly. If warfarin is initiated as monotherapy during an acute thrombotic illness, a paradoxical exacerbation of hypercoagulability increases the likelihood of thrombosis. Overlapping UFH, LMWH, fondaparinux, or parenteral direct thrombin inhibitors with warfarin for at least 5 days will nullify the early procoagulant effect of warfarin.

WARFARIN DOSING In an average-size adult, warfarin is often initiated in a dose of 5 mg. The prothrombin time is standardized by calculating the international normalized ratio (INR), which assesses the anticoagulant effect of warfarin (Chap. 78). The target INR is usually 2.5, with a range of 2.0–3.0.

The warfarin dose is usually titrated empirically to achieve the target INR. Proper dosing is difficult because hundreds of drug-drug and drug-food interactions affect warfarin metabolism. Increasing age and systemic illness reduce the required warfarin dose. Pharmacogenomics may provide more precise initial dosing of warfarin. *CYP2C9* variant alleles impair the hydroxylation of S-warfarin, thereby lowering the dose requirement. Variants in the gene encoding the vitamin K epoxide reductase complex 1 (*VKORC1*) can predict whether patients require low, moderate, or high warfarin doses.

Centralized anticoagulation clinics have improved the efficacy and safety of warfarin dosing. Patients can self-monitor their INR with a home point-of-care fingerstick machine and can occasionally be taught to self-dose their warfarin.

Novel Oral Anticoagulants Novel oral anticoagulants are administered in a fixed dose, establish effective anticoagulation within hours of ingestion, require no laboratory coagulation monitoring, and have few of the drug-drug or drug-food interactions that make warfarin so difficult to dose. Rivaroxaban, a factor Xa inhibitor, is approved for treatment of acute DVT and acute PE as monotherapy, without a parenteral "bridging" anticoagulant. Apixaban is likely to receive similar approval for oral monotherapy. Dabigatran, a direct thrombin inhibitor, and edoxaban, a factor Xa inhibitor, are likely to be approved for treatment of VTE after an initial course of parenteral anticoagulation.

Complications of Anticoagulants The most serious adverse effect of anticoagulation is hemorrhage. For life-threatening or intracranial hemorrhage due to heparin or LMWH, protamine sulfate can be administered. Heparin-induced thrombocytopenia is less common with LMWH than with UFH. There is no specific reversal agent for bleeding caused by fondaparinux, direct thrombin inhibitors, or factor Xa inhibitors.

Major bleeding from warfarin is best managed with prothrombin complex concentrate. With serious but non–life-threatening bleeding, fresh-frozen plasma or intravenous vitamin K can be used. Recombinant human coagulation factor VIIa (rFVIIa) is an off-label option to manage catastrophic bleeding from warfarin, but prothrombin complex concentrate is a better choice. Oral vitamin K is effective for managing minor bleeding or an excessively high INR in the absence of bleeding.

Duration of Anticoagulation For DVT isolated to an upper extremity or calf that has been provoked by surgery, trauma, estrogen, or an indwelling central venous catheter or pacemaker, 3 months of anticoagulation usually suffice. For an initial episode of provoked proximal leg DVT or PE, 3 to 6 months of anticoagulation are considered sufficient. For patients with cancer and VTE, prescribe LMWH as monotherapy without warfarin and continue anticoagulation indefinitely unless the patient is rendered cancer-free.

Among patients with idiopathic, unprovoked VTE, the recurrence rate is high after cessation of anticoagulation. VTE that occurs during long-haul air travel is considered unprovoked. Unprovoked VTE may be caused by an exacerbation of an underlying inflammatory state and can be conceptualized as a chronic illness, with latent periods between flares of recurrent episodes. American College of Chest Physicians (ACCP) guidelines recommend considering anticoagulation for an indefinite duration with a target INR between 2 and 3 for patients with idiopathic VTE. An alternative approach after the first 6 months of anticoagulation is to reduce the intensity of anticoagulation and to lower the target INR range to between 1.5 and 2.

Counterintuitively, the presence of genetic mutations such as heterozygous factor V Leiden and prothrombin gene mutation does not appear to increase the risk of recurrent VTE. However, patients with antiphospholipid antibody syndrome may warrant indefinite-duration anticoagulation, even if the initial VTE was provoked by trauma or surgery.

INFERIOR VENA CAVAL (IVC) FILTERS

The two principal indications for insertion of an IVC filter are (1) active bleeding that precludes anticoagulation and (2) recurrent venous thrombosis despite intensive anticoagulation. Prevention of recurrent PE in patients with right heart failure who are not candidates for fibrinolysis and prophylaxis of extremely high-risk patients are "softer" indications for filter placement. The filter itself may fail by permitting the passage of small-to medium-size clots. Large thrombi may embolize to the pulmonary arteries via collateral veins that develop. A more common complication is caval thrombosis with marked bilateral leg swelling.

Paradoxically, by providing a nidus for clot formation, filters increase the DVT rate, even though they usually prevent PE (over the short term). Retrievable filters can now be placed for patients with an anticipated temporary bleeding disorder or for patients at temporary high risk of PE, such as individuals undergoing bariatric surgery who have a prior history of perioperative PE. The filters can be retrieved up to several months after insertion unless thrombus forms and is trapped within the filter. The retrievable filter becomes permanent if it remains in place or if, for technical reasons such as rapid endothelialization, it cannot be removed.

MANAGEMENT OF MASSIVE PE

For patients with massive PE and hypotension, replete volume with 500 mL of normal saline. Additional fluid should be infused with extreme caution because excessive fluid administration exacerbates RV wall stress, causes more profound RV ischemia, and worsens LV compliance and filling by causing further interventricular septal shift toward the LV. Dopamine and dobutamine are first-line inotropic agents for treatment of PE-related shock. Maintain a low threshold for initiating these pressors. Often, a "trial-and-error" approach works best; other agents that may be effective include norepinephrine, vasopressin, or phenylephrine.

FIBRINOLYSIS

Successful fibrinolytic therapy rapidly reverses right heart failure and may result in a lower rate of death and recurrent PE by (1) dissolving much of the anatomically obstructing pulmonary arterial thrombus, (2) preventing the continued release of serotonin and other neurohumoral factors that exacerbate pulmonary hypertension, and (3) lysing much of the source of the thrombus in the pelvic or deep leg veins, thereby decreasing the likelihood of recurrent PE.

The preferred fibrinolytic regimen is 100 mg of recombinant tissue plasminogen activator (tPA) administered as a continuous peripheral intravenous infusion over 2 h. The sooner thrombolysis is administered, the more effective it is. However, this approach can be used for at least 14 days after the PE has occurred.

Contraindications to fibrinolysis include intracranial disease, recent surgery, and trauma. The overall major bleeding rate is about 10%, including a 1–3% risk of intracranial hemorrhage. Careful screening of patients for contraindications to fibrinolytic therapy (Chap. 295) is the best way to minimize bleeding risk.

The only Food and Drug Administration–approved indication for PE fibrinolysis is massive PE. For patients with submassive PE, who have preserved systolic blood pressure but moderate or severe RV dysfunction, use of fibrinolysis remains controversial. Results of a 1006-patient European multicentered randomized trial of submassive PE, using the thrombolytic agent tenecteplase, were published in 2014. Death or hemodynamic collapse within 7 days of randomization was reduced by 56% in the tenecteplase group. However, hemorrhagic stroke occurred in 2% of tenecteplase patients versus 0.2% in patients who only received heparin.

PHARMACOMECHANICAL CATHETER-DIRECTED THERAPY

Many patients have relative contraindications to full-dose thrombolysis. Pharmacomechanical catheter-directed therapy usually combines physical fragmentation or pulverization of thrombus with catheter-directed low-dose thrombolysis. Mechanical techniques include catheter maceration and intentional embolization of clot more distally, suction thrombectomy, rheolytic hydrolysis, and low-energy ultrasound-facilitated thrombolysis. The dose of alteplase can be markedly reduced, usually to a range of 20 to 25 mg instead of the peripheral intravenous systemic dose of 100 mg.

PULMONARY EMBOLECTOMY

The risk of major hemorrhage with systemically administered fibrinolysis has prompted a renaissance of interest in surgical embolectomy, an operation that had almost become extinct. More rapid referral before the onset of irreversible multisystem organ failure and improved surgical technique have resulted in a high survival rate.

PULMONARY THROMBOENDARTERECTOMY

Chronic thromboembolic pulmonary hypertension develops in 2–4% of acute PE patients. Therefore, PE patients who have initial pulmonary hypertension (usually diagnosed with Doppler echocardiography) should be followed up at about 6 weeks with a repeat echocardiogram to determine whether pulmonary arterial pressure has normalized. Patients impaired by dyspnea due to chronic thromboembolic pulmonary hypertension should be considered for pulmonary thromboendarterectomy, which, if successful, can markedly reduce, and sometimes even cure, pulmonary hypertension (Chap. 304). The operation requires median sternotomy, cardiopulmonary bypass, deep hypothermia, and periods of hypothermic circulatory arrest. The mortality rate at experienced centers is approximately 5%. Inoperable patients should be managed with pulmonary vasodilator therapy.

EMOTIONAL SUPPORT

Patients with VTE may feel overwhelmed when they learn that they are suffering from PE or DVT. Some have never previously encountered serious cardiovascular illness. They wonder whether they will be able to adapt to the new limitations imposed by anticoagulation. They worry about the health of their families and the genetic implications of their illness. Those who are advised to discontinue anticoagulation may feel especially vulnerable about the potential for suffering recurrent VTE. At Brigham and Woman's Hospital, a physician-nurse–facilitated PE support group was initiated to address these concerns and has met monthly for more than 20 years.

PREVENTION OF VTE

Prevention of DVT and PE (Table 300-4) is of paramount importance because VTE is difficult to detect and poses a profound medical and economic burden. Low-dose UFH or LMWH is the most common form of in-hospital prophylaxis. Computerized reminder systems can increase the use of preventive measures and, at Brigham and Women's Hospital, have reduced the symptomatic VTE rate by more than 40%. Audits of hospitals to ensure that prophylaxis protocols are being used will also increase utilization of preventive measures. Duration of prophylaxis is an important consideration. Extended-duration prophylaxis has not been shown to be both effective and safe in medically ill patients after hospital discharge in separate large trials that have tested enoxaparin, apixaban, and rivaroxaban. There is an ongoing trial of a novel oral anticoagulant, betrixaban, for extended-duration VTE prophylaxis in medically ill patients.

TABLE 300-4 PREVENTION OF VENOUS THROMBOEMBOLISM AMONG HOSPITALIZED PATIENTS

Condition	Prophylaxis Strategy
High-risk nonorthopedic surgery	Unfractionated heparin 5000 units SC bid or tid Enoxaparin 40 mg daily Dalteparin 2500 or 5000 units daily
Cancer surgery, including gynecologic cancer surgery	Enoxaparin 40 mg daily, consider 1 month of prophylaxis
Major orthopedic surgery	Warfarin (target INR 2.0–3.0) Enoxaparin 40 mg daily Enoxaparin 30 mg bid Dalteparin 2500 or 5000 units daily Fondaparinux 2.5 mg daily Rivaroxaban 10 mg daily Aspirin 81–325 mg daily Dabigatran 220 mg daily (not in the United States) Apixaban 2.5 mg bid (not in the United States) Intermittent pneumatic compression (with or without pharmacologic prophylaxis)
Medically ill patients, especially if immobilized, with a history of prior VTE, with an indwelling central venous catheter, or with cancer (but without active gastroduodenal ulcer, major bleeding within 3 months, or platelet count <50,000)	Unfractionated heparin 5000 units bid or tid Enoxaparin 40 mg daily Dalteparin 2500 or 5000 units daily Fondaparinux 2.5 mg daily
Anticoagulation contraindicated	Intermittent pneumatic compression devices (but whether graduated compression stockings are effective in medical patients is controversial)

Patients who have undergone total hip or knee replacement or cancer surgery will benefit from extended pharmacologic VTE prophylaxis after hospital discharge. For hip replacement or extensive cancer surgery, the duration of prophylaxis is usually at least 1 month.

301 Diseases of the Aorta

Mark A. Creager, Joseph Loscalzo

The aorta is the conduit through which blood ejected from the left ventricle is delivered to the systemic arterial bed. In adults, its diameter is approximately 3 cm at the origin and in the ascending portion, 2.5 cm in the descending portion in the thorax, and 1.8–2 cm in the abdomen. The aortic wall consists of a thin intima composed of endothelium, subendothelial connective tissue, and an internal elastic lamina; a thick tunica media composed of smooth muscle cells and extracellular matrix; and an adventitia composed primarily of connective tissue enclosing the vasa vasorum and nervi vascularis. In addition to the conduit function of the aorta, its viscoelastic and compliant properties serve a buffering function. The aorta is distended during systole to allow a portion of the stroke volume and elastic energy to be stored, and it recoils during diastole so that blood continues to flow to the periphery. Owing to its continuous exposure to high pulsatile pressure and shear stress, the aorta is particularly prone to injury and disease resulting from mechanical trauma. The aorta is also more prone to rupture than is any other vessel, especially with the development of aneurysmal dilation, since its wall tension, as governed by Laplace's law (i.e., proportional to the product of pressure and radius), will be increased.

CONGENITAL ANOMALIES OF THE AORTA

Congenital anomalies of the aorta usually involve the aortic arch and its branches. Symptoms such as dysphagia, stridor, and cough may occur if an anomaly causes a ring around or otherwise compresses the esophagus or trachea. Anomalies associated with symptoms include double aortic arch, origin of the right subclavian artery distal to the left subclavian artery, and right-sided aortic arch with an aberrant left subclavian artery. A Kommerell's diverticulum is an anatomic remnant of a right aortic arch. Most congenital anomalies of the aorta do not cause symptoms and are detected during catheter-based procedures. The diagnosis of suspected congenital anomalies of the aorta typically is confirmed by computed tomographic (CT) or magnetic resonance (MR) angiography. Surgery is used to treat symptomatic anomalies.

AORTIC ANEURYSM

An *aneurysm* is defined as a pathologic dilation of a segment of a blood vessel. A *true aneurysm* involves all three layers of the vessel wall and is distinguished from a *pseudoaneurysm*, in which the intimal and medial layers are disrupted and the dilated segment of the aorta is lined by adventitia only and, at times, by perivascular clot. Aneurysms also may be classified according to their gross appearance. A *fusiform aneurysm* affects the entire circumference of a segment of the vessel, resulting in a diffusely dilated artery. In contrast, a *saccular aneurysm* involves only a portion of the circumference, resulting in an outpouching of the vessel wall. Aortic aneurysms also are classified according to location, i.e., abdominal versus thoracic. Aneurysms of the descending thoracic aorta are usually contiguous with infradiaphragmatic aneurysms and are referred to as *thoracoabdominal aortic aneurysms.*

ETIOLOGY

Aortic aneurysms result from conditions that cause degradation or abnormal production of the structural components of the aortic wall: elastin and collagen. The causes of aortic aneurysms may be broadly categorized as degenerative disorders, genetic or developmental diseases, vasculitis, infections, and trauma (Table 301-1). Inflammation, oxidative stress, proteolysis, and biomechanical wall stress contribute to the degenerative processes that characterize most aneurysms of the abdominal and descending thoracic aorta. These are mediated by B cell and T cell lymphocytes, macrophages, inflammatory cytokines, and matrix metalloproteinases that degrade elastin and collagen and alter the tensile strength and ability of the aorta to accommodate pulsatile stretch. The associated histopathology demonstrates destruction of elastin and collagen, decreased vascular smooth muscle, in-growth of new blood vessels, and inflammation. Factors associated with degenerative aortic aneurysms include aging, cigarette smoking, hypercholesterolemia, hypertension, and male sex.

TABLE 301-1 DISEASES OF THE AORTA: ETIOLOGY AND ASSOCIATED FACTORS

Aortic aneurysm
Degenerative
Aging
Cigarette smoking
Hypercholesterolemia
Hypertension
Atherosclerosis
Genetic or developmental
Marfan's syndrome
Loeys-Dietz syndrome
Ehlers-Danlos syndrome type IV
Turner's syndrome
Familial
Bicuspid aortic valve
Chronic aortic dissection
Aortitis (see below)
Infective (see below)
Trauma
Acute aortic syndromes (aortic dissection, acute intramural hematoma, penetrating atherosclerotic ulcer)
Degenerative disorders (see above)
Genetic/developmental disorders (see above)
Hypertension
Aortitis (see below)
Pregnancy
Trauma
Aortic occlusion
Atherosclerosis
Thromboembolism
Aortitis
Vasculitis
Takayasu's arteritis
Giant cell arteritis
Rheumatic
HLA-B27–associated spondyloarthropathies
Behçet's syndrome
Cogan's syndrome
Idiopathic aortitis
Infective
Syphilis
Tuberculosis
Mycotic (*Salmonella*, staphylococcal, streptococcal, fungal)

The most common pathologic condition associated with degenerative aortic aneurysms is *atherosclerosis.* Many patients with aortic aneurysms have coexisting risk factors for atherosclerosis (Chap. 291e), as well as atherosclerosis in other blood vessels.

Medial degeneration, previously designated *cystic medial necrosis,* is the histopathologic term used to describe the degeneration of collagen and elastic fibers in the tunica media of the aorta as well as the loss of medial cells that are replaced by multiple clefts of mucoid material, such as proteoglycans. Medial degeneration characteristically affects the proximal aorta, results in circumferential weakness and dilation, and leads to the development of fusiform aneurysms involving the ascending aorta and the sinuses of Valsalva. This condition is particularly prevalent in patients with Marfan's syndrome, Loeys-Dietz syndrome, Ehlers-Danlos syndrome type IV (Chap. 427), hypertension, congenital bicuspid aortic valves, and familial thoracic aortic aneurysm syndromes; sometimes it appears as an isolated condition in patients without any other apparent disease.

Familial clusterings of aortic aneurysms occur in 20% of patients, suggesting a hereditary basis for the disease. Mutations of the gene that encodes fibrillin-1 are present in patients with Marfan's syndrome. Fibrillin-1 is an important component of extracellular microfibrils, which support the architecture of elastic fibers and other connective tissue. Deficiency of fibrillin-1 in the extracellular matrix leads to excessive signaling by transforming growth factor β (TGF-β). Loeys-Dietz syndrome is caused by mutations in the genes that encode TGF-β receptors 1 (*TGFBR1*) and 2 (*TGFBR2*). Increased signaling by TGF-β and mutations of *TGFBR1* and *TGFBR2* may cause thoracic aortic aneurysms. Mutations of type III procollagen have been implicated in Ehlers-Danlos type IV syndrome. Mutations of *SMAD3*, which encodes a downstream signaling protein involved with TGF binding to its receptors, have been described in a syndrome of thoracic aortic aneurysm; craniofacial, skeletal, and cutaneous anomalies; and osteoarthritis. Mutations of the genes encoding the smooth muscle–specific alpha-actin (*ACTA2*), smooth muscle cell–specific myosin heavy chain 11 (*MHC11*), and myosin light chain kinase (*MYLK*) and mutations of *TGFBR2* and *SMAD3* have been reported in some patients with nonsyndromic familial thoracic aortic aneurysms.

The infectious causes of aortic aneurysms include syphilis, tuberculosis, and other bacterial infections. *Syphilis* (Chap. 206) is a relatively uncommon cause of aortic aneurysm. Syphilitic periaortitis and mesoaortitis damage elastic fibers, resulting in thickening and weakening of the aortic wall. Approximately 90% of syphilitic aneurysms are located in the ascending aorta or aortic arch. *Tuberculous aneurysms* (Chap. 202) typically affect the thoracic aorta and result from direct extension of infection from hilar lymph nodes or contiguous abscesses as well as from bacterial seeding. Loss of aortic wall elasticity results from granulomatous destruction of the medial layer. A *mycotic aneurysm* is a rare condition that develops as a result of staphylococcal, streptococcal, *Salmonella*, or other bacterial or fungal infections of the aorta, usually at an atherosclerotic plaque. These aneurysms are usually saccular. Blood cultures are often positive and reveal the nature of the infective agent.

Vasculitides associated with aortic aneurysm include Takayasu's arteritis and giant cell arteritis, which may cause aneurysms of the aortic arch and descending thoracic aorta. Spondyloarthropathies such as ankylosing spondylitis, rheumatoid arthritis, psoriatic arthritis, relapsing polychondritis, and reactive arthritis (formerly known as Reiter's syndrome) are associated with dilation of the ascending aorta. Aortic aneurysms occur in patients with Behçet's syndrome (Chap. 387), Cogan's syndrome, and IgG4-related systemic disease. Aortic aneurysms also result from idiopathic aortitis. *Traumatic aneurysms* may occur after penetrating or nonpenetrating chest trauma and most commonly affect the descending thoracic aorta just beyond the site of insertion of the ligamentum arteriosum. Chronic aortic dissections are associated with weakening of the aortic wall that may lead to the development of aneurysmal dilatation.

THORACIC AORTIC ANEURYSMS

The clinical manifestations and natural history of thoracic aortic aneurysms depend on their location. Medial degeneration is the most common pathology associated with ascending aortic aneurysms, whereas atherosclerosis is the condition most frequently associated with aneurysms of the descending thoracic aorta. The average growth rate of thoracic aneurysms is 0.1–0.2 cm per year. Thoracic aortic aneurysms associated with Marfan's syndrome or aortic dissection may expand at a greater rate. The risk of rupture is related to the size of the aneurysm and the presence of symptoms, ranging approximately from 2–3% per year for thoracic aortic aneurysms <4.0 cm in diameter to 7% per year for those >6 cm in diameter. Most thoracic aortic aneurysms are asymptomatic; however, compression or erosion of adjacent tissue by aneurysms may cause symptoms such as chest pain, shortness of breath, cough, hoarseness, and dysphagia. Aneurysmal dilation of the ascending aorta may cause congestive heart failure as a consequence of aortic regurgitation, and compression of the superior vena cava may produce congestion of the head, neck, and upper extremities.

A chest x-ray may be the first test that suggests the diagnosis of a thoracic aortic aneurysm (Fig. 301-1). Findings include widening

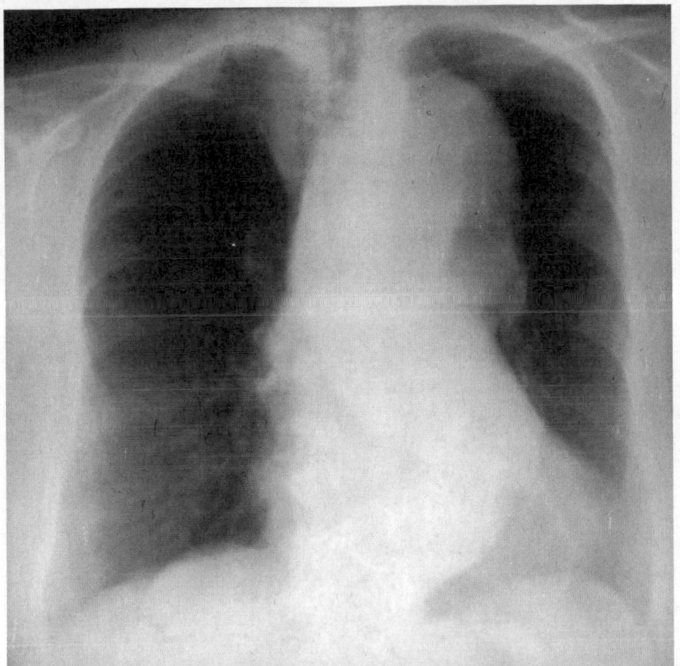

FIGURE 301-1 A chest x-ray of a patient with a thoracic aortic aneurysm.

of the mediastinal shadow and displacement or compression of the trachea or left main stem bronchus. Echocardiography, particularly transesophageal echocardiography, can be used to assess the proximal ascending aorta and descending thoracic aorta. Contrast-enhanced CT, magnetic resonance imaging (MRI), and conventional invasive aortography are sensitive and specific tests for assessment of aneurysms of the thoracic aorta and involvement of branch vessels (Fig. 301-2). In asymptomatic patients whose aneurysms are too small to justify surgery, noninvasive testing with either contrast-enhanced CT or MRI should be performed at least every 6–12 months to monitor expansion.

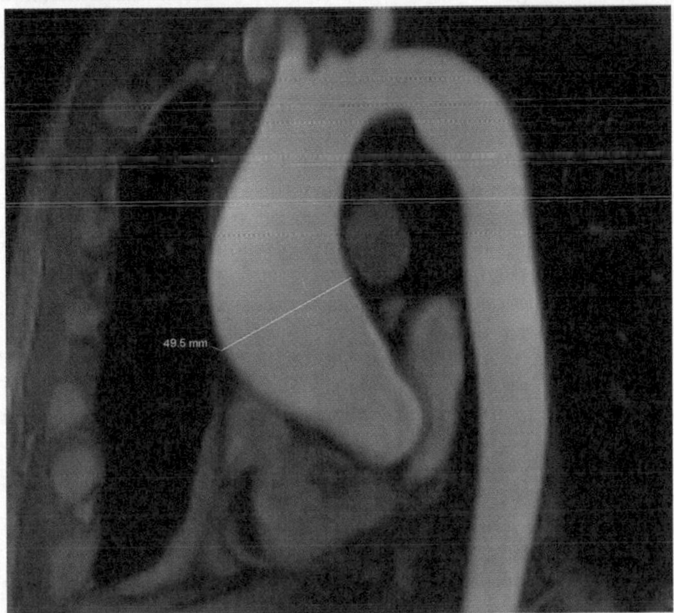

FIGURE 301-2 A magnetic resonance angiogram demonstrating a fusiform aneurysm of the ascending thoracic aorta. *(Courtesy of Dr. Michael Steigner, Brigham and Women's Hospital, Boston, MA, with permission.)*

TREATMENT THORACIC AORTIC ANEURYSMS

β-Adrenergic blockers currently are recommended for patients with thoracic aortic aneurysms, particularly those with Marfan's syndrome, who have evidence of aortic root dilatation to reduce the rate of further expansion. Additional medical therapy should be given as necessary to control hypertension. Recent studies indicate that angiotensin receptor antagonists and angiotensin-converting enzyme inhibitors reduce the rate of aortic dilation in patients with Marfan's syndrome by blocking TGF-β signaling; clinical outcome trials of this treatment approach are in progress. Operative repair with placement of a prosthetic graft is indicated in patients with symptomatic ascending thoracic aortic aneurysms and for most asymptomatic aneurysms when the ascending aortic diameter is >5.5 cm. In patients with Marfan's syndrome or bicuspid aortic valve, ascending thoracic aortic aneurysms of 4–5 cm should be considered for surgery. Operative repair is indicated for patients with descending thoracic aortic aneurysms when the diameter is >6 cm, and endovascular repair should be considered if feasible when the diameter is >5.5 cm. Repair is also recommended when the diameter of an aneurysm has increased >1 cm per year.

ABDOMINAL AORTIC ANEURYSMS

Abdominal aortic aneurysms occur more frequently in males than in females, and the incidence increases with age. Abdominal aortic aneurysms ≥4.0 cm may affect 1–2% of men older than 50 years. At least 90% of all abdominal aortic aneurysms >4.0 cm are related to atherosclerotic disease, and most of these aneurysms are below the level of the renal arteries. Prognosis is related to both the size of the aneurysm and the severity of coexisting coronary artery and cerebrovascular disease. The risk of rupture increases with the size of the aneurysm: the 5-year risk for aneurysms <5 cm is 1–2%, whereas it is 20–40% for aneurysms >5 cm in diameter. The formation of mural thrombi within aneurysms may predispose to peripheral embolization.

An abdominal aortic aneurysm commonly produces no symptoms. It usually is detected on routine examination as a palpable, pulsatile, expansile, and nontender mass, or it is an incidental finding observed on an abdominal imaging study performed for other reasons. As abdominal aortic aneurysms expand, however, they may become painful. Some patients complain of strong pulsations in the abdomen; others experience pain in the chest, lower back, or scrotum. Aneurysmal pain is usually a harbinger of rupture and represents a medical emergency. More often, acute rupture occurs without any prior warning, and this complication is always life-threatening. Rarely, there is leakage of the aneurysm with severe pain and tenderness. Acute pain and hypotension occur with rupture of the aneurysm, which requires an emergency operation.

Abdominal radiography may demonstrate the calcified outline of the aneurysm; however, about 25% of aneurysms are not calcified and cannot be visualized by x-ray imaging. An abdominal ultrasound can delineate the transverse and longitudinal dimensions of an abdominal aortic aneurysm and may detect mural thrombus. Abdominal ultrasound is useful for serial documentation of aneurysm size and can be used to screen patients at risk for developing an aortic aneurysm. In one large study, ultrasound screening of men age 65–74 years was associated with a risk reduction in aneurysm-related death of 42%. For this reason, screening by ultrasonography is recommended for men age 65–75 years who have ever smoked. In addition, siblings or offspring of persons with abdominal aortic aneurysms, as well as individuals with thoracic aortic or peripheral arterial aneurysms, should be considered for screening for abdominal aortic aneurysms. CT with contrast and MRI are accurate noninvasive tests to determine the location and size of abdominal aortic aneurysms and to plan endovascular or open surgical repair (Fig. 301-3). Contrast aortography may be used for the evaluation of patients with aneurysms, but the procedure carries a small risk of complications such as bleeding, allergic reactions, and atheroembolism. Since the presence of mural thrombi may reduce the luminal size, aortography may underestimate the diameter of an aneurysm.

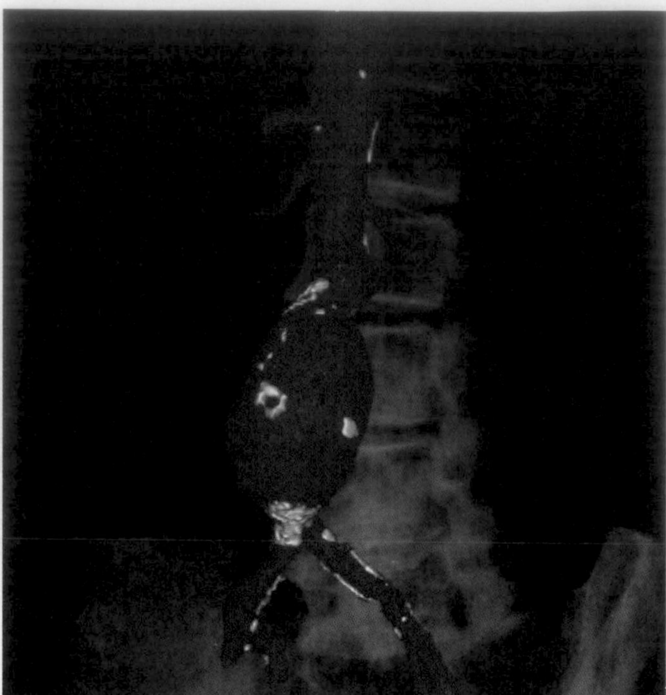
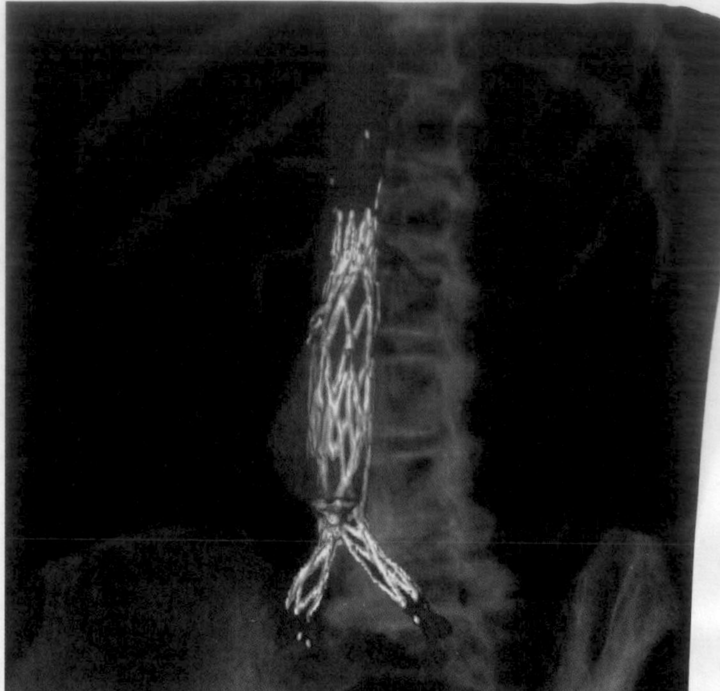

FIGURE 301-3 A computed tomographic angiogram depicting a fusiform abdominal aortic aneurysm before (*left*) and after (*right*) treatment with a bifurcated stent graft. *(Courtesy of Drs. Elizabeth George and Frank Rybicki, Brigham and Women's Hospital, Boston, MA, with permission.)*

TREATMENT ABDOMINAL AORTIC ANEURYSMS

Operative repair of the aneurysm with insertion of a prosthetic graft or endovascular placement of an aortic stent graft (Fig. 301-3) is indicated for abdominal aortic aneurysms of any size that are expanding rapidly or are associated with symptoms. For asymptomatic aneurysms, abdominal aortic aneurysm repair is indicated if the diameter is >5.5 cm. In randomized trials of patients with abdominal aortic aneurysms <5.5 cm, there was no difference in the long-term (5- to 8-year) mortality rate between those followed with ultrasound surveillance and those undergoing elective surgical repair. Thus, serial noninvasive follow-up of smaller aneurysms (<5 cm) is an alternative to immediate repair. The decision to perform an open surgical operation or endovascular repair is based in part on the vascular anatomy and comorbid conditions. Endovascular repair of abdominal aortic aneurysms has a lower short-term morbidity rate but a comparable long-term mortality rate with open surgical reconstruction. Long-term surveillance with CT or MR aortography is indicated after endovascular repair to detect leaks and possible aneurysm expansion.

In surgical candidates, careful preoperative cardiac and general medical evaluations (followed by appropriate therapy for complicating conditions) are essential. Preexisting coronary artery disease, congestive heart failure, pulmonary disease, diabetes mellitus, and advanced age add to the risk of surgery. β-Adrenergic blockers decrease perioperative cardiovascular morbidity and mortality. With careful preoperative cardiac evaluation and postoperative care, the operative mortality rate approximates 1–2%. After acute rupture, the mortality rate of emergent operation is 45–50%. Endovascular repair with stent placement is an alternative approach to treat ruptured aneurysms and may be associated with a lower mortality rate.

ACUTE AORTIC SYNDROMES

The four major acute aortic syndromes are aortic rupture (discussed earlier), aortic dissection, intramural hematoma, and penetrating atherosclerotic ulcer. Aortic dissection is caused by a circumferential or, less frequently, transverse tear of the intima. It often occurs along the right lateral wall of the ascending aorta where the hydraulic shear stress is high. Another common site is the descending thoracic aorta just below the ligamentum arteriosum. The initiating event is either a primary intimal tear with secondary dissection into the media or a medial hemorrhage that dissects into and disrupts the intima. The pulsatile aortic flow then dissects along the elastic lamellar plates of the aorta and creates a false lumen. The dissection usually propagates distally down the descending aorta and into its major branches, but it may propagate proximally. Distal propagation may be limited by atherosclerotic plaque. In some cases, a secondary distal intimal disruption occurs, resulting in the reentry of blood from the false to the true lumen.

There are at least two important pathologic and radiologic variants of aortic dissection: intramural hematoma without an intimal flap and penetrating atherosclerotic ulcer. Acute intramural hematoma is thought to result from rupture of the vasa vasorum with hemorrhage into the wall of the aorta. Most of these hematomas occur in the descending thoracic aorta. Acute intramural hematomas may progress to dissection and rupture. Penetrating atherosclerotic ulcers are caused by erosion of a plaque into the aortic media, are usually localized, and are not associated with extensive propagation. They are found primarily in the middle and distal portions of the descending thoracic aorta and are associated with extensive atherosclerotic disease. The ulcer can erode beyond the internal elastic lamina, leading to medial hematoma, and may progress to false aneurysm formation or rupture.

Several classification schemes have been developed for thoracic aortic dissections. DeBakey and colleagues initially classified aortic dissections as type I, in which an intimal tear occurs in the ascending aorta but involves the descending aorta as well; type II, in which the dissection is limited to the ascending aorta; and type III, in which the intimal tear is located in the descending aorta with distal propagation of the dissection (Fig. 301-4). Another classification (Stanford) is [illegible] of type A, in which the dissection involves the ascending aorta (pr[illegible] mal dissection), and type B, in which it is limited to the arch an[illegible] descending aorta (distal dissection). From a management stand[illegible] classification of aortic dissections and intramural hematomas int[illegible] A or B is more practical and useful, since DeBakey types I and [illegible] managed in a similar manner.

The factors that predispose to aortic dissection include thos[illegible] ciated with medial degeneration and others that increase aorti[illegible] stress (Table 301-1). Systemic hypertension is a coexisting condi[illegible]

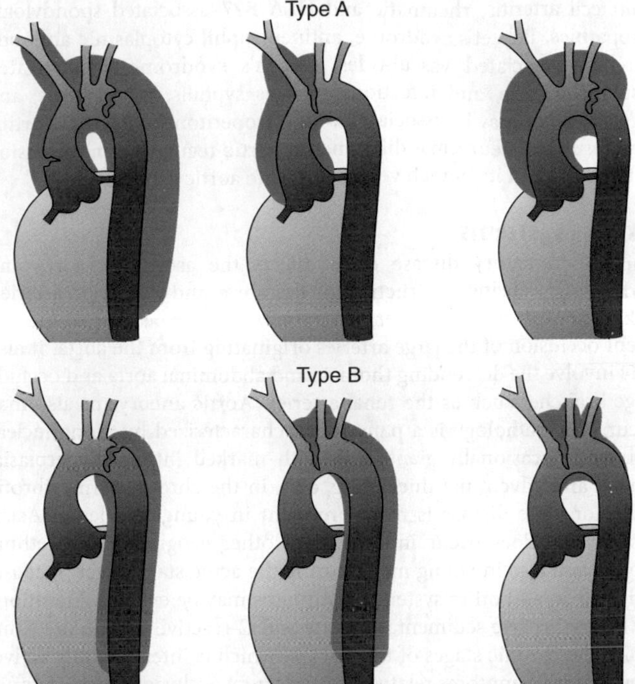

FIGURE 301-4 Classification of aortic dissections. Stanford classification: Type A dissections (*top*) involve the ascending aorta independent of site of tear and distal extension; type B dissections (*bottom*) involve transverse and/or descending aorta without involvement of the ascending aorta. DeBakey classification: Type I dissection involves ascending to descending aorta (*top left*); type II dissection is limited to ascending or transverse aorta, without descending aorta (*top center + top right*); type III dissection involves descending aorta only (*bottom left*). *(From DC Miller, in RM Doroghazi, EE Slater [eds]: Aortic Dissection. New York, McGraw-Hill, 1983, with permission.)*

70% of patients. Aortic dissection is the major cause of morbidity and mortality in patients with Marfan's syndrome (Chap. 427) or Loeys-Dietz syndrome, and similarly may affect patients with Ehlers-Danlos syndrome. The incidence also is increased in patients with inflammatory aortitis (i.e., Takayasu's arteritis, giant cell arteritis), congenital aortic valve anomalies (e.g., bicuspid valve), coarctation of the aorta, and a history of aortic trauma. In addition, the risk of dissection is increased in otherwise normal women during the third trimester of pregnancy. Aortic dissection also may occur as a consequence of weight lifting, cocaine use, or deceleration injury.

CLINICAL MANIFESTATIONS

The peak incidence of aortic dissection is in the sixth and seventh decades. Men are more affected than women by a ratio of 2:1. The presentations of aortic dissection and its variants are the consequences of intimal tear, dissecting hematoma, occlusion of involved arteries, and compression of adjacent tissues. Acute aortic dissection presents with the sudden onset of pain (Chap. 19), which often is described as very severe and tearing and is associated with diaphoresis. The pain may be localized to the front or back of the chest, often the interscapular region, and typically migrates with propagation of the dissection. Other symptoms include syncope, dyspnea, and weakness. Physical findings may include hypertension or hypotension, loss of pulses, aortic regurgitation, pulmonary edema, and neurologic findings due to carotid artery obstruction (hemiplegia, hemianesthesia) or spinal cord ischemia (paraplegia). Bowel ischemia, hematuria, and myocardial ischemia have all been observed. These clinical manifestations reflect complications resulting from the dissection occluding the major arteries. Furthermore, clinical manifestations may result from the compression of adjacent structures (e.g., superior cervical ganglia, superior vena cava, bronchus, esophagus) by the expanding dissection, causing aneurysmal dilation, and include Horner's syndrome, superior vena cava syndrome, hoarseness, dysphagia, and airway compromise. Hemopericardium and cardiac tamponade may complicate a type A lesion with retrograde dissection. Acute aortic regurgitation is an important and common (>50%) complication of proximal dissection. It is the outcome of either a circumferential tear that widens the aortic root or a disruption of the annulus by a dissecting hematoma that tears a leaflet(s) or displaces it, inferior to the line of closure. Signs of aortic regurgitation include bounding pulses, a wide pulse pressure, a diastolic murmur often radiating along the right sternal border, and evidence of congestive heart failure. The clinical manifestations depend on the severity of the regurgitation.

In dissections involving the ascending aorta, the chest x-ray often reveals a widened superior mediastinum. A pleural effusion (usually left-sided) also may be present. This effusion is typically serosanguineous and not indicative of rupture unless accompanied by hypotension and falling hematocrit. In dissections of the descending thoracic aorta, a widened mediastinum may be observed on chest x-ray. In addition, the descending aorta may appear to be wider than the ascending portion. An electrocardiogram that shows no evidence of myocardial ischemia is helpful in distinguishing aortic dissection from myocardial infarction. Rarely, the dissection involves the right or, less commonly, left coronary ostium and causes acute myocardial infarction.

The diagnosis of aortic dissection can be established by noninvasive techniques such as echocardiography, CT, and MRI. Aortography is used less commonly because of the accuracy of these noninvasive techniques. Transthoracic echocardiography can be performed simply and rapidly and has an overall sensitivity of 60–85% for aortic dissection. For diagnosing proximal ascending aortic dissections, its sensitivity exceeds 80%; it is less useful for detecting dissection of the arch and descending thoracic aorta. Transesophageal echocardiography requires greater skill and patient cooperation but is very accurate in identifying dissections of the ascending and descending thoracic aorta but not the arch, achieving 98% sensitivity and approximately 90% specificity. Echocardiography also provides important information regarding the presence and severity of aortic regurgitation and pericardial effusion. CT and MRI are both highly accurate in identifying the intimal flap and the extent of the dissection and involvement of major arteries; each has a sensitivity and specificity >90%. They are useful in recognizing intramural hemorrhage and penetrating ulcers. The relative utility of transesophageal echocardiography, CT, and MRI depends on the availability and expertise in individual institutions as well as on the hemodynamic stability of the patient, with CT and MRI obviously less suitable for unstable patients.

TREATMENT AORTIC DISSECTION

Medical therapy should be initiated as soon as the diagnosis is considered. The patient should be admitted to an intensive care unit for hemodynamic monitoring. Unless hypotension is present, therapy should be aimed at reducing cardiac contractility and systemic arterial pressure, and thus shear stress. For acute dissection, unless contraindicated, β-adrenergic blockers should be administered parenterally, using intravenous propranolol, metoprolol, or the short-acting esmolol to achieve a heart rate of approximately 60 beats/min. This should be accompanied by sodium nitroprusside infusion to lower systolic blood pressure to ≤120 mmHg. Labetalol (Chap. 298), a drug with both β- and α-adrenergic blocking properties, also may be used as a parenteral agent in acute therapy for dissection.

The calcium channel antagonists verapamil and diltiazem may be used intravenously if nitroprusside or β-adrenergic blockers cannot be employed. The addition of a parenteral angiotensin-converting enzyme (ACE) inhibitor such as enalaprilat to a β-adrenergic blocker also may be considered. Isolated use of a direct vasodilator such as hydralazine is contraindicated because these agents can increase hydraulic shear and may propagate the dissection.

Emergent or urgent surgical correction is the preferred treatment for acute ascending aortic dissections and intramural hematomas (type A) and for complicated type B dissections, including those characterized by propagation, compromise of major aortic branches, impending rupture, or continued pain. Surgery involves excision of the intimal flap, obliteration of the false lumen, and placement of an interposition graft. A composite valve-graft conduit is used if the aortic valve is disrupted. The overall in-hospital mortality rate after surgical treatment of patients with aortic dissection is reported to be 15–25%. The major causes of perioperative mortality and morbidity include myocardial infarction, paraplegia, renal failure, tamponade, hemorrhage, and sepsis. Endoluminal stent grafts may be considered in selected patients. Other transcatheter techniques, such as fenestration of the intimal flaps and stenting of narrowed branch vessels to increase flow to compromised organs, are used in selected patients. For uncomplicated and stable distal dissections and intramural hematomas (type B), medical therapy is the preferred treatment. The in-hospital mortality rate of medically treated patients with type B dissection is 10–20%. Long-term therapy for patients with aortic dissection and intramural hematomas (with or without surgery) consists of control of hypertension and reduction of cardiac contractility with the use of beta blockers plus other antihypertensive agents, such as ACE inhibitors or calcium antagonists. Patients with chronic type B dissection and intramural hematomas should be followed on an outpatient basis every 6–12 months with contrast-enhanced CT or MRI to detect propagation or expansion. Patients with Marfan's syndrome are at high risk for postdissection complications. The long-term prognosis for patients with treated dissections is generally good with careful follow-up; the 10-year survival rate is approximately 60%.

CHRONIC ATHEROSCLEROTIC OCCLUSIVE DISEASE

Atherosclerosis may affect the thoracic and abdominal aorta. Occlusive aortic disease caused by atherosclerosis usually is confined to the distal abdominal aorta below the renal arteries. Frequently the disease extends to the iliac arteries (Chap. 302). Claudication characteristically involves the buttocks, thighs, and calves and may be associated with impotence in males (Leriche's syndrome). The severity of the symptoms depends on the adequacy of collaterals. With sufficient collateral blood flow, a complete occlusion of the abdominal aorta may occur without the development of ischemic symptoms. The physical findings include the absence of femoral and other distal pulses bilaterally and the detection of an audible bruit over the abdomen (usually at or below the umbilicus) and the common femoral arteries. Atrophic skin, loss of hair, and coolness of the lower extremities usually are observed. In advanced ischemia, rubor on dependency and pallor on elevation can be seen.

The diagnosis usually is established by physical examination and noninvasive testing, including leg pressure measurements, Doppler velocity analysis, pulse volume recordings, and duplex ultrasonography. The anatomy may be defined by MRI, CT, or conventional aortography, typically performed when one is considering revascularization. Catheter-based endovascular or operative treatment is indicated in patients with lifestyle-limiting or debilitating symptoms of claudication and patients with critical limb ischemia.

ACUTE AORTIC OCCLUSION

Acute occlusion in the distal abdominal aorta constitutes a medical emergency because it threatens the viability of the lower extremities; it usually results from an occlusive (saddle) embolus that almost always originates from the heart. Rarely, acute occlusion may occur as the result of in situ thrombosis in a preexisting severely narrowed segment of the aorta.

The clinical picture is one of acute ischemia of the lower extremities. Severe rest pain, coolness, and pallor of the lower extremities and the absence of distal pulses bilaterally are the usual manifestations. Diagnosis should be established rapidly by MRI, CT, or aortography. Emergency thrombectomy or revascularization is indicated.

AORTITIS

Aortitis, a term referring to inflammatory disease of the aorta, may be caused by large vessel vasculitides such as Takayasu's arteritis and giant cell arteritis, rheumatic and HLA-B27–associated spondyloarthropathies, Behçet's syndrome, antineutrophil cytoplasmic antibody (ANCA)–associated vasculitides, Cogan's syndrome, IgG4-related systemic disease, and infections such as syphilis, tuberculosis, and *Salmonella,* or may be associated with retroperitoneal fibrosis. Aortitis may result in aneurysmal dilation and aortic regurgitation, occlusion of the aorta and its branch vessels, or acute aortic syndromes.

TAKAYASU'S ARTERITIS

This inflammatory disease often affects the ascending aorta and aortic arch, causing obstruction of the aorta and its major arteries. Takayasu's arteritis is also termed *pulseless disease* because of the frequent occlusion of the large arteries originating from the aorta. It also may involve the descending thoracic and abdominal aorta and occlude large branches such as the renal arteries. Aortic aneurysms also may occur. The pathology is a panarteritis characterized by mononuclear cells and occasionally giant cells, with marked intimal hyperplasia, medial and adventitial thickening, and, in the chronic form, fibrotic occlusion. The disease is most prevalent in young females of Asian descent but does occur in women of other geographic and ethnic origins and also in young men. During the acute stage, fever, malaise, weight loss, and other systemic symptoms may be evident. Elevations of the erythrocyte sedimentation rate and C-reactive protein are common. The chronic stages of the disease, which is intermittently active, present with symptoms related to large artery occlusion, such as upper extremity claudication, cerebral ischemia, and syncope. The process is progressive, and there is no definitive therapy. Glucocorticoids and immunosuppressive agents are effective in some patients during the acute phase. Surgical bypass or endovascular intervention of a critically stenotic artery may be necessary.

GIANT CELL ARTERITIS

(See also Chap. 385) This vasculitis occurs in older individuals and affects women more often than men. Primarily large and medium-size arteries are affected. The pathology is that of focal granulomatous lesions involving the entire arterial wall; it may be associated with polymyalgia rheumatica. Obstruction of medium-size arteries (e.g., temporal and ophthalmic arteries) and major branches of the aorta and the development of aortitis and aortic regurgitation are important complications of the disease. High-dose glucocorticoid therapy may be effective when given early.

RHEUMATIC AORTITIS

Rheumatoid arthritis (Chap. 380), ankylosing spondylitis (Chap. 384), psoriatic arthritis (Chap. 384), reactive arthritis (formerly known as Reiter's syndrome) (Chap. 384), relapsing polychondritis, and inflammatory bowel disorders may all be associated with aortitis involving the ascending aorta. The inflammatory lesions usually involve the ascending aorta and may extend to the sinuses of Valsalva, the mitral valve leaflets, and adjacent myocardium. The clinical manifestations are aneurysm, aortic regurgitation, and involvement of the cardiac conduction system.

IDIOPATHIC AORTITIS

Idiopathic abdominal aortitis is characterized by adventitial and periaortic inflammation with thickening of the aortic wall. It is associated with abdominal aortic aneurysms and idiopathic retroperitoneal fibrosis. Affected individuals may present with vague constitutional symptoms, fever, and abdominal pain. Retroperitoneal fibrosis can cause ureteral obstruction and hydronephrosis. Glucocorticoids and immunosuppressive agents may reduce the inflammation.

INFECTIVE AORTITIS

Infective aortitis may result from direct invasion of the aortic wall by bacterial pathogens such as *Staphylococcus*, *Streptococcus*, and *Salmonella* or by fungi. These bacteria cause aortitis by infecting the aorta at sites of atherosclerotic plaque. Bacterial proteases lead to degradation of collagen, and the ensuing destruction of the aortic wall leads to the formation of a saccular aneurysm referred to as a mycotic aneurysm. Mycotic aneurysms have a predilection for the suprarenal abdominal aorta. The pathologic characteristics of the aortic wall include acute and chronic inflammation, abscesses, hemorrhage, and necrosis. Mycotic aneurysms typically affect the elderly and occur in men three times more frequently than in women. Patients may present with fever, sepsis, and chest, back, or abdominal pain; there may have been a preceding diarrheal illness. Blood cultures are positive in the majority of patients. Both CT and MRI are useful to diagnose mycotic aneurysms. Treatment includes antibiotic therapy and surgical removal of the affected part of the aorta and revascularization of the lower extremities with grafts placed in uninfected tissue.

Syphilitic aortitis is a late manifestation of luctic infection (Chap. 206) that usually affects the proximal ascending aorta, particularly the aortic root, resulting in aortic dilation and aneurysm formation. Syphilitic aortitis occasionally may involve the aortic arch or the descending aorta. The aneurysms may be saccular or fusiform and are usually asymptomatic, but compression of and erosion into adjacent structures may result in symptoms; rupture also may occur.

The initial lesion is an obliterative endarteritis of the vasa vasorum, especially in the adventitia. This is an inflammatory response to the invasion of the adventitia by the spirochetes. Destruction of the aortic media occurs as the spirochetes spread into this layer, usually via the lymphatics accompanying the vasa vasorum. Destruction of collagen and elastic tissues leads to dilation of the aorta, scar formation, and calcification. These changes account for the characteristic radiographic appearance of linear calcification of the ascending aorta.

The disease typically presents as an incidental chest radiographic finding 15–30 years after initial infection. Symptoms may result from aortic regurgitation, narrowing of coronary ostia due to syphilitic aortitis, compression of adjacent structures (e.g., esophagus), or rupture. Diagnosis is established by a positive serologic test, i.e., rapid plasmin reagin (RPR) or fluorescent treponemal antibody. Treatment includes penicillin and surgical excision and repair.

302 Arterial Diseases of the Extremities

Mark A. Creager, Joseph Loscalzo

PERIPHERAL ARTERY DISEASE

Peripheral artery disease (PAD) is defined as a clinical disorder in which there is a stenosis or occlusion in the aorta or the arteries of the limbs. Atherosclerosis is the leading cause of PAD in patients >40 years old. Other causes include thrombosis, embolism, vasculitis, fibromuscular dysplasia, entrapment, cystic adventitial disease, and trauma. The highest prevalence of atherosclerotic PAD occurs in the sixth and seventh decades of life. As in patients with atherosclerosis of the coronary and cerebral vasculature, there is an increased risk of developing PAD in cigarette smokers and in persons with diabetes mellitus, hypercholesterolemia, hypertension, or renal insufficiency.

Pathology (See also Chap. 291e) Segmental lesions that cause stenosis or occlusion are usually localized to large and medium-size vessels. The pathology of the lesions includes atherosclerotic plaques with calcium deposition, thinning of the media, patchy destruction of muscle and elastic fibers, fragmentation of the internal elastic lamina, and thrombi composed of platelets and fibrin. The primary sites of involvement are the abdominal aorta and iliac arteries (30% of symptomatic patients), the femoral and popliteal arteries (80–90% of patients), and the more distal vessels, including the tibial and peroneal arteries (40–50% of patients). Atherosclerotic lesions occur preferentially at arterial branch points, which are sites of increased turbulence, altered shear stress, and intimal injury. Involvement of the distal vasculature is most common in elderly individuals and patients with diabetes mellitus.

Clinical Evaluation Fewer than 50% of patients with PAD are symptomatic, although many have a slow or impaired gait. The most common *symptom* is intermittent claudication, which is defined as a pain, ache, cramp, numbness, or a sense of fatigue in the muscles; it occurs during exercise and is relieved by rest. The site of claudication is distal to the location of the occlusive lesion. For example, buttock, hip, thigh, and calf discomfort occurs in patients with aortoiliac disease, whereas calf claudication develops in patients with femoral-popliteal disease. Symptoms are far more common in the lower than in the upper extremities because of the higher incidence of obstructive lesions in the former region. In patients with severe arterial occlusive disease in whom resting blood flow cannot accommodate basal nutritional needs of the tissues, critical limb ischemia may develop. Patients complain of rest pain or a feeling of cold or numbness in the foot and toes. Frequently, these symptoms occur at night when the legs are horizontal and improve when the legs are in a dependent position. With severe ischemia, rest pain may be persistent.

Important *physical findings* of PAD include decreased or absent pulses distal to the obstruction, the presence of bruits over the narrowed artery, and muscle atrophy. With more severe disease, hair loss, thickened nails, smooth and shiny skin, reduced skin temperature, and pallor or cyanosis are common physical signs. In patients with critical limb ischemia, ulcers or gangrene may occur. Elevation of the legs and repeated flexing of the calf muscles produce pallor of the soles of the feet, whereas rubor, secondary to reactive hyperemia, may develop when the legs are dependent. The time required for rubor to develop or for the veins in the foot to fill when the patient's legs are transferred from an elevated to a dependent position is related to the severity of the ischemia and the presence of collateral vessels. Patients with severe ischemia may develop peripheral edema because they keep their legs in a dependent position much of the time. Ischemic neuropathy can result in numbness and hyporeflexia.

Noninvasive Testing The history and physical examination are often sufficient to establish the diagnosis of PAD. An objective assessment of the presence and severity of disease is obtained by noninvasive techniques. Arterial pressure can be recorded noninvasively in the legs by placement of sphygmomanometric cuffs at the ankles and the use of a Doppler device to auscultate or record blood flow from the dorsalis pedis and posterior tibial arteries. Normally, systolic blood pressure in the legs and arms is similar. Indeed, ankle pressure may be slightly higher than arm pressure due to pulse-wave amplification. In the presence of hemodynamically significant stenoses, the systolic blood pressure in the leg is decreased. Thus, the ratio of the ankle and brachial artery pressures (termed the *ankle:brachial index*, or ABI) is 1.00–1.40 in normal individuals. ABI values of 0.91–0.99 are considered "borderline," and those <0.90 are abnormal and diagnostic of PAD. ABIs >1.40 indicate noncompressible arteries secondary to vascular calcification.

Other noninvasive tests include segmental pressure measurements, segmental pulse volume recordings, duplex ultrasonography (which combines B-mode imaging and Doppler flow velocity waveform analysis examination), transcutaneous oximetry, and stress testing (usually using a treadmill). Placement of pneumatic cuffs enables assessment of systolic pressure along the legs. The presence of pressure gradients between sequential cuffs provides evidence of the presence and location of hemodynamically significant stenoses. In addition, the amplitude of the pulse volume contour becomes blunted in the presence of significant PAD. Duplex ultrasonography is used to image and detect stenotic lesions in native arteries and bypass grafts.

Treadmill testing allows the physician to assess functional limitations objectively. Decline of the ABI immediately after exercise provides further support for the diagnosis of PAD in patients with equivocal symptoms and findings on examination.

Magnetic resonance angiography (MRA), computed tomographic angiography (CTA), and conventional catheter-based angiography should not be used for routine diagnostic testing but are performed before potential revascularization (Fig. 302-1). Each test is useful in defining the anatomy to assist planning for endovascular and surgical revascularization procedures.

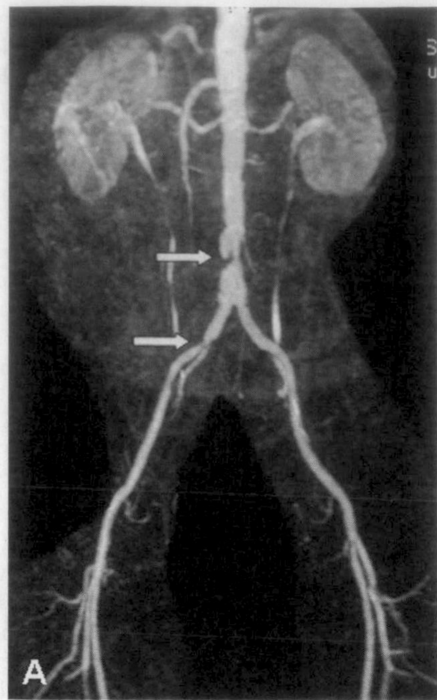

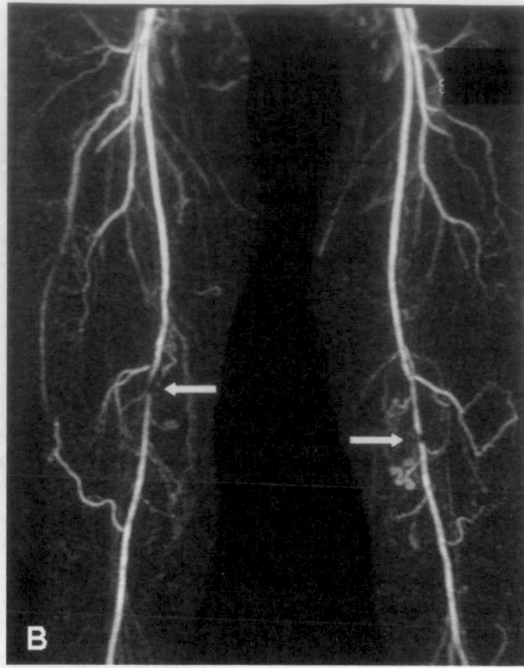

FIGURE 302-1 Magnetic resonance angiography of a patient with intermittent claudication, showing stenoses of the distal abdominal aorta and right iliac common iliac artery (***A***) and stenoses of the right and left superficial femoral arteries (***B***). *(Courtesy of Dr. Edwin Gravereaux, with permission.)*

Prognosis The natural history of patients with PAD is influenced primarily by the extent of coexisting coronary artery and cerebrovascular disease. Approximately one-third to one-half of patients with symptomatic PAD have evidence of coronary artery disease (CAD) based on clinical presentation and electrocardiogram, and over one-half have significant CAD by coronary angiography. Patients with PAD have a 15–30% 5-year mortality rate and a two- to sixfold increased risk of death from coronary heart disease. Mortality rates are highest in those with the most severe PAD. Measurement of ABI is useful for detecting PAD and identifying persons at risk for future atherothrombotic events. The likelihood of symptomatic progression of PAD is lower than the chance of succumbing to CAD. Approximately 75–80% of nondiabetic patients who present with mild to moderate claudication remain symptomatically stable. Deterioration is likely to occur in the remainder, with approximately 1–2% of the group ultimately developing critical limb ischemia each year. Approximately 25–30% of patients with critical limb ischemia undergo amputation within 1 year. The prognosis is worse in patients who continue to smoke cigarettes or have diabetes mellitus.

TREATMENT PERIPHERAL ARTERY DISEASE

Patients with PAD should receive therapies to reduce the risk of associated cardiovascular events, such as myocardial infarction and death, and to improve limb symptoms, prevent progression to critical limb ischemia, and preserve limb viability. Risk factor modification and antiplatelet therapy should be initiated to improve cardiovascular outcomes. The importance of discontinuing cigarette smoking cannot be overemphasized. The physician must assume a major role in this lifestyle modification. Counseling and adjunctive drug therapy with the nicotine patch, bupropion, or varenicline increase smoking cessation rates and reduce recidivism. It is important to control blood pressure in hypertensive patients. Angiotensin-converting enzyme inhibitors may reduce the risk of cardiovascular events in patients with symptomatic PAD. β-Adrenergic blockers do not worsen claudication and may be used to treat hypertension, especially in patients with coexistent CAD. Treatment of hypercholesterolemia with statins is advocated to reduce the risk of myocardial infarction, stroke, and death. The 2013 ACC/AHA Guideline on the Treatment of Blood Cholesterol to Reduce Atherosclerotic Cardiovascular Risk in Adults recommends high intensity statin treatment in patients with atherosclerotic disorders, including peripheral artery disease. Platelet inhibitors, including aspirin and clopidogrel, reduce the risk of adverse cardiovascular events in patients with atherosclerosis and are recommended for patients with symptomatic PAD, including those with intermittent claudication or critical limb ischemia or prior lower extremity revascularization. Dual antiplatelet therapy with both aspirin and clopidogrel is not more effective than aspirin alone in reducing cardiovascular morbidity and mortality rates in patients with PAD. The anticoagulant warfarin is as effective as antiplatelet therapy in preventing adverse cardiovascular events but causes more major bleeding; therefore, it is not indicated to improve outcomes in patients with chronic PAD.

Therapies for intermittent claudication and critical limb ischemia include supportive measures, medications, nonoperative interventions, and surgery. Supportive measures include meticulous care of the feet, which should be kept clean and protected against excessive drying with moisturizing creams. Well-fitting and protective shoes are advised to reduce trauma. Elastic support hose should be avoided, as it reduces blood flow to the skin. In patients with critical limb ischemia, shock blocks under the head of the bed together with a canopy over the feet may improve perfusion pressure and ameliorate some of the rest pain.

Patients with claudication should be encouraged to exercise regularly and at progressively more strenuous levels. Supervised exercise training programs for 30- to 45-min sessions, three to five times per week for at least 12 weeks, prolong walking distance. Patients also should be advised to walk until nearly maximum claudication discomfort occurs and then rest until the symptoms resolve before resuming ambulation. The beneficial effect of supervised exercise training on walking performance in patients with claudication often is similar to or greater than that realized after a revascularization procedure. Pharmacologic treatment of PAD has not been as successful as the medical treatment of CAD (Chap. 293). In particular, vasodilators as a class have not proved to be beneficial. During exercise, peripheral vasodilation occurs distal to sites of significant arterial stenoses. As a result, perfusion pressure falls, often to levels lower than that generated in the interstitial tissue by the exercising muscle. Drugs such as α-adrenergic blocking agents, calcium channel antagonists, and other vasodilators have not been shown to be effective in patients with PAD.

Cilostazol, a phosphodiesterase inhibitor with vasodilator and antiplatelet properties, increases claudication distance by 40–60% and improves measures of quality of life. The mechanism of action accounting for its beneficial effects is not known. Pentoxifylline, a substituted xanthine derivative, increases blood flow to the microcirculation and enhances tissue oxygenation. Although several placebo-controlled studies have found that pentoxifylline increases the duration of exercise in patients with claudication, its efficacy has not been confirmed in all clinical trials. Statins and angiotensin-converting enzyme inhibitors appear promising for treatment of intermittent claudication in initial clinical trials, but more studies are needed to confirm the efficacy of each class of drugs. There is no definitive medical therapy for critical limb ischemia, although several studies have suggested that long-term parenteral administration of vasodilator prostaglandins decreases pain and facilitates healing of ulcers. Enthusiasm for therapy with angiogenic growth factors abated when clinical trials of intramuscular gene transfer of DNA encoding vascular endothelial growth factor, fibroblast growth factor, hepatocyte growth factor, or hypoxia-inducible factor 1α failed to demonstrate improvement in symptoms or outcomes in patients with intermittent claudication or critical limb ischemia. Clinical trials assessing the ability of bone marrow–derived vascular progenitor cells to promote angiogenesis and preserve limb viability in patients with critical limb ischemia are ongoing.

REVASCULARIZATION

Revascularization procedures, including catheter-based and surgical interventions, are usually indicated for patients with disabling, progressive, or severe symptoms of intermittent claudication despite medical therapy and for those with critical limb ischemia. MRA, CTA, or conventional angiography should be performed to assess vascular anatomy in patients who are being considered for revascularization. Nonoperative interventions include percutaneous transluminal angiography (PTA) and stent placement (Chap. 296e). PTA and stenting of the iliac artery are associated with higher success rates than are PTA and stenting of the femoral and popliteal arteries. Approximately 90–95% of iliac PTAs are initially successful, and the 3-year patency rate is >75%. Patency rates may be higher if a stent is placed in the iliac artery. The initial success rates for femoral-popliteal PTA and stenting are approximately 80%, with 60% 3-year patency rates. Patency rates are influenced by the severity of pretreatment stenoses; the prognosis of occlusive lesions is worse than that of nonocclusive stenotic lesions. The role of drug-eluting stents and drug-coated balloons in PAD is under investigation.

Several operative procedures are available for treating patients with aortoiliac and femoral-popliteal artery disease. The preferred operative procedure depends on the location and extent of the obstruction(s) and the general medical condition of the patient. Operative procedures for aortoiliac disease include aortobifemoral bypass, axillofemoral bypass, femoro-femoral bypass, and aortoiliac endarterectomy. The most frequently used procedure is the aortobifemoral bypass using knitted Dacron grafts. Immediate graft patency approaches 99%, and 5- and 10-year graft patency rates in survivors are >90% and 80%, respectively. Operative complications include myocardial infarction and stroke, infection of the graft, peripheral embolization, and sexual dysfunction from interruption of autonomic nerves in the pelvis. The operative mortality rate ranges from 1–3%, mostly due to ischemic heart disease.

Operative therapy for femoral-popliteal artery disease includes in situ and reverse autogenous saphenous vein bypass grafts, placement of polytetrafluoroethylene (PTFE) or other synthetic grafts, and thromboendarterectomy. The operative mortality rate ranges from 1–3%. The long-term patency rate depends on the type of graft used, the location of the distal anastomosis, and the patency of runoff vessels beyond the anastomosis. Patency rates of femoral-popliteal saphenous vein bypass grafts approach 90% at 1 year and 70–80% at 5 years. Five-year patency rates of infrapopliteal saphenous vein bypass grafts are 60–70%. In contrast, 5-year patency rates of infrapopliteal PTFE grafts are <30%.

Preoperative cardiac risk assessment may identify individuals who are especially likely to experience an adverse cardiac event during the perioperative period. Patients with angina, prior myocardial infarction, ventricular ectopy, heart failure, or diabetes are among those at increased risk. Stress testing with treadmill exercise (if feasible), radionuclide myocardial perfusion imaging, or echocardiography permits further stratification of risk in these patients (Chap. 296e). Patients with abnormal test results require close supervision and adjunctive management with anti-ischemic medications. β-Adrenergic blockers and statins reduce the risk of postoperative cardiovascular complications. Coronary angiography and coronary artery revascularization compared with optimal medical therapy do not improve outcomes in most patients undergoing peripheral vascular surgery, but cardiac catheterization should be considered in patients with unstable angina and angina refractory to medical therapy as well as those suspected of having left main or three-vessel CAD.

FIBROMUSCULAR DYSPLASIA

Fibromuscular dysplasia is a hyperplastic disorder that affects medium-size and small arteries. It occurs predominantly in females and usually involves the renal and carotid arteries but can affect extremity vessels such as the iliac and subclavian arteries. The histologic classification includes intimal fibroplasia (also classified as focal), medial dysplasia (multifocal), and adventitial hyperplasia. Medial dysplasia is subdivided into medial fibroplasia, perimedial fibroplasia, and medial hyperplasia. Medial fibroplasia is the most common type and is characterized by alternating areas of thinned media and fibromuscular ridges. The internal elastic lamina usually is preserved. The iliac arteries are the limb arteries most likely to be affected by fibromuscular dysplasia. It is identified angiographically by a "string of beads" appearance caused by thickened fibromuscular ridges contiguous with thin, less involved portions of the arterial wall, which is typical of medial fibroplasia. When limb vessels are involved, clinical manifestations are similar to those for atherosclerosis, including claudication and rest pain. PTA and surgical reconstruction have been beneficial in patients with debilitating symptoms or threatened limbs.

THROMBOANGIITIS OBLITERANS

Thromboangiitis obliterans (Buerger's disease) is an inflammatory occlusive vascular disorder involving small and medium-size arteries and veins in the distal upper and lower extremities. Cerebral, visceral, and coronary vessels may be affected rarely. This disorder develops most frequently in men <40 years of age. The prevalence is higher in Asians and individuals of Eastern European descent. Although the cause of thromboangiitis obliterans is not known, there is a definite relationship to cigarette smoking in patients with this disorder.

In the initial stages of thromboangiitis obliterans, polymorphonuclear leukocytes infiltrate the walls of the small and medium-size arteries and veins. The internal elastic lamina is preserved, and a cellular, inflammatory thrombus develops in the vascular lumen. As the disease progresses, mononuclear cells, fibroblasts, and giant cells replace the neutrophils. Later stages are characterized by perivascular fibrosis, organized thrombus, and recanalization.

The clinical features of thromboangiitis obliterans often include a triad of claudication of the affected extremity, Raynaud's phenomenon, and migratory superficial vein thrombophlebitis. Claudication usually is confined to the calves and feet or the forearms and hands because this disorder primarily affects distal vessels. In the presence of severe digital ischemia, trophic nail changes, painful ulcerations, and gangrene may develop at the tips of the fingers or toes. The physical examination shows normal brachial and popliteal pulses but reduced or absent radial, ulnar, and/or tibial pulses. MRA, CTA, and conventional arteriography are helpful in making the diagnosis. Smooth, tapering segmental lesions in the distal vessels are characteristic, as are collateral vessels at sites of vascular occlusion. Proximal atherosclerotic disease is usually absent. The diagnosis can be confirmed by excisional biopsy and pathologic examination of an involved vessel.

There is no specific treatment except abstention from tobacco. The prognosis is worse in individuals who continue to smoke, but results are discouraging even in those who stop smoking. Arterial bypass of the larger vessels may be used in selected instances, as well as local debridement, depending on the symptoms and severity of ischemia. Antibiotics may be useful; anticoagulants and glucocorticoids are not helpful. If these measures fail, amputation may be required.

VASCULITIS

Other vasculitides may affect the arteries that supply the upper and lower extremities. Takayasu's arteritis and giant cell (temporal) arteritis are discussed in Chap. 385.

ACUTE LIMB ISCHEMIA

Acute limb ischemia occurs when arterial occlusion results in the sudden cessation of blood flow to an extremity. The severity of ischemia and the viability of the extremity depend on the location and extent of the occlusion and the presence and subsequent development of collateral blood vessels. Principal causes of acute arterial occlusion include embolism, thrombus in situ, arterial dissection, and trauma.

The most common sources of arterial emboli are the heart, aorta, and large arteries. Cardiac disorders that cause thromboembolism include atrial fibrillation, both chronic and paroxysmal; acute myocardial infarction; ventricular aneurysm; cardiomyopathy; infectious and marantic endocarditis; thrombi associated with prosthetic heart valves; and atrial myxoma. Emboli to the distal vessels may also originate from proximal sites of atherosclerosis and aneurysms of the aorta and large vessels. Less frequently, an arterial occlusion results paradoxically from a venous thrombus that has entered the systemic circulation via a patent foramen ovale or another septal defect. Arterial emboli tend to lodge at vessel bifurcations because the vessel caliber decreases at those sites; in the lower extremities, emboli lodge most frequently in the femoral artery, followed by the iliac artery, aorta, and popliteal and tibioperoneal arteries.

Acute arterial thrombosis in situ occurs most frequently in atherosclerotic vessels at the site of an atherosclerotic plaque or aneurysm and in arterial bypass grafts. Trauma to an artery may disrupt continuity of blood flow and cause acute limb ischemia via formation of an acute arterial thrombus or by disruption of an artery's integrity and extravasation of blood. Arterial occlusion may complicate arterial punctures and placement of catheters; it also may result from arterial dissection if the intimal flap obstructs the artery. Less common causes include thoracic outlet compression syndrome, which causes subclavian artery occlusion, and entrapment of the popliteal artery by abnormal placement of the medial head of the gastrocnemius muscle. Polycythemia and hypercoagulable disorders (Chaps. 131 and 141) are also associated with acute arterial thrombosis.

CLINICAL FEATURES

The symptoms of an acute arterial occlusion depend on the location, duration, and severity of the obstruction. Often, severe pain, paresthesia, numbness, and coldness develop in the involved extremity within 1 hour. Paralysis may occur with severe and persistent ischemia. Physical findings include loss of pulses distal to the occlusion, cyanosis or pallor, mottling, decreased skin temperature, muscle stiffening, loss of sensation, weakness, and/or absent deep tendon reflexes. If acute arterial occlusion occurs in the presence of an adequate collateral circulation, as is often the case in acute graft occlusion, the symptoms and findings may be less impressive. In this situation, the patient complains about an abrupt decrease in the distance walked before claudication occurs or of modest pain and paresthesia. Pallor and coolness are evident, but sensory and motor functions generally are preserved. The diagnosis of acute limb ischemia is usually apparent from the clinical presentation. In most circumstances, MRA, CTA, or catheter-based arteriography is used to confirm the diagnosis and demonstrate the location and extent of arterial occlusion.

TREATMENT ACUTE LIMB ISCHEMIA

Once the diagnosis is made, the patient should be anticoagulated with intravenous heparin to prevent propagation of the clot. In cases of severe ischemia of recent onset, particularly when limb viability is jeopardized, immediate intervention to ensure reperfusion is indicated. Catheter-directed thrombolysis/thrombectomy, surgical thromboembolectomy, and arterial bypass procedures are used to restore blood flow to the ischemic extremity promptly, particularly when a large proximal vessel is occluded.

Intraarterial thrombolytic therapy with recombinant tissue plasminogen activator, reteplase, or tenecteplase is most effective when acute arterial occlusion is recent (<2 weeks) and caused by a thrombus in an atherosclerotic vessel, arterial bypass graft, or occluded stent. Thrombolytic therapy is also indicated when the patient's overall condition contraindicates surgical intervention or when smaller distal vessels are occluded, thus preventing surgical access. Meticulous observation for hemorrhagic complications is required during intraarterial thrombolytic therapy. Another endovascular approach to thrombus removal is percutaneous mechanical thrombectomy using devices that employ hydrodynamic forces or rotating baskets to fragment and remove the clot. These treatments may be used alone but usually are used in conjunction with pharmacologic thrombolysis. Surgical revascularization is preferred when restoration of blood flow must occur within 24 h to prevent limb loss or when symptoms of occlusion have been present for more than 2 weeks. Amputation is performed when the limb is not viable, as characterized by loss of sensation, paralysis, and the absence of Doppler-detected blood flow in both arteries and veins.

If the limb is not in jeopardy, a more conservative approach that includes observation and administration of anticoagulants may be taken. Anticoagulation prevents recurrent embolism and reduces the likelihood of thrombus propagation; it can be initiated with intravenous heparin and followed by oral warfarin. Recommended doses are the same as those used for deep vein thrombosis (Chap. 300). Emboli resulting from infective endocarditis, the presence of prosthetic heart valves, or atrial myxoma often require surgical intervention to remove the cause.

ATHEROEMBOLISM

Atheroembolism is another cause of limb ischemia. In this condition, multiple small deposits of fibrin, platelets, and cholesterol debris embolize from proximal atherosclerotic lesions or aneurysmal sites. Large protruding aortic atheromas are a source of emboli that may lead to limb ischemia, as well as stroke and renal insufficiency. Atheroembolism may occur after intraarterial procedures. Since atheroemboli to limbs tend to lodge in the small vessels of the muscle and skin and may not occlude the large vessels, distal pulses usually remain palpable. Patients complain of acute pain and tenderness at the site of embolization. Digital vascular occlusion may result in ischemia and the "blue toe" syndrome; digital necrosis and gangrene may develop (Fig. 302-2). Localized areas of tenderness, pallor, and livedo reticularis (see below) occur at sites of emboli. Skin or muscle biopsy may demonstrate cholesterol crystals.

Ischemia resulting from atheroemboli is notoriously difficult to treat. Usually neither surgical revascularization procedures nor thrombolytic therapy is helpful because of the multiplicity, composition, and distal location of the emboli. There is limited evidence that antithrombotic therapy with platelet inhibitors or anticoagulants prevents atheroembolism. Statins may stabilize plaque and potentially reduce the risk of atheroembolism. Surgical intervention to remove or bypass the atherosclerotic vessel or aneurysm that causes the recurrent atheroemboli may be necessary.

THORACIC OUTLET COMPRESSION SYNDROME

This is a symptom complex resulting from compression of the neurovascular bundle (artery, vein, or nerves) at the thoracic outlet as it courses through the neck and shoulder. Cervical ribs, abnormalities of

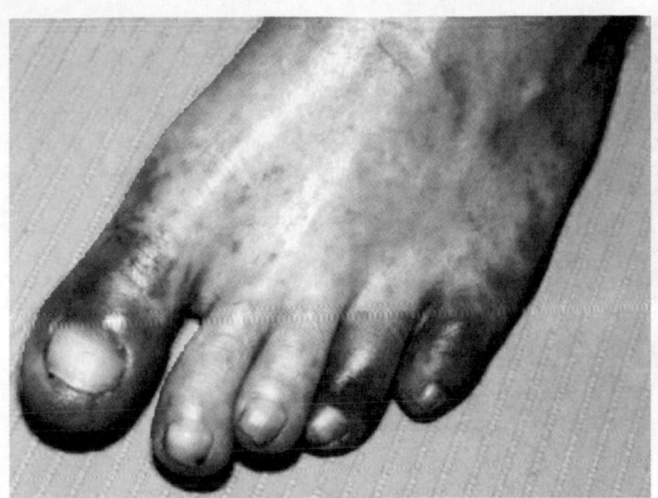

FIGURE 302-2 Atheroembolism causing cyanotic discoloration and impending necrosis of the toes ("blue toe" syndrome).

the scalenus anticus muscle, proximity of the clavicle to the first rib, or abnormal insertion of the pectoralis minor muscle may compress the subclavian artery, subclavian vein, and brachial plexus as these structures pass from the thorax to the arm. Depending on the structures affected, thoracic outlet compression syndrome is divided into arterial, venous, and neurogenic forms. Patients with neurogenic thoracic outlet compression may develop shoulder and arm pain, weakness, and paresthesias. Patients with arterial compression may experience claudication, Raynaud's phenomenon, and even ischemic tissue loss and gangrene. Venous compression may cause thrombosis of the subclavian and axillary veins; this is often associated with effort and is referred to as *Paget-Schroetter syndrome.*

APPROACH TO THE PATIENT
Thoracic Outlet Compression Syndrome

Examination of a patient with arterial thoracic outlet compression syndrome is often normal unless provocative maneuvers are performed. Occasionally, distal pulses are decreased or absent and digital cyanosis and ischemia may be evident.

Several maneuvers that support the diagnosis of arterial thoracic outlet compression syndrome may be used to precipitate symptoms, cause a subclavian artery bruit, and diminish arm pulses. These maneuvers include the abduction and external rotation test, in which the affected arm is abducted by 90° and the shoulder is externally rotated; the scalene maneuver (extension of the neck and rotation of the head to the side of the symptoms); the costoclavicular maneuver (posterior rotation of shoulders); and the hyperabduction maneuver (raising the arm 180°). A chest x-ray will indicate the presence of cervical ribs. Duplex ultrasonography, MRA, and contrast angiography can be performed during provocative maneuvers to demonstrate thoracic outlet compression of the subclavian artery. Neurophysiologic tests such as the electromyogram, nerve conduction studies, and somatosensory evoked potentials may be abnormal if the brachial plexus is involved, but the diagnosis of neurogenic thoracic outlet syndrome is not necessarily excluded if these tests are normal owing to their low sensitivity.

Most patients can be managed conservatively. They should be advised to avoid the positions that cause symptoms. Many patients benefit from shoulder girdle exercises. Surgical procedures such as removal of the first rib and resection of the scalenus anticus muscle are necessary occasionally for relief of symptoms or treatment of ischemia.

POPLITEAL ARTERY ENTRAPMENT

Popliteal artery entrapment typically affects young athletic men and women when the gastrocnemius or popliteus muscle compresses the popliteal artery and causes intermittent claudication. Thrombosis, embolism, or popliteal artery aneurysm may occur. The pulse examination may be normal unless provocative maneuvers such as ankle dorsiflexion and plantar flexion are performed. The diagnosis is confirmed by duplex ultrasound, CTA, MRA, or conventional angiography. Treatment involves surgical release of the popliteal artery or vascular reconstruction.

POPLITEAL ARTERY ANEURYSM

Popliteal artery aneurysms are the most common peripheral artery aneurysms. Approximately 50% are bilateral. Patients with popliteal artery aneurysms often have aneurysms of other arteries, especially the aorta. The most common clinical presentation is limb ischemia secondary to thrombosis or embolism. Rupture occurs less frequently. Other complications include compression of the adjacent popliteal vein or peroneal nerve. Popliteal artery aneurysm can be detected by palpation and confirmed by duplex ultrasonography. Repair is indicated for symptomatic aneurysms or when the diameter exceeds 2–3 cm, owing to the risk of thrombosis, embolism, or rupture.

ARTERIOVENOUS FISTULA

Abnormal communications between an artery and a vein, bypassing the capillary bed, may be congenital or acquired. Congenital arteriovenous fistulas are a result of persistent embryonic vessels that fail to differentiate into arteries and veins; they may be associated with birthmarks, can be located in almost any organ of the body, and frequently occur in the extremities. Acquired arteriovenous fistulas either are created to provide vascular access for hemodialysis or occur as a result of a penetrating injury such as a gunshot or knife wound or as complications of arterial catheterization or surgical dissection. An uncommon cause of arteriovenous fistula is rupture of an arterial aneurysm into a vein.

The clinical features depend on the location and size of the fistula. Frequently, a pulsatile mass is palpable, and a thrill and a bruit lasting throughout systole and diastole are present over the fistula. With long-standing fistulas, clinical manifestations of chronic venous insufficiency, including peripheral edema; large, tortuous varicose veins; and stasis pigmentation become apparent because of the high venous pressure. Evidence of ischemia may occur in the distal portion of the extremity. Skin temperature is higher over the arteriovenous fistula. Large arteriovenous fistulas may result in an increased cardiac output with consequent cardiomegaly and high output heart failure (Chap. 279).

The diagnosis is often evident from the physical examination. Compression of a large arteriovenous fistula may cause reflex slowing of the heart rate (Nicoladoni-Branham sign). Duplex ultrasonography may detect an arteriovenous fistula, especially one that affects the femoral artery and vein at the site of catheter access. CTA and conventional angiography can confirm the diagnosis and are useful in demonstrating the site and size of the arteriovenous fistula.

Management of arteriovenous fistulas may involve surgery, radiotherapy, or embolization. Congenital arteriovenous fistulas are often difficult to treat because the communications may be numerous and extensive, and new communications frequently develop after ligation of the most obvious ones. Many of these lesions are best treated conservatively using elastic support hose to reduce the consequences of venous hypertension. Occasionally, embolization with autologous material, such as fat or muscle, or with hemostatic agents, such as gelatin sponges or silicon spheres, is used to obliterate the fistula. Acquired arteriovenous fistulas are usually amenable to surgical treatment that involves division or excision of the fistula. Occasionally, autogenous or synthetic grafting is necessary to reestablish continuity of the artery and vein.

RAYNAUD'S PHENOMENON

Raynaud's phenomenon is characterized by episodic digital ischemia, manifested clinically by the sequential development of digital blanching, cyanosis, and rubor of the fingers or toes after cold exposure

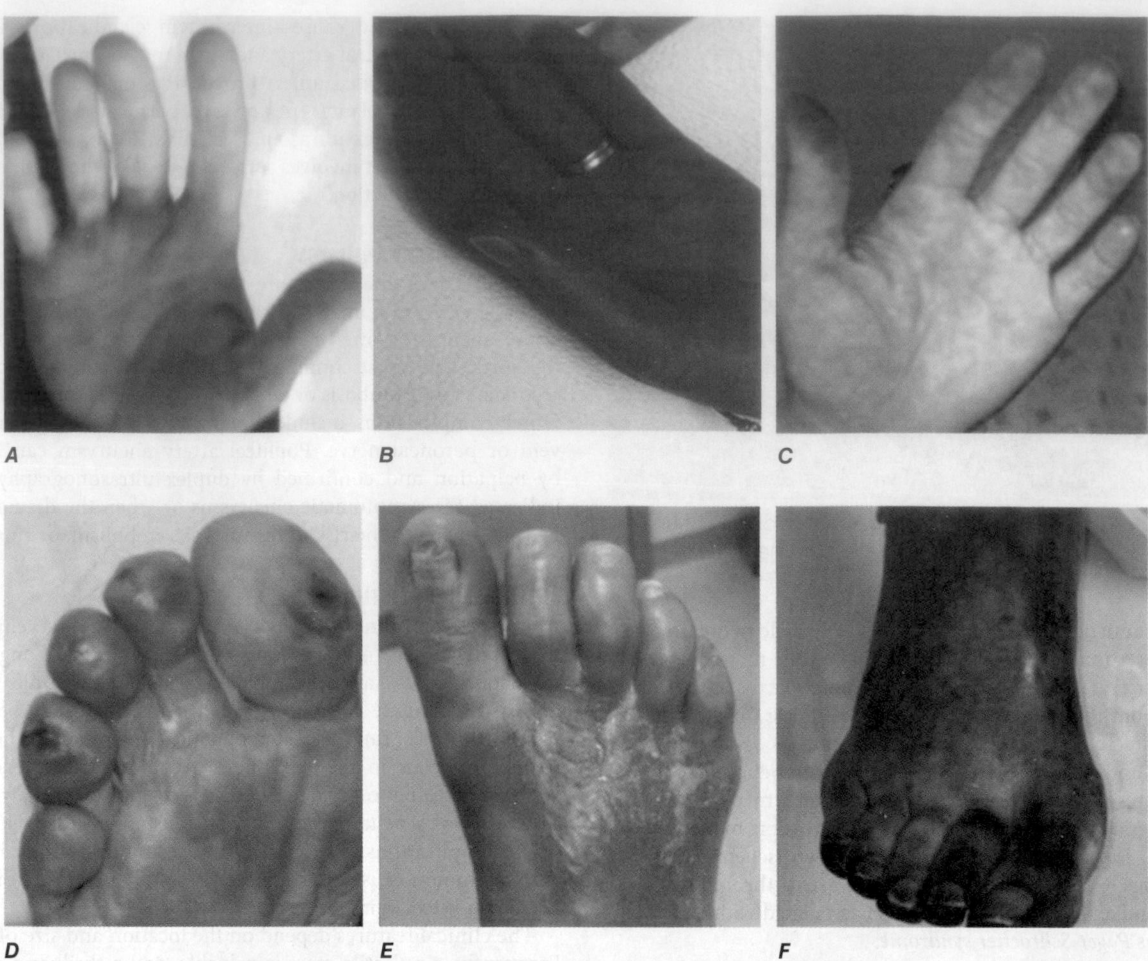

FIGURE 302-3 Vascular diseases associated with temperature: (*A*) Raynaud's phenomenon; (*B*) acrocyanosis; (*C*) livedo reticularis; (*D*) pernio; (*E*) erythromelalgia; and (*F*) frostbite.

and subsequent rewarming. Emotional stress may also precipitate Raynaud's phenomenon. The color changes are usually well demarcated and are confined to the fingers or toes. Typically, one or more digits will appear white when the patient is exposed to a cold environment or touches a cold object (Fig. 302-3*A*). The blanching, or pallor, represents the ischemic phase of the phenomenon and results from vasospasm of digital arteries. During the ischemic phase, capillaries and venules dilate, and cyanosis results from the deoxygenated blood that is present in these vessels. A sensation of cold or numbness or paresthesia of the digits often accompanies the phases of pallor and cyanosis.

With rewarming, the digital vasospasm resolves, and blood flow into the dilated arterioles and capillaries increases dramatically. This "reactive hyperemia" imparts a bright red color to the digits. In addition to rubor and warmth, patients often experience a throbbing, painful sensation during the hyperemic phase. Although the triphasic color response is typical of Raynaud's phenomenon, some patients may develop only pallor and cyanosis; others may experience only cyanosis.

Raynaud's phenomenon is broadly separated into two categories: idiopathic, termed primary Raynaud's phenomenon, and secondary Raynaud's phenomenon, which is associated with other disease states or known causes of vasospasm (Table 302-1).

Primary Raynaud's Phenomenon This appellation is applied when the secondary causes of Raynaud's phenomenon have been excluded. Over 50% of patients with Raynaud's phenomenon have the primary form. Women are affected about five times more often than men, and the age of presentation is usually between 20 and 40 years. The fingers are involved more frequently than the toes. Initial episodes may involve only one or two fingertips, but subsequent attacks may involve the entire finger and may include all the fingers. The toes are affected in 40% of patients. Although vasospasm of the toes usually occurs in patients with symptoms in the fingers, it may happen alone. Rarely, the earlobes, the tip of the nose, and the penis are involved. Raynaud's phenomenon occurs frequently in patients who also have migraine headaches or variant angina. These associations suggest that there may be a common predisposing cause for the vasospasm.

Results of physical examination are often entirely normal; the radial, ulnar, and pedal pulses are normal. The fingers and toes may

TABLE 302-1 CLASSIFICATION OF RAYNAUD'S PHENOMENON

Primary or idiopathic Raynaud's phenomenon
Secondary Raynaud's phenomenon
Collagen vascular diseases: scleroderma, systemic lupus erythematosus, rheumatoid arthritis, dermatomyositis, polymyositis, mixed connective tissue disease, Sjögren's syndrome
Arterial occlusive diseases: atherosclerosis of the extremities, thromboangiitis obliterans, acute arterial occlusion, thoracic outlet syndrome
Pulmonary hypertension
Neurologic disorders: intervertebral disk disease, syringomyelia, spinal cord tumors, stroke, poliomyelitis, carpal tunnel syndrome, complex regional pain syndrome
Blood dyscrasias: cold agglutinins, cryoglobulinemia, cryofibrinogenemia, myeloproliferative disorders, lymphoplasmacytic lymphoma
Trauma: vibration injury, hammer hand syndrome, electric shock, cold injury, typing, piano playing
Drugs and toxins: ergot derivatives, methysergide, β-adrenergic receptor blockers, bleomycin, vinblastine, cisplatin, gemcitabine, vinyl chloride

be cool between attacks and may perspire excessively. Thickening and tightening of the digital subcutaneous tissue (*sclerodactyly*) develop in 10% of patients. Angiography of the digits for diagnostic purposes is not indicated.

In general, patients with primary Raynaud's disease have milder clinical manifestations. Fewer than 1% of these patients lose a part of a digit. After the diagnosis is made, the disease improves spontaneously in approximately 15% of patients and progresses in about 30%.

Secondary Causes of Raynaud's Phenomenon Raynaud's phenomenon occurs in 80–90% of patients with systemic sclerosis (scleroderma) and is the presenting symptom in 30% (Chap. 382). It may be the only symptom of scleroderma for many years. Abnormalities of the digital vessels may contribute to the development of Raynaud's phenomenon in this disorder. Ischemic fingertip ulcers may develop and progress to gangrene and autoamputation. About 20% of patients with systemic lupus erythematosus (SLE) have Raynaud's phenomenon (Chap. 378). Occasionally, persistent digital ischemia develops and may result in ulcers or gangrene. In most severe cases, the small vessels are occluded by a proliferative endarteritis. Raynaud's phenomenon occurs in about 30% of patients with dermatomyositis or polymyositis (Chap. 388). It frequently develops in patients with rheumatoid arthritis and may be related to the intimal proliferation that occurs in the digital arteries.

Atherosclerosis of the extremities is a common cause of Raynaud's phenomenon in men >50 years. Thromboangiitis obliterans is an uncommon cause of Raynaud's phenomenon but should be considered in young men, particularly those who are cigarette smokers. The development of cold-induced pallor in these disorders may be confined to one or two digits of the involved extremity. Occasionally, Raynaud's phenomenon may follow acute occlusion of large and medium-size arteries by a thrombus or embolus. Embolization of atheroembolic debris may cause digital ischemia. The latter situation often involves one or two digits and should not be confused with Raynaud's phenomenon. In patients with thoracic outlet compression syndrome, Raynaud's phenomenon may result from diminished intravascular pressure, stimulation of sympathetic fibers in the brachial plexus, or a combination of both. Raynaud's phenomenon occurs in patients with primary pulmonary hypertension (Chap. 304); this is more than coincidental and may reflect a neurohumoral abnormality that affects both the pulmonary and digital circulations.

A variety of blood dyscrasias may be associated with Raynaud's phenomenon. Cold-induced precipitation of plasma proteins, hyperviscosity, and aggregation of red cells and platelets may occur in patients with cold agglutinins, cryoglobulinemia, or cryofibrinogenemia. Hyperviscosity syndromes that accompany myeloproliferative disorders and lymphoplasmacytic lymphoma (Waldenström's macroglobulinemia) should also be considered in the initial evaluation of patients with Raynaud's phenomenon.

Raynaud's phenomenon occurs often in patients whose vocations require the use of vibrating hand tools, such as chain saws or jackhammers. The frequency of Raynaud's phenomenon also seems to be increased in pianists and keyboard operators. Electric shock injury to the hands or frostbite may lead to the later development of Raynaud's phenomenon.

Several drugs have been causally implicated in Raynaud's phenomenon. They include ergot preparations, methysergide, β-adrenergic receptor antagonists, and the chemotherapeutic agents bleomycin, vinblastine, cisplatin, and gemcitabine.

TREATMENT RAYNAUD'S PHENOMENON

Most patients with Raynaud's phenomenon experience only mild and infrequent episodes. These patients need reassurance and should be instructed to dress warmly and avoid unnecessary cold exposure. In addition to gloves and mittens, patients should protect the trunk, head, and feet with warm clothing to prevent cold-induced reflex vasoconstriction. Tobacco use is contraindicated.

Drug treatment should be reserved for severe cases. Dihydropyridine calcium channel antagonists such as nifedipine, isradipine, felodipine, and amlodipine decrease the frequency and severity of Raynaud's phenomenon. Diltiazem may be considered but is less effective. The postsynaptic α_1-adrenergic antagonist prazosin has been used with favorable responses; doxazosin and terazosin may also be effective. Phosphodiesterase type 5 inhibitors such as sildenafil and tadalafil may improve symptoms in patients with secondary Raynaud's phenomenon, as occurs with systemic sclerosis. Digital sympathectomy is helpful in some patients who are unresponsive to medical therapy.

ACROCYANOSIS

In this condition, there is arterial vasoconstriction and secondary dilation of the capillaries and venules with resulting persistent cyanosis of the hands and, less frequently, the feet. Cyanosis may be intensified by exposure to a cold environment. Acrocyanosis may be categorized as primary or secondary to an underlying condition. In primary acrocyanosis, women are affected much more frequently than men, and the age of onset is usually <30 years. Generally, patients are asymptomatic but seek medical attention because of the discoloration. The prognosis is favorable, and pain, ulcers, and gangrene do not occur. Examination reveals normal pulses, peripheral cyanosis, and moist palms (Fig. 302-3*B*). Trophic skin changes and ulcerations do *not* occur. The disorder can be distinguished from Raynaud's phenomenon because it is persistent and not episodic, the discoloration extends proximally from the digits, and blanching does not occur. Ischemia secondary to arterial occlusive disease can usually be excluded by the presence of normal pulses. Central cyanosis and decreased arterial oxygen saturation are not present. Patients should be reassured and advised to dress warmly and avoid cold exposure. Pharmacologic intervention is not indicated.

Secondary acrocyanosis may result from hypoxemia, vasopressor medications, connective tissue diseases, atheroembolism, antiphospholipid antibodies, cold agglutinins, or cryoglobulins and is associated with anorexia nervosa and postural orthostatic tachycardia syndrome. Treatment should be directed at the underlying disorder.

LIVEDO RETICULARIS

In this condition, localized areas of the extremities develop a mottled or rete (netlike) appearance of reddish to blue discoloration (Fig. 302-3*C*). The mottled appearance may be more prominent after cold exposure. There are primary and secondary forms of livedo reticularis. The primary, or idiopathic, form of this disorder may be benign or associated with ulcerations. The benign form occurs more frequently in women than in men, and the most common age of onset is the third decade. Patients with the benign form are usually asymptomatic and seek attention for cosmetic reasons. These patients should be reassured and advised to avoid cold environments. No drug treatment is indicated. Primary livedo reticularis with ulceration is also called *atrophie blanche en plaque*. The ulcers are painful and may take months to heal. Secondary livedo reticularis can occur with atheroembolism (see above), SLE and other vasculitides, anticardiolipin antibodies, hyperviscosity, cryoglobulinemia, and Sneddon's syndrome (ischemic stroke and livedo reticularis). Rarely, skin ulcerations develop.

PERNIO (CHILBLAINS)

Pernio is a vasculitic disorder associated with exposure to cold; acute forms have been described. Raised erythematous lesions develop on the lower part of the legs and feet in cold weather (Fig. 302-3*D*). They are associated with pruritus and a burning sensation, and they may blister and ulcerate. Pathologic examination demonstrates angiitis characterized by intimal proliferation and perivascular infiltration of mononuclear and polymorphonuclear leukocytes. Giant cells may be present in the subcutaneous tissue. Patients should avoid exposure to cold, and ulcers should be kept clean and protected with sterile dressings. Sympatholytic drugs and dihydropyridine calcium channel antagonists may be effective in some patients.

ERYTHROMELALGIA

This disorder is characterized by burning pain and erythema of the extremities (Fig. 302-3*E*). The feet are involved more frequently than the hands, and males are affected more frequently than females. Erythromelalgia may occur at any age but is most common in middle age. It may be primary (also termed erythermalgia) or secondary. Mutations in the *SCN9A* gene, which encodes the Nav1.7 voltage-gated sodium channel expressed in sensory and sympathetic nerves, has been described in inherited forms of erythromelalgia. The most common causes of secondary erythromelalgia are myeloproliferative disorders such as polycythemia vera and essential thrombocytosis. Less common causes include drugs, such as calcium channel blockers, bromocriptine, and pergolide; neuropathies; connective tissue diseases such as SLE; and paraneoplastic syndromes. Patients complain of burning in the extremities that is precipitated by exposure to a warm environment and aggravated by a dependent position. The symptoms are relieved by exposing the affected area to cool air or water or by elevation. Erythromelalgia can be distinguished from ischemia secondary to peripheral arterial disorders because the peripheral pulses are present. There is no specific treatment; aspirin may produce relief in patients with erythromelalgia secondary to myeloproliferative disease. Treatment of associated disorders in secondary erythromelalgia may be helpful.

FROSTBITE

In this condition, tissue damage results from severe environmental cold exposure or from direct contact with a very cold object. Tissue injury results from both freezing and vasoconstriction. Frostbite usually affects the distal aspects of the extremities or exposed parts of the face, such as the ears, nose, chin, and cheeks. Superficial frostbite involves the skin and subcutaneous tissue. Patients experience pain or paresthesia, and the skin appears white and waxy. After rewarming, there is cyanosis and erythema, wheal-and-flare formation, edema, and superficial blisters. Deep frostbite involves muscle, nerves, and deeper blood vessels. It may result in edema of the hand or foot, vesicles and bullae, tissue necrosis, and gangrene (Fig. 302-3*F*).

Initial treatment is rewarming, performed in an environment where reexposure to freezing conditions will not occur. Rewarming is accomplished by immersion of the affected part in a water bath at temperatures of 40°–44°C (104°–111°F). Massage, application of ice water, and extreme heat are contraindicated. The injured area should be cleansed with soap or antiseptic, and sterile dressings should be applied. Analgesics are often required during rewarming. Antibiotics are used if there is evidence of infection. The efficacy of sympathetic blocking drugs is not established. After recovery, the affected extremity may exhibit increased sensitivity to cold.

303 Chronic Venous Disease and Lymphedema

Mark A. Creager, Joseph Loscalzo

CHRONIC VENOUS DISEASE

Chronic venous diseases range from telangiectasias and reticular veins, to varicose veins, to chronic venous insufficiency with edema, skin changes, and ulceration. This section of the chapter will focus on identification and treatment of varicose veins and chronic venous insufficiency, since these problems are encountered frequently by the internist. The estimated prevalence of varicose veins in the United States is approximately 15% in men and 30% in women. Chronic venous insufficiency with edema affects approximately 7.5% of men and 5% of women, and the prevalence increases with age ranging from 2% among those less than 50 years of age to 10% of those 70 years of age. Approximately 20% of patients with chronic venous insufficiency develop venous ulcers.

VENOUS ANATOMY

Veins in the extremities can be broadly classified as either superficial or deep. The superficial veins are located between the skin and deep fascia. In the legs, these include the great and small saphenous veins and their tributaries. The great saphenous vein is the longest vein in the body. It originates on the medial side of the foot and ascends anterior to the medial malleolus and then along the medial side of the calf and thigh, and drains into the common femoral vein. The small saphenous vein originates on the dorsolateral aspect of the foot, ascends posterior to the lateral malleolus and along the posterolateral aspect of the calf, and drains into the popliteal vein. The deep veins of the leg accompany the major arteries. There are usually paired peroneal, anterior tibial, and posterior tibial veins in the calf, which converge to form the popliteal vein. Soleal tributary veins drain into the posterior tibial or peroneal veins, and gastrocnemius tributary veins drain into the popliteal vein. The popliteal vein ascends in the thigh as the femoral vein. The confluence of the femoral vein and deep femoral vein form the common femoral vein, which ascends in the pelvis as the external iliac and then common iliac vein, which converges with the contralateral common iliac vein at the inferior vena cava. Perforating veins connect the superficial and deep systems in the legs at multiple locations, normally allowing blood to flow from the superficial to deep veins. In the arms, the superficial veins include the basilic, cephalic, and median cubital veins and their tributaries. The basilic and cephalic veins course along the medial and lateral aspects of the arm, respectively, and these are connected via the median cubital vein in the antecubital fossa. The deep veins of the arms accompany the major arteries and include the radial, ulnar, brachial, axillary, and subclavian veins. The subclavian vein converges with the internal jugular vein to form the brachiocephalic vein, which joins the contralateral brachiocephalic vein to form the superior vena cava. Bicuspid valves are present throughout the venous system to direct the flow of venous blood centrally.

Pathophysiology of Chronic Venous Disease *Varicose veins* are dilated, bulging, tortuous superficial veins, measuring at least 3 mm in diameter. The smaller and less tortuous reticular veins are dilated intradermal veins, which appear blue-green, measure 1 to 3 mm in diameter, and do not protrude from the skin surface. Telangiectasias, or spider veins, are small, dilated veins, less than 1 mm in diameter, located near the skin surface, and form blue, purple, or red linear, branching, or spider-web patterns.

Varicose veins can be categorized as primary or secondary. Primary varicose veins originate in the superficial system and result from defective structure and function of the valves of the saphenous veins, intrinsic weakness of the vein wall, and high intraluminal pressure. Approximately one-half of these patients have a family history of varicose veins. Other factors associated with primary varicose veins include aging, pregnancy, hormonal therapy, obesity, and prolonged standing. Secondary varicose veins result from venous hypertension, associated with deep venous insufficiency or deep venous obstruction, and incompetent perforating veins that cause enlargement of superficial veins. Arteriovenous fistulas also cause varicose veins in the affected limb.

Chronic venous insufficiency is a consequence of incompetent veins in which there is venous hypertension and extravasation of fluid and blood elements into the tissue of the limb. It may occur in patients with varicose veins but usually is caused by disease in the deep veins. It also is categorized as primary or secondary. Primary deep venous insufficiency is a consequence of an intrinsic structural or functional abnormality in the vein wall or venous valves leading to valvular reflux. Secondary deep venous insufficiency is caused by obstruction and/or valvular incompetence from previous deep vein thrombosis (Chap. 300). Deep venous insufficiency occurs following deep vein thrombosis, as the delicate valve leaflets become thickened and contracted and can no longer prevent retrograde flow of blood and the vein itself becomes rigid and thick walled. Although most veins recanalize after an episode of thrombosis, the large proximal veins may remain occluded. Secondary incompetence develops in distal valves because high pressures distend the vein and separate the leaflets. Other causes of secondary deep venous insufficiency include May-Thurner syndrome, where the left iliac vein is occluded or stenosed by extrinsic compression from the overlapping right common iliac artery; arteriovenous fistulas resulting in increased venous pressure; congenital deep vein agenesis or hypoplasia; and venous malformations as may occur in Klippel-Trénaunay-Weber and Parkes-Weber syndromes.

Clinical Presentation Patients with venous varicosities are often asymptomatic but still concerned about the cosmetic appearance of their legs. Superficial venous thrombosis may be a recurring problem, and, rarely, a varicosity ruptures and bleeds. Symptoms in patients with varicose veins or venous insufficiency, when they occur, include a dull ache, throbbing or heaviness, or pressure sensation in the legs typically after prolonged standing; these symptoms usually are relieved with leg elevation. Additional symptoms may include cramping, burning, pruritus, leg swelling, and skin ulceration.

The legs are examined in both the supine and standing positions. Visual inspection and palpation of the legs in the standing position confirm the presence of varicose veins. The location and extent of the varicose veins should be noted. Edema, stasis dermatitis, and skin ulceration near the ankle may be present if there is superficial venous insufficiency and venous hypertension. Findings of deep venous insufficiency include increased leg circumference, venous varicosities, edema, and skin changes. The edema, which is usually pitting, may be confined to the ankles, extend above the ankles to the knees, or involve the thighs in severe cases. Over time, the edema may become less pitting and more indurated. Dermatologic findings associated with venous stasis include hyperpigmentation, erythema, eczema, lipodermatosclerosis, *atrophie blanche,* and a phlebectasia corona. Lipodermatosclerosis is the combination of induration, hemosiderin deposition, and inflammation, and typically occurs in the lower part of the leg just above the ankle. Atrophie blanche is a white patch of scar tissue, often with focal telangiectasias and a hyperpigmented border; it usually develops near the medial malleolus. A phlebectasia corona is a fan-shaped pattern of intradermal veins near the ankle or on the foot. Skin ulceration may occur near the medial and lateral malleoli. A venous ulcer is often shallow and characterized by an irregular border, a base of granulation tissue, and the presence of exudate (Fig. 303-1).

Bedside maneuvers can be used to distinguish primary varicose veins from secondary varicose veins caused by deep venous insufficiency. With the contemporary use of venous ultrasound (see below), however, these maneuvers are employed infrequently. The Brodie-Trendelenburg test is used to determine whether varicose veins are secondary to deep venous insufficiency. As the patient is lying supine, the leg is elevated and the veins allowed to empty. Then, a tourniquet is placed on the proximal part of the thigh and the patient is asked to stand. Filling of the varicose veins within 30 s indicates that the varicose veins are caused by deep venous insufficiency and incompetent perforating veins. Primary varicose veins with superficial venous insufficiency are the likely diagnosis if venous refilling occurs promptly after tourniquet removal. The Perthes test assesses the possibility of deep venous obstruction. A tourniquet is placed on the midthigh after the patient has stood, and the varicose veins are filled. The patient is then instructed to walk for 5 min. A patent deep venous system and competent perforating veins enable the superficial veins below the tourniquet to collapse. Deep venous obstruction is likely to be present if the superficial veins distend further with walking.

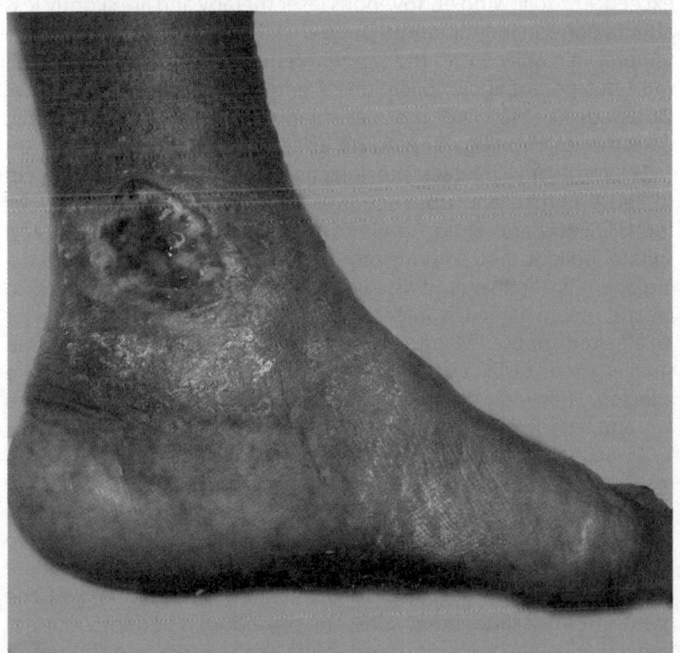

FIGURE 303-1 Venous insufficiency with active venous ulcer near the medial malleolus. *(Courtesy of Dr. Steven Dean, with permission.)*

Differential Diagnosis The duration of leg edema helps to distinguish chronic venous insufficiency from acute deep vein thrombosis. Lymphedema, as discussed later in this chapter, is often confused with chronic venous insufficiency, and both may occur together. Other disorders that cause leg swelling should be considered and excluded when evaluating a patient with presumed venous insufficiency. Bilateral leg swelling occurs in patients with congestive heart failure, hypoalbuminemia secondary to nephrotic syndrome or severe hepatic disease, myxedema caused by hypothyroidism or pretibial myxedema associated with Graves' disease, and with drugs such as dihydropyridine calcium channel blockers and thiazolidinediones. Unilateral causes of leg swelling also include ruptured leg muscles, hematomas secondary to trauma, and popliteal cysts. Cellulitis may cause erythema and swelling of the affected limb. Leg ulcers may be caused by severe peripheral artery disease and critical limb ischemia; neuropathies, particularly those associated with diabetes; and less commonly, skin cancer, vasculitis, or rarely as a complication of hydroxyurea. The location and characteristics of venous ulcers help to differentiate these from other causes.

Classification of Chronic Venous Disease The CEAP (clinical, etiologic, anatomic, pathophysiologic) classification schema incorporates the range of symptoms and signs of chronic venous disease to characterize its severity. It also broadly categorizes the etiology as congenital, primary, or secondary; identifies the affected veins as superficial, deep, or perforating; and characterizes the pathophysiology as reflux, obstruction, both, or neither (Table 303-1).

Diagnostic Testing The principal diagnostic test to evaluate patients with chronic venous disease is venous duplex ultrasonography. A venous duplex ultrasound examination uses a combination of B-mode imaging and spectral Doppler to detect the presence of venous obstruction and venous reflux in superficial and deep veins. Color-assisted Doppler ultrasound is useful to visualize venous flow patterns. Obstruction may be diagnosed by absence of flow, the presence of an echogenic thrombus within the vein, or failure of the vein to collapse when a compression maneuver is applied by the sonographer, the last implicating the presence of an intraluminal thrombus. Venous reflux is detected by prolonged reversal of venous flow direction during a Valsalva maneuver, particularly for the common femoral vein or saphenofemoral junction, or after compression and release of a cuff placed on the limb distal to the area being interrogated.

Some vascular laboratories use air or strange gauge plethysmography to assess the severity of venous reflux and complement findings from the venous ultrasound examination. Venous volume and venous refilling time are measured when the legs are placed in a dependent position and after calf exercise to quantify the severity of venous reflux and the efficiency of the calf muscle pump to affect venous return.

Magnetic resonance, computed tomographic, and conventional venography are rarely required to determine the cause and plan treatment for chronic venous insufficiency unless there is suspicion for pathology that might warrant intervention. These modalities are used to identify obstruction or stenosis of the inferior vena cava and iliofemoral veins, as may occur in patients with previous proximal

TABLE 303-1 CEAP (CLINICAL, ETIOLOGIC, ANATOMIC, PATHOPHYSIOLOGIC) CLASSIFICATION

Clinical Classification
C0 No visible or palpable signs of venous disease
C1 Telangiectasias, reticular veins
C2 Varicose veins
C3 Edema without skin changes
C4 Skin changes, including pigmentation, eczema, lipodermatosclerosis, and atrophie blanche
C5 Healed venous ulcer
C6 Active venous ulcer
Etiologic Classification
Ec Congenital
Ep Primary
Es Secondary (postthrombotic)
En No venous etiology identified
Anatomic Classification
As Superficial veins
Ap Perforator veins
Ad Deep veins
An No venous location identified
Pathophysiologic Classification
Pr Reflux
Po Obstruction
Pr,o Reflux and obstruction
Pn No venous pathophysiology identifiable

Source: B Eklöf et al: J Vasc Surg 40:1248, 2004.

deep vein thrombosis; occlusion of inferior vena cava filters; extrinsic compression from tumors; and May-Thurner syndrome.

TREATMENT CHRONIC VENOUS DISEASE

SUPPORTIVE MEASURES

Varicose veins usually are treated with conservative measures. Symptoms often decrease when the legs are elevated periodically, prolonged standing is avoided, and elastic support hose are worn. External compression with elastic stockings or stretch bandages provides a counterbalance to the hydrostatic pressure in the veins. Although compression garments may improve symptoms, they do not prevent progression of varicose veins. Graduated compression stockings with pressures of 20–30 mmHg are suitable for most patients with simple varicose veins, although pressures of 30–40 mmHg may be required for patients with manifestations of venous insufficiency such as edema and ulcers.

Patients with chronic venous insufficiency also should be advised to avoid prolonged standing or sitting; frequent leg elevation is helpful. Graded compression therapy consisting of stockings or multilayered compression bandages is the standard of care for advanced chronic venous insufficiency characterized by edema, skin changes, or venous ulcers defined as CEAP clinical class C3–C6. Graduated compression stockings of 30–40 mmHg are more effective than lesser grades for healing venous ulcers. The length of stocking depends on the distribution of edema. Calf-length stockings are tolerated better by most patients, particularly elderly patients; for patients with varicose veins or edema extending to the thigh, thigh-length stockings or panty hose should be considered. Overweight and obese patients should be advised to lose weight via caloric restriction and exercise.

In addition to a compression bandage or stocking, patients with venous ulcers also may be treated with low adherent absorbent dressings that take up exudates while maintaining a moist environment. Other types of dressings include hydrocolloid (an adhesive dressing comprised of polymers such as carboxymethylcellulose that absorbs exudates by forming a gel), hydrogel (a nonabsorbent dressing comprising over 80% water or glycerin that moisturizes wounds), foam (an absorbent dressing made with polymers such as polyurethane), and alginate (an absorbent, biodegradable dressing that is derived from seaweed), but there is little evidence that these are more effective than low adherent absorbent dressings. The choice of specific dressing depends on the amount of drainage, presence of infection, and integrity of the skin surrounding the ulcer. Antibiotics are not indicated unless the ulcer is infected. The multilayered compression bandage or graduated compression garment is then put over the dressing.

MEDICAL THERAPIES

There are no drugs approved by the U.S. Food and Drug Administration for the treatment of chronic venous insufficiency. Diuretics may reduce edema, but at the risk of volume depletion and compromise in renal function. Topical steroids may be used for a short period of time to treat inflammation associated with stasis dermatitis. Several herbal supplements, such as horse chestnut seed extract (aescin); flavonoids including diosmin, hesperidin, or the two combined as micronized purified flavonoid fraction; and French maritime pine bark extract, are touted to have venoconstrictive and anti-inflammatory properties. Although meta-analyses have suggested that aescin reduces edema, pruritus, and pain and that micronized purified flavonoid fraction in conjunction with compression therapy facilitates venous ulcer healing, there is insufficient evidence to recommend the general use of these substances in patients with chronic venous insufficiency.

INTERVENTIONAL AND SURGICAL THERAPIES

Ablative procedures, including endovenous thermal ablation, sclerotherapy, and surgery, are used to treat varicose veins in selected patients who have persistent symptoms, great saphenous vein incompetency, and complications of venous insufficiency including dermatitis, edema, and ulcers. Ablative therapy may also be indicated for cosmetic reasons.

Endovenous thermal ablation procedures of the saphenous veins include endovenous laser therapy and radiofrequency ablation. To ablate the great saphenous vein, a catheter is placed percutaneously and advanced from the level of the knee to just below the saphenofemoral junction via ultrasound guidance. Thermal energy is then delivered as the catheter is pulled back. The heat injures the endothelium and media and promotes thrombosis and fibrosis, resulting in venous occlusion. Average 1- and 5-year occlusion rates exceed 90% following endovenous laser therapy and are slightly less after radiofrequency ablation. Deep vein thrombosis of the common femoral vein adjacent to the saphenofemoral junction is an uncommon but potential complication of endovenous thermal ablation. Other adverse effects of thermal ablation procedures include pain, paresthesias, bruising, hematoma, and hyperpigmentation.

Sclerotherapy involves the injection of a chemical into a vein to cause fibrosis and obstruction. Sclerosing agents approved by the U.S. Food and Drug Administration include sodium tetradecyl sulfate, polidocanol, sodium morrhuate, and glycerin. The sclerosing agent is administered as a liquid or mixed with air or CO_2/O_2 to create a foam. It first is injected into the great saphenous vein or its affected tributaries, often with ultrasound guidance. Thereafter, smaller more distal veins and incompetent perforating veins are injected. Following completion of the procedure, elastic bandages are applied, or 30–40 mmHg compression stockings are worn for 1–2 weeks. Average 1- and 5-year occlusion rates are 81% and 74%, respectively, following sclerotherapy. Complications are uncommon and include deep vein thrombosis, hematomas, damage to adjacent saphenous or sural nerves, and infection. Anaphylaxis is a very rare but severe complication.

Surgical therapy usually involves ligation and stripping of the great and small saphenous veins. The procedure is performed under general anesthesia. Incisions are made at the groin and the upper calf. The great saphenous vein is ligated below the saphenofemoral junction, and a wire is inserted into the great saphenous vein and advanced distally. The proximal part of the great saphenous vein is secured to the wire and retrieved, i.e., stripped, via the calf incision. Stripping of the great saphenous vein below the knee and stripping of the small saphenous vein usually are not performed because of the respective risks of saphenous and sural nerve injury. Complications of great saphenous vein ligation and stripping include deep vein thrombosis, bleeding, hematoma, infection, and nerve injury. Recurrent varicose veins occur in up to 50% patients by 5 years, due to technical failures, deep venous insufficiency, and incompetent perforating veins.

Stab phlebectomy is another surgical treatment for of varicose veins. A small incision is made alongside the varicose vein, and it is avulsed by means of a forceps or hook. This procedure may be performed in conjunction with saphenous vein ligation and stripping or thermal ablation. Subfascial endoscopic perforator surgery (SEPS) uses endoscopy to identify and occlude incompetent perforating veins. It also may be performed along with other ablative procedures.

Endovascular interventions, surgical bypass, and reconstruction of the valves of the deep veins are performed when feasible to treat patients with advanced chronic venous insufficiency who have not responded to other therapies. Catheter-based interventions, usually involving placement of endovenous stents, may be considered to treat some patients with chronic occlusions of the iliac veins. Technical success rates exceed 85% in most series, and long-term patency is achieved in approximately 75% of these patients. Iliocaval bypass, femoroiliac venous bypass, and femorofemoral crossover venous bypass are procedures used occasionally to treat iliofemoral vein occlusion; saphenopopliteal vein bypass can be used to treat chronic femoropopliteal vein obstruction. Long-term patency rates for venous bypass procedures generally exceed 60% and are associated with improvement in symptoms. Surgical reconstruction of the valves of the deep veins and valve transfer procedures are used to treat valvular incompetence. Valvuloplasty involves tightening the valve by commissural apposition. With valve transfer procedures, a segment of vein with a competent valve, such as a brachial or axillary vein, or adjacent saphenous or deep femoral vein, is inserted as an interposition graft in the incompetent vein. Both valvuloplasty and vein transfer operations result in ulcer healing in the majority of patients, although success rates are somewhat better with valvuloplasty.

Lymphedema Lymphedema is a chronic condition caused by impaired transport of lymph and characterized by swelling of one or more limbs and occasionally the trunk and genitalia. Fluid accumulates in interstitial tissues when there is an imbalance between lymph production and lymph absorption, a process governed in large part by Starling forces. Deficiency, reflux, or obstruction of lymph vessels perturbs the ability of the lymphatic system to reabsorb proteins that had been filtered by blood vessels, and the tissue osmotic load promotes interstitial accumulation of water. Persistent lymphedema leads to inflammatory and immune responses characterized by infiltration of mononuclear cells, fibroblasts, and adipocytes, leading to adipose and collagen deposition in the skin and subcutaneous tissues.

Lymphatic Anatomy Lymphatic capillaries are blind-ended tubes formed by a single layer of endothelial cells. The absent or widely fenestrated basement membrane of lymphatic capillaries allows access to interstitial proteins and particles. Lymphatic capillaries merge to form microlymphatic precollector vessels, which contain few smooth muscle cells. The precollector vessels drain into collecting lymphatic vessels, which comprise endothelial cells, a basement membrane, smooth muscle, and bileaflet valves. The collecting lymphatic vessels in term merge to form larger lymphatic conduits. Analogous to venous anatomy, there are superficial and deep lymphatic vessels in the legs, which communicate at the popliteal and inguinal lymph nodes. Pelvic lymphatic vessels drain into the thoracic duct, which ascends from the abdomen to the thorax and connects with the left brachiocephalic vein. Lymph is propelled centrally by the phasic contractile activity of lymphatic smooth muscle and facilitated by the contractions of contiguous skeletal muscle. The presence of lymphatic valves ensures unidirectional flow.

Etiology Lymphedema may be categorized as primary or secondary (Table 303-2). The prevalence of primary lymphedema is approximately 1.15 per 100,000 persons less than 20 years of age. Females are affected more frequently than males. Primary lymphedema may be caused by agenesis, hypoplasia, hyperplasia, or obstruction of the lymphatic vessels. There are three clinical subtypes: congenital lymphedema, which appears shortly after birth; lymphedema praecox, which has its onset at the time of puberty; and lymphedema tarda, which usually begins after age 35. Familial forms of congenital lymphedema (Milroy's disease) and lymphedema praecox (Meige's disease) may be inherited in an autosomal dominant manner with variable penetrance; autosomal or sex-linked recessive forms are less common. Mutations in genes expressing vascular endothelial growth factor receptor 3 (VEGFR3), which is a determinant of lymphangiogenesis, have been described in patients with Milroy's disease. A mutation on chromosome 15q is associated with the cholestasis-lymphedema syndrome. A mutation in the *FOXC2* gene, which encodes a transcription factor

TABLE 303-2 CAUSES OF LYMPHEDEMA

Primary
Sporadic (no identified cause)
Genetic disorders
Milroy's disease
Meige's disease
Lymphedema-distichiasis syndrome
Cholestasis-lymphedema
Hypotrichosis-lymphedema-telangiectasia
Turner's syndrome
Klinefelter's syndrome
Trisomy 13, 18, or 21
Noonan's syndrome
Klippel-Trénaunay syndrome
Parkes-Weber syndrome
Hennekam's syndrome
Yellow nail syndrome
Intestinal lymphangiectasia syndrome
Lymphangiomyomatosis
Neurofibromatosis type 1
Secondary
Infection
Bacterial lymphangitis (*Streptococcus pyogenes, Staphylococcus aureus*)
Lymphogranuloma venereum (*Chlamydia trachomatis*)
Filariasis (*Wucheria bancrofti, Brugia malayi, B. timori*)
Tuberculosis
Neoplastic infiltration of lymph nodes
Lymphoma
Prostate
Others
Surgery or irradiation of axillary or inguinal lymph nodes for treatment of cancer
Iatrogenic
Lymphatic division (during peripheral bypass surgery, varicose vein surgery, or harvesting of saphenous veins)
Miscellaneous
Contact dermatitis
Rheumatoid arthritis
Pregnancy
Factitious

that interacts with a signaling pathway involved in the development of lymphatic vessels, has been reported in patients with the lymphedema-distichiasis syndrome, in which lymphedema praecox occurs in patients who also have a double row of eyelashes. A mutation of *SOX18*, a transcription factor upstream of lymphatic endothelial cell differentiation, has been described in patients with lymphedema, alopecia, and telangiectasias (hypotrichosis, lymphedema, telangiectasia syndrome). Patients with a chromosomal aneuploidy, such as Turner's syndrome, Klinefelter's syndrome, or trisomy 18, 13, or 21, may develop lymphedema. Syndromic vascular anomalies associated with lymphedema include Klippel-Trénaunay syndrome, Parkes-Weber syndrome, and Hennekam's syndrome. Other disorders associated with lymphedema include Noonan's syndrome, yellow nail syndrome, intestinal lymphangiectasia syndrome, lymphangiomyomatosis, and neurofibromatosis type 1.

Secondary lymphedema is an acquired condition that results from damage to or obstruction of previously normal lymphatic channels. Recurrent episodes of bacterial lymphangitis, usually caused by streptococci, are a very common cause of lymphedema. The most common cause of secondary lymphedema worldwide is lymphatic filariasis, affecting approximately 129 million children and adults worldwide and causing lymphedema and elephantiasis in 14 million of these affected individuals (Chap. 258). Recurrent bacterial lymphangitis by *Streptococcus* may result in chronic lymphedema. Other infectious causes include lymphogranuloma venereum and tuberculosis. In developed countries, the most common secondary cause of lymphedema is surgical excision or irradiation of axillary and inguinal lymph nodes for treatment of cancers, such as breast, cervical, endometrial, and prostate cancer, sarcomas, and malignant melanoma. Lymphedema of the arm occurs in 13% of breast cancer patients after axillary node dissection and in 22% after both surgery and radiotherapy. Lymphedema of the leg affects approximately 15% of patients with cancer after inguinal lymph node dissection. Tumors, such as prostate cancer and lymphoma, also can infiltrate and obstruct lymphatic vessels. Less common causes include contact dermatitis, rheumatoid arthritis, pregnancy, and self-induced or factitious lymphedema after application of tourniquets.

Clinical Presentation Lymphedema is generally a painless condition, but patients may experience a chronic dull, heavy sensation in the leg, and most often they are concerned about the appearance of the leg. Lymphedema of the lower extremity initially involves the foot and gradually progresses up the leg so that the entire limb becomes edematous (Fig. 303-2). In the early stages, the edema is soft and pits easily with pressure. Over time, subcutaneous adipose tissue accumulates, the limb enlarges further and loses its normal contour, and the toes appear square. Thickening of the skin is detected by Stemmer's sign, which is the inability to tent the skin at the base of the toes. Peau d'orange is a term used to describe dimpling of the skin, resembling that of an orange peel, caused by lymphedema. In the chronic stages, the edema no longer pits and the limb acquires a woody texture as the tissues become indurated and fibrotic. The International Society of Lymphology describes four clinical stages of lymphedema (Table 303-3).

Differential Diagnosis Lymphedema should be distinguished from other disorders that cause unilateral leg swelling, such as deep vein thrombosis and chronic venous insufficiency. In the latter condition, the edema is softer, and there is often evidence of a stasis dermatitis, hyperpigmentation, and superficial venous varicosities, as described earlier. Other causes of leg swelling that resemble lymphedema are myxedema and lipedema. Lipedema usually occurs in women and is caused by accumulation of adipose tissue in the leg from the thigh to the ankle with sparing of the feet.

Diagnostic Testing The evaluation of patients with lymphedema should include diagnostic studies to clarify the cause. Abdominal and pelvic ultrasound and computed tomography (CT) can be used to detect obstructing lesions such as neoplasms. Magnetic resonance imaging (MRI) of the affected limb may reveal a honeycomb pattern characteristic of lymphedema in the epifascial compartment and identify enlarged lymphatic channels and lymph nodes. MRI also is useful to distinguish lymphedema from lipedema. Lymphoscintigraphy and lymphangiography are rarely indicated, but either can be used to confirm the diagnosis or differentiate primary from secondary lymphedema. Lymphoscintigraphy involves the injection of radioactively labeled technetium-containing colloid into the distal subcutaneous tissue of the affected extremity, which is imaged with a scintigraphic camera to visualize lymphatic vessels and lymph nodes. Findings indicative of primary lymphedema include absent or delayed filling of the lymphatic vessels or dermal back flow caused by lymphatic reflux. Findings of secondary lymphedema include dilated lymphatic vessels distal to an area of obstruction. In lymphangiography, iodinated radiocontrast material is injected into a distal lymphatic vessel that has been isolated and cannulated. In primary lymphedema, lymphatic channels are absent, hypoplastic, or ectatic. In secondary lymphedema, lymphatic channels often appear dilated beneath the level of obstruction.

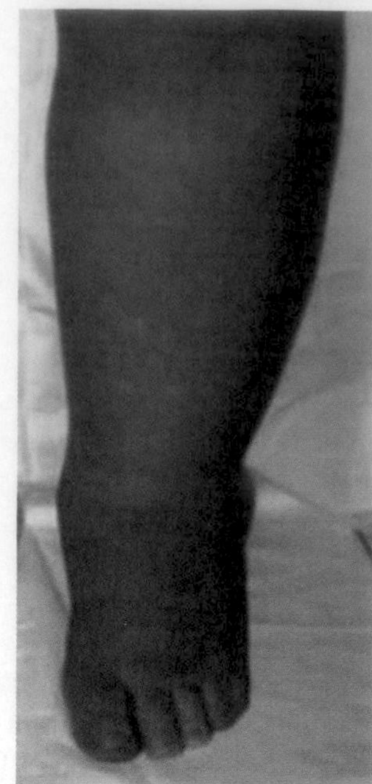
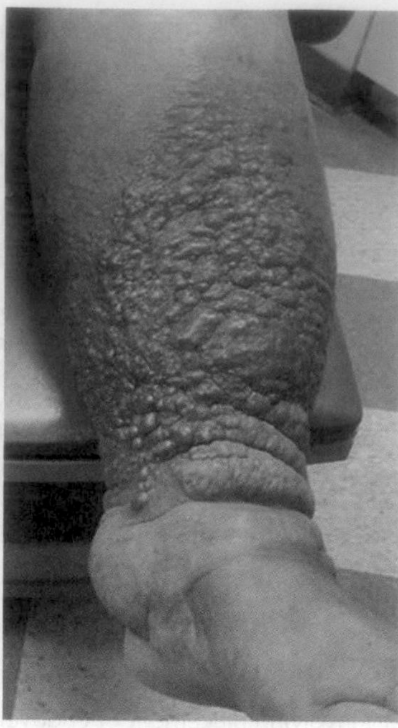

A B

FIGURE 303-2 ***A.*** Lymphedema characterized by swelling of the leg, nonpitting edema, and squaring of the toes. *(Courtesy of Dr. Marie Gerhard-Herman, with permission.)* ***B.*** Advanced chronic stage of lymphedema illustrating the woody appearance of the leg with acanthosis and verrucous overgrowths. *(Courtesy of Dr. Jeffrey Olin, with permission.)*

TABLE 303-3 STAGES OF LYMPHEDEMA

Stage 0 (or Ia)
A latent or subclinical condition where swelling is not evident despite impaired lymph transport. It may exist for months or years before overt edema occurs.
Stage I
Early accumulation of fluid relatively high in protein content that subsides with limb elevation. Pitting may occur. An increase in proliferating cells may also be seen.
Stage II
Limb elevation alone rarely reduces tissue swelling, and pitting is manifest. Late in stage II, the limb may or may not pit as excess fat and fibrosis supervene.
Stage III
Lymphostatic elephantiasis where pitting can be absent and trophic skin changes such as acanthosis, further deposition of fat and fibrosis, and warty overgrowths have developed.

Source: Adapted from The 2013 Consensus Document of the International Society of Lymphology: Lymphology 46:1, 2013.

The complexities of lymphatic cannulation and the risk of lymphangitis associated with the contrast agent limit the utility of lymphangiography. A novel technique of optical imaging with a near-infrared fluorescence dye may enable quantitative imaging of lymph flow.

TREATMENT LYMPHEDEMA

Patients with lymphedema of the lower extremities must be instructed to take meticulous care of their feet to prevent recurrent lymphangitis. Skin hygiene is important, and emollients can be used to prevent drying. Prophylactic antibiotics are often helpful, and fungal infection should be treated aggressively. Patients should be encouraged to participate in physical activity; frequent leg elevation can reduce the amount of edema. Psychosocial support is indicated to assist patients cope with anxiety or depression related to body image, self-esteem, functional disability, and fear of limb loss.

Physical therapy, including massage to facilitate lymphatic drainage, may be helpful. The type of massage used in decongestive physiotherapy for lymphedema involves mild compression of the skin of the affected extremity to dilate the lymphatic channels and enhance lymphatic motility. Multilayered, compressive bandages are applied after each massage session to reduce recurrent edema. After optimal reduction in limb volume by decongestive physiotherapy, patients can be fitted with graduated compression hose. Occasionally, intermittent pneumatic compression devices can be applied at home to facilitate reduction of the edema. Diuretics are contraindicated and may cause depletion of intravascular volume and metabolic abnormalities.

Liposuction in conjunction with decongestive physiotherapy may be considered to treat lymphedema, particularly postmastectomy lymphedema. Other surgical interventions are rarely used and often not successful in ameliorating lymphedema. Microsurgical lymphaticovenous anastomotic procedures have been performed to rechannel lymph flow from obstructed lymphatic vessels into the venous system. Limb reduction procedures to resect subcutaneous tissue and excessive skin are performed occasionally in severe cases of lymphedema to improve mobility.

Therapeutic lymphangiogenesis has been studied in rodent models of lymphedema, but not as yet in humans. Overexpression of vascular endothelial growth factor (VEGF) C generates new lymphatic vessels and improves lymphedema in a murine model of primary lymphedema, and administration of recombinant VEGF-C or VEGF-D stimulated lymphatic growth in preclinical models of postsurgical lymphedema. Clinical trials in patients with lymphedema are required to determine efficacy of gene transfer (cell-based) therapies for lymphedema.

304 Pulmonary Hypertension

Aaron B. Waxman, Joseph Loscalzo

Pulmonary hypertension (PH) is a spectrum of diseases involving the pulmonary vasculature, and is defined as an elevation in pulmonary arterial pressures (mean pulmonary artery pressure >22 mmHg). Pulmonary arterial hypertension (PAH) is a relatively rare form of PH and is characterized by symptoms of dyspnea, chest pain, and syncope. If left untreated, the disease carries a high mortality rate, with the most common cause of death being decompensated right heart failure. There have been significant advances in this field in regard to understanding the pathogenesis, diagnosis, and classification of PAH. Despite these significant advances, there is still a substantial delay in diagnosis of up to 2 years. In many cases, patients whose primary complaint is dyspnea on exertion are frequently misdiagnosed with more common diseases such as asthma or chronic obstructive pulmonary disease. The availability of newer drugs has resulted in a radical change in the management of this disease with significant improvement in both quality of life and mortality. A delay in diagnosis results in an obvious delay in the initiation of appropriate treatment. Clinicians should be able to recognize the signs and symptoms of PH and to complete a systematic workup in patients suspected of having it. In this way, early diagnosis, prompt treatment, and improved outcomes for patients become achievable.

PATHOBIOLOGY

Vasoconstriction, vascular proliferation, thrombosis, and inflammation appear to underlie the development of PAH (Fig. 304-1). In long-standing PH, intimal proliferation and fibrosis, medial hypertrophy, and in situ thrombosis characterize the pathologic findings in the pulmonary vasculature. Vascular remodeling at earlier stages may be confined to the small pulmonary arteries. As the disease advances, intimal proliferation and pathologic remodeling progress, resulting in decreased compliance and increased elastance of the pulmonary vasculature. The outcome is a progressive increase in the right ventricular afterload or total pulmonary vascular resistance (PVR) and, thus, right ventricular work. In subjects with moderate to severe pulmonary vascular disease with significantly increased PVR, as the resting PVR increases, there will be a corresponding increase in mean pulmonary artery pressure (PAP) until the cardiac output (CO) is compromised and starts to fall. With a decline in CO, the PAP will fall. As CO declines as a result of increased afterload and decreased contractility, tachycardia is a compensatory response. Tachycardia decreases filling time and, thus, preload, and results in a reduced fraction of stroke volume available to distend the pulmonary vascular tree.

Abnormalities in multiple molecular pathways and genes that regulate the pulmonary vascular endothelial and smooth muscle cells have been identified (Table 304-1). These abnormalities include decreased expression of the voltage-regulated potassium channel, mutations in the bone morphogenetic protein receptor-2, increased tissue factor expression, overactivation of the serotonin transporter, hypoxia-induced activation of hypoxia-inducible factor-1α, and activation of nuclear factor of activated T cells. As a result, there is a decrease in apoptosis of the smooth muscle cells and the emergence of apoptosis-resistant endothelial cells that promote their accumulation and can obliterate the vascular lumen. In addition, thrombin deposition in the pulmonary vasculature from the prothrombotic state that develops as an independent abnormality or as a result of endothelial dysfunction may amplify vascular cell proliferation and the obliterative arteriopathy.

DIAGNOSIS AND CLASSIFICATION

The diagnosis of PH can be missed without a reasonable index of suspicion. Dyspnea is the most common presenting symptom, but this complaint is far from specific for the diagnosis of PH. PH symptoms are insidious and overlap considerably with many common conditions, including asthma and other lung disease and cardiac disease. The symptoms of PH are often nonspecific and variable. Most patients will present with dyspnea and/or fatigue, whereas edema, chest pain, presyncope, and frank syncope are less common and associated with more advanced disease. On examination, there may be evidence of right ventricular failure with elevated jugular venous pressure, lower extremity edema, and ascites. Additionally, the cardiovascular examination may reveal an accentuated P_2 component of the second heart sound, a right-sided S_3 or S_4, and a holosystolic tricuspid regurgitant murmur. It is also important to seek signs of the diseases that are often concurrent with PH: clubbing may be seen in some chronic lung diseases, sclerodactyly and telangiectasia may signify scleroderma, and crackles and systemic hypertension may be clues to left-sided systolic or diastolic heart failure.

Once clinical suspicion is raised, a systematic approach to diagnosis and assessment is essential. An echocardiogram with (if indicated) a *bubble study* is the most important screening test. Echocardiography is important for the diagnosis of PH and often essential for determining the cause. All forms of PH may demonstrate a hypertrophied and

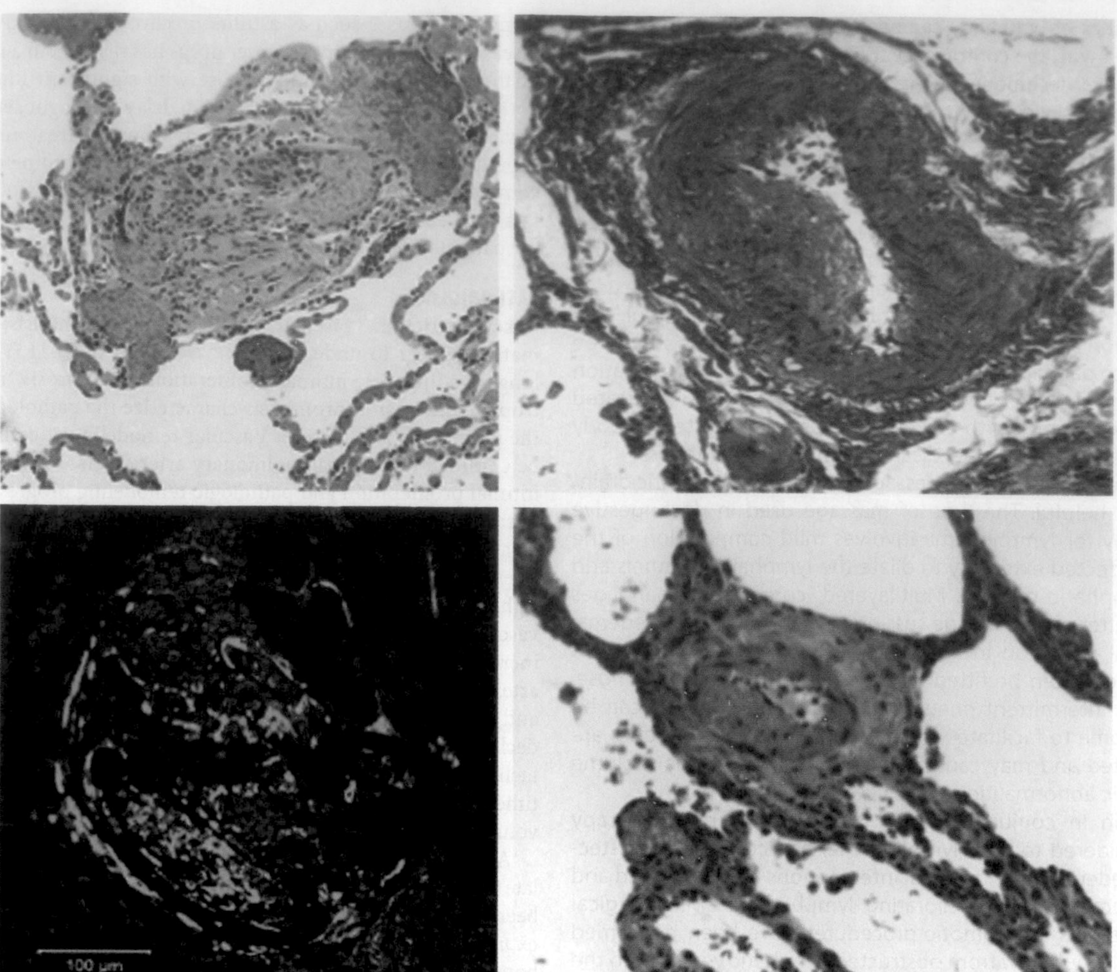

FIGURE 304-1 The *left panels* show examples of plexogenic pulmonary arteriopathy. These are obstructive and proliferative lesions of the small muscular pulmonary arteries, composed primarily of endothelial cells with intermixed inflammatory cells, myofibroblasts, and connective tissue components. The *lower left panel* demonstrates proliferating cells (red PCNA stained cells). *Panels on the right* demonstrate medial hypertrophy of muscular pulmonary arteries. *(Photographs on the left are courtesy of Dr. Stephen Archer, Queen's University School of Medicine, Kingston, Ontario, Canada.)*

dilated right ventricle (Fig. 304-2) with elevated estimated pulmonary artery systolic pressure. Important additional information can be gleaned about specific etiologies of PH such as valvular disease, left ventricular systolic and diastolic function, intracardiac shunts, and other cardiac diseases.

Although the accuracy of Doppler echocardiography is often debated, a high-quality echocardiogram that is absolutely normal may obviate the need for further evaluation for PH. An echocardiogram is a screening test, whereas invasive hemodynamic monitoring is the gold standard for diagnosis and assessment of disease severity. With a normal echocardiogram, there may still be some concern for PH; this is particularly true if there is unexplained dyspnea or hypoxemia. In this setting, it is reasonable to proceed to right heart catheterization for definitive diagnosis. Alternatively, if the patient has a reasonable functional capacity, a cardiopulmonary exercise test may help to identify a true physiologic limitation as well as differentiate between cardiac and pulmonary causes of dyspnea. If this test is normal, there is no indication for a right heart catheterization. If a cardiovascular limitation to exercise is found, a right heart catheterization should be pursued.

If the echocardiogram or cardiopulmonary exercise test (CPET) suggests PH and the diagnosis is confirmed by catheterization, a reasonable effort must be made to establish the etiology because this will largely determine the therapeutic approach. A stepwise approach to evaluation is outlined below.

Chest imaging and lung function tests are essential because lung disease is an important cause of PH. A sign of PH that may be evident on chest x-ray include enlargement of the central pulmonary arteries associated with "vascular pruning," a relative paucity of peripheral vessels (Fig. 304-3). Cardiomegaly, with specific evidence of right atrial and ventricular enlargement, can often be observed. The chest x-ray may also demonstrate significant interstitial lung disease or suggest hyperinflation from obstructive lung disease, which may be the underlying cause or contributor to the development of PH. High-resolution computed tomography (CT) may provide additional useful information. Classic findings of PH on CT include those found on chest x-ray: enlarged pulmonary arteries (Fig. 304-4), peripheral pruning of the small vessels, and enlarged right ventricle and atrium. However, high-resolution CT may also reveal signs of venous congestion including centrilobular ground-glass infiltrate and thickened septal lines. In the absence of left heart disease, these findings suggest pulmonary veno-occlusive disease, a rare cause of PAH that can be quite challenging to diagnose.

CT angiograms are commonly used to evaluate acute thromboembolic disease and have demonstrated excellent sensitivity and specificity for that purpose. Ventilation-perfusion ($\dot{V}/\dot{Q}$) scanning has traditionally been used for screening because of its high sensitivity and its role in qualifying patients for surgical intervention. The role of CT angiograms in the diagnosis of chronic thromboembolic pulmonary hypertension (CTEPH) remains controversial, even with the advent of spiral CT. Although a negative $\dot{V}/\dot{Q}$ virtually rules out CTEPH, some cases may be missed through the use of CT angiograms.

Pulmonary function tests are an important component of the evaluation. Although an isolated reduction in DL_{CO} is the classic finding in PAH, results of pulmonary function tests may also suggest restrictive or obstructive lung diseases as the cause of dyspnea or PH. The 6-minute walk test

TABLE 304-1 COMPONENTS OF THE PATHOGENESIS OF PULMONARY ARTERIAL HYPERTENSION

Alterations in regulators of proliferation
- Growth factors
  - Platelet-derived growth factor
  - Fibroblast growth factor
  - Vascular endothelial growth factor
  - Epidermal growth factor
- Transforming growth factor β (TGF-β)
- Bone morphogenetic protein
- Transcription factors
- Matrix metalloproteinases
- Cytokines
- Chemokines
- Mitochondria

Alterations in inflammatory mediators
- Altered T cell subsets
- Monocytes and macrophages
- Interleukin (IL) 1β
- IL-6
- MCP-1
- RANTES
- Fractalkine

Alterations in vascular tone
- Endothelin
- Nitric oxide
- Serotonin
- Prostaglandin
- K^+ channels
- Ca^{2+} channels

Hypoxia-induced remodeling
- HIF-1α
- ROS
- Mitochondria

TGF-β signaling
- BMPR2
- ALK1
- Endoglin
- Smad9
- TGF-β1

Abbreviations: PDGF, platelet-derived growth factor; EGF, epidermal-derived growth factor; FGF, fetal-derived growth factor; VEGF, vascular endothelial-derived growth factor; MCP-1, monocyte chemoattractant protein-1; IL, interleukin.

is also important to evaluate the degree of exertional hypoxemia and limitation and to monitor progression and response to therapy.

Sleep-disordered breathing is another important cause of PH, but a sleep study is generally necessary only when indicated by the patient's history. Nocturnal desaturation is a common finding in PH, even in the absence of sleep-disordered breathing. Thus, all patients should undergo nocturnal oximetry screening, regardless of whether classic symptoms of obstructive sleep apnea or obesity-hypoventilation syndrome are observed. Laboratory tests that are important for screening include an HIV test when clinically indicated. In addition, all patients should have antinuclear antibodies, rheumatoid factor, and scl-70 antibodies assessed to screen for the most common rheumatologic diseases associated with PH if clinically indicated. Liver function and hepatitis serology tests are important to screen for underlying liver disease. Finally, there is an increasing role for brain natriuretic peptide (BNP) testing in the diagnosis and management of PH. BNP and the N-terminus of its propeptide (NT-proBNP) correlate with right ventricular function, hemodynamic severity, and functional status in PAH.

Right heart catheterization with pulmonary vasodilator testing remains the gold standard both to establish the diagnosis of PH and to enable selection of appropriate medical therapy. The definition of precapillary PH or PAH requires (1) an increased mean pulmonary artery pressure (mPAP ≥25 mmHg); (2) a pulmonary capillary wedge pressure (PCWP), left atrial pressure, or left ventricular end-diastolic pressure ≤15 mmHg; and (3) PVR >3 Wood units. Postcapillary PH is differentiated from precapillary PH by a PCWP of ≥15 mmHg; this is further differentiated into passive, based on a transpulmonary gradient <12 mmHg, or reactive, based on a transpulmonary gradient >12 mmHg and an increased PVR. In either case, the CO may be normal or reduced.

Vasodilators with a short duration of action, such as inhaled nitric oxide, inhaled epoprostenol, or intravenous adenosine, are preferred for vasodilator testing. A decrease in mPAP by ≥10 mmHg to an absolute level of ≤40 mmHg without a decrease in CO is defined as a positive pulmonary vasodilator response, and responders are considered for long-term treatment with calcium channel blockers (CCBs). Less than 12% of patients are deemed vasoreactive during testing, and even fewer exhibit long-term responsiveness to CCBs. Acute vasodilator-induced reductions in PVR and mPAP predict better long-term survival even among patients not treated with CCBs. The need for invasive hemodynamic measurements to diagnose PH accurately poses an additional problem when evaluating older patients. Physicians are often reluctant to refer older patients for invasive procedures. However, the diagnosis of PH is increasing in the older population, at least in part because of increased awareness of this disease in the elderly and increased use of screening echocardiograms. Furthermore, the increased availability of oral and less complicated therapeutic options has encouraged the referral of older patients for evaluation and treatment.

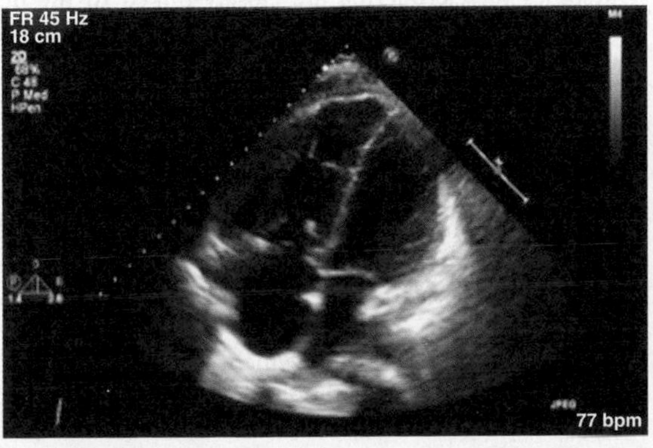

A

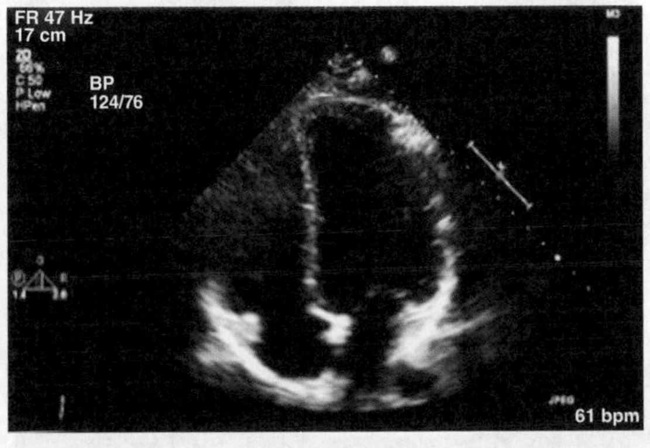

B

FIGURE 304-2 ***A.*** Representative echocardiogram showing the apical four-chamber view from a patient with pulmonary hypertension demonstrating an enlarged right atrium and ventricle with some compression of the left side of the heart. ***B.*** Same echocardiographic view showing a normal echocardiogram.

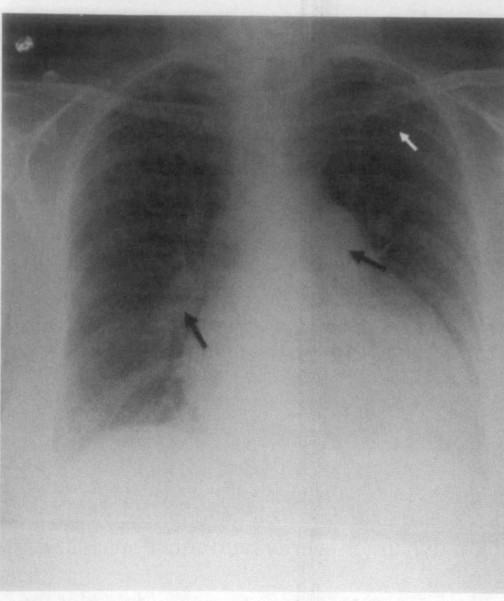

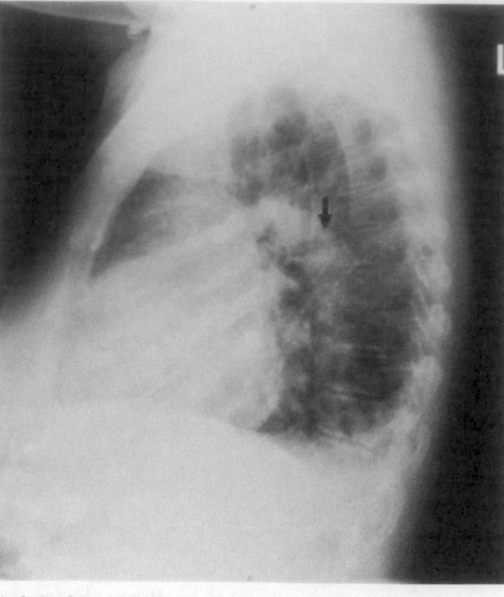

FIGURE 304-3 Posteroanterior (*left*) and lateral (*right*) chest radiograph showing enlarged pulmonary arteries (*black arrows*) and pruning of the distal pulmonary vasculature (*white arrow*) commonly seen with advanced pulmonary arterial hypertension.

PULMONARY HYPERTENSION AS A COMORBID DISEASE

PAH is just one of a number of disease classifications that affect the pulmonary vascular bed. PH was previously classified as primary or secondary, but as understanding of the various contributing diseases has increased, classification systems have attempted to group these diseases by clinical features to aid in diagnosis. The World Health Organization (WHO) formulated a clinical classification of the various manifestations of PH, of which PAH is a subgroup, according to similarities in pathophysiologic mechanisms and clinical presentation. PH is a diverse mix of pathologies in which the only unifying theme is elevated PAP relative to left atrial pressure. The categorization of PH was designed by convenience for the purpose of facilitating novel treatments to be tested across different presentations and is not based on a molecular understanding of the pathology and is not a guide for management decisions.

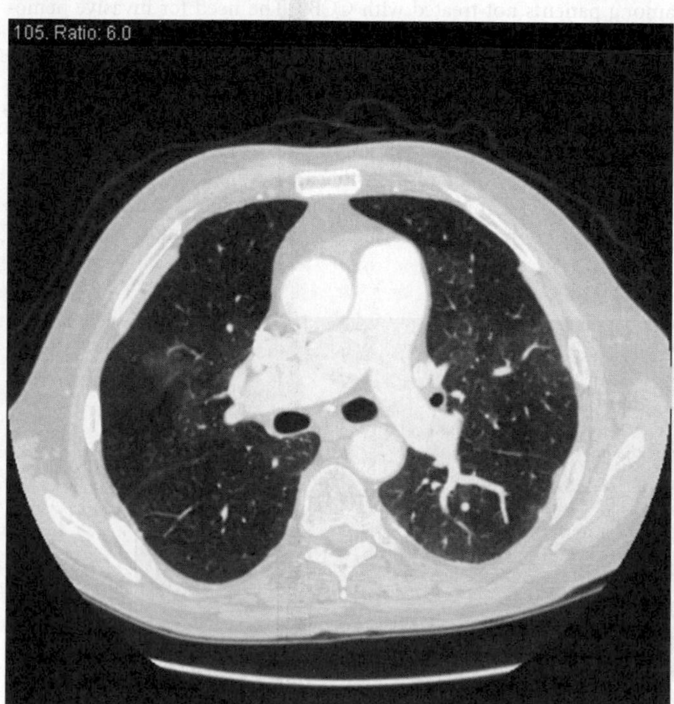

FIGURE 304-4 Representative computed tomography scan of the chest demonstrating enlarged main pulmonary arteries. There is also a mosaic pattern evident in both lungs.

The current classification system, last revised in 2013 during the Fifth World Symposium on Pulmonary Hypertension, recognizes five categories of PH, including PAH, PH due to left heart disease, PH due to chronic lung disease, PH associated with chronic thromboemboli, and a group of miscellaneous diseases that only rarely cause PH.

Pulmonary Arterial Hypertension WHO Group I PH, pulmonary arterial hypertension (PAH), is a relatively rare cause of PH. PAH includes a group of diseases that result in pulmonary arterial precapillary remodeling marked by intimal fibrosis, increased medial thickness, pulmonary arteriolar occlusion, and classic plexiform lesions. PAH is defined as a sustained elevation in resting mPAP ≥25 mmHg, PVR>240 dyne·s/cm^5, and PCWP or left ventricle end-diastolic pressure of ≤15 mmHg based on a right heart catheterization. With a normal PCWP and an elevated mPAP, these diseases demonstrate an increased transpulmonary gradient (mPAP – PCWP); in addition, the PVR is elevated.

Idiopathic pulmonary arterial hypertension (IPAH) is a progressive disease that leads to right heart failure and death. It is typically seen in young women. The National Institutes of Health registry, the first large registry of patients with PAH, reported that the average age at diagnosis was 36 years, with only 9% of patients with IPAH over the age of 60 at diagnosis. However, the more current clinical data suggest that the patient demographics are changing. The Pulmonary Hypertension Connection registry found that the average age of diagnosis for IPAH was 45 years, with 8.5% of patients older than 70 years at diagnosis. This finding is supported by data from the Registry to Evaluate Early and Long-Term PAH Disease Management (REVEAL), the largest cohort of PAH to date, which reported that the average age at diagnosis of IPAH was 44.9±0.6 years.

Other forms of PAH that deserve specific consideration in patients are those associated with HIV, connective tissue disease, and portal hypertension. Although HIV is a rare cause of PAH, this form of PAH is indistinguishable from IPAH and is an important cause of mortality in the HIV-infected population. Importantly, there is no correlation between the stage of HIV infection and the development of PAH.

Among connective tissue diseases, the prevalence of PAH has been established only for systemic sclerosis, especially in those with limited cutaneous scleroderma. Although the average age of scleroderma onset is 30 to 50 years old, patients who eventually develop scleroderma-associated PAH tend to be older at the time of scleroderma diagnosis. Outcomes of scleroderma are closely linked to the development of PAH and are associated with a poor prognosis, although modern therapies have improved outcomes.

Portopulmonary hypertension occurs in 2–10% of patients with established portal hypertension. Its occurrence appears to be independent of the cause of liver disease and is observed in patients with nonhepatic causes of portal hypertension. A hyperdynamic circulatory state is common, as in most patients with advanced liver disease; however, the same pulmonary vascular remodeling observed in other forms of PAH is seen in the pulmonary vascular bed in portopulmonary hypertension. It is important to distinguish this process from hepatopulmonary syndrome, which can also manifest with dyspnea and hypoxemia but is pathophysiologically distinct from portopulmonary hypertension in that abnormal vasodilation of the pulmonary vasculature leads to intrapulmonary shunting.

Pulmonary Hypertension Associated with Left Heart Disease WHO Group II PH includes patients with left heart systolic failure, aortic and mitral valve disease, and heart failure with preserved ejection fraction (HFpEF). PH can develop as a result of all of these conditions. The hallmark of Group II PH (i.e., PH due to left heart disease) is elevated left atrial pressure with resulting pulmonary venous hypertension. In general, the transpulmonary gradient and PVR remain normal. Although this phenomenon is well described in both left-sided valvular disease and left-sided systolic heart failure, studies suggest that HFpEF may carry a higher overall risk of PH.

Whatever the cause of elevated left atrial pressure (i.e., systolic or diastolic heart failure or valvular disease), the increased pulmonary venous pressure indirectly leads to a rise in pulmonary arterial pressure. The presence of PH portends a poor prognosis in all forms of heart failure. In particular, chronic pulmonary venous hypertension may lead to a reactive pulmonary arterial vasculopathy, seen as an elevated transpulmonary gradient (>12 mmHg) and elevated PVR (>3 Wood units). Pathologically, this process is marked by pulmonary arteriolar remodeling with intimal fibrosis and medial hyperplasia akin to that seen in PAH.

Pulmonary Hypertension Associated with Lung Disease Intrinsic lung disease is the second most common cause of PH, although its actual prevalence is difficult to ascertain. PH has been observed in both chronic obstructive lung disease and interstitial lung disease. It can also be seen in diseases with mixed obstructive/restrictive physiology: bronchiectasis, cystic fibrosis, mixed obstructive restrictive disease marked by fibrosis in the lower lung zones, and emphysema predominantly in the upper lung zones. As in patients with left heart disease, PH associated with chronic lung disease is usually modest; however, some of these patients appear to have PH "out of proportion" to their parenchymal lung disease, suggesting intrinsic pulmonary arterial disease. These patients typically have more severe PH, with results of pulmonary function tests demonstrating a very low DL_{CO}.

Although PH is described in most forms of interstitial lung disease, it has been most extensively studied in idiopathic pulmonary fibrosis; however, the individual studies have been small. Early echocardiographic data suggested that the prevalence of PH in interstitial lung diseases was high, but invasive hemodynamic monitoring suggests that the incidence is considerably lower than originally believed. The diagnosis of PH portends poor outcome in pulmonary fibrosis.

Also included in Group III PH is sleep-disordered breathing. Sleep apnea has long been associated with PH. However, PH associated with sleep-disordered breathing is generally mild.

Pulmonary Hypertension Associated with Chronic Thromboembolic Disease The development of PH after chronic thromboembolic obstruction of the pulmonary arteries is well described, but its incidence is not known. The incidence of PH after a single pulmonary embolic event is thought to be quite low and likely increases following recurrent embolism. The risk factors for developing CTEPH are unclear. Many patients have no history of clinical venous thromboembolism. The pathogenesis of CTEPH is poorly understood. Obstruction of the proximal pulmonary vasculature is important and often the dominant factor; however, additional pulmonary vascular remodeling occurs. Approximately 10–15% of patients will develop a disease very similar clinically and pathologically to PAH after resection of the proximal thrombus.

OTHER DISORDERS AFFECTING THE PULMONARY VASCULATURE

Sarcoidosis Patients with sarcoidosis can develop PH as a result of lung involvement. Consequently, patients with sarcoidosis who present with progressive dyspnea and PH require a thorough evaluation. Although the majority of sarcoidosis patients with PH generally do not respond to therapy for PAH, a subset of patients with sarcoidosis and severe PH do have a beneficial response to therapy.

Sickle Cell Disease Cardiovascular system abnormalities are prominent in the clinical spectrum of sickle cell disease, including PH. The etiology is multifactorial, including hemolysis, hypoxemia, thromboembolism, chronic high CO, and chronic liver disease. The presence of PH in patients with sickle cell disease is rare.

Schistosomiasis Globally, schistosomiasis is one of the most common causes of PH. The development of PH occurs in the setting of hepatosplenic disease and portal hypertension. Studies suggest that inflammation from the infection triggers the pulmonary vascular changes that occur. The diagnosis is confirmed by finding the parasite ova in the urine or stool of patients with symptoms, which can be difficult. The efficacy of therapies directed toward PH in these patients is unknown.

PHARMACOLOGIC TREATMENT OF PAH

PH was a consistently fatal condition with no effective medical treatment options before 1996; however, since that time, there has been an upsurge in the development of novel therapeutic agents for PAH. There are several approved agents for PAH, including prostacyclin and prostacyclin analogues, phosphodiesterase-5 inhibitors, a soluble guanylyl cyclase stimulator, and endothelin receptor antagonists, that have improved the outlook dramatically. Although there is no cure for PAH, current pharmacologic therapies improve morbidity and, in some cases, mortality.

PROSTANOIDS

In PAH, endothelial dysfunction and platelet activation cause an imbalance of arachidonic acid metabolites with reduced prostacyclin levels and increased thromboxane A_2 production. Prostacyclin (PGI_2) activates cyclic adenosine monophosphate (cAMP)-dependent pathways that mediate vasodilation. PGI_2 also has antiproliferative effects on vascular smooth muscle and inhibits platelet aggregation. Protein levels of prostacyclin synthase are decreased in pulmonary arteries of patients with PAH. This imbalance of mediators is addressed by the exogenous administration of prostanoids as therapy in advanced PAH.

Epoprostenol was the first prostanoid available for the management of PAH. Epoprostenol delivered as a continuous intravenous infusion improves functional capacity and survival in PAH. The efficacy of epoprostenol in WHO functional class 3 and 4 PAH patients was demonstrated in a clinical trial that showed improved quality of life, mPAP, PVR, 6-minute walk distance (6MWD), and mortality. Treprostinil has a longer half-life than epoprostenol (~4 h vs ~6 min), which allows for continuous subcutaneous and intravenous administration. Treprostinil has been shown to improve pulmonary hemodynamics, symptoms, exercise capacity, and survival in PAH.

Inhaled prostacyclins provide the beneficial effects of infused prostacyclin therapy without the inconvenience and side effects (risk of infection and infusion site reactions) of infusion catheters. Both inhaled iloprost and treprostinil have been approved for patients with WHO class 3 and 4 PAH. The main advantage of treprostinil is less frequent administration. Inhaled formulations can be efficacious in moderately symptomatic patients with PAH and may be appropriate when used in combination with an oral medication. Phosphodiesterase-5 (PDE5) inhibitors (e.g., sildenafil) increase cyclic guanosine monophosphate (cGMP) levels and activate cGMP-dependent signaling pathways that also mediate vasodilation and platelet inhibition. Thus, the addition of a PDE5 inhibitor augments the pulmonary hemodynamic and functional capacity benefits of prostanoids in PAH.

Endothelin Receptor Antagonists Endothelin receptor antagonists (ERAs) target endothelin-1 (ET-1), a potent endogenous vasoconstrictor and vascular smooth muscle mitogen that is elevated in PAH patients. Endothelin levels are increased coincident with increased PVR and mPAP and decreased CO and 6MWD.

ERAs block the binding of ET-1 to either endothelin receptor A (ET-A) and/or B (ET-B). ET-A receptors found on pulmonary artery smooth muscle cells mediate vasoconstriction. In the normal pulmonary vasculature, ET-B receptors are found on endothelial cells and mediate vasodilation via production of prostacyclin and nitric oxide as well as ET-1 clearance. Three ERAs approved for use in the United States are bosentan and macitentan both, nonselective receptor antagonists, and ambrisentan, a selective ET-A receptor antagonist.

Studies have shown that both bosentan and macitentan improve hemodynamics and exercise capacity and delay clinical worsening.

TABLE 304-2 FDA-APPROVED THERAPIES FOR THE TREATMENT OF PAH

Generic Name	Route of Administration	Drug Class	Indication
Epoprostenol	IV	Prostacyclin derivative	Treatment of PAH to improve exercise capacity
Iloprost	Inhaled	Prostacyclin derivative	Treatment of PAH to improve a composite endpoint consisting of exercise tolerance, symptoms (NYHA Class), and lack of deterioration
Treprostinil	IV or SC	Prostacyclin derivative	Treatment of PAH to diminish symptoms associated with exercise
Treprostinil	Inhaled	Prostacyclin derivative	Treatment of PAH to improve exercise ability
Treprostinil	Oral	Prostacyclin derivative	Treatment of PAH to improve exercise ability
Bosentan	Oral	Non-selective endothelin receptor antagonist	Treatment of PAH to improve exercise capacity and to decrease clinical worsening
Ambrisentan	Oral	Endothelin receptor antagonist	Treatment of PAH to improve exercise capacity and delay clinical worsening
Macitentan	Oral	Non-selective endothelin antagonist	Treatment of PAH to improve exercise capacity and delay clinical worsening
Sildenafil	Oral	PDE5 inhibitor	Treatment of PAH to improve exercise capacity and delay clinical worsening
Tadalafil	Oral	PDE5 inhibitor	Treatment of PAH to improve exercise ability
Riociguat	Oral	Soluble guanylyl cyclase stimulator	Treatment of PAH to improve exercise capacity and delay clinical worsening

Abbreviations: FDA, U.S. Food and Drug Administration; NYHA, New York Heart Association; PAH, pulmonary arterial hypertension; PDE5, phosphodiesterase-5.

The randomized, placebo-controlled, phase III Bosentan Randomized Trial of Endothelin Antagonist Therapy (BREATHE)-1 comparing bosentan with placebo demonstrated improved symptoms, 6MWD, and WHO functional class. The Endothelin Antagonist Trial in Mildly Symptomatic Pulmonary Arterial Hypertension Patients (EARLY) comparing bosentan with placebo demonstrated improved PVR and 6MWD.

Several studies, including the phase III, placebo-controlled Ambrisentan in Pulmonary Arterial Hypertension-1 (ARIES-1) trial, suggest that ambrisentan improves exercise tolerance, WHO functional class, hemodynamics, and quality of life in patients with PAH. There are no trial data to evaluate whether the selective ET-A receptor antagonism of ambrisentan has any advantage over the nonselective ET receptor antagonism of bosentan.

Phosphodiesterase Type-5 Inhibitors Nitric oxide derived from endothelial cells activates guanylyl cyclase, which, in turn, generates cGMP in vascular smooth muscle cells and platelets. cGMP is a second messenger that induces vasodilation through relaxation of the arterial smooth muscle cells and inhibits platelet activation. PDE5 enzymes metabolize cGMP. Therefore, cGMP PDE5 inhibitors prolong the vasodilatory effect of nitric oxide, especially within the pulmonary arterial bed where high concentrations of cGMP are found. There are currently two PDE5 inhibitors used for the treatment of PAH, sildenafil and tadalafil. Both agents have been shown to improve hemodynamics and 6MWD. Recently, the oral soluble guanylyl cyclase stimulator, riociguat, was approved for the treatment of both PAH and CTEPH.

Unmet and Future Research Needs in Pulmonary Hypertension Presently there are only three classes of therapy for patients with PAH, and even with therapy, the median survival for a person with PAH is only 5–6 years (Table 304-2). Although there are five subtypes of PH, current approved therapies only address one subtype. Not only do we need to expand the treatment options for patients with PAH, we also need to develop effective therapies for all patients with PH. Limited survival is, in part, a result of delay in diagnosis. Improved awareness among clinicians and patients could lead to more timely diagnosis that will affect the response to therapy and survival. PH needs to be diagnosed in a timely manner so that therapy can be initiated as soon as possible. Patients should also have the option of referral to a specialty center that focuses on treatment of patients with pulmonary vascular disease, which will ensure their access to state-of-the-art care and a multidisciplinary approach to care. Finally, there need to be continued efforts at developing new therapies that target the increasingly complex and overlapping pathways involved in the various forms of PH.

SECTION 1 DIAGNOSIS OF RESPIRATORY DISORDERS

305 Approach to the Patient with Disease of the Respiratory System

Patricia A. Kritek, Augustine M. K. Choi

The majority of diseases of the respiratory system fall into one of three major categories: (1) obstructive lung diseases; (2) restrictive disorders; and (3) abnormalities of the vasculature. Obstructive lung diseases are most common and primarily include disorders of the airways, such as asthma, chronic obstructive pulmonary disease (COPD), bronchiectasis, and bronchiolitis. Diseases resulting in restrictive pathophysiology include parenchymal lung diseases, abnormalities of the chest wall and pleura, and neuromuscular disease. Disorders of the pulmonary vasculature include pulmonary embolism, pulmonary hypertension, and pulmonary veno-occlusive disease. Although many specific diseases fall into these major categories, both infective and neoplastic processes can affect the respiratory system and result in myriad pathologic findings, including those listed in the three categories above (Table 305-1).

Disorders can also be grouped according to gas exchange abnormalities, including hypoxemic, hypercarbic, or combined impairment. However, many diseases of the lung do not manifest as gas exchange abnormalities.

As with the evaluation of most patients, the approach to a patient with disease of the respiratory system begins with a thorough history and a focused physical examination. Many patients will subsequently undergo pulmonary function testing, chest imaging, blood and sputum analysis, a variety of serologic or microbiologic studies, and diagnostic procedures, such as bronchoscopy. This stepwise approach is discussed in detail below.

TABLE 305-1 CATEGORIES OF RESPIRATORY DISEASE

Category	Examples
Obstructive lung disease	Asthma
	Chronic obstructive pulmonary disease (COPD)
	Bronchiectasis
	Bronchiolitis
Restrictive pathophysiology—parenchymal disease	Idiopathic pulmonary fibrosis (IPF)
	Asbestosis
	Desquamative interstitial pneumonitis (DIP)
	Sarcoidosis
Restrictive pathophysiology—neuromuscular weakness	Amyotrophic lateral sclerosis (ALS)
	Guillain-Barré syndrome
Restrictive pathophysiology—chest wall/pleural disease	Kyphoscoliosis
	Ankylosing spondylitis
	Chronic pleural effusions
Pulmonary vascular disease	Pulmonary embolism
	Pulmonary arterial hypertension (PAH)
Malignancy	Bronchogenic carcinoma (non-small-cell and small-cell)
	Metastatic disease
Infectious diseases	Pneumonia
	Bronchitis
	Tracheitis

HISTORY

Dyspnea and Cough The cardinal symptoms of respiratory disease are dyspnea and cough (Chaps. 47e and 48). Dyspnea has many causes, some of which are not predominantly due to lung pathology. The words a patient uses to describe shortness of breath can suggest certain etiologies for dyspnea. Patients with obstructive lung disease often complain of "chest tightness" or "inability to get a deep breath," whereas patients with congestive heart failure more commonly report "air hunger" or a sense of suffocation.

The tempo of onset and the duration of a patient's dyspnea are likewise helpful in determining the etiology. Acute shortness of breath is usually associated with sudden physiologic changes, such as laryngeal edema, bronchospasm, myocardial infarction, pulmonary embolism, or pneumothorax. Patients with COPD and idiopathic pulmonary fibrosis (IPF) experience a gradual progression of dyspnea on exertion, punctuated by acute exacerbations of shortness of breath. In contrast, most asthmatics have normal breathing the majority of the time with recurrent episodes of dyspnea that are usually associated with specific triggers, such as an upper respiratory tract infection or exposure to allergens.

Specific questioning should focus on factors that incite dyspnea as well as on any intervention that helps resolve the patient's shortness of breath. Asthma is commonly exacerbated by specific triggers, although this can also be true of COPD. Many patients with lung disease report dyspnea on exertion. Determining the degree of activity that results in shortness of breath gives the clinician a gauge of the patient's degree of disability. Many patients adapt their level of activity to accommodate progressive limitation. For this reason, it is important, particularly in older patients, to delineate the activities in which they engage and how these activities have changed over time. Dyspnea on exertion is often an early symptom of underlying lung or heart disease and warrants a thorough evaluation.

Cough generally indicates disease of the respiratory system. The clinician should inquire about the duration of the cough, whether or not it is associated with sputum production, and any specific triggers that induce it. Acute cough productive of phlegm is often a symptom of infection of the respiratory system, including processes affecting the upper airway (e.g., sinusitis, tracheitis), the lower airways (e.g., bronchitis, bronchiectasis), and the lung parenchyma (e.g., pneumonia). Both the quantity and quality of the sputum, including whether it is blood-streaked or frankly bloody, should be determined. Hemoptysis warrants an evaluation as delineated in Chap. 48.

Chronic cough (defined as that persisting for >8 weeks) is commonly associated with obstructive lung diseases, particularly asthma and chronic bronchitis, as well as "nonrespiratory" diseases, such as gastroesophageal reflux and postnasal drip. Diffuse parenchymal lung diseases, including IPF, frequently present as a persistent, nonproductive cough. As with dyspnea, all causes of cough are not respiratory in origin, and assessment should encompass a broad differential, including cardiac and gastrointestinal diseases as well as psychogenic causes.

Additional Symptoms Patients with respiratory disease may report wheezing, which is suggestive of airways disease, particularly asthma. Hemoptysis can be a symptom of a variety of lung diseases, including infections of the respiratory tract, bronchogenic carcinoma, and pulmonary embolism. In addition, chest pain or discomfort is often thought to be respiratory in origin. As the lung parenchyma is not innervated with pain fibers, pain in the chest from respiratory disorders usually results from either diseases of the parietal pleura (e.g., pneumothorax) or pulmonary vascular diseases (e.g., pulmonary hypertension). As many diseases of the lung can result in strain on the right side of the heart, patients may also present with symptoms of cor pulmonale, including abdominal bloating or distention and pedal edema (Chap. 279).

Additional History A thorough social history is an essential component of the evaluation of patients with respiratory disease. All patients should be asked about current or previous cigarette smoking, as this exposure is associated with many diseases of the respiratory system, most notably COPD and bronchogenic lung cancer but also a variety of diffuse parenchymal lung diseases (e.g., desquamative interstitial pneumonitis and pulmonary Langerhans cell histiocytosis). For most disorders, longer duration and greater intensity of exposure to cigarette smoke increases the risk of disease. There is growing evidence that "second-hand smoke" is also a risk factor for respiratory tract pathology; for this reason, patients should be asked about parents, spouses, or housemates who smoke. Possible inhalational exposures should be explored, including those at the work place (e.g., asbestos, wood smoke) and those associated with leisure (e.g., excrement from pet birds) (Chap. 311). Travel predisposes to certain infections of the respiratory tract, most notably the risk of tuberculosis. Potential exposure to fungi found in specific geographic regions or climates (e.g., *Histoplasma capsulatum*) should be explored.

Associated symptoms of fever and chills should raise the suspicion of infective etiologies, both pulmonary and systemic. A comprehensive review of systems may suggest rheumatologic or autoimmune disease presenting with respiratory tract manifestations. Questions should focus on joint pain or swelling, rashes, dry eyes, dry mouth, or constitutional symptoms. In addition, carcinomas from a variety of primary sources commonly metastasize to the lung and cause respiratory symptoms. Finally, therapy for other conditions, including both irradiation and medications, can result in diseases of the chest.

Physical Examination The clinician's suspicion of respiratory disease often begins with a patient's vital signs. The respiratory rate is often informative, whether elevated (tachypnea) or depressed (hypopnea). In addition, pulse oximetry should be measured, as many patients with respiratory disease have hypoxemia, either at rest or with exertion. The classic structure of the respiratory examination proceeds through inspection, percussion, palpation, and auscultation as described below. Often, however, auscultatory findings will lead the clinician to perform further percussion or palpation in order to clarify these findings.

The first step of the physical examination is inspection. Patients with respiratory disease may be in distress, often using accessory muscles of respiration to breathe. Severe kyphoscoliosis can result in restrictive pathophysiology. Inability to complete a sentence in conversation is generally a sign of severe impairment and should result in an expedited evaluation of the patient.

Percussion of the chest is used to establish diaphragm excursion and lung size. In the setting of decreased breath sounds, percussion is used to distinguish between pleural effusions (dull to percussion) and pneumothorax (hyper-resonant note).

The role of palpation is limited in the respiratory examination. Palpation can demonstrate subcutaneous air in the setting of barotrauma. It can also be used as an adjunctive assessment to determine whether an area of decreased breath sounds is due to consolidation (increased tactile fremitus) or a pleural effusion (decreased tactile fremitus).

The majority of the manifestations of respiratory disease present as abnormalities of auscultation. Wheezes are a manifestation of airway obstruction. While most commonly a sign of asthma, peribronchial edema in the setting of congestive heart failure can also result in diffuse wheezes, as can any other process that causes narrowing of small airways. For this reason, clinicians must take care not to attribute all wheezing to asthma.

Rhonchi are a manifestation of obstruction of medium-sized airways, most often with secretions. In the acute setting, this manifestation may be a sign of viral or bacterial bronchitis. Chronic rhonchi suggest bronchiectasis or COPD. Stridor, a high-pitched, focal inspiratory wheeze, usually heard over the neck, is a manifestation of upper airway obstruction and should prompt expedited evaluation of the patient, as it can precede complete upper airway obstruction and respiratory failure.

Crackles, or rales, are commonly a sign of alveolar disease. A variety of processes that fill the alveoli with fluid may result in crackles. Pneumonia can cause focal crackles. Pulmonary edema is associated with crackles, generally more prominent at the bases. Interestingly, diseases that result in fibrosis of the interstitium (e.g., IPF) also result in crackles often sounding like Velcro being ripped apart. Although some clinicians make a distinction between "wet" and "dry" crackles, this distinction has not been shown to be a reliable way to differentiate among etiologies of respiratory disease.

One way to help distinguish between crackles associated with alveolar fluid and those associated with interstitial fibrosis is to assess for egophony. *Egophony* is the auscultation of the sound "AH" instead of "EEE" when a patient phonates "EEE." This change in note is due to abnormal sound transmission through consolidated parenchyma and is present in pneumonia but not in IPF. Similarly, areas of alveolar filling have increased whispered *pectoriloquy* as well as transmission of larger-airway sounds (i.e., bronchial breath sounds in a lung zone where vesicular breath sounds are expected).

The lack or diminution of breath sounds can also help determine the etiology of respiratory disease. Patients with emphysema often have a quiet chest with diffusely decreased breath sounds. A pneumothorax or pleural effusion may present with an area of absent breath sounds.

Other Systems Pedal edema, if symmetric, may suggest cor pulmonale; if asymmetric, it may be due to deep venous thrombosis and associated pulmonary embolism. Jugular venous distention may also be a sign of volume overload associated with right heart failure. *Pulsus paradoxus* is an ominous sign in a patient with obstructive lung disease, as it is associated with significant negative intrathoracic (pleural) pressures required for ventilation and impending respiratory failure.

As stated earlier, rheumatologic disease may manifest primarily as lung disease. Owing to this association, particular attention should be paid to joint and skin examination. Clubbing can be found in many lung diseases, including cystic fibrosis, IPF, and lung cancer. Cyanosis is seen in hypoxemic respiratory disorders that result in >5 g of deoxygenated hemoglobin/dL.

DIAGNOSTIC EVALUATION

The sequence of studies is dictated by the clinician's differential diagnosis, as determined by the history and physical examination. Acute respiratory symptoms are often evaluated with multiple tests performed at the same time in order to diagnose any life-threatening diseases rapidly (e.g., pulmonary embolism or multilobar pneumonia). In contrast, chronic dyspnea and cough can be evaluated in a more protracted, stepwise fashion.

Pulmonary Function Testing (See also Chap. 307) The initial pulmonary function test obtained is spirometry. This study is an effort-dependent test used to assess for obstructive pathophysiology as seen in asthma, COPD, and bronchiectasis. A diminished-forced expiratory volume in 1 sec (FEV_1)/forced vital capacity (FVC) (often defined as <70% of the predicted value) is diagnostic of obstruction. In addition to measuring FEV_1 and FVC, the clinician should examine the flow-volume loop (which is effort-independent). A plateau of the inspiratory and expiratory curves suggests large-airway obstruction in extrathoracic and intrathoracic locations, respectively.

Spirometry with symmetric decreases in FEV_1 and FVC warrants further testing, including measurement of lung volumes and the diffusion capacity of the lung for carbon monoxide (D_LCO). A total lung capacity <80% of the predicted value for a patient's age, race, sex, and height defines restrictive pathophysiology. Restriction can result from parenchymal disease, neuromuscular weakness, or chest wall or pleural diseases. Restriction with impaired gas exchange, as indicated by a decreased D_LCO, suggests parenchymal lung disease. Additional testing, such as measurements of maximal expiratory pressure and maximal inspiratory pressure, can help diagnose neuromuscular weakness. Normal spirometry, normal lung volumes, and a low D_LCO should prompt further evaluation for pulmonary vascular disease.

Arterial blood gas testing is often helpful in assessing respiratory disease. Hypoxemia, while usually apparent with pulse oximetry, can be further evaluated with the measurement of arterial PO_2 and the calculation of an alveolar gas and arterial blood oxygen tension difference ($[A–a]DO_2$). Patients with diseases that cause ventilation-perfusion mismatch or shunt physiology have an increased $(A–a) DO_2$ at rest. Arterial blood gas testing also allows the measurement of arterial PCO_2. Hypercarbia can accompany severe airway obstruction (e.g., COPD) or progressive restrictive physiology, as in patients with neuromuscular weakness.

Chest Imaging (See Chap. 308e) Most patients with disease of the respiratory system undergo imaging of the chest as part of the initial evaluation. Clinicians should generally begin with a plain chest radiograph, preferably posterior-anterior and lateral films. Several findings, including opacities of the parenchyma, blunting of the costophrenic angles, mass lesions, and volume loss, can be very helpful in determining an etiology. However, many diseases of the respiratory system, particularly those of the airways and pulmonary vasculature, are associated with a normal chest radiograph.

CT of the chest is often performed subsequently and allows better delineation of parenchymal processes, pleural disease, masses or nodules, and large airways. If the test includes administration of contrast, the pulmonary vasculature can be assessed with particular utility for determination of pulmonary emboli. Intravenous contrast also allows lymph nodes to be delineated in greater detail.

FURTHER STUDIES

Depending on the clinician's suspicion, a variety of other studies may be done. Concern about large-airway lesions may warrant bronchoscopy. This procedure may also be used to sample the alveolar space with bronchoalveolar lavage or to obtain nonsurgical lung biopsies. Blood testing may include assessment for hypercoagulable states in the setting of pulmonary vascular disease, serologic testing for infectious or rheumatologic disease, or assessment of inflammatory markers or leukocyte counts (e.g., eosinophils). Sputum evaluation for malignant cells or microorganisms may be appropriate. An echocardiogram to assess right- and left-sided heart function is often obtained. Finally, at times, a surgical lung biopsy is needed to diagnose certain diseases of the respiratory system. All of these studies will be guided by the preceding history, physical examination, pulmonary function testing, and chest imaging.

306e Disturbances of Respiratory Function

Edward T. Naureckas, Julian Solway

This is a digital-only chapter. It is available on the DVD that accompanies this book, as well as on Access Medicine/Harrison's Online, and the eBook and "app" editions of HPIM 19e.

The primary functions of the respiratory system—to oxygenate blood and eliminate carbon dioxide—require virtual contact between blood and fresh air, which facilitates diffusion of respiratory gases between blood and gas. This process occurs in the lung alveoli, where blood flowing through alveolar wall capillaries is separated from alveolar gas by an extremely thin membrane of flattened endothelial and epithelial cells, across which respiratory gases diffuse and equilibrate. Blood flow through the lung is unidirectional via a continuous vascular path, along which venous blood absorbs oxygen from and loses CO_2 to inspired gas. The path for airflow, in contrast, reaches a dead end at the alveolar walls; thus the alveolar space must be ventilated tidally, with inflow of fresh gas and outflow of alveolar gas alternating periodically at the respiratory rate (RR). To provide an enormous alveolar surface area (typically 70 m^2) for blood-gas diffusion within the modest volume of a thoracic cavity (typically 7 L), nature has distributed both blood flow and ventilation among millions of tiny alveoli through multigenerational branching of both pulmonary arteries and bronchial airways. As a consequence of variations in tube lengths and calibers along these pathways as well as the effects of gravity, tidal pressure fluctuations, and anatomic constraints from the chest wall, the alveoli vary in their relative ventilations and perfusions. Not surprisingly, for the lung to be most efficient in exchanging gas, the fresh gas ventilation of a given alveolus must be matched to its perfusion.

307 Diagnostic Procedures in Respiratory Disease

Anne L. Fuhlbrigge, Augustine M. K. Choi

The diagnostic modalities available for assessing the patient with suspected or known respiratory system disease include imaging studies and techniques for acquiring biologic specimens, some of which involve direct visualization of part of the respiratory system. Methods to characterize the functional changes developing as a result of disease, including pulmonary function tests and measurements of gas exchange, are discussed in Chap. 306e.

IMAGING STUDIES

ROUTINE RADIOGRAPHY

Routine chest radiography, including both posteroanterior (PA) and lateral views, is an integral part of the diagnostic evaluation of diseases involving the pulmonary parenchyma, the pleura, and, to a lesser extent, the airways and the mediastinum (see Chaps. 305 and 308e). Lateral decubitus views are useful for determining whether pleural abnormalities represent freely flowing fluid, whereas apical lordotic views can visualize disease at the lung apices better than the standard PA view. Portable equipment is often used for acutely ill patients who cannot be transported to a radiology suite but are more difficult to interpret owing to several limitations: (1) the single anteroposterior (AP) projection obtained; (2) variability in over- and underexposure of film; (3) a shorter focal spot-film distance leading to lack of edge sharpness and loss of fine detail; and (4) magnification of the cardiac silhouette and other anterior structures by the AP projection. Common radiographic patterns and their clinical correlates are reviewed in Chap. 308e.

Advances in computer technology have allowed the development of digital or computed radiography, which has several benefits: (1) immediate availability of the images; (2) significant postprocessing analysis of images to improve diagnostic information; and (3) ability to store images electronically and to transfer them within or between health care systems.

ULTRASOUND

Diagnostic ultrasound (US) produces images using echoes or reflection of the US beam from interfaces between tissues with differing acoustic properties. US is nonionizing and safe to perform on pregnant patients and children. It can detect and localize pleural abnormalities and is a quick and effective way of guiding percutaneous needle biopsy of peripheral lung, pleural, or chest wall lesions. US is also helpful in identifying septations within loculated collections and can facilitate placement of a needle for sampling of pleural liquid (i.e., for thoracentesis), improving the yield and safety of the procedure. Bedside availability makes it valuable in the intensive care setting. Real-time imaging can be used to assess the movement of the diaphragm. Because US energy is rapidly dissipated in air, it is not useful for evaluation of the pulmonary parenchyma and cannot be used if there is any aerated lung between the US probe and the abnormality of interest.

Endobronchial US, in which the US probe is passed through a bronchoscope, is a valuable adjunct to bronchoscopy, allowing identification and localization of pathology adjacent to airway walls or within the mediastinum.

NUCLEAR MEDICINE TECHNIQUES

Nuclear imaging depends on the selective uptake of various compounds by organs of the body. In thoracic imaging, these compounds are concentrated by one of three mechanisms: blood pool or compartmentalization (e.g., within the heart), physiologic incorporation (e.g., bone or thyroid) and capillary blockage (e.g., lung scan). Radioactive isotopes can be administered by either the IV or inhaled routes or both. When injected intravenously, albumin macroaggregates labeled with technetium-99m (^{99m}Tc) become lodged in pulmonary capillaries; the distribution of the trapped radioisotope follows the distribution of blood flow. When inhaled, radiolabeled xenon gas can be used to demonstrate the distribution of ventilation. Using these techniques, ventilation-perfusion lung scanning was a commonly used technique for the evaluation of pulmonary embolism. Pulmonary thromboembolism produces one or more regions of ventilation-perfusion mismatch (i.e., regions in which there is a defect in perfusion that follows the distribution of a vessel and that is not accompanied by a corresponding defect in ventilation [Chap. 300]). However, with advances in computed tomography (CT) scanning, scintigraphic imaging has been largely replaced by CT angiography in patients with suspected pulmonary embolism.

Another common use of ventilation-perfusion scans is in patients with impaired lung function, who are being considered for lung resection. Many patients with bronchogenic carcinoma have coexisting chronic obstructive pulmonary disease (COPD), and the question arises as to whether or not a patient can tolerate lung resection. The distribution of the isotope(s) can be used to assess the regional distribution of blood flow and ventilation, allowing the physician to estimate the level of postoperative lung function.

COMPUTED TOMOGRAPHY

CT offers several advantages over routine chest radiography (Figs. 307-1*A*, *B* and 307-2*A*, *B*; see also Figs. 315-3, 315-4, and 322-4). First, the use of cross-sectional images allows distinction between densities that would be superimposed on plain radiographs. Second, CT is far better than routine radiographic studies at characterizing tissue density and providing accurate size assessment of lesions.

CT is particularly valuable in assessing hilar and mediastinal disease (often poorly characterized by plain radiography), in identifying and characterizing disease adjacent to the chest wall or spine (including pleural disease), and in identifying areas of fat density or calcification in pulmonary nodules (Fig. 307-2). Its utility in the assessment of mediastinal disease has made CT an important tool in the staging of lung cancer (Chap. 107). With the additional use of contrast material, CT also makes it possible to distinguish vascular from nonvascular structures, which is particularly important in distinguishing lymph nodes and masses from vascular structures primarily in the mediastinum, and vascular disorders such as pulmonary embolism.

In high-resolution CT (HRCT), the thickness of individual cross-sectional images is ~1–2 mm, rather than the usual 7–10 mm in conventional CT. The visible detail on HRCT scans allows better recognition of subtle parenchymal and airway disease, thickened interlobular septa, ground-glass opacification, small nodules, and the abnormally thickened or dilated airways seen in bronchiectasis. Using HRCT, characteristic patterns are recognized for many interstitial lung diseases such as lymphangitic carcinoma, idiopathic pulmonary fibrosis, sarcoidosis, and eosinophilic granuloma. However, there is debate about the settings in which the presence of a characteristic pattern on HRCT eliminates the need for obtaining lung tissue to make a diagnosis.

Helical CT and Multidetector CT Helical scanning is currently the standard method for thoracic CT. Helical CT technology results in faster scans with improved contrast enhancement and thinner collimation. Images are obtained during a single breath-holding maneuver that allows less motion artifact and collection of continuous data over a larger volume of lung than is possible with conventional CT. Data from the imaging procedure can be reconstructed in coronal or sagittal planes (Fig. 307-3*A*), as well as the traditional cross-sectional (axial) view.

Further refinements in detector technology have allowed production of scanners with additional detectors along the scanning axis (*z*-axis). These *multidetector CT* (MDCT) scanners can obtain multiple slices in a single rotation that are thinner and can be acquired in a shorter period of time. This results in enhanced resolution and

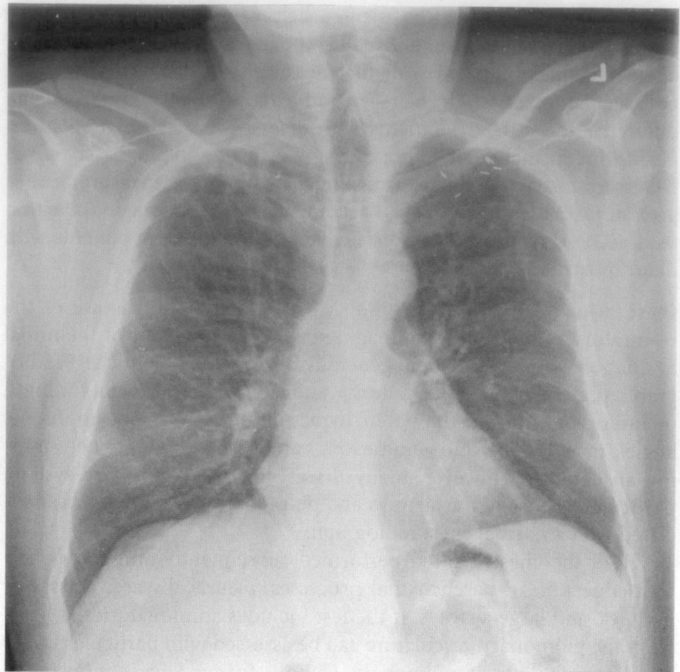

A

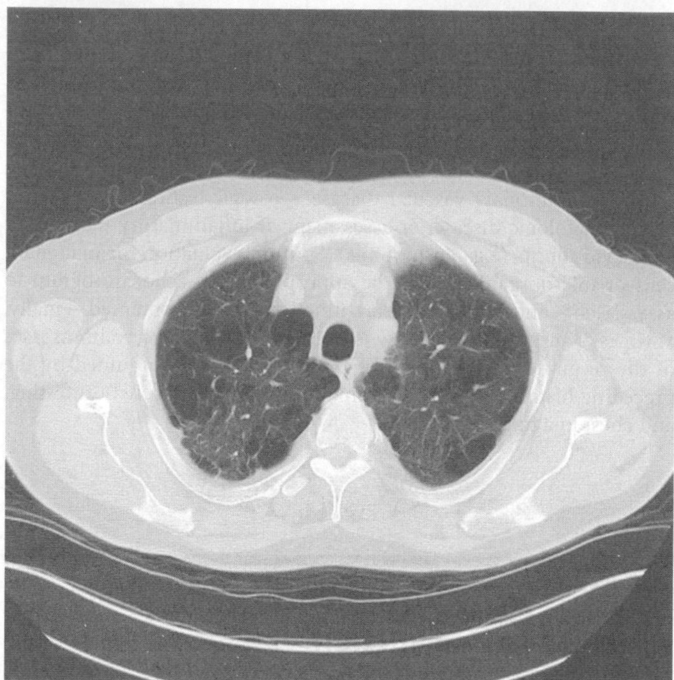

B

FIGURE 307-1 Chest x-ray (*A*) and computed tomography (CT) scan (*B*) from a patient with emphysema. The extent and distribution of emphysema are not well appreciated on plain film but clearly evident on the CT scan obtained.

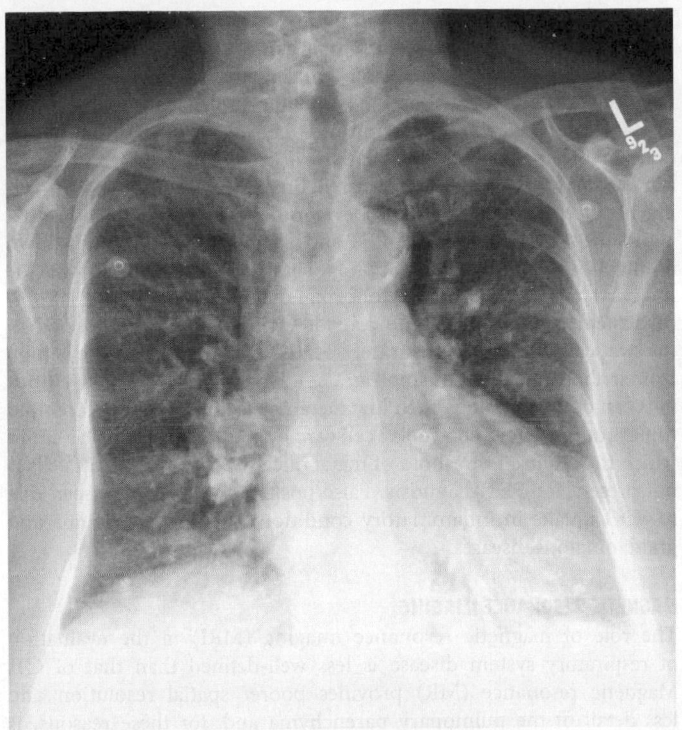

A

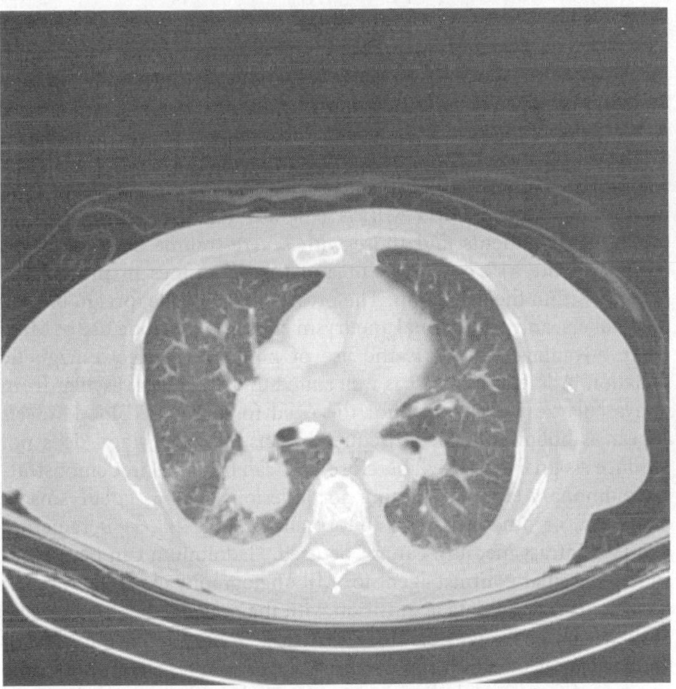

B

FIGURE 307-2 Chest x-ray (*A*) and computed tomography (CT) scan (*B*) demonstrating a right lower-lobe mass. The mass is not well appreciated on the plain film because of the hilar structures and known calcified adenopathy. CT is superior to plain radiography for the detection of abnormal mediastinal densities and the distinction of masses from adjacent vascular structures.

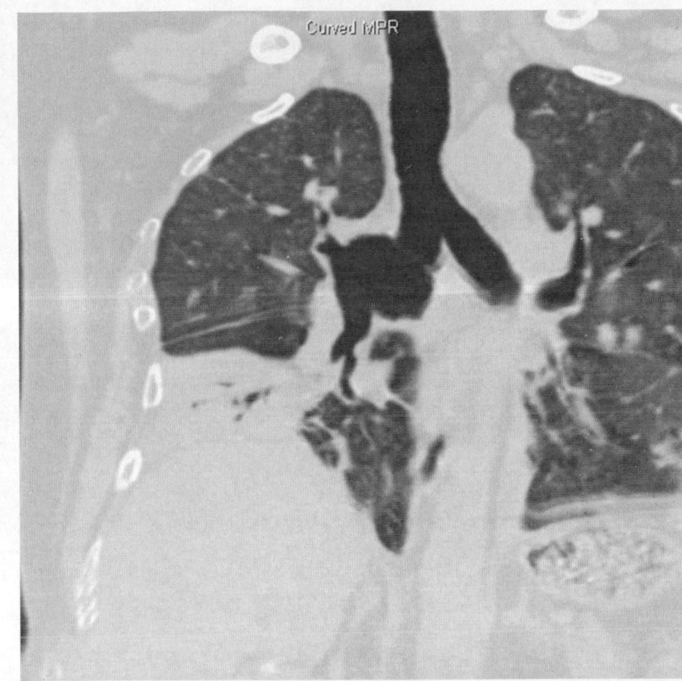

A

B

FIGURE 307-3 Spiral computed tomography (CT) with reconstruction of images in planes other than axial view. Spiral CT in a lung transplant patient with a dehiscence and subsequent aneurysm of the anastomosis. CT images were reconstructed in the sagittal view (***A***) and using digital subtraction to view images of the airways only (***B***), which demonstrate the exact location and extent of the abnormality.

increased image reconstruction ability. As the technology has progressed, higher numbers (currently up to 64) of detectors are used to produce clearer final images. MDCT allows for even shorter breath holds, which are beneficial for all patients but especially children, the elderly, and the critically ill. However, it should be noted that despite the advantages of MDCT, there is an increase in radiation dose compared to single-detector CT to consider.

In MDCT, the additional detectors along the *z*-axis result in improved use of the contrast bolus. This and the faster scanning times and increased resolution have all led to improved imaging of the pulmonary vasculature and the ability to detect segmental and subsegmental emboli. CT pulmonary angiography (CTPA) also allows simultaneous detection of parenchymal abnormalities that may be contributing to a patient's clinical presentation. Secondary to these

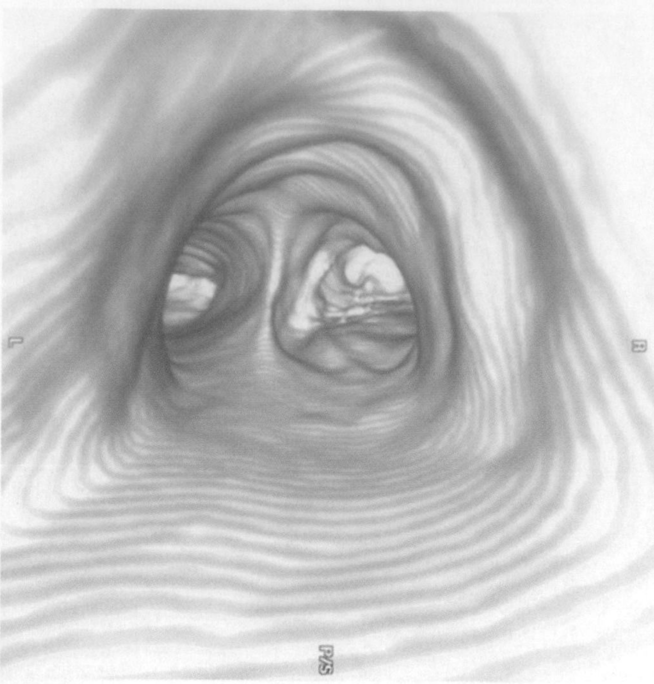

FIGURE 307-4 Virtual bronchoscopic image of the trachea. The view projected is one that would be obtained from the trachea looking down to the carina. The left and right main stem airways are seen bifurcating from the carina.

advantages and increasing availability, CTPA has rapidly become the test of choice for many clinicians in the evaluation of pulmonary embolism; compared with pulmonary angiography, it is considered equal in terms of accuracy and with less associated risks.

VIRTUAL BRONCHOSCOPY

The three-dimensional (3D) image of the thorax obtained by MDCT can be digitally stored, reanalyzed, and displayed as 3D reconstructions of the airways down to the sixth to seventh generation. Using these reconstructions, a "virtual" bronchoscopy can be performed (Fig. 307-4). Virtual bronchoscopy has been proposed as an adjunct to conventional bronchoscopy in several clinical situations: It can allow accurate assessment of the extent and length of an airway stenosis, including the airway distal to the narrowing; it can provide useful information about the relationship of the airway abnormality to adjacent mediastinal structures; and it allows preprocedure planning for therapeutic bronchoscopy to help ensure the appropriate equipment is available for the procedure.

Virtual bronchoscopy can be used to help target the area of peripheral lung for endobronchial lung volume reduction surgery that is being used in the management of pulmonary emphysema. The extent of emphysema in each segmental region together with other anatomic details may help in choosing the most appropriate subsegments. However, software packages for the generation of virtual bronchoscopic images are relatively early in development, and their utilization and potential impact on patient care are still unknown. Electromagnetic navigational bronchoscopy systems (EMN or ENB) using virtual bronchoscopy have been developed to allow accurate navigation to peripheral pulmonary target lesions, using technology similar to a car global positioning system (GPS) unit.

POSITRON EMISSION TOMOGRAPHIC SCANNING

Positron emission tomographic (PET) scanning is commonly used to identify malignant lesions in the lung, based on their increased uptake and metabolism of glucose. The technique involves injection of a radiolabeled glucose analogue, [^{18}F]-fluoro-2-deoxyglucose (FDG), which is taken up by metabolically active malignant cells. However, FDG is trapped within the cells following phosphorylation, and the unstable [^{18}F] decays by emission of positrons, which can be detected by a specialized PET camera or by a gamma camera that has been adapted for imaging of positron-emitting nuclides. This technique has been used in the evaluation of solitary pulmonary nodules and in staging lung cancer. Detection or exclusion of mediastinal lymph node involvement and identification of extrathoracic disease can be achieved. The limited anatomical definition of radionuclide imaging has been improved by the development of hybrid imaging that allows the superimposition of PET and CT images, a technique known as functional–anatomical mapping. Hybrid PET/CT scans provide images that help pinpoint the abnormal metabolic activity to anatomical structures seen on CT and provide more accurate diagnoses than the two scans performed separately. FDG-PET can differentiate benign from malignant lesions as small as 1 cm. However, false-negative findings can occur in lesions with low metabolic activity such as carcinoid tumors and bronchioloalveolar cell carcinomas, or in lesions <1 cm in which the required threshold of metabolically active malignant cells is not present for PET diagnosis. False-positive results can be seen due to FDG uptake in inflammatory conditions such as pneumonia and granulomatous diseases.

MAGNETIC RESONANCE IMAGING

The role of magnetic resonance imaging (MRI) in the evaluation of respiratory system disease is less well-defined than that of CT. Magnetic resonance (MR) provides poorer spatial resolution and less detail of the pulmonary parenchyma and, for these reasons, is currently not considered a substitute for CT in imaging the thorax. However, the use of hyperpolarized gas in conjunction with MR has led to the investigational use of MR for imaging the lungs, particularly in obstructive lung disease. In addition, imaging performed during an inhalation and exhalation can provide dynamic information on lung function. Of note, MR examinations are difficult to obtain among several subgroups of patients. Patients who cannot lie still or who cannot lie on their backs may have MRIs that are of poor quality; some tests require patients to hold their breaths for 15–25 seconds at a time in order to get good MRIs. MRI is generally avoided in unstable and/or ventilated patients and those with severe trauma because of the hazards of the MR environment and the difficulties in monitoring patients within the MR room. The presence of metallic foreign bodies, pacemakers, and intracranial aneurysm clips also preclude use of MRI.

An advantage of MR is the use of nonionizing electromagnetic radiation. Additionally, MR is well suited to distinguish vascular from nonvascular structures without the need for contrast. Blood vessels appear as hollow tubular structures because flowing blood does not produce a signal on MRI. Therefore, MR can be useful in demonstrating pulmonary emboli, defining aortic lesions such as aneurysms or dissection, or other vascular abnormalities (Fig. 307-5) if radiation and IV contrast medium cannot be used. Gadolinium can be used as an intravascular contrast agent for MR angiography (MRA); however, synchronization of data acquisition with the peak arterial bolus is one of the major challenges of MRA. The flow of contrast medium from the peripheral injection site to the vessel of interest is affected by a number of factors including heart rate, stroke volume, and the presence of proximal stenotic lesions.

PULMONARY ANGIOGRAPHY

The pulmonary arterial system can be visualized by pulmonary angiography, in which radiopaque contrast medium is injected through a catheter placed in the pulmonary artery. When performed in cases of pulmonary embolism, pulmonary angiography demonstrates the consequences of an intravascular thrombus—either a defect in the lumen of a vessel (a filling defect) or an abrupt termination (cutoff) of the vessel. Other, less common indications for pulmonary angiography include visualization of a suspected pulmonary arteriovenous malformation and assessment of pulmonary arterial invasion by a neoplasm. The risks associated with modern arteriography are small, generally of greatest concern in patients with severe pulmonary hypertension or chronic kidney disease. With advances in CT scanning, MDCT

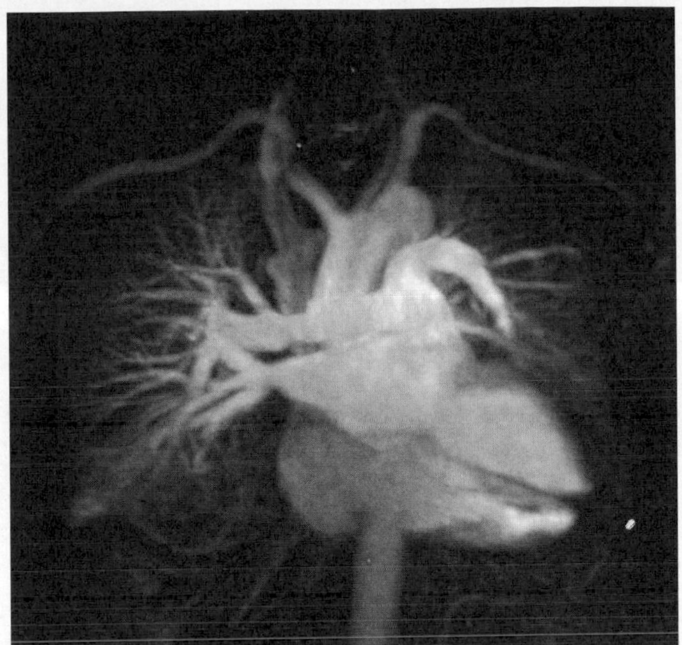

FIGURE 307-5 Magnetic resonance angiography image of the vasculature of a patient after lung transplant. The image demonstrates the detailed view of the vasculature that can be obtained using digital subtraction techniques. Images from a patient after lung transplant show the venous and arterial anastomosis on the right; a slight narrowing is seen at the site of the anastomosis, which is considered within normal limits and not suggestive of obstruction.

angiography (MDCTA) is replacing conventional angiography for the diagnosis of pulmonary embolism.

MEDICAL TECHNIQUES FOR OBTAINING BIOLOGIC SPECIMENS

COLLECTION OF SPUTUM

Sputum can be collected either by spontaneous expectoration or induced (after inhalation of an irritating aerosol such as hypertonic saline). *Sputum induction* is used either because sputum is not spontaneously being produced or because of an expected higher yield of certain types of findings. Because sputum consists mainly of secretions from the tracheobronchial tree rather than the upper airway, the finding of alveolar macrophages and other inflammatory cells is consistent with a lower respiratory tract origin of the sample, whereas the presence of squamous epithelial cells in a "sputum" sample indicates contamination by secretions from the upper airways.

In addition to processing for routine bacterial pathogens by Gram's method and culture, sputum can be processed for a variety of other pathogens, including staining and culture for mycobacteria or fungi, culture for viruses, and staining for *Pneumocystis jiroveci.* In the specific case of sputum obtained for evaluation of *P. jiroveci* pneumonia, for example, sputum should be collected by induction rather than spontaneous expectoration, and an immunofluorescent stain should be used to detect the organisms. Traditional stains and cultures are now also being supplemented in some cases by immunologic techniques and by molecular biologic methods, including the use of polymerase chain reaction amplification and DNA probes. Cytologic staining of sputum for malignant cells, using the traditional Papanicolaou method, allows noninvasive evaluation for suspected lung cancer.

PERCUTANEOUS NEEDLE ASPIRATION (TRANSTHORACIC)

A needle can be inserted through the chest wall into a pulmonary lesion to obtain an aspirate or tissue core for cytologic/histologic or microbiologic analysis. Aspiration can be performed to obtain a diagnosis or to decompress and/or drain a fluid collection. The procedure is usually carried out under CT or ultrasound guidance to assist positioning of the needle and assure localization in the lesion. The low potential risk of this procedure (intrapulmonary bleeding or creation of a pneumothorax with collapse of the underlying lung) in experienced hands is usually acceptable compared with the information obtained. However, a limitation of the technique is sampling error due to the small size of the tissue sample. Thus, findings other than a specific cytologic or microbiologic diagnosis are of limited clinical value.

THORACENTESIS

Sampling of pleural liquid by thoracentesis is commonly performed for diagnostic purposes or, in the case of a large effusion, for palliation of dyspnea. Diagnostic sampling, either by blind needle aspiration or after localization by US, allows the collection of liquid for microbiologic and cytologic studies. Analysis of the fluid obtained for its cellular composition and chemical constituents allows classification of the effusion and can help with diagnosis and treatment (Chap. 316).

BRONCHOSCOPY

Bronchoscopy is the process of direct visualization of the tracheobronchial tree. Although bronchoscopy is now performed almost exclusively with flexible fiberoptic instruments, rigid bronchoscopy, generally performed in an operating room on a patient under general anesthesia, still has a role in selected circumstances, primarily because of a larger suction channel and the fact that the patient can be ventilated through the bronchoscope channel. These situations include the retrieval of a foreign body and the suctioning of a massive hemorrhage, for which the small suction channel of the bronchoscope may be insufficient.

FLEXIBLE FIBEROPTIC BRONCHOSCOPY

This outpatient procedure is usually performed in an awake but sedated patient (conscious sedation). The bronchoscope is passed through either the mouth or the nose, between the vocal cords, and into the trachea. The ability to flex the scope makes it possible to visualize virtually all airways to the level of subsegmental bronchi. The bronchoscopist is able to identify endobronchial pathology, including tumors, granulomas, bronchitis, foreign bodies, and sites of bleeding. Samples from airway lesions can be taken by several methods, including washing, brushing, and biopsy. Washing involves instillation of sterile saline through a channel of the bronchoscope and onto the surface of a lesion. A portion of the liquid is collected by suctioning through the bronchoscope, and the recovered material can be analyzed for cells (cytology) or organisms (by standard stains and cultures). Brushing or biopsy of the surface of the lesion, using a small brush or biopsy forceps at the end of a long cable inserted through a channel of the bronchoscope, allows recovery of cellular material or tissue for analysis by standard cytologic and histopathologic methods.

The bronchoscope can be used to sample material not only from the regions that can be directly visualized (i.e., the airways) but also from the more distal pulmonary parenchyma. With the bronchoscope wedged into a subsegmental airway, aliquots of sterile saline can be instilled through the scope, allowing sampling of cells and organisms from alveolar spaces. This procedure, called *bronchoalveolar lavage,* has been particularly useful for the recovery of organisms such as *P. jiroveci.*

Brushing and biopsy of the distal lung parenchyma can also be performed with the same instruments that are used for endobronchial sampling. These instruments can be passed through the scope into small airways. When biopsies are performed, the forceps penetrate the airway wall, allowing biopsy of peribronchial alveolar tissue. This procedure, called *transbronchial biopsy,* is used when there is either relatively diffuse disease or a localized lesion of adequate size. With the aid of fluoroscopic imaging, the bronchoscopist is able to determine not only whether and when the instrument is in the area of abnormality, but also the proximity of the instrument to the pleural surface. If the forceps are too close to the pleural surface, there is a risk of violating the visceral pleura and creating a pneumothorax; the other potential complication of transbronchial biopsy is pulmonary hemorrhage. The incidence of these complications is less than several percent.

TRANSBRONCHIAL NEEDLE ASPIRATION (TBNA)

Another procedure involves use of a hollow-bore needle passed through the bronchoscope for sampling of tissue adjacent to the trachea or a large bronchus. The needle is passed through the airway wall (transbronchial), and cellular material can be aspirated from mass lesions or enlarged lymph nodes, generally in a search for malignant cells. Mediastinoscopy has been considered the gold standard for mediastinal staging; however, transbronchial needle aspiration (TBNA) allows sampling from the lungs and surrounding lymph nodes without the need for surgery or general anesthesia.

ENDOBRONCHIAL ULTRASOUND (EBUS)–TRANSBRONCHIAL NEEDLE ASPIRATION (TBNA)

Further advances in needle aspiration techniques have been accomplished with the development of endobronchial ultrasound (EBUS). The technology uses an ultrasonic bronchoscope fitted with a probe that allows for needle aspiration of mediastinal and hilar lymph nodes guided by real-time US images. EBUS allows sampling of mediastinal lymph nodes and masses under direct vision to better identify and localize peribronchial and mediastinal pathology and offers access to more difficult-to-reach areas and smaller lymph nodes in the staging of malignancies. EBUS-TBNA has the potential to access the same paratracheal and subcarinal lymph node stations as mediastinoscopy, but also extends out to the hilar lymph nodes (levels 10 and 11). The usefulness of EBUS for clinical indications other than lung cancer is improving and has been recommended in the evaluation of mediastinal masses of unknown origin early in the diagnostic process.

EMERGING BRONCHOSCOPIC TECHNIQUES

Emerging techniques that can be performed using bronchoscopy include video/autofluorescence bronchoscopy (AFB), narrow band imaging (NBI), optical coherence tomography (OCT), and endomicroscopy using confocal fluorescent laser microscopy (CFM). AFB uses bronchoscopy with an additional light source to screen high-risk individuals and identify premalignant lesions (airway dysplasia) and carcinoma in situ. NBI capitalizes on the increased absorption of blue and green wavelengths of light by hemoglobin to enhance the visibility of vessels of the mucosa and differentiate between inflammatory versus malignant mucosal lesions. CFM uses a blue laser to induce fluorescence, and its high degree of resolution provides a real-time view of living tissue at an almost histologic resolution. OCT uses near-infrared light source and has spatial resolution advantages over CT and MRI. It can penetrate the airway wall up to three times deeper than CFM and is less susceptible to motion artifacts from cardiac pulsation and respiratory movements. However, careful assessment is required before these methods find a place in the evaluation strategy of early lung cancer and other lung diseases.

THERAPEUTIC BRONCHOSCOPY

The bronchoscope may provide the opportunity for treatment as well as diagnosis. A central role of the interventional pulmonology (IP) physician is the performance of therapeutic bronchoscopy. For example, an aspirated foreign body may be retrieved with an instrument passed through the bronchoscope (either flexible or rigid), and bleeding may be controlled with a balloon catheter similarly introduced. Newer interventional techniques performed through a bronchoscope include methods for achieving and maintaining patency of airways that are partially or completely occluded, especially by tumors. These techniques include laser therapy, cryotherapy, argon plasma coagulation, electrocautery, balloon bronchoplasty and dilation, and stent placement. Many IP physicians are also trained in performing percutaneous tracheotomy.

MEDICAL THORACOSCOPY

Medical thoracoscopy (or pleuroscopy) focuses on the diagnosis of pleural-based problems. The procedure is performed with a conventional rigid or a semi-rigid pleuroscope (similar in design to a bronchoscope and enabling the operator to inspect the pleural surface, sample and/or drain pleural fluid, or perform targeted biopsies of the parietal pleura). Medical thoracoscopy can be performed in the endoscopy suite or operating room with the patient under conscious sedation and local anesthesia. In contrast, video-assisted thoracoscopic surgery (VATS) requires general anesthesia and is only performed in the operating room. A common diagnostic indication for medical thoracoscopy is the evaluation of a pleural effusion or biopsy of presumed parietal pleural carcinomatosis. It can also be used to place a chest tube under visual guidance, or perform chemical or talc pleurodesis, a therapeutic intervention to prevent a recurrent pleural effusion (usually malignant) or recurrent pneumothorax.

The increasing availability of advanced bronchoscopic and pleuroscopic techniques has motivated the development of IP programs. IP can be defined as "the art and science of medicine as related to the performance of diagnostic and invasive therapeutic procedures, that which require additional training and expertise beyond that which required in a standard pulmonary medicine training program." IP physicians provide alternatives to surgery for patients with a wide variety of thoracic disorders and problems.

SURGICAL TECHNIQUES FOR OBTAINING BIOLOGIC SPECIMENS

Evaluation and diagnosis of disorders of the chest commonly involve collaboration between pulmonologists and thoracic surgeons. Although procedures such as mediastinoscopy, VATS, and thoracotomy are performed by thoracic surgeons, there is overlap in many minimally invasive techniques that can be performed by a pulmonologist, an interventional pulmonologist, or a thoracic surgeon.

MEDIASTINOSCOPY AND MEDIASTINOTOMY

Proper staging of lung cancer is of paramount concern when determining a treatment regimen. Although CT and PET scanning are useful for determining the size and nature of mediastinal lymph nodes as part of the staging of lung cancer, tissue biopsy and histopathologic examination are often critical for the diagnosis of mediastinal masses or enlarged mediastinal lymph nodes. The two major surgical procedures used to obtain specimens from masses or nodes in the mediastinum are mediastinoscopy (via a suprasternal approach) and mediastinotomy (via a parasternal approach). Both procedures are performed under general anesthesia by a qualified surgeon. In the case of suprasternal mediastinoscopy, a rigid mediastinoscope is inserted at the suprasternal notch and passed into the mediastinum along a pathway just anterior to the trachea. Tissue can be obtained with biopsy forceps passed through the scope, sampling masses or nodes that are in a paratracheal or pretracheal position (levels 2R, 2L, 3, 4R, 4L). Aortopulmonary lymph nodes (levels 5, 6) are not accessible by this route and thus are commonly sampled by parasternal mediastinotomy (the Chamberlain procedure). This approach involves a parasternal incision and dissection directly down to a mass or node that requires biopsy.

As an alternative to surgery, a bronchoscope can be used to perform TBNA to obtain tissue from the mediastinum, and, when combined with EBUS, can allow access to the same lymph node stations associated with mediastinoscopy, but also extend access out to the hilar lymph nodes (levels 10, 11). Finally, endoscopic ultrasound (EUS)–fine-needle aspiration (FNA) is a second procedure that complements EBUS-FNA in the staging of lung cancer. EUS-FNA is performed via the esophagus and is ideally suited for sampling lymph nodes in the posterior mediastinum (levels 7, 8, 9). Because US imaging cannot penetrate air-filled spaces, the area directly anterior to the trachea cannot accurately be assessed and is a "blind spot" for EUS-FNA. However, EBUS-FNA can visualize the anterior lymph nodes and can complement EUS-FNA. The combination of EUS-FNA and EBUS-FNA is a technique that is becoming an alternative to surgery for staging the mediastinum in thoracic malignancies.

VIDEO-ASSISTED THORACOSCOPIC SURGERY

VATS has become a standard technique for the diagnosis and management of pleural as well as parenchymal lung disease. This procedure is performed in the operating room using single-lung ventilation with double-lumen endotracheal intubation and involves the passage of a rigid scope with a distal lens through a trocar inserted into the pleura. A high-quality image is shown on a monitor screen, allowing the operator to manipulate instruments passed into the pleural space through separate small intercostal incisions. With these instruments the operator can biopsy lesions of the pleura under direct visualization. In addition, this procedure is now used commonly to biopsy peripheral lung tissue or to remove peripheral nodules for both diagnostic and therapeutic purposes. This much less invasive procedure has largely supplanted the traditional "open lung biopsy" performed via thoracotomy. The decision to use a VATS technique versus performing an open thoracotomy is made by the thoracic surgeon and is based on whether a patient can tolerate the single-lung ventilation that is required to allow adequate visualization of the lung. With further advances in instrumentation and experience, VATS can be used to perform procedures previously requiring thoracotomy, including stapled lung biopsy, resection of pulmonary nodules, lobectomy, pneumonectomy, pericardial window, or other standard thoracic surgical procedures, but allows them to be performed in a minimally invasive manner.

THORACOTOMY

Although frequently replaced by VATS, thoracotomy remains an option for the diagnostic sampling of lung tissue. It provides the largest amount of material, and it can be used to biopsy and/or excise lesions that are too deep or too close to vital structures for removal by VATS. The choice between VATS and thoracotomy needs to be made on a case-by-case basis.

308e Atlas of Chest Imaging

Patricia A. Kritek, John J. Reilly, Jr.

This is a digital-only chapter. It is available on the DVD that accompanies this book, as well as on Access Medicine/Harrison's Online, and the eBook and "app" editions of HPIM 19e.

This atlas of chest imaging is a collection of interesting chest radiographs and computed tomograms (CTs) of the chest. The readings of the films are meant to be illustrative of specific, major findings. The associated text is not intended as a comprehensive assessment of the images.

SECTION 2 DISEASES OF THE RESPIRATORY SYSTEM

309 Asthma

Peter J. Barnes

Asthma is a syndrome characterized by airflow obstruction that varies markedly, both spontaneously and with treatment. Asthmatics harbor a special type of inflammation in the airways that makes them more responsive than nonasthmatics to a wide range of triggers, leading to excessive narrowing with consequent reduced airflow and symptomatic wheezing and dyspnea. Narrowing of the airways is usually reversible, but in some patients with chronic asthma there may be an element of irreversible airflow obstruction. The increasing global prevalence of asthma, the large burden it now imposes on patients, and the high health care costs have led to extensive research into its mechanisms and treatment.

PREVALENCE

Asthma is one of the most common chronic diseases globally and currently affects approximately 300 million people worldwide. The prevalence of asthma has risen in affluent countries over the last 30 years but now appears to have stabilized, with approximately 10–12% of adults and 15% of children affected by the disease. In developing countries where the prevalence of asthma had been much lower, there is a rising prevalence, which is associated with increased urbanization. The prevalence of atopy and other allergic diseases has also increased over the same time, suggesting that the reasons for the increase are likely to be systemic rather than confined to the lungs. Most patients with asthma in affluent countries are atopic, with allergic sensitization to the house dust mite *Dermatophagoides pteronyssinus* and other environmental allergens, such as animal fur and pollens.

Asthma can present at any age, with a peak age of 3 years. In childhood, twice as many males as females are asthmatic, but by adulthood the sex ratio has equalized. Long-term studies that have followed children until they reach the age of 40 years suggest that many with asthma become asymptomatic during adolescence but that asthma returns in some during adult life, particularly in those with persistent symptoms and severe asthma. Adults with asthma, including those with onset during adulthood, rarely become permanently asymptomatic. The severity of asthma does not vary significantly within a given patient; those with mild asthma rarely progress to more severe disease, whereas those with severe asthma usually have severe disease at the onset.

Deaths from asthma are uncommon, and in many affluent countries have been steadily declining over the last decade. A rise in asthma mortality seen in several countries during the 1960s was associated with increased use of short-acting inhaled β_2-adrenergic agonists (as rescue therapy), but there is now compelling evidence that the more widespread use of inhaled corticosteroids (ICS) in patients with persistent asthma is responsible for the decrease in mortality in recent years. Major risk factors for asthma deaths are poorly controlled disease with frequent use of bronchodilator inhalers, lack of or poor compliance with ICS therapy, and previous admissions to hospital with near-fatal asthma.

It has proved difficult to agree on a definition of asthma, but there is good agreement on the description of the clinical syndrome and disease pathology. Until the etiologic mechanisms of the disease are better understood, it will be difficult to provide an accurate definition.

RISK FACTORS AND TRIGGERS

Asthma is a heterogeneous disease with interplay between genetic and environmental factors. Several risk factors that predispose to asthma have been identified (Table 309-1). These should be distinguished from triggers, which are environmental factors that worsen asthma in a patient with established disease.

Atopy Atopy is the major risk factor for asthma, and nonatopic individuals have a very low risk of developing asthma. Patients with asthma commonly suffer from other atopic diseases, particularly allergic rhinitis, which may be found in over 80% of asthmatic patients, and atopic dermatitis (eczema). Atopy may be found in 40–50% of the population in affluent countries, with only a proportion of atopic

TABLE 309-1 RISK FACTORS AND TRIGGERS INVOLVED IN ASTHMA

Endogenous Factors	Environmental Factors
Genetic predisposition	Indoor allergens
Atopy	Outdoor allergens
Airway hyperresponsiveness	Occupational sensitizers
Gender	Passive smoking
Ethnicity	Respiratory infections
Obesity	Diet
Early viral infections	Acetaminophen (paracetamol)
Triggers	
Allergens	
Upper respiratory tract viral infections	
Exercise and hyperventilation	
Cold air	
Sulfur dioxide and irritant gases	
Drugs (β blockers, aspirin)	
Stress	
Irritants (household sprays, paint fumes)	

individuals becoming asthmatic. This observation suggests that some other environmental or genetic factor(s) predispose to the development of asthma in atopic individuals. The allergens that lead to sensitization are usually proteins that have protease activity, and the most common allergens are derived from house dust mites, cat and dog fur, cockroaches (in inner cities), grass and tree pollens, and rodents (in laboratory workers). Atopy is due to the genetically determined production of specific IgE antibody, with many patients showing a family history of allergic diseases.

Genetic Predisposition The familial association of asthma and a high degree of concordance for asthma in identical twins indicate a genetic predisposition to the disease; however, whether or not the genes predisposing to asthma are similar or in addition to those predisposing to atopy is not yet clear. It now seems likely that different genes may also contribute to asthma specifically, and there is increasing evidence that the severity of asthma is also genetically determined. Genetic screens with classical linkage analysis and single-nucleotide polymorphisms of various candidate genes indicate that asthma is polygenic, with each gene identified having a small effect that is often not replicated in different populations. This observation suggests that the interaction of many genes is important, and these may differ in different populations. The most consistent findings have been associations with polymorphisms of genes on chromosome 5q, including the T helper 2 (T_H2) cells interleukin (IL)-4, IL-5, IL-9, and IL-13, which are associated with atopy. There is increasing evidence for a complex interaction between genetic polymorphisms and environmental factors that will require very large population studies to unravel. Novel genes that have been associated with asthma, including *ADAM-33*, and *DPP-10*, have also been identified by positional cloning, but their function in disease pathogenesis is not yet clear. Recent genome-wide association studies have identified further novel genes, such as *ORMDL3*, although their functional role is not yet clear. Genetic polymorphisms may also be important in determining the response to asthma therapy. For example, the Arg-Gly-16 variant in the β_2-receptor has been associated with reduced response to β_2-agonists, and repeats of an Sp1 recognition sequence in the promoter region of 5-lipoxygenase may affect the response to antileukotrienes. However, these effects are small and inconsistent and do not yet have any implications for asthma therapy.

It is likely that environmental factors in early life determine which atopic individuals become asthmatic. The increasing prevalence of asthma, particularly in developing countries, over the last few decades also indicates the importance of environmental mechanisms interacting with a genetic predisposition.

Infections Although viral infections (especially rhinovirus) are common triggers of asthma exacerbations, it is uncertain whether they play a role in etiology. There is some association between respiratory syncytial virus infection in infancy and the development of asthma, but the specific pathogenesis is difficult to elucidate because this infection is very common in children. Atypical bacteria, such as *Mycoplasma* and *Chlamydophila*, have been implicated in the mechanism of severe asthma, but thus far, the evidence is not very convincing of a true association.

The observation that allergic sensitization and asthma were less common in children with older siblings first suggested that lower levels of infection may be a factor in affluent societies that increase the risks of asthma. This "hygiene hypothesis" proposes that lack of infections in early childhood preserves the T_H2 cell bias at birth, whereas exposure to infections and endotoxin results in a shift toward a predominant protective T_H1 immune response. Children brought up on farms who are exposed to a high level of endotoxin are less likely to develop allergic sensitization than children raised on dairy farms. Intestinal parasite infection, such as hookworm, may also be associated with a reduced risk of asthma. Although there is considerable epidemiologic support for the hygiene hypothesis, it cannot account for the parallel increase in T_H1-driven diseases such as diabetes mellitus over the same period.

Diet The role of dietary factors is controversial. Observational studies have shown that diets low in antioxidants such as vitamin C and vitamin A, magnesium, selenium, and omega-3 polyunsaturated fats (fish oil) or high in sodium and omega-6 polyunsaturated fats are associated with an increased risk of asthma. Vitamin D deficiency may also predispose to the development of asthma. However, interventional studies with supplementary diets have not supported an important role for these dietary factors. Obesity is also an independent risk factor for asthma, particularly in women, but the mechanisms are thus far unknown.

Air Pollution Air pollutants, such as sulfur dioxide, ozone, and diesel particulates, may trigger asthma symptoms, but the role of different air pollutants in the etiology of the disease is much less certain. Most evidence argues against an important role for air pollution because asthma is no more prevalent in cities with a high ambient level of traffic pollution than in rural areas with low levels of pollution. Asthma had a much lower prevalence in East Germany compared to West Germany despite a much higher level of air pollution, but since reunification, these differences have decreased as eastern Germany has become more affluent. Indoor air pollution may be more important with exposure to nitrogen oxides from cooking stoves and exposure to passive cigarette smoke. There is some evidence that maternal smoking is a risk factor for asthma, but it is difficult to dissociate this association from an increased risk of respiratory infections.

Allergens Inhaled allergens are common triggers of asthma symptoms and have also been implicated in allergic sensitization. Exposure to house dust mites in early childhood is a risk factor for allergic sensitization and asthma, but rigorous allergen avoidance has not shown any evidence for a reduced risk of developing asthma. The increase in house dust mites in centrally heated poorly ventilated homes with fitted carpets has been implicated in the increasing prevalence of asthma in affluent countries. Domestic pets, particularly cats, have also been associated with allergic sensitization, but early exposure to cats in the home may be protective through the induction of tolerance.

Occupational Exposure Occupational asthma is relatively common and may affect up to 10% of young adults. Over 300 sensitizing agents have been identified. Chemicals such as toluene diisocyanate and trimellitic anhydride, may lead to sensitization independent of atopy. Individuals may also be exposed to allergens in the workplace such as small animal allergens in laboratory workers and fungal amylase in wheat flour in bakers. Occupational asthma may be suspected when symptoms improve during weekends and holidays.

Obesity Asthma occurs more frequently in obese people (body mass index >30 kg/m^2) and is often more difficult to control. Although mechanical factors may contribute, it may also be linked to the proinflammatory adipokines and reduced anti-inflammatory adipokines that are released from fat stores.

Other Factors Several other factors have been implicated in the etiology of asthma, including lower maternal age, duration of breast-feeding, prematurity and low birthweight, and inactivity, but are unlikely to contribute to the recent global increase in asthma prevalence. There is also an association with acetaminophen (paracetamol) consumption in childhood, which may be linked to increased oxidative stress.

Intrinsic Asthma A minority of asthmatic patients (approximately 10%) have negative skin tests to common inhalant allergens and normal serum concentrations of IgE. These patients, with nonatopic or intrinsic asthma, usually show later onset of disease (adult-onset asthma), commonly have concomitant nasal polyps, and may be aspirin-sensitive. They usually have more severe, persistent asthma. Little is understood about mechanism, but the immunopathology in bronchial biopsies and sputum appears to be identical to that found in atopic asthma. There is recent evidence for increased local production of IgE in the airways, suggesting that there may be common IgE-mediated mechanisms; staphylococcal enterotoxins, which serve as "superantigens," have been implicated.

Asthma Triggers Several stimuli trigger airway narrowing, wheezing, and dyspnea in asthmatic patients. Although a previous view held that these stimuli should be avoided, the triggering of asthma by these stimuli is now seen as evidence for poor control and an indicator of the need to increase controller (preventive) therapy.

ALLERGENS Inhaled allergens activate mast cells with bound IgE directly leading to the immediate release of bronchoconstrictor mediators, resulting in the early response that is reversed by bronchodilators. Often, experimental allergen challenge is followed by a late response when there is airway edema and an acute inflammatory response with increased eosinophils and neutrophils that are not very reversible with bronchodilators. The most common allergens to trigger asthma are *Dermatophagoides* species, and environmental exposure leads to low-grade chronic symptoms that are perennial. Other perennial allergens are derived from cats and other domestic pets, as well as cockroaches. Other allergens, including grass pollen, ragweed, tree pollen, and fungal spores, are seasonal. Pollens usually cause allergic rhinitis rather than asthma, but in thunderstorms, the pollen grains are disrupted and the particles that may be released can trigger severe asthma exacerbations (thunderstorm asthma).

VIRUS INFECTIONS Upper respiratory tract virus infections such as rhinovirus, respiratory syncytial virus, and coronavirus are the most common triggers of acute severe exacerbations and may invade epithelial cells of the lower as well as the upper airways. The mechanism whereby these viruses cause exacerbations is poorly understood, but there is an increase in airway inflammation with increased numbers of eosinophils and neutrophils. There is evidence for reduced production of type I interferons by epithelial cells from asthmatic patients, resulting in increased susceptibility to these viral infections and a greater inflammatory response.

PHARMACOLOGIC AGENTS Several drugs may trigger asthma. Beta-adrenergic blockers commonly acutely worsen asthma, and their use may be fatal. The mechanisms are not clear, but are likely mediated through increased cholinergic bronchoconstriction. All β blockers need to be avoided, and even selective β_2 blockers or topical application (e.g., timolol eye drops) may be dangerous. Angiotensin-converting enzyme inhibitors are theoretically detrimental as they inhibit breakdown of kinins, which are bronchoconstrictors; however, they rarely worsen asthma, and the characteristic cough is no more frequent in asthmatics than in nonasthmatics. Aspirin may worsen asthma in some patients (aspirin-sensitive asthma is discussed below under "Special Considerations").

EXERCISE Exercise is a common trigger of asthma, particularly in children. The mechanism is linked to hyperventilation, which results in increased osmolality in airway lining fluid and triggers mast cell mediator release, resulting in bronchoconstriction. Exercise-induced asthma (EIA) typically begins after exercise has ended and resolves spontaneously within about 30 min. EIA is worse in cold, dry climates than in hot, humid conditions. It is, therefore, more common in sports activities such as cross-country running in cold weather, overland skiing, and ice hockey than in swimming. It may be prevented by prior administration of β_2-agonists and antileukotrienes, but is best prevented by regular treatment with ICSs, which reduce the population of surface mast cells required for this response.

PHYSICAL FACTORS Cold air and hyperventilation may trigger asthma through the same mechanisms as exercise. Laughter may also be a trigger. Many patients report worsening of asthma in hot weather and when the weather changes. Some asthmatics become worse when exposed to strong smells or perfumes, but the mechanism of this response is uncertain.

FOOD AND DIET There is little evidence that allergic reactions to food lead to increased asthma symptoms, despite the belief of many patients that their symptoms are triggered by particular food constituents. Exclusion diets are usually unsuccessful at reducing the frequency of episodes. Some foods such as shellfish and nuts may induce anaphylactic reactions that may include wheezing. Patients with aspirin-induced asthma may benefit from a salicylate-free diet, but these are difficult to maintain. Certain food additives may trigger asthma. Metabisulfite, which is used as a food preservative, may trigger asthma through the release of sulfur dioxide gas in the stomach. Tartrazine, a yellow food-coloring agent, was believed to be a trigger for asthma, but there is little convincing evidence for this.

AIR POLLUTION Increased ambient levels of sulfur dioxide, ozone, and nitrogen oxides are associated with increased asthma symptoms.

OCCUPATIONAL FACTORS Several substances found in the workplace may act as sensitizing agents, as discussed above, but may also act as triggers of asthma symptoms. Occupational asthma is characteristically associated with symptoms at work with relief on weekends and holidays. If removed from exposure within the first 6 months of symptoms, there is usually complete recovery. More persistent symptoms lead to irreversible airway changes, and thus, early detection and avoidance are important.

HORMONES Some women show premenstrual worsening of asthma, which can occasionally be very severe. The mechanisms are not completely understood, but are related to a fall in progesterone and in severe cases may be improved by treatment with high doses of progesterone or gonadotropin-releasing factors. Thyrotoxicosis and hypothyroidism can both worsen asthma, although the mechanisms are uncertain.

GASTROESOPHAGEAL REFLUX Gastroesophageal reflux is common in asthmatic patients because it is increased by bronchodilators. Although acid reflux might trigger reflex bronchoconstriction, it rarely causes asthma symptoms, and antireflux therapy usually fails to reduce asthma symptoms in most patients.

STRESS Many asthmatics report worsening of symptoms with stress. Psychological factors can induce bronchoconstriction through cholinergic reflex pathways. Paradoxically, very severe stress such as bereavement usually does not worsen, and may even improve, asthma symptoms.

PATHOPHYSIOLOGY

Asthma is associated with a specific chronic inflammation of the mucosa of the lower airways. One of the main aims of treatment is to reduce this inflammation.

Pathology The pathology of asthma has been revealed through examining the lungs of patients who have died of asthma and from bronchial biopsies. The airway mucosa is infiltrated with activated eosinophils and T lymphocytes, and there is activation of mucosal mast cells. The degree of inflammation is poorly related to disease severity and may even be found in atopic patients without asthma symptoms. This inflammation is usually reduced by treatment with ICS. There are also structural changes in the airways (described as remodeling). A characteristic finding is thickening of the basement membrane due to subepithelial collagen deposition. This feature is also found in patients with eosinophilic bronchitis presenting as cough who do not have asthma and is, therefore, likely to be a marker of eosinophilic inflammation in the airway as eosinophils release fibrogenic mediators. The epithelium is often shed or friable, with reduced attachments to the airway wall and increased numbers of epithelial cells in the lumen. The airway wall itself may be thickened and edematous, particularly in fatal asthma. Another common finding in fatal asthma is occlusion of the airway lumen by a mucous plug, which is comprised of mucous glycoproteins secreted from goblet cells and plasma proteins from leaky bronchial vessels (Fig. 309-1). There is also vasodilation and increased numbers of blood vessels (angiogenesis). Direct observation by bronchoscopy indicates that the airways may be narrowed, erythematous, and edematous. The pathology of asthma is remarkably uniform in different phenotypes of asthma, including atopic (extrinsic), nonatopic (intrinsic), occupational, aspirin-sensitive, and pediatric asthma. These pathologic changes are found in all airways, but do not extend to the lung parenchyma; peripheral airway inflammation is found particularly in patients with severe asthma. The involvement of airways may be patchy, and this is consistent with bronchographic findings of uneven narrowing of the airways.

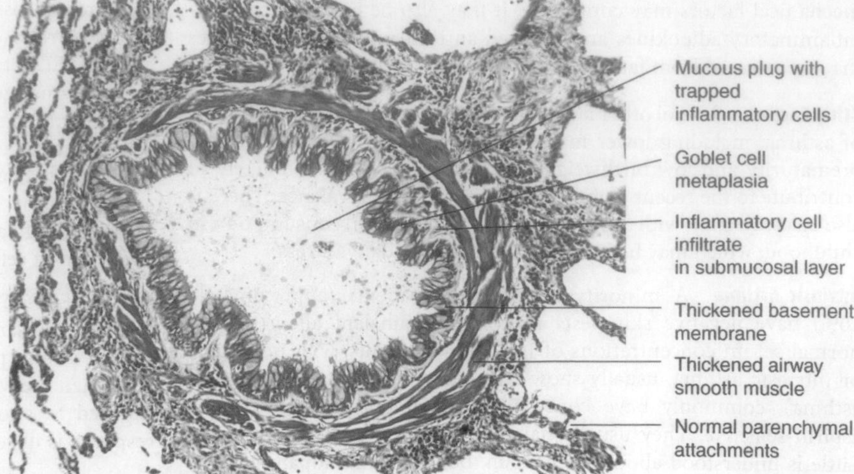

FIGURE 309-1 Histopathology of a small airway in fatal asthma. The lumen is occluded with a mucous plug, there is goblet cell metaplasia, and the airway wall is thickened, with an increase in basement membrane thickness and airway smooth muscle. *(Courtesy of Dr. J. Hogg, University of British Colombia.)*

Airway Inflammation There is inflammation in the respiratory mucosa from the trachea to terminal bronchioles, but with a predominance in the bronchi (cartilaginous airways); however, it is still uncertain as to how inflammatory cells interact and how inflammation translates into the symptoms of asthma (Fig. 309-2). There is good evidence that the specific pattern of airway inflammation in asthma is associated with airway hyperresponsiveness (AHR), the physiologic abnormality of asthma, which is correlated with variable airflow obstruction. The pattern of inflammation in asthma is characteristic of allergic diseases, with similar inflammatory cells seen in the nasal mucosa in rhinitis. However, an indistinguishable pattern of inflammation is found in intrinsic asthma, and this may reflect local rather than systemic IgE production. Although most attention has focused on the acute inflammatory changes seen in asthma, this is a chronic condition, with inflammation persisting over many years in most patients. The mechanisms involved in persistence of inflammation in asthma are still poorly understood. Superimposed on this chronic inflammatory state are acute inflammatory episodes, which correspond to exacerbations of asthma. Although the common pattern of inflammation in asthma is characterized by eosinophil infiltration, some patients with severe asthma show a neutrophilic pattern of inflammation that is less sensitive to corticosteroids. However, many inflammatory cells are involved in asthma with no key cell that is predominant (Fig. 309-3).

MAST CELLS Mast cells are important in initiating the acute bronchoconstrictor responses to allergens and several other indirectly acting stimuli, such as exercise and hyperventilation (via osmolality changes), as well as fog. Activated mucosal mast cells are found at the airway surface in asthma patients and also in the airway smooth-muscle layer, whereas this is not seen in normal subjects or patients with eosinophilic bronchitis. Mast cells are activated by allergens through an IgE-dependent mechanism, and binding of specific IgE to mast cells renders them more sensitive to activation by physical stimuli such as osmolality. The importance of IgE in the pathophysiology of asthma has been highlighted by clinical studies with humanized anti-IgE antibodies, which inhibit IgE-mediated effects, reduce asthma symptoms, and reduce exacerbations. There are, however, uncertainties about the role of mast cells in more chronic allergic inflammatory events. Mast cells release several bronchoconstrictor mediators, including histamine, prostaglandin D_2, and cysteinyl-leukotrienes, but also several cytokines, chemokines, growth factors, and neurotrophins.

MACROPHAGES AND DENDRITIC CELLS Macrophages, which are derived from blood monocytes, may traffic into the airways in asthma and may be activated by allergens via low-affinity IgE receptors ($Fc_\varepsilon RII$). Macrophages have the capacity to initiate a type of inflammatory response via the release of a certain pattern of cytokines, but these cells also release anti-inflammatory mediators (e.g., IL-10), and thus, their roles in asthma are uncertain. Dendritic cells are specialized macrophage-like cells in the airway epithelium, which are the major antigen-presenting cells. Dendritic cells take up allergens, process them to peptides, and migrate to local lymph nodes where they present the allergenic peptides to uncommitted T lymphocytes to program the production of allergen-specific T cells. Immature dendritic cells in the respiratory tract promote T_H2 cell differentiation and require cytokines, such as IL-12 and tumor necrosis factor α (TNF-α), to promote the normally preponderant T_H1 response. The cytokine thymic stromal lymphopoietin (TSLP) released from epithelial cells in asthmatic patients instructs dendritic cells to release chemokines that attract T_H2 cells into the airways.

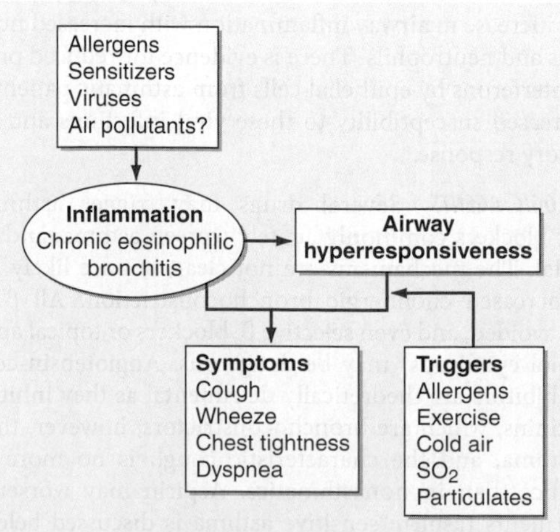

FIGURE 309-2 Inflammation in the airways of asthmatic patients leads to airway hyperresponsiveness and symptoms. SO_2, sulfur dioxide.

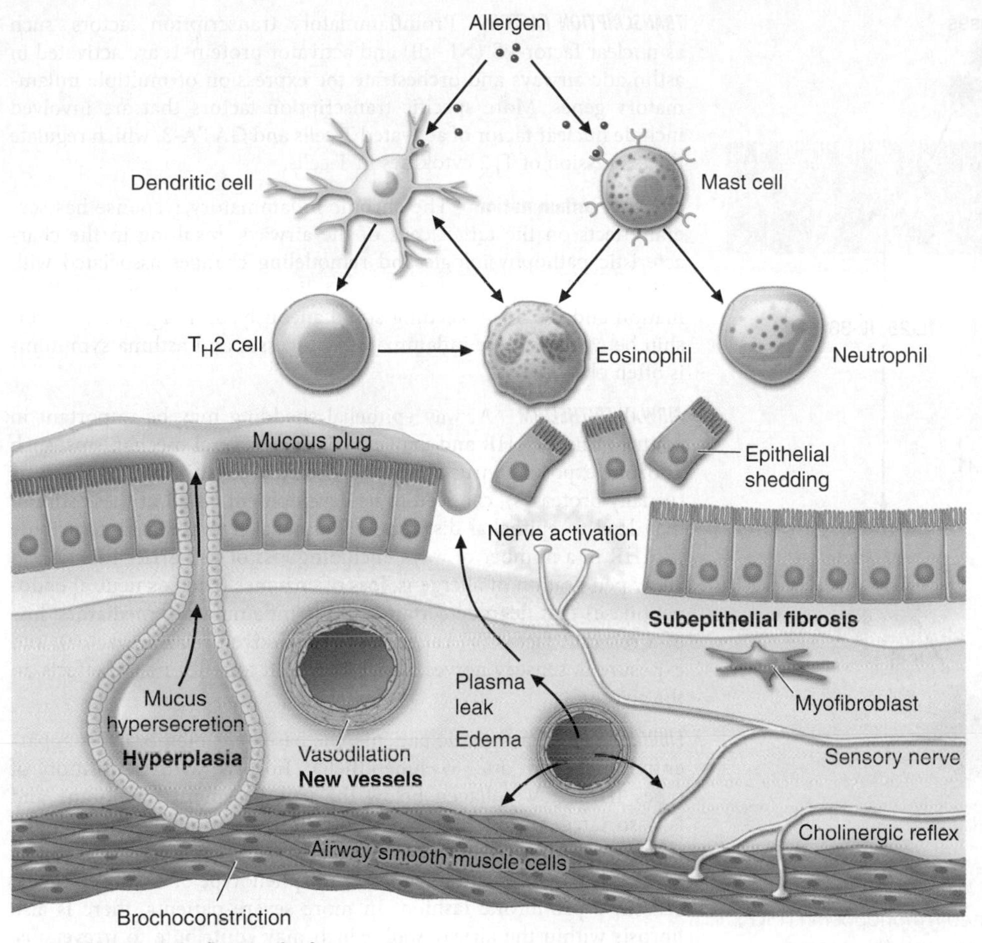

FIGURE 309-3 The pathophysiology of asthma is complex with participation of several interacting inflammatory cells, which result in acute and chronic inflammatory effects on the airway.

EOSINOPHILS Eosinophil infiltration is a characteristic feature of asthmatic airways. Allergen inhalation results in a marked increase in activated eosinophils in the airways at the time of the late reaction. Eosinophils are linked to the development of AHR through the release of basic proteins and oxygen-derived free radicals. Eosinophil recruitment involves adhesion of eosinophils to vascular endothelial cells in the airway circulation due to interaction between adhesion molecules, migration into the submucosa under the direction of chemokines, and their subsequent activation and prolonged survival. Blocking antibodies to IL-5 causes a profound and prolonged reduction in circulating and sputum eosinophils, but is not associated with reduced AHR or asthma symptoms, although in selected patients with steroid-resistant airway eosinophils, there is a reduction in exacerbations. Eosinophils may be important in release of growth factors involved in airway remodeling and in exacerbations but probably not in AHR.

NEUTROPHILS Increased numbers of activated neutrophils are found in sputum and airways of some patients with severe asthma and during exacerbations, although there is a proportion of patients even with mild or moderate asthma who have a predominance of neutrophils. The roles of neutrophils in asthma that are resistant to the anti-inflammatory effects of corticosteroids are currently unknown.

T LYMPHOCYTES T lymphocytes play a very important role in coordinating the inflammatory response in asthma through the release of specific patterns of cytokines, resulting in the recruitment and survival of eosinophils and in the maintenance of a mast cell population in the airways. The naïve immune system and the immune system of asthmatics are skewed to express the T_H2 phenotype, whereas in normal airways, T_H1 cells predominate. T_H2 cells, through the release of IL-5, are associated with eosinophilic inflammation and, through the release of IL-4 and IL-13, are associated with increased IgE formation. Recently, bronchial biopsies have demonstrated a preponderance of natural killer CD4+ T lymphocytes that express high levels of IL-4. Regulatory T cells play an important role in determining the expression of other T cells, and there is evidence for a reduction in a certain subset of regulatory T cells (CD4+CD25+) in asthma that is associated with increased T_H2 cells. Recently, innate T cells (ILC2) without T cell receptors have been identified that release T_H2 cytokines and are regulated by epithelial cytokines, such as IL-25 and IL-33.

STRUCTURAL CELLS Structural cells of the airways, including epithelial cells, fibroblasts, and airway smooth-muscle cells, are also important sources of inflammatory mediators, such as cytokines and lipid mediators, in asthma. Indeed, because structural cells far outnumber inflammatory cells, they may become the major sources of mediators driving chronic inflammation in asthmatic airways. In addition, epithelial cells may have key roles in translating inhaled environmental signals into an airway inflammatory response and are probably major target cells for ICS.

Inflammatory Mediators Multiple inflammatory mediators have been implicated in asthma, and they may have a variety of effects on the airways that account for the pathologic features of asthma (Fig. 309-4). Mediators such as histamine, prostaglandin D_2, and cysteinyl-leukotrienes contract airway smooth muscle, increase microvascular leakage, increase airway mucus secretion, and attract other inflammatory cells. Because each mediator has many effects, the role of individual mediators in the pathophysiology of asthma is not yet clear. Although the multiplicity of mediators makes it unlikely that preventing the synthesis or action of a single mediator will have a major impact in clinical asthma, recent clinical studies with antileukotrienes suggest that cysteinyl-leukotrienes have clinically important effects.

CYTOKINES Multiple cytokines regulate the chronic inflammation of asthma. The T_H2 cytokines IL-4, IL-5, and IL-13 mediate allergic inflammation, whereas proinflammatory cytokines, such as TNF-α and IL-1β, amplify the inflammatory response and play a role in more

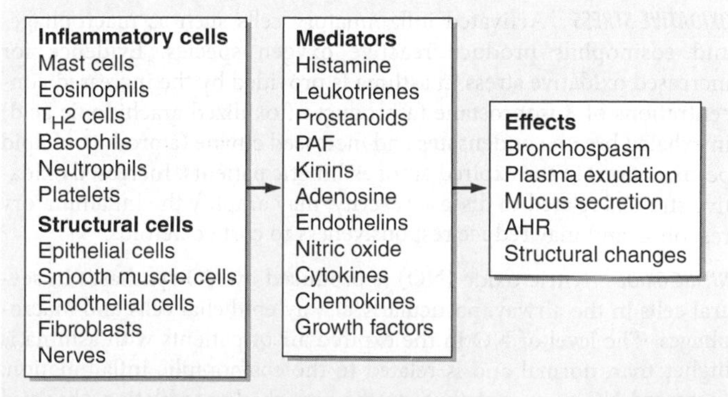

FIGURE 309-4 Many cells and mediators are involved in asthma and lead to several effects on the airways. AHR, airway hyperresponsiveness; PAF, platelet-activating factor.

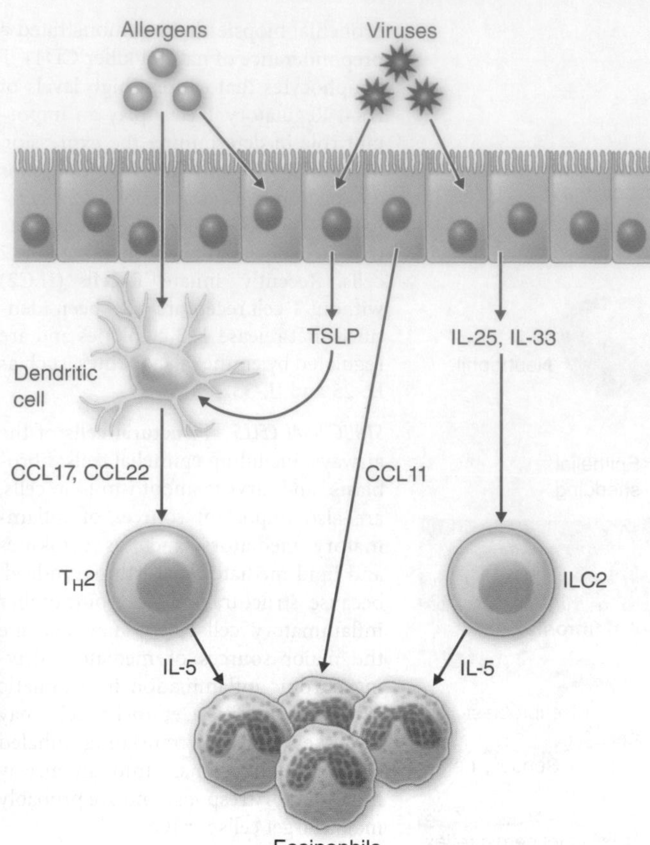

FIGURE 309-5 T lymphocytes in asthma. Allergen interacts with dendritic cells and releases thymus stimulated lymphopoeitin (TSLP), which stimulates activated dendritic cells to release the chemokines CCL17 and CCL22, which attract T helper 2 (T_H2) lymphocytes. Allergens and viral infection may release interleukin (IL)-25 and -33, which recruit and activate type 2 innate lymphoid cells (ILC2). Both T_H2 and ILC2 cells release IL-5 and epithelial cells release CCL11 (eotaxin), which together lead to recruitment of eosinophils into the airways.

severe disease. TSLP is an upstream cytokine released from epithelial cells of asthmatics that orchestrates the release of chemokines that selectively attract T_H2 cells. Some cytokines such as IL-10 and IL-12 are anti-inflammatory and may be deficient in asthma.

CHEMOKINES Chemokines are involved in attracting inflammatory cells from the bronchial circulation into the airways. Eotaxin (CCL11) is selectively attractant to eosinophils via CCR3 and is expressed by epithelial cells of asthmatics, whereas CCL17 (TARC) and CCL22 (MDC) from epithelial cells attract T_H2 cells via CCR4 (Fig. 309-5).

OXIDATIVE STRESS Activated inflammatory cells such as macrophages and eosinophils produce reactive oxygen species. Evidence for increased oxidative stress in asthma is provided by the increased concentrations of 8-isoprostane (a product of oxidized arachidonic acid) in exhaled breath condensates and increased ethane (a product of lipid peroxidation) in the expired air of asthmatic patients. Increased oxidative stress is related to disease severity, may amplify the inflammatory response, and may reduce responsiveness to corticosteroids.

NITRIC OXIDE Nitric oxide (NO) is produced by NO synthases in several cells in the airway, particularly airway epithelial cells and macrophages. The level of NO in the expired air of patients with asthma is higher than normal and is related to the eosinophilic inflammation. Increased NO may contribute to the bronchial vasodilation observed in asthma. Fractional exhaled NO (F_ENO) is increasingly used in the diagnosis and monitoring of asthmatic inflammation, although it is not yet used routinely in clinical practice.

TRANSCRIPTION FACTORS Proinflammatory transcription factors, such as nuclear factor-κB (NF-κB) and activator protein-1, are activated in asthmatic airways and orchestrate the expression of multiple inflammatory genes. More specific transcription factors that are involved include nuclear factor of activated T cells and GATA-3, which regulate the expression of T_H2 cytokines in T cells.

Effects of Inflammation The chronic inflammatory response has several effects on the target cells of the airways, resulting in the characteristic pathophysiologic and remodeling changes associated with asthma. Asthma may be regarded as a disease with continuous inflammation and repair proceeding simultaneously, although the relationship between chronic inflammatory processes and asthma symptoms is often obscure.

AIRWAY EPITHELIUM Airway epithelial shedding may be important in contributing to AHR and may explain how several mechanisms, such as ozone exposure, virus infections, chemical sensitizers, and allergens (usually proteases), can lead to its development, as all of these stimuli may lead to epithelial disruption. Epithelial damage may contribute to AHR in a number of ways, including loss of its barrier function to allow penetration of allergens; loss of enzymes (such as neutral endopeptidase) that degrade certain peptide inflammatory mediators; loss of a relaxant factor (so called epithelial-derived relaxant factor); and exposure of sensory nerves, which may lead to reflex neural effects on the airway.

FIBROSIS In all asthmatic patients, the basement membrane is apparently thickened due to subepithelial fibrosis with deposition of types III and V collagen below the true basement membrane and is associated with eosinophil infiltration, presumably through the release of profibrotic mediators such as transforming growth factor-β. Mechanical manipulations can alter the phenotype of airway epithelial cells in a profibrotic fashion. In more severe patients, there is also fibrosis within the airway wall, which may contribute to irreversible narrowing of the airways.

AIRWAY SMOOTH MUSCLE In vitro airway smooth muscle from asthmatic patients usually shows no increased responsiveness to constrictors. Reduced responsiveness to β-agonists has also been reported in postmortem or surgically removed bronchi from asthmatics, although the number of β-receptors is not reduced, suggesting that β-receptors have been uncoupled. These abnormalities of airway smooth muscle may be secondary to the chronic inflammatory process. Inflammatory mediators may modulate the ion channels that serve to regulate the resting membrane potential of airway smooth-muscle cells, thus altering the level of excitability of these cells. In asthmatic airways there is also a characteristic hypertrophy and hyperplasia of airway smooth muscle, which is presumably the result of stimulation of airway smooth-muscle cells by various growth factors such as platelet-derived growth factor (PDGF) or endothelin-1 released from inflammatory or epithelial cells.

VASCULAR RESPONSES There is increased airway mucosal blood flow in asthma, which may contribute to airway narrowing. There is an increase in the number of blood vessels in asthmatic airways as a result of angiogenesis in response to growth factors, particularly vascular endothelial growth factor. Microvascular leakage from postcapillary venules in response to inflammatory mediators is observed in asthma, resulting in airway edema and plasma exudation into the airway lumen.

MUCUS HYPERSECRETION Increased mucus secretion contributes to the viscid mucous plugs that occlude asthmatic airways, particularly in fatal asthma. There is hyperplasia of submucosal glands that are confined to large airways and of increased numbers of epithelial goblet cells. IL-13 induces mucus hypersecretion in experimental models of asthma.

NEURAL REGULATION Various defects in autonomic neural control may contribute to AHR in asthma, but these are likely to be secondary to the disease, rather than primary defects. Cholinergic pathways, through the release of acetylcholine acting on muscarinic receptors, cause bronchoconstriction and may be activated reflexly in asthma.

Inflammatory mediators may activate sensory nerves, resulting in reflex cholinergic bronchoconstriction or release of inflammatory neuropeptides. Inflammatory products may also sensitize sensory nerve endings in the airway epithelium such that the nerves become hyperalgesic. Neurotrophins, which may be released from various cell types in airways, including epithelial cells and mast cells, may cause proliferation and sensitization of airway sensory nerves. Airway nerves may also release neurotransmitters, such as substance P, which have inflammatory effects.

Airway Remodeling Several changes in the structure of the airway are characteristically found in asthma, and these may lead to irreversible narrowing of the airways. Population studies have shown a greater decline in lung function over time than in normal subjects; however, most patients with asthma preserve normal or near-normal lung function throughout life if appropriately treated.

The accelerated decline in lung function occurs in a smaller proportion of asthmatics, and these are usually patients with more severe disease. There is some evidence that the early use of ICS may reduce the decline in lung function. The characteristic structural changes are increased airway smooth muscle, fibrosis, angiogenesis, and mucus hyperplasia.

Physiology Limitation of airflow is due mainly to bronchoconstriction, but airway edema, vascular congestion, and luminal occlusion with exudate may contribute. This results in a reduction in forced expiratory volume in 1 second (FEV_1), FEV_1/forced vital capacity (FVC) ratio, and peak expiratory flow (PEF), as well as an increase in airway resistance. Early closure of peripheral airway results in lung hyperinflation (air trapping) and increased residual volume, particularly during acute exacerbations and in severe persistent asthma. In more severe asthma, reduced ventilation and increased pulmonary blood flow result in mismatching of ventilation and perfusion and in bronchial hyperemia. Ventilatory failure is very uncommon, even in patients with severe asthma, and arterial PCO_2 tends to be low due to increased ventilation.

Airway Hyperresponsiveness AHR is the characteristic physiologic abnormality of asthma and describes the excessive bronchoconstrictor response to multiple inhaled triggers that would have no effect on normal airways. The increase in AHR is linked to the frequency of asthma symptoms, and, thus, an important aim of therapy is to reduce AHR. Increased bronchoconstrictor responsiveness is seen with *direct* bronchoconstrictors such as histamine and methacholine, which contract airway smooth muscle, but is characteristically also seen with many *indirect* stimuli, which release bronchoconstrictors from mast cells or activate sensory nerves. Most of the triggers for asthma symptoms appear to act indirectly, including allergens, exercise, hyperventilation, fog (via mast cell activation), irritant dusts, and sulfur dioxide (via a cholinergic reflex).

CLINICAL FEATURES AND DIAGNOSIS

The characteristic symptoms of asthma are wheezing, dyspnea, and coughing, which are variable, both spontaneously and with therapy. Symptoms may be worse at night, and patients typically awake in the early morning hours. Patients may report difficulty in filling their lungs with air. There is increased mucus production in some patients, with typically tenacious mucus that is difficult to expectorate. There may be increased ventilation and use of accessory muscles of ventilation. Prodromal symptoms may precede an attack, with itching under the chin, discomfort between the scapulae, or inexplicable fear (impending doom).

Typical physical signs are inspiratory, and to a greater extent expiratory, rhonchi throughout the chest, and there may be hyperinflation. Some patients, particularly children, may present with a predominant nonproductive cough (cough-variant asthma). There may be no abnormal physical findings when asthma is under control.

DIAGNOSIS

The diagnosis of asthma is usually apparent from the symptoms of variable and intermittent airways obstruction, but must be confirmed by objective measurements of lung function.

Lung Function Tests Simple spirometry confirms airflow limitation with a reduced FEV_1, FEV_1/FVC ratio, and PEF (Fig. 309-6). Reversibility is demonstrated by a >12% and 200-mL increase in FEV_1 15 min after an inhaled short-acting β_2-agonist or in some patients by a 2- to 4-week trial of oral corticosteroids (OCS) (prednisone or prednisolone 30–40 mg daily). Measurements of PEF twice daily may confirm the diurnal variations in airflow obstruction. Flow-volume loops show reduced peak flow and reduced maximum expiratory flow. Further lung function tests are rarely necessary, but whole-body plethysmography shows increased airway resistance and may show increased total lung capacity and residual volume. Gas diffusion is usually normal, but there may be a small increase in gas transfer in some patients.

Airway Responsiveness The increased AHR is normally measured by methacholine or histamine challenge with calculation of the provocative concentration that reduces FEV_1 by 20% (PC_{20}). This is rarely useful in clinical practice, but can be used in the differential diagnosis of chronic cough and when the diagnosis is in doubt in the setting of normal pulmonary function tests. Occasionally exercise testing is done to demonstrate the postexercise bronchoconstriction if there is a predominant history of EIA. Allergen challenge is rarely necessary and should only be undertaken by a specialist if specific occupational agents are to be identified.

Hematologic Tests Blood tests are not usually helpful. Total serum IgE and specific IgE to inhaled allergens (radioallergosorbent test [RAST]) may be measured in some patients.

Imaging Chest roentgenography is usually normal but in more severe patients may show hyperinflated lungs. In exacerbations, there may be evidence of a pneumothorax. Lung shadowing usually indicates pneumonia or eosinophilic infiltrates in patients with bronchopulmonary aspergillosis. High-resolution computed tomography (CT) may show areas of bronchiectasis in patients with severe asthma, and there may be thickening of the bronchial walls, but these changes are not diagnostic of asthma.

Skin Tests Skin prick tests to common inhalant allergens (house dust mite, cat fur, grass pollen) are positive in allergic asthma and negative

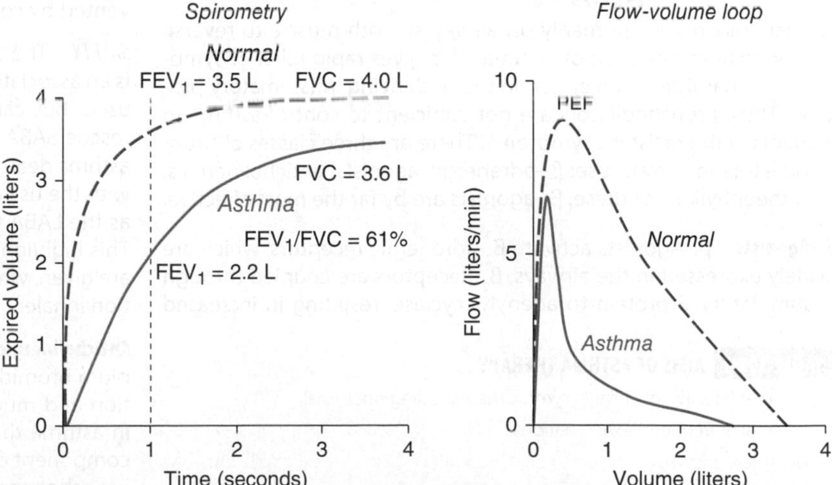

FIGURE 309-6 Spirometry and flow-volume loop in asthmatic compared to normal subject. There is a reduction in forced expiratory volume in 1 second (FEV_1) but less reduction in forced vital capacity (FVC), giving a reduced FEV_1/FVC ratio (<70%). The flow-volume loop shows reduced peak expiratory flow and a typical scalloped appearance indicating widespread airflow obstruction.

in intrinsic asthma, but are not helpful in diagnosis. Positive skin responses may be useful in persuading patients to undertake allergen avoidance measures.

Exhaled Nitric Oxide F_ENO is now being used as a noninvasive test to measure airway inflammation. The typically elevated levels in asthma are reduced by ICS, so this may be a test of compliance with therapy. It may also be useful in demonstrating insufficient anti-inflammatory therapy and may be useful in down-titrating ICS. However, studies in unselected patients have not convincingly demonstrated improved clinical outcomes, and it may be necessary to select patients who are poorly controlled.

Differential Diagnosis It is usually not difficult to differentiate asthma from other conditions that cause wheezing and dyspnea. Upper airway obstruction by a tumor or laryngeal edema can mimic severe asthma, but patients typically present with stridor localized to large airways. The diagnosis is confirmed by a flow-volume loop that shows a reduction in inspiratory as well as expiratory flow, and bronchoscopy to demonstrate the site of upper airway narrowing. Persistent wheezing in a specific area of the chest may indicate endobronchial obstruction with a foreign body. Left ventricular failure may mimic the wheezing of asthma, but basilar crackles are present in contrast to asthma. Vocal chord dysfunction may mimic asthma and is thought to be an hysterical conversion syndrome.

Eosinophilic pneumonias and systemic vasculitis, including Churg-Strauss syndrome and polyarteritis nodosa, may be associated with wheezing. Chronic obstructive pulmonary disease (COPD) is usually easy to differentiate from asthma as symptoms show less variability, never completely remit, and show much less (or no) reversibility to bronchodilators. Approximately 10% of COPD patients have features of asthma, with increased sputum eosinophils and a response to OCSs; these patients probably have both diseases concomitantly.

TREATMENT ASTHMA

The treatment of asthma is straightforward, and the majority of patients are now managed by internists and family doctors with effective and safe therapies. There are several aims of therapy (Table 309-2). Most emphasis has been placed on drug therapy, but several nonpharmacologic approaches have also been used. The main drugs for asthma can be divided into bronchodilators, which give rapid relief of symptoms mainly through relaxation of airway smooth muscle, and controllers, which inhibit the underlying inflammatory process.

BRONCHODILATOR THERAPIES

Bronchodilators act primarily on airway smooth muscle to reverse the bronchoconstriction of asthma. This gives rapid relief of symptoms but has little or no effect on the underlying inflammatory process. Thus, bronchodilators are not sufficient to control asthma in patients with persistent symptoms. There are three classes of bronchodilators in current use: β_2-adrenergic agonists, anticholinergics, and theophylline; of these, β_2-agonists are by far the most effective.

β_2-Agonists β_2-Agonists activate β_2-adrenergic receptors, which are widely expressed in the airways. β_2-Receptors are coupled through a stimulatory G protein to adenylyl cyclase, resulting in increased intracellular cyclic adenosine monophosphate (AMP), which relaxes smooth-muscle cells and inhibits certain inflammatory cells, particularly mast cells.

MODE OF ACTION The primary action of β_2-agonists is to relax airway smooth-muscle cells of all airways, where they act as functional antagonists, reversing and preventing contraction of airway smooth-muscle cells by all known bronchoconstrictors. This generalized action is likely to account for their great efficacy as bronchodilators in asthma. There are also additional nonbronchodilator effects that may be clinically useful, including inhibition of mast cell mediator release, reduction in plasma exudation, and inhibition of sensory nerve activation. Inflammatory cells express small numbers of β_2-receptors, but these are rapidly downregulated with β_2-agonist activation so that, in contrast to corticosteroids, there are no effects on inflammatory cells in the airways and there is no reduction in AHR.

CLINICAL USE β_2-Agonists are usually given by inhalation to reduce side effects. Short-acting β_2-agonists (SABAs) such as albuterol and terbutaline have a duration of action of 3–6 h. They have a rapid onset of bronchodilatation and are, therefore, used as needed for symptom relief. Increased use of SABA indicates that asthma is not controlled. They are also useful in preventing EIA if taken prior to exercise. SABAs are used in high doses by nebulizer or via a metered-dose inhaler with a spacer. Long-acting β_2-agonists (LABAs) include salmeterol and formoterol, both of which have a duration of action over 12 h and are given twice daily by inhalation; indacaterol is given once daily. LABAs have replaced the regular use of SABAs, but LABAs should not be given in the absence of ICS therapy because they do not control the underlying inflammation. They do, however, improve asthma control and reduce exacerbations when added to ICS, which allows asthma to be controlled at lower doses of corticosteroids. This observation has led to the widespread use of fixed-combination inhalers that contain a corticosteroid and a LABA, which have proved to be highly effective in the control of asthma.

SIDE EFFECTS Adverse effects are not usually a problem with β_2-agonists when given by inhalation. The most common side effects are muscle tremor and palpitations, which are seen more commonly in elderly patients. There is a small fall in plasma potassium due to increased uptake by skeletal muscle cells, but this effect does not usually cause any clinical problem.

TOLERANCE Tolerance is a potential problem with any agonist given chronically, but although there is downregulation of β_2-receptors, this does not reduce the bronchodilator response because there is a large receptor reserve in airway smooth-muscle cells. By contrast, mast cells become rapidly tolerant, but their tolerance may be prevented by concomitant administration of ICS.

SAFETY The safety of β_2-agonists has been an important issue. There is an association between asthma mortality and the amount of SABA used, but careful analysis demonstrates that the increased use of rescue SABA reflects poor asthma control, which is a risk factor for asthma death. The slight excess in mortality that has been associated with the use of LABA is related to the lack of use of concomitant ICS, as the LABA therapy fails to suppress the underlying inflammation. This highlights the importance of always using an ICS when LABAs are given, which is most conveniently achieved by using a combination inhaler.

Anticholinergics Muscarinic receptor antagonists such as ipratropium bromide prevent cholinergic nerve-induced bronchoconstriction and mucus secretion. They are less effective than β_2-agonists in asthma therapy because they inhibit only the cholinergic reflex component of bronchoconstriction, whereas β_2-agonists prevent all bronchoconstrictor mechanisms. Anticholinergics, including once-daily tiotropium bromide, may be used as an additional bronchodilator in patients with asthma that is not controlled by ICS and LABA combinations. High doses may be given by nebulizer in treating acute severe asthma but should only be given following β_2-agonists, because they have a slower onset of bronchodilatation.

TABLE 309-2 AIMS OF ASTHMA THERAPY

- Minimal (ideally no) chronic symptoms, including nocturnal
- Minimal (infrequent) exacerbations
- No emergency visits
- Minimal (ideally no) use of a required β_2-agonist
- No limitations on activities, including exercise
- Peak expiratory flow circadian variation <20%
- (Near) normal peak expiratory flow
- Minimal (or no) adverse effects from medicine

Side effects are not usually a problem because there is little or no systemic absorption. The most common side effect is dry mouth; in elderly patients, urinary retention and glaucoma may also be observed.

Theophylline Theophylline was widely prescribed as an oral bronchodilator several years ago, especially because it was inexpensive. It has now fallen out of favor because side effects are common and inhaled β_2-agonists are much more effective as bronchodilators. The bronchodilator effect is due to inhibition of phosphodiesterases in airway smooth-muscle cells, which increases cyclic AMP, but doses required for bronchodilatation commonly cause side effects that are mediated mainly by phosphodiesterase inhibition. There is increasing evidence that theophylline at lower doses has anti-inflammatory effects, and these are likely to be mediated through different molecular mechanisms. Theophylline activates the key nuclear enzyme histone deacetylase-2 (HDAC2), which is a critical mechanism for switching off activated inflammatory genes and may, therefore, reduce corticosteroid insensitivity in severe asthma.

CLINICAL USE Oral theophylline is usually given as a slow-release preparation once or twice daily because this gives more stable plasma concentrations than normal theophylline tablets. It may be used as an additional bronchodilator in patients with severe asthma when plasma concentrations of 10–20 mg/L are required, although these concentrations are often associated with side effects. Low doses of theophylline, giving plasma concentrations of 5–10 mg/L, have additive effects to ICS and are particularly useful in patients with severe asthma. Indeed, withdrawal of theophylline from these patients may result in marked deterioration in asthma control. At low doses, the drug is well tolerated. IV aminophylline (a soluble salt of theophylline) was used for the treatment of severe asthma but has now been largely replaced by high doses of inhaled SABA, which are more effective and have fewer side effects. Aminophylline is occasionally used (via slow IV infusion) in patients with severe exacerbations that are refractory to SABA.

SIDE EFFECTS Oral theophylline is well absorbed and is largely inactivated in the liver. Side effects are related to plasma concentrations; measurement of plasma theophylline may be useful in determining the correct dose. The most common side effects are nausea, vomiting, and headaches and are due to phosphodiesterase inhibition. Diuresis and palpitations may also occur, and at high concentrations, cardiac arrhythmias, epileptic seizures, and death may occur due to adenosine A_1-receptor antagonism. Theophylline side effects are related to plasma concentration and are rarely observed at plasma concentrations below 10 mg/L. Theophylline is metabolized by CYP450 in the liver, and thus, plasma concentrations may be elevated by drugs that block CYP450 such as erythromycin and allopurinol. Other drugs may also reduce clearance by other mechanisms leading to increased plasma concentrations (Table 309-3).

TABLE 309-3 FACTORS AFFECTING CLEARANCE OF THEOPHYLLINE

Increased Clearance
• Enzyme induction (rifampicin, phenobarbitone, ethanol)
• Smoking (tobacco, marijuana)
• High-protein, low-carbohydrate diet
• Barbecued meat
• Childhood
Decreased Clearance
• Enzyme inhibition (cimetidine, erythromycin, ciprofloxacin, allopurinol, zileuton, zafirlukast)
• Congestive heart failure
• Liver disease
• Pneumonia
• Viral infection and vaccination
• High-carbohydrate diet
• Old age

CONTROLLER THERAPIES

Inhaled Corticosteroids ICSs are by far the most effective controllers for asthma, and their early use has revolutionized asthma therapy.

MODE OF ACTION ICSs are the most effective anti-inflammatory agents used in asthma therapy, reducing inflammatory cell numbers and their activation in the airways. ICSs reduce eosinophils in the airways and sputum and the numbers of activated T lymphocytes and surface mast cells in the airway mucosa. These effects may account for the reduction in AHR that is seen with chronic ICS therapy.

The molecular mechanism of action of corticosteroids involves several effects on the inflammatory process. The major effect of corticosteroids is to switch off the transcription of multiple activated genes that encode inflammatory proteins such as cytokines, chemokines, adhesion molecules, and inflammatory enzymes. This effect involves several mechanisms, including inhibition of the transcription factor NF-κB, but an important mechanism is recruitment of HDAC2 to the inflammatory gene complex, which reverses the histone acetylation associated with increased gene transcription. Corticosteroids also activate anti-inflammatory genes, such as mitogen-activated protein (MAP) kinase phosphatase-1, and increase the expression of β_2-receptors. Most of the metabolic and endocrine side effects of corticosteroids are also mediated through transcriptional activation.

CLINICAL USE ICSs are by far the most effective controllers in the management of asthma and are beneficial in treating asthma of any severity and age. ICSs are usually given twice daily, but some may be effective once daily in mildly symptomatic patients. ICSs rapidly improve the symptoms of asthma, and lung function improves over several days. They are effective in preventing asthma symptoms, such as EIA and nocturnal exacerbations, but also prevent severe exacerbations. ICSs reduce AHR, but maximal improvement may take several months of therapy. Early treatment with ICS appears to prevent irreversible changes in airway function that occur with chronic asthma. Withdrawal of ICS results in slow deterioration of asthma control, indicating that they suppress inflammation and symptoms, but do not cure the underlying condition. ICSs are now given as first-line therapy for patients with persistent asthma, but if they do not control symptoms at low doses, it is usual to add a LABA as the next step.

SIDE EFFECTS Local side effects include hoarseness (dysphonia) and oral candidiasis, which may be reduced with the use of a large-volume spacer device. There has been concern about systemic side effects from lung absorption, but many studies have demonstrated that ICS have minimal systemic effects (Fig. 309-7). At the highest recommended doses, there may be some suppression of plasma and urinary cortisol concentrations, but there is no convincing evidence that long-term treatment leads to impaired growth in children or to osteoporosis in adults. Indeed effective control of asthma with ICS reduces the number of courses of OCS that are needed and, thus, reduces systemic exposure to ICS.

Systemic Corticosteroids Corticosteroids are used intravenously (hydrocortisone or methylprednisolone) for the treatment of acute severe asthma, although several studies now show that OCSs are as effective and easier to administer. A course of OCS (usually prednisone or prednisolone 30–45 mg once daily for 5–10 days) is used to treat acute exacerbations of asthma; no tapering of the dose is needed. Approximately 1% of asthma patients may require maintenance treatment with OCS; the lowest dose necessary to maintain control needs to be determined. Systemic side effects, including truncal obesity, bruising, osteoporosis, diabetes, hypertension, gastric ulceration, proximal myopathy, depression, and cataracts, may be a major problem, and steroid-sparing therapies may be considered if side effects are a significant problem. If patients require maintenance treatment with OCS, it is important to monitor bone density so that preventive treatment with bisphosphonates or estrogen in postmenopausal women may be initiated if bone density is low.

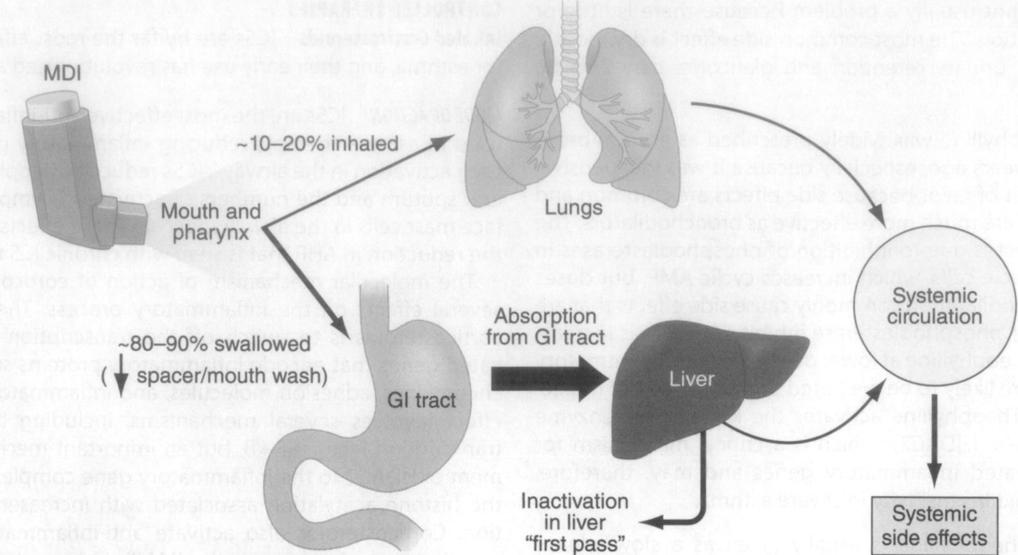

FIGURE 309-7 Pharmacokinetics of inhaled corticosteroids. GI, gastrointestinal; MDI, metered-dose inhaler.

Intramuscular triamcinolone acetonide is a depot preparation that is occasionally used in noncompliant patients, but proximal myopathy is a major problem with this therapy.

Antileukotrienes Cysteinyl-leukotrienes are potent bronchoconstrictors, cause microvascular leakage, and increase eosinophilic inflammation through the activation of cys-LT_1-receptors. These inflammatory mediators are produced predominantly by mast cells and, to a lesser extent, eosinophils in asthma. Antileukotrienes, such as montelukast, block cys-LT_1-receptors and provide modest clinical benefit in asthma. They are less effective than ICS in controlling asthma and have less effect on airway inflammation, but are useful as an add-on therapy in some patients not controlled with low doses of ICS, although less effective than LABA. They are given orally once or twice daily and are well tolerated. Some patients show a better response than others to antileukotrienes, but this has not been convincingly linked to any genomic differences in the leukotriene pathway.

Cromones Cromolyn sodium and nedocromil sodium are asthma controller drugs that appear to inhibit mast cell and sensory nerve activation and are, therefore, effective in blocking trigger-induced asthma such as EIA and allergen- and sulfur dioxide–induced symptoms. Cromones have relatively little benefit in the long-term control of asthma due to their short duration of action (at least four times daily by inhalation). They are very safe and were popular in the treatment of childhood asthma, although now low doses of ICS are preferred because they are more effective and have a proven safety profile.

Steroid-Sparing Therapies Various immunomodulatory treatments have been used to reduce the requirement for OCS in patients with severe asthma who have serious side effects with this therapy. Methotrexate, cyclosporin A, azathioprine, gold, and IV gamma globulin have all been used as steroid-sparing therapies, but none of these treatments has any long-term benefit, and each is associated with a relatively high risk of side effects.

Anti-IgE Omalizumab is a blocking antibody that neutralizes circulating IgE without binding to cell-bound IgE and, thus, inhibits IgE-mediated reactions. This treatment has been shown to reduce the number of exacerbations in patients with severe asthma and may improve asthma control. However, the treatment is very expensive and is only suitable for highly selected patients who are not controlled on maximal doses of inhaler therapy and have a circulating IgE within a specified range. Patients should be given a 3- to 4-month trial of therapy to show objective benefit. Omalizumab is usually given as a subcutaneous injection every 2–4 weeks and appears not to have significant side effects, although anaphylaxis is very occasionally seen.

Immunotherapy Specific immunotherapy using injected extracts of pollens or house dust mites has not been very effective in controlling asthma and may cause anaphylaxis. Side effects may be reduced by sublingual dosing. It is not recommended in most asthma treatment guidelines because of lack of evidence of clinical efficacy.

Alternative Therapies Nonpharmacologic treatments, including hypnosis, acupuncture, chiropraxis, breathing control, yoga, and speleotherapy, may be popular with some patients. However, placebo-controlled studies have shown that each of these treatments lacks efficacy and cannot be recommended. However, they are not detrimental and may be used as long as conventional pharmacologic therapy is continued.

Future Therapies It has proved very difficult to discover novel pharmaceutical therapies, particularly because current therapy with corticosteroids and β_2-agonists is so effective in the majority of patients. There is, however, a need for the development of new therapies for patients with refractory asthma who have side effects with systemic corticosteroids. Antagonists of specific mediators have little or no benefit in asthma, apart from antileukotrienes, which have rather weak effects, presumably reflecting the fact that multiple mediators are involved. Blocking antibodies against IL-5 may reduce exacerbations in highly selected patients who have sputum eosinophils despite high doses of corticosteroids, whereas anti-TNF-α antibodies are not effective in severe asthma. Novel anti-inflammatory treatments that are in clinical development include inhibitors of phosphodiesterase-4, NF-κB, and p38 MAP kinase. However, these drugs, which act on signal transduction pathways common to many cells, are likely to have troublesome side effects, necessitating their delivery by inhalation. Safer and more effective immunotherapy using T cell peptide fragments of allergens or DNA vaccination is also being investigated. Bacterial products, such as CpG oligonucleotides that stimulate T_H1 immunity or regulatory T cells, are also currently under evaluation.

MANAGEMENT OF CHRONIC ASTHMA

There are several aims of chronic therapy in asthma (Table 309-2). It is important to establish the diagnosis objectively using spirometry or PEF measurements at home. Triggers that worsen asthma control, such as allergens or occupational agents, should be avoided, whereas triggers, such as exercise and fog, which result in transient symptoms, provide an indication that more controller therapy is needed. It is important to assess asthma control, determined by

TABLE 309-4 ASTHMA CONTROL

Characteristic	Controlled (all of the following)	Partly Controlled	Uncontrolled
Daytime symptoms	None (≤2/week)	>2/week	Three or more features of partly controlled
Limitation of activities	None	Any	
Nocturnal symptoms/awakening	None	Any	
Need for reliever/rescue treatment	None (≤2/week)	>2/week	
Lung function (PEF or FEV_1)	Normal	<80% predicted or personal best (if known)	

Abbreviations: FEV_1, forced expiratory volume in 1 s; PEF, peak expiratory flow.

symptoms, night awakening, need for reliever inhalers, limitation of activity, and lung function (Table 309-4). Avoidance of side effects and expense of medications are also important. There are several validated questionnaires for quantifying asthma control, such as the Asthma Quality of Life Questionnaire (AQLQ) and Asthma Control Test (ACT).

Stepwise Therapy For patients with mild, intermittent asthma, a short-acting β_2-agonist is all that is required (Fig. 309-8). However, use of a reliever medication more than twice a week indicates the need for regular controller therapy. The treatment of choice for all patients is an ICS given twice daily. It is usual to start with an intermediate dose (e.g., 200 μg bid of beclomethasone dipropionate [BDP]) or equivalent and to decrease the dose if symptoms are controlled after 3 months. If symptoms are not controlled, a LABA should be added, which is most conveniently given by switching to a combination inhaler. The dose of controller should be adjusted accordingly, as judged by the need for a rescue inhaler. Low doses of theophylline or an antileukotriene may also be considered as an add-on therapy, but these are less effective than LABA. In patients with severe asthma, low-dose oral theophylline is also helpful, and when there is irreversible airway narrowing, the long-acting anticholinergic tiotropium bromide may be tried. If asthma is not controlled despite the maximal recommended dose of inhaled therapy, it is important to check compliance and inhaler technique. In these patients, maintenance treatment with an OCS may be needed, and the lowest dose that maintains control should be used. Occasionally omalizumab may be tried in steroid-dependent asthmatics who are not well controlled. Once asthma is controlled, it is important to slowly decrease therapy in order to find the optimal dose to control symptoms.

Education Patients with asthma need to understand how to use their medications and the difference between reliever and controller therapies. Education may improve compliance, particularly with ICS. All patients should be taught how to use their inhalers correctly. In particular, they need to understand how to recognize worsening of asthma and how to step up therapy. Written action plans have been shown to reduce hospital admissions and morbidity rates in adults and children, and are recommended particularly in patients with unstable disease who have frequent exacerbations.

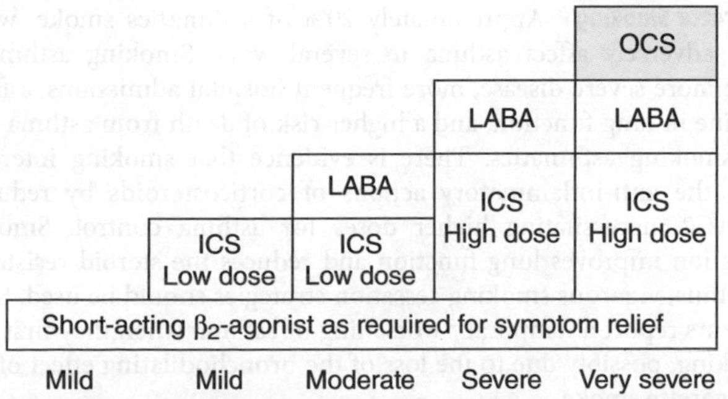

FIGURE 309-8 Stepwise approach to asthma therapy according to the severity of asthma and ability to control symptoms. ICS, inhaled corticosteroids; LABA, long-acting β_2-agonist; OCS, oral corticosteroid.

ACUTE SEVERE ASTHMA

Exacerbations of asthma are feared by patients and may be life threatening. One of the main aims of controller therapy is to prevent exacerbations; in this respect, ICS and combination inhalers are very effective.

Clinical Features Patients are aware of increasing chest tightness, wheezing, and dyspnea that are often not or poorly relieved by their usual reliever inhaler. In severe exacerbations, patients may be so breathless that they are unable to complete sentences and may become cyanotic. Examination usually shows increased ventilation, hyperinflation, and tachycardia. Pulsus paradoxus may be present, but this is rarely a useful clinical sign. There is a marked fall in spirometric values and PEF. Arterial blood gases on air show hypoxemia, and PCO_2 is usually low due to hyperventilation. A normal or rising PCO_2 is an indication of impending respiratory failure and requires immediate monitoring and therapy. A chest roentgenogram is not usually informative but may show pneumonia or pneumothorax.

TREATMENT ACUTE SEVERE ASTHMA

A high concentration of oxygen should be given by face mask to achieve oxygen saturation of >90%. The mainstay of treatment are high doses of SABA given either by nebulizer or via a metered-dose inhaler with a spacer. In severely ill patients with impending respiratory failure, IV β_2-agonists may be given. A nebulized anticholinergic may be added if there is not a satisfactory response to β_2-agonists alone, as there are additive effects. In patients who are refractory to inhaled therapies, a slow infusion of aminophylline may be effective, but it is important to monitor blood levels, especially if patients have already been treated with oral theophylline. Magnesium sulfate given intravenously or by nebulizer is effective when added to inhaled β_2-agonists, and is relatively well tolerated but is not routinely recommended. Prophylactic intubation may be indicated for impending respiratory failure, when the PCO_2 is normal or rises. For patients with respiratory failure, it is necessary to intubate and institute ventilation. These patients may benefit from an anesthetic such as halothane if they have not responded to conventional bronchodilators. Sedatives should never be given because they may depress ventilation. Antibiotics should not be used routinely unless there are signs of pneumonia.

SPECIAL CONSIDERATIONS

Refractory Asthma Although most patients with asthma are easily controlled with appropriate medication, a small proportion of patients (approximately 5–10% of asthmatics) are difficult to control despite maximal inhaled therapy. Some of these patients will require maintenance treatment with OCS. In managing these patients, it is important to investigate and correct any mechanisms that may be aggravating asthma. There are two major patterns of difficult asthma: some patients have persistent symptoms and poor lung function, despite appropriate therapy, whereas others may have normal or near-normal lung function but intermittent, severe (sometimes life-threatening) exacerbations.

MECHANISMS The most common reason for poor control of asthma is noncompliance with medication, particularly ICS. Compliance with ICS may be low because patients do not feel any immediate clinical benefit or may be concerned about side effects. Compliance with ICS is difficult to monitor because there are no useful plasma measurements that can be made, but measuring the fractional excretion of induced NO (F_ENO) may identify the problem. Compliance may be improved by giving the ICS as a combination with a LABA that gives symptom relief. Compliance with OCS may be measured by suppression of plasma cortisol and the expected concentration of prednisone/prednisolone in the plasma. There are several factors that may make asthma more difficult to control, including exposure to high, ambient levels of allergens or unidentified occupational agents. Severe rhinosinusitis may make asthma more difficult to control; upper airway disease should be vigorously treated. Drugs such as beta-adrenergic blockers, aspirin, and other cyclooxygenase (COX) inhibitors may worsen asthma. Some women develop severe premenstrual worsening of asthma, which is unresponsive to corticosteroids and requires treatment with progesterone or gonadotropin-releasing factors. Few systemic diseases make asthma more difficult to control, but hyper- and hypothyroidism may increase asthma symptoms and should be investigated if suspected.

Bronchial biopsy studies in refractory asthma may show the typical eosinophilic pattern of inflammation, whereas others have a predominantly neutrophilic pattern. There may be an increase in T_H1 cells, T_H17 cells, and CD8 lymphocytes compared to mild asthma and increased expression of TNF-α. Structural changes in the airway, including fibrosis, angiogenesis, and airway smooth-muscle thickening, are more commonly seen in these patients.

Corticosteroid-Resistant Asthma A few patients with asthma show a poor response to corticosteroid therapy and may have various molecular abnormalities that impair the anti-inflammatory action of corticosteroids. Complete resistance to corticosteroids is extremely uncommon and affects less than 1 in 1000 patients. It is defined by a failure to respond to a high dose of oral prednisone/prednisolone (40 mg once daily over 2 weeks), ideally with a 2-week run-in with matched placebo. More common is reduced responsiveness to corticosteroids where control of asthma requires OCS (corticosteroid-dependent asthma). In patients with poor responsiveness to corticosteroids, there is a reduction in the response of circulating monocytes and lymphocytes to the anti-inflammatory effects of corticosteroids in vitro and reduced skin blanching in response to topical corticosteroids. There are several mechanisms that have been described, including an increase in the alternatively spliced form of the glucocorticoid receptor (GR)-β, an abnormal pattern of histone acetylation in response to corticosteroids, a defect in IL-10 production, and a reduction in HDAC2 activity (as in COPD). These observations suggest that there are likely to be heterogeneous mechanisms for corticosteroid resistance; whether these mechanisms are genetically determined has yet to be decided.

Brittle Asthma Some patients show chaotic variations in lung function despite taking appropriate therapy. Some show a persistent pattern of variability and may require oral corticosteroids or, at times, continuous infusion of β_2-agonists (type 1 brittle asthma), whereas others have generally normal or near-normal lung function but precipitous, unpredictable falls in lung function that may result in death (type 2 brittle asthma). These latter patients are difficult to manage because they do not respond well to corticosteroids, and the worsening of asthma does not reverse well with inhaled bronchodilators. The most effective therapy is subcutaneous epinephrine, which suggests that the worsening is likely to be a localized airway anaphylactic reaction with edema. In some of these patients, there may be allergy to specific foods. These patients should be taught to self-administer epinephrine and should carry a medical warning accordingly.

TREATMENT REFRACTORY ASTHMA

Refractory asthma is difficult to control, by definition. It is important to check compliance and the correct use of inhalers and to identify and eliminate any underlying triggers. Low doses of theophylline may be helpful in some patients, and theophylline withdrawal has been found to worsen in many patients. Most of these patients will require maintenance treatment with oral corticosteroids, and the minimal dose that achieves satisfactory control should be determined by careful dose titration. Steroid-sparing therapies are rarely effective. In some patients with allergic asthma, omalizumab is effective, particularly when there are frequent exacerbations. Anti-TNF therapy is not effective in severe asthma and should not be used. A few patients may benefit from infusions of β_2-agonists. New therapies are needed for these patients, who currently consume a disproportionate amount of health care spending.

Aspirin-Sensitive Asthma A small proportion (1–5%) of asthmatics become worse with aspirin and other COX inhibitors, although this is much more commonly seen in severe cases and in patients with frequent hospital admission. Aspirin-sensitive asthma is a well-defined phenotype of asthma that is usually preceded by perennial rhinitis and nasal polyps in nonatopic patients with a late onset of the disease. Aspirin, even in small doses, characteristically provokes rhinorrhea, conjunctival injection, facial flushing, and wheezing. There is a genetic predisposition to increased production of cysteinyl-leukotrienes with functional polymorphism of *cys*-leukotriene C_4 synthase. Asthma is triggered by COX inhibitors but is persistent even in their absence. All nonselective COX inhibitors should be avoided, but selective COX2 inhibitors are safe to use when an anti-inflammatory analgesic is needed. Aspirin-sensitive asthma responds to usual therapy with ICS. Although antileukotrienes should be effective in these patients, they are no more effective than in allergic asthma. Occasionally, aspirin desensitization is necessary, but this should only be undertaken in specialized centers.

Asthma in the Elderly Asthma may start at any age, including in elderly patients. The principles of management are the same as in other asthmatics, but side effects of therapy may be a problem, including muscle tremor with β_2-agonists and more systemic side effects with ICS. Comorbidities are more frequent in this age group, and interactions with drugs such as β_2-blockers, COX inhibitors, and agents that may affect theophylline metabolism need to be considered. COPD is more likely in elderly patients and may coexist with asthma. A trial of OCS may be very useful in documenting the steroid responsiveness of asthma.

Pregnancy Approximately one-third of asthmatic patients who are pregnant improve during the course of a pregnancy, one-third deteriorate, and one-third are unchanged. It is important to maintain good control of asthma because poor control may have adverse effects on fetal development. Compliance may be a problem because there is often concern about the effects of antiasthma medications on fetal development. The drugs that have been used for many years in asthma therapy have now been shown to be safe and without teratogenic potential. These drugs include SABA, ICS, and theophylline; there is less safety information about newer classes of drugs such as LABA, antileukotrienes, and anti-IgE. If an OCS is needed, it is better to use prednisone rather than prednisolone because it cannot be converted to the active prednisolone by the fetal liver, thus protecting the fetus from systemic effects of the corticosteroid. There is no contraindication to breast-feeding when patients are using these drugs.

Cigarette Smoking Approximately 20% of asthmatics smoke, which may adversely affect asthma in several ways. Smoking asthmatics have more severe disease, more frequent hospital admissions, a faster decline in lung function, and a higher risk of death from asthma than nonsmoking asthmatics. There is evidence that smoking interferes with the anti-inflammatory actions of corticosteroids by reducing HDAC2, necessitating higher doses for asthma control. Smoking cessation improves lung function and reduces the steroid resistance, and thus, vigorous smoking cessation strategies should be used. Some patients report a temporary worsening of asthma when they first stop smoking, possibly due to the loss of the bronchodilating effect of NO in cigarette smoke.

Surgery If asthma is well controlled, there is no contraindication to general anesthesia and intubation. Patients who are treated with OCS will have adrenal suppression and should be treated with an increased dose of OCS immediately prior to surgery. Patients with FEV_1 <80%

of their normal levels should also be given a boost of OCS prior to surgery. High-maintenance doses of corticosteroids may be a contraindication to surgery because of increased risks of infection and delayed wound healing.

Bronchopulmonary Aspergillosis Bronchopulmonary aspergillosis (BPA) is uncommon and results from an allergic pulmonary reaction to inhaled spores of *Aspergillus fumigatus* and, occasionally, other *Aspergillus* species. A skin prick test to *A. fumigatus* is always positive, whereas serum *Aspergillus* precipitins are low or undetectable. Characteristically, there are fleeting eosinophilic infiltrates in the lungs, particularly in the upper lobes. Airways become blocked with mucoid plugs rich in eosinophils, and patients may cough up brown plugs and have hemoptysis. BPA may result in bronchiectasis, particularly affecting central airways, if not suppressed by corticosteroids. Asthma is controlled in the usual way by ICS, but it is necessary to give a course of OCS if any sign of worsening or pulmonary shadowing is found. Treatment with the oral antifungal itraconazole is beneficial in preventing exacerbations.

310 Hypersensitivity Pneumonitis and Pulmonary Infiltrates with Eosinophilia

Praveen Akuthota, Michael E. Wechsler

HYPERSENSITIVITY PNEUMONITIS

INTRODUCTION AND DEFINITION

Hypersensitivity pneumonitis (HP), also referred to as extrinsic allergic alveolitis, is a pulmonary disease that occurs due to inhalational exposure to a variety of antigens leading to an inflammatory response of the alveoli and small airways. Systemic manifestations such as fever and fatigue can accompany respiratory symptoms. Although sensitization to an inhaled antigen as manifested by specific circulating IgG antibodies is necessary for the development of HP, sensitization alone is not sufficient as a defining characteristic, because many sensitized individuals do not develop HP. The incidence and prevalence of HP are variable, depending on geography, occupation, avocation, and environment of the cohort being studied. As yet unexplained is the decreased risk of developing HP in smokers.

OFFENDING ANTIGENS

HP can be caused by any of a large list of potential offending inhaled antigens (Table 310-1). The various antigens and environmental conditions described to be associated with HP give rise to an expansive list of monikers given to specific forms of HP. Antigens derived from fungal, bacterial, mycobacterial, bird-derived, and chemical sources have all been implicated in causing HP.

Categories of individuals at particular risk in the United States include farmers, bird owners, industrial workers, and hot tub users. Farmer's lung occurs as a result of exposure to one of several possible sources of bacterial or fungal antigens such as grain, moldy hay, or silage. Potential offending antigens include thermophilic actinomycetes or *Aspergillus* species. Bird fancier's lung (also referred to by names corresponding to specific birds) must be considered in patients who give a history of keeping birds in their home and is precipitated by exposure to antigens derived from feathers, droppings, and serum proteins. Occupational exposure to birds may also cause HP, as is seen in poultry worker's lung. Chemical worker's lung is provoked by exposure to occupational chemical antigens such as diphenylmethane diisocyanate and toluene diisocyanate. Mycobacteria may cause HP rather than frank infection, a phenomenon observed in hot tub lung and in HP due to metalworking fluid.

TABLE 310-1 EXAMPLES OF HYPERSENSITIVITY PNEUMONITIS

Disease	Antigen	Source
Farming/Food Processing		
Farmer's lung	Thermophilic actinomycetes (e.g., *Saccharopolyspora rectivirgula*); fungus	Grain, moldy hay, silage
Bagassosis	Thermophilic actinomycetes	Sugarcane
Cheese washer's lung	*Penicillium casei; Aspergillus clavatus*	Cheese
Coffee worker's lung	Coffee bean dust	Coffee beans
Malt worker's lung	*Aspergillus* species	Barley
Miller's lung	*Sitophilus granarius* (wheat weevil)	Wheat flour
Mushroom worker's lung	Thermophilic actinomycetes; mushroom spores	Mushrooms
Potato riddler's lung	Thermophilic actinomycetes; *Aspergillus* species	Moldy hay around potatoes
Tobacco grower's lung	*Aspergillus* species	Tobacco
Wine maker's lung	*Botrytis cinerea*	Grapes
Birds and Other Animals		
Bird fancier's lung (also named by specific bird exposures)	Proteins derived by parakeets, pigeons, budgerigars	Bird feathers, droppings, serum proteins
Duck fever	Duck feathers, serum proteins	Ducks
Fish meal worker's lung	Fish meal dust	Fish meal
Furrier's lung	Dust from animal furs	Animal furs
Laboratory worker's lung	Rat urine, serum, fur	Laboratory rats
Pituitary snuff taker's lung	Animal proteins	Pituitary snuff from bovine and porcine sources
Poultry worker's lung	Chicken serum proteins	Chickens
Turkey handling disease	Turkey serum proteins	Turkeys
Other Occupational and Environmental Exposures		
Chemical worker's lung	Isocyanates	Polyurethane foam, varnish, lacquer
Detergent worker's lung	*Bacillus subtilis* enzymes	Detergent
Hot tub lung	*Cladosporium* species; *Mycobacterium avium* complex	Contaminated water, mold on ceiling
Humidifier fever (and air conditioner lung)	Several microorganisms including: *Aureobasidium pullulans; Candida albicans*; thermophilic actinomycetes; *Mycobacterium* species; *Klebsiella oxytoca; Naegleria gruberi*	Humidifiers and air conditioners (contaminated water)
Machine operator's lung	*Pseudomonas* species; *Mycobacteria* species	Metal working fluid
Sauna taker's lung	*Aureobasidium* species; other antigens	Sauna water
Suberosis	*Penicillium glabrum; Chrysonilia sitophila*	Cork dust
Summer-type pneumonitis	*Trichosporon cutaneum*	House dust mites, bird droppings
Woodworker's lung	*Alternaria* species; *Bacillus subtilis*	Oak, cedar, pine, mahogany dusts

PATHOPHYSIOLOGY

The pathophysiology of HP has not been characterized in depth on an immunologic level, although it has been established that HP is an immune-mediated condition that occurs in response to inhaled antigens that are small enough to deposit in distal airways and alveoli. From a lymphocyte perspective, HP has been categorized as a condition with a T_H1 inflammatory pattern. However, emerging evidence suggests that T_H17 lymphocyte subsets may be involved in the pathogenesis of the disease as well. Although the presence of precipitating IgG antibodies against specific antigens in HP suggests a prominent role for adaptive immunity in the pathophysiology of HP, innate immune mechanisms may also make an important contribution. This is highlighted by the observation that Toll-like receptors and downstream signaling proteins such as MyD88 are activated in HP. Although no clear genetic basis for HP has been established, in specific cohorts, polymorphisms in genes involved in antigen processing and presentation, including TAP1 and major histocompatibility complex type II, have been observed.

CLINICAL PRESENTATION

Given the heterogeneity among patients, variability in offending antigens, and differences in the intensity and duration of exposure to antigen, the presentation of HP is accordingly variable. Although these categories are not fully satisfactory in capturing this variability, HP has been traditionally categorized as having *acute, subacute, and chronic* forms. Acute HP usually manifests itself 4–8 h following exposure to the inciting antigen, often intense in nature. Systemic symptoms, including fevers, chills, and malaise, are prominent and are accompanied by dyspnea. Symptoms resolve within hours to days if no further exposure to the offending antigen occurs. In subacute HP resulting from ongoing antigen exposure, the onset of respiratory and systemic symptoms is typically more gradual over the course of weeks. A similar presentation may occur as a culmination of intermittent episodes of acute HP. Although respiratory impairment may be quite severe, antigen avoidance generally results in resolution of the symptoms, although with a slower time course, on the order of weeks to months, than that seen with acute HP. Chronic HP can present with an even more gradual onset of symptoms than subacute HP, with progressive dyspnea, cough, fatigue, weight loss, and clubbing of the digits. The insidious onset of symptoms and frequent lack of an anteceding episode of acute HP make diagnosing chronic HP a challenge. Unlike with the other forms of HP, there can be an irreversible component to the respiratory impairment that is not responsive to removal of the responsible antigen from the patient's environment. The disease progression to hypoxemic respiratory failure can mirror that seen in idiopathic pulmonary fibrosis (IPF). Fibrotic lung disease is a potential feature of chronic HP due to exposure to bird antigens, whereas an emphysematous phenotype may be seen in farmer's lung.

The categories of acute, subacute, and chronic HP are not completely sufficient in classifying HP. The HP Study Group found on cluster analysis that a cohort of HP patients is best described in bipartite fashion, with one group featuring recurrent systemic signs and symptoms and the other featuring more severe respiratory findings.

Concordant with the variability in the presentation of HP is the observed variability in outcome. HP that has not progressed to chronic lung disease has a more favorable outcome with likely resolution if antigen avoidance can be achieved. However, chronic HP resulting in lung fibrosis has a poorer prognosis, with patients with chronic pigeon breeder's lung having demonstrated a similar mortality as seen in IPF.

DIAGNOSIS

Although there is no set of universally accepted criteria for arriving at a diagnosis of HP, diagnosis depends foremost on establishing a history of exposure to an offending antigen that correlates with respiratory and systemic symptoms. A careful occupational and home exposure history should be taken and may be supplemented if necessary by a clinician visit to the work or home environment. Specific inquiries will be influenced by geography and the occupation of the patient. When HP is suspected by history, the additional workup is aimed at establishing an immunologic and physiologic response to inhalational antigen exposure with chest imaging, pulmonary function testing, serologic studies, bronchoscopy, and, on occasion, lung biopsy.

Chest Imaging Chest x-ray findings in HP are nonspecific and can even lack any discernible abnormalities. In cases of acute and subacute HP, findings may be transient and can include ill-defined micronodular opacities or hazy ground-glass airspace opacities. Findings on chest x-ray will often resolve with removal from the offending antigen, although the time course of resolution may vary. With chronic HP, the abnormalities seen on the chest radiograph are frequently more fibrotic in nature and may be difficult to distinguish from IPF.

With the wide availability of high-resolution computed tomography (HRCT), this modality has become a common component in the diagnostic workup for HP. Although the HRCT may be normal in acute forms of HP, this may be due to lack of temporal correlation between exposure to the offending antigen and obtaining the imaging. Additionally, because of the transient nature of acute HP, HRCT is not always performed. In subacute forms of the disease, ground-glass airspace opacities are characteristic, as is the presence of centrilobular nodules. Expiratory images may show areas of air trapping that are likely caused by involvement of the small airways (Fig. 310-1). Reticular changes and traction bronchiectasis can be observed in chronic HP. Subpleural honeycombing similar to that seen in IPF may be present in advanced cases, although unlike in IPF, the lung bases are frequently spared.

Pulmonary Function Testing (PFT) Either restrictive or obstructive PFTs can be present in HP, so the pattern of PFT change is not useful in establishing the diagnosis of HP. However, obtaining PFTs is of use in characterizing the physiologic impairment of an individual patient and in gauging the response to antigen avoidance and/or corticosteroid therapy. Diffusion capacity for carbon monoxide may be significantly impaired, particularly in cases of chronic HP with fibrotic pulmonary parenchymal changes.

Serum Precipitins Assaying for precipitating IgG antibodies against specific antigens can be a useful adjunct in the diagnosis of HP. However, the presence of an immunologic response alone is not sufficient for establishing the diagnosis, because many asymptomatic individuals with high levels of exposure to antigen may display serum precipitins, as has been observed in farmers and in pigeon breeders. It should also be noted that panels that test for several specific serum

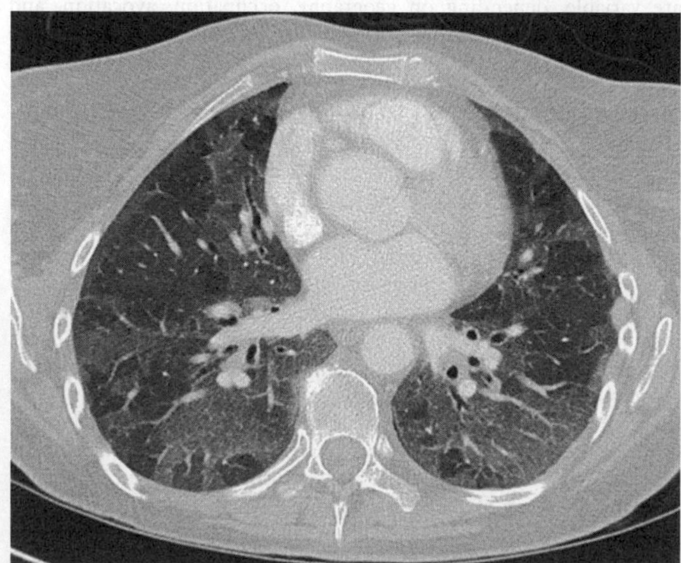

FIGURE 310-1 Chest computed tomography scan of a patient with subacute hypersensitivity pneumonitis in which scattered regions of ground-glass infiltrates in a mosaic pattern consistent with air trapping are seen bilaterally. This patient had bird fancier's lung. *(Courtesy of TJ Gross; with permission.)*

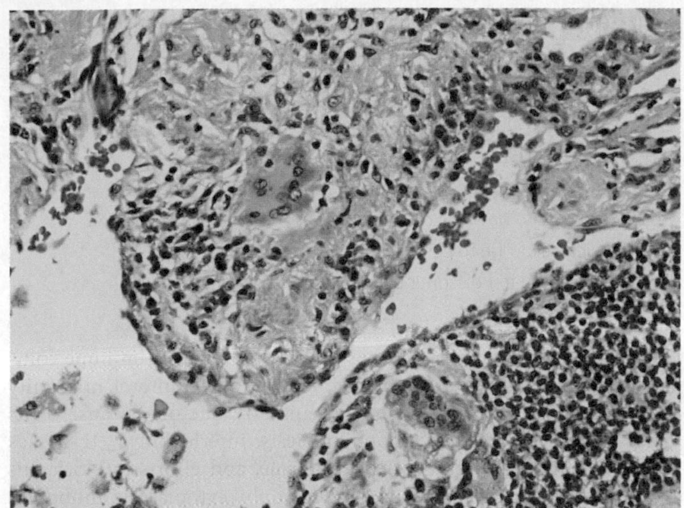

FIGURE 310-2 Open-lung biopsy from a patient with subacute hypersensitivity pneumonitis demonstrating a loose, nonnecrotizing granuloma made up of histiocytes and multinucleated giant cells. Peribronchial inflammatory infiltrate made up of lymphocytes and plasma cells is also seen. *(Courtesy of TJ Gross; with permission.)*

precipitins often provide false-negative results, because they represent an extremely limited proportion of the universe of potential offending environmental antigens.

Bronchoscopy Bronchoscopy with bronchoalveolar lavage (BAL) may be used in the evaluation of HP. Although not a specific finding, BAL lymphocytosis is characteristic of HP. However, in active smokers, a lower threshold should be used to establish BAL lymphocytosis, because smoking will result in lower lymphocyte percentages. Most cases of HP have a CD4+/CD8+ lymphocyte ratio of less than 1, but again, this is not a specific finding and has limited utility in the diagnosis of HP.

Lung Biopsy Tissue samples may be obtained by a bronchoscopic approach using transbronchial biopsy, or more architecturally preserved specimens may be obtained by a surgical approach (video-assisted thoracoscopy or open approach). As is the case with BAL, histologic specimens are not absolutely necessary to establish the diagnosis of HP, but they can be useful in the correct clinical context. A common histologic feature in HP is the presence of noncaseating granulomas in the vicinity of small airways (Fig. 310-2). As opposed to pulmonary sarcoidosis, in which noncaseating granulomas are well defined, the granulomas seen in HP are loose and poorly defined in nature. Within the alveolar spaces and in the interstitium, a mixed cellular infiltrate with a lymphocytic predominance is observed that is frequently patchy in distribution. Bronchiolitis with the presence of organizing exudate is also often observed. Fibrosis may be present as well, particularly as the disease progresses to its chronic form. Fibrotic changes may be focal but can be diffuse and severe with honeycombing in advanced cases, similar to findings in IPF.

Clinical Prediction Rule Although not meant as a set of validated diagnostic criteria, a clinical prediction rule for predicting the presence of HP has been published by the HP Study Group. They identified six statistically significant predictors for HP, the strongest of which was exposure to an antigen known to cause HP. Other predictive criteria were the presence of serum precipitins, recurrent symptoms, symptoms occurring 4–8 h after antigen exposure, crackles on inspiration, and weight loss.

DIFFERENTIAL DIAGNOSIS

Differentiating HP from other conditions that cause a similar constellation of respiratory and systemic symptoms requires an increased index of suspicion based on obtaining a history of possible exposure to an offending antigen. Presentations of acute or subacute HP can be mistaken for respiratory infection. In cases of chronic disease, HP must be differentiated from interstitial lung disease, such as IPF or nonspecific interstitial pneumonitis (NSIP); this can be a difficult task even with lung biopsy. Given the presence of pulmonary infiltrates and noncaseating granulomas on biopsy, sarcoidosis is also a consideration in the differential diagnosis of HP. Unlike in HP, however, hilar adenopathy may be prominent on chest x-ray, organs other than the lung may be involved, and noncaseating granulomas in pathologic specimens tend to be well formed. Other inhalational syndromes, such as organic toxic dust syndrome (OTDS), can be misdiagnosed as HP. OTDS occurs with exposure to organic dusts, including those produced by grains or mold silage, but neither requires prior antigen sensitization nor is characterized by positive serum precipitins.

TREATMENT HYPERSENSITIVITY PNEUMONITIS

The mainstay of treatment for HP is antigen avoidance. A careful exposure history must be obtained to attempt to identify the potential offending antigen and to identify the location where a patient is exposed. Once a potential antigen and location are identified, efforts should be made to modify the environment to minimize patient exposure. This may be accomplished with measures such as removal of birds, removal of molds, and improved ventilation. Personal protective equipment including respirators and ventilated helmets can be used but may not provide adequate protection for sensitized individuals. In some cases, fully avoiding specific environments may be necessary, although such a recommendation must be balanced against the effects to an individual's lifestyle or occupation. It is not uncommon for patients with HP due to exposure to household birds to be unwilling to remove them from the home.

Because acute HP is generally a self-limited disease after a discrete exposure to an offending antigen, pharmacologic therapy is generally not necessary. However, in so-called subacute and chronic forms of the disease, there is a role for glucocorticoid therapy. In patients with particularly severe symptoms as a result of subacute HP, antigen avoidance may be insufficient after establishing the diagnosis. Although glucocorticoids do not change the long-term outcome in these patients, they can accelerate the resolution of symptoms. While there is significant variability in the approach to glucocorticoid therapy by individual clinicians, prednisone therapy can be initiated at 0.5–1 mg/kg of ideal body weight per day (not to exceed 60 mg/d or alternative glucocorticoid equivalent) over a duration of 1–2 weeks, followed by a taper over the next 2–6 weeks. In chronic HP, a similar trial of corticosteroids may be used, although a variable component of fibrotic disease may be irreversible.

GLOBAL CONSIDERATIONS

As the ever-expanding list of antigens and exposures associated with the development of HP suggests, populations at risk for HP will vary globally based on specifics of local occupational, avocational, and environmental factors. Specific examples of geographically limited HP include summer-type pneumonitis seen in Japan and suberosis seen in cork workers in Portugal and Spain.

PULMONARY INFILTRATES WITH EOSINOPHILIA

Although eosinophils are normal constituents of the lungs, there are several pulmonary eosinophilic syndromes that are characterized by pulmonary infiltrates on imaging along with an increased number of eosinophils in lung tissue, in sputum, and/or in BAL fluid, with resultant increased respiratory symptoms and the potential for systemic manifestations. Because the eosinophil plays such an important role in each of these syndromes, it is often difficult to distinguish between them, but there are important clinical and pathologic differences as well as differences in prognosis and treatment paradigms.

CLASSIFYING PULMONARY INFILTRATES WITH EOSINOPHILIA AND GENERAL APPROACH

Because there are so many different diagnoses associated with pulmonary infiltrates with eosinophilia, the first step in classifying pulmonary

TABLE 310-2 PULMONARY INFILTRATES WITH EOSINOPHILIA

Primary Pulmonary Eosinophilic Disorders
Acute eosinophilic pneumonia
Chronic eosinophilic pneumonia
Eosinophilic granulomatosis with polyangiitis (Churg-Strauss syndrome)
Hypereosinophilic syndrome
Pulmonary Disorders of Known Cause Associated with Eosinophilia
Asthma and eosinophilic bronchitis
Allergic bronchopulmonary aspergillosis
Bronchocentric granulomatosis
Drug/toxin reaction
Infection (Table 310-4)
Parasitic/helminthic disease
Nonparasitic infection
Lung Diseases Associated with Eosinophilia
Cryptogenic organizing pneumonia
Hypersensitivity pneumonitis
Idiopathic pulmonary fibrosis
Pulmonary Langerhans cell granulomatosis
Malignant Neoplasms Associated with Eosinophilia
Leukemia
Lymphoma
Lung cancer
Adenocarcinoma of various organs
Squamous cell carcinoma of various organs
Systemic Disease Associated with Eosinophilia
Postradiation pneumonitis
Rheumatoid arthritis
Sarcoidosis
Sjögren's syndrome

eosinophilic syndromes is distinguishing between primary pulmonary eosinophilic lung disorders and those with eosinophilia that are secondary to a specific cause such as a drug reaction, an infection, a malignancy, or another pulmonary condition such as asthma. Table 310-2 lists primary and secondary pulmonary eosinophilic disorders.

For each patient, a detailed history is of utmost importance and can help elucidate what the underlying disease is. Details regarding onset, timing, and precipitants of specific symptoms can help discern one diagnosis from another. History regarding pharmacologic, occupational, and environmental exposures is instructive, and family and travel history are crucial. In addition to details about the sinuses and lungs, it is important to inquire about systemic manifestations and assess for physical findings of cardiac, gastrointestinal (GI), neurologic, dermatologic, and genitourinary involvement, all of which may give clues to specific diagnoses. Once the details from history and physical are teased out, laboratory testing (including measurements of blood eosinophils, cultures, and markers of inflammation), spirometry and radiographic imaging can help distinguish between different diseases. Often, however, BAL, transbronchial, or open lung biopsies are required. In many cases, biopsies or noninvasive diagnostic studies of other organs (e.g., echocardiogram, electromyogram, or bone marrow biopsy) can be helpful.

PATHOPHYSIOLOGY

Pathologically, the pulmonary eosinophilic syndromes are characterized by tissue infiltration by eosinophils (Fig. 310-2). In eosinophilic granulomatosis with polyangiitis (EGPA), extravascular granulomas and necrotizing vasculitis may occur in the lungs, as well as in the heart, skin, muscle, liver, spleen, and kidneys, and may be associated with fibrinoid necrosis and thrombosis.

The exact etiology of the various pulmonary eosinophilic syndromes is unknown; however, it is felt that these syndromes result from dysregulated eosinophilopoiesis or an autoimmune process because of the prominence of allergic features and the presence of immune complexes, heightened T cell immunity, and altered humoral immunity as evidenced by elevated IgE and rheumatoid factor. Because of its integral involvement in eosinophilopoiesis, interleukin 5 (IL-5) has been hypothesized to play an etiologic role, and efforts to block this cytokine are being investigated. Antineutrophil cytoplasmic antibodies (ANCAs) are present in about half of patients with EGPA; binding of ANCAs to vascular walls likely contributes to vascular inflammation and injury as well as chemotaxis of inflammatory cells.

TABLE 310-3 DIAGNOSTIC CRITERIA OF ACUTE EOSINOPHILIC PNEUMONIA

Criteria
Acute febrile illness with respiratory manifestations of <1 month in duration
Hypoxemic respiratory failure
Diffuse pulmonary infiltrates on chest x-ray
Bronchoalveolar lavage eosinophilia >25%
Absence of parasitic, fungal, or other infection
Absence of drugs known to cause pulmonary eosinophilia
Quick clinical response to corticosteroids
Failure to relapse after discontinuation of corticosteroids

ACUTE EOSINOPHILIC PNEUMONIA

Acute eosinophilic pneumonia is a syndrome characterized by fevers, acute respiratory failure that often requires mechanical ventilation, diffuse pulmonary infiltrates, and pulmonary eosinophilia in a previously healthy individual (Table 310-3).

Clinical Features and Etiology At presentation, acute eosinophilic pneumonia is often mistaken for acute lung injury or acute respiratory distress syndrome (ARDS), until a BAL is performed and reveals >25% eosinophils. Although the predominant symptoms of acute eosinophilic pneumonia are cough, dyspnea, malaise, myalgias, night sweats, and pleuritic chest pain, physical exam findings include high fevers, basilar rales, and rhonchi on forced expiration. Acute eosinophilic pneumonia most often affects males between age 20 and 40 with no history of asthma. Although no clear etiology has been identified, several case reports have linked acute eosinophilic pneumonia to recent initiation of tobacco smoking or exposure to other environmental stimuli including dust from indoor renovations.

In addition to a suggestive history, the key to establishing a diagnosis of acute eosinophilic pneumonia is the presence of >25% eosinophilia on BAL fluid. While lung biopsies show eosinophilic infiltration with acute and organizing diffuse alveolar damage, it is generally not necessary to proceed to biopsy to establish a diagnosis. Although patients present with an elevated white blood cell count, in contrast to other pulmonary eosinophilic syndromes, acute eosinophilic pneumonia is often not associated with peripheral eosinophilia upon presentation. However, between 7 and 30 days of disease onset, peripheral eosinophilia often occurs with mean eosinophil counts of 1700. Erythrocyte sedimentation rate (ESR), C-reactive protein, and IgE levels are high but nonspecific, whereas HRCT is always abnormal with bilateral random patchy ground-glass or reticular opacities, and small pleural effusions in as many as two-thirds of patients. Pleural fluid is characterized by a high pH with marked eosinophilia.

Clinical Course and Response to Therapy Although some patients improve spontaneously, most patients require admission to an intensive care unit and respiratory support with either invasive (intubation) or noninvasive mechanical ventilation. However, what distinguishes acute eosinophilic pneumonia from both other cases of acute lung injury as well as some of the other pulmonary eosinophilic syndromes is the absence of organ dysfunction or multisystem organ failure other than respiratory failure. One of the characteristic features of acute eosinophilic pneumonia is the high degree of corticosteroid responsiveness and the excellent prognosis. Another distinguishing feature of acute eosinophilic pneumonia is that complete clinical and radiographic recovery without recurrence or residual sequelae occurs in almost all patients within several weeks of initiation of therapy.

CHRONIC EOSINOPHILIC PNEUMONIA

In contrast to acute eosinophilic pneumonia, chronic eosinophilic pneumonia is a more indolent syndrome that is characterized by pulmonary infiltrates and eosinophilia in both the tissue and blood. Most patients are female nonsmokers with a mean age of 45, and patients do not usually develop the acute respiratory failure and significant hypoxemia appreciated in acute eosinophilic pneumonia. Similar to EGPA, a majority have asthma, with many having a history of allergies.

Patients present with a subacute illness over weeks to months, with cough, low-grade fevers, progressive dyspnea, weight loss, wheezing, malaise, and night sweats, and a chest x-ray with migratory bilateral peripheral or pleural-based opacities. Although this "photographic negative pulmonary edema" appearance on chest x-ray and chest CT is pathognomonic of chronic eosinophilic pneumonia, less than 25% of patients present with this finding. Other radiographic findings include atelectasis, pleural effusions, lymphadenopathy, and septal line thickening.

Almost 90% of patients have peripheral eosinophilia, with mean eosinophil counts of over 30% of total white blood cell count. BAL eosinophilia is also an important distinguishing feature with mean BAL eosinophil counts of close to 60%. Both peripheral and BAL eosinophilia are very responsive to treatment with corticosteroids. Other laboratory features of chronic eosinophilic pneumonia include increased ESR, C-reactive protein, platelets, and IgE. Lung biopsy is also often not required to establish a diagnosis, but may show accumulation of eosinophils and histiocytes in the lung parenchyma and interstitium, as well as cryptogenic organizing pneumonia, but with minimal fibrosis. Nonrespiratory manifestations are uncommon, but arthralgias, neuropathy, and skin and GI symptoms have all been reported; their presence may suggest EGPA or hypereosinophilic syndrome. Another similarity is the rapid response to corticosteroids with quick resolution of peripheral and BAL eosinophilia and improvement in symptoms. In contrast to acute eosinophilic pneumonia, though, over 50% of patients relapse, and many require prolonged courses of corticosteroids for months to years.

EOSINOPHILIC GRANULOMATOSIS WITH POLYANGIITIS (EGPA)

Previously known as allergic angiitis granulomatosis or Churg-Strauss syndrome, this complex syndrome is characterized by eosinophilic vasculitis that may involve multiple organ systems including the lungs, heart, skin, GI tract, and nervous system. Although EGPA is characterized by peripheral and pulmonary eosinophilia with infiltrates on chest x-ray, the primary features that distinguish EGPA from other pulmonary eosinophilic syndromes are the presence of eosinophilic vasculitis in the setting of asthma and involvement of multiple end organs (a feature it shares with hypereosinophilic syndrome). Although perceived to be quite rare, in the last few years, there has appeared to be an increased incidence of this disease, particularly in association with various asthma therapies.

The primary features of EGPA include asthma, peripheral eosinophilia, neuropathy, pulmonary infiltrates, paranasal sinus abnormality, and presence of eosinophilic vasculitis. It typically occurs in several phases. The prodromal phase is characterized by asthma and allergic rhinitis, and usually begins when the individual is in his or her twenties or thirties, typically persisting for many years. The eosinophilic infiltrative phase is characterized by peripheral eosinophilia and eosinophilic tissue infiltration of various organs including the lungs and GI tract. The third phase is the vasculitic phase and may be associated with constitutional signs and symptoms including fever, weight loss, malaise, and fatigue. The mean age at diagnosis is 48 years, with a range of 14 to 74 years; the average length of time between diagnosis of asthma and vasculitis is 9 years.

Similar to other pulmonary eosinophilic syndromes, constitutional symptoms are very common in EGPA and include weight loss of 10–20 lb, fevers, and diffuse myalgias and migratory polyarthralgias. Myositis may be present with evidence of vasculitis on muscle biopsies. In contrast to the eosinophilic pneumonias, EGPA involves many organ systems including the lungs, skin, nerves, heart, GI tract, and kidneys.

Symptoms and Clinical Manifestations • ***RESPIRATORY*** Most EGPA patients have asthma that arises later in life and in individuals who have no family history of atopy. The asthma can often be severe, and oral corticosteroids are often required to control symptoms but may lead to suppression of vasculitic symptoms. In addition to the more common symptoms of cough, dyspnea, sinusitis, and allergic rhinitis, alveolar hemorrhage and hemoptysis may also occur.

NEUROLOGIC Over three-fourths of EGPA patients have neurologic manifestations. Mononeuritis multiplex most commonly involves the peroneal nerve, but also involves the ulnar, radial, internal popliteal, and occasionally, cranial nerves. Cerebral hemorrhage and infarction may also occur and are important causes of death. Despite treatment, neurologic sequelae often do not completely resolve.

DERMATOLOGIC Approximately half of EGPA patients develop dermatologic manifestations. These include palpable purpura, skin nodules, urticarial rashes, and livedo.

CARDIOVASCULAR Granulomas, vasculitis, and widespread myocardial damage may be found on biopsy or at autopsy, and cardiomyopathy and heart failure may be seen in up to half of all patients but are often at least partially reversible. Acute pericarditis, constrictive pericarditis, myocardial infarction, and other electrocardiographic changes all may occur. The heart is a primary target organ in EGPA, and cardiac involvement often portends a worse prognosis.

GI GI symptoms are common in EGPA and likely represent an eosinophilic gastroenteritis characterized by abdominal pain, diarrhea, GI bleeding, and colitis. Ischemic bowel, pancreatitis, and cholecystitis have also been reported in association with EGPA and usually portend a worse prognosis.

RENAL Renal involvement is more common than once thought, and approximately 25% of patients have some degree of renal involvement. This may include proteinuria, glomerulonephritis, renal insufficiency, and rarely, renal infarct.

Lab Abnormalities Systemic eosinophilia is the hallmark laboratory finding in patients with EGPA and reflects the likely pathogenic role that the eosinophil plays in this disease. Eosinophilia greater than 10% is one of the defining features of this illness and may be as high as 75% of the peripheral white blood cell count. It is present at the time of diagnosis in over 80% of patients but may respond quickly (often within 24 h) to initiation of systemic corticosteroid therapy. Even in the absence of systemic eosinophilia, tissue eosinophilia may be present.

Although not specific to EGPA, ANCAs are present in up to two-thirds of patients, mostly with a perinuclear staining pattern. Nonspecific lab abnormalities that may be present in patients with EGPA include a marked elevation in ESR, a normochromic normocytic anemia, an elevated IgE, hypergammaglobulinemia, and positive rheumatoid factor and antinuclear antibodies (ANA). Although BAL often reveals significant eosinophilia, this may be seen in other eosinophilic lung diseases. Similarly, PFT often reveals an obstructive defect similar to asthma.

Radiographic Features Chest x-ray abnormalities are extremely common in EGPA and consist of bilateral, nonsegmental, patchy infiltrates that often migrate and may be interstitial or alveolar in appearance. Reticulonodular and nodular disease without cavitation can be seen, as can pleural effusions and hilar adenopathy. The most common CT findings include bilateral ground-glass opacity and airspace consolidation that is predominantly subpleural. Other CT findings include bronchial wall thickening, hyperinflation, interlobular septal thickening, lymph node enlargement, and pericardial and pleural effusions. Angiography may be used diagnostically and may show signs of vasculitis in the coronary, central nervous system, and peripheral vasculature.

Treatment and Prognosis of EGPA Most patients diagnosed with EGPA have previously been diagnosed with asthma, rhinitis, and sinusitis, and have received treatment with inhaled or systemic corticosteroids.

Because these agents are also the initial treatment of choice for EGPA patients, institution of these therapies in patients with EGPA who are perceived to have severe asthma may delay the diagnosis of EGPA because signs of vasculitis may be masked. Corticosteroids dramatically alter the course of EGPA: up to 50% of those who are untreated die within 3 months of diagnosis, whereas treated patients have a 6-year survival of over 70%. Common causes of death include heart failure, cerebral hemorrhage, renal failure, and GI bleeding. Recent data suggest that clinical remission may be obtained in over 90% of patients treated; approximately 25% of those patients may relapse, often due to corticosteroid tapering, with a rising eosinophil count heralding the relapse. Myocardial, GI, and renal involvement most often portend a poor prognosis. In such cases, treatment with higher doses of corticosteroids or the addition of cytotoxic agents such as cyclophosphamide is often warranted. Although survival does not differ between those treated or untreated with cyclophosphamide, cyclophosphamide is associated with a reduced incidence of relapse and an improved clinical response to treatment. Other therapies that have been used successfully in the management of EGPA include azathioprine, methotrexate, intravenous gamma globulin, and interferon α. Plasma exchange has not been shown to provide any additional benefit. Recent studies examining the efficacy of anti-IL-5 therapy have shown promise.

HYPEREOSINOPHILIC SYNDROMES

Hypereosinophilic syndromes (HES) constitute a heterogeneous group of disease entities manifest by persistent eosinophilia >1500 eosinophils/μL in association with end organ damage or dysfunction, in the absence of secondary causes of eosinophilia. In addition to familial, undefined, and overlap syndromes with incomplete criteria, the predominant HES subtypes are the myeloproliferative and lymphocytic variants. The myeloproliferative variant may be divided into three subgroups: (1) chronic eosinophilic leukemia with demonstrable cytogenetic abnormalities and/or blasts on peripheral smear; (2) the platelet-derived growth factor receptor α (PDGFRα)–associated HES, attributed to a constitutively activated tyrosine kinase fusion protein (Fip1L1-PDGFRα) due to a chromosomal deletion on 4q12; this variant is often responsive to imatinib; and (3) the FIP1-negative variant associated with clonal eosinophilia and at least four of the following: dysplastic peripheral eosinophils, increased serum vitamin B_{12}, increased tryptase, anemia, thrombocytopenia, splenomegaly, bone marrow cellularity >80%, spindle-shaped mast cells, and myelofibrosis.

Extrapulmonary Manifestations of HES More common in men than in women, HES occurs between the ages of 20 and 50 and is characterized by significant extrapulmonary involvement, including infiltration of the heart, GI tract, kidney, liver, joints, and skin. Cardiac involvement includes myocarditis and/or endomyocardial fibrosis, as well as a restrictive cardiomyopathy.

Pulmonary Manifestations of HES Similar to the other pulmonary eosinophilic syndromes, these HES are manifest by high levels of blood, BAL, and tissue eosinophilia. Lung involvement occurs in 40% of these patients and is characterized by cough and dyspnea, as well as pulmonary infiltrates. Although it is often difficult to discern the pulmonary infiltrates and effusions seen on chest x-ray from pulmonary edema resulting from cardiac involvement, CT scan findings include interstitial infiltrates, ground-glass opacities, and small nodules. HES are typically not associated with ANCA or elevated IgE.

Course and Response to Therapy Unlike the other pulmonary eosinophilic syndromes, less than half of patients with these HES respond to corticosteroids as first-line therapy. Although other treatment options include hydroxyurea, cyclosporine, and interferon, the tyrosine kinase inhibitor imatinib has emerged as an important therapeutic option for patients with the myeloproliferative variant. Anti-IL-5 therapy with mepolizumab also holds promise for these patients and is currently being investigated.

ALLERGIC BRONCHOPULMONARY ASPERGILLOSIS

Allergic bronchopulmonary aspergillosis (ABPA) is an eosinophilic pulmonary disorder that occurs in response to allergic sensitization to antigens from *Aspergillus* species fungi. The predominant clinical presentation of ABPA is an asthmatic phenotype, often accompanied by cough with production of brownish plugs of mucus. ABPA has also been well described as a complication of cystic fibrosis. A workup for ABPA may be beneficial in patients who carry a diagnosis of asthma but have proven refractory to usual therapy. ABPA is a distinct diagnosis from simple asthma, characterized by prominent peripheral eosinophilia and elevated circulating levels of IgE (>417 IU/mL). Establishing a diagnosis of ABPA also requires establishing sensitivity to *Aspergillus* antigens by skin test reactivity, positive serum precipitins for *Aspergillus*, and/or direct measurement of circulating specific IgG and IgE to *Aspergillus*. Central bronchiectasis is described as a classic finding on chest imaging in ABPA but is not necessary for making a diagnosis. Other possible findings on chest imaging include patchy infiltrates and evidence of mucus impaction.

Systemic glucocorticoids may be used in the treatment of ABPA that is persistently symptomatic despite the use of inhaled therapies for asthma. Courses of glucocorticoids should be tapered over 3–6 months, and their use must be balanced against the risks of prolonged steroid therapy. Antifungal agents such as fluconazole and voriconazole given over a 4-month course reduce the antigenic stimulus in ABPA and may therefore modulate disease activity in selected patients. The use of monoclonal antibody against IgE (omalizumab) has been described in treating severe ABPA, particularly in individuals with ABPA as a complication of cystic fibrosis.

ABPA-like syndromes have been reported as a result to sensitization to several non-*Aspergillus* species fungi. However, these conditions are substantially rarer than ABPA, which may be present in a significant proportion of patients with refractory asthma.

INFECTIOUS PROCESSES

Infectious etiologies of pulmonary eosinophilia are largely due to helminths and are of particular importance in the evaluation of pulmonary eosinophilia in tropical environments and in the developing world (Table 310-4). These infectious conditions may also be considered in recent travelers to endemic regions. Loffler syndrome refers to transient pulmonary infiltrates with eosinophilia that occurs in response to passage of helminthic larvae through the lungs, most

TABLE 310-4 INFECTIOUS CAUSES OF PULMONARY EOSINOPHILIA

Löffler Syndrome
Ascaris
Hookworm
Schistosomiasis
Heavy Parasite Burden
Strongyloidiasis
Direct Pulmonary Penetration
Paragonimiasis
Visceral larval migrans
Immunologic Response to Organisms in Lungs
Filariasis
Dirofilariasis
Cystic Disease
Echinococcus
Cysticercosis
Other Nonparasitic
Coccidioidomycosis
Basidiobolomycosis
Paracoccidioidomycosis
Tuberculosis

Source: Adapted from P Akuthota, PF Weller: Clin Microbiol Rev 25:649, 2012.

commonly larvae of *Ascaris* species (roundworm). Symptoms are generally self-limited and may include dyspnea, cough, wheeze, and hemoptysis. Loffler syndrome may also occur in response to hookworm infection with *Ancylostoma duodenale* or *Necator americanus.* Chronic *Strongyloides stercoralis* infection can lead to recurrent respiratory symptoms with peripheral eosinophilia between flares. In immunocompromised hosts, including patients on glucocorticoids, a severe, potentially fatal, hyperinfection syndrome can result from *Strongyloides* infection. Paragonimiasis, filariasis, and visceral larval migrans can all cause pulmonary eosinophilia as well.

DRUGS AND TOXINS

A host of medications are associated with the development of pulmonary infiltrates with peripheral eosinophilia. Therefore, drug reaction must always be included in the differential diagnosis of pulmonary eosinophilia. Although the list of medications associated with pulmonary eosinophilia is ever expanding, common culprits include nonsteroidal anti-inflammatory medications and systemic antibiotics, most specifically nitrofurantoin. Additionally, various and diverse environmental exposures such as particulate metals, scorpion stings, and inhalational drugs of abuse may also cause pulmonary eosinophilia. Radiation therapy for breast cancer has been linked with eosinophilic pulmonary infiltration as well. The mainstay of treatment is removal of the offending exposure, although glucocorticoids may be necessary if respiratory symptoms are severe.

GLOBAL CONSIDERATIONS

In the United States, drug-induced eosinophilic pneumonias are the most common cause of eosinophilic pulmonary infiltrates. A travel history or evidence of recent immigration should prompt the consideration of parasite-associated disorders. Tropical eosinophilia is usually caused by filarial infection; however, eosinophilic pneumonias also occur with other parasites such as *Ascaris* spp., *Ancylostoma* spp., *Toxocara* spp., and *Strongyloides stercoralis.* Tropical eosinophilia due to *Wuchereria bancrofti* or *Wuchereria malayi* occurs most commonly in southern Asia, Africa, and South America and is treated successfully with diethylcarbamazine. In the United States, *Strongyloides* is endemic to the southeastern and Appalachian regions.

ACKNOWLEDGMENTS

We acknowledge the contributions of Dr. Alicia K. Gerke and Dr. Gary W. Hunninghake to the previous edition of this chapter.

311 Occupational and Environmental Lung Disease

John R. Balmes, Frank E. Speizer

Occupational and environmental lung diseases are difficult to distinguish from those of nonenvironmental origin. Virtually all major categories of pulmonary disease can be caused by environmental agents, and environmentally related disease usually presents clinically in a manner indistinguishable from that of disease not caused by such agents. In addition, the etiology of many diseases may be multifactorial; occupational and environmental factors may interact with other factors (such as smoking and genetic risk). It is often only after a careful exposure history is taken that the underlying workplace or general environmental exposure is uncovered.

Why is knowledge of occupational or environmental etiology so important? Patient management and prognosis are affected significantly by such knowledge. For example, patients with occupational asthma or hypersensitivity pneumonitis often cannot be managed adequately without cessation of exposure to the offending agent. Establishment of cause may have significant legal and financial implications for a patient who no longer can work in his or her usual job. Other exposed people may be identified as having the disease or prevented from getting it. In addition, new associations between exposure and disease may be identified (e.g., nylon flock worker's lung disease and diacetyl-induced bronchiolitis obliterans).

Although the exact proportion of lung disease due to occupational and environmental factors is unknown, a large number of individuals are at risk. For example, 15–20% of the burden of adult asthma and chronic obstructive pulmonary disease (COPD) has been estimated to be due to occupational factors.

HISTORY AND EXPOSURE ASSESSMENT

The patient's history is of paramount importance in assessing any potential occupational or environmental exposure. Inquiry into specific work practices should include questions about the specific contaminants involved, the presence of visible dusts, chemical odors, the size and ventilation of workspaces, the use of respiratory protective equipment, and whether co-workers have similar complaints. The temporal association of exposure at work and symptoms may provide clues to occupation-related disease. In addition, the patient must be questioned about alternative sources of exposure to potentially toxic agents, including hobbies, home characteristics, exposure to secondhand smoke, and proximity to traffic or industrial facilities. Short-term and long-term exposures to potential toxic agents in the distant past also must be considered.

Workers in the United States have the right to know about potential hazards in their workplaces under federal Occupational Safety and Health Administration (OSHA) regulations. Employers must provide specific information about potential hazardous agents in products being used through Material Safety Data Sheets as well as training in personal protective equipment and environmental control procedures. However, the introduction of new processes and/or new chemical compounds may change exposure significantly, and often only the employee on the production line is aware of the change. For the physician caring for a patient with a suspected work-related illness, a visit to the work site can be very instructive. Alternatively, an affected worker can request an inspection by OSHA. If reliable environmental sampling data are available, that information should be used in assessing a patient's exposure. Because many of the chronic diseases result from exposure over many years, current environmental measurements should be combined with work histories to arrive at estimates of past exposure.

PULMONARY FUNCTION TESTS AND CHEST IMAGING

Exposures to inorganic and organic dusts can cause interstitial lung disease that presents with a restrictive pattern and a decreased diffusing capacity (Chap. 306e). Similarly, exposures to a number of organic dusts or chemical agents may result in occupational asthma or COPD that is characterized by airway obstruction. Measurement of change in forced expiratory volume (FEV_1) before and after a working shift can be used to detect an acute bronchoconstrictive response.

The chest radiograph is useful in detecting and monitoring the pulmonary response to mineral dusts, certain metals, and organic dusts capable of inducing hypersensitivity pneumonitis. The International Labour Organisation (ILO) International Classification of Radiographs of Pneumoconioses classifies chest radiographs by the nature and size of opacities seen and the extent of involvement of the parenchyma. In general, small rounded opacities are seen in silicosis or coal worker's pneumoconiosis, and small linear opacities are seen in asbestosis. Although useful for epidemiologic studies and screening large numbers of workers, the ILO system can be problematic when applied to an individual worker's chest radiograph. With dusts causing rounded opacities, the degree of involvement on the chest radiograph may be extensive, whereas pulmonary function may be only minimally impaired. In contrast, in pneumoconiosis causing linear, irregular opacities like those seen in asbestosis, the radiograph may lead to underestimation of the severity of the impairment until relatively late in the disease. For patients with a history of asbestos exposure, conventional computed tomography (CT) is more sensitive for the detection of pleural thickening, and high-resolution CT (HRCT) improves the detection of asbestosis.

Other procedures that may be of use in identifying the role of environmental exposures in causing lung disease include skin prick testing or specific IgE antibody titers for evidence of immediate hypersensitivity to agents capable of inducing occupational asthma (flour antigens in bakers), specific IgG precipitating antibody titers for agents capable of causing hypersensitivity pneumonitis (pigeon antigen in bird handlers), and assays for specific cell-mediated immune responses (beryllium lymphocyte proliferation testing in nuclear workers or tuberculin skin testing in health care workers). Sometimes a bronchoscopy to obtain transbronchial biopsies of lung tissue may be required for histologic diagnosis (chronic beryllium disease). Rarely, video-assisted thoracoscopic surgery to obtain a larger sample of lung tissue may be required to determine the specific diagnosis of environmentally induced lung disease (hypersensitivity pneumonitis or giant cell interstitial pneumonitis due to cobalt exposure).

DETERMINANTS OF INHALATIONAL EXPOSURE

The chemical and physical characteristics of inhaled agents affect both the dose and the site of deposition in the respiratory tract. Water-soluble gases such as ammonia and sulfur dioxide are absorbed in the lining fluid of the upper and proximal airways and thus tend to produce irritative and bronchoconstrictive responses. In contrast, nitrogen dioxide and phosgene, which are less soluble, may penetrate to the bronchioles and alveoli in sufficient quantities to produce acute chemical pneumonitis.

Particle size of air contaminants must also be considered. Because of their settling velocities in air, particles >10–15 μm in diameter do not penetrate beyond the nose and throat. Particles <10 μm in size are deposited below the larynx. These particles are divided into three size fractions on the basis of their size characteristics and sources. Particles ~2.5–10 μm (coarse-mode fraction) contain crustal elements such as silica, aluminum, and iron. These particles mostly deposit relatively high in the tracheobronchial tree. Although the total mass of an ambient sample is dominated by these larger respirable particles, the number of particles, and therefore the surface area on which potential toxic agents can deposit and be carried to the lower airways, is dominated by particles <2.5 μm (fine-mode fraction). These fine particles are created primarily by the burning of fossil fuels or high-temperature industrial processes resulting in condensation products from gases, fumes, or vapors. The smallest particles, those <0.1 μm in size, represent the ultrafine fraction and make up the largest number of particles; they tend to remain in the airstream and deposit in the lung only on a random basis as they come into contact with the alveolar walls. If they do deposit, however, particles of this size range may penetrate into the circulation and be carried to extrapulmonary sites. New technologies create particles of this size ("nanoparticles") for use in many commercial applications. Besides the size characteristics of particles and the solubility of gases, the actual chemical composition, mechanical properties, and immunogenicity or infectivity of inhaled material determine in large part the nature of the diseases found among exposed persons.

OCCUPATIONAL EXPOSURES AND PULMONARY DISEASE

Table 311-1 provides broad categories of exposure in the workplace and diseases associated with chronic exposure in those industries.

ASBESTOS-RELATED DISEASES

Asbestos is a generic term for several different mineral silicates, including chrysolite, amosite, anthophyllite, and crocidolite. In addition to workers involved in the production of asbestos products (mining, milling, and manufacturing), many workers in the shipbuilding and construction trades, including pipe fitters and boilermakers, were occupationally exposed because asbestos was widely used during the twentieth century for its thermal and electrical insulation properties. Asbestos also was used in the manufacture of fire-resistant textiles, in cement and floor tiles, and in friction materials such as brake and clutch linings.

TABLE 311-1 CATEGORIES OF OCCUPATIONAL EXPOSURE AND ASSOCIATED RESPIRATORY CONDITIONS

Occupational Exposures	Nature of Respiratory Responses	Comment
Inorganic Dusts		
Asbestos: mining, processing, construction, ship repair	Fibrosis (asbestosis), pleural disease, cancer, mesothelioma	Virtually all new mining and construction with asbestos done in developing countries
Silica: mining, stone cutting, sandblasting, quarrying	Fibrosis (silicosis), progressive massive fibrosis (PMF), cancer, tuberculosis, chronic obstructive pulmonary disease (COPD)	Improved protection in United States; persistent risk in developing countries
Coal dust: mining	Fibrosis (coal worker's pneumoconiosis), PMF, COPD	Risk persists in certain areas of United States, increasing in countries where new mines open
Beryllium: processing alloys for high-tech industries	Acute pneumonitis (rare), chronic granulomatous disease, lung cancer (highly suspect)	Risk in high-tech industries persists
Other metals: aluminum, chromium, cobalt, nickel, titanium, tungsten carbide, or "hard metal" (contains cobalt)	Wide variety of conditions from acute pneumonitis to lung cancer and asthma	New diseases appear with new process development
Organic Dusts		
Cotton dust: milling, processing	Byssinosis (an asthma-like syndrome), chronic bronchitis, COPD	Increasing risk in developing countries with drop in United States as jobs shift overseas
Grain dust: elevator agents, dock workers, milling, bakers	Asthma, chronic bronchitis, COPD	Risk shifting more to migrant labor pool
Other agricultural dusts: fungal spores, vegetable products, insect fragments, animal dander, bird and rodent feces, endotoxins, microorganisms, pollens	Hypersensitivity pneumonitis (farmer's lung), asthma, chronic bronchitis	Important in migrant labor pool but also resulting from in-home exposures
Toxic chemicals: wide variety of industries; see Table 311-2	Asthma, chronic bronchitis, COPD, hypersensitivity pneumonitis, pneumoconiosis, and cancer	Reduced risk with recognized hazards; increasing risk for developing countries where controlled labor practices are less stringent
Other respiratory environmental agents: uranium and radon daughters, secondhand tobacco smoke, polycyclic aromatic hydrocarbons (PAHs), biomass smoke, diesel exhaust, welding fumes, wood finishing	Occupational exposures estimated to contribute to up to 10% of all lung cancers; chronic bronchitis, COPD, and fibrosis	In-home exposures important; in developing countries, biomass smoke is a major risk factor for COPD among women

Exposure to asbestos is not limited to persons who directly handle the material. Cases of asbestos-related diseases have been encountered in individuals with only bystander exposure, such as painters and electricians who worked alongside insulation workers in a shipyard. Community exposure resulted from the use of asbestos-containing mine and mill tailings as landfill, road surface, and playground material (e.g., Libby, MT, the site of a vermiculite mine in which the ore was contaminated with asbestos). Finally, exposure can occur from the disturbance of naturally occurring asbestos (e.g., from increasing residential development in the foothills of the Sierra Mountains in California).

Asbestos has largely been replaced in the developed world with synthetic mineral fibers such as fiberglass and refractory ceramic fibers, but it continues to be used in the developing world. The major health effects from exposure to asbestos are pleural and pulmonary fibrosis, cancers of the respiratory tract, and pleural and peritoneal mesothelioma.

Asbestosis is a diffuse interstitial fibrosing disease of the lung that is directly related to the intensity and duration of exposure. The disease resembles other forms of diffuse interstitial fibrosis (Chap. 315). Usually, exposure has taken place for at least 10 years before the disease becomes manifest. The mechanisms by which asbestos fibers induce lung fibrosis are not completely understood but are known to involve oxidative injury due to the generation of reactive oxygen species by the transition metals on the surface of the fibers as well as from cells engaged in phagocytosis.

Past exposure to asbestos is specifically indicated by pleural plaques on chest radiographs, which are characterized by either thickening or calcification along the parietal pleura, particularly along the lower lung fields, the diaphragm, and the cardiac border. Without additional manifestations, pleural plaques imply only exposure, not pulmonary impairment. Benign pleural effusions also may occur. The fluid is typically a serous or bloody exudate. The effusion may be slowly progressive or may resolve spontaneously.

Irregular or linear opacities that usually are first noted in the lower lung fields are the chest radiographic hallmark of asbestosis. An indistinct heart border or a "ground-glass" appearance in the lung fields may be seen. HRCT may show distinct changes of subpleural curvilinear lines 5–10 mm in length that appear to be parallel to the pleural surface (Fig. 311-1).

Pulmonary function testing in asbestosis reveals a restrictive pattern with a decrease in both lung volumes and diffusing capacity. There may also be evidence of mild airflow obstruction (due to peribronchiolar fibrosis).

Because no specific therapy is available for asbestosis, supportive care is the same as that given to any patient with diffuse interstitial fibrosis of any cause. In general, newly diagnosed cases will have resulted from exposures that occurred many years before.

Lung cancer (Chap. 107) is the most common cancer associated with asbestos exposure. The excess frequency of lung cancer (all histologic types) in asbestos workers is associated with a minimum latency of 15–19 years between first exposure and development of the disease. Persons with more exposure are at greater risk of disease. In addition, there is a significant interactive effect of smoking and asbestos exposure that results in greater risk than what would be expected from the additive effect of each factor.

Mesotheliomas (Chap. 316), both pleural and peritoneal, are also associated with asbestos exposure. In contrast to lung cancers, these tumors do not appear to be associated with smoking. Relatively short-term asbestos exposures of ≤1–2 years, occurring up to 40 years in the past, have been associated with the development of mesotheliomas (an observation that emphasizes the importance of obtaining a complete environmental exposure history). Although the risk of mesothelioma is much less than that of lung cancer among asbestos-exposed workers, over 2000 cases were reported in the United States per year at the start of the twenty-first century.

Because epidemiologic studies have shown that >80% of mesotheliomas may be associated with asbestos exposure, documented mesothelioma in a patient with occupational or environmental exposure to asbestos may be compensable.

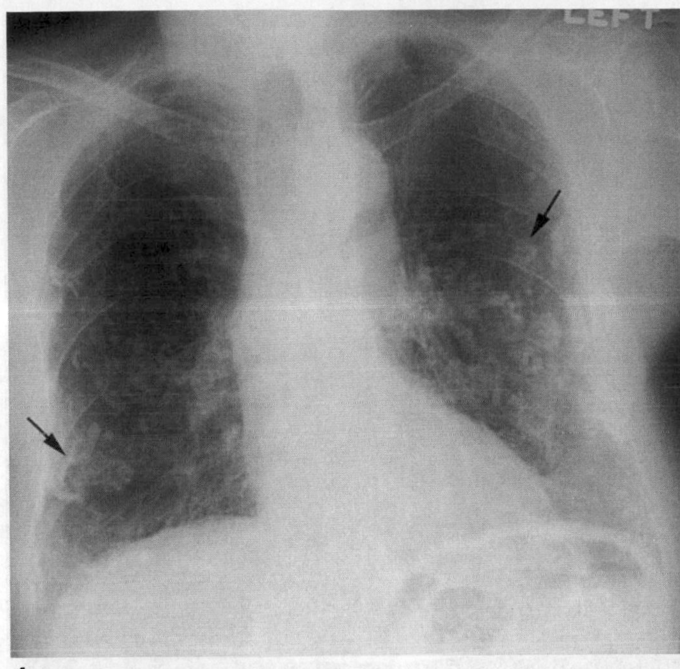

A

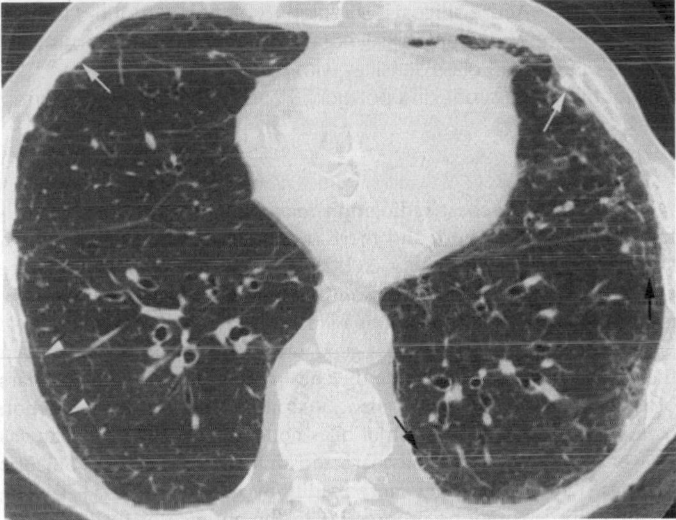

B

FIGURE 311-1 Asbestosis. *A.* Frontal chest radiograph shows bilateral calcified pleural plaques consistent with asbestos-related pleural disease. Poorly defined linear and reticular abnormalities are seen in the lower lobes bilaterally. ***B.*** Axial high-resolution computed tomography of the thorax obtained through the lung bases shows bilateral, subpleural reticulation (*black arrows*), representing fibrotic lung disease due to asbestosis. Subpleural lines are also present (*arrowheads*), characteristic of, though not specific for, asbestosis. Calcified pleural plaques representing asbestos-related pleural disease (*white arrows*) are also evident.

SILICOSIS

Despite being one of the oldest known occupational pulmonary hazards, *free silica* (SiO_2), or crystalline quartz, is still a major cause of disease. The major occupational exposures include mining; stonecutting; sand blasting; glass and cement manufacturing; foundry work; packing of silica flour; and quarrying, particularly of granite. Most often, pulmonary fibrosis due to silica exposure (silicosis) occurs in a dose-response fashion after many years of exposure.

Workers heavily exposed through sandblasting in confined spaces, tunneling through rock with a high quartz content (15–25%), or the manufacture of abrasive soaps may develop acute silicosis with as little as 10 months of exposure. The clinical and pathologic features of acute silicosis are similar to those of pulmonary alveolar proteinosis

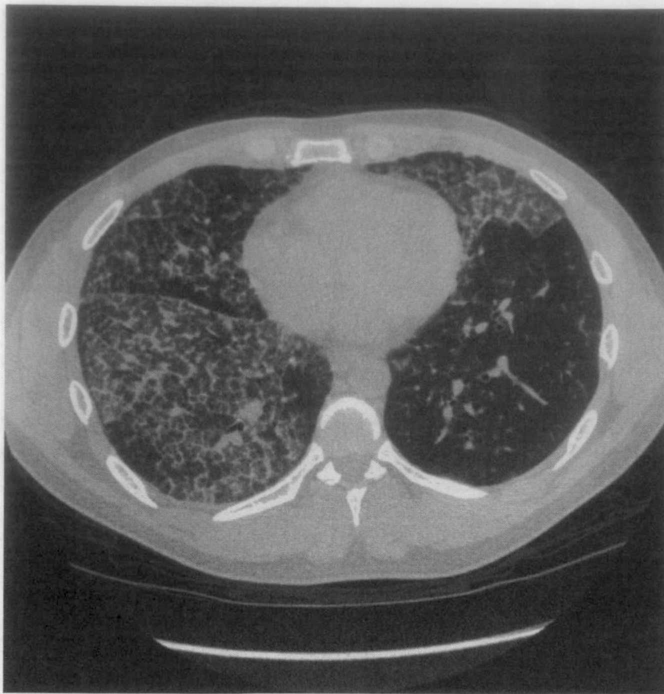

FIGURE 311-2 Acute silicosis. This high-resolution computed tomography scan shows multiple small nodules consistent with silicosis but also diffuse ground-glass densities with thickened intralobular and interlobular septa producing polygonal shapes. This has been referred to as "crazy paving."

(Chap. 315). The chest radiograph may show profuse miliary infiltration or consolidation, and there is a characteristic HRCT pattern known as "crazy paving" (Fig. 311-2). The disease may be quite severe and progressive despite the discontinuation of exposure. Whole-lung lavage may provide symptomatic relief and slow the progression.

With long-term, less intense exposure, small rounded opacities in the upper lobes may appear on the chest radiograph after 15–20 years of exposure, usually without associated impairment of lung function (*simple silicosis*). Calcification of hilar nodes may occur in as many as 20% of cases and produces a characteristic "eggshell" pattern. Silicotic nodules may be identified more readily by HRCT (Fig. 311-3). The nodular fibrosis may be progressive in the absence of further exposure, with coalescence and formation of nonsegmental conglomerates of irregular masses >1 cm in diameter (*complicated silicosis*). These masses can become quite large, and when this occurs, the term *progressive massive fibrosis* (PMF) is applied. Significant functional impairment with both restrictive and obstructive components may be associated with PMF.

Because silica is cytotoxic to alveolar macrophages, patients with silicosis are at greater risk of acquiring lung infections that involve these cells as a primary defense (*Mycobacterium tuberculosis*, atypical mycobacteria and fungi). Because of the increased risk of active tuberculosis, the recommended treatment of latent tuberculosis in these patients is longer. Another potential clinical complication of silicosis is autoimmune connective tissue disorders such as rheumatoid arthritis and scleroderma. In addition, there are sufficient epidemiologic data that the International Agency for Research on Cancer lists silica as a probable lung carcinogen.

Other, less hazardous silicates include fuller's earth, kaolin, mica, diatomaceous earths, silica gel, soapstone, carbonate dusts, and cement dusts. The production of fibrosis in workers exposed to these agents is believed to be related either to the free silica content of these dusts or, for substances that contain no free silica, to the potentially large dust loads to which these workers may be exposed. Some silicates, including *talc* and *vermiculite*, may be contaminated with asbestos. Fibrosis of lung or pleura, lung cancer, and mesothelioma have been associated with chronic exposure to talc and vermiculite dusts.

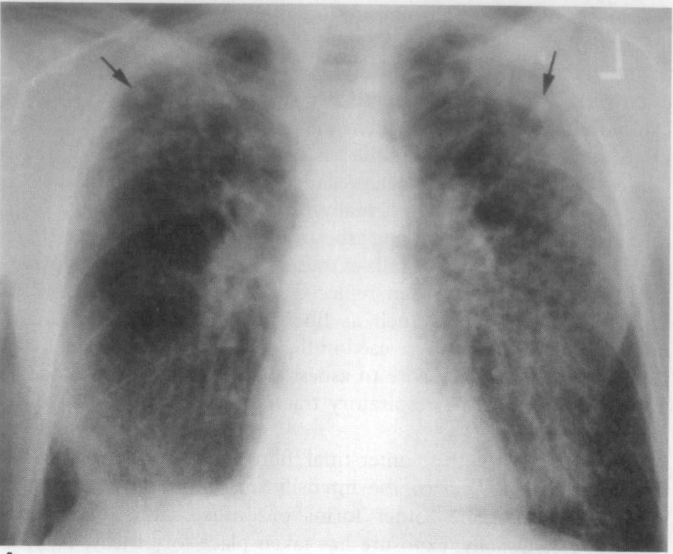

A

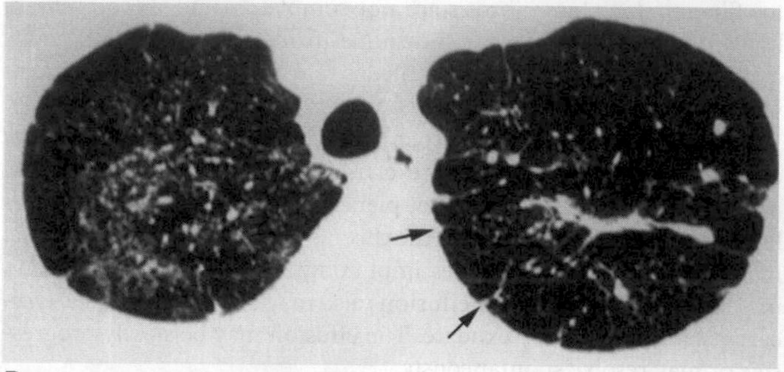

B

FIGURE 311-3 Chronic silicosis. *A.* Frontal chest radiograph in a patient with silicosis shows variably sized, poorly defined nodules (*arrows*) predominating in the upper lobes. ***B.*** Axial thoracic computed tomography image through the lung apices shows numerous small nodules, more pronounced in the right upper lobe. A number of the nodules are subpleural in location (*arrows*).

COAL WORKER'S PNEUMOCONIOSIS (CWP)

Occupational exposure to *coal dust* can lead to CWP, which has enormous social, economic, and medical significance in every nation in which coal mining is an important industry. Simple radiographically identified CWP is seen in ~10% of all coal miners and in as many as 50% of anthracite miners with more than 20 years of work on the coal face. The prevalence of disease is lower in workers in bituminous coal mines.

With prolonged exposure to coal dust (i.e., 15–20 years), small, rounded opacities similar to those of silicosis may develop. As in silicosis, the presence of these nodules (*simple CWP*) usually is not associated with pulmonary impairment. In addition to CWP, coal dust can cause chronic bronchitis and COPD (Chap. 314). The effects of coal dust are additive to those of cigarette smoking.

Complicated CWP is manifested by the appearance on the chest radiograph of nodules ≥1 cm in diameter generally confined to the upper half of the lungs. As in silicosis, this condition can progress to PMF that is accompanied by severe lung function deficits and associated with premature mortality. Despite improvements in technology to protect coal miners, cases of PMF still occur in the United States at a disturbing rate.

Caplan syndrome (Chap. 380), first described in coal miners but subsequently in patients with silicosis, is the combination of pneumoconiotic nodules and seropositive rheumatoid arthritis. Silica has immunoadjuvant properties and is often present in anthracitic coal dust.

CHRONIC BERYLLIUM DISEASE

Beryllium is a lightweight metal with tensile strength, good electrical conductivity, and value in the control of nuclear reactions through its ability to quench neutrons. Although beryllium may produce an acute pneumonitis, it is far more commonly associated with a chronic granulomatous inflammatory disease that is similar to sarcoidosis (Chap. 390). Unless one inquires specifically about occupational exposures to beryllium in the manufacture of alloys, ceramics, or high-technology electronics in a patient with sarcoidosis, one may miss entirely the etiologic relationship to the occupational exposure. What distinguishes chronic beryllium disease (CBD) from sarcoidosis is evidence of a specific cell-mediated immune response (i.e., delayed hypersensitivity) to beryllium.

The test that usually provides this evidence is the beryllium lymphocyte proliferation test (BeLPT). The BeLPT compares the in vitro proliferation of lymphocytes from blood or bronchoalveolar lavage in the presence of beryllium salts with that of unstimulated cells. Proliferation is usually measured by lymphocyte uptake of radiolabeled thymidine.

Chest imaging findings are similar to those of sarcoidosis (nodules along septal lines) except that hilar adenopathy is somewhat less common. As with sarcoidosis, pulmonary function test results may show restrictive and/or obstructive ventilatory deficits and decreased diffusing capacity. With early disease, both chest imaging studies and pulmonary function tests may be normal. Fiberoptic bronchoscopy with transbronchial lung biopsy usually is required to make the diagnosis of CBD. In a beryllium-sensitized individual, the presence of noncaseating granulomas or monocytic infiltration in lung tissue establishes the diagnosis. Accumulation of beryllium-specific CD4+ T cells occurs in the granulomatous inflammation seen on lung biopsy. Susceptibility to CBD is highly associated with human leukocyte antigen DP (HLA-DP) alleles that have a glutamic acid in position 69 of the β chain.

OTHER METALS

Aluminum and titanium dioxide have been rarely associated with a sarcoid-like reaction in lung tissue. Exposure to dust containing tungsten carbide, also known as "hard metal," may produce giant cell interstitial pneumonitis. Cobalt is a constituent of tungsten carbide and is the likely etiologic agent of both the interstitial pneumonitis and the occupational asthma that may occur. The most common exposures to tungsten carbide occur in tool and dye, saw blade, and drill bit manufacture. Diamond polishing may also involve exposure to cobalt dust. In patients with interstitial lung disease, one should always inquire about exposure to metal fumes and/or dusts. Especially when sarcoidosis appears to be the diagnosis, one should always consider possible CBD.

OTHER INORGANIC DUSTS

Most of the inorganic dusts discussed thus far are associated with the production of either dust macules or interstitial fibrotic changes in the lung. Other inorganic and organic dusts (see categories in Table 311-1), along with some of the dusts previously discussed, are associated with chronic mucus hypersecretion (chronic bronchitis), with or without reduction of expiratory flow rates. Cigarette smoking is the major cause of these conditions, and any effort to attribute some component of the disease to occupational and environmental exposures must take cigarette smoking into account. Most studies suggest an additive effect of dust exposure and smoking. The pattern of the irritant dust effect is similar to that of cigarette smoking, suggesting that small airway inflammation may be the initial site of pathologic response in those cases and continued exposure may lead to chronic bronchitis and COPD.

ORGANIC DUSTS

Some of the specific diseases associated with organic dusts are discussed in detail in the chapters on asthma (Chap. 309) and hypersensitivity pneumonitis (Chap. 310). Many of these diseases are named for the specific setting in which they are found, e.g., farmer's lung, malt worker's disease, and mushroom worker's disease. Often the temporal relation of symptoms to exposure furnishes the best evidence for the diagnosis. Three occupational exposures are singled out for discussion here because they affect the largest proportions of workers.

Cotton Dust (Byssinosis) Workers occupationally exposed to cotton dust (but also to flax, hemp, or jute dust) in the production of yarns for textiles and rope making are at risk for an asthma-like syndrome known as byssinosis. Exposure occurs throughout the manufacturing process but is most pronounced in the portions of the factory involved with the treatment of the cotton before spinning, i.e., blowing, mixing, and carding (straightening of fibers). The risk of byssinosis is associated with both cotton dust and endotoxin levels in the workplace environment.

Byssinosis is characterized clinically as occasional (early-stage) and then regular (late-stage) chest tightness toward the end of the first day of the workweek ("Monday chest tightness"). Exposed workers may show a significant drop in FEV_1 over the course of a Monday workshift. Initially the symptoms do not recur on subsequent days of the week. However, in 10–25% of workers, the disease may be progressive, with chest tightness recurring or persisting throughout the workweek. After >10 years of exposure, workers with recurrent symptoms are more likely to have an obstructive pattern on pulmonary function testing. The highest grades of impairment generally are seen in smokers.

Dust exposure can be reduced by the use of exhaust hoods, general increases in ventilation, and wetting procedures, but respiratory protective equipment may be required during certain operations. Regular surveillance of pulmonary function in cotton dust–exposed workers using spirometry before and after the workshift is required by OSHA. All workers with persistent symptoms or significantly reduced levels of pulmonary function should be moved to areas of lower risk of exposure.

Grain Dust Worldwide, many farmers and workers in grain storage facilities are exposed to grain dust. The presentation of obstructive airway disease in grain dust–exposed workers is virtually identical to the characteristic findings in cigarette smokers, i.e., persistent cough, mucus hypersecretion, wheeze and dyspnea on exertion, and reduced FEV_1 and FEV_1/FVC (forced vital capacity) ratio (Chap. 306e).

Dust concentrations in grain elevators vary greatly but can be >10,000 μg/m³ with many particles in the respirable size range. The effect of grain dust exposure is additive to that of cigarette smoking, with ~50% of workers who smoke having symptoms. Smoking grain dust–exposed workers are more likely to have obstructive ventilatory deficits on pulmonary function testing. As in byssinosis, endotoxin may play a role in grain dust–induced chronic bronchitis and COPD.

Farmer's Lung This condition results from exposure to moldy hay containing spores of thermophilic actinomycetes that produce a hypersensitivity pneumonitis (Chap. 310). A patient with acute farmer's lung presents 4–8 h after exposure with fever, chills, malaise, cough, and dyspnea without wheezing. The history of exposure is obviously essential to distinguish this disease from influenza or pneumonia with similar symptoms. In the chronic form of the disease, the history of repeated attacks after similar exposure is important in differentiating this syndrome from other causes of patchy fibrosis (e.g., sarcoidosis).

A wide variety of other organic dusts are associated with the occurrence of hypersensitivity pneumonitis (Chap. 310). For patients who present with hypersensitivity pneumonitis, specific and careful inquiry about occupations, hobbies, and other home environmental exposures is necessary to uncover the source of the etiologic agent.

TOXIC CHEMICALS

Exposure to toxic chemicals affecting the lung generally involves gases and vapors. A common accident is one in which the victim is trapped in a confined space where the chemicals have accumulated to harmful levels. In addition to the specific toxic effects of the chemical, the victim often sustains considerable anoxia, which can play a dominant role in determining whether the individual survives.

Table 311-2 lists a variety of toxic agents that can produce acute and sometimes life-threatening reactions in the lung. All these agents in sufficient concentrations have been demonstrated, at least in animal studies, to affect the lower airways and disrupt alveolar architecture, either acutely or as a result of chronic exposure. Some of these agents may be generated acutely in the environment (see below).

TABLE 311-2 SELECTED COMMON TOXIC CHEMICAL AGENTS THAT AFFECT THE LUNG

Agent(s)	Selected Exposures	Acute Effects from High or Accidental Exposure	Chronic Effects from Relatively Low Exposure
Acid anhydrides	Manufacture of resin esters, polyester resins, thermoactivated adhesives	Nasal irritation, cough	Asthma, chronic bronchitis, hypersensitivity pneumonitis
Acid fumes: H_2SO_4, HNO_3	Manufacture of fertilizers, chlorinated organic compounds, dyes, explosives, rubber products, metal etching, plastics	Mucous membrane irritation, followed by chemical pneumonitis 2–3 days later	Bronchitis and suggestion of mildly reduced pulmonary function in children with lifelong residential exposure to high levels
Acrolein and other aldehydes	By-product of burning plastics, woods, tobacco smoke	Mucous membrane irritant, decrease in lung function	Upper respiratory tract irritation
Ammonia	Refrigeration; petroleum refining; manufacture of fertilizers, explosives, plastics, and other chemicals	Same as for acid fumes, but bronchiectasis also has been reported	Upper respiratory tract irritation, chronic bronchitis
Cadmium fumes	Smelting, soldering, battery production	Mucous membrane irritant, acute respiratory distress syndrome (ARDS)	Chronic obstructive pulmonary disease (COPD)
Formaldehyde	Manufacture of resins, leathers, rubber, metals, and woods; laboratory workers, embalmers; emission from urethane foam insulation	Same as for acid fumes	Nasopharyngeal cancer
Halides and acid salts (Cl, Br, F)	Bleaching in pulp, paper, textile industry; manufacture of chemical compounds; synthetic rubber, plastics, disinfectant, rocket fuel, gasoline	Mucous membrane irritation, pulmonary edema; possible reduced forced vital capacity (FVC) 1–2 years after exposure	Upper respiratory tract irritation, epistaxis, tracheobronchitis
Hydrogen sulfide	By-product of many industrial processes, oil, other petroleum processes and storage	Increase in respiratory rate followed by respiratory arrest, lactic acidosis, pulmonary edema, death	Conjunctival irritation, chronic bronchitis, recurrent pneumonitis
Isocyanates (TDI, HDI, MDI)	Production of polyurethane foams, plastics, adhesives, surface coatings	Mucous membrane irritation, dyspnea, cough, wheeze, pulmonary edema	Upper respiratory tract irritation, cough, asthma, hypersensitivity pneumonitis, reduced lung function
Nitrogen dioxide	Silage, metal etching, explosives, rocket fuels, welding, by-product of burning fossil fuels	Cough, dyspnea, pulmonary edema may be delayed 4–12 h; possible result from acute exposure: bronchiolitis obliterans in 2–6 weeks	Emphysema in animals, ? chronic bronchitis, associated with reduced lung function in children with lifelong residential exposure
Ozone	Arc welding, flour bleaching, deodorizing, emissions from copying equipment, photochemical air pollutant	Mucous membrane irritant, pulmonary hemorrhage and edema, reduced pulmonary function transiently in children and adults, and increased hospitalization with exposure to summer haze	Excess cardiopulmonary mortality rates
Phosgene	Organic compound, metallurgy, volatilization of chlorine-containing compounds	Delayed onset of bronchiolitis and pulmonary edema	Chronic bronchitis
Sulfur dioxide	Manufacture of sulfuric acid, bleaches, coating of nonferrous metals, food processing, refrigerant, burning of fossil fuels, wood pulp industry	Mucous membrane irritant, epistaxis, bronchospasm (especially in people with asthma)	Chronic bronchitis

Abbreviations: HDI, hexamethylene diisocyanate; MDI, methylene diphenyl diisocyanate; TDI, toluene diisocyanate.

Firefighters and fire victims are at risk of *smoke inhalation*, an important cause of acute cardiorespiratory failure. Smoke inhalation kills more fire victims than does thermal injury. Carbon monoxide poisoning with resulting significant hypoxemia can be life-threatening (**Chap. 473e**). Synthetic materials (plastic, polyurethanes), when burned, may release a variety of other toxic agents (such as cyanide and hydrochloric acid), and this must be considered in evaluating smoke inhalation victims. Exposed victims may have some degree of lower respiratory tract inflammation and/or pulmonary edema.

Exposure to certain highly reactive, low-molecular-weight agents used in the manufacture of synthetic polymers, paints, and coatings (*diisocyanates* in polyurethanes, *aromatic amines* and *acid anhydrides* in epoxies) is associated with a high risk of occupational asthma. Although this occupational asthma manifests clinically as if sensitization has occurred, an IgE antibody–mediated mechanism is not necessarily involved. Hypersensitivity pneumonitis–like reactions also have been described in diisocyanate and acid anhydride–exposed workers.

Fluoropolymers such as Teflon, which at normal temperatures produce no reaction, become volatilized upon heating. The inhaled agents cause a characteristic syndrome of fever, chills, malaise, and occasionally mild wheezing, leading to the diagnosis of *polymer fume fever*. A similar self-limited, influenza-like syndrome—*metal fume fever*—results from acute exposure to fumes containing zinc oxide, typically from welding of galvanized steel. These inhalational fever syndromes may begin several hours after work and resolve within 24 h, only to return on repeated exposure.

Two other agents have been associated with potentially severe lung disease. Occupational exposure to nylon flock has been shown to induce a lymphocytic bronchiolitis, and workers exposed to diacetyl, which is used to provide "butter" flavor in the manufacture of microwave popcorn and other foods, have developed bronchiolitis obliterans (**Chap. 315**).

World Trade Center Disaster A consequence of the attack on the World Trade Center (WTC) on September 11, 2001, was relatively heavy exposure of a large number of firefighters and other rescue workers to the dust generated by the collapse of the buildings. Environmental monitoring and chemical characterization of WTC dust has revealed a wide variety of potentially toxic constituents, although much of the dust was pulverized cement. Possibly because of the high alkalinity of WTC dust, significant cough, wheeze, and phlegm production occurred among firefighters and cleanup crews. New cough and wheeze syndromes also occurred among local residents. Heavier exposure to WTC dust among New York City firefighters was associated with accelerated decline of lung function over the first year after the disaster. More recently, concerns have been raised about risk of interstitial lung disease, especially of a granulomatous nature.

OCCUPATIONAL RESPIRATORY CARCINOGENS

Exposures at work have been estimated to contribute to 10% of all lung cancer cases. In addition to asbestos, other agents either proven or suspected to be respiratory carcinogens include acrylonitrile, arsenic compounds, beryllium, bis(chloromethyl) ether, chromium (hexavalent), formaldehyde (nasal), isopropanol (nasal sinuses), mustard gas, nickel carbonyl (nickel smelting), polycyclic aromatic hydrocarbons (coke oven emissions and diesel exhaust), secondhand tobacco smoke, silica (both mining and processing), talc (possible asbestos contamination in both mining and milling), vinyl chloride (sarcomas), wood (nasal cancer only), and uranium. Workers at risk of radiation-related lung cancer include not only those involved in mining or processing uranium but also those exposed in underground mining operations of other ores where radon daughters may be emitted from rock formations.

ASSESSMENT OF DISABILITY

Disability is the term used to describe the decreased ability to work due to the effects of a medical condition. Physicians are generally able to assess physiologic dysfunction, or *impairment*, but the rating of disability for compensation of loss of income also involves nonmedical factors such as the education and employability of the individual. The disability rating scheme differs with the compensation-granting agency. For example, the U.S. Social Security Administration requires that an individual be unable to do any work (i.e., *total* disability) before he or she will receive income replacement payments. Many state workers' compensation systems allow for payments for *partial* disability. In the Social Security scheme, no determination of cause is done, whereas work-relatedness must be established in workers' compensation systems.

For respiratory impairment rating, resting pulmonary function tests (spirometry and diffusing capacity) are used as the initial assessment tool, with cardiopulmonary exercise testing (to assess maximal oxygen consumption) used if the results of the resting tests do not correlate with the patient's symptoms. Methacholine challenge (to assess airway reactivity) can also be useful in patients with asthma who have normal spirometry when evaluated. Some compensation agencies (e.g., Social Security) have proscribed disability classification schemes based on pulmonary function test results. When no specific scheme is proscribed, the *Guidelines of the American Medical Association* should be used.

GENERAL ENVIRONMENTAL EXPOSURES

OUTDOOR AIR POLLUTION

In 1971, the U.S. government established national air quality standards for several pollutants believed to be responsible for excess cardiorespiratory diseases. Primary standards regulated by the U.S. Environmental Protection Agency (EPA) designed to protect the public health with an adequate margin of safety exist for sulfur dioxide, particulates matter, nitrogen dioxide, ozone, lead, and carbon monoxide. Standards for each of these pollutants are updated regularly through an extensive review process conducted by the EPA. (For details on current standards, go to *http://www.epa.gov/air/criteria.html.*)

Pollutants are generated from both stationary sources (power plants and industrial complexes) and mobile sources (motor vehicles), and none of the regulated pollutants occurs in isolation. Furthermore, pollutants may be changed by chemical reactions after being emitted. For example, sulfur dioxide and particulate matter emissions from a coal-fired power plant may react in air to produce acid sulfates and aerosols, which can be transported long distances in the atmosphere. Oxides of nitrogen and volatile organic compounds from automobile exhaust react with sunlight to produce ozone. Although originally thought to be confined to Los Angeles, photochemically derived pollution ("smog") is now known to be a problem throughout the United States and in many other countries. Both acute and chronic effects of these exposures have been documented in large population studies.

The symptoms and diseases associated with air pollution are the same as conditions commonly associated with cigarette smoking. In addition, decreased growth of lung function and asthma have been associated with chronic exposure to only modestly elevated levels of traffic-related gases and respirable particles. Multiple population-based time-series studies within cities have demonstrated excess health care utilization for asthma and other cardiopulmonary conditions as well as increased mortality rates. Cohort studies comparing cities that have relatively high levels of particulate exposures with less polluted communities suggest excess morbidity and mortality rates from cardiopulmonary conditions in long-term residents of the former. The strong epidemiologic evidence that fine particulate matter is a risk factor for cardiovascular morbidity and mortality has prompted toxicologic investigations into the underlying mechanisms. The inhalation of fine particles from combustion sources probably generates oxidative stress followed by local injury and inflammation in the lungs that in turn lead to autonomic and systemic inflammatory responses that can induce endothelial dysfunction and/or injury. Recent research findings on the health effects of air pollutants has led to stricter U.S. ambient air quality standards for ozone, oxides of nitrogen, and particulate matter as well as greater emphasis on publicizing pollution alerts to encourage individuals with significant cardiopulmonary impairment to stay indoors during high-pollution episodes.

INDOOR EXPOSURES

Secondhand tobacco smoke (Chap. 470), radon gas, wood smoke, and other biologic agents generated indoors must be considered. Several studies have shown that the respirable particulate load in any household is directly proportional to the number of cigarette smokers living in that home. Increases in prevalence of respiratory illnesses, especially asthma, and reduced levels of pulmonary function measured with simple spirometry have been found in the children of smoking parents in a number of studies. Recent meta-analyses for lung cancer and cardiopulmonary diseases, combining data from multiple secondhand tobacco smoke epidemiologic studies, suggest an ~25% increase in relative risk for each condition, even after adjustment for major potential confounders.

Exposure to *radon gas* in homes is a risk factor for lung cancer. The main radon product (radon-222) is a gas that results from the decay series of uranium-238, with the immediate precursor being radium-226. The amount of radium in earth materials determines how much radon gas will be emitted. Levels associated with excess lung cancer risk may be present in as many as 10% of the houses in the United States. When smokers reside in the home, the problem is potentially greater, because the molecular size of radon particles allows them to attach readily to smoke particles that are inhaled. Fortunately, technology is available for assessing and reducing the level of exposure.

Other indoor exposures of concern are bioaerosols that contain antigenic material (fungi, cockroaches, dust mites, and pet danders) associated with an increased risk of atopy and asthma. Indoor chemical agents include strong cleaning agents (bleach, ammonia), formaldehyde, perfumes, pesticides, and oxides of nitrogen from gas appliances. Nonspecific responses associated with "tight-building syndrome," perhaps better termed "building-associated illness," in which no particular agent has been implicated, have included a wide variety of complaints, among them respiratory symptoms that are relieved only by avoiding exposure in the building in question. The degree to which "smells" and other sensory stimuli are involved in the triggering of potentially incapacitating psychological or physical responses has yet to be determined, and the long-term consequences of such environmental exposures are unknown.

GLOBAL CONSIDERATIONS

Indoor exposure to *biomass smoke* (wood, dung, crop residues, charcoal) is estimated to be responsible for >4% of worldwide disability-adjusted life-years (DALYs) lost, due to acute lower respiratory infections in children, COPD and lung cancer in women, and cardiovascular disease among men. This burden of disease places indoor exposure to biomass smoke as the leading environmental hazard for poor health and the third most important risk factor overall.

Almost one-half of the world's population uses biomass fuel for cooking, heating, or baking. This occurs predominantly in the rural areas of developing countries. Because many families burn biomass fuels in open stoves, which are highly inefficient, and inside homes with poor ventilation, women and young children are exposed on a daily basis to high levels of smoke. In these homes, 24-h mean levels

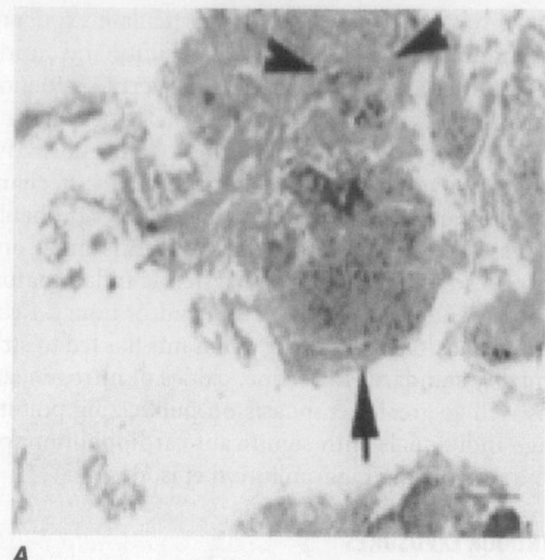

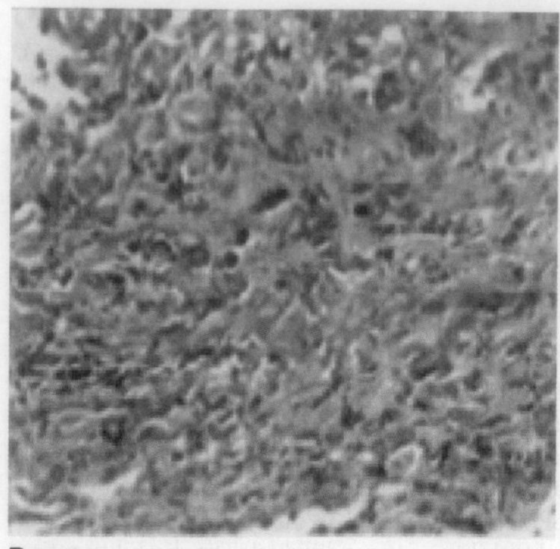

FIGURE 311-4 Histopathologic features of biomass smoke–induced interstitial lung disease. ***A.*** Anthracitic pigment is seen accumulating along alveolar septae (*arrowheads*) and within a pigmented dust macule (*single arrow*). ***B.*** A high-power photomicrograph contains a mixture of fibroblasts and carbon-laden macrophages.

of fine particulate matter, a component of biomass smoke, have been reported to be 2–30 times higher than the National Ambient Air Quality Standards set by the U.S. EPA.

Epidemiologic studies have consistently shown associations between exposure to biomass smoke and both chronic bronchitis and COPD, with odds ratios ranging between 3 and 10 and increasing with longer exposures. In addition to the common occupational exposure to biomass smoke of women in developing countries, men from such countries may be occupationally exposed. Because of increased migration to the United States from developing countries, clinicians need to be aware of the chronic respiratory effects of exposure to biomass smoke, which can include interstitial lung disease (Fig. 311-4). Evidence is beginning to emerge that improved stoves with chimneys can reduce biomass smoke–induced respiratory illness in both children and women.

312 Bronchiectasis

Rebecca M. Baron, Miriam Baron Barshak

Bronchiectasis refers to an irreversible airway dilation that involves the lung in either a focal or a diffuse manner and that classically has been categorized as cylindrical or tubular (the most common form), varicose, or cystic.

ETIOLOGY

Bronchiectasis can arise from infectious or noninfectious causes (Table 312-1). Clues to the underlying etiology are often provided by the pattern of lung involvement. *Focal bronchiectasis* refers to bronchiectatic changes in a localized area of the lung and can be a consequence of obstruction of the airway—either extrinsic (e.g., due to compression by adjacent lymphadenopathy or parenchymal tumor mass) or intrinsic (e.g., due to an airway tumor or aspirated foreign body, a scarred/stenotic airway, or bronchial atresia from congenital underdevelopment of the airway). *Diffuse bronchiectasis* is characterized by widespread bronchiectatic changes throughout the lung and often arises from an underlying systemic or infectious disease process.

More pronounced involvement of the upper lung fields is most common in cystic fibrosis (CF) and is also observed in postradiation fibrosis, corresponding to the lung region encompassed by the radiation port. Bronchiectasis with predominant involvement of the lower lung fields usually has its source in chronic recurrent aspiration (e.g., due to esophageal motility disorders like those in scleroderma), end-stage fibrotic lung disease (e.g., traction bronchiectasis from idiopathic

TABLE 312-1 MAJOR ETIOLOGIES OF BRONCHIECTASIS AND PROPOSED WORKUP

Pattern of Lung Involvement	Etiology by Category (Examples)	Workup
Focal	Obstruction (aspirated foreign body, tumor mass)	Chest imaging (chest x-ray and/or chest computed tomography); bronchoscopy
Diffuse	Infection (bacterial, nontuberculous mycobacterial)	Sputum Gram's stain/culture; stains/cultures for acid-fast bacilli and fungi. If no pathogen is identified, consider bronchoscopy with bronchoalveolar lavage.
	Immunodeficiency (hypogammaglobulinemia, HIV infection, bronchiolitis obliterans after lung transplantation)	Complete blood count with differential; immunoglobulin measurement; HIV testing
	Genetic causes (cystic fibrosis, Kartagener's syndrome, α_1 antitrypsin deficiency)	Measurement of chloride levels in sweat (for cystic fibrosis), α_1 antitrypsin levels; nasal or respiratory tract brush/biopsy (for dyskinetic/immotile cilia syndrome); genetic testing
	Autoimmune or rheumatologic causes (rheumatoid arthritis, Sjögren's syndrome, inflammatory bowel disease); immune-mediated disease (allergic bronchopulmonary aspergillosis)	Clinical examination with careful joint exam, serologic testing (e.g., for rheumatoid factor). Consider workup for allergic bronchopulmonary aspergillosis, especially in patients with refractory asthma.[a]
	Recurrent aspiration	Test of swallowing function and general neuromuscular strength
	Miscellaneous (yellow nail syndrome, traction bronchiectasis from postradiation fibrosis or idiopathic pulmonary fibrosis)	Guided by clinical condition
	Idiopathic	Exclusion of other causes

[a]Skin testing for *Aspergillus* reactivity; measurement of serum precipitins for *Aspergillus*, serum IgE levels, serum eosinophils, etc.

pulmonary fibrosis), or recurrent immunodeficiency-associated infections (e.g., hypogammaglobulinemia). Bronchiectasis resulting from infection by nontuberculous mycobacteria (NTM), most commonly the *Mycobacterium avium-intracellulare* complex (MAC), often preferentially affects the midlung fields. Congenital causes of bronchiectasis with predominant midlung field involvement include the dyskinetic/immotile cilia syndrome. Finally, predominant involvement of the central airways is reported in association with allergic bronchopulmonary aspergillosis (ABPA), in which an immune-mediated reaction to *Aspergillus* damages the bronchial wall. Congenital causes of central airway–predominant bronchiectasis resulting from cartilage deficiency include tracheobronchomegaly (Mounier-Kuhn syndrome) and Williams-Campbell syndrome.

In many cases, the etiology of bronchiectasis is not determined. In case series, as many as 25–50% of patients referred for bronchiectasis have idiopathic disease.

EPIDEMIOLOGY

The overall reported prevalence of bronchiectasis in the United States has recently increased, but the epidemiology of bronchiectasis varies greatly with the underlying etiology. For example, patients born with CF often develop significant clinical bronchiectasis in late adolescence or early adulthood, although atypical presentations of CF in adults in their thirties and forties are also possible. In contrast, bronchiectasis resulting from MAC infection classically affects nonsmoking women >50 years of age. In general, the incidence of bronchiectasis increases with age. Bronchiectasis is more common among women than among men.

In areas where tuberculosis is prevalent, bronchiectasis more frequently occurs as a sequela of granulomatous infection. Focal bronchiectasis can arise from extrinsic compression of the airway by enlarged granulomatous lymph nodes and/or from development of intrinsic obstruction as a result of erosion of a calcified lymph node through the airway wall (e.g., broncholithiasis). Especially in reactivated tuberculosis, parenchymal destruction from infection can result in areas of more diffuse bronchiectasis. Apart from cases associated with tuberculosis, an increased incidence of non-CF bronchiectasis with an unclear underlying mechanism has been reported as a significant problem in developing nations. It has been suggested that the high incidence of malnutrition in certain areas may predispose to immune dysfunction and development of bronchiectasis.

PATHOGENESIS AND PATHOLOGY

The most widely cited mechanism of infectious bronchiectasis is the "vicious cycle hypothesis," in which susceptibility to infection and poor mucociliary clearance result in microbial colonization of the bronchial tree. Some organisms, such as *Pseudomonas aeruginosa*, exhibit a particular propensity for colonizing damaged airways and evading host defense mechanisms. Impaired mucociliary clearance can result from inherited conditions such as CF or dyskinetic cilia syndrome, and it has been proposed that a single severe infection (e.g., pneumonia caused by *Bordetella pertussis* or *Mycoplasma pneumoniae*) can result in significant airway damage and poor secretion clearance. The presence of the microbes incites continued chronic inflammation, with consequent damage to the airway wall, continued impairment of secretion and microbial clearance, and ongoing propagation of the infectious/inflammatory cycle. Moreover, it has been proposed that mediators released directly from bacteria can interfere with mucociliary clearance.

Classic studies of the pathology of bronchiectasis from the 1950s demonstrated significant small-airway wall inflammation and larger-airway wall destruction as well as dilation, with loss of elastin, smooth muscle, and cartilage. It has been proposed that inflammatory cells in the small airways release proteases and other mediators, such as reactive oxygen species and proinflammatory cytokines, that damage the larger-airway walls. Furthermore, the ongoing inflammatory process in the smaller airways results in airflow obstruction. It is thought that antiproteases, such as α_1 antitrypsin, play an important role in neutralizing the damaging effects of neutrophil elastase and in enhancing bacterial killing. Bronchiectasis and emphysema have been observed in patients with α_1 antitrypsin deficiency.

Proposed mechanisms for noninfectious bronchiectasis include immune-mediated reactions that damage the bronchial wall (e.g., those associated with systemic autoimmune conditions such as Sjögren's syndrome and rheumatoid arthritis). *Traction bronchiectasis* refers to dilated airways arising from parenchymal distortion as a result of lung fibrosis (e.g., postradiation fibrosis or idiopathic pulmonary fibrosis).

CLINICAL MANIFESTATIONS

The most common clinical presentation is a persistent productive cough with ongoing production of thick, tenacious sputum. Physical findings often include crackles and wheezing on lung auscultation, and some patients with bronchiectasis exhibit clubbing of the digits. Mild to moderate airflow obstruction is often detected on pulmonary function tests, overlapping with that seen at presentation with other conditions, such as chronic obstructive pulmonary disease (COPD). Acute exacerbations of bronchiectasis are usually characterized by changes in the nature of sputum production, with increased volume and purulence. However, typical signs and symptoms of lung infection, such as fever and new infiltrates, may not be present.

DIAGNOSIS

The diagnosis is usually based on presentation with a persistent chronic cough and sputum production accompanied by consistent radiographic features. Although chest radiographs lack sensitivity, the presence of "tram tracks" indicating dilated airways is consistent with bronchiectasis. Chest computed tomography (CT) is more specific for bronchiectasis and is the imaging modality of choice for confirming the diagnosis. CT findings include airway dilation (detected as parallel "tram tracks" or as the "signet-ring sign"—a cross-sectional area of the airway with a diameter at least 1.5 times that of the adjacent vessel), lack of bronchial tapering (including the presence of tubular structures within 1 cm from the pleural surface), bronchial wall thickening in dilated airways, inspissated secretions (e.g., the "tree-in-bud" pattern), or cysts emanating from the bronchial wall (especially pronounced in cystic bronchiectasis; Fig. 312-1).

APPROACH TO THE PATIENT: Bronchiectasis

The evaluation of a patient with bronchiectasis entails elicitation of a clinical history, chest imaging, and a workup to determine the underlying etiology. Evaluation of focal bronchiectasis almost always requires bronchoscopy to exclude airway obstruction by an underlying mass or foreign body. A workup for diffuse bronchiectasis includes analysis for the major etiologies (Table 312-1), with an initial focus on excluding CF. Pulmonary function testing is an important component of a functional assessment of the patient.

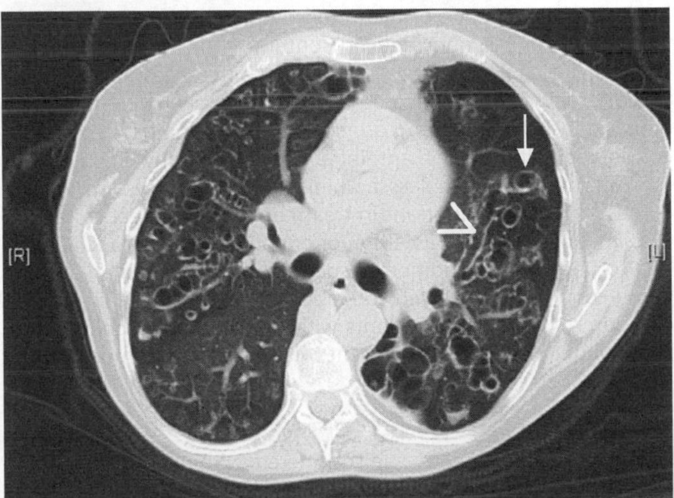

FIGURE 312-1 Representative chest computed tomography (CT) image of severe bronchiectasis. This patient's CT demonstrates many severely dilated airways, seen both longitudinally (*arrowhead*) and in cross-section (*arrow*).

TREATMENT BRONCHIECTASIS

Treatment of infectious bronchiectasis is directed at the control of active infection and improvements in secretion clearance and bronchial hygiene so as to decrease the microbial load within the airways and minimize the risk of repeated infections.

ANTIBIOTIC TREATMENT

Antibiotics targeting the causative or presumptive pathogen (with *Haemophilus influenzae* and *P. aeruginosa* isolated commonly) should be administered in acute exacerbations, usually for a minimum of 7–10 days and perhaps for as long as 14 days. Decisions about treatment of NTM infection can be difficult, given that these organisms can be colonizers as well as pathogens and the prolonged treatment course often is not well tolerated. Consensus guidelines have advised that diagnostic criteria for true clinical infection with NTM should be considered in patients with symptoms and radiographic findings of lung disease who have at least two sputum samples positive on culture; at least one bronchoalveolar lavage (BAL) fluid sample positive on culture; a biopsy sample displaying histopathologic features of NTM infection (e.g., granuloma or a positive stain for acid-fast bacilli) along with one positive sputum culture; or a pleural fluid sample (or a sample from another sterile extrapulmonary site) positive on culture. MAC strains are the most common NTM pathogens, and the recommended regimen for HIV-negative patients includes a macrolide combined with rifampin and ethambutol. Consensus guidelines also recommend macrolide susceptibility testing for clinically significant MAC isolates.

BRONCHIAL HYGIENE

The numerous approaches used to enhance secretion clearance in bronchiectasis include hydration and mucolytic administration, aerosolization of bronchodilators and hyperosmolar agents (e.g., hypertonic saline), and chest physiotherapy (e.g., postural drainage, traditional mechanical chest percussion via hand clapping to the chest, or use of devices such as an oscillatory positive expiratory pressure flutter valve or a high-frequency chest wall oscillation vest). Pulmonary rehabilitation and a regular exercise program may assist with secretion clearance as well as with other aspects of bronchiectasis, including improved exercise capacity and quality of life. The mucolytic dornase (DNase) is recommended routinely in CF-related bronchiectasis but not in non-CF bronchiectasis, given concerns about lack of efficacy and potential harm in the non-CF population.

ANTI-INFLAMMATORY THERAPY

It has been proposed that control of the inflammatory response may be of benefit in bronchiectasis, and relatively small-scale trials have yielded evidence of alleviated dyspnea, decreased need for inhaled β-agonists, and reduced sputum production with inhaled glucocorticoids. However, no significant differences in lung function or bronchiectasis exacerbation rates have been observed. Risks of immunosuppression and adrenal suppression must be carefully considered with use of anti-inflammatory therapy in infectious bronchiectasis. Nevertheless, administration of oral/systemic glucocorticoids may be important in treatment of bronchiectasis due to certain etiologies, such as ABPA, or of noninfectious bronchiectasis due to underlying conditions, especially that in which an autoimmune condition is believed to be active (e.g., rheumatoid arthritis or Sjögren's syndrome). Patients with ABPA may also benefit from a prolonged course of treatment with the oral antifungal agent itraconazole.

REFRACTORY CASES

In select cases, surgery can be considered, with resection of a focal area of suppuration. In advanced cases, lung transplantation can be considered.

COMPLICATIONS

In more severe cases of infectious bronchiectasis, recurrent infections and repeated courses of antibiotics can lead to microbial resistance to antibiotics. In certain cases, combinations of antibiotics that have their own independent toxicity profiles may be necessary to treat resistant organisms.

Recurrent infections can result in injury to superficial mucosal vessels, with bleeding and, in severe cases, life-threatening hemoptysis. Management of massive hemoptysis usually requires intubation to stabilize the patient, identification of the source of bleeding, and protection of the nonbleeding lung. Control of bleeding often necessitates bronchial artery embolization and, in severe cases, surgery.

PROGNOSIS

Outcomes of bronchiectasis can vary widely with the underlying etiology and may also be influenced by the frequency of exacerbations and (in infectious cases) the specific pathogens involved. In one study, the decline of lung function in patients with non-CF bronchiectasis was similar to that in patients with COPD, with the forced expiratory volume in 1 s (FEV_1) declining by 50–55 mL per year as opposed to 20–30 mL per year for healthy controls.

PREVENTION

Reversal of an underlying immunodeficient state (e.g., by administration of gamma globulin for immunoglobulin-deficient patients) and vaccination of patients with chronic respiratory conditions (e.g., influenza and pneumococcal vaccines) can decrease the risk of recurrent infections. Patients who smoke should be counseled about smoking cessation.

After resolution of an acute infection in patients with recurrences (e.g., ≥3 episodes per year), the use of suppressive antibiotics to minimize the microbial load and reduce the frequency of exacerbations has been proposed, although there is less consensus with regard to this approach in non-CF-associated bronchiectasis than in patients with CF-related bronchiectasis. Possible suppressive treatments include (1) administration of an oral antibiotic (e.g., ciprofloxacin) daily for 1–2 weeks per month; (2) use of a rotating schedule of oral antibiotics (to minimize the risk of development of drug resistance); (3) administration of a macrolide antibiotic (see below) daily or three times per week (with mechanisms of possible benefit related to non-antimicrobial properties, such as anti-inflammatory effects and reduction of gram-negative bacillary biofilms); (4) inhalation of aerosolized antibiotics (e.g., tobramycin inhalation solution) by select patients on a rotating schedule (e.g., 30 days on, 30 days off), with the goal of decreasing the microbial load without eliciting the side effects of systemic drug administration; and (5) intermittent administration of IV antibiotics (e.g., "clean-outs") for patients with more severe bronchiectasis and/or resistant pathogens. In relation to macrolide therapy (point 3 above), a number of double-blind, placebo-controlled, randomized trials have recently been published in non-CF bronchiectasis and support a benefit of long-term macrolides (6–12 months of azithromycin or erythromycin) in decreasing rates of bronchiectasis exacerbation, mucus production, and decline in lung function. However, two of these studies also reported increased macrolide resistance in commensal pathogens, dampening enthusiasm for universal use of macrolides in this setting and raising the question of whether there might be select non-CF bronchiectasis patients with higher morbidity for whom benefits of long-term macrolides might outweigh the risks of emergence of antibiotic resistance. In particular, development of macrolide-resistant NTM is a significant concern, making treatment of that pathogen much more difficult. Therefore, it is advised to rule out NTM infection before chronic macrolide therapy is considered.

In addition, ongoing consistent attention to bronchial hygiene can promote secretion clearance and decrease the microbial load in the airways.

313 Cystic Fibrosis

Eric J. Sorscher

CLINICAL FEATURES

Cystic fibrosis (CF) is an autosomal recessive exocrinopathy affecting multiple epithelial tissues. The gene product responsible for CF (the cystic fibrosis transmembrane conductance regulator [CFTR]) serves as an anion channel in the apical (luminal) plasma membranes of epithelial cells and regulates volume and composition of exocrine secretion. An increasingly sophisticated understanding of CFTR molecular genetics and membrane protein biochemistry has facilitated CF drug discovery, with a number of new agents advancing through the clinical testing phase.

Respiratory Manifestations The major morbidity and mortality associated with CF is attributable to respiratory compromise, characterized by copious hyperviscous and adherent pulmonary secretions that obstruct small and medium-sized airways. CF airway secretions are exceedingly difficult to clear, and a complex bacterial flora that includes *Staphylococcus aureus, Haemophilus influenzae*, and *Pseudomonas aeruginosa* (among other pathogens) is routinely cultured from CF sputum. Robust pulmonary inflammation in the setting of inspissated mucus and chronic bacterial infection leads to collateral tissue injury and further aggravates respiratory decline. Organisms such as *P. aeruginosa* exhibit a stereotypic mode of pathogenesis; a sentinel and early colonization event often engenders lifelong pulmonary infection by the same genetic strain. Over the course of many years, *P. aeruginosa* evolves in CF lungs to adopt a mucoid phenotype (attributable to release of alginate exoproduct) that confers selective advantage for the pathogen and poor prognosis for the host. Infection with other bacterial organisms such as *Burkholderia cepacia* also indicates a less favorable pulmonary outlook. Strategies to eradicate organisms such as *P. aeruginosa* early in the pathogenesis cascade have been successful and are thought to improve prognosis significantly if sustained.

Pancreatic Findings The complete name of the disease, *cystic fibrosis of the pancreas*, refers to profound tissue destruction of the exocrine pancreas, with fibrotic scarring and/or fatty replacement, cyst proliferation, loss of acinar tissue, and ablation of normal pancreatic architecture. As in the lung, tenacious exocrine secretions (sometimes termed *concretions*) obstruct pancreatic ducts and impair production and flow of digestive enzymes to the duodenum. The sequelae of exocrine pancreatic insufficiency include chronic malabsorption, poor growth, fat-soluble vitamin insufficiency, high levels of serum immunoreactive trypsinogen (a diagnostic test used in newborn screening), and loss of pancreatic islet cell mass. CF-related diabetes mellitus is a manifestation in over 30% of adults with the disease and is likely multifactorial in nature (attributable to progressive destruction of the endocrine pancreas, insulin resistance due to stress hormones, and other factors).

Other Organ System Damage As in CF lung and pancreas, thick and tenacious secretions compromise numerous other exocrine tissues. Obstruction of intrahepatic bile ducts and parenchymal fibrosis are commonly observed in pathologic specimens, with multilobular cirrhosis in 4–15% of patients with CF and significant hepatic insufficiency as a resulting manifestation among adults. Contents of the intestinal lumen are often difficult to excrete, leading to meconium ileus (a presentation in approximately 10–20% of newborns with CF) or distal intestinal obstructive syndrome in older individuals. Men typically exhibit complete involution of the vas deferens and infertility (despite functioning spermatogenesis), and approximately 99% of males with CF are infertile. The etiology of this dramatic anatomic defect in the male genitourinary system is not understood but may represent a developmental abnormality secondary to secretory obstruction of the vas. Abnormalities of female reproductive tract secretions are likely contributors to an increased incidence of infertility among women with CF. Radiographic evidence of sinusitis occurs in most CF patients and is associated with pathogens similar to those recovered from lower airways, suggesting that the sinus may serve as a reservoir for bacterial seeding.

PATHOGENESIS

Cystic Fibrosis Transmembrane Conductance Regulator (CFTR) CFTR is an integral membrane protein that functions as an epithelial anion channel. The ~1480-amino-acid molecule encodes a passive conduit for chloride and bicarbonate transport across plasma membranes of epithelial tissues, with direction of ion flow dependent on the electrochemical driving force. Gating of CFTR involves conformational cycling between an open and closed configuration and is augmented by hydrolysis of adenosine triphosphate (ATP). Anion flux mediated by CFTR does not involve active transport against a concentration gradient but utilizes the energy provided from ATP hydrolysis as a central feature of ion channel mechanochemistry and gating.

CFTR is situated in the apical plasma membranes of acinar and other epithelial cells where it regulates the amount and composition of secretion by exocrine glands. In numerous epithelia, chloride and bicarbonate release is followed passively by the flow of water, allowing for mobilization and clearance of exocrine products. Along respiratory mucosa, CFTR is necessary to provide sufficient depth of the periciliary fluid layer (PCL), allowing normal ciliary extension and mucociliary transport. CFTR-deficient airway cells exhibit depleted PCL, causing ciliary collapse and failure to clear overlying mucus (Video 313-1). In airway submucosal glands, CFTR is highly expressed in acini and may participate both in the formation of mucus and extrusion of glandular secretion onto the airway surface (Fig. 313-1). In other exocrine glands characterized by abrogated mucus transport (e.g., pancreatic acini and ducts, bile canaliculi, intestinal lumen), similar pathogenic mechanisms have been implicated. In these tissues, a driving force for apical chloride and/or bicarbonate secretion is believed to promote CFTR-mediated fluid and electrolyte release into the lumen, which confers proper rheology of mucins and other exocrine products. Failure of this mechanism disrupts normal hydration and transport of glandular secretion and is widely viewed as a proximate cause of ductular obstruction, with concomitant tissue injury.

Pulmonary Inflammation and Remodeling The CF airway is characterized by an aggressive, unrelenting, neutrophilic inflammatory response with release of proteases and oxidants leading to airway remodeling and bronchiectasis. Intense pulmonary inflammation is largely driven by chronic respiratory infection. Macrophages resident in CF lungs augment elaboration of proinflammatory cytokines, which contribute to innate and adaptive immune reactivity. CFTR-dependent abnormalities of airway surface fluid composition (e.g., pH) have been reported as contributors to impaired bacterial killing in CF lungs. The role of CFTR as a direct mediator of inflammatory responsiveness and/or pulmonary remodeling represents an important and topical area of investigation.

MOLECULAR GENETICS

DNA sequencing of *CFTR* from patients (and others) worldwide has revealed almost 2000 allelic variants; however, only about 10% of these have been well-characterized as disease-causing mutations. Distinguishing the single nucleotide transversions or other polymorphisms with causal relevance often presents a significant challenge. The CFTR2 resource (*www.cftr2.org/*) delineates gene variants with a clear etiologic role.

CFTR defects known to elicit disease are often categorized based on molecular mechanism. For example, the common F508del mutation (nomenclature denotes omission of a single phenylalanine residue [F] at CFTR position 508) leads to a folding abnormality recognized by cellular quality control pathways. CFTR encoding F508del retains partial ion channel function, but protein maturation is arrested in the endoplasmic reticulum, and CFTR fails to arrive at the plasma membrane. Instead, F508del CFTR is misrouted and undergoes endoplasmic reticulum–associated degradation via the proteasome. CFTR mutations that disrupt protein maturation are termed class II defects and are by far the most common genetic abnormalities. F508del alone accounts for ~70% of defective *CFTR* alleles in the United States, where

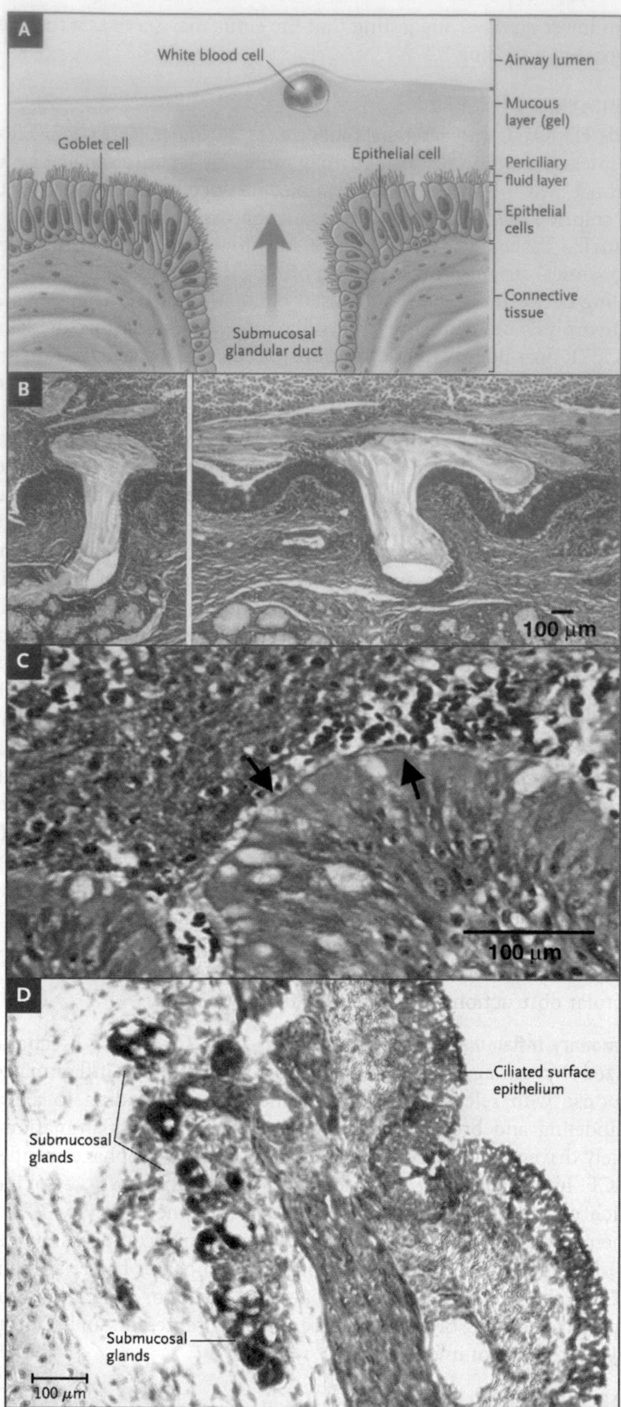

FIGURE 313-1 Extrusion of mucus secretion onto the epithelial surface of airways in cystic fibrosis. ***A.*** Schematic of the surface epithelium and supporting glandular structure of the human airway. ***B.*** The submucosal glands of a patient with cystic fibrosis are filled with mucus, and mucopurulent debris overlies the airway surfaces, essentially burying the epithelium. ***C.*** A higher magnification view of a mucus plug tightly adhering to the airway surface, with *arrows* indicating the interface between infected and inflamed secretions and the underlying epithelium to which the secretions adhere. (Both ***B*** and ***C*** were stained with hematoxylin and eosin, with the colors modified to highlight structures.) Infected secretions obstruct airways and, over time, dramatically disrupt the normal architecture of the lung. ***D.*** CFTR is expressed in surface epithelium and serous cells at the base of submucosal glands in a porcine lung sample, as shown by the dark staining, signifying binding by CFTR antibodies to epithelial structures (aminoethylcarbazole detection of horseradish peroxidase with hematoxylin counterstain). *(From SM Rowe, S Miller, EJ Sorscher: N Engl J Med 352:1992, 2005.)*

approximately 90% of individuals with CF carry at least one F508del mutation.

Other gene defects include CFTR ion channels properly trafficked to the apical cell surface but unable to open and/or gate. Such channel proteins include G551D (a glycine to aspartic acid replacement at CFTR position 551), which leads to an inability to transport Cl^- or HCO_3^- in the presence of ATP (a class III abnormality). Individuals with at least one G551D allele represent 4–5% of CF patients in North America. *CFTR* nonsense alleles such as G542X, R553X, and W1282X (premature termination codon replaces glycine, arginine, or tryptophan at positions 542, 553, or 1282, respectively) are among the common class I defects, in addition to large deletions or other major disruptions of the gene. The W1282X mutation, for example, is prevalent among individuals of Ashkenazi descent and is a predominant CF genotype in Israel. Additional categories of *CFTR* mutation include defects in the ion channel pore (class IV), RNA splicing (class V), and increased plasma membrane turnover (class VI) (Fig. 313-2).

DIAGNOSIS

The diagnosis of CF is based in part on clinical symptoms, family history, or positive newborn screening. *CFTR* mutation analysis together with sweat electrolyte measurements represent cardinal diagnostic tests. DNA-based evaluation typically surveys numerous disease-associated mutations; panels that identify 20–80 gene defects are

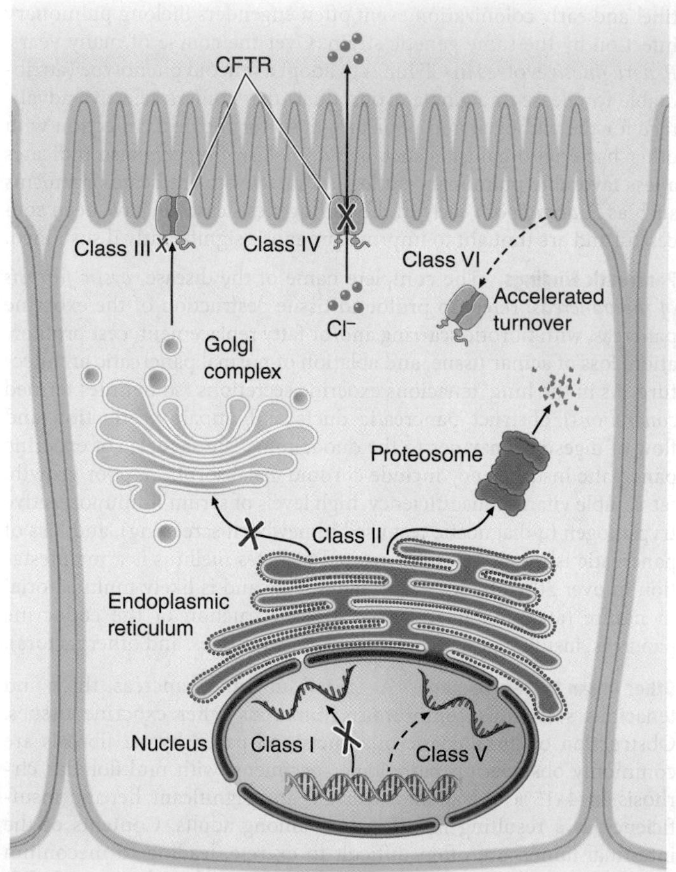

FIGURE 313-2 Categories of *CFTR* mutations. Classes of defects in the *CFTR* gene include the absence of synthesis (class I); defective protein maturation and premature degradation (class II); disordered gating/regulation, such as diminished adenosine triphosphate (ATP) binding and hydrolysis (class III); defective conductance through the ion channel pore (class IV); a reduced number of *CFTR* transcripts due to a promoter or splicing abnormality (class V); and accelerated turnover from the cell surface (class VI). *(From SM Rowe, S Miller, EJ Sorscher: N Engl J Med 352:1992, 2005.)*

available through commercial sources. For difficult cases, complete *CFTR* exonic sequencing together with analysis of splice junctions and key regulatory elements can be obtained. Sweat electrolytes following pilocarpine iontophoresis comprise an invaluable diagnostic measurement, with levels of chloride markedly elevated in CF compared to non-CF individuals. The sweat test result is highly specific and served as the mainstay of diagnosis for many decades prior to availability of *CFTR* genotyping. Notably, hyperviscosity of eccrine sweat is not a clinical feature of the disease. Sweat ducts function to reabsorb chloride from a primary sweat secretion produced by the glandular coil. Malfunction of CFTR leads to diminished chloride uptake from the ductular lumen, and sweat emerges on the skin with markedly elevated levels of chloride. For the unusual situation in which both *CFTR* genotype and sweat electrolytes are inconclusive, in vivo measurement of ion transport across the nasal airways can serve as a specific test for CF and is used by a number of referral centers. For example, elevated (sodium-dependent) transepithelial charge separation across airway epithelial tissue and failure of isoproterenol-dependent chloride secretion (via CFTR) represent bioelectric findings highly specific for the disease. Measurements of CFTR activity in excised rectal mucosal biopsies can also be obtained.

COMPLEXITY OF A CF PHENOTYPE

CF classically presents in childhood with chronic productive cough, malabsorption including steatorrhea, and failure to thrive. The disease is most common among whites (~1 in 3300 live births) and much less frequent among African-American (~1 in 15,000) or Asian populations (~1 in 33,000). Several "severe" defects that impair CFTR activity (including F508del, G551D, and truncation alleles) are predictive of pancreatic insufficiency, which is clinically evident in 80–90% of individuals with CF. These few specific genotype-phenotype correlations notwithstanding, genotype is, in general, a poor predictor of overall respiratory prognosis.

A spectrum of CFTR-related diseases with features resembling classic CF has been well described. In addition to multiorgan involvement, forme frustes, such as isolated congenital bilateral absence of the vas deferens or pancreatitis (without other organ system findings), are strongly associated with *CFTR* mutations in at least one allele. Although CF is a classic monogenic disease, the importance of non-*CFTR* gene modifiers and proteins that regulate ion flux, inflammatory pathways, and airway remodeling has been increasingly appreciated as influencing clinical course. For example, the magnitude of transepithelial sodium reabsorption in CF airways, which helps control periciliary fluid depth and composition, is strongly influenced by CFTR and represents a molecular target for disease intervention.

THERAPEUTICS DIRECTED TOWARD CF SEQUELAE

Standard care for outpatients with CF is intensive, with regimens that include exogenous pancreatic enzymes taken with meals, nutritional supplementation, anti-inflammatory medication, bronchodilators, and chronic or periodic administration of oral or aerosolized antibiotics (e.g., as maintenance therapy for patients with *P. aeruginosa*). Recombinant DNAse aerosols (degraded DNA strands that contribute to mucus viscosity) and nebulized hypertonic saline (serves to augment PCL depth, activate mucociliary clearance, and mobilize inspissated airway secretions) are administered routinely. Chest physiotherapy several times each day is a standard means to promote clearance of airway mucus. Among older individuals with CF, malabsorption, chronic inflammation, and endocrine abnormalities can lead to poor bone mineralization, requiring treatment with vitamin D, calcium, and other measures. The time, complexity, and expense of home care are considerable and take a significant toll on patients and their families.

Severe respiratory exacerbation is commonly managed by hospital admission for frequent chest physiotherapy and parenteral antibiotics directed against serious (and often multiply resistant) bacterial pathogens. Aggressive intervention in this setting can restore a large component of lung function, but ongoing and cumulative loss of pulmonary reserve reflects the natural history of the disease. Poor prognostic indicators such as sputum culture containing *B. cepacia*, mucoid *P. aeruginosa*, or atypical mycobacteria are rigorously monitored in the CF patient population. An increasing incidence of methicillin-resistant *S. aureus* has also been observed, although the clinical significance of this finding has not been fully elucidated. Typical inpatient antibiotic coverage includes combination drug therapy with an aminoglycoside and β-lactam for up to 14 days. Maximal improvement in lung function is often achieved by 8–10 days in this setting. Many families elect parenteral antibiotic treatment at home, and additional studies are needed to evaluate specific drug combinations, duration of therapy, and home versus inpatient management. Other CF respiratory sequelae that may require hospitalization include hemoptysis and pneumothorax. Hypersensitivity to *Aspergillus* (allergic bronchopulmonary aspergillosis) occurs in approximately 5% of individuals with the disease and should be suspected in the absence of a response to conventional treatment.

Lung transplantation remains a viable therapeutic option in the setting of end-stage CF pulmonary failure, with 5-year postoperative survival rates on the order of 50–60%. Determining the optimal timing for surgery presents a substantial challenge, particularly because overall prognosis for individuals with severe lung disease is sometimes difficult to predict, and mortality associated with transplantation is significant (1-year survival rates of approximately 80%). Forced expiratory volume in 1 s (FEV_1) measurements less than 30% predicted, together with an assortment of other clinical features, are often used as thresholds for entry onto transplantation lists, although waiting periods for healthy donor lungs can be quite protracted. Based on clinical outcome and limited access to healthy donor lungs, many CF patients and their families do not pursue this option.

CFTR MODULATION

Potentiation of Mutant CFTR Gating A massive effort directed toward high-throughput drug analysis of large compound libraries (containing millions of individual agents) has identified novel and promising approaches to CF therapy. The approved compound ivacaftor, for example, robustly potentiates CFTR channel opening and stimulates ion transport. Ivacaftor overcomes the G551D CFTR gating defect, and individuals carrying this mutation exhibit dramatic improvement in lung function, weight gain, and other clinical parameters after only a few weeks of oral therapy. Remarkably, sweat chloride values are significantly improved with this treatment in patients with G551D CFTR. No clinical intervention of any sort has previously been shown to normalize the CF sweat chloride abnormality. Long-term studies of the drug in patients with G551D CFTR are ongoing. Ivacaftor has been viewed as the harbinger of a new era for CF therapeutics directed at treating the most fundamental causes of the disease.

Correction of the F508del Processing Abnormality Advancement of new drugs that address specific CFTR defects in protein folding and maturation has been bolstered by clinical studies of F508del rescue in combination with ivacaftor. So-called "corrector" molecules (as distinct from CFTR gating "potentiators" such as ivacaftor) discovered through compound library screening are suitable for promoting cell surface localization of the F508del protein. Significant improvement in pulmonary function of F508del homozygous individuals has been achieved with potentiator/corrector combination therapy in early clinical trials, and several candidate molecules are under evaluation.

Personalized Molecular Therapies The advent of modulators with robust clinical impact has engendered new optimism regarding care of patients with CF. It is clear that future interventions will be tailored to specific genotypic abnormalities. Drug screening campaigns and other research programs have identified agents capable of suppressing CFTR nonsense alleles, augmenting potentiator activity, and promoting F508del correction. Efforts to apply these compounds in a fashion that will benefit CF subjects carrying a single copy of F508del (i.e., with a distinct or unusual *CFTR* mutation on the second allele) comprise an essential priority for the future. Progress in CF drug discovery is emblematic of what might be accomplished in other refractory genetic diseases using an approach grounded in molecular mechanism and unbiased compound library screening.

As a direct result of advances in basic research, new therapies have transformed CF from a disease typically leading to death in early childhood to a condition with frequent survival well into the fourth decade of life. It has also become increasingly clear that specified approaches to patient management can have an impact on overall prognosis. For example, standardization of clinical intervention throughout the United States has led to remarkable benefit among the CF population. Well-defined measures for outpatient care are now established, including thresholds for hospital admission, antibiotic regimens, nutritional guidelines, periodicity of diagnostic tests, and other clinical parameters. These therapeutic recommendations have become standardized throughout approximately 110 specialized CF care centers and 55 affiliated programs. The initiative has improved endpoints such as weight gain, body mass index, and pulmonary function. Information regarding standardized protocols for CF therapy can be accessed at (*www.cff.org/treatments/cfcareguidelines/*) or through a number of excellent reviews.

Newborn screening for CF is now universal throughout the United States, most of the Canadian provinces, Australia, New Zealand, and much of Europe, and will facilitate early CF intervention. Based on data indicating that early nutritional and other therapies can be beneficial, newborn diagnosis is expected to significantly promote health in the CF population. Export of quality control measures and novel therapeutics worldwide has become an increasing imperative. For example, median survival of individuals with CF is less than 20 years in much of Central and South America (compared to ~40 years in the United States and Canada), and efforts to apply state-of-the-art management to underdiagnosed and underserved CF patient populations are expected to improve outcome and mitigate CF health disparities in the future.

VIDEO 313-1 Initial video sequences describe establishment of the normal periciliary fluid layer bathing the surface airway epithelium, with spheres representing chloride and bicarbonate ions secreted through CFTR and across the apical (mucosal) respiratory surface. Later video sequences depict failure of CFTR anion transport and resulting depletion of the periciliary layer, "plastering" of cilia against the mucosal surface, and accumulation of mucus in the airway with resulting bacterial infection. *(Video courtesy of the Cystic Fibrosis Foundation.)*

314 Chronic Obstructive Pulmonary Disease

John J. Reilly, Jr., Edwin K. Silverman, Steven D. Shapiro

Chronic obstructive pulmonary disease (COPD) is defined as a disease state characterized by airflow limitation that is not fully reversible (*http://www.goldcopd.com/*). COPD includes *emphysema,* an anatomically defined condition characterized by destruction and enlargement of the lung alveoli; *chronic bronchitis,* a clinically defined condition with chronic cough and phlegm; and *small airways disease,* a condition in which small bronchioles are narrowed. COPD is present only if chronic airflow obstruction occurs; chronic bronchitis *without* chronic airflow obstruction is *not* included within COPD.

COPD is the third leading cause of death and affects >10 million persons in the United States. COPD is also a disease of increasing public health importance around the world. Estimates suggest that COPD will rise from the sixth to the third most common cause of death worldwide by 2020.

PATHOGENESIS

Airflow limitation, the major physiologic change in COPD, can result from both small airway obstruction and emphysema. As described below, small airways may become narrowed by cells (hyperplasia and accumulation), mucus, and fibrosis. Of note, activation of transforming growth factor β (TGF-β) contributes to airway fibrosis, while lack of TGF-β may contribute to parenchymal inflammation and emphysema. Largely due to greater similarity of animal air spaces than airways to humans, we know more about mechanisms involved in emphysema than small airway obstruction.

The dominant paradigm of the pathogenesis of emphysema comprises four interrelated events (Fig. 314-1): (1) Chronic exposure to cigarette smoke leads to inflammatory and immune cell recruitment within the terminal air spaces of the lung. (2) These inflammatory cells release elastolytic and other proteinases that damage the extracellular matrix of the lung. (3) Structural cell death (endothelial and epithelial cells) occurs directly through oxidant-induced cigarette smoke damage and senescence as well as indirectly via proteolytic loss of matrix attachment. (4) Ineffective repair of elastin and other extracellular matrix components result in air space enlargement that defines pulmonary emphysema.

THE ELASTASE:ANTIELASTASE HYPOTHESIS

Elastin, the principal component of elastic fibers, is a highly stable component of the extracellular matrix that is critical to the integrity of the lung. The elastase:antielastase hypothesis proposed in the mid-1960s states that the balance of elastin-degrading enzymes and their inhibitors determines the susceptibility of the lung to destruction resulting in air space enlargement. This hypothesis was based on the clinical observation that patients with genetic deficiency in α_1 antitrypsin (α_1AT), the inhibitor of the serine proteinase neutrophil elastase, were at increased risk of emphysema, and that instillation of elastases, including neutrophil elastase, into experimental animals results in emphysema. The elastase:antielastase hypothesis remains a prevailing mechanism for the development of emphysema. However, a complex

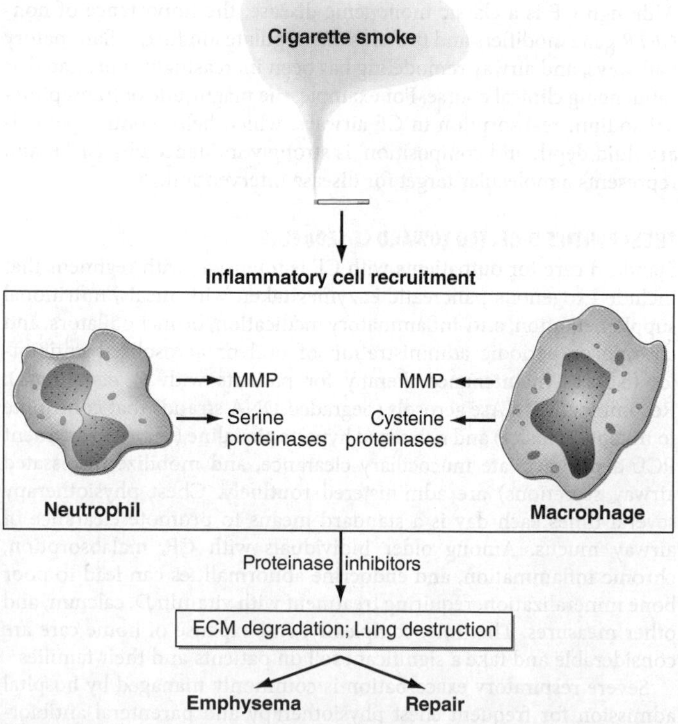

FIGURE 314-1 Pathogenesis of emphysema. Upon long-term exposure to cigarette smoke, inflammatory cells are recruited to the lung; they release proteinases in excess of inhibitors, and if repair is abnormal, this leads to air space destruction and enlargement or emphysema. ECM, extracellular matrix; MMP, matrix metalloproteinase.

network of immune and inflammatory cells and additional proteinases that contribute to emphysema have subsequently been identified.

INFLAMMATION AND EXTRACELLULAR MATRIX PROTEOLYSIS

Upon exposure to oxidants from cigarette smoke, macrophages and epithelial cells become activated, producing proteinases and chemokines that attract other inflammatory and immune cells. One mechanism of macrophage activation occurs via oxidant-induced inactivation of histone deacetylase-2, shifting the balance toward acetylated or loose chromatin, exposing nuclear factor-κB sites, and resulting in transcription of matrix metalloproteinases, proinflammatory cytokines such as interleukin 8 (IL-8), and tumor necrosis factor α (TNF-α); this leads to neutrophil recruitment. CD8+ T cells are also recruited in response to cigarette smoke and release interferon-inducible protein-10 (IP-10, CXCL-7), which in turn leads to macrophage production of macrophage elastase (matrix metalloproteinase-12 [MMP-12]). Matrix metalloproteinases and serine proteinases, most notably neutrophil elastase, work together by degrading the inhibitor of the other, leading to lung destruction. Proteolytic cleavage products of elastin also serve as a macrophage chemokine, fueling this destructive positive feedback loop.

Autoimmune mechanisms may promote the progression of disease. Increased B cells and lymphoid follicles are present in patients, particularly those with advanced disease. Antibodies have been found against elastin fragments as well; IgG autoantibodies with avidity for pulmonary epithelium and the potential to mediate cytotoxicity have been detected.

Concomitant cigarette smoke–induced loss of cilia in the airway epithelium and impaired macrophage phagocytosis predispose to bacterial infection with neutrophilia. In end-stage lung disease, long after smoking cessation, there remains an exuberant inflammatory response, suggesting that mechanisms of cigarette smoke–induced inflammation that initiate the disease differ from mechanisms that sustain inflammation after smoking cessation.

Cell Death Cigarette smoke oxidant-mediated structural cell death occurs via a variety of mechanisms including rt801 inhibition of mammalian target of rapamycin (mTOR), leading to cell death as well as inflammation and proteolysis. Involvement of mTOR and other senescence markers has led to the recent concept that emphysema resembles premature aging of the lung. Uptake of apoptotic cells by macrophages results in production of growth factors and dampens inflammation, promoting lung repair. Cigarette smoke impairs macrophage uptake of apoptotic cells, limiting repair.

Ineffective Repair The ability of the adult lung to repair damaged alveoli appears limited. It is unlikely that the process of septation that is responsible for alveologenesis during lung development can be reinitiated. The capacity of stem cells to repopulate the lung is under active investigation. It appears difficult for an adult human to completely restore an appropriate extracellular matrix, particularly functional elastic fibers.

PATHOLOGY

Cigarette smoke exposure may affect the large airways, small airways (≤2 mm diameter), and alveoli. Changes in large airways cause cough and sputum, while changes in small airways and alveoli are responsible for physiologic alterations. Emphysema and small airway pathology are both present in most persons with COPD; however, they do not appear to be mechanistically related to each other, and their relative contributions to obstruction vary from one person to another.

LARGE AIRWAY

Cigarette smoking often results in mucus gland enlargement and goblet cell hyperplasia, leading to cough and mucus production that define chronic bronchitis, but these abnormalities are not related to airflow limitation. Goblet cells not only increase in number but in extent through the bronchial tree. Bronchi also undergo squamous metaplasia, predisposing to carcinogenesis and disrupting mucociliary clearance. Although not as prominent as in asthma, patients may have smooth-muscle hypertrophy and bronchial hyperreactivity leading to airflow limitation. Neutrophil influx has been associated with purulent sputum of upper respiratory tract infections. Independent of its proteolytic activity, neutrophil elastase is among the most potent secretagogues identified.

SMALL AIRWAYS

The major site of increased resistance in most individuals with COPD is in airways ≤2 mm diameter. Characteristic cellular changes include goblet cell metaplasia, with these mucus-secreting cells replacing surfactant-secreting Clara cells. Smooth-muscle hypertrophy may also be present. These abnormalities may cause luminal narrowing by fibrosis, excess mucus, edema, and cellular infiltration. Reduced surfactant may increase surface tension at the air-tissue interface, predisposing to airway narrowing or collapse. Respiratory bronchiolitis with mononuclear inflammatory cells collecting in distal airway tissues may cause proteolytic destruction of elastic fibers in the respiratory bronchioles and alveolar ducts where the fibers are concentrated as rings around alveolar entrances. Narrowing and drop-out of small airways precede the onset of emphysematous destruction.

LUNG PARENCHYMA

Emphysema is characterized by destruction of gas exchanging air spaces, i.e., the respiratory bronchioles, alveolar ducts, and alveoli. Their walls become perforated and later obliterated with coalescence of small distinct air spaces into abnormal and much larger air spaces. Macrophages accumulate in respiratory bronchioles of essentially all young smokers. Bronchoalveolar lavage fluid from such individuals contains roughly five times as many macrophages as lavage from nonsmokers. In smokers' lavage fluid, macrophages comprise >95% of the total cell count, and neutrophils, nearly absent in nonsmokers' lavage, account for 1–2% of the cells. T lymphocytes, particularly CD8+ cells, are also increased in the alveolar space of smokers.

Emphysema is classified into distinct pathologic types, the most important being centriacinar and panacinar. *Centriacinar emphysema*, the type most frequently associated with cigarette smoking, is characterized by enlarged air spaces found (initially) in association with respiratory bronchioles. Centriacinar emphysema is usually most prominent in the upper lobes and superior segments of lower lobes and is often quite focal. *Panacinar emphysema* refers to abnormally large air spaces evenly distributed within and across acinar units. Panacinar emphysema is usually observed in patients with α_1AT deficiency, which has a predilection for the lower lobes.

PATHOPHYSIOLOGY

Persistent reduction in forced expiratory flow rates is the most typical finding in COPD. Increases in the residual volume and the residual volume/total lung capacity ratio, nonuniform distribution of ventilation, and ventilation-perfusion mismatching also occur.

AIRFLOW OBSTRUCTION

Airflow limitation, also known as airflow obstruction, is typically determined by spirometry, which involves forced expiratory maneuvers after the subject has inhaled to total lung capacity. Key parameters obtained from spirometry include the volume of air exhaled within the first second of the forced expiratory maneuver (FEV_1) and the total volume of air exhaled during the entire spirometric maneuver (forced vital capacity [FVC]). Patients with airflow obstruction related to COPD have a chronically reduced ratio of FEV_1/FVC. In contrast to asthma, the reduced FEV_1 in COPD seldom shows large responses to inhaled bronchodilators, although improvements up to 15% are common. Asthma patients can also develop chronic (not fully reversible) airflow obstruction.

Airflow during forced exhalation is the result of the balance between the elastic recoil of the lungs promoting flow and the resistance of the airways limiting flow. In normal lungs, as well as in lungs affected by COPD, maximal expiratory flow diminishes as the lungs empty because the lung parenchyma provides progressively less elastic recoil and because the cross-sectional area of the airways falls, raising the resistance to airflow. The decrease in flow coincident with decreased lung volume is readily apparent on the expiratory limb of a flow-volume curve. In the early stages of COPD, the abnormality in airflow is only evident at lung volumes at or below the functional residual capacity (closer to residual volume), appearing as a scooped-out lower part of the descending limb of the flow-volume curve. In more advanced disease, the entire curve has decreased expiratory flow compared to normal.

HYPERINFLATION

Lung volumes are also routinely assessed in pulmonary function testing. In COPD there is often "air trapping" (increased residual volume and increased ratio of residual volume to total lung capacity) and progressive hyperinflation (increased total lung capacity) late in the disease. Hyperinflation of the thorax during tidal breathing preserves maximum expiratory airflow, because as lung volume increases, elastic recoil pressure increases, and airways enlarge so that airway resistance decreases.

Despite compensating for airway obstruction, hyperinflation can push the diaphragm into a flattened position with a number of adverse effects. First, by decreasing the zone of apposition between the diaphragm and the abdominal wall, positive abdominal pressure during inspiration is not applied as effectively to the chest wall, hindering rib cage movement and impairing inspiration. Second, because the muscle fibers of the flattened diaphragm are shorter than those of a more normally curved diaphragm, they are less capable of generating inspiratory pressures than normal. Third, the flattened diaphragm (with increased radius of curvature, *r*) must generate greater tension (*t*) to develop the transpulmonary pressure (*p*) required to produce tidal breathing. This follows from Laplace's law, $p = 2t/r$. Also, because the thoracic cage is distended beyond its normal resting volume, during tidal breathing the inspiratory muscles must do work to overcome the resistance of the thoracic cage to further inflation instead of gaining the normal assistance from the chest wall recoiling outward toward its resting volume.

GAS EXCHANGE

Although there is considerable variability in the relationships between the FEV_1 and other physiologic abnormalities in COPD, certain generalizations may be made. The partial pressure of oxygen in arterial blood Pao_2 usually remains near normal until the FEV_1 is decreased to ~50% of predicted, and even much lower FEV_1 values can be associated with a normal Pao_2, at least at rest. An elevation of arterial level of carbon dioxide ($Paco_2$) is not expected until the FEV_1 is <25% of predicted and even then may not occur. Pulmonary hypertension severe enough to cause cor pulmonale and right ventricular failure due to COPD typically occurs in individuals who have marked decreases in FEV_1 (<25% of predicted) and chronic hypoxemia (Pao_2 <55 mmHg); however, recent evidence suggests that some patients will develop significant pulmonary hypertension independent of COPD severity (Chap. 304).

Nonuniform ventilation and ventilation-perfusion mismatching are characteristic of COPD, reflecting the heterogeneous nature of the disease process within the airways and lung parenchyma. Physiologic studies are consistent with multiple parenchymal compartments having different rates of ventilation due to regional differences in compliance and airway resistance. Ventilation-perfusion mismatching accounts for essentially all of the reduction in Pao_2 that occurs in COPD; shunting is minimal. This finding explains the effectiveness of modest elevations of inspired oxygen in treating hypoxemia due to COPD and therefore the need to consider problems other than COPD when hypoxemia is difficult to correct with modest levels of supplemental oxygen.

RISK FACTORS

CIGARETTE SMOKING

By 1964, the Advisory Committee to the Surgeon General of the United States had concluded that cigarette smoking was a major risk factor for mortality from chronic bronchitis and emphysema. Subsequent longitudinal studies have shown accelerated decline in FEV_1 in a dose-response relationship to the intensity of cigarette smoking, which is typically expressed as pack-years (average number of packs of cigarettes smoked per day multiplied by the total number of years of smoking). This dose-response relationship between reduced pulmonary function and cigarette smoking intensity accounts for the higher prevalence rates of COPD with increasing age. The historically higher rate of smoking among males is the likely explanation for the higher prevalence of COPD among males; however, the prevalence of COPD among females is increasing as the gender gap in smoking rates has diminished in the past 50 years.

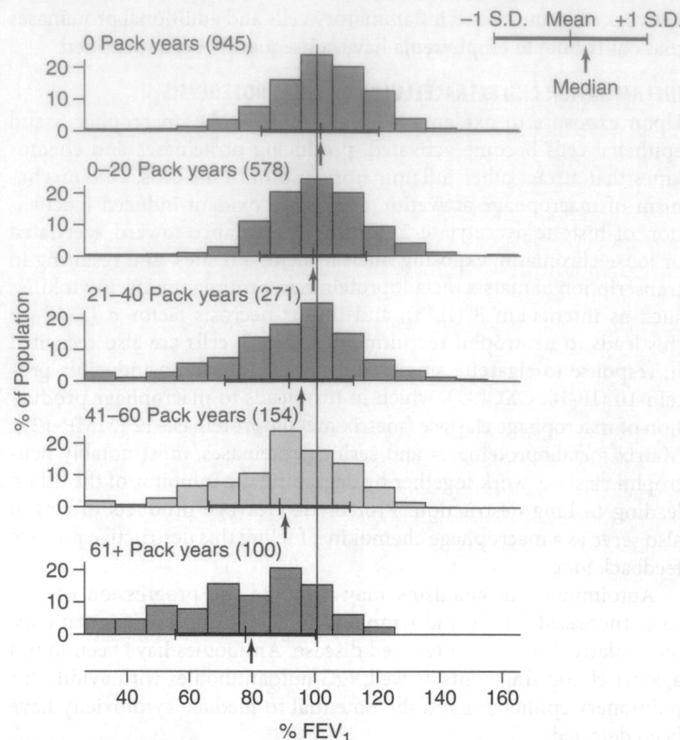

FIGURE 314-2 Distributions of forced expiratory volume in 1 s (FEV_1) values in a general population sample, stratified by pack-years of smoking. Means, medians, and ±1 standard deviation of percent predicted FEV_1 are shown for each smoking group. Although a dose-response relationship between smoking intensity and FEV_1 was found, marked variability in pulmonary function was observed among subjects with similar smoking histories. *(From B Burrows et al: Am Rev Respir Dis 115:95, 1977; with permission.)*

Although the causal relationship between cigarette smoking and the development of COPD has been absolutely proved, there is considerable variability in the response to smoking. Although pack-years of cigarette smoking is the most highly significant predictor of FEV_1 (Fig. 314-2), only 15% of the variability in FEV_1 is explained by pack-years. This finding suggests that additional environmental and/or genetic factors contribute to the impact of smoking on the development of airflow obstruction.

Although cigar and pipe smoking may also be associated with the development of COPD, the evidence supporting such associations is less compelling, likely related to the lower dose of inhaled tobacco by-products during cigar and pipe smoking.

AIRWAY RESPONSIVENESS AND COPD

A tendency for increased bronchoconstriction in response to a variety of exogenous stimuli, including methacholine and histamine, is one of the defining features of asthma (Chap. 309). However, many patients with COPD also share this feature of airway hyperresponsiveness. The considerable overlap between persons with asthma and those with COPD in airway responsiveness, airflow obstruction, and pulmonary symptoms led to the formulation of the Dutch hypothesis. This suggests that asthma, chronic bronchitis, and emphysema are variations of the same basic disease, which is modulated by environmental and genetic factors to produce these pathologically distinct entities. The alternative British hypothesis contends that asthma and COPD are fundamentally different diseases: Asthma is viewed as largely an allergic phenomenon, whereas COPD results from smoking-related inflammation and damage. Determination of the validity of the Dutch hypothesis versus the British hypothesis awaits identification of all of the genetic predisposing factors for asthma and/or COPD, as well as the interactions between these postulated genetic factors and environmental risk factors.

Longitudinal studies that compared airway responsiveness at the beginning of the study to subsequent decline in pulmonary function have demonstrated that increased airway responsiveness is clearly a significant predictor of subsequent decline in pulmonary function. Thus, airway hyperresponsiveness is a risk factor for COPD.

RESPIRATORY INFECTIONS

The impact of adult respiratory infections on decline in pulmonary function is controversial, but significant long-term reductions in pulmonary function are not typically seen following an episode of bronchitis or pneumonia. The impact of the effects of childhood respiratory illnesses on the subsequent development of COPD has been difficult to assess due to a lack of adequate longitudinal data. Thus, although respiratory infections are important causes of exacerbations of COPD, the association of both adult and childhood respiratory infections with the development and progression of COPD remains to be proven.

OCCUPATIONAL EXPOSURES

Increased respiratory symptoms and airflow obstruction have been suggested to result from exposure to dust and fumes at work. Several specific occupational exposures, including coal mining, gold mining, and cotton textile dust, have been suggested as risk factors for chronic airflow obstruction. Although nonsmokers in these occupations can develop some reductions in FEV_1, the importance of dust exposure as a risk factor for COPD, independent of cigarette smoking, is not certain for most of these exposures. However, among coal miners, coal mine dust exposure was a significant risk factor for emphysema in both smokers and nonsmokers. In most cases, the magnitude of these occupational exposures on COPD risk is likely substantially less important than the effect of cigarette smoking.

AMBIENT AIR POLLUTION

Some investigators have reported increased respiratory symptoms in those living in urban compared to rural areas, which may relate to increased pollution in the urban settings. However, the relationship of air pollution to chronic airflow obstruction remains unproved. Prolonged exposure to smoke produced by biomass combustion—a common mode of cooking in some countries—also appears to be a significant risk factor for COPD among women in those countries. However, in most populations, ambient air pollution is a much less important risk factor for COPD than cigarette smoking.

PASSIVE, OR SECOND-HAND, SMOKING EXPOSURE

Exposure of children to maternal smoking results in significantly reduced lung growth. In utero, tobacco smoke exposure also contributes to significant reductions in postnatal pulmonary function. Although passive smoke exposure has been associated with reductions in pulmonary function, the importance of this risk factor in the development of the severe pulmonary function reductions in COPD remains uncertain.

GENETIC CONSIDERATIONS

Although cigarette smoking is the major environmental risk factor for the development of COPD, the development of airflow obstruction in smokers is highly variable. Severe α_1AT deficiency is a proven genetic risk factor for COPD; there is increasing evidence that other genetic determinants also exist.

α_1 Antitrypsin Deficiency Many variants of the protease inhibitor (PI or SERPINA1) locus that encodes α_1AT have been described. The common M allele is associated with normal α_1AT levels. The S allele, associated with slightly reduced α_1AT levels, and the Z allele, associated with markedly reduced α_1AT levels, also occur with frequencies of >1% in most white populations. Rare individuals inherit null alleles, which lead to the absence of any α_1AT production through a heterogeneous collection of mutations. Individuals with two Z alleles or one Z and one null allele are referred to as Pi^Z, which is the most common form of severe α_1AT deficiency.

Although only approximately 1% of COPD patients are found to have severe α_1AT deficiency as a contributing cause of COPD, these patients demonstrate that genetic factors can have a profound influence on the susceptibility for developing COPD. Pi^Z individuals often develop early-onset COPD, but the ascertainment bias in the published series of Pi^Z individuals—which have usually included many Pi^Z subjects who were tested for α_1AT deficiency because they had COPD—means that the fraction of Pi^Z individuals who will develop COPD and the age-of-onset distribution for the development of COPD in Pi^Z subjects remain unknown. Approximately 1 in 3000 individuals in the United States inherits severe α_1AT deficiency, but only a small minority of these individuals has been identified. The clinical laboratory test used most frequently to screen for α_1AT deficiency is measurement of the immunologic level of α_1AT in serum (see "Laboratory Findings").

A significant percentage of the variability in pulmonary function among Pi^Z individuals is explained by cigarette smoking; cigarette smokers with severe α_1AT deficiency are more likely to develop COPD at early ages. However, the development of COPD in Pi^Z subjects, even among current or ex-smokers, is not absolute. Among Pi^Z nonsmokers, impressive variability has been noted in the development of airflow obstruction. Asthma and male gender also appear to increase the risk of COPD in Pi^Z subjects. Other genetic and/or environmental factors likely contribute to this variability.

Specific treatment in the form of α_1AT augmentation therapy is available for severe α_1AT deficiency as a weekly IV infusion (see "Treatment," below).

The risk of lung disease in heterozygous Pi^{MZ} individuals, who have intermediate serum levels of α_1AT (~60% of Pi^{MM} levels), is controversial. Several recent large studies have suggested that Pi^{MZ} subjects are at slightly increased risk for the development of airflow obstruction, but it remains unclear if all Pi^{MZ} subjects are at slightly increased risk for COPD or if a subset of Pi^{MZ} subjects are at substantially increased risk for COPD due to other genetic or environmental factors.

Other Genetic Risk Factors Studies of pulmonary function measurements performed in general population samples have suggested that genetic factors other than PI type influence variation in pulmonary function. Familial aggregation of airflow obstruction within families of COPD patients has also been demonstrated.

Association studies have compared the distribution of variants in candidate genes hypothesized to be involved in the development of COPD in COPD patients and control subjects. However, the results have been quite inconsistent, often due to underpowered studies. However, a well-powered association study comprising 8300 patients and 7 separate cohorts found that a minor allele single nucleotide polymorphism (SNP) of *MMP12* (rs2276109) associated with decreased MMP12 expression has a positive effect on lung function in children with asthma and in adult smokers. Recent genome-wide association studies have identified several COPD susceptibility loci, including a region near the hedgehog interacting protein (*HHIP*) gene on chromosome 4, a cluster of genes on chromosome 15 (including components of the nicotinic acetylcholine receptor), and a region within a gene of unknown function (*FAM13A*). A regulatory SNP upstream from the *HHIP* gene has been identified as one potential functional variant; the specific genetic determinants in the other genomic regions have yet to be definitively identified.

NATURAL HISTORY

The effects of cigarette smoking on pulmonary function appear to depend on the intensity of smoking exposure, the timing of smoking exposure during growth, and the baseline lung function of the individual; other environmental factors may have similar effects. Most individuals follow a steady trajectory of increasing pulmonary function with

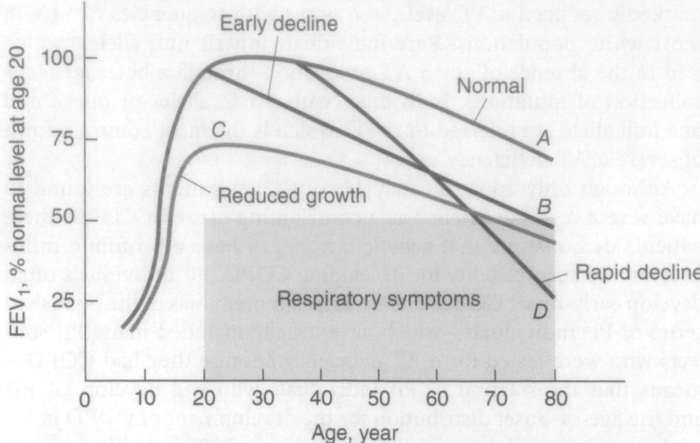

FIGURE 314-3 Hypothetical tracking curves of forced expiratory volume in 1 s (FEV_1) for individuals throughout their life spans. The normal pattern of growth and decline with age is shown by curve *A*. Significantly reduced FEV_1 (<65% of predicted value at age 20) can develop from a normal rate of decline after a reduced pulmonary function growth phase (curve *C*), early initiation of pulmonary function decline after normal growth (curve *B*), or accelerated decline after normal growth (curve *D*). *(From B Rijcken: Doctoral dissertation, p 133, University of Groningen, 1991; with permission.)*

growth during childhood and adolescence, followed by a gradual decline with aging. Individuals appear to track in their quantile of pulmonary function based on environmental and genetic factors that put them on different tracks. The risk of eventual mortality from COPD is closely associated with reduced levels of FEV_1. A graphic depiction of the natural history of COPD is shown as a function of the influences on tracking curves of FEV_1 in Fig. 314-3. Death or disability from COPD can result from a normal rate of decline after a reduced growth phase (curve *C*), an early initiation of pulmonary function decline after normal growth (curve *B*), or an accelerated decline after normal growth (curve *D*). The rate of decline in pulmonary function can be modified by changing environmental exposures (i.e., quitting smoking), with smoking cessation at an earlier age providing a more beneficial effect than smoking cessation after marked reductions in pulmonary function have already developed. Genetic factors likely contribute to the level of pulmonary function achieved during growth and to the rate of decline in response to smoking and potentially to other environmental factors as well.

CLINICAL PRESENTATION

HISTORY

The three most common symptoms in COPD are cough, sputum production, and exertional dyspnea. Many patients have such symptoms for months or years before seeking medical attention. Although the development of airflow obstruction is a gradual process, many patients date the onset of their disease to an acute illness or exacerbation. A careful history, however, usually reveals the presence of symptoms prior to the acute exacerbation. The development of exertional dyspnea, often described as increased effort to breathe, heaviness, air hunger, or gasping, can be insidious. It is best elicited by a careful history focused on typical physical activities and how the patient's ability to perform them has changed. Activities involving significant arm work, particularly at or above shoulder level, are particularly difficult for patients with COPD. Conversely, activities that allow the patient to brace the arms and use accessory muscles of respiration are better tolerated. Examples of such activities include pushing a shopping cart or walking on a treadmill. As COPD advances, the principal feature is worsening dyspnea on exertion with increasing intrusion on the ability to perform vocational or avocational activities. In the most advanced stages, patients are breathless doing simple activities of daily living.

Accompanying worsening airflow obstruction is an increased frequency of exacerbations (described below). Patients may also develop resting hypoxemia and require institution of supplemental oxygen.

PHYSICAL FINDINGS

In the early stages of COPD, patients usually have an entirely normal physical examination. Current smokers may have signs of active smoking, including an odor of smoke or nicotine staining of fingernails. In patients with more severe disease, the physical examination is notable for a prolonged expiratory phase and may include expiratory wheezing. In addition, signs of hyperinflation include a barrel chest and enlarged lung volumes with poor diaphragmatic excursion as assessed by percussion. Patients with severe airflow obstruction may also exhibit use of accessory muscles of respiration, sitting in the characteristic "tripod" position to facilitate the actions of the sternocleidomastoid, scalene, and intercostal muscles. Patients may develop cyanosis, visible in the lips and nail beds.

Although traditional teaching is that patients with predominant emphysema, termed "pink puffers," are thin and noncyanotic at rest and have prominent use of accessory muscles, and patients with chronic bronchitis are more likely to be heavy and cyanotic ("blue bloaters"), current evidence demonstrates that most patients have elements of both bronchitis and emphysema and that the physical examination does not reliably differentiate the two entities.

Advanced disease may be accompanied by cachexia, with significant weight loss, bitemporal wasting, and diffuse loss of subcutaneous adipose tissue. This syndrome has been associated with both inadequate oral intake and elevated levels of inflammatory cytokines (TNF-α). Such wasting is an independent poor prognostic factor in COPD. Some patients with advanced disease have paradoxical inward movement of the rib cage with inspiration (Hoover's sign), the result of alteration of the vector of diaphragmatic contraction on the rib cage as a result of chronic hyperinflation.

Signs of overt right heart failure, termed *cor pulmonale,* are relatively infrequent since the advent of supplemental oxygen therapy.

Clubbing of the digits is not a sign of COPD, and its presence should alert the clinician to initiate an investigation for causes of clubbing. In this population, the development of lung cancer is the most likely explanation for newly developed clubbing.

LABORATORY FINDINGS

The hallmark of COPD is airflow obstruction (discussed above). Pulmonary function testing shows airflow obstruction with a reduction in FEV_1 and FEV_1/FVC (Chap. 306e). With worsening disease severity, lung volumes may increase, resulting in an increase in total lung capacity, functional residual capacity, and residual volume. In patients with emphysema, the diffusing capacity may be reduced, reflecting the lung parenchymal destruction characteristic of the disease. The degree of airflow obstruction is an important prognostic factor in COPD and is the basis for the Global Initiative for Lung Disease (GOLD) severity classification (Table 314-1). More recently it has been shown that a multifactorial index incorporating airflow obstruction, exercise performance, dyspnea, and body mass index is a better predictor of mortality rate than pulmonary function alone. In 2011, the GOLD added an additional classification system incorporating symptoms and exacerbation history; the utility of this system remains to be defined.

Arterial blood gases and oximetry may demonstrate resting or exertional hypoxemia. Arterial blood gases provide additional information

TABLE 314-1 GOLD CRITERIA FOR SEVERITY OF AIRFLOW OBSTRUCTION IN COPD

GOLD Stage	Severity	Spirometry
I	Mild	FEV_1/FVC <0.7 and FEV_1 ≥80% predicted
II	Moderate	FEV_1/FVC <0.7 and FEV_1 ≥50% but <80% predicted
III	Severe	FEV_1/FVC <0.7 and FEV_1 ≥30% but <50% predicted
IV	Very severe	FEV_1/FVC <0.7 and FEV_1 <30% predicted

Abbreviations: COPD, chronic obstructive pulmonary disease; GOLD, Global Initiative for Lung Disease.

Source: From the Global Strategy for Diagnosis, Management and Prevention of COPD 2014, © Global Initiative for Chronic Obstructive Lung Disease (GOLD), all rights reserved. Available from *http://www.goldcopd.org.*

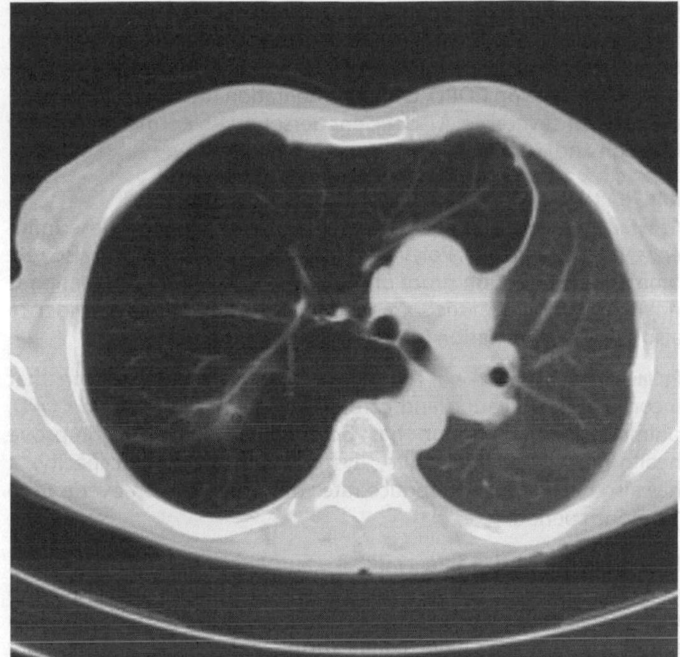

FIGURE 314-4 Chest computed tomography scan of a patient with chronic obstructive pulmonary disease who underwent a left single-lung transplant. Note the reduced parenchymal markings in the right lung (*left side of figure*) as compared to the left lung, representing emphysematous destruction of the lung, and mediastinal shift to the left, indicative of hyperinflation.

about alveolar ventilation and acid-base status by measuring arterial P_{CO_2} and pH. The change in pH with P_{CO_2} is 0.08 units/10 mmHg acutely and 0.03 units/10 mmHg in the chronic state. Knowledge of the arterial pH therefore allows the classification of ventilatory failure, defined as P_{CO_2} >45 mmHg, into acute or chronic conditions. The arterial blood gas is an important component of the evaluation of patients presenting with symptoms of an exacerbation. An elevated hematocrit suggests the presence of chronic hypoxemia, as does the presence of signs of right ventricular hypertrophy.

Radiographic studies may assist in the classification of the type of COPD. Obvious bullae, paucity of parenchymal markings, or hyperlucency suggests the presence of emphysema. Increased lung volumes and flattening of the diaphragm suggest hyperinflation but do not provide information about chronicity of the changes. Computed tomography (CT) scan is the current definitive test for establishing the presence or absence of emphysema in living subjects (Fig. 314-4). From a practical perspective, the CT scan currently does little to influence therapy of COPD except in individuals considering surgical therapy for their disease (described below) and as screening for lung cancer.

Recent guidelines have suggested testing for α_1AT deficiency in all subjects with COPD or asthma with chronic airflow obstruction. Measurement of the serum α_1AT level is a reasonable initial test. For subjects with low α_1AT levels, the definitive diagnosis of α_1AT deficiency requires protease inhibitor (PI) type determination. This is typically performed by isoelectric focusing of serum, which reflects the genotype at the PI locus for the common alleles and many of the rare PI alleles as well. Molecular genotyping of DNA can be performed for the common PI alleles (M, S, and Z).

TREATMENT CHRONIC OBSTRUCTIVE PULMONARY DISEASE

STABLE PHASE COPD

Only three interventions—smoking cessation, oxygen therapy in chronically hypoxemic patients, and lung volume reduction surgery in selected patients with emphysema—have been demonstrated to influence the natural history of patients with COPD. There is currently suggestive, but not definitive, evidence that the use of inhaled glucocorticoids may alter mortality rate (but not lung function). All other current therapies are directed at improving symptoms and decreasing the frequency and severity of exacerbations. The institution of these therapies should involve an assessment of symptoms, potential risks, costs, and benefits of therapy. This should be followed by an assessment of response to therapy, and a decision should be made whether or not to continue treatment.

PHARMACOTHERAPY

Smoking Cessation (See also Chap. 470) It has been shown that middle-aged smokers who were able to successfully stop smoking experienced a significant improvement in the rate of decline in pulmonary function, returning to annual changes similar to that of nonsmoking patients. Thus, all patients with COPD should be strongly urged to quit smoking and educated about the benefits of quitting. An emerging body of evidence demonstrates that combining pharmacotherapy with traditional supportive approaches considerably enhances the chances of successful smoking cessation. There are three principal pharmacologic approaches to the problem: bupropion; nicotine replacement therapy available as gum, transdermal patch, lozenge, inhaler, and nasal spray; and varenicline, a nicotinic acid receptor agonist/antagonist. Current recommendations from the U.S. Surgeon General are that all adult, nonpregnant smokers considering quitting be offered pharmacotherapy, in the absence of any contraindication to treatment.

Bronchodilators In general, bronchodilators are used for symptomatic benefit in patients with COPD. The inhaled route is preferred for medication delivery because the incidence of side effects is lower than that seen with the use of parenteral medication delivery.

Anticholinergic Agents Ipratropium bromide improves symptoms and produces acute improvement in FEV_1. Tiotropium, a long-acting anticholinergic, has been shown to improve symptoms and reduce exacerbations. Studies of both ipratropium and tiotropium have failed to demonstrate that either influences the rate of decline in FEV_1. In a large randomized clinical trial, there was a trend toward reduced mortality rate in the tiotropium-treated patients that approached, but did not reach, statistical significance. Side effects are minor, and a trial of inhaled anticholinergics is recommended in symptomatic patients with COPD. Recent retrospective analyses raised the possibility that anticholinergic use is associated with increased cardiovascular events in the COPD population. This was not demonstrated in a large, prospective randomized trial of tiotropium.

Beta Agonists These provide symptomatic benefit. The main side effects are tremor and tachycardia. Long-acting inhaled β agonists, such as salmeterol or formoterol, have benefits comparable to ipratropium bromide. Their use is more convenient than short-acting agents. The addition of a β agonist to inhaled anticholinergic therapy has been demonstrated to provide incremental benefit. A recent report in asthma suggests that those patients, particularly African Americans, using a long-acting β agonist without concomitant inhaled corticosteroids have an increased risk of deaths from respiratory causes. The applicability of these data to patients with COPD is unclear.

Inhaled Glucocorticoids Although a recent trial demonstrated an apparent benefit from the regular use of inhaled glucocorticoids on the rate of decline of lung function, a number of other well-designed randomized trials have not. Patients studied included those with mild to severe airflow obstruction and current and ex-smokers. Patients with significant acute response to inhaled β agonists were excluded from many of these trials, which may impact the generalizability of the findings. Their use has been associated with increased rates of oropharyngeal candidiasis and an increased rate of loss of bone density. Available data suggest that inhaled glucocorticoids reduce exacerbation frequency by ~25%. The impact of inhaled corticosteroids on mortality rates in COPD is controversial. A meta-analysis and several retrospective studies suggest a mortality benefit, but in a recently published randomized trial, differences in mortality rate approached, but did not reach, conventional criteria for statistical significance. A trial of inhaled glucocorticoids should be considered in patients with frequent exacerbations, defined as two or more per year, and in patients who demonstrate a significant amount of acute reversibility in response to inhaled bronchodilators.

Oral Glucocorticoids The chronic use of oral glucocorticoids for treatment of COPD is not recommended because of an unfavorable benefit/risk ratio. The chronic use of oral glucocorticoids is associated with significant side effects, including osteoporosis, weight gain, cataracts, glucose intolerance, and increased risk of infection. A recent study demonstrated that patients tapered off chronic low-dose prednisone (~10 mg/d) did not experience any adverse effect on the frequency of exacerbations, health-related quality of life, or lung function. On average, patients lost ~4.5 kg (~10 lb) when steroids were withdrawn.

Theophylline Theophylline produces modest improvements in expiratory flow rates and vital capacity and a slight improvement in arterial oxygen and carbon dioxide levels in patients with moderate to severe COPD. Nausea is a common side effect; tachycardia and tremor have also been reported. Monitoring of blood theophylline levels is typically required to minimize toxicity. The selective phosphodiesterase 4 (PDE4) inhibitor roflumilast has been demonstrated to reduce exacerbation frequency in COPD patients with chronic bronchitis and a prior history of exacerbations; its effects on airflow obstruction and symptoms are modest.

Antibiotics As outlined below, there are strong data implicating bacterial infection as a precipitant of a substantial portion of exacerbations. Early trials of prophylactic or suppressive antibiotics, given either seasonally or year round, failed to show a positive impact on exacerbation occurrence. More recently, a randomized clinical trial of azithromycin, chosen for both its anti-inflammatory and antimicrobial properties, administered daily to subjects with a history of exacerbation in the past 6 months demonstrated a reduced exacerbation frequency and longer time to first exacerbation in the macrolide-treated cohort (hazard ratio, 0.73).

Oxygen Supplemental O_2 is the only pharmacologic therapy demonstrated to unequivocally decrease mortality rates in patients with COPD. For patients with resting hypoxemia (resting O_2 saturation ≤88% or <90% with signs of pulmonary hypertension or right heart failure), the use of O_2 has been demonstrated to have a significant impact on mortality rate. Patients meeting these criteria should be on continual oxygen supplementation because the mortality benefit is proportional to the number of hours per day oxygen is used. Various delivery systems are available, including portable systems that patients may carry to allow mobility outside the home.

Supplemental O_2 is commonly prescribed for patients with exertional hypoxemia or nocturnal hypoxemia. Although the rationale for supplemental O_2 in these settings is physiologically sound, the benefits of such therapy are not well substantiated.

Other Agents *N*-acetyl cysteine has been used in patients with COPD for both its mucolytic and antioxidant properties. A prospective trial failed to find any benefit with respect to decline in lung function or prevention of exacerbations. Specific treatment in the form of IV α_1AT augmentation therapy is available for individuals with severe α_1AT deficiency. Despite sterilization procedures for these blood-derived products and the absence of reported cases of viral infection from therapy, some physicians recommend hepatitis B vaccination prior to starting augmentation therapy. Although biochemical efficacy of α_1AT augmentation therapy has been shown, a randomized controlled trial of α_1AT augmentation therapy has not definitively established the efficacy of augmentation therapy in reducing decline of pulmonary function. Eligibility for α_1AT augmentation therapy requires a serum α_1AT level <11 μ*M* (approximately 50 mg/dL). Typically, Pi^Z individuals will qualify, although other rare types associated with severe deficiency (e.g., null-null) are also eligible. Because only a fraction of individuals with severe α_1AT deficiency will develop COPD, α_1AT augmentation therapy is not recommended for severely α_1AT-deficient persons with normal pulmonary function and a normal chest CT scan.

NONPHARMACOLOGIC THERAPIES

General Medical Care Patients with COPD should receive the influenza vaccine annually. Polyvalent pneumococcal vaccine is also recommended, although proof of efficacy in this patient population is not definitive. Similar recommendations and limitations of evidence also exist for vaccination for *Bordetella pertussis*.

Pulmonary Rehabilitation This refers to a treatment program that incorporates education and cardiovascular conditioning. In COPD, pulmonary rehabilitation has been demonstrated to improve health-related quality of life, dyspnea, and exercise capacity. It has also been shown to reduce rates of hospitalization over a 6- to 12-month period.

Lung Volume Reduction Surgery (LVRS) Surgery to reduce the volume of lung in patients with emphysema was first introduced with minimal success in the 1950s and was reintroduced in the 1990s. Patients are excluded if they have significant pleural disease, a pulmonary artery systolic pressure >45 mmHg, extreme deconditioning, congestive heart failure, or other severe comorbid conditions. Patients with an FEV_1 <20% of predicted and either diffusely distributed emphysema on CT scan or diffusing capacity of lung for carbon monoxide (DL_{CO}) <20% of predicted have an increased mortality rate after the procedure and thus are not candidates for LVRS.

The National Emphysema Treatment trial demonstrated that LVRS offers both a mortality benefit and a symptomatic benefit in certain patients with emphysema. The anatomic distribution of emphysema and post-rehabilitation exercise capacity are important prognostic characteristics. Patients with upper lobe–predominant emphysema and a low post-rehabilitation exercise capacity are most likely to benefit from LVRS.

Lung Transplantation **(See also Chap. 320e)** COPD is currently the second leading indication for lung transplantation (Fig. 314-4). Current recommendations are that candidates for lung transplantation should have severe disability despite maximal medical therapy and be free of comorbid conditions such as liver, renal, or cardiac disease. In contrast to LVRS, the anatomic distribution of emphysema and the presence of pulmonary hypertension are not contraindications to lung transplantation.

EXACERBATIONS OF COPD

Exacerbations are a prominent feature of the natural history of COPD. Exacerbations are episodes of increased dyspnea and cough and change in the amount and character of sputum. They may or may not be accompanied by other signs of illness, including fever, myalgias, and sore throat. Self-reported health-related quality of life correlates with frequency of exacerbations more closely than it does with the degree of airflow obstruction. Economic analyses have shown that >70% of COPD-related health care expenditures go to emergency department visits and hospital care; this translates to >$10 billion annually in the United States. The frequency of exacerbations increases as airflow obstruction increases; patients with moderate to severe airflow obstruction (GOLD stage III or IV; Table 314-1) on average have one to three episodes per year. However, some individuals with very severe airflow obstruction do not have frequent exacerbations; the history of prior exacerbations is a strong predictor of future exacerbations. Recently, an elevated ratio of the diameter of the pulmonary artery to aorta on chest CT has been associated with increased risk of COPD exacerbations.

The approach to the patient experiencing an exacerbation includes an assessment of the severity of the patient's illness, both acute and chronic components; an attempt to identify the precipitant of the exacerbation; and the institution of therapy.

Precipitating Causes and Strategies to Reduce Frequency of Exacerbations A variety of stimuli may result in the final common pathway of airway inflammation and increased symptoms that are characteristic of COPD exacerbations. Studies suggest that acquiring a new strain of bacteria is associated with increased near-term risk of exacerbation and that bacterial infection/superinfection is involved in over 50% of exacerbations. Viral respiratory infections are present in approximately one-third of COPD exacerbations. In a significant minority of instances (20–35%), no specific precipitant can be identified.

The role of pharmacotherapy in reducing exacerbation frequency is less well studied. Chronic oral glucocorticoids are not recommended for this purpose. Inhaled glucocorticoids reduce the frequency of exacerbations by 25–30% in most analyses. The use of inhaled glucocorticoids should be considered in patients with frequent exacerbations or those who have an asthmatic component, i.e., significant reversibility on pulmonary function testing or marked symptomatic improvement after inhaled bronchodilators. Similar magnitudes of reduction have been reported for anticholinergic and long-acting β-agonist therapy. The influenza vaccine has been shown to reduce exacerbation rates in patients with COPD. As outlined above, daily azithromycin administered to subjects with COPD and an exacerbation history reduces exacerbation frequency.

Patient Assessment An attempt should be made to establish the severity of the exacerbation as well as the severity of preexisting COPD. The more severe either of these two components, the more likely that the patient will require hospital admission. The history should include quantification of the degree of dyspnea by asking about breathlessness during activities of daily living and typical activities for the patient. The patient should be asked about fever; change in character of sputum; any ill contacts; and associated symptoms such as nausea, vomiting, diarrhea, myalgias, and chills. Inquiring about the frequency and severity of prior exacerbations can provide important information.

The physical examination should incorporate an assessment of the degree of distress of the patient. Specific attention should be focused on tachycardia, tachypnea, use of accessory muscles, signs of perioral or peripheral cyanosis, the ability to speak in complete sentences, and the patient's mental status. The chest examination should establish the presence or absence of focal findings, degree of air movement, presence or absence of wheezing, asymmetry in the chest examination (suggesting large airway obstruction or pneumothorax mimicking an exacerbation), and the presence or absence of paradoxical motion of the abdominal wall.

Patients with severe underlying COPD, who are in moderate or severe distress, or those with focal findings should have a chest x-ray. Approximately 25% of x-rays in this clinical situation will be abnormal, with the most frequent findings being pneumonia and congestive heart failure. Patients with advanced COPD, those with a history of hypercarbia, those with mental status changes (confusion, sleepiness), or those in significant distress should have an arterial blood-gas measurement. The presence of hypercarbia, defined as a P_{CO_2} >45 mmHg, has important implications for treatment (discussed below). In contrast to its utility in the management of exacerbations of asthma, measurement of pulmonary function has not been demonstrated to be helpful in the diagnosis or management of exacerbations of COPD.

There are no definitive guidelines concerning the need for inpatient treatment of exacerbations. Patients with respiratory acidosis and hypercarbia, significant hypoxemia, or severe underlying disease or those whose living situation is not conducive to careful observation and the delivery of prescribed treatment should be admitted to the hospital.

ACUTE EXACERBATIONS

Bronchodilators Typically, patients are treated with an inhaled β agonist, often with the addition of an anticholinergic agent. These may be administered separately or together, and the frequency of administration depends on the severity of the exacerbation. Patients are often treated initially with nebulized therapy, as such treatment is often easier to administer in older patients or to those in respiratory distress. It has been shown, however, that conversion to metered-dose inhalers is effective when accompanied by education and training of patients and staff. This approach has significant economic benefits and also allows an easier transition to outpatient care. The addition of methylxanthines (such as theophylline) to this regimen can be considered, although convincing proof of its efficacy is lacking. If added, serum levels should be monitored in an attempt to minimize toxicity.

Antibiotics Patients with COPD are frequently colonized with potential respiratory pathogens, and it is often difficult to identify conclusively a specific species of bacteria responsible for a particular clinical event. Bacteria frequently implicated in COPD exacerbations include *Streptococcus pneumoniae, Haemophilus influenzae,* and *Moraxella catarrhalis.* In addition, *Mycoplasma pneumoniae* or *Chlamydia pneumoniae* are found in 5–10% of exacerbations. The choice of antibiotic should be based on local patterns of antibiotic susceptibility of the above pathogens as well as the patient's clinical condition. Most practitioners treat patients with moderate or severe exacerbations with antibiotics, even in the absence of data implicating a specific pathogen.

Glucocorticoids Among patients admitted to the hospital, the use of glucocorticoids has been demonstrated to reduce the length of stay, hasten recovery, and reduce the chance of subsequent exacerbation or relapse for a period of up to 6 months. One study demonstrated that 2 weeks of glucocorticoid therapy produced benefit indistinguishable from 8 weeks of therapy. The GOLD guidelines recommend 30–40 mg of oral prednisolone or its equivalent for a period of 10–14 days. Hyperglycemia, particularly in patients with preexisting diagnosis of diabetes, is the most frequently reported acute complication of glucocorticoid treatment.

Oxygen Supplemental O_2 should be supplied to keep arterial saturations ≥90%. Hypoxemic respiratory drive plays a small role in patients with COPD. Studies have demonstrated that in patients with both acute and chronic hypercarbia, the administration of supplemental O_2 does not reduce minute ventilation. It does, in some patients, result in modest increases in arterial P_{CO_2}, chiefly by altering ventilation-perfusion relationships within the lung. This should not deter practitioners from providing the oxygen needed to correct hypoxemia.

Mechanical Ventilatory Support The initiation of noninvasive positive-pressure ventilation (NIPPV) in patients with respiratory failure, defined as Pa_{CO_2} >45 mmHg, results in a significant reduction in mortality rate, need for intubation, complications of therapy, and hospital length of stay. Contraindications to NIPPV include cardiovascular instability, impaired mental status or inability to cooperate, copious secretions or the inability to clear secretions, craniofacial abnormalities or trauma precluding effective fitting of mask, extreme obesity, or significant burns.

Invasive (conventional) mechanical ventilation via an endotracheal tube is indicated for patients with severe respiratory distress despite initial therapy, life-threatening hypoxemia, severe hypercarbia and/or acidosis, markedly impaired mental status, respiratory arrest, hemodynamic instability, or other complications. The goal of mechanical ventilation is to correct the aforementioned conditions. Factors to consider during mechanical ventilatory support include the need to provide sufficient expiratory time in patients with severe airflow obstruction and the presence of auto-PEEP (positive end-expiratory pressure), which can result in patients having to generate significant respiratory effort to trigger a breath during a demand mode of ventilation. The mortality rate of patients requiring mechanical ventilatory support is 17–30% for that particular hospitalization. For patients age >65 admitted to the intensive care unit for treatment, the mortality rate doubles over the next year to 60%, regardless of whether mechanical ventilation was required.

315 Interstitial Lung Diseases

Talmadge E. King, Jr.

Patients with interstitial lung diseases (ILDs) come to medical attention mainly because of the onset of progressive exertional dyspnea or a persistent nonproductive cough. Hemoptysis, wheezing, and chest pain may be present. Often, the identification of interstitial opacities on chest x-ray focuses the diagnostic approach on one of the ILDs.

ILDs represent a large number of conditions that involve the parenchyma of the lung—the alveoli, the alveolar epithelium, the capillary endothelium, and the spaces between those structures—as well as the perivascular and lymphatic tissues. The disorders in this heterogeneous group are classified together because of similar clinical, roentgenographic, physiologic, or pathologic manifestations. These disorders often are associated with considerable rates of morbidity and mortality, and there is little consensus regarding the best management of most of them.

ILDs have been difficult to classify because >200 known individual diseases are characterized by diffuse parenchymal lung involvement, either as the primary condition or as a significant part of a multiorgan process, as may occur in the connective tissue diseases (CTDs). One useful approach to classification is to separate the ILDs into two groups based on the major underlying histopathology: (1) those associated with predominant inflammation and fibrosis and (2) those with a predominantly granulomatous reaction in interstitial or vascular areas (Table 315-1). Each of these groups can be subdivided further according to whether the cause is known or unknown. For each ILD there may be an acute phase, and there is usually a chronic one as well. Rarely, some are recurrent, with intervals of subclinical disease.

Sarcoidosis (Chap. 390), idiopathic pulmonary fibrosis (IPF), and pulmonary fibrosis associated with CTDs (Chaps. 378, 382, 388, and 427) are the most common ILDs of unknown etiology. Among the ILDs of known cause, the largest group includes occupational and environmental exposures, especially the inhalation of inorganic dusts, organic dusts, and various fumes or gases (Chap. 311). A multidisciplinary approach—requiring close communication between clinician, radiologist, and when appropriate, pathologist—is often required to make the diagnosis. High-resolution computed tomography (HRCT) scanning improves the diagnostic accuracy and may eliminate the need for tissue examination in many cases, especially in IPF. For other forms, tissue examination, usually obtained by thoracoscopic lung biopsy, is critical to confirmation of the diagnosis.

PATHOGENESIS

The ILDs are nonmalignant disorders and are not caused by identified infectious agents. The precise pathway(s) leading from injury to fibrosis is not known. Although there are multiple initiating agent(s) of injury, the immunopathogenic responses of lung tissue are limited, and the mechanisms of repair have common features (Fig. 315-1).

As mentioned above, the two major histopathologic patterns are a granulomatous pattern and a pattern in which inflammation and fibrosis predominate.

Granulomatous Lung Disease This process is characterized by an accumulation of T lymphocytes, macrophages, and epithelioid cells organized into discrete structures (granulomas) in the lung parenchyma. The granulomatous lesions can progress to fibrosis. Many patients with granulomatous lung disease remain free of severe impairment of lung function or, when symptomatic, improve after treatment. The main differential diagnosis is between sarcoidosis (Chap. 390) and hypersensitivity pneumonitis (Chap. 310).

Inflammation and Fibrosis The initial insult is an injury to the epithelial surface that causes inflammation in the air spaces and alveolar walls. If the disease becomes chronic, inflammation spreads to adjacent portions of the interstitium and vasculature and eventually causes interstitial fibrosis. Important histopathologic patterns found in the ILDs include usual interstitial pneumonia (UIP), nonspecific interstitial [...] respiratory bronchiolitis/desquamative interstitial pneu[...]nizing pneumonia, diffuse alveolar damage (acute or or[...] lymphocytic interstitial pneumonia. The development [...] scarring (fibrosis) of alveolar walls, airways, or vasculat[...] feared outcome in all of these conditions because it is [...]sive and leads to significant derangement of ventilato[...] gas exchange.

TABLE 315-1 MAJOR CATEGORIES OF ALVEOLAR AND INTERSTITIAL INFLAMMATORY LUNG DISEASE

Lung Response: Alveolitis, Interstitial Inflammation, and Fibrosis	
Known Cause	
Asbestos	Residual of acute respiratory distress syndrome
Fumes, gases	Smoking-related
Drugs (antibiotics, amiodarone, gold) and chemotherapy drugs	Desquamative interstitial pneumonia
Radiation	Respiratory bronchiolitis–associated interstitial lung disease
Aspiration pneumonia	Pulmonary Langerhans cell granulomatosis
Unknown Cause	
Idiopathic interstitial pneumonias	Pulmonary alveolar proteinosis
Idiopathic pulmonary fibrosis (usual interstitial pneumonia)	Lymphocytic infiltrative disorders (lymphocytic interstitial pneumonitis associated with connective tissue disease)
Acute interstitial pneumonia (diffuse alveolar damage)	Eosinophilic pneumonias
Cryptogenic organizing pneumonia	Lymphangioleiomyomatosis
Nonspecific interstitial pneumonia	Inherited diseases
Idiopathic lymphocytic interstitial pneumonia	Tuberous sclerosis, neurofibromatosis, Niemann-Pick disease, Gaucher disease, Hermansky-Pudlak syndrome
Rare and ill-defined entities	
Idiopathic pleuroparenchymal fibroelastosis	
Acute fibrinous and organizing pneumonia	
Bronchiolocentric patterns of interstitial pneumonia	
Connective tissue diseases	Gastrointestinal or liver diseases (Crohn disease, primary biliary cirrhosis, chronic active hepatitis, ulcerative colitis)
Systemic lupus erythematosus, rheumatoid arthritis, ankylosing spondylitis, systemic sclerosis, Sjögren syndrome, polymyositis-dermatomyositis	
Pulmonary hemorrhage syndromes	Graft-versus-host disease (bone marrow transplantation; solid organ transplantation)
Goodpasture syndrome, idiopathic pulmonary hemosiderosis, isolated pulmonary capillaritis	
Amyloidosis	
Lung Response: Granulomatous	
Known Cause	
Hypersensitivity pneumonitis (organic dusts)	Inorganic dusts: beryllium, silica
Unknown Cause	
Sarcoidosis	Bronchocentric granulomatosis
Granulomatous vasculitides	Lymphomatoid granulomatosis
Granulomatosis with polyangiitis (Wegener)	
Eosinophilic granulomatosis with polyangiitis (Churg-Strauss)	

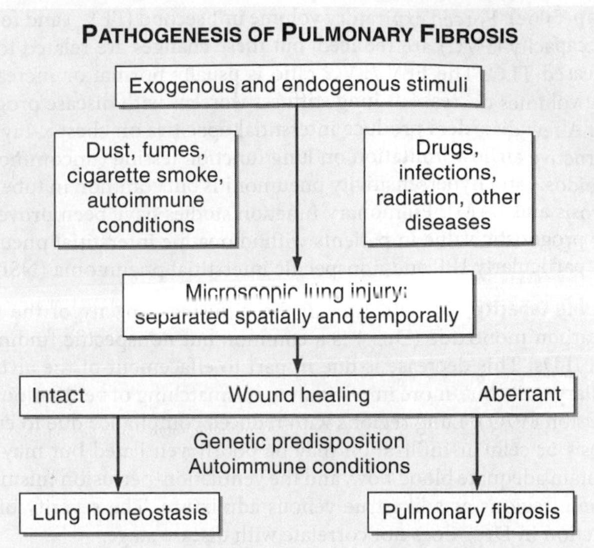

FIGURE 315-1 Proposed mechanism for the pathogenesis of pulmonary fibrosis. The lung is naturally exposed to repetitive injury from a variety of exogenous and endogenous stimuli. Several local and systemic factors (e.g., fibroblasts, circulating fibrocytes, chemokines, growth factors, and clotting factors) contribute to tissue healing and functional recovery. Dysregulation of this intricate network through genetic predisposition, autoimmune conditions, or superimposed diseases can lead to aberrant wound healing, with the result of pulmonary fibrosis. Alternatively, excessive injury to the lung may overwhelm even intact reparative mechanisms and lead to pulmonary fibrosis. *(From S Garantziotis et al: J Clin Invest 114:319, 2004.)*

HISTORY

Duration of Illness *Acute presentation* (days to weeks), although unusual, occurs with allergy (drugs, fungi, helminths), acute interstitial pneumonia (AIP), eosinophilic pneumonia, and hypersensitivity pneumonitis. These conditions may be confused with atypical pneumonias because of diffuse alveolar opacities on chest x-ray. *Subacute presentation* (weeks to months) may occur in all ILDs but is seen especially in sarcoidosis, drug-induced ILDs, the alveolar hemorrhage syndromes, cryptogenic organizing pneumonia (COP), and the acute immunologic pneumonia that complicates systemic lupus erythematosus (SLE) or polymyositis. In most ILDs, the symptoms and signs form a *chronic presentation* (months to years). Examples include IPF, sarcoidosis, pulmonary Langerhans cell histiocytosis (PLCH), pneumoconioses, and CTDs. *Episodic presentations* are unusual and include eosinophilic pneumonia, hypersensitivity pneumonitis, COP, vasculitides, pulmonary hemorrhage, and Churg-Strauss syndrome.

Age Most patients with sarcoidosis, ILD associated with CTD, lymphangioleiomyomatosis (LAM), PLCH, and inherited forms of ILD (familial IPF, Gaucher disease, Hermansky-Pudlak syndrome) present between the ages of 20 and 40 years. Most patients with IPF are older than 60 years.

Gender LAM and pulmonary involvement in tuberous sclerosis occur exclusively in premenopausal women. In addition, ILD in Hermansky-Pudlak syndrome and in the CTDs is more common in women; an exception is ILD in rheumatoid arthritis (RA), which is more common in men. IPF is more common in men. Because of occupational exposures, pneumoconioses also occur more frequently in men.

Family History Familial lung fibrosis has been associated with mutations in the surfactant protein C gene, the surfactant protein A2 gene, telomerase reverse transcriptase (*TERT*), telomerase RNA component (*TERC*), and the promoter of a mucin gene (*MUC5B*). Familial lung fibrosis is characterized by several patterns of interstitial pneumonia, including nonspecific interstitial pneumonia, desquamative interstitial pneumonia, and UIP. Older age, male sex, and a history of cigarette smoking have been identified as risk factors for familial lung fibrosis. Family associations (with an autosomal dominant pattern) have been identified in tuberous sclerosis and neurofibromatosis. Familial clustering has been identified increasingly in sarcoidosis. The genes responsible for several rare ILDs have been identified, i.e., alveolar microlithiasis, Gaucher disease, Hermansky-Pudlak syndrome, and Niemann-Pick disease, along with the genes for surfactant homeostasis in pulmonary alveolar proteinosis and for control of cell growth and differentiation in LAM.

Smoking History Two-thirds to 75% of patients with IPF and familial lung fibrosis have a history of smoking. Patients with PLCH, respiratory bronchiolitis/desquamative interstitial pneumonia (DIP), Goodpasture syndrome, respiratory bronchiolitis, and pulmonary alveolar proteinosis are usually current or former smokers.

Occupational and Environmental History A strict chronologic listing of the patient's lifelong employment must be sought, including specific duties and known exposures. In hypersensitivity pneumonitis (see Fig. 310-1), respiratory symptoms, fever, chills, and an abnormal chest roentgenogram are often temporally related to a hobby (pigeon breeder's disease) or to the workplace (farmer's lung) (Chap. 310). Symptoms may diminish or disappear after the patient leaves the site of exposure for several days; similarly, symptoms may reappear when the patient returns to the exposure site.

Other Important Past History Parasitic infections may cause pulmonary eosinophilia, and therefore a travel history should be taken in patients with known or suspected ILD. History of risk factors for HIV infection should be elicited because several processes may occur at the time of initial presentation or during the clinical course, e.g., HIV infection, organizing pneumonia, AIP, lymphocytic interstitial pneumonitis, and diffuse alveolar hemorrhage.

Respiratory Symptoms and Signs Dyspnea is a common and prominent complaint in patients with ILD, especially the idiopathic interstitial pneumonias, hypersensitivity pneumonitis, COP, sarcoidosis, eosinophilic pneumonias, and PLCH. Some patients, especially those with sarcoidosis, silicosis, PLCH, hypersensitivity pneumonitis, lipoid pneumonia, or lymphangitis carcinomatosis, may have extensive parenchymal lung disease on chest imaging studies without significant dyspnea, especially early in the course of the illness. Wheezing is an uncommon manifestation of ILD but has been described in patients with chronic eosinophilic pneumonia, Churg-Strauss syndrome, respiratory bronchiolitis, and sarcoidosis. Clinically significant chest pain is uncommon in most ILDs. However, substernal discomfort is common in sarcoidosis. Sudden worsening of dyspnea, especially if associated with acute chest pain, may indicate a spontaneous pneumothorax, which occurs in PLCH, tuberous sclerosis, LAM, and neurofibromatosis. Frank hemoptysis and blood-streaked sputum are rarely presenting manifestations of ILD but can be seen in the diffuse alveolar hemorrhage (DAH) syndromes, LAM, tuberous sclerosis, and the granulomatous vasculitides. Fatigue and weight loss are common in all ILDs.

PHYSICAL EXAMINATION

The findings are usually not specific. Most commonly, physical examination reveals tachypnea and bibasilar end-inspiratory dry crackles, which are common in most forms of ILD associated with inflammation but are less likely to be heard in the granulomatous lung diseases. Crackles may be present in the absence of radiographic abnormalities on the chest radiograph. Scattered late inspiratory high-pitched rhonchi—so-called inspiratory squeaks—are heard in patients with bronchiolitis. The cardiac examination is usually normal except in the middle or late stages of the disease, when findings of pulmonary hypertension and cor pulmonale may become evident (Chap. 304). Cyanosis and clubbing of the digits occur in some patients with advanced disease.

LABORATORY

Antinuclear antibodies and anti-immunoglobulin antibodies (rheumatoid factors) are identified in some patients, even in the absence of a defined CTD. A raised lactate dehydrogenase (LDH) level is a nonspecific finding common to ILDs. Elevation of the serum level of angiotensin-converting enzyme is common in ILDs, especially sarcoidosis. Serum precipitins confirm exposure when hypersensitivity pneumonitis is suspected, although they are not diagnostic of the process. Antineutrophil cytoplasmic or anti-basement membrane antibodies are useful if vasculitis is suspected. The electrocardiogram is usually normal unless pulmonary hypertension is present; then it demonstrates right-axis deviation, right ventricular hypertrophy, or right atrial enlargement or hypertrophy. Echocardiography also reveals right ventricular dilation and/or hypertrophy in the presence of pulmonary hypertension.

CHEST IMAGING STUDIES

Chest X-Ray ILD may be first suspected on the basis of an abnormal chest radiograph, which most commonly reveals a bibasilar reticular pattern. A nodular or mixed pattern of alveolar filling and increased reticular markings also may be present. Subgroups of ILDs exhibit nodular opacities with a predilection for the upper lung zones (sarcoidosis, PLCH, chronic hypersensitivity pneumonitis, silicosis, beryllіosis, RA [necrobiotic nodular form], ankylosing spondylitis). The chest x-ray correlates poorly with the clinical or histopathologic stage of the disease. The radiographic finding of honeycombing correlates with pathologic findings of small cystic spaces and progressive fibrosis; when present, it portends a poor prognosis. In most cases, the chest radiograph is nonspecific and usually does not allow a specific diagnosis.

Computed Tomography HRCT is superior to the plain chest x-ray for early detection and confirmation of suspected ILD (Fig. 315-2). In addition, HRCT allows better assessment of the extent and distribution of disease, and it is especially useful in the investigation of patients with a normal chest radiograph. Coexisting disease is often best recognized on HRCT scanning, e.g., mediastinal adenopathy, carcinoma, or emphysema. In the appropriate clinical setting, HRCT may be sufficiently characteristic to preclude the need for lung biopsy in IPF, sarcoidosis, hypersensitivity pneumonitis, asbestosis, lymphangitic carcinoma, and PLCH. When a lung biopsy is required, HRCT scanning is useful for determining the most appropriate area from which biopsy samples should be taken.

PULMONARY FUNCTION TESTING

Spirometry and Lung Volumes Measurement of lung function is important in assessing the extent of pulmonary involvement in patients with ILD. Most forms of ILD produce a restrictive defect with reduced total lung capacity (TLC), functional residual capacity, and residual volume

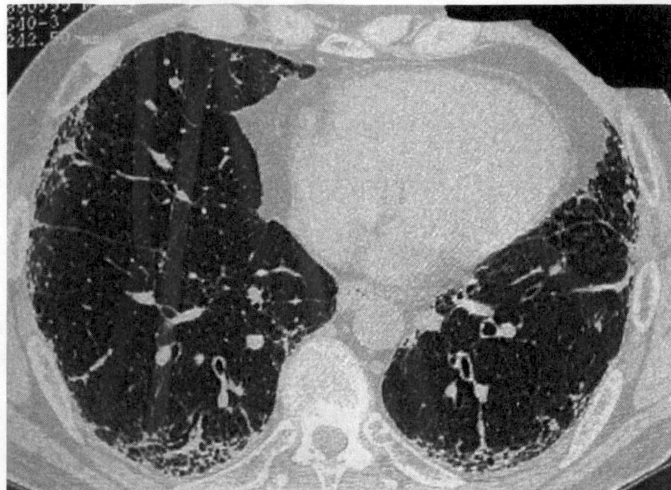

FIGURE 315-2 **Idiopathic pulmonary fibrosis.** High-resolution computed tomography image shows bibasal, peripheral predominant reticular abnormality with traction bronchiectasis and honeycombing. The lung biopsy showed the typical features of usual interstitial pneumonia.

(Chap. 306e). Forced expiratory volume in 1 second (FEV_1) and forced vital capacity (FVC) are reduced, but these changes are related to the decreased TLC. The FEV_1/FVC ratio is usually normal or increased. Lung volumes decrease as lung stiffness worsens with disease progression. A few disorders produce interstitial opacities on chest x-ray and obstructive airflow limitation on lung function testing (uncommon in sarcoidosis and hypersensitivity pneumonitis but common in tuberous sclerosis and LAM). Pulmonary function studies have been proved to have prognostic value in patients with idiopathic interstitial pneumonias, particularly IPF and nonspecific interstitial pneumonia (NSIP).

Diffusing Capacity A reduction in the diffusing capacity of the lung for carbon monoxide (DL_{CO}) is a common but nonspecific finding in most ILDs. This decrease is due in part to effacement of the alveolar capillary units but, more important, to mismatching of ventilation and perfusion ($\dot{V}/\dot{Q}$). Lung regions with reduced compliance due to either fibrosis or cellular infiltration may be poorly ventilated but may still maintain adequate blood flow, and the ventilation-perfusion mismatch in these regions acts like true venous admixture. The severity of the reduction in DL_{CO} does not correlate with disease stage.

Arterial Blood Gas The resting arterial blood gas may be normal or reveal hypoxemia (secondary to a mismatching of ventilation to perfusion) and respiratory alkalosis. A normal arterial O_2 tension (or saturation by oximetry) at rest does not rule out significant hypoxemia during exercise or sleep. Carbon dioxide (CO_2) retention is rare and is usually a manifestation of end-stage disease.

CARDIOPULMONARY EXERCISE TESTING

Because hypoxemia at rest is not always present and because severe exercise-induced hypoxemia may go undetected, it is useful to perform exercise testing with measurement of arterial blood gases to detect abnormalities of gas exchange. Arterial oxygen desaturation, a failure to decrease dead space appropriately with exercise (i.e., a high V_D/V_T [dead space/tidal volume] ratio [Chap. 306e]), and an excessive increase in respiratory rate with a lower than expected recruitment of tidal volume provide useful information about physiologic abnormalities and extent of disease. Serial assessment of resting and exercise gas exchange is an excellent method for following disease activity and responsiveness to treatment, especially in patients with IPF. Increasingly, the 6-min walk test is used to obtain a global evaluation of submaximal exercise capacity in patients with ILD. The walk distance and level of oxygen desaturation tend to correlate with the patient's baseline lung function and mirror the patient's clinical course.

FIBEROPTIC BRONCHOSCOPY AND BRONCHOALVEOLAR LAVAGE (BAL)

In selected diseases (e.g., sarcoidosis, hypersensitivity pneumonitis, DAH syndrome, cancer, pulmonary alveolar proteinosis), cellular analysis of BAL fluid may be useful in narrowing the differential diagnostic possibilities among various types of ILD (Table 315-2). The role of BAL in defining the stage of disease and assessment of disease progression or response to therapy remains poorly understood, and the usefulness of BAL in the clinical assessment and management remains to be established.

TISSUE AND CELLULAR EXAMINATION

Lung biopsy is the most effective method for confirming the diagnosis and assessing disease activity. The findings may identify a more treatable process than originally suspected, particularly chronic hypersensitivity pneumonitis, COP, respiratory bronchiolitis–associated ILD, or sarcoidosis. Biopsy should be obtained before the initiation of treatment. A definitive diagnosis avoids confusion and anxiety later in the clinical course if the patient does not respond to therapy or experiences serious side effects from it.

Fiberoptic bronchoscopy with multiple transbronchial lung biopsies (four to eight biopsy samples) is often the initial procedure of choice, especially when sarcoidosis, lymphangitic carcinomatosis, eosinophilic pneumonia, Goodpasture syndrome, or infection is suspected. If a specific diagnosis is not made by transbronchial biopsy, surgical lung biopsy by video-assisted thoracic surgery or open thoracotomy is

TABLE 315-2 DIAGNOSTIC VALUE OF BRONCHOALVEOLAR LAVAGE IN INTERSTITIAL LUNG DISEASE	
Condition	**Bronchoalveolar Lavage Finding**
Sarcoidosis	Lymphocytosis; CD4:CD8 ratio >3.5 most specific of diagnosis
Hypersensitivity pneumonitis	Marked lymphocytosis (>50%)
Organizing pneumonia	Foamy macrophages; mixed pattern of increased cells characteristic; decreased CD4:CD8 ratio
Eosinophilic lung disease	Eosinophils >25%
Diffuse alveolar bleeding	Hemosiderin-laden macrophages, red blood cells
Diffuse alveolar damage, drug toxicity	Atypical hyperplastic type II pneumocytes
Opportunistic infections	*Pneumocystis carinii,* fungi, cytomegalovirus-transformed cells
Lymphangitic carcinomatosis, alveolar cell carcinoma, pulmonary lymphoma	Malignant cells
Alveolar proteinosis	Milky effluent, foamy macrophages and lipoproteinaceous intraalveolar material (periodic acid–Schiff stain–positive)
Lipoid pneumonia	Fat globules in macrophages
Pulmonary Langerhans cell histiocytosis	Increased CD1+ Langerhans cells, electron microscopy demonstrating Birbeck granule in lavaged macrophage (expensive and difficult to perform)
Asbestos-related pulmonary disease	Dust particles, ferruginous bodies
Berylliosis	Positive lymphocyte transformation test to beryllium
Silicosis	Dust particles by polarized light microscopy
Lipoidosis	Accumulation of specific lipopigment in alveolar macrophages

indicated. Adequate-sized biopsies from multiple sites, usually from two lobes, should be obtained. Relative contraindications to lung biopsy include serious cardiovascular disease, honeycombing and other roentgenographic evidence of diffuse end stage disease, severe pulmonary dysfunction, and other major operative risks, especially in the elderly.

TREATMENT INTERSTITIAL LUNG DISEASE

Although the course of ILD is variable, progression is common and often insidious. All treatable possibilities should be carefully considered. Because therapy does not reverse fibrosis, the major goals of treatment are permanent removal of the offending agent, when known, and early identification and aggressive suppression of the acute and chronic inflammatory process, thereby reducing further lung damage. Hypoxemia (Pa_{O_2} <55 mmHg) at rest and/or with exercise should be managed with supplemental oxygen. Management of cor pulmonale may be required as the disease progresses (Chaps. 280 and 304). Pulmonary rehabilitation has been shown to improve the quality of life in patients with ILD.

DRUG THERAPY

Glucocorticoids are the mainstay of therapy for suppression of the inflammation present in ILD, but the success rate is low. There have been no placebo-controlled trials of glucocorticoids in ILD, and so there is no direct evidence that steroids improve survival in many of the diseases for which they are commonly used. Glucocorticoid therapy is recommended for symptomatic ILD patients with eosinophilic pneumonias, COP, CTD, sarcoidosis, hypersensitivity pneumonitis, acute inorganic dust exposures, acute radiation pneumonitis, DAH, and drug-induced ILD. In organic dust disease, glucocorticoids are recommended for both the acute and chronic stages.

The optimal dose and proper length of therapy with glucocorticoids in the treatment of most ILDs are not known. A common starting dose is prednisone, 0.5–1 mg/kg in a once-daily oral dose (based on the patient's lean body weight). This dose is continued for 4–12 weeks, at which time the patient is reevaluated. If the patient is stable or improved, the dose is tapered to 0.25–0.5 mg/kg and is maintained at this level for an additional 4–12 weeks, depending on the course. Rapid tapering or a shortened course of glucocorticoid treatment can result in recurrence. If the patient's condition continues to decline on glucocorticoids, a second agent (see below) often is added and the prednisone dose is lowered to or maintained at 0.25 mg/kg per day.

Cyclophosphamide, azathioprine (1–2 mg/kg lean body weight per day), and mycophenolate mofetil, with or without glucocorticoids, have been tried with variable success in IPF, vasculitis, progressive systemic sclerosis, and other ILDs. An objective response usually requires at least 8–12 weeks to occur. In situations in which these drugs have failed or could not be tolerated, other agents, including methotrexate and cyclosporine, have been tried. However, their role in the treatment of ILDs remains to be determined.

Many cases of ILD are chronic and irreversible despite the therapy discussed above, and lung transplantation may then be considered (Chap. 320e).

INDIVIDUAL FORMS OF INTERSTITIAL LUNG DISEASE

IDIOPATHIC PULMONARY FIBROSIS

IPF is the most common form of idiopathic interstitial pneumonia. Separating IPF from other forms of lung fibrosis is an important step in the evaluation of all patients presenting with ILD. IPF has a distinctly poor response to therapy and a bad prognosis.

Clinical Manifestations Exertional dyspnea, a nonproductive cough, and inspiratory crackles with or without digital clubbing may be present on physical examination. HRCT lung scans typically show patchy, predominantly basilar, subpleural reticular opacities, often associated with traction bronchiectasis and honeycombing (Fig. 315-2). A definite UIP pattern on HRCT is highly accurate for the presence of a UIP pattern on surgical lung biopsy. Atypical findings that should suggest an alternative diagnosis include extensive ground-glass abnormality, nodular opacities, upper or midzone predominance, and prominent hilar or mediastinal lymphadenopathy. Pulmonary function tests often reveal a restrictive pattern, a reduced DL_{CO}, and arterial hypoxemia that is exaggerated or elicited by exercise.

Histologic Findings Confirmation of the presence of the UIP pattern on histologic examination is essential to confirm this diagnosis. Transbronchial biopsies are not helpful in making the diagnosis of UIP, and surgical biopsy usually is required. The histologic hallmark and chief diagnostic criterion of UIP is a heterogeneous appearance at low magnification with alternating areas of normal lung, interstitial inflammation, foci of proliferating fibroblasts, dense collagen fibrosis, and honeycomb changes. These histologic changes affect the peripheral, subpleural parenchyma most severely. The interstitial inflammation is usually patchy and consists of a lymphoplasmacytic infiltrate in the alveolar septa, associated with hyperplasia of type 2 pneumocytes. The fibrotic zones are composed mainly of dense collagen, although scattered foci of proliferating fibroblasts are a consistent finding. The extent of fibroblastic proliferation is predictive of disease progression. Areas of honeycomb change are composed of cystic fibrotic air spaces that frequently are lined by bronchiolar epithelium and filled with mucin. Smooth-muscle hyperplasia is commonly seen in areas of fibrosis and honeycomb change. A fibrotic pattern with some features similar to UIP may be found in the chronic stage of several specific disorders, such as pneumoconioses (e.g., asbestosis), radiation injury, certain drug-induced lung diseases (e.g., nitrofurantoin), chronic aspiration, sarcoidosis, chronic hypersensitivity pneumonitis, organized chronic eosinophilic pneumonia, and PLCH. Commonly, other histopathologic features are present in these situations, thus allowing separation of these lesions from the UIP-like pattern. Consequently, the term *usual interstitial pneumonia* is used for patients in whom the lesion is idiopathic and not associated with another condition.

TREATMENT MANAGEMENT ISSUES IN PATIENTS WITH IPF

Untreated patients with IPF show continued progression of their disease and have a high mortality rate. There is no effective therapy for IPF. Thalidomide appears to improve cough in patients with IPF. Chronic microaspiration secondary to gastroesophageal reflux may play a role in the pathogenesis and natural history of IPF. Gastroesophageal reflux (GER) therapy may be of benefit in IPF. In patients with IPF, treatment with the three-drug regimen of prednisone, azathioprine, and *N*-acetylcysteine (NAC) or warfarin (in IPF patients who lacked other indications for anticoagulation) has been shown to increase the risks of hospitalization and death.

Patients with IPF and coexisting emphysema (combined pulmonary fibrosis and emphysema [CPFE]) are more likely to require long-term oxygen therapy and develop pulmonary hypertension and may have a more dismal outcome than those without emphysema.

Patients with IPF may have acute deterioration secondary to infections, pulmonary embolism, or pneumothorax. Heart failure and ischemic heart disease are common problems in patients with IPF, accounting for nearly one-third of deaths. These patients also commonly experience an accelerated phase of rapid clinical decline that is associated with a poor prognosis (so-called acute exacerbations of IPF). These acute exacerbations are defined by worsening of dyspnea within a few days to 4 weeks; newly developing diffuse ground-glass abnormality and/or consolidation superimposed on a background reticular or honeycomb pattern consistent with the UIP pattern; worsening hypoxemia; and absence of infectious pneumonia, heart failure, and sepsis. The rate of these acute exacerbations ranges from 10–57%, apparently depending on the length of follow-up. During these episodes, the histopathologic pattern of diffuse alveolar damage is often found on the background of UIP. No therapy has been found to be effective in the management of acute exacerbations of IPF. Often mechanical ventilation is required, but it is usually not successful, with a hospital mortality rate of up to three-fourths of patients. In those who survive, a recurrence of acute exacerbation is common and usually results in death at those times.

Patients should be referred early for lung transplant because of the unpredictability of disease progression (e.g., acute exacerbations) (Chap. 320e).

NONSPECIFIC INTERSTITIAL PNEUMONIA

This condition defines a subgroup of the idiopathic interstitial pneumonias that can be distinguished clinically and pathologically from UIP, DIP, AIP, and COP. Importantly, many cases with this histopathologic pattern occur in the context of an underlying disorder, such as a CTD, drug-induced ILD, or chronic hypersensitivity pneumonitis.

Clinical Manifestations Patients with idiopathic NSIP have clinical, serologic, radiographic, and pathologic characteristics highly suggestive of autoimmune disease and meet the criteria for undifferentiated CTD. Idiopathic NSIP is a subacute restrictive process with a presentation similar to that of IPF but usually at a younger age, most commonly in women who have never smoked. It is often associated with a febrile illness. HRCT shows bilateral, subpleural ground-glass opacities, often associated with lower lobe volume loss (Fig. 315-3). Patchy areas of airspace consolidation and reticular abnormalities may be present, but honeycombing is unusual.

Histologic Findings The key histopathologic feature of NSIP is the uniformity of interstitial involvement across the biopsy section, and this may be predominantly cellular or fibrosing. There is less temporal and spatial heterogeneity than in UIP, and little or no honeycombing is found. The cellular variant is rare.

Treatment The majority of patients with NSIP have a good prognosis (5-year mortality rate estimated at <15%), with most showing improvement after treatment with glucocorticoids, often used in combination with azathioprine or mycophenolate mofetil.

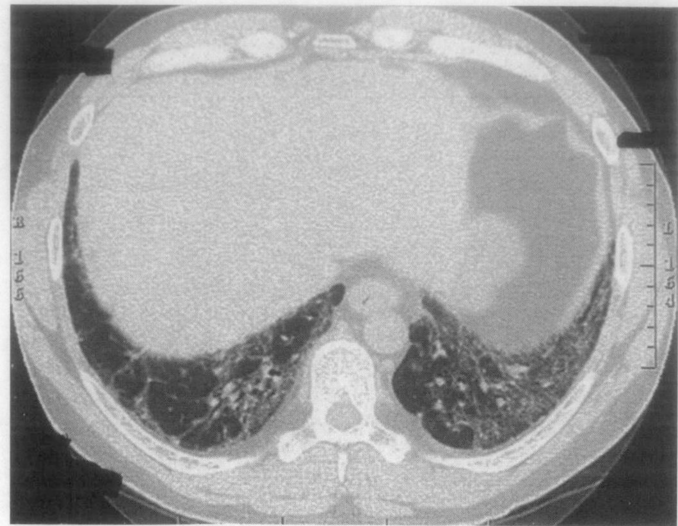

FIGURE 315-3 Nonspecific interstitial pneumonia. High-resolution computed tomography through the lower lung shows volume loss with extensive ground-glass abnormality, reticular abnormality, and traction bronchiectasis. There is sparing on the lung immediately adjacent to the pleura. Histology showed a combination of inflammation and mild fibrosis.

ACUTE INTERSTITIAL PNEUMONIA (HAMMAN-RICH SYNDROME)

Clinical Manifestations AIP is a rare, fulminant form of lung injury characterized histologically by diffuse alveolar damage on lung biopsy. Most patients are older than 40 years. AIP is similar in presentation to the acute respiratory distress syndrome (ARDS) (Chap. 322) and probably corresponds to the subset of cases of idiopathic ARDS. The onset is usually abrupt in a previously healthy individual. A prodromal illness, usually lasting 7–14 days before presentation, is common. Fever, cough, and dyspnea are common manifestations at presentation. Diffuse, bilateral, air-space opacification is present on the chest radiograph. HRCT scans show bilateral, patchy, symmetric areas of ground-glass attenuation. Bilateral areas of air-space consolidation also may be present. A predominantly subpleural distribution may be seen.

Histologic Findings The diagnosis of AIP requires the presence of a clinical syndrome of idiopathic ARDS and pathologic confirmation of organizing diffuse alveolar damage. Therefore, lung biopsy is required to confirm the diagnosis.

Treatment Most patients have moderate to severe hypoxemia and develop respiratory failure. Mechanical ventilation is often required. The mortality rate is high (>60%), with most patients dying within 6 months of presentation. Recurrences have been reported. However, those who recover often have substantial improvement in lung function. The main treatment is supportive. It is not clear that glucocorticoid therapy is effective.

CRYPTOGENIC ORGANIZING PNEUMONIA

Clinical Manifestations COP is a clinicopathologic syndrome of unknown etiology. The onset is usually in the fifth and sixth decades. The presentation may be of a flulike illness with cough, fever, malaise, fatigue, and weight loss. Inspiratory crackles are frequently present on examination. Pulmonary function is usually impaired, with a restrictive defect and arterial hypoxemia being most common. The roentgenographic manifestations are distinctive, revealing bilateral, patchy, or diffuse alveolar opacities in the presence of normal lung volume. Recurrent and migratory pulmonary opacities are common. HRCT shows areas of air-space consolidation, ground-glass opacities, small nodular opacities, and bronchial wall thickening and dilation. These changes occur more frequently in the periphery of the lung and in the lower lung zone.

Histologic Findings Lung biopsy shows granulation tissue within small airways, alveolar ducts, and airspaces, with chronic inflammation in the surrounding alveoli. Foci of organizing pneumonia are a nonspecific reaction to lung injury found adjacent to other pathologic processes or as a component of other primary pulmonary disorders (e.g., cryptococcosis, granulomatosis with polyangiitis [Wegener], lymphoma, hypersensitivity pneumonitis, and eosinophilic pneumonia). Consequently, the clinician must carefully reevaluate any patient found to have this histopathologic lesion to rule out these possibilities.

Treatment Glucocorticoid therapy induces clinical recovery in two-thirds of patients. A few patients have rapidly progressive courses with fatal outcomes despite glucocorticoids.

ILD ASSOCIATED WITH CIGARETTE SMOKING

Desquamative Interstitial Pneumonia • *CLINICAL MANIFESTATIONS* DIP is a rare but distinct clinical and pathologic entity found almost exclusively in cigarette smokers. The histologic hallmark is the extensive accumulation of macrophages in intraalveolar spaces with minimal interstitial fibrosis. The peak incidence is in the fourth and fifth decades. Most patients present with dyspnea and cough. Lung function testing shows a restrictive pattern with reduced DL_{CO} and arterial hypoxemia. The chest x-ray and HRCT scans usually show diffuse hazy opacities.

HISTOLOGIC FINDINGS A diffuse and uniform accumulation of macrophages in the alveolar spaces is the hallmark of DIP. The macrophages contain golden, brown, or black pigment of tobacco smoke. There may be mild thickening of the alveolar walls by fibrosis and scanty inflammatory cell infiltration.

TREATMENT Clinical recognition of DIP is important because the process is associated with a better prognosis (10-year survival rate is ~70%) in response to smoking cessation. There are no clear data showing that systemic glucocorticoids are effective in DIP.

Respiratory Bronchiolitis–Associated ILD • *CLINICAL MANIFESTATIONS* Respiratory bronchiolitis–associated ILD (RB-ILD) is considered to be a subset of DIP and is characterized by the accumulation of macrophages in peribronchial alveoli. The clinical presentation is similar to that of DIP. Crackles are often heard on chest examination and occur throughout inspiration; sometimes they continue into expiration. The process is best seen on HRCT lung scanning, which shows bronchial wall thickening, centrilobular nodules, ground-glass opacity, and emphysema with air trapping. There is a spectrum of CT features in asymptomatic smokers (and elderly asymptomatic individuals) that may not necessarily represent clinically relevant disease.

HISTOLOGIC FINDINGS The histologic findings in RB-ILD include alveolar macrophage accumulation in respiratory bronchioles, with a variable chronic inflammatory cell infiltrate in bronchiolar and surrounding alveolar walls and occasional peribronchial alveolar septal fibrosis. The pulmonary parenchyma may show presence of smoking-related emphysema.

TREATMENT RB-ILD appears to resolve in most patients after smoking cessation alone.

Pulmonary Langerhans Cell Histiocytosis • *CLINICAL MANIFESTATIONS* This is a rare, smoking-related, diffuse lung disease that primarily affects men between the ages of 20 and 40 years. The clinical presentation varies from an asymptomatic state to a rapidly progressive condition. The most common clinical manifestations at presentation are cough, dyspnea, chest pain, weight loss, and fever. Pneumothorax occurs in ~25% of patients. Hemoptysis and diabetes insipidus are rare manifestations. The radiographic features vary with the stage of the disease. The combination of ill-defined or stellate nodules (2–10 mm in diameter), reticular or nodular opacities, bizarre-shaped upper zone cysts, preservation of lung volume, and sparing of the costophrenic angles are characteristics of PLCH. HRCT that reveals a combination of nodules and thin-walled cysts is virtually diagnostic of PLCH. The most common pulmonary function abnormality is a markedly reduced DL_{CO}, although varying degrees of restrictive disease, airflow limitation, and diminished exercise capacity may occur.

HISTOLOGIC FINDINGS The characteristic histopathologic finding in PLCH is the presence of nodular sclerosing lesions that contain Langerhans cells accompanied by mixed cellular infiltrates. The nodular lesions are poorly defined and are distributed in a bronchiolocentric fashion with intervening normal lung parenchyma. As the disease advances, fibrosis progresses to involve adjacent lung tissue, leading to pericicatricial air space enlargement, which accounts for the concomitant cystic changes.

TREATMENT Discontinuance of smoking is the key treatment, resulting in clinical improvement in one-third of patients. Most patients with PLCH experience persistent or progressive disease. Death due to respiratory failure occurs in ~10% of patients.

ILD ASSOCIATED WITH CONNECTIVE TISSUE DISORDERS

Clinical findings suggestive of a CTD (musculoskeletal pain, weakness, fatigue, fever, joint pain or swelling, photosensitivity, Raynaud's phenomenon, pleuritis, dry eyes, dry mouth) should be sought in any patient with ILD. The CTDs may be difficult to rule out since the pulmonary manifestations occasionally precede the more typical systemic manifestations by months or years. The most common form of pulmonary involvement is the nonspecific interstitial pneumonia histopathologic pattern. However, determining the precise nature of lung involvement in most of the CTDs is difficult due to the high incidence of lung involvement caused by disease-associated complications of esophageal dysfunction (predisposing to aspiration and secondary infections), respiratory muscle weakness (atelectasis and secondary infections), complications of therapy (opportunistic infections), and associated malignancies. For the majority of CTDs, with the exception of progressive system sclerosis, recommended initial treatment for ILD includes oral glucocorticoids often in association with an immunosuppressive agent (usually oral or intravenous cyclophosphamide or oral azathioprine) or mycophenolate mofetil.

Progressive Systemic Sclerosis (PSS) • *CLINICAL MANIFESTATIONS* (See also Chap. 382) Clinical evidence of ILD is present in about one-half of patients with PSS, and pathologic evidence in three-quarters. Pulmonary function tests show a restrictive pattern and impaired diffusing capacity, often before any clinical or radiographic evidence of lung disease appears. The HRCT features of lung disease in PSS range from predominant ground-glass attenuation to a predominant reticular pattern and are mostly similar to idiopathic NSIP.

HISTOLOGIC FINDINGS NSIP is the histopathologic pattern in most patients (~75%); the UIP pattern is rare (<10%).

TREATMENT Therapy is similar to that in idiopathic NSIP. UIP in PSS has a better outcome than IPF. The most widely used initial treatment regimen is low-dose glucocorticoid therapy and an immunosuppressive agent, usually oral or pulse cyclophosphamide. There are no convincing data showing this regime to be efficacious, and there is concern that the risk of renal crisis rises substantially with corticosteroids. Pulmonary vascular disease alone or in association with pulmonary fibrosis, pleuritis, or recurrent aspiration pneumonitis is strikingly resistant to current modes of therapy.

Rheumatoid Arthritis • *CLINICAL MANIFESTATIONS* (See also Chap. 380) ILD associated with RA is more common in men. Pulmonary manifestations of RA include pleurisy with or without effusion, ILD in up to 20% of cases, necrobiotic nodules (nonpneumoconiotic intrapulmonary rheumatoid nodules) with or without cavities, Caplan syndrome (rheumatoid pneumoconiosis), pulmonary hypertension secondary to rheumatoid pulmonary vasculitis, organized pneumonia, and upper airway obstruction due to cricoarytenoid arthritis.

HISTOLOGIC FINDINGS There are two primary histopathologic patterns of ILD that are observed in patients with ILD associated with RA: NSIP pattern and UIP pattern.

TREATMENT Little data exist to support the management of ILD in RA. Initial treatment of rheumatoid ILD, if required, is typically with oral glucocorticoids, which should be tried for 1–3 months. The potential benefit of anti-tumor necrosis factor α (TNF-α) therapy has been clouded by concerns about the development of a rapid and occasionally fatal lung disease in patients with RA-associated ILD treated with anti-TNF-α therapy.

Systemic Lupus Erythematosus • *CLINICAL MANIFESTATIONS* (See also Chap. 378) Lung disease is a common complication in SLE. Pleuritis with or without effusion is the most common pulmonary manifestation. Other lung manifestations include the following: atelectasis, diaphragmatic dysfunction with loss of lung volumes, pulmonary vascular disease, pulmonary hemorrhage, uremic pulmonary edema, infectious pneumonia, and organized pneumonia. Acute lupus pneumonitis characterized by pulmonary capillaritis leading to alveolar hemorrhage is uncommon. Chronic, progressive ILD is uncommon (<10%). It is important to exclude pulmonary infection. Although pleuropulmonary involvement may not be evident clinically, pulmonary function testing, particularly DL_{CO}, reveals abnormalities in many patients with SLE.

HISTOLOGIC FINDINGS The most common pathologic patterns seen include NSIP, UIP, LIP, and, on occasion, organizing pneumonia and amyloidosis.

TREATMENT There have been no controlled trials of treatment for ILD in SLE. Treatment involves the use of a glucocorticoid, either alone or, more often, in combination with an additional immunomodulating agent.

Polymyositis and Dermatomyositis (PM/DM) • *CLINICAL MANIFESTATIONS* (See also Chap. 388) ILD occurs in ~10% of patients with PM/DM. Diffuse reticular or nodular opacities with or without an alveolar component occur radiographically, with a predilection for the lung bases (NSIP pattern). ILD occurs more commonly in the subgroup of patients with an anti-Jo-1 antibody that is directed to histidyl tRNA synthetase. Weakness of respiratory muscles contributing to aspiration pneumonia may be present. A rapidly progressive illness characterized by diffuse alveolar damage may cause respiratory failure.

HISTOLOGIC FINDINGS NSIP predominates over UIP, organizing pneumonia, or other patterns of interstitial pneumonia.

TREATMENT The optimal treatment is unknown. The most widely used initial treatment is oral glucocorticoids. Fulminant disease may require high-dose intravenous methylprednisolone (1.0 g/d) for 3–5 days.

Sjögren Syndrome • *CLINICAL MANIFESTATIONS* (See also Chap. 383) General dryness and lack of airway secretion cause the major problems of hoarseness, cough, and bronchitis.

HISTOLOGIC FINDINGS Lung biopsy is frequently required to establish a precise pulmonary diagnosis. Fibrotic NSIP is most common. Lymphocytic interstitial pneumonitis, lymphoma, pseudolymphoma, bronchiolitis, and bronchiolitis obliterans are associated with this condition.

TREATMENT Glucocorticoids have been used in the management of ILD associated with Sjögren syndrome with some degree of clinical success.

DRUG-INDUCED ILD

Clinical Manifestations Many classes of drugs have the potential to induce diffuse ILD, which is manifest most commonly as exertional dyspnea and nonproductive cough. A detailed history of the medications taken by the patient is needed to identify drug-induced disease, including over-the-counter medications, oily nose drops, and petroleum products (mineral oil). In most cases, the pathogenesis is unknown, although a combination of direct toxic effects of the drug (or its metabolite) and indirect inflammatory and immunologic events are likely. The onset of the illness may be abrupt and fulminant, or it may be insidious, extending over weeks to months. The drug may have been taken for several years before a reaction develops (e.g., amiodarone), or the lung disease may occur weeks to years after the drug has been discontinued (e.g., carmustine). The extent and severity of disease are usually dose-related.

Histologic Findings The patterns of lung injury vary widely and depend on the agent.

Treatment Treatment consists of discontinuation of any possible offending drug and supportive care.

EOSINOPHILIC PNEUMONIA

(See Chap. 310)

PULMONARY ALVEOLAR PROTEINOSIS (PAP)

Clinical Manifestations Although not strictly an ILD, PAP resembles and is therefore considered with these conditions. It has been proposed that a defect in macrophage function, more specifically an impaired ability to process surfactant, may play a role in the pathogenesis of PAP. PAP is an autoimmune disease with a neutralizing antibody of immunoglobulin G isotype against granulocyte-macrophage colony-stimulating factor (GM-CSF). These findings suggest that neutralization of GM-CSF bioactivity by the antibody causes dysfunction of alveolar macrophages, which results in reduced surfactant clearance. There are three distinct classes of PAP: acquired (>90% of all cases), congenital, and secondary. *Congenital PAP* is transmitted in an autosomal recessive manner and is caused by homozygosity for a frameshift mutation (121ins2) in the *SP-B* gene, which leads to an unstable SP-B mRNA, reduced protein levels, and secondary disturbances of SP-C processing. *Secondary PAP* is rare among adults and is caused by lysinuric protein intolerance, acute silicosis and other inhalational syndromes, immunodeficiency disorders, and malignancies (almost exclusively of hematopoietic origin) and hematopoietic disorders.

The typical age of presentation is 30–50 years, and males predominate. The clinical presentation is usually insidious and is manifested by progressive exertional dyspnea, fatigue, weight loss, and low-grade fever. A nonproductive cough is common, but occasionally expectoration of "chunky" gelatinous material may occur. Polycythemia, hypergammaglobulinemia, and increased LDH levels are common. Markedly elevated serum levels of lung surfactant proteins A and D have been found in PAP. In the absence of any known secondary cause of PAP, an elevated serum anti-GM-CSF titer is highly sensitive and specific for the diagnosis of acquired PAP. BAL fluid levels of anti-GM-CSF antibodies correlate better with the severity of PAP than do serum titers. Radiographically, bilateral symmetric alveolar opacities located centrally in middle and lower lung zones result in a "bat-wing" distribution. HRCT shows a ground-glass opacification and thickened intralobular structures and interlobular septa.

Histologic Findings This diffuse disease is characterized by the accumulation of an amorphous, periodic acid–Schiff–positive lipoproteinaceous material in the distal air spaces. There is little or no lung inflammation, and the underlying lung architecture is preserved.

Treatment Whole-lung lavage(s) through a double-lumen endotracheal tube provides relief to many patients with dyspnea or progressive hypoxemia and also may provide long-term benefit.

PULMONARY LYMPHANGIOLEIOMYOMATOSIS

Clinical Manifestations Pulmonary LAM is a rare condition that afflicts premenopausal women and should be suspected in young women with "emphysema," recurrent pneumothorax, or chylous pleural effusion. It is often misdiagnosed as asthma or chronic obstructive pulmonary disease. Whites are affected much more commonly than are members of other racial groups. The disease accelerates during pregnancy and abates after oophorectomy. Common complaints at presentation are dyspnea, cough, and chest pain. Hemoptysis may be life threatening. Spontaneous pneumothorax occurs in 50% of patients; it may be bilateral and necessitate pleurodesis. Meningioma and renal angiomyolipomas (hamartomas), characteristic findings in the genetic disorder tuberous sclerosis, are also common in patients with LAM. Chylothorax, chyloperitoneum (chylous ascites), chyluria, and chylopericardium are other complications. Pulmonary function testing usually reveals an obstructive or mixed obstructive-restrictive pattern, and gas exchange is often abnormal. HRCT shows thin-walled cysts surrounded by normal lung without zonal predominance.

Histologic Findings Pathologically, LAM is characterized by the proliferation of atypical pulmonary interstitial smooth muscle and cyst formation. The immature-appearing smooth-muscle cells react with monoclonal antibody HMB45, which recognizes a 100-kDa glycoprotein (gp100) originally found in human melanoma cells.

Treatment Progression is common, with a median survival of 8–10 years from diagnosis. No therapy is of proven benefit in LAM. Sirolimus, an inhibitor of the mammalian target of rapamycin (mTOR), appears to be an active agent for LAM. After 12 months, it stabilized lung function (FVC, FEV_1, and functional residual capacity) and was associated with a reduction in symptoms and improvement in quality of life. Adverse effects (e.g., mucositis, diarrhea, nausea, hypercholesterolemia, acneiform rash, peripheral edema) were more common in the sirolimus group, but serious adverse effects were not increased. Subjects were followed off sirolimus for an additional 12 months, during which time pulmonary function declined at the same rate as in the placebo group. Progesterone and luteinizing hormone–releasing hormone analogues have been used. Oophorectomy is no longer recommended, and estrogen-containing drugs should be discontinued. Lung transplantation offers the only hope for cure despite reports of recurrent disease in the transplanted lung.

SYNDROMES OF ILD WITH DIFFUSE ALVEOLAR HEMORRHAGE

Clinical Manifestations The clinical onset is often abrupt, with cough, fever, and dyspnea. Severe respiratory distress requiring ventilatory support may be evident at initial presentation. Although hemoptysis is expected, it can be absent at the time of presentation in one-third of the cases. For patients without hemoptysis, new alveolar opacities, a falling hemoglobin level, and hemorrhagic BAL fluid point to the diagnosis. The chest radiograph is nonspecific and most commonly shows new patchy or diffuse alveolar opacities. Recurrent episodes of DAH may lead to pulmonary fibrosis, resulting in interstitial opacities on the chest radiograph. An elevated white blood cell count and falling hematocrit are common. Evidence for impaired renal function caused by focal segmental necrotizing glomerulonephritis, usually with crescent formation, also may be present. Varying degrees of hypoxemia may occur and are often severe enough to require ventilatory support. DL_{CO} may be increased, resulting from the increased hemoglobin within the alveoli compartment.

Histologic Findings Injury to arterioles, venules, and the alveolar septal (alveolar wall or interstitial) capillaries can result in hemoptysis secondary to disruption of the alveolar-capillary basement membrane. This results in bleeding into the alveolar spaces, which characterizes DAH. Pulmonary capillaritis, characterized by a neutrophilic infiltration of the alveolar septae, may lead to necrosis of these structures, loss of capillary structural integrity, and the pouring of red blood cells into the alveolar space. Fibrinoid necrosis of the interstitium and red blood cells within the interstitial space are sometimes seen. Bland pulmonary hemorrhage (i.e., DAH without inflammation of the alveolar structures) also may occur.

Evaluation of either lung or renal tissue by immunofluorescent techniques indicates an absence of immune complexes (pauci-immune) in granulomatosis with polyangiitis (Wegener), microscopic polyangiitis, pauci-immune glomerulonephritis, and isolated pulmonary capillaritis. A granular pattern is found in the CTDs, particularly SLE, and a characteristic linear deposition is found in Goodpasture syndrome. Granular deposition of IgA-containing immune complexes is present in Henoch-Schönlein purpura.

Treatment The mainstay of therapy for the DAH associated with systemic vasculitis, CTD, Goodpasture syndrome, and isolated pulmonary capillaritis is IV methylprednisolone, 0.5–2 g daily in divided doses for up to 5 days, followed by a gradual tapering, and then maintenance on an oral preparation. Prompt initiation of therapy is important, particularly in the face of renal insufficiency, because early initiation of therapy has the best chance of preserving renal function. The decision to start other immunosuppressive therapy (cyclophosphamide or azathioprine) acutely depends on the severity of illness.

Goodpasture Syndrome • ***CLINICAL MANIFESTATIONS*** Pulmonary hemorrhage and glomerulonephritis are features in most patients with this disease. Autoantibodies to renal glomerular and lung alveolar basement membranes are present. This syndrome can present and recur as DAH without an associated glomerulonephritis. In such cases, circulating anti-basement membrane antibody is often absent, and the only way to establish the diagnosis is by demonstrating linear immunofluorescence in lung tissue.

HISTOLOGIC FINDINGS The underlying histology may be bland hemorrhage or DAH associated with capillaritis.

TREATMENT Plasmapheresis has been recommended as adjunctive treatment.

INHERITED DISORDERS ASSOCIATED WITH ILD

Pulmonary opacities and respiratory symptoms typical of ILD can develop in related family members and in several inherited diseases. These diseases include the phakomatoses, tuberous sclerosis and neurofibromatosis (Chap. 118), and the lysosomal storage diseases, Niemann-Pick disease and Gaucher disease (Chap. 432e). The Hermansky-Pudlak syndrome is an autosomal recessive disorder in which granulomatous colitis and ILD may occur. It is characterized by oculocutaneous albinism, bleeding diathesis secondary to platelet dysfunction, and the accumulation of a chromolipid, lipofuscin material in cells of the reticuloendothelial system. A fibrotic pattern is found on lung biopsy, but the alveolar macrophages may contain cytoplasmic ceroid-like inclusions.

ILD WITH A GRANULOMATOUS RESPONSE IN LUNG TISSUE OR VASCULAR STRUCTURES

Inhalation of organic dusts, which cause hypersensitivity pneumonitis, or of inorganic dust, such as silica, which elicits a granulomatous inflammatory reaction leading to ILD, produces diseases of known etiology (Table 315-1) that are discussed in Chaps. 310 and 311. Sarcoidosis (Chap. 390) is prominent among granulomatous diseases of unknown cause in which ILD is an important feature.

Granulomatous Vasculitides (See also Chap. 385) The granulomatous vasculitides are characterized by pulmonary angiitis (i.e., inflammation and necrosis of blood vessels) with associated granuloma formation (i.e., infiltrates of lymphocytes, plasma cells, epithelioid cells, or histiocytes, with or without the presence of multinucleated giant cells, sometimes with tissue necrosis). The lungs are almost always involved, although any organ system may be affected. Granulomatosis with polyangiitis (Wegener) and Eosinophilic granulomatosis with polyangiitis (Churg-Strauss) primarily affect the lung but are associated with a systemic vasculitis as well. The granulomatous vasculitides generally limited to the lung include necrotizing sarcoid granulomatosis and benign lymphocytic angiitis and granulomatosis. Granulomatous infection and pulmonary angiitis due to irritating embolic material (e.g., talc) are important known causes of pulmonary vasculitis.

LYMPHOCYTIC INFILTRATIVE DISORDERS

This group of disorders features lymphocyte and plasma cell infiltration of the lung parenchyma. The disorders either are benign or can behave as low-grade lymphomas. Included is angioimmunoblastic lymphadenopathy with dysproteinemia, a rare lymphoproliferative disorder characterized by diffuse lymphadenopathy, fever, hepatosplenomegaly, and hemolytic anemia, with ILD in some cases.

Lymphocytic Interstitial Pneumonitis This rare form of ILD occurs in adults, some of whom have an autoimmune disease or dysproteinemia. It has been reported in patients with Sjögren syndrome and HIV infection.

Lymphomatoid Granulomatosis • *CLINICAL MANIFESTATIONS* Pulmonary lymphomatoid granulomatosis generally presents predominantly in men between the ages of 30 and 50, although patients can be affected at any age. The effects of race and geography on disease incidence are not known, although a higher diagnosis rate is reported in Western countries. Although it may affect virtually any organ, it is most frequently characterized by pulmonary (>90%), skin, and central nervous system involvement. The most common presenting symptoms and signs include cough, fever, rash/nodules, malaise, weight loss, neurologic abnormalities, dyspnea, and chest pain.

HISTOLOGIC FINDINGS This multisystem disorder of unknown etiology is an angiocentric malignant (T cell) lymphoma characterized by a polymorphic lymphoid infiltrate, an angiitis, and granulomatosis.

TREATMENT The clinical course of lymphomatoid granulomatosis ranges from remission without treatment to death from malignant lymphoma within 2 years. The choice of a treatment strategy should be based upon the presence of symptoms, history of using an inciting medication, extent of extrapulmonary involvement, and careful assessment of the histopathologic grade of the lesion. Referral to a hematology oncology specialist for consultation is recommended.

BRONCHOCENTRIC GRANULOMATOSIS

Clinical Manifestations Rather than a specific clinical entity, bronchocentric granulomatosis (BG) is a descriptive histologic term that is applied to an uncommon and nonspecific pathologic response to a variety of airway injuries. There is evidence that BG is caused by a hypersensitivity reaction to *Aspergillus* or other fungi in patients with asthma. About one-half of the patients described have had chronic asthma with severe wheezing and peripheral blood eosinophilia. In patients with asthma, BG probably represents one pathologic manifestation of allergic bronchopulmonary aspergillosis or another allergic mycosis. In patients without asthma, BG has been associated with RA and a variety of infections, including tuberculosis, echinococcosis, histoplasmosis, coccidioidomycosis, and nocardiosis. The chest roentgenogram reveals irregularly shaped nodular or mass lesions with ill-defined margins, which are usually unilateral and solitary, with upper lobe predominance.

Histologic Findings Bronchocentric granulomatosis is characterized by peribronchial and peribronchiolar necrotizing granulomatous inflammation. Destruction of airway walls and adjacent parenchyma leads to granulomatous replacement of mucosa and submucosa by palisading, epithelioid, and multinucleated histiocytes. Bronchocentric granulomatosis does not typically involve the pulmonary arteries.

Treatment Glucocorticoids are the treatment of choice, often with an excellent outcome, although recurrences may occur as therapy is tapered or stopped.

GLOBAL CONSIDERATIONS

Limited epidemiologic data exist describing the prevalence or incidence of ILD in the general population. With a few exceptions, e.g., sarcoidosis and certain occupational and environmental exposures, there appear to be no significant differences in the prevalence or incidence of ILD among various populations. For sarcoidosis, there are important environmental, racial, and genetic differences (Chap. 390).

316 Disorders of the Pleura

Richard W. Light

PLEURAL EFFUSION

The pleural space lies between the lung and the chest wall and normally contains a very thin layer of fluid, which serves as a coupling system. A pleural effusion is present when there is an excess quantity of fluid in the pleural space.

Etiology Pleural fluid accumulates when pleural fluid formation exceeds pleural fluid absorption. Normally, fluid enters the pleural space from the capillaries in the parietal pleura and is removed via the lymphatics in the parietal pleura. Fluid also can enter the pleural space from the interstitial spaces of the lung via the visceral pleura or from the peritoneal cavity via small holes in the diaphragm. The lymphatics have the capacity to absorb 20 times more fluid than is formed normally. Accordingly, a pleural effusion may develop when there is excess pleural fluid formation (from the interstitial spaces of the lung, the parietal pleura, or the peritoneal cavity) or when there is decreased fluid removal by the lymphatics.

Diagnostic Approach Patients suspected of having a pleural effusion should undergo chest imaging to diagnose its extent. Chest ultrasound has replaced the lateral decubitus x-ray in the evaluation of suspected pleural effusions and as a guide to thoracentesis. When a patient is found to have a pleural effusion, an effort should be made to determine the cause (Fig. 316-1). The first step is to determine whether the effusion is a transudate or an exudate. A *transudative pleural effusion* occurs when *systemic factors* that influence the formation and absorption of pleural fluid are altered. The leading causes of transudative pleural effusions in the United States are left ventricular failure and cirrhosis. An *exudative pleural effusion* occurs when *local factors* that influence the formation and absorption of pleural fluid are altered. The leading causes of exudative pleural effusions are bacterial pneumonia, malignancy, viral infection, and pulmonary embolism. The primary reason for making this differentiation is that additional diagnostic procedures are indicated with exudative effusions to define the cause of the local disease.

Transudative and exudative pleural effusions are distinguished by measuring the lactate dehydrogenase (LDH) and protein levels in the pleural fluid. Exudative pleural effusions meet at least one of the following criteria, whereas transudative pleural effusions meet none:

1. Pleural fluid protein/serum protein >0.5
2. Pleural fluid LDH/serum LDH >0.6
3. Pleural fluid LDH more than two-thirds the normal upper limit for serum

These criteria misidentify ~25% of transudates as exudates. If one or more of the exudative criteria are met and the patient is clinically thought to have a condition producing a transudative effusion, the difference between the protein levels in the serum and the pleural fluid should be measured. If this gradient is >31 g/L (3.1 g/dL), the exudative categorization by these criteria can be ignored because almost all such patients have a transudative pleural effusion.

If a patient has an exudative pleural effusion, the following tests on the pleural fluid should be obtained: description of the appearance of the fluid, glucose level, differential cell count, microbiologic studies, and cytology.

Effusion Due to Heart Failure The most common cause of pleural effusion is left ventricular failure. The effusion occurs because the increased amounts of fluid in the lung interstitial spaces exit in part across the visceral pleura; this overwhelms the capacity of the lymphatics in the parietal pleura to remove fluid. In patients with heart failure,

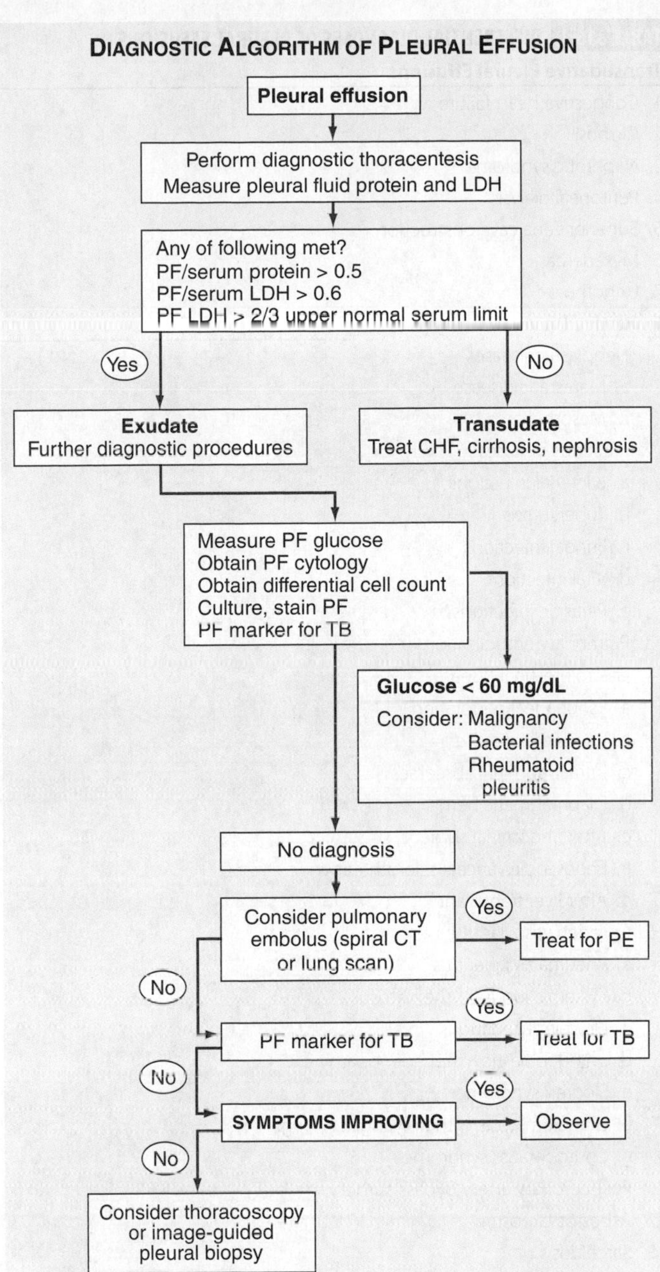

FIGURE 316-1 Approach to the diagnosis of pleural effusions. CHF, congestive heart failure; CT, computed tomography; LDH, lactate dehydrogenase; PE, pulmonary embolism; PF, pleural fluid; TB, tuberculosis.

a diagnostic thoracentesis should be performed if the effusions are not bilateral and comparable in size, if the patient is febrile, or if the patient has pleuritic chest pain to verify that the patient has a transudative effusion. Otherwise the patient's heart failure is treated. If the effusion persists despite therapy, a diagnostic thoracentesis should be performed. A pleural fluid N-terminal pro-brain natriuretic peptide (NT-proBNP) >1500 pg/mL is virtually diagnostic that the effusion is secondary to congestive heart failure.

Hepatic Hydrothorax Pleural effusions occur in ~5% of patients with cirrhosis and ascites. The predominant mechanism is the direct movement of peritoneal fluid through small openings in the diaphragm into the pleural space. The effusion is usually right-sided and frequently is large enough to produce severe dyspnea.

Parapneumonic Effusion Parapneumonic effusions are associated with bacterial pneumonia, lung abscess, or bronchiectasis and are probably the most common cause of exudative pleural effusion in the United States. *Empyema* refers to a grossly purulent effusion.

Patients with aerobic bacterial pneumonia and pleural effusion present with an acute febrile illness consisting of chest pain, sputum production, and leukocytosis. Patients with anaerobic infections present with a subacute illness with weight loss, a brisk leukocytosis, mild anemia, and a history of some factor that predisposes them to aspiration.

The possibility of a parapneumonic effusion should be considered whenever a patient with bacterial pneumonia is initially evaluated. The presence of free pleural fluid can be demonstrated with a lateral decubitus radiograph, computed tomography (CT) of the chest, or ultrasound. If the free fluid separates the lung from the chest wall by >10 mm, a therapeutic thoracentesis should be performed. Factors indicating the likely need for a procedure more invasive than a thoracentesis (in increasing order of importance) include the following:

1. Loculated pleural fluid
2. Pleural fluid pH <7.20
3. Pleural fluid glucose <3.3 mmol/L (<60 mg/dL)
4. Positive Gram stain or culture of the pleural fluid
5. Presence of gross pus in the pleural space

If the fluid recurs after the initial therapeutic thoracentesis and if any of these characteristics are present, a repeat thoracentesis should be performed. If the fluid cannot be completely removed with the therapeutic thoracentesis, consideration should be given to inserting a chest tube and instilling the combination of a fibrinolytic agent (e.g., tissue plasminogen activator, 10 mg) and deoxyribonuclease (5 mg) or performing a thoracoscopy with the breakdown of adhesions. Decortication should be considered when these measures are ineffective.

Effusion Secondary to Malignancy Malignant pleural effusions secondary to metastatic disease are the second most common type of exudative pleural effusion. The three tumors that cause ~75% of all malignant pleural effusions are lung carcinoma, breast carcinoma, and lymphoma. Most patients complain of dyspnea, which is frequently out of proportion to the size of the effusion. The pleural fluid is an exudate, and its glucose level may be reduced if the tumor burden in the pleural space is high.

The diagnosis usually is made via cytology of the pleural fluid. If the initial cytologic examination is negative, thoracoscopy is the best next procedure if malignancy is strongly suspected. At the time of thoracoscopy, a procedure such as pleural abrasion should be performed to effect a pleurodesis. An alternative to thoracoscopy is CT- or ultrasound-guided needle biopsy of pleural thickening or nodules. Patients with a malignant pleural effusion are treated symptomatically for the most part, since the presence of the effusion indicates disseminated disease and most malignancies associated with pleural effusion are not curable with chemotherapy. The only symptom that can be attributed to the effusion itself is dyspnea. If the patient's lifestyle is compromised by dyspnea and if the dyspnea is relieved with a therapeutic thoracentesis, one of the following procedures should be considered: (1) insertion of a small indwelling catheter or (2) tube thoracostomy with the instillation of a sclerosing agent such as doxycycline (500 mg).

Mesothelioma Malignant mesotheliomas are primary tumors that arise from the mesothelial cells that line the pleural cavities; most are related to asbestos exposure. Patients with mesothelioma present with chest pain and shortness of breath. The chest radiograph reveals a pleural effusion, generalized pleural thickening, and a shrunken hemithorax. The diagnosis is usually established with image-guided needle biopsy or thoracoscopy.

Effusion Secondary to Pulmonary Embolization The diagnosis most commonly overlooked in the differential diagnosis of a patient with an undiagnosed pleural effusion is pulmonary embolism. Dyspnea is the most common symptom. The pleural fluid is almost always an exudate. The diagnosis is established by spiral CT scan or pulmonary arteriography (Chap. 300). Treatment of a patient with a pleural effusion secondary to pulmonary embolism is the same as it is for any patient with pulmonary emboli. If the pleural effusion increases in size after anticoagulation, the patient probably has recurrent emboli or another complication, such as a hemothorax or a pleural infection.

Tuberculous Pleuritis (See also Chap. 202) In many parts of the world, the most common cause of an exudative pleural effusion is tuberculosis (TB), but tuberculous effusions are relatively uncommon in the United States. Tuberculous pleural effusions usually are associated with primary TB and are thought to be due primarily to a hypersensitivity reaction to tuberculous protein in the pleural space. Patients with tuberculous pleuritis present with fever, weight loss, dyspnea, and/or pleuritic chest pain. The pleural fluid is an exudate with predominantly small lymphocytes. The diagnosis is established by demonstrating high levels of TB markers in the pleural fluid (adenosine deaminase >40 IU/L or interferon γ >140 pg/mL). Alternatively, the diagnosis can be established by culture of the pleural fluid, needle biopsy of the pleura, or thoracoscopy. The recommended treatments of pleural and pulmonary TB are identical (Chap. 202).

Effusion Secondary to Viral Infection Viral infections are probably responsible for a sizable percentage of undiagnosed exudative pleural effusions. In many series, no diagnosis is established for ~20% of exudative effusions, and these effusions resolve spontaneously with no long-term residua. The importance of these effusions is that one should not be too aggressive in trying to establish a diagnosis for the undiagnosed effusion, particularly if the patient is improving clinically.

Chylothorax A chylothorax occurs when the thoracic duct is disrupted and chyle accumulates in the pleural space. The most common cause of chylothorax is trauma (most frequently thoracic surgery), but it also may result from tumors in the mediastinum. Patients with chylothorax present with dyspnea, and a large pleural effusion is present on the chest radiograph. Thoracentesis reveals milky fluid, and biochemical analysis reveals a triglyceride level that exceeds 1.2 mmol/L (110 mg/dL). Patients with chylothorax and no obvious trauma should have a lymphangiogram and a mediastinal CT scan to assess the mediastinum for lymph nodes. The treatment of choice for most chylothoraxes is insertion of a chest tube plus the administration of octreotide. If these modalities fail, a pleuroperitoneal shunt should be placed unless the patient has chylous ascites. Alternative treatments are ligation of the thoracic duct and percutaneous transabdominal thoracic duct blockage. Patients with chylothoraxes should not undergo prolonged tube thoracostomy with chest tube drainage because this will lead to malnutrition and immunologic incompetence.

Hemothorax When a diagnostic thoracentesis reveals bloody pleural fluid, a hematocrit should be obtained on the pleural fluid. If the hematocrit is more than one-half of that in the peripheral blood, the patient is considered to have a hemothorax. Most hemothoraxes are the result of trauma; other causes include rupture of a blood vessel or tumor. Most patients with hemothorax should be treated with tube thoracostomy, which allows continuous quantification of bleeding. If the bleeding emanates from a laceration of the pleura, apposition of the two pleural surfaces is likely to stop the bleeding. If the pleural hemorrhage exceeds 200 mL/h, consideration should be given to thoracoscopy or thoracotomy.

Miscellaneous Causes of Pleural Effusion There are many other causes of pleural effusion (Table 316-1). Key features of some of these conditions are as follows: If the pleural fluid amylase level is elevated, the diagnosis of esophageal rupture or pancreatic disease is likely. If the patient is febrile, has predominantly polymorphonuclear cells in the pleural fluid, and has no pulmonary parenchymal abnormalities, an intraabdominal abscess should be considered.

The diagnosis of an asbestos pleural effusion is one of exclusion. Benign ovarian tumors can produce ascites and a pleural effusion (Meigs' syndrome), as can the ovarian hyperstimulation syndrome. Several drugs can cause pleural effusion; the associated fluid is usually eosinophilic. Pleural effusions commonly occur after coronary artery bypass surgery. Effusions occurring within the first weeks are typically left-sided and bloody, with large numbers of eosinophils, and respond to one or two therapeutic thoracenteses. Effusions occurring after the first few weeks are typically left-sided and clear yellow, with predominantly small lymphocytes, and tend to recur. Other medical manipulations that induce pleural effusions include abdominal

TABLE 316-1 DIFFERENTIAL DIAGNOSES OF PLEURAL EFFUSIONS

Transudative Pleural Effusions

1. Congestive heart failure
2. Cirrhosis
3. Nephrotic syndrome
4. Peritoneal dialysis
5. Superior vena cava obstruction
6. Myxedema
7. Urinothorax

Exudative Pleural Effusions

1. Neoplastic diseases
   a. Metastatic disease
   b. Mesothelioma
2. Infectious diseases
   a. Bacterial infections
   b. Tuberculosis
   c. Fungal infections
   d. Viral infections
   e. Parasitic infections
3. Pulmonary embolization
4. Gastrointestinal disease
   a. Esophageal perforation
   b. Pancreatic disease
   c. Intraabdominal abscesses
   d. Diaphragmatic hernia
   e. After abdominal surgery
   f. Endoscopic variceal sclerotherapy
   g. After liver transplant
5. Collagen vascular diseases
   a. Rheumatoid pleuritis
   b. Systemic lupus erythematosus
   c. Drug-induced lupus
   d. Immunoblastic lymphadenopathy
   e. Sjögren syndrome
   f. Granulomatosis with polyangiitis (Wegener)
   g. Churg-Strauss syndrome
6. Post-coronary artery bypass surgery
7. Asbestos exposure
8. Sarcoidosis
9. Uremia
10. Meigs' syndrome
11. Yellow nail syndrome
12. Drug-induced pleural disease
    a. Nitrofurantoin
    b. Dantrolene
    c. Methysergide
    d. Bromocriptine
    e. Procarbazine
    f. Amiodarone
    g. Dasatinib
13. Trapped lung
14. Radiation therapy
15. Post-cardiac injury syndrome
16. Hemothorax
17. Iatrogenic injury
18. Ovarian hyperstimulation syndrome
19. Pericardial disease
20. Chylothorax

surgery; radiation therapy; liver, lung, or heart transplantation; and the intravascular insertion of central lines.

PNEUMOTHORAX

Pneumothorax is the presence of gas in the pleural space. A *spontaneous pneumothorax* is one that occurs without antecedent trauma to the thorax. A *primary spontaneous pneumothorax* occurs in the absence of underlying lung disease, whereas a *secondary pneumothorax* occurs in its presence. A *traumatic pneumothorax* results from penetrating or nonpenetrating chest injuries. A *tension pneumothorax* is a pneumothorax in which the pressure in the pleural space is positive throughout the respiratory cycle.

Primary Spontaneous Pneumothorax Primary spontaneous pneumothoraxes are usually due to rupture of apical pleural blebs, small cystic spaces that lie within or immediately under the visceral pleura. Primary spontaneous pneumothoraxes occur almost exclusively in smokers; this suggests that these patients have subclinical lung disease. Approximately one-half of patients with an initial primary spontaneous pneumothorax will have a recurrence. The initial recommended treatment for primary spontaneous pneumothorax is simple aspiration. If the lung does not expand with aspiration or if the patient has a recurrent pneumothorax, thoracoscopy with stapling of blebs and pleural abrasion is indicated. Thoracoscopy or thoracotomy with pleural abrasion is almost 100% successful in preventing recurrences.

Secondary Pneumothorax Most secondary pneumothoraxes are due to chronic obstructive pulmonary disease, but pneumothoraxes have been reported with virtually every lung disease. Pneumothorax in patients with lung disease is more life-threatening than it is in normal individuals because of the lack of pulmonary reserve in these patients. Nearly all patients with secondary pneumothorax should be treated with tube thoracostomy. Most should also be treated with thoracoscopy or thoracotomy with the stapling of blebs and pleural abrasion. If the patient is not a good operative candidate or refuses surgery, pleurodesis should be attempted by the intrapleural injection of a sclerosing agent such as doxycycline.

Traumatic Pneumothorax Traumatic pneumothoraxes can result from both penetrating and nonpenetrating chest trauma. Traumatic pneumothoraxes should be treated with tube thoracostomy unless they are very small. If a hemopneumothorax is present, one chest tube should be placed in the superior part of the hemithorax to evacuate the air and another should be placed in the inferior part of the hemithorax to remove the blood. Iatrogenic pneumothorax is a type of traumatic pneumothorax that is becoming more common. The leading causes are transthoracic needle aspiration, thoracentesis, and the insertion of central intravenous catheters. Most can be managed with supplemental oxygen or aspiration, but if these measures are unsuccessful, a tube thoracostomy should be performed.

Tension Pneumothorax This condition usually occurs during mechanical ventilation or resuscitative efforts. The positive pleural pressure is life-threatening both because ventilation is severely compromised and because the positive pressure is transmitted to the mediastinum, resulting in decreased venous return to the heart and reduced cardiac output.

Difficulty in ventilation during resuscitation or high peak inspiratory pressures during mechanical ventilation strongly suggest the diagnosis. The diagnosis is made by physical examination showing an enlarged hemithorax with no breath sounds, hyperresonance to percussion, and shift of the mediastinum to the contralateral side. Tension pneumothorax must be treated as a medical emergency. If the tension in the pleural space is not relieved, the patient is likely to die from inadequate cardiac output or marked hypoxemia. A large-bore needle should be inserted into the pleural space through the second anterior intercostal space. If large amounts of gas escape from the needle after insertion, the diagnosis is confirmed. The needle should be left in place until a thoracostomy tube can be inserted.

317 Disorders of the Mediastinum

Richard W. Light

The mediastinum is the region between the pleural sacs. It is separated into three compartments (Table 317-1). The *anterior mediastinum* extends from the sternum anteriorly to the pericardium and brachiocephalic vessels posteriorly. It contains the thymus gland, the anterior mediastinal lymph nodes, and the internal mammary arteries and veins. The *middle mediastinum* lies between the anterior and posterior mediastina and contains the heart; the ascending and transverse arches of the aorta; the venae cavae; the brachiocephalic arteries and veins; the phrenic nerves; the trachea, the main bronchi, and their contiguous lymph nodes; and the pulmonary arteries and veins. The *posterior mediastinum* is bounded by the pericardium and trachea anteriorly and the vertebral column posteriorly. It contains the descending thoracic aorta, the esophagus, the thoracic duct, the azygos and hemiazygos veins, and the posterior group of mediastinal lymph nodes.

MEDIASTINAL MASSES

The first step in evaluating a mediastinal mass is to place it in one of the three mediastinal compartments, since each has different characteristic lesions (Table 317-1). The most common lesions in the anterior mediastinum are thymomas, lymphomas, teratomatous neoplasms, and thyroid masses. The most common masses in the middle mediastinum are vascular masses, lymph node enlargement from metastases or granulomatous disease, and pleuropericardial and bronchogenic cysts. In the posterior mediastinum, neurogenic tumors, meningoceles, meningomyeloceles, gastroenteric cysts, and esophageal diverticula are commonly found.

Computed tomography (CT) scanning is the most valuable imaging technique for evaluating mediastinal masses and is the only imaging technique that should be done in most instances. Barium studies of the gastrointestinal tract are indicated in many patients with posterior mediastinal lesions, because hernias, diverticula, and achalasia are readily diagnosed in this manner. An iodine-131 scan can efficiently establish the diagnosis of intrathoracic goiter.

A definite diagnosis can be obtained with mediastinoscopy or anterior mediastinotomy in many patients with masses in the anterior or middle mediastinal compartments. A diagnosis can be established without thoracotomy via percutaneous fine-needle aspiration biopsy or endoscopic transesophageal or endobronchial ultrasound-guided biopsy of mediastinal masses in most cases. An alternative way to establish the diagnosis is video-assisted thoracoscopy. In many cases, the diagnosis can be established and the mediastinal mass removed with video-assisted thoracoscopy.

ACUTE MEDIASTINITIS

Most cases of acute mediastinitis either are due to esophageal perforation or occur after median sternotomy for cardiac surgery. Patients with esophageal rupture are acutely ill with chest pain and dyspnea due to the mediastinal infection. The esophageal rupture can occur spontaneously or as a complication of esophagoscopy or the insertion of a Blakemore tube. Appropriate treatment consists of exploration of the mediastinum with primary repair of the esophageal tear and drainage of the pleural space and the mediastinum.

The incidence of mediastinitis after median sternotomy is 0.4–5.0%. Patients most commonly present with wound drainage. Other presentations include sepsis and a widened mediastinum. The diagnosis usually is established with mediastinal needle aspiration. Treatment includes immediate drainage, debridement, and parenteral antibiotic therapy, but the mortality rate still exceeds 20%.

CHRONIC MEDIASTINITIS

The spectrum of chronic mediastinitis ranges from granulomatous inflammation of the lymph nodes in the mediastinum to fibrosing

TABLE 317-1 THE THREE COMPARTMENTS OF THE MEDIASTINUM

	Anterior Compartment	Middle Compartment	Posterior Compartment
Anatomical boundaries	Manubrium and sternum anteriorly, pericardium, aorta, and brachiocephalic vessels posteriorly	Anterior mediastinum anteriorly, posterior mediastinum posteriorly	Pericardium and trachea anteriorly; vertebral column posteriorly
Contents	Thymus gland, anterior mediastinal lymph nodes, internal mammary arteries and veins	Pericardium, heart, ascending and transverse arch of aorta, superior and inferior vena cavae, brachiocephalic arteries and veins, phrenic nerves, trachea, and main bronchi and their contiguous lymph nodes, pulmonary arteries, and veins	Descending thoracic aorta, esophagus, thoracic duct, azygos and hemiazygos veins, sympathetic chains, and the posterior group of mediastinal lymph nodes
Common abnormalities	Thymoma, lymphomas, teratomatous neoplasms, thyroid masses, parathyroid masses, mesenchymal tumors, giant lymph node hyperplasia, hernia through foramen of Morgagni	Metastatic lymph node enlargement, granulomatous lymph node enlargement, pleuropericardial cysts, bronchogenic cysts, masses of vascular origin	Neurogenic tumors, meningocele, meningomyelocele, gastroenteric cysts, esophageal diverticula, hernia through foramen of Bochdalek, extramedullary hematopoiesis

mediastinitis. Most cases are due to histoplasmosis or tuberculosis, but sarcoidosis, silicosis, and other fungal diseases are at times causative. Patients with granulomatous mediastinitis are usually asymptomatic. Those with fibrosing mediastinitis usually have signs of compression of a mediastinal structure such as the superior vena cava or large airways, phrenic or recurrent laryngeal nerve paralysis, or obstruction of the pulmonary artery or proximal pulmonary veins. Other than antituberculous therapy for tuberculous mediastinitis, no medical or surgical therapy has been demonstrated to be effective for mediastinal fibrosis.

PNEUMOMEDIASTINUM

In this condition, there is gas in the interstices of the mediastinum. The three main causes are (1) alveolar rupture with dissection of air into the mediastinum; (2) perforation or rupture of the esophagus, trachea, or main bronchi; and (3) dissection of air from the neck or the abdomen into the mediastinum. Typically, there is severe substernal chest pain with or without radiation into the neck and arms. The physical examination usually reveals subcutaneous emphysema in the suprasternal notch and *Hamman's sign*, which is a crunching or clicking noise synchronous with the heartbeat and is best heard in the left lateral decubitus position. The diagnosis is confirmed with the chest radiograph. Usually no treatment is required, but the mediastinal air will be absorbed faster if the patient inspires high concentrations of oxygen. If mediastinal structures are compressed, the compression can be relieved with needle aspiration.

318 Disorders of Ventilation

John F. McConville, Babak Mokhlesi, Julian Solway

DEFINITION AND PHYSIOLOGY

In health the arterial level of carbon dioxide (Pa_{CO_2}) is maintained between 37 and 43 mmHg at sea level. All disorders of ventilation result in abnormal measurements of Pa_{CO_2}. This chapter reviews chronic ventilatory disorders.

The continuous production of C_{O_2} by cellular metabolism necessitates its efficient elimination by the respiratory system. The relationship between C_{O_2} production and Pa_{CO_2} is described by the equation: $Pa_{CO_2} = (k)\ (\dot{V}_{CO_2})/\dot{V}A$, where $\dot{V}_{CO_2}$ represents the carbon dioxide production, k is a constant, and $\dot{V}A$ is fresh gas alveolar ventilation (Chap. 306e). $\dot{V}A$ can be calculated as minute ventilation × (1 – Vd/Vt), where the dead space fraction Vd/Vt represents the portion of a tidal breath that remains within the conducting airways at the conclusion of inspiration and so does not contribute to alveolar ventilation. As such, all disturbances of Pa_{CO_2} must reflect altered C_{O_2} production, minute ventilation, or dead space fraction.

Diseases that alter $\dot{V}_{CO_2}$ are often acute (e.g., sepsis, burns, or pyrexia), and their contribution to ventilatory abnormalities and/or respiratory failure is reviewed elsewhere. Chronic ventilatory disorders typically involve inappropriate levels of minute ventilation or increased dead space fraction. Characterization of these disorders requires a review of the normal respiratory cycle.

The spontaneous cycle of inspiration and expiration is automatically generated in the brainstem. Two groups of neurons located within the medulla are particularly important: the dorsal respiratory group (DRG) and the ventral respiratory column (VRC). These neurons have widespread projections including the descending projections into the contralateral spinal cord where they perform many functions. They initiate activity in the phrenic nerve/diaphragm, project to the upper airway muscle groups and spinal respiratory neurons, and innervate the intercostal and abdominal muscles that participate in normal respiration. The DRG acts as the initial integration site for many of the afferent nerves relaying information about Pa_{O_2}, Pa_{CO_2}, pH, and blood pressure from the carotid and aortic chemoreceptors and baroreceptors to the central nervous system (CNS). In addition, the vagus nerve relays information from stretch receptors and juxtapulmonary-capillary receptors in the lung parenchyma and chest wall to the DRG. The respiratory rhythm is generated within the VRC as well as the more rostrally located parafacial respiratory group (pFRG), which is particularly important for the generation of active expiration. One particularly important area within the VRC is the so-called pre-Bötzinger complex. This area is responsible for the generation of various forms of inspiratory activity, and lesioning of the pre-Bötzinger complex leads to the complete cessation of breathing. The neural output of these medullary respiratory networks can be voluntarily suppressed or augmented by input from higher brain centers and the autonomic nervous system. During normal sleep, there is an attenuated response to hypercapnia and hypoxemia, resulting in mild nocturnal hypoventilation that corrects upon awakening.

Once neural input has been delivered to the respiratory pump muscles, normal gas exchange requires an adequate amount of respiratory muscle strength to overcome the elastic and resistive loads of the respiratory system (Fig. 318-1*A*) (Chap. 306e). In health, the strength of the respiratory muscles readily accomplishes this, and normal respiration continues indefinitely. Reduction in respiratory drive or neuromuscular competence or substantial increase in respiratory load can diminish minute ventilation, resulting in hypercapnia (Fig. 318-1*B*). Alternatively, if normal respiratory muscle strength is coupled with excessive respiratory drive, then alveolar hyperventilation ensues and leads to hypocapnia (Fig. 318-1*C*).

HYPOVENTILATION

CLINICAL FEATURES

Diseases that reduce minute ventilation or increase dead space fall into four major categories: parenchymal lung and chest wall disease, sleep-disordered breathing, neuromuscular disease, and respiratory drive disorders (Fig. 318-1*B*). The clinical manifestations of hypoventilation

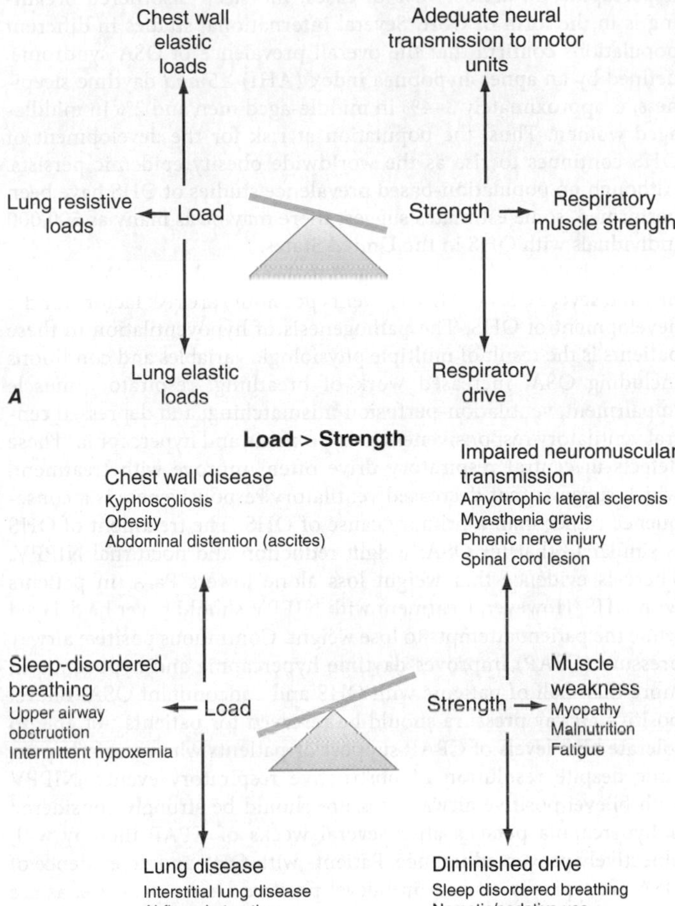

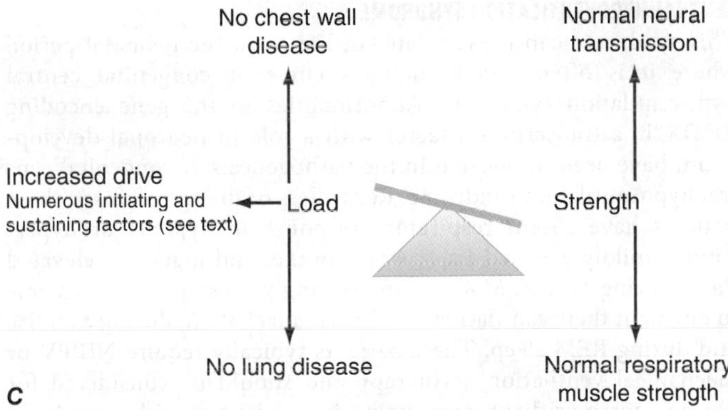

FIGURE 318-1 Examples of balance between respiratory system strength and load. ***A.*** Excess respiratory muscle strength in health. ***B.*** Load greater than strength. ***C.*** Increased drive with acceptable strength.

syndromes are nonspecific (Table 318-1) and vary depending on the severity of hypoventilation, the rate at which hypercapnia develops, the degree of compensation for respiratory acidosis, and the underlying disorder. Patients with parenchymal lung or chest wall disease typically present with shortness of breath and diminished exercise tolerance. Episodes of increased dyspnea and sputum production are hallmarks of obstructive lung diseases such as chronic obstructive pulmonary disease, whereas progressive dyspnea and cough are common in interstitial lung diseases. Excessive daytime somnolence, poor-quality sleep, and snoring are common among patients with sleep-disordered breathing. Sleep disturbance and orthopnea are also described in

TABLE 318-1 SIGNS AND SYMPTOMS OF HYPOVENTILATION

Dyspnea during activities of daily living
Orthopnea in diseases affecting diaphragm function
Poor-quality sleep
Daytime hypersomnolence
Early morning headaches
Anxiety
Impaired cough in neuromuscular diseases

neuromuscular disorders. As neuromuscular weakness progresses, the respiratory muscles, including the diaphragm, are placed at a mechanical disadvantage in the supine position due to the upward movement of the abdominal contents. New-onset orthopnea is frequently a sign of reduced respiratory muscle force generation. More commonly, however, extremity weakness or bulbar symptoms develop prior to sleep disturbance in neuromuscular diseases such as amyotrophic lateral sclerosis (ALS) or muscular dystrophy. Patients with respiratory drive disorders do not have symptoms distinguishable from other causes of chronic hypoventilation.

The clinical course of patients with chronic hypoventilation from neuromuscular or chest wall disease follows a characteristic sequence: an asymptomatic stage where daytime Pa_{O_2} and Pa_{CO_2} are normal followed by nocturnal hypoventilation, initially during rapid eye movement (REM) sleep and later in non-REM sleep. Finally, if vital capacity drops further, daytime hypercapnia develops. Symptoms can develop at any point along this time course and often depend on the pace of respiratory muscle functional decline. Regardless of cause, the hallmark of all alveolar hypoventilation syndromes is an increase in alveolar P_{CO_2} (PA_{CO_2}) and therefore in Pa_{CO_2}. The resulting respiratory acidosis eventually leads to a compensatory increase in plasma bicarbonate concentration. The increase in PA_{CO_2} results in an obligatory decrease in PA_{O_2}, often resulting in hypoxemia. If severe, the hypoxemia manifests clinically as cyanosis and can stimulate erythropoiesis and thus induce secondary erythrocytosis. The combination of chronic hypoxemia and hypercapnia may also induce pulmonary vasoconstriction, leading eventually to pulmonary hypertension, right ventricular hypertrophy, and right heart failure.

DIAGNOSIS

Elevated plasma bicarbonate in the absence of volume depletion is suggestive of hypoventilation. An arterial blood gas demonstrating elevated Pa_{CO_2} with a normal pH confirms chronic alveolar hypoventilation. The subsequent evaluation to identify an etiology should initially focus on whether the patient has lung disease or chest wall abnormalities. Physical examination, imaging studies (chest x-ray and/or computed tomography [CT] scan), and pulmonary function tests are sufficient to identify most lung/chest wall disorders leading to hypercapnia. If these evaluations are unrevealing, then the clinician should screen for obesity hypoventilation syndrome (OHS), the most frequent sleep disorder leading to chronic hypoventilation, which is typically accompanied by obstructive sleep apnea (OSA). Several screening tools have been developed to identify patients at risk for OSA. The Berlin Questionnaire has been validated in a primary care setting and identifies patients likely to have OSA. The Epworth Sleepiness Scale (ESS) and the STOP-Bang questionnaires have not been validated in outpatient primary care settings but are quick and easy to use. The ESS measures daytime sleepiness, with a score of ≥10 identifying individuals who warrant additional investigation. The STOP-Bang survey has been used in preoperative clinics to identify patients at risk of having OSA. In this population, it has 93% sensitivity and 90% negative predictive value.

If the ventilatory apparatus (lungs, airways, chest wall) is not responsible for chronic hypercapnia, then the focus should shift to respiratory drive and neuromuscular disorders. There is an attenuated increase in minute ventilation in response to elevated C_{O_2} and/or low O_2 in respiratory drive disorders. These diseases are difficult to diagnose and should be suspected when patients with hypercapnia are found to have normal respiratory muscle strength, normal pulmonary function, and normal alveolar-arterial P_{O_2} difference. Hypoventilation is more marked during sleep in patients with respiratory drive defects, and polysomnography often reveals central apneas, hypopneas, or hypoventilation. Brain imaging (CT scan or magnetic resonance imaging [MRI]) can sometimes identify structural abnormalities in the pons or medulla that result in hypoventilation. Chronic narcotic use or significant hypothyroidism can depress the central respiratory drive and lead to chronic hypercapnia as well.

Respiratory muscle weakness has to be profound before lung volumes are compromised and hypercapnia develops. Typically physical examination reveals decreased strength in major muscle groups prior to the development of hypercapnia. Measurement of maximum inspiratory and expiratory pressures or forced vital capacity (FVC) can be used to monitor for respiratory muscle involvement in diseases with progressive muscle weakness. These patients also have increased risk for sleep-disordered breathing, including hypopneas, central and obstructive apneas, and hypoxemia. Nighttime oximetry and capnometry during polysomnography are helpful in better characterizing sleep disturbances in this patient population.

TREATMENT HYPOVENTILATION

Nocturnal noninvasive positive-pressure ventilation (NIPPV) has been used successfully in the treatment of hypoventilation and apneas, both central and obstructive, in patients with neuromuscular and chest wall disorders. Nocturnal NIPPV has been shown to improve daytime hypercapnia, prolong survival, and improve health-related quality of life when daytime hypercapnia is documented. ALS guidelines recommend consideration of nocturnal NIPPV if symptoms of hypoventilation exist *and* one of the following criteria is present: Pa_{CO_2} ≥45 mmHg; nocturnal oximetry demonstrates oxygen saturation ≤88% for 5 consecutive min; maximal inspiratory pressure <60 cmH_2O; FVC <50% predicted; or sniff nasal pressure <40 cmH_2O. However, at present, there is inconclusive evidence to support preemptive nocturnal NIPPV use in all patients with neuromuscular and chest wall disorders who demonstrate nocturnal but not daytime hypercapnia. Nevertheless, at some point, the institution of full-time ventilatory support with either pressure or volume-preset modes is required in progressive neuromuscular disorders. There is less evidence to direct the timing of this decision, but ventilatory failure requiring mechanical ventilation and chest infections related to ineffective cough are frequent triggers for the institution of full-time ventilatory support.

Treatment of chronic hypoventilation from lung or neuromuscular diseases should be directed at the underlying disorder. Pharmacologic agents that stimulate respiration, such as medroxyprogesterone and acetazolamide, have been poorly studied in chronic hypoventilation and should not replace treatment of the underlying disease process. Regardless of the cause, excessive metabolic alkalosis should be corrected, because plasma bicarbonate levels elevated out of proportion for the degree of chronic respiratory acidosis can result in additional hypoventilation. When indicated, administration of supplemental oxygen is effective in attenuating hypoxemia, polycythemia, and pulmonary hypertension. However, in some patients, supplemental oxygen can worsen hypercapnia.

Phrenic nerve or diaphragm pacing is a potential therapy for patients with hypoventilation from high cervical spinal cord lesions or respiratory drive disorders. Prior to surgical implantation, patients should have nerve conduction studies to ensure normal bilateral phrenic nerve function. Small case series suggest that effective diaphragmatic pacing can improve quality of life in these patients.

HYPOVENTILATION SYNDROMES

OBESITY HYPOVENTILATION SYNDROME

The diagnosis of OHS requires body mass index (BMI) ≥30 kg/m² and chronic daytime alveolar hypoventilation, defined as Pa_{CO_2} ≥45 mmHg at sea level in the absence of other known causes of hypercapnia. In almost 90% of cases, the sleep-disordered breathing is in the form of OSA. Several international studies in different populations confirm that the overall prevalence of OSA syndrome, defined by an apnea-hypopnea index (AHI) ≥5 *and* daytime sleepiness, is approximately 3–4% in middle-aged men and 2% in middle-aged women. Thus, the population at risk for the development of OHS continues to rise as the worldwide obesity epidemic persists. Although no population-based prevalence studies of OHS have been performed, some estimates suggest there may be as many as 500,000 individuals with OHS in the United States.

Some, but not all, studies suggest that severe obesity (BMI >40 kg/m²) and severe OSA (AHI >30 events per hour) are risk factors for the development of OHS. The pathogenesis of hypoventilation in these patients is the result of multiple physiologic variables and conditions including OSA, increased work of breathing, respiratory muscle impairment, ventilation-perfusion mismatching, and depressed central ventilatory responsiveness to hypoxemia and hypercapnia. These defects in central respiratory drive often improve with treatment, which suggests that decreased ventilatory responsiveness is a consequence rather than a primary cause of OHS. The treatment of OHS is similar to that for OSA: weight reduction and nocturnal NIPPV. There is evidence that weight loss alone lowers Pa_{CO_2} in patients with OHS. However, treatment with NIPPV should never be delayed while the patient attempts to lose weight. Continuous positive airway pressure (CPAP) improves daytime hypercapnia and hypoxemia in more than half of patients with OHS and concomitant OSA. Bilevel positive airway pressure should be reserved for patients not able to tolerate high levels of CPAP support or patients who remain hypoxemic despite resolution of obstructive respiratory events. NIPPV with bilevel positive airway pressure should be strongly considered if hypercapnia persists after several weeks of CPAP therapy with objectively proven adherence. Patients with OHS and no evidence of OSA are typically started on bilevel positive airway pressure, as are patients presenting with acute decompensated OHS. Finally, comorbid conditions that impair ventilation, such as chronic obstructive pulmonary disease, should be aggressively treated in conjunction with coexisting OHS.

CENTRAL HYPOVENTILATION SYNDROME

This syndrome can present later in life or in the neonatal period where it is often called Ondine's curse or congenital central hypoventilation syndrome. Abnormalities in the gene encoding PHOX2b, a transcription factor with a role in neuronal development, have been implicated in the pathogenesis of congenital central hypoventilation syndrome. Regardless of the age of onset, these patients have absent respiratory response to hypoxia or hypercapnia, mildly elevated Pa_{CO_2} while awake, and markedly elevated Pa_{CO_2} during non-REM sleep. Interestingly these patients are able to augment their ventilation and "normalize" Pa_{CO_2} during exercise and during REM sleep. These patients typically require NIPPV or mechanical ventilation as therapy and should be considered for phrenic nerve or diaphragmatic pacing at centers with experience performing these procedures.

HYPERVENTILATION

CLINICAL FEATURES

Hyperventilation is defined as ventilation in excess of metabolic requirements (CO_2 production) leading to a reduction in Pa_{CO_2}. The physiology of patients with chronic hyperventilation is poorly understood, and there is no typical clinical presentation. Symptoms can include dyspnea, paresthesias, tetany, headache, dizziness, visual disturbances, and atypical chest pain. Because symptoms can be so diverse, patients with chronic hyperventilation present to a variety of health care providers, including internists, neurologists, psychologists, psychiatrists, and pulmonologists.

It is helpful to think of hyperventilation as having initiating and sustaining factors. Some investigators believe that an initial event leads to increased alveolar ventilation and a drop in Pa_{CO_2}

to ~20 mmHg. The ensuing onset of chest pain, breathlessness, paresthesia, or altered consciousness can be alarming. The resultant increase in minute volume to relieve these acute symptoms only serves to exacerbate symptoms that are often misattributed by the patient and health care workers to cardiopulmonary disorders. An unrevealing evaluation for causes of these symptoms often results in patients being anxious and fearful of additional attacks. It is important to note that **anxiety disorders and panic attacks are *not* synonymous with hyperventilation**. Anxiety disorders can be both an initiating and sustaining factor in the pathogenesis of chronic hyperventilation, but these are not necessary for the development of chronic hypocapnia.

DIAGNOSIS

Respiratory symptoms associated with acute hyperventilation can be the initial manifestation of systemic illnesses such as diabetic ketoacidosis. Causes of acute hyperventilation need to be excluded before a diagnosis of chronic hyperventilation is considered. Arterial blood gas sampling that demonstrates a compensated respiratory alkalosis with a near normal pH, low Pa_{CO_2}, and low calculated bicarbonate is necessary to confirm chronic hyperventilation. Other causes of respiratory alkalosis, such as mild asthma, need to be diagnosed and treated before chronic hyperventilation can be considered. A high index of suspicion is required because increased minute ventilation can be difficult to detect on physical examination. Once chronic hyperventilation is established, a sustained 10% increase in alveolar ventilation is enough to perpetuate hypocapnia. This increase can be accomplished with subtle changes in the respiratory pattern, such as occasional sigh breaths or yawning two to three times per minute.

TREATMENT HYPERVENTILATION

There are few well-controlled treatment studies of chronic hyperventilation due to its diverse features and the lack of a universally accepted diagnostic process. Clinicians often spend considerable time identifying initiating factors, excluding alternative diagnoses, and discussing the patient's concerns and fears. In some patients, reassurance and frank discussion about hyperventilation can be liberating. Identifying and eliminating habits that perpetuate hypocapnia, such as frequent yawning or sigh breathing, can be helpful. Some evidence suggests that breathing exercises and diaphragmatic retraining may be beneficial for some patients. The evidence for using medications to treat hyperventilation is scant. Beta blockers may be helpful in patients with sympathetically mediated symptoms such as palpitations and tremors.

ACKNOWLEDGMENT

We would like to acknowledge Eliot A. Phillipson for earlier versions of this chapter and Jan-Marino Ramirez for his careful critique and helpful suggestions.

319 Sleep Apnea

Andrew Wellman, Susan Redline

Obstructive sleep apnea/hypopnea syndrome (OSAHS) and central sleep apnea (CSA) are both classified as sleep-related breathing disorders. OSAHS and CSA share some risk factors and physiological bases but also have unique features. Each disorder is associated with impaired ventilation during sleep and disruption of sleep, and each diagnosis requires careful elicitation of the patient's history, physical examination, and physiological testing. OSAHS, the more common disorder, causes daytime sleepiness, impairs daily function, and is a major contributor to cardiovascular disease in adults and to behavioral problems in children. CSA is less common and may occur in combination with obstructive sleep apnea, as a primary condition, or secondary to a medical condition or medication. CSA impairs overnight gas exchange and may result in symptoms of either insomnia or excessive sleepiness.

OBSTRUCTIVE SLEEP APNEA/HYPOPNEA SYNDROME (OSAHS)

Definition OSAHS is defined on the basis of nocturnal and daytime symptoms as well as sleep study findings. Diagnosis requires the patient to have (1) either symptoms of nocturnal breathing disturbances (snoring, snorting, gasping, or breathing pauses during sleep) or daytime sleepiness or fatigue that occurs despite sufficient opportunities to sleep and is unexplained by other medical problems; and (2) five or more episodes of obstructive apnea or hypopnea per hour of sleep (the apnea-hypopnea index [AHI], calculated as the number of episodes divided by the number of hours of sleep) documented during a sleep study. OSAHS also may be diagnosed in the absence of symptoms if the AHI is above 15. Each episode of apnea or hypopnea represents a reduction in breathing for at least 10 sec. OSAHS is often identified when associated with a ≥3% drop in oxygen saturation and/or a brain cortical arousal. OSAHS severity is based on the frequency of breathing disturbances (AHI), the amount of oxygen desaturation with respiratory events, the duration of apneas and hypopneas, the degree of sleep fragmentation, and the level of daytime sleepiness.

Pathophysiology During inspiration, intraluminal pharyngeal pressure becomes increasingly negative, creating a "suctioning" force. Because the pharyngeal airway has no bone or cartilage, airway patency is dependent on the stabilizing influence of the pharyngeal dilator muscles. Although these muscles are continuously activated during wakefulness, neuromuscular output declines with sleep onset. In patients with a collapsible airway, the reduction in neuromuscular output results in transient episodes of pharyngeal collapse (manifesting as an "apnea") or near collapse (manifesting as a "hypopnea"). The episodes of collapse are terminated when ventilatory reflexes are activated and cause arousal, thus stimulating an increase in neuromuscular activity and opening of the airway. The airway may collapse at various levels: the soft palate (most common), tongue base, lateral pharyngeal walls, and/or epiglottis (Fig. 319-1). OSAHS may be most

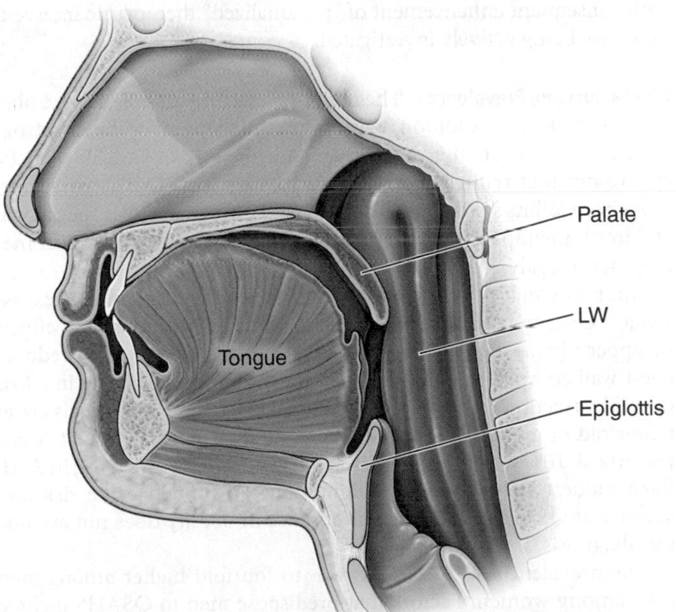

FIGURE 319-1 Common sites of airway collapse. For example, the palate, tongue, and/or epiglottis (Ep) can be posteriorly displaced, and the lateral pharyngeal walls (LW) can collapse.

severe during REM (rapid eye movement) sleep, when neuromuscular output to the skeletal muscles is particularly low, and in the supine position due to gravitational forces.

Individuals with a small pharyngeal lumen require relatively high levels of neuromuscular innervation to maintain patency during wakefulness and thus are predisposed to excessive airway collapsibility during sleep. The airway lumen may be narrowed with enlargement of soft tissue structures (tongue, palate, and uvula) due to fat deposition, increased lymphoid tissue, or genetic variation. Craniofacial factors such as mandibular retroposition or micrognathia, reflecting genetic variation or developmental influences, also can reduce lumen dimensions. In addition, lung volumes influence the caudal traction on the pharynx and consequently the stiffness of the pharyngeal wall. Accordingly, low lung volume in the recumbent position, which is particularly pronounced in the obese, contributes to collapse. A high degree of nasal resistance (e.g., due to nasal septal deviation or polyps) can contribute to airway collapse by increasing the negative intraluminal suction pressure. High-level nasal resistance also may trigger mouth opening during sleep, which breaks the seal between the tongue and the teeth and allows the tongue to fall posteriorly and occlude the airway.

Pharyngeal muscle activation is integrally linked to ventilatory drive. Thus, factors related to ventilatory control, particularly ventilatory sensitivity, arousal threshold, and neuromuscular responses to CO_2, contribute to the pathogenesis of OSAHS. A buildup in CO_2 during sleep activates both the diaphragm and the pharyngeal muscles, which stiffen the upper airway and can counteract inspiratory suction pressures and maintain airway patency to an extent that depends on the anatomic predisposition to collapse. However, pharyngeal collapse can occur when the ventilatory control system is overly sensitive to CO_2, with resultant wide fluctuations in ventilation and ventilatory drive and in upper airway instability. Moreover, increasing levels of CO_2 during sleep result in central nervous system arousal, causing the individual to move from a deeper to a lighter level of sleep or to awaken. A low arousal threshold (i.e., awaken to a low level of CO_2 or ventilatory drive) can preempt the CO_2-mediated process of pharyngeal muscle compensation and prevent airway stabilization. A high arousal threshold, conversely, may prevent appropriate termination of apneas, prolonging apnea duration and oxyhemoglobin desaturation severity. Finally, any impairment in the ability of the muscles to compensate during sleep can contribute to collapse of the pharynx. The relative contributions of risk factors vary among individuals. Approaches to the measurement of these factors in clinical settings, with consequent enhancement of "personalized" therapeutic interventions, are being actively investigated.

Risk Factors and Prevalence The major risk factors for OSAHS are obesity and male sex. Additional risk factors include mandibular retrognathia and micrognathia, a positive family history of OSAHS, genetic syndromes that reduce upper airway patency (e.g., Down syndrome, Treacher-Collins syndrome), adenotonsillar hypertrophy (especially in children), menopause (in women), and various endocrine syndromes (e.g., acromegaly, hypothyroidism).

Approximately 40–60% of cases of OSAHS are attributable to excess weight. Obesity predisposes to OSAHS through the narrowing effects of upper airway fat on the pharyngeal lumen. Obesity also reduces chest wall compliance and decreases lung volumes, resulting in a loss of caudal traction on upper airway structures. Obese individuals are at a fourfold or greater risk for OSAHS than their normal-weight counterparts. A 10% weight gain is associated with a >30% increase in AHI. Even modest weight loss or weight gain can influence the risk and severity of OSAHS. However, the absence of obesity does not exclude this diagnosis.

The prevalence of OSAHS is two- to fourfold higher among men than among women. Factors that predispose men to OSAHS include android patterns of obesity (resulting in upper-airway fat deposition) and relatively great pharyngeal length, which exacerbates collapsibility. Premenopausal women are relatively protected from OSAHS by the influence of sex hormones on ventilatory drive. The decline in sex differences in older age is associated with an increased OSAHS prevalence in women after menopause.

Variations in craniofacial morphology that reduce the size of the posterior airway space increase OSAHS risk. The contribution of hard-tissue structural features to OSAHS is most evident in nonobese patients. Identification of features such as retrognathia can influence therapeutic decision-making.

OSAHS has a strong genetic basis, as evidenced by its significant familial aggregation and heritability. For a first-degree relative of a patient with OSAHS, the odds ratio of having OSAHS is approximately twofold higher than that for someone without an affected relative.

OSAHS prevalence varies with age, from 2–15% among middle-aged adults to >20% among elderly individuals. There is a peak due to lymphoid hypertrophy among children between the ages of 3 and 8 years; with airway growth and lymphoid tissue regression during later childhood, prevalence declines. Then, as obesity prevalence increases in middle life and women enter menopause, OSAHS again increases.

The prevalence of OSAHS may be especially high among patients with diabetes or hypertension. Individuals of Asian ancestry appear to be at increased risk of OSAHS at relatively low levels of body mass index, possibly because of the influence of craniofacial risk factors that narrow the nasopharynx. In the United States, African Americans, especially children and young adults, are at higher risk for OSAHS than their Caucasian counterparts. In a majority of adults with OSAHS, the disorder is undiagnosed.

Course of the Disorder The precise onset of OSAHS is usually hard to identify. A person may snore for many years, often beginning in childhood, before OSAHS is identified. Weight gain may precipitate an increase in symptoms, which in turn may lead the patient to pursue an evaluation. OSAHS may become less severe with weight loss, particularly after bariatric surgery. Marked increases and decreases in the AHI are uncommon unless accompanied by weight change.

APPROACH TO THE PATIENT: **Obstructive Sleep Apnea/Hypopnea Syndrome (OSAHS)**

An evaluation for OSAHS should be considered in patients with symptoms of OSAHS and one or more risk factors. Screening also should be considered in patients who report symptoms consistent with OSAHS and who are at high risk for OSAHS-related morbidities, such as hypertension, diabetes mellitus, and cardiac and cerebrovascular diseases.

SYMPTOMS AND HISTORY

When possible, a sleep history should be obtained in the presence of a bed partner. Snoring is the most common complaint; however, its absence does not exclude the diagnosis, as pharyngeal collapse may occur without tissue vibration. Gasping or snorting during sleep may also be reported, reflecting termination of individual apneas with abrupt airway opening. Dyspnea is unusual, and its absence generally distinguishes OSAHS from paroxysmal nocturnal dyspnea, nocturnal asthma, and acid reflux with laryngospasm. Patients also may describe frequent awakening or sleep disruption, which is more common among women and older adults. The most common daytime symptom is sleepiness. This symptom can be difficult to elicit and may be hard to distinguish from exercise-related fatigue, deconditioning, and malaise. In contrast to true sleepiness, the latter symptoms generally improve with rest. Other symptoms include a dry mouth, nocturnal heartburn, diaphoresis of the chest and neck, nocturia, morning headaches, trouble concentrating, irritability, and mood disturbances. Several questionnaires that evaluate snoring frequency, self-reported apneas, and daytime sleepiness can facilitate OSAHS screening. The predictive ability of a questionnaire can be enhanced by a consideration of whether the patient is male or has risk factors such as obesity or hypertension.

PHYSICAL FINDINGS

Physical findings often reflect the etiologic factors for the disorder as well as comorbid conditions, particularly vascular disease. On examination, patients may exhibit hypertension and regional (central) obesity, as indicated by a large waist and neck circumference. The oropharynx may reveal a small orifice with crowding due to an enlarged tongue, a low-lying soft palate with a bulky uvula, large tonsils, a high arched palate, and/or micro/retrognathia. Since high-level nasal resistance can increase pharyngeal collapsibility, the nasal cavity should be inspected for polyps, septal deviation, and other signs of obstruction. Because patients with heart failure are at increased risk for both OSAHS and CSA, a careful cardiac examination should be conducted to detect possible left- or right-sided cardiac dysfunction. Evidence of cor pulmonale suggests severe OSAHS or a comorbid cardiopulmonary condition. A neurologic evaluation is needed to evaluate for conditions such as neuromuscular and cerebrovascular diseases, which increase OSAHS risk.

LABORATORY FINDINGS

Diagnostic Findings Since symptoms and signs do not accurately predict the severity of sleep-related breathing disturbances, specific diagnosis and categorization of OSAHS severity require objective measurement of breathing during the period of sleep. The gold standard for diagnosis of OSAHS is an overnight polysomnogram (PSG). A negative in-laboratory PSG rules out OSAHS except in unusual circumstances—e.g., with insufficient REM sleep or supine sleep. Home sleep tests that record only a few respiratory and cardiac channels commonly are used as a cost-effective means for diagnosing patients without significant comorbidity who have a high pretest probability of OSAHS. However, a home study may yield a false-negative result if sleep time is not accurately estimated, and further evaluation may therefore be required.

The key physiological information collected during a sleep study for OSAHS assessment includes measurement of breathing (changes in airflow, respiratory excursion), oxygenation (hemoglobin oxygen saturation), body position, and cardiac rhythm. In addition, PSGs and some home sleep studies measure sleep continuity and sleep stages (by electroencephalography, chin electromyography, and electro-oculography), limb movements (by leg sensors), and snoring intensity. This information is used to quantify the frequency and subtypes of abnormal respiratory events during sleep as well as associated changes in oxygen saturation, arousals, and sleep stage distributions. Tables 319-1 and 319-2 define the respiratory events scored and the severity guidelines employed during a sleep study. Figure 319-2 shows examples of sleep-related respiratory events. A typical sleep study report provides quantitative data such as the AHI and the profile of oxygen saturation over the night (mean, nadir, time at low levels). Reports may also include the respiratory disturbance index, which includes the number of respiratory effort–related arousals in addition to the number of apneas plus hypopneas. In-laboratory PSG also quantifies sleep latency (time from "lights off" to first sleep onset), sleep efficiency (percentage of time asleep relative to time in bed), arousal index (number of cortical arousals per hour of sleep), time in each sleep stage, and periodic limb movement index. OSAHS severity can be further characterized according to the degree of sleep fragmentation associated with respiratory disturbances. Relevant metrics include the frequency of cortical micro-arousals or awakenings per sleep hour, reduction in sleep continuity (low sleep efficiency), reduction of time in deeper stages of sleep (stage N3 and REM sleep) and increases in light sleep (stage N1). The detection of autonomic arousals, such as surges in blood pressure, changes in heart rate, and abnormalities in cardiac rhythm, also provides relevant information on OSAHS severity.

TABLE 319-1 RESPIRATORY EVENT DEFINITIONS

- *Apnea:* Cessation of airflow for ≥10 sec during sleep, accompanied by:
  - Persistent respiratory effort (obstructive apneas, Fig. 319-2*A*), or
  - Absence of respiratory effort (central apneas, Fig. 319-2*B*)
- *Hypopnea:* A ≥30% reduction in airflow for at least 10 sec during sleep that is accompanied by either a ≥3% desaturation or an arousal (Fig. 319-2*C*)
- *Respiratory effort–related arousal (RERA):* A partially obstructed breath that does not meet the criteria for hypopnea but provides evidence of increasing inspiratory effort (usually through pleural pressure monitoring) punctuated by an arousal (Fig. 319-2*D*)
- *Flow-limited breath:* A partially obstructed breath, typically within a hypopnea or RERA, identified by a flattened or "scooped-out" inspiratory flow shape **(Fig. 319-3)**

TABLE 319-2 OBSTRUCTIVE SLEEP APNEA/HYPOPNEA SYNDROME (OSAHS): QUANTIFICATION AND SEVERITY SCALE

- *Apnea-hypopnea index (AHI):*[a] Number of apneas plus hypopneas per hour of sleep
- *Respiratory disturbance index (RDI):* Number of apneas plus hypopneas plus RERAs per hour of sleep
- *Mild OSAHS:* AHI of 5–14 events/h
- *Moderate OSAHS:* AHI of 15–29 events/h
- *Severe OSAHS:* AHI of ≥30 events/h

[a]Each level of AHI can be further quantified by level of sleepiness and associated hypoxemia.

Other Laboratory Findings Various imaging studies, including cephalometric radiography, MRI, CT, and fiberoptic endoscopy, can be used to identify anatomic risk factors for OSAHS. Cardiac testing may yield evidence of impaired systolic or diastolic ventricular function or abnormal cardiac structure. Overnight blood pressure monitoring often displays a "non-dipping" pattern (absence of the typical 10-mmHg fall during sleep from blood pressure while awake). Arterial blood gas measurements made during wakefulness are usually normal. Waking hypoxemia or hypercarbia suggests coexisting lung disease or hypoventilation syndrome. Patients with severe nocturnal hypoxemia may have elevated hemoglobin values. A multiple sleep latency test or a maintenance of wakefulness test can be useful in quantifying sleepiness and helping to distinguish OSAHS from narcolepsy.

Health Consequences and Comorbidities OSAHS is a major contributor to cardiac, cerebrovascular, and metabolic disorders as well as to premature death. It is the most common medical cause of daytime sleepiness and negatively influences quality of life. This broad range of health effects is attributable to the impact of sleep fragmentation, cortical arousal, and intermittent hypoxemia on vascular, cardiac, metabolic, and neurologic functions. OSAHS-related respiratory events stimulate sympathetic overactivity, leading to acute blood pressure surges during sleep, endothelial damage, and nocturnal as well as daytime hypertension. OSAHS-related hypoxemia also stimulates release of acute-phase proteins and reactive oxygen species that exacerbate insulin resistance and lipolysis and cause an augmented prothrombotic and proinflammatory state. Inspiratory effort against an occluded airway causes large intrathoracic negative pressure swings, altering cardiac preload and afterload and resulting in cardiac remodeling and reduced cardiac function. Hypoxemia and sympathetic-parasympathetic imbalance also may cause electrical remodeling of the heart and myocyte injury.

HYPERTENSION OSAHS can raise blood pressure to prehypertensive and hypertensive ranges, increase the prevalence of a non-dipping overnight blood pressure pattern, and increase the risk of resistant hypertension. Elevations in blood pressure are due to augmented sympathetic nervous system activation as well as alterations in the rennin–angiotensin–aldosterone system and fluid balance. Treatment of OSAHS with nocturnal continuous positive airway pressure (CPAP) has been shown to reduce 24-h ambulatory blood pressure. Although the overall impact of CPAP on blood pressure levels is relatively modest (averaging 2–4 mmHg), larger improvements are observed among patients with high AHIs and sleepiness.

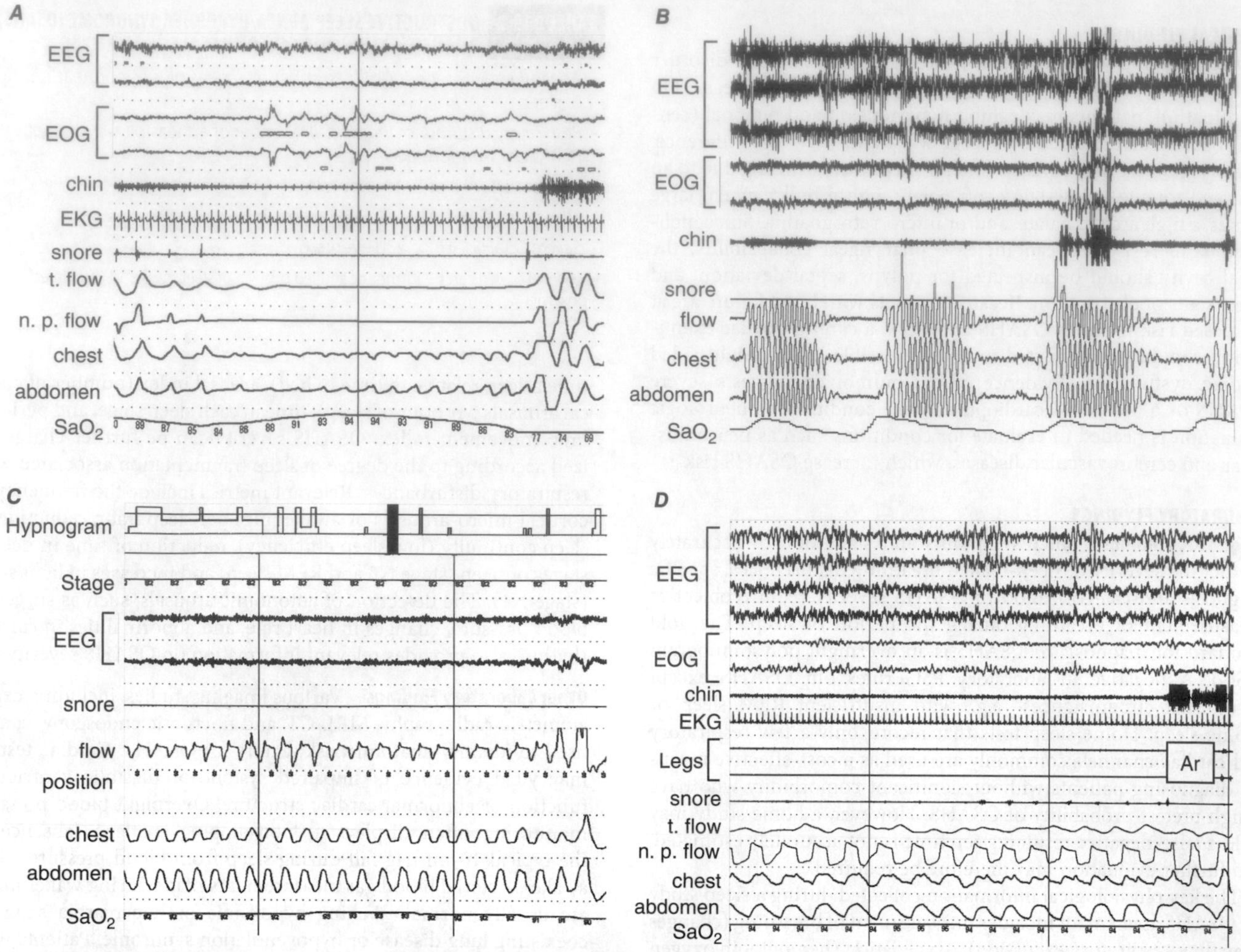

FIGURE 319-2 ***A.*** Obstructive apnea. There are 30 sec of no airflow, as shown in the nasal pressure (n. p. flow) and thermistor-measured flow (t. flow). Note the presence of chest-abdomen motion, indicating respiratory effort against an occluded airway. ***B.*** Central apnea in a patient with Cheyne-Stokes respiration due to congestive heart failure. The flat chest-abdomen tracings indicate the absence of inspiratory effort during the central apneas. ***C.*** Hypopnea. Partial obstruction of the pharyngeal airway can limit ventilation, leading to desaturation (a mild decrease in this patient, from 93% to 90%) and arousal. ***D.*** Respiratory effort–related arousal (RERA). Minimal flow reduction terminated by an arousal (Ar) without desaturation constitutes a RERA. EEG, electroencephalogram; EOG, electro-oculogram; EKG, electrocardiogram.

CARDIOVASCULAR, CEREBROVASCULAR, AND METABOLIC DISEASES Among the most serious health consequences of OSAHS is its impact on cardiac and metabolic functions. Strong epidemiologic evidence indicates that OSAHS significantly increases the risk of coronary artery disease, heart failure with and without reduced ejection fraction, atrial and ventricular arrhythmias, atherosclerosis and coronary artery disease, stroke, and diabetes. Treatment of OSAHS has been shown to reduce several markers of cardiovascular risk, improve insulin resistance, decrease the recurrence rate of atrial fibrillation, and improve various outcomes in patients with active cardiovascular disease. Large-scale trials are under way to evaluate the role of OSAHS treatment in reducing cardiac event rates and in prolonging the survival of patients with cardiac disease.

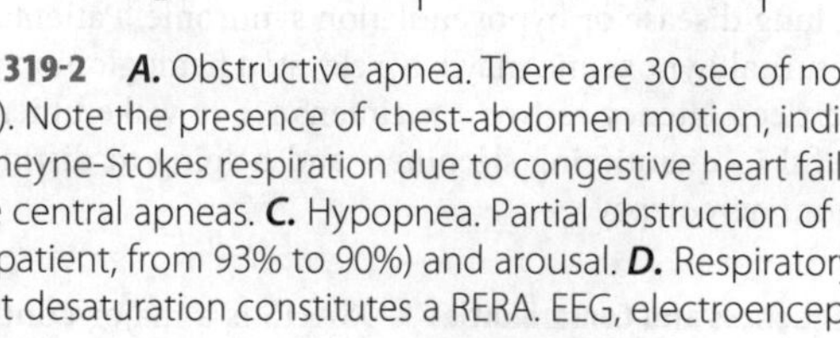

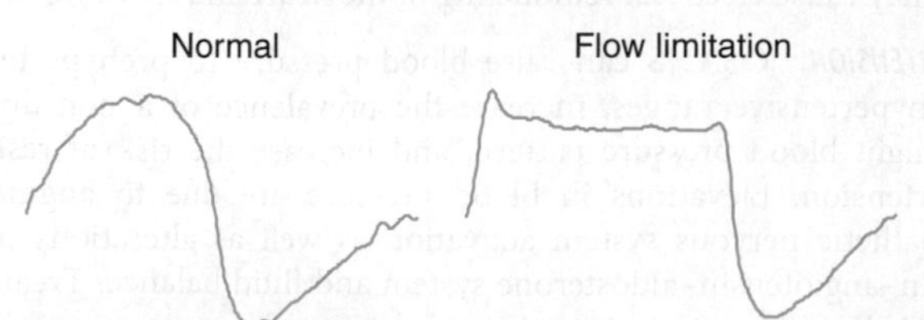

FIGURE 319-3 Example of flow limitation. The inspiratory flow pattern in a patent airway is rounded and peaks in the middle. In contrast, a partially obstructed airway exhibits an early peak followed by mid-inspiratory flattening, yielding a scooped-out appearance.

SLEEPINESS More than 50% of patients with moderate to severe OSAHS report daytime sleepiness. Patients with OSAHS symptoms have a twofold increased risk of occupational accidents. Individuals with elevated AHIs are involved in motor vehicle crashes as much as seven times more often than persons with normal AHIs. Randomized controlled trials have shown that treatment of OSAHS with nasal CPAP therapy alleviates sleepiness as measured by either questionnaire or objective testing. However, the degree of improvement varies widely. Residual sleepiness may be due to several factors, including suboptimal treatment adherence, insufficient sleep time, other sleep disorders, or prior hypoxic-mediated damage in brain areas involved in alertness. Visceral adipose tissue, whose amounts are increased in patients with OSAHS, releases somnogenic cytokines that may contribute to sleepiness. Thus, even after treatment, it is important to assess and monitor patients for residual sleepiness and to evaluate the necessity of optimizing treatment adherence, improving sleep patterns, and identifying other disorders contributing to sleepiness.

QUALITY OF LIFE AND MOOD Reductions in health-related quality of life are common in patients with OSAHS, with the largest decrements on the physical and vitality subscales. Treatment with CPAP often results in improvement in these patient-reported outcomes. Depression, in particular symptoms of somatic depression (irritability, fatigue, lack of energy) is commonly reported in OSAHS.

TREATMENT OBSTRUCTIVE SLEEP APNEA/HYPOPNEA SYNDROME (OSAHS)

A comprehensive approach to the management of OSAHS is needed to reduce risk factors and comorbidities. The clinician should seek to identify and address lifestyle and behavioral factors as well as comorbidities that may be exacerbating OSAHS. As appropriate, treatment should aim to reduce weight; optimize sleep duration (7–9 hours); regulate sleep schedules (with similar bedtimes and wake times across the week); encourage the patient to avoid sleeping in the supine position; treat nasal allergies; increase physical activity; eliminate alcohol ingestion within 3 h of bedtime; and minimize use of sedating medications. Patients should be counseled to avoid drowsy driving.

CPAP is the standard medical therapy with the highest level of evidence for efficacy. Delivered through a nasal or nasal-oral mask, CPAP works as a mechanical splint to hold the airway open, thus maintaining airway patency during sleep. An overnight CPAP titration study, performed either in a laboratory or with a home "autotitrating" device, is required to determine the optimal pressure setting that reduces the number of apneas/hypopneas during sleep, improves gas exchange, and reduces arousals. Rates of adherence to CPAP treatment are highly variable (average, 50–80%) and may be improved with support by a skilled health care team who can address side effects (Table 319-3). Despite the limitations of CPAP, controlled studies have demonstrated its beneficial effect on blood pressure, alertness, mood, and insulin sensitivity. Uncontrolled studies also indicate a favorable effect on cardiovascular outcomes, cardiac ejection fraction, atrial fibrillation recurrence, and mortality risk.

Oral appliances for OSAHS work by advancing the mandible, thus opening the airway by repositioning the lower jaw and pulling the tongue forward. These devices generally work better when customized for patient use; maximal adaptation can take several weeks. Efficacy studies show that these devices can reduce the AHI by ≥50% in two-thirds of individuals, although these data are based largely on patients with mild OSAHS. Side effects of oral appliances include temporomandibular joint pain and tooth movement. Oral appliances are most often used for treating patients with mild OSAHS or patients who do not tolerate CPAP. However, since adherence to the use of oral appliances sometimes exceeds CPAP adherence, these devices are under investigation for treatment of more severe disease.

Upper airway surgery for OSAHS is less effective than CPAP and is mostly reserved for the treatment of patients who snore, have mild OSAHS, and cannot tolerate CPAP. Uvulopalatopharyngoplasty (removal of the uvula and the margin of the soft palate) is the most common surgery and, although results vary greatly, has a success rate similar to or slightly lower than treatment with oral appliances. Upper airway surgery is less effective in severe OSAHS and in obese patients. Success rates may be higher for multilevel surgery (involving more than one site/structure) performed by an experienced surgeon, but the selection of patients is an important factor and relies on careful targeting of culprit areas for surgical resection. Bariatric surgery is an option for obese patients with OSAHS and can improve not only OSAHS but also other obesity-associated health conditions. Other procedures that can decrease snoring but have minimal effects on OSAHS include injection of the soft palate (resulting in stiffening), radiofrequency ablation, laser-assisted uvulopalatoplasty, and palatal implants.

Supplemental oxygen can improve oxygen saturation, but there is little evidence that it improves OSAHS symptoms or the AHI.

TABLE 319-3 SIDE EFFECTS OF CONTINUOUS POSITIVE AIRWAY PRESSURE (CPAP) AND THEIR TREATMENTS

Side Effect	Treatment
Nasal congestion	Provide heated humidification, administer saline/steroid nasal sprays
Claustrophobia	Change mask interface (e.g., to nasal prongs), promote habituation (i.e., practice breathing on CPAP while awake)
Difficulty exhaling	Temporarily reduce pressure, provide bilevel positive airway pressure
Bruised nasal ridge	Change mask interface, provide protective padding
Aerophagia	Administer antacids

CENTRAL SLEEP APNEA

CSA, which is less common than OSAHS, may occur in isolation or, more often, in combination with obstructive events in the form of "mixed" apneas. CSA is often caused by an increased sensitivity to pCO_2, which leads to an unstable breathing pattern that manifests as hyperventilation alternating with apnea. A prolonged circulation delay between the pulmonary capillaries and carotid chemoreceptors is also a contributing cause; thus individuals with congestive heart failure are at risk for CSA. With prolonged circulation delay, there is a crescendo-decrescendo breathing pattern known as *Cheyne-Stokes respiration* (Fig. 319–2B). Other risk factors for CSA include opioid medications (which appear to have a dose-dependent effect on CSA) and hypoxia (e.g., breathing at high altitude). In some individuals, CPAP—particularly at high pressures—seems to induce central apnea; this condition is referred to as *complex sleep apnea.* Rarely, CSA may be caused by blunted chemosensitivity due to congenital disorders (congenital central hypoventilation syndrome) or acquired factors. Treatment of CSA is difficult and depends on the underlying cause. Limited data suggest that supplemental oxygen can reduce the frequency of central apneas, particularly in patients with hypoxemia. Cheyne-Stokes respiration is treated by optimizing therapy for heart failure and, in some cases, using CPAP with or without supplemental oxygen. *Adaptive servoventilation*, a form of ventilatory support that dynamically changes inspiratory support levels across periods of apnea and hypopnea, can minimize large fluctuations in PCO_2 that produce central apnea and can be effective for the treatment of CSA.

320e Lung Transplantation

Elbert P. Trulock

This is a digital-only chapter. It is available on the DVD that accompanies this book, as well as on Access Medicine/Harrison's Online, and the eBook and "app" editions of HPIM 19e.

Lung transplantation is a therapeutic consideration for many patients with nonmalignant end-stage lung disease, and it prolongs survival and improves quality of life in appropriately selected recipients. Since 1985 almost 40,000 procedures have been recorded worldwide, and since 2009 more than 3000 transplants have been reported annually.

SECTION 1 RESPIRATORY CRITICAL CARE

321 Approach to the Patient with Critical Illness

John P. Kress, Jesse B. Hall

The care of critically ill patients requires a thorough understanding of pathophysiology and centers initially on the resuscitation of patients at the extremes of physiologic deterioration. This resuscitation is often fast-paced and occurs early, without a detailed awareness of the patient's chronic medical problems. While physiologic stabilization is taking place, intensivists attempt to gather important background medical information to supplement the real-time assessment of the patient's current physiologic conditions. Numerous tools are available to assist intensivists in the accurate assessment of pathophysiology and management of incipient organ failure, offering a window of opportunity for diagnosing and treating underlying disease(s) in a stabilized patient. Indeed, the use of invasive interventions such as mechanical ventilation and renal replacement therapy is commonplace in the intensive care unit (ICU). An appreciation of the risks and benefits of such aggressive and often invasive interventions is vital to ensure an optimal outcome. Nonetheless, intensivists must recognize when a patient's chances for recovery are remote or nonexistent and must counsel and comfort dying patients and their significant others. Critical care physicians often must redirect the goals of care from resuscitation and cure to comfort when the resolution of an underlying illness is not possible.

ASSESSMENT OF ILLNESS SEVERITY

In the ICU, illnesses are frequently categorized by degree of severity. Numerous severity-of-illness (SOI) scoring systems have been developed and validated over the past three decades. Although these scoring systems have been validated as tools to assess populations of critically ill patients, their utility in predicting individual patient outcomes is not clear. SOI scoring systems are important for defining populations of critically ill patients. Such systematic scoring allows effective comparison of groups of patients enrolled in clinical trials. In verifying a purported benefit of therapy, investigators must be confident that different groups involved in a clinical trial have similar illness severities. SOI scores are also useful in guiding hospital administrative policies, directing the allocation of resources such as nursing and ancillary care and assisting in assessments of quality of ICU care over time. Scoring system validations are based on the premise that age, chronic medical illnesses, and derangements from normal physiology are associated with increased mortality rates. All existing SOI scoring systems are derived from patients who have already been admitted to the ICU.

SOI scoring systems cannot be used to predict survival in individual patients. No established scoring systems that purport to direct clinicians' decision-making regarding criteria for admission to an ICU are available, although such models are being developed. Thus the use of SOI scoring systems to direct therapy and clinical decision-making cannot be recommended at present. Instead, these tools should be used as a source of important data to complement clinical bedside decision-making.

The most commonly utilized scoring systems are the APACHE (Acute Physiology and Chronic Health Evaluation) and the SAPS (Simplified Acute Physiology Score) systems.

THE APACHE II SCORING SYSTEM

The APACHE II system is the most commonly used SOI scoring system in North America. Age, type of ICU admission (after elective surgery vs. nonsurgical or after emergency surgery), chronic health problems, and 12 physiologic variables (the worst values for each in the first 24 h after ICU admission) are used to derive a score. The predicted hospital mortality rate is derived from a formula that takes into account the APACHE II score, the need for emergency surgery, and a weighted, disease-specific diagnostic category (Table 321-1). The relationship between APACHE II score and mortality risk is illustrated in Fig. 321-1. Updated versions of the APACHE scoring system (APACHE III and APACHE IV) have been published.

THE SAPS SCORING SYSTEM

The SAPS II score, used more frequently in Europe than in the United States, was derived in a manner similar to the APACHE score. This score is not disease specific but rather incorporates three underlying disease variables: AIDS, metastatic cancer, and hematologic malignancy. SAPS 3, which utilizes a 1-h rather than a 24-h window for measuring physiologic derangement scores, was developed in 2005.

SHOCK

See also Chap. 324.

INITIAL EVALUATION

Shock, a common condition necessitating ICU admission or occurring in the course of critical care, is defined by the presence of multisystem end-organ hypoperfusion. Clinical indicators include reduced mean arterial pressure (MAP), tachycardia, tachypnea, cool skin and extremities, acute altered mental status, and oliguria. Hypotension is usually, though not always, present. The end result of multiorgan hypoperfusion is tissue hypoxia, often with accompanying lactic acidosis. Since the MAP is the product of cardiac output and systemic vascular resistance (SVR), reductions in blood pressure can be caused by decreases in cardiac output and/or SVR. Accordingly, once shock is contemplated, the initial evaluation of a hypotensive patient should include an early bedside assessment of the adequacy of cardiac output (Fig. 321-2). Clinical evidence of *diminished* cardiac output includes a narrow pulse pressure—a marker that correlates with stroke volume—and cool extremities with delayed capillary refill. Signs of *increased* cardiac output include a widened pulse pressure (particularly with a reduced diastolic pressure), warm extremities with bounding pulses, and rapid capillary refill. If a hypotensive patient has clinical signs of increased cardiac output, it can be inferred that the reduced blood pressure is from decreased SVR.

In hypotensive patients with signs of reduced cardiac output, an assessment of intravascular volume status is appropriate. A hypotensive patient with decreased intravascular volume status may have a history suggesting hemorrhage or other volume losses (e.g., vomiting, diarrhea, polyuria). Although evidence of a reduced jugular venous pressure (JVP) is often sought, static measures of right atrial pressure do not predict fluid responsiveness reliably; the *change* in right atrial pressure as a function of spontaneous respiration is a better predictor of fluid responsiveness (Fig. 321-3). Patients with fluid-responsive (i.e., hypovolemic) shock also may manifest large changes in pulse pressure as a function of respiration during mechanical ventilation (Fig. 321-4). A hypotensive patient with increased intravascular volume and cardiac dysfunction may have S_3 and/or S_4 gallops on examination, increased JVP, extremity edema, and crackles on lung auscultation. The chest x-ray may show cardiomegaly, widening of the vascular pedicle, Kerley B lines, and pulmonary edema. Chest pain and electrocardiographic changes consistent with ischemia may be noted (Chap. 326).

In hypotensive patients with clinical evidence of increased cardiac output, a search for causes of decreased SVR is appropriate. The

TABLE 321-1 CALCULATION OF ACUTE PHYSIOLOGY AND CHRONIC HEALTH EVALUATION II (APACHE II) SCORE[a]

Acute Physiology Score

Score	*4*	*3*	*2*	*1*	*0*	*1*	*2*	*3*	*4*
Rectal temperature (°C)	≥41	39.0–40.9		38.5–38.9	36.0–38.4	34.0–35.9	32.0–33.9	30.0–31.9	≤29.9
Mean blood pressure (mmHg)	≥160	130–159	110–129		70–109		50–69		≤49
Heart rate (beats/min)	≥180	140–179	110–139		70–109		55–69	40–54	≤39
Respiratory rate (breaths/min)	≥50	35–49		25–34	12–24	10–11	6–9		≤5
Arterial pH	≥7.70	7.60–7.69		7.50–7.59	7.33–7.49		7.25–7.32	7.15–7.24	<7.15
Oxygenation									
If FI_{O_2} > 0.5, use (A – a) D_{O_2}	≥500	350–499	200–349		<200				
If FI_{O_2} ≤ 0.5, use Pa_{O_2}					>70	61–70		55–60	<55
Serum sodium (meq/L)	≥180	160–179	155–159	150–154	130–149		120–129	111–119	≤110
Serum potassium (meq/L)	≥7.0	6.0–6.9		5.5–5.9	3.5–5.4	3.0–3.4	2.5–2.9		<2.5
Serum creatinine (mg/dL)	≥3.5	2.0–3.4	1.5–1.9		0.6–1.4		<0.6		
Hematocrit (%)	≥60		50–59.9	46–49.9	30–45.9		20–29.9		<20
WBC count (10^3/mL)	≥40		20–39.9	15–19.9	3–14.9		1–2.9		<1

Glasgow Coma Score[b,c]

Eye Opening	*Verbal (Nonintubated)*	*Verbal (Intubated)*	*Motor Activity*
4—Spontaneous	5—Oriented and talks	5—Seems able to talk	6—Verbal command
3—Verbal stimuli	4—Disoriented and talks	3—Questionable ability to talk	5—Localizes to pain
2—Painful stimuli	3—Inappropriate words	1—Generally unresponsive	4—Withdraws from pain
1—No response	2—Incomprehensible sounds		3—Decorticate
	1—No response		2—Decerebrate
			1—No response

Points Assigned to Age and Chronic Disease

Age, Years	*Score*
<45	0
45–54	2
55–64	3
65–74	5
≥75	6

Chronic Health (History of Chronic Conditions)[d]	*Score*
None	0
If patient is admitted after elective surgery	2
If patient is admitted after emergency surgery or for reason other than after elective surgery	5

[a]The APACHE II score is the sum of the acute physiology score (vital signs, oxygenation, laboratory values), the Glasgow coma score, age, and chronic health points. The worst values during the first 24 h in the ICU should be used. [b]Glasgow coma score (GCS) = eye-opening score + verbal (intubated or nonintubated) score + motor score. [c]For GCS component of acute physiology score, subtract GCS from 15 to obtain points assigned. [d]Hepatic: cirrhosis with portal hypertension or encephalopathy; cardiovascular: class IV angina (at rest or with minimal self-care activities); pulmonary: chronic hypoxemia or hypercapnia, polycythemia, ventilator dependence; renal: chronic peritoneal or hemodialysis; immune: immunocompromised host.

Abbreviations: (A – a) D_{O_2}, alveolar-arterial oxygen difference; FI_{O_2}, fraction of inspired oxygen; Pa_{O_2}, partial pressure of oxygen; WBC, white blood cell count.

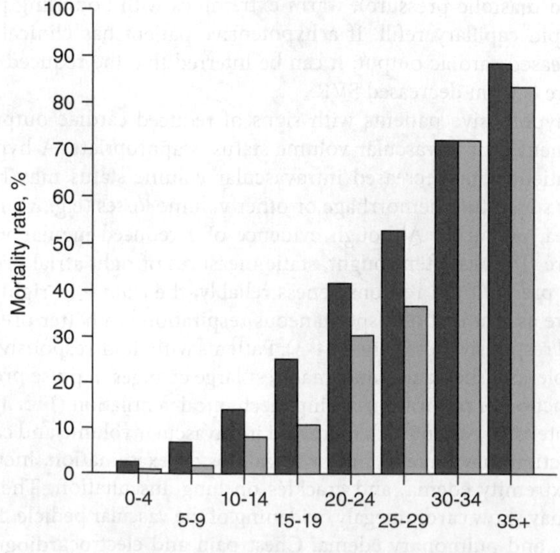

FIGURE 321-1 APACHE II survival curve. Blue, nonoperative; green, postoperative.

most common cause of high-cardiac-output hypotension is sepsis (Chap. 325). Other causes include liver failure, severe pancreatitis, burns and other trauma that elicit the systemic inflammatory response syndrome (SIRS), anaphylaxis, thyrotoxicosis, and peripheral arteriovenous shunts.

In summary, the most common categories of shock are hypovolemic, cardiogenic, and high-cardiac-output with decreased SVR (high-output hypotension). Certainly more than one category can occur simultaneously (e.g., hypovolemic and septic shock).

The initial assessment of a patient in shock should take only a few minutes. It is important that aggressive resuscitation is instituted on the basis of the initial assessment, particularly since early resuscitation from septic and cardiogenic shock may improve survival (see below). If the initial bedside assessment yields equivocal or confounding data, more objective assessments such as echocardiography and/or invasive vascular monitoring may be useful. The goal of early resuscitation is to reestablish adequate tissue perfusion and thus to prevent or minimize end-organ injury.

MECHANICAL VENTILATORY SUPPORT

(See also Chap. 323) During the initial resuscitation of patients in shock, principles of advanced cardiac life support should be followed.

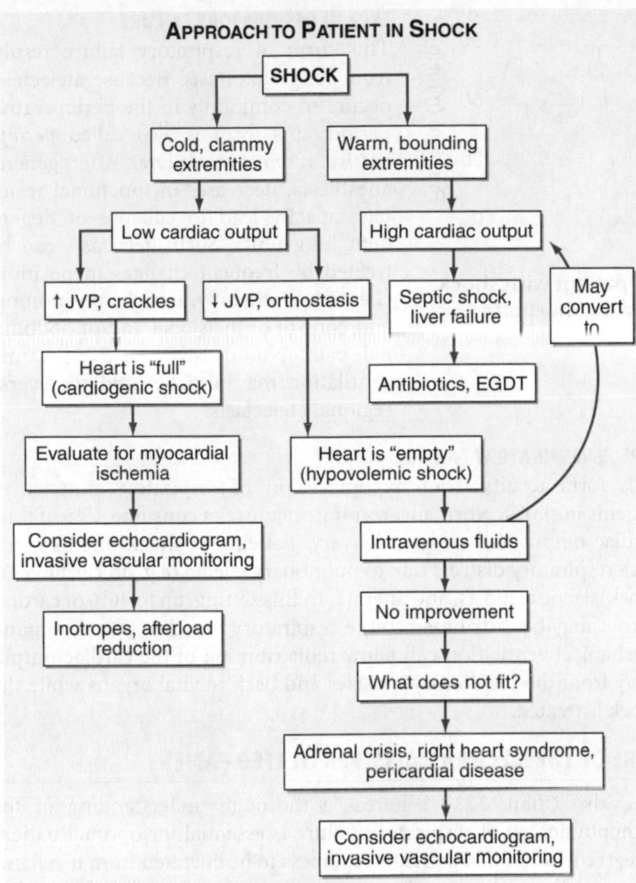

FIGURE 321-2 Approach to the patient in shock. EGDT, early goal-directed therapy; JVP, jugular venous pulse.

As such patients may be obtunded and unable to protect the airway, an early assessment of the airway is mandatory. Early intubation and mechanical ventilation often are required. Reasons for the institution of endotracheal intubation and mechanical ventilation include acute hypoxemic respiratory failure and ventilatory failure, which frequently accompany shock. Acute hypoxemic respiratory failure may occur in patients with cardiogenic shock and pulmonary edema (Chap. 326) as well as in those who are in septic shock with pneumonia or acute respiratory distress syndrome (ARDS) (Chaps. 322 and 325). Ventilatory failure often occurs as a consequence of an increased load on the respiratory system in the form of acute metabolic (often lactic) acidosis or decreased lung compliance due to pulmonary edema. Inadequate perfusion to respiratory muscles in the setting of shock may be another reason for early intubation and mechanical ventilation. Normally, the respiratory muscles receive a very small percentage of the cardiac output. However, in patients who are in shock with respiratory distress, the percentage of cardiac output dedicated to respiratory muscles may increase by tenfold or more. Lactic acid production from inefficient respiratory muscle activity presents an additional ventilatory load.

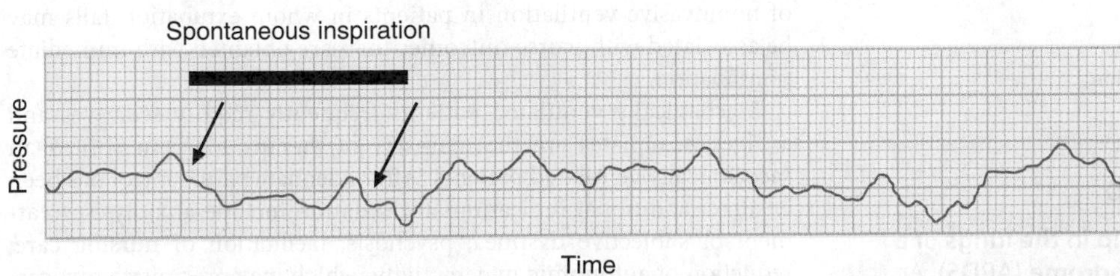

FIGURE 321-3 Right atrial pressure change during spontaneous respiration in a patient with shock whose cardiac output will increase in response to intravenous fluid administration. The right atrial pressure decreases from 7 mmHg to 4 mmHg. The horizontal bar marks the time of spontaneous inspiration.

Mechanical ventilation may relieve the work of breathing and allow redistribution of a limited cardiac output to other vital organs. Patients demonstrate respiratory distress by an inability to speak full sentences, accessory use of respiratory muscles, paradoxical abdominal muscle activity, extreme tachypnea (>40 breaths/min), and decreasing respiratory rate despite an increasing drive to breathe. When patients with shock are treated with mechanical ventilation, a major goal is for the ventilator to assume all or the majority of the work of breathing, facilitating a state of minimal respiratory muscle work. With the institution of mechanical ventilation for shock, further declines in MAP are frequently seen. The reasons include impeded venous return from positive-pressure ventilation, reduced endogenous catecholamine secretion once the stress associated with respiratory failure abates, and the actions of drugs used to facilitate endotracheal intubation (e.g., propofol, opiates). Accordingly, hypotension should be anticipated during endotracheal intubation. Because many of these patients may be fluid responsive, IV volume administration should be considered. Figure 321-2 summarizes the diagnosis and treatment of different types of shock For further discussion of individual forms of shock, see Chaps. 324, 325, and 326.

RESPIRATORY FAILURE

Respiratory failure is one of the most common reasons for ICU admission. In some ICUs, ≥75% of patients require mechanical ventilation during their stay. Respiratory failure can be categorized mechanistically on the basis of pathophysiologic derangements in respiratory function.

TYPE I: ACUTE HYPOXEMIC RESPIRATORY FAILURE

This type of respiratory failure occurs with alveolar flooding and subsequent intrapulmonary shunt physiology. Alveolar flooding may be a consequence of pulmonary edema, pneumonia, or alveolar hemorrhage. Pulmonary edema can be further categorized as occurring due to elevated pulmonary microvascular pressures, as seen in heart failure and intravascular volume overload or ARDS ("low-pressure pulmonary edema," Chap. 322). This syndrome is defined by acute onset (≤1 week) of bilateral opacities on chest imaging that are not fully explained by cardiac failure or fluid overload and of shunt physiology requiring positive end-expiratory pressure (PEEP). Type I respiratory failure occurs in clinical settings such as sepsis, gastric aspiration, pneumonia, near-drowning, multiple blood transfusions, and pancreatitis. The mortality rate among patients with ARDS was traditionally very high (50–70%), although changes in patient care have led to mortality rates closer to 30% (see below).

For many years, physicians have suspected that mechanical ventilation of patients with ARDS may propagate lung injury. Cyclical collapse and reopening of alveoli may be partly responsible for this adverse effect. As seen in Fig. 321-5, the pressure-volume relationship of the lung in ARDS is not linear. Alveoli may collapse at very low lung volumes. Animal studies have suggested that stretching and overdistention of injured alveoli during mechanical ventilation can further injure the lung. Concern over this alveolar overdistention, termed *ventilator-induced "volutrauma,"* led to a multicenter, randomized, prospective trial comparing traditional ventilator strategies for ARDS (large tidal volume: 12 mL/kg of ideal body weight) with a low tidal volume (6 mL/kg of ideal body weight). This study showed a dramatic reduction in mortality rate in the low-tidal-volume group from that in the high-tidal-volume group (31% versus 39.8%). In addition, a "fluid-conservative" management strategy (maintaining a low central venous pressure [CVP] or pulmonary capillary wedge pressure [PCWP]) is associated with fewer days of mechanical ventilation than a "fluid-liberal" strategy (maintaining a relatively high CVP or PCWP) in ARDS.

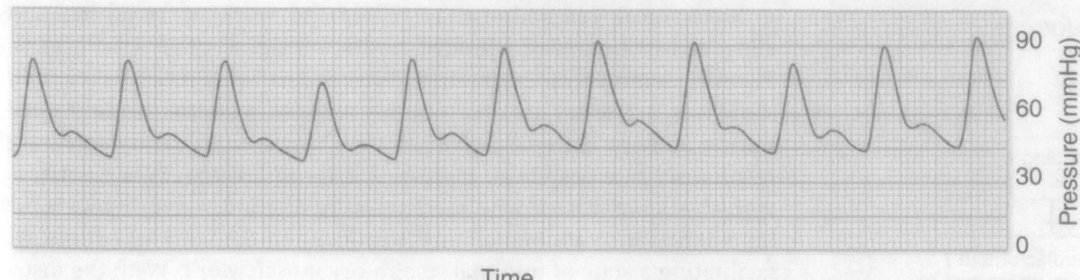

FIGURE 321-4 Pulse pressure change during mechanical ventilation in a patient with shock whose cardiac output will increase in response to intravenous fluid administration. The pulse pressure (systolic minus diastolic blood pressure) changes during mechanical ventilation in a patient with septic shock.

TYPE II RESPIRATORY FAILURE

This type of respiratory failure is a consequence of alveolar hypoventilation and results from the inability to eliminate carbon dioxide effectively. Mechanisms are categorized by impaired central nervous system (CNS) drive to breathe, impaired strength with failure of neuromuscular function in the respiratory system, and increased load(s) on the respiratory system. Reasons for diminished CNS drive to breathe include drug overdose, brainstem injury, sleep-disordered breathing, and severe hypothyroidism. Reduced strength can be due to impaired neuromuscular transmission (e.g., myasthenia gravis, Guillain-Barré syndrome, amyotrophic lateral sclerosis) or respiratory muscle weakness (e.g., myopathy, electrolyte derangements, fatigue).

The overall load on the respiratory system can be subclassified into resistive loads (e.g., bronchospasm), loads due to reduced lung compliance (e.g., alveolar edema, atelectasis, intrinsic positive end-expiratory pressure [auto-PEEP]—see below), loads due to reduced chest wall compliance (e.g., pneumothorax, pleural effusion, abdominal distention), and loads due to increased minute ventilation requirements (e.g., pulmonary embolus with increased dead-space fraction, sepsis).

The mainstays of therapy for type II respiratory failure are directed at reversing the underlying cause(s) of ventilatory failure. Noninvasive positive-pressure ventilation with a tight-fitting facial or nasal mask, with avoidance of endotracheal intubation, often stabilizes these patients. This approach has been shown to be beneficial in treating patients with exacerbations of chronic obstructive pulmonary disease; it has been tested less extensively in other kinds of respiratory failure but may be attempted nonetheless in the absence of contraindications (hemodynamic instability, inability to protect the airway, respiratory arrest).

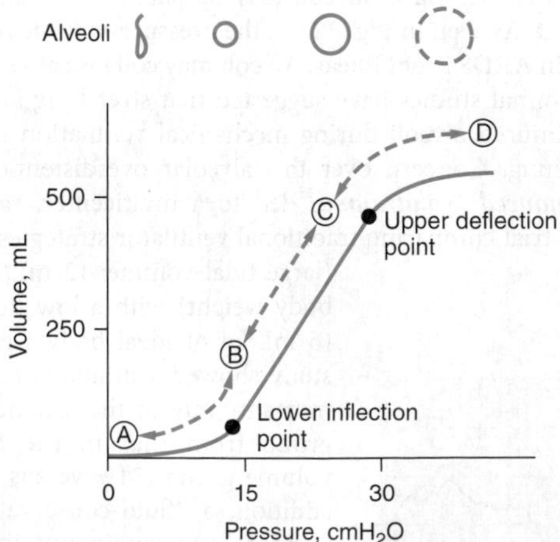

FIGURE 321-5 Pressure-volume relationship in the lungs of a patient with acute respiratory distress syndrome (ARDS). At the lower inflection point, collapsed alveoli begin to open and lung compliance changes. At the upper deflection point, alveoli become overdistended. The shape and size of alveoli are illustrated at the top of the figure.

TYPE III RESPIRATORY FAILURE

This form of respiratory failure results from lung atelectasis. Because atelectasis occurs so commonly in the perioperative period, this form is also called *perioperative respiratory failure.* After general anesthesia, decreases in functional residual capacity lead to collapse of dependent lung units. Such atelectasis can be treated by frequent changes in position, chest physiotherapy, upright positioning, and control of incisional and/or abdominal pain. Noninvasive positive-pressure ventilation may also be used to reverse regional atelectasis.

TYPE IV RESPIRATORY FAILURE

This form results from hypoperfusion of respiratory muscles in patients in shock. Normally, respiratory muscles consume <5% of total cardiac output and oxygen delivery. Patients in shock often experience respiratory distress due to pulmonary edema (e.g., in cardiogenic shock), lactic acidosis, and anemia. In this setting, up to 40% of cardiac output may be distributed to the respiratory muscles. Intubation and mechanical ventilation can allow redistribution of the cardiac output away from the respiratory muscles and back to vital organs while the shock is treated.

CARE OF THE MECHANICALLY VENTILATED PATIENT

(See also Chap. 323) Whereas a thorough understanding of the pathophysiology of respiratory failure is essential for optimal patient care, recognition of a patient's readiness to be liberated from mechanical ventilation is likewise important. Several studies have shown that daily spontaneous breathing trials can identify patients who are ready for extubation. Accordingly, all intubated, mechanically ventilated patients should undergo daily screening of respiratory function. If oxygenation is stable (i.e., Pa_{O_2}/FI_{O_2} [partial pressure of oxygen/fraction of inspired oxygen] >200 and PEEP ≤5 cmH_2O), cough and airway reflexes are intact, and no vasopressor agents or sedatives are being administered, the patient has passed the screening test and should undergo a spontaneous breathing trial. This trial consists of a period of breathing through the endotracheal tube without ventilator support (both continuous positive airway pressure [CPAP] of 5 cmH_2O and an open T-piece breathing system can be used) for 30–120 min. The spontaneous breathing trial is declared a failure and stopped if *any* of the following occur: (1) respiratory rate >35/min for >5 min, (2) O_2 saturation <90%, (3) heart rate >140/min or a 20% increase or decrease from baseline, (4) systolic blood pressure <90 mmHg or >180 mmHg, or (5) increased anxiety or diaphoresis. If, at the end of the spontaneous breathing trial, none of the above events has occurred and the ratio of the respiratory rate and tidal volume in liters (f/V_T) is <105, the patient can be extubated. Such protocol-driven approaches to patient care can have an important impact on the duration of mechanical ventilation and ICU stay. In spite of such a careful approach to liberation from mechanical ventilation, up to 10% of patients develop respiratory distress after extubation and may require resumption of mechanical ventilation. Many of these patients will require reintubation. The use of noninvasive ventilation in patients in whom extubation fails may be associated with worse outcomes than are obtained with immediate reintubation.

Mechanically ventilated patients frequently require sedatives and analgesics. Opiates are the mainstay of therapy for pain control in mechanically ventilated patients. After adequate pain control has been ensured, additional indications for sedation include anxiolysis; treatment of subjective dyspnea; psychosis; facilitation of nursing care; reduction of autonomic hyperactivity, which may precipitate myocardial ischemia; and reduction of total O_2 consumption (V_{O_2}).

Neuromuscular blocking agents are occasionally needed to facilitate mechanical ventilation in patients with profound ventilator dyssynchrony despite optimal sedation, particularly in the setting of severe

ARDS. Use of these agents may result in prolonged weakness—a myopathy known as the *postparalytic syndrome*. For this reason, neuromuscular blocking agents typically are used as a last resort when aggressive sedation fails to achieve patient-ventilator synchrony. Because neuromuscular blocking agents result in pharmacologic paralysis without altering mental status, sedative-induced amnesia is mandatory when these agents are administered.

Amnesia can be achieved reliably with benzodiazepines such as lorazepam and midazolam as well as the the IV anesthetic agent propofol. Outside the setting of pharmacologic paralysis, few data support the idea that amnesia is mandatory in all patients who require intubation and mechanical ventilation. Since many of these critically patients have impaired hepatic and renal function, sedatives and opiates may accumulate when given for prolonged periods. A nursing protocol–driven approach to sedation of mechanically ventilated patients or daily interruption of sedative infusions paired with daily spontaneous breathing trials has been shown to prevent excessive drug accumulation and shorten the duration of both mechanical ventilation and ICU stay.

MULTIORGAN SYSTEM FAILURE

Multiorgan system failure, which is commonly associated with critical illness, is defined by the simultaneous presence of physiologic dysfunction and/or failure of two or more organs. Typically, this syndrome occurs in the setting of severe sepsis, shock of any kind, severe inflammatory conditions such as pancreatitis, and trauma. The fact that multiorgan system failure occurs commonly in the ICU is a testament to our current ability to stabilize and support single-organ failure. The ability to support single-organ failure aggressively (e.g., by mechanical ventilation or by renal replacement therapy) has reduced rates of early mortality in critical illness. As a result, it is uncommon for critically ill patients to die in the initial stages of resuscitation. Instead, many patients succumb to critical illness later in the ICU stay, after the initial presenting problem has been stabilized.

Although there is debate regarding specific definitions of organ failure, several general principles governing the syndrome of multiorgan system failure apply. First, organ failure, no matter how it is defined, must persist beyond 24 h. Second, mortality risk increases with the accrual of failing organs. Third, the prognosis worsens with increased duration of organ failure. These observations remain true across various critical care settings (e.g., medical versus surgical). SIRS is a common basis for multiorgan system failure. Although infection is a common cause of SIRS, "sterile" triggers such as pancreatitis, trauma, and burns often are invoked to explain multiorgan system failure.

MONITORING IN THE ICU

Because respiratory failure and circulatory failure are common in critically ill patients, monitoring of the respiratory and cardiovascular systems is undertaken frequently. Evaluation of respiratory gas exchange is routine in critical illness. The "gold standard" remains arterial blood-gas analysis, in which pH, PaO_2, partial pressure of carbon dioxide (PCO_2), and O_2 saturation are measured directly. With arterial blood-gas analysis, the two main functions of the lung—oxygenation of arterial blood and elimination of CO_2—can be assessed directly. In fact, the blood pH, which has a profound effect on the drive to breathe, can be assessed only by such sampling. Although sampling of arterial blood is generally safe, it may be painful and cannot provide continuous information. In light of these limitations, noninvasive monitoring of respiratory function is often employed.

PULSE OXIMETRY

The most commonly utilized noninvasive technique for monitoring respiratory function, pulse oximetry takes advantage of differences in the absorptive properties of oxygenated and deoxygenated hemoglobin. At wavelengths of 660 nm, oxyhemoglobin reflects light more effectively than does deoxyhemoglobin, whereas the reverse is true in the infrared spectrum (940 nm). A pulse oximeter passes both wavelengths of light through a perfused digit such as a finger, and the relative intensity of light transmission at these two wavelengths is recorded. From this information, the relative percentage of oxyhemoglobin is derived. Since arterial pulsations produce phasic changes in the intensity of transmitted light, the pulse oximeter is designed to detect only light of alternating intensity. This feature allows distinction of arterial and venous blood O_2 saturations.

RESPIRATORY SYSTEM MECHANICS

Respiratory system mechanics can be measured in patients during mechanical ventilation (Chap. 323). When volume-controlled modes of mechanical ventilation are used, accompanying airway pressures can easily be measured as long as the patient is passive. The peak airway pressure is determined by two variables: airway resistance and respiratory system compliance. At the end of inspiration, inspiratory flow can be stopped transiently. This end-inspiratory pause (*plateau pressure*) is a static measurement, affected only by respiratory system compliance and not by airway resistance. Therefore, during volume-controlled ventilation, the difference between the peak (airway resistance + respiratory system compliance) and plateau (respiratory system compliance only) airway pressures provides a quantitative assessment of airway resistance. Accordingly, during volume-controlled ventilation, patients with increases in airway resistance typically have increased peak airway pressures as well as abnormally high gradients between peak and plateau airway pressures (typically >15 cmH_2O) at an inspiratory flow rate of 1 L/sec. The compliance of the respiratory system is defined by the change in pressure of the respiratory system per unit change in volume.

The respiratory system can be divided into two components: the lungs and the chest wall. Normally, respiratory system compliance is ~100 mL/cmH_2O. Pathophysiologic processes such as pleural effusions, pneumothorax, and increased abdominal girth all reduce chest wall compliance. Lung compliance may be reduced by pneumonia, pulmonary edema, interstitial lung disease, or auto-PEEP. Accordingly, patients with abnormalities in compliance of the respiratory system (lungs and/or chest wall) typically have elevated peak *and* plateau airway pressures but a normal gradient between these two pressures. Auto PEEP occurs when there is insufficient time for emptying of alveoli before the next inspiratory cycle. Since the alveoli have not decompressed completely, alveolar pressure remains positive at the end of exhalation (*functional residual capacity*). This phenomenon results most commonly from critical narrowing of distal airways in disease processes such as asthma and COPD. Auto-PEEP with resulting alveolar overdistention may result in diminished lung compliance, reflected by abnormally increased plateau airway pressures. Modern mechanical ventilators allow breath-to-breath display of pressure and flow, permitting detection of problems such as patient-ventilator dyssynchrony, airflow obstruction, and auto-PEEP (Fig. 321-6).

CIRCULATORY STATUS

Oxygen delivery (Q_{O_2}) is a function of cardiac output and the content of O_2 in the arterial blood (Ca_{O_2}). The Ca_{O_2} is determined by the hemoglobin concentration, the arterial hemoglobin saturation, and dissolved O_2 not bound to hemoglobin. For normal adults:

$$\begin{aligned} Q_{O_2} &= 50\ \text{dL/min} \times (1.39 \times 15\ \text{g/dL [hemoglobin concentration]} \\ &\quad \times 1.0\ \text{[hemoglobin \% saturation]} + 0.0031 \times 100\ [\text{Pa}_{O_2}]) \\ &= 50\ \text{dL/min (cardiac output)} \times 21.6\ \text{mL } O_2 \text{ per dL blood } (\text{Ca}_{O_2}) \\ &= 1058\ \text{mL } O_2 \text{ per min} \end{aligned}$$

It is apparent that nearly all of the O_2 delivered to tissues is bound to hemoglobin and that the dissolved O_2 (Pa_{O_2}) contributes very little to O_2 content in arterial blood or to O_2 delivery. Normally, the content of O_2 in mixed venous blood ($C\bar{v}_{O_2}$) is 15.76 mL/dL since the mixed venous blood is 75% saturated. Therefore, the normal tissue extraction ratio for O_2 is $Ca_{O_2} - C\bar{v}_{O_2}/Ca_{O_2}$ ([21.16–15.76]/21.16) or ~25%. A pulmonary artery catheter allows measurements of O_2 delivery and the O_2 extraction ratio.

Information on the mixed venous O_2 saturation allows assessment of global tissue perfusion. A reduced mixed venous O_2 saturation may be caused by inadequate cardiac output, reduced hemoglobin concentration, and/or reduced arterial O_2 saturation. An abnormally high V_{O_2} may also lead to a reduced mixed venous O_2 saturation if O_2 delivery is

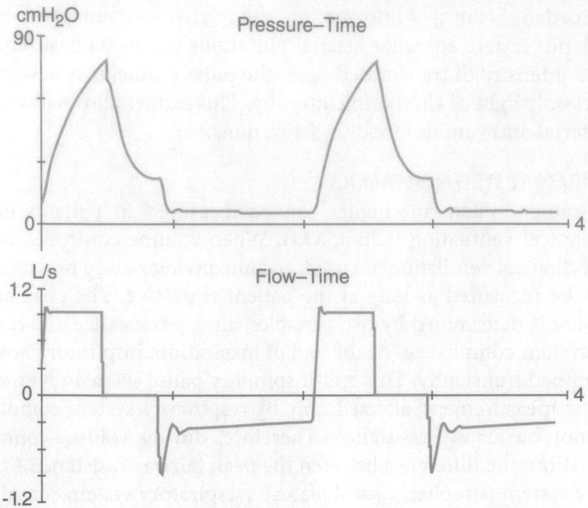

FIGURE 321-6 Increased airway resistance with auto-PEEP. The top waveform (airway pressure vs. time) shows a large difference between the peak airway pressure (80 cmH_2O) and the plateau airway pressure (20 cmH_2O). The bottom waveform (flow vs. time) demonstrates airflow throughout expiration (reflected by the flow tracing on the negative portion of the abscissa) that persists up to the next inspiratory effort.

not concomitantly increased. Abnormally increased V_{O_2} in peripheral tissues may be caused by problems such as fever, agitation, shivering, and thyrotoxicosis.

The pulmonary artery catheter originally was designed as a tool to guide therapy for acute myocardial infarction but has been used in the ICU for evaluation and treatment of a variety of other conditions, such as ARDS, septic shock, congestive heart failure, and acute renal failure. This device has never been validated as a tool associated with reduction in morbidity and mortality rates. Indeed, despite numerous prospective studies, mortality or morbidity rate benefits associated with use of the pulmonary artery catheter have never been reported in any setting. Accordingly, it appears that routine pulmonary artery catheterization is not indicated as a means of monitoring and characterizing circulatory status in most critically ill patients.

Static measurements of circulatory parameters (e.g., CVP, PCWP) do not provide reliable information on the circulatory status of critically ill patients. In contrast, dynamic assessments measuring the impact of breathing on the circulation are more reliable predictors of responsiveness to IV fluid administration. A decrease in CVP of >1 mmHg during inspiration in a spontaneously breathing patient may predict an increase in cardiac output after IV fluid administration. Similarly, a changing pulse pressure during mechanical ventilation has been shown to predict an increase in cardiac output after IV fluid administration in patients with septic shock.

PREVENTION OF COMPLICATIONS OF CRITICAL ILLNESS

SEPSIS IN THE CRITICAL CARE UNIT

(See also Chap. 325) Sepsis, defined as the presence of SIRS in the setting of known or suspected infection, is a significant problem in the care of critically ill patients, who often progress to severe sepsis with the failure of one or more organs. Sepsis is the leading cause of death in noncoronary ICUs in the United States, with case rates expected to increase as the population ages and a higher percentage of people are vulnerable to infection.

NOSOCOMIAL INFECTIONS IN THE ICU

Many therapeutic interventions in the ICU are invasive and predispose patients to infectious complications. These interventions include endotracheal intubation, indwelling vascular catheters, transurethral bladder catheters, and other catheters placed into sterile body cavities (e.g., tube thoracostomy, percutaneous intraabdominal drainage catheterization). The longer such devices remain in place, the more prone to these infections patients become. For example, ventilator-associated pneumonia correlates strongly with the duration of intubation and mechanical ventilation. Therefore, an important aspect of preventive care is the timely removal of invasive devices as soon as they are no longer needed. Moreover, multidrug-resistant organisms are commonplace in the ICU.

Infection control is critical in the ICU. Care bundles, which include measures such as frequent hand washing, are effective but underutilized strategies. Other components of care bundles, such as protective isolation of patients colonized or infected by drug-resistant organisms, are also commonly used. Silver-coated endotracheal tubes reportedly reduce the incidence of ventilator-associated pneumonia. Studies evaluating multifaceted, evidence-based strategies to decrease catheter-related bloodstream infections have shown improved outcomes with strict adherence to measures such as hand washing, full-barrier precautions during catheter insertion, chlorhexidine skin preparation, avoidance of the femoral site, and timely catheter removal.

DEEP VENOUS THROMBOSIS (DVT)

(See also Chap. 300) All ICU patients are at high risk for this complication because of their predilection for immobility. Therefore, all should receive some form of prophylaxis against DVT. The most commonly employed forms of prophylaxis are subcutaneous low-dose heparin injections and sequential compression devices for the lower extremities. Observational studies report an alarming incidence of DVTs despite the use of these standard prophylactic regimens. Furthermore, heparin prophylaxis may result in heparin-induced thrombocytopenia, another nosocomial complication in critically ill patients.

Low-molecular-weight heparins such as enoxaparin are more effective than unfractionated heparin for DVT prophylaxis in high-risk patients (e.g., those undergoing orthopedic surgery) and are associated with a lower incidence of heparin-induced thrombocytopenia. Fondaparinux, a selective factor Xa inhibitor, is even more effective than enoxaparin in high-risk orthopedic patients.

STRESS ULCERS

Prophylaxis against stress ulcers is frequently administered in most ICUs; typically, histamine-2 antagonists or proton pump inhibitors are given. Available data suggest that high-risk patients, such as those with coagulopathy, shock, or respiratory failure requiring mechanical ventilation, benefit from such prophylactic treatment.

NUTRITION AND GLYCEMIC CONTROL

These are important issues that may be associated with respiratory failure, impaired wound healing, and dysfunctional immune response in critically ill patients. Early enteral feeding is reasonable, though no data are available to suggest that this treatment improves patient outcome per se. Certainly, enteral feeding, if possible, is preferred over parenteral nutrition, which is associated with numerous complications, including hyperglycemia, fatty liver, cholestasis, and sepsis. When parenteral feeding is necessary to supplement enteral nutrition, delaying this intervention until day 8 in the ICU results in better recovery and fewer ICU-related complications. Tight glucose control is an area of controversy in critical care. Although one study showed a significant mortality benefit when glucose levels were aggressively normalized in a large group of surgical ICU patients, more recent data for a large population of both medical and surgical ICU patients suggested that tight glucose control resulted in increased rates of mortality.

ICU-ACQUIRED WEAKNESS

ICU-acquired weakness occurs frequently in patients who survive critical illness, particularly those with SIRS and/or sepsis. Both neuropathies and myopathies have been described, most commonly after ~1 week in the ICU. The mechanisms behind ICU-acquired weakness syndromes are poorly understood. Intensive insulin therapy may reduce polyneuropathy in critical illness. Very early physical and occupational therapy in mechanically ventilated patients reportedly results in significant improvements in functional independence at hospital discharge as well as in reduced durations of mechanical ventilation and delirium.

ANEMIA

Studies have shown that most ICU patients are anemic as a result of chronic inflammation. Phlebotomy also contributes to ICU anemia. A large multicenter study involving patients in many different ICU settings challenged the conventional notion that a hemoglobin level of 100 g/L (10 g/dL) is needed in critically ill patients, with similar outcomes noted in those whose transfusion trigger was 7 g/dL. Red blood cell transfusion is associated with impairment of immune function and increased risk of infections as well as of ARDS and volume overload, all of which may explain the findings in this study. Recently, a conservative transfusion strategy enhanced survival among patients with active upper gastrointestinal hemorrhage.

ACUTE RENAL FAILURE

(See also Chap. 334) Acute renal failure occurs in a significant percentage of critically ill patients. The most common underlying etiology is acute tubular necrosis, usually precipitated by hypoperfusion and/or nephrotoxic agents. Currently, no pharmacologic agents are available for prevention of renal injury in critical illness. Studies have shown convincingly that low-dose dopamine is *not* effective in protecting the kidneys from acute injury.

NEUROLOGIC DYSFUNCTION IN CRITICALLY ILL PATIENTS

DELIRIUM

(See also Chaps. 34 and 328) This state is defined by (1) an acute onset of changes or fluctuations in mental status, (2) inattention, (3) disorganized thinking, and (4) an altered level of consciousness (i.e., a state other than alertness). Delirium is reported to occur in a wide range of mechanically ventilated ICU patients and can be detected by the Confusion Assessment Method (CAM)-ICU or the Intensive Care Delirium Screening Checklist. These tools are used to ask patients to answer simple questions and perform simple tasks and can be used readily at the bedside. The differential diagnosis of delirium in ICU patients is broad and includes infectious etiologies (including sepsis), medications (particularly sedatives and analgesics), drug withdrawal, metabolic/electrolyte derangements, intracranial pathology (e.g., stroke, intracranial hemorrhage), seizures, hypoxia, hypertensive crisis, shock, and vitamin deficiencies (particularly thiamine). Patients with ICU delirium have increases in length of hospital stay, time on mechanical ventilation, cognitive impairment at hospital discharge, and 6-month mortality rate. Interventions to reduce ICU delirium are limited. The sedative dexmedetomidine has been less strongly associated with ICU delirium than midazolam. In addition, as mentioned above, very early physical and occupational therapy in mechanically ventilated patients has been demonstrated to reduce delirium.

ANOXIC CEREBRAL INJURY

(See also Chap. 330) This condition is common after cardiac arrest and often results in severe and permanent brain injury in survivors. Active cooling of patients after cardiac arrest has been shown to improve neurologic outcomes. Therefore, patients who present to the ICU after circulatory arrest from ventricular fibrillation or pulseless ventricular tachycardia should be actively cooled to achieve a core body temperature of 32–34°C.

STROKE

(See also Chap. 446) Stroke is a common cause of neurologic critical illness. Hypertension must be managed carefully, since abrupt reductions in blood pressure may be associated with further brain ischemia and injury. Acute ischemic stroke treated with tissue plasminogen activator (tPA) has an improved neurologic outcome when treatment is given within 3 h of onset of symptoms. The mortality rate is not reduced when tPA is compared with placebo, despite the improved neurologic outcome. The risk of cerebral hemorrhage is significantly higher in patients given tPA. No benefit is seen when tPA therapy is given beyond 3 h after symptom onset. Heparin has not been convincingly shown to improve outcomes in patients with acute ischemic stroke. Decompressive craniectomy is a surgical procedure that relieves increased intracranial pressure in the setting of space-occupying brain lesions or brain swelling from stroke; available evidence suggests that this procedure may improve survival among select patients (≤55 years or age), albeit at a cost of increased disability for some.

SUBARACHNOID HEMORRHAGE

(See also Chap. 446) Subarachnoid hemorrhage may occur secondary to aneurysm rupture and is often complicated by cerebral vasospasm, re-bleeding, and hydrocephalus. Vasospasm can be detected by either transcranial Doppler assessment or cerebral angiography; it is typically treated with the calcium channel blocker nimodipine, aggressive IV fluid administration, and therapy aimed at increasing blood pressure, typically with vasoactive drugs such as phenylephrine. The IV fluids and vasoactive drugs (hypertensive hypervolemic therapy) are used to overcome the cerebral vasospasm. Early surgical clipping or endovascular coiling of aneurysms is advocated to prevent complications related to re-bleeding. Hydrocephalus, typically heralded by a decreased level of consciousness, may require ventriculostomy drainage.

STATUS EPILEPTICUS

(See also Chap. 445) Recurrent or relentless seizure activity is a medical emergency. Cessation of seizure activity is required to prevent irreversible neurologic injury. Lorazepam is the most effective benzodiazepine for treating status epilepticus and is the treatment of choice for controlling seizures acutely. Phenytoin or fosphenytoin should be given concomitantly since lorazepam has a short half-life. Other drugs, such as gabapentin, carbamazepine, and phenobarbital, should be reserved for patients with contraindications to phenytoin (e.g., allergy or pregnancy) or ongoing seizures despite phenytoin.

BRAIN DEATH

(See also Chap. 330) Although deaths of critically ill patients usually are attributable to irreversible cessation of circulatory and respiratory function, a diagnosis of death also may be established by irreversible cessation of all functions of the entire brain, including the brainstem, even if circulatory and respiratory functions remain intact on artificial life support. Such a diagnosis requires demonstration of the absence of cerebral function (no response to any external stimulus) and brainstem functions (e.g., unreactive pupils, lack of ocular movement in response to head turning or ice-water irrigation of ear canals, positive apnea test [no drive to breathe]). Absence of brain function must have an established cause and be permanent without possibility of recovery; a sedative effect, hypothermia, hypoxemia, neuromuscular paralysis, and severe hypotension must be ruled out. If there is uncertainty about the cause of coma, studies of cerebral blood flow and electroencephalography should be performed.

WITHHOLDING OR WITHDRAWING CARE

(See also Chap. 10) Withholding or withdrawal of care occurs commonly in the ICU setting. The Task Force on Ethics of the Society of Critical Care Medicine reported that it is ethically sound to withhold or withdraw care if a patient or the patient's surrogate makes such a request or if the physician judges that the goals of therapy are not achievable. Since all medical treatments are justified by their expected benefits, the loss of such an expectation justifies the act of withdrawing or withholding such treatment; these two actions are judged to be fundamentally similar. An underlying stipulation derived from this report is that an informed patient should have his or her wishes respected with regard to life-sustaining therapy. Implicit in this stipulation is the need to ensure that patients are thoroughly and accurately informed regarding the plausibility and expected results of various therapies.

The act of informing patients and/or surrogate decision-makers is the responsibility of the physician and other health care providers. If a patient or surrogate desires therapy deemed futile by the treating physician, the physician is not obligated ethically to provide such treatment. Rather, arrangements may be made to transfer the patient's care to another care provider. Whether the decision to withdraw life support should be initiated by the physician or left to surrogate decision-makers alone is not clear. One study reported that slightly more than half of surrogate decision-makers preferred to receive such a recommendation, whereas the rest did not. Critical care providers should meet regularly with patients and/or surrogates to discuss prognosis when the withholding or withdrawal of care is being considered. After a consensus among caregivers has been reached, this information should be relayed to the patient and/or surrogate decision-maker. If a decision to withhold or withdraw life-sustaining care for a patient has been made, aggressive attention to analgesia and anxiolysis is needed.

322 Acute Respiratory Distress Syndrome

Bruce D. Levy, Augustine M. K. Choi

Acute respiratory distress syndrome (ARDS) is a clinical syndrome of severe dyspnea of rapid onset, hypoxemia, and diffuse pulmonary infiltrates leading to respiratory failure. ARDS is caused by diffuse lung injury from many underlying medical and surgical disorders. The lung injury may be direct, as occurs in toxic inhalation, or indirect, as occurs in sepsis (Table 322-1). The clinical features of ARDS are listed in Table 322-2. By expert consensus, ARDS is defined by three categories based on the degrees of hypoxemia (Table 322-2). These stages of mild, moderate, and severe ARDS are associated with mortality risk and with the duration of mechanical ventilation in survivors.

The annual incidence of ARDS is estimated to be as high as 60 cases/100,000 population. Approximately 10% of all intensive care unit (ICU) admissions involve patients with acute respiratory failure; ~20% of these patients meet the criteria for ARDS.

ETIOLOGY

While many medical and surgical illnesses have been associated with the development of ARDS, most cases (>80%) are caused by a relatively small number of clinical disorders: severe sepsis syndrome and/or bacterial pneumonia (~40–50%), trauma, multiple transfusions, aspiration of gastric contents, and drug overdose. Among patients with trauma, the most frequently reported surgical conditions in ARDS are pulmonary contusion, multiple bone fractures, and chest wall trauma/flail chest, whereas head trauma, near-drowning, toxic inhalation, and burns are rare causes. The risks of developing ARDS are increased in patients with more than one predisposing medical or surgical condition.

Several other clinical variables have been associated with the development of ARDS. These include older age, chronic alcohol abuse, metabolic acidosis, and severity of critical illness. Trauma patients with an Acute Physiology and Chronic Health Evaluation (APACHE) II score ≥16 (Chap. 321) have a 2.5-fold increased risk of developing ARDS, and those with a score >20 have an incidence of ARDS that is more than threefold greater than the incidence among those with APACHE II scores ≤9.

TABLE 322-1 CLINICAL DISORDERS COMMONLY ASSOCIATED WITH ARDS

Direct Lung Injury	Indirect Lung Injury
Pneumonia	Sepsis
Aspiration of gastric contents	Severe trauma
Pulmonary contusion	Multiple bone fractures
Near-drowning	Flail chest
Toxic inhalation injury	Head trauma
	Burns
	Multiple transfusions
	Drug overdose
	Pancreatitis
	Postcardiopulmonary bypass

TABLE 322-2 DIAGNOSTIC CRITERIA FOR ARDS

Severity: Oxygenation	Onset	Chest Radiograph	Absence of Left Atrial Hypertension
Mild: 200 mmHg < Pao_2/Fio_2 ≤ 300 mmHg *Moderate:* 100 mmHg < Pao_2/Fio_2 ≤ 200 mmHg *Severe:* Pao_2/Fio_2 ≤ 100 mmHg	Acute	Bilateral alveolar or interstitial infiltrates	PCWP ≤18 mmHg *or* no clinical evidence of increased left atrial pressure

Abbreviations: ARDS, acute respiratory distress syndrome; Fio_2, inspired O_2 percentage; Pao_2, arterial partial pressure of O_2; PCWP, pulmonary capillary wedge pressure.

CLINICAL COURSE AND PATHOPHYSIOLOGY

The natural history of ARDS is marked by three phases—exudative, proliferative, and fibrotic—that each have characteristic clinical and pathologic features (Fig. 322-1).

Exudative Phase In this phase (Fig. 322-2), alveolar capillary endothelial cells and type I pneumocytes (alveolar epithelial cells) are injured, with consequent loss of the normally tight alveolar barrier to fluid and macromolecules. Edema fluid that is rich in protein accumulates in the interstitial and alveolar spaces. Significant concentrations of cytokines (e.g., interleukin 1, interleukin 8, and tumor necrosis factor α) and lipid mediators (e.g., leukotriene B_4) are present in the lung in this acute phase. In response to proinflammatory mediators, leukocytes (especially neutrophils) traffic into the pulmonary interstitium and alveoli. In addition, condensed plasma proteins aggregate in the air spaces with cellular debris and dysfunctional pulmonary surfactant to form hyaline membrane whorls. Pulmonary vascular injury also occurs early in ARDS, with vascular obliteration by microthrombi and fibrocellular proliferation (Fig. 322-3).

Alveolar edema predominantly involves *dependent* portions of the lung, with diminished aeration and atelectasis. Collapse of large sections of dependent lung markedly decreases lung compliance. Consequently, intrapulmonary shunting and hypoxemia develop and the work of breathing increases, leading to dyspnea. The pathophysiologic alterations in alveolar spaces are exacerbated by microvascular occlusion that results in reductions in pulmonary arterial blood flow to ventilated portions of the lung (and thus in increased dead space) and in pulmonary hypertension. Thus, in addition to severe hypoxemia, hypercapnia secondary to an increase in pulmonary dead space is prominent in early ARDS.

The exudative phase encompasses the first 7 days of illness after exposure to a precipitating ARDS risk factor, with the patient experiencing the onset of respiratory symptoms. Although usually presenting within 12–36 h after the initial insult, symptoms can be delayed by 5–7 days. Dyspnea develops, with a sensation of rapid shallow breathing

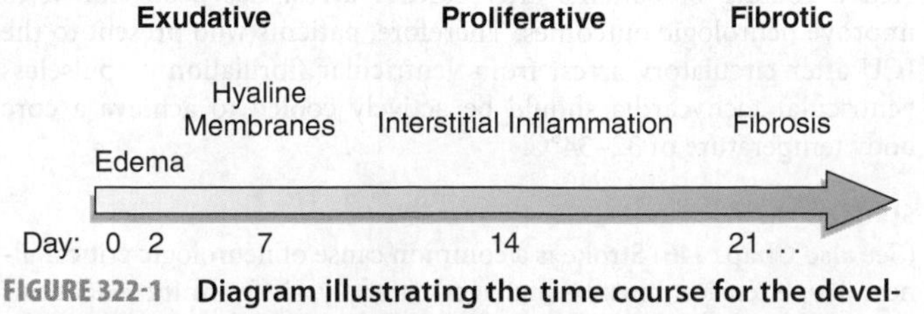

FIGURE 322-1 Diagram illustrating the time course for the development and resolution of ARDS. The exudative phase is notable for early alveolar edema and neutrophil-rich leukocytic infiltration of the lungs, with subsequent formation of hyaline membranes from diffuse alveolar damage. Within 7 days, a proliferative phase ensues with prominent interstitial inflammation and early fibrotic changes. Approximately 3 weeks after the initial pulmonary injury, most patients recover. However, some patients enter the fibrotic phase, with substantial fibrosis and bullae formation.

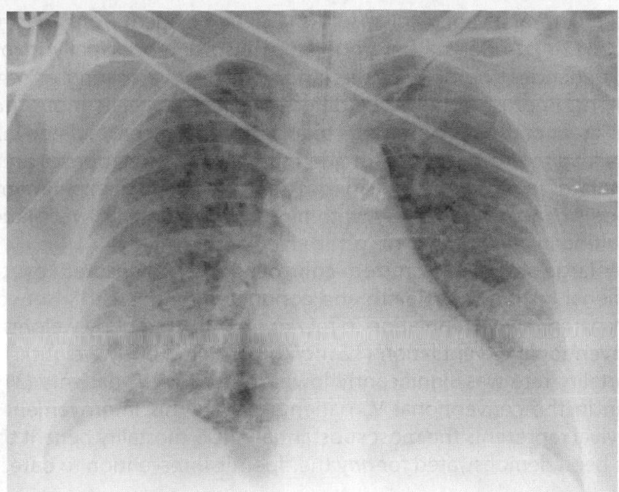

FIGURE 322-2 A representative anteroposterior chest x-ray in the exudative phase of ARDS shows diffuse interstitial and alveolar infiltrates that can be difficult to distinguish from left ventricular failure.

and an inability to get enough air. Tachypnea and increased work of breathing result frequently in respiratory fatigue and ultimately in respiratory failure. Laboratory values are generally nonspecific and are primarily indicative of underlying clinical disorders. The chest radiograph usually reveals alveolar and interstitial opacities involving at least three-quarters of the lung fields (Fig. 322-2). While characteristic for ARDS, these radiographic findings are not specific and can be indistinguishable from cardiogenic pulmonary edema (Chap. 326). Unlike the latter, however, the chest x-ray in ARDS rarely shows cardiomegaly, pleural effusions, or pulmonary vascular redistribution. Chest CT in ARDS reveals extensive heterogeneity of lung involvement (Fig. 322-4).

Because the early features of ARDS are nonspecific, alternative diagnoses must be considered. In the differential diagnosis of ARDS, the most common disorders are cardiogenic pulmonary edema, diffuse pneumonia, and alveolar hemorrhage. Less common diagnoses to consider include acute interstitial lung diseases (e.g., acute interstitial pneumonitis; Chap. 315), acute immunologic injury (e.g., hypersensitivity pneumonitis; Chap. 310), toxin injury (e.g., radiation pneumonitis; Chap. 263), and neurogenic pulmonary edema (Chap. 47e).

Proliferative Phase This phase of ARDS usually lasts from day 7 to day 21. Most patients recover rapidly and are liberated from mechanical

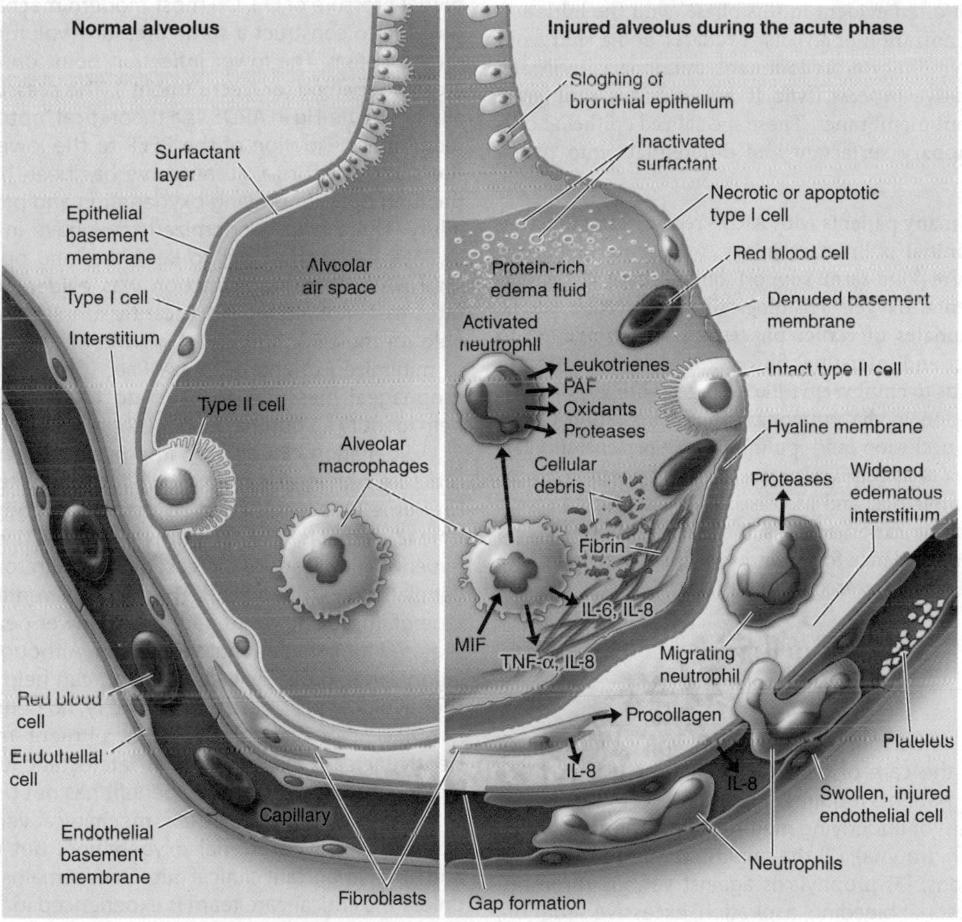

FIGURE 322-3 The normal alveolus (*left*) and the injured alveolus in the acute phase of acute lung injury and the acute respiratory distress syndrome (*right*). In the acute phase of the syndrome (*right*), there is sloughing of both the bronchial and alveolar epithelial cells, with the formation of protein-rich hyaline membranes on the denuded basement membrane. Neutrophils are shown adhering to the injured capillary endothelium and transmigrating through the interstitium into the air space, which is filled with protein-rich edema fluid. In the air space, an alveolar macrophage is secreting cytokines—i.e., interleukins 1, 6, 8, and 10 (IL-1, -6, -8, and -10) and tumor necrosis factor α (TNF-α)—that act locally to stimulate chemotaxis and activate neutrophils. Macrophages also secrete other cytokines, including IL-1, -6, and -10. IL-1 can also stimulate the production of extracellular matrix by fibroblasts. Neutrophils can release oxidants, proteases, leukotrienes, and other proinflammatory molecules, such as platelet-activating factor (PAF). A number of antiinflammatory mediators are also present in the alveolar milieu, including the IL-1-receptor antagonist, soluble TNF-α receptor, autoantibodies to IL-8, and cytokines such as IL-10 and IL-11 (not shown). The influx of protein-rich edema fluid into the alveolus has led to the inactivation of surfactant. MIF, macrophage inhibitory factor. *(From LB Ware, MA Matthay: N Engl J Med 342:1334, 2000, with permission.)*

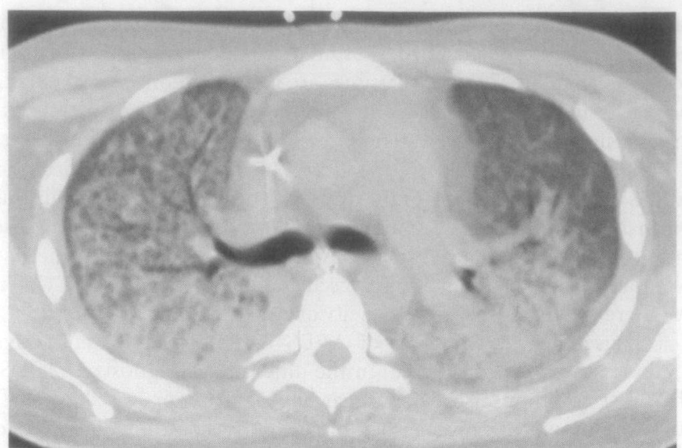

FIGURE 322-4 A representative CT scan of the chest during the exudative phase of ARDS, in which *dependent* alveolar edema and atelectasis predominate.

ventilation during this phase. Despite this improvement, many patients still experience dyspnea, tachypnea, and hypoxemia. Some patients develop progressive lung injury and early changes of pulmonary fibrosis during the proliferative phase. Histologically, the first signs of resolution are often evident in this phase, with the initiation of lung repair, the organization of alveolar exudates, and a shift from a neutrophil- to a lymphocyte-predominant pulmonary infiltrate. As part of the reparative process, type II pneumocytes proliferate along alveolar basement membranes. These specialized epithelial cells synthesize new pulmonary surfactant and differentiate into type I pneumocytes.

Fibrotic Phase While many patients with ARDS recover lung function 3–4 weeks after the initial pulmonary injury, some enter a fibrotic phase that may require long-term support on mechanical ventilators and/or supplemental oxygen. Histologically, the alveolar edema and inflammatory exudates of earlier phases are now converted to extensive alveolar-duct and interstitial fibrosis. Marked disruption of acinar architecture leads to emphysema-like changes, with large bullae. Intimal fibroproliferation in the pulmonary microcirculation causes progressive vascular occlusion and pulmonary hypertension. The physiologic consequences include an increased risk of pneumothorax, reductions in lung compliance, and increased pulmonary dead space. Patients in this late phase experience a substantial burden of excess morbidity. Lung biopsy evidence for pulmonary fibrosis in any phase of ARDS is associated with increased mortality risk.

TREATMENT ACUTE RESPIRATORY DISTRESS SYNDROME

GENERAL PRINCIPLES

Recent reductions in ARDS mortality rates are largely the result of general advances in the care of critically ill patients (Chap. 321). Thus, caring for these patients requires close attention to (1) the recognition and treatment of underlying medical and surgical disorders (e.g., sepsis, aspiration, trauma); (2) the minimization of procedures and their complications; (3) prophylaxis against venous thromboembolism, gastrointestinal bleeding, aspiration, excessive sedation, and central venous catheter infections; (4) prompt recognition of nosocomial infections; and (5) provision of adequate nutrition.

MANAGEMENT OF MECHANICAL VENTILATION

(See also Chap. 323) Patients meeting clinical criteria for ARDS frequently become fatigued from increased work of breathing and progressive hypoxemia, requiring mechanical ventilation for support.

Ventilator-Induced Lung Injury Despite its life-saving potential, mechanical ventilation can aggravate lung injury. Experimental models have demonstrated that ventilator-induced lung injury appears to require two processes: repeated alveolar overdistention and recurrent alveolar collapse. As is clearly evident from chest CT (Fig. 322-4), ARDS is a heterogeneous disorder, principally involving dependent portions of the lung with relative sparing of other regions. Because compliance differs in affected versus more "normal" areas of the lung, attempts to fully inflate the consolidated lung may lead to overdistention of and injury to the more normal areas. Ventilator-induced injury can be demonstrated in experimental models of acute lung injury, with high-tidal-volume (V_T) ventilation resulting in additional, synergistic alveolar damage.

A large-scale, randomized controlled trial sponsored by the National Institutes of Health and conducted by the ARDS Network compared low V_T ventilation (6 mL/kg of predicted body weight) to conventional V_T ventilation (12 mL/kg predicted body weight). The mortality rate was significantly lower in the low V_T patients (31%) than in the conventional V_T patients (40%). This improvement in survival represents the most substantial ARDS-mortality benefit that has been demonstrated for *any* therapeutic intervention to date.

Prevention of Alveolar Collapse In ARDS, the presence of alveolar and interstitial fluid and the loss of surfactant can lead to a marked reduction of lung compliance. Without an increase in end-expiratory pressure, significant alveolar collapse can occur at end-expiration, with consequent impairment of oxygenation. In most clinical settings, positive end-expiratory pressure (PEEP) is empirically set to minimize F_{IO_2} (inspired O_2 percentage) and maximize Pa_{O_2} (arterial partial pressure of O_2). On most modern mechanical ventilators, it is possible to construct a static pressure–volume curve for the respiratory system. The lower inflection point on the curve represents alveolar opening (or "recruitment"). The pressure at this point, usually 12–15 mmHg in ARDS, is a theoretical "optimal PEEP" for alveolar recruitment. Titration of the PEEP to the lower inflection point on the static pressure–volume curve has been hypothesized to keep the lung open, improving oxygenation and protecting against lung injury. Three large randomized trials have investigated the utility of PEEP-based strategies to keep the lung open. In all three trials, improvement in lung function was evident but overall mortality rates were not altered significantly. Until more data become available on the clinical utility of high PEEP, it is advisable to set PEEP to minimize F_{IO_2} and optimize Pa_{O_2} (Chap. 323). Measurement of esophageal pressures to estimate transpulmonary pressure may help identify an optimal PEEP in some cases.

Oxygenation can also be improved by increasing mean airway pressure with *inverse-ratio ventilation*. In this technique, the inspiratory time (*I*) is lengthened so that it is longer than the expiratory time (*E*)— that is, *I:E* > 1:1. With diminished time to exhale, dynamic hyperinflation leads to increased end-expiratory pressure, similar to ventilator-prescribed PEEP. This mode of ventilation has the advantage of improving oxygenation with lower peak pressures than are required for conventional ventilation. Although inverse-ratio ventilation can improve oxygenation and can help reduce F_{IO_2} to ≤0.60, thus avoiding possible oxygen toxicity, no benefit in ARDS mortality risk has been demonstrated. Recruitment maneuvers that transiently increase PEEP to "recruit" atelectatic lung can also increase oxygenation, but a mortality benefit has not been established.

In several randomized trials, mechanical ventilation in the prone position improved arterial oxygenation, but its effect on survival and other important clinical outcomes remains uncertain. Moreover, unless the critical-care team is experienced in "proning," repositioning critically ill patients can be hazardous, leading to accidental endotracheal extubation, loss of central venous catheters, and orthopedic injury.

OTHER STRATEGIES IN MECHANICAL VENTILATION

Several additional mechanical-ventilation strategies that use specialized equipment have been tested in ARDS patients; most of these approaches have had mixed or disappointing results in adults. *High-frequency ventilation* (HFV) entails ventilating at extremely high respiratory rates (5–20 cycles per second) and low V_Ts (1–2 mL/kg). Use of *partial liquid ventilation* (PLV) with perfluorocarbon—an inert, high-density liquid that easily solubilizes oxygen and carbon dioxide—has yielded promising preliminary results, enhancing pulmonary function in patients with ARDS, but also has provided no survival benefit. *Lung-replacement therapy with extracorporeal membrane oxygenation* (ECMO), which provides a clear survival benefit in neonatal respiratory distress syndrome, may also have utility in selected adult patients with ARDS.

Data supporting the efficacy of "adjunctive" ventilator therapies (e.g., high PEEP, inverse ratio ventilation, recruitment maneuvers, prone positioning, HFV, ECMO, and PLV) remain incomplete. Accordingly, these modalities are reserved for use as rescue rather than primary therapies.

FLUID MANAGEMENT

(See also Chap. 321) Increased pulmonary vascular permeability leading to interstitial and alveolar edema fluid rich in protein is a central feature of ARDS. In addition, impaired vascular integrity augments the normal increase in extravascular lung water that occurs with increasing left atrial pressure. Maintaining a low left atrial filling pressure minimizes pulmonary edema and prevents further decrements in arterial oxygenation and lung compliance; improves pulmonary mechanics; shortens ICU stay and the duration of mechanical ventilation; and is associated with a lower mortality rate in both medical and surgical ICU patients. Thus, aggressive attempts to reduce left atrial filling pressures with fluid restriction and diuretics should be an important aspect of ARDS management, limited only by hypotension and hypoperfusion of critical organs such as the kidneys.

NEUROMUSCULAR BLOCKADE

In severe ARDS, sedation alone can be inadequate for the patient-ventilator synchrony required for lung-protective ventilation. This clinical problem was recently addressed in a multicenter, randomized, placebo-controlled trial of early neuromuscular blockade (with cisatracurium besylate) for 48 h. In severe ARDS, early neuromuscular blockade increased the rate of survival and ventilator-free days without increasing ICU-acquired paresis. These promising findings support the early administration of neuromuscular blockade if needed to facilitate mechanical ventilation in severe ARDS; however, these results must be replicated prior to their widespread application in clinical practice.

GLUCOCORTICOIDS

Many attempts have been made to treat both early and late ARDS with glucocorticoids, with the goal of reducing potentially deleterious pulmonary inflammation. Few studies have shown any benefit. Current evidence does *not* support the use of high-dose glucocorticoids in the care of ARDS patients.

OTHER THERAPIES

Clinical trials of surfactant replacement and multiple other medical therapies have proved disappointing. Inhaled nitric oxide and inhaled epoprostenol sodium can transiently improve oxygenation but do not improve survival or decrease time on mechanical ventilation.

RECOMMENDATIONS

Many clinical trials have been undertaken to improve the outcome of patients with ARDS; most have been unsuccessful in modifying the natural history. While results of large clinical trials must be judiciously applied to *individual* patients, evidence-based recommendations are summarized in **Table 322-3**, and an algorithm for the initial therapeutic goals and limits in ARDS management is provided in **Fig. 322-5**.

PROGNOSIS

Mortality Recent mortality estimates for ARDS range from 26% to 44%. There is substantial variability, but a trend toward improved ARDS outcomes appears evident. Of interest, mortality in ARDS is largely attributable to nonpulmonary causes, with sepsis and nonpulmonary organ failure accounting for >80% of deaths. Thus, improvement in survival is likely secondary to advances in the care of septic/infected patients and those with multiple organ failure **(Chap. 321)**.

The major risk factors for ARDS mortality are nonpulmonary. Advanced age is an important risk factor. Patients >75 years of age have a substantially higher mortality risk (~60%) than those <45 (~20%). Moreover, patients >60 years of age with ARDS and sepsis have a threefold higher mortality risk than those <60. Other risk factors include preexisting organ dysfunction from chronic medical illness—in particular, chronic liver disease, cirrhosis, chronic alcohol abuse, chronic immunosuppression, sepsis, chronic renal disease, failure of any nonpulmonary organ, and increased APACHE III scores **(Chap. 321)**. Patients with ARDS arising from direct lung injury (including pneumonia, pulmonary contusion, and aspiration;

TABLE 322-3 EVIDENCE-BASED RECOMMENDATIONS FOR ARDS THERAPIES

Treatment	Recommendation[a]
Mechanical ventilation	
Low tidal volume	A
Minimized left atrial filling pressures	B
High-PEEP or "open lung"	C
Prone position	C
Recruitment maneuvers	C
High-frequency ventilation	D
ECMO	C
Early neuromuscular blockade	A
Glucocorticoid treatment	D
Surfactant replacement, inhaled NO, inhaled epoprostenol, and other anti-inflammatory therapy (e.g., ketoconazole, PGE1, NSAIDs)	D

[a]Key: A, recommended therapy based on strong clinical evidence from randomized clinical trials; B, recommended therapy based on supportive but limited clinical data; C, recommended only as alternative therapy on the basis of indeterminate evidence; D, not recommended on the basis of clinical evidence against efficacy of therapy.

Abbreviations: ARDS, acute respiratory distress syndrome; ECMO, extracorporeal membrane oxygenation; NO, nitric oxide; NSAIDs, nonsteroidal anti-inflammatory drugs; PEEP, positive end-expiratory pressure; PGE1, prostaglandin E_1.

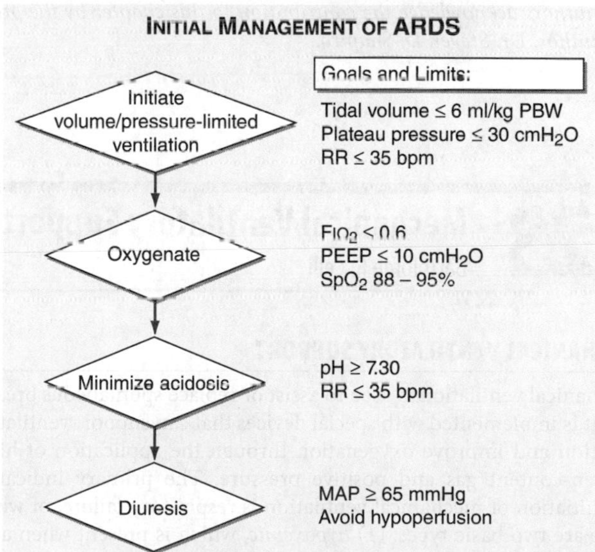

FIGURE 322-5 Algorithm for the initial management of ARDS. Clinical trials have provided evidence-based therapeutic goals for a stepwise approach to the early mechanical ventilation, oxygenation, and correction of acidosis and diuresis of critically ill patients with ARDS. FIO_2, inspired O_2 percentage; MAP, mean arterial pressure; PBW, predicted body weight; PEEP, positive end expiratory pressure; RR, respiratory rate; SpO_2, arterial oxyhemoglobin saturation measured by pulse oximetry.

Table 322-1) are nearly twice as likely to die as those with indirect causes of lung injury, while surgical and trauma patients with ARDS—especially those without direct lung injury—have a higher survival rate than other ARDS patients.

An early (within 24 h of presentation) elevation in pulmonary dead space (>0.60) and severe arterial hypoxemia (Pao_2/Fio_2, <100 mmHg) predict increased mortality risk from ARDS; however, there is surprisingly little additional value in predicting ARDS mortality from other measures of the severity of lung injury, including the level of PEEP (≥10 cm H_2O), respiratory system compliance (≤40 mL/cm H_2O), the extent of alveolar infiltrates on chest radiography, and the corrected expired volume per minute (≥10 L/min).

Functional Recovery in ARDS Survivors While it is common for patients with ARDS to experience prolonged respiratory failure and remain dependent on mechanical ventilation for survival, it is a testament to the resolving powers of the lung that the majority of patients recover nearly normal lung function. Patients usually recover maximal lung function within 6 months. One year after endotracheal extubation, more than one-third of ARDS survivors have normal spirometry values and diffusion capacity. Most of the remaining patients have only mild abnormalities in pulmonary function. Unlike mortality risk, recovery of lung function is strongly associated with the extent of lung injury in early ARDS. Low static respiratory compliance, high levels of required PEEP, longer durations of mechanical ventilation, and high lung injury scores are all associated with less recovery of pulmonary function. Of note, when physical function is assessed 5 years after ARDS, exercise limitation and decreased physical quality of life are often documented despite normal or nearly normal pulmonary function. When caring for ARDS survivors, it is important to be aware of the potential for a substantial burden of psychological problems in patients and family caregivers, including significant rates of depression and posttraumatic stress disorder.

WEBSITES

ARDS Support Center for patient-oriented education: *www.ards.org*
NHLBI ARDS Clinical Trials information: *www.ardsnet.org*
ARDS Foundation: *www.ardsusa.org*

Acknowledgment

The authors acknowledge the contribution to this chapter by the previous author, Dr. Steven D. Shapiro.

323 Mechanical Ventilatory Support

Bartolome R. Celli

MECHANICAL VENTILATORY SUPPORT

Mechanical ventilation is used to assist or replace spontaneous breathing. It is implemented with special devices that can support ventilatory function and improve oxygenation through the application of high-oxygen-content gas and positive pressure. The primary indication for initiation of mechanical ventilation is respiratory failure, of which there are two basic types: (1) *hypoxemic*, which is present when arterial O_2 saturation (Sao_2) <90% occurs despite an increased inspired O_2 fraction and usually results from ventilation-perfusion mismatch or shunt; and (2) *hypercarbic*, which is characterized by elevated arterial carbon dioxide partial pressure (PCO_2) values (usually >50 mmHg) resulting from conditions that decrease minute ventilation or increase physiologic dead space such that alveolar ventilation is inadequate to meet metabolic demands. When respiratory failure is chronic, neither of the two types is obligatorily treated with mechanical ventilation, but when it is acute, mechanical ventilation may be lifesaving.

INDICATIONS

The most common reasons for instituting mechanical ventilation are acute respiratory failure with hypoxemia (acute respiratory distress syndrome, heart failure with pulmonary edema, pneumonia, sepsis, complications of surgery and trauma), which accounts for ~65% of all ventilated cases, and hypercarbic ventilatory failure—e.g., due to coma (15%), exacerbations of chronic obstructive pulmonary disease (COPD; 13%), and neuromuscular diseases (5%). The primary objectives of mechanical ventilation are to decrease the work of breathing, thus avoiding respiratory muscle fatigue, and to reverse life-threatening hypoxemia and progressive respiratory acidosis.

In some cases, mechanical ventilation is used as an adjunct to other forms of therapy. For example, it is used to reduce cerebral blood flow in patients with increased intracranial pressure. Mechanical ventilation also is used frequently in conjunction with endotracheal intubation for airway protection to prevent aspiration of gastric contents in otherwise unstable patients during gastric lavage for suspected drug overdose or during gastrointestinal endoscopy. In critically ill patients, intubation and mechanical ventilation may be indicated before the performance of essential diagnostic or therapeutic studies if it appears that respiratory failure may occur during those maneuvers.

TYPES OF MECHANICAL VENTILATION

There are two basic methods of mechanical ventilation: noninvasive ventilation (NIV) and invasive (or conventional mechanical) ventilation (MV).

Noninvasive Ventilation NIV has gained acceptance because it is effective in certain conditions, such as acute or chronic respiratory failure, and is associated with fewer complications—namely, pneumonia and tracheolaryngeal trauma. NIV usually is provided with a tight-fitting face mask or nasal mask similar to the masks traditionally used for treatment of sleep apnea. NIV has proved highly effective in patients with respiratory failure arising from acute exacerbations of chronic obstructive pulmonary disease. It is most frequently implemented as bilevel positive airway pressure ventilation or pressure-support ventilation. Both modes, which apply a preset positive pressure during inspiration and a lower pressure during expiration at the mask, are well tolerated by a conscious patient and optimize patient-ventilator synchrony. The major limitation to the widespread application of NIV has been patient intolerance: the tight-fitting mask required for NIV can cause both physical and psychological discomfort. In addition, NIV has had limited success in patients with acute hypoxemic respiratory failure, for whom endotracheal intubation and conventional MV remain the ventilatory method of choice.

The most important group of patients who benefit from a trial of NIV are those with exacerbations of COPD and respiratory acidosis (pH <7.35). Experience from several randomized trials has shown that, in patients with ventilatory failure characterized by blood pH levels between 7.25 and 7.35, NIV is associated with low failure rates (15–20%) and good outcomes (as judged by intubation rate, length of stay in intensive care, and—in some series—mortality rates). In more severely ill patients with a blood pH <7.25, the rate of NIV failure is inversely related to the severity of respiratory acidosis, with higher failure rates as the pH decreases. In patients with milder acidosis (pH >7.35), NIV is not better than conventional treatment that includes controlled oxygen delivery and pharmacotherapy for exacerbations of COPD (systemic glucocorticoids, bronchodilators, and, if needed, antibiotics).

Despite its benign outcomes, NIV is not useful in the majority of cases of respiratory failure and is contraindicated in patients with the conditions listed in Table 323-1. NIV can delay lifesaving ventilatory support in those cases and, in fact, can actually result in aspiration or hypoventilation. Once NIV is initiated, patients should be monitored; a reduction in respiratory frequency and a decrease in the use of accessory muscles (scalene, sternomastoid, and intercostals) are good clinical indicators of adequate therapeutic benefit. Arterial blood gases should be determined at least within hours of the initiation of therapy to ensure that NIV is having the desired effect. Lack of benefit within

TABLE 323-1 CONTRAINDICATIONS FOR NONINVASIVE VENTILATION

Cardiac or respiratory arrest
Severe encephalopathy
Severe gastrointestinal bleed
Hemodynamic instability
Unstable angina and myocardial infarction
Facial surgery or trauma
Upper airway obstruction
High-risk aspiration and/or inability to protect airways
Inability to clear secretions

that time frame should alert the physician to the possible need for conventional MV.

Conventional Mechanical Ventilation Conventional MV is implemented once a cuffed tube is inserted into the trachea to allow conditioned gas (warmed, oxygenated, and humidified) to be delivered to the airways and lungs at pressures above atmospheric pressure. Care should be taken during intubation to avoid brain-damaging hypoxia. In most cases, the administration of mild sedation may facilitate the procedure. Opiates and benzodiazepines are good choices but can have a deleterious effect on hemodynamics in patients with depressed cardiac function or low systemic vascular resistance. Morphine can promote histamine release from tissue mast cells and may worsen bronchospasm in patients with asthma; fentanyl, sufentanil, and alfentanil are acceptable alternatives. Ketamine may increase systemic arterial pressure and has been associated with hallucinatory responses. The shorter-acting agents etomidate and propofol have been used for both induction and maintenance of anesthesia in ventilated patients because they have fewer adverse hemodynamic effects, but both are significantly more expensive than older agents. Great care must be taken to avoid the use of neuromuscular paralysis during intubation of patients with renal failure, tumor lysis syndrome, crush injuries, medical conditions associated with elevated serum potassium levels, and muscular dystrophy syndromes, in particular, the use of agents whose mechanism of action includes depolarization at the neuromuscular junction, such as succinylcholine chloride, must be avoided.

PRINCIPLES OF MECHANICAL VENTILATION

Once the patient has been intubated, the basic goals of MV are *to optimize oxygenation while avoiding ventilator-induced lung injury due to overstretch and collapse/re-recruitment*. This concept, known as the "protective ventilatory strategy" (see below and Fig. 323-1) is supported by evidence linking high airway pressures and volumes and overstretching of the lung as well as collapse/re-recruitment to poor clinical outcomes (barotrauma and volume trauma). Although normalization of pH through elimination of CO_2 is desirable, the risk of lung damage associated with the large volume and high pressures needed to achieve this goal has led to the acceptance of permissive hypercapnia. This condition is well tolerated when care is taken to avoid excess acidosis by pH buffering.

MODES OF VENTILATION

Mode refers to the manner in which ventilator breaths are triggered, cycled, and limited. The *trigger*, either an inspiratory effort or a time-based signal, defines what the ventilator senses to initiate an assisted breath. *Cycle* refers to the factors that determine the end of inspiration. For example, in volume-cycled ventilation, inspiration ends when a specific tidal volume is delivered. Other types of cycling include pressure cycling and time cycling. The *limiting factors* are operator-specified values, such as airway pressure, that are monitored by transducers internal to the ventilator circuit throughout the respiratory cycle; if the specified values are exceeded, inspiratory flow is terminated, and the ventilator circuit is vented to atmospheric pressure or the specified pressure at the end of expiration (positive end-expiratory pressure, or PEEP). Most patients are ventilated with assist-control ventilation,

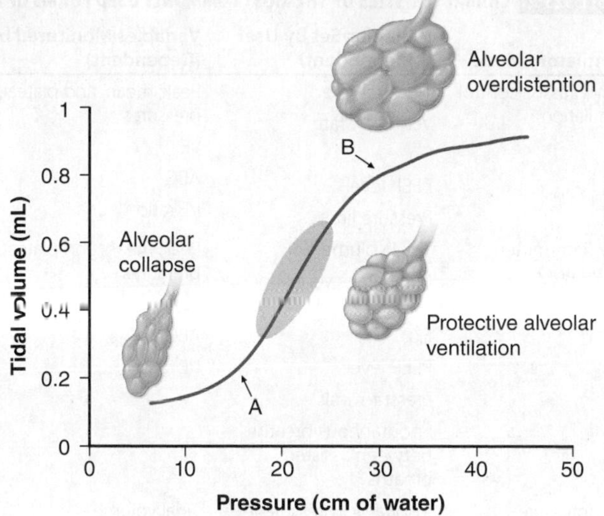

FIGURE 323-1 Hypothetical pressure-volume curve of the lung in a patient undergoing mechanical ventilation. Alveoli tend to close if the distending pressure falls below the lower inflection point (***A***), whereas they overstretch if the pressure within them is higher than that of the upper inflection point (***B***). Collapse and opening of ventilated alveoli are associated with poor outcomes in patients with acute respiratory failure. Protective ventilation (*purple shaded area*), using a lower tidal volume (6 mL/kg of ideal body weight) and maintaining positive end-expiratory pressure to prevent overstretching and collapse/opening of alveoli, has resulted in improved survival rates among patients receiving mechanical ventilatory support.

intermittent mandatory ventilation, or pressure-support ventilation, with the latter two modes often used simultaneously (Table 323-2).

Assist-Control Ventilation (ACMV) ACMV is the most widely used mode of ventilation. In this mode, an inspiratory cycle is initiated either by the patient's inspiratory effort or, if none is detected within a specified time window, by a timer signal within the ventilator. Every breath delivered, whether patient- or timer-triggered, consists of the operator-specified tidal volume. Ventilatory rate is determined either by the patient or by the operator-specified backup rate, whichever is of higher frequency. ACMV is commonly used for initiation of mechanical ventilation because it ensures a backup minute ventilation in the absence of an intact respiratory drive and allows for synchronization of the ventilator cycle with the patient's inspiratory effort.

Problems can arise when ACMV is used in patients with tachypnea due to nonrespiratory or nonmetabolic factors, such as anxiety, pain, and airway irritation. Respiratory alkalemia may develop and trigger myoclonus or seizures. Dynamic hyperinflation leading to increased intrathoracic pressures (so-called auto-PEEP) may occur if the patient's respiratory mechanics are such that inadequate time is available for complete exhalation between inspiratory cycles. Auto-PEEP can limit venous return, decrease cardiac output, and increase airway pressures, predisposing to barotrauma.

Intermittent Mandatory Ventilation (IMV) With this mode, the operator sets the number of mandatory breaths of fixed volume to be delivered by the ventilator; between those breaths, the patient can breathe spontaneously. In the most frequently used synchronized mode (SIMV), mandatory breaths are delivered in synchrony with the patient's inspiratory efforts at a frequency determined by the operator. If the patient fails to initiate a breath, the ventilator delivers a fixed-tidal-volume breath and resets the internal timer for the next inspiratory cycle. SIMV differs from ACMV in that only a preset number of breaths are ventilator-assisted.

SIMV allows patients with an intact respiratory drive to exercise inspiratory muscles between assisted breaths; thus it is useful for both supporting and weaning intubated patients. SIMV may be difficult to

TABLE 323-2 CHARACTERISTICS OF THE MOST COMMONLY USED FORMS OF MECHANICAL VENTILATION

Ventilatory Mode	Variables Set by User (Independent)	Variables Monitored by User (Dependent)	Trigger Cycle Limit	Advantages	Disadvantages
ACMV (assist-control ventilation)	Tidal volume Ventilator rate FIO_2 PEEP level Pressure limit	Peak, mean, and plateau airway pressures VE ABG I/E ratio	Patient effort Timer Pressure limit	Patient control Guaranteed ventilation	Potential hyperventilation Barotrauma and volume trauma Every effective breath generates a ventilator volume
IMV (intermittent mandatory ventilation)	Tidal volume Mandatory ventilator rate FIO_2 PEEP level Pressure limit Spontaneous breaths between assisted breaths	Peak, mean, and plateau airway pressures VE ABG I/E ratio	Patient effort Timer Pressure limit	Patient control Comfort from spontaneous breaths Guaranteed ventilation	Potential dysynchrony Potential hypoventilation
PSV (pressure-support ventilation)	Inspiratory pressure level FIO_2 PEEP Pressure limit	Tidal volume Respiratory rate VE ABG	Pressure limit Inspiratory flow	Patient control Comfort Assures synchrony	No timer backup Potential hypoventilation
NIV (noninvasive ventilation)	Inspiratory and expiratory pressure level FIO_2	Tidal volume Respiratory rate VE ABG	Pressure limit Inspiratory flow	Patient control	Mask interface may cause discomfort and facial bruising Leaks are common Hypoventilation

Abbreviations: ABG, arterial blood gases; FIO_2, fraction of inspired oxygen; PEEP, positive end-expiratory pressure; I/E, inspiratory to expiratory time ratio; VE, minute ventilation.

use in patients with tachypnea because they may attempt to exhale during the ventilator-programmed inspiratory cycle. Consequently, the airway pressure may exceed the inspiratory pressure limit, the ventilator-assisted breath will be aborted, and minute volume may drop below that programmed by the operator. In this setting, if the tachypnea represents a response to respiratory or metabolic acidosis, a change in ACMV will increase minute ventilation and help normalize the pH while the underlying process is further evaluated and treated.

Pressure-Support Ventilation (PSV) This form of ventilation is patient-triggered, flow-cycled, and pressure-limited. It provides graded assistance and differs from the other two modes in that the operator sets the pressure level (rather than the volume) to augment every spontaneous respiratory effort. The level of pressure is adjusted by observing the patient's respiratory frequency. During PSV, the inspiration is terminated when inspiratory airflow falls below a certain level; in most ventilators, this flow rate cannot be adjusted by the operator. With PSV, patients receive ventilator assistance only when the ventilator detects an inspiratory effort. PSV is often used in combination with SIMV to ensure volume-cycled backup for patients whose respiratory drive is depressed. PSV is well tolerated by most patients who are being weaned from MV; PSV parameters can be set to provide full ventilatory support and can be withdrawn to load the respiratory muscles gradually.

Other Modes of Ventilation There are other modes of ventilation, each with its own acronym and each with specific modifications of the manner and duration in which pressure is applied to the airway and lungs and of the interaction between the mechanical assistance provided by the ventilator and the patient's respiratory effort. Although their use in acute respiratory failure is limited, the following modes have been used with varying levels of enthusiasm and adoption.

PRESSURE-CONTROL VENTILATION (PCV) This form of ventilation is time-triggered, time-cycled, and pressure-limited. A specified pressure is imposed at the airway opening throughout inspiration. Since the inspiratory pressure is specified by the operator, tidal volume and inspiratory flow rate are *dependent*, rather than *independent*, variables and are not operator-specified. PCV is the preferred mode of ventilation for patients in whom it is desirable to regulate peak airway pressures, such as those with preexisting barotrauma, and for post-thoracic surgery patients, in whom the shear forces across a fresh suture line should be limited. When PCV is used, minute ventilation is altered through changes in rate or in the pressure-control value, with consequent changes in tidal volume.

INVERSE-RATIO VENTILATION (IRV) This mode is a variant of PCV that incorporates the use of a prolonged inspiratory time with the appropriate shortening of the expiratory time. IRV has been used in patients with severe hypoxemic respiratory failure. This approach increases mean distending pressures without increasing peak airway pressures. It is thought to work in conjunction with PEEP to open collapsed alveoli and improve oxygenation. However, no clinical-trial data have shown that IRV improves outcomes.

CONTINUOUS POSITIVE AIRWAY PRESSURE (CPAP) CPAP is not a true support mode of ventilation because all ventilation occurs through the patient's spontaneous efforts. The ventilator provides fresh gas to the breathing circuit with each inspiration and sets the circuit to a constant, operator-specified pressure. CPAP is used to assess extubation potential in patients who have been effectively weaned and who require little ventilatory support and in patients with intact respiratory system function who require an endotracheal tube for airway protection.

Nonconventional Ventilatory Strategies Several nonconventional strategies have been evaluated for their ability to improve oxygenation and reduce mortality rates in patients with advanced hypoxemic respiratory failure. These strategies include high-frequency oscillatory ventilation (HFOV), airway pressure release ventilation (APRV), extracorporeal membrane oxygenation (ECMO), and partial liquid ventilation (PLV) using perfluorocarbons. Although case reports and small uncontrolled cohort studies have shown benefit, randomized controlled trials have failed to demonstrate consistent improvements in outcome with most of these strategies. A recent randomized trial of ECMO documented positive outcomes, but the technique remains controversial because older studies failed to document positive results. Currently, these approaches should be thought of as "salvage" techniques and considered for patients with hypoxemia refractory to conventional therapy. Prone positioning of patients with refractory hypoxemia has also been explored because, in theory, lying prone should improve ventilation-perfusion matching. Several randomized trials in patients with acute lung injury did not demonstrate a survival advantage with prone positioning despite demonstration of a transient physiologic benefit. The administration of nitric oxide gas, which has bronchodilator and pulmonary vasodilator effects when delivered through the airways and improves arterial oxygenation in many patients with advanced hypoxemic respiratory failure, also failed to improve outcomes in these patients with acute lung injury.

The design of new ventilator modes reflect attempts to improve patient-ventilator synchrony—a major practical issue during MV—by allowing patients to trigger the ventilator with their own effort while also incorporating flow algorithms that terminate the cycles once certain preset criteria are reached; this approach has greatly improved patient comfort. New modes of ventilation that synchronize not only the timing but also the levels of assistance to match the patient's effort have been developed. Proportional assist ventilation (PAV) and neurally adjusted ventilatory-assist ventilation (NAV) are two modes that are designed to deliver assisted breaths through algorithms incorporating not only pressure, volume, and time but also overall respiratory resistance as well as compliance (in the case of PAV) and neural activation of the diaphragm (in the case of NAV). Although these modes enhance patient-ventilator synchrony, their practical use in the everyday management of patients undergoing MV needs further study.

PROTECTIVE VENTILATORY STRATEGY

Whichever mode of MV is used in acute respiratory failure, the evidence from several important controlled trials indicates that a protective ventilation approach guided by the following principles (and summarized in Fig. 323-1) is safe and offers the best chance of a good outcome: (1) Set a target tidal volume close to 6 mL/kg of ideal body weight. (2) Prevent plateau pressure (static pressure in the airway at the end of inspiration) exceeding 30 cm H_2O. (3) Use the lowest possible fraction of inspired oxygen (FIO_2) to keep the SaO_2 at ≥90%. (4) Adjust the PEEP to maintain alveolar patency while preventing overdistention and closure/reopening. With the application of these techniques, the mortality rate among patients with acute hypoxemic respiratory failure has decreased to ~30% from close to 50% a decade ago.

PATIENT MANAGEMENT

Once the patient has been stabilized with respect to gas exchange, definitive therapy for the underlying process responsible for respiratory failure is initiated. Subsequent modifications in ventilator therapy must be provided in parallel with changes in the patient's clinical status. As improvement in respiratory function is noted, the first priority is to reduce the level of mechanical ventilatory support. Patients on full ventilatory support should be monitored frequently, with the goal of switching to a mode that allows for weaning as soon as possible. Protocols and guidelines that can be applied by paramedical personnel when physicians are not readily available have proved to be of value in shortening ventilator and intensive care unit (ICU) time, with very good outcomes. Patients whose condition continues to deteriorate after ventilatory support is initiated may require increased O_2, PEEP, or one of the alternative modes of ventilation.

GENERAL SUPPORT DURING VENTILATION

Patients for whom mechanical ventilation has been initiated usually require sedation and analgesia to maintain an acceptable level of comfort. Often, this treatment consists of a combination of a benzodiazepine and an opiate administered intravenously. Medications commonly used for this purpose include lorazepam, midazolam, diazepam, morphine, and fentanyl. Oversedation must be avoided in the ICU because most (but not all) studies show that daily interruption of sedation in patients with improved ventilatory status results in a shorter time on the ventilator and a shorter ICU stay.

Immobilized patients receiving mechanical ventilatory support are at risk for deep venous thrombosis and decubitus ulcers. Venous thrombosis should be prevented with the use of subcutaneous heparin and/or pneumatic compression boots. Fractionated low-molecular-weight heparin appears to be equally effective for this purpose. To help prevent decubitus ulcers, frequent changes in body position and the use of soft mattress overlays and air mattresses are employed. Prophylaxis against diffuse gastrointestinal mucosal injury is indicated for patients undergoing MV. Histamine-receptor (H_2-receptor) antagonists, antacids, and cytoprotective agents such as sucralfate have all been used for this purpose and appear to be effective. Nutritional support by enteral feeding through either a nasogastric or an orogastric tube should be initiated and maintained whenever possible. Delayed gastric emptying is common in critically ill patients taking sedative medications but often responds to promotility agents such as metoclopramide. Parenteral nutrition is an alternative to enteral nutrition in patients with severe gastrointestinal pathology who need prolonged MV.

COMPLICATIONS OF MECHANICAL VENTILATION

Endotracheal intubation and mechanical ventilation have direct and indirect effects on the lung and upper airways, the cardiovascular system, and the gastrointestinal system. Pulmonary complications include barotrauma, nosocomial pneumonia, oxygen toxicity, tracheal stenosis, and deconditioning of respiratory muscles. Barotrauma and volutrauma overdistend and disrupt lung tissue; may be clinically manifest by interstitial emphysema, pneumomediastinum, subcutaneous emphysema, or pneumothorax; and can result in the liberation of cytokines from overdistended tissues, further promoting tissue injury. Clinically significant pneumothorax requires tube thoracostomy. Intubated patients are at high risk for ventilator-associated pneumonia as a result of aspiration from the upper airways through small leaks around the endotracheal tube cuff; the most common organisms responsible for this condition are *Pseudomonas aeruginosa*, enteric gram-negative rods, and *Staphylococcus aureus*. Given the high associated mortality rates, early initiation of empirical antibiotics directed against likely pathogens is recommended. *Hypotension* resulting from elevated intrathoracic pressures with decreased venous return is almost always responsive to intravascular volume repletion. In patients who are judged to have respiratory failure on the basis of alveolar edema but in whom the cardiac or pulmonary origin of the edema is unclear, hemodynamic monitoring with a pulmonary arterial catheter may be of value in helping to clarify the cause of the edema. Gastrointestinal effects of positive-pressure ventilation include stress ulceration and mild to moderate cholestasis.

WEANING FROM MECHANICAL VENTILATION

The Decision to Wean It is important to consider discontinuation of mechanical ventilation once the underlying respiratory disease begins to reverse. Although the predictive capacities of multiple clinical and physiologic variables have been explored, the consensus from a ventilatory weaning task force cites the following conditions as indicating amenability to weaning: (1) Lung injury is stable or resolving. (2) Gas exchange is adequate, with low PEEP/FIO_2 (<8 cmH_2O) and FIO_2(<0.5). (3) Hemodynamic variables are stable, and the patient is no longer receiving vasopressors). (4) The patient is capable of initiating spontaneous breaths. A "wean screen" based on these variables should be done at least daily. If the patient is deemed capable of beginning to wean, the recommendation is to perform a spontaneous breathing trial (SBT), whose value is supported by several randomized trials (Fig. 323-2). The SBT involves an integrated patient assessment during spontaneous breathing with little or no ventilatory support. The SBT is usually implemented with a T-piece using 1–5 cmH_2O CPAP with 5–7 cmH_2O or PSV from the ventilator to offset resistance from the endotracheal tube. Once it is determined that the patient can breathe spontaneously, a decision must be made about the removal of the artificial airway, which should be undertaken only when it is concluded that the patient has the ability to protect the airway, is able to cough and clear

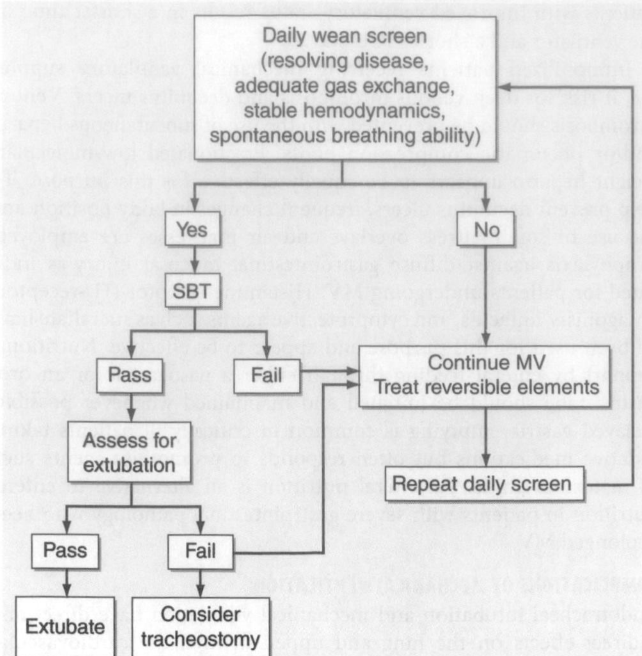

FIGURE 323-2 Flow chart to guide the daily approach to management of patients being considered for weaning off mechanical ventilation (MV). If attempts at extubation fail, a tracheostomy should be considered. SBT, spontaneous breathing trial.

secretions, and is alert enough to follow commands. In addition, other factors must be taken into account, such as the possible difficulty of replacing the tube if that maneuver is required. If upper airway difficulty is suspected, an evaluation using a "cuff-leak" test (assessing the presence of air movement around a deflated endotracheal tube cuff) is supported by some internists. Despite all precautions, ~10–15% of extubated patients require reintubation. Several studies suggest that NIV can be used to obviate reintubation, particularly in patients with ventilatory failure secondary to COPD exacerbation; in this setting, earlier extubation with the use of prophylactic NIV has yielded good results. The use of NIV to facilitate weaning in respiratory failure of other etiologies is not currently indicated.

Prolonged Mechanical Ventilation and Tracheostomy From 5% to 13% of patients undergoing MV will go on to require prolonged MV (>21 days). In these instances, critical care personnel must decide whether and when to perform a tracheostomy. This decision is individualized and is based on the risk and benefits of tracheostomy and prolonged intubation as well as the patient's preferences and expected outcomes. A tracheostomy is thought to be more comfortable, to require less sedation, and to provide a more secure airway and may also reduce weaning time. However, tracheostomy carries the risk of complications, which occur in 5–40% of these procedures and include bleeding, cardiopulmonary arrest, hypoxia, structural damage, pneumothorax, pneumomediastinum, and wound infection. In patients with long-term tracheostomy, complex complications include tracheal stenosis, granulation, and erosion of the innominate artery. In general, if a patient needs MV for more than 10–14 days, a tracheostomy, planned under optimal conditions, is indicated. Whether it is completed at the bedside or as an operative procedure depends on local resources and experience. Some 5–10% of patients are deemed unable to wean in the ICU. These patients may benefit from transfer to special units where a multidisciplinary approach, including nutrition optimization, physical therapy with rehabilitation, and slower weaning methods (including SIMV with PSV), results in successful weaning rates of up to 30%. Unfortunately, close to 2% of ventilated patients may ultimately become dependent on ventilatory support to maintain life. Most of these patients remain in chronic care institutions, although some with strong social, economic, and family support may live a relatively fulfilling life with at-home ventilation.

SECTION 2 SHOCK AND CARDIAC ARREST

324 Approach to the Patient with Shock

Ronald V. Maier

Shock is the clinical syndrome that results from inadequate tissue perfusion. Irrespective of cause, the hypoperfusion-induced imbalance between the delivery of and requirements for oxygen and substrate leads to cellular dysfunction. The cellular injury created by the inadequate delivery of oxygen and substrates also induces the production and release of damage-associated molecular patterns (DAMPs or "danger signals") and inflammatory mediators that further compromise perfusion through functional and structural changes within the microvasculature. This leads to a vicious cycle in which impaired perfusion is responsible for cellular injury that causes maldistribution of blood flow, further compromising cellular perfusion; the latter ultimately causes multiple organ failure (MOF) and, if the process is not interrupted, leads to death. The clinical manifestations of shock are also the result, in part, of autonomic neuroendocrine responses to hypoperfusion as well as the breakdown in organ function induced by severe cellular dysfunction (Fig. 324-1).

When very severe and/or persistent, inadequate oxygen delivery leads to irreversible cell injury, only rapid restoration of oxygen delivery can reverse the progression of the shock state. The fundamental approach to management, therefore, is to recognize overt and impending shock in a timely fashion and to intervene emergently to restore perfusion. Doing so often requires the expansion or reexpansion of intravascular blood volume. Control of any inciting pathologic process (e.g., continued hemorrhage, impairment of cardiac function, or infection) must occur simultaneously.

Clinical shock is usually accompanied by hypotension (i.e., a mean arterial pressure [MAP] <60 mmHg in previously normotensive persons). Multiple classification schemes have been developed in an attempt to synthesize the seemingly dissimilar processes leading to shock. Strict adherence to a classification scheme may be difficult from a clinical standpoint because of the frequent combination of two or more causes of shock in any individual patient, but the classification shown in Table 324-1 provides a useful reference point from which to discuss and further delineate the underlying processes.

PATHOGENESIS AND ORGAN RESPONSE

MICROCIRCULATION

Normally when cardiac output falls, systemic vascular resistance rises to maintain a level of systemic pressure that is adequate for perfusion of the heart and brain at the expense of other tissues such as muscle, skin, and especially the gastrointestinal (GI) tract. Systemic vascular resistance is determined primarily by the luminal diameter of arterioles. The metabolic rates of the heart and brain are high, and their stores of energy substrate are low. These organs are critically dependent on a

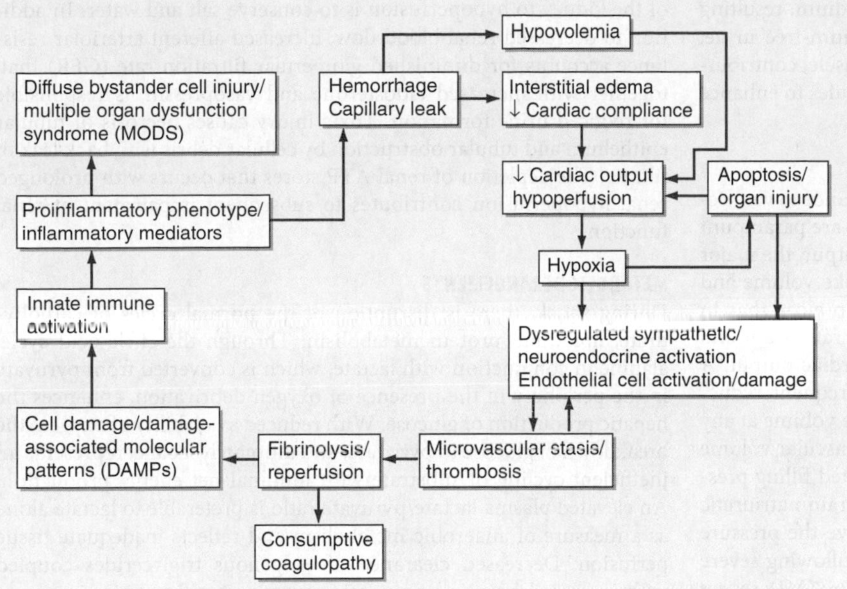

FIGURE 324-1 Shock-induced vicious cycle.

continuous supply of oxygen and nutrients, and neither tolerates severe ischemia for more than brief periods (minutes). Autoregulation (i.e., the maintenance of blood flow over a wide range of perfusion pressures) is critical in sustaining cerebral and coronary perfusion despite significant hypotension. However, when MAP drops to ≤60 mmHg, blood flow to these organs falls, and their function deteriorates.

Arteriolar vascular smooth muscle has both α- and β-adrenergic receptors. The α_1 receptors mediate vasoconstriction, while the β_2 receptors mediate vasodilation. Efferent sympathetic fibers release norepinephrine, which acts primarily on α_1 receptors as one of the most fundamental compensatory responses to reduced perfusion pressure. Other constrictor substances that are increased in most forms of shock include angiotensin II, vasopressin, endothelin 1, and thromboxane A_2. Both norepinephrine and epinephrine are released by the adrenal medulla, and the concentrations of these catecholamines in the bloodstream rise. Circulating vasodilators in shock include prostacyclin (prostaglandin [PG] I_2), nitric oxide (NO), and, importantly, products of local metabolism such as adenosine that match flow to the tissue's metabolic needs. The balance between these various vasoconstrictors and vasodilators influences the microcirculation and determines local perfusion.

Transport to cells depends on microcirculatory flow; capillary permeability; the diffusion of oxygen, carbon dioxide, nutrients, and products of metabolism through the interstitium; and the exchange of these products across cell membranes. Impairment of the microcirculation that is central to the pathophysiologic responses in the late stages of all forms of shock results in the derangement of cellular metabolism that is ultimately responsible for organ failure.

The endogenous response to mild or moderate hypovolemia is an attempt at restitution of intravascular volume through alterations in hydrostatic pressure and osmolarity. Constriction of arterioles leads to reductions in both the capillary hydrostatic pressure and the number of capillary beds perfused, thereby limiting the capillary surface area across which filtration occurs. When filtration is reduced while intravascular oncotic pressure remains constant or rises, there is net

TABLE 324-1 CLASSIFICATION OF SHOCK

Hypovolemic	Septic
Traumatic	Hyperdynamic (early)
Cardiogenic	Hypodynamic (late)
Intrinsic	Neurogenic
Compressive	Hypoadrenal

reabsorption of fluid into the vascular bed, in accord with Starling's law of capillary interstitial liquid exchange. Metabolic changes (including hyperglycemia and elevations in the products of glycolysis, lipolysis, and proteolysis) raise extracellular osmolarity, leading to an osmotic gradient that increases interstitial and intravascular volume at the expense of intracellular volume.

CELLULAR RESPONSES

Interstitial transport of nutrients is impaired in shock, leading to a decline in intracellular high energy phosphate stores. Mitochondrial dysfunction and uncoupling of oxidative phosphorylation are the most likely causes for decreased amounts of adenosine triphosphate (ATP). As a consequence, there is an accumulation of hydrogen ions, lactate, reactive oxygen species, and other products of anaerobic metabolism. As shock progresses, these vasodilator metabolites override vasomotor tone, causing further hypotension and hypoperfusion. Dysfunction of cell membranes is thought to represent a common end-stage pathophysiologic pathway in the various forms of shock. Normal cellular transmembrane potential falls, and there is an associated increase in intracellular sodium and water, leading to cell swelling that interferes further with microvascular perfusion. In a preterminal event, homeostasis of calcium via membrane channels is lost with flooding of calcium into the cytosol and concomitant extracellular hypocalcemia. There is also evidence for a widespread but selective apoptotic (programmed cell death) loss of cells, contributing to organ and immune failure.

NEUROENDOCRINE RESPONSE

Hypovolemia, hypotension, and hypoxia are sensed by baroreceptors and chemoreceptors that contribute to an autonomic response that attempts to restore blood volume, maintain central perfusion, and mobilize metabolic substrates. Hypotension disinhibits the vasomotor center, resulting in increased adrenergic output and reduced vagal activity. Release of norepinephrine from adrenergic neurons induces significant peripheral and splanchnic vasoconstriction, a major contributor to the maintenance of central organ perfusion, while reduced vagal activity increases the heart rate and cardiac output. Loss of vagal activity is also recognized to upregulate the innate immune inflammatory response. The effects of circulating epinephrine released by the adrenal medulla in shock are largely metabolic, causing increased glycogenolysis and gluconeogenesis and reduced pancreatic insulin release. However, epinephrine also inhibits production and release of inflammatory mediators through stimulation of β-adrenergic receptors on innate immune cells.

Severe pain or other stresses cause the hypothalamic release of adrenocorticotropic hormone (ACTH). This stimulates cortisol secretion that contributes to decreased peripheral uptake of glucose and amino acids, enhances lipolysis, and increases gluconeogenesis. Increased pancreatic secretion of glucagon during stress accelerates hepatic gluconeogenesis and further elevates blood glucose concentration. These hormonal actions act synergistically to increase blood glucose for both selective tissue metabolism and the maintenance of blood volume. Many critically ill patients have recently been shown to exhibit low plasma cortisol levels and an impaired response to ACTH stimulation, which is linked to a decrease in survival. The importance of the cortisol response to stress is illustrated by the profound circulatory collapse that occurs in patients with adrenocortical insufficiency (Chap. 406).

Renin release is increased in response to adrenergic discharge and reduced perfusion of the juxtaglomerular apparatus in the kidney. Renin induces the formation of angiotensin I that is then converted to angiotensin II by the angiotensin converting enzyme; angiotensin II is an extremely potent vasoconstrictor and stimulator of aldosterone release by the adrenal cortex and of vasopressin by the posterior pituitary. Aldosterone contributes to the maintenance of intravascular volume by enhancing renal tubular reabsorption of sodium, resulting in the excretion of a low-volume, concentrated, sodium-free urine. Vasopressin has a direct action on vascular smooth muscle, contributing to vasoconstriction, and acts on the distal renal tubules to enhance water reabsorption.

CARDIOVASCULAR RESPONSE

Three variables—ventricular filling (preload), the resistance to ventricular ejection (afterload), and myocardial contractility—are paramount in controlling stroke volume (Chap. 265e). Cardiac output, the major determinant of tissue perfusion, is the product of stroke volume and heart rate. Hypovolemia leads to decreased ventricular preload that, in turn, reduces the stroke volume. An increase in heart rate is a useful but limited compensatory mechanism to maintain cardiac output. A shock-induced reduction in myocardial compliance is frequent, reducing ventricular end-diastolic volume and, hence, stroke volume at any given ventricular filling pressure. Restoration of intravascular volume may return stroke volume to normal but only at elevated filling pressures. Increased filling pressures stimulate release of brain natriuretic peptide (BNP) to secrete sodium and volume to relieve the pressure on the heart. Levels of BNP correlate with outcome following severe stress. In addition, sepsis, ischemia, myocardial infarction (MI), severe tissue trauma, hypothermia, general anesthesia, prolonged hypotension, and acidemia may all also impair myocardial contractility and reduce the stroke volume at any given ventricular end-diastolic volume. The resistance to ventricular ejection is significantly influenced by the systemic vascular resistance, which is elevated in most forms of shock. However, resistance is decreased in the early hyperdynamic stage of septic shock or neurogenic shock (Chap. 325), thereby initially allowing the cardiac output to be maintained or elevated.

The venous system contains nearly two-thirds of the total circulating blood volume, most in the small veins, and serves as a dynamic reservoir for autoinfusion of blood. Active venoconstriction as a consequence of α-adrenergic activity is an important compensatory mechanism for the maintenance of venous return and, therefore, of ventricular filling during shock. By contrast, venous dilation, as occurs in neurogenic shock, reduces ventricular filling and hence stroke volume and potentially cardiac output.

PULMONARY RESPONSE

The response of the pulmonary vascular bed to shock parallels that of the systemic vascular bed, and the relative increase in pulmonary vascular resistance, particularly in septic shock, may exceed that of the systemic vascular resistance, leading to right heart failure. Shock-induced tachypnea reduces tidal volume and increases both dead space and minute ventilation. Relative hypoxia and the subsequent tachypnea induce a respiratory alkalosis. Recumbency and involuntary restriction of ventilation secondary to pain reduce functional residual capacity and may lead to atelectasis. Shock and, in particular, resuscitation-induced reactive oxygen species (oxidant radical) generation are recognized as major causes of acute lung injury and subsequent acute respiratory distress syndrome (ARDS; Chap. 322). These disorders are characterized by noncardiogenic pulmonary edema secondary to diffuse pulmonary capillary endothelial and alveolar epithelial injury, hypoxemia, and bilateral diffuse pulmonary infiltrates. Hypoxemia results from perfusion of underventilated and nonventilated alveoli. Loss of surfactant and lung volume in combination with increased interstitial and alveolar edema reduces lung compliance. The work of breathing and the oxygen requirements of respiratory muscles increase.

RENAL RESPONSE

Acute kidney injury (Chap. 334), a serious complication of shock and hypoperfusion, occurs less frequently than heretofore because of early aggressive volume repletion. Acute tubular necrosis is now more frequently seen as a result of the interactions of shock, sepsis, the administration of nephrotoxic agents (such as aminoglycosides and angiographic contrast media), and rhabdomyolysis; the latter may be particularly severe in skeletal muscle trauma. The physiologic response of the kidney to hypoperfusion is to conserve salt and water. In addition to decreased renal blood flow, increased afferent arteriolar resistance accounts for diminished glomerular filtration rate (GFR) that, together with increased aldosterone and vasopressin, is responsible for reduced urine formation. Toxic injury causes necrosis of tubular epithelium and tubular obstruction by cellular debris with back leak of filtrate. The depletion of renal ATP stores that occurs with prolonged renal hypoperfusion contributes to subsequent impairment of renal function.

METABOLIC DERANGEMENTS

During shock, there is disruption of the normal cycles of carbohydrate, lipid, and protein metabolism. Through the citric acid cycle, alanine in conjunction with lactate, which is converted from pyruvate in the periphery in the presence of oxygen deprivation, enhances the hepatic production of glucose. With reduced availability of oxygen, the breakdown of glucose to pyruvate, and ultimately lactate, represents an inefficient cycling of substrate with minimal net energy production. An elevated plasma lactate/pyruvate ratio is preferable to lactate alone as a measure of anaerobic metabolism and reflects inadequate tissue perfusion. Decreased clearance of exogenous triglycerides coupled with increased hepatic lipogenesis causes a significant rise in serum triglyceride concentrations. There is increased protein catabolism as energy substrate, a negative nitrogen balance, and, if the process is prolonged, severe muscle wasting.

INFLAMMATORY RESPONSES

Activation of an extensive network of proinflammatory mediator pathways by the innate immune system plays a significant role in the progression of shock and contributes importantly to the development of multiple organ injury, multiple organ dysfunction (MOD), and MOF (Fig. 324-2). In those surviving the acute insult, there is a prolonged endogenous counterregulatory response to "turn off" or balance the excessive proinflammatory response. If balance is restored, the patient does well. If the response is excessive, adaptive immunity is suppressed and the patient is highly susceptible to secondary nosocomial infections, which may then drive the inflammatory response and lead to delayed MOF.

Multiple humoral mediators are activated during shock and tissue injury. The complement cascade, activated through both the classic and alternate pathways, generates the anaphylatoxins C3a and C5a (Chap. 372e). Direct complement fixation to injured tissues can progress to the C5-C9 attack complex, causing further cell damage. Activation of the coagulation cascade (Chap. 141) causes microvascular thrombosis, with subsequent fibrinolysis leading to repeated episodes of ischemia and reperfusion. Components of the coagulation system (e.g., thrombin) are potent proinflammatory mediators that cause expression of adhesion molecules on endothelial cells and activation of neutrophils, leading to microvascular injury. Coagulation also activates the kallikrein-kininogen cascade, contributing to hypotension.

Eicosanoids are vasoactive and immunomodulatory products of arachidonic acid metabolism that include cyclooxygenase-derived prostaglandins (PGs) and thromboxane A_2, as well as lipoxygenase-derived leukotrienes and lipoxins. Thromboxane A_2 is a potent vasoconstrictor that contributes to the pulmonary hypertension and acute tubular necrosis of shock. PGI_2 and PGE_2 are potent vasodilators that enhance capillary permeability and edema formation. The cysteinyl leukotrienes LTC_4 and LTD_4 are pivotal mediators of the vascular sequelae of anaphylaxis, as well as of shock states resulting from sepsis or tissue injury. LTB_4 is a potent neutrophil chemoattractant and secretagogue that stimulates the formation of reactive oxygen species. Platelet-activating factor, an ether-linked, arachidonyl-containing phospholipid mediator, causes pulmonary vasoconstriction, bronchoconstriction, systemic vasodilation, increased capillary permeability, and the priming of macrophages and neutrophils to produce enhanced levels of inflammatory mediators.

Tumor necrosis factor α (TNF-α), produced by activated macrophages, reproduces many components of the shock state, including

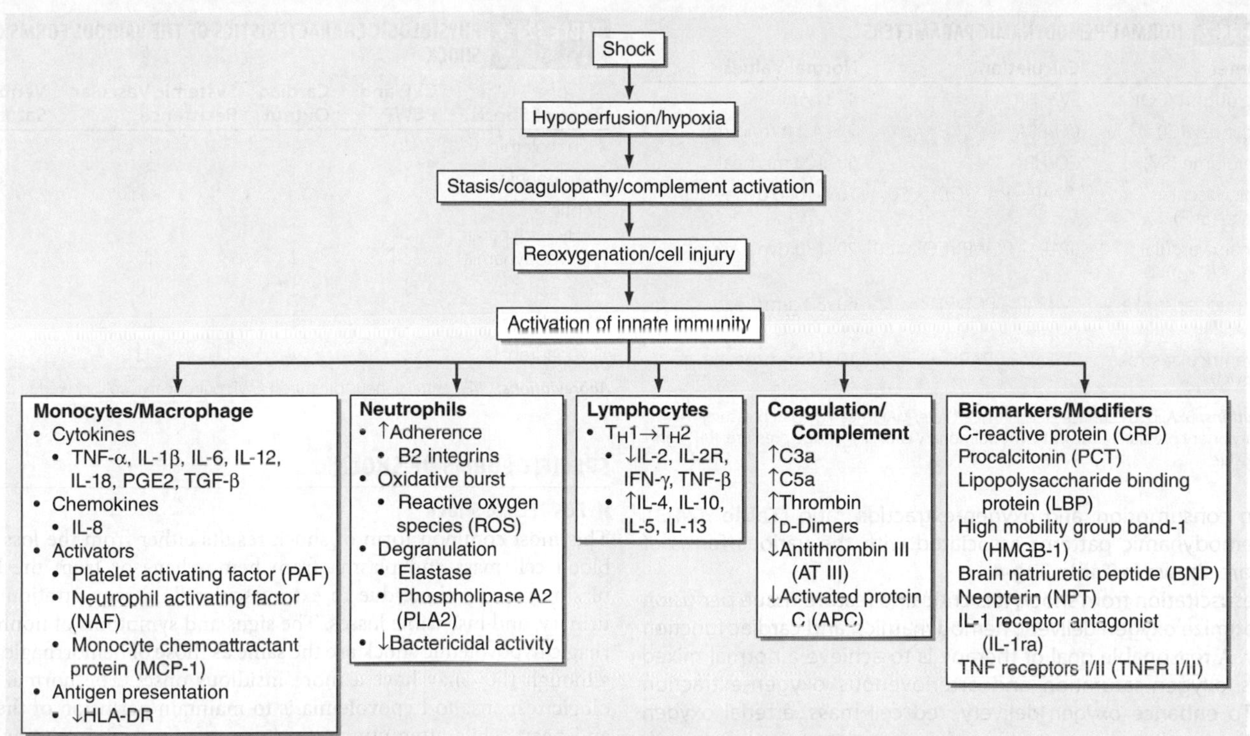

FIGURE 324-2 A schematic of the host immunoinflammatory response to shock. IFN, interferon; IL, interleukin; PG, prostaglandin; TGF, tumor growth factor; TNF, tumor necrosis factor.

hypotension, lactic acidosis, and respiratory failure. Interleukin 1β (IL-1β), originally defined as "endogenous pyrogen" and produced by tissue-fixed macrophages, is critical to the inflammatory response. Both are significantly elevated immediately following trauma and shock. IL-6, also produced predominantly by the macrophage, has a slightly delayed peak response but is the best single predictor of prolonged recovery and development of MOF following shock. Chemokines such as IL-8 are potent neutrophil chemoattractants and activators that upregulate adhesion molecules on the neutrophil to enhance aggregation, adherence, and damage to the vascular endothelium. While the endothelium normally produces low levels of NO, the inflammatory response stimulates the inducible isoform of NO synthase (iNOS), which is overexpressed and produces toxic nitroxyl and oxygen-derived free radicals that contribute to the hyperdynamic cardiovascular response and tissue injury in sepsis.

Multiple inflammatory cells, including neutrophils, macrophages, and platelets, are major contributors to inflammation-induced injury. Margination of activated neutrophils in the microcirculation is a common pathologic finding in shock, causing secondary injury due to the release of toxic oxygen radicals, lipases (primarily PLA_2), and proteases. Release of high levels of reactive oxygen intermediates/species (ROI/ROS) rapidly consumes endogenous essential antioxidants and generates diffuse oxygen radical damage. Newer efforts to control ischemia/reperfusion injury include treatment with carbon monoxide, hydrogen sulfide, or other agents to reduce oxidant stress. Tissue-fixed macrophages produce virtually all major mediators of the inflammatory response and orchestrate the progression and duration of the inflammatory response. A major source of activation of the monocyte/macrophage is through the highly conserved membrane toll-like receptors (TLRs) that recognize DAMPs, such as HMGB-1, and pathogen-associated molecular patterns (PAMPs), such as endotoxins released following tissue injury, and by pathogenic microbial organisms, respectively. TLRs also appear important in the chronic inflammation seen in Crohn's disease, ulcerative colitis, and transplant rejection. The variability in individual responses is a genetic predisposition that, in part, is due to variants in genetic sequences affecting the function and production of various inflammatory mediators.

TREATMENT SHOCK

MONITORING

Patients in shock require care in an intensive care unit (ICU). Careful and continuous assessment of the physiologic status is necessary. Arterial pressure through an indwelling line, pulse, and respiratory rate should be monitored continuously; a Foley catheter should be inserted to follow urine flow; and mental status should be assessed frequently. Sedated patients should be allowed to awaken ("drug holiday") daily to assess their neurologic status and to shorten duration of ventilator support.

There is ongoing debate as to the indications for using the flow-directed pulmonary artery catheter (PAC; Swan-Ganz catheter) in the ICU. A recent Cochrane analysis showed that the use of a PAC did not alter mortality, length of stay, or cost for adult ICU patients. Most patients in the ICU can be safely managed without the use of a PAC. However, in shock with significant ongoing blood loss, fluid shifts, and underlying cardiac dysfunction, a PAC may be useful. The PAC is placed percutaneously via the subclavian or jugular vein through the central venous circulation and right heart into the pulmonary artery. There are ports both proximal in the right atrium and distal in the pulmonary artery to provide access for infusions and for cardiac output measurements. Right atrial and pulmonary artery pressures (PAPs) are measured, and the pulmonary capillary wedge pressure (PCWP) serves as an approximation of the left atrial pressure. Normal hemodynamic parameters and their derivation are summarized in **Table 272-2** and **Table 324-2**.

Cardiac output is determined by the thermodilution technique, and high-resolution thermistors can also be used to determine right ventricular end-diastolic volume to monitor further the response of the right heart to fluid resuscitation. A PAC with an oximeter port offers the additional advantage of online monitoring of the mixed venous oxygen saturation, an important index of overall tissue perfusion. Systemic and pulmonary vascular resistances are calculated as the ratio of the pressure drop across these vascular beds to the cardiac output **(Chap. 272)**. Determinations of oxygen content in arterial and venous blood, together with cardiac output and hemoglobin concentration, allow calculation of oxygen delivery,

TABLE 324-2 NORMAL HEMODYNAMIC PARAMETERS

Parameter	Calculation	Normal Values
Cardiac output (CO)	SV × HR	4–8 L/min
Cardiac index (CI)	CO/BSA	2.6–4.2 (L/min)/m^2
Stroke volume (SV)	CO/HR	50–100 mL/beat
Systemic vascular resistance (SVR)	([MAP – RAP]/CO) × 80	700–1600 dynes·s/cm^5
Pulmonary vascular resistance (PVR)	([PAP_m – PCWP]/CO) × 80	20–130 dynes·s/cm^5
Left ventricular stroke work (LVSW)	SV(MAP – PCWP) × 0.0136	60–80 g-m/beat
Right ventricular stroke work (RVSW)	SV(PAP_m – RAP)	10–15 g-m/beat

Abbreviations: BSA, body surface area; HR, heart rate; MAP, mean arterial pressure; PAP_m, pulmonary artery pressure—mean; PCWP, pulmonary capillary wedge pressure; RAP, right atrial pressure.

oxygen consumption, and oxygen-extraction ratio (**Table 324-3**). The hemodynamic patterns associated with the various forms of shock are shown in **Table 324-4**.

In resuscitation from shock, it is critical to restore tissue perfusion and optimize oxygen delivery, hemodynamics, and cardiac function rapidly. A reasonable goal of therapy is to achieve a normal mixed venous oxygen-saturation and arteriovenous oxygen-extraction ratio. To enhance oxygen delivery, red cell mass, arterial oxygen saturation, and cardiac output may be augmented singly or simultaneously. An increase in oxygen delivery not accompanied by an increase in oxygen consumption implies that oxygen availability is adequate and that oxygen consumption is not flow dependent. Conversely, an elevation of oxygen consumption with increased delivery implies that the oxygen supply was inadequate. However, cautious interpretation is required due to the link among increased oxygen delivery, cardiac work, and oxygen consumption. A reduction in systemic vascular resistance accompanying an increase in cardiac output indicates that compensatory vasoconstriction is reversing due to improved tissue perfusion. The determination of stepwise expansion of blood volume on cardiac performance allows identification of the optimum preload (Starling's law). An algorithm for the resuscitation of the patient in shock is shown in **Fig. 324-3**.

TABLE 324-3 OXYGEN TRANSPORT CALCULATIONS

Parameter	Calculation	Normal Values
Oxygen-carrying capacity of hemoglobin		1.39 mL/g
Plasma O_2 concentration		Po_2 × 0.0031
Arterial O_2 concentration (Cao_2)	1.39 Sao_2 + 0.0031 Pao_2	20 vol%
Venous O_2 concentration (Cvo_2)	1.39 Svo_2 + 0.0031 Pvo_2	15.5 vol%
Arteriovenous O_2 difference (Cao_2 – Cvo_2)	1.39 (Sao_2 – Svo_2) + 0.0031 (Pao_2 – Pvo_2)	3.5 vol%
Oxygen delivery (Do_2)	Cao_2 × CO (L/min) × 10 (dL/L) 1.39 Sao_2 × CO × 10	800–1600 mL/min
Oxygen uptake (Vo_2)	(Cao_2 – Cvo_2) × CO × 10 1.39 (Sao_2 – Svo_2) × CO × 10	150–400 mL/min
Oxygen delivery index (Do_2I)	Do_2/BSA	520–720 (mL/min)/m^2
Oxygen uptake index (Vo_2I)	Vo_2/BSA	115–165 (mL/min)/m^2
Oxygen extraction ratio (O_2ER)	[1 – ($\dot{V}o_2$/$\dot{D}o_2$)] × 100	22–32%

Abbreviations: BSA, body surface area; CO, cardiac output; Po_2, partial pressure of oxygen; Pao_2, partial pressure of oxygen in arterial blood; Pvo_2, partial pressure of oxygen in venous blood; Sao_2, saturation of hemoglobin with oxygen in arterial blood; Svo_2, saturation of hemoglobin with oxygen in venous blood.

TABLE 324-4 PHYSIOLOGIC CHARACTERISTICS OF THE VARIOUS FORMS OF SHOCK

Type of Shock	CVP and PCWP	Cardiac Output	Systemic Vascular Resistance	Venous O_2 Saturation
Hypovolemic	↓	↓	↑	↓
Cardiogenic	↑	↓	↑	↓
Septic				
Hyperdynamic	↓↑	↑	↓	↑
Hypodynamic	↓↑	↓	↑	↓↑
Traumatic	↓	↓↑	↑↓	↓
Neurogenic	↓	↓	↓	↓
Hypoadrenal	↓	↓	=↓	↓

Abbreviations: CVP, central venous pressure; PCWP, pulmonary capillary wedge pressure.

SPECIFIC FORMS OF SHOCK

HYPOVOLEMIC SHOCK

This most common form of shock results either from the loss of red blood cell mass and plasma from hemorrhage or from the loss of plasma volume alone due to extravascular fluid sequestration or GI, urinary, and insensible losses. The signs and symptoms of nonhemorrhagic hypovolemic shock are the same as those of hemorrhagic shock, although they may have a more insidious onset. The normal physiologic response to hypovolemia is to maintain perfusion of the brain and heart while attempting to restore an effective circulating blood volume. There is an increase in sympathetic activity, hyperventilation, collapse of venous capacitance vessels, release of stress hormones, and an attempt to replace the loss of intravascular volume through the recruitment of interstitial and intracellular fluid and by reduction of urine output.

Mild hypovolemia (≤20% of the blood volume) generates mild tachycardia but relatively few external signs, especially in a supine young patient (**Table 324-5**). With moderate hypovolemia (~20–40% of the blood volume), the patient becomes increasingly anxious and tachycardic; although normal blood pressure may be maintained in the supine position, there may be significant postural hypotension and tachycardia. If hypovolemia is severe (≥40% of the blood volume), the classic signs of shock appear; the blood pressure declines and becomes unstable even in the supine position, and the patient develops marked tachycardia, oliguria, and agitation or confusion. Perfusion of the central nervous system is well maintained until shock becomes severe. Hence, mental obtundation is an ominous clinical sign. The transition from mild to severe hypovolemic shock can be insidious or extremely rapid. If severe shock is not reversed rapidly, especially in elderly patients and those with comorbid illnesses, death is imminent. A very narrow time frame separates the derangements found in severe shock that can be reversed with aggressive resuscitation from those of progressive decompensation and irreversible cell injury.

Diagnosis Hypovolemic shock is readily diagnosed when there are signs of hemodynamic instability and the source of volume loss is obvious. The diagnosis is more difficult when the source of blood loss is occult, as into the GI tract, or when plasma volume alone is depleted. Even after acute hemorrhage, hemoglobin and hematocrit values do not change until compensatory fluid shifts have occurred or exogenous fluid is administered. Thus, an initial normal hematocrit does not disprove the presence of significant blood loss. Plasma losses cause hemoconcentration, and free water loss leads to hypernatremia. These findings should suggest the presence of hypovolemia.

It is essential to distinguish between hypovolemic and cardiogenic shock (**Chap. 326**) because, although both may respond to volume initially, definitive therapy differs significantly. Both forms are associated with a reduced cardiac output and a compensatory sympathetic mediated response characterized by tachycardia and elevated systemic vascular resistance. However, the findings in cardiogenic shock of jugular venous distention, rales, and an S_3 gallop distinguish it from hypovolemic shock and signify that ongoing volume expansion is undesirable and may cause further organ dysfunction.

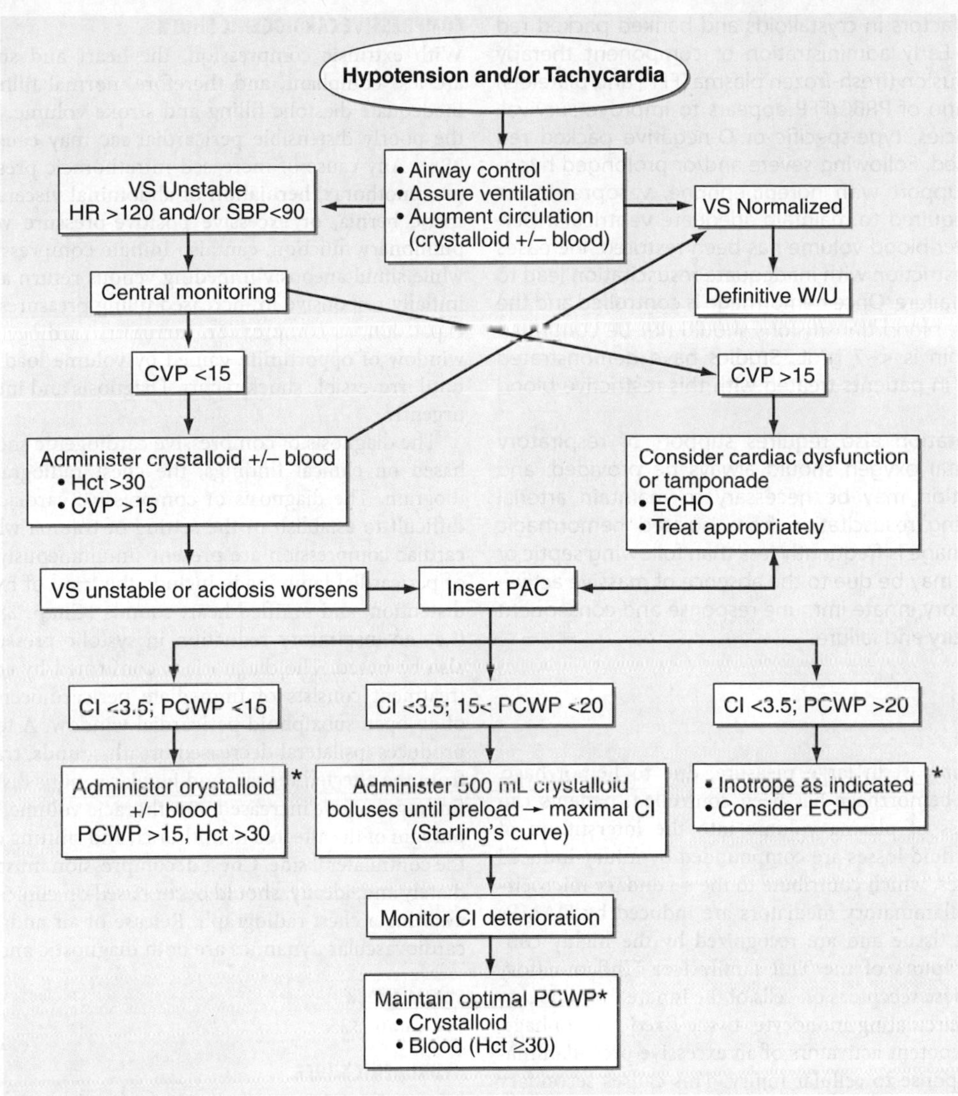

FIGURE 324-3 An algorithm for the resuscitation of the patient in shock. *Monitor Svo_2, SVRI, and RVEDVI as additional markers of correction for perfusion and hypovolemia. Consider age-adjusted CI. CI, cardiac index in (L/min) per m²; CVP, central venous pressure; ECHO, echocardiogram; Hct, hematocrit; HR, heart rate; PAC, pulmonary artery catheter; PCWP, pulmonary capillary wedge pressure in mmHg; RVEDVI, right ventricular end-diastolic volume index; SBP, systolic blood pressure; Svo_2, saturation of hemoglobin with O_2 in venous blood; SVRI, systemic vascular resistance index; VS, vital signs; W/U, workup.

TREATMENT HYPOVOLEMIC SHOCK

Initial resuscitation requires rapid reexpansion of the circulating intravascular blood volume along with interventions to control ongoing losses. In accordance with Starling's law (**Chap. 265e**), stroke volume and cardiac output rise with the increase in preload. After resuscitation, the compliance of the ventricles may remain reduced due to increased interstitial fluid in the myocardium.

TABLE 324-5 HYPOVOLEMIC SHOCK

Mild (<20% Blood Volume)	Moderate (20–40% Blood Volume)	Severe (>40% Blood Volume)
Cool extremities	Same, plus:	Same, plus:
Increased capillary refill time	Tachycardia	Hemodynamic instability
Diaphoresis	Tachypnea	Marked tachycardia
Collapsed veins	Oliguria	Hypotension
Anxiety	Postural changes	Mental status deterioration (coma)

Therefore, elevated filling pressures are frequently required to maintain adequate ventricular performance.

Volume resuscitation is initiated with the rapid infusion of either isotonic saline (although care must be taken to avoid hyperchloremic acidosis from loss of bicarbonate buffering capacity and replacement with excess chloride) or a balanced salt solution such as Ringer's lactate (being cognizant of the presence of potassium and potential renal dysfunction) through large-bore intravenous lines. Data, particularly on severe traumatic brain injury (TBI), regarding benefits of small volumes of hypertonic saline that more rapidly restore blood pressure are variable but tend to show improved survival thought to be linked to immunomodulation. No distinct benefit from the use of colloid has been demonstrated, and in trauma patients, it is associated with a higher mortality particularly in patients with TBI. The infusion of 2–3 L of salt solution over 20–30 min should restore normal hemodynamic parameters. Continued hemodynamic instability implies that shock has not been reversed and/or there are significant ongoing blood or other volume losses. Continuing acute blood loss with hemoglobin concentrations declining to ≤100 g/L (10 g/dL) should initiate blood transfusion preferably as fully cross-matched, recently banked (<14 days old) blood. Resuscitated patients are often coagulopathic due to deficient clotting factors in crystalloids and banked packed red blood cells (PRBCs). Early administration of component therapy during massive transfusion (fresh-frozen plasma [FFP] and platelets) approaching a 1:1 ratio of PRBC/FFP appears to improve survival. In extreme emergencies, type-specific or O-negative packed red cells may be transfused. Following severe and/or prolonged hypovolemia, inotropic support with norepinephrine, vasopressin, or dopamine may be required to maintain adequate ventricular performance *but only after* blood volume has been restored. Increases in peripheral vasoconstriction with inadequate resuscitation lead to tissue loss and organ failure. Once hemorrhage is controlled and the patient has stabilized, blood transfusions should not be continued unless the hemoglobin is <~7 g/dL. Studies have demonstrated an increased survival in patients treated with this restrictive blood transfusion protocol.

Successful resuscitation also requires support of respiratory function. Supplemental oxygen should always be provided, and endotracheal intubation may be necessary to maintain arterial oxygenation. Following resuscitation from isolated hemorrhagic shock, end-organ damage is frequently less than following septic or traumatic shock. This may be due to the absence of massive activation of the inflammatory innate immune response and consequent nonspecific organ injury and failure.

TRAUMATIC SHOCK

Shock following trauma is, in large measure, due to hemorrhage. However, even when hemorrhage has been controlled, patients can continue to suffer loss of plasma volume into the interstitium of injured tissues. These fluid losses are compounded by injury-induced inflammatory responses, which contribute to the secondary microcirculatory injury. Proinflammatory mediators are induced by DAMPs released from injured tissue and are recognized by the highly conserved membrane receptors of the TLR family (see "Inflammatory Responses" above). These receptors on cells of the innate immune system, particularly the circulating monocyte, tissue-fixed macrophage, and dendritic cell, are potent activators of an excessive proinflammatory phenotype in response to cellular injury. This causes secondary tissue injury and maldistribution of blood flow, intensifying tissue ischemia and leading to multiple organ system failure. In addition, direct structural injury to the heart, chest, or head can also contribute to shock. For example, pericardial tamponade or tension pneumothorax impairs ventricular filling, whereas myocardial contusion depresses myocardial contractility.

TREATMENT TRAUMATIC SHOCK

Inability of the patient to maintain a systolic blood pressure ≥90 mmHg after trauma-induced hypovolemia is associated with a mortality rate up to ~50%. To prevent this decompensation of homeostatic mechanisms, therapy must be promptly administered.

The initial management of the seriously injured patient requires attention to the "ABCs" of resuscitation: assurance of an *airway* (A), adequate ventilation (*breathing*, B), and establishment of an adequate blood volume to support the *circulation* (C). Control of ongoing hemorrhage requires immediate attention. Early stabilization of fractures, debridement of devitalized or contaminated tissues, and evacuation of hematomata all reduce the subsequent inflammatory response to the initial insult and minimize damaged tissue release of DAMPs and subsequent diffuse organ injury. Supplementation of depleted endogenous antioxidants also reduces subsequent organ failure and mortality.

CARDIOGENIC SHOCK

See Chap. 326.

COMPRESSIVE CARDIOGENIC SHOCK

With extrinsic compression, the heart and surrounding structures are less compliant, and therefore, normal filling pressures generate inadequate diastolic filling and stroke volume. Blood or fluid within the poorly distensible pericardial sac may cause tamponade (Chap. 288). Any cause of increased intrathoracic pressure, such as tension pneumothorax, herniation of abdominal viscera through a diaphragmatic hernia, or excessive positive-pressure ventilation to support pulmonary function, can also initiate compressive cardiogenic shock while simultaneously impeding venous return and preload. Although initially responsive to increased filling pressures produced by volume expansion, as compression increases, cardiogenic shock recurs. The window of opportunity gained by volume loading may be very brief until irreversible shock recurs. Diagnosis and intervention must occur urgently.

The diagnosis of compressive cardiogenic shock is most frequently based on clinical findings, the chest radiograph, and an echocardiogram. The diagnosis of compressive cardiac shock may be more difficult to establish in the setting of trauma when hypovolemia and cardiac compression are present simultaneously. The classic findings of pericardial tamponade include the triad of hypotension, neck vein distention, and muffled heart sounds (Chap. 288). Pulsus paradoxus (i.e., an inspiratory reduction in systolic pressure >10 mmHg) may also be noted. The diagnosis is confirmed by echocardiography, and treatment consists of immediate pericardiocentesis or the creation of an open subxiphoid pericardial window. A tension pneumothorax produces ipsilateral decreased breath sounds, tracheal deviation away from the affected thorax, and jugular venous distention. Radiographic findings include increased intrathoracic volume, depression of the diaphragm of the affected hemithorax, and shifting of the mediastinum to the contralateral side. Chest decompression must be carried out immediately and, ideally, should occur based on clinical findings rather than awaiting a chest radiograph. Release of air and restoration of normal cardiovascular dynamics are both diagnostic and therapeutic.

SEPTIC SHOCK

See Chap. 325.

NEUROGENIC SHOCK

Interruption of sympathetic vasomotor input after a high cervical spinal cord injury, inadvertent cephalad migration of spinal anesthesia, or devastating head injury may result in neurogenic shock. In addition to arteriolar dilation, venodilation causes pooling in the venous system, which decreases venous return and cardiac output. The extremities are often warm, in contrast to the usual sympathetic vasoconstriction-induced coolness in hypovolemic or cardiogenic shock. Treatment involves a simultaneous approach to the relative hypovolemia and to the loss of vasomotor tone. Excessive volumes of fluid may be required to restore normal hemodynamics if given alone. Once hemorrhage has been ruled out, norepinephrine or a pure α-adrenergic agent (phenylephrine) may be necessary to augment vascular resistance and maintain an adequate MAP.

HYPOADRENAL SHOCK

(See also Chap. 406) The normal host response to the stress of illness, operation, or trauma requires that the adrenal glands hypersecrete cortisol in excess of that normally required. Hypoadrenal shock occurs in settings in which unrecognized adrenal insufficiency complicates the host response to the stress induced by acute illness or major surgery. Adrenocortical insufficiency may occur as a consequence of the chronic administration of high doses of exogenous glucocorticoids. In addition, recent studies have shown that critical illness, including trauma and sepsis, may also induce a relative hypoadrenal state. Other, less common causes include adrenal insufficiency secondary to idiopathic atrophy, use of etomidate for intubation, tuberculosis, metastatic disease, bilateral hemorrhage, and amyloidosis. The shock produced by adrenal insufficiency is characterized by loss of homeostasis with reductions in systemic vascular resistance, hypovolemia, and reduced cardiac output. The diagnosis of adrenal insufficiency may be established by means of an ACTH stimulation test.

TREATMENT HYPOADRENAL SHOCK

In the persistently hemodynamically unstable patient, dexamethasone sodium phosphate, 4 mg, should be given intravenously. This agent is preferred if empiric therapy is required because, unlike hydrocortisone, it does not interfere with the ACTH stimulation test. If the diagnosis of absolute or relative adrenal insufficiency is established as shown by nonresponse to corticotropin stimulation (cortisol ≤9 μg/dL change after stimulation), the patient has a reduced risk of death if treated with hydrocortisone, 100 mg every 6–8 h, and tapered as the patient achieves hemodynamic stability. Simultaneous volume resuscitation and pressor support are required. The need for simultaneous mineralocoid is unclear.

ADJUNCTIVE THERAPIES

The sympathomimetic amines dobutamine, dopamine, and norepinephrine are widely used in the treatment of all forms of shock. Dobutamine is inotropic with simultaneous afterload reduction, thus minimizing cardiac-oxygen consumption increases as cardiac output increases. Dopamine is an inotropic and chronotropic agent that also supports vascular resistance in those whose blood pressure will not tolerate peripheral vascular dilation. Norepinephrine primarily supports blood pressure through vasoconstriction and increases myocardial oxygen consumption while placing marginally perfused tissues, such as extremities and splanchnic organs, at risk for ischemia or necrosis, but it is also inotropic without significant chronotropy. Arginine-vasopressin (antidiuretic hormone) is being used increasingly to increase afterload and may better protect vital organ blood flow and prevent pathologic vasodilation.

REWARMING

Hypothermia is a frequent adverse consequence of massive volume resuscitation (Chap. 478e). The infusion of large volumes of refrigerated blood products and room temperature crystalloid solutions can rapidly drop core temperatures if fluid is not run through warming devices. Hypothermia may depress cardiac contractility and thereby further impair cardiac output and oxygen delivery/utilization. Hypothermia, particularly temperatures <35°C (<95°F), directly impairs the coagulation pathway, sometimes causing a significant coagulopathy. Rapid rewarming to >35°C (>95°F) significantly decreases the requirement for blood products and produces an improvement in cardiac function. The most effective method for rewarming is endovascular countercurrent warmers through femoral vein cannulation. This process does not require a pump and can rewarm a patient from 30° to 35°C (86° to 95°F) in 30–60 min.

325 Severe Sepsis and Septic Shock

Robert S. Munford

DEFINITIONS

(Table 325-1) Animals mount both local and systemic responses to microbes that traverse their epithelial barriers and enter underlying tissues. Fever or hypothermia, leukocytosis or leukopenia, tachypnea, and tachycardia are cardinal signs of the systemic response. To date, attempts to devise precise definitions for the harmful systemic reaction to infection ("sepsis") have not resulted in a clinically useful level of specificity, in part because the systemic responses to infection, trauma, and other major stresses can be so similar. In general, when an infectious etiology is proven or strongly suspected and the response results in hypofunction of uninfected organs, the term *sepsis* (or *severe sepsis*) should be used. *Septic shock* refers to sepsis accompanied by hypotension that cannot be corrected by the infusion of fluids.

TABLE 325-1 DEFINITIONS USED TO DESCRIBE THE CONDITION OF SEPTIC PATIENTS

Bacteremia	Presence of bacteria in blood, as evidenced by positive blood cultures
Signs of possibly harmful systemic response	Two or more of the following conditions: (1) fever (oral temperature >38°C [>100.4°F]) or hypothermia (<36°C [<96.8°F]); (2) tachypnea (>24 breaths/min); (3) tachycardia (heart rate >90 beats/min); (4) leukocytosis (>12,000/μL), leukopenia (<4000/μL), or >10% bands
Sepsis (or severe sepsis)	The harmful host response to infection; systemic response to proven or suspected infection plus some degree of organ hypofunction, i.e.: 1. *Cardiovascular:* Arterial systolic blood pressure ≤90 mmHg or mean arterial pressure ≤70 mmHg that responds to administration of IV fluid 2. *Renal:* Urine output <0.5 mL/kg per hour for 1 h despite adequate fluid resuscitation 3. *Respiratory:* Pa_{O_2}/F_{IO_2} ≤250 or, if the lung is the only dysfunctional organ, ≤200 4. *Hematologic:* Platelet count <80,000/μL or 50% decrease in platelet count from highest value recorded over previous 3 days 5. *Unexplained metabolic acidosis:* A pH ≤7.30 or a base deficit ≥5.0 mEq/L and a plasma lactate level >1.5 times upper limit of normal for reporting lab
Septic shock	Sepsis with hypotension (arterial blood pressure <90 mmHg systolic, or 40 mmHg less than patient's normal blood pressure) for at least 1 h despite adequate fluid resuscitation[a] *or* Need for vasopressors to maintain systolic blood pressure ≥90 mmHg *or* mean arterial pressure ≥70 mmHg
Refractory septic shock	Septic shock that lasts for >1 h and does not respond to fluid or pressor administration

[a]Fluid resuscitation is considered adequate when the pulmonary artery wedge pressure is ≥12 mmHg or the central venous pressure is ≥8 mmHg.

ETIOLOGY

The systemic response to any class of microorganism can be harmful. Microbial invasion of the bloodstream is not essential because local inflammation can also elicit distant organ dysfunction and hypotension. In fact, blood cultures yield bacteria or fungi in only ~20–40% of cases of severe sepsis and 40–70% of cases of septic shock. In a prevalence study of 14,414 patients in intensive care units (ICUs) from 75 countries in 2007, 51% of patients were considered infected. Respiratory infection was most common (64%). Microbiologic results were positive in 70% of individuals considered infected; of the isolates, 62% were gram-negative bacteria (*Pseudomonas* species and *Escherichia coli* were most common), 47% were gram-positive bacteria (*Staphylococcus aureus* was most common), and 19% were fungi (*Candida* species). This distribution is similar to that reported a decade earlier from eight academic centers in the United States (Table 325-2). In patients whose blood cultures are negative, the etiologic agent is often established by culture or microscopic examination of infected material from a local site; specific identification of microbial DNA or RNA in blood or tissue samples is also used. In some case series, a majority of patients with a clinical picture of severe sepsis or septic shock have had negative microbiologic data.

TABLE 325-2 MICROORGANISMS INVOLVED IN EPISODES OF SEVERE SEPSIS AT EIGHT ACADEMIC MEDICAL CENTERS

Microorganisms	Episodes with Bloodstream Infection, % (*n* = 436)	Episodes with Documented Infection but No Bloodstream Infection, % (*n* = 430)	Total Episodes, % (*n* = 866)
Gram-negative bacteria[a]	35	44	40
Gram-positive bacteria[b]	40	24	31
Fungi	7	5	6
Polymicrobial	11	21	16
Classic pathogens[c]	<5	<5	<5

[a]Enterobacteriaceae, pseudomonads, *Haemophilus* spp., other gram-negative bacteria. [b]*Staphylococcus aureus*, coagulase-negative staphylococci, enterococci, *Streptococcus pneumoniae*, other streptococci, other gram-positive bacteria. [c]Such as *Neisseria meningitidis, S. pneumoniae, Haemophilus influenzae*, and *Streptococcus pyogenes*.

Source: Adapted from KE Sands et al: JAMA 278:234, 1997.

EPIDEMIOLOGY

Severe sepsis is a contributing factor in >200,000 deaths per year in the United States. The incidence of severe sepsis and septic shock has increased over the past 30 years, and the annual number of cases is now >750,000 (~3 per 1000 population). Approximately two-thirds of the cases occur in patients with significant underlying illness. Sepsis-related incidence and mortality rates increase with age and preexisting comorbidity. The rising incidence of severe sepsis in the United States has been attributable to the aging of the population, the increasing longevity of patients with chronic diseases, and the relatively high frequency with which sepsis has occurred in patients with AIDS. The widespread use of immunosuppressive drugs, indwelling catheters, and mechanical devices has also played a role. In the aforementioned international ICU prevalence study, the case–fatality rate among infected patients (33%) greatly exceeded that among uninfected patients (15%).

Invasive bacterial infections are prominent causes of death around the world, particularly among young children. In sub-Saharan Africa, for example, careful screening for positive blood cultures found that community-acquired bacteremia accounted for at least one-fourth of deaths of children >1 year of age. Nontyphoidal *Salmonella* species, *Streptococcus pneumoniae, Haemophilus influenzae*, and *E. coli* were the most commonly isolated bacteria. Bacteremic children often had HIV infection or were severely malnourished.

PATHOPHYSIOLOGY

Sepsis is triggered most often by bacteria or fungi that do not ordinarily cause systemic disease in immunocompetent hosts (Table 325-2). To survive within the human body, these microbes often exploit acquired deficiencies in host defenses, indwelling catheters or other foreign matter, or obstructed fluid drainage conduits. Microbial pathogens, in contrast, can circumvent innate defenses because they (1) lack molecules that can be recognized by host receptors (see below) or (2) elaborate toxins or other virulence factors. In both cases, the body can mount a vigorous inflammatory reaction that results in sepsis or septic shock yet fails to kill the invaders. The septic response may also be induced by microbial exotoxins that act as superantigens (e.g., toxic shock syndrome toxin 1; Chap. 172) as well as by many pathogenic viruses.

Host Mechanisms for Sensing Microbes Animals have exquisitely sensitive mechanisms for recognizing and responding to certain highly conserved microbial molecules. Recognition of the lipid A moiety of lipopolysaccharide (LPS, also called *endotoxin*; Chap. 145e) is the best-studied example. A host protein (LPS-binding protein) binds lipid A and transfers the LPS to CD14 on the surfaces of monocytes, macrophages, and neutrophils. LPS then is passed to MD-2, a small receptor protein that is bound to Toll-like receptor (TLR) 4 to form a molecular complex that transduces the LPS recognition signal to the interior of the cell. This signal rapidly triggers the production and release of mediators, such as tumor necrosis factor (TNF; see below), that amplify the LPS signal and transmit it to other cells and tissues. Bacterial peptidoglycan and lipopeptides elicit responses in animals that are generally similar to those induced by LPS, although they interact with different TLRs. Having numerous TLR-based receptor complexes (10 different TLRs have been identified in humans) allows animals to recognize many conserved microbial molecules; others include lipopeptides (TLR2/1, TLR2/6), flagellin (TLR5), undermethylated DNA CpG sequences (TLR9), single-stranded RNA (TLR7, 8), and double-stranded RNA (TLR3). The ability of some TLRs to serve as receptors for host ligands (e.g., hyaluronans, heparan sulfate, saturated fatty acids, high-mobility group box 1) raises the possibility that they also play a role in producing noninfectious sepsis-like states. Other host pattern-recognition proteins that are important for sensing microbes include the intracellular NOD1 and NOD2 proteins, which recognize discrete fragments of bacterial peptidoglycan; the inflammasome, which senses some pathogens and produces interleukin (IL) 1β and IL-18; early complement components (principally in the alternative pathway); mannose-binding lectin and C-reactive protein, which activate the classic complement pathway; and Dectin-1 and complement receptor 3, which sense fungal β-glucan.

A host's ability to recognize certain microbial molecules may influence both the potency of its own defenses and the pathogenesis of severe sepsis. For example, MD-2–TLR4 best senses LPS that has a bisphosphorylated, hexaacyl lipid A moiety (i.e., one with two phosphates and six fatty acyl chains). Most of the commensal aerobic and facultatively anaerobic gram-negative bacteria that trigger severe sepsis and shock (including *E. coli, Klebsiella*, and *Enterobacter*) make this lipid A structure. When they invade human hosts, often through breaks in an epithelial barrier, they are typically confined to the subepithelial tissue by a localized inflammatory response. Bacteremia, if it occurs, is intermittent and low grade because these bacteria are efficiently cleared from the bloodstream by TLR4-expressing Kupffer cells and splenic macrophages. These mucosal commensals seem to induce severe sepsis most often by triggering severe local tissue inflammation rather than by circulating within the bloodstream. One exception is *Neisseria meningitidis*. Its hexaacyl LPS seems to be shielded from host recognition by its polysaccharide capsule. This protection may allow meningococci to transit undetected from the nasopharyngeal mucosa into the bloodstream, where they can infect vascular endothelial cells and release large amounts of endotoxin and DNA. Host recognition of lipid A may nonetheless influence pathogenesis, as meningococci that produce pentaacyl LPS were isolated from the blood of patients with less severe coagulopathy than was found in patients whose isolates produced hexaacyl lipid A; underacylated *N. meningitidis* LPS has also been found in many isolates from patients with chronic meningococcemia. In contrast, gram-negative bacteria that make lipid A with fewer than six acyl chains (*Yersinia pestis, Francisella tularensis, Vibrio vulnificus, Pseudomonas aeruginosa*, and *Burkholderia pseudomallei*, among others) are poorly recognized by MD-2–TLR4. When these bacteria enter the body, they may initially induce relatively little inflammation. When they do trigger severe sepsis, it is often after they have multiplied to high density in tissues and blood. The importance of LPS recognition in disease pathogenesis was demonstrated by engineering of a virulent strain of *Y. pestis* that makes tetraacyl LPS at 37°C to produce hexaacyl LPS; unlike its virulent parent, the mutant strain stimulated local inflammation and was rapidly cleared from tissues. These findings were subsequently replicated in *F. tularensis*. For at least one large class of microbes—gram-negative aerobic bacteria—the pathogenesis of sepsis thus depends, at least in part, on whether the bacterium's major signal molecule, LPS, can be sensed by the host.

Local and Systemic Host Responses to Invading Microbes Recognition of microbial molecules by tissue phagocytes triggers the production and/or release of numerous host molecules (cytokines, chemokines, prostanoids, leukotrienes, and others) that increase blood flow to the infected tissue (*rubor*), enhance the permeability of local blood vessels (*tumor*), recruit neutrophils and other cells to the site of infection (*calor*), and elicit pain (*dolor*). These reactions are familiar elements of local inflammation, the body's frontline innate immune mechanism for eliminating microbial invaders. Systemic responses are activated by neural and/or humoral communication with the hypothalamus and brainstem; these responses enhance local defenses by increasing blood flow to the infected area, augmenting the number of circulating neutrophils, and elevating blood levels of numerous molecules (such as the microbial recognition proteins discussed above) that have anti-infective functions.

CYTOKINES AND OTHER MEDIATORS Cytokines can exert endocrine, paracrine, and autocrine effects (Chap. 372e). TNF-α stimulates leukocytes and vascular endothelial cells to release other cytokines (as well as additional TNF-α), to express cell-surface molecules that enhance neutrophil endothelial adhesion at sites of infection, and to increase prostaglandin and leukotriene production. Whereas blood levels of TNF-α are not elevated in individuals with localized infections, they increase in most patients with severe sepsis or septic shock. Moreover, IV infusion of TNF-α can elicit fever, tachycardia, hypotension, and other responses. In animals, larger doses of TNF-α induce shock and death.

Although TNF-α is a central mediator, it is only one of many proinflammatory molecules that contribute to innate host defense. Chemokines, most prominently IL-8 and IL-17, attract circulating neutrophils to the infection site. IL-1β exhibits many of the same activities as TNF-α. TNF-α, IL-1β, interferon γ, IL-12, IL-17, and other proinflammatory cytokines probably interact synergistically with one another and with additional mediators. The nonlinearity and multiplicity of these interactions have made it difficult to interpret the roles played by individual mediators in both tissues and blood.

COAGULATION FACTORS Intravascular thrombosis, a hallmark of the local inflammatory response, may help wall off invading microbes and prevent infection and inflammation from spreading to other tissues. IL-6 and other mediators promote intravascular coagulation initially by inducing blood monocytes and vascular endothelial cells to express tissue factor (Chap. 78). When tissue factor is expressed on cell surfaces, it binds to factor VIIa to form an active complex that can convert factors X and IX to their enzymatically active forms. The result is activation of both extrinsic and intrinsic clotting pathways, culminating in the generation of fibrin. Clotting is also favored by impaired function of the protein C–protein S inhibitory pathway and depletion of antithrombin and proteins C and S, whereas fibrinolysis is reduced by increases in plasma levels of plasminogen activator inhibitor 1. Thus, there may be a striking propensity toward intravascular fibrin deposition, thrombosis, and bleeding; this propensity has been most apparent in patients with intravascular endothelial infections such as meningococcemia (Chap. 180). Evidence points to tissue factor–expressing microparticles derived from leukocytes as a potential trigger for intravascular coagulation. The contact system is activated during sepsis but contributes more to the development of hypotension than to that of disseminated intravascular coagulation (DIC).

Neutrophil extracellular traps (NETs) are produced when neutrophils, stimulated by microbial agonists or IL-8, release granule proteins and chromatin to form an extracellular fibrillar matrix. NETs kill bacteria and fungi with antimicrobial granule proteins (e.g., elastase) and histones. It has been reported that NETs can form within hepatic sinusoids in animals injected with large amounts of LPS, and platelets can induce NET formation without killing neutrophils. A role played by NETs in organ hypofunction during sepsis has been proposed but not established.

CONTROL MECHANISMS Elaborate control mechanisms operate within both local sites of inflammation and the systemic compartment.

Local control mechanisms Host recognition of invading microbes within subepithelial tissues typically ignites immune responses that rapidly kill the invaders and then subside to allow tissue recovery. The forces that put out the fire and clean up the battleground include molecules that neutralize or inactivate microbial signals. Among these molecules are intracellular factors (e.g., suppressor of cytokine signaling 3 and IL-1 receptor–associated kinase 3) that diminish the production of proinflammatory mediators by neutrophils and macrophages; anti-inflammatory cytokines (IL-10, IL-4); and molecules derived from essential polyunsaturated fatty acids (lipoxins, resolvins, and protectins) that promote tissue restoration. Enzymatic inactivation of microbial signal molecules (e.g., LPS) may be required to restore homeostasis; a leukocyte enzyme, acyloxyacyl hydrolase, has been shown to prevent prolonged inflammation in mice by inactivating LPS.

Systemic control mechanisms The signaling apparatus that links microbial recognition to cellular responses in tissues is less active in the blood. For example, whereas LPS-binding protein plays a role in recognizing LPS, in plasma it also prevents LPS signaling by transferring LPS molecules into plasma lipoprotein particles that sequester the lipid A moiety so that it cannot interact with cells. At the high concentrations found in blood, LPS-binding protein also inhibits monocyte responses to LPS, and the soluble (circulating) form of CD14 strips off LPS that has bound to monocyte surfaces.

Systemic responses to infection also diminish cellular responses to microbial molecules. Circulating levels of cortisol and anti-inflammatory cytokines (e.g., IL-6 and IL-10) increase even in patients with minor infections. Glucocorticoids inhibit cytokine synthesis by monocytes in vitro; the increase in blood cortisol levels that occurs early in the systemic response presumably plays a similarly inhibitory role. Epinephrine inhibits the TNF-α response to endotoxin infusion in humans while augmenting and accelerating the release of IL-10; prostaglandin E_2 has a similar "reprogramming" effect on the responses of circulating monocytes to LPS and other bacterial agonists. Cortisol, epinephrine, IL-10, and C-reactive protein reduce the ability of neutrophils to attach to vascular endothelium, favoring their demargination and thus contributing to leukocytosis while preventing neutrophil-endothelial adhesion in uninflamed organs. Studies in rodents have found that macrophage cytokine synthesis is inhibited by acetylcholine that is produced by choline acetyltransferase–secreting CD4+ T cells in response to stimulation by norepinephrine, whereas acetylcholine-producing B cells reduce neutrophil infiltration into tissues. Several lines of evidence thus suggest that the body's neuroendocrine responses to injury and infection normally prevent inflammation within organs distant from a site of infection. There is also evidence that these responses may be immunosuppressive.

IL-6 plays important roles in the systemic compartment. Released by many different cell types, IL-6 is an important stimulus to the hypothalamic-pituitary-adrenal axis, is the major procoagulant cytokine, and is a principal inducer of the acute-phase response, which increases the blood concentrations of numerous molecules that have anti-infective, procoagulant, or anti-inflammatory actions. Blood levels of IL-1 receptor antagonist often greatly exceed those of circulating IL-1β, for example, and this excess may inhibit the binding of IL-1β to its receptors. High levels of soluble TNF receptors neutralize TNF-α that enters the circulation. Other acute-phase proteins are protease inhibitors or antioxidants; these may neutralize potentially harmful molecules released from neutrophils and other inflammatory cells. Increased hepatic production of hepcidin (stimulated largely by IL-6) promotes the sequestration of iron in hepatocytes, intestinal epithelial cells, and erythrocytes; this effect reduces iron acquisition by invading microbes while contributing to the normocytic, normochromic anemia associated with inflammation.

It may thus be said that both local and systemic responses to infectious agents benefit the host in important ways. Most of these responses and the molecules responsible for them have been highly conserved during animal evolution and therefore may be adaptive.

Elucidating how they become maladaptive and contribute to lethality remains a major challenge for sepsis research.

Organ Dysfunction and Shock As the body's responses to infection intensify, the mixture of circulating cytokines and other molecules becomes very complex: elevated blood levels of more than 60 molecules have been found in patients with septic shock. Although high concentrations of both pro- and anti-inflammatory molecules are found, the net mediator balance in the plasma of these extremely sick patients seems to be anti-inflammatory. For example, blood leukocytes from patients with severe sepsis are often hyporesponsive to agonists such as LPS. In patients with severe sepsis, persistence of leukocyte hyporesponsiveness has been associated with an increased risk of dying; at this time, the most predictive biomarker is a decrease in the expression of HLA-DR (class II) molecules on the surfaces of circulating monocytes, a response that seems to be induced by cortisol and/or IL-10. Apoptotic death of B cells, follicular dendritic cells, and CD4+ T lymphocytes also may contribute significantly to the immunosuppressive state.

ENDOTHELIAL INJURY Given the vascular endothelium's important roles in regulating vascular tone, vascular permeability, and coagulation, many investigators have favored widespread vascular endothelial injury as the major mechanism for multiorgan dysfunction. In keeping with this idea, one study found high numbers of vascular endothelial cells in the peripheral blood of septic patients. Leukocyte-derived mediators and platelet-leukocyte-fibrin thrombi may contribute to vascular injury, but the vascular endothelium also seems to play an active role. Stimuli such as TNF-α induce vascular endothelial cells to produce and release cytokines, procoagulant molecules, platelet-activating factor, nitric oxide, and other mediators. In addition, regulated cell-adhesion molecules promote the adherence of neutrophils to endothelial cells. Although these responses can attract phagocytes to infected sites and activate their antimicrobial arsenals, endothelial cell activation can also promote increased vascular permeability, microvascular thrombosis, DIC, and hypotension.

Tissue oxygenation may decrease as the number of functional capillaries is reduced by luminal obstruction due to swollen endothelial cells, decreased deformability of circulating erythrocytes, leukocyte-platelet-fibrin thrombi, or compression by edema fluid. On the other hand, studies using orthogonal polarization spectral imaging of the microcirculation in the tongue found that sepsis-associated derangements in capillary flow could be reversed by applying acetylcholine to the surface of the tongue or by giving nitroprusside intravenously; these observations suggest a neuroendocrine basis for the loss of capillary filling. Oxygen utilization by tissues may also be impaired by changes (possibly induced by nitric oxide) that decrease oxidative phosphorylation and ATP production while increasing glycolysis. The local accumulation of lactic acid, a consequence of increased glycolysis, may decrease extracellular pH and contribute to the slowdown in cellular metabolism that occurs within affected tissues.

Remarkably, poorly functioning "septic" organs usually appear normal at autopsy. There is typically very little necrosis or thrombosis, and apoptosis is largely confined to lymphoid organs and the gastrointestinal tract. Moreover, organ function usually returns to normal if patients recover. These points suggest that organ dysfunction during severe sepsis has a basis that is principally biochemical, not structural.

SEPTIC SHOCK The hallmark of septic shock is a decrease in peripheral vascular resistance that occurs despite increased levels of vasopressor catecholamines. Before this vasodilatory phase, many patients experience a period during which oxygen delivery to tissues is compromised by myocardial depression, hypovolemia, and other factors. During this "hypodynamic" period, the blood lactate concentration is elevated and central venous oxygen saturation is low. Fluid administration is usually followed by the hyperdynamic vasodilatory phase, during which cardiac output is normal (or even high) and oxygen consumption declines despite adequate oxygen delivery. The blood lactate level may be normal or increased, and normalization of central venous oxygen saturation may reflect improved oxygen delivery, decreased oxygen uptake by tissues, or left-to-right shunting.

Prominent hypotensive molecules include nitric oxide, β-endorphin, bradykinin, platelet-activating factor, and prostacyclin. Agents that inhibit the synthesis or action of each of these mediators can prevent or reverse endotoxic shock in animals. However, in clinical trials, neither a platelet-activating factor receptor antagonist nor a bradykinin antagonist improved survival rates among patients with septic shock, and a nitric oxide synthase inhibitor, L-N^G-methylarginine HCl, actually increased the mortality rate.

Severe Sepsis: A Single Pathogenesis? In some cases, circulating bacteria and their products almost certainly elicit multiorgan dysfunction and hypotension by directly stimulating inflammatory responses within the vasculature. In patients with fulminant meningococcemia, for example, mortality rates have correlated directly with blood levels of endotoxin and bacterial DNA and with the occurrence of DIC (Chap. 180). In most patients infected with other gram-negative bacteria, in contrast, circulating bacteria or bacterial molecules may reflect uncontrolled infection at a local tissue site and have little or no direct impact on distant organs; in these patients, inflammatory mediators or neural signals arising from the local site seem to be the key triggers for severe sepsis and septic shock. In a large series of patients with positive blood cultures, the risk of developing severe sepsis was strongly related to the site of primary infection: bacteremia arising from a pulmonary or abdominal source was eightfold more likely to be associated with severe sepsis than was bacteremic urinary tract infection, even after the investigators controlled for age, the kind of bacteria isolated from the blood, and other factors. A third pathogenesis may be represented by severe sepsis due to superantigen-producing *S. aureus* or *Streptococcus pyogenes*; the T cell activation induced by these toxins produces a cytokine profile that differs substantially from that elicited by gram-negative bacterial infection. Further evidence for different pathogenetic pathways has come from observations that the pattern of mRNA expression in peripheral-blood leukocytes from children with sepsis is different for gram-positive, gram-negative, and viral pathogens.

The pathogenesis of severe sepsis thus may differ according to the infecting microbe, the ability of the host's innate defense mechanisms to sense and respond to it, the site of the primary infection, the presence or absence of immune defects, and the prior physiologic status of the host. Genetic factors are probably important as well, yet despite much study very few allelic polymorphisms have been associated with sepsis severity in more than one or two analyses. Further studies in this area are needed.

CLINICAL MANIFESTATIONS

The manifestations of the septic response are superimposed on the symptoms and signs of the patient's underlying illness and primary infection. The rate at which severe sepsis develops may differ from patient to patient, and there are striking individual variations in presentation. For example, some patients with sepsis are normo- or hypothermic; the absence of fever is most common in neonates, in elderly patients, and in persons with uremia or alcoholism.

Hyperventilation, producing respiratory alkalosis, is often an early sign of the septic response. Disorientation, confusion, and other manifestations of encephalopathy may also develop early on, particularly in the elderly and in individuals with preexisting neurologic impairment. Focal neurologic signs are uncommon, although preexisting focal deficits may become more prominent.

Hypotension and DIC predispose to acrocyanosis and ischemic necrosis of peripheral tissues, most commonly the digits. Cellulitis, pustules, bullae, or hemorrhagic lesions may develop when hematogenous bacteria or fungi seed the skin or underlying soft tissue. Bacterial toxins may also be distributed hematogenously and elicit diffuse cutaneous reactions. On occasion, skin lesions may suggest specific pathogens. When sepsis is accompanied by cutaneous petechiae or purpura, infection with *N. meningitidis* (or, less commonly, *H. influenzae*) should be suspected (see Fig. 25e-42); in a patient who has been bitten by a tick while in an endemic area, petechial lesions also suggest Rocky Mountain spotted fever (see Fig. 211-1). A cutaneous lesion seen almost exclusively in neutropenic patients is ecthyma gangrenosum, often caused by *P. aeruginosa*. This bullous lesion surrounded by edema undergoes central hemorrhage and necrosis (see Fig. 189-1).

Histopathologic examination shows bacteria in and around the wall of a small vessel, with little or no neutrophilic response. Hemorrhagic or bullous lesions in a septic patient who has recently eaten raw oysters suggest *V. vulnificus* bacteremia, whereas such lesions in a patient who has recently sustained a dog bite may indicate bloodstream infection due to *Capnocytophaga canimorsus* or *Capnocytophaga cynodegmi*. Generalized erythroderma in a septic patient suggests the toxic shock syndrome due to *S. aureus* or *S. pyogenes*.

Gastrointestinal manifestations such as nausea, vomiting, diarrhea, and ileus may suggest acute gastroenteritis. Stress ulceration can lead to upper gastrointestinal bleeding. Cholestatic jaundice, with elevated levels of serum bilirubin (mostly conjugated) and alkaline phosphatase, may precede other signs of sepsis. Hepatocellular or canalicular dysfunction appears to underlie most cases, and the results of hepatic function tests return to normal with resolution of the infection. Prolonged or severe hypotension may induce acute hepatic injury or ischemic bowel necrosis.

Many tissues may be unable to extract oxygen normally from the blood, so that anaerobic metabolism occurs despite near-normal mixed venous oxygen saturation. Blood lactate levels rise early because of increased glycolysis as well as impaired clearance of the resulting lactate and pyruvate by the liver and kidneys. The blood glucose concentration often increases, particularly in patients with diabetes, although impaired gluconeogenesis and excessive insulin release on occasion produce hypoglycemia. The cytokine-driven acute-phase response inhibits the synthesis of transthyretin while enhancing the production of C-reactive protein, fibrinogen, and complement components. Protein catabolism is often markedly accelerated. Serum albumin levels decline as a result of decreased hepatic synthesis and the movement of albumin into interstitial spaces.

MAJOR COMPLICATIONS

Cardiopulmonary Complications Ventilation-perfusion mismatching produces a fall in arterial Po_2 early in the course. Increasing alveolar epithelial injury and capillary permeability result in increased pulmonary water content, which decreases pulmonary compliance and interferes with oxygen exchange. In the absence of pneumonia or heart failure, progressive diffuse pulmonary infiltrates and arterial hypoxemia occurring within 1 week of a known insult indicate the development of mild acute respiratory distress syndrome (ARDS) (200 mmHg $< Pao_2/Fio_2 \leq 300$ mmHg), moderate ARDS (100 mmHg $< Pao_2/Fio_2 \leq 200$ mmHg), or severe ARDS ($Pao_2/Fio_2 \leq 100$ mmHg). Acute lung injury or ARDS develops in ~50% of patients with severe sepsis or septic shock. Respiratory muscle fatigue can exacerbate hypoxemia and hypercapnia. An elevated pulmonary capillary wedge pressure (>18 mmHg) suggests fluid volume overload or cardiac failure rather than ARDS. Pneumonia caused by viruses or by *Pneumocystis* may be clinically indistinguishable from ARDS.

Sepsis-induced hypotension (see "Septic Shock," above) usually results initially from a generalized maldistribution of blood flow and blood volume and from hypovolemia that is due, at least in part, to diffuse capillary leakage of intravascular fluid. Other factors that may decrease effective intravascular volume include dehydration from antecedent disease or insensible fluid losses, vomiting or diarrhea, and polyuria. During early septic shock, systemic vascular resistance is usually elevated and cardiac output may be low. After fluid repletion, in contrast, cardiac output typically increases and systemic vascular resistance falls. Indeed, normal or increased cardiac output and decreased systemic vascular resistance distinguish septic shock from cardiogenic, extracardiac obstructive, and hypovolemic shock; other processes that can produce this combination include anaphylaxis, beriberi, cirrhosis, and overdoses of nitroprusside or narcotics.

Depression of myocardial function, manifested as increased end-diastolic and systolic ventricular volumes with a decreased ejection fraction, develops within 24 h in most patients with severe sepsis. Cardiac output is maintained despite the low ejection fraction because ventricular dilation permits a normal stroke volume. In survivors, myocardial function returns to normal over several days. Although myocardial dysfunction may contribute to hypotension, refractory hypotension is usually due to low systemic vascular resistance, and death most often results from refractory shock or the failure of multiple organs rather than from cardiac dysfunction per se.

Adrenal Insufficiency The diagnosis of adrenal insufficiency may be very difficult in critically ill patients. Whereas a plasma cortisol level of ≤15 μg/mL (≤10 μg/mL if the serum albumin concentration is <2.5 mg/dL) indicates adrenal insufficiency (inadequate production of cortisol), many experts now feel that the adrenocorticotropic hormone (CoSyntropin®) stimulation test is not useful for detecting less profound degrees of corticosteroid deficiency in patients who are critically ill. The concept of critical illness–related corticosteroid insufficiency (CIRCI) was proposed to encompass the different mechanisms that may produce corticosteroid activity that is inadequate for the severity of a patient's illness. Although CIRCI may result from structural damage to the adrenal gland, it is more commonly due to reversible dysfunction of the hypothalamic-pituitary axis or to tissue corticosteroid resistance resulting from abnormalities of the glucocorticoid receptor or increased conversion of cortisol to cortisone. The major clinical manifestation of CIRCI is hypotension that is refractory to fluid replacement and requires pressor therapy. Some classic features of adrenal insufficiency, such as hyponatremia and hyperkalemia, are usually absent; others, such as eosinophilia and modest hypoglycemia, may sometimes be found. Specific etiologies include fulminant *N. meningitidis* bacteremia, disseminated tuberculosis, AIDS (with cytomegalovirus, *Mycobacterium avium-intracellulare*, or *Histoplasma capsulatum* disease), or the prior use of drugs that diminish glucocorticoid production, such as glucocorticoids, megestrol, etomidate, or ketoconazole.

Renal Complications Oliguria, azotemia, proteinuria, and nonspecific urinary casts are frequently found. Many patients are inappropriately polyuric; hyperglycemia may exacerbate this tendency. Most renal failure is due to acute tubular necrosis induced by hypovolemia, arterial hypotension, or toxic drugs, although some patients also have glomerulonephritis, renal cortical necrosis, or interstitial nephritis. Drug-induced renal damage may greatly complicate therapy, particularly when hypotensive patients are given aminoglycoside antibiotics. Nosocomial sepsis following acute renal injury is associated with a high mortality rate.

Coagulopathy Although thrombocytopenia occurs in 10–30% of patients, the underlying mechanisms are not understood. Platelet counts are usually very low (<50,000/μL) in patients with DIC; these low counts may reflect diffuse endothelial injury or microvascular thrombosis, yet thrombi have only infrequently been found on biopsy of septic organs.

Neurologic Complications Delirium (acute encephalopathy) is often an early manifestation of sepsis. Depending on the diagnostic criteria used, it occurs in 10–70% of septic patients at some point during the hospital course. When the septic illness lasts for weeks or months, "critical illness" polyneuropathy may prevent weaning from ventilatory support and produce distal motor weakness. Electrophysiologic studies are diagnostic. Guillain-Barré syndrome, metabolic disturbances, and toxin activity must be ruled out. Recent studies have documented long-term cognitive loss in survivors of severe sepsis.

Immunosuppression Patients with severe sepsis often become profoundly immunosuppressed. Manifestations include loss of delayed-type hypersensitivity reactions to common antigens, failure to control the primary infection, and increased risk for secondary infections (e.g., by opportunists such as *Stenotrophomonas maltophilia*, *Acinetobacter calcoaceticus-baumannii*, and *Candida albicans*). Approximately one-third of patients experience reactivation of herpes simplex virus, varicella-zoster virus, or cytomegalovirus infections; the latter are thought to contribute to adverse outcomes in some instances.

LABORATORY FINDINGS

Abnormalities that occur early in the septic response may include leukocytosis with a left shift, thrombocytopenia, hyperbilirubinemia, and proteinuria. Leukopenia may develop. The neutrophils may contain toxic granulations, Döhle bodies, or cytoplasmic vacuoles. As the septic response becomes more severe, thrombocytopenia worsens (often with prolonged thrombin time, decreased fibrinogen, and the presence of D-dimers, suggesting DIC), azotemia and hyperbilirubinemia become more prominent, and levels of aminotransferases rise. Active hemolysis suggests clostridial bacteremia, malaria, a drug reaction, or DIC; in the case of DIC, microangiopathic changes may be seen on a blood smear.

During early sepsis, hyperventilation induces respiratory alkalosis. With respiratory muscle fatigue and the accumulation of lactate, metabolic acidosis (with increased anion gap) typically supervenes. Evaluation of arterial blood gases reveals hypoxemia that is initially correctable with supplemental oxygen but whose later refractoriness to 100% oxygen inhalation indicates right-to-left shunting. The chest radiograph may be normal or may show evidence of underlying pneumonia, volume overload, or the diffuse infiltrates of ARDS. The electrocardiogram may show only sinus tachycardia or nonspecific ST–T wave abnormalities.

Most diabetic patients with sepsis develop hyperglycemia. Severe infection may precipitate diabetic ketoacidosis that may exacerbate hypotension (Chap. 417). Hypoglycemia occurs rarely and may indicate adrenal insufficiency. The serum albumin level declines as sepsis continues. Hypocalcemia is rare.

DIAGNOSIS

There is no specific diagnostic test for sepsis. Diagnostically sensitive findings in a patient with suspected or proven infection include fever or hypothermia, tachypnea, tachycardia, and leukocytosis or leukopenia (Table 325-1); acutely altered mental status, thrombocytopenia, an elevated blood lactate level, respiratory alkalosis, or hypotension also should suggest the diagnosis. The systemic response can be quite variable, however. In one study, 36% of patients with severe sepsis had a normal temperature, 40% had a normal respiratory rate, 10% had a normal pulse rate, and 33% had normal white blood cell counts. Moreover, the systemic responses of uninfected patients with other conditions may be similar to those characteristic of sepsis. Examples include pancreatitis, burns, trauma, adrenal insufficiency, pulmonary embolism, dissecting or ruptured aortic aneurysm, myocardial infarction, occult hemorrhage, cardiac tamponade, postcardiopulmonary bypass syndrome, anaphylaxis, tumor-associated lactic acidosis, and drug overdose.

Definitive etiologic diagnosis requires identification of the causative microorganism from blood or a local site of infection. At least two blood samples should be obtained (from two different venipuncture sites) for culture; in a patient with an indwelling catheter, one sample should be collected from each lumen of the catheter and another via venipuncture. In many cases, blood cultures are negative; this result can reflect prior antibiotic administration, the presence of slow-growing or fastidious organisms, or the absence of microbial invasion of the bloodstream. In these cases, Gram's staining and culture of material from the primary site of infection or from infected cutaneous lesions may help establish the microbial etiology. Identification of microbial DNA in peripheral blood or tissue samples by polymerase chain reaction may also be definitive. The skin and mucosae should be examined carefully and repeatedly for lesions that might yield diagnostic information. With overwhelming bacteremia (e.g., pneumococcal sepsis in splenectomized individuals; fulminant meningococcemia; or infection with *V. vulnificus*, *B. pseudomallei*, or *Y. pestis*), microorganisms are sometimes visible on buffy coat smears of peripheral blood.

TREATMENT SEVERE SEPSIS AND SEPTIC SHOCK

Patients in whom sepsis is suspected must be managed expeditiously. This task is best accomplished by personnel who are experienced in the care of the critically ill. Successful management requires urgent measures to treat the infection, to provide hemodynamic and respiratory support, and to remove or drain infected tissues. These measures should be initiated within 1 h of the patient's presentation with severe sepsis or septic shock. Rapid assessment and diagnosis are therefore essential.

ANTIMICROBIAL AGENTS

Antimicrobial chemotherapy should be started as soon as samples of blood and other relevant sites have been obtained for culture. A large retrospective review of patients who developed septic shock found that the interval between the onset of hypotension and the administration of appropriate antimicrobial chemotherapy was the major determinant of outcome; a delay of as little as 1 h was associated with lower survival rates. Use of "inappropriate" antibiotics, defined on the basis of local microbial susceptibilities and published guidelines for empirical therapy (see below), was associated with fivefold lower survival rates, even among patients with negative cultures.

It is therefore very important to promptly initiate empirical antimicrobial therapy that is effective against both gram-positive and gram-negative bacteria (Table 325-3). Maximal recommended doses of antimicrobial drugs should be given intravenously, with adjustment for impaired renal function when necessary. Available information about patterns of antimicrobial susceptibility among bacterial isolates from the community, the hospital, and the patient should be taken into account. When culture results become available, the regimen can often be simplified because a single antimicrobial agent is usually adequate for the treatment of a known pathogen. Meta-analyses have concluded that, with one exception, combination antimicrobial therapy is not superior to monotherapy for treating gram-negative bacteremia; the exception is that aminoglycoside monotherapy for *P. aeruginosa* bacteremia is less effective than the combination of an aminoglycoside with an antipseudomonal β-lactam agent. Empirical antifungal therapy should be strongly considered if the septic patient is already receiving broad-spectrum antibiotics or parenteral nutrition, has been neutropenic for ≥5 days, has had a long-term central venous catheter in place, or has been hospitalized in an ICU for a prolonged period. The chosen antimicrobial regimen should be reconsidered daily in order to provide maximal efficacy with minimal resistance, toxicity, and cost.

Most patients require antimicrobial therapy for at least 1 week. The duration of treatment is typically influenced by factors such as the site of tissue infection, the adequacy of surgical drainage, the patient's underlying disease, and the antimicrobial susceptibility of the microbial isolate(s). The absence of an identified microbial pathogen is not necessarily an indication for discontinuing antimicrobial therapy because "appropriate" antimicrobial regimens seem to be beneficial in both culture-negative and culture-positive cases.

REMOVAL OF THE SOURCE OF INFECTION

Removal or drainage of a focal source of infection is essential. In one series, a focus of ongoing infection was found in ~80% of surgical ICU patients who died of severe sepsis or septic shock. Sites of occult infection should be sought carefully, particularly in the lungs, abdomen, and urinary tract. Indwelling IV or arterial catheters should be removed and the tip rolled over a blood agar plate for quantitative culture; after antibiotic therapy has been initiated, a new catheter should be inserted at a different site. Foley and drainage catheters should be replaced. The possibility of paranasal sinusitis (often caused by gram-negative bacteria) should be considered if the patient has undergone nasal intubation or has an indwelling nasogastric or feeding tube. Even in patients without abnormalities on chest radiographs, computed tomography (CT) of the chest may identify unsuspected parenchymal, mediastinal, or pleural disease. In the neutropenic patient, cutaneous sites of tenderness and erythema, particularly in the perianal region, must be carefully sought. In patients with sacral or ischial decubitus ulcers, it is important to exclude pelvic or other soft tissue pus collections with CT or magnetic resonance imaging (MRI). In patients with severe sepsis arising from the urinary tract, sonography or CT should be used to rule out ureteral obstruction, perinephric abscess, and renal abscess. Sonographic or CT imaging of the upper abdomen may disclose

TABLE 325-3 INITIAL ANTIMICROBIAL THERAPY FOR SEVERE SEPSIS WITH NO OBVIOUS SOURCE IN ADULTS WITH NORMAL RENAL FUNCTION

Clinical Condition	Antimicrobial Regimens (Intravenous Therapy)
Immunocompetent adult	The many acceptable regimens include (1) piperacillin-tazobactam (3.375 g q4–6h); (2) imipenem-cilastatin (0.5 g q6h), ertapenem (1 g q24h), or meropenem (1 g q8h); or (3) cefepime (2 g q12h). If the patient is allergic to β-lactam agents, use ciprofloxacin (400 mg q12h) or levofloxacin (500–750 mg q12h) plus clindamycin (600 mg q8h). Vancomycin (15 mg/kg q12h) should be added to each of the above regimens.
Neutropenia (<500 neutrophils/μL)	Regimens include (1) imipenem-cilastatin (0.5 g q6h) or meropenem (1 g q8h) or cefepime (2 g q8h) or (2) piperacillin-tazobactam (3.375 g q4h) plus tobramycin (5–7 mg/kg q24h). Vancomycin (15 mg/kg q12h) should be added if the patient has an indwelling vascular catheter, has received quinolone prophylaxis, or has received intensive chemotherapy that produces mucosal damage; if staphylococci are suspected; if the institution has a high incidence of MRSA infections; or if there is a high prevalence of MRSA isolates in the community. Empirical antifungal therapy with an echinocandin (for caspofungin: a 70-mg loading dose, then 50 mg daily), voriconazole (6 mg/kg q12h for 2 doses, then 3 mg/kg q12h), or a lipid formulation of amphotericin B should be added if the patient is hypotensive, has been receiving broad-spectrum antibacterial drugs, or remains febrile 5 days after initiation of empirical antibacterial therapy.
Splenectomy	Cefotaxime (2 g q6–8h) or ceftriaxone (2 g q12h) should be used. If the local prevalence of cephalosporin-resistant pneumococci is high, add vancomycin. If the patient is allergic to β-lactam drugs, vancomycin (15 mg/kg q12h) plus either moxifloxacin (400 mg q24h) or levofloxacin (750 mg q24h) should be used.
IV drug user	Vancomycin (15 mg/kg q12h) is essential.
AIDS	Cefepime alone (2 g q8h) or piperacillin-tazobactam (3.375 g q4h) plus tobramycin (5–7 mg/kg q24h) should be used. If the patient is allergic to β-lactam drugs, ciprofloxacin (400 mg q12h) or levofloxacin (750 mg q12h) plus vancomycin (15 mg/kg q12h) plus tobramycin should be used.

Abbreviation: MRSA, methicillin-resistant *Staphylococcus aureus.*

Source: Adapted in part from DN Gilbert et al: *The Sanford Guide to Antimicrobial Therapy*, 43rd ed, 2013.

evidence of cholecystitis, bile duct dilation, and pus collections in the liver, subphrenic space, or spleen.

HEMODYNAMIC, RESPIRATORY, AND METABOLIC SUPPORT

The primary goals are to restore adequate oxygen and substrate delivery to the tissues as quickly as possible and to improve tissue oxygen utilization and cellular metabolism. Adequate organ perfusion is thus essential. Circulatory adequacy is assessed by measurement of arterial blood pressure and monitoring of parameters such as mentation, urine output, and skin perfusion. Indirect indices of oxygen delivery and consumption, such as central venous oxygen saturation, may also be useful. Initial management of hypotension should include the administration of IV fluids, typically beginning with 1–2 L of normal saline over 1–2 h. To avoid pulmonary edema, the central venous pressure should be maintained at 8–12 cmH_2O. The urine output rate should be kept at >0.5 mL/kg per hour by continuing fluid administration; a diuretic such as furosemide may be used if needed. In about one-third of patients, hypotension and organ hypoperfusion respond to fluid resuscitation; a reasonable goal is to maintain a mean arterial blood pressure of >65 mmHg (systolic pressure >90 mmHg). If these guidelines cannot be met by volume infusion, vasopressor therapy is indicated (**Chap. 326**). Titrated doses of norepinephrine should be administered through a central catheter. If myocardial dysfunction produces elevated cardiac filling pressures and low cardiac output, inotropic therapy with dobutamine is recommended. Dopamine is rarely used.

In patients with septic shock, plasma vasopressin levels increase transiently but then decrease dramatically. Early studies found that vasopressin infusion can reverse septic shock in some patients, reducing or eliminating the need for catecholamine pressors. Although vasopressin may benefit patients who require less norepinephrine, its role in the treatment of septic shock seems to be a minor one overall.

CIRCI (see "Adrenal Insufficiency," above) should be strongly considered in patients who develop hypotension that does not respond to fluid replacement therapy. Hydrocortisone (50 mg IV every 6 h) should be given; if clinical improvement occurs over 24–48 h, most experts would continue hydrocortisone therapy for 5–7 days before slowly tapering and discontinuing it. Meta-analyses of recent clinical trials have concluded that hydrocortisone therapy hastens recovery from sepsis-induced hypotension without increasing long-term survival.

Ventilator therapy is indicated for progressive hypoxemia, hypercapnia, neurologic deterioration, or respiratory muscle failure. Sustained tachypnea (respiratory rate, >30 breaths/min) is frequently a harbinger of impending respiratory collapse; mechanical ventilation is often initiated to ensure adequate oxygenation, to divert blood from the muscles of respiration, to prevent aspiration of oropharyngeal contents, and to reduce the cardiac afterload. The results of recent studies favor the use of low tidal volumes (6 mL/kg of ideal body weight, or as low as 4 mL/kg if the plateau pressure exceeds 30 cmH_2O). Patients undergoing mechanical ventilation require careful sedation, with daily interruptions; elevation of the head of the bed helps to prevent nosocomial pneumonia. Stress-ulcer prophylaxis with a histamine H_2-receptor antagonist may decrease the risk of gastrointestinal hemorrhage in ventilated patients.

Erythrocyte transfusion is generally recommended when the blood hemoglobin level decreases to ≤7 g/dL, with a target level of 9 g/dL in adults. Erythropoietin is not used to treat sepsis-related anemia. Bicarbonate is sometimes administered for severe metabolic acidosis (arterial pH <7.2), but there is little evidence that it improves either hemodynamics or the response to vasopressor hormones. DIC, if complicated by major bleeding, should be treated with transfusion of fresh-frozen plasma and platelets. Successful treatment of the underlying infection is essential to reverse both acidosis and DIC. Patients who are hypercatabolic and have acute renal failure may benefit greatly from intermittent hemodialysis or continuous veno-venous hemofiltration.

GENERAL SUPPORT

In patients with prolonged severe sepsis (i.e., that lasting more than 2 or 3 days), nutritional supplementation may reduce the impact of protein hypercatabolism; the available evidence favors the enteral delivery route. Prophylactic heparinization to prevent deep venous thrombosis is indicated for patients who do not have active bleeding or coagulopathy; when heparin is contraindicated, compression stockings or an intermittent compression device should be used. Recovery is also assisted by prevention of skin breakdown, nosocomial infections, and stress ulcers.

The role of tight control of the blood glucose concentration in recovery from critical illness has been addressed in numerous controlled trials. Meta-analyses of these trials have concluded that use of insulin to lower blood glucose levels to 100–120 mg/dL is potentially harmful and does not improve survival rates. Most experts now recommend using insulin only if it is needed to maintain the blood glucose concentration below ~180 mg/dL. Patients receiving intravenous insulin must be monitored frequently (every 1–2 h) for hypoglycemia.

OTHER MEASURES

Despite aggressive management, many patients with severe sepsis or septic shock die. Numerous interventions have been tested for their ability to improve survival rates among patients with severe sepsis. The list includes endotoxin-neutralizing proteins, inhibitors of cyclooxygenase or nitric oxide synthase, anticoagulants, polyclonal immunoglobulins, glucocorticoids, a phospholipid emulsion, and antagonists to TNF-α, IL-1, platelet-activating factor, and bradykinin. Unfortunately, none of these agents has improved rates of survival among patients with severe sepsis/septic shock in more than one large-scale, randomized, placebo-controlled clinical trial. Many factors have contributed to this lack of reproducibility, including (1) heterogeneity of the patient populations studied, the primary infection sites, the preexisting illnesses, and the inciting microbes; and (2) the nature of the "standard" therapy also used. A dramatic example of this problem was seen in a trial of tissue factor pathway inhibitor. Whereas the drug appeared to improve survival rates after 722 patients had been studied ($p = .006$), it did not do so in the next 1032 patients, and the overall result was negative. This inconsistency argues that the results of a clinical trial may not apply to individual patients, even within a carefully selected patient population. It also suggests that, at a minimum, a sepsis intervention should show a significant survival benefit in more than one placebo-controlled, randomized clinical trial before it is accepted as routine clinical practice. In one attempt to reduce patient heterogeneity in clinical trials, experts have called for changes that would restrict these trials to patients who have similar underlying diseases (e.g., major trauma) and inciting infections (e.g., pneumonia). Other investigators have proposed using specific biomarkers, such as IL-6 levels in blood or the expression of HLA-DR on peripheral-blood monocytes, to identify the patients most likely to benefit from certain interventions.

Recombinant activated protein C (aPC) was the first immunomodulatory drug to be approved by the U.S. Food and Drug Administration (FDA) for the treatment of patients with severe sepsis or septic shock. Approval was based on the results of a single randomized controlled trial in which the drug was given within 24 h of the patient's first sepsis-related organ dysfunction; the 28-day survival rate was significantly higher among aPC recipients who were very sick (APACHE II score, ≥25) before infusion of the protein than among placebo-treated controls. Subsequent trials failed to show a benefit of aPC treatment in patients who were less sick (APACHE II score, <25) or in children, and, a decade after its licensure by the FDA, the drug was withdrawn from the market when a European trial failed to confirm its efficacy in adults with sepsis. Agents in ongoing or planned clinical trials include intravenous immunoglobulin, a polymyxin B hemofiltration column, and granulocyte-macrophage colony-stimulating factor, which has been reported to restore monocyte immunocompetence in patients with sepsis-associated immunosuppression.

A careful retrospective analysis found that the apparent efficacy of all sepsis therapeutics studied to date has been greatest among the patients at greatest risk of dying before treatment; conversely, use of many of these drugs has been associated with increased mortality rates among patients who are less ill. It is possible that neutralizing one of many different mediators may help patients who are very sick, whereas disrupting the mediator balance may be harmful to patients whose adaptive defense mechanisms are working well. This analysis suggests that if more aggressive early resuscitation improves survival rates among sicker patients, it will become more difficult to obtain additional benefit from other therapies; that is, if an intervention improves patients' risk status, moving them into a "less severe illness" category, it will be harder to show that adding another agent to the therapeutic regimen is beneficial.

THE SURVIVING SEPSIS CAMPAIGN

An international consortium has advocated "bundling" of multiple therapeutic maneuvers into a unified algorithmic approach that will become the standard of care for severe sepsis. In theory, such a strategy would improve care by mandating measures that seem to bring maximal benefit, such as the rapid administration of appropriate antimicrobial therapy, fluids, and blood pressure support. Caution may be engendered by the fact that three of the key elements of the initial algorithm were eventually withdrawn for lack of evidence; moreover, the benefit of the current sepsis bundles has not been established in randomized controlled clinical trials.

PROGNOSIS

Approximately 20–35% of patients with severe sepsis and 40–60% of patients with septic shock die within 30 days. Others die within the ensuing 6 months. Late deaths often result from poorly controlled infection, immunosuppression, complications of intensive care, failure of multiple organs, or the patient's underlying disease. Case–fatality rates are similar for culture-positive and culture-negative severe sepsis. Prognostic stratification systems such as APACHE II indicate that factoring in the patient's age, underlying condition, and various physiologic variables can yield useful estimates of the risk of dying of severe sepsis. Age and prior health status are probably the most important risk factors (Fig. 325-1). In patients with no known preexisting morbidity, the case–fatality rate remains <10% until the fourth decade of life, after which it gradually increases to >35% in the very elderly. Death is significantly more likely in severely septic patients with preexisting illness. Septic shock is also a strong predictor of

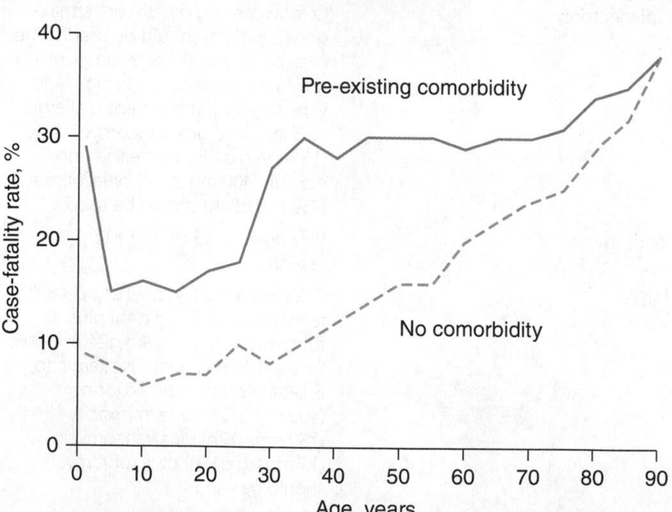

FIGURE 325-1 Influence of age and prior health status on outcome of severe sepsis. With modern therapy, fewer than 10% of previously healthy young individuals (below 35 years of age) die with severe sepsis; the case–fatality rate then increases slowly through middle and old age. The most commonly identified etiologic agents in patients who die are *Staphylococcus aureus*, *Streptococcus pyogenes*, *Streptococcus pneumoniae*, and *Neisseria meningitidis*. Individuals with preexisting comorbidities are at greater risk of dying of severe sepsis at any age. The etiologic agents in these cases are likely to be *S. aureus*, *Pseudomonas aeruginosa*, various Enterobacteriaceae, enterococci, or fungi. *(Adapted from DC Angus et al: Crit Care Med 29:1303, 2001.)*

both short- and long-term mortality. Cognitive impairment may be significant in survivors, particularly those who are elderly.

PREVENTION

Prevention offers the best opportunity to reduce morbidity and mortality from severe sepsis. In developed countries, most episodes of severe sepsis and septic shock are complications of nosocomial infections. These cases might be prevented by reducing the number of invasive procedures undertaken, by limiting the use (and duration of use) of indwelling vascular and bladder catheters, by reducing the incidence and duration of profound neutropenia (<500 neutrophils/μL), and by more aggressively treating localized nosocomial infections. Indiscriminate use of antimicrobial agents and glucocorticoids should be avoided, and optimal infection-control measures (Chap. 168) should be used. Studies indicate that 50–70% of patients who develop nosocomial severe sepsis or septic shock have experienced a less severe stage of the septic response on at least one previous day in the hospital. Research is needed to identify patients at increased risk and to develop adjunctive agents that can modulate the septic response before organ dysfunction or hypotension occurs.

326 Cardiogenic Shock and Pulmonary Edema

Judith S. Hochman, David H. Ingbar

Cardiogenic shock and pulmonary edema are life-threatening conditions that should be treated as medical emergencies. The most common joint etiology is severe left ventricular (LV) dysfunction that leads to pulmonary congestion and/or systemic hypoperfusion (Fig. 326-1). The pathophysiology of pulmonary edema and shock is discussed in Chaps. 47e and 324, respectively.

CARDIOGENIC SHOCK

Cardiogenic shock (CS) is characterized by systemic hypoperfusion due to severe depression of the cardiac index (<2.2 [L/min]/m^2) and sustained systolic arterial hypotension (<90 mmHg) despite an elevated filling pressure (pulmonary capillary wedge pressure [PCWP] >18 mmHg). It is associated with in-hospital mortality rates >50%. The major causes of CS are listed in Table 326-1. Circulatory failure based on cardiac dysfunction may be caused by primary myocardial failure, most commonly secondary to acute myocardial infarction (MI) (Chap. 295), and less frequently by cardiomyopathy or myocarditis (Chap. 287), cardiac tamponade (Chap. 288), or critical valvular heart disease (Chap. 283).

Incidence The rate of CS complicating acute MI was 20% in the 1960s, stayed at ~8% for >20 years, but decreased to 5–7% in the first decade of this millennium largely due to increasing use of early reperfusion therapy for acute MI. Shock is more common with ST elevation MI (STEMI) than with non-ST elevation MI (Chap. 295).

LV failure accounts for ~80% of cases of CS complicating acute MI. Acute severe mitral regurgitation (MR), ventricular septal rupture (VSR), predominant right ventricular (RV) failure, and free wall rupture or tamponade account for the remainder.

Pathophysiology CS is characterized by a vicious circle in which depression of myocardial contractility, usually due to ischemia, results in reduced cardiac output and arterial blood pressure (BP), which result in hypoperfusion of the myocardium and further ischemia and depression of cardiac output (Fig. 326-1). Systolic myocardial dysfunction reduces stroke volume and, together with diastolic dysfunction, leads to elevated LV end-diastolic pressure and PCWP as well as to pulmonary congestion. Reduced coronary perfusion leads to worsening ischemia and progressive myocardial dysfunction and a rapid

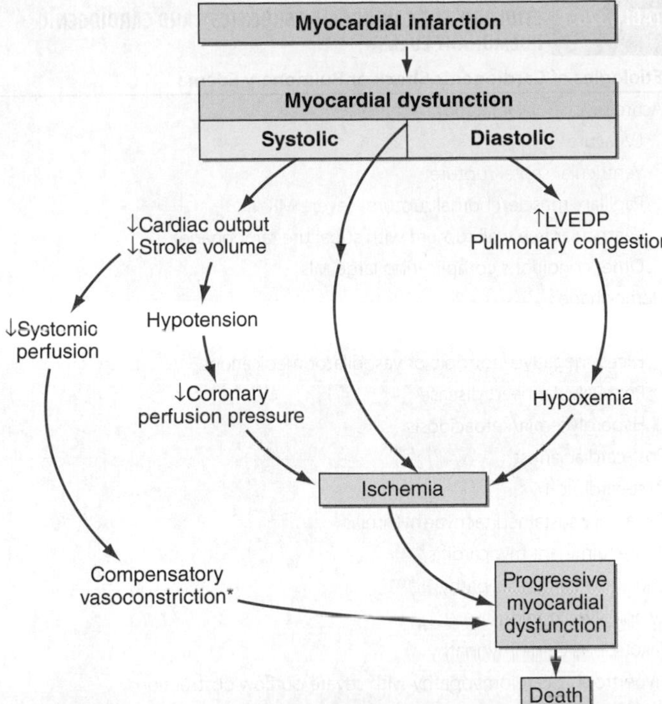

FIGURE 326-1 Pathophysiology of cardiogenic shock. Systolic and diastolic myocardial dysfunction results in a reduction in cardiac output and often pulmonary congestion. Systemic and coronary hypoperfusion occur, resulting in progressive ischemia. Although a number of compensatory mechanisms are activated in an attempt to support the circulation, these compensatory mechanisms may become maladaptive and produce a worsening of hemodynamics. *Release of inflammatory cytokines after myocardial infarction may lead to inducible nitric oxide expression, excess nitric oxide, and inappropriate vasodilation. This causes further reduction in systemic and coronary perfusion. A vicious spiral of progressive myocardial dysfunction occurs that ultimately results in death if it is not interrupted. LVEDP, left ventricular end-diastolic pressure. *(From SM Hollenberg et al: Ann Intern Med 131:47, 1999.)*

downward spiral, which, if uninterrupted, is often fatal. A systemic inflammatory response syndrome may accompany large infarctions and shock. Inflammatory cytokines, inducible nitric oxide synthase, and excess nitric oxide and peroxynitrite may contribute to the genesis of CS as they do to that of other forms of shock (Chap. 324). Lactic acidosis and hypoxemia from CS contribute to the vicious circle by worsening myocardial ischemia and hypotension. Severe acidosis reduces the efficacy of endogenous and exogenously administered catecholamines. Refractory sustained ventricular or atrial tachyarrhythmias can cause or exacerbate CS.

Patient Profile Older age, female sex, prior MI, diabetes, anterior MI location, and extensive coronary artery stenoses are associated with an increased risk of CS complicating MI. Shock associated with a first inferior MI should prompt a search for a mechanical cause. CS may rarely occur in the absence of significant stenosis, as seen in LV apical ballooning/Takotsubo's cardiomyopathy.

Timing Shock is present on admission in only one-quarter of patients who develop CS complicating MI; one-quarter develop it rapidly thereafter, within 6 h of MI onset. Another quarter develop shock later on the first day. Subsequent onset of CS may be due to reinfarction, marked infarct expansion, or a mechanical complication.

Diagnosis Due to the unstable condition of these patients, supportive therapy must be initiated simultaneously with diagnostic evaluation (Fig. 326-2). A focused history and physical examination should be performed, blood specimens sent to the laboratory, and an electrocardiogram (ECG) and chest x-ray obtained.

TABLE 326-1 ETIOLOGIES OF CARDIOGENIC SHOCK (CS)[a] AND CARDIOGENIC PULMONARY EDEMA

Etiologies of Cardiogenic Shock or Pulmonary Edema
Acute myocardial infarction/ischemia
LV failure
Ventricular septal rupture
Papillary muscle/chordal rupture–severe MR
Ventricular free wall rupture with subacute tamponade
Other conditions complicating large MIs
Hemorrhage
Infection
Excess negative inotropic or vasodilator medications
Prior valvular heart disease
Hyperglycemia/ketoacidosis
Post-cardiac arrest
Post-cardiotomy
Refractory sustained tachyarrhythmias
Acute fulminant myocarditis
End-stage cardiomyopathy
LV apical ballooning
Takotsubo's cardiomyopathy
Hypertrophic cardiomyopathy with severe outflow obstruction
Aortic dissection with aortic insufficiency or tamponade
Severe valvular heart disease
Critical aortic or mitral stenosis
Acute severe aortic regurgitation or mitral regurgitation
Toxic/metabolic
β blocker or calcium channel antagonist overdose
Other Etiologies of Cardiogenic Shock[b]
RV failure due to:
Acute myocardial infarction
Acute cor pulmonale
Refractory sustained bradyarrhythmias
Pericardial tamponade
Toxic/metabolic
Severe acidosis, severe hypoxemia

[a]The etiologies of CS are listed. Most of these can cause pulmonary edema instead of shock or pulmonary edema with CS. [b]These cause CS but not pulmonary edema.

Abbreviations: LV, left ventricular; MI, myocardial infarction; MR, mitral regurgitation; RV, right ventricular; VSR, ventricular septal rupture.

Echocardiography is an invaluable diagnostic tool in patients with suspected CS.

CLINICAL FINDINGS Most patients have dyspnea and appear pale, apprehensive, and diaphoretic, and mental status may be altered. The pulse is typically weak and rapid, often in the range of 90–110 beats/min, or severe bradycardia due to high-grade heart block may be present. Systolic BP is reduced (<90 mmHg or ≥30 mmHg below baseline) with a narrow pulse pressure (<30 mmHg), but occasionally BP may be maintained by very high systemic vascular resistance. Tachypnea, Cheyne-Stokes respirations, and jugular venous distention may be present. There is typically a weak apical pulse and soft S_1, and an S_3 gallop may be audible. Acute, severe MR and VSR usually are associated with characteristic systolic murmurs (Chap. 295). Rales are audible in most patients with LV failure. Oliguria is common.

LABORATORY FINDINGS The white blood cell count is typically elevated with a left shift. Renal function is initially unchanged, but blood urea nitrogen and creatinine rise progressively. Hepatic transaminases may be markedly elevated due to liver hypoperfusion. The lactic acid level is elevated. Arterial blood gases usually demonstrate hypoxemia and anion gap metabolic acidosis, which may be compensated by respiratory alkalosis. Cardiac markers, creatine phosphokinase and its MB fraction, and troponins I and T are typically markedly elevated.

ELECTROCARDIOGRAM In CS due to acute MI with LV failure, Q waves and/or >2-mm ST elevation in multiple leads or left bundle branch block are usually present. More than one-half of all infarcts associated with shock are anterior. Global ischemia due to severe left main stenosis usually is accompanied by severe (e.g., >3 mm) ST depressions in multiple leads.

CHEST ROENTGENOGRAM The chest x-ray typically shows pulmonary vascular congestion and often pulmonary edema, but these findings may be absent in up to a third of patients. The heart size is usually normal when CS results from a first MI but is enlarged when it occurs in a patient with a previous MI.

ECHOCARDIOGRAM A two-dimensional echocardiogram with color-flow Doppler (Chap. 270e) should be obtained promptly in patients with suspected CS to help define its etiology. Doppler mapping demonstrates a left-to-right shunt in patients with VSR and the severity of MR when the latter is present. Proximal aortic dissection with aortic regurgitation or tamponade may be visualized, or evidence for pulmonary embolism may be obtained (Chap. 300).

PULMONARY ARTERY CATHETERIZATION The use of pulmonary artery (Swan-Ganz) catheters in patients with established or suspected CS is controversial (Chaps. 272 and 321). Their use is generally recommended for measurement of filling pressures and cardiac output to confirm the diagnosis and to optimize the use of IV fluids, inotropic agents, and vasopressors in persistent shock (Table 326-2). O_2 saturation measurement from right atrial, RV, and pulmonary arterial blood samples can rule out a left-to-right shunt. In CS, low mixed venous O_2 saturations and elevated arteriovenous (AV) O_2 differences reflect low cardiac index and high fractional O_2 extraction. However, when sepsis accompanies CS, AV O_2 differences may not be elevated (Chap. 324). The PCWP is elevated. Use of sympathomimetic amines may return these measurements and the systemic BP to normal. Systemic vascular resistance may be low, normal, or elevated in CS. Equalization of right- and left-sided filling pressures (right atrial and PCWP) suggests cardiac tamponade as the cause of CS (Chap. 288).

LEFT HEART CATHETERIZATION AND CORONARY ANGIOGRAPHY Measurement of LV pressure and definition of the coronary anatomy provide useful information and are indicated in most patients with CS complicating MI. Cardiac catheterization should be performed when there is a plan and capability for immediate coronary intervention (see below) or when a definitive diagnosis has not been made by other tests.

TREATMENT ACUTE MYOCARDIAL INFARCTION

GENERAL MEASURES

(Fig. 326-2) In addition to the usual treatment of acute MI (**Chap. 295**), initial therapy is aimed at maintaining adequate systemic and coronary perfusion by raising systemic BP with vasopressors and adjusting volume status to a level that ensures optimum LV filling pressure. There is interpatient variability, but the values that generally are associated with adequate perfusion are systolic BP ~90 mmHg or mean BP >60 mmHg and PCWP >20 mmHg. Hypoxemia and acidosis must be corrected; most patients require ventilatory support (see "Pulmonary Edema," below). Negative inotropic agents should be discontinued and the doses of renally cleared medications adjusted. Hyperglycemia should be controlled with insulin. Bradyarrhythmias may require transvenous pacing. Recurrent ventricular tachycardia or rapid atrial fibrillation may require immediate treatment (**Chap. 276**).

VASOPRESSORS

Various IV drugs may be used to augment BP and cardiac output in patients with CS. All have important disadvantages, and none has been shown to change the outcome in patients with established shock. *Norepinephrine* is a potent vasoconstrictor and inotropic stimulant that is useful for patients with CS. As first line of therapy norepinephrine was associated with fewer adverse events, including arrhythmias, compared to a dopamine randomized trial of patients

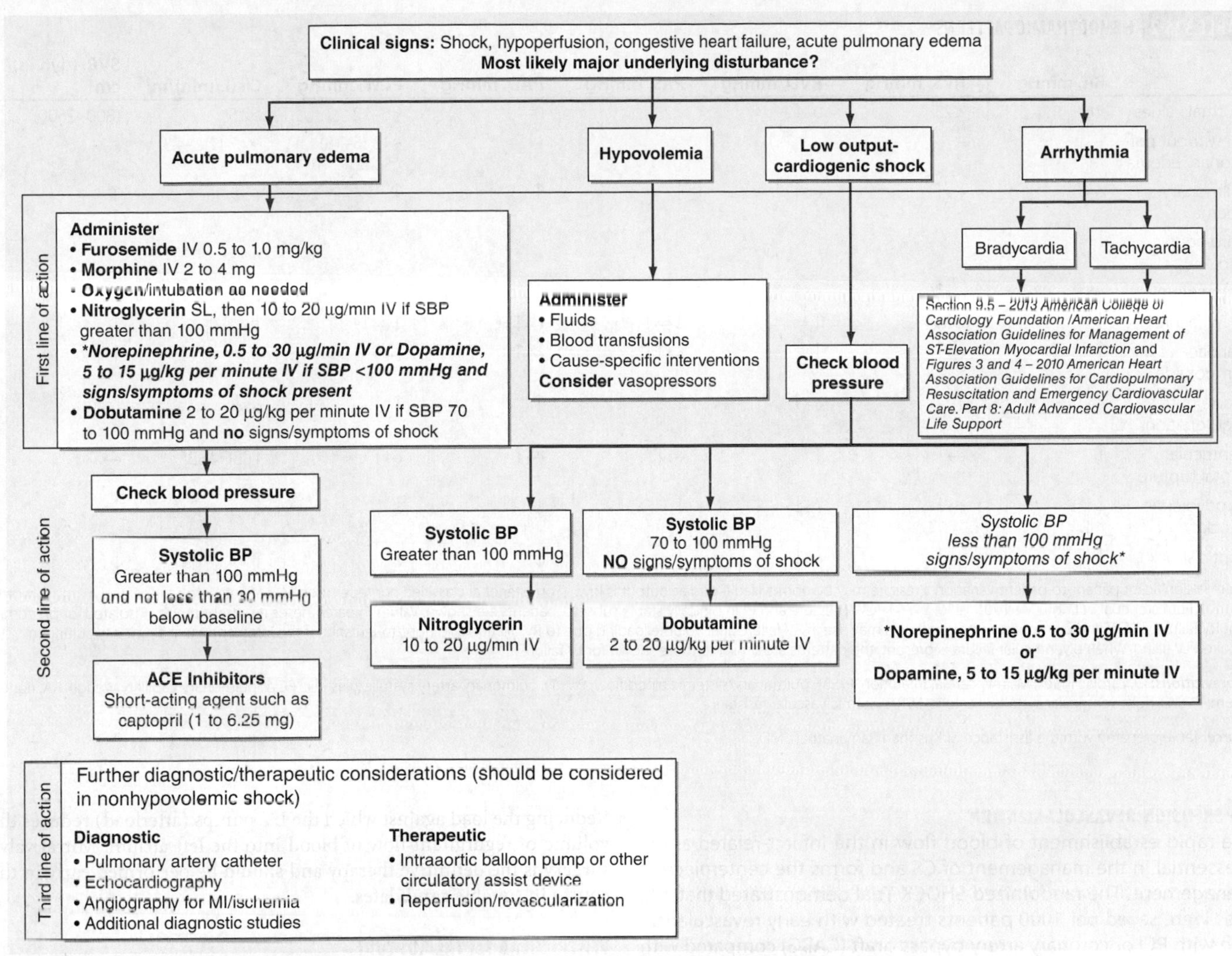
Clinical signs: Shock, hypoperfusion, congestive heart failure, acute pulmonary edema
Most likely major underlying disturbance?
Acute pulmonary edema
Hypovolemia
Low output-cardiogenic shock
Arrhythmia
Bradycardia
Tachycardia
First line of action
Administer
• Furosemide IV 0.5 to 1.0 mg/kg
• Morphine IV 2 to 4 mg
• Oxygen/intubation as needed
• Nitroglycerin SL, then 10 to 20 μg/min IV if SBP greater than 100 mmHg
• *Norepinephrine, 0.5 to 30 μg/min IV or Dopamine, 5 to 15 μg/kg per minute IV if SBP <100 mmHg and signs/symptoms of shock present
• Dobutamine 2 to 20 μg/kg per minute IV if SBP 70 to 100 mmHg and no signs/symptoms of shock
Administer
• Fluids
• Blood transfusions
• Cause-specific interventions
Consider vasopressors
Check blood pressure
Section 9.5 – 2013 American College of Cardiology Foundation /American Heart Association Guidelines for Management of ST-Elevation Myocardial Infarction and Figures 3 and 4 – 2010 American Heart Association Guidelines for Cardiopulmonary Resuscitation and Emergency Cardiovascular Care. Part 8: Adult Advanced Cardiovascular Life Support
Second line of action
Check blood pressure
Systolic BP Greater than 100 mmHg and not less than 30 mmHg below baseline
ACE Inhibitors Short-acting agent such as captopril (1 to 6.25 mg)
Systolic BP Greater than 100 mmHg
Nitroglycerin 10 to 20 μg/min IV
Systolic BP 70 to 100 mmHg NO signs/symptoms of shock
Dobutamine 2 to 20 μg/kg per minute IV
Systolic BP less than 100 mmHg signs/symptoms of shock*
*Norepinephrine 0.5 to 30 μg/min IV or Dopamine, 5 to 15 μg/kg per minute IV
Third line of action
Further diagnostic/therapeutic considerations (should be considered in nonhypovolemic shock)
Diagnostic
• Pulmonary artery catheter
• Echocardiography
• Angiography for MI/ischemia
• Additional diagnostic studies
Therapeutic
• Intraaortic balloon pump or other circulatory assist device
• Reperfusion/revascularization

FIGURE 326-2 The emergency management of patients with cardiogenic shock, acute pulmonary edema, or both is outlined. *Furosemide: <0.5 mg/kg for new-onset acute pulmonary edema without hypervolemia; 1 mg/kg for acute on chronic volume overload, renal insufficiency. †For management of bradycardia and tachycardia, see **Chaps. 274 and 276**. Additional information can also be found in Section 9.5 of the 2013 American College of Cardiology Foundation/American Heart Association Guidelines for Management of ST-Elevation Myocardial Infarction and Figures 3 and 4 of the 2010 American Heart Association Guidelines for Cardiopulmonary Resuscitation and Emergency Cardiovascular Care. Part 8: Adult Advanced Cardiovascular Life Support. *Indicates modification from published guidelines. ACE, angiotensin-converting enzyme; BP, blood pressure; MI, myocardial infarction. *(Modified from Guidelines 2000 for Cardiopulmonary Resuscitation and Emergency Cardiovascular Care. Part 7: The era of reperfusion: Section 1: Acute coronary syndromes [acute myocardial infarction]. The American Heart Association in collaboration with the International Liaison Committee on Resuscitation. Circulation 102:I172, 2000.)*

with several etiologies of circulatory shock. Although it did not significantly improve survival compared to dopamine, its relative safety suggests that norepinephrine is reasonable as initial vasopressor therapy. Norepinephrine should be started at a dose of 2 to 4 μg/min and titrated upward as necessary. If systemic perfusion or systolic pressure cannot be maintained at >90 mmHg with a dose of 15 μg/min, it is unlikely that a further increase will be beneficial.

Dopamine has varying hemodynamic effects based on the dose; at low doses (≤ 2 μg/kg per min), it dilates the renal vascular bed, although its outcome benefits at this low dose have not been demonstrated conclusively; at moderate doses (2–10 μg/kg per min), it has positive chronotropic and inotropic effects as a consequence of β-adrenergic receptor stimulation. At higher doses, a vasoconstrictor effect results from α-receptor stimulation. It is started at an infusion rate of 2–5 μg/kg per min, and the dose is increased every 2–5 min to a maximum of 20–50 μg/kg per min. *Dobutamine* is a synthetic sympathomimetic amine with positive inotropic action and minimal positive chronotropic activity at low doses (2.5 μg/kg per min) but moderate chronotropic activity at higher doses. Although the usual dose is up to 10 μg/kg per min, its vasodilating activity precludes its use when a vasoconstrictor effect is required.

MECHANICAL CIRCULATORY SUPPORT

Circulatory assist devices can be placed percutaneously or surgically and can be used to support the left, right, or both ventricles. Venoarterial extracorporeal membrane oxygenation (VA ECMO, a pump in combination with an oxygenator) may be used when respiratory failure accompanies biventricular failure. Temporary percutaneous devices can be used as a bridge to surgically implanted devices in community hospital settings or when neurologic status is uncertain. The most commonly used device is an intraaortic balloon pump (IABP), which is inserted into the aorta via the femoral artery and provides temporary hemodynamic support. However, routine IABP use in conjunction with early revascularization (predominantly with percutaneous coronary intervention [PCI]) did not reduce 30-day mortality in the IABP-SHOCK II trial. Although other percutaneous devices, including VA ECMO, result in better hemodynamic support compared to IABP, the effects on clinical outcomes are unknown. Surgically implanted devices can support the circulation as bridging therapy for cardiac transplant candidates or as destination therapy **(Chap. 281)**. Assist devices should be used selectively in suitable patients in consultation with advanced heart failure specialists.

TABLE 326-2 HEMODYNAMIC PATTERNS[a]

	RA, mmHg	RVS, mmHg	RVD, mmHg	PAS, mmHg	PAD, mmHg	PCW, mmHg	CI, (L/min)/m^2	SVR, (dyn · s)/cm^5
Normal values	<6	<25	0–12	<25	0–12	<6–12	≥2.5	(800–1600)
MI without pulmonary edema[b]	–	–	–	–	–	~13 (5–18)	~2.7 (2.2–4.3)	–
Pulmonary edema	↔↑	↔↑	↔↑	↑	↑	↑	↔↓	↑
Cardiogenic shock								
LV failure	↔↑	↔↑	↔↑	↔↑	↑	↑	↓	↔↑
RV failure[c]	↑	↓↔↑[d]	↑	↓↔↑[d]	↔↓↑[d]	↓↔↑[d]	↓	↑
Cardiac tamponade	↑	↔↑	↑	↔↑	↔↑	↔↑	↓	↑
Acute mitral regurgitation	↔↑	↑	↔↑	↑	↑	↑	↔↓	↔↑
Ventricular septal rupture	↑	↔↑	↑	↔↑	↔↑	↔↑	↑PBF ↓SBF	↔↑
Hypovolemic shock	↓	↔↓	↔↓	↓	↓	↓	↓	↑
Septic shock	↓	↔↓	↔↓	↓	↓	↓	↑	↓

[a]There is significant patient-to-patient variation. Pressure may be normalized if cardiac output is low. [b]Forrester et al classified nonreperfused MI patients into four hemodynamic subsets. (From JS Forrester et al: N Engl J Med 295:1356, 1976.) PCW pressure and CI in clinically stable subset 1 patients are shown. Values in parentheses represent range. [c]"Isolated" or predominant RV failure. [d]PCW and pulmonary artery pressures may rise in RV failure after volume loading due to RV dilation and right-to-left shift of the interventricular septum, resulting in impaired LV filling. When biventricular failure is present, the patterns are similar to those shown for LV failure.

Abbreviations: CI, cardiac index; MI, myocardial infarction; P/SBF, pulmonary/systemic blood flow; PAS/D, pulmonary artery systolic/diastolic; PCW, pulmonary capillary wedge; RA, right atrium; RVS/D, right ventricular systolic/diastolic; SVR, systemic vascular resistance.

Source: Table prepared with the assistance of Krishnan Ramanathan, MD.

REPERFUSION-REVASCULARIZATION

The rapid establishment of blood flow in the infarct-related artery is essential in the management of CS and forms the centerpiece of management. The randomized SHOCK Trial demonstrated that 132 lives were saved per 1000 patients treated with early revascularization with PCI or coronary artery bypass graft (CABG) compared with initial medical therapy including IABP with fibrinolytics followed by delayed revascularization. The benefit is seen across the risk strata and is sustained up to 11 years after an MI. Early revascularization with PCI or CABG is recommended in candidates suitable for aggressive care.

Prognosis Within this high-risk condition, there is a wide range of expected death rates based on age, severity of hemodynamic abnormalities, severity of the clinical manifestations of hypoperfusion, and the performance of early revascularization.

SHOCK SECONDARY TO RIGHT VENTRICULAR INFARCTION

Although transient hypotension is common in patients with RV infarction and inferior MI (Chap. 295), persistent CS due to RV failure accounts for only 3% of CS complicating MI. The salient features of RV shock are absence of pulmonary congestion, high right atrial pressure (which may be seen only after volume loading), RV dilation and dysfunction, only mildly or moderately depressed LV function, and predominance of single-vessel proximal right coronary artery occlusion. Management includes IV fluid administration to optimize right atrial pressure (10–15 mmHg); avoidance of excess fluids, which cause a shift of the interventricular septum into the LV; sympathomimetic amines; the early reestablishment of infarct-artery flow; and assist devices.

MITRAL REGURGITATION

(See also Chap. 295) Acute severe MR due to papillary muscle dysfunction and/or rupture may complicate MI and result in CS and/or pulmonary edema. This complication most often occurs on the first day, with a second peak several days later. The diagnosis is confirmed by echo-Doppler. Rapid stabilization with IABP is recommended, with administration of dobutamine as needed to raise cardiac output. Reducing the load against which the LV pumps (afterload) reduces the volume of regurgitant flow of blood into the left atrium. Mitral valve surgery is the definitive therapy and should be performed early in the course in suitable candidates.

VENTRICULAR SEPTAL RUPTURE

(See also Chap. 295) Echo-Doppler demonstrates shunting of blood from the left to the right ventricle and may visualize the opening in the interventricular septum. Timing and management are similar to those for MR with IABP support and surgical correction for suitable candidates.

FREE WALL RUPTURE

Myocardial rupture is a dramatic complication of STEMI that is most likely to occur during the first week after the onset of symptoms; its frequency increases with the age of the patient. The clinical presentation typically is a sudden loss of pulse, blood pressure, and consciousness but sinus rhythm on ECG (pulseless electrical activity) due to cardiac tamponade (Chap. 288). Free wall rupture may also result in CS due to subacute tamponade when the pericardium temporarily seals the rupture sites. Definitive surgical repair is required.

ACUTE FULMINANT MYOCARDITIS

(See also Chap. 287) Myocarditis can mimic acute MI with ST deviation or bundle branch block on the ECG and marked elevation of cardiac markers. Acute myocarditis causes CS in a small proportion of cases. These patients are typically younger than those with CS due to acute MI and often do not have typical ischemic chest pain. Echocardiography usually shows global LV dysfunction. Initial management is the same as for CS complicating acute MI (Fig. 326-2) but does not involve coronary revascularization. Endomyocardial biopsy is recommended to determine the diagnosis and need for immunosuppressives for entities such as giant cell myocarditis. Refractory CS can be managed with assist devices with or without ECMO.

PULMONARY EDEMA

The etiologies and pathophysiology of pulmonary edema are discussed in Chap. 47e.

Diagnosis Acute pulmonary edema usually presents with the rapid onset of dyspnea at rest, tachypnea, tachycardia, and severe hypoxemia. Crackles and wheezing due to alveolar flooding and airway compression from peribronchial cuffing may be audible. Release of endogenous catecholamines often causes hypertension.

It is often difficult to distinguish between cardiogenic and noncardiogenic causes of acute pulmonary edema. *Echocardiography* may identify systolic and diastolic ventricular dysfunction and valvular lesions. Electrocardiographic ST elevation and evolving Q waves are usually diagnostic of acute MI and should prompt immediate institution of MI protocols and coronary artery reperfusion therapy (Chap. 295). Brain natriuretic peptide levels, when substantially elevated, support heart failure as the etiology of acute dyspnea with pulmonary edema (Chap. 279).

The use of a *Swan-Ganz catheter* permits measurement of PCWP and helps differentiate high-pressure (cardiogenic) from normal-pressure (noncardiogenic) causes of pulmonary edema. Pulmonary artery catheterization is indicated when the etiology of the pulmonary edema is uncertain, when edema is refractory to therapy, or when it is accompanied by hypotension. Data derived from use of a catheter often alter the treatment plan, but no impact on mortality rates has been demonstrated.

TREATMENT PULMONARY EDEMA

The treatment of pulmonary edema depends on the specific etiology. As an acute, life-threatening condition, a number of measures must be applied immediately to support the circulation, gas exchange, and lung mechanics. Simultaneously, conditions that frequently complicate pulmonary edema, such as infection, acidemia, anemia, and acute kidney dysfunction, must be corrected.

SUPPORT OF OXYGENATION AND VENTILATION

Patients with acute cardiogenic pulmonary edema generally have an identifiable cause of acute LV failure—such as arrhythmia, ischemia/infarction, or myocardial decompensation (Chap. 279)—that may be rapidly treated, with improvement in gas exchange. In contrast, noncardiogenic edema usually resolves much less quickly, and most patients require mechanical ventilation.

Oxygen Therapy Support of oxygenation is essential to ensure adequate O_2 delivery to peripheral tissues, including the heart.

Positive-Pressure Ventilation Pulmonary edema increases the work of breathing and the O_2 requirements of this work, imposing a significant physiologic stress on the heart. When oxygenation or ventilation is not adequate in spite of supplemental O_2, positive-pressure ventilation by face or nasal mask or by endotracheal intubation should be initiated. Noninvasive ventilation (Chap. 323) can rest the respiratory muscles, improve oxygenation and cardiac function, and reduce the need for intubation. In refractory cases, mechanical ventilation can relieve the work of breathing more completely than can noninvasive ventilation. Mechanical ventilation with positive end-expiratory pressure can have multiple beneficial effects on pulmonary edema: (1) decreases both preload and afterload, thereby improving cardiac function; (2) redistributes lung water from the intraalveolar to the extraalveolar space, where the fluid interferes less with gas exchange; and (3) increases lung volume to avoid atelectasis.

REDUCTION OF PRELOAD

In most forms of pulmonary edema, the quantity of extravascular lung water is determined by both the PCWP and the intravascular volume status.

Diuretics The "loop diuretics" furosemide, bumetanide, and torsemide are effective in most forms of pulmonary edema, even in the presence of hypoalbuminemia, hyponatremia, or hypochloremia. Furosemide is also a venodilator that rapidly reduces preload before any diuresis, and is the diuretic of choice. The initial dose of furosemide should be ≤0.5 mg/kg, but a higher dose (1 mg/kg) is required in patients with renal insufficiency, chronic diuretic use, or hypervolemia or after failure of a lower dose.

Nitrates Nitroglycerin and isosorbide dinitrate act predominantly as venodilators but have coronary vasodilating properties as well. They are rapid in onset and effective when administered by a variety of routes. Sublingual nitroglycerin (0.4 mg × 3 every 5 min) is first-line therapy for acute cardiogenic pulmonary edema. If pulmonary edema persists in the absence of hypotension, sublingual may be followed by IV nitroglycerin, commencing at 5–10 μg/min. IV nitroprusside (0.1–5 μg/kg per min) is a potent venous and arterial vasodilator. It is useful for patients with pulmonary edema and hypertension but is not recommended in states of reduced coronary artery perfusion. It requires close monitoring and titration using an arterial catheter for continuous BP measurement.

Morphine Given in 2- to 4-mg IV boluses, morphine is a transient venodilator that reduces preload while relieving dyspnea and anxiety. These effects can diminish stress, catecholamine levels, tachycardia, and ventricular afterload in patients with pulmonary edema and systemic hypertension.

Angiotensin-Converting Enzyme (ACE) Inhibitors ACE inhibitors reduce both afterload and preload and are recommended for hypertensive patients. A low dose of a short-acting agent may be initiated and followed by increasing oral doses. In acute MI with heart failure, ACE inhibitors reduce short- and long-term mortality rates.

Other Preload-Reducing Agents IV recombinant brain natriuretic peptide (nesiritide) is a potent vasodilator with diuretic properties and is effective in the treatment of cardiogenic pulmonary edema. It should be reserved for refractory patients and is not recommended in the setting of ischemia or MI.

Physical Methods In nonhypotensive patients, venous return can be reduced by use of the sitting position with the legs dangling along the side of the bed.

Inotropic and Inodilator Drugs The sympathomimetic amines dopamine and dobutamine (see above) are potent inotropic agents. The bipyridine phosphodiesterase-3 inhibitors (inodilators), such as milrinone (50 μg/kg followed by 0.25–0.75 μg/kg per min), stimulate myocardial contractility while promoting peripheral and pulmonary vasodilation. Such agents are indicated in patients with cardiogenic pulmonary edema and severe LV dysfunction.

Digitalis Glycosides Once a mainstay of treatment because of their positive inotropic action (Chap. 279), digitalis glycosides are rarely used at present. However, they may be useful for control of ventricular rate in patients with rapid atrial fibrillation or flutter and LV dysfunction, because they do not have the negative inotropic effects of other drugs that inhibit atrioventricular nodal conduction.

Intraaortic Balloon Counterpulsation IABP or other LV-assist devices (Chap. 281) may help relieve cardiogenic pulmonary edema and are indicated when refractory pulmonary edema results from the etiologies discussed in the CS section, especially in preparation for surgical repair.

Treatment of Tachyarrhythmias and Atrial-Ventricular Resynchronization (See also Chap. 277) Sinus tachycardia or atrial fibrillation can result from elevated left atrial pressure and sympathetic stimulation. Tachycardia itself can limit LV filling time and raise left atrial pressure further. Although relief of pulmonary congestion will slow the sinus rate or ventricular response in atrial fibrillation, a primary tachyarrhythmia may require cardioversion. In patients with reduced LV function and without atrial contraction or with lack of synchronized atrioventricular contraction, placement of an atrioventricular sequential pacemaker should be considered (Chap. 274).

Stimulation of Alveolar Fluid Clearance A variety of drugs can stimulate alveolar epithelial ion transport and upregulate the clearance of alveolar solute and water, but this strategy has not been proven beneficial in clinical trials thus far.

Risk of Iatrogenic Cardiogenic Shock In the treatment of pulmonary edema, vasodilators lower BP, and their use, particularly in combination, may lead to hypotension, coronary artery hypoperfusion, and shock (Fig. 326-1). In general, patients with a *hypertensive* response to pulmonary edema tolerate and benefit from these medications. In normotensive patients, low doses of single agents should be instituted sequentially, as needed.

Acute Coronary Syndromes (See also Chap. 295) Acute STEMI complicated by pulmonary edema is associated with in-hospital mortality rates of 20–40%. After immediate stabilization, coronary artery blood flow must be reestablished rapidly. When available, primary PCI is preferable; alternatively, a fibrinolytic agent should be administered. Early coronary angiography and revascularization by PCI or CABG also are indicated for patients with non-ST elevation acute coronary syndrome. Assist devices may be used selectively as noted for refractory pulmonary edema.

Extracorporeal Membrane Oxygenation For patients with acute, severe noncardiogenic edema with a potential rapidly reversible cause, ECMO may be considered as a temporizing supportive measure to achieve adequate gas exchange. Usually venovenous ECMO is used in this setting.

Unusual Types of Edema Specific etiologies of pulmonary edema may require particular therapy. Reexpansion pulmonary edema can develop after removal of longstanding pleural space air or fluid. These patients may develop hypotension or oliguria resulting from rapid fluid shifts into the lung. Diuretics and preload reduction are contraindicated, and intravascular volume repletion often is needed while supporting oxygenation and gas exchange.

High-altitude pulmonary edema often can be prevented by use of dexamethasone, calcium channel–blocking drugs, or long-acting inhaled β_2-adrenergic agonists. Treatment includes descent from altitude, bed rest, oxygen, and, if feasible, inhaled nitric oxide; nifedipine may also be effective.

For pulmonary edema resulting from upper airway obstruction, recognition of the obstructing cause is key, because treatment then is to relieve or bypass the obstruction.

327 Cardiovascular Collapse, Cardiac Arrest, and Sudden Cardiac Death

Robert J. Myerburg, Agustin Castellanos

OVERVIEW AND DEFINITIONS

Sudden cardiac death (SCD) is defined *as natural death due to cardiac causes* in a person who may or may not have previously recognized heart disease but in whom the time and mode of death are *unexpected*. The term "sudden," in the context of SCD, is defined for most clinical and epidemiologic purposes as *1 h or less* between a change in clinical status heralding the onset of the terminal clinical event and the cardiac arrest itself. One exception is unwitnessed deaths, in which pathologists may expand the temporal definition to 24 h after the victim was last seen to be alive and stable.

Another exception is the variable interval between cardiac arrest and biological death that results from community-based interventions, following which victims may remain biologically alive for days or even weeks after a cardiac arrest that has resulted in irreversible central nervous system damage. Confusion in terms can be avoided by adhering strictly to definitions of cardiovascular collapse, cardiac arrest, and death (Table 327-1). Although cardiac arrest is often potentially reversible by appropriate and timely interventions, death is biologically, legally, and literally an absolute and irreversible event. Biological death may be delayed by interventions, but the relevant pathophysiologic event remains the sudden and unexpected cardiac arrest. Accordingly, for statistical purposes, deaths that occur during hospitalization or within 30 days after resuscitated cardiac arrest are counted as sudden deaths.

The majority of natural deaths are caused by cardiac disorders. However, it is common for underlying heart diseases—often far advanced—to go unrecognized before the fatal event. As a result, up to two-thirds of all SCDs occur as the first clinical expression of previously undiagnosed disease or in patients with known heart disease, the extent of which suggests low individual risk. The magnitude of sudden *cardiac* death as a public health problem is highlighted by the estimate that ~50% of all cardiac deaths are sudden and unexpected, accounting for a total SCD burden estimated to range from <200,000 to >450,000 deaths each year in the United States. SCD is a direct consequence of cardiac arrest, which may be reversible if addressed promptly. Because resuscitation techniques and emergency rescue systems are available to respond to victims of out-of-hospital cardiac arrest, which was uniformly fatal in the past, understanding the SCD problem has practical clinical importance.

CLINICAL DEFINITION OF FORMS OF CARDIOVASCULAR COLLAPSE

Cardiovascular collapse is a general term connoting loss of sufficient cerebral blood flow to maintain consciousness due to acute dysfunction of the heart and/or peripheral vasculature. It may be caused by vasodepressor syncope (vasovagal syncope, postural hypotension with syncope, neurocardiogenic syncope; Chap. 27), a transient severe bradycardia, or cardiac arrest. The latter is distinguished from the transient forms of cardiovascular collapse in that it usually requires an active intervention to restore spontaneous blood flow. In contrast, vasodepressor syncope and other primary bradyarrhythmic syncopal events are transient and non-life-threatening, with spontaneous return of consciousness.

In the past, the most common electrical mechanism for cardiac arrest was ventricular fibrillation (VF) or pulseless sustained ventricular tachycardia (PVT). These were the initial rhythms recorded in 60–80% of cardiac arrests, with VF being the far more common of the two. Severe persistent bradyarrhythmias, asystole, and pulseless electrical activity (PEA; organized electrical activity, unusually slow, without mechanical response, formerly called electromechanical dissociation [EMD]) caused another 20–30%. Currently, asystole has emerged as the most common mechanism recorded at initial contact (45–50% of cases). PEA accounts for 20–25%, and VF is now present on initial contact in 25–35%. Undoubtedly, a significant proportion of the asystole cases began as VF and deteriorated to asystole because of long response times, but there are data suggesting an absolute reduction in VF as well. Acute low cardiac output states, having a precipitous onset, also may present clinically as a cardiac arrest. These hemodynamic causes include massive acute pulmonary emboli, internal blood loss from a ruptured aortic aneurysm, intense anaphylaxis, and cardiac rupture with tamponade after myocardial infarction (MI).

ETIOLOGY, INITIATING EVENTS, AND CLINICAL EPIDEMIOLOGY

Clinical, epidemiologic, and pathologic studies have provided information on the underlying *structural substrates* in victims of SCD and identified subgroups at high risk for SCD. In addition, studies of clinical physiology have begun to identify *transient functional factors* that may convert a long-standing underlying structural abnormality from a stable to an unstable state, leading to the onset of cardiac arrest (Table 327-2).

Cardiac disorders constitute the most common causes of sudden *natural* death. After an initial peak incidence of sudden death between birth and 6 months of age (sudden infant death syndrome [SIDS]), the incidence of sudden death declines sharply and remains low through childhood and adolescence. Among adolescents and young adults, the incidence of SCD is approximately 1 per 100,000 population per year. The incidence begins to increase in adults over age 30 years, reaching a second peak in the age range of 45–75 years, when it approximates 1–2 per 1000 per year among the unselected adult population. Increasing

TABLE 327-1 DISTINCTION BETWEEN CARDIOVASCULAR COLLAPSE, CARDIAC ARREST, AND DEATH

Term	Definition	Qualifiers	Mechanisms
Cardiovascular collapse	Sudden loss of effective blood flow due to cardiac and/or peripheral vascular factors that may reverse spontaneously (e.g., neurocardiogenic syncope, vasovagal syncope) or require interventions (e.g., cardiac arrest)	Nonspecific term: includes cardiac arrest and its consequences and transient events that characteristically revert spontaneously	Same as "Cardiac Arrest," plus vasodepressor syncope or other causes of transient loss of blood flow
Cardiac arrest	Abrupt cessation of cardiac mechanical function, which may be reversible by a prompt intervention but will lead to death in its absence	Rare spontaneous reversions; likelihood of successful intervention relates to mechanism of arrest, clinical setting, and prompt return of circulation	Ventricular fibrillation, ventricular tachycardia, asystole, bradycardia, pulseless electrical activity, noncardiac mechanical factors (e.g., pulmonary embolism)
Sudden cardiac death	Sudden, irreversible cessation of all biological functions	None	

Source: Modified from RJ Myerburg, A Castellanos: Cardiac arrest and sudden cardiac death, in P Libby et al (eds): *Braunwald's Heart Disease*, 8th ed. Philadelphia, Saunders, 2008.

TABLE 327-2 CARDIAC ARREST AND SUDDEN CARDIAC DEATH

Structural Substrates and Causes

- I. Coronary heart disease
  - A. Coronary artery abnormalities
    - 1. Chronic atherosclerotic lesions
    - 2. Active lesions (plaque fissuring, platelet aggregation, acute thrombosis)
    - 3. Anomalous coronary artery anatomy
  - B. Myocardial infarction
    - 1. Healed
    - 2. Acute
- II. Myocardial hypertrophy
  - A. Secondary
  - B. Hypertrophic cardiomyopathy
    - 1. Obstructive
    - 2. Nonobstructive
- III. Dilated cardiomyopathy—primary muscle disease
- IV. Inflammatory and infiltrative disorders
  - A. Myocarditis
  - B. Noninfectious inflammatory diseases
  - C. Infiltrative diseases
- V. Valvular heart disease
- VI. Electrophysiologic abnormalities, structural
  - A. Anomalous pathways in Wolff-Parkinson-White syndrome
  - B. Conducting system disease
- VII. Inherited disorders associated with electrophysiologic abnormalities (congenital long QT syndromes, right ventricular dysplasia, Brugada syndrome, catecholaminergic polymorphic ventricular tachycardia, etc.)

Triggers for Expression of Cardiac Arrest

- I. Alterations of coronary blood flow
  - A. Transient ischemia
  - B. Reperfusion after ischemia
- II. Low cardiac output states
  - A. Heart failure
    - 1. Chronic
    - 2. Acute decompensation
  - B. Shock
- III. Systemic metabolic abnormalities
  - A. Electrolyte imbalance (e.g., hypokalemia)
  - B. Hypoxemia, acidosis
- IV. Neurologic disturbances
  - A. Autonomic fluctuations: central, neural, humoral
  - B. Receptor function
- V. Toxic responses
  - A. Proarrhythmic drug effects
  - B. Cardiac toxins (e.g., cocaine, digitalis intoxication)
  - C. Drug interactions

age within this range is associated with increasing risk for sudden *cardiac* death (Fig. 327-1A). From 1 to 13 years of age, only one of five sudden *natural* deaths is due to cardiac causes. Between 14 and 21 years of age, the proportion increases to 30%, and it rises to 88% in the middle-aged and elderly.

Young and middle-aged men and women have different susceptibilities to SCD, but the sex differences decrease and ultimately disappear with advancing age. The difference in risk for SCD parallels the differences in age-related risks for other manifestations of coronary heart disease (CHD) between men and women. As the gender gap for manifestations of CHD closes in the sixth to eighth decades of life, the excess risk of SCD in males progressively narrows. Despite the lower incidence among younger women, coronary risk factors such as cigarette smoking, diabetes, hyperlipidemia, and hypertension are highly influential, and SCD remains an important clinical and epidemiologic problem. The incidence of SCD among the African-American population appears to be higher than it is among the white population; the reasons remain uncertain.

Genetic factors contribute to the risk of acquiring CHD, and a genetic basis for its expression as SCD is being explored. A genetic hypothesis for at least part of the SCD risk is supported by data suggesting a familial predisposition to SCD as a specific form of expression of CHD. A parental history of SCD as a first cardiac event increases the probability that an acute coronary event in the offspring will express similarly. In a number of less common syndromes, such as hypertrophic cardiomyopathy, congenital long QT interval syndromes, right ventricular dysplasia, and the syndrome of right bundle branch block and nonischemic ST-segment elevations (Brugada syndrome), and other more rare syndromes, there is a specific inherited risk of ventricular arrhythmias and SCD (Chap. 277).

The etiologic structural substrates and functional factors contributing to expression of the SCD syndrome are listed in Table 327-2. Worldwide, and especially in Western cultures, coronary atherosclerotic heart disease is the most common structural abnormality associated with SCD in middle-aged and older adults. Up to 80% of all SCDs in the United States are due to the consequences of coronary atherosclerosis. The nonischemic cardiomyopathies (dilated and hypertrophic, collectively; Chap. 273e) account for another 10–15% of SCDs, and all the remaining diverse etiologies cause only 5–10% of all SCDs. The inherited arrhythmia syndromes (see above and Table 327-2) are proportionally more common causes in adolescents and young adults. For some of these syndromes, such as hypertrophic cardiomyopathy (Chap. 287), the risk of SCD increases significantly after the onset of puberty.

Transient ischemia in a previously scarred or hypertrophied heart, hemodynamic and fluid and electrolyte disturbances, fluctuations in autonomic nervous system activity, and transient electrophysiologic changes caused by drugs or other chemicals (e.g., proarrhythmia) have all been implicated as mechanisms responsible for the transition from electrophysiologic stability to instability. In addition, reperfusion of ischemic myocardium may cause transient electrophysiologic instability and arrhythmias.

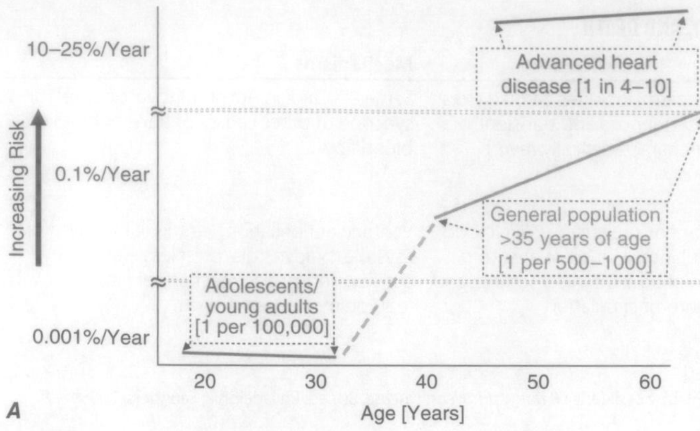

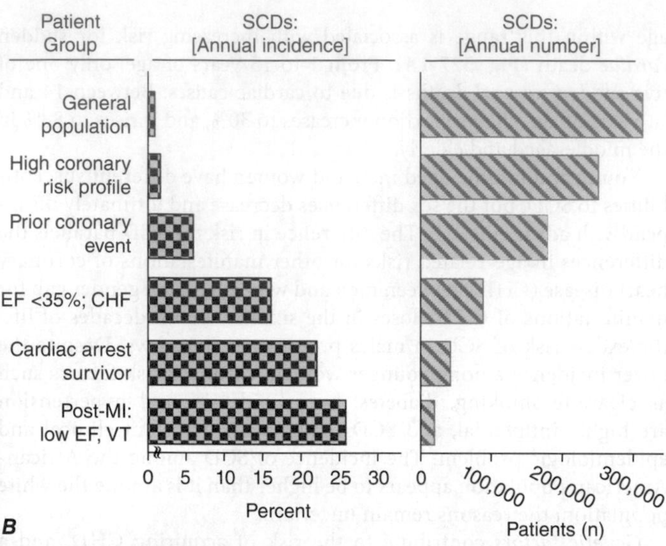

FIGURE 327-1 ***Panel A*** demonstrates age-related risk for sudden cardiac death (SCD). For the general population age 35 years and older, SCD risk is 0.1–0.2% per year (1 per 500–1000 population). Among the general population of adolescents and adults younger than age 30 years, the overall risk of SCD is 1 per 100,000 population, or 0.001% per year. The risk of SCD increases dramatically beyond age 35 years. The greatest rate of increase is between 40 and 65 years (vertical axis is discontinuous). Among patients older than 30 years of age, with advanced structural heart disease and markers of high risk for cardiac arrest, the event rate may exceed 25% per year, and age-related risk attenuates. *(Modified from RJ Myerburg, A Castellanos: Cardiac arrest and sudden cardiac death, in P Libby et al [eds]: Braunwald's Heart Disease, 8th ed. Philadelphia, Saunders, 2008.)* ***Panel B*** demonstrates the incidence of SCD in population subgroups and the relation of total number of events per year to incidence figures. Approximations of subgroup incidence figures and the related population pool from which they are derived are presented. Approximately 50% of all cardiac deaths are sudden and unexpected. The incidence bars on the left (percent/year) indicate the approximate percentage of sudden and nonsudden deaths in each of the population subgroups indicated, ranging from the lowest percentage in unselected adult populations (0.1–2% per year) to the highest percentage in patients with severe left ventricular dysfunction and heart failure (approximately 25% per year). The bars on the right indicate the total number of events per year in each of these groups with the population impact size of each of the subgroups. The highest risk categories identify the smallest number of total annual events, and the lowest incidence category accounts for the largest number of events per year. CHF, congestive heart failure; EF, ejection fraction; MI, myocardial infarction; VT, ventricular tachycardia. *(After RJ Myerburg et al: Circulation 85:2, 1992.)*

PATHOLOGY

Data from postmortem examinations of SCD victims parallel the clinical observations on the prevalence of CHD as the major structural etiologic factor. More than 80% of SCD victims have pathologic findings of CHD. The pathologic description often includes a combination of long-standing, extensive atherosclerosis of the epicardial coronary arteries and unstable coronary artery lesions, which include various permutations of eroded, fissured, or ruptured plaques; platelet aggregates; hemorrhage; and/or thrombosis. As many as 70–75% of males who die suddenly have preexisting healed MIs, whereas only 20–30% have recent acute MIs, despite the prevalence of unstable plaques and thrombi. The latter suggests transient ischemia as the mechanism of onset. Regional or global left ventricular (LV) hypertrophy often coexists with prior MIs.

PREDICTION AND PREVENTION OF CARDIAC ARREST AND SUDDEN CARDIAC DEATH

SCD accounts for approximately one-half the total number of cardiovascular deaths. As shown in Fig. 327-1*B*, the very-high-risk subgroups consist of more focused populations at higher risk of cardiac arrest or SCD, with better individual prediction, but the representation of such subgroups within the overall population burden of SCD is small. This is indicated by the absolute number of events ("events per year"), in contrast to the percentage per year in the subgroup. To achieve a major population impact, effective prevention of underlying diseases and the development of new epidemiologic and clinical probes that will allow better individual risk prediction by identifying specific high-risk subgroups within the large general populations are needed.

Strategies for predicting and preventing SCD are classified as primary and secondary. *Primary prevention* refers to the attempt to identify individual patients at specific risk for SCD and institute preventive strategies. *Secondary prevention* refers to measures taken to prevent recurrent cardiac arrest or death in individuals who have survived a prior cardiac arrest.

The effectiveness of the prevention strategies currently used depends on the magnitude of risk among the various population subgroups. Because the annual incidence of SCD among the unselected adult population is limited to approximately 1 per 1000 population per year (Fig. 327-1) and ~50% of all SCDs due to coronary artery disease occur as the first clinical manifestation of the disease (Fig. 327-2*A*), the only currently practical strategies are profiling for risk of developing CHD and risk factor control (Fig. 327-2*B*). The most powerful long-term risk factors include age, cigarette smoking, elevated serum cholesterol, diabetes mellitus, elevated blood pressure, LV hypertrophy, and nonspecific electrocardiographic abnormalities. Markers of inflammation (e.g., levels of C-reactive protein) that may predict plaque destabilization have been added to risk classifications. The presence of multiple risk factors progressively increases incidence, but not sufficiently or specifically enough to warrant therapies targeted to potentially fatal arrhythmias (Fig. 327-1*A*). However, recent studies suggesting familial clustering of SCD associated with a first acute coronary syndrome offer hope that genetic markers for specific risk may be forthcoming.

After coronary artery disease has been identified in a patient, additional strategies for risk profiling become available (Fig. 327-2*B*), but the majority of SCDs occur among the large unselected groups rather than in the specific high-risk subgroups that become evident among populations with established disease (compare events per year with percentage per year in Fig. 327-1*B*). After a major cardiovascular event, such as acute MI, recent onset of heart failure, or survival after out-of-hospital cardiac arrest, the highest risk of death occurs during the initial 6–18 months after the event and then plateaus toward the baseline risk associated with the extent of underlying disease. However, many of the early deaths are nonsudden, diluting the potential benefit of strategies targeted specifically to SCD. Thus, although post-MI beta blocker therapy has an identifiable benefit for both early SCD and nonsudden mortality risk, a total mortality benefit for implantable cardioverter-defibrillator (ICD) therapy early after MI has not been observed.

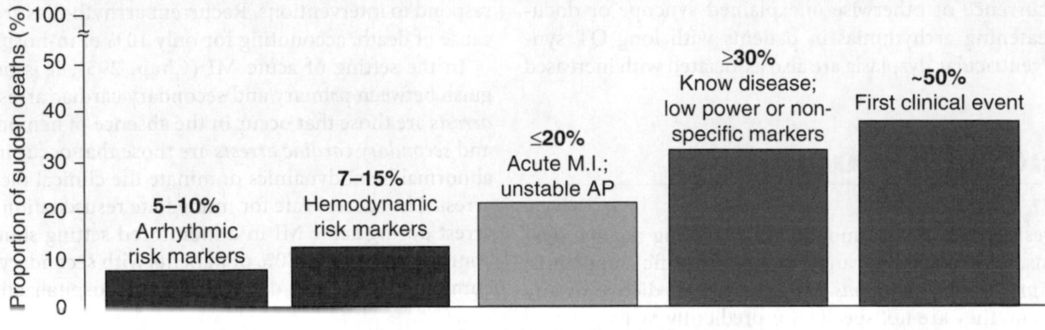

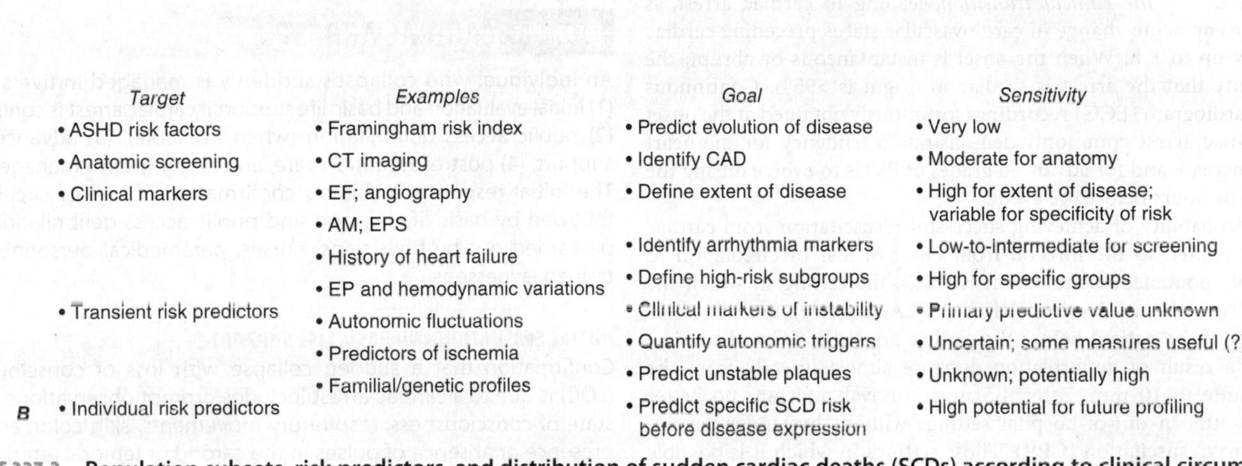

FIGURE 327-2 Population subsets, risk predictors, and distribution of sudden cardiac deaths (SCDs) according to clinical circumstances. ***A.*** The population subset with high-risk arrhythmia markers in conjunction with low ejection fraction is a group at high risk of SCD but accounts for <10% of the total SCD burden attributable to coronary artery disease. In contrast, 50% of all SCD victims present with SCD as the first and only manifestation of underlying disease, and up to 30% have known disease but are considered relatively low risk because of the absence of high-risk markers. ***B.*** Profiling for individual prediction and prevention of SCD is difficult. The highest absolute numbers of events occur among the general population who may have risk factors for coronary heart disease or expressions of disease that do not predict high risk. This results in a low sensitivity for predicting and preventing SCD. New approaches that include epidemiologic modeling of transient risk factors and genetic predictors of individual patient risk offer hope for greater sensitivity in the future. AM, ambulatory monitoring; AP, angina pectoris; ASHD, arteriosclerotic heart disease; CAD, coronary artery disease; CT, computed tomography; EF, ejection fraction; EP, electrophysiologic; EPS, electrophysiologic study; MI, myocardial infarction. *(Modified from RJ Myerburg: J Cardiovasc Electrophysiol 12:369–381, 2001.)*

Among patients in the acute, convalescent, and chronic phases of MI (Chap. 295), subgroups at high absolute risk of SCD can be identified. During the acute phase, the potential risk of cardiac arrest from onset through the first 48 h used to be as high as 15%, but is now reported in the range of 2.3–4.4% because of early patient awareness of the significance of symptoms and the availability of emergency revascularization strategies. Those who survive acute-phase VF are not at continuing risk for recurrent cardiac arrest indexed to that event. During the convalescent phase after MI (3 days to ~6 weeks), an episode of sustained ventricular tachycardia (VT) or VF, which is usually associated with a large infarct, predicts a natural history mortality risk of >25% at 12 months. At least one-half of the deaths are sudden. Aggressive intervention techniques may reduce this incidence.

During the chronic phase after MI, the longer-term risk for total mortality and SCD mortality is predicted by a number of factors (Fig. 327-2*B*). The most important for both SCD and nonsudden death is the extent of myocardial damage sustained as a result of the acute MI. This is measured by the magnitude of reduction of the ejection fraction (EF) and/or the occurrence of heart failure. Various studies have demonstrated that ventricular arrhythmias identified by ambulatory monitoring contribute significantly to this risk, especially in patients with an EF <40%. In addition, inducibility of VT or VF during electrophysiologic testing of patients who have ambient ventricular arrhythmias (premature ventricular contractions [PVCs] and nonsustained VT) and an EF <35% is a strong predictor of SCD risk. Patients in this subgroup are now considered candidates for ICDs (see below). Risk falls off sharply with EFs >35% and the absence of ambient arrhythmias after MI, and conversely is high with EFs <30% even without the ambient arrhythmia markers.

The cardiomyopathies (dilated and hypertrophic, Chap. 287) are the second most common category of diseases associated with risk of SCD (Table 327-2). Some risk factors have been identified, largely related to extent of disease, presence of heart failure, documented ventricular arrhythmias, and syncope thought to be due to arrhythmias. The less common causes of SCD include valvular heart disease (primarily aortic) and inflammatory and infiltrative disorders of the myocardium. The latter include viral myocarditis, sarcoidosis, and amyloidosis.

Among adolescents and young adults, rare inherited disorders such as hypertrophic cardiomyopathy, the long QT interval syndromes, right ventricular dysplasia, and the Brugada syndrome have received attention as important causes of SCD, as has acute myocarditis and other less common acquired diseases. Among the subgroup of young competitive athletes, the incidence of SCD may be higher than it is for the general adolescent and young adult population, perhaps up to 1 in 75,000–100,000. Hypertrophic cardiomyopathy (Chap. 287) is the most common cause in the United States.

Secondary prevention strategies should be applied to survivors of cardiac arrest that was not associated with an acute MI or other controllable transient risk factors, such as certain drug exposures and correctable electrolyte imbalances. Multivessel coronary artery disease and dilated cardiomyopathy, especially with markedly reduced left ventricular EF, predict a high risk of recurrence of cardiac arrest or SCD and are indications for specific interventions, such as ICDs (see below). The occurrence of otherwise unexplained syncope or documented life-threatening arrhythmias in patients with long QT syndromes or right ventricular dysplasia are also associated with increased risk of SCD.

CLINICAL CHARACTERISTICS OF CARDIAC ARREST

PRODROME, ONSET, ARREST, DEATH

SCD may be presaged by days to months of increasing angina, dyspnea, palpitations, easy fatigability, and other nonspecific complaints. However, these *prodromal symptoms* are generally predictive of any major cardiac event; they are not specific for predicting SCD.

The *onset of the clinical transition*, leading to cardiac arrest, is defined as an acute change in cardiovascular status preceding cardiac arrest by up to 1 h. When the onset is instantaneous or abrupt, the probability that the arrest is cardiac in origin is >95%. Continuous electrocardiogram (ECG) recordings fortuitously obtained at the onset of a cardiac arrest commonly demonstrate a tendency for the heart rate to increase and for advanced grades of PVCs to evolve during the minutes or hours before the event.

The probability of achieving successful resuscitation from cardiac arrest is related to the interval from onset of loss of circulation to return of spontaneous circulation (ROSC), the setting in which the event occurs, the mechanism (VF, VT, PEA, asystole), and the clinical status of the patient before the cardiac arrest. ROSC and survival rates as a result of defibrillation decrease almost linearly from the first minute to 10 min. After 4-5 min, survival rates are no better than 25–30% in out-of-hospital settings without bystander cardiopulmonary resuscitation (CPR). Those settings in which it is possible to institute prompt CPR followed by prompt defibrillation provide a better chance of a successful outcome. The outcome in intensive care units and other in-hospital environments is heavily influenced by the patient's preceding clinical status. The immediate outcome is good for cardiac arrest occurring in the intensive care unit in the presence of an acute cardiac event or transient metabolic disturbance, but survival among patients with far-advanced chronic cardiac disease or advanced noncardiac diseases (e.g., renal failure, pneumonia, sepsis, diabetes, cancer) is low and not much better in the in-hospital setting. Survival rates after unexpected cardiac arrest in unmonitored areas in a hospital do not differ from witnessed out-of-hospital arrests. Since implementation of community response systems, survival from out-of-hospital cardiac arrest has improved, although it still remains low, under most circumstances. Survival probabilities in public sites exceed those in the home environment, where the majority of cardiac arrests occur.

The success rate for initial resuscitation and survival to hospital discharge after an out-of-hospital cardiac arrest depends heavily on the mechanism of the event. When the mechanism is pulseless VT, the outcome is best; VF is the next most successful; and asystole and PEA, now the most common mechanisms, generate dismal outcome statistics. Advanced age also adversely influences the chances of successful resuscitation.

The probability of *progression to biologic death* is a function of the mechanism of cardiac arrest and the length of the delay before interventions. VF without CPR within the first 4–6 min has a poor outcome even if defibrillation is successful because of secondary brain damage; the prompt interposition of bystander CPR (basic life support; see below) improves outcome at any point along the time scale, especially when followed by early successful defibrillation. However, there are few survivors among patients who had no life support activities for the first 8 min after onset. Evaluations of deployment of automatic external defibrillators (AEDs) in communities (e.g., police vehicles, large buildings, airports, and stadiums) are beginning to generate encouraging data, but the data for home deployment has been have been less impressive.

Death during the hospitalization after a successfully resuscitated cardiac arrest relates closely to the severity of central nervous system injury. Anoxic encephalopathy and infections subsequent to prolonged respirator dependence account for 60% of the deaths. Another 30% occur as a consequence of low cardiac output states that fail to respond to interventions. Recurrent arrhythmias are the least common cause of death, accounting for only 10% of in-hospital deaths.

In the setting of acute MI (Chap. 295), it is important to distinguish between primary and secondary cardiac arrests. *Primary cardiac arrests* are those that occur in the absence of hemodynamic instability, and *secondary cardiac arrests* are those that occur in patients in whom abnormal hemodynamics dominate the clinical picture before cardiac arrest. The success rate for immediate resuscitation in primary cardiac arrest during acute MI in a monitored setting should exceed 90%. In contrast, as many as 70% of patients with secondary cardiac arrest succumb immediately or during the same hospitalization.

TREATMENT CARDIAC ARREST

An individual who collapses suddenly is managed in five stages: (1) initial evaluation and basic life support if cardiac arrest is confirmed, (2) public access defibrillation (when available), (3) advanced life support, (4) postresuscitation care, and (5) long-term management. The initial response, including confirmation of loss of circulation, followed by basic life support and public access defibrillation, can be carried out by physicians, nurses, paramedical personnel, and trained laypersons.

INITIAL EVALUATION AND BASIC LIFE SUPPORT

Confirmation that a sudden collapse with loss of consciousness (LOC) is due to a cardiac arrest includes prompt observations of the state of consciousness, respiratory movements, skin color, and the presence or absence of pulses in the carotid or femoral arteries. For lay responders, the pulse check is no longer recommended because it is unreliable. As soon as a cardiac arrest is suspected, confirmed, or even considered to be impending, calling an emergency rescue system (e.g., 911) is the immediate priority. With the development of AEDs that are easily used by nonconventional emergency responders, an additional layer for response has evolved (see below).

Careful attention to the respiratory status after abrupt LOC is important. Although normal breathing or tachypnea after LOC makes cardiac arrest less likely, gasping respiratory movements may persist during a true cardiac arrest, and their presence should not deter appropriate responses. In fact, continued gasping is considered a good prognostic sign for successful outcome. It is also important to observe for severe stridor with a persistent pulse as a clue to aspiration of a foreign body or food. If this is suspected, a Heimlich maneuver (see below) may dislodge the obstructing body. A precordial blow, or "thump," delivered firmly with a clenched fist to the junction of the middle and lower thirds of the sternum may occasionally revert VT or VF, but there is concern about converting VT to VF. Therefore, it is recommended to use precordial thumps as a life support technique only when monitoring and defibrillation are available. This conservative application of the technique remains controversial.

The third action during the initial response is to clear the airway. The head is tilted back and the chin lifted so that the oropharynx can be explored to clear the airway. Dentures or foreign bodies are removed, and the Heimlich maneuver is performed if there is reason to suspect that a foreign body is lodged in the oropharynx. If respiratory arrest precipitating cardiac arrest is suspected, a second precordial thump is delivered after the airway is cleared.

Basic life support, more popularly known as CPR, is intended to maintain organ perfusion until definitive interventions can be instituted. The initial and primary element of CPR is maintenance of perfusion until spontaneous circulation can be restored. Closed chest cardiac compression maintains a pump function by sequential filling and emptying of the chambers, with competent valves maintaining forward direction of flow. The palm of one hand is placed over the lower sternum, with the heel of the other resting on the dorsum of the lower hand. The sternum is depressed, with the arms remaining straight, at a rate of 100 per minute. Sufficient force is applied to depress the sternum 4–5 cm, and relaxation is abrupt.

Until recently, providing ventilation of the lungs by mouth-to-mouth respiration was used if no specific rescue equipment was immediately available (e.g., plastic oropharyngeal airways, esophageal obturators, masked Ambu bag). However, ventilatory support during CPR has yielded to evidence that continuous chest compressions ("hands only" CPR) results in better outcomes. Compressions are interrupted only for single shocks from an AED when available, with 2 min of CPR between each single shock.

AUTOMATED EXTERNAL DEFIBRILLATION (AED)

AEDs that are easily used by nonconventional responders, such as nonparamedic firefighters, police officers, ambulance drivers, trained security guards, and minimally trained or untrained laypersons, have been developed. This advance has inserted another level of response into the cardiac arrest paradigm. A number of studies have demonstrated that AED use by nonconventional responders in strategic response systems and public access lay responders can improve cardiac arrest survival rates. The rapidity with which defibrillation/cardioversion is achieved is an important element for successful resuscitation, both for ROSC and for protection of the central nervous system. Chest compressions should be carried out while the defibrillator is being charged. As soon as a diagnosis of VF or VT is established, a biphasic waveform shock of 150–200 J (360 J if a monophasic waveform device is used) should be delivered. If 5 min has elapsed between collapse and first contact with the victim, there is some evidence that 60–90 s of CPR before the first shock may improve probability of survival without neurologic damage. If the initial shock does not successfully revert VT or VF, chest compression at a rate of 100 per minute is resumed for 2 min, and then a second shock is delivered. Multiple shocks given in sequence are no longer recommended, in order to minimize interruptions of chest compressions. This sequence is continued until personnel capable of, and equipped for, advanced life support are available, although not much data support the notion that shocks and chest compressions alone will revert VF after three shocks have failed.

ADVANCED CARDIAC LIFE SUPPORT (ACLS)

ACLS is intended to achieve and maintain organ perfusion and adequate ventilation, control cardiac arrhythmias, and stabilize blood pressure and cardiac output. The activities carried out to achieve these goals include (1) defibrillation/cardioversion and/or pacing, (2) intubation with an endotracheal tube, and (3) insertion of an intravenous line.

As in basic life support, the major emphasis during ACLS is minimizing interruptions of chest compressions until ROSC is achieved. After two or three unsuccessful defibrillation attempts, epinephrine, 1 mg IV, is given and attempts to defibrillate are repeated. The dose of epinephrine may be repeated after intervals of 3–5 min (Fig. 327-3A). Vasopressin (a single 40-unit dose given IV) has been suggested as an alternative to epinephrine.

If the patient is less than fully conscious upon reversion or if two or three attempts fail, prompt intubation, ventilation, and arterial blood gas analysis should be carried out. Ventilation with O_2 (room air if O_2 is not immediately available) may promptly reverse hypoxemia and acidosis. Quantitative waveform capnography is now recommended for confirmation and monitoring of endotracheal tube placement. A patient who is persistently acidotic after successful defibrillation and intubation or had acidosis prior to arrest, may be

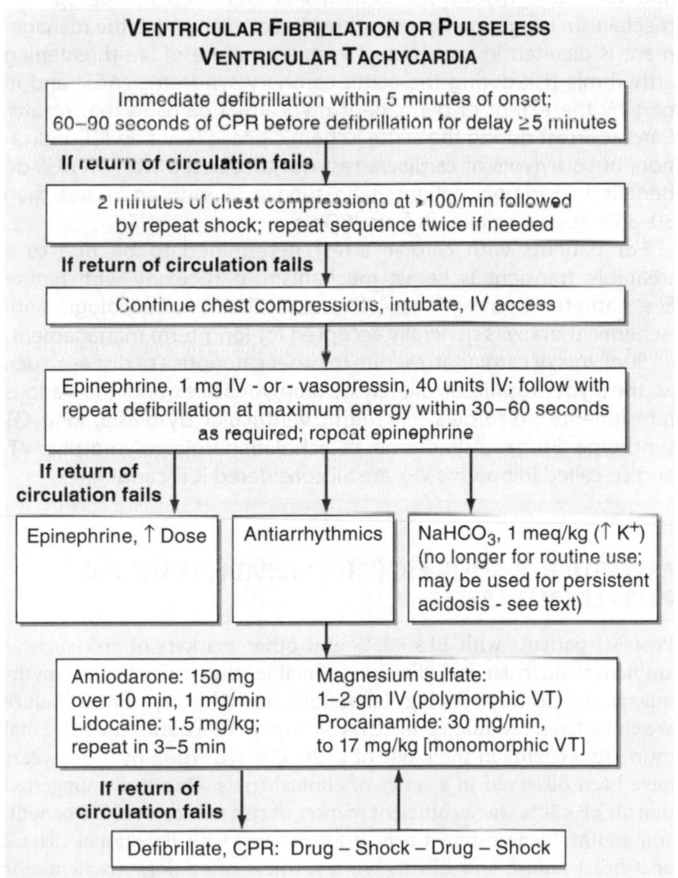

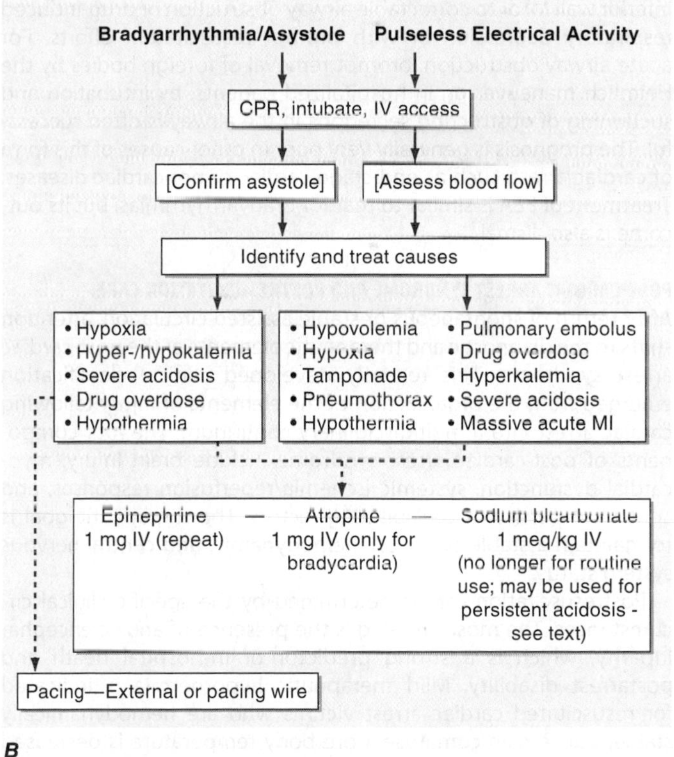

FIGURE 327-3 ***A.*** The algorithm of ventricular fibrillation or pulseless ventricular tachycardia begins with and initial defibrillate on attempt. If a single shock fails to restore a pulse, it is followed by 2 min of cardiopulmonary resuscitation (CPR; chest compressions), followed by another single shock. After three such sequences, epinephrine and then antiarrhythmic drugs are added to the protocol. See text for details. ***B.*** The algorithms for bradyarrhythmia/asystole (*left*) or pulseless electrical activity (*right*) are dominated first by continued life support and a search for reversible causes. Subsequent therapy is nonspecific and is accompanied by a low success rate. See text for details. MI, myocardial infarction; VT, ventricular tachycardia.

given 1 meq/kg $NaHCO_3$ initially and an additional 50% of the dose repeated every 10–15 min. However, it should not be used routinely.

After initial unsuccessful defibrillation attempts or with persistent/recurrent electrical instability, antiarrhythmic therapy should be instituted. Intravenous amiodarone has emerged as the initial treatment of choice (150 mg over 10 min, followed by 1 mg/min for up to 6 h and 0.5 mg/min thereafter) (Fig. 327-3*A*). For cardiac arrest due to VF in the early phase of an acute coronary syndrome, a bolus of 1 mg/kg of lidocaine may be given intravenously as an alternative, and the dose may be repeated in 2 min. It also may be tried in patients in whom amiodarone is unsuccessful. Intravenous procainamide (loading infusion of 100 mg/5 min to a total dose of 500–800 mg, followed by continuous infusion at 2–5 mg/min) is now rarely used in this setting but may be tried for persisting, hemodynamically stable arrhythmias. Intravenous calcium gluconate is no longer considered safe or necessary for routine administration. It is used only in patients in whom acute hyperkalemia is known to be the triggering event for resistant VF, in the presence of known hypocalcemia, or in patients who have received toxic doses of calcium channel antagonists.

Cardiac arrest due to bradyarrhythmias or asystole (B/A cardiac arrest) is managed differently (**Fig. 327-3*B***). The patient is promptly intubated, CPR is continued, and an attempt is made to control hypoxemia and acidosis and identify other reversible causes. Epinephrine may be given intravenously or by an intraosseous route. Atropine is no longer considered effective for asystole or PEA, but can be used for bradyarrhythmias. External pacing devices are used to attempt to establish a regular rhythm when atropine fails for a bradyarrhythmia, but chronotropic agents given intravenously are now recognized as an equally effective alternative.

The success rate may be good when B/A arrest is due to acute inferior wall MI or to correctable airway obstruction or drug-induced respiratory depression or with prompt resuscitation efforts. For acute airway obstruction, prompt removal of foreign bodies by the Heimlich maneuver or, in hospitalized patients, by intubation and suctioning of obstructing secretions in the airway is often successful. The prognosis is generally very poor in other causes of this form of cardiac arrest, such as end-stage cardiac or noncardiac diseases. Treatment of PEA is similar to that for bradyarrhythmias, but its outcome is also dismal.

POST-CARDIAC ARREST SYNDROME AND POSTRESUSCITATION CARE

After return of spontaneous or stable assisted circulation, attention shifts to the diagnostic and therapeutic elements of the post-cardiac arrest syndrome. This recently developed clinical classification emerged from the organization of the elements of injury following cardiac arrest into a multidisciplinary continuum. The four components of post-cardiac arrest syndrome include brain injury, myocardial dysfunction, systemic ischemia/reperfusion responses, and control of persistent precipitating factors. The therapeutic goal is to maintain a stable electrical, hemodynamic, and central nervous system status.

Postresuscitation care is determined by the specific clinical circumstances. The most pressing is the presence of anoxic encephalopathy, which is a strong predictor of in-hospital death and postarrest disability. Mild therapeutic hypothermia is indicated for resuscitated cardiac arrest victims who are hemodynamically stable, but remain comatose. Core body temperature is decreased to 32–34°C, by several available techniques (external and/or internal [core]), as soon as practical after resuscitation and maintained for a minimum of 12–24 h. By reducing metabolic demands and cerebral edema, this intervention improves probability of survival with better neurologic outcome.

Primary VF in acute MI (not accompanied by low-output states) (**Chap. 295**) is generally very responsive to life support techniques and easily controlled after the initial event. In the in-hospital setting, respirator support is usually not necessary or is needed for only a short time, and hemodynamics stabilize promptly after defibrillation or cardioversion. In *secondary VF* in acute MI (those events in which hemodynamic abnormalities predispose to the potentially fatal arrhythmia), resuscitative efforts are less often successful, and in patients who are successfully resuscitated, the recurrence rate is high. The clinical picture and outcome are dominated by hemodynamic instability and the ability to control hemodynamic dysfunction. Bradyarrhythmias, asystole, and PEA are commonly secondary events in hemodynamically unstable patients.

The outcome after in-hospital cardiac arrest associated with noncardiac diseases is poor, and in the few successfully resuscitated patients, the postresuscitation course is dominated by the nature of the underlying disease. Patients with end-stage cancer, renal failure, acute central nervous system disease, and uncontrolled infections, as a group, have a survival rate of <10% after in-hospital cardiac arrest. Some major exceptions are patients with transient airway obstruction, electrolyte disturbances, proarrhythmic effects of drugs, and severe metabolic abnormalities, most of whom may have a good chance of survival if they can be resuscitated promptly and stabilized while the transient abnormalities are being corrected.

LONG-TERM MANAGEMENT AFTER SURVIVAL OF OUT-OF-HOSPITAL CARDIAC ARREST

Patients who survive cardiac arrest without irreversible damage to the central nervous system and who achieve hemodynamic stability should have diagnostic testing to define appropriate therapeutic interventions for their long-term management. This approach is driven by the fact that survival after out-of-hospital cardiac arrest is followed by a 10–25% mortality rate during the first 2 years after the event, and there are data suggesting that significant survival benefits can be achieved by prescription of an ICD.

Among patients in whom an acute ST elevation MI or transient and reversible myocardial ischemia is identified as the specific mechanism triggering an out-of-hospital cardiac arrest, the management is dictated in part by the transient nature of life-threatening arrhythmia risk during the acute coronary syndrome (ACS) and in part by the extent of permanent myocardial damage that results. Cardiac arrest during the acute ischemic phase is not an ICD indication, but survivors of cardiac arrest not associated with an ACS do benefit. In addition, patients who survive MI with an EF less than 30–35% appear to benefit from ICDs.

For patients with cardiac arrest determined to be due to a treatable transient ischemic mechanism, particularly with higher EFs, catheter interventional, surgical, and/or pharmacologic anti-ischemic therapy is generally accepted for long-term management.

Survivors of cardiac arrest due to other categories of disease, such as the hypertrophic or dilated cardiomyopathies and the various rare inherited disorders (e.g., right ventricular dysplasia, long QT syndrome, Brugada syndrome, catecholaminergic polymorphic VT, and so-called idiopathic VF), are all considered ICD candidates.

PREVENTION OF SCD IN HIGH-RISK INDIVIDUALS WITHOUT PRIOR CARDIAC ARREST

Post-MI patients with EFs <35% and other markers of risk such as ambient ventricular arrhythmias, inducible ventricular tachyarrhythmias in the electrophysiology laboratory, and a history of heart failure are considered candidates for ICDs 40 days or more after the MI. Total mortality benefits in the range of a 20–35% reduction over 2–5 years have been observed in a series of clinical trials. One study suggested that an EF <30% was a sufficient marker of risk to indicate ICD benefit, and another demonstrated benefit for patients with Functional Class 2 or 3 heart failure and EFs ≤35%, regardless of etiology (ischemic or nonischemic) or the presence of ambient or induced arrhythmias (**Chaps. 277 and 279**). For patients with newly diagnosed heart failure and an EF <35%, the required delay between diagnosis and institution of medical therapy, and subsequent implantation of an ICD, is 90 days. In general, there appears to be a gradient of increasing ICD benefit with EFs ranging lower than the threshold indications. However, patients with very low EFs (e.g., <20%) may receive less benefit.

Decision making for primary prevention in disorders other than coronary artery disease and dilated cardiomyopathy is generally driven by observational data and judgment based on clinical observations. Controlled clinical trials providing evidence-based indicators for ICDs are lacking for these smaller population subgroups. In general, for the rare disorders listed above, indicators of arrhythmic risk such as syncope, documented ventricular tachyarrhythmias, aborted cardiac arrest, or a family history of premature SCD in some conditions, and a number of other clinical or ECG markers, may be used as indicators for ICDs.

SECTION 3 NEUROLOGIC CRITICAL CARE

328 Coma

Allan H. Ropper

Coma is among the most common and striking problems in general medicine. It accounts for a substantial portion of admissions to emergency wards and occurs on all hospital services. It demands immediate attention and requires an organized approach.

There is a continuum of states of reduced alertness, the most severe form being coma, defined as a deep sleeplike state from which the patient cannot be aroused. Stupor refers to a higher degree of arousability in which the patient can be transiently awakened by vigorous stimuli, accompanied by motor behavior that leads to avoidance of uncomfortable or aggravating stimuli. Drowsiness, which is familiar to all persons, simulates light sleep and is characterized by easy arousal and the persistence of alertness for brief periods. Drowsiness and stupor are usually accompanied by some degree of confusion (Chap. 34). A precise narrative description of the level of arousal and of the type of responses evoked by various stimuli as observed at the bedside is preferable to ambiguous terms such as lethargy, semicoma, or obtundation.

Several conditions that render patients unresponsive and simulate coma are considered separately because of their special significance. The vegetative state signifies an awake-appearing but nonresponsive state in a patient who has emerged from coma. In the vegetative state, the eyelids may open, giving the appearance of wakefulness. Respiratory and autonomic functions are retained. Yawning, coughing, swallowing, and limb and head movements persist, and the patient may follow visually presented objects, but there are few, if any, meaningful responses to the external and internal environment—in essence, an "awake coma." The term *vegetative* is unfortunate because it is subject to misinterpretation. There are always accompanying signs that indicate extensive damage in both cerebral hemispheres, e.g., decerebrate or decorticate limb posturing and absent responses to visual stimuli (see below). In the closely related but less severe minimally conscious state, the patient displays rudimentary vocal or motor behaviors, often spontaneous, but some in response to touch, visual stimuli, or command. Cardiac arrest with cerebral hypoperfusion and head injuries are the most common causes of the vegetative and minimally conscious states (Chaps. 327 and 330). The prognosis for regaining mental faculties once the vegetative state has supervened for several months is very poor, and after a year, almost nil; hence the term *persistent vegetative state*. Most reports of dramatic recovery, when investigated carefully, are found to yield to the usual rules for prognosis, but there have been rare instances in which recovery has occurred to a severely disabled condition and, in rare childhood cases, to an even better state. The possibility of incorrectly attributing meaningful behavior to patients in the vegetative and minimally conscious states creates inordinate problems and anguish. On the other hand, the question of whether these patients lack any capability for cognition has been reopened by functional imaging studies that have demonstrated, in a small proportion of posttraumatic cases, meaningful cerebral activation in response to verbal and other stimuli.

Apart from the above conditions, several syndromes that affect alertness are prone to be misinterpreted as stupor or coma. Akinetic mutism refers to a partially or fully awake state in which the patient is able to form impressions and think, as demonstrated by later recounting of events, but remains virtually immobile and mute. The condition results from damage in the regions of the medial thalamic nuclei or the frontal lobes (particularly lesions situated deeply or on the orbitofrontal surfaces) or from extreme hydrocephalus. The term abulia describes a milder form of akinetic mutism characterized by mental and physical slowness and diminished ability to initiate activity. It is also usually the result of damage to the frontal lobes and its connections (Chap. 36).

Catatonia is a curious hypomobile and mute syndrome that occurs as part of a major psychosis, usually schizophrenia or major depression. Catatonic patients make few voluntary or responsive movements, although they blink, swallow, and may not appear distressed. There are nonetheless signs that the patient is responsive, although it may take ingenuity on the part of the examiner to demonstrate them. For example, eyelid elevation is actively resisted, blinking occurs in response to a visual threat, and the eyes move concomitantly with head rotation, all of which are inconsistent with the presence of a brain lesion causing unresponsiveness. It is characteristic but not invariable in catatonia for the limbs to retain the postures in which they have been placed by the examiner ("waxy flexibility," or catalepsy). With recovery, patients often have some memory of events that occurred during their catatonic stupor. Catatonia is superficially similar to akinetic mutism, but clinical evidence of cerebral damage such as Babinski signs and hypertonicity of the limbs is lacking. The special problem of coma in brain death is discussed below.

The locked-in state describes yet another type of pseudocoma in which an awake patient has no means of producing speech or volitional movement but retains voluntary vertical eye movements and lid elevation, thus allowing the patient to signal with a clear mind. The pupils are normally reactive. Such individuals have written entire treatises using Morse code. The usual cause is an infarction or hemorrhage of the ventral pons that transects all descending motor (corticospinal and corticobulbar) pathways. A similar awake but de-efferented state occurs as a result of total paralysis of the musculature in severe cases of Guillain-Barré syndrome (Chap. 460), critical illness neuropathy (Chap. 330), and pharmacologic neuromuscular blockade.

THE ANATOMY AND PHYSIOLOGY OF COMA

Almost all instances of diminished alertness can be traced to widespread abnormalities of the cerebral hemispheres or to reduced activity of a special thalamocortical alerting system termed the reticular activating system (RAS). The proper functioning of this system, its ascending projections to the cortex, and the cortex itself are required to maintain alertness and coherence of thought. It follows that the principal causes of coma are (1) lesions that damage the RAS in the upper midbrain or its projections; (2) destruction of large portions of both cerebral hemispheres; or (3) suppression of reticulocerebral function by drugs, toxins, or metabolic derangements such as hypoglycemia, anoxia, uremia, and hepatic failure.

The proximity of the RAS to midbrain structures that control pupillary function and eye movements permits clinical localization of the cause of coma in many cases. Pupillary enlargement with loss of light reaction and loss of vertical and adduction movements of the eyes suggests that the lesion is in the upper brainstem where the nuclei subserving these functions reside. Conversely, preservation of pupillary light reactivity and of eye movements absolves the upper brainstem and indicates that widespread structural lesions or metabolic suppression of the cerebral hemispheres is responsible for coma.

Coma Due to Cerebral Mass Lesions and Herniations In addition to the fixed restriction of the skull, the cranial cavity is separated into compartments by infoldings of the dura. The two cerebral hemispheres are separated by the falx, and the anterior and posterior fossae by the tentorium. Herniation refers to displacement of brain tissue by an overlying or adjacent mass into a contiguous compartment that it normally does not occupy. Coma and many of its associated signs can be attributed to these tissue shifts, and certain clinical features are characteristic of specific configurations of herniation (Fig. 328-1). They are in essence "false localizing" signs because they derive from compression of brain structures at a distance from the mass.

In the most common form of herniation, brain tissue is displaced from the supratentorial to the infratentorial compartment through the tentorial opening; this is referred to as transtentorial herniation. Uncal transtentorial herniation refers to impaction of the anterior medial temporal gyrus (the uncus) into the tentorial opening just anterior to and adjacent to the midbrain (Fig. 328-1*A*). The uncus compresses the third nerve as the nerve traverses the subarachnoid space, causing enlargement of the ipsilateral pupil (the fibers subserving parasympathetic pupillary function are located peripherally in the nerve). The coma that follows is due to compression of the midbrain against the opposite tentorial edge by the displaced parahippocampal gyrus (Fig. 328-2). Lateral displacement of the midbrain may compress the opposite cerebral peduncle against the tentorial edge, producing a Babinski sign and hemiparesis contralateral to the hemiparesis that resulted from the mass (the Kernohan-Woltman sign). Herniation may also compress the anterior and posterior cerebral arteries as they pass over the tentorial reflections, with resultant brain infarction. The distortions may also entrap portions of the ventricular system, resulting in hydrocephalus.

Central transtentorial herniation denotes a symmetric downward movement of the thalamic structures through the tentorial opening with compression of the upper midbrain (Fig. 328-1*B*). Miotic pupils and drowsiness are the heralding signs, in contrast to a unilaterally

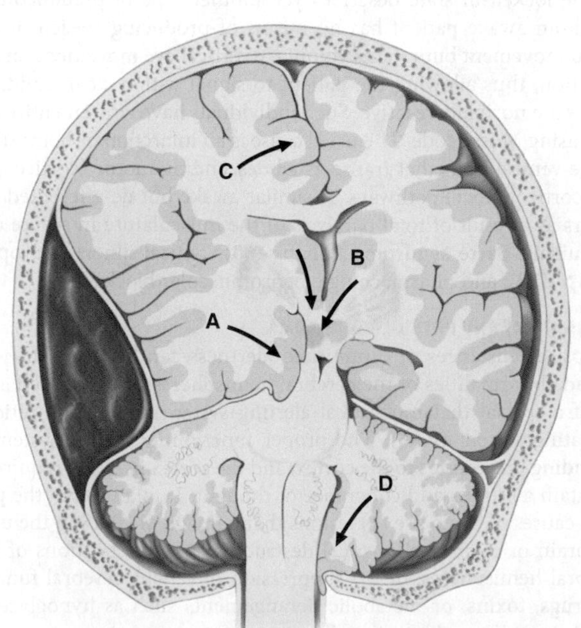

FIGURE 328-1 Types of cerebral herniation: (*A*) uncal; (*B*) central; (*C*) transfalcial; and (*D*) foraminal.

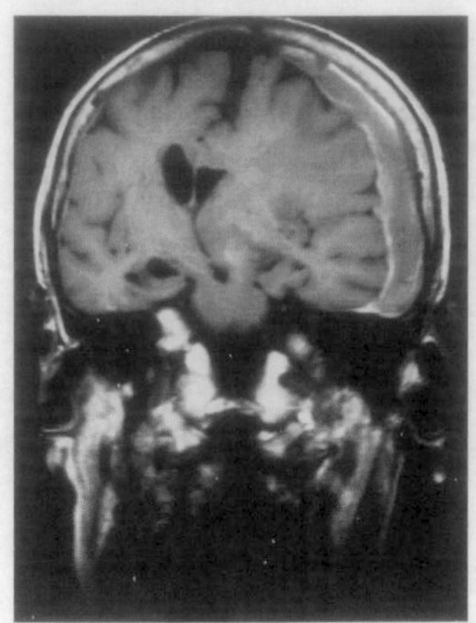

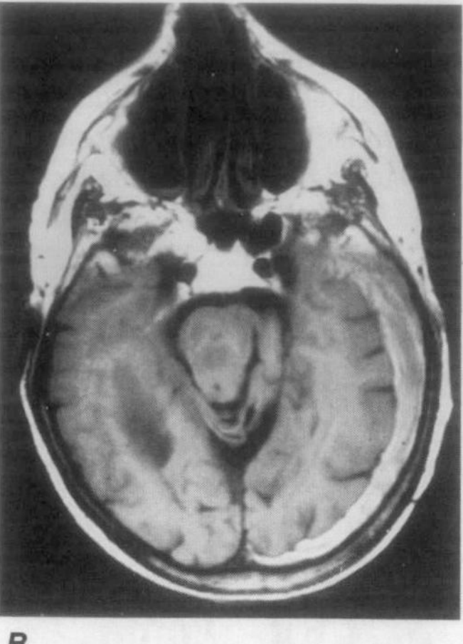

A *B*

FIGURE 328-2 Coronal (*A*) and axial (*B*) magnetic resonance images from a stuporous patient with a left third nerve palsy as a result of a large left-sided subdural hematoma (seen as a gray-white rim). The upper midbrain and lower thalamic regions are compressed and displaced horizontally away from the mass, and there is transtentorial herniation of the medial temporal lobe structures, including the uncus anteriorly. The lateral ventricle opposite to the hematoma has become enlarged as a result of compression of the third ventricle.

enlarged pupil of the uncal syndrome. Both uncal and central transtentorial herniations cause progressive compression of the brainstem, with initial damage to the midbrain, then the pons, and finally the medulla. The result is an approximate sequence of neurologic signs that corresponds to each affected level. Other forms of herniation are transfalcial herniation (displacement of the cingulate gyrus under the falx and across the midline, Fig. 328-1*C*) and foraminal herniation (downward forcing of the cerebellar tonsils into the foramen magnum, Fig. 328-1*D*), which causes compression of the medulla, respiratory arrest, and death.

A direct relationship between the various configurations of transtentorial herniation and coma is not always found. Drowsiness and stupor can occur with moderate horizontal displacement of the diencephalon (thalamus), before transtentorial herniation is evident. This lateral shift may be quantified on axial images of computed tomography (CT) and magnetic resonance imaging (MRI) scans (Fig. 328-2). In cases of acutely enlarging masses, horizontal displacement of the pineal calcification of 3–5 mm is generally associated with drowsiness, 6–8 mm with stupor, and >9 mm with coma. Intrusion of the medial temporal lobe into the tentorial opening is also apparent on MRI and CT scans as obliteration of the cisterna that surrounds the upper brainstem.

Coma due to Metabolic Disorders Many systemic metabolic abnormalities cause coma by interrupting the delivery of energy substrates (e.g., oxygen, glucose) or by altering neuronal excitability (drugs and alcohol, anesthesia, and epilepsy). The metabolic abnormalities that produce coma may, in milder forms, induce an acute confusional state. Thus, in metabolic encephalopathies, clouded consciousness and coma are in a continuum.

Cerebral neurons are fully dependent on cerebral blood flow (CBF) and the delivery of oxygen and glucose. CBF is ~75 mL per 100 g/min in gray matter and 30 mL per 100 g/min in white matter (mean ~55 mL per 100 g/min); oxygen consumption is 3.5 mL per 100 g/min, and glucose utilization is 5 mg per 100 g/min. Brain stores of glucose are able to provide energy for ~2 min after blood flow is interrupted, and oxygen stores last 8–10 s after the cessation of blood flow. Simultaneous hypoxia and ischemia exhaust glucose more rapidly. The electroencephalogram (EEG) rhythm in these circumstances becomes diffusely slowed, typical of metabolic encephalopathies, and as substrate delivery worsens, eventually brain electrical activity ceases.

Unlike hypoxia-ischemia, which causes neuronal destruction, most metabolic disorders such as hypoglycemia, hyponatremia, hyperosmolarity, hypercapnia, hypercalcemia, and hepatic and renal failure cause only minor neuropathologic changes. The reversible effects of these conditions on the brain are not understood but may result from impaired energy supplies, changes in ion fluxes across neuronal membranes, and neurotransmitter abnormalities. For example, the high ammonia concentration of hepatic coma interferes with cerebral energy metabolism and with the Na^+, K^+-ATPase pump, increases the number and size of astrocytes, and causes increased concentrations of potentially toxic products of ammonia metabolism; it may also affect neurotransmitters, including the production of putative "false" neurotransmitters that are active at receptor sites. Apart from hyperammonemia, which of these mechanisms is of critical importance is not clear. The mechanism of the encephalopathy of renal failure is also not known. Unlike ammonia, urea does not produce central nervous system (CNS) toxicity, and a multifactorial causation has been proposed for the encephalopathy, including increased permeability of the blood-brain barrier to toxic substances such as organic acids and an increase in brain calcium and cerebrospinal fluid (CSF) phosphate content.

Coma and seizures are common accompaniments of large shifts in sodium and water balance in the brain. These changes in osmolarity arise from systemic medical disorders, including diabetic ketoacidosis, the nonketotic hyperosmolar state, and hyponatremia from any cause (e.g., water intoxication, excessive secretion of antidiuretic hormone, or atrial natriuretic peptides). Sodium levels <125 mmol/L induce confusion, and levels <115 mmol/L are typically associated with coma and convulsions. In hyperosmolar coma, the serum osmolarity is generally >350 mosmol/L. Hypercapnia depresses the level of consciousness in proportion to the rise in carbon dioxide (CO_2) tension in the blood. In all of these metabolic encephalopathies, the degree of neurologic change depends to a large extent on the rapidity with which the serum changes occur. The pathophysiology of other metabolic encephalopathies such as those due to hypercalcemia, hypothyroidism, vitamin B_{12} deficiency, and hypothermia are incompletely understood but must reflect derangements of CNS biochemistry, membrane function, or neurotransmitters.

Epileptic Coma Generalized electrical seizures are associated with coma, even in the absence of motor convulsions (nonconvulsive status epilepticus). The self-limited coma that follows a seizure, the postictal state, may be due to exhaustion of energy reserves or effects of locally toxic molecules that are the by-product of seizures. The postictal state produces continuous, generalized slowing of the background EEG activity similar to that of metabolic encephalopathies.

Toxic (Including Drug-Induced) Coma This common class of encephalopathy is in large measure reversible and leaves no residual damage provided there has not been cardiorespiratory failure. Many drugs and toxins are capable of depressing nervous system function. Some produce coma by affecting both the brainstem nuclei, including the RAS, and the cerebral cortex. The combination of cortical and brainstem signs, which occurs in certain drug overdoses, may lead to an incorrect diagnosis of structural brainstem disease. Overdose of medications that have atropinic actions produces signs such as dilated pupils, tachycardia, and dry skin; opiate overdose produces pinpoint pupils <1 mm in diameter.

Coma due to Widespread Damage to the Cerebral Hemispheres This category, comprising a number of unrelated disorders, results from widespread structural cerebral damage that simulates a metabolic disorder of the cortex. Hypoxia-ischemia is perhaps the best characterized and one in which it is not possible initially to distinguish the acute reversible effects of oxygen deprivation of the brain from the subsequent effects of anoxic neuronal damage. Similar widespread cerebral damage may be produced by disorders that occlude small blood vessels throughout the brain; examples include cerebral malaria, thrombotic thrombocytopenic purpura, and hyperviscosity. Diffuse white matter damage from cranial trauma or inflammatory demyelinating diseases can cause a similar coma syndrome.

APPROACH TO THE PATIENT: Coma

A video examination of the comatose patient is shown in Chap. 329e.

Acute respiratory and cardiovascular problems should be attended to prior to neurologic assessment. In most instances, a complete medical evaluation, except for vital signs, funduscopy, and examination for nuchal rigidity, may be deferred until the neurologic evaluation has established the severity and nature of coma. **The approach to the patient with coma from cranial trauma is discussed in Chap. 457e.**

HISTORY

The cause of coma may be immediately evident as in cases of trauma, cardiac arrest, or observed drug ingestion. In the remainder, certain points are useful: (1) the circumstances and rapidity with which neurologic symptoms developed; (2) the antecedent symptoms (confusion, weakness, headache, fever, seizures, dizziness, double vision, or vomiting); (3) the use of medications, drugs, or alcohol; and (4) chronic liver, kidney, lung, heart, or other medical disease. Direct interrogation of family, observers, and ambulance technicians on the scene, in person or by telephone, is an important part of the evaluation when possible.

GENERAL PHYSICAL EXAMINATION

Fever suggests a systemic infection, bacterial meningitis, encephalitis, heat stroke, neuroleptic malignant syndrome, malignant hyperthermia due to anesthetics, or anticholinergic drug intoxication. Only rarely is fever attributable to a lesion that has disturbed hypothalamic temperature-regulating centers ("central fever"). A slight elevation in temperature may follow vigorous convulsions. Hypothermia is observed with exposure that attends alcohol, barbiturate, sedative, or phenothiazine intoxication; hypoglycemia; peripheral circulatory failure; or extreme hypothyroidism. Hypothermia itself causes coma when the temperature is <31°C (87.8°F). Tachypnea may indicate systemic acidosis or pneumonia or, rarely, infiltration of the brain with lymphoma. Aberrant respiratory patterns that reflect brainstem disorders are discussed below. Marked hypertension suggests hypertensive encephalopathy or cerebral hemorrhage or head injury. Hypotension is characteristic of coma from alcohol or barbiturate intoxication, internal hemorrhage, myocardial infarction, sepsis, profound hypothyroidism, or Addisonian crisis. The funduscopic examination can detect subarachnoid hemorrhage (subhyaloid hemorrhages), hypertensive encephalopathy (exudates, hemorrhages, vessel-crossing changes, papilledema), and increased intracranial pressure (ICP) (papilledema). Cutaneous petechiae suggest thrombotic thrombocytopenic purpura, meningococcemia, or a bleeding diathesis associated with an intracerebral hemorrhage. Cyanosis and reddish or anemic skin coloration are other indications of an underlying systemic disease or carbon monoxide as responsible for the coma.

NEUROLOGIC EXAMINATION

The patient should be observed without intervention by the examiner. Tossing about in the bed, reaching up toward the face, crossing legs, yawning, swallowing, coughing, or moaning reflect a drowsy state that is close to normal awakeness. Lack of restless movements on one side or an outturned leg suggests a hemiplegia. Intermittent twitching movements of a foot, finger, or facial muscle may be the only sign of seizures. Multifocal myoclonus almost always indicates a metabolic disorder, particularly uremia, anoxia, drug intoxication (especially with lithium or haloperidol), or a prion disease (Chap. 453e). In a drowsy and confused patient, bilateral asterixis is a certain sign of metabolic encephalopathy or drug intoxication.

Decorticate rigidity and decerebrate rigidity, or "posturing," describe stereotyped arm and leg movements occurring spontaneously or elicited by sensory stimulation. Flexion of the elbows and wrists and supination of the arm (decorticate posturing) suggests bilateral damage rostral to the midbrain, whereas extension of the elbows and wrists with pronation (decerebrate posturing) indicates damage to motor tracts in the midbrain or caudal diencephalon. The less frequent combination of arm extension with leg flexion or flaccid legs is associated with lesions in the pons. These concepts have been adapted from animal work and cannot be applied with precision to coma in humans. In fact, acute and widespread disorders of any type, regardless of location, frequently cause limb extension, and almost all extensor posturing becomes predominantly flexor as time passes.

LEVEL OF AROUSAL

A sequence of increasingly intense stimuli is used to determine the threshold for arousal and the motor response of each side of the body. The results of testing may vary from minute to minute, and serial examinations are useful. Tickling the nostrils with a cotton wisp is a moderate stimulus to arousal—all but deeply stuporous and comatose patients will move the head away and arouse to some degree. An even greater degree of responsiveness is present if the patient uses his hand to remove an offending stimulus. Pressure on the knuckles or bony prominences and pinprick stimulation are humane forms of noxious stimuli; pinching the skin causes unsightly ecchymoses and is generally not necessary but may be useful in eliciting abduction withdrawal movements of the limbs. Posturing in response to noxious stimuli indicates severe damage to the corticospinal system, whereas abduction-avoidance movement of a limb is usually purposeful and denotes an intact corticospinal system. Posturing may also be unilateral and coexist with purposeful limb movements, reflecting incomplete damage to the motor system.

BRAINSTEM REFLEXES

Assessment of brainstem function is essential to localization of the lesion in coma (Fig. 328-3). The brainstem reflexes that are examined are pupillary size and reaction to light, spontaneous and elicited eye movements, corneal responses, and the respiratory pattern. As a rule, coma due to bilateral hemispheral disease preserves these brainstem activities, particularly the pupillary reactions and eye movements. However, the presence of abnormal brainstem signs does not always indicate that the primary lesion is in the brainstem because hemispheral masses can cause secondary brainstem damage by the earlier described transtentorial herniations.

Pupillary Signs Pupillary reactions are examined with a bright, diffuse light (preferably not an ophthalmoscope, which illuminates only a limited part of the retina). Reactive and round pupils of midsize (2.5–5 mm) essentially exclude midbrain damage, either primary or secondary to compression. A response to light may be difficult to appreciate in pupils <2 mm in diameter, and bright room lighting mutes pupillary reactivity. One enlarged and poorly reactive pupil (>6 mm) signifies compression or stretching of the third nerve from the effects of a cerebral mass above. Enlargement of the pupil contralateral to a hemispheral mass may occur but is infrequent. An oval and slightly eccentric pupil is a transitional sign that accompanies early midbrain–third nerve compression. The most extreme pupillary sign, bilaterally dilated and unreactive pupils, indicates severe midbrain damage, usually from compression by a supratentorial mass. Ingestion of drugs with anticholinergic activity, the use of mydriatic eye drops, and direct ocular trauma are among the causes of misleading pupillary enlargement.

Unilateral miosis in coma has been attributed to dysfunction of sympathetic efferents originating in the posterior hypothalamus and descending in the tegmentum of the brainstem to the cervical cord. It is therefore of limited localizing value but is an occasional finding in patients with a large cerebral hemorrhage that affects the thalamus. Reactive and bilaterally small (1–2.5 mm) but not pinpoint pupils are seen in metabolic encephalopathies or in deep bilateral hemispheral lesions such as hydrocephalus or thalamic

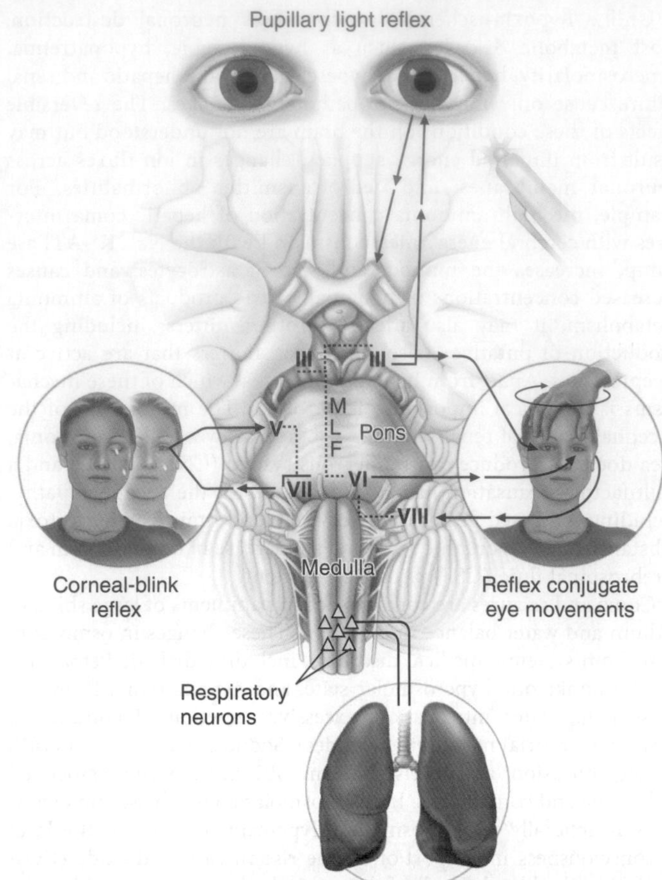

FIGURE 328-3 Examination of brainstem reflexes in coma. Midbrain and third nerve function are tested by pupillary reaction to light, pontine function by spontaneous and reflex eye movements and corneal responses, and medullary function by respiratory and pharyngeal responses. Reflex conjugate, horizontal eye movements are dependent on the medial longitudinal fasciculus (MLF) interconnecting the sixth and contralateral third nerve nuclei. Head rotation (oculocephalic reflex) or caloric stimulation of the labyrinths (oculovestibular reflex) elicits contraversive eye movements (for details see text).

hemorrhage. Even smaller reactive pupils (<1 mm) characterize narcotic or barbiturate overdoses but also occur with extensive pontine hemorrhage. The response to naloxone and the presence of reflex eye movements (see below) assist in distinguishing between these.

Ocular Movements The eyes are first observed by elevating the lids and observing the resting position and spontaneous movements of the globes. Lid tone, tested by lifting the eyelids and noting their resistance to opening and the speed of closure, is progressively reduced as unresponsiveness progresses. Horizontal divergence of the eyes at rest is normal in drowsiness. As coma deepens, the ocular axes may become parallel again.

Spontaneous eye movements in coma often take the form of conjugate horizontal roving. This finding alone exonerates damage in the midbrain and pons and has the same significance as normal reflex eye movements (see below). Conjugate horizontal ocular deviation to one side indicates damage to the pons on the opposite side or, alternatively, to the frontal lobe on the same side. This phenomenon is summarized by the following maxim: *The eyes look toward a hemispheral lesion and away from a brainstem lesion.* Seizures also drive the eyes to one side but usually with superimposed clonic movements of the globes. The eyes may occasionally turn paradoxically away from the side of a deep hemispheral lesion ("wrong-way eyes"). The eyes turn down and inward with thalamic and upper midbrain lesions, typically thalamic hemorrhage.

"Ocular bobbing" describes brisk downward and slow upward movements of the eyes associated with loss of horizontal eye movements and is diagnostic of bilateral pontine damage, usually from thrombosis of the basilar artery. "Ocular dipping" is a slower, arrhythmic downward movement followed by a faster upward movement in patients with normal reflex horizontal gaze; it usually indicates diffuse cortical anoxic damage.

The oculocephalic reflexes, elicited by moving the head from side to side or vertically and observing eye movements in the direction opposite to the head movement, depend on the integrity of the ocular motor nuclei and their interconnecting tracts that extend from the midbrain to the pons and medulla (Fig. 328-3). The movements, called somewhat inappropriately "doll's eyes" (which refers more accurately to the reflex elevation of the eyelids with flexion of the neck), are normally suppressed in the awake patient. The ability to elicit them therefore reflects both reduced cortical influence on the brainstem and intact brainstem pathways, indicating that coma is caused by a lesion or dysfunction in the cerebral hemispheres. The opposite, an absence of reflex eye movements, usually signifies damage within the brainstem but can result from overdoses of certain drugs. In this circumstance, normal pupillary size and light reaction distinguishes most drug-induced comas from structural brainstem damage.

Thermal, or "caloric," stimulation of the vestibular apparatus (oculovestibular response) provides a more intense stimulus for the oculocephalic reflex but provides essentially the same information. The test is performed by irrigating the external auditory canal with cool water in order to induce convection currents in the labyrinths. After a brief latency, the result is tonic deviation of both eyes to the side of cool-water irrigation and nystagmus in the opposite direction. (The acronym "COWS" has been used to remind generations of medical students of the direction of nystagmus "cold water opposite, warm water same.") The loss of induced conjugate ocular movements indicates brainstem damage. The presence of corrective nystagmus indicates that the frontal lobes are functioning and connected to the brainstem; thus catatonia or hysterical coma is likely.

By touching the cornea with a wisp of cotton, a response consisting of brief bilateral lid closure is normally observed. The corneal reflex depends on the integrity of pontine pathways between the fifth (afferent) and both seventh (efferent) cranial nerves; in conjunction with reflex eye movements, it is a useful test of pontine function. CNS-depressant drugs diminish or eliminate the corneal responses soon after reflex eye movements are paralyzed but before the pupils become unreactive to light. The corneal (and pharyngeal) response may be lost for a time on the side of an acute hemiplegia.

Respiratory Patterns These are of less localizing value in comparison to other brainstem signs. Shallow, slow, but regular breathing suggests metabolic or drug depression. Cheyne-Stokes respiration in its typical cyclic form, ending with a brief apneic period, signifies bihemispheral damage or metabolic suppression and commonly accompanies light coma. Rapid, deep (Kussmaul) breathing usually implies metabolic acidosis but may also occur with pontomesencephalic lesions. Agonal gasps are the result of lower brainstem (medullary) damage and are recognized as the terminal respiratory pattern of severe brain damage. A number of other cyclic breathing variations have been described but are of lesser significance.

LABORATORY STUDIES AND IMAGING

The studies that are most useful in the diagnosis of coma are chemical-toxicologic analysis of blood and urine, cranial CT or MRI, EEG, and CSF examination. Arterial blood gas analysis is helpful in patients with lung disease and acid-base disorders. The metabolic aberrations commonly encountered in clinical practice are usually exposed by measurement of electrolytes, glucose, calcium, osmolarity, and renal (blood urea nitrogen) and hepatic (NH_3) function. Toxicologic analysis may be necessary in any case of acute coma where the diagnosis is not immediately clear. However, the presence of exogenous drugs or toxins, especially alcohol, does not exclude the possibility that other factors, particularly head trauma, are also contributing to the clinical state. An ethanol level of 43 mmol/L (0.2 g/dL) in nonhabituated patients generally causes impaired mental activity; a level of >65 mmol/L (0.3 g/dL) is associated with stupor. The development of tolerance may allow the chronic alcoholic to remain awake at levels >87 mmol/L (0.4 g/dL).

The availability of CT and MRI has focused attention on causes of coma that are detectable by imaging (e.g., hemorrhage, tumor, or hydrocephalus). Resorting primarily to this approach, although at times expedient, is imprudent because most cases of coma (and confusion) are metabolic or toxic in origin. Furthermore, the notion that a normal CT scan excludes an anatomic lesion as the cause of coma is erroneous. Bilateral hemisphere infarction, acute brainstem infarction, encephalitis, meningitis, mechanical shearing of axons as a result of closed head trauma, sagittal sinus thrombosis, and subdural hematoma isodense to adjacent brain are some of the disorders that may not be detected. Nevertheless, if the source of coma remains unknown, a scan should be obtained.

The EEG (Chap. 442e) is useful in metabolic or drug-induced states but is rarely diagnostic. However, it is the essential test to reveal coma that is due to clinically unrecognized, nonconvulsive seizures, and shows fairly characteristic patterns in herpesvirus encephalitis and prion (Creutzfeldt-Jakob) disease. The EEG may be further helpful in disclosing generalized slowing of the background activity, a reflection of the severity of an encephalopathy. Predominant high-voltage slowing (δ or triphasic waves) in the frontal regions is typical of metabolic coma, as from hepatic failure, and widespread fast (β) activity implicates sedative drugs (e.g., benzodiazepines). A special pattern of "alpha coma," defined by widespread, variable 8- to 12-Hz activity, superficially resembles the normal α rhythm of waking but, unlike normal α activity, is not altered by environmental stimuli. Alpha coma results from pontine or diffuse cortical damage and is associated with a poor prognosis. Normal α activity on the EEG, which is suppressed by stimulating the patient, also alerts the clinician to the locked-in syndrome or to hysteria or catatonia. Still, the most important use of EEG recordings in coma is to reveal clinically inapparent epileptic discharges.

Lumbar puncture is performed less frequently than in the past for coma diagnosis because neuroimaging effectively excludes intracerebral and extensive subarachnoid hemorrhage. However, examination of the CSF remains indispensable in the diagnosis of meningitis and encephalitis. For patients with an altered level of consciousness, it is generally recommended that an imaging study be performed prior to lumbar puncture to exclude a large intracranial mass lesion. Blood culture and antibiotic administration usually precede the imaging study if meningitis is suspected (Chap. 164).

DIFFERENTIAL DIAGNOSIS OF COMA

(Table 328-1) The causes of coma can be divided into three broad categories: those cases without focal neurologic signs (e.g., metabolic and toxic encephalopathies); meningitis syndromes, characterized by fever or stiff neck and an excess of cells in the spinal fluid (e.g., bacterial meningitis, subarachnoid hemorrhage, encephalitis); and diseases associated with prominent focal signs (e.g., stroke, cerebral hemorrhage). Conditions that cause sudden coma include drug ingestion, cerebral hemorrhage, trauma, cardiac arrest, epilepsy, and basilar artery occlusion from an embolism. Coma that appears subacutely is usually related to a preexisting medical or neurologic problem or, less often, to secondary brain swelling surrounding a mass such as tumor or cerebral infarction.

The diagnosis of coma due to cerebrovascular disease can be difficult (Chap. 446). The most common diseases are (1) basal ganglia and thalamic hemorrhage (acute but not instantaneous onset, vomiting, headache, hemiplegia, and characteristic eye signs); (2) pontine hemorrhage (sudden onset, pinpoint pupils, loss of reflex eye movements and corneal responses, ocular bobbing, posturing, and hyperventilation); (3) cerebellar hemorrhage (occipital headache, vomiting, gaze paresis, and inability to stand and walk); (4) basilar artery thrombosis (neurologic prodrome or warning spells, diplopia, dysarthria, vomiting, eye movement and corneal response abnormalities, and asymmetric limb paresis); and (5) subarachnoid hemorrhage (precipitous

TABLE 328-1 DIFFERENTIAL DIAGNOSIS OF COMA

1. Diseases that cause no focal or lateralizing neurologic signs, usually with normal brainstem functions; CT scan and cellular content of the CSF are normal
   a. Intoxications: alcohol, sedative drugs, opiates, etc.
   b. Metabolic disturbances: anoxia, hyponatremia, hypernatremia, hypercalcemia, diabetic acidosis, nonketotic hyperosmolar hyperglycemia, hypoglycemia, uremia, hepatic coma, hypercarbia, Addisonian crisis, hypo- and hyperthyroid states, profound nutritional deficiency
   c. Severe systemic infections: pneumonia, septicemia, typhoid fever, malaria, Waterhouse-Friderichsen syndrome
   d. Shock from any cause
   e. Postseizure states, status epilepticus, nonconvulsive status epilepticus
   f. Hypertensive encephalopathy, eclampsia
   g. Severe hyperthermia, hypothermia
   h. Concussion
   i. Acute hydrocephalus
2. Diseases that cause meningeal irritation with or without fever, and with an excess of WBCs or RBCs in the CSF, usually without focal or lateralizing cerebral or brainstem signs; CT or MRI shows no mass lesion
   a. Subarachnoid hemorrhage from ruptured aneurysm, arteriovenous malformation, trauma
   b. Acute bacterial meningitis
   c. Viral encephalitis
   d. Miscellaneous: fat embolism, cholesterol embolism, carcinomatous and lymphomatous meningitis, etc.
3. Diseases that cause focal brainstem or lateralizing cerebral signs, with or without changes in the CSF; CT and MRI are abnormal
   a. Hemispheral hemorrhage (basal ganglionic, thalamic) or infarction (large middle cerebral artery territory) with secondary brainstem compression
   b. Brainstem infarction due to basilar artery thrombosis or embolism
   c. Brain abscess, subdural empyema
   d. Epidural and subdural hemorrhage, brain contusion
   e. Brain tumor with surrounding edema
   f. Cerebellar and pontine hemorrhage and infarction
   g. Widespread traumatic brain injury
   h. Metabolic coma (see above) with preexisting focal damage
   i. Miscellaneous: Cortical vein thrombosis, herpes simplex encephalitis, multiple cerebral emboli due to bacterial endocarditis, acute hemorrhagic leukoencephalitis, acute disseminated (postinfectious) encephalomyelitis, thrombotic thrombocytopenic purpura, cerebral vasculitis, gliomatosis cerebri, pituitary apoplexy, intravascular lymphoma, etc.

Abbreviations: CSF, cerebrospinal fluid; CT, computed tomography; MRI, magnetic resonance imaging; RBCs, red blood cells; WBCs, white blood cells.

coma after sudden severe headache and vomiting). The most common stroke, infarction in the territory of the middle cerebral artery, does not cause coma, but edema surrounding large infarctions may expand over several days and cause coma from mass effect.

The syndrome of acute hydrocephalus accompanies many intracranial diseases, particularly subarachnoid hemorrhage. It is characterized by headache and sometimes vomiting that may progress quickly to coma with extensor posturing of the limbs, bilateral Babinski signs, small unreactive pupils, and impaired oculocephalic movements in the vertical direction.

The majority of medical causes of coma can be established without a neuroimaging study but if the history and examination do not indicate the cause of coma, CT or MRI is needed. Sometimes imaging results can be misleading such as when small subdural hematomas or old strokes are found, but the patient's coma is due to intoxication.

BRAIN DEATH

This is a state of irreversible cessation of all cerebral function with preservation of cardiac activity and maintenance of respiratory and somatic function by artificial means. It is the only type of brain damage recognized as equivalent to death. Criteria have been advanced for the diagnosis of brain death, and it is essential to adhere to standards endorsed by the local medical community. Ideal criteria are simple, can be assessed at the bedside, and allow no chance of diagnostic error. They contain three essential elements: (1) widespread cortical destruction that is reflected by deep coma and unresponsiveness to all forms of stimulation; (2) global brainstem damage demonstrated by absent pupillary light reaction and by the loss of oculovestibular and corneal reflexes; and (3) destruction of the medulla, manifested by complete and irreversible apnea. The heart rate is invariant and does not accelerate to atropine. Diabetes insipidus is usually present but may only develop hours or days after the other clinical signs of brain death. The pupils are usually midsized but may be enlarged; they should not, however, be small. Loss of deep tendon reflexes is not required because the spinal cord remains functional. Babinski signs are generally absent and the toe response is instead, often flexor.

Demonstration that apnea is due to structural medullary damage requires that the Pco_2 be high enough to stimulate respiration during a test of spontaneous breathing. Apnea testing can be done safely by the use of diffusion oxygenation prior to removing the ventilator. This is accomplished by preoxygenation with 100% oxygen, which is then sustained during the test by oxygen administered through a tracheal cannula. CO_2 tension increases ~0.3–0.4 kPa/min (2–3 mmHg/min) during apnea. At the end of a period of observation, typically several minutes, arterial Pco_2 should be at least >6.6–8.0 kPa (50–60 mmHg) for the test to be valid. Apnea is confirmed if no respiratory effort has been observed in the presence of a sufficiently elevated Pco_2. Other techniques, including the administration of CO_2 to accelerate the test, are used in special circumstances. The apnea test is usually stopped if there is serious cardiovascular instability.

An isoelectric EEG may be used as a confirmatory test for total cerebral damage. Radionuclide brain scanning, cerebral angiography, or transcranial Doppler measurements may also be included to demonstrate the absence of CBF, but they have not been as extensively correlated with pathologic changes.

The possibility of profound drug-induced or hypothermic depression of the nervous system must be excluded, and some period of observation, usually 6–24 h, is desirable, during which the clinical signs of brain death are sustained. It is advisable to delay clinical testing for at least 24 h if a cardiac arrest has caused brain death or if the inciting disease is not known.

Although it is largely accepted in Western society that the respirator can be disconnected from a brain-dead patient and that organ donation is subsequently possible, problems frequently arise because of poor communication and inadequate preparation of the family by the physician. Reasonable medical practice, ideally with the agreement of the family, also allows the removal of support or transfer out of an intensive care unit of patients who are not brain dead but whose neurologic conditions are nonetheless hopeless.

TREATMENT COMA

The immediate goal in a comatose patient is prevention of further nervous system damage. Hypotension, hypoglycemia, hypercalcemia, hypoxia, hypercapnia, and hyperthermia should be corrected rapidly. An oropharyngeal airway is adequate to keep the pharynx open in a drowsy patient who is breathing normally. Tracheal intubation is indicated if there is apnea, upper airway obstruction, hypoventilation, or emesis, or if the patient is liable to aspirate because of coma. Mechanical ventilation is required if there is hypoventilation or a need to induce hypocapnia in order to lower ICP. IV access is established, and naloxone and dextrose are administered if narcotic overdose or hypoglycemia is a possibility; thiamine is given along with glucose to avoid provoking Wernicke's disease in malnourished patients. In cases of suspected basilar thrombosis with brainstem ischemia, IV heparin or a thrombolytic agent is often used, after cerebral hemorrhage has been excluded by a neuroimaging study. Physostigmine may awaken patients with anticholinergic-type drug overdose but should be used only with careful monitoring; many physicians believe that it should only be used to treat anticholinergic overdose–associated cardiac arrhythmias. The use of benzodiazepine antagonists offers some prospect of improvement after overdose of soporific drugs and has transient benefit in hepatic encephalopathy. Certain other toxic and drug-induced comas have specific treatments such as fomepizole for ethylene glycol ingestion.

Administration of hypotonic intravenous solutions should be monitored carefully in any serious acute brain illness because of the potential for exacerbating brain swelling. Cervical spine injuries must not be overlooked, particularly before attempting intubation or evaluation of oculocephalic responses. Fever and meningismus indicate an urgent need for examination of the CSF to diagnose meningitis. If the lumbar puncture in a case of suspected meningitis is delayed, an antibiotic such as a third-generation cephalosporin may be administered, preferably after obtaining blood cultures. The management of raised ICP is discussed in Chap. 330.

PROGNOSIS

One hopes to avoid the difficult outcome of a patient who is left severely disabled or vegetative. Children and young adults may have ominous early clinical findings such as abnormal brainstem reflexes and yet recover; temporization in offering a prognosis in this group of patients is wise. Metabolic comas have a far better prognosis than traumatic ones. All systems for estimating prognosis in adults should be taken as approximations, and medical judgments must be tempered by factors such as age, underlying systemic disease, and general medical condition. In an attempt to collect prognostic information from large numbers of patients with head injury, the Glasgow Coma Scale was devised; empirically, it has predictive value in cases of brain trauma (see Table 457e-2). For anoxic and metabolic coma, clinical signs such as the pupillary and motor responses after 1 day, 3 days, and 1 week have been shown to have predictive value. Other studies suggest that the absence of corneal responses may have the most discriminative value. The absence of the cortical waves of the somatosensory evoked potentials has also proved a strong indicator of poor outcome in coma from any cause.

The uniformly poor outcome of the prolonged vegetative state has already been mentioned, but recent reports that a small number of such patients display consistent cortical activation on functional MRI in response to salient stimuli have begun to alter the perception of the possible internal mental milieu of such individuals. These findings do not change the poor prognosis. For example, in one series, about 10% of vegetative patients after traumatic brain injury could activate their frontal or temporal lobes in response to requests by an examiner to imagine certain visuospatial tasks. In one case, a rudimentary form of communication could be established. There are also reports in exceptional patients of improvement in cognitive function with the implantation of thalamic-stimulating electrodes. It is prudent to avoid generalizations from these findings.

329e Examination of the Comatose Patient

S. Andrew Josephson

This is a digital-only chapter. It is available on the DVD that accompanies this book, as well as on Access Medicine/Harrison's Online, and the eBook and "app" editions of HPIM 19e.

This chapter features a video illustrating the examination of a comatose patient. Proper techniques are demonstrated and supplemented with a discussion of interpretation of findings and implications for management. Also included is an overview of coma and its anatomic basis.

330 Neurologic Critical Care, Including Hypoxic-Ischemic Encephalopathy, and Subarachnoid Hemorrhage

J. Claude Hemphill, III, Wade S. Smith, Daryl R. Gress

Life-threatening neurologic illness may be caused by a primary disorder affecting any region of the neuraxis or may occur as a consequence of a systemic disorder such as hepatic failure, multisystem organ failure, or cardiac arrest (Table 330-1). Neurologic critical care focuses on preservation of neurologic tissue and prevention of secondary brain injury caused by ischemia, hemorrhage, edema, herniation, and elevated intracranial pressure (ICP). Management of other organ systems proceeds concurrently and may need to be modified in order to maintain the overall focus on neurologic issues.

PATHOPHYSIOLOGY

Brain Edema Swelling, or edema, of brain tissue occurs with many types of brain injury. The two principal types of edema are vasogenic and cytotoxic. *Vasogenic edema* refers to the influx of fluid and solutes into the brain through an incompetent blood-brain barrier (BBB). In the normal cerebral vasculature, endothelial tight junctions associated with astrocytes create an impermeable barrier (the BBB), through which access into the brain interstitium is dependent upon specific transport mechanisms. The BBB may be compromised in ischemia, trauma, infection, and metabolic derangements. *Vasogenic edema* results from abnormal permeability of the BBB, and typically develops rapidly following injury. *Cytotoxic edema* results from cellular swelling, membrane breakdown, and ultimately cell death. Clinically significant brain edema usually represents a combination of vasogenic and cytotoxic components. Edema can lead to increased ICP as well as tissue shifts and brain displacement or herniation from focal processes (Chap. 328). These tissue shifts can cause injury by mechanical distention and compression in addition to the ischemia of impaired perfusion consequent to the elevated ICP.

Ischemic Cascade and Cellular Injury When delivery of substrates, principally oxygen and glucose, is inadequate to sustain cellular function, a series of interrelated biochemical reactions known as the *ischemic cascade* is initiated (see Fig. 446-2). The release of excitatory amino acids, especially glutamate, leads to influx of calcium and sodium ions, which disrupt cellular homeostasis. An increased intracellular calcium concentration may activate proteases and lipases, which then lead to lipid peroxidation and free radical–mediated cell membrane injury. Cytotoxic edema ensues, and ultimately necrotic cell death and tissue infarction occur. This pathway to irreversible cell death is common to ischemic stroke, global cerebral ischemia, and traumatic brain injury.

Penumbra refers to areas of ischemic brain tissue that have not yet undergone irreversible infarction, implying that these regions are potentially salvageable if ischemia can be reversed. Factors that may exacerbate ischemic brain injury include systemic hypotension and hypoxia, which further reduce substrate delivery to vulnerable brain tissue, and fever, seizures, and hyperglycemia, which can increase cellular metabolism, outstripping compensatory processes. Clinically, these events are known as *secondary brain insults* because they lead to exacerbation of the primary brain injury. Prevention, identification, and treatment of secondary brain insults are fundamental goals of management.

An alternative pathway of cellular injury is *apoptosis*. This process implies programmed cell death, which may occur in the setting of ischemic stroke, global cerebral ischemia, traumatic brain injury, and possibly intracerebral hemorrhage. Apoptotic cell death can be distinguished histologically from the necrotic cell death of ischemia and is mediated through a different set of biochemical pathways; apoptotic

TABLE 330-1 NEUROLOGIC DISORDERS IN CRITICAL ILLNESS

Localization Along Neuroaxis	Syndrome
Central Nervous System	
Brain: Cerebral hemispheres	Global encephalopathy
	Delirium
	Sepsis
	Organ failure—hepatic, renal
	Medication related—sedatives, hypnotics, analgesics, H_2 blockers, antihypertensives
	Drug overdose
	Electrolyte disturbance—hyponatremia, hypoglycemia
	Hypotension/hypoperfusion
	Hypoxia
	Meningitis
	Subarachnoid hemorrhage
	Wernicke's disease
	Seizure—postictal or nonconvulsive status
	Hypertensive encephalopathy
	Hypothyroidism—myxedema
	Focal deficits
	Ischemic stroke
	Tumor
	Abscess, subdural empyema
	Intraparenchymal hemorrhage
	Subdural/epidural hematoma
Brainstem/cerebellum	Mass effect and compression
	Basilar artery thrombosis
	Intraparenchymal hemorrhage
	Central pontine myelinolysis
Spinal cord	Mass effect and compression
	Disk herniation
	Epidural hematoma
	Ischemia—hypotension/embolic
	Epidural abscess
	Trauma
	Myelitis
Peripheral Nervous System	
Peripheral nerve	
Axonal	Critical illness polyneuropathy
	Neuromuscular blocking agent complications
	Metabolic disturbances, uremia, hyperglycemia
	Medication effects—chemotherapeutic, antiretroviral
Demyelinating	Guillain-Barré syndrome
	Chronic inflammatory demyelinating polyneuropathy
Neuromuscular junction	Prolonged effect of neuromuscular blockade
	Medication effects—aminoglycosides
	Myasthenia gravis, Lambert-Eaton syndrome, botulism
Muscle	Critical illness myopathy
	Cachectic myopathy
	Acute necrotizing myopathy
	Thick-filament myopathy
	Electrolyte disturbances—hypokalemia/hyperkalemia, hypophosphatemia
	Rhabdomyolysis

cell death occurs without cerebral edema and therefore is often not seen on brain imaging. At present, interventions for prevention and treatment of apoptotic cell death remain less well defined than those for ischemia. Excitotoxicity and mechanisms of cell death are discussed in more detail in Chap. 444e.

Cerebral Perfusion and Autoregulation Brain tissue requires constant perfusion in order to ensure adequate delivery of substrate. The hemodynamic response of the brain has the capacity to preserve perfusion across a wide range of systemic blood pressures. Cerebral perfusion pressure (CPP), defined as the mean systemic arterial pressure (MAP) minus the ICP, provides the driving force for circulation across the capillary beds of the brain. *Autoregulation* refers to the physiologic response whereby cerebral blood flow (CBF) is regulated via alterations in cerebrovascular resistance in order to maintain perfusion over wide physiologic changes such as neuronal activation or changes in hemodynamic function. If systemic blood pressure drops, cerebral perfusion is preserved through vasodilation of arterioles in the brain; likewise, arteriolar vasoconstriction occurs at high systemic pressures to prevent hyperperfusion, resulting in fairly constant perfusion across a wide range of systemic blood pressures (Fig. 330-1). At the extreme limits of MAP or CPP (high or low), flow becomes directly related to perfusion pressure. These autoregulatory changes occur in the microcirculation and are mediated by vessels below the resolution of those seen on angiography. CBF is also strongly influenced by pH and Pa_{CO_2}. CBF increases with hypercapnia and acidosis and decreases with hypocapnia and alkalosis because of pH related changes in cerebral vascular resistance. This forms the basis for the use of hyperventilation to lower ICP, and this effect on ICP is mediated through a decrease in both CBF and intracranial blood volume. Cerebral autoregulation is a complex process critical to the normal homeostatic functioning of the brain, and this process may be disordered focally and unpredictably in disease states such as traumatic brain injury and severe focal cerebral ischemia.

Cerebrospinal Fluid and Intracranial Pressure The cranial contents consist essentially of brain, cerebrospinal fluid (CSF), and blood. CSF is produced principally in the choroid plexus of each lateral ventricle, exits the brain via the foramens of Luschka and Magendie, and flows over the cortex to be absorbed into the venous system along the superior sagittal sinus. In adults, approximately 150 mL of CSF are contained within the ventricles and surrounding the brain and spinal cord; the cerebral blood volume is also ~150 mL. The bony skull offers excellent protection for the brain but allows little tolerance for additional volume. Significant

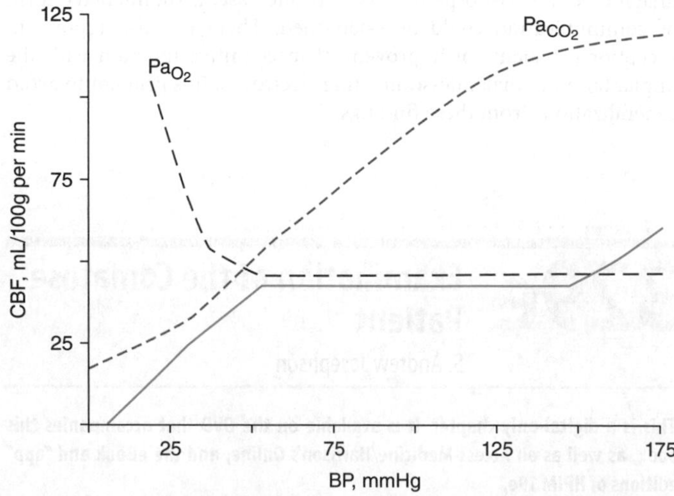

FIGURE 330-1 Autoregulation of cerebral blood flow (*solid line*). Cerebral perfusion is constant over a wide range of systemic blood pressure. Perfusion is increased in the setting of hypoxia or hypercarbia. BP, blood pressure; CBF, cerebral blood flow. *(Reprinted with permission from HM Shapiro: Anesthesiology 43:447, 1975. Copyright 1975, Lippincott Company.).*

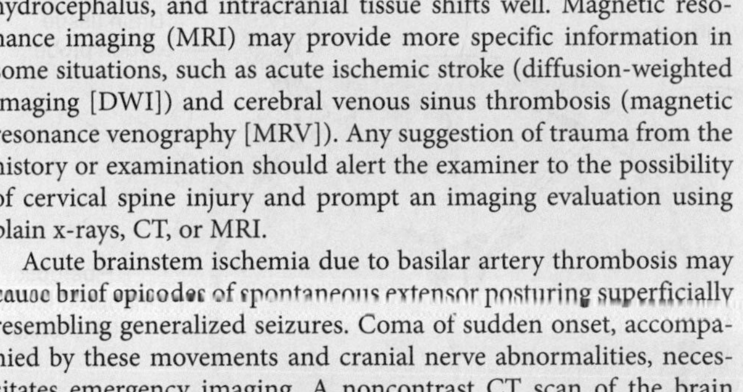

FIGURE 330-2 Ischemia and vasodilatation. Reduced cerebral perfusion pressure (CPP) leads to increased ischemia, vasodilation, increased intracranial pressure (ICP), and further reductions in CPP, a cycle leading to further neurologic injury. CBV, cerebral blood volume; CMR, cerebral metabolic rate; CSF, cerebrospinal fluid; SABP, systolic arterial blood pressure. *(Adapted from MJ Rosner et al: J Neurosurg 83:949, 1995; with permission.)*

increases in volume eventually result in increased ICP. Obstruction of CSF outflow, edema of cerebral tissue, or increases in volume from tumor or hematoma may increase ICP. Elevated ICP diminishes cerebral perfusion and can lead to tissue ischemia. Ischemia in turn may lead to vasodilation via autoregulatory mechanisms designed to restore cerebral perfusion. However, vasodilation also increases cerebral blood volume, which in turn then increases ICP, lowers CPP, and provokes further ischemia (Fig. 330-2). This vicious cycle is commonly seen in traumatic brain injury, massive intracerebral hemorrhage, and large hemispheric infarcts with significant tissue shifts.

APPROACH TO THE PATIENT: Severe Central Nervous System Dysfunction

Critically ill patients with severe central nervous system (CNS) dysfunction require rapid evaluation and intervention in order to limit primary and secondary brain injury. Initial neurologic evaluation should be performed concurrent with stabilization of basic respiratory, cardiac, and hemodynamic parameters. Significant barriers may exist to neurologic assessment in the critical care unit, including endotracheal intubation and the use of sedative or paralytic agents to facilitate procedures.

An impaired level of consciousness is common in critically ill patients. The essential first task in assessment is to determine whether the cause of dysfunction is related to a diffuse, usually metabolic, process or whether a focal, usually structural, process is implicated. Examples of diffuse processes include metabolic encephalopathies related to organ failure, drug overdose, or hypoxia-ischemia. Focal processes include ischemic and hemorrhagic stroke and traumatic brain injury, especially with intracranial hematomas. Because these two categories of disorders have fundamentally different causes, treatments, and prognoses, the initial focus is on making this distinction rapidly and accurately. The approach to the comatose patient is discussed in Chap. 328; etiologies are listed in Table 328-1.

Minor focal deficits may be present on the neurologic examination in patients with metabolic encephalopathies. However, the finding of prominent focal signs such as pupillary asymmetry, hemiparesis, gaze palsy, or paraplegia should suggest the possibility of a structural lesion. All patients with a decreased level of consciousness associated with focal findings should undergo an urgent neuroimaging procedure, as should all patients with coma of unknown etiology. Computed tomography (CT) scanning is usually the most appropriate initial study because it can be performed quickly in critically ill patients and demonstrates hemorrhage, hydrocephalus, and intracranial tissue shifts well. Magnetic resonance imaging (MRI) may provide more specific information in some situations, such as acute ischemic stroke (diffusion-weighted imaging [DWI]) and cerebral venous sinus thrombosis (magnetic resonance venography [MRV]). Any suggestion of trauma from the history or examination should alert the examiner to the possibility of cervical spine injury and prompt an imaging evaluation using plain x-rays, CT, or MRI.

Acute brainstem ischemia due to basilar artery thrombosis may cause brief episodes of spontaneous extensor posturing superficially resembling generalized seizures. Coma of sudden onset, accompanied by these movements and cranial nerve abnormalities, necessitates emergency imaging. A noncontrast CT scan of the brain may reveal a hyperdense basilar artery indicating thrombus in the vessel, and subsequent CT or MR angiography can assess basilar artery patency.

Other diagnostic studies are best used in specific circumstances, usually when neuroimaging studies fail to reveal a structural lesion and the etiology of the altered mental state remains uncertain. Electroencephalography (EEG) can be important in the evaluation of critically ill patients with severe brain dysfunction. The EEG of metabolic encephalopathy typically reveals generalized slowing. One of the most important uses of EEG is to help exclude inapparent seizures, especially nonconvulsive status epilepticus. Untreated continuous or frequently recurrent seizures may cause neuronal injury, making the diagnosis and treatment of seizures crucial in this patient group. Lumbar puncture (LP) may be necessary to exclude infectious or inflammatory processes, and an elevated opening pressure may be an important clue to cerebral venous sinus thrombosis. In patients with coma or profound encephalopathy, it is preferable to perform a neuroimaging study prior to LP. If bacterial meningitis is suspected, an LP may be performed first or antibiotics may be empirically administered before the diagnostic studies are completed. Standard laboratory evaluation of critically ill patients should include assessment of serum electrolytes (especially sodium and calcium), glucose, renal and hepatic function, complete blood count, and coagulation. Serum or urine toxicology screens should be performed in patients with encephalopathy of unknown cause. EEG, LP, and other specific laboratory tests are most useful when the mechanism of the altered level of consciousness is uncertain; they are not routinely performed in clear-cut cases of stroke or traumatic brain injury.

Monitoring of ICP can be an important tool in selected patients. In general, patients who should be considered for ICP monitoring are those with primary neurologic disorders, such as stroke or traumatic brain injury, who are at significant risk for secondary brain injury due to elevated ICP and decreased CPP. Included are patients with the following: severe traumatic brain injury (Glasgow Coma Scale [GCS] score ≤8 [see Table 457e-2]); large tissue shifts from supratentorial ischemic or hemorrhagic stroke; or hydrocephalus from subarachnoid hemorrhage (SAH), intraventricular hemorrhage, or posterior fossa stroke. An additional disorder in which ICP monitoring can add important information is fulminant hepatic failure, in which elevated ICP may be treated with barbiturates or, eventually, liver transplantation. In general, ventriculostomy is preferable to ICP monitoring devices that are placed in the brain parenchyma, because ventriculostomy allows CSF drainage as a method of treating elevated ICP. However, parenchymal ICP monitoring is most appropriate for patients with diffuse edema and small ventricles (which may make ventriculostomy placement more difficult) or any degree of coagulopathy (in which ventriculostomy carries a higher risk of hemorrhagic complications) (Fig 330-3).

Treatment of Elevated ICP Elevated ICP may occur in a wide range of disorders, including head trauma, intracerebral hemorrhage, SAH with hydrocephalus, and fulminant hepatic failure. Because CSF and blood volume can be redistributed initially, by the time

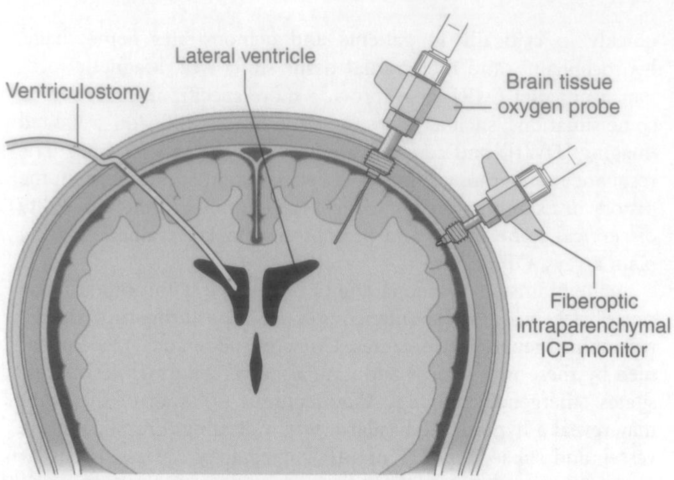

FIGURE 330-3 Intracranial pressure and brain tissue oxygen monitoring. A ventriculostomy allows for drainage of cerebrospinal fluid to treat elevated intracranial pressure (ICP). Fiberoptic ICP and brain tissue oxygen monitors are usually secured using a screwlike skull bolt. Cerebral blood flow and microdialysis probes (not shown) may be placed in a manner similar to the brain tissue oxygen probe.

elevated ICP occurs, intracranial compliance is severely impaired. At this point, any small increase in the volume of CSF, intravascular blood, edema, or a mass lesion may result in a significant increase in ICP and a decrease in cerebral perfusion. This is a fundamental mechanism of secondary ischemic brain injury and constitutes an emergency that requires immediate attention. In general, ICP should be maintained at <20 mmHg and CPP should be maintained at ≥60 mmHg.

Interventions to lower ICP are ideally based on the underlying mechanism responsible for the elevated ICP (Table 330-2). For

TABLE 330-2 STEPWISE APPROACH TO TREATMENT OF ELEVATED INTRACRANIAL PRESSURE (ICP)[a]

Insert ICP monitor—ventriculostomy versus parenchymal device

General goals: maintain ICP <20 mmHg and CPP ≥60 mmHg. For ICP >20–25 mmHg for >5 min:

1. Elevate head of the bed; midline head position
2. Drain CSF via ventriculostomy (if in place)
3. Osmotherapy—mannitol 25–100 g q4h as needed (maintain serum osmolality <320 mosmol) or hypertonic saline (30 mL, 23.4% NaCl bolus)
4. Glucocorticoids—dexamethasone 4 mg q6h for vasogenic edema from tumor, abscess (avoid glucocorticoids in head trauma, ischemic and hemorrhagic stroke)
5. Sedation (e.g., morphine, propofol, or midazolam); add neuromuscular paralysis if necessary (patient will require endotracheal intubation and mechanical ventilation at this point, if not before)
6. Hyperventilation—to $PaCO_2$ 30–35 mmHg (short-term use or skip this step)
7. Pressor therapy—phenylephrine, dopamine, or norepinephrine to maintain adequate MAP to ensure CPP ≥60 mmHg (maintain euvolemia to minimize deleterious systemic effects of pressors). May adjust target CPP in individual patients based on autoregulation status.
8. Consider second-tier therapies for refractory elevated ICP
   a. Decompressive craniectomy
   b. High-dose barbiturate therapy ("pentobarb coma")
   c. Hypothermia to 33°C

[a]Throughout ICP treatment algorithm, consider repeat head computed tomography to identify mass lesions amenable to surgical evacuation. May alter order of steps based on directed treatment to specific cause of elevated ICP.

Abbreviations: CPP, cerebral perfusion pressure; CSF, cerebrospinal fluid; MAP, mean arterial pressure; $PaCO_2$, arterial partial pressure of carbon dioxide.

example, in hydrocephalus from SAH, the principal cause of elevated ICP is impairment of CSF drainage. In this setting, ventricular drainage of CSF is likely to be sufficient and most appropriate. In head trauma and stroke, cytotoxic edema may be most responsible, and the use of osmotic agents such as mannitol or hypertonic saline becomes an appropriate early step. As described above, elevated ICP may cause tissue ischemia, and, if cerebral autoregulation is intact, the resulting vasodilation can lead to a cycle of worsening ischemia. Paradoxically, administration of vasopressor agents to increase mean arterial pressure may actually lower ICP by improving perfusion, thereby allowing autoregulatory vasoconstriction as ischemia is relieved and ultimately decreasing intracranial blood volume.

Early signs of elevated ICP include drowsiness and a diminished level of consciousness. Neuroimaging studies may reveal evidence of edema and mass effect. Hypotonic IV fluids should be avoided, and elevation of the head of the bed is recommended. Patients must be carefully observed for risk of aspiration and compromise of the airway as the level of alertness declines. Coma and unilateral pupillary changes are late signs and require immediate intervention. Emergent treatment of elevated ICP is most quickly achieved by intubation and hyperventilation, which causes vasoconstriction and reduces cerebral blood volume. To avoid provoking or worsening cerebral ischemia, hyperventilation, if used at all, is best administered only for short periods of time until a more definitive treatment can be instituted. Furthermore, the effects of hyperventilation on ICP are short-lived, often lasting only for several hours because of the buffering capacity of the cerebral interstitium, and rebound elevations of ICP may accompany abrupt discontinuation of hyperventilation. As the level of consciousness declines to coma, the ability to follow the neurologic status of the patient by examination lessens and measurement of ICP assumes greater importance. If a ventriculostomy device is in place, direct drainage of CSF to reduce ICP is possible. Finally, high-dose barbiturates, decompressive hemicraniectomy, and hypothermia are sometimes used for refractory elevations of ICP, although these have significant side effects and have not been proven to improve outcome.

Secondary Brain Insults Patients with primary brain injuries, whether due to trauma or stroke, are at risk for ongoing secondary ischemic brain injury. Because secondary brain injury can be a major determinant of a poor outcome, strategies for minimizing secondary brain insults are an integral part of the critical care of all patients. Although elevated ICP may lead to secondary ischemia, most secondary brain injury is mediated through other clinical events that exacerbate the ischemic cascade already initiated by the primary brain injury. Episodes of secondary brain insults are usually not associated with apparent neurologic worsening. Rather, they lead to cumulative injury limiting eventual recovery, which manifests as a higher mortality rate or worsened long-term functional outcome. Thus, close monitoring of vital signs is important, as is early intervention to prevent secondary ischemia. Avoiding hypotension and hypoxia is critical, as significant hypotensive events (systolic blood pressure <90 mmHg) as short as 10 min in duration have been shown to adversely influence outcome after traumatic brain injury. Even in patients with stroke or head trauma who do not require ICP monitoring, close attention to adequate cerebral perfusion is warranted. Hypoxia (pulse oximetry saturation <90%), particularly in combination with hypotension, also leads to secondary brain injury. Likewise, fever and hyperglycemia both worsen experimental ischemia and have been associated with worsened clinical outcome after stroke and head trauma. Aggressive control of fever with a goal of normothermia is warranted but may be difficult to achieve with antipyretic medications and cooling blankets. The value of newer surface or intravascular temperature control devices for the management of refractory fever is under investigation. The use of IV insulin infusion is encouraged for control of hyperglycemia because this allows better regulation of serum glucose levels than SC insulin. A reasonable goal is to maintain the serum glucose level at <10.0 mmol/L (<180 mg/dL), although episodes of hypoglycemia appear equally detrimental and the optimal targets remain uncertain. New cerebral monitoring tools that allow continuous evaluation of brain tissue oxygen tension, CBF, and metabolism (via microdialysis) may further improve the management of secondary brain injury.

CRITICAL CARE DISORDERS OF THE CENTRAL NERVOUS SYSTEM

HYPOXIC-ISCHEMIC ENCEPHALOPATHY

This occurs from lack of delivery of oxygen to the brain because of extreme hypotension (hypoxia-ischemia) or hypoxia due to respiratory failure. Causes include myocardial infarction, cardiac arrest, shock, asphyxiation, paralysis of respiration, and carbon monoxide or cyanide poisoning. In some circumstances, hypoxia may predominate. Carbon monoxide and cyanide poisoning are sometimes termed *histotoxic hypoxia* because they cause a direct impairment of the respiratory chain.

Clinical Manifestations Mild degrees of pure hypoxia, such as occur at high altitudes, cause impaired judgment, inattentiveness, motor incoordination, and, at times, euphoria. However, with hypoxia-ischemia, such as occurs with circulatory arrest, consciousness is lost within seconds. If circulation is restored within 3–5 min, full recovery may occur, but if hypoxia ischemia lasts beyond 3–5 min, some degree of permanent cerebral damage usually results. Except in extreme cases, it may be difficult to judge the precise degree of hypoxia-ischemia, and some patients make a relatively full recovery after even 8–10 min of global cerebral ischemia. The brain is more tolerant to pure hypoxia than it is to hypoxia-ischemia. For example, a Pa_{O_2} as low as 20 mmHg (2.7 kPa) can be well tolerated if it develops gradually and normal blood pressure is maintained, whereas short durations of very low or absent cerebral circulation usually result in permanent impairment.

Clinical examination at different time points after a hypoxic-ischemic insult (especially cardiac arrest) is useful in assessing prognosis for long-term neurologic outcome. The prognosis is better for patients with intact brainstem function, as indicated by normal pupillary light responses and intact oculocephalic (doll's eyes), oculovestibular (caloric), and corneal reflexes. Absence of these reflexes and the presence of persistently dilated pupils that do not react to light are grave prognostic signs. A low likelihood of a favorable outcome from hypoxic-ischemic coma is strongly suggested by an absent pupillary light reflex or extensor or absent motor response to pain on day 3 following the injury, excluding patients with metabolic disturbances and those treated with high-dose barbiturates or hypothermia, which confound interpretation of these signs. Electrophysiologically, the bilateral absence of the N20 component of the somatosensory evoked potential (SSEP) in the first several days also conveys a poor prognosis. A very elevated serum level (>33 μg/L) of the biochemical marker neuron-specific enolase (NSE) is indicative of brain damage after resuscitation from cardiac arrest and predicts a poor outcome. However, at present, SSEPs and NSE levels may be difficult to obtain in a timely fashion, with SSEP testing requiring substantial expertise in interpretation and NSE measurements not yet standardized. Recent studies suggest that the administration of mild hypothermia after cardiac arrest (see "Treatment") may affect the time points when these clinical and electrophysiologic predictors become reliable in identifying patients with a very low likelihood of clinically meaningful recovery. For example, the false-positive rate for incorrect prediction of poor neurologic outcome may be as high as 21% (95% confidence interval [CI] 8–43%) for patients treated with mild hypothermia who exhibit 3-day motor function no better than extensor posturing. Long-term consequences of hypoxic-ischemic encephalopathy include persistent coma or a vegetative state (Chap. 328), dementia, visual agnosia (Chap. 36), parkinsonism, choreoathetosis, cerebellar ataxia, myoclonus, seizures, and an amnestic state, which may be a consequence of selective damage to the hippocampus.

Pathology Principal histologic findings are extensive multifocal or diffuse laminar cortical necrosis (Fig. 330-4), with frequent involvement of the hippocampus. The hippocampal CA1 neurons are vulnerable to even brief episodes of hypoxia-ischemia, perhaps explaining why selective persistent memory deficits may occur after brief cardiac arrest. Scattered small areas of infarction or neuronal loss may be present in the basal ganglia, hypothalamus, or brainstem. In some cases, extensive bilateral thalamic scarring may affect pathways that mediate arousal, and this pathology may be responsible for the persistent vegetative state. A specific form of hypoxic-ischemic encephalopathy, so-called watershed infarcts, occurs at the distal territories between the major cerebral arteries and can cause cognitive deficits, including visual agnosia, and weakness that is greater in proximal than in distal muscle groups.

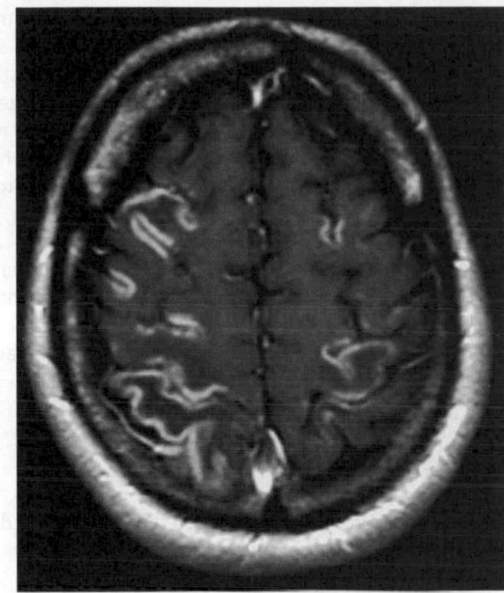

FIGURE 330-4 Cortical laminar necrosis in hypoxic-ischemic encephalopathy. T1-weighted postcontrast magnetic resonance imaging shows cortical enhancement in a watershed distribution consistent with laminar necrosis.

Diagnosis Diagnosis is based on the history of a hypoxic-ischemic event such as cardiac arrest. Blood pressure <70 mmHg systolic or Pa_{O_2} <40 mmHg is usually necessary, although both absolute levels and duration of exposure are important determinants of cellular injury. Carbon monoxide intoxication can be confirmed by measurement of carboxyhemoglobin and is suggested by a cherry red color of the venous blood and skin, although the latter is an inconsistent clinical finding.

TREATMENT HYPOXIC-ISCHEMIC ENCEPHALOPATHY

Treatment should be directed at restoration of normal cardiorespiratory function. This includes securing a clear airway, ensuring adequate oxygenation and ventilation, and restoring cerebral perfusion, whether by cardiopulmonary resuscitation, fluid, pressors, or cardiac pacing. Hypothermia may target the neuronal cell injury cascade and has substantial neuroprotective properties in experimental models of brain injury. In two trials, mild hypothermia (33°C) improved functional outcome in patients who remained comatose after resuscitation from a cardiac arrest. Treatment was initiated within minutes of cardiac resuscitation and continued for 12 h in one study and 24 h in the other. Potential complications of hypothermia include coagulopathy and an increased risk of infection. Based on these studies, the International Liaison Committee on Resuscitation issued the following advisory statement: "Unconscious adult patients with spontaneous circulation after out-of-hospital cardiac arrest should be cooled to 32°–34°C for 12–24 h when the initial rhythm was ventricular fibrillation. Such cooling may also be beneficial for other rhythms or in-hospital cardiac arrest."

Severe carbon monoxide intoxication may be treated with hyperbaric oxygen. Anticonvulsants may be needed to control seizures, although these are not usually given prophylactically. Posthypoxic myoclonus may respond to oral administration of clonazepam at doses of 1.5–10 mg daily or valproate at doses of 300–1200 mg daily in divided doses. Myoclonic status epilepticus within 24 h after a primary circulatory arrest generally portends a very poor prognosis, even if seizures are controlled.

Carbon monoxide and cyanide intoxication can also cause a delayed encephalopathy. Little clinical impairment is evident when the patient first regains consciousness, but a parkinsonian syndrome characterized by akinesia and rigidity without tremor may develop. Symptoms can worsen over months, accompanied by increasing evidence of damage in the basal ganglia as seen on both CT and MRI.

METABOLIC ENCEPHALOPATHIES

Altered mental states, variously described as confusion, delirium, disorientation, and encephalopathy, are present in many patients with severe illness in an intensive care unit (ICU). Older patients are particularly vulnerable to delirium, a confusional state characterized by disordered perception, frequent hallucinations, delusions, and sleep disturbance. This is often attributed to medication effects, sleep deprivation, pain, and anxiety. The presence of delirium is associated with worsened outcome in critically ill patients, even in those without an identifiable CNS pathology such as stroke or brain trauma. In these patients, the cause of delirium is often multifactorial, resulting from organ dysfunction, sepsis, and especially the use of medications given to treat pain, agitation, or anxiety. Critically ill patients are often treated with a variety of sedative and analgesic medications, including opiates, benzodiazepines, neuroleptics, and sedative-anesthetic medications, such as propofol. In critically ill patients requiring sedation, use of the centrally acting α_2 agonist dexmedetomidine may reduce delirium and shorten the duration of mechanical ventilation compared to the use of benzodiazepines such as lorazepam or midazolam. The presence of family members in the ICU may also help to calm and orient agitated patients, and in severe cases, low doses of neuroleptics (e.g., haloperidol 0.5–1 mg) can be useful. Current strategies focus on limiting the use of sedative medications when this can be done safely.

In the ICU setting, several metabolic causes of an altered level of consciousness predominate. Hypercarbic encephalopathy can present with headache, confusion, stupor, or coma. Hypoventilation syndrome occurs most frequently in patients with a history of chronic CO_2 retention who are receiving oxygen therapy for emphysema or chronic pulmonary disease (Chap. 318). The elevated $Paco_2$ leading to CO_2 narcosis may have a direct anesthetic effect, and cerebral vasodilation from increased $Paco_2$ can lead to increased ICP. Hepatic encephalopathy is suggested by asterixis and can occur in chronic liver failure or acute fulminant hepatic failure. Both hyperglycemia and hypoglycemia can cause encephalopathy, as can hypernatremia and hyponatremia. Confusion, impairment of eye movements, and gait ataxia are the hallmarks of acute Wernicke's disease (see below).

SEPSIS-ASSOCIATED ENCEPHALOPATHY

Pathogenesis In patients with sepsis, the systemic response to infectious agents leads to the release of circulating inflammatory mediators that appear to contribute to encephalopathy. Critical illness, in association with the systemic inflammatory response syndrome (SIRS), can lead to multisystem organ failure. This syndrome can occur in the setting of apparent sepsis, severe burns, or trauma, even without clear identification of an infectious agent. Many patients with critical illness, sepsis, or SIRS develop encephalopathy without obvious explanation. This condition is broadly termed *sepsis-associated encephalopathy*. Although the specific mediators leading to neurologic dysfunction remain uncertain, it is clear that the encephalopathy is not simply the result of metabolic derangements of multiorgan failure. The cytokines tumor necrosis factor, interleukin (IL)-1, IL-2, and IL-6 are thought to play a role in this syndrome.

Diagnosis Sepsis-associated encephalopathy presents clinically as a diffuse dysfunction of the brain without prominent focal findings. Confusion, disorientation, agitation, and fluctuations in level of alertness are typical. In more profound cases, especially with hemodynamic compromise, the decrease in level of alertness can be more prominent, at times resulting in coma. Hyperreflexia and frontal release signs such as a grasp or snout reflex (Chap. 36) can be seen. Abnormal movements such as myoclonus, tremor, or asterixis can occur. Sepsis-associated encephalopathy is quite common, occurring in the majority of patients with sepsis and multisystem organ failure. Diagnosis is often difficult because of the multiple potential causes of neurologic dysfunction in critically ill patients and requires exclusion of structural, metabolic, toxic, and infectious (e.g., meningitis or encephalitis) causes. The mortality rate of patients with sepsis-associated encephalopathy severe enough to produce coma approaches 50%, although this principally reflects the severity of the underlying critical illness and is not a direct result of the encephalopathy. Patients dying from severe sepsis or septic shock may have elevated levels of the serum brain injury biomarker S-100β and neuropathologic findings of neuronal apoptosis and cerebral ischemic injury. Successful treatment of the underlying critical illness almost always results in substantial improvement of the encephalopathy. However, although severe disability to the level of chronic vegetative or minimally conscious states is uncommon, long-term cognitive dysfunction clinically similar to dementia is being increasingly recognized in some survivors.

CENTRAL PONTINE MYELINOLYSIS

This disorder typically presents in a devastating fashion as quadriplegia and pseudobulbar palsy. Predisposing factors include severe underlying medical illness or nutritional deficiency; most cases are associated with rapid correction of hyponatremia or with hyperosmolar states. The pathology consists of demyelination without inflammation in the base of the pons, with relative sparing of axons and nerve cells. MRI is useful in establishing the diagnosis (Fig. 330-5) and may also identify partial forms that present as confusion, dysarthria, and/or disturbances of conjugate gaze without quadriplegia. Occasional cases present with lesions outside of the brainstem. Therapeutic guidelines for the restoration of severe hyponatremia should aim for gradual correction, i.e., by ≤10 mmol/L (10 meq/L) within 24 h and 20 mmol/L (20 meq/L) within 48 h.

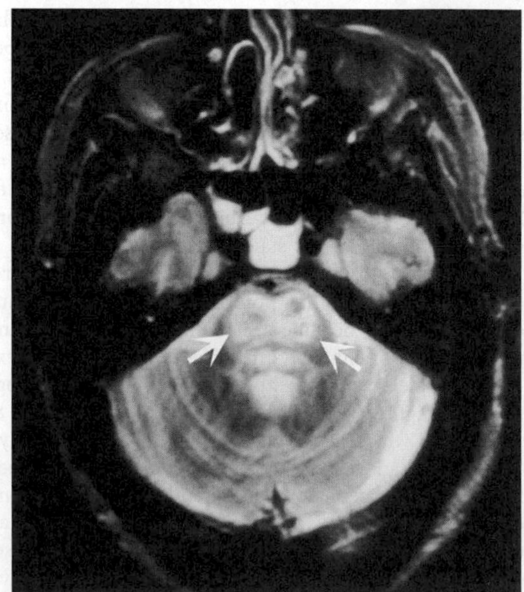

FIGURE 330-5 Central pontine myelinolysis. Axial T2-weighted magnetic resonance scan through the pons reveals a symmetric area of abnormal high signal intensity within the basis pontis (*arrows*).

WERNICKE'S DISEASE

Wernicke's disease is a common and preventable disorder due to a deficiency of thiamine (Chap. 96e). In the United States, alcoholics account for most cases, but patients with malnutrition due to hyperemesis, starvation, renal dialysis, cancer, AIDS, or rarely gastric surgery are also at risk. The characteristic clinical triad is that of ophthalmoplegia, ataxia, and global confusion. However, only one-third of patients with acute Wernicke's disease present with the classic clinical triad. Most patients are profoundly disoriented, indifferent, and inattentive, although rarely they have an agitated delirium related to ethanol withdrawal. If the disease is not treated, stupor, coma, and death may ensue. Ocular motor abnormalities include horizontal nystagmus on lateral gaze, lateral rectus palsy (usually bilateral), conjugate gaze palsies, and rarely ptosis. Gait ataxia probably results from a combination of polyneuropathy, cerebellar involvement, and vestibular paresis. The pupils are usually spared, but they may become miotic with advanced disease.

Wernicke's disease is usually associated with other manifestations of nutritional disease, such as polyneuropathy. Rarely, amblyopia or myelopathy occurs. Tachycardia and postural hypotension may be related to impaired function of the autonomic nervous system or to the coexistence of cardiovascular beriberi. Patients who recover show improvement in ocular palsies within hours after the administration of thiamine, but horizontal nystagmus may persist. Ataxia improves more slowly than the ocular motor abnormalities. Approximately half recover incompletely and are left with a slow, shuffling, wide-based gait and an inability to tandem walk. Apathy, drowsiness, and confusion improve more gradually. As these symptoms recede, an amnestic state with impairment in recent memory and learning may become more apparent (*Korsakoff's psychosis*). Korsakoff's psychosis is frequently persistent; the residual mental state is characterized by gaps in memory, confabulation, and disordered temporal sequencing.

Pathology Periventricular lesions surround the third ventricle, aqueduct, and fourth ventricle, with petechial hemorrhages in occasional acute cases and atrophy of the mammillary bodies in most chronic cases. There is frequently endothelial proliferation, demyelination, and some neuronal loss. These changes may be detected by MRI scanning (Fig. 330-6). The amnestic defect is related to lesions in the dorsal medial nuclei of the thalamus.

Pathogenesis Thiamine is a cofactor of several enzymes, including transketolase, pyruvate dehydrogenase, and α-ketoglutarate dehydrogenase. Thiamine deficiency produces a diffuse decrease in cerebral glucose utilization and results in mitochondrial damage. Glutamate accumulates due to impairment of α-ketoglutarate dehydrogenase activity and, in combination with the energy deficiency, may result in excitotoxic cell damage.

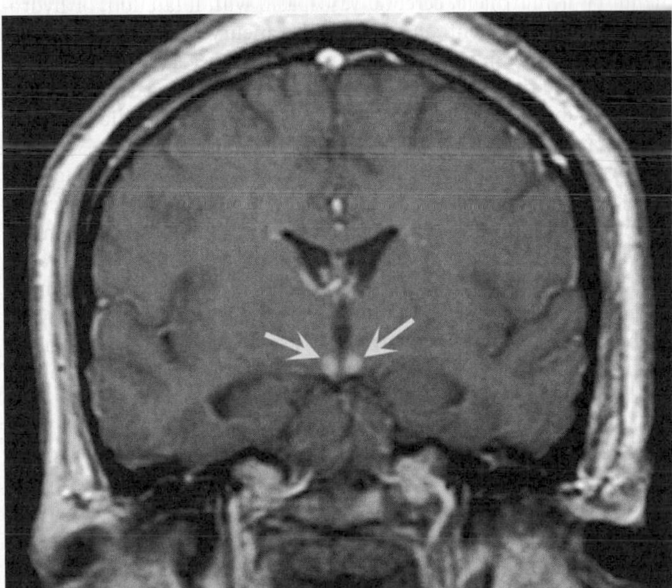

FIGURE 330-6 Wernicke's disease. Coronal T1-weighted postcontrast magnetic resonance imaging reveals abnormal enhancement of the mammillary bodies (*arrows*), typical of acute Wernicke's encephalopathy.

TREATMENT WERNICKE'S DISEASE

Wernicke's disease is a medical emergency and requires immediate administration of thiamine, in a dose of 100 mg either IV or IM. The dose should be given daily until the patient resumes a normal diet and should be begun prior to treatment with IV glucose solutions. Larger doses, 100 mg four times a day or more, have been advocated by some. Glucose infusions may precipitate Wernicke's disease in a previously unaffected patient or cause a rapid worsening of an early form of the disease. For this reason, thiamine should be administered to all alcoholic patients requiring parenteral glucose.

CRITICAL CARE DISORDERS OF THE PERIPHERAL NERVOUS SYSTEM

Critical illness with disorders of the peripheral nervous system (PNS) arises in two contexts: (1) primary neurologic diseases that require critical care interventions such as intubation and mechanical ventilation, and (2) secondary PNS manifestations of systemic critical illness, often involving multisystem organ failure. The former include acute polyneuropathies such as Guillain-Barré syndrome (Chap. 460), neuromuscular junction disorders including myasthenia gravis (Chap. 461) and botulism (Chap. 178), and primary muscle disorders such as polymyositis (Chap. 462e). The latter result either from the systemic disease itself or as a consequence of interventions.

General principles of respiratory evaluation in patients with PNS involvement, regardless of cause, include assessment of pulmonary mechanics, such as maximal inspiratory force (MIF) and vital capacity (VC), and evaluation of strength of bulbar muscles. Regardless of the cause of weakness, endotracheal intubation should be considered when the MIF falls to <–25 cmH_2O or the VC is <1 L. Also, patients with severe palatal weakness may require endotracheal intubation in order to prevent acute upper airway obstruction or recurrent aspiration. Arterial blood gases and oxygen saturation from pulse oximetry are used to follow patients with potential respiratory compromise from PNS dysfunction. However, intubation and mechanical ventilation should be undertaken based on clinical assessment rather than waiting until oxygen saturation drops or CO_2 retention develops from hypoventilation. Noninvasive mechanical ventilation may be considered initially in lieu of endotracheal intubation but is generally insufficient in patients with severe bulbar weakness or ventilatory failure with hypercarbia. Principles of mechanical ventilation are discussed in Chap. 323.

NEUROPATHY

Although encephalopathy may be the most obvious neurologic dysfunction in critically ill patients, dysfunction of the PNS is also quite common. It is typically present in patients with prolonged critical illnesses lasting several weeks and involving sepsis; clinical suspicion is aroused when there is failure to wean from mechanical ventilation despite improvement of the underlying sepsis and critical illness. *Critical illness polyneuropathy* refers to the most common PNS complication related to critical illness; it is seen in the setting of prolonged critical illness, sepsis, and multisystem organ failure. Neurologic findings include diffuse weakness, decreased reflexes, and distal sensory loss. Electrophysiologic studies demonstrate a diffuse, symmetric, distal axonal sensorimotor neuropathy, and pathologic studies have confirmed axonal degeneration. The precise mechanism of critical illness polyneuropathy remains unclear, but circulating factors such as cytokines, which are associated with sepsis and SIRS, are thought to play a role. It has been reported that up to 70% of patients with the sepsis syndrome have some degree of neuropathy, although far fewer have a clinical syndrome profound enough to cause severe respiratory muscle weakness requiring prolonged mechanical ventilation or resulting in failure to wean. Aggressive glycemic control with insulin infusions appears to decrease the risk of critical illness polyneuropathy. Treatment is otherwise supportive, with specific intervention directed at treating the underlying illness. Although spontaneous recovery is usually seen, the time course may extend over weeks to months and necessitate long-term ventilatory support and care even after the underlying critical illness has resolved.

DISORDERS OF NEUROMUSCULAR TRANSMISSION

A defect in neuromuscular transmission may be a source of weakness in critically ill patients. Botulism (Chap. 178) may be acquired by ingesting botulinum toxin from improperly stored food or may arise from an anaerobic abscess from *Clostridium botulinum* (wound botulism). Infants can present with generalized weakness from gut-derived *Clostridium* infection, especially if they are fed honey. Diplopia and dysphagia are early signs of foodborne botulism. Treatment is mostly supportive, although use of antitoxin early in the course may limit the duration of the neuromuscular blockade. General ICU care is similar to patients with Guillain-Barré syndrome or myasthenia gravis with focused care to avoid ulcer formation at pressure points, deep venous thromboprophylaxis, and infection prevention. Public health officers should be rapidly informed when the diagnosis is made to prevent further exposure to others from the tainted food or source of wound botulism (such as injection drug use).

Undiagnosed myasthenia gravis (Chap. 461) may be a consideration in weak ICU patients; however, persistent weakness secondary to impaired neuromuscular junction transmission is almost always due to administration of drugs. A number of medications impair neuromuscular transmission; these include antibiotics, especially aminoglycosides, and beta-blocking agents. In the ICU, the nondepolarizing neuromuscular blocking agents (nd-NMBAs), also known as muscle relaxants, are most commonly responsible. Included in this group of drugs are such agents as pancuronium, vecuronium, rocuronium, and cisatracurium. They are often used to facilitate mechanical ventilation or other critical care procedures, but with prolonged use persistent neuromuscular blockade may result in weakness even after discontinuation of these agents hours or days earlier. Risk factors for this prolonged action of neuromuscular blocking agents include female sex, metabolic acidosis, and renal failure.

Prolonged neuromuscular blockade does not appear to produce permanent damage to the PNS. Once the offending medications are discontinued, full strength is restored, although this may take days. In general, the lowest dose of neuromuscular blocking agent should be used to achieve the desired result and, when these agents are used in the ICU, a peripheral nerve stimulator should be used to monitor neuromuscular junction function.

MYOPATHY

Critically ill patients, especially those with sepsis, frequently develop muscle weakness and wasting, often in the face of seemingly adequate nutritional support. *Critical illness myopathy* is an overall term that describes several different discrete muscle disorders that may occur in critically ill patients. The assumption has been that a catabolic myopathy may develop as a result of multiple factors, including elevated cortisol and catecholamine release and other circulating factors induced by the SIRS. In this syndrome, known as *cachectic myopathy*, serum creatine kinase levels and electromyography (EMG) are normal. Muscle biopsy shows type II fiber atrophy. Panfascicular muscle fiber necrosis may also occur in the setting of profound sepsis. This less common *acute necrotizing intensive care myopathy* is characterized clinically by weakness progressing to a profound level over just a few days. There may be associated elevations in serum creatine kinase and urine myoglobin. Both EMG and muscle biopsy may be normal initially but eventually show abnormal spontaneous activity and panfascicular necrosis with an accompanying inflammatory reaction. Acute rhabdomyolysis can occur from alcohol ingestion or from compartment syndromes.

A *thick-filament myopathy* may occur in the setting of glucocorticoid and nd-NMBA use. The most frequent scenario in which this is encountered is the asthmatic patient who requires high-dose glucocorticoids and nd-NMBA to facilitate mechanical ventilation. This muscle disorder is not due to prolonged action of nd-NMBAs at the neuromuscular junction but, rather, is an actual myopathy with muscle damage; it has occasionally been described with high-dose glucocorticoid use or sepsis alone. Clinically this syndrome is most often recognized when a patient fails to wean from mechanical ventilation despite resolution of the primary pulmonary process. Pathologically, there may be loss of thick (myosin) filaments. Thick-filament critical illness myopathy has a good prognosis. If patients survive their underlying critical illness, the myopathy invariably improves and most patients return to normal. However, because this syndrome is a result of true muscle damage, not just prolonged blockade at the neuromuscular junction, this process may take weeks or months, and tracheotomy with prolonged ventilatory support may be necessary. Some patients do have residual long-term weakness, with atrophy and fatigue limiting ambulation. At present, it is unclear how to prevent this myopathic complication, except by avoiding use of nd-NMBAs, a strategy not always possible. Monitoring with a peripheral nerve stimulator can help to avoid the overuse of these agents. However, this is more likely to prevent the complication of prolonged neuromuscular junction blockade than it is to prevent this myopathy.

SUBARACHNOID HEMORRHAGE

Subarachnoid hemorrhage (SAH) renders the brain critically ill from both primary and secondary brain insults. Excluding head trauma, the most common cause of SAH is rupture of a saccular aneurysm. Other causes include bleeding from a vascular malformation (arteriovenous malformation or dural arteriovenous fistula) and extension into the subarachnoid space from a primary intracerebral hemorrhage. Some idiopathic SAHs are localized to the perimesencephalic cisterns and are benign; they probably have a venous or capillary source, and angiography is unrevealing.

SACCULAR ("BERRY") ANEURYSM

Autopsy and angiography studies have found that about 2% of adults harbor intracranial aneurysms, for a prevalence of 4 million persons in the United States; the aneurysm will rupture, producing SAH, in 25,000–30,000 cases per year. For patients who arrive alive at hospital, the mortality rate over the next month is about 45%. Of those who survive, more than half are left with major neurologic deficits as a result of the initial hemorrhage, cerebral vasospasm with infarction, or hydrocephalus. If the patient survives but the aneurysm is not obliterated, the rate of rebleeding is about 20% in the first 2 weeks, 30% in the first month, and about 3% per year afterward. Given these alarming figures, the major therapeutic emphasis is on preventing the predictable early complications of the SAH.

Unruptured, asymptomatic aneurysms are much less dangerous than a recently ruptured aneurysm. The annual risk of rupture for aneurysms <10 mm in size is ~0.1%, and for aneurysms ≥10 mm in size is ~0.5–1%; the surgical morbidity rate far exceeds these percentages. Because of the longer length of exposure to risk of rupture, younger patients with aneurysms >10 mm in size may benefit from prophylactic treatment. As with the treatment of asymptomatic carotid stenosis, this risk-benefit ratio strongly depends on the complication rate of treatment.

Giant aneurysms, those >2.5 cm in diameter, occur at the same sites (see below) as small aneurysms and account for 5% of cases. The three most common locations are the terminal internal carotid artery, middle cerebral artery (MCA) bifurcation, and top of the basilar artery. Their risk of rupture is ~6% in the first year after identification and may remain high indefinitely. They often cause symptoms by compressing the adjacent brain or cranial nerves.

Mycotic aneurysms are usually located distal to the first bifurcation of major arteries of the circle of Willis. Most result from infected emboli due to bacterial endocarditis causing septic degeneration of arteries and subsequent dilation and rupture. Whether these lesions should be sought and repaired prior to rupture or left to heal spontaneously with antibiotic treatment is controversial.

Pathophysiology Saccular aneurysms occur at the bifurcations of the large- to medium-sized intracranial arteries; rupture is into the subarachnoid space in the basal cisterns and often into the parenchyma of the adjacent brain. Approximately 85% of aneurysms occur in the anterior circulation, mostly on the circle of Willis. About 20% of patients have multiple aneurysms, many at mirror sites bilaterally. As an aneurysm develops, it typically forms a neck with a dome. The length of the neck and the size of the dome vary greatly and are important factors in planning neurosurgical obliteration or endovascular embolization. The arterial internal elastic lamina disappears at the base of the neck. The media thins, and connective tissue replaces smooth-muscle cells. At the site of rupture (most often the dome), the wall thins, and the tear that allows bleeding is often ≤0.5 mm long. Aneurysm size and site are important in predicting risk of rupture. Those >7 mm in diameter and those at the top of the basilar artery and at the origin of the posterior communicating artery are at greater risk of rupture.

Clinical Manifestations Most unruptured intracranial aneurysms are completely asymptomatic. Symptoms are usually due to rupture and resultant SAH, although some unruptured aneurysms present with mass effect on cranial nerves or brain parenchyma. At the moment of aneurysmal rupture with major SAH, the ICP suddenly rises. This may account for the sudden transient loss of consciousness that occurs in nearly half of patients. Sudden loss of consciousness may be preceded by a brief moment of excruciating headache, but most patients first complain of headache upon regaining consciousness. In 10% of cases, aneurysmal bleeding is severe enough to cause loss of consciousness for several days. In ~45% of cases, severe headache associated with exertion is the presenting complaint. The patient often calls the headache "the worst headache of my life"; however, the most important characteristic is sudden onset. Occasionally, these ruptures may present as headache of only moderate intensity or as a change in the patient's usual headache pattern. The headache is usually generalized, often with neck stiffness, and vomiting is common.

Although sudden headache in the absence of focal neurologic symptoms is the hallmark of aneurysmal rupture, focal neurologic deficits may occur. Anterior communicating artery or MCA bifurcation aneurysms may rupture into the adjacent brain or subdural space and form a hematoma large enough to produce mass effect. The deficits that result can include hemiparesis, aphasia, and abulia.

Occasionally, prodromal symptoms suggest the location of a progressively enlarging unruptured aneurysm. A third cranial nerve palsy, particularly when associated with pupillary dilation, loss of ipsilateral (but retained contralateral) light reflex, and focal pain above or behind the eye, may occur with an expanding aneurysm at the junction of the posterior communicating artery and the internal carotid artery. A sixth nerve palsy may indicate an aneurysm in the cavernous sinus, and visual field defects can occur with an expanding supraclinoid carotid or anterior cerebral artery aneurysm. Occipital and posterior cervical pain may signal a posterior inferior cerebellar artery or anterior inferior cerebellar artery aneurysm (Chap. 446). Pain in or behind the eye and in the low temple can occur with an expanding MCA aneurysm. Thunderclap headache is a variant of migraine that simulates an SAH. Before concluding that a patient with sudden, severe headache has thunderclap migraine, a definitive workup for aneurysm or other intracranial pathology is required.

Aneurysms can undergo small ruptures and leaks of blood into the subarachnoid space, so-called *sentinel bleeds*. Sudden unexplained headache at any location should raise suspicion of SAH and be investigated, because a major hemorrhage may be imminent.

The initial clinical manifestations of SAH can be graded using the Hunt-Hess or World Federation of Neurosurgical Societies classification schemes (Table 330-3). For ruptured aneurysms, prognosis for good outcomes falls as the grade increases. For example, it is unusual for a Hunt-Hess grade 1 patient to die if the aneurysm is treated, but the mortality rate for grade 4 and 5 patients may be as high as 80%.

TABLE 330-3 GRADING SCALES FOR SUBARACHNOID HEMORRHAGE

Grade	Hunt-Hess Scale	World Federation of Neurosurgical Societies (WFNS) Scale
1	Mild headache, normal mental status, no cranial nerve or motor findings	GCS[a] score 15, no motor deficits
2	Severe headache, normal mental status, may have cranial nerve deficit	GCS score 13–14, no motor deficits
3	Somnolent, confused, may have cranial nerve or mild motor deficit	GCS score 13–14, with motor deficits
4	Stupor, moderate to severe motor deficit, may have intermittent reflex posturing	GCS score 7–12, with or without motor deficits
5	Coma, reflex posturing or flaccid	GCS score 3–6, with or without motor deficits

[a]Glasgow Coma Scale; see **Table 457e-1**.

Delayed Neurologic Deficits There are four major causes of delayed neurologic deficits: rerupture, hydrocephalus, vasospasm, and hyponatremia.

1. *Rerupture.* The incidence of rerupture of an untreated aneurysm in the first month following SAH is ~30%, with the peak in the first 7 days. Rerupture is associated with a 60% mortality rate and poor outcome. Early treatment eliminates this risk.
2. *Hydrocephalus.* Acute hydrocephalus can cause stupor and coma and can be mitigated by placement of an external ventricular drain. More often, subacute hydrocephalus may develop over a few days or weeks and causes progressive drowsiness or slowed mentation (abulia) with incontinence. Hydrocephalus is differentiated from cerebral vasospasm with a CT scan, CT angiogram, transcranial Doppler (TCD) ultrasound, or conventional x-ray angiography. Hydrocephalus may clear spontaneously or require temporary ventricular drainage. Chronic hydrocephalus may develop weeks to months after SAH and manifest as gait difficulty, incontinence, or impaired mentation. Subtle signs may be a lack of initiative in conversation or a failure to recover independence.
3. *Vasospasm.* Narrowing of the arteries at the base of the brain following SAH causes symptomatic ischemia and infarction in ~30% of patients and is the major cause of delayed morbidity and death. Signs of ischemia appear 4–14 days after the hemorrhage, most often at 7 days. The severity and distribution of vasospasm determine whether infarction will occur.
4. Delayed vasospasm is believed to result from direct effects of clotted blood and its breakdown products on the arteries within the subarachnoid space. In general, the more blood that surrounds the arteries, the greater the chance of symptomatic vasospasm. Spasm of major arteries produces symptoms referable to the appropriate vascular territory (Chap. 446). All of these focal symptoms may present abruptly, fluctuate, or develop over a few days. In most cases, focal spasm is preceded by a decline in mental status.
5. Vasospasm can be detected reliably with conventional x-ray angiography, but this invasive procedure is expensive and carries the risk of stroke and other complications. TCD ultrasound is based on the principle that the velocity of blood flow within an artery will rise as the lumen diameter is narrowed. By directing the probe along the MCA and proximal anterior cerebral artery (ACA), carotid terminus, and vertebral and basilar arteries on a daily or every-other-day basis, vasospasm can be reliably detected and treatments initiated to prevent cerebral ischemia (see below). CT angiography is another method that can detect vasospasm.
6. Severe cerebral edema in patients with infarction from vasospasm may increase the ICP enough to reduce cerebral perfusion pressure. Treatment may include mannitol, hyperventilation, and hemicraniectomy; moderate hypothermia may have a role as well.
7. *Hyponatremia.* Hyponatremia may be profound and can develop quickly in the first 2 weeks following SAH. There is both natriuresis and volume depletion with SAH, so that patients become both hyponatremic and hypovolemic. Both atrial natriuretic peptide and brain natriuretic peptide have a role in producing this "cerebral

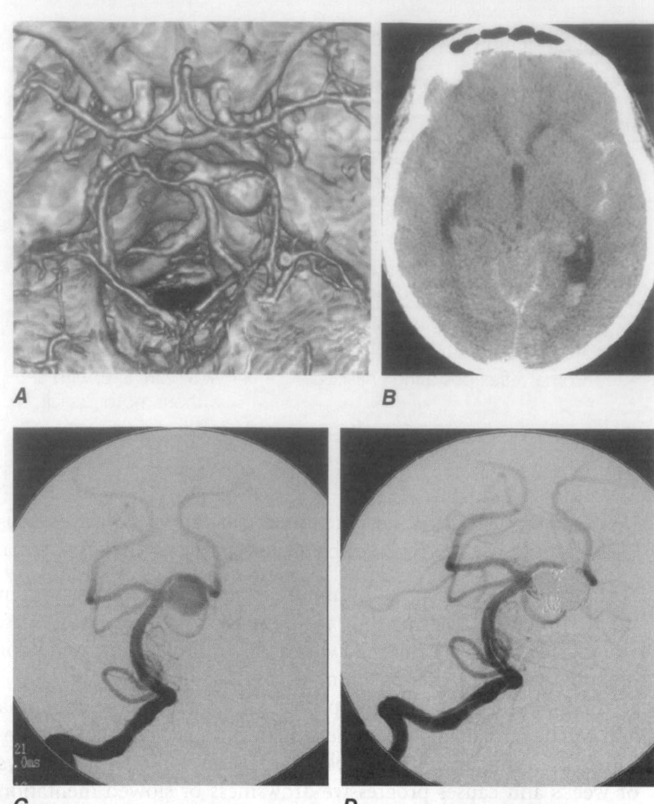

FIGURE 330-7 Subarachnoid hemorrhage. ***A.*** Computed tomography (CT) angiography revealing an aneurysm of the left superior cerebellar artery. ***B.*** Noncontrast CT scan at the level of the third ventricle revealing subarachnoid blood (*bright*) in the left sylvian fissure and within the left lateral ventricle. ***C.*** Conventional anteroposterior x-ray angiogram of the right vertebral and basilar artery showing the large aneurysm. ***D.*** Conventional angiogram following coil embolization of the aneurysm, whereby the aneurysm body is filled with platinum coils delivered through a microcatheter navigated from the femoral artery into the aneurysm neck.

salt-wasting syndrome." Typically, it clears over the course of 1–2 weeks and, in the setting of SAH, should not be treated with free-water restriction as this may increase the risk of stroke (see below).

Laboratory Evaluation and Imaging (Fig. 330-7) The hallmark of aneurysmal rupture is blood in the CSF. More than 95% of cases have enough blood to be visualized on a high-quality noncontrast CT scan obtained within 72 h. If the scan fails to establish the diagnosis of SAH and no mass lesion or obstructive hydrocephalus is found, a lumbar puncture should be performed to establish the presence of subarachnoid blood. Lysis of the red blood cells and subsequent conversion of hemoglobin to bilirubin stains the spinal fluid yellow within 6–12 h. This xanthochromic spinal fluid peaks in intensity at 48 h and lasts for 1–4 weeks, depending on the amount of subarachnoid blood.

The extent and location of subarachnoid blood on a noncontrast CT scan help locate the underlying aneurysm, identify the cause of any neurologic deficit, and predict delayed vasospasm. A high incidence of symptomatic vasospasm in the MCA and ACA has been found when early CT scans show subarachnoid clots >5 × 3 mm in the basal cisterns, or layers of blood >1 mm thick in the cerebral fissures. CT scans less reliably predict vasospasm in the vertebral, basilar, or posterior cerebral arteries.

Lumbar puncture prior to an imaging procedure is indicated only if a CT scan is not available at the time of the suspected SAH. Once the diagnosis of hemorrhage from a ruptured saccular aneurysm is suspected, four-vessel conventional x-ray angiography (both carotids and both vertebrals) is generally performed to localize and define the anatomic details of the aneurysm and to determine if other unruptured aneurysms exist (Fig. 330-7*C*). At some centers, the ruptured aneurysm can be treated using endovascular techniques at the time of the initial angiogram as a way to expedite treatment and minimize the number of invasive procedures. CT angiography is an alternative method for locating the aneurysm and may be sufficient to plan definitive therapy.

Close monitoring (daily or twice daily) of electrolytes is important because hyponatremia can occur precipitously during the first 2 weeks following SAH (see above).

The electrocardiogram (ECG) frequently shows ST-segment and T-wave changes similar to those associated with cardiac ischemia. A prolonged QRS complex, increased QT interval, and prominent "peaked" or deeply inverted symmetric T waves are usually secondary to the intracranial hemorrhage. There is evidence that structural myocardial lesions produced by circulating catecholamines and excessive discharge of sympathetic neurons may occur after SAH, causing these ECG changes and a reversible cardiomyopathy sufficient to cause shock or congestive heart failure. Echocardiography reveals a pattern of regional wall motion abnormalities that follow the distribution of sympathetic nerves rather than the major coronary arteries, with relative sparing of the ventricular wall apex. The sympathetic nerves themselves appear to be injured by direct toxicity from the excessive catecholamine release. An asymptomatic troponin elevation is common. Serious ventricular dysrhythmias occurring in-hospital are unusual.

TREATMENT SUBARACHNOID HEMORRHAGE

Early aneurysm repair prevents rerupture and allows the safe application of techniques to improve blood flow (e.g., induced hypertension) should symptomatic vasospasm develop. An aneurysm can be "clipped" by a neurosurgeon or "coiled" by an endovascular surgeon. Surgical repair involves placing a metal clip across the aneurysm neck, thereby immediately eliminating the risk of rebleeding. This approach requires craniotomy and brain retraction, which is associated with neurologic morbidity. Endovascular techniques involve placing platinum coils, or other embolic material, within the aneurysm via a catheter that is passed from the femoral artery. The aneurysm is packed tightly to enhance thrombosis and over time is walled off from the circulation (**Fig. 330-7*D***). There have been two prospective randomized trials of surgery versus endovascular treatment for ruptured aneurysms: the first was the International Subarachnoid Aneurysm Trial (ISAT), which was terminated early when 24% of patients treated with endovascular therapy were dead or dependent at 1 year compared to 31% treated with surgery, a significant 23% relative reduction. After 5 years, risk of death was lower in the coiling group, although the proportion of survivors who were independent was the same in both groups. Risk of rebleeding was low, but more common in the coiling group. These results favoring coiling at 1 year were confirmed in a second trial, although the differences in functional outcome were no longer significant at 3 years. Because some aneurysms have a morphology that is not amenable to endovascular treatment, surgery remains an important treatment option. Centers that combine both endovascular and neurosurgical expertise likely offer the best outcomes for patients, and there are reliable data showing that specialized aneurysm treatment centers can improve mortality rates.

The medical management of SAH focuses on protecting the airway, managing blood pressure before and after aneurysm treatment, preventing rebleeding prior to treatment, managing vasospasm, treating hydrocephalus, treating hyponatremia, limiting secondary brain insults, and preventing pulmonary embolus (PE).

Intracranial hypertension following aneurysmal rupture occurs secondary to subarachnoid blood, parenchymal hematoma, acute hydrocephalus, or loss of vascular autoregulation. Patients who are stuporous should undergo emergent ventriculostomy to measure ICP and to treat high ICP in order to prevent cerebral ischemia. Medical therapies designed to combat raised ICP (e.g., osmotic therapy and sedation) can also be used as needed. High ICP refractory to treatment is a poor prognostic sign.

Prior to definitive treatment of the ruptured aneurysm, care is required to maintain adequate cerebral perfusion pressure while avoiding excessive elevation of arterial pressure. If the patient is alert, it is reasonable to lower the systolic blood pressure to below 160 mmHg using nicardipine, labetalol, or esmolol. If the patient has a depressed level of consciousness, ICP should be measured and the cerebral perfusion pressure targeted to 60–70 mmHg. If headache or neck pain is severe, mild sedation and analgesia are prescribed. Extreme sedation is avoided if possible because it can obscure the ability to clinically detect changes in neurologic status. Adequate hydration is necessary to avoid a decrease in blood volume predisposing to brain ischemia.

Seizures are uncommon at the onset of aneurysmal rupture. The quivering, jerking, and extensor posturing that often accompany loss of consciousness with SAH are probably related to the sharp rise in ICP rather than seizures. However, anticonvulsants are sometimes given as prophylactic therapy because a seizure could theoretically promote rebleeding.

Glucocorticoids may help reduce the head and neck ache caused by the irritative effect of the subarachnoid blood. There is no good evidence that they reduce cerebral edema, are neuroprotective, or reduce vascular injury, and their routine use therefore is not recommended.

Antifibrinolytic agents are not routinely prescribed but may be considered in patients in whom aneurysm treatment cannot proceed immediately. They are associated with a reduced incidence of aneurysmal rerupture but may also increase the risk of delayed cerebral infarction and deep vein thrombosis (DVT). Several recent studies suggest that a shorter duration of use (until the aneurysm is secured or for the first 3 days) may decrease rerupture and be safer than found in earlier studies of longer duration treatment.

Vasospasm remains the leading cause of morbidity and mortality following aneurysmal SAH. Treatment with the calcium channel antagonist nimodipine (60 mg PO every 4 h) improves outcome, perhaps by preventing ischemic injury rather than reducing the risk of vasospasm. Nimodipine can cause significant hypotension in some patients, which may worsen cerebral ischemia in patients with vasospasm. Symptomatic cerebral vasospasm can also be treated by increasing the cerebral perfusion pressure by raising mean arterial pressure through plasma volume expansion and the judicious use of IV vasopressor agents, usually phenylephrine or norepinephrine. Raised perfusion pressure has been associated with clinical improvement in many patients, but high arterial pressure may promote rebleeding in unprotected aneurysms. Treatment with induced hypertension and hypervolemia generally requires monitoring of arterial and central venous pressures; it is best to infuse pressors through a central venous line as well. Volume expansion helps prevent hypotension and augments cardiac output.

If symptomatic vasospasm persists despite optimal medical therapy, intraarterial vasodilators and percutaneous transluminal angioplasty are considered. Vasodilatation by direct angioplasty appears to be permanent, allowing hypertensive therapy to be tapered sooner. The pharmacologic vasodilators (verapamil and nicardipine) do not last more than about 24 h, and therefore multiple treatments may be required until the subarachnoid blood is reabsorbed. Although intraarterial papaverine is an effective vasodilator, there is evidence that papaverine may be neurotoxic, so its use should generally be avoided.

Acute hydrocephalus can cause stupor or coma. It may clear spontaneously or require temporary ventricular drainage. When chronic hydrocephalus develops, ventricular shunting is the treatment of choice.

Free-water restriction is contraindicated in patients with SAH at risk for vasospasm because hypovolemia and hypotension may occur and precipitate cerebral ischemia. Many patients continue to experience a decline in serum sodium despite receiving parenteral fluids containing normal saline. Frequently, supplemental oral salt coupled with normal saline will mitigate hyponatremia, but often patients also require intravenous hypertonic saline. Care must be taken not to correct serum sodium too quickly in patients with marked hyponatremia of several days' duration, as central pontine myelinolysis may occur.

All patients should have pneumatic compression stockings applied to prevent pulmonary embolism. Unfractionated heparin administered subcutaneously for DVT prophylaxis can be initiated immediately following endovascular treatment and within days following craniotomy with surgical clipping and is a useful adjunct to pneumatic compression stockings. Treatment of pulmonary embolus depends on whether the aneurysm has been treated and whether or not the patient has had a craniotomy. Systemic anticoagulation with heparin is contraindicated in patients with ruptured and untreated aneurysms. It is a relative contraindication following craniotomy for several days, and it may delay thrombosis of a coiled aneurysm. If DVT or PE occurs within the first days following craniotomy, use of an inferior vena cava filter may be considered to prevent additional pulmonary emboli, whereas systemic anticoagulation with heparin is preferred following successful endovascular treatment.

SECTION 4 ONCOLOGIC EMERGENCIES

331 Oncologic Emergencies

Rasim Gucalp, Janice P. Dutcher

Emergencies in patients with cancer may be classified into three groups: pressure or obstruction caused by a space-occupying lesion, metabolic or hormonal problems (paraneoplastic syndromes, Chap. 121), and treatment-related complications.

STRUCTURAL-OBSTRUCTIVE ONCOLOGIC EMERGENCIES

SUPERIOR VENA CAVA SYNDROME

Superior vena cava syndrome (SVCS) is the clinical manifestation of superior vena cava (SVC) obstruction, with severe reduction in venous return from the head, neck, and upper extremities. Malignant tumors, such as lung cancer, lymphoma, and metastatic tumors, are responsible for the majority of SVCS cases. With the expanding use of intravascular devices (e.g., permanent central venous access catheters, pacemaker/defibrillator leads), the prevalence of benign causes of SVCS is increasing now, accounting for at least 40% of cases. Lung cancer, particularly of small-cell and squamous cell histologies, accounts for approximately 85% of all cases of malignant origin. In young adults, malignant lymphoma is a leading cause of SVCS. Hodgkin's lymphoma involves the mediastinum more commonly than other lymphomas but rarely causes SVCS. When SVCS is noted in a young man with a mediastinal mass, the differential diagnosis is lymphoma versus primary mediastinal germ cell tumor. Metastatic cancers to the mediastinal lymph nodes, such as testicular and breast carcinomas, account for a small proportion of cases. Other causes include benign tumors, aortic aneurysm, thyromegaly, thrombosis, and fibrosing mediastinitis from prior irradiation, histoplasmosis, or Behçet's syndrome. SVCS as the initial manifestation of Behçet's syndrome may be due to inflammation of the SVC associated with thrombosis.

Patients with SVCS usually present with neck and facial swelling (especially around the eyes), dyspnea, and cough. Other symptoms include hoarseness, tongue swelling, headaches, nasal congestion, epistaxis, hemoptysis, dysphagia, pain, dizziness, syncope, and lethargy. Bending forward or lying down may aggravate the symptoms. The characteristic physical findings are dilated neck veins; an increased number of collateral veins covering the anterior chest wall; cyanosis; and edema of the face, arms, and chest. Facial swelling and plethora are typically exacerbated when the patient is supine. More severe cases include proptosis, glossal and laryngeal edema, and obtundation. The clinical picture is milder if the obstruction is located above the azygos vein. Symptoms are usually progressive, but in some cases, they may improve as collateral circulation develops.

Signs and symptoms of cerebral and/or laryngeal edema, though rare, are associated with a poorer prognosis and require urgent evaluation. Seizures are more likely related to brain metastases than to cerebral edema from venous occlusion. Patients with small-cell lung cancer and SVCS have a higher incidence of brain metastases than those without SVCS.

Cardiorespiratory symptoms at rest, particularly with positional changes, suggest significant airway and vascular obstruction and limited physiologic reserve. Cardiac arrest or respiratory failure can occur, particularly in patients receiving sedatives or undergoing general anesthesia.

Rarely, esophageal varices may develop. These are "downhill" varices based on the direction of blood flow from cephalad to caudad (in contrast to "uphill" varices associated with caudad to cephalad flow from portal hypertension). If the obstruction to the SVC is proximal to the azygous vein, varices develop in the upper one-third of the esophagus. If the obstruction involves or is distal to the azygous vein, varices occur in the entire length of the esophagus. Variceal bleeding may be a late complication of chronic SVCS.

Superior vena cava obstruction may lead to bilateral breast edema with bilateral enlarged breast. Unilateral breast dilatation may be seen as a consequence of axillary or subclavian vein blockage.

The diagnosis of SVCS is a clinical one. The most significant chest radiographic finding is widening of the superior mediastinum, most commonly on the right side. Pleural effusion occurs in only 25% of patients, often on the right side. The majority of these effusions are exudative and occasionally chylous. However, a normal chest radiograph is still compatible with the diagnosis if other characteristic findings are present. Computed tomography (CT) provides the most reliable view of the mediastinal anatomy. The diagnosis of SVCS requires diminished or absent opacification of central venous structures with prominent collateral venous circulation. Magnetic resonance imaging (MRI) has no advantages over CT. Invasive procedures, including bronchoscopy, percutaneous needle biopsy, mediastinoscopy, and even thoracotomy, can be performed by a skilled clinician without any major risk of bleeding. Endobronchial or esophageal ultrasound-guided needle aspiration may establish the diagnosis safely. For patients with a known cancer, a detailed workup usually is not necessary, and appropriate treatment may be started after obtaining a CT scan of the thorax. For those with no history of malignancy, a detailed evaluation is essential to rule out benign causes and determine a specific diagnosis to direct the appropriate therapy.

TREATMENT SUPERIOR VENA CAVA SYNDROME

The one potentially life-threatening complication of a superior mediastinal mass is tracheal obstruction. Upper airway obstruction demands emergent therapy. Diuretics with a low-salt diet, head elevation, and oxygen may produce temporary symptomatic relief. Glucocorticoids may be useful at shrinking lymphoma masses; they are of no benefit in patients with lung cancer.

Radiation therapy is the primary treatment for SVCS caused by non-small-cell lung cancer and other metastatic solid tumors. Chemotherapy is effective when the underlying cancer is small-cell carcinoma of the lung, lymphoma, or germ cell tumor. SVCS recurs in 10–30% of patients; it may be palliated with the use of intravascular self-expanding stents (Fig. 331-1). Early stenting may be necessary in patients with severe symptoms; however, the prompt increase in venous return after stenting may precipitate heart failure and pulmonary edema. Other complications of stent placement include hematoma at the insertion site, SVC perforation, stent migration in the right ventricle, stent fracture, and pulmonary embolism. Surgery may provide immediate relief for patients in whom a benign process is the cause.

Clinical improvement occurs in most patients, although this improvement may be due to the development of adequate collateral circulation. The mortality associated with SVCS does not relate to caval obstruction but rather to the underlying cause.

SVCS AND CENTRAL VENOUS CATHETERS IN ADULTS

The use of long-term central venous catheters has become common practice in patients with cancer. Major vessel thrombosis may occur. In these cases, catheter removal should be combined with anticoagulation to prevent embolization. SVCS in this setting, if detected early, can be treated by fibrinolytic therapy without sacrificing the catheter. The routine use of low-dose warfarin or low-molecular-weight heparin to prevent thrombosis related to permanent central venous access catheters in cancer patients is not recommended.

PERICARDIAL EFFUSION/TAMPONADE

Malignant pericardial disease is found at autopsy in 5–10% of patients with cancer, most frequently with lung cancer, breast cancer, leukemias, and lymphomas. Cardiac tamponade as the initial presentation of extrathoracic malignancy is rare. The origin is not malignancy in about 50% of cancer patients with symptomatic pericardial disease, but it can be related to irradiation, drug-induced pericarditis, hypothyroidism, idiopathic pericarditis, infection, or autoimmune diseases. Two types of radiation pericarditis occur: an acute inflammatory, effusive pericarditis occurring within months of irradiation, which usually resolves spontaneously, and a chronic effusive pericarditis that may appear up to 20 years after radiation therapy and is accompanied by a thickened pericardium.

Most patients with pericardial metastasis are asymptomatic. However, the common symptoms are dyspnea, cough, chest pain, orthopnea, and weakness. Pleural effusion, sinus tachycardia, jugular venous distention, hepatomegaly, peripheral edema, and cyanosis are the most frequent physical findings. Relatively specific diagnostic findings, such as paradoxical pulse, diminished heart sounds, pulsus alternans (pulse waves alternating between those of greater and lesser amplitude with successive beats), and friction rub are less common than with nonmalignant pericardial disease. Chest radiographs and electrocardiogram (ECG) reveal abnormalities in 90% of patients, but half of these abnormalities are nonspecific. Echocardiography is the most helpful diagnostic test. Pericardial fluid may be serous, serosanguineous, or hemorrhagic, and cytologic examination of pericardial fluid is diagnostic in most patients. Measurements of tumor markers in the pericardial fluid are not helpful in the diagnosis of malignant pericardial fluid. Pericardioscopy (not widely available) with targeted pericardial and epicardial biopsy may differentiate neoplastic and benign pericardial disease. A combination of cytology, pericardial and epicardial biopsy, and guided pericardioscopy gives the best diagnostic yield. CT scan findings of irregular pericardial thickening and mediastinal lymphadenopathy suggest this is a malignant pericardial effusion. Cancer patients with pericardial effusion containing malignant cells on cytology have a very poor survival, about 7 weeks.

TREATMENT PERICARDIAL EFFUSION/TAMPONADE

Pericardiocentesis with or without the introduction of sclerosing agents, the creation of a pericardial window, complete pericardial stripping, cardiac irradiation, or systemic chemotherapy are effective treatments. Acute pericardial tamponade with life-threatening hemodynamic instability requires immediate drainage of fluid. This

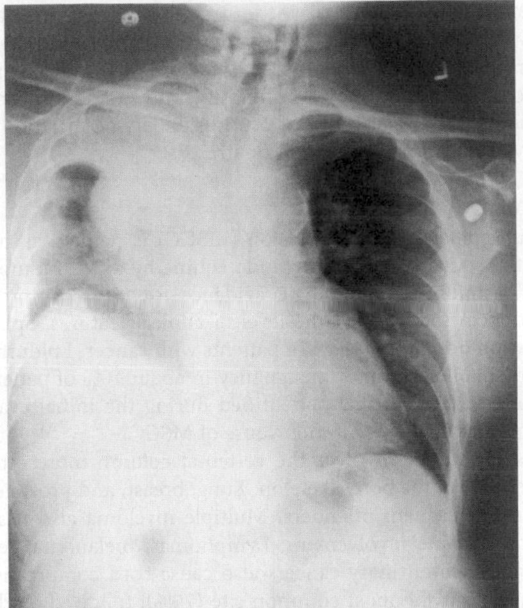

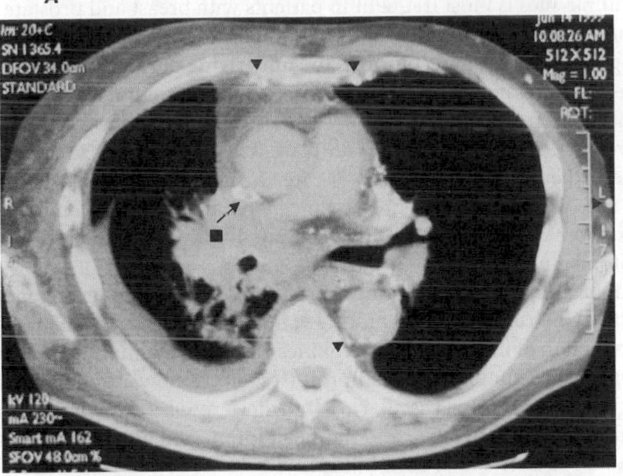

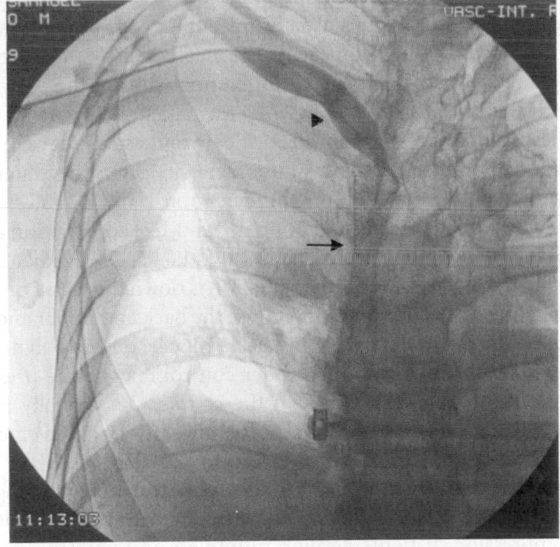

FIGURE 331–1 Superior vena cava syndrome (SVCS). ***A.*** Chest radiographs of a 59-year-old man with recurrent SVCS caused by non-small-cell lung cancer showing right paratracheal mass with right pleural effusion. ***B.*** Computed tomography of same patient demonstrating obstruction of the superior vena cava with thrombosis (*arrow*) by the lung cancer (*square*) and collaterals (*arrowheads*). ***C.*** Balloon angioplasty (*arrowhead*) with Wallstent (arrow) in same patient.

can be quickly achieved by pericardiocentesis. The recurrence rate after percutaneous catheter drainage is about 20%. Sclerotherapy (pericardial instillation of bleomycin, mitomycin C, or tetracycline) may decrease recurrences. Alternatively, subxiphoid pericardiotomy can be performed in 45 min under local anesthesia. Thoracoscopic pericardial fenestration can be employed for benign causes; however, 60% of malignant pericardial effusions recur after this procedure. In a subset of patients, drainage of the pericardial effusion is paradoxically followed by worsening hemodynamic instability. This so-called "postoperative low cardiac output syndrome" occurs in up to 10% of patients undergoing surgical drainage and carries poor short-term survival.

INTESTINAL OBSTRUCTION

Intestinal obstruction and reobstruction are common problems in patients with advanced cancer, particularly colorectal or ovarian carcinoma. However, other cancers, such as lung or breast cancer and melanoma, can metastasize within the abdomen, leading to intestinal obstruction. Metastatic disease from colorectal, ovarian, pancreatic, gastric, and occasionally breast cancer can lead to peritoneal carcinomatosis, with infiltration of the omentum and peritoneal surface, thus limiting bowel motility. Typically, obstruction occurs at multiple sites in peritoneal carcinomatosis. Melanoma has a predilection to involve the small bowel; this involvement may be isolated, and resection may result in prolonged survival. Intestinal pseudoobstruction is caused by infiltration of the mesentery or bowel muscle by tumor, involvement of the celiac plexus, or paraneoplastic neuropathy in patients with small-cell lung cancer. Paraneoplastic neuropathy is associated with IgG antibodies reactive to neurons of the myenteric and submucosal plexuses of the jejunum and stomach. Ovarian cancer can lead to authentic luminal obstruction or to pseudoobstruction that results when circumferential invasion of a bowel segment arrests the forward progression of peristaltic contractions.

The onset of obstruction is usually insidious. Pain is the most common symptom and is usually colicky in nature. Pain can also be due to abdominal distention, tumor masses, or hepatomegaly. Vomiting can be intermittent or continuous. Patients with complete obstruction usually have constipation. Physical examination may reveal abdominal distention with tympany, ascites, visible peristalsis, high-pitched bowel sounds, and tumor masses. Erect plain abdominal films may reveal multiple air-fluid levels and dilation of the small or large bowel. Acute cecal dilation to >12–14 cm is considered a surgical emergency because of the high likelihood of rupture. CT scan is useful in defining the extent of disease and the exact nature of the obstruction and differentiating benign from malignant causes of obstruction in patients who have undergone surgery for malignancy. Malignant obstruction is suggested by a mass at the site of obstruction or prior surgery, adenopathy, or an abrupt transition zone and irregular bowel thickening at the obstruction site. Benign obstruction is more likely when CT shows mesenteric vascular changes, a large volume of ascites, or a smooth transition zone and smooth bowel thickening at the obstruction site. In challenging patients with obstructive symptoms, particularly low-grade small-bowel obstruction (SBO), CT enteroclysis often can help establish the diagnosis by providing distention of small-bowel loops. In this technique, water-soluble contrast is infused through a nasoenteric tube into the duodenum or proximal small bowel followed by CT images. The prognosis for the patient with cancer who develops intestinal obstruction is poor; median survival is 3–4 months. About 25–30% of patients are found to have intestinal obstruction due to causes other than cancer. Adhesions from previous operations are a common benign cause. Ileus induced by vinca alkaloids, narcotics, or other drugs is another reversible cause.

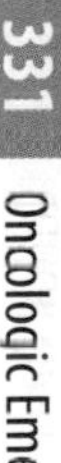

TREATMENT INTESTINAL OBSTRUCTION

The management of intestinal obstruction in patients with advanced malignancy depends on the extent of the underlying malignancy, options for further antineoplastic therapy, estimated life expectancy, the functional status of the major organs, and the extent of the obstruction. The initial management should include surgical evaluation. Operation is not always successful and may lead to further complications with a substantial mortality rate (10–20%). Laparoscopy can diagnose and treat malignant bowel obstruction in some cases. Self-expanding metal stents placed in the gastric outlet, duodenum, proximal jejunum, colon, or rectum may palliate obstructive symptoms at those sites without major surgery. Patients known to have advanced intraabdominal malignancy should receive a prolonged course of conservative management, including nasogastric decompression. Percutaneous endoscopic or surgical gastrostomy tube placement is an option for palliation of nausea and vomiting, the so-called "venting gastrostomy." Treatment with antiemetics, antispasmodics, and analgesics may allow patients to remain outside the hospital. Octreotide may relieve obstructive symptoms through its inhibitory effect on gastrointestinal secretion. Glucocorticoids have anti-inflammatory effects and may help the resolution of bowel obstruction. They also have antiemetic effects.

URINARY OBSTRUCTION

Urinary obstruction may occur in patients with prostatic or gynecologic malignancies, particularly cervical carcinoma; metastatic disease from other primary sites such as carcinomas of the breast, stomach, lung, colon, and pancreas; or lymphomas. Radiation therapy to pelvic tumors may cause fibrosis and subsequent ureteral obstruction. Bladder outlet obstruction is usually due to prostate and cervical cancers and may lead to bilateral hydronephrosis and renal failure.

Flank pain is the most common symptom. Persistent urinary tract infection, persistent proteinuria, or hematuria in patients with cancer should raise suspicion of ureteral obstruction. Total anuria and/or anuria alternating with polyuria may occur. A slow, continuous rise in the serum creatinine level necessitates immediate evaluation. Renal ultrasound is the safest and cheapest way to identify hydronephrosis. The function of an obstructed kidney can be evaluated by a nuclear scan. CT scan can reveal the point of obstruction and identify a retroperitoneal mass or adenopathy.

TREATMENT URINARY OBSTRUCTION

Obstruction associated with flank pain, sepsis, or fistula formation is an indication for immediate palliative urinary diversion. Internal ureteral stents can be placed under local anesthesia. Percutaneous nephrostomy offers an alternative approach for drainage. The placement of a nephrostomy is associated with a significant rate of pyelonephritis. In the case of bladder outlet obstruction due to malignancy, a suprapubic cystostomy can be used for urinary drainage. An aggressive intervention with invasive approaches to improve the obstruction should be weighed against the likelihood of antitumor response, and the ability to reverse renal insufficiency should be evaluated.

MALIGNANT BILIARY OBSTRUCTION

This common clinical problem can be caused by a primary carcinoma arising in the pancreas, ampulla of Vater, bile duct, or liver or by metastatic disease to the periductal lymph nodes or liver parenchyma. The most common metastatic tumors causing biliary obstruction are gastric, colon, breast, and lung cancers. Jaundice, light-colored stools, dark urine, pruritus, and weight loss due to malabsorption are usual symptoms. Pain and secondary infection are uncommon in malignant biliary obstruction. Ultrasound, CT scan, or percutaneous transhepatic or endoscopic retrograde cholangiography will identify the site and nature of the biliary obstruction.

TREATMENT MALIGNANT BILIARY OBSTRUCTION

Palliative intervention is indicated only in patients with disabling pruritus resistant to medical treatment, severe malabsorption, or infection. Stenting under radiographic control, surgical bypass, or radiation therapy with or without chemotherapy may alleviate the obstruction. The choice of therapy should be based on the site of obstruction (proximal vs distal), the type of tumor (sensitive to radiotherapy, chemotherapy, or neither), and the general condition of the patient. In the absence of pruritus, biliary obstruction may be a largely asymptomatic cause of death.

SPINAL CORD COMPRESSION

Malignant spinal cord compression (MSCC) is defined as compression of the spinal cord and/or cauda equina by an extradural tumor mass. The minimum radiologic evidence for cord compression is indentation of the theca at the level of clinical features. Spinal cord compression occurs in 5–10% of patients with cancer. Epidural tumor is the first manifestation of malignancy in about 10% of patients. The underlying cancer is usually identified during the initial evaluation; lung cancer is the most common cause of MSCC.

Metastatic tumor involves the vertebral column more often than any other part of the bony skeleton. Lung, breast, and prostate cancer are the most frequent offenders. Multiple myeloma also has a high incidence of spine involvement. Lymphomas, melanoma, renal cell cancer, and genitourinary cancers also cause cord compression. The thoracic spine is the most common site (70%), followed by the lumbosacral spine (20%) and the cervical spine (10%). Involvement of multiple sites is most frequent in patients with breast and prostate carcinoma. Cord injury develops when metastases to the vertebral body or pedicle enlarge and compress the underlying dura. Another cause of cord compression is direct extension of a paravertebral lesion through the intervertebral foramen. These cases usually involve a lymphoma, myeloma, or pediatric neoplasm. Parenchymal spinal cord metastasis due to hematogenous spread is rare. Intramedullary metastases can be seen in lung cancer, breast cancer, renal cancer, melanoma, and lymphoma and are frequently associated with brain metastases and leptomeningeal disease.

Expanding extradural tumors induce injury through several mechanisms. Obstruction of the epidural venous plexus leads to edema. Local production of inflammatory cytokines enhances blood flow and edema formation. Compression compromises blood flow, leading to ischemia. Production of vascular endothelial growth factor is associated with spinal cord hypoxia and has been implicated as a potential cause of damage after spinal cord injury.

The most common initial symptom in patients with spinal cord compression is localized back pain and tenderness due to involvement of vertebrae by tumor. Pain is usually present for days or months before other neurologic findings appear. It is exacerbated by movement and by coughing or sneezing. It can be differentiated from the pain of disk disease by the fact that it worsens when the patient is supine. Radicular pain is less common than localized back pain and usually develops later. Radicular pain in the cervical or lumbosacral areas may be unilateral or bilateral. Radicular pain from the thoracic roots is often bilateral and is described by patients as a feeling of tight, band-like constriction around the thorax and abdomen. Typical cervical radicular pain radiates down the arm; in the lumbar region, the radiation is down the legs. *Lhermitte's sign*, a tingling or electric sensation down the back and upper and lower limbs upon flexing or extending the neck, may be an early sign of cord compression. Loss of bowel or bladder control may be the presenting symptom but usually occurs late in the course. Occasionally patients present with ataxia of gait without motor and sensory involvement due to involvement of the spinocerebellar tract.

On physical examination, pain induced by straight leg raising, neck flexion, or vertebral percussion may help to determine the level of cord compression. Patients develop numbness and paresthesias in the extremities or trunk. Loss of sensibility to pinprick is as common as loss of sensibility to vibration or position. The upper limit of the zone of sensory loss is often one or two vertebrae below the site of compression. Motor findings include weakness, spasticity, and abnormal muscle stretching. An extensor plantar reflex reflects significant compression. Deep tendon reflexes may be brisk. Motor and sensory loss usually precedes sphincter disturbance. Patients with autonomic dysfunction may present with decreased anal tonus, decreased perineal sensibility, and a distended bladder. The absence of the anal wink reflex or the bulbocavernosus reflex confirms cord involvement. In doubtful cases, evaluation of postvoiding urinary residual volume can be helpful. A residual volume of >150 mL suggests bladder dysfunction. Autonomic dysfunction is an unfavorable prognostic factor. Patients with progressive neurologic symptoms should have frequent neurologic examinations and rapid therapeutic intervention. Other illnesses that may mimic cord compression include osteoporotic vertebral collapse, disk disease, pyogenic abscess or vertebral tuberculosis, radiation myelopathy, neoplastic leptomeningitis, benign tumors, epidural hematoma, and spinal lipomatosis.

Cauda equina syndrome is characterized by low back pain; diminished sensation over the buttocks, posterior-superior thighs, and perineal area in a saddle distribution; rectal and bladder dysfunction; sexual impotence; absent bulbocavernous, patellar, and Achilles' reflexes; and variable amount of lower-extremity weakness. This reflects compression of nerve roots as they form the cauda equina after leaving the spinal cord. The majority of cauda equine tumors are primary tumors of glial or nerve sheath origin; metastases are very rare.

Patients with cancer who develop back pain should be evaluated for spinal cord compression as quickly as possible (Fig. 331-2). Treatment is more often successful in patients who are ambulatory and still have sphincter control at the time treatment is initiated. Patients should have a neurologic examination and plain films of the spine. Those whose physical examination suggests cord compression should receive dexamethasone (6 mg intravenously every 6 h), starting immediately.

Erosion of the pedicles (the "winking owl" sign) is the earliest radiologic finding of vertebral tumor. Other radiographic changes include increased intrapedicular distance, vertebral destruction, lytic or sclerotic lesions, scalloped vertebral bodies, and vertebral body collapse. Vertebral collapse is not a reliable indicator of the presence of tumor; about 20% of cases of vertebral collapse, particularly those in older patients and postmenopausal women, are due not to cancer but to osteoporosis. Also, a normal appearance on plain films of the spine does not exclude the diagnosis of cancer. The role of bone scans in the detection of cord compression is not clear; this method is sensitive but less specific than spinal radiography.

The full-length image of the cord provided by MRI is the imaging procedure of choice. Multiple epidural metastases are noted in 25% of patients with cord compression, and their presence influences treatment plans. On T1-weighted images, good contrast is noted between the cord, cerebrospinal fluid, and extradural lesions. Owing to its sensitivity in demonstrating the replacement of bone marrow by tumor, MRI can show which parts of a vertebra are involved by tumor. MRI also visualizes intraspinal extradural masses compressing the cord. T2-weighted images are most useful for the demonstration of intramedullary pathology. Gadolinium-enhanced MRI can help to delineate intramedullary disease. MRI is as good as or better than myelography plus postmyelogram CT scan in detecting metastatic epidural disease with cord compression. Myelography should be reserved for patients who have poor MRIs or who cannot undergo MRI promptly. CT scan in conjunction with myelography enhances the detection of small areas of spinal destruction.

In patients with cord compression and an unknown primary tumor, a simple workup including chest radiography, mammography, measurement of prostate specific antigen, and abdominal CT usually reveals the underlying malignancy.

TREATMENT SPINAL CORD COMPRESSION

The treatment of patients with spinal cord compression is aimed at relief of pain and restoration/preservation of neurologic function (Fig. 331-2). Management of MSCC requires a multidisciplinary approach.

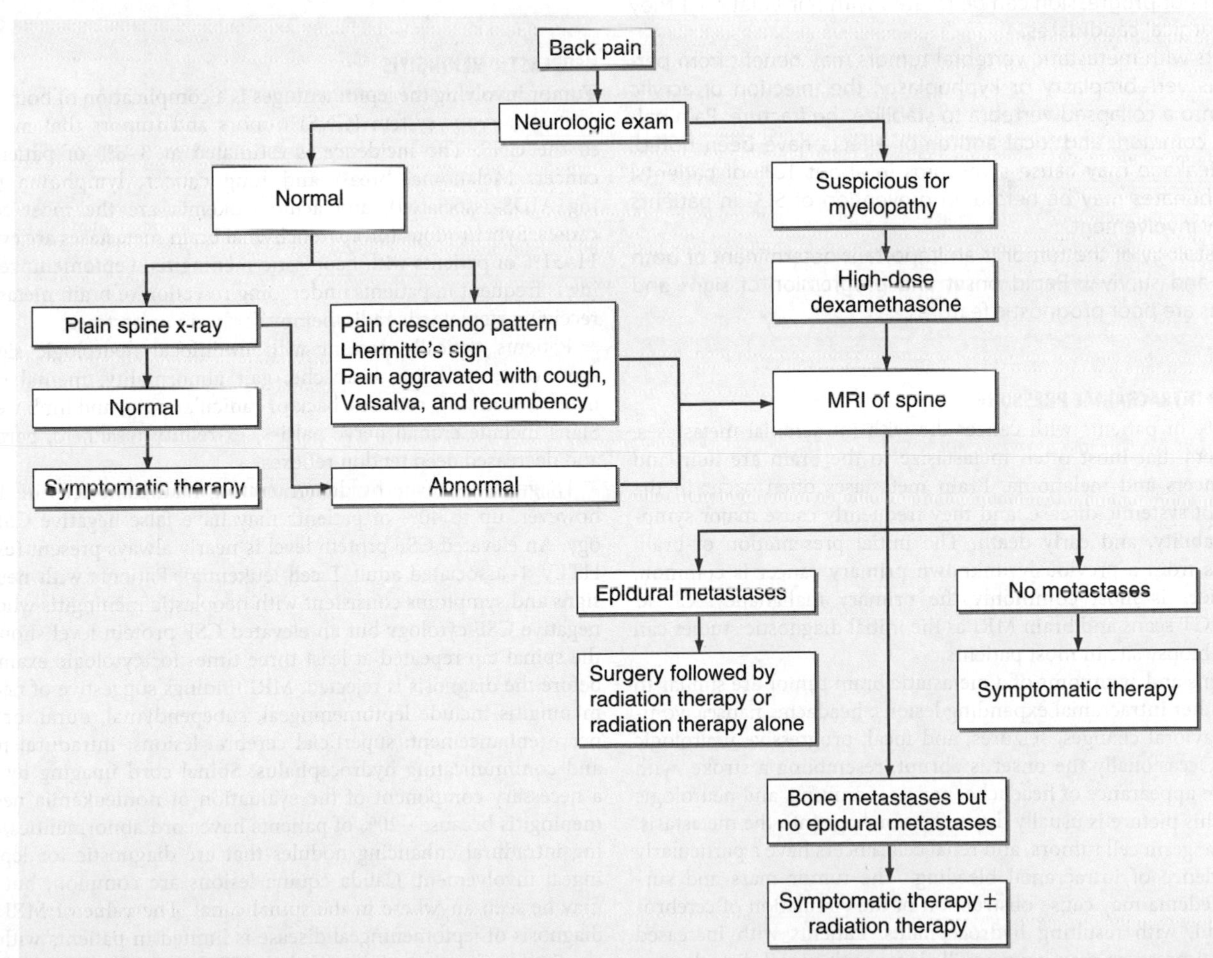

FIGURE 331-2 **Management of cancer patients with back pain.**

Radiation therapy plus glucocorticoids is generally the initial treatment of choice for most patients with spinal cord compression. Up to 75% of patients treated when still ambulatory remain ambulatory, but only 10% of patients with paraplegia recover walking capacity. Indications for surgical intervention include unknown etiology, failure of radiation therapy, a radioresistant tumor type (e.g., melanoma or renal cell cancer), pathologic fracture dislocation, and rapidly evolving neurologic symptoms. Laminectomy is done for tissue diagnosis and for the removal of posteriorly localized epidural deposits in the absence of vertebral body disease. Because most cases of epidural spinal cord compression are due to anterior or anterolateral extradural disease, resection of the anterior vertebral body along with the tumor, followed by spinal stabilization, has achieved good results. A randomized trial showed that patients who underwent an operation followed by radiotherapy (within 14 days) retained the ability to walk significantly longer than those treated with radiotherapy alone. Surgically treated patients also maintained continence and neurologic function significantly longer than patients in the radiation group. The length of survival was not significantly different in the two groups, although there was a trend toward longer survival in the surgery group. The study drew some criticism for the poorer than expected results in the patients who did not go to surgery. The benefit of surgery over radiotherapy decreased in patients over age 65 years. However, patients should be evaluated for surgery if they are expected to survive longer than 3 months. Conventional radiotherapy has a role after surgery. Chemotherapy may have a role in patients with chemosensitive tumors who have had prior radiotherapy to the same region and who are not candidates for surgery. Most patients with prostate cancer who develop cord compression have already had hormonal therapy; however, for those who have not, androgen deprivation is combined with surgery and radiotherapy. Patients who previously received radiotherapy for MSCC with an in-field tumor progression can be treated with reirradiation if they are not surgical candidates.

Patients with metastatic vertebral tumors may benefit from percutaneous vertebroplasty or kyphoplasty, the injection of acrylic cement into a collapsed vertebra to stabilize the fracture. Pain palliation is common, and local antitumor effects have been noted. Cement leakage may cause symptoms in about 10% of patients. Bisphosphonates may be helpful in prevention of SCC in patients with bony involvement.

The histology of the tumor is an important determinant of both recovery and survival. Rapid onset and progression of signs and symptoms are poor prognostic features.

INCREASED INTRACRANIAL PRESSURE

About 25% of patients with cancer die with intracranial metastases. The cancers that most often metastasize to the brain are lung and breast cancers and melanoma. Brain metastases often occur in the presence of systemic disease, and they frequently cause major symptoms, disability, and early death. The initial presentation of brain metastases from a previously unknown primary cancer is common. Lung cancer is most commonly the primary malignancy. Chest/abdomen CT scans and brain MRI as the initial diagnostic studies can identify a biopsy site in most patients.

The signs and symptoms of a metastatic brain tumor are similar to those of other intracranial expanding lesions: headache, nausea, vomiting, behavioral changes, seizures, and focal, progressive neurologic changes. Occasionally the onset is abrupt, resembling a stroke, with the sudden appearance of headache, nausea, vomiting, and neurologic deficits. This picture is usually due to hemorrhage into the metastasis. Melanoma, germ cell tumors, and renal cell cancers have a particularly high incidence of intracranial bleeding. The tumor mass and surrounding edema may cause obstruction of the circulation of cerebrospinal fluid, with resulting hydrocephalus. Patients with increased intracranial pressure may have papilledema with visual disturbances and neck stiffness. As the mass enlarges, brain tissue may be displaced through the fixed cranial openings, producing various herniation syndromes.

CT scan and MRI are equally effective in the diagnosis of brain metastases. CT scan with contrast should be used as a screening procedure. The CT scan shows brain metastases as multiple enhancing lesions of various sizes with surrounding areas of low-density edema. If a single lesion or no metastases are visualized by contrast-enhanced CT, MRI of the brain should be performed. Gadolinium-enhanced MRI is more sensitive than CT at revealing meningeal involvement and small lesions, particularly in the brainstem or cerebellum.

Intracranial hypertension ("pseudotumor cerebri") secondary to tretinoin therapy has been reported.

TREATMENT INCREASED INTRACRANIAL PRESSURE

Dexamethasone is the best initial treatment for all symptomatic patients with brain metastases. Patients with multiple lesions should usually receive whole-brain radiation. Patients with a single brain metastasis and with controlled extracranial disease may be treated with surgical excision followed by whole-brain radiation therapy, especially if they are younger than 60 years. Radioresistant tumors should be resected if possible. Stereotactic radiosurgery (SRS) is recommended in patients with a limited number of brain metastases (one to four) who have stable, systemic disease or reasonable systemic treatment options and for patients who have a small number of metastatic lesions in whom whole-brain radiation therapy has failed. With a gamma knife or linear accelerator, multiple small, well-collimated beams of ionizing radiation destroy lesions seen on MRI. Some patients with increased intracranial pressure associated with hydrocephalus may benefit from shunt placement. If neurologic deterioration is not reversed with medical therapy, ventriculotomy to remove cerebrospinal fluid (CSF) or craniotomy to remove tumors or hematomas may be necessary.

NEOPLASTIC MENINGITIS

Tumor involving the leptomeninges is a complication of both primary central nervous system (CNS) tumors and tumors that metastasize to the CNS. The incidence is estimated at 3–8% of patients with cancer. Melanoma, breast and lung cancer, lymphoma (including AIDS-associated), and acute leukemia are the most common causes. Synchronous intraparenchymal brain metastases are evident in 11–31% of patients with neoplastic meningitis. Leptomeningeal seeding is frequent in patients undergoing resection of brain metastases or receiving stereotactic radiotherapy for brain metastases.

Patients typically present with multifocal neurologic signs and symptoms, including headache, gait abnormality, mental changes, nausea, vomiting, seizures, back or radicular pain, and limb weakness. Signs include cranial nerve palsies, extremity weakness, paresthesia, and decreased deep tendon reflexes.

Diagnosis is made by demonstrating malignant cells in the CSF; however, up to 40% of patients may have false-negative CSF cytology. An elevated CSF protein level is nearly always present (except in HTLV-1–associated adult T cell leukemia). Patients with neurologic signs and symptoms consistent with neoplastic meningitis who have a negative CSF cytology but an elevated CSF protein level should have the spinal tap repeated at least three times for cytologic examination before the diagnosis is rejected. MRI findings suggestive of neoplastic meningitis include leptomeningeal, subependymal, dural, or cranial nerve enhancement; superficial cerebral lesions; intradural nodules; and communicating hydrocephalus. Spinal cord imaging by MRI is a necessary component of the evaluation of nonleukemia neoplastic meningitis because ~20% of patients have cord abnormalities, including intradural enhancing nodules that are diagnostic for leptomeningeal involvement. Cauda equina lesions are common, but lesions may be seen anywhere in the spinal canal. The value of MRI for the diagnosis of leptomeningeal disease is limited in patients with hematopoietic malignancy. Radiolabeled CSF flow studies are abnormal in up to 70% of patients with neoplastic meningitis; ventricular outlet obstruction, abnormal flow in the spinal canal, or impaired flow over the cerebral convexities may affect distribution of intrathecal chemotherapy, resulting in decreased efficacy or increased toxicity. Radiation therapy may correct CSF flow abnormalities before use of intrathecal chemotherapy. Neoplastic meningitis can also lead to intracranial hypertension and hydrocephalus. Placement of a ventriculoperitoneal shunt may effectively palliate symptoms in these patients.

The development of neoplastic meningitis usually occurs in the setting of uncontrolled cancer outside the CNS; thus, prognosis is poor (median survival 10–12 weeks). However, treatment of the neoplastic meningitis may successfully alleviate symptoms and control the CNS spread.

TREATMENT NEOPLASTIC MENINGITIS

Intrathecal chemotherapy, usually methotrexate, cytarabine, or thiotepa, is delivered by lumbar puncture or by an intraventricular reservoir (Ommaya). An extended-release preparation of cytarabine (Depocyte) has a longer half-life and is more effective than other formulations. Among solid tumors, breast cancer responds best to therapy. Epidermal growth factor receptor (EGFR) tyrosine kinase inhibitors (TKIs) may be effective in non-small-cell lung cancer patients with *EGFR* mutations and leptomeningeal involvement. Patients with neoplastic meningitis from either acute leukemia or lymphoma may be cured of their CNS disease if the systemic disease can be eliminated.

SEIZURES

Seizures occurring in a patient with cancer can be caused by the tumor itself, by metabolic disturbances, by radiation injury, by cerebral infarctions, by chemotherapy-related encephalopathies, or by CNS infections. Metastatic disease to the CNS is the most common cause of seizures in patients with cancer. However, seizures occur more frequently in primary brain tumors than in metastatic brain lesions. Seizures are a presenting symptom of CNS metastasis in 6–29% of cases. Approximately 10% of patients with CNS metastasis eventually develop seizures. Tumors that affect the frontal, temporal, and parietal lobes are more commonly associated with seizures than are occipital lesions. The presence of frontal lesions correlates with early seizures, and the presence of hemispheric symptoms increases the risk for late seizures. Both early and late seizures are uncommon in patients with posterior fossa and sellar lesions. Seizures are common in patients with CNS metastases from melanoma and low-grade primary brain tumors. Very rarely, cytotoxic drugs such as etoposide, busulfan, ifosfamide, and chlorambucil cause seizures. Another cause of seizures related to drug therapy is reversible posterior leukoencephalopathy syndrome (RPLS). RPLS is associated rarely with administration of cisplatin, 5-fluorouracil, bleomycin, vinblastine, vincristine, etoposide, paclitaxel, ifosfamide, cyclophosphamide, doxorubicin, cytarabine, methotrexate, oxaliplatin, cyclosporine, tacrolimus, and vascular endothelial growth factor inhibitors including bevacizumab, aflibercept, sunitinib, sorafenib, pazopanib, and axitinib. RPLS occurs in patients undergoing allogeneic bone marrow or solid-organ transplantation. RPLS is characterized by headache, altered consciousness, generalized seizures, visual disturbances, hypertension, and posterior cerebral white matter vasogenic edema on CT/MRI. Seizures may begin focally but are typically generalized.

TREATMENT SEIZURES

Patients in whom seizures due to CNS metastases have been demonstrated should receive anticonvulsive treatment with phenytoin or levetiracetam. If this is not effective, valproic acid can be added. Prophylactic anticonvulsant therapy is not recommended. In postcraniotomy patients, prophylactic antiepileptic drugs should be withdrawn during the first week after surgery. Most antiseizure medications including phenytoin induce cytochrome P450 (CYP450), which alters the metabolism of many antitumor agents, including irinotecan, taxanes, and etoposide as well as molecular targeted agents, including imatinib, gefitinib, erlotinib, tipifarnib, sorafenib, sunitinib, temsirolimus, everolimus, and vemurafenib. Levetiracetam and topiramate are anticonvulsant agents not metabolized by the hepatic CYP450 system and do not alter the metabolism of antitumor agents. They have become the preferred drugs. Surgical resection and other antitumor treatments such as radiotherapy and chemotherapy may improve seizure control.

PULMONARY AND INTRACEREBRAL LEUKOSTASIS

Hyperleukocytosis and the leukostasis syndrome associated with it is a potentially fatal complication of acute leukemia (particularly myeloid leukemia) that can occur when the peripheral blast cell count is >100,000/mL. The frequency of hyperleukocytosis is 5–13% in acute myeloid leukemia (AML) and 10–30% in acute lymphoid leukemia; however, leukostasis is rare in lymphoid leukemia. At such high blast cell counts, blood viscosity is increased, blood flow is slowed by aggregates of tumor cells, and the primitive myeloid leukemic cells are capable of invading through the endothelium and causing hemorrhage. Brain and lung are most commonly affected. Patients with brain leukostasis may experience stupor, headache, dizziness, tinnitus, visual disturbances, ataxia, confusion, coma, or sudden death. On examination, papilledema, retinal vein distension, retinal hemorrhages, and focal deficit may be present. Administration of 600 cGy of whole-brain irradiation can protect against this complication and can be followed by rapid institution of antileukemic therapy. Hydroxyurea, 3–5 g, can rapidly reduce a high blast cell count while the accurate diagnostic workup is in progress. Pulmonary leukostasis may present as respiratory distress and hypoxemia, and progress to respiratory failure. Chest radiographs may be normal but usually show interstitial or alveolar infiltrates. Hyperleukocytosis rarely may cause acute leg ischemia, renal vein thrombosis, myocardial ischemia, bowel infraction, and priapism. Arterial blood gas results should be interpreted cautiously. Rapid consumption of plasma oxygen by the markedly increased number of white blood cells can cause spuriously low arterial oxygen tension. Pulse oximetry is the most accurate way of assessing oxygenation in patients with hyperleukocytosis. Leukapheresis may be helpful in decreasing circulating blast counts. Treatment of the leukemia can result in pulmonary hemorrhage from lysis of blasts in the lung, called *leukemic cell lysis pneumopathy*. Intravascular volume depletion and unnecessary blood transfusions may increase blood viscosity and worsen the leukostasis syndrome. Leukostasis is very rarely a feature of the high white cell counts associated with chronic lymphoid or chronic myeloid leukemia.

When acute promyelocytic leukemia is treated with differentiating agents like tretinoin and arsenic trioxide, cerebral or pulmonary leukostasis may occur as tumor cells differentiate into mature neutrophils. This complication can be largely avoided by using cytotoxic chemotherapy or arsenic together with the differentiating agents.

HEMOPTYSIS

Hemoptysis may be caused by nonmalignant conditions, but lung cancer accounts for a large proportion of cases. Up to 20% of patients with lung cancer have hemoptysis some time in their course. Endobronchial metastases from carcinoid tumors, breast cancer, colon cancer, kidney cancer, and melanoma may also cause hemoptysis. The volume of bleeding is often difficult to gauge. Massive hemoptysis is defined as >200–600 mL of blood produced in 24 h. However, any hemoptysis should be considered massive if it threatens life. When respiratory difficulty occurs, hemoptysis should be treated emergently. The first priorities are to maintain the airway, optimize oxygenation, and stabilize the hemodynamic status. If the bleeding side is known, the patient should be placed in a lateral decubitus position, with the bleeding side down to prevent aspiration into the unaffected lung, and given supplemental oxygen. If large-volume bleeding continues or the airway is compromised, the patient should be intubated and undergo emergency bronchoscopy. If the site of bleeding is detected, either the patient undergoes a definitive surgical procedure or the lesion is treated with a neodymium:yttrium-aluminum-garnet (Nd:YAG) laser, argon plasma coagulation, or electrocautery. In stable patients, multidetector CT angiography delineates bronchial and nonbronchial systemic arteries and identifies the source of bleeding and underlying pathology with high sensitivity. Massive hemoptysis usually originates from the high-pressure bronchial circulation. Bronchial artery embolization is considered a first-line definite procedure for managing hemoptysis. Bronchial artery embolization may control brisk bleeding in 75–90% of patients, permitting the definitive surgical procedure to be done more safely.

Embolization without definitive surgery is associated with rebleeding in 20–50% of patients. Recurrent hemoptysis usually responds to a second embolization procedure. A postembolization syndrome characterized by pleuritic pain, fever, dysphagia, and leukocytosis may occur; it lasts 5–7 days and resolves with symptomatic treatment. Bronchial or esophageal wall necrosis, myocardial infarction, and spinal cord infarction are rare complications. Surgery, as a salvage strategy, is indicated after failure of embolization and is associated with better survival when performed in a nonurgent setting.

Pulmonary hemorrhage with or without hemoptysis in hematologic malignancies is often associated with fungal infections, particularly *Aspergillus* sp. After granulocytopenia resolves, the lung infiltrates in aspergillosis may cavitate and cause massive hemoptysis. Thrombocytopenia and coagulation defects should be corrected, if possible. Surgical evaluation is recommended in patients with aspergillosis-related cavitary lesions.

Bevacizumab, an antibody to vascular endothelial growth factor (VEGF) that inhibits angiogenesis, has been associated with life-threatening hemoptysis in patients with non-small-cell lung cancer, particularly of squamous cell histology. Non-small-cell lung cancer patients with cavitary lesions or previous hemoptysis (≥2.5 mL) within the past 3 months have higher risk for pulmonary hemorrhage.

AIRWAY OBSTRUCTION

Airway obstruction refers to a blockage at the level of the mainstem bronchi or above. It may result either from intraluminal tumor growth or from extrinsic compression of the airway. The most common cause of malignant upper airway obstruction is invasion from an adjacent primary tumor, most commonly lung cancer, followed by esophageal, thyroid, and mediastinal malignancies including lymphomas. Extrathoracic primary tumors such as renal, colon, or breast cancer can cause airway obstruction through endobronchial and/or mediastinal lymph node metastases. Patients may present with dyspnea, hemoptysis, stridor, wheezing, intractable cough, postobstructive pneumonia, or hoarseness. Chest radiographs usually demonstrate obstructing lesions. CT scans reveal the extent of tumor. Cool, humidified oxygen, glucocorticoids, and ventilation with a mixture of helium and oxygen (Heliox) may provide temporary relief. If the obstruction is proximal to the larynx, a tracheostomy may be lifesaving. For more distal obstructions, particularly intrinsic lesions incompletely obstructing the airway, bronchoscopy with mechanical debulking and dilatation or ablational treatments including laser treatment, photodynamic therapy, argon plasma coagulation, electrocautery, or stenting can produce immediate relief in most patients (Fig. 331-3). However, radiation therapy (either external-beam irradiation or brachytherapy) given together with glucocorticoids may also open the airway. Symptomatic extrinsic compression may be palliated by stenting. Patients with primary airway tumors such as squamous cell carcinoma, carcinoid tumor, adenocystic carcinoma, or non-small-cell lung cancer, if resectable, should have surgery.

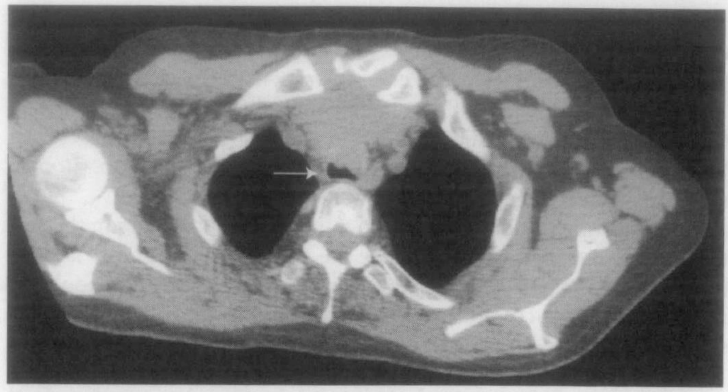

A

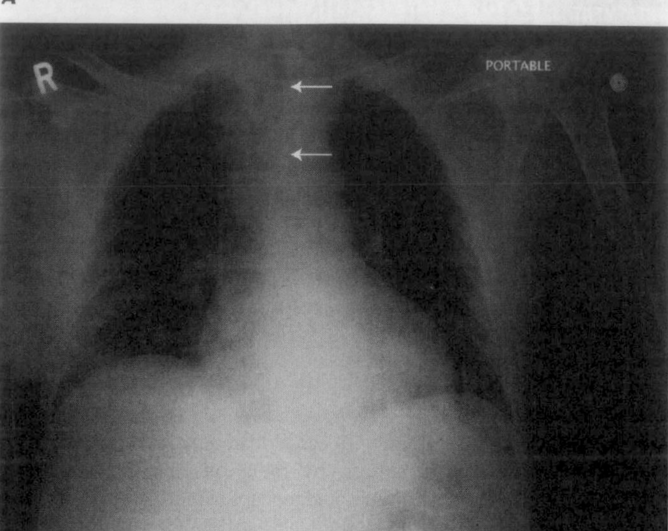

B

FIGURE 331-3 Airway obstruction. ***A.*** Computed tomography scan of a 62-year-old man with tracheal obstruction caused by renal carcinoma showing paratracheal mass with tracheal invasion/obstruction (*arrow*). ***B.*** Chest x-ray of same patient after stent (*arrows*) placement.

METABOLIC EMERGENCIES

HYPERCALCEMIA

Hypercalcemia is the most common paraneoplastic syndrome. Its pathogenesis and management are discussed fully in Chaps. 121 and 424.

SYNDROME OF INAPPROPRIATE SECRETION OF ANTIDIURETIC HORMONE (SIADH)

Hyponatremia is a common electrolyte abnormality in cancer patients, and SIADH is the most common cause among patients with cancer. SIADH is discussed fully in Chaps. 121 and 401e.

LACTIC ACIDOSIS

Lactic acidosis is a rare and potentially fatal metabolic complication of cancer. Lactic acidosis associated with sepsis and circulatory failure is a common preterminal event in many malignancies. Lactic acidosis in the absence of hypoxemia may occur in patients with leukemia, lymphoma, or solid tumors. In some cases, hypoglycemia also is present. Extensive involvement of the liver by tumor is often present. In most cases, decreased metabolism and increased production by the tumor both contribute to lactate accumulation. Tumor cell overexpression of certain glycolytic enzymes and mitochondrial dysfunction can contribute to its increased lactate production. HIV-infected patients have an increased risk of aggressive lymphoma; lactic acidosis that occurs in such patients may be related either to the rapid growth of the tumor or from toxicity of nucleoside reverse transcriptase inhibitors. Symptoms of lactic acidosis include tachypnea, tachycardia, change of mental status, and hepatomegaly. The serum level of lactic acid may reach 10–20 mmol/L (90–180 mg/dL). Treatment is aimed at the underlying disease. *The danger from lactic acidosis is from the acidosis, not the lactate.* Sodium bicarbonate should be added if acidosis is very severe or if hydrogen ion production is very rapid and uncontrolled. Other treatment options include renal replacement therapy, such as hemodialysis, and thiamine replacement. The prognosis is poor regardless of the treatment offered.

HYPOGLYCEMIA

Persistent hypoglycemia is occasionally associated with tumors other than pancreatic islet cell tumors. Usually these tumors are large; tumors of mesenchymal origin, hepatomas, or adrenocortical tumors may cause hypoglycemia. Mesenchymal tumors are usually located in the retroperitoneum or thorax. Obtundation, confusion, and behavioral aberrations occur in the postabsorptive period and may precede the diagnosis of the tumor. These tumors often secrete incompletely processed insulin-like growth factor II (IGF-II), a hormone capable of activating insulin receptors and causing hypoglycemia. Tumors secreting incompletely processed big IGF-II are characterized by an increased IGF-II to IGF-I ratio, suppressed insulin and C-peptide level, and inappropriately low growth hormone and β-hydroxybutyrate concentrations. Rarely, hypoglycemia is due to insulin secretion by a non-islet cell carcinoma. The development of hepatic dysfunction from liver metastases and increased glucose consumption by the tumor can contribute to hypoglycemia. If the tumor cannot be resected, hypoglycemia symptoms may be relieved by the administration of glucose, glucocorticoids, or glucagon.

Hypoglycemia can be artifactual; hyperleukocytosis from leukemia, myeloproliferative diseases, leukemoid reactions, or colony-stimulating factor treatment can increase glucose consumption in the test tube after blood is drawn, leading to pseudohypoglycemia.

ADRENAL INSUFFICIENCY

In patients with cancer, adrenal insufficiency may go unrecognized because the symptoms, such as nausea, vomiting, anorexia, and orthostatic hypotension, are nonspecific and may be mistakenly attributed to progressive cancer or to therapy. Primary adrenal insufficiency may develop owing to replacement of both glands by metastases (lung, breast, colon, or kidney cancer; lymphoma), to removal of both glands, or to hemorrhagic necrosis in association with sepsis or anticoagulation. Impaired adrenal steroid synthesis occurs in patients being treated for cancer with mitotane, ketoconazole, or aminoglutethimide or undergoing rapid reduction in glucocorticoid therapy. Rarely, metastatic replacement causes primary adrenal insufficiency as the first manifestation of an occult malignancy. Metastasis to the pituitary or hypothalamus is found at autopsy in up to 5% of patients with cancer, but associated secondary adrenal insufficiency is rare. On the other hand, ipilimumab, an anti-CTLA-4 antibody used for treatment of malignant melanoma, may cause autoimmunity including autoimmune-like enterocolitis, hypophysitis, and hepatitis. Autoimmune hypophysitis may present with headache, visual field defects, and pituitary hormone deficiencies manifesting as hypopituitarism, adrenal insufficiency (including adrenal crisis), or hypothyroidism. Anti-CTLA-4-associated hypophysitis symptoms occur at an average of 6–12 weeks after initiation of therapy. The treatment of severe autoimmune toxicity is glucocorticoids. Almost all patients with hypophysitis respond to withdrawal of ipilimumab and glucocorticoid therapy in several days. However, pituitary dysfunction may resolve or may be permanent, requiring long-term therapy and thyroid and testosterone replacement. Peripheral Addison's disease can also be observed with anti-CTLA-4 antibodies. Megestrol acetate, used to manage cancer and HIV-related cachexia, may suppress plasma levels of cortisol and adrenocorticotropic hormone (ACTH). Patients taking megestrol may develop adrenal insufficiency, and even those whose adrenal dysfunction is not symptomatic may have inadequate adrenal reserve if they become seriously ill. Paradoxically, some patients may develop Cushing's syndrome and/or hyperglycemia because of the glucocorticoid-like activity of megestrol acetate. Cranial irradiation for childhood brain tumors may affect the hypothalamus-pituitary-adrenal axis, resulting in secondary adrenal insufficiency.

Acute adrenal insufficiency is potentially lethal. Treatment of suspected adrenal crisis is initiated after the sampling of serum cortisol and ACTH levels (Chap. 406).

TREATMENT-RELATED EMERGENCIES

TUMOR LYSIS SYNDROME

Tumor lysis syndrome (TLS) is characterized by hyperuricemia, hyperkalemia, hyperphosphatemia, and hypocalcemia and is caused by the destruction of a large number of rapidly proliferating neoplastic cells. Acidosis may also develop. Acute renal failure occurs frequently.

TLS is most often associated with the treatment of Burkitt's lymphoma, acute lymphoblastic leukemia, and other rapidly proliferating lymphomas, but it also may be seen with chronic leukemias and, rarely, with solid tumors. This syndrome has been seen in patients with chronic lymphocytic leukemia after treatment with nucleosides like fludarabine. TLS has been observed with administration of glucocorticoids, hormonal agents such as letrozole and tamoxifen, and monoclonal antibodies such as rituximab and gemtuzumab. TLS usually occurs during or shortly (1–5 days) after chemotherapy. Rarely, spontaneous necrosis of malignancies causes TLS.

Hyperuricemia may be present at the time of chemotherapy. Effective treatment kills malignant cells and leads to increased serum uric acid levels from the turnover of nucleic acids. Owing to the acidic local environment, uric acid can precipitate in the tubules, medulla, and collecting ducts of the kidney, leading to renal failure. Lactic acidosis and dehydration may contribute to the precipitation of uric acid in the renal tubules. The finding of uric acid crystals in the urine is strong evidence for uric acid nephropathy. The ratio of urinary uric acid to urinary creatinine is >1 in patients with acute hyperuricemic nephropathy and <1 in patients with renal failure due to other causes.

Hyperphosphatemia, which can be caused by the release of intracellular phosphate pools by tumor lysis, produces a reciprocal depression in serum calcium, which causes severe neuromuscular irritability and tetany. Deposition of calcium phosphate in the kidney and hyperphosphatemia may cause renal failure. Potassium is the principal intracellular cation, and massive destruction of malignant cells may lead to hyperkalemia. Hyperkalemia in patients with renal failure may rapidly become life-threatening by causing ventricular arrhythmias and sudden death.

The likelihood that TLS will occur in patients with Burkitt's lymphoma is related to the tumor burden and renal function. Hyperuricemia and high serum levels of lactate dehydrogenase (LDH >1500 U/L), both of which correlate with total tumor burden, also correlate with the risk of TLS. In patients at risk for TLS, pretreatment evaluations should include a complete blood count, serum chemistry evaluation, and urine analysis. High leukocyte and platelet counts may artificially elevate potassium levels ("pseudohyperkalemia") due to lysis of these cells after the blood is drawn. In these cases, plasma potassium instead of serum potassium should be followed. In pseudohyperkalemia, no electrocardiographic abnormalities are present. In patients with abnormal baseline renal function, the kidneys and retroperitoneal area should be evaluated by sonography and/or CT to rule out obstructive uropathy. Urine output should be watched closely.

TREATMENT TUMOR LYSIS SYNDROME

Recognition of risk and prevention are the most important steps in the management of this syndrome (Fig. 331-4). The standard preventive approach consists of allopurinol, urinary alkalinization, and aggressive hydration. Urinary alkalization with sodium bicarbonate is controversial. It increases uric acid solubility, but decreases calcium phosphate solubility. If it is used, it should be discontinued when hyperphosphatemia develops. Intravenous allopurinol may be given in patients who cannot tolerate oral therapy. In some cases, uric acid levels cannot be lowered sufficiently with the standard preventive approach. Rasburicase (recombinant urate oxidase) can be effective in these instances, particularly when renal failure is present. Urate oxidase is missing from primates and catalyzes the conversion of poorly soluble uric acid to readily soluble allantoin. Rasburicase acts rapidly, decreasing uric acid levels within hours; however, it may cause hypersensitivity reactions such as bronchospasm, hypoxemia, and hypotension. Rasburicase should also be administered to high-risk patients for TLS prophylaxis. Rasburicase is contraindicated in patients with glucose-6-phosphate dehydrogenase deficiency who are unable to break down hydrogen peroxide, an end product of the urate oxidase reaction. Rasburicase is known to cause ex vivo enzymatic degradation of uric acid in test tube at room temperature. This leads to spuriously low uric acid levels

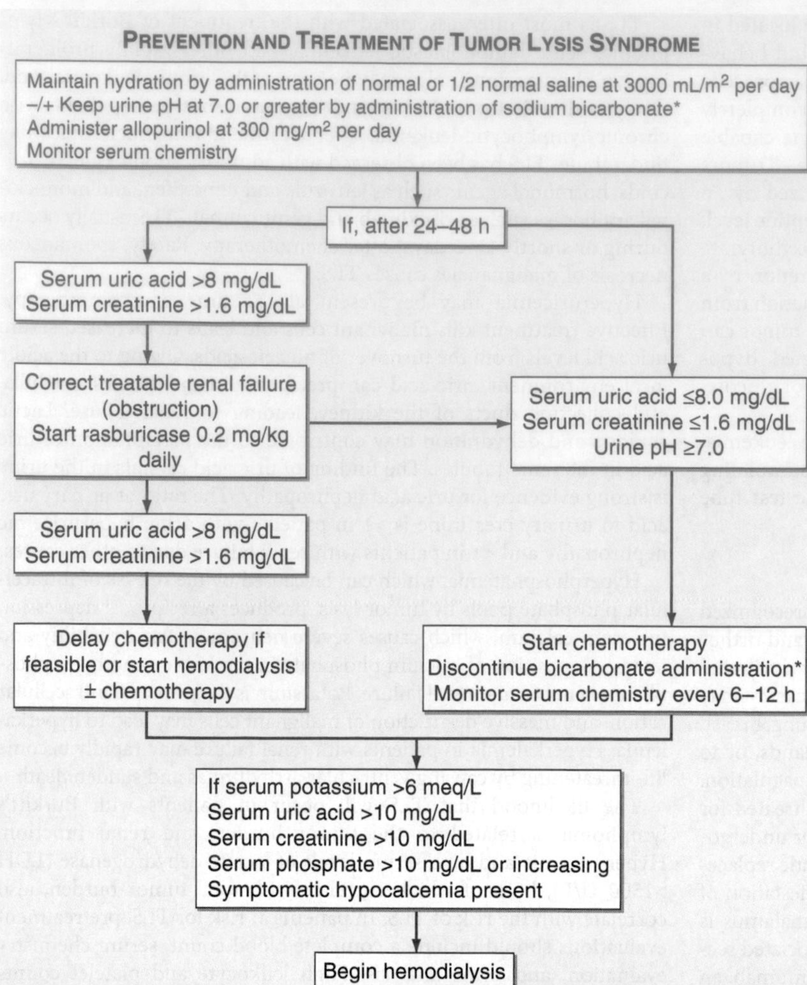
PREVENTION AND TREATMENT OF TUMOR LYSIS SYNDROME
Maintain hydration by administration of normal or 1/2 normal saline at 3000 mL/m2 per day
–/+ Keep urine pH at 7.0 or greater by administration of sodium bicarbonate*
Administer allopurinol at 300 mg/m2 per day
Monitor serum chemistry
If, after 24–48 h
Serum uric acid >8 mg/dL
Serum creatinine >1.6 mg/dL
Correct treatable renal failure (obstruction)
Start rasburicase 0.2 mg/kg daily
Serum uric acid ≤8.0 mg/dL
Serum creatinine ≤1.6 mg/dL
Urine pH ≥7.0
Serum uric acid >8 mg/dL
Serum creatinine >1.6 mg/dL
Delay chemotherapy if feasible or start hemodialysis ± chemotherapy
Start chemotherapy
Discontinue bicarbonate administration*
Monitor serum chemistry every 6–12 h
If serum potassium >6 meq/L
Serum uric acid >10 mg/dL
Serum creatinine >10 mg/dL
Serum phosphate >10 mg/dL or increasing
Symptomatic hypocalcemia present
Begin hemodialysis

FIGURE 331-4 Management of patients at high risk for the tumor lysis syndrome. *See text.

during laboratory monitoring of the patient with TLS. Samples must be cooled immediately to deactivate the urate oxidase. Despite aggressive prophylaxis, TLS and/or oliguric or anuric renal failure may occur. Care should be taken to prevent worsening of symptomatic hypocalcemia by induction of alkalosis during bicarbonate infusion. Administration of sodium bicarbonate may also lead to urinary precipitation of calcium phosphate, which is less soluble at alkaline pH. Dialysis is often necessary and should be considered early in the course. Hemodialysis is preferred. Hemofiltration offers a gradual, continuous method of removing cellular by-products and fluid. The prognosis is excellent, and renal function recovers after the uric acid level is lowered to ≤10 mg/dL.

HUMAN ANTIBODY INFUSION REACTIONS

The initial infusion of human or humanized antibodies (e.g., rituximab, gemtuzumab, trastuzumab, alemtuzumab, panitumumab, brentuximab vedotin) is associated with fever, chills, nausea, asthenia, and headache in up to half of treated patients. Bronchospasm and hypotension occur in 1% of patients. Severe manifestations including pulmonary infiltrates, acute respiratory distress syndrome, and cardiogenic shock occur rarely. Laboratory manifestations include elevated hepatic aminotransferase levels, thrombocytopenia, and prolongation of prothrombin time. The pathogenesis is thought to be activation of immune effector processes (cells and complement) and release of inflammatory cytokines, such as tumor necrosis factor α, interferon gamma, interleukin 6, and interleukin 10 (cytokine release syndrome [CRS]). Although its origins are not completely understood, CRS is believed to be due to activation of a variety of cell types including monocytes/macrophages and T and B lymphocytes. Severe reactions from rituximab have occurred with high numbers (>50 × 10^9 lymphocytes) of circulating cells bearing the target antigen (CD20) and have been associated with a rapid fall in circulating tumor cells, mild electrolyte evidence of TLS, and very rarely, death. In addition, increased liver enzymes, D-dimer, and LDH and prolongation of the prothrombin time may occur. Diphenhydramine, hydrocortisone, and acetaminophen can often prevent or suppress the infusion-related symptoms. If they occur, the infusion is stopped and restarted at half the initial infusion rate after the symptoms have abated. Severe CRS may require intensive support for acute respiratory distress syndrome (ARDS) and resistant hypotension.

HEMOLYTIC-UREMIC SYNDROME

Hemolytic-uremic syndrome (HUS) and, less commonly, thrombotic thrombocytopenic purpura (TTP) (Chap. 341) may rarely occur after treatment with antineoplastic drugs, including mitomycin, gemcitabine, cisplatin, and bleomycin, and with VEGF inhibitors. It occurs most often in patients with gastric, lung, colorectal, pancreatic, and breast carcinoma. In one series, 35% of patients were without evident cancer at the time this syndrome appeared. Secondary HUS/TTP has also been reported as a rare but sometimes fatal complication of bone marrow transplantation.

HUS usually has its onset 4–8 weeks after the last dose of chemotherapy, but it is not rare to detect it several months later. HUS is characterized by microangiopathic hemolytic anemia, thrombocytopenia, and renal failure. Dyspnea, weakness, fatigue, oliguria, and purpura are also common initial symptoms and findings. Systemic hypertension and pulmonary edema frequently occur. Severe hypertension, pulmonary edema, and rapid worsening of hemolysis and renal function may occur after a blood or blood product transfusion. Cardiac findings include atrial arrhythmias, pericardial friction rub, and pericardial effusion. Raynaud's phenomenon is part of the syndrome in patients treated with bleomycin.

Laboratory findings include severe to moderate anemia associated with red blood cell fragmentation and numerous schistocytes on peripheral smear. Reticulocytosis, decreased plasma haptoglobin, and an LDH level document hemolysis. The serum bilirubin level is usually normal or slightly elevated. The Coombs' test is negative. The white cell count is usually normal, and thrombocytopenia (<100,000/μL) is almost always present. Most patients have a normal coagulation profile, although some have mild elevations in thrombin time and in levels of fibrin degradation products. The serum creatinine level is elevated at presentation and shows a pattern of subacute worsening within weeks of the initial azotemia. The urinalysis reveals hematuria, proteinuria, and granular or hyaline casts; and circulating immune complexes may be present.

The basic pathologic lesion appears to be deposition of fibrin in the walls of capillaries and arterioles, and these deposits are similar to those seen in HUS due to other causes. These microvascular abnormalities involve mainly the kidneys and rarely occur in other organs. The pathogenesis of cancer treatment–related HUS is not completely understood, but probably the most important factor is endothelial damage. Primary forms of HUS/TTP are related to a decrease in processing of von Willebrand factor by a protease called ADAMTS13.

The case fatality rate is high; most patients die within a few months. There is no consensus on the optimal treatment for chemotherapy-induced HUS. Treatment modalities for HUS/TTP including immunocomplex removal (plasmapheresis, immunoadsorption, or exchange transfusion), antiplatelet/anticoagulant therapies, immunosuppressive therapies, and plasma exchange have varying degrees of success. The outcome with plasma exchange is generally poor, as in many other cases of secondary TTP. Rituximab is successfully used in patients with chemotherapy-induced HUS as well as in ADAMTS13-deficient TTP.

NEUTROPENIA AND INFECTION

These remain the most common serious complications of cancer therapy. They are covered in detail in Chap. 104.

PULMONARY INFILTRATES

Patients with cancer may present with dyspnea associated with diffuse interstitial infiltrates on chest radiographs. Such infiltrates may be due to progression of the underlying malignancy, treatment-related toxicities, infection, and/or unrelated diseases. The cause may be multifactorial; however, most commonly they occur as a consequence of treatment. Infiltration of the lung by malignancy has been described in patients with leukemia, lymphoma, and breast and other solid cancers. Pulmonary lymphatics may be involved diffusely by neoplasm (pulmonary lymphangitic carcinomatosis), resulting in a diffuse increase in interstitial markings on chest radiographs. The patient is often mildly dyspneic at the onset, but pulmonary failure develops over a period of weeks. In some patients, dyspnea precedes changes on the chest radiographs and is accompanied by a nonproductive cough. This syndrome is characteristic of solid tumors. In patients with leukemia, diffuse microscopic neoplastic peribronchial and peribronchiolar infiltration is frequent but may be asymptomatic. However, some patients present with diffuse interstitial infiltrates, an alveolar capillary block syndrome, and respiratory distress. In these situations, glucocorticoids can provide symptomatic relief, but specific chemotherapy should always be started promptly.

Several cytotoxic agents, such as bleomycin, methotrexate, busulfan, nitrosoureas, gemcitabine, mitomycin, vinorelbine, docetaxel, paclitaxel, fludarabine, pentostatin, and ifosfamide may cause pulmonary damage. The most frequent presentations are interstitial pneumonitis, alveolitis, and pulmonary fibrosis. Some cytotoxic agents, including methotrexate and procarbazine, may cause an acute hypersensitivity reaction. Cytosine arabinoside has been associated with noncardiogenic pulmonary edema. Administration of multiple cytotoxic drugs, as well as radiotherapy and preexisting lung disease, may potentiate the pulmonary toxicity. Supplemental oxygen may potentiate the effects of drugs and radiation injury. Patients should always be managed with the lowest FIO2 that is sufficient to maintain hemoglobin saturation.

The onset of symptoms may be insidious, with symptoms including dyspnea, nonproductive cough, and tachycardia. Patients may have bibasilar crepitant rales, end-inspiratory crackles, fever, and cyanosis. The chest radiograph generally shows an interstitial and sometimes an intraalveolar pattern that is strongest at the lung bases and may be symmetric. A small effusion may occur. Hypoxemia with decreased carbon monoxide diffusing capacity is always present. Glucocorticoids may be helpful in patients in whom pulmonary toxicity is related to radiation therapy or to chemotherapy. Treatment is otherwise supportive.

Molecular targeted agents, imatinib, erlotinib, and gefitinib are potent inhibitors of tyrosine kinases. These drugs may cause interstitial lung disease (ILD). In the case of gefitinib, preexisting fibrosis, poor performance status, and prior thoracic irradiation are independent risk factors; this complication has a high fatality rate. In Japan, incidence of interstitial lung disease associated with gefitinib was about 4.5% compared to 0.5% in the United States. Temsirolimus and everolimus, both esters a derivative of rapamycin, are agents that block the effects of mammalian target of rapamycin (mTOR), an enzyme that has an important role in regulating the synthesis of proteins that control cell division. It may cause ground-glass opacities in the lung with or without diffuse interstitial disease and lung parenchymal consolidation. Patients may be asymptomatic with only radiologic findings or may be symptomatic. Symptoms include cough, dyspnea, and/or hypoxemia, and sometimes patients present with systemic symptoms such as fever and fatigue. The incidence of everolimus-induced interstitial lung disease also appears to be higher in Japanese patients. Treatment includes dose reduction or withdrawal and, in some cases, the addition of glucocorticoids.

Radiation pneumonitis and/or fibrosis is a relatively frequent side effect of thoracic radiation therapy. It may be acute or chronic. Radiation-induced lung toxicity is a function of the irradiated lung volume, dose per fraction, and radiation dose. The larger the irradiated lung field, the higher is the risk for radiation pneumonitis. The use of concurrent chemoradiation, particularly regimens including paclitaxel, increases pulmonary toxicity. Radiation pneumonitis usually develops 2–6 months after completion of radiotherapy. The clinical syndrome, which varies in severity, consists of dyspnea, cough with scanty sputum, low-grade fever, and an initial hazy infiltrate on chest radiographs. The infiltrate and tissue damage usually are confined to the radiation field. The patients subsequently may develop a patchy alveolar infiltrate and air bronchograms, which may progress to acute respiratory failure that is sometimes fatal. A lung biopsy may be necessary to make the diagnosis. Asymptomatic infiltrates found incidentally after radiation therapy need not be treated. However, prednisone should be administered to patients with fever or other symptoms. The dosage should be tapered slowly after the resolution of radiation pneumonitis, because abrupt withdrawal of glucocorticoids may cause an exacerbation of pneumonia. Delayed radiation fibrosis may occur years after radiation therapy and is signaled by dyspnea on exertion. Often it is mild, but it can progress to chronic respiratory failure. Therapy is supportive.

Classical radiation pneumonitis that leads to pulmonary fibrosis is due to radiation-induced production of local cytokines such as platelet-derived growth factor β, tumor necrosis factor, interleukins, and transforming growth factor β in the radiation field. An immunologically mediated sporadic radiation pneumonitis occurs in about 10% of patients; bilateral alveolitis mediated by T cells results in infiltrates outside the radiation field. This form of radiation pneumonitis usually resolves without sequelae.

Pneumonia is a common problem in patients undergoing treatment for cancer. Bacterial pneumonia typically causes a localized infiltrate on chest radiographs. Therapy is tailored to the causative organism. When diffuse interstitial infiltrates appear in a febrile patient, the differential diagnosis is extensive and includes pneumonia due to infection with *Pneumocystis carinii*; viral infections including cytomegalovirus, adenovirus, herpes simplex virus, herpes zoster, respiratory syncytial virus, or intracellular pathogens such as *Mycoplasma* and *Legionella*; effects of drugs or radiation; tumor progression; nonspecific pneumonitis; and fungal disease. Detection of opportunistic pathogens in pulmonary infections is still a challenge. Diagnostic tools include chest radiographs, CT scans, bronchoscopy with bronchoalveolar lavage, brush cytology, transbronchial biopsy, fine-needle aspiration, and open lung biopsy. In addition to the culture, evaluation of bronchoalveolar lavage fluid for *P. carinii* by polymerase chain reaction (PCR) and serum galactomannan test improve the diagnostic yield. Patients with cancer who are neutropenic and have fever and local infiltrates on chest radiograph should be treated initially with broad-spectrum antibiotics. A new or persistent focal infiltrate not responding to broad-spectrum antibiotics argues for initiation of empiric antifungal therapy. When diffuse bilateral infiltrates develop in patients with febrile neutropenia, broad-spectrum antibiotics plus trimethoprim-sulfamethoxazole, with or without erythromycin, should be initiated. Addition of an antiviral agent is necessary in some settings, such as patients undergoing allogeneic hematopoietic stem cell transplantation. If the patient does not improve in 4 days, open lung biopsy is the procedure of choice. Bronchoscopy with bronchoalveolar lavage may be used in patients who are poor candidates for surgery.

In patients with pulmonary infiltrates who are afebrile, heart failure and multiple pulmonary emboli are in the differential diagnosis.

NEUTROPENIC ENTEROCOLITIS

Neutropenic enterocolitis (typhlitis) is the inflammation and necrosis of the cecum and surrounding tissues that may complicate the treatment

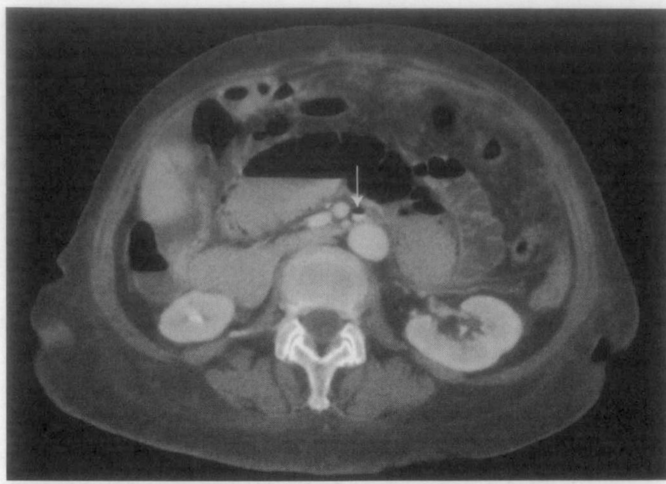

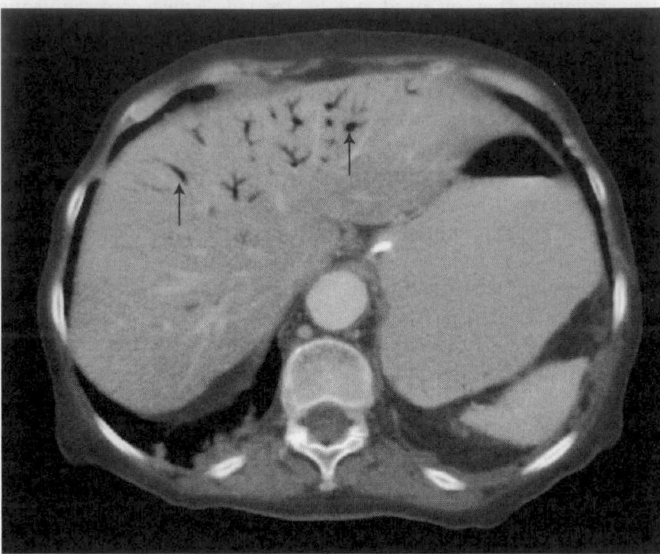

FIGURE 331-5 Abdominal computed tomography (CT) scans of a 72-year-old woman with neutropenic enterocolitis secondary to chemotherapy. ***A.*** Air in inferior mesenteric vein (*arrow*) and bowel wall with pneumatosis intestinalis. ***B.*** CT scan of upper abdomen demonstrating air in portal vein (*arrows*).

of acute leukemia. Nevertheless, it may involve any segment of the gastrointestinal tract including small intestine, appendix, and colon. This complication has also been seen in patients with other forms of cancer treated with taxanes, 5-fluorouracil, irinotecan, vinorelbine, cisplatin, carboplatin, and high-dose chemotherapy (Fig. 331-5). It also has been reported in patients with AIDS, aplastic anemia, cyclic neutropenia, idiosyncratic drug reactions involving antibiotics, and immunosuppressive therapies. The patient develops right lower quadrant abdominal pain, often with rebound tenderness and a tense, distended abdomen, in a setting of fever and neutropenia. Watery diarrhea (often containing sloughed mucosa) and bacteremia are common, and bleeding may occur. Plain abdominal films are generally of little value in the diagnosis; CT scan may show marked bowel wall thickening, particularly in the cecum, with bowel wall edema, mesenteric stranding, and ascites, and may help to differentiate neutropenic colitis from other abdominal disorders such as appendicitis, diverticulitis, and *Clostridium difficile*–associated colitis in this high-risk population. Patients with bowel wall thickness >10 mm on ultrasonogram have higher mortality rates. However, bowel wall thickening is significantly more prominent in patients with *C. difficile* colitis. Pneumatosis intestinalis is a more specific finding, seen only in those with neutropenic enterocolitis and ischemia. The combined involvement of the small and large bowel suggests a diagnosis of neutropenic enterocolitis. Rapid institution of broad-spectrum antibiotics, bowel rest, and nasogastric suction may reverse the process. Use of myeloid growth factors improved outcome significantly. Surgical intervention is reserved for severe cases of neutropenic enterocolitis with evidence of perforation, peritonitis, gangrenous bowel, or gastrointestinal hemorrhage despite correction of any coagulopathy.

C. difficile colitis is increasing in incidence. Newer strains of *C. difficile* produce about 20 times more of toxins A and B compared to previously studied strains. *C. difficile* risk is also increased with chemotherapy. Antibiotic coverage for *C. difficile* should be added if pseudomembranous colitis cannot be excluded.

HEMORRHAGIC CYSTITIS

Hemorrhagic cystitis can develop in patients receiving cyclophosphamide or ifosfamide. Both drugs are metabolized to acrolein, which is a strong chemical irritant that is excreted in the urine. Prolonged contact or high concentrations may lead to bladder irritation and hemorrhage. Symptoms include gross hematuria, frequency, dysuria, burning, urgency, incontinence, and nocturia. The best management is prevention. Maintaining a high rate of urine flow minimizes exposure. In addition, 2-mercaptoethanesulfonate (mesna) detoxifies the metabolites and can be coadministered with the instigating drugs. Mesna usually is given three times on the day of ifosfamide administration in doses that are each 20% of the total ifosfamide dose. If hemorrhagic cystitis develops, the maintenance of a high urine flow may be sufficient supportive care. If conservative management is not effective, irrigation of the bladder with a 0.37–0.74% formalin solution for 10 min stops the bleeding in most cases. N-Acetylcysteine may also be an effective irrigant. Prostaglandin (carboprost) can inhibit the process. In extreme cases, ligation of the hypogastric arteries, urinary diversion, or cystectomy may be necessary.

Hemorrhagic cystitis also occurs in patients who undergo bone marrow transplantation (BMT). In the BMT setting, early-onset hemorrhagic cystitis is related to drugs in the treatment regimen (e.g., cyclophosphamide), and late-onset hemorrhagic cystitis is usually due to the polyoma virus BKV or adenovirus type 11. BKV load in urine alone or in combination with acute graft-versus-host disease correlates with development of hemorrhagic cystitis. Viral causes are usually detected by PCR-based diagnostic tests. Treatment of viral hemorrhagic cystitis is largely supportive, with reduction in doses of immunosuppressive agents, if possible. No antiviral therapy is approved, although cidofovir is reported to be effective in a small series. Hyperbaric oxygen therapy has been used successfully in patients with BKV-associated and cyclophosphamide-induced hemorrhagic cystitis during hematopoietic stem cell transplantation, as well as in hemorrhagic radiation cystitis.

HYPERSENSITIVITY REACTIONS TO ANTINEOPLASTIC DRUGS

Many antineoplastic drugs may cause hypersensitivity reaction. These reactions are unpredictable and potentially life-threatening. Most reactions occur during or within hours of parenteral drug administration. Taxanes, platinum compounds, asparaginase, etoposide, procarbazine, and biologic agents, including rituximab, bevacizumab, trastuzumab, gemtuzumab, cetuximab, and alemtuzumab, are more commonly associated with acute hypersensitivity reactions than are other agents. Acute hypersensitivity reactions to some drugs, such as taxanes, occur during the first or second dose administered. Hypersensitivity to platinum compounds occurs after prolonged exposure. Skin testing may identify patients with high risk for hypersensitivity after carboplatin exposure. Premedication with histamine H_1 and H_2 receptor antagonists and glucocorticoids reduces the incidence of hypersensitivity reaction to taxanes, particularly paclitaxel. Despite premedication, hypersensitivity reactions may still occur. In these cases, rapid desensitization in the intensive care unit setting or re-treatment may be attempted with care, but the use of alternative agents may be required. Candidate patients for desensitization include those who have mild to severe hypersensitivity type I, with mast cell–mediated and IgE-dependent reactions occurring during a chemotherapy infusion or shortly thereafter.

332e Cellular and Molecular Biology of the Kidney

Alfred L. George, Jr., Eric G. Neilson

This is a digital-only chapter. It is available on the DVD that accompanies this book, as well as on Access Medicine/Harrison's Online, and the eBook and "app" editions of HPIM 19e.

The kidney is one of the most highly differentiated organs in the body. At the conclusion of embryologic development, nearly 30 different cell types form a multitude of filtering capillaries and segmented nephrons enveloped by a dynamic interstitium. This cellular diversity modulates a variety of complex physiologic processes. Endocrine functions, the regulation of blood pressure and intraglomerular hemodynamics, solute and water transport, acid-base balance, and removal of drug metabolites are all accomplished by intricate mechanisms of renal response. This breadth of physiology hinges on the clever ingenuity of nephron architecture that evolved as complex organisms came out of water to live on land.

333e Adaptation of the Kidney to Injury

Joseph V. Bonventre

This is a digital-only chapter. It is available on the DVD that accompanies this book, as well as on Access Medicine/Harrison's Online, and the eBook and "app" editions of HPIM 19e.

Many years ago Claude Bernard (1878) introduced the concepts of *milieu extérieur* (the environment where an organism lives) and a *milieu intérieur* (the environment in which the tissues of that organism live). He argued that the milieu intérieur varied very little and that there were vital mechanisms that functioned to maintain this internal environment constant. Walter B. Cannon later extended these concepts by recognizing that the constancy of the internal state, which he termed the *homeostatic state*, was evidence of physiologic mechanisms that act to maintain this minimal variability. In higher animals, the plasma is maintained remarkably constant in composition both within an individual and among individuals. The kidney plays a vital role in this constancy. The kidney changes the composition of the urine to maintain electrolyte and acid-base balance and can produce hormones that can maintain constancy of blood hemoglobin and mineral metabolism. When the kidney is injured, the remaining functional mass responds and attempts to continue to maintain the milieu intérieur. It is remarkable how well the residual nephrons can perform in this task so that in many cases homeostasis is maintained until the glomerular filtration rate (GFR) drops to very low levels. At this point, the functional tissue can no longer compensate. In this chapter, we will discuss a number of these compensatory adaptations that the kidney makes in response to injury in an attempt to protect itself and protect the milieu intérieur. A theme that permeates, however, is that these adaptive processes can often be maladaptive and contribute to enhanced renal dysfunction, facilitating a positive feedback process that is inherently unstable.

334 Acute Kidney Injury

Sushrut S. Waikar, Joseph V. Bonventre

Acute kidney injury (AKI), previously known as acute renal failure, is characterized by the sudden impairment of kidney function resulting in the retention of nitrogenous and other waste products normally cleared by the kidneys. AKI is not a single disease but, rather, a designation for a heterogeneous group of conditions that share common diagnostic features: specifically, an increase in the blood urea nitrogen (BUN) concentration and/or an increase in the plasma or serum creatinine (SCr) concentration, often associated with a reduction in urine volume. It is important to recognize that AKI is a clinical diagnosis and not a structural one. A patient may have AKI without injury to the kidney parenchyma. AKI can range in severity from asymptomatic and transient changes in laboratory parameters of glomerular filtration rate (GFR), to overwhelming and rapidly fatal derangements in effective circulating volume regulation and electrolyte and acid-base composition of the plasma.

EPIDEMIOLOGY

AKI complicates 5–7% of acute care hospital admissions and up to 30% of admissions to the intensive care unit, particularly in the setting of diarrheal illnesses, infectious diseases like malaria and leptospirosis, and natural disasters such as earthquakes. The incidence of AKI has grown by more than fourfold in the United States since 1988 and is estimated to have a yearly incidence of 500 per 100,000 population, higher than the yearly incidence of stroke. AKI is associated with a markedly increased risk of death in hospitalized individuals, particularly in those admitted to the ICU where in-hospital mortality rates may exceed 50%. AKI increases the risk for the development or worsening of chronic kidney disease. Patients who survive and recover from an episode of severe AKI requiring dialysis are at increased risk for the later development of dialysis-requiring end-stage kidney disease. AKI may be community-acquired or hospital-acquired. Common causes of community-acquired AKI include volume depletion, adverse effects of medications, and obstruction of the urinary tract. The most common clinical settings for hospital-acquired AKI are sepsis, major surgical procedures, critical illness involving heart or liver failure, intravenous iodinated contrast administration, and nephrotoxic medication administration.

AKI IN THE DEVELOPING WORLD

AKI is also a major medical complication in the developing world, where the epidemiology differs from that in developed countries due to differences in demographics, economics, geography, and comorbid disease burden. While certain features of AKI are common to both—particularly since urban centers of some developing countries increasingly resemble those in the developed world—many etiologies for AKI are region-specific such as envenomations from snakes, spiders, caterpillars, and bees; infectious causes such as malaria and leptospirosis; and crush injuries and resultant rhabdomyolysis from earthquakes.

ETIOLOGY AND PATHOPHYSIOLOGY

The causes of AKI have traditionally been divided into three broad categories: prerenal azotemia, intrinsic renal parenchymal disease, and postrenal obstruction (Fig. 334-1).

PRERENAL AZOTEMIA

Prerenal azotemia (from "azo," meaning nitrogen, and "-emia") is the most common form of AKI. It is the designation for a rise in SCr or BUN concentration due to inadequate renal plasma flow and intraglomerular hydrostatic pressure to support normal glomerular

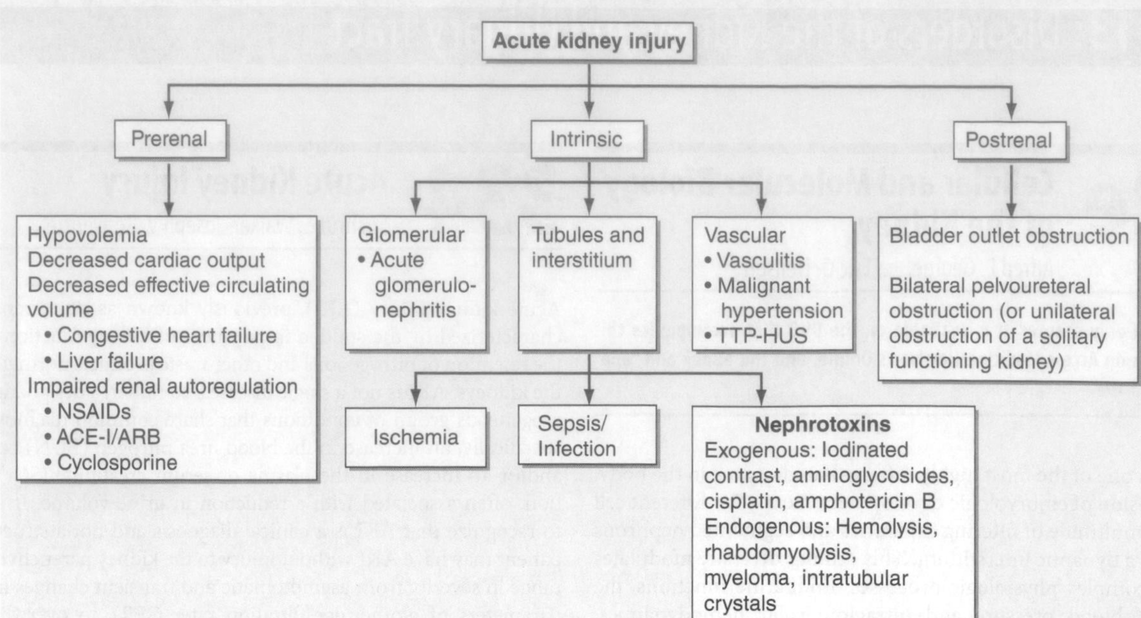

FIGURE 334-1 Classification of the major causes of acute kidney injury. ACE-I, angiotensin-converting enzyme inhibitor-I; ARB, angiotensin receptor blocker; NSAIDs, nonsteroidal anti-inflammatory drugs; TTP-HUS, thrombotic thrombocytopenic purpura–hemolytic-uremic syndrome.

filtration. The most common clinical conditions associated with prerenal azotemia are hypovolemia, decreased cardiac output, and medications that interfere with renal autoregulatory responses such as nonsteroidal anti-inflammatory drugs (NSAIDs) and inhibitors of angiotensin II (Fig. 334-2). Prerenal azotemia may coexist with other forms of intrinsic AKI associated with processes acting directly on the renal parenchyma. Prolonged periods of prerenal azotemia may lead to ischemic injury, often termed acute tubular necrosis (ATN). By definition, prerenal azotemia involves no parenchymal damage to the kidney and is rapidly reversible once intraglomerular hemodynamics are restored.

Normal GFR is maintained in part by the relative resistances of the afferent and efferent renal arterioles, which determine the glomerular plasma flow and the transcapillary hydraulic pressure gradient that drive glomerular ultrafiltration. Mild degrees of hypovolemia and reductions in cardiac output elicit compensatory renal physiologic changes. Because renal blood flow accounts for 20% of the cardiac output, renal vasoconstriction and salt and water reabsorption occur as homeostatic responses to decreased effective circulating volume or cardiac output in order to maintain blood pressure and increase intravascular volume to sustain perfusion to the cerebral and coronary vessels. Mediators of this response include angiotensin II, norepinephrine, and vasopressin (also termed antidiuretic hormone). Glomerular filtration can be maintained despite reduced renal blood flow by angiotensin II–mediated renal efferent vasoconstriction, which maintains glomerular capillary hydrostatic pressure closer to normal and thereby prevents marked reductions in GFR if renal blood flow reduction is not excessive.

In addition, a myogenic reflex within the afferent arteriole leads to dilation in the setting of low perfusion pressure, thereby maintaining glomerular perfusion. Intrarenal biosynthesis of vasodilator prostaglandins (prostacyclin, prostaglandin E_2), kallikrein and kinins, and possibly nitric oxide (NO) also increase in response to low renal perfusion pressure. Autoregulation is also accomplished by tubuloglomerular feedback, in which decreases in solute delivery to the macula densa (specialized cells within the distal tubule) elicit dilation of the juxtaposed afferent arteriole in order to maintain glomerular perfusion, a mechanism mediated, in part, by NO. There is a limit, however, to the ability of these counterregulatory mechanisms to maintain GFR in the face of systemic hypotension. Even in healthy adults, renal autoregulation usually fails once the systolic blood pressure falls below 80 mmHg.

A number of factors determine the robustness of the autoregulatory response and the risk of prerenal azotemia. Atherosclerosis, long-standing hypertension, and older age can lead to hyalinosis and myointimal hyperplasia, causing structural narrowing of the intrarenal arterioles and impaired capacity for renal afferent vasodilation. In chronic kidney disease, renal afferent vasodilation may be operating at maximal capacity in order to maximize GFR in response to reduced functional renal mass. Drugs can affect the compensatory changes evoked to maintain GFR. NSAIDs inhibit renal prostaglandin production, limiting renal afferent vasodilation. Angiotensin-converting enzyme (ACE) inhibitors and angiotensin receptor blockers (ARBs) limit renal efferent vasoconstriction; this effect is particularly pronounced in patients with bilateral renal artery stenosis or unilateral renal artery stenosis (in the case of a solitary functioning kidney) because renal efferent vasoconstriction is needed to maintain GFR due to low renal perfusion. The combined use of NSAIDs with ACE inhibitors or ARBs poses a particularly high risk for developing prerenal azotemia.

Many individuals with advanced cirrhosis exhibit a unique hemodynamic profile that resembles prerenal azotemia despite total-body volume overload. Systemic vascular resistance is markedly reduced due to primary arterial vasodilation in the splanchnic circulation, resulting ultimately in activation of vasoconstrictor responses similar to those seen in hypovolemia. AKI is a common complication in this setting, and it can be triggered by volume depletion and spontaneous bacterial peritonitis. A particularly poor prognosis is seen in the case of type 1 hepatorenal syndrome, in which AKI without an alternate cause (e.g., shock and nephrotoxic drugs) persists despite volume administration and withholding of diuretics. Type 2 hepatorenal syndrome is a less severe form characterized mainly by refractory ascites.

INTRINSIC AKI

The most common causes of intrinsic AKI are sepsis, ischemia, and nephrotoxins, both endogenous and exogenous (Fig. 334-3). In many cases, prerenal azotemia advances to tubular injury. Although classically termed "acute tubular necrosis," human biopsy confirmation of tubular necrosis is, in general, often lacking in cases of sepsis and ischemia; indeed, processes such as inflammation, apoptosis, and altered regional perfusion may be important contributors pathophysiologically. Other causes of intrinsic AKI are less common and can be conceptualized anatomically according to the major site of renal parenchymal damage: glomeruli, tubulointerstitium, and vessels.

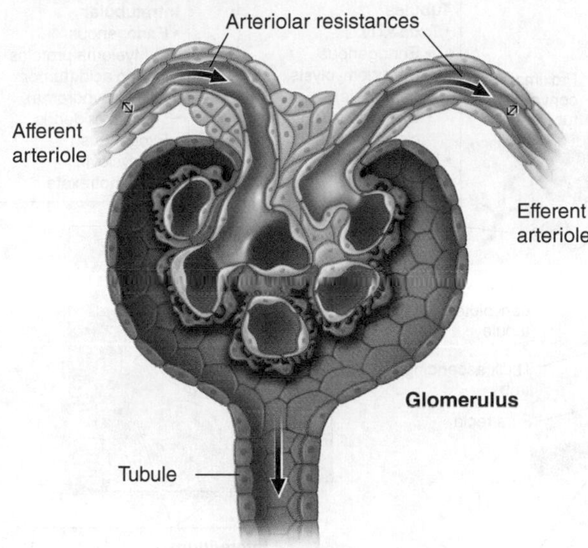

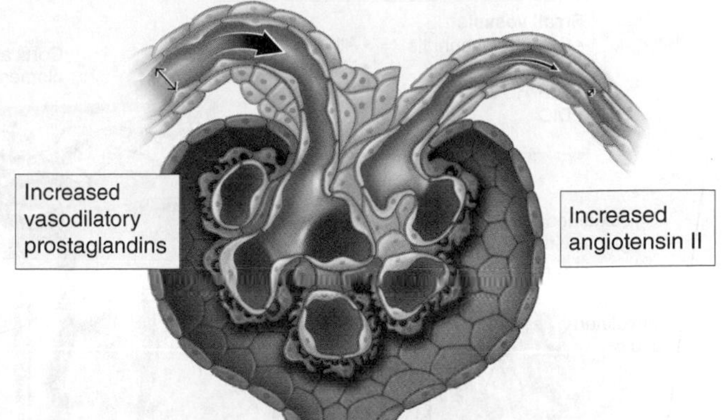

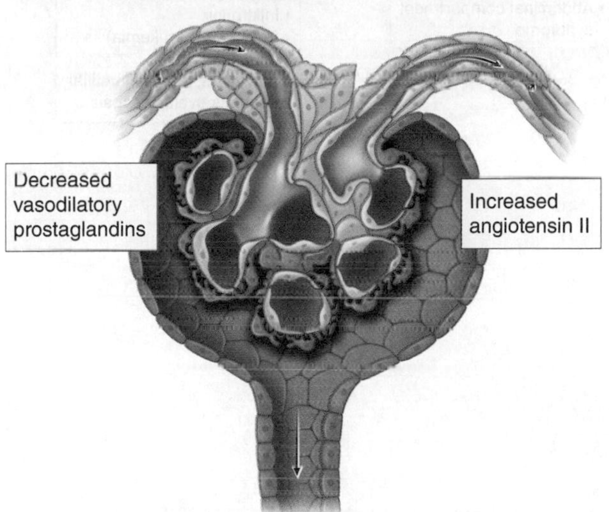

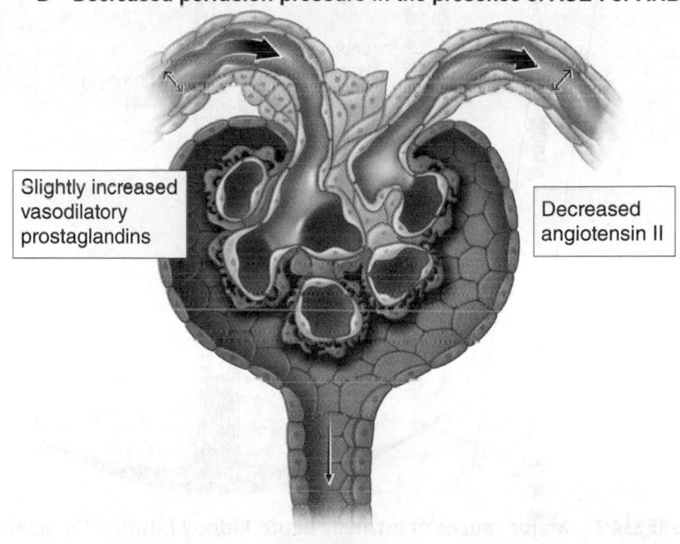

FIGURE 334-2 Intrarenal mechanisms for autoregulation of the glomerular filtration rate (GFR) under decreased perfusion pressure and reduction of the GFR by drugs. *A.* Normal conditions and a normal GFR. ***B.*** Reduced perfusion pressure within the autoregulatory range. Normal glomerular capillary pressure is maintained by afferent vasodilatation and efferent vasoconstriction. ***C.*** Reduced perfusion pressure with a nonsteroidal anti-inflammatory drug (NSAID). Loss of vasodilatory prostaglandins increases afferent resistance; this causes the glomerular capillary pressure to drop below normal values and the GFR to decrease. ***D.*** Reduced perfusion pressure with an angiotensin-converting enzyme inhibitor (ACE-I) or an angiotensin receptor blocker (ARB). Loss of angiotensin II action reduces efferent resistance; this causes the glomerular capillary pressure to drop below normal values and the GFR to decrease. *(From JG Abuelo: N Engl J Med 357:797-805, 2007; with permission.)*

SEPSIS-ASSOCIATED AKI

In the United States, more than 700,000 cases of sepsis occur each year. AKI complicates more than 50% of cases of severe sepsis and greatly increases the risk of death. Sepsis is also a very important cause of AKI in the developing world. Decreases in GFR with sepsis can occur even in the absence of overt hypotension, although most cases of severe AKI typically occur in the setting of hemodynamic collapse requiring vasopressor support. While there is clearly tubular injury associated with AKI in sepsis as manifest by the presence of tubular debris and casts in the urine, postmortem examinations of kidneys from individuals with severe sepsis suggest that other factors, perhaps related to inflammation, mitochondrial dysfunction, and interstitial edema, must be considered in the pathophysiology of sepsis-induced AKI.

The hemodynamic effects of sepsis—arising from generalized arterial vasodilation, mediated in part by cytokines that upregulate the expression of inducible NO synthase in the vasculature—can lead to a reduction in GFR. The operative mechanisms may be excessive efferent arteriole vasodilation, particularly early in the course of sepsis, or renal vasoconstriction from activation of the sympathetic nervous system, the renin-angiotensin-aldosterone system, vasopressin, and endothelin. Sepsis may lead to endothelial damage, which results in microvascular thrombosis, activation of reactive oxygen species, and leukocyte adhesion and migration, all of which may injure renal tubular cells.

ISCHEMIA-ASSOCIATED AKI

Healthy kidneys receive 20% of the cardiac output and account for 10% of resting oxygen consumption, despite constituting only 0.5% of the human body mass. The kidneys are also the site of one of the most hypoxic regions in the body, the renal medulla. The outer medulla is particularly vulnerable to ischemic damage because of the

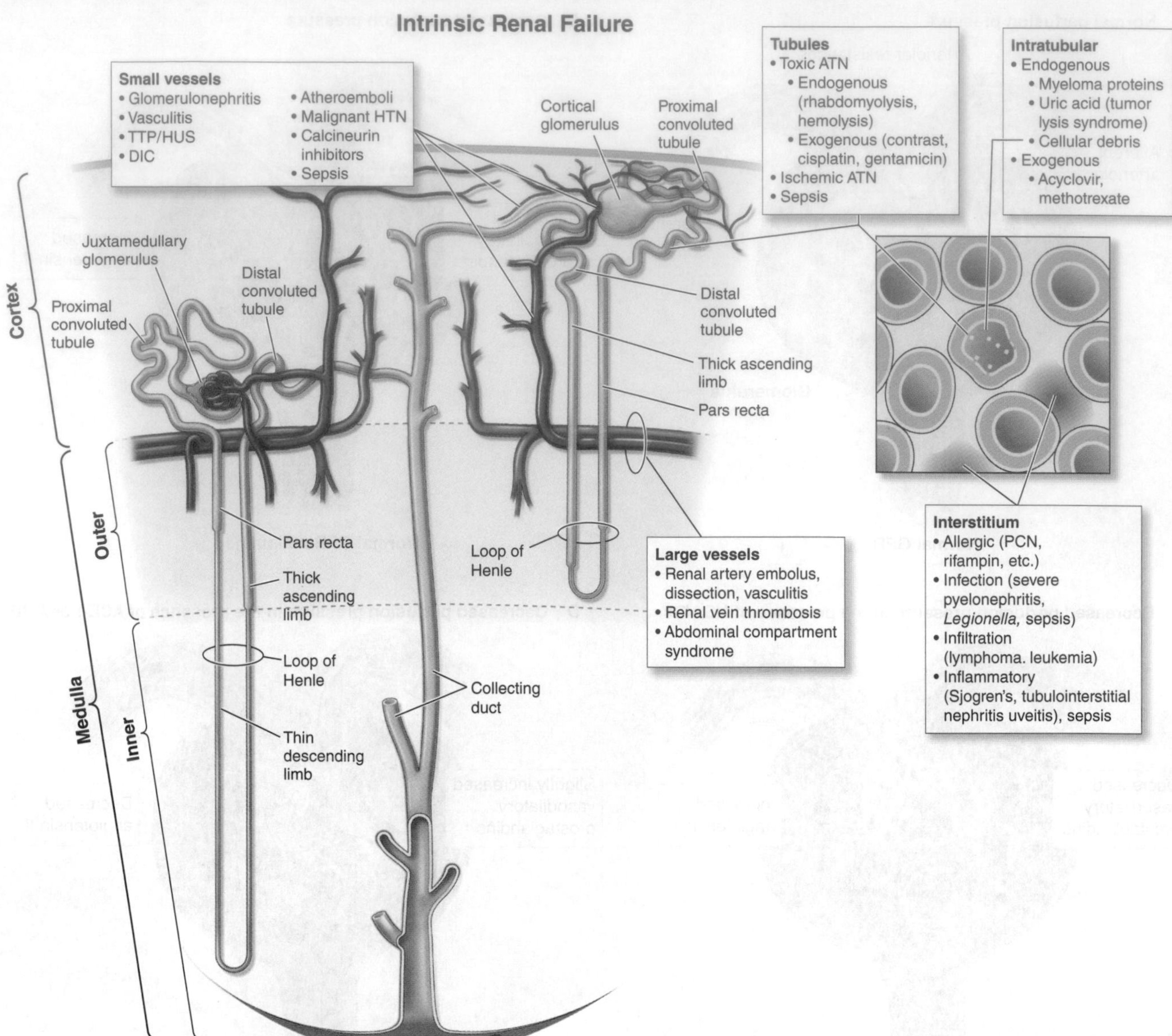

FIGURE 334-3 Major causes of intrinsic acute kidney injury. ATN, acute tubular necrosis; DIC, disseminated intravascular coagulation; HTN, hypertension; PCN, penicillin; TTP/HUS, thrombotic thrombocytopenic purpura/hemolytic-uremic syndrome; TINU, tubulointerstitial nephritis-uveitis.

architecture of the blood vessels that supply oxygen and nutrients to the tubules. Enhanced leukocyte-endothelial interactions in the small vessels lead to inflammation and reduced local blood flow to the metabolically very active S3 segment of the proximal tubule, which depends on oxidative metabolism for survival. Ischemia alone in a normal kidney is usually not sufficient to cause severe AKI, as evidenced by the relatively low risk of severe AKI even after total interruption of renal blood flow during suprarenal aortic clamping or cardiac arrest. Clinically, AKI more commonly develops when ischemia occurs in the context of limited renal reserve (e.g., chronic kidney disease or older age) or coexisting insults such as sepsis, vasoactive or nephrotoxic drugs, rhabdomyolysis, or the systemic inflammatory states associated with burns and pancreatitis. Prerenal azotemia and ischemia-associated AKI represent a continuum of the manifestations of renal hypoperfusion. Persistent preglomerular vasoconstriction may be a common underlying cause of the reduction in GFR seen in AKI; implicated factors for vasoconstriction include activation of tubuloglomerular feedback from enhanced delivery of solute to the macula densa following proximal tubule injury, increased basal vascular tone and reactivity to vasoconstrictive agents, and decreased vasodilator responsiveness. Other contributors to low GFR include backleak of filtrate across damaged and denuded tubular epithelium and mechanical obstruction of tubules from necrotic debris (Fig. 334-4).

Postoperative AKI Ischemia-associated AKI is a serious complication in the postoperative period, especially after major operations involving significant blood loss and intraoperative hypotension. The procedures most commonly associated with AKI are cardiac surgery with cardiopulmonary bypass (particularly for combined valve and bypass procedures), vascular procedures with aortic cross clamping, and intraperitoneal procedures. Severe AKI requiring dialysis occurs in approximately 1% of cardiac and vascular surgery procedures. The risk of severe AKI has been less well studied for major intraperitoneal procedures but appears to be of comparable magnitude. Common risk factors for postoperative AKI include underlying chronic kidney disease, older age, diabetes mellitus, congestive heart failure, and emergency procedures. The pathophysiology of AKI following cardiac surgery is multifactorial. Major AKI risk factors are common in the population undergoing cardiac surgery. The use of nephrotoxic agents including iodinated contrast for cardiac imaging prior to surgery may increase the risk of AKI. Cardiopulmonary bypass is a unique hemodynamic state characterized by nonpulsatile flow and exposure of the circulation to extracorporeal circuits. Longer duration of cardiopulmonary bypass is a risk factor for AKI. In addition to ischemic

Pathophysiology of Ischemic Acute Renal Failure

MICROVASCULAR (Glomerular, Medullary)		TUBULAR
↑ Vasoconstriction *in response to*: endothelin, adenosine, angiotensin II, thromboxane A2, leukotrienes, sympathetic nerve activity	↓O_2	Cytoskeletal breakdown
↓ Vasodilation *in response to*: nitric oxide, PGE_2, acetylcholine, bradykinin		Loss of polarity
↑ Endothelial and vascular smooth muscle cell structural damage	← Inflammatory and vasoactive mediators	Apoptosis and necrosis
↑ Leukocyte-endothelial adhesion, vascular obstruction, leukocyte activation, and inflammation		Desquamation of viable and necrotic cells
		Tubular obstruction
		Backleak

FIGURE 334-4 Interacting microvascular and tubular events contributing to the pathophysiology of ischemic acute kidney injury. PGE_2, prostaglandin E_2. *(From JV Bonventre, JM Weinberg: J Am Soc Nephrol 14:2199, 2003.)*

injury from sustained hypoperfusion, cardiopulmonary bypass may cause AKI through a number of mechanisms including extracorporeal circuit activation of leukocytes and inflammatory processes, hemolysis with resultant pigment nephropathy (see below), and aortic injury with resultant atheroemboli. AKI from atheroembolic disease, which can also occur following percutaneous catheterization of the aorta, or spontaneously, is due to cholesterol crystal embolization resulting in partial or total occlusion of multiple small arteries within the kidney. Over time, a foreign body reaction can result in intimal proliferation, giant cell formation, and further narrowing of the vascular lumen, accounting for the generally subacute (over a period of weeks rather than days) decline in renal function.

Burns and Acute Pancreatitis Extensive fluid losses into the extravascular compartments of the body frequently accompany severe burns and acute pancreatitis. AKI is an ominous complication of burns, affecting 25% of individuals with more than 10% total body surface area involvement. In addition to severe hypovolemia resulting in decreased cardiac output and increased neurohormonal activation, burns and acute pancreatitis both lead to dysregulated inflammation and an increased risk of sepsis and acute lung injury, all of which may facilitate the development and progression of AKI. Individuals undergoing massive fluid resuscitation for trauma, burns, and acute pancreatitis can also develop the abdominal compartment syndrome, where markedly elevated intraabdominal pressures, usually higher than 20 mmHg, lead to renal vein compression and reduced GFR.

Diseases of the Microvasculature Leading to Ischemia Microvascular causes of AKI include the thrombotic microangiopathies (antiphospholipid antibody syndrome, radiation nephritis, malignant nephrosclerosis, and thrombotic thrombocytopenic purpura/hemolytic-uremic syndrome [TTP-HUS]), scleroderma, and atheroembolic disease. Large-vessel diseases associated with AKI include renal artery dissection, thromboembolism, thrombosis, and renal vein compression or thrombosis.

NEPHROTOXIN-ASSOCIATED AKI

The kidney has very high susceptibility to nephrotoxicity due to extremely high blood perfusion and concentration of circulating substances along the nephron where water is reabsorbed and in the medullary interstitium; this results in high-concentration exposure of toxins to tubular, interstitial, and endothelial cells. Nephrotoxic injury occurs in response to a number of pharmacologic compounds with diverse structures, endogenous substances, and environmental exposures. All structures of the kidney are vulnerable to toxic injury, including the tubules, interstitium, vasculature, and collecting system. As with other forms of AKI, risk factors for nephrotoxicity include older age, chronic kidney disease (CKD), and prerenal azotemia. Hypoalbuminemia may increase the risk of some forms of nephrotoxin-associated AKI due to increased free circulating drug concentrations.

Contrast Agents Iodinated contrast agents used for cardiovascular and computed tomography (CT) imaging are a leading cause of AKI. The risk of AKI, or "contrast nephropathy," is negligible in those with normal renal function but increases markedly in the setting of CKD, particularly diabetic nephropathy. The most common clinical course of contrast nephropathy is characterized by a rise in SCr beginning 24–48 h following exposure, peaking within 3–5 days, and resolving within 1 week. More severe, dialysis-requiring AKI is uncommon except in the setting of significant preexisting CKD, often in association with congestive heart failure or other coexisting causes for ischemia-associated AKI. Patients with multiple myeloma and renal disease are particularly susceptible. Low fractional excretion of sodium and relatively benign urinary sediment without features of tubular necrosis (see below) are common findings. Contrast nephropathy is thought to occur from a combination of factors, including (1) hypoxia in the renal outer medulla due to perturbations in renal microcirculation and occlusion of small vessels; (2) cytotoxic damage to the tubules directly or via the generation of oxygen free radicals, especially because the concentration of the agent within the tubule is markedly increased; and (3) transient tubule obstruction with precipitated contrast material. Other diagnostic agents implicated as a cause of AKI are high-dose gadolinium used for magnetic resonance imaging (MRI) and oral sodium phosphate solutions used as bowel purgatives.

Antibiotics Several antimicrobial agents are commonly associated with AKI. *Aminoglycosides and amphotericin B* both cause tubular necrosis. Nonoliguric AKI (i.e., without a significant reduction in urine volume) accompanies 10–30% of courses of aminoglycoside antibiotics, even when plasma levels are in the therapeutic range. Aminoglycosides are freely filtered across the glomerulus and then accumulate within the renal cortex, where concentrations can greatly exceed those of the plasma. AKI typically manifests after 5–7 days of therapy and can present even after the drug has been discontinued. Hypomagnesemia is a common finding.

Amphotericin B causes renal vasoconstriction from an increase in tubuloglomerular feedback as well as direct tubular toxicity mediated by reactive oxygen species. Nephrotoxicity from amphotericin B is dose and duration dependent. This drug binds to tubular membrane cholesterol and introduces pores. Clinical features of amphotericin B nephrotoxicity include polyuria, hypomagnesemia, hypocalcemia, and nongap metabolic acidosis.

Vancomycin may be associated with AKI, particularly when trough levels are high, but a causal relationship with AKI has not been definitively established. *Acyclovir* can precipitate in tubules and cause AKI by tubular obstruction, particularly when given as an intravenous bolus at high doses (500 mg/m^2) or in the setting of hypovolemia. *Foscarnet*, *pentamidine*, *tenofovir*, and *cidofovir* are also frequently associated with AKI due to tubular toxicity. AKI secondary to acute interstitial nephritis can occur as a consequence of exposure to many antibiotics, including *penicillins*, *cephalosporins*, *quinolones*, *sulfonamides*, and *rifampin*.

Chemotherapeutic Agents *Cisplatin* and *carboplatin* are accumulated by proximal tubular cells and cause necrosis and apoptosis. Intensive hydration regimens have reduced the incidence of cisplatin nephrotoxicity, but it remains a dose-limiting toxicity. *Ifosfamide* may cause hemorrhagic cystitis and tubular toxicity, manifested as type II renal tubular acidosis (Fanconi's syndrome), polyuria, hypokalemia, and a modest decline in GFR. Antiangiogenesis agents, such as *bevacizumab*, can cause proteinuria and hypertension via injury to the glomerular microvasculature (thrombotic microangiopathy). Other antineoplastic agents such as mitomycin C and gemcitabine may cause thrombotic microangiopathy with resultant AKI.

Toxic Ingestions Ethylene glycol, present in automobile antifreeze, is metabolized to oxalic acid, glycolaldehyde, and glyoxylate, which may cause AKI through direct tubular injury. Diethylene glycol is an industrial agent that has been the cause of outbreaks of severe AKI around the world due to adulteration of pharmaceutical preparations. The metabolite 2-hydroxyethoxyacetic acid (HEAA) is thought to be responsible for tubular injury. Melamine contamination of foodstuffs has led to nephrolithiasis and AKI, either through intratubular obstruction or possibly direct tubular toxicity. Aristolochic acid was found to be the cause of "Chinese herb nephropathy" and "Balkan nephropathy" due to contamination of medicinal herbs or farming. The list of environmental toxins is likely to grow and contribute to a better understanding of previously catalogued "idiopathic" chronic tubular interstitial disease, a common diagnosis in both the developed and developing world.

Endogenous Toxins AKI may be caused by a number of endogenous compounds, including myoglobin, hemoglobin, uric acid, and myeloma light chains. Myoglobin can be released by injured muscle cells, and hemoglobin can be released during massive hemolysis leading to pigment nephropathy. Rhabdomyolysis may result from traumatic crush injuries, muscle ischemia during vascular or orthopedic surgery, compression during coma or immobilization, prolonged seizure activity, excessive exercise, heat stroke or malignant hyperthermia, infections, metabolic disorders (e.g., hypophosphatemia, severe hypothyroidism), and myopathies (drug-induced, metabolic, or inflammatory). Pathogenic factors for AKI include intrarenal vasoconstriction, direct proximal tubular toxicity, and mechanical obstruction of the distal nephron lumen when myoglobin or hemoglobin precipitates with Tamm-Horsfall protein (uromodulin, the most common protein in urine and produced in the thick ascending limb of the loop of Henle), a process favored by acidic urine. Tumor lysis syndrome may follow initiation of cytotoxic therapy in patients with high-grade lymphomas and acute lymphoblastic leukemia; massive release of uric acid (with serum levels often exceeding 15 mg/dL) leads to precipitation of uric acid in the renal tubules and AKI (Chap. 331). Other features of tumor lysis syndrome include hyperkalemia and hyperphosphatemia. The tumor lysis syndrome can also occasionally occur spontaneously or with treatment for solid tumors or multiple myeloma. Myeloma light chains can also cause AKI by direct tubular toxicity and by binding to Tamm-Horsfall protein to form obstructing intratubular casts. Hypercalcemia, which can also be seen in multiple myeloma, may cause AKI by intense renal vasoconstriction and volume depletion.

Allergic Acute Tubulointerstitial Disease and Other Causes of Intrinsic AKI While many of the ischemic and toxic causes of AKI previously described result in tubulointerstitial disease, many drugs are also associated with the development of an allergic response characterized by an inflammatory infiltrate and often peripheral and urinary eosinophilia. AKI may be caused by severe infections and infiltrative diseases. Diseases of the glomeruli or vasculature can lead to AKI by compromising blood flow within the renal circulation. Glomerulonephritis and vasculitis are less common causes of AKI. It is particularly important to recognize these diseases early because they require timely treatment with immunosuppressive agents or therapeutic plasma exchange.

POSTRENAL ACUTE KIDNEY INJURY

(See also Chap. 343) Postrenal AKI occurs when the normally unidirectional flow of urine is acutely blocked either partially or totally, leading to increased retrograde hydrostatic pressure and interference with glomerular filtration. Obstruction to urinary flow may be caused by functional or structural derangements anywhere from the renal pelvis to the tip of the urethra (Fig. 334-5). Normal urinary flow rate

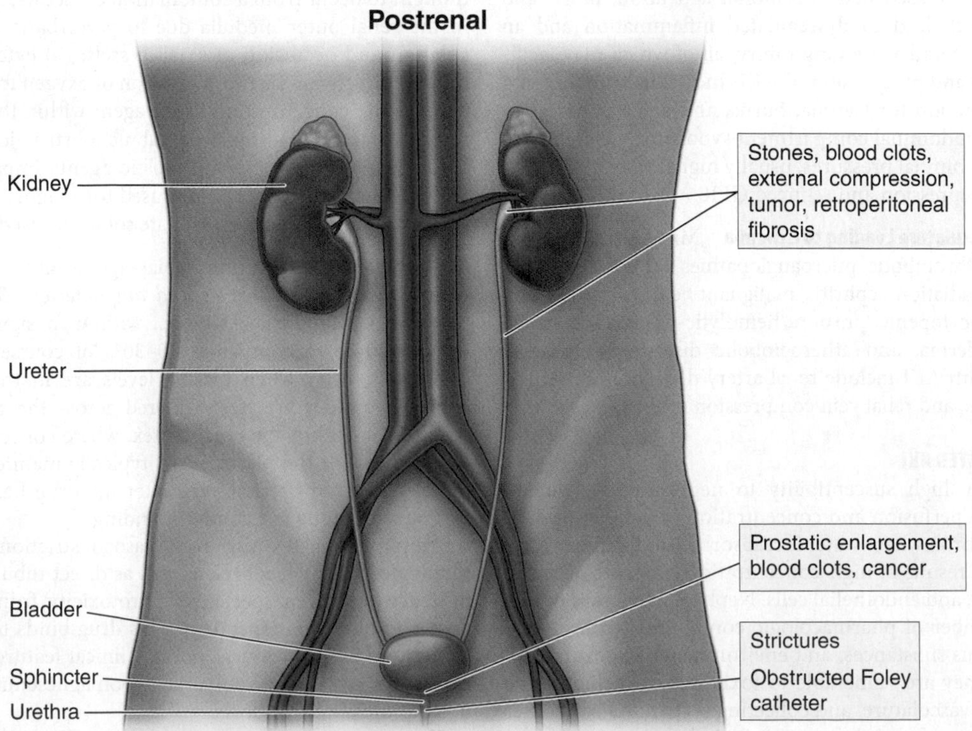

FIGURE 334-5 Anatomic sites and causes of obstruction leading to postrenal acute kidney injury.

does not rule out the presence of partial obstruction, because the GFR is normally two orders of magnitude higher than the urinary flow rate. For AKI to occur in healthy individuals, obstruction must affect both kidneys unless only one kidney is functional, in which case unilateral obstruction can cause AKI. Unilateral obstruction may cause AKI in the setting of significant underlying CKD or, in rare cases, from reflex vasospasm of the contralateral kidney. Bladder neck obstruction is a common cause of postrenal AKI and can be due to prostate disease (benign prostatic hypertrophy or prostate cancer), neurogenic bladder, or therapy with anticholinergic drugs. Obstructed Foley catheters can cause postrenal AKI if not recognized and relieved. Other causes of lower tract obstruction are blood clots, calculi, and urethral strictures. Ureteric obstruction can occur from intraluminal obstruction (e.g., calculi, blood clots, sloughed renal papillae), infiltration of the ureteric wall (e.g., neoplasia), or external compression (e.g., retroperitoneal fibrosis, neoplasia, abscess, or inadvertent surgical damage). The pathophysiology of postrenal AKI involves hemodynamic alterations triggered by an abrupt increase in intratubular pressures. An initial period of hyperemia from afferent arteriolar dilation is followed by intrarenal vasoconstriction from the generation of angiotensin II, thromboxane A2, and vasopressin, and a reduction in NO production. Reduced GFR is due to underperfusion of glomeruli and, possibly, changes in the glomerular ultrafiltration coefficient.

DIAGNOSTIC EVALUATION (TABLE 334-1)

The presence of AKI is usually inferred by an elevation in the SCr concentration. AKI is currently defined by a rise from baseline of at least 0.3 mg/dL within 48 h or at least 50% higher than baseline within 1 week, or a reduction in urine output to less than 0.5 mL/kg per hour for longer than 6 h. It is important to recognize that given this definition, some patients with AKI will not have tubular or glomerular damage (e.g., prerenal azotemia). The distinction between AKI and CKD is important for proper diagnosis and treatment. The distinction is straightforward when a recent baseline SCr concentration is available, but more difficult in the many instances in which the baseline is unknown. In such cases, clues suggestive of CKD can come from radiologic studies (e.g., small, shrunken kidneys with cortical thinning on renal ultrasound, or evidence of renal osteodystrophy) or laboratory tests such as normocytic anemia in the absence of blood loss or secondary hyperparathyroidism with hyperphosphatemia and hypocalcemia, consistent with CKD. No set of tests, however, can rule out AKI superimposed on CKD because AKI is a frequent complication in patients with CKD, further complicating the distinction. Serial blood tests showing continued substantial rise of SCr represents clear evidence of AKI. Once the diagnosis of AKI is established, its cause needs to be determined.

HISTORY AND PHYSICAL EXAMINATION

The clinical context, careful history taking, and physical examination often narrow the differential diagnosis for the cause of AKI. Prerenal azotemia should be suspected in the setting of vomiting, diarrhea, glycosuria causing polyuria, and several medications including diuretics, NSAIDs, ACE inhibitors, and ARBs. Physical signs of orthostatic hypotension, tachycardia, reduced jugular venous pressure, decreased skin turgor, and dry mucous membranes are often present in prerenal azotemia. A history of prostatic disease, nephrolithiasis, or pelvic or paraaortic malignancy would suggest the possibility of postrenal AKI. Whether or not symptoms are present early during obstruction of the urinary tract depends on the location of obstruction. Colicky flank pain radiating to the groin suggests acute ureteric obstruction. Nocturia and urinary frequency or hesitancy can be seen in prostatic disease. Abdominal fullness and suprapubic pain can accompany massive bladder enlargement. Definitive diagnosis of obstruction requires radiologic investigations.

A careful review of all medications is imperative in the evaluation of an individual with AKI. Not only are medications frequently a cause of AKI, but doses of administered medications must be adjusted for estimated GFR. Idiosyncratic reactions to a wide variety of medications can lead to allergic interstitial nephritis, which may be accompanied by fever, arthralgias, and a pruritic erythematous rash. The absence of systemic features of hypersensitivity, however, does not exclude the diagnosis of interstitial nephritis.

AKI accompanied by palpable purpura, pulmonary hemorrhage, or sinusitis raises the possibility of systemic vasculitis with glomerulonephritis. Atheroembolic disease can be associated with livedo reticularis and other signs of emboli to the legs. A tense abdomen should prompt consideration of acute abdominal compartment syndrome, which requires measurement of bladder pressure. Signs of limb ischemia may be clues to the diagnosis of rhabdomyolysis.

URINE FINDINGS

Complete anuria early in the course of AKI is uncommon except in the following situations: complete urinary tract obstruction, renal artery occlusion, overwhelming septic shock, severe ischemia (often with cortical necrosis), or severe proliferative glomerulonephritis or vasculitis. A reduction in urine output (oliguria, defined as <400 mL/24 h) usually denotes more severe AKI (i.e., lower GFR) than when urine output is preserved. Oliguria is associated with worse clinical outcomes. Preserved urine output can be seen in nephrogenic diabetes insipidus characteristic of longstanding urinary tract obstruction, tubulointerstitial disease, or nephrotoxicity from cisplatin or aminoglycosides, among other causes. Red or brown urine may be seen with or without gross hematuria; if the color persists in the supernatant after centrifugation, then pigment nephropathy from rhabdomyolysis or hemolysis should be suspected.

The urinalysis and urine sediment examination are invaluable tools, but they require clinical correlation because of generally limited sensitivity and specificity (Fig. 334-6) (Chap. 62e). In the absence of preexisting proteinuria from CKD, AKI from ischemia or nephrotoxins leads to mild proteinuria (<1 g/d). Greater proteinuria in AKI suggests damage to the glomerular ultrafiltration barrier or excretion of myeloma light chains; the latter are not detected with conventional urine dipsticks (which detect albumin) and require the sulfosalicylic acid test or immunoelectrophoresis. Atheroemboli can cause a variable degree of proteinuria. Extremely heavy proteinuria ("nephrotic range," >3.5 g/d) can occasionally be seen in glomerulonephritis, vasculitis, or interstitial nephritis (particularly from NSAIDs). AKI can also complicate cases of minimal change disease, a cause of the nephrotic syndrome (Chap. 332e). If the dipstick is positive for hemoglobin but few red blood cells are evident in the urine sediment, then rhabdomyolysis or hemolysis should be suspected.

Prerenal azotemia may present with hyaline casts or an unremarkable urine sediment exam. Postrenal AKI may also lead to an unremarkable sediment, but hematuria and pyuria may be seen depending on the cause of obstruction. AKI from ATN due to ischemic injury, sepsis, or certain nephrotoxins has characteristic urine sediment findings: pigmented "muddy brown" granular casts and tubular epithelial cell casts. These findings may be absent in more than 20% of cases, however. Glomerulonephritis may lead to dysmorphic red blood cells or red blood cell casts. Interstitial nephritis may lead to white blood cell casts. The urine sediment findings overlap somewhat in glomerulonephritis and interstitial nephritis, and a diagnosis is not always possible on the basis of the urine sediment alone. Urine eosinophils have a limited role in differential diagnosis; they can be seen in interstitial nephritis, pyelonephritis, cystitis, atheroembolic disease, or glomerulonephritis. Crystalluria may be important diagnostically. The finding of oxalate crystals in AKI should prompt an evaluation for ethylene glycol toxicity. Abundant uric acid crystals may be seen in the tumor lysis syndrome.

BLOOD LABORATORY FINDINGS

Certain forms of AKI are associated with characteristic patterns in the rise and fall of SCr. Prerenal azotemia typically leads to modest rises in SCr that return to baseline with improvement in hemodynamic status. Contrast nephropathy leads to a rise in SCr within 24–48 h, peak within 3–5 days, and resolution within 5–7 days. In comparison, atheroembolic disease usually manifests with more subacute rises in

TABLE 334-1 MAJOR CAUSES, CLINICAL FEATURES, AND DIAGNOSTIC STUDIES FOR PRERENAL AND INTRINSIC ACUTE KIDNEY INJURY

Etiology	Clinical Features	Laboratory Features	Comments
Prerenal azotemia	History of poor fluid intake or fluid loss (hemorrhage, diarrhea, vomiting, sequestration into extravascular space); NSAID/ACE-I/ARB; heart failure; evidence of volume depletion (tachycardia, absolute or postural hypotension, low jugular venous pressure, dry mucous membranes), decreased effective circulatory volume (cirrhosis, heart failure)	BUN/creatinine ratio above 20, FeNa <1%, hyaline casts in urine sediment, urine specific gravity >1.018, urine osmolality >500 mOsm/kg	Low FeNa, high specific gravity and osmolality may not be seen in the setting of CKD, diuretic use; BUN elevation out of proportion to creatinine may alternatively indicate upper GI bleed or increased catabolism. Response to restoration of hemodynamics is most diagnostic.
Sepsis-associated AKI	Sepsis, sepsis syndrome, or septic shock. Overt hypotension not always seen in mild to moderate AKI	Positive culture from normally sterile body fluid; urine sediment often contains granular casts, renal tubular epithelial cell casts	FeNa may be low (<1%), particularly early in the course, but is usually >1% with osmolality <500 mOsm/kg
Ischemia-associated AKI	Systemic hypotension, often superimposed upon sepsis and/or reasons for limited renal reserve such as older age, CKD	Urine sediment often contains granular casts, renal tubular epithelial cell casts. FeNa typically >1%.	
Nephrotoxin-Associated AKI: Endogenous			
Rhabdomyolysis	Traumatic crush injuries, seizures, immobilization	Elevated myoglobin, creatine kinase; urine heme positive with few red blood cells	FeNa may be low (<1%)
Hemolysis	Recent blood transfusion with transfusion reaction	Anemia, elevated LDH, low haptoglobin	FeNa may be low (<1%); evaluation for transfusion reaction
Tumor lysis	Recent chemotherapy	Hyperphosphatemia, hypocalcemia, hyperuricemia	
Multiple myeloma	Age >60 years, constitutional symptoms, bone pain	Monoclonal spike in urine or serum electrophoresis; low anion gap; anemia	Bone marrow or renal biopsy can be diagnostic
Nephrotoxin-Associated AKI: Exogenous			
Contrast nephropathy	Exposure to iodinated contrast	Characteristic course is rise in SCr within 1–2 d, peak within 3–5 d, recovery within 7 d	FeNa may be low (<1%)
Tubular injury	Aminoglycoside antibiotics, cisplatin, tenofovir, zoledronate, ethylene glycol, aristolochic acid, and melamine (to name a few)	Urine sediment often contains granular casts, renal tubular epithelial cell casts. FeNa typically >1%.	Can be oliguric or nonoliguric
Interstitial nephritis	Recent medication exposure; can have fever, rash, arthralgias	Eosinophilia, sterile pyuria; often nonoliguric	Urine eosinophils have limited diagnostic accuracy; systemic signs of drug reaction often absent; kidney biopsy may be helpful
Other Causes of Intrinsic AKI			
Glomerulonephritis/vasculitis	Variable (**Chap. 338**) features include skin rash, arthralgias, sinusitis (AGBM disease), lung hemorrhage (AGBM, ANCA, lupus), recent skin infection or pharyngitis (poststreptococcal)	ANA, ANCA, AGBM antibody, hepatitis serologies, cryoglobulins, blood culture, decreased complement levels, ASO titer (abnormalities of these tests depending on etiology)	Kidney biopsy may be necessary
Interstitial nephritis	Nondrug-related causes include tubulointerstitial nephritis-uveitis (TINU) syndrome, *Legionella* infection	Eosinophilia, sterile pyuria; often nonoliguric	Urine eosinophils have limited diagnostic accuracy; kidney biopsy may be necessary
TTP/HUS	Neurologic abnormalities and/or AKI; recent diarrheal illness; use of calcineurin inhibitors; pregnancy or postpartum; spontaneous	Schistocytes on peripheral blood smear, elevated LDH, anemia, thrombocytopenia	"Typical HUS" refers to AKI with a diarrheal prodrome, often due to Shiga toxin released from *Escherichia coli* or other bacteria; "atypical HUS" is due to inherited or acquired complement dysregulation. "TTP-HUS" refers to sporadic cases in adults. Diagnosis may involve screening for ADAMTS13 activity, Shiga toxin–producing *E. coli*, genetic evaluation of complement regulatory proteins, and kidney biopsy.
Atheroembolic disease	Recent manipulation of the aorta or other large vessels; may occur spontaneously or after anticoagulation; retinal plaques, palpable purpura, livedo reticularis, GI bleed	Hypocomplementemia, eosinophiluria (variable), variable amounts of proteinuria	Skin or kidney biopsy can be diagnostic
Postrenal AKI	History of kidney stones, prostate disease, obstructed bladder catheter, retroperitoneal or pelvic neoplasm	No specific findings other than AKI; may have pyuria or hematuria	Imaging with computed tomography or ultrasound

Abbreviations: ACE-I, angiotensin-converting enzyme inhibitor-I; AGBM, antiglomerular basement membrane; AKI, acute kidney injury; ANA, antinuclear antibody; ANCA, antineutrophilic cytoplasmic antibody; ARB, angiotensin receptor blocker; ASO, antistreptolysin O; BUN, blood urea nitrogen; CKD, chronic kidney disease; FeNa, fractional excretion of sodium; GI, gastrointestinal; LDH, lactate dehydrogenase; NSAID, nonsteroidal anti-inflammatory drug; TTP/HUS, thrombotic thrombocytopenic purpura/hemolytic-uremic syndrome.

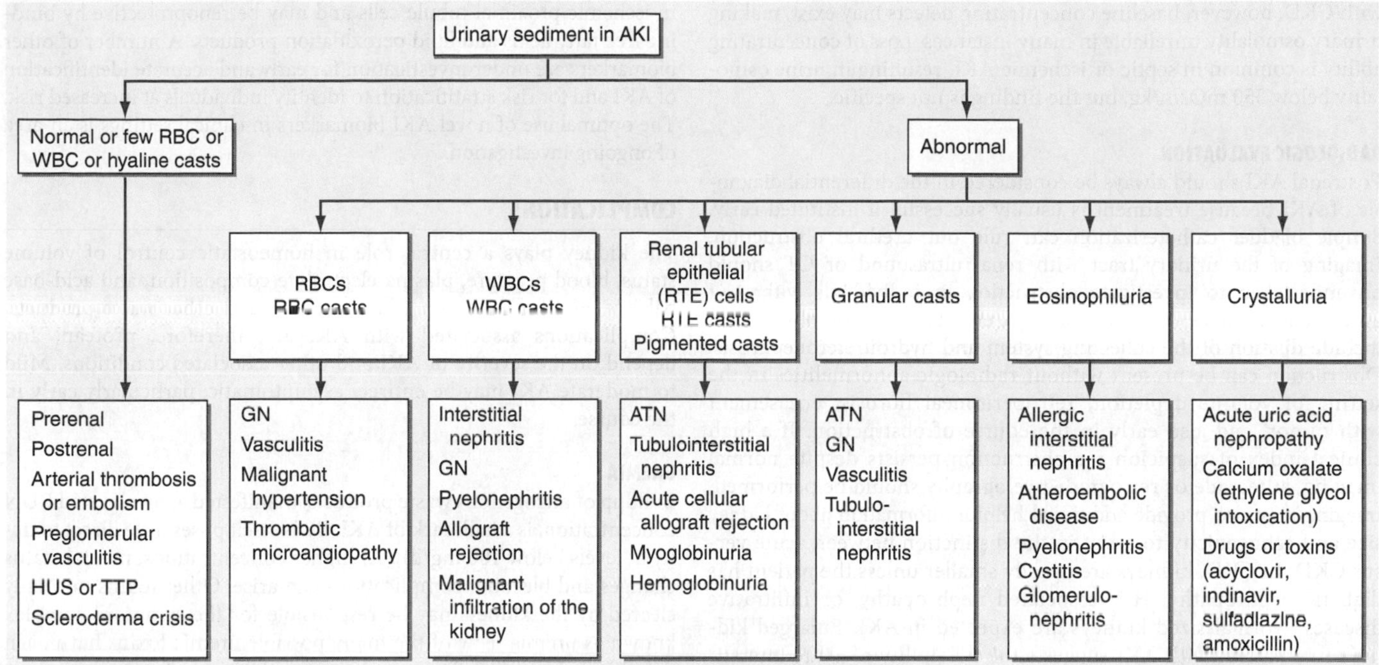

FIGURE 334-6 Interpretation of urinary sediment findings in acute kidney injury (AKI). ATN, acute tubular necrosis; GN, glomerulonephritis; HUS, hemolytic-uremic syndrome; RBCs, red blood cells; RTE, renal tubular epithelial; TTP, thrombotic thrombocytopenic purpura; WBCs, white blood cells. *(Adapted from L Yang, JV Bonventre: Diagnosis and clinical evaluation of acute kidney injury. In Comprehensive Nephrology, 4th ed. J Floege et al [eds]. Philadelphia, Elsevier, 2010.)*

SCr, although severe AKI with rapid increases in SCr can occur in this setting. With many of the epithelial cell toxins such as aminoglycoside antibiotics and cisplatin, the rise in SCr is characteristically delayed for 3–5 days to 2 weeks after initial exposure.

A complete blood count may provide diagnostic clues. Anemia is common in AKI and is usually multifactorial in origin. It is not related to an effect of AKI solely on production of red blood cells because this effect in isolation takes longer to manifest. Peripheral eosinophilia can accompany interstitial nephritis, atheroembolic disease, polyarteritis nodosa, and Churg-Strauss vasculitis. Severe anemia in the absence of bleeding may reflect hemolysis, multiple myeloma, or thrombotic microangiopathy (e.g., HUS or TTP). Other laboratory findings of thrombotic microangiopathy include thrombocytopenia, schistocytes on peripheral blood smear, elevated lactate dehydrogenase level, and low haptoglobin content. Evaluation of patients suspected of having TTP-HUS includes measurement of levels of the von Willebrand factor cleaving protease (ADAMTS13) and testing for Shiga toxin–producing *Escherichia coli*. "Atypical HUS" constitutes the majority of adult cases of HUS; genetic testing is important because it is estimated that 60–70% of atypical HUS patients have mutations in genes encoding proteins that regulate the alternative complement pathway.

AKI often leads to hyperkalemia, hyperphosphatemia, and hypocalcemia. Marked hyperphosphatemia with accompanying hypocalcemia, however, suggests rhabdomyolysis or the tumor lysis syndrome. Creatine phosphokinase levels and serum uric acid are elevated in rhabdomyolysis, while tumor lysis syndrome shows normal or marginally elevated creatine kinase and markedly elevated serum uric acid. The anion gap may be increased with any cause of uremia due to retention of anions such as phosphate, hippurate, sulfate, and urate. The co-occurrence of an increased anion gap and an osmolal gap may suggest ethylene glycol poisoning, which may also cause oxalate crystalluria. Low anion gap may provide a clue to the diagnosis of multiple myeloma due to the presence of unmeasured cationic proteins. Laboratory blood tests helpful for the diagnosis of glomerulonephritis and vasculitis include depressed complement levels and high titers of antinuclear antibodies (ANAs), antineutrophilic cytoplasmic antibodies (ANCAs), antiglomerular basement membrane (AGBM) antibodies, and cryoglobulins.

RENAL FAILURE INDICES

Several indices have been used to help differentiate prerenal azotemia from intrinsic AKI when the tubules are malfunctioning. The low tubular flow rate and increased renal medullary recycling of urea seen in prerenal azotemia may cause a disproportionate elevation of the BUN compared to creatinine. Other causes of disproportionate BUN elevation need to be kept in mind, however, including upper gastrointestinal bleeding, hyperalimentation, increased tissue catabolism, and glucocorticoid use.

The fractional excretion of sodium (FeNa) is the fraction of the filtered sodium load that is reabsorbed by the tubules, and is a measure of both the kidney's ability to reabsorb sodium as well as endogenously and exogenously administered factors that affect tubular reabsorption. As such, it depends on sodium intake, effective intravascular volume, GFR, diuretic intake, and intact tubular reabsorptive mechanisms. With prerenal azotemia, the FeNa may be below 1%, suggesting avid tubular sodium reabsorption. In patients with CKD, a FeNa significantly above 1% can be present despite a superimposed prerenal state. The FeNa may also be above 1% despite hypovolemia due to treatment with diuretics. Low FeNa is often seen early in glomerulonephritis and other disorders and, hence, should not be taken as prima facie evidence of prerenal azotemia. Low FeNa is therefore suggestive, but not synonymous, with effective intravascular volume depletion, and should not be used as the sole guide for volume management. The response of urine output to crystalloid or colloid fluid administration may be both diagnostic and therapeutic in prerenal azotemia. In ischemic AKI, the FeNa is frequently above 1% because of tubular injury and resultant inability to reabsorb sodium. Several causes of ischemia-associated and nephrotoxin-associated AKI can present with FeNa below 1%, however, including sepsis (often early in the course), rhabdomyolysis, and contrast nephropathy.

The ability of the kidney to produce a concentrated urine is dependent upon many factors and reliant on good tubular function in multiple regions of the kidney. In the patient not taking diuretics and with good baseline kidney function, urine osmolality may be above 500 mOsm/kg in prerenal azotemia, consistent with an intact medullary gradient and elevated serum vasopressin levels causing water reabsorption resulting in concentrated urine. In elderly patients and those with CKD, however, baseline concentrating defects may exist, making urinary osmolality unreliable in many instances. Loss of concentrating ability is common in septic or ischemic AKI, resulting in urine osmolality below 350 mOsm/kg, but the finding is not specific.

RADIOLOGIC EVALUATION

Postrenal AKI should always be considered in the differential diagnosis of AKI because treatment is usually successful if instituted early. Simple bladder catheterization can rule out urethral obstruction. Imaging of the urinary tract with renal ultrasound or CT should be undertaken to investigate obstruction in individuals with AKI unless an alternate diagnosis is apparent. Findings of obstruction include dilation of the collecting system and hydroureteronephrosis. Obstruction can be present without radiologic abnormalities in the setting of volume depletion, retroperitoneal fibrosis, encasement with tumor, and also early in the course of obstruction. If a high clinical index of suspicion for obstruction persists despite normal imaging, antegrade or retrograde pyelography should be performed. Imaging may also provide additional helpful information about kidney size and echogenicity to assist in the distinction between acute versus CKD. In CKD, kidneys are usually smaller unless the patient has diabetic nephropathy, HIV-associated nephropathy, or infiltrative diseases. Normal sized kidneys are expected in AKI. Enlarged kidneys in a patient with AKI suggests the possibility of acute interstitial nephritis. Vascular imaging may be useful if venous or arterial obstruction is suspected, but the risks of contrast administration should be kept in mind. MRI with gadolinium-based contrast agents should be avoided if possible in severe AKI due to the possibility of inducing nephrogenic system fibrosis, a rare but serious complication seen most commonly in patients with end-stage renal disease.

KIDNEY BIOPSY

If the cause of AKI is not apparent based on the clinical context, physical examination, laboratory studies, and radiologic evaluation, kidney biopsy should be considered. The kidney biopsy can provide definitive diagnostic and prognostic information about acute kidney disease and CKD. The procedure is most often used in AKI when prerenal azotemia, postrenal AKI, and ischemic or nephrotoxic AKI have been deemed unlikely, and other possible diagnoses are being considered such as glomerulonephritis, vasculitis, interstitial nephritis, myeloma kidney, HUS and TTP, and allograft dysfunction. Kidney biopsy is associated with a risk of bleeding, which can be severe and organ- or life-threatening in patients with thrombocytopenia or coagulopathy.

NOVEL BIOMARKERS

BUN and creatinine are functional biomarkers of glomerular filtration rather than tissue injury biomarkers and, therefore, may be suboptimal for the diagnosis of actual parenchymal kidney damage. BUN and creatinine are also relatively slow to rise after kidney injury. Several novel kidney injury biomarkers have been investigated and show promise for earlier and accurate diagnosis of AKI. *Kidney injury molecule-1* (KIM-1) is a type 1 transmembrane protein that is abundantly expressed in proximal tubular cells injured by ischemia or nephrotoxins such as cisplatin. KIM-1 is not expressed in appreciable quantities in the absence of tubular injury or in extrarenal tissues. KIM-1's functional role may be to confer phagocytic properties to tubular cells, enabling them to clear debris from the tubular lumen after kidney injury. KIM-1 can be detected shortly after ischemic or nephrotoxic injury in the urine and, therefore, may be an easily tested biomarker in the clinical setting. *Neutrophil gelatinase associated lipocalin* (NGAL, also known as lipocalin-2 or siderocalin) is another novel biomarker of AKI. NGAL was first discovered as a protein in granules of human neutrophils. NGAL can bind to iron siderophore complexes and may have tissue-protective effects in the proximal tubule. NGAL is highly upregulated after inflammation and kidney injury and can be detected in the plasma and urine within 2 h of cardiopulmonary bypass–associated AKI. Other candidate biomarkers of AKI include interleukin (IL) 18, a proinflammatory cytokine of the IL-1 superfamily that may mediate ischemic proximal tubular injury, and L-type fatty acid binding protein, which is expressed in ischemic proximal tubule cells and may be renoprotective by binding free fatty acids and lipid peroxidation products. A number of other biomarkers are under investigation for early and accurate identification of AKI and for risk stratification to identify individuals at increased risk. The optimal use of novel AKI biomarkers in clinical settings is an area of ongoing investigation.

COMPLICATIONS

The kidney plays a central role in homeostatic control of volume status, blood pressure, plasma electrolyte composition, and acid-base balance, and for excretion of nitrogenous and other waste products. Complications associated with AKI are, therefore, protean, and depend on the severity of AKI and other associated conditions. Mild to moderate AKI may be entirely asymptomatic, particularly early in the course.

UREMIA

Buildup of nitrogenous waste products, manifested as an elevated BUN concentration, is a hallmark of AKI. BUN itself poses little direct toxicity at levels below 100 mg/dL. At higher concentrations, mental status changes and bleeding complications can arise. Other toxins normally cleared by the kidney may be responsible for the symptom complex known as uremia. Few of the many possible uremic toxins have been definitively identified. The correlation of BUN and SCr concentrations with uremic symptoms is extremely variable, due in part to differences in urea and creatinine generation rates across individuals.

HYPERVOLEMIA AND HYPOVOLEMIA

Expansion of extracellular fluid volume is a major complication of oliguric and anuric AKI, due to impaired salt and water excretion. The result can be weight gain, dependent edema, increased jugular venous pressure, and pulmonary edema; the latter can be life threatening. Pulmonary edema can also occur from volume overload and hemorrhage in pulmonary renal syndromes. AKI may also induce or exacerbate acute lung injury characterized by increased vascular permeability and inflammatory cell infiltration in lung parenchyma. Recovery from AKI can sometimes be accompanied by polyuria, which, if untreated, can lead to significant volume depletion. The polyuric phase of recovery may be due to an osmotic diuresis from retained urea and other waste products as well as delayed recovery of tubular reabsorptive functions.

HYPONATREMIA

Administration of excessive hypotonic crystalloid or isotonic dextrose solutions can result in hypoosmolality and hyponatremia, which, if severe, can cause neurologic abnormalities, including seizures.

HYPERKALEMIA

Abnormalities in plasma electrolyte composition can be mild or life threatening. Frequently the most concerning complication of AKI is hyperkalemia. Marked hyperkalemia is particularly common in rhabdomyolysis, hemolysis, and tumor lysis syndrome due to release of intracellular potassium from damaged cells. Potassium affects the cellular membrane potential of cardiac and neuromuscular tissues. Muscle weakness may be a symptom of hyperkalemia. The more serious complication of hyperkalemia is due to effects on cardiac conduction, leading to potentially fatal arrhythmias.

ACIDOSIS

Metabolic acidosis, usually accompanied by an elevation in the anion gap, is common in AKI, and can further complicate acid-base and potassium balance in individuals with other causes of acidosis, including sepsis, diabetic ketoacidosis, or respiratory acidosis.

HYPERPHOSPHATEMIA AND HYPOCALCEMIA

AKI can lead to hyperphosphatemia, particularly in highly catabolic patients or those with AKI from rhabdomyolysis, hemolysis, and tumor lysis syndrome. Metastatic deposition of calcium phosphate can lead to hypocalcemia. AKI-associated hypocalcemia may also arise from derangements in the vitamin D–parathyroid hormone–fibroblast growth factor-23 axis. Hypocalcemia is often asymptomatic but can lead to perioral paresthesias, muscle cramps, seizures, carpopedal spasms, and prolongation of the QT interval on electrocardiography. Calcium levels should be corrected for the degree of hypoalbuminemia, if present, or ionized calcium levels should be followed. Mild, asymptomatic hypocalcemia does not require treatment.

BLEEDING

Hematologic complications of AKI include anemia and bleeding, both of which are exacerbated by coexisting disease processes such as sepsis, liver disease, and disseminated intravascular coagulation. Direct hematologic effects from AKI-related uremia include decreased erythropoiesis and platelet dysfunction.

INFECTIONS

Infections are a common precipitant of AKI and also a dreaded complication of AKI. Impaired host immunity has been described in end-stage renal disease and may be operative in severe AKI.

CARDIAC COMPLICATIONS

The major cardiac complications of AKI are arrhythmias, pericarditis, and pericardial effusion.

MALNUTRITION

AKI is often a severely hypercatabolic state, and therefore, malnutrition is a major complication.

TREATMENT ACUTE KIDNEY INJURY

PREVENTION AND TREATMENT

The management of individuals with and at risk for AKI varies according to the underlying cause (Table 334-2). Common to all are several principles. Optimization of hemodynamics, correction of fluid and electrolyte imbalances, discontinuation of nephrotoxic medications, and dose adjustment of administered medications are all critical. Common causes of AKI such as sepsis and ischemic ATN do not yet have specific therapies once injury is established, but meticulous clinical attention is needed to support the patient until (if) AKI resolves. The kidney possesses remarkable capacity to repair itself after even severe, dialysis-requiring AKI. However, many patients with AKI do not recover fully and may remain dialysis dependent. It has become increasingly apparent that AKI predisposes to accelerated progression of CKD, and CKD is an important risk factor for AKI.

Prerenal Azotemia Prevention and treatment of prerenal azotemia require optimization of renal perfusion. The composition of replacement fluids should be targeted to the type of fluid lost. Severe acute blood loss should be treated with packed red blood cells. Isotonic crystalloid and/or colloid should be used for less severe acute hemorrhage or plasma loss in the case of burns and pancreatitis. Crystalloid solutions are less expensive and probably equally efficacious as colloid solutions. Hydroxyethyl starch solutions increase the risk of severe AKI and are contraindicated. Crystalloid has been reported to be preferable to albumin in the setting of traumatic brain injury. Isotonic crystalloid (e.g., 0.9% saline) or colloid should be used for volume resuscitation in severe hypovolemia, whereas hypotonic crystalloids (e.g., 0.45% saline) suffice for less severe hypovolemia. Excessive chloride administration from 0.9% saline may lead to hyperchloremic metabolic acidosis and may impair GFR. Bicarbonate-containing solutions (e.g., dextrose water with 150 mEq sodium bicarbonate) should be used if metabolic acidosis is a concern.

Optimization of cardiac function in AKI may require use of inotropic agents, preload- and afterload-reducing agents, antiarrhythmic drugs, and mechanical aids such as an intraaortic balloon pump. Invasive hemodynamic monitoring to guide therapy may be necessary.

Cirrhosis and Hepatorenal Syndrome Fluid management in individuals with cirrhosis, ascites, and AKI is challenging because of the frequent difficulty in ascertaining intravascular volume status. Administration of intravenous fluids as a volume challenge may be required diagnostically as well as therapeutically. Excessive volume administration may, however, result in worsening ascites and pulmonary compromise in

TABLE 334-2 MANAGEMENT OF ACUTE KIDNEY INJURY

General Issues

1. Optimization of systemic and renal hemodynamics through volume resuscitation and judicious use of vasopressors
2. Elimination of nephrotoxic agents (e.g., ACE inhibitors, ARBs, NSAIDs, aminoglycosides) if possible
3. Initiation of renal replacement therapy when indicated

Specific Issues

1. Nephrotoxin-specific
   a. Rhabdomyolysis: aggressive intravenous fluids; consider forced alkaline diuresis
   b. Tumor lysis syndrome: aggressive intravenous fluids and allopurinol or rasburicase
2. Volume overload
   a. Salt and water restriction
   b. Diuretics
   c. Ultrafiltration
3. Hyponatremia
   a. Restriction of enteral free water intake, minimization of hypotonic intravenous solutions including those containing dextrose
   b. Hypertonic saline is rarely necessary in AKI. Vasopressin antagonists are generally not needed
4. Hyperkalemia
   a. Restriction of dietary potassium intake
   b. Discontinuation of potassium-sparing diuretics, ACE inhibitors, ARBs, NSAIDs
   c. Loop diuretics to promote urinary potassium loss
   d. Potassium binding ion-exchange resin (sodium polystyrene sulfonate)
   e. Insulin (10 units regular) and glucose (50 mL of 50% dextrose) to promote entry of potassium intracellularly
   f. Inhaled beta-agonist therapy to promote entry of potassium intracellularly
   g. Calcium gluconate or calcium chloride (1 g) to stabilize the myocardium
5. Metabolic acidosis
   a. Sodium bicarbonate (if pH <7.2 to keep serum bicarbonate >15 mmol/L)
   b. Administration of other bases, e.g., THAM
   c. Renal replacement therapy
6. Hyperphosphatemia
   a. Restriction of dietary phosphate intake
   b. Phosphate binding agents (calcium acetate, sevelamer hydrochloride, aluminum hydroxide—taken with meals)
7. Hypocalcemia
   a. Calcium carbonate or calcium gluconate if symptomatic
8. Hypermagnesemia
   a. Discontinue Mg^{2+} containing antacids
9. Hyperuricemia
   a. Acute treatment is usually not required except in the setting of tumor lysis syndrome (see above)
10. Nutrition
    a. Sufficient protein and calorie intake (20–30 kcal/kg per day) to avoid negative nitrogen balance. Nutrition should be provided via the enteral route if possible.
11. Drug dosing
    a. Careful attention to dosages and frequency of administration of drugs, adjustment for degree of renal failure
    b. Note that serum creatinine concentration may overestimate renal function in the non–steady state characteristic of patients with AKI

Abbreviations: ACE, angiotensin-converting enzyme; ARBs, angiotensin receptor blocker; NSAIDs, nonsteroidal anti-inflammatory drug; THAM, tris (hydroxymethyl) aminomethane.

the setting of hepatorenal syndrome or AKI due to superimposed spontaneous bacterial peritonitis. Peritonitis should be ruled out by culture of ascitic fluid. Albumin may prevent AKI in those treated with antibiotics for spontaneous bacterial peritonitis. The definitive treatment of the hepatorenal syndrome is orthotopic liver transplantation. Bridge therapies that have shown promise include terlipressin (a vasopressin analog), combination therapy with octreotide (a somatostatin analog) and midodrine (an α_1-adrenergic agonist), and norepinephrine, in combination with intravenous albumin (25–50 g, maximum 100 g/d).

Intrinsic AKI Several agents have been tested and have failed to show benefit in the treatment of acute tubular injury. These include atrial natriuretic peptide, low-dose dopamine, endothelin antagonists, loop diuretics, calcium channel blockers, α-adrenergic receptor blockers, prostaglandin analogs, antioxidants, antibodies against leukocyte adhesion molecules, and insulin-like growth factor, among many others. Most studies have enrolled patients with severe and well-established AKI, and treatment may have been initiated too late. Novel kidney injury biomarkers may provide an opportunity to test agents earlier in the course of AKI.

AKI due to acute glomerulonephritis or vasculitis may respond to immunosuppressive agents and/or plasmapheresis (Chap. 332e). Allergic interstitial nephritis due to medications requires discontinuation of the offending agent. Glucocorticoids have been used, but not tested in randomized trials, in cases where AKI persists or worsens despite discontinuation of the suspected medication. AKI due to scleroderma (scleroderma renal crisis) should be treated with ACE inhibitors. Idiopathic TTP-HUS is a medical emergency and should be treated promptly with plasma exchange. Pharmacologic blockade of complement activation may be effective in atypical HUS.

Early and aggressive volume repletion is mandatory in patients with rhabdomyolysis, who may initially require 10 L of fluid per day. Alkaline fluids (e.g., 75 mmol/L sodium bicarbonate added to 0.45% saline) may be beneficial in preventing tubular injury and cast formation, but carry the risk of worsening hypocalcemia. Diuretics may be used if fluid repletion is adequate but unsuccessful in achieving urinary flow rates of 200–300 mL/h. There is no specific therapy for established AKI in rhabdomyolysis, other than dialysis in severe cases or general supportive care to maintain fluid and electrolyte balance and tissue perfusion. Careful attention must be focused on calcium and phosphate status because of precipitation in damaged tissue and release when the tissue heals.

Postrenal AKI Prompt recognition and relief of urinary tract obstruction can forestall the development of permanent structural damage induced by urinary stasis. The site of obstruction defines the treatment approach. Transurethral or suprapubic bladder catheterization may be all that is needed initially for urethral strictures or functional bladder impairment. Ureteric obstruction may be treated by percutaneous nephrostomy tube placement or ureteral stent placement. Relief of obstruction is usually followed by an appropriate diuresis for several days. In rare cases, severe polyuria persists due to tubular dysfunction and may require continued administration of intravenous fluids and electrolytes for a period of time.

SUPPORTIVE MEASURES

Volume Management Hypervolemia in oliguric or anuric AKI may be life threatening due to acute pulmonary edema, especially because many patients have coexisting pulmonary disease, and AKI likely increases pulmonary vascular permeability. Fluid and sodium should be restricted, and diuretics may be used to increase the urinary flow rate. There is no evidence that increasing urine output itself improves the natural history of AKI, but diuretics may help to avoid the need for dialysis in some cases. In severe cases of volume overload, furosemide may be given as a bolus (200 mg) followed by an intravenous drip (10–40 mg/h), with or without a thiazide diuretic. In decompensated heart failure, stepped diuretic therapy was found to be superior to ultrafiltration in preserving renal function. Diuretic therapy should be stopped if there is no response. Dopamine in low doses may transiently increase salt and water excretion by the kidney in prerenal states, but clinical trials have failed to show any benefit in patients with intrinsic AKI. Because of the risk of arrhythmias and potential bowel ischemia, it has been argued that the risks of dopamine outweigh the benefits in the treatment or prevention of AKI.

Electrolyte and Acid-Base Abnormalities The treatment of dysnatremias and hyperkalemia is described in Chap. 63. Metabolic acidosis is generally not treated unless severe (pH <7.20 and serum bicarbonate <15 mmol/L). Acidosis can be treated with oral or intravenous sodium bicarbonate (Chap. 66), but overcorrection should be avoided because of the possibility of metabolic alkalosis, hypocalcemia, hypokalemia, and volume overload. Hyperphosphatemia is common in AKI and can usually be treated by limiting intestinal absorption of phosphate using phosphate binders (calcium carbonate, calcium acetate, lanthanum, sevelamer, or aluminum hydroxide). Hypocalcemia does not usually require therapy unless symptoms are present. Ionized calcium should be monitored rather than total calcium when hypoalbuminemia is present.

Malnutrition Protein energy wasting is common in AKI, particularly in the setting of multisystem organ failure. Inadequate nutrition may lead to starvation ketoacidosis and protein catabolism. Excessive nutrition may increase the generation of nitrogenous waste and lead to worsening azotemia. Total parenteral nutrition requires large volumes of fluid administration and may complicate efforts at volume control. According to the Kidney Disease Improving Global Outcomes (KDIGO) guidelines, patients with AKI should achieve a total energy intake of 20–30 kcal/kg per day. Protein intake should vary depending on the severity of AKI: 0.8–1.0 g/kg per day in noncatabolic AKI without the need for dialysis; 1.0–1.5 g/kg per day in patients on dialysis; and up to a maximum of 1.7 g/kg per day if hypercatabolic and receiving continuous renal replacement therapy. Trace elements and water-soluble vitamins should also be supplemented in AKI patients treated with dialysis and continuous renal replacement therapy.

Anemia The anemia seen in AKI is usually multifactorial and is not improved by erythropoiesis-stimulating agents, due to their delayed onset of action and the presence of bone marrow resistance in critically ill patients. Uremic bleeding may respond to desmopressin or estrogens, but may require dialysis for treatment in the case of long-standing or severe uremia. Gastrointestinal prophylaxis with proton pump inhibitors or histamine (H_2) receptor blockers is required. Venous thromboembolism prophylaxis is important and should be tailored to the clinical setting; low-molecular-weight heparins and factor Xa inhibitors have unpredictable pharmacokinetics in severe AKI and should be avoided.

Dialysis Indications and Modalities (See also Chap. 336) Dialysis is indicated when medical management fails to control volume overload, hyperkalemia, or acidosis; in some toxic ingestions; and when there are severe complications of uremia (asterixis, pericardial rub or effusion, encephalopathy, uremic bleeding). The timing of dialysis is still a matter of debate. Late initiation of dialysis carries the risk of avoidable volume, electrolyte, and metabolic complications of AKI. On the other hand, initiating dialysis too early may unnecessarily expose individuals to intravenous lines and invasive procedures, with the attendant risks of infection, bleeding, procedural complications, and hypotension. The initiation of dialysis should not await the development of a life-threatening complication of renal failure. Many nephrologists initiate dialysis for AKI empirically when the BUN exceeds a certain value (e.g., 100 mg/dL) in patients without clinical signs of recovery of kidney function. The available modes for renal replacement therapy in AKI require either access to the peritoneal cavity (for peritoneal dialysis) or the large blood vessels (for hemodialysis, hemofiltration, and other hybrid procedures). Small solutes are removed across a semipermeable membrane down their concentration gradient ("diffusive" clearance) and/or along with the movement of plasma water ("convective" clearance). The choice of modality is often dictated by the immediate availability of technology and the expertise of medical staff. Peritoneal dialysis is performed through a temporary intraperitoneal catheter. It is rarely used in the United States for AKI in adults but has enjoyed widespread use internationally, particularly when hemodialysis technology is not available. Dialysate solution is instilled into and removed from the peritoneal cavity at regular intervals in order to achieve diffusive and convective clearance of solutes across the peritoneal membrane; ultrafiltration of water is achieved by the presence of an osmotic gradient across the peritoneal membrane achieved by high concentrations of dextrose in the dialysate solution. Because of its continuous nature, it is often better tolerated than intermittent procedures like hemodialysis in hypotensive patients. Peritoneal dialysis may not be sufficient for hypercatabolic patients due to inherent limitations in dialysis efficacy.

Hemodialysis can be used intermittently or continuously and can be done through convective clearance, diffusive clearance, or a combination of the two. Vascular access is through the femoral, internal jugular, or subclavian veins. Hemodialysis is an intermittent procedure that removes solutes through diffusive and convective clearance. Hemodialysis is typically performed 3–4 h per day, three to four times per week, and is the most common form of renal replacement therapy for AKI. One of the major complications of hemodialysis is hypotension, particularly in the critically ill.

Continuous intravascular procedures were developed in the early 1980s to treat hemodynamically unstable patients without inducing the rapid shifts of volume, osmolarity, and electrolytes characteristic of intermittent hemodialysis. Continuous renal replacement therapy (CRRT) can be performed by convective clearance (continuous venovenous hemofiltration [CVVH]), in which large volumes of plasma water (and accompanying solutes) are forced across the semipermeable membrane by means of hydrostatic pressure; the plasma water is then replaced by a physiologic crystalloid solution. CRRT can also be performed by diffusive clearance (continuous venovenous hemodialysis [CVVHD]), a technology similar to hemodialysis except at lower blood flow and dialysate flow rates. A hybrid therapy combines both diffusive and convective clearance (continuous venovenous hemodiafiltration [CVVHDF]). To achieve some of the advantages of CRRT without the need for 24-h staffing of the procedure, some physicians favor slow low-efficiency dialysis (SLED) or extended daily dialysis (EDD). In this therapy, blood flow and dialysate flow are higher than in CVVHD, but the treatment time is reduced to 12 h or less.

The optimal dose of dialysis for AKI is not clear. Daily intermittent hemodialysis and high-dose CRRT do not confer a demonstrable survival or renal recovery advantage, but care should be taken to avoid undertreatment. Studies have failed to show that continuous therapies are superior to intermittent therapies. If available, CRRT is often preferred in patients with severe hemodynamic instability, cerebral edema, or significant volume overload.

OUTCOME AND PROGNOSIS

The development of AKI is associated with a significantly increased risk of in-hospital and long-term mortality, longer length of stay, and increased costs. Prerenal azotemia, with the exception of the cardiorenal and hepatorenal syndromes, and postrenal azotemia carry a better prognosis than most cases of intrinsic AKI. The kidneys may recover even after severe, dialysis-requiring AKI. Survivors of an episode of AKI requiring temporary dialysis, however, are at extremely high risk for progressive CKD, and up to 10% may develop end-stage renal disease. Postdischarge care under the supervision of a nephrologist for aggressive secondary prevention of kidney disease is prudent. Patients with AKI are more likely to die prematurely after they leave the hospital even if their kidney function has recovered.

335 Chronic Kidney Disease

Joanne M. Bargman, Karl Skorecki

Chronic kidney disease (CKD) encompasses a spectrum of different pathophysiologic processes associated with abnormal kidney function and a progressive decline in glomerular filtration rate (GFR). Figure 335-1 provides a recently updated classification, in which stages of CKD are stratified by both estimated GFR and the degree of albuminuria, in order to predict risk of progression of CKD. Previously, CKD had been staged solely by the GFR. However, the risk of worsening of kidney function is closely linked to the amount of albuminuria, and so it has been incorporated into the classification.

The pathophysiologic processes, adaptations, clinical presentations, assessment, and therapeutic interventions associated with CKD will be the focus of this chapter. The dispiriting term *end-stage renal disease* represents a stage of CKD where the accumulation of toxins, fluid, and electrolytes normally excreted by the kidneys results in the *uremic syndrome*. This syndrome leads to death unless the toxins are removed by renal replacement therapy, using dialysis or kidney transplantation. These interventions are discussed in Chaps. 336 and 337. *End-stage renal disease* will be supplanted in this chapter by the term *stage 5 CKD*.

PATHOPHYSIOLOGY OF CHRONIC KIDNEY DISEASE

The pathophysiology of CKD involves two broad sets of mechanisms of damage: (1) initiating mechanisms specific to the underlying etiology (e.g., genetically determined abnormalities in kidney development or integrity, immune complex deposition and inflammation in certain types of glomerulonephritis, or toxin exposure in certain diseases of the renal tubules and interstitium) and (2) a set of progressive mechanisms, involving hyperfiltration and hypertrophy of the remaining viable nephrons, that are a common consequence following long-term reduction of renal mass, irrespective of underlying etiology (Chap. 333e). The responses to reduction in nephron number are mediated by vasoactive hormones, cytokines, and growth factors. Eventually, these short-term adaptations of hypertrophy and hyperfiltration become maladaptive as the increased pressure and flow within the nephron predisposes to distortion of glomerular architecture, abnormal podocyte function, and disruption of the filtration barrier leading to sclerosis and dropout of the remaining nephrons (Fig. 335-2). Increased intrarenal activity of the renin-angiotensin system (RAS) appears to contribute both to the initial adaptive hyperfiltration and to the subsequent maladaptive hypertrophy and sclerosis. This process explains why a reduction in renal mass from an isolated insult may lead to a progressive decline in renal function over many years (Fig. 335-3).

IDENTIFICATION OF RISK FACTORS AND STAGING OF CKD

It is important to identify factors that increase the risk for CKD, even in individuals with normal GFR. Risk factors include small for gestation birth weight, childhood obesity, hypertension, diabetes mellitus, autoimmune disease, advanced age, African ancestry, a family history of kidney disease, a previous episode of acute kidney injury, and the presence of proteinuria, abnormal urinary sediment, or structural abnormalities of the urinary tract.

Many rare inherited forms of CKD follow a Mendelian inheritance pattern, often as part of a systemic syndrome, with the most common in this category being autosomal dominant polycystic kidney disease. In addition, recent research in the genetics of predisposition to common complex diseases (Chap. 82) has revealed DNA sequence variants at a number of genetic loci that are associated with common forms of CKD. A striking example is the finding of allelic versions of the *APOL1* gene, of West African population ancestry, which contributes to the several-fold higher frequency of certain common etiologies of nondiabetic CKD (e.g., focal segmental glomerulosclerosis) observed among African and Hispanic Americans. The prevalence in West African populations seems to have arisen as an evolutionary adaptation conferring protection from tropical pathogens. As in other common diseases

Prognosis of CKD by GFR and albuminuria categories: KDIGO 2012

GFR categories (ml/min/1.73 m²) description and range			Persistent albuminuria categories description and range: A1	A2	A3
			Normal to mildly increased	Moderately increased	Severely increased
			<30 mg/g <3 mg/mmol	30–300 mg/g 3–30 mg/mmol	>300 mg/g >30 mg/mmol
G1	Normal or high	≥90			
G2	Mildly decreased	60–89			
G3a	Mildly to moderately decreased	45–59			
G3b	Moderately to severely decreased	30–44			
G4	Severely decreased	15–29			
G5	Kidney failure	<15			

FIGURE 335-1 Kidney Disease Improving Global Outcome (KDIGO) classification of chronic kidney disease (CKD). Gradation of color from green to red corresponds to increasing risk and progression of CKD. GFR, glomerular filtration rate. *(Reproduced with permission from Kidney Int Suppl 3:5-14, 2013.)*

with a heritable component, an environmental trigger (such as a viral pathogen) is required to transform genetic risk into disease.

To stage CKD, it is necessary to estimate the GFR rather than relying on serum creatinine concentration (Table 335-1). Many laboratories now report an estimated GFR, or eGFR, using one of these equations.

The normal annual mean decline in GFR with age from the peak GFR (~120 mL/min per 1.73 m^2) attained during the third decade of life is ~1 mL/min per year per 1.73 m^2, reaching a mean value of 70 mL/min per 1.73 m^2 at age 70. Although reduced GFR occurs with human aging, the lower GFR signifies a true loss of kidney function, with all of the implications that apply to the corresponding stage of CKD. The mean GFR is lower in women than in men. For example, a woman in her 80s with a normal serum creatinine may have a GFR of just 50 mL/min per 1.73 m^2. Thus, even a mild elevation in serum creatinine concentration (e.g., 130 μmol/L [1.5 mg/dL]) often signifies a substantial reduction in GFR in most individuals.

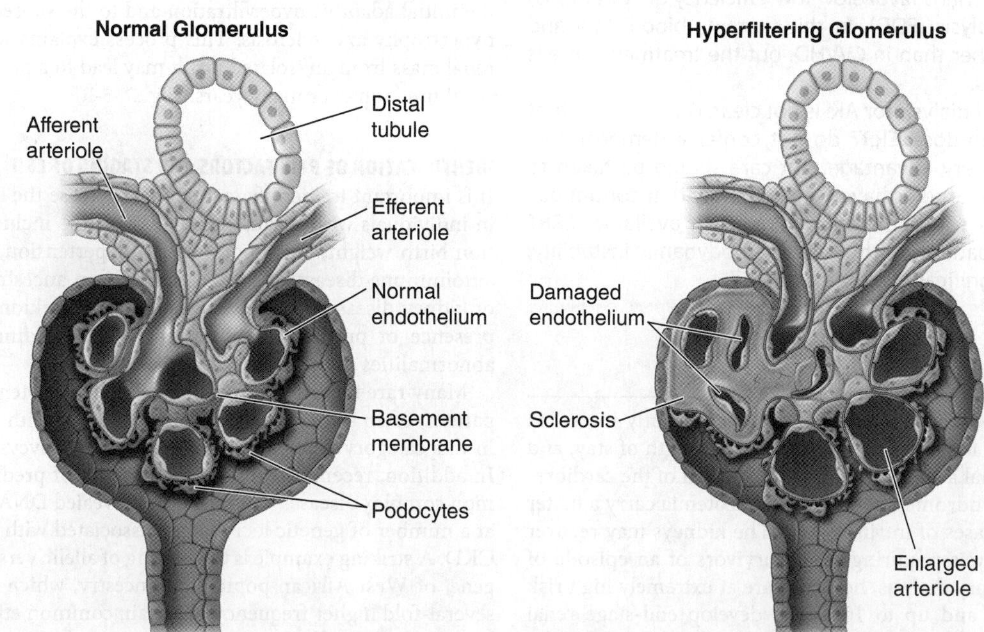

FIGURE 335-2 ***Left:*** Schema of the normal glomerular architecture. ***Right:*** Secondary glomerular changes associated with a reduction in nephron number, including enlargement of capillary lumens and focal adhesions, which are thought to occur consequent to compensatory hyperfiltration and hypertrophy in the remaining nephrons. *(Modified from JR Ingelfinger: N Engl J Med 348:99, 2003.)*

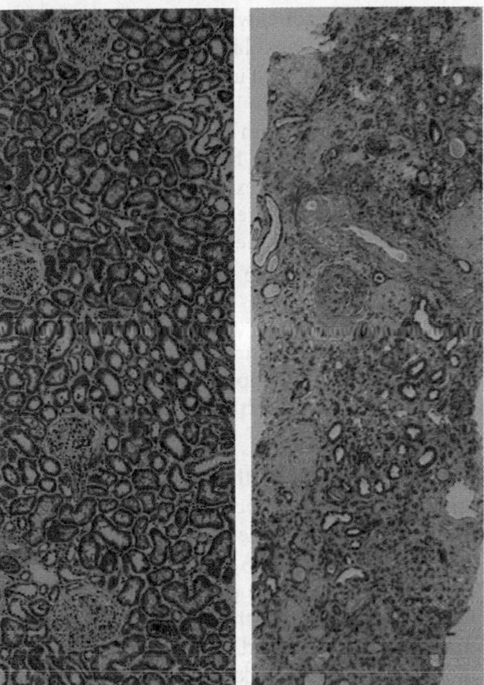

FIGURE 335-3 ***Left:*** Low-power photomicrograph of a normal kidney showing normal glomeruli and healthy tubulointerstitium without fibrosis. ***Right:*** Low-power photomicrograph of chronic kidney disease with sclerosis of many glomeruli and severe tubulointerstitial fibrosis (Masson trichrome, ×40 magnification). *(Slides courtesy of the late Dr. Andrew Herzenberg.)*

The equations for estimating GFR are valid only if the patient is in steady state, that is, the serum creatinine is neither rising nor falling over days.

Measurement of albuminuria is also helpful for monitoring nephron injury and the response to therapy in many forms of CKD, especially chronic glomerular diseases. Although an accurate 24-h urine collection is the standard for measurement of albuminuria, the measurement of protein-to-creatinine ratio in a spot first-morning urine sample is often more practical to obtain and correlates well, but not perfectly, with 24-h urine collections. *Microalbuminuria* (Fig. 335-1, stage A2) refers to the excretion of amounts of albumin too small to detect by urinary dipstick or conventional measures of urine protein. It is a good screening test for early detection of renal disease, and may be a marker for the presence of microvascular disease in general. If a patient has a large amount of excreted albumin, there is no reason to test for microalbuminuria.

Stages 1 and 2 CKD are usually not associated with any symptoms arising from the decrement in GFR. If the decline in GFR progresses to stages 3 and 4, clinical and laboratory complications of CKD become more prominent. Virtually all organ systems are affected, but the most evident complications include anemia and associated easy fatigability; decreased appetite with progressive malnutrition; abnormalities in calcium, phosphorus, and mineral-regulating hormones, such as $1,25(OH)_2D_3$ (calcitriol), parathyroid hormone (PTH), and fibroblast growth factor 23 (FGF-23); and abnormalities in sodium, potassium, water, and acid-base homeostasis. Many patients, especially the elderly, will have eGFR values compatible with stage 2 or 3 CKD. However, the majority of these patients will show no further deterioration of renal function. The primary care physician is advised to recheck kidney function, and if it is stable and not associated with proteinuria, the patient can usually be managed in this setting. However, if there is evidence of decline of GFR, uncontrolled hypertension, or proteinuria, referral to a nephrologist is appropriate. If the patient progresses to stage 5 CKD, toxins accumulate such that patients usually experience a marked disturbance in their activities of daily living, well-being, nutritional status, and water and electrolyte homeostasis, eventuating in the *uremic syndrome.*

TABLE 335-1 RECOMMENDED EQUATIONS FOR ESTIMATION OF GLOMERULAR FILTRATION RATE (GFR) USING SERUM CREATININE CONCENTRATION (S_{CR}), AGE, SEX, RACE, AND BODY WEIGHT

1. Equation from the Modification of Diet in Renal Disease study
Estimated GFR (mL/min per 1.73 m^2) = $1.86 \times (S_{Cr})^{-1.154} \times (\text{age})^{-0.203}$
Multiply by 0.742 for women
Multiply by 1.21 for African ancestry
2. CKD-EPI equation
GFR = $141 \times \min(S_{Cr}/\kappa, 1)^{\alpha} \times \max(S_{Cr}/\kappa, 1)^{-1.209} \times 0.993^{Age}$
Multiply by 1.018 for women
Multiply by 1.159 for African ancestry
where S_{Cr} is serum creatinine in mg/dL, κ is 0.7 for females and 0.9 for males, α is −0.329 for females and −0.411 for males, min indicates the minimum of S_{Cr}/κ or 1, and max indicates the maximum of S_{Cr}/κ or 1.

Abbreviation: CKD-EPI, Chronic Kidney Disease Epidemiology Collaboration.

ETIOLOGY AND EPIDEMIOLOGY

It has been estimated from population survey data that at least 6% of the adult population in the United States has CKD at stages 1 and 2. An additional 4.5% of the U.S. population is estimated to have stages 3 and 4 CKD. Table 335-2 lists the five most frequent categories of causes of CKD, cumulatively accounting for greater than 90% of the CKD disease burden worldwide. The relative contribution of each category varies among different geographic regions. The most frequent cause of CKD in North America and Europe is diabetic nephropathy, most often secondary to type 2 diabetes mellitus. Patients with newly diagnosed CKD often also present with hypertension. When no overt evidence for a primary glomerular or tubulointerstitial kidney disease process is present, CKD is often attributed to hypertension. However, it is now appreciated that such individuals can be considered in two categories. The first includes patients with a silent primary glomerulopathy, such as focal segmental glomerulosclerosis, without the overt nephrotic or nephritic manifestations of glomerular disease (Chap. 338). The second includes patients in whom progressive nephrosclerosis and hypertension is the renal correlate of a systemic vascular disease, often also involving large- and small-vessel cardiac and cerebral pathology. This latter combination is especially common in the elderly, in whom chronic renal ischemia as a cause of CKD may be underdiagnosed. The increasing incidence of CKD in the elderly has been ascribed, in part, to decreased mortality rate from the cardiac and cerebral complications of atherosclerotic vascular disease, enabling a greater segment of the population to eventually manifest the renal component of generalized vascular disease. Nevertheless, it should be appreciated that the vast majority of such patients with early stages of CKD will succumb to the cardiovascular and cerebrovascular consequences of the vascular disease before they can progress to the most advanced stages of CKD. Indeed, even a minor decrement in GFR or the presence of albuminuria is now recognized as a major risk factor for cardiovascular disease.

PATHOPHYSIOLOGY AND BIOCHEMISTRY OF UREMIA

Although serum urea and creatinine concentrations are used to measure the excretory capacity of the kidneys, accumulation of these two molecules themselves does not account for the many symptoms and signs that characterize the uremic syndrome in advanced renal failure.

TABLE 335-2 LEADING CATEGORIES OF ETIOLOGIES OF CKD[a]

- Diabetic nephropathy
- Glomerulonephritis
- Hypertension-associated CKD (includes vascular and ischemic kidney disease and primary glomerular disease with associated hypertension)
- Autosomal dominant polycystic kidney disease
- Other cystic and tubulointerstitial nephropathy

[a]Relative contribution of each category varies with geographic region and race.

Hundreds of toxins that accumulate in renal failure have been implicated in the uremic syndrome. These include water-soluble, hydrophobic, protein-bound, charged, and uncharged compounds. Additional categories of nitrogenous excretory products include guanidino compounds, urates and hippurates, products of nucleic acid metabolism, polyamines, myoinositol, phenols, benzoates, and indoles. It is thus evident that the serum concentrations of urea and creatinine should be viewed as being readily measured, but incomplete, surrogate markers for these compounds, and monitoring the levels of urea and creatinine in the patient with impaired kidney function represents a vast oversimplification of the uremic state.

The uremic syndrome and the disease state associated with advanced renal impairment involve more than renal excretory failure. A host of metabolic and endocrine functions normally performed by the kidneys is also impaired or suppressed, and this results in anemia, malnutrition, and abnormal metabolism of carbohydrates, fats, and proteins. Furthermore, plasma levels of many hormones, including PTH, FGF-23, insulin, glucagon, steroid hormones including vitamin D and sex hormones, and prolactin, change with CKD as a result of reduced excretion, decreased degradation, or abnormal regulation. Finally, CKD is associated with worsening systemic inflammation. Elevated levels of C-reactive protein are detected along with other acute-phase reactants, whereas levels of so-called negative acute-phase reactants, such as albumin and fetuin, decline with progressive reduction in GFR. Thus, the inflammation associated with CKD is important in the *malnutrition-inflammation-atherosclerosis/calcification syndrome*, which contributes in turn to the acceleration of vascular disease and comorbidity associated with advanced kidney disease.

In summary, the pathophysiology of the uremic syndrome can be divided into manifestations in three spheres of dysfunction: (1) those consequent to the accumulation of toxins that normally undergo renal excretion, including products of protein metabolism; (2) those consequent to the loss of other kidney functions, such as fluid and electrolyte homeostasis and hormone regulation; and (3) progressive systemic inflammation and its vascular and nutritional consequences.

CLINICAL AND LABORATORY MANIFESTATIONS OF CHRONIC KIDNEY DISEASE AND UREMIA

Uremia leads to disturbances in the function of virtually every organ system. Chronic dialysis can reduce the incidence and severity of many of these disturbances, so that the overt and florid manifestations of uremia have largely disappeared in the modern health setting. However, even optimal dialysis therapy is not completely effective as renal replacement therapy, because some disturbances resulting from impaired kidney function fail to respond to dialysis.

FLUID, ELECTROLYTE, AND ACID-BASE DISORDERS

Sodium and Water Homeostasis In most patients with stable CKD, the total-body content of sodium and water is modestly increased, although this may not be apparent on clinical examination. With normal renal function, the tubular reabsorption of filtered sodium and water is adjusted so that urinary excretion matches intake. Many forms of kidney disease (e.g., glomerulonephritis) disrupt this balance such that dietary intake of sodium exceeds its urinary excretion, leading to sodium retention and attendant extracellular fluid volume (ECFV) expansion. This expansion may contribute to hypertension, which itself can accelerate the nephron injury. As long as water intake does not exceed the capacity for water clearance, the ECFV expansion will be isotonic and the patient will have a normal plasma sodium concentration (Chap. 333e). Hyponatremia is not commonly seen in CKD patients but, when present, often responds to water restriction. The patient with ECFV expansion (peripheral edema, sometimes hypertension poorly responsive to therapy) should be counseled regarding salt restriction. Thiazide diuretics have limited utility in stages 3–5 CKD, such that administration of loop diuretics, including furosemide, bumetanide, or torsemide, may also be needed. Resistance to loop diuretics in CKD often mandates use of higher doses than those used in patients with more normal kidney function. The combination of loop diuretics with metolazone, which inhibits the sodium chloride co-transporter of the distal convoluted tubule, can promote renal salt excretion. Diuretic resistance with intractable edema and hypertension in advanced CKD may serve as an indication to initiate dialysis.

In addition to problems with salt and water excretion, some patients with CKD may instead have impaired renal conservation of sodium and water. When an extrarenal cause for fluid loss, such as gastrointestinal (GI) loss, is present, these patients may be prone to ECFV depletion because of the inability of the failing kidney to reclaim filtered sodium adequately. Furthermore, depletion of ECFV, whether due to GI losses or overzealous diuretic therapy, can further compromise kidney function through underperfusion, or a "prerenal" basis, leading to acute-on-chronic kidney failure. In this setting, cautious volume repletion with normal saline may return the ECFV to normal and restore renal function to baseline without having to intervene with dialysis.

Potassium Homeostasis In CKD, the decline in GFR is not necessarily accompanied by a parallel decline in urinary potassium excretion, which is predominantly mediated by aldosterone-dependent secretion in the distal nephron. Another defense against potassium retention in these patients is augmented potassium excretion in the GI tract. Notwithstanding these two homeostatic responses, hyperkalemia may be precipitated in certain settings. These include increased dietary potassium intake, protein catabolism, hemolysis, hemorrhage, transfusion of stored red blood cells, and metabolic acidosis. In addition, a host of medications can inhibit renal potassium excretion and lead to hyperkalemia. The most important medications in this respect include the RAS inhibitors and spironolactone and other potassium-sparing diuretics such as amiloride, eplerenone, and triamterene.

Certain causes of CKD can be associated with earlier and more severe disruption of potassium-secretory mechanisms in the distal nephron, out of proportion to the decline in GFR. These include conditions associated with hyporeninemic hypoaldosteronism, such as diabetes, and renal diseases that preferentially affect the distal nephron, such as obstructive uropathy and sickle cell nephropathy.

Hypokalemia is not common in CKD and usually reflects markedly reduced dietary potassium intake, especially in association with excessive diuretic therapy or concurrent GI losses. The use of potassium supplements and potassium-sparing diuretics may be risky in patients with impaired renal function, and should be constantly reevaluated as GFR declines.

Metabolic Acidosis Metabolic acidosis is a common disturbance in advanced CKD. The majority of patients can still acidify the urine, but they produce less ammonia and, therefore, cannot excrete the normal quantity of protons in combination with this urinary buffer. Hyperkalemia, if present, further depresses ammonia production. The combination of hyperkalemia and hyperchloremic metabolic acidosis is often present, even at earlier stages of CKD (stages 1–3), in patients with diabetic nephropathy or in those with predominant tubulointerstitial disease or obstructive uropathy; this is a non-anion-gap metabolic acidosis.

With worsening renal function, the total urinary net daily acid excretion is usually limited to 30–40 mmol, and the anions of retained organic acids can then lead to an anion-gap metabolic acidosis. Thus, the non-anion-gap metabolic acidosis that can be seen in earlier stages of CKD may be complicated by the addition of an anion-gap metabolic acidosis as CKD progresses. In most patients, the metabolic acidosis is mild; the pH is rarely <7.35 and can usually be corrected with oral sodium bicarbonate supplementation. Animal and human studies have suggested that even modest degrees of metabolic acidosis may be associated with the development of protein catabolism. Alkali supplementation may attenuate the catabolic state and possibly slow CKD progression and accordingly is recommended when the serum bicarbonate concentration falls below 20–23 mmol/L. The concomitant sodium load mandates careful attention to volume status and the need for diuretic agents.

TREATMENT FLUID, ELECTROLYTE, AND ACID-BASE DISORDERS

Dietary salt restriction and the use of loop diuretics, occasionally in combination with metolazone, may be needed to maintain euvolemia. In contrast, overzealous salt restriction or diuretic use can lead to ECFV depletion and precipitate a further decline in GFR. The rare patient with salt-losing nephropathy may require a sodium-rich diet or salt supplementation. Water restriction is indicated only if there is a problem with hyponatremia. Intractable ECFV expansion, despite dietary salt restriction and diuretic therapy, may be an indication to start renal replacement therapy. Hyperkalemia often responds to dietary restriction of potassium, the use of kaliuretic diuretics, and avoidance of both potassium supplements (including occult sources, such as dietary salt substitutes) and potassium-retaining medications (especially angiotensin-converting enzyme [ACE] inhibitors or angiotensin receptor blockers [ARBs]). Kaliuretic diuretics promote urinary potassium excretion, whereas potassium-binding resins, such as calcium resonium or sodium polystyrene, can promote potassium loss through the GI tract and may reduce the incidence of hyperkalemia. Intractable hyperkalemia is an indication (although uncommon) to consider institution of dialysis in a CKD patient. The renal tubular acidosis and subsequent anion-gap metabolic acidosis in progressive CKD will respond to alkali supplementation, typically with sodium bicarbonate. Recent studies suggest that this replacement should be considered when the serum bicarbonate concentration falls below 20–23 mmol/L to avoid the protein catabolic state seen with even mild degrees of metabolic acidosis and to slow the progression of CKD.

DISORDERS OF CALCIUM AND PHOSPHATE METABOLISM

The principal complications of abnormalities of calcium and phosphate metabolism in CKD occur in the skeleton and the vascular bed, with occasional severe involvement of extraosseous soft tissues. It is likely that disorders of bone turnover and disorders of vascular and soft tissue calcification are related to each other (Fig. 335-3).

Bone Manifestations of CKD The major disorders of bone disease can be classified into those associated with high bone turnover with increased PTH levels (including osteitis fibrosa cystica, the classic lesion of secondary hyperparathyroidism) and low bone turnover with low or normal PTH levels (adynamic bone disease and osteomalacia).

The pathophysiology of secondary hyperparathyroidism and the consequent high-turnover bone disease is related to abnormal mineral metabolism through the following events: (1) declining GFR leads to reduced excretion of phosphate and, thus, phosphate retention; (2) the retained phosphate stimulates increased synthesis of both FGF-23 by osteocytes and PTH and stimulates growth of parathyroid gland mass; and (3) decreased levels of ionized calcium, resulting from suppression of calcitriol production by FGF-23 and by the failing kidney, as well as phosphate retention, also stimulate PTH production. Low calcitriol levels contribute to hyperparathyroidism, both by leading to hypocalcemia and also by a direct effect on PTH gene transcription. These changes start to occur when the GFR falls below 60 mL/min.

FGF-23 is part of a family of phosphatonins that promotes renal phosphate excretion. Recent studies have shown that levels of this hormone, secreted by osteocytes, increase early in the course of CKD, even before phosphate retention and hyperphosphatemia. FGF-23 may defend normal serum phosphorus in at least three ways: (1) increased renal phosphate excretion; (2) stimulation of PTH, which also increases renal phosphate excretion; and (3) suppression of the formation of $1,25(OH)_2D_3$, leading to diminished phosphorus absorption from the GI tract. Interestingly, high levels of FGF-23 are also an independent risk factor for left ventricular hypertrophy and mortality in CKD, dialysis, and renal transplant patients. Moreover, elevated levels of FGF-23 may indicate the need for therapeutic intervention (e.g., phosphate restriction), even when serum phosphate levels are within the normal range.

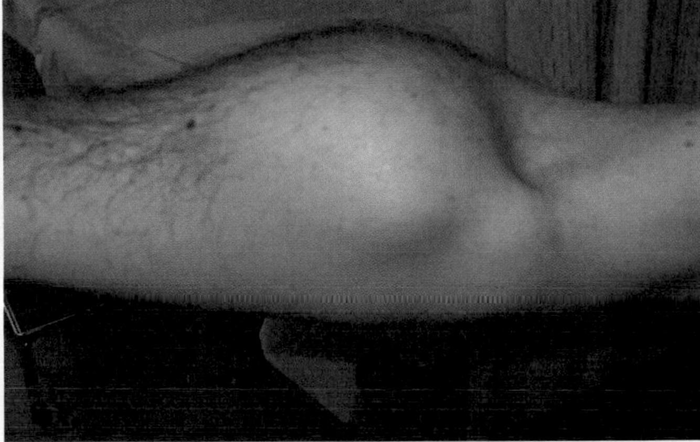

FIGURE 335-4 Tumoral calcinosis. This patient was on hemodialysis for many years and was nonadherent to dietary phosphorus restriction or the use of phosphate binders. He was chronically severely hyperphosphatemic. He developed an enlarging painful mass on his arm that was extensively calcified.

Hyperparathyroidism stimulates bone turnover and leads to *osteitis fibrosa cystica*. Bone histology shows abnormal osteoid, bone and bone marrow fibrosis, and in advanced stages, the formation of bone cysts, sometimes with hemorrhagic elements so that they appear brown in color, hence the term *brown tumor*. Clinical manifestations of severe hyperparathyroidism include bone pain and fragility, brown tumors, compression syndromes, and erythropoietin resistance in part related to the bone marrow fibrosis. Furthermore, PTH itself is considered a uremic toxin, and high levels are associated with muscle weakness, fibrosis of cardiac muscle, and nonspecific constitutional symptoms.

Low-turnover bone disease can be grouped into two categories—adynamic bone disease and osteomalacia. Adynamic bone disease is increasing in prevalence, especially among diabetics and the elderly. It is characterized by reduced bone volume and mineralization and may result from excessive suppression of PTH production, chronic inflammation, or both. Suppression of PTH can result from the use of vitamin D preparations or from excessive calcium exposure in the form of calcium-containing phosphate binders or high-calcium dialysis solutions. Complications of adynamic bone disease include an increased incidence of fracture and bone pain and an association with increased vascular and cardiac calcification. Occasionally the calcium will precipitate in the soft tissues into large concretions termed "tumoral calcinosis" (Fig. 335-4).

Calcium, Phosphorus, and the Cardiovascular System Recent epidemiologic evidence has shown a strong association between hyperphosphatemia and increased cardiovascular mortality rate in patients with stage 5 CKD and even in patients with earlier stages of CKD. Hyperphosphatemia and hypercalcemia are associated with increased vascular calcification, but it is unclear whether the excessive mortality rate is mediated by this mechanism. Studies using computed tomography (CT) and electron-beam CT scanning show that CKD patients have calcification of the media in coronary arteries and even heart valves that appear to be orders of magnitude greater than that in patients without renal disease. The magnitude of the calcification is proportional to age and hyperphosphatemia and is also associated with low PTH levels and low bone turnover. It is possible that in patients with advanced kidney disease, ingested calcium cannot be deposited in bones with low turnover and, therefore, is deposited at extraosseous sites, such as the vascular bed and soft tissues. It is interesting in this regard that there is also an association between osteoporosis and vascular calcification in the general population. Finally, hyperphosphatemia can induce a change in gene expression in vascular cells to an osteoblast-like profile, leading to vascular calcification and even ossification.

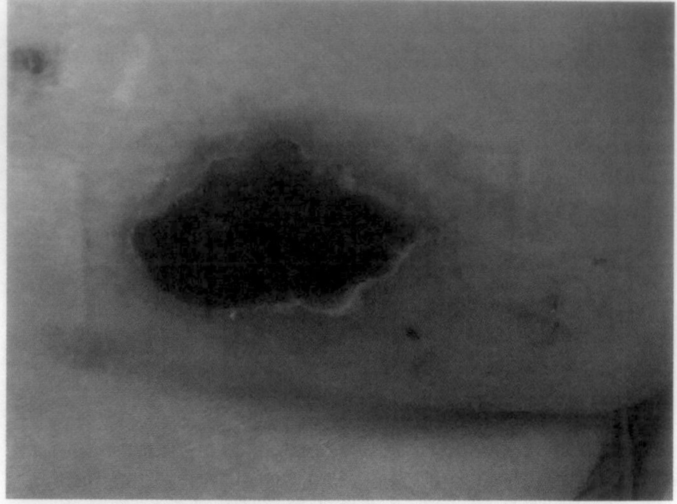

FIGURE 335-5 Calciphylaxis. This peritoneal dialysis patient was on chronic warfarin therapy for atrial fibrillation. She noticed a small painful nodule on the abdomen that was followed by progressive skin necrosis and ulceration of the anterior abdominal wall. She was treated with hyperbaric oxygen, intravenous thiosulfate, and discontinuation of warfarin, with slow resolution of the ulceration.

Other Complications of Abnormal Mineral Metabolism Calciphylaxis (calcific uremic arteriolopathy) is a devastating condition seen almost exclusively in patients with advanced CKD. It is heralded by livedo reticularis and advances to patches of ischemic necrosis, especially on the legs, thighs, abdomen, and breasts (Fig. 335-5). Pathologically, there is evidence of vascular occlusion in association with extensive vascular and soft tissue calcification. It appears that this condition is increasing in incidence. Originally it was ascribed to severe abnormalities in calcium and phosphorus control in dialysis patients, usually associated with advanced hyperparathyroidism. However, more recently, calciphylaxis has been seen with increasing frequency in the absence of severe hyperparathyroidism. Other etiologies have been suggested, including the increased use of oral calcium as a phosphate binder. Warfarin is commonly used in hemodialysis patients, and one of the effects of warfarin therapy is to decrease the vitamin K–dependent regeneration of matrix GLA protein. This latter protein is important in preventing vascular calcification. Thus, warfarin treatment is considered a risk factor for calciphylaxis, and if a patient develops this syndrome, this medication should be discontinued and replaced with alternative forms of anticoagulation.

TREATMENT DISORDERS OF CALCIUM AND PHOSPHATE METABOLISM

The optimal management of secondary hyperparathyroidism and osteitis fibrosa is prevention. Once the parathyroid gland mass is very large, it is difficult to control the disease. Careful attention should be paid to the plasma phosphate concentration in CKD patients, who should be counseled on a low-phosphate diet as well as the appropriate use of phosphate-binding agents. These are agents that are taken with meals and complex the dietary phosphate to limit its GI absorption. Examples of phosphate binders are calcium acetate and calcium carbonate. A major side effect of calcium-based phosphate binders is calcium accumulation and hypercalcemia, especially in patients with low-turnover bone disease. Sevelamer and lanthanum are non-calcium-containing polymers that also function as phosphate binders; they do not predispose CKD patients to hypercalcemia and may attenuate calcium deposition in the vascular bed.

Calcitriol exerts a direct suppressive effect on PTH secretion and also indirectly suppresses PTH secretion by raising the concentration of ionized calcium. However, calcitriol therapy may result in hypercalcemia and/or hyperphosphatemia through increased GI absorption of these minerals. Certain analogues of calcitriol are available (e.g., paricalcitol) that suppress PTH secretion with less attendant hypercalcemia.

Recognition of the role of the extracellular calcium-sensing receptor has led to the development of calcimimetic agents that enhance the sensitivity of the parathyroid cell to the suppressive effect of calcium. This class of drug, which includes cinacalcet, produces a dose-dependent reduction in PTH and plasma calcium concentration in some patients.

Current National Kidney Foundation Kidney Disease Outcomes Quality Initiative guidelines recommend a target PTH level between 150 and 300 pg/mL, recognizing that very low PTH levels are associated with adynamic bone disease and possible consequences of fracture and ectopic calcification.

CARDIOVASCULAR ABNORMALITIES

Cardiovascular disease is the leading cause of morbidity and mortality in patients at every stage of CKD. The incremental risk of cardiovascular disease in those with CKD compared to the age- and sex-matched general population ranges from 10- to 200-fold, depending on the stage of CKD. Between 30 and 45% of patients reaching stage 5 CKD already have advanced cardiovascular complications. As a result, most patients with CKD succumb to cardiovascular disease (Fig. 335-6) before ever reaching stage 5 CKD. Thus, the focus of patient care in earlier CKD stages should be directed to prevention of cardiovascular complications.

Ischemic Vascular Disease The presence of any stage of CKD is a major risk factor for ischemic cardiovascular disease, including occlusive coronary, cerebrovascular, and peripheral vascular disease. The increased prevalence of vascular disease in CKD patients derives from both traditional ("classic") and nontraditional (CKD-related) risk factors. Traditional risk factors include hypertension, hypervolemia, dyslipidemia, sympathetic overactivity, and hyperhomocysteinemia. The CKD-related risk factors comprise anemia, hyperphosphatemia, hyperparathyroidism, increased FGF-23, sleep apnea, and generalized inflammation. The inflammatory state associated with a reduction in kidney function is reflected in increased circulating acute-phase reactants, such as inflammatory cytokines and C-reactive protein, with a corresponding fall in the "negative acute-phase reactants," such as serum albumin and fetuin. The inflammatory state appears to accelerate vascular occlusive disease, and low levels of fetuin may permit more rapid vascular calcification, especially in the face of hyperphosphatemia. Other abnormalities seen in CKD may augment

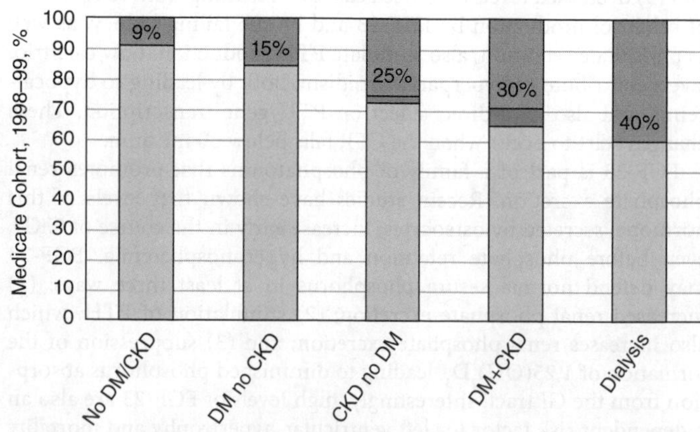

FIGURE 335-6 U.S. Renal Data System showing increased likelihood of dying rather than starting dialysis or reaching stage 5 chronic kidney disease (CKD). [1], Death; [2], ESRD; [3], event-free. DM; diabetes mellitus. *(Adapted from RN Foley et al: J Am Soc Nephrol 16:489-495, 2005.)*

myocardial ischemia, including left ventricular hypertrophy and microvascular disease. In addition, hemodialysis, with its attendant episodes of hypotension and hypovolemia, may further aggravate coronary ischemia and repeatedly stun the myocardium. Interestingly, however, the largest increment in cardiovascular mortality rate in dialysis patients is not necessarily directly associated with documented acute myocardial infarction but, instead, presents with congestive heart failure and all of its manifestations and sudden death.

Cardiac troponin levels are frequently elevated in CKD without evidence of acute ischemia. The elevation complicates the diagnosis of acute myocardial infarction in this population. Serial measurements may be needed, and if the level is unchanged, it is possible that there is no acute myocardial ischemia. Therefore, the trend in levels over the hours after presentation may be more informative than a single, elevated level. Interestingly, consistently elevated levels are an independent prognostic factor for adverse cardiovascular events in this population.

Heart Failure Abnormal cardiac function secondary to myocardial ischemia, left ventricular hypertrophy, and frank cardiomyopathy, in combination with the salt and water retention that can be seen with CKD, often results in heart failure or even pulmonary edema. Heart failure can be a consequence of diastolic or systolic dysfunction, or both. A form of "low-pressure" pulmonary edema can also occur in advanced CKD, manifesting as shortness of breath and a "bat wing" distribution of alveolar edema fluid on the chest x-ray. This finding can occur even in the absence of ECFV overload and is associated with normal or mildly elevated pulmonary capillary wedge pressure. This process has been ascribed to increased permeability of alveolar capillary membranes as a manifestation of the uremic state, and it responds to dialysis. Other CKD-related risk factors, including anemia and sleep apnea, may contribute to the risk of heart failure.

Hypertension and Left Ventricular Hypertrophy Hypertension is one of the most common complications of CKD. It usually develops early during the course of CKD and is associated with adverse outcomes, including the development of ventricular hypertrophy and a more rapid loss of renal function. Many studies have shown a relationship between the level of blood pressure and the rate of progression of diabetic and nondiabetic kidney disease. Left ventricular hypertrophy and dilated cardiomyopathy are among the strongest risk factors for cardiovascular morbidity and mortality in patients with CKD and are thought to be related primarily, but not exclusively, to prolonged hypertension and ECFV overload. In addition, anemia and the placement of an arteriovenous fistula for hemodialysis can generate a high cardiac output state and consequent heart failure.

The absence of hypertension may signify poor left ventricular function. Indeed, in epidemiologic studies of dialysis patients, low blood pressure actually carries a worse prognosis than does high blood pressure. This mechanism, in part, accounts for the "reverse causation" seen in dialysis patients, wherein the presence of traditional risk factors, such as hypertension, hyperlipidemia, and obesity, appear to portend a better prognosis. Importantly, these observations derive from cross-sectional studies of late-stage CKD patients and should not be interpreted to discourage appropriate management of these risk factors in CKD patients, especially at early stages. In contrast to the general population, it is possible that in late-stage CKD, low blood pressure, reduced body mass index, and hypolipidemia indicate the presence of an advanced malnutrition-inflammation state, with poor prognosis.

The use of exogenous erythropoiesis-stimulating agents can increase blood pressure and the requirement for antihypertensive drugs. Chronic ECFV overload is also a contributor to hypertension, and improvement in blood pressure can often be seen with the use of dietary sodium restriction, diuretics, and fluid removal with dialysis. Nevertheless, because of activation of the RAS and other disturbances in the balance of vasoconstrictors and vasodilators, some patients remain hypertensive despite careful attention to ECFV status.

TREATMENT CARDIOVASCULAR ABNORMALITIES

MANAGEMENT OF HYPERTENSION

The overarching goal of hypertension therapy in CKD is to prevent the extrarenal complications of high blood pressure, such as cardiovascular disease and stroke. Although a clear-cut generalizable benefit in slowing progression of CKD remains as yet unproven, the benefit for cardiac and neurologic health is compelling. In all patients with CKD, blood pressure should be controlled to levels recommended by national guideline panels. In CKD patients with diabetes or proteinuria >1 g per 24 h, blood pressure should be reduced to 130/80 mmHg, if achievable without prohibitive adverse effects. Salt restriction should be the first line of therapy. When volume management alone is not sufficient, the choice of antihypertensive agent is similar to that in the general population. ACE inhibitors and ARBs appear to slow the rate of decline of kidney function in a manner that extends beyond reduction of systemic arterial pressure and that involves correction of the intraglomerular hyperfiltration and hypertension involved in progression of CKD described above. Occasionally, introduction of ACE inhibitors and ARBs can actually precipitate an episode of acute kidney injury, especially when used in combination in patients with ischemic renovascular disease. The use of ACE inhibitors and ARBs may also be complicated by the development of hyperkalemia. Often the concomitant use of a kaliuretic diuretic, such as metolazone, can improve potassium excretion in addition to improving blood pressure control. Potassium-sparing diuretics should be used with caution or avoided altogether in most patients.

MANAGEMENT OF CARDIOVASCULAR DISEASE

There are many strategies available to treat the traditional and nontraditional risk factors in CKD patients. Although these have proved effective in the general population, there is little evidence for their benefit in patients with advanced CKD, especially those on dialysis. Certainly hypertension, elevated serum levels of homocysteine, and dyslipidemia promote atherosclerotic disease and are treatable complications of CKD. Renal disease complicated by nephrotic syndrome is associated with a very atherogenic lipid profile and hypercoagulability, which increases the risk of occlusive vascular disease. Because diabetes mellitus and hypertension are the two most frequent causes of advanced CKD, it is not surprising that cardiovascular disease is the most frequent cause of death in dialysis patients. The role of "inflammation" may be quantitatively more important in patients with kidney disease, and the treatment of more traditional risk factors may result in only modest success. However, modulation of traditional risk factors may be the only weapon in the therapeutic armamentarium for these patients until the nature of inflammation in CKD and its treatment are better understood.

Lifestyle changes, including regular exercise, should be advocated. Hyperlipidemia in patients with CKD should be managed according to national guidelines. If dietary measures are not sufficient, preferred lipid-lowering medications, such as statins, should be used. Again, the use of these agents has not been of proven benefit for patients with advanced CKD.

Pericardial Disease Chest pain with respiratory accentuation, accompanied by a friction rub, is diagnostic of pericarditis. Classic electrocardiographic abnormalities include PR-interval depression and diffuse ST-segment elevation. Pericarditis can be accompanied by pericardial effusion that is seen on echocardiography and can rarely lead to tamponade. However, the pericardial effusion can be asymptomatic, and pericarditis can be seen without significant effusion.

Pericarditis is observed in advanced uremia, and with the advent of timely initiation of dialysis, is not as common as it once was. It is now more often observed in underdialyzed, nonadherent patients than in those starting dialysis.

TREATMENT PERICARDIAL DISEASE

Uremic pericarditis is an absolute indication for the urgent initiation of dialysis or for intensification of the dialysis prescription in those already receiving dialysis. Because of the propensity to hemorrhage in pericardial fluid, hemodialysis should be performed without heparin. A pericardial drainage procedure should be considered in patients with recurrent pericardial effusion, especially with echocardiographic signs of impending tamponade. Nonuremic causes of pericarditis and effusion include viral, malignant, tuberculous, and autoimmune etiologies. It may also be seen after myocardial infarction and as a complication of treatment with the antihypertensive drug minoxidil.

HEMATOLOGIC ABNORMALITIES

Anemia A normocytic, normochromic anemia is observed as early as stage 3 CKD and is almost universal by stage 4. The primary cause in patients with CKD is insufficient production of erythropoietin (EPO) by the diseased kidneys. Additional factors are reviewed in Table 335-3.

The anemia of CKD is associated with a number of adverse pathophysiologic consequences, including decreased tissue oxygen delivery and utilization, increased cardiac output, ventricular dilation, and ventricular hypertrophy. Clinical manifestations include fatigue and diminished exercise tolerance, angina, heart failure, decreased cognition and mental acuity, and impaired host defense against infection. In addition, anemia may play a role in growth restriction in children with CKD. Although many studies in CKD patients have found that anemia and resistance to exogenous erythropoietic-stimulating agents (ESA) are associated with a poor prognosis, the relative contribution to a poor outcome of the low hematocrit itself, versus inflammation as a cause of the anemia and ESA resistance, remains unclear.

TREATMENT ANEMIA

The availability of recombinant human ESA has been one of the most significant advances in the care of renal patients since the introduction of dialysis and renal transplantation. The routine use of these recombinant hormones has obviated the need for regular blood transfusions in severely anemic CKD patients, thus dramatically reducing the incidence of transfusion-associated infections and iron overload. Frequent blood transfusions in dialysis patients also lead to the development of alloantibodies that can sensitize the patient to donor kidney antigens and make renal transplantation more problematic.

Adequate bone marrow iron stores should be available before treatment with ESA is initiated. Iron supplementation is usually essential to ensure an optimal response to ESA in patients with CKD because the demand for iron by the marrow frequently exceeds the amount of iron that is immediately available for erythropoiesis (measured by percent transferrin saturation), as well as the amount in iron stores (measured by serum ferritin). For the CKD patient not yet on dialysis or the patient treated with peritoneal dialysis, oral iron supplementation should be attempted. If there is GI intolerance, the patient may have to undergo IV iron infusion. For patients on hemodialysis, IV iron can be administered during dialysis, keeping in mind that iron therapy can increase the susceptibility to bacterial infections. In addition to iron, an adequate supply of other major substrates and cofactors for red cell production must be ensured, including vitamin B_{12} and folate. Anemia resistant to recommended doses of ESA in the face of adequate iron stores may be due to some combination of the following: acute or chronic inflammation, inadequate dialysis, severe hyperparathyroidism, chronic blood loss or hemolysis, chronic infection, or malignancy. Blood transfusions increase the risk of hepatitis, iron overload, and transplant sensitization; they should be avoided unless the anemia fails to respond to ESA and the patient is symptomatic.

Randomized, controlled trials of ESA in CKD have failed to show an improvement in cardiovascular outcomes with this therapy. Indeed, there has been an indication that the use of ESA in CKD may be associated with an increased risk of stroke in those with type 2 diabetes, an increase in thromboembolic events, and perhaps a faster progression to the need for dialysis. Therefore, any benefit in terms of improvement of anemic symptoms needs to be balanced against the potential cardiovascular risk. Although further studies are needed, it is quite clear that complete normalization of the hemoglobin concentration has not been demonstrated to be of incremental benefit to CKD patients. Current practice is to target a hemoglobin concentration of 100–115 g/L.

TABLE 335-3 CAUSES OF ANEMIA IN CKD

Relative deficiency of erythropoietin
Diminished red blood cell survival
Bleeding diathesis
Iron deficiency
Hyperparathyroidism/bone marrow fibrosis
Chronic inflammation
Folate or vitamin B_{12} deficiency
Hemoglobinopathy
Comorbid conditions: hypo-/hyperthyroidism, pregnancy, HIV-associated disease, autoimmune disease, immunosuppressive drugs

Abnormal Hemostasis Patients with later stages of CKD may have a prolonged bleeding time, decreased activity of platelet factor III, abnormal platelet aggregation and adhesiveness, and impaired prothrombin consumption. Clinical manifestations include an increased tendency to bleeding and bruising, prolonged bleeding from surgical incisions, menorrhagia, and GI bleeding. Interestingly, CKD patients also have a greater susceptibility to thromboembolism, especially if they have renal disease that includes nephrotic-range proteinuria. The latter condition results in hypoalbuminemia and renal loss of anticoagulant factors, which can lead to a thrombophilic state.

TREATMENT ABNORMAL HEMOSTASIS

Abnormal bleeding time and coagulopathy in patients with renal failure may be reversed temporarily with desmopressin (DDAVP), cryoprecipitate, IV conjugated estrogens, blood transfusions, and ESA therapy. Optimal dialysis will usually correct a prolonged bleeding time.

Given the coexistence of bleeding disorders and a propensity to thrombosis that is unique in the CKD patient, decisions about anticoagulation that have a favorable risk-benefit profile in the general population may not be applicable to the patient with advanced CKD. One example is warfarin anticoagulation for atrial fibrillation; the decision to anticoagulate should be made on an individual basis in the CKD patient because there appears to be a greater risk of bleeding complications.

Certain anticoagulants, such as fractionated low-molecular-weight heparin, may need to be avoided or dose-adjusted in these patients, with monitoring of factor Xa activity where available. It is often more prudent to use conventional unfractionated heparin, titrated to the measured partial thromboplastin time, in hospitalized patients requiring an alternative to warfarin anticoagulation. The new classes of oral anticoagulants are all, in part, renally eliminated and need dose adjustment in the face of decreased GFR (Chap. 143).

NEUROMUSCULAR ABNORMALITIES

Central nervous system (CNS), peripheral, and autonomic neuropathy as well as abnormalities in muscle structure and function are all well-recognized complications of CKD. Subtle clinical manifestations of uremic neuromuscular disease usually become evident at stage 3 CKD. Early manifestations of CNS complications include mild disturbances in memory and concentration and sleep disturbance. Neuromuscular irritability, including hiccups, cramps, and twitching, becomes evident at later stages. In advanced untreated kidney failure, asterixis, myoclonus, seizures, and coma can be seen.

Peripheral neuropathy usually becomes clinically evident after the patient reaches stage 4 CKD, although electrophysiologic and histologic evidence occurs earlier. Initially, sensory nerves are involved more than motor, lower extremities more than upper, and distal parts of the extremities more than proximal. The "restless leg syndrome" is characterized by ill-defined sensations of sometimes debilitating discomfort in the legs and feet relieved by frequent leg movement. If dialysis is not instituted soon after onset of sensory abnormalities, motor involvement follows, including muscle weakness. Evidence of peripheral neuropathy without another cause (e.g., diabetes mellitus) is an indication for starting renal replacement therapy. Many of the complications described above will resolve with dialysis, although subtle nonspecific abnormalities may persist.

GASTROINTESTINAL AND NUTRITIONAL ABNORMALITIES

Uremic fetor, a urine-like odor on the breath, derives from the breakdown of urea to ammonia in saliva and is often associated with an unpleasant metallic taste (dysgeusia). Gastritis, peptic disease, and mucosal ulcerations at any level of the GI tract occur in uremic patients and can lead to abdominal pain, nausea, vomiting, and GI bleeding. These patients are also prone to constipation, which can be worsened by the administration of calcium and iron supplements. The retention of uremic toxins also leads to anorexia, nausea, and vomiting.

Protein restriction may be useful to decrease nausea and vomiting; however, it may put the patient at risk for malnutrition and should be carried out, if possible, in consultation with a registered dietitian specializing in the management of CKD patients. Protein-energy malnutrition, a consequence of low protein and caloric intake, is common in advanced CKD and is often an indication for initiation of renal replacement therapy. Metabolic acidosis and the activation of inflammatory cytokines can promote protein catabolism. Assessment for protein-energy malnutrition should begin at stage 3 CKD. A number of indices are useful in this assessment and include dietary history, including food diary and subjective global assessment; edema-free body weight; and measurement of urinary protein nitrogen appearance. Dual-energy x-ray absorptiometry is now widely used to estimate lean body mass versus ECFV. Adjunctive tools include clinical signs, such as skinfold thickness, mid-arm muscle circumference, and additional laboratory tests such as serum pre-albumin and cholesterol levels. Nutritional guidelines for patients with CKD are summarized in the "Treatment" section.

ENDOCRINE-METABOLIC DISTURBANCES

Glucose metabolism is impaired in CKD, as evidenced by a slowing of the rate at which blood glucose levels decline after a glucose load. However, fasting blood glucose is usually normal or only slightly elevated, and the mild glucose intolerance does not require specific therapy. Because the kidney contributes to insulin removal from the circulation, plasma levels of insulin are slightly to moderately elevated in most uremic patients, both in the fasting and postprandial states. Because of this diminished renal degradation of insulin, patients on insulin therapy may need progressive reduction in dose as their renal function worsens. Many hypoglycemic agents, including the gliptins, require dose reduction in renal failure, and some, such as metformin, are contraindicated when the GFR is less than half of normal.

In women with CKD, estrogen levels are low, and menstrual abnormalities, infertility, and inability to carry pregnancies to term are common. When the GFR has declined to ~40 mL/min, pregnancy is associated with a high rate of spontaneous abortion, with only ~20% of pregnancies leading to live births, and pregnancy may hasten the progression of the kidney disease itself. Women with CKD who are contemplating pregnancy should consult first with a nephrologist in conjunction with an obstetrician specializing in high-risk pregnancy. Men with CKD have reduced plasma testosterone levels, and sexual dysfunction and oligospermia may supervene. Sexual maturation may be delayed or impaired in adolescent children with CKD, even among those treated with dialysis. Many of these abnormalities improve or reverse with intensive dialysis or with successful renal transplantation.

DERMATOLOGIC ABNORMALITIES

Abnormalities of the skin are prevalent in progressive CKD. Pruritus is quite common and one of the most vexing manifestations of the uremic state. In advanced CKD, even on dialysis, patients may become more pigmented, and this is felt to reflect the deposition of retained pigmented metabolites, or *urochromes*. Although many of the cutaneous abnormalities improve with dialysis, pruritus is often tenacious. The first lines of management are to rule out unrelated skin disorders, such as scabies, and to treat hyperphosphatemia, which can cause itch. Local moisturizers, mild topical glucocorticoids, oral antihistamines, and ultraviolet radiation have been reported to be helpful.

A skin condition unique to CKD patients called *nephrogenic fibrosing dermopathy* consists of progressive subcutaneous induration, especially on the arms and legs. The condition is similar to scleromyxedema and is seen very rarely in patients with CKD who have been exposed to the magnetic resonance contrast agent gadolinium. Current recommendations are that patients with CKD stage 3 (GFR 30–59 mL/min) should minimize exposure to gadolinium, and those with CKD stages 4–5 (GFR <30 mL/min) should avoid the use of gadolinium agents unless it is medically necessary. Concomitant liver disease appears to be a risk factor. However, no patient should be denied an imaging investigation that is critical to management, and under such circumstances, rapid removal of gadolinium by hemodialysis (even in patients not yet receiving renal replacement therapy) shortly after the procedure may mitigate this sometimes devastating complication.

EVALUATION AND MANAGEMENT OF PATIENTS WITH CKD

INITIAL APPROACH

History and Physical Examination Symptoms and overt signs of kidney disease are often subtle or absent until renal failure supervenes. Thus, the diagnosis of kidney disease often surprises patients and may be a cause of skepticism and denial. Particular aspects of the history that are germane to renal disease include a history of hypertension (which can cause CKD or more commonly be a consequence of CKD), diabetes mellitus, abnormal urinalyses, and problems with pregnancy such as preeclampsia or early pregnancy loss. A careful drug history should be elicited: patients may not volunteer use of analgesics, for example. Other drugs to consider include nonsteroidal anti-inflammatory agents, cyclooxygenase-2 (COX-2) inhibitors, antimicrobials, chemotherapeutic agents, antiretroviral agents, proton pump inhibitors, phosphate-containing bowel cathartics, and lithium. In evaluating the uremic syndrome, questions about appetite, weight loss, nausea, hiccups, peripheral edema, muscle cramps, pruritus, and restless legs are especially helpful. A careful family history of kidney disease, together with assessment of manifestations in other organ systems such as auditory, visual, and integumentary, may lead to the diagnosis of a heritable form of CKD (e.g., Alport or Fabry disease, cystinosis) or shared environmental exposure to nephrotoxic agents (e.g., heavy metals, aristolochic acid). It should be noted that clustering of CKD, sometimes of different etiologies, is often observed within families.

The physical examination should focus on blood pressure and target organ damage from hypertension. Thus, funduscopy and precordial examination (left ventricular heave, a fourth heart sound) should be carried out. Funduscopy is important in the diabetic patient, because it may show evidence of diabetic retinopathy, which is associated with nephropathy. Other physical examination manifestations of CKD include edema and sensory polyneuropathy. The finding of asterixis or a pericardial friction rub not attributable to other causes usually signifies the presence of the uremic syndrome.

Laboratory Investigation Laboratory studies should focus on a search for clues to an underlying causative or aggravating disease process and on the degree of renal damage and its consequences. Serum and urine protein electrophoresis, looking for multiple myeloma, should be obtained in all patients >35 years with unexplained CKD, especially if there is associated anemia and elevated, or even inappropriately normal, serum calcium concentration in the face of renal insufficiency. In the presence of glomerulonephritis, autoimmune diseases such as lupus and underlying infectious etiologies such as hepatitis B and C and HIV should be tested. Serial measurements of renal function should be obtained to determine the pace of renal deterioration and ensure that the disease is truly chronic rather than acute or subacute and hence potentially reversible. Serum concentrations of calcium, phosphorus, vitamin D, and PTH should be measured to evaluate metabolic bone disease. Hemoglobin concentration, iron, vitamin B_{12}, and folate should also be evaluated. A 24-h urine collection may be helpful, because protein excretion >300 mg may be an indication for therapy with ACE inhibitors or ARBs.

Imaging Studies The most useful imaging study is a renal ultrasound, which can verify the presence of two kidneys, determine if they are symmetric, provide an estimate of kidney size, and rule out renal masses and evidence of obstruction. Because it takes time for kidneys to shrink as a result of chronic disease, the finding of bilaterally small kidneys supports the diagnosis of CKD of long-standing duration, with an irreversible component of scarring. If the kidney size is normal, it is possible that the renal disease is acute or subacute. The exceptions are diabetic nephropathy (where kidney size is increased at the onset of diabetic nephropathy before CKD supervenes), amyloidosis, and HIV nephropathy, where kidney size may be normal in the face of CKD. Polycystic kidney disease that has reached some degree of renal failure will almost always present with enlarged kidneys with multiple cysts (Chap. 339). A discrepancy >1 cm in kidney length suggests either a unilateral developmental abnormality or disease process or renovascular disease with arterial insufficiency affecting one kidney more than the other. The diagnosis of renovascular disease can be undertaken with different techniques, including Doppler sonography, nuclear medicine studies, or CT or magnetic resonance imaging (MRI) studies. If there is a suspicion of reflux nephropathy (recurrent childhood urinary tract infection, asymmetric renal size with scars on the renal poles), a voiding cystogram may be indicated. However, in most cases, by the time the patient has CKD, the reflux has resolved, and even if still present, repair does not improve renal function. Radiographic contrast imaging studies are not particularly helpful in the investigation of CKD. Intravenous or intraarterial dye should be avoided where possible in the CKD patient, especially with diabetic nephropathy, because of the risk of radiographic contrast dye–induced renal failure. When unavoidable, appropriate precautionary measures include avoidance of hypovolemia at the time of contrast exposure, minimization of the dye load, and choice of radiographic contrast preparations with the least nephrotoxic potential. Additional measures thought to attenuate contrast-induced worsening of renal function include judicious administration of sodium bicarbonate–containing solutions and *N* -acetylcysteine.

Kidney Biopsy In the patient with bilaterally small kidneys, renal biopsy is not advised because (1) it is technically difficult and has a greater likelihood of causing bleeding and other adverse consequences, (2) there is usually so much scarring that the underlying disease may not be apparent, and (3) the window of opportunity to render disease-specific therapy has passed. Other contraindications to renal biopsy include uncontrolled hypertension, active urinary tract infection, bleeding diathesis (including ongoing anticoagulation), and severe obesity. Ultrasound-guided percutaneous biopsy is the favored approach, but a surgical or laparoscopic approach can be considered, especially in the patient with a single kidney where direct visualization and control of bleeding are crucial. In the CKD patient in whom a kidney biopsy is indicated (e.g., suspicion of a concomitant or superimposed active process such as interstitial nephritis or in the face of accelerated loss of GFR), the bleeding time should be measured, and if increased, desmopressin should be administered immediately prior to the procedure.

A brief run of hemodialysis (without heparin) may also be considered prior to renal biopsy to normalize the bleeding time.

ESTABLISHING THE DIAGNOSIS AND ETIOLOGY OF CKD

The most important initial diagnostic step is to distinguish newly diagnosed CKD from acute or subacute renal failure, because the latter two conditions may respond to targeted therapy. Previous measurements of serum creatinine concentration are particularly helpful in this regard. Normal values from recent months or even years suggest that the current extent of renal dysfunction could be more acute, and hence reversible, than might otherwise be appreciated. In contrast, elevated serum creatinine concentration in the past suggests that the renal disease represents a chronic process. Even if there is evidence of chronicity, there is the possibility of a superimposed acute process (e.g., ECFV depletion, urinary infection or obstruction, or nephrotoxin exposure) supervening on the chronic condition. If the history suggests multiple systemic manifestations of recent onset (e.g., fever, polyarthritis, rash), it should be assumed that renal insufficiency is part of an acute systemic illness.

Although renal biopsy can usually be performed in early CKD (stages 1–3), it is not always indicated. For example, in a patient with a history of type 1 diabetes mellitus for 15–20 years with retinopathy, nephrotic-range proteinuria, and absence of hematuria, the diagnosis of diabetic nephropathy is very likely and biopsy is usually not necessary. However, if there were some other finding not typical of diabetic nephropathy, such as hematuria or white blood cell casts, or absence of diabetic retinopathy, some other disease may be present and a biopsy may be indicated.

In the absence of a clinical diagnosis, renal biopsy may be the only recourse to establish an etiology in early-stage CKD. However, as noted above, once the CKD is advanced and the kidneys are small and scarred, there is little utility and significant risk in attempting to arrive at a specific diagnosis. Genetic testing is increasingly entering the repertoire of diagnostic tests, since the patterns of injury and kidney morphologic abnormalities often reflect overlapping causal mechanisms, whose origins can sometimes be attributed to a genetic predisposition or cause.

TREATMENT CHRONIC KIDNEY DISEASE

Treatments aimed at specific causes of CKD are discussed elsewhere. Among others, these include optimized glucose control in diabetes mellitus, immunosuppressive agents for glomerulonephritis, and emerging specific therapies to retard cystogenesis in polycystic kidney disease. The optimal timing of both specific and nonspecific therapy is usually well before there has been a measurable decline in GFR and certainly before CKD is established. It is helpful to measure sequentially and plot the rate of decline of GFR in all patients. Any acceleration in the rate of decline should prompt a search for superimposed acute or subacute processes that may be reversible. These include ECFV depletion, uncontrolled hypertension, urinary tract infection, new obstructive uropathy, exposure to nephrotoxic agents (such as nonsteroidal anti-inflammatory drugs [NSAIDs] or radiographic dye), and reactivation or flare of the original disease, such as lupus or vasculitis.

SLOWING THE PROGRESSION OF CKD

There is variation in the rate of decline of GFR among patients with CKD. However, the following interventions should be considered in an effort to stabilize or slow the decline of renal function.

Reducing Intraglomerular Hypertension and Proteinuria Increased intraglomerular filtration pressures and glomerular hypertrophy develop as a response to loss of nephron number from different kidney diseases. This response is maladaptive, as it promotes the ongoing decline of kidney function even if the inciting process has been treated or spontaneously resolved. Control of glomerular hypertension is important in slowing the progression of CKD. Moreover, elevated blood pressure increases proteinuria by increasing its flux across the glomerular capillaries. Conversely, the renoprotective effect of antihypertensive medications is gauged through the consequent reduction of proteinuria. Thus, the more effective a given treatment is in lowering protein excretion, the greater the subsequent impact on protection from decline in GFR. This observation is the basis for the treatment guideline establishing 130/80 mmHg as the target blood pressure in proteinuric CKD patients.

ACE inhibitors and ARBs inhibit the angiotensin-induced vasoconstriction of the efferent arterioles of the glomerular microcirculation. This inhibition leads to a reduction in both intraglomerular filtration pressure and proteinuria. Several controlled studies have shown that these drugs are effective in slowing the progression of renal failure in patients with advanced stages of both diabetic and nondiabetic CKD. This slowing in progression of CKD is strongly associated with the proteinuria-lowering effect. In the absence of an antiproteinuric response with either agent alone, combined treatment with both ACE inhibitors and ARBs has been considered. The combination is associated with a greater reduction in proteinuria compared to either agent alone. Insofar as reduction in proteinuria is a surrogate for improved renal outcome, the combination would appear to be advantageous. However, there is a greater incidence of acute kidney injury and adverse cardiac events from such combination therapy. It is uncertain, therefore, whether the ACE inhibitor plus ARB therapy can be advised routinely. Adverse effects from these agents include cough and angioedema with ACE inhibitors and anaphylaxis and hyperkalemia with either class. A progressive increase in serum creatinine concentration with these agents may suggest the presence of renovascular disease within the large or small arteries. Development of these side effects may mandate the use of second-line antihypertensive agents instead of the ACE inhibitors or ARBs. Among the calcium channel blockers, diltiazem and verapamil may exhibit superior antiproteinuric and renoprotective effects compared to the dihydropyridines. At least two different categories of response can be considered: one in which progression is strongly associated with systemic and intraglomerular hypertension and proteinuria (e.g., diabetic nephropathy, glomerular diseases) and in which ACE inhibitors and ARBs are likely to be the first choice; and another in which proteinuria is mild or absent initially (e.g., adult polycystic kidney disease and other tubulointerstitial diseases), where the contribution of intraglomerular hypertension is less prominent and other antihypertensive agents can be useful for control of systemic hypertension.

SLOWING THE PROGRESSION OF DIABETIC NEPHROPATHY

See Chap. 418.

MANAGING OTHER COMPLICATIONS OF CHRONIC KIDNEY DISEASE

Medication Dose Adjustment Although the loading dose of most drugs is not affected by CKD because no renal elimination is used in the calculation, the maintenance doses of many drugs will need to be adjusted. For those agents in which >70% excretion is by a nonrenal route, such as hepatic elimination, dose adjustment may not be needed. Some drugs that should be avoided include metformin, meperidine, and oral hypoglycemics that are eliminated by the kidney. NSAIDs should be avoided because of the risk of further worsening of kidney function. Many antibiotics, antihypertensives, and antiarrhythmics may require a reduction in dosage or change in the dose interval. Several online Web-based databases for dose adjustment of medications according to stage of CKD or estimated GFR are available (e.g., *http://www.globalrph.com/renaldosing2.htm*). Nephrotoxic radiocontrast agents and gadolinium should be avoided or used according to strict guidelines when medically necessary as described above.

PREPARATION FOR RENAL REPLACEMENT THERAPY (See also Chap. 337)

Temporary relief of symptoms and signs of impending uremia, such as anorexia, nausea, vomiting, lassitude, and pruritus, may sometimes be achieved with protein restriction. However, this carries a significant risk of malnutrition, and thus plans for more long-term management should be in place.

Maintenance dialysis and kidney transplantation have extended the lives of hundreds of thousands of patients with CKD worldwide. Clear indications for initiation of renal replacement therapy for patients with CKD include uremic pericarditis, encephalopathy, intractable muscle cramping, anorexia, and nausea not attributable to reversible causes such as peptic ulcer disease, evidence of malnutrition, and fluid and electrolyte abnormalities, principally hyperkalemia or ECFV overload, that are refractory to other measures.

Recommendations for the Optimal Time for Initiation of Renal Replacement Therapy Because of the individual variability in the severity of uremic symptoms and renal function, it is ill-advised to assign an arbitrary urea nitrogen or creatinine level to the need to start dialysis. Moreover, patients may become accustomed to chronic uremia and deny symptoms, only to find that they feel better with dialysis and realize in retrospect how poorly they were feeling before its initiation.

Previous studies suggested that starting dialysis before the onset of severe symptoms and signs of uremia was associated with prolongation of survival. This led to the concept of "healthy" start and is congruent with the philosophy that it is better to keep patients feeling well all along rather than allowing them to become ill with uremia before trying to return them to better health with dialysis or transplantation. Although recent studies have not confirmed an association of early-start dialysis with improved patient survival, there may be merit in this approach for some patients. On a practical level, advanced preparation may help to avoid problems with the dialysis process itself (e.g., a poorly functioning fistula for hemodialysis or malfunctioning peritoneal dialysis catheter) and, thus, preempt the morbidity associated with resorting to the insertion of temporary hemodialysis access with its attendant risks of sepsis, bleeding, thrombosis, and association with accelerated mortality.

Patient Education Social, psychological, and physical preparation for the transition to renal replacement therapy and the choice of the optimal initial modality are best accomplished with a gradual approach involving a multidisciplinary team. Along with conservative measures discussed in the sections above, it is important to prepare patients with an intensive educational program, explaining the likelihood and timing of initiation of renal replacement therapy and the various forms of therapy available, and the option of nondialytic maximum conservative care. The more knowledgeable that patients are about hemodialysis (both in-center and home-based), peritoneal dialysis, and kidney transplantation, the easier and more appropriate will be their decisions. Patients who are provided with educational programs are more likely to choose home-based dialysis therapy. This approach is of societal benefit because home-based therapy is less expensive and is associated with improved quality of life. The educational programs should be commenced no later than stage 4 CKD so that the patient has sufficient time and cognitive function to learn the important concepts, make informed choices, and implement preparatory measures for renal replacement therapy.

Exploration of social support is also important. In those who may perform home dialysis or undergo preemptive renal transplantation, early education of family members for selection and preparation of a home dialysis helper or a biologically or emotionally related potential living kidney donor should occur long before the onset of symptomatic renal failure.

Kidney transplantation (Chap. 337) offers the best potential for complete rehabilitation, because dialysis replaces only a small fraction of the kidneys' filtration function and none of the other renal functions, including endocrine and anti-inflammatory effects. Generally, kidney transplantation follows a period of dialysis treatment, although preemptive kidney transplantation (usually from a living donor) can be carried out if it is certain that the renal failure is irreversible.

IMPLICATIONS FOR GLOBAL HEALTH

In contrast to the natural decline and successful eradication of many devastating infectious diseases, there is rapid growth in the prevalence of metabolic and vascular disease in developing countries. Diabetes mellitus is becoming increasingly prevalent in these countries, perhaps due in part to change in dietary habits, diminished physical activity, and weight gain. Therefore, it follows that there will be a proportionate increase in vascular and renal disease. Health care agencies must plan for improved screening for early detection, prevention, and treatment plans in these nations and must start considering options for improved availability of renal replacement therapies.

336 Dialysis in the Treatment of Renal Failure

Kathleen D. Liu, Glenn M. Chertow

Dialysis may be required for the treatment of either acute or chronic kidney disease. The use of continuous renal replacement therapies (CRRTs) and slow low-efficiency dialysis (SLED) is specific to the management of acute renal failure and is discussed in Chap. 334. These modalities are performed continuously (CRRT) or over 6–12 h per session (SLED), in contrast to the 3–4 h of an intermittent hemodialysis session. Advantages and disadvantages of CRRT and SLED are discussed in Chap. 334.

Peritoneal dialysis is rarely used in developed countries for the treatment of acute renal failure because of the increased risk of infection and (as will be discussed in more detail below) less efficient clearance per unit of time. The focus of this chapter will be on the use of peritoneal and hemodialysis for end-stage renal disease (ESRD).

With the widespread availability of dialysis, the lives of hundreds of thousands of patients with ESRD have been prolonged. In the United States alone, there are now approximately 615,000 patients with ESRD, the vast majority of whom require dialysis. The incidence rate for ESRD is 357 cases per million population per year. The incidence of ESRD is disproportionately higher in African Americans (940 per million population per year) as compared with white Americans (280 per million population per year). In the United States, the leading cause of ESRD is diabetes mellitus, currently accounting for nearly 45% of newly diagnosed cases of ESRD. Approximately 30% of patients have ESRD that has been attributed to hypertension, although it is unclear whether in these cases hypertension is the cause or a consequence of vascular disease or other unknown causes of kidney failure. Other prevalent causes of ESRD include glomerulonephritis, polycystic kidney disease, and obstructive uropathy.

Globally, mortality rates for patients with ESRD are lowest in Europe and Japan but very high in the developing world because of the limited availability of dialysis. In the United States, the mortality rate of patients on dialysis has decreased slightly but remains extremely high, with a 5-year survival rate of approximately 35–40%. Deaths are due mainly to cardiovascular diseases and infections (approximately 40 and 10% of deaths, respectively). Older age, male sex, nonblack race, diabetes mellitus, malnutrition, and underlying heart disease are important predictors of death.

TREATMENT OPTIONS FOR ESRD PATIENTS

Commonly accepted criteria for initiating patients on maintenance dialysis include the presence of uremic symptoms, the presence of hyperkalemia unresponsive to conservative measures, persistent extracellular volume expansion despite diuretic therapy, acidosis refractory to medical therapy, a bleeding diathesis, and a creatinine clearance or estimated glomerular filtration rate (GFR) below 10 mL/min per 1.73 m^2 (see Chap. 335 for estimating equations). Timely referral to a nephrologist for advanced planning and creation of a dialysis access, education about ESRD treatment options, and management of the complications of advanced chronic kidney disease (CKD), including hypertension, anemia, acidosis, and secondary hyperparathyroidism, are advisable. Recent data have suggested that a sizable fraction of ESRD cases result following episodes of acute renal failure, particularly among persons with underlying CKD. Furthermore, there is no benefit to initiating dialysis preemptively at a GFR of 10–14 mL/min per 1.73 m^2 compared to initiating dialysis for symptoms of uremia.

In ESRD, treatment options include hemodialysis (in center or at home); peritoneal dialysis, as either continuous ambulatory peritoneal dialysis (CAPD) or continuous cyclic peritoneal dialysis (CCPD); or transplantation (Chap. 337). Although there are significant geographic variations and differences in practice patterns, hemodialysis remains the most common therapeutic modality for ESRD (>90% of patients) in the United States. In contrast to hemodialysis, peritoneal dialysis is continuous, but much less efficient, in terms of solute clearance. Although no large-scale clinical trials have been completed comparing outcomes among patients randomized to either hemodialysis or peritoneal dialysis, outcomes associated with both therapies are similar in most reports, and the decision of which modality to select is often based on personal preferences and quality-of-life considerations.

HEMODIALYSIS

Hemodialysis relies on the principles of solute diffusion across a semipermeable membrane. Movement of metabolic waste products takes place down a concentration gradient from the circulation into the dialysate. The rate of diffusive transport increases in response to several factors, including the magnitude of the concentration gradient, the membrane surface area, and the mass transfer coefficient of the membrane. The latter is a function of the porosity and thickness of the membrane, the size of the solute molecule, and the conditions of flow on the two sides of the membrane. According to laws of diffusion, the larger the molecule, the slower is its rate of transfer across the membrane. A small molecule, such as urea (60 Da), undergoes substantial clearance, whereas a larger molecule, such as creatinine (113 Da), is cleared less efficiently. In addition to diffusive clearance, movement of waste products from the circulation into the dialysate may occur as a result of ultrafiltration. Convective clearance occurs because of solvent drag, with solutes being swept along with water across the semipermeable dialysis membrane.

THE DIALYZER

There are three essential components to hemodialysis: the dialyzer, the composition and delivery of the dialysate, and the blood delivery system (Fig. 336-1). The dialyzer is a plastic chamber with the ability to perfuse blood and dialysate compartments simultaneously at very high flow rates. The hollow-fiber dialyzer is the most common in use in the United States. These dialyzers are composed of bundles of capillary tubes through which blood circulates while dialysate travels on the outside of the fiber bundle. The majority of dialyzers now manufactured in the United States are "biocompatible" synthetic membranes derived from polysulfone or related compounds (versus older cellulose "bioincompatible" membranes that activated the complement cascade). The frequency of reprocessing and reuse of hemodialyzers and blood lines varies across the world. In general, as the cost of disposable supplies has decreased, their use has increased. Formaldehyde, peracetic acid–hydrogen peroxide, glutaraldehyde, and bleach have all been used as reprocessing agents.

DIALYSATE

The potassium concentration of dialysate may be varied from 0 to 4 mmol/L depending on the predialysis serum potassium concentration. The usual dialysate calcium concentration is 1.25 mmol/L (2.5 meq/L), although modification may be required in selected settings (e.g., higher dialysate calcium concentrations may be used in patients with hypocalcemia associated with secondary hyperparathyroidism or following parathyroidectomy). The usual dialysate sodium concentration is 136–140 mmol/L. In patients who frequently develop hypotension during their dialysis run, "sodium modeling" to counterbalance urea-related osmolar gradients is often used. With sodium modeling, the dialysate sodium concentration is gradually lowered from the range of 145–155 mmol/L to isotonic concentrations (136–140 mmol/L) near the end of the dialysis treatment, typically declining either in steps or in a linear or exponential fashion. Higher dialysate sodium concentrations and sodium modeling may predispose patients to positive sodium balance and increased thirst; thus, these strategies to ameliorate intradialytic hypotension may be undesirable in hypertensive patients or in patients with large interdialytic weight gains. Because patients are exposed to approximately 120 L of water during each dialysis treatment, water used for the dialysate is subjected to filtration, softening, deionization, and, ultimately, reverse osmosis to remove microbiologic contaminants and dissolved ions.

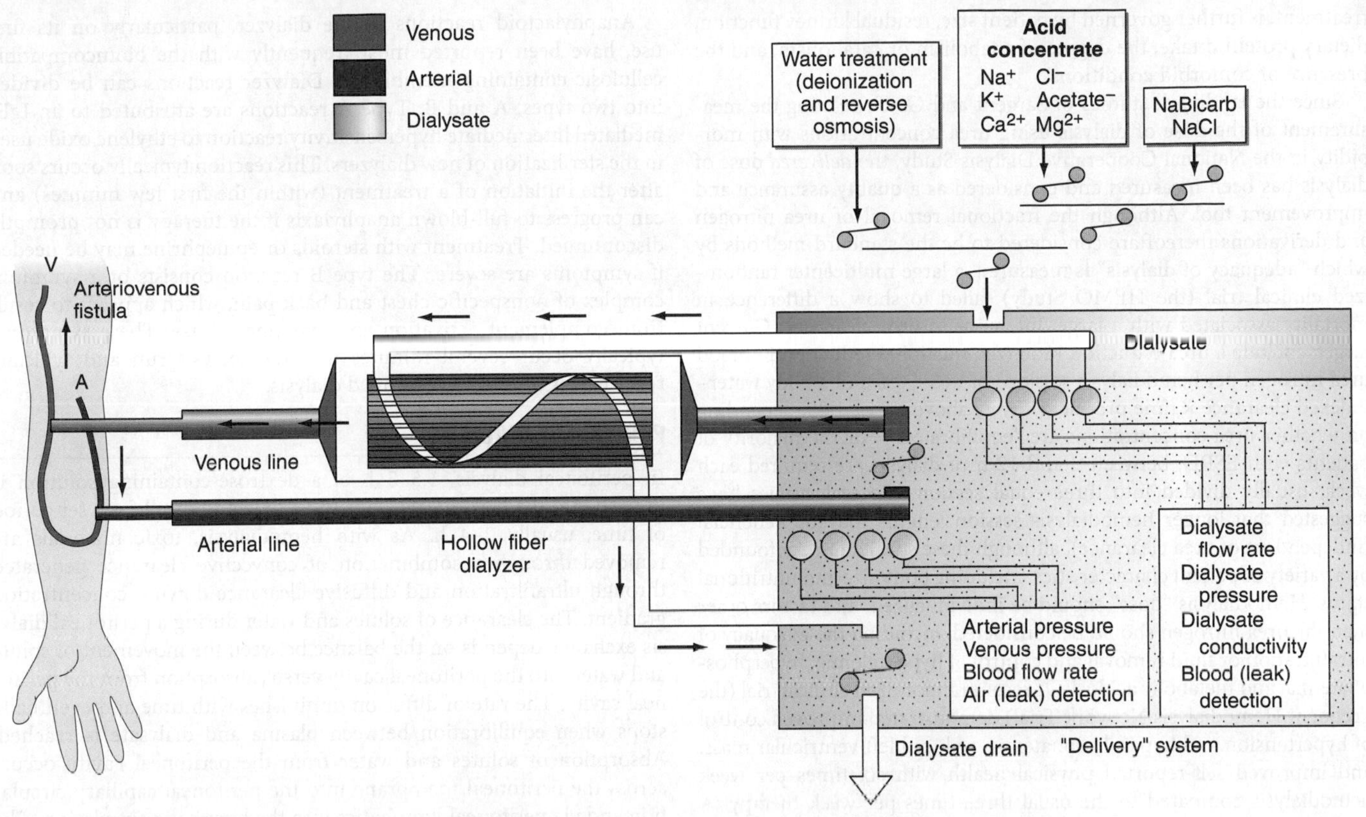

FIGURE 336-1 Schema for hemodialysis. A, artery; V, vein.

BLOOD DELIVERY SYSTEM

The blood delivery system is composed of the extracorporeal circuit and the dialysis access. The dialysis machine consists of a blood pump, dialysis solution delivery system, and various safety monitors. The blood pump moves blood from the access site, through the dialyzer, and back to the patient. The blood flow rate may range from 250–500 mL/min, depending on the type and integrity of the vascular access. Negative hydrostatic pressure on the dialysate side can be manipulated to achieve desirable fluid removal or *ultrafiltration*. Dialysis membranes have different ultrafiltration coefficients (i.e., mL removed/min per mmHg) so that along with hydrostatic changes, fluid removal can be varied. The dialysis solution delivery system dilutes the concentrated dialysate with water and monitors the temperature, conductivity, and flow of dialysate.

DIALYSIS ACCESS

The fistula, graft, or catheter through which blood is obtained for hemodialysis is often referred to as a *dialysis access*. A native fistula created by the anastomosis of an artery to a vein (e.g., the Brescia-Cimino fistula, in which the cephalic vein is anastomosed end-to-side to the radial artery) results in arterialization of the vein. This facilitates its subsequent use in the placement of large needles (typically 15 gauge) to access the circulation. Although fistulas have the highest long-term patency rate of all dialysis access options, fistulas are created in a minority of patients in the United States. Many patients undergo placement of an arteriovenous graft (i.e., the interposition of prosthetic material, usually polytetrafluoroethylene, between an artery and a vein) or a tunneled dialysis catheter. In recent years, nephrologists, vascular surgeons, and health care policy makers in the United States have encouraged creation of arteriovenous fistulas in a larger fraction of patients (the "fistula first" initiative). Unfortunately, even when created, arteriovenous fistulas may not mature sufficiently to provide reliable access to the circulation, or they may thrombose early in their development.

Grafts and catheters tend to be used among persons with smaller-caliber veins or persons whose veins have been damaged by repeated venipuncture, or after prolonged hospitalization. The most important complication of arteriovenous grafts is thrombosis of the graft and graft failure, due principally to intimal hyperplasia at the anastomosis between the graft and recipient vein. When grafts (or fistulas) fail, catheter-guided angioplasty can be used to dilate stenoses; monitoring of venous pressures on dialysis and of access flow, although not routinely performed, may assist in the early recognition of impending vascular access failure. In addition to an increased rate of access failure, grafts and (in particular) catheters are associated with much higher rates of infection than fistulas.

Intravenous large-bore catheters are often used in patients with acute and chronic kidney disease. For persons on maintenance hemodialysis, tunneled catheters (either two separate catheters or a single catheter with two lumens) are often used when arteriovenous fistulas and grafts have failed or are not feasible due to anatomic considerations. These catheters are tunneled under the skin; the tunnel reduces bacterial translocation from the skin, resulting in a lower infection rate than with nontunneled temporary catheters. Most tunneled catheters are placed in the internal jugular veins; the external jugular, femoral, and subclavian veins may also be used.

Nephrologists, interventional radiologists, and vascular surgeons generally prefer to avoid placement of catheters into the subclavian veins; while flow rates are usually excellent, subclavian stenosis is a frequent complication and, if present, will likely prohibit permanent vascular access (i.e., a fistula or graft) in the ipsilateral extremity. Infection rates may be higher with femoral catheters. For patients with multiple vascular access complications and no other options for permanent vascular access, tunneled catheters may be the last "lifeline" for hemodialysis. Translumbar or transhepatic approaches into the inferior vena cava may be required if the superior vena cava or other central veins draining the upper extremities are stenosed or thrombosed.

GOALS OF DIALYSIS

The hemodialysis procedure consists of pumping heparinized blood through the dialyzer at a flow rate of 300–500 mL/min, while dialysate flows in an opposite *counter-current* direction at 500–800 mL/min. The efficiency of dialysis is determined by blood and dialysate flow through the dialyzer as well as dialyzer characteristics (i.e., its efficiency in removing solute). The *dose* of dialysis, which is currently defined as a derivation of the fractional urea clearance during a single treatment, is further governed by patient size, residual kidney function, dietary protein intake, the degree of anabolism or catabolism, and the presence of comorbid conditions.

Since the landmark studies of Sargent and Gotch relating the measurement of the dose of dialysis using urea concentrations with morbidity in the National Cooperative Dialysis Study, the *delivered* dose of dialysis has been measured and considered as a quality assurance and improvement tool. Although the fractional removal of urea nitrogen and derivations thereof are considered to be the standard methods by which "adequacy of dialysis" is measured, a large multicenter randomized clinical trial (the HEMO Study) failed to show a difference in mortality associated with a large difference in urea clearance. Current targets include a urea reduction ratio (the fractional reduction in blood urea nitrogen per hemodialysis session) of >65–70% and a body water–indexed clearance × time product (KT/V) above 1.2 or 1.05, depending on whether urea concentrations are "equilibrated." For the majority of patients with ESRD, between 9 and 12 h of dialysis are required each week, usually divided into three equal sessions. Several studies have suggested that longer hemodialysis session lengths may be beneficial (independent of urea clearance), although these studies are confounded by a variety of patient characteristics, including body size and nutritional status. Hemodialysis "dose" should be individualized, and factors other than the urea nitrogen should be considered, including the adequacy of ultrafiltration or fluid removal and control of hyperkalemia, hyperphosphatemia, and metabolic acidosis. A recent randomized clinical trial (the Frequent Hemodialysis Network Trial) demonstrated improved control of hypertension and hyperphosphatemia, reduced left ventricular mass, and improved self-reported physical health with six times per week hemodialysis compared to the usual three times per week therapy. A companion trial in which frequent nocturnal hemodialysis was compared to conventional hemodialysis at home showed no significant effect on left ventricular mass or self-reported physical health. Finally, an evaluation of the U.S. Renal Data System registry showed a significant increase in mortality and hospitalization for heart failure after the longer interdialytic interval that occurs over the dialysis "weekend."

COMPLICATIONS DURING HEMODIALYSIS

Hypotension is the most common acute complication of hemodialysis, particularly among patients with diabetes mellitus. Numerous factors appear to increase the risk of hypotension, including excessive ultrafiltration with inadequate compensatory vascular filling, impaired vasoactive or autonomic responses, osmolar shifts, overzealous use of antihypertensive agents, and reduced cardiac reserve. Patients with arteriovenous fistulas and grafts may develop high-output cardiac failure due to shunting of blood through the dialysis access; on rare occasions, this may necessitate ligation of the fistula or graft. Because of the vasodilatory and cardiodepressive effects of acetate, its use as the buffer in dialysate was once a common cause of hypotension. Since the introduction of bicarbonate-containing dialysate, dialysis-associated hypotension has become less common. The management of hypotension during dialysis consists of discontinuing ultrafiltration, the administration of 100–250 mL of isotonic saline or 10 mL of 23% saturated hypertonic saline, or administration of salt-poor albumin. Hypotension during dialysis can frequently be prevented by careful evaluation of the dry weight and by ultrafiltration modeling, such that more fluid is removed at the beginning rather than the end of the dialysis procedure. Additional maneuvers include the performance of sequential ultrafiltration followed by dialysis, cooling of the dialysate during dialysis treatment, and avoiding heavy meals during dialysis. Midodrine, an oral selective α_1 adrenergic agent, has been advocated by some practitioners, although there is insufficient evidence of its safety and efficacy to support its routine use.

Muscle cramps during dialysis are also a common complication. The etiology of dialysis-associated cramps remains obscure. Changes in muscle perfusion because of excessively rapid volume removal (e.g., >10–12 mL/kg per hour) or targeted removal below the patient's estimated dry weight often precipitate dialysis-associated cramps. Strategies that may be used to prevent cramps include reducing volume removal during dialysis, ultrafiltration profiling, and the use of sodium modeling (see above).

Anaphylactoid reactions to the dialyzer, particularly on its first use, have been reported most frequently with the bioincompatible cellulosic-containing membranes. Dialyzer reactions can be divided into two types, A and B. Type A reactions are attributed to an IgE-mediated intermediate hypersensitivity reaction to ethylene oxide used in the sterilization of new dialyzers. This reaction typically occurs soon after the initiation of a treatment (within the first few minutes) and can progress to full-blown anaphylaxis if the therapy is not promptly discontinued. Treatment with steroids or epinephrine may be needed if symptoms are severe. The type B reaction consists of a symptom complex of nonspecific chest and back pain, which appears to result from complement activation and cytokine release. These symptoms typically occur several minutes into the dialysis run and typically resolve over time with continued dialysis.

PERITONEAL DIALYSIS

In peritoneal dialysis, 1.5–3 L of a dextrose-containing solution is infused into the peritoneal cavity and allowed to dwell for a set period of time, usually 2–4 h. As with hemodialysis, toxic materials are removed through a combination of convective clearance generated through ultrafiltration and diffusive clearance down a concentration gradient. The clearance of solutes and water during a peritoneal dialysis exchange depends on the balance between the movement of solute and water into the peritoneal cavity versus absorption from the peritoneal cavity. The rate of diffusion diminishes with time and eventually stops when equilibration between plasma and dialysate is reached. Absorption of solutes and water from the peritoneal cavity occurs across the peritoneal membrane into the peritoneal capillary circulation and via peritoneal lymphatics into the lymphatic circulation. The rate of peritoneal solute transport varies from patient to patient and may be altered by the presence of infection (peritonitis), drugs, and physical factors such as position and exercise.

FORMS OF PERITONEAL DIALYSIS

Peritoneal dialysis may be carried out as CAPD, CCPD, or a combination of both. In CAPD, dialysate is manually infused into the peritoneal cavity and exchanged three to five times during the day. A nighttime dwell is frequently instilled at bedtime and remains in the peritoneal cavity through the night. In CCPD, exchanges are performed in an automated fashion, usually at night; the patient is connected to an automated cycler that performs a series of exchange cycles while the patient sleeps. The number of exchange cycles required to optimize peritoneal solute clearance varies by the peritoneal membrane characteristics; as with hemodialysis, solute clearance should be tracked to ensure dialysis "adequacy."

Peritoneal dialysis solutions are available in volumes typically ranging from 1.5 to 3 L. The major difference between the dialysate used for peritoneal dialysis rather than hemodialysis is that the hypertonicity of peritoneal dialysis solutions drives solute and fluid removal, whereas solute removal in hemodialysis depends on concentration gradients, and fluid removal requires transmembrane pressure. Typically, dextrose at varying concentrations contributes to the hypertonicity of peritoneal dialysate. Icodextrin is a nonabsorbable carbohydrate that can be used in place of dextrose. Studies have demonstrated more efficient ultrafiltration with icodextrin than with dextrose-containing solutions. Icodextrin is typically used as the "last fill" for patients on CCPD or for the longest dwell in patients on CAPD. The most common additives to peritoneal dialysis solutions are heparin to prevent obstruction of the dialysis catheter lumen with fibrin and antibiotics during an episode of acute peritonitis. Insulin may also be added in patients with diabetes mellitus.

ACCESS TO THE PERITONEAL CAVITY

Access to the peritoneal cavity is obtained through a peritoneal catheter. Catheters used for maintenance peritoneal dialysis are flexible, being made of silicone rubber with numerous side holes at the distal end. These catheters usually have two Dacron cuffs. The scarring that occurs around the cuffs anchors the catheter and seals it from bacteria tracking from the skin surface into the peritoneal cavity; it also prevents the external leakage of fluid from the peritoneal cavity. The cuffs are placed in the preperitoneal plane and ~2 cm from the skin surface.

The *peritoneal equilibrium test* is a formal evaluation of peritoneal membrane characteristics that measures the transfer rates of creatinine and glucose across the peritoneal membrane. Patients are classified as low, low–average, high–average, and high transporters. Patients with rapid equilibration (i.e., high transporters) tend to absorb more glucose and lose efficiency of ultrafiltration with long daytime dwells. High transporters also tend to lose larger quantities of albumin and other proteins across the peritoneal membrane. In general, patients with rapid transporting characteristics require more frequent, shorter dwell time exchanges, nearly always obligating use of a cycler. Slower (low and low–average) transporters tend to do well with fewer exchanges. The efficiency of solute clearance also depends on the volume of dialysate infused. Larger volumes allow for greater solute clearance, particularly with CAPD in patients with low and low–average transport characteristics.

As with hemodialysis, the optimal dose of peritoneal dialysis is unknown. Several observational studies have suggested that higher rates of urea and creatinine clearance (the latter generally measured in liters per week) are associated with lower mortality rates and fewer uremic complications. However, a randomized clinical trial (Adequacy of Peritoneal Dialysis in Mexico [ADEMEX]) failed to show a significant reduction in mortality or complications with a relatively large increment in urea clearance. In general, patients on peritoneal dialysis do well when they retain residual kidney function. The rates of technique failure increase with years on dialysis and have been correlated with loss of residual function to a greater extent than loss of peritoneal membrane capacity. For some patients in whom CCPD does not provide sufficient solute clearance, a hybrid approach can be adopted where one or more daytime exchanges are added to the CCPD regimen. Although this approach can enhance solute clearance and prolong a patient's capacity to remain on peritoneal dialysis, the burden of the hybrid approach can be overwhelming.

COMPLICATIONS DURING PERITONEAL DIALYSIS

The major complications of peritoneal dialysis are peritonitis, catheter-associated nonperitonitis infections, weight gain and other metabolic disturbances, and residual uremia (especially among patients with no residual kidney function).

Peritonitis typically develops when there has been a break in sterile technique during one or more of the exchange procedures. Peritonitis is usually defined by an elevated peritoneal fluid leukocyte count (100/μL, of which at least 50% are polymorphonuclear neutrophils); these cut-offs are lower than in spontaneous bacterial peritonitis because of the presence of dextrose in peritoneal dialysis solutions and rapid bacterial proliferation in this environment without antibiotic therapy. The clinical presentation typically consists of pain and cloudy dialysate, often with fever and other constitutional symptoms. The most common culprit organisms are gram-positive cocci, including *Staphylococcus*, reflecting the origin from the skin. Gram-negative rod infections are less common; fungal and mycobacterial infections can be seen in selected patients, particularly after antibacterial therapy. Most cases of peritonitis can be managed either with intraperitoneal or oral antibiotics, depending on the organism; many patients with peritonitis do not require hospitalization. In cases where peritonitis is due to hydrophilic gram-negative rods (e.g., *Pseudomonas* sp.) or yeast, antimicrobial therapy is usually not sufficient, and catheter removal is required to ensure complete eradication of infection. Nonperitonitis catheter-associated infections (often termed *tunnel infections*) vary widely in severity. Some cases can be managed with local antibiotic or silver nitrate administration, whereas others are severe enough to require parenteral antibiotic therapy and catheter removal.

Peritoneal dialysis is associated with a variety of metabolic complications. Albumin and other proteins can be lost across the peritoneal membrane in concert with the loss of metabolic wastes. Hypoproteinemia obligates a higher dietary protein intake in order to maintain nitrogen balance. Hyperglycemia and weight gain are also common complications of peritoneal dialysis. Several hundred calories in the form of dextrose are absorbed each day, depending on the concentration employed. Peritoneal dialysis patients, particularly those with diabetes mellitus, are then prone to other complications of insulin resistance, including hypertriglyceridemia. On the positive side, the continuous nature of peritoneal dialysis usually allows for a more liberal diet, due to continuous removal of potassium and phosphorus—two major dietary components whose accumulation can be hazardous in ESRD.

LONG-TERM OUTCOMES IN ESRD

Cardiovascular disease constitutes the major cause of death in patients with ESRD. Cardiovascular mortality and event rates are higher in dialysis patients than in patients after transplantation, although rates are extraordinarily high in both populations. The underlying cause of cardiovascular disease is unclear but may be related to shared risk factors (e.g., diabetes mellitus, hypertension, atherosclerotic and arteriosclerotic vascular disease), chronic inflammation, massive changes in extracellular volume (especially with high interdialytic weight gains), inadequate treatment of hypertension, dyslipidemia, anemia, dystrophic vascular calcification, hyperhomocysteinemia, and, perhaps, alterations in cardiovascular dynamics during the dialysis treatment. Few studies have targeted cardiovascular risk reduction in ESRD patients; none have demonstrated consistent benefit. Two clinical trials of statin agents in ESRD demonstrated significant reductions in low-density lipoprotein (LDL) cholesterol concentrations, but no significant reductions in death or cardiovascular events (Die Deutsche Diabetes Dialyse Studie [4D] and A Study to Evaluate the Use of Rosuvastatin in Subjects on Regular Hemodialysis [AURORA]). The Study of Heart and Renal Protection (SHARP), which included patients on dialysis- and non-dialysis-requiring CKD, showed a 17% reduction in the rate of major cardiovascular events or cardiovascular death with simvastatin-ezetimibe treatment. Most experts recommend conventional cardioprotective strategies (e.g., lipid-lowering agents, aspirin, inhibitors of the renin-angiotensin-aldosterone system, and β-adrenergic antagonists) in dialysis patients based on the patients' cardiovascular risk profile, which appears to be increased by more than an order of magnitude relative to persons unaffected by kidney disease. Other complications of ESRD include a high incidence of infection, progressive debility and frailty, protein-energy malnutrition, and impaired cognitive function.

GLOBAL PERSPECTIVE

The incidence of ESRD is increasing worldwide with longer life expectancies and improved care of infectious and cardiovascular diseases. The management of ESRD varies widely by country and within country by region, and it is influenced by economic and other major factors. In general, peritoneal dialysis is more commonly performed in poorer countries owing to its lower expense and the high cost of establishing in-center hemodialysis units.

337 Transplantation in the Treatment of Renal Failure

Jamil Azzi, Edgar L. Milford, Mohamed H. Sayegh, Anil Chandraker

Transplantation of the human kidney is the treatment of choice for advanced chronic renal failure. Worldwide, tens of thousands of these procedures have been performed with more than 180,000 patients bearing functioning kidney transplants in the United States today. When azathioprine and prednisone initially were used as immunosuppressive drugs in the 1960s, the results with properly matched familial donors were superior to those with organs from deceased donors: 75–90% compared with 50–60% graft survival rates at 1 year. During the 1970s and 1980s, the success rate at the 1-year mark for deceased-donor

TABLE 337-1 DEFINITION OF AN EXPANDED CRITERIA DONOR AND A NON-HEART-BEATING DONOR (DONATION AFTER CARDIAC DEATH)

Expanded Criteria Donor (ECD)
Deceased donor >60 years
Deceased donor >50 years and hypertension and creatinine >1.5 mg/dL
Deceased donor >50 years and hypertension and death caused by cerebrovascular accident (CVA)
Deceased donor >50 years and death caused by CVA and creatinine >1.5 mg/dL
Donation after Cardiac Death[a] (DCD)
I: Brought in dead
II: Unsuccessful resuscitation
III: Awaiting cardiac arrest
IV: Cardiac arrest after brainstem death
V: Cardiac arrest in a hospital patient

[a]Kidneys can be used for transplantation from categories II–V but are commonly only used from categories III and IV. The survival of these kidneys has not been shown to be inferior to that of deceased-donor kidneys.

Note: Kidneys can be both ECD and DCD. ECD kidneys have been shown to have a poorer survival, and there is a separate shorter waiting list for ECD kidneys. They are generally used for patients for whom the benefits of being transplanted earlier outweigh the associated risks of using an ECD kidney.

transplants rose progressively. Currently, deceased-donor grafts have a 92% 1-year survival and living-donor grafts have a 96% 1-year survival. Although there has been improvement in long-term survival, it has not been as impressive as the short-term survival, and currently the "average" ($t_{1/2}$) life expectancy of a living-donor graft is around 20 years and that of a deceased-donor graft is close to 14 years.

Mortality rates after transplantation are highest in the first year and are age-related: 2% for ages 18–34 years, 3% for ages 35–49 years, and 6.8% for ages ≥50–60 years. These rates compare favorably with those in the chronic dialysis population even after risk adjustments for age, diabetes, and cardiovascular status. Although the loss of kidney transplant due to acute rejection is currently rare, most allografts succumb at varying rates to a chronic process consisting of interstitial fibrosis, tubular atrophy, vasculopathy, and glomerulopathy, the pathogenesis of which is incompletely understood. Overall, transplantation returns most patients to an improved lifestyle and an improved life expectancy compared with patients on dialysis.

RECENT ACTIVITY AND RESULTS

In 2011, there were more than 11,835 deceased-donor kidney transplants and 5772 living-donor transplants in the United States, with the ratio of deceased to living donors remaining stable over the last few years. The backlog of patients with end-stage renal disease (ESRD) has been increasing every year, and it always lags behind the number of available donors. As the number of patients with end-stage kidney disease increases, the demand for kidney transplants continues to increase. In 2011, there were 55,371 active adult candidates on the waiting list, and less than 18,000 patients were transplanted. This imbalance is set to worsen over the coming years with the predicted increased rates of obesity and diabetes worldwide. In an attempt to increase utilization of deceased-donor kidneys and reduce discard rates of organs, criteria for the use of so-called expanded criteria donor (ECD) kidneys and kidneys from donors after cardiac death (DCD) have been developed (Table 337-1). ECD kidneys are usually used for older patients who are expected to fare less well on dialysis.

The overall results of transplantation are presented in Table 337-2 as the survival of grafts and of patients. At the 1-year mark, graft survival is higher for living-donor recipients, most likely because those grafts are not subject to as much ischemic injury. The more effective drugs now in use for immunosuppression have almost equalized the risk of graft rejection in all patients for the first year. At 5 and 10 years, however, there has been a steeper decline in survival of those with deceased-donor kidneys.

RECIPIENT SELECTION

There are few absolute contraindications to renal transplantation. The transplant procedure is relatively noninvasive, as the organ is placed in the inguinal fossa without entering the peritoneal cavity. Recipients without perioperative complications often can be discharged from the hospital in excellent condition within 5 days of the operation.

Virtually all patients with ESRD who receive a transplant have a higher life expectancy than do risk-matched patients who remain on dialysis. Even though diabetic patients and older candidates have a higher mortality rate than other transplant recipients, their survival is improved with transplantation compared with those remaining on dialysis. This global benefit of transplantation as a treatment modality poses substantial ethical issues for policy makers, as the number of deceased kidneys available is far from sufficient to meet the current needs of the candidates. The current standard of care is that the candidate should have a life expectancy of >5 years to be put on a deceased organ wait list. Even for living donation, the candidate should have >5 years of life expectancy. This standard has been established because the benefits of kidney transplantation over dialysis are realized only after a perioperative period in which the mortality rate is higher in transplanted patients than in dialysis patients with comparable risk profiles.

All candidates must have a thorough risk-versus-benefit evaluation before being approved for transplantation. In particular, an aggressive approach to diagnosis of correctable coronary artery disease, presence of latent or indolent infection (HIV, hepatitis B or C, tuberculosis), and neoplasm should be a routine part of the candidate workup. Most transplant centers consider overt AIDS and active hepatitis absolute contraindications to transplantation because of the high risk of opportunistic infection. Some centers are now transplanting individuals with hepatitis and even HIV infection under strict protocols to determine whether the risks and benefits favor transplantation over dialysis.

Among the few absolute "immunologic" contraindications to transplantation is the presence of antibodies against the donor kidney at the time of the anticipated transplant that can cause hyperacute rejection. Those harmful antibodies include natural antibodies against the ABO blood group antigens and antibodies against human leukocyte antigen (HLA) class I (A, B, C) or class II (DR) antigens. These antibodies are routinely excluded by proper screening of the candidate's ABO compatibility and direct cytotoxic cross-matching of candidate serum with lymphocytes of the donor.

TISSUE TYPING AND CLINICAL IMMUNOGENETICS

Matching for antigens of the HLA major histocompatibility gene complex (Chap. 373e) is an important criterion for selection of donors for renal allografts. Each mammalian species has a single chromosomal

TABLE 337-2 MEAN RATES OF GRAFT AND PATIENT SURVIVAL FOR KIDNEYS TRANSPLANTED IN THE UNITED STATES FROM 1998 TO 2008[a]

	1-Year Follow-Up		5-Year Follow-Up		10-Year Follow-Up	
	Grafts, %	Patients, %	Grafts, %	Patients, %	Grafts, %	Patients, %
Deceased donor	92	96	72	84	46	64
Living donor	96	99	81	91	59	77

[a]All patients transplanted are included, and the follow-up unadjusted survival data from the 1-, 5-, and 10-year periods are presented to show the attrition rates over time within the two types of organ donors.

Source: Data from Summary Tables, 2009 Annual Reports, Scientific Registry of Transplant Recipients.

region that encodes the strong, or major, transplantation antigens, and this region on the human sixth chromosome is called *HLA*. HLA antigens have been classically defined by serologic techniques, but methods to define specific nucleotide sequences in genomic DNA are increasingly being used. Other "minor" antigens may play crucial roles, in addition to the ABH(O) blood groups and endothelial antigens that are not shared with lymphocytes. The Rh system is not expressed on graft tissue. Evidence for designation of HLA as the genetic region that encodes major transplantation antigens comes from the success rate in living related donor renal and bone marrow transplantation, with superior results in HLA-identical sibling pairs. Nevertheless, 5% of HLA-identical renal allografts are rejected, often within the first weeks after transplantation. These failures represent states of prior sensitization to non-HLA antigens. Non-HLA minor antigens are relatively weak when initially encountered and are, therefore, suppressible by conventional immunosuppressive therapy. Once priming has occurred, however, secondary responses are much more refractory to treatment.

DONOR SELECTION

Donors can be deceased or volunteer living donors. When first-degree relatives are donors, graft survival rates at 1 year are 5–7% greater than those for deceased-donor grafts. The 5-year survival rates still favor a partially matched (3/6 HLA mismatched) family donor over a randomly selected cadaver donor. In addition, living donors provide the advantage of immediate availability. For both living and deceased donors, the 5-year outcomes are poor if there is a complete (6/6) HLA mismatch.

The survival rate of living unrelated renal allografts is as high as that of perfectly HLA-matched cadaver renal transplants and comparable to that of kidneys from living relatives. This outcome is probably a consequence of both short cold ischemia time and the extra care taken to document that the condition and renal function of the donor are optimal before proceeding with a living unrelated donation. It is illegal in the United States to purchase organs for transplantation.

Living volunteer donors should be cleared of any medical conditions that may cause morbidity and mortality after kidney transplantation. Concern has been expressed about the potential risk to a volunteer kidney donor of premature renal failure after several years of increased blood flow and hyperfiltration per nephron in the remaining kidney. There are a few reports of the development of hypertension, proteinuria, and even lesions of focal segmental sclerosis in donors over long-term follow-up. It is also desirable to consider the risk of development of type 1 diabetes mellitus in a family member who is a potential donor to a diabetic renal failure patient. Anti-insulin and anti-islet cell antibodies should be measured and glucose tolerance tests should be performed in such donors to exclude a prediabetic state. Selective renal arteriography should be performed on donors to rule out the presence of multiple or abnormal renal arteries, because the surgical procedure is difficult and the ischemic time of the transplanted kidney is long when there are vascular abnormalities. Transplant surgeons are now using a laparoscopic method to isolate and remove the living donor's kidney. This operation has the advantage of less evident surgical scars, and, because there is less tissue trauma, the laparoscopic donors have a substantially shorter hospital stay and less discomfort than those who have the traditional surgery.

Deceased donors should be free of malignant neoplastic disease, hepatitis, and HIV due to possible transmission to the recipient, although there is increasing interest in using hepatitis C– and HIV-positive organs in previously infected recipients. Increased risk of graft failure exists when the donor is elderly or has renal failure and when the kidney has a prolonged period of ischemia and storage.

In the United States, there is a coordinated national system of regulations, allocation support, and outcomes analysis for kidney transplantation called the Organ Procurement Transplant Network. It is now possible to remove deceased-donor kidneys and maintain them for up to 48 h on cold pulsatile perfusion or with simple flushing and cooling. This approach permits adequate time for typing, cross-matching, transportation, and selection problems to be solved.

PRESENSITIZATION

A positive cytotoxic cross-match of recipient serum with donor T lymphocytes indicates the presence of preformed donor-specific anti-HLA class I antibodies and is usually predictive of an acute vasculitic event termed *hyperacute rejection*. This finding, along with ABO incompatibility, represents the only absolute immunologic contraindication for kidney transplantation. Recently, more tissue typing laboratories have shifted to a flow cytometric–based cross-match assay, which detects the presence of anti-HLA antibodies that are not necessarily detected on a cytotoxic cross-match assay and may not be an absolute contraindication to transplantation. The known sources of such sensitization are blood transfusion, a prior transplant, pregnancy, and vaccination/infection. Patients sustained by dialysis often show fluctuating antibody titers and specificity patterns. At the time of assignment of a cadaveric kidney, cross-matches are performed with at least a current serum. Previously analyzed antibody specificities and additional cross-matches are performed accordingly. Flow cytometry detects binding of anti-HLA antibodies of a candidate's serum by a recipient's lymphocytes. This highly sensitive test can be useful for avoidance of accelerated, and often untreatable, early graft rejection in patients receiving second or third transplants.

For the purposes of cross-matching, donor T lymphocytes, which express class I but not class II antigens, are used as targets for detection of anti–class I (HLA-A and -B) antibodies that are expressed on all nucleated cells. Preformed anti–class II (HLA-DR and -DQ) antibodies against the donor also carry a higher risk of graft loss, particularly in recipients who have suffered early loss of a prior kidney transplant. B lymphocytes, which express both class I and class II antigens, are used as targets in these assays.

Some non-HLA antigens restricted in expression to endothelium and monocytes have been described, but clinical relevance is not well established. A series of minor histocompatibility antigens do not elicit antibodies, and sensitization to these antigens is detectable only by cytotoxic T cells, an assay too cumbersome for routine use.

Desensitization before transplantation by reducing the level of anti-donor antibodies using plasmapheresis and administration of pooled immunoglobulin, or both, has been useful in reducing the risk of hyperacute rejection following transplantation.

IMMUNOLOGY OF REJECTION

Both cellular and humoral (antibody-mediated) effector mechanisms can play roles in kidney transplant rejection.

Cellular rejection is mediated by lymphocytes that respond to HLA antigens expressed within the organ. The CD4+ lymphocyte responds to class II (HLA-DR) incompatibility by proliferating and releasing proinflammatory cytokines that augment the proliferative response of the immune system. CD8+ cytotoxic lymphocyte precursors respond primarily to class I (HLA-A, -B) antigens and mature into cytotoxic effector cells that cause organ damage through direct contact and lysis of donor target cells. Full T cell activation requires not only T cell receptor binding to the alloantigens presented by self or donor HLA molecules (indirect and direct presentation, respectively), but also engaging costimulatory molecules such as CD28 on T cells and CD80 and CD86 ligands on antigen-presenting cells (Fig. 337-1). Signaling through both of these pathways induces activation of the kinase activity of calcineurin, which, in turn, activates transcription factors, leading to upregulation of multiple genes, including interleukin 2 (IL-2) and interferon gamma. IL-2 signals through the target of rapamycin (TOR) to induce cell proliferation in an autocrine fashion. There is evidence that non-HLA antigens can also play a role in renal transplant rejection episodes. Recipients who receive a kidney from an HLA-identical sibling can have rejection episodes and require maintenance immunosuppression, whereas identical twin transplants require no immunosuppression. There are documented non-HLA antigens, such as an endothelial-specific antigen system with limited polymorphism and a tubular antigen, which can act as targets of humoral or cellular rejection responses, respectively.

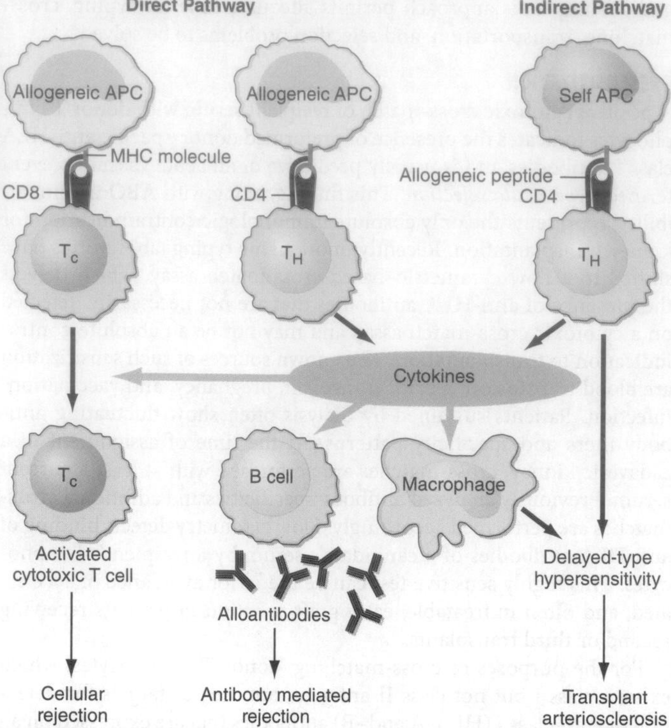

FIGURE 337-1 Recognition pathways for major histocompatibility complex (MHC) antigens. Graft rejection is initiated by CD4 helper T lymphocytes (T_H) having antigen receptors that bind to specific complexes of peptides and MHC class II molecules on antigen-presenting cells (APC). In transplantation, in contrast to other immunologic responses, there are two sets of T cell clones involved in rejection. In the direct pathway, the class II MHC of donor allogeneic APCs is recognized by CD4 T_H cells that bind to the intact MHC molecule, and class I MHC allogeneic cells are recognized by CD8 T cells. The latter generally proliferate into cytotoxic cells (T_C). In the indirect pathway, the incompatible MHC molecules are processed into peptides that are presented by the self-APCs of the recipient. The indirect, but not the direct, pathway is the normal physiologic process in T cell recognition of foreign antigens. Once T_H cells are activated, they proliferate and, by secretion of cytokines and direct contact, exert strong helper effects on macrophages, T_C, and B cells. *(From MH Sayegh, LH Turka: N Engl J Med, 338:1813, 1998. Copyright 1998, Massachusetts Medical Society. All rights reserved.)*

IMMUNOSUPPRESSIVE TREATMENT

Immunosuppressive therapy, as currently available, generally suppresses all immune responses, including those to bacteria, fungi, and even malignant tumors. In general, all clinically useful drugs are more selective to primary than to memory immune responses. Agents to suppress the immune response are classically divided into induction and maintenance agents and will be discussed in the following paragraphs. Those currently in clinical use are listed in Table 337-3.

INDUCTION THERAPY

Induction therapy is currently given to most kidney transplant recipients in the United States at the time of transplant to reduce the risk of early acute rejection and to minimize or eliminate the use of either steroids or calcineurin inhibitors and their associated toxicities. Induction therapy consists of antibodies that could be monoclonal or polyclonal and depletional or nondepletional.

Depleting Agents Peripheral human lymphocytes, thymocytes, or lymphocytes from spleens or thoracic duct fistulas are injected into horses, rabbits, or goats to produce antilymphocyte serum, from which the globulin fraction is then separated, resulting in antithymocyte globulin. Those polyclonal antibodies induce lymphocyte depletion, and the immune system may take several months to recover.

Monoclonal antibodies against defined lymphocyte subsets offer a more precise and standardized form of therapy. Alemtuzumab is directed to the CD52 protein, widely distributed on immune cells such as B and T cells, natural killer cells, macrophages, and some granulocytes.

Nondepleting Agents Another approach to more selective therapy is to target the 55-kDa alpha chain of the IL-2 receptor, which is expressed only on T cells that have been recently activated. This approach is used as prophylaxis for acute rejection in the immediate posttransplant period and is effective at decreasing the early acute rejection rate with few adverse side effects.

The next step in the evolution of this therapeutic strategy, which has already been achieved in the short term in small numbers of immunologically well-matched patients, is the elimination of all maintenance immunosuppression therapy.

MAINTENANCE THERAPY

All kidney transplant recipients should receive maintenance immunosuppressive therapies except identical twins. The most frequently used combination is triple therapy with prednisone, a calcineurin inhibitor, and an antimetabolite; mammalian TOR (mTOR) inhibitors can replace one of the last two agents. More recently, the U.S. Food and Drug Administration (FDA) approved a new costimulatory blocking antibody, belatacept, as a new strategy to prevent long-term calcineurin inhibitor toxicity.

Antimetabolites *Azathioprine*, an analogue of mercaptopurine, was for two decades the keystone to immunosuppressive therapy in humans, but has given way to more effective agents. This agent can inhibit synthesis of DNA, RNA, or both. Azathioprine is administered in doses of 1.5–2 mg/kg per day. Reduction in the dose is required because of leukopenia and occasionally thrombocytopenia. Excessive amounts of azathioprine may also cause jaundice, anemia, and alopecia. If it is essential to administer allopurinol concurrently, the azathioprine dose must be reduced. Because inhibition of xanthine oxidase delays degradation, this combination is best avoided.

Mycophenolate mofetil or *mycophenolate sodium*, both of which are metabolized to mycophenolic acid, is now used in place of azathioprine in most centers. It has a similar mode of action and a mild degree of gastrointestinal toxicity but produces less bone marrow suppression. Its advantage is its increased potency in preventing or reversing rejection.

Steroids *Glucocorticoids* are important adjuncts to immunosuppressive therapy. Among all the agents employed, prednisone has effects that are easiest to assess, and in large doses it is usually effective for the reversal of rejection. In general, 200–300 mg prednisone is given immediately before or at the time of transplantation, and the dose is reduced to 30 mg within a week. The side effects of the glucocorticoids, particularly impairment of wound healing and predisposition to infection, make it desirable to taper the dose as rapidly as possible in the immediate postoperative period. Many centers now have protocols for early discontinuance or avoidance of steroids because of long-term adverse effects on bone, skin, and glucose metabolism. For treatment of acute rejection, methylprednisolone, 0.5–1 g IV, is administered immediately upon diagnosis of beginning rejection and continued once daily for 3 days. Such "pulse" doses are not effective in chronic rejection. Most patients whose renal function is stable after 6 months or a year do not require large doses of prednisone; maintenance doses of 5–10 mg/d are the rule. A major effect of steroids is preventing the release of IL-6 and IL-1 by monocytes-macrophages.

Calcineurin Inhibitors *Cyclosporine* is a fungal peptide with potent immunosuppressive activity. It acts on the calcineurin pathway to block transcription of mRNA for IL-2 and other proinflammatory cytokines, thereby inhibiting T cell proliferation. Although it works alone, cyclosporine is more effective in conjunction with glucocorticoids and mycophenolate. Clinical results with tens of thousands of renal transplants have been impressive. Among its toxic effects (nephrotoxicity, hepatotoxicity, hirsutism, tremor, gingival hyperplasia,

TABLE 337-3 MAINTENANCE IMMUNOSUPPRESSIVE DRUGS

Agent	Pharmacology	Mechanisms	Side Effects
Glucocorticoids	Increased bioavailability with hypoalbuminemia and liver disease; prednisone/prednisolone generally used	Binds cytosolic receptors and heat shock proteins. Blocks transcription of IL-1, -2, -3, -6, TNF-α, and IFN-γ	Hypertension, glucose intolerance, dyslipidemia, osteoporosis
Cyclosporine (CsA)	Lipid-soluble polypeptide, variable absorption, microemulsion more predictable	Trimolecular complex with cyclophilin and calcineurin → block in cytokine (e.g., IL-2) production; however, stimulates TGF-β production	Nephrotoxicity, hypertension, dyslipidemia, glucose intolerance, hirsutism/hyperplasia of gums
Tacrolimus	Macrolide, well absorbed	Trimolecular complex with FKBP-12 and calcineurin → block in cytokine (e.g., IL-2) production; may stimulate TGF-β production	Similar to CsA, but hirsutism/hyperplasia of gums unusual and diabetes more likely
Azathioprine	Mercaptopurine analogue	Hepatic metabolites inhibit purine synthesis	Marrow suppression (WBC > RBC > platelets)
Mycophenolate mofetil/sodium	Metabolized to mycophenolic acid	Inhibits purine synthesis via inosine monophosphate dehydrogenase	Diarrhea/cramps; dose-related liver and marrow suppression is uncommon
Sirolimus/everolimus	Macrolide, poor oral bioavailability	Complexes with FKBP-12 and then blocks p70 S6 kinase in the IL-2 receptor pathway for proliferation	Hyperlipidemia, thrombocytopenia
Belatacept	Fusion protein, intravenous injections	Binds CD80 and CD86, prevents CD28 binding and T cell activation	Posttransplant lymphoproliferative disease

Abbreviations: FKBP-12, FK506 binding protein 12; IFN, interferon; IL, interleukin; RBC, red blood cells; TGF, transforming growth factor; TNF, tumor necrosis factor; WBC, white blood cells.

diabetes), only nephrotoxicity presents a serious management problem and is further discussed below.

Tacrolimus (previously called FK506) is a fungal macrolide that has the same mode of action as cyclosporine as well as a similar side effect profile; it does not, however, produce hirsutism or gingival hyperplasia. De novo diabetes mellitus is more common with tacrolimus. The drug was first used in liver transplantation and may substitute for cyclosporine entirely or as an alternative in renal patients whose rejections are poorly controlled by cyclosporine.

mTOR Inhibitors *Sirolimus* (previously called rapamycin) is another fungal macrolide but has a different mode of action; i.e., it inhibits T cell growth factor signaling pathways, preventing the response to IL-2 and other cytokines. Sirolimus can be used in conjunction with cyclosporine or tacrolimus, or with mycophenolic acid, to avoid the use of calcineurin inhibitors.

Everolimus is another mTOR inhibitor with similar mechanism of action as sirolimus but with better bioavailability.

Belatacept *Belatacept* is a fusion protein that binds costimulatory ligands (CD80 and CD86) present on antigen-presenting cells, interrupting their binding to CD28 on T cells. This inhibition leads to T cell anergy and apoptosis. *Belatacept* is FDA approved for kidney transplant recipients and is given monthly as an intravenous infusion.

CLINICAL COURSE AND MANAGEMENT OF THE RECIPIENT

Adequate hemodialysis should be performed within 48 h of surgery, and care should be taken that the serum potassium level is not markedly elevated so that intraoperative cardiac arrhythmias can be averted. The diuresis that commonly occurs postoperatively must be carefully monitored. In some instances, it may be massive, reflecting the inability of ischemic tubules to regulate sodium and water excretion; with large diureses, massive potassium losses may occur. Most chronically uremic patients have some excess of extracellular fluid, and it is useful to maintain an expanded fluid volume in the immediate postoperative period. Acute tubular necrosis (ATN) due to ischemia may cause immediate oliguria or may follow an initial short period of graft function. Recovery usually occurs within 3 weeks, although periods as long as 6 weeks have been reported. Superimposition of rejection on ATN is common, and the differential diagnosis may be difficult without a graft biopsy. Cyclosporine therapy prolongs ATN, and some patients do not diurese until the dose is reduced drastically. Many centers avoid starting cyclosporine for the first several days, using antilymphocyte globulin (ALG) or a monoclonal antibody along with mycophenolic acid and prednisone until renal function is established. Figure 337-2 illustrates an algorithm followed by many transplant centers for early posttransplant management of recipients at high or low risk of early renal dysfunction.

THE REJECTION EPISODE

Early diagnosis of rejection allows prompt institution of therapy to preserve renal function and prevent irreversible damage. Clinical evidence of rejection is rarely characterized by fever, swelling, and tenderness over the allograft. Rejection may present only with a rise in serum creatinine, with or without a reduction in urine volume. The focus should be on ruling out other causes of functional deterioration.

Doppler ultrasonography may be useful in ascertaining changes in the renal vasculature and in renal blood flow. Thrombosis of the renal vein occurs rarely; it may be reversible if it is caused by technical factors and intervention is prompt. Diagnostic ultrasound is the procedure of choice to rule out urinary obstruction or to confirm the presence of perirenal collections of urine, blood, or lymph. A rise in the serum creatinine level is a late marker of rejection, but it may be the only sign. Novel biomarkers are needed for early noninvasive detection of allograft rejection.

Calcineurin inhibitors (cyclosporine and tacrolimus) have an afferent arteriolar constrictor effect on the kidney and may produce permanent vascular and interstitial injury after sustained high-dose therapy. This action will lead to a deterioration in renal function difficult to distinguish from rejection without a renal biopsy. Interstitial fibrosis, isometric tubular vacuolization, and thickening of arteriolar walls are suggestive of this side effect, but not diagnostic. Hence, if no rejection is detected on the biopsy, serum creatinine may respond to a reduction in dose. However, if rejection activity is present in the biopsy, appropriate therapy is indicated. The first rejection episode is usually treated with IV administration of methylprednisolone, 500–1000 mg daily for 3 days. Failure to respond is an indication for antibody therapy, usually with antithymocyte globulin.

Evidence of antibody-mediated injury is present when endothelial injury and deposition of complement component c4d is detected by fluorescence labeling. This is usually accompanied by detection of the antibody in the recipient blood. The prognosis is poor, and aggressive use of plasmapheresis, immunoglobulin infusions, anti-CD20 monoclonal antibody (rituximab) to target B lymphocytes, bortezomib to target antibody-producing plasma cells, and eculizumab to inhibit complement is indicated.

MANAGEMENT PROBLEMS

The typical times after transplantation when the most common opportunistic infections occur are shown in Table 337-4. Prophylaxis for cytomegalovirus (CMV) and *Pneumocystis jiroveci* pneumonia is given for 6–12 months after transplantation.

The signs and symptoms of infection may be masked or distorted. Fever without obvious cause is common, and only after days or weeks may it become apparent that it has a viral or fungal origin. Bacterial infections are most common during the first month after transplantation.

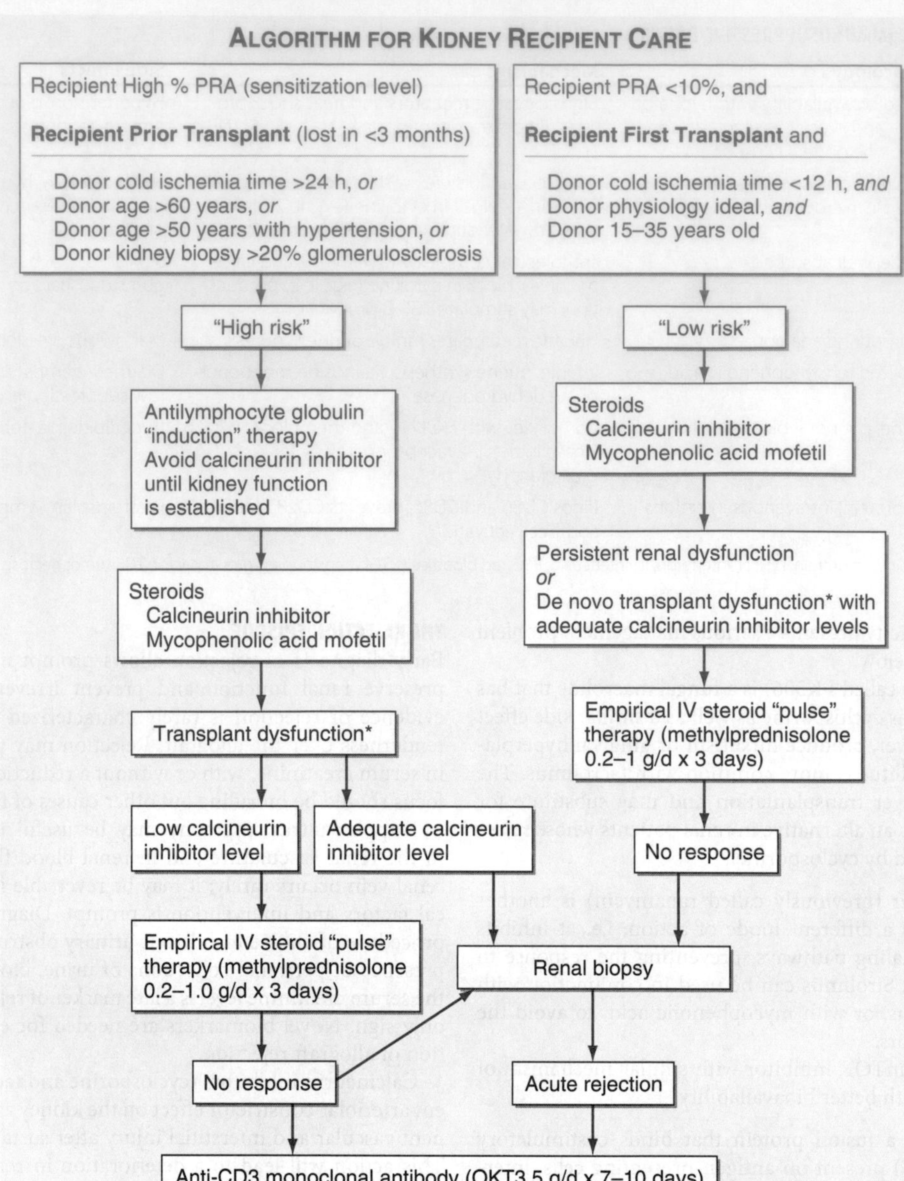

FIGURE 337-2 A typical algorithm for early posttransplant care of a kidney recipient. If any of the recipient or donor "high-risk" factors exist, more aggressive management is called for. Low-risk patients can be treated with a standard immunosuppressive regimen. Patients at higher risk of rejection or early ischemic and nephrotoxic transplant dysfunction are often induced with an antilymphocyte globulin to provide more potent early immunosuppression or to spare calcineurin nephrotoxicity. *When there is early transplant dysfunction, prerenal, obstructive, and vascular causes must be ruled out by ultrasonographic examination. The panel reactive antibody (PRA) is a quantitation of how much antibody is present in a candidate against a panel of cells representing the distribution of antigens in the donor pool.

TABLE 337-4 THE MOST COMMON OPPORTUNISTIC INFECTIONS IN RENAL TRANSPLANT RECIPIENTS

Peritransplant (<1 month)	Late (>6 months)
Wound infections	*Aspergillus*
Herpesvirus	*Nocardia*
Oral candidiasis	BK virus (polyoma)
Urinary tract infection	Herpes zoster
Early (1–6 months)	Hepatitis B
Pneumocystis jiroveci	Hepatitis C
Cytomegalovirus	
Legionella	
Listeria	
Hepatitis B	
Hepatitis C	

The importance of blood cultures in such patients cannot be overemphasized because systemic infection without obvious foci is common. Particularly ominous are rapidly occurring pulmonary lesions, which may result in death within 5 days of onset. When these lesions become apparent, immunosuppressive agents should be discontinued, except for maintenance doses of prednisone.

Aggressive diagnostic procedures, including transbronchial and open-lung biopsy, are frequently indicated. In the case of *P. jiroveci* (Chap. 244) infection, trimethoprim-sulfamethoxazole (TMP-SMX) is the treatment of choice; amphotericin B has been used effectively in systemic fungal infections. Prophylaxis against *P. jiroveci* with daily or alternate-day low-dose TMP-SMX is very effective. Involvement of the oropharynx with *Candida* (Chap. 240) may be treated with local nystatin. Tissue-invasive fungal infections require treatment with systemic agents such as fluconazole. Small doses (a total of 300 mg) of amphotericin given over a period of 2 weeks may be effective in fungal infections refractory to fluconazole. Macrolide antibiotics, especially ketoconazole and erythromycin, and some calcium channel blockers (diltiazem, verapamil) compete with calcineurin inhibitors for P450 catabolism and cause elevated levels of these immunosuppressive drugs. Analeptics, such as phenytoin and carbamazepine, will increase catabolism to result in low levels. *Aspergillus* (Chap. 241), *Nocardia* (Chap. 199), and especially CMV (Chap. 219) infections also occur.

CMV is a common and dangerous DNA virus in transplant recipients. It does not generally appear until the end of the first posttransplant month. Active CMV infection is sometimes associated, or occasionally confused, with rejection episodes. Patients at highest risk for severe CMV disease are those without anti-CMV antibodies who receive a graft from a CMV antibody–positive donor (15% mortality). Valganciclovir is a cost-effective and bioavailable oral form of ganciclovir that has been proved effective in both prophylaxis and treatment of CMV disease. Early diagnosis in a febrile patient with clinical suspicion of CMV disease can be made by determining CMV viral load in the blood. A rise in IgM antibodies to CMV is also diagnostic. Culture of CMV from blood may be less sensitive. Tissue invasion of CMV is common in the gastrointestinal tract and lungs. CMV retinopathy occurs late in the course, if untreated. Treatment of active CMV disease with valganciclovir is always indicated. In many patients immune to CMV, viral activation can occur with major immunosuppressive regimens.

The polyoma group (BK, JC, SV40) is another class of DNA viruses that can become dormant in kidneys and can be activated by immunosuppression. When reactivation occurs with BK, there is a 50% chance of progressive fibrosis and loss of the graft within 1 year by the activated virus. Risk of infection is associated with the overall degree of immunosuppression rather than the individual immunosuppressive drugs used. Renal biopsy is necessary for the diagnosis. There have been variable results with leflunomide, cidofovir, and quinolone antibiotics (which are effective against polyoma helicase), but it is most important to reduce the immunosuppressive load.

The complications of glucocorticoid therapy are well known and include gastrointestinal bleeding, impairment of wound healing, osteoporosis, diabetes mellitus, cataract formation, and hemorrhagic pancreatitis. The treatment of unexplained jaundice in transplant patients should include cessation or reduction of immunosuppressive drugs if hepatitis or drug toxicity is suspected. Therapy in such circumstances often does not result in rejection of a graft, at least for several weeks. Acyclovir is effective in therapy for herpes simplex virus infections.

CHRONIC LESIONS OF THE TRANSPLANTED KIDNEY

Although 1-year transplant survival is excellent, most recipients experience progressive decline in kidney function over time thereafter. Chronic renal transplant dysfunction can be caused by recurrent disease, hypertension, cyclosporine or tacrolimus nephrotoxicity, chronic immunologic rejection, secondary focal glomerulosclerosis, or a combination of these pathophysiologies. Chronic vascular changes with intimal proliferation and medial hypertrophy are commonly found. Control of systemic and intrarenal hypertension with angiotensin-converting enzyme (ACE) inhibitors is thought to have a beneficial influence on the rate of progression of chronic renal transplant dysfunction. Renal biopsy can distinguish subacute cellular rejection from recurrent disease or secondary focal sclerosis.

MALIGNANCY

The incidence of tumors in patients on immunosuppressive therapy is 5–6%, or approximately 100 times greater than that in the general population in the same age range. The most common lesions are cancer of the skin and lips and carcinoma in situ of the cervix, as well as lymphomas such as non-Hodgkin's lymphoma. The risks are increased in proportion to the total immunosuppressive load administered and the time elapsed since transplantation. Surveillance for skin and cervical cancers is necessary.

OTHER COMPLICATIONS

Both chronic dialysis and renal transplant patients have a higher incidence of death from myocardial infarction and stroke than does the population at large, and this is particularly true in diabetic patients. Contributing factors are the use of glucocorticoids and sirolimus and hypertension. Recipients of renal transplants have a high prevalence of coronary artery and peripheral vascular diseases. The percentage of deaths from these causes has been slowly rising as the numbers of transplanted diabetic patients and the average age of all recipients increase. More than 50% of renal recipient mortality is attributable to cardiovascular disease. In addition to strict control of blood pressure and blood lipid levels, close monitoring of patients for indications of further medical or surgical intervention is an important part of management.

Hypertension may be caused by (1) native kidney disease, (2) rejection activity in the transplant, (3) renal artery stenosis if an end-to-end anastomosis was constructed with an iliac artery branch, and (4) renal calcineurin inhibitor toxicity, which may improve with reduction in dose. Whereas ACE inhibitors may be useful, calcium channel blockers are more frequently used initially. Amelioration of hypertension to the range of 120–130/70–80 mmHg should be the goal in all patients.

Hypercalcemia after transplantation may indicate failure of hyperplastic parathyroid glands to regress. Aseptic necrosis of the head of the femur is probably due to preexisting hyperparathyroidism, with aggravation by glucocorticoid treatment. With improved management of calcium and phosphorus metabolism during chronic dialysis, the incidence of parathyroid-related complications has fallen dramatically. Persistent hyperparathyroid activity may require subtotal parathyroidectomy.

Although most transplant patients have robust production of erythropoietin and normalization of hemoglobin, *anemia* is commonly seen in the posttransplant period. Often the anemia is attributable to bone marrow–suppressant immunosuppressive medications such as azathioprine, mycophenolic acid, and sirolimus. Gastrointestinal bleeding is a common side effect of high-dose and long-term steroid administration. Many transplant patients have creatinine clearances of 30–50 mL/min and can be considered in the same way as other patients with chronic renal insufficiency for anemia management, including supplemental erythropoietin.

Chronic hepatitis, particularly when due to hepatitis B virus, can be a progressive, fatal disease over a decade or so. Patients who are persistently hepatitis B surface antigen–positive are at higher risk, according to some studies, but the presence of hepatitis C virus is also a concern when one embarks on a course of immunosuppression in a transplant recipient.

338 Glomerular Diseases

Julia B. Lewis, Eric G. Neilson

Two human kidneys harbor nearly 1.8 million glomerular capillary tufts. Each glomerular tuft resides within Bowman's space. The capsule circumscribing this space is lined by parietal epithelial cells that transition into tubular epithelia forming the proximal nephron or migrate into the tuft to replenish podocytes. The glomerular capillary tuft derives from an afferent arteriole that forms a branching capillary bed embedded in mesangial matrix (Fig. 338-1). This capillary network funnels into an efferent arteriole, which passes filtered blood into cortical peritubular capillaries or medullary vasa recta that supply and exchange with a folded tubular architecture. Hence the glomerular capillary tuft, fed and drained by arterioles, represents an arteriolar portal system. Fenestrated endothelial cells resting on a glomerular basement membrane (GBM) line glomerular capillaries. Delicate foot processes extending from epithelial podocytes shroud the outer surface of these capillaries, and podocytes interconnect to each other by slit-pore membranes forming a selective filtration barrier.

The glomerular capillaries filter 120–180 L/d of plasma water containing various solutes for reclamation or discharge by downstream

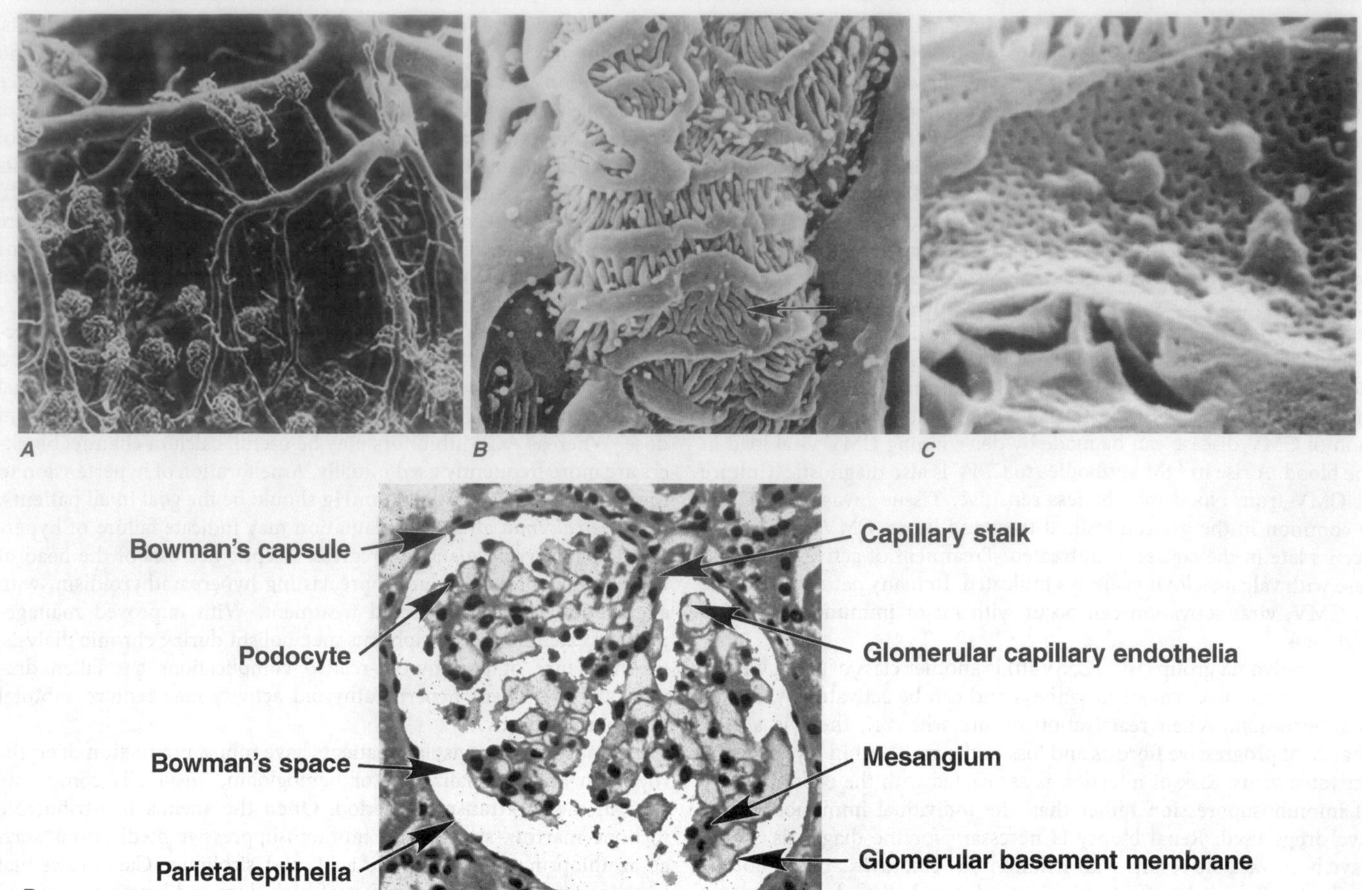

FIGURE 338-1 Glomerular architecture. ***A.*** The glomerular capillaries form from a branching network of renal arteries, arterioles, leading to an afferent arteriole, glomerular capillary bed (tuft), and a draining efferent arteriole. *(From VH Gattone II et al: Hypertension 5:8, 1983.)* ***B.*** Scanning electron micrograph of podocytes that line the outer surface of the glomerular capillaries (*arrow* shows foot process). ***C.*** Scanning electron micrograph of the fenestrated endothelia lining the glomerular capillary. ***D.*** The various normal regions of the glomerulus on light microscopy. *(A–C: Courtesy of Dr. Vincent Gattone, Indiana University; with permission.)*

tubules. Most large proteins and all cells are excluded from filtration by a physicochemical barrier governed by pore size and negative electrostatic charge. The mechanics of filtration and reclamation are quite complicated for many solutes (Chap. 325). For example, in the case of serum albumin, the glomerulus is an imperfect barrier. Although albumin has a negative charge, which would tend to repel the negatively charged GBM, it only has a physical radius of 3.6 nm, while pores in the GBM and slit-pore membranes have a radius of 4 nm. Consequently, variable amounts of albumin inevitably cross the filtration barrier to be reclaimed by megalin and cubilin receptors along the proximal tubule. Remarkably, humans with normal nephrons excrete on average 8–10 mg of albumin in daily voided urine, approximately 20–60% of total excreted protein. This amount of albumin, and other proteins, can rise to gram quantities following glomerular injury.

The breadth of diseases affecting the glomerulus is expansive because the glomerular capillaries can be injured in a variety of ways, producing many different lesions. Some order to this vast subject is brought by grouping all of these diseases into a smaller number of clinical syndromes.

PATHOGENESIS OF GLOMERULAR DISEASE

There are many forms of glomerular disease with pathogenesis variably linked to the presence of genetic mutations, infection, toxin exposure, autoimmunity, atherosclerosis, hypertension, emboli, thrombosis, or diabetes mellitus. Even after careful study, however, the cause often remains unknown, and the lesion is called *idiopathic*. Specific or unique features of pathogenesis are mentioned with the description of each of the glomerular diseases later in this chapter.

Some glomerular diseases result from genetic mutations producing familial disease or a founder effect: congenital nephrotic syndrome from mutations in *NPHS1* (nephrin) and *NPHS2* (podocin) affect the slit-pore membrane at birth, and *TRPC6* cation channel mutations produce *focal segmental glomerulosclerosis (FSGS)* in adulthood; polymorphisms in the gene encoding apolipoprotein L1, *APOL1*, are a major risk for nearly 70% of African Americans with nondiabetic end-stage renal disease, particularly FSGS; mutations in complement factor H associate with *membranoproliferative glomerulonephritis (MPGN)* or *atypical hemolytic uremic syndrome (aHUS)*, type II partial lipodystrophy from mutations in genes encoding lamin A/C, or PPARγ cause a metabolic syndrome associated with MPGN, which is sometimes accompanied by dense deposits and C3 nephritic factor; Alport's syndrome, from mutations in the genes encoding for the α3, α4, or α5 chains of type IV collagen, produces *split-basement membranes* with *glomerulosclerosis;* and lysosomal storage diseases, such as α-galactosidase A deficiency causing Fabry's disease and *N* -acetylneuraminic acid hydrolase deficiency causing nephrosialidosis, produce FSGS.

Systemic hypertension and atherosclerosis can produce pressure stress, ischemia, or lipid oxidants that lead to *chronic glomerulosclerosis. Malignant hypertension* can quickly complicate glomerulosclerosis with fibrinoid necrosis of arterioles and glomeruli, thrombotic microangiopathy, and acute renal failure. *Diabetic nephropathy* is an acquired sclerotic injury associated with thickening of the GBM secondary to the long-standing effects of hyperglycemia, advanced glycosylation end products, and reactive oxygen species.

Inflammation of the glomerular capillaries is called *glomerulonephritis.* Most glomerular or mesangial antigens involved in *immune-mediated glomerulonephritis* are unknown (Fig. 338-2). Glomerular epithelial or mesangial cells may shed or express epitopes that mimic other immunogenic proteins made elsewhere in the body. Bacteria, fungi, and viruses can directly infect the kidney producing their own antigens. Autoimmune diseases like idiopathic *membranous glomerulonephritis (MGN)* or MPGN are confined to the kidney, whereas systemic inflammatory diseases like *lupus nephritis* or *granulomatosis with polyangiitis (Wegener's)* spread to the kidney, causing secondary glomerular injury. *Antiglomerular basement membrane disease* producing Goodpasture's syndrome primarily injures both the lung and kidney because of the narrow distribution of the α3 NC1 domain of type IV collagen that is the target antigen.

Local activation of Toll-like receptors on glomerular cells, deposition of immune complexes, or complement injury to glomerular structures induces mononuclear cell infiltration, which subsequently leads to an adaptive immune response attracted to the kidney by local release of chemokines. Neutrophils, macrophages, and T cells are drawn by chemokines into the glomerular tuft, where they react with antigens and epitopes on or near somatic cells or their structures, producing more cytokines and proteases that damage the mesangium, capillaries, and/or the GBM. While the adaptive immune response is similar to that of other tissues, early T cell activation plays an important role in the mechanism of glomerulonephritis. Antigens presented by class II major histocompatibility complex (MHC) molecules on macrophages and dendritic cells in conjunction with associative recognition molecules engage the CD4/8 T cell repertoire.

Mononuclear cells by themselves can injure the kidney, but autoimmune events that damage glomeruli classically produce a humoral immune response. *Poststreptococcal glomerulonephritis, lupus nephritis,* and idiopathic *membranous nephritis* typically are associated with immune deposits along the GBM, while anti-GBM antibodies produce the linear binding of anti-GBM disease. Preformed circulating

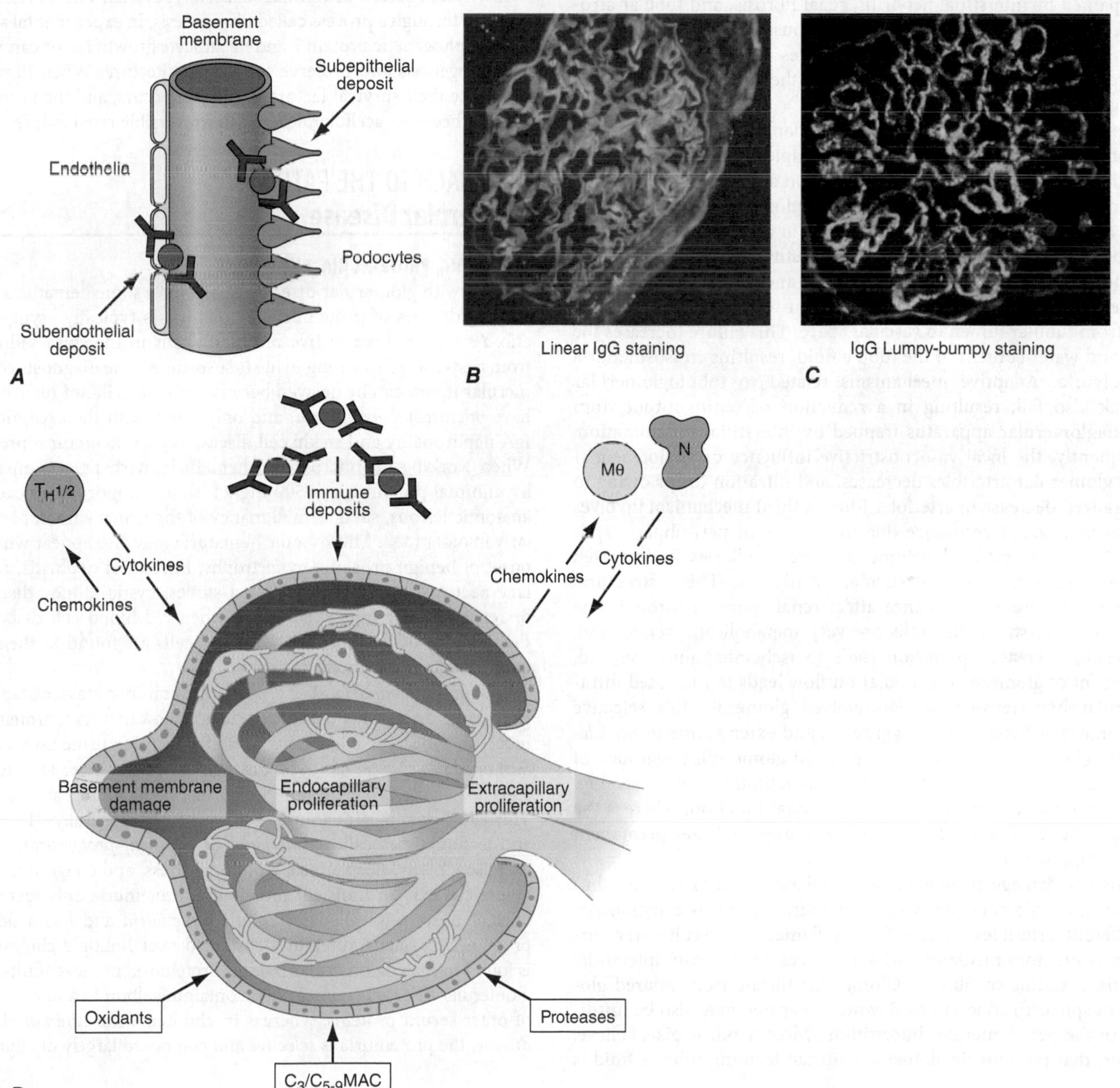

FIGURE 338-2 The glomerulus is injured by a variety of mechanisms. ***A.*** Preformed immune deposits can precipitate from the circulation and collect along the glomerular basement membrane (GBM) in the subendothelial space or can form in situ along the subepithelial space. ***B.*** Immunofluorescent staining of glomeruli with labeled anti-IgG demonstrating linear staining from a patient with anti-GBM disease or immune deposits from a patient with membranous glomerulonephritis. ***C.*** The mechanisms of glomerular injury have a complicated pathogenesis. Immune deposits and complement deposition classically draw macrophages and neutrophils into the glomerulus. T lymphocytes may follow to participate in the injury pattern as well. ***D.*** Amplification mediators as locally derived oxidants and proteases expand this inflammation, and, depending on the location of the target antigen and the genetic polymorphisms of the host, basement membranes are damaged with either endocapillary or extracapillary proliferation.

immune complexes can precipitate along the subendothelial side of the GBM, while other immune deposits form in situ on the subepithelial side. These latter deposits accumulate when circulating autoantibodies find their antigen trapped along the subepithelial edge of the GBM. Immune deposits in the glomerular mesangium may result from the deposition of preformed circulating complexes or in situ antigen-antibody interactions. Immune deposits stimulate the release of local proteases and activate the complement cascade, producing C_{5-9} attack complexes. In addition, local oxidants damage glomerular structures, producing proteinuria and effacement of the podocytes. Overlapping etiologies or pathophysiologic mechanisms can produce similar glomerular lesions, suggesting that downstream molecular and cellular responses often converge toward common patterns of injury.

PROGRESSION OF GLOMERULAR DISEASE

Persistent glomerulonephritis that worsens renal function is always accompanied by interstitial nephritis, renal fibrosis, and tubular atrophy (see Fig. 62e-27). What is not so obvious, however, is that renal failure in glomerulonephritis best correlates histologically with the appearance of tubulointerstitial nephritis rather than with the type of inciting glomerular injury.

Loss of renal function due to interstitial damage is explained hypothetically by several mechanisms. The simplest explanation is that urine flow is impeded by tubular obstruction as a result of interstitial inflammation and fibrosis. Thus, obstruction of the tubules with debris or by extrinsic compression results in aglomerular nephrons. A second mechanism suggests that interstitial changes, including interstitial edema or fibrosis, alter tubular and vascular architecture and thereby compromise the normal tubular transport of solutes and water from tubular lumen to vascular space. This failure increases the solute and water content of the tubule fluid, resulting in isosthenuria and polyuria. Adaptive mechanisms related to tubuloglomerular feedback also fail, resulting in a reduction of renin output from the juxtaglomerular apparatus trapped by interstitial inflammation. Consequently, the local vasoconstrictive influence of angiotensin II on the glomerular arterioles decreases, and filtration drops owing to a generalized decrease in arteriolar tone. A third mechanism involves changes in vascular resistance due to damage of peritubular capillaries. The cross-sectional volume of these capillaries is decreased by interstitial inflammation, edema, or fibrosis. These structural alterations in vascular resistance affect renal function through two mechanisms. First, tubular cells are very metabolically active, and, as a result, decreased perfusion leads to ischemic injury. Second, impairment of glomerular arteriolar outflow leads to increased intraglomerular hypertension in less-involved glomeruli; this selective intraglomerular hypertension aggravates and extends *mesangial sclerosis* and *glomerulosclerosis* to less-involved glomeruli. Regardless of the exact mechanism, early *acute tubulointerstitial nephritis* (see Fig. 62e-27) suggests potentially recoverable renal function, whereas the development of *chronic interstitial fibrosis* prognosticates permanent loss (see Fig. 62e-30).

Persistent damage to glomerular capillaries spreads to the tubulointerstitium in association with proteinuria. There is a hypothesis that efferent arterioles leading from inflamed glomeruli carry forward inflammatory mediators, which induces downstream interstitial nephritis, resulting in fibrosis. Glomerular filtrate from injured glomerular capillaries adherent to Bowman's capsule may also be misdirected to the periglomerular interstitium. Most nephrologists believe, however, that proteinuric glomerular filtrate forming tubular fluid is the primary route to downstream tubulointerstitial injury, although none of these hypotheses are mutually exclusive.

The simplest explanation for the effect of proteinuria on the development of interstitial nephritis is that increasingly severe proteinuria, carrying activated cytokines and lipoproteins producing reactive oxygen species, triggers a downstream inflammatory cascade in and around epithelial cells lining the tubular nephron. These effects induce T lymphocyte and macrophage infiltrates in the interstitial spaces along with fibrosis and tubular atrophy.

Tubules disaggregate following direct damage to their basement membranes, leading to epithelial-mesenchymal transitions forming more interstitial fibroblasts at the site of injury. Transforming growth factor β (TGF-β), fibroblast growth factor 2 (FGF-2), hypoxemia-inducible factor 1α (HIF-1α), and platelet-derived growth factor (PDGF) are particularly active in this transition. With persistent nephritis, fibroblasts multiply and lay down tenascin and a fibronectin scaffold for the polymerization of new interstitial collagen types I/III. These events form scar tissue through a process called fibrogenesis. In experimental studies, bone morphogenetic protein 7 and hepatocyte growth factor can reverse early fibrogenesis and preserve tubular architecture. When fibroblasts outdistance their survival factors, apoptoses occurs, and the permanent renal scar becomes acellular, leading to irreversible renal failure.

APPROACH TO THE PATIENT: Glomerular Disease

HEMATURIA, PROTEINURIA, AND PYURIA

Patients with glomerular disease usually have some hematuria with varying degrees of proteinuria. Hematuria is typically asymptomatic. As few as three to five red blood cells in the spun sediment from first-voided morning urine is suspicious. The diagnosis of glomerular injury can be delayed because patients will not realize they have *microscopic hematuria,* and only rarely with the exception of IgA nephropathy and sickle cell disease is *gross hematuria* present. When working up microscopic hematuria, perhaps accompanied by minimal proteinuria (<500 mg/24 h), it is important to exclude anatomic lesions, such as malignancy of the urinary tract, particularly in older men. Microscopic hematuria may also appear with the onset of benign prostatic hypertrophy, interstitial nephritis, papillary necrosis, hypercalciuria, renal stones, cystic kidney diseases, or renal vascular injury. However, when red blood cell casts (see Fig. 62e-34) or dysmorphic red blood cells are found in the sediment, glomerulonephritis is likely.

Sustained proteinuria >1–2 g/24 h is also commonly associated with glomerular disease. Patients often will not know they have proteinuria unless they become edematous or notice foaming urine on voiding. *Sustained proteinuria* has to be distinguished from lesser amounts of so-called *benign proteinuria* in the normal population (Table 338-1). This latter class of proteinuria is nonsustained, generally <1 g/24 h, and is sometimes called *functional* or *transient proteinuria.* Fever, exercise, obesity, sleep apnea, emotional stress, and congestive heart failure can explain transient proteinuria. Proteinuria only seen with upright posture is called *orthostatic proteinuria* and has a benign prognosis. Isolated proteinuria sustained over multiple clinic visits is found in many glomerular lesions. Proteinuria in most adults with glomerular disease is *nonselective,* containing albumin and a mixture of other serum proteins, whereas in children with *minimal change disease,* the proteinuria is *selective* and composed largely of albumin.

TABLE 338-1 URINE ASSAYS FOR ALBUMINURIA/PROTEINURIA

	24-Hour Albumin[a] (mg/24 h)	Albumin[a] /Creatinine Ratio (mg/g)	Dipstick Proteinuria	24-Hour Urine Protein[b] (mg/24 h)
Normal	8–10	<30	–	<150
Microalbuminuria	30–300	30–300	–/Trace/1+	–
Proteinuria	>300	>300	Trace–3+	>150

[a]Albumin detected by radioimmunoassay. [b]Albumin represents 20–60% of the total protein excreted in the urine.

Some patients with inflammatory glomerular disease, such as acute poststreptococcal glomerulonephritis or MPGN, have *pyuria* characterized by the presence of considerable numbers of leukocytes. This latter finding has to be distinguished from urine infected with bacteria.

CLINICAL SYNDROMES

Various forms of glomerular injury can also be parsed into several distinct syndromes on clinical grounds (Table 338-2). These syndromes, however, are not always mutually exclusive. There is an *acute nephritic syndrome* producing 1–2 g/24 h of proteinuria,

TABLE 338-2 PATTERNS OF CLINICAL GLOMERULONEPHRITIS

Glomerular Syndromes	Proteinuria	Hematuria	Vascular Injury
Acute Nephritic Syndromes			
Poststreptococcal glomerulonephritis[a]	+/++	++/+++	–
Subacute bacterial endocarditis[a]	+/++	++	–
Lupus nephritis[a]	+/++	++/+++	+
Antiglomerular basement membrane disease[a]	++	++/+++	–
IgA nephropathy[a]	+/++	+++[c]	–
ANCA small-vessel vasculitis[a]			
Granulomatosis with polyangiitis (Wegener's)	+/++	++/+++	++++
Microscopic polyangiitis	+/++	++/+++	++++
Churg-Strauss syndrome	+/++	++/+++	++++
Henoch-Schönlein purpura[a]	+/++	++/+++	++++
Cryoglobulinemia[a]	+/++	++/+++	++++
Membranoproliferative glomerulonephritis[a]	++	++/+++	–
Mesangioproliferative glomerulonephritis	+	+/++	–
Pulmonary-Renal Syndromes			
Goodpasture's syndrome[a]	++	++/+++	–
ANCA small-vessel vasculitis[a]			
Granulomatosis with polyangiitis (Wegener's)	+/++	++/+++	++++
Microscopic polyangiitis	+/++	++/+++	++++
Churg-Strauss syndrome	+/++	++/+++	++++
Henoch-Schönlein purpura[a]	+/++	++/+++	++++
Cryoglobulinemia[a]	+/++	++/+++	++++
Nephrotic Syndromes			
Minimal change disease	++++	–	–
Focal segmental glomerulosclerosis	+++/++++	+	–
Membranous glomerulonephritis	++++	+	–
Diabetic nephropathy	++/++++	–/+	–
AL and AA amyloidosis	+++/++++	+	+/++
Light chain deposition disease	+++	+	–
Fibrillary-immunotactoid disease	+++/++++	+	+
Fabry's disease	+	+	–
Basement Membrane Syndromes			
Anti-GBM disease[a]	++	++/+++	–
Alport's syndrome	++	++	–
Thin basement membrane disease	+	++	–
Nail-patella syndrome	++/+++	++	–
Glomerular Vascular Syndromes			
Atherosclerotic nephropathy	+	+	+++
Hypertensive nephropathy[b]	+/++	+/++	++
Cholesterol emboli	+/++	++	+++
Sickle cell disease	+/++	+++[c]	+++
Thrombotic microangiopathies	++	++	+++
Antiphospholipid syndrome	++	++	+++
ANCA small-vessel vasculitis[a]			
Granulomatosis with polyangiitis (Wegener's)	+/++	++/+++	++++
Microscopic polyangiitis	+/++	++/+++	++++
Churg-Strauss syndrome	+++	++/+++	++++
Henoch-Schönlein purpura[a]	+/++	++/+++	++++
Cryoglobulinemia[a]	+/++	++/+++	++++
AL and AA amyloidosis	+++/++++	+	+/++

(Continued)

TABLE 338-2 PATTERNS OF CLINICAL GLOMERULONEPHRITIS (*CONTINUED*)

Infectious Disease–Associated Syndromes			
Poststreptococcal glomerulonephritis[a]	+/++	++/+++	–
Subacute bacterial endocarditis[a]	+/++	++	–
HIV	+++	+/++	–
Hepatitis B and C	+++	+/++	–
Syphilis	+++	+	–
Leprosy	+++	+	–
Malaria	+++	+/++	–
Schistosomiasis	+++	+/++	–

[a]Can present as rapidly progressive glomerulonephritis (RPGN); sometimes called crescentic glomerulonephritis. [b]Can present as a malignant hypertensive crisis producing an aggressive fibrinoid necrosis in arterioles and small arteries with microangiopathic hemolytic anemia. [c]Can present with gross hematuria.

Abbreviations: AA, amyloid A; AL, amyloid L; ANCA, antineutrophil cytoplasmic antibodies; GBM, glomerular basement membrane.

hematuria with red blood cell casts, pyuria, hypertension, fluid retention, and a rise in serum creatinine associated with a reduction in glomerular filtration. If glomerular inflammation develops slowly, the serum creatinine will rise gradually over many weeks, but if the serum creatinine rises quickly, particularly over a few days, acute nephritis is sometimes called *rapidly progressive glomerulonephritis* (RPGN); the histopathologic term *crescentic glomerulonephritis* is the pathologic equivalent of the clinical presentation of RPGN. When patients with RPGN present with lung hemorrhage from Goodpasture's syndrome, antineutrophil cytoplasmic antibodies (ANCA)-associated small-vessel vasculitis, lupus erythematosus, or cryoglobulinemia, they are often diagnosed as having a *pulmonary-renal syndrome. Nephrotic syndrome* describes the onset of heavy proteinuria (>3.0 g/24 h), hypertension, hypercholesterolemia, hypoalbuminemia, edema/anasarca, and microscopic hematuria; if only large amounts of proteinuria are present without clinical manifestations, the condition is sometimes called *nephrotic-range proteinuria.* The glomerular filtration rate (GFR) in these patients may initially be normal or, rarely, higher than normal, but with persistent hyperfiltration and continued nephron loss, it typically declines over months to years. Patients with a *basement membrane syndrome* either have genetically abnormal basement membranes (Alport's syndrome) or an autoimmune response to basement membrane collagen IV (Goodpasture's syndrome) associated with microscopic hematuria, mild to heavy proteinuria, and hypertension with variable elevations in serum creatinine. *Glomerular–vascular syndrome* describes patients with vascular injury producing hematuria and moderate proteinuria. Affected individuals can have vasculitis, thrombotic microangiopathy, antiphospholipid syndrome, or, more commonly, a systemic disease such as atherosclerosis, cholesterol emboli, hypertension, sickle cell anemia, and autoimmunity. *Infectious disease–associated syndrome* is most important if one has a global perspective. Save for subacute bacterial endocarditis in the Western Hemisphere, malaria and schistosomiasis may be the most common causes of glomerulonephritis throughout the world, closely followed by HIV and chronic hepatitis B and C. These infectious diseases produce a variety of inflammatory reactions in glomerular capillaries, ranging from nephrotic syndrome to acute nephritic injury, and urinalyses that demonstrate a combination of hematuria and proteinuria.

These six general categories of syndromes are usually determined at the bedside with the help of a history and physical examination, blood chemistries, renal ultrasound, and urinalysis. These initial studies help frame further diagnostic workup that typically involves testing of the serum for the presence of various proteins (HIV and hepatitis B and C antigens), antibodies (anti-GBM, antiphospholipid, antistreptolysin O [ASO], anti-DNAse, antihyaluronidase, ANCA, anti-DNA, cryoglobulins, anti-HIV, and anti-hepatitis B and C antibodies) or depletion of complement components (C_3 and C_4). The bedside history and physical examination can also help determine whether the glomerulonephritis is isolated to the kidney (*primary glomerulonephritis*) or is part of a systemic disease (*secondary glomerulonephritis*).

When confronted with an abnormal urinalysis and elevated serum creatinine, with or without edema or congestive heart failure, one must consider whether the glomerulonephritis is *acute* or *chronic.* This assessment is best made by careful history (last known urinalysis or serum creatinine during pregnancy or insurance physical, evidence of infection, or use of medication or recreational drugs); the size of the kidneys on renal ultrasound examination; and how the patient feels at presentation. Chronic glomerular disease often presents with decreased kidney size. Patients who quickly develop renal failure are fatigued and weak and often have uremic symptoms associated with nausea, vomiting, fluid retention, and somnolence. Primary glomerulonephritis presenting with renal failure that has progressed slowly, however, can be remarkably asymptomatic, as are patients with acute glomerulonephritis without much loss in renal function. Once this initial information is collected, selected patients who are clinically stable, have adequate blood clotting parameters, and are willing and able to receive treatment are encouraged to have a renal biopsy.

RENAL PATHOLOGY

A renal biopsy in the setting of glomerulonephritis quickly identifies the type of glomerular injury and often suggests a course of treatment. The biopsy is processed for light microscopy using stains for *hematoxylin and eosin (H&E)* to assess cellularity and architecture, *periodic acid–Schiff (PAS)* to stain carbohydrate moieties in the membranes of the glomerular tuft and tubules, *Jones-methenamine silver* to enhance basement membrane structure, *Congo red* for amyloid deposits, and *Masson's trichrome* to identify collagen deposition and assess the degree of glomerulosclerosis and interstitial fibrosis. Biopsies are also processed for direct immunofluorescence using conjugated antibodies against IgG, IgM, and IgA to detect the presence of "lumpy-bumpy" immune deposits or "linear" IgG or IgA antibodies bound to GBM, antibodies against trapped complement proteins (C_3 and C_4), or specific antibodies against a relevant antigen. High-resolution electron microscopy can clarify the principal location of immune deposits and the status of the basement membrane.

Each region of a renal biopsy is assessed separately. By light microscopy, glomeruli (at least 10 and ideally 20) are reviewed individually for discrete lesions; <50% involvement is considered *focal,* and >50% is *diffuse.* Injury in each glomerular tuft can be *segmental,* involving a portion of the tuft, or *global,* involving most of the glomerulus. Glomeruli having *proliferative* characteristics show increased cellularity. When cells in the capillary tuft proliferate, it is called *endocapillary,* and when cellular proliferation extends into Bowman's space, it is called *extracapillary. Synechiae* are formed when epithelial podocytes attach to Bowman's capsule in the setting of glomerular injury; *crescents,* which in some cases may be the extension of synechiae, develop when fibrocellular/fibrin collections fill all or part of Bowman's space; and *sclerotic* glomeruli show acellular, amorphous accumulations of proteinaceous material throughout the tuft with loss of functional capillaries and normal mesangium. Since *age-related glomerulosclerosis* is common in adults, one can estimate the background percentage of sclerosis by dividing the patient's age in half and subtracting 10. Immunofluorescent and electron microscopy can detect the presence and location of *subepithelial, subendothelial, or mesangial* immune deposits, or *reduplication* or *splitting* of the basement membrane. In the other regions of the biopsy, the vasculature surrounding glomeruli and tubules can show *angiopathy, vasculitis,* the presence of *fibrils,* or *thrombi.* The tubules can be assessed for adjacency to one another; separation can be the result of edema, tubular dropout, or collagen deposition resulting from interstitial fibrosis. Interstitial fibrosis is an ominous sign of irreversibility and progression to renal failure.

ACUTE NEPHRITIC SYNDROMES

Acute nephritic syndromes classically present with hypertension, hematuria, red blood cell casts, pyuria, and mild to moderate proteinuria. Extensive inflammatory damage to glomeruli causes a fall in GFR and eventually produces uremic symptoms with salt and water retention, leading to edema and hypertension.

POSTSTREPTOCOCCAL GLOMERULONEPHRITIS

Poststreptococcal glomerulonephritis is prototypical for *acute endocapillary proliferative glomerulonephritis.* The incidence of poststreptococcal glomerulonephritis has dramatically decreased in developed countries and in these locations is typically sporadic. Acute poststreptococcal glomerulonephritis in underdeveloped countries is epidemic and usually affects children between the ages of 2 and 14 years, but in developed countries is more typical in the elderly, especially in association with debilitating conditions. It is more common in males, and the familial or cohabitant incidence is as high as 40%. Skin and throat infections with particular M types of streptococci (nephritogenic strains) antedate glomerular disease; M types 47, 49, 55, 2, 60, and 57 are seen following impetigo and M types 1, 2, 4, 3, 25, 49, and 12 with pharyngitis. Poststreptococcal glomerulonephritis due to impetigo develops 2–6 weeks after skin infection and 1–3 weeks after streptococcal pharyngitis.

The renal biopsy in poststreptococcal glomerulonephritis demonstrates hypercellularity of mesangial and endothelial cells, glomerular infiltrates of polymorphonuclear leukocytes, granular subendothelial immune deposits of IgG, IgM, C_3, C_4, and C_{5-9}, and subepithelial deposits (which appear as "humps") (see Fig. 62e-6). (See Glomerular Schematic 1.) Poststreptococcal glomerulonephritis is an immune-mediated disease involving putative streptococcal antigens, circulating immune complexes, and activation of complement in association with cell-mediated injury. Many candidate antigens have been proposed over the years; candidates from nephritogenic streptococci of interest at the moment are: a cationic cysteine proteinase known as streptococcal pyrogenic exotoxin B (SPEB) that is generated by proteolysis of a zymogen precursor (zSPEB), and NAPlr, the nephritis-associated plasmin receptor. These two antigens have biochemical affinity for plasmin, bind as complexes facilitated by this relationship, and activate the alternate complement pathway. The nephritogenic antigen, SPEB, has been demonstrated inside the subepithelial "humps" on biopsy.

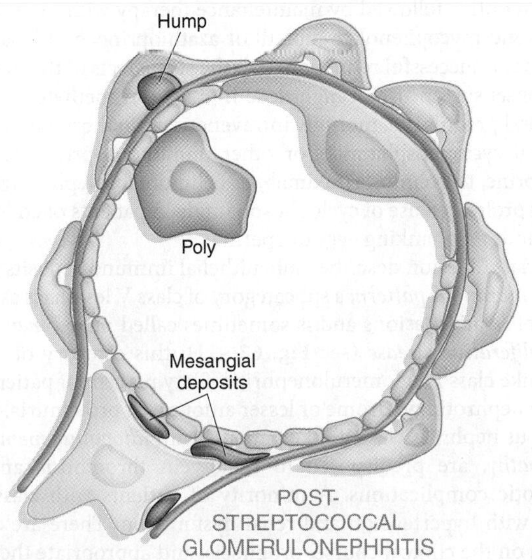

The classic presentation is an acute nephritic picture with hematuria, pyuria, red blood cell casts, edema, hypertension, and oliguric renal failure, which may be severe enough to appear as RPGN. Systemic symptoms of headache, malaise, anorexia, and flank pain (due to swelling of the renal capsule) are reported in as many as 50% of cases. Five percent of children and 20% of adults have proteinuria in the nephrotic range. In the first week of symptoms, 90% of patients will have a depressed CH_{50} and decreased levels of C_3 with normal levels of C_4. Positive rheumatoid factor (30–40%), cryoglobulins and circulating immune complexes (60–70%), and ANCA against myeloperoxidase (10%) are also reported. Positive cultures for streptococcal infection are inconsistently present (10–70%), but increased titers of ASO (30%), anti-DNAse, (70%), or antihyaluronidase antibodies (40%) can help confirm the diagnosis. Consequently, the diagnosis of poststreptococcal glomerulonephritis rarely requires a renal biopsy. A subclinical disease is reported in some series to be four to five times as common as clinical nephritis, and these latter cases are characterized by asymptomatic microscopic hematuria with low serum C_3 complement levels.

Treatment is supportive, with control of hypertension, edema, and dialysis as needed. Antibiotic treatment for streptococcal infection should be given to all patients and their cohabitants. There is no role for immunosuppressive therapy, even in the setting of crescents. Recurrent poststreptococcal glomerulonephritis is rare despite repeated streptococcal infections. Early death is rare in children but does occur in the elderly. Overall, the prognosis is good, with permanent renal failure being very uncommon, less than 1% in children. Complete resolution of the hematuria and proteinuria in the majority of children occurs within 3–6 weeks of the onset of nephritis but 3–10% of children may have persistent microscopic hematuria, nonnephrotic proteinuria, or hypertension. The prognosis in elderly patients is worse with a high incidence of azotemia (up to 60%), nephrotic-range proteinuria, and end-stage renal disease.

SUBACUTE BACTERIAL ENDOCARDITIS

Endocarditis-associated glomerulonephritis is typically a complication of subacute bacterial endocarditis, particularly in patients who remain untreated for a long time, have negative blood cultures, or have right-sided endocarditis. Glomerulonephritis is unusual in acute bacterial endocarditis because it takes 10–14 days to develop immune complex–mediated injury, by which time the patient has been treated, often with emergent surgery. Grossly, the kidneys in subacute bacterial endocarditis have subcapsular hemorrhages with a "flea-bitten" appearance, and microscopy on renal biopsy reveals focal proliferation around foci of necrosis associated with abundant mesangial, subendothelial, and subepithelial immune deposits of IgG, IgM, and C_3. Patients who present with a clinical picture of RPGN have crescents. Embolic infarcts or septic abscesses may also be present. The pathogenesis hinges on the renal deposition of circulating immune complexes in the kidney with complement activation. Patients present with gross or microscopic hematuria, pyuria, and mild proteinuria or, less commonly, RPGN with rapid loss of renal function. A normocytic anemia, elevated erythrocyte sedimentation rate, hypocomplementemia, high titers of rheumatoid factor, type III cryoglobulins, circulating immune complexes, and ANCAs may be present. Levels of serum creatinine may be elevated at diagnosis, but with modern therapy there is little progression to chronic renal failure. Primary treatment is eradication of the infection with 4–6 weeks of antibiotics, and if accomplished expeditiously, the prognosis for renal recovery is good. ANCA-associated vasculitis sometimes accompanies or is confused with subacute bacterial endocarditis (SBE) and should be ruled out, as the treatment is different.

As variants of persistent bacterial infection in blood-associated glomerulonephritis, postinfectious glomerulonephritis can occur in patients with ventriculoatrial and ventriculoperitoneal shunts; pulmonary, intraabdominal, pelvic, or cutaneous infections; and infected vascular prostheses. In developed countries, a significant proportion of cases afflict adults, especially the immunocompromised, and the predominant organism is *Staphylococcus*. The clinical presentation of these conditions is variable and includes proteinuria, microscopic hematuria, acute renal failure, and hypertension. Serum complement levels are low, and there may be elevated levels of C-reactive proteins, rheumatoid factor, antinuclear antibodies, and cryoglobulins. Renal lesions include membranoproliferative glomerulonephritis (MPGN), diffuse proliferative and exudative glomerulonephritis (DPGN), or mesangioproliferative glomerulonephritis, sometimes leading to RPGN. Treatment focuses on eradicating the infection, with most patients treated as if they have endocarditis. The prognosis is guarded.

LUPUS NEPHRITIS

Lupus nephritis is a common and serious complication of systemic lupus erythematosus (SLE) and most severe in African-American female adolescents. Thirty to 50% of patients will have clinical manifestations of renal disease at the time of diagnosis, and 60% of adults and 80% of children develop renal abnormalities at some point in the course of their disease. Lupus nephritis results from the deposition of circulating immune complexes, which activate the complement cascade leading to complement-mediated damage, leukocyte infiltration, activation of procoagulant factors, and release of various cytokines. In situ immune complex formation following glomerular binding of nuclear antigens, particularly necrotic nucleosomes, also plays a role in renal injury. The presence of antiphospholipid antibodies may also trigger a thrombotic microangiopathy in a minority of patients.

The clinical manifestations, course of disease, and treatment of lupus nephritis are closely linked to renal pathology. The most common clinical sign of renal disease is proteinuria, but hematuria, hypertension, varying degrees of renal failure, and active urine sediment with red blood cell casts can all be present. Although significant renal pathology can be found on biopsy even in the absence of major abnormalities in the urinalysis, most nephrologists do not biopsy patients until the urinalysis is convincingly abnormal. The extrarenal manifestations of lupus are important in establishing a firm diagnosis of systemic lupus because, while serologic abnormalities are common in lupus nephritis, they are not diagnostic. Anti-dsDNA antibodies that fix complement correlate best with the presence of renal disease. Hypocomplementemia is common in patients with acute lupus nephritis (70–90%) and declining complement levels may herald a flare. Although urinary biomarkers of lupus nephritis are being identified to assist in predicting renal flares, renal biopsy is the only reliable method of identifying the morphologic variants of lupus nephritis.

The World Health Organization (WHO) workshop in 1974 first outlined several distinct patterns of lupus-related glomerular injury; these were modified in 1982. In 2004 the International Society of Nephrology in conjunction with the Renal Pathology Society again updated the classification. This latest version of lesions seen on biopsy (Table 338-3) best defines clinicopathologic correlations, provides valuable prognostic information, and forms the basis for modern treatment recommendations. Class I nephritis describes normal glomerular histology by any technique or normal light microscopy with minimal mesangial deposits on immunofluorescent or electron microscopy. Class II designates mesangial immune complexes with *mesangial proliferation*. Both class I and II lesions are typically associated with minimal renal manifestation and normal renal function; nephrotic syndrome is rare. Patients with lesions limited to the renal mesangium have an excellent prognosis and generally do not need therapy for their lupus nephritis.

The subject of lupus nephritis is presented under acute nephritic syndromes because of the aggressive and important proliferative lesions seen in class III–V renal disease. Class III describes *focal lesions with proliferation or scarring,* often involving only a segment of the glomerulus (see Fig. 62e-12). Class III lesions have the most varied course. Hypertension, an active urinary sediment, and proteinuria are common with nephrotic-range proteinuria in 25–33% of patients. Elevated serum creatinine is present in 25% of patients. Patients with mild proliferation involving a small percentage of glomeruli respond well to therapy with steroids alone, and fewer than 5% progress to renal failure over 5 years. Patients with more severe proliferation involving a greater percentage of glomeruli have a far worse prognosis and lower remission rates. Treatment of those patients is the same as that for class IV lesions. Many nephrologists believe that class III lesions are simply an early presentation of class IV disease. Others believe severe class III disease is a discrete lesion requiring aggressive therapy. Class IV describes *global, diffuse proliferative lesions* involving the vast majority of glomeruli. Patients with class IV lesions commonly have high anti-DNA antibody titers, low serum complement, hematuria, red blood cell casts, proteinuria, hypertension, and decreased renal function; 50% of patients have nephrotic-range proteinuria. Patients with crescents on biopsy often have a rapidly progressive decline in renal function (see Fig. 62e-12). Without treatment, this aggressive lesion has the worst renal prognosis. However, if a remission—defined as a return to near-normal renal function and proteinuria ≤330 mg/dL per day—is achieved with treatment, renal outcomes are excellent. Current evidence suggests that inducing a remission with administration of high-dose steroids and either cyclophosphamide or mycophenolate mofetil for 2–6 months, followed by maintenance therapy with lower doses of steroids and mycophenolate mofetil or azathioprine, best balances the likelihood of successful remission with the side effects of therapy. There is no consensus on use of high-dose intravenous methylprednisolone versus oral prednisone, monthly intravenous cyclophosphamide versus daily oral cyclophosphamide, or other immunosuppressants such as cyclosporine, tacrolimus, rituximab, or belimumab. Nephrologists tend to avoid prolonged use of cyclophosphamide in patients of childbearing age without first banking eggs or sperm.

The class V lesion describes subepithelial immune deposits producing a *membranous pattern;* a subcategory of class V lesions is associated with proliferative lesions and is sometimes called *mixed membranous and proliferative disease* (see Fig. 62e-11); this category of injury is treated like class IV glomerulonephritis. Sixty percent of patients present with nephrotic syndrome or lesser amounts of proteinuria. Patients with lupus nephritis class V, like patients with *idiopathic membranous nephropathy,* are predisposed to renal-vein thrombosis and other thrombotic complications. A minority of patients with class V will present with hypertension and renal dysfunction. There are conflicting data on the clinical course, prognosis, and appropriate therapy for

TABLE 338-3 CLASSIFICATION FOR LUPUS NEPHRITIS

Class I	Minimal mesangial	Normal histology with mesangial deposits
Class II	Mesangial proliferation	Mesangial hypercellularity with expansion of the mesangial matrix
Class III	Focal nephritis	Focal endocapillary ± extracapillary proliferation with focal subendothelial immune deposits and mild mesangial expansion
Class IV	Diffuse nephritis	Diffuse endocapillary ± extracapillary proliferation with diffuse subendothelial immune deposits and mesangial alterations
Class V	Membranous nephritis	Thickened basement membranes with diffuse subepithelial immune deposits; may occur with class III or IV lesions and is sometimes called mixed membranous and proliferative nephritis
Class VI	Sclerotic nephritis	Global sclerosis of nearly all glomerular capillaries

Note: Revised in 2004 by the International Society of Nephrology-Renal Pathology Society Study Group.

patients with class V disease, which may reflect the heterogeneity of this group of patients. Patients with severe nephrotic syndrome, elevated serum creatinine, and a progressive course will probably benefit from therapy with steroids in combination with other immunosuppressive agents. Therapy with inhibitors of the renin-angiotensin system also may attenuate the proteinuria. Antiphospholipid antibodies present in lupus may result in glomerular microthromboses and complicate the course in up to 20% of lupus nephritis patients. The renal prognosis is worse even with anticoagulant therapy.

Patients with any of the above lesions also can transform to another lesion; hence patients often require reevaluation, including repeat renal biopsy. Lupus patients with class VI lesions have greater than 90% *sclerotic glomeruli* and end-stage renal disease with interstitial fibrosis. As a group, approximately 20% of patients with lupus nephritis will reach end-stage disease, requiring dialysis or transplantation. Systemic lupus tends to become quiescent once there is renal failure, perhaps due to the immunosuppressant effects of uremia. However, patients with lupus nephritis have a markedly increased mortality compared with the general population. Renal transplantation in renal failure from lupus, usually performed after approximately 6 months of inactive disease, results in allograft survival rates comparable to patients transplanted for other reasons.

ANTIGLOMERULAR BASEMENT MEMBRANE DISEASE

Patients who develop autoantibodies directed against glomerular basement antigens frequently develop a glomerulonephritis termed *antiglomerular basement membrane (anti-GBM) disease.* When they present with lung hemorrhage and glomerulonephritis, they have a pulmonary-renal syndrome called *Goodpasture's syndrome.* The target epitopes for this autoimmune disease lie in the quaternary structure of α3 NC1 domain of collagen IV. Indeed, anti-GBM disease may be considered an autoimmune "conformeropathy" that involves the perturbation of quaternary structure of the α 345NC1 hexamer. MHC-restricted T cells initiate the autoantibody response because humans are not tolerant to the epitopes created by this quaternary structure. The epitopes are normally sequestered in the collagen IV hexamer and can be exposed by infection, smoking, oxidants, or solvents. Goodpasture's syndrome appears in two age groups: in young men in their late twenties and in men and women in their sixties and seventies. Disease in the younger age group is usually explosive, with hemoptysis, a sudden fall in hemoglobin, fever, dyspnea, and hematuria. Hemoptysis is largely confined to smokers, and those who present with lung hemorrhage as a group do better than older populations who have prolonged, asymptomatic renal injury; presentation with oliguria is often associated with a particularly bad outcome. The performance of an urgent kidney biopsy is important in suspected cases of Goodpasture's syndrome to confirm the diagnosis and assess prognosis. Renal biopsies typically show *focal or segmental necrosis* that later, with aggressive destruction of the capillaries by cellular proliferation, leads to crescent formation in Bowman's space (see Fig. 62e-14). As these lesions progress, there is concomitant interstitial nephritis with fibrosis and tubular atrophy.

The presence of anti-GBM antibodies and complement is recognized on biopsy by linear immunofluorescent staining for IgG (rarely IgA). In testing serum for anti-GBM antibodies, it is particularly important that the α3 NC1 domain of collagen IV alone be used as the target. This is because nonnephritic antibodies against the α1 NC1 domain are seen in paraneoplastic syndromes and cannot be discerned from assays that use whole basement membrane fragments as the binding target. Between 10 and 15% of sera from patients with Goodpasture's syndrome also contain ANCA antibodies against myeloperoxidase. This subset of patients has a vasculitis-associated variant, which has a surprisingly good prognosis with treatment. Prognosis at presentation is worse if there are >50% crescents on renal biopsy with advanced fibrosis, if serum creatinine is >5–6 mg/dL, if oliguria is present, or if there is a need for acute dialysis. Although frequently attempted, most of these latter patients will not respond to plasmapheresis and steroids. Patients with advanced renal failure who present with hemoptysis should still be treated for their lung hemorrhage, as it responds to plasmapheresis and can be lifesaving. Treated patients with less severe disease typically respond to 8–10 treatments of plasmapheresis accompanied by oral prednisone and cyclophosphamide in the first 2 weeks. Kidney transplantation is possible, but because there is risk of recurrence, experience suggests that patients should wait for 6 months and until serum antibodies are undetectable.

IgA NEPHROPATHY

Berger first described the glomerulonephritis now termed *IgA nephropathy.* It is classically characterized by episodic hematuria associated with the deposition of IgA in the mesangium. IgA nephropathy is one of the most common forms of glomerulonephritis worldwide. There is a male preponderance, a peak incidence in the second and third decades of life, and rare familial clustering. There are geographic differences in the prevalence of IgA nephropathy, with 30% prevalence along the Asian and Pacific Rim and 20% in southern Europe, compared to a much lower prevalence in northern Europe and North America. It was initially hypothesized that variation in detection, in part, accounted for regional differences. With clinical care in nephrology becoming more uniform, this variation in prevalence more likely reflects true differences among racial and ethnic groups.

IgA nephropathy is predominantly a sporadic disease but susceptibility to it has been shown uncommonly to have a genetic component depending on geography and the existence of "founder effects." Familial forms of IgA nephropathy are more common in northern Italy and eastern Kentucky. No single causal gene has been identified. Clinical and laboratory evidence suggests close similarities between Henoch-Schönlein purpura and IgA nephropathy. Henoch-Schönlein purpura is distinguished clinically from IgA nephropathy by prominent systemic symptoms, a younger age (<20 years old), preceding infection, and abdominal complaints. Deposits of IgA are also found in the glomerular mesangium in a variety of systemic diseases, including chronic liver disease, Crohn's disease, gastrointestinal adenocarcinoma, chronic bronchiectasis, idiopathic interstitial pneumonia, dermatitis herpetiformis, mycosis fungoides, leprosy, ankylosing spondylitis, relapsing polychondritis, and Sjögren's syndrome. IgA deposition in these entities is not usually associated with clinically significant glomerular inflammation or renal dysfunction and thus is not called IgA nephropathy.

IgA nephropathy is an immune complex–mediated glomerulonephritis defined by the presence of diffuse mesangial IgA deposits often associated with mesangial hypercellularity. (See Glomerular Schematic 2.) IgM, IgG, C_3, or immunoglobulin light chains may be codistributed with IgA. IgA deposited in the mesangium is typically polymeric and of the IgA1 subclass, the pathogenic significance of which is not clear. Abnormalities have been described in IgA production by plasma cells, particularly secretory IgA; in IgA clearance, predominately by the liver; in mesangial IgA clearance and receptors for IgA; and in growth factor and cytokine-mediated events. Currently, however, abnormalities in the *O* -glycosylation of the hinge region of IgA seem to best account for the pathogenesis of sporadic IgA nephropathy. Despite the presence of elevated serum IgA levels in 20–50% of patients, IgA deposition in skin biopsies in 15–55% of patients, or elevated levels of secretory IgA and IgA-fibronectin complexes, a renal biopsy is necessary to confirm the diagnosis. Although the immunofluorescent pattern of IgA on renal biopsy defines IgA nephropathy in the proper clinical context, a variety of histologic lesions may be seen on light microscopy (see Fig. 62e-8), including DPGN; *segmental sclerosis;* and, rarely, *segmental necrosis with cellular crescent formation,* which typically presents as RPGN.

The two most common presentations of IgA nephropathy are recurrent episodes of macroscopic hematuria during or immediately following an upper respiratory infection often accompanied by proteinuria or persistent asymptomatic microscopic hematuria. Nephrotic syndrome is uncommon. Proteinuria can also first appear late in the course of the disease. Rarely patients present with acute renal failure and a rapidly progressive clinical picture. IgA nephropathy is a benign disease for the majority of patients, and 5–30% of patients may go into a complete remission, with others having hematuria but well

Glomerular schematic 2

Mesangial deposits plus more mesangial cells

IgA NEPHROPATHY

preserved renal function. In the minority of patients who have progressive disease, progression is slow, with renal failure seen in only 25–30% of patients with IgA nephropathy over 20–25 years. This risk varies considerably among populations. Cumulatively, risk factors for the loss of renal function identified thus far account for less than 50% of the variation in observed outcome but include the presence of hypertension or proteinuria, the absence of episodes of macroscopic hematuria, male sex, older age of onset, and extensive glomerulosclerosis or interstitial fibrosis on renal biopsy. Several analyses in large populations of patients found persistent proteinuria for 6 months or longer to have the greatest predictive power for adverse renal outcomes.

There is no agreement on optimal treatment. Both large studies that include patients with multiple glomerular diseases and small studies of patients with IgA nephropathy support the use of angiotensin-converting enzyme (ACE) inhibitors in patients with proteinuria or declining renal function. Tonsillectomy, steroid therapy, and fish oil have all been suggested in small studies to benefit select patients with IgA nephropathy. When presenting as RPGN, patients typically receive steroids, cytotoxic agents, and plasmapheresis.

ANCA SMALL-VESSEL VASCULITIS

A group of patients with small-vessel vasculitis (arterioles, capillaries, and venules; rarely small arteries) and glomerulonephritis have serum ANCA; the antibodies are of two types, anti-proteinase 3 (PR3) or anti-myeloperoxidase (MPO) (Chap. 385); Lamp-2 antibodies have also been reported experimentally as potentially pathogenic. ANCA are produced with the help of T cells and activate leukocytes and monocytes, which together damage the walls of small vessels. Endothelial injury also attracts more leukocytes and extends the inflammation. Granulomatosis with polyangiitis, microscopic polyangiitis, and Churg-Strauss syndrome belong to this group because they are ANCA-positive and have a *pauci-immune glomerulonephritis* with few immune complexes in small vessels and glomerular capillaries. Patients with any of these three diseases can have any combination of the above serum antibodies, but anti-PR3 antibodies are more common in granulomatosis with polyangiitis and anti-MPO antibodies are more common in microscopic polyangiitis or Churg-Strauss. Although each of these diseases has some unique clinical features, most features do not predict relapse or progression, and as a group, they are generally treated in the same way. Since mortality is high without treatment, virtually all patients receive urgent treatment. Induction therapy usually includes some combination of plasmapheresis, methylprednisolone, and cyclophosphamide. Monthly "pulse" IV cyclophosphamide to induce remission of ANCA-associated vasculitis is as effective as daily oral cyclophosphamide but may be associated with increased relapses. Steroids are tapered soon after acute inflammation subsides, and patients are maintained on cyclophosphamide or azathioprine for up to a year to minimize the risk of relapse. Benefit with using mycophenolate mofetil or rituximab has not been proven.

Granulomatosis with Polyangiitis Patients with this disease classically present with fever, purulent rhinorrhea, nasal ulcers, sinus pain, polyarthralgias/arthritis, cough, hemoptysis, shortness of breath, microscopic hematuria, and 0.5–1 g/24 h of proteinuria; occasionally there may be cutaneous purpura and mononeuritis multiplex. Presentation without renal involvement is termed *limited granulomatosis with polyangiitis,* although some of these patients will show signs of renal injury later. Chest x-ray often reveals nodules and persistent infiltrates, sometimes with cavities. Biopsy of involved tissue will show a small-vessel vasculitis and adjacent noncaseating granulomas. Renal biopsies during active disease demonstrate *segmental necrotizing glomerulonephritis* without immune deposits (see Fig. 62e-13). The disease is more common in patients exposed to silica dust and those with α_1-antitrypsin deficiency, which is an inhibitor of PR3. Relapse after achieving remission is common and is more common in patients with granulomatosis with polyangiitis than the other ANCA-associated vasculitis, necessitating diligent follow-up care. Although associated with an unacceptable high mortality rate without treatment, the greatest threat to patients, especially elderly patients in the first year of therapy, is from adverse events, which are often secondary to treatment, rather than active vasculitis.

Microscopic Polyangiitis Clinically, these patients look somewhat similar to those with granulomatosis with polyangiitis, except they rarely have significant lung disease or destructive sinusitis. The distinction is made on biopsy, where the vasculitis in microscopic polyangiitis is without granulomas. Some patients will also have injury limited to the capillaries and venules.

Churg-Strauss Syndrome When small-vessel vasculitis is associated with peripheral eosinophilia, cutaneous purpura, mononeuritis, asthma, and allergic rhinitis, a diagnosis of Churg-Strauss syndrome is considered. Hypergammaglobulinemia, elevated levels of serum IgE, or the presence of rheumatoid factor sometimes accompanies the allergic state. Lung inflammation, including fleeting cough and pulmonary infiltrates, often precedes the systemic manifestations of disease by years; lung manifestations are rarely absent. A third of patients may have exudative pleural effusions associated with eosinophils. Small-vessel vasculitis and *focal segmental necrotizing glomerulonephritis* can be seen on renal biopsy, usually absent eosinophils or granulomas. The cause of Churg-Strauss syndrome is autoimmune, but the inciting factors are unknown.

MEMBRANOPROLIFERATIVE GLOMERULONEPHRITIS

MPGN is sometimes called *mesangiocapillary glomerulonephritis* or *lobar glomerulonephritis*. It is an immune-mediated glomerulonephritis characterized by thickening of the GBM with mesangioproliferative changes; 70% of patients have hypocomplementemia. MPGN is rare in African Americans, and idiopathic disease usually presents in childhood or young adulthood. MPGN is subdivided pathologically into type I, type II, and type III disease. *Type I MPGN* is commonly associated with persistent hepatitis C infections, autoimmune diseases like lupus or cryoglobulinemia, or neoplastic diseases (Table 338-4). *Types II and III MPGN* are usually idiopathic, except in patients with complement factor H deficiency, in the presence of C_3 nephritic factor and/or in partial lipodystrophy producing type II disease, or complement receptor deficiency in type III disease. MPGN has been proposed to be reclassified into immunoglobulin-mediated disease (driven by the classical complement pathway) and non–immunoglobulin-mediated disease (driven by the alternative complement pathway).

TABLE 338-4 MEMBRANOPROLIFERATIVE GLOMERULONEPHRITIS

Type I Disease (Most Common)
Idiopathic
Subacute bacterial endocarditis
Systemic lupus erythematosus
Hepatitis C ± cryoglobulinemia
Mixed cryoglobulinemia
Hepatitis B
Cancer: Lung, breast, and ovary (germinal)
Type II Disease (Dense Deposit Disease)
Idiopathic
C_3 nephritic factor–associated
Partial lipodystrophy
Type III Disease
Idiopathic
Complement receptor deficiency

Type I MPGN, the most proliferative of the three types, shows mesangial proliferation with lobular segmentation on renal biopsy and mesangial interposition between the capillary basement membrane and endothelial cells, producing a double contour sometimes called *tram-tracking* (see Fig. 62e-9). (See Glomerular Schematic 3.) Subendothelial deposits with low serum levels of C_3 are typical, although 50% of patients have normal levels of C_3 and occasional intramesangial deposits. Low serum C_3 and a dense thickening of the GBM containing ribbons of dense deposits and C_3 characterize type II MPGN, sometimes called *dense deposit disease* (see Fig. 62e-10). Classically, the glomerular tuft has a lobular appearance; intramesangial deposits are rarely present and subendothelial deposits are generally absent. Proliferation in type III MPGN is less common than the other two types and is often focal; mesangial interposition is rare, and subepithelial deposits can occur along widened segments of the GBM that appear laminated and disrupted.

Type I MPGN is secondary to glomerular deposition of circulating immune complexes or their in situ formation. Types II and III MPGN may be related to "nephritic factors," which are autoantibodies that stabilize C_3 convertase and allow it to activate serum C_3. MPGN can also result from acquired or genetic abnormalities in the alternative complement pathway. Patients with MPGN present with proteinuria, hematuria, and pyuria (30%); systemic symptoms of fatigue and malaise that are most common in children with type I disease; or an acute nephritic picture with RPGN and a speedy deterioration in renal function in up to 25% of patients. Low serum C_3 levels are common. Fifty percent of patients with MPGN develop end-stage disease 10 years after diagnosis, and 90% have renal insufficiency after 20 years. Nephrotic syndrome, hypertension, and renal insufficiency all predict poor outcome. In the presence of proteinuria, treatment with inhibitors of the renin-angiotensin system is prudent. Evidence for treatment with dipyridamole, Coumadin (warfarin), or cyclophosphamide is not strongly established. There is some evidence supporting the efficacy of treatment of *primary MPGN* with steroids, particularly in children, as well as reports of efficacy with plasma exchange and other immunosuppressive drugs. If defects in the complement pathway are found, treatment with eculizumab is of hypothetical but unproven benefit. In *secondary MPGN,* treating the associated infection, autoimmune disease, or neoplasms is of demonstrated benefit. In particular, pegylated interferon and ribavirin are useful in reducing viral load. Although all primary renal diseases can recur over time in transplanted renal allografts, patients with MPGN are well known to be at risk for not only a histologic recurrence but also a clinically significant recurrence with loss of graft function.

Glomerular schematic 3

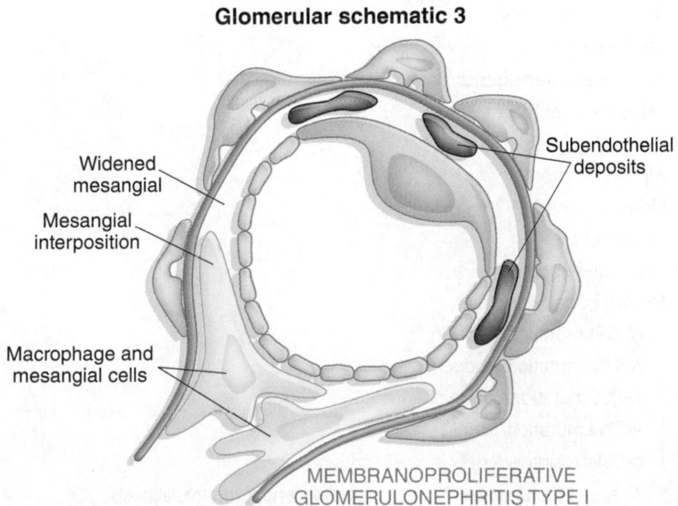

MESANGIOPROLIFERATIVE GLOMERULONEPHRITIS

Mesangioproliferative glomerulonephritis is characterized by expansion of the mesangium, sometimes associated with mesangial hypercellularity; thin, single contoured capillary walls; and mesangial immune deposits. Clinically, it can present with varying degrees of proteinuria and, commonly, hematuria. Mesangioproliferative disease may be seen in IgA nephropathy, *Plasmodium falciparum* malaria, resolving postinfectious glomerulonephritis, and class II nephritis from lupus, all of which can have a similar histologic appearance. With these secondary entities excluded, the diagnosis of *primary mesangioproliferative glomerulonephritis* is made in less than 15% of renal biopsies. As an immune-mediated renal lesion with deposits of IgM, C1q, and C_3, the clinical course is variable. Patients with isolated hematuria may have a very benign course, and those with heavy proteinuria occasionally progress to renal failure. There is little agreement on treatment, but some clinical reports suggest benefit from use of inhibitors of the renin-angiotensin system, steroid therapy, and even cytotoxic agents.

NEPHROTIC SYNDROME

Nephrotic syndrome classically presents with heavy proteinuria, minimal hematuria, hypoalbuminemia, hypercholesterolemia, edema, and hypertension. If left undiagnosed or untreated, some of these syndromes will progressively damage enough glomeruli to cause a fall in GFR, producing renal failure. Multiple studies have noted that the higher the 24-h urine protein excretion, the more rapid is the decline in GFR.

Therapies for various causes of nephrotic syndrome are noted under individual disease headings below. In general, all patients with hypercholesterolemia secondary to nephrotic syndrome should be treated with lipid-lowering agents because they are at increased risk for cardiovascular disease. Edema secondary to salt and water retention can be controlled with the judicious use of diuretics, avoiding intravascular volume depletion. Venous complications secondary to the hypercoagulable state associated with nephrotic syndrome can be treated with anticoagulants. The losses of various serum binding proteins, such as thyroid-binding globulin, lead to alterations in functional tests. Lastly, proteinuria itself is hypothesized to be nephrotoxic, and treatment of proteinuria with inhibitors of the renin-angiotensin system can lower urinary protein excretion.

MINIMAL CHANGE DISEASE

Minimal change disease (MCD), sometimes known as *nil lesion,* causes 70–90% of nephrotic syndrome in childhood but only 10–15% of nephrotic syndrome in adults. Minimal change disease usually presents as a primary renal disease but can be associated with several other conditions, including Hodgkin's disease, allergies, or use of nonsteroidal anti-inflammatory agents; significant interstitial nephritis often accompanies cases associated with nonsteroidal drug use. Minimal change disease on renal biopsy shows no obvious glomerular lesion by light microscopy and is negative for deposits by immunofluorescent microscopy, or occasionally shows small amounts of IgM in the mesangium

Glomerular schematic 4

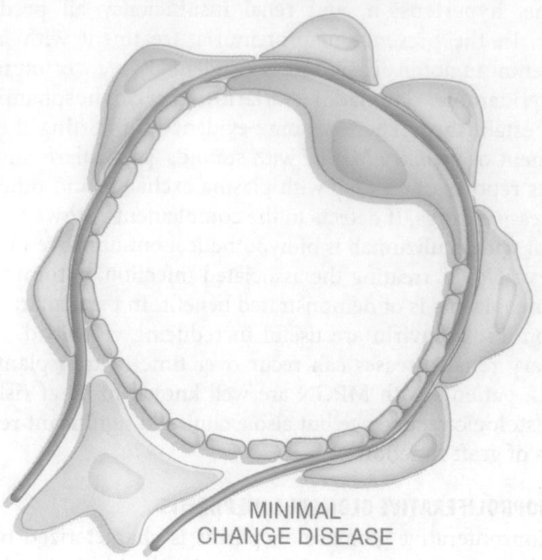

(see Fig. 62e-1). (See Glomerular Schematic 4.) Electron microscopy, however, consistently demonstrates an effacement of the foot process supporting the epithelial podocytes with weakening of slit-pore membranes. The pathophysiology of this lesion is uncertain. Most agree there is a circulating cytokine, perhaps related to a T cell response that alters capillary charge and podocyte integrity. The evidence for cytokine-related immune injury is circumstantial and is suggested by the presence of preceding allergies, altered cell-mediated immunity during viral infections, and the high frequency of remissions with steroids.

Minimal change disease presents clinically with the abrupt onset of edema and nephrotic syndrome accompanied by acellular urinary sediment. Average urine protein excretion reported in 24 h is 10 g with severe hypoalbuminemia. Less common clinical features include hypertension (30% in children, 50% in adults), microscopic hematuria (20% in children, 33% in adults), atopy or allergic symptoms (40% in children, 30% in adults), and decreased renal function (<5% in children, 30% in adults). The appearance of acute renal failure in adults is often seen more commonly in patients with low serum albumin and intrarenal edema (nephrosarca) that is responsive to intravenous albumin and diuretics. This presentation must be distinguished from acute renal failure secondary to hypovolemia. Acute tubular necrosis and interstitial inflammation are also reported. In children, the abnormal urine principally contains albumin with minimal amounts of higher-molecular-weight proteins, and is sometimes called *selective proteinuria*. Although up to 30% of children have a spontaneous remission, all children today are treated with steroids; only children who are nonresponders are biopsied in this setting. Primary responders are patients who have a complete remission (<0.2 mg/24 h of proteinuria) after a single course of prednisone; steroid-dependent patients relapse as their steroid dose is tapered. Frequent relapsers have two or more relapses in the 6 months following taper, and steroid-resistant patients fail to respond to steroid therapy. Adults are not considered steroid-resistant until after 4 months of therapy. Ninety to 95% of children will develop a complete remission after 8 weeks of steroid therapy, and 80–85% of adults will achieve complete remission, but only after a longer course of 20–24 weeks. Patients with steroid resistance may have FSGS on repeat biopsy. Some hypothesize that if the first renal biopsy does not have a sample of deeper corticomedullary glomeruli, then the correct diagnosis of FSGS may be missed.

Relapses occur in 70–75% of children after the first remission, and early relapse predicts multiple subsequent relapses, as do high levels of basal proteinuria. The frequency of relapses decreases after puberty. There is an increased risk of relapse following the rapid tapering of steroids in all groups. Relapses are less common in adults but are more resistant to subsequent therapy. Prednisone is first-line therapy, either given daily or on alternate days. Other immunosuppressive drugs, such as cyclophosphamide, chlorambucil, and mycophenolate mofetil, are saved for frequent relapsers, steroid-dependent patients, or steroid-resistant patients. Cyclosporine can induce remission, but relapse is also common when cyclosporine is withdrawn. The long-term prognosis in adults is less favorable when acute renal failure or steroid resistance occurs.

FOCAL SEGMENTAL GLOMERULOSCLEROSIS

Focal segmental glomerulosclerosis (FSGS) refers to a pattern of renal injury characterized by segmental glomerular scars that involve some but not all glomeruli; the clinical findings of FSGS largely manifest as proteinuria. When the secondary causes of FSGS are eliminated (Table 338-5), the remaining patients are considered to have primary FSGS. The incidence of this disease is increasing, and it now represents up to one-third of cases of nephrotic syndrome in adults and one-half of cases of nephrotic syndrome in African Americans, in whom it is seen more commonly. The pathogenesis of FSGS is probably multifactorial. Possible mechanisms include a T cell–mediated circulating permeability factor, increased soluble urokinase receptor levels, TGF-β–mediated cellular proliferation and matrix synthesis, and podocyte abnormalities associated with genetic mutations. Risk polymorphisms at the *APOL1* locus encoding apolipoprotein L1 expressed in podocytes substantially explain the increased burden of FSGS among African Americans with or without HIV-associated disease.

The pathologic changes of FSGS are most prominent in glomeruli located at the corticomedullary junction (see Fig. 62e-2), so if the renal biopsy specimen is from superficial tissue, the lesions can be missed, which sometimes leads to a misdiagnosis of MCD. In addition to focal and segmental scarring, other variants have been described, including cellular lesions with *endocapillary hypercellularity* and heavy proteinuria; *collapsing glomerulopath y* (see Fig. 62e-3) with segmental or global glomerular collapse and a rapid decline in renal function; a hilar stalk lesion (see Fig. 62e-4); or the *glomerular tip lesion* (see Fig. 62e-5), which may have a better prognosis. (See Glomerular Schematic 5.)

FSGS can present with hematuria, hypertension, any level of proteinuria, or renal insufficiency. Nephrotic-range proteinuria, African-American race, and renal insufficiency are associated with a poor outcome, with 50% of patients reaching renal failure in 6–8 years. FSGS rarely remits spontaneously, but treatment-induced remission of proteinuria significantly improves prognosis. Treatment of patients with *primary FSGS* should include inhibitors of the renin-angiotensin system. Based on retrospective studies, patients with nephrotic-range proteinuria can be treated with steroids but respond far less often and

TABLE 338-5 FOCAL SEGMENTAL GLOMERULOSCLEROSIS

Primary focal segmental glomerulosclerosis
Secondary focal segmental glomerulosclerosis
Viruses: HIV/hepatitis B/parvovirus
Hypertensive nephropathy
Reflux nephropathy
Cholesterol emboli
Drugs: Heroin/analgesics/pamidronate
Oligomeganephronia
Renal dysgenesis
Alport's syndrome
Sickle cell disease
Lymphoma
Radiation nephritis
Familial podocytopathies
NPHS1 mutation/nephrin
NPHS2 mutation/podocin
TRPC6 mutation/cation channel
ACTN4 mutation/actinin
α-Galactosidase A deficiency/Fabry's disease
N-acetylneuraminic acid hydrolase deficiency/nephrosialidosis

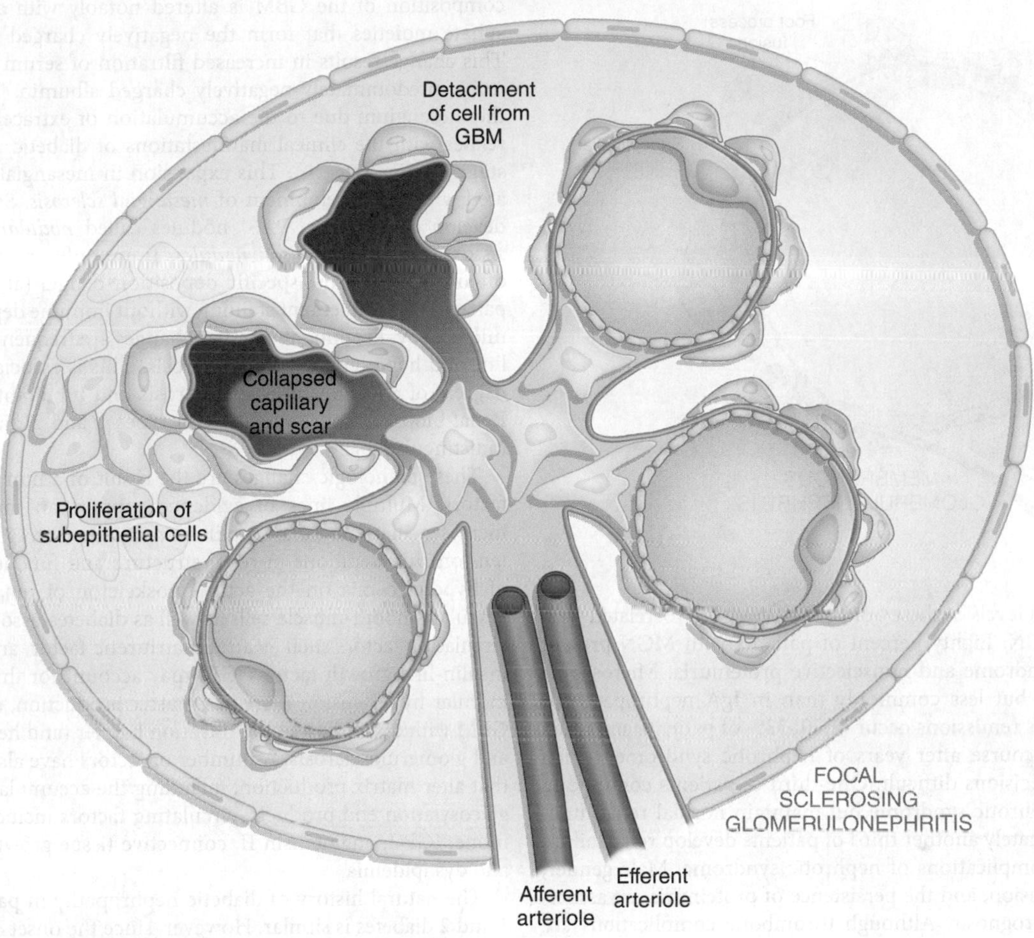

after a longer course of therapy than patients with MCD. Proteinuria remits in only 20–45% of patients receiving a course of steroids over 6–9 months. Limited evidence suggests the use of cyclosporine in steroid-responsive patients helps ensure remissions. Relapse frequently occurs after cessation of cyclosporine therapy, and cyclosporine itself can lead to a deterioration of renal function due to its nephrotoxic effects. A role for other agents that suppress the immune system has not been established. Primary FSGS recurs in 25–40% of patients given allografts at end-stage disease, leading to graft loss in half of those cases. The treatment of *secondary FSGS* typically involves treating the underlying cause and controlling proteinuria. There is no role for steroids or other immunosuppressive agents in secondary FSGS.

MEMBRANOUS GLOMERULONEPHRITIS

Membranous glomerulonephritis (MGN), or *membranous nephropathy* as it is sometimes called, accounts for approximately 30% of cases of nephrotic syndrome in adults, with a peak incidence between the ages of 30 and 50 years and a male to female ratio of 2:1. It is rare in childhood and the most common cause of nephrotic syndrome in the elderly. In 25–30% of cases, MGN is associated with a malignancy (solid tumors of the breast, lung, colon), infection (hepatitis B, malaria, schistosomiasis), or rheumatologic disorders like lupus or rarely rheumatoid arthritis (Table 338-6).

Uniform thickening of the basement membrane along the peripheral capillary loops is seen by light microscopy on renal biopsy (see Fig. 62e-7); this thickening needs to be distinguished from that seen in diabetes and amyloidosis. (See Glomerular Schematic 6.) Immunofluorescence demonstrates diffuse granular deposits of IgG and C_3, and electron microscopy typically reveals electron-dense subepithelial deposits. While different stages (I–V) of progressive membranous lesions have been described, some published analyses indicate the degree of tubular atrophy or interstitial fibrosis is more predictive of progression than is the stage of glomerular disease. The presence of subendothelial deposits or the presence of tubuloreticular inclusions strongly points to a diagnosis of membranous lupus nephritis, which may precede the extrarenal manifestations of lupus. Work in Heyman nephritis, an animal model of MGN, suggests that glomerular lesions result from in situ formation of immune complexes with megalin receptor–associated protein as the putative antigen. This antigen is not found in human podocytes. Human antibodies have been described against neutral endopeptidase expressed by podocytes in infants whose mothers lack this protein. In most adults, autoantibodies against the M-type phospholipase A_2 receptor (PLA_2R) circulate and bind to a conformational epitope present in the receptor on human podocytes, producing in situ deposits characteristic of idiopathic membranous nephropathy. Other renal diseases and secondary membranous nephropathy do not appear to involve such

TABLE 338-6 MEMBRANOUS GLOMERULONEPHRITIS

Primary/idiopathic membranous glomerulonephritis
Secondary membranous glomerulonephritis
Infection: Hepatitis B and C, syphilis, malaria, schistosomiasis, leprosy, filariasis
Cancer: Breast, colon, lung, stomach, kidney, esophagus, neuroblastoma
Drugs: Gold, mercury, penicillamine, nonsteroidal anti-inflammatory agents, probenecid
Autoimmune diseases: Systemic lupus erythematosus, rheumatoid arthritis, primary biliary cirrhosis, dermatitis herpetiformis, bullous pemphigoid, myasthenia gravis, Sjögren's syndrome, Hashimoto's thyroiditis
Other systemic diseases: Fanconi's syndrome, sickle cell anemia, diabetes, Crohn's disease, sarcoidosis, Guillain-Barré syndrome, Weber-Christian disease, angiofollicular lymph node hyperplasia

Glomerular schematic 6

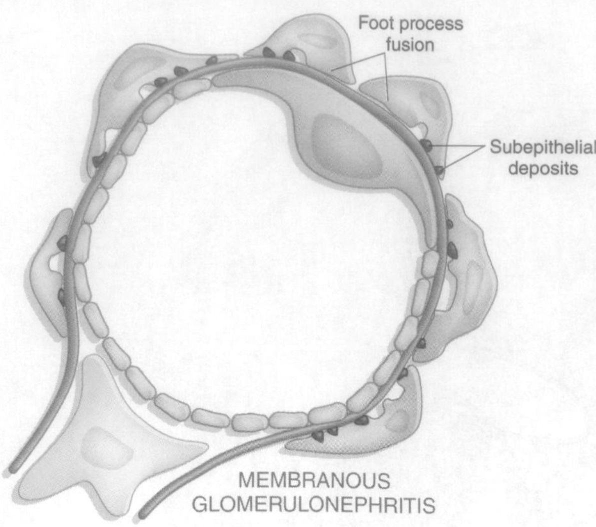

autoantibodies and levels of these autoantibodies have correlated with the severity of MGN. Eighty percent of patients with MGN present with nephrotic syndrome and nonselective proteinuria. Microscopic hematuria is seen but less commonly than in IgA nephropathy or FSGS. Spontaneous remissions occur in 20–33% of patients and often occur late in the course after years of nephrotic syndrome, which make treatment decisions difficult. One-third of patients continue to have relapsing nephrotic syndrome but maintain normal renal function, and approximately another third of patients develop renal failure or die from the complications of nephrotic syndrome. Male gender, older age, hypertension, and the persistence of proteinuria are associated with worse prognosis. Although thrombotic complications are a feature of all nephrotic syndromes, MGN has the highest reported incidences of renal vein thrombosis, pulmonary embolism, and deep vein thrombosis. Prophylactic anticoagulation is controversial but has been recommended for patients with severe or prolonged proteinuria in the absence of risk factors for bleeding.

In addition to the treatment of edema, dyslipidemia, and hypertension, inhibition of the renin-angiotensin system is recommended. Therapy with immunosuppressive drugs is also recommended for patients with primary MGN and persistent proteinuria (>3.0 g/24 h). The choice of immunosuppressive drugs for therapy is controversial, but current recommendations are to treat with steroids and cyclophosphamide, chlorambucil, mycophenolate mofetil, or cyclosporine. In patients who relapse or fail to respond to this therapy, the use of rituximab, an anti-CD20 antibody directed at B cells, or synthetic adrenocorticotropic hormone may be considered.

DIABETIC NEPHROPATHY

Diabetic nephropathy is the single most common cause of chronic renal failure in the United States, accounting for 45% of patients receiving renal replacement therapy, and is a rapidly growing problem worldwide. The dramatic increase in the number of patients with diabetic nephropathy reflects the epidemic increase in obesity, metabolic syndrome, and type 2 diabetes mellitus. Approximately 40% of patients with types 1 or 2 diabetes develop nephropathy, but due to the higher prevalence of type 2 diabetes (90%) compared to type 1 (10%), the majority of patients with diabetic nephropathy have type 2 disease. Renal lesions are more common in African-American, Native American, Polynesian, and Maori populations. Risk factors for the development of diabetic nephropathy include hyperglycemia, hypertension, dyslipidemia, smoking, a family history of diabetic nephropathy, and gene polymorphisms affecting the activity of the renin-angiotensin-aldosterone axis.

Within 1–2 years after the onset of clinical diabetes, morphologic changes appear in the kidney. Thickening of the GBM is a sensitive indicator for the presence of diabetes but correlates poorly with the presence or absence of clinically significant nephropathy. The composition of the GBM is altered notably with a loss of heparan sulfate moieties that form the negatively charged filtration barrier. This change results in increased filtration of serum proteins into the urine, predominately negatively charged albumin. The expansion of the mesangium due to the accumulation of extracellular matrix correlates with the clinical manifestations of diabetic nephropathy (see stages in Fig. 62e-20). This expansion in mesangial matrix is associated with the development of *mesangial sclerosis.* Some patients also develop eosinophilic, PAS$^+$ nodules called *nodular glomerulosclerosis* or *Kimmelstiel-Wilson nodules.* Immunofluorescence microscopy often reveals the nonspecific deposition of IgG (at times in a linear pattern) or complement staining without immune deposits on electron microscopy. Prominent vascular changes are frequently seen with hyaline and hypertensive arteriosclerosis. This is associated with varying degrees of chronic glomerulosclerosis and tubulointerstitial changes. Renal biopsies from patients with types 1 and 2 diabetes are largely indistinguishable.

These pathologic changes are the result of a number of postulated factors. Multiple lines of evidence support an important role for increases in glomerular capillary pressure (intraglomerular hypertension) in alterations in renal structure and function. Direct effects of hyperglycemia on the actin cytoskeleton of renal mesangial and vascular smooth-muscle cells as well as diabetes-associated changes in circulating factors such as atrial natriuretic factor, angiotensin II, and insulin-like growth factor (IGF) may account for this. Sustained glomerular hypertension increases matrix production, alterations in the GBM with disruption in the filtration barrier (and hence proteinuria), and glomerulosclerosis. A number of factors have also been identified that alter matrix production, including the accumulation of advanced glycosylation end products, circulating factors including growth hormone, IGF-I, angiotensin II, connective tissue growth factor, TGF-β, and dyslipidemia.

The natural history of diabetic nephropathy in patients with types 1 and 2 diabetes is similar. However, since the onset of type 1 diabetes is readily identifiable and the onset of type 2 diabetes is not, a patient newly diagnosed with type 2 diabetes may present with *advanced diabetic nephropathy.* At the onset of diabetes, renal hypertrophy and glomerular hyperfiltration are present. The degree of glomerular hyperfiltration correlates with the subsequent risk of clinically significant nephropathy. In the approximately 40% of patients with diabetes who develop diabetic nephropathy, the earliest manifestation is an increase in albuminuria detected by sensitive radioimmunoassay (Table 338-1). Albuminuria in the range of 30–300 mg/24 h is called *microalbuminuria.* Microalbuminuria appears 5–10 years after the onset of diabetes. It is currently recommended to test patients with type 1 disease for microalbuminuria 5 years after diagnosis of diabetes and yearly thereafter and, because the time of onset of type 2 diabetes is often unknown, to test type 2 patients at the time of diagnosis of diabetes and yearly thereafter.

Patients with small increases in albuminuria increase their levels of urinary albumin excretion, typically reaching dipstick positive levels of proteinuria (>300 mg albuminuria) 5–10 years after the onset of early albuminuria. Microalbuminuria is a potent risk factor for cardiovascular events and death in patients with type 2 diabetes. Many patients with type 2 diabetes and microalbuminuria succumb to cardiovascular events before they progress to proteinuria or renal failure. Proteinuria in frank diabetic nephropathy can be variable, ranging from 500 mg to 25 g/24 h, and is often associated with nephrotic syndrome. More than 90% of patients with type 1 diabetes and nephropathy have diabetic retinopathy, so the absence of retinopathy in type 1 patients with proteinuria should prompt consideration of a diagnosis other than diabetic nephropathy; only 60% of patients with type 2 diabetes with nephropathy have diabetic retinopathy. There is a significant correlation between the presence of retinopathy and the presence of Kimmelstiel-Wilson nodules (see Fig. 62e-20). Also, characteristically, patients with advanced diabetic nephropathy have normal to enlarged kidneys, in contrast to other glomerular diseases where kidney size is usually decreased. Using the above epidemiologic and clinical data, and in the absence of other clinical or serologic data suggesting another disease, diabetic nephropathy is usually diagnosed without a renal biopsy. After the onset of proteinuria, renal function inexorably declines, with 50% of patients reaching renal failure over another 5–10 years; thus, from the earliest stages of microalbuminuria, it usually takes 10–20 years to reach end-stage renal disease. Once renal failure appears, however, survival on dialysis is shorter for patients with diabetes compared to other dialysis patients. Survival is best for patients with type 1 diabetes who receive a transplant from a living related donor.

Good evidence supports the benefits of blood sugar and blood pressure control as well as inhibition of the renin-angiotensin system in retarding the progression of diabetic nephropathy. In patients with type 1 diabetes, intensive control of blood sugar clearly prevents the development or progression of diabetic nephropathy. The evidence for benefit of intensive blood glucose control in patients with type 2 diabetes is less certain, with current studies reporting conflicting results.

Controlling systemic blood pressure decreases renal and cardiovascular adverse events in this high-risk population. The vast majority of patients with diabetic nephropathy require three or more antihypertensive drugs to achieve this goal. Drugs that inhibit the renin-angiotensin system, independent of their effects on systemic blood pressure, have been shown in numerous large clinical trials to slow the progression of diabetic nephropathy at early (microalbuminuria) and late (proteinuria with reduced glomerular filtration) stages, independent of any effect they may have on systemic blood pressure. Since angiotensin II increases efferent arteriolar resistance and, hence, glomerular capillary pressure, one key mechanism for the efficacy of ACE inhibitors or angiotensin receptor blockers (ARBs) is reducing glomerular hypertension. Patients with type 1 diabetes for 5 years who develop albuminuria or declining renal function should be treated with ACE inhibitors. Patients with type 2 diabetes and microalbuminuria or proteinuria may be treated with ACE inhibitors or ARBs. Evidence suggests increased risk for cardiovascular adverse events in some patients with a combination of two drugs (ACE inhibitors, ARBs, renin inhibitors, or aldosterone antagonists) that suppress several components of the renin-angiotensin system.

GLOMERULAR DEPOSITION DISEASES

Plasma cell dyscrasias producing excess light chain immunoglobulin sometimes lead to the formation of glomerular and tubular deposits that cause heavy proteinuria and renal failure; the same is true for the accumulation of serum amyloid A protein fragments seen in several inflammatory diseases. This broad group of proteinuric patients has *glomerular deposition disease*.

Light Chain Deposition Disease The biochemical characteristics of nephrotoxic light chains produced in patients with light chain malignancies often confer a specific pattern of renal injury; that of either *cast nephropathy* (see Fig. 62e-17), which causes renal failure but not heavy proteinuria or amyloidosis, or light chain deposition disease (see Fig. 62e-16), which produces nephrotic syndrome with renal failure. These latter patients produce kappa light chains that do not have the biochemical features necessary to form amyloid fibrils. Instead, they self-aggregate and form granular deposits along the glomerular capillary and mesangium, tubular basement membrane, and Bowman's capsule. When predominant in glomeruli, nephrotic syndrome develops, and about 70% of patients progress to dialysis. Light-chain deposits are not fibrillar and do not stain with Congo red, but they are easily detected with anti–light chain antibody using immunofluorescence or as granular deposits on electron microscopy. A combination of the light chain rearrangement, self-aggregating properties at neutral pH, and abnormal metabolism probably contribute to the deposition. Treatment for light chain deposition disease is treatment of the primary disease and, if possible, autologous stem cell transplantation.

Renal Amyloidosis Most *renal amyloidosis* is either the result of primary fibrillar deposits of immunoglobulin light chains known as amyloid L (AL), or secondary to fibrillar deposits of serum amyloid A (AA) protein fragments (Chap. 137). Even though both occur for different reasons, their clinicopathophysiology is quite similar and will be discussed together. Amyloid infiltrates the liver, heart, peripheral nerves, carpal tunnel, upper pharynx, and kidney, producing restrictive cardiomyopathy, hepatomegaly, macroglossia, and heavy proteinuria sometimes associated with renal vein thrombosis. In systemic AL amyloidosis, also called *primary amyloidosis*, light chains produced in excess by clonal plasma cell dyscrasias are made into fragments by macrophages so they can self-aggregate at acid pH. A disproportionate number of these light chains (75%) are of the *lambda* class. About 10% of these patients have overt myeloma with lytic bone lesions and infiltration of the bone marrow with >30% plasma cells; nephrotic syndrome is common, and about 20% of patients progress to dialysis. AA amyloidosis is sometimes called *secondary amyloidosis* and also presents as nephrotic syndrome. It is due to deposition of β-pleated sheets of serum amyloid A protein, an acute phase reactant whose physiologic functions include cholesterol transport, immune cell attraction, and metalloproteases activation. Forty percent of patients with AA amyloid have rheumatoid arthritis, and another 10% have ankylosing spondylitis or psoriatic arthritis; the rest derive from other lesser causes. Less common in Western countries but more common in Mediterranean regions, particularly in Sephardic and Iraqi Jews, is familial Mediterranean fever (FMF). FMF is caused by a mutation in the gene encoding pyrin, whereas Muckle-Wells syndrome, a related disorder, results from a mutation in cryopyrin; both proteins are important in the apoptosis of leukocytes early in inflammation; such proteins with pyrin domains are part of a new pathway called the *inflammasome*. Receptor mutations in tumor necrosis factor receptor 1 (TNFR1) associated periodic syndrome also produce chronic inflammation and secondary amyloidosis. Fragments of serum amyloid A protein increase and self-aggregate by attaching to receptors for advanced glycation end products in the extracellular environment; nephrotic syndrome is common, and about 40–60% of patients progress to dialysis. AA and AL amyloid fibrils are detectable with Congo red or in more detail with electron microscopy (see Fig. 62e-15). Currently developed serum free light chain nephelometry assays are useful in the early diagnosis and follow-up of disease progression. Biopsy of involved liver or kidney is diagnostic 90% of the time when the pretest probability is high; abdominal fat pad aspirates are positive about 70% of the time, but apparently less so when looking for AA amyloid. Amyloid deposits are distributed along blood vessels and in the mesangial regions of the kidney. The treatment for primary amyloidosis, melphalan and autologous hematopoietic stem cell transplantation, can delay the course of disease in about 30% of patients. Secondary amyloidosis is also relentless unless the primary disease can be controlled. Some new drugs in development that disrupt the formation of fibrils may be available in the future.

Fibrillary-Immunotactoid Glomerulopathy Fibrillary-immunotactoid glomerulopathy is a rare (<1.0% of renal biopsies), morphologically defined disease characterized by glomerular accumulation of nonbranching randomly arranged fibrils. Some classify amyloid and nonamyloid fibril-associated renal diseases all as fibrillary glomerulopathies with immunotactoid glomerulopathy reserved for nonamyloid fibrillary disease not associated with a systemic illness. Others define fibrillary glomerulonephritis as a nonamyloid fibrillary disease with fibrils 12–24 nm and immunotactoid glomerulonephritis with fibrils >30 nm. In either case, fibrillar/microtubular deposits of oligoclonal or oligotypic immunoglobulins and complement appear in the mesangium and along the glomerular capillary wall. Congo red stains are negative. The cause of this "nonamyloid" glomerulopathy is mostly idiopathic; reports of immunotactoid glomerulonephritis describe an occasional association with chronic lymphocytic leukemia or B cell lymphoma. Both disorders appear in adults in the fourth decade with moderate to heavy proteinuria, hematuria, and a wide variety of histologic lesions, including DPGN, MPGN, MGN, or mesangioproliferative glomerulonephritis. Nearly half of patients develop renal failure over a few years. There is no consensus on treatment of this uncommon disorder. The disease has been reported to recur following renal transplantation in a minority of cases.

FABRY'S DISEASE

Fabry's disease is an X-linked inborn error of globotriaosylceramide metabolism secondary to deficient lysosomal α-galactosidase A activity, resulting in excessive intracellular storage of globotriaosylceramide. Affected organs include the vascular endothelium, heart, brain, and kidneys. Classically, Fabry's disease presents in childhood in males with acroparesthesias, angiokeratoma, and hypohidrosis. Over time male patients develop cardiomyopathy, cerebrovascular disease, and renal injury, with an average age of death around 50 years of age. Hemizygotes with hypomorphic mutations sometimes present in the fourth to sixth decade with single-organ involvement. Rarely, dominant-negative α-galactosidase A mutations or female heterozygotes with unfavorable X inactivation present with mild single-organ involvement. Rare females develop severe manifestations including renal failure but do so later in life than males. Renal biopsy reveals enlarged glomerular visceral epithelial cells packed with small clear vacuoles containing globotriaosylceramide; vacuoles may also be found in parietal and tubular epithelia (see Fig. 62e-18). These vacuoles of electron-dense materials in parallel arrays (zebra bodies) are easily seen on electron microscopy. Ultimately, renal biopsies reveal FSGS. The nephropathy of Fabry's disease typically presents in the third decade as mild to moderate proteinuria, sometimes with microscopic hematuria or nephrotic syndrome. Urinalysis may reveal oval fat bodies and birefringent glycolipid globules under polarized light (Maltese cross). Renal biopsy is necessary for definitive diagnosis. Progression to renal failure occurs by the fourth or fifth decade. Treatment with inhibitors of the renin-angiotensin system is recommended. Treatment with recombinant α-galactosidase A clears microvascular endothelial deposits of globotriaosylceramide from the kidneys, heart, and skin. In patients with advanced organ involvement, progression of disease occurs despite enzyme replacement therapy. Variable responses to enzyme therapy may be due to the occurrence of neutralizing antibodies or differences in uptake of the enzyme. Graft and patient survival following renal transplantation in patients with Fabry's are similar to other causes of end-stage renal disease.

PULMONARY-RENAL SYNDROMES

Several diseases can present with catastrophic hemoptysis and glomerulonephritis associated with varying degrees of renal failure. The usual causes include Goodpasture's syndrome, granulomatosis with polyangiitis, microscopic polyangiitis, Churg-Strauss vasculitis, and, rarely, Henoch-Schönlein purpura or cryoglobulinemia. Each of these diseases can also present without hemoptysis and are discussed in detail earlier in "Acute Nephritic Syndromes." (See Glomerular Schematic 7.) Pulmonary bleeding in this setting is life-threatening and often results in airway intubation, and acute renal failure requires dialysis. Diagnosis is difficult initially because biopsies and serologic testing take time. Treatment with plasmapheresis and methylprednisolone is often empirical and temporizing until results of testing are available.

BASEMENT MEMBRANE SYNDROMES

All kidney epithelia, including podocytes, rest on basement membranes assembled into a planar surface through the interweaving of collagen IV with laminins, nidogen, and sulfated proteoglycans. Structural abnormalities in GBM associated with hematuria are characteristic of several familial disorders related to the expression of collagen IV genes. The extended family of collagen IV contains six chains, which are expressed in different tissues at different stages of embryonic development. All epithelial basement membranes early in human development are composed of interconnected triple-helical protomers rich in α1.α1.α2(IV) collagen. Some specialized tissues undergo a developmental switch replacing α1.α1.α2(IV) protomers with an α3.α4.α5(IV) collagen network; this switch occurs in the kidney (glomerular and tubular basement membrane), lung, testis, cochlea, and eye, while an

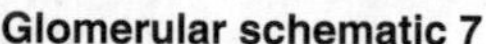
Glomerular schematic 7

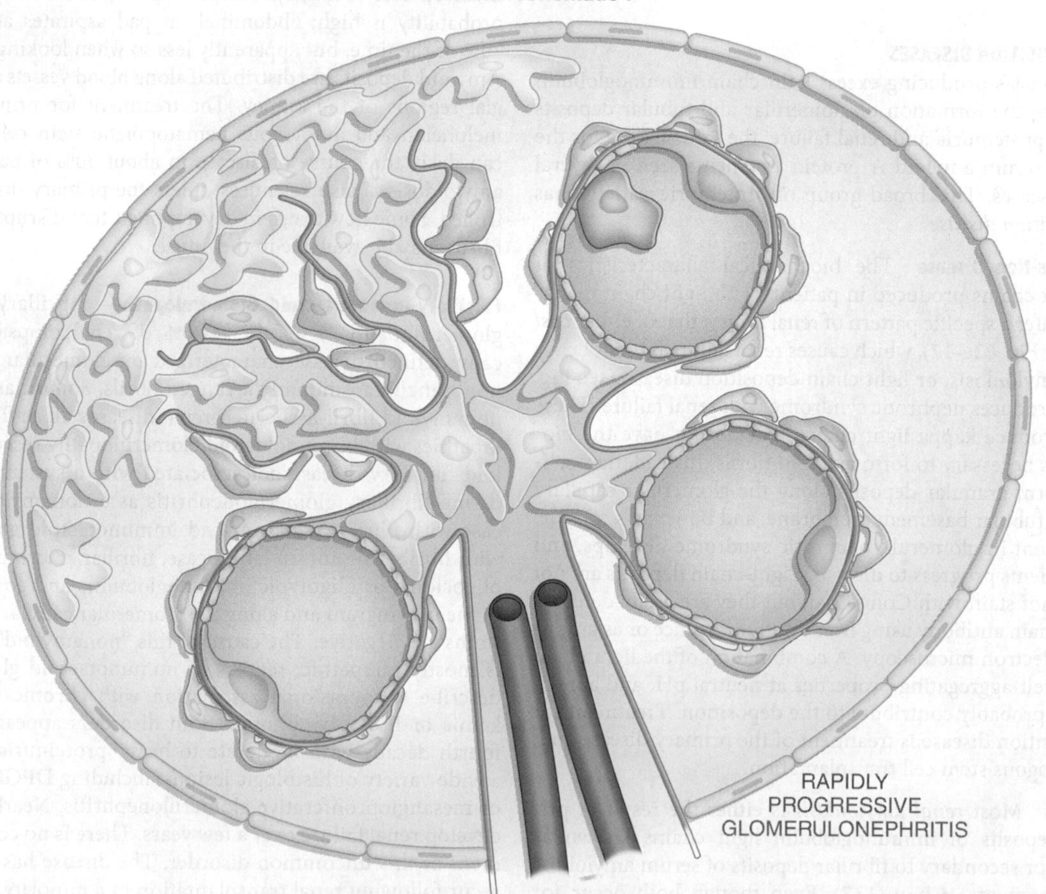

α5.α5.α6(IV) network appears in skin, smooth muscle, and esophagus and along Bowman's capsule in the kidney. This switch probably occurs because the α3.α4.α5(IV) network is more resistant to proteases and ensures the structural longevity of critical tissues. When basement membranes are the target of glomerular disease, they produce moderate proteinuria, some hematuria, and progressive renal failure.

ANTI-GBM DISEASE

Autoimmune disease where antibodies are directed against the α3 NC1 domain of collagen IV produces an *anti-GBM disease* often associated with RPGN and/or a pulmonary-renal syndrome called *Goodpasture's syndrome*. Discussion of this disease is covered earlier in "Acute Nephritic Syndromes."

ALPORT'S SYNDROME

Classically, patients with Alport's syndrome develop hematuria, thinning and splitting of the GBMs, mild proteinuria (<1–2 g/24 h), which appears late in the course, followed by chronic glomerulosclerosis leading to renal failure in association with sensorineural deafness. Some patients develop lenticonus of the anterior lens capsule, "dot and fleck" retinopathy, and rarely, mental retardation or leiomyomatosis. Approximately 85% of patients with Alport's syndrome have an X-linked inheritance of mutations in the α5(IV) collagen chain on chromosome Xq22–24. Female carriers have variable penetrance depending on the type of mutation or the degree of mosaicism created by X inactivation. Fifteen percent of patients have autosomal recessive disease of the α3(IV) or α4(IV) chains on chromosome 2q35–37. Rarely, some kindred have an autosomal dominant inheritance of dominant-negative mutations in α3(IV) or α4(IV) chains.

Pedigrees with the X-linked syndrome are quite variable in their rate and frequency of tissue damage leading to organ failure. Seventy percent of patients have the juvenile form with nonsense or missense mutations, reading frame shifts, or large deletions and generally develop renal failure and sensorineural deafness by age 30. Patients with splice variants, exon skipping, or missense mutations of α-helical glycines generally deteriorate after the age of 30 (adult form) with mild or late deafness. Early severe deafness, lenticonus, or proteinuria suggests a poorer prognosis. Usually females from X-linked pedigrees have only microhematuria, but up to 25% of carrier females have been reported to have more severe renal manifestations. Pedigrees with the autosomal recessive form of the disease have severe early disease in both females and males with asymptomatic parents.

Clinical evaluation should include a careful eye examination and hearing tests. However, the absence of extrarenal symptoms does not rule out the diagnosis. Since α5(IV) collagen is expressed in the skin, some X-linked Alport's patients can be diagnosed with a skin biopsy revealing the lack of the α5(IV) collagen chain on immunofluorescent analysis. Patients with mutations in α3(IV) or α4(IV) require a renal biopsy. Genetic testing can be used for the diagnosis of Alport's syndrome and the demonstration of the mode of inheritance. Early in their disease, Alport's patients typically have thin basement membranes on renal biopsy (see Fig. 62e-19), which thicken over time into multilamellations surrounding lucent areas that often contain granules of varying density—the so-called split basement membrane. In any Alport's kidney, there are areas of thinning mixed with splitting of the GBM. Tubules drop out, glomeruli scar, and the kidney eventually succumbs to interstitial fibrosis. All affected members of a family with X-linked Alport's syndrome should be identified and followed, including mothers of affected males. Primary treatment is control of systemic hypertension and use of ACE inhibitors to slow renal progression. Although patients who receive renal allografts usually develop anti-GBM antibodies directed toward the collagen epitopes absent in their native kidney, overt Goodpasture's syndrome is rare and graft survival is good.

THIN BASEMENT MEMBRANE DISEASE

Thin basement membrane disease (TBMD) characterized by persistent or recurrent hematuria is not typically associated with proteinuria, hypertension, or loss of renal function or extrarenal disease. Although not all cases are familial (perhaps a founder effect), it usually presents in childhood in multiple family members and is also called *benign familial hematuria*. Cases of TBMD have genetic defects in type IV collagen but in contrast to Alport behave as an autosomal dominant disorder that in ~40% of families segregates with the *COL(IV) α3/COL(IV) α4* loci. Mutations in these loci can result in a spectrum of disease ranging from TBMD to autosomal dominant or recessive Alport's. The GBM shows diffuse thinning compared to normal values for the patient's age in otherwise normal biopsies (see Fig. 62e-19). The vast majority of patients have a benign course.

NAIL PATELLA SYNDROME

Patients with nail-patella syndrome develop iliac horns on the pelvis and dysplasia of the dorsal limbs involving the patella, elbows, and nails, variably associated with neural-sensory hearing impairment, glaucoma, and abnormalities of the GBM and podocytes, leading to hematuria, proteinuria, and FSGS. The syndrome is autosomal dominant, with haploinsufficiency for the *LIM* homeodomain transcription factor LMX1B; pedigrees are extremely variable in the penetrance for all features of the disease. LMX1B regulates the expression of genes encoding α3 and α4 chains of collagen IV, interstitial type III collagen, podocin, and CD2AP that help form the slit-pore membranes connecting podocytes. Mutations in the LIM domain region of *LMX1B* associate with glomerulopathy, and renal failure appears in as many as 30% of patients. Proteinuria or isolated hematuria is discovered throughout life, but usually by the third decade, and is inexplicably more common in females. On renal biopsy there is lucent damage to the lamina densa of the GBM, an increase in collagen III fibrils along glomerular capillaries and in the mesangium, and damage to the slit-pore membrane, producing heavy proteinuria not unlike that seen in congenital nephrotic syndrome. Patients with renal failure do well with transplantation.

GLOMERULAR-VASCULAR SYNDROMES

A variety of diseases result in classic vascular injury to the glomerular capillaries. Most of these processes also damage blood vessels elsewhere in the body. The group of diseases discussed here lead to vasculitis, renal endothelial injury, thrombosis, ischemia, and/or lipid-based occlusions.

ATHEROSCLEROTIC NEPHROPATHY

Aging in the developed world is commonly associated with the occlusion of coronary and systemic blood vessels. The reasons for this include obesity, insulin resistance, smoking, hypertension, and diets rich in lipids that deposit in the arterial and arteriolar circulation, producing local inflammation and fibrosis of small blood vessels. When the renal arterial circulation is involved, the glomerular microcirculation is damaged, leading to *chronic nephrosclerosis*. Patients with GFRs <60 mL/min have more cardiovascular events and hospitalizations than those with higher filtration rates. Several aggressive lipid disorders can accelerate this process, but most of the time atherosclerotic progression to chronic nephrosclerosis is associated with poorly controlled hypertension. Approximately 10% of glomeruli are normally sclerotic by age 40, rising to 20% by age 60 and 30% by age 80. Serum lipid profiles in humans are greatly affected by *apolipoprotein E* polymorphisms; the E4 allele is accompanied by increases in serum cholesterol and is more closely associated with atherogenic profiles in patients with renal failure. Mutations in E2 alleles, particularly in Japanese patients, produce a specific renal abnormality called *lipoprotein glomerulopathy* associated with glomerular lipoprotein thrombi and capillary dilation.

HYPERTENSIVE NEPHROSCLEROSIS

Uncontrolled systemic hypertension causes permanent damage to the kidneys in about 6% of patients with elevated blood pressure. As many as 27% of patients with end-stage kidney disease have hypertension as a primary cause. Although there is not a clear correlation between the extent or duration of hypertension and the risk of end-organ damage, *hypertensive nephrosclerosis* is fivefold more frequent in African Americans than whites. Risk alleles associated with *APOL1*, a functional gene for apolipoprotein L1 expressed in podocytes substantially explains the increased burden of end-stage renal disease among African Americans. Associated risk factors for progression to end-stage kidney disease include increased age, male gender, race, smoking, hypercholesterolemia, duration of hypertension, low birth weight, and preexisting renal injury. Kidney biopsies in patients with hypertension, microhematuria, and moderate proteinuria demonstrate arteriolosclerosis, chronic nephrosclerosis, and interstitial fibrosis in the absence of immune deposits (see Fig. 62e-21). Today, based on a careful history, physical examination, urinalysis, and some serologic testing, the diagnosis of chronic nephrosclerosis is usually inferred without a biopsy. Treating hypertension is the best way to avoid progressive renal failure; most guidelines recommend lowering blood pressure to <130/80 mmHg if there is preexisting diabetes or kidney disease. In the presence of kidney disease, most patients begin antihypertensive therapy with two drugs, classically a thiazide diuretic and an ACE inhibitor; most will require three drugs. There is strong evidence in African Americans with hypertensive nephrosclerosis that therapy initiated with an ACE inhibitor can slow the rate of decline in renal function independent of effects on systemic blood pressure. Malignant acceleration of hypertension complicates the course of chronic nephrosclerosis, particularly in the setting of scleroderma or cocaine use (see Fig. 62e-24). The hemodynamic stress of malignant hypertension leads to fibrinoid necrosis of small blood vessels, thrombotic microangiography, a nephritic urinalysis, and acute renal failure. In the setting of renal failure, chest pain, or papilledema, the condition is treated as a hypertensive emergency. Slightly lowering the blood pressure often produces an immediate reduction in GFR that improves as the vascular injury attenuates and autoregulation of blood vessel tone is restored.

CHOLESTEROL EMBOLI

Aging patients with clinical complications from atherosclerosis sometimes shower cholesterol crystals into the circulation—either spontaneously or, more commonly, following an endovascular procedure with manipulation of the aorta—or with use of systemic anticoagulation. Spontaneous emboli may shower acutely or shower subacutely and somewhat more silently. Irregular emboli trapped in the microcirculation produce ischemic damage that induces an inflammatory reaction. Depending on the location of the atherosclerotic plaques releasing these cholesterol fragments, one may see cerebral transient ischemic attacks; livedo reticularis in the lower extremities; Hollenhorst plaques in the retina with visual field cuts; necrosis of the toes; and acute glomerular capillary injury leading to *focal segmental glomerulosclerosis* sometimes associated with hematuria, mild proteinuria, and loss of renal function, which typically progresses over a few years. Occasional patients have fever, eosinophilia, or eosinophiluria. A skin biopsy of an involved area may be diagnostic. Since tissue fixation dissolves the cholesterol, one typically sees only residual, biconvex clefts in involved vessels (see Fig. 62e-22). There is no therapy to reverse embolic occlusions, and steroids do not help. Controlling blood pressure and lipids and cessation of smoking are usually recommended for prevention.

SICKLE CELL DISEASE

Although individuals with SA-hemoglobin are usually asymptomatic, most will gradually develop hyposthenuria due to subclinical infarction of the renal medulla, thus predisposing them to volume depletion. There is an unexpectedly high prevalence of sickle trait among dialysis patients who are African American. Patients with homozygous SS-sickle cell disease develop chronic vasoocclusive disease in many organs. Polymers of deoxygenated SS-hemoglobin distort the shape of red blood cells. These cells attach to endothelia and obstruct small blood vessels, producing frequent and painful sickle cell crises over time. Vessel occlusions in the kidney produce glomerular hypertension, FSGS, interstitial nephritis, and renal infarction associated with hyposthenuria, microscopic hematuria, and even gross hematuria; some patients also present with MPGN. Renal function can be overestimated due to the increased tubular secretion of creatinine seen in many patients with SS-sickle cell. By the second or third decade of life, persistent vasoocclusive disease in the kidney leads to varying degrees of renal failure, and some patients end up on dialysis. Treatment is directed to reducing the frequency of painful crises and administering ACE inhibitors in the hope of delaying a progressive decline in renal function. In sickle cell patients undergoing renal transplantation, renal graft survival is comparable to African Americans in the general transplant population.

THROMBOTIC MICROANGIOPATHIES

Thrombotic thrombocytopenic purpura (TTP) and *hemolytic-uremic syndrome* (HUS) represent a spectrum of thrombotic microangiopathies. Thrombotic thrombocytopenic purpura and hemolytic-uremic syndrome share the general features of idiopathic thrombocytopenic purpura, hemolytic anemia, fever, renal failure, and neurologic disturbances. When patients, particularly children, have more evidence of renal injury, their condition tends to be called HUS. In adults with neurologic disease, it is considered to be TTP. In adults there is often a mixture of both, which is why they are often referred to as having TTP/HUS. On examination of kidney tissue, there is evidence of *glomerular capillary endotheliosis* associated with platelet thrombi, damage to the capillary wall, and formation of fibrin material in and around glomeruli (see Fig. 62e-23). These tissue findings are similar to what is seen in preeclampsia/HELLP (*h*emolysis, *e*levated *l*iver enzymes, and *l*ow *p*latelet count syndrome), malignant hypertension, and the antiphospholipid syndrome. TTP/HUS is also seen in pregnancy; with the use of oral contraceptives or quinine; in renal *t*ransplant patients given OKT3 for rejection; in patients taking the calcineurin inhibitors, cyclosporine and tacrolimus, or in patients taking the antiplatelet agents, ticlopidine and clopidogrel; or following HIV infection.

Although there is no agreement on how much they share a final common pathophysiology, two general groups of patients are recognized: childhood HUS associated with enterohemorrhagic diarrhea and TTP/HUS in adults. Childhood HUS is caused by a toxin released by *Escherichia coli* 0157:H7 and occasionally by *Shigella dysenteriae.* This shiga toxin (verotoxin) directly injures endothelia, enterocytes, and renal cells, causing apoptosis, platelet clumping, and intravascular hemolysis by binding to the glycolipid receptors (Gb3). These receptors are more abundant along endothelia in children compared to adults. Shiga toxin also inhibits the endothelial production of ADAMTS13. In familial cases of adult TTP/HUS, there is a genetic deficiency of the ADAMTS13 metalloprotease that cleaves large multimers of von Willebrand's factor. Absent ADAMTS13, these large multimers cause platelet clumping and intravascular hemolysis. An antibody to ADAMTS13 is found in many sporadic cases of adult TTP/HUS, but not all; many patients also have antibodies to the thrombospondin receptor on selected endothelial cells in small vessels or increased levels of plasminogen-activator inhibitor 1 (PAI-1). Some children with complement protein deficiencies express atypical HUS (aHUS), which can be treated with liver transplant. The treatment of adult TTP/HUS is daily plasmapheresis, which can be lifesaving. Plasmapheresis is given until the platelet count rises, but in relapsing patients it normally is continued well after the platelet count improves, and in resistant patients twice-daily exchange may be helpful. Most patients respond within 2 weeks of daily plasmapheresis. Since TTP/HUS often has an autoimmune basis, there is an anecdotal role in relapsing patients for using splenectomy, steroids, immunosuppressive drugs, bortezomib, or rituximab, an anti-CD20 antibody. Patients with childhood HUS from infectious diarrhea are not given antibiotics, because antibiotics are thought to accelerate the release of the toxin and the diarrhea is usually self-limited. No intervention appears superior to supportive therapy in children with postdiarrheal HUS.

ANTIPHOSPHOLIPID ANTIBODY SYNDROME (SEE CHAP. 379)

GLOBAL CONSIDERATIONS

INFECTIOUS DISEASE–ASSOCIATED SYNDROMES

A number of infectious diseases will injure the glomerular capillaries as part of a systemic reaction producing an immune response or from direct infection of renal tissue. Evidence of this immune response is collected by glomeruli in the form of immune deposits that damage the kidney, producing moderate proteinuria and hematuria. A high prevalence of many of these infectious diseases in undeveloped countries results in infection-associated renal disease being the most common cause of glomerulonephritis in many parts of the world.

Poststreptococcal Glomerulonephritis This form of glomerulonephritis is one of the classic complications of streptococcal infection. The discussion of this disease can be found earlier, in the section "Acute Nephritic Syndromes."

Subacute Bacterial Endocarditis Renal injury from persistent bacteremia absent the continued presence of a foreign body, regardless of cause, is treated presumptively as if the patient has endocarditis. The discussion of this disease can be found earlier, in the section "Acute Nephritic Syndromes."

Human Immunodeficiency Virus Renal disease is an important complication of HIV disease. The risk of development of end-stage renal disease is much higher in HIV-infected African Americans than in HIV-infected whites. About 50% of HIV-infected patients with kidney disease have HIV-associated nephropathy (HIVAN) on biopsy. The lesion in HIVAN is FSGS, characteristically revealing a collapsing glomerulopathy (see Fig. 62e-3) with visceral epithelial cell swelling, microcystic dilatation of renal tubules, and tubuloreticular inclusion. Renal epithelial cells express replicating HIV virus, but host immune responses also play a role in the pathogenesis. MPGN and DPGN have also been reported but more commonly in HIV-infected whites and in patients coinfected with hepatitis B or C. HIV-associated TTP has also been reported. Other renal lesions include DPGN, IgA nephropathy, and MCD. Renal biopsy may be indicated to distinguish between these lesions.

HIV patients with FSGS typically present with nephrotic-range proteinuria and hypoalbuminemia, but unlike patients with other etiologies for nephrotic syndrome, they do not commonly have hypertension, edema, or hyperlipidemia. Renal ultrasound also reveals large, echogenic kidneys despite the finding that renal function in some patients declines rapidly. Treatment with inhibitors of the renin-angiotensin system decreases the proteinuria. Effective antiretroviral therapy benefits both the patient and the kidney and improves survival of HIV-infected patients with chronic kidney disease (CKD) or end-stage renal disease. In HIV-infected patients not yet on therapy, the presence of HIVAN is an indication to initiate therapy. Following the introduction of antiretroviral therapy, survival on dialysis for the HIV-infected patient has improved dramatically. Renal transplantations in HIV-infected patients without detectable viral loads or histories of opportunistic infections provide a better survival benefit over dialysis. Following transplantation, patient and graft survival are similar to the general transplant population despite frequent rejections.

Hepatitis B and C Typically infected patients present with microscopic hematuria, nonnephrotic or nephrotic-range proteinuria, and hypertension. There is a close association between hepatitis B infection and polyarteritis nodosa with vasculitis appearing generally in the first 6 months following infection. Renal manifestations include renal artery aneurysms, renal infarction, and ischemic scars. Alternatively, the hepatitis B carrier state can produce a MGN that is more common in children than adults, or MPGN that is more common in adults than in children. Renal histology is indistinguishable from idiopathic MGN or type I MPGN. Viral antigens are found in the renal deposits. There are no good treatment guidelines, but interferon α-2b and lamivudine have been used to some effect in small studies. Children have a good prognosis, with 60–65% achieving spontaneous remission within 4 years. In contrast, 30% of adults have renal insufficiency and 10% have renal failure 5 years after diagnosis.

Up to 30% of patients with chronic hepatitis C infection have some renal manifestations. Patients often present with type II mixed cryoglobulinemia, nephrotic syndrome, microscopic hematuria, abnormal liver function tests, depressed C3 levels, anti–hepatitis C virus (HCV) antibodies, and viral RNA in the blood. The renal lesions most commonly seen, in order of decreasing frequency, are *cryoglobulinemic glomerulonephritis, MGN,* and *type I MPGN.* Treatment with pegylated interferon and ribavirin is typical to reduce the viral load.

Other Viruses Other viral infections are occasionally associated with glomerular lesions, but cause and effect are not well established. These viral infections and their respective glomerular lesions include: cytomegalovirus producing MPGN; influenza and anti-GBM disease; measles-associated endocapillary proliferative glomerulonephritis, with measles antigen in the capillary loops and mesangium; parvovirus causing mild proliferative or mesangioproliferative glomerulonephritis or FSGS; mumps and mesangioproliferative glomerulonephritis; Epstein-Barr virus producing MPGN, diffuse proliferative nephritis, or IgA nephropathy; dengue hemorrhagic fever causing endocapillary proliferative glomerulonephritis; and coxsackievirus producing *focal glomerulonephritis* or DPGN.

Syphilis Secondary syphilis, with rash and constitutional symptoms, develops weeks to months after the chancre first appears and occasionally presents with the nephrotic syndrome from MGN caused by subepithelial immune deposits containing treponemal antigens. Other lesions have also rarely been described including interstitial syphilitic nephritis. The diagnosis is confirmed with nontreponemal and treponemal tests for *Treponema pallidum*. The renal lesion responds to treatment with penicillin or an alternative drug, if allergic. Additional testing for other sexually transmitted diseases is an important part of disease management.

Leprosy Despite aggressive eradication programs, approximately 400,000 new cases of leprosy appear annually worldwide. The diagnosis is best made in patients with multiple skin lesions accompanied by sensory loss in affected areas, using skin smears showing paucibacillary or multibacillary infection (WHO criteria). Leprosy is caused by infection with *Mycobacterium leprae* and can be classified by Ridley-Jopling criteria into various types: tuberculoid, borderline tuberculoid, mid-borderline and borderline lepromatous, and lepromatous. Renal involvement in leprosy is related to the quantity of bacilli in the body, and the kidney is one of the target organs during splanchnic localization. In some series, all cases with borderline lepromatous and lepromatous types of leprosy have various forms of renal involvement including FSGS, mesangioproliferative glomerulonephritis, or renal amyloidosis; much less common are the renal lesions of DPGN and MPGN. Treatment of the infection can cause remission of the renal disease.

Malaria There are 300–500 million incident cases of malaria each year worldwide, and the kidney is commonly involved. Glomerulonephritis is due to immune complexes containing malarial antigens that are implanted in the glomerulus. In malaria from *P. falciparum,* mild proteinuria is associated with subendothelial deposits, mesangial deposits, and mesangioproliferative glomerulonephritis that usually resolve with treatment. In quartan malaria from infection with *Plasmodium malariae,* children are more commonly affected and renal involvement is more severe. Transient proteinuria and microscopic hematuria can resolve with treatment of the infection. However, resistant nephrotic syndrome with progression to renal failure over 3–5 years does happen, as <50% of patients respond to steroid therapy. Affected patients with nephrotic syndrome have thickening of the glomerular capillary walls, with subendothelial deposits of IgG, IgM, and C_3 associated with a sparse membranoproliferative lesion. The rare mesangioproliferative glomerulonephritis reported with *Plasmodium vivax* or *Plasmodium ovale* typically has a benign course.

Schistosomiasis Schistosomiasis affects more than 300 million people worldwide and primarily involves the urinary and gastrointestinal tracts. Glomerular involvement varies with the specific strain of schistosomiasis; *Schistosoma mansoni* is most commonly associated with clinical renal disease, and the glomerular lesions can be classified: Class I is a *mesangioproliferative glomerulonephritis;* class II is an *extracapillary proliferative glomerulonephritis;* class III is a *membranoproliferative glomerulonephritis;* class IV is a *focal segmental glomerulonephritis;* and class V is *amyloidosis*. Classes I–II often remit with treatment of the infection, but classes III and IV lesions are associated with IgA immune deposits and progress despite antiparasitic and/or immunosuppressive therapy.

Other Parasites Renal involvement with toxoplasmosis infections is rare. When it occurs, patients present with nephrotic syndrome and have a histologic picture of MPGN. Fifty percent of patients with leishmaniasis will have mild to moderate proteinuria and microscopic hematuria, but renal insufficiency is rare. Acute DPGN, MGN, and mesangioproliferative glomerulonephritis have all been observed on biopsy. Filariasis and trichinosis are caused by nematodes and are sometimes associated with glomerular injury presenting with proteinuria, hematuria, and a variety of histologic lesions that typically resolve with eradication of the infection.

339 Polycystic Kidney Disease and Other Inherited Disorders of Tubule Growth and Development

Jing Zhou, Martin R. Pollak

The polycystic kidney diseases are a group of genetically heterogeneous disorders and a leading cause of kidney failure. The autosomal dominant form of polycystic kidney disease (ADPKD) is the most common life-threatening monogenic disease, affecting 12 million people worldwide. The autosomal recessive form of polycystic kidney disease (ARPKD) is rarer but affects the pediatric population. Kidney cysts are often seen in a wide range of syndromic diseases. Recent studies have shown that defects in the structure or function of the primary cilia may underlie this group of genetic diseases collectively termed *ciliopathies* (Table 339-1).

AUTOSOMAL DOMINANT POLYCYSTIC KIDNEY DISEASE

Etiology and Pathogenesis (Fig. 339-1) ADPKD is characterized by progressive formation of epithelial-lined cysts in the kidney. Although cysts only occur in 5% of the tubules in the kidney, the enormous growth of these cysts ultimately leads to the loss of normal surrounding tissues and loss of renal function. The cellular defects in ADPKD that have been known for a long time are increased cell proliferation and fluid secretion, decreased cell differentiation, and abnormal extracellular matrix. ADPKD is caused by mutations in *PKD1* and *PKD2*, which, respectively, code for polycystin-1 (PC1) and polycystin-2 (PC2). PC1 is a large 11-transmembrane protein that functions like a G protein–coupled receptor. PC2 is a calcium-permeable six-transmembrane protein that structurally belongs to the transient receptor potential (TRP) cation channel family. PC1 and PC2 are widely expressed in almost all tissues and organs. PC1 expression is high in development and low in the adult, whereas PC2 expression is relatively constant. PC1 and PC2 are found on the primary cilium, a hair-like structure present on the apical membrane of a cell, in addition to the cell membranes and cell-cell junctions of tubular epithelial cells. Defects in the primary cilia are linked to a wide spectrum of human diseases, collectively termed ciliopathies. The most common phenotype shared by many ciliopathies is kidney cysts. PC1 and PC2 bind to each other via their respective C-terminal tails to form a receptor-channel complex and regulate each other's function. The PC1/2 protein complex serves as a mechanosensor or chemical sensor and regulates calcium and G-protein signaling. The PC1/2 protein complex may also directly regulate a number of cellular functions including the cell cycle, the actin cytoskeleton, planar cell polarity (PCP), and cell migration. This protein complex has also been implicated in regulating a number of signaling pathways, including Wnt, mammalian target of rapamycin (mTOR), STAT3, cMET, phosphoinositide 3-kinase (PI3K)/AKT, G protein–coupled receptor (GPCR), and epidermal growth factor receptor (EGFR), as well as in the localization and activity of cystic fibrosis transmembrane conductance (CFTR). One hypothesis is

TABLE 339-1 INHERITED DISEASES COMMONLY ASSOCIATED WITH A CYSTIC PHENOTYPE

Disease	Mode of Inheritance	Renal Abnormalities	Other Clinical Features	Genes
Autosomal dominant polycystic kidney disease	AD	Cortical and medullary cysts	Liver, pancreatic cysts, hypertension, subarachnoid hemorrhage	*PKD1, PKD2*
Autosomal recessive polycystic kidney disease	AR	Distal and collecting duct cysts	Oligohydramnios if severe, hypertension, ascending cholangitis, liver fibrosis	*PKHD1*
Medullary cystic kidney	AD	Small fibrotic kidneys; medullary cysts	In adults, gout	*MCKD1, MCKD2/UMOD*
Nephronophthisis	AR	Small fibrotic kidneys; medullary cysts	Growth retardation, anemia (visual loss, liver fibrosis, cerebellar ataxia if associated with another syndrome)	*NPHP1-4, IQCB1, CEP290, GLIS2, RPGRIP1L, NEK8, SDCCAG8, TMEM67, TTC21B*
Senior-Løken syndrome	AR	Renal cysts	Juvenile nephronophthisis, Leber's amaurosis	*NPHP1-6, SDCCAG8*
Leber's congenital amaurosis	AR	Renal cysts	Visual impairment in first year of life, pigmentary retinopathy	*GUCY2D, RPE65, LCA3-14* (including *LCA10, CEP290*)
Meckel-Gruber syndrome	AR	Cortical and medullary cysts	CNS anomalies, polydactyly, congenital heart defects	*MKS1, TMEM216, TMEM67, CEP290, RPGRIP1L, CC2D2A, TCTN2, B9D1, B9D2, NPHP3*
Bardet-Biedl syndrome	AR	Renal cysts	Obesity, polydactyly, retinitis pigmentosa, anosmia, congenital heart defects, mental retardation	*BBS1, 2, ARL6, BBS4,5, MKKS, BBS7, TTC8, BBS9, 10, TRIM32, BBS12, MKS1, CEP290, C2ORF86*; modifiers *MKS1, MKS3, CCDC28B*
Oral-facial-digital syndrome type I	AR	Renal cysts	Oral cavity, face, and digit anomalies; CNS abnormalities; cystic kidney disease; X-linked with male lethality, primary ciliary dyskinesia	*OFD1*
Cranioectodermal dysplasia (Sensenbrenner's syndrome)	AR	Renal cysts	Skeletal dysplasia, thoracic deformities, polydactyly, renal cysts, retinitis pigmentosa	*IFT80*
Tuberous sclerosis	AD	Renal cysts	Angiomyolipomas, renal cell carcinoma, facial angiofibromas, CNS hamartomas	*TSC1, TSC2*
Von Hippel-Lindau disease	AD	Renal cysts	Renal cell carcinoma, retinal angiomas, CNS hemangioblastomas, pheochromocytomas	*VHL*

Abbreviations: AD, autosomal dominant; AR, autosomal recessive; CNS, central nervous system.

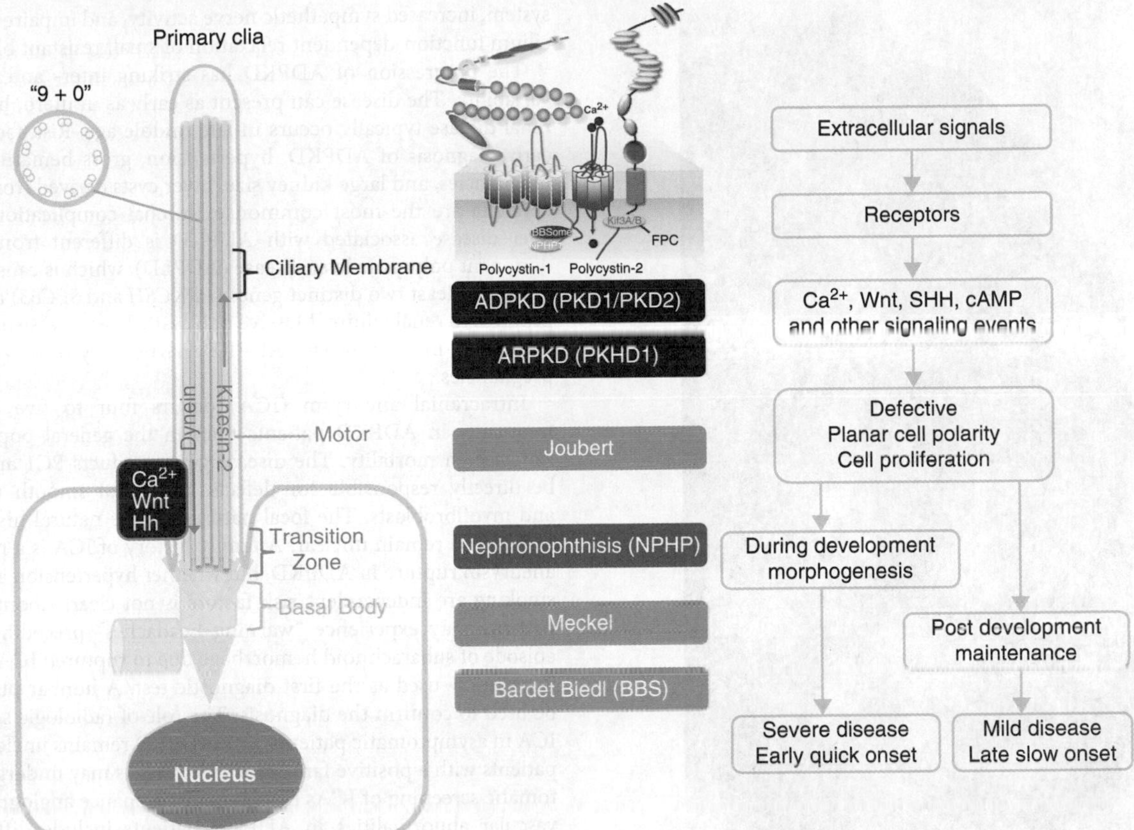

FIGURE 339-1 Scheme of the primary cilium and cystic kidney disease proteins. ***Left.*** A scheme of the primary cilium. Primary cilia share a "9+0" organization of microtubule doublets. Proteins are transported into the cilium by motor protein kinesin 2 and transported out of the cilium by dynein. The cilium is connected to the basal body through the transition zone. ***Middle.*** Topology of autosomal dominant polycystic kidney disease (ADPKD) and autosomal recessive polycystic kidney disease (ARPKD) proteins polycystin-1, polycystin-2, and fibrocystin/polyductin (FPC) are shown. PC1 also interacts with other proteins such as components of the BBSome and NPHP1. PC2 and FPC both interact with kinesin 2 (KIF 3A/B). Localization of disease proteins in the cilium, the transition zone, and the basal body is color coded. ***Right.*** Potential disease mechanisms due to cilium-mediated signaling events.

that loss of ciliary function of PC1 and PC2 leads to reduced calcium signaling and a subsequent increase of adenylyl cyclase activity and decrease of phosphodiesterase activity, which, in turn, causes increased cellular cyclic AMP (cAMP). Increased cAMP promotes protein kinase A activity, among other effectors, and, in turn, leads to cyst growth by promoting proliferation and fluid secretion of cyst-lining cells through chloride and aquaporin channels in ADPKD kidneys.

Genetic Considerations ADPKD is inherited as an autosomal dominant trait with complete penetrance but variable expressivity. The disease affects all ethnic groups worldwide with an estimated prevalence of 1:1000 to 1:400. Only half of the patients with ADPKD are clinically diagnosed during their lifetime. ADPKD is genetically heterogeneous. The first disease gene (*PKD1*) was localized to the region of the α-globin gene on chromosome 16p13 in 1985, and a second disease gene (*PKD2*) locus was mapped to chromosome 4q21-q23 in 1993. Mutations of *PKD1* and *PKD2* are responsible for ~85% and ~15% of ADPKD cases, respectively. However, patients with *PKD2* mutations may be higher than 15% because they tend to have milder clinical disease and, as a result, may be underdiagnosed. Embryonic lethality of *Pkd1* and *Pkd2* knockout mice suggests that human homozygotes may be lethal and thus not clinically recognized.

PKD1 is comprised of 46 exons occupying ~52 kb of genomic DNA. It produces an ~14-kb transcript that encodes PC1, a protein of ~4300 amino acids. A feature of the *PKD1* gene is that the 5′ three-quarters of *PKD1* have been duplicated at six other sites on chromosome 16p, and many of them produce mRNA transcripts, which provides a major challenge for genetic analysis of the duplicated region. *PKD2* is a single-copy gene with 15 exons producing an ~5.3-kb mRNA transcript that encodes PC2, a protein of 968 amino acids. The presence of additional genes for ADPKD was suggested based on several families linked to neither *PKD1* nor *PKD2* genes. However, careful analyses have excluded the existence of a third ADPKD gene.

In ADPKD patients, every cell carries a germline mutant allele of either *PKD1* or *PKD2*. However, cysts develop in only a small fraction of the nephrons. Cysts are thought to originate from clonal growth of single cells that have received a somatic "second hit" mutation in the "normal" allele of the *PKD1* or *PKD2* gene. Accumulating evidence in mouse models now shows that partial loss of function of the second allele of *Pkd1* in a proliferative environment is sufficient for cystogenesis, suggesting that a critical amount of *PKD1* is needed in a cell. Somatic inactivation of the second allele of *Pkd1* in adult mice results in very slow onset of cyst development in the kidney, but a "third hit," such as an additional genetic or epigenetic event, the inactivation of a growth-suppressor gene, the activation of a growth-promoting gene(s), or an event like renal injury that activates the developmental program, may promote rapid cyst formation.

Clinical Manifestations ADPKD is characterized by the progressive bilateral formation of renal cysts. Focal renal cysts are typically detected in affected subjects before 30 years of age. Hundreds to thousands of cysts are usually present in the kidneys of most patients in the fifth decade (Fig. 339-2). Enlarged kidneys can each reach a fourfold increase in length and weigh up to 20 times the normal weight. The clinical presentations of ADPKD are highly variable. Although many patients are asymptomatic until the fourth to fifth decade of life and are diagnosed by incidental discoveries of hypertension or abdominal masses, back or flank pain is a frequent symptom in ~60% of patients with ADPKD. The pain may result from renal cyst infection, hemorrhage, or nephrolithiasis. Gross hematuria resulting from cyst rupture occurs in ~40% of patients during the course of their disease, and many of them will have recurrent episodes. Flank pain and hematuria

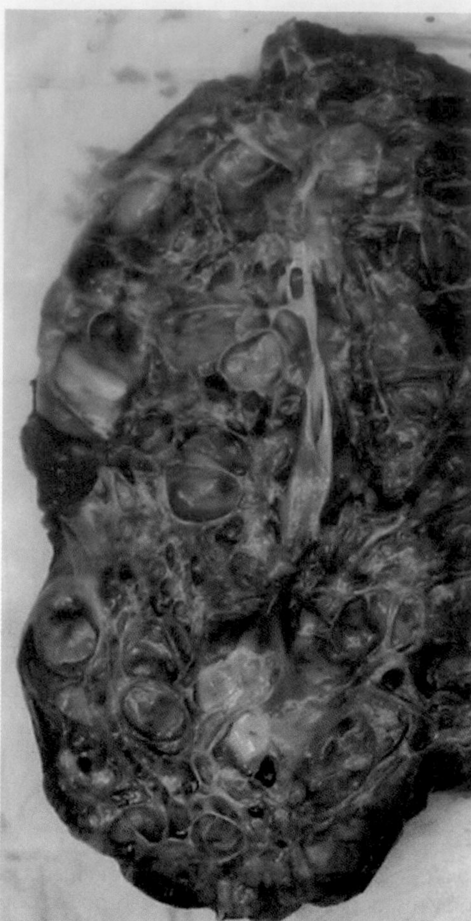

FIGURE 339-2 Photograph showing a kidney from a patient with autosomal dominant polycystic kidney disease. The kidney has been cut open to expose the parenchyma and internal aspects of cysts.

may coexist if the cyst that ruptures is connected with the collecting system. Proteinuria is usually a minor feature of ADPKD. Infection is the second most common cause of death for patients with ADPKD. Up to half of patients with ADPKD will have one or more episodes of renal infection during their lifetime. An infected cyst and acute pyelonephritis are the most common renal infections often due to gram-negative bacteria, which are associated with fever and flank pain, with or without bacteremia. These complications and renal insufficiency often correlate with structural abnormality of the renal parenchyma. Kidney stones occur in ~20% of patients with ADPKD. Different from the general population, more than half of the stones in patients with ADPKD are composed of uric acid, with the remainder due to calcium oxalate. Distal acidification defects, abnormal ammonium transport, low urine pH, and hypocitraturia may be important in the pathogenesis of renal stones in ADPKD. Renal cell carcinoma is a rare complication of ADPKD with no apparent increased frequency compared to the general population. However, in ADPKD, these tumors are more often bilateral at presentation, multicentric, and sarcomatoid in type. Radiologic imaging is often not helpful in distinguishing cyst infection and cyst hemorrhage because of their complexity. Computed tomography (CT) scan and magnetic resonance imaging (MRI) are often useful in distinguishing a malignancy from a complex cyst. Cardiovascular complications are the major cause of mortality in patients with ADPKD. Hypertension is common and typically occurs before any reduction in glomerular filtration rate (GFR). Hypertension is a risk factor for both cardiovascular and kidney disease progression in ADPKD. Notably, some normotensive patients with ADPKD may also have left ventricular hypertrophy. Hypertension in ADPKD may result from the increased activation of the renin-angiotensin-aldosterone system, increased sympathetic nerve activity, and impaired endothelial cilium function-dependent relaxation of small resistant blood vessels.

The progression of ADPKD has striking inter- and intrafamilial variability. The disease can present as early as in utero, but end-stage renal disease typically occurs in late middle age. Risk factors include early diagnosis of ADPKD, hypertension, gross hematuria, multiple pregnancies, and large kidney size. Liver cysts derived from the biliary epithelia are the most common extrarenal complication. Polycystic liver disease associated with ADPKD is different from autosomal dominant polycystic liver disease (ADPLD), which is caused by mutations in at least two distinct genes (*PRKCSH* and *SEC63*) and does not progress to renal failure. Massive polycystic liver disease occurs almost exclusively in women with ADPKD, particularly those with multiple pregnancies.

Intracranial aneurysm (ICA) occurs four to five times more frequently in ADPKD patients than in the general population and causes high mortality. The disease gene products PC1 and PC2 may be directly responsible for defects in arterial smooth muscle cells and myofibroblasts. The focal nature and the natural history of ICA in ADPKD remain unclear. A family history of ICA is a risk factor of aneurysm rupture in ADPKD, but whether hypertension and cigarette smoking are independent risk factors is not clear. About 20–50% of patients may experience "warning headaches" preceding the index episode of subarachnoid hemorrhage due to ruptured ICA. A CT scan is generally used as the first diagnostic test. A lumbar puncture may be used to confirm the diagnosis. The role of radiologic screening for ICA in asymptomatic patients with ADPKD remains unclear. ADPKD patients with a positive family history of ICAs may undergo presymptomatic screening of ICAs by magnetic resonance angiography. Other vascular abnormalities in ADPKD patients include diffuse arterial dolichoectasias of the anterior and posterior cerebral circulation, which can predispose to arterial dissection and stroke. Mitral valve prolapse occurs in up to 30% of patients with ADPKD, and tricuspid valve prolapse is less common. Other valvular abnormalities occurring with increased frequency in ADPKD patients include insufficiency of the mitral, aortic, and tricuspid valves. Most patients are asymptomatic, but some may progress and require valve replacement. The prevalence of colonic diverticulae and abdominal wall hernias is also increased in ADPKD patients.

Diagnosis Diagnosis is typically made from a positive family history consistent with autosomal dominant inheritance and multiple kidney cysts bilaterally. Renal ultrasonography is often used for presymptomatic screening of at-risk subjects and for evaluation of potential living-related kidney donors from ADPKD families. The presence of *at least two renal cysts (unilateral or bilateral)* is sufficient for diagnosis among at-risk subjects between 15 and 29 years of age with a sensitivity of 96% and specificity of 100%. The presence of *at least two cysts in each kidney* and the presence *at least four cysts in each kidney* are required for the diagnosis of at-risk subjects age 30 to 59 years and age 60 years or older, respectively, with a sensitivity of 100% and specificity of 100%. This is because there is an increased frequency of developing simple renal cysts with age. Conversely, in subjects between age 30 and 59 years, the absence of *at least two cysts in each kidney*, which is associated with a false-negative rate of 0%, can be used for disease exclusion. These criteria have a lower sensitivity for patients with a *PKD2* mutation because of a late onset of ADPKD2. CT scan and T2-weighted MRI, with and without contrast enhancement, are more sensitive than ultrasonography and can detect cysts of smaller size. However, a CT scan exposes the patient to radiation and radiocontrast, which may cause serious allergic reactions and nephrotoxicity in patients with renal insufficiency. T2-weighted MRI, with gadolinium as a contrast agent, has minimal renal toxicity and can detect cysts of only 2–3 mm in diameter. However, a large majority of cysts may still be below the detection level. Genetic testing by linkage analyses and mutational analyses is available for ambiguous cases. Because of the large size of the *PKD1* gene and the presence of multiple highly homologous pseudogenes, mutational analysis of the *PKD1* gene is difficult and costly. Application of new technologies, such as paired-end next-generation sequencing with multiplexing individually bar-coded long-range polymerase chain reaction libraries, may reduce the costs and improve the sensitivity for clinical genetic testing.

TREATMENT AUTOSOMAL DOMINANT POLYCYSTIC KIDNEY DISEASE

No specific treatment to prevent cyst growth or the decline of renal function has been approved by U.S. Food and Drug Administration. Blood pressure control to a target of 140/90 mmHg is recommended according to the guidelines from the eighth report of the Joint National Committee on Prevention, Detection, Evaluation, and Treatment of High Blood Pressure (JNC VIII report) for reducing cardiovascular complications in ADPKD and renal disease progression. More rigorous blood pressure control does not equal greater clinical benefits. Maintaining a target systolic blood pressure to 110 mmHg in patients with moderate or advanced disease may increase the risk of renal disease progression by reducing renal blood flow. Lipid-soluble antibiotics against common gram-negative enteric organisms, such as trimethoprim-sulfamethoxazole, quinolones, and chloramphenicol, are preferred for cyst infection because most renal cysts are not connected to glomerular filtration and antibiotics that are capable of penetrating the cyst walls are likely to be more effective. Treatment often requires 4–6 weeks. The treatment of kidney stones in ADPKD includes standard measures such as analgesics for pain relief and hydration to ensure adequate urine flow. Management of chronic flank, back, or abdominal pain due to renal enlargement may include both pharmacologic (nonnarcotic and narcotic analgesics) and nonpharmacologic measures (transcutaneous electrical nerve stimulation, acupuncture, and biofeedback). Occasionally, surgical decompression of cysts may be necessary. More than half of ADPKD patients eventually require peritoneal dialysis, hemodialysis, or kidney transplantation. Peritoneal dialysis may not be suitable for some patients with massively enlarged polycystic kidneys due to the small intraabdominal space for efficient peritoneal exchange of fluid and solutes and increased chance of abdominal hernia and back pain. Patients with very large polycystic kidneys and recurrent renal cyst infection may require pretransplant nephrectomy or bilateral nephrectomy to accommodate the allograft and reduce the pain.

Specific treatment strategies for ADPKD have focused on slowing renal disease progression and lowering cardiovascular risk. For the latter, the main approach is to control blood pressure by inhibiting the renin-angiotensin-aldosterone system. The ongoing HALT PKD trial was set to evaluate the impact of intensive blockade of the renin-angiotensin-aldosterone system and levels of blood pressure control on progressive renal disease. Most approaches target the slowing of renal disease progression by inhibiting cell proliferation and fluid secretion. Several clinical trials have been conducted targeting cell proliferation, including studies on sirolimus and everolimus, inhibitors of the mTOR pathway; OPC31260 and tolvaptan, which inhibit cAMP pathways by antagonizing the activation of vasopressin V2 receptor (V2R) in collecting ducts and reduce cell proliferation by decreasing renal cAMP levels; and somatostatin analogues, which reduce cAMP levels by binding to several GPCRs. Both the V2R antagonists and somatostatin analogues appear to slow the decline of renal function, although with some side effects such as liver function impairment, polydipsia, and diarrhea. A combination of different growth inhibitors may enhance efficacy and reduce side effects. Additional preclinical studies in animal models include the use of inhibitors to nonreceptor tyrosine kinase Src, B-raf, cyclin-dependent kinase (CDK), transcription factors STAT3 and STAT6 (pyrimethamine and leflunomide), purinergic receptors, hepatocyte growth factor receptor, and glucosylceramide, and agonists to peroxisome proliferator activated receptor-γ (PPARγ receptors (thiazolidodinediones).

AUTOSOMAL RECESSIVE POLYCYSTIC KIDNEY DISEASE

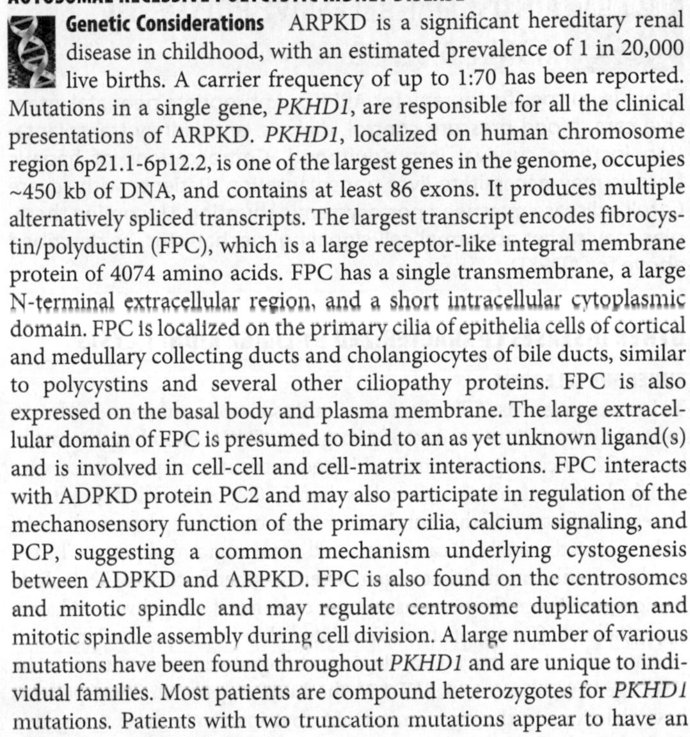

Genetic Considerations ARPKD is a significant hereditary renal disease in childhood, with an estimated prevalence of 1 in 20,000 live births. A carrier frequency of up to 1:70 has been reported. Mutations in a single gene, *PKHD1*, are responsible for all the clinical presentations of ARPKD. *PKHD1*, localized on human chromosome region 6p21.1-6p12.2, is one of the largest genes in the genome, occupies ~450 kb of DNA, and contains at least 86 exons. It produces multiple alternatively spliced transcripts. The largest transcript encodes fibrocystin/polyductin (FPC), which is a large receptor-like integral membrane protein of 4074 amino acids. FPC has a single transmembrane, a large N-terminal extracellular region, and a short intracellular cytoplasmic domain. FPC is localized on the primary cilia of epithelia cells of cortical and medullary collecting ducts and cholangiocytes of bile ducts, similar to polycystins and several other ciliopathy proteins. FPC is also expressed on the basal body and plasma membrane. The large extracellular domain of FPC is presumed to bind to an as yet unknown ligand(s) and is involved in cell-cell and cell-matrix interactions. FPC interacts with ADPKD protein PC2 and may also participate in regulation of the mechanosensory function of the primary cilia, calcium signaling, and PCP, suggesting a common mechanism underlying cystogenesis between ADPKD and ARPKD. FPC is also found on the centrosomes and mitotic spindle and may regulate centrosome duplication and mitotic spindle assembly during cell division. A large number of various mutations have been found throughout *PKHD1* and are unique to individual families. Most patients are compound heterozygotes for *PKHD1* mutations. Patients with two truncation mutations appear to have an earlier onset of the disease.

Clinical Features Classic ARPKD is generally diagnosed in utero or within the neonatal period and characterized by greatly enlarged echogenic kidneys in diseased fetuses. Reduced fetal urine production may contribute to oligohydramnios and pulmonary hypoplasia. About 30% of affected neonates die shortly after birth due to respiratory insufficiency. Close to 60% of mortality occurs within the first month of life. In the classic group, most patients are born with renal insufficiency and ESRD. However, infants often have a transient improvement in their GFR; death from renal insufficiency at this stage is rare. Some patients are diagnosed after the neonatal stage and form the older group. Morbidity and mortality in this group often involve systemic hypertension, progressive renal insufficiency, and liver manifestations. The hallmarks of ARPKD liver disease are biliary dysgenesis due to a primary ductal plate malformation with associated periportal fibrosis, namely congenital hepatic fibrosis (CHF) and dilatation of intrahepatic bile ducts (Caroli's disease). CHF and Caroli's disease can then lead to portal hypertension exhibiting hepatosplenomegaly, variceal bleeding, and cholangitis. Some patients with the diagnosis of ARPKD at 1 year of age with nephromegaly exhibit slowly declining renal function over 20 years with only minimally enlarged kidneys at ESRD and markedly atrophic kidneys following renal transplantation. The slow progression of renal disease is likely due to increasing fibrosis rather than the development of cysts. Systemic hypertension is common in all ARPKD patients, even those with normal renal function.

Diagnosis Ultrasonography, CT, and MRI all can be used for diagnosis. Ultrasonography reveals large, echogenic kidneys with poor corticomedullary differentiation. The diagnosis can be made in utero after 24 weeks of gestation in severe cases. Macrocysts generally are not common at birth in ARPKD patients. The absence of renal cysts in either parent, particularly if they are more than 40 years of age on ultrasonography, helps distinguish ARPKD from ADPKD in older patients. Clinical, laboratory, or radiographic evidence of hepatic fibrosis, hepatic pathology demonstrating characteristic ductal plate abnormalities, family history of affected siblings, or parental consanguinity suggestive of autosomal recessive inheritance is helpful. The lack of mutational hotspots and the large and complex genomic structure of *PKHD1* make molecular diagnosis difficult; however, presymptomatic screening of other at-risk members in a family with already identified ARPKD mutations is straightforward and inexpensive.

TREATMENT AUTOSOMAL RECESSIVE POLYCYSTIC KIDNEY DISEASE

There is no specific therapy for ARPKD. Appropriate neonatal intensive care, blood pressure control, dialysis, and kidney transplantation increase survival into adulthood. Complications of hepatic fibrosis may necessitate liver transplantation. Patients with severe Caroli's disease may need portosystemic shunting. Upcoming therapies may target abnormal cell signaling mechanisms, as described above for ADPKD.

OTHER DISEASES CHARACTERIZED BY LARGE KIDNEY CYSTS

TUBEROUS SCLEROSIS

Tuberous sclerosis (TS) is a rare autosomal dominant syndrome caused by mutations in one of two genes, *TSC1*, encoding hamartin, or, *TSC2*, encoding tuberin. Published estimates of prevalence vary widely, but it certainly occurs in less than 1:5000 births. Kidney cysts are a frequent feature of this condition, as are two other abnormalities of kidney growth, renal cell carcinoma and renal angiomyolipomas. TS is a syndrome affecting multiple organ systems. Other features of TS include benign growths in the nervous system, eyes, heart, lung, liver, and skin. Essentially all TS patients have associated skin lesions, and a large proportion of patients have neurologic and cognitive manifestations. The *TSC2* gene is adjacent to *PKD1* in the human genome. Some patients have deletions in their genomic DNA that inactivate these two genes. Such individuals may have manifestations of both ADPKD and TS.

The most common kidney finding in TS is the presence of angiomyolipomas. These growths tend to be multiple and bilateral. Although they are usually benign, they may bleed. Surgical removal is often recommended as a prophylactic measure in people with angiomyolipomas larger than 4 cm in diameter. The cysts in TS are radiographically similar to those seen in ADPKD. In contrast to ADPKD, there is a clearly increased risk of renal cell carcinoma in TS patients. Regular periodic imaging is recommended in TS patients with kidney involvement to screen for the development of renal cell carcinoma.

Although not common, TS may lead to significant chronic kidney disease (CKD) and progress to end-stage kidney failure. Patients with TS and CKD typically have an unremarkable urine sediment and only minimal to mild amounts of proteinuria.

Mechanistically, the *TSC1* and *TSC2* gene products tuberin and hamartin interact physically. This protein complex is localized to the base of the cilia and inhibits intracellular signaling processes mediated by mTOR, leading to abnormal growth in a number of tissues. Investigation of mTOR inhibitors as therapy for TS is ongoing.

VON HIPPEL-LINDAU DISEASE

Von Hippel-Lindau disease (VHL) is an inherited cancer syndrome with renal manifestations. VHL is an autosomal dominant condition caused by mutations in the VHL tumor-suppressor gene. VHL is localized to the primary cilia and is necessary for the formation of primary cilia. Like many autosomal dominant cancer syndromes, VHL is recessive at the cellular level: a somatic mutation in the second VHL allele leads to loss of VHL in the cell and abnormal growth. Kidney manifestations of VHL include multiple bilateral kidney cysts and renal cell carcinomas. Kidney cysts and carcinoma affect the majority of VHL patients. Nonrenal features of VHL include pheochromocytomas, cerebellar hemangioblastomas, and retinal hemangiomas.

Annual screening of the kidneys by imaging with CT or MRI is recommended for early detection of renal cell carcinomas. Increasingly, nephron-sparing surgical approaches are being used for removal of cancerous lesions in order to preserve kidney function.

OTHER INHERITED DISEASES OF TUBULE GROWTH AND DEVELOPMENT

ADPKD is by far the most common adult-onset, single-gene form of kidney disease. The large cysts that are sometimes seen in VHL and TS are similar in appearance to the cysts seen in ADPKD. A variety of other inherited disorders affecting primarily tubule and renal interstitial function can lead to CKD and eventual end-stage kidney disease in the absence of large tubule-derived cysts.

Inherited diseases affecting the tubulointerstitial compartment of the kidney can lead to secondary glomerular stress and glomerulosclerosis with some degree of concomitant proteinuria. Similarly, disorders of glomerular function will typically lead to secondary interstitial fibrosis and tubule atrophy. From a clinical perspective, therefore, distinguishing between a genetic disease of the renal tubules and a disease of the glomerulus may not be easy, particularly in the absence of a gross phenotype such as large kidney cysts.

MEDULLARY CYSTIC KIDNEY DISEASE (AUTOSOMAL DOMINANT INTERSTITIAL KIDNEY DISEASE)

The medullary cystic kidney diseases (MCKD) are autosomal dominant disorders. Despite the nosology, kidney cysts are not invariably present. Older literature often grouped MCKD together with the childhood-onset disorders known as the nephronophthises, but these are distinct clinical and genetic entities.

Medullary Cystic Kidney Disease Type I Patients with MCKD type I (MCKD I) have mutations in the mucin 1 gene *MUC1*. In contrast to MCKD type II (MCKD II) patients, individuals with MCKD I do not have elevated uric acid levels. The disease-causing *MUC1* mutations that have been reported all alter a repeat region within the *MUC1* gene, leading to a large "neoprotein" fragment that may lead to toxic effects on the kidney tubule.

Clinically, patients with MCKD I exhibit slowly progressive CKD in adulthood, with only minimal amounts of increased urine protein and occasional renal cysts seen on ultrasound examination. Kidney histology shows tubulointerstitial fibrosis and tubular atrophy. The mechanisms by which *MUC1* mutations cause human kidney disease are not known.

Medullary Cystic Kidney Disease Type II MCKD II is caused by mutations in the *UMOD* gene, which encodes the protein uromodulin, also known as Tamm-Horsfall protein. Uromodulin is also found on the centrosome, the mitotic spindle, and the primary cilia; it colocalizes with nephrocystin-1 and KIF3A on the cilia. *UMOD* mutations also cause the conditions that have been referred to as familial juvenile hyperuricemic nephropathy (HNFJ1) and glomerulocystic kidney disease (GCKD), although it is not clear that these different names represent clearly distinct disorders. The term *uromodulin-associated kidney disease* (UAKD) has been suggested as a better name for MCKD II and the various other related *UMOD*-associated diseases. Despite the name, kidney cysts are not a common feature of MCKD II. MCKD II should be suspected clinically in patients with a family history of late-onset kidney disease, benign urine sediments, absence of significant proteinuria, and hyperuricemia. Large genome-wide association studies have suggested that certain common noncoding sequence variants in *UMOD* are associated with a moderately increased risk of CKD in the general population.

Other Forms of Familial Tubulointerstitial Kidney Disease A small number of families have been identified with autosomal dominant tubulointerstitial kidney disease and hyperuricemia who lack *UMOD* mutations. Some of these families carry disease-segregating mutations in the renin gene *REN*. There are other families who lack mutations in *UMOD*, *MUC1*, or *REN*. Thus, mutations in other yet-to-be identified genes are able to produce similar interstitial kidney disease, both with and without hyperuricemia.

Kidney biopsies in patients with any of the various forms of MCKD typically show interstitial fibrosis. These histologic features are not diagnostic of any particular genetic entity, and the specific diagnosis must be made by other means. Genetic tests for alterations in specific genes are increasingly available in the clinical setting.

Patients with autosomal dominant interstitial kidney disease, *UMOD* or *REN* mutations, or hyperuricemia and gout should be treated similarly to others with these findings, with uric acid–lowering agents, such allopurinol or febuxostat.

NEPHRONOPHTHISIS

A large and growing number of genetically distinct but related autosomal recessive disorders are referred to as nephronophthises. These should not be confused with the adult-onset autosomal dominant medullary cystic kidney diseases discussed above, despite the often confusing nomenclature seen in older medical literature. Nephronophthisis is quite rare but is nevertheless the most common inherited childhood form of kidney failure requiring kidney replacement therapy.

Like ADPKD and ARPKD, the various genetically heterogeneous entities that fall under the category of nephronophthisis (NPHP) are disorders of ciliary function. Mutations in a very large number of genes have been identified that lead to NPHP under an autosomal recessive pattern of inheritance. The various forms of NPHP share common features, including tubulointerstitial fibrosis, corticomedullary cysts, and progressive CKD, leading to renal failure. Proteinuria is absent or mild, and the urine sediment is not active.

NPHP is often divided into infantile, juvenile, and adolescent forms. The juvenile form is the most frequent and usually caused by mutations in the *NPHP2* gene. The infantile form, usually caused by *NPHP2* mutations, is associated with end-stage kidney failure in early childhood. Patients with the adolescent form of NPHP typically develop end-stage kidney failure in early adulthood. The products of the NPHP genes are referred to as nephrocystins. *NPHP1* through *NPHP16* have been reported; some are referred to by other names as well.

NPHP can present as an isolated finding or be part of several multiorgan syndromes. Neurologic abnormalities are present in a significant number of patients. Bone and liver abnormities are seen in some NPHP patients. Senior-Løken syndrome is defined by the presence of NPHP with retinitis pigmentosa. Joubert's syndrome is defined by multiple neurologic findings, including hypoplasia of the cerebellar vermis. Some forms of this genetically heterogeneous syndrome include NPHP as a component.

The multisystem disease Bardet-Biedl syndrome (BBS) is defined clinically by a spectrum of features, including truncal obesity, cognitive impairment, retinal dystrophy, polydactyly, developmental urogenital abnormalities, and kidney cysts. The kidney phenotype is NPHP-like, with small cysts deriving from the tubules, tubulointerstitial and often secondary glomerular disease, and urine concentrating defects. There are 18 BBS genes cloned. BBS follows autosomal recessive inheritance. Like ADPKD, ARPKD, and NPHP, BBS is a disease of abnormal ciliary function.

The multiple genes and gene products (nephrocystins) that are responsible for NPHP are expressed in cilia, basal bodies, and the centrosomes of kidney tubule cells. It has been hypothesized that all of the NPHP gene defects lead to a clinical phenotype by interfering with the regulation of PCP.

There are no specific clinical tests that define NPHP. Genetic diagnosis is possible but cumbersome because of the large number of genes that can be responsible. There are no specific therapies for NPHP. Rather, therapy is aimed at treating signs of these diseases as well as the systemic abnormalities seen with all CKDs. Chronic dialysis or kidney transplantation is eventually required for NPHP-affected individuals.

KARYOMEGALIC TUBULOINTERSTITIAL NEPHRITIS

Karyomegalic tubulointerstitial nephritis is an exceptionally rare form of kidney disease with adult-onset progressive kidney failure. Kidney biopsy shows chronic tubulointerstitial nephritis, as well as interstitial fibrosis. This is a recessive disorder caused by inheritance of two mutant copies of the *FAN1* gene. *FAN1* encodes a component of a DNA repair machinery complex. Individuals with two mutant *FAN1* genes are genetically sensitized to the effect of DNA damage. Kidney histology shows karyomegaly in addition to the nonspecific findings of interstitial fibrosis and tubular atrophy.

MEDULLARY SPONGE KIDNEY

Medullary sponge kidney (MSK) is often grouped together with inherited disorders of the kidney affecting tubule growth and development, although it is usually a sporadic finding rather than an inherited phenotype. MSK is caused by developmental malformation and cystic dilatation of the renal collecting ducts. The medullary cysts seen in this entity can be quite variable in size.

MSK is usually a benign entity. The diagnosis of MSK is often made incidentally. In the past, the diagnosis of MSK was often made by intravenous pyelography (IVP). CT scans, which have replaced IVPs for much routine kidney imaging, are not as sensitive in detecting MSK.

MSK is associated with an increased frequency of calcium phosphate and calcium oxalate kidney stones. Altered flow characteristics in the kidney tubules may lead to the development of formation of a nidus for stone formation. Kidney stones in this group are treated the same as are kidney stones in the general population. MSK patients also often exhibit reduced kidney concentrating ability and an increased frequency of urinary tract infections.

CONGENITAL ABNORMALITIES OF THE KIDNEY AND URINARY TRACT

The structural abnormalities known as the congenital abnormalities of the kidney and urinary tract (CAKUTs) are a group of etiologically and phenotypically heterogeneous disorders. Some form of CAKUT is estimated to occur in up to 1 in 500 live births. Specific abnormalities classified as part of the CAKUT spectrum include kidney hypoplasia, kidney agenesis, ureteropelvic junction obstruction, and vesicoureteral reflux.

CAKUT can be the cause of clinically significant problems in both adults and children. However, it is a major contributor to kidney failure in children, accounting for more than one-third of end-stage kidney disease in this group.

CAKUT is typically a sporadic finding but can also cluster in families. Familial forms can be observed as parts of multisystem developmental syndromes. A growing list of specific genes have been identified, which when mutated lead to syndromic forms of CAKUT. For example, the branchio-oto-renal syndrome, characterized by developmental abnormalities in the neck, ears, and kidney, can be caused by mutations in the *EYA1* and *SIX1* genes. Mutations in the *PAX2* transcription factor gene can cause the autosomal dominant renal coloboma syndrome, characterized by optic nerve malformations and hypoplastic kidneys.

In many instances, CAKUT is caused by environmental influences rather than genetic alterations. For example, renal tubular dysgenesis, defined by altered tubule development, can be caused by prenatal exposure to angiotensin-converting enzyme inhibitors or angiotensin receptor blockers.

MITOCHONDRIAL DISEASE

Inherited disorders of the mitochondrial genome (discussed elsewhere in this text [Chap. 85e]) commonly affect kidney function. Thirteen of the genes involved in encoding components of the mitochondrial respiratory chain are located on the mitochondrial genome that is inherited maternally. The remainder of these components is encoded by the nuclear genome. These defects of oxidative phosphorylation may affect multiple organs and tissues.

Neuromuscular disease is the best recognized part of this complex phenotype. Kidney disease is now recognized as a common component as well. Tubulointerstitial disease may be seen on kidney biopsy, and progression to kidney failure may occur. Glomerular involvement, manifest as proteinuria and glomerulosclerosis, can also develop. Changes in proximal tubule activity are the most common renal phenotype. Patients may have several defects in proximal tubule transport, including the Fanconi syndrome. Some patients may also have acidosis, hypophosphatemic rickets, hypercalciuria, glycosuria, and tubular proteinuria. Decreased urine concentrating ability is common.

GLOBAL CONSIDERATIONS

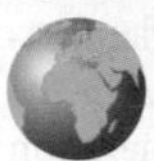

The disorders discussed above are all seen worldwide. In addition, a previously unrecognized epidemic of kidney disease is leading to very high rates of kidney failure in and near the western coast of Central America. This Mesoamerican nephropathy is particularly common in Nicaragua and El Salvador. Mesoamerican nephropathy patients do not have significant proteinuria, suggesting that this is a disease of the kidney tubules and interstitium. The cause is unknown, but some have suggested that a combination of toxic environmental factors and heat stress underlies the development of this kidney disease, which has a striking male predominance. However, the fact that, in many families, a large fraction of the men are affected with kidney disease has suggested that a strong genetic component may be involved as well.

340 Tubulointerstitial Diseases of the Kidney

Laurence H. Beck, David J. Salant

Inflammation or fibrosis of the renal interstitium and atrophy of the tubular compartment are common consequences of diseases that target the glomeruli or vasculature. Distinct from these secondary phenomena, however, are a group of disorders that primarily affect the tubules and interstitium, with relative sparing of the glomeruli and renal vessels. Such disorders are conveniently divided into acute and chronic tubulointerstitial nephritis (TIN) (Table 340-1).

Acute TIN most often presents with acute renal failure (Chap. 334). The acute nature of this group of disorders may be caused by aggressive inflammatory infiltrates that lead to tissue edema, tubular cell injury, and compromised tubular flow, or by frank obstruction of the tubules with casts, cellular debris, or crystals. There is sometimes flank pain due to distention of the renal capsule. Urinary sediment is often active with leukocytes and cellular casts, but depends on the exact nature of the disorder in question.

The clinical features of chronic TIN are more indolent and may manifest with disorders of tubular function, including polyuria from impaired concentrating ability (nephrogenic diabetes insipidus), defective proximal tubular reabsorption leading to features of Fanconi's syndrome (glycosuria, phosphaturia, aminoaciduria, hypokalemia, and type II renal tubular acidosis [RTA] from bicarbonaturia), or non-anion-gap metabolic acidosis and hyperkalemia (type IV RTA) due to impaired ammoniagenesis, as well as progressive azotemia (rising creatinine and blood urea nitrogen [BUN]). There is often modest proteinuria (rarely >2 g/d) attributable to decreased tubular reabsorption of filtered proteins; however, nephrotic-range albuminuria may occur in some conditions due to the development of secondary focal segmental glomerulosclerosis (FSGS). Renal ultrasonography may reveal changes of "medical renal disease," such as increased echogenicity of the renal parenchyma with loss of corticomedullary differentiation, prominence of the renal pyramids, and cortical scarring in some conditions. The predominant pathology in chronic TIN is interstitial fibrosis with patchy mononuclear cell infiltration and widespread tubular atrophy, luminal dilation, and thickening of tubular basement membranes. Because of the nonspecific nature of the histopathology, biopsy specimens rarely provide a specific diagnosis. Thus, diagnosis relies on careful analysis of history, drug or toxin exposure, associated symptoms, and imaging studies.

TABLE 340-1 CLASSIFICATION OF THE CAUSES OF TUBULOINTERSTITIAL DISEASES OF THE KIDNEY

Acute Tubulointerstitial Disorders

Acute Interstitial Nephritis

Therapeutic agents

- Antibiotics (β-lactams, sulfonamides, quinolones, vancomycin, erythromycin, linezolid, minocycline, rifampin, ethambutol, acyclovir)
- Nonsteroidal anti-inflammatory drugs, COX-2 inhibitors
- Diuretics (rarely thiazides, loop diuretics, triamterene)
- Anticonvulsants (phenytoin, valproate, carbamazepine, phenobarbital)
- Miscellaneous (proton pump inhibitors, H_2 blockers, captopril, mesalazine, indinavir, allopurinol, lenalidomide)

Infection

- Bacteria (*Streptococcus, Staphylococcus, Legionella, Salmonella, Brucella, Yersinia, Corynebacterium diphtheriae*)
- Viruses (EBV, CMV, hantavirus, polyomavirus, HIV)
- Miscellaneous (*Leptospira, Rickettsia, Mycoplasma, Histoplasma*)

Autoimmune

- Tubulointerstitial nephritis with uveitis (TINU)
- Sjögren's syndrome
- Systemic lupus erythematosus
- Granulomatous interstitial nephritis
- IgG4-related systemic disease
- Idiopathic autoimmune interstitial nephritis

Acute obstructive disorders

- Light chain cast nephropathy ("myeloma kidney")
- Acute phosphate nephropathy
- Acute urate nephropathy

Chronic Tubulointerstitial Disorders

- Vesicoureteral reflux/reflux nephropathy
- Sickle cell disease
- Chronic exposure to toxins or therapeutic agents
- Analgesics, especially those containing phenacetin
- Lithium
- Heavy metals (lead, cadmium)
- Aristolochic acid (Chinese herbal and Balkan endemic nephropathies)
- Calcineurin inhibitors (cyclosporine, tacrolimus)

Metabolic Disturbances

- Hypercalcemia and/or nephrocalcinosis
- Hyperuricemia
- Prolonged hypokalemia
- Hyperoxaluria
- Cystinosis (see Chap. 339)

Cystic and Hereditary Disorders (see Chap. 339)

- Polycystic kidney disease
- Nephronophthisis
- Adult medullary cystic disease
- Medullary sponge kidney

Miscellaneous

- Aging
- Chronic glomerulonephritis
- Chronic urinary tract obstruction
- Ischemia and vascular disease
- Radiation nephritis (rare)

Abbreviations: CMV, cytomegalovirus; COX, cyclooxygenase; EBV, Epstein-Barr virus.

ACUTE INTERSTITIAL NEPHRITIS

In 1897, Councilman reported on eight cases of acute interstitial nephritis (AIN) in the Medical and Surgical Reports of the Boston City Hospital; three as a postinfectious complication of scarlet fever and two from diphtheria. Later, he described the lesion as "an acute inflammation of the kidney characterized by cellular and fluid exudation in the interstitial tissue, accompanied by, but not dependant on, degeneration of the epithelium; the exudation is not purulent in character, and the lesions may be both diffuse and focal." Today AIN is far more often encountered as an allergic reaction to a drug (Table 340-1). Immune-mediated AIN may also occur as part of a known autoimmune syndrome, but in some cases there is no identifiable cause despite features suggestive of an immunologic etiology (Table 340-1).

ALLERGIC INTERSTITIAL NEPHRITIS

Although biopsy-proven AIN accounts for no more than ~15% of cases of unexplained acute renal failure, this is likely a substantial underestimate of the true incidence. This is because potentially offending medications are more often identified and empirically discontinued in a patient noted to have a rising serum creatinine, without the benefit of a renal biopsy to establish the diagnosis of AIN.

Clinical Features The classic presentation of AIN, namely, fever, rash, peripheral eosinophilia, and oliguric renal failure occurring after 7–10 days of treatment with methicillin or another β-lactam antibiotic, is the exception rather than the rule. More often, patients are found incidentally to have a rising serum creatinine or present with symptoms attributable to acute renal failure (Chap. 334). Atypical reactions can occur, most notably nonsteroidal anti-inflammatory drug (NSAID)-induced AIN, in which fever, rash, and eosinophilia are rare, but acute renal failure with heavy proteinuria is common. A particularly severe and rapid-onset AIN may occur upon reintroduction of rifampin after a drug-free period. More insidious reactions to the agents listed in Table 340-1 may lead to progressive tubulointerstitial damage. Examples include proton pump inhibitors and, rarely, sulfonamide and 5-aminosalicylate (mesalazine and sulfasalazine) derivatives and antiretrovirals.

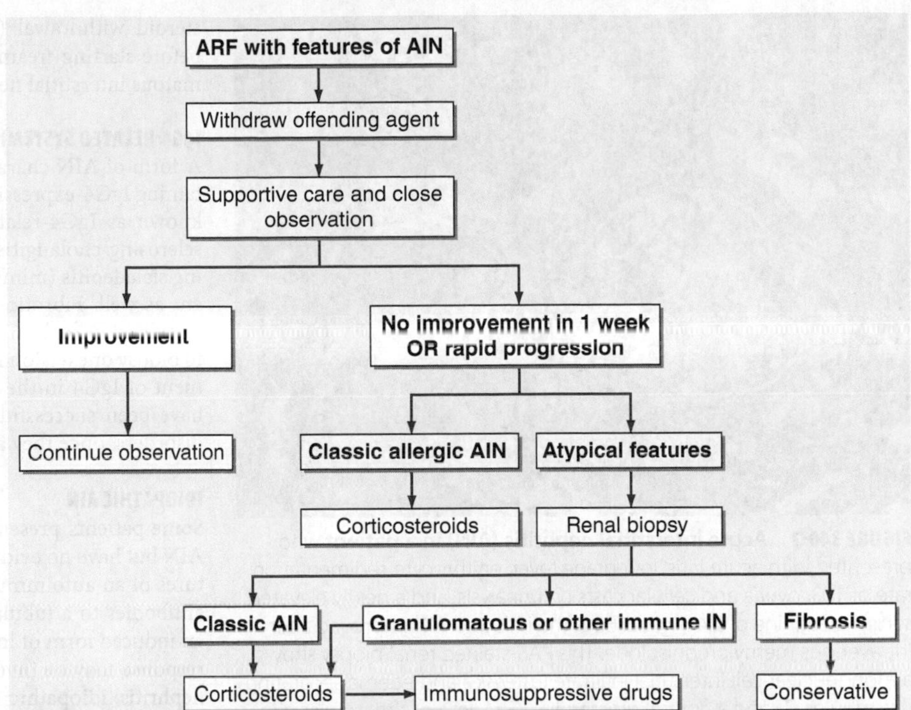

FIGURE 340-1 Algorithm for the treatment of allergic and other immune-mediated acute interstitial nephritis (AIN). ARF, acute renal failure; IN, interstitial nephritis. See text for immunosuppressive drugs used for refractory or relapsing AIN. *(Modified from S Reddy, DJ Salant: Ren Fail 20:829, 1998.)*

Diagnosis Finding otherwise unexplained renal failure with or without oliguria and exposure to a potentially offending agent usually points to the diagnosis. Peripheral blood eosinophilia adds supporting evidence but is present in only a minority of patients. Urinalysis reveals pyuria with white blood cell casts and hematuria. Urinary eosinophils are neither sensitive nor specific for AIN; therefore, testing is not recommended. Renal biopsy is generally not required for diagnosis but reveals extensive interstitial and tubular infiltration of leukocytes, including eosinophils.

TREATMENT ALLERGIC INTERSTITIAL NEPHRITIS

Discontinuation of the offending agent often leads to reversal of the renal injury. However, depending on the duration of exposure and degree of tubular atrophy and interstitial fibrosis that has occurred, the renal damage may not be completely reversible. Glucocorticoid therapy may accelerate renal recovery, but does not appear to impact long-term renal survival. It is best reserved for those cases with severe renal failure in which dialysis is imminent or if renal function continues to deteriorate despite stopping the offending drug (Fig. 340-1 and Table 340-2).

SJÖGREN'S SYNDROME

Sjögren's syndrome is a systemic autoimmune disorder that primarily targets the exocrine glands, especially the lacrimal and salivary glands, and thus results in symptoms, such as dry eyes and mouth, that constitute the "sicca syndrome" (Chap. 383). Tubulointerstitial nephritis with a predominant lymphocytic infiltrate is the most common renal manifestation of Sjögren's syndrome and can be associated with distal RTA, nephrogenic diabetes insipidus, and moderate renal failure. Diagnosis is strongly supported by positive serologic testing for anti-Ro (SS-A) and anti-La (SS-B) antibodies. A large proportion of patients with Sjögren's syndrome also have polyclonal hypergammaglobulinemia. Treatment is initially with glucocorticoids, although patients may require maintenance therapy with azathioprine or mycophenolate mofetil to prevent relapse (Fig. 340-1 and Table 340-2).

TUBULOINTERSTITIAL NEPHRITIS WITH UVEITIS (TINU)

TINU is a systemic autoimmune disease of unknown etiology. It accounts for fewer than 5% of all cases of AIN, affects females three times more often than males, and has a median age of onset of 15 years. Its hallmark feature, in addition to a lymphocyte-predominant interstitial nephritis (Fig. 340-2), is a painful anterior uveitis, often bilateral and accompanied by blurred vision and photophobia. Diagnosis is

TABLE 340-2 INDICATIONS FOR CORTICOSTEROIDS AND IMMUNOSUPPRESSIVES IN INTERSTITIAL NEPHRITIS

Absolute Indications
• Sjögren's syndrome
• Sarcoidosis
• SLE interstitial nephritis
• Adults with TINU
• Idiopathic and other granulomatous interstitial nephritis
Relative Indications
• Drug-induced or idiopathic AIN with:
Rapid progression of renal failure
Diffuse infiltrates on biopsy
Impending need for dialysis
Delayed recovery
• Children with TINU
• Postinfectious AIN with delayed recovery (?)

Abbreviations: AIN, acute interstitial nephritis; SLE, systemic lupus erythematosus; TINU, tubulointerstitial nephritis with uveitis.

Source: Modified from S Reddy, DJ Salant: Ren Fail 20:829, 1998.

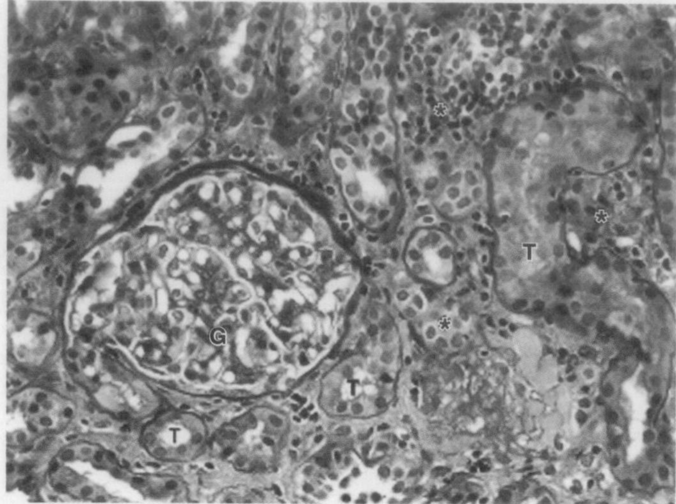

FIGURE 340-2 Acute interstitial nephritis (AIN) in a patient who presented with acute iritis, low-grade fever, erythrocyte sedimentation rate of 103, pyuria and cellular casts on urinalysis, and a newly elevated serum creatinine of 2.4 mg/dL. Both the iritis and AIN improved after intravenous methylprednisolone. This PAS-stained renal biopsy shows a mononuclear cell interstitial infiltrate (*asterisks*) and edema separating the tubules (T) and a normal glomerulus (G). Some of the tubules contain cellular debris and infiltrating inflammatory cells. The findings in this biopsy are indistinguishable from those that would be seen in a case of drug-induced AIN. PAS, Periodic acid–Schiff.

often confounded by the fact that the ocular symptoms precede or accompany the renal disease in only one-third of cases. Additional extrarenal features include fever, anorexia, weight loss, abdominal pain, and arthralgia. The presence of such symptoms as well as elevated creatinine, sterile pyuria, mild proteinuria, features of Fanconi's syndrome, and elevated erythrocyte sedimentation rate should raise suspicion for this disorder. Serologies suggestive of the more common autoimmune diseases are usually negative, and TINU is often a diagnosis of exclusion after other causes of uveitis and renal disease, such as Sjögren's syndrome, Behçet's disease, sarcoidosis, and systemic lupus erythematosus, have been considered. Clinical symptoms are typically self-limited in children, but are more apt to follow a relapsing course in adults. The renal and ocular manifestations generally respond well to oral glucocorticoids, although maintenance therapy with agents such as methotrexate, azathioprine, or mycophenolate may be necessary to prevent relapses (Fig. 340-1 and Table 340-2).

SYSTEMIC LUPUS ERYTHEMATOSUS

An interstitial mononuclear cell inflammatory reaction often accompanies the glomerular lesion in most cases of class III or IV lupus nephritis (Chap. 338), and deposits of immune complexes can be identified in tubule basement membranes in about 50% of cases. Occasionally, however, the tubulointerstitial inflammation predominates and may manifest with azotemia and type IV RTA rather than features of glomerulonephritis.

GRANULOMATOUS INTERSTITIAL NEPHRITIS

Some patients may present with features of AIN but follow a protracted and relapsing course. Renal biopsy in such patients reveals a more chronic inflammatory infiltrate with granulomas and multinucleated giant cells. Most often, no associated disease or cause is found; however, some of these cases may have or subsequently develop the pulmonary, cutaneous, or other systemic manifestations of *sarcoidosis* such as hypercalcemia. Most patients experience some improvement in renal function if treated early with glucocorticoids before the development of significant interstitial fibrosis and tubular atrophy (Table 340-2). Other immunosuppressive agents may be required for those who relapse frequently upon steroid withdrawal. Other immunosuppressive agents may be required for those who relapse frequently upon steroid withdrawal (Fig. 340-1). Tuberculosis should be ruled out before starting treatment because this too is a rare cause of granulomatous interstitial nephritis.

IgG4-RELATED SYSTEMIC DISEASE

A form of AIN characterized by a dense inflammatory infiltrate containing IgG4-expressing plasma cells can occur as a part of a syndrome known as IgG4-related systemic disease. Autoimmune pancreatitis, sclerosing cholangitis, retroperitoneal fibrosis, and a chronic sclerosing sialadenitis (mimicking Sjögren's syndrome) may variably be present as well. Fibrotic lesions that form pseudotumors in the affected organs soon replace the initial inflammatory infiltrates and often lead to biopsy or excision for fear of true malignancy. Although the involvement of IgG4 in the pathogenesis is not understood, glucocorticoids have been successfully used as first-line treatment in this group of disorders, once they are correctly diagnosed.

IDIOPATHIC AIN

Some patients present with typical clinical and histologic features of AIN but have no evidence of drug exposure or clinical or serologic features of an autoimmune disease. The presence in some cases of autoantibodies to a tubular antigen, similar to that identified in rats with an induced form of interstitial nephritis, suggests that an autoimmune response may be involved. Like TINU and granulomatous interstitial nephritis, idiopathic AIN is responsive to glucocorticoid therapy but may follow a relapsing course requiring maintenance treatment with another immunosuppressive agent (Fig. 340-1 and Table 340-2).

INFECTION-ASSOCIATED AIN

AIN may also occur as a local inflammatory reaction to microbial infection (Table 340-1) and should be distinguished from acute bacterial pyelonephritis (Chap. 162). Acute bacterial pyelonephritis does not generally cause acute renal failure unless it affects both kidneys or causes septic shock. Presently, infection-associated AIN is most often seen in immunocompromised patients, particularly renal transplant recipients with reactivation of polyomavirus BK (Chaps. 169 and 337).

CRYSTAL DEPOSITION DISORDERS AND OBSTRUCTIVE TUBULOPATHIES

Acute renal failure may occur when crystals of various types are deposited in tubular cells and interstitium or when they obstruct tubules. Oliguric acute renal failure, often accompanied by flank pain from tubular obstruction, may occur in patients treated with sulfadiazine for toxoplasmosis, indinavir and atazanavir for HIV, and intravenous acyclovir for severe herpesvirus infections. Urinalysis reveals "sheaf of wheat" sulfonamide crystals, individual or parallel clusters of needle-shaped indinavir crystals, or red-green birefringement needle-shaped crystals of acyclovir. This adverse effect is generally precipitated by hypovolemia and is reversible with saline volume repletion and drug withdrawal. Distinct from the obstructive disease, a frank AIN from indinavir crystal deposition has also been reported.

Acute tubular obstruction is also the cause of oliguric renal failure in patients with *acute urate nephropathy*. It typically results from severe hyperuricemia from tumor lysis syndrome in patients with lympho- or myeloproliferative disorders treated with cytotoxic agents, but also may occur spontaneously before the treatment has been initiated (Chap. 331). Uric acid crystallization in the tubules and collecting system leads to partial or complete obstruction of the collecting ducts, renal pelvis, or ureter. A dense precipitate of birefringent uric acid crystals is found in the urine, usually in association with microscopic or gross hematuria. Prophylactic allopurinol reduces the risk of uric acid nephropathy but is of no benefit once tumor lysis has occurred. Once oliguria has developed, attempts to increase tubular flow and solubility of uric acid with alkaline diuresis may be of some benefit; however, emergent treatment with hemodialysis or rasburicase, a recombinant urate oxidase, is usually required to rapidly lower uric acid levels and restore renal function.

Calcium oxalate crystal deposition in tubular cells and interstitium may lead to permanent renal dysfunction in patients who survive ethylene glycol intoxication, in patients with enteric hyperoxaluria from ileal resection or small-bowel bypass surgery, and in patients with hereditary hyperoxaluria (Chap. 342). *Acute phosphate nephropathy* is an uncommon but serious complication of oral Phospho-soda used as a laxative or for bowel preparation for colonoscopy. It results from calcium phosphate crystal deposition in tubules and interstitium and occurs especially in subjects with underlying renal impairment and hypovolemia. Consequently, Phospho-soda should be avoided in patients with chronic kidney disease.

LIGHT CHAIN CAST NEPHROPATHY

Patients with multiple myeloma may develop acute renal failure in the setting of hypovolemia, infection, or hypercalcemia or after exposure to NSAIDs or radiographic contrast media. The diagnosis of light chain cast nephropathy (LCCN)—commonly known as *myeloma kidney*—should be considered in patients who fail to recover when the precipitating factor is corrected or in any elderly patient with otherwise unexplained acute renal failure.

In this disorder, filtered monoclonal immunoglobulin light chains (Bence-Jones proteins) form intratubular aggregates with secreted Tamm-Horsfall protein in the distal tubule. Casts, in addition to obstructing the tubular flow in affected nephrons, incite a giant cell or foreign body reaction and can lead to tubular rupture, resulting in interstitial fibrosis (Fig. 340-3). Although LCCN generally occurs in patients with known multiple myeloma and a large plasma cell burden, the disorder should also be considered as a possible diagnosis in patients who have known monoclonal gammopathy even in the absence of frank myeloma. Filtered monoclonal light chains may also cause less pronounced renal manifestations in the absence of obstruction, due to direct toxicity to proximal tubular cells and intracellular crystal formation. This may result in isolated tubular disorders such as RTA or full Fanconi's syndrome.

Diagnosis Clinical clues to the diagnosis include anemia, bone pain, hypercalcemia, and an abnormally narrow anion gap due to hypoalbuminemia and hypergammaglobulinemia. Urinary dipsticks detect albumin but not immunoglobulin light chains; however, laboratory detection of increased amounts of protein in a spot urine specimen and a negative dipstick result are highly suggestive that the urine contains Bence-Jones protein. Serum and urine should both be sent for protein electrophoresis and for immunofixation for the detection and identification of a potential monoclonal band. A sensitive method is available to detect urine and serum free light chains.

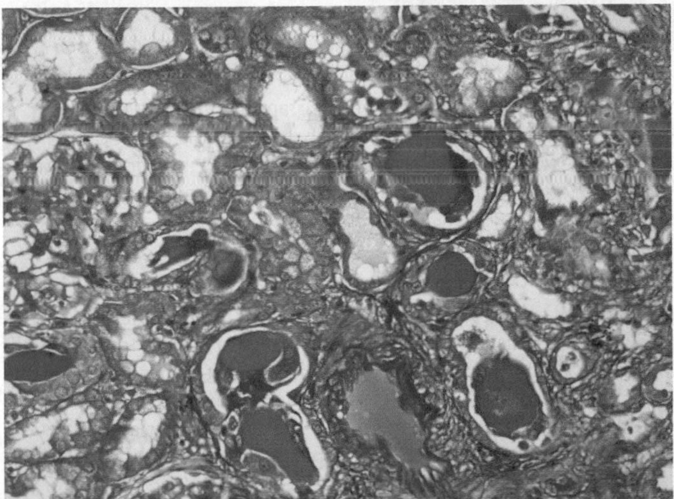

FIGURE 340-3 Histologic appearance of myeloma cast nephropathy. A hematoxylin-eosin–stained kidney biopsy shows many atrophic tubules filled with eosinophilic casts (consisting of Bence-Jones protein), which are surrounded by giant cell reactions. *(Courtesy of Dr. Michael N. Koss, University of Southern California Keck School of Medicine; with permission.)*

TREATMENT LIGHT CHAIN CAST NEPHROPATHY

The goals of treatment are to correct precipitating factors such as hypovolemia and hypercalcemia, discontinue potential nephrotoxic agents, and treat the underlying plasma cell dyscrasia (Chap. 136); plasmapheresis to remove light chains is of questionable value for LCCN.

LYMPHOMATOUS INFILTRATION OF THE KIDNEY

Interstitial infiltration by malignant B lymphocytes is a common autopsy finding in patients dying of chronic lymphocytic leukemia and non-Hodgkin's lymphoma; however, this is usually an incidental finding. Rarely, such infiltrates may cause massive enlargement of the kidneys and oliguric acute renal failure. Although high-dose glucocorticoids and subsequent chemotherapy often result in recovery of renal function, the prognosis in such cases is generally poor.

CHRONIC TUBULOINTERSTITIAL DISEASES

Improved occupational and public health measures, together with the banning of over-the-counter phenacetin-containing analgesics, has led to a dramatic decline in the incidence of chronic interstitial nephritis (CIN) from heavy metal—particularly lead and cadmium—exposure and analgesic nephropathy in North America. Today, CIN is most often the result of renal ischemia or secondary to a primary glomerular disease (Chap. 338). Other important forms of CIN are the result of developmental anomalies or inherited diseases such as reflux nephropathy or sickle cell nephropathy and may not be recognized until adolescence or adulthood. Although it is impossible to reverse damage that has already occurred, further deterioration may be prevented or at least slowed in such cases by treating glomerular hypertension, a common denominator in the development of secondary FSGS and progressive loss of functioning nephrons. Therefore, awareness and early detection of patients at risk may prevent them from developing end-stage renal disease (ESRD).

VESICOURETERAL REFLUX AND REFLUX NEPHROPATHY

Reflux nephropathy is the consequence of vesicoureteral reflux (VUR) or other urologic anomalies in early childhood. It was previously called *chronic pyelonephritis* because it was believed to result from recurrent urinary tract infections (UTIs) in childhood. VUR stems from abnormal retrograde urine flow from the bladder into one or both ureters and kidneys because of mislocated and incompetent ureterovesical valves (Fig. 340-4). Although high-pressure sterile reflux may impair normal growth of the kidneys, when coupled with recurrent UTIs in early childhood, the result is patchy interstitial scarring and tubular atrophy. Loss of functioning nephrons leads to hypertrophy of the remnant glomeruli and eventual secondary FSGS. Reflux nephropathy often goes unnoticed until early adulthood when chronic kidney disease is detected during routine evaluation or during pregnancy. Affected adults are frequently asymptomatic, but may give a history of prolonged bed-wetting or recurrent UTIs during childhood, and exhibit variable renal insufficiency, hypertension, mild to moderate proteinuria, and unremarkable urine sediment. When both kidneys are affected, the disease often progresses inexorably over several years to ESRD, despite the absence of ongoing urinary infections or reflux. A single affected kidney may go undetected, except for the presence of hypertension. Renal ultrasound in adults characteristically shows asymmetric small kidneys with irregular outlines, thinned cortices, and regions of compensatory hypertrophy (Fig. 340-4).

TREATMENT VESICOURETERAL REFLUX AND REFLUX NEPHROPATHY

Maintenance of sterile urine in childhood has been shown to limit scarring of the kidneys. Surgical reimplantation of the ureters into the bladder to restore competency is indicated in young children with persistent high-grade reflux but is ineffective and is

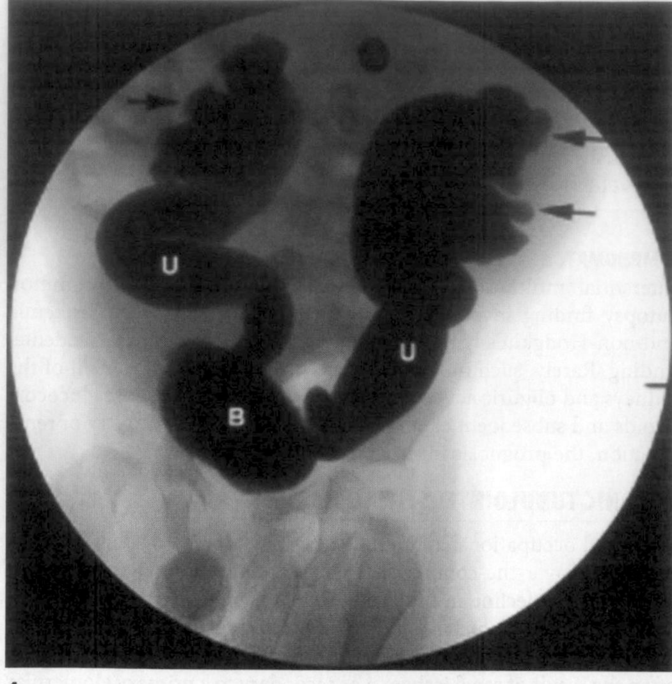

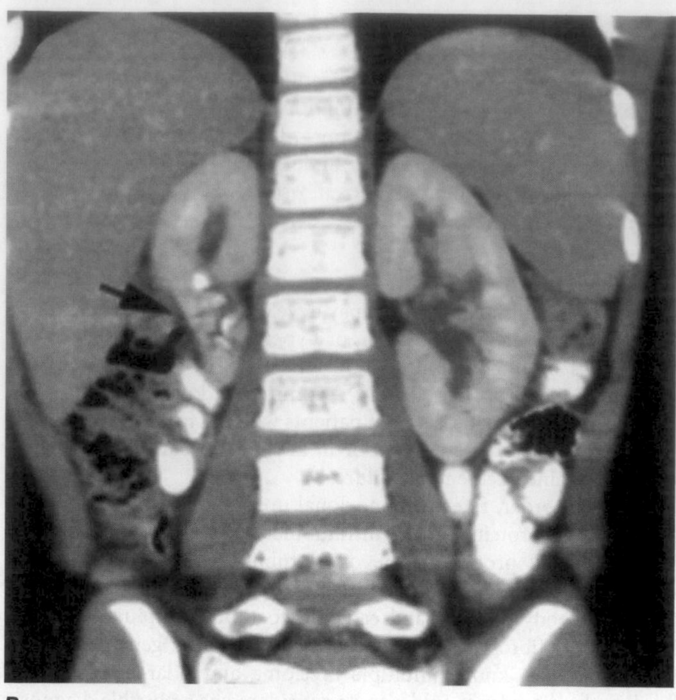

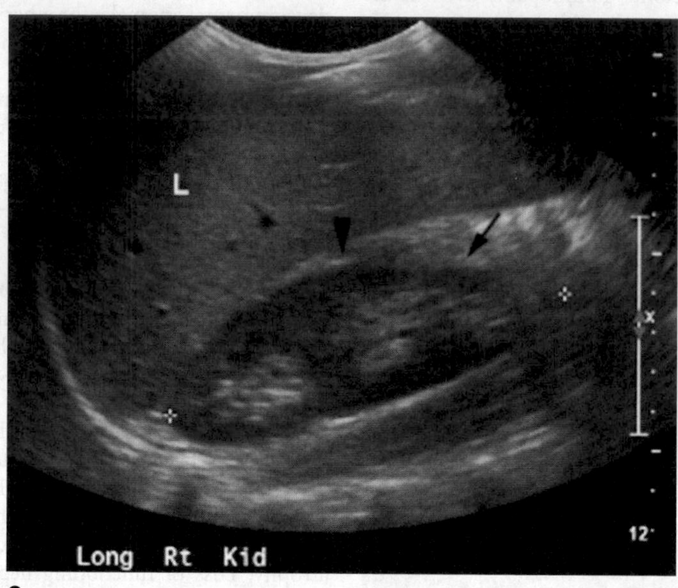

FIGURE 340-4 Radiographs of vesicoureteral reflux (VUR) and reflux nephropathy. ***A.*** Voiding cystourethrogram in a 7-month-old baby with bilateral high-grade VUR evidenced by clubbed calyces (*arrows*) and dilated tortuous ureters (U) entering the bladder (B). ***B.*** Abdominal computed tomography scan (coronal plane reconstruction) in a child showing severe scarring of the lower portion of the right kidney (*arrow*). ***C.*** Sonogram of the right kidney showing loss of parenchyma at the lower pole due to scarring (*arrow*) and hypertrophy of the mid-region (*arrowhead*). *(Courtesy of Dr. George Gross, University of Maryland Medical Center; with permission.)*

not indicated in adolescents or adults after scarring has occurred. Aggressive control of blood pressure with an angiotensin-converting enzyme inhibitor (ACEI) or angiotensin receptor blocker (ARB) and other agents is effective in reducing proteinuria and may significantly forestall further deterioration of renal function.

SICKLE CELL NEPHROPATHY

The pathogenesis and clinical manifestations of sickle cell nephropathy are described in Chap. 341. Evidence of tubular injury may be evident in childhood and early adolescence in the form of polyuria due to decreased concentrating ability or type IV renal tubular acidosis years before there is significant nephron loss and proteinuria from secondary FSGS. Early recognition of these subtle renal abnormalities or development of microalbuminuria in a child with sickle cell disease may warrant consultation with a nephrologist and/or therapy with low-dose ACEIs. Papillary necrosis may result from ischemia due to sickling of red cells in the relatively hypoxemic and hypertonic medullary vasculature and present with gross hematuria and ureteric obstruction by sloughed ischemic papillae (Table 340-3).

TUBULOINTERSTITIAL ABNORMALITIES ASSOCIATED WITH GLOMERULONEPHRITIS

Primary glomerulopathies are often associated with damage to tubules and interstitium. This may occasionally be due to the same pathologic process affecting the glomerulus and tubulointerstitium, as is the case with immune-complex deposition in lupus nephritis. More often, however, chronic tubulointerstitial changes occur as a secondary

TABLE 340-3 MAJOR CAUSES OF PAPILLARY NECROSIS

Analgesic nephropathy
Sickle cell nephropathy
Diabetes with urinary tract infection
Prolonged NSAID use (rare)

Abbreviation: NSAID, nonsteroidal anti-inflammatory drug.

consequence of prolonged glomerular dysfunction. Potential mechanisms by which glomerular disease might cause tubulointerstitial injury include proteinuria-mediated damage to the epithelial cells, activation of tubular cells by cytokines and complement, or reduced peritubular blood flow leading to downstream tubulointerstitial ischemia, especially in the case of glomeruli that are globally obsolescent due to severe glomerulonephritis. It is often difficult to discern the initial cause of injury by renal biopsy in a patient who presents with advanced renal disease in this setting.

ANALGESIC NEPHROPATHY

Analgesic nephropathy results from the long-term use of compound analgesic preparations containing phenacetin (banned in the United States since 1983), aspirin, and caffeine. In its classic form, analgesic nephropathy is characterized by renal insufficiency, papillary necrosis (Table 340-3) attributable to the presumed concentration of the drug to toxic levels in the inner medulla, and a radiographic constellation of small, scarred kidneys with papillary calcifications best appreciated by computed tomography (Fig. 340-5). Patients may also have polyuria due to impaired concentrating ability and non-anion-gap metabolic acidosis from tubular damage. Shedding of a sloughed necrotic papilla can cause gross hematuria and ureteric colic due to ureteral obstruction. Individuals with ESRD as a result of analgesic nephropathy are at increased risk of a urothelial malignancy compared to patients with other causes of renal failure. Recent cohort studies in individuals with normal baseline renal function suggest that the moderate chronic use of current analgesic preparations available in the United States, including acetaminophen and NSAIDs, does not seem to cause the constellation of findings known as analgesic nephropathy, although volume-depleted individuals and those with chronic kidney disease are at higher risk of NSAID-related renal toxicity. Nonetheless, it is recommended that heavy users of acetaminophen and NSAIDs be screened for evidence of renal disease.

ARISTOLOCHIC ACID NEPHROPATHY

Two seemingly unrelated forms of CIN, Chinese herbal nephropathy and Balkan endemic nephropathy, have recently been linked by the underlying etiologic agent aristolochic acid and are now collectively termed aristolochic acid nephropathy (AAN). In Chinese herbal nephropathy, first described in the early 1990s in young women taking traditional Chinese herbal preparations as part of a weight-loss regimen, one of the offending agents has been identified as aristolochic acid, a known carcinogen from the plant *Aristolochia*. Multiple *Aristolochia* species have been used in traditional herbal remedies for centuries and continue to be available despite official bans on their use in many countries. Molecular evidence has also implicated aristolochic acid in Balkan endemic nephropathy, a chronic tubulointerstitial nephritis found primarily in towns along the tributaries of the Danube River and first described in the 1950s. Although the exact route of exposure is not known with certainty, contamination of local grain preparations with the seeds of *Aristolochia* species seems most likely. Aristolochic acid, after prolonged exposure, produces renal interstitial fibrosis with a relative paucity of cellular infiltrates. The urine sediment is bland, with rare leukocytes and only mild proteinuria. Anemia may be disproportionately severe relative to the level of renal dysfunction. Definitive diagnosis of AAN requires two of the following three features: characteristic histology on kidney biopsy; confirmation of aristolochic acid ingestion; and detection of aristolactam-DNA adducts in kidney or urinary tract tissue. These latter lesions represent a molecular signature of aristolochic acid–derived DNA damage and often consist of characteristic A:T-to-T:A transversions. Due to this mutagenic activity, AAN is associated with a very high incidence of upper urinary tract urothelial cancers, with risk related to cumulative dose. Surveillance with computed tomography, ureteroscopy, and urine cytology is warranted, and consideration should be given to bilateral nephroureterectomy once a patient has reached ESRD.

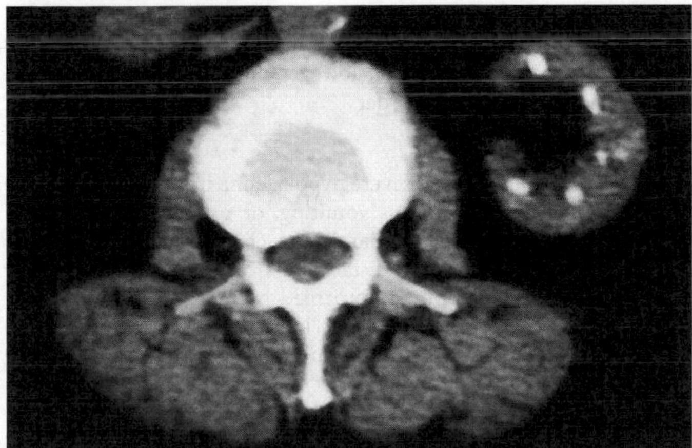

FIGURE 340-5 Radiologic appearance of analgesic nephropathy. A noncontrast computed tomography scan shows an atrophic left kidney with papillary calcifications in a garland pattern. *(Reprinted by permission from Macmillan Publishers, Ltd., MM Elseviers et al: Kidney International 48:1316, 1995.)*

KARYOMEGALIC INTERSTITIAL NEPHRITIS

Karyomegalic interstitial nephritis is an unusual form of slowly progressive chronic kidney disease with mild proteinuria, interstitial fibrosis, tubular atrophy, and oddly enlarged nuclei of proximal tubular epithelial cells. It has been linked to mutations in *FAN1*, a nuclease involved in DNA repair, which may render carriers of the mutation susceptible to environmental DNA-damaging agents.

LITHIUM-ASSOCIATED NEPHROPATHY

The use of lithium salts for the treatment of manic-depressive illness may have several renal sequelae, the most common of which is nephrogenic diabetes insipidus manifesting as polyuria and polydipsia. Lithium accumulates in principal cells of the collecting duct by entering through the epithelial sodium channel (ENaC), where it inhibits glycogen synthase kinase 3β and downregulates vasopressin-regulated aquaporin water channels. Less frequently, chronic tubulointerstitial nephritis develops after prolonged (>10–20 years) lithium use and is most likely to occur in patients who have experienced repeated episodes of toxic lithium levels. Findings on renal biopsy include interstitial fibrosis and tubular atrophy that are out of proportion to the degree of glomerulosclerosis or vascular disease, a sparse lymphocytic infiltrate, and small cysts or dilation of the distal tubule and collecting duct that are highly characteristic of this disorder. The degree of interstitial fibrosis correlates with both duration and cumulative dose of lithium. Individuals with lithium-associated nephropathy are typically asymptomatic, with minimal proteinuria, few urinary leukocytes, and normal blood pressure. Some patients develop more severe proteinuria due to secondary FSGS, which may contribute to further loss of renal function.

TREATMENT LITHIUM-ASSOCIATED NEPHROPATHY

Renal function should be followed regularly in patients taking lithium, and caution should be exercised in patients with underlying renal disease. The use of amiloride to inhibit lithium entry via ENaC has been effective to prevent and treat lithium-induced nephrogenic diabetes insipidus, but it is not clear if it will prevent lithium-induced CIN. Once lithium-associated nephropathy is detected, the discontinuation of lithium in attempt to forestall further renal deterioration can be problematic, as lithium is an effective mood stabilizer that is often incompletely substituted by other agents. Furthermore, despite discontinuation of lithium, chronic renal disease in such patients is often irreversible and can slowly progress to ESRD. The most prudent approach is to monitor lithium levels frequently and adjust dosing to avoid toxic levels (preferably <1 meq/L). This is especially important because lithium is cleared less effectively as renal function declines. In patients who develop significant proteinuria, ACEI or ARB treatment should be initiated.

CALCINEURIN-INHIBITOR NEPHROTOXICITY

The calcineurin inhibitor (CNI) immunosuppressive agents cyclosporine and tacrolimus can cause both acute and chronic renal injury. Acute forms can result from vascular causes such as vasoconstriction or the development of thrombotic microangiopathy, or can be due to a toxic tubulopathy. Chronic CNI-induced renal injury is typically seen in solid organ (including heart-lung and liver) transplant recipients and manifests with a slow but irreversible reduction of glomerular filtration rate, with mild proteinuria and arterial hypertension. Hyperkalemia is a relatively common complication and is caused, in part, by tubular resistance to aldosterone. The histologic changes in renal tissue include patchy interstitial fibrosis and tubular atrophy, often in a "striped" pattern. In addition, the intrarenal vasculature often demonstrates hyalinosis, and focal glomerulosclerosis can be present as well. Similar changes may occur in patients receiving CNIs for autoimmune diseases, although the doses are generally lower than those used for organ transplantation. Dose reduction or CNI avoidance appears to mitigate the chronic tubulointerstitial changes, but may increase the risk of rejection and graft loss.

HEAVY METAL (LEAD) NEPHROPATHY

Heavy metals, such as lead or cadmium, can lead to a chronic tubulointerstitial process after prolonged exposure. The disease entity is no longer commonly diagnosed, because such heavy metal exposure has been greatly reduced due to the known health risks from lead and the consequent removal of lead from most commercial products and fuels. Nonetheless, occupational exposure is possible in workers involved in the manufacture or destruction of batteries, removal of lead paint, or manufacture of alloys and electrical equipment (cadmium) in countries where industrial regulation is less stringent. In addition, ingestion of moonshine whiskey distilled in lead-tainted containers has been one of the more frequent sources of lead exposure.

Early signs of chronic lead intoxication are attributable to proximal tubule dysfunction, particularly hyperuricemia as a result of diminished urate secretion. The triad of "saturnine gout," hypertension, and renal insufficiency should prompt a practitioner to ask specifically about lead exposure. Unfortunately, evaluating lead burden is not as straightforward as ordering a blood test; the preferred methods involve measuring urinary lead after infusion of a chelating agent or by radiographic fluoroscopy of bone. Several recent studies have shown an association between chronic low-level lead exposure and decreased renal function, although either of these two factors may have been the primary event. In those patients who have CIN of unclear origin and an elevated total body lead burden, repeated treatments of lead chelation therapy have been shown to slow the decline in renal function.

METABOLIC DISORDERS

Disorders leading to excessively high or low levels of certain electrolytes and products of metabolism can also lead to chronic kidney disease if untreated.

CHRONIC URIC ACID NEPHROPATHY

The constellation of pathologic findings that represent *gouty nephropathy* are very uncommon nowadays and are more of historical interest than clinical importance, as gout is typically well managed with allopurinol and other agents. However, there is emerging evidence that hyperuricemia is an independent risk factor for the development of chronic kidney disease, perhaps through endothelial damage. The complex interactions of hyperuricemia, hypertension, and renal failure are still incompletely understood.

Presently, gouty nephropathy is most likely to be encountered in patients with severe tophaceous gout and prolonged hyperuricemia from a hereditary disorder of purine metabolism (Chap. 431e). This should be distinguished from juvenile hyperuricemic nephropathy, a form of medullary cystic kidney disease caused by mutations in uromodulin (UMOD) (Chap. 339). Histologically, the distinctive feature of gouty nephropathy is the presence of crystalline deposits of uric acid and monosodium urate salts in the kidney parenchyma. These deposits not only cause intrarenal obstruction but also incite an inflammatory response, leading to lymphocytic infiltration, foreign-body giant cell reaction, and eventual fibrosis, especially in the medullary and papillary regions of the kidney. Since patients with gout frequently suffer from hypertension and hyperlipidemia, degenerative changes of the renal arterioles may constitute a striking feature of the histologic abnormality, out of proportion to the other morphologic defects. Clinically, gouty nephropathy is an insidious cause of chronic kidney disease. Early in its course, glomerular filtration rate may be near normal, often despite morphologic changes in medullary and cortical interstitium, proteinuria, and diminished urinary concentrating ability. Treatment with allopurinol and urine alkalinization is generally effective in preventing uric acid nephrolithiasis and the consequences of recurrent kidney stones; however, gouty nephropathy may be intractable to such measures. Furthermore, the use of allopurinol in asymptomatic hyperuricemia has not been consistently shown to improve renal function.

HYPERCALCEMIC NEPHROPATHY

(See also Chap. 424) Chronic hypercalcemia, as occurs in primary hyperparathyroidism, sarcoidosis, multiple myeloma, vitamin D intoxication, or metastatic bone disease, can cause tubulointerstitial disease and progressive renal failure. The earliest lesion is a focal degenerative change in renal epithelia, primarily in collecting ducts, distal tubules, and loops of Henle. Tubular cell necrosis leads to nephron obstruction and stasis of intrarenal urine, favoring local precipitation of calcium salts and infection. Dilation and atrophy of tubules eventually occur, as do interstitial fibrosis, mononuclear leukocyte infiltration, and interstitial calcium deposition (nephrocalcinosis). Calcium deposition may also occur in glomeruli and the walls of renal arterioles.

Clinically, the most striking defect is an inability to maximally concentrate the urine, due to reduced collecting duct responsiveness to arginine vasopressin and defective transport of sodium and chloride in the loop of Henle. Reductions in both glomerular filtration rate and renal blood flow can occur, both in acute and in prolonged hypercalcemia. Eventually, uncontrolled hypercalcemia leads to severe tubulointerstitial damage and overt renal failure. Abdominal x-rays may demonstrate nephrocalcinosis as well as nephrolithiasis, the latter due to the hypercalciuria that often accompanies hypercalcemia.

Treatment consists of reducing the serum calcium concentration toward normal and correcting the primary abnormality of calcium metabolism (Chap. 424). Renal dysfunction of acute hypercalcemia may be completely reversible. Gradual progressive renal insufficiency related to chronic hypercalcemia, however, may not improve even with correction of the calcium disorder.

HYPOKALEMIC NEPHROPATHY

Patients with prolonged and severe hypokalemia from chronic laxative or diuretic abuse, surreptitious vomiting, or primary aldosteronism may develop a reversible tubular lesion characterized by vacuolar degeneration of proximal and distal tubular cells. Eventually, tubular atrophy and cystic dilation accompanied by interstitial fibrosis may ensue, leading to irreversible chronic kidney disease. Timely correction of the hypokalemia will prevent further progression, but persistent hypokalemia can cause ESRD.

GLOBAL PERSPECTIVE

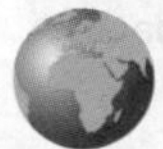

The causes of acute and chronic interstitial nephritis vary widely across the globe. Analgesic nephropathy continues to be seen in countries where phenacetin-containing compound analgesic preparations are readily available. Adulterants in unregulated herbal and traditional medicaments pose a threat of toxic interstitial nephritis, as exemplified by aristolochic acid contamination of herbal slimming preparations. Contamination of food sources with toxins, such as the recent outbreak of nephrolithiasis and acute renal failure from melamine contamination of infant milk formula, poses a continuing risk. Large-scale exposure to aristolochic acid remains prevalent in many Asian countries where traditional herbal medicine use is common. Although industrial exposure to lead and cadmium has largely disappeared as a cause of chronic interstitial nephritis in developed nations, it remains a risk for nephrotoxicity in countries where such exposure is less well controlled. New endemic forms of chronic kidney disease continue to be described, such as the nephropathy found among Pacific coastal plantation workers in Central America, which may be related to repetitive heat exposure and fluid losses.

341 Vascular Injury to the Kidney

Nelson Leung, Stephen C. Textor

The renal circulation is complex and is characterized by a highly perfused arteriolar network, reaching cortical glomerular structures adjacent to lower-flow vasa recta that descend into medullary segments. Disorders of the larger vessels, including renal artery stenosis and atheroembolic disease, are discussed elsewhere (Chap. 354). This chapter examines primary disorders of the renal microvessels, many of which are associated with thrombosis and hemolysis.

THROMBOTIC MICROANGIOPATHY

Thrombotic microangiopathy (TMA) is characterized by injured endothelial cells that are thickened, swollen, or detached mainly from arterioles and capillaries. Platelet and hyaline thrombi causing partial or complete occlusion are integral to the histopathology of TMA. TMA is usually the result of microangiopathic hemolytic anemia (MAHA), with its typical features of thrombocytopenia and schistocytes. In the kidney, TMA is characterized by swollen endocapillary cells (endotheliosis), fibrin thrombi, platelet plugs, arterial intimal fibrosis, and a membranoproliferative pattern. Fibrin thrombi may extend into the arteriolar vascular pole, producing glomerular collapse and at times cortical necrosis. In kidneys that recover from acute TMA, secondary focal segmental glomerulosclerosis may be seen. Diseases associated with this lesion include thrombotic thrombocytopenic purpura (TTP), hemolytic-uremic syndrome (HUS), malignant hypertension, scleroderma renal crisis, antiphospholipid syndrome, preeclampsia/HELLP (hemolysis, elevated liver enzymes, low platelet count) syndrome, HIV infection, and radiation nephropathy.

HEMOLYTIC-UREMIC SYNDROME/THROMBOTIC THROMBOCYTOPENIC PURPURA

HUS and TTP are the prototypes for MAHA. Historically, HUS and TTP were distinguished mainly by their clinical and epidemiologic differences. TTP develops more commonly in adults and was thought to include neurologic involvement more often. HUS occurs more commonly in children, particularly when associated with hemorrhagic diarrhea. However, atypical HUS (aHUS) can first appear in adulthood, and better testing has revealed that neurologic involvement is as common in HUS as in TTP. Accordingly, HUS and TTP now should be differentiated and treated according to their specific pathophysiologic features.

Hemolytic-Uremic Syndrome HUS is loosely defined by the presence of MAHA and renal impairment. At least four variants are recognized. The most common is Shiga toxin–producing *Escherichia coli* (STEC) HUS, which is also known as D$^+$HUS or enterohemorrhagic *E. coli* (EHEC) HUS. Most cases involve children <5 years of age, but adults also are susceptible, as evidenced by a 2011 outbreak in northern Europe. Diarrhea, often bloody, precedes MAHA within 1 week in >80% of cases. Abdominal pain, cramping, and vomiting are frequent, whereas fever is typically absent. Neurologic symptoms, including dysphasia, hyperreflexia, blurred vision, memory deficits, encephalopathy, perseveration, and agraphia, often develop, especially in adults. Seizures and cerebral infarction can occur in severe cases. STEC HUS is caused by the Shiga toxins (Stx1 and Stx2), which are also referred to as *verotoxins.* These toxins are produced by certain strains of *E. coli* and *Shigella dysenteriae.* In the United States and Europe, the most common STEC strain is O157:H7, but HUS due to other strains (O157/H$^-$, O111:H$^-$, O26:H11/H$^-$, O145:H28, and O104:H4) has occurred. After entry into the circulation, Shiga toxin binds to the glycolipid surface receptor globotriaosylceramide (Gb3), which is richly expressed on cells of the renal microvasculature. Upon binding, the toxin enters the cells, inducing inflammatory cytokines (interleukin 8 [IL-8], monocyte chemotactic protein 1 [MCP-1], and stromal cell–derived factor 1 [SDF-1]) and chemokine receptors (CXCR4 and CXCR7); this action results in platelet aggregation and the microangiopathic process. *Streptococcus pneumoniae* can also cause HUS. Certain strains produce a neuraminidase that cleaves the N-acetylneuraminic acid moieties covering the Thomsen-Friedenreich antigen on platelets and endothelial cells. Exposure of this normally cryptic antigen to preformed IgM results in severe MAHA.

Atypical HUS is the result of congenital complement dysregulation. The affected patients have the low C3 and normal C4 levels characteristic of alternative pathway activation. Factor H deficiency, the most common defect, has been linked to families with aHUS. Factor H competes with factor B to prevent the formation of C3bBb and acts as a cofactor for factor I, which proteolytically degrades C3b. More than 70 mutations of the factor H gene have been identified. Most are missense mutations that produce abnormalities in the C-terminus region, affecting its binding to C3b but not its concentration. Other mutations result in low levels or the complete absence of the protein. Deficiencies in other complement-regulatory proteins, such as factor I, factor B, membrane cofactor protein (CD46), C3, complement factor H–related protein 1 (CFHR1), CFHR3, CFHR5, and thrombomodulin, have also been reported. Finally, an autoimmune variant of aHUS has been discovered. DEAP (deficient for CFHR protein and positive for factor H autoantibody) HUS occurs when an autoantibody to factor H is formed. DEAP HUS is often associated with a deletion of an 84-kb fragment of the chromosome that encodes for CFHR1 and CFHR3. The autoantibody blocks the binding of factor H to C3b and surface-bound C3 convertase.

Thrombotic Thrombocytopenic Purpura Traditionally, TTP is characterized by the pentad: MAHA, thrombocytopenia, neurologic symptoms, fever, and renal failure. The pathophysiology of TTP involves the accumulation of ultra-large multimers of von Willebrand factor as a result of the absence or markedly decreased activity (<5–10%) of the plasma protease ADAMTS13, a disintegrin and metalloproteinase with a thrombospondin type 1 motif, member 13. These ultra-large multimers form clots and shear erythrocytes, resulting in MAHA; however, the absence of ADAMTS13 alone may not itself produce TTP. Often, an additional trigger (such as infection, surgery, pancreatitis, or pregnancy) is required to initiate clinical TTP.

Data from the Oklahoma TTP/HUS Registry suggest an incidence rate of 11.3 cases/10^6 patients in the United States. The median age of onset is 40 years. The incidence is more than nine times higher among blacks than among non-blacks. Like that of systemic lupus erythematosus, the incidence of TTP is nearly three times higher among women than among men. If untreated, TTP has a mortality rate exceeding 90%. Even with modern therapy, 20% of patients die within the first month from complications of microvascular thrombosis.

The classic form of TTP is idiopathic TTP, which is usually the result of a deficiency in ADAMTS13. While TTP had traditionally been associated with infection, malignancy, and intense inflammation (e.g., pancreatitis), ADAMTS13 activity usually is not decreased in these conditions. In idiopathic TTP, the formation of an autoantibody to ADAMTS13 (IgG or IgM) either increases its clearance or inhibits its activity. Upshaw-Schülman syndrome is a hereditary condition characterized by congenital deficiency of ADAMTS13. TTP in these patients can start within the first weeks of life but in some instances may not present until the patient is several years of age. Both environmental and genetic factors are thought to influence the development of TTP. Plasma transfusion is an effective strategy for prevention and treatment.

Drug-induced TMA is a recognized complication of treatment with some chemotherapeutic agents, immunosuppressive agents, antiplatelet agents, and quinine. Two different mechanisms have been described. Endothelial damage (pathologically similar to that in HUS) is the main cause of the TMA that develops in association with chemotherapeutic agents (e.g., mitomycin C, gemcitabine) and immunosuppressive agents (cyclosporine, tacrolimus, and sirolimus). This process is usually dose-dependent. Alternatively, TMA may develop as a result of drug-induced autoantibodies. This form is less likely to be dose-dependent and can, in fact, occur after a single dose in patients with previous exposure. Ticlopidine produces TTP by inducing an autoantibody to ADAMTS13, but ADAMTS13 deficiency is found in fewer than half of patients with clopidogrel-associated TTP. Quinine appears to induce autoantibodies to granulocytes, lymphocytes, endothelial cells, and platelet glycoprotein IbB/IX or IIb/IIIa complexes, but not to ADAMTS13. Quinine-associated TTP is more common among women. TMA has been reported with drugs that inhibit vascular endothelial growth factor, such as bevacizumab; the mechanism is not completely understood.

TREATMENT HUS/TTP

Treatment should be based on pathophysiology. Autoantibody-mediated TTP and DEAP HUS respond to plasma exchange or plasmapheresis. In addition to removing the autoantibodies, plasma exchange with fresh-frozen plasma replaces ADAMTS13. Twice-daily plasma exchanges with administration of vincristine and rituximab may be effective in refractory cases. Plasma infusion is usually sufficient to replace the ADAMTS13 in Upshaw-Schülman syndrome. Plasma exchange should be considered if larger volumes are necessary. Drug-induced TMA secondary to endothelial damage typically does not respond to plasma exchange and is treated primarily by discontinuing use of the agent and providing supportive care. Similarly, STEC HUS should be treated with supportive measures. Plasma exchange has not been found to be effective. Antimotility agents and antibiotics increase the incidence of HUS among children, but azithromycin was recently found to decrease the duration of bacterial shedding by adults. Eculizumab is a monoclonal antibody to C5 that is approved for use in aHUS, for which ongoing therapy may be necessary. Plasma infusion/exchange may play a role in aHUS by replacing complement-regulatory proteins. Antibiotics and washed red cells should be given in neuraminidase-associated HUS, and plasmapheresis may be helpful. However, plasma and whole-blood transfusion should be avoided since these products contain IgM, which may exacerbate MAHA. Finally, combined factor H and ADAMTS13 deficiency have been reported. The affected patients are generally less responsive to plasma infusion, a result illustrating the complexity of the management of these cases.

HEMATOPOIETIC STEM CELL TRANSPLANTATION–ASSOCIATED THROMBOTIC MICROANGIOPATHY (HSCT-TMA)

HSCT-TMA develops after HSCT, with an incidence of 8.2%. Etiologic factors include conditioning regimens, immunosuppression, infections, and graft-versus-host disease. Other risk factors include female sex and human leukocyte antigen (HLA)–mismatched donor grafts. HSCT-TMA usually occurs within the first 100 days of HSCT. Table 341-1 lists definitions of HSCT-TMA currently used for clinical trials. Diagnosis may be difficult since thrombocytopenia, anemia, and renal insufficiency are common after HSCT. HSCT-TMA carries a high mortality rate (75% within 3 months). The majority of patients have >5% ADAMTS13 activity, and plasma exchange is beneficial in <50% of patients. Discontinuation of calcineurin inhibitors and substitution with daclizumab (antibody to the IL-2 receptor) are recommended. Treatment with rituximab and defibrotide may also be helpful.

TABLE 341-1 CRITERIA FOR ESTABLISHING MICROANGIOPATHIC KIDNEY INJURY ASSOCIATED WITH HEMATOPOIETIC STEM CELL TRANSPLANTATION

International Working Group	Blood and Marrow Transplant Clinical Trials Network Toxicity Committee
>4% schistocytes in the blood	RBC fragmentation and at least 2 schistocytes per high-power field
De novo, prolonged, or progressive thrombocytopenia	Concurrent increase in LDH concentration above baseline
A sudden and persistent increase in LDH concentration	Negative direct and indirect Coombs test
Decrease in hemoglobin level or increased RBC transfusion requirement	Concurrent renal and/or neurologic dysfunction without other explanations
Decrease in haptoglobin concentration	

Note: These features underscore the need to identify pathways of hemolysis and thrombocytopenia that accompany deterioration of kidney function.

Abbreviations: LDH, lactate dehydrogenase; RBC, red blood cell.

HIV-RELATED TMA

HIV-related TMA is a complication encountered mainly before widespread use of highly active antiretroviral therapy. It is seen in patients with advanced AIDS and low CD4+ T cell counts although it can be the first manifestation of HIV infection. The presence of MAHA, thrombocytopenia, and renal failure are suggestive, but renal biopsy is required for diagnosis since other renal diseases are also associated with HIV infection. Thrombocytopenia may prohibit renal biopsy in some patients. The mechanism of injury is unclear, although HIV can induce apoptosis in endothelial cells. ADAMTS13 activity is not reduced in these patients. Cytomegalovirus co-infection may also be a risk factor. Effective antiviral therapy is key, while plasma exchange should be limited to patients who have evidence of TTP.

RADIATION NEPHROPATHY

Either local or total body irradiation can produce microangiopathic injury. The kidney is one of the most radiosensitive organs, and injury can result with as little as 4–5 Gy. Such injury is characterized by renal insufficiency, proteinuria, and hypertension usually developing ≥6 months after radiation exposure. Renal biopsy reveals classic TMA with damage to glomerular, tubular, and vascular cells, but systemic evidence of MAHA is uncommon. Because of its high incidence after allogeneic HSCT, radiation nephropathy is often referred to as *bone marrow transplant nephropathy*. No specific therapy is available, although observational evidence supports renin-angiotensin system blockade.

SCLERODERMA (PROGRESSIVE SYSTEMIC SCLEROSIS)

Kidney involvement is common (up to 52%) in patients with widespread scleroderma, with 20% of cases resulting directly from scleroderma renal crisis. Other renal manifestations in scleroderma include transient (prerenal) or medication-related forms of acute kidney injury (e.g., associated with *D*-penicillamine, nonsteroidal anti-inflammatory drugs, or cyclosporine). Scleroderma renal crisis occurs in 12% of patients with diffuse systemic sclerosis but in only 2% of those with limited systemic sclerosis. Scleroderma renal crisis is the most severe manifestation of renal involvement, and is characterized by accelerated hypertension, a rapid decline in renal function, nephrotic proteinuria, and hematuria. Retinopathy and encephalopathy may accompany the hypertension. Salt and water retention with microvascular injury can lead to pulmonary edema. Cardiac manifestations, including myocarditis, pericarditis, and arrhythmias, denote an especially poor prognosis. Although MAHA is present in more half of patients, coagulopathy is rare.

The renal lesion in scleroderma renal crisis is characterized by arcuate artery intimal and medial proliferation with luminal narrowing.

This lesion is described as "onion-skinning" and can be accompanied by glomerular collapse due to reduced blood flow. Histologically, scleroderma renal crisis is indistinguishable from malignant hypertension, with which it can coexist. Fibrinoid necrosis and thrombosis are common. Before the availability of angiotensin-converting enzyme (ACE) inhibitors, the mortality rate for scleroderma renal crisis was >90% at 1 month. Introduction of renin-angiotensin system blockade has lowered the mortality rate to 30% at 3 years. Nearly two-thirds of patients with scleroderma renal crisis may require dialysis support, with recovery of renal function in 50% (median time, 1 year). Glomerulonephritis and vasculitis associated with antineutrophil cytoplasmic antibodies and systemic lupus erythematosus have been described in patients with scleroderma. An association has been found with a speckled pattern of antinuclear antibodies and with antibodies to RNA polymerases I and III. Anti-U3-RNP may identify young patients at risk for scleroderma renal crisis. Anticentromere antibody, in contrast, is a negative predictor of this disorder. Because of the overlap between scleroderma renal crisis and other autoimmune disorders, a renal biopsy is recommended for patients with atypical renal involvement, especially if hypertension is absent.

Treatment with ACE inhibition is the first-line therapy unless contraindicated. The goal of therapy is to reduce systolic and diastolic blood pressure by 20 mmHg and 10 mmHg, respectively, every 24 h until blood pressure is normal. Additional antihypertensive therapy may be given once the dose of drug for ACE inhibition is maximized. Both ACE inhibitors and angiotensin II receptor antagonists are effective, although data suggest that treatment with ACE inhibitors is superior. ACE inhibition alone does not prevent scleroderma renal crisis, but it does reduce the impact of hypertension. Intravenous iloprost has been used in Europe for blood pressure management and improvement of renal perfusion. Kidney transplantation is not recommended for 2 years after the start of dialysis since delayed recovery may occur.

ANTIPHOSPHOLIPID SYNDROME

Antiphospholipid syndrome (Chap. 379) can be either primary or secondary to systemic lupus erythematosus. It is characterized by a predisposition to systemic thrombosis (arterial and venous) and fetal morbidity mediated by antiphospholipid antibodies—mainly anticardiolipin antibodies (IgG, IgM, or IgA), lupus anticoagulant, or anti-β-2 glycoprotein I antibodies (antiβ2GPI). Patients with both anticardiolipin antibodies and antiβ2GPI appear to have the highest risk of thrombosis. The vascular compartment within the kidney is the main site of renal involvement. Arteriosclerosis is commonly present in the arcuate and intralobular arteries. In the intralobular arteries, fibrous intimal hyperplasia characterized by intimal thickening secondary to intense myofibroblastic intimal cellular proliferation with extracellular matrix deposition is frequently seen along with onion-skinning. Arterial and arteriolar fibrous and fibrocellular occlusions are present in more than two-thirds of biopsy samples. Cortical necrosis and focal cortical atrophy may result from vascular occlusion. TMA is commonly present in renal biopsies, although signs of MAHA and platelet consumption are usually absent. TMA is especially common in the catastrophic variant of antiphospholipid syndrome. In patients with secondary antiphospholipid syndrome, other glomerulopathies may be present, including membranous nephropathy, minimal change disease, focal segmental glomerulosclerosis, and pauci-immune crescentic glomerulonephritis.

Large vessels can be involved in antiphospholipid syndrome and may form the proximal nidus near the ostium for thrombosis of the renal artery. Renal vein thrombosis can occur and should be suspected in patients with lupus anticoagulant who develop nephrotic-range proteinuria. Progression to end-stage renal disease can occur, and a thrombosis may form in the vascular access and the renal allografts. Hypertension is common. Treatment entails lifelong anticoagulation. Glucocorticoids may be beneficial in accelerated hypertension. Immunosuppression and plasma exchange may be helpful for catastrophic episodes of antiphospholipid syndrome but by themselves do not reduce recurrent thrombosis.

HELLP SYNDROME

HELLP (hemolysis, elevated liver enzymes, low platelets) syndrome is a dangerous complication of pregnancy associated with microvascular injury. Occurring in 0.2–0.9% of all pregnancies and in 10–20% of women with severe preeclampsia, this syndrome carries a mortality rate of 7.4–34%. Most commonly developing in the third trimester, 10% of cases occur before week 27 and 30% post-partum. Although a strong association exists between HELLP syndrome and preeclampsia, nearly 20% of cases are not preceded by recognized preeclampsia. Risk factors include abnormal placentation, family history, and elevated levels of fetal mRNA for FLT1 (vascular endothelial growth factor receptor 1) and endoglin. Patients with HELLP syndrome have higher levels of inflammatory markers (C-reactive protein, IL-1Ra, and IL-6) and soluble HLA-DR than do those with preeclampsia alone.

Renal failure occurs in half of patients with HELLP syndrome, although the etiology is not well understood. Limited data suggest that renal failure is the result of both preeclampsia and acute tubular necrosis. Renal histologic findings are those of TMA with endothelial cell swelling and occlusion of the capillary lumens, but luminal thrombi are typically absent. However, thrombi become more common in severe eclampsia and HELLP syndrome. Although renal failure is common, the organ that defines this syndrome is the liver. Subcapsular hepatic hematomas sometimes produce spontaneous rupture of the liver and can be life threatening. Neurologic complications such as cerebral infarction, cerebral and brainstem hemorrhage, and cerebral edema are other potentially life-threatening complications. Nonfatal complications include placental abruption, permanent vision loss due to Purtscher-like (hemorrhagic and vaso-occlusive vasculopathy) retinopathy, pulmonary edema, bleeding, and fetal demise.

Many features are shared by HELLP syndrome and MAHA. Diagnosis of HELLP syndrome is complicated by the fact that aHUS and TTP also can be triggered by pregnancy. Patients with antiphospholipid syndrome also have an elevated risk of HELLP syndrome. A history of MAHA before pregnancy is of diagnostic value. Serum levels of ADAMTS13 activity are reduced (by 30–60%) in HELLP syndrome but not to the levels seen in TTP (<5%). Determination of the ratio of lactate dehydrogenase to aspartate aminotransferase may be helpful; this ratio is 13:1 in patients with HELLP syndrome and preeclampsia as opposed to 29:1 in patients without preeclampsia. Other markers, such as antithrombin III (decreased in HELLP syndrome but not in TTP) and D-dimer (elevated in HELLP syndrome but not in TTP), may also be useful. HELLP syndrome usually resolves spontaneously after delivery, although a small percentage of HELLP cases occur post partum. Glucocorticoids may decrease inflammatory markers, although two randomized controlled trials failed to show much benefit. Plasma exchange should be considered if hemolysis is refractory to glucocorticoids and/or delivery, especially if TTP has not been ruled out.

SICKLE CELL NEPHROPATHY

Renal complications in sickle cell disease result from occlusion of the vasa recta in the renal medulla. The low partial pressure of oxygen and high osmolarity predispose to hemoglobin S polymerization and erythrocyte sickling. Sequelae include hyposthenuria, hematuria, and papillary necrosis (which can also occur in sickle trait). The kidney responds by increases in blood flow and glomerular filtration rate mediated by prostaglandins. This dependence on prostaglandins may explain the greater reduction of glomerular filtration rate by nonsteroidal anti-inflammatory drugs in these patients than in others. The glomeruli are typically enlarged. Intracapillary fragmentation and phagocytosis of sickled erythrocytes are thought to be responsible for the membranoproliferative glomerulonephritis–like lesion, and focal segmental glomerulosclerosis is seen in more advanced cases. Proteinuria is present in 20–30%, and nephrotic-range proteinuria is associated with progression to renal failure. ACE inhibitors reduce proteinuria, although data are lacking on prevention of renal failure. Patients with sickle cell disease are also more prone to acute renal failure. The cause is thought to reflect microvascular occlusion associated with nontraumatic rhabdomyolysis, high fever, infection, and generalized sickling. Chronic kidney disease is present in 12–20% of patients. Despite the frequency of renal disease, hypertension is uncommon in patients with sickle cell disease.

RENAL VEIN THROMBOSIS

Renal vein thrombosis either can present with flank pain, tenderness, hematuria, rapid decline in renal function, and proteinuria or can be silent. Occasionally, renal vein thrombosis is identified during a workup for pulmonary embolism. The left renal vein is more commonly involved, and two-thirds of cases are bilateral. Etiologies can be divided into three broad categories: endothelial damage, venous stasis, and hypercoagulability. Homocystinuria, endovascular intervention, and surgery can produce vascular endothelial damage. Dehydration, which is more common among male patients, is a common cause of stasis in the pediatric population. Stasis also can result from compression and kinking of the renal veins from retroperitoneal processes such as retroperitoneal fibrosis and abdominal neoplasms. Thrombosis can occur throughout the renal circulation, including the renal veins, with antiphospholipid antibody syndrome. Renal vein thrombosis can also be secondary to nephrotic syndrome, particularly membranous nephropathy. Other hypercoagulable states less commonly associated with renal vein thrombosis include proteins C and S, antithrombin deficiency, factor V Leiden, disseminated malignancy, and oral contraceptives. Severe nephrotic syndrome may also predispose patients to renal vein thrombosis.

Diagnostic screening can be performed with Doppler ultrasonography, which is more sensitive than ultrasonography alone. CT angiography is nearly 100% sensitive. Magnetic resonance angiography is another option but is more expensive. Treatment for renal vein thrombosis consists of anticoagulation and therapy for the underlying cause. Endovascular thrombolysis may be considered in severe cases. Occasionally, nephrectomy may be undertaken for life-threatening complications. Vena caval filters are often used to prevent migration of thrombi.

342 Nephrolithiasis

Gary C. Curhan

Nephrolithiasis, or kidney stone disease, is a common, painful, and costly condition. Each year, billions of dollars are spent on nephrolithiasis-related activity, with the majority of expenditures on surgical treatment of existing stones. While a stone may form due to crystallization of lithogenic factors in the upper urinary tract, it can subsequently move into the ureter and cause renal colic. Although nephrolithiasis is rarely fatal, patients who have had renal colic report that it is the worst pain they have ever experienced. The evidence on which to base clinical recommendations is not as strong as desired; nonetheless, most experts agree that the recurrence of most, if not all, types of stones can be prevented with careful evaluation and targeted recommendations. Preventive treatment may be lifelong; therefore, an in-depth understanding of this condition must inform the implementation of tailored interventions that are most appropriate for and acceptable to the patient.

There are various types of kidney stones. It is clinically important to identify the stone type, which informs prognosis and selection of the optimal preventive regimen. Calcium oxalate stones are most common (~75%); next, in order, are calcium phosphate (~15%), uric acid (~8%), struvite (~1%), and cystine (<1%) stones. Many stones are a mixture of crystal types (e.g., calcium oxalate and calcium phosphate) and also contain protein in the stone matrix. Rarely, stones are composed of medications, such as acyclovir, indinavir, and triamterene.

Infectious stones, if not appropriately treated, can have devastating consequences and lead to end-stage renal disease. Consideration should be given to teaching practitioners strategies to prevent stone recurrence and its related morbidity.

EPIDEMIOLOGY

Nephrolithiasis is a global disease. Data suggest an increasing prevalence, likely due to Westernization of lifestyle habits (e.g., dietary changes, increasing body mass index). National Health and Nutrition Examination Survey data for 2007–2010 indicate that up to 19% of men and 9% of women will develop at least one stone during their lifetime. The prevalence is ~50% lower among black individuals than among whites. The incidence of nephrolithiasis (i.e., the rate at which previously unaffected individuals develop their first stone) also varies by age, sex, and race. Among white men, the peak annual incidence is ~3.5 cases/1000 at age 40 and declines to ~2 cases/1000 by age 70. Among white women in their thirties, the annual incidence is ~2.5 cases/1000; the figure decreases to ~1.5/1000 at age 50 and beyond. In addition to the medical costs associated with nephrolithiasis, this condition also has a substantial economic impact, as those affected are often of working age. Once an individual has had a stone, the prevention of a recurrence is essential. Published recurrence rates vary by the definitions and diagnostic methods used. Some reports have relied on symptomatic events, while others have been based on imaging. Most experts agree that radiographic evidence of a second stone should be considered to represent a recurrence, even if the stone has not yet caused symptoms.

ASSOCIATED MEDICAL CONDITIONS

Nephrolithiasis is a systemic disorder. Several conditions predispose to stone formation, including gastrointestinal malabsorption (e.g., Crohn's disease, gastric bypass surgery), primary hyperparathyroidism, obesity, type 2 diabetes mellitus, and distal renal tubular acidosis. A number of other medical conditions are more likely to be present in individuals with a history of nephrolithiasis, including hypertension, gout, cholelithiasis, reduced bone mineral density, and chronic kidney disease.

Individuals with medullary sponge kidney (MSK), a condition designated by an anatomic description, often have metabolic abnormalities, such as higher levels of urine calcium and lower levels of urine citrate, and are more likely to form calcium phosphate stones. As intravenous urography is now rarely used, the diagnosis of MSK has become less frequent. Fortunately, the diagnosis of MSK does not change either the evaluation or the treatment recommendations; thus, it is not essential in pursuing the diagnosis of nephrolithiasis.

Although nephrolithiasis does not directly cause upper urinary tract infections (UTIs), a UTI in the setting of an obstructing stone is a urologic emergency ("pus under pressure") and requires urgent intervention to reestablish drainage.

PATHOGENESIS

In the consideration of the processes involved in crystal formation, it is helpful to view urine as a complex solution. A clinically useful concept is *supersaturation* (the point at which the concentration product exceeds the solubility product). However, even though the urine in most individuals is supersaturated with respect to one or more types of crystals, the presence of inhibitors of crystallization prevents the majority of the population from continuously forming stones. The most clinically important inhibitor of calcium-containing stones is urine citrate. While supersaturation is a calculated value (rather than being directly measured) and does not perfectly predict stone formation, it is a useful guide as it integrates the multiple factors that are measured in a 24-h urine collection.

Recent studies have changed the paradigm for the site of initiation of stone formation. Renal biopsies of stone formers have revealed calcium phosphate in the renal interstitium. It is hypothesized that this calcium phosphate extends down to the papilla and erodes through the papillary epithelium, where it provides a site for deposition of calcium oxalate and calcium phosphate crystals. The majority of calcium oxalate stones grow on calcium phosphate at the tip of the renal papilla (*Randall's plaque*). Thus, the process of stone formation may begin years before a clinically detectable stone is identified. The processes involved in interstitial deposition are under active investigation.

RISK FACTORS

Risk factors for nephrolithiasis can be categorized as dietary, nondietary, or urinary.These risk factors vary by stone type and by clinical characteristics.

Dietary Risk Factors Patients who develop stones often change their diet; therefore, studies that retrospectively assess diet may be hampered by recall bias. Some studies have examined the relation between diet and changes in the lithogenic composition of the urine, often using calculated supersaturation. However, the composition of the urine does not perfectly predict risk, and not all components that modify risk are included in the calculation of supersaturation. Thus, dietary associations are best investigated by prospective studies that examine actual stone formation as the outcome. Dietary factors that are associated with an increased risk of nephrolithiasis include animal protein, oxalate, sodium, sucrose, and fructose. Dietary factors associated with a lower risk include calcium, potassium, and phytate.

CALCIUM The role of dietary calcium deserves special attention. Although in the past dietary calcium had been suspected of increasing the risk of stone disease, several prospective observational studies and a randomized controlled trial have demonstrated that higher dietary calcium intake is related to a *lower* risk of stone formation. The reduction in risk associated with higher calcium intake may be due to a reduction in intestinal absorption of dietary oxalate that results in lower urine oxalate. Low calcium intake is contraindicated as it increases the risk of stone formation and may contribute to lower bone density in stone formers.

Despite similar bioavailability, supplemental calcium may increase the risk of stone formation. The discrepancy between the risks from dietary calcium and calcium supplements may be due to the timing of supplemental calcium intake or to higher total calcium consumption leading to higher urinary calcium excretion.

OXALATE Urinary oxalate is derived from both endogenous production and absorption of dietary oxalate. Owing to its low and often variable bioavailability, much of the oxalate in food may not be readily absorbed. However, absorption may be higher in stone formers. Although observational studies demonstrate that dietary oxalate is only a weak risk factor for stone formation, urinary oxalate is a strong risk factor for calcium oxalate stone formation, and efforts to avoid high oxalate intake should thus be beneficial.

OTHER NUTRIENTS Several other nutrients have been studied and implicated in stone formation. Higher intake of animal protein may lead to increased excretion of calcium and uric acid as well as to decreased urinary excretion of citrate, all of which increase the risk of stone formation. Higher sodium and sucrose intake increases calcium excretion independent of calcium intake. Higher potassium intake decreases calcium excretion, and many potassium-rich foods increase urinary citrate excretion due to their alkali content. Other dietary factors that have been inconsistently associated with lower stone risk include magnesium and phytate.

Vitamin C supplements are associated with an increased risk of calcium oxalate stone formation, possibly because of raised levels of oxalate in urine. Thus, calcium oxalate stone formers should be advised to avoid vitamin C supplements. Although high doses of supplemental vitamin B_6 may be beneficial in selected patients with type 1 primary hyperoxaluria, the benefit of supplemental vitamin B_6 in other patients is uncertain.

FLUIDS AND BEVERAGES The risk of stone formation increases as urine volume decreases. When the urine output is less than 1 L/d, the risk of stone formation more than doubles. Fluid intake is the main determinant of urine volume, and the importance of fluid intake in preventing stone formation has been demonstrated in observational studies and in a randomized controlled trial. Observational studies have found that coffee, tea, beer, and wine are associated with a reduced risk of stone formation. Sugar-sweetened carbonated beverage consumption may increase risk.

Nondietary Risk Factors Age, race, body size, and environment are important risk factors for nephrolithiasis. The incidence of stone disease is highest in middle-aged white men, but stones can form in infants as well as in the elderly. There is geographic variability, with the highest prevalence in the southeastern United States. Weight gain increases the risk of stone formation, and the increasing prevalence of nephrolithiasis in the United States may be due in part to the increasing prevalence of obesity. Environmental and occupational influences that may lead to lower urine volume, such as working in a hot environment or lack of ready access to water or a bathroom, are important considerations.

Urinary Risk Factors • *URINE VOLUME* As mentioned above, lower urine volume results in increased concentrations of lithogenic factors and is a common and readily modifiable risk factor. A randomized trial has demonstrated the effectiveness of elevated fluid intake in increasing urine volume and reducing the risk of stone recurrence.

URINE CALCIUM Higher urine calcium excretion increases the likelihood of formation of calcium oxalate and calcium phosphate stones. While the term *hypercalciuria* is often used, there is no widely accepted cutoff that distinguishes between normal and abnormal urine calcium excretion. In fact, the relation between urine calcium and stone risk appears to be continuous; thus the use of an arbitrary threshold should be avoided. Levels of urine calcium excretion are higher in individuals with a history of nephrolithiasis; however, the mechanisms remain poorly understood. Greater gastrointestinal calcium absorption is one important contributor, and greater bone turnover (with a resultant reduction in bone mineral density) may be another. Primary renal calcium loss, with lower serum calcium concentrations and elevated serum levels of parathyroid hormone (PTH) (and a normal 25-hydroxy vitamin D level), is rare.

URINE OXALATE Higher urine oxalate excretion increases the likelihood of calcium oxalate stone formation. As for urine calcium, no definition for "abnormal" urine oxalate excretion is widely accepted. Given that the relation between urine oxalate and stone risk is continuous, simple dichotomization of urine oxalate excretion is not helpful in assessing risk. The two sources of urine oxalate are endogenous generation and dietary intake. Dietary oxalate is the major contributor and also the source that can be modified. Notably, higher dietary calcium intake reduces gastrointestinal oxalate absorption and thereby reduces urine oxalate.

URINE CITRATE Urine citrate is a natural inhibitor of calcium-containing stones; thus, lower urine citrate excretion increases the risk of stone formation. Citrate reabsorption is influenced by the intracellular pH of proximal tubular cells. Metabolic acidosis will lead to a reduction in citrate excretion by increasing reabsorption of filtered citrate. However, a notable proportion of patients have lower urine citrate for reasons that remain unclear.

URINE URIC ACID Higher urine levels of uric acid—a risk factor for uric acid stone formation—are found in individuals with excess purine consumption and rare genetic conditions that lead to overproduction of uric acid. This characteristic does not appear to be associated with the risk of calcium oxalate stone formation.

URINE pH Urine pH influences the solubility of some crystal types. Uric acid stones form only when the urine pH is consistently ≤5.5 or lower, whereas calcium phosphate stones are more likely to form when the urine pH is ≥6.5 or higher. Cystine is more soluble at higher urine pH. Calcium oxalate stones are not influenced by urine pH.

Genetic Risk Factors The risk of nephrolithiasis is more than twofold greater in individuals with a family history of stone disease. This association is likely due to a combination of genetic predisposition and similar environmental exposures. While a number of monogenic disorders cause nephrolithiasis, the genetic contributors to common forms of stone disease remain to be determined.

The two most common and well-characterized rare monogenic disorders that lead to stone formation are primary hyperoxaluria and cystinuria. *Primary hyperoxaluria* is an autosomal recessive disorder that causes excessive endogenous oxalate generation by the liver, with consequent calcium oxalate stone formation and crystal deposition in organs. Intraparenchymal calcium oxalate deposition in the kidney can eventually lead to renal failure. *Cystinuria* is an autosomal recessive disorder that causes abnormal reabsorption of filtered dibasic amino acids. The excessive urinary excretion of cystine, which is poorly soluble, leads to cystine stone formation. Cystine stones are visible on plain radiographs and often manifest as staghorn calculi or multiple bilateral stones. Repeat episodes of obstruction and instrumentation can cause chronic renal impairment.

APPROACH TO THE PATIENT: Nephrolithiasis

At present, there are no widely accepted, evidence-based guidelines for the evaluation and treatment of nephrolithiasis. However, there are standard approaches to patients with acute and chronic presentations that can reasonably guide the clinical evaluation.

It typically requires weeks to months (and often much longer) for a kidney stone to grow to a clinically detectable size. Although the passage of a stone is a dramatic event, stone formation and growth are characteristically clinically silent. A stone can remain asymptomatic in the kidney for years or even decades before signs (e.g., hematuria) or symptoms (e.g., pain) become apparent. Thus, it is important to remember that the onset of symptoms, typically attributable to a stone moving into the ureter, does not provide insight into when the stone actually formed. The factors that induce stone movement are unknown.

Clinical Presentation and Differential Diagnosis There are two common presentations for individuals with an acute stone event: renal colic and painless gross hematuria. *Renal colic* is a misnomer because pain typically does not subside completely; rather, it varies in intensity. When a stone moves into the ureter, the discomfort often begins with a sudden onset of unilateral flank pain. The intensity of the pain can increase rapidly, and there are no alleviating factors. This pain, which is accompanied often by nausea and occasionally by vomiting, may radiate, depending on the location of the stone. If the stone lodges in the upper part of the ureter, pain may radiate anteriorly; if the stone is in the lower part of the ureter, pain can radiate to the ipsilateral testicle in men or the ipsilateral labium in women. Occasionally, a patient has gross hematuria without pain.

Other diagnoses may be confused with acute renal colic. If the stone is lodged at the right ureteral pelvic junction, symptoms may mimic those of acute cholecystitis. If the stone blocks the ureter as it crosses over the right pelvic brim, symptoms may mimic acute appendicitis, whereas blockage at the left pelvic brim may be confused with acute diverticulitis. If the stone lodges in the ureter at the ureterovesical junction, the patient may experience urinary urgency and frequency. In female patients, the latter symptoms may lead to an incorrect diagnosis of bacterial cystitis; the urine will contain red and white blood cells, but the urine culture will be negative. An obstructing stone with proximal infection may present as acute pyelonephritis. A UTI in the setting of ureteral obstruction is a medical emergency that requires immediate restoration of drainage by placement of either a ureteral stent or a percutaneous nephrostomy tube. Other conditions to consider in the differential diagnosis include muscular or skeletal pain, *herpes zoster*, duodenal ulcer, abdominal aortic aneurysm, gynecologic conditions, ureteral stricture, and ureteral obstruction by materials other than a stone, such as a blood clot or sloughed papilla. Extraluminal processes can lead to ureteral compression and obstruction; however, because of the gradual onset, these conditions do not typically present with renal colic.

Diagnosis and Intervention Serum chemistry findings are typically normal, but the white blood cell count may be elevated. Examination of the urine sediment will usually reveal red and white blood cells and occasionally crystals (Fig. 342-1). The absence of hematuria does not exclude a stone, particularly when urine flow is completely obstructed by a stone.

The diagnosis is often made on the basis of the history, physical examination, and urinalysis. Thus, it may not be necessary to wait for radiographic confirmation before treating the symptoms. The diagnosis is confirmed by an appropriate imaging study—preferably helical CT, which is highly sensitive, allows visualization of uric acid stones (traditionally considered "radiolucent"), and is able to avoid radiocontrast (Fig. 342-2). Helical CT detects stones as small as 1 mm that may be missed by other imaging modalities. Typically, helical CT reveals a ureteral stone or evidence of recent passage (e.g., perinephric stranding or hydronephrosis), whereas a plain abdominal radiograph (kidney/ureter/bladder, or KUB) can miss a stone in the ureter or kidney, even if it is radiopaque, and does not provide information on obstruction. Abdominal ultrasound offers the advantage of avoiding radiation and provides

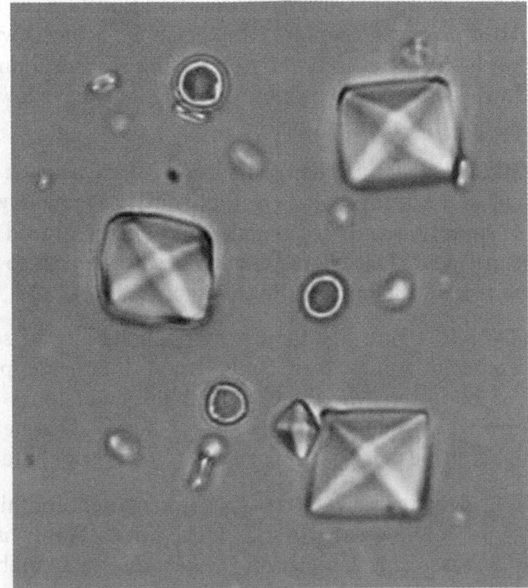

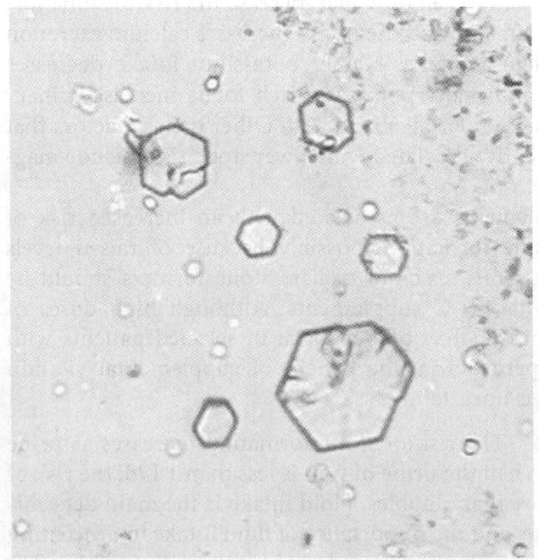

FIGURE 342-1 Urine sediment from a patient with calcium oxalate stones (*left*) and a patient with cystine stones (*right*). Calcium oxalate dihydrate crystals are bipyramidally shaped, and cystine crystals are hexagonal. *(Left panel image courtesy of Dr. John Lieske, Mayo Clinic.)*

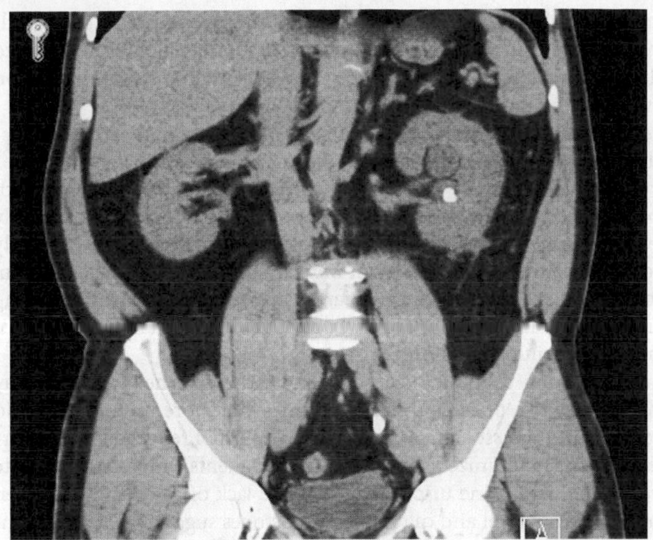

FIGURE 342-2 Coronal noncontrast CT image from a patient who presented with left-sided renal colic. An obstructing calculus, present in the distal left ureter at the level of S1, measures 10 mm in maximal dimension. There is severe left hydroureteronephrosis and associated left perinephric fat stranding. In addition, there is a non-obstructing 6-mm left renal calculus in the interpolar region. *(Image courtesy of Dr. Stuart Silverman, Brigham and Women's Hospital.)*

information on hydronephrosis, but it is not as sensitive as CT and images only the kidney and possibly the proximal segment of the ureter; thus most ureteral stones are not detectable by ultrasound.

Many patients who experience their first episode of colic seek emergent medical care. Randomized trials have demonstrated that parenterally administered nonsteroidal anti-inflammatory drugs (such as ketorolac) are just as effective as opioids in relieving symptoms and have fewer side effects. Excessive fluid administration has not been shown to be beneficial; therefore, the goal should be to maintain euvolemia. If the pain can be adequately controlled and the patient is able to take fluids orally, hospitalization can be avoided. Use of an alpha-blocker may increase the rate of spontaneous stone passage.

Urologic intervention should be postponed unless there is evidence of UTI, a low probability of spontaneous stone passage (e.g., a stone measuring ≥6 mm or an anatomic abnormality), or intractable pain. A ureteral stent may be placed cystoscopically, but this procedure typically requires general anesthesia, and the stent can be quite uncomfortable, may cause gross hematuria, and may increase the risk of UTI.

If an intervention is indicated, the selection of the most appropriate intervention is determined by the size, location, and composition of the stone; the urinary tract anatomy; and the experience of the urologist. Extracorporeal shockwave lithotripsy, the least invasive option, uses shock waves generated outside the body to fragment the stone. An endourologic approach can remove a stone by basket extraction or laser fragmentation. For large upper-tract stones, percutaneous nephrostolithotomy has the highest likelihood of rendering the patient stone-free. Advances in urologic approaches and instruments have nearly eliminated the need for open surgical procedures such as ureterolithotomy or pyelolithotomy.

Evaluation for Stone Prevention More than half of first-time stone formers will have a recurrence within 10 years. A careful evaluation is indicated to identify predisposing factors, which can then be modified to reduce the risk of new stone formation. It is appropriate to proceed with an evaluation even after the first stone because recurrences are common and are usually preventable with inexpensive lifestyle modifications or other treatments.

History A detailed history, obtained from the patient and from a thorough review of medical records, should include the number and frequency of episodes (distinguishing stone passage from stone formation) and previous imaging studies, interventions, evaluations, and treatments. Inquiries about the patient's medical history should cover UTIs, bariatric surgery, gout, hypertension, and diabetes mellitus. A family history of stone disease may reveal a genetic predisposition. A complete list of current prescription and over-the-counter medications as well as vitamin and mineral supplements is essential. The review of systems should focus on identifying possible etiologic factors related to low urine volume (e.g., high insensible losses; low fluid intake) and gastrointestinal malabsorption as well as on ascertaining how frequently the patient voids during the day and overnight.

A large body of compelling evidence has demonstrated the important role of diet in stone disease. Thus, the dietary history should encompass information on usual dietary habits (meals and snacks), calcium intake, consumption of high-oxalate foods (spinach, rhubarb, potatoes), and fluid intake (including specific beverages typically consumed).

Physical Examination The physical examination should assess weight, blood pressure, costovertebral angle tenderness, and lower-extremity edema as well as signs of other systemic conditions such as primary hyperparathyroidism and gout.

Laboratory Evaluation If not recently measured, the following serum levels should be determined: electrolytes (to uncover hypokalemia or renal tubular acidosis), creatinine, calcium, and uric acid. The PTH level should be measured if indicated by high-normal or elevated serum and urine calcium concentrations. Often, 25-hydroxy vitamin D is measured in concert with PTH to investigate the possible role of secondarily elevated PTH levels in the setting of vitamin D insufficiency.

The urinalysis, including examination of the sediment, can provide useful information. In individuals with asymptomatic residual renal stones, red and white blood cells are frequently present in urine. If there is concern about the possibility of an infection, a urine culture should be performed. The sediment may also reveal crystals (Fig. 342-1), which may help identify the stone type and also provide prognostic information, as crystalluria is a strong risk factor for new stone formation.

The results from 24-h urine collections serve as the cornerstone on which therapeutic recommendations are based. Recommendations on lifestyle modification should be deferred until urine collection is complete. As a baseline assessment, patients should collect at least two 24-h urine samples while consuming their usual diet and usual volume of fluid. The following factors should be measured: total volume, calcium, oxalate, citrate, uric acid, sodium, potassium, phosphorus, pH, and creatinine. When available, the calculated supersaturation is also informative. There is substantial day-to-day variability in the 24-h excretion of many relevant factors; therefore, obtaining values from two collections is important before committing a patient to long-term lifestyle changes or medication. The interpretation of the 24-h urine results should take into account that the collections are usually performed on a weekend day when the patient is staying at home; an individual's habits may differ dramatically (beneficially or detrimentally) at work or outside the home. Specialized testing, such as calcium loading or restriction, is not recommended as it does not influence clinical recommendations.

Stone composition analysis is essential if a stone or fragment is available; patients should be encouraged to retrieve passed stones. The stone type cannot be determined with certainty from 24-h urine results.

Imaging The "gold standard" diagnostic test is helical CT without contrast. If not already performed during an acute episode, a CT should be considered to definitively establish the baseline stone burden. A suboptimal imaging study may not detect a residual stone that, if subsequently passed, would be mistaken for a new stone. In this instance, the preventive medical regimen might be unnecessarily changed as the result of a preexisting stone.

Recommendations for follow-up imaging should be tailored to the individual patient. While CT provides the best information, the radiation dose is substantially higher than from other modalities; therefore, CT should be performed only if the results will lead to a change in clinical recommendations. Although they are less sensitive, renal ultrasound or a KUB exam are typically used to minimize radiation exposure, with recognition of the limitations.

Prevention of New Stone Formation Recommendations for preventing stone formation depend on the stone type and the results of metabolic evaluation. After remediable secondary causes of stone formation (e.g., primary hyperparathyroidism) are excluded, the focus should turn to modification of the urine composition to reduce the risk of new stone formation. The urinary constituents are continuous variables, and the associated risk is continuous; thus, there is no definitive threshold. Dichotomization into "normal" and "abnormal" can be misleading and should be avoided.

For all stone types, consistently diluted urine reduces the likelihood of crystal formation. The urine volume should be at least 2 L/d. Because of differences in insensible fluid losses and fluid intake from food sources, the required total fluid intake will vary from person to person. Rather than specify how much to drink, it is more helpful to educate patients about how much *more* they need to drink in light of their 24-h urine volume. For example, if the daily urine volume is 1.5 L, then the patient should be advised to drink at least 0.5 L more per day in order to increase the urine volume to the goal of 2 L/day.

RECOMMENDATIONS FOR SPECIFIC STONE TYPES

Calcium Oxalate Risk factors for calcium oxalate stones include higher urine calcium, higher urine oxalate, and lower urine citrate. This stone type is insensitive to pH in the physiologic range.

Individuals with higher urine calcium excretion tend to absorb a higher percentage of ingested calcium. Nevertheless, dietary calcium restriction is not beneficial and, in fact, is likely to be harmful (see "Dietary Risk Factors," above). In a randomized trial in men with high urine calcium and recurrent calcium oxalate stones, a diet containing 1200 mg of calcium and a low intake of sodium and animal protein significantly reduced subsequent stone formation from that with a low-calcium diet (400 mg/d). Excessive calcium intake (>1200 mg/d) should be avoided.

A thiazide diuretic, in doses higher than those used to treat hypertension, can substantially lower urine calcium excretion. Several randomized controlled trials have demonstrated that thiazide diuretics can reduce calcium oxalate stone recurrence by ~50%. When a thiazide is prescribed, dietary sodium restriction is essential to obtain the desired reduction in urinary calcium excretion. While bisphosphonates may reduce urine calcium excretion in some individuals, there are no data on whether this class of medication can reduce stone formation; therefore, bisphosphonates cannot be recommended solely for stone prevention at present.

A reduction in urine oxalate will in turn reduce the supersaturation of calcium oxalate. In patients with the common form of nephrolithiasis, avoiding high-dose vitamin C supplements is the only known strategy that reduces endogenous oxalate production.

Oxalate is a metabolic end product; therefore, any dietary oxalate that is absorbed will be excreted in the urine. Reducing absorption of exogenous oxalate involves two approaches. First, the avoidance of foods that contain high amounts of oxalate, such as spinach, rhubarb, and potatoes, is prudent. However, extreme oxalate restriction has not been demonstrated to reduce stone recurrence and could be harmful to overall health, given other health benefits of many foods that are erroneously considered to be high in oxalate. Controversy exists regarding the most clinically relevant measure of the oxalate content of foods (e.g., bioavailability). Notably, the absorption of oxalate is reduced by higher calcium intake; therefore, individuals with higher-than-desired urinary oxalate should be counseled to consume adequate calcium. Oxalate absorption can be influenced by the intestinal microbiota, depending on the presence of oxalate-degrading bacteria. Currently, however, there are no available therapies to alter the microbiota that beneficially affect urinary oxalate excretion over the long term.

Citrate is a natural inhibitor of calcium oxalate and calcium phosphate stones. Higher-level consumption of foods rich in alkali (i.e., fruits and vegetables) can increase urine citrate. For patients with lower urine citrate in whom dietary modification does not adequately increase urine citrate, the addition of supplemental alkali (typically potassium citrate) will lead to an increase in urinary citrate excretion. Sodium salts, such as sodium bicarbonate, while successful in raising urine citrate, are typically avoided due to the adverse effects of sodium on urine calcium excretion.

Past reports suggested that higher levels of urine uric acid may increase the risk of calcium oxalate stones, but more recent studies do not support this association. However, allopurinol reduced stone recurrence in one randomized controlled trial in patients with calcium oxalate stones and high urine uric acid levels. The lack of association between urine uric acid level and calcium oxalate stones suggests that a different mechanism underlies the observed beneficial effect of allopurinol.

Additional dietary modifications may be beneficial in reducing stone recurrence. Restriction of nondairy animal protein (e.g., meat, chicken, seafood) is a reasonable approach and may result in higher excretion of citrate and lower excretion of calcium. In addition, reducing sodium intake to <2.5 g/d may decrease urinary excretion of calcium. Sucrose and fructose intake should be minimized.

For adherence to a dietary pattern that is more manageable for patients than manipulating individual nutrients, the DASH (Dietary Approaches to Stop Hypertension) diet provides an appropriate and readily available option. Randomized trials have conclusively shown the DASH diet to reduce blood pressure. At present, only data from observational studies are available, but these demonstrate a strong and consistent inverse association between the DASH diet and risk of stone formation.

Calcium Phosphate Calcium phosphate stones share risk factors with calcium oxalate stones, including higher concentrations of urine calcium and lower concentrations of urine citrate, but additional factors deserve attention. Higher urine phosphate levels and higher urine pH (typically ≥6.5) are associated with an increased likelihood of calcium phosphate stone formation. Calcium phosphate stones are more common in patients with distal renal tubular acidosis and primary hyperparathyroidism.

There are no randomized trials on which to base preventive recommendations for calcium phosphate stone formers, so the interventions are focused on modification of the recognized risk factors. Thiazide diuretics (with sodium restriction) may be used to reduce urine calcium, as described above for calcium oxalate stones. In patients with low urine citrate levels, alkali supplements (e.g., potassium citrate) may be used to increase these concentrations. However, the urine pH of these patients should be monitored carefully because supplemental alkali can raise urine pH, thereby potentially increasing the risk of stone formation. Reduction of dietary phosphate may be beneficial by reducing urine phosphate excretion.

Uric Acid The two main risk factors for uric acid stones are persistently low urine pH and higher uric acid excretion. Urine pH is the predominant influence on uric acid solubility; therefore, the mainstay of prevention of uric acid stone formation entails increasing urine pH. While acidifying the urine is not easily done, alkalinizing the urine can be readily achieved by increasing the intake of foods rich in alkali (e.g., fruits and vegetables) and reducing the intake of foods that produce acid (e.g., animal flesh). If necessary, supplementation with bicarbonate or citrate salts (preferably potassium citrate) can be used to reach the recommended pH goal of 6 to 7 throughout the day and night.

Urine uric acid excretion is determined by uric acid generation. Uric acid is the end product of purine metabolism; thus reduced consumption of purine-containing foods can lower urine uric acid excretion. It is noteworthy that the serum uric acid level is dependent on the fractional excretion of uric acid and therefore does not provide information on urine uric acid excretion. For example, an individual with high uric acid generation and concurrent high fractional excretion of uric acid will have high urine uric acid excretion with a normal (or even low) serum uric acid level. If alkalinization of the urine alone is not successful and if dietary modifications do not reduce urine uric acid sufficiently, then the use of a xanthine oxidase inhibitor, such as allopurinol or febuxostat, can reduce urine uric acid excretion by 40–50%.

Cystine Cystine excretion is not easily modified. Long-term dietary cystine restriction is not feasible and is unlikely to be successful; thus the focus for cystine stone prevention is on increasing cystine solubility. This goal may be achieved by treatment with medication that covalently binds to cystine (tiopronin and penicillamine) and a medication that raises urine pH. Tiopronin is the preferred choice due to its better adverse event profile. The preferred alkalinizing agent is potassium citrate as sodium salts may increase cystine excretion. As with all stone types, and especially in patients with cystinuria, maintaining a high urine volume is an essential component of the preventive regimen.

Struvite Struvite stones, also known as *infection stones* or *triple-phosphate stones*, form only when the upper urinary tract is infected with urease-producing bacteria such as *Proteus mirabilis, Klebsiella pneumoniae*, or *Providencia* species. Urease produced by these bacteria hydrolyzes urea and may elevate the urine pH to a supraphysiologic level (>8.0). Struvite stones may grow quickly and fill the renal pelvis (*staghorn calculi*).

Struvite stones require complete removal by a urologist. New stone formation can be avoided by the prevention of UTIs. In patients with recurrent upper UTIs (e.g., some individuals with surgically altered urinary drainage or spinal cord injury), the urease inhibitor acetohydroxamic acid can be considered; however, this agent should be used with caution because of potential side effects.

LONG-TERM FOLLOW-UP

In general, the preventive regimens described above do not cure the underlying pathophysiologic process. Thus these recommendations typically need to be followed for the patient's lifetime, and it is essential to tailor recommendations in a way that is acceptable to the patient. Because the memory of the acute stone event fades and patients often return to old habits (e.g., insufficient fluid intake), long-term follow-up is important to ensure that the preventive regimen has been implemented and has resulted in the desired reduction in the risk of new stone formation.

Follow-up imaging should be planned thoughtfully. Many patients with recurrent episodes of renal colic that lead to emergency room visits often undergo repeat CT studies. While CT does provide the best information, the radiation dose is substantially higher than that with plain abdominal radiography (KUB). Small stones may be missed by KUB, and ultrasound has a limited ability to determine size and number of stones. Minimizing radiation exposure should be a goal of the long-term follow-up plan and must be balanced against the gain in diagnostic information.

343 Urinary Tract Obstruction

Julian L. Seifter

Obstruction to the flow of urine, with attendant stasis and elevation in urinary tract pressure, impairs renal and urinary conduit functions and is a common cause of acute and chronic kidney disease (obstructive nephropathy). With early relief of obstruction, the defects in function usually disappear completely. However, chronic obstruction may produce permanent loss of renal mass (renal atrophy) and excretory capability, as well as enhanced susceptibility to local infection and stone formation. Early diagnosis and prompt therapy are, therefore, essential to minimize the otherwise devastating effects of obstruction on kidney structure and function.

ETIOLOGY

Obstruction to urine flow can result from *intrinsic* or *extrinsic mechanical blockade* as well as from *functional defects* not associated with fixed occlusion of the urinary drainage system. Mechanical obstruction can occur at any level of the urinary tract, from the renal calyces to the external urethral meatus. Normal points of narrowing, such as the ureteropelvic and ureterovesical junctions, bladder neck, and urethral meatus, are common sites of obstruction. When obstruction is above the level of the bladder, unilateral dilatation of the ureter (*hydroureter*) and renal pyelocalyceal system (*hydronephrosis*) occurs; lesions at or below the level of the bladder cause bilateral involvement.

Common forms of obstruction are listed in Table 343-1. Childhood causes include *congenital malformations*, such as narrowing of the ureteropelvic junction and abnormal insertion of the ureter into the bladder, the most common cause. Vesicoureteral reflux in the absence of urinary tract infection or bladder neck obstruction often resolves with age. Reinsertion of the ureter into the bladder is indicated if reflux is severe and unlikely to improve spontaneously, if renal function deteriorates, or if urinary tract infections recur despite chronic antimicrobial therapy. Vesicoureteral reflux may cause prenatal hydronephrosis and, if severe, can lead to recurrent urinary infections and renal scarring in childhood. Posterior urethral valves are the most common cause of bilateral hydronephrosis in boys. In adults, urinary tract obstruction (UTO) is due mainly to *acquired defects*. Pelvic tumors, calculi, and urethral stricture predominate. Ligation of, or injury to, the ureter during pelvic or colonic surgery can lead to hydronephrosis which, if unilateral, may remain undetected. Obstructive uropathy may also result from extrinsic neoplastic (carcinoma of

TABLE 343-1 COMMON MECHANICAL CAUSES OF URINARY TRACT OBSTRUCTION

Ureter	Bladder Outlet	Urethra
Congenital		
Ureteropelvic junction narrowing or obstruction	Bladder neck obstruction	Posterior urethral valves
Ureterovesical junction narrowing or obstruction and reflux	Ureterocele	Anterior urethral valves
		Stricture
Ureterocele		Meatal stenosis
Retrocaval ureter		Phimosis
Acquired Intrinsic Defects		
Calculi	Benign prostatic hyperplasia	Stricture
Inflammation		Tumor
Infection	Cancer of prostate	Calculi
Trauma	Cancer of bladder	Trauma
Sloughed papillae	Calculi	Phimosis
Tumor	Diabetic neuropathy	
Blood clots	Spinal cord disease	
	Anticholinergic drugs and α-adrenergic antagonists	
Acquired Extrinsic Defects		
Pregnant uterus	Carcinoma of cervix, colon	Trauma
Retroperitoneal fibrosis		
Aortic aneurysm	Trauma	
Uterine leiomyomata		
Carcinoma of uterus, prostate, bladder, colon, rectum		
Lymphoma		
Pelvic inflammatory disease, endometriosis		
Accidental surgical ligation		

cervix or colon) or inflammatory disorders. Lymphomas and pelvic or colonic neoplasms with retroperitoneal involvement are causes of ureteral obstruction. As many as 50% of men over 40 years old may have lower urinary tract symptoms associated with benign prostatic hypertrophy, but these symptoms may occur without bladder outlet obstruction.

Functional impairment of urine flow occurs when voiding is altered by abnormal pontine or sacral centers of micturition control. It may be asymptomatic or associated with lower urinary tract symptoms such as frequency, urgency, urge and postmicturition incontinence, nocturia, straining to void, slow stream, hesitancy, or a feeling of incomplete emptying. A history should be sought for trauma, back injury, surgery, diabetes, neurologic or psychiatric conditions, and medications. Causes include neurogenic bladder, often with adynamic ureter, and vesicoureteral reflux. Reflux in children may result in severe unilateral or bilateral hydroureter and hydronephrosis. Urinary retention may be the consequence of α-adrenergic and anticholinergic agents, as well as opiates. Hydronephrosis in pregnancy is due to relaxational effects of progesterone on smooth muscle of the renal pelvis, as well as ureteral compression by the enlarged uterus.

Diagnostic tools to identify anatomic obstruction include urinary flow measurements and a postvoid residual. Cystourethroscopy and urodynamic studies may be reserved for the symptomatic patient to assess the filling phase (cystometry), pressure-volume relationship of the bladder, bladder compliance, and capacity. Pressure-flow analysis evaluates bladder contractility and bladder outlet resistance during voiding. Bladder obstruction is characterized by high pressures in women, whereas in men, a diagnosis of bladder outlet obstruction is based on flow rate and voiding pressures. A voiding cystourethrogram may be useful in evaluating incomplete emptying and bladder neck and urethral pathology.

CLINICAL FEATURES AND PATHOPHYSIOLOGY

The pathophysiology and clinical features of UTO are summarized in Table 343-2. *Pain*, the symptom that most commonly leads to medical attention, is due to distention of the collecting system or renal capsule. Pain severity is influenced more by the rate at which distention develops than by the degree of distention. Acute supravesical obstruction, as from a stone lodged in a ureter (Chap. 342), is associated with excruciating pain, known as *renal colic*. This pain often radiates to the lower abdomen, testes, or labia. By contrast, more insidious causes of obstruction, such as chronic narrowing of the ureteropelvic junction, may produce little or no pain and yet result in total destruction of the affected kidney. Flank pain that occurs only with micturition is pathognomonic of vesicoureteral reflux.

Obstruction of urine flow results in an increase in hydrostatic pressures proximal to the site of obstruction. It is this buildup of pressure that leads to the accompanying pain, the distention of the collecting system in the kidney, and elevated intratubular pressures that initiate tubular dysfunction. As the increased hydrostatic pressure is expressed in the urinary space of the glomeruli, further filtration decreases or stops completely.

Azotemia develops when overall excretory function is impaired, often in the setting of bladder outlet obstruction, bilateral renal pelvic or ureteric obstruction, or unilateral disease in a patient with a solitary functioning kidney. Complete bilateral obstruction should be suspected when acute renal failure is accompanied by anuria. Any patient with renal failure otherwise unexplained, or with a history of nephrolithiasis, hematuria, diabetes mellitus, prostatic enlargement, pelvic surgery, trauma, or tumor should be evaluated for UTO.

In the acute setting, partial, bilateral obstruction may mimic prerenal azotemia with concentrated urine and sodium retention. However, with more prolonged obstruction, symptoms of *polyuria* and *nocturia* commonly accompany partial UTO and result from diminished renal concentrating ability. Impairment of transcellular salt reabsorption in the proximal tubule, medullary thick ascending limb of Henle, and collecting duct cells is due to downregulation of transport proteins including the Na^+, K^+ adenosine triphosphatase (ATPase), NaK_2Cl cotransporter (NKCC) in the thick ascending limb, and the epithelial Na^+ channel (ENaC) in collecting duct cells. Consequences include failure to produce urine free of salt (natriuresis) and loss of medullary hypertonicity producing a urinary concentrating defect. In addition to direct effects on renal transport mechanisms, increased prostaglandin E_2 (PGE_2) (due to induction of cyclooxygenase-2 [COX-2]), angiotensin II (with its downregulation of Na^+ transporters), and atrial or B-type natriuretic peptides (ANP or BNP) (due to volume expansion in the azotemic patient) contribute to the decreased salt reabsorption along the nephron.

Dysregulation of aquaporin-2 water channels in the collecting duct contributes to the polyuria. The defect usually does not improve with administration of vasopressin and is therefore a form of acquired nephrogenic diabetes insipidus.

Wide fluctuations in urine output in a patient with azotemia should always raise the possibility of intermittent or partial UTO. If fluid intake is inadequate, severe dehydration and hypernatremia may develop. However, as with other causes of poor renal function, excesses of salt and water intake may result in edema and hyponatremia.

Partial bilateral UTO often results in *acquired distal renal tubular acidosis, hyperkalemia*, and *renal salt wasting*. The H^+-ATPase, situated on the apical membrane of the intercalated cells of the collecting duct, is critical for distal H^+ secretion. The trafficking of intracellular H^+ pumps from the cytoplasm to the cell membrane is disrupted in UTO. The decreased function of the ENaC, in the apical membrane of neighboring collecting duct principal cells, contributes to decreased Na^+ reabsorption (salt-wasting), decreased electronegativity of the tubule lumen, and therefore decreased K^+ secretion via K^+ channels (hyperkalemia) and H^+ secretion via the H^+-ATPases (distal renal tubular acidosis [RTA]). Proximal tubule ammoniagenesis, important to the elimination of H^+ as NH_4^+, is impaired. These defects in tubule function are often accompanied by renal tubulointerstitial damage. Azotemia with hyperkalemia and metabolic acidosis should prompt consideration of UTO.

The renal interstitium becomes edematous and infiltrated with mononuclear inflammatory cells early in UTO. Later, interstitial fibrosis and atrophy of the papillae and medulla occur and precede these processes in the cortex. The increase in angiotensin II noted in UTO contributes to the inflammatory response and fibroblast accumulation through mechanisms involving profibrotic cytokines. With time, this process leads to chronic kidney damage.

TABLE 343-2 PATHOPHYSIOLOGY OF BILATERAL URETERAL OBSTRUCTION

Hemodynamic Effects	Tubule Effects	Clinical Features
Acute		
↑ Renal blood flow ↓ GFR ↓ Medullary blood flow ↑ Vasodilator prostaglandins, nitric oxide	↑ Ureteral and tubule pressures ↑ Reabsorption of Na^+, urea, water	Pain (capsule distention) Azotemia Oliguria or anuria
Chronic		
↓ Renal blood flow ↓↓ GFR ↑ Vasoconstrictor prostaglandins ↑ Renin-angiotensin production	↓ Medullary osmolarity ↓ Concentrating ability Structural damage; parenchymal atrophy ↓ Transport functions for Na^+, K^+, H^+	Azotemia Hypertension AVP-insensitive polyuria Natriuresis Hyperkalemic, hyperchloremic acidosis
Release of Obstruction		
Slow ↑ in GFR (variable)	↓ Tubule pressure ↑ Solute load per nephron (urea, NaCl) Natriuretic factors present	Postobstructive diuresis Potential for volume depletion and electrolyte imbalance due to losses of Na^+, K^+, PO_4^{2-}, Mg^{2+}, and water

Abbreviations: AVP, arginine vasopressin; GFR, glomerular filtration rate.

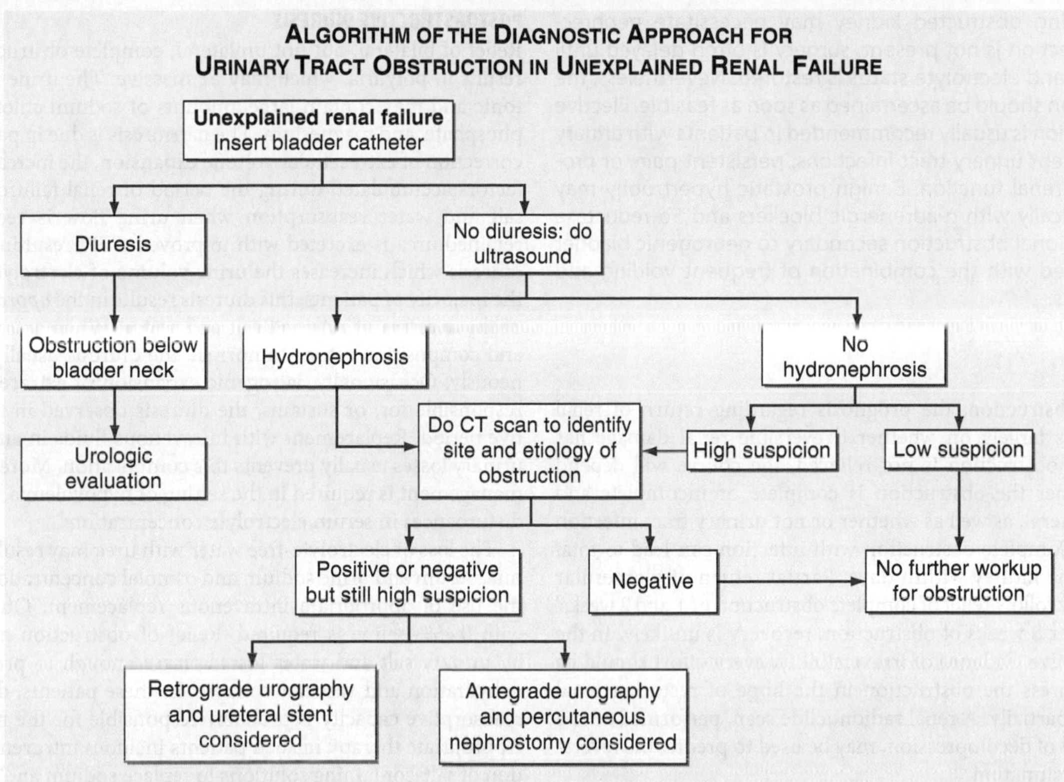

FIGURE 343-1 Diagnostic approach for urinary tract obstruction in unexplained renal failure. CT, computed tomography.

UTO must always be considered in patients with urinary tract infections or urolithiasis. Urinary stasis encourages the growth of organisms. Urea-splitting bacteria are associated with magnesium ammonium phosphate (struvite) calculi. *Hypertension* is frequent in acute and subacute unilateral obstruction and is usually a consequence of increased release of renin by the involved kidney. Chronic kidney disease from bilateral UTO, often associated with extracellular volume expansion, may result in significant hypertension. *Erythrocytosis*, an infrequent complication of obstructive uropathy, is secondary to increased erythropoietin production.

DIAGNOSIS

A history of difficulty in voiding, pain, infection, or change in urinary volume is common. Evidence for distention of the kidney or urinary bladder can often be obtained by palpation and percussion of the abdomen. A careful rectal and genital examination may reveal enlargement or nodularity of the prostate, abnormal rectal sphincter tone, or a rectal or pelvic mass.

Urinalysis may reveal hematuria, pyuria, and bacteriuria. The urine sediment is often normal, even when obstruction leads to marked azotemia and extensive structural damage. An abdominal scout film may detect nephrocalcinosis or a radiopaque stone. As indicated in Fig. 343-1, if UTO is suspected, a bladder catheter should be inserted. Abdominal ultrasonography should be performed to evaluate renal and bladder size, as well as pyelocalyceal contour. Ultrasonography is approximately 90% specific and sensitive for detection of hydronephrosis. False-positive results are associated with diuresis, renal cysts, or the presence of an extrarenal pelvis, a normal congenital variant. Congenital ureteropelvic junction (UPJ) obstruction may be mistaken for renal cystic disease. Hydronephrosis may be absent on ultrasound when obstruction is less than 48 h in duration or associated with volume contraction, staghorn calculi, retroperitoneal fibrosis, or infiltrative renal disease. Duplex Doppler ultrasonography may detect an increased resistive index in urinary obstruction.

Recent advances in technology have led to alternatives and have largely replaced the once standard intravenous urogram in the further evaluation of UTO. The high-resolution multidetector row computed tomography (CT) scan in particular has advantages of visualizing the retroperitoneum, as well as identifying both intrinsic and extrinsic sites of obstruction. Noncontrast CT scans improve visualization of the urinary tract in the patient with renal impairment and are safer for patients at risk for contrast nephropathy. Magnetic resonance urography is a promising technique but, at this time, not superior to the CT scan and carries the risk of certain gadolinium agents in patients with renal insufficiency, i.e., nephrogenic systemic fibrosis. The intravenous urogram may define the site of obstruction and demonstrate dilatation of the calyces, renal pelvis, and ureter above the obstruction. The ureter may be tortuous in chronic obstruction. Radionuclide scans are able to give differential renal function but give less anatomic detail than CT or intravenous urography (IVU).

To facilitate visualization of a suspected lesion in a ureter or renal pelvis, *retrograde* or *antegrade urography* should be attempted. These procedures do not carry risk of contrast-induced acute renal failure in patients with renal insufficiency. The retrograde approach involves catheterization of the involved ureter under cystoscopic control, whereas the antegrade technique necessitates percutaneous placement of a catheter into the renal pelvis. Although the antegrade approach may provide immediate decompression of a unilateral obstructing lesion, many urologists initially attempt the retrograde approach unless the catheterization is unsuccessful.

Voiding cystourethrography is of value in the diagnosis of vesicoureteral reflux and bladder neck and urethral obstructions. Postvoiding films reveal residual urine. Endoscopic visualization by the urologist often permits precise identification of lesions involving the urethra, prostate, bladder, and ureteral orifices.

TREATMENT URINARY TRACT OBSTRUCTION

UTO complicated by infection requires immediate relief of obstruction to prevent development of generalized sepsis and progressive renal damage. Sepsis necessitates prompt urologic intervention. Drainage may be achieved by nephrostomy, ureterostomy, or ureteral, urethral, or suprapubic catheterization. Prolonged antibiotic treatment may be necessary. Chronic or recurrent infections in a poorly functioning obstructed kidney may necessitate nephrectomy. When infection is not present, surgery is often delayed until acid-base, fluid, and electrolyte status is restored. Nevertheless, the site of obstruction should be ascertained as soon as feasible. Elective relief of obstruction is usually recommended in patients with urinary retention, recurrent urinary tract infections, persistent pain, or progressive loss of renal function. Benign prostatic hypertrophy may be treated medically with α-adrenergic blockers and 5α-reductase inhibitors. Functional obstruction secondary to neurogenic bladder may be decreased with the combination of frequent voiding and cholinergic drugs.

PROGNOSIS

With relief of obstruction, the prognosis regarding return of renal function depends largely on whether irreversible renal damage has occurred. When obstruction is not relieved, the course will depend mainly on whether the obstruction is complete or incomplete and bilateral or unilateral, as well as whether or not urinary tract infection is also present. Complete obstruction with infection can lead to total destruction of the kidney within days. Partial return of glomerular filtration rate may follow relief of complete obstruction of 1 and 2 weeks' duration, but after 8 weeks of obstruction, recovery is unlikely. In the absence of definitive evidence of irreversibility, every effort should be made to decompress the obstruction in the hope of restoring renal function at least partially. A renal radionuclide scan, performed after a prolonged period of decompression, may be used to predict the reversibility of renal dysfunction.

POSTOBSTRUCTIVE DIURESIS

Relief of bilateral, but not unilateral, complete obstruction commonly results in polyuria, which may be massive. The urine is usually hypotonic and may contain large amounts of sodium chloride, potassium, phosphate, and magnesium. The natriuresis is due in part to the normal correction of extracellular volume expansion, the increase in natriuretic factors accumulated during the period of renal failure, and depressed salt and water reabsorption when urine flow is reestablished. The retained urea is excreted with improved GFR, resulting in an osmotic diuresis which increases the urine volume of electrolyte-free water. In the majority of patients, this diuresis results in the *appropriate* excretion of the excesses of retained salt and water. When extracellular volume and composition return to normal, the diuresis usually abates spontaneously. Occasionally, iatrogenic expansion of extracellular volume is responsible for, or sustains, the diuresis observed in the postobstructive period. Replacement with intravenous fluids in amounts less than urinary losses usually prevents this complication. More aggressive fluid management is required in the setting of hypovolemia, hypotension, or disturbances in serum electrolyte concentrations.

The loss of electrolyte-free water with urea may result in hypernatremia. Serum and urine sodium and osmolal concentrations should guide the use of appropriate intravenous replacement. Often replacement with 0.45% saline is required. Relief of obstruction may be followed by urinary salt and water losses severe enough to provoke profound dehydration and vascular collapse. In these patients, decreased tubule reabsorptive capacity is probably responsible for the marked diuresis. Appropriate therapy in such patients includes intravenous administration of salt-containing solutions to replace sodium and volume deficits.

SECTION 1 DISORDERS OF THE ALIMENTARY TRACT

344 Approach to the Patient with Gastrointestinal Disease

William L. Hasler, Chung Owyang

ANATOMIC CONSIDERATIONS

The gastrointestinal (GI) tract extends from the mouth to the anus and is composed of several organs with distinct functions. Specialized independently controlled thickened sphincters that assist in gut compartmentalization separate the organs. The gut wall is organized into well-defined layers that contribute to functional activities in each region. The mucosa is a barrier to luminal contents or a site for transfer of fluids or nutrients. Gut smooth muscle in association with the enteric nervous system mediates propulsion from one region to the next. Many GI organs possess a serosal layer that provides a supportive foundation but that also permits external input.

Interactions with other organ systems serve the needs both of the gut and the body. Pancreaticobiliary conduits deliver bile and enzymes into the duodenum. A rich vascular supply is modulated by GI tract activity. Lymphatic channels assist in gut immune activities. Intrinsic gut wall nerves provide the basic controls for propulsion and fluid regulation. Extrinsic neural input provides volitional or involuntary control to degrees that are specific for each gut region.

FUNCTIONS OF THE GASTROINTESTINAL TRACT

The GI tract serves two main functions—assimilating nutrients and eliminating waste. The gut anatomy is organized to serve these functions. In the mouth, food is processed, mixed with salivary amylase, and delivered to the gut lumen. The esophagus propels the bolus into the stomach; the lower esophageal sphincter prevents oral reflux of gastric contents. The esophageal mucosa has a protective squamous histology, which does not permit significant diffusion or absorption. Propulsive esophageal activities are exclusively aboral and coordinate with relaxation of the upper and lower esophageal sphincters on swallowing.

The stomach furthers food preparation by triturating and mixing the bolus with pepsin and acid. Gastric acid also sterilizes the upper gut. The proximal stomach serves a storage function by relaxing to accommodate the meal. The distal stomach exhibits phasic contractions that propel solid food residue against the pylorus, where it is repeatedly propelled proximally for further mixing before it is emptied into the duodenum. Finally, the stomach secretes intrinsic factor for vitamin B_{12} absorption.

The small intestine serves most of the nutrient absorptive function of the gut. The intestinal mucosa exhibits villus architecture to provide maximal surface area for absorption and is endowed with specialized enzymes and transporters. Triturated food from the stomach mixes with pancreatic juice and bile in the duodenum to facilitate digestion. Pancreatic juice contains the main enzymes for carbohydrate, protein, and fat digestion as well as bicarbonate to optimize the pH for activation of these enzymes. Bile secreted by the liver and stored in the gallbladder is essential for intestinal lipid digestion. The proximal intestine is optimized for rapid absorption of nutrient breakdown products and most minerals, whereas the ileum is better suited for absorption of vitamin B_{12} and bile acids. The small intestine also aids in waste elimination. Bile contains by-products of erythrocyte degradation, toxins, metabolized and unmetabolized medications, and cholesterol. Motor function of the small intestine delivers indigestible food residue and sloughed enterocytes into the colon for further processing. The small intestine terminates in the ileocecal junction, a sphincteric structure that prevents coloileal reflux and maintains small-intestinal sterility.

The colon prepares the waste material for controlled evacuation. The colonic mucosa dehydrates the stool, decreasing daily fecal volumes from 1000–1500 mL delivered from the ileum to 100–200 mL expelled from the rectum. The colonic lumen possesses a dense bacterial colonization that ferments undigested carbohydrates and short-chain fatty acids. Whereas transit times in the esophagus are on the order of seconds and times in the stomach and small intestine range from minutes to a few hours, propagation through the colon takes more than 1 day in most individuals. Colonic motor patterns exhibit a to-and-fro character that facilitates slow fecal desiccation. The proximal colon serves to mix and absorb fluid, while the distal colon exhibits peristaltic contractions and mass actions that function to expel the stool. The colon terminates in the anus, a structure with volitional and involuntary controls to permit retention of the fecal bolus until it can be released in a socially convenient setting.

EXTRINSIC MODULATION OF GUT FUNCTION

GI function is modified by influences outside of the gut. Unlike other organ systems, the gut is in continuity with the outside environment. Thus, protective mechanisms are vigilant against deleterious effects of foods, medications, toxins, and infectious organisms. Mucosal immune mechanisms include chronic lymphocyte and plasma cell populations in the epithelial layer and lamina propria backed up by lymph node chains to prevent noxious agents from entering the circulation. Antimicrobial peptides secreted by Paneth cells in the intestine further contribute to the defense mechanisms against pathogens in the lumen. All substances absorbed into the bloodstream are filtered through the liver via the portal venous circulation. In the liver, many drugs and toxins are detoxified by a variety of mechanisms. Although intrinsic nerves control most basic gut activities, extrinsic neural input modulates many functions. Two activities under voluntary control are swallowing and defecation. Many normal GI reflexes involve extrinsic vagus or splanchnic nerve pathways. The brain-gut axis further alters function in regions not under volitional regulation. As an example, stress has potent effects on gut motor, secretory, and sensory functions.

OVERVIEW OF GASTROINTESTINAL DISEASES

GI diseases develop as a result of abnormalities within or outside of the gut and range in severity from those that produce mild symptoms and no long-term morbidity to those with intractable symptoms or adverse outcomes. Diseases may be localized to one organ or exhibit diffuse involvement at many sites.

CLASSIFICATION OF GI DISEASES

GI diseases are manifestations of alterations in nutrient assimilation or waste evacuation or in the activities supporting these main functions.

Impaired Digestion and Absorption Diseases of the stomach, intestine, biliary tree, and pancreas can disrupt digestion and absorption. The most common intestinal maldigestion syndrome, lactase deficiency, produces gas and diarrhea after ingestion of dairy products and has no adverse outcomes. Other intestinal enzyme deficiencies produce similar symptoms after ingestion of other simple sugars. Conversely, celiac disease, bacterial overgrowth, infectious enteritis, Crohn's ileitis, and radiation damage, which affect digestion and/or absorption more diffusely, produce anemia, dehydration, electrolyte disorders, or malnutrition. Gastric hypersecretory conditions such as Zollinger-Ellison syndrome damage the intestinal mucosa, impair pancreatic enzyme activation, and accelerate transit due to excess gastric acid. Biliary obstruction from stricture or neoplasm impairs fat digestion. Impaired pancreatic enzyme release in chronic pancreatitis or pancreatic cancer decreases intraluminal digestion and can lead to malnutrition.

Altered Secretion Selected GI diseases result from dysregulation of gut secretion. Gastric acid hypersecretion occurs in Zollinger-Ellison syndrome, G cell hyperplasia, retained antrum syndrome, and some individuals with duodenal ulcers. Conversely, patients with atrophic gastritis or pernicious anemia release little or no gastric acid. Inflammatory and infectious small-intestinal and colonic diseases produce fluid loss through impaired absorption or enhanced secretion. Common intestinal and colonic hypersecretory conditions cause diarrhea and include acute bacterial or viral infection, chronic *Giardia* or cryptosporidia infections, small-intestinal bacterial overgrowth, bile salt diarrhea, microscopic colitis, diabetic diarrhea, and abuse of certain laxatives. Less common causes include large colonic villus adenomas and endocrine neoplasias with tumor overproduction of secretagogue transmitters like vasoactive intestinal polypeptide.

Altered Gut Transit Impaired gut transit may be secondary to mechanical obstruction. Esophageal occlusion often results from acid-induced stricture or neoplasm. Gastric outlet obstruction develops from peptic ulcer disease or gastric cancer. Small-intestinal obstruction most commonly results from adhesions but may also occur with Crohn's disease, radiation- or drug-induced strictures, and less likely malignancy. The most common cause of colonic obstruction is colon cancer, although inflammatory strictures develop in patients with inflammatory bowel disease, after certain infections such as diverticulitis, or with some drugs.

Retardation of propulsion also develops from disordered motor function. Achalasia is characterized by impaired esophageal body peristalsis and incomplete lower esophageal sphincter relaxation. Gastroparesis is the symptomatic delay in gastric emptying of meals due to impaired gastric motility. Intestinal pseudoobstruction causes marked delays in small-bowel transit due to enteric nerve or intestinal smooth-muscle injury. Slow-transit constipation is produced by diffusely impaired colonic propulsion. Constipation also is produced by outlet abnormalities such as rectal prolapse, intussusception, or dyssynergia—a failure of anal or puborectalis relaxation upon attempted defecation.

Disorders of rapid propulsion are less common than those with delayed transit. Rapid gastric emptying occurs in postvagotomy dumping syndrome, with gastric hypersecretion, and in some cases of functional dyspepsia and cyclic vomiting syndrome. Exaggerated intestinal or colonic motor patterns may be responsible for diarrhea in irritable bowel syndrome. Accelerated transit with hyperdefecation is noted in hyperthyroidism.

Immune Dysregulation Many inflammatory GI conditions are consequences of altered gut immune function. The mucosal inflammation of celiac disease results from dietary ingestion of gluten-containing grains. Some patients with food allergy also exhibit altered immune populations. Eosinophilic esophagitis and eosinophilic gastroenteritis are inflammatory disorders with prominent mucosal eosinophils. Ulcerative colitis and Crohn's disease are disorders of uncertain etiology that produce mucosal injury primarily in the lower gut. The microscopic colitides, lymphocytic and collagenous colitis, exhibit colonic subepithelial infiltrates without visible mucosal damage. Bacterial, viral, and protozoal organisms may produce ileitis or colitis in selected patient populations.

Impaired Gut Blood Flow Different GI regions are at variable risk for ischemic damage from impaired blood flow. Rare cases of gastroparesis result from blockage of the celiac and superior mesenteric arteries. More commonly encountered are intestinal and colonic ischemia that are consequences of arterial embolus, arterial thrombosis, venous thrombosis, or hypoperfusion from dehydration, sepsis, hemorrhage, or reduced cardiac output. These may produce mucosal injury, hemorrhage, or even perforation. Chronic ischemia may result in intestinal stricture. Some cases of radiation enterocolitis exhibit reduced mucosal blood flow.

Neoplastic Degeneration All GI regions are susceptible to malignant degeneration to varying degrees. In the United States, colorectal cancer is most common and usually presents after age 50 years. Worldwide, gastric cancer is prevalent especially in certain Asian regions. Esophageal cancer develops with chronic acid reflux or after an extensive alcohol or tobacco use history. Small-intestinal neoplasms are rare and occur with underlying inflammatory disease. Anal cancers arise after prior anal infection or inflammation. Pancreatic and biliary cancers elicit severe pain, weight loss, and jaundice and have poor prognoses. Hepatocellular carcinoma usually arises in the setting of chronic viral hepatitis or cirrhosis secondary to other causes. Most GI cancers exhibit carcinomatous histology; however, lymphomas and other cell types also are observed.

Disorders Without Obvious Organic Abnormalities The most common GI disorders show no abnormalities on biochemical or structural testing and include irritable bowel syndrome, functional dyspepsia, functional chest pain, and functional heartburn. These disorders exhibit altered gut motor function; however, the pathogenic relevance of these abnormalities is uncertain. Exaggerated visceral sensory responses to noxious stimulation may cause discomfort in these disorders. Symptoms in other patients result from altered processing of visceral pain sensations in the central nervous system. Functional bowel patients with severe symptoms may exhibit significant emotional disturbances on psychometric testing. Subtle immunologic defects may contribute to functional symptoms as well.

Genetic Influences Although many GI diseases result from environmental factors, others exhibit hereditary components. Family members of inflammatory bowel disease patients show a genetic predisposition to disease development themselves. Colonic and esophageal malignancies arise in certain inherited disorders. Rare genetic dysmotility syndromes are described. Familial clustering is even observed in the functional bowel disorders, although this may be secondary learned familial illness behavior rather than a true hereditary factor.

SYMPTOMS OF GASTROINTESTINAL DISEASE

The most common GI symptoms are abdominal pain, heartburn, nausea and vomiting, altered bowel habits, GI bleeding, and jaundice (Table 344-1). Others are dysphagia, anorexia, weight loss, fatigue, and extraintestinal symptoms.

Abdominal Pain Abdominal pain results from GI disease and extraintestinal conditions involving the genitourinary tract, abdominal wall, thorax, or spine. Visceral pain generally is midline in location and vague in character, whereas parietal pain is localized and precisely described. Common inflammatory diseases with pain include peptic ulcer, appendicitis, diverticulitis, inflammatory bowel disease, and infectious enterocolitis. Other intraabdominal causes of pain include gallstone disease and pancreatitis. Noninflammatory visceral sources include mesenteric ischemia and neoplasia. The most common causes of abdominal pain are irritable bowel syndrome and functional dyspepsia.

Heartburn Heartburn, a burning substernal sensation, is reported intermittently by at least 40% of the population. Classically, heartburn is felt to result from excess gastroesophageal reflux of acid. However, some cases exhibit normal esophageal acid exposure and may result from reflux of nonacidic material or heightened sensitivity of esophageal mucosal nerves.

Nausea and Vomiting Nausea and vomiting are caused by GI diseases, medications, toxins, acute and chronic infection, endocrine disorders, labyrinthine conditions, and central nervous system disease. The best-characterized GI etiologies relate to mechanical obstruction of the upper gut; however, disorders of propulsion including gastroparesis and intestinal pseudoobstruction also elicit prominent symptoms. Nausea and vomiting also are commonly reported by patients with

TABLE 344-1 COMMON CAUSES OF COMMON GASTROINTESTINAL (GI) SYMPTOMS

Abdominal Pain	Nausea and Vomiting	Diarrhea	GI Bleeding	Obstructive Jaundice
Appendicitis	Medications	Infection	Ulcer disease	Bile duct stones
Gallstone disease	GI obstruction	Poorly absorbed sugars	Esophagitis	Cholangiocarcinoma
Pancreatitis	Motor disorders	Inflammatory bowel disease	Varices	Cholangitis
Diverticulitis	Functional bowel disorder	Microscopic colitis	Vascular lesions	Sclerosing cholangitis
Ulcer disease	Enteric infection	Functional bowel disorder	Neoplasm	Ampullary stenosis
Esophagitis	Pregnancy	Celiac disease	Diverticula	Ampullary carcinoma
GI obstruction	Endocrine disease	Pancreatic insufficiency	Hemorrhoids	Pancreatitis
Inflammatory bowel disease	Motion sickness	Hyperthyroidism	Fissures	Pancreatic tumor
Functional bowel disorder	Central nervous system disease	Ischemia	Inflammatory bowel disease	
Vascular disease		Endocrine tumor	Infectious colitis	
Gynecologic causes				
Renal stone				

irritable bowel syndrome and functional disorders of the upper gut (including chronic idiopathic nausea and functional vomiting).

Altered Bowel Habits Altered bowel habits are common complaints of patients with GI disease. Constipation is reported as infrequent defecation, straining with defecation, passage of hard stools, or a sense of incomplete fecal evacuation. Causes of constipation include obstruction, motor disorders of the colon, medications, and endocrine diseases such as hypothyroidism and hyperparathyroidism. Diarrhea is reported as frequent defecation, passage of loose or watery stools, fecal urgency, or a similar sense of incomplete evacuation. The differential diagnosis of diarrhea is broad and includes infections, inflammatory causes, malabsorption, and medications. Irritable bowel syndrome produces constipation, diarrhea, or an alternating bowel pattern. Fecal mucus is common in irritable bowel syndrome, whereas pus characterizes inflammatory disease. Steatorrhea develops with malabsorption.

GI Bleeding Hemorrhage may develop from any gut organ. Most commonly, upper GI bleeding presents with melena or hematemesis, whereas lower GI bleeding produces passage of bright red or maroon stools. However, briskly bleeding upper sites can elicit voluminous red rectal bleeding, whereas slowly bleeding ascending colon sites may produce melena. Chronic slow GI bleeding may present with iron deficiency anemia. The most common upper GI causes of bleeding are ulcer disease, gastroduodenitis, and esophagitis. Other etiologies include portal hypertensive causes, malignancy, tears across the gastroesophageal junction, and vascular lesions. The most prevalent lower GI sources of hemorrhage include hemorrhoids, anal fissures, diverticula, ischemic colitis, and arteriovenous malformations. Other causes include neoplasm, inflammatory bowel disease, infectious colitis, drug-induced colitis, and other vascular lesions.

Jaundice Jaundice results from prehepatic, intrahepatic, or posthepatic disease. Posthepatic causes of jaundice include biliary diseases, such as choledocholithiasis, acute cholangitis, primary sclerosing cholangitis, other strictures, and neoplasm, and pancreatic disorders, such as acute and chronic pancreatitis, stricture, and malignancy.

Other Symptoms Other symptoms are manifestations of GI disease. Dysphagia, odynophagia, and unexplained chest pain suggest esophageal disease. A globus sensation is reported with esophagopharyngeal conditions, but also occurs with functional GI disorders. Weight loss, anorexia, and fatigue are nonspecific symptoms of neoplastic, inflammatory, gut motility, pancreatic, small-bowel mucosal, and psychiatric conditions. Fever is reported with inflammatory illness, but malignancies also evoke febrile responses. GI disorders also produce extraintestinal symptoms. Inflammatory bowel disease is associated with hepatobiliary dysfunction, skin and eye lesions, and arthritis. Celiac disease may present with dermatitis herpetiformis. Jaundice can produce pruritus. Conversely, systemic diseases can have GI consequences. Systemic lupus may cause gut ischemia, presenting with pain or bleeding. Overwhelming stress or severe burns may lead to gastric ulcer formation.

EVALUATION OF THE PATIENT WITH GASTROINTESTINAL DISEASE

Evaluation of the patient with GI disease begins with a careful history and examination. Subsequent investigation with a variety of tools designed to test gut structure or function are indicated in selected cases. Some patients exhibit normal findings on diagnostic testing. In these individuals, validated symptom profiles are used to confidently diagnose a functional bowel disorder.

HISTORY

The history of the patient with suspected GI disease has several components. Symptom timing suggests specific etiologies. Symptoms of short duration commonly result from acute infection, toxin exposure, or abrupt inflammation or ischemia. Long-standing symptoms point to underlying chronic inflammatory or neoplastic conditions or functional bowel disorders. Symptoms from mechanical obstruction, ischemia, inflammatory bowel disease, and functional bowel disorders are worsened by meals. Conversely, ulcer symptoms may be relieved by eating or antacids. Symptom patterns and duration may suggest underlying etiologies. Ulcer pain occurs at intermittent intervals lasting weeks to months, whereas biliary colic has a sudden onset and lasts up to several hours. Pain from acute inflammation as with acute pancreatitis is severe and persists for days to weeks. Meals elicit diarrhea in some cases of inflammatory bowel disease and irritable bowel syndrome. Defecation relieves discomfort in inflammatory bowel disease and irritable bowel syndrome. Functional bowel disorders are exacerbated by stress. Sudden awakening from sound sleep suggests organic rather than functional disease. Diarrhea from malabsorption usually improves with fasting, whereas secretory diarrhea persists without oral intake.

Symptom relation to other factors narrows the list of diagnostic possibilities. Obstructive symptoms with prior abdominal surgery raise concern for adhesions, whereas loose stools after gastrectomy or gallbladder excision suggest dumping syndrome or postcholecystectomy diarrhea. Symptom onset after travel prompts a search for enteric infection. Medications may produce pain, altered bowel habits, or GI bleeding. Lower GI bleeding likely results from neoplasms, diverticula, or vascular lesions in an older person and from anorectal abnormalities or inflammatory bowel disease in a younger individual. Celiac disease is prevalent in people of northern European descent, whereas inflammatory bowel disease is more common in certain Jewish populations. A sexual history may raise concern for sexually transmitted diseases or immunodeficiency.

For more than two decades, working groups have been convened to devise symptom criteria to improve the confident diagnosis of functional bowel disorders and to minimize the numbers of unnecessary diagnostic tests performed. The most widely accepted symptom-based criteria are the Rome criteria. When tested against findings of structural investigations, the Rome criteria exhibit diagnostic specificities exceeding 90% for many of the functional bowel disorders.

PHYSICAL EXAMINATION

The physical exam complements information from the history. Abnormal vital signs provide diagnostic clues and determine the need for acute intervention. Fever suggests inflammation or neoplasm. Orthostasis is found with significant blood loss, dehydration, sepsis, or autonomic neuropathy. Skin, eye, or joint findings may point to specific diagnoses. Neck exam with swallowing assessment evaluates dysphagia. Cardiopulmonary disease may present with abdominal pain or nausea; thus lung and cardiac exams are important. Pelvic examination tests for a gynecologic source of abdominal pain. Rectal exam may detect blood, indicating gut mucosal injury or neoplasm or a palpable inflammatory mass in appendicitis. Metabolic conditions and gut motor disorders have associated peripheral neuropathy.

Inspection of the abdomen may reveal distention from obstruction, tumor, or ascites or vascular abnormalities with liver disease. Ecchymoses develop with severe pancreatitis. Auscultation can detect bruits or friction rubs from vascular disease or hepatic tumors. Loss of bowel sounds signifies ileus, whereas high-pitched, hyperactive sounds characterize intestinal obstruction. Percussion assesses liver size and can detect shifting dullness from ascites. Palpation assesses for hepatosplenomegaly as well as neoplastic or inflammatory masses. Abdominal exam is helpful in evaluating unexplained pain. Intestinal ischemia elicits severe pain but little tenderness. Patients with visceral pain may exhibit generalized discomfort, whereas those with parietal pain or peritonitis have directed pain, often with involuntary guarding, rigidity, or rebound. Patients with musculoskeletal abdominal wall pain may note tenderness exacerbated by Valsalva or straight-leg lift maneuvers.

TOOLS FOR PATIENT EVALUATION

Laboratory, radiographic, and functional tests can assist in diagnosis of suspected GI disease. The GI tract also is amenable to internal evaluation with upper and lower endoscopy and to examination of luminal contents. Histopathologic exams of GI tissues complement these tests.

Laboratory Selected laboratory tests facilitate the diagnosis of GI disease. Iron-deficiency anemia suggests mucosal blood loss, whereas vitamin B_{12} deficiency results from small-intestinal, gastric, or pancreatic disease. Either also can result from inadequate oral intake. Leukocytosis and increased sedimentation rates and C-reactive protein levels are found in inflammatory conditions, whereas leukopenia is seen in viremic illness. Severe vomiting or diarrhea elicits electrolyte disturbances, acid-base abnormalities, and elevated blood urea nitrogen. Pancreaticobiliary or liver disease is suggested by elevated pancreatic or liver chemistries. Thyroid chemistries, cortisol, and calcium levels are obtained to exclude endocrinologic causes of GI symptoms. Pregnancy testing is considered for women with unexplained nausea. Serologic tests can screen for celiac disease, inflammatory bowel disease, rheumatologic diseases like lupus or scleroderma, and paraneoplastic dysmotility syndromes. Hormone levels are obtained for suspected endocrine neoplasia. Intraabdominal malignancies produce other tumor markers including the carcinoembryonic antigen CA 19-9 and α-fetoprotein. Blood testing also monitors medication therapy in some diseases, as with thiopurine metabolite levels in inflammatory bowel disease. Other body fluids are sampled under certain circumstances. Ascitic fluid is analyzed for infection, malignancy, or findings of portal hypertension. Cerebrospinal fluid is obtained for suspected central nervous system causes of vomiting. Urine samples screen for carcinoid, porphyria, and heavy metal intoxication.

Luminal Contents Luminal contents can be examined for diagnostic clues. Stool samples are cultured for bacterial pathogens, examined for leukocytes and parasites, or tested for *Giardia* antigen. Duodenal aspirates can be examined for parasites or cultured for bacterial overgrowth. Fecal fat is quantified in possible malabsorption. Stool electrolytes can be measured in diarrheal conditions. Laxative screens are done when laxative abuse is suspected. Gastric acid is quantified to rule out Zollinger-Ellison syndrome. Esophageal pH testing is done for refractory symptoms of acid reflux, whereas impedance techniques assess for nonacidic reflux. Pancreatic juice is analyzed for enzyme or bicarbonate content to exclude pancreatic exocrine insufficiency.

Endoscopy The gut is accessible with endoscopy, which can provide the diagnosis of the causes of bleeding, pain, nausea and vomiting, weight loss, altered bowel function, and fever. Table 344-2 lists the most common indications for the major endoscopic procedures. Upper endoscopy evaluates the esophagus, stomach, and duodenum, whereas colonoscopy assesses the colon and distal ileum. Upper endoscopy is advocated as the initial structural test performed in patients with suspected ulcer disease, esophagitis, neoplasm, malabsorption, and Barrett's metaplasia because of its ability to directly visualize as well as biopsy the abnormality. Colonoscopy is the procedure of choice for colon cancer screening and surveillance as well as diagnosis of colitis secondary to infection, ischemia, radiation, and inflammatory bowel disease. Sigmoidoscopy examines the colon up to the splenic flexure and is currently used to exclude distal colonic inflammation or obstruction in young patients not at significant risk for colon cancer. For elusive GI bleeding secondary to arteriovenous malformations or superficial ulcers, small-intestinal examination is performed with push enteroscopy, capsule endoscopy, or double-balloon enteroscopy. Capsule endoscopy also can visualize small-intestinal Crohn's disease in individuals with negative barium radiography. Endoscopic retrograde cholangiopancreaticography (ERCP) provides diagnoses of pancreatic and biliary disease. Endoscopic ultrasound is useful for evaluating extent of disease in GI malignancy as well as exclusion of choledocholithiasis, evaluation of pancreatitis, drainage of pancreatic pseudocysts, and assessment of anal continuity.

Radiography/Nuclear Medicine Radiographic tests evaluate diseases of the gut and extraluminal structures. Oral or rectal contrast agents like barium provide mucosal definition from the esophagus to the rectum. Contrast radiography also assesses gut transit and pelvic floor dysfunction. Barium swallow is the initial procedure for evaluation of dysphagia to exclude subtle rings or strictures and assess for achalasia, whereas small-bowel contrast radiology reliably diagnoses intestinal tumors and Crohn's ileitis. Contrast enemas are performed when colonoscopy is unsuccessful or contraindicated. Ultrasound and computed tomography (CT) evaluate regions not accessible by endoscopy or contrast studies, including the liver, pancreas, gallbladder, kidneys, and retroperitoneum. These tests are useful for diagnosis of mass lesions, fluid collections, organ enlargement, and, in the case of ultrasound, gallstones. CT and magnetic resonance (MR) colonography are being evaluated as alternatives to colonoscopy for colon cancer screening. MR imaging assesses the pancreaticobiliary ducts to exclude neoplasm, stones, and sclerosing cholangitis, and the liver to characterize benign and malignant tumors. Specialized CT or MR enterography can assess intensity of inflammatory bowel disease. Angiography excludes mesenteric ischemia and determines spread of malignancy. Angiographic techniques also access the biliary tree in obstructive jaundice. CT and MR techniques can be used to screen for mesenteric occlusion, thereby limiting exposure to angiographic dyes. Positron emission tomography can facilitate distinguishing malignant from benign disease in several organ systems.

Scintigraphy both evaluates structural abnormalities and quantifies luminal transit. Radionuclide bleeding scans localize bleeding sites in patients with brisk hemorrhage so that therapy with endoscopy, angiography, or surgery may be directed. Radiolabeled leukocyte scans can search for intraabdominal abscesses not visualized on CT. Biliary scintigraphy is complementary to ultrasound in the assessment of cholecystitis. Scintigraphy to quantify esophageal and gastric emptying is well established, whereas techniques to measure small-intestinal or colonic transit are less widely used.

Histopathology Gut mucosal biopsies obtained at endoscopy evaluate for inflammatory, infectious, and neoplastic disease. Deep rectal biopsies assist with diagnosis of Hirschsprung's disease or amyloid. Liver

TABLE 344-2 COMMON INDICATIONS FOR ENDOSCOPY

Upper Endoscopy	Colonoscopy	Endoscopic Retrograde Cholangiopancreatography	Endoscopic Ultrasound	Capsule Endoscopy	Double-Balloon Endoscopy
Dyspepsia despite treatment	Cancer screening	Jaundice	Staging of malignancy	Obscure gastrointestinal (GI) bleeding	Ablation of small-intestinal bleeding sources
Dyspepsia with signs of organic disease	Lower GI bleeding	Postbiliary surgery complaints	Characterize and biopsy submucosal mass	Suspected Crohn's disease of the small intestine	Biopsy of suspicious small-intestinal masses/ulcers
Refractory vomiting	Anemia	Cholangitis	Bile duct stones		
Dysphagia	Diarrhea	Gallstone pancreatitis	Chronic pancreatitis		
Upper GI bleeding	Polypectomy	Pancreatic/biliary/ampullary tumor	Drain pseudocyst		
Anemia	Obstruction	Unexplained pancreatitis	Anal continuity		
Weight loss	Biopsy radiologic abnormality	Pancreatitis with unrelenting pain			
Malabsorption	Cancer surveillance: family history prior polyp/cancer, colitis	Fistulas			
Biopsy radiologic abnormality	Palliate neoplasm	Biopsy radiologic abnormality			
Polypectomy	Remove foreign body	Pancreaticobiliary drainage			
Place gastrostomy	Place stent across stenosis	Sample bile			
Barrett's surveillance		Sphincter of Oddi manometry			
Palliate neoplasm					
Sample duodenal tissue/fluid					
Remove foreign body					
Endoscopic mucosal resection or ablation of dysplastic Barrett's mucosa					
Place stent across stenosis					

biopsy is indicated in cases with abnormal liver chemistries, in unexplained jaundice, following liver transplant to exclude rejection, and to characterize the degree of inflammation in patients with chronic viral hepatitis prior to initiating antiviral therapy. Biopsies obtained during CT or ultrasound can evaluate for other intraabdominal conditions not accessible by endoscopy.

Functional Testing Tests of gut function provide important data when structural testing is nondiagnostic. In addition to gastric acid and pancreatic function testing, functional testing of motor activity is provided by manometric techniques. Esophageal manometry is useful for suspected achalasia, whereas small-intestinal manometry tests for pseudoobstruction. A wireless motility capsule is now available to measure transit and contractile activity in the stomach, small intestine, and colon in a single test. Anorectal manometry with balloon expulsion testing is used for unexplained incontinence or constipation from outlet dysfunction. Anorectal manometry and electromyography also assess anal function in fecal incontinence. Biliary manometry tests for sphincter of Oddi dysfunction with unexplained biliary pain. Measurement of breath hydrogen while fasting and after oral mono- or oligosaccharide challenge can screen for carbohydrate intolerance and small-intestinal bacterial overgrowth.

TREATMENT GASTROINTESTINAL DISEASE

Management options for the patient with GI disease depend on the cause of symptoms. Available treatments include modifications in dietary intake, medications, interventional endoscopy or radiology techniques, surgery, and therapies directed to external influences.

NUTRITIONAL MANIPULATION

Dietary modifications for GI disease include treatments that only reduce symptoms, therapies that correct pathologic defects, and measures that replace normal food intake with enteral or parenteral formulations. Changes that improve symptoms but do not reverse an organic abnormality include lactose restriction for lactase deficiency, liquid meals in gastroparesis, carbohydrate restrictions with dumping syndrome, and low-FODMAP (fermentable oligo-di-monosaccharides and polyols) diets in irritable bowel syndrome. The gluten-free diet for celiac disease exemplifies a modification that serves as primary therapy to reduce mucosal inflammation. Enteral medium-chain triglycerides replace normal fats in short-gut syndrome or severe ileal disease. Perfusion of liquid meals through a gastrostomy is performed in those who cannot swallow safely. Enteral feeding through a jejunostomy is considered for gastric dysmotility syndromes that preclude feeding into the stomach. Intravenous hyperalimentation is used for individuals with generalized gut malfunction who cannot tolerate or who cannot be sustained with enteral nutrition.

PHARMACOTHERAPY

Several medications are available to treat GI diseases. Considerable health care resources are expended on over-the-counter remedies. Many prescription drug classes are offered as short-term or continuous therapy of GI illness. A plethora of alternative treatments have gained popularity in GI conditions for which traditional therapies provide incomplete relief.

Over-the-Counter Agents Over-the-counter agents are reserved for mild GI symptoms. Antacids and histamine H_2 antagonists decrease symptoms in gastroesophageal reflux and dyspepsia, whereas antiflatulents and adsorbents reduce gaseous symptoms. More potent acid inhibitors such as proton pump inhibitors are now available over the counter for treatment of chronic gastroesophageal reflux disease (GERD). Fiber supplements, stool softeners, enemas, and laxatives are used for constipation. Laxatives are categorized as stimulants, osmotic agents (including isotonic preparations containing polyethylene glycol), and poorly absorbed sugars. Nonprescription antidiarrheal agents include bismuth subsalicylate, kaolin-pectin combinations, and loperamide. Supplemental enzymes include lactase pills for lactose intolerance and bacterial α-galactosidase to treat excess gas. In general, use of a nonprescription preparation for more than a short time for chronic persistent symptoms should be supervised by a health care provider.

Prescription Drugs Prescription drugs for GI diseases are a major focus of attention from pharmaceutical companies. Potent acid suppressants, including drugs that inhibit the proton pump, are advocated for acid reflux when over-the-counter preparations are inadequate. Cytoprotective agents rarely are used for upper gut ulcers. Prokinetic drugs stimulate GI propulsion in gastroparesis and pseudoobstruction. Prosecretory drugs are prescribed for constipation refractory to other agents. Prescription antidiarrheals include opiate drugs, anticholinergic antispasmodics, tricyclics, bile acid binders, and serotonin antagonists. Antispasmodics and antidepressants also are useful for functional abdominal pain, whereas narcotics are used for pain control in organic conditions such as disseminated malignancy and chronic pancreatitis. Antiemetics in several classes reduce nausea and vomiting. Potent pancreatic enzymes decrease malabsorption and pain from pancreatic disease. Antisecretory drugs such as the somatostatin analogue octreotide treat hypersecretory states. Antibiotics treat ulcer disease secondary to *Helicobacter pylori*, infectious diarrhea, diverticulitis, intestinal bacterial overgrowth, and Crohn's disease. Some cases of irritable bowel syndrome (especially those with diarrhea) respond to nonabsorbable antibiotic therapy. Anti-inflammatory and immunosuppressive drugs are used in ulcerative colitis, Crohn's disease, microscopic colitis, refractory celiac disease, and gut vasculitis. Chemotherapy with or without radiotherapy is offered for GI malignancies. Most GI carcinomas respond poorly to such therapy, whereas lymphomas may be cured with such intervention.

Alternative Therapies Alternative treatments are marketed to treat selected GI symptoms. Ginger, acupressure, and acustimulation have been advocated for nausea, whereas pyridoxine has been investigated for nausea of first-trimester pregnancy. Probiotics containing active bacterial cultures are used as adjuncts in some cases of infectious diarrhea and irritable bowel syndrome. Probiotics that selectively nourish benign commensal bacteria may ultimately show benefit in functional disorders as well. Low-potency pancreatic enzyme preparations are sold as general digestive aids but have little evidence to support their efficacy.

ENTERIC THERAPIES/INTERVENTIONAL ENDOSCOPY AND RADIOLOGY

Simple luminal interventions are commonly performed for GI diseases. Nasogastric tube suction decompresses the upper gut in ileus or mechanical obstruction. Nasogastric lavage of saline or water in the patient with upper GI hemorrhage determines the rate of bleeding and helps evacuate blood prior to endoscopy. Enteral feedings can be initiated through a nasogastric or nasoenteric tube. Enemas relieve fecal impaction or assist in gas evacuation in acute colonic pseudoobstruction. A rectal tube can be left in place to vent the distal colon in colonic pseudoobstruction and other colonic distention disorders.

In addition to its diagnostic role, endoscopy has therapeutic capabilities in certain settings. Cautery techniques can stop hemorrhage from ulcers, vascular malformations, and tumors. Injection with vasoconstrictor substances or sclerosants is used for bleeding ulcers, vascular malformations, varices, and hemorrhoids. Endoscopic encirclement of varices and hemorrhoids with constricting bands stops hemorrhage from these sites, whereas endoscopically placed clips can occlude arterial bleeding sites. Endoscopy can remove polyps or debulk lumen-narrowing malignancies. Endoscopic mucosal resection and radiofrequency techniques can remove or ablate some cases of Barrett's esophagus with dysplasia. Endoscopic sphincterotomy of the ampulla of Vater relieves symptoms of choledocholithiasis. Obstructions of the gut lumen and pancreaticobiliary tree are relieved by endoscopic dilatation or placement of plastic or expandable metal stents. In cases of acute colonic pseudoobstruction, colonoscopy is used to withdraw luminal gas. Finally, endoscopy is commonly used to insert feeding tubes.

Radiologic measures also are useful in GI disease. Angiographic embolization or vasoconstriction decreases bleeding from sites not amenable to endoscopic intervention. Dilatation or stenting with fluoroscopic guidance relieves luminal strictures. Contrast enemas can reduce volvulus and evacuate air in acute colonic pseudoobstruction. CT and ultrasound help drain abdominal fluid collections, in many cases obviating the need for surgery. Percutaneous transhepatic cholangiography relieves biliary obstruction when ERCP is contraindicated. Lithotripsy can fragment gallstones in patients who are not candidates for surgery. In some instances, radiologic approaches offer advantages over endoscopy for gastroenterostomy placement. Finally, central venous catheters for parenteral nutrition may be placed using radiographic techniques.

SURGERY

Surgery is performed to cure disease, control symptoms without cure, maintain nutrition, or palliate unresectable neoplasm. Medication-unresponsive ulcerative colitis, diverticulitis, cholecystitis, appendicitis, and intraabdominal abscess are curable with surgery, whereas only symptom control without cure is possible with Crohn's disease. Surgery is mandated for ulcer complications such as bleeding, obstruction, or perforation and intestinal obstructions that persist after conservative care. Fundoplication of the gastroesophageal junction is performed for severe ulcerative esophagitis and drug-refractory symptomatic acid reflux. Achalasia responds to operations to relieve lower esophageal sphincter pressure. Operations for motor disorders have been introduced including implanted electrical stimulators for gastroparesis and electrical devices and artificial sphincters for fecal incontinence. Surgery may be needed to place a jejunostomy for long-term enteral feedings. The threshold for performing surgery depends on the clinical setting. In all cases, the benefits of operation must be weighed against the potential for postoperative complications.

THERAPY DIRECTED TO EXTERNAL INFLUENCES

In some conditions, GI symptoms respond to treatments directed outside the gut. Psychological therapies including psychotherapy, behavior modification, hypnosis, and biofeedback have shown efficacy in functional bowel disorders. Patients with significant psychological dysfunction and those with little response to treatments targeting the gut are likely to benefit from this form of therapy.

345 Gastrointestinal Endoscopy

Louis Michel Wong Kee Song, Mark Topazian

Gastrointestinal endoscopy has been attempted for over 200 years, but the introduction of semirigid gastroscopes in the middle of the twentieth century marked the dawn of the modern endoscopic era. Since then, rapid advances in endoscopic technology have led to dramatic changes in the diagnosis and treatment of many digestive diseases. Innovative endoscopic devices and new endoscopic treatment modalities continue to expand the use of endoscopy in patient care.

Current flexible endoscopes provide an electronic video image generated by a charge-coupled device in the tip of the endoscope. Operator controls permit deflection of the endoscope tip; fiberoptic bundles or light-emitting diodes bring light to the tip of the endoscope; and working channels allow washing, suctioning, and the passage of instruments. Progressive changes in the diameter and stiffness of endoscopes have improved the ease and patient tolerance of endoscopy.

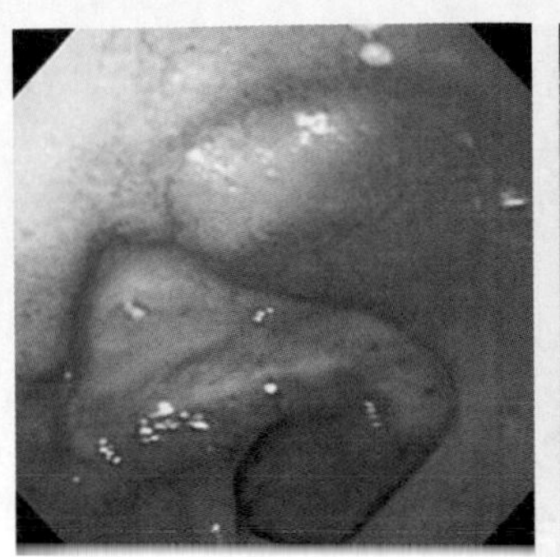

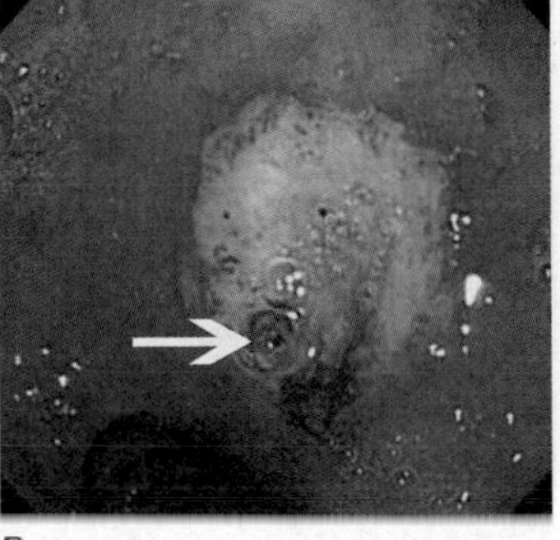

A B

FIGURE 345-1 Duodenal ulcers. ***A.*** Ulcer with a clean base. ***B.*** Ulcer with a visible vessel (*arrow*) in a patient with recent hemorrhage.

ENDOSCOPIC PROCEDURES

UPPER ENDOSCOPY

Upper endoscopy, also referred to as esophagogastroduodenoscopy (EGD), is performed by passing a flexible endoscope through the mouth into the esophagus, stomach, and duodenum. The procedure is the best method for examining the upper gastrointestinal mucosa. While the upper gastrointestinal radiographic series has similar accuracy for diagnosis of duodenal ulcer (Fig. 345-1), EGD is superior for detection of gastric ulcers (Fig. 345-2) and flat mucosal lesions such as Barrett's esophagus (Fig. 345-3), and it permits directed biopsy and endoscopic therapy. Intravenous conscious sedation is given to most patients in the United States to ease the anxiety and discomfort of the procedure, although in many countries EGD is routinely performed with topical pharyngeal anesthesia only. Patient tolerance of unsedated EGD is improved by the use of an ultrathin, 5-mm diameter endoscope that can be passed transorally or transnasally.

COLONOSCOPY

Colonoscopy is performed by passing a flexible colonoscope through the anal canal into the rectum and colon. The cecum is reached in >95% of cases, and the terminal ileum can often be examined. Colonoscopy is the gold standard for imaging the colonic mucosa. Colonoscopy has greater sensitivity than barium enema for colitis (Fig. 345-4), polyps (Fig. 345-5), and cancer (Fig. 345-6). Computed tomography (CT) colonography is an emerging technology that rivals the accuracy of colonoscopy for detection of some polyps and cancer, although it may not be sensitive for the detection of flat lesions, such as serrated polyps (Fig. 345-7). Conscious sedation is usually given before colonoscopy in the United States, although a willing patient and a skilled examiner can complete the procedure without sedation in many cases.

FLEXIBLE SIGMOIDOSCOPY

Flexible sigmoidoscopy is similar to colonoscopy, but visualizes only the rectum and a variable portion of the left colon, typically to 60 cm from the anal verge. This procedure causes abdominal cramping, but it is brief and is usually performed without sedation. Flexible sigmoidoscopy is primarily used for evaluation of diarrhea and rectal outlet bleeding.

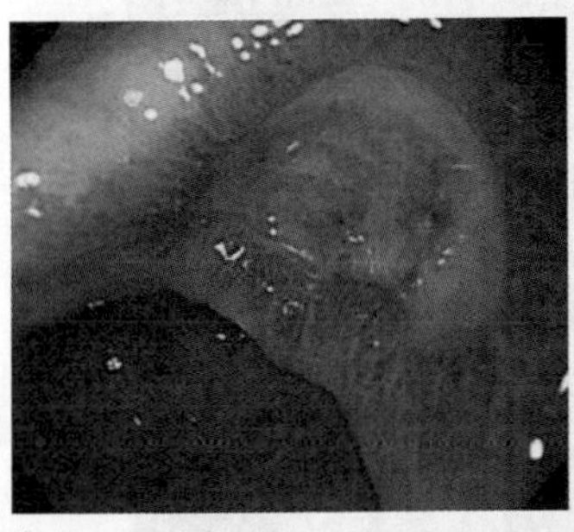

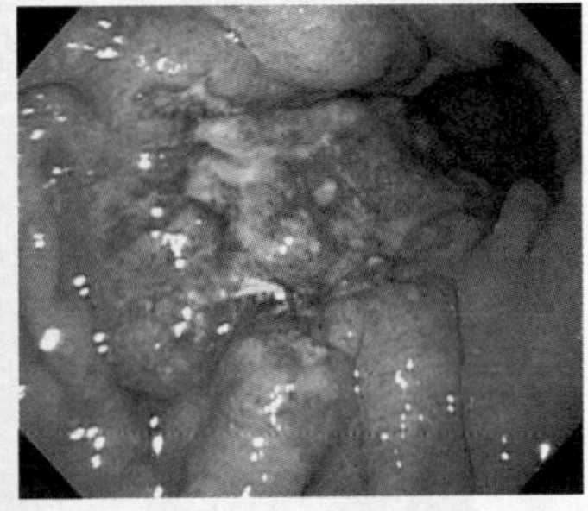

A B

FIGURE 345-2 Gastric ulcers. ***A.*** Benign gastric ulcer. ***B.*** Malignant gastric ulcer involving greater curvature of stomach.

SMALL-BOWEL ENDOSCOPY

Three endoscopic techniques are currently used to evaluate the small intestine, most often in patients presenting with presumed small-bowel bleeding. For *capsule endoscopy*, the patient swallows a disposable capsule that contains a complementary metal oxide silicon (CMOS) chip camera. Color still images (Fig. 345-8) are transmitted wirelessly to an external receiver at several frames per second until the capsule's battery is exhausted or it is passed into the toilet. Capsule endoscopy enables visualization of the small-bowel mucosa beyond the reach of a conventional endoscope and, at present, is solely a diagnostic procedure.

Push enteroscopy is performed with a long endoscope similar in design to an upper endoscope. The enteroscope is pushed down the small bowel, sometimes with the help of a stiffening overtube that extends from the mouth to the small intestine. The proximal to mid-jejunum is usually reached, and the instrument channel of the endoscope allows for biopsy or endoscopic therapy.

Deeper insertion into the small bowel can be accomplished by *single-* or *double-balloon enteroscopy* or *spiral enteroscopy* (Fig. 345-9). These instruments enable pleating of the small intestine onto an overtube (see Video 346e-1). With balloon-assisted enteroscopy, the entire intestinal tract can be visualized in some patients when both the oral and anal routes of insertion are used. Biopsies and endoscopic therapy can be performed throughout the visualized small bowel (Fig. 345-10).

ENDOSCOPIC RETROGRADE CHOLANGIOPANCREATOGRAPHY (ERCP)

During ERCP a side-viewing endoscope is passed through the mouth to the duodenum, the ampulla of Vater is identified and cannulated with a thin plastic catheter, and radiographic contrast material is injected into the bile duct and pancreatic duct under fluoroscopic guidance (Fig. 345-11). When indicated, the sphincter of Oddi can be opened using the technique of endoscopic sphincterotomy (Fig. 345-12). Stones can be retrieved from the ducts (see Video 346e-15), biopsies can be performed, strictures can be dilated and/or stented (Fig. 345-13), and ductal leaks can be stented (Fig. 345-14). ERCP is often performed for therapy but remains important in diagnosis, especially for sphincter of Oddi dysfunction and for tissue sampling of ductal strictures.

ENDOSCOPIC ULTRASOUND (EUS)

EUS utilizes high-frequency ultrasound transducers incorporated into the tip of a flexible endoscope. Ultrasound images are obtained of the gut wall and adjacent organs, vessels, and lymph nodes. By sacrificing depth of ultrasound penetration and bringing the ultrasound transducer close to the area of interest via endoscopy, high-resolution images are obtained. EUS provides the most accurate preoperative local staging of esophageal, pancreatic, and rectal malignancies (Fig. 345-15), although it does not detect most distant metastases. EUS is also useful for diagnosis of bile duct stones, gallbladder disease, submucosal gastrointestinal lesions, and chronic pancreatitis. Fine-needle aspirates and core biopsies of masses and lymph nodes in the posterior mediastinum, abdomen, pancreas, retroperitoneum, and pelvis can be obtained under EUS guidance (Fig. 345-16). EUS-guided therapeutic procedures are increasingly performed, including drainage of abscesses, pseudocysts, and pancreatic necrosis into the gut lumen (see Video 346e-2), celiac plexus neurolysis for treatment of pancreatic pain, ethanol ablation of pancreatic neuroendocrine tumors, treatment of gastrointestinal hemorrhage, and drainage of obstructed biliary and pancreatic ducts.

NATURAL ORIFICE TRANSLUMINAL ENDOSCOPIC SURGERY (NOTES)

NOTES is an evolving collection of endoscopic methods that entail passage of an endoscope or its accessories into or through the wall of the gastrointestinal tract to perform diagnostic or therapeutic

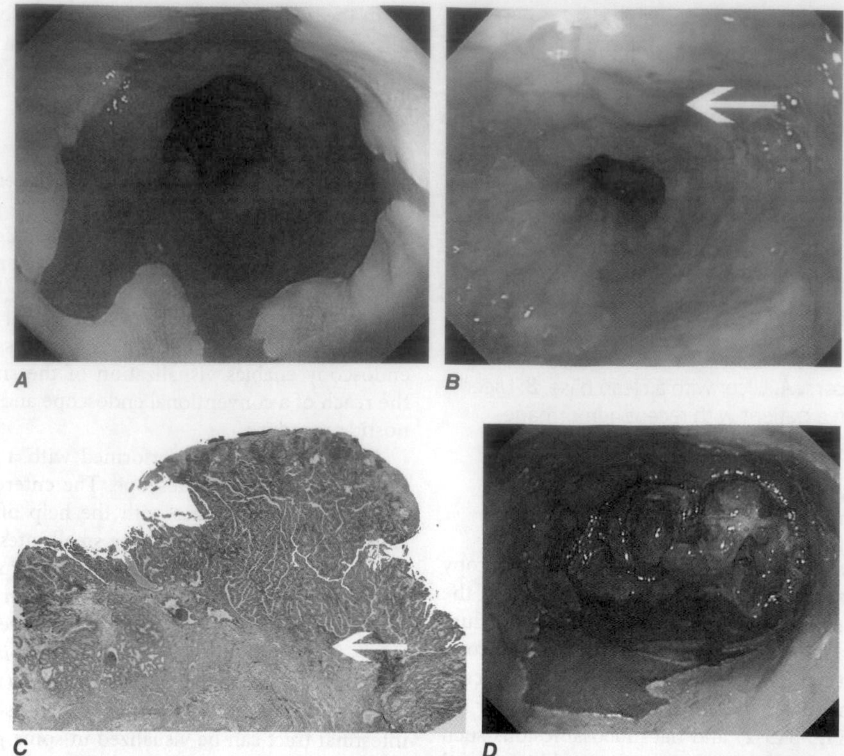

FIGURE 345-3 Barrett's esophagus. ***A.*** Pink tongues of Barrett's mucosa extending proximally from the gastroesophageal junction. ***B.*** Barrett's esophagus with a suspicious nodule (*arrow*) identified during endoscopic surveillance. ***C.*** Histologic finding of intramucosal adenocarcinoma in the endoscopically resected nodule. Tumor extends into the esophageal submucosa (*arrow*). ***D.*** Barrett's esophagus with locally advanced adenocarcinoma.

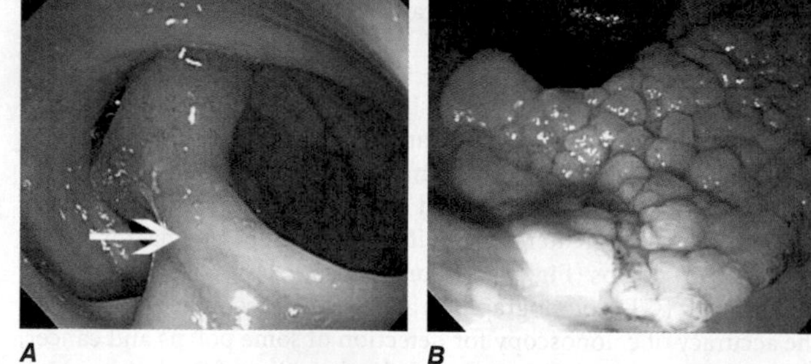

FIGURE 345-5 Colonic polyps. ***A.*** Pedunculated colon polyp on a thick stalk covered with normal mucosa (*arrow*). ***B.*** Sessile rectal polyp.

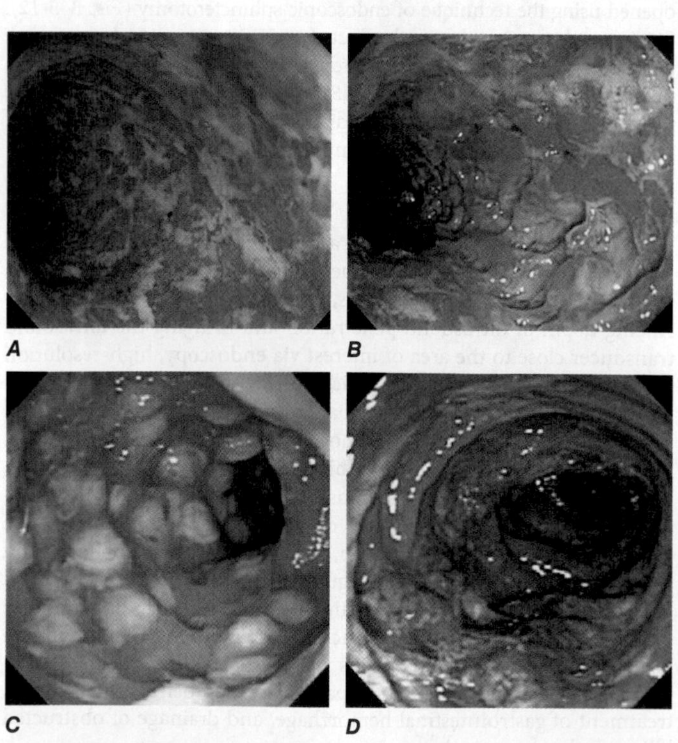

FIGURE 345-4 Causes of colitis. ***A.*** Chronic ulcerative colitis with diffuse ulcerations and exudates. ***B.*** Severe Crohn's colitis with deep ulcers. ***C.*** Pseudomembranous colitis with yellow, adherent pseudomembranes. ***D.*** Ischemic colitis with patchy mucosal edema, subepithelial hemorrhage, and cyanosis.

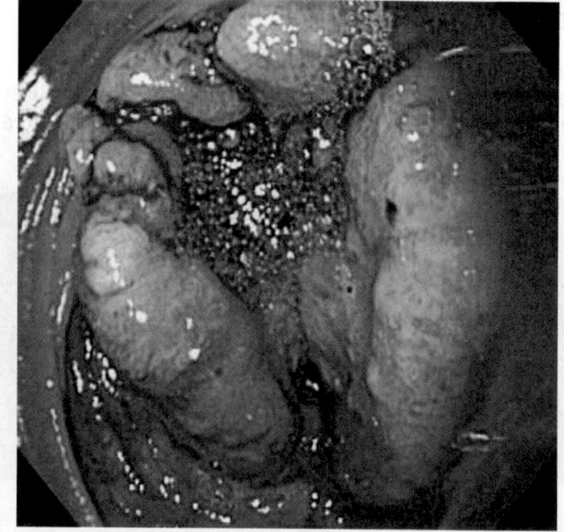

FIGURE 345-6 Colon adenocarcinoma growing into the lumen.

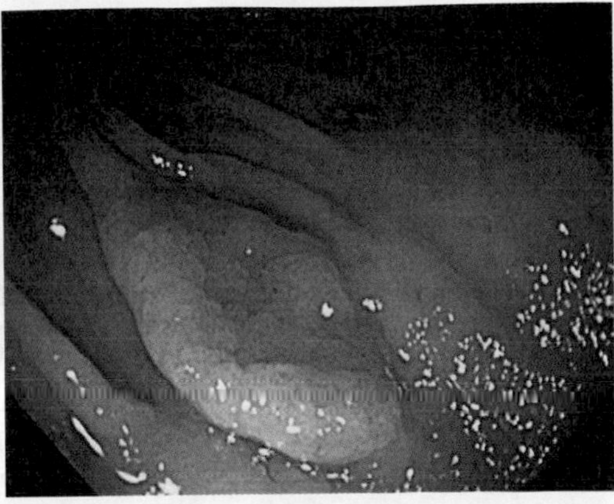

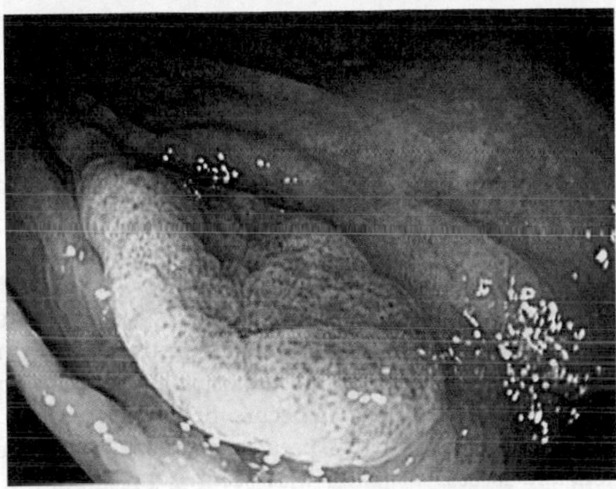

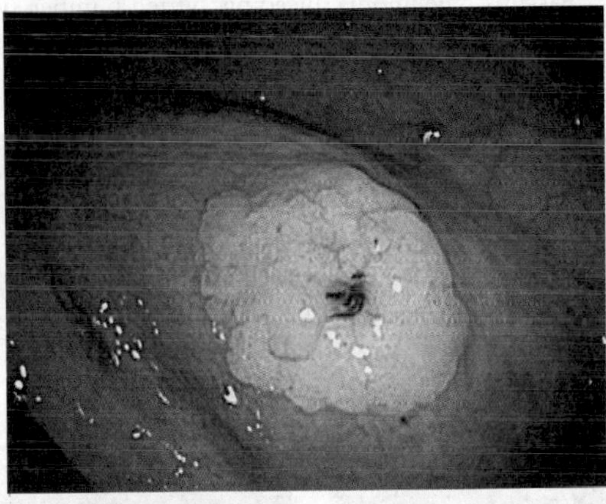

FIGURE 345-7 Flat serrated polyp in the cecum. ***A.*** Appearance of the lesion under conventional white-light imaging. ***B.*** Mucosal patterns and boundary of the lesion enhanced with narrow band imaging. ***C.*** Submucosal lifting of the lesion with dye (methylene blue) injection prior to resection.

interventions. Some NOTES procedures, such as percutaneous endoscopic gastrostomy (PEG) or endoscopic necrosectomy of pancreatic necrosis, are well-established clinical procedures (see Video 346e-2); others, such as per-oral endoscopic myotomy (POEM) and endoscopic full-thickness resection of gastrointestinal mural lesions (Fig. 345-17, see Video 346e-3), are emerging as viable clinical therapeutic options; and still others, such as endoscopic appendectomy, cholecystectomy, and tubal ligation, are in development, and their ultimate clinical application is presently unclear. NOTES is currently an area of intense innovation and endoscopic research.

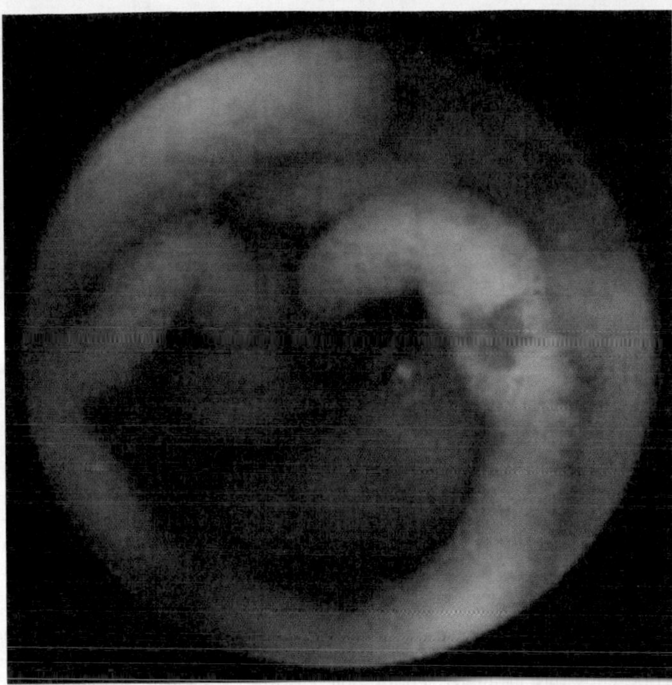

FIGURE 345-8 Capsule endoscopy image of jejunal vascular ectasia.

ENDOSCOPIC RESECTION AND CLOSURE TECHNIQUES

Endoscopic mucosal resection (EMR) (see Video 346e-4) and endoscopic submucosal dissection (ESD) (Fig. 345-18, see Video 346e-5) are two commonly used techniques for the resection of benign and early-stage malignant gastrointestinal neoplasms. In addition to providing larger specimens for more accurate histopathologic assessment and diagnosis, these techniques can be potentially

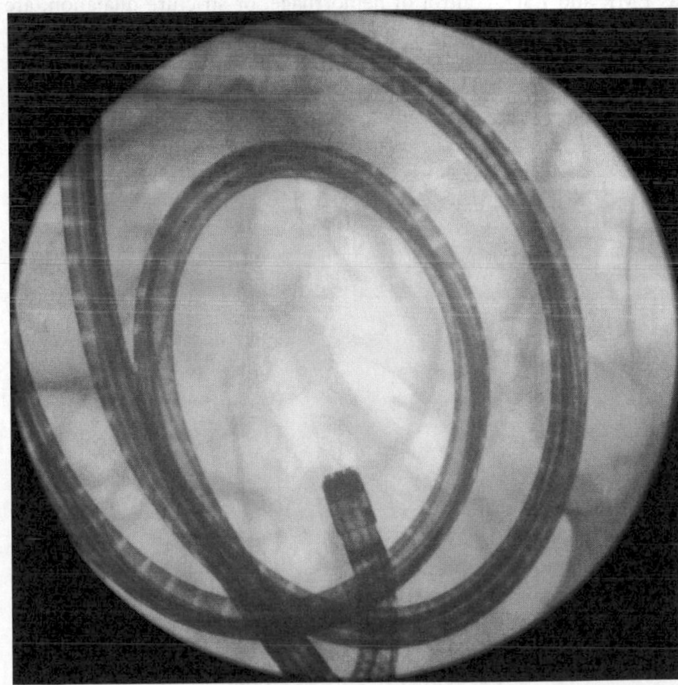

FIGURE 345-9 Radiograph of a double-balloon enteroscope in the small intestine.

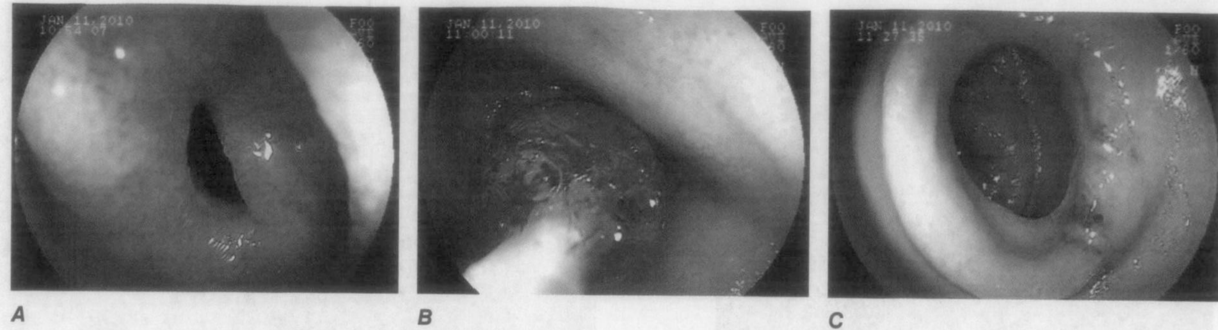

FIGURE 345-10 Nonsteroidal anti-inflammatory drug (NSAID)–induced proximal ileal stricture diagnosed by double-balloon endoscopy. ***A.*** Ileal stricture causing obstructive symptoms. ***B.*** Balloon dilatation of the ileal stricture. ***C.*** Appearance of stricture after dilatation.

curative for certain dysplastic lesions and focal intramucosal carcinomas involving the esophagus, stomach, and colon. Several devices are also available for closure of EMR and ESD defects, as well as gastrointestinal fistulas and perforations. Endoscopic clips deployed through the working channel of an endoscope have been used for many years to treat bleeding lesions, but the development of more robust over-the-scope clips has facilitated endoscopic closure of gastrointestinal fistulas and perforations not previously amenable to endoscopic therapy (see Video 346e-6). Endoscopic suturing is also feasible, and the technique can be used to close perforations and large defects (Fig. 345-19, see Video 346e-7), anastomotic leaks, and fistulas. Other potential indications for endoscopic suturing include stent fixation to prevent its migration (Fig. 345-20), and endoscopic bariatric procedures. These technologies are likely to have an expanding role in patient care.

RISKS OF ENDOSCOPY

Medications used during conscious sedation may cause respiratory depression or allergic reactions. All endoscopic procedures carry some risk of bleeding and gastrointestinal perforation. The risk is small with diagnostic upper endoscopy and colonoscopy (<1:1000 procedures), but ranges from 0.5 to 5% when therapeutic procedures, such as EMR and ESD, control of hemorrhage, or stricture dilatation, are performed. Bleeding and perforation are rare adverse events with flexible sigmoidoscopy. The risk of adverse events for diagnostic EUS (without needle aspiration) is similar to that for diagnostic upper endoscopy.

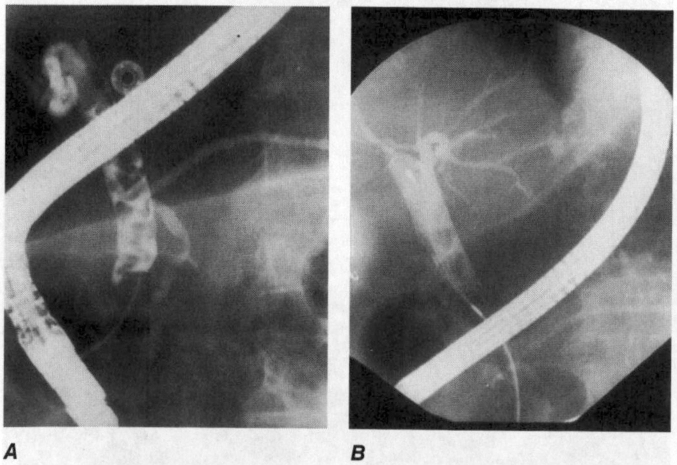

FIGURE 345-11 Endoscopic retrograde cholangiopancreatography (ERCP) for bile duct stones with cholangitis. ***A.*** Faceted bile duct stones are demonstrated in the common bile duct. ***B.*** After endoscopic sphincterotomy, the stones are extracted with a Dormia basket. A small abscess communicates with the left hepatic duct.

Infectious complications are uncommon with most endoscopic procedures. Some procedures carry a higher incidence of postprocedure bacteremia, and prophylactic antibiotics may be indicated (Table 345-1). Management of antithrombotic agents prior to endoscopic procedures should take into account the procedural risk of hemorrhage, the agent, and the patient condition, as summarized in Table 345-2.

ERCP carries additional risks. Pancreatitis occurs in about 5% of patients undergoing the procedure and in up to 30% of patients with sphincter of Oddi dysfunction. Young anicteric patients with normal ducts are at increased risk. Post-ERCP pancreatitis is usually mild and self-limited, but may result in prolonged hospitalization, surgery, diabetes, or death when severe. Bleeding occurs in 1% of endoscopic sphincterotomies. Ascending cholangitis, pseudocyst infection, retroperitoneal perforation, and abscess formation may occur as a result of ERCP.

Percutaneous gastrostomy tube placement during EGD is associated with a 10–15% incidence of adverse events, most often wound infections. Fasciitis, pneumonia, bleeding, buried bumper syndrome, and colonic injury may result from gastrostomy tube placement.

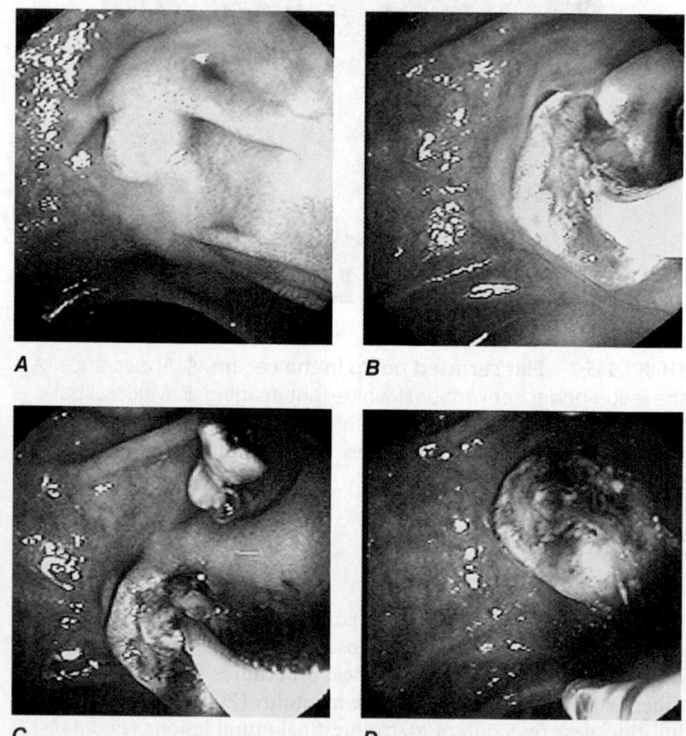

FIGURE 345-12 Endoscopic sphincterotomy. ***A.*** A normal-appearing ampulla of Vater. ***B.*** Sphincterotomy is performed with electrocautery. ***C.*** Bile duct stones are extracted with a balloon catheter. ***D.*** Final appearance of the sphincterotomy.

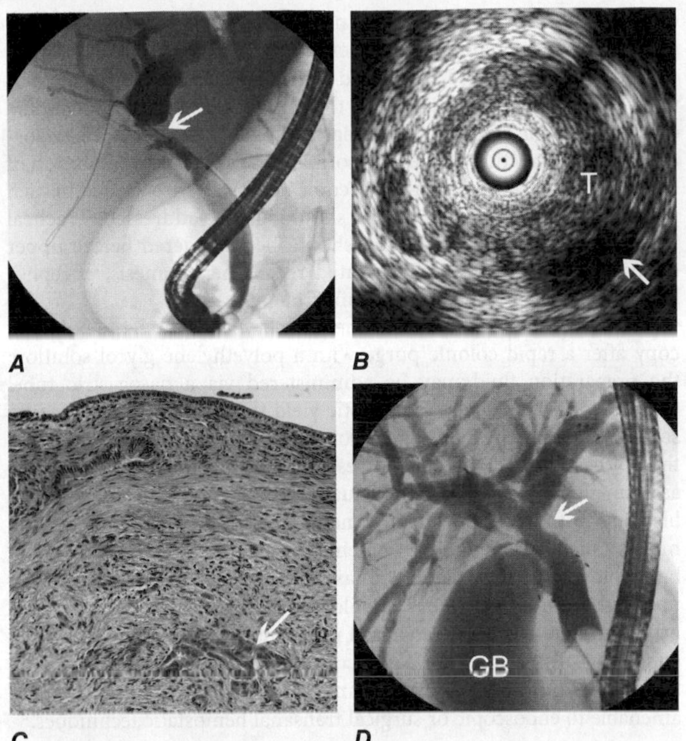

FIGURE 345-13 Endoscopic diagnosis, staging, and palliation of hilar cholangiocarcinoma. ***A.*** Endoscopic retrograde cholangiopancreatography (ERCP) in a patient with obstructive jaundice demonstrates a malignant-appearing stricture of the biliary confluence extending into the left and right intrahepatic ducts. ***B.*** Intraductal ultrasound of the biliary stricture demonstrates marked bile duct wall thickening due to tumor (T) with partial encasement of the hepatic artery (*arrow*). ***C.*** Intraductal biopsy obtained during ERCP demonstrates malignant cells infiltrating the submucosa of the bile duct wall (*arrow*). ***D.*** Endoscopic placement of bilateral self-expanding metal stents (*arrow*) relieves the biliary obstruction. GB, gallbladder. *(Image C courtesy of Dr. Thomas Smyrk; with permission.)*

URGENT ENDOSCOPY

ACUTE GASTROINTESTINAL HEMORRHAGE

Endoscopy is an important diagnostic and therapeutic technique for patients with acute gastrointestinal hemorrhage. Although gastrointestinal bleeding stops spontaneously in most cases, some patients will have persistent or recurrent hemorrhage that may be life-threatening. Clinical predictors of rebleeding help identify patients most likely

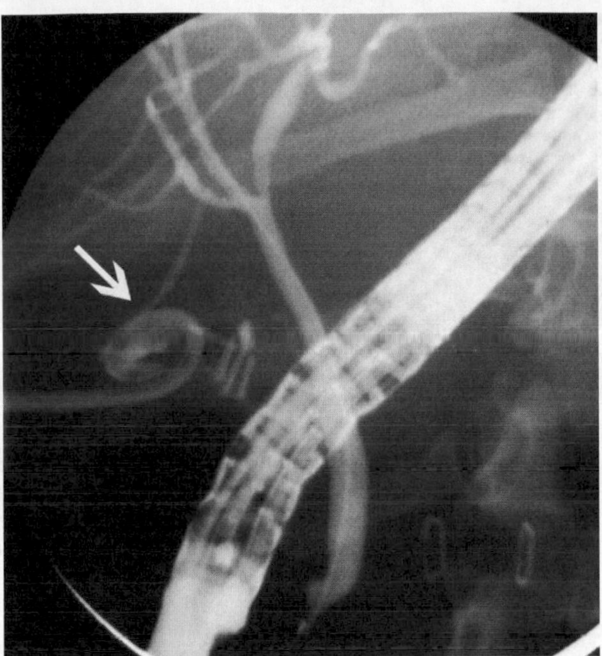

FIGURE 345-14 Bile leak (*arrow*) from a duct of Luschka after laparoscopic cholecystectomy. Contrast leaks from a small right intrahepatic duct into the gallbladder fossa and then flows into the pigtail of a percutaneous drainage catheter.

to benefit from urgent endoscopy and endoscopic, angiographic, or surgical hemostasis.

Initial Evaluation The initial evaluation of the bleeding patient focuses on the severity of hemorrhage as reflected by the postural vital signs, the frequency of hematemesis or melena, and (in some cases) findings on nasogastric lavage. Decreases in hematocrit and hemoglobin lag behind the clinical course and are not reliable gauges of the magnitude of acute bleeding. This initial evaluation, completed well before the bleeding source is confidently identified, guides immediate supportive care of the patient, triage to the ward or intensive care unit, and timing of endoscopy. The severity of the initial hemorrhage is the most important indication for urgent endoscopy, since a large initial bleed increases the likelihood of ongoing or recurrent bleeding. Patients with resting hypotension or orthostatic change in vital signs, repeated hematemesis, or bloody nasogastric aspirate that does not clear with large-volume lavage, or those requiring blood transfusions, should be considered for urgent endoscopy. In addition, patients with cirrhosis, coagulopathy, or respiratory or renal failure and those over 70 years of age are more likely to have significant rebleeding.

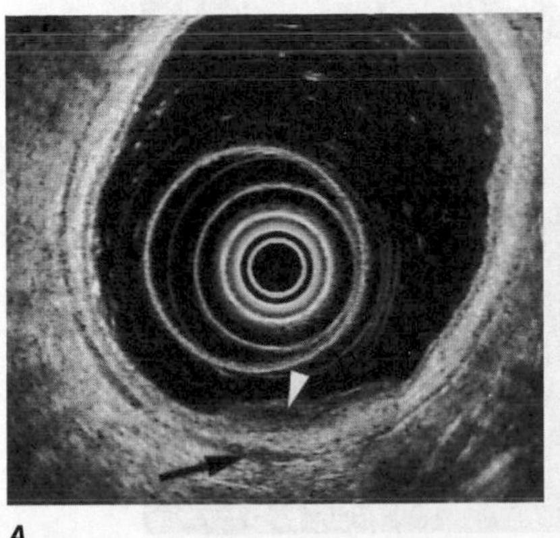

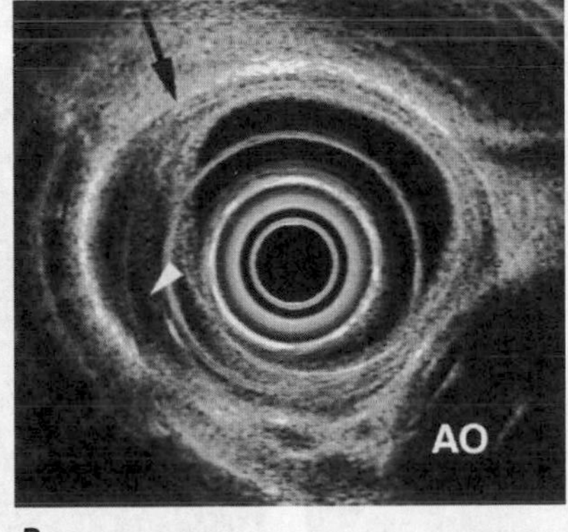

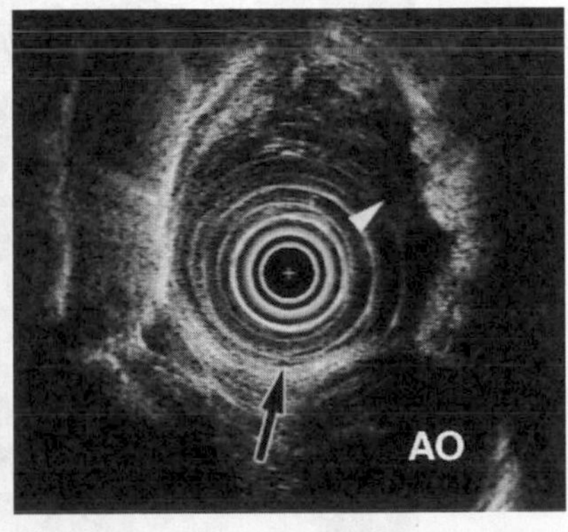

FIGURE 345-15 Local staging of gastrointestinal cancers with endoscopic ultrasound. In each example, the *white arrowhead* marks the primary tumor and the *black arrow* indicates the muscularis propria of the intestinal wall. ***A.*** T1 gastric cancer. The tumor does not invade the mp. ***B.*** T2 esophageal cancer. The tumor invades the muscularis propria. ***C.*** T3 esophageal cancer. The tumor extends through the muscularis propria into the surrounding tissue and focally abuts the aorta. AO, aorta.

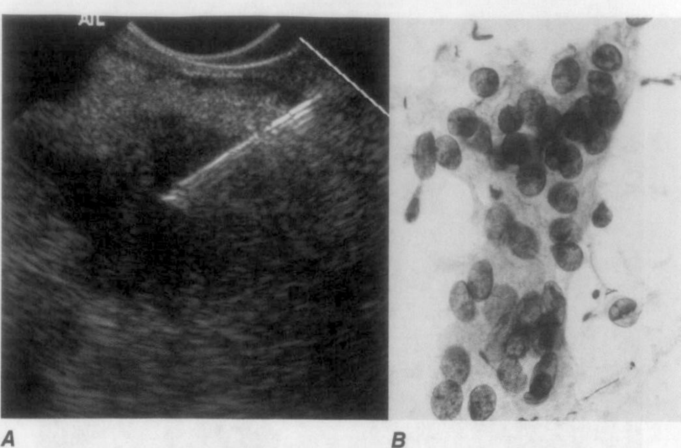

FIGURE 345-16 Endoscopic ultrasound (EUS)–guided fine-needle aspiration (FNA). ***A.*** Ultrasound image of a 22-gauge needle passed through the duodenal wall and positioned in a hypoechoic pancreatic head mass. ***B.*** Micrograph of aspirated malignant cells. *(Image B courtesy of Dr. Michael R. Henry; with permission.)*

Bedside evaluation also suggests an upper or lower gastrointestinal source of bleeding in most patients. Over 90% of patients with melena are bleeding proximal to the ligament of Treitz, and about 85% of patients with hematochezia are bleeding from the colon. Melena can result from bleeding in the small bowel or right colon, especially in older patients with slow colonic transit. Conversely, some patients with massive hematochezia may be bleeding from an upper gastrointestinal source, such as a gastric Dieulafoy lesion or duodenal ulcer, with rapid intestinal transit. Early upper endoscopy should be considered in such patients.

Endoscopy should be performed after the patient has been resuscitated with intravenous fluids and transfusions, as necessary. Marked coagulopathy or thrombocytopenia is usually treated before endoscopy, since correction of these abnormalities may lead to resolution of bleeding, and techniques for endoscopic hemostasis are limited in such patients. Metabolic derangements should also be addressed. Tracheal intubation for airway protection should be considered before upper endoscopy in patients with repeated recent hematemesis, encephalopathy, and suspected variceal hemorrhage.

Most patients with significant hematochezia can undergo colonoscopy after a rapid colonic purge with a polyethylene glycol solution; the preparation fluid may be administered via a nasogastric tube. Colonoscopy has a higher diagnostic yield than radionuclide bleeding scans or angiography in lower gastrointestinal bleeding, and endoscopic therapy can be applied in some cases. In a minority of cases, endoscopic assessment is hindered by poor visualization due to persistent vigorous bleeding with recurrent hemodynamic instability, and other techniques (such as angiography or emergent subtotal colectomy) must be employed. In such patients, massive bleeding originating from an upper gastrointestinal source should also be considered and excluded by upper endoscopy. The anal and rectal mucosa should be visualized endoscopically early in the course of massive rectal bleeding, because bleeding lesions in or close to the anal canal may be identified that are amenable to endoscopic or surgical transanal hemostatic techniques.

Peptic Ulcer The endoscopic appearance of peptic ulcers provides useful prognostic information and guides the need for endoscopic therapy in patients with acute hemorrhage (Fig. 345-21). A clean-based ulcer is associated with a low risk (3–5%) of rebleeding; patients with melena and a clean-based ulcer are often discharged home from the emergency

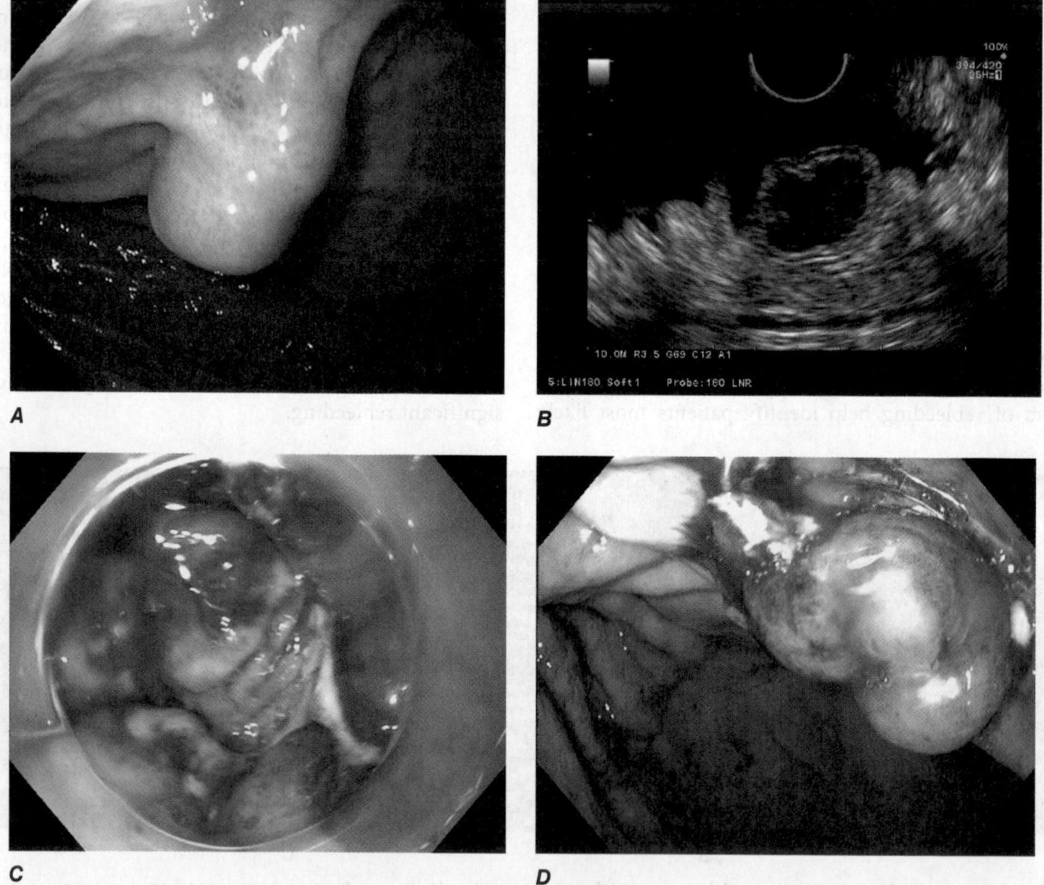

FIGURE 345-17 Endoscopic full-thickness resection of a gastrointestinal stromal tumor. ***A.*** Subepithelial lesion in the proximal stomach. ***B.*** Hypoechoic lesion arising from the fourth layer (muscularis propria) at endoscopic ultrasound. ***C.*** Full-thickness resection defect. ***D.*** Closure of defect using an over-the-scope clip.

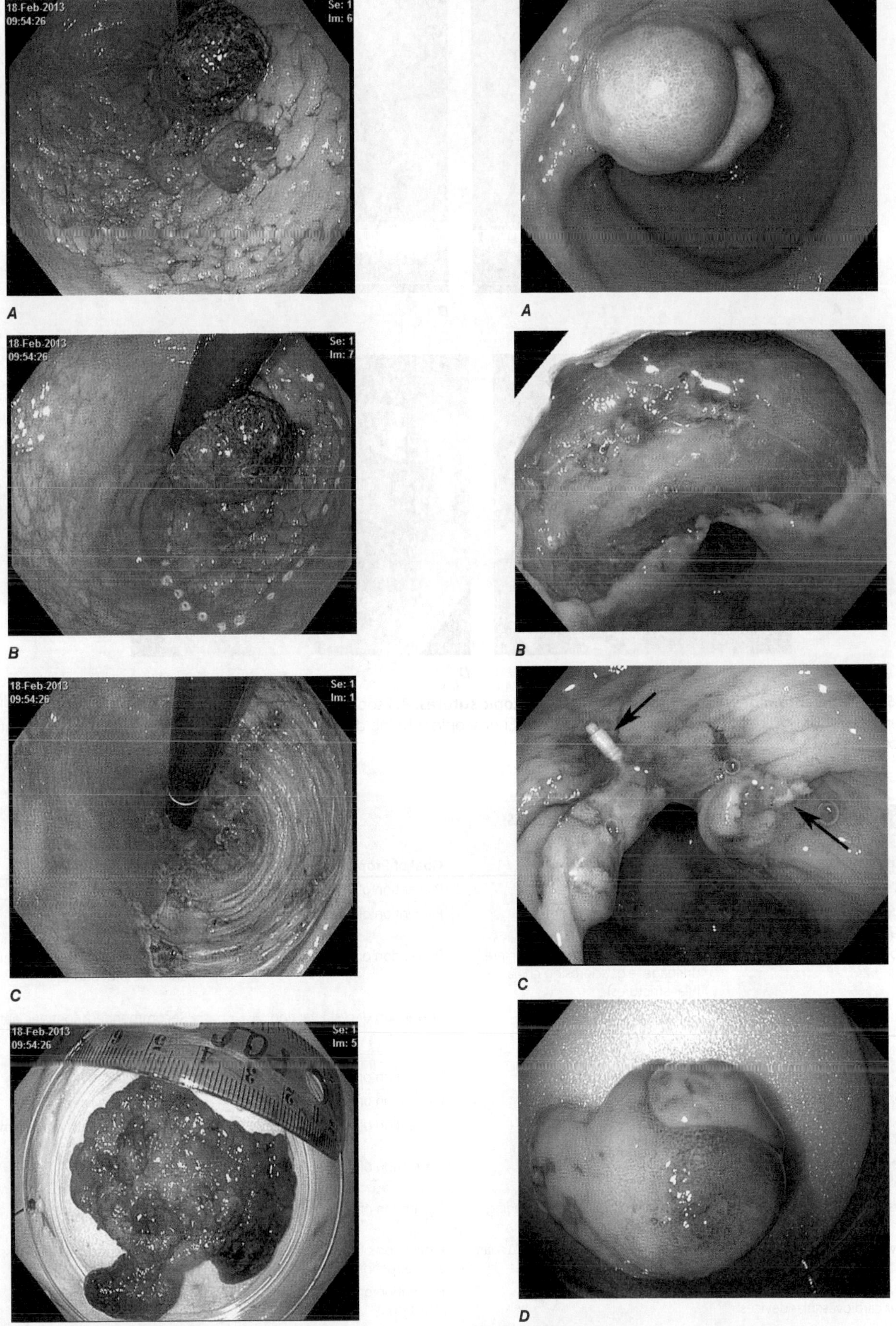

FIGURE 345-18 Endoscopic submucosal dissection. ***A.*** Large flat distal rectal adenoma with central lobulation. ***B.*** Marking the periphery of the lesion with coagulation dots. ***C.*** Rectal defect following endoscopic submucosal dissection. ***D.*** Specimen resected en bloc.

FIGURE 345-19 Closure of large defect using an endoscopic suturing device. ***A.*** Ulcerated inflammatory fibroid polyp in the antrum. ***B.*** Large defect following endoscopic submucosal dissection of the lesion. ***C.*** Closure of the defect using endoscopic sutures (*arrows*). ***D.*** Resected specimen.

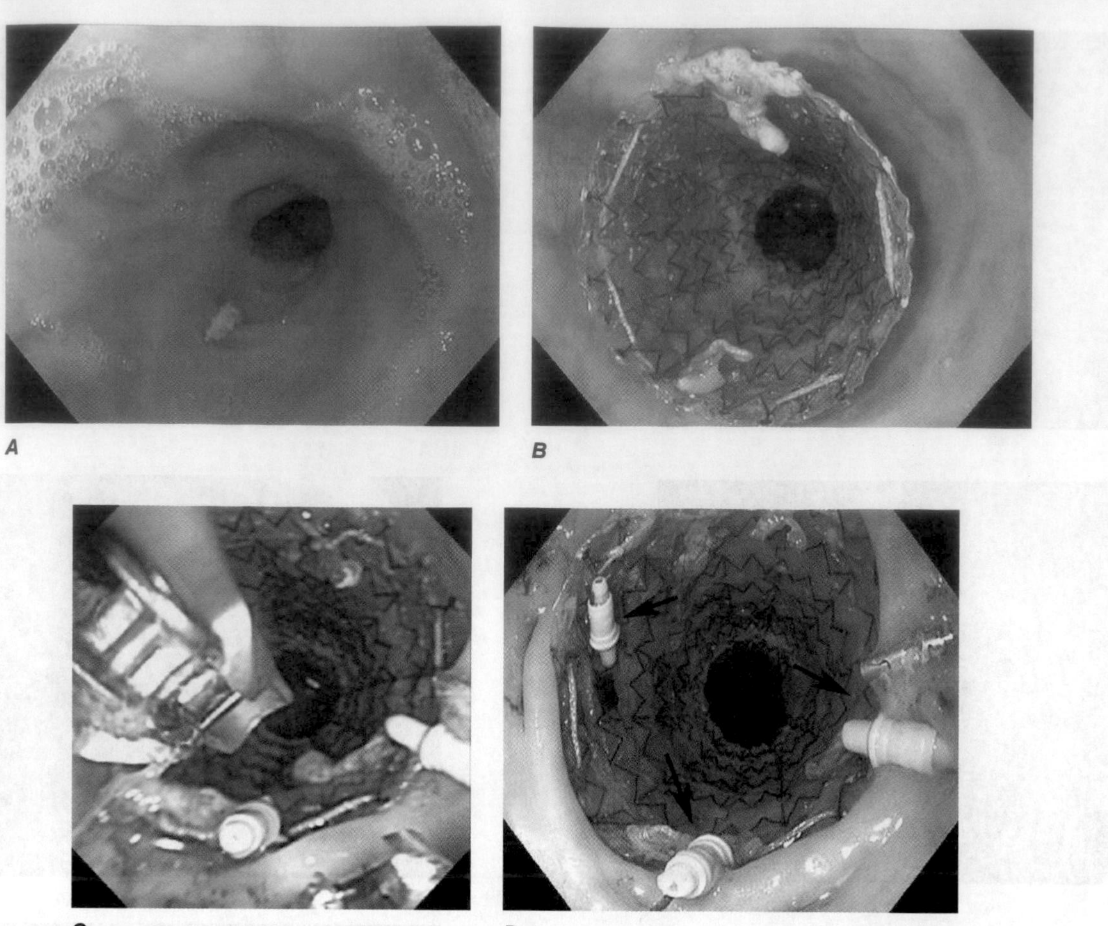

FIGURE 345-20 Prevention of stent migration using endoscopic sutures. ***A.*** Esophagogastric anastomotic stricture refractory to balloon dilation. ***B.*** Temporary placement of covered esophageal stent. ***C.*** Endoscopic suturing device to anchor stent to esophageal wall. ***D.*** Stent fixation with endoscopic sutures (*arrows*).

TABLE 345-1 ANTIBIOTIC PROPHYLAXIS FOR ENDOSCOPIC PROCEDURES

Patient Condition	Procedure Contemplated	Goal of Prophylaxis	Periprocedural Antibiotic Prophylaxis
All cardiac conditions	Any endoscopic procedure	Prevention of infective endocarditis	Not indicated
Bile duct obstruction in the absence of cholangitis	ERCP with complete drainage	Prevention of cholangitis	Not recommended
Bile duct obstruction in absence of cholangitis	ERCP with anticipated incomplete drainage (e.g., sclerosing cholangitis, hilar strictures)	Prevention of cholangitis	Recommended; continue antibiotics after the procedure
Sterile pancreatic fluid collection (e.g., pseudocyst, necrosis), which communicates with pancreatic duct	ERCP	Prevention of cyst infection	Recommended; continue antibiotics after the procedure
Sterile pancreatic fluid collection	Transmural drainage	Prevention of cyst infection	Recommended
Solid lesion along upper GI tract	EUS-FNA	Prevention of local infection	Not recommended[a]
Solid lesion along lower GI tract	EUS-FNA	Prevention of local infection	Insufficient data to make firm recommendation[b]
Cystic lesions along GI tract (including mediastinum)	EUS-FNA	Prevention of cyst infection	Recommended
All patients	Percutaneous endoscopic feeding tube placement	Prevention of peristomal infection	Recommended
Cirrhosis with acute GI bleeding	Required for all such patients, regardless of endoscopic procedures	Prevention of infectious complications and reduction of mortality	Recommended, upon admission[c]
Synthetic vascular graft and other nonvalvular cardiovascular devices	Any endoscopic procedure	Prevention of graft and device infection	Not recommended[d]
Prosthetic joints	Any endoscopic procedure	Prevention of septic arthritis	Not recommended[e]

[a]Low rates of bacteremia and local infection. [b]Endoscopists may choose on a case-by-case basis. [c]Risk for bacterial infection associated with cirrhosis and GI bleeding is well established. [d]No reported cases of infection associated with endoscopy. [e]Very low risk of infection.

Abbreviations: ERCP, endoscopic retrograde cholangiopancreatography; EUS-FNA, endoscopic ultrasound–fine-needle aspiration; GI, gastrointestinal.

Source: Adapted from S Banerjee et al: Gastrointest Endosc 67:719, 2008; with permission from Elsevier.

TABLE 345-2 MANAGEMENT OF ANTITHROMBOTIC DRUGS BEFORE ENDOSCOPIC PROCEDURES

Drug	Bleeding Risk of Procedure	Management	Interval Between Last Dose and Procedure	Comments
Warfarin	Low[a]	Continue	N/A	Ensure that INR is not supratherapeutic
	High[b]	Discontinue	3–7 days (usually 5), INR should be ≤1.5 for procedure	Consider bridging therapy with heparin[c]
New oral anticoagulants (dabigatran, rivaroxaban, apixaban)	Low[a]	Continue	N/A	
	High[b]	Discontinue	Varies from 1 to 5 days, depending on the drug and the patient's renal function	Bridging therapy generally unnecessary
Heparin	Low[a]	Continue	N/A	
	High[b]	Discontinue	4-6 h for unfractionated heparin	Skip one dose if using low-molecular-weight heparin
Aspirin	Any	Continue	N/A	Low-dose aspirin does not substantially increase the risk of endoscopic procedures
Aspirin with dipyridamole	Low[a]	Continue	N/A	
	High[b]	Discontinue	2–7 days	Consider continuing aspirin monotherapy
Thienopyridines	Low[a]	Continue	N/A	
	High[b]	Discontinue	5 days (clopidogrel or ticagrelor), 7 days (prasugrel), 10–14 days (ticlopidine)	Consider bridging therapy with aspirin

[a]Low-risk endoscopic procedures include esophagogastroduodenoscopy (EGD) or colonoscopy with or without biopsy, endoscopic ultrasound (EUS) without fine-needle aspiration (FNA), and endoscopic retrograde cholangiopancreatography (ERCP) with stent exchange. [b]High-risk endoscopic procedures include EGD or colonoscopy with dilation, polypectomy, or thermal ablation; percutaneous endoscopic gastrostomy; EUS with FNA; and ERCP with sphincterotomy or pseudocyst drainage. [c]Bridging therapy with heparin may be considered for patients discontinuing warfarin who are at high risk for thromboembolism, including those with mitral valve replacement or aortic valve replacement with other risk factors; those with nonvalvular atrial fibrillation with a history of stroke, embolic event, cardiac thrombus, or $CHADS_2$ score ≥4; and those with venous thromboembolism within the past 3 months or severe underlying thrombophilia.

Source: TH Baron et al: N Engl J Med 368:2113, 2013; MA Anderson et al: Gastrointest Endosc 70:1060, 2009; MJ Zuckerman et al: Gastrointest Endosc 61:189, 2005.

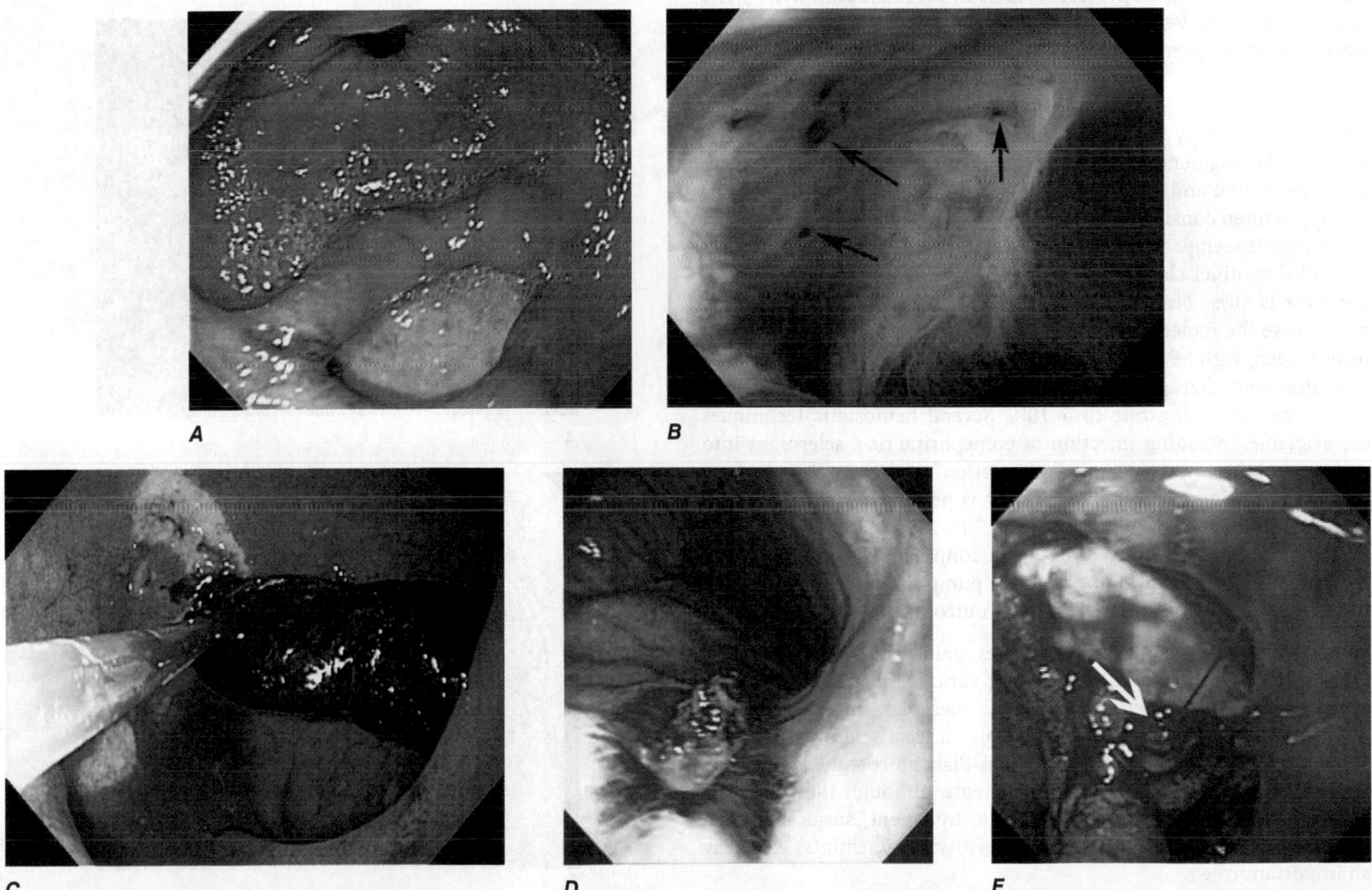

FIGURE 345-21 Stigmata of hemorrhage in peptic ulcers. ***A.*** Gastric antral ulcer with a clean base. ***B.*** Duodenal ulcer with flat pigmented spots (*arrows*). ***C.*** Duodenal ulcer with a dense adherent clot. ***D.*** Gastric ulcer with a pigmented protuberance/visible vessel. ***E.*** Duodenal ulcer with active spurting (*arrow*).

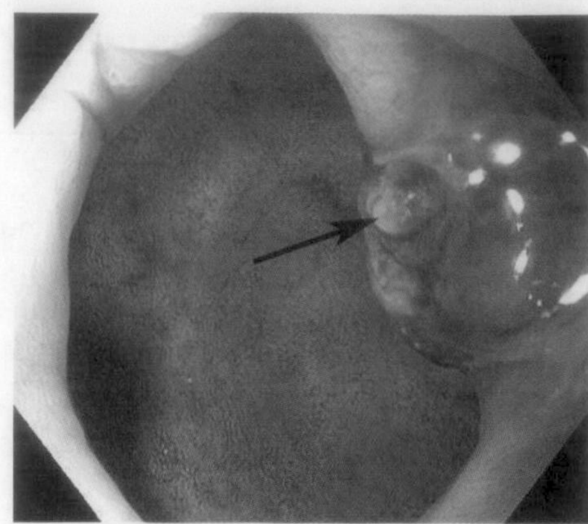

A

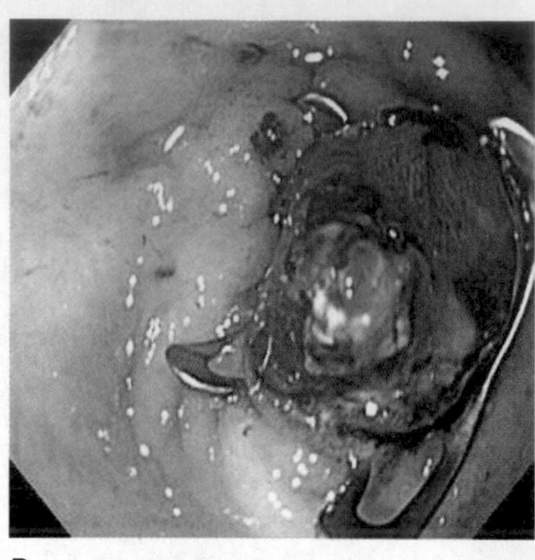

B

FIGURE 345-22 Endoscopic hemostasis of ulcer bleeding. ***A.*** Pyloric channel ulcer with visible vessel (*arrow*). ***B.*** Ulcer hemostasis with placement of an over-the-scope clip.

room or endoscopy suite if they are young, reliable, and otherwise healthy. Flat pigmented spots and adherent clots covering the ulcer base have a 10% and 20% risk of rebleeding, respectively. Endoscopic therapy is often considered for an ulcer with an adherent clot. When a fibrin plug is seen protruding from a vessel wall in the base of an ulcer (so-called sentinel clot or visible vessel), the risk of rebleeding from the ulcer is 40%. This finding generally leads to endoscopic therapy to decrease the rebleeding rate. Occasionally, active spurting from an ulcer is seen, with >90% risk of ongoing bleeding without therapy.

Endoscopic therapy of ulcers with high-risk stigmata typically lowers the rebleeding rate to 5–10%. Several hemostatic techniques are available, including injection of epinephrine or a sclerosant into and around the vessel, "coaptive coagulation" of the vessel in the base of the ulcer using a thermal probe that is pressed against the site of bleeding, placement of hemoclips (Fig. 345-22), or a combination of these modalities (see Video 346e-8). In conjunction with endoscopic therapy, the administration of a proton pump inhibitor decreases the risk of rebleeding and improves patient outcome.

Varices Two complementary strategies guide therapy of bleeding varices: local treatment of the bleeding varices and treatment of the underlying portal hypertension. Local therapies, including endoscopic variceal band ligation, endoscopic variceal sclerotherapy, and balloon tamponade with a Sengstaken-Blakemore tube, effectively control acute hemorrhage in most patients, although therapies that decrease portal pressure (pharmacologic treatment, surgical shunts, or radiologically placed intrahepatic portosystemic shunts) also play an important role.

Endoscopic variceal ligation (EVL) is indicated for the prevention of a first bleed (primary prophylaxis) from large esophageal varices (Figs. 345-23 and 24), particularly in patients in whom beta blockers are contraindicated or not tolerated. EVL is also the preferred endoscopic therapy for control of active esophageal variceal bleeding and for subsequent eradication of esophageal varices (secondary prophylaxis). During EVL, a varix is suctioned into a cap fitted on the end of the endoscope, and a rubber band is released from the cap, ligating the varix (Fig. 345-24, see Video 346e-9). EVL controls acute hemorrhage in up to 90% of patients. Complications of EVL, such as postbanding ulcer bleeding and esophageal stenosis, are uncommon. Endoscopic variceal sclerotherapy (EVS) involves the injection of a sclerosing, thrombogenic solution into or next to esophageal varices. EVS also controls acute hemorrhage in most patients, but it is generally used as salvage therapy when band ligation fails because of its higher complication rate compared to EVL. These techniques are used when varices are actively bleeding during endoscopy or (more commonly) when

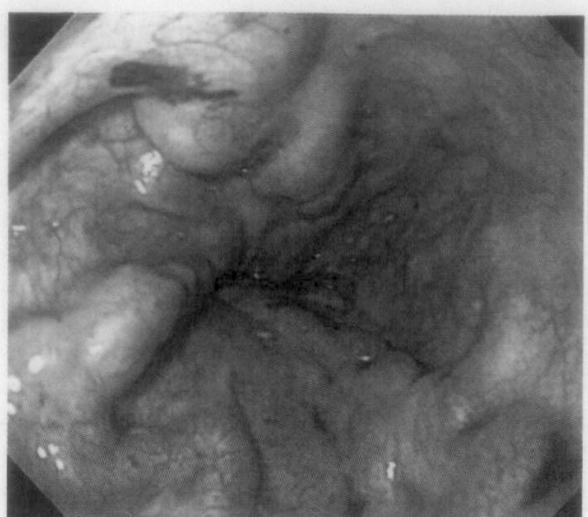

FIGURE 345-23 Esophageal varices.

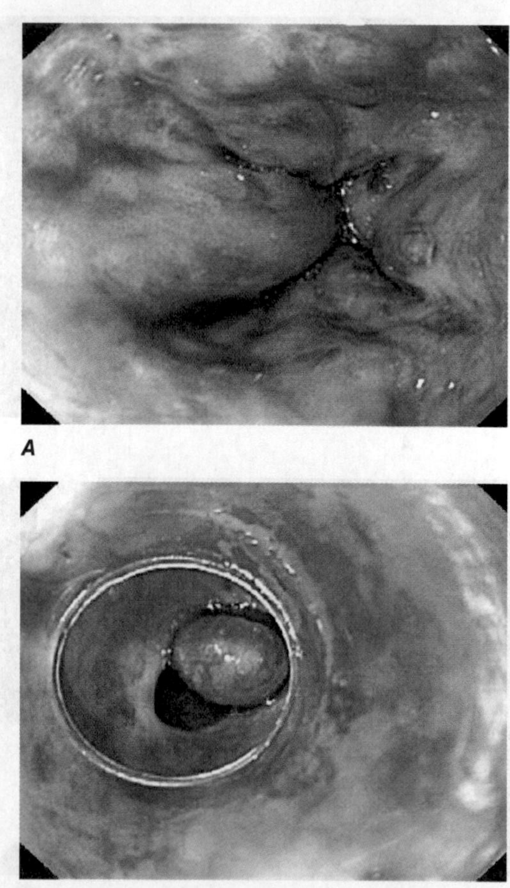

A

B

FIGURE 345-24 Endoscopic band ligation of esophageal varices. ***A.*** Large esophageal varices with stigmata of recent bleeding. ***B.*** Band ligation of varices.

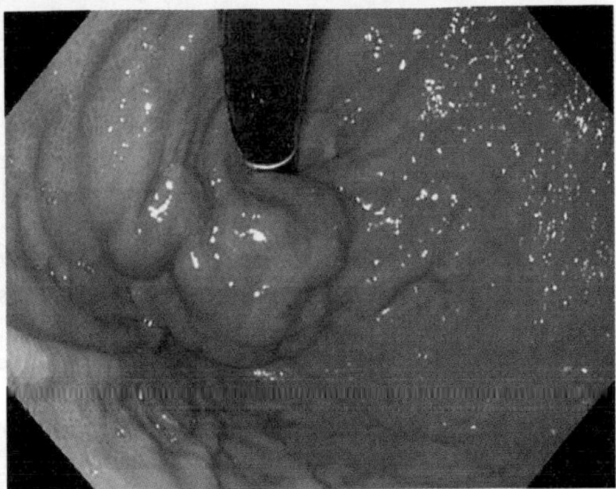

A

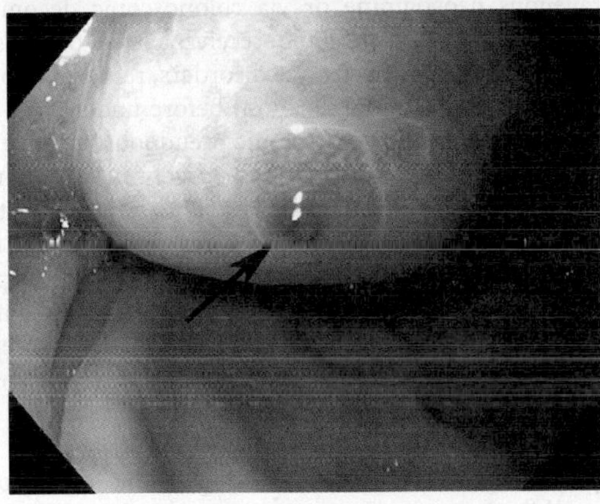

B

FIGURE 345-25 Gastric varices. *A.* Large gastric fundal varices. ***B.*** Stigmata of recent bleeding from the same gastric varices (*arrow*).

varices are the only identifiable cause of acute hemorrhage. Bleeding from large gastric fundic varices (Fig. 345-25) is best treated with endoscopic cyanoacrylate ("glue") injection (see Video 346e-10), because EVL or EVS of these varices is associated with a high rebleeding rate. Complications of cyanoacrylate injection include infection and glue embolization to other organs, such as the lungs, brain, and spleen.

After treatment of the acute hemorrhage, an elective course of endoscopic therapy can be undertaken with the goal of eradicating esophageal varices and preventing rebleeding months to years later. However, this chronic therapy is less successful, preventing long-term rebleeding in ~50% of patients. Pharmacologic therapies that decrease portal pressure have similar efficacy, and the two modalities may be combined.

Dieulafoy's Lesion This lesion, also called *persistent caliber artery*, is a large-caliber arteriole that runs immediately beneath the gastrointestinal mucosa and bleeds through a pinpoint mucosal erosion (Fig. 345-26). Dieulafoy's lesion is seen most commonly on the lesser curvature of the proximal stomach, causes impressive arterial hemorrhage, and may be difficult to diagnose; it is often recognized only after repeated endoscopy for recurrent bleeding. Endoscopic therapy, such as thermal coagulation or band ligation, is typically effective for control of bleeding and ablation of the underlying vessel once the lesion has been identified (see Video 346e-11). Rescue therapies, such as angiographic embolization or surgical oversewing, are considered in situations where endoscopic therapy has failed.

Mallory-Weiss Tear A Mallory-Weiss tear is a linear mucosal rent near or across the gastroesophageal junction that is often associated with retching or vomiting (Fig. 345-27). When the tear disrupts a submucosal arteriole, brisk hemorrhage may result. Endoscopy is the best method of diagnosis, and an actively bleeding tear can be treated endoscopically with epinephrine injection, coaptive coagulation, band ligation, or hemoclips (see Video 346e-12). Unlike peptic ulcer, a Mallory-Weiss tear with a nonbleeding sentinel clot in its base rarely rebleeds and thus does not necessitate endoscopic therapy.

Vascular Ectasias Vascular ectasias are flat mucosal vascular anomalies that are best diagnosed by endoscopy. They usually cause slow intestinal blood loss and occur either in a sporadic fashion or in a well-defined pattern of distribution (e.g., gastric antral vascular ectasia [GAVE] or "watermelon stomach") (Fig. 345-28). Cecal vascular ectasias, GAVE, and radiation-induced rectal ectasias are often responsive to local endoscopic ablative therapy, such as argon plasma coagulation (see Video 346e-13). Patients with diffuse small-bowel vascular ectasias (associated with chronic renal failure and with hereditary hemorrhagic telangiectasia) may continue to bleed despite endoscopic treatment of easily accessible lesions by conventional endoscopy. These patients may benefit from deep enteroscopy with endoscopic therapy, pharmacologic treatment with octreotide or estrogen/progesterone therapy, or intraoperative enteroscopy.

Colonic Diverticula Diverticula form where nutrient arteries penetrate the muscular wall of the colon en route to the colonic mucosa (Fig. 345-29). The artery found in the base of a diverticulum may bleed, causing painless and impressive hematochezia. Colonoscopy is indicated in patients with hematochezia and suspected diverticular hemorrhage, because other causes of bleeding (such as vascular ectasias, colitis, and colon cancer) must be excluded. In addition, an actively bleeding diverticulum may be seen and treated during colonoscopy (Fig. 345-30, see Video 346e-14).

GASTROINTESTINAL OBSTRUCTION AND PSEUDOOBSTRUCTION

Endoscopy is useful for evaluation and treatment of some forms of gastrointestinal obstruction. An important exception is small-bowel obstruction due to surgical adhesions, which is generally not diagnosed or treated endoscopically. Esophageal, gastroduodenal, and colonic obstruction or pseudoobstruction can all be diagnosed and often managed endoscopically.

Acute Esophageal Obstruction

Esophageal obstruction by impacted food (Fig. 345-31) or an ingested foreign body is a potentially life-threatening event and represents an endoscopic emergency. Left untreated, the patient may develop esophageal ulceration, ischemia, and perforation. Patients with persistent esophageal obstruction often have hypersalivation and are usually

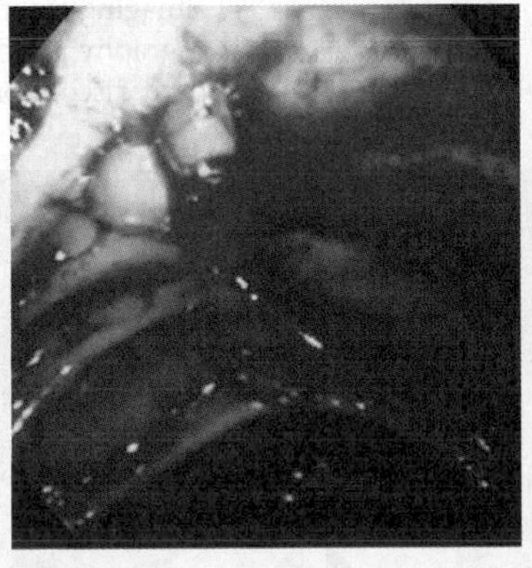

A

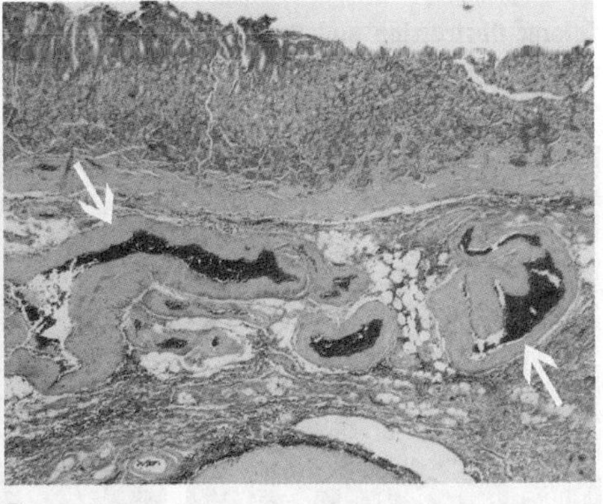

B

FIGURE 345-26 Dieulafoy's lesion. *A.* Actively spurting jejunal Dieulafoy's lesion. There is no underlying mucosal lesion. ***B.*** Histology of a gastric Dieulafoy's lesion. A persistent caliber artery (*arrows*) is present in the gastric submucosa, immediately beneath the mucosa.

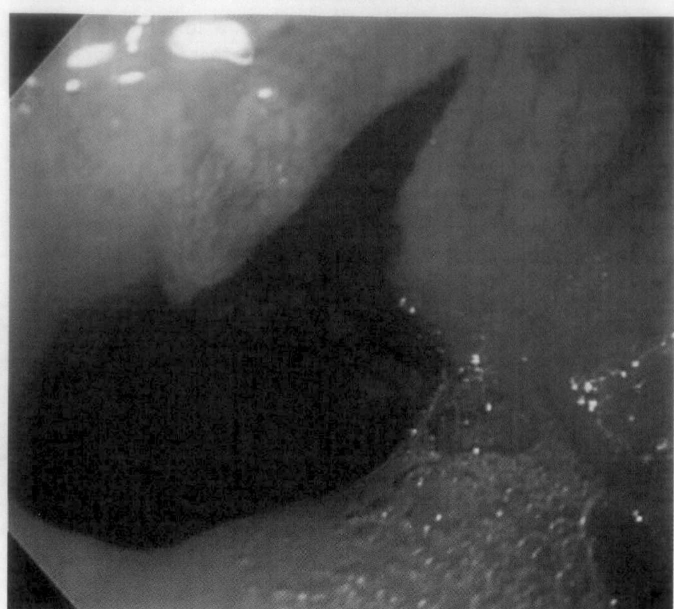

FIGURE 345-27 Mallory-Weiss tear at the gastroesophageal junction.

unable to swallow water; endoscopy is generally the best initial test in such patients, because endoscopic removal of the obstructing material is usually possible, and the presence of an underlying esophageal pathology can often be determined. Radiographs of the chest and neck should be considered before endoscopy in patients with fever, obstruction for ≥24 h, or ingestion of a sharp object, such as a fishbone. Radiographic contrast studies interfere with subsequent endoscopy and are not advisable in most patients with a clinical picture of esophageal obstruction. Sips of a carbonated beverage, sublingual nifedipine or nitrates, or intravenous glucagon may resolve an esophageal food impaction, but in most patients, an underlying web, ring, or stricture is present and endoscopic removal of the obstructing food bolus is necessary.

Gastric Outlet Obstruction Obstruction of the gastric outlet is commonly caused by gastric, duodenal, or pancreatic malignancy or chronic peptic ulceration with stenosis of the pylorus (Fig. 345-32). Patients vomit partially digested food many hours after eating. Gastric decompression with a nasogastric tube and subsequent lavage for removal of retained material is the first step in treatment. The diagnosis can then be confirmed with a saline load test, if desired. Endoscopy is useful for diagnosis and treatment. Patients with benign pyloric stenosis may be treated with endoscopic balloon dilatation of the pylorus, and a course of endoscopic dilatation results in long-term relief of symptoms in about 50% of patients. Malignant gastric outlet obstruction can be relieved with endoscopically placed expandable stents in patients with inoperable malignancy (Fig. 345-33).

Colonic Obstruction and Pseudoobstruction These both present with abdominal distention and discomfort; tympany; and a dilated, air-filled colon on plain abdominal radiography. The radiographic appearance can be characteristic of a particular condition, such as sigmoid volvulus (Fig. 345-34). Both structural obstruction and pseudoobstruction may lead to colonic perforation if left untreated. Acute colonic pseudoobstruction is a form of colonic ileus that is usually attributable to electrolyte disorders, narcotic and anticholinergic medications, immobility (as after surgery), and retroperitoneal hemorrhage or mass. Multiple causative factors are often present. Colonoscopy, water-soluble contrast enema, or CT may be used to assess for an obstructing lesion and differentiate obstruction from pseudoobstruction. One of these diagnostic studies should be strongly considered if the patient does not have clear risk factors for pseudoobstruction, if radiographs do not show air in the rectum, or if the patient fails to improve when underlying causes of pseudoobstruction have been addressed. The risk of cecal perforation in pseudoobstruction rises when the cecal diameter exceeds 12 cm, and decompression of the colon may be achieved using intravenous neostigmine or via colonoscopic decompression (Fig. 345-35). Most patients should receive a trial of conservative therapy (with correction of electrolyte disorders, removal of offending medications, and increased mobilization) before undergoing an invasive decompressive procedure for colonic pseudoobstruction.

Colonic obstruction is an indication for urgent intervention. In the past, emergent diverting colostomy was usually performed with a subsequent second operation after bowel preparation to treat the underlying cause of obstruction. Colonoscopic placement of an expandable stent is now a widely used alternative that can relieve malignant colonic obstruction without emergency surgery and permit bowel preparation for an elective one-stage operation (Fig. 345-36, see Video 346e-15).

ACUTE BILIARY OBSTRUCTION

The steady, severe pain that occurs when a gallstone acutely obstructs the common bile duct often brings patients to a hospital. The diagnosis of a ductal stone is suspected when the patient is jaundiced or when serum liver tests or pancreatic enzyme levels are elevated; it is confirmed by EUS, magnetic resonance cholangiography (MRCP), or direct cholangiography (performed endoscopically, percutaneously, or during surgery). ERCP is currently the primary means of diagnosing and treating common bile duct stones in most hospitals in the United States (Figs. 345-11 and 345-12).

Bile Duct Imaging Whereas transabdominal ultrasound diagnoses only a minority of bile duct stones, MRCP and EUS are >90% accurate and have an important role in diagnosis. Examples of these modalities are shown in Fig. 345-37.

If the suspicion for a bile duct stone is high and urgent treatment is required (as in a patient with obstructive jaundice and biliary sepsis), ERCP is the procedure of choice, because it remains the gold standard for diagnosis and allows for immediate treatment (see Video 346e-16). If a persistent bile duct stone is relatively unlikely (as in a patient with gallstone pancreatitis), ERCP may be supplanted by less invasive imaging techniques, such as EUS, MRCP, or intraoperative cholangiography performed during cholecystectomy, sparing patients the risk and discomfort of ERCP.

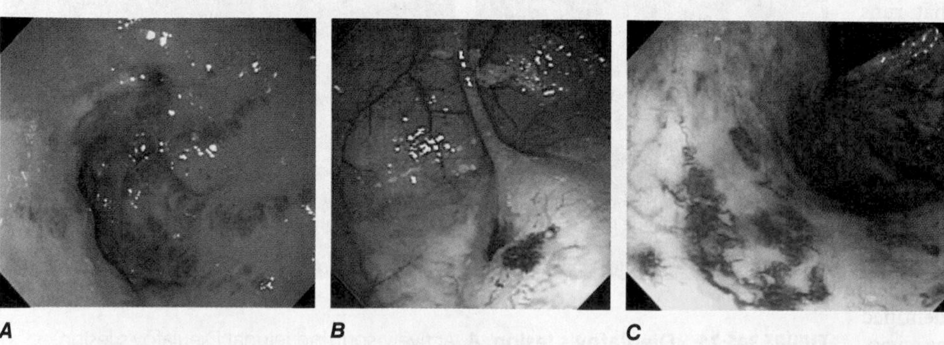

FIGURE 345-28 Gastrointestinal vascular ectasias. ***A.*** Gastric antral vascular ectasia ("watermelon stomach") characterized by stripes of prominent flat or raised vascular ectasias. ***B.*** Cecal vascular ectasias. ***C.*** Radiation-induced vascular ectasias of the rectum in a patient previously treated for prostate cancer.

Ascending Cholangitis Charcot's triad of jaundice, abdominal pain, and fever is present in about 70% of patients with ascending cholangitis and biliary sepsis. These patients are managed initially with fluid resuscitation and intravenous antibiotics. Abdominal ultrasound is often performed to assess for gallbladder stones and bile duct dilation. However, the bile duct may not be dilated early in the course of acute biliary obstruction. Medical management usually improves the patient's clinical status, providing a window of approximately 24 h during which biliary drainage should be established, typically by ERCP. Undue delay

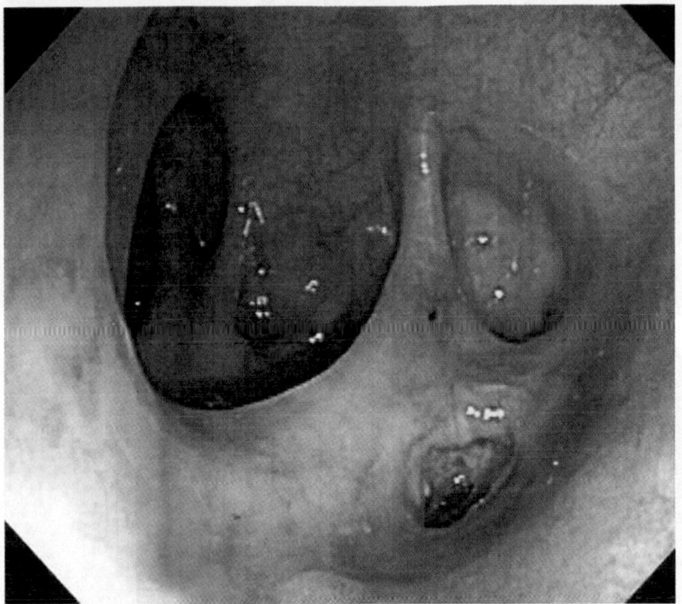

FIGURE 345-29 **Colonic diverticula.**

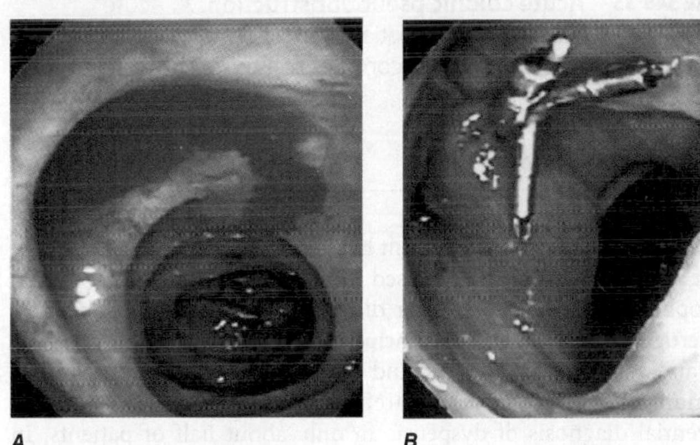

FIGURE 345-30 **Diverticular hemorrhage.** ***A.*** Actively bleeding sigmoid diverticulum. ***B.*** Hemostasis achieved using endoscopic clips.

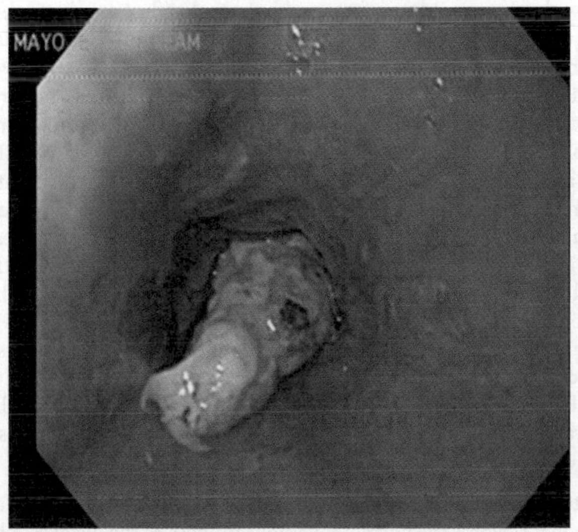

FIGURE 345-31 **Esophageal food** (meat) impaction.

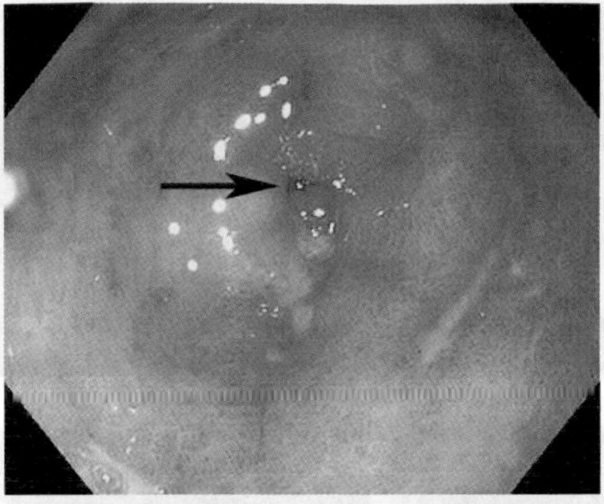

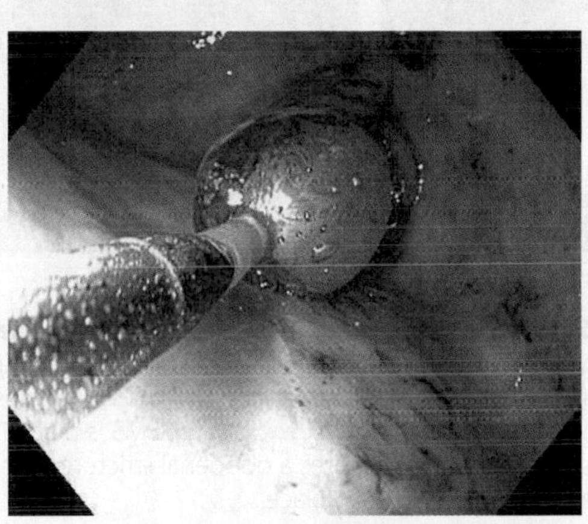

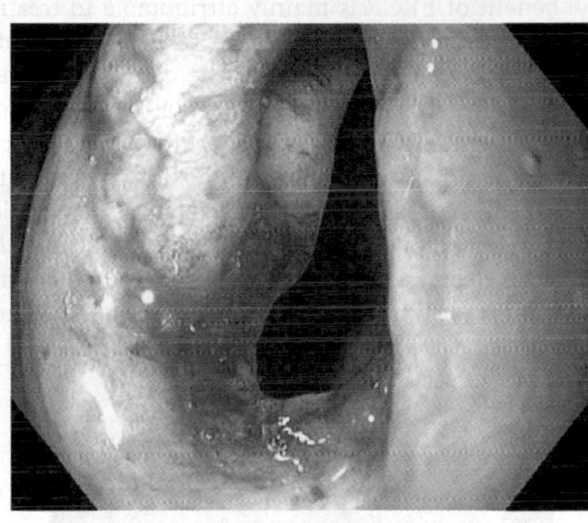

FIGURE 345-32 **Gastric outlet obstruction due to pyloric stenosis.** ***A.*** Sequela of nonsteroidal anti-inflammatory drug (NSAID)–induced ulcer disease with severe stenosis of the pylorus (*arrow*). ***B.*** Balloon dilation of the stenosis. ***C.*** Appearance of pyloric ring after dilation.

can result in recrudescence of overt sepsis and increased morbidity and mortality rates. In addition to Charcot's triad, the additional presence of shock and confusion (Reynolds's pentad) is associated with high mortality rate and should prompt urgent intervention to restore biliary drainage.

Gallstone Pancreatitis Gallstones may cause acute pancreatitis as they pass through the ampulla of Vater. The occurrence of gallstone pancreatitis usually implies passage of a stone into the duodenum, and only about 20% of patients harbor a persistent stone in the ampulla or the common bile duct. Retained stones are more common in patients with jaundice, rising serum liver tests following hospitalization, severe pancreatitis, or superimposed ascending cholangitis.

Urgent ERCP decreases the morbidity rate of gallstone pancreatitis in a subset of patients with retained bile duct stones. It is unclear

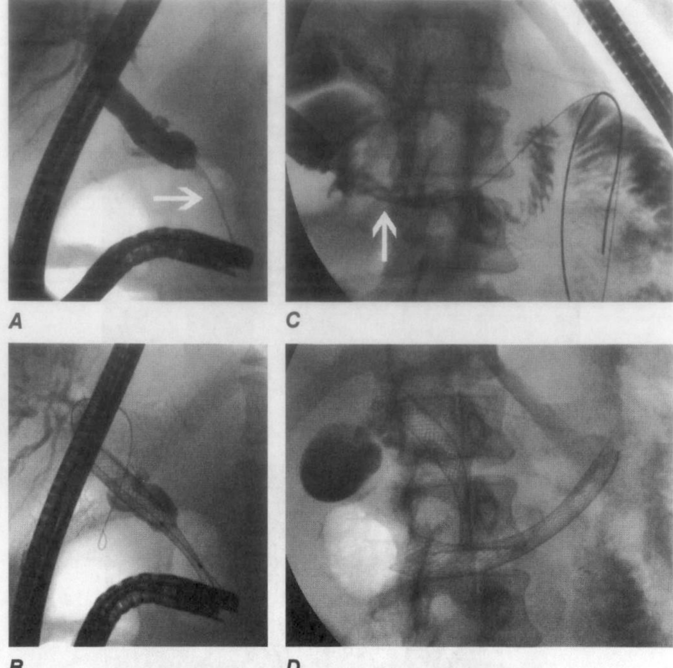

FIGURE 345-33 Biliary and duodenal self-expanding metal stents (SEMS) for obstruction caused by pancreatic cancer. *A.* Endoscopic retrograde cholangiopancreatography (ERCP) demonstrates a distal bile duct stricture (*arrow*). ***B.*** A biliary SEMS is placed. ***C.*** Contrast injection demonstrates a duodenal stricture (*arrow*). ***D.*** Biliary and duodenal SEMS in place.

whether the benefit of ERCP is mainly attributable to treatment and prevention of ascending cholangitis or to relief of pancreatic ductal obstruction. ERCP is warranted early in the course of gallstone pancreatitis if ascending cholangitis is suspected, especially in a jaundiced patient. Urgent ERCP may also benefit patients predicted to have severe pancreatitis using a clinical index of severity, such as the Glasgow or Ranson score. Because the benefit of ERCP is limited to patients with a retained bile duct stone, a strategy of initial MRCP or EUS for diagnosis decreases the utilization of ERCP in gallstone pancreatitis and improves clinical outcomes by limiting the occurrence of ERCP-related adverse events.

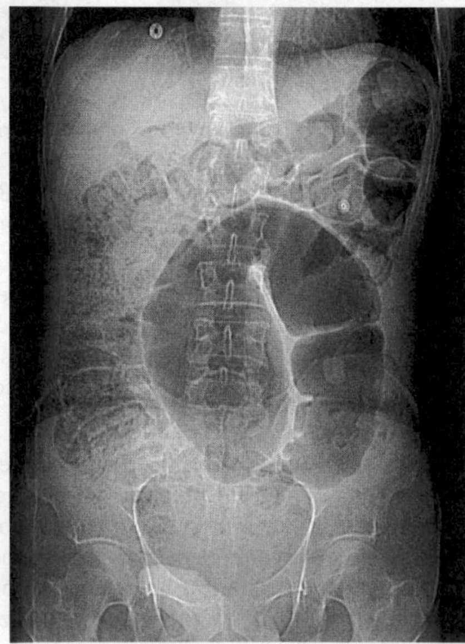

FIGURE 345-34 Sigmoid volvulus with the characteristic radiologic appearance of a "bent inner tube."

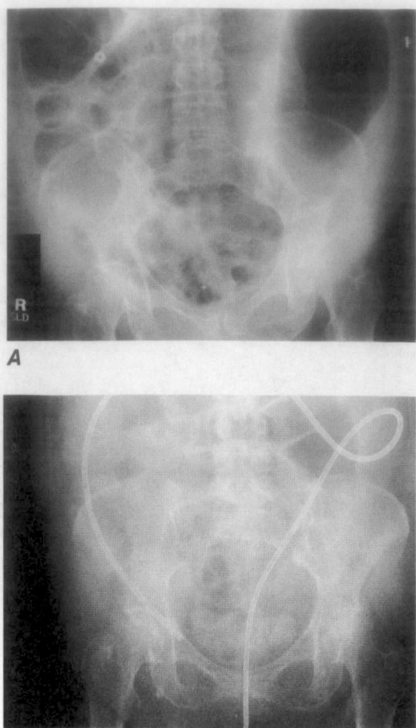

FIGURE 345-35 Acute colonic pseudoobstruction. *A.* Acute colonic dilatation occurring in a patient soon after knee surgery. ***B.*** Colonoscopic placement of decompression tube with marked improvement in colonic dilatation.

ELECTIVE ENDOSCOPY

DYSPEPSIA

Dyspepsia is a chronic or recurrent burning discomfort or pain in the upper abdomen that may be caused by diverse processes such as gastroesophageal reflux, peptic ulcer disease, and "nonulcer dyspepsia," a heterogeneous category that includes disorders of motility, sensation, and somatization. Gastric and esophageal malignancies are less common causes of dyspepsia. Careful history-taking allows accurate differential diagnosis of dyspepsia in only about half of patients. In the remainder, endoscopy can be a useful diagnostic tool, especially in patients whose symptoms are not resolved by an empirical trial of symptomatic treatment. Endoscopy should be performed at the outset in patients with dyspepsia and alarm features, such as weight loss or iron-deficiency anemia.

GASTROESOPHAGEAL REFLUX DISEASE (GERD)

When classic symptoms of gastroesophageal reflux are present, such as water brash and substernal heartburn, presumptive diagnosis and empirical treatment are often sufficient. Endoscopy is a sensitive test for diagnosis of esophagitis (Fig. 345-38), but will miss nonerosive reflux disease (NERD) because some patients have symptomatic reflux without esophagitis. The most sensitive test for diagnosis of GERD is 24-h ambulatory pH monitoring. Endoscopy is indicated in patients with reflux symptoms refractory to antisecretory therapy; in those with alarm symptoms, such as dysphagia, weight loss, or gastrointestinal bleeding; and in those with recurrent dyspepsia after treatment that is not clearly due to reflux on clinical grounds alone. Endoscopy should be considered in patients with long-standing (≥10 years) GERD, because they have a sixfold increased risk of harboring Barrett's esophagus compared to a patient with <1 year of reflux symptoms. Patients with Barrett's esophagus (Fig. 345-3) generally undergo a surveillance program of periodic endoscopy with biopsies to detect dysplasia or early carcinoma.

Barrett's Esophagus Barrett's esophagus is specialized columnar metaplasia that replaces the normal squamous mucosa of the distal esophagus in some persons with GERD. Barrett's epithelium is a major risk factor

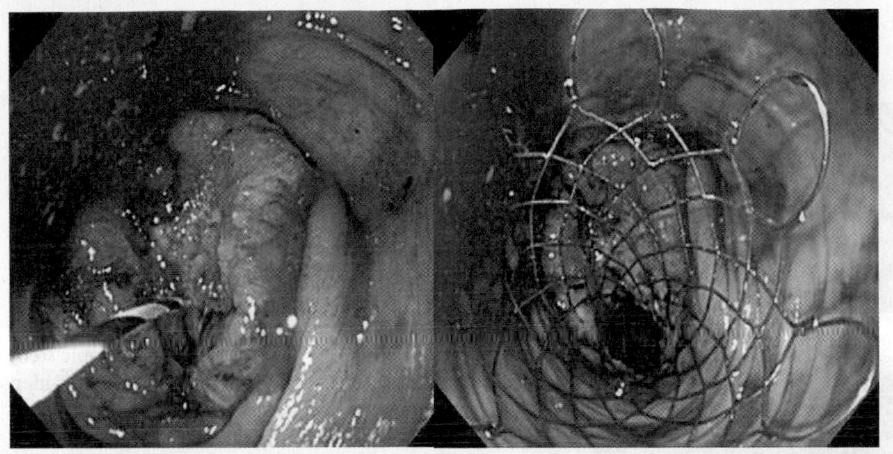
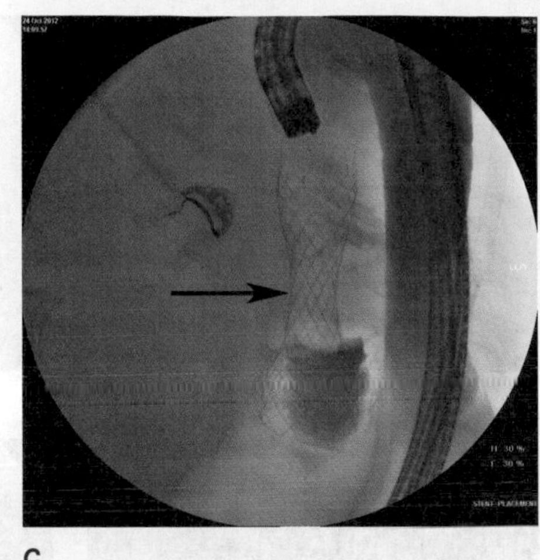

FIGURE 345-36 Obstructing colonic carcinoma. ***A.*** Colonic adenocarcinoma causing marked luminal narrowing of the distal transverse colon. ***B.*** Endoscopic placement of a self-expandable metal stent. ***C.*** Radiograph of expanded stent across the obstructing tumor with a residual waist (*arrow*).

for adenocarcinoma of the esophagus and is readily detected endoscopically, due to proximal displacement of the squamocolumnar junction (Fig. 345-3). A screening EGD for Barrett's esophagus should be considered in patients with a chronic (≥10 year) history of GERD symptoms. Endoscopic biopsy is the gold standard for confirmation of Barrett's esophagus and for dysplasia or cancer arising in Barrett's mucosa.

PEPTIC ULCER

Peptic ulcer classically causes epigastric gnawing or burning, often occurring nocturnally and promptly relieved by food or antacids. Although endoscopy is the most sensitive diagnostic test for peptic ulcer, it is not a cost-effective strategy in young patients with ulcer-like dyspeptic symptoms unless endoscopy is available at low cost. Patients with suspected peptic ulcer should be evaluated for *Helicobacter pylori* infection. Serology (past or present infection), urea breath testing (current infection), and stool tests are noninvasive and less costly than endoscopy with biopsy. Patients with alarm symptoms and those with persistent symptoms despite treatment should undergo endoscopy to exclude gastric malignancy and other etiologies.

NONULCER DYSPEPSIA

Nonulcer dyspepsia may be associated with bloating and, unlike peptic ulcer, tends not to remit and recur. Most patients describe marginal relief on acid-reducing, prokinetic, or anti-*Helicobacter* therapy, and are referred for endoscopy to exclude a refractory ulcer and assess for other causes. Although endoscopy is useful for excluding other diagnoses, its impact on the treatment of patients with nonulcer dyspepsia is limited.

DYSPHAGIA

About 50% of patients presenting with difficulty swallowing have a mechanical obstruction; the remainder has a motility disorder, such as achalasia or diffuse esophageal spasm. Careful history-taking often points to a presumptive diagnosis and leads to the appropriate use of diagnostic tests. Esophageal strictures (Fig. 345-39) typically cause progressive dysphagia, first for solids, then for liquids; motility disorders often cause intermittent dysphagia for both solids and liquids. Some underlying disorders have characteristic historic features: Schatzki's ring (Fig. 345-40) causes episodic dysphagia for solids, typically at the beginning of a meal; oropharyngeal motor disorders typically present with difficulty initiating deglutition (*transfer dysphagia*) and nasal reflux or coughing with swallowing; and achalasia may cause nocturnal regurgitation of undigested food.

When mechanical obstruction is suspected, endoscopy is a useful initial diagnostic test, because it permits immediate biopsy and/or dilatation of strictures, masses, or rings. The presence of linear furrows and multiple corrugated rings throughout a narrowed esophagus (*feline esophagus*) should raise suspicion for eosinophilic esophagitis, an increasingly recognized cause for recurrent dysphagia and food impaction (Fig. 345-41). Blind or forceful passage of an endoscope may lead to perforation in a patient with stenosis of the cervical esophagus or a Zenker's diverticulum, but gentle passage of an endoscope under direct visual guidance is reasonably safe. Endoscopy can miss a subtle stricture or ring in some patients.

When transfer dysphagia is evident or an esophageal motility disorder is suspected, esophageal radiography and/or a video-swallow study

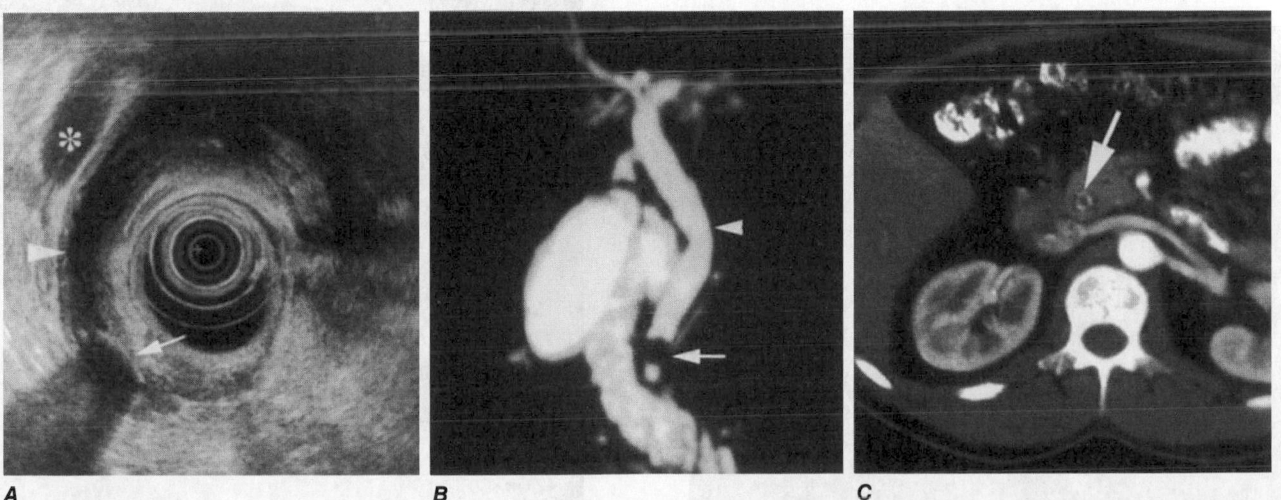

FIGURE 345-37 Methods of bile duct imaging. *Arrows* mark bile duct stones. *Arrowheads* indicate the common bile duct, and the *asterisk* marks the portal vein. ***A.*** Endoscopic ultrasound (EUS). ***B.*** Magnetic resonance cholangiopancreatography (MRCP). ***C.*** Helical computed tomography (CT).

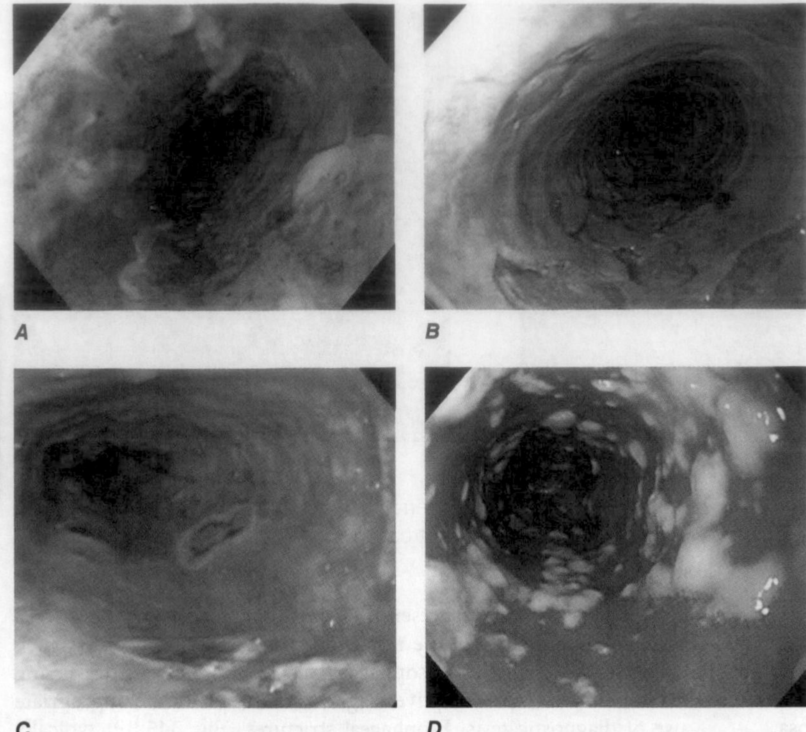

FIGURE 345-38 Causes of esophagitis. ***A.*** Severe reflux esophagitis with mucosal ulceration and friability. ***B.*** Cytomegalovirus esophagitis. ***C.*** Herpes simplex virus esophagitis with target-type shallow ulcerations. ***D.*** *Candida* esophagitis with white plaques adherent to the esophageal mucosa.

are the best initial diagnostic tests. The oropharyngeal swallowing mechanism, esophageal peristalsis, and the lower esophageal sphincter can all be assessed. In some disorders, subsequent esophageal manometry may also be important for diagnosis.

TREATMENT OF MALIGNANCIES

Endoscopy plays an important role in the treatment of gastrointestinal malignancies. Early-stage malignancies limited to the superficial layers of the gastrointestinal mucosa may be resected using the techniques of endoscopic mucosal resection (EMR) (see Video 346e-4) or endoscopic submucosal dissection (ESD) (see Video 346e-5). Photodynamic therapy (PDT) and radiofrequency ablation (RFA) are effective modalities for ablative treatment of high-grade dysplasia and intramucosal cancer in Barrett's esophagus. Gastrointestinal stromal tumors can be removed en bloc by endoscopic full-thickness resection (see Video 346e-3). In general, endoscopic techniques offer the advantage of a minimally invasive approach to treatment, but rely on other imaging techniques (such as CT, magnetic resonance imaging [MRI], positron emission tomography [PET], and EUS) to exclude distant metastases or locally advanced disease better treated by surgery or other modalities. The decision to treat an early-stage gastrointestinal malignancy endoscopically is often made in collaboration with a surgeon and/or oncologist.

Endoscopic palliation of gastrointestinal malignancies relieves symptoms and in many cases prolongs survival. Malignant obstruction can be relieved by endoscopic stent placement (Figs. 345-13, 345-33, and 345-36; see Video 346e-15), and malignant gastrointestinal bleeding can often be palliated endoscopically as well. EUS-guided celiac plexus neurolysis may relieve pancreatic cancer pain.

ANEMIA AND OCCULT BLOOD IN THE STOOL

Iron-deficiency anemia may be attributed to poor iron absorption (as in celiac sprue) or, more commonly, chronic blood loss. Intestinal bleeding should be strongly suspected in men and postmenopausal women with iron-deficiency anemia, and colonoscopy is indicated in such patients, even in the absence of detectable occult blood in the stool. Approximately 30% will have large colonic polyps, 10% will have colorectal cancer, and a few additional patients will have colonic vascular lesions. When a convincing source of blood loss is not found in the colon, upper gastrointestinal endoscopy should be considered; if no lesion is found, duodenal biopsies should be obtained to exclude sprue (Fig. 345-42). Small-bowel evaluation with capsule endoscopy (Fig. 345-43), CT or magnetic resonance (MR) enterography, or balloon-assisted enteroscopy may be appropriate if both EGD and colonoscopy are unrevealing.

Tests for occult blood in the stool detect hemoglobin or the heme moiety and are most sensitive for colonic blood loss, although they will also detect larger amounts of upper gastrointestinal bleeding. Patients over age 50 with occult blood in normal-appearing stool should undergo colonoscopy to diagnose or exclude colorectal neoplasia. The diagnostic yield is lower than in iron-deficiency anemia. Whether upper endoscopy is also indicated depends on the patient's symptoms.

The small intestine may be the source of chronic intestinal bleeding, especially if colonoscopy and upper endoscopy are not diagnostic. The utility of small-bowel evaluation varies with the clinical setting and is most important in patients in whom bleeding causes chronic or recurrent anemia. In contrast to the low diagnostic yield

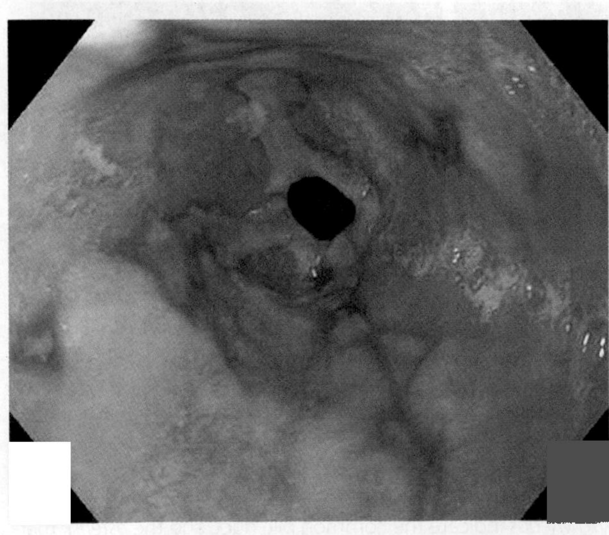

FIGURE 345-39 Peptic esophageal stricture associated with esophagitis.

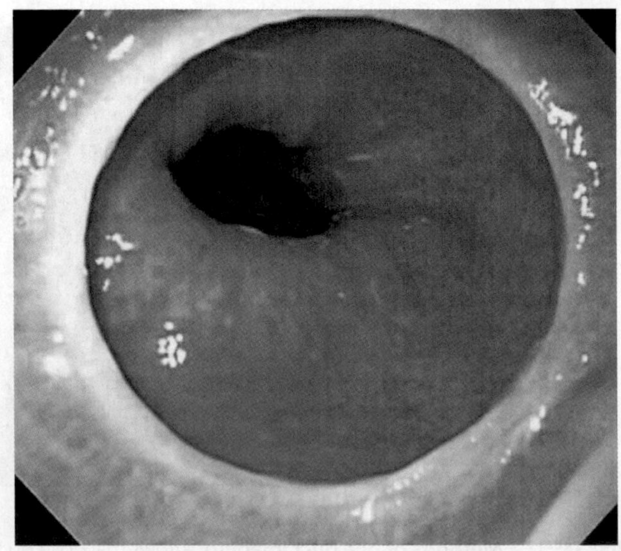

FIGURE 345-40 Schatzki's ring at the gastroesophageal junction.

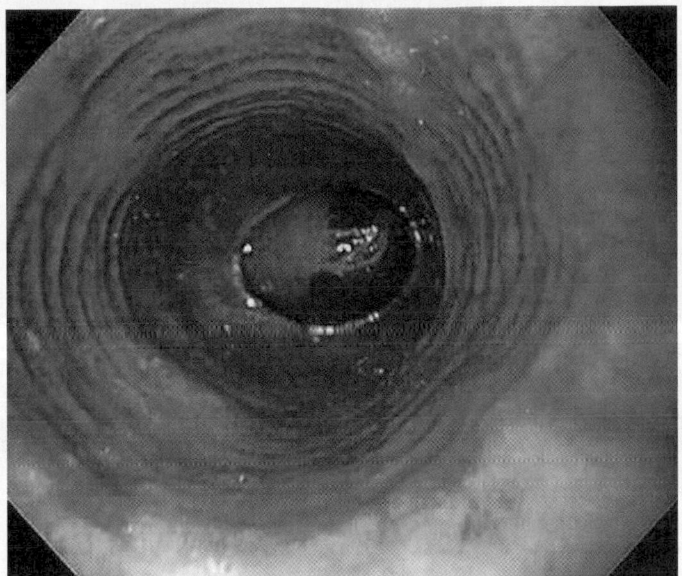

FIGURE 345-41 Eosinophilic esophagitis with multiple circular rings of the esophagus creating a corrugated appearance, and an impacted grape at the narrowed esophagogastric junction. The diagnosis requires biopsy with histologic finding of > 15–20 eosinophils per high-power field.

of small-bowel radiography, positive findings on capsule endoscopy are seen in 50–70% of patients with suspected small intestinal bleeding. The most common finding is mucosal vascular ectasias. CT or MR enterography accurately detects small-bowel masses and inflammation and is also useful for initial small-bowel evaluation. Deep enteroscopy may follow capsule endoscopy for biopsy of lesions or to provide specific therapy, such as argon plasma coagulation of vascular ectasias (Fig. 345-44).

COLORECTAL CANCER SCREENING

The majority of colon cancers develop from preexisting colonic adenomas, and colorectal cancer can be largely prevented by the detection and removal of adenomatous polyps (see Video 346e-17). The choice of screening strategy for an asymptomatic person depends on personal and family history. Individuals with inflammatory bowel disease, a history of colorectal polyps or cancer, family members with adenomatous polyps or cancer, or certain familial cancer syndromes (Fig. 345-45)

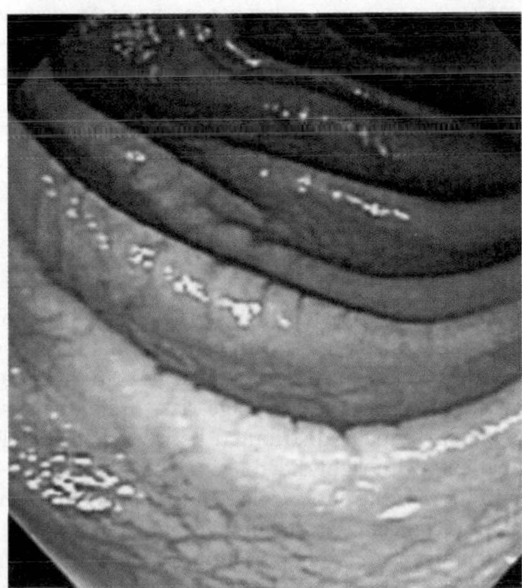

FIGURE 345-42 Scalloped duodenal folds in a patient with celiac sprue.

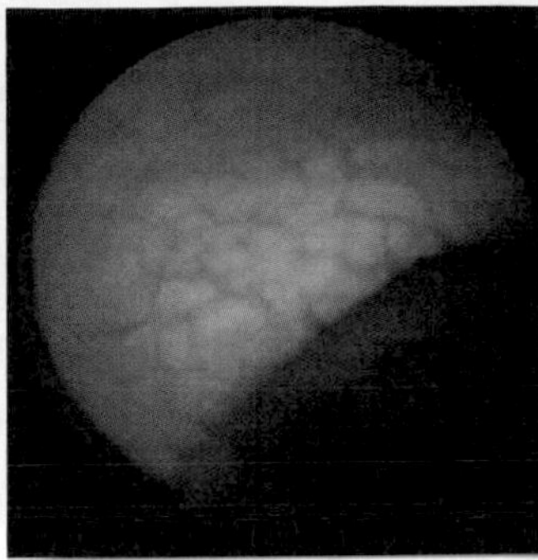

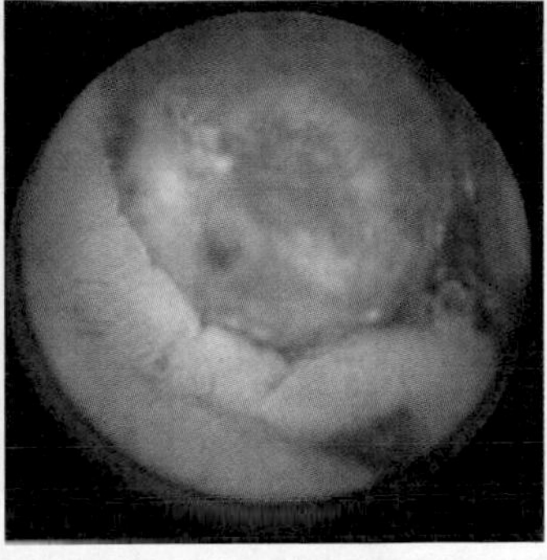

FIGURE 345-43 Capsule endoscopy images of a mildly scalloped jejunal fold (*left*) and an ileal tumor (*right*) in a patient with celiac sprue. *(Images courtesy of Dr. Elizabeth Rajan; with permission.)*

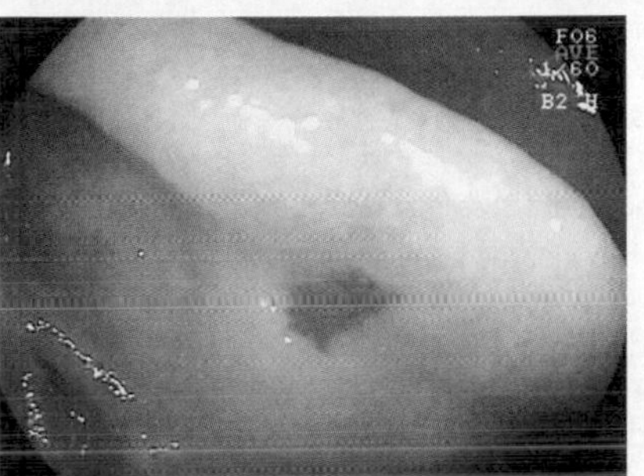

A

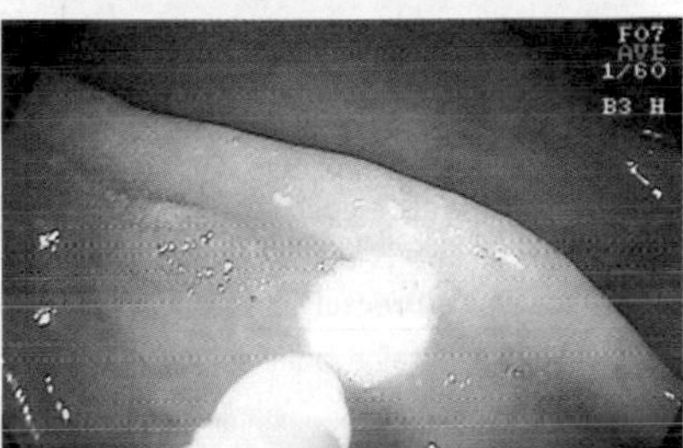

B

FIGURE 345-44 ***A.*** Mid-jejunal vascular ectasia identified by double-balloon endoscopy. ***B.*** Ablation of vascular ectasia with argon plasma coagulation.

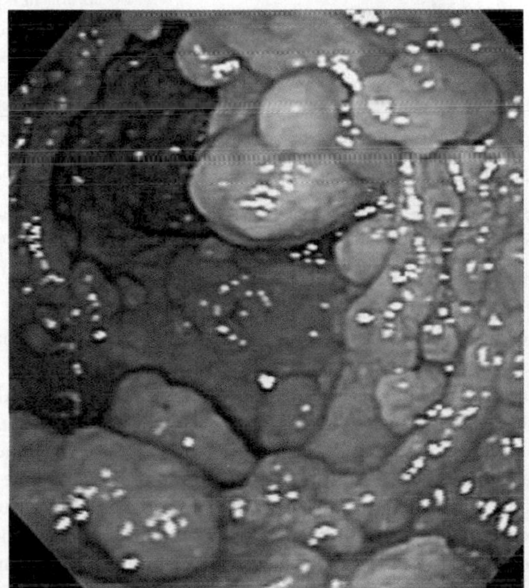

FIGURE 345-45 Innumerable colon polyps of various sizes in a patient with familial adenomatous polyposis syndrome.

TABLE 345-3 COLORECTAL CANCER SCREENING STRATEGIES

	Choices/Recommendations	Comments
Average-Risk Patients		
Asymptomatic individuals ≥50 years of age (≥45 years of age for African Americans)	Colonoscopy every 10 years[a]	Preferred cancer prevention strategy
	Annual fecal immunochemical test (FIT) or fecal occult blood test (FOBT), multiple take-home specimen cards	Cancer detection strategy; fails to detect most polyps; colonoscopy if results are positive
	Computed tomography (CT) colonography every 5 years	Colonoscopy if results are positive
	Flexible sigmoidoscopy every 5 years	Fails to detect proximal colon polyps and cancers
	Double-contrast barium enema every 5 years	Less sensitive than colonoscopy or CT colonography; misses some cancers and polyps
Personal History of Polyps or Colorectal Cancer		
1 or 2 small (<1 cm) adenomas with low-grade dysplasia	Repeat colonoscopy in 5–10 years	Assuming complete polyp resection; interval may vary based on prior history, family history
3 to 9 adenomas, or any high-risk adenoma[b]	Repeat colonoscopy in 3 years; subsequent colonoscopy based on findings	Assuming complete polyp resection
≥10 adenomas	Repeat colonoscopy in <3 years based on clinical judgment	Consider evaluation for FAP or HNPCC; see recommendations below
Piecemeal removal of a sessile polyp	Exam in 2–6 months to verify complete removal	
Small (<1 cm) hyperplastic polyps of sigmoid and rectum	Repeat colonoscopy in 10 years	Those with hyperplastic polyposis syndrome merit more frequent follow-up
Sessile serrated adenoma/polyp <10 mm, without dysplasia	Repeat colonoscopy in 5 years	
Sessile serrated adenoma/polyp ≥10 mm or with dysplasia, or ≥2 serrated polyps	Repeat colonoscopy in 3 years	Serrated polyposis syndrome merits more frequent follow-up
Incompletely removed serrated polyp ≥1 cm	Exam in 2–6 months to verify complete removal	
Colon cancer	Evaluate entire colon around the time of resection, then repeat colonoscopy in 1 year	Subsequent colonoscopy in 3 years if the 1-year exam is normal
Inflammatory Bowel Disease		
Long-standing (>8 years) ulcerative pancolitis or Crohn's colitis, or left-sided ulcerative colitis of >15 years in duration	Colonoscopy with biopsies every 1–3 years	
Family History of Polyps or Colorectal Cancer		
First-degree relatives with only small tubular adenomas	Same as average risk	
Single first-degree relative with CRC or advanced adenoma at age ≥60 years	Colonoscopy every 10 years starting at age 40	
Single first-degree relative with CRC or advanced adenoma at age <60 years, OR two first-degree relatives with CRC or advanced adenomas at any age	Colonoscopy every 5 years beginning at age 40 years or 10 years younger than age at diagnosis of the youngest affected relative, whichever is earlier	
FAP	Sigmoidoscopy or colonoscopy annually, beginning at age 10–12 years	Consider genetic counseling and testing
HNPCC	Colonoscopy every 2 years beginning at age 20–25 years (or 10 years younger than the youngest affected first-degree relative) until age 40, then annually thereafter	Consider histologic evaluation for microsatellite instability in tumor specimens of patients who meet Bethesda criteria; consider genetic counseling and testing

[a]Assumes good colonic preparation and complete exam to cecum. [b]High-risk adenoma: any adenoma ≥1 cm in size or containing high-grade dysplasia or villous features.

Abbreviations: CRC, colorectal cancer; FAP, familial adenomatous polyposis; HNPCC, hereditary nonpolyposis colorectal cancer.

Source: Adapted from DA Lieberman et al: Gastroenterology 143:844, 2012; B Levin et al: CA Cancer J Clin 58:130, 2008; American Cancer Society Guidelines (*http://www.cancer.org/cancer/colonandrectumcancer/moreinformation/colonandrectumcancerearlydetection/colorectal-cancer-early-detection-acs-recommendations*), accessed November 15, 2013.

are at increased risk for colorectal cancer. An individual without these factors is generally considered at average risk.

Screening strategies are summarized in Table 345-3. Although stool tests for occult blood have been shown to decrease mortality rate from colorectal cancer, they do not detect some cancers and many polyps, and direct visualization of the colon is a more effective screening strategy. Either sigmoidoscopy or colonoscopy may be used for cancer screening in asymptomatic average-risk individuals. The use of sigmoidoscopy was based on the historical finding that the majority of colorectal cancers occurred in the rectum and left colon and that patients with right-sided colon cancers had left-sided polyps. Over the past several decades, however, the distribution of colon cancers has changed in the United States, with proportionally fewer rectal and left-sided cancers than in the past. Large American studies of colonoscopy for screening of average-risk individuals show that cancers are roughly equally distributed between left and right colon and half of patients with right-sided lesions have no polyps in the left colon. Visualization of the entire colon thus appears to be the optimal strategy for colorectal cancer screening and prevention.

Virtual colonoscopy (VC) is a radiologic technique that images the colon with CT following rectal insufflation of the colonic lumen. Computer rendering of CT images generates an electronic display of

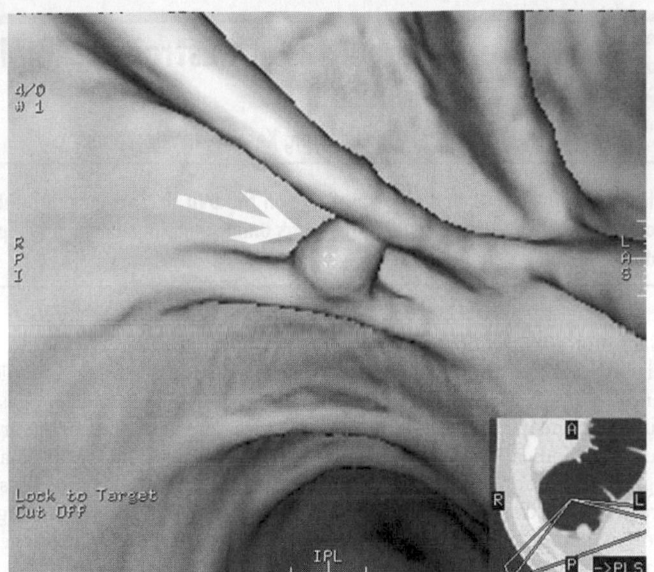

FIGURE 345-46 Virtual colonoscopy image of a colon polyp *(arrow). (Image courtesy of Dr. Jeff Fidler; with permission.)*

a virtual "flight" along the colonic lumen, simulating colonoscopy (Fig. 345-46). Comparative studies of virtual and routine colonoscopy have shown conflicting results, but technical refinements have improved the performance characteristics of VC. The use of VC for colorectal cancer screening may become more widespread in the future, particularly at institutions with demonstrated skill with this technique. Findings detected during virtual colonoscopy often require subsequent conventional colonoscopy for confirmation and treatment.

DIARRHEA

Most cases of diarrhea are acute, self-limited, and due to infections or medication. Chronic diarrhea (lasting >6 weeks) is more often due to a primary inflammatory, malabsorptive, or motility disorder; is less likely to resolve spontaneously; and generally requires diagnostic evaluation. Patients with chronic diarrhea or severe, unexplained acute diarrhea often undergo endoscopy if stool tests for pathogens are unrevealing. The choice of endoscopic testing depends on the clinical setting.

Patients with colonic symptoms and findings such as bloody diarrhea, tenesmus, fever, or leukocytes in stool generally undergo sigmoidoscopy or colonoscopy to assess for colitis (Fig. 345-4). Sigmoidoscopy is an appropriate initial test in most patients. Conversely, patients with symptoms and findings suggesting small-bowel disease, such as large-volume watery stools, substantial weight loss, and malabsorption of iron, calcium, or fat, may undergo upper endoscopy with duodenal aspirates for assessment of bacterial overgrowth and biopsies for assessment of mucosal diseases, such as celiac sprue.

Many patients with chronic diarrhea do not fit either of these patterns. In the setting of a long-standing history of alternating constipation and diarrhea dating to early adulthood, without findings such as blood in the stool or anemia, a diagnosis of irritable bowel syndrome may be made without direct visualization of the bowel. Steatorrhea and upper abdominal pain may prompt evaluation of the pancreas rather than the gut. Patients whose chronic diarrhea is not easily categorized often undergo initial colonoscopy to examine the entire colon and terminal ileum for inflammatory or neoplastic disease (Fig. 345-47).

MINOR HEMATOCHEZIA

Bright red blood passed with or on formed brown stool usually has a rectal, anal, or distal sigmoid source (Fig. 345-48). Patients with even trivial amounts of hematochezia should be investigated with flexible sigmoidoscopy and anoscopy to exclude polyps or cancers in the distal colon. Patients reporting red blood on the toilet tissue only, without blood in the toilet or on the stool, are generally bleeding from a lesion

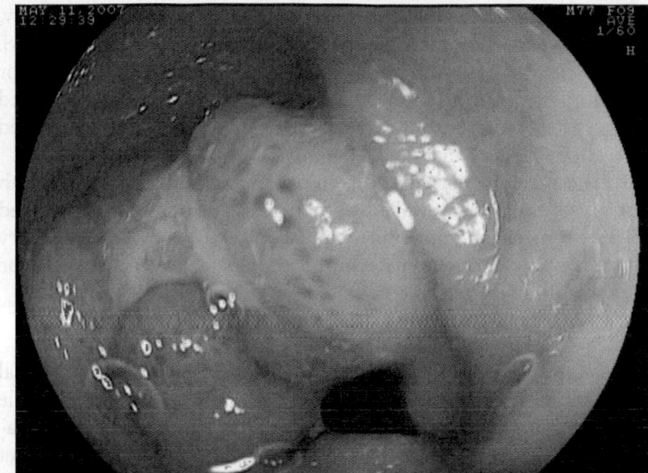

FIGURE 345-47 Ulcerated ileal carcinoid tumor.

in the anal canal. Careful external inspection, digital examination, and proctoscopy with anoscopy are sufficient for diagnosis in most cases.

PANCREATITIS

About 20% of patients with pancreatitis have no identified cause after routine clinical investigation (including a review of medication and alcohol use, measurement of serum triglyceride and calcium levels, abdominal ultrasonography, and CT). Endoscopic assessment leads to a specific diagnosis in the majority of such patients, often altering clinical management. Endoscopic investigation is particularly appropriate if the patient has had more than one episode of pancreatitis.

Microlithiasis, or the presence of microscopic crystals in bile, is a leading cause of previously unexplained acute pancreatitis and is sometimes seen during abdominal ultrasonography as layering sludge or flecks of floating, echogenic material in the gallbladder. Gallbladder bile can be obtained for microscopic analysis by administering a cholecystokinin analogue during endoscopy, causing contraction of the gallbladder. Bile is suctioned from the duodenum as it drains from the papilla, and the darkest fraction is examined for cholesterol crystals or bilirubinate granules. The combination of EUS of the gallbladder and bile microscopy is probably the most sensitive means of diagnosing microlithiasis.

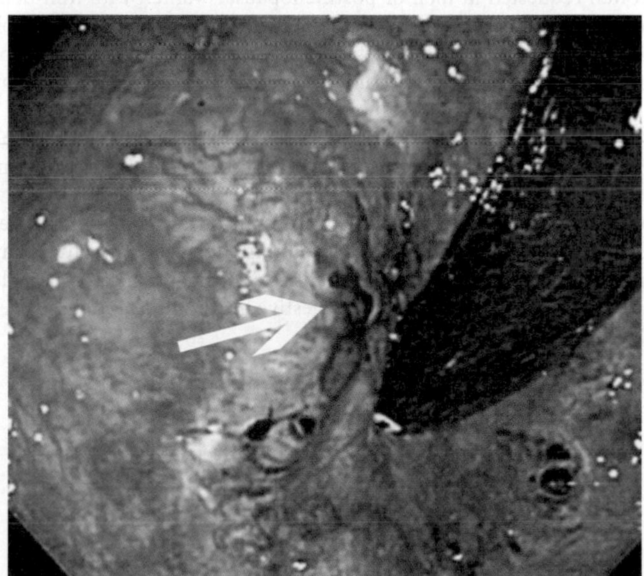

FIGURE 345-48 Internal hemorrhoids with bleeding *(arrow)* as seen on a retroflexed view of the rectum.

Previously undetected chronic pancreatitis, pancreatic malignancy, or pancreas divisum may be diagnosed by either ERCP or EUS. Sphincter of Oddi dysfunction or stenosis is a potential cause for pancreatitis and can be diagnosed by manometric studies performed during ERCP. Autoimmune pancreatitis may require EUS-guided pancreatic biopsy for histologic diagnosis.

Severe pancreatitis often results in pancreatic fluid collections. Both pseudocysts and areas of walled-off pancreatic necrosis can be drained into the stomach or duodenum endoscopically, using transpapillary and transmural endoscopic techniques. Pancreatic necrosis can be treated by direct endoscopic necrosectomy (see Video 346e-2).

CANCER STAGING

Local staging of esophageal, gastric, pancreatic, bile duct, and rectal cancers can be obtained with EUS (Fig. 345-15). EUS with fine-needle aspiration (Fig. 345-16) currently provides the most accurate preoperative assessment of local tumor and nodal staging, but it does not detect most distant metastases. Details of the local tumor stage can guide treatment decisions including resectability and need for neoadjuvant therapy. EUS with transesophageal needle biopsy may also be used to assess the presence of non-small-cell lung cancer in mediastinal nodes.

OPEN-ACCESS ENDOSCOPY

Direct scheduling of endoscopic procedures by primary care physicians without preceding gastroenterology consultation, or *open-access endoscopy*, is common. When the indications for endoscopy are clear-cut and appropriate, the procedural risks are low, and the patient understands what to expect, open-access endoscopy streamlines patient care and decreases costs.

Patients referred for open-access endoscopy should have a recent history, physical examination, and medication review. A copy of such an evaluation should be available when the patient comes to the endoscopy suite. Patients with unstable cardiovascular or respiratory conditions should not be referred directly for open-access endoscopy. Patients with particular conditions and undergoing certain procedures should be prescribed prophylactic antibiotics prior to endoscopy (Table 345-1). In addition, patients taking anticoagulants and/or antiplatelet drugs may require adjustment of these agents before endoscopy based on the procedure risk for bleeding and condition risk for a thromboembolic event (Table 345-2).

Common indications for open-access EGD include dyspepsia resistant to a trial of appropriate therapy; dysphagia; gastrointestinal bleeding; and persistent anorexia or early satiety. Open-access colonoscopy is often requested in men or postmenopausal women with iron-deficiency anemia, in patients over age 50 with occult blood in the stool, in patients with a previous history of colorectal adenomatous polyps or cancer, and for colorectal cancer screening. Flexible sigmoidoscopy is commonly performed as an open-access procedure.

When patients are referred for open-access colonoscopy, the primary care provider may need to choose a colonic preparation. Commonly used oral preparations include polyethylene glycol lavage solution, with or without citric acid. A "split-dose" regimen improves the quality of colonic preparation. Sodium phosphate purgatives may cause fluid and electrolyte abnormalities and renal toxicity, especially in patients with renal failure or congestive heart failure and those over 70 years of age.

346e Video Atlas of Gastrointestinal Endoscopy

Louis Michel Wong Kee Song, Mark Topazian

This is a digital-only chapter. It is available on the DVD that accompanies this book, as well as on Access Medicine/Harrison's Online, and the eBook and "app" editions of HPIM 19e.

Gastrointestinal endoscopy is an increasingly important method for diagnosis and treatment of disease. This atlas demonstrates endoscopic findings in a variety of gastrointestinal infectious, inflammatory, vascular, and neoplastic conditions. Cancer screening and prevention are common indications for gastrointestinal endoscopy, and the premalignant conditions of Barrett's esophagus and colonic polyps are illustrated. Endoscopic treatment modalities for gastrointestinal bleeding, polyps, and biliary stones are demonstrated in video clips. The images shown in this atlas are also found in Chap. 345 of the book.

347 Diseases of the Esophagus

Peter J. Kahrilas, Ikuo Hirano

ESOPHAGEAL STRUCTURE AND FUNCTION

The esophagus is a hollow, muscular tube coursing through the posterior mediastinum joining the hypopharynx to the stomach with a sphincter at each end. It functions to transport food and fluid between these ends, otherwise remaining empty. The physiology of swallowing, esophageal motility, and oral and pharyngeal dysphagia are described in Chap. 53. Esophageal diseases can be manifested by impaired function or pain. Key functional impairments are swallowing disorders and excessive gastroesophageal reflux. Pain, sometimes indistinguishable from cardiac chest pain, can result from inflammation, infection, dysmotility, or neoplasm.

SYMPTOMS OF ESOPHAGEAL DISEASE

The clinical history remains central to the evaluation of esophageal symptoms. A thoughtfully obtained history will often expedite management. Important details include weight gain or loss, gastrointestinal bleeding, dietary habits including the timing of meals, smoking, and alcohol consumption. The major esophageal symptoms are heartburn, regurgitation, chest pain, dysphagia, odynophagia, and globus sensation.

Heartburn (pyrosis), the most common esophageal symptom, is characterized by a discomfort or burning sensation behind the sternum that arises from the epigastrium and may radiate toward the neck. Heartburn is an intermittent symptom, most commonly experienced after eating, during exercise, and while lying recumbent. The discomfort is relieved with drinking water or antacid but can occur frequently interfering with normal activities including sleep. The association between heartburn and gastroesophageal reflux disease (GERD) is so strong that empirical therapy for GERD has become accepted management. However, the term "heartburn" is often misused and/or referred to with other terms such as "indigestion" or "repeating," making it important to clarify the intended meaning.

Regurgitation is the effortless return of food or fluid into the pharynx without nausea or retching. Patients report a sour or burning fluid in the throat or mouth that may also contain undigested food particles. Bending, belching, or maneuvers that increase intraabdominal pressure can provoke regurgitation. A clinician needs to discriminate among regurgitation, vomiting, and rumination. *Vomiting* is preceded by nausea and accompanied by retching. *Rumination* is a behavior in which recently swallowed food is regurgitated and then reswallowed repetitively for up to an hour. Although there is some linkage between rumination and mental deficiency, the behavior is also exhibited by unimpaired individuals who sometimes even find it pleasurable.

Chest pain is a common esophageal symptom with characteristics similar to cardiac pain, sometimes making this distinction difficult. Esophageal pain is usually experienced as a pressure type sensation in the mid chest, radiating to the mid back, arms, or jaws. The similarity to cardiac pain is likely because the two organs share a nerve plexus and the nerve endings in the esophageal wall have poor discriminative ability among stimuli. Esophageal distention or even chemostimulation (e.g., with acid) will often be perceived as chest pain. Gastroesophageal reflux is the most common cause of esophageal chest pain.

Esophageal *dysphagia* (Chap. 53) is often described as a feeling of food "sticking" or even lodging in the chest. Important distinctions are between uniquely solid food dysphagia as opposed to liquid and solid, episodic versus constant dysphagia, and progressive versus static dysphagia. If the dysphagia is for liquids as well as solid food, it suggests a motility disorder such as achalasia. Conversely, uniquely solid food dysphagia is suggestive of a stricture, ring, or tumor. Of note, a patient's localization of food hang-up in the esophagus is notoriously imprecise. Approximately 30% of distal esophageal obstructions are perceived as cervical dysphagia. In such instances, the absence of concomitant symptoms generally associated with oropharyngeal dysphagia such as aspiration, nasopharyngeal regurgitation, cough, drooling, or obvious neuromuscular compromise should suggest an esophageal etiology.

Odynophagia is pain either caused by or exacerbated by swallowing. Although typically considered distinct from dysphagia, odynophagia may manifest concurrently with dysphagia. Odynophagia is more common with pill or infectious esophagitis than with reflux esophagitis and should prompt a search for these entities. When odynophagia does occur in GERD, it is likely related to an esophageal ulcer or deep erosion.

Globus sensation, alternatively labeled "globus hystericus," is the perception of a lump or fullness in the throat that is felt irrespective of swallowing. Although such patients are frequently referred for an evaluation of dysphagia, globus sensation is often relieved by the act of swallowing. As implied by its alternative name (globus hystericus), globus sensation often occurs in the setting of anxiety or obsessive-compulsive disorders. Clinical experience teaches that it is often attributable to GERD.

Water brash is excessive salivation resulting from a vagal reflex triggered by acidification of the esophageal mucosa. This is not a common symptom. Afflicted individuals will describe the unpleasant sensation of the mouth rapidly filling with salty thin fluid, often in the setting of concomitant heartburn.

DIAGNOSTIC STUDIES

ENDOSCOPY

Endoscopy, also known as esophagogastroduodenoscopy (EGD), is the most useful test for the evaluation of the proximal gastrointestinal tract. Modern instruments produce high-quality, color images of the esophageal, gastric, and duodenal lumen. Endoscopes also have an instrumentation channel through which biopsy forceps, injection catheters for local delivery of therapeutic agents, balloon dilators, or hemostatic devices can be used. The key advantages of endoscopy over barium radiography are: (1) increased sensitivity for the detection of mucosal lesions, (2) vastly increased sensitivity for the detection of abnormalities mainly identifiable by color such as Barrett's metaplasia or vascular lesions, (3) the ability to obtain biopsy specimens for histologic examination of suspected abnormalities, and (4) the ability to dilate strictures during the examination. The main disadvantages of endoscopy are cost and the utilization of sedatives or anesthetics.

RADIOGRAPHY

Contrast radiography of the esophagus, stomach, and duodenum can demonstrate reflux of the contrast media, hiatal hernia, mucosal granularity, erosions, ulcerations, and strictures. The sensitivity of radiography compared with endoscopy for detecting reflux esophagitis reportedly ranges from 22–95%, with higher grades of esophagitis (i.e., ulceration or stricture) exhibiting greater detection rates. Conversely, the sensitivity of barium radiography for detecting esophageal strictures is greater than that of endoscopy, especially when the study is done in conjunction with barium-soaked bread or a 13-mm barium tablet. Barium studies also provide an assessment of esophageal function and morphology that may be undetected on endoscopy. Tracheoesophageal fistula, altered postsurgical anatomy, and extrinsic esophageal compression are conditions where radiographic imaging complements endoscopic assessment. Hypopharyngeal pathology and disorders of the cricopharyngeus muscle are better appreciated on radiographic examination than with endoscopy, particularly with rapid sequence or video fluoroscopic recording. The major shortcoming of barium radiography is that it rarely obviates the need for endoscopy. Either a positive or a negative study is usually followed by an endoscopic evaluation either to obtain biopsies, provide therapy, or clarify findings in the case of a positive examination or to add a level of certainty in the case of a negative one.

ENDOSCOPIC ULTRASOUND

Endoscopic ultrasound (EUS) instruments combine an endoscope with an ultrasound transducer to create a transmural image of the tissue surrounding the endoscope tip. The key advantage of EUS over alternative radiologic imaging techniques is much greater resolution attributable to the proximity of the ultrasound transducer to the area being examined. Available devices can provide either radial imaging (360-degree, cross-sectional) or a curved linear image that can guide fine-needle aspiration of imaged structures such as lymph nodes or tumors. Major esophageal applications of EUS are to stage esophageal cancer, to evaluate dysplasia in Barrett's esophagus, and to assess submucosal lesions.

ESOPHAGEAL MANOMETRY

Esophageal manometry, or motility testing, entails positioning a pressure-sensing catheter within the esophagus and then observing the contractility following test swallows. The upper and lower esophageal sphincters appear as zones of high pressure that relax on swallowing, while the intersphincteric esophagus exhibits peristaltic contractions. Manometry is used to diagnose motility disorders (achalasia, diffuse esophageal spasm) and to assess peristaltic integrity prior to the surgery for reflux disease. Technologic advances have enhanced esophageal manometry as high-resolution esophageal pressure topography (Fig. 347-1). Manometry can also be combined with intraluminal impedance monitoring. Impedance recordings use a catheter with a series of paired electrodes. Esophageal luminal contents in contact with the electrodes decrease (liquid) or increase (air) the impedance signal, allowing detection of anterograde or retrograde esophageal bolus transit.

REFLUX TESTING

GERD is often diagnosed in the absence of endoscopic esophagitis, which would otherwise define the disease. This occurs in the settings of partially treated disease, an abnormally sensitive esophageal mucosa, or without obvious explanation. In such instances, reflux

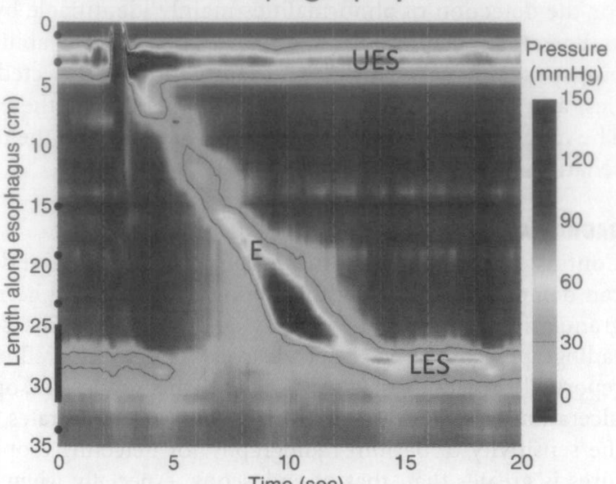

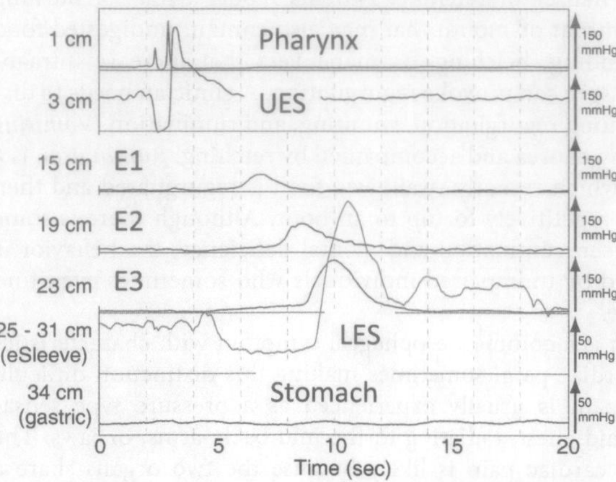

FIGURE 347-1 High-resolution esophageal pressure topography (*right*) and conventional manometry (*left*) of a normal swallow. E, esophageal body; LES, lower esophageal sphincter; UES, upper esophageal sphincter.

testing can demonstrate excessive esophageal exposure to refluxed gastric juice, the physiologic abnormality of GERD. This can be done by ambulatory 24- to 48-h esophageal pH recording using either a wireless pH-sensitive transmitter that is anchored to the esophageal mucosa or a transnasally positioned wire electrode with the tip stationed in the distal esophagus. Either way, the outcome is expressed as the percentage of the day that the pH was less than 4 (indicative of recent acid reflux), with values exceeding 5% indicative of GERD. Reflux testing is useful with atypical symptoms or an inexplicably poor response to therapy. Intraluminal impedance monitoring can be added to pH monitoring to detect reflux events irrespective of whether or not they are acidic, potentially increasing the sensitivity of the study.

STRUCTURAL DISORDERS

HIATAL HERNIA

Hiatus hernia is a herniation of viscera, most commonly the stomach, into the mediastinum through the esophageal hiatus of the diaphragm. Four types of hiatus hernia are distinguished with type I, or sliding hiatal hernia, comprising at least 95% of the overall total. A sliding hiatal hernia is one in which the gastroesophageal junction and gastric cardia translocate cephalad as a result of weakening of the phrenoesophageal ligament attaching the gastroesophageal junction to the diaphragm at the hiatus and dilatation of the diaphragmatic hiatus. The incidence of sliding hernia increases with age. True to its name, sliding hernias enlarge with increased intraabdominal pressure, swallowing, and respiration. Conceptually, sliding hernias are the result of wear and tear: increased intraabdominal pressure from abdominal obesity, pregnancy, etc., along with hereditary factors predisposing to the condition. The main significance of sliding hernias is the propensity of affected individuals to have GERD.

Types II, III, and IV hiatal hernias are all subtypes of paraesophageal hernia in which the herniation into the mediastinum includes a visceral structure other than the gastric cardia. With type II and III paraesophageal hernias, the gastric fundus also herniates with the distinction being that in type II, the gastroesophageal junction remains fixed at the hiatus, whereas type III is a combined sliding and paraesophageal hernia. With type IV hiatal hernias, viscera other than the stomach herniate into the mediastinum, most commonly the colon. With type II and III paraesophageal hernias, the stomach inverts as it herniates and large paraesophageal hernias can lead to an upside down stomach, gastric volvulus, and even strangulation of the stomach. Because of this risk, surgical repair is often advocated for large paraesophageal hernias.

RINGS AND WEBS

A lower esophageal mucosal ring, also called a *B ring*, is a thin membranous narrowing at the squamocolumnar mucosal junction (Fig. 347-2). Its origin is unknown, but B rings are demonstrable in about 10–15% of the general population and are usually asymptomatic. When the lumen diameter is less than 13 mm, distal rings are usually associated with episodic solid food dysphagia and are called *Schatzki rings*. Patients typically present older than 40 years, consistent with an acquired rather than congenital origin. Schatzki ring is one of the most common causes of intermittent food impaction, also known as "steakhouse syndrome" because meat is a typical instigator. Symptomatic rings are easily treated by dilation.

Web-like constrictions higher in the esophagus can be of congenital or inflammatory origin. Asymptomatic cervical esophageal webs are demonstrated in about 10% of people and typically originate along the anterior aspect of the esophagus. When circumferential, they can

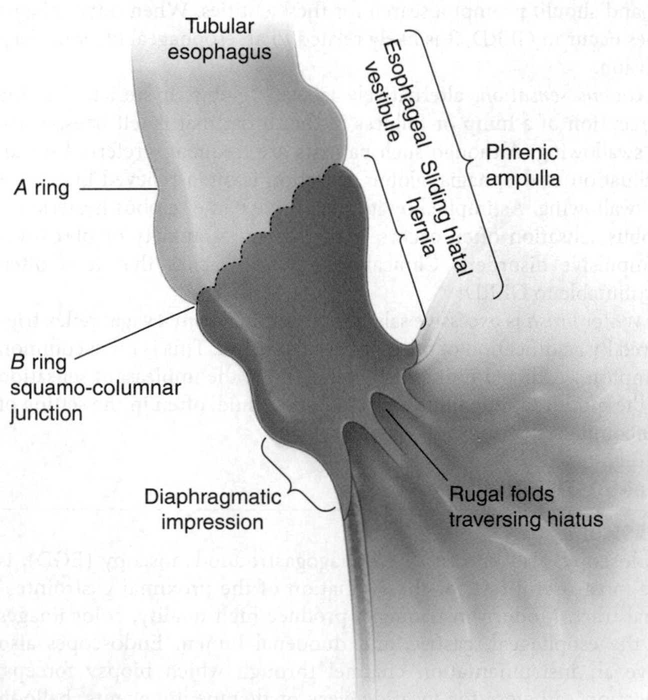

FIGURE 347-2 Radiographic anatomy of the gastroesophageal junction.

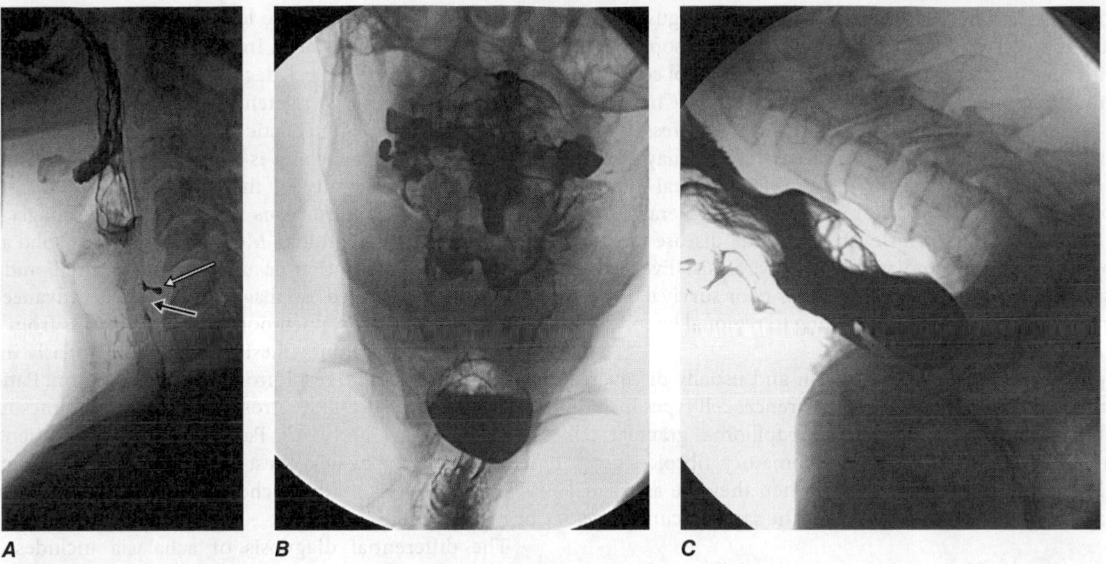

FIGURE 347-3 Examples of small (*A*) and large (*B, C*) Zenker's diverticula arising from Killian's triangle in the distal hypopharynx. Smaller diverticula are evident only during the swallow, whereas larger ones retain food and fluid.

cause intermittent dysphagia to solids similar to Schatzki rings and are similarly treated with dilatation. The combination of symptomatic proximal esophageal webs and iron-deficiency anemia in middle-aged women constitutes Plummer-Vinson syndrome.

DIVERTICULA

Esophageal diverticula are categorized by location with the most common being epiphrenic, hypopharyngeal (Zenker's), and midesophageal. Epiphrenic and Zenker's diverticula are false diverticula involving herniation of the mucosa and submucosa through the muscular layer of the esophagus. These lesions result from increased intraluminal pressure associated with distal obstruction. In the case of Zenker's, the obstruction is a stenotic cricopharyngeus muscle (upper esophageal sphincter), and the hypopharyngeal herniation most commonly occurs in an area of natural weakness proximal to the cricopharyngeus known as *Killian's triangle* (Fig. 347-3). Small Zenker's diverticula are usually asymptomatic, but when they enlarge sufficiently to retain food and saliva they can be associated with dysphagia, halitosis, and aspiration. Treatment is by surgical diverticulectomy and cricopharyngeal myotomy or a marsupialization procedure in which an endoscopic stapling device is used to divide the cricopharyngeus.

Epiphrenic diverticula are usually associated with achalasia or a distal esophageal stricture. Midesophageal diverticula may be caused by traction from adjacent inflammation (classically tuberculosis) in which case they are true diverticula involving all layers of the esophageal wall, or by pulsion associated with esophageal motor disorders. Midesophageal and epiphrenic diverticula are usually asymptomatic until they enlarge sufficiently to retain food and cause dysphagia and regurgitation. Symptoms attributable to the diverticula tend to correlate more with the underlying esophageal disorder than the size of the diverticula. Large diverticula can be removed surgically, usually in conjunction with a myotomy if the underlying cause is achalasia. Diffuse intramural esophageal diverticulosis is a rare entity that results from dilatation of the excretory ducts of submucosal esophageal glands (Fig. 347-4). Esophageal candidiasis and proximal esophageal strictures are commonly found in association with this disorder.

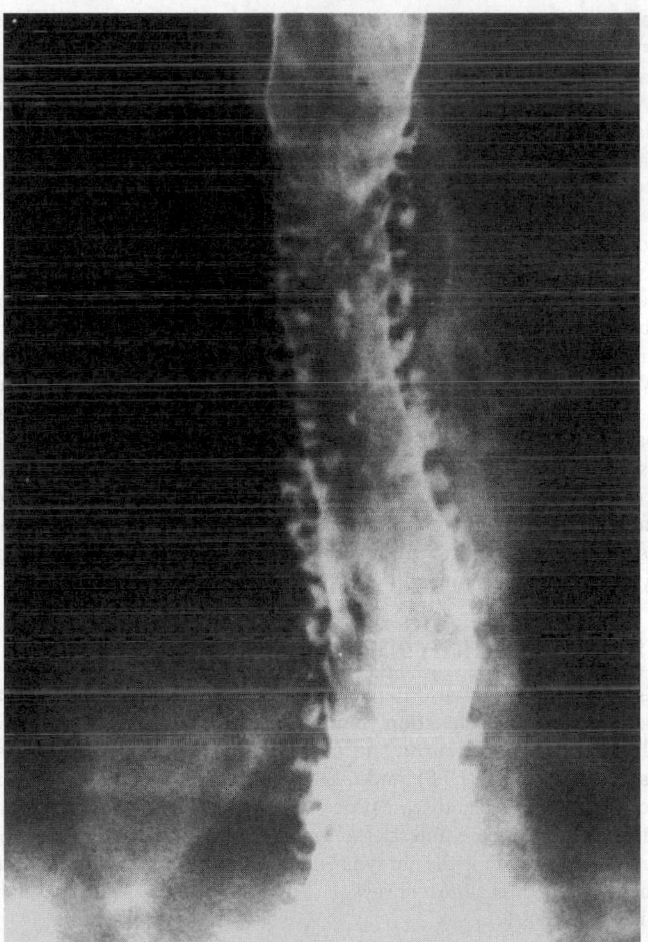

FIGURE 347-4 Intramural esophageal pseudodiverticulosis associated with chronic obstruction. Invaginations of contrast into the esophageal wall outline deep esophageal glands.

TUMORS

Esophageal cancer occurs in about 4.5:100,000 people in the United States with the associated mortality being only slightly less at 4.4:100,000. It is about 10 times less common than colorectal cancer but kills about one-quarter as many patients. These statistics emphasize both the rarity and lethality of esophageal cancer. One notable trend is the shift of dominant esophageal cancer type from squamous cell to adenocarcinoma, strongly linked to reflux disease and Barrett's metaplasia. Other distinctions between cell types are the predilection for adenocarcinoma to affect the distal esophagus in white males and squamous cell to affect the more proximal esophagus in black males with the added risk factors of smoking, alcohol consumption, caustic injury, and human papilloma virus infection (Chap. 109).

The typical presentation of esophageal cancer is of progressive solid food dysphagia and weight loss. Associated symptoms may include odynophagia, iron deficiency, and, with midesophageal tumors, hoarseness from left recurrent laryngeal nerve injury. Generally, these are indications of locally invasive or even metastatic disease manifest by tracheoesophageal fistulas and vocal cord paralysis. Even when detected as a small lesion, esophageal cancer has poor survival because of the abundant esophageal lymphatics leading to regional lymph node metastases.

Benign esophageal tumors are uncommon and usually discovered incidentally. In decreasing frequency of occurrence, cell types include leiomyoma, fibrovascular polyps, squamous papilloma, granular cell tumors, lipomas, neurofibromas, and inflammatory fibroid polyps. These generally become symptomatic only when they are associated with dysphagia and merit removal only under the same circumstances.

CONGENITAL ANOMALIES

The most common congenital esophageal anomaly is esophageal atresia, occurring in about 1 in 5000 live births. Atresia can occur in several permutations, the common denominator being developmental failure of fusion between the proximal and distal esophagus associated with a tracheoesophageal fistula, most commonly with the distal segment excluded. Alternatively, there can be an H-type configuration in which esophageal fusion has occurred, but with a tracheoesophageal fistula. Esophageal atresia is usually recognized and corrected surgically within the first few days of life. Later life complications include dysphagia from anastomotic strictures or absent peristalsis and reflux, which can be severe. Less common developmental anomalies include congenital esophageal stenosis, webs, and duplications.

Dysphagia can also result from congenital abnormalities that cause extrinsic compression of the esophagus. In dysphagia lusoria, the esophagus is compressed by an aberrant right subclavian artery arising from the descending aorta and passing behind the esophagus. Alternatively vascular rings may surround and constrict the esophagus.

Heterotopic gastric mucosa, also known as an esophageal inlet patch, is a focus of gastric type epithelium in the proximal cervical esophagus; the estimated prevalence is 4.5%. The inlet patch is thought to result from incomplete replacement of embryonic columnar epithelium with squamous epithelium. The majority of inlet patches are asymptomatic, but acid production can occur as most contain fundic type gastric epithelium with parietal cells.

ESOPHAGEAL MOTILITY DISORDERS

Esophageal motility disorders are diseases attributable to esophageal neuromuscular dysfunction commonly associated with dysphagia, chest pain, or heartburn. The major entities are achalasia, diffuse esophageal spasm (DES), and GERD. Motility disorders can also be secondary to broader disease processes as is the case with pseudoachalasia, Chagas' disease, and scleroderma. Not included in this discussion are diseases affecting the pharynx and proximal esophagus, the impairment of which is almost always part of a more global neuromuscular disease process.

ACHALASIA

Achalasia is a rare disease caused by loss of ganglion cells within the esophageal myenteric plexus with a population incidence of about 1:100,000 and usually presenting between age 25 and 60. With longstanding disease, aganglionosis is noted. The disease involves both excitatory (cholinergic) and inhibitory (nitric oxide) ganglionic neurons. Functionally, inhibitory neurons mediate deglutitive lower esophageal sphincter (LES) relaxation and the sequential propagation of peristalsis. Their absence leads to impaired deglutitive LES relaxation and absent peristalsis. Increasing evidence suggests that the ultimate cause of ganglion cell degeneration in achalasia is an autoimmune process attributable to a latent infection with human herpes simplex virus 1 combined with genetic susceptibility.

Long-standing achalasia is characterized by progressive dilatation and sigmoid deformity of the esophagus with hypertrophy of the LES. Clinical manifestations may include dysphagia, regurgitation, chest pain, and weight loss. Most patients report solid and liquid food dysphagia. Regurgitation occurs when food, fluid, and secretions are retained in the dilated esophagus. Patients with advanced achalasia are at risk for bronchitis, pneumonia, or lung abscess from chronic regurgitation and aspiration. Chest pain is frequent early in the course of achalasia, thought to result from esophageal spasm. Patients describe a squeezing, pressure-like retrosternal pain, sometimes radiating to the neck, arms, jaw, and back. Paradoxically, some patients complain of heartburn that may be a chest pain equivalent. Treatment of achalasia is less effective in relieving chest pain than it is in relieving dysphagia or regurgitation.

The differential diagnosis of achalasia includes DES, Chagas' disease, and pseudoachalasia. Chagas' disease is endemic in areas of central Brazil, Venezuela, and northern Argentina and spread by the bite of the reduviid (kissing) bug that transmits the protozoan, *Trypanosoma cruzi*. The chronic phase of the disease develops years after infection and results from destruction of autonomic ganglion cells throughout the body, including the heart, gut, urinary tract, and respiratory tract. Tumor infiltration, most commonly seen with carcinoma in the gastric fundus or distal esophagus, can mimic idiopathic achalasia. The resultant "pseudoachalasia" accounts for up to 5% of suspected cases and is more likely with advanced age, abrupt onset of symptoms (<1 year), and weight loss. Hence, endoscopy is a necessary part of the evaluation of achalasia. When the clinical suspicion for pseudoachalasia is high and endoscopy nondiagnostic, computed tomography (CT) scanning or EUS may be of value. Rarely, pseudoachalasia can result from a paraneoplastic syndrome with circulating antineuronal antibodies.

Achalasia is diagnosed by barium swallow x-ray and/or esophageal manometry; endoscopy has a relatively minor role other than to exclude pseudoachalasia. The barium swallow x-ray appearance is of a dilated esophagus with poor emptying, an air-fluid level, and tapering at the LES giving it a beak-like appearance (Fig. 347-5). Occasionally, an epiphrenic diverticulum is observed. In long-standing achalasia, the esophagus may assume a sigmoid configuration. The diagnostic criteria for achalasia with esophageal manometry are impaired LES relaxation and absent peristalsis. High-resolution manometry has somewhat advanced this diagnosis; three subtypes of achalasia are differentiated based on the pattern of pressurization in the nonperistaltic esophagus (Fig. 347-6). Because manometry identifies early disease before esophageal dilatation and food retention, it is the most sensitive diagnostic test.

There is no known way of preventing or reversing achalasia. Therapy is directed at reducing LES pressure so that gravity and esophageal pressurization promote esophageal emptying. Peristalsis rarely, if ever, recovers. However, in many instances, remnants of peristalsis masked by esophageal pressurization and dilatation prior to therapy are demonstrable following effective treatment. LES pressure can be reduced by pharmacologic therapy, pneumatic balloon dilatation, or surgical myotomy. No large, controlled trials of the therapeutic alternatives exist, and the optimal approach is debated. Pharmacologic therapies are relatively ineffective but are often used as temporizing therapies. Nitrates or calcium channel blockers are administered before eating, advising caution because of their effects on blood pressure. Botulinum toxin, injected into the LES under endoscopic guidance, inhibits acetylcholine release from nerve endings and improves dysphagia in about 66% of cases for at least 6 months. Sildenafil and alternative phosphodiesterase inhibitors effectively decrease LES pressure, but practicalities limit their clinical use in achalasia.

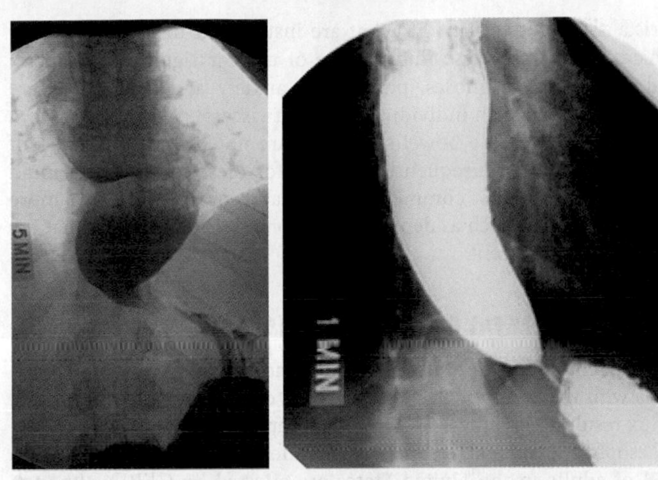

FIGURE 347-5 Achalasia with esophageal dilatation, tapering at the gastroesophageal junction, and an air-fluid level within the esophagus. The example on the *left* shows sigmoid deformity with very advanced disease.

The only durable therapies for achalasia are pneumatic dilatation and Heller myotomy. Pneumatic dilatation, with a reported efficacy ranging from 32–98%, is an endoscopic technique using a noncompliant, cylindrical balloon dilator positioned across the LES and inflated to a diameter of 3–4 cm. The major complication is perforation with a reported incidence of 0.5–5%. The most common surgical procedure for achalasia is laparoscopic Heller myotomy, usually performed in conjunction with an antireflux procedure (partial fundoplication); good to excellent results are reported in 62–100% of cases. A European randomized controlled trial demonstrated an equivalent response rate of approximately 90% for both pneumatic dilation and laparoscopic Heller myotomy at 2-year follow-up. Occasionally, patients with advanced disease fail to respond to pneumatic dilatation or Heller myotomy. In such refractory cases, esophageal resection with gastric pull-up or interposition of a segment of transverse colon may be the only option other than gastrostomy feeding.

An endoscopic approach to LES myotomy has been introduced, referred to as per oral esophageal myotomy. This technique involves the creation of a tunnel within the esophageal wall through which the circular muscle of the LES and distal esophagus are transected with electrocautery. Short-term studies of efficacy have been favorable. Potential advantages over the conventional laparoscopic approach include avoidance of surgical disruption of the diaphragmatic hiatus and more rapid recovery.

In untreated or inadequately treated achalasia, esophageal dilatation predisposes to stasis esophagitis. Prolonged stasis esophagitis is the likely explanation for the association between achalasia and esophageal squamous cell cancer. Tumors develop after years of achalasia, usually in the setting of a greatly dilated esophagus with the overall squamous cell cancer risk increased 17-fold compared to controls.

DIFFUSE ESOPHAGEAL SPASM (DES)

DES is manifested by episodes of dysphagia and chest pain attributable to abnormal esophageal contractions with normal deglutitive LES relaxation. Beyond that, there is little consensus. The pathophysiology and natural history of DES are ill defined. Radiographically, DES has been characterized by tertiary contractions or a "corkscrew esophagus" (Fig. 347-7), but in many instances, these abnormalities are actually indicative of achalasia. Manometrically, a variety of defining features have been proposed including uncoordinated ("spastic") activity in the distal esophagus, spontaneous and repetitive contractions, or high-amplitude and prolonged contractions. The current consensus, derived from high-resolution manometry studies, is to define spasm by the occurrence of contractions in the distal esophagus with short latency relative to the time of the pharyngeal contraction, a dysfunction indicative of impairment of inhibitory myenteric plexus neurons.

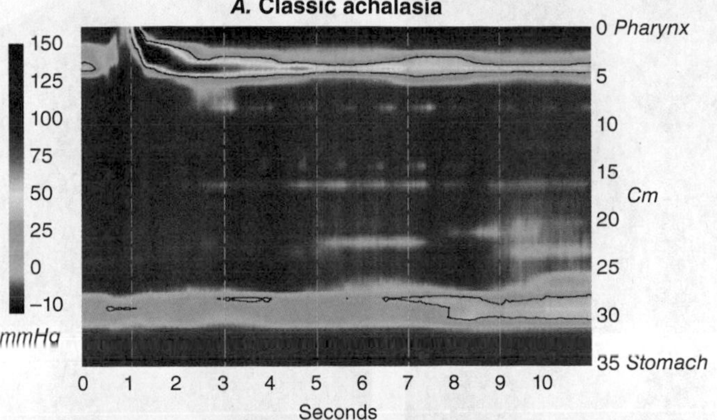

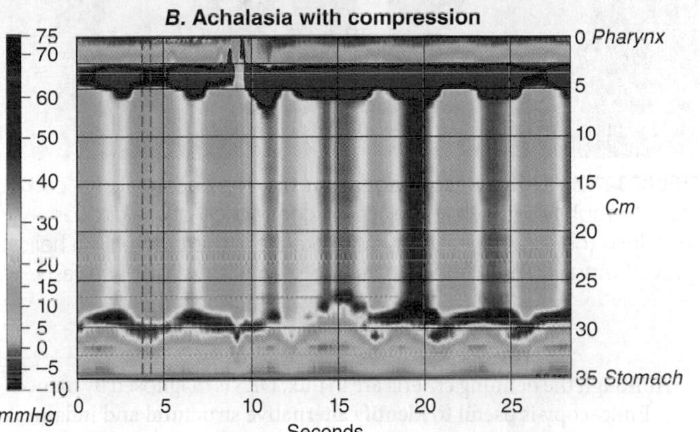

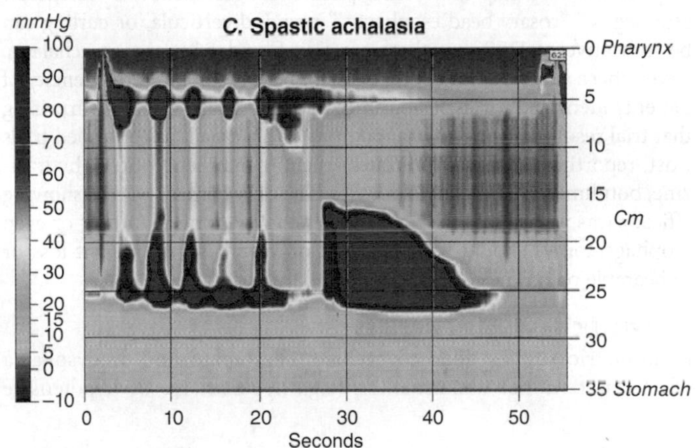

FIGURE 347-6 Three subtypes of achalasia: classic (*A*), with esophageal compression (*B*), and spastic achalasia (*C*) imaged with pressure topography. All are characterized by impaired lower esophageal sphincter (LES) relaxation and absent peristalsis. However, classic achalasia has minimal pressurization of the esophageal body, whereas substantial fluid pressurization is observed in achalasia with esophageal compression, and spastic esophageal contractions are observed with spastic achalasia.

When defined in this restrictive fashion (Fig. 347-8), DES is actually much less common than achalasia.

Esophageal chest pain closely mimics angina pectoris. Features suggesting esophageal pain include pain that is nonexertional, prolonged, interrupts sleep, meal-related, relieved with antacids, and accompanied by heartburn, dysphagia, or regurgitation. However, all of these features exhibit overlap with cardiac pain, which still must be the primary consideration. Furthermore, even within the spectrum of esophageal diseases, both chest pain and dysphagia are also characteristic of peptic or infectious esophagitis. Only after these more common entities have been excluded by evaluation and/or treatment should a diagnosis of DES be pursued.

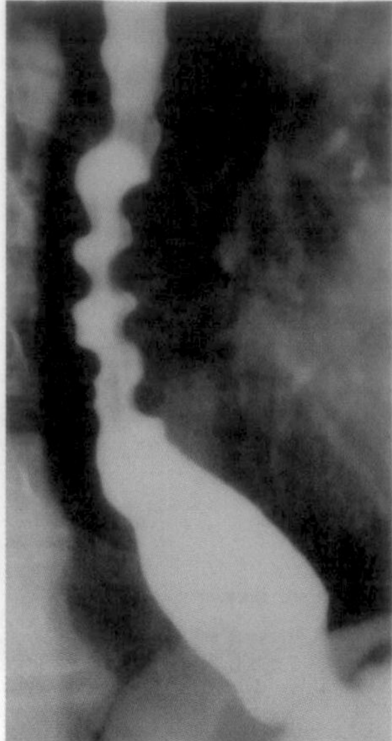

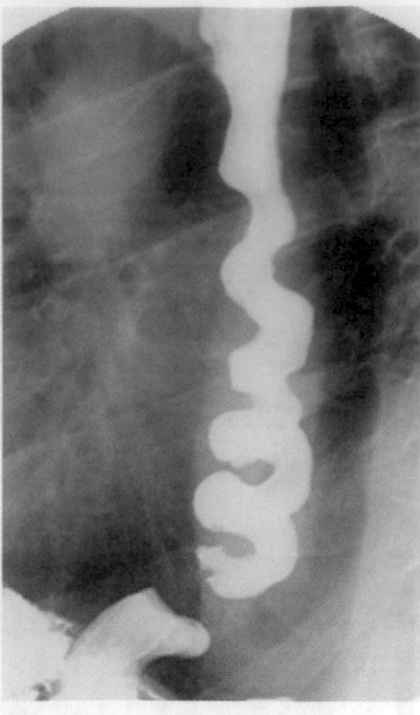

FIGURE 347-7 Diffuse esophageal spasm. The characteristic "corkscrew" esophagus results from spastic contraction of the circular muscle in the esophageal wall; more precisely, this is actually a helical array of muscle. These findings are also seen with spastic achalasia.

Although the defining criteria are in flux, DES is diagnosed by manometry. Endoscopy is useful to identify alternative structural and inflammatory lesions that may cause chest pain. Radiographically, a "corkscrew esophagus," "rosary bead esophagus," pseudodiverticula, or curling can be indicative of DES, but these are also found with spastic achalasia. Given these vagaries of defining DES, and the resultant heterogeneity of patients identified for inclusion in therapeutic trials, it is not surprising that trial results have been disappointing. Only small, uncontrolled trials exist, reporting response to nitrates, calcium channel blockers, hydralazine, botulinum toxin, and anxiolytics. The only controlled trial showing efficacy was with an anxiolytic. Surgical therapy (long myotomy or even esophagectomy) should be considered only with severe weight loss or unbearable pain. These indications are extremely rare.

NONSPECIFIC MANOMETRIC FINDINGS

Manometric studies done to evaluate chest pain and/or dysphagia often report minor abnormalities (e.g., hypertensive or hypotensive peristalsis, hypertensive LES) that are insufficient to diagnose either achalasia or DES. These findings are of unclear significance. Reflux and psychiatric diagnoses, particularly anxiety and depression, are common among such individuals. A lower visceral pain threshold and symptoms of irritable bowel syndrome are noted in more than half of such patients. Consequently, therapy for these individuals should either target the most common esophageal disorder, GERD, or more global conditions such as depression or somatization neurosis that are found to be coexistent.

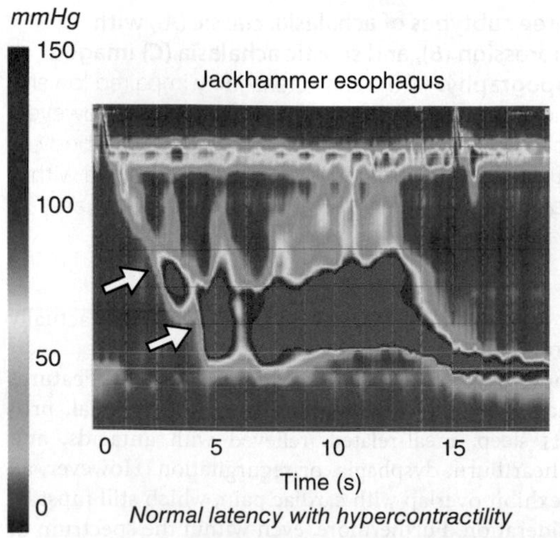

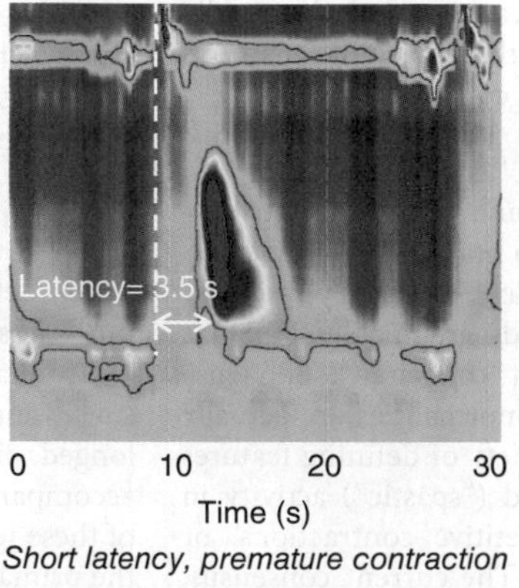

FIGURE 347-8 Esophageal pressure topography of the two major variants of esophageal spasm: jackhammer esophagus (*left*) and diffuse esophageal spasm (*right*). Jackhammer esophagus is defined by the extraordinarily vigorous and repetitive contractions with normal peristaltic onset and normal latency of the contraction. Diffuse esophageal spasm is similar but primarily defined by a short latency (premature) contraction.

GASTROESOPHAGEAL REFLUX DISEASE (GERD)

The current conception of GERD is to encompass a family of conditions with the commonality that they are caused by gastroesophageal reflux resulting in either troublesome symptoms or an array of potential esophageal and extraesophageal manifestations. It is estimated that 15% of adults in the United States are affected by GERD, although such estimates are based only on population studies of self-reported chronic heartburn. With respect to the esophagus, the spectrum of injury includes esophagitis, stricture, Barrett's esophagus, and adenocarcinoma (Fig. 347-9). Of particular concern is the rising incidence of esophageal adenocarcinoma, an epidemiologic trend that parallels the increasing incidence of GERD. There were about 8000 incident cases of esophageal adenocarcinoma in the United States in 2013 (half of all esophageal cancers); it is estimated that this disease burden has increased two- to sixfold in the last 20 years.

PATHOPHYSIOLOGY

The best-defined subset of GERD patients, albeit a minority overall, have esophagitis. Esophagitis occurs when refluxed gastric acid and pepsin cause necrosis of the esophageal mucosa causing erosions and ulcers. Note that some degree of gastroesophageal reflux is normal, physiologically intertwined with the mechanism of belching (transient LES relaxation), but esophagitis results from excessive reflux, often accompanied by impaired clearance of the refluxed gastric juice. Restricting reflux to that which is physiologically intended depends on the anatomic and physiologic integrity of the esophagogastric junction, a complex sphincter comprised of both the LES and the surrounding crural diaphragm. Three dominant mechanisms of esophagogastric junction incompetence are recognized: (1) transient LES relaxations (a vagovagal reflex in which LES relaxation is elicited by gastric distention), (2) LES hypotension, or (3) anatomic distortion of the esophagogastric junction inclusive of hiatus hernia. Of note, the third factor, esophagogastric junction anatomic disruption, is both significant unto itself and also because it interacts with the first two mechanisms. Transient LES relaxations account for about 90% of reflux in normal subjects or GERD patients without hiatus hernia, but patients with hiatus hernia have a more heterogeneous mechanistic profile. Factors tending to exacerbate reflux regardless of mechanism are abdominal obesity, pregnancy, gastric hypersecretory states, delayed gastric emptying, disruption of esophageal peristalsis, and gluttony.

After acid reflux, peristalsis returns the refluxed fluid to the stomach and acid clearance is completed by titration of the residual acid by bicarbonate contained in swallowed saliva. Consequently, two causes of prolonged acid clearance are impaired peristalsis and reduced salivation. Impaired peristaltic emptying can be attributable to disrupted peristalsis or superimposed reflux associated with a hiatal hernia. With superimposed reflux, fluid retained within a sliding hiatal hernia refluxes back into the

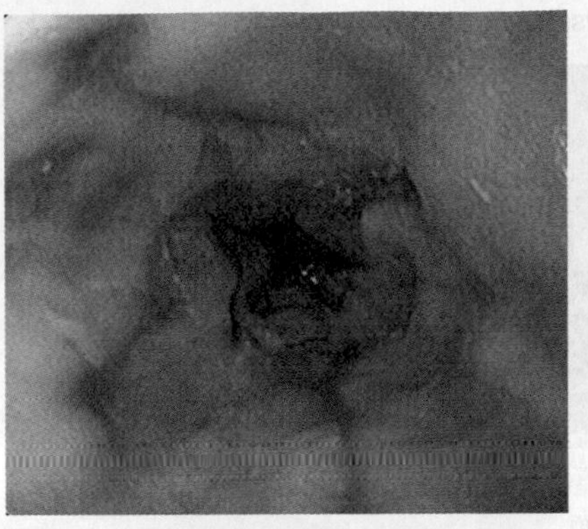

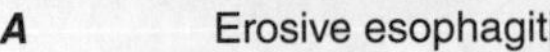

A Erosive esophagitis

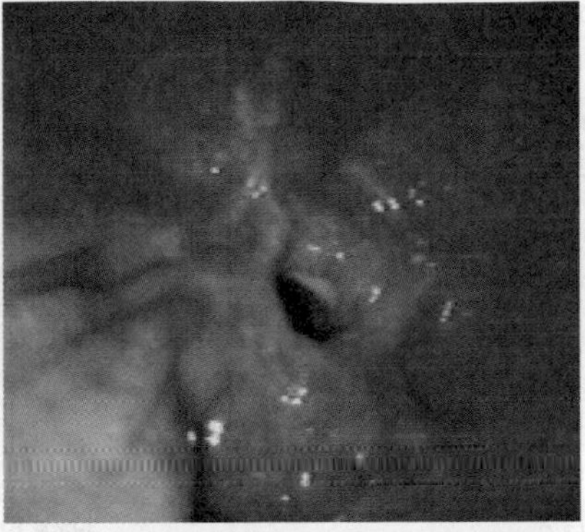

B Esophageal stricture with chronic erosive esophagitis

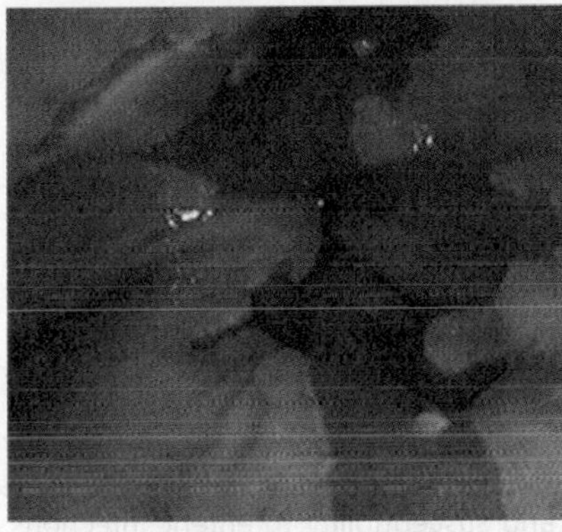

C Barrett's esophagus

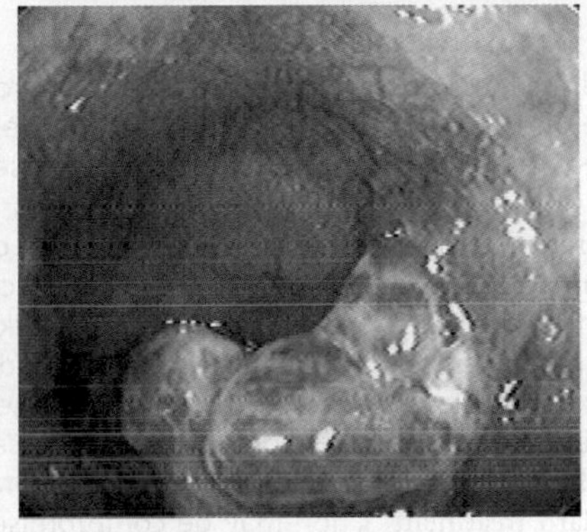

D Esophageal adenocarcinoma with Barrett's esophagus

FIGURE 347-9 Endoscopic appearance of (*A*) peptic esophagitis, (*B*) a peptic stricture, (*C*) Barrett's metaplasia, and (*D*) adenocarcinoma developing within an area of Barrett's esophagus.

esophagus during swallow-related LES relaxation, a phenomenon that does not normally occur.

Inherent in the pathophysiologic model of GERD is that gastric juice is harmful to the esophageal epithelium. However, gastric acid hypersecretion is usually not a dominant factor in the development of esophagitis. An obvious exception is with Zollinger-Ellison syndrome, which is associated with severe esophagitis in about 50% of patients. Another caveat is with chronic *Helicobacter pylori* gastritis, which may have a protective effect by inducing atrophic gastritis with concomitant hypoacidity. Pepsin, bile, and pancreatic enzymes within gastric secretions can also injure the esophageal epithelium, but their noxious properties are either lessened without an acidic environment or dependent on acidity for activation. Bile warrants attention because it persists in refluxate despite acid-suppressing medications. Bile can transverse the cell membrane, imparting severe cellular injury in a weakly acidic environment, and has also been invoked as a cofactor in the pathogenesis of Barrett's metaplasia and adenocarcinoma. Hence, the causticity of gastric refluxate extends beyond hydrochloric acid.

SYMPTOMS

Heartburn and regurgitation are the typical symptoms of GERD. Somewhat less common are dysphagia and chest pain. In each case, multiple potential mechanisms for symptom genesis operate that extend beyond the basic concepts of mucosal erosion and activation of afferent sensory nerves. Specifically, hypersensitivity and functional pain are increasingly recognized as cofactors. Nonetheless, the dominant clinical strategy is empirical treatment with acid inhibitors, reserving further evaluation for those who fail to respond. Important exceptions to this are patients with chest pain or persistent dysphagia, each of which may be indicative of more morbid conditions. With chest pain, cardiac disease must be carefully considered. In the case of persistent dysphagia, chronic reflux can lead to the development of a peptic stricture or adenocarcinoma, each of which benefits from early detection and/or specific therapy.

Extraesophageal syndromes with an established association to GERD include chronic cough, laryngitis, asthma, and dental erosions. A multitude of other conditions including pharyngitis, chronic bronchitis, pulmonary fibrosis, chronic sinusitis, cardiac arrhythmias, sleep apnea, and recurrent aspiration pneumonia have proposed associations with GERD. However, in both cases, it is important to emphasize the word *association* as opposed to *causation*. In many instances, the disorders likely coexist because of shared pathogenetic mechanisms rather than strict causality. Potential mechanisms for extraesophageal GERD manifestations are either regurgitation with direct contact between the refluxate and supraesophageal structures or via a vagovagal reflex wherein reflux activation of esophageal afferent nerves triggers efferent vagal reflexes such as bronchospasm, cough, or arrhythmias.

DIFFERENTIAL DIAGNOSIS

Although generally quite characteristic, symptoms from GERD need to be distinguished from symptoms related to infectious, pill, or eosinophilic esophagitis, peptic ulcer disease, dyspepsia, biliary colic, coronary artery disease, and esophageal motility disorders. It is especially important that coronary artery disease be given early consideration because of its potentially lethal implications. The remaining elements of the differential diagnosis can be addressed by endoscopy, upper gastrointestinal series, or biliary tract ultrasonography as appropriate. The distinction among etiologies of esophagitis is usually easily made by endoscopy with mucosal biopsies, which are necessary to evaluate for infection or eosinophilic inflammation. In terms of endoscopic appearance, infectious esophagitis is diffuse and tends to involve the proximal esophagus far more frequently than does reflux esophagitis. The ulcerations seen in peptic esophagitis are usually solitary and distal, whereas infectious ulcerations are punctate and diffuse. Eosinophilic esophagitis characteristically exhibits multiple esophageal rings, linear furrows, or white punctate exudate. Esophageal ulcerations from pill esophagitis are usually singular and deep at points of luminal narrowing, especially near the carina, with sparing of the distal esophagus.

COMPLICATIONS

The complications of GERD are related to chronic esophagitis (bleeding and stricture) and the relationship between GERD and esophageal adenocarcinoma. However, both esophagitis and peptic strictures have become increasingly rare in the era of potent antisecretory medications. Conversely, the most severe histologic consequence of GERD is Barrett's metaplasia with the associated risk of esophageal adenocarcinoma, and the incidence of these lesions has increased, not decreased, in the era of potent acid suppression. Barrett's metaplasia, endoscopically recognized by tongues of reddish mucosa extending proximally from the gastroesophageal junction (Fig. 347-9) or histopathologically by the finding of specialized columnar metaplasia, is associated with a substantially increased risk for development of esophageal adenocarcinoma.

Barrett's metaplasia can progress to adenocarcinoma through the intermediate stages of low- and high-grade dysplasia (Fig. 347-10). Owing to this risk, areas of Barrett's and especially any included areas of mucosal irregularity should be extensively biopsied. The rate of cancer development is estimated at 0.1–0.3% per year, but vagaries in definitional criteria and of the extent of Barrett's metaplasia requisite to establish the diagnosis have contributed to variability and inconsistency in this risk assessment. The group at greatest risk is obese white males in their sixth decade of life. However, despite common practice, the utility of endoscopic screening and surveillance programs intended

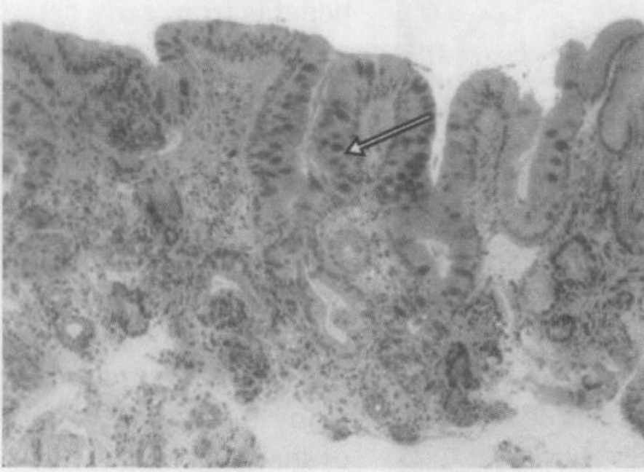

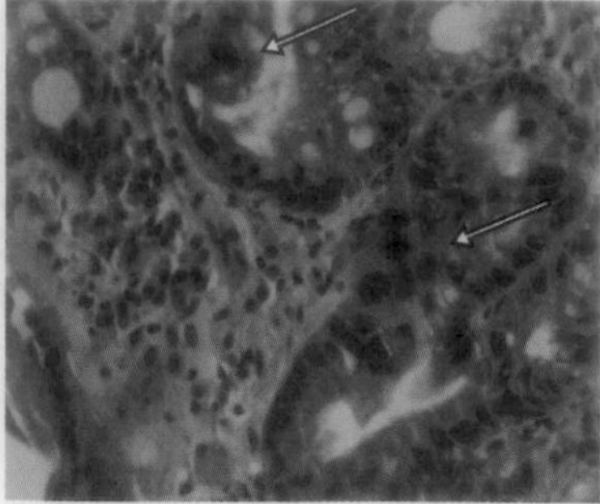

FIGURE 347-10 Histopathology of Barrett's metaplasia and Barrett's with high-grade dysplasia. H&E, hematoxylin and eosin.

to control the adenocarcinoma risk has not been established. Also of note, no high-level evidence confirms that aggressive antisecretory therapy or antireflux surgery causes regression of Barrett's esophagus or prevents adenocarcinoma.

Although the management of Barrett's esophagus remains controversial, the finding of dysplasia in Barrett's, particularly high-grade dysplasia, mandates further intervention. In addition to the high rate of progression to adenocarcinoma, there is also a high prevalence of unrecognized coexisting cancer with high-grade dysplasia. Nonetheless, treatment remains controversial. Esophagectomy, intensive endoscopic surveillance, and mucosal ablation have all been advocated. Currently, esophagectomy is the gold standard treatment for high-grade dysplasia in an otherwise healthy patient with minimal surgical risk. However, esophagectomy has a mortality ranging from 3–10%, along with substantial morbidity. That, along with increasing evidence of the effectiveness of endoscopic therapy with purpose-built radiofrequency ablation devices, has led many to favor this therapy as a preferable management strategy.

TREATMENT GASTROESOPHAGEAL REFLUX DISEASE (GERD)

Lifestyle modifications are routinely advocated as GERD therapy. Broadly speaking, these fall into three categories: (1) avoidance of foods that reduce LES pressure, making them "refluxogenic" (these commonly include fatty foods, alcohol, spearmint, peppermint, tomato-based foods, and possibly coffee and tea); (2) avoidance of acidic foods that are inherently irritating; and (3) adoption of behaviors to minimize reflux and/or heartburn. In general, minimal evidence supports the efficacy of these measures. However, clinical experience dictates that subsets of patients are benefitted by specific recommendations, based on their unique history and symptom profile. A patient with sleep disturbance from nighttime heartburn is likely to benefit from elevation of the head of the bed and avoidance of eating before retiring, but those recommendations are superfluous for a patient without nighttime symptoms. The most broadly applicable recommendation is for weight reduction. Even though the benefit with respect to reflux cannot be assured, the strong epidemiologic relationship between body mass index and GERD and the secondary health gains of weight reduction are beyond dispute.

The dominant pharmacologic approach to GERD management is with inhibitors of gastric acid secretion, and abundant data support the effectiveness of this approach. Pharmacologically reducing the acidity of gastric juice does not prevent reflux, but it ameliorates reflux symptoms and allows esophagitis to heal. The hierarchy of effectiveness among pharmaceuticals parallels their antisecretory potency. Proton pump inhibitors (PPIs) are more efficacious than histamine$_2$ receptor antagonists (H_2RAs), and both are superior to placebo. No major differences exist among PPIs, and only modest gain is achieved by increased dosage.

Paradoxically, the perceived frequency and severity of heartburn correlate poorly with the presence or severity of esophagitis. When GERD treatments are assessed in terms of resolving heartburn, both efficacy and differences among pharmaceuticals are less clear-cut than with the objective of healing esophagitis. Although the same overall hierarchy of effectiveness exists, observed efficacy rates are lower and vary widely, likely reflecting patient heterogeneity.

Reflux symptoms tend to be chronic, irrespective of esophagitis. Thus, a common management strategy is indefinite treatment with PPIs or H_2RAs as necessary for symptom control. The side effects of PPI therapy are generally minimal. Vitamin B_{12} and iron absorption may be compromised and susceptibility to enteric infections, particularly *Clostridium difficile* colitis, increased with treatment. Population studies have also suggested a slight increased risk of bone fracture with chronic PPI use suggesting an impairment of calcium absorption, but prospective studies have failed to corroborate this. Nonetheless, as with any medication, PPI dosage should be minimized to that necessary for the clinical indication.

Laparoscopic Nissen fundoplication, wherein the proximal stomach is wrapped around the distal esophagus to create an antireflux barrier, is a surgical alternative to the management of chronic GERD. Just as with PPI therapy, evidence on the utility of fundoplication is strongest for treating esophagitis, and controlled trials suggest similar efficacy to PPI therapy. However, the benefits of fundoplication must be weighed against potential deleterious effects, including surgical morbidity and mortality, postoperative dysphagia, failure or breakdown requiring reoperation, an inability to belch, and increased bloating, flatulence, and bowel symptoms after surgery.

EOSINOPHILIC ESOPHAGITIS

Eosinophilic esophagitis (EoE) is increasingly recognized in adults and children around the world. Current prevalence estimates identified 4–6 cases per 10,000 with a predilection for white males. The increasing prevalence of EoE is attributable to a combination of an increasing incidence and a growing recognition of the condition. There is also an incompletely understood, but important, overlap between EoE and GERD that confuses diagnosis of the disease.

EoE is diagnosed based on the combination of typical esophageal symptoms and esophageal mucosal biopsies demonstrating squamous epithelial eosinophil-predominant inflammation. Alternative etiologies of esophageal eosinophilia include GERD, drug hypersensitivity, connective tissue disorders, hypereosinophilic syndrome, and infection. Current evidence indicates that EoE is an immunologic disorder induced by antigen sensitization in susceptible individuals. Dietary factors play an important role in both the pathogenesis and treatment of EoE. Aeroallergens may also contribute, but the evidence is weaker. The natural history of EoE is unclear, but an increased risk of esophageal stricture development paralleling the duration of untreated disease has been noted.

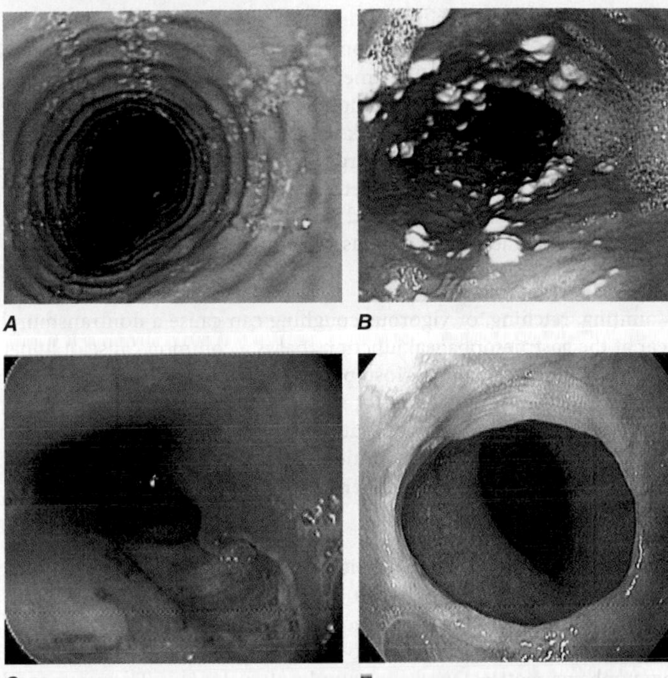

FIGURE 347-11 Endoscopic features of (*A*) eosinophilic esophagitis (EoE), (*B*) *Candida* esophagitis, (*C*) giant ulcer associated with HIV, (*D*) and a Schatzki ring.

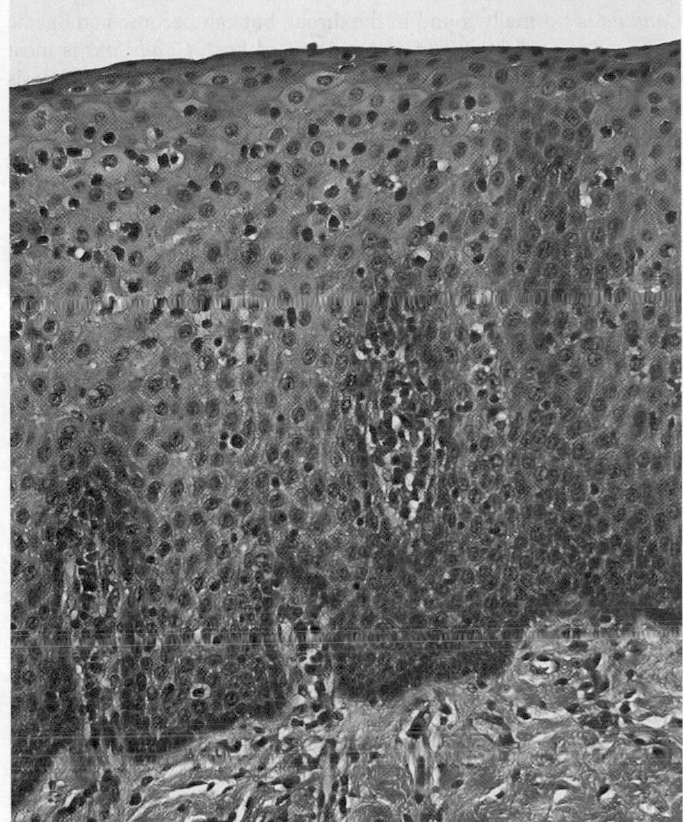

FIGURE 347-12 Histopathology of eosinophilic esophagitis (EoE) showing infiltration of the esophageal squamous epithelium with eosinophils. Additional features of basal cell hyperplasia and lamina propria fibrosis are present. Eosinophilic inflammation can also be seen with gastroesophageal reflux disease.

EoE should be strongly considered in children and adults with dysphagia and esophageal food impactions. In preadolescent children, symptom presentations of EoE include chest or abdominal pain, nausea, vomiting, and food aversion. Other symptoms in adults may include atypical chest pain and heartburn, particularly heartburn that is refractory to PPI therapy. An atopic history of food allergy, asthma, eczema, or allergic rhinitis is present in the majority of patients. Peripheral blood eosinophilia is demonstrable in up to 50% of patients, but the specificity of this finding is problematic in the setting of concomitant atopy. The characteristic endoscopic esophageal findings are loss of vascular markings (edema), multiple esophageal rings, longitudinally oriented furrows, and punctate exudate (Fig. 347-11). Histologic confirmation is made with the demonstration of esophageal mucosal eosinophilia (greatest density ±15 eosinophils per high-power field) (Fig. 347-12). Complications of EoE include esophageal stricture, narrow-caliber esophagus, food impaction, and esophageal perforation.

The goals of EoE management are symptom control and the prevention of complications. Once esophageal eosinophilia is demonstrated, patients typically undergo a trial of PPI therapy as a practical means of excluding a contribution of GERD to the esophageal mucosal inflammation. PPI-responsive esophageal eosinophilia, characterized by elimination of mucosal eosinophilia, occurs in 30–50% of cases of suspected EoE. Patients with persistent symptoms and eosinophilic inflammation following PPI therapy are subsequently considered for EoE treatments such as elimination diets or swallowed topical glucocorticoids. Elemental formula diets are a highly effective therapy that have primarily been studied in children but are limited by palatability. Notably, allergy testing by means of either serum IgE or skin prick testing has demonstrated poor sensitivity and specificity in the identification of foods that incite the esophageal inflammatory response. Allergy testing combining skin prick and atopy patch testing has been effective in children with EoE, but additional validation is needed. Empiric elimination of common food allergies (milk, wheat, egg, soy, nuts, and seafood) followed by systematic reintroduction has been an effective diet therapy in both children and adults with EoE. The intent of the elimination diet approach is the identification of a single food trigger or a small number of food triggers. Swallowed, topical glucocorticoids (fluticasone propionate or budesonide) are highly effective, but recurrence of disease is common following the cessation of therapy. Systemic glucocorticoids are reserved for severely afflicted patients refractory to less morbid treatments. Esophageal dilation is very effective at relieving dysphagia in patients with fibrostenosis. Dilation should be approached conservatively because of the risk of deep, esophageal mural laceration or perforation in the stiff-walled esophagus that is characteristic of the disease.

INFECTIOUS ESOPHAGITIS

With the increased use of immunosuppression for organ transplantation as well as chronic inflammatory diseases and chemotherapy along with the AIDS epidemic, infections with *Candida* species, herpesvirus, and cytomegalovirus (CMV) have become relatively common. Although rare, infectious esophagitis also occurs among the nonimmunocompromised, with herpes simplex and *Candida albicans* being the most common pathogens. Among AIDS patients, infectious esophagitis becomes more common as the CD4 count declines; cases are rare with a CD4 count >200 and common when <100. HIV itself may also be associated with a self-limited syndrome of acute esophageal ulceration with oral ulcers and a maculopapular skin rash at the time of seroconversion. Additionally, some patients with advanced disease have deep, persistent esophageal ulcers treated with oral glucocorticoids or thalidomide. However, with the widespread use of protease inhibitors, a reduction in these HIV complications has been noted.

Regardless of the infectious agent, odynophagia is a characteristic symptom of infectious esophagitis; dysphagia, chest pain, and hemorrhage are also common. Odynophagia is uncommon with reflux esophagitis, so its presence should always raise suspicion of an alternative etiology.

CANDIDA ESOPHAGITIS

Candida is normally found in the throat, but can become pathogenic and produce esophagitis in a compromised host; *C. albicans* is most common. *Candida* esophagitis also occurs with esophageal stasis secondary to esophageal motor disorders and diverticula. Patients complain of odynophagia and dysphagia. If oral thrush is present, empirical therapy is appropriate, but co-infection is common, and persistent symptoms should lead to prompt endoscopy with biopsy, which is the most useful diagnostic evaluation. *Candida* esophagitis has a characteristic appearance of white plaques with friability. Rarely, *Candida* esophagitis is complicated by bleeding, perforation, stricture, or systemic invasion. Oral fluconazole (200–400 mg on the first day, followed by 100–200 mg daily) for 14–21 days is the preferred treatment. Patients refractory to fluconazole may respond to itraconazole, voriconazole, or posaconazole. Alternatively, poorly responsive patients or those who cannot swallow medications can be treated with an intravenous echinocandin (caspofungin 50 mg daily for 7–21 days).

HERPETIC ESOPHAGITIS

Herpes simplex virus type 1 or 2 may cause esophagitis. Vesicles on the nose and lips may coexist and are suggestive of a herpetic etiology. Varicella-zoster virus can also cause esophagitis in children with chickenpox or adults with zoster. The characteristic endoscopic findings are vesicles and small, punched-out ulcerations. Because herpes simplex infections are limited to squamous epithelium, biopsies from the ulcer margins are most likely to reveal the characteristic ground-glass nuclei, eosinophilic Cowdry's type A inclusion bodies, and giant cells. Culture or polymerase chain reaction (PCR) assays are helpful to identify acyclovir-resistant strains. Acyclovir (200 mg orally five times a day for 7–10 days) can be used for immunocompetent hosts, although the disease is typically self-limited after a 1- to 2-week period in such patients. Immunocompromised patients are treated with acyclovir (400 mg orally five times a day for 14–21 days), famciclovir (500 mg orally three times a day), or valacyclovir (1 g orally three times a day). In patients with severe odynophagia, intravenous acyclovir, 5 mg/kg every 8 h for 7–14 days, reduces this morbidity.

CYTOMEGALOVIRUS

CMV esophagitis occurs primarily in immunocompromised patients, particularly organ transplant recipients. CMV is usually activated from a latent stage. Endoscopically, CMV lesions appear as serpiginous ulcers in an otherwise normal mucosa, particularly in the distal esophagus. Biopsies from the ulcer bases have the greatest diagnostic yield for finding the pathognomonic large nuclear or cytoplasmic inclusion bodies. Immunohistology with monoclonal antibodies to CMV and in situ hybridization tests are useful for early diagnosis. Data on therapy for CMV esophagitis are limited. Treatment studies of CMV gastrointestinal disease have demonstrated effectiveness of both ganciclovir (5 mg/kg every 12 h intravenously) and foscarnet (90 mg/kg every 12 h intravenously). Valganciclovir (900 mg two times a day), an oral formulation of ganciclovir, can also be used. Therapy is continued until healing, which may take 3–6 weeks. Maintenance therapy may be needed for patients with relapsing disease.

MECHANICAL TRAUMA AND IATROGENIC INJURY

ESOPHAGEAL PERFORATION

Most cases of esophageal perforation are from instrumentation of the esophagus or trauma. Alternatively, forceful vomiting or retching can lead to spontaneous rupture at the gastroesophageal junction (Boerhaave's syndrome). More rarely, corrosive esophagitis or neoplasms lead to perforation. Instrument perforation from endoscopy or nasogastric tube placement typically occurs in the hypopharynx or at the gastroesophageal junction. Perforation may also occur at the site of a stricture in the setting of endoscopic food disimpaction or esophageal dilation. Esophageal perforation causes pleuritic retrosternal pain that can be associated with pneumomediastinum and subcutaneous emphysema. Mediastinitis is a major complication of esophageal perforation, and prompt recognition is key to optimizing outcome. CT of the chest is most sensitive in detecting mediastinal air. Esophageal perforation is confirmed by a contrast swallow, usually Gastrografin followed by thin barium. Treatment includes nasogastric suction and parenteral broad-spectrum antibiotics with prompt surgical drainage and repair in noncontained leaks. Conservative therapy with NPO status and antibiotics without surgery may be appropriate in cases of contained perforation that are detected early. Endoscopic clipping or stent placement may be indicated in nonoperated iatrogenic perforations or nonoperable cases such as perforated tumors.

MALLORY-WEISS TEAR

Vomiting, retching, or vigorous coughing can cause a nontransmural tear at the gastroesophageal junction that is a common cause of upper gastrointestinal bleeding. Most patients present with hematemesis. Antecedent vomiting is anticipated but not always evident. Bleeding usually abates spontaneously, but protracted bleeding may respond to local epinephrine or cauterization therapy, endoscopic clipping, or angiographic embolization. Surgery is rarely needed.

RADIATION ESOPHAGITIS

Radiation esophagitis can complicate treatment for thoracic cancers, especially breast and lung, with the risk proportional to radiation dosage. Radiosensitizing drugs such as doxorubicin, bleomycin, cyclophosphamide, and cisplatin also increase the risk. Dysphagia and odynophagia may last weeks to months after therapy. The esophageal mucosa becomes erythematous, edematous, and friable. Submucosal fibrosis and degenerative tissue changes and stricturing may occur years after the radiation exposure. Radiation exposure in excess of 5000 cGy has been associated with increased risk of esophageal stricture. Treatment for acute radiation esophagitis is supportive. Chronic strictures are managed with esophageal dilation.

CORROSIVE ESOPHAGITIS

Caustic esophageal injury from ingestion of alkali or, less commonly, acid can be accidental or from attempted suicide. Absence of oral injury does not exclude possible esophageal involvement. Thus, early endoscopic evaluation is recommended to assess and grade the injury to the esophageal mucosa. Severe corrosive injury may lead to esophageal perforation, bleeding, stricture, and death. Glucocorticoids have not been shown to improve the clinical outcome of acute corrosive esophagitis and are not recommended. Healing of more severe grades of caustic injury is commonly associated with severe stricture formation and often requires repeated dilatation.

PILL ESOPHAGITIS

Pill-induced esophagitis occurs when a swallowed pill fails to traverses the entire esophagus and lodges within the lumen. Generally, this is attributed to poor "pill taking habits": inadequate liquid with the pill or lying down immediately after taking a pill. The most common location for the pill to lodge is in the mid-esophagus near the crossing of the aorta or carina. Extrinsic compression from these structures halts the movement of the pill or capsule. Since initially reported in 1970, more than 1000 cases of pill esophagitis have been reported, suggesting that this is not an unusual occurrence. A wide variety of medications are implicated with the most common being doxycycline, tetracycline, quinidine, phenytoin, potassium chloride, ferrous sulfate, nonsteroidal anti-inflammatory drugs (NSAIDs), and bisphosphonates. However, virtually any pill can result in pill esophagitis if taken carelessly.

Typical symptoms of pill esophagitis are the sudden onset of chest pain and odynophagia. Characteristically, the pain will develop over a period of hours or will awaken the individual from sleep. A classic history in the setting of ingestion of recognized pill offenders obviates the need for diagnostic testing in most patients. When endoscopy is performed, localized ulceration or inflammation is evident. Histologically, acute inflammation is typical. Chest CT imaging will sometimes reveal esophageal thickening consistent with transmural inflammation. Although the condition usually resolves within days to weeks, symptoms may persist for months and stricture can develop in severe cases. No specific therapy is known to hasten the healing process, but antisecretory medications are frequently prescribed to remove concomitant reflux as an aggravating factor. When healing results in stricture formation, dilation is indicated.

FOREIGN BODIES AND FOOD IMPACTION

Food or foreign bodies may lodge in the esophagus causing complete obstruction, which in turn can cause an inability to handle secretions (foaming at the mouth) and severe chest pain. Food impaction may occur due to stricture, carcinoma, Schatzki ring, eosinophilic esophagitis, or simply inattentive eating. If it does not spontaneously resolve, impacted food can be dislodged endoscopically. Use of meat tenderizer enzymes to facilitate passage of a meat bolus is discouraged because of potential esophageal injury. Glucagon (1 mg IV) is sometimes tried before endoscopic dislodgement. After emergent treatment, patients should be evaluated for potential causes of the impaction with treatment rendered as indicated.

ESOPHAGEAL MANIFESTATIONS OF SYSTEMIC DISEASE

SCLERODERMA AND COLLAGEN VASCULAR DISEASES

Scleroderma esophagus (hypotensive LES and absent esophageal peristalsis) was initially described as a manifestation of scleroderma or other collagen vascular diseases and thought to be specific for these disorders. However, this nomenclature subsequently proved unfortunate and has been discarded because an estimated half of qualifying patients do not have an identifiable systemic disease, and reflux disease is often the only identifiable association. When scleroderma esophagus occurs as a manifestation of a collagen vascular disease, the histopathologic findings are of infiltration and destruction of the esophageal muscularis propria with collagen deposition and fibrosis. The pathogenesis of absent peristalsis and LES hypotension in the absence of a collagen vascular disease is unknown. Regardless of the underlying cause, the manometric abnormalities predispose patients to severe GERD due to inadequate LES barrier function combined with poor esophageal clearance of refluxed acid. Dysphagia may also be manifest but is generally mild and alleviated by eating in an upright position and using liquids to facilitate solid emptying.

DERMATOLOGIC DISEASES

A host of dermatologic disorders (pemphigus vulgaris, bullous pemphigoid, cicatricial pemphigoid, Behçet's syndrome, and epidermolysis bullosa) can affect the oropharynx and esophagus, particularly the proximal esophagus with blisters, bullae, webs, and strictures. Glucocorticoid treatment is usually effective. Erosive lichen planus, Stevens-Johnson syndrome, and graft-versus-host disease can also involve the esophagus. Esophageal dilatation may be necessary to treat strictures.

348 Peptic Ulcer Disease and Related Disorders

John Del Valle

PEPTIC ULCER DISEASE

Burning epigastric pain exacerbated by fasting and improved with meals is a symptom complex associated with peptic ulcer disease (PUD). An *ulcer* is defined as disruption of the mucosal integrity of the stomach and/or duodenum leading to a local defect or excavation due to active inflammation. Ulcers occur within the stomach and/or duodenum and are often chronic in nature. Acid peptic disorders are very common in the United States, with 4 million individuals (new cases and recurrences) affected per year. Lifetime prevalence of PUD in the United States is ~12% in men and 10% in women. PUD significantly affects quality of life by impairing overall patient well-being and contributing substantially to work absenteeism. Moreover, an estimated 15,000 deaths per year occur as a consequence of complicated PUD. The financial impact of these common disorders has been substantial, with an estimated burden on direct and indirect health care costs of ~$6 billion per year in the United States, with $3 billion spent on hospitalizations, $2 billion on physician office visits, and $1 billion in decreased productivity and days lost from work.

GASTRIC PHYSIOLOGY

Despite the constant attack on the gastroduodenal mucosa by a host of noxious agents (acid, pepsin, bile acids, pancreatic enzymes, drugs, and bacteria), integrity is maintained by an intricate system that provides mucosal defense and repair.

Gastric Anatomy The gastric epithelial lining consists of rugae that contain microscopic gastric pits, each branching into four or five gastric glands made up of highly specialized epithelial cells. The makeup of gastric glands varies with their anatomic location. Glands within the gastric cardia comprise <5% of the gastric gland area and contain mucous and endocrine cells. The 75% of gastric glands are found within the oxyntic mucosa and contain mucous neck, parietal, chief, endocrine, enterochromaffin, and enterochromaffin-like (ECL) cells (Fig. 348-1). Pyloric glands contain mucous and endocrine cells (including gastrin cells) and are found in the antrum.

The parietal cell, also known as the oxyntic cell, is usually found in the neck, or isthmus, or in the oxyntic gland. The resting, or unstimulated, parietal cell has prominent cytoplasmic tubulovesicles and intracellular canaliculi containing short microvilli along its apical surface (Fig. 348-2). H^+,K^+-adenosine triphosphatase (ATPase) is expressed in the tubulovesicle membrane; upon cell stimulation, this membrane, along with apical membranes, transforms into a dense network of apical intracellular canaliculi containing long microvilli. Acid secretion, a

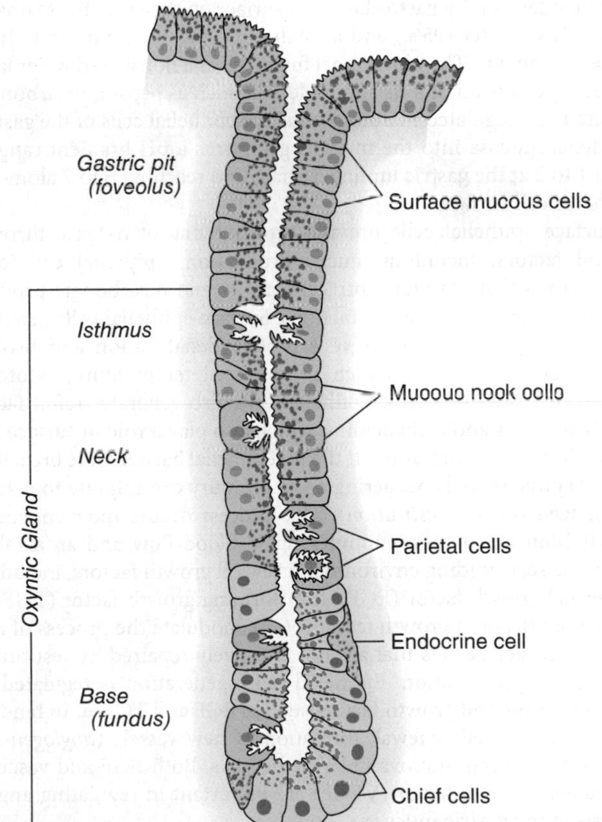

FIGURE 348-1 Diagrammatic representation of the oxyntic gastric gland. *(Adapted from S Ito, RJ Winchester: J Cell Biol 16:541, 1963. doi:10.1083/jcb.16.3.541. © 1963 Ito and Winchester.)*

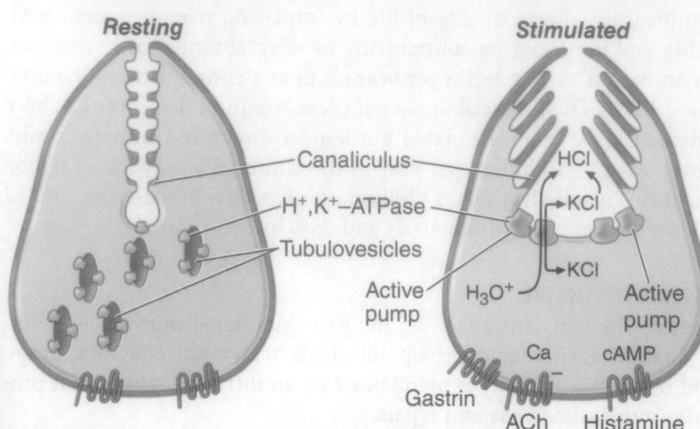

FIGURE 348-2 Gastric parietal cell undergoing transformation after secretagogue-mediated stimulation. cAMP, cyclic adenosine monophosphate. *(Adapted from SJ Hersey, G Sachs: Physiol Rev 75:155, 1995.)*

process requiring high energy, occurs at the apical canalicular surface. Numerous mitochondria (30–40% of total cell volume) generate the energy required for secretion.

Gastroduodenal Mucosal Defense The gastric epithelium is under constant assault by a series of endogenous noxious factors, including hydrochloric acid (HCl), pepsinogen/pepsin, and bile salts. In addition, a steady flow of exogenous substances such as medications, alcohol, and bacteria encounter the gastric mucosa. A highly intricate biologic system is in place to provide defense from mucosal injury and to repair any injury that may occur.

The mucosal defense system can be envisioned as a three-level barrier, composed of preepithelial, epithelial, and subepithelial elements (Fig. 348-3). The first line of defense is a mucus-bicarbonate-phospholipid layer, which serves as a physicochemical barrier to multiple molecules, including hydrogen ions. Mucus is secreted in a regulated fashion by gastroduodenal surface epithelial cells. It consists primarily of water (95%) and a mixture of phospholipids and glycoproteins (mucin). The mucous gel functions as a nonstirred water layer impeding diffusion of ions and molecules such as pepsin. Bicarbonate, secreted in a regulated manner by surface epithelial cells of the gastroduodenal mucosa into the mucous gel, forms a pH gradient ranging from 1 to 2 at the gastric luminal surface and reaching 6 to 7 along the epithelial cell surface.

Surface epithelial cells provide the next line of defense through several factors, including mucus production, epithelial cell ionic transporters that maintain intracellular pH and bicarbonate production, and intracellular tight junctions. Surface epithelial cells generate heat shock proteins that prevent protein denaturation and protect cells from certain factors such as increased temperature, cytotoxic agents, or oxidative stress. Epithelial cells also generate trefoil factor family peptides and cathelicidins, which also play a role in surface cell protection and regeneration. If the preepithelial barrier were breached, gastric epithelial cells bordering a site of injury can migrate to restore a damaged region (*restitution*). This process occurs independent of cell division and requires uninterrupted blood flow and an alkaline pH in the surrounding environment. Several growth factors, including epidermal growth factor (EGF), transforming growth factor (TGF) α, and basic fibroblast growth factor (FGF), modulate the process of restitution. Larger defects that are not effectively repaired by restitution require cell proliferation. Epithelial cell regeneration is regulated by prostaglandins and growth factors such as EGF and TGF-α. In tandem with epithelial cell renewal, formation of new vessels (*angiogenesis*) within the injured microvascular bed occurs. Both FGF and vascular endothelial growth factor (VEGF) are important in regulating angiogenesis in the gastric mucosa.

An elaborate microvascular system within the gastric submucosal layer is the key component of the subepithelial defense/repair system, providing HCO_3^-, which neutralizes the acid generated by the parietal cell. Moreover, this microcirculatory bed provides an adequate supply of micronutrients and oxygen while removing toxic metabolic by-products.

Prostaglandins play a central role in gastric epithelial defense/repair (Fig. 348-4). The gastric mucosa contains abundant levels of prostaglandins that regulate the release of mucosal bicarbonate and mucus, inhibit parietal cell secretion, and are important in maintaining mucosal blood flow and epithelial cell restitution. Prostaglandins are derived from esterified arachidonic acid, which is formed from phospholipids (cell membrane) by the action of phospholipase A_2. A key enzyme that controls the rate-limiting step in prostaglandin synthesis is cyclooxygenase (COX), which is present in two isoforms (COX-1, COX-2), each having distinct characteristics regarding structure, tissue distribution, and expression. COX-1 is expressed in a host of tissues, including the stomach, platelets, kidneys, and endothelial cells. This isoform is expressed in a constitutive manner and plays an important role in maintaining the integrity of renal function, platelet aggregation, and gastrointestinal (GI) mucosal integrity. In contrast, the expression of COX-2 is inducible by inflammatory stimuli, and it is expressed in macrophages, leukocytes, fibroblasts, and synovial cells. The beneficial effects of nonsteroidal anti-inflammatory drugs (NSAIDs) on tissue inflammation are due to inhibition of COX-2; the toxicity of these drugs (e.g., GI mucosal ulceration and renal dysfunction) is related to inhibition of the COX-1 isoform. The highly COX-2–selective NSAIDs have the potential to provide the beneficial effect of decreasing tissue inflammation while minimizing toxicity in the GI tract. Selective COX-2 inhibitors have had adverse effects on the cardiovascular system, leading to increased risk of myocardial infarction. Therefore, the U.S. Food and Drug Administration (FDA) has removed two of these agents (valdecoxib and rofecoxib) from the market (see below).

Nitric oxide (NO) is important in the maintenance of gastric mucosal integrity. The key enzyme NO synthase is constitutively expressed in the mucosa and contributes to cytoprotection by stimulating gastric mucus, increasing mucosal blood flow, and maintaining epithelial cell barrier function. The central nervous system (CNS) and hormonal factors also play a role in regulating mucosal defense through multiple pathways (Fig. 348-3).

Physiology of Gastric Secretion Hydrochloric acid and pepsinogen are the two principal gastric secretory products capable of inducing mucosal injury. Gastric acid and pepsinogen play a physiologic role in protein digestion; absorption of iron, calcium, magnesium, and vitamin B_{12}; and killing ingested bacteria. Acid secretion should be viewed as occurring under basal and stimulated conditions. Basal acid production occurs in a circadian pattern, with highest levels occurring during the night and lowest levels during the morning hours. Cholinergic input via the vagus nerve and histaminergic input from local gastric sources are the principal contributors to basal acid secretion. Stimulated gastric acid secretion occurs primarily in three phases based on the site where the signal originates (cephalic, gastric, and intestinal). Sight, smell, and taste of food are the components of the cephalic phase, which stimulates gastric secretion via the vagus nerve. The gastric phase is activated once food enters the stomach. This component of secretion is driven by nutrients (amino acids and amines) that directly stimulate the G cell to release gastrin, which in turn activates the parietal cell via direct and indirect mechanisms. Distention of the stomach wall also leads to gastrin release and acid production. The last phase of gastric acid secretion is initiated as food enters the intestine and is mediated by luminal distention and nutrient assimilation. A series of pathways that inhibit gastric acid production are also set into motion during these phases. The GI hormone somatostatin is released from endocrine cells found in the gastric mucosa (D cells) in response to HCl. Somatostatin can inhibit acid production by both direct (parietal cell) and indirect mechanisms (decreased histamine release from ECL cells and gastrin release from G cells). Additional neural (central and peripheral) and humoral (amylin, atrial natriuretic peptide [ANP], cholecystokinin, ghrelin, interleukin 11 [IL-11], obestatin, secretin, and serotonin) factors play a role in counterbalancing acid secretion. Under physiologic circumstances, these phases occur simultaneously. Ghrelin, the appetite-regulating hormone expressed in Gr cells in the

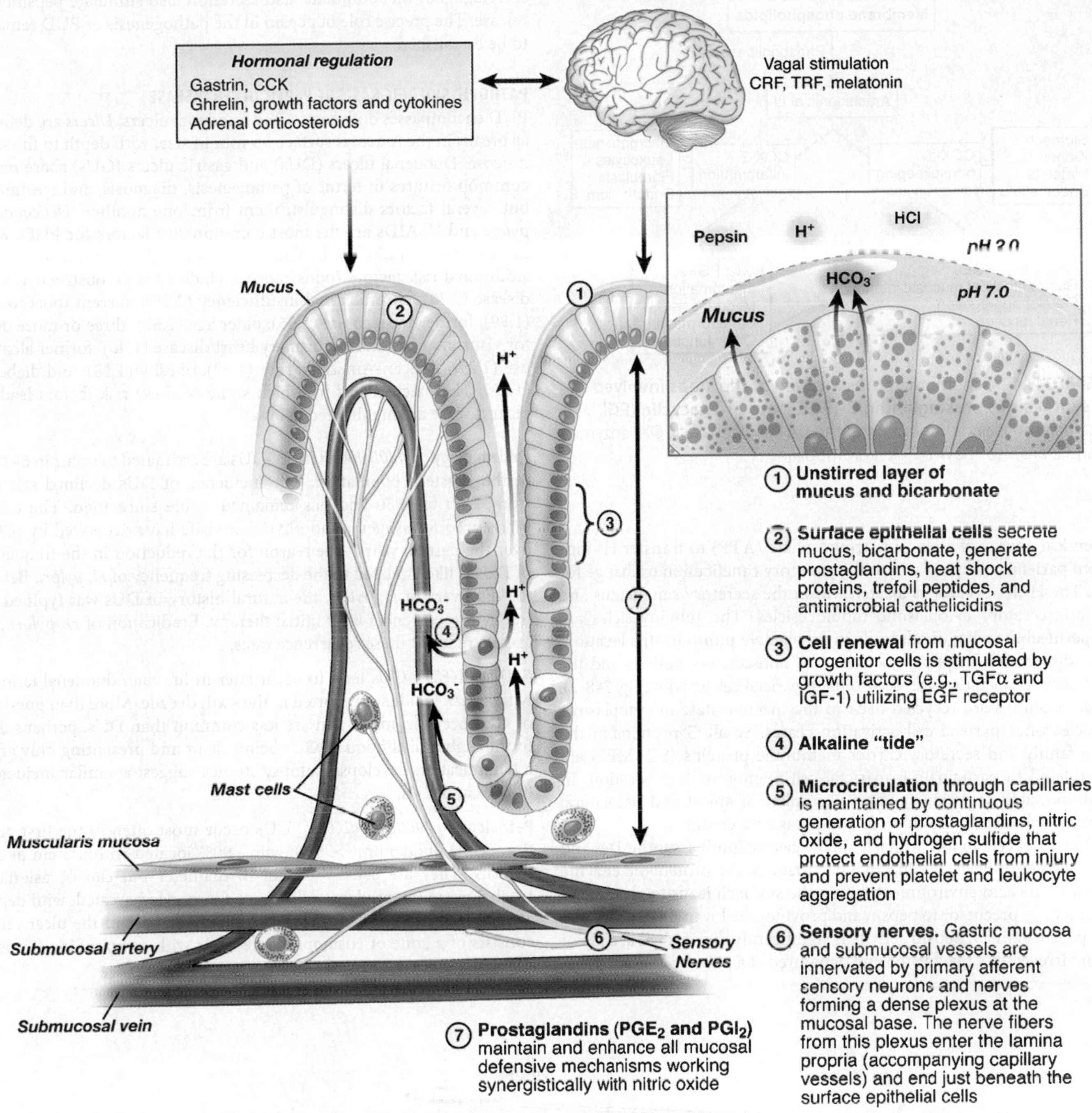

CNS
Hormonal regulation
Gastrin, CCK
Ghrelin, growth factors and cytokines
Adrenal corticosteroids
Vagal stimulation
CRF, TRF, melatonin
Pepsin
H+
HCl
pH 2.0
HCO3-
pH 7.0
Mucus
Mucus
H+
HCO3-
H+
H+
HCO3-
Mast cells
Muscularis mucosa
Submucosal artery
Submucosal vein
Sensory Nerves
1 Unstirred layer of mucus and bicarbonate
2 Surface epithelial cells secrete mucus, bicarbonate, generate prostaglandins, heat shock proteins, trefoil peptides, and antimicrobial cathelicidins
3 Cell renewal from mucosal progenitor cells is stimulated by growth factors (e.g., TGFα and IGF-1) utilizing EGF receptor
4 Alkaline "tide"
5 Microcirculation through capillaries is maintained by continuous generation of prostaglandins, nitric oxide, and hydrogen sulfide that protect endothelial cells from injury and prevent platelet and leukocyte aggregation
6 Sensory nerves. Gastric mucosa and submucosal vessels are innervated by primary afferent sensory neurons and nerves forming a dense plexus at the mucosal base. The nerve fibers from this plexus enter the lamina propria (accompanying capillary vessels) and end just beneath the surface epithelial cells
7 Prostaglandins (PGE2 and PGI2) maintain and enhance all mucosal defensive mechanisms working synergistically with nitric oxide

FIGURE 348-3 Components involved in providing gastroduodenal mucosal defense and repair. CCK, cholecystokinin; CRF, corticotropin-releasing factor; EGF, epidermal growth factor; HCl, hydrochloride; IGF, insulin-like growth factor; TGFα, transforming growth factor α; TRF, thyrotropin releasing factor. *(Modified and updated from Tarnawski A. Cellular and molecular mechanisms of mucosal defense and repair. In: Yoshikawa T, Arakawa T. Bioregulation and Its Disorders in the Gastrointestinal Tract. Tokyo, Japan: Blackwell Science, 1998:3–17.)*

stomach, may increase gastric acid secretion through stimulation of histamine release from ECL cells, but this remains to be confirmed.

The acid-secreting parietal cell is located in the oxyntic gland, adjacent to other cellular elements (ECL cell, D cell) important in the gastric secretory process (Fig. 348-5). This unique cell also secretes intrinsic factor (IF) and IL-11. The parietal cell expresses receptors for several stimulants of acid secretion, including histamine (H_2), gastrin (cholecystokinin B/gastrin receptor), and acetylcholine (muscarinic, M_3). Binding of histamine to the H_2 receptor leads to activation of adenylate cyclase and an increase in cyclic adenosine monophosphate (AMP). Activation of the gastrin and muscarinic receptors results in activation of the protein kinase C/phosphoinositide signaling pathway. Each of these signaling pathways in turn regulates a series of downstream kinase cascades that control the acid-secreting pump, H^+,K^+-ATPase. The discovery that different ligands and their corresponding receptors lead to activation of different signaling pathways explains the potentiation of acid secretion that occurs when histamine and gastrin or acetylcholine are combined. More importantly, this observation explains why blocking one receptor type (H_2) decreases acid secretion stimulated by agents that activate a different pathway (gastrin, acetylcholine). Parietal cells also express receptors for ligands that inhibit acid production (prostaglandins, somatostatin, and EGF). Histamine also stimulates gastric acid secretion indirectly by activating the histamine H_3 receptor on D-cells, which inhibits somatostatin release.

The enzyme H^+,K^+-ATPase is responsible for generating the large concentration of H^+. It is a membrane-bound protein that consists of two subunits, α and β. The active catalytic site is found within the α subunit; the function of the β subunit is unclear. This enzyme uses the

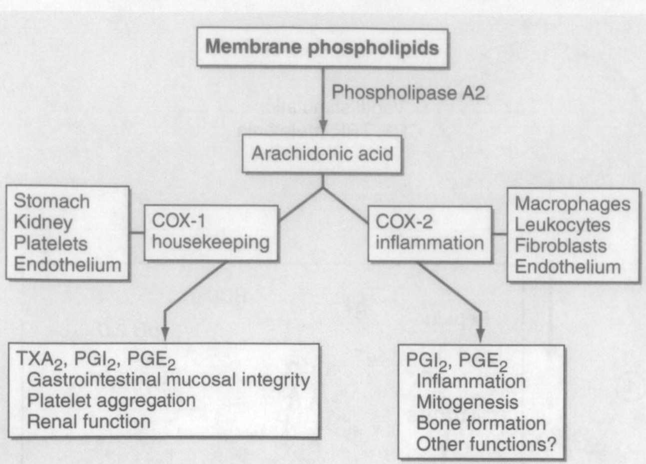

FIGURE 348-4 Schematic representation of the steps involved in synthesis of prostaglandin E_2 (PGE_2) and prostacyclin (PGI_2). Characteristics and distribution of the cyclooxygenase (COX) enzymes 1 and 2 are also shown. TXA_2, thromboxane A_2.

chemical energy of adenosine triphosphate (ATP) to transfer H^+ ions from parietal cell cytoplasm to the secretory canaliculi in exchange for K^+. The H^+,K^+-ATPase is located within the secretory canaliculus and in nonsecretory cytoplasmic tubulovesicles. The tubulovesicles are impermeable to K^+, which leads to an inactive pump in this location. The distribution of pumps between the nonsecretory vesicles and the secretory canaliculus varies according to parietal cell activity (Fig. 348-2). Proton pumps are recycled back to the inactive state in cytoplasmic vesicles once parietal cell activation ceases. Small G proteins of the Rab family and secretory carrier membrane proteins (SCAMPS) are postulated to participate in parietal cell membrane translocation. In addition, acid secretion requires a number of apical and basolateral parietal cell membrane chloride and potassium channels.

The chief cell, found primarily in the gastric fundus, synthesizes and secretes pepsinogen, the inactive precursor of the proteolytic enzyme pepsin. The acid environment within the stomach leads to cleavage of the inactive precursor to pepsin and provides the low pH (<2) required for pepsin activity. Pepsin activity is significantly diminished at a pH of 4 and irreversibly inactivated and denatured at a pH of ≥7. Many of the secretagogues that stimulate acid secretion also stimulate pepsinogen release. The precise role of pepsin in the pathogenesis of PUD remains to be established.

PATHOPHYSIOLOGIC BASIS OF PEPTIC ULCER DISEASE

PUD encompasses both gastric and duodenal ulcers. *Ulcers* are defined as breaks in the mucosal surface >5 mm in size, with depth to the submucosa. Duodenal ulcers (DUs) and gastric ulcers (GUs) share many common features in terms of pathogenesis, diagnosis, and treatment, but several factors distinguish them from one another. *Helicobacter pylori* and NSAIDs are the most common risk factors for PUD, with estimated odds ratios in the United States of 3.7 and 3.3, respectively. Additional risk factors (odds ratio) include chronic obstructive lung disease (2.34), chronic renal insufficiency (2.29), current tobacco use (1.99), former tobacco use (1.55), older age (1.67), three or more doctor visits in a year (1.49), coronary heart disease (1.46), former alcohol use (1.29), African-American race (1.20), obesity (1.18), and diabetes (1.13). The mechanisms by which some of these risk factors lead to ulcer disease are highlighted below.

Epidemiology • ***DUODENAL ULCERS*** DUs are estimated to occur in 6–15% of the Western population. The incidence of DUs declined steadily from 1960 to 1980 and has remained stable since then. The death rates, need for surgery, and physician visits have decreased by >50% over the past 30 years. The reason for the reduction in the frequency of DUs is likely related to the decreasing frequency of *H. pylori*. Before the discovery of *H. pylori*, the natural history of DUs was typified by frequent recurrences after initial therapy. Eradication of *H. pylori* has greatly reduced these recurrence rates.

GASTRIC ULCERS GUs tend to occur later in life than duodenal lesions, with a peak incidence reported in the sixth decade. More than one-half of GUs occur in males and are less common than DUs, perhaps due to the higher likelihood of GUs being silent and presenting only after a complication develops. Autopsy studies suggest a similar incidence of DUs and GUs.

Pathology • ***DUODENAL ULCERS*** DUs occur most often in the first portion of the duodenum (>95%), with ~90% located within 3 cm of the pylorus. They are usually ≤1 cm in diameter but can occasionally reach 3–6 cm (giant ulcer). Ulcers are sharply demarcated, with depth at times reaching the muscularis propria. The base of the ulcer often consists of a zone of eosinophilic necrosis with surrounding fibrosis. Malignant DUs are extremely rare.

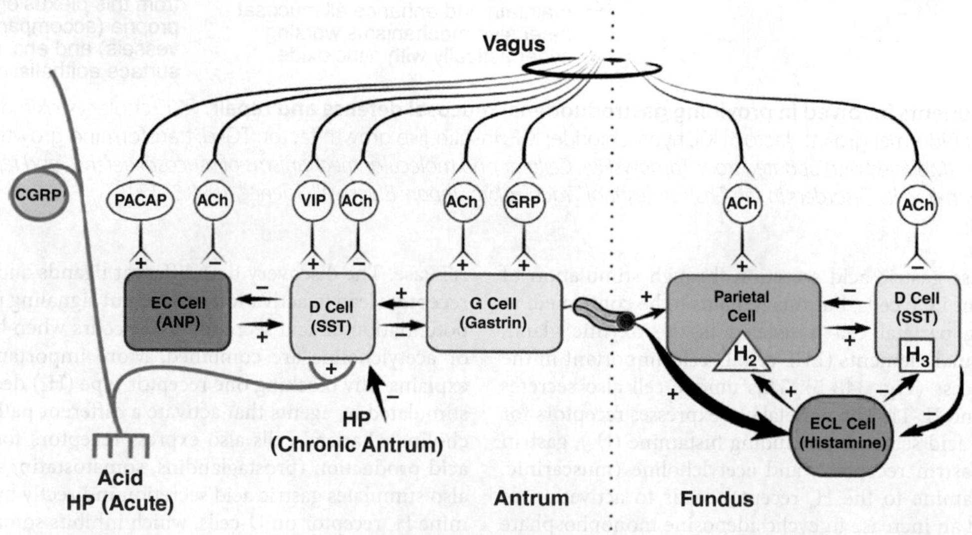

FIGURE 348-5 Regulation of gastric acid secretion at the cellular level. ACh, acetylcholine; ANP, atrial natriuretic peptide; CGRP, calcitonin gene-related peptide; EC, enterochromaffin; ECL, enterochromaffin-like; GRP, gastrin-releasing peptide; PACAP, pituitary adenylate-cyclase activating peptide; SST, somatostatin; VIP, vasoactive intestinal peptide.

GASTRIC ULCERS In contrast to DUs, GUs can represent a malignancy and should be biopsied upon discovery. Benign GUs are most often found distal to the junction between the antrum and the acid secretory mucosa. Benign GUs are quite rare in the gastric fundus and are histologically similar to DUs. Benign GUs associated with *H. pylori* are also associated with antral gastritis. In contrast, NSAID-related GUs are not accompanied by chronic active gastritis but may instead have evidence of a chemical gastropathy, typified by foveolar hyperplasia, edema of the lamina propria, and epithelial regeneration in the absence of *H. pylori*. Extension of smooth-muscle fibers into the upper portions of the mucosa, where they are not typically found, may also occur.

Pathophysiology • *DUODENAL ULCERS* *H. pylori* and NSAID-induced injury account for the majority of DUs. Many acid secretory abnormalities have been described in DU patients. Of these, average basal and nocturnal gastric acid secretion appears to be increased in DU patients as compared to controls; however, the level of overlap between DU patients and control subjects is substantial. The reason for this altered secretory process is unclear, but *H. pylori* infection may contribute. Bicarbonate secretion is significantly decreased in the duodenal bulb of patients with an active DU as compared to control subjects. *H. pylori* infection may also play a role in this process (see below).

GASTRIC ULCERS As in DUs, the majority of GUs can be attributed to either *H. pylori* or NSAID-induced mucosal damage. GUs that occur in the prepyloric area or those in the body associated with a DU or a duodenal scar are similar in pathogenesis to DUs. Gastric acid output (basal and stimulated) tends to be normal or decreased in GU patients. When GUs develop in the presence of minimal acid levels, impairment of mucosal defense factors may be present. GUs have been classified based on their location: Type I occur in the gastric body and tend to be associated with low gastric acid production; type II occur in the antrum and gastric acid can vary from low to normal; type III occur within 3 cm of the pylorus and are commonly accompanied by DUs and normal or high gastric acid production; and type IV are found in the cardia and are associated with low gastric acid production.

H. PYLORI AND ACID PEPTIC DISORDERS Gastric infection with the bacterium *H. pylori* accounts for the majority of PUD (Chap. 188). This organism also plays a role in the development of gastric mucosa-associated lymphoid tissue (MALT) lymphoma and gastric adenocarcinoma. Although the entire genome of *H. pylori* has been sequenced, it is still not clear how this organism, which resides in the stomach, causes ulceration in the duodenum, or whether its eradication will lead to a decrease in gastric cancer.

The bacterium The bacterium, initially named *Campylobacter pyloridis,* is a gram-negative microaerophilic rod found most commonly in the deeper portions of the mucous gel coating the gastric mucosa or between the mucous layer and the gastric epithelium. It may attach to gastric epithelium but under normal circumstances does not appear to invade cells. It is strategically designed to live within the aggressive environment of the stomach. It is S-shaped (~0.5–3 μm in size) and contains multiple sheathed flagella. Initially, *H. pylori* resides in the antrum but, over time, migrates toward the more proximal segments of the stomach. The organism is capable of transforming into a coccoid form, which represents a dormant state that may facilitate survival in adverse conditions. The genome of *H. pylori* (1.65 million base pairs) encodes ~1500 proteins. Among this multitude of proteins there are factors that are essential determinants of *H. pylori*–mediated pathogenesis and colonization such as the outer membrane protein (Hop proteins), urease, and the vacuolating cytotoxin (Vac A). Moreover, the majority of *H. pylori* strains contain a genomic fragment that encodes the cag pathogenicity island (cag-PAI). Several of the genes that make up cag-PAI encode components of a type IV secretion island that translocates Cag A into host cells. Once in the cell, Cag A activates a series of cellular events important in cell growth and cytokine production. *H. pylori* also has extensive genetic diversity that in turn enhances its ability to promote disease. The first step in infection by *H. pylori* is dependent on the bacteria's motility and its ability to produce urease. Urease produces ammonia from urea, an essential step in alkalinizing the surrounding pH. Additional bacterial factors include catalase, lipase, adhesins, platelet-activating factor, and pic B (induces cytokines). Multiple strains of *H. pylori* exist and are characterized by their ability to express several of these factors (Cag A, Vac A, etc.). It is possible that the different diseases related to *H. pylori* infection can be attributed to different strains of the organism with distinct pathogenic features.

Epidemiology The prevalence of *H. pylori* varies throughout the world and depends largely on the overall standard of living in the region. In developing parts of the world, 80% of the population may be infected by the age of 20, whereas the prevalence is 20–50% in industrialized countries. In contrast, in the United States this organism is rare in childhood. The overall prevalence of *H. pylori* in the United States is ~30%, with individuals born before 1950 having a higher rate of infection than those born later. About 10% of Americans <30 years of age are colonized with the bacteria. The rate of infection with *H. pylori* in industrialized countries has decreased substantially in recent decades. The steady increase in the prevalence of *H. pylori* noted with increasing age is due primarily to a cohort effect, reflecting higher transmission during a period in which the earlier cohorts were children. It has been calculated through mathematical models that improved sanitation during the latter half of the nineteenth century dramatically decreased transmission of *H. pylori*. Moreover, with the present rate of intervention, the organism will be ultimately eliminated from the United States. Two factors that predispose to higher colonization rates include poor socioeconomic status and less education. These factors, not race, are responsible for the rate of *H. pylori* infection in blacks and Hispanic Americans being double the rate seen in whites of comparable age. Other risk factors for *H. pylori* infection are (1) birth or residence in a developing country, (2) domestic crowding, (3) unsanitary living conditions, (4) unclean food or water, and (5) exposure to gastric contents of an infected individual.

Transmission of *H. pylori* occurs from person to person, following an oral-oral or fecal-oral route. The risk of *H. pylori* infection is declining in developing countries. The rate of infection in the United States has fallen by >50% when compared to 30 years ago.

Pathophysiology *H. pylori* infection is virtually always associated with a chronic active gastritis, but only 10–15% of infected individuals develop frank peptic ulceration. The basis for this difference is unknown, but is likely due to a combination of host and bacterial factors some of which are outlined below. Initial studies suggested that >90% of all DUs were associated with *H. pylori*, but *H. pylori* is present in only 30–60% of individuals with GUs and 50–70% of patients with DUs. The pathophysiology of ulcers not associated with *H. pylori* or NSAID ingestion (or the rare Zollinger-Ellison syndrome [ZES]) is becoming more relevant as the incidence of *H. pylori* is dropping, particularly in the Western world (see below).

The particular end result of *H. pylori* infection (gastritis, PUD, gastric MALT lymphoma, gastric cancer) is determined by a complex interplay between bacterial and host factors (Fig. 348-6).

1. *Bacterial factors: H. pylori* is able to facilitate gastric residence, induce mucosal injury, and avoid host defense. Different strains of *H. pylori* produce different virulence factors. A specific region of the bacterial genome, the pathogenicity island (cag-PAI), encodes the virulence factors Cag A and pic B. Vac A also contributes to pathogenicity, although it is not encoded within the pathogenicity island. These virulence factors, in conjunction with additional bacterial constituents, can cause mucosal damage, in part through their ability to target the host immune cells. For example, Vac A targets human CD4 T cells, inhibiting their proliferation and in addition can disrupt normal function of B cells, CD8 T cells, macrophages, and mast cells. Multiple studies have demonstrated that *H. pylori* strains that are cag-PAI positive are associated with a higher risk of PUD, premalignant gastric lesions, and gastric cancer than are strains that lack the cag-PAI. In addition, *H. pylori* may directly inhibit parietal cell H^+,K^+-ATPase activity through a

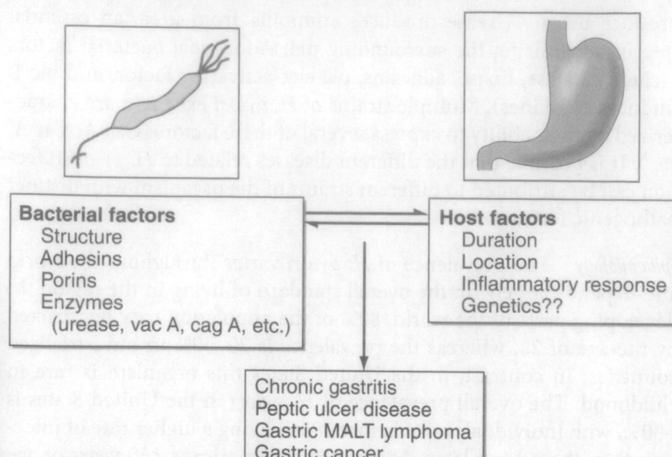

FIGURE 348-6 Outline of the bacterial and host factors important in determining *H. pylori*–induced gastrointestinal disease. MALT, mucosal-associated lymphoid tissue.

Cag A–dependent mechanism, leading in part to the low acid production observed after acute infection with the organism. Urease, which allows the bacteria to reside in the acidic stomach, generates NH_3, which can damage epithelial cells. The bacteria produce surface factors that are chemotactic for neutrophils and monocytes, which in turn contribute to epithelial cell injury (see below). *H. pylori* makes proteases and phospholipases that break down the glycoprotein lipid complex of the mucous gel, thus reducing the efficacy of this first line of mucosal defense. *H. pylori* expresses adhesins (OMPs like BabA), which facilitate attachment of the bacteria to gastric epithelial cells. Although lipopolysaccharide (LPS) of gram-negative bacteria often plays an important role in the infection, *H. pylori* LPS has low immunologic activity compared to that of other organisms. It may promote a smoldering chronic inflammation.

2. *Host factors:* Studies in twins suggest that there may be genetic predisposition to acquire *H. pylori.* The inflammatory response to *H. pylori* includes recruitment of neutrophils, lymphocytes (T and B), macrophages, and plasma cells. The pathogen leads to local injury by binding to class II major histocompatibility complex (MHC) molecules expressed on gastric epithelial cells, leading to cell death (*apoptosis*). Moreover, bacterial strains that encode cag-PAI can introduce Cag A into the host cells, leading to further cell injury and activation of cellular pathways involved in cytokine production and repression of tumor-suppressor genes. Elevated concentrations of multiple cytokines are found in the gastric epithelium of *H. pylori*–infected individuals, including interleukin (IL) 1α/β, IL-2, IL-6, IL-8, tumor necrosis factor (TNF) α, and interferon (IFN) γ. *H. pylori* infection also leads to both a mucosal and a systemic humoral response, which does not lead to eradication of the bacteria but further compounds epithelial cell injury. Additional mechanisms by which *H. pylori* may cause epithelial cell injury include (1) activated neutrophil-mediated production of reactive oxygen or nitrogen species and enhanced epithelial cell turnover and (2) apoptosis related to interaction with T cells (T helper 1, or T_H1, cells) and IFN-γ. Finally, the human stomach can be colonized by a host of commensal organisms that may affect the likelihood of *H. pylori*–mediated mucosal injury.

The reason for *H. pylori*–mediated duodenal ulceration remains unclear. Studies suggest that *H. pylori* associated with duodenal ulceration may be more virulent. In addition, certain specific bacterial factors such as the DU-promoting gene A (*dupA*), may be associated with the development of DUs. Another potential contributing factor is that gastric metaplasia in the duodenum of DU patients, which may be due to high acid exposure (see below), permits *H. pylori* to bind to it and produce local injury secondary to the host response. Another hypothesis is that *H. pylori* antral infection could lead to increased

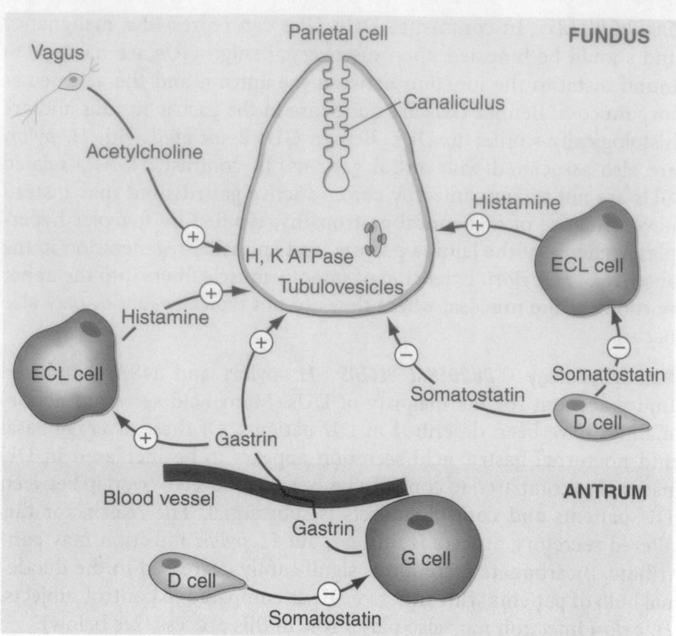

FIGURE 348-7 Summary of potential mechanisms by which *H. pylori* may lead to gastric secretory abnormalities. D, somatostatin cell; ECL, enterochromaffin-like cell; G, G cell. *(Adapted from J Calam et al: Gastroenterology 113:543, 1997.)*

acid production, increased duodenal acid, and mucosal injury. Basal and stimulated (meal, gastrin-releasing peptide [GRP]) gastrin release are increased in *H. pylori*–infected individuals, and somatostatin-secreting D cells may be decreased. *H. pylori* infection might induce increased acid secretion through both direct and indirect actions of *H. pylori* and proinflammatory cytokines (IL-8, TNF, and IL-1) on G, D, and parietal cells (Fig. 348-7). GUs, in contrast, are associated with *H. pylori*–induced pangastritis and normal or low gastric acid secretion. *H. pylori* infection has also been associated with decreased duodenal mucosal bicarbonate production. Data supporting and contradicting each of these interesting theories have been demonstrated. Thus, the mechanism by which *H. pylori* infection of the stomach leads to duodenal ulceration remains to be established.

In summary, the final effect of *H. pylori* on the GI tract is variable and determined by microbial and host factors. The type and distribution of gastritis correlate with the ultimate gastric and duodenal pathology observed. Specifically, the presence of antral-predominant gastritis is associated with DU formation; gastritis involving primarily the corpus predisposes to the development of GUs, gastric atrophy, and ultimately gastric carcinoma (Fig. 348-8).

NSAID-INDUCED DISEASE

Epidemiology NSAIDs represent a group of the most commonly used medications in the United States. More than 30 billion over-the-counter tablets and over 100 million prescriptions are sold yearly in the United States alone. In fact, after the introduction of COX-2 inhibitors in the year 2000, the number of prescriptions written for NSAIDs was >111 million at a cost of $4.8 billion. Side effects and complications due to NSAIDs are considered the most common drug-related toxicities in the United States. The spectrum of NSAID-induced morbidity ranges from nausea and dyspepsia (prevalence reported as high as 50–60%) to a serious GI complication such as endoscopy-documented peptic ulceration (15–30% of individuals taking NSAIDs regularly) complicated by bleeding or perforation in as many as 1.5% of users per year. It is estimated that NSAID-induced GI bleeding accounts for 60,000–120,000 hospital admissions per year, and deaths related to NSAID-induced toxicity may be as high as 16,000 per year in the United States. Approximately 4–5% of patients develop symptomatic ulcers within 1 year. Unfortunately, dyspeptic symptoms do not correlate with NSAID-induced pathology. Over 80% of patients with serious NSAID-related complications did not have preceding dyspepsia.

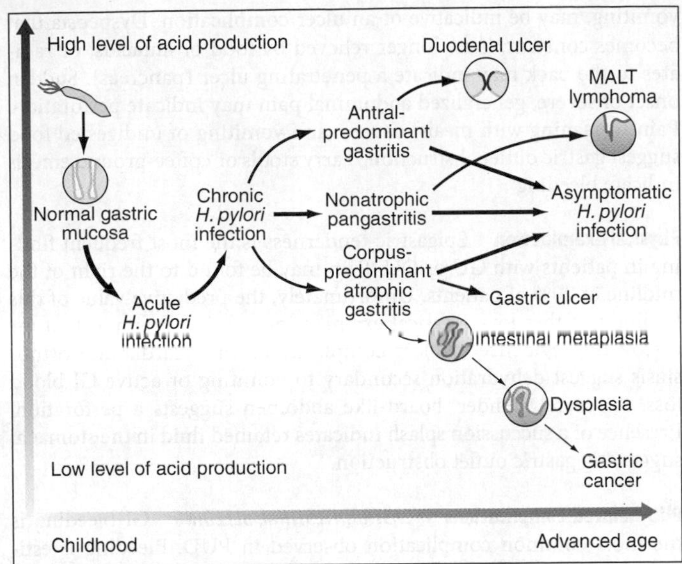

FIGURE 348-8 Natural history of *H. pylori* infection. MALT, mucosal-associated lymphoid tissue. *(Used with permission from S Suerbaum, P Michetti: N Engl J Med 347:1175, 2002.)*

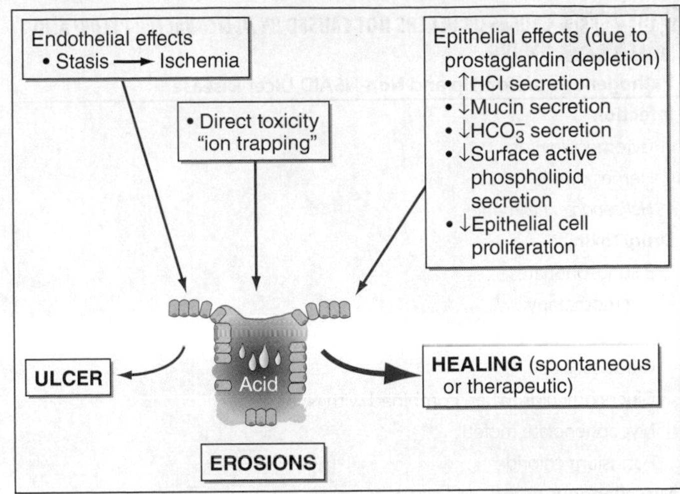

FIGURE 348-9 Mechanisms by which nonsteroidal anti-inflammatory drugs may induce mucosal injury. *(Adapted from J Scheiman et al: J Clin Outcomes Management 3:23, 1996. Copyright 2003 Turner White Communications, Inc., www.turner-white.com. Used with permission.)*

In view of the lack of warning signs, it is important to identify patients who are at increased risk for morbidity and mortality related to NSAID usage. Even 75 mg/d of aspirin may lead to serious GI ulceration; thus, no dose of NSAID is completely safe. In fact, the incidence of mucosal injury (ulcers and erosions) in patients taking low-dose aspirin (75–325 mg) has been estimated to range from as low as 8% to as high as 60%. It appears that *H. pylori* infection increases the risk of PUD-associated GI bleeding in chronic users of low-dose aspirin. Established risk factors include advanced age, history of ulcer, concomitant use of glucocorticoids, high-dose NSAIDs, multiple NSAIDs, concomitant use of anticoagulants, clopidogrel, and serious or multisystem disease. Possible risk factors include concomitant infection with *H. pylori*, cigarette smoking, and alcohol consumption.

Pathophysiology Prostaglandins play a critical role in maintaining gastroduodenal mucosal integrity and repair. It therefore follows that interruption of prostaglandin synthesis can impair mucosal defense and repair, thus facilitating mucosal injury via a systemic mechanism. Animal studies have demonstrated that neutrophil adherence to the gastric microcirculation plays an essential role in the initiation of NSAID-induced mucosal injury. A summary of the pathogenetic pathways by which systemically administered NSAIDs may lead to mucosal injury is shown in Fig. 348-9. Single nucleotide polymorphisms (SNPs) have been found in several genes, including those encoding certain subtypes of cytochrome P450 (see below), interleukin-1β (*IL-1β*), angiotensinogen (*AGT*), and an organic ion transporting polypeptide (*SLCO1B1*), but these findings need confirmation in larger scale studies.

Injury to the mucosa also occurs as a result of the topical encounter with NSAIDs. Aspirin and many NSAIDs are weak acids that remain in a nonionized lipophilic form when found within the acid environment of the stomach. Under these conditions, NSAIDs migrate across lipid membranes of epithelial cells, leading to cell injury once trapped intracellularly in an ionized form. Topical NSAIDs can also alter the surface mucous layer, permitting back diffusion of H^+ and pepsin, leading to further epithelial cell damage. Moreover, enteric-coated or buffered preparations are also associated with risk of peptic ulceration.

The interplay between *H. pylori* and NSAIDs in the pathogenesis of PUD is complex. Meta-analysis supports the conclusion that each of these aggressive factors is independent and synergistic risk factors for PUD and its complications such as GI bleeding. For example, eradication of *H. pylori* reduces the likelihood of GI complications in high-risk individuals to levels observed in individuals with average risk of NSAID-induced complications.

PATHOGENETIC FACTORS UNRELATED TO H. PYLORI AND NSAIDs IN ACID PEPTIC DISEASE Cigarette smoking has been implicated in the pathogenesis of PUD. Not only have smokers been found to have ulcers more frequently than do nonsmokers, but smoking appears to decrease healing rates, impair response to therapy, and increase ulcer-related complications such as perforation. The mechanism responsible for increased ulcer diathesis in smokers is unknown. Theories have included altered gastric emptying, decreased proximal duodenal bicarbonate production, increased risk for *H. pylori* infection, and cigarette-induced generation of noxious mucosal free radicals. Genetic predisposition may play a role in ulcer development. First-degree relatives of DU patients are three times as likely to develop an ulcer; however, the potential role of *H. pylori* infection in contacts is a major consideration. Increased frequencies of blood group O and of the nonsecretor status have also been implicated as genetic risk factors for peptic diathesis. However, *H. pylori* preferentially binds to group O antigens. Additional genetic factors have been postulated to predispose certain individuals to developing PUD and/or upper GI bleeding. Specifically, genes encoding the NSAID-metabolizing enzymes cytochrome P450 2C9 and 2C8 (CYP2C9 and CYP2C8) are potential susceptibility genes for NSAID-induced PUD, but unfortunately, the studies have not been consistent in demonstrating this association. In a United Kingdom study, the *CYP2C19*17* gain-of-function polymorphism was associated with PUD in a Caucasian cohort, irrespective of ulcer etiology. These findings need to be confirmed in broader studies. Psychological stress has been thought to contribute to PUD, but studies examining the role of psychological factors in its pathogenesis have generated conflicting results. Although PUD is associated with certain personality traits (neuroticism), these same traits are also present in individuals with nonulcer dyspepsia (NUD) and other functional and organic disorders.

Diet has also been thought to play a role in peptic diseases. Certain foods and beverages can cause dyspepsia, but no convincing studies indicate an association between ulcer formation and a specific diet. Specific chronic disorders have been shown to have a strong association with PUD: (1) advanced age, (2) chronic pulmonary disease, (3) chronic renal failure, (4) cirrhosis, (5) nephrolithiasis, (6) α_1-antitrypsin deficiency, and (7) systemic mastocytosis. Disorders with a possible association are (1) hyperparathyroidism, (2) coronary artery disease, (3) polycythemia vera, (4) chronic pancreatitis, (5) former alcohol use, (6) obesity, (7) African-American race, and (8) three or more doctor visits in a year.

Multiple factors play a role in the pathogenesis of PUD. The two predominant causes are *H. pylori* infection and NSAID ingestion. PUD

TABLE 348-1 CAUSES OF ULCERS NOT CAUSED BY *HELICOBACTER PYLORI* AND NSAIDs

Pathogenesis of Non-Hp and Non-NSAID Ulcer Disease
Infection
Cytomegalovirus
Herpes simplex virus
Helicobacter heilmannii
Drug/Toxin
Bisphosphonates
Chemotherapy
Clopidogrel
Crack cocaine
Glucocorticoids (when combined with NSAIDs)
Mycophenolate mofetil
Potassium chloride
Miscellaneous
Basophilia in myeloproliferative disease
Duodenal obstruction (e.g., annular pancreas)
Infiltrating disease
Ischemia
Radiation therapy
Eosinophilic infiltration
Sarcoidosis
Crohn's disease
Idiopathic hypersecretory state

Abbreviations: Hp, *H. pylori*; NSAIDs, nonsteroidal anti-inflammatory drugs.

not related to *H. pylori* or NSAIDs is increasing. Other less common causes of PUD are shown in Table 348-1. These etiologic agents should be considered as the incidence of *H. pylori* is decreasing. Independent of the inciting or injurious agent, peptic ulcers develop as a result of an imbalance between mucosal protection/repair and aggressive factors. Gastric acid plays an important role in mucosal injury.

CLINICAL FEATURES

History Abdominal pain is common to many GI disorders, including DU and GU, but has a poor predictive value for the presence of either DU or GU. Up to 10% of patients with NSAID-induced mucosal disease can present with a complication (bleeding, perforation, and obstruction) without antecedent symptoms. Despite this poor correlation, a careful history and physical examination are essential components of the approach to a patient suspected of having peptic ulcers.

Epigastric pain described as a burning or gnawing discomfort can be present in both DU and GU. The discomfort is also described as an ill-defined, aching sensation or as hunger pain. The typical pain pattern in DU occurs 90 minutes to 3 hours after a meal and is frequently relieved by antacids or food. Pain that awakes the patient from sleep (between midnight and 3 A.M.) is the most discriminating symptom, with two-thirds of DU patients describing this complaint. Unfortunately, this symptom is also present in one-third of patients with NUD (see below). Elderly patients are less likely to have abdominal pain as a manifestation of PUD and may instead present with a complication such as ulcer bleeding or perforation. The pain pattern in GU patients may be different from that in DU patients, where discomfort may actually be precipitated by food. Nausea and weight loss occur more commonly in GU patients. Endoscopy detects ulcers in <30% of patients who have dyspepsia.

The mechanism for development of abdominal pain in ulcer patients is unknown. Several possible explanations include acid-induced activation of chemical receptors in the duodenum, enhanced duodenal sensitivity to bile acids and pepsin, or altered gastroduodenal motility.

Variation in the intensity or distribution of the abdominal pain, as well as the onset of associated symptoms such as nausea and/or vomiting, may be indicative of an ulcer complication. Dyspepsia that becomes constant, is no longer relieved by food or antacids, or radiates to the back may indicate a penetrating ulcer (pancreas). Sudden onset of severe, generalized abdominal pain may indicate perforation. Pain worsening with meals, nausea, and vomiting of undigested food suggest gastric outlet obstruction. Tarry stools or coffee-ground emesis indicate bleeding.

Physical examination Epigastric tenderness is the most frequent finding in patients with GU or DU. Pain may be found to the right of the midline in 20% of patients. Unfortunately, the predictive value of this finding is rather low. Physical examination is critically important for discovering evidence of ulcer complication. Tachycardia and orthostasis suggest dehydration secondary to vomiting or active GI blood loss. A severely tender, board-like abdomen suggests a perforation. Presence of a succussion splash indicates retained fluid in the stomach, suggesting gastric outlet obstruction.

PUD-Related Complications • *GASTROINTESTINAL BLEEDING* GI bleeding is the most common complication observed in PUD. Bleeding is estimated to occur in 19.4–57 per 100,000 individuals in a general population or in approximately 15% of patients. Bleeding and complications of ulcer disease occur more often in individuals >60 years of age. The 30-day mortality rate is as high as 5–10%. The higher incidence in the elderly is likely due to the increased use of NSAIDs in this group. In addition, up to 80% of the mortality in PUD-related bleeding is due to nonbleeding causes such as multiorgan failure (24%), pulmonary complications (24%), and malignancy (34%).

Up to 20% of patients with ulcer-related hemorrhage bleed without any preceding warning signs or symptoms.

PERFORATION The second most common ulcer-related complication is perforation, being reported in as many as 6–7% of PUD patients with an estimated 30-day mortality of over 20%. As in the case of bleeding, the incidence of perforation in the elderly appears to be increasing secondary to increased use of NSAIDs. *Penetration* is a form of perforation in which the ulcer bed tunnels into an adjacent organ. DUs tend to penetrate posteriorly into the pancreas, leading to pancreatitis, whereas GUs tend to penetrate into the left hepatic lobe. Gastrocolic fistulas associated with GUs have also been described.

GASTRIC OUTLET OBSTRUCTION Gastric outlet obstruction is the least common ulcer-related complication, occurring in 1–2% of patients. A patient may have relative obstruction secondary to ulcer-related inflammation and edema in the peripyloric region. This process often resolves with ulcer healing. A fixed, mechanical obstruction secondary to scar formation in the peripyloric areas is also possible. The latter requires endoscopic (balloon dilation) or surgical intervention. Signs and symptoms relative to mechanical obstruction may develop insidiously. New onset of early satiety, nausea, vomiting, increase of postprandial abdominal pain, and weight loss should make gastric outlet obstruction a possible diagnosis.

Differential Diagnosis The list of GI and non-GI disorders that can mimic ulceration of the stomach or duodenum is quite extensive. The most commonly encountered diagnosis among patients seen for upper abdominal discomfort is NUD. NUD, also known as *functional dyspepsia* or *essential dyspepsia,* refers to a group of heterogeneous disorders typified by upper abdominal pain without the presence of an ulcer. Dyspepsia has been reported to occur in up to 30% of the U.S. population. Up to 60% of patients seeking medical care for dyspepsia have a negative diagnostic evaluation. The etiology of NUD is not established, and the potential role of *H. pylori* in NUD remains controversial.

Several additional disease processes that may present with "ulcer-like" symptoms include proximal GI tumors, gastroesophageal reflux, vascular disease, pancreaticobiliary disease (biliary colic, chronic pancreatitis), and gastroduodenal Crohn's disease.

Diagnostic Evaluation In view of the poor predictive value of abdominal pain for the presence of a gastroduodenal ulcer and the multiple disease

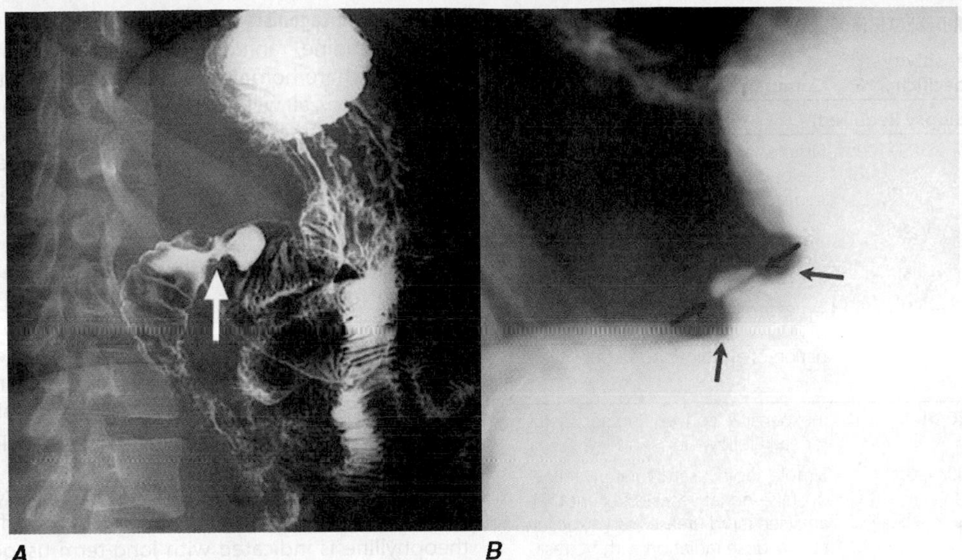

FIGURE 348-10 **Barium study demonstrating (*A*) a benign duodenal ulcer and (*B*) a benign gastric ulcer.**

processes that can mimic this disease, the clinician is often confronted with having to establish the presence of an ulcer. Documentation of an ulcer requires either a radiographic (barium study) or an endoscopic procedure. However, a large percentage of patients with symptoms suggestive of an ulcer have NUD; testing for *H. pylori* and antibiotic therapy (see below) is appropriate for individuals who are otherwise healthy and <45 years of age, before embarking on a diagnostic evaluation (Chap. 54).

Barium studies of the proximal GI tract are still occasionally used as a first test for documenting an ulcer. The sensitivity of older single-contrast barium meals for detecting a DU is as high as 80%, with a double-contrast study providing detection rates as high as 90%. Sensitivity for detection is decreased in small ulcers (<0.5 cm), with presence of previous scarring, or in postoperative patients. A DU appears as a well-demarcated crater, most often seen in the bulb (Fig. 348-10*A*). A GU may represent benign or malignant disease. Typically, a benign GU also appears as a discrete crater with radiating mucosal folds originating from the ulcer margin (Fig. 348-10*B*). Ulcers >3 cm in size or those associated with a mass are more often malignant. Unfortunately, up to 8% of GUs that appear to be benign by radiographic appearance are malignant by endoscopy or surgery. Radiographic studies that show a GU must be followed by endoscopy and biopsy.

Endoscopy provides the most sensitive and specific approach for examining the upper GI tract (Fig. 348-11). In addition to permitting direct visualization of the mucosa, endoscopy facilitates photographic documentation of a mucosal defect and tissue biopsy to rule out malignancy (GU) or *H. pylori*. Endoscopic examination is particularly helpful in identifying lesions too small to detect by radiographic examination, for evaluation of atypical radiographic abnormalities, or to determine if an ulcer is a source of blood loss.

Although the methods for diagnosing *H. pylori* are outlined in Chap. 181, a brief summary will be included here (Table 348-2). Several biopsy urease tests have been developed (PyloriTek, CLOtest, Hpfast, Pronto Dry) that have a sensitivity and specificity of >90–95%. Several noninvasive methods for detecting this organism have been developed. Three types of studies routinely used include serologic testing, the ^{13}C- or ^{14}C-urea breath test, and the fecal *H. pylori* (Hp) antigen test. A urinary Hp antigen test, as well as a refined monoclonal antibody stool antigen test, appears promising.

Occasionally, specialized testing such as serum gastrin and gastric acid analysis or sham feeding may be needed in individuals with complicated or refractory PUD (see "Zollinger-Ellison Syndrome [ZES]," below). Screening for aspirin or NSAIDs (blood or urine) may also be necessary in refractory *H. pylori*–negative PUD patients.

TREATMENT PEPTIC ULCER DISEASE

Before the discovery of *H. pylori,* the therapy of PUD was centered on the old dictum by Schwartz of "no acid, no ulcer." Although acid secretion is still important in the pathogenesis of PUD, eradication of *H. pylori* and therapy/prevention of NSAID-induced disease is the mainstay of treatment. A summary of commonly used drugs for treatment of acid peptic disorders is shown in Table 348-3.

ACID-NEUTRALIZING/INHIBITORY DRUGS

Antacids Before we understood the important role of histamine in stimulating parietal cell activity, neutralization of secreted acid with antacids constituted the main form of therapy for peptic

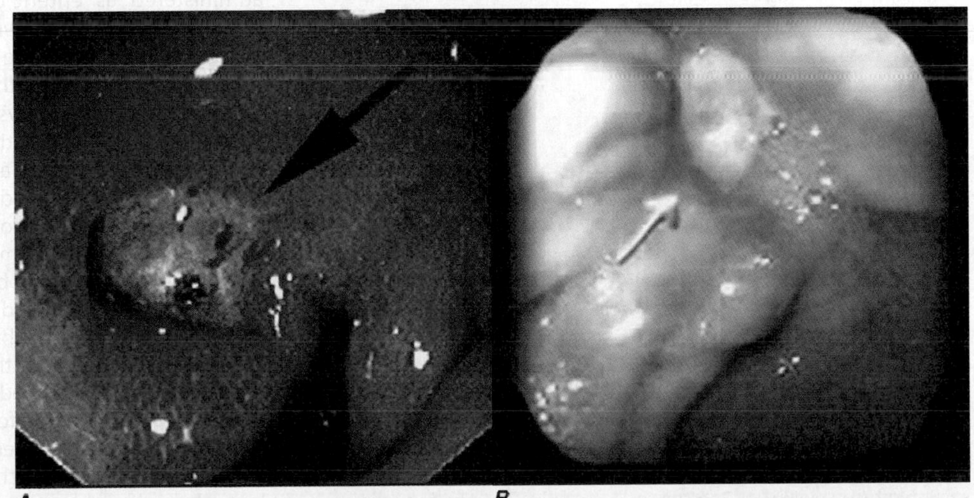

FIGURE 348-11 **Endoscopy demonstrating (*A*) a benign duodenal ulcer and (*B*) a benign gastric ulcer.**

TABLE 348-2 TESTS FOR DETECTION OF *H. PYLORI*

Test	Sensitivity/ Specificity, %	Comments
Invasive (Endoscopy/Biopsy Required)		
Rapid urease	80–95/95–100	Simple, false negative with recent use of PPIs, antibiotics, or bismuth compounds
Histology	80–90/>95	Requires pathology processing and staining; provides histologic information
Culture	—/—	Time-consuming, expensive, dependent on experience; allows determination of antibiotic susceptibility
Noninvasive		
Serology	>80/>90	Inexpensive, convenient; not useful for early follow-up
Urea breath test	>90/>90	Simple, rapid; useful for early follow-up; false negatives with recent therapy (see rapid urease test); exposure to low-dose radiation with ^{14}C test
Stool antigen	>90/>90	Inexpensive, convenient

Abbreviation: PPIs, proton pump inhibitors.

ulcers. They are now rarely, if ever, used as the primary therapeutic agent but instead are often used by patients for symptomatic relief of dyspepsia. The most commonly used agents are mixtures of aluminum hydroxide and magnesium hydroxide. Aluminum hydroxide can produce constipation and phosphate depletion; magnesium hydroxide may cause loose stools. Many of the commonly used antacids (e.g., Maalox, Mylanta) have a combination of both aluminum and magnesium hydroxide in order to avoid these side effects. The magnesium-containing preparation should not be used in chronic renal failure patients because of possible hypermagnesemia, and aluminum may cause chronic neurotoxicity in these patients.

Calcium carbonate and sodium bicarbonate are potent antacids with varying levels of potential problems. The long-term use of calcium carbonate (converts to calcium chloride in the stomach) can lead to milk-alkali syndrome (hypercalcemia, hyperphosphatemia with possible renal calcinosis and progression to renal insufficiency). Sodium bicarbonate may induce systemic alkalosis.

TABLE 348-3 DRUGS USED IN THE TREATMENT OF PEPTIC ULCER DISEASE

Drug Type/Mechanism	Examples	Dose
Acid-suppressing drugs		
Antacids	Mylanta, Maalox, Tums, Gaviscon	100–140 meq/L 1 and 3 h after meals and hs
H_2 receptor antagonists	Cimetidine	400 mg bid
	Ranitidine	300 mg hs
	Famotidine	40 mg hs
	Nizatidine	300 mg hs
Proton pump inhibitors	Omeprazole	20 mg/d
	Lansoprazole	30 mg/d
	Rabeprazole	20 mg/d
	Pantoprazole	40 mg/d
	Esomeprazole	20 mg/d
	Dexlansoprazole	30 mg/d
Mucosal protective agents		
Sucralfate	Sucralfate	1 g qid
Prostaglandin analogue	Misoprostol	200 μg qid
Bismuth-containing compounds	Bismuth subsalicylate (BSS)	See anti-*H. pylori* regimens (Table 348-4)

Abbreviation: hs, at bedtime (*hora somni*).

H_2 Receptor Antagonists Four of these agents are presently available (cimetidine, ranitidine, famotidine, and nizatidine), and their structures share homology with histamine. Although each has different potency, all will significantly inhibit basal and stimulated acid secretion to comparable levels when used at therapeutic doses. Moreover, similar ulcer-healing rates are achieved with each drug when used at the correct dosage. Presently, this class of drug is often used for treatment of active ulcers (4–6 weeks) in combination with antibiotics directed at eradicating *H. pylori* (see below).

Cimetidine was the first H_2 receptor antagonist used for the treatment of acid peptic disorders. The initial recommended dosing profile for cimetidine was 300 mg qid. Subsequent studies have documented the efficacy of using 800 mg at bedtime for treatment of active ulcer, with healing rates approaching 80% at 4 weeks. Cimetidine may have weak antiandrogenic side effects resulting in reversible gynecomastia and impotence, primarily in patients receiving high doses for prolonged periods of time (months to years, as in ZES). In view of cimetidine's ability to inhibit cytochrome P450, careful monitoring of drugs such as warfarin, phenytoin, and theophylline is indicated with long-term usage. Other rare reversible adverse effects reported with cimetidine include confusion and elevated levels of serum aminotransferases, creatinine, and serum prolactin. Ranitidine, famotidine, and nizatidine are more potent H_2 receptor antagonists than cimetidine. Each can be used once a day at bedtime for ulcer prevention, which was commonly done before the discovery of *H. pylori* and the development of proton pump inhibitors (PPIs). Patients may develop tolerance to H_2 blockers, a rare event with PPIs (see below). Comparable nighttime dosing regimens are ranitidine 300 mg, famotidine 40 mg, and nizatidine 300 mg.

Additional rare, reversible systemic toxicities reported with H_2 receptor antagonists include pancytopenia, neutropenia, anemia, and thrombocytopenia, with a prevalence rate varying from 0.01–0.2%. Cimetidine and ranitidine (to a lesser extent) can bind to hepatic cytochrome P450; famotidine and nizatidine do not.

Proton Pump (H^+,K^+-ATPase) Inhibitors Omeprazole, esomeprazole, lansoprazole, rabeprazole, and pantoprazole are substituted benzimidazole derivatives that covalently bind and irreversibly inhibit H^+,K^+-ATPase. Esomeprazole, one of the newest members of this drug class, is the S-enantiomer of omeprazole, which is a racemic mixture of both S- and R-optical isomers. The R-isomer of lansoprazole, dexlansoprazole, is the most recent PPI approved for clinical use. Its reported advantage is a dual delayed-release system, aimed at improving treatment of gastroesophageal reflux disease (GERD). These are the most potent acid inhibitory agents available. Omeprazole and lansoprazole are the PPIs that have been used for the longest time. Both are acid-labile and are administered as enteric-coated granules in a sustained-release capsule that dissolves within the small intestine at a pH of 6. Lansoprazole is available in an orally disintegrating tablet that can be taken with or without water, an advantage for individuals who have significant dysphagia. Absorption kinetics are similar to the capsule. In addition, a lansoprazole-naproxen combination preparation that has been made available is targeted at decreasing NSAID-related GI injury (see below). Omeprazole is available as nonenteric-coated granules mixed with sodium bicarbonate in a powder form that can be administered orally or via gastric tube. The sodium bicarbonate has two purposes: to protect the omeprazole from acid degradation and to promote rapid gastric alkalinization and subsequent proton pump activation, which facilitates rapid action of the PPI. Pantoprazole and rabeprazole are available as enteric-coated tablets. Pantoprazole is also available as a parenteral formulation for intravenous use. These agents are lipophilic compounds; upon entering the parietal cell, they are protonated and trapped within the acid environment of the tubulovesicular and canalicular system. These agents potently inhibit all phases of gastric acid secretion. Onset of action is rapid, with a maximum acid inhibitory effect between 2 and 6 h after administration and duration of inhibition lasting up to 72–96 h. With repeated daily dosing, progressive acid inhibitory effects are observed, with basal and secretagogue-stimulated acid production being inhibited by >95% after 1 week of therapy. The half-life of PPIs is ~18 h; thus, it can take between 2 and 5 days for gastric acid secretion to return to normal levels once these drugs have been discontinued. Because the pumps need to be activated for these agents to be effective, their efficacy is maximized if they are administered before a meal (except for the immediate-release formulation of omeprazole) (e.g., in the morning before breakfast). Mild to moderate hypergastrinemia has been observed in patients taking these drugs. Carcinoid tumors developed in some animals given the drugs preclinically; however, extensive experience has failed to demonstrate gastric carcinoid tumor development in humans. Serum gastrin levels return to normal levels within 1–2 weeks after drug cessation. Rebound gastric acid hypersecretion has been described in *H. pylori*–negative individuals after discontinuation of PPIs. It occurs even after relatively short-term usage (2 months) and may last for up to 2 months after the PPI has been discontinued. The mechanism involves gastrin-induced hyperplasia and hypertrophy of histamine-secreting ECL cells. The clinical relevance of this observation is that individuals may have worsening symptoms of GERD or dyspepsia upon stopping the PPI. Gradual tapering of the PPI and switching to an H_2 receptor antagonist may prevent this from occurring. *H. pylori*–induced inflammation and concomitant decrease in acid production may explain why this does not occur in *H. pylori*–positive patients. IF production is also inhibited, but vitamin B_{12}-deficiency anemia is uncommon, probably because of the large stores of the vitamin. As with any agent that leads to significant hypochlorhydria, PPIs may interfere with absorption of drugs such as ketoconazole, ampicillin, iron, and digoxin. Hepatic cytochrome P450 can be inhibited by the earlier PPIs (omeprazole, lansoprazole). Rabeprazole, pantoprazole, and esomeprazole do not appear to interact significantly with drugs metabolized by the cytochrome P450 system. The overall clinical significance of this observation is not definitely established. Caution should be taken when using theophylline, warfarin, diazepam, atazanavir, and phenytoin concomitantly with PPIs. Long-term acid suppression, especially with PPIs, has been associated with a higher incidence of community-acquired pneumonia as well as community and hospital acquired *Clostridium difficile*–associated disease. These observations require confirmation but should alert the practitioner to take caution when recommending these agents for long-term use, especially in elderly patients at risk for developing pneumonia or *C. difficile* infection. A population-based study revealed that long-term use of PPIs was associated with the development of hip fractures in older women. The absolute risk of fracture remained low despite an observed increase associated with the dose and duration of acid suppression. The mechanism for this observation is not clear, and this finding must be confirmed before making broad recommendations regarding the discontinuation of these agents in patients who benefit from them. Long-term use of PPIs has also been implicated in the development of iron and magnesium deficiency, but here again, the studies are limited and inconclusive. PPIs may exert a negative effect on the antiplatelet effect of clopidogrel. Although the evidence is mixed and inconclusive, a small increase in mortality and readmission rate for coronary events was seen in patients receiving a PPI while on clopidogrel in earlier studies. Subsequently, three meta-analyses reported an inverse correlation between clopidogrel and PPI use; therefore, the influence of this drug interaction on mortality is not clearly established. The mechanism involves the competition of the PPI and clopidogrel with the same cytochrome P450 (CYP2C19). Whether this is a class effect of PPIs is unclear; there appears to be at least a theoretical advantage of pantoprazole over the other PPIs, but this has not been confirmed. This drug interaction is particularly relevant in light of the common use of aspirin and clopidogrel for prevention of coronary events and the efficacy of PPIs in preventing GI bleeding in these patients. The FDA has made several recommendations while awaiting further evidence to clarify the impact of PPI therapy on clopidogrel use. Health care providers should continue to prescribe clopidogrel to patients who require it and should reevaluate the need for starting or continuing treatment with a PPI. From a practical standpoint, additional recommendations to consider include the following: Patients taking clopidogrel with aspirin, especially with other GI risk factors for bleeding, should receive GI protective therapy. Although high-dose H_2 blockers have been considered an option, these do not appear to be as effective as PPIs. If PPIs are to be given, some have recommended that there be a 12-h separation between administration of the PPI and clopidogrel to minimize competition of the two agents with the involved cytochrome P450. One option is to give the PPI 30 min before breakfast and the clopidogrel at bedtime. Insufficient data are available to firmly recommend one PPI over another. Patients 65 years of age or older have a higher risk for some of the long-term side effects of PPIs highlighted above, in part due to the higher prevalence of concomitant chronic diseases. It is therefore important to carefully select individuals, especially among the elderly, who need long-term PPI therapy and discontinue it in those individuals who do not need it.

Two new formulations of acid inhibitory agents are being developed. Tenatoprazole is a PPI containing an imidazopyridine ring instead of a benzimidazole ring, which promotes irreversible proton pump inhibition. This agent has a longer half-life than the other PPIs and may be beneficial for inhibiting nocturnal acid secretion, which has significant relevance in GERD. A second new class of agents is the potassium-competitive acid pump antagonists (P-CABs). These compounds inhibit gastric acid secretion via potassium competitive binding of the H^+,K^+-ATPase.

CYTOPROTECTIVE AGENTS

Sucralfate Sucralfate is a complex sucrose salt in which the hydroxyl groups have been substituted by aluminum hydroxide and sulfate. This compound is insoluble in water and becomes a viscous paste within the stomach and duodenum, binding primarily to sites of active ulceration. Sucralfate may act by several mechanisms: serving as a physicochemical barrier, promoting a trophic action by binding growth factors such as EGF, enhancing prostaglandin synthesis, stimulating mucus and bicarbonate secretion, and enhancing mucosal defense and repair. Toxicity from this drug is rare, with constipation being most common (2–3%). It should be avoided in patients with chronic renal insufficiency to prevent aluminum induced neurotoxicity. Hypophosphatemia and gastric bezoar formation have also been reported rarely. Standard dosing of sucralfate is 1 g qid.

Bismuth-Containing Preparations Sir William Osler considered bismuth-containing compounds the drug of choice for treating PUD. The resurgence in the use of these agents is due to their effect against *H. pylori*. Colloidal bismuth subcitrate (CBS) and bismuth subsalicylate (BSS, Pepto-Bismol) are the most widely used preparations. The mechanism by which these agents induce ulcer healing is unclear. Adverse effects with short term use include black stools, constipation, and darkening of the tongue. Long-term use with high doses, especially with the avidly absorbed CBS, may lead to neurotoxicity. These compounds are commonly used as one of the agents in an anti-*H. pylori* regimen (see below).

Prostaglandin Analogues In view of their central role in maintaining mucosal integrity and repair, stable prostaglandin analogues were developed for the treatment of PUD. The mechanism by which this rapidly absorbed drug provides its therapeutic effect is through enhancement of mucosal defense and repair. The most common toxicity noted with this drug is diarrhea (10–30% incidence). Other major toxicities include uterine bleeding and contractions; misoprostol is contraindicated in women who may be pregnant, and women of childbearing age must be made clearly aware of this potential drug toxicity. The standard therapeutic dose is 200 μg qid.

Miscellaneous Drugs A number of drugs including anticholinergic agents and tricyclic antidepressants were used for treating acid peptic disorders, but in light of their toxicity and the development of potent antisecretory agents, these are rarely, if ever, used today.

THERAPY OF *H. PYLORI*

The physician's goal in treating PUD is to provide relief of symptoms (pain or dyspepsia), promote ulcer healing, and ultimately prevent ulcer recurrence and complications. The greatest influence of understanding the role of *H. pylori* in peptic disease has been the ability to prevent recurrence. Documented eradication of *H. pylori* in patients with PUD is associated with a dramatic decrease in ulcer recurrence to <10–20% as compared to 59% in GU patients and 67% in DU patients when the organism is not eliminated. Eradication of the organism may lead to diminished recurrent ulcer bleeding. The effect of its eradication on ulcer perforation is unclear.

Extensive effort has been made in determining who of the many individuals with *H. pylori* infection should be treated. The common conclusion arrived at by multiple consensus conferences around the world is that *H. pylori* should be eradicated in patients with documented PUD. This holds true independent of time of presentation (first episode or not), severity of symptoms, presence of confounding factors such as ingestion of NSAIDs, or whether the ulcer is in remission. Some have advocated treating patients with a history of documented PUD who are found to be *H. pylori*–positive by serology or breath testing. Over one-half of patients with gastric MALT lymphoma experience complete remission of the tumor in response to *H. pylori* eradication. The Maastricht IV/Florence Consensus Report recommends a test-and-treat approach for patients with uninvestigated dyspepsia if the local incidence of *H. pylori* is greater than 20%. In addition, recommendations from this consensus report include testing and eradicating *H. pylori* in patients who will be using NSAIDs (including low-dose aspirin) on a long-term basis, especially if there is a prior history of PUD. These individuals will require continued PPI treatment as well as eradication treatment, because eradication of the organism alone does not eliminate the risk of gastroduodenal ulcers in patients already receiving long-term NSAIDs. Treating patients with NUD to prevent gastric cancer or patients with GERD requiring long-term acid suppression remains controversial. Guidelines from the American College of Gastroenterology suggest eradication of *H. pylori* in patients who have undergone resection of early gastric cancer. The Maastricht IV/Florence Consensus Report also evaluated *H. pylori* treatment in gastric cancer prevention and recommends that eradication should be considered in the following situations: first-degree relatives of family members with gastric cancer; patients with previous gastric neoplasm treated by endoscopic or subtotal resection; individuals with a risk of gastritis (severe pangastritis or body-predominant gastritis) or severe atrophy; patients with gastric acid inhibition for more than 1 year; individuals with strong environmental risk factors for gastric cancer (heavy smoking; high exposure to dust, coal, quartz, or cement; and/or work in quarries); and *H. pylori*–positive patients with a fear of gastric cancer.

Multiple drugs have been evaluated in the therapy of *H. pylori*. No single agent is effective in eradicating the organism. Combination therapy for 14 days provides the greatest efficacy, although regimens based on sequential administration of antibiotics also appear promising (see below). A shorter administration course (7–10 days), although attractive, has not proved as successful as the 14-day regimens. The agents used with the greatest frequency include amoxicillin, metronidazole, tetracycline, clarithromycin, and bismuth compounds.

Suggested treatment regimens for *H. pylori* are outlined in Table 348-4. Choice of a particular regimen will be influenced by several factors, including efficacy, patient tolerance, existing antibiotic resistance, and cost of the drugs. The aim for initial eradication rates should be 85–90%. Dual therapy (PPI plus amoxicillin, PPI plus clarithromycin, ranitidine bismuth citrate [Tritec] plus clarithromycin) is not recommended in view of studies demonstrating eradication rates of <80–85%. The combination of bismuth, metronidazole, and tetracycline was the first triple regimen found effective against *H. pylori*. The combination of two antibiotics plus either a PPI, H_2 blocker, or bismuth compound has comparable success rates. Addition of acid suppression assists in providing early symptom relief and enhances bacterial eradication.

TABLE 348-4 REGIMENS RECOMMENDED FOR ERADICATION OF *H. PYLORI* INFECTION

Drug	Dose
Triple Therapy	
1. Bismuth subsalicylate *plus*	2 tablets qid
Metronidazole *plus*	250 mg qid
Tetracycline[a]	500 mg qid
2. Ranitidine bismuth citrate *plus*	400 mg bid
Tetracycline *plus*	500 mg bid
Clarithromycin or metronidazole	500 mg bid
3. Omeprazole (lansoprazole) *plus*	20 mg bid (30 mg bid)
Clarithromycin *plus*	250 or 500 mg bid
Metronidazole[b] *or*	500 mg bid
Amoxicillin[c]	1 g bid
Quadruple Therapy	
Omeprazole (lansoprazole)	20 mg (30 mg) daily
Bismuth subsalicylate	2 tablets qid
Metronidazole	250 mg qid
Tetracycline	500 mg qid

[a]Alternative: use prepacked Helidac (see text). [b]Alternative: use prepacked Prevpac (see text). [c]Use either metronidazole or amoxicillin, not both.

Triple therapy, although effective, has several drawbacks, including the potential for poor patient compliance and drug-induced side effects. Compliance is being addressed by simplifying the regimens so that patients can take the medications twice a day. Simpler (dual therapy) and shorter regimens (7 and 10 days) are not as effective as triple therapy for 14 days. Two anti-*H. pylori* regimens are available in prepackaged formulation: Prevpac (lansoprazole, clarithromycin, and amoxicillin) and Helidac (BSS, tetracycline, and metronidazole). The contents of the Prevpac are to be taken twice per day for 14 days, whereas Helidac constituents are taken four times per day with an antisecretory agent (PPI or H_2 blocker), also for at least 14 days. Clarithromycin-based triple therapy should be avoided in settings where *H. pylori* resistance to this agent exceeds 15–20%.

Side effects have been reported in up to 20–30% of patients on triple therapy. Bismuth may cause black stools, constipation, or darkening of the tongue. The most feared complication with amoxicillin is pseudomembranous colitis, but this occurs in <1–2% of patients. Amoxicillin can also lead to antibiotic-associated diarrhea, nausea, vomiting, skin rash, and allergic reaction. Concomitant use of probiotics may ameliorate some of the antibiotic side effects (see below). Tetracycline has been reported to cause rashes and, very rarely, hepatotoxicity and anaphylaxis.

One important concern with treating patients who may not need therapy is the potential for development of antibiotic-resistant strains. The incidence and type of antibiotic-resistant *H. pylori* strains vary worldwide. Strains resistant to metronidazole, clarithromycin, amoxicillin, and tetracycline have been described, with the latter two being uncommon. Antibiotic-resistant strains are the most common cause for treatment failure in compliant patients. Unfortunately, in vitro resistance does not predict outcome in patients. Culture and sensitivity testing of *H. pylori* is not performed routinely. Although resistance to metronidazole has been found in as many as 30% of isolates in North America and 80% in developing countries, triple therapy is effective in eradicating the organism in >50% of patients infected with a resistant strain. Clarithromycin resistance is seen in 13% of individuals in the United States, with resistance to amoxicillin being <1% and resistance to both metronidazole and clarithromycin in the 5% range.

Failure of *H. pylori* eradication with triple therapy in a compliant patient is usually due to infection with a resistant organism. Quadruple therapy (Table 348-4), where clarithromycin is substituted for metronidazole (or vice versa), should be the next step. The combination of pantoprazole, amoxicillin, and rifabutin for 10 days has also been used successfully (86% cure rate) in patients infected with resistant strains. Additional regimens considered for second-line therapy include levofloxacin-based triple therapy (levofloxacin, amoxicillin, PPI) for 10 days and furazolidone-based triple therapy (furazolidone, amoxicillin, PPI) for 14 days. Unfortunately, there is no universally accepted treatment regimen recommended for patients who have failed two courses of antibiotics. If eradication is still not achieved in a compliant patient, then culture and sensitivity of the organism should be considered. Additional factors that may lower eradication rates include the patient's country of origin (higher in Northeast Asia than other parts of Asia or Europe) and cigarette smoking. In addition, meta-analysis suggests that even the most effective regimens (quadruple therapy including PPI, bismuth, tetracycline, and metronidazole and triple therapy including PPI, clarithromycin, and amoxicillin) may have suboptimal eradication rates (<80%), thus demonstrating the need for the development of more efficacious treatments.

In view of the observation that 15–25% of patients treated with first-line therapy may still remain infected with the organism, new approaches to treatment have been explored. One promising approach is sequential therapy. Regimens examined consist of 5 days of amoxicillin and a PPI, followed by an additional 5 days of PPI plus tinidazole and clarithromycin or levofloxacin. One promising regimen that has the benefit of being shorter in duration, easier to take, and less expensive is 5 days of concomitant therapy (PPI twice daily, amoxicillin 1 g twice daily, levofloxacin 500 mg twice daily, and tinidazole 500 mg twice daily). Initial studies have demonstrated eradication rates of >90% with good patient tolerance. Confirmation of these findings and applicability of this approach in the United States are needed, although some experts are recommending abandoning clarithromycin-based triple therapy in the United States for the concomitant therapy or the alternative sequential therapies highlighted above.

Innovative non–antibiotic-mediated approaches have been explored in an effort to improve eradication rates of *H. pylori*. Pretreatment of patients with *N*-acetylcysteine as a mucolytic agent to destroy the *H. pylori* biofilm and therefore impair antibiotic resistance has been examined, but more studies are needed to confirm the applicability of this approach. In vitro studies suggest that certain probiotics like *Lactobacillus* or its metabolites can inhibit *H. pylori*. Administration of probiotics has been attempted in several clinical studies in an effort to maximize antibiotic-mediated eradication with varying results. Overall, it appears that the use of certain probiotics, such as *Lactobacillus* spp., *Saccharomyces* spp., *Bifidobacterium* spp., and *Bacillus clausii*, did not alter eradication rates but importantly decreased antibiotic-associated side effects including nausea, dysgeusia, diarrhea, and abdominal discomfort/pain, resulting in enhanced tolerability of *H. pylori* therapies. Additional studies are needed to confirm the potential benefits of probiotics in this setting.

Reinfection after successful eradication of *H. pylori* is rare in the United States (<1% per year). If recurrent infection occurs within the first 6 months after completing therapy, the most likely explanation is recrudescence as opposed to reinfection.

THERAPY OF NSAID-RELATED GASTRIC OR DUODENAL INJURY

Medical intervention for NSAID-related mucosal injury includes treatment of an active ulcer and primary prevention of future injury. Recommendations for the treatment and primary prevention of NSAID-related mucosal injury are listed in Table 348-5. Ideally, the injurious agent should be stopped as the first step in the therapy of an active NSAID-induced ulcer. If that is possible, then treatment with one of the acid inhibitory agents (H_2 blockers, PPIs) is indicated. Cessation of NSAIDs is not always possible because of the patient's severe underlying disease. Only PPIs can heal GUs or DUs, independent of whether NSAIDs are discontinued.

TABLE 348-5 RECOMMENDATIONS FOR TREATMENT OF NSAID-RELATED MUCOSAL INJURY

Clinical Setting	Recommendation
Active ulcer	
NSAID discontinued	H_2 receptor antagonist or PPI
NSAID continued	PPI
Prophylactic therapy	Misoprostol
	PPI
	Selective COX-2 inhibitor
H. pylori infection	Eradication if active ulcer present or there is a past history of peptic ulcer disease

Abbreviations: COX-2, isoenzyme of cyclooxygenase; NSAID, nonsteroidal anti-inflammatory drug; PPI, proton pump inhibitor.

The approach to primary prevention has included avoiding the agent, using the lowest possible dose of the agent, using NSAIDs that are theoretically less injurious, using newer topical NSAID preparations, and/or using concomitant medical therapy to prevent NSAID-induced injury. Several nonselective NSAIDs that are associated with a lower likelihood of GI toxicity include diclofenac, aceclofenac, and ibuprofen, although the beneficial effect may be eliminated if higher dosages of the agents are used. Primary prevention of NSAID-induced ulceration can be accomplished by misoprostol (200 μg qid) or a PPI. High-dose H_2 blockers (famotidine, 40 mg bid) have also shown some promise in preventing endoscopically documented ulcers, although PPIs are superior. The highly selective COX-2 inhibitors, celecoxib and rofecoxib, are 100 times more selective inhibitors of COX-2 than standard NSAIDs, leading to gastric or duodenal mucosal injury that is comparable to placebo; their utilization led to an increase in cardiovascular events and withdrawal from the market. Additional caution was engendered when the CLASS study demonstrated that the advantage of celecoxib in preventing GI complications was offset when low-dose aspirin was used simultaneously. Therefore, gastric protection therapy is required in individuals taking COX-2 inhibitors and aspirin prophylaxis. Finally, much of the work demonstrating the benefit of COX-2 inhibitors and PPIs on GI injury has been performed in individuals of average risk; it is unclear if the same level of benefit will be achieved in high-risk patients. For example, concomitant use of warfarin and a COX-2 inhibitor was associated with rates of GI bleeding similar to those observed in patients taking nonselective NSAIDs. A combination of factors, including withdrawal of the majority of COX-2 inhibitors from the market, the observation that low-dose aspirin appears to diminish the beneficial effect of COX-2 selective inhibitors, and the growing use of aspirin for prophylaxis of cardiovascular events, have significantly altered the approach to gastric protective therapy during the use of NSAIDs. A set of guidelines for the approach to the use of NSAIDs was published by the American College of Gastroenterology and is shown in Table 348-6. Individuals who are not at risk for cardiovascular events, do not use aspirin, and are without risk for GI complications can receive nonselective NSAIDs without gastric protection. In those without cardiovascular risk factors but with a high potential risk (prior GI bleeding or multiple GI risk factors) for NSAID-induced GI toxicity, cautious use of a selective COX-2 inhibitor and co-therapy with misoprostol or high-dose PPI are recommended. Individuals at moderate GI risk without cardiac risk factors can be treated with a COX-2 inhibitor alone or with a nonselective NSAID with misoprostol or a PPI. Individuals with cardiovascular risk factors, who require low-dose aspirin and have low potential for NSAID-induced toxicity, should be considered for a non-NSAID agent or use of a traditional NSAID in combination with gastric protection, if warranted. Finally, individuals with cardiovascular and GI risks who require aspirin must be considered for non-NSAID therapy, but if that is not an option, then gastric protection with any type of NSAID must be considered. Any patient, regardless

TABLE 348-6 GUIDE TO NSAID THERAPY

	No/Low NSAID GI Risk	NSAID GI Risk
No CV risk (no aspirin)	Traditional NSAID	Coxib *or* Traditional NSAID + PPI *or* misoprostol Consider non-NSAID therapy
CV risk (consider aspirin)	Traditional NSAID + PPI *or* misoprostol if GI risk warrants gastroprotection Consider non-NSAID therapy	A gastroprotective agent must be added if a traditional NSAID is prescribed Consider non-NSAID therapy

Abbreviations: CV, cardiovascular; GI, gastrointestinal; NSAID, nonsteroidal anti-inflammatory drug; PPI, proton pump inhibitor.

Source: Adapted from AM Fendrick: Am J Manag Care 10:740, 2004. Reproduced with permission of INTELLISPHERE, LLC via Copyright Clearance Center.

of risk status, who is being considered for long-term traditional NSAID therapy, should also be considered for *H. pylori* testing and treatment if positive. Assuring the use of GI protective agents with NSAIDs is difficult, even in high-risk patients. This is in part due to underprescribing of the appropriate protective agent; other times the difficulty is related to patient compliance. The latter may be due to patients forgetting to take multiple pills or preferring not to take the extra pill, especially if they have no GI symptoms. Several NSAID gastroprotective-containing combination pills are now commercially available, including double-dose famotidine with ibuprofen, diclofenac with misoprostol, and naproxen with esomeprazole. Although initial studies suggested improved compliance and a cost advantage when taking these combination drugs, their clinical benefit over the use of separate pills has not been established. Efforts continue toward developing safer NSAIDs, including NO–releasing NSAIDs, hydrogen sulfide–releasing NSAIDs, dual COX/5-LOX inhibitors, NSAID prodrugs, or agents that can effectively sequester unbound NSAIDs without interfering with their efficacy.

APPROACH AND THERAPY: SUMMARY

Controversy continues regarding the best approach to the patient who presents with dyspepsia (**Chap. 54**). The discovery of *H. pylori* and its role in pathogenesis of ulcers has added a new variable to the equation. Previously, if a patient <50 years of age presented with dyspepsia and without alarming signs or symptoms suggestive of an ulcer complication or malignancy, an empirical therapeutic trial with acid suppression was commonly recommended. Although this approach is practiced by some today, an approach presently gaining approval for the treatment of patients with dyspepsia is outlined in **Fig. 348-12**. The referral to a gastroenterologist is for the potential need of endoscopy and subsequent evaluation and treatment if the endoscopy is negative.

Once an ulcer (GU or DU) is documented, the main issue at stake is whether *H. pylori* or an NSAID is involved. With *H. pylori* present, independent of the NSAID status, triple therapy is recommended for 14 days, followed by continued acid-suppressing drugs (H_2 receptor antagonist or PPIs) for a total of 4–6 weeks. Selection of patients for documentation of *H. pylori* eradication (organisms gone at least 4 weeks after completing antibiotics) is an area of some debate. The test of choice for documenting eradication is the laboratory-based validated monoclonal stool antigen test or a urea breath test (UBT). The patient must be off antisecretory agents when being tested for eradication of *H. pylori* with UBT or stool antigen. Serologic testing is not useful for the purpose of documenting eradication because antibody titers fall slowly and often do not become undetectable. Two approaches toward documentation of eradication exist: (1) Test for eradication only in individuals with a complicated course or in individuals who are frail or with multisystem disease who would do poorly with an ulcer recurrence, and (2) test all patients for

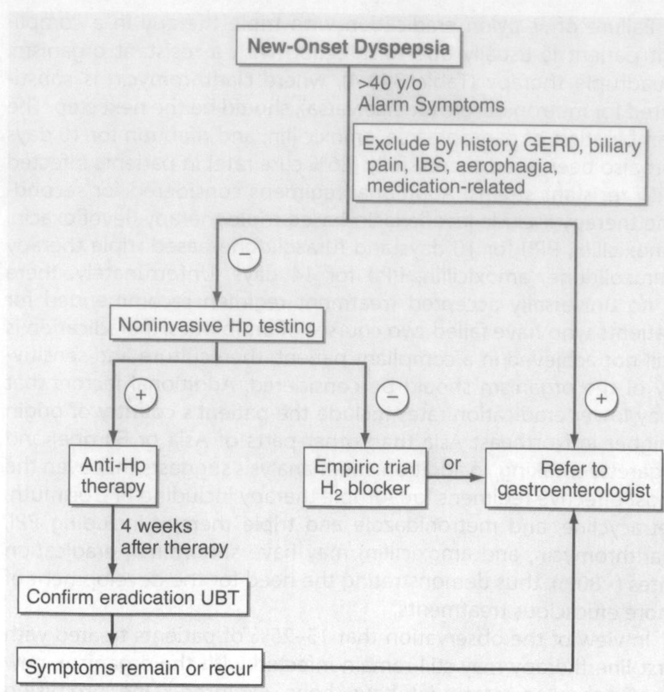

FIGURE 348-12 Overview of new-onset dyspepsia. GERD, gastroesophageal reflux disease; Hp, *Helicobacter pylori*; IBS, irritable bowel syndrome; UBT, urea breath test. *(Adapted from BS Anand and DY Graham: Endoscopy 31:215, 1999.)*

successful eradication. Some recommend that patients with complicated ulcer disease, or who are frail, should be treated with long-term acid suppression, thus making documentation of *H. pylori* eradication a moot point. In view of this discrepancy in practice, it would be best to discuss with the patient the different options available.

Several issues differentiate the approach to a GU versus a DU. GUs, especially of the body and fundus, have the potential of being malignant. Multiple biopsies of a GU should be taken initially; even if these are negative for neoplasm, repeat endoscopy to document healing at 8–12 weeks should be performed, with biopsy if the ulcer is still present. About 70% of GUs eventually found to be malignant undergo significant (usually incomplete) healing. Repeat endoscopy is warranted in patients with DU if symptoms persist despite medical therapy or a complication is suspected.

The majority (>90%) of GUs and DUs heal with the conventional therapy outlined above. A GU that fails to heal after 12 weeks and a DU that does not heal after 8 weeks of therapy should be considered refractory. Once poor compliance and persistent *H. pylori* infection have been excluded, NSAID use, either inadvertent or surreptitious, must be excluded. In addition, cigarette smoking must be eliminated. For a GU, malignancy must be meticulously excluded. Next, consideration should be given to a gastric acid hypersecretory state such as ZES (see "Zollinger-Ellison Syndrome," below) or the idiopathic form, which can be excluded with gastric acid analysis. Although a subset of patients have gastric acid hypersecretion of unclear etiology as a contributing factor to refractory ulcers, ZES should be excluded with a fasting gastrin or secretin stimulation test (see below). More than 90% of refractory ulcers (either DUs or GUs) heal after 8 weeks of treatment with higher doses of PPI (omeprazole, 40 mg/d; lansoprazole 30–60 mg/d). This higher dose is also effective in maintaining remission. Surgical intervention may be a consideration at this point; however, other rare causes of refractory ulcers must be excluded before recommending surgery. Rare etiologies of refractory ulcers that may be diagnosed by gastric or duodenal biopsies include ischemia, Crohn's disease, amyloidosis, sarcoidosis, lymphoma, eosinophilic gastroenteritis, or infection (cytomegalovirus [CMV], tuberculosis, or syphilis).

SURGICAL THERAPY

Surgical intervention in PUD can be viewed as being either elective, for treatment of medically refractory disease, or as urgent/emergent, for the treatment of an ulcer-related complication. The development of pharmacologic and endoscopic approaches for the treatment of peptic disease and its complications has led to a substantial decrease in the number of operations needed for this disorder with a drop of over 90% for elective ulcer surgery over the last four decades. Refractory ulcers are an exceedingly rare occurrence. Surgery is more often required for treatment of an ulcer-related complication.

Hemorrhage is the most common ulcer-related complication, occurring in ~15–25% of patients. Bleeding may occur in any age group but is most often seen in older patients (sixth decade or beyond). The majority of patients stop bleeding spontaneously, but endoscopic therapy (Chap. 345) is necessary in some. Parenterally and orally administered PPIs also decrease ulcer rebleeding in patients who have undergone endoscopic therapy. Patients unresponsive or refractory to endoscopic intervention will require surgery (~5% of transfusion-requiring patients).

Free peritoneal perforation occurs in ~2–3% of DU patients. As in the case of bleeding, up to 10% of these patients will not have antecedent ulcer symptoms. Concomitant bleeding may occur in up to 10% of patients with perforation, with mortality being increased substantially. Peptic ulcer can also penetrate into adjacent organs, especially with a posterior DU, which can penetrate into the pancreas, colon, liver, or biliary tree.

Pyloric channel ulcers or DUs can lead to gastric outlet obstruction in ~2–3% of patients. This can result from chronic scarring or from impaired motility due to inflammation and/or edema with pylorospasm. Patients may present with early satiety, nausea, vomiting of undigested food, and weight loss. Conservative management with nasogastric suction, intravenous hydration/nutrition, and antisecretory agents is indicated for 7–10 days with the hope that a functional obstruction will reverse. If a mechanical obstruction persists, endoscopic intervention with balloon dilation may be effective. Surgery should be considered if all else fails.

SPECIFIC OPERATIONS FOR DUODENAL ULCERS

Surgical treatment was originally designed to decrease gastric acid secretion. Operations most commonly performed include (1) vagotomy and drainage (by pyloroplasty, gastroduodenostomy, or gastrojejunostomy), (2) highly selective vagotomy (which does not require a drainage procedure), and (3) vagotomy with antrectomy. The specific procedure performed is dictated by the underlying circumstances: elective versus emergency, the degree and extent of duodenal ulceration, the etiology of the ulcer (*H. pylori*, NSAIDs, malignancy), and the expertise of the surgeon. Moreover, the trend has been toward a dramatic decrease in the need for surgery for treatment of refractory PUD, and when needed, minimally invasive and anatomy-preserving operations are preferred.

Vagotomy is a component of each of these procedures and is aimed at decreasing acid secretion through ablating cholinergic input to the stomach. Unfortunately, both truncal and selective vagotomy (preserves the celiac and hepatic branches) result in gastric atony despite successful reduction of both basal acid output (BAO; decreased by 85%) and maximal acid output (MAO; decreased by 50%). Drainage through pyloroplasty or gastroduodenostomy is required in an effort to compensate for the vagotomy-induced gastric motility disorder. This procedure has an intermediate complication rate and a 10% ulcer recurrence rate. To minimize gastric dysmotility, highly selective vagotomy (also known as parietal cell, super-selective, or proximal vagotomy) was developed. Only the vagal fibers innervating the portion of the stomach that contains parietal cells is transected, thus leaving fibers important for regulating gastric motility intact. Although this procedure leads to an immediate decrease in both BAO and stimulated acid output, acid secretion recovers over time. By the end of the first postoperative year, basal and stimulated acid output are ~30 and 50%, respectively, of preoperative levels. Ulcer recurrence rates are higher with highly selective vagotomy (≥10%), although the overall complication rates are the lowest of the three procedures.

The procedure that provides the lowest rates of ulcer recurrence (1%) but has the highest complication rate is vagotomy (truncal or selective) in combination with antrectomy. Antrectomy is aimed at eliminating an additional stimulant of gastric acid secretion, gastrin. Two principal types of reanastomoses are used after antrectomy: gastroduodenostomy (Billroth I) or gastrojejunostomy (Billroth II) (Fig. 348-13). Although Billroth I is often preferred over II, severe duodenal inflammation or scarring may preclude its performance. Prospective, randomized studies confirm that partial gastrectomy followed by Roux-en-Y reconstruction leads to a significantly better clinical, endoscopic, and histologic outcome than Billroth II reconstruction.

Of these procedures, highly selective vagotomy may be the one of choice in the elective setting, except in situations where ulcer recurrence rates are high (prepyloric ulcers and those refractory to medical therapy). Selection of vagotomy and antrectomy may be more appropriate in these circumstances.

These procedures have been traditionally performed by standard laparotomy. The advent of laparoscopic surgery has led several surgical teams to successfully perform highly selective vagotomy, truncal vagotomy/pyloroplasty, and truncal vagotomy/antrectomy through this approach. An increase in the number of laparoscopic procedures for treatment of PUD has occurred. Laparoscopic repair of perforated peptic ulcers is safe, feasible for the experienced surgeon and is associated with decreased postoperative pain, although it does take longer than an open approach. Moreover, no difference between the two approaches is noted in postoperative complications or length of hospital stay.

Specific Operations for Gastric Ulcers The location and the presence of a concomitant DU dictate the operative procedure performed for a GU. Antrectomy (including the ulcer) with a Billroth I

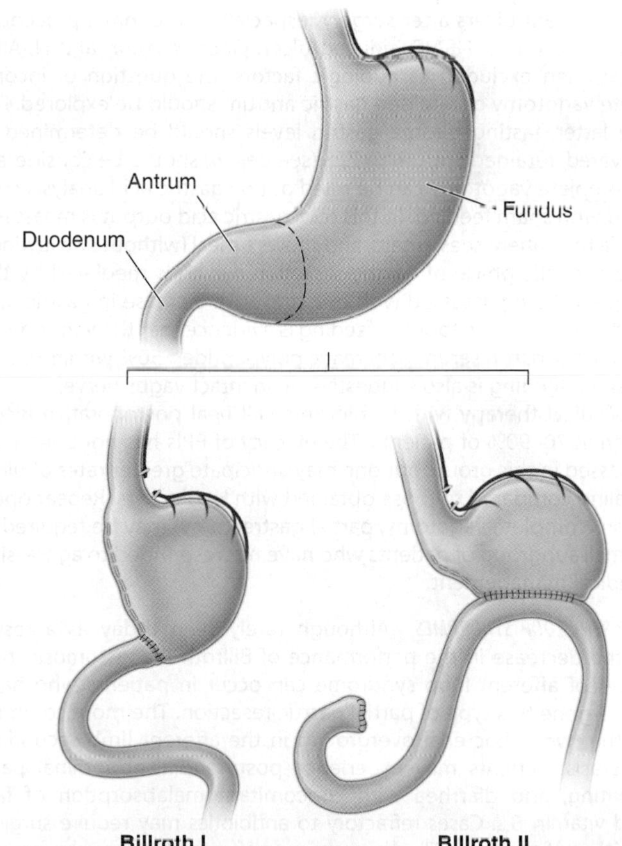

FIGURE 348-13 Schematic representation of Billroth I and II procedures.

anastomosis is the treatment of choice for an antral ulcer. Vagotomy is performed only if a DU is present. Although ulcer excision with vagotomy and drainage procedure has been proposed, the higher incidence of ulcer recurrence makes this a less desirable approach. Ulcers located near the esophagogastric junction may require a more radical approach, a subtotal gastrectomy with a Roux-en-Y esophagogastrojejunostomy (Csendes' procedure). A less aggressive approach, including antrectomy, intraoperative ulcer biopsy, and vagotomy (Kelling-Madlener procedure), may be indicated in fragile patients with a high GU. Ulcer recurrence approaches 30% with this procedure.

Surgery-Related Complications Complications seen after surgery for PUD are related primarily to the extent of the anatomic modification performed. Minimal alteration (highly selective vagotomy) is associated with higher rates of ulcer recurrence and less GI disturbance. More aggressive surgical procedures have a lower rate of ulcer recurrence but a greater incidence of GI dysfunction. Overall, morbidity and mortality related to these procedures are quite low. Morbidity associated with vagotomy and antrectomy or pyloroplasty is ≤5%, with mortality ~1%. Highly selective vagotomy has lower morbidity and mortality rates of 1 and 0.3%, respectively.

In addition to the potential early consequences of any intraabdominal procedure (bleeding, infection, thromboembolism), gastroparesis, duodenal stump leak, and efferent loop obstruction can be observed.

RECURRENT ULCERATION The risk of ulcer recurrence is directly related to the procedure performed. Ulcers that recur after partial gastric resection tend to develop at the anastomosis (stomal or marginal ulcer). Epigastric abdominal pain is the most frequent presenting complaint (>90%). Severity and duration of pain tend to be more progressive than observed with DUs before surgery.

Ulcers may recur for several reasons, including incomplete vagotomy, inadequate drainage, retained antrum, and, less likely, persistent or recurrent *H. pylori* infection. ZES should have been excluded preoperatively. Surreptitious use of NSAIDs is an important reason for recurrent ulcers after surgery, especially if the initial procedure was done for an NSAID-induced ulcer. Once *H. pylori* and NSAIDs have been excluded as etiologic factors, the question of incomplete vagotomy or retained gastric antrum should be explored. For the latter, fasting plasma gastrin levels should be determined. If elevated, retained antrum or ZES (see below) should be considered. Incomplete vagotomy can be ruled out by gastric acid analysis coupled with sham feeding. In this test, gastric acid output is measured while the patient sees, smells, and chews a meal (without swallowing). The cephalic phase of gastric secretion, which is mediated by the vagus, is being assessed with this study. An increase in gastric acid output in response to sham feeding is evidence that the vagus nerve is intact. A rise in serum pancreatic polypeptide >50% within 30 min of sham feeding is also suggestive of an intact vagus nerve.

Medical therapy with H_2 blockers will heal postoperative ulceration in 70–90% of patients. The efficacy of PPIs has not been fully assessed in this group, but one may anticipate greater rates of ulcer healing compared to those obtained with H_2 blockers. Repeat operation (complete vagotomy, partial gastrectomy) may be required in a small subgroup of patients who have not responded to aggressive medical management.

AFFERENT LOOP SYNDROMES Although rarely seen today as a result of the decrease in the performance of Billroth II anastomosis, two types of afferent loop syndrome can occur in patients who have undergone this type of partial gastric resection. The more common of the two is bacterial overgrowth in the afferent limb secondary to stasis. Patients may experience postprandial abdominal pain, bloating, and diarrhea with concomitant malabsorption of fats and vitamin B_{12}. Cases refractory to antibiotics may require surgical revision of the loop. The less common afferent loop syndrome can present with severe abdominal pain and bloating that occur 20–60 min after meals. Pain is often followed by nausea and vomiting of bile-containing material. The pain and bloating may improve after emesis. The cause of this clinical picture is theorized to be incomplete drainage of bile and pancreatic secretions from an afferent loop that is partially obstructed. Cases refractory to dietary measures may need surgical revision or conversion of the Billroth II anastomosis to a Roux-en-Y gastrojejunostomy.

DUMPING SYNDROME Dumping syndrome consists of a series of vasomotor and GI signs and symptoms and occurs in patients who have undergone vagotomy and drainage (especially Billroth procedures). Two phases of dumping, early and late, can occur. Early dumping takes place 15–30 min after meals and consists of crampy abdominal discomfort, nausea, diarrhea, belching, tachycardia, palpitations, diaphoresis, light-headedness, and, rarely, syncope. These signs and symptoms arise from the rapid emptying of hyperosmolar gastric contents into the small intestine, resulting in a fluid shift into the gut lumen with plasma volume contraction and acute intestinal distention. Release of vasoactive GI hormones (vasoactive intestinal polypeptide, neurotensin, motilin) is also theorized to play a role in early dumping.

The late phase of dumping typically occurs 90 min to 3 h after meals. Vasomotor symptoms (light-headedness, diaphoresis, palpitations, tachycardia, and syncope) predominate during this phase. This component of dumping is thought to be secondary to hypoglycemia from excessive insulin release.

Dumping syndrome is most noticeable after meals rich in simple carbohydrates (especially sucrose) and high osmolarity. Ingestion of large amounts of fluids may also contribute. Up to 50% of postvagotomy and drainage patients will experience dumping syndrome to some degree early on. Signs and symptoms often improve with time, but a severe protracted picture can occur in up to 1% of patients.

Dietary modification is the cornerstone of therapy for patients with dumping syndrome. Small, multiple (six) meals devoid of simple carbohydrates coupled with elimination of liquids during meals is important. Antidiarrheals and anticholinergic agents are complementary to diet. Guar and pectin, which increase the viscosity of intraluminal contents, may be beneficial in more symptomatic individuals. Acarbose, an α-glucosidase inhibitor that delays digestion of ingested carbohydrates, has also been shown to be beneficial in the treatment of the late phases of dumping. The somatostatin analogue octreotide has been successful in diet-refractory cases. This drug is administered subcutaneously (50 μg tid), titrated according to clinical response. A long-acting depot formulation of octreotide can be administered once every 28 days and provides symptom relief comparable to the short-acting agent. In addition, patient weight gain and quality of life appear to be superior with the long-acting form.

POSTVAGOTOMY DIARRHEA Up to 10% of patients may seek medical attention for the treatment of postvagotomy diarrhea. This complication is most commonly observed after truncal vagotomy, which is rarely performed today. Patients may complain of intermittent diarrhea that occurs typically 1–2 h after meals. Occasionally the symptoms may be severe and relentless. This is due to a motility disorder from interruption of the vagal fibers supplying the luminal gut. Other contributing factors may include decreased absorption of nutrients (see below), increased excretion of bile acids, and release of luminal factors that promote secretion. Diphenoxylate or loperamide is often useful in symptom control. The bile salt–binding agent cholestyramine may be helpful in severe cases. Surgical reversal of a 10-cm segment of jejunum may yield a substantial improvement in bowel frequency in a subset of patients.

BILE REFLUX GASTROPATHY A subset of post–partial gastrectomy patients who present with abdominal pain, early satiety, nausea, and vomiting will have mucosal erythema of the gastric remnant as the only finding. Histologic examination of the gastric mucosa reveals minimal inflammation but the presence of epithelial cell injury. This clinical picture is categorized as bile or alkaline reflux gastropathy/gastritis. Although reflux of bile is implicated as the reason for this disorder, the mechanism is unknown. Prokinetic agents, cholestyramine, and sucralfate have been somewhat effective treatments. Severe refractory symptoms may require using either nuclear scanning with ^{99m}Tc-HIDA to document reflux or an alkaline challenge test, where 0.1 *N* NaOH is infused into the stomach in an effort to reproduce the patient's symptoms. Surgical diversion of pancreaticobiliary secretions away from the gastric remnant with a Roux-en-Y gastrojejunostomy consisting of a long (50–60 cm) Roux limb has been used in severe cases. Bilious vomiting improves, but early satiety and bloating may persist in up to 50% of patients.

MALDIGESTION AND MALABSORPTION Weight loss can be observed in up to 60% of patients after partial gastric resection. Patients can experience a 10% loss of body weight, which stabilizes 3 months postoperatively. A significant component of this weight reduction is due to decreased oral intake. However, mild steatorrhea can also develop. Reasons for maldigestion/malabsorption include decreased gastric acid production, rapid gastric emptying, decreased food dispersion in the stomach, reduced luminal bile concentration, reduced pancreatic secretory response to feeding, and rapid intestinal transit.

Decreased serum vitamin B_{12} levels can be observed after partial gastrectomy. This is usually not due to deficiency of IF, since a minimal amount of parietal cells (source of IF) are removed during antrectomy. Reduced vitamin B_{12} may be due to competition for the vitamin by bacterial overgrowth or inability to split the vitamin from its protein-bound source due to hypochlorhydria.

Iron-deficiency anemia may be a consequence of impaired absorption of dietary iron in patients with a Billroth II gastrojejunostomy. Absorption of iron salts is normal in these individuals; thus, a favorable response to oral iron supplementation can be anticipated. Folate deficiency with concomitant anemia can also develop in these patients. This deficiency may be secondary to decreased absorption or diminished oral intake.

Malabsorption of vitamin D and calcium resulting in osteoporosis and osteomalacia is common after partial gastrectomy and gastrojejunostomy (Billroth II). Osteomalacia can occur as a late complication in up to 25% of post–partial gastrectomy patients. Bone fractures occur twice as commonly in men after gastric surgery as in a control population. It may take years before x-ray findings demonstrate diminished bone density. Elevated alkaline phosphatase, reduced serum calcium, bone pain, and pathologic fractures may be seen in patients with osteomalacia. The high incidence of these abnormalities in this subgroup of patients justifies treating them with vitamin D and calcium supplementation indefinitely. Therapy is especially important in females. Copper deficiency has also been reported in patients undergoing surgeries that bypass the duodenum, where copper is primarily absorbed. Patients may present with a rare syndrome that includes ataxia, myelopathy, and peripheral neuropathy.

GASTRIC ADENOCARCINOMA The incidence of adenocarcinoma in the gastric stump is increased 15 years after resection. Some have reported a four- to fivefold increase in gastric cancer 20–25 years after resection. The pathogenesis is unclear but may involve alkaline reflux, bacterial proliferation, or hypochlorhydria. The role of endoscopic screening is not clear, and most guidelines do not support its use.

ADDITIONAL COMPLICATIONS Reflux esophagitis and a higher incidence of gallstones and cholecystitis have been reported to patients undergoing subtotal gastrectomy. The latter is thought to be due to decreased gallbladder contractility associated with vagotomy and bypass of the duodenum, leading to decreased postprandial release of cholecystokinin.

RELATED CONDITIONS

ZOLLINGER–ELLISON SYNDROME

Severe peptic ulcer diathesis secondary to gastric acid hypersecretion due to unregulated gastrin release from a non-β cell endocrine tumor (gastrinoma) defines the components of ZES. Initially, ZES was typified by aggressive and refractory ulceration in which total gastrectomy provided the only chance for enhancing survival. Today it can be cured by surgical resection in up to 40% of patients.

Epidemiology The incidence of ZES varies from 0.1–1% of individuals presenting with PUD. Males are more commonly affected than females, and the majority of patients are diagnosed between ages 30 and 50. Gastrinomas are classified into sporadic tumors (more common) and those associated with multiple endocrine neoplasia (MEN) type 1 (see below). The widespread availability and use of PPIs has led to a decreased patient referral for gastrinoma evaluation, delay in diagnosis, and an increase in false-positive diagnoses of ZES. In fact, diagnosis may be delayed for 6 or more years after symptoms consistent with ZES are displayed.

Pathophysiology Hypergastrinemia originating from an autonomous neoplasm is the driving force responsible for the clinical manifestations in ZES. Gastrin stimulates acid secretion through gastrin receptors on parietal cells and by inducing histamine release from ECL cells. Gastrin also has a trophic action on gastric epithelial cells. Longstanding hypergastrinemia leads to markedly increased gastric acid secretion through both parietal cell stimulation and increased parietal cell mass. The increased gastric acid output leads to peptic ulcer diathesis, erosive esophagitis, and diarrhea.

Tumor Distribution Although early studies suggested that the vast majority of gastrinomas occurred within the pancreas, a significant number of these lesions are extrapancreatic. Over 80% of these tumors are found within the hypothetical gastrinoma triangle (confluence of the cystic and common bile ducts superiorly, junction of the second and third portions of the duodenum inferiorly, and junction of the neck and body of the pancreas medially). Duodenal tumors constitute the most common nonpancreatic lesion; between 50 and 75% of gastrinomas are found here. Duodenal tumors are smaller, slower growing, and less likely to metastasize than pancreatic lesions. Less common extrapancreatic sites include stomach, bones, ovaries, heart, liver, and lymph nodes. More than 60% of tumors are considered malignant, with up to 30–50% of patients having multiple lesions or metastatic disease at presentation. Histologically, gastrin-producing cells appear well-differentiated, expressing markers typically found in endocrine neoplasms (chromogranin, neuron-specific enolase).

Clinical Manifestations Gastric acid hypersecretion is responsible for the signs and symptoms observed in patients with ZES. Peptic ulcer is the most common clinical manifestation, occurring in >90% of gastrinoma patients. Initial presentation and ulcer location (duodenal bulb) may be indistinguishable from common PUD. Clinical situations that should create suspicion of gastrinoma are ulcers in unusual locations (second part of the duodenum and beyond), ulcers refractory to standard medical therapy, ulcer recurrence after acid-reducing surgery, ulcers presenting with frank complications (bleeding, obstruction, and perforation), or ulcers in the absence of *H. pylori* or NSAID ingestion. Symptoms of esophageal origin are present in up to two-thirds of patients with ZES, with a spectrum ranging from mild esophagitis to frank ulceration with stricture and Barrett's mucosa.

Diarrhea, the next most common clinical manifestation, is found in up to 50% of patients. Although diarrhea often occurs concomitantly with acid peptic disease, it may also occur independent of an ulcer. Etiology of the diarrhea is multifactorial, resulting from marked volume overload to the small bowel, pancreatic enzyme inactivation by acid, and damage of the intestinal epithelial surface by acid. The epithelial damage can lead to a mild degree of maldigestion and malabsorption of nutrients. The diarrhea may also have a secretory component due to the direct stimulatory effect of gastrin on enterocytes or the co-secretion of additional hormones from the tumor such as vasoactive intestinal peptide.

Gastrinomas can develop in the presence of MEN 1 syndrome (Chaps. 113 and 408) in ~25% of patients. This autosomal dominant disorder involves primarily three organ sites: the parathyroid glands (80–90%), pancreas (40–80%), and pituitary gland (30–60%). The syndrome is caused by inactivating mutations of the *MEN1* tumor suppressor gene found on the long arm of chromosome 11q13. The gene encodes for Menin, which has an important role in DNA replication and transcriptional regulation. A genetic diagnosis is obtained by sequencing of the *MEN1* gene, which can reveal mutations in 70–90% of typical MEN 1 cases. A family may have an unknown mutation, making a genetic diagnosis impossible, and therefore certain individuals will require a clinical diagnosis, which is determined by whether a patient has tumors in two of the three endocrine organs (parathyroid, pancreas/duodenum, or pituitary) or has a family history of MEN 1 and one of the endocrine organ tumors. In view of the stimulatory effect of calcium on gastric secretion, the hyperparathyroidism and hypercalcemia seen in MEN 1 patients may have a direct effect on ulcer disease. Resolution of hypercalcemia by parathyroidectomy reduces gastrin and gastric acid output in gastrinoma patients. An additional distinguishing feature in ZES patients with MEN 1 is the higher incidence of gastric carcinoid tumor development (as compared to patients with sporadic gastrinomas). ZES presents and is diagnosed earlier in MEN 1 patients, and they have a more indolent course as compared to patients with sporadic gastrinoma. Gastrinomas tend to be smaller, multiple, and located in the duodenal wall more often than is seen in patients with sporadic ZES. Establishing the diagnosis of MEN 1 is critical in order to provide genetic counseling to the patient and his or her family and also to determine the recommended surgical approach.

Diagnosis Biochemical measurements of gastrin and acid secretion in patients suspected of ZES play an important role is establishing this rare diagnosis. Often, patients suspected of having ZES will be treated with a PPI in an effort to ameliorate symptoms and decrease the likelihood of possible acid-related complications. The presence of the PPI, which will lower acid secretion and potentially elevate fasting gastrin levels in normal individuals, will make the diagnostic approach in these individuals somewhat difficult. Significant morbidity related to peptic diathesis has been described when stopping PPIs in gastrinoma patients; therefore, a systematic approach in stopping these agents is warranted (see below). The first step in the evaluation of a patient suspected of having ZES is to obtain a fasting gastrin level. A list of clinical scenarios that should arouse suspicion regarding this diagnosis is shown in Table 348-7. Fasting gastrin levels obtained using a dependable assay are usually <150 pg/mL. A normal fasting gastrin, on two separate occasions, especially if the patient is on a PPI, virtually excludes this diagnosis. Virtually all gastrinoma patients will have a gastrin level >150–200 pg/mL. Measurement of fasting gastrin should be repeated to confirm the clinical suspicion. Some of the commercial biochemical assays used for measuring serum gastrin may be inaccurate. Variable specificity of the antibodies used have led to both false-positive and false-negative fasting gastrin levels, placing in jeopardy the ability to make an accurate diagnosis of ZES.

Multiple processes can lead to an elevated fasting gastrin level, the most frequent of which are gastric hypochlorhydria and achlorhydria, with or without pernicious anemia. Gastric acid induces feedback inhibition of gastrin release. A decrease in acid production will subsequently lead to failure of the feedback inhibitory pathway, resulting in net hypergastrinemia. Gastrin levels will thus be high in patients using antisecretory agents for the treatment of acid peptic disorders and dyspepsia. *H. pylori* infection can also cause hypergastrinemia. Additional causes of elevated gastrin include retained gastric antrum; G cell hyperplasia; gastric outlet obstruction; renal insufficiency; massive small-bowel obstruction; and conditions such as rheumatoid arthritis, vitiligo, diabetes mellitus, and pheochromocytoma. Although a fasting gastrin >10 times normal is highly suggestive of ZES, two-thirds of patients will have fasting gastrin levels that overlap with levels found in the more common disorders outlined above, especially if a PPI is being taken by the patient. The effect of the PPI on gastrin levels and acid secretion will linger several days after stopping the PPI; therefore, it should be stopped for a minimum of 7 days before testing. During this period, the patient should be placed on a histamine H_2 antagonist, such as famotidine, twice to three times per day. Although this type of agent has a short-term effect on gastrin and acid secretion, it needs to be stopped 24 h before repeating fasting gastrin levels or performing some the tests highlighted below. The patient may take antacids for the final day, stopping them approximately 12 h before testing is performed. Heightened awareness of complications related to gastric acid hypersecretion during the period of PPI cessation is critical.

The next step in establishing a biochemical diagnosis of gastrinoma is to assess acid secretion. Nothing further needs to be done if decreased acid output in the absence of a PPI is observed. A pH can be measured on gastric fluid obtained either during endoscopy or through nasogastric aspiration; a pH <3 is suggestive of a gastrinoma, but a pH >3 is not helpful in excluding the diagnosis. In those situations where the pH is >3, formal gastric acid analysis should be performed if available. Normal BAO in nongastric surgery patients is typically <5 meq/h. A BAO >15 meq/h in the presence of hypergastrinemia is considered pathognomonic of ZES, but up to 12% of patients with common PUD may have elevated BAO to a lesser degree that can overlap with levels seen in ZES patients. In an effort to improve the sensitivity and specificity of gastric secretory studies, a BAO/MAO ratio was established using pentagastrin infusion as a way to maximally stimulate acid production, with a BAO/MAO ratio >0.6 being highly suggestive of ZES. Pentagastrin is no longer available in the United States, making measurement of MAO virtually impossible. An endoscopic method for measuring gastric acid output has been developed but requires further validation.

Gastrin provocative tests have been developed in an effort to differentiate between the causes of hypergastrinemia and are especially helpful in patients with indeterminate acid secretory studies. The tests are the secretin stimulation test and the calcium infusion study. The most sensitive and specific gastrin provocative test for the diagnosis of gastrinoma is the secretin study. An increase in gastrin of ≥120 pg within 15 min of secretin injection has a sensitivity and specificity of >90% for ZES. PPI-induced hypochlorhydria or achlorhydria may lead to a false-positive secretin test; thus, this agent must be stopped for 1 week before testing.

The calcium infusion study is less sensitive and specific than the secretin test, which, coupled with it being a more cumbersome study with greater potential for adverse effects, relegates it to rare utilization in the cases where the patient's clinical characteristics are highly suggestive of ZES but the secretin stimulation is inconclusive.

TABLE 348-7 WHEN TO OBTAIN A FASTING SERUM GASTRIN LEVEL

Multiple ulcers
Ulcers in unusual locations; associated with severe esophagitis; resistant to therapy with frequent recurrences; in the absence of nonsteroidal anti-inflammatory drug ingestion or *H. pylori* infection
Ulcer patients awaiting surgery
Extensive family history for peptic ulcer disease
Postoperative ulcer recurrence
Basal hyperchlorhydria
Unexplained diarrhea or steatorrhea
Hypercalcemia
Family history of pancreatic islet, pituitary, or parathyroid tumor
Prominent gastric or duodenal folds

Tumor Localization Once the biochemical diagnosis of gastrinoma has been confirmed, the tumor must be located. Multiple imaging studies have been used in an effort to enhance tumor localization (Table 348-8). The broad range of sensitivity is due to the variable success rates achieved by the different investigative groups. Endoscopic ultrasound (EUS) permits imaging of the pancreas with a high degree of resolution (<5 mm). This modality is particularly helpful in excluding small neoplasms within the pancreas and in assessing the presence of surrounding lymph nodes and vascular involvement, but it is not very sensitive for finding duodenal lesions. Several types of endocrine tumors express cell-surface receptors for somatostatin. This permits the localization of gastrinomas by measuring the uptake of the stable somatostatin analogue ^{111}In-pentreotide (OctreoScan) with sensitivity and specificity rates of >85%.

TABLE 348-8 SENSITIVITY OF IMAGING STUDIES IN ZOLLINGER-ELLISON SYNDROME

	Sensitivity, %	
Study	**Primary Gastrinoma**	**Metastatic Gastrinoma**
Ultrasound	21–28	14
CT scan	55–70	>85
Selective angiography	35–68	33–86
Portal venous sampling	70–90	N/A
SASI	55–78	41
MRI	55–70	>85
OctreoScan	67–86	80–100
EUS	80–100	N/A

Abbreviations: CT, computed tomography; EUS, endoscopic ultrasonography; MRI, magnetic resonance imaging; N/A, not applicable; OctreoScan, imaging with ^{111}In-pentreotide; SASI, selective arterial secretin injection.

Up to 50% of patients have metastatic disease at diagnosis. Success in controlling gastric acid hypersecretion has shifted the emphasis of therapy toward providing a surgical cure. Detecting the primary tumor and excluding metastatic disease are critical in view of this paradigm shift. Once a biochemical diagnosis has been confirmed, the patient should first undergo an abdominal computed tomography (CT) scan, magnetic resonance imaging (MRI), or OctreoScan (depending on availability) to exclude metastatic disease. In addition, the positron emitter ^{68}Ga has been used to label somatostatin analogues for positron emission tomography (PET) with some success. In addition, hybrid scanners combining CT scan with PET scan are also available in certain specialized centers. Once metastatic disease has been excluded, an experienced endocrine surgeon may opt for exploratory laparotomy with intraoperative ultrasound or transillumination. In other centers, careful examination of the peripancreatic area with EUS, accompanied by endoscopic exploration of the duodenum for primary tumors, will be performed before surgery. Selective arterial secretin injection may be a useful adjuvant for localizing tumors in a subset of patients. The extent of the diagnostic and surgical approach must be carefully balanced with the patient's overall physiologic condition and the natural history of a slow-growing gastrinoma.

TREATMENT ZOLLINGER-ELLISON SYNDROME

Treatment of functional endocrine tumors is directed at ameliorating the signs and symptoms related to hormone overproduction, curative resection of the neoplasm, and attempts to control tumor growth in metastatic disease.

PPIs are the treatment of choice and have decreased the need for total gastrectomy. Initial PPI doses tend to be higher than those used for treatment of GERD or PUD. The initial dose of omeprazole, lansoprazole, rabeprazole, or esomeprazole should be in the range of 60 mg in divided doses in a 24-h period. Dosing can be adjusted to achieve a BAO <10 meq/h (at the drug trough) in surgery-naive patients and to <5 meq/h in individuals who have previously undergone an acid-reducing operation. Although the somatostatin analogue has inhibitory effects on gastrin release from receptor-bearing tumors and inhibits gastric acid secretion to some extent, PPIs have the advantage of reducing parietal cell activity to a greater degree. Despite this, octreotide may be considered as adjunctive therapy to the PPI in patients with tumors that express somatostatin receptors and have peptic symptoms that are difficult to control with high-dose PPI.

The ultimate goal of surgery would be to provide a definitive cure. Improved understanding of tumor distribution has led to immediate cure rates as high as 60% with 10-year disease-free intervals as high as 34% in sporadic gastrinoma patients undergoing surgery. A positive outcome is highly dependent on the experience of the surgical team treating these rare tumors. Surgical therapy of gastrinoma patients with MEN 1 remains controversial because of the difficulty in rendering these patients disease-free with surgery. In contrast to the encouraging postoperative results observed in patients with sporadic disease, only 6% of MEN 1 patients are disease free 5 years after an operation. Moreover, in contrast to patients with sporadic ZES, the clinical course of MEN 1 patients is benign and rarely leads to disease-related mortality, recommending that early surgery be deferred. Some groups suggest surgery only if a clearly identifiable, nonmetastatic lesion is documented by structural studies. Others advocate a more aggressive approach, where all patients free of hepatic metastasis are explored and all detected tumors in the duodenum are resected; this is followed by enucleation of lesions in the pancreatic head, with a distal pancreatectomy to follow. The outcome of the two approaches has not been clearly defined. Laparoscopic surgical interventions may provide attractive approaches in the future but currently seem to be of some limited benefit in patients with gastrinoma because a significant percentage of the tumors may be extrapancreatic and difficult to localize with a laparoscopic approach. Finally, patients selected for surgery should be individuals whose health status would lead them to tolerate a more aggressive operation and obtain the long-term benefits from such aggressive surgery, which are often witnessed after 10 years.

Therapy of metastatic endocrine tumors in general remains suboptimal; gastrinomas are no exception. In light of the observation that in many instances tumor growth is indolent and that many individuals with metastatic disease remain relatively stable for significant periods of time, many advocate not instituting systemic tumor-targeted therapy until evidence of tumor progression or refractory symptoms not controlled with PPIs are noted. Medical approaches, including biological therapy (IFN-α, long-acting somatostatin analogues, peptide receptor radionuclides), systemic chemotherapy (streptozotocin, 5-fluorouracil, and doxorubicin), and hepatic artery embolization, may lead to significant toxicity without a substantial improvement in overall survival. ^{111}In pentetreotide has been used in the therapy of metastatic neuroendocrine tumors; further studies are needed. Several novel therapies are being explored, including radiofrequency ablation or cryoablation of liver lesions and use of agents that block the vascular endothelial growth receptor pathway (bevacizumab, sunitinib) or the mammalian target of rapamycin (Chap. 113).

Surgical approaches, including debulking surgery and liver transplantation for hepatic metastasis, have also produced limited benefit.

The overall 5- and 10-year survival rates for gastrinoma patients are 62–75% and 47–53%, respectively. Individuals with the entire tumor resected or those with a negative laparotomy have 5- and 10-year survival rates >90%. Patients with incompletely resected tumors have 5- and 10-year survival rates of 43% and 25%, respectively. Patients with hepatic metastasis have <20% survival at 5 years. Favorable prognostic indicators include primary duodenal wall tumors, isolated lymph node tumor, the presence of MEN 1, and undetectable tumor upon surgical exploration. Poor outcome is seen in patients with shorter disease duration; higher gastrin levels (>10,000 pg/mL); large pancreatic primary tumors (>3 cm); metastatic disease to lymph nodes, liver, and bone; and Cushing's syndrome. Rapid growth of hepatic metastases is also predictive of poor outcome.

STRESS-RELATED MUCOSAL INJURY

Patients suffering from shock, sepsis, massive burns, severe trauma, or head injury can develop acute erosive gastric mucosal changes or frank ulceration with bleeding. Classified as stress-induced gastritis or ulcers, injury is most commonly observed in the acid-producing (fundus and body) portions of the stomach. The most common presentation is GI bleeding, which is usually minimal but can occasionally be life threatening. Respiratory failure requiring mechanical ventilation and underlying coagulopathy are risk factors for bleeding, which tends to occur 48–72 h after the acute injury or insult.

Histologically, stress injury does not contain inflammation or *H. pylori*; thus, "gastritis" is a misnomer. Although elevated gastric acid secretion may be noted in patients with stress ulceration after head trauma (Cushing's ulcer) and severe burns (Curling's ulcer), mucosal ischemia, breakdown of the normal protective barriers of the stomach, systemic release of cytokines, poor GI motility, and oxidative stress also play an important role in the pathogenesis. Acid must contribute to injury in view of the significant drop in bleeding noted when acid inhibitors are used as prophylaxis for stress gastritis.

Improvement in the general management of intensive care unit patients has led to a significant decrease in the incidence of GI bleeding due to stress ulceration. The estimated decrease in bleeding is from 20–30% to <5%. This improvement has led to some debate regarding the need for prophylactic therapy. The high mortality associated with stress-induced clinically important GI bleeding (>40%) and the limited benefit of medical (endoscopic, angiographic) and surgical therapy in a patient with hemodynamically compromising bleeding associated with stress ulcer/gastritis support the use of preventive measures in high-risk patients (mechanically ventilated, coagulopathy, multiorgan failure, or severe burns). Maintenance of gastric pH >3.5 with continuous infusion of H_2 blockers or liquid antacids administered every 2–3 h are viable options. Tolerance to the H_2 blocker is likely to develop; thus, careful monitoring of the gastric pH and dose adjustment are important if H_2 blockers are used. Sucralfate slurry (1 g every 4–6 h) has also been somewhat successful but requires a gastric tube and may lead to constipation and aluminum toxicity. Sucralfate use in endotracheal intubated patients has also been associated with aspiration pneumonia. Meta-analysis comparing H_2 blockers with PPIs for the prevention of stress-associated clinically important and overt GI bleeding demonstrates superiority of the latter without increasing the risk of nosocomial infections, increasing mortality, or prolonging intensive care unit length of stay. Therefore, PPIs are the treatment of choice for stress prophylaxis. Oral PPI is the best option if the patient can tolerate enteral administration. Pantoprazole is available as an intravenous formulation for individuals in whom enteral administration is not possible. If bleeding occurs despite these measures, endoscopy, intra-arterial vasopressin, and embolization are options. If all else fails, then surgery should be considered. Although vagotomy and antrectomy may be used, the better approach would be a total gastrectomy, which has an exceedingly high mortality rate in this setting.

GASTRITIS

The term *gastritis* should be reserved for histologically documented inflammation of the gastric mucosa. Gastritis is not the mucosal erythema seen during endoscopy and is not interchangeable with "dyspepsia." The etiologic factors leading to gastritis are broad and heterogeneous. Gastritis has been classified based on time course (acute vs chronic), histologic features, and anatomic distribution or proposed pathogenic mechanism (Table 348-9).

The correlation between the histologic findings of gastritis, the clinical picture of abdominal pain or dyspepsia, and endoscopic findings noted on gross inspection of the gastric mucosa is poor. Therefore, there is no typical clinical manifestation of gastritis.

Acute Gastritis The most common causes of acute gastritis are infectious. Acute infection with *H. pylori* induces gastritis. However, *H. pylori* acute gastritis has not been extensively studied. It is reported as presenting with sudden onset of epigastric pain, nausea, and vomiting, and limited mucosal histologic studies demonstrate a marked infiltrate of neutrophils with edema and hyperemia. If not treated, this picture will evolve into one of chronic gastritis. Hypochlorhydria lasting for up to 1 year may follow acute *H. pylori* infection.

Bacterial infection of the stomach or phlegmonous gastritis is a rare, potentially life-threatening disorder characterized by marked and diffuse acute inflammatory infiltrates of the entire gastric wall, at times accompanied by necrosis. Elderly individuals, alcoholics, and AIDS patients may be affected. Potential iatrogenic causes include polypectomy and mucosal injection with India ink. Organisms associated with this entity include streptococci, staphylococci, *Escherichia coli, Proteus,* and *Haemophilus* species. Failure of supportive measures and antibiotics may result in gastrectomy.

TABLE 348-9 CLASSIFICATION OF GASTRITIS

I. Acute gastritis
   A. Acute *H. pylori* infection
   B. Other acute Infectious gastritides
      1. Bacterial (other than *H. pylori*)
      2. *H. heilmannii*
      3. Phlegmonous
      4. Mycobacterial
      5. Syphilitic
      6. Viral
      7. Parasitic
      8. Fungal
II. Chronic atrophic gastritis
   A. Type A: Autoimmune, body-predominant
   B. Type B: *H. pylori*–related, antral-predominant
   C. Indeterminate
III. Uncommon forms of gastritis
   A. Lymphocytic
   B. Eosinophilic
   C. Crohn's disease
   D. Sarcoidosis
   E. Isolated granulomatous gastritis
   F. Russell body gastritis

Other types of infectious gastritis may occur in immunocompromised individuals such as AIDS patients. Examples include herpetic (herpes simplex) or CMV gastritis. The histologic finding of intranuclear inclusions would be observed in the latter.

Chronic Gastritis Chronic gastritis is identified histologically by an inflammatory cell infiltrate consisting primarily of lymphocytes and plasma cells, with very scant neutrophil involvement. Distribution of the inflammation may be patchy, initially involving superficial and glandular portions of the gastric mucosa. This picture may progress to more severe glandular destruction, with atrophy and metaplasia. Chronic gastritis has been classified according to histologic characteristics. These include superficial atrophic changes and gastric atrophy. The association of atrophic gastritis with the development of gastric cancer has led to the development of endoscopic and serologic markers of severity. Some of these include gross inspection and classification of mucosal abnormalities during standard endoscopy, magnification endoscopy, endoscopy with narrow band imaging and/or autofluorescence imaging, and measurement of several serum biomarkers including pepsinogen I and II levels, gastrin-17, and anti-*H. pylori* serologies. The clinical utility of these tools is currently being explored.

The early phase of chronic gastritis is *superficial gastritis.* The inflammatory changes are limited to the lamina propria of the surface mucosa, with edema and cellular infiltrates separating intact gastric glands. The next stage is *atrophic gastritis.* The inflammatory infiltrate extends deeper into the mucosa, with progressive distortion and destruction of the glands. The final stage of chronic gastritis is *gastric atrophy.* Glandular structures are lost, and there is a paucity of inflammatory infiltrates. Endoscopically, the mucosa may be substantially thin, permitting clear visualization of the underlying blood vessels.

Gastric glands may undergo morphologic transformation in chronic gastritis. Intestinal metaplasia denotes the conversion of gastric glands to a small intestinal phenotype with small-bowel mucosal glands containing goblet cells. The metaplastic changes may vary in distribution from patchy to fairly extensive gastric involvement. Intestinal metaplasia is an important predisposing factor for gastric cancer (Chap. 109).

Chronic gastritis is also classified according to the predominant site of involvement. Type A refers to the body-predominant form (autoimmune), and type B is the antral-predominant form (*H. pylori*–related).

This classification is artificial in view of the difficulty in distinguishing between these two entities. The term *AB gastritis* has been used to refer to a mixed antral/body picture.

TYPE A GASTRITIS The less common of the two forms involves primarily the fundus and body, with antral sparing. Traditionally, this form of gastritis has been associated with pernicious anemia (Chap. 128) in the presence of circulating antibodies against parietal cells and IF; thus, it is also called *autoimmune gastritis. H. pylori* infection can lead to a similar distribution of gastritis. The characteristics of an autoimmune picture are not always present.

Antibodies to parietal cells have been detected in >90% of patients with pernicious anemia and in up to 50% of patients with type A gastritis. The parietal cell antibody is directed against H^+,K^+-ATPase. T cells are also implicated in the injury pattern of this form of gastritis. A subset of patients infected with *H. pylori* develop antibodies against H^+,K^+-ATPase, potentially leading to the atrophic gastritis pattern seen in some patients infected with this organism. The mechanism is thought to involve molecular mimicry between *H. pylori* LPS and H^+,K^+-ATPase.

Parietal cell antibodies and atrophic gastritis are observed in family members of patients with pernicious anemia. These antibodies are observed in up to 20% of individuals over age 60 and in ~20% of patients with vitiligo and Addison's disease. About one-half of patients with pernicious anemia have antibodies to thyroid antigens, and about 30% of patients with thyroid disease have circulating antiparietal cell antibodies. Anti-IF antibodies are more specific than parietal cell antibodies for type A gastritis, being present in ~40% of patients with pernicious anemia. Another parameter consistent with this form of gastritis being autoimmune in origin is the higher incidence of specific familial histocompatibility haplotypes such as HLA-B8 and HLA-DR3.

The parietal cell–containing gastric gland is preferentially targeted in this form of gastritis, and achlorhydria results. Parietal cells are the source of IF, the lack of which will lead to vitamin B_{12} deficiency and its sequelae (megaloblastic anemia, neurologic dysfunction).

Gastric acid plays an important role in feedback inhibition of gastrin release from G cells. Achlorhydria, coupled with relative sparing of the antral mucosa (site of G cells), leads to hypergastrinemia. Gastrin levels can be markedly elevated (>500 pg/mL) in patients with pernicious anemia. ECL cell hyperplasia with frank development of gastric carcinoid tumors may result from gastrin trophic effects. Hypergastrinemia and achlorhydria may also be seen in nonpernicious anemia–associated type A gastritis.

TYPE B GASTRITIS Type B, or antral-predominant, gastritis is the more common form of chronic gastritis. *H. pylori* infection is the cause of this entity. Although described as "antral-predominant," this is likely a misnomer in view of studies documenting the progression of the inflammatory process toward the body and fundus of infected individuals. The conversion to a pangastritis is time-dependent and estimated to require 15–20 years. This form of gastritis increases with age, being present in up to 100% of persons over age 70. Histology improves after *H. pylori* eradication. The number of *H. pylori* organisms decreases dramatically with progression to gastric atrophy, and the degree of inflammation correlates with the level of these organisms. Early on, with antral-predominant findings, the quantity of *H. pylori* is highest and a dense chronic inflammatory infiltrate of the lamina propria is noted, accompanied by epithelial cell infiltration with polymorphonuclear leukocytes (Fig. 348-14).

Multifocal atrophic gastritis, gastric atrophy with subsequent metaplasia, has been observed in chronic *H. pylori*–induced gastritis. This may ultimately lead to development of gastric adenocarcinoma (Fig. 348-8; Chap. 109). *H. pylori* infection is now considered an independent risk factor for gastric cancer. Worldwide epidemiologic studies have documented a higher incidence of *H. pylori* infection in patients with adenocarcinoma of the stomach as compared to control subjects. Seropositivity for *H. pylori* is associated with a three- to sixfold increased risk of gastric cancer. This risk may be as high as ninefold after adjusting for the inaccuracy of serologic testing in the elderly. The mechanism by which *H. pylori* infection leads to cancer

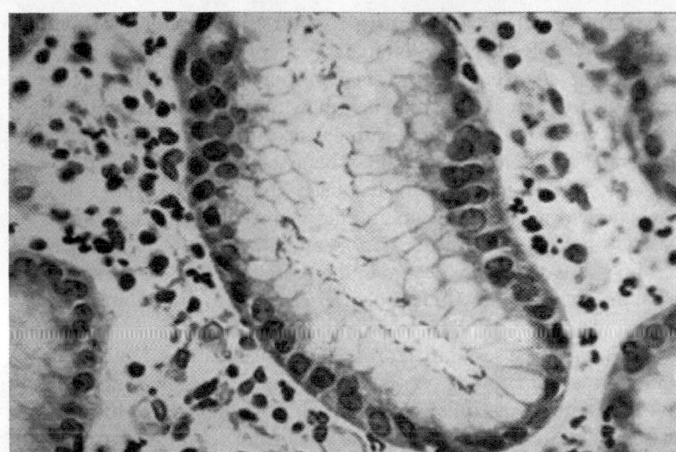

FIGURE 348-14 Chronic gastritis and *H. pylori* organisms. Steiner silver stain of superficial gastric mucosa showing abundant darkly stained microorganisms layered over the apical portion of the surface epithelium. Note that there is no tissue invasion.

is unknown, but it appears to be related to the chronic inflammation induced by the organism. Eradication of *H. pylori* as a general preventative measure for gastric cancer is being evaluated but is not yet recommended.

Infection with *H. pylori* is also associated with development of a low-grade B cell lymphoma, gastric MALT lymphoma (Chap. 134). The chronic T cell stimulation caused by the infection leads to production of cytokines that promote the B cell tumor. The tumor should be initially staged with a CT scan of the abdomen and EUS. Tumor growth remains dependent on the presence of *H. pylori,* and its eradication is often associated with complete regression of the tumor. The tumor may take more than a year to regress after treating the infection. Such patients should be followed by EUS every 2–3 months. If the tumor is stable or decreasing in size, no other therapy is necessary. If the tumor grows, it may have become a high-grade B cell lymphoma. When the tumor becomes a high-grade aggressive lymphoma histologically, it loses responsiveness to *H. pylori* eradication.

TREATMENT CHRONIC GASTRITIS

Treatment in chronic gastritis is aimed at the sequelae and not the underlying inflammation. Patients with pernicious anemia will require parenteral vitamin B_{12} supplementation on a long-term basis. Eradication of *H. pylori* is often recommended even if PUD or a low-grade MALT lymphoma is not present.

Miscellaneous Forms of Gastritis *Lymphocytic gastritis* is characterized histologically by intense infiltration of the surface epithelium with lymphocytes. The infiltrative process is primarily in the body of the stomach and consists of mature T cells and plasmacytes. The etiology of this form of chronic gastritis is unknown. It has been described in patients with celiac sprue, but whether there is a common factor associating these two entities is unknown. No specific symptoms suggest lymphocytic gastritis. A subgroup of patients have thickened folds noted on endoscopy. These folds are often capped by small nodules that contain a central depression or erosion; this form of the disease is called *varioliform gastritis. H. pylori* probably plays no significant role in lymphocytic gastritis. Therapy with glucocorticoids or sodium cromoglycate has obtained unclear results.

Marked eosinophilic infiltration involving any layer of the stomach (mucosa, muscularis propria, and serosa) is characteristic of *eosinophilic gastritis.* Affected individuals will often have circulating eosinophilia with clinical manifestation of systemic allergy. Involvement may range from isolated gastric disease to diffuse eosinophilic gastroenteritis. Antral involvement predominates, with prominent edematous folds being observed on endoscopy. These prominent antral folds can lead to outlet obstruction. Patients can present with epigastric discomfort, nausea, and vomiting. Treatment with glucocorticoids has been successful.

Several systemic disorders may be associated with *granulomatous gastritis.* Gastric involvement has been observed in Crohn's disease. Involvement may range from granulomatous infiltrates noted only on gastric biopsies to frank ulceration and stricture formation. Gastric Crohn's disease usually occurs in the presence of small-intestinal disease. Several rare infectious processes can lead to granulomatous gastritis, including histoplasmosis, candidiasis, syphilis, and tuberculosis. Other unusual causes of this form of gastritis include sarcoidosis, idiopathic granulomatous gastritis, and eosinophilic granulomas involving the stomach. Establishing the specific etiologic agent in this form of gastritis can be difficult, at times requiring repeat endoscopy with biopsy and cytology. Occasionally, a surgically obtained full-thickness biopsy of the stomach may be required to exclude malignancy.

Russell body gastritis (RBG) is a mucosal lesion of unknown etiology that has a pseudotumoral endoscopic appearance. Histologically, it is defined by the presence of numerous plasma cells containing Russell bodies (RBs) that express kappa and lambda light chains. Only 10 cases have been reported, and 7 of these have been associated with *H. pylori* infection. The lesion can be confused with a neoplastic process, but it is benign in nature, and the natural history of the lesion is not known. There have been cases of resolution of the lesion when *H. pylori* was eradicated.

MÉNÉTRIER'S DISEASE

Ménétrier's disease (MD) is a very rare gastropathy characterized by large, tortuous mucosal folds. MD has an average age of onset of 40–60 years with a male predominance. The differential diagnosis of large gastric folds includes ZES, malignancy (lymphoma, infiltrating carcinoma), infectious etiologies (CMV, histoplasmosis, syphilis, tuberculosis), gastritis polyposa profunda, and infiltrative disorders such as sarcoidosis. MD is most commonly confused with large or multiple gastric polyps (prolonged PPI use) or familial polyposis syndromes. The mucosal folds in MD are often most prominent in the body and fundus, sparing the antrum. Histologically, massive foveolar hyperplasia (hyperplasia of surface and glandular mucous cells) and a marked reduction in oxyntic glands and parietal cells and chief cells are noted. This hyperplasia produces the prominent folds observed. The pits of the gastric glands elongate and may become extremely dilated and tortuous. Although the lamina propria may contain a mild chronic inflammatory infiltrate including eosinophils and plasma cells, MD is not considered a form of gastritis. The etiology of this unusual clinical picture in children is often CMV, but the etiology in adults is unknown. Overexpression of the growth factor TGF-α has been demonstrated in patients with MD. The overexpression of TGF-α in turn results in overstimulation of the epidermal growth factor receptor (EGFR) pathway and increased proliferation of mucus cells, resulting in the observed foveolar hyperplasia.

The clinical presentation in adults is usually insidious and progressive. Epigastric pain, nausea, vomiting, anorexia, peripheral edema, and weight loss are signs and symptoms in patients with MD. Occult GI bleeding may occur, but overt bleeding is unusual and, when present, is due to superficial mucosal erosions. In fact, bleeding is more often seen in one of the common mimics of MD, gastric polyposis. Twenty to 100% of patients (depending on time of presentation) develop a protein-losing gastropathy due to hypersecretion of gastric mucus accompanied by hypoalbuminemia and edema. Gastric acid secretion is usually reduced or absent because of the decreased parietal cells. Large gastric folds are readily detectable by either radiographic (barium meal) or endoscopic methods. Endoscopy with deep mucosal biopsy, preferably full thickness with a snare technique, is required to establish the diagnosis and exclude other entities that may present similarly. A nondiagnostic biopsy may lead to a surgically obtained full-thickness biopsy to exclude malignancy. Although MD is considered premalignant by some, the risk of neoplastic progression is not defined. Complete blood count, serum gastrin, serum albumin, CMV and *H. pylori* serology, and pH testing of gastric aspirate during endoscopy should be included as part of the initial evaluation of patients with large gastric folds.

TREATMENT MÉNÉTRIER'S DISEASE

Medical therapy with anticholinergic agents, prostaglandins, PPIs, prednisone, somatostatin analogues (octreotide) and H_2 receptor antagonists yields varying results. Ulcers should be treated with a standard approach. The discovery that MD is associated with overstimulation of the EGFR pathway has led to the successful use of the EGF inhibitory antibody, cetuximab, in these patients. Specifically, four of seven patients who completed a 1-month trial with this agent demonstrated near complete histologic remission and improvement in symptoms. Cetuximab is now considered the first-line treatment for MD, leaving total gastrectomy for severe disease with persistent and substantial protein loss despite therapy with this agent.

349 Disorders of Absorption

Henry J. Binder

Disorders of absorption constitute a broad spectrum of conditions with multiple etiologies and varied clinical manifestations. Almost all of these clinical problems are associated with *diminished* intestinal absorption of one or more dietary nutrients and are often referred to as the *malabsorption syndrome.* This term is not ideal as it represents a pathophysiologic state, does *not* provide an etiologic explanation for the underlying problem, and should not be considered an adequate final diagnosis. The only clinical conditions in which absorption is *increased* are hemochromatosis and Wilson's disease, in which absorption of iron and copper, respectively, is elevated.

Most malabsorption syndromes are associated with *steatorrhea*, an increase in stool fat excretion to >6% of dietary fat intake. Some malabsorption disorders are not associated with steatorrhea: primary lactase deficiency, a congenital absence of the small-intestinal brush border disaccharidase enzyme lactase, is associated with lactose "malabsorption," and pernicious anemia is associated with a marked decrease in intestinal absorption of cobalamin (vitamin B_{12}) due to an absence of gastric parietal-cell intrinsic factor, which is required for cobalamin absorption.

Disorders of absorption must be included in the differential diagnosis of diarrhea (Chap. 55). First, diarrhea is frequently associated with and/or is a consequence of the diminished absorption of one or more dietary nutrients. The diarrhea may be secondary either to the intestinal process that is responsible for the steatorrhea or to steatorrhea per se. Thus, celiac disease (see below) is associated with both extensive morphologic changes in the small-intestinal mucosa and reduced absorption of several dietary nutrients; in contrast, the diarrhea of steatorrhea is the result of the effect of nonabsorbed dietary fatty acids on intestinal (usually colonic) ion transport. For example, oleic acid and ricinoleic acid (a bacterially hydroxylated fatty acid that is also the active ingredient in castor oil, a widely used laxative) induce active colonic Cl ion secretion, most likely secondary to increasing intracellular Ca. In addition, diarrhea per se may result in mild steatorrhea (<11 g of fat excretion while on a 100-g fat diet). Second, most patients will indicate that they have diarrhea, not that they have fat malabsorption. Third, many intestinal disorders that have diarrhea as a prominent symptom (e.g., ulcerative colitis, traveler's diarrhea secondary to an enterotoxin produced by *Escherichia coli*) do not necessarily have diminished absorption of any dietary nutrient.

Diarrhea as a *symptom* (i.e., when the term is used by patients to describe their bowel movement pattern) may reflect a decrease in stool consistency, an increase in stool volume, an increase in number of bowel movements, or any combination of these three changes. In contrast, diarrhea as a *sign* is a quantitative increase in stool water or weight of >200–225 mL or g per 24 h when a Western-type diet is consumed. Individuals consuming a diet with higher fiber content may normally have a stool weight of up to 400 g/24 h. Thus, the clinician must clarify what an individual patient means by diarrhea. Some 10% of patients referred to gastroenterologists for further evaluation of unexplained diarrhea do not have an increase in stool water when this variable is determined quantitatively. Such patients may have small, frequent, somewhat loose bowel movements with stool urgency that is indicative of proctitis but do not have an increase in stool weight or volume.

It is also critical to establish whether a patient's diarrhea is secondary to diminished absorption of one or more dietary nutrients rather than being due to small- and/or large-intestinal fluid and electrolyte secretion. The former has often been termed *osmotic diarrhea*, while the latter has been referred to as *secretory diarrhea*. Unfortunately, both secretory and osmotic elements can be present simultaneously in the same disorder; thus, this distinction is not always precise. Nonetheless, two studies—determination of stool electrolytes and observation of the effect of a fast on stool output—can help make this distinction.

The demonstration of the effect of prolonged (>24 h) fasting on stool output can suggest that a *dietary nutrient* is responsible for the individual's diarrhea. Secretory diarrhea associated with enterotoxin-induced traveler's diarrhea would not be affected by prolonged fasting, as enterotoxin-induced stimulation of intestinal fluid and electrolyte secretion is not altered by eating. In contrast, diarrhea secondary to lactose malabsorption in primary lactase deficiency would undoubtedly cease during a prolonged fast. Thus, a substantial decrease in stool output by a fasting patient during quantitative stool collection lasting at least 24 h is presumptive evidence that the diarrhea is related to malabsorption of a dietary nutrient. The persistence of stool output during fasting indicates that the diarrhea is likely secretory and that its cause is *not* a dietary nutrient. Either a luminal (e.g., *E. coli* enterotoxin) or a circulating (e.g., vasoactive intestinal peptide) secretagogue could be responsible for unaltered persistence of a patient's diarrhea during a prolonged fast. The observed effects of fasting can be compared and correlated with stool electrolyte and osmolality determinations.

Measurement of stool electrolytes and osmolality requires comparison of Na^+ and K^+ concentrations in liquid stool with the osmolality of the stool in order to determine the presence or absence of a so-called stool osmotic gap. The following formula is used:

$$2 \times (\text{stool } [Na^+] + \text{stool } [K^+]) \leq \text{stool osmolality}$$

The cation concentrations are doubled to estimate stool anion concentrations. The presence of a significant osmotic gap suggests the presence in stool water of a substance (or substances) other than Na/K/anions that is presumably responsible for the patient's diarrhea. Originally, stool osmolality was measured, but it is almost invariably greater than the required 290–300 mosmol/kg H_2O, reflecting bacterial degradation of nonabsorbed carbohydrate either immediately before defecation or in the stool jar while specimen awaits chemical analysis, even when the stool is refrigerated. As a result, the stool osmolality should be assumed to be 300 mosmol/kg H_2O. A low stool osmolality (<290 mosmol/kg H_2O) reflects the addition of either dilute urine or water, indicating either collection of urine and stool together or so-called factitious diarrhea, a form of Münchausen's syndrome. When the calculated difference in the formula above is >50, an osmotic gap exists; its presence suggests that the diarrhea is due to a nonabsorbed dietary nutrient—e.g., a fatty acid and/or a carbohydrate. When this difference is <25, it is presumed that a dietary nutrient is not responsible for the diarrhea. Since elements of both osmotic diarrhea (i.e., due to malabsorption of a dietary nutrient) and secretory diarrhea may be present, this distinction at times is less clear-cut at the bedside than when used as a teaching example. Ideally, the presence of an osmotic gap will be associated with a marked decrease in stool output during a prolonged fast, while an osmotic gap will likely be absent in an individual whose stool output is not reduced substantially during a period of fasting.

NUTRIENT DIGESTION AND ABSORPTION

The lengths of the small intestine and the colon are ~300 cm and ~80 cm, respectively. However, the effective functional surface area is ~600-fold greater than that of a hollow tube as a result of folds, villi (in the small intestine), and microvilli. The functional surface area of the small intestine is somewhat greater than that of a doubles tennis court. In addition to nutrient digestion and absorption, the intestinal epithelia have several other functions:

1. *Barrier and immune defense.* The intestine is exposed to a large number of potential antigens and enteric and invasive microorganisms, and it is extremely effective at preventing the entry of almost all of these agents. The intestinal mucosa also synthesizes and secretes secretory IgA.
2. *Fluid and electrolyte absorption and secretion.* The intestine absorbs ~7–8 L of fluid daily, a volume comprising dietary fluid intake (1–2 L/d) and salivary, gastric, pancreatic, biliary, and intestinal fluid (6–7 L/d). Several stimuli, especially bacteria and bacterial enterotoxins, induce fluid and electrolyte secretion that may lead to diarrhea (Chap. 160).
3. *Synthesis and secretion of several proteins.* The intestinal mucosa is a major site for the production of proteins, including apolipoproteins.
4. *Production of several bioactive amines and peptides.* The intestine is one of the largest endocrine organs in the body and produces several amines (e.g., 5-hydroxytryptophan) and peptides that serve as paracrine and hormonal mediators of intestinal function.

The small and large intestines are distinct anatomically (villi are present in the small intestine but are absent in the colon) and functionally (nutrient digestion and absorption take place in the small intestine but not in the colon). No precise anatomic characteristics separate duodenum, jejunum, and ileum, although certain nutrients are absorbed exclusively in specific areas of the small intestine. However, villous cells in the small intestine (surface epithelial cells in the colon) and crypt cells have distinct anatomic and functional characteristics. Intestinal epithelial cells are continuously renewed; new proliferating epithelial cells at the base of the crypt migrate over 48–72 h to the tip of the villus (or surface of the colon), where they exist as well-developed epithelial cells with digestive and absorptive function. This high rate of cell turnover explains the relatively rapid resolution of diarrhea and other digestive-tract side effects during chemotherapy as new cells not exposed to these toxic agents are produced. Equally important is the paradigm of separation of villous/surface cell and crypt cell functions. Digestive hydrolytic enzymes are present primarily in the brush border of villous epithelial cells. Absorptive and secretory functions are also separate: villous/surface cells are primarily, but not exclusively, the site for absorptive function, while secretory function is located in crypts of both the small and large intestines.

Nutrients, minerals, and vitamins are absorbed by one or more active-transport mechanisms. These mechanisms are energy dependent and are mediated by membrane transport proteins. These processes will result in the *net* movement of a substance against or in the absence of an electrochemical concentration gradient. Intestinal absorption of amino acids and monosaccharides (e.g., glucose) is also a specialized form of active transport—*secondary active transport*. The movement of actively transported nutrients against a concentration gradient is Na^+ dependent and is due to a Na^+ gradient across the apical membrane. The Na^+ gradient is maintained by Na^+,K^+-adenosine triphosphatase (ATPase), the so-called Na^+ pump located on the basolateral membrane, which extrudes Na^+ and maintains low intracellular [Na] as well as the Na^+ gradient across the apical membrane. As a result, active glucose absorption and glucose-stimulated Na^+ absorption require both the apical membrane transport protein SGLT1 and the basolateral Na^+,K^+-ATPase. In addition to exhibiting Na^+ for its absorption, glucose stimulates Na^+ and fluid absorption; this effect is the physiologic basis of oral rehydration therapy for the treatment of diarrhea (Chap. 55). The mechanisms of intestinal fluid and electrolyte absorption and secretion are discussed in Chap. 55.

Although the intestinal epithelial cells are crucial mediators of absorption and of ion and water flow, the several cell types in the lamina propria (e.g., mast cells, macrophages, myofibroblasts) and the enteric nervous system interact with the epithelium to regulate mucosal cell function. Intestinal function results from the integrated responses and interactions of intestinal epithelial cells and intestinal muscle.

ENTEROHEPATIC CIRCULATION OF BILE ACIDS

Bile acids are not present in the diet but are synthesized in the liver by a series of enzymatic steps that also represent cholesterol catabolism. Indeed, interruption of the enterohepatic circulation of bile acids can reduce serum cholesterol levels by 10% before a new steady state is established. Bile acids are either primary or secondary. Primary bile acids are synthesized in the liver from cholesterol, and secondary bile acids are synthesized from primary bile acids in the intestine by colonic bacterial enzymes. The two primary bile acids in humans are cholic acid and chenodeoxycholic acid; the two most abundant secondary bile acids are deoxycholic acid and lithocholic acid. The liver synthesizes ~500 mg of bile acids daily; the bile acids are conjugated to either taurine or glycine (to form tauroconjugated and glycoconjugated bile acids, respectively) and are secreted into the duodenum in bile. The primary functions of bile acids are (1) to promote bile flow, (2) to solubilize cholesterol and phospholipid in the gallbladder by mixed micelle formation, and (3) to enhance dietary lipid digestion and absorption by forming mixed micelles in the proximal small intestine.

Bile acids are primarily absorbed by an active, Na^+-dependent process that takes place exclusively in the ileum; to a lesser extent, they are absorbed by non-carrier-mediated transport processes in the jejunum, ileum, and colon. Conjugated bile acids that enter the colon are deconjugated by colonic bacterial enzymes. The unconjugated bile acids are rapidly absorbed by nonionic diffusion. Colonic bacterial enzymes also dehydroxylate bile acids to secondary bile acids.

Bile acids absorbed from the intestine return to the liver via the portal vein and are then re-secreted (Fig. 349-1). Bile acid synthesis is largely autoregulated by 7α-hydroxylase, the initial enzyme in cholesterol degradation. A decrease in the volume of bile acids returning to the liver from the intestine is associated with an increase in bile acid synthesis/cholesterol catabolism, which helps keep the bile-acid pool size relatively constant. However, the capacity to increase bile acid synthesis is limited to ~2- to 2.5-fold (see below). The bile-acid pool size is ~4 g. The pool is circulated via the enterohepatic circulation about twice during each meal, or six to eight times during a 24-h period. A relatively small quantity of bile acids is not absorbed and is excreted in stool daily; this fecal loss is matched by hepatic bile-acid synthesis.

Defects in any of the steps in enterohepatic circulation of bile acids can result in a decrease in the duodenal concentration of conjugated bile acids and consequently in the development of steatorrhea. Thus, steatorrhea can be caused by abnormalities in bile acid synthesis and excretion, their physical state in the intestinal lumen, and reabsorption (Table 349-1).

Synthesis Decreased bile acid synthesis and steatorrhea have been demonstrated in chronic liver disease, but steatorrhea often is not a major component of illness in these patients.

Secretion Although bile acid secretion may be reduced or absent in biliary obstruction, steatorrhea is rarely a significant medical problem in these patients. In contrast, primary biliary cirrhosis represents a defect in canalicular excretion of organic anions, including bile acids, and not infrequently is associated with steatorrhea and its consequences (e.g., chronic bone disease). Thus, the osteopenia/osteomalacia and other chronic bone abnormalities often present in patients with primary biliary cirrhosis and other cholestatic syndromes are secondary to steatorrhea that then leads to calcium and vitamin D malabsorption as well as to the effects of cholestasis (e.g., bile acids and inflammatory cytokines).

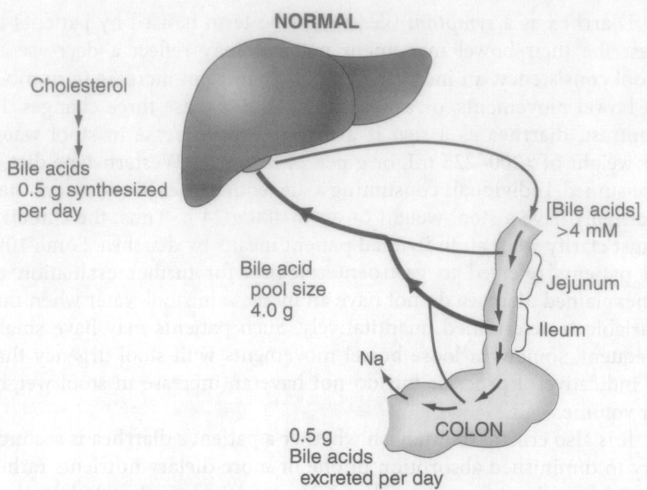

FIGURE 349-1 Schematic representation of the enterohepatic circulation of bile acids. Bile acid synthesis is cholesterol catabolism and occurs in the liver. Bile acids are secreted in bile and are stored in the gallbladder between meals and at night. Food in the duodenum induces the release of cholecystokinin, a potent stimulus for gallbladder contraction resulting in bile acid entry into the duodenum. Bile acids are primarily absorbed via an Na-dependent transport process that is located only in the ileum. A relatively small quantity of bile acids (~500 mg) is not absorbed in a 24-h period and is lost in stool. Fecal bile acid losses are matched by bile acid synthesis. The bile acid pool (the total amount of bile acids in the body) is ~4 g and is circulated twice during each meal or six to eight times in a 24-h period.

Maintenance of Conjugated Bile Acids In bacterial overgrowth syndromes associated with diarrhea, steatorrhea, and macrocytic anemia, a colonic type of bacterial flora is increased in the small intestine. Steatorrhea is primarily a result of the decrease in conjugated bile acids secondary to their deconjugation by colonic-type bacteria. Two complementary explanations account for the resulting impairment of micelle formation: (1) Unconjugated bile acids are rapidly absorbed in the jejunum by nonionic diffusion, and the result is a reduced concentration of duodenal bile acids. (2) The critical micellar concentration (CMC) of unconjugated bile acids is higher than that of conjugated bile acids; therefore, unconjugated bile acids are less effective than conjugated bile acids in micelle formation.

Reabsorption Ileal dysfunction caused by either Crohn's disease or surgical resection results in a decrease in bile acid reabsorption in the ileum and an *increase* in the delivery of bile acids to the large intestine. The resulting clinical consequences—diarrhea with or without steatorrhea—are determined by the *degree* of ileal dysfunction and the *response* of the enterohepatic circulation to bile acid losses (Table 349-2). Patients with limited ileal disease or resection often have diarrhea but not steatorrhea. The diarrhea, a result of stimulation of active Cl secretion by bile acids in the colon, has been called *bile acid diarrhea* or *choleretic enteropathy* and responds promptly to cholestyramine, an anion-binding resin. Steatorrhea does not develop because hepatic synthesis of bile acids increases to compensate for

TABLE 349-1 DEFECTS IN ENTEROHEPATIC CIRCULATION OF BILE ACIDS

Process	Pathophysiologic Defect	Disease Example
Synthesis	Decreased hepatic function	Cirrhosis
Biliary secretion	Altered canalicular function	Primary biliary cirrhosis
Maintenance of conjugated bile acids	Bacterial overgrowth	Jejunal diverticulosis
Reabsorption	Abnormal ileal function	Crohn's disease

TABLE 349-2 COMPARISON OF BILE ACID AND FATTY ACID DIARRHEA

	Bile Acid Diarrhea	Fatty Acid Diarrhea
Extent of ileal disease	Limited	Extensive
Ileal bile-acid absorption	Reduced	Reduced
Fecal bile-acid excretion	Increased	Increased
Fecal bile-acid loss compensated by hepatic synthesis	Yes	No
Bile-acid pool size	Normal	Reduced
Intraduodenal (bile acid)	Normal	Reduced
Steatorrhea	None or mild	>20 g
Response to cholestyramine	Yes	No
Response to low-fat diet	No	Yes

the rate of fecal bile-acid losses, resulting in maintenance of both the bile-acid pool size and the intraduodenal concentrations of bile acids. In contrast, patients with greater degrees of ileal disease and/or resection often have diarrhea and steatorrhea that do not respond to cholestyramine. In this situation, ileal disease is also associated with increased volumes of bile acids entering the colon; however, hepatic synthesis can no longer increase sufficiently to maintain the bile-acid pool size. As a consequence, the intraduodenal concentration of bile acids is reduced to less than the CMC, and the result is impaired micelle formation and steatorrhea. This second situation is often called *fatty acid diarrhea.* Cholestyramine may not be effective (and may even exacerbate the diarrhea by further depleting the intraduodenal bile-acid concentration); however, a low-fat diet to reduce fatty acid entry into the colon can be effective. Two clinical features—the length of the ileal section removed and the degree of steatorrhea—can predict whether an individual patient will respond to cholestyramine. Unfortunately, these predictors are imperfect, and a therapeutic trial of cholestyramine is often necessary to establish whether an individual patient will benefit from cholestyramine. Table 349-2 contrasts the characteristics of bile acid diarrhea (small ileal dysfunction) and fatty acid diarrhea (large ileal dysfunction).

Bile acid diarrhea can also occur in the absence of ileal inflammation and/or resection and is characterized by an abnormal ^{75}SeHCAT retention study and reduced ileal release of fibroblast growth factor 19, a negative regulator of bile acid synthesis, with a consequent increase in bile acid synthesis and secretion that exceeds ileal bile-acid absorption. The diarrhea in these patients also responds to cholestyramine.

LIPIDS

Steatorrhea is caused by one or more defects in the digestion and absorption of dietary fat. The average intake of dietary fat in the United States is ~120–150 g/d, and fat absorption is linear to dietary fat intake. The total load of fat presented to the small intestine is considerably greater, as substantial amounts of lipid are secreted in bile each day (see "Enterohepatic Circulation of Bile Acids," above). Three types of fatty acids compose fats: long-chain fatty acids (LCFAs), medium-chain fatty acids (MCFAs), and short-chain fatty acids (SCFAs) (Table 349-3). Dietary fat is exclusively composed of long-chain triglycerides (LCTs)—i.e., glycerol that is bound via ester linkages to three LCFAs. While the majority of dietary LCFAs have carbon chain lengths of 16 or 18, all fatty acids of carbon chain length >12 are metabolized in the same manner; saturated and unsaturated fatty acids are handled identically.

Assimilation of dietary lipid requires three integrated processes: (1) an intraluminal, or digestive, phase; (2) a mucosal, or absorptive, phase; and (3) a delivery, or postabsorptive, phase. An abnormality at any site involved in these processes can cause steatorrhea (Table 349-4). Therefore, it is essential that any patient with steatorrhea be evaluated to identify the specific physiologic defect in overall lipid digestion/absorption, as therapy will be determined by the specific etiology.

The digestive phase has two components, *lipolysis* and *micelle formation.* Although dietary lipid is in the form of LCTs, the intestinal mucosa does not absorb triglycerides; they must first be hydrolyzed (Fig. 349-2). The initial step in lipid digestion is the formation of emulsions of finely dispersed lipid, which is accomplished by mastication and gastric contractions. Lipolysis, the hydrolysis of triglycerides to free fatty acids, monoglycerides, and glycerol by lipase, is initiated in the stomach by lingual and gastric lipases that have a pH optimum of 4.5–6.0. About 20–30% of total lipolysis occurs in the stomach. Lipolysis is completed in the duodenum and jejunum by pancreatic lipase, which is inactivated by a pH <7.0. Pancreatic lipolysis is greatly enhanced by the presence of a second pancreatic enzyme, colipase, which facilitates the movement of lipase to the triglyceride.

TABLE 349-3 COMPARISON OF DIFFERENT TYPES OF FATTY ACIDS

	Long-Chain	Medium-Chain	Short-Chain
Carbon chain length	>12	8–12	<8
Present in diet	In large amounts	In small amounts	No
Origin	In diet as triglycerides	Only in small amounts in diet as triglycerides	Bacterial degradation in colon of nonabsorbed carbohydrate to fatty acids
Primary site of absorption	Small intestine	Small intestine	Colon
Requires pancreatic lipolysis	Yes	No	No
Requires micelle formation	Yes	No	No
Present in stool	Minimal	No	Substantial

Impaired lipolysis can lead to steatorrhea and can occur in the presence of pancreatic insufficiency due to chronic pancreatitis in adults or cystic fibrosis in children and adolescents. Normal lipolysis can be maintained by ~5% of maximal pancreatic lipase secretion; thus, steatorrhea is a late manifestation of these disorders. A reduction in intraduodenal pH can also result in altered lipolysis, as pancreatic lipase is inactivated at pH <7. Thus, ~15% of patients who have gastrinoma (Chap. 348), with substantial increases in gastric acid secretion from ectopic production of gastrin (usually from an islet cell adenoma), have diarrhea, and some have steatorrhea believed to be secondary to acid inactivation of pancreatic lipase. Similarly, patients who have chronic pancreatitis (with reduced lipase secretion) often have a decrease in pancreatic bicarbonate secretion, which will also result in a lowering of intraduodenal pH and inactivation of endogenous pancreatic lipase or of therapeutically administered lipase.

Overlying the microvillus membrane of the small intestine is the so-called unstirred water layer, a relatively stagnant aqueous phase that must be traversed by the products of lipolysis that are primarily water insoluble. Water-soluble mixed micelles provide a mechanism

TABLE 349-4 DEFECTS IN LIPID DIGESTION AND ABSORPTION IN STEATORRHEA

Phase, Process	Pathophysiologic Defect	Disease Example
Digestive		
Lipolysis formation	Decreased lipase secretion	Chronic pancreatitis
Micelle formation	Decreased intraduodenal bile acids	See Table 349-1
Absorptive		
Mucosal uptake and re-esterification	Mucosal dysfunction	Celiac disease
Postabsorptive		
Chylomicron formation	Absent betalipoproteins	Abetalipoproteinemia
Delivery from intestine	Abnormal lymphatics	Intestinal lymphangiectasia

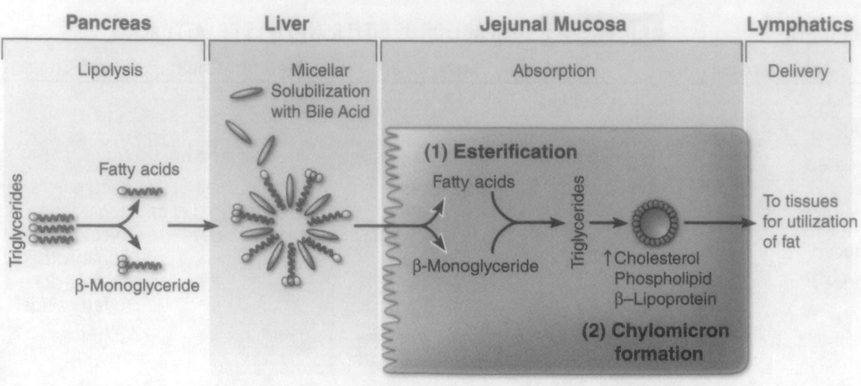

FIGURE 349-2 Schematic representation of lipid digestion and absorption. Dietary lipid is in the form of long-chain triglycerides. The overall process can be divided into (1) a digestive phase that includes both lipolysis and micelle formation requiring pancreatic lipase and conjugated bile acids, respectively, in the duodenum; (2) an absorptive phase for mucosal uptake and re-esterification; and (3) a postabsorptive phase that includes chylomicron formation and exit from the intestinal epithelial cell via lymphatics. *(Courtesy of John M. Dietschy, MD; with permission.)*

by which the water-insoluble products of lipolysis can reach the luminal plasma membrane of villous epithelial cells—the site for lipid absorption. Mixed micelles are molecular aggregates composed of fatty acids, monoglycerides, phospholipids, cholesterol, and conjugated bile acids. These mixed micelles are formed when the concentration of conjugated bile acids is greater than its CMC, which differs among the several bile acids present in the small-intestinal lumen. Conjugated bile acids, synthesized in the liver and excreted into the duodenum in bile, are regulated by the enterohepatic circulation (see above). Steatorrhea can result from impaired movement of fatty acids across the unstirred aqueous fluid layer in two situations: (1) an increase in the relative thickness of the unstirred water layer that occurs in bacterial overgrowth syndromes (see below) secondary to functional stasis (e.g., scleroderma); and (2) a decrease in the *duodenal* concentration of conjugated bile acids below the CMC, resulting in impaired micelle formation. Thus, steatorrhea can be caused by one or more defects in the enterohepatic circulation of bile acids.

Uptake and re-esterification constitute the *absorptive phase* of lipid digestion/absorption. Although passive diffusion has been thought to be responsible, a carrier-mediated process may mediate fatty acid and monoglyceride uptake. Regardless of the uptake process, fatty acids and monoglycerides are re-esterified by a series of enzymatic steps in the endoplasmic reticulum to form triglycerides, in which lipid exits from the intestinal epithelial cell. Impaired lipid absorption as a result of mucosal inflammation (e.g., celiac disease) and/or intestinal resection can also lead to steatorrhea.

The re-esterified triglycerides require the formation of *chylomicrons* to permit their exit from the small-intestinal epithelial cell and their delivery to the liver via the lymphatics. Chylomicrons are composed of β-lipoprotein and contain triglycerides, cholesterol, cholesterol esters, and phospholipids and enter the lymphatics, not the portal vein. Defects in the *postabsorptive phase* of lipid digestion/absorption can also result in steatorrhea, but these disorders are uncommon. Abetalipoproteinemia, or acanthocytosis, is a rare disorder of impaired synthesis of β-lipoprotein associated with abnormal erythrocytes (acanthocytes), neurologic problems, and steatorrhea (Chap. 421). Lipolysis, micelle formation, and lipid uptake are all normal in patients with abetalipoproteinemia, but the re-esterified triglyceride cannot exit the epithelial cell because of the failure to produce chylomicrons. Small-intestinal biopsy samples obtained from these rare patients in the postprandial state reveal lipid-laden small-intestinal epithelial cells that become perfectly normal in appearance after a 72- to 96-h fast. Similarly, abnormalities of intestinal lymphatics (e.g., intestinal lymphangiectasia) may also be associated with steatorrhea as well as protein loss (see below). Steatorrhea can result from defects at any of the several steps in lipid digestion/absorption.

The mechanism of lipid digestion/absorption outlined above is limited to *dietary* lipid, which is almost exclusively in the form of LCTs (Table 349-3). Medium-chain triglycerides (MCTs), composed of fatty acids with carbon chain lengths of 8–12, are present in large amounts in coconut oil and are used as a nutritional supplement. MCTs can be digested and absorbed by a pathway different from that involved in LCT digestion and absorption; at one time, MCTs held promise as an important treatment for steatorrhea of almost all etiologies. Unfortunately, they have been less therapeutically effective than expected because, for reasons that are not completely understood, their use often is not associated with an increase in body weight.

In contrast to LCTs, MCTs do not require pancreatic lipolysis as they can be absorbed intact by the intestinal epithelial cell. Further, micelle formation is not necessary for the absorption of MCTs (or MCFAs, if hydrolyzed by pancreatic lipase). MCTs are absorbed more efficiently than LCTs for the following reasons: (1) The rate of absorption is greater for MCTs than for LCFAs. (2) After absorption, MCFAs are not re-esterified. (3) After absorption, MCTs are hydrolyzed to MCFAs. (4) MCTs do not require chylomicron formation to exit intestinal epithelial cells. (5) The route of MCT exit is via the portal vein and not via lymphatics. Thus, the absorption of MCTs is greater than that of LCTs in pancreatic insufficiency, conditions with reduced intraduodenal bile acid concentrations, small-intestinal mucosal disease, abetalipoproteinemia, and intestinal lymphangiectasia.

SCFAs are not dietary lipids but are synthesized by colonic bacterial enzymes from nonabsorbed carbohydrate and are the anions present at the highest concentration in stool (80–130 m*M*). The SCFAs in stool are primarily acetate, propionate, and butyrate, whose carbon chain lengths are 2, 3, and 4, respectively. Butyrate is the primary nutrient for colonic epithelial cells, and its deficiency can be associated with one or more colitides. SCFAs conserve calories and carbohydrate: carbohydrates that are not completely absorbed in the small intestine will not be absorbed in the large intestine because of the absence of both disaccharidases and SGLT1, the transport protein that mediates monosaccharide absorption. In contrast, SCFAs are rapidly absorbed and stimulate colonic NaCl and fluid absorption. Most antibiotic-associated diarrhea not caused by *Clostridium difficile* is due to antibiotic suppression of the colonic microbiota, with a resulting decrease in SCFA production. As *C. difficile* accounts for only ~15–20% of all antibiotic-associated diarrhea, a relative decrease in colonic production of SCFA is likely the cause of most antibiotic-associated diarrhea.

The clinical manifestations of steatorrhea are a consequence both of the underlying disorder responsible for its development and of steatorrhea per se. Depending on the degree of steatorrhea and the level of dietary intake, significant fat malabsorption may lead to weight loss. Steatorrhea per se can be responsible for diarrhea; if the primary cause of the steatorrhea has not been identified, a low-fat diet can often ameliorate the diarrhea by decreasing fecal fat excretion. Steatorrhea is commonly associated with fat-soluble vitamin deficiency, which requires replacement with water-soluble preparations of these vitamins.

Disorders of absorption may also be associated with malabsorption of other dietary nutrients— most often carbohydrates—with or without a decrease in dietary lipid digestion and absorption. Therefore, knowledge of the mechanisms of digestion and absorption of carbohydrates, proteins, and other minerals and vitamins is useful in the evaluation of patients with altered intestinal nutrient absorption.

TABLE 349-5 PRIMARY LACTASE DEFICIENCY IN ADULT ETHNIC GROUPS

Ethnic Group	Prevalence of Lactase Deficiency, %
Northern European	5–15
Mediterranean	60–85
African black	85–100
American black	45–80
American white	10–25
Native American	50–95
Mexican American	40–75
Asian	90–100

Source: From FJ Simoons: Am J Dig Dis 23:963, 1978.

CARBOHYDRATES

Carbohydrates in the diet are present in the form of starch, disaccharides (sucrose and lactose), and glucose. Carbohydrates are absorbed only in the small intestine and only in the form of monosaccharides. Therefore, before their absorption, starch and disaccharides must first be digested by pancreatic amylase and intestinal brush border disaccharidases to monosaccharides. Monosaccharide absorption occurs by a Na-dependent process mediated by the brush border transport protein SGLT1.

Lactose malabsorption is the only clinically important disorder of carbohydrate absorption. Lactose, the disaccharide present in milk, requires digestion by brush border lactase to its two constituent monosaccharides, glucose and galactose. Lactase is present in almost all species in the postnatal period but then disappears throughout the animal kingdom, except in humans. Lactase activity persists in many individuals throughout life. Two different types of lactase deficiency exist—primary and secondary. In *primary lactase deficiency*, a genetically determined decrease or absence of lactase is noted, while all other aspects of both intestinal absorption and brush border enzymes are normal. In a number of nonwhite groups, primary lactase deficiency is common in adulthood. In fact, Northern European and North American whites are the only groups to maintain small-intestinal lactase activity throughout adult life. Table 349-5 presents the incidence of primary lactase deficiency in several ethnic groups. Lactase persistence in adults is an abnormality due to a defect in the regulation of its maturation. In contrast, *secondary lactase deficiency* occurs in association with small-intestinal mucosal disease, with abnormalities in both structure and function of other brush border enzymes and transport processes. Secondary lactase deficiency is often seen in celiac disease.

As lactose digestion is rate-limiting compared to glucose/galactose absorption, lactase deficiency is associated with significant lactose malabsorption. Some individuals with lactose malabsorption develop symptoms such as diarrhea, abdominal pain, cramps, and/or flatus. Most individuals with primary lactase deficiency do not have symptoms. Since lactose intolerance may be associated with symptoms suggestive of irritable bowel syndrome, persistence of such symptoms in an individual who exhibits lactose intolerance while on a strict lactose-free diet suggests that the person's symptoms were related to irritable bowel syndrome.

The development of symptoms of lactose intolerance is related to several factors:

1. *Amount of lactose in the diet.*
2. *Rate of gastric emptying.* Symptoms are more likely when gastric emptying is rapid than when it is slower. Therefore, skim milk is more likely to be associated with symptoms of lactose intolerance than whole milk, as the rate of gastric emptying after skim milk intake is more rapid. Similarly, diarrhea following subtotal gastrectomy is often a result of lactose intolerance, as gastric emptying is accelerated in patients with a gastrojejunostomy.
3. *Small-intestinal transit time.* Although the small and large intestines both contribute to the development of symptoms, many symptoms of lactase deficiency are related to the interaction of colonic bacteria and nonabsorbed lactose. More rapid small-intestinal transit makes symptoms more likely.
4. *Colonic compensation by production of SCFAs from nonabsorbed lactose.* Reduced levels of colonic microflora, which can follow antibiotic use, are associated with increased symptoms after lactose ingestion, especially in a lactase-deficient individual.

Glucose-galactose or monosaccharide malabsorption may also be associated with diarrhea and is due to a congenital absence of SGLT1. Diarrhea develops when individuals with this disorder ingest carbohydrates that contain actively transported monosaccharides (e.g., glucose, galactose) but not when they ingest monosaccharides that are not actively transported (e.g., fructose). Fructose is absorbed by the brush border transport protein GLUT 5, a facilitated diffusion process that is not Na-dependent and is distinct from SGLT1. In contrast, some individuals develop diarrhea as a result of the consumption of large quantities of sorbitol, a sugar used in diabetic candy; sorbitol is only minimally absorbed because of the absence of an intestinal absorptive transport mechanism for this sugar.

PROTEINS

Protein is present in food almost exclusively as polypeptides and requires extensive hydrolysis to di- and tripeptides and amino acids before absorption. Proteolysis occurs in both the stomach and the small intestine; it is mediated by pepsin, which is secreted as pepsinogen by gastric chief cells, and by trypsinogen and other peptidases from pancreatic acinar cells. The proenzymes pepsinogen and trypsinogen must be activated to pepsin (by pepsin at a pH <5) and to trypsin (by the intestinal brush border enzyme enterokinase and subsequently by trypsin), respectively. Proteins are absorbed by separate transport systems for di- and tripeptides and for different types of amino acids—e.g., neutral and dibasic. Alterations in either protein or amino acid digestion and absorption are rarely observed clinically, even in the presence of extensive small-intestinal mucosal inflammation. However, three rare genetic disorders involve protein digestion/absorption: (1) *Enterokinase deficiency* is due to an absence of the brush border enzyme that converts the proenzyme trypsinogen to trypsin and is associated with diarrhea, growth retardation, and hypoproteinemia. (2) *Hartnup's syndrome*, a defect in neutral amino acid transport, is characterized by a pellagra-like rash and neuropsychiatric symptoms. (3) *Cystinuria*, a defect in dibasic amino acid transport, is associated with renal calculi and chronic pancreatitis.

APPROACH TO THE PATIENT: Malabsorption

The clues provided by the history, symptoms, and initial preliminary observations will serve to limit extensive, ill-focused, and expensive laboratory and imaging studies. For example, a clinician evaluating a patient who has symptoms suggestive of malabsorption and who has recently undergone extensive small-intestinal resection for mesenteric ischemia should direct the initial assessment almost exclusively to defining whether a short-bowel syndrome might explain the entire clinical picture. Similarly, the development of a pattern of bowel movements suggestive of steatorrhea in a patient with long-standing alcohol abuse and chronic pancreatitis should prompt an assessment of pancreatic exocrine function.

The classic picture of malabsorption is rarely seen today in most parts of the United States. As a consequence, diseases with malabsorption must be suspected in individuals who have less severe symptoms and signs and subtle evidence of the altered absorption of only a *single* nutrient rather than obvious evidence of the malabsorption of multiple nutrients.

Although diarrhea can be caused by changes in fluid and electrolyte movement in either the small or the large intestine, dietary nutrients are absorbed almost exclusively in the small intestine.

Therefore, the demonstration of diminished absorption of a dietary nutrient provides unequivocal evidence for small-intestinal disease, although colonic dysfunction may also be present (e.g., Crohn's disease may involve both the small and large intestines). Dietary nutrient absorption may be segmental or diffuse along the small intestine and is site specific. Thus, for example, calcium, iron, and folic acid are exclusively absorbed by active-transport processes in the proximal small intestine, especially the duodenum; in contrast, the active-transport mechanisms for both cobalamin and bile acids are operative only in the ileum. Therefore, in an individual who years previously has had an intestinal resection, the details of which are not presently available, a presentation with evidence of calcium, folic acid, and/or iron malabsorption but without cobalamin deficiency makes it likely that the duodenum and proximal jejunum, but not the ileum, were resected.

Some nutrients—e.g., glucose, amino acids, and lipids—are absorbed throughout the small intestine, although their rate of absorption is greater in the proximal than in the distal segments. However, after segmental resection of the small intestine, the remaining segments undergo both morphologic and functional "adaptation" to enhance absorption. Such adaptation is secondary to the presence of luminal nutrients and hormonal stimuli and may not be complete in humans for several months after resection. Adaptation is critical for the survival of individuals who have undergone massive resection of the small intestine and/or colon.

Establishing the diagnosis of steatorrhea and identifying its specific cause are often quite difficult. The "gold standard" remains a timed, quantitative stool-fat determination. From a practical standpoint, stool collections are invariably difficult and often incomplete, as nobody wants to handle stool. A qualitative test—Sudan III staining—has long been available to document an increase in stool fat. This test is rapid and inexpensive but, as a qualitative test, does not establish the degree of fat malabsorption and is best used as a preliminary screening study. Many of the blood, breath, and isotopic tests that have been developed (1) do not directly measure fat absorption; (2) exhibit excellent sensitivity when steatorrhea is obvious and severe but poor sensitivity when steatorrhea is mild (e.g., assays for stool chymotrypsin and elastase, which can potentially distinguish pancreatic from nonpancreatic etiologies of steatorrhea); or (3) have not survived the transition from the research laboratory to commercial application.

Nevertheless, routine laboratory studies (i.e., complete blood count, prothrombin time, serum protein determination, alkaline phosphatase) may suggest dietary nutrient depletion, especially deficiencies of iron, folate, cobalamin, and vitamins D and K. Additional studies include measurement of serum carotene, cholesterol, albumin, iron, folate, and cobalamin levels. The serum carotene level can also be reduced if the patient's dietary intake of leafy vegetables is poor.

If steatorrhea and/or altered absorption of other nutrients is suspected, then history, clinical observations, and laboratory testing can help detect deficiency of a nutrient, especially of a fat-soluble vitamin (A, D, E, or K). Thus, evidence of metabolic bone disease with elevated alkaline phosphatase concentrations and/or reduced serum calcium levels suggests vitamin D malabsorption. A deficiency of vitamin K is suggested by an elevated prothrombin time in an individual without liver disease who is not taking anticoagulants. Macrocytic anemia leads to an evaluation for possible cobalamin or folic acid malabsorption. Iron-deficiency anemia in the absence of occult bleeding from the gastrointestinal tract in either a male patient or a nonmenstruating female patient requires an evaluation for iron malabsorption and the exclusion of celiac disease, as iron is absorbed exclusively in the proximal small intestine.

At times, however, a timed (72-h) quantitative stool collection, preferably while the patient is on a defined diet, must be undertaken in order to determine stool fat content and establish the diagnosis of steatorrhea. The presence of steatorrhea then requires further assessment to identify the pathophysiologic process(es) responsible for the defect in dietary lipid digestion/absorption (Table 349-4). Other studies include the Schilling test (Chap. 350e), the D-xylose test, duodenal mucosal biopsy, small-intestinal radiologic examination, and tests of pancreatic exocrine function.

THE SCHILLING TEST

This test (Chap. 350e) is performed to determine the cause of cobalamin malabsorption. An understanding of the physiology and pathophysiology of cobalamin absorption is very valuable, enhancing comprehension of aspects of gastric, pancreatic, and ileal function. Unfortunately, the Schilling test has not been available commercially in the United States for the past few years.

URINARY D-XYLOSE TEST

The urinary D-xylose test for carbohydrate absorption provides an assessment of proximal small-intestinal mucosal function. D-Xylose, a pentose, is absorbed almost exclusively in the proximal small intestine. The D-xylose test is usually performed by administering 25 g of D-xylose and collecting urine for 5 h. An abnormal test (excretion of <4.5 g) primarily reflects duodenal/jejunal mucosal disease. The D-xylose test can also be abnormal in patients with blind loop syndrome (as a consequence primarily of an abnormal intestinal mucosa) and, as a false-positive study, in patients with large collections of fluid in a third space (i.e., ascites, pleural fluid). The ease of obtaining a mucosal biopsy of the small intestine by endoscopy and the false-negative rate of the D-xylose test have led to its diminished use. When small-intestinal mucosal disease is suspected, a small-intestinal mucosal biopsy should be performed.

RADIOLOGIC EXAMINATION

Radiologic examination of the small intestine using barium contrast (small-bowel series or study) can provide important information in the evaluation of the patient with presumed or suspected malabsorption. This study is most often performed in conjunction with an examination of the esophagus, stomach, and duodenal bulb. Because insufficient barium is given to the patient to permit an adequate examination of the small-intestinal mucosa, especially in the ileum, many gastrointestinal radiologists alter the procedure by performing either a small-bowel series in which a large amount of barium is given by mouth, without concurrent examination of the esophagus and stomach, or an enteroclysis study in which a large amount of barium is introduced into the duodenum via a fluoroscopically placed tube. In addition, many of the diagnostic features initially described by radiologists to denote the presence of small-intestinal disease (e.g., flocculation, segmentation) are rarely seen with current barium suspensions. Nonetheless, in skilled hands, barium contrast examination of the small intestine can yield important information. For example, with extensive mucosal disease, intestinal dilation can be seen as a dilution of barium from increased intestinal fluid secretion (Fig. 349-3). A normal barium contrast study does *not* exclude the possibility of small-intestinal disease. However, a small-bowel series remains useful in the search for anatomic abnormalities, such as strictures and fistulas (as in Crohn's disease) or blind loop syndrome (e.g., multiple jejunal diverticula) and to define the extent of a previous surgical resection. Other imaging studies that assess the integrity of small-intestinal morphology are CT enterography and magnetic resonance enterography. Capsule endoscopy and double-balloon enteroscopy are other useful aids in the diagnostic assessment of small-intestinal pathology.

BIOPSY OF SMALL-INTESTINAL MUCOSA

A small-intestinal mucosal biopsy is essential in the evaluation of a patient with documented steatorrhea or chronic diarrhea (i.e., that lasting >3 weeks) (Chap. 55). The ready availability of endoscopic equipment to examine the stomach and duodenum has led to its almost uniform use as the preferred method of obtaining

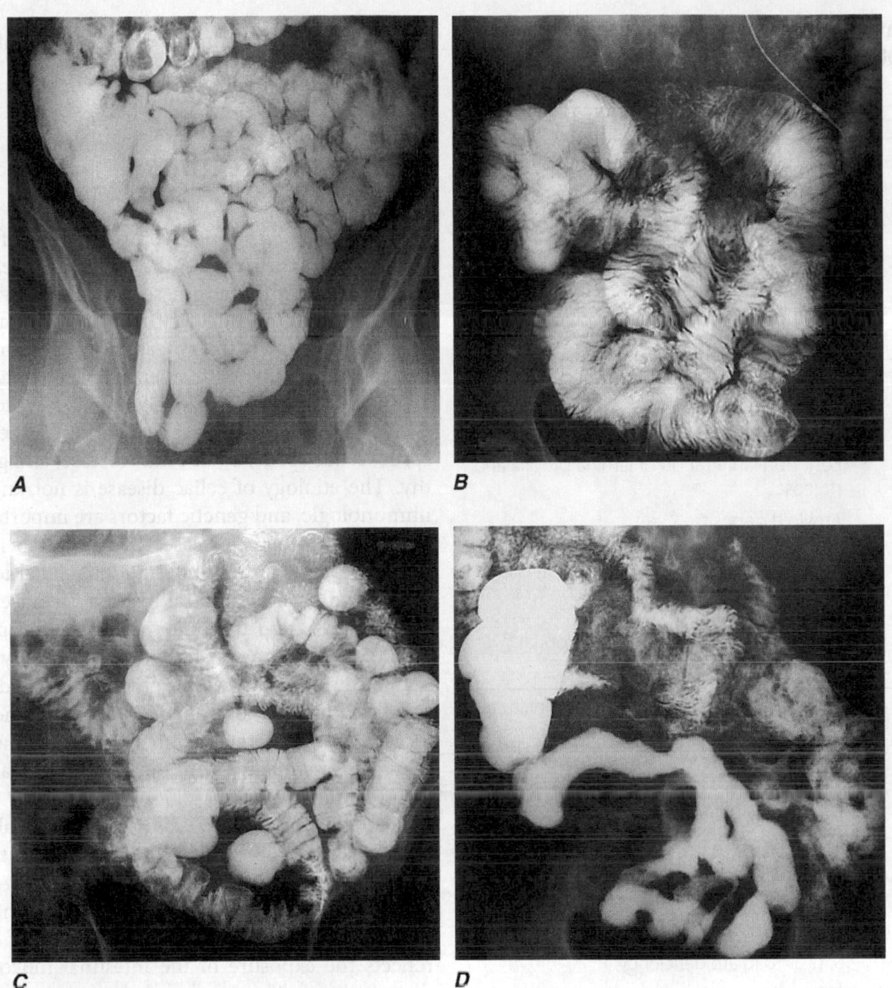

FIGURE 349-3 Barium contrast small-intestinal radiologic examinations. ***A.*** Normal individual. ***B.*** Celiac sprue. ***C.*** Jejunal diverticulosis. ***D.*** Crohn's disease. *(Courtesy of Morton Burrell, MD, Yale University; with permission.)*

histologic material from the proximal small-intestinal mucosa. The primary indications for a small-intestinal biopsy are evaluation of a patient (1) either with documented or suspected steatorrhea or with chronic diarrhea, and (2) with diffuse or focal abnormalities of the small intestine defined on a small-intestinal series. Lesions seen on small-bowel biopsy can be classified into three categories (Table 349-6):

1. *Diffuse, specific lesions.* Relatively few diseases associated with altered nutrient absorption have specific histopathologic abnormalities on small-intestinal mucosal biopsy, and these diseases are uncommon. *Whipple's disease* is characterized by the presence of periodic acid–Schiff (PAS)–positive macrophages in the lamina propria; the bacilli that are also present may require electron microscopic examination for identification (Fig. 349-4). *Abetalipoproteinemia* is characterized by a normal mucosal appearance except for the presence of mucosal absorptive cells that contain lipid postprandially and disappear after a prolonged period of either fat-free intake or fasting. *Immune globulin deficiency* is associated with a variety of histopathologic findings on small-intestinal mucosal biopsy. The characteristic feature is the absence of or substantial reduction in the number of plasma cells in the lamina propria; the mucosal architecture may be either perfectly normal or flat (i.e., villous atrophy). As patients with immune globulin deficiency are often infected with *Giardia lamblia, Giardia* trophozoites may also be seen in the biopsy.
2. *Patchy, specific lesions.* Several diseases feature an abnormal small-intestinal mucosa with a patchy distribution. As a result, biopsy samples obtained randomly or in the absence of endoscopically visualized abnormalities may not reveal diagnostic features. Intestinal *lymphoma* can at times be diagnosed on mucosal biopsy by the identification of malignant lymphoma cells in the lamina propria and submucosa (Chap. 134). Dilated lymphatics in the submucosa and sometimes in the lamina propria indicate *lymphangiectasia* associated with hypoproteinemia secondary to protein loss into the intestine. *Eosinophilic gastroenteritis* comprises a heterogeneous group of disorders with a spectrum of presentations and symptoms, with an eosinophilic infiltrate of the lamina propria, and with or without peripheral eosinophilia. The patchy nature of the infiltrate and its presence in the submucosa often lead to an absence of histopathologic findings on mucosal biopsy. As the involvement of the duodenum in *Crohn's disease* is also submucosal and not necessarily continuous, mucosal biopsies are not the most direct approach to the diagnosis of duodenal Crohn's disease (Chap. 351). Amyloid deposition can be identified by Congo Red staining in some patients with *amyloidosis* involving the duodenum (Chap. 136).
3. *Diffuse, nonspecific lesions. Celiac disease* presents with a characteristic mucosal appearance on duodenal/proximal jejunal mucosal biopsy that is *not* diagnostic of the disease. The diagnosis of celiac disease is established by clinical, histologic, and immunologic responses to a gluten-free diet. *Tropical sprue* (see below) is associated with histologic findings similar to those of celiac disease after a tropical or subtropical exposure but does not respond to gluten restriction; most often symptoms improve with antibiotics and folate administration.

TABLE 349-6 DISEASES THAT CAN BE DIAGNOSED BY SMALL-INTESTINAL MUCOSAL BIOPSIES

Lesions	Pathologic Findings
Diffuse, Specific	
Whipple's disease	Lamina propria includes macrophages containing material positive on periodic acid–Schiff staining
Agammaglobulinemia	No plasma cells; either normal or absent villi ("flat mucosa")
Abetalipoproteinemia	Normal villi; epithelial cells vacuolated with fat postprandially
Patchy, Specific	
Intestinal lymphoma	Malignant cells in lamina propria and submucosa
Intestinal lymphangiectasia	Dilated lymphatics; clubbed villi
Eosinophilic gastroenteritis	Eosinophil infiltration of lamina propria and mucosa
Amyloidosis	Amyloid deposits
Crohn's disease	Noncaseating granulomas
Infection by one or more microorganisms (see text)	Specific organisms
Mastocytosis	Mast cell infiltration of lamina propria
Diffuse, Nonspecific	
Celiac disease	Short or absent villi; mononuclear infiltrate; epithelial cell damage; hypertrophy of crypts
Tropical sprue	Similar to celiac disease
Bacterial overgrowth	Patchy damage to villi; lymphocyte infiltration
Folate deficiency	Short villi; decreased mitosis in crypts; megalocytosis
Vitamin B_{12} deficiency	Similar to folate deficiency
Radiation enteritis	Similar to folate deficiency
Zollinger-Ellison syndrome	Mucosal ulceration and erosion from acid
Protein-calorie malnutrition	Villous atrophy; secondary bacterial overgrowth
Drug-induced enteritis	Variable histology

Several microorganisms can be identified in small-intestinal biopsy samples, establishing a correct diagnosis. At times, the biopsy is performed specifically to diagnose infection (e.g., Whipple's disease or giardiasis). In most other instances, the infection is detected incidentally during the workup for diarrhea or other abdominal symptoms. Many of these infections occur in immunocompromised patients with diarrhea; the etiologic agents include *Cryptosporidium, Isospora belli,* microsporidia, *Cyclospora, Toxoplasma,* cytomegalovirus, adenovirus, *Mycobacterium avium-intracellulare,* and *G. lamblia.* In immunocompromised patients, when *Candida, Aspergillus, Cryptococcus,* or *Histoplasma* organisms are seen on duodenal biopsy, their presence generally reflects systemic infection. Apart from Whipple's disease and infections in the immunocompromised host, small-bowel biopsy is seldom used as the primary mode of diagnosis of infection. Even giardiasis is more easily diagnosed by stool antigen studies and/or duodenal aspiration than by duodenal biopsy.

Patients with steatorrhea require assessment of *pancreatic exocrine function,* which is often abnormal in chronic pancreatitis. The secretin test that collects pancreatic secretions by duodenal intubation following intravenous administration of secretin is the only test that directly measures pancreatic exocrine function but is available only at a few specialized centers. Endoscopic approaches (endoscopic retrograde cholangiopancreatography, endoscopic ultrasound) provide an excellent assessment of pancreatic duct anatomy but do *not* assess exocrine function (Chap. 370).

Table 349-7 summarizes the results of the D-xylose test, the Schilling test, and small-intestinal mucosal biopsy in patients with steatorrhea of various etiologies.

SPECIFIC DISEASE ENTITIES

CELIAC DISEASE

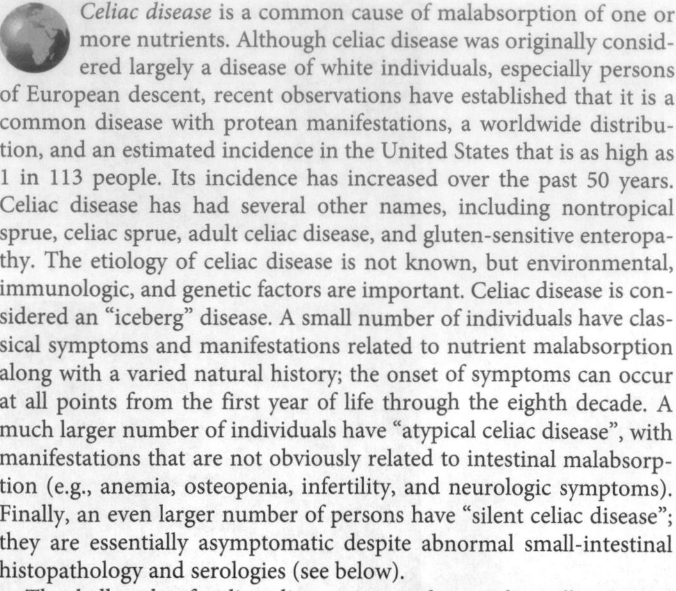

Celiac disease is a common cause of malabsorption of one or more nutrients. Although celiac disease was originally considered largely a disease of white individuals, especially persons of European descent, recent observations have established that it is a common disease with protean manifestations, a worldwide distribution, and an estimated incidence in the United States that is as high as 1 in 113 people. Its incidence has increased over the past 50 years. Celiac disease has had several other names, including nontropical sprue, celiac sprue, adult celiac disease, and gluten-sensitive enteropathy. The etiology of celiac disease is not known, but environmental, immunologic, and genetic factors are important. Celiac disease is considered an "iceberg" disease. A small number of individuals have classical symptoms and manifestations related to nutrient malabsorption along with a varied natural history; the onset of symptoms can occur at all points from the first year of life through the eighth decade. A much larger number of individuals have "atypical celiac disease", with manifestations that are not obviously related to intestinal malabsorption (e.g., anemia, osteopenia, infertility, and neurologic symptoms). Finally, an even larger number of persons have "silent celiac disease"; they are essentially asymptomatic despite abnormal small-intestinal histopathology and serologies (see below).

The hallmark of celiac disease is an abnormal small-intestinal biopsy (Fig. 349-4) and the response of the condition (including symptoms and histologic changes on small-intestinal biopsy) to the elimination of gluten from the diet. The histologic changes have a proximal-to-distal intestinal distribution of severity, which probably reflects the exposure of the intestinal mucosa to varied amounts of dietary gluten. The symptoms do not necessarily correlate with histologic changes, especially as many newly diagnosed patients with celiac disease may be asymptomatic or only minimally symptomatic (often with no gastrointestinal symptoms).

The symptoms of celiac disease may appear with the introduction of cereals into an infant's diet, although spontaneous remissions often occur during the second decade of life that may be either permanent or followed by the reappearance of symptoms over several years. Alternatively, the symptoms of celiac disease may first become evident at almost any age throughout adulthood. In many patients, frequent spontaneous remissions and exacerbations occur. The symptoms range from significant malabsorption of multiple nutrients, with diarrhea, steatorrhea, weight loss, and the consequences of nutrient depletion (i.e., anemia and metabolic bone disease), to the absence of gastrointestinal symptoms despite evidence of the depletion of a single nutrient (e.g., iron or folate deficiency, osteomalacia, edema from protein loss). Asymptomatic relatives of patients with celiac disease have been identified as having this disease either by small-intestinal biopsy or by serologic studies (e.g., antiendomysial antibodies, tissue transglutaminase [tTG], deamidated gliadin peptide). The availability of these "celiac serologies" has led to a substantial increase in the frequency of diagnosis of celiac disease, and the diagnosis is now being made primarily in patients without "classic" symptoms but with atypical and subclinical presentations.

Etiology The etiology of celiac disease is not known, but environmental, immunologic, and genetic factors all appear to contribute to the disease. One *environmental* factor is the clear association of the disease with gliadin, a component of gluten that is present in wheat, barley, and rye. In addition to the role of gluten restriction in treatment, the instillation of gluten into both the normal-appearing rectum and the distal ileum of patients with celiac disease results in morphologic changes within hours.

An *immunologic* component in the pathogenesis of celiac disease is critical and involves both adaptive and innate immune responses. Serum

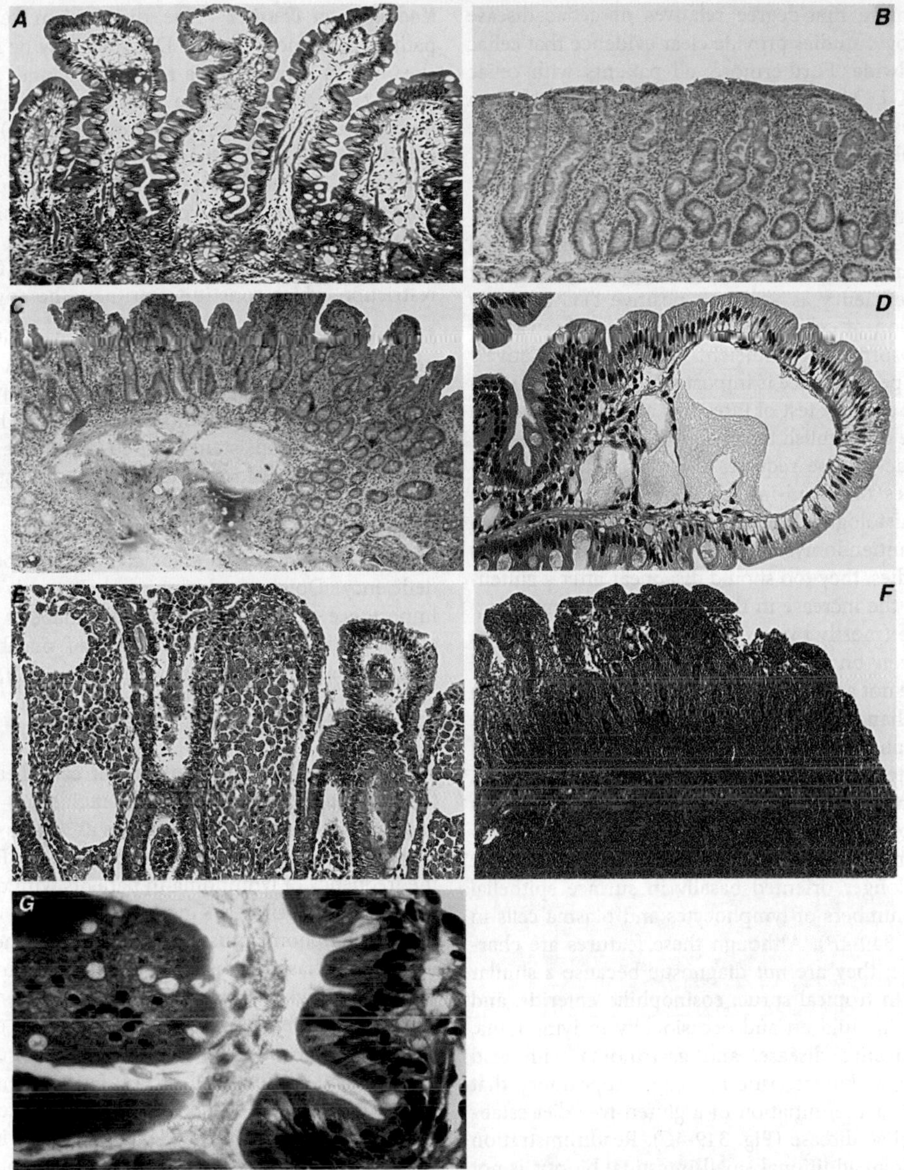

FIGURE 349-4 Small-intestinal mucosal biopsies. ***A.*** Normal individual. ***B.*** Untreated celiac sprue. ***C.*** Treated celiac sprue. ***D.*** Intestinal lymphangiectasia. ***E.*** Whipple's disease. ***F.*** Lymphoma. ***G.*** Giardiasis. *(Courtesy of Marie Robert, MD, Yale University; with permission.)*

antibodies—IgA antigliadin, antiendomysial, and anti-tTG antibodies—are present, but it is not known whether such antibodies are primary or secondary to the tissue damage. The presence of antiendomysial antibody is 90–95% sensitive and 90–95% specific; the antigen recognized by antiendomysial antibody is tTG, which deaminates gliadin, which is presented to HLA-DQ2 or HLA-DQ8 (see below). Antibody studies are frequently used to identify patients with celiac disease; patients with these antibodies should undergo duodenal biopsy. This autoantibody has not been linked to a pathogenetic mechanism (or mechanisms) responsible for celiac disease. Nonetheless, this antibody is useful in establishing the true prevalence of celiac disease in the general population. A 4-week course of treatment with prednisolone induces a remission in a patient with celiac disease who continues to eat gluten and converts the "flat" abnormal duodenal biopsy to a more normal-appearing one. In addition, gliadin peptides interact with gliadin-specific T cells that mediate tissue injury and induce the release of one or more cytokines (e.g., interferon γ) that cause tissue injury.

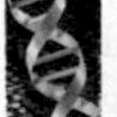

Genetic factor(s) are also involved in celiac disease. The incidence of symptomatic celiac disease varies widely in different population groups (high among whites, low among blacks and

TABLE 349-7 RESULTS OF DIAGNOSTIC STUDIES IN STEATORRHEA OF VARIOUS ETIOLOGIES

	D-Xylose Test	Schilling Test	Duodenal Mucosal Biopsy
Chronic pancreatitis	Normal	50% abnormal; if abnormal, normal with pancreatic enzyme treatment	Normal
Bacterial overgrowth syndromes	Normal or only modestly abnormal	Often abnormal; if abnormal, normal after antibiotic treatment	Usually normal
Ileal disease	Normal	Abnormal	Normal
Celiac disease	Decreased	Normal	Abnormal: probably "flat"
Intestinal lymphangiectasiaia	Normal	Normal	Abnormal: "dilated lymphatics"

Asians) and is 10% among first-degree relatives of celiac disease patients. However, serologic studies provide clear evidence that celiac disease is present worldwide. Furthermore, all patients with celiac disease express the HLA-DQ2 or HLA-DQ8 allele, although only a minority of people expressing DQ2/DQ8 have celiac disease. Absence of DQ2/DQ8 excludes the diagnosis of celiac disease.

Diagnosis A small-intestinal biopsy is required to establish a diagnosis of celiac disease (Fig. 349-4). A biopsy should be performed when patients have symptoms and laboratory findings suggestive of nutrient malabsorption and/or deficiency as well as a positive tTG antibody test. Since the presentation of celiac disease is often subtle, without overt evidence of malabsorption or nutrient deficiency, a relatively low threshold for biopsy performance is important. It is more prudent to perform a biopsy than another test of intestinal absorption that can never completely exclude or establish this diagnosis.

The diagnosis of celiac disease requires the detection of characteristic histologic changes on small-intestinal biopsy together with a prompt clinical and histologic response after the institution of a gluten-free diet. If IgA antiendomysial or tTG antibodies have been detected in serologic studies, they too should disappear after a gluten-free diet is started. With the increase in the number of patients diagnosed with celiac disease (mostly by serologic studies), the spectrum of histologic changes seen on duodenal biopsy has increased and includes findings that are not as severe as the classic changes shown in Fig. 349-4. The classic changes seen on duodenal/jejunal biopsy are restricted to the mucosa and include (1) an increase in the number of intraepithelial lymphocytes; (2) absence or a reduced height of villi, which causes a flat appearance with increased crypt cell proliferation resulting in crypt hyperplasia and loss of villous structure, with consequent villous, but not mucosal, atrophy; (3) a cuboidal appearance and nuclei that are no longer oriented basally in surface epithelial cells; and (4) increased numbers of lymphocytes and plasma cells in the lamina propria (Fig. 349-4*B*). Although these features are characteristic of celiac disease, they are *not* diagnostic because a similar appearance can develop in tropical sprue, eosinophilic enteritis, and milk-protein intolerance in children and occasionally in lymphoma, bacterial overgrowth, Crohn's disease, and gastrinoma with acid hypersecretion. However, a characteristic histologic appearance that reverts toward normal after the initiation of a gluten-free diet establishes the diagnosis of celiac disease (Fig. 349-4*C*). Readministration of gluten, with or without an additional small-intestinal biopsy, is not necessary.

A number of patients exhibit *gluten sensitivity*; i.e., they have gastrointestinal symptoms that respond to gluten restriction but do not have celiac disease. The basis for such gluten sensitivity is not known.

Failure to Respond to Gluten Restriction The most common cause of persistent symptoms in a patient who fulfills all the criteria for the diagnosis of celiac disease is *continued intake of gluten*. Gluten is ubiquitous, and a significant effort must be made to exclude all gluten from the diet. Use of rice flour in place of wheat flour is very helpful, and several support groups provide important aid to patients with celiac disease and to their families. More than 90% of patients who have the characteristic findings of celiac disease respond to complete dietary gluten restriction. The remainder constitute a heterogeneous group (whose condition is often called *refractory celiac disease* or *refractory sprue*) that includes some patients who (1) respond to restriction of other dietary protein (e.g., soy); (2) respond to glucocorticoid treatment; (3) are "temporary" (i.e., whose clinical and morphologic findings disappear after several months or years); or (4) fail to respond to all measures and have a fatal outcome, with or without documented complications of celiac disease, such as the development of intestinal T cell lymphoma or autoimmune enteropathy.

Therapeutic approaches that do not include a gluten-free diet are being developed and include the use of peptidases to inactivate toxic gliadin peptides and of small molecules to block toxic peptide uptake across intestinal tight junctions.

Mechanism of Diarrhea The diarrhea in celiac disease has several pathogenetic mechanisms. Diarrhea may be secondary to (1) steatorrhea, which is primarily a result of changes in jejunal mucosal function; (2) secondary lactase deficiency, a consequence of changes in jejunal brush border enzymatic function; (3) bile acid malabsorption resulting in bile acid–induced fluid secretion in the colon (in cases with more extensive disease involving the ileum); and (4) endogenous fluid secretion resulting from crypt hyperplasia. Celiac disease patients with more severe involvement may improve temporarily with *dietary lactose and fat restriction* while awaiting the full effects of total gluten restriction, which constitutes primary therapy.

Associated Diseases Celiac disease is associated with dermatitis herpetiformis (DH), but this association has not been explained. Patients with DH have characteristic papulovesicular lesions that respond to dapsone. Almost all patients with DH have histologic changes in the small intestine consistent with celiac disease, although usually much milder and less diffuse in distribution. Most patients with DH have mild or no gastrointestinal symptoms. In contrast, relatively few patients with celiac disease have DH.

Celiac disease is also associated with diabetes mellitus type 1, IgA deficiency, Down syndrome, and Turner's syndrome. The clinical importance of the association with diabetes is that, although severe watery diarrhea without evidence of malabsorption is most often diagnosed as "diabetic diarrhea" (Chap. 417), assay of antiendomysial antibodies and/or a small-intestinal biopsy must be considered to exclude celiac disease.

Complications The most important complication of celiac disease is the development of cancer. The incidences of both gastrointestinal and nongastrointestinal neoplasms as well as intestinal lymphoma are elevated among patients with celiac disease. For unexplained reasons, the frequency of lymphoma in patients with celiac disease is higher in Ireland and the United Kingdom than in the United States. The possibility of lymphoma must be considered whenever a patient with celiac disease who has previously done well on a gluten-free diet is no longer responsive to gluten restriction or a patient who presents with clinical and histologic features consistent with celiac disease does not respond to a gluten-free diet. Other complications of celiac disease include the development of intestinal ulceration independent of lymphoma and so-called refractory sprue (see above) and collagenous sprue. In *collagenous sprue*, a layer of collagen-like material is present beneath the basement membrane; patients with collagenous sprue generally do not respond to a gluten-free diet and often have a poor prognosis.

TROPICAL SPRUE

Tropical sprue is a poorly understood syndrome that affects both expatriates and natives in certain but not all tropical areas and is manifested by chronic diarrhea, steatorrhea, weight loss, and nutritional deficiencies, including those of both folate and cobalamin. This disease affects 5–10% of the population in some tropical areas.

Chronic diarrhea in a tropical environment is most often caused by infectious agents, including *G. lamblia, Yersinia enterocolitica, C. difficile, Cryptosporidium parvum*, and *Cyclospora cayetanensis*. Tropical sprue should not be entertained as a possible diagnosis until the presence of cysts and trophozoites has been excluded in three stool samples. Chronic infections of the gastrointestinal tract and diarrhea in patients with or without AIDS are discussed in Chaps. 160, 161, and 226.

The small-intestinal mucosa of individuals living in tropical areas is not identical to that of individuals who reside in temperate climates. In residents of tropical areas, biopsies reveal a mild alteration of villous architecture with a modest increase in mononuclear cells in the lamina propria, which on occasion can be as severe as that seen in celiac disease. These changes are observed both in native residents and in expatriates living in tropical regions and are usually associated with mild decreases in absorptive function, but they revert to "normal" when an individual moves or returns to a temperate area. Some have suggested that the changes seen in tropical enteropathy and in tropical sprue represent different ends of the spectrum of a single entity, but convincing evidence to support this concept is lacking.

Etiology Because tropical sprue responds to antibiotics, the consensus is that it may be caused by one or more infectious agents. Nonetheless, the etiology and pathogenesis of tropical sprue are uncertain. First, its occurrence is not evenly distributed in all tropical areas; rather, it is found in specific locations, including southern India, the Philippines, and several Caribbean islands (e.g., Puerto Rico, Haiti), but is rarely observed in Africa, Jamaica, or Southeast Asia. Second, an occasional individual does not develop symptoms of tropical sprue until long after having left an endemic area. For this reason, celiac disease (often referred to as celiac sprue) was originally called *nontropical sprue* to distinguish it from tropical sprue. Third, multiple microorganisms have been identified in jejunal aspirates, with relatively little consistency among studies. *Klebsiella pneumoniae, Enterobacter cloacae*, and *E. coli* have been implicated in some studies of tropical sprue, while other studies have favored a role for a toxin produced by one or more of these bacteria. Fourth, the incidence of tropical sprue appears to have decreased substantially during the past two or three decades, perhaps in relation to improved sanitation in many tropical countries during this time. Some have speculated that the reduced occurrence is attributable to the wider use of antibiotics in acute diarrhea, especially in travelers to tropical areas from temperate countries. Fifth, the role of folic acid deficiency in the pathogenesis of tropical sprue requires clarification. Folic acid is absorbed exclusively in the duodenum and proximal jejunum, and most patients with tropical sprue have evidence of folate malabsorption and depletion. Although folate deficiency can cause changes in small-intestinal mucosa that are corrected by folate replacement, several earlier studies reporting that tropical sprue could be cured by folic acid did not provide an explanation for the "insult" that was initially responsible for folate malabsorption.

The clinical pattern of tropical sprue varies in different areas of the world (e.g., India vs. Puerto Rico). Not infrequently, individuals in southern India initially report the occurrence of acute enteritis before the development of steatorrhea and malabsorption. In contrast, in Puerto Rico, a more insidious onset of symptoms and a more dramatic response to antibiotics are seen than in some other locations. Tropical sprue in different areas of the world may not be the same disease, and similar clinical entities may have different etiologies.

Diagnosis The diagnosis of tropical sprue is best based on an abnormal small-intestinal mucosal biopsy in an individual with chronic diarrhea and evidence of malabsorption who is either residing or has recently lived in a tropical country. The small-intestinal biopsy in tropical sprue does not reveal pathognomonic features but resembles, and can often be indistinguishable from, that seen in celiac disease (Fig. 349-4). The biopsy sample in tropical sprue has less villous architectural alteration and more mononuclear cell infiltrate in the lamina propria. In contrast to those of celiac disease, the histologic features of tropical sprue manifest with a similar degree of severity throughout the small intestine, and a gluten-free diet does not result in either clinical or histologic improvement in tropical sprue.

TREATMENT TROPICAL SPRUE

Broad-spectrum antibiotics and folic acid are most often curative, especially if the patient leaves the tropical area and does not return. Tetracycline should be used for up to 6 months and may be associated with improvement within 1–2 weeks. Folic acid alone induces hematologic remission as well as improvement in appetite, weight gain, and some morphologic changes in small-intestinal biopsy. Because of marked folate deficiency, folic acid is most often given together with antibiotics.

SHORT-BOWEL SYNDROME

Short-bowel syndrome is a descriptive term for the myriad clinical problems that follow resection of various lengths of small intestine or, on rare occasions, are congenital (e.g., microvillous inclusion disease). The factors that determine both the type and degree of symptoms include (1) the specific segment (jejunum vs. ileum) resected, (2) the length of the resected segment, (3) the integrity of the ileocecal valve, (4) whether any large intestine has also been removed, (5) residual disease in the remaining small and/or large intestine (e.g., Crohn's disease, mesenteric artery disease), and (6) the degree of adaptation in the remaining intestine. Short-bowel syndrome can occur in persons of any age, from neonates to the elderly.

Three different situations in adults mandate intestinal resection: (1) mesenteric vascular disease, including atherosclerosis, thrombotic phenomena, and vasculitides; (2) primary mucosal and submucosal disease (e.g., Crohn's disease); and (3) operations without preexisting small-intestinal disease (e.g., after trauma).

After resection of the small intestine, the residual intestine undergoes adaptation of both structure and function that may last for up to 6–12 months. Continued intake of dietary nutrients and calories is required to stimulate adaptation via direct contact with the intestinal mucosa, the release of one or more intestinal hormones, and pancreatic and biliary secretions. Thus, enteral nutrition with calorie administration must be maintained, especially in the early postoperative period, even if an extensive intestinal resection requiring parenteral nutrition (PN) has been performed. The subsequent ability of such patients to absorb nutrients will not be known for several months, until adaptation is complete.

Multiple factors besides the absence of intestinal mucosa (required for lipid, fluid, and electrolyte absorption) contribute to diarrhea and steatorrhea in these patients. Removal of the ileum, and especially the ileocecal valve, is often associated with more severe diarrhea than jejunal resection. Without part or all of the ileum, diarrhea can be caused by an increase in bile acids entering the colon; these acids stimulate colonic fluid and electrolyte secretion. Absence of the ileocecal valve is also associated with a decrease in intestinal transit time and bacterial overgrowth from the colon. The presence of the colon (or a major portion) is associated with substantially less diarrhea and a lower likelihood of *intestinal failure* (an inability to maintain nutrition without parenteral support) as a result of fermentation of nonabsorbed carbohydrates to SCFAs. The latter are absorbed in the colon and stimulate Na and water absorption, improving overall fluid balance. Lactose intolerance as a result of the removal of lactase-containing mucosa as well as gastric hypersecretion may also contribute to the diarrhea.

In addition to diarrhea and/or steatorrhea, a range of nonintestinal symptoms is observed in some patients. The frequency of renal calcium oxalate calculi increases significantly in patients with a small-intestinal resection and an intact colon; this greater frequency is due to an increase in oxalate absorption by the large intestine, with subsequent *enteric hyperoxaluria*. Two possible mechanisms for the increase in oxalate absorption in the colon have been suggested: (1) increased bile acids and fatty acids that augment colonic mucosal permeability, resulting in enhanced oxalate absorption; and (2) increased fatty acids that bind calcium, resulting in an enhanced amount of soluble oxalate that is then absorbed. Since oxalate is high in relatively few foods (e.g., spinach, rhubarb, tea), dietary restrictions alone do not constitute adequate treatment. Cholestyramine (an anion-binding resin) and calcium have proved useful in reducing hyperoxaluria. Similarly, an increase in cholesterol gallstones is related to a decrease in the bile-acid pool size, which results in the generation of cholesterol supersaturation in gallbladder bile. Gastric hypersecretion of acid occurs in many patients after large resections of the small intestine. The etiology is unclear but may be related to either reduced hormonal inhibition of acid secretion or increased gastrin levels due to reduced small-intestinal catabolism of circulating gastrin. The resulting gastric acid secretion may be an important factor contributing to diarrhea and steatorrhea. A reduced pH in the duodenum can inactivate pancreatic lipase and/or precipitate duodenal bile acids, thereby increasing steatorrhea, and an increase in gastric secretion can create a volume overload relative to the reduced small-intestinal absorptive capacity. Inhibition of gastric acid secretion with proton pump inhibitors can help reduce diarrhea and steatorrhea, but only for the first 6 months.

TREATMENT SHORT-BOWEL SYNDROME

Treatment of short-bowel syndrome depends on the severity of symptoms and on whether the individual is able to maintain caloric and electrolyte balance with oral intake alone. Initial treatment includes judicious use of opiates (including codeine) to reduce stool output and to establish an effective diet. If the colon is in situ, the initial diet should be low in fat and high in carbohydrate in order to minimize diarrhea from fatty acid stimulation of colonic fluid secretion. MCTs (see Table 349-3), a low-lactose diet, and various soluble fiber–containing diets should also be tried. In the absence of an ileocecal valve, possible bacterial overgrowth must be considered and treated. If gastric acid hypersecretion is contributing to diarrhea and steatorrhea, a proton pump inhibitor may be helpful. Usually none of these therapeutic approaches provides an instant solution, but each can contribute to the reduction of disabling diarrhea.

The patient's vitamin and mineral status must also be monitored; replacement therapy should be initiated if indicated. Fat-soluble vitamins, folate, cobalamin, calcium, iron, magnesium, and zinc are the most critical factors to monitor on a regular basis. If these approaches are not successful, home PN is an established therapy that can be maintained for many years. Small-intestinal transplantation is becoming established as a possible approach for individuals with extensive intestinal resection who cannot be maintained without PN—i.e., those with intestinal failure. A recombinant analogue of glucagon-like peptide 2 (GLP-2; teduglutide) is approved for use in patients with PN-dependent short-bowel syndrome on the basis of its ability to increase intestinal growth and improve absorption.

BACTERIAL OVERGROWTH SYNDROMES

Bacterial overgrowth syndromes comprise a group of disorders with diarrhea, steatorrhea, and macrocytic anemia whose common feature is the proliferation of colonic-type bacteria within the small intestine. This bacterial proliferation is due to stasis caused by impaired peristalsis (*functional stasis*), changes in intestinal anatomy (*anatomic stasis*), or direct communication between the small and large intestine. These conditions have also been referred to as *stagnant bowel syndrome* or *blind loop syndrome.*

Pathogenesis The manifestations of bacterial overgrowth syndromes are a direct consequence of the presence of increased amounts of a colonic-type bacterial flora, such as *E. coli* or *Bacteroides*, in the small intestine. *Macrocytic anemia* is due to cobalamin—not folate—deficiency. Most bacteria require cobalamin for growth, and increasing concentrations of bacteria use up the relatively small amounts of dietary cobalamin. *Steatorrhea* is due to impaired micelle formation as a consequence of a reduced intraduodenal concentration of conjugated bile acids and the presence of unconjugated bile acids. Certain bacteria, including *Bacteroides*, deconjugate conjugated bile acids to unconjugated bile acids. Unconjugated bile acids are absorbed more rapidly than conjugated bile acids; as a result, the intraduodenal concentration of bile acids is reduced. In addition, the CMC of unconjugated bile acids is higher than that of conjugated bile acids, and the result is a decrease in micelle formation. *Diarrhea* is due, at least in part, to steatorrhea, when it is present. However, some patients manifest diarrhea *without* steatorrhea, and it is assumed that the colonic-type bacteria in these patients are producing one or more bacterial enterotoxins that are responsible for fluid secretion and diarrhea.

Etiology The etiology of these different disorders is bacterial proliferation in the small-intestinal lumen secondary to anatomic or functional stasis or to a communication between the relatively sterile small intestine and the colon, with its high levels of aerobic and anaerobic bacteria. Several examples of *anatomic* stasis have been identified: (1) one or more diverticula (both duodenal and jejunal) (Fig. 294-3*C*); (2) fistulas and strictures related to Crohn's disease (Fig. 349-3*D*); (3) a proximal duodenal afferent loop following subtotal gastrectomy and gastrojejunostomy; (4) a bypass of the intestine (e.g., a jejunoileal bypass for obesity); and (5) dilation at the site of a previous intestinal anastomosis. These anatomic derangements are often associated with the presence of a segment (or segments) of intestine out of continuity of propagated peristalsis, with consequent stasis and bacterial proliferation. Bacterial overgrowth syndromes can also occur in the *absence* of an anatomic blind loop when *functional* stasis is present. Impaired peristalsis and bacterial overgrowth in the absence of a blind loop occur in scleroderma, where motility abnormalities exist in both the esophagus and the small intestine (Chap. 382). Functional stasis and bacterial overgrowth can also develop in association with diabetes mellitus and in the small intestine when a direct connection exists between the small and large intestines, including an ileocolonic resection, or occasionally after an enterocolic anastomosis that permits entry of bacteria into the small intestine as a result of bypassing the ileocecal valve.

Diagnosis The diagnosis may be suspected from the combination of a low serum cobalamin level and an elevated serum folate level, as enteric bacteria frequently produce folate compounds that are absorbed in the duodenum. Ideally, the bacterial overgrowth syndromes are diagnosed by the demonstration of increased levels of aerobic and/or anaerobic colonic-type bacteria in a jejunal aspirate obtained by intubation. However, this specialized test is rarely available. Breath hydrogen testing with administration of lactulose (a nondigestible disaccharide) has also been used to detect bacterial overgrowth. The Schilling test can diagnose bacterial overgrowth (see Chap. 350e) but is not available routinely. Often the diagnosis is suspected clinically and confirmed by the response to treatment.

TREATMENT BACTERIAL OVERGROWTH SYNDROMES

Primary treatment should be directed, if at all possible, to the surgical correction of an anatomic blind loop. In the absence of functional stasis, it is important to define the anatomic relationships responsible for stasis and bacterial overgrowth. For example, bacterial overgrowth secondary to strictures, one or more diverticula, or a proximal afferent loop can potentially be cured by surgical correction of the anatomic state. In contrast, the functional stasis of scleroderma or certain anatomic stasis states (e.g., multiple jejunal diverticula) cannot be corrected surgically, and these conditions should be treated with broad-spectrum antibiotics. Tetracycline used to be the initial drug of choice; because of increasing resistance, however, other antibiotics, such as metronidazole, amoxicillin/clavulanic acid, rifaximin and cephalosporins, have been employed. The antibiotic should be given for ~3 weeks or until symptoms remit. Although the natural history of these conditions is chronic, antibiotics should not be given continuously. Symptoms usually remit within 2–3 weeks of initial antibiotic therapy. Treatment need not be repeated until symptoms recur. For frequent recurrences, several treatment strategies exist, but the use of antibiotics for 1 week per month, whether or not symptoms are present, is often most effective.

Unfortunately, therapy for bacterial overgrowth syndromes is largely empirical, with an absence of clinical trials on which to base rational decisions regarding antibiotic choice, treatment duration, and/or the best approach to therapy for recurrences. Bacterial overgrowth may also occur as a component of another chronic disease, such as Crohn's disease, radiation enteritis, or short-bowel syndrome. Treatment of the bacterial overgrowth in these settings will not cure the underlying problem but may be very important in ameliorating a subset of clinical problems that are related to bacterial overgrowth.

WHIPPLE'S DISEASE

Whipple's disease is a chronic multisystemic disease associated with diarrhea, steatorrhea, weight loss, arthralgia, and central nervous system (CNS) and cardiac problems; it is caused by the bacterium *Tropheryma whipplei.* Until the identification of *T. whipplei* by polymerase chain reaction, the hallmark of Whipple's disease had been the presence of PAS-positive macrophages in the small intestine (Fig. 349-4*E*) and other organs with evidence of disease.

Etiology *T. whipplei*, a small (50–500 nm) gram-positive bacillus in the group Actinobacteria, has low virulence but high infectivity. Symptoms of Whipple's disease are relatively minimal compared to the bacterial burden in multiple tissues.

Clinical presentation The onset of Whipple's disease is insidious and is characterized by diarrhea, steatorrhea, abdominal pain, weight loss, migratory large-joint arthropathy, and fever as well as ophthalmologic and CNS symptoms. Dementia is a relatively late symptom and an extremely poor prognostic sign, especially in patients who experience relapse after the induction of a remission with antibiotics. For unexplained reasons, the disease occurs primarily in middle-aged white men. The steatorrhea in these patients is generally believed to be secondary to both small-intestinal mucosal injury and lymphatic obstruction due to the increased number of PAS-positive macrophages in the lamina propria of the small intestine.

Diagnosis The diagnosis of Whipple's disease is suggested by a multisystemic disease in a patient with diarrhea and steatorrhea. Tissue biopsy of the small intestine and/or other organs that may be involved (e.g., liver, lymph nodes, heart, eyes, CNS, or synovial membranes), given the patient's symptoms, is the primary approach. The presence of PAS-positive macrophages containing the characteristic small bacilli is suggestive of this diagnosis. However, *T. whipplei*–containing macrophages can be confused with PAS-positive macrophages containing *M. avium* complex, which may be a cause of diarrhea in AIDS. The presence of the *T. whipplei* bacillus outside of macrophages is a more important indicator of active disease than is their presence within the macrophages. *T. whipplei* has now been successfully grown in culture.

TREATMENT WHIPPLE'S DISEASE

The treatment for Whipple's disease is prolonged use of antibiotics. The current regimen of choice is double-strength trimethoprim-sulfamethoxazole for ~1 year. PAS-positive macrophages can persist after successful treatment, and the presence of bacilli outside of macrophages is indicative of persistent infection or an early sign of recurrence. Recurrence of disease activity, especially with dementia, is an extremely poor prognostic sign and requires an antibiotic that crosses the blood-brain barrier. If trimethoprim-sulfamethoxazole is not tolerated, chloramphenicol is an appropriate second choice.

PROTEIN-LOSING ENTEROPATHY

Protein-losing enteropathy is not a specific disease but rather a group of gastrointestinal and nongastrointestinal disorders with hypoproteinemia and edema in the absence of either proteinuria or defects in protein synthesis (e.g., chronic liver disease). These diseases are characterized by excess protein loss into the gastrointestinal tract. Normally, ~10% of total protein catabolism occurs via the gastrointestinal tract. Evidence of increased protein loss into the gastrointestinal tract is found in more than 65 different diseases, which can be classified into three groups: (1) mucosal ulceration, such that the protein loss primarily represents exudation across damaged mucosa (e.g., ulcerative colitis, gastrointestinal carcinomas, and peptic ulcer); (2) nonulcerated mucosa, but with evidence of mucosal damage so that the protein loss represents loss across epithelia with altered permeability (e.g., celiac disease and Ménétrier's disease in the small intestine and stomach, respectively); and (3) lymphatic dysfunction, representing either primary lymphatic disease or lymphatic disease secondary to partial lymphatic obstruction that may occur as a result of enlarged lymph nodes or cardiac disease.

Diagnosis The diagnosis of protein-losing enteropathy is suggested by peripheral edema and low serum albumin and globulin levels in the absence of renal and hepatic disease. An individual with protein-losing enteropathy only rarely has selective loss of *only* albumin or *only* globulins. Therefore, marked reduction of serum albumin with normal serum globulins should not initiate an evaluation for protein-losing enteropathy but should suggest renal and/or hepatic disease. Likewise, reduced serum globulins with normal serum albumin levels are more likely a result of reduced globulin synthesis rather than enhanced globulin loss into the intestine. An increase in protein loss into the gastrointestinal tract has been documented by the administration of one of several radiolabeled proteins and its quantitation in stool during a 24- or 48-h period. Unfortunately, none of these radiolabeled proteins is available for routine clinical use. α_1-Antitrypsin, a protein that accounts for ~4% of total serum proteins and is resistant to proteolysis, can be used to detect enhanced rates of serum protein loss into the intestinal tract but cannot be used to assess gastric protein loss because of its degradation in an acid milieu. α_1-Antitrypsin clearance is measured by determining stool volume as well as both stool and plasma α_1-antitrypsin concentrations. In addition to the loss of protein via abnormal and distended lymphatics, peripheral lymphocytes may be lost via lymphatics, with consequent relative lymphopenia. Thus, lymphopenia in a patient with hypoproteinemia indicates increased loss of protein into the gastrointestinal tract.

Patients with increased protein loss into the gastrointestinal tract from lymphatic obstruction often have steatorrhea and diarrhea. The steatorrhea is a result of altered lymphatic flow as lipid-containing chylomicrons exit from intestinal epithelial cells via intestinal lymphatics (Table 349-4; Fig. 349-4). In the absence of mechanical or anatomic lymphatic obstruction, intrinsic intestinal lymphatic dysfunction—with or without lymphatic dysfunction in the peripheral extremities—has been designated *intestinal lymphangiectasia.* Similarly, ~50% of individuals with intrinsic peripheral lymphatic disease (Milroy's disease) also have intestinal lymphangiectasia and hypoproteinemia. Other than steatorrhea and enhanced protein loss into the gastrointestinal tract, all other aspects of intestinal absorptive function are normal in intestinal lymphangiectasia.

Other Causes Patients who appear to have idiopathic protein-losing enteropathy without evidence of gastrointestinal disease should be examined for cardiac disease—especially right-sided valvular disease and chronic pericarditis (Chaps. 284 and 288). On occasion, hypoproteinemia can be the only presenting manifestation in these two types of heart disease. Ménétrier's disease (also called *hypertrophic gastropathy*) is an uncommon entity that involves the body and fundus of the stomach and is characterized by large gastric folds, reduced gastric acid secretion, and, at times, enhanced protein loss into the stomach.

TREATMENT PROTEIN-LOSING ENTEROPATHY

As excess protein loss into the gastrointestinal tract is most often secondary to a specific disease, treatment should be directed primarily to the underlying disease process and not to the hypoproteinemia. For example, if significant hypoproteinemia with resulting peripheral edema is secondary to celiac disease or ulcerative colitis, a gluten-free diet and mesalamine, respectively, would be the initial therapy. When enhanced protein loss is secondary to lymphatic obstruction, it is critical to establish the nature of this obstruction. Identification of mesenteric nodes or lymphoma may be possible by imaging studies. Similarly, it is important to exclude cardiac disease as a cause of protein-losing enteropathy, either by echosonography or, on occasion, by a right-heart catheterization.

The increased protein loss that occurs in intestinal lymphangiectasia is a result of distended lymphatics associated with lipid malabsorption. The hypoproteinemia is treated with a low-fat diet and the administration of MCTs (Table 349-3), which do not exit from the intestinal epithelial cells via lymphatics but are delivered to the body via the portal vein.

TABLE 349-8 CLASSIFICATION OF MALABSORPTION SYNDROMES

Inadequate digestion
- Postgastrectomy[a]
- Deficiency or inactivation of pancreatic lipase
  - Exocrine pancreatic insufficiency
    - Chronic pancreatitis
    - Pancreatic carcinoma
    - Cystic fibrosis
    - Pancreatic insufficiency—congenital or acquired
- Gastrinoma—acid inactivation of lipasea
- Drugs—orlistat

Reduced intraduodenal bile acid concentration/impaired micelle formation
- Liver disease
  - Parenchymal liver disease
  - Cholestatic liver disease
- Bacterial overgrowth in small intestine:

Anatomic stasis	Functional stasis
Afferent loop	Diabetes[a]
Stasis/blind	Scleroderma[a]
Loop/strictures/fistulae	Intestinal pseudo-obstruction

- Interrupted enterohepatic circulation of bile salts
  - Ileal resection
  - Crohn's diseasea
- Drugs (binding or precipitating bile salts)—neomycin, cholestyramine, calcium carbonate

Impaired mucosal absorption/mucosal loss or defect
- Intestinal resection or bypass[a]
- Inflammation, infiltration, or infection:

Crohn's disease[a]	Celiac disease
Amyloidosis	Collagenous sprue
Scleroderma[a]	Whipple's disease[a]
Lymphoma[a]	Radiation enteritis[a]
Eosinophilic enteritis	Folate and vitamin B_{12} deficiency
Mastocytosis	Infections—giardiasis
Tropical sprue	Graft versus host disease

- Genetic disorders
  - Disaccharidase deficiency
  - Agammaglobulinemia
  - Abetalipoproteinemia
  - Hartnup's disease
  - Cystinuria

Impaired nutrient delivery to and/or from intestine:

Lymphatic obstruction	Circulatory disorders
Lymphoma[a]	Congestive heart failure
Lymphangiectasia	Constrictive pericarditis
	Mesenteric artery atherosclerosis
	Vasculitis

Endocrine and metabolic disorders
- Diabetes[a]
- Hypoparathyroidism
- Adrenal insufficiency
- Hyperthyroidism
- Carcinoid syndrome

[a]Malabsorption caused by more than one mechanism.

TABLE 349-9 PATHOPHYSIOLOGY OF CLINICAL MANIFESTATIONS OF MALABSORPTION DISORDERS

Symptom or Sign	Mechanism
Weight loss/malnutrition	Anorexia, malabsorption of nutrients
Diarrhea	Impaired absorption or secretion of water and electrolytes; colonic fluid secretion secondary to unabsorbed dihydroxy bile acids and fatty acids
Flatus	Bacterial fermentation of unabsorbed carbohydrate
Glossitis, cheilosis, stomatitis	Deficiency of iron, vitamin B_{12}, folate, and vitamin A
Abdominal pain	Bowel distention or inflammation, pancreatitis
Bone pain	Calcium, vitamin D malabsorption, protein deficiency, osteoporosis
Tetany, paresthesia	Calcium and magnesium malabsorption
Weakness	Anemia, electrolyte depletion (particularly K^+)
Azotemia, hypotension	Fluid and electrolyte depletion
Amenorrhea, decreased libido	Protein depletion, decreased calories, secondary hypopituitarism
Anemia	Impaired absorption of iron, folate, vitamin B_{12}
Bleeding	Vitamin K malabsorption, hypoprothrombinemia
Night blindness/xerophthalmia	Vitamin A malabsorption
Peripheral neuropathy	Vitamin B_{12} and thiamine deficiency
Dermatitis	Deficiency of vitamin A, zinc, and essential fatty acid

SUMMARY

The many conditions that can produce malabsorption are classified by their pathophysiology in Table 349-8. The pathophysiology of the various clinical manifestations of malabsorption is summarized in Table 349-9.

350e The Schilling Test

Henry J. Binder

This is a digital-only chapter. It is available on the DVD that accompanies this book, as well as on Access Medicine/Harrison's Online, and the eBook and "app" editions of HPIM 19e.

The Schilling test is performed to determine the cause of cobalamin malabsorption. Unfortunately, this test has not been available commercially in the United States for the last few years. Since an understanding of the physiology and pathophysiology of cobalamin absorption is very valuable in enhancing one's understanding of aspects of gastric, pancreatic, and ileal function, discussion of the Schilling test is provided as supplemental information to Chap. 349. Because cobalamin absorption requires multiple steps, including gastric, pancreatic, and ileal processes, the Schilling test also can be used to assess the integrity of the organs involved in those processes (Chap. 128).

351 Inflammatory Bowel Disease

Sonia Friedman, Richard S. Blumberg

Inflammatory bowel disease (IBD) is an immune-mediated chronic intestinal condition. Ulcerative colitis (UC) and Crohn's disease (CD) are the two major types of IBD.

GLOBAL CONSIDERATIONS: EPIDEMIOLOGY

The incidence and prevalence of IBD are highest in Westernized nations, with UC incidence estimates ranging from 0.6 to 24.3 per 100,000 in Europe, 0 to 19.2 per 100,000 in North America, and 0.1 to 6.3 per 100,000 in the Middle East and Asia and CD estimates ranging from 0.3 to 12.7 per 100,000 in Europe, 0 to 20.2 per 100,000 in North America, and 0.04 to 5.0 per 100,000 in the Middle East and Asia (Table 351-1). For prevalence rates, the UC estimates range from 4.9 to 505 per 100,000 in Europe, 37.5 to 248.6 per 100,000 in North America, and 4.9 to 168.3 per 100,000 in the Middle East and Asia, and the CD estimates range from 0.6 to 322 per 100,000 in Europe, 16.7 to 318.5 per 100,000 in North America, and 0.88 to 67.9 per 100,000 in Asia and the Middle East. The highest reported incidence rates are in Canada (19.2 per 100,000 for UC and 20.2 per 100,000 for CD), with approximately 0.6% of the Canadian population having IBD. Countries in the Pacific, including New Zealand and Australia, which share many possible environmental risk factors and similar genetic background as northwest Europe and North America, have high incidence rates of IBD.

In countries that are becoming more Westernized, including China, South Korea, India, Lebanon, Iran, Thailand, and countries in the French West Indies and North Africa, IBD appears to be emerging, emphasizing the importance of environmental factors in disease pathogenesis. In Japan, the prevalence of CD has risen rapidly from 2.9 cases per 100,000 in 1986 to 13.5 per 100,000 in 1998, whereas in South Korea, the prevalence of UC has quadrupled from 7.6 per 100,000 in 1997 to 30.9 per 100,000 in 2005. In Hong Kong, the prevalence of UC almost tripled from 2.3 in 1997 to 6.3 per 100,000 over a 9-year period. In Singapore, the prevalence of CD increased from 1.3 in 1990 to 7.2 per 100,000 in 2004. In China the number of cases of UC has increased by fourfold between 1981–1990 and 1991–2000.

Increasing immigration to Western societies also has an impact on the incidence and prevalence of IBD. The prevalence of UC among southern Asians who immigrated to the United Kingdom (UK) was higher in comparison to the European UK population (17 cases per 100,000 persons vs 7 per 100,000). Spanish patients who emigrated within Europe, but not those who immigrated to Latin America, developed IBD more frequently than controls. Individuals who have immigrated to Westernized countries and then returned to their country of birth also continue to demonstrate an increased risk of developing IBD.

TABLE 351-1 EPIDEMIOLOGY OF IBD

	Ulcerative Colitis	Crohn's Disease
Incidence (North America) per person-years	0–19.2 per 100,000	0–20.2 per 100,000
Age of onset	Second to fourth decades and seventh to ninth decades	Second to fourth decades and seventh to ninth decades
Ethnicity	Jewish > non-Jewish white > African American > Hispanic > Asian	
Female/male ratio	0.51–1.58	0.34–1.65
Smoking	May prevent disease (odds ratio 0.58)	May cause disease (odds ratio 1.76)
Oral contraceptives	No increased risk	Odds ratio 1.4
Appendectomy	Protective (risk reduction of 13–26%)	Not protective
Monozygotic twins	6–18% concordance	38–58% concordance
Dizygotic twins	0–2% concordance	4% concordance
Antibiotic use in the first year of life	2.9× the risk of developing childhood IBD	

Abbreviation: IBD, inflammatory bowel disease.

Peak incidence of UC and CD is in the second to fourth decades, with 78% of CD studies and 51% of UC studies reporting the highest incidence among those age 20–29 years old. A second modest rise in incidence occurs between the seventh and ninth decades of life. The female-to-male ratio ranges from 0.51 to 1.58 for UC studies and 0.34 to 1.65 for CD studies, suggesting that the diagnosis of IBD is not gender specific. The greatest incidence of IBD is among white and Jewish people, but the incidence of IBD in Hispanic and Asian people is increasing, as noted above. Urban areas have a higher prevalence of IBD than rural areas, and high socioeconomic classes have a higher prevalence than lower socioeconomic classes.

Epidemiologic studies have identified a number of potential environmental factors that are associated with disease risk (Fig. 351-1). In Caucasian populations, smoking is an important risk factor in IBD with opposite effects on UC (odds ratio [OR] 0.58) and CD (OR 1.76), whereas in other ethnic groups with different genetic susceptibility, smoking may play a lesser role. There is a protective effect of previous appendectomy with confirmed appendicitis (reduction of 13–26%), particularly at a young age, on the development of UC across different geographical regions and populations. There is a modest association with the development of CD. Oral contraceptive use is associated with the risk of CD (OR 1.4). The association between oral contraceptive use and UC is limited to women with a history of smoking. There is an association between antibiotic use and the development of childhood IBD with children who received one or more dispensations of antibiotics during the first year of life having a 2.9-fold increase in the risk of developing IBD during childhood. Breastfeeding may also protect against the development of IBD. These factors are consistent with the rapid increase in IBD incidence recently noted during the first decade of life. Infectious gastroenteritis with pathogens (e.g., *Salmonella*, *Shigella*, *Campylobacter* spp., *Clostridium difficile*) increases IBD risk by two- to threefold. Diets high in animal protein, sugars, sweets, oils, fish and shellfish, and dietary fat, especially ω-6 fatty acids, and low in ω-3 fatty acids have been implicated in increasing the risk of IBD.

IBD is a familial disease in 5–10% of patients (Fig. 351-2). Some of these patients may exhibit early-onset disease during the first decade of life and, in CD, a concordance of anatomic site and clinical type within families. In the remainder of patients, IBD is observed in the absence of a family history (i.e., sporadic disease). If a patient has IBD, the lifetime risk that a first-degree relative will be affected is ~10%. If two parents have IBD, each child has a 36% chance of being affected. In twin studies, 38–58% of monozygotic twins are concordant for CD and 6–18% are concordant for UC, whereas 4% of dizygotic twins are concordant for CD and 0–2% are concordant for UC in Swedish and Danish cohorts. The risks of developing IBD are higher in first-degree relatives of Jewish versus non-Jewish patients: 7.8% versus 5.2% for CD and 4.5% versus 1.6% for UC.

GLOBAL CONSIDERATIONS: IBD PHENOTYPES

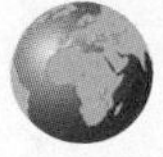

There are racial differences in IBD location and behavior that may reflect underlying genetic variations and have important implications for diagnosis and management of disease. For example, African-American patients are more likely than non-Hispanic whites to develop esophagogastroduodenal CD, colorectal disease, and perianal disease and are less likely to have ileal involvement. They are also at higher risk for uveitis and sacroiliitis. Hispanics have a higher prevalence of perianal CD and erythema nodosum and a more proximal extent of disease. Fistulizing CD has been reported in nearly one-third of Hispanic patients, up to one-quarter of African-American patients, and up to one-half of Asian patients. Both African-American

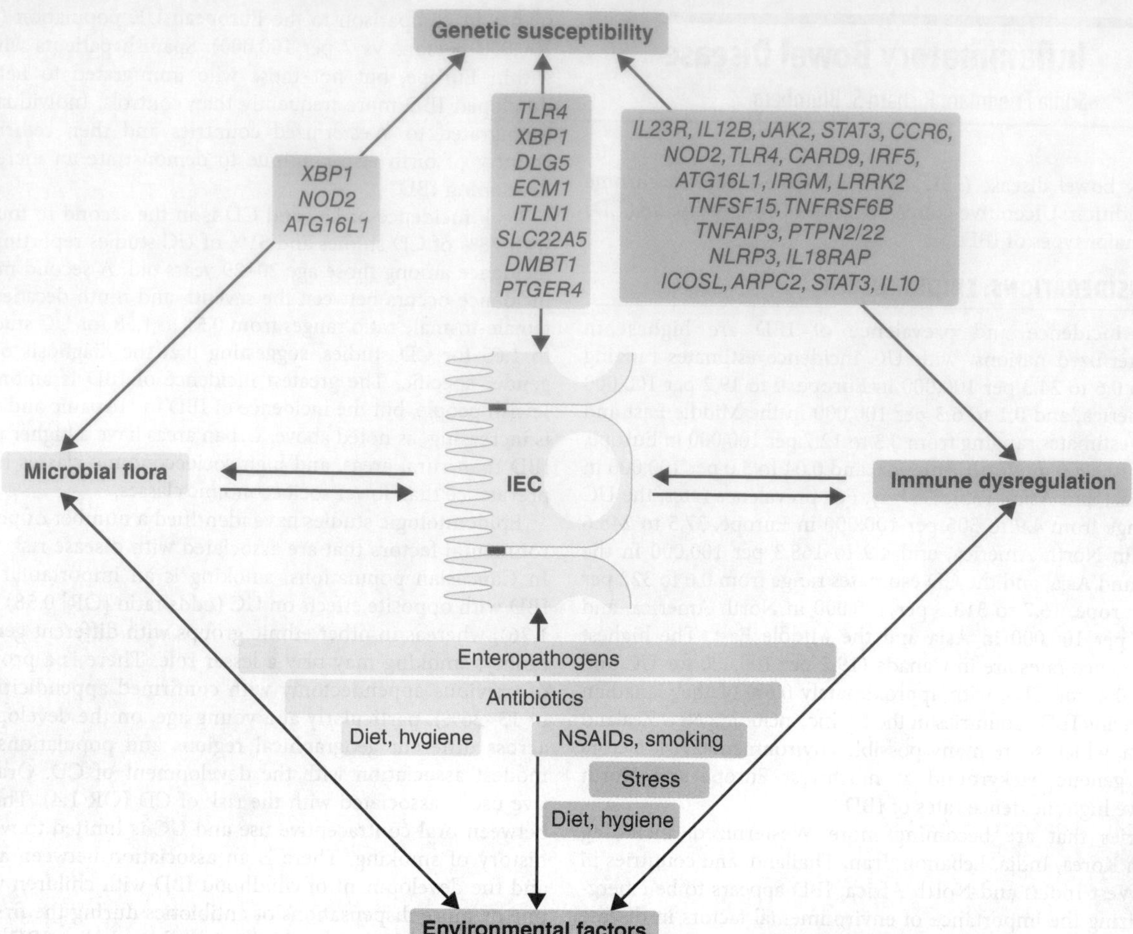

FIGURE 351-1 Pathogenesis of inflammatory bowel disease (IBD). In IBD, the tridirectional relationship between the commensal flora (microbiota), intestinal epithelial cells (IEC), and mucosal immune system is dysregulated, leading to chronic inflammation. Each of these three factors is affected by genetic and environmental factors that determine risk for the disease. NSAIDs, nonsteroidal anti-inflammatory drugs. *(Adapted from A Kaser et al: Annu Rev Immunol 28:573, 2010.)*

and Hispanic CD patients, but not UC patients, had a lower prevalence of family history of IBD than their white counterparts. There are few data on all aspects of disease in Hispanics, in the incidence and prevalence of IBD in African Americans, and in Asians with IBD outside Asia. These ethnic variations implicate the importance of different genetic and/or environmental factors in the pathogenesis of this disorder.

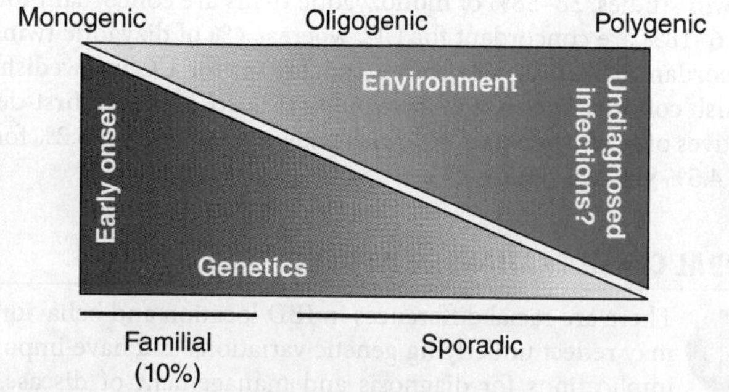

FIGURE 351-2 A model for the syndromic nature of inflammatory bowel disease. Genetic and environmental factors variably influence the development and phenotypic manifestations of IBD. At the one extreme, IBD is a exemplified as a simple Mendelian disorder as observed in "early-onset IBD" due to single gene defects such as *IL10*, *IL10RA*, and *IL10RB*; and at the other extreme, it may be exemplified by as yet to be described emerging infectious diseases. *(Adapted from A Kaser et al: Dig Dis 28:395, 2010.)*

ETIOLOGY AND PATHOGENESIS

Under physiologic conditions, homeostasis normally exists between the commensal microbiota, epithelial cells that line the interior of the intestines (intestinal epithelial cells [IECs]) and immune cells within the tissues (Fig. 351-1). A consensus hypothesis is that each of these three major host compartments that function together as an integrated "supraorganism" (microbiota, IECs, and immune cells) are affected by specific environmental (e.g., smoking, antibiotics, enteropathogens) and genetic factors that, in a susceptible host, cumulatively and interactively disrupt homeostasis, which in so doing culminates in a chronic state of dysregulated inflammation; that is IBD. Although chronic activation of the mucosal immune system may represent an appropriate response to an infectious agent, a search for such an agent has thus far been unrewarding in IBD. As such, IBD is currently considered an inappropriate immune response to the endogenous (autocthonous) commensal microbiota within the intestines, with or without some component of autoimmunity. Importantly, the normal, uninflamed intestines contain a large number of immune cells that are in a unique state of activation, in which the gut is restrained from full immunologic responses to the commensal microbiota and dietary antigens by very powerful regulatory pathways that function within the immune system (e.g., T regulatory cells that express the FoxP3 transcription factor and suppress inflammation). During the course of infections or other environmental stimuli in the normal host, full activation of the gut-associated lymphoid tissues occurs but is rapidly superseded by dampening of the immune response and tissue repair. In IBD such processes may not be regulated normally.

GENETIC CONSIDERATIONS

The genetic underpinning of IBD is known from its occurrence in the context of several genetic syndromes and the development of severe, refractory IBD in early life in the setting of single gene defects that affect the immune system (Table 351-2). In addition, IBD has a familial origin in at least 10% of afflicted individuals (Fig. 351-2). In the majority of patients, IBD is considered to be a polygenic disorder that gives rise to multiple clinical subgroups within UC and CD. A variety of genetic approaches including candidate gene studies, linkage analysis, and genome-wide association studies (GWASs) that focus on the identification of disease-associated, single-nucleotide polymorphisms (SNPs) within the human genome and, more recently, whole-genome sequencing have elucidated many of the genetic factors that affect risk for these diseases. GWASs have, to date, identified 163 genetic loci with 100 of these loci observed to be associated with both disease phenotypes (Table 351-3). The remainder are specific for either CD (30 loci) or UC (20 loci). These genetic similarities account for the overlapping immunopathogenesis and consequently epidemiologic observations of both diseases in the same families and similarities in response to therapies. Because the specific causal variants for each identified gene or locus are largely unknown, it is not clear whether the similarities in the genetic risk factors associated with CD and UC that are observed are shared at structural or functional levels. The risk conferred by each identified gene or locus is unequal and generally small, such that only ~20% of the genetic variance is considered to be explained by the current genetic information. Further, many of the genetic risk factors identified are also observed to be associated with risk for other immune-mediated diseases, suggesting that related immunogenetic pathways are involved in the pathogenesis of multiple different disorders accounting for the common responsiveness to similar types of biologic therapies (e.g., anti–tumor necrosis factor therapies) and possibly the simultaneous occurrence of these disorders. The diseases and the genetic risk factors that are shared with IBD include rheumatoid arthritis (*TNFAIP3*), psoriasis (*IL23R, IL12B*), ankylosing spondylitis (*IL23R*), type 1 diabetes mellitus (*IL10, PTPN2*), asthma (*ORMDL3*), and systemic lupus erythematosus (*TNFAIP3, IL10*) among others.

The genetic factors defined to date that are recognized to mediate risk for IBD have highlighted the importance of several common mechanisms of disease (Table 351-3). These include the following: those genes that are associated with fundamental cell biologic processes such as endoplasmic reticulum (ER) and metabolic stress (e.g., *XBP1, ORMDL3, OCTN*), which serve to regulate the secretory activity of cells involved in responses to the commensal microbiota such as Paneth and goblet cells and the manner in which intestinal cells respond to the metabolic products of bacteria; those associated with innate immunity and autophagy (e.g., *NOD2, ATG16L1, IRGM, JAK2, STAT3*) that function in innate immune cells (both parenchymal and hematopoietic) to respond to and effectively clear bacteria, mycobacteria, and viruses; those that are associated with the regulation of adaptive immunity (e.g., *IL23R, IL12B, IL10, PTPN2*), which regulate the balance between inflammatory and anti-inflammatory (regulatory) cytokines; and, finally, those that are involved in the development and resolution of inflammation (e.g., *MST1, CCR6, TNFAIP3, PTGER4*) and ultimately leukocyte recruitment and inflammatory mediator production. Some of these loci are associated with specific subtypes of disease such as the association between *NOD2* polymorphisms and fibrostenosing CD or *ATG16L1* and fistulizing disease, especially within the ileum. However, the clinical utility of these genetic risk factors for the diagnosis or determination of prognosis and therapeutic responses remains to be defined.

TABLE 351-2 PRIMARY GENETIC DISORDERS ASSOCIATED WITH IBD

Name	Genetic Association	Phenotype
Turner's syndrome	Loss of part or all of X chromosome	Associated with UC and colonic CD
Hermansky-Pudlak	Autosomal recessive chromosome 10q23	Granulomatous colitis, oculocutaneous albinism, platelet dysfunction, pulmonary fibrosis
Wiskott-Aldrich syndrome (WAS)	X-linked recessive disorder, loss of WAS protein function	Colitis, immunodeficiency, severely dysfunctional platelets, and thrombocytopenia
Glycogen storage disease	Deficiency of the glucose-6-phosphate transport protein type B1	Granulomatous colitis, presents in infancy with hypoglycemia, growth failure, hepatomegaly, and neutropenia
Immune dysregulation polyendocrinopathy, enteropathy X-linked (IPEX)	Loss of FoxP3 transcription factor and T regulatory cell function	UC-like autoimmune enteropathy, with endocrinopathy (neonatal type 1 diabetes or thyroiditis), dermatitis
Early-onset IBD	Deficient IL-10 and IL-10 receptor function	Severe, refractory IBD in early life

Abbreviations: CD, Crohn's disease; IBD, inflammatory bowel disease; IL, interleukin; UC, ulcerative colitis.

COMMENSAL MICROBIOTA AND IBD

The endogenous commensal microbiota within the intestines plays a central role in the pathogenesis of IBD. Humans are born sterile and acquire their commensal microbiota initially from the mother during egress through the birth canal and subsequently from environmental sources. A stable configuration of up to 1000 species of bacteria that achieves a biomass of approximately 10^{12} colony-forming units per gram of feces is achieved by 3 years of age, which likely persists into adult life, with each individual human possessing a unique combination of species. In addition, the intestines contain other microbial life forms including archae, viruses, and protists. The microbiota is thus considered as a critical and sustaining component of the organism. The establishment and maintenance of the intestinal microbiota composition and function is under the control of host (e.g., immune and epithelial responses), environmental (e.g., diet and antibiotics), and likely genetic (e.g., *NOD2*) factors (Fig. 351-1). In turn, the microbiota, through its structural components and metabolic activity, has major influences on the epithelial and immune function of the host, which, through epigenetic effects, may have durable consequences. During early life when the commensal microbiota is being established, these microbial effects on the host may be particularly important in determining later life risk for IBD. Specific components of the microbiota can promote or protect from disease. The commensal microbiota in patients with both UC and CD is demonstrably different from nonafflicted individuals, a state of dysbiosis, suggesting the presence of microorganisms that drive disease (e.g., Proteobacteria such as enteroinvasive and adherent *Escherichia coli*) and to which the immune response is directed and/or the loss of microorganisms that hinder inflammation (e.g., Firmicutes such as *Faecalibacterium prausnitzii*). Many of the changes in the commensal microbiota occur as a consequence of the inflammation. In addition, agents that alter the intestinal microbiota such as metronidazole, ciprofloxacin, and elemental diets, may improve CD. CD may also respond to fecal diversion, demonstrating the ability of luminal contents to exacerbate disease.

DEFECTIVE IMMUNE REGULATION IN IBD

The mucosal immune system is normally unreactive to luminal contents due to oral (mucosal) tolerance. When soluble antigens are administered orally rather than subcutaneously or intramuscularly, antigen-specific nonresponsiveness is induced. Multiple mechanisms are involved in the induction of oral tolerance and include deletion or anergy of antigen-reactive T cells or induction of CD4+ T cells that suppress gut inflammation (e.g., T regulatory cells expressing the FoxP3 transcription factor) that secrete anti-inflammatory cytokines such as interleukin (IL) 10, IL-35, and transforming growth factor β (TGF-β). Oral tolerance may be responsible for the lack of immune responsiveness to dietary antigens and the commensal microbiota

TABLE 351-3 EXAMPLES OF GENETIC LOCI ASSOCIATED WITH CD AND/OR UC

Chromosome	Putative Gene	Gene Name	Protein Function	CD	UC
ER Stress and Metabolism					
5q31	*SLC22A5*	Solute carrier family 22, member 5	β carnitine transporter	+	
7p21	*AGR2*	Anterior gradient 2	ER stress	+	+
17q21	*ORMDL3*	Orosomucoid related member 1-like 3	ER stress and lipid synthesis	+	+
22q12	*XBP1*	X-box binding protein 1	ER stress	+	+
1q23	*ITLN1*	Intelectin 1	Bacterial binding	+	
2q37	*ATG16L1*	ATG16 autophagy related 16-like 1	Autophagy	+	
5q33	*IRGM*	Immunity-related GTPase family, M	Autophagy	+	
9p24	*JAK2*	Janus kinase 2	IL-6R and IL-23R signaling	+	+
12q12	*LRRK2*	Leucine-rich repeat kinase 2	Autophagy?	+	
16q12	*NOD2*	Nucleotide-binding oligomerization domain containing 2	Bacterial sensing and autophagy activation	+	
17q21	*STAT3*	Signal transducer and activator of transcription 3	IL-6R, IL-23R, and IL-10R signaling	+	+
Adaptive Immunity					
1p31	*IL23R*	Interleukin 23 receptor	Th17 cell stimulation	+	+
1q32	*IL10*	Interleukin 10	Treg-associated cytokine		+
5q33	*IL12B*	Interleukin 12B	IL-12 p40 chain of IL-12/IL-23	+	+
18p11	*PTPN2*	Protein tyrosine phosphatase, nonreceptor type 2	T cell regulation	+	
Inflammation					
3p21	*MST1*	Macrophage stimulating 1	Macrophage activation	+	+
5p13	*PTGER4*	Prostaglandin E receptor 4	PGE_2 receptor	+	+
6q23	*TNFAIP3*	Tumor necrosis factor, alpha-induced protein 3 (A20)	Toll-like receptor regulation	+	
6q27	*CCR6*	Chemokine (C-C motif) receptor 6	Dendritic cell migration	+	

Abbreviations: CD, Crohn's disease; ER, endoplasmic reticulum; GTPase, guanosine triphosphatase; IL, interleukin; PGE_2, prostaglandin E_2; UC, ulcerative colitis.

Source: Adapted from A Kaser et al: Ann Rev Immunol 28:573, 2010; B Khor et al: Nature 474:307, 2011; and L Jostins et al: Nature 491:119, 2012.

in the intestinal lumen. In IBD this suppression of inflammation is altered, leading to uncontrolled inflammation. The mechanisms of this regulated immune suppression are incompletely known.

Gene knockout ($^{-/-}$) or transgenic (Tg) mouse models of IBD, which include those that are directed at genes demonstrated to be associated with risk for the human disease, have revealed that deleting specific cytokines (e.g., IL-2, IL-10, TGF-β) or their receptors, deleting molecules associated with T cell antigen recognition (e.g., T cell antigen receptors), or interfering with IEC barrier function and the regulation of responses to commensal bacteria (e.g., XBP1, N-cadherin, mucus glycoprotein, or nuclear factor-κB [NF-κB]) leads to spontaneous colitis or enteritis. In the majority of circumstances, intestinal inflammation in these animal models requires the presence of the commensal microbiota. Thus, a variety of specific alterations can lead to immune activation by commensal microbiota and inflammation directed at the intestines in mice. How these relate to human IBD remains to be defined, but they are consistent with inappropriate responses of the genetically susceptible host to the commensal microbiota.

In both UC and CD, an inflammatory pathway thus likely emerges from the genetic predisposition that is associated with inappropriate innate immune and epithelial sensing and reactivity to commensal bacteria that secrete inflammatory mediators together with inadequate regulatory pathways that lead to activated CD4+ and $CD8^+$ T cells within the epithelium and lamina propria that altogether secrete excessive quantities of inflammatory cytokines relative to anti-inflammatory cytokines. Some cytokines activate other inflammatory cells (macrophages and B cells), and others act indirectly to recruit other lymphocytes, inflammatory leukocytes, and mononuclear cells from the bloodstream into the gut through interactions between homing receptors on leukocytes (e.g., α4β7 integrin) and addressins on vascular endothelium (e.g., MadCAM1). Consistent with this, neutralization of tumor necrosis factor (TNF) or α4β7 integrin demonstrate therapeutic efficacy in IBD. CD4+ T helper (T_H) cells that promote inflammation are of three major types, all of which may be associated with colitis in animal models and perhaps humans: T_H1 cells (secrete interferon [IFN] γ), T_H2 cells (secrete IL-4, IL-5, IL-13), and T_H17 cells (secrete IL-17, IL-21). T_H1 cells induce transmural granulomatous inflammation that resembles CD; T_H2 cells, and related natural killer T cells that secrete IL-13, induce superficial mucosal inflammation resembling UC in animal models; and T_H17 cells may be responsible for neutrophilic recruitment. However, neutralization of the cytokines produced by these cells, such as IFN-γ or IL-17, has yet to show efficacy in therapeutic trials. Each of these T cell subsets cross-regulate each other. The T_H1 cytokine pathway is initiated by IL-12, a key cytokine in the pathogenesis of experimental models of mucosal inflammation. IL-4 and IL-23, together with IL-6 and TGF-β, induce T_H2 and T_H17 cells, respectively, and IL-23 inhibits the suppressive function of regulatory T cells. Activated macrophages secrete TNF and IL-6. These characteristics of the immune response in IBD explain the beneficial therapeutic effects of antibodies to block proinflammatory cytokines or the signaling by their receptors (e.g., anti-TNF, anti-IL-12, anti-IL-23, anti-IL-6, or Janus kinase [JAK] inhibitors) or molecules associated with leukocyte recruitment (e.g., anti-α4β7), or the use of cytokines that inhibit inflammation and promote regulatory T cells (e.g., IL-10) or promote intestinal barrier function and may be beneficial to humans with intestinal inflammation.

THE INFLAMMATORY CASCADE IN IBD

Once initiated in IBD by abnormal innate immune sensing of bacteria by parenchymal cells (e.g., IECs) and hematopoietic cells (e.g., dendritic cells), the immune inflammatory response is perpetuated by T cell activation. A sequential cascade of inflammatory mediators extends the response; each step is a potential target for therapy. Inflammatory cytokines such as IL-1, IL-6, and TNF have diverse effects on tissues. They promote fibrogenesis, collagen production, activation of tissue metalloproteinases, and the production of other inflammatory mediators; they also activate the coagulation cascade in local blood vessels (e.g., increased production of von Willebrand's factor). These cytokines are normally produced in response to infection but are usually turned off or inhibited at the appropriate time to limit tissue damage. In IBD their activity is not regulated, resulting in an imbalance between the proinflammatory and anti-inflammatory mediators. Therapies such as the 5-aminosalicylic acid (5-ASA) compounds and glucocorticoids are potent inhibitors of these inflammatory mediators through inhibition of transcription factors such as NF-κB that regulate their expression.

PATHOLOGY

ULCERATIVE COLITIS: MACROSCOPIC FEATURES

UC is a mucosal disease that usually involves the rectum and extends proximally to involve all or part of the colon. About 40–50% of patients have disease limited to the rectum and rectosigmoid, 30–40% have disease extending beyond the sigmoid but not involving the whole colon, and 20% have a total colitis. Proximal spread occurs in continuity without areas of uninvolved mucosa. When the whole colon is involved, the inflammation extends 2–3 cm into the terminal ileum in 10–20% of patients. The endoscopic changes of *backwash ileitis* are superficial and mild and are of little clinical significance. Although variations in macroscopic activity may suggest skip areas, biopsies from normal-appearing mucosa are usually abnormal. Thus, it is important to obtain multiple biopsies from apparently uninvolved mucosa, whether proximal or distal, during endoscopy. One caveat is that effective medical therapy can change the appearance of the mucosa such that either skip areas or the entire colon can be microscopically normal.

With mild inflammation, the mucosa is erythematous and has a fine granular surface that resembles sandpaper. In more severe disease, the mucosa is hemorrhagic, edematous, and ulcerated (Fig. 351-3). In long-standing disease, inflammatory polyps (pseudopolyps) may be present as a result of epithelial regeneration. The mucosa may appear normal in remission, but in patients with many years of disease it appears atrophic and featureless, and the entire colon becomes narrowed and shortened. Patients with fulminant disease can develop a toxic colitis or megacolon where the bowel wall thins and the mucosa is severely ulcerated; this may lead to perforation.

ULCERATIVE COLITIS: MICROSCOPIC FEATURES

Histologic findings correlate well with the endoscopic appearance and clinical course of UC. The process is limited to the mucosa and superficial submucosa, with deeper layers unaffected except in fulminant disease. In UC, two major histologic features suggest chronicity and help distinguish it from infectious or acute self-limited colitis. First, the crypt architecture of the colon is distorted; crypts may be bifid and reduced in number, often with a gap between the crypt bases and the muscularis mucosae. Second, some patients have basal plasma cells and multiple basal lymphoid aggregates. Mucosal vascular congestion, with edema and focal hemorrhage, and an inflammatory cell infiltrate of neutrophils, lymphocytes, plasma cells, and macrophages may be present.

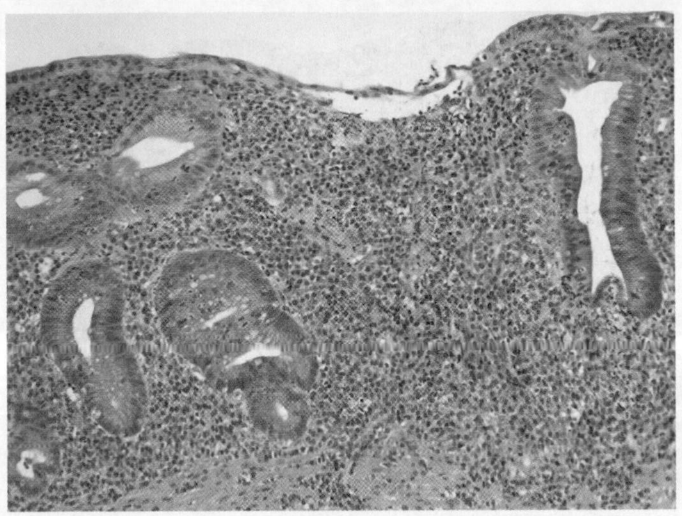

FIGURE 351-4 Medium-power view of colonic mucosa in ulcerative colitis showing diffuse mixed inflammation, basal lymphoplasmacytosis, crypt atrophy and irregularity, and superficial erosion. These features are typical of chronic active ulcerative colitis. *(Courtesy of Dr. R. Odze, Division of Gastrointestinal Pathology, Department of Pathology, Brigham and Women's Hospital, Boston, Massachusetts; with permission.)*

The neutrophils invade the epithelium, usually in the crypts, giving rise to cryptitis and, ultimately, to crypt abscesses (Fig. 351-4). Ileal changes in patients with backwash ileitis include villous atrophy and crypt regeneration with increased inflammation, increased neutrophil and mononuclear inflammation in the lamina propria, and patchy cryptitis and crypt abscesses.

CROHN'S DISEASE: MACROSCOPIC FEATURES

CD can affect any part of the gastrointestinal (GI) tract from the mouth to the anus. Some 30–40% of patients have small bowel disease alone, 40–55% have disease involving both the small and large intestines, and 15–25% have colitis alone. In the 75% of patients with small intestinal disease, the terminal ileum is involved in 90%. Unlike UC, which almost always involves the rectum, the rectum is often spared in CD. CD is segmental with skip areas in the midst of diseased intestine (Fig. 351-5). Perirectal fistulas, fissures, abscesses, and anal stenosis are present in one-third of patients with CD, particularly those with

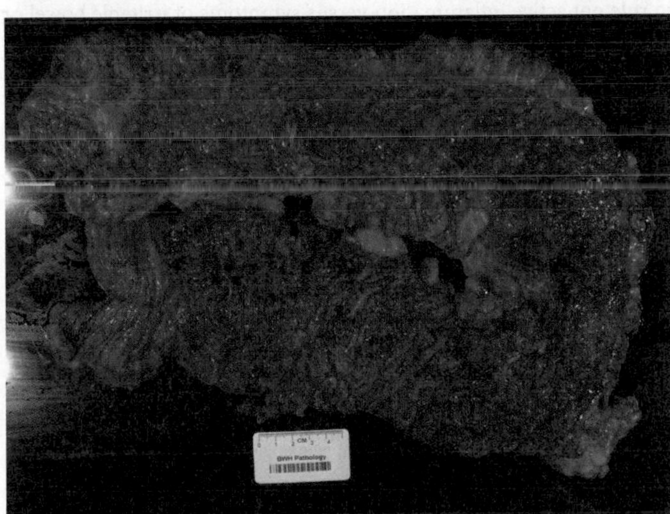

FIGURE 351-3 Ulcerative colitis. Diffuse (nonsegmental) mucosal disease, with broad areas of ulceration. The bowel wall is not thickened, and there is no cobblestoning. *(Courtesy of Dr. R. Odze, Division of Gastrointestinal Pathology, Department of Pathology, Brigham and Women's Hospital, Boston, Massachusetts; with permission.)*

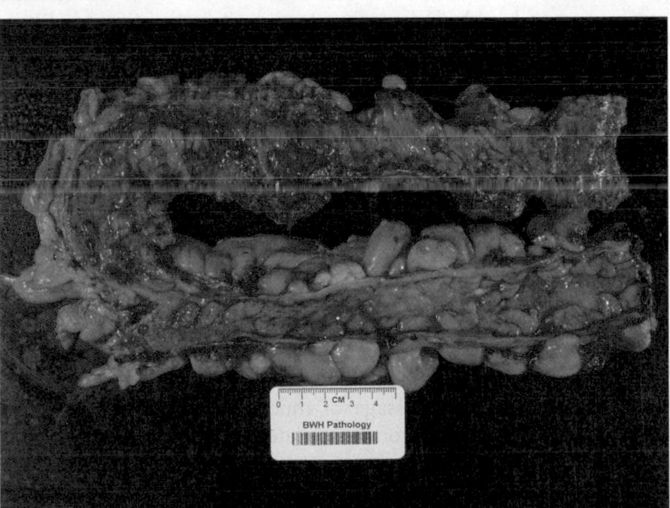

FIGURE 351-5 Crohn's disease of the colon showing thickening of the wall, with stenosis, linear serpiginous ulcers and cobblestoning of the mucosa. *(Courtesy of Dr. R Odze, Division of Gastrointestinal Pathology, Department of Pathology, Brigham and Women's Hospital, Boston, Massachusetts; with permission.)*

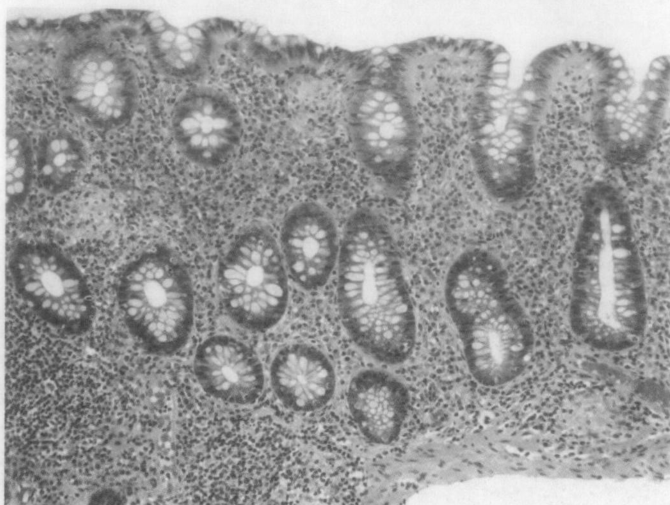

FIGURE 351-6 Medium-power view of Crohn's colitis showing mixed acute and chronic inflammation, crypt atrophy, and multiple small epithelioid granulomas in the mucosa. *(Courtesy of Dr. R Odze, Division of Gastrointestinal Pathology, Department of Pathology, Brigham and Women's Hospital, Boston, Massachusetts; with permission.)*

colonic involvement. Rarely, CD may also involve the liver and the pancreas.

Unlike UC, CD is a transmural process. Endoscopically, aphthous or small superficial ulcerations characterize mild disease; in more active disease, stellate ulcerations fuse longitudinally and transversely to demarcate islands of mucosa that frequently are histologically normal. This "cobblestone" appearance is characteristic of CD, both endoscopically and by barium radiography. As in UC, pseudopolyps can form in CD.

Active CD is characterized by focal inflammation and formation of fistula tracts, which resolve by fibrosis and stricturing of the bowel. The bowel wall thickens and becomes narrowed and fibrotic, leading to chronic, recurrent bowel obstructions. Projections of thickened mesentery encase the bowel ("creeping fat"), and serosal and mesenteric inflammation promotes adhesions and fistula formation.

CROHN'S DISEASE: MICROSCOPIC FEATURES

The earliest lesions are aphthoid ulcerations and focal crypt abscesses with loose aggregations of macrophages, which form noncaseating granulomas in all layers of the bowel wall (Fig. 351-6). Granulomas can be seen in lymph nodes, mesentery, peritoneum, liver, and pancreas. Although granulomas are a pathognomonic feature of CD, they are rarely found on mucosal biopsies. Surgical resection reveals granulomas in about one-half of cases. Other histologic features of CD include submucosal or subserosal lymphoid aggregates, particularly away from areas of ulceration, gross and microscopic skip areas, and transmural inflammation that is accompanied by fissures that penetrate deeply into the bowel wall and sometimes form fistulous tracts or local abscesses.

CLINICAL PRESENTATION

ULCERATIVE COLITIS

Signs and Symptoms The major symptoms of UC are diarrhea, rectal bleeding, tenesmus, passage of mucus, and crampy abdominal pain. The severity of symptoms correlates with the extent of disease. Although UC can present acutely, symptoms usually have been present for weeks to months. Occasionally, diarrhea and bleeding are so intermittent and mild that the patient does not seek medical attention.

Patients with proctitis usually pass fresh blood or blood-stained mucus, either mixed with stool or streaked onto the surface of a normal or hard stool. They also have tenesmus, or urgency with a feeling of incomplete evacuation, but rarely have abdominal pain. With proctitis or proctosigmoiditis, proximal transit slows, which

TABLE 351-4 ULCERATIVE COLITIS: DISEASE PRESENTATION

	Mild	Moderate	Severe
Bowel movements	<4 per day	4–6 per day	>6 per day
Blood in stool	Small	Moderate	Severe
Fever	None	<37.5°C mean (<99.5°F)	>37.5°C mean (>99.5°F)
Tachycardia	None	<90 mean pulse	>90 mean pulse
Anemia	Mild	>75%	≤75%
Sedimentation rate	<30 mm		>30 mm
Endoscopic appearance	Erythema, decreased vascular pattern, fine granularity	Marked erythema, coarse granularity, absent vascular markings, contact bleeding, no ulcerations	Spontaneous bleeding, ulcerations

may account for the constipation commonly seen in patients with distal disease.

When the disease extends beyond the rectum, blood is usually mixed with stool or grossly bloody diarrhea may be noted. Colonic motility is altered by inflammation with rapid transit through the inflamed intestine. When the disease is severe, patients pass a liquid stool containing blood, pus, and fecal matter. Diarrhea is often nocturnal and/or postprandial. Although severe pain is not a prominent symptom, some patients with active disease may experience vague lower abdominal discomfort or mild central abdominal cramping. Severe cramping and abdominal pain can occur with severe attacks of the disease. Other symptoms in moderate to severe disease include anorexia, nausea, vomiting, fever, and weight loss.

Physical signs of proctitis include a tender anal canal and blood on rectal examination. With more extensive disease, patients have tenderness to palpation directly over the colon. Patients with a toxic colitis have severe pain and bleeding, and those with megacolon have hepatic tympany. Both may have signs of peritonitis if a perforation has occurred. The classification of disease activity is shown in Table 351-4.

Laboratory, Endoscopic, and Radiographic Features Active disease can be associated with a rise in acute-phase reactants (C-reactive protein [CRP]), platelet count, and erythrocyte sedimentation rate (ESR), and a decrease in hemoglobin. Fecal lactoferrin is a highly sensitive and specific marker for detecting intestinal inflammation. Fecal calprotectin levels correlate well with histologic inflammation, predict relapses, and detect pouchitis. Both fecal lactoferrin and calprotectin are becoming an integral part of IBD management and are used frequently to rule out active inflammation versus symptoms of irritable bowel or bacterial overgrowth. In severely ill patients, the serum albumin level will fall rather quickly. Leukocytosis may be present but is not a specific indicator of disease activity. Proctitis or proctosigmoiditis rarely causes a rise in CRP. Diagnosis relies on the patient's history; clinical symptoms; negative stool examination for bacteria, *C. difficile* toxin, and ova and parasites; sigmoidoscopic appearance (see Fig. 345-4A); and histology of rectal or colonic biopsy specimens.

Sigmoidoscopy is used to assess disease activity and is usually performed before treatment. If the patient is not having an acute flare, colonoscopy is used to assess disease extent and activity (Fig. 351-7). Endoscopically mild disease is characterized by erythema, decreased vascular pattern, and mild friability. Moderate disease is characterized by marked erythema, absent vascular pattern, friability and erosions, and severe disease by spontaneous bleeding and ulcerations. Histologic features change more slowly than clinical features but can also be used to grade disease activity.

The earliest radiologic change of UC seen on single-contrast barium enema is a fine mucosal granularity. With increasing severity, the mucosa becomes thickened, and superficial ulcers are seen. Deep ulcerations can appear as "collar-button" ulcers, which indicate that the ulceration has penetrated the mucosa. Haustral folds may be normal in mild disease, but as activity progresses they become edematous and thickened. Loss of haustration can occur, especially in patients

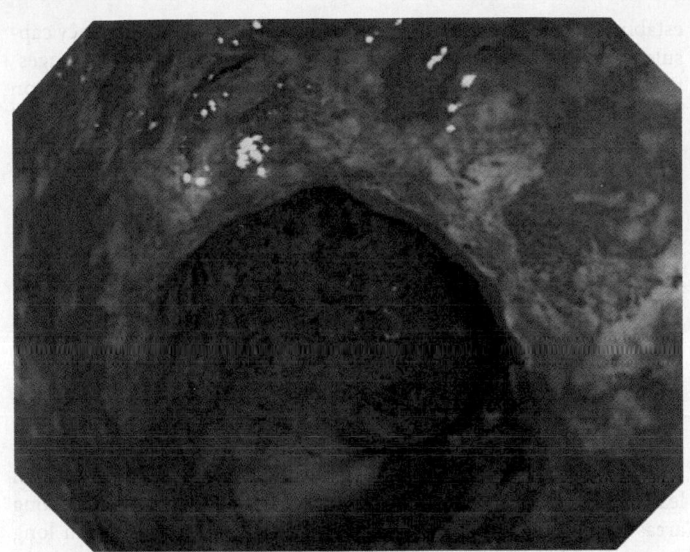

FIGURE 351-7 Colonoscopy with acute ulcerative colitis: severe colon inflammation with erythema, friability, and exudates. *(Courtesy of Dr. M. Hamilton, Gastroenterology Division, Department of Medicine, Brigham and Women's Hospital, Boston, Massachusetts; with permission.)*

with long-standing disease. In addition, the colon becomes shortened and narrowed. Polyps in the colon may be postinflammatory polyps or pseudopolyps, adenomatous polyps, or carcinoma.

Computed tomography (CT) scanning or magnetic resonance imaging (MRI) is not as helpful as endoscopy in making the diagnosis of UC, but typical findings include mild mural thickening (<1.5 cm), inhomogeneous wall density, absence of small bowel thickening, increased perirectal and presacral fat, target appearance of the rectum, and adenopathy.

Complications Only 15% of patients with UC present initially with catastrophic illness. Massive hemorrhage occurs with severe attacks of disease in 1% of patients, and treatment for the disease usually stops the bleeding. However, if a patient requires 6–8 units of blood within 24–48 h, colectomy is indicated. *Toxic megacolon* is defined as a transverse or right colon with a diameter of >6 cm, with loss of haustration in patients with severe attacks of UC. It occurs in about 5% of attacks and can be triggered by electrolyte abnormalities and narcotics. About 50% of acute dilations will resolve with medical therapy alone, but urgent colectomy is required for those that do not improve. Perforation is the most dangerous of the local complications, and the physical signs of peritonitis may not be obvious, especially if the patient is receiving glucocorticoids. Although perforation is rare, the mortality rate for perforation complicating a toxic megacolon is about 15%. In addition, patients can develop a toxic colitis and such severe ulcerations that the bowel may perforate without first dilating.

Strictures occur in 5–10% of patients and are always a concern in UC because of the possibility of underlying neoplasia. Although benign strictures can form from the inflammation and fibrosis of UC, strictures that are impassable with the colonoscope should be presumed malignant until proven otherwise. A stricture that prevents passage of the colonoscope is an indication for surgery. UC patients occasionally develop anal fissures, perianal abscesses, or hemorrhoids, but the occurrence of extensive perianal lesions should suggest CD.

CROHN'S DISEASE

Signs and Symptoms Although CD usually presents as acute or chronic bowel inflammation, the inflammatory process evolves toward one of two patterns of disease: a fibrostenotic obstructing pattern or a penetrating fistulous pattern, each with different treatments and prognoses. The site of disease influences the clinical manifestations.

ILEOCOLITIS Because the most common site of inflammation is the terminal ileum, the usual presentation of ileocolitis is a chronic history of recurrent episodes of right lower quadrant pain and diarrhea. Sometimes the initial presentation mimics acute appendicitis with pronounced right lower quadrant pain, a palpable mass, fever, and leukocytosis. Pain is usually colicky; it precedes and is relieved by defecation. A low-grade fever is usually noted. High-spiking fever suggests intraabdominal abscess formation. Weight loss is common—typically 10–20% of body weight—and develops as a consequence of diarrhea, anorexia, and fear of eating.

An inflammatory mass may be palpated in the right lower quadrant of the abdomen. The mass is composed of inflamed bowel, adherent and indurated mesentery, and enlarged abdominal lymph nodes. Extension of the mass can cause obstruction of the right ureter or bladder inflammation, manifested by dysuria and fever. Edema, bowel wall thickening, and fibrosis of the bowel wall within the mass account for the radiographic "string sign" of a narrowed intestinal lumen.

Bowel obstruction may take several forms. In the early stages of disease, bowel wall edema and spasm produce intermittent obstructive manifestations and increasing symptoms of postprandial pain. Over several years, persistent inflammation gradually progresses to fibrostenotic narrowing and stricture. Diarrhea will decrease and be replaced by chronic bowel obstruction. Acute episodes of obstruction occur as well, precipitated by bowel inflammation and spasm or sometimes by impaction of undigested food or medication. These episodes usually resolve with intravenous fluids and gastric decompression.

Severe inflammation of the ileocecal region may lead to localized wall thinning, with microperforation and fistula formation to the adjacent bowel, the skin, or the urinary bladder, or to an abscess cavity in the mesentery. Enterovesical fistulas typically present as dysuria or recurrent bladder infections or, less commonly, as pneumaturia or fecaluria. Enterocutaneous fistulas follow tissue planes of least resistance, usually draining through abdominal surgical scars. Enterovaginal fistulas are rare and present as dyspareunia or as a feculent or foul-smelling, often painful vaginal discharge. They are unlikely to develop without a prior hysterectomy.

JEJUNOILEITIS Extensive inflammatory disease is associated with a loss of digestive and absorptive surface, resulting in malabsorption and steatorrhea. Nutritional deficiencies can also result from poor intake and enteric losses of protein and other nutrients. Intestinal malabsorption can cause anemia, hypoalbuminemia, hypocalcemia, hypomagnesemia, coagulopathy, and hyperoxaluria with nephrolithiasis in patients with an intact colon. Many patients need to take oral and often intravenous iron. Vertebral fractures are caused by a combination of vitamin D deficiency, hypocalcemia, and prolonged glucocorticoid use. Pellagra from niacin deficiency can occur in extensive small-bowel disease, and malabsorption of vitamin B_{12} can lead to megaloblastic anemia and neurologic symptoms. Other important nutrients to measure and replete if low are folate and vitamins A, E, and K. Levels of minerals such as zinc, selenium, copper, and magnesium are often low in patients with extensive small-bowel inflammation or resections, and these should be repleted as well. Most patients should take a daily multivitamin, calcium, and vitamin D supplements.

Diarrhea is characteristic of active disease; its causes include (1) bacterial overgrowth in obstructive stasis or fistulization, (2) bile-acid malabsorption due to a diseased or resected terminal ileum, and (3) intestinal inflammation with decreased water absorption and increased secretion of electrolytes.

COLITIS AND PERIANAL DISEASE Patients with colitis present with low-grade fevers, malaise, diarrhea, crampy abdominal pain, and sometimes hematochezia. Gross bleeding is not as common as in UC and appears in about one-half of patients with exclusively colonic disease. Only 1–2% bleed massively. Pain is caused by passage of fecal material through narrowed and inflamed segments of the large bowel. Decreased rectal compliance is another cause for diarrhea in Crohn's colitis patients. Toxic megacolon is rare but may be seen with severe inflammation and short duration disease.

Stricturing can occur in the colon in 4–16% of patients and produce symptoms of bowel obstruction. If the endoscopist is unable to traverse a stricture in Crohn's colitis, surgical resection should be considered, especially if the patient has symptoms of chronic obstruction.

Colonic disease may fistulize into the stomach or duodenum, causing feculent vomiting, or to the proximal or mid-small bowel, causing malabsorption by "short circuiting" and bacterial overgrowth. Ten percent of women with Crohn's colitis will develop a rectovaginal fistula.

Perianal disease affects about one-third of patients with Crohn's colitis and is manifested by incontinence, large hemorrhoidal tags, anal strictures, anorectal fistulae, and perirectal abscesses. Not all patients with perianal fistula will have endoscopic evidence of colonic inflammation.

GASTRODUODENAL DISEASE Symptoms and signs of upper GI tract disease include nausea, vomiting, and epigastric pain. Patients usually have an *Helicobacter pylori*–negative gastritis. The second portion of the duodenum is more commonly involved than the bulb. Fistulas involving the stomach or duodenum arise from the small or large bowel and do not necessarily signify the presence of upper GI tract involvement. Patients with advanced gastroduodenal CD may develop a chronic gastric outlet obstruction.

Laboratory, Endoscopic, and Radiographic Features Laboratory abnormalities include elevated ESR and CRP. In more severe disease, findings include hypoalbuminemia, anemia, and leukocytosis.

Endoscopic features of CD include rectal sparing, aphthous ulcerations, fistulas, and skip lesions. Colonoscopy allows examination and biopsy of mass lesions or strictures and biopsy of the terminal ileum. Upper endoscopy is useful in diagnosing gastroduodenal involvement in patients with upper tract symptoms. Ileal or colonic strictures may be dilated with balloons introduced through the colonoscope. Strictures ≤4 cm and those at anastomotic sites respond better to endoscopic dilation. The perforation rate is as high as 10%. Most endoscopists dilate only fibrotic strictures and not those associated with active inflammation. Wireless capsule endoscopy (WCE) allows direct visualization of the entire small-bowel mucosa (Fig. 351-8). The diagnostic yield of detecting lesions suggestive of active CD is higher with WCE than CT or magnetic resonance (MR) enterography or small-bowel series. WCE cannot be used in the setting of a small-bowel stricture. Capsule retention occurs in <1% of patients with suspected CD, but retention rates of 4–6% are seen in patients with established CD. It is helpful to give the patient with CD a patency capsule, which is made of barium and starts to dissolve 30 h after ingestion. An abdominal x-ray can be taken at around 30 h after ingestion to see if the capsule is still present in the small bowel, which would indicate a stricture.

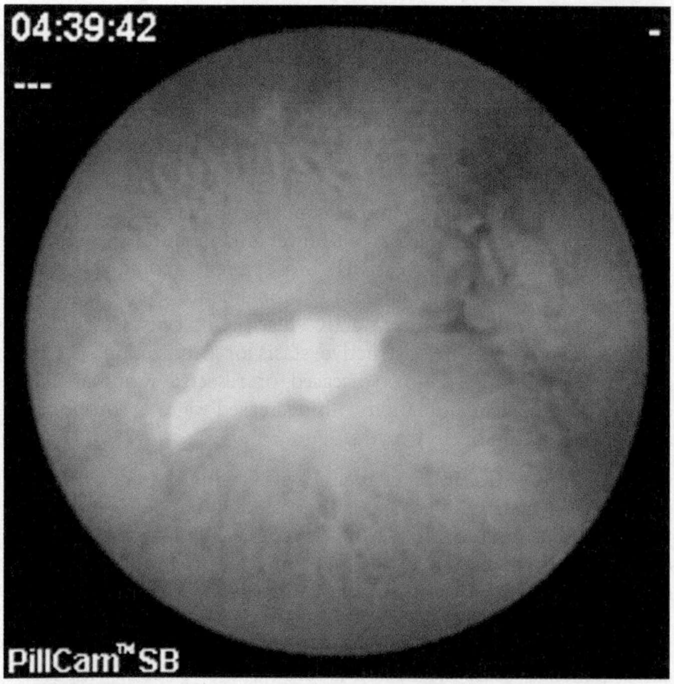

FIGURE 351-8 Wireless capsule endoscopy image in a patient with Crohn's disease of the ileum shows ulcerations and narrowing of the intestinal lumen. *(Courtesy of Dr. S. Reddy, Gastroenterology Division, Department of Medicine, Brigham and Women's Hospital, Boston, Massachusetts; with permission.)*

In CD, early radiographic findings in the small bowel include thickened folds and aphthous ulcerations. "Cobblestoning" from longitudinal and transverse ulcerations most frequently involves the small bowel. In more advanced disease, strictures, fistulas, inflammatory masses, and abscesses may be detected. The earliest macroscopic findings of colonic CD are aphthous ulcers. These small ulcers are often multiple and separated by normal intervening mucosa. As the disease progresses, aphthous ulcers become enlarged, deeper, and occasionally connected to one another, forming longitudinal stellate, serpiginous, and linear ulcers (see Fig. 345-4*B*).

The transmural inflammation of CD leads to decreased luminal diameter and limited distensibility. As ulcers progress deeper, they can lead to fistula formation. The radiographic "string sign" represents long areas of circumferential inflammation and fibrosis, resulting in long segments of luminal narrowing. The segmental nature of CD results in wide gaps of normal or dilated bowel between involved segments.

Both CT and MRI of the small bowel can be performed by enterography (CTE or MRE), using oral and IV contrast, as well as enteroclysis. Although institutional preference guides technique selection, CTE and MRE tend to be preferred over enteroclysis due to ease and patient preference. Although CTE, MRE, and small-bowel follow-through (SBFT) have been shown to be equally accurate in the identification of active small-bowel inflammation, CTE and MRE have been shown to be superior to SBFT in the detection of extraluminal complications, including fistulas, sinus tracts, and abscesses. Currently, the use of CT scans is more common than MRI due to institutional availability and expertise. However, MRI is thought to offer superior soft tissue contrast and has the added advantage of avoiding radiation exposure changes (Figs. 351-9 and 351-10). The lack of ionizing radiation is particularly appealing in younger patients and when monitoring response to therapy where serial images will be obtained. Either CTE or MRE is the first-line test for the evaluation of suspected CD and its complications. Pelvic MRI is superior to CT for demonstrating pelvic lesions such as ischiorectal abscesses and perianal fistulae (Fig. 351-11).

Complications Because CD is a transmural process, serosal adhesions develop that provide direct pathways for fistula formation and reduce the incidence of free perforation. Perforation occurs in 1–2% of patients, usually in the ileum but occasionally in the jejunum or as a complication of toxic megacolon. The peritonitis of free perforation, especially colonic, may be fatal. Intraabdominal and pelvic abscesses occur in 10–30% of patients with CD at some time in the course of their illness. CT-guided percutaneous drainage of the abscess is standard therapy. Despite adequate drainage, most patients need resection of the offending bowel segment. Percutaneous drainage has an especially high failure rate in abdominal wall abscesses. Systemic glucocorticoid therapy increases the risk of intraabdominal and pelvic abscesses in CD patients who have never had an operation. Other complications include intestinal obstruction in 40%, massive hemorrhage, malabsorption, and severe perianal disease.

Serologic Markers Patients with CD show a wide variation in the way they present and progress over time. Some patients present with mild disease activity and do well with generally safe and mild medications, but many others exhibit more severe disease and can develop serious complications that will require surgery. Current and developing biologic therapies can help halt progression of disease and give patients with moderate to severe CD a better quality of life. There are potential risks of biologic therapies such as infection and malignancy, and it would be optimal to determine at the time of diagnosis which patients will require more aggressive medical therapy. This same argument holds true for UC patients as well.

Subsets of patients with differing immune responses to microbial antigens have been described, and serology is often tested for

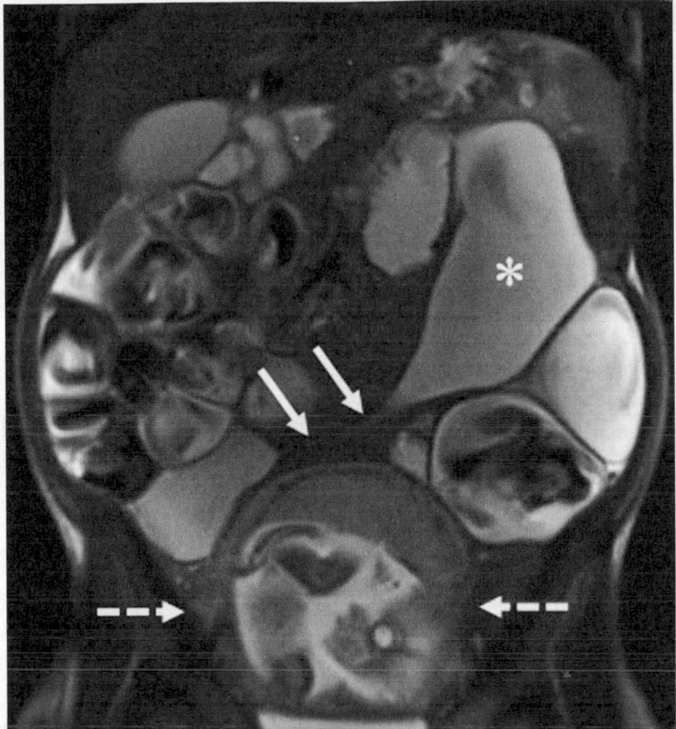

FIGURE 351-9 A coronal magnetic resonance image was obtained using a half Fourier single-shot T2-weighted acquisition with fat saturation in a 27-year-old pregnant (23 weeks' gestation) woman. The patient had Crohn's disease and was maintained on 6-mercaptopurine and prednisone. She presented with abdominal pain, distension, vomiting, and small-bowel obstruction. The image reveals a 7- to 10-cm long stricture at the terminal ileum (*white arrows*) causing obstruction and significant dilatation of the proximal small bowel (*white asterisk*). A fetus is seen in the uterus (*dashed white arrows*). *(Courtesy of Drs. J. F. B. Chick and P. B. Shyn, Abdominal Imaging and Intervention, Department of Radiology, Brigham and Women's Hospital, Harvard Medical School, Boston, Massachusetts; with permission.)*

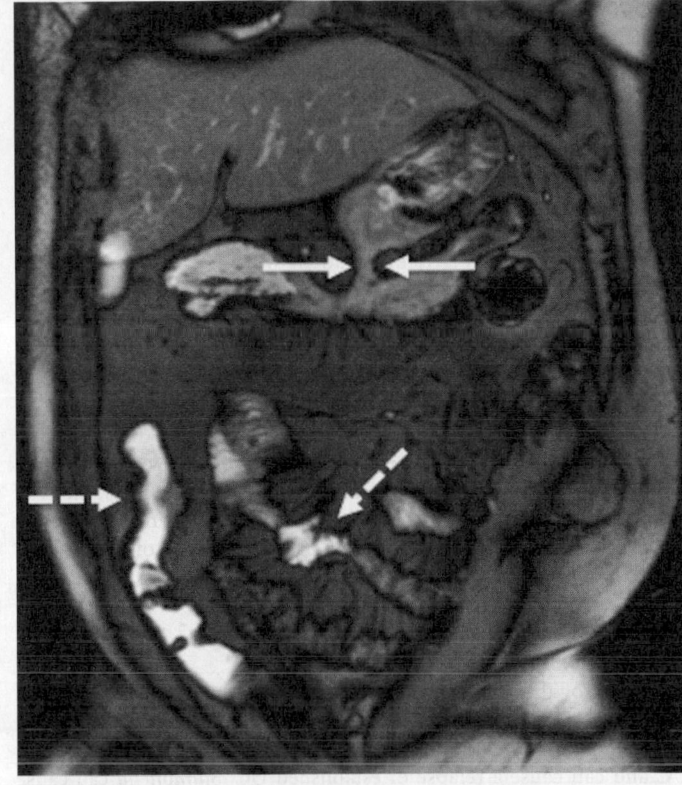

FIGURE 351-10 A coronal balanced, steady-state, free precession, T2-weighted image with fat saturation was obtained in a 32-year-old man with Crohn's disease and prior episodes of bowel obstruction, fistulas, and abscesses. He was being treated with 6-mercaptopurine and presented with abdominal distention and diarrhea. The image demonstrates a new gastrocolic fistula (*solid white arrows*). Multifocal involvement of the small bowel and terminal ileum is also present (*dashed white arrows*). *(Courtesy of Drs. J. F. B. Chick and P. B. Shyn, Abdominal Imaging and Intervention, Department of Radiology, Brigham and Women's Hospital, Harvard Medical School, Boston, Massachusetts; with permission.)*

perinuclear antineutrophil cytoplasmic antibodies (pANCAs) and anti-*Saccharomyces cerevisiae* antibodies (ASCAs). Unfortunately, these serologic markers are only marginally useful in helping to make the diagnosis of UC or CD and in predicting the course of disease. For success in diagnosing IBD and in differentiating between CD and UC, the efficacy of these serologic tests depends on the prevalence of IBD in a specific population. pANCA positivity is found in about 60–70% of UC patients and 5–10% of CD patients; 5–15% of first-degree relatives of UC patients are pANCA positive, whereas only 2–3% of the general population is pANCA positive. Sixty to 70% of CD patients, 10–15% of UC patients, and up to 5% of non-IBD controls are ASCA positive. In a patient population with a combined prevalence of UC and CD of 62%, pANCA/ASCA serology showed a sensitivity of 64% and a specificity of 94%. Positive and negative predictive values (PPVs and NPVs) for pANCA/ASCA also vary based on the prevalence of IBD in a given population. For the patient population with a prevalence of IBD of 62%, the PPV is 94%, and the NPV is 63%.

Other serologic tests include antibodies to *Escherichia coli* outer membrane porin protein C (OmpC), which is found in 55% of CD patients; antibodies to I_2, a homologue of the bacterial transcription factor families from a *Pseudomonas fluorescens*–associated sequence that is found in 50–54% of CD patients; and anti-flagellin (anti-CBir1) antibodies, which have been identified in approximately 50% of CD patients.

Children with CD positive for all four immune responses (ASCA+, OmpC+, I_2+, and anti-Cbir1+) may have more aggressive disease and a shorter time to progression to internal perforating

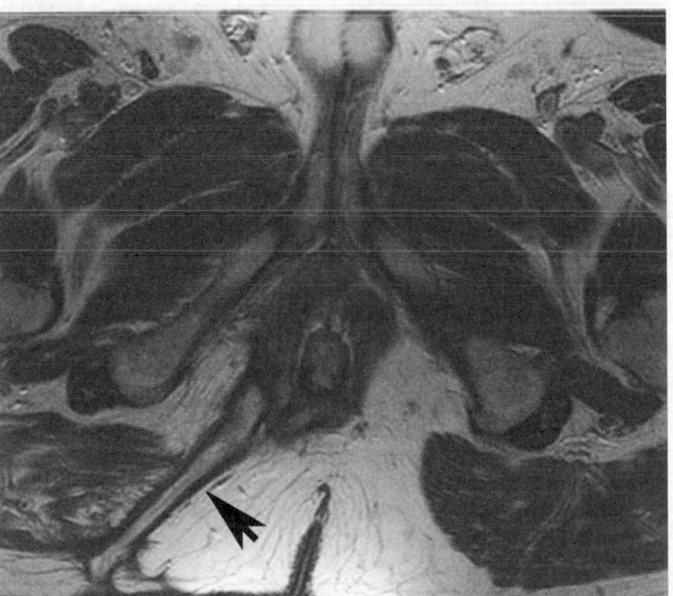

FIGURE 351-11 Axial T2-weighted magnetic resonance image obtained in a 37-year-old man with Crohn's disease shows a linear fluid-filled perianal fistula (*arrow*) in the right ischioanal fossa. *(Courtesy of Dr. K. Mortele, Gastrointestinal Radiology, Department of Radiology, Brigham and Women's Hospital, Boston, Massachusetts; with permission.)*

and/or stricturing disease. However, larger prospective studies in both children and adults have not yet been performed and compared to CRP or other markers.

Clinical factors described at diagnosis are more helpful than serologies at predicting the natural history of CD. The initial requirements for glucocorticoid use, an age at diagnosis below 40 years and the presence of perianal disease at diagnosis, have been shown to be independently associated with subsequent disabling CD after 5 years. Except in special circumstances (such as before consideration of an ileoanal pouch anastomosis [IPAA] in a patient with indeterminate colitis), serologic markers have only minimal clinical utility.

DIFFERENTIAL DIAGNOSIS OF UC AND CD

UC and CD have similar features to many other diseases. In the absence of a key diagnostic test, a combination of features is used (Table 351-5). Once a diagnosis of IBD is made, distinguishing between UC and CD is impossible initially in up to 15% of cases. These are termed *indeterminate colitis*. Fortunately, in most cases, the true nature of the underlying colitis becomes evident later in the course of the patient's disease. Approximately 5% (range 1–20%) of colon resection specimens are difficult to classify as either UC or CD because they exhibit overlapping histologic features.

INFECTIOUS DISEASES

Infections of the small intestines and colon can mimic CD or UC. They may be bacterial, fungal, viral, or protozoal in origin (Table 351-6). *Campylobacter* colitis can mimic the endoscopic appearance of severe UC and can cause a relapse of established UC. *Salmonella* can cause watery or bloody diarrhea, nausea, and vomiting. Shigellosis causes watery diarrhea, abdominal pain, and fever followed by rectal tenesmus and by the passage of blood and mucus per rectum. All three are usually self-limited, but 1% of patients infected with *Salmonella* become asymptomatic carriers. *Yersinia enterocolitica* infection occurs mainly in the terminal ileum and causes mucosal ulceration, neutrophil invasion, and thickening of the ileal wall. Other bacterial infections that may mimic IBD include *C. difficile*, which presents with watery diarrhea, tenesmus, nausea, and vomiting; and *E. coli*, three categories of which can cause colitis. These are enterohemorrhagic, enteroinvasive, and enteroadherent *E. coli*, all of which can cause bloody diarrhea and abdominal tenderness. Diagnosis of bacterial colitis is made by sending stool specimens for bacterial culture and *C. difficile* toxin analysis. Gonorrhea, *Chlamydia*, and syphilis can also cause proctitis.

GI involvement with mycobacterial infection occurs primarily in the immunosuppressed patient but may occur in patients with normal immunity. Distal ileal and cecal involvement predominates, and patients present with symptoms of small-bowel obstruction and a tender abdominal mass. The diagnosis is made most directly by colonoscopy with biopsy and culture. *Mycobacterium avium-intracellulare* complex infection occurs in advanced stages of HIV infection and in other immunocompromised states; it usually manifests as a systemic infection with diarrhea, abdominal pain, weight loss, fever, and malabsorption. Diagnosis is established by acid-fast smear and culture of mucosal biopsies.

Although most of the patients with viral colitis are immunosuppressed, cytomegalovirus (CMV) and herpes simplex proctitis may occur in immunocompetent individuals. CMV occurs most commonly in the esophagus, colon, and rectum but may also involve the small intestine. Symptoms include abdominal pain, bloody diarrhea, fever, and weight loss. With severe disease, necrosis and perforation can occur. Diagnosis is made by identification of characteristic intranuclear inclusions in mucosal cells on biopsy. Herpes simplex infection of the GI tract is limited to the oropharynx, anorectum, and perianal areas. Symptoms include anorectal pain, tenesmus, constipation, inguinal adenopathy, difficulty with urinary voiding, and sacral paresthesias. Diagnosis is made by rectal biopsy with identification of characteristic cellular inclusions and viral culture. HIV itself can cause diarrhea, nausea, vomiting, and anorexia. Small intestinal biopsies show partial villous atrophy; small bowel bacterial overgrowth and fat malabsorption may also be noted.

TABLE 351-5 DIFFERENT CLINICAL, ENDOSCOPIC, AND RADIOGRAPHIC FEATURES

	Ulcerative Colitis	Crohn's Disease
Clinical		
Gross blood in stool	Yes	Occasionally
Mucus	Yes	Occasionally
Systemic symptoms	Occasionally	Frequently
Pain	Occasionally	Frequently
Abdominal mass	Rarely	Yes
Significant perineal disease	No	Frequently
Fistulas	No	Yes
Small intestinal obstruction	No	Frequently
Colonic obstruction	Rarely	Frequently
Response to antibiotics	No	Yes
Recurrence after surgery	No	Yes
Endoscopic		
Rectal sparing	Rarely	Frequently
Continuous disease	Yes	Occasionally
"Cobblestoning"	No	Yes
Granuloma on biopsy	No	Occasionally
Radiographic		
Small bowel significantly abnormal	No	Yes
Abnormal terminal ileum	No	Yes
Segmental colitis	No	Yes
Asymmetric colitis	No	Yes
Stricture	Occasionally	Frequently

TABLE 351-6 DISEASES THAT MIMIC IBD

Bacterial	Mycobacterial	Viral
Infectious Etiologies		
Salmonella	Tuberculosis	Cytomegalovirus
Shigella	*Mycobacterium avium*	Herpes simplex
Toxigenic		HIV
Escherichia coli	**Parasitic**	**Fungal**
Campylobacter	Amebiasis	Histoplasmosis
Yersinia	*Isospora*	*Candida*
Clostridium difficile	*Trichuris trichiura*	*Aspergillus*
Gonorrhea	Hookworm	
Chlamydia trachomatis	*Strongyloides*	
Noninfectious Etiologies		
Inflammatory	**Neoplastic**	**Drugs and Chemicals**
Appendicitis	Lymphoma	NSAIDs
Diverticulitis	Metastatic	Phosphosoda
Diversion colitis	Carcinoma	Cathartic colon
Collagenous/lymphocytic colitis	Carcinoma of the ileum	Gold
		Oral contraceptives
Ischemic colitis	Carcinoid	Cocaine
Radiation colitis/enteritis	Familial polyposis	Ipilimumab
Solitary rectal ulcer syndrome		Mycophenolate mofetil
Eosinophilic gastroenteritis		
Neutropenic colitis		
Behçet's syndrome		
Graft-versus-host disease		

Abbreviation: IBD, inflammatory bowel disease; NSAIDs, nonsteroidal anti-inflammatory drugs.

Protozoan parasites include *Isospora belli,* which can cause a self-limited infection in healthy hosts but causes a chronic profuse, watery diarrhea, and weight loss in AIDS patients. *Entamoeba histolytica* or related species infect about 10% of the world's population; symptoms include abdominal pain, tenesmus, frequent loose stools containing blood and mucus, and abdominal tenderness. Colonoscopy reveals focal punctate ulcers with normal intervening mucosa; diagnosis is made by biopsy or serum amebic antibodies. Fulminant amebic colitis is rare but has a mortality rate of >50%.

Other parasitic infections that may mimic IBD include hookworm (*Necator americanus*), whipworm (*Trichuris trichiura*), and *Strongyloides stercoralis*. In severely immunocompromised patients, *Candida* or *Aspergillus* can be identified in the submucosa. Disseminated histoplasmosis can involve the ileocecal area.

NONINFECTIOUS DISEASES

Diverticulitis can be confused with CD clinically and radiographically. Both diseases cause fever, abdominal pain, tender abdominal mass, leukocytosis, elevated ESR, partial obstruction, and fistulas. Perianal disease or ileitis on small-bowel series favors the diagnosis of CD. Significant endoscopic mucosal abnormalities are more likely in CD than in diverticulitis. Endoscopic or clinical recurrence following segmental resection favors CD. Diverticular-associated colitis is similar to CD, but mucosal abnormalities are limited to the sigmoid and descending colon.

Ischemic colitis is commonly confused with IBD. The ischemic process can be chronic and diffuse, as in UC, or segmental, as in CD. Colonic inflammation due to ischemia may resolve quickly or may persist and result in transmural scarring and stricture formation. Ischemic bowel disease should be considered in the elderly following abdominal aortic aneurysm repair or when a patient has a hypercoagulable state or a severe cardiac or peripheral vascular disorder. Patients usually present with sudden onset of left lower quadrant pain, urgency to defecate, and the passage of bright red blood per rectum. Endoscopic examination often demonstrates a normal-appearing rectum and a sharp transition to an area of inflammation in the descending colon and splenic flexure.

The effects of radiotherapy on the GI tract can be difficult to distinguish from IBD. Acute symptoms can occur within 1–2 weeks of starting radiotherapy. When the rectum and sigmoid are irradiated, patients develop bloody, mucoid diarrhea and tenesmus, as in distal UC. With small-bowel involvement, diarrhea is common. Late symptoms include malabsorption and weight loss. Stricturing with obstruction and bacterial overgrowth may occur. Fistulas can penetrate the bladder, vagina, or abdominal wall. Flexible sigmoidoscopy reveals mucosal granularity, friability, numerous telangiectasias, and occasionally discrete ulcerations. Biopsy can be diagnostic.

Solitary rectal ulcer syndrome is uncommon and can be confused with IBD. It occurs in persons of all ages and may be caused by impaired evacuation and failure of relaxation of the puborectalis muscle. Single or multiple ulcerations may arise from anal sphincter overactivity, higher intrarectal pressures during defecation, and digital removal of stool. Patients complain of constipation with straining and pass blood and mucus per rectum. Other symptoms include abdominal pain, diarrhea, tenesmus, and perineal pain. Ulceration as large as 5 cm in diameter is usually seen anteriorly or anterior-laterally 3–15 cm from the anal verge. Biopsies can be diagnostic.

Several types of colitis are associated with nonsteroidal anti-inflammatory drugs (NSAIDs), including de novo colitis, reactivation of IBD, and proctitis caused by use of suppositories. Most patients with NSAID-related colitis present with diarrhea and abdominal pain, and complications include stricture, bleeding, obstruction, perforation, and fistulization. Withdrawal of these agents is crucial, and in cases of reactivated IBD, standard therapies are indicated.

There are complications of two drugs used in a hospital setting that mimic IBD. The first is ipilimumab, a drug that targets cytotoxic T lymphocyte antigen 4 (CTLA-4) and reverses T cell inhibition and is used to treat metastatic melanoma; ipilimumab has an incidence of IBD in 0.0017 cases per 100 person-years. Ipilimumab-induced colitis is typically treated with glucocorticoids or infliximab. The second is mycophenolate mofetil (MMF), an immunosuppressive agent commonly used to prevent posttransplant rejection. The colitis associated with MMF is common and can occur in more than one-third of patients taking the drug. Treatment is dose reduction or cessation of the drug.

THE ATYPICAL COLITIDES

Two atypical colitides—collagenous colitis and lymphocytic colitis—have completely normal endoscopic appearances. Collagenous colitis has two main histologic components: increased subepithelial collagen deposition and colitis with increased intraepithelial lymphocytes. The female to male ratio is 9:1, and most patients present in the sixth or seventh decades of life. The main symptom is chronic watery diarrhea. Treatments range from sulfasalazine or mesalamine and diphenoxylate/atropine (Lomotil) to bismuth to budesonide to prednisone or azathioprine/6-mercaptopurine for refractory disease. Risk factors include smoking; use of NSAIDs, proton pump inhibitors, or beta blockers; and a history of autoimmune disease.

Lymphocytic colitis has features similar to collagenous colitis, including age at onset and clinical presentation, but it has almost equal incidence in men and women and no subepithelial collagen deposition on pathologic section. However, intraepithelial lymphocytes are increased. Use of sertraline (but not beta blockers) is an additional risk factor. The frequency of celiac disease is increased in lymphocytic colitis and ranges from 9 to 27%. Celiac disease should be excluded in all patients with lymphocytic colitis, particularly if diarrhea does not respond to conventional therapy. Treatment is similar to that of collagenous colitis with the exception of a gluten-free diet for those who have celiac disease.

Diversion colitis is an inflammatory process that arises in segments of the large intestine that are excluded from the fecal stream. It usually occurs in patients with ileostomy or colostomy when a mucus fistula or a Hartmann's pouch has been created. Clinically, patients have mucus or bloody discharge from the rectum. Erythema, granularity, friability, and, in more severe cases, ulceration can be seen on endoscopy. Histopathology shows areas of active inflammation with foci of cryptitis and crypt abscesses. Crypt architecture is normal, which differentiates it from UC. It may be impossible to distinguish from CD. Short-chain fatty acid enemas may help in diversion colitis, but the definitive therapy is surgical reanastomosis.

EXTRAINTESTINAL MANIFESTATIONS

Up to one-third of IBD patients have at least one extraintestinal disease manifestation.

DERMATOLOGIC

Erythema nodosum (EN) occurs in up to 15% of CD patients and 10% of UC patients. Attacks usually correlate with bowel activity; skin lesions develop after the onset of bowel symptoms, and patients frequently have concomitant active peripheral arthritis. The lesions of EN are hot, red, tender nodules measuring 1–5 cm in diameter and are found on the anterior surface of the lower legs, ankles, calves, thighs, and arms. Therapy is directed toward the underlying bowel disease.

Pyoderma gangrenosum (PG) is seen in 1–12% of UC patients and less commonly in Crohn's colitis. Although it usually presents after the diagnosis of IBD, PG may occur years before the onset of bowel symptoms, run a course independent of the bowel disease, respond poorly to colectomy, and even develop years after proctocolectomy. It is usually associated with severe disease. Lesions are commonly found on the dorsal surface of the feet and legs but may occur on the arms, chest, stoma, and even the face. PG usually begins as a pustule and then spreads concentrically to rapidly undermine healthy skin. Lesions then ulcerate, with violaceous edges surrounded by a margin of erythema. Centrally, they contain necrotic tissue with blood and exudates. Lesions may be single or multiple and grow as large as 30 cm. They are sometimes very difficult to treat and often require IV antibiotics, IV glucocorticoids, dapsone, azathioprine, thalidomide, IV cyclosporine, or infliximab.

Other dermatologic manifestations include pyoderma vegetans, which occurs in intertriginous areas; pyostomatitis vegetans, which involves the mucous membranes; Sweet syndrome, a neutrophilic dermatosis; and metastatic CD, a rare disorder defined by cutaneous granuloma formation. Psoriasis affects 5–10% of patients with IBD and is unrelated to bowel activity consistent with the potential shared immunogenetic basis of these diseases. Perianal skin tags are found in 75–80% of patients with CD, especially those with colon involvement. Oral mucosal lesions, seen often in CD and rarely in UC, include aphthous stomatitis and "cobblestone" lesions of the buccal mucosa.

RHEUMATOLOGIC

Peripheral arthritis develops in 15–20% of IBD patients, is more common in CD, and worsens with exacerbations of bowel activity. It is asymmetric, polyarticular, and migratory and most often affects large joints of the upper and lower extremities. Treatment is directed at reducing bowel inflammation. In severe UC, colectomy frequently cures the arthritis.

Ankylosing spondylitis (AS) occurs in about 10% of IBD patients and is more common in CD than UC. About two-thirds of IBD patients with AS express the HLA-B27 antigen. The AS activity is not related to bowel activity and does not remit with glucocorticoids or colectomy. It most often affects the spine and pelvis, producing symptoms of diffuse low-back pain, buttock pain, and morning stiffness. The course is continuous and progressive, leading to permanent skeletal damage and deformity. Anti-TNF therapy reduces spinal inflammation and improves functional status and quality of life.

Sacroiliitis is symmetric, occurs equally in UC and CD, is often asymptomatic, does not correlate with bowel activity, and does not always progress to AS. Other rheumatic manifestations include hypertrophic osteoarthropathy, pelvic/femoral osteomyelitis, and relapsing polychondritis.

OCULAR

The incidence of ocular complications in IBD patients is 1–10%. The most common are conjunctivitis, anterior uveitis/iritis, and episcleritis. Uveitis is associated with both UC and Crohn's colitis, may be found during periods of remission, and may develop in patients following bowel resection. Symptoms include ocular pain, photophobia, blurred vision, and headache. Prompt intervention, sometimes with systemic glucocorticoids, is required to prevent scarring and visual impairment. Episcleritis is a benign disorder that presents with symptoms of mild ocular burning. It occurs in 3–4% of IBD patients, more commonly in Crohn's colitis, and is treated with topical glucocorticoids.

HEPATOBILIARY

Hepatic steatosis is detectable in about one-half of the abnormal liver biopsies from patients with CD and UC; patients usually present with hepatomegaly. Fatty liver usually results from a combination of chronic debilitating illness, malnutrition, and glucocorticoid therapy. Cholelithiasis occurs in 10–35% of CD patients with ileitis or ileal resection. Gallstone formation is caused by malabsorption of bile acids, resulting in depletion of the bile salt pool and the secretion of lithogenic bile.

Primary sclerosing cholangitis (PSC) is a disorder characterized by both intrahepatic and extrahepatic bile duct inflammation and fibrosis, frequently leading to biliary cirrhosis and hepatic failure; approximately 5% of patients with UC have PSC, but 50–75% of patients with PSC have IBD. PSC occurs less often in patients with CD. Although it can be recognized after the diagnosis of IBD, PSC can be detected earlier or even years after proctocolectomy. Consistent with this, the immunogenetic basis for PSC appears to be overlapping but distinct from UC based on GWAS, although both IBD and PSC are commonly pANCA positive. Most patients have no symptoms at the time of diagnosis; when symptoms are present, they consist of fatigue, jaundice, abdominal pain, fever, anorexia, and malaise. The traditional gold standard diagnostic test is endoscopic retrograde cholangiopancreatography (ERCP), but magnetic resonance cholangiopancreatography (MRCP) is also sensitive and specific. MRCP is reasonable as an initial diagnostic test in children and can visualize irregularities, multifocal strictures, and dilatations of all levels of the biliary tree. In patients with PSC, both ERCP and MRCP demonstrate multiple bile duct strictures alternating with relatively normal segments.

The bile acid ursodeoxycholic acid (ursodiol) may reduce alkaline phosphatase and serum aminotransferase levels, but histologic improvement has been marginal. High doses (25–30 mg/kg per day) may decrease the risk of colorectal dysplasia and cancer in patients with UC and PSC. Endoscopic stenting may be palliative for cholestasis secondary to bile duct obstruction. Patients with symptomatic disease develop cirrhosis and liver failure over 5–10 years and eventually require liver transplantation. PSC patients have a 10–15% lifetime risk of developing cholangiocarcinoma and then cannot be transplanted. Patients with IBD and PSC are at increased risk of colon cancer and should be surveyed yearly by colonoscopy and biopsy.

In addition, cholangiography is normal in a small percentage of patients who have a variant of PSC known as *small duct primary sclerosing cholangitis*. This variant (sometimes referred to as "pericholangitis") is probably a form of PSC involving small-caliber bile ducts. It has similar biochemical and histologic features to classic PSC. It appears to have a significantly better prognosis than classic PSC, although it may evolve into classic PSC. Granulomatous hepatitis and hepatic amyloidosis are much rarer extraintestinal manifestations of IBD.

UROLOGIC

The most frequent genitourinary complications are calculi, ureteral obstruction, and ileal bladder fistulas. The highest frequency of nephrolithiasis (10–20%) occurs in patients with CD following small bowel resection. Calcium oxalate stones develop secondary to hyperoxaluria, which results from increased absorption of dietary oxalate. Normally, dietary calcium combines with luminal oxalate to form insoluble calcium oxalate, which is eliminated in the stool. In patients with ileal dysfunction, however, nonabsorbed fatty acids bind calcium and leave oxalate unbound. The unbound oxalate is then delivered to the colon, where it is readily absorbed, especially in the presence of inflammation.

METABOLIC BONE DISORDERS

Low bone mass occurs in 3–30% of IBD patients. The risk is increased by glucocorticoids, cyclosporine, methotrexate, and total parenteral nutrition (TPN). Malabsorption and inflammation mediated by IL-1, IL-6, TNF, and other inflammatory mediators also contribute to low bone density. An increased incidence of hip, spine, wrist, and rib fractures has been noted: 36% in CD and 45% in UC. The absolute risk of an osteoporotic fracture is about 1% per person per year. Fracture rates, particularly in the spine and hip, are highest among the elderly (age >60). One study noted an OR of 1.72 for vertebral fracture and an OR of 1.59 for hip fracture. The disease severity predicted the risk of a fracture. Only 13% of IBD patients who had a fracture were on any kind of antifracture treatment. Up to 20% of bone mass can be lost per year with chronic glucocorticoid use. The effect is dosage-dependent. Budesonide may also suppress the pituitary-adrenal axis and thus carries a risk of causing osteoporosis.

Osteonecrosis is characterized by death of osteocytes and adipocytes and eventual bone collapse. The pain is aggravated by motion and swelling of the joints. It affects the hips more often than knees and shoulders, and in one series, 4.3% of patients developed osteonecrosis within 6 months of starting glucocorticoids. Diagnosis is made by bone scan or MRI, and treatment consists of pain control, cord decompression, osteotomy, and joint replacement.

THROMBOEMBOLIC DISORDERS

Patients with IBD have an increased risk of both venous and arterial thrombosis even if the disease is not active. Factors responsible for the hypercoagulable state have included abnormalities of the platelet-endothelial interaction, hyperhomocysteinemia, alterations in the coagulation cascade, impaired fibrinolysis, involvement of tissue factor-bearing microvesicles, disruption of the normal coagulation system by autoantibodies, and a genetic predisposition. A spectrum of vasculitides involving small, medium, and large vessels has also been observed.

OTHER DISORDERS

More common cardiopulmonary manifestations include endocarditis, myocarditis, pleuropericarditis, and interstitial lung disease. A secondary or reactive amyloidosis can occur in patients with long-standing IBD, especially in patients with CD. Amyloid material is deposited systemically and can cause diarrhea, constipation, and renal failure. The renal disease can be successfully treated with colchicine. Pancreatitis is a rare extraintestinal manifestation of IBD and results from duodenal fistulas; ampullary CD; gallstones; PSC; drugs such as 6-mercaptopurine, azathioprine, or, very rarely, 5-ASA agents; autoimmune pancreatitis; and primary CD of the pancreas.

TREATMENT INFLAMMATORY BOWEL DISEASE TREATMENT

5-ASA AGENTS

The mainstay of therapy for mild to moderate UC is sulfasalazine and the other 5-ASA agents. These agents are effective at inducing and maintaining remission in UC. They may have a limited role in inducing remission in CD but no clear role in maintenance of CD. Newer sulfa-free aminosalicylate preparations deliver increased amounts of the pharmacologically active ingredient of sulfasalazine (5-ASA, mesalamine) to the site of active bowel disease while limiting systemic toxicity. Peroxisome proliferator activated receptor γ (PPAR γ) may mediate 5-ASA therapeutic action by decreasing nuclear localization of NF-κB. Sulfa-free aminosalicylate formulations include alternative azo-bonded carriers, 5-ASA dimers, and delayed-release and controlled-release preparations. Each has the same efficacy as sulfasalazine when equimolar concentrations are used.

Sulfasalazine was originally developed to deliver both antibacterial (sulfapyridine) and anti-inflammatory (5-ASA) therapy into the connective tissues of joints and the colonic mucosa. The molecular structure provides a convenient delivery system to the colon by allowing the intact molecule to pass through the small intestine after only partial absorption and to be broken down in the colon by bacterial azo reductases that cleave the azo bond linking the sulfa and 5-ASA moieties. Sulfasalazine is effective treatment for mild to moderate UC and is occasionally used in Crohn's colitis, but its high rate of side effects limits its use. Although sulfasalazine is more effective at higher doses, at 6 or 8 g/d up to 30% of patients experience allergic reactions or intolerable side effects such as headache, anorexia, nausea, and vomiting that are attributable to the sulfapyridine moiety. Hypersensitivity reactions, independent of sulfapyridine levels, include rash, fever, hepatitis, agranulocytosis, hypersensitivity pneumonitis, pancreatitis, worsening of colitis, and reversible sperm abnormalities. Sulfasalazine can also impair folate absorption, and patients should be given folic acid supplements.

Balsalazide contains an azo bond binding mesalamine to the carrier molecule 4-aminobenzoyl-β-alanine; it is effective in the colon.

Olsalazine is composed of two 5-ASA radicals linked by an azo bond, which is split in the colon by bacterial reduction, and two 5-ASA molecules are released. Olsalazine is similar in effectiveness to sulfasalazine in treating UC, but up to 17% of patients experience nonbloody diarrhea caused by increased secretion of fluid in the small bowel.

Delzicol and Asacol HD (high dose) are enteric-coated forms of mesalamine with the 5-ASA being released at pH >7. They disintegrate with complete breakup of the tablet occurring in many different parts of the gut ranging from the small intestine to the splenic flexure; they have increased gastric residence when taken with a meal. Asacol has recently been discontinued and replaced with Delzicol, which lacks dibutyl phthalate (DBP), an inactive ingredient in Asacol's enteric coating. DBP has been associated with adverse effects on the male reproductive system in animals at very high doses. Asacol HD with the same chemical in its coating is still on the market, but the human doses of DBP are within acceptable limits of toxicity.

Lialda is a once-a-day formulation of mesalamine (Multi-Matrix System [MMX]) designed to release mesalamine in the colon. The MMX technology incorporates mesalamine into a lipophilic matrix within a hydrophilic matrix encapsulated in a polymer resistant to degradation at a low pH (<7) to delay release throughout the colon. The safety profile appears to be comparable to other 5-ASA formulations.

Apriso is a formulation containing encapsulated mesalamine granules that delivers mesalamine to the terminal ileum and colon via a proprietary extended-release mechanism (Intellicor). The outer coating (Eudragit L) dissolves at a pH >6. In addition, there is a polymer matrix core that aids in sustained release throughout the colon. Because Lialda and Apriso are given once daily, an anticipated benefit is improved compliance compared with two to four daily doses required for other mesalamine preparations.

Pentasa is another mesalamine formulation that uses an ethylcellulose coating to allow water absorption into small beads containing the mesalamine. Water dissolves the 5-ASA, which then diffuses out of the bead into the lumen. Disintegration of the capsule occurs in the stomach. The microspheres then disperse throughout the entire GI tract from the small intestine through the distal colon in both fasted and fed conditions.

Salofalk® Granu-Stix, an unencapsulated version of mesalamine, has been in use in Europe for induction and maintenance of remission for several years.

Appropriate doses of the 5-ASA compounds are shown in **Table 351-7**. Some 50–75% of patients with mild to moderate UC improve when treated with 5-ASA doses equivalent to 2 g/d of

TABLE 351-7 ORAL 5-ASA PREPARATIONS

Preparation	Formulation	Delivery	Dosing Per Day
Azo-Bond			
Sulfasalazine (500 mg) (Azulfidine)	Sulfapyridine-5-ASA	Colon	3–6 g (acute) 2–4 g (maintenance)
Olsalazine (250 mg) (Dipentum)	5-ASA–5-ASA	Colon	1–3 g
Balsalazide (750 mg) (Colazal)	Aminobenzoyl-alanine–5-ASA	Colon	6.75–9 g
Delayed-Release			
Mesalamine (400, 800 mg) (Delzicol, Asacol HD)	Eudragit S (pH 7)	Distal ileum-colon	2.4–4.8 g (acute) 1.6–4.8 g (maintenance)
Mesalamine (1.2 g) (Lialda)	MMX mesalamine (SPD476)	Ileum-colon	2.4–4.8 g
Controlled-Release			
Mesalamine (250, 500, 1000 mg) (Pentasa)	Ethylcellulose microgranules	Stomach-colon	2–4 g (acute) 1.5–4 g (maintenance)
Delayed- and Extended-Release			
Mesalamine (0.375 g) (Apriso)	Intellicor extended-release mechanism	Ileum-colon	1.5 g (maintenance)

mesalamine; the dose response continues up to at least 4.8 g/d. As a general rule, 5-ASA agents act within 2–4 weeks. 5-ASA doses equivalent to 1.5–4 g/d of mesalamine maintain remission in 50–75% of patients with UC.

More common side effects of the 5-ASA medications include headaches, nausea, hair loss, and abdominal pain. Rare side effects of the 5-ASA medications include renal impairment, hematuria, pancreatitis, and paradoxical worsening of colitis. Renal function tests and urinalysis should be checked yearly.

Topical *Rowasa* enemas are composed of mesalamine and are effective in mild-to-moderate distal UC. Clinical response occurs in up to 80% of UC patients with colitis distal to the splenic flexure. Combination therapy with mesalamine in both oral and enema form is more effective than either treatment alone for both distal and extensive UC.

Canasa suppositories composed of mesalamine are effective in treating proctitis.

GLUCOCORTICOIDS

The majority of patients with moderate to severe UC benefit from oral or parenteral glucocorticoids. Prednisone is usually started at doses of 40–60 mg/d for active UC that is unresponsive to 5-ASA therapy. Parenteral glucocorticoids may be administered as hydrocortisone, 300 mg/d, or methylprednisolone, 40–60 mg/d. A new glucocorticoid for UC, budesonide (Uceris), is released entirely in the colon and has minimal to no glucocorticoid side effects. The dose is 9 mg/d for 8 weeks, and no taper is required. Topically applied glucocorticoids are also beneficial for distal colitis and may serve as an adjunct in those who have rectal involvement plus more proximal disease. Hydrocortisone enemas or foam may control active disease, although they have no proven role as maintenance therapy. These glucocorticoids are significantly absorbed from the rectum and can lead to adrenal suppression with prolonged administration. Topical 5-ASA therapy is more effective than topical steroid therapy in the treatment of distal UC.

Glucocorticoids are also effective for treatment of moderate to severe CD and induce a 60–70% remission rate compared to a 30% placebo response. The systemic effects of standard glucocorticoid formulations have led to the development of more potent formulations that are less well-absorbed and have increased first-pass metabolism. Controlled ileal-release budesonide has been nearly equal to prednisone for ileocolonic CD with fewer glucocorticoid side effects. Budesonide is used for 2–3 months at a dose of 9 mg/d, and then tapered. Budesonide 6 mg/d is effective in reducing relapse rates at 3–6 months but not at 12 months in CD patients with a medically induced remission.

Glucocorticoids play no role in maintenance therapy in either UC or CD. Once clinical remission has been induced, they should be tapered according to the clinical activity, normally at a rate of no more than 5 mg/week. They can usually be tapered to 20 mg/d within 4–5 weeks but often take several months to be discontinued altogether. The side effects are numerous, including fluid retention, abdominal striae, fat redistribution, hyperglycemia, subcapsular cataracts, osteonecrosis, osteoporosis, myopathy, emotional disturbances, and withdrawal symptoms. Most of these side effects, aside from osteonecrosis, are related to the dose and duration of therapy.

ANTIBIOTICS

Antibiotics have no role in the treatment of active or quiescent UC. However, pouchitis, which occurs in about a third of UC patients after colectomy and IPAA, usually responds to treatment with metronidazole and/or ciprofloxacin.

Metronidazole is effective in active inflammatory, fistulous, and perianal CD and may prevent recurrence after ileal resection. The most effective dose is 15–20 mg/kg per day in three divided doses; it is usually continued for several months. Common side effects include nausea, metallic taste, and disulfiram-like reaction. Peripheral neuropathy can occur with prolonged administration (several months) and on rare occasions is permanent despite discontinuation. *Ciprofloxacin* (500 mg bid) is also beneficial for inflammatory, perianal, and fistulous CD but has been associated with Achilles tendinitis and rupture. Both ciprofloxacin and metronidazole antibiotics can be used as first-line drugs for short periods of time in active inflammatory, fistulizing, and perianal CD.

AZATHIOPRINE AND 6-MERCAPTOPURINE

Azathioprine and 6-mercaptopurine (6-MP) are purine analogues commonly employed in the management of glucocorticoid-dependent IBD. Azathioprine is rapidly absorbed and converted to 6-MP, which is then metabolized to the active end product, thioinosinic acid, an inhibitor of purine ribonucleotide synthesis and cell proliferation. These agents also inhibit the immune response. Efficacy can be seen as early as 3–4 weeks but can take up to 4–6 months. Adherence can be monitored by measuring the levels of 6-thioguanine and 6-methylmercaptopurine, end products of 6-MP metabolism. Azathioprine (2–3 mg/kg per day) and 6-MP (1–1.5 mg/kg per day) have been used successfully as glucocorticoid-sparing agents in up to two-thirds of UC and CD patients previously unable to be weaned from glucocorticoids. They are also used as maintenance therapy in UC and CD and for treating active perianal disease and fistulas in CD. In addition, 6-MP or azathioprine is effective for postoperative prophylaxis of CD.

Although azathioprine and 6-MP are usually well tolerated, pancreatitis occurs in 3–4% of patients, typically presents within the first few weeks of therapy, and is completely reversible when the drug is stopped. Other side effects include nausea, fever, rash, and hepatitis. Bone marrow suppression (particularly leukopenia) is dose-related and often delayed, necessitating regular monitoring of the complete blood cell count (CBC). Additionally, 1 in 300 individuals lacks thiopurine methyltransferase, the enzyme responsible for drug metabolism to inactive end-products (6-methylmercaptopurine); an additional 11% of the population are heterozygotes with intermediate enzyme activity. Both are at increased risk of toxicity because of increased accumulation of active 6-thioguanine metabolites. Although 6-thioguanine and 6-methylmercaptopurine levels can be followed to determine correct drug dosing and reduce toxicity, weight-based dosing is an acceptable alternative. CBCs and liver function tests should be monitored frequently regardless of dosing strategy. IBD patients treated with azathioprine/6-MP are at approximately a fourfold increased risk of developing a lymphoma. This increased risk could be a result of the medications, the underlying disease, or both.

METHOTREXATE

Methotrexate (MTX) inhibits dihydrofolate reductase, resulting in impaired DNA synthesis. Additional anti-inflammatory properties may be related to decreased IL-1 production. Intramuscular (IM) or subcutaneous (SC) MTX (25 mg/week) is effective in inducing remission and reducing glucocorticoid dosage; 15 mg/week is effective in maintaining remission in active CD. Potential toxicities include leukopenia and hepatic fibrosis, necessitating periodic evaluation of CBCs and liver enzymes. The role of liver biopsy in patients on long-term MTX is uncertain but is probably limited to those with increased liver enzymes. Hypersensitivity pneumonitis is a rare but serious complication of therapy.

CYCLOSPORINE

Cyclosporine (CSA) is a lipophilic peptide with inhibitory effects on both the cellular and humoral immune systems. CSA blocks the production of IL-2 by T helper lymphocytes. CSA binds to cyclophilin, and this complex inhibits calcineurin, a cytoplasmic phosphatase enzyme involved in the activation of T cells. CSA also indirectly inhibits B cell function by blocking helper T cells. CSA has a more rapid onset of action than 6-MP and azathioprine.

CSA is most effective when given at 2–4 mg/kg per day IV in severe UC that is refractory to IV glucocorticoids, with 82% of patients responding. CSA can be an alternative to colectomy. The long-term success of oral CSA is not as dramatic, but if patients are started on 6-MP or azathioprine at the time of hospital discharge, remission can be maintained. For the 2 mg/kg dose, levels as measured by monoclonal radioimmunoassay or by the high-performance liquid chromatography assay should be maintained between 150 and 350 ng/mL.

CSA may cause significant toxicity; renal function should be monitored frequently. Hypertension, gingival hyperplasia, hypertrichosis, paresthesias, tremors, headaches, and electrolyte abnormalities are common side effects. Creatinine elevation calls for dose reduction or discontinuation. Seizures may also complicate therapy, especially if the patient is hypomagnesemic or if serum cholesterol levels are <3.1 mmol/L (<120 mg/dL). Opportunistic infections, most notably *Pneumocystis carinii* pneumonia, may occur with combination immunosuppressive treatment; prophylaxis should be given. Major adverse events occurred in 15% of patients in one large study, including nephrotoxicity not responding to dose adjustment, serious infections, seizures, anaphylaxis, and death of two patients. This high incidence suggests that vigorous monitoring by experienced clinicians at tertiary care centers may be required. To compare IV cyclosporine versus infliximab, a large trial was conducted in Europe by the GETAID group. The results indicated identical 7-day response rates between cyclosporine 2 mg/kg (with doses adjusted for levels of 150–250 ng/mL) and infliximab 5 mg/kg, with both groups achieving response rates of 85%. Serious infections occurred in 5 of 55 cyclosporine patients and 4 of 56 infliximab patients. Response rates were similar in the two groups at day 98 among patients treated with oral cyclosporine versus infliximab at the usual induction dose and maintenance dose regimen (40% and 46%, respectively). In light of data showing equal efficacy of CSA and infliximab in severe UC, more physicians are relying on infliximab rather than CSA in these patients.

TACROLIMUS

Tacrolimus is a macrolide antibiotic with immunomodulatory properties similar to CSA. It is 100 times as potent as CSA and is not dependent on bile or mucosal integrity for absorption. These pharmacologic properties enable tacrolimus to have good oral absorption despite proximal small bowel Crohn's involvement. It has shown efficacy in children with refractory IBD and in adults with extensive involvement of the small bowel. It is also effective in adults with glucocorticoid-dependent or refractory UC and CD as well as refractory fistulizing CD.

BIOLOGIC THERAPIES

Biologic therapy was traditionally reserved for moderately to severely ill patients with CD who had failed other therapies. However, it is now commonly given as an initial therapy for patients with moderate to severe CD in order to prevent future disease complications. Patients who respond to biologic therapies enjoy an improvement in clinical symptoms; a better quality of life; less disability, fatigue, and depression; and fewer surgeries and hospitalizations.

Anti-TNF Therapies The first biologic therapy approved for CD was *infliximab*, a chimeric IgG1 antibody against TNF-α, which is now also approved for treatment of moderately to severely active UC. Of active CD patients refractory to glucocorticoids, 6-MP, or 5-ASA, 65% will respond to IV infliximab (5 mg/kg); one-third will enter complete remission. The ACCENT I (A Crohn's Disease Clinical Trial Evaluating Infliximab in a New Long-Term Treatment Regimen) study showed that of the patients who experience an initial response, 40% will maintain remission for at least 1 year with repeated infusions of infliximab every 8 weeks.

Infliximab is also effective in CD patients with refractory perianal and enterocutaneous fistulas, with the ACCENT II trial showing a 68% response rate (50% reduction in fistula drainage) and a 50% complete remission rate. Reinfusion, typically every 8 weeks, is necessary to continue therapeutic benefits in many patients.

The SONIC (Study of Biologic and Immunomodulator-Naive Patients with Crohn's Disease) trial compared infliximab plus azathioprine, infliximab alone, and azathioprine alone in immunomodulator- and biologic-naive patients with moderate to severe CD. At 1 year, the infliximab plus azathioprine group had a glucocorticoid-free remission rate of 46% compared with 35% for infliximab alone and 24% for azathioprine alone. There was also complete mucosal healing at week 26 with the combined approach relative to either infliximab or azathioprine alone (44% vs 30% vs 17%). The adverse events were equal between groups.

Two large trials of infliximab in moderate to severe UC also showed efficacy with a response rate of 37–49%, with about one-fifth of patients maintaining remission after 54 weeks. Dosing for UC and CD are identical, with induction dosing at 0, 2, and 6 weeks and every 8 weeks thereafter. There is a similar study to SONIC in patients with moderate to severe UC. After 16 weeks of therapy, UC patients taking azathioprine plus infliximab had a glucocorticoid-free remission rate of 40% compared to 24% (article now published) and 22% of those on azathioprine and infliximab alone, respectively. This is even further evidence for "top-down" or more aggressive therapy for both moderate to severe CD and UC.

Adalimumab is a recombinant human monoclonal IgG1 antibody containing only human peptide sequences and is injected subcutaneously. Adalimumab binds TNF and neutralizes its function by blocking the interaction between TNF and its cell-surface receptor. Therefore, it seems to have a similar mechanism of action to infliximab but with less immunogenicity. Adalimumab has been approved for treatment of moderate to severe CD. CHARM (Crohn's Trial of the Fully Human Adalimumab for Remission Maintenance) is an adalimumab maintenance study in patients who responded to adalimumab induction therapy. About 50% of the patients in this trial were previously treated with infliximab. Remission rates ranged from 42–48% of infliximab naïve patients at 1 year compared with remission rates of 31–34% in patients who had previously received infliximab. Another trial showed a remission rate of 21% at 4 weeks in patients who had initially responded to and then failed infliximab. In clinical practice, the remission rate in patients taking adalimumab increases with a dose increase to 40 mg weekly instead of every other week. Adalimumab is now also approved for the treatment of moderately to severely active UC.

Certolizumab pegol is a pegylated form of an anti-TNF Fab portion of an antibody administered SC once monthly. SC certolizumab pegol was effective for induction of clinical response in patients with active inflammatory CD. In the PRECISE II (Pegylated Antibody Fragment Evaluation in Crohn's Disease) trial of maintenance therapy with certolizumab in patients who responded to certolizumab induction, the results were similar to the CHARM trial. At week 26, the subgroup of patients who were infliximab naïve had a response of 69% as compared to 44% in patients who had previously received infliximab.

Golimumab is another fully human IgG1 antibody against TNF-α and is currently approved for the treatment of moderately to severely active UC. All of the patients in the golimumab trial were infliximab-naive. Like adalimumab and certolizumab, golimumab is injected SC.

Side Effects of Anti-TNF Therapies • *DEVELOPMENT OF ANTIBODIES* The development of antibodies to infliximab (ATIs) is associated with an increased risk of infusion reactions and a decreased response to treatment. Current practice does not include giving on-demand or episodic infusions in contrast to periodic (every 8 week) infusions because patients are most likely to develop ATIs. ATIs are generally present when the quality of response or the response duration to infliximab infusion decreases. Decreasing the dosing intervals or increasing the dosage to 10 mg/kg may restore the efficacy. There are commercial assays for both infliximab and adalimumab antibodies and trough levels to determine optimal dosing. If a patient has high ATIs and a low trough level of infliximab, it is best to switch to another anti-TNF therapy. Most acute infusion reactions and serum sickness can be managed with glucocorticoids and antihistamines. Some reactions can be serious and would necessitate a change in therapy, especially if a patient has ATIs.

NON-HODGKIN'S LYMPHOMA (NHL) The baseline risk of NHL in CD patients is 2:10,000, which is slightly higher than in the general population.

Azathioprine and/or 6-MP therapy increases the risk to about 4:10,000. The highest risk for thiopurine-associated NHL is in patients over 65 years old, with a moderate risk in those between the ages of 50 and 65. Anti-TNF therapy increases the risk to approximately 6:10,000.

HEPATOSPLENIC T CELL LYMPHOMA (HSTCL) HSTCL is a nearly universally fatal lymphoma in patients with or without CD. In patients with CD, events reported to the Food and Drug Administration Adverse Event Reporting System (FDA AERS) and search of PubMed and Embase published case reports demonstrate a total of 37 unique cases. Eighty-six percent of the patients were male, with a median age of 26 years. Patients had CD for a mean of 10 years before the diagnosis of HSTCL. Thirty-six cases had used either 6-MP or azathioprine, and 28 cases had used infliximab. Of these 28 cases, 27 had also used 6-MP or azathioprine. The other case had a history of both infliximab and adalimumab exposure.

SKIN LESIONS New-onset psoriasiform skin lesions develop in nearly 5% of IBD patients treated with anti-TNF therapy. Most often, these can be treated topically, and rarely, anti-TNF therapy must be decreased, switched, or stopped. The risk of melanoma is increased almost twofold with anti-TNF and not thiopurine use. The risk of nonmelanoma skin cancer is increased with thiopurines and biologics, especially with 1 year of follow-up or greater. Patients on these medications should have a skin check at least once a year.

INFECTIONS All of the anti-TNF drugs are associated with an increased risk of infections, particularly reactivation of latent tuberculosis and opportunistic fungal infections including disseminated histoplasmosis and coccidioidomycosis. It is recommended that patients have a purified protein derivative (PPD) or a QuantiFERON-TB gold test as well as a chest x-ray before initiation of anti-TNF therapy. Patients over 65 have a higher rate of infections and death on infliximab or adalimumab than those younger than 65 years of age.

OTHER Acute liver injury due to reactivation of hepatitis B virus and to autoimmune effects and cholestasis has been reported. Rarely, infliximab and the other anti-TNF drugs have been associated with optic neuritis, seizures, new onset or exacerbation of clinical symptoms, and radiographic evidence of central nervous system demyelinating disorders, including multiple sclerosis. They may exacerbate symptoms in patients with New York Heart Association functional class III/IV heart failure.

ANTI-INTEGRINS Integrins are expressed on the cell surface of leukocytes and serve as mediators of leukocyte adhesion to vascular endothelium. α4-Integrin along with its β1 or β7 subunit interact with endothelial ligands termed adhesion molecules. Interaction between α4β7 and mucosal addressin cellular adhesion molecule (MAdCAM-1) is important in lymphocyte trafficking to gut mucosa.

Natalizumab is a recombinant humanized IgG4 antibody against α4-integrin that has been shown to be effective in induction and maintenance of patients with CD. It has been approved since February 2008 for the treatment of patients with CD refractory or intolerant to anti-TNF therapy. The rates of response and remission at 3 months are about 60% and 40%, respectively, with a sustained remission rate of about 40% at 36 weeks.

One case of progressive multifocal leukoencephalopathy (PML) after eight infusions of natalizumab was observed among 1043 patients in the clinical trials for CD, and two patients developed PML in the multiple sclerosis (MS) trials after a median of 120 weeks. There were 410 postmarketing cases of PML, 408 in MS and 2 in CD. The most important risk factor for development of PML is exposure to the John Cunningham (JC) polyomavirus, seen in 50–55% of the adult population. The other two risk factors for development of PML are longer duration of treatment, especially beyond 2 years, and prior treatment with an immunosuppressant medication. Patients with all three risk factors have an estimated risk of 11:1000.

The FDA approved a commercial enzyme-linked immunosorbent assay (ELISA) kit to assay anti-JC viral antibodies (Stratify JCV Antibody ELISA; Focus Diagnostics, Cypress, CA) in early 2012. The test is 99% accurate in stratifying risk of PML. It is recommended that all patients be tested prior to initiating natalizumab therapy. JC virus serologies are then measured every 6 months because 1–2% of patients will seroconvert yearly. All patients taking natalizumab and their providers must be enrolled in the TOUCH (Tysabri Outreach Unified Commitment for Health) pharmacovigilance program. Natalizumab is administered IV, 300 mg every 4 weeks. Labeling requirements mandate that it not be used in combination with any immunosuppressant medications.

Vedolizumab, another leukocyte trafficking inhibitor, is indicated for patients who have had an inadequate response or lost response to, or were intolerant of a TNF blocker or immunomodulator; or had an inadequate response or were intolerant to, or demonstrated dependence on glucocorticoids. It is an option for patients who are JC antibody positive since it does not cross the blood-brain barrier. Vedolizumab is a monoclonal antibody directed against α4β7 integrin specifically and has the ability to convey gut-selective immunosuppression.

THERAPIES IN DEVELOPMENT

Ustekinumab, a fully human IgG1 monoclonal antibody, blocks the biologic activity of IL-12 and IL-23 through their common p40 subunit by inhibiting the interaction of these cytokines with their receptors on T cells, natural killer cells, and antigen presenting cells. It shows efficacy in moderate to severe CD in clinical trials.

Tofacitinib is an oral inhibitor of Janus kinases 1, 3, and, to a lesser extent, 2. It is expected to block signaling involving common gamma chain–containing cytokines including IL-2, IL-4, IL-7, IL-9, IL-15, and IL-21. These cytokines are integral to lymphocyte activation, function, and proliferation. It is effective in moderate to severe UC in clinical trials.

NUTRITIONAL THERAPIES

Dietary antigens may stimulate the mucosal immune response. Patients with active CD respond to bowel rest, along with TPN. Bowel rest and TPN are as effective as glucocorticoids at inducing remission of active CD but are not effective as maintenance therapy. Enteral nutrition in the form of elemental or peptide-based preparations is also as effective as glucocorticoids or TPN, but these diets are not palatable. Enteral diets may provide the small intestine with nutrients vital to cell growth and do not have the complications of TPN. In contrast to CD, dietary intervention does not reduce inflammation in UC. Standard medical management of UC and CD is shown in Fig. 351-12.

SURGICAL THERAPY

Ulcerative Colitis Nearly one-half of patients with extensive chronic UC undergo surgery within the first 10 years of their illness. The indications for surgery are listed in Table 351-8. Morbidity is about 20% for elective, 30% for urgent, and 40% for emergency proctocolectomy. The risks are primarily hemorrhage, contamination and sepsis, and neural injury. The operation of choice is an ileoanal J pouch anastomosis (IPAA).

Because UC is a mucosal disease, the rectal mucosa can be dissected and removed down to the dentate line of the anus or about 2 cm proximal to this landmark. The ileum is fashioned into a pouch that serves as a neorectum. This ileal pouch is then sutured circumferentially to the anus in an end-to-end fashion. If performed carefully, this operation preserves the anal sphincter and maintains continence. The overall operative morbidity is 10%, with the major complication being bowel obstruction. Pouch failure necessitating conversion to permanent ileostomy occurs in 5–10% of patients. Some inflamed rectal mucosa is usually left behind, and thus endoscopic surveillance is necessary. Primary dysplasia of the ileal mucosa of the pouch has occurred rarely.

Patients with IPAA usually have about 6–10 bowel movements a day. On validated quality-of-life indices, they report better performance in sports and sexual activities than ileostomy patients. The most frequent complication of IPAA is pouchitis in about 30–50%

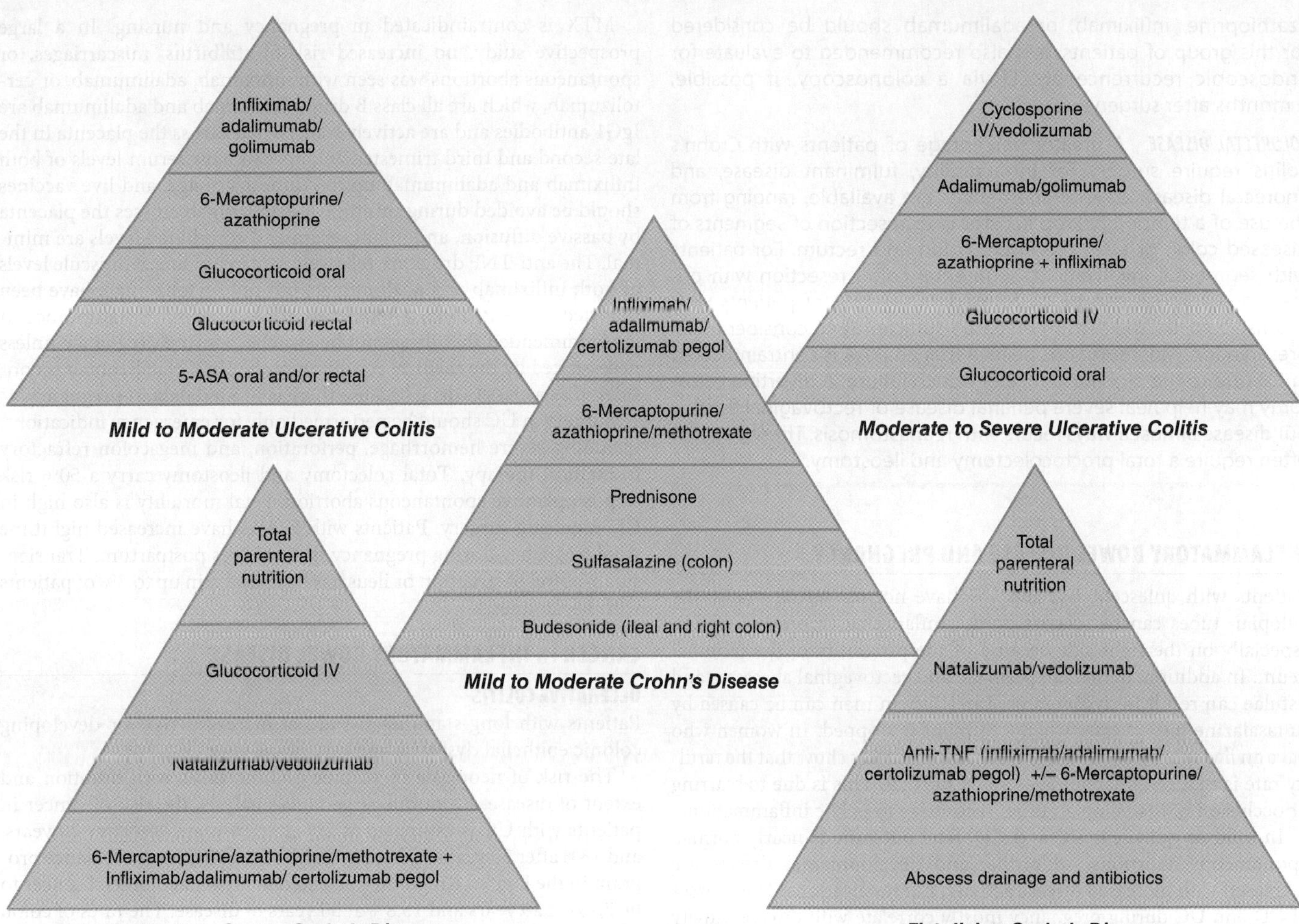

FIGURE 351-12 Medical management of inflammatory bowel disease. 5-ASA, 5-aminosalicylic acid; CD, Crohn's disease; UC, ulcerative colitis.

of patients with UC. This syndrome consists of increased stool frequency, watery stools, cramping, urgency, nocturnal leakage of stool, arthralgias, malaise, and fever. Pouch biopsies may distinguish true pouchitis from underlying CD. Although pouchitis usually responds to antibiotics, 3–5% of patients remain refractory and may require glucocorticoids, immunomodulators, anti-TNF therapy, or even pouch removal. A highly concentrated probiotic preparation with four strains of *Lactobacillus,* three strains of *Bifidobacterium,* and one strain of *Streptococcus salivarius* can prevent the recurrence of pouchitis when taken daily.

TABLE 351-8 INDICATIONS FOR SURGERY

Ulcerative Colitis	Crohn's Disease
Intractable disease	Small Intestine
Fulminant disease	Stricture and obstruction unresponsive to medical therapy
Toxic megacolon	Massive hemorrhage
Colonic perforation	Refractory fistula
Massive colonic hemorrhage	Abscess
Extracolonic disease	Colon and rectum
Colonic obstruction	Intractable disease
Colon cancer prophylaxis	Fulminant disease
Colon dysplasia or cancer	Perianal disease unresponsive to medical therapy
	Refractory fistula
	Colonic obstruction
	Cancer prophylaxis
	Colon dysplasia or cancer

Crohn's Disease Most patients with CD require at least one operation in their lifetime. The need for surgery is related to duration of disease and the site of involvement. Patients with small-bowel disease have an 80% chance of requiring surgery. Those with colitis alone have a 50% chance. Surgery is an option only when medical treatment has failed or complications dictate its necessity. The indications for surgery are shown in Table 351-8.

SMALL INTESTINAL DISEASE Because CD is chronic and recurrent, with no clear surgical cure, as little intestine as possible is resected. Current surgical alternatives for treatment of obstructing CD include resection of the diseased segment and strictureplasty. Surgical resection of the diseased segment is the most frequently performed operation, and in most cases, primary anastomosis can be done to restore continuity. If much of the small bowel has already been resected and the strictures are short, with intervening areas of normal mucosa, strictureplasties should be done to avoid a functionally insufficient length of bowel. The strictured area of intestine is incised longitudinally and the incision sutured transversely, thus widening the narrowed area. Complications of strictureplasty include prolonged ileus, hemorrhage, fistula, abscess, leak, and restricture.

There is evidence that mesalamine, nitroimidazole antibiotics, 6-MP/azathioprine, infliximab, and adalimumab are all superior to placebo for the prevention of postoperative recurrence of CD. Mesalamine is the least effective, and the side effects of the nitroimidazole antibiotics limit their use. Risk factors for early recurrence of disease include cigarette smoking, penetrating disease (internal fistulas, abscesses, or other evidence of penetration through the wall of the bowel), early recurrence since a previous surgery, multiple surgeries, and a young age at the time of the first surgery. Aggressive postoperative treatment with 6-MP/

azathioprine, infliximab, or adalimumab should be considered for this group of patients. It is also recommended to evaluate for endoscopic recurrence of CD via a colonoscopy, if possible, 6 months after surgery.

COLORECTAL DISEASE A greater percentage of patients with Crohn's colitis require surgery for intractability, fulminant disease, and anorectal disease. Several alternatives are available, ranging from the use of a temporary loop ileostomy to resection of segments of diseased colon or even the entire colon and rectum. For patients with segmental involvement, segmental colon resection with primary anastomosis can be performed. In 20–25% of patients with extensive colitis, the rectum is spared sufficiently to consider rectal preservation. Most surgeons believe that an IPAA is contraindicated in CD due to the high incidence of pouch failure. A diverting colostomy may help heal severe perianal disease or rectovaginal fistulas, but disease almost always recurs with reanastomosis. These patients often require a total proctocolectomy and ileostomy.

INFLAMMATORY BOWEL DISEASE AND PREGNANCY

Patients with quiescent UC and CD have normal fertility rates; the fallopian tubes can be scarred by the inflammatory process of CD, especially on the right side because of the proximity of the terminal ileum. In addition, perirectal, perineal, and rectovaginal abscesses and fistulae can result in dyspareunia. Infertility in men can be caused by sulfasalazine but reverses when treatment is stopped. In women who have an ileoanal J pouch anastomosis, most studies show that the fertility rate is reduced to about 50–80% of normal. This is due to scarring or occlusion of the fallopian tubes secondary to pelvic inflammation.

In mild or quiescent UC and CD, fetal outcome is nearly normal. Spontaneous abortions, stillbirths, and developmental defects are increased with increased disease activity, not medications. The courses of CD and UC during pregnancy mostly correlate with disease activity at the time of conception. Patients should be in remission for 6 months before conceiving. Most CD patients can deliver vaginally, but cesarean delivery may be the preferred route of delivery for patients with anorectal and perirectal abscesses and fistulas to reduce the likelihood of fistulas developing or extending into the episiotomy scar. Unless they desire multiple children, UC patients with an IPAA should consider a cesarean delivery due to an increased risk of future fecal incontinence.

Sulfasalazine, Lialda, Apriso, Delzicol, and balsalazide are safe for use in pregnancy and nursing with the caveat that additional folate supplementation must be given with sulfasalazine. Asacol HD and olsalazine are considered by the FDA to be class C agents in pregnancy and thus not recommended. Topical 5-ASA agents are also safe during pregnancy and nursing. Glucocorticoids are generally safe for use during pregnancy and are indicated for patients with moderate to severe disease activity. The amount of glucocorticoids received by the nursing infant is minimal. The safest antibiotics to use for CD in pregnancy for short periods of time (weeks, not months) are ampicillin and cephalosporins. Metronidazole can be used in the second or third trimester. Ciprofloxacin causes cartilage lesions in immature animals and should be avoided because of the absence of data on its effects on growth and development in humans.

6-MP and azathioprine pose minimal or no risk during pregnancy, but experience is limited. If the patient cannot be weaned from the drug or has an exacerbation that requires 6-MP/azathioprine during pregnancy, she should continue the drug with informed consent. Breast milk has been shown to contain negligible levels of 6-MP/azathioprine when measured in a limited number of patients.

Little data exist on CSA in pregnancy. In a small number of patients with severe IBD treated with IV CSA during pregnancy, 80% of pregnancies were successfully completed without development of renal toxicity or congenital malformations. However, because of the lack of data, CSA should probably be avoided unless the patient would otherwise require surgery.

MTX is contraindicated in pregnancy and nursing. In a large prospective study, no increased risk of stillbirths, miscarriages, or spontaneous abortions was seen with infliximab, adalimumab, or certolizumab, which are all class B drugs. Infliximab and adalimumab are IgG1 antibodies and are actively transported across the placenta in the late second and third trimester. Infants can have serum levels of both infliximab and adalimumab up to 7 months of age, and live vaccines should be avoided during this time. Certolizumab crosses the placenta by passive diffusion, and infant serum and cord blood levels are minimal. The anti-TNF drugs are relatively safe in nursing. Miniscule levels of both infliximab and adalimumab, but not certolizumab, have been reported in breast milk. These levels are of no clinical significance. It is recommended that drugs not be switched during pregnancy unless necessitated by the medical condition of the IBD. Natalizumab is considered as a class C drug because there is limited data in pregnancy.

Surgery in UC should be performed only for emergency indications, including severe hemorrhage, perforation, and megacolon refractory to medical therapy. Total colectomy and ileostomy carry a 50% risk of postoperative spontaneous abortion. Fetal mortality is also high in CD requiring surgery. Patients with IPAAs have increased nighttime stool frequency during pregnancy that resolves postpartum. Transient small-bowel obstruction or ileus has been noted in up to 8% of patients with ileostomies.

CANCER IN INFLAMMATORY BOWEL DISEASE

ULCERATIVE COLITIS

Patients with long-standing UC are at increased risk for developing colonic epithelial dysplasia and carcinoma (Fig. 351-13).

The risk of neoplasia in chronic UC increases with duration and extent of disease. From one large meta-analysis, the risk of cancer in patients with UC is estimated at 2% after 10 years, 8% after 20 years, and 18% after 30 years of disease. Data from a 30-year surveillance program in the United Kingdom calculated the risk of colorectal cancer to be 7.7% at 20 years and 15.8% at 30 years of disease. The rates of colon cancer are higher than in the general population, and colonoscopic surveillance is the standard of care.

Annual or biennial colonoscopy with multiple biopsies is recommended for patients with >8–10 years of extensive colitis (greater than one-third of the colon involved) or 12–15 years of proctosigmoiditis (less than one-third but more than just the rectum) and has been widely used to screen and survey for subsequent dysplasia and carcinoma. Risk factors for cancer in UC include long-duration disease, extensive disease, family history of colon cancer, PSC, a colon stricture, and the presence of postinflammatory pseudopolyps on colonoscopy.

CROHN'S DISEASE

Risk factors for developing cancer in Crohn's colitis are long-duration and extensive disease, bypassed colon segments, colon strictures, PSC,

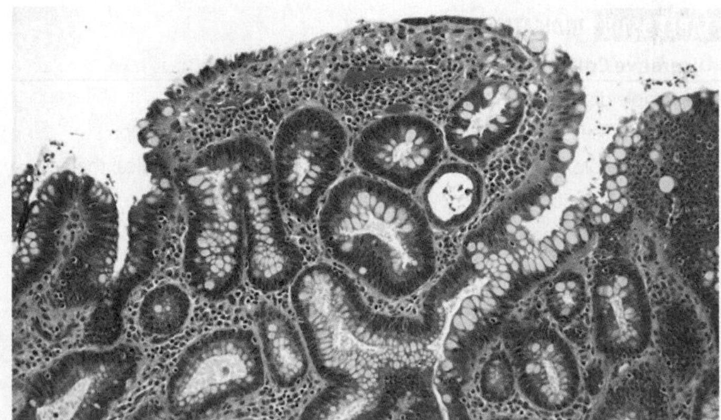

FIGURE 351-13 Medium-power view of low-grade dysplasia in a patient with chronic ulcerative colitis. Low-grade dysplastic crypts are interspersed among regenerating crypts. *(Courtesy of Dr. R. Odze, Division of Gastrointestinal Pathology, Department of Pathology, Brigham and Women's Hospital, Boston, Massachusetts; with permission.)*

and family history of colon cancer. The cancer risks in CD and UC are probably equivalent for similar extent and duration of disease. In the CESAME study, a prospective observational cohort of IBD patients in France, the standardized incidence ratios of colorectal cancer were 2.2 for all IBD patients (95% confidence interval [CI], 1.5–3.0; $p < .001$) and 7.0 for patients with long-standing extensive colitis (both Crohn's and UC) (95% CI, 4.4–10.5; $p < .001$). Thus, the same endoscopic surveillance strategy used for UC is recommended for patients with chronic Crohn's colitis. A pediatric colonoscope can be used to pass narrow strictures in CD patients, but surgery should be considered in symptomatic patients with impassable strictures.

MANAGEMENT OF DYSPLASIA AND CANCER

Dysplasia can be flat or polypoid. If flat high-grade dysplasia is encountered on colonoscopic surveillance, the usual treatment is colectomy for UC and either colectomy or segmental resection for CD. If flat low-grade dysplasia is found (Fig. 351-13), most investigators recommend immediate colectomy. Adenomas may occur coincidently in UC and CD patients with chronic colitis and can be removed endoscopically provided that biopsies of the surrounding mucosa are free of dysplasia. High-definition and high-magnification colonoscopes and dye sprays have increased the rate of dysplasia detection.

IBD patients are also at greater risk for other malignancies. Patients with CD may have an increased risk of non-Hodgkin's lymphoma, leukemia, and myelodysplastic syndromes. Severe, chronic, complicated perianal disease in CD patients may be associated with an increased risk of cancer in the lower rectum and anal canal (squamous cell cancers). Although the absolute risk of small-bowel adenocarcinoma in CD is low (2.2% at 25 years in one study), patients with long-standing, extensive, small-bowel disease should consider screening.

352 Irritable Bowel Syndrome

Chung Owyang

Irritable bowel syndrome (IBS) is a functional bowel disorder characterized by abdominal pain or discomfort and altered bowel habits in the absence of detectable structural abnormalities. No clear diagnostic markers exist for IBS; thus the diagnosis of the disorder is based on clinical presentation. In 2006, the Rome II criteria for the diagnosis of IBS were revised (Table 352-1). Throughout the world, about 10–20% of adults and adolescents have symptoms consistent with IBS, and most studies show a female predominance. IBS symptoms tend to come and go over time and often overlap with other functional disorders such as fibromyalgia, headache, backache, and genitourinary symptoms. Severity of symptoms varies and can significantly impair quality of life, resulting in high health care costs. Advances in basic, mechanistic, and clinical investigations have improved our understanding of this disorder and its physiologic and psychosocial determinants. Altered gastrointestinal (GI) motility, visceral hyperalgesia, disturbance of brain-gut interaction, abnormal central processing, autonomic and hormonal events, genetic and environmental factors, and psychosocial disturbances are variably involved, depending on the individual. This progress may result in improved methods of treatment.

TABLE 352-1 DIAGNOSTIC CRITERIA FOR IRRITABLE BOWEL SYNDROME[a]

Recurrent abdominal pain or discomfort[b] at least 3 days per month in the last 3 months associated with two or more of the following:

1. Improvement with defecation
2. Onset associated with a change in frequency of stool
3. Onset associated with a change in form (appearance) of stool

[a]Criteria fulfilled for the last 3 months with symptom onset at least 6 months prior to diagnosis. [b]Discomfort means an uncomfortable sensation not described as pain. In pathophysiology research and clinical trials, a pain/discomfort frequency of at least 2 days a week during screening evaluation is required for subject eligibility.

Source: Adapted from GF Longstreth et al: Gastroenterology 130:1480, 2006.

CLINICAL FEATURES

IBS is a disorder that affects all ages, although most patients have their first symptoms before age 45. Older individuals have a lower reporting frequency. Women are diagnosed with IBS two to three times as often as men and make up 80% of the population with severe IBS. As indicated in Table 352-1, pain or abdominal discomfort is a key symptom for the diagnosis of IBS. These symptoms should be improved with defecation and/or have their onset associated with a change in frequency or form of stool. Painless diarrhea or constipation does not fulfill the diagnostic criteria to be classified as IBS. Supportive symptoms that are not part of the diagnostic criteria include defecation straining, urgency or a feeling of incomplete bowel movement, passing mucus, and bloating.

Abdominal Pain According to the current IBS diagnostic criteria, abdominal pain or discomfort is a prerequisite clinical feature of IBS. Abdominal pain in IBS is highly variable in intensity and location. It is frequently episodic and crampy, but it may be superimposed on a background of constant ache. Pain may be mild enough to be ignored or it may interfere with daily activities. Despite this, malnutrition due to inadequate caloric intake is exceedingly rare with IBS. Sleep deprivation is also unusual because abdominal pain is almost uniformly present only during waking hours. However, patients with severe IBS frequently wake repeatedly during the night; thus, nocturnal pain is a poor discriminating factor between organic and functional bowel disease. Pain is often exacerbated by eating or emotional stress and improved by passage of flatus or stools. In addition, female patients with IBS commonly report worsening symptoms during the premenstrual and menstrual phases.

Altered Bowel Habits Alteration in bowel habits is the most consistent clinical feature in IBS. The most common pattern is constipation alternating with diarrhea, usually with one of these symptoms predominating. At first, constipation may be episodic, but eventually it becomes continuous and increasingly intractable to treatment with laxatives. Stools are usually hard with narrowed caliber, possibly reflecting excessive dehydration caused by prolonged colonic retention and spasm. Most patients also experience a sense of incomplete evacuation, thus leading to repeated attempts at defecation in a short time span. Patients whose predominant symptom is constipation may have weeks or months of constipation interrupted with brief periods of diarrhea. In other patients, diarrhea may be the predominant symptom. Diarrhea resulting from IBS usually consists of small volumes of loose stools. Most patients have stool volumes of <200 mL. Nocturnal diarrhea does not occur in IBS. Diarrhea may be aggravated by emotional stress or eating. Stool may be accompanied by passage of large amounts of mucus. Bleeding is not a feature of IBS unless hemorrhoids are present, and malabsorption or weight loss does not occur.

Bowel pattern subtypes are highly unstable. In a patient population with ~33% prevalence rates of IBS-diarrhea predominant (IBS-D), IBS-constipation predominant (IBS-C), and IBS-mixed (IBS-M) forms, 75% of patients change subtypes and 29% switch between IBS-C and IBS-D over 1 year. The heterogeneity and variable natural history of bowel habits in IBS increase the difficulty of conducting pathophysiology studies and clinical trials.

Gas and Flatulence Patients with IBS frequently complain of abdominal distention and increased belching or flatulence, all of which they attribute to increased gas. Although some patients with these symptoms actually may have a larger amount of gas, quantitative measurements reveal that most patients who complain of increased gas generate no more than a normal amount of intestinal gas. Most IBS patients have impaired transit and tolerance of intestinal gas loads. In addition, patients with IBS tend to reflux gas from the distal to the more proximal intestine, which may explain the belching.

Some patients with bloating may also experience visible distention with increase in abdominal girth. Both symptoms are more common among female patients and in those with higher overall Somatic Symptom Checklist scores. IBS patients who experienced bloating alone have been shown to have lower thresholds for pain and desire to defecate compared to those with concomitant distention irrespective of bowel habit. When patients were grouped according to sensory threshold, hyposensitive individuals had distention significantly more than those with hypersensitivity and this was observed more in the constipation subgroup. This suggests that the pathogenesis of bloating and distention may not be the same.

Upper Gastrointestinal Symptoms Between 25 and 50% of patients with IBS complain of dyspepsia, heartburn, nausea, and vomiting. This suggests that other areas of the gut apart from the colon may be involved. Prolonged ambulant recordings of small-bowel motility in patients with IBS show a high incidence of abnormalities in the small bowel during the diurnal (waking) period; nocturnal motor patterns are not different from those of healthy controls. The overlap between dyspepsia and IBS is great. The prevalence of IBS is higher among patients with dyspepsia (31.7%) than among those who reported no symptoms of dyspepsia (7.9%). Conversely, among patients with IBS, 55.6% reported symptoms of dyspepsia. In addition, the functional abdominal symptoms can change over time. Those with predominant dyspepsia or IBS can flux between the two. Although the prevalence of functional gastrointestinal disorders is stable over time, the turnover in symptom status is high. Many episodes of symptom disappearance are due to subjects changing symptoms rather than total symptom resolution. Thus it is conceivable that functional dyspepsia and IBS are two manifestations of a single, more extensive digestive system disorder. Furthermore, IBS symptoms are prevalent in noncardiac chest pain patients, suggesting overlap with other functional gut disorders.

PATHOPHYSIOLOGY

The pathogenesis of IBS is poorly understood, although roles of abnormal gut motor and sensory activity, central neural dysfunction, psychological disturbances, mucosal inflammation, stress, and luminal factors have been proposed.

Gastrointestinal Motor Abnormalities Studies of colonic myoelectrical and motor activity under unstimulated conditions have not shown consistent abnormalities in IBS. In contrast, colonic motor abnormalities are more prominent under stimulated conditions in IBS. IBS patients may exhibit increased rectosigmoid motor activity for up to 3 h after eating. Similarly, inflation of rectal balloons both in IBS-D and IBS-C patients leads to marked and prolonged distention-evoked contractile activity. Recordings from the transverse, descending, and sigmoid colon showed that the motility index and peak amplitude of high-amplitude propagating contractions (HAPCs) in diarrhea-prone IBS patients were greatly increased compared to those in healthy subjects and were associated with rapid colonic transit and accompanied by abdominal pain.

Visceral Hypersensitivity As with studies of motor activity, IBS patients frequently exhibit exaggerated sensory responses to visceral stimulation. The frequency of perceptions of food intolerance is at least twofold more common than in the general population. Postprandial pain has been temporally related to entry of the food bolus into the cecum in 74% of patients. On the other hand, prolonged fasting in IBS patients is often associated with significant improvement in symptoms. Rectal balloon inflation produces nonpainful and painful sensations at lower volumes in IBS patients than in healthy controls without altering rectal tension, suggestive of visceral afferent dysfunction in IBS. Similar studies show gastric and esophageal hypersensitivity in patients with nonulcer dyspepsia and noncardiac chest pain, raising the possibility that these conditions have a similar pathophysiologic basis. Lipids lower the thresholds for the first sensation of gas, discomfort, and pain in IBS patients. Hence, postprandial symptoms in IBS patients may be explained in part by a nutrient-dependent exaggerated sensory component of the gastrocolonic response. In contrast to enhanced gut sensitivity, IBS patients do not exhibit heightened sensitivity elsewhere in the body. Thus, the afferent pathway disturbances in IBS appear to be selective for visceral innervation with sparing of somatic pathways. The mechanisms responsible for visceral hypersensitivity are still under investigation. It has been proposed that these exaggerated responses may be due to (1) increased end-organ sensitivity with recruitment of "silent" nociceptors; (2) spinal hyperexcitability with activation of nitric oxide and possibly other neurotransmitters; (3) endogenous (cortical and brainstem) modulation of caudad nociceptive transmission; and (4) over time, the possible development of long-term hyperalgesia due to development of neuroplasticity, resulting in permanent or semipermanent changes in neural responses to chronic or recurrent visceral stimulation (Table 352-2).

TABLE 352-2 PROPOSED MECHANISMS FOR VISCERAL HYPERSENSITIVITY

End-organ sensitivity	Long-term hyperalgesia
"Silent" nociceptors	Tonic cortical regulation
CNS modulation	Neuroplasticity
Cortex	
Brainstem	

Abbreviation: CNS, central nervous system.

Central Neural Dysregulation The role of central nervous system (CNS) factors in the pathogenesis of IBS is strongly suggested by the clinical association of emotional disorders and stress with symptom exacerbation and the therapeutic response to therapies that act on cerebral cortical sites. Functional brain imaging studies such as magnetic resonance imaging (MRI) have shown that in response to distal colonic stimulation, the mid-cingulate cortex—a brain region concerned with attention processes and response selection—shows greater activation in IBS patients. Modulation of this region is associated with changes in the subjective unpleasantness of pain. In addition, IBS patients also show preferential activation of the prefrontal lobe, which contains a vigilance network within the brain that increases alertness. These may represent a form of cerebral dysfunction leading to the increased perception of visceral pain.

Abnormal Psychological Features Abnormal psychiatric features are recorded in up to 80% of IBS patients, especially in referral centers; however, no single psychiatric diagnosis predominates. Most of these patients demonstrated exaggerated symptoms in response to visceral distention, and this abnormality persists even after exclusion of psychological factors.

Psychological factors influence pain thresholds in IBS patients, as stress alters sensory thresholds. An association between prior sexual or physical abuse and development of IBS has been reported. Abuse is associated with greater pain reporting, psychological distress, and poor health outcome. Brain functional MRI studies show greater activation of the posterior and middle dorsal cingulate cortex, which is implicated in affect processing in IBS patients with a past history of sexual abuse.

Thus, patients with IBS frequently demonstrate increased motor reactivity of the colon and small bowel to a variety of stimuli and altered visceral sensation associated with lowered sensation thresholds. These may result from CNS–enteric nervous system dysregulation (Fig. 352-1).

Postinfectious IBS IBS may be induced by GI infection. In an investigation of 544 patients with confirmed bacterial gastroenteritis, one-quarter developed IBS subsequently. Conversely, about a third of IBS patients experienced an acute "gastroenteritis-like" illness at the onset of their chronic IBS symptomatology. This group of "postinfective" IBS occurs more commonly in females and affects younger rather than older patients. Risk factors for developing postinfectious IBS include, in order of importance, prolonged duration of initial illness, toxicity of infecting bacterial strain, smoking, mucosal markers of inflammation, female gender, depression, hypochondriasis, and adverse life events in the preceding 3 months. Age older than 60 years might protect against postinfectious IBS, whereas treatment with antibiotics has been

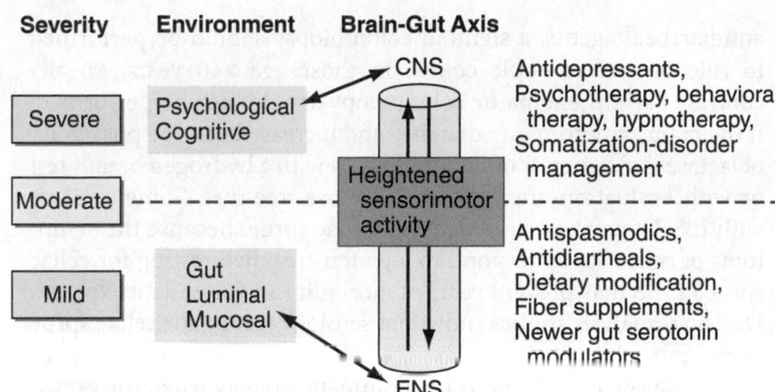

FIGURE 352-1 Therapeutic targets for irritable bowel syndrome. Patients with mild to moderate symptoms usually have intermittent symptoms that correlate with altered gut physiology. Treatments include gut-acting pharmacologic agents such as antispasmodics, antidiarrheals, fiber supplements, and gut serotonin modulators. Patients who have severe symptoms usually have constant pain and psychosocial difficulties. This group of patients is best managed with antidepressants and other psychosocial treatments. CNS, central nervous system; ENS, enteric nervous system.

associated with increased risk. The microbes involved in the initial infection are *Campylobacter*, *Salmonella*, and *Shigella*. Those patients with *Campylobacter* infection who are toxin-positive are more likely to develop postinfective IBS. Increased rectal mucosal enteroendocrine cells, T lymphocytes, and increased gut permeability are acute changes following *Campylobacter* enteritis that could persist for more than a year and may contribute to postinfective IBS.

Immune Activation and Mucosal Inflammation Some patients with IBS display persistent signs of low-grade mucosal inflammation with activated lymphocytes, mast cells, and enhanced expression of proinflammatory cytokines. These abnormalities may contribute to abnormal epithelial secretion and visceral hypersensitivity. There is increasing evidence that some members of the superfamily of transient receptor potential (TRP) cation channels such as TRPV1 (vanilloid) channels are central to the initiation and persistence of visceral hypersensitivity. Mucosal inflammation can lead to increased expression of TRPV1 in the enteric nervous system. Enhanced expression of TRPV1 channels in the sensory neurons of the gut has been observed in IBS, and such expression appears to correlate with visceral hypersensitivity and abdominal pain. Interestingly, clinical studies have also shown increased intestinal permeability in patients with IBS-D. Psychological stress and anxiety can increase the release of proinflammatory cytokine, and this in turn may alter intestinal permeability. This provides a functional link between psychological stress, immune activation, and symptom generation in patients with IBS.

Altered Gut Flora A high prevalence of small intestinal bacterial overgrowth in IBS patients has been noted based on positive lactulose hydrogen breath test. This finding, however, has been challenged by a number of other studies that found no increased incidence of bacterial overgrowth based on jejunal aspirate culture. Abnormal H_2 breath test can occur because of small-bowel rapid transit and may lead to erroneous interpretation. Hence, the role of testing for small intestinal bacterial overgrowth in IBS patients remains unclear.

Studies using culture-independent approaches such as 16S rRNA gene-based analysis found significant differences between the molecular profile of the fecal microbiota of IBS patients and that of healthy subjects. IBS patients had decreased proportions of the genera *Bifidobacterium* and *Lactobacillus* and increased ratios of Firmicutes:Bacteroidetes. It has been speculated that these changes may be related to stress and diet. A temporary reduction in lactobacilli has been reported in animal models of early-life stress. On the other hand, Firmicutes is the dominant phylum in adults consuming a diet high in animal fat and protein. However, it is still unclear whether such changes in fecal microbiota are causal, consequential, or merely the result of constipation and diarrhea. In addition, the stability of the change in the microbiota needs to be determined.

Abnormal Serotonin Pathways The serotonin (5-HT)-containing enterochromaffin cells in the colon are increased in a subset of IBS-D patients compared to healthy individuals or patients with ulcerative colitis. Furthermore, postprandial plasma 5-HT levels were significantly higher in this group of patients compared to healthy controls. Because serotonin plays an important role in the regulation of GI motility and visceral perception, the increased release of serotonin may contribute to the postprandial symptoms of these patients and provides a rationale for the use of serotonin antagonists in the treatment of this disorder.

APPROACH TO THE PATIENT: Irritable Bowel Syndrome

Because IBS is a disorder for which no pathognomonic abnormalities have been identified, its diagnosis relies on recognition of positive clinical features and elimination of other organic diseases. Symptom-based criteria have been developed for the purpose of differentiating patients with IBS from those with organic diseases. These include the Manning, Rome I, Rome II, and Rome III criteria (Table 352-1). The diagnostic values of these criteria are shown in Table 352-3. In a validation study, Rome III performed less well than either the Rome I and II criteria and all criteria studied to date showed positive predictive values of <50%, which underscores the need for developing diagnostic strategies for IBS that are more cost-effective than the current approaches. A careful history and physical examination are frequently helpful in establishing the diagnosis. Clinical features suggestive of IBS include the following: recurrence of lower abdominal pain with altered bowel habits over a period of time without progressive deterioration, onset of symptoms during periods of stress or emotional upset, absence of other systemic symptoms such as fever and weight loss, and small-volume stool without any evidence of blood.

On the other hand, the appearance of the disorder for the first time in old age, progressive course from time of onset, persistent diarrhea after a 48-h fast, and presence of nocturnal diarrhea or steatorrheal stools argue against the diagnosis of IBS.

TABLE 352-3 SENSITIVITY, SPECIFICITY, POSITIVE AND NEGATIVE PREDICTIVE VALUES, AND POSITIVE AND NEGATIVE LIKELIHOOD RATIOS FOR THE ROME AND MANNING CRITERIA FOR IRRITABLE BOWEL SYNDROME[a]

	Sensitivity, % (95% CI)	Specificity, % (95% CI)	Positive Predictive Value, % (95% CI)	Negative Predictive Value, % (95% CI)	Positive Likelihood Ratio (95% CI)	Negative Likelihood Ratio (95% CI)
Rome III criteria	17.4 (13.9–21.5)	95.6 (94.4–96.5)	49.6 (42.0–58.7)	82.1 (80.0–83.6)	3.92 (2.85–5.38)	0.86 (0.83–0.91)
Rome II criteria	23.3 (19.4–27.8)	94.5 (93.2–95.5)	51.7 (44.9–59.5)	82.9 (80.8–84.4)	4.21 (3.20–5.53)	0.81 (0.77–0.86)
Rome I criteria	24.3 (20.3–28.8)	93.9 (92.6–95.0)	50.5 (44.0–58.1)	83.0 (80.9–84.4)	4.01 (3.08–5.22)	0.81 (0.76–0.85)
Manning criteria (3 criteria)	13.7 (10.6–17.6)	97.1 (96.1–97.8)	54.1 (45.3–64.6)	81.6 (79.6–83.1)	4.66 (3.18–6.82)	0.89 (0.85–0.93)

[a]Excluding individuals reporting lower gastrointestinal alarm symptoms from the definition of irritable bowel syndrome.

Source: Adapted from AC Ford et al: Gastroenterology 145:1262, 2013.

Because the major symptoms of IBS—abdominal pain, abdominal bloating, and alteration in bowel habits—are common complaints of many GI organic disorders, the list of differential diagnoses is a long one. The quality, location, and timing of pain may be helpful to suggest specific disorders. Pain due to IBS that occurs in the epigastric or periumbilical area must be differentiated from biliary tract disease, peptic ulcer disorders, intestinal ischemia, and carcinoma of the stomach and pancreas. If pain occurs mainly in the lower abdomen, the possibility of diverticular disease of the colon, inflammatory bowel disease (including ulcerative colitis and Crohn's disease), and carcinoma of the colon must be considered. Postprandial pain accompanied by bloating, nausea, and vomiting suggests gastroparesis or partial intestinal obstruction. Intestinal infestation with *Giardia lamblia* or other parasites may cause similar symptoms. When diarrhea is the major complaint, the possibility of lactase deficiency, laxative abuse, malabsorption, celiac sprue, hyperthyroidism, inflammatory bowel disease, and infectious diarrhea must be ruled out. On the other hand, constipation may be a side effect of many different drugs, such as anticholinergic, antihypertensive, and antidepressant medications. Endocrinopathies such as hypothyroidism and hypoparathyroidism must also be considered in the differential diagnosis of constipation, particularly if other systemic signs or symptoms of these endocrinopathies are present. In addition, acute intermittent porphyria and lead poisoning may present in a fashion similar to IBS, with painful constipation as the major complaint. These possibilities are suspected on the basis of their clinical presentations and are confirmed by appropriate serum and urine tests.

Few tests are required for patients who have typical IBS symptoms and no alarm features. Unnecessary investigations may be costly and even harmful. The American Gastroenterological Association has delineated factors to be considered when determining the aggressiveness of the diagnostic evaluation. These include the duration of symptoms, the change in symptoms over time, the age and sex of the patient, the referral status of the patient, prior diagnostic studies, a family history of colorectal malignancy, and the degree of psychosocial dysfunction. Thus, a younger individual with mild symptoms requires a minimal diagnostic evaluation, while an older person or an individual with rapidly progressive symptoms should undergo a more thorough exclusion of organic disease. Most patients should have a complete blood count and sigmoidoscopic examination; in addition, stool specimens should be examined for ova and parasites in those who have diarrhea. In patients with persistent diarrhea not responding to simple antidiarrheal agents, a sigmoid colon biopsy should be performed to rule out microscopic colitis. In those age >40 years, an air-contrast barium enema or colonoscopy should also be performed. If the main symptoms are diarrhea and increased gas, the possibility of lactase deficiency should be ruled out with a hydrogen breath test or with evaluation after a 3-week lactose-free diet. Some patients with IBS-D may have undiagnosed celiac sprue. Because the symptoms of celiac sprue respond to a gluten-free diet, testing for celiac sprue in IBS may prevent years of morbidity and attendant expense. Decision-analysis studies show that serology testing for celiac sprue in patients with IBS-D has an acceptable cost when the prevalence of celiac sprue is >1% and is the dominant strategy when the prevalence is >8%. In patients with concurrent symptoms of dyspepsia, upper GI radiographs or esophagogastroduodenoscopy may be advisable. In patients with postprandial right upper quadrant pain, an ultrasonogram of the gallbladder should be obtained. Laboratory features that argue against IBS include evidence of anemia, elevated sedimentation rate, presence of leukocytes or blood in stool, and stool volume >200–300 mL/d. These findings would necessitate other diagnostic considerations.

TREATMENT IRRITABLE BOWEL SYNDROME

PATIENT COUNSELING AND DIETARY ALTERATIONS

Reassurance and careful explanation of the functional nature of the disorder and of how to avoid obvious food precipitants are important first steps in patient counseling and dietary change. Occasionally, a meticulous dietary history may reveal substances (such as coffee, disaccharides, legumes, and cabbage) that aggravate symptoms. Excessive fructose and artificial sweeteners, such as sorbitol or mannitol, may cause diarrhea, bloating, cramping, or flatulence. As a therapeutic trial, patients should be encouraged to eliminate any foodstuffs that appear to produce symptoms. However patients should avoid nutritionally depleted diets. A diet low in fermentable oligosaccharides, disaccharides, monosaccharides, and polyols (FODMAPs) (Table 352-4) has been shown to be helpful in IBS patients. FODMAPs are poorly absorbed by the small intestine and fermented by bacteria in the colon to produce gas and osmotically active carbohydrates. Clinical studies demonstrate that in IBS patients, ingestion of FODMAPs such as lactose, fructose, or sorbitol, alone or in combination, produce gut symptoms such as gas and diarrhea. On the other hand, a randomized controlled study showed that a diet low in FODMAPs reduced symptoms in IBS patients. This

TABLE 352-4 SOME COMMON FOOD SOURCES OF FODMAPs

Food Type	Free Fructose	Lactose	Fructans	Galacto-oligosaccharides	Polyols
Fruits	Apple, cherry, mango, pear, watermelon		Peach, persimmon, watermelon		Apple, apricot, pear, avocado, blackberries, cherry, nectarine, plum, prune
Vegetables	Asparagus, artichokes, sugar snap peas		Artichokes, beetroot, Brussels sprout, chicory, fennel, garlic, leek, onion, peas		Cauliflower, mushroom, snow peas
Grains and cereals			Wheat, rye, barley		
Nuts and seeds			Pistachios		
Milk and milk products		Milk, yogurt, ice cream, custard, soft cheeses			
Legumes			Legumes, lentils, chickpeas	Legumes, chickpeas, lentils	
Other	Honey, high-fructose corn syrup		Chicory drinks		
Food additives			Inulin, FOS		Sorbitol, mannitol, maltitol, xylitol, isomalt

Abbreviations: FODMAPs, fermentable oligosaccharides, disaccharides, monosaccharides, and polyols; FOS, fructo-oligosaccharides

Source: Adapted from PR Gibson et al: Am J Gastroenterol 107:657, 2012.

approach may be used in diarrhea-predominant IBS patients with severe gas and bloating. Durable adherence can be expected in up to 75% of patients.

Stool-Bulking Agents High-fiber diets and bulking agents, such as bran or hydrophilic colloid, are frequently used in treating IBS. The water-holding action of fibers may contribute to increased stool bulk because of the ability of fiber to increase fecal output of bacteria. Fiber also speeds up colonic transit in most persons. In diarrhea-prone patients, whole-colonic transit is faster than average; however, dietary fiber can delay transit. Furthermore, because of their hydrophilic properties, stool-bulking agents bind water and thus prevent both excessive hydration and dehydration of stool. The latter observation may explain the clinical experience that a high-fiber diet relieves diarrhea in some IBS patients. Fiber supplementation with psyllium has been shown to reduce perception of rectal distention, indicating that fiber may have a positive effect on visceral afferent function.

The beneficial effects of dietary fiber on colonic physiology suggest that dietary fiber should be an effective treatment for IBS patients, but controlled trials of dietary fiber have produced variable results. This is not surprising since IBS is a heterogeneous disorder, with some patients being constipated and other having predominant diarrhea. Most investigations report increases in stool weight, decreases in colonic transit times, and improvement in constipation. Others have noted benefits in patients with alternating diarrhea and constipation, pain, and bloating. However, most studies observe no responses in patients with diarrhea- or pain-predominant IBS. It is possible that different fiber preparations may have dissimilar effects on selected symptoms in IBS. A cross-over comparison of different fiber preparations found that psyllium produced greater improvements in stool pattern and abdominal pain than bran. Furthermore, psyllium preparations tend to produce less bloating and distention. Despite the equivocal data regarding efficacy, most gastroenterologists consider stool-bulking agents worth trying in patients with IBS-C. Fiber should be started at a nominal dose and slowly titrated up as tolerated over the course of several weeks to a targeted dose of 20–30 g of total dietary and supplementary fiber per day. Even when used judiciously, fiber can exacerbate bloating, flatulence, constipation, and diarrhea.

Antispasmodics Clinicians have observed that anticholinergic drugs may provide temporary relief for symptoms such as painful cramps related to intestinal spasm. Although controlled clinical trials have produced mixed results, evidence generally supports beneficial effects of anticholinergic drugs for pain. A meta-analysis of 26 double-blind clinical trials of antispasmodic agents in IBS reported better global improvement (62%) and abdominal pain reductions (64%) compared to placebo (35% and 45%, respectively), suggesting efficacy in some patients. The drugs are most effective when prescribed in anticipation of predictable pain. Physiologic studies demonstrate that anticholinergic drugs inhibit the gastrocolic reflex; hence, postprandial pain is best managed by giving antispasmodics 30 min before meals so that effective blood levels are achieved shortly before the anticipated onset of pain. Most anticholinergics contain natural belladonna alkaloids, which may cause xerostomia, urinary hesitancy and retention, blurred vision, and drowsiness. They should be used in the elderly with caution. Some physicians prefer to use synthetic anticholinergics such as dicyclomine that have less effect on mucous membrane secretions and produce fewer undesirable side effects.

Antidiarrheal Agents Peripherally acting opiate-based agents are the initial therapy of choice for IBS-D. Physiologic studies demonstrate increases in segmenting colonic contractions, delays in fecal transit, increases in anal pressures, and reductions in rectal perception with these drugs. When diarrhea is severe, especially in the painless diarrhea variant of IBS, small doses of loperamide, 2–4 mg every 4–6 h up to a maximum of 12 g/d, can be prescribed. These agents are less addictive than paregoric, codeine, or tincture of opium. In general, the intestines do not become tolerant of the antidiarrheal effect of opiates, and increasing doses are not required to maintain antidiarrheal potency. These agents are most useful if taken before anticipated stressful events that are known to cause diarrhea. However, not infrequently, a high dose of loperamide may cause cramping because of increases in segmenting colonic contractions. Another antidiarrheal agent that may be used in IBS patients is the bile acid binder cholestyramine resin.

Antidepressant Drugs In addition to their mood-elevating effects, antidepressant medications have several physiologic effects that suggest they may be beneficial in IBS. In IBS-D patients, the tricyclic antidepressant imipramine slows jejunal migrating motor complex transit propagation and delays orocecal and whole-gut transit, indicative of a motor inhibitory effect. Some studies also suggest that tricyclic agents may alter visceral afferent neural function.

A number of studies indicate that tricyclic antidepressants may be effective in some IBS patients. In a 2-month study of desipramine, abdominal pain improved in 86% of patients compared to 59% given placebo. Another study of desipramine in 28 IBS patients showed improvement in stool frequency, diarrhea, pain, and depression. When stratified according to the predominant symptoms, improvements were observed in IBS-D patients, with no improvement being noted in IBS-C patients. The beneficial effects of the tricyclic compounds in the treatment of IBS appear to be independent of their effects on depression. The therapeutic benefits for the bowel symptoms occur faster and at a lower dosage. The efficacy of antidepressant agents in other chemical classes in the management of IBS is less well evaluated. In contrast to tricyclic agents, the selective serotonin reuptake inhibitor (SSRI) paroxetine accelerates orocecal transit, raising the possibility that this drug class may be useful in IBS-C patients. The SSRI citalopram blunts perception of rectal distention and reduces the magnitude of the gastrocolonic response in healthy volunteers. A small placebo-controlled study of citalopram in IBS patients reported reductions in pain. However, these findings could not be confirmed in another randomized controlled trial that showed that citalopram at 20 mg/d for 4 weeks was not superior to placebo in treating nondepressed IBS patients. Hence, the efficacy of SSRIs in the treatment of IBS needs further confirmation.

Antiflatulence Therapy The management of excessive gas is seldom satisfactory, except when there is obvious aerophagia or disaccharidase deficiency. Patients should be advised to eat slowly and not chew gum or drink carbonated beverages. Bloating may decrease if an associated gut syndrome such as IBS or constipation is improved. If bloating is accompanied by diarrhea and worsens after ingesting dairy products, fresh fruits, vegetables, or juices, further investigation or a dietary exclusion trial may be worthwhile. Avoiding flatogenic foods, exercising, losing excess weight, and taking activated charcoal are safe but unproven remedies. Data regarding the use of surfactants such as simethicone are conflicting. Antibiotics may help in a subgroup of IBS patients with predominant symptoms of bloating. Beano, an over-the-counter oral β-glycosidase solution, may reduce rectal passage of gas without decreasing bloating and pain. Pancreatic enzymes reduce bloating, gas, and fullness during and after high-calorie, high-fat meal ingestion.

Modulation of Gut Flora Antibiotic treatment benefits a subset of IBS patients. In a double-blind, randomized, placebo-controlled study, neomycin dosed at 500 mg twice daily for 10 days was more effective than placebo at improving symptom scores among IBS patients. The nonabsorbed oral antibiotic rifaximin is the most thoroughly studied antibiotic for the treatment of IBS. In a double-blind, placebo-controlled study, patients receiving rifaximin at a dose of 550 mg two times daily for 2 weeks experienced substantial improvement of global IBS symptoms over placebo. Rifaximin is the only antibiotic with demonstrated sustained benefit beyond therapy cessation in IBS patients. The drug has a favorable safety and tolerability profile compared with systemic antibiotics. A systematic review and meta-analysis of five studies of IBS patients found that rifaximin is more effective than placebo for global symptoms and bloating (odds ratio 1.57) with a number needed to treat (NNT) of

10.2. The modest therapeutic gain was similar to that yielded by other current available therapies for IBS. However, currently there are still insufficient data to recommend routine use of this antibiotic in the treatment of IBS.

Because altered colonic flora may contribute to the pathogenesis of IBS, this has led to great interest in using probiotics to naturally alter the flora. A meta-analysis of 10 probiotic studies in IBS patients found significant relief of pain and bloating with the use of *Bifidobacterium breve, B. longum*, and *Lactobacillus acidophilus* species compared to placebo. However, there was no change in stool frequency or consistency. Large-scale studies of well-phenotyped IBS patients are needed to establish the efficacy of these probiotics.

Serotonin Receptor Agonist and Antagonists Serotonin receptor antagonists have been evaluated as therapies for IBS-D. Serotonin acting on 5-HT_3 receptors enhances the sensitivity of afferent neurons projecting from the gut. In humans, a 5-HT_3 receptor antagonist such as alosetron reduces perception of painful visceral stimulation in IBS. It also induces rectal relaxation, increases rectal compliance, and delays colonic transit. Meta-analysis of 14 randomized controlled trials of alosetron or cilansetron showed that these antagonists are more effective than placebo in achieving global improvement in IBS symptoms and relief of abdominal pain and discomfort. These agents are more likely to cause constipation in IBS patients with diarrhea alternating with constipation. Also, 0.2% of patients using 5-HT_3 antagonists developed ischemic colitis versus none in the control group. In postrelease surveillance, 84 cases of ischemic colitis were observed, including 44 cases that required surgery and 4 deaths. As a consequence, the medication was voluntarily withdrawn by the manufacturer in 2000. Alosetron has been reintroduced under a new risk-management program where patients have to sign a patient-physician agreement. This has significantly limited its usage.

Novel 5-HT_4 receptor agonists such as tegaserod exhibit prokinetic activity by stimulating peristalsis. In IBS patients with constipation, tegaserod accelerated intestinal and ascending colon transit. Clinical trials involving >4000 IBS-C patients reported reductions in discomfort and improvements in constipation and bloating, compared to placebo. Diarrhea is the major side effect. However, tegaserod has been withdrawn from the market; a meta-analysis revealed an increase in serious cardiovascular events.

Chloride Channel Activators Lubiprostone is a bicyclic fatty acid that stimulates chloride channels in the apical membrane of intestinal epithelial cells. Chloride secretion induces passive movement of sodium and water into the bowel lumen and improves bowel function. Oral lubiprostone was effective in the treatment of patients with constipation-predominant IBS in large phase II and phase III randomized, double-blinded, placebo-controlled multicenter trials. Responses were significantly greater in patients receiving lubiprostone 8 μg twice daily for 3 months than in those receiving placebo. In general, the drug was quite well tolerated. The major side effects are nausea and diarrhea. Lubiprostone is a new class of compounds for treatment of chronic constipation with or without IBS.

Guanylate Cyclase-C Agonist Linaclotide is a minimally absorbed 14-amino-acid peptide guanylate cyclase-C (GC-C) agonist that binds to and activates GC-C on the luminal surface of intestinal epithelium. Activation of GC-C results in generation of cyclic guanosine monophosphate (cGMP), which triggers secretion of fluid, sodium, and bicarbonate. In animal models, linaclotide accelerates GI transit and reduces visceral nociception. The analgesic action of linaclotide appears to be mediated by cGMP acting on afferent pain fibers innervating the GI tract. A phase III, double-blind, controlled trial showed that linaclotide, 290 μg given once daily, significantly improved abdominal pain, bloating, and spontaneous bowel movement. The only significant side effect was diarrhea, which occurred in 4.5% of the patients. The drug has been approved for treatment of constipation in IBS-C patients.

TABLE 352-5 SPECTRUM OF SEVERITY IN IBS

	Mild	Moderate	Severe
Clinical Features			
Prevalence	70%	25%	5%
Correlations with gut physiology	+++	++	+
Symptoms constant	0	+	+++
Psychosocial difficulties	0	+	+++
Health care issues	+	++	+++
Practice type	Primary	Specialty	Referral

SUMMARY

The treatment strategy of IBS depends on the severity of the disorder (Table 352-5). Most IBS patients have mild symptoms. They are usually cared for in primary care practices, have little or no psychosocial difficulties, and do not seek health care often. Treatment usually involves education, reassurance, and dietary/lifestyle changes. A smaller portion have moderate symptoms that are usually intermittent and correlate with altered gut physiology, e.g., worsened with eating or stress and relieved by defecation. For IBS-D patients, treatments include gut-acting pharmacologic agents such as antispasmodics, antidiarrheals, bile acid binders, and the newer gut serotonin modulators (Table 352-6). In IBS-C patients, increased fiber intake and the use of osmotic agents such as polyethylene glycol may achieve satisfactory results. For patients with more severe constipation, a chloride channel opener (lubiprostone) or GC-C agonist (linaclotide) may be considered. For IBS patients with predominant gas and bloating, a low-FODMAP diet may provide significant relief. Some patients may benefit from probiotics and rifaximin treatment. A small proportion of IBS patients have severe and refractory symptoms, are usually seen in referral centers, and frequently have constant pain and psychosocial difficulties (Fig. 352-1). This group of patients is best managed with antidepressants and other psychological treatments (Table 352-6).

TABLE 352-6 POSSIBLE DRUGS FOR A DOMINANT SYMPTOM IN IBS

Symptom	Drug	Dose
Diarrhea	Loperamide	2–4 mg when necessary/ maximum 12 g/d
	Cholestyramine resin	4 g with meals
	Alosetron[a]	0.5–1 mg bid (for severe IBS, women)
Constipation	Psyllium husk	3–4 g bid with meals, then adjust
	Methylcellulose	2 g bid with meals, then adjust
	Calcium polycarbophil	1 g qd to qid
	Lactulose syrup	10–20 g bid
	70% sorbitol	15 mL bid
	Polyethylene glycol 3350	17 g in 250 mL water qd
	Lubiprostone (Amitiza)	24 mg bid
	Magnesium hydroxide	30–60 mL qd
	Linaclotide	290 μg qd
Abdominal pain	Smooth-muscle relaxant	qd to qid ac
	Tricyclic antidepressants	Start 25–50 mg hs, then adjust
	Selective serotonin reuptake inhibitors	Begin small dose, increase as needed
Gas and bloating	Low FODMAP diet	
	Probiotics	qd
	Rifaximin	550 mg bid

[a]Available only in the United States.

Abbreviation: FODMAP, fermentable oligosaccharides, disaccharides, monosaccharides, and polyols.

Source: Adapted from GF Longstreth et al: Gastroenterology 130:1480, 2006.

353 Diverticular Disease and Common Anorectal Disorders

Rizwan Ahmed, Susan L. Gearhart

DIVERTICULAR DISEASE

Incidence and Epidemiology In the United States, diverticulosis affects 70% of the population above the age of 80. Fortunately, only 20% of patients with diverticulosis develop symptomatic disease, 1–2% require hospitalization, and <1% will require surgery. Diverticular disease has become the fifth most costly gastrointestinal disorder in the United States. Previously overlooked, the majority of patients with diverticular disease report a lower health-related quality of life and more depression as compared to matched controls, thus adding to health care costs. Formerly, diverticular disease was confined to developed countries; however, with the adoption of westernized diets in underdeveloped countries, diverticulosis is on the rise across the globe. Immigrants to the United States develop diverticular disease at the same rate as U.S. natives. Although the prevalence among females and males is similar, males tend to present at a younger age. The mean age at presentation of the disease is 59 years and is now shifting to affect younger populations.

Anatomy and Pathophysiology Two types of diverticula occur in the intestine: true and false (or pseudo diverticula). A true diverticulum is a saclike herniation of the entire bowel wall, whereas a pseudo diverticulum involves only a protrusion of the mucosa and submucosa through the muscularis propria of the colon (Fig. 353-1). The type of diverticulum affecting the colon is the pseudodiverticulum. Diverticula commonly affect the left and sigmoid colon; the rectum is always spared. However, in Asian populations, 70% of diverticula are seen in the right colon and cecum as well. *Diverticulitis* is inflammation of a diverticulum. Previous understanding of the pathogenesis of diverticulosis attributed a low-fiber diet as the sole culprit, and onset of diverticulitis would occur acutely when these diverticula become obstructed. However, evidence now suggests that the pathogenesis is more complex and multifactorial. The diverticula occur at the point where the nutrient artery, or *vasa recti*, penetrates through the muscularis propria, resulting in a break in the integrity of the colonic wall. This anatomic restriction may be a result of the relative high-pressure zone within the muscular sigmoid colon. Thus, higher-amplitude contractions combined with constipated, high-fat-content stool within the sigmoid lumen in an area of weakness in the colonic wall results in the creation of these diverticula. Consequently, the vasa recti is either compressed or eroded, leading to either perforation or bleeding. Chronic low-grade inflammation is thought to play a key role. Furthermore, better understanding of the gut microbiota suggests that dysbiosis is an important aspect of disease.

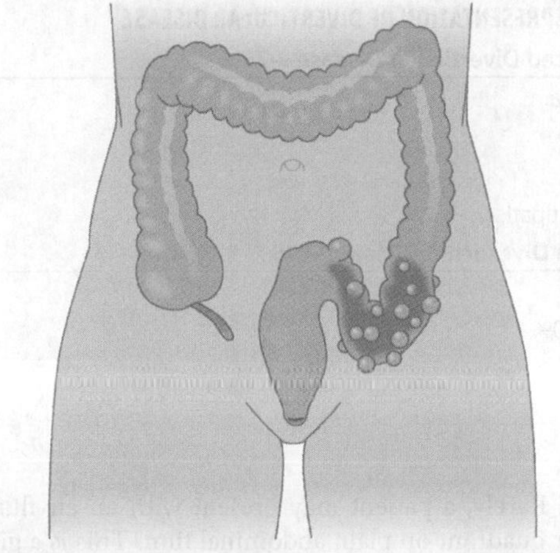

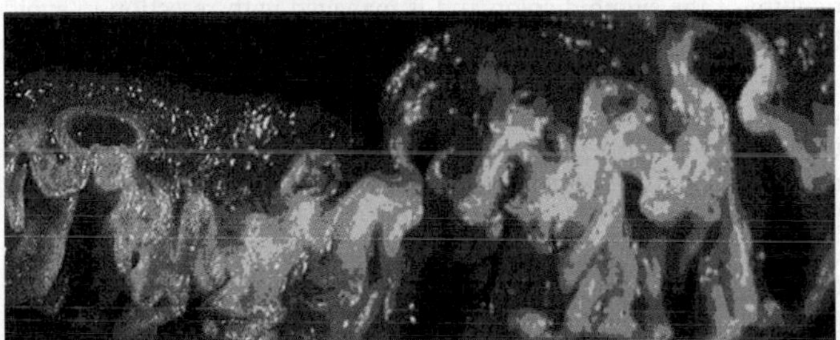

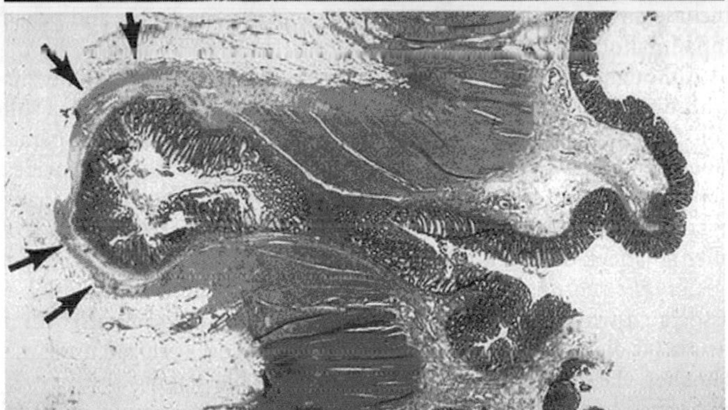

FIGURE 353-1 Gross and microscopic view of sigmoid diverticular disease. *Arrows* mark an inflamed diverticulum with the diverticular wall made up only of mucosa.

Presentation, Evaluation, and Management of Diverticular Bleeding Hemorrhage from a colonic diverticulum is the most common cause of hematochezia in patients >60 years, yet only 20% of patients with diverticulosis will have gastrointestinal bleeding. Patients at increased risk for bleeding tend to be hypertensive, have atherosclerosis, and regularly use aspirin and nonsteroidal anti-inflammatory agents. Most bleeds are self-limited and stop spontaneously with bowel rest. The lifetime risk of rebleeding is 25%.

Initial localization of diverticular bleeding may include colonoscopy, multiplanar computed tomography (CT) angiogram, or nuclear medicine tagged red cell scan. If the patient is stable, ongoing bleeding is best managed by angiography. If mesenteric angiography can localize the bleeding site, the vessel can be occluded successfully with a coil in 80% of cases. The patient can then be followed closely with repetitive colonoscopy, if necessary, looking for evidence of colonic ischemia. Alternatively, a segmental resection of the colon can be undertaken to eliminate the risk of further bleeding. This may be advantageous in patients on chronic anticoagulation. However, with highly selective coil embolization, the rate of colonic ischemia is <10% and the risk of acute rebleeding is <25%. Long-term results (40 months) indicate that more than 50% of patients with acute diverticular bleeds treated with highly selective angiography have had definitive treatment. As another alternative, a selective infusion of vasopressin can be given to stop the hemorrhage, although this has been associated with significant complications, including myocardial infarction and intestinal ischemia. Furthermore, bleeding recurs in 50% of patients once the infusion is stopped.

If the patient is unstable or has had a 6-unit bleed within 24 h, current recommendations are that surgery should be performed. If the bleeding has been localized, a segmental resection can be performed. If the site of bleeding has not been definitively identified, a subtotal colectomy may be required. In patients without severe comorbidities, surgical resection can be performed with a primary anastomosis. A higher anastomotic leak rate has been reported in patients who received >10 units of blood.

Presentation, Evaluation, and Staging of Diverticulitis Acute uncomplicated diverticulitis characteristically presents with fever, anorexia, left lower quadrant abdominal pain, and obstipation (Table 353-1). In <25% of cases, patients may present with generalized peritonitis indicating the presence of a diverticular perforation. If a pericolonic abscess has formed, the patient may have abdominal distention and signs of localized peritonitis. Laboratory investigations will demonstrate a

TABLE 353-1 PRESENTATION OF DIVERTICULAR DISEASE

Uncomplicated Diverticular Disease—75%
Abdominal pain
Fever
Leukocytosis
Anorexia/obstipation
Complicated Diverticular Disease—25%
Abscess 16%
Perforation 10%
Stricture 5%
Fistula 2%

leukocytosis. Rarely, a patient may present with an air-fluid level in the left lower quadrant on plain abdominal film. This is a giant diverticulum of the sigmoid colon and is managed with resection to avoid impending perforation.

The diagnosis of diverticulitis is best made on CT with the following findings: sigmoid diverticula, thickened colonic wall >4 mm, and inflammation within the periodic fat ± the collection of contrast material or fluid. In 16% of patients, an abdominal abscess may be present. Symptoms of irritable bowel syndrome (Chap. 352) may mimic those of diverticulitis. Therefore, suspected diverticulitis that does not meet CT criteria or is not associated with a leukocytosis or fever is not diverticular disease. Other conditions that can mimic diverticular disease include an ovarian cyst, endometriosis, acute appendicitis, and pelvic inflammatory disease.

Although the benefit of colonoscopy in the evaluation of patients with diverticular disease has been called into question, its use is still considered important in the exclusion of colorectal cancer. The parallel epidemiology of colorectal cancer and diverticular disease provides enough concern for an endoscopic evaluation before operative management. Therefore, a colonoscopy should be performed ~6 weeks after an attack of diverticular disease.

Complicated diverticular disease is defined as diverticular disease associated with an abscess or perforation and less commonly with a fistula (Table 353-1). Perforated diverticular disease is staged using the Hinchey classification system (Fig. 353-2). This staging system was developed to predict outcomes following the surgical management of complicated diverticular disease. In complicated diverticular disease with fistula formation, common locations include cutaneous, vaginal, or vesicle fistulas. These conditions present with either passage of stool through the skin or vagina or the presence of air in the urinary stream (pneumaturia). Colovaginal fistulas are more common in women who have undergone a hysterectomy.

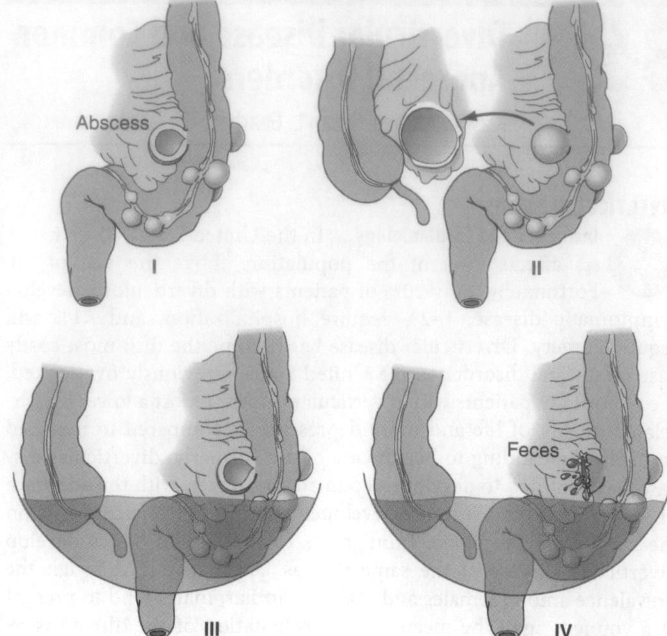

FIGURE 353-2 Hinchey classification of diverticulitis. Stage I: Perforated diverticulitis with a confined paracolic abscess. Stage II: Perforated diverticulitis that has closed spontaneously with distant abscess formation. Stage III: Noncommunicating perforated diverticulitis with fecal peritonitis (the diverticular neck is closed off, and therefore, contrast will not freely expel on radiographic images). Stage IV: Perforation and free communication with the peritoneum, resulting in fecal peritonitis.

TREATMENT DIVERTICULAR DISEASE

MEDICAL MANAGEMENT

Asymptomatic diverticular disease discovered on imaging studies or at the time of colonoscopy is best managed by diet alterations. Patients should be instructed to eat a fiber-enriched diet that includes 30 g of fiber each day. Supplementary fiber products such as Metamucil, Fibercon, or Citrucel are useful. The incidence of complicated diverticular disease appears to be increased in patients who smoke. Therefore, patients should be encouraged to refrain from smoking. The historical recommendation to avoid eating nuts is not based on more than anecdotal data.

Symptomatic uncomplicated diverticular disease with confirmation of inflammation and infection within the colon should be treated initially with antibiotics and bowel rest. Nearly 75% of patients hospitalized for acute diverticulitis will respond to nonoperative treatment with a suitable antimicrobial regimen. The current recommended antimicrobial coverage is trimethoprim/sulfamethoxazole or ciprofloxacin and metronidazole targeting aerobic gram-negative rods and anaerobic bacteria. Unfortunately, these agents do not cover enterococci, and the addition of ampicillin to this regimen for nonresponders is recommended. Alternatively, single-agent therapy with a third-generation penicillin such as IV piperacillin or oral penicillin/clavulanic acid may be effective. The usual course of antibiotics is 7–10 days, although this length of time is being investigated. Patients should remain on a limited diet until their pain resolves.

Once the acute attack has resolved, the mainstay medical management of diverticular disease to prevent symptoms has evolved. Newer directions are targeted at colonic inflammation and dysbiosis. Diverticular disease is now considered a functional bowel disorder associated with low-grade inflammation. Therefore, the use of anti-inflammatory medications such as mesalazine has become popular. Patients treated with mesalazine have a decreased recurrence of symptomatic disease. Randomized trials of anti-inflammatory medications are ongoing.

Treatment strategies targeting dysbiosis in diverticular disease are also beneficial. Use of the polymerase chain reaction (PCR) on stool specimens from consumers of a high-fiber diet has shown different bacterial content than stool of consumers of a low-fiber, high-fat diet. Probiotics are being increasingly used by gastroenterologists for multiple bowel disorders and have been shown to prevent recurrence of diverticulitis. Specifically probiotics containing *Lactobacillus acidophilus* and *Bifidobacterium* strains have been shown to be beneficial. Furthermore, rifaximin (a poorly absorbed broad-spectrum antibiotic), when compared to fiber alone, is associated with 30% less frequent recurrent symptoms from uncomplicated diverticular disease.

SURGICAL MANAGEMENT

Preoperative risk factors influencing postoperative mortality rates include higher American Society of Anesthesiologists (ASA) physical status class (Table 353-2) and preexisting organ failure. In patients who are low risk (ASA P1 and P2), surgical therapy can be offered to those who do not rapidly improve on medical therapy. For uncomplicated diverticular disease, medical therapy can be continued beyond two attacks without an increased risk of perforation requiring a

TABLE 353-2	AMERICAN SOCIETY OF ANESTHESIOLOGISTS PHYSICAL STATUS CLASSIFICATION SYSTEM
P1	A normal healthy patient
P2	A patient with mild systemic disease
P3	A patient with severe systemic disease
P4	A patient with severe systemic disease that is a constant threat to life
P5	A moribund patient who is not expected to survive without the operation
P6	A declared brain-dead patient whose organs are being removed for donor purposes

colostomy. However, patients on immunosuppressive therapy, in chronic renal failure, or with a collagen-vascular disease have a fivefold greater risk of perforation during recurrent attacks. Surgical therapy is indicated in all low-surgical-risk patients with complicated diverticular disease.

The goals of surgical management of diverticular disease include controlling sepsis, eliminating complications such as fistula or obstruction, removing the diseased colonic segment, and restoring intestinal continuity. These goals must be obtained while minimizing morbidity rate, length of hospitalization, and cost in addition to maximizing survival and quality of life. Table 353-3 lists the operations most commonly indicated based on the Hinchey classification and the predicted morbidity and mortality rates. Surgical objectives include removal of the diseased sigmoid down to the rectosigmoid junction. Failure to do this may result in recurrent disease. The current options for uncomplicated diverticular disease include an open sigmoid resection or a laparoscopic sigmoid resection. The benefits of laparoscopic resection over open surgical techniques include early discharge (by at least 1 day), less narcotic use, less postoperative complications, and an earlier return to work.

The options for the surgical management of complicated diverticular disease (Fig. 353-3) include the following: (1) proximal diversion of the fecal stream with an ileostomy or colostomy and sutured omental patch with drainage, (2) resection with colostomy and mucous fistula or closure of distal bowel with formation of a Hartmann's pouch, (3) resection with anastomosis (coloproctostomy), or (4) resection with anastomosis and diversion (coloproctostomy with loop ileostomy or colostomy). Laparoscopic techniques have been used for complicated diverticular disease; however, higher conversion rates to open techniques have been reported.

Patients with Hinchey stages I and II disease are managed with percutaneous drainage followed by resection with anastomosis about 6 weeks later. Current guidelines put forth by the American Society of Colon and Rectal Surgeons suggest, in addition to antibiotic therapy, CT-guided percutaneous drainage of diverticular abscesses that are greater than 3 cm and have a well-defined wall. Abscesses that are less than 3 cm may resolve with antibiotic therapy alone. Contraindications to percutaneous drainage are no percutaneous access route, pneumoperitoneum, and fecal peritonitis.

TABLE 353-3 OUTCOME FOLLOWING SURGICAL THERAPY FOR COMPLICATED DIVERTICULAR DISEASE

Hinchey Stage	Operative Procedure	Anastomotic Leak Rate, %	Overall Morbidity Rate, %
I	Resection with primary anastomosis without diverting stoma	3.8	22
II	Resection with primary anastomosis +/– diversion	3.8	30
III	Hartmann's procedure vs diverting colostomy and omental pedal graft	—	0 vs. 6 mortality
IV	Hartmann's procedure vs diverting colostomy and omental pedicle graft	—	6 vs. 2 mortality

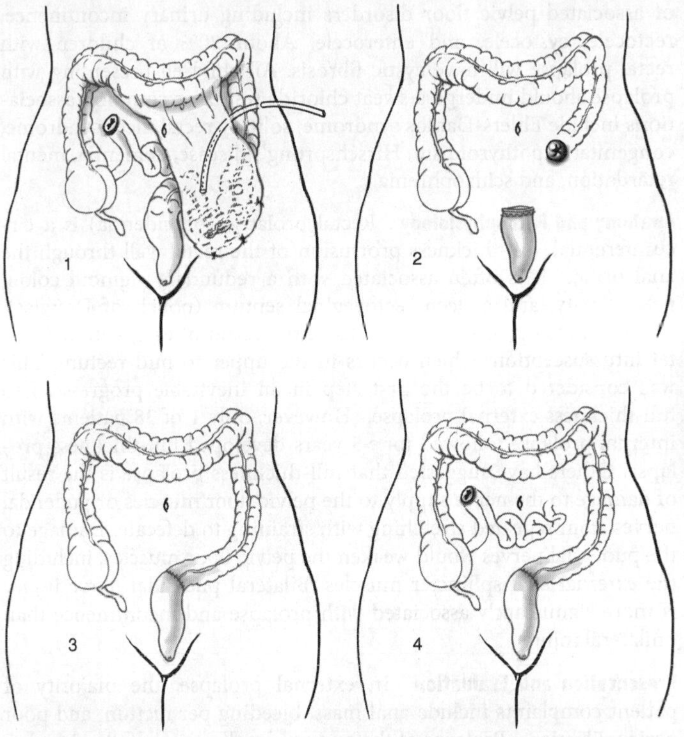

FIGURE 353-3 Methods of surgical management of complicated diverticular disease. *(1)* Drainage, omental pedicle graft, and proximal diversion. *(2)* Hartmann's procedure. *(3)* Sigmoid resection with coloproctostomy. *(4)* Sigmoid resection with coloproctostomy and proximal diversion.

Urgent operative intervention is undertaken if patients develop generalized peritonitis, and most will need to be managed with a Hartmann's procedure (resection of the sigmoid colon with end colostomy and rectal stump). In selected cases, nonoperative therapy may be considered. In one nonrandomized study, nonoperative management of isolated paracolic abscesses (Hinchey stage I) was associated with only a 20% recurrence rate at 2 years. More than 80% of patients with distant abscesses (Hinchey stage II) required surgical resection for recurrent symptoms.

Hinchey stage III disease is managed with a Hartmann's procedure or with primary anastomosis and proximal diversion. If the patient has significant comorbidities, making operative intervention risky, a limited procedure including intraoperative peritoneal lavage (irrigation), omental patch to the oversewn perforation, and proximal diversion of the fecal stream with either an ileostomy or transverse colostomy can be performed. No anastomosis of any type should be attempted in Hinchey stage IV disease. A limited approach to these patients is associated with a decreased mortality rate.

Recurrent Symptoms Recurrent abdominal symptoms following surgical resection for diverticular disease occur in 10% of patients. Recurrent diverticular disease develops in patients following inadequate surgical resection. A retained segment of diseased rectosigmoid colon is associated with twice the incidence of recurrence. The presence of irritable bowel syndrome may also cause recurrence of initial symptoms. Patients undergoing surgical resection for presumed diverticulitis and symptoms of chronic abdominal cramping and irregular loose bowel movements consistent with irritable bowel syndrome have poorer functional outcomes.

COMMON DISEASES OF THE ANORECTUM

RECTAL PROLAPSE (PROCIDENTIA)

Incidence and Epidemiology Rectal prolapse is six times more common in women than in men. The incidence of rectal prolapse peaks in women >60 years. Women with rectal prolapse have a higher incidence of associated pelvic floor disorders including urinary incontinence, rectocele, cystocele, and enterocele. About 20% of children with rectal prolapse will have cystic fibrosis. All children presenting with prolapse should undergo a sweat chloride test. Less common associations include Ehlers-Danlos syndrome, solitary rectal ulcer syndrome, congenital hypothyroidism, Hirschsprung's disease, dementia, mental retardation, and schizophrenia.

Anatomy and Pathophysiology Rectal prolapse (procidentia) is a circumferential, full-thickness protrusion of the rectal wall through the anal orifice. It is often associated with a redundant sigmoid colon, pelvic laxity, and a deep rectovaginal septum (pouch of Douglas). Initially, rectal prolapse was felt to be the result of early internal rectal intussusception, which occurs in the upper to mid rectum. This was considered to be the first step in an inevitable progression to full-thickness external prolapse. However, only 1 of 38 patients with internal prolapse followed for >5 years developed full-thickness prolapse. Others have suggested that full-thickness prolapse is the result of damage to the nerve supply to the pelvic floor muscles or pudendal nerves from repeated stretching with straining to defecate. Damage to the pudendal nerves would weaken the pelvic floor muscles, including the external anal sphincter muscles. Bilateral pudendal nerve injury is more significantly associated with prolapse and incontinence than unilateral injury.

Presentation and Evaluation In external prolapse, the majority of patient complaints include anal mass, bleeding per rectum, and poor perianal hygiene. Prolapse of the rectum usually occurs following defecation and will spontaneously reduce or require the patient to manually reduce the prolapse. Constipation occurs in ~30–67% of patients with rectal prolapse. Differing degrees of fecal incontinence occur in 50–70% of patients. Patients with internal rectal prolapse will present with symptoms of both constipation and incontinence. Other associated findings include outlet obstruction (anismus) in 30%, colonic inertia in 10%, and solitary rectal ulcer syndrome in 12%.

Office evaluation is best performed after the patient has been given an enema, which enables the prolapse to protrude. An important distinction should be made between full-thickness rectal prolapse and isolated mucosal prolapse associated with hemorrhoidal disease (Fig. 353-4). Mucosal prolapse is known for radial grooves rather than circumferential folds around the anus and is due to increased laxity of the connective tissue between the submucosa and underlying muscle of the anal canal. The evaluation of prolapse should also include cystoproctography and colonoscopy. These examinations evaluate for associated pelvic floor disorders and rule out a malignancy or a polyp as the lead point for prolapse. If rectal prolapse is associated with chronic constipation, the patient should undergo a defecating proctogram and a sitzmark study. This will evaluate for the presence of anismus or colonic inertia. Anismus is the result of attempting to defecate against a closed pelvic floor and is also known as *nonrelaxing puborectalis*. This can be seen when straightening of the rectum fails to occur on fluoroscopy while the patient is attempting to defecate. In colonic inertia, a sitzmark study will demonstrate retention of >20% of markers on abdominal x-ray 5 days after swallowing. For patients with fecal incontinence, endoanal ultrasound and manometric evaluation, including pudendal nerve testing of their anal sphincter muscles, may be performed before surgery for prolapse (see "Fecal Incontinence," below).

TREATMENT RECTAL PROLAPSE

The medical approach to the management of rectal prolapse is limited and includes stool-bulking agents or fiber supplementation to ease the process of evacuation. Surgical correction of rectal prolapse is the mainstay of therapy. Two approaches are commonly considered, transabdominal and transperineal. Transabdominal approaches have been associated with lower recurrence rates, but some patients with significant comorbidities are better served by a transperineal approach.

Common transperineal approaches include a transanal proctectomy (Altmeier procedure), mucosal proctectomy (Delorme procedure), or placement of a Tirsch wire encircling the anus. The goal of the transperineal approach is to remove the redundant rectosigmoid colon. Common transabdominal approaches include presacral suture or mesh rectopexy (Ripstein) with (Frykman-Goldberg) or without resection of the redundant sigmoid. Colon resection, in general, is reserved for patients with constipation and outlet obstruction. Ventral rectopexy is an effective method of abdominal repair of full-thickness prolapse that does not require sigmoid resection (see description below). This repair may have improved functional results over other abdominal repairs. Transabdominal procedures can be performed effectively with laparoscopic and, more recently, robotic techniques without increased incidence of recurrence. The goal of the transabdominal approach is to restore normal anatomy by removing redundant bowel and reattaching the supportive tissue of the rectum to the presacral fascia. The final alternative is abdominal proctectomy with end-sigmoid colostomy. If total colonic inertia is present, as defined by a history of constipation and a positive sitzmark study, a subtotal colectomy with an ileosigmoid or rectal anastomosis may be required at the time of rectopexy.

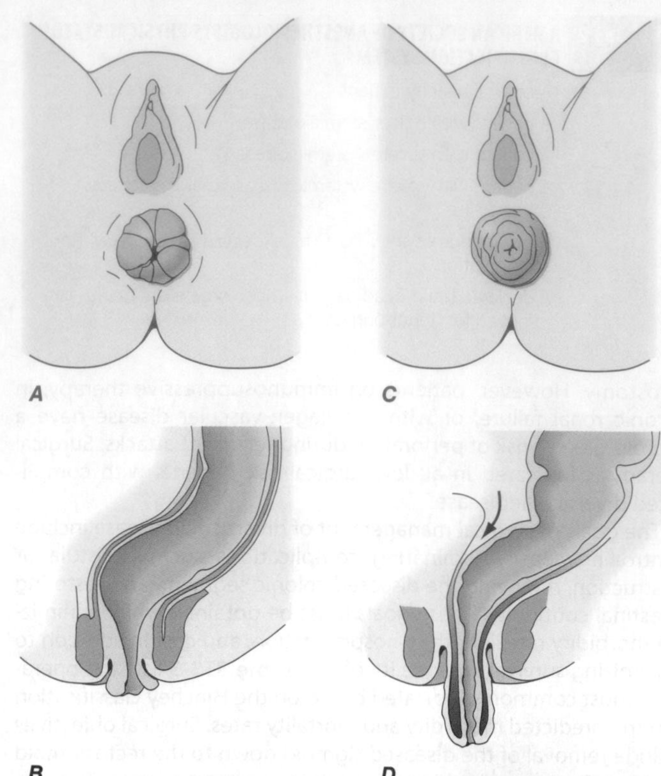

FIGURE 353-4 Degrees of rectal prolapse. Mucosal prolapse only (***A, B,*** sagittal view). Full-thickness prolapse associated with redundant rectosigmoid and deep pouch of Douglas (***C, D,*** sagittal view).

Previously, the presence of internal rectal prolapse identified on imaging studies has been considered a nonsurgical disorder and biofeedback was recommended. However, only one-third of patients will have successful resolution of symptoms from biofeedback. Two surgical procedures more effective than biofeedback are the Stapled Transanal Rectal Resection (STARR) and the Laparoscopic Ventral Rectopexy (LVR). The STARR procedure (Fig. 353-5) is performed through the anus in patients with internal prolapse. A circular stapling device is inserted through the anus; the internal prolapse is identified and ligated with the stapling device. LVR (Fig. 353-6) is performed through an abdominal approach. An opening in the peritoneum is created on the left side of the rectosigmoid junction, and this opening continues down anterior on the rectum into the pouch of Douglas. No rectal mobilization is performed, thus avoiding any autonomic nerve injury. Mesh is secured to the anterior and lateral portion of the rectum, the vaginal fornix,

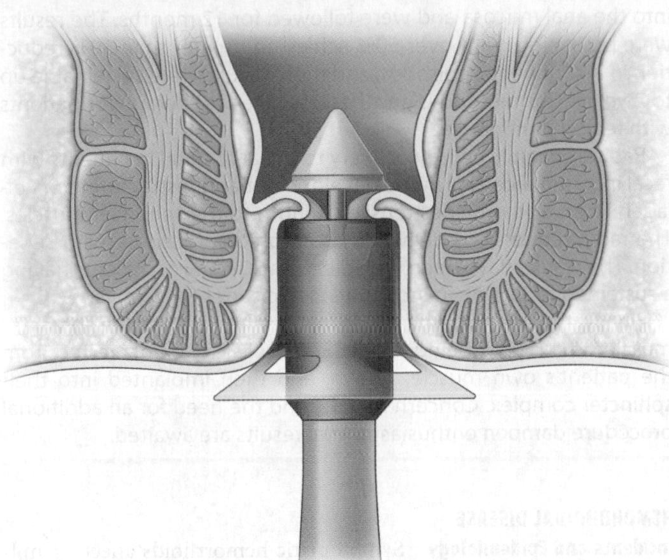

FIGURE 353-5 Stapled transanal rectal resection. Schematic of placement of the circular stapling device.

and the sacral promontory, allowing for closure of the rectovaginal septum and correction of the internal prolapse. In both procedures, recurrence at 1 year was low (<10%) and symptoms improved in more than three-fourths of patients.

FECAL INCONTINENCE

Incidence and Epidemiology Fecal incontinence is the involuntary passage of fecal material for at least 1 month in an individual with a developmental age of at least 4 years. The prevalence of fecal incontinence in the United States is 0.5–11%. The majority of patients are women and above the age of 65. A higher incidence of incontinence is seen among parous women. One-half of patients with fecal incontinence also suffer from urinary incontinence. The majority of incontinence is a result of obstetric injury to the pelvic floor, either while carrying a fetus or during the delivery. An anatomic sphincter defect may occur in up to 32% of women following childbirth regardless of visible damage to the perineum. Risk factors at the time of delivery include prolonged labor, the use of forceps, and the need for an episiotomy. Symptoms of incontinence can present after two or more decades following obstetric injury. Medical conditions known to contribute to the development of fecal incontinence are listed in Table 353-4.

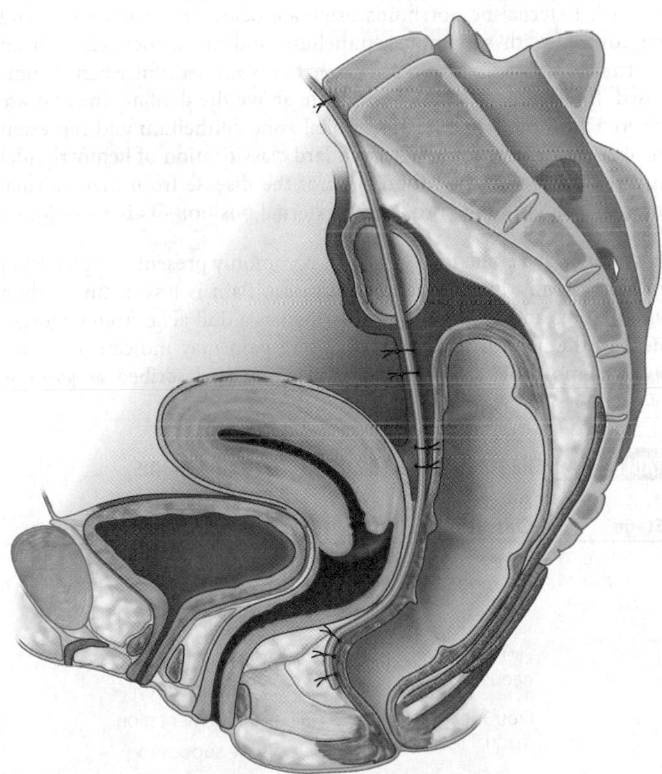

FIGURE 353-6 Laparoscopic ventral rectopexy (LVR). To reduce the internal prolapse and close any rectovaginal septal defect, the pouch of Douglas is opened and mesh is secured to the anterolateral rectum, vaginal fornix, and sacrum. *(From A D'Hoore et al: Br J Surg 91:1500, 2004.)*

TABLE 353-4 MEDICAL CONDITIONS THAT CONTRIBUTE TO SYMPTOMS OF FECAL INCONTINENCE

Neurologic Disorders
• Dementia
• Brain tumor
• Stroke
• Multiple sclerosis
• Tabes dorsalis
• Cauda equina lesions
Skeletal Muscle Disorders
• Myasthenia gravis
• Myopathies, muscular dystrophy
Miscellaneous
• Hypothyroidism
• Irritable bowel syndrome
• Diabetes
• Severe diarrhea
• Scleroderma

Anatomy and Pathophysiology The anal sphincter complex is made up of the internal and external anal sphincter. The internal sphincter is smooth muscle and a continuation of the circular fibers of the rectal wall. It is innervated by the intestinal myenteric plexus and is therefore not under voluntary control. The external anal sphincter is formed in continuation with the levator ani muscles and is under voluntary control. The pudendal nerve supplies motor innervation to the external anal sphincter. Obstetric injury may result in tearing of the muscle fibers anteriorly at the time of the delivery. This results in an obvious anterior defect on endoanal ultrasound. Injury may also be the result of stretching of the pudendal nerves during pregnancy or delivery of the fetus through the birth canal.

Presentation and Evaluation Patients may suffer with varying degrees of fecal incontinence. Minor incontinence includes incontinence to flatus and occasional seepage of liquid stool. Major incontinence is frequent inability to control solid waste. As a result of fecal incontinence, patients suffer from poor perianal hygiene. Beyond the immediate problems associated with fecal incontinence, these patients are often withdrawn and suffer from depression. For this reason, quality-of-life measures are an important component in the evaluation of patients with fecal incontinence.

The evaluation of fecal incontinence should include a thorough history and physical exam including digital rectal examination (DRE). Weak sphincter tone on DRE and loss of the "anal wink" reflex (S1-level control) may indicate a neurogenic dysfunction. Perianal scars may represent surgical injury. Other studies helpful in the diagnosis of fecal incontinence include anal manometry, pudendal nerve terminal motor latency (PNTML), and endoanal ultrasound. Centers that care for patients with fecal incontinence will have an anorectal physiology laboratory that uses standardized methods of evaluating anorectal physiology. Anorectal manometry (ARM) measures resting and squeeze pressures within the anal canal using an intraluminal water-perfused catheter. Current methods of ARM include use of a three-dimensional, high-resolution system with a 12-catheter perfusion system, which allows physiologic delineation of anatomic abnormalities.

Pudendal nerve studies evaluate the function of the nerves innervating the anal canal using a finger electrode placed in the anal canal. Stretch injuries to these nerves will result in a delayed response of the sphincter muscle to a stimulus, indicating a prolonged latency. Finally, endoanal ultrasound will evaluate the extent of the injury to the sphincter muscles before surgical repair. Unfortunately, all of these investigations are user-dependent, and very few studies demonstrate that these studies predict outcome following an intervention. Magnetic resonance imaging (MRI) has been used, but its routine use for imaging in fecal incontinence is not well established.

Rarely does a pelvic floor disorder exist alone. The majority of patients with fecal incontinence will have some degree of urinary incontinence. Similarly, fecal incontinence is a part of the spectrum of pelvic organ prolapse. For this reason, patients may present with symptoms of obstructed defecation as well as fecal incontinence. Careful evaluation including dynamic MRI or cinedefecography should be performed to search for other associated defects. Surgical repair of incontinence without attention to other associated defects may decrease the success of the repair.

TREATMENT FECAL INCONTINENCE

Medical management of fecal incontinence includes strategies to bulk up the stool, which help in increasing fecal sensation. These include fiber supplementation, loperamide, diphenoxylate, and bile acid binders. These agents harden the stool and delay frequency of bowel movements and are helpful in patients with minimal to mild symptoms. Furthermore, patients can be offered a form of physical therapy called biofeedback. This therapy helps strengthen the external sphincter muscle while training the patient to relax with defecation to avoid unnecessary straining and further injury to the sphincter muscles. Biofeedback has had variable success and is dependent on the motivation of the patient. At a minimum, biofeedback is risk free and safe. Most patients will have some improvement. For this reason, it should be incorporated into the initial recommendation to all patients with fecal incontinence.

The "gold standard" for the treatment of fecal incontinence with an isolated sphincter defect has been the overlapping sphincteroplasty. The external anal sphincter muscle and scar tissue as well as any identifiable internal sphincter muscle are dissected free from the surrounding adipose and connective tissue and then an overlapping repair is performed in an attempt to rebuild the muscular ring and restore its function. Long-term results following overlapping sphincteroplasty show about a 50% failure rate over 5 years. Poorer outcome has been seen in patients with prolonged pudendal nerve terminal motor latency.

Sacral neuromodulation, collagen-enhancing injectables, radiofrequency therapy, and the artificial bowel sphincter are other options. Sacral nerve stimulation and the artificial bowel sphincter are both adaptations of procedures developed for the management of urinary incontinence. Sacral nerve stimulation is ideally suited for patients with intact but weak anal sphincters. A temporary nerve stimulator is placed on the third sacral nerve. If there is at least a 50% improvement in symptoms, a permanent nerve stimulator is placed under the skin. The artificial bowel sphincter is a cuff and reservoir apparatus that allows for manual inflation of a cuff placed around the anus, increasing anal tone. This allows the patient to manually close off the anal canal until defecation is necessary. Long-term results for sacral stimulation have been promising, with nearly 80% of patients having a reduction in incontinence episodes by at least 50%. This reduction has been sustainable in studies out to 5 years. Unfortunately, the artificial bowel sphincter has been associated with a 30% infection rate. Accordingly, implantation is performed less often.

Collagen-enhancing injectables have been around for several years. The largest open trial involved 115 incontinent patients treated with nonanimal stabilized hyaluronic acid (NASHA/DX) gel. In this study, patients underwent injections of NASHA/DX (Solesta) into the anal mucosa and were followed for 12 months. The results were promising, with over 50% achieving greater than 50% reduction in incontinence episodes, and these results were sustainable up to 2 years. This method is another less invasive therapy for patients with fecal incontinence.

Radiofrequency energy delivery to the anal canal in patients with fecal incontinence aids in the development and restructuring of collagen fibers and provides tensile strength to the sphincter muscles. The radiofrequency is delivered as an office procedure with sedation. The results have been variable, with 20–50% of patients having a sustained reduction in incontinence episodes for 5 years.

Finally, the use of stem cells to increase the bulk of the sphincter muscles is currently being tested. Stem cells can be harvested from the patient's own muscle, grown, and then implanted into their sphincter complex. Concern for cost and the need for an additional procedure dampen enthusiasm. Trial results are awaited.

HEMORRHOIDAL DISEASE

Incidence and Epidemiology Symptomatic hemorrhoids affect >1 million individuals in the Western world per year. The prevalence of hemorrhoidal disease is not selective for age or sex. However, age is known to be a risk factor. The prevalence of hemorrhoidal disease is less in underdeveloped countries. The typical low-fiber, high-fat Western diet is associated with constipation and straining and the development of symptomatic hemorrhoids.

Anatomy and Pathophysiology Hemorrhoidal cushions are a normal part of the anal canal. The vascular structures contained within this tissue aid in continence by preventing damage to the sphincter muscle. Three main hemorrhoidal complexes traverse the anal canal—the left lateral, the right anterior, and the right posterior. Engorgement and straining lead to prolapse of this tissue into the anal canal. Over time, the anatomic support system of the hemorrhoidal complex weakens, exposing this tissue to the outside of the anal canal where it is susceptible to injury. Hemorrhoids are commonly classified as external or internal. External hemorrhoids originate below the dentate line and are covered with squamous epithelium and are associated with an internal component. External hemorrhoids are painful when thrombosed. Internal hemorrhoids originate above the dentate line and are covered with mucosa and transitional zone epithelium and represent majority of hemorrhoids. The standard classification of hemorrhoidal disease is based on the progression of the disease from their normal internal location to the prolapsing external position (Table 353-5).

Presentation and Evaluation Patients commonly present to a physician for two reasons: bleeding and protrusion. Pain is less common than with fissures and, if present, is described as a dull ache from engorgement of the hemorrhoidal tissue. Severe pain may indicate a thrombosed hemorrhoid. Hemorrhoidal bleeding is described as painless

TABLE 353-5 THE STAGING AND TREATMENT OF HEMORRHOIDS

Stage	Description of Classification	Treatment
I	Enlargement with bleeding	Fiber supplementation Cortisone suppository Sclerotherapy
II	Protrusion with spontaneous reduction	Fiber supplementation Cortisone suppository
III	Protrusion requiring manual reduction	Fiber supplementation Cortisone suppository Banding Operative hemorrhoidectomy
IV	Irreducible protrusion	Fiber supplementation Cortisone suppository Operative hemorrhoidectomy

bright red blood seen either in the toilet or upon wiping. Occasional patients can present with significant bleeding, which may be a cause of anemia; however, the presence of a colonic neoplasm must be ruled out in anemic patients. Patients who present with a protruding mass complain about inability to maintain perianal hygiene and are often concerned about the presence of a malignancy.

The diagnosis of hemorrhoidal disease is made on physical examination. Inspection of the perianal region for evidence of thrombosis or excoriation is performed, followed by a careful digital examination. Anoscopy is performed paying particular attention to the known position of hemorrhoidal disease. The patient is asked to strain. If this is difficult for the patient, the maneuver can be performed while sitting on a toilet. The physician is notified when the tissue prolapses. It is important to differentiate the circumferential appearance of a full-thickness rectal prolapse from the radial nature of prolapsing hemorrhoids (see "Rectal Prolapse," above). The stage and location of the hemorrhoidal complexes are defined.

TREATMENT HEMORRHOIDAL DISEASE

The treatment for bleeding hemorrhoids is based on the stage of the disease (Table 353-5). In all patients with bleeding, the possibility of other causes must be considered. In young patients without a family history of colorectal cancer, the hemorrhoidal disease may be treated first and a colonoscopic examination performed if the bleeding continues. Older patients who have not had colorectal cancer screening should undergo colonoscopy or flexible sigmoidoscopy.

With rare exceptions, the acutely thrombosed hemorrhoid can be excised within the first 72 h by performing an elliptical excision. Sitz baths, fiber, and stool softeners are prescribed. Additional therapy for bleeding hemorrhoids includes the office procedures of banding and sclerotherapy. Sensation begins at the dentate line; therefore, banding or sclerotherapy can be performed without discomfort in the office. Bands are placed around the engorged tissue, causing ischemia and fibrosis. This aids in fixing the tissue proximally in the anal canal. Patients may complain of a dull ache for 24 h following band application. During sclerotherapy, 1–2 mL of a sclerosant (usually sodium tetradecyl sulfate) is injected using a 25-gauge needle into the submucosa of the hemorrhoidal complex. Care must be taken not to inject the anal canal circumferentially, or stenosis may occur.

For surgical management of hemorrhoidal disease, excisional hemorrhoidectomy, transhemorrhoidal dearterialization (THD), or stapled hemorrhoidectomy ("the procedure for prolapse or hemorrhoids" [PPH]) is the procedure of choice. All surgical methods of management are equally effective in the treatment of symptomatic third- and fourth-degree hemorrhoids. However, because the sutured hemorrhoidectomy involves the removal of redundant tissue down to the anal verge, unpleasant anal skin tags are removed as well. The stapled hemorrhoidectomy is associated with less discomfort; however, this procedure does not remove anal skin tags. THD uses ultrasound guidance to ligate the blood supply to the anal tissue, hence reducing hemorrhoidal engorgement. No procedures on hemorrhoids should be done in patients who are immunocompromised or who have active proctitis. Furthermore, emergent hemorrhoidectomy for bleeding hemorrhoids is associated with a higher complication rate.

Acute complications associated with the treatment of hemorrhoids include pain, infection, recurrent bleeding, and urinary retention. Care should be taken to place bands properly and to avoid overhydration in patients undergoing operative hemorrhoidectomy. Late complications include fecal incontinence as a result of injury to the sphincter during the dissection. Anal stenosis may develop from overzealous excision, with loss of mucosal skin bridges for reepithelialization. Finally, an *ectropion* (prolapse of rectal mucosa from the anal canal) may develop. Patients with an ectropion complain of a "wet" anus as a result of inability to prevent soiling once the rectal mucosa is exposed below the dentate line.

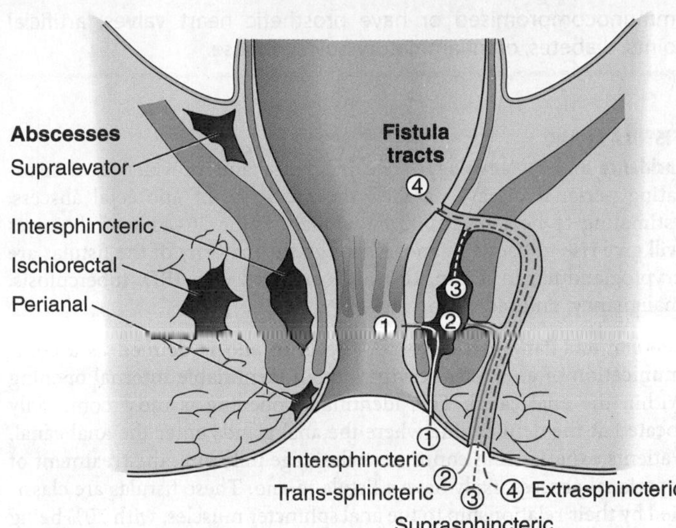

FIGURE 353-7 Common locations of anorectal abscess (*left*) and fistula in ano (***right***).

ANORECTAL ABSCESS

Incidence and Epidemiology The development of a perianal abscess is more common in men than women by a ratio of 3:1. The peak incidence is in the third to fifth decade of life. Perianal pain associated with the presence of an abscess accounts for 15% of office visits to a colorectal surgeon. The disease is more prevalent in immunocompromised patients such as those with diabetes, hematologic disorders, or inflammatory bowel disease and persons who are HIV positive. These disorders should be considered in patients with recurrent perianal infections.

Anatomy and Pathophysiology An anorectal abscess is an abnormal fluid-containing cavity in the anorectal region. Anorectal abscess results from an infection involving the glands surrounding the anal canal. Normally, these glands release mucus into the anal canal, which aids in defecation. When stool accidentally enters the anal glands, the glands become infected and an abscess develops. Anorectal abscesses are perianal in 40–50% of patients, ischiorectal in 20–25%, intersphincteric in 2–5%, and supralevator in 2.5% (Fig. 353-7).

Presentation and Evaluation Perianal pain and fever are the hallmarks of an abscess. Patients may have difficulty voiding and have blood in the stool. A prostatic abscess may present with similar complaints, including dysuria. Patients with a prostatic abscess will often have a history of recurrent sexually transmitted diseases. On physical examination, a large fluctuant area is usually readily visible. Routine laboratory evaluation shows an elevated white blood cell count. Diagnostic procedures are rarely necessary unless evaluating a recurrent abscess. A CT scan or MRI has an accuracy of 80% in determining incomplete drainage. If there is a concern about the presence of inflammatory bowel disease, a rigid or flexible sigmoidoscopic examination may be done at the time of drainage to evaluate for inflammation within the rectosigmoid region. A more complete evaluation for Crohn's disease would include a full colonoscopy and small-bowel series.

TREATMENT ANORECTAL ABSCESS

As with all abscesses, the "gold standard" is drainage. Office drainage of an uncomplicated anorectal abscess may suffice. A small incision close to the anal verge is made, and a Mallenkot drain is advanced into the abscess cavity. For patients who have a complicated abscess or who are diabetic or immunocompromised, drainage should be performed in an operating room under anesthesia. These patients are at greater risk for developing necrotizing fasciitis. There is limited role of antibiotics in management of anorectal abscesses. The antibiotics are only warranted in patients who are immunocompromised or have prosthetic heart valves, artificial joints, diabetes, or inflammatory bowel disease.

FISTULA IN ANO

Incidence and Epidemiology The incidence and prevalence of fistulating perianal disease parallels the incidence of anorectal abscess, estimating to be 1 in 10,000 individuals. Some 30–40% of abscesses will give rise to fistula in ano. Although the majority of the fistulas are cryptoglandular in origin, 10% are associated with IBD, tuberculosis, malignancy, and radiation.

Anatomy and Pathophysiology A fistula in ano is defined as a communication of an abscess cavity with an identifiable internal opening within the anal canal. This identifiable opening is most commonly located at the dentate line where the anal glands enter the anal canal. Patients experiencing continuous drainage following the treatment of a perianal abscess likely have a fistula in ano. These fistulas are classified by their relationship to the anal sphincter muscles, with 70% being intersphincteric, 23% transsphincteric, 5% suprasphincteric, and 2% extrasphincteric (Fig. 353-7).

Presentation and Evaluation A patient with a fistula in ano will complain of constant drainage from the perianal region associated with a firm mass. The drainage may increase with defecation. Perianal hygiene is difficult to maintain. Examination under anesthesia is the best way to evaluate a fistula. At the time of the examination, anoscopy is performed to look for an internal opening. Diluted hydrogen peroxide will aid in identifying such an opening. In lieu of anesthesia, MRI with an endoanal coil will also identify tracts in 80% of the cases. After drainage of an abscess with insertion of a Mallenkot catheter, a fistulagram through the catheter can be obtained in search of an occult fistula tract. Goodsall's rule states that a posterior external fistula will enter the anal canal in the posterior midline, whereas an anterior fistula will enter at the nearest crypt. A fistula exiting >3 cm from the anal verge may have a complicated upward extension and may not obey Goodsall's rule.

TREATMENT FISTULA IN ANO

A newly diagnosed draining fistula is best managed with placement of a seton, a vessel loop or silk tie placed through the fistula tract, which maintains the tract open and quiets down the surrounding inflammation that occurs from repeated blockage of the tract. Once the inflammation is less, the exact relationship of the fistula tract to the anal sphincters can be ascertained. A simple fistulotomy can be performed for intersphincteric and low (less than one-third of the muscle) transsphincteric fistulas without compromising continence. For a higher transsphincteric fistula, an anorectal advancement flap in combination with a drainage catheter or fibrin glue may be used. Very long (>2 cm) and narrow tracts respond better to fibrin glue than shorter tracts. Simple ligation of the internal fistula tract (LIFT procedure) has also been used in the management of simple fistula with good success.

Patients should be maintained on stool-bulking agents, nonnarcotic pain medication, and sitz baths following surgery for a fistula. Early complications from these procedures include urinary retention and bleeding. Later complications are rare (<10%) and include temporary and permanent incontinence. Recurrence is 0–18% following fistulotomy and 20–30% following anorectal advancement flap and the LIFT procedure,

ANAL FISSURE

Incidence and Epidemiology Anal fissures occur at all ages but are more common in the third through the fifth decades. A fissure is the most common cause of rectal bleeding in infancy. The prevalence is equal in males and females. It is associated with constipation, diarrhea, infectious etiologies, perianal trauma, and Crohn's disease.

Anatomy and Pathophysiology Trauma to the anal canal occurs following defecation. This injury occurs in the anterior or, more commonly, the posterior anal canal. Irritation caused by the trauma to the anal canal results in an increased resting pressure of the internal sphincter. The blood supply to the sphincter and anal mucosa enters laterally. Therefore, increased anal sphincter tone results in a relative ischemia in the region of the fissure and leads to poor healing of the anal injury. A fissure that is not in the posterior or anterior position should raise suspicion for other causes, including tuberculosis, syphilis, Crohn's disease, and malignancy.

Presentation and Evaluation A fissure can be easily diagnosed on history alone. The classic complaint is pain, which is strongly associated with defecation and is relentless. The bright red bleeding that can be associated with a fissure is less extensive than that associated with hemorrhoids. On examination, most fissures are located in either the posterior or anterior position. A lateral fissure is worrisome because it may have a less benign nature, and systemic disorders should be ruled out. A chronic fissure is indicated by the presence of a hypertrophied anal papilla at the proximal end of the fissure and a sentinel pile or skin tag at the distal end. Often the circular fibers of the hypertrophied internal sphincter are visible within the base of the fissure. If anal manometry is performed, elevation in anal resting pressure and a sawtooth deformity with paradoxical contractions of the sphincter muscles are pathognomonic.

TREATMENT ANAL FISSURE

The management of the acute fissure is conservative. Stool softeners for those with constipation, increased dietary fiber, topical anesthetics, glucocorticoids, and sitz baths are prescribed and will heal 60–90% of fissures. Chronic fissures are those present for >6 weeks. These can be treated with modalities aimed at decreasing the anal canal resting pressure including nifedipine or nitroglycerin ointment applied three times a day and botulinum toxin type A, up to 20 units, injected into the internal sphincter on each side of the fissure. Surgical management includes anal dilatation and lateral internal sphincterotomy. Usually, one-third of the internal sphincter muscle is divided; it is easily identified because it is hypertrophied. Recurrence rates from medical therapy are higher, but this is offset by a risk of incontinence following sphincterotomy. Lateral internal sphincterotomy may lead to incontinence more commonly in women.

ACKNOWLEDGMENT

We would like to thank Cory Sandore for providing some illustrations for this chapter. Gregory Bulkley, MD, contributed to this chapter in an earlier edition and some of that material has been retained here.

354 Mesenteric Vascular Insufficiency

Rizwan Ahmed, Mahmoud Malas

INTESTINAL ISCHEMIA

INCIDENCE AND EPIDEMIOLOGY

Intestinal ischemia occurs when splanchnic perfusion fails to meet the metabolic demands of the intestines, resulting in ischemic tissue injury. Mesenteric ischemia affects 2–3 people per 100,000, and the incidence of mesenteric ischemia is bound to increase in the aging population. Delay in diagnosis and management results in a high mortality, and prompt interventions may be life-saving. Intestinal ischemia is further classified based on etiology, which dictates management: (1) arteriocclusive mesenteric ischemia, (2) nonocclusive mesenteric ischemia, and (3) mesenteric venous thrombosis.

Risk factors for arteriocclusive mesenteric ischemia are generally acute in onset and include atrial fibrillation, recent myocardial infarction, valvular heart disease, and recent cardiac or vascular catheterization, all of which result in embolic clots reaching the mesenteric circulation. Nonocclusive mesenteric ischemia, also known as "intestinal angina," is generally more insidious and most often seen in the aging population affected by atherosclerotic disease. Patients with chronic atherosclerotic disease could also suffer an acute insult from emboli leading to complete occlusion. Nonocclusive mesenteric ischemia is also seen in patients receiving high-dose vasopressor infusions, patients with cardiogenic or septic shock, and patients with cocaine overdose. Nonocclusive mesenteric ischemia is the most prevalent gastrointestinal disease complicating cardiovascular surgery. The incidence of ischemic colitis following elective aortic repair is 5–9%, and the incidence triples in patients following emergent repair. Mesenteric venous thrombosis is less common and is associated with the presence of a hypercoagulable state including protein C or S deficiency, antithrombin III deficiency, polycythemia vera, and carcinoma.

ANATOMY AND PATHOPHYSIOLOGY

The blood supply to the intestines is depicted in Fig. 354-1. To prevent ischemic injury, extensive collateralization occurs between major mesenteric trunks and branches of the mesenteric arcades. Collateral vessels within the small bowel are numerous and meet within the duodenum and the bed of the pancreas. Collateral vessels within the colon meet at the splenic flexure and descending/sigmoid colon. These areas, which are inherently at risk for decreased blood flow, are known as *Griffiths' point* and *Sudeck's point*, respectively, and are the most common locations for colonic ischemia (Fig. 354-1, shaded areas). The splanchnic circulation can receive up to 30% of the cardiac output. Protective responses to prevent intestinal ischemia include abundant

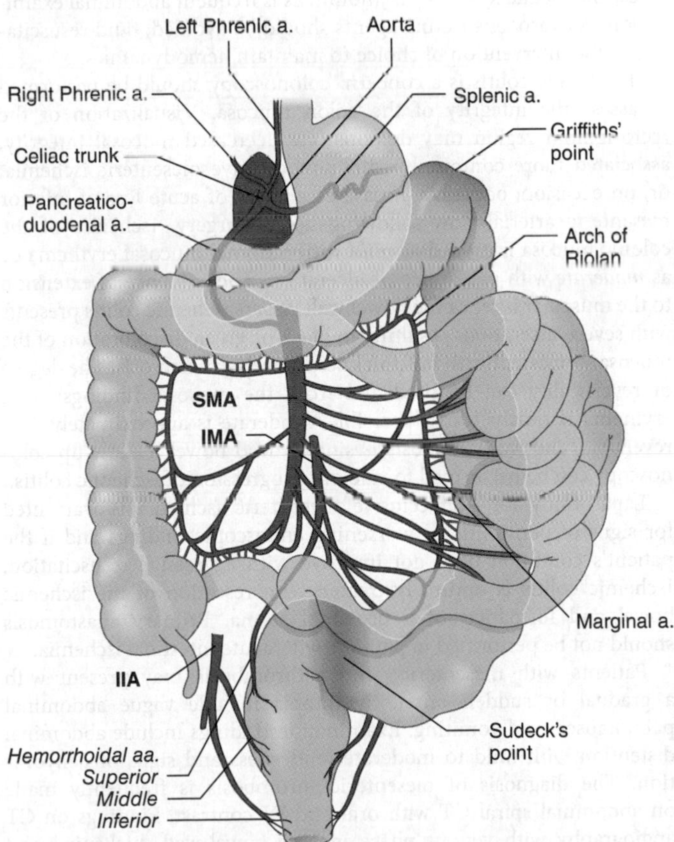

FIGURE 354-1 Blood supply to the intestines includes the celiac artery, superior mesenteric artery (SMA), inferior mesenteric artery (IMA), and branches of the internal iliac artery (IIA). Griffiths' and Sudeck's points, indicated by shaded areas, are watershed areas within the colonic blood supply and common locations for ischemia.

collateralization, autoregulation of blood flow, and the ability to increase oxygen extraction from the blood.

Occlusive ischemia is a result of disruption of blood flow by an embolus or progressive thrombosis in a major artery supplying the intestine. Emboli originate from the heart in more than 75% of cases and lodge preferentially in the superior mesenteric artery just distal to the origin of the middle colic artery. Progressive thrombosis of at least two of the major vessels supplying the intestine is required for the development of chronic intestinal angina. Nonocclusive ischemia is disproportionate mesenteric vasoconstriction (arteriolar vasospasm) in response to a severe physiologic stress such as shock. If left untreated, early mucosal stress ulceration will progress to full-thickness injury. Even in the early stages of ischemia, there is translocation of bacteria across the intestinal mucosa, resulting in bacteremia that can lead to sepsis.

PRESENTATION, EVALUATION, AND MANAGEMENT

Intestinal ischemia remains one of the most challenging diagnoses. The mortality rate is greater than 50%. The most significant indicator of survival is the timeliness of diagnosis and treatment. An overview of diagnosis and management of each form of intestinal ischemia is given in Table 354-1.

Acute mesenteric ischemia resulting from arterial embolus or thrombosis presents with severe acute, nonremitting abdominal pain strikingly out of proportion to the physical findings. Associated symptoms may include nausea and vomiting, transient diarrhea, anorexia, and bloody stools. With the exception of minimal abdominal distention and hypoactive bowel sounds, early abdominal examination is unimpressive. Later findings will demonstrate peritonitis and cardiovascular collapse. In the evaluation of acute intestinal ischemia, routine laboratory tests should be obtained, including complete blood count, serum chemistry, coagulation profile, arterial blood gas, amylase, lipase, lactic acid, blood type and cross match, and cardiac enzymes. Regardless of the need for urgent surgery, emergent admission to a monitored bed or intensive care unit is recommended for resuscitation and further evaluation. If the diagnosis of intestinal ischemia is being considered, consultation with a surgical service is necessary. Often the decision to operate is made on a high index of suspicion from the history and physical exam despite normal laboratory findings.

Other diagnostic modalities that may be useful in diagnosis but should not delay surgical therapy include electrocardiogram (ECG), echocardiogram, abdominal radiographs, computed tomography (CT), and mesenteric angiography. More recently, mesentery duplex scanning and visible light spectroscopy during colonoscopy have been demonstrated to be beneficial. The ECG may demonstrate an arrhythmia, indicating the possible source of the emboli. A plain abdominal film may show evidence of free intraperitoneal air, indicating a perforated viscus and the need for emergent exploration. Earlier features of intestinal ischemia seen on abdominal radiographs include bowel-wall edema, known as "thumbprinting." If the ischemia progresses, air can be seen within the bowel wall (*pneumatosis intestinalis*) and within the portal venous system. Other features include calcifications of the aorta and its tributaries, indicating atherosclerotic disease. With the administration of oral and IV contrast, dynamic CT angiography with three-dimensional reconstruction is a highly sensitive test for intestinal ischemia. In acute embolic disease, mesenteric angiography is best performed intraoperatively. A mesenteric duplex scan demonstrating a high peak velocity of flow in the superior mesenteric artery (SMA) is associated with an approximately 80% positive predictive value of mesenteric ischemia. More significantly, a negative duplex scan virtually precludes the diagnosis of mesenteric ischemia. Duplex imaging serves as a screening test; further investigations with angiography are needed. The biggest limitation of duplex scanning is body habitus; in obese patients, imaging is poor yield. However, in patients with chronic disease, "food fear" often leads to a decreased appetite and therefore less abdominal fat, and duplex imaging is very high yield. The endoscopic techniques using visible light spectroscopy can be used in the diagnosis of chronic ischemia. When suspecting mesenteric ischemia involving the colon, performing an endoscopy to evaluate up to the splenic

TABLE 354-1 OVERVIEW OF THE MANAGEMENT OF ACUTE INTESTINAL ISCHEMIA

Condition	Key to Early Diagnosis	Treatment of Underlying Cause	Treatment of Specific Lesion	Treatment of Systemic Consequence
Arterioocclusive mesenteric ischemia 1. Arterial embolus	Computed tomography (CT) angiography Early laparotomy	Anticoagulation Cardioversion Proximal thrombectomy	Laparotomy Embolectomy Vascular bypass Assess viability and resect dead bowel	Ensure hydration Give antibiotics Reverse acidosis Optimize oxygen delivery Avoid vasoconstrictors
2. Arterial thrombosis	Duplex ultrasound Angiography	Anticoagulation Hydration	Endovascular approach: thrombolysis, angioplasty and stenting Endarterectomy/thrombectomy or vascular bypass Assess viability and resect dead bowel	Give antibiotics Reverse acidosis Optimize oxygen delivery Support cardiac output Avoid vasoconstrictors
Mesenteric venous thrombosis Venous thrombosis	Spiral CT Angiography with venous phase	Anticoagulation Massive hydration	Anticoagulation ± laparotomy/thrombectomy/catheter-directed thrombolysis Assess viability and resect dead bowel	Give antibiotics Reverse acidosis Optimize oxygen delivery Support cardiac output Avoid vasoconstrictors
Nonocclusive mesenteric ischemia	Vasospasm: Angiography Hypoperfusion: Spiral CT or colonoscopy	Ensure hydration Support cardiac output Avoid vasoconstrictors	Vasospasm Intraarterial vasodilators Hypoperfusion Delayed laparotomy Assess viability and resect dead bowel	Ensure hydration Give antibiotics Reverse acidosis Optimize oxygen delivery Support cardiac output Avoid vasoconstrictors

Source: Modified from GB Bulkley, in JL Cameron (ed): *Current Surgical Therapy*, 2nd ed. Toronto, BC Decker, 1986.

flexure is high yield. This is often an excellent diagnostic tool in patients with chronic renal insufficiency who cannot tolerate IV contrast.

The "gold standard" for the diagnosis of acute arterial occlusive disease is angiography, and management is laparotomy. Surgical exploration should not be delayed if suspicion of acute occlusive mesenteric ischemia is high or evidence of clinical deterioration or frank peritonitis is present. The goal of operative exploration is to resect compromised bowel and restore blood supply. The entire length of the small and large bowel beginning at the ligament of Treitz should be evaluated. The pattern of intestinal ischemia may indicate the level of arterial occlusion. In the case of SMA occlusion where the embolus usually lies just proximal to the origin of the middle colic artery, the proximal jejunum is often spared while the remainder of the small bowel to the transverse colon will be ischemic. The surgical management of acute mesenteric ischemia of the small bowel is embolectomy via arteriotomy; a small incision is made in the artery through which the clot is retrieved. Another way to manage acute thrombosis is thrombolysis therapy and angioplasty, with stent placement. However, this approach is more commonly applied to treat chronic mesenteric ischemia. If this is unsuccessful, a bypass from the aorta or iliac artery to the SMA is performed.

Nonocclusive or vasospastic mesenteric ischemia presents with generalized abdominal pain, anorexia, bloody stools, and abdominal distention. Often these patients are obtunded, and physical findings may not assist in the diagnosis. The presence of a leukocytosis, metabolic acidosis, elevated amylase or creatinine phosphokinase levels, and/or lactic acidosis is useful in support of the diagnosis of advanced intestinal ischemia; however, these markers may not be indicative of either reversible ischemia or frank necrosis. Investigational markers for intestinal ischemia include D-dimer, glutathione *S*-transferase, platelet-activating factor (PAF), and mucosal pH monitoring. Regardless of the need for urgent surgery, emergent admission to a monitored bed or intensive care unit is recommended for resuscitation and further evaluation. Early manifestations of intestinal ischemia include fluid sequestration within the bowel wall leading to a loss of interstitial volume. Aggressive fluid resuscitation may be necessary. To optimize oxygen delivery, nasal O_2 and blood transfusions may be given. Broad-spectrum antibiotics should be given to provide sufficient coverage for enteric pathogens, including gram-negative and anaerobic organisms. Frequent monitoring of the patient's vital signs, urine output, blood gases, and lactate levels is paramount, as is frequent abdominal examination. All vasoconstricting agents should be avoided; fluid resuscitation is the intervention of choice to maintain hemodynamics.

If ischemic colitis is a concern, colonoscopy should be performed to assess the integrity of the colon mucosa. Visualization of the rectosigmoid region may demonstrate decreased mucosal integrity, associated more commonly with nonocclusive mesenteric ischemia, or, on occasion, occlusive disease as a result of acute loss of inferior mesenteric arterial flow following aortic surgery. Ischemia of the colonic mucosa is graded as *mild* with minimal mucosal erythema or as *moderate* with pale mucosal ulcerations and evidence of extension to the muscular layer of the bowel wall. *Severe* ischemic colitis presents with severe ulcerations resulting in black or green discoloration of the mucosa, consistent with full-thickness bowel-wall necrosis. The degree of reversibility can be predicted from the mucosal findings: mild erythema is nearly 100% reversible, moderate is approximately 50% reversible, and frank necrosis is simply dead bowel. Follow-up colonoscopy can be performed to rule out progression of ischemic colitis.

Laparotomy for nonocclusive mesenteric ischemia is warranted for signs of peritonitis or worsening endoscopic findings and if the patient's condition does not improve with aggressive resuscitation. Ischemic colitis is optimally treated with resection of the ischemic bowel and formation of a proximal stoma. Primary anastomosis should not be performed in patients with acute intestinal ischemia.

Patients with mesenteric venous thrombosis may present with a gradual or sudden onset. Symptoms include vague abdominal pain, nausea, and vomiting. Examination findings include abdominal distention with mild to moderate tenderness and signs of dehydration. The diagnosis of mesenteric thrombosis is frequently made on abdominal spiral CT with oral and IV contrast. Findings on CT angiography with venous phase include bowel-wall thickening and ascites. Intravenous contrast will demonstrate a delayed arterial phase and clot within the superior mesenteric vein. The goal of management is to optimize hemodynamics and correct electrolyte abnormalities with massive fluid resuscitation. Intravenous antibiotics as well as anticoagulation should be initiated. If laparotomy is performed and mesenteric venous thrombosis is suspected, heparin anticoagulation is immediately initiated, and compromised bowel is resected. Of all acute intestinal disorders, mesenteric venous insufficiency is associated with the best prognosis.

Chronic intestinal ischemia presents with intestinal angina or postprandial abdominal pain associated with need for increased blood flow to the intestine following meals. Patients report abdominal cramping and pain following ingestion of a meal. Weight loss and chronic diarrhea may also be noted. Abdominal pain without weight loss is not chronic mesenteric angina. Physical examination will often reveal a malnourished patient with an abdominal bruit as well as other manifestations of atherosclerosis. Duplex ultrasound evaluation of the mesenteric vessels has gained in popularity. It is important to perform the test fasting because the presence of increased bowel gas prevents adequate visualization of flow disturbances within the vessels or the lack of a vasodilation response to feeding during the test. This tool is frequently used as a screening test for patients with symptoms suggestive of chronic mesenteric ischemia. The gold standard for confirmation of mesenteric arterial occlusion is mesenteric angiography. Evaluation with mesenteric angiography allows for identification and possible intervention for the treatment of atherosclerosis within the vessel lumen and will also evaluate the patency of remaining mesenteric vessels. The use of mesenteric angiography may be limited in the presence of renal failure or contrast allergy. Magnetic resonance angiography is an alternative if the administration of contrast dye is contraindicated.

The management of chronic intestinal ischemia includes medical management of atherosclerotic disease by exercise, cessation of smoking, and antiplatelet and lipid-lowering medications. A full cardiac evaluation should be performed before intervention on chronic mesenteric ischemia. Newer endovascular procedures may avoid an operative intervention in selected patient populations. Angioplasty with endovascular stenting in the treatment of chronic mesenteric ischemia is associated with an 80% long-term success rate. In patients requiring surgical exploration, the approach used is determined by findings of the mesenteric angiogram. The entire length of the small and large bowel should be evaluated, beginning at the ligament of Treitz. Restoration of blood flow at the time of laparotomy is accomplished with mesenteric vessel endarterectomy or bypass.

Determination of intestinal viability intraoperatively in patients with suspected intestinal ischemia can be challenging. After revascularization, the bowel wall should be observed for return of a pink color and peristalsis. Palpation of major arterial mesenteric vessels can be performed, as well as applying a Doppler flowmeter to the antimesenteric border of the bowel wall, but neither is a definitive indicator of viability. In equivocal cases, 1 g of IV sodium fluorescein is administered, and the pattern of bowel reperfusion is observed under ultraviolet illumination with a standard (3600 A) Wood's lamp. An area of nonfluorescence >5 mm in diameter suggests nonviability. If doubt persists, reexploration performed 24–48 h following surgery will allow demarcation of nonviable bowel. Primary intestinal anastomosis in patients with ischemic bowel is always worrisome; thus, delayed bowel reconstruction and reanastomosis should be deferred to the time of second-look laparotomy.

Acknowledgments

We thank Cory Sandore for providing the illustration for this chapter. Susan Gearhart contributed to this chapter in the 18th edition.

355 Acute Intestinal Obstruction

Danny O. Jacobs

EPIDEMIOLOGY

Morbidity and mortality from acute intestinal obstruction have been decreasing over the past several decades. Nevertheless, the diagnosis can still be challenging, and the type of complications that patients suffer has not changed significantly. The extent of mechanical obstruction is typically described as partial, high-grade, or complete—generally correlating with the risk of complications and the urgency with which the underlying disease process must be addressed. Obstruction is also commonly described as being either "simple" or, alternatively, "strangulated" if vascular insufficiency and intestinal ischemia are evident.

Acute intestinal obstruction occurs either *mechanically* from blockage or from intestinal dysmotility when there is no blockage. In the latter instance, the abnormality is described as being *functional*. Mechanical bowel obstruction may be caused by extrinsic processes, intrinsic abnormalities of the bowel wall, or intraluminal abnormalities (Table 355-1). Within each of these broad categories are many diseases that can impede intestinal propulsion. Intrinsic diseases that can cause intestinal obstruction are usually congenital, inflammatory, neoplastic, or traumatic in origin, although intussusception and radiation injury can also be etiologic. Primary small-bowel cancers rarely cause acute obstruction.

Acute intestinal obstruction accounts for approximately 1–3 % of all hospitalizations and a quarter of all urgent or emergent general surgery admissions. Approximately 80% of cases involve the small bowel, and about one-third of these patients show evidence of significant ischemia. The mortality rate for patients with strangulation who are operated on within 24–30 h of the onset of symptoms is approximately 8% but triples shortly thereafter.

Extrinsic diseases most commonly cause mechanical obstruction of the small intestine. In the United States and Europe, almost all cases are caused by postoperative adhesions (>50%), carcinomatosis, or herniation of the anterior abdominal wall. Carcinomatosis most often originates from the ovary, pancreas, stomach, or colon, although rarely, metastasis from distant organs like the breast and skin can occur. Adhesions are responsible for >90% of cases of early postoperative obstruction that require intervention.

Operations of the lower abdomen, including appendectomy and colorectal and gynecologic procedures, are especially likely to create

TABLE 355-1 MOST COMMON CAUSES OF ACUTE INTESTINAL OBSTRUCTION

Extrinsic Disease
Adhesions (especially due to previous abdominal surgery), internal or external hernias, neoplasms (including carcinomatosis and extraintestinal malignancies, mostly commonly ovarian), endometriosis or intraperitoneal abscesses, and idiopathic sclerosis
Intrinsic Disease
Congenital (e.g., malrotation, atresia, stenosis, intestinal duplication, cyst formation, and congenital bands—the latter rarely in adults)
Inflammation (e.g., inflammatory bowel disease, especially Crohn's disease, but also diverticulitis, radiation, tuberculosis, lymphogranuloma venereum, and schistosomiasis)
Neoplasia (note: primary small-bowel cancer is rare; obstructive colon cancer may mimic small-bowel obstruction if the ileocecal valve is incompetent)
Traumatic (e.g., hematoma formation, anastomotic strictures)
Other, including intussusception (where the lead point is typically a polyp or tumor in adults), volvulus, obstruction of duodenum by superior mesenteric artery, radiation or ischemic injury, and aganglionosis, which is Hirschsprung's disease
Intraluminal Abnormalities
Bezoars, feces, foreign bodies including inspissated barium, gallstones (entering the lumen via a cholecystoenteric fistula), enteroliths

TABLE 355-2 ACUTE SMALL-INTESTINAL AND COLONIC OBSTRUCTION INCIDENCES

Cause	Incidence
Postoperative adhesions	>50%
Neoplasms	~20%
Hernias (especially ventral or internal types, where the risk of strangulation is increased)	~10%
Inflammatory bowel disease, other inflammation (obstruction may resolve if acute inflammation and edema subside)	~5%
Intussusception, volvulus, other miscellaneous diseases	<15%

adhesions that can cause bowel obstruction (Table 355-2). Overall, small-bowel obstruction is slightly more common in women. The risk of internal herniation is increased by abdominal procedures such as laparoscopic or open Roux-en-Y gastric bypass. Although laparoscopic procedures may generate fewer postoperative adhesions compared with open surgery, the risk of obstructive adhesion formation is not eliminated.

In many patients who are successfully treated for adhesive small-bowel obstruction, obstruction will recur. The rate varies according to how patients were initially managed. Approximately 20% of patients who were treated conservatively and between 5 and 30% of patients who were managed operatively will require readmission within 10 years.

Volvulus, which occurs when bowel twists on its mesenteric axis, can cause partial or complete obstruction and vascular insufficiency. The sigmoid colon is most commonly affected, accounting for approximately two-thirds of all cases of volvulus and 4% of all cases of large-bowel obstruction. The cecum and terminal ileum can also volvulize, or the cecum alone may be involved as a cecal bascule. Risk factors include institutionalization, the presence of neuropsychiatric conditions requiring psychotropic medication, chronic constipation, and aging; patients typically present in their seventies or eighties. Colonic volvulus is more common in Eastern Europe, Russia, and Africa than it is in the United States. It is rare for adhesions or hernias to obstruct the colon. Cancer of the descending colon and rectum is responsible for approximately two-thirds of all cases, followed by diverticulitis and volvulus.

Functional obstruction, also known as *ileus* and *pseudo-obstruction*, is present when dysmotility prevents intestinal contents from being propelled distally and no mechanical blockage exists. Ileus that occurs after intraabdominal surgery is the most commonly identified form of functional bowel obstruction, although there are many other causes (Table 355-3). Although postoperative ileus is most often transient, it is the most common reason why hospital discharge is delayed. Pseudo-obstruction of the colon, also known as Ogilvie's syndrome, is a relatively rare disease. Some patients with Ogilvie's syndrome have colonic dysmotility due to abnormalities of their autonomic nervous system that may be inherited.

TABLE 355-3 MOST COMMON CAUSES OF ILEUS (FUNCTIONAL OR PSEUDO-OBSTRUCTION OF THE INTESTINE)

Intraabdominal procedures, lumbar spinal injuries, or surgical procedures on the lumbar spine and pelvis
Metabolic or electrolyte abnormalities, especially hypokalemia and hypomagnesemia, but also hyponatremia, uremia, and severe hyperglycemia
Drugs such as opiates, antihistamines, and some psychotropic (e.g., haloperidol, tricyclic antidepressants) and anticholinergic agents
Intestinal ischemia
Intraabdominal or retroperitoneal inflammation or hemorrhage
Lower lobe pneumonias
Intraoperative radiation (likely due to muscle damage)
Systemic sepsis
Hyperparathyroidism
Pseudo-obstruction (Ogilvie's syndrome)
Ileus secondary to hereditary or acquired visceral myopathies and neuropathies that disrupt myocellular neural coordination
Some collagen vascular diseases such as lupus erythematosus or scleroderma

PATHOPHYSIOLOGY

The manifestations of acute intestinal obstruction depend on the nature of the underlying disease process, its location, and changes in blood flow (Fig. 355-1). Increased intestinal contractility, which occurs proximally and distal to the obstruction, is a characteristic response. Subsequently, intestinal peristalsis slows as the intestine or stomach proximal to the point of obstruction dilates and fills with gastrointestinal secretions and swallowed air. Although swallowed air is the primary contributor to intestinal distension, intraluminal air may also accumulate from fermentation, local carbon dioxide production, and altered gaseous diffusion.

Intraluminal dilation also increases intraluminal pressure. When luminal pressure exceeds venous pressure, venous and lymphatic drainage is impeded. Edema ensues, and the bowel wall proximal to the site of blockage may become hypoxemic. Epithelial necrosis can be identified within 12 h of obstruction. Ultimately, arterial blood supply may become so compromised that full-thickness ischemia, necrosis, and perforation result. Stasis increases the bacteria counts within the jejunum and ileum. The most commonly cultured intraluminal organisms are *Escherichia coli*, *Streptococcus faecalis*, and *Klebsiella*, which may also be recovered from mesenteric lymph nodes and other more distant sites.

Other manifestations depend on the degree of hypovolemia, the patient's metabolic response, and the presence or absence of associated intestinal ischemia. Inflammatory edema eventually increases the production of reactive oxygen species and activates neutrophils and macrophages, which accumulate within the bowel wall. Their accumulation, along with changes in innate immunity, disrupts secretory and neuromotor processes. Dehydration is caused by loss of the normal intestinal absorptive capacity as well as fluid accumulation in the gastric or intestinal wall and intraperitoneally.

Anorexia and emesis tend to exacerbate intravascular volume depletion. In the worst case scenario that is most commonly identified after distal obstruction, emesis leads to losses of gastric potassium, hydrogen, and chloride, while dehydration stimulates proximal renal tubule bicarbonate reabsorption. Intraperitoneal fluid accumulation, especially in patients with severe distal bowel obstruction, may increase intraabdominal pressure enough to elevate the diaphragm and inhibit respiration and to impede systemic venous return and promote vascular instability. Severe hemodynamic compromise may elicit a systemic inflammatory response and generalized microvascular leakage.

Closed-loop obstruction results when the proximal and distal openings of a given bowel segment are both occluded, e.g., due to volvulus or a hernia. It is the most common precursor for strangulation, but not every closed loop strangulates. The risk of vascular insufficiency, systemic inflammation, hemodynamic compromise, and irreversible intestinal ischemia is much greater in patients with closed-loop obstruction. Pathologic changes may occur more rapidly, and emergency intervention is indicated. Irreversible bowel ischemia progresses to transmural necrosis even if the obstruction is relieved. It is also important to remember that patients with high-grade distal colonic obstruction who have competent ileocecal valves may present with closed-loop obstruction. In the latter instance, the cecum may progressively dilate such that ischemic necrosis results in cecal perforation. This risk is generally greatest when the cecal diameter exceeds 12 cm, as informed by Laplace's law. Patients with distal colonic obstruction whose ileocecal valves are incompetent tend to present later in the course of disease and mimic patients with distal small-bowel obstruction.

HISTORY AND PHYSICAL FINDINGS

Even though the presenting signs and symptoms can be misleading, many patients with acute obstruction can be accurately diagnosed after a thorough history and physical examination is performed. Early

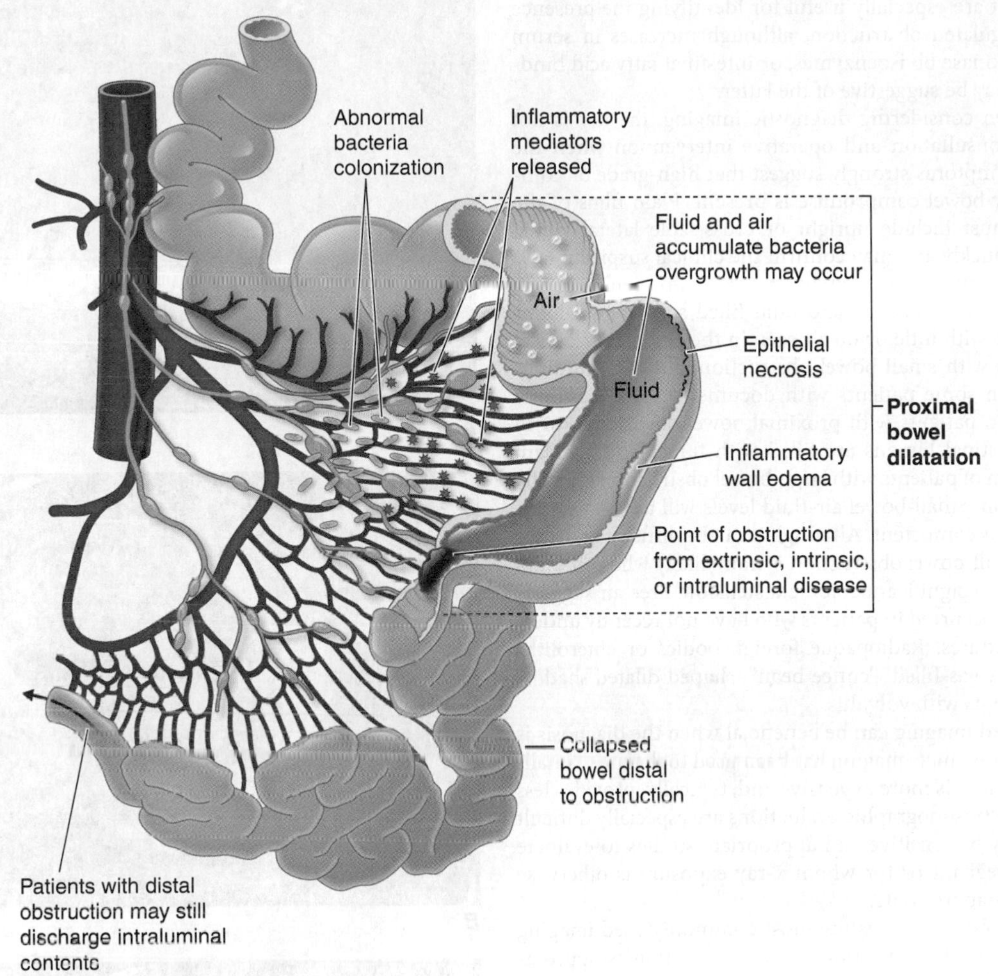

FIGURE 355-1 Pathophysiologic changes of small-bowel obstruction.

recognition allows earlier treatment that decreases the risk of progression or other excess morbidity. Small-bowel obstruction with strangulation can be especially difficult to diagnosis promptly.

The cardinal signs are colicky abdominal pain, abdominal distention, emesis, and obstipation. More intraluminal fluid accumulates in patients with distal obstruction, which typically leads to greater distention, more discomfort, and delayed emesis. This emesis is feculent when there is bacterial overgrowth. Patients with more proximal obstruction commonly present with less abdominal distention but more pronounced vomiting. Elements of the history that might be helpful include any prior history of surgery, including herniorrhaphy, as well as any history of cancer or inflammatory bowel disease.

Most patients, even with simple obstruction, appear to be critically ill. Many may be oliguric, hypotensive, and tachycardic because of severe intravascular volume depletion. Fever is worrisome for strangulation or systemic inflammatory changes. Bowel sounds and bowel functional activity are notoriously difficult to interpret. Classically, many patients with early small-bowel obstruction will have high-pitched, "musical" tinkling bowel sounds and peristaltic "rushes" known as borborygmi. Later in the course of disease, the bowel sounds may be absent or hypoactive as peristaltic activity decreases. This is in contrast to the common findings in patients with ileus or pseudo-obstruction where bowel sounds are typically absent or hypoactive from the beginning. Lastly, patients with partial blockage may continue to pass flatus and stool, and those with complete blockage may evacuate bowel contents present downstream beyond their obstruction.

All surgical incisions should be examined. The presence of a tender abdominal or groin mass strongly suggests that an incarcerated hernia may be the cause of obstruction. The presence of tenderness should increase the concern about the presence of complications such as ischemia, necrosis, or peritonitis. Severe pain with localization or signs of peritoneal irritation is suspicious for strangulated or closed-loop obstruction. It is important to remember that the discomfort may be out of proportion to physical findings mimicking the complaints of patients with acute mesenteric ischemia. Every patient should have a rectal examination. Patients with colonic volvulus present with the classic manifestations of closed-loop obstruction: severe abdominal pain, vomiting, and obstipation. Asymmetrical abdominal distension and a tympanic mass may be evident.

Patients with ileus or pseudo-obstruction may have signs and symptoms similar to those of bowel obstruction. Although abdominal distention is present, colicky abdominal pain is typically absent, and patients may not have nausea or emesis. Ongoing, regular discharge of stool or flatus can sometimes help distinguish patients with ileus from those with complete mechanical bowel obstruction.

LABORATORY AND IMAGING STUDIES

Laboratory testing should include a complete blood count and serum electrolyte and creatinine measurements. Serial assessments are often useful. Mild hemoconcentration and slight elevation of the white blood cell count commonly occur after simple bowel obstruction. Emesis and dehydration may cause hypokalemia, hypochloremia, elevated blood urea nitrogen–to–creatinine ratios, and metabolic alkalosis. Patients may be hyponatremic on admission because many have attempted to rehydrate themselves with hypotonic fluids. The presence of guaiac-positive stools and iron-deficiency anemia are strongly suggestive of malignancy.

Higher white blood cell counts with the presence of immature forms or the presence of metabolic acidosis are worrisome for severe volume depletion or ischemic necrosis and sepsis. At this time, there are no laboratory tests that are especially useful for identifying the presence of simple or strangulated obstruction, although increases in serum D-lactate, creatine kinase bb isoenzymes, or intestinal fatty acid binding protein levels may be suggestive of the latter.

In all cases, when considering diagnostic imaging, the key is not to delay surgical consultation and operative intervention when the patient's signs or symptoms strongly suggest that high-grade or complete obstruction or bowel compromise is present. Plain films of the abdomen, which must include upright or cross-table lateral views, can be completed quickly and may confirm the clinical suspicion 60% of the time. Interpretation immediately after operation is difficult. A "staircasing" pattern of dilated air and fluid-filled small-bowel loops >2.5 cm in diameter with little or no air seen in the colon are classical findings in patients with small-bowel obstruction, although findings may be equivocal in some patients with documented disease. Little bowel gas appears in patients with proximal bowel obstruction or in patients whose intestinal lumens are filled with fluid. Upright plain films of the abdomen of patients with large-bowel obstruction typically show colon dilatation. Small-bowel air-fluid levels will not be obvious if the ileocecal valve is competent. Although it can be difficult to distinguish from ileus, small-bowel obstruction is more likely when air-fluid levels are seen without significant colonic distension. Free air suggests that perforation has occurred in patients who have not recently undergone surgical procedures. Radiopaque foreign bodies or enteroliths may be visualized. A gas-filled, "coffee bean"–shaped dilated shadow may be seen in patients with volvulus.

More sophisticated imaging can be beneficial when the diagnosis is unclear. Magnetic resonance imaging has been used to diagnose small-bowel obstruction, but it is more expensive and, typically, provides less spatial resolution. Ultrasonographic evaluations are especially difficult to interpret but may be sensitive and appropriate studies to evaluate patients who are pregnant or for whom x-ray exposure is otherwise contraindicated or inappropriate.

Computed tomography (CT) is the most commonly used imaging modality. Its sensitivity for detecting bowel obstruction is approximately 95% (78–100%) in patients with high-grade obstruction, with a specificity of 96% and an accuracy of ≥95%. Its accuracy in diagnosing closed-loop obstruction is much lower (60%). Examples of some CT images are reproduced in Fig. 355-2. It may also provide useful information regarding location or identify particular circumstances where surgical intervention is needed urgently. Patients who have evidence of contrast appearing within the cecum within 4–24 h of oral administration can be expected to improve with high sensitivity and specificity (~95% each). For example, contrast studies may demonstrate a "bird's beak," a "c-loop," or "whorl" deformity on CT imaging at the site where twisting obstructs the lumen when a colonic volvulus is present.

CT imaging with enteral and IV contrast can also identify ischemia. Altered bowel wall enhancement is the most specific early finding, but its sensitivity is low. Mesenteric venous gas, pneumoperitoneum, and pneumatosis intestinalis are late findings indicating the presence of bowel necrosis. CT scanning after a water-soluble contrast enema may help distinguish ileus or pseudo-obstruction from distal large-bowel obstruction in patients who present with evidence of small-bowel and colonic distention. CT enteroclysis can accurately identify neoplasia as a cause of bowel obstruction. Contrast enemas or colonoscopies are almost always needed to identify causes of acute colonic obstruction.

Barium studies are generally contraindicated in patients with firm evidence of complete or high-grade bowel obstruction, especially when they present acutely. Barium should never be given orally to a patient with possible obstruction until that diagnosis has been excluded. In every other case, such investigations should only be performed in exceptional circumstances and with great caution because patients with significant obstruction may develop barium concretions as an additional source of blockage and some who would have otherwise recovered will require operative intervention. Barium opacification also renders cross-sectional imaging studies or angiography uninterpretable.

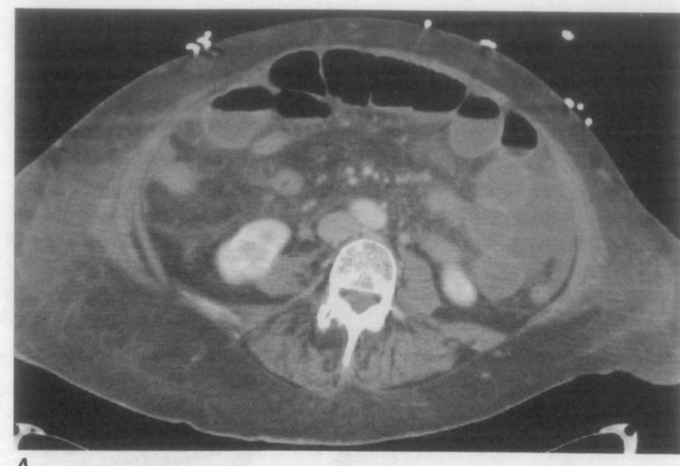

A

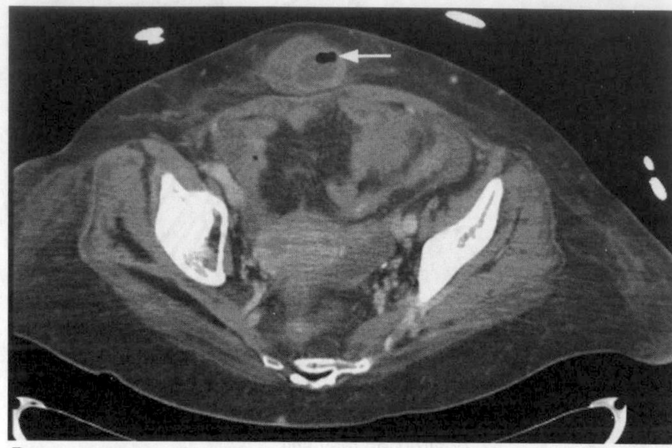

B

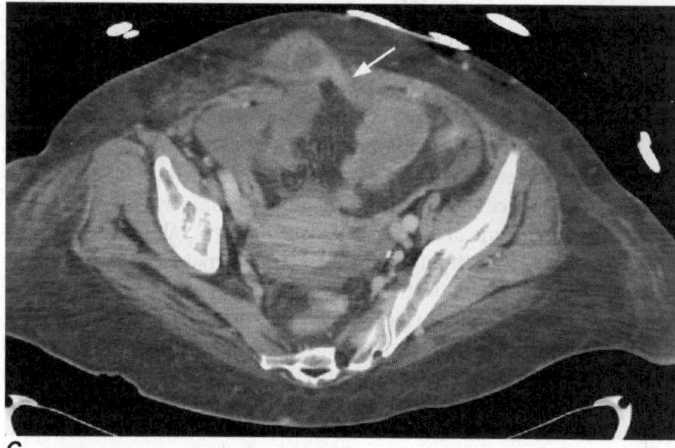

C

FIGURE 355-2 Computed tomography with oral and intravenous contrast demonstrating (***A***) evidence of small-bowel dilatation with air-fluid levels consistent with a small-bowel obstruction; (***B***) a partial small-bowel obstruction from an incarcerated ventral hernia (*arrow*); and (***C***) decompressed bowel seen distal to the hernia (*arrow*). *(From W Silen: Acute intestinal obstruction, in DL Longo et al [eds]: Harrison's Principles of Internal Medicine, 18th ed. New York, McGraw-Hill, 2012.)*

TREATMENT ACUTE INTESTINAL OBSTRUCTION

An improved understanding of the pathophysiology of bowel obstruction and the importance of fluid resuscitation, electrolyte repletion, intestinal decompression, and the selected use of antibiotics have likely contributed to a reduction in the mortality from acute bowel obstruction. Every patient should be stabilized as quickly as possible. Nasogastric tube suction decompresses the stomach, minimizes further distention from swallowed air, improves patient comfort, and reduces the risk of aspiration. Urine output should be assessed using a Foley catheter. In some cases, for example, in patients with cardiac disease, central venous pressures should be monitored. The use of antibiotics is controversial, although prophylactic administration is warranted if surgery is required. Complete bowel obstruction is an indication for intervention. Stenting may be possible and warranted for some patients with high-grade obstruction due to unresectable stage IV malignancy. Stenting may also allow elective mechanical bowel preparation before surgery is undertaken. Because treatment options are so variable, it is helpful to make as precise a diagnosis as possible preoperatively.

ILEUS

Patients with ileus are treated supportively with intravenous fluids and nasogastric decompression while any underlying pathology is treated. Pharmacologic therapy is not yet proven to be efficacious or cost-effective. However, peripherally active μ-opioid receptor antagonists (e.g., alvimopan and methylnaltrexone) may accelerate gastrointestinal recovery in some patients who have undergone abdominal surgery.

COLONIC PSEUDO-OBSTRUCTION (OGILVIE'S DISEASE)

Neostigmine is an acetylcholinsterase inhibitor that increases cholinergic (parasympathetic) activity, which can stimulate colonic motility. Some studies have shown it to be moderately effective in alleviating acute colonic pseudo-obstruction. It is the most common therapeutic approach and can be used once it is certain that there is no mechanical obstruction. Cardiac monitoring is required, and atropine should be immediately available. Intravenous administration induces defecation and flatus within 10 min in the majority of patients who will respond. Sympathetic blockade by epidural anesthesia can successfully ameliorate pseudo-obstruction in some patients.

VOLVULUS

Patients with sigmoid volvulus can often be decompressed using a flexible tube inserted through a rigid proctoscope or using a flexible sigmoidoscope. Successful decompression results in sudden release of gas and fluid with evidence of decreased abdominal distension and allows definitive correction to be scheduled electively. Cecal volvulus most often requires laparotomy or laparoscopic correction.

INTRAOPERATIVE STRATEGIES

Approximately 60–80% of selected patients with mechanical bowel obstruction can be successfully treated conservatively. Indeed, most cases of radiation-induced obstruction should also be managed nonoperatively if possible. In most circumstances, early consultation with a general surgeon is prudent when there is concern about strangulation obstruction or other abnormality that needs to be addressed urgently. Deterioration signifies a need for intervention. At this time, the decision as to whether the patient can continue to be treated nonoperatively can only be based on clinical judgment, although, as described earlier, imaging studies can sometimes be helpful. The frequency of major complications after operation ranges from 12 to 47%, with greater risk being attributed to resection therapies and the patient's overall health. Risk is increased for patients with American Society of Anesthesiologists (ASA) class III or higher.

At operation, dilation proximal to the site of blockage with distal collapse is a defining feature of bowel obstruction. Intraoperative strategies depend on the underlying problem and range from lysis of adhesions to resection with or without diverting ostomy to primary resection with anastomosis. Resection is warranted when there is concern about the bowel's viability after the obstructive process is relieved. Laparoscopic approaches can be useful for patients with early obstruction when extensive adhesions are not expected to be present. Some patients with high-grade obstruction secondary to malignant disease that is not amendable to resection will benefit from bypass procedures.

ADULT INTUSSUSCEPTION AND GALLSTONE ILEUS

Primary resection is prudent. Careful manual reduction of any involved bowel may limit the amount of intestine that needs to be removed. A proximal ostomy may be required if unprepped colon is involved. Only 60% of patients with gallstone ileus obstruct in the ileum. The most common site of intestinal obstruction in patients with gallstone "ileus" is the ileum (60% of patients). The gallstone enters the intestinal tract most often via a cholecystoduodenal fistula. It can usually be removed by operative enterolithotomy. Addressing the gallbladder disease during urgent or emergent surgery is not recommended.

POSTOPERATIVE BOWEL OBSTRUCTION

Early postoperative mechanical bowel obstruction is that which occurs within the first 6 weeks of operation. Most are partial and can be expected to resolve spontaneously. It tends to respond and behave differently from classic mechanical bowel obstruction and may be very difficult to distinguish from postoperative ileus. A higher index of suspicion for a definitive site of obstruction is warranted for patients who undergo laparoscopic surgical procedures. Patients who first had ileus and then subsequently develop obstructive symptoms after an initial return of normal bowel function are more likely to have true postoperative small-bowel obstruction. The longer it takes for a patient's obstructive symptoms to resolve after hospitalization, the more likely the patient is to require surgical intervention.

Acknowledgment

The wisdom and expertise of Dr. William Silen are gratefully acknowledged.

356 Acute Appendicitis and Peritonitis

Danny O. Jacobs

ACUTE APPENDICITIS

INCIDENCE AND EPIDEMIOLOGY

Appendicitis occurs more frequently in Westernized societies. Although its incidence is decreasing for uncertain reasons, acute appendicitis remains the most common emergency general surgical disease affecting the abdomen, with a rate of approximately 100 per 100,000 person-years in Europe and the Americas or about 11 cases per 10,000 people annually. Approximately 9% of men and 7% of women will experience an episode during their lifetime. Appendicitis occurs most commonly in 10- to 19-year-olds, although the average age at diagnosis appears to be gradually increasing, as is the frequency of the disease in African Americans, Asians, and Native Americans. Overall, 70% of patients are less than 30 years old and most are men; the male-to-female ratio is 1.4:1.

One of the more common complications and most important causes of excess morbidity and mortality is perforation, whether it is contained and localized or unconstrained within the peritoneal cavity. In contrast to the trend observed for appendicitis and appendectomy, the incidence of perforated appendicitis (~20 cases per 100,000 person-years) is increasing. The explanation for this phenomenon is unknown. Approximately 20% of all patients have evidence of perforation at presentation, but the percentage risk is much higher in patients under 5 or over 65 years of age.

PATHOGENESIS OF APPENDICITIS AND APPENDICEAL PERFORATION

Appendicitis was first described in 1886 by Reginald Fitz. Its etiology is still not completely understood. Fecaliths, incompletely digested food residue, lymphoid hyperplasia, intraluminal scarring, tumors, bacteria, viruses, and inflammatory bowel disease have all been associated with inflammation of the appendix and appendicitis.

Although not proven, obstruction of the appendiceal lumen is believed to be an important step in the development of appendicitis. In some cases, obstruction leads to bacterial overgrowth and luminal distension, with an increase in intraluminal pressure that can inhibit the flow of lymph and blood in some cases. Then, vascular thrombosis and ischemic necrosis with perforation of the distal appendix may occur. Any perforation that occurs near the base of the appendix should raise concerns about another disease process. Most patients who will perforate do so before they are evaluated by surgeons.

Appendiceal fecaliths (or appendicoliths) are found in approximately 50% of patients with gangrenous appendicitis who perforate but are rarely identified in those who have simple disease. As mentioned earlier, the incidence of perforated, but not simple, appendicitis is increasing. The rate of perforated and nonperforated appendicitis is correlated in men but not in women. Together these observations suggest that the underlying pathophysiologic processes are different and that simple appendicitis does not always progress to perforation. Furthermore, some cases of simple acute appendicitis may resolve spontaneously or with antibiotic therapy, and recurrent disease is remotely possible. The relative frequency of these events is unknown.

When perforation occurs, the resultant leak may be contained by the omentum or other surrounding tissues to form an abscess. Free perforation normally causes severe peritonitis. These patients may also develop infective suppurative thrombosis of the portal vein and its tributaries along with intrahepatic abscesses. The prognosis of the very unfortunate patients who develop this dreaded complication is very poor.

CLINICAL MANIFESTATIONS

More refined approaches to diagnosis, supportive care, and surgical intervention are likely responsible for the remarkable decrease in the risk of mortality from simple appendicitis to currently less than 1%. Nevertheless, it is still important to identify patients who might have appendicitis as early as possible to minimize their risk of developing complications. Patients who have had symptoms for more than 48 h are more likely to perforate.

Appendicitis should be included in the differential diagnosis of abdominal pain for every patient in any age group unless it is certain that the organ has been previously removed (Table 356-1).

The appendix's anatomical location, which varies, directly influences how the patient presents for care. Where the appendix can be "found" ranges from local differences in how the appendiceal body and tip lie relative to its attachment to the cecum (Figs. 356-1 and 356-2), to where the appendix is actually situated in the peritoneal cavity—for example, from its typical location in the right lower quadrant, to the pelvis, right flank, right upper quadrant (as may be observed during

TABLE 356-1 SOME CONDITIONS THAT MIMIC APPENDICITIS

Crohn's disease	Meckel's diverticulitis
Cholecystitis or other gallbladder disease	Mittelschmerz
	Mesenteric adenitis
Diverticulitis	Omental torsion
Ectopic pregnancy	Pancreatitis
Endometriosis	Lower lobe pneumonia
Gastroenteritis or colitis	Pelvic inflammatory disease
Gastric or duodenal ulceration	Ruptured ovarian cyst or other cystic disease of the ovaries
Hepatitis	
Kidney disease, including nephrolithiasis	Small-bowel obstruction
	Urinary tract infection
Liver abscess	

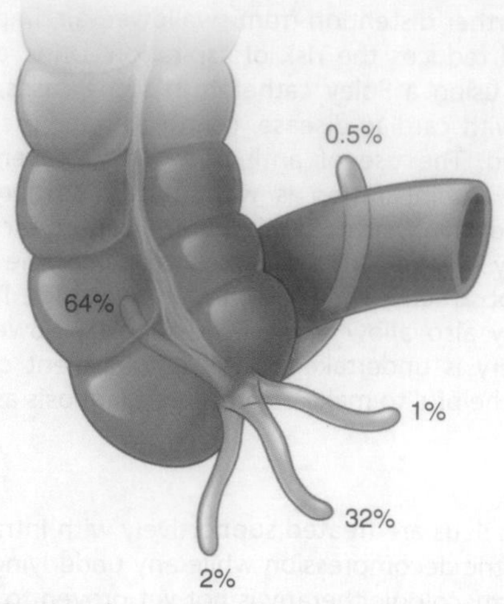

FIGURE 356-1 Regional anatomical variations of the appendix.

pregnancy), or even the left side of the abdomen for patients with malrotation or who have severely redundant colons.

Because the differential diagnosis of appendicitis is so extensive, deciding if a patient has appendicitis can be difficult (Table 356-2). Soliciting an appropriate history requires detecting symptoms that might suggest alternative diagnoses. Patients with appendicitis may not have any abdominal discomfort early in the disease process. Furthermore, many patients may not present with the classically described history or physical findings.

What is the classic history? Nonspecific complaints occur first. Patients may notice changes in bowel habits or malaise and vague, perhaps intermittent, crampy, abdominal pain in the epigastric or periumbilical region. The pain subsequently migrates to the right lower quadrant over 12–24 h, where it is sharper and can be definitively localized as transmural inflammation when the appendix irritates the parietal peritoneum. Parietal peritoneal irritation may be associated with local muscle rigidity and stiffness. Patients with appendicitis

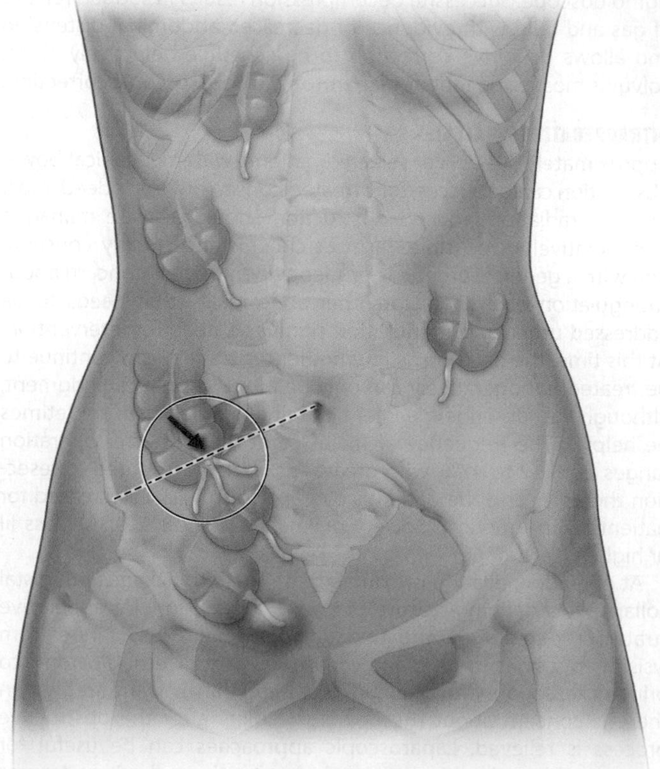

FIGURE 356-2 Locations of the appendix and cecum.

TABLE 356-2 RELATIVE FREQUENCY OF COMMON PRESENTING SYMPTOMS	
Symptoms	**Frequency**
Abdominal pain	>95%
Anorexia	>70%
Constipation	4–16%
Diarrhea	4–16%
Fever	10–20%
Migration of pain to right lower quadrant	50–60%
Nausea	>65%
Vomiting	50–75%

will most often observe that their nausea, if present, followed the development of abdominal pain, which can help distinguish them from patients with gastroenteritis, for example, where nausea occurs first. Emesis, if present, also occurs after the onset of pain and is typically mild and scant. Thus, timing of the onset of symptoms and the characteristics of the patient's pain and any associated findings must be rigorously assessed. Anorexia is so common that the diagnosis of appendicitis should be questioned in its absence.

Arriving at the correct diagnosis is even more challenging when the appendix is not located in the right lower quadrant, in women of childbearing age, and in the very young or elderly. Because the differential diagnosis of appendicitis is so broad, often the key question to answer expeditiously is whether the patient has appendicitis or some other condition that requires immediate operative intervention. A major concern is that the likelihood of a delay in diagnosis is greater if the appendix is unusually positioned. All patients should undergo a rectal examination. An inflamed appendix located behind the cecum or below the pelvic brim may prompt very little tenderness of the anterior abdominal wall.

Patients with pelvic appendicitis are more likely to present with dysuria, urinary frequency, diarrhea, or tenesmus. They may only experience pain in the suprapubic region on palpation or on rectal or pelvic examination. A pelvic examination in women is mandatory to rule out conditions affecting urogynecologic organs that can cause abdominal pain and mimic appendicitis such as pelvic inflammatory disease, ectopic pregnancy, and ovarian torsion. The relative frequencies of some presenting signs are displayed in Table 356-3.

Patients with simple appendicitis normally only appear mildly ill with a pulse and temperature that are usually only slightly above normal. The provider should be concerned about other disease processes beside appendicitis or the presence of complications such as perforation, phlegmon, or abscess formation if the temperature is >38.3°C (~101°F) and if there are rigors.

Patients with appendicitis will be found to lie quite still to avoid peritoneal irritation caused by movement, and some will report discomfort caused by a bumpy car ride on the way to the hospital or clinic, coughing, sneezing, or other actions that replicate a Valsalva maneuver. The entire abdomen should be examined systematically starting in an area where the patient does not report discomfort if

TABLE 356-3 RELATIVE FREQUENCY OF SOME PRESENTING SIGNS	
Signs	**Frequency (%)**
Abdominal tenderness	>95%
Right lower quadrant tenderness	>90%
Rebound tenderness	30–70%
Rectal tenderness	30–40%
Cervical motion tenderness	30%
Rigidity	~10%
Psoas sign	3–5%
Obturator sign	5–10%
Rovsing's sign	5%
Palpable mass	<5%

TABLE 356-4 CLASSIC SIGNS OF APPENDICITIS IN PATIENTS WITH ABDOMINAL PAIN	
Maneuver	**Findings**
Rovsing's sign	Palpating in the left lower quadrant causes pain in the right lower quadrant
Obturator sign	Internal rotation of the hip causes pain, suggesting the possibility of an inflamed appendix located in the pelvis
Iliopsoas sign	Extending the right hip causes pain along posterolateral back and hip, suggesting retrocecal appendicitis

possible. Classically, maximal tenderness is identified in the right lower quadrant at or near McBurney's point, which is located approximately one-third of the way along a line originating at the anterior iliac spine and running to the umbilicus. Gentle pressure in the left lower quadrant may elicit pain in the right lower quadrant if the appendix is located there. This is Rovsing's sign (Table 356-4). Evidence of parietal peritoneal irritation is often best elicited by gentle abdominal percussion, jiggling the patient's gurney or bed, or mildly bumping the feet.

Atypical presentation and pain patterns are common, especially in the very old or the very young. Diagnosing appendicitis in children can be especially challenging because they tend to respond so dramatically to stimulation and obtaining an accurate history may be difficult. In addition, it is important to remember that the smaller omentum found in children may be less likely to wall off an appendiceal perforation. Observing the child in a quiet surrounding may be helpful.

Signs and symptoms of appendicitis can be subtle in the elderly who may not react as vigorously to appendicitis as younger people. Pain, if noticed, may be minimal and have originated in the right lower quadrant or, otherwise, where the appendix is located. It may never have been noticed to be intermittent, or there may only be significant discomfort with deep palpation. Nausea, anorexia, and emesis may be the predominant complaints. The rare patient may even present with signs and symptoms of distal bowel obstruction secondary to appendiceal inflammation and phlegmon or abscess formation.

LABORATORY TESTING

Laboratory testing does not identify patients with appendicitis but can help the clinician work through the differential diagnosis. The white blood cell count is only mildly to moderately elevated in approximately 70% of patients with simple appendicitis (with a leukocytosis of 10,000–18,000 cells/μL). A "left shift" toward immature polymorphonuclear leukocytes is present in >95% of cases. A sickle cell preparation may be prudent to obtain in those of African, Spanish, Mediterranean, or Indian ancestry. Serum amylase and lipase levels should be measured.

Urinalysis is indicated to help exclude genitourinary conditions that may mimic acute appendicitis, but a few red or white blood cells may be present as a nonspecific finding. However, an inflamed appendix that abuts the ureter or bladder may cause sterile pyuria or hematuria. Every woman of childbearing age should have a pregnancy test. Cervical cultures are indicated if pelvic inflammatory disease is suspected. Anemia and guaiac-positive stools should raise concern about the presence of other diseases or complications such as cancer.

IMAGING

Plain films of the abdomen are rarely helpful and so are not routinely obtained unless the clinician is worried about other conditions such as intestinal obstruction, perforated viscus, or ureterolithiasis. Less than 5% of patients will present with an opaque fecalith in the right lower quadrant. The presence of a fecalith is not diagnostic of appendicitis, although its presence in an appropriate location where the patient complains of pain is suggestive.

The effectiveness of ultrasonography as a tool to diagnosis appendicitis is highly operator dependent. Even in very skilled hands, the appendix may not be visualized. Its overall sensitivity is 0.86, with a

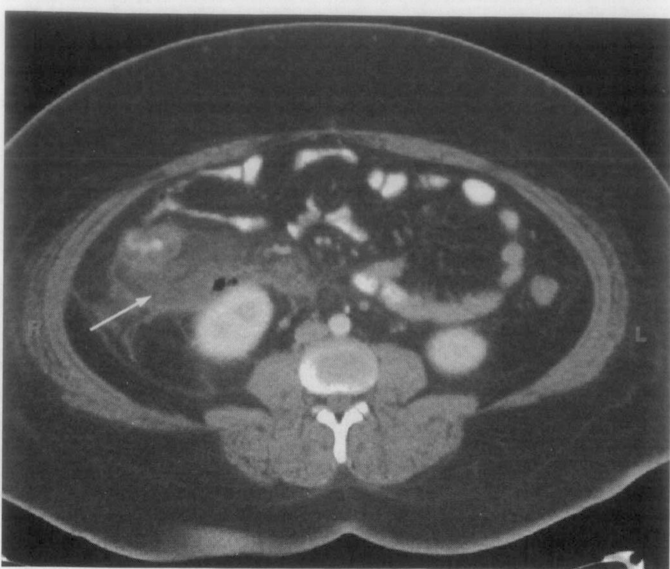

FIGURE 356-3 Computed tomography with oral and intravenous contrast of acute appendicitis. There is thickening of the wall of the appendix and periappendiceal stranding (*arrow*).

specificity of 0.81. Ultrasonography, especially intravaginal techniques, appears to be most useful for identifying pelvic pathology in women. Ultrasonographic findings suggesting the presence of appendicitis include wall thickening, an increased appendiceal diameter, and the presence of free fluid.

The sensitivity and specificity of computed tomography (CT) are 0.94 and 0.95, respectively. Thus, CT imaging, given its high negative predictive value, may be helpful if the diagnosis is in doubt, although studies performed early in the course of disease may not have any typical radiographic findings. Suggestive findings on CT examination include dilatation >6 mm with wall thickening, a lumen that does not fill with enteric contrast, and fatty tissue stranding or air surrounding the appendix, which suggests inflammation (Figs. 356-3 and 356-4). The presence of luminal air or contrast is not consistent with a diagnosis of appendicitis. Furthermore, nonvisualization of the appendix is a nonspecific finding that should not be used to rule out the presence of appendiceal or periappendiceal inflammation.

SPECIAL PATIENT POPULATIONS

Appendicitis in the most common extrauterine general surgical emergency observed during pregnancy. Early symptoms of appendicitis such as nausea and anorexia may be overlooked. Diagnosing appendicitis in pregnant patients may be especially difficult because as the uterus enlarges the appendix may be pushed higher along the right flank even to the right upper quadrant or because the gravid uterus may obscure typical physical findings. Ultrasonography may facilitate early diagnosis. A high index of suspicion is required because of the effects of unrecognized and untreated appendicitis on the fetus. For example, the fetal mortality rate is four times greater (from 5 to 20%) in patients with perforation.

Immunocompromised patients may present with only mild tenderness and may have many other disease processes in their differential diagnosis, including atypical infections from mycobacteria, *Cytomegalovirus*, or other fungi. Enterocolitis is a concern and may be present in patients who present with abdominal pain, fever, and neutropenia due to chemotherapy. CT imaging may be very helpful, although it is important not to be overly cautious and delay operative intervention for those patients who are believed to have appendicitis.

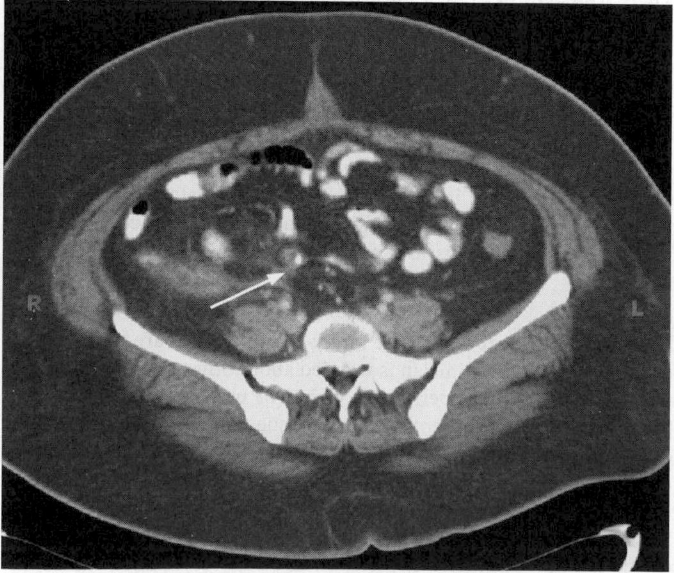

FIGURE 356-4 Appendiceal fecalith (*arrow*).

TREATMENT ACUTE APPENDICITIS

In the absence of contraindications, a patient who has a strongly suggestive medical history and physical examination with supportive laboratory findings should undergo appendectomy urgently. In this instance, imaging studies are not required. In patients in whom the evaluation is suggestive but not convincing, imaging and further study are appropriate. Pelvic ultrasonography is indicated in women of childbearing age. Thereafter, CT may accurately indicate the presence of appendicitis or other intraabdominal processes that warrant intervention. Whenever the diagnosis is uncertain, it is prudent to observe the patient and repeat the abdominal examination over 6–8 h. Any evidence of progression is an indication for operation. Narcotics can be given to patients with severe discomfort, especially if the first abdominal examination is completed before drugs are administered.

All patients should be fully prepared for surgery and have any fluid and electrolyte abnormalities corrected. Either laparoscopic or open appendectomy is a satisfactory choice for patients with uncomplicated appendicitis. Management of those who present with a mass representing a phlegmon or abscess can be more difficult. Such patients are best served by treatment with broad-spectrum antibiotics, drainage if there is an abscess >3 cm in diameter, and parenteral fluids and bowel rest if they appear to respond to conservative management. The appendix can then be more safely removed 6–12 weeks later when inflammation has diminished.

Laparoscopic appendectomy now accounts for approximately 60% of all appendectomies. Laparoscopic appendectomy is associated with less postoperative pain and, possibly, a shorter length of stay and faster return to normal activity. Patients who undergo laparoscopic appendectomy also appear to have fewer wound infections, although the risk of intraabdominal abscess formation may be higher. A laparoscopic approach may also be useful when the exact diagnosis is uncertain, yet direct visualization and exploration of the abdomen are needed. A laparoscopic approach may also facilitate exposure in those who are very obese. A thorough examination of the abdomen is indicated if the appendix appears normal at operation, which can be expected to occur in up to 15–20% of cases.

Absent complications, most patients can be discharged within 24–40 h of operation. The most common postoperative complications are fever and leukocytosis. Continuation of these findings beyond 5 days should raise concern for the presence of an intraabdominal abscess. The mortality rate for uncomplicated, nonperforated appendicitis is 0.1–0.5%, which approximates the overall risk of general anesthesia. The mortality rate for perforated appendicitis or other complicated disease is much higher, ranging from 3% overall to a high as 15% in the elderly.

ACUTE PERITONITIS

Acute peritonitis, or inflammation of the visceral and parietal peritoneum, is most often but not always infectious in origin, resulting from perforation of a hollow viscus. This is called *secondary peritonitis*, as opposed to *primary* or *spontaneous peritonitis*, when a specific intraabdominal source cannot be identified. In either instance, the inflammation can be localized or diffuse.

ETIOLOGY

Infective organisms may contaminate the peritoneal cavity after spillage from a hollow viscus, because of a penetrating wound of the abdominal wall, or because of the introduction of a foreign object like a peritoneal dialysis catheter or port that becomes infected. Secondary peritonitis most commonly results from perforation of the appendix, colonic diverticuli, or the stomach and duodenum. It may also occur as a complication of bowel infarction or incarceration, cancer, inflammatory bowel disease, and intestinal obstruction or volvulus. Conditions that may cause secondary bacterial peritonitis and their mechanisms are listed in Table 356-5. Over 90% of the cases of primary or spontaneous bacterial peritonitis occur in patients with ascites or hypoproteinemia (<1 g/L).

TABLE 356-5 CONDITIONS LEADING TO SECONDARY BACTERIAL PERITONITIS

Bowel Perforation	Perforation or Leakage of Other Organs
Appendicitis trauma (blunt or penetrating)	Biliary leakage (e.g., after liver biopsy)
Anastomotic leakage	Cholecystitis
Adhesion	Intraperitoneal bleeding
Diverticulitis	Pancreatitis
Iatrogenic (including endoscopic perforation)	Salpingitis
Ingested foreign body	Traumatic or other rupture of urinary bladder
Inflammation	
Intussusception	**Loss of peritoneal integrity**
Neoplasms	Intraperitoneal chemotherapy
Obstruction	Iatrogenic (e.g., postoperative foreign body)
Peptic ulcer disease	Perinephric abscess
Strangulated hernia	Peritoneal dialysis or other indwelling devices
Vascular (including ischemia or embolus)	Trauma

Aseptic peritonitis is most commonly caused by the abnormal presence of physiologic fluids like gastric juice, bile, pancreatic enzymes, blood, or urine. It can also be caused by the effects of normally sterile foreign bodies like surgical sponges or instruments. More rarely, it occurs as a complication of systemic diseases like lupus erythematosus, porphyria, and familial Mediterranean fever. The chemical irritation caused by stomach acid and activated pancreatic enzymes is extreme and secondary bacterial infection may occur.

CLINICAL FEATURES

The cardinal signs and symptoms of peritonitis are acute, typically severe, abdominal pain with tenderness and fever. How the patient's complaints of pain are manifested depends on their overall physical health and whether the inflammation is diffuse or localized. Elderly and immunosuppressed patients may not respond as aggressively to the irritation. Diffuse, generalized peritonitis is most often recognized as diffuse abdominal tenderness with local guarding, rigidity, and other evidence of parietal peritoneal irritation. Physical findings may only be identified in a specific region of the abdomen if the intraperitoneal inflammatory process is limited or otherwise contained as may occur in patients with uncomplicated appendicitis or diverticulitis. Bowel sounds are usually absent to hypoactive.

Most patients present with tachycardia and signs of volume depletion with hypotension. Laboratory testing typically reveals a significant leukocytosis, and patients may be severely acidotic. Radiographic studies may show dilatation of the bowel and associated bowel wall edema. Free air, or other evidence of leakage, requires attention and could represent a surgical emergency. In stable patients in whom ascites is present, diagnostic paracentesis is indicated, where the fluid is tested for protein and lactate dehydrogenase and the cell count is measured.

THERAPY AND PROGNOSIS

Whereas mortality rates can be less than 10% for reasonably healthy patients with relatively uncomplicated, localized peritonitis, mortality rates >40% have been reported for the elderly or immunocompromised. Successful treatment depends on correcting any electrolyte abnormalities, restoration of fluid volume and stabilization of the cardiovascular system, appropriate antibiotic therapy, and surgical correction of any underlying abnormalities.

ACKNOWLEDGMENT

The wisdom and expertise of Dr. William Silen is gratefully acknowledged in this updated chapter on acute appendicitis and peritonitis.

SECTION 2 LIVER AND BILIARY TRACT DISEASE

357 Approach to the Patient with Liver Disease

Marc G. Ghany, Jay H. Hoofnagle

A diagnosis of liver disease usually can be made accurately by careful elicitation of the patient's history, physical examination, and application of a few laboratory tests. In some circumstances, radiologic examinations are helpful or, indeed, diagnostic. Liver biopsy is considered the criterion standard in evaluation of liver disease but is now needed less for diagnosis than for grading and staging of disease. This chapter provides an introduction to diagnosis and management of liver disease, briefly reviewing the structure and function of the liver; the major clinical manifestations of liver disease; and the use of clinical history, physical examination, laboratory tests, imaging studies, and liver biopsy.

LIVER STRUCTURE AND FUNCTION

The liver is the largest organ of the body, weighing 1–1.5 kg and representing 1.5–2.5% of the lean body mass. The size and shape of the liver vary and generally match the general body shape—long and lean or squat and square. This organ is located in the right upper quadrant of the abdomen under the right lower rib cage against the diaphragm and projects for a variable extent into the left upper quadrant. It is held in place by ligamentous attachments to the diaphragm, peritoneum, great vessels, and upper gastrointestinal organs. The liver receives a dual blood supply; ~20% of the blood flow is oxygen-rich blood from the hepatic artery, and 80% is nutrient-rich blood from the portal vein arising from the stomach, intestines, pancreas, and spleen.

The majority of cells in the liver are hepatocytes, which constitute two-thirds of the organ's mass. The remaining cell types are Kupffer cells (members of the reticuloendothelial system), stellate (Ito or fat-storing) cells, endothelial and blood vessel cells, bile ductular cells, and cells of supporting structures. Viewed by light microscopy, the liver appears to be organized in lobules, with portal areas at the periphery and central veins in the center of each lobule. However, from a functional point of view, the liver is organized into acini, with both hepatic arterial and portal venous blood entering the acinus from the portal areas (zone 1) and then flowing through the sinusoids to the terminal hepatic veins (zone 3); the intervening hepatocytes constitute zone 2. The advantage of viewing the acinus as the physiologic unit of the liver is that this perspective helps to explain the morphologic patterns and zonality of many vascular and biliary diseases not explained by the lobular arrangement.

Portal areas of the liver consist of small veins, arteries, bile ducts, and lymphatics organized in a loose stroma of supporting matrix and small amounts of collagen. Blood flowing into the portal areas is distributed through the sinusoids, passing from zone 1 to zone 3 of the acinus and draining into the terminal hepatic veins ("central veins"). Secreted bile flows in the opposite direction—i.e., in a counter-current pattern from zone 3 to zone 1. The sinusoids are lined by unique endothelial cells that have prominent fenestrae of variable sizes, allowing the free flow of plasma but not of cellular elements. The plasma is thus in direct contact with hepatocytes in the subendothelial space of Disse.

Hepatocytes have distinct polarity. The basolateral side of the hepatocyte lines the space of Disse and is richly lined with microvilli; it exhibits endocytotic and pinocytotic activity, with passive and active uptake of nutrients, proteins, and other molecules. The apical pole of the hepatocyte forms the canalicular membranes through which bile components are secreted. The canaliculi of hepatocytes form a fine network, which fuses into the bile ductular elements near the portal areas. Kupffer cells usually lie within the sinusoidal vascular space and represent the largest group of fixed macrophages in the body. The stellate cells are located in the space of Disse but are not usually prominent unless activated, when they produce collagen and matrix. Red blood cells stay in the sinusoidal space as blood flows through the lobules, but white blood cells can migrate through or around endothelial cells into the space of Disse and from there to portal areas, where they can return to the circulation through lymphatics.

Hepatocytes perform numerous and vital roles in maintaining homeostasis and health. These functions include the synthesis of most essential serum proteins (albumin, carrier proteins, coagulation factors, many hormonal and growth factors), the production of bile and its carriers (bile acids, cholesterol, lecithin, phospholipids), the regulation of nutrients (glucose, glycogen, lipids, cholesterol, amino acids), and the metabolism and conjugation of lipophilic compounds (bilirubin, anions, cations, drugs) for excretion in the bile or urine. Measurement of these activities to assess liver function is complicated by the multiplicity and variability of these functions. The most commonly used liver "function" tests are measurements of serum bilirubin, serum albumin, and prothrombin time. The serum bilirubin level is a measure of hepatic conjugation and excretion; the serum albumin level and prothrombin time are measures of protein synthesis. Abnormalities of bilirubin, albumin, and prothrombin time are typical of hepatic dysfunction. Frank liver failure is incompatible with life, and the functions of the liver are too complex and diverse to be subserved by a mechanical pump; a dialysis membrane; or a concoction of infused hormones, proteins, and growth factors.

TABLE 357-1 LIVER DISEASES

Inherited hyperbilirubinemia
- Gilbert's syndrome
- Crigler-Najjar syndrome, types I and II
- Dubin-Johnson syndrome
- Rotor syndrome

Viral hepatitis
- Hepatitis A
- Hepatitis B
- Hepatitis C
- Hepatitis D
- Hepatitis E
- Others (Epstein-Barr virus [mononucleosis] herpesvirus, adenovirus hepatitis)
- Cryptogenic hepatitis

Immune and autoimmune liver diseases
- Primary biliary cirrhosis
- Autoimmune hepatitis
- Sclerosing cholangitis
- Overlap syndromes
- Graft-versus-host disease
- Allograft rejection

Genetic liver diseases
- α_1 Antitrypsin deficiency
- Hemochromatosis
- Wilson's disease
- Benign recurrent intrahepatic cholestasis
- Progressive familial intrahepatic cholestasis, types I–III
- Others (galactosemia, tyrosinemia, cystic fibrosis, Newman-Pick disease, Gaucher's disease)

Alcoholic liver disease
- Acute fatty liver
- Acute alcoholic hepatitis
- Laënnec's cirrhosis

Nonalcoholic fatty liver
- Steatosis
- Steatohepatitis

Acute fatty liver of pregnancy

Liver involvement in systemic diseases
- Sarcoidosis
- Amyloidosis
- Glycogen storage diseases
- Celiac disease
- Tuberculosis
- *Mycobacterium avium-intracellulare* infection

Cholestatic syndromes
- Benign postoperative cholestasis
- Jaundice of sepsis
- Total parenteral nutrition–induced jaundice
- Cholestasis of pregnancy
- Cholangitis and cholecystitis
- Extrahepatic biliary obstruction (stone, stricture, cancer)
- Biliary atresia
- Caroli's disease
- Cryptosporidiosis

Drug-induced liver disease
- Hepatocellular patterns (isoniazid, acetaminophen)
- Cholestatic patterns (methyltestosterone)
- Mixed patterns (sulfonamides, phenytoin)
- Micro- and macrovesicular steatosis (methotrexate, fialuridine)

Vascular injury
- Veno-occlusive disease
- Budd-Chiari syndrome
- Ischemic hepatitis
- Passive congestion
- Portal vein thrombosis
- Nodular regenerative hyperplasia

Mass lesions
- Hepatocellular carcinoma
- Cholangiocarcinoma
- Adenoma
- Focal nodular hyperplasia
- Metastatic tumors
- Abscess
- Cysts
- Hemangioma

LIVER DISEASES

While there are many causes of liver disease (Table 357-1), these disorders generally present clinically in a few distinct patterns and are usually classified as hepatocellular, cholestatic (obstructive), or mixed. In *hepatocellular diseases* (such as viral hepatitis and alcoholic liver disease), features of liver injury, inflammation, and necrosis predominate. In *cholestatic diseases* (such as gallstone or malignant obstruction, primary biliary cirrhosis, and some drug-induced liver diseases), features of inhibition of bile flow predominate. In a mixed pattern, features of both hepatocellular and cholestatic injury are present (such as in cholestatic forms of viral hepatitis and many drug-induced liver diseases). The pattern of onset and prominence of symptoms can rapidly suggest a diagnosis, particularly if major risk factors are considered, such as the age and sex of the patient and a history of exposure or risk behaviors.

Typical presenting symptoms of liver disease include jaundice, fatigue, itching, right-upper-quadrant pain, nausea, poor appetite, abdominal distention, and intestinal bleeding. At present, however, many patients are diagnosed with liver disease who have no symptoms and who have been found to have abnormalities in biochemical liver tests as a part of a routine physical examination or screening for blood donation or for insurance or employment. The wide availability of batteries of liver tests makes it relatively simple to demonstrate the presence of liver injury as well as to rule it out in someone in whom liver disease is suspected.

Evaluation of patients with liver disease should be directed at (1) establishing the etiologic diagnosis, (2) estimating disease severity (*grading*), and (3) establishing the disease stage (*staging*). *Diagnosis* should focus on the category of disease (hepatocellular, cholestatic, or mixed injury) as well as on the specific etiologic diagnosis. *Grading* refers to assessment of the severity or activity of disease—active or inactive as well as mild, moderate, or severe. *Staging* refers to estimation of the point in the course of the natural history of the disease, whether early or late; or precirrhotic, cirrhotic, or end-stage. This chapter introduces general, salient concepts in the evaluation of patients with liver disease that help lead to the diagnoses discussed in subsequent chapters.

CLINICAL HISTORY

The clinical history should focus on the symptoms of liver disease—their nature, patterns of onset, and progression—and on potential risk factors for liver disease. The manifestations of liver disease include constitutional symptoms such as fatigue, weakness, nausea, poor appetite, and malaise and the more liver-specific symptoms of jaundice, dark urine, light stools, itching, abdominal pain, and bloating. Symptoms can also suggest the presence of cirrhosis, end-stage liver disease, or complications of cirrhosis such as portal hypertension. Generally, the constellation of symptoms and their patterns of onset rather than a specific symptom points to an etiology.

Fatigue is the most common and most characteristic symptom of liver disease. It is variously described as lethargy, weakness, listlessness, malaise, increased need for sleep, lack of stamina, and poor energy. The fatigue of liver disease typically arises after activity or exercise and is rarely present or severe after adequate rest; i.e., it is "afternoon" rather than "morning" fatigue. Fatigue in liver disease is often intermittent and variable in severity from hour to hour and day to day. In some patients, it may not be clear whether fatigue is due to the liver disease or to other problems such as stress, anxiety, sleep disturbance, or a concurrent illness.

Nausea occurs with more severe liver disease and may accompany fatigue or be provoked by smelling food odors or eating fatty foods. Vomiting can occur but is rarely persistent or prominent. Poor appetite with weight loss occurs frequently in acute liver disease but is rare in chronic disease except when cirrhosis is present and advanced. Diarrhea is uncommon in liver disease except with severe jaundice, in which a lack of bile acids reaching the intestine can lead to steatorrhea.

Right-upper-quadrant discomfort or ache ("liver pain") occurs in many liver diseases and is usually marked by tenderness over the liver area. The pain arises from stretching or irritation of Glisson's capsule, which surrounds the liver and is rich in nerve endings. Severe pain is most typical of gallbladder disease, liver abscess, and severe veno-occlusive disease but is also an occasional accompaniment of acute hepatitis.

Itching occurs with acute liver disease, appearing early in obstructive jaundice (from biliary obstruction or drug-induced cholestasis) and somewhat later in hepatocellular disease (acute hepatitis). Itching also occurs in chronic liver diseases—typically the cholestatic forms such as primary biliary cirrhosis and sclerosing cholangitis, in which it is often the presenting symptom, preceding the onset of jaundice. However, itching can occur in any liver disease, particularly once cirrhosis develops.

Jaundice is the hallmark symptom of liver disease and perhaps the most reliable marker of severity. Patients usually report darkening of the urine before they notice scleral icterus. Jaundice is rarely detectable with a bilirubin level <43 μmol/L (2.5 mg/dL). With severe cholestasis, there will also be lightening of the color of the stools and steatorrhea. Jaundice without dark urine usually indicates indirect (unconjugated) hyperbilirubinemia and is typical of hemolytic anemia and the genetic disorders of bilirubin conjugation, the common and benign form being Gilbert's syndrome and the rare and severe form being Crigler-Najjar syndrome. Gilbert's syndrome affects up to 5% of the general population; the jaundice in this condition is more noticeable after fasting and with stress.

Major risk factors for liver disease that should be sought in the clinical history include details of alcohol use, medication use (including herbal compounds, birth control pills, and over-the-counter medications), personal habits, sexual activity, travel, exposure to jaundiced or other high-risk persons, injection drug use, recent surgery, remote or recent transfusion of blood or blood products, occupation, accidental exposure to blood or needlestick, and familial history of liver disease.

For assessing the risk of viral hepatitis, a careful history of sexual activity is of particular importance and should include the number of lifetime sexual partners and, for men, a history of having sex with men. Sexual exposure is a common mode of spread of hepatitis B but is rare for hepatitis C. A family history of hepatitis, liver disease, and liver cancer is also important. Maternal-infant transmission occurs with both hepatitis B and C. Vertical spread of hepatitis B can now be prevented by passive and active immunization of the infant at birth. Vertical spread of hepatitis C is uncommon, but there are no reliable means of prevention. Transmission is more common among HIV-coinfected mothers and is also linked to prolonged and difficult labor and delivery, early rupture of membranes, and internal fetal monitoring. A history of injection drug use, even in the remote past, is of great importance in assessing the risk for hepatitis B and C. Injection drug use is now the single most common risk factor for hepatitis C. Transfusion with blood or blood products is no longer an important risk factor for acute viral hepatitis. However, blood transfusions received before the introduction of sensitive enzyme immunoassays for antibody to hepatitis C virus in 1992 is an important risk factor for chronic hepatitis C. Blood transfusion before 1986, when screening for antibody to hepatitis B core antigen was introduced, is also a risk factor for hepatitis B. Travel to a developing area of the world, exposure to persons with jaundice, and exposure to young children in day-care centers are risk factors for hepatitis A. Tattooing and body piercing (for hepatitis B and C) and eating shellfish (for hepatitis A) are frequently mentioned but are actually types of exposure that quite rarely lead to the acquisition of hepatitis.

Hepatitis E is one of the more common causes of jaundice in Asia and Africa but is uncommon in developed nations. Recently, non-travel-related (*autochthonous*) cases of hepatitis E have been described in developed countries, including the United States. These cases appear to be due to strains of hepatitis E virus that are endemic in swine and some wild animals (genotypes 3 and 4). While occasional cases are associated with eating raw or undercooked pork or game (deer and wild boars), most cases of hepatitis E occur without known exposure, predominantly in elderly man without typical risk factors for viral hepatitis. Hepatitis E infection can become chronic in immunosuppressed individuals (such as transplant recipients, patients receiving chemotherapy, or patients with HIV infection), in whom it presents with abnormal serum enzymes in the absence of markers of hepatitis B or C.

A history of alcohol intake is important in assessing the cause of liver disease and also in planning management and recommendations. In the United States, for example, at least 70% of adults drink alcohol to some degree, but significant alcohol intake is less common; in population-based surveys, only 5% of individuals have more than two drinks per day, the average drink representing 11–15 g of alcohol. Alcohol consumption associated with an increased rate of alcoholic liver disease is probably more than two drinks (22–30 g) per day in women and three drinks (33–45 g) in men. Most patients with alcoholic cirrhosis have a much higher daily intake and have drunk excessively for ≥10 years before onset of liver disease. In assessing alcohol intake, the history should also focus on whether alcohol abuse or dependence is present. Alcoholism is usually defined by the behavioral patterns and consequences of alcohol intake, not by the amount. *Abuse* is defined by a repetitive pattern of drinking alcohol that has adverse effects on social, family, occupational, or health status. *Dependence* is defined by alcohol-seeking behavior, despite its adverse effects. Many

TABLE 357-2 CAGE QUESTIONS[a]

Acronym	Question
C	Have you ever felt you ought to cut down on your drinking?
A	Have people annoyed you by criticizing your drinking?
G	Have you ever felt guilty or bad about your drinking?
E	Have you ever had a drink first thing in the morning to steady your nerves or get rid of a hangover (eye-opener)?

[a]One "yes" response should raise suspicion of an alcohol use problem, and more than one is a strong indication of abuse or dependence.

alcoholics demonstrate both dependence and abuse, and dependence is considered the more serious and advanced form of alcoholism. A clinically helpful approach to diagnosis of alcohol dependence and abuse is the use of the CAGE questionnaire (Table 357-2), which is recommended for all medical history-taking.

Family history can be helpful in assessing liver disease. Familial causes of liver disease include Wilson's disease; hemochromatosis and α_1 antitrypsin deficiency; and the more uncommon inherited pediatric liver diseases—i.e., familial intrahepatic cholestasis, benign recurrent intrahepatic cholestasis, and Alagille syndrome. Onset of severe liver disease in childhood or adolescence in conjunction with a family history of liver disease or neuropsychiatric disturbance should lead to investigation for Wilson's disease. A family history of cirrhosis, diabetes, or endocrine failure and the appearance of liver disease in adulthood suggests hemochromatosis and should prompt investigation of iron status. Abnormal iron studies in adult patients warrant genotyping of the *HFE* gene for the C282Y and H63D mutations typical of genetic hemochromatosis. In children and adolescents with iron overload, other non-*HFE* causes of hemochromatosis should be sought. A family history of emphysema should provoke investigation of α_1 antitrypsin levels and, if levels are low, for protease inhibitor (Pi) genotype.

PHYSICAL EXAMINATION

The physical examination rarely uncovers evidence of liver dysfunction in a patient without symptoms or laboratory findings, nor are most signs of liver disease specific to one diagnosis. Thus, the physical examination complements rather than replaces the need for other diagnostic approaches. In many patients, the physical examination is normal unless the disease is acute or severe and advanced. Nevertheless, the physical examination is important in that it can yield the first evidence of hepatic failure, portal hypertension, and liver decompensation. In addition, the physical examination can reveal signs—related either to risk factors or to associated diseases or findings—that point to a specific diagnosis.

Typical physical findings in liver disease are icterus, hepatomegaly, hepatic tenderness, splenomegaly, spider angiomata, palmar erythema, and excoriations. Signs of advanced disease include muscle wasting, ascites, edema, dilated abdominal veins, hepatic fetor, asterixis, mental confusion, stupor, and coma. In male patients with cirrhosis, particularly that related to alcohol use, signs of hyperestrogenemia such as gynecomastia, testicular atrophy, and loss of male-pattern hair distribution may be found.

Icterus is best appreciated when the sclera is inspected under natural light. In fair-skinned individuals, a yellow tinge to the skin may be obvious. In dark-skinned individuals, examination of the mucous membranes below the tongue can demonstrate jaundice. Jaundice is rarely detectable if the serum bilirubin level is <43 μmol/L (2.5 mg/dL) but may remain detectable below this level during recovery from jaundice (because of protein and tissue binding of conjugated bilirubin).

Spider angiomata and palmar erythema occur in both acute and chronic liver disease; these manifestations may be especially prominent in persons with cirrhosis but can develop in normal individuals and are frequently found during pregnancy. Spider angiomata are superficial, tortuous arterioles and—unlike simple telangiectases—typically fill from the center outward. Spider angiomata occur only on the arms, face, and upper torso; they can be pulsatile and may be difficult to detect in dark-skinned individuals.

Hepatomegaly is not a highly reliable sign of liver disease because of variability in the liver's size and shape and the physical impediments to assessment of liver size by percussion and palpation. Marked hepatomegaly is typical of cirrhosis, veno-occlusive disease, infiltrative disorders such as amyloidosis, metastatic or primary cancers of the liver, and alcoholic hepatitis. Careful assessment of the liver edge may also reveal unusual firmness, irregularity of the surface, or frank nodules. Perhaps the most reliable physical finding in the liver examination is hepatic tenderness. Discomfort when the liver is touched or pressed upon should be carefully sought with percussive comparison of the right and left upper quadrants.

Splenomegaly, which occurs in many medical conditions, can be a subtle but significant physical finding in liver disease. The availability of ultrasound methods for assessment of the spleen allows confirmation of the physical finding.

Signs of advanced liver disease include muscle wasting and weight loss as well as hepatomegaly, bruising, ascites, and edema. Ascites is best appreciated by attempts to detect shifting dullness by careful percussion. Ultrasound examination will confirm the finding of ascites in equivocal cases. Peripheral edema can occur with or without ascites. In patients with advanced liver disease, other factors frequently contribute to edema formation, including hypoalbuminemia, venous insufficiency, heart failure, and medications.

Hepatic failure is defined as the occurrence of signs or symptoms of hepatic encephalopathy in a person with severe acute or chronic liver disease. The first signs of hepatic encephalopathy can be subtle and nonspecific—change in sleep patterns, change in personality, irritability, and mental dullness. Thereafter, confusion, disorientation, stupor, and eventually coma supervene. In acute liver failure, excitability and mania may be present. Physical findings include asterixis and flapping tremors of the body and tongue. *Fetor hepaticus* refers to the slightly sweet, ammoniacal odor that can develop in patients with liver failure, particularly if there is portal-venous shunting of blood around the liver. Other causes of coma and disorientation should be excluded, mainly electrolyte imbalances, sedative use, and renal or respiratory failure. The appearance of hepatic encephalopathy during acute hepatitis is the major criterion for diagnosis of fulminant hepatitis and indicates a poor prognosis. In chronic liver disease, encephalopathy is usually triggered by a medical complication such as gastrointestinal bleeding, over-diuresis, uremia, dehydration, electrolyte imbalance, infection, constipation, or use of narcotic analgesics.

A helpful measure of hepatic encephalopathy is a careful mental-status examination and use of the trail-making test, which consists of a series of 25 numbered circles that the patient is asked to connect as rapidly as possible using a pencil. The normal range for the connect-the-dot test is 15–30 sec; it is considerably longer in patients with early hepatic encephalopathy. Other tests include drawing of abstract objects or comparison of a signature to previous examples. More sophisticated testing—e.g., with electroencephalography and visual evoked potentials—can detect mild forms of encephalopathy but are rarely clinically useful.

Other signs of advanced liver disease include umbilical hernia from ascites, hydrothorax, prominent veins over the abdomen, and *caput medusa*, a condition that consists of collateral veins radiating from the umbilicus and results from recanulation of the umbilical vein. Widened pulse pressure and signs of a hyperdynamic circulation can occur in patients with cirrhosis as a result of fluid and sodium retention, increased cardiac output, and reduced peripheral resistance. Patients with long-standing cirrhosis and portal hypertension are prone to develop the hepatopulmonary syndrome, which is defined by the triad of liver disease, hypoxemia, and pulmonary arteriovenous shunting. The hepatopulmonary syndrome is characterized by platypnea and orthodeoxia: shortness of breath and oxygen desaturation that occur paradoxically upon the assumption of an upright position. Measurement of oxygen saturation by pulse oximetry is a reliable screening test for hepatopulmonary syndrome.

Several skin disorders and changes are common in liver disease. Hyperpigmentation is typical of advanced chronic cholestatic diseases such as primary biliary cirrhosis and sclerosing cholangitis. In these same conditions, xanthelasma and tendon xanthomata occur as a result of retention and high serum levels of lipids and cholesterol. Slate-gray pigmentation of the skin is also seen with hemochromatosis if iron levels are high for a prolonged period. Mucocutaneous vasculitis with palpable purpura, especially on the lower extremities, is typical of cryoglobulinemia of chronic hepatitis C but can also occur in chronic hepatitis B.

Some physical signs point to specific liver diseases. Kayser-Fleischer rings occur in Wilson's disease and consist of a golden-brown copper pigment deposited in Descemet's membrane at the periphery of the cornea; they are best seen by slit-lamp examination. Dupuytren contracture and parotid enlargement are suggestive of chronic alcoholism and alcoholic liver disease. In metastatic liver disease or primary hepatocellular carcinoma, signs of cachexia and wasting as well as firm hepatomegaly and a hepatic bruit may be prominent.

DIAGNOSIS OF LIVER DISEASE

The major causes of liver disease and key diagnostic features are outlined in Table 357-3, and an algorithm for evaluation of the patient with suspected liver disease is shown in Fig. 357-1. Specifics of diagnosis are discussed in later chapters. The most common causes of acute liver disease are viral hepatitis (particularly hepatitis A, B, and C), drug-induced liver injury, cholangitis, and alcoholic liver disease. Liver biopsy usually is not needed in the diagnosis and management of acute liver disease, exceptions being situations where the diagnosis remains unclear despite thorough clinical and laboratory investigation. Liver biopsy can be helpful in diagnosing drug-induced liver disease and acute alcoholic hepatitis.

The most common causes of chronic liver disease, in general order of frequency, are chronic hepatitis C, alcoholic liver disease, nonalcoholic steatohepatitis, chronic hepatitis B, autoimmune hepatitis, sclerosing cholangitis, primary biliary cirrhosis, hemochromatosis, and Wilson's disease. Hepatitis E virus is a rare cause of chronic hepatitis, with cases occurring mostly in persons who are immunosuppressed or immunodeficient. Strict diagnostic criteria have not been developed for most liver diseases, but liver biopsy plays an important role in the diagnosis of autoimmune hepatitis, primary biliary cirrhosis, nonalcoholic and alcoholic steatohepatitis, and Wilson's disease (with a quantitative hepatic copper level in the last instance).

TABLE 357-3 IMPORTANT DIAGNOSTIC TESTS IN COMMON LIVER DISEASES

Disease	Diagnostic Test
Hepatitis A	Anti-HAV IgM
Hepatitis B	
Acute	HBsAg and anti-HBc IgM
Chronic	HBsAg and HBeAg and/or HBV DNA
Hepatitis C	Anti-HCV and HCV RNA
Hepatitis D (delta)	HBsAg and anti-HDV
Hepatitis E	Anti-HEV IgM and HEV RNA
Autoimmune hepatitis	ANA or SMA, elevated IgG levels, and compatible histology
Primary biliary cirrhosis	Mitochondrial antibody, elevated IgM levels, and compatible histology
Primary sclerosing cholangitis	P-ANCA, cholangiography
Drug-induced liver disease	History of drug ingestion
Alcoholic liver disease	History of excessive alcohol intake and compatible histology
Nonalcoholic steatohepatitis	Ultrasound or CT evidence of fatty liver and compatible histology
α_1 Antitrypsin disease	Reduced α_1 antitrypsin levels, phenotype PiZZ or PiSZ
Wilson's disease	Decreased serum ceruloplasmin and increased urinary copper; increased hepatic copper level
Hemochromatosis	Elevated iron saturation and serum ferritin; genetic testing for *HFE* gene mutations
Hepatocellular cancer	Elevated α-fetoprotein level (to >500 ng/mL); ultrasound or CT image of mass

Abbreviations: HAV, HBV, HCV, HDV, HEV: hepatitis A, B, C, D, E virus; HBsAg, hepatitis B surface antigen; anti-HBc, antibody to hepatitis B core (antigen); HBeAg, hepatitis B e antigen; ANA, antinuclear antibody; SMA, smooth-muscle antibody; P-ANCA, peripheral antineutrophil cytoplasmic antibody.

Laboratory Testing Diagnosis of liver disease is greatly aided by the availability of reliable and sensitive tests of liver injury and function. A typical battery of blood tests used for initial assessment of liver disease includes measurement of levels of serum alanine and aspartate aminotransferases, alkaline phosphatase, direct and total serum bilirubin and albumin, and prothrombin time. The pattern of abnormalities generally points to hepatocellular versus cholestatic liver disease and helps determine whether the disease is acute or chronic and whether cirrhosis and hepatic failure are present. On the basis of these results, further testing over time may be necessary. Other laboratory tests may be helpful, such as γ-glutamyl transpeptidase to define whether alkaline phosphatase elevations are due to liver disease; hepatitis serology to define the type of viral hepatitis; and autoimmune markers to diagnose primary biliary cirrhosis (antimitochondrial antibody), sclerosing cholangitis (peripheral antineutrophil cytoplasmic antibody), and autoimmune hepatitis (antinuclear, smooth-muscle, and liver-kidney microsomal antibody). A simple delineation of laboratory abnormalities and common liver diseases is given in Table 357-3.

The use and interpretation of liver function tests are summarized in Chap. 358.

Diagnostic Imaging Great advances have been made in hepatobiliary imaging, although no method is adequately accurate in demonstrating underlying cirrhosis. Of the many modalities available for imaging the liver, ultrasound, CT, and MRI are the most commonly employed and are complementary to one another. In general, ultrasound and CT are highly sensitive for detecting biliary duct dilation and are the first-line options for investigating cases of suspected obstructive jaundice. All three modalities can detect a fatty liver, which appears bright on imaging studies. Modifications of CT and MRI can be used to quantify liver fat, and this information may ultimately be valuable in monitoring therapy in patients with fatty liver disease. Magnetic resonance cholangiopancreatography (MRCP) and endoscopic retrograde cholangiopancreatography (ERCP) are the procedures of choice for visualization of the biliary tree. MRCP offers several advantages over ERCP: there is no need for contrast media or ionizing radiation, images can be acquired faster, the procedure is less operator dependent, and it carries no risk of pancreatitis. MRCP is superior to ultrasound and CT for detecting choledocholithiasis but is less specific. MRCP is useful in the diagnosis of bile duct obstruction and congenital biliary abnormalities, but ERCP is more valuable in evaluating ampullary lesions and primary sclerosing cholangitis. ERCP permits biopsy, direct visualization of the ampulla and common bile duct, and intraductal ultrasonography. It also provides several therapeutic options in patients with obstructive jaundice, such as sphincterotomy, stone extraction, and placement of nasobiliary catheters and biliary stents. Doppler ultrasound and MRI are used to assess hepatic vasculature and hemodynamics and to monitor surgically or radiologically placed vascular shunts, including transjugular intrahepatic portosystemic shunts. Multidetector or spiral CT and MRI with contrast-enhancement are the procedures of choice for the identification and evaluation of hepatic masses, the staging of liver tumors, and preoperative assessment. With regard to mass lesions, the sensitivity of hepatic imaging continues to increase; unfortunately, specificity remains a problem, and often two and sometimes three studies are needed before a diagnosis can be reached. Recently, ultrasound transient elastography has been approved for the measurement of hepatic stiffness—providing an indirect assessment of cirrhosis; this technique can eliminate the need for liver biopsy if the only indication is the assessment of disease stage. Magnetic resonance elastography is now undergoing evaluation for its ability to detect different degrees of hepatic fibrosis. Studies are ongoing to determine whether hepatic elastography is an appropriate means of monitoring fibrosis and disease progression. Finally, interventional radiologic techniques allow the biopsy of solitary lesions, the radiofrequency

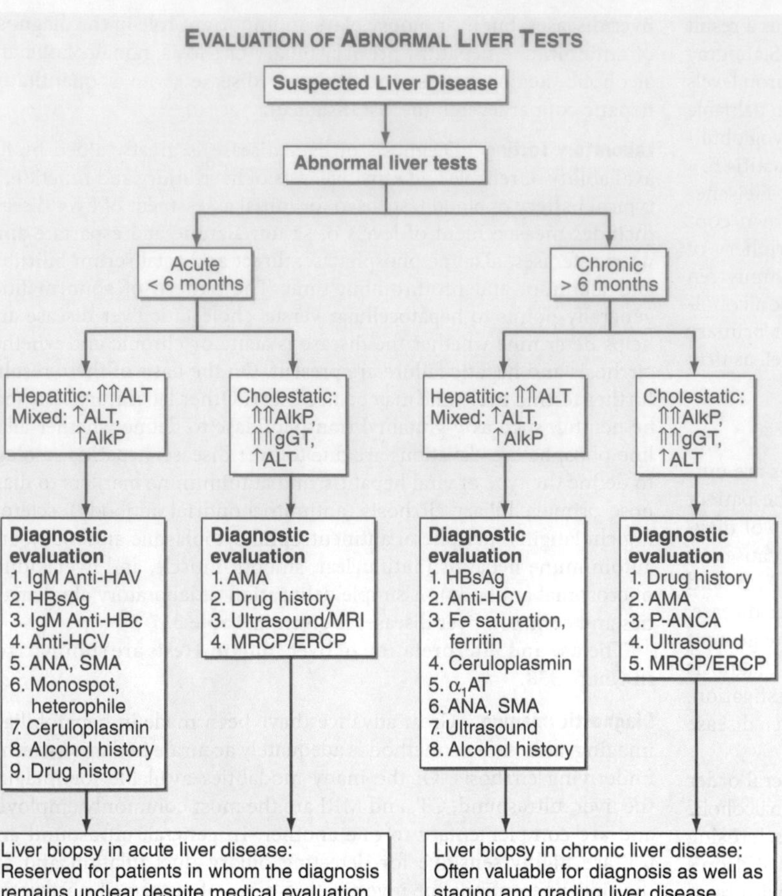

FIGURE 357-1 Algorithm for evaluation of abnormal liver tests. For patients with suspected liver disease, an appropriate approach to evaluation is initial routine liver testing—e.g., measurement of serum bilirubin, albumin, alanine aminotransferase (ALT), aspartate aminotransferase (AST), and alkaline phosphatase (AlkP). These results (sometimes complemented by testing of γ-glutamyl transpeptidase; gGT) will establish whether the pattern of abnormalities is hepatic, cholestatic, or mixed. In addition, the duration of symptoms or abnormalities will indicate whether the disease is acute or chronic. If the disease is acute and if history, laboratory tests, and imaging studies do not reveal a diagnosis, liver biopsy is appropriate to help establish the diagnosis. If the disease is chronic, liver biopsy can be helpful not only for diagnosis but also for grading of the activity and staging the progression of disease. This approach is generally applicable to patients without immune deficiency. In patients with HIV infection or recipients of bone marrow or solid organ transplants, the diagnostic evaluation should also include evaluation for opportunistic infections (e.g., with adenovirus, cytomegalovirus, *Coccidioides*, hepatitis E virus) as well as for vascular and immunologic conditions (veno-occlusive disease, graft-versus-host disease). HAV, hepatitis A virus; HCV, hepatitis C virus; HBsAg, hepatitis B surface antigen; anti-HBc, antibody to hepatitis B core (antigen); ANA, antinuclear antibody; SMA, smooth-muscle antibody; MRCP, magnetic resonance cholangiopancreatography; ERCP, endoscopic retrograde cholangiopancreatography; α_1AT, α_1 antitrypsin; AMA; antimitochondrial antibody; P-ANCA, peripheral antineutrophil cytoplasmic antibody.

ablation and chemoembolization of cancerous lesions, the insertion of drains into hepatic abscesses, the measurement of portal pressure, and the creation of vascular shunts in patients with portal hypertension. Which modality to use depends on factors such as availability, cost, and experience of the radiologist with each technique.

Liver Biopsy Liver biopsy remains the criterion standard in the evaluation of patients with liver disease, particularly chronic liver disease. Liver biopsy is necessary for diagnosis in selected instances but is more often useful for assessment of the severity (grade) and stage of liver damage, prediction of prognosis, and monitoring of the response to treatment. The size of the liver biopsy sample is an important determinant of reliability; a length of 1.5–2 cm is necessary for accurate assessment of fibrosis. In the future, noninvasive means of assessing disease activity (batteries of blood tests) and fibrosis (elastography and fibrosis markers) may replace liver biopsy for the staging and grading of disease.

GRADING AND STAGING OF LIVER DISEASE

Grading refers to an assessment of the severity or activity of liver disease, whether acute or chronic; active or inactive; and mild, moderate, or severe. Liver biopsy is the most accurate means of assessing severity, particularly in chronic liver disease. Serum aminotransferase levels serve as convenient and noninvasive markers for disease activity but do not always reliably reflect disease severity. Thus, normal serum aminotransferase levels in patients with hepatitis B surface antigen in serum may indicate the inactive carrier state or may reflect mild chronic hepatitis B or hepatitis B with fluctuating disease activity. Serum testing for hepatitis B e antigen and hepatitis B virus DNA can help sort out these different patterns, but these markers can also fluctuate and change over time. Similarly, in chronic hepatitis C, serum aminotransferase levels can be normal despite moderate disease activity. Finally, in both alcoholic and nonalcoholic steatohepatitis, aminotransferase levels are quite unreliable in reflecting severity. In these conditions, liver biopsy is helpful in guiding management and identifying appropriate therapy, particularly if treatment is difficult, prolonged, and expensive, as is often the case in chronic viral hepatitis. Of the several well-verified numerical scales for grading activity in chronic liver disease, the most commonly used are the histology activity index and the Ishak histology scale.

Liver biopsy is also the most accurate means of assessing stage of disease as early or advanced, precirrhotic, and cirrhotic. Staging of disease pertains largely to chronic liver diseases in which progression to cirrhosis and end-stage disease can occur but may require years or decades. Clinical features, biochemical tests, and hepatic imaging studies are helpful in assessing stage but generally become abnormal only in the middle to late stages of cirrhosis. Noninvasive tests that suggest advanced fibrosis include mild elevations of bilirubin, prolongation of prothrombin time, slight decreases in serum albumin, and mild thrombocytopenia (which is often the first indication of worsening fibrosis). Combinations of blood test results have been used to create models for predicting advanced liver disease, but these models are not reliable enough to use on a regular basis and only separate advanced from early disease. Recently, elastography and noninvasive breath tests using ^{13}C-labeled compounds have been proposed as a means of detecting early stages of fibrosis and liver dysfunction, but their reliability and reproducibility remain to be proven. Thus, at present, mild to moderate stages of hepatic fibrosis are detectable only by liver biopsy. In the assessment of stage, the degree of fibrosis is usually used as the quantitative measure. The amount of fibrosis is generally staged on a scale of 0 to 4+ (Metavir scale) or 0 to 6+ (Ishak scale). The importance of staging relates primarily to prognosis and to optimal management of complications. Patients with cirrhosis are candidates for screening and surveillance for esophageal varices and hepatocellular carcinoma. Patients without advanced fibrosis need not undergo screening.

Cirrhosis can also be staged clinically. A reliable staging system is the modified Child-Pugh classification, with a scoring system of 5–15: scores of 5 and 6 represent Child-Pugh class A (consistent with "compensated cirrhosis"), scores of 7–9 represent class B, and scores of 10–15 represent class C (Table 357-4). This scoring system was initially devised to stratify patients into risk groups before portal

TABLE 357-4 CHILD-PUGH CLASSIFICATION OF CIRRHOSIS

		Points Toward Total Score		
Factor	**Units**	**1**	**2**	**3**
Serum bilirubin	μmol/L	<34	34–51	>51
	mg/dL	<2.0	2.0–3.0	>3.0
Serum albumin	g/L	>35	30–35	<30
	g/dL	>3.5	3.0–3.5	<3.0
Prothrombin time	seconds prolonged	<4	4–6	>6
	INR[a]	<1.7	1.7–2.3	>2.3
Ascites		None	Easily controlled	Poorly controlled
Hepatic encephalopathy		None	Minimal	Advanced

[a]International normalized ratio.

Note: The Child-Pugh score is calculated by adding the scores for the five factors and can range from 5 to 15. The resulting Child-Pugh class can be A (a score of 5–6), B (7–9), or C (≥10). Decompensation indicates cirrhosis, with a Child-Pugh score of ≥7 (class B). This level has been the accepted criterion for listing a patient for liver transplantation.

decompressive surgery. The Child-Pugh score is a reasonably reliable predictor of survival in many liver diseases and predicts the likelihood of major complications of cirrhosis, such as bleeding from varices and spontaneous bacterial peritonitis. This classification scheme was used to assess prognosis in cirrhosis and to provide standard criteria for listing a patient as a candidate for liver transplantation (Child-Pugh class B). Recently, the Child-Pugh system has been replaced by the Model for End-Stage Liver Disease (MELD) system for the latter purpose. The MELD score is a prospectively derived system designed to predict the prognosis of patients with liver disease and portal hypertension. This score is calculated from three noninvasive variables: the prothrombin time expressed as the international normalized ratio (INR), the serum bilirubin level, and the serum creatinine concentration. *(http://optn.transplant.hrsa.gov/resources/MeldPeldCalculator.asp?index=98).*

The MELD system provides a more objective means of assessing disease severity and has less center-to-center variation than the Child-Pugh score as well as a wider range of values. MELD is currently used to establish priority listing for liver transplantation in the United States. A similar system, PELD (pediatric end-stage liver disease), is based on bilirubin, INR, serum albumin, age, and nutritional status and is used for children <12 years of age.

Thus, liver biopsy is helpful not only in diagnosis but also in management of chronic liver disease and assessment of prognosis. Because liver biopsy is an invasive procedure and not without complications, it should be used only when it will contribute materially to decisions about management and therapy.

NONSPECIFIC ISSUES IN THE MANAGEMENT OF PATIENTS WITH LIVER DISEASE

Specifics on the management of different forms of acute or chronic liver disease are supplied in subsequent chapters, but certain issues are applicable to any patient with liver disease. These issues include advice regarding alcohol use, medication use, vaccination, and surveillance for complications of liver disease. Alcohol should be used sparingly, if at all, by patients with liver disease. Abstinence from alcohol should be encouraged for all patients with alcohol-related liver disease, patients with cirrhosis, and patients receiving interferon-based therapy for hepatitis B or C. With regard to vaccinations, all patients with liver disease should receive hepatitis A vaccine, and those with risk factors should receive hepatitis B vaccine as well. Influenza and pneumococcal vaccination should also be encouraged, with adherence to the recommendations of the Centers for Disease Control and Prevention. Patients with liver disease should exercise caution in using any medications other than those that are most necessary. Drug-induced hepatotoxicity can mimic many forms of liver disease and can cause exacerbations of chronic hepatitis and cirrhosis; drugs should be suspected in any situation in which the cause of exacerbation is unknown. Finally, consideration should be given to surveillance for complications of chronic liver disease such as variceal hemorrhage and hepatocellular carcinoma. Cirrhosis warrants upper endoscopy to assess the presence of varices, and the patient should receive chronic therapy with beta blockers or should be offered endoscopic obliteration if large varices are found. Moreover, cirrhosis warrants screening and long-term surveillance for development of hepatocellular carcinoma. While the optimal regimen for such surveillance has not been established, an appropriate approach is ultrasound of the liver at 6- to 12-month intervals.

358 Evaluation of Liver Function

Daniel S. Pratt

Several biochemical tests are useful in the evaluation and management of patients with hepatic dysfunction. These tests can be used to (1) detect the presence of liver disease, (2) distinguish among different types of liver disorders, (3) gauge the extent of known liver damage, and (4) follow the response to treatment.

Liver tests have shortcomings. They can be normal in patients with serious liver disease and abnormal in patients with diseases that do not affect the liver. Liver tests rarely suggest a specific diagnosis; rather, they suggest a general category of liver disease, such as hepatocellular or cholestatic, which then further directs the evaluation.

The liver carries out thousands of biochemical functions, most of which cannot be easily measured by blood tests. Laboratory tests measure only a limited number of these functions. In fact, many tests, such as the aminotransferases or alkaline phosphatase, do not measure liver function at all. Rather, they detect liver cell damage or interference with bile flow. Thus, no one test enables the clinician to accurately assess the liver's total functional capacity.

To increase both the sensitivity and the specificity of laboratory tests in the detection of liver disease, it is best to use them as a battery. Tests usually employed in clinical practice include the bilirubin, aminotransferases, alkaline phosphatase, albumin, and prothrombin time tests. When more than one of these tests provide abnormal findings or the findings are persistently abnormal on serial determinations, the probability of liver disease is high. When all test results are normal, the probability of missing occult liver disease is low.

When evaluating patients with liver disorders, it is helpful to group these tests into general categories as outlined below.

TESTS BASED ON DETOXIFICATION AND EXCRETORY FUNCTIONS

Serum Bilirubin (See also Chap. 58) Bilirubin, a breakdown product of the porphyrin ring of heme-containing proteins, is found in the blood in two fractions—conjugated and unconjugated. The unconjugated fraction, also termed the *indirect fraction*, is insoluble in water and is bound to albumin in the blood. The conjugated (direct) bilirubin fraction is water soluble and can therefore be excreted by the kidney. When measured by modifications of the original van den Bergh method, normal values of total serum bilirubin are reported between 1 and 1.5 mg/dL with 95% of a normal population falling between 0.2 and 0.9 mg/dL. If the direct-acting fraction is less than 15% of the total, the bilirubin can be considered to all be indirect. The most frequently reported upper limit of normal for conjugated bilirubin is 0.3 mg/dL.

Elevation of the unconjugated fraction of bilirubin is rarely due to liver disease. An isolated elevation of unconjugated bilirubin is seen primarily in hemolytic disorders and in a number of genetic conditions such as Crigler-Najjar and Gilbert's syndromes (Chap. 58). Isolated unconjugated hyperbilirubinemia (bilirubin elevated but <15% direct) should prompt a workup for hemolysis (Fig. 358-1). In the absence of hemolysis, an isolated, unconjugated hyperbilirubinemia in an otherwise healthy patient can be attributed to Gilbert's syndrome, and no further evaluation is required.

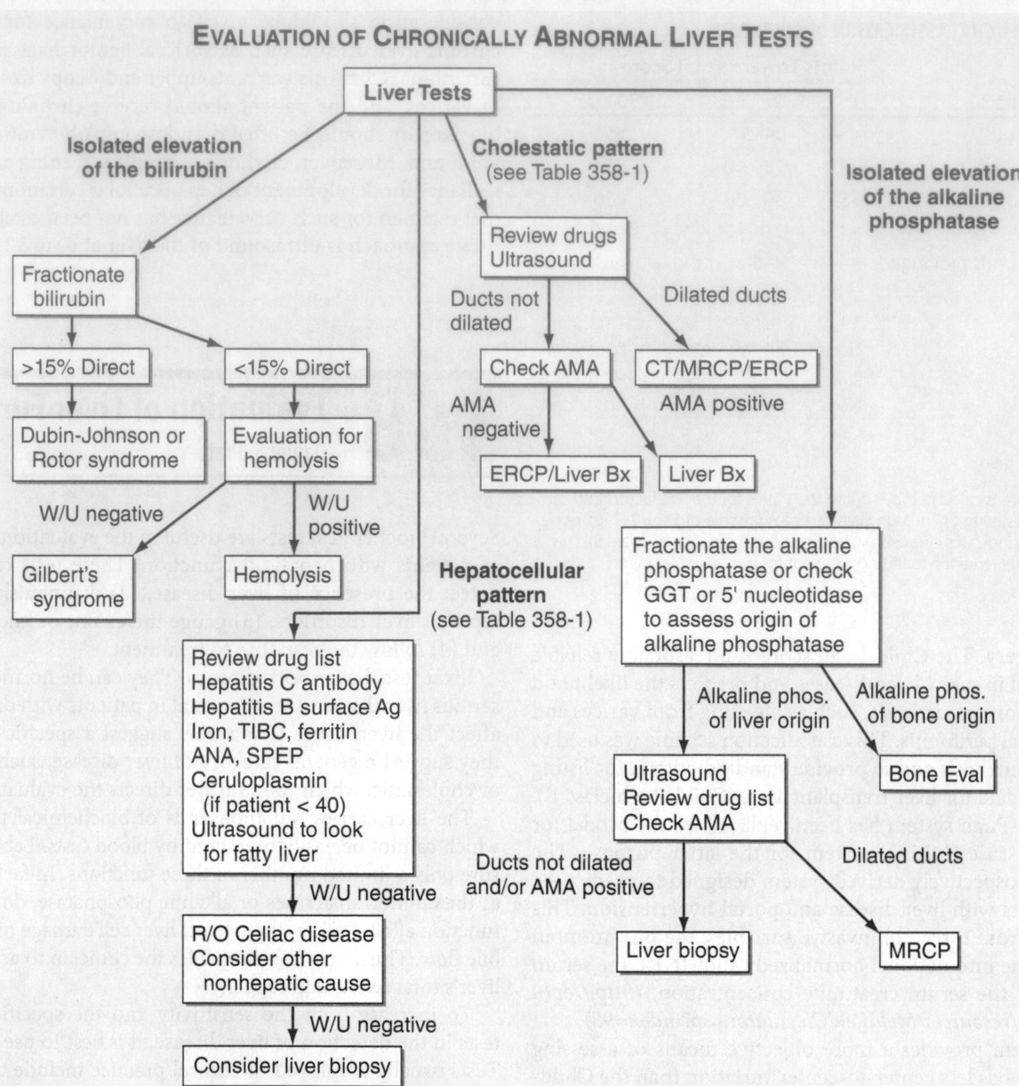

FIGURE 358-1 Algorithm for the evaluation of chronically abnormal liver tests. AMA, antimitochondrial antibody; ANA, antinuclear antibody; Bx, biopsy; CT, computed tomography; ERCP, endoscopic retrograde cholangiopancreatography; GGT, γ glutamyl transpeptidase; MRCP, magnetic resonance cholangiopancreatography; R/O, rule out; SPEP, serum protein electrophoresis; TIBC, total iron-binding capacity; W/U, workup.

In contrast, conjugated hyperbilirubinemia almost always implies liver or biliary tract disease. The rate-limiting step in bilirubin metabolism is not conjugation of bilirubin, but rather the transport of conjugated bilirubin into the bile canaliculi. Thus, elevation of the conjugated fraction may be seen in any type of liver disease. In most liver diseases, both conjugated and unconjugated fractions of the bilirubin tend to be elevated. Except in the presence of a purely unconjugated hyperbilirubinemia, fractionation of the bilirubin is rarely helpful in determining the cause of jaundice.

Although the degree of elevation of the serum bilirubin has not been critically assessed as a prognostic marker, it is important in a number of conditions. In viral hepatitis, the higher the serum bilirubin, the greater is the hepatocellular damage. Total serum bilirubin correlates with poor outcomes in alcoholic hepatitis. It is also a critical component of the Model for End-Stage Liver Disease (MELD) score, a tool used to estimate survival of patients with end-stage liver disease and assess operative risk of patients with cirrhosis. An elevated total serum bilirubin in patients with drug-induced liver disease indicates more severe injury.

Urine Bilirubin Unconjugated bilirubin always binds to albumin in the serum and is not filtered by the kidney. Therefore, any bilirubin found in the urine is conjugated bilirubin; the presence of bilirubinuria implies the presence of liver disease. A urine dipstick test can theoretically give the same information as fractionation of the serum bilirubin. This test is almost 100% accurate. Phenothiazines may give a false-positive reading with the Ictotest tablet. In patients recovering from jaundice, the urine bilirubin clears prior to the serum bilirubin.

Blood Ammonia Ammonia is produced in the body during normal protein metabolism and by intestinal bacteria, primarily those in the colon. The liver plays a role in the detoxification of ammonia by converting it to urea, which is excreted by the kidneys. Striated muscle also plays a role in detoxification of ammonia, where it is combined with glutamic acid to form glutamine. Patients with advanced liver disease typically have significant muscle wasting, which likely contributes to hyperammonemia in these patients. Some physicians use the blood ammonia for detecting encephalopathy or for monitoring hepatic synthetic function, although its use for either of these indications has problems. There is very poor correlation between either the presence or the severity of acute encephalopathy and elevation of blood ammonia; it can be occasionally useful for identifying occult liver disease in patients with mental status changes. There is also a poor correlation of the blood serum ammonia and hepatic function. The ammonia can be elevated in patients with severe portal hypertension and portal blood shunting around the liver even in the presence of normal or near-normal hepatic function. Elevated arterial ammonia levels have been shown to correlate with outcome in fulminant hepatic failure.

Serum Enzymes The liver contains thousands of enzymes, some of which are also present in the serum in very low concentrations. These enzymes have no known function in the serum and behave like other serum proteins. They are distributed in the plasma and in interstitial fluid and have characteristic half-lives, which are usually measured in days. Very little is known about the catabolism of serum enzymes, although they are probably cleared by cells in the reticuloendothelial system. The elevation of a given enzyme activity in the serum is thought to primarily reflect its increased rate of entrance into serum from damaged liver cells.

Serum enzyme tests can be grouped into three categories: (1) enzymes whose elevation in serum reflects damage to hepatocytes, (2) enzymes whose elevation in serum reflects cholestasis, and (3) enzyme tests that do not fit precisely into either pattern.

ENZYMES THAT REFLECT DAMAGE TO HEPATOCYTES The aminotransferases (transaminases) are sensitive indicators of liver cell injury and are most helpful in recognizing acute hepatocellular diseases such as hepatitis. They include aspartate aminotransferase (AST) and alanine aminotransferase (ALT). AST is found in the liver, cardiac muscle, skeletal muscle, kidneys, brain, pancreas, lungs, leukocytes, and erythrocytes in decreasing order of concentration. ALT is found primarily in the liver and is therefore a more specific indicator of liver injury. The aminotransferases are normally present in the serum in low concentrations. These enzymes are released into the blood in greater amounts when there is damage to the liver cell membrane resulting in increased permeability. Liver cell necrosis is not required for the release of the aminotransferases, and there is a poor correlation between the degree of liver cell damage and the level of the aminotransferases. Thus, the absolute elevation of the aminotransferases is of no prognostic significance in acute hepatocellular disorders.

The normal range for aminotransferases varies widely among laboratories, but generally ranges from 10–40 IU/L. The interlaboratory variation in normal range is due to technical reasons; no reference standards exist to establish upper limits of normal for ALT and AST. Some have recommended revisions of normal limits of the aminotransferases to adjust for sex and body mass index, but others have noted the potential costs and unclear benefits of implementing this change.

Any type of liver cell injury can cause modest elevations in the serum aminotransferases. Levels of up to 300 IU/L are nonspecific and may be found in any type of liver disorder. Minimal ALT elevations in asymptomatic blood donors rarely indicate severe liver disease; studies have shown that fatty liver disease is the most likely explanation. Striking elevations—i.e., aminotransferases >1000 IU/L—occur almost exclusively in disorders associated with extensive hepatocellular injury such as (1) viral hepatitis, (2) ischemic liver injury (prolonged hypotension or acute heart failure), or (3) toxin- or drug-induced liver injury.

The pattern of the aminotransferase elevation can be helpful diagnostically. In most acute hepatocellular disorders, the ALT is higher than or equal to the AST. Whereas the AST:ALT ratio is typically <1 in patients with chronic viral hepatitis and nonalcoholic fatty liver disease, a number of groups have noted that as cirrhosis develops, this ratio rises to >1. An AST:ALT ratio >2:1 is suggestive, whereas a ratio >3:1 is highly suggestive, of alcoholic liver disease. The AST in alcoholic liver disease is rarely >300 IU/L, and the ALT is often normal. A low level of ALT in the serum is due to an alcohol-induced deficiency of pyridoxal phosphate.

The aminotransferases are usually not greatly elevated in obstructive jaundice. One notable exception occurs during the acute phase of biliary obstruction caused by the passage of a gallstone into the common bile duct. In this setting, the aminotransferases can briefly be in the 1000–2000 IU/L range. However, aminotransferase levels decrease quickly, and the liver function tests rapidly evolve into those typical of cholestasis.

ENZYMES THAT REFLECT CHOLESTASIS The activities of three enzymes—alkaline phosphatase, 5′-nucleotidase, and γ-glutamyl transpeptidase (GGT)—are usually elevated in cholestasis. Alkaline phosphatase and 5′-nucleotidase are found in or near the bile canalicular membrane of hepatocytes, whereas GGT is located in the endoplasmic reticulum and in bile duct epithelial cells. Reflecting its more diffuse localization in the liver, GGT elevation in serum is less specific for cholestasis than are elevations of alkaline phosphatase or 5′-nucleotidase. Some have advocated the use of GGT to identify patients with occult alcohol use. Its lack of specificity makes its use in this setting questionable.

The normal serum alkaline phosphatase consists of many distinct isoenzymes found in the liver; bone; placenta; and, less commonly, small intestine. Patients over age 60 can have a mildly elevated alkaline phosphatase (1–1.5 times normal), whereas individuals with blood types O and B can have an elevation of the serum alkaline phosphatase after eating a fatty meal due to the influx of intestinal alkaline phosphatase into the blood. It is also nonpathologically elevated in children and adolescents undergoing rapid bone growth because of bone alkaline phosphatase, and late in normal pregnancies due to the influx of placental alkaline phosphatase.

Elevation of liver-derived alkaline phosphatase is not totally specific for cholestasis, and a less than threefold elevation can be seen in almost any type of liver disease. Alkaline phosphatase elevations greater than four times normal occur primarily in patients with cholestatic liver disorders, infiltrative liver diseases such as cancer and amyloidosis, and bone conditions characterized by rapid bone turnover (e.g., Paget's disease). In bone diseases, the elevation is due to increased amounts of the bone isoenzymes. In liver diseases, the elevation is almost always due to increased amounts of the liver isoenzyme.

If an elevated serum alkaline phosphatase is the only abnormal finding in an apparently healthy person, or if the degree of elevation is higher than expected in the clinical setting, identification of the source of elevated isoenzymes is helpful (Fig. 358-1). This problem can be approached in two ways. First, and most precise, is the fractionation of the alkaline phosphatase by electrophoresis. The second, best substantiated, and most available approach involves the measurement of serum 5′-nucleotidase or GGT. These enzymes are rarely elevated in conditions other than liver disease.

In the absence of jaundice or elevated aminotransferases, an elevated alkaline phosphatase of liver origin often, but not always, suggests early cholestasis and, less often, hepatic infiltration by tumor or granulomata. Other conditions that cause isolated elevations of the alkaline phosphatase include Hodgkin's disease, diabetes, hyperthyroidism, congestive heart failure, amyloidosis, and inflammatory bowel disease.

The level of serum alkaline phosphatase elevation is not helpful in distinguishing between intrahepatic and extrahepatic cholestasis. There is essentially no difference among the values found in obstructive jaundice due to cancer, common duct stone, sclerosing cholangitis, or bile duct stricture. Values are similarly increased in patients with intrahepatic cholestasis due to drug-induced hepatitis; primary biliary cirrhosis; rejection of transplanted livers; and, rarely, alcohol-induced steatohepatitis. Values are also greatly elevated in hepatobiliary disorders seen in patients with AIDS (e.g., AIDS cholangiopathy due to cytomegalovirus or cryptosporidial infection and tuberculosis with hepatic involvement).

TESTS THAT MEASURE BIOSYNTHETIC FUNCTION OF THE LIVER

Serum Albumin Serum albumin is synthesized exclusively by hepatocytes. Serum albumin has a long half-life: 18–20 days, with ~4% degraded per day. Because of this slow turnover, the serum albumin is not a good indicator of acute or mild hepatic dysfunction; only minimal changes in the serum albumin are seen in acute liver conditions such as viral hepatitis, drug-related hepatotoxicity, and obstructive jaundice. In hepatitis, albumin levels <3 g/dL should raise the possibility of chronic liver disease. Hypoalbuminemia is more common in chronic liver disorders such as cirrhosis and usually reflects severe liver damage and decreased albumin synthesis. One exception is the patient with ascites in whom synthesis may be normal or even increased, but levels are low because of the increased volume of distribution. However, hypoalbuminemia is not specific for liver disease and may occur in protein malnutrition of any cause, as well as protein-losing enteropathies, nephrotic syndrome, and chronic infections that are associated with prolonged increases in levels of serum interleukin 1 and/or tumor necrosis factor, cytokines that inhibit albumin synthesis. Serum albumin should not be measured for screening in patients in whom there is no suspicion of liver disease. A general medical clinic study of consecutive patients in whom no indications were present for albumin measurement showed that although 12% of patients had abnormal test results, the finding was of clinical importance in only 0.4%.

Serum Globulins Serum globulins are a group of proteins made up of γ globulins (immunoglobulins) produced by B lymphocytes and α and β globulins produced primarily in hepatocytes. γ globulins are increased in chronic liver disease, such as chronic hepatitis and cirrhosis. In cirrhosis, the increased serum γ globulin concentration is due to the increased synthesis of antibodies, some of which are directed against intestinal bacteria. This occurs because the cirrhotic liver fails to clear bacterial antigens that normally reach the liver through the hepatic circulation.

Increases in the concentration of specific isotypes of γ globulins are often helpful in the recognition of certain chronic liver diseases. Diffuse polyclonal increases in IgG levels are common in autoimmune hepatitis; increases >100% should alert the clinician to this possibility. Increases in the IgM levels are common in primary biliary cirrhosis, whereas increases in the IgA levels occur in alcoholic liver disease.

COAGULATION FACTORS

With the exception of factor VIII, which is produced by vascular endothelial cells, the blood clotting factors are made exclusively in hepatocytes. Their serum half-lives are much shorter than albumin, ranging from 6 h for factor VII to 5 days for fibrinogen. Because of their rapid turnover, measurement of the clotting factors is the single best acute measure of hepatic synthetic function and helpful in both diagnosis and assessing the prognosis of acute parenchymal liver disease. Useful for this purpose is the *serum prothrombin time*, which collectively measures factors II, V, VII, and X. Biosynthesis of factors II, VII, IX, and X depends on vitamin K. The international normalized ratio (INR) is used to express the degree of anticoagulation on warfarin therapy. The INR standardizes prothrombin time measurement according to the characteristics of the thromboplastin reagent used in a particular lab, which is expressed as an International Sensitivity Index (ISI); the ISI is then used in calculating the INR.

The prothrombin time may be elevated in hepatitis and cirrhosis as well as in disorders that lead to vitamin K deficiency such as obstructive jaundice or fat malabsorption of any kind. Marked prolongation of the prothrombin time, >5 s above control and not corrected by parenteral vitamin K administration, is a poor prognostic sign in acute viral hepatitis and other acute and chronic liver diseases. The INR, along with the total serum bilirubin and creatinine, are components of the MELD score, which is used as a measure of hepatic decompensation and to allocate organs for liver transplantation.

OTHER DIAGNOSTIC TESTS

Although tests may direct the physician to a category of liver disease, additional radiologic testing and procedures are often necessary to make the proper diagnosis, as shown in Fig. 358-1. The most commonly used ancillary tests are reviewed here, as are the noninvasive tests available for assessing hepatic fibrosis.

Percutaneous Liver Biopsy Percutaneous biopsy of the liver is a safe procedure that can be easily performed at the bedside with local anesthesia and ultrasound guidance. Liver biopsy is of proven value in the following situations: (1) hepatocellular disease of uncertain cause, (2) prolonged hepatitis with the possibility of autoimmune hepatitis, (3) unexplained hepatomegaly, (4) unexplained splenomegaly, (5) hepatic filling defects by radiologic imaging, (6) fever of unknown origin, (7) and staging of malignant lymphoma. Liver biopsy is most accurate in disorders causing diffuse changes throughout the liver and is subject to sampling error in focal infiltrative disorders such as hepatic metastases. Liver biopsy should not be the initial procedure in the diagnosis of cholestasis. The biliary tree should first be assessed for signs of obstruction. Contraindications to performing a percutaneous liver biopsy include significant ascites and prolonged INR. Under these circumstances, the biopsy can be performed via the transjugular approach.

TABLE 358-1 LIVER TEST PATTERNS IN HEPATOBILIARY DISORDERS

Type of Disorder	Bilirubin	Aminotransferases	Alkaline Phosphatase	Albumin	Prothrombin Time
Hemolysis/Gilbert's syndrome	Normal to 86 μmol/L (5 mg/dL) 85% due to indirect fractions No bilirubinuria	Normal	Normal	Normal	Normal
Acute hepatocellular necrosis (viral and drug hepatitis, hepatotoxins, acute heart failure)	Both fractions may be elevated Peak usually follows aminotransferases Bilirubinuria	Elevated, often >500 IU, ALT > AST	Normal to <3× normal elevation	Normal	Usually normal. If >5× above control and not corrected by parenteral vitamin K, suggests poor prognosis
Chronic hepatocellular disorders	Both fractions may be elevated Bilirubinuria	Elevated, but usually <300 IU	Normal to <3× normal elevation	Often decreased	Often prolonged Fails to correct with parenteral vitamin K
Alcoholic hepatitis, cirrhosis	Both fractions may be elevated Bilirubinuria	AST:ALT >2 suggests alcoholic hepatitis or cirrhosis	Normal to <3× normal elevation	Often decreased	Often prolonged Fails to correct with parenteral vitamin K
Intra- and extrahepatic cholestasis	Both fractions may be elevated	Normal to moderate elevation	Elevated, often >4× normal elevation	Normal, unless chronic	Normal If prolonged, will correct with parenteral vitamin K
(Obstructive jaundice)	Bilirubinuria	Rarely >500 IU		Normal	Normal
Infiltrative diseases (tumor, granulomata); partial bile duct obstruction	Usually normal	Normal to slight elevation	Elevated, often >4× normal elevation Fractionate, or confirm liver origin with 5′-nucleotidase or γ glutamyl transpeptidase		

Noninvasive Tests to Detect Hepatic Fibrosis Although liver biopsy is the standard for the assessment of hepatic fibrosis, noninvasive measures of hepatic fibrosis have been developed and show promise. These measures include multiparameter tests aimed at detecting and staging the degree of hepatic fibrosis and imaging techniques. FibroTest (marketed as FibroSure in the United States) is the best evaluated of the multiparameter blood tests. The test incorporates haptoglobin, bilirubin, GGT, apolipoprotein A-I, and α2-macroglobulin and has been found to have high positive and negative predictive values for diagnosing advanced fibrosis in patients with chronic hepatitis C, chronic hepatitis B, and alcoholic liver disease and patients taking methotrexate for psoriasis. Transient elastography (TE), marketed as FibroScan, and magnetic resonance elastography (MRE) both have gained U.S. Food and Drug Administration approval for use in the management of patients with liver disease. TE uses ultrasound waves to measure hepatic stiffness noninvasively. TE has been shown to be accurate for identifying advanced fibrosis in patients with chronic hepatitis C, primary biliary cirrhosis, hemochromatosis, nonalcoholic fatty liver disease, and recurrent chronic hepatitis after liver transplantation. MRE has been found to be superior to TE for staging liver fibrosis in patients with a variety of chronic liver diseases, but requires access to a magnetic resonance imaging scanner.

Ultrasonography Ultrasonography is the first diagnostic test to use in patients whose liver tests suggest cholestasis, to look for the presence of a dilated intrahepatic or extrahepatic biliary tree or to identify gallstones. In addition, it shows space-occupying lesions within the liver, enables the clinician to distinguish between cystic and solid masses, and helps direct percutaneous biopsies. Ultrasound with Doppler imaging can detect the patency of the portal vein, hepatic artery, and hepatic veins and determine the direction of blood flow. This is the first test ordered in patients suspected of having Budd-Chiari syndrome.

USE OF LIVER TESTS

As previously noted, the best way to increase the sensitivity and specificity of laboratory tests in the detection of liver disease is to employ a battery of tests that includes the aminotransferases, alkaline phosphatase, bilirubin, albumin, and prothrombin time along with the judicious use of the other tests described in this chapter. Table 358-1 shows how patterns of liver tests can lead the clinician to a category of disease that will direct further evaluation. However, it is important to remember that no single set of liver tests will necessarily provide a diagnosis. It is often necessary to repeat these tests on several occasions over days to weeks for a diagnostic pattern to emerge. Figure 358-1 is an algorithm for the evaluation of chronically abnormal liver tests.

GLOBAL CONSIDERATIONS

The tests and principles presented in this chapter are applicable worldwide. The causes of liver test abnormalities vary according to region. In developing nations, infectious diseases are more commonly the etiology of abnormal serum liver tests than in developed nations.

Acknowledgment

This chapter represents a revised version of a chapter in previous editions of Harrison's in which Marshall M. Kaplan was a co-author.

359 The Hyperbilirubinemias

Allan W. Wolkoff

BILIRUBIN METABOLISM

The details of bilirubin metabolism are presented in Chap. 58. However, the hyperbilirubinemias are best understood in terms of perturbations of specific aspects of bilirubin metabolism and transport, and these will be briefly reviewed here as depicted in Fig. 359-1.

Bilirubin is the end product of heme degradation. Some 70–90% of bilirubin is derived from degradation of the hemoglobin of senescent red blood cells. Bilirubin produced in the periphery is transported to the liver within the plasma, where, due to its insolubility in aqueous solutions, it is tightly bound to albumin. Under normal circumstances, bilirubin is removed from the circulation rapidly and efficiently by hepatocytes. Transfer of bilirubin from blood to bile involves four distinct but interrelated steps (Fig. 359-1).

1. *Hepatocellular uptake:* Uptake of bilirubin by the hepatocyte has carrier-mediated kinetics. Although a number of candidate bilirubin transporters have been proposed, the actual transporter remains elusive.
2. *Intracellular binding:* Within the hepatocyte, bilirubin is kept in solution by binding as a nonsubstrate ligand to several of the glutathione-S-transferases, formerly called ligandins.
3. *Conjugation:* Bilirubin is conjugated with one or two glucuronic acid moieties by a specific UDP-glucuronosyltransferase to form bilirubin mono- and diglucuronide, respectively. Conjugation disrupts the internal hydrogen bonding that limits aqueous solubility of bilirubin, and the resulting glucuronide conjugates are highly soluble in water. Conjugation is obligatory for excretion of bilirubin across the bile canalicular membrane into bile. The UDP-glucuronosyltransferases have been classified into gene families based on the degree of homology among the mRNAs for the various isoforms. Those that conjugate bilirubin and certain

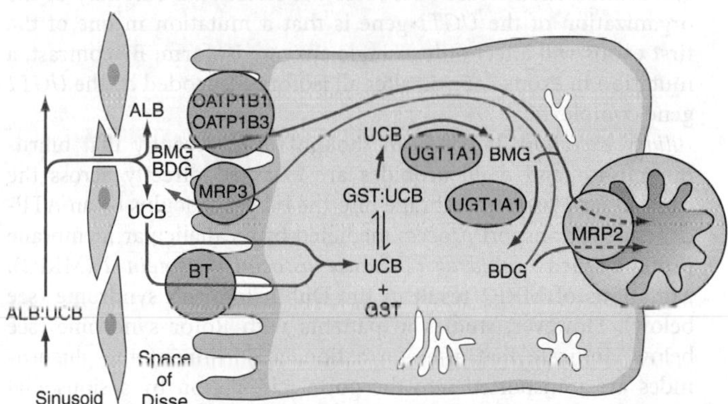

FIGURE 359-1 Hepatocellular bilirubin transport. Albumin-bound bilirubin in sinusoidal blood passes through endothelial cell fenestrae to reach the hepatocyte surface, entering the cell by both facilitated and simple diffusional processes. Within the cell, it is bound to glutathione-S-transferases and conjugated by bilirubin-UDP-glucuronosyltransferase (UGT1A1) to mono- and diglucuronides, which are actively transported across the canalicular membrane into the bile. In addition to this direct excretion of bilirubin glucuronides, a portion are transported into the portal circulation by MRP3 and subjected to reuptake into the hepatocyte by OATP1B1 and OATP1B3. ALB, albumin; BDG, bilirubin diglucuronide; BMG, bilirubin monoglucuronide; BT, proposed bilirubin transporter; GST, glutathione-S-transferase; MRP2 and MRP3, multidrug resistance–associated proteins 2 and 3; OATP1B1 and OATP1B3, organic anion transport proteins 1B1 and 1B3; UCB, unconjugated bilirubin; UGT1A1, bilirubin-UDP-glucuronosyltransferase.

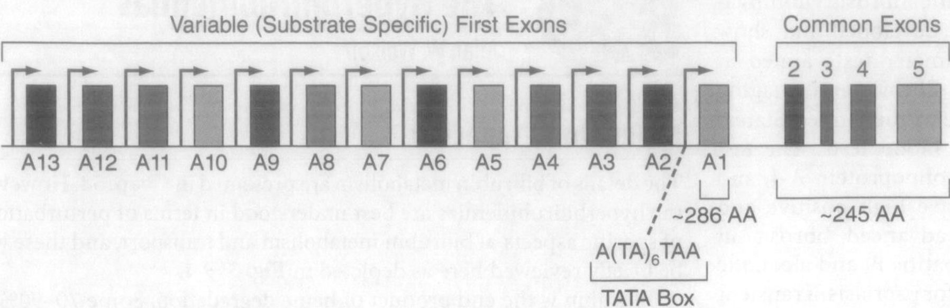

FIGURE 359-2 Structural organization of the human *UGT1* gene complex. This large complex on chromosome 2 contains at least 13 substrate-specific first exons (A1, A2, etc.). Since four of these are pseudogenes, nine UGT1 isoforms with differing substrate specificities are expressed. Each exon 1 has its own promoter and encodes the amino-terminal substrate-specific ~286 amino acids of the various *UGT1*-encoded isoforms, and common exons 2–5 that encode the 245 carboxyl-terminal amino acids common to all of the isoforms. mRNAs for specific isoforms are assembled by splicing a particular first exon such as the bilirubin-specific exon A1 to exons 2 to 5. The resulting message encodes a complete enzyme, in this particular case bilirubin-UDP-glucuronosyltransferase (UGT1A1). Mutations in a first exon affect only a single isoform. Those in exons 2–5 affect all enzymes encoded by the UGT1 complex.

other substrates have been designated the *UGT1* family. These are expressed from a single gene complex by alternative promoter usage. This gene complex contains multiple substrate-specific first exons, designated A1, A2, etc. (Fig. 359-2), each with its own promoter and each encoding the amino-terminal half of a specific isoform. In addition, there are four common exons (exons 2–5) that encode the shared carboxyl-terminal half of all of the *UGT1* isoforms. The various first exons encode the specific aglycone substrate binding sites for each isoform, while the shared exons encode the binding site for the sugar donor, UDP-glucuronic acid, and the transmembrane domain. Exon A1 and the four common exons, collectively designated the UGT1A1 gene (Fig. 359-2), encode the physiologically critical enzyme bilirubin-UDP-glucuronosyltransferase (UGT1A1). A functional corollary of the organization of the *UGT1* gene is that a mutation in one of the first exons will affect only a single enzyme isoform. By contrast, a mutation in exons 2–5 will alter all isoforms encoded by the *UGT1* gene complex.

4. *Biliary excretion:* It has been thought until recently that bilirubin mono- and diglucuronides are excreted directly across the canalicular plasma membrane into the bile canaliculus by an ATP-dependent transport process mediated by a canalicular membrane protein called *multidrug resistance–associated protein 2* (MRP2). Mutations of MRP2 result in the Dubin-Johnson syndrome (see below). However, studies in patients with Rotor syndrome (see below) indicate that after formation, a portion of the glucuronides are transported into the portal circulation by a sinusoidal membrane protein called *multidrug resistance–associated protein 3* (MRP3) and subjected to reuptake into the hepatocyte by the sinusoidal membrane uptake transporters *organic anion transport protein 1B1* (OATP1B1) and OATP1B3.

EXTRAHEPATIC ASPECTS OF BILIRUBIN DISPOSITION

Bilirubin in the Gut Following secretion into bile, conjugated bilirubin reaches the duodenum and passes down the gastrointestinal tract without reabsorption by the intestinal mucosa. An appreciable fraction is converted by bacterial metabolism in the gut to the water-soluble colorless compound urobilinogen. Urobilinogen undergoes enterohepatic cycling. Urobilinogen not taken up by the liver reaches the systemic circulation, from which some is cleared by the kidneys. Unconjugated bilirubin ordinarily does not reach the gut except in neonates or, by ill-defined alternative pathways, in the presence of severe unconjugated hyperbilirubinemia (e.g., Crigler-Najjar syndrome, type I [CN-I]). Unconjugated bilirubin that reaches the gut is partly reabsorbed, amplifying any underlying hyperbilirubinemia. Recent reports suggest that oral administration of calcium phosphate with or without the lipase inhibitor orlistat may be an efficient means to interrupt bilirubin enterohepatic cycling to reduce serum bilirubin levels in this situation. Although orlistat administration for 4–6 weeks to 16 patients with Crigler-Najjar syndrome was associated with a 10–20% decrease in serum bilirubin in 7 patients, the cost and side effects (i.e., diarrhea) may obviate the small benefit achievable with this treatment.

Renal Excretion of Bilirubin Conjugates Unconjugated bilirubin is not excreted in urine, as it is too tightly bound to albumin for effective glomerular filtration and there is no tubular mechanism for its renal secretion. In contrast, the bilirubin conjugates are readily filtered at the glomerulus and can appear in urine in disorders characterized by increased bilirubin conjugates in the circulation.

DISORDERS OF BILIRUBIN METABOLISM LEADING TO UNCONJUGATED HYPERBILIRUBINEMIA

INCREASED BILIRUBIN PRODUCTION

Hemolysis Increased destruction of erythrocytes leads to increased bilirubin turnover and unconjugated hyperbilirubinemia; the hyperbilirubinemia is usually modest in the presence of normal liver function. In particular, the bone marrow is only capable of a sustained eightfold increase in erythrocyte production in response to a hemolytic stress. Therefore, hemolysis alone cannot result in a sustained hyperbilirubinemia of more than ~68 μmol/L (4 mg/dL). Higher values imply concomitant hepatic dysfunction. When hemolysis is the only abnormality in an otherwise healthy individual, the result is a purely unconjugated hyperbilirubinemia, with the direct-reacting fraction as measured in a typical clinical laboratory being ≤15% of the total serum bilirubin. In the presence of systemic disease, which may include a degree of hepatic dysfunction, hemolysis may produce a component of conjugated hyperbilirubinemia in addition to an elevated unconjugated bilirubin concentration. Prolonged hemolysis may lead to the precipitation of bilirubin salts within the gallbladder or biliary tree, resulting in the formation of gallstones in which bilirubin, rather than cholesterol, is the major component. Such pigment stones may lead to acute or chronic cholecystitis, biliary obstruction, or any other biliary tract consequence of calculous disease.

Ineffective Erythropoiesis During erythroid maturation, small amounts of hemoglobin may be lost at the time of nuclear extrusion, and a fraction of developing erythroid cells is destroyed within the marrow. These processes normally account for a small proportion of bilirubin that is produced. In various disorders, including thalassemia major, megaloblastic anemias due to folate or vitamin B_{12} deficiency, congenital erythropoietic porphyria, lead poisoning, and various congenital and acquired dyserythropoietic anemias, the fraction of total bilirubin production derived from ineffective erythropoiesis is increased, reaching as much as 70% of the total. This may be sufficient to produce modest degrees of unconjugated hyperbilirubinemia.

Miscellaneous Degradation of the hemoglobin of extravascular collections of erythrocytes, such as those seen in massive tissue infarctions or large hematomas, may lead transiently to unconjugated hyperbilirubinemia.

DECREASED HEPATIC BILIRUBIN CLEARANCE

Decreased Hepatic Uptake Decreased hepatic bilirubin uptake is believed to contribute to the unconjugated hyperbilirubinemia of Gilbert syndrome (GS), although the molecular basis for this finding remains unclear (see below). Several drugs, including flavaspidic acid, novobiocin, and rifampin, as well as various cholecystographic contrast agents, have been reported to inhibit bilirubin uptake. The resulting unconjugated hyperbilirubinemia resolves with cessation of the medication.

Impaired Conjugation • *PHYSIOLOGIC NEONATAL JAUNDICE* Bilirubin produced by the fetus is cleared by the placenta and eliminated by the maternal liver. Immediately after birth, the neonatal liver must assume responsibility for bilirubin clearance and excretion. However, many hepatic physiologic processes are incompletely developed at birth. Levels of UGT1A1 are low, and alternative excretory pathways allow passage of unconjugated bilirubin into the gut. Since the intestinal flora that convert bilirubin to urobilinogen are also undeveloped, an enterohepatic circulation of unconjugated bilirubin ensues. As a consequence, most neonates develop mild unconjugated hyperbilirubinemia between days 2 and 5 after birth. Peak levels are typically <85–170 μmol/L (5–10 mg/dL) and decline to normal adult concentrations within 2 weeks, as mechanisms required for bilirubin disposition mature. Prematurity, often associated with more profound immaturity of hepatic function and hemolysis, can result in higher levels of unconjugated hyperbilirubinemia. A rapidly rising unconjugated bilirubin concentration, or absolute levels >340 μmol/L (20 mg/dL), puts the infant at risk for bilirubin encephalopathy, or kernicterus. Under these circumstances, bilirubin crosses an immature blood-brain barrier and precipitates in the basal ganglia and other areas of the brain. The consequences range from appreciable neurologic deficits to death. Treatment options include phototherapy, which converts bilirubin into water-soluble photoisomers that are excreted directly into bile, and exchange transfusion. The canalicular mechanisms responsible for bilirubin excretion are also immature at birth, and their maturation may lag behind that of UGT1A1; this can lead to transient conjugated neonatal hyperbilirubinemia, especially in infants with hemolysis.

ACQUIRED CONJUGATION DEFECTS A modest reduction in bilirubin conjugating capacity may be observed in advanced hepatitis or cirrhosis. However, in this setting, conjugation is better preserved than other aspects of bilirubin disposition, such as canalicular excretion. Various drugs, including pregnanediol, novobiocin, chloramphenicol, and gentamicin, may produce unconjugated hyperbilirubinemia by inhibiting UGT1A1 activity. Bilirubin conjugation may be inhibited by certain fatty acids that are present in breast milk but not serum of mothers whose infants have excessive neonatal hyperbilirubinemia (*breast milk jaundice*). Alternatively, there may be increased enterohepatic circulation of bilirubin in these infants. A recent study has correlated epidermal growth factor (EGF) content of breast milk with elevated bilirubin levels in these infants; however, a cause-and-effect relationship remains to be established. The pathogenesis of breast milk jaundice appears to differ from that of transient familial neonatal hyperbilirubinemia (Lucey-Driscoll syndrome), in which there is a UGT1A1 inhibitor in maternal serum.

HEREDITARY DEFECTS IN BILIRUBIN CONJUGATION

Three familial disorders characterized by differing degrees of unconjugated hyperbilirubinemia have long been recognized. The defining clinical features of each are described below (Table 359-1). While these disorders have been recognized for decades to reflect differing degrees of deficiency in the ability to conjugate bilirubin, recent advances in the molecular biology of the *UGT1* gene complex have elucidated their interrelationships and clarified previously puzzling features.

Crigler-Najjar Syndrome, Type I CN-I is characterized by striking unconjugated hyperbilirubinemia of about 340–765 μmol/L (20–45 mg/dL) that appears in the neonatal period and persists for life. Other conventional hepatic biochemical tests such as serum aminotransferases and alkaline phosphatase are normal, and there is no evidence of hemolysis. Hepatic histology is also essentially normal except for the occasional presence of bile plugs within canaliculi. Bilirubin glucuronides are virtually absent from the bile, and there is no detectable constitutive expression of UGT1A1 activity in hepatic tissue. Neither UGT1A1 activity nor the serum bilirubin concentration responds to administration of phenobarbital or other enzyme inducers. In the absence of conjugation, unconjugated bilirubin accumulates in plasma, from which it is eliminated very slowly by alternative pathways that include direct passage into the bile and small intestine. These account for the small amounts of urobilinogen found in feces. No bilirubin is found in the urine. First described in 1952, the disorder is rare (estimated prevalence, 0.6–1.0 per million). Many patients are from geographically or socially isolated communities in which consanguinity is common, and pedigree analyses show an autosomal recessive pattern of inheritance. The majority of patients (type IA) exhibit defects in the glucuronide conjugation of a spectrum of substrates in addition to bilirubin, including various drugs and other xenobiotics. These individuals have mutations in one of the common exons (2–5) of the *UGT1* gene (Fig. 359-2). In a smaller subset (type IB), the defect is limited largely to bilirubin conjugation, and the causative mutation is in the bilirubin-specific exon A1. Estrogen glucuronidation is mediated by UGT1A1 and is defective in all CN-I patients. More than 30 different genetic lesions of *UGT1A1* responsible for CN-I have been identified,

TABLE 359-1 PRINCIPAL DIFFERENTIAL CHARACTERISTICS OF GILBERT AND CRIGLER-NAJJAR SYNDROMES

	Crigler-Najjar Syndrome		
Feature	**Type I**	**Type II**	**Gilbert Syndrome**
Total serum bilirubin, μmol/L (mg/dL)	310–755 (usually >345) (18–45 [usually >20])	100–430 (usually ≤345) (6–25 [usually ≤20])	Typically ≤70 μmol/L (≤4 mg/dL) in absence of fasting or hemolysis
Routine liver tests	Normal	Normal	Normal
Response to phenobarbital	None	Decreases bilirubin by >25%	Decreases bilirubin to normal
Kernicterus	Usual	Rare	No
Hepatic histology	Normal	Normal	Usually normal; increased lipofuscin pigment in some
Bile characteristics			
Color	Pale or colorless	Pigmented	Normal dark color
Bilirubin fractions	>90% unconjugated	Largest fraction (mean: 57%) monoconjugates	Mainly diconjugates but monoconjugates increased (mean: 23%)
Bilirubin UDP-glucuronosyltransferase activity	Typically absent; traces in some patients	Markedly reduced: 0–10% of normal	Reduced: typically 10–33% of normal
Inheritance (all autosomal)	Recessive	Predominantly recessive	Promoter mutation: recessive Missense mutations: 7 of 8 dominant; 1 reportedly recessive

including deletions, insertions, alterations in intron splice donor and acceptor sites, exon skipping, and point mutations that introduce premature stop codons or alter critical amino acids. Their common feature is that they all encode proteins with absent or, at most, traces of bilirubin-UDP-glucuronosyltransferase enzymatic activity.

Prior to the availability of phototherapy, most patients with CN-I died of bilirubin encephalopathy (*kernicterus*) in infancy or early childhood. A few lived as long as early adult life without overt neurologic damage, although more subtle testing usually indicated mild but progressive brain damage. In the absence of liver transplantation, death eventually supervened from late-onset bilirubin encephalopathy, which often followed a nonspecific febrile illness. Although isolated hepatocyte transplantation has been used in a small number of cases of CN-I, early liver transplantation (Chap. 368) remains the best hope to prevent brain injury and death.

Crigler-Najjar Syndrome, Type II (CN-II) This condition was recognized as a distinct entity in 1962 and is characterized by marked unconjugated hyperbilirubinemia in the absence of abnormalities of other conventional hepatic biochemical tests, hepatic histology, or hemolysis. It differs from CN-I in several specific ways (Table 359-1): (1) Although there is considerable overlap, average bilirubin concentrations are lower in CN-II; (2) accordingly, CN-II is only infrequently associated with kernicterus; (3) bile is deeply colored, and bilirubin glucuronides are present, with a striking, characteristic increase in the proportion of monoglucuronides; (4) UGT1A1 in liver is usually present at reduced levels (typically ≤10% of normal) but may be undetectable by older, less sensitive assays; and (5) while typically detected in infancy, hyperbilirubinemia was not recognized in some cases until later in life and, in one instance, at age 34. As with CN-I, most CN-II cases exhibit abnormalities in the conjugation of other compounds, such as salicylamide and menthol, but in some instances, the defect appears limited to bilirubin. Reduction of serum bilirubin concentrations by >25% in response to enzyme inducers such as phenobarbital distinguishes CN-II from CN-I, although this response may not be elicited in early infancy and often is not accompanied by measurable UGT1A1 induction. Bilirubin concentrations during phenobarbital administration do not return to normal but are typically in the range of 51–86 μmol/L (3–5 mg/dL). Although the incidence of kernicterus in CN-II is low, instances have occurred, not only in infants but also in adolescents and adults, often in the setting of an intercurrent illness, fasting, or another factor that temporarily raises the serum bilirubin concentration above baseline and reduces serum albumin levels. For this reason, phenobarbital therapy is widely recommended, a single bedtime dose often sufficing to maintain clinically safe serum bilirubin concentrations.

Over 77 different mutations in the *UGT1* gene have been identified as causing CN-I or CN-II. It was found that missense mutations are more common in CN-II patients, as would be expected in this less severe phenotype. Their common feature is that they encode for a bilirubin-UDP-glucuronosyltransferase with markedly reduced, but detectable, enzymatic activity. The spectrum of residual enzyme activity explains the spectrum of phenotypic severity of the resulting hyperbilirubinemia. Molecular analysis has established that a large majority of CN-II patients are either homozygotes or compound heterozygotes for CN-II mutations and that individuals carrying one mutated and one entirely normal allele have normal bilirubin concentrations.

Gilbert Syndrome (GS) This syndrome is characterized by mild unconjugated hyperbilirubinemia, normal values for standard hepatic biochemical tests, and normal hepatic histology other than a modest increase of lipofuscin pigment in some patients. Serum bilirubin concentrations are most often <51 μmol/L (<3 mg/dL), although both higher and lower values are frequent. The clinical spectrum of hyperbilirubinemia fades into that of CN-II at serum bilirubin concentrations of 86–136 μmol/L (5–8 mg/dL). At the other end of the scale, the distinction between mild cases of GS and a normal state is often blurred. Bilirubin concentrations may fluctuate substantially in any given individual, and at least 25% of patients will exhibit temporarily normal values during prolonged follow-up. More elevated values are associated with stress, fatigue, alcohol use, reduced caloric intake, and intercurrent illness, while increased caloric intake or administration of enzyme-inducing agents produces lower bilirubin levels. GS is most often diagnosed at or shortly after puberty or in adult life during routine examinations that include multichannel biochemical analyses. UGT1A1 activity is typically reduced to 10–35% of normal, and bile pigments exhibit a characteristic increase in bilirubin monoglucuronides. Studies of radiobilirubin kinetics indicate that hepatic bilirubin clearance is reduced to an average of one-third of normal. Administration of phenobarbital normalizes both the serum bilirubin concentration and hepatic bilirubin clearance; however, failure of UGT1A1 activity to improve in many such instances suggests the possible coexistence of an additional defect. Compartmental analysis of bilirubin kinetic data suggests that GS patients have a defect in bilirubin uptake as well as in conjugation. Defect(s) in the hepatic uptake of other organic anions that at least partially share an uptake mechanism with bilirubin, such as sulfobromophthalein and indocyanine green (ICG), are observed in a minority of patients. The metabolism and transport of bile acids that do not utilize the bilirubin uptake mechanism are normal. The magnitude of changes in the serum bilirubin concentration induced by provocation tests such as 48 hours of fasting or the IV administration of nicotinic acid have been reported to be of help in separating GS patients from normal individuals. Other studies dispute this assertion. Moreover, on theoretical grounds, the results of such studies should provide no more information than simple measurements of the baseline serum bilirubin concentration. Family studies indicate that GS and hereditary hemolytic anemias such as hereditary spherocytosis, glucose-6-phosphate dehydrogenase deficiency, and β-thalassemia trait sort independently. Reports of hemolysis in up to 50% of GS patients are believed to reflect better case finding, since patients with both GS and hemolysis have higher bilirubin concentrations, and are more likely to be jaundiced, than patients with either defect alone.

GS is common, with many series placing its prevalence at ≥8%. Males predominate over females by reported ratios ranging from 1.5:1 to >7:1. However, these ratios may have a large artifactual component since normal males have higher mean bilirubin levels than normal females, but the diagnosis of GS is often based on comparison to normal ranges established in men. The high prevalence of GS in the general population may explain the reported frequency of mild unconjugated hyperbilirubinemia in liver transplant recipients. The disposition of most xenobiotics metabolized by glucuronidation appears to be normal in GS, as is oxidative drug metabolism in the majority of reported studies. The principal exception is the metabolism of the antitumor agent irinotecan (CPT-11), whose active metabolite (SN-38) is glucuronidated specifically by bilirubin-UDP-glucuronosyltransferase. Administration of CPT-11 to patients with GS has resulted in several toxicities, including intractable diarrhea and myelosuppression. Some reports also suggest abnormal disposition of menthol, estradiol benzoate, acetaminophen, tolbutamide, and rifamycin SV. Although some of these studies have been disputed, and there have been no reports of clinical complications from use of these agents in GS, prudence should be exercised in prescribing them, or any agents metabolized primarily by glucuronidation, in this condition. It should also be noted that the HIV protease inhibitors indinavir and atazanavir (Chap. 226) can inhibit UGT1A1, resulting in hyperbilirubinemia that is most pronounced in patients with preexisting GS.

Most older pedigree studies of GS were consistent with autosomal dominant inheritance with variable expressivity. However, studies of the *UGT1* gene in GS have indicated a variety of molecular genetic bases for the phenotypic picture and several different patterns of inheritance. Studies in Europe and the United States found that nearly all patients had normal coding regions for UGT1A1 but were homozygous for the insertion of an extra TA (i.e., $A[TA]_7TAA$ rather than $A[TA]_6TAA$) in the promoter region of the first exon. This appeared to be necessary, but not sufficient, for clinically expressed GS, since 15% of normal controls were also homozygous for this variant. While normal by standard criteria, these individuals had somewhat higher bilirubin concentrations than the rest of the controls studied. Heterozygotes for this abnormality had bilirubin concentrations identical to those homozygous for the normal A[TA]$_6$TAA allele. The prevalence of the A[TA]$_7$TAA allele in a general Western population is 30%, in which case 9% would be homozygotes. This is slightly higher than the prevalence of GS based on purely phenotypic parameters. It was suggested that additional variables, such as mild hemolysis or a defect in bilirubin uptake, might be among the factors enhancing phenotypic expression of the defect.

Phenotypic expression of GS due solely to the A[TA]$_7$TAA promoter abnormality is inherited as an autosomal recessive trait. A number of CN-II kindreds have been identified in whom there is also an allele containing a normal coding region but the A[TA]$_7$TAA promoter abnormality. CN-II heterozygotes who have the A[TA]$_6$TAA promoter are phenotypically normal, whereas those with the A[TA]$_7$TAA promoter express the phenotypic picture of GS. GS in such kindreds may also result from homozygosity for the A[TA]$_7$TAA promoter abnormality. Seven different missense mutations in the *UGT1* gene that reportedly cause GS with dominant inheritance have been found in Japanese individuals. Another Japanese patient with mild unconjugated hyperbilirubinemia was homozygous for a missense mutation in exon 5. GS in her family appeared to be recessive. Missense mutations causing GS have not been reported outside of certain Asian populations.

DISORDERS OF BILIRUBIN METABOLISM LEADING TO MIXED OR PREDOMINANTLY CONJUGATED HYPERBILIRUBINEMIA

In hyperbilirubinemia due to acquired liver disease (e.g., acute hepatitis, common bile duct stone), there are usually elevations in the serum concentrations of both conjugated and unconjugated bilirubin. Although biliary tract obstruction or hepatocellular cholestatic injury may present on occasion with a predominantly conjugated hyperbilirubinemia, it is generally not possible to differentiate intrahepatic from extrahepatic causes of jaundice based on the serum levels or relative proportions of unconjugated and conjugated bilirubin. The major reason for determining the amounts of conjugated and unconjugated bilirubin in the serum is for the initial differentiation of hepatic parenchymal and obstructive disorders (mixed conjugated and unconjugated hyperbilirubinemia) from the inheritable and hemolytic disorders discussed above that are associated with unconjugated hyperbilirubinemia.

FAMILIAL DEFECTS IN HEPATIC EXCRETORY FUNCTION

Dubin-Johnson Syndrome (DJS) This benign, relatively rare disorder is characterized by low-grade, predominantly conjugated hyperbilirubinemia (Table 359-2). Total bilirubin concentrations are typically between 34 and 85 μmol/L (2 and 5 mg/dL) but on occasion can be in the normal range or as high as 340–430 μmol/L (20–25 mg/dL) and can fluctuate widely in any given patient. The degree of hyperbilirubinemia may be increased by intercurrent illness, oral contraceptive use, and pregnancy. Because the hyperbilirubinemia is due to a predominant rise in conjugated bilirubin, bilirubinuria is characteristically present. Aside from elevated serum bilirubin levels, other routine laboratory tests are normal. Physical examination is usually normal except for jaundice, although an occasional patient may have hepatosplenomegaly.

Patients with DJS are usually asymptomatic, although some may have vague constitutional symptoms. These latter patients have usually undergone extensive and often unnecessary diagnostic examinations for unexplained jaundice and have high levels of anxiety. In women, the condition may be subclinical until the patient becomes pregnant or receives oral contraceptives, at which time chemical hyperbilirubinemia becomes frank jaundice. Even in these situations, other routine liver function tests, including serum alkaline phosphatase and transaminase activities, are normal.

A cardinal feature of DJS is the accumulation in the lysosomes of centrilobular hepatocytes of dark, coarsely granular pigment. As a result, the liver may be grossly black in appearance. This pigment is thought to be derived from epinephrine metabolites that are not excreted normally. The pigment may disappear during bouts of viral hepatitis, only to reaccumulate slowly after recovery.

Biliary excretion of a number of anionic compounds is compromised in DJS. These include various cholecystographic agents, as well as sulfobromophthalein (Bromsulphalein, BSP), a synthetic dye formerly used in a test of liver function. In this test, the rate of disappearance of BSP from plasma was determined following bolus IV administration. BSP is conjugated with glutathione in the hepatocyte; the resulting conjugate is normally excreted rapidly into the bile canaliculus. Patients with DJS exhibit characteristic rises in plasma concentrations at 90 minutes after injection, due to reflux of conjugated BSP into the circulation from the hepatocyte. Dyes such as ICG that are taken up by hepatocytes but are not further metabolized prior to biliary excretion do not show this reflux phenomenon. Continuous BSP infusion studies suggest a reduction in the time to maximum plasma concentration (t_{max}) for biliary excretion. Bile acid disposition, including hepatocellular uptake and biliary excretion, is normal in DJS. These patients have normal serum and biliary bile acid concentrations and do not have pruritus.

By analogy with findings in several mutant rat strains, the selective defect in biliary excretion of bilirubin conjugates and certain other classes of organic compounds, but not of bile acids, that characterizes DJS in humans was found to reflect defective expression of MRP2, an ATP-dependent canalicular membrane transporter. Several different mutations in the *MRP2* gene produce the Dubin-Johnson phenotype, which has an autosomal recessive pattern of inheritance. Although

TABLE 359-2 PRINCIPAL DIFFERENTIAL CHARACTERISTICS OF INHERITABLE DISORDERS OF BILE CANALICULAR FUNCTION

	DJS	Rotor	PFIC1	BRIC1	PFIC2	BRIC2	PFIC3
Gene	*ABCCA*	*SLCO1B1/SLCO1B3*	*ATP8B1*	*ATP8B1*	*ABCB11*	*ABCB11*	*ABCB4*
Protein	MRP2	OATP1B1/1B3	FIC1	FIC1	BSEP	BSEP	MDR3
Cholestasis	No	No	Yes	Episodic	Yes	Episodic	Yes
Serum γ-GT	Normal	Normal	Normal	Normal	Normal	Normal	↑↑
Serum bile acids	Normal	Normal	↑↑	↑↑ during episodes	↑↑	↑↑ during episodes	↑↑
Clinical features	Mild conjugated hyperbilirubinemia; otherwise normal liver function; dark pigment in liver; characteristic pattern of urinary coproporphyrins	Mild conjugated hyperbilirubinemia; otherwise normal liver function; liver without abnormal pigmentation	Severe cholestasis beginning in childhood	Recurrent episodes of cholestasis beginning at any age	Severe cholestasis beginning in childhood	Recurrent episodes of cholestasis beginning at any age	Severe cholestasis beginning in childhood; decreased phospholipids in bile

Abbreviations: BRIC, benign recurrent intrahepatic cholestasis; BSEP, bile salt excretory protein; DJS, Dubin-Johnson syndrome; γ-GT, γ-glutamyltransferase; MRP2, multidrug resistance–associated protein 2; OATP1A/1B, organic anion transport proteins 1B1 and 1B3; PFIC, progressive familial intrahepatic cholestasis; ↑↑, increased.

MRP2 is undoubtedly important in the biliary excretion of conjugated bilirubin, the fact that this pigment is still excreted in the absence of MRP2 suggests that other, as yet uncharacterized, transport proteins may serve in a secondary role in this process.

Patients with DJS also have a diagnostic abnormality in urinary coproporphyrin excretion. There are two naturally occurring coproporphyrin isomers, I and III. Normally, ~75% of the coproporphyrin in urine is isomer III. In urine from DJS patients, total coproporphyrin content is normal, but >80% is isomer I. Heterozygotes for the syndrome show an intermediate pattern. The molecular basis for this phenomenon remains unclear.

Rotor Syndrome This benign, autosomal recessive disorder is clinically similar to DJS (Table 359-2), although it is seen even less frequently. A major phenotypic difference is that the liver in patients with Rotor syndrome has no increased pigmentation and appears totally normal. The only abnormality in routine laboratory tests is an elevation of total serum bilirubin, due to a predominant rise in conjugated bilirubin. This is accompanied by bilirubinuria. Several additional features differentiate Rotor syndrome from DJS. In Rotor syndrome, the gallbladder is usually visualized on oral cholecystography, in contrast to the nonvisualization that is typical of DJS. The pattern of urinary coproporphyrin excretion also differs. The pattern in Rotor syndrome resembles that of many acquired disorders of hepatobiliary function, in which coproporphyrin I, the major coproporphyrin isomer in bile, refluxes from the hepatocyte back into the circulation and is excreted in urine. Thus, total urinary coproporphyrin excretion is substantially increased in Rotor syndrome, in contrast to the normal levels seen in DJS. Although the fraction of coproporphyrin I in urine is elevated, it is usually <70% of the total, compared with ≥80% in DJS. The disorders also can be distinguished by their patterns of BSP excretion. Although clearance of BSP from plasma is delayed in Rotor syndrome, there is no reflux of conjugated BSP back into the circulation as seen in DJS. Kinetic analysis of plasma BSP infusion studies suggests the presence of a defect in intrahepatocellular storage of this compound. This has never been demonstrated directly. Recent studies indicate that the molecular basis of Rotor syndrome results from simultaneous deficiency of the plasma membrane transporters OATP1B1 and OATP1B3. This results in reduced reuptake of conjugated bilirubin that has been pumped out of the cell into the portal circulation by MRP3 (Fig. 359-1).

Benign Recurrent Intrahepatic Cholestasis (BRIC) This rare disorder is characterized by recurrent attacks of pruritus and jaundice. The typical episode begins with mild malaise and elevations in serum aminotransferase levels, followed rapidly by rises in alkaline phosphatase and conjugated bilirubin and onset of jaundice and itching. The first one or two episodes may be misdiagnosed as acute viral hepatitis. The cholestatic episodes, which may begin in childhood or adulthood, can vary in duration from several weeks to months, followed by a complete clinical and biochemical resolution. Intervals between attacks may vary from several months to years. Between episodes, physical examination is normal, as are serum levels of bile acids, bilirubin, transaminases, and alkaline phosphatase. The disorder is familial and has an autosomal recessive pattern of inheritance. BRIC is considered a benign disorder in that it does not lead to cirrhosis or end-stage liver disease. However, the episodes of jaundice and pruritus can be prolonged and debilitating, and some patients have undergone liver transplantation to relieve the intractable and disabling symptoms. Treatment during the cholestatic episodes is symptomatic; there is no specific treatment to prevent or shorten the occurrence of episodes.

A gene termed *FIC1* was recently identified and found to be mutated in patients with BRIC. Curiously, this gene is expressed strongly in the small intestine but only weakly in the liver. The protein encoded by *FIC1* shows little similarity to those that have been shown to play a role in bile canalicular excretion of various compounds. Rather, it appears to be a member of a P-type ATPase family that transports aminophospholipids from the outer to the inner leaflet of a variety of cell membranes. Its relationship to the pathobiology of this disorder remains unclear. A second phenotypically identical form of BRIC, termed BRIC type 2, has been described resulting from mutations in the bile salt excretory protein (BSEP), the protein that is defective in progressive familial intrahepatic cholestasis type 2 (Table 359-2). How some mutations in this protein result in the episodic BRIC phenotype is unknown.

Progressive Familial Intrahepatic Cholestasis (FIC) This name is applied to three phenotypically related syndromes (Table 359-2). Progressive FIC type 1 (Byler disease) presents in early infancy as cholestasis that may be initially episodic. However, in contrast to BRIC, Byler disease progresses to malnutrition, growth retardation, and end-stage liver disease during childhood. This disorder is also a consequence of a *FIC1* mutation. The functional relationship of the FIC1 protein to the pathogenesis of cholestasis in these disorders is unknown. Two other types of progressive FIC (types 2 and 3) have been described. Progressive FIC type 2 is associated with a mutation in the protein originally named *sister of p-glycoprotein*, now known as *bile salt excretory protein*, which is the major bile canalicular exporter of bile acids. As noted above, some mutations of this protein are associated with BRIC type 2, rather than the progressive FIC type 2 phenotype. Progressive FIC type 3 has been associated with a mutation of MDR3, a protein that is essential for normal hepatocellular excretion of phospholipids across the bile canaliculus. Although all three types of progressive FIC have similar clinical phenotypes, only type 3 is associated with high serum levels of γ-glutamyltransferase activity. In contrast, activity of this enzyme is normal or only mildly elevated in symptomatic BRIC and progressive FIC types 1 and 2.

360 Acute Viral Hepatitis

Jules L. Dienstag

Acute viral hepatitis is a systemic infection affecting the liver predominantly. Almost all cases of acute viral hepatitis are caused by one of five viral agents: hepatitis A virus (HAV), hepatitis B virus (HBV), hepatitis C virus (HCV), the HBV-associated delta agent or hepatitis D virus (HDV), and hepatitis E virus (HEV). All these human hepatitis viruses are RNA viruses, except for hepatitis B, which is a DNA virus but replicates like a retrovirus. Although these agents can be distinguished by their molecular and antigenic properties, all types of viral hepatitis produce clinically similar illnesses. These range from asymptomatic and inapparent to fulminant and fatal acute infections common to all types, on the one hand, and from subclinical persistent infections to rapidly progressive chronic liver disease with cirrhosis and even hepatocellular carcinoma, common to the bloodborne types (HBV, HCV, and HDV), on the other.

VIROLOGY AND ETIOLOGY

Hepatitis A HAV is a nonenveloped 27-nm, heat-, acid-, and ether-resistant RNA virus in the *Hepatovirus* genus of the picornavirus family (Fig. 360-1). Its virion contains four capsid polypeptides, designated VP1 to VP4, which are cleaved posttranslationally from the polyprotein product of a 7500-nucleotide genome. Inactivation of viral activity can be achieved by boiling for 1 min, by contact with formaldehyde and chlorine, or by ultraviolet irradiation. Despite nucleotide sequence variation of up to 20% among isolates of HAV, and despite the recognition of four genotypes affecting humans, all strains of this virus are immunologically indistinguishable and belong to one serotype. Hepatitis A has an incubation period of ~4 weeks. Its replication is limited to the liver, but the virus is present in the liver, bile, stools, and blood during the late incubation period and acute preicteric/presymptomatic phase of illness. Despite slightly longer persistence of virus in the liver, fecal shedding, viremia, and infectivity diminish rapidly once jaundice becomes apparent. HAV can be cultivated reproducibly in vitro.

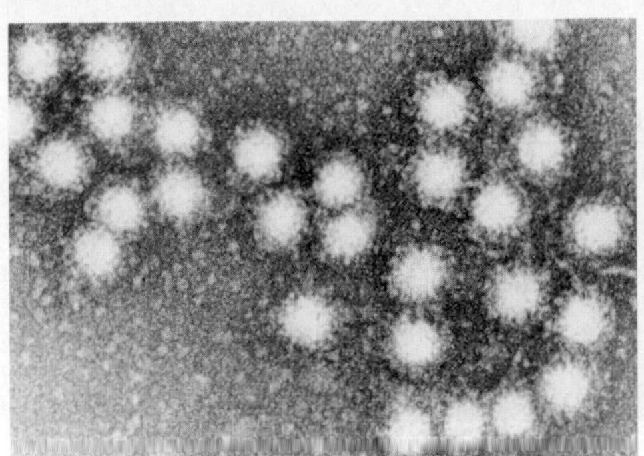

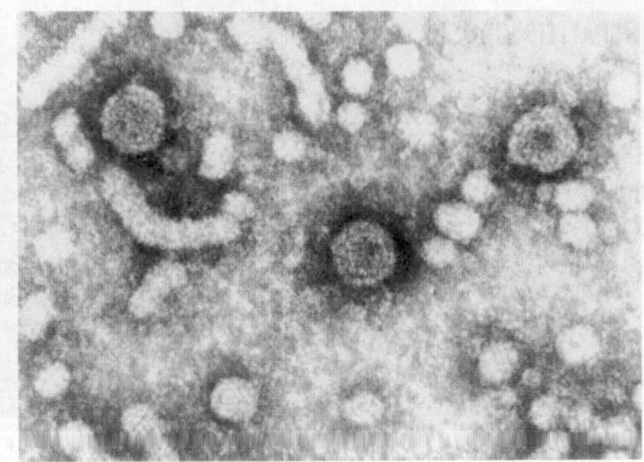

FIGURE 360-1 Electron micrographs of hepatitis A virus particles and serum from a patient with hepatitis B. ***Left:*** 27-nm hepatitis A virus particles purified from stool of a patient with acute hepatitis A and aggregated by antibody to hepatitis A virus. ***Right:*** Concentrated serum from a patient with hepatitis B, demonstrating the 42-nm virions, tubular forms, and spherical 22-nm particles of hepatitis B surface antigen. 132,000×. (Hepatitis D resembles 42-nm virions of hepatitis B but is smaller, 35–37 nm; hepatitis E resembles hepatitis A virus but is slightly larger, 32–34 nm; hepatitis C has been visualized as a 55-nm particle.)

Antibodies to HAV (anti-HAV) can be detected during acute illness when serum aminotransferase activity is elevated and fecal HAV shedding is still occurring. This early antibody response is predominantly of the IgM class and persists for several (~3) months, rarely for 6–12 months. During convalescence, however, anti-HAV of the IgG class becomes the predominant antibody (Fig. 360-2). Therefore, the diagnosis of hepatitis A is made during acute illness by demonstrating anti-HAV of the IgM class. After acute illness, anti-HAV of the IgG class remains detectable indefinitely, and patients with serum anti-HAV are immune to reinfection. Neutralizing antibody activity parallels the appearance of anti-HAV, and the IgG anti-HAV present in immune globulin accounts for the protection it affords against HAV infection.

Hepatitis B HBV is a DNA virus with a remarkably compact genomic structure; despite its small, circular, 3200-bp size, HBV DNA codes for four sets of viral products with a complex, multiparticle structure. HBV achieves its genomic economy by relying on an efficient strategy of encoding proteins from four overlapping genes: S, C, P, and X (Fig. 360-3), as detailed below. Once thought to be unique among viruses, HBV is now recognized as one of a family of animal viruses, hepadnaviruses (hepatotropic DNA viruses), and is classified as hepadnavirus type 1. Similar viruses infect certain species of woodchucks, ground and tree squirrels, and Pekin ducks, to mention the most carefully characterized. Like HBV, all have the same distinctive three morphologic forms, have counterparts to the envelope and nucleocapsid virus antigens of HBV, replicate in the liver but exist in extrahepatic sites, contain their own endogenous DNA polymerase, have partially double-strand and partially single-strand genomes, are associated with acute and chronic hepatitis and hepatocellular carcinoma, and rely on a replicative strategy unique among DNA viruses but typical of retroviruses. Instead of DNA replication directly from a DNA template, hepadnaviruses rely on reverse transcription (effected by the DNA polymerase) of minus-strand DNA from a "pregenomic" RNA intermediate. Then plus-strand DNA is transcribed from the minus-strand DNA template by the DNA-dependent DNA polymerase and converted in the hepatocyte nucleus to a covalently closed circular DNA, which serves as a template for messenger RNA and pregenomic RNA. Viral proteins are translated by the messenger RNA, and the proteins and genome are packaged into virions and secreted from the hepatocyte. Although HBV is difficult to cultivate in vitro in the conventional sense from clinical material, several cell lines have been transfected with HBV DNA. Such transfected cells support in vitro replication of the intact virus and its component proteins.

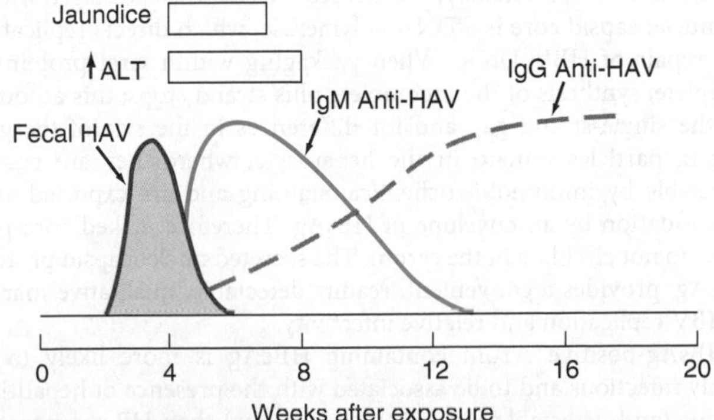

FIGURE 360-2 Scheme of typical clinical and laboratory features of hepatitis A virus (HAV). ALT, alanine aminotransferase.

VIRAL PROTEINS AND PARTICLES Of the three particulate forms of HBV (Table 360-1), the most numerous are the 22-nm particles, which appear as spherical or long filamentous forms; these are antigenically indistinguishable from the outer surface or envelope protein of HBV and are thought to represent excess viral envelope protein. Outnumbered in serum by a factor of 100 or 1000 to 1 compared with the spheres and tubules are large, 42-nm, double-shelled spherical particles, which represent the intact hepatitis B virion (Fig. 360-1). The envelope protein expressed on the outer surface of the virion and on the smaller spherical and tubular structures is referred to as *hepatitis B surface antigen* (HBsAg). The concentration of HBsAg and virus particles in the blood may reach 500 μg/mL and 10 trillion particles per milliliter, respectively. The envelope protein, HBsAg, is the product of the S gene of HBV.

Envelope HBsAg subdeterminants include a common group-reactive antigen, *a*, shared by all HBsAg isolates and one of several subtype-specific antigens—*d* or *y*, *w* or *r* —as well as other specificities. Hepatitis B isolates fall into one of at least eight subtypes and ten

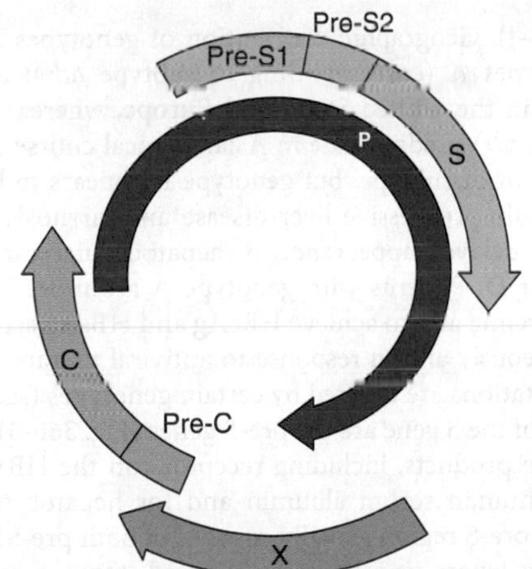

FIGURE 360-3 Compact genomic structure of hepatitis B virus (HBV). This structure, with overlapping genes, permits HBV to code for multiple proteins. The S gene codes for the "major" envelope protein, HBsAg. Pre-S1 and pre-S2, upstream of S, combine with S to code for two larger proteins, "middle" protein, the product of pre-S2 + S, and "large" protein, the product of pre-S1 + pre-S2 + S. The largest gene, P, codes for DNA polymerase. The C gene codes for two nucleocapsid proteins, HBeAg, a soluble, secreted protein (initiation from the pre-C region of the gene), and HBcAg, the intracellular core protein (initiation after pre-C). The X gene codes for HBxAg, which can transactivate the transcription of cellular and viral genes; its clinical relevance is not known, but it may contribute to carcinogenesis by binding to p53.

TABLE 360-1 NOMENCLATURE AND FEATURES OF HEPATITIS VIRUSES

Hepatitis Type	Virus Particle, nm	Morphology	Genome[a]	Classification	Antigen(s)	Antibodies	Remarks
HAV	27	Icosahedral nonenveloped	7.5-kb RNA, linear, ss, +	Hepatovirus	HAV	Anti-HAV	Early fecal shedding Diagnosis: IgM anti-HAV Previous infection: IgG anti-HAV
HBV	42	Double-shelled virion (surface and core) spherical	3.2-kb DNA, circular, ss/ds	Hepadnavirus	HBsAg HBcAg HBeAg	Anti-HBs Anti-HBc Anti-HBe	Bloodborne virus; carrier state Acute diagnosis: HBsAg, IgM anti-HBc Chronic diagnosis: IgG anti-HBc, HBsAg Markers of replication: HBeAg, HBV DNA Liver, lymphocytes, other organs
	27	Nucleocapsid core			HBcAg HBeAg	Anti-HBc Anti-HBe	Nucleocapsid contains DNA and DNA polymerase; present in hepatocyte nucleus; HBcAg does not circulate; HBeAg (soluble, nonparticulate) and HBV DNA circulate—correlate with infectivity and complete virions
	22	Spherical and filamentous; represents excess virus coat material			HBsAg	Anti-HBs	HBsAg detectable in >95% of patients with acute hepatitis B; found in serum, body fluids, hepatocyte cytoplasm; anti-HBs appears following infection—protective antibody
HCV	Approx. 50–80	Enveloped	9.4-kb RNA, linear, ss, +	Hepacivirus	HCV C100-3 C33c C22-3 NS5	Anti-HCV	Bloodborne agent, formerly labeled non-A, non-B hepatitis Acute diagnosis: anti-HCV (C33c, C22-3, NS5), HCV RNA Chronic diagnosis: anti-HCV (C100-3, C33c, C22-3, NS5) and HCV RNA; cytoplasmic location in hepatocytes
HDV	35–37	Enveloped hybrid particle with HBsAg coat and HDV core	1.7-kb RNA, circular, ss, –	Resembles viroids and plant satellite viruses (genus Deltavirus)	HBsAg HDAg	Anti-HBs Anti-HDV	Defective RNA virus, requires helper function of HBV (hepadnaviruses); HDV antigen (HDAg) present in hepatocyte nucleus Diagnosis: anti-HDV, HDV RNA; HBV/HDV co-infection—IgM anti-HBc and anti-HDV; HDV superinfection—IgG anti-HBc and anti-HDV
HEV	32–34	Nonenveloped icosahedral	7.6-kb RNA, linear, ss, +	Hepevirus	HEV antigen	Anti-HEV	Agent of enterically transmitted hepatitis; rare in United States; occurs in Asia, Mediterranean countries, Central America Diagnosis: IgM/IgG anti-HEV (assays not routinely available); virus in stool, bile, hepatocyte cytoplasm

[a]ss, single-strand; ss/ds, partially single-strand, partially double-strand; –, minus-strand; +, plus-strand.

Note: See text for abbreviations.

genotypes (A–J). Geographic distribution of genotypes and subtypes varies; genotypes A (corresponding to subtype *adw*) and D (*ayw*) predominate in the United States and Europe, whereas genotypes B (*adw*) and C (*adr*) predominate in Asia. Clinical course and outcome are independent of subtype, but genotype B appears to be associated with less rapidly progressive liver disease and cirrhosis and a lower likelihood, or delayed appearance, of hepatocellular carcinoma than genotype C or D. Patients with genotype A are more likely to clear circulating viremia and to achieve HBeAg and HBsAg seroconversion, both spontaneously and in response to antiviral therapy. In addition, "precore" mutations are favored by certain genotypes (see below).

Upstream of the S gene are the pre-S genes (Fig. 360-3), which code for pre-S gene products, including receptors on the HBV surface for polymerized human serum albumin and for hepatocyte membrane proteins. The pre-S region actually consists of both pre-S1 and pre-S2. Depending on where translation is initiated, three potential HBsAg gene products are synthesized. The protein product of the S gene is HBsAg (*major protein*), the product of the S region plus the adjacent pre-S2 region is the *middle protein*, and the product of the pre-S1 plus pre-S2 plus S regions is the *large protein*. Compared with the smaller spherical and tubular particles of HBV, complete 42-nm virions are enriched in the large protein. Both pre-S proteins and their respective antibodies can be detected during HBV infection, and the period of pre-S antigenemia appears to coincide with other markers of virus replication, as detailed below; however, pre-S proteins have little clinical relevance and are not included in routine serologic testing repertoires.

The intact 42-nm virion contains a 27-nm nucleocapsid core particle. Nucleocapsid proteins are coded for by the C gene. The antigen expressed on the surface of the nucleocapsid core is *hepatitis B core antigen* (HBcAg), and its corresponding antibody is anti-HBc. A third HBV antigen is *hepatitis B e antigen* (HBeAg), a soluble, nonparticulate, nucleocapsid protein that is immunologically distinct from intact HBcAg but is a product of the same C gene. The C gene has two initiation codons, a precore and a core region (Fig. 360-3). If translation is initiated at the precore region, the protein product is HBeAg, which has a signal peptide that binds it to the smooth endoplasmic reticulum, the secretory apparatus of the cell, leading to its secretion into the circulation. If translation begins at the core region, HBcAg is the protein product; it has no signal peptide, it is not secreted, but it assembles into nucleocapsid particles, which bind to and incorporate RNA, and which, ultimately, contain HBV DNA. Also packaged within the nucleocapsid core is a DNA polymerase, which directs replication and repair of HBV DNA. When packaging within viral proteins is complete, synthesis of the incomplete plus strand stops; this accounts for the single-strand gap and for differences in the size of the gap. HBcAg particles remain in the hepatocyte, where they are readily detectable by immunohistochemical staining and are exported after encapsidation by an envelope of HBsAg. Therefore, naked core particles do not circulate in the serum. The secreted nucleocapsid protein, HBeAg, provides a convenient, readily detectable, qualitative marker of HBV replication and relative infectivity.

HBsAg-positive serum containing HBeAg is more likely to be highly infectious and to be associated with the presence of hepatitis B virions (and detectable HBV DNA, see below) than HBeAg-negative or anti-HBe-positive serum. For example, HBsAg-positive mothers who are HBeAg-positive almost invariably (>90%) transmit hepatitis

B infection to their offspring, whereas HBsAg-positive mothers with anti-HBe rarely (10–15%) infect their offspring.

Early during the course of acute hepatitis B, HBeAg appears transiently; its disappearance may be a harbinger of clinical improvement and resolution of infection. Persistence of HBeAg in serum beyond the first 3 months of acute infection may be predictive of the development of chronic infection, and the presence of HBeAg during chronic hepatitis B tends to be associated with ongoing viral replication, infectivity, and inflammatory liver injury (except during the early decades after perinatally acquired HBV infection; see below).

The third and largest of the HBV genes, the P gene (Fig. 360-3), codes for HBV DNA polymerase; as noted above, this enzyme has both DNA-dependent DNA polymerase and RNA-dependent reverse transcriptase activities. The fourth gene, X, codes for a small, nonparticulate protein, *hepatitis B x antigen* (HBxAg), that is capable of transactivating the transcription of both viral and cellular genes (Fig. 360-3). In the cytoplasm, HBxAg effects calcium release (possibly from mitochondria), which activates signal-transduction pathways that lead to stimulation of HBV reverse transcription and HBV DNA replication. Such transactivation may enhance the replication of HBV, leading to the clinical association observed between the expression of HBxAg and antibodies to it in patients with severe chronic hepatitis and hepatocellular carcinoma. The transactivating activity can enhance the transcription and replication of other viruses besides HBV, such as HIV. Cellular processes transactivated by X include the human interferon γ gene and class I major histocompatibility genes; potentially, these effects could contribute to enhanced susceptibility of HBV-infected hepatocytes to cytolytic T cells. The expression of X can also induce programmed cell death (apoptosis). The clinical relevance of HBxAg is limited, however, and testing for it is not part of routine clinical practice.

SEROLOGIC AND VIROLOGIC MARKERS After a person is infected with HBV, the first virologic marker detectable in serum within 1–12 weeks, usually between 8 and 12 weeks, is HBsAg (Fig. 360-4). Circulating HBsAg precedes elevations of serum aminotransferase activity and clinical symptoms by 2–6 weeks and remains detectable during the entire icteric or symptomatic phase of acute hepatitis B and beyond. In typical cases, HBsAg becomes undetectable 1–2 months after the onset of jaundice and rarely persists beyond 6 months. After HBsAg disappears, antibody to HBsAg (anti-HBs) becomes detectable in serum and remains detectable indefinitely thereafter. Because HBcAg is intracellular and, when in the serum, sequestered within an HBsAg coat, naked core particles do not circulate in serum, and therefore, HBcAg is not detectable routinely in the serum of patients with HBV infection. By contrast, anti-HBc is readily demonstrable in serum, beginning within the first 1–2 weeks after the appearance of HBsAg and preceding detectable levels of anti-HBs by weeks to months.

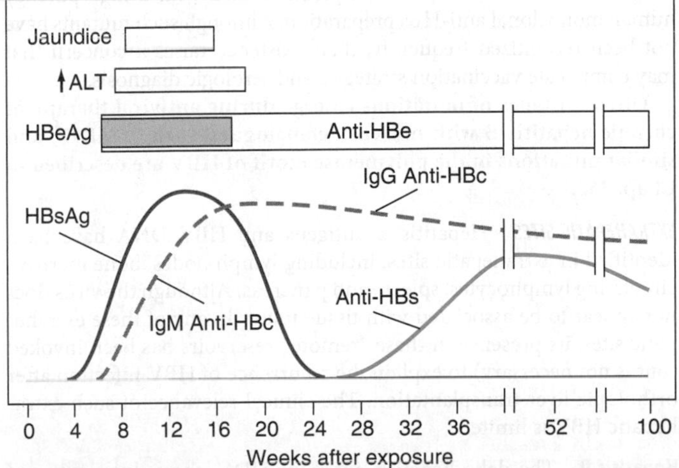

FIGURE 360-4 Scheme of typical clinical and laboratory features of acute hepatitis B. ALT, alanine aminotransferase.

Because variability exists in the time of appearance of anti-HBs after HBV infection, occasionally a gap of several weeks or longer may separate the disappearance of HBsAg and the appearance of anti-HBs. During this "gap" or "window" period, anti-HBc may represent the only serologic evidence of current or recent HBV infection, and blood containing anti-HBc in the absence of HBsAg and anti-HBs has been implicated in transfusion-associated hepatitis B. In part because the sensitivity of immunoassays for HBsAg and anti-HBs has increased, however, this window period is rarely encountered. In some persons, years after HBV infection, anti-HBc may persist in the circulation longer than anti-HBs. Therefore, isolated anti-HBc does not necessarily indicate active virus replication; most instances of isolated anti-HBc represent hepatitis B infection in the remote past. Rarely, however, isolated anti-HBc represents low-level hepatitis B viremia, with HBsAg below the detection threshold, and, occasionally, isolated anti-HBc represents a cross-reacting or false-positive immunologic specificity. Recent and remote HBV infections can be distinguished by determination of the immunoglobulin class of anti-HBc. Anti-HBc of the IgM class (IgM anti-HBc) predominates during the first 6 months after acute infection, whereas IgG anti-HBc is the predominant class of anti-HBc beyond 6 months. Therefore, patients with current or recent acute hepatitis B, including those in the anti-HBc window, have IgM anti-HBc in their serum. In patients who have recovered from hepatitis B in the remote past as well as those with chronic HBV infection, anti-HBc is predominantly of the IgG class. Infrequently, in ≤1–5% of patients with acute HBV infection, levels of HBsAg are too low to be detected; in such cases, the presence of IgM anti-HBc establishes the diagnosis of acute hepatitis B. When isolated anti-HBc occurs in the rare patient with chronic hepatitis B whose HBsAg level is below the sensitivity threshold of contemporary immunoassays (a low-level carrier), anti-HBc is of the IgG class. Generally, in persons who have recovered from hepatitis B, anti-HBs and anti-HBc persist indefinitely.

The temporal association between the appearance of anti-HBs and resolution of HBV infection as well as the observation that persons with anti-HBs in serum are protected against reinfection with HBV suggests that *anti-HBs is the protective antibody*. Therefore, strategies for prevention of HBV infection are based on providing susceptible persons with circulating anti-HBs (see below). Occasionally, in ~10% of patients with chronic hepatitis B, low-level, low-affinity anti-HBs can be detected. This antibody is directed against a subtype determinant different from that represented by the patient's HBsAg; its presence is thought to reflect the stimulation of a related clone of antibody-forming cells, but it has no clinical relevance and does not signal imminent clearance of hepatitis B. These patients with HBsAg and such nonneutralizing anti-HBs should be categorized as having chronic HBV infection.

The other readily detectable serologic marker of HBV infection, HBeAg, appears concurrently with or shortly after HBsAg. Its appearance coincides temporally with high levels of virus replication and reflects the presence of circulating intact virions and detectable HBV DNA (with the notable exception of patients with precore mutations who cannot synthesize HBeAg—see "Molecular Variants"). Pre-S1 and pre-S2 proteins are also expressed during periods of peak replication, but assays for these gene products are not routinely available. In self-limited HBV infections, HBeAg becomes undetectable shortly after peak elevations in aminotransferase activity, before the disappearance of HBsAg, and anti-HBe then becomes detectable, coinciding with a period of relatively lower infectivity (Fig. 360-4). Because markers of HBV replication appear transiently during acute infection, testing for such markers is of little clinical utility in typical cases of acute HBV infection. In contrast, markers of HBV replication provide valuable information in patients with protracted infections.

Departing from the pattern typical of acute HBV infections, in chronic HBV infection, HBsAg remains detectable beyond 6 months, anti-HBc is primarily of the IgG class, and anti-HBs is either undetectable or detectable at low levels (see "Laboratory Features") (Fig. 360-5). During early chronic HBV infection, HBV DNA can be detected both in serum and in hepatocyte nuclei, where it is present in free or episomal form. This relatively highly *replicative stage* of HBV infection is

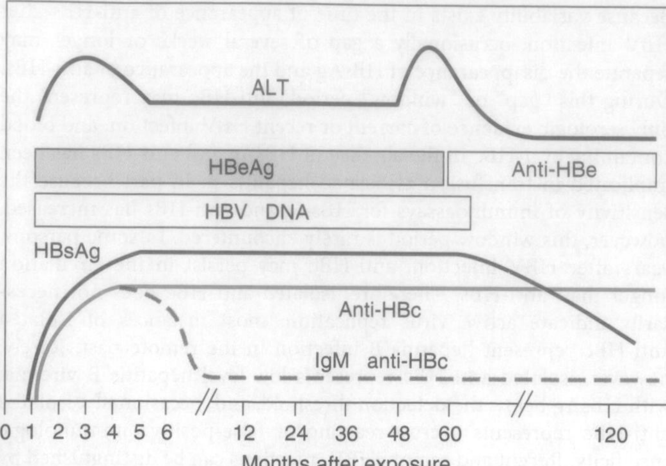

FIGURE 360-5 Scheme of typical laboratory features of wild-type chronic hepatitis B. HBeAg and hepatitis B virus (HBV) DNA can be detected in serum during the relatively *replicative phase* of chronic infection, which is associated with infectivity and liver injury. Seroconversion from the replicative phase to the relatively *nonreplicative phase* occurs at a rate of ~10% per year and is heralded by an acute hepatitis–like elevation of alanine aminotransferase (ALT) activity; during the nonreplicative phase, infectivity and liver injury are limited. In HBeAg-negative chronic hepatitis B associated with mutations in the precore region of the HBV genome, replicative chronic hepatitis B occurs in the absence of HBeAg.

the time of maximal infectivity and liver injury; HBeAg is a qualitative marker and HBV DNA a quantitative marker of this replicative phase, during which all three forms of HBV circulate, including intact virions. Over time, the relatively replicative phase of chronic HBV infection gives way to a relatively *nonreplicative phase.* This occurs at a rate of ~10% per year and is accompanied by seroconversion from HBeAg to anti-HBe. In many cases, this seroconversion coincides with a transient, usually mild, acute hepatitis-like elevation in aminotransferase activity, believed to reflect cell-mediated immune clearance of virus-infected hepatocytes. In the nonreplicative phase of chronic infection, when HBV DNA is demonstrable in hepatocyte nuclei, it tends to be integrated into the host genome. In this phase, only spherical and tubular forms of HBV, *not intact virions,* circulate, and liver injury tends to subside. Most such patients would be characterized as *inactive HBV carriers.* In reality, the designations *replicative* and *nonreplicative* are only relative; even in the so-called nonreplicative phase, HBV replication can be detected at levels of approximately $\leq 10^3$ virions with highly sensitive amplification probes such as the polymerase chain reaction (PCR); below this replication threshold, liver injury and infectivity of HBV are limited to negligible. Still, the distinctions are pathophysiologically and clinically meaningful. Occasionally, nonreplicative HBV infection converts back to replicative infection. Such spontaneous reactivations are accompanied by reexpression of HBeAg and HBV DNA, and sometimes of IgM anti-HBc, as well as by exacerbations of liver injury. Because high-titer IgM anti-HBc can reappear during acute exacerbations of chronic hepatitis B, relying on IgM anti-HBc versus IgG anti-HBc to distinguish between acute and chronic hepatitis B infection, respectively, may not always be reliable; in such cases, patient history is invaluable in helping to distinguish de novo acute hepatitis B infection from acute exacerbation of chronic hepatitis B infection.

MOLECULAR VARIANTS Variation occurs throughout the HBV genome, and clinical isolates of HBV that do not express typical viral proteins have been attributed to mutations in individual or even multiple gene locations. For example, variants have been described that lack nucleocapsid proteins (commonly), envelope proteins (very rarely), or both. Two categories of naturally occurring HBV variants have attracted the most attention. One of these was identified initially in Mediterranean countries among patients with severe chronic HBV infection and detectable HBV DNA but with anti-HBe instead of HBeAg. These patients were found to be infected with an HBV mutant that contained an alteration in the precore region rendering the virus incapable of encoding HBeAg. Although several potential mutation sites exist in the pre-C region, the region of the C gene necessary for the expression of HBeAg (see "Virology and Etiology"), the most commonly encountered in such patients is a single base substitution, from G to A in the second to last codon of the pre-C gene at nucleotide 1896. This substitution results in the replacement of the TGG tryptophan codon by a stop codon (TAG), which prevents the translation of HBeAg. Another mutation, in the core-promoter region, prevents transcription of the coding region for HBeAg and yields an HBeAg-negative phenotype. Patients with such mutations in the precore region and who are unable to secrete HBeAg may have severe liver disease that progresses more rapidly to cirrhosis, or alternatively, they are identified clinically later in the course of the natural history of chronic hepatitis B, when the disease is more advanced. Both "wild-type" HBV and precore-mutant HBV can coexist in the same patient, or mutant HBV may arise late during wild-type HBV infection. In addition, clusters of fulminant hepatitis B in Israel and Japan were attributed to common-source infection with a precore mutant. Fulminant hepatitis B in North America and western Europe, however, occurs in patients infected with wild-type HBV, in the absence of precore mutants, and both precore mutants and other mutations throughout the HBV genome occur commonly, even in patients with typical, self-limited, milder forms of HBV infection. HBeAg-negative chronic hepatitis with mutations in the precore region is now the most frequently encountered form of hepatitis B in Mediterranean countries and in Europe. In the United States, where HBV genotype A (less prone to G1896A mutation) is prevalent, precore-mutant HBV is much less common; however, as a result of immigration from Asia and Europe, the proportion of HBeAg-negative hepatitis B–infected individuals has increased in the United States, and they now represent approximately 30–40% of patients with chronic hepatitis B. Characteristic of such HBeAg-negative chronic hepatitis B are lower levels of HBV DNA (usually $\leq 10^5$ IU/mL) and one of several patterns of aminotransferase activity—persistent elevations, periodic fluctuations above the normal range, and periodic fluctuations between the normal and elevated range.

The second important category of HBV mutants consists of *escape mutants,* in which a single amino acid substitution, from glycine to arginine, occurs at position 145 of the immunodominant *a* determinant common to all HBsAg subtypes. This HBsAg alteration leads to a critical conformational change that results in a loss of neutralizing activity by anti-HBs. This specific HBV/*a* mutant has been observed in two situations, active and passive immunization, in which humoral immunologic pressure may favor evolutionary change ("escape") in the virus—in a small number of hepatitis B vaccine recipients who acquired HBV infection despite the prior appearance of neutralizing anti-HBs and in HBV-infected liver transplant recipients treated with a high-potency human monoclonal anti-HBs preparation. Although such mutants have not been recognized frequently, their existence raises a concern that may complicate vaccination strategies and serologic diagnosis.

Different types of mutations emerge during antiviral therapy of chronic hepatitis B with nucleoside analogues; such "YMDD" and similar mutations in the polymerase motif of HBV are described in Chap. 362.

EXTRAHEPATIC SITES Hepatitis B antigens and HBV DNA have been identified in extrahepatic sites, including lymph nodes, bone marrow, circulating lymphocytes, spleen, and pancreas. Although the virus does not appear to be associated with tissue injury in any of these extrahepatic sites, its presence in these "remote" reservoirs has been invoked (but is not necessary) to explain the recurrence of HBV infection after orthotopic liver transplantation. The clinical relevance of such extrahepatic HBV is limited.

Hepatitis D The delta hepatitis agent, or HDV, the only member of the genus *Deltavirus,* is a defective RNA virus that co-infects with and requires the helper function of HBV (or other hepadnaviruses) for its replication and expression. Slightly smaller than HBV, HDV is a formalin-sensitive, 35- to 37-nm virus with a hybrid structure. Its nucleocapsid expresses HDV antigen (HDAg), which bears no antigenic homology with any of the HBV antigens, and contains the virus genome. The HDV core is "encapsidated" by an outer envelope of HBsAg, indistinguishable from that of HBV except in its relative compositions of major, middle, and large HBsAg component proteins. The genome is a small, 1700-nucleotide, circular, single-strand RNA of negative polarity that is nonhomologous with HBV DNA (except for a small area of the polymerase gene) but that has features and the rolling circle model of replication common to genomes of plant satellite viruses or viroids. HDV RNA contains many areas of internal complementarity; therefore, it can fold on itself by internal base pairing to form an unusual, very stable, rodlike structure that contains a very stable, self-cleaving and self-ligating ribozyme. HDV RNA requires host RNA polymerase II for its replication in the hepatocyte nucleus via RNA-directed RNA synthesis by transcription of genomic RNA to a complementary antigenomic (plus strand) RNA; the antigenomic RNA, in turn, serves as a template for subsequent genomic RNA synthesis effected by host RNA polymerase I. HDV RNA has only one open reading frame, and HDAg, a product of the antigenomic strand, is the only known HDV protein; HDAg exists in two forms: a small, 195-amino-acid species, which plays a role in facilitating HDV RNA replication, and a large, 214-amino-acid species, which appears to suppress replication but is required for assembly of the antigen into virions. HDV antigens have been shown to bind directly to RNA polymerase II, resulting in stimulation of transcription. Although complete hepatitis D virions and liver injury require the cooperative helper function of HBV, intracellular replication of HDV RNA can occur without HBV. Genomic heterogeneity among HDV isolates has been described; however, pathophysiologic and clinical consequences of this genetic diversity have not been recognized. The clinical spectrum of hepatitis D is common to all eight genotypes identified, the predominant of which is genotype 1.

HDV can either infect a person simultaneously with HBV (*co-infection*) or superinfect a person already infected with HBV (*super-infection*); when HDV infection is transmitted from a donor with one HBsAg subtype to an HBsAg-positive recipient with a different subtype, HDV assumes the HBsAg subtype of the recipient, rather than the donor. Because HDV relies absolutely on HBV, the duration of HDV infection is determined by the duration of (and cannot outlast) HBV infection. HDV replication tends to suppress HBV replication; therefore, patients with hepatitis D tend to have lower levels of HBV replication. HDV antigen is expressed primarily in hepatocyte nuclei and is occasionally detectable in serum. During acute HDV infection, anti-HDV of the IgM class predominates, and 30–40 days may elapse after symptoms appear before anti-HDV can be detected. In self-limited infection, anti-HDV is low-titer and transient, rarely remaining detectable beyond the clearance of HBsAg and HDV antigen. In chronic HDV infection, anti-HDV circulates in high titer, and both IgM and IgG anti-HDV can be detected. HDV antigen in the liver and HDV RNA in serum and liver can be detected during HDV replication.

Hepatitis C Hepatitis C virus, which, before its identification was labeled "non-A, non-B hepatitis," is a linear, single-strand, positive-sense, 9600-nucleotide RNA virus, the genome of which is similar in organization to that of flaviviruses and pestiviruses; HCV is the only member of the genus *Hepacivirus* in the family Flaviviridae. The HCV genome contains a single, large open reading frame (gene) that codes for a virus polyprotein of ~3000 amino acids, which is cleaved after translation to yield 10 viral proteins. The 5′ end of the genome consists of an untranslated region (containing an internal ribosomal entry site, IRES) adjacent to the genes for three structural proteins, the nucleocapsid core protein, C, and two structural envelope glycoproteins, E1 and E2. The 5′ untranslated region and core gene are highly conserved among genotypes, but the envelope proteins are coded for by the hypervariable region, which varies from isolate to isolate and may allow the virus to evade host immunologic containment directed at accessible virus-envelope proteins. The 3′ end of the genome also includes an untranslated region and contains the genes for seven nonstructural (NS) proteins, p7, NS2, NS3, NS4A, NS4B, NS5A, and NS5B. p7 is a membrane ion channel protein necessary for efficient assembly and release of HCV. The NS2 cysteine protease cleaves NS3 from NS2, and the NS3-4A serine protease cleaves all the downstream proteins from the polyprotein. Important NS proteins involved in virus replication include the NS3 helicase; NS3-4A serine protease; the multifunctional membrane-associated phosphoprotein NS5A, an essential component of the viral replication membranous web (along with NS4B); and the NS5B RNA-dependent RNA polymerase (Fig. 360-6). Because HCV does not replicate via a DNA intermediate, it does not integrate into the host genome. Because HCV tends to circulate in relatively low titer, 10^3–10^7 virions/mL, visualization of the 50 to 80 nm virus particles remains difficult. Still, the replication rate of HCV is very high, 10^{12} virions per day; its half-life is 2.7 h. The chimpanzee is a helpful but cumbersome animal model. Although a robust, reproducible, small animal model is lacking, HCV replication has been documented in an immunodeficient mouse model containing explants of human liver and in transgenic mouse and rat models. Although in vitro replication is difficult, replicons in hepatocellular carcinoma–derived cell lines support replication of genetically manipulated, truncated, or full-length HCV RNA (but not intact virions); infectious pseudotyped retroviral HCV particles have been shown to yield functioning envelope proteins. In 2005, complete replication of HCV and intact 55-nm virions were described in cell culture systems. HCV entry into the hepatocyte occurs via the nonliver-specific CD81 receptor and the liver-specific tight junction protein claudin-1. A growing list of additional host receptors to which HCV binds on cell entry includes occludin, low-density lipoprotein receptors, glycosaminoglycans, scavenger receptor B1, and epidermal growth factor receptor, among others. Relying on the same assembly and secretion pathway as low-density and very-low-density lipoproteins, HCV is a lipoviroparticle and masquerades as a lipoprotein, which may limit its visibility to the adaptive immune system and which may explain its ability to evade immune containment and clearance. After viral entry and uncoating, translation is initiated by the IRES on the endoplasmic reticulum

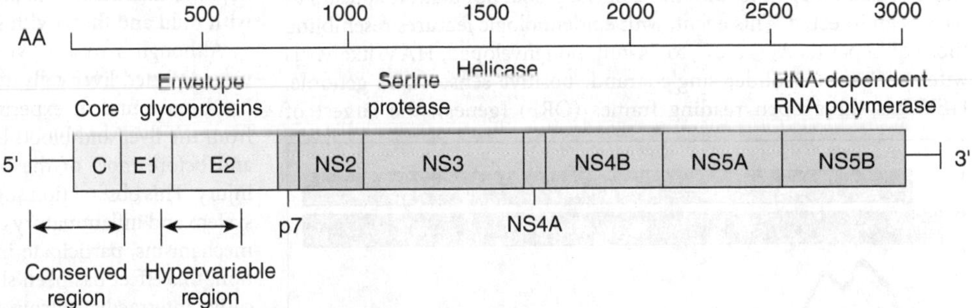

FIGURE 360-6 Organization of the hepatitis C virus genome and its associated, 3000-amino-acid (AA) proteins. The three structural genes at the 5′ end are the core region, C, which codes for the nucleocapsid, and the envelope regions, E1 and E2, which code for envelope glycoproteins. The 5′ untranslated region and the C region are highly conserved among isolates, whereas the envelope domain E2 contains the hypervariable region. At the 3′ end are seven nonstructural (NS) regions—p7, a membrane protein adjacent to the structural proteins that appears to function as an ion channel; NS2, which codes for a cysteine protease; NS3, which codes for a serine protease and an RNA helicase; NS4 and NS4B; NS5A, a multifunctional membrane-associated phosphoprotein, an essential component of the viral replication membranous web; and NS5B, which codes for an RNA-dependent RNA polymerase. After translation of the entire polyprotein, individual proteins are cleaved by both host and viral proteases.

membrane, and the HCV polyprotein is cleaved during translation and posttranslationally by host cellular proteases as well as HCV NS2-3 and NS3-4A proteases. Host cofactors involved in HCV replication include cyclophilin A, which binds to NS5A and yields conformational changes required for viral replication, and liver-specific host microRNA miR-122.

At least six distinct major genotypes (and a minor genotype 7), as well as >50 subtypes within genotypes, of HCV have been identified by nucleotide sequencing. Genotypes differ from one another in sequence homology by ≥30%, and subtypes differ by approximately 20%. Because divergence of HCV isolates within a genotype or subtype and within the same host may vary insufficiently to define a distinct genotype, these intragenotypic differences are referred to as *quasispecies* and differ in sequence homology by only a few percent. The genotypic and quasispecies diversity of HCV, resulting from its high mutation rate, interferes with effective humoral immunity. Neutralizing antibodies to HCV have been demonstrated, but they tend to be short lived, and HCV infection does not induce lasting immunity against reinfection with different virus isolates or even the same virus isolate. Thus, neither *heterologous* nor *homologous* immunity appears to develop commonly after acute HCV infection. Some HCV genotypes are distributed worldwide, whereas others are more geographically confined (see "Epidemiology and Global Features"). In addition, differences exist among genotypes in responsiveness to antiviral therapy but not in pathogenicity or clinical progression (except for genotype 3, in which hepatic steatosis and clinical progression are more likely).

Currently available, third-generation immunoassays, which incorporate proteins from the core, NS3, and NS5 regions, detect anti-HCV antibodies during acute infection. The most sensitive indicator of HCV infection is the presence of HCV RNA, which requires molecular amplification by PCR or transcription-mediated amplification (TMA) (Fig. 360-7). To allow standardization of the quantification of HCV RNA among laboratories and commercial assays, HCV RNA is reported as international units (IUs) per milliliter; quantitative assays with a broad dynamic range are available that allow detection of HCV RNA with a sensitivity as low as 5 IU/mL. HCV RNA can be detected within a few days of exposure to HCV—well before the appearance of anti-HCV—and tends to persist for the duration of HCV infection. Application of sensitive molecular probes for HCV RNA has revealed the presence of replicative HCV in peripheral blood lymphocytes of infected persons; however, as is the case for HBV in lymphocytes, the clinical relevance of HCV lymphocyte infection is not known.

Hepatitis E Previously labeled *epidemic* or *enterically transmitted non-A, non-B hepatitis*, HEV is an enterically transmitted virus that causes clinically apparent hepatitis primarily in India, Asia, Africa, and Central America; in those geographic areas, HEV is the most common cause of acute hepatitis; one-third of the global population appears to have been infected. This agent, with epidemiologic features resembling those of hepatitis A, is a 27- to 34-nm, nonenveloped, HAV-like virus with a 7200-nucleotide, single-strand, positive-sense RNA genome. HEV has three open reading frames (ORF) (genes), the largest of which, *ORF1*, encodes nonstructural proteins involved in virus replication. A middle-sized gene, *ORF2*, encodes the nucleocapsid protein, the major nonstructural protein, and the smallest, *ORF3*, encodes a structural protein whose function remains undetermined. All HEV isolates appear to belong to a single serotype, despite genomic heterogeneity of up to 25% and the existence of five genotypes, only four of which have been detected in humans; genotypes 1 and 2 appear to be more virulent, whereas genotypes 3 and 4 are more attenuated and account for subclinical infections. Contributing to the perpetuation of this virus are animal reservoirs, most notably in swine. No genomic or antigenic homology, however, exists between HEV and HAV or other picornaviruses; and HEV, although resembling caliciviruses, is sufficiently distinct from any known agent to merit its own classification as a unique genus, *Hepevirus*, within the family Hepeviridae. The virus has been detected in stool, bile, and liver and is excreted in the stool during the late incubation period. Both IgM anti-HEV during early acute infection and IgG anti-HEV predominating after the first 3 months can be detected. Currently, availability and reliability of serologic/virologic testing for HEV infection is limited but can be done in specialized laboratories (e.g., the Centers for Disease Control and Prevention).

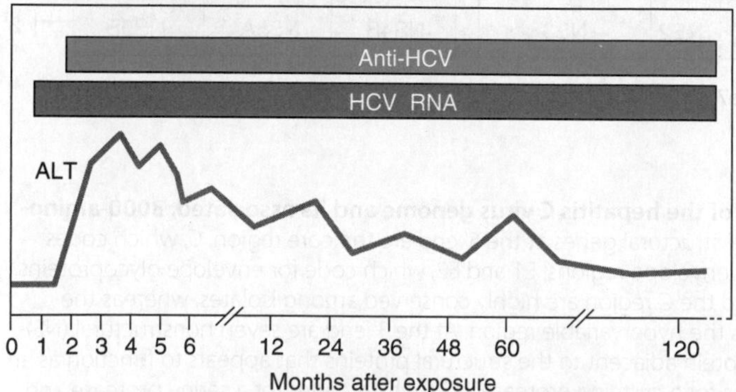

FIGURE 360-7 Scheme of typical laboratory features during acute hepatitis C progressing to chronicity. Hepatitis C virus (HCV) RNA is the first detectable event, preceding alanine aminotransferase (ALT) elevation and the appearance of anti-HCV.

PATHOGENESIS

Under ordinary circumstances, none of the hepatitis viruses is known to be directly cytopathic to hepatocytes. Evidence suggests that the clinical manifestations and outcomes after acute liver injury associated with viral hepatitis are determined by the immunologic responses of the host. Among the viral hepatitides, the immunopathogenesis of hepatitis B and C has been studied most extensively.

Hepatitis B For HBV, the existence of inactive hepatitis B carriers with normal liver histology and function suggests that the virus is not directly cytopathic. The fact that patients with defects in cellular immune competence are more likely to remain chronically infected rather than to clear HBV supports the role of cellular immune responses in the pathogenesis of hepatitis B–related liver injury. The model that has the most experimental support involves cytolytic T cells sensitized specifically to recognize host and hepatitis B viral antigens on the liver cell surface. Nucleocapsid proteins (HBcAg and possibly HBeAg), present on the cell membrane in minute quantities, are the viral target antigens that, with host antigens, invite cytolytic T cells to destroy HBV-infected hepatocytes. Differences in the robustness and broad polyclonality of CD8+ cytolytic T cell responsiveness; in the level of HBV-specific helper CD4+ T cells; in attenuation, depletion, and exhaustion of virus-specific T cells; in viral T cell epitope escape mutations that allow the virus to evade T cell containment; and in the elaboration of antiviral cytokines by T cells have been invoked to explain differences in outcomes between those who recover after acute hepatitis and those who progress to chronic hepatitis, or between those with mild and those with severe (fulminant) acute HBV infection.

Although a robust cytolytic T cell response occurs and eliminates virus-infected liver cells during acute hepatitis B, >90% of HBV DNA has been found in experimentally infected chimpanzees to disappear from the liver and blood before maximal T cell infiltration of the liver and before most of the biochemical and histologic evidence of liver injury. This observation suggests that components of the innate immune system and inflammatory cytokines, independent of cytopathic antiviral mechanisms, participate in the early immune response to HBV infection; this effect has been shown to represent elimination of HBV replicative intermediates from the cytoplasm and covalently closed circular viral DNA from the nucleus of infected hepatocytes. In turn, the innate immune response to HBV infection is mediated largely by natural killer (NK) cell cytotoxicity, activated by immunosuppressive cytokines (e.g., interleukin [IL] 10 and transforming growth factor [TGF] β), reduced signals from inhibitory receptor expression (e.g., major histocompatibility complex), or increased signals from activating receptor expression on infected hepatocytes. In addition, NK cells reduce helper CD4+ cells, which results in reduced CD8+ cells and exhaustion of the virus-specific T cell response to HBV infection. Ultimately, HBV-HLA-specific cytolytic T cell responses of the adaptive immune system are felt to be responsible for recovery from HBV infection.

Debate continues over the relative importance of viral and host factors in the pathogenesis of HBV-associated liver injury and its outcome. As noted above, precore genetic mutants of HBV have been associated with the more severe outcomes of HBV infection (severe chronic and fulminant hepatitis), suggesting that, under certain circumstances, relative pathogenicity is a property of the virus, not the host. The fact that concomitant HDV and HBV infections are associated with more severe liver injury than HBV infection alone and the fact that cells transfected in vitro with the gene for HDV antigen express HDV antigen and then become necrotic in the absence of any immunologic influences are also consistent with a viral effect on pathogenicity. Similarly, in patients who undergo liver transplantation for end-stage chronic hepatitis B, occasionally, rapidly progressive liver injury appears in the new liver. This clinical pattern is associated with an unusual histologic pattern in the new liver, *fibrosing cholestatic hepatitis*, which, ultrastructurally, appears to represent a choking of the cell with overwhelming quantities of HBsAg. This observation suggests that, under the influence of the potent immunosuppressive agents required to prevent allograft rejection, HBV may have a direct cytopathic effect on liver cells, independent of the immune system.

Although the precise mechanism of liver injury in HBV infection remains elusive, studies of nucleocapsid proteins have shed light on the profound immunologic tolerance to HBV of babies born to mothers with highly replicative (HBeAg-positive), chronic HBV infection. In HBeAg-expressing transgenic mice, in utero exposure to HBeAg, which is sufficiently small to traverse the placenta, induces T cell tolerance to both nucleocapsid proteins. This, in turn, may explain why, when infection occurs so early in life, immunologic clearance does not occur, and protracted, lifelong infection ensues.

An important distinction should be drawn between HBV infection acquired at birth, common in endemic areas, such as East Asia, and infection acquired in adulthood, common in the West. Infection in the neonatal period is associated with the acquisition of high-level immunologic tolerance to HBV and absence of an acute hepatitis illness, but the almost invariable establishment of chronic, often lifelong infection. Neonatally acquired HBV infection can culminate decades later in cirrhosis and hepatocellular carcinoma (see "Complications and Sequelae"). In contrast, when HBV infection is acquired during adolescence or early adulthood, the host immune response to HBV-infected hepatocytes tends to be robust, an acute hepatitis-like illness is the rule, and failure to recover is the exception. After adulthood-acquired infection, chronicity is uncommon, and the risk of hepatocellular carcinoma is very low. Based on these observations, some authorities categorize HBV infection into an "immunotolerant" phase, an "immunoreactive" phase, and an "inactive" phase. This somewhat simplistic formulation does not apply at all to the typical adult in the West with self-limited acute hepatitis B, in whom no period of immunologic tolerance occurs. Even among those with neonatally acquired HBV infection, in whom immunologic tolerance is established definitively, intermittent bursts of hepatic necroinflammatory activity punctuate the early decades of life during which liver injury appears to be quiescent (labeled by some as the "immunotolerant" phase). In addition, even when clinically apparent liver injury and progressive fibrosis emerge during later decades (the so-called immunoreactive, or immunointolerant, phase), the level of immunologic tolerance to HBV remains substantial. More accurately, in patients with neonatally acquired HBV infection, a dynamic equilibrium exists between tolerance and intolerance, the outcome of which determines the clinical expression of chronic infection. Persons infected as neonates tend to have a relatively higher level of immunologic tolerance during the early decades of life and a relatively lower level (but only rarely a loss) of tolerance in the later decades of life.

Hepatitis C Cell-mediated immune responses and elaboration by T cells of antiviral cytokines contribute to the multicellular innate and adaptive immune responses involved in the containment of infection and pathogenesis of liver injury associated with hepatitis C. The fact that HCV is so efficient in evading these immune mechanisms is a testament to its highly evolved ability to disrupt host immune responses at multiple levels. After exposure to HCV, the host cell identifies viral product motifs (pattern recognition receptors) that distinguish the virus from "self," resulting in the elaboration of interferons and other cytokines that result in activation of innate and adaptive immune responses. Intrahepatic HLA class I restricted cytolytic T cells directed at nucleocapsid, envelope, and nonstructural viral protein antigens have been demonstrated in patients with chronic hepatitis C; however, such virus-specific cytolytic T cell responses do not correlate adequately with the degree of liver injury or with recovery. Yet, a consensus has emerged supporting a role in the pathogenesis of HCV-associated liver injury of virus-activated CD4+ helper T cells that stimulate, via the cytokines they elaborate, HCV-specific CD8+ cytotoxic T cells. These responses appear to be more robust (higher in number, more diverse in viral antigen specificity, more functionally effective, and more long lasting) in those who recover from HCV than in those who have chronic infection. Contributing to chronic infection are a CD4+ proliferative defect that results in rapid contraction of CD4+ responses, mutations in CD8+ T cell–targeted viral epitopes that allow HCV to escape immune-mediated clearance, and upregulation of inhibitory receptors on functionally impaired, exhausted T cells. Although attention has focused on adaptive immunity, HCV proteins have been shown to interfere with innate immunity by resulting in blocking of type 1 interferon responses and inhibition of interferon signaling and effector molecules in the interferon signaling cascade. Several HLA alleles have been linked with self-limited hepatitis C, the most convincing of which is the CC haplotype of the *IL28B* gene, which codes for interferon λ3, a component of innate immune antiviral defense. The *IL28B* association is even stronger when combined with HLA class II *DQB1*03:01*. The link between non-CC *IL28B* polymorphisms and failure to clear HCV infection has been explained by a chromosome 19q13.13 frameshift variant upstream of *IL28B*, the ΔG polymorphism of which creates an ORF in a novel interferon gene (*IFN-λ4*) associated with impaired HCV clearance. Also shown to contribute to limiting HCV infection are NK cells of the innate immune system that function when HLA class I molecules required for successful adaptive immunity are underexpressed. Both peripheral and intrahepatic NK cell cytotoxicity are dysfunctional in persistent HCV infection. Adding to the complexity of the immune response, HCV core, NS4B, and NS5B have been shown to suppress the immunoregulatory nuclear factor (NF)-κB pathway, resulting in reduced antiapoptotic proteins and a resultant increased vulnerability to tumor necrosis factor (TNF) α–mediated cell death. Patients with hepatitis C and unfavorable (non-CC, associated with reduced HCV clearance) *IL28B* alleles have been shown to have depressed NK cell/innate immune function. Of note, the emergence of substantial viral quasispecies diversity and HCV sequence variation allow the virus to evade attempts by the host to contain HCV infection by both humoral and cellular immunity.

Finally, cross-reactivity between viral antigens (HCV NS3 and NS5A) and host autoantigens (cytochrome P450 2D6) has been invoked to explain the association between hepatitis C and a subset of patients with autoimmune hepatitis and antibodies to liver-kidney microsomal (LKM) antigen (anti LKM) (Chap. 362).

EXTRAHEPATIC MANIFESTATIONS

Immune complex–mediated tissue damage appears to play a pathogenetic role in the extrahepatic manifestations of acute hepatitis B. The occasional prodromal serum sickness–like syndrome observed in acute hepatitis B appears to be related to the deposition in tissue blood vessel walls of HBsAg-anti-HBs circulating immune complexes, leading to activation of the complement system and depressed serum complement levels.

In patients with chronic hepatitis B, other types of immune-complex disease may be seen. Glomerulonephritis with the nephrotic syndrome is observed occasionally; HBsAg, immunoglobulin, and C3 deposition has been found in the glomerular basement membrane. Whereas generalized vasculitis (polyarteritis nodosa) develops in considerably fewer than 1% of patients with chronic HBV infection, 20–30% of patients with polyarteritis nodosa have HBsAg in serum (Chap. 385). In these patients, the affected small- and medium-size arterioles contain

HBsAg, immunoglobulins, and complement components. Another extrahepatic manifestation of viral hepatitis, essential mixed cryoglobulinemia (EMC), was reported initially to be associated with hepatitis B. The disorder is characterized clinically by arthritis, cutaneous vasculitis (palpable purpura), and occasionally, glomerulonephritis and serologically by the presence of circulating cryoprecipitable immune complexes of more than one immunoglobulin class (Chaps. 338 and 385). Many patients with this syndrome have chronic liver disease, but the association with HBV infection is limited; instead, a substantial proportion has chronic HCV infection, with circulating immune complexes containing HCV RNA. Immune-complex glomerulonephritis is another recognized extrahepatic manifestation of chronic hepatitis C.

PATHOLOGY

The typical morphologic lesions of all types of viral hepatitis are similar and consist of panlobular infiltration with mononuclear cells, hepatic cell necrosis, hyperplasia of Kupffer cells, and variable degrees of cholestasis. Hepatic cell regeneration is present, as evidenced by numerous mitotic figures, multinucleated cells, and "rosette" or "pseudoacinar" formation. The mononuclear infiltration consists primarily of small lymphocytes, although plasma cells and eosinophils occasionally are present. Liver cell damage consists of hepatic cell degeneration and necrosis, cell dropout, ballooning of cells, and acidophilic degeneration of hepatocytes (forming so-called Councilman or apoptotic bodies). Large hepatocytes with a ground-glass appearance of the cytoplasm may be seen in chronic but not in acute HBV infection; these cells contain HBsAg and can be identified histochemically with orcein or aldehyde fuchsin. In uncomplicated viral hepatitis, the reticulin framework is preserved.

In hepatitis C, the histologic lesion is often remarkable for a relative paucity of inflammation, a marked increase in activation of sinusoidal lining cells, lymphoid aggregates, the presence of fat (more frequent in genotype 3 and linked to increased fibrosis), and, occasionally, bile duct lesions in which biliary epithelial cells appear to be piled up without interruption of the basement membrane. Occasionally, microvesicular steatosis occurs in hepatitis D. In hepatitis E, a common histologic feature is marked cholestasis. A cholestatic variant of slowly resolving acute hepatitis A also has been described.

A more severe histologic lesion, *bridging hepatic necrosis*, also termed *subacute* or *confluent necrosis* or *interface hepatitis*, is observed occasionally in acute hepatitis. "Bridging" between lobules results from large areas of hepatic cell dropout, with collapse of the reticulin framework. Characteristically, the bridge consists of condensed reticulum, inflammatory debris, and degenerating liver cells that span adjacent portal areas, portal to central veins, or central vein to central vein. This lesion had been thought to have prognostic significance; in many of the originally described patients with this lesion, a subacute course terminated in death within several weeks to months, or severe chronic hepatitis and cirrhosis developed; however, the association between bridging necrosis and a poor prognosis in patients with acute hepatitis has not been upheld. Therefore, although demonstration of this lesion in patients with chronic hepatitis has prognostic significance (Chap. 362), its demonstration during acute hepatitis is less meaningful, and liver biopsies to identify this lesion are no longer undertaken routinely in patients with acute hepatitis. In *massive hepatic necrosis* (fulminant hepatitis, "acute yellow atrophy"), the striking feature at postmortem examination is the finding of a small, shrunken, soft liver. Histologic examination reveals massive necrosis and dropout of liver cells of most lobules with extensive collapse and condensation of the reticulin framework. When histologic documentation is required in the management of fulminant or very severe hepatitis, a biopsy can be done by the angiographically guided transjugular route, which permits the performance of this invasive procedure in the presence of severe coagulopathy.

Immunohistochemical and electron-microscopic studies have localized HBsAg to the cytoplasm and plasma membrane of infected liver cells. In contrast, HBcAg predominates in the nucleus, but, occasionally, scant amounts are also seen in the cytoplasm and on the cell membrane. HDV antigen is localized to the hepatocyte nucleus, whereas HAV, HCV, and HEV antigens are localized to the cytoplasm.

EPIDEMIOLOGY AND GLOBAL FEATURES

Before the availability of serologic tests for hepatitis viruses, all viral hepatitis cases were labeled either as "infectious" or "serum" hepatitis. Modes of transmission overlap, however, and *a clear distinction among the different types of viral hepatitis cannot be made solely on the basis of clinical or epidemiologic features* (Table 360-2). The most accurate means to distinguish the various types of viral hepatitis involves specific serologic testing.

Hepatitis A *This agent is transmitted almost exclusively by the fecal-oral route.* Person-to-person spread of HAV is enhanced by poor personal hygiene and overcrowding; large outbreaks as well as sporadic cases have been traced to contaminated food, water, milk, frozen raspberries and strawberries, green onions imported from Mexico, and shellfish. Intrafamily and intrainstitutional spread are also common. Early epidemiologic observations supported a predilection for hepatitis A to occur in late fall and early winter. In temperate zones, epidemic waves have been recorded every 5–20 years as new segments of nonimmune population appeared; however, in developed countries, the incidence of hepatitis A has been declining, presumably as a function of improved sanitation, and these cyclic patterns are no longer observed. No HAV carrier state has been identified after acute hepatitis A; perpetuation of the virus in nature depends presumably on nonepidemic, inapparent subclinical infection, ingestion of contaminated food or water in, or imported from, endemic areas, and/or contamination linked to environmental reservoirs.

In the general population, anti-HAV, a marker for previous HAV infection, increases in prevalence as a function of increasing age and of decreasing socioeconomic status. In the 1970s, serologic evidence of prior hepatitis A infection occurred in ~40% of urban populations in the United States, most of whose members never recalled having had a symptomatic case of hepatitis. In subsequent decades, however, the prevalence of anti-HAV has been declining in the United States. In developing countries, exposure, infection, and subsequent immunity are almost universal in childhood. As the frequency of subclinical childhood infections declines in developed countries, a susceptible cohort of adults emerges. Hepatitis A tends to be more symptomatic in adults; therefore, paradoxically, as the frequency of HAV infection declines, the likelihood of clinically apparent, even severe, HAV illnesses increases in the susceptible adult population. Travel to endemic areas is a common source of infection for adults from nonendemic areas. More recently recognized epidemiologic foci of HAV infection include child care centers, neonatal intensive care units, promiscuous men who have sex with men, injection drug users, and unvaccinated close contacts of newly arrived international adopted children, most of whom emanate from countries with intermediate-to-high hepatitis A endemicity. Although hepatitis A is rarely bloodborne, several outbreaks have been recognized in recipients of clotting-factor concentrates. In the United States, the introduction of hepatitis A vaccination programs among children from high-incidence states has resulted in a >70% reduction in the annual incidence of new HAV infections and has shifted the burden of new infections from children to young adults. In the most recent, 1999–2006 U.S. Public Health Service National Health and Nutrition Examination Survey (NHANES), the prevalence of anti-HAV in the U.S. population was 35%, representing (compared to the 1988–1994 survey) a stable frequency of infection and natural immunity in adults >19 years old but an increase in vaccine-induced immunity for children age 6–19 years.

Hepatitis B Percutaneous inoculation has long been recognized as a major route of hepatitis B transmission, but the outmoded designation "serum hepatitis" is an inaccurate label for the epidemiologic spectrum of HBV infection. As detailed below, most of the hepatitis transmitted by blood transfusion is not caused by HBV; moreover, in approximately two-thirds of patients with acute type B hepatitis, no history of an identifiable percutaneous exposure can be elicited. We now recognize that many cases of hepatitis B result from less obvious modes of nonpercutaneous or covert percutaneous transmission. HBsAg has been identified in almost every body fluid from

TABLE 360-2 CLINICAL AND EPIDEMIOLOGIC FEATURES OF VIRAL HEPATITIS

Feature	HAV	HBV	HCV	HDV	HEV
Incubation (days)	15–45, mean 30	30–180, mean 60–90	15–160, mean 50	30–180, mean 60–90	14–60, mean 40
Onset	Acute	Insidious or acute	Insidious	Insidious or acute	Acute
Age preference	Children, young adults	Young adults (sexual and percutaneous), babies, toddlers	Any age, but more common in adults	Any age (similar to HBV)	Epidemic cases: young adults (20–40 years); sporadic cases: older adults (>60)
Transmission					
Fecal-oral	+++	–	–	–	+++
Percutaneous	Unusual	+++	+++	+++	–
Perinatal	–	+++	±[a]	+	–
Sexual	±	++	±[a]	++	–
Clinical					
Severity	Mild	Occasionally severe	Moderate	Occasionally severe	Mild
Fulminant	0.1%	0.1–1%	0.1%	5–20%[b]	1–2%[e]
Progression to chronicity	None	Occasional (1–10%) (90% of neonates)	Common (85%)	Common[d]	None[f]
Carrier	None	0.1–30%[c]	1.5–3.2%	Variable[g]	None
Cancer	None	+ (neonatal infection)	+	±	None
Prognosis	Excellent	Worse with age, debility	Moderate	Acute, good Chronic, poor	Good
Prophylaxis	Ig, inactivated vaccine	HBIG, recombinant vaccine	None	HBV vaccine (none for HBV carriers)	Vaccine
Therapy	None	Interferon Lamivudine Adefovir Pegylated interferon Entecavir Telbivudine Tenofovir	Pegylated interferon plus ribavirin, telaprevir, boceprevir	Pegylated interferon ±	None[h]

[a]Primarily with HIV co-infection and high-level viremia in index case; risk ~5%. [b]Up to 5% in acute HBV/HDV co-infection; up to 20% in HDV superinfection of chronic HBV infection. [c]Varies considerably throughout the world and in subpopulations within countries; see text. [d]In acute HBV/HDV co-infection, the frequency of chronicity is the same as that for HBV; in HDV superinfection, chronicity is invariable. [e]10–20% in pregnant women. [f]Except as observed in immunosuppressed liver allograft recipients or other immunosuppressed hosts. [g]Common in Mediterranean countries; rare in North America and western Europe. [h]Anecdotal reports and retrospective studies suggest that pegylated interferon and/or ribavirin are effective in treating chronic hepatitis E, observed in immunocompromised persons.

Abbreviation: HBIG, hepatitis B immunoglobulin. See text for other abbreviations.

infected persons, and at least some of these body fluids—most notably semen and saliva—are infectious, albeit less so than serum, when administered percutaneously or nonpercutaneously to experimental animals. Among the nonpercutaneous modes of HBV transmission, oral ingestion has been documented as a potential but inefficient route of exposure. By contrast, the two nonpercutaneous routes considered to have the greatest impact are intimate (especially sexual) contact and perinatal transmission.

In sub-Saharan Africa, intimate contact among toddlers is considered instrumental in contributing to the maintenance of the high frequency of hepatitis B in the population. Perinatal transmission occurs primarily in infants born to mothers with chronic hepatitis B or (rarely) mothers with acute hepatitis B during the third trimester of pregnancy or during the early postpartum period. Perinatal transmission is uncommon in North America and western Europe but occurs with great frequency and is the most important mode of HBV perpetuation in East Asia and developing countries. Although the precise mode of perinatal transmission is unknown, and although ~10% of infections may be acquired in utero, epidemiologic evidence suggests that most infections occur approximately at the time of delivery and are not related to breast-feeding. The likelihood of perinatal transmission of HBV correlates with the presence of HBeAg and high-level viral replication; 90% of HBeAg-positive mothers but only 10–15% of anti-HBe-positive mothers transmit HBV infection to their offspring. In most cases, acute infection in the neonate is clinically asymptomatic, but the child is very likely to remain chronically infected.

The >350–400 million HBsAg carriers in the world constitute the main reservoir of hepatitis B in human beings. Whereas serum HBsAg is infrequent (0.1–0.5%) in normal populations in the United States and western Europe, a prevalence of up to 5–20% has been found in East Asia and in some tropical countries; in persons with Down's syndrome, lepromatous leprosy, leukemia, Hodgkin's disease, or polyarteritis nodosa; in patients with chronic renal disease on hemodialysis; and in injection drug users.

Other groups with high rates of HBV infection include spouses of acutely infected persons; sexually promiscuous persons (especially promiscuous men who have sex with men); health care workers exposed to blood; persons who require repeated transfusions especially with pooled blood-product concentrates (e.g., hemophiliacs); residents and staff of custodial institutions for the developmentally handicapped; prisoners; and, to a lesser extent, family members of chronically infected patients. In volunteer blood donors, the prevalence of anti-HBs, a reflection of previous HBV infection, ranges from 5–10%, but the prevalence is higher in lower socioeconomic strata, older age groups, and persons—including those mentioned above—exposed to blood products. Because of highly sensitive virologic screening of donor blood, the risk of acquiring HBV infection from a blood transfusion is 1 in 230,000.

Prevalence of infection, modes of transmission, and human behavior conspire to mold geographically different epidemiologic patterns of HBV infection. In East Asia and Africa, hepatitis B, a disease of the newborn and young children, is perpetuated by a cycle of maternal-neonatal spread. In North America and western Europe, hepatitis B is primarily a disease of adolescence and early adulthood, the time of life when intimate sexual contact and recreational and occupational percutaneous exposures tend to occur. To some degree, however, this dichotomy between high-prevalence and low-prevalence geographic regions has been minimized by immigration from high-prevalence to low-prevalence areas. The introduction of hepatitis B vaccine in the early 1980s and adoption of universal childhood vaccination policies in many countries resulted in a dramatic, ~90% decline in the incidence of new HBV infections in those countries as well as in the dire

TABLE 360-3 HIGH-RISK POPULATIONS FOR WHOM HBV INFECTION SCREENING IS RECOMMENDED

Persons born in countries/regions with a high (≥8%) and intermediate (≥2%) prevalence of HBV infection including immigrants and adopted children and including persons born in the United States who were not vaccinated as infants and whose parents emigrated from areas of high HBV endemicity
Household and sexual contacts of persons with hepatitis B
Babies born to HBsAg-positive mothers
Persons who have used injection drugs
Persons with multiple sexual contacts or a history of sexually transmitted disease
Men who have sex with men
Inmates of correctional facilities
Persons with elevated alanine or aspartate aminotransferase levels
Blood/plasma/organ/tissue/semen donors
Persons with HCV or HIV infection
Hemodialysis patients
Pregnant women
Persons who are the source of blood or body fluids that would be an indication for postexposure prophylaxis (e.g., needlestick, mucosal exposure, sexual assault)
Persons who require immunosuppressive or cytotoxic therapy (including anti–tumor necrosis factor α therapy for rheumatologic or inflammatory bowel disorders)

consequences of chronic infection, including hepatocellular carcinoma. Populations and groups for whom HBV infection screening is recommended are listed in Table 360-3.

Hepatitis D Infection with HDV has a worldwide distribution, but two epidemiologic patterns exist. In Mediterranean countries (northern Africa, southern Europe, the Middle East), HDV infection is endemic among those with hepatitis B, and the disease is transmitted predominantly by nonpercutaneous means, especially close personal contact. In nonendemic areas, such as the United States and northern Europe, HDV infection is confined to persons exposed frequently to blood and blood products, primarily injection drug users and hemophiliacs. HDV infection can be introduced into a population through drug users or by migration of persons from endemic to nonendemic areas. Thus, patterns of population migration and human behavior facilitating percutaneous contact play important roles in the introduction and amplification of HDV infection. Occasionally, the migrating epidemiology of hepatitis D is expressed in explosive outbreaks of severe hepatitis, such as those that have occurred in remote South American villages as well as in urban centers in the United States. Ultimately, such outbreaks of hepatitis D—either of co-infections with acute hepatitis B or of superinfections in those already infected with HBV—may blur the distinctions between endemic and nonendemic areas. On a global scale, HDV infection declined at the end of the 1990s. Even in Italy, an HDV-endemic area, public health measures introduced to control HBV infection resulted during the 1990s in a 1.5%/year reduction in the prevalence of HDV infection. Still, the frequency of HDV infection during the first decade of the twenty-first century has not fallen below levels reached during the 1990s; the reservoir has been sustained by survivors infected during 1970–1980 and recent immigrants from still-endemic to less-endemic countries.

Hepatitis C Routine screening of blood donors for HBsAg and the elimination of commercial blood sources in the early 1970s reduced the frequency of, but did not eliminate, transfusion-associated hepatitis. During the 1970s, the likelihood of acquiring hepatitis after transfusion of voluntarily donated, HBsAg-screened blood was ~10% per patient (up to 0.9% per unit transfused); 90–95% of these cases were classified, based on serologic exclusion of hepatitis A and B, as "non-A, non-B" hepatitis. For patients requiring transfusion of pooled products, such as clotting factor concentrates, the risk was even higher, up to 20–30%.

During the 1980s, voluntary self-exclusion of blood donors with risk factors for AIDS and then the introduction of donor screening for anti-HIV reduced further the likelihood of transfusion-associated hepatitis to <5%. During the late 1980s and early 1990s, the introduction first of "surrogate" screening tests for non-A, non-B hepatitis (alanine aminotransferase [ALT] and anti-HBc, both shown to identify blood donors with a higher likelihood of transmitting non-A, non-B hepatitis to recipients) and, subsequently, after the discovery of HCV, first-generation immunoassays for anti-HCV reduced the frequency of transfusion-associated hepatitis even further. A prospective analysis of transfusion-associated hepatitis conducted between 1986 and 1990 showed that the frequency of transfusion-associated hepatitis at one urban university hospital fell from a baseline of 3.8% per patient (0.45% per unit transfused) to 1.5% per patient (0.19% per unit) after the introduction of surrogate testing and to 0.6% per patient (0.03% per unit) after the introduction of first-generation anti-HCV assays. The introduction of second-generation anti-HCV assays reduced the frequency of transfusion-associated hepatitis C to almost imperceptible levels—1 in 100,000—and these gains were reinforced by the application of third-generation anti-HCV assays and of automated PCR testing of donated blood for HCV RNA, which has resulted in a reduction in the risk of transfusion-associated HCV infection to 1 in 2.3 million transfusions.

In addition to being transmitted by transfusion, hepatitis C can be transmitted by other percutaneous routes, such as injection drug use. In addition, this virus can be transmitted by occupational exposure to blood, and the likelihood of infection is increased in hemodialysis units. Although the frequency of transfusion-associated hepatitis C fell as a result of blood-donor screening, the overall frequency of hepatitis C remained the same until the early 1990s, when the overall frequency fell by 80%, in parallel with a reduction in the number of new cases in injection drug users. After the exclusion of anti-HCV-positive plasma units from the donor pool, rare, sporadic instances have occurred of hepatitis C among recipients of immunoglobulin (Ig) preparations for intravenous (but not intramuscular) use.

Serologic evidence for HCV infection occurs in 90% of patients with a history of transfusion-associated hepatitis (almost all occurring before 1992, when second-generation HCV screening tests were introduced); hemophiliacs and others treated with clotting factors; injection drug users; 60–70% of patients with sporadic "non-A, non-B" hepatitis who lack identifiable risk factors; 0.5% of volunteer blood donors; and, in a survey conducted in the United States between 1999 and 2002, 1.6% of the general population in the United States, which translates into 4.1 million persons (3.2 million with viremia), the majority of whom are unaware of their infections. Moreover, such population surveys do not include higher-risk groups such as incarcerated prisoners and active injection drug users, indicating that the actual prevalence is even higher. Comparable frequencies of HCV infection occur in most countries around the world, with 170 million persons infected worldwide, but extraordinarily high prevalences of HCV infection occur in certain countries such as Egypt, where >20% of the population (as high as 50% in persons born prior to 1960) in some cities is infected. The high frequency in Egypt is attributable to contaminated equipment used for medical procedures and unsafe injection practices in the 1950s to 1980s (during a campaign to eradicate schistosomiasis with intravenous tartar emetic). In the United States, African Americans and Mexican Americans have higher frequencies of HCV infection than whites. Between 1988 and 1994, 30- to 40-year-old adult males had the highest prevalence of HCV infection; however, in a survey conducted between 1999 and 2002, the peak age decile had shifted to those age 40–49 years; an increase in hepatitis C–related mortality has paralleled this secular trend, increasing since 1995 predominantly in the 45- to 65-year age group. Thus, despite an 80% reduction in new HCV infections during the 1990s, the prevalence of HCV infection in the population was sustained by an aging cohort that had acquired their infections three to four decades earlier, during the 1960s and 1970s, as a result predominantly of self-inoculation with recreational drugs. As death resulting from HIV infection fell after 1999, age-adjusted mortality associated with HCV infection surpassed that of HIV infection in 2007; >70% of HCV-associated deaths occurred in the "baby boomer" cohort born between 1945 and 1965. Compared to the 1.6%

prevalence of HCV infection in the population at large, the prevalence in the 1945–1965 birth cohort was 3.2%, representing three-quarters of all infected persons. Therefore, in 2012, the Centers for Disease Control and Prevention recommended that all persons born between 1945 and 1965 be screened for hepatitis C, without ascertainment of risk, a recommendation shown to be cost-effective and predicted to identify 800,000 infected persons. Because of the availability of highly effective antiviral therapy, such screening would have the potential to avert 200,000 cases of cirrhosis and 47,000 cases of hepatocellular carcinoma and to prevent 120,000 hepatitis-related deaths.

Hepatitis C accounts for 40% of chronic liver disease, is the most frequent indication for liver transplantation, and is estimated to account for 8000–10,000 deaths per year in the United States. The distribution of HCV genotypes varies in different parts of the world. Worldwide, genotype 1 is the most common. In the United States, genotype 1 accounts for 70% of HCV infections, whereas genotypes 2 and 3 account for the remaining 30%; among African Americans, the frequency of genotype 1 is even higher (i.e., 90%). Genotype 4 predominates in Egypt; genotype 5 is localized to South Africa, genotype 6 to Hong Kong, and genotype 7 to Central Africa. Most asymptomatic blood donors found to have anti-HCV and ~20–30% of persons with reported cases of acute hepatitis C do not fall into a recognized risk group; however, many such blood donors do recall risk associated behaviors when questioned carefully.

As a bloodborne infection, HCV potentially can be transmitted sexually and perinatally; however, both of these modes of transmission are inefficient for hepatitis C. Although 10–15% of patients with acute hepatitis C report having potential sexual sources of infection, most studies have failed to identify sexual transmission of this agent. The chances of sexual and perinatal transmission have been estimated to be ~5% but shown in a prospective study to be only 1% between monogamous sexual partners, well below comparable rates for HIV and HBV infections. Moreover, sexual transmission appears to be confined to such subgroups as persons with multiple sexual partners and sexually transmitted diseases. Breast-feeding does not increase the risk of HCV infection between an infected mother and her infant. Infection of health workers is not dramatically higher than among the general population; however, health workers are more likely to acquire HCV infection through accidental needle punctures, the efficiency of which is ~3%. Infection of household contacts is rare as well.

Besides persons born between 1945 and 1965, other groups with an increased frequency of HCV infection are listed in Table 360-4. In immunosuppressed individuals, levels of anti-HCV may be undetectable, and a diagnosis may require testing for HCV RNA. Although new acute cases of hepatitis C are rare, newly diagnosed cases are common among otherwise healthy persons who experimented briefly with injection drugs, as noted above, three or four decades earlier. Such instances usually remain unrecognized for years, until unearthed by laboratory screening for routine medical examinations, insurance applications, and attempted blood donation. Although, overall, the annual incidence of new HCV infections has continued to fall, the rate of new infections has been increasing since 2002 in a new cohort of young injection drug users, age 15–24 years (accounting for more than two-thirds of all acute cases), who, unlike older cohorts, had not learned to take precautions to prevent bloodborne infections.

TABLE 360-4 HIGH-RISK POPULATIONS FOR WHOM HCV-INFECTION SCREENING IS RECOMMENDED

Persons born between 1945 and 1965
Persons who have ever used injection drugs
Persons with HIV infection
Hemophiliacs treated with clotting factor concentrates prior to 1987
Persons who have ever undergone long-term hemodialysis
Persons with unexplained elevations of aminotransferase levels
Transfusion or transplantation recipients prior to July 1992
Recipients of blood or organs from a donor found to be positive for hepatitis C
Children born to women with hepatitis C
Health care, public safety, and emergency medical personnel following needle injury or mucosal exposure to HCV-contaminated blood
Sexual partners of persons with hepatitis C infection

Hepatitis E This type of hepatitis, identified in India, Asia, Africa, the Middle East, and Central America, resembles hepatitis A in its primarily enteric mode of spread. The commonly recognized cases occur after contamination of water supplies such as after monsoon flooding, but sporadic, isolated cases occur. An epidemiologic feature that distinguishes HEV from other enteric agents is the rarity of secondary person-to-person spread from infected persons to their close contacts. Large waterborne outbreaks in endemic areas are linked to genotypes 1 and 2, arise in populations that are immune to HAV, favor young adults, and account for antibody prevalences of 30–80%. In nonendemic areas of the world, such as the United States, clinically apparent acute hepatitis E is extremely rare; however, during the 1988–1994 NHANES survey conducted by the U.S. Public Health Service, the prevalence of anti-HEV was 21%, reflecting subclinical infections, infection with genotypes 3 and 4, predominantly in older males (>60 years). In nonendemic areas, HEV accounts hardly at all for cases of sporadic hepatitis; however, cases imported from endemic areas have been found in the United States. Evidence supports a zoonotic reservoir for HEV primarily in swine, which may account for the mostly subclinical infections in nonendemic areas.

CLINICAL AND LABORATORY FEATURES

Symptoms and Signs Acute viral hepatitis occurs after an incubation period that varies according to the responsible agent. Generally, incubation periods for hepatitis A range from 15–45 days (mean, 4 weeks), for hepatitis B and D from 30–180 days (mean, 8–12 weeks), for hepatitis C from 15–160 days (mean, 7 weeks), and for hepatitis E from 14–60 days (mean, 5–6 weeks). The *prodromal symptoms* of acute viral hepatitis are systemic and quite variable. Constitutional symptoms of anorexia, nausea and vomiting, fatigue, malaise, arthralgias, myalgias, headache, photophobia, pharyngitis, cough, and coryza may precede the onset of jaundice by 1–2 weeks. The nausea, vomiting, and anorexia are frequently associated with alterations in olfaction and taste. A low-grade fever between 38° and 39°C (100°–102°F) is more often present in hepatitis A and E than in hepatitis B or C, except when hepatitis B is heralded by a serum sickness–like syndrome; rarely, a fever of 39.5°–40°C (103°–104°F) may accompany the constitutional symptoms. Dark urine and clay-colored stools may be noticed by the patient from 1–5 days before the onset of clinical jaundice.

With the onset of *clinical jaundice*, the constitutional prodromal symptoms usually diminish, but in some patients, mild weight loss (2.5–5 kg) is common and may continue during the entire icteric phase. The liver becomes enlarged and tender and may be associated with right upper quadrant pain and discomfort. Infrequently, patients present with a cholestatic picture, suggesting extrahepatic biliary obstruction. Splenomegaly and cervical adenopathy are present in 10–20% of patients with acute hepatitis. Rarely, a few spider angiomas appear during the icteric phase and disappear during convalescence. During the *recovery phase*, constitutional symptoms disappear, but usually some liver enlargement and abnormalities in liver biochemical tests are still evident. The duration of the posticteric phase is variable, ranging from 2–12 weeks, and is usually more prolonged in acute hepatitis B and C. Complete clinical and biochemical recovery is to be expected 1–2 months after all cases of hepatitis A and E and 3–4 months after the onset of jaundice in three-quarters of uncomplicated, self-limited cases of hepatitis B and C (among healthy adults, acute hepatitis B is self-limited in 95–99%, whereas hepatitis C is self-limited in only ~15%). In the remainder, biochemical recovery may be delayed. A substantial proportion of patients with viral hepatitis never become icteric.

Infection with HDV can occur in the presence of acute or chronic HBV infection; the duration of HBV infection determines the duration of HDV infection. When acute HDV and HBV infection occur simultaneously, clinical and biochemical features may be indistinguishable from those of HBV infection alone, although occasionally they are more severe. As opposed to patients with *acute* HBV infection, patients with *chronic* HBV infection can support HDV replication indefinitely, as when acute HDV infection occurs in the presence of a nonresolving acute HBV infection or, more commonly, when acute hepatitis D is superimposed on underlying chronic hepatitis B. In such cases, the HDV superinfection appears as a clinical exacerbation or an episode resembling acute viral hepatitis in someone already chronically infected with HBV. Superinfection with HDV in a patient with chronic hepatitis B often leads to clinical deterioration (see below).

In addition to superinfections with other hepatitis agents, acute hepatitis-like clinical events in persons with chronic hepatitis B may accompany spontaneous HBeAg to anti-HBe seroconversion or spontaneous reactivation (i.e., reversion from relatively nonreplicative to replicative infection). Such reactivations can occur as well in therapeutically immunosuppressed patients with chronic HBV infection when cytotoxic/immunosuppressive drugs are withdrawn; in these cases, restoration of immune competence is thought to allow resumption of previously checked cell-mediated immune cytolysis of HBV-infected hepatocytes. Occasionally, acute clinical exacerbations of chronic hepatitis B may represent the emergence of a precore mutant (see "Virology and Etiology"), and the subsequent course in such patients may be characterized by periodic exacerbations. Cytotoxic chemotherapy can lead to reactivation of chronic hepatitis C as well, and anti-TNF-α therapy can lead to reactivation of both hepatitis B and C.

Laboratory Features The serum aminotransferases aspartate aminotransferase (AST) and alanine aminotransferase (ALT) (previously designated SGOT and SGPT) increase to a variable degree during the prodromal phase of acute viral hepatitis and precede the rise in bilirubin level (Figs. 360-2 and 360-4). The level of these enzymes, however, does not correlate well with the degree of liver cell damage. Peak levels vary from 400–4000 IU or more; these levels are usually reached at the time the patient is clinically icteric and diminish progressively during the recovery phase of acute hepatitis. The diagnosis of anicteric hepatitis is based on clinical features and on aminotransferase elevations.

Jaundice is usually visible in the sclera or skin when the serum bilirubin value is >43 μmol/L (2.5 mg/dL). When jaundice appears, the serum bilirubin typically rises to levels ranging from 85–340 μmol/L (5–20 mg/dL). The serum bilirubin may continue to rise despite falling serum aminotransferase levels. In most instances, the total bilirubin is equally divided between the conjugated and unconjugated fractions. Bilirubin levels >340 μmol/L (20 mg/dL) extending and persisting late into the course of viral hepatitis are more likely to be associated with severe disease. In certain patients with underlying hemolytic anemia, however, such as glucose-6-phosphate dehydrogenase deficiency and sickle cell anemia, a high serum bilirubin level is common, resulting from superimposed hemolysis. In such patients, bilirubin levels >513 μmol/L (30 mg/dL) have been observed and are not necessarily associated with a poor prognosis.

Neutropenia and lymphopenia are transient and are followed by a relative lymphocytosis. Atypical lymphocytes (varying between 2 and 20%) are common during the acute phase. Measurement of the prothrombin time (PT) is important in patients with acute viral hepatitis, because a prolonged value may reflect a severe hepatic synthetic defect, signify extensive hepatocellular necrosis, and indicate a worse prognosis. Occasionally, a prolonged PT may occur with only mild increases in the serum bilirubin and aminotransferase levels. Prolonged nausea and vomiting, inadequate carbohydrate intake, and poor hepatic glycogen reserves may contribute to hypoglycemia noted occasionally in patients with severe viral hepatitis. Serum alkaline phosphatase may be normal or only mildly elevated, whereas a fall in serum albumin is uncommon in uncomplicated acute viral hepatitis. In some patients, mild and transient steatorrhea has been noted, as well as slight microscopic hematuria and minimal proteinuria.

A diffuse but mild elevation of the γ globulin fraction is common during acute viral hepatitis. Serum IgG and IgM levels are elevated in about one-third of patients during the acute phase of viral hepatitis, but the serum IgM level is elevated more characteristically during acute hepatitis A. During the acute phase of viral hepatitis, antibodies to smooth muscle and other cell constituents may be present, and low titers of rheumatoid factor, nuclear antibody, and heterophile antibody can also be found occasionally. In hepatitis C and D, antibodies to LKM may occur; however, the species of LKM antibodies in the two types of hepatitis are different from each other as well as from the LKM antibody species characteristic of autoimmune hepatitis type 2 (Chap. 362). The autoantibodies in viral hepatitis are nonspecific and can also be associated with other viral and systemic diseases. In contrast, virus-specific antibodies, which appear during and after hepatitis virus infection, are serologic markers of diagnostic importance.

As described above, serologic tests are available routinely with which to establish a diagnosis of hepatitis A, B, D, and C. Tests for fecal or serum HAV are not routinely available. Therefore, a diagnosis of hepatitis A is based on detection of IgM anti-HAV during acute illness (Fig. 360-2). Rheumatoid factor can give rise to false-positive results in this test.

A diagnosis of HBV infection can usually be made by detection of HBsAg in serum. Infrequently, levels of HBsAg are too low to be detected during acute HBV infection, even with contemporary, highly sensitive immunoassays. In such cases, the diagnosis can be established by the presence of IgM anti-HBc.

The titer of HBsAg bears little relation to the severity of clinical disease. Indeed, an inverse correlation exists between the serum concentration of HBsAg and the degree of liver cell damage. For example, titers are highest in immunosuppressed patients, lower in patients with chronic liver disease (but higher in mild chronic than in severe chronic hepatitis), and very low in patients with acute fulminant hepatitis. These observations suggest that, in hepatitis B, the degree of liver cell damage and the clinical course are related to variations in the patient's immune response to HBV rather than to the amount of circulating HBsAg. In immunocompetent persons, however, a correlation exists between markers of HBV *replication* and liver injury (see below).

Another important serologic marker in patients with hepatitis B is HBeAg. Its principal clinical usefulness is as an indicator of relative infectivity. Because HBeAg is invariably present during early acute hepatitis B, HBeAg testing is indicated primarily in chronic infection.

In patients with hepatitis B surface antigenemia of unknown duration (e.g., blood donors found to be HBsAg-positive) testing for IgM anti-HBc may be useful to distinguish between acute or recent infection (IgM anti-HBc-positive) and chronic HBV infection (IgM anti-HBc-negative, IgG anti-HBc-positive). A false-positive test for IgM anti-HBc may be encountered in patients with high-titer rheumatoid factor. Also, IgM anti-HBc may be reexpressed during acute reactivation of chronic hepatitis B.

Anti-HBs is rarely detectable in the presence of HBsAg in patients with *acute* hepatitis B, but 10–20% of persons with *chronic* HBV infection may harbor low-level anti-HBs. This antibody is directed not against the common group determinant, *a*, but against the heterotypic subtype determinant (e.g., HBsAg of subtype *ad* with anti-HBs of subtype *y*). In most cases, this serologic pattern cannot be attributed to infection with two different HBV subtypes, and the presence of this antibody is not a harbinger of imminent HBsAg clearance. When such antibody is detected, its presence is of no recognized clinical significance (see "Virology and Etiology").

After immunization with hepatitis B vaccine, which consists of HBsAg alone, anti-HBs is the only serologic marker to appear. The commonly encountered serologic patterns of hepatitis B and their interpretations are summarized in Table 360-5. Tests for the detection of HBV DNA in liver and serum are now available. Like HBeAg, serum HBV DNA is an indicator of HBV replication, but tests for HBV DNA are more sensitive and quantitative. First-generation hybridization assays for HBV DNA had a sensitivity of 10^5–10^6 virions/mL, a relative threshold below which infectivity and liver injury are limited and HBeAg is usually undetectable. Currently, testing for HBV DNA has shifted from insensitive hybridization assays to amplification assays (e.g., the PCR-based assay, which can detect as few as 10 or 100 virions/mL); among the commercially available PCR assays, the most useful are those with the highest sensitivity (5–10 IU/mL) and the largest dynamic range (10^0–10^9 IU/mL). With increased sensitivity,

TABLE 360-5 COMMONLY ENCOUNTERED SEROLOGIC PATTERNS OF HEPATITIS B INFECTION

HBsAg	Anti-HBs	Anti-HBc	HBeAg	Anti-HBe	Interpretation
+	−	IgM	+	−	Acute hepatitis B, high infectivity[a]
+	−	IgG	+	−	Chronic hepatitis B, high infectivity
+	−	IgG	−	+	1. Late acute or chronic hepatitis B, low infectivity 2. HBeAg-negative ("precore-mutant") hepatitis B (chronic or, rarely, acute)
+	+	+	+/−	+/−	1. HBsAg of one subtype and heterotypic anti-HBs (common) 2. Process of seroconversion from HBsAg to anti-HBs (rare)
−	−	IgM	+/−	+/−	1. Acute hepatitis B[a] 2. Anti-HBc "window"
	−	IgG	−	+/−	1. Low-level hepatitis B carrier 2. Hepatitis B in remote past
−	+	IgG	−	+/−	Recovery from hepatitis B
−	+	−	−	−	1. Immunization with HBsAg (after vaccination) 2. Hepatitis B in the remote past (?) 3. False-positive

[a]IgM anti-HBc may reappear during acute reactivation of chronic hepatitis B.

Note: See text for abbreviations.

amplification assays remain reactive well below the current 10^3–10^4 IU/mL threshold for infectivity and liver injury. These markers are useful in following the course of HBV replication in patients with chronic hepatitis B receiving antiviral chemotherapy (Chap. 362). Except for the early decades of life after perinatally acquired HBV infection (see above), in immunocompetent adults with chronic hepatitis B, a general correlation exists between the level of HBV replication, as reflected by the level of serum HBV DNA, and the degree of liver injury. High-serum HBV DNA levels, increased expression of viral antigens, and necroinflammatory activity in the liver go hand in hand unless immunosuppression interferes with cytolytic T cell responses to virus-infected cells; reduction of HBV replication with antiviral drugs tends to be accompanied by an improvement in liver histology. Among patients with chronic hepatitis B, high levels of HBV DNA increase the risk of cirrhosis, hepatic decompensation, and hepatocellular carcinoma (see "Complications and Sequelae").

In patients with hepatitis C, an episodic pattern of aminotransferase elevation is common. A specific serologic diagnosis of hepatitis C can be made by demonstrating the presence in serum of anti-HCV. When contemporary immunoassays are used, anti-HCV can be detected in acute hepatitis C during the initial phase of elevated aminotransferase activity and remains detectable after recovery (rare) and during chronic infection (common). Nonspecificity can confound immunoassays for anti-HCV, especially in persons with a low prior probability of infection, such as volunteer blood donors, or in persons with circulating rheumatoid factor, which can bind nonspecifically to assay reagents; testing for HCV RNA can be used in such settings to distinguish between true-positive and false-positive anti-HCV determinations. Assays for HCV RNA are the most sensitive tests for HCV infection and represent the "gold standard" in establishing a diagnosis of hepatitis C. HCV RNA can be detected even before acute elevation of aminotransferase activity and before the appearance of anti-HCV in patients with acute hepatitis C. In addition, HCV RNA remains detectable indefinitely, continuously in most but intermittently in some, in patients with chronic hepatitis C (detectable as well in some persons with normal liver tests, i.e., inactive carriers). In the very small minority of patients with hepatitis C who lack anti-HCV, a diagnosis can be supported by detection of HCV RNA. If all these tests are negative and the patient has a well-characterized case of hepatitis after percutaneous exposure to blood or blood products, a diagnosis of hepatitis caused by an unidentified agent can be entertained.

Amplification techniques are required to detect HCV RNA, and two types are available. One is a branched-chain complementary DNA (bDNA) assay, in which the detection signal (a colorimetrically detectable enzyme bound to a complementary DNA probe) is amplified. The other involves target amplification (i.e., synthesis of multiple copies of the viral genome) by PCR or TMA, in which the viral RNA is reverse transcribed to complementary DNA and then amplified by repeated cycles of DNA synthesis. Both can be used as quantitative assays and a measurement of relative "viral load"; PCR and TMA, with a sensitivity of 10–10^2 IU/mL, are more sensitive than bDNA, with a sensitivity of 10^3 IU/mL; assays are available with a wide dynamic range (10–10^7 IU/mL). Determination of HCV RNA level is not a reliable marker of disease severity or prognosis but is helpful in predicting relative responsiveness to antiviral therapy. The same is true for determinations of HCV genotype (Chap. 362).

A proportion of patients with hepatitis C have isolated anti-HBc in their blood, a reflection of a common risk in certain populations of exposure to multiple bloodborne hepatitis agents. The anti-HBc in such cases is almost invariably of the IgG class and usually represents HBV infection in the remote past (HBV DNA undetectable); it rarely represents current HBV infection with low-level virus carriage.

The presence of HDV infection can be identified by demonstrating intrahepatic HDV antigen or, more practically, an anti-HDV seroconversion (a rise in titer of anti-HDV or de novo appearance of anti-HDV). Circulating HDV antigen, also diagnostic of acute infection, is detectable only briefly, if at all. Because anti-HDV is often undetectable once HBsAg disappears, retrospective serodiagnosis of acute self-limited, simultaneous HBV and HDV infection is difficult. Early diagnosis of acute infection may be hampered by a delay of up to 30–40 days in the appearance of anti-HDV.

When a patient presents with acute hepatitis and has HBsAg and anti-HDV in serum, determination of the class of anti-HBc is helpful in establishing the relationship between infection with HBV and HDV. Although IgM anti-HBc does not distinguish *absolutely* between acute and chronic HBV infection, its presence is a reliable indicator of recent infection and its absence a reliable indicator of infection in the remote past. In simultaneous acute HBV and HDV infections, IgM anti-HBc will be detectable, whereas in acute HDV infection superimposed on chronic HBV infection, anti-HBc will be of the IgG class. Tests for the presence of HDV RNA are useful for determining the presence of ongoing HDV replication and relative infectivity.

The serologic/virologic course of events during acute hepatitis E is entirely analogous to that of acute hepatitis A, with brief fecal shedding of virus and viremia and an early IgM anti-HEV response that predominates during approximately the first 3 months but is eclipsed thereafter by long-lasting IgG anti-HEV. Diagnostic tests of varying reliability for hepatitis E are commercially available but used routinely primarily outside the United States; in the United States, diagnostic serologic/virologic assays can be performed at the Centers for Disease Control and Prevention or other specialized reference laboratories.

Liver biopsy is rarely necessary or indicated in acute viral hepatitis, except when the diagnosis is questionable or when clinical evidence suggests a diagnosis of chronic hepatitis.

A diagnostic algorithm can be applied in the evaluation of cases of acute viral hepatitis. A patient with acute hepatitis should undergo four serologic tests, HBsAg, IgM anti-HAV, IgM anti-HBc, and anti-HCV (Table 360-6). The presence of HBsAg, with or without IgM anti-HBc, represents HBV infection. If IgM anti-HBc is present, the HBV infection is considered acute; if IgM anti-HBc is absent, the HBV infection is considered chronic. A diagnosis of acute hepatitis B can be made in

TABLE 360-6 SIMPLIFIED DIAGNOSTIC APPROACH IN PATIENTS PRESENTING WITH ACUTE HEPATITIS

Serologic Tests of Patient's Serum				
HBsAg	IgM Anti-HAV	IgM Anti-HBc	Anti-HCV	Diagnostic Interpretation
+	−	+	−	Acute hepatitis B
+	−	−	−	Chronic hepatitis B
+	+	−	−	Acute hepatitis A superimposed on chronic hepatitis B
+	+	+	−	Acute hepatitis A and B
−	+	−	−	Acute hepatitis A
−	+	+	−	Acute hepatitis A and B (HBsAg below detection threshold)
−	−	+	−	Acute hepatitis B (HBsAg below detection threshold)
−	−	−	+	Acute hepatitis C

Note: See text for abbreviations.

the absence of HBsAg when IgM anti-HBc is detectable. A diagnosis of acute hepatitis A is based on the presence of IgM anti-HAV. If IgM anti-HAV coexists with HBsAg, a diagnosis of simultaneous HAV and HBV infections can be made; if IgM anti-HBc (with or without HBsAg) is detectable, the patient has simultaneous acute hepatitis A and B, and if IgM anti-HBc is undetectable, the patient has acute hepatitis A superimposed on chronic HBV infection. The presence of anti-HCV supports a diagnosis of acute hepatitis C. Occasionally, testing for HCV RNA or repeat anti-HCV testing later during the illness is necessary to establish the diagnosis. Absence of all serologic markers is consistent with a diagnosis of "non-A, non-B, non-C" hepatitis, if the epidemiologic setting is appropriate.

In patients with chronic hepatitis, initial testing should consist of HBsAg and anti-HCV. Anti-HCV supports and HCV RNA testing establishes the diagnosis of chronic hepatitis C. If a serologic diagnosis of chronic hepatitis B is made, testing for HBeAg and anti-HBe is indicated to evaluate relative infectivity. Testing for HBV DNA in such patients provides a more quantitative and sensitive measure of the level of virus replication and, therefore, is very helpful during antiviral therapy (Chap. 362). In patients with chronic hepatitis B and normal aminotransferase activity in the absence of HBeAg, serial testing over time is often required to distinguish between inactive carriage and HBeAg-negative chronic hepatitis B with fluctuating virologic and necroinflammatory activity. In persons with hepatitis B, testing for anti-HDV is useful in those with severe and fulminant disease, with severe chronic disease, with chronic hepatitis B and acute hepatitis-like exacerbations, with frequent percutaneous exposures, and from areas where HDV infection is endemic.

PROGNOSIS

Virtually all previously healthy patients with hepatitis A recover completely with no clinical sequelae. Similarly, in acute hepatitis B, 95–99% of previously healthy adults have a favorable course and recover completely. Certain clinical and laboratory features, however, suggest a more complicated and protracted course. Patients of advanced age and with serious underlying medical disorders may have a prolonged course and are more likely to experience severe hepatitis. Initial presenting features such as ascites, peripheral edema, and symptoms of hepatic encephalopathy suggest a poorer prognosis. In addition, a prolonged PT, low serum albumin level, hypoglycemia, and very high serum bilirubin values suggest severe hepatocellular disease. Patients with these clinical and laboratory features deserve prompt hospital admission. The case fatality rate in hepatitis A and B is very low (~0.1%) but is increased by advanced age and underlying debilitating disorders. Among patients ill enough to be hospitalized for acute hepatitis B, the fatality rate is 1%. Hepatitis C is less severe during the acute phase than hepatitis B and is more likely to be anicteric; fatalities are rare, but the precise case fatality rate is not known. In outbreaks of waterborne hepatitis E in India and Asia, the case fatality rate is 1–2% and up to 10–20% in pregnant women. Contributing to fulminant hepatitis E in endemic countries are instances of acute hepatitis E superimposed on underlying chronic liver disease ("acute-on-chronic" liver disease). Patients with simultaneous acute hepatitis B and hepatitis D do not necessarily experience a higher mortality rate than do patients with acute hepatitis B alone; however, in several outbreaks of acute simultaneous HBV and HDV infection among injection drug users, the case fatality rate was ~5%. When HDV superinfection occurs in a person with chronic hepatitis B, the likelihood of fulminant hepatitis and death is increased substantially. Although the case fatality rate for hepatitis D is not known definitively, in outbreaks of severe HDV superinfection in isolated populations with a high hepatitis B carrier rate, a mortality rate >20% has been recorded.

COMPLICATIONS AND SEQUELAE

A small proportion of patients with hepatitis A experience *relapsing hepatitis* weeks to months after apparent recovery from acute hepatitis. Relapses are characterized by recurrence of symptoms, aminotransferase elevations, occasionally jaundice, and fecal excretion of HAV. Another unusual variant of acute hepatitis A is *cholestatic hepatitis*, characterized by protracted cholestatic jaundice and pruritus. Rarely, liver test abnormalities persist for many months, even up to a year. Even when these complications occur, hepatitis A remains self-limited and does not progress to chronic liver disease. During the prodromal phase of acute hepatitis B, a serum sickness–like syndrome characterized by arthralgia or arthritis, rash, angioedema, and rarely, hematuria and proteinuria may develop in 5–10% of patients. This syndrome occurs before the onset of clinical jaundice, and these patients are often diagnosed erroneously as having rheumatologic diseases. The diagnosis can be established by measuring serum aminotransferase levels, which are almost invariably elevated, and serum HBsAg. As noted above, EMC is an immune-complex disease that can complicate chronic hepatitis C and is part of a spectrum of B cell lymphoproliferative disorders, which, in rare instances, can evolve to B cell lymphoma (Chap. 134). Attention has been drawn as well to associations between hepatitis C and such cutaneous disorders as porphyria cutanea tarda and lichen planus. A mechanism for these associations is unknown. Finally, related to the reliance of HCV on lipoprotein secretion and assembly pathways and on interactions of HCV with glucose metabolism, HCV infection may be complicated by hepatic steatosis, hypercholesterolemia, insulin resistance (and other manifestations of the metabolic syndrome), and type 2 diabetes mellitus; both hepatic steatosis and insulin resistance appear to accelerate hepatic fibrosis and blunt responsiveness to antiviral therapy (Chap. 362).

The most feared complication of viral hepatitis is *fulminant hepatitis* (massive hepatic necrosis); fortunately, this is a rare event. Fulminant hepatitis is seen primarily in hepatitis B, D, and E, but rare fulminant cases of hepatitis A occur primarily in older adults and in persons with underlying chronic liver disease, including, according to some reports, chronic hepatitis B and C. Hepatitis B accounts for >50% of fulminant cases of viral hepatitis, a sizable proportion of which are associated with HDV infection and another proportion with underlying chronic hepatitis C. Fulminant hepatitis is hardly ever seen in hepatitis C, but hepatitis E, as noted above, can be complicated by fatal fulminant hepatitis in 1–2% of all cases and in up to 20% of cases in pregnant women. Patients usually present with signs and symptoms of encephalopathy that may evolve to deep coma. The liver is usually small and the PT excessively prolonged. The combination of rapidly shrinking liver size, rapidly rising bilirubin level, and marked prolongation of the PT, even as aminotransferase levels fall, together with clinical signs of confusion, disorientation, somnolence, ascites, and edema, indicates that the patient has hepatic failure with encephalopathy. Cerebral edema is common; brainstem compression, gastrointestinal bleeding, sepsis, respiratory failure, cardiovascular collapse, and renal failure are terminal events. The mortality rate is exceedingly high (>80% in patients with deep coma), but patients who survive may have a complete biochemical and histologic recovery. If a donor liver can be located in time, liver transplantation may be life-saving in patients with fulminant hepatitis (Chap. 368).

Documenting the disappearance of HBsAg after apparent clinical recovery from acute hepatitis B is particularly important. Before laboratory methods were available to distinguish between acute hepatitis and acute hepatitis-like exacerbations (*spontaneous reactivations*) of chronic hepatitis B, observations suggested that ~10% of previously healthy patients remained HBsAg-positive for >6 months after the onset of clinically apparent acute hepatitis B. One-half of these persons cleared the antigen from their circulations during the next several years, but the other 5% remained chronically HBsAg-positive. More recent observations suggest that the true rate of chronic infection after clinically apparent acute hepatitis B is as low as 1% in normal, immunocompetent, young adults. Earlier, higher estimates may have been confounded by inadvertent inclusion of acute exacerbations in chronically infected patients; these patients, chronically HBsAg-positive before exacerbation, were unlikely to seroconvert to HBsAg-negative thereafter. Whether the rate of chronicity is 10% or 1%, such patients have IgG anti-HBc in serum; anti-HBs is either undetected or detected at low titer against the opposite subtype specificity of the antigen (see "Laboratory Features"). These patients may (1) be inactive carriers; (2) have low-grade, mild chronic hepatitis; or (3) have moderate to severe chronic hepatitis with or without cirrhosis. The likelihood of remaining chronically infected after acute HBV infection is especially high among neonates, persons with Down's syndrome, chronically hemodialyzed patients, and immunosuppressed patients, including persons with HIV infection.

Chronic hepatitis is an important late complication of acute hepatitis B occurring in a small proportion of patients with acute disease but more common in those who present with chronic infection without having experienced an acute illness, as occurs typically after neonatal infection or after infection in an immunosuppressed host (Chap. 362). The following clinical and laboratory features suggest progression of acute hepatitis to chronic hepatitis: (1) lack of complete resolution of clinical symptoms of anorexia, weight loss, fatigue, and the persistence of hepatomegaly; (2) the presence of bridging/interface or multilobular hepatic necrosis on liver biopsy during protracted, severe acute viral hepatitis; (3) failure of the serum aminotransferase, bilirubin, and globulin levels to return to normal within 6–12 months after the acute illness; and (4) the persistence of HBeAg for >3 months or HBsAg for >6 months after acute hepatitis.

Although acute hepatitis D infection does not increase the likelihood of chronicity of simultaneous acute hepatitis B, hepatitis D has the potential for contributing to the severity of chronic hepatitis B. Hepatitis D superinfection can transform inactive or mild chronic hepatitis B into severe, progressive chronic hepatitis and cirrhosis; it also can accelerate the course of chronic hepatitis B. Some HDV superinfections in patients with chronic hepatitis B lead to fulminant hepatitis. As defined in longitudinal studies over three decades, the annual rates of cirrhosis and hepatocellular carcinoma in patients with chronic hepatitis D are 4% and 2.8%, respectively. Although HDV and HBV infections are associated with severe liver disease, mild hepatitis and even inactive carriage have been identified in some patients, and the disease may become indolent beyond the early years of infection.

After acute HCV infection, the likelihood of remaining chronically *infected* approaches 85–90%. Although many patients with chronic hepatitis C have no symptoms, cirrhosis may develop in as many as 20% within 10–20 years of acute illness; in some series of cases reported by referral centers, cirrhosis has been reported in as many as 50% of patients with chronic hepatitis C. Although chronic hepatitis C accounts for at least 40% of cases of chronic liver disease and of patients undergoing liver transplantation for end-stage liver disease in the United States and Europe, in the majority of patients with chronic hepatitis C, morbidity and mortality are limited during the initial 20 years after the onset of infection. Progression of chronic hepatitis C may be influenced by advanced age of acquisition, long duration of infection, immunosuppression, coexisting excessive alcohol use, concomitant hepatic steatosis, other hepatitis virus infection, or HIV coinfection. In fact, instances of severe and rapidly progressive chronic hepatitis B and C are being recognized with increasing frequency in patients with HIV infection (Chap. 226). In contrast, neither HAV nor HEV causes chronic liver disease in immunocompetent hosts; however, cases of chronic hepatitis E have been observed in immunosuppressed organ-transplant recipients, persons receiving cytotoxic chemotherapy, and persons with HIV infection.

Rare complications of viral hepatitis include pancreatitis, myocarditis, atypical pneumonia, aplastic anemia, transverse myelitis, and peripheral neuropathy. Persons with chronic hepatitis B, particularly those infected in infancy or early childhood and especially those with HBeAg and/or high-level HBV DNA, have an enhanced risk of hepatocellular carcinoma. The risk of hepatocellular carcinoma is increased as well in patients with chronic hepatitis C, almost exclusively in patients with cirrhosis, and almost always after at least several decades usually after three decades of disease (Chap. 111). In children, hepatitis B may present rarely with anicteric hepatitis, a nonpruritic papular rash of the face, buttocks, and limbs, and lymphadenopathy (papular acrodermatitis of childhood or Gianotti-Crosti syndrome).

Rarely, autoimmune hepatitis (Chap. 362) can be triggered by a bout of otherwise self-limited acute hepatitis, as reported after acute hepatitis A, B, and C.

DIFFERENTIAL DIAGNOSIS

Viral diseases such as infectious mononucleosis; those due to cytomegalovirus, herpes simplex, and coxsackieviruses; and toxoplasmosis may share certain clinical features with viral hepatitis and cause elevations in serum aminotransferase and, less commonly, in serum bilirubin levels. Tests such as the differential heterophile and serologic tests for these agents may be helpful in the differential diagnosis if HBsAg, anti-HBc, IgM anti-HAV, and anti-HCV determinations are negative. Aminotransferase elevations can accompany almost any systemic viral infection; other rare causes of liver injury confused with viral hepatitis are infections with *Leptospira, Candida, Brucella, Mycobacteria,* and *Pneumocystis*. A complete drug history is particularly important because many drugs and certain anesthetic agents can produce a picture of either acute hepatitis or cholestasis (Chap. 361). Equally important is a past history of unexplained "repeated episodes" of acute hepatitis. This history should alert the physician to the possibility that the underlying disorder is chronic hepatitis. Alcoholic hepatitis must also be considered, but usually the serum aminotransferase levels are not as markedly elevated, and other stigmata of alcoholism may be present. The finding on liver biopsy of fatty infiltration, a neutrophilic inflammatory reaction, and "alcoholic hyaline" would be consistent with alcohol-induced rather than viral liver injury. Because acute hepatitis may present with right upper quadrant abdominal pain, nausea and vomiting, fever, and icterus, it is often confused with acute cholecystitis, common duct stone, or ascending cholangitis. Patients with acute viral hepatitis may tolerate surgery poorly; therefore, it is important to exclude this diagnosis, and in confusing cases, a percutaneous liver biopsy may be necessary before laparotomy. Viral hepatitis in the elderly is often misdiagnosed as obstructive jaundice resulting from a common duct stone or carcinoma of the pancreas. Because acute hepatitis in the elderly may be quite severe and the operative mortality high, a thorough evaluation including biochemical tests, radiographic studies of the biliary tree, and even liver biopsy may be necessary to exclude primary parenchymal liver disease. Another clinical constellation that may mimic acute hepatitis is right ventricular failure with passive hepatic congestion or hypoperfusion syndromes, such as those associated with shock, severe hypotension, and severe left ventricular failure. Also included in this general category is any disorder that interferes with venous return to the heart, such as right atrial myxoma, constrictive pericarditis, hepatic vein occlusion (Budd-Chiari syndrome), or venoocclusive disease. Clinical features are usually sufficient to distinguish among these vascular disorders and viral hepatitis. Acute fatty liver of pregnancy, cholestasis of pregnancy, eclampsia, and the HELLP (*h* emolysis, *e* levated *l* iver tests, and *l* ow *p* latelets) syndrome can be confused with viral hepatitis during pregnancy. Very rarely, malignancies metastatic to the liver can mimic acute or even fulminant viral hepatitis. Occasionally, genetic or metabolic liver disorders (e.g., Wilson's disease, α_1 antitrypsin deficiency) and nonalcoholic fatty liver disease are confused with acute viral hepatitis.

TREATMENT ACUTE VIRAL HEPATITIS

In hepatitis B, among previously healthy adults who present with clinically apparent acute hepatitis, recovery occurs in ~99%; therefore, antiviral therapy is not likely to improve the rate of recovery and is not required. In rare instances of severe acute hepatitis B, treatment with a nucleoside analogue at oral doses used to treat chronic hepatitis B (Chap. 362) has been attempted successfully. Although clinical trials have not been done to establish the efficacy or duration of this approach, most authorities would recommend institution of antiviral therapy with a nucleoside analogue (entecavir or tenofovir, the most potent and least resistance-prone agents) for severe, but not mild–moderate, acute hepatitis B. Treatment should continue until 3 months after HBsAg seroconversion or 6 months after HBeAg seroconversion.

In typical cases of acute hepatitis C, recovery is rare, progression to chronic hepatitis is the rule, and meta-analyses of small clinical trials suggest that antiviral therapy with interferon α monotherapy (3 million units SC three times a week) is beneficial, reducing the rate of chronicity considerably by inducing sustained responses in 30–70% of patients. In a German multicenter study of 44 patients with acute symptomatic hepatitis C, initiation of intensive interferon α therapy (5 million units SC daily for 4 weeks, then three times a week for another 20 weeks) within an average of 3 months after infection resulted in a sustained virologic response rate of 98%. Although treatment of acute hepatitis C is recommended, the optimum regimen, duration of therapy, and time to initiate therapy remain to be determined. Many authorities now opt for a 24-week course (beginning within 2–3 months after onset) of long-acting pegylated interferon plus the nucleoside analogue ribavirin, although the value of adding ribavirin has not been demonstrated (see Chap. 362 for doses). Patients with jaundice and women are more likely to recover from acute hepatitis C, and now that genetic markers associated with spontaneous recovery (*IL28B* CC haplotype) versus persistence (non-CC haplotypes) have been defined, such genetic testing can help determine the need for and immediacy of treating acute hepatitis C—maintaining a high threshold for treating patients with CC and a very low threshold for early intervention in patients with non-CC genotypes. Protease inhibitor–based antiviral therapy with telaprevir or boceprevir, now approved for chronic hepatitis C, genotype 1 (Chap. 362), has not been approved for acute hepatitis C. Moreover, given the high efficacy of pegylated interferon–based therapy for acute hepatitis C, in all likelihood, the addition of a protease inhibitor would add costs and side effects without incremental efficacy. When, however, after 2014, all-oral, brief-duration, low-resistance antiviral regimens replace the current standard of care, the new approaches will be applied to acute hepatitis C and, potentially (pending the outcome of clinical trials), could even be used immediately after exposure (e.g., occupational) to prevent infection and the onset of hepatitis. Because of the marked reduction over the past two decades in the frequency of acute hepatitis C, opportunities to identify and treat patients with acute hepatitis C are rare, except in injection drug users and health workers who sustain hepatitis C–contaminated needle sticks. After such occupational accidents, when monitoring for ALT elevations and the presence of HCV RNA identifies acute hepatitis C (risk only ~3%), therapy should be initiated.

Notwithstanding these specific therapeutic considerations, in most cases of typical acute viral hepatitis, specific treatment generally is not necessary. Although hospitalization may be required for clinically severe illness, most patients do not require hospital care. Forced and prolonged bed rest is not essential for full recovery, but many patients will feel better with restricted physical activity. A high-calorie diet is desirable, and because many patients may experience nausea late in the day, the major caloric intake is best tolerated in the morning. Intravenous feeding is necessary in the acute stage if the patient has persistent vomiting and cannot maintain oral intake. Drugs capable of producing adverse reactions such as cholestasis and drugs metabolized by the liver should be avoided. If severe pruritus is present, the use of the bile salt–sequestering resin cholestyramine is helpful. Glucocorticoid therapy has no value in acute viral hepatitis, even in severe cases associated with *bridging necrosis*, and may be deleterious, even increasing the risk of chronicity (e.g., of acute hepatitis B).

Physical isolation of patients with hepatitis to a single room and bathroom is rarely necessary except in the case of fecal incontinence for hepatitis A and E or uncontrolled, voluminous bleeding for hepatitis B (with or without concomitant hepatitis D) and hepatitis C. Because most patients hospitalized with hepatitis A excrete little, if any, HAV, the likelihood of HAV transmission from these patients during their hospitalization is low. Therefore, burdensome *enteric precautions are no longer recommended*. Although gloves should be worn when the bed pans or fecal material of patients with hepatitis A are handled, these precautions do not represent a departure from sensible procedure and contemporary universal precautions for all hospitalized patients. For patients with hepatitis B and hepatitis C, emphasis should be placed on blood precautions (i.e., avoiding direct, ungloved hand contact with blood and other body fluids). Enteric precautions are unnecessary. The importance of simple hygienic precautions such as hand washing cannot be overemphasized. Universal precautions that have been adopted for all patients apply to patients with viral hepatitis. Hospitalized patients may be discharged following substantial symptomatic improvement, a significant downward trend in the serum aminotransferase and bilirubin values, and a return to normal of the PT. Mild aminotransferase elevations should not be considered contraindications to the gradual resumption of normal activity.

In *fulminant hepatitis*, the goal of therapy is to support the patient by maintenance of fluid balance, support of circulation and respiration, control of bleeding, correction of hypoglycemia, and treatment of other complications of the comatose state in anticipation of liver regeneration and repair. Protein intake should be restricted, and oral lactulose or neomycin administered. Glucocorticoid therapy has been shown in controlled trials to be ineffective. Likewise, exchange transfusion, plasmapheresis, human cross-circulation, porcine liver cross-perfusion, hemoperfusion, and extracorporeal liver-assist devices have not been proven to enhance survival. Meticulous intensive care that includes prophylactic antibiotic coverage is the one factor that does appear to improve survival. Orthotopic liver transplantation is resorted to with increasing frequency, with excellent results, in patients with fulminant hepatitis (Chap. 368).

PROPHYLAXIS

Because application of therapy for acute viral hepatitis is limited and because antiviral therapy for chronic viral hepatitis is cumbersome, costly, and not effective in all patients (Chap. 362), emphasis is placed on prevention through immunization. The prophylactic approach differs for each of the types of viral hepatitis. In the past, immunoprophylaxis relied exclusively on passive immunization with antibody-containing globulin preparations purified by cold ethanol fractionation from the plasma of hundreds of normal donors. Currently, for hepatitis A, B, and E, active immunization with vaccines is the preferable approach to prevention.

Hepatitis A Both passive immunization with IG and active immunization with killed vaccines are available. All preparations of IG contain anti-HAV concentrations sufficient to be protective. When administered before exposure or during the early incubation period, IG is effective in preventing clinically apparent hepatitis A. For postexposure prophylaxis of intimate contacts (household, sexual, institutional) of persons with hepatitis A, the administration of 0.02 mL/kg is recommended as early after exposure as possible; it may be effective even when administered as late as 2 weeks after exposure. Prophylaxis is not necessary for those who have already received hepatitis A vaccine, for casual contacts (office, factory, school, or hospital), for most elderly persons, who are very likely to be immune, or for those known to have anti-HAV in their serum. In day care centers, recognition of hepatitis A in children or staff should provide a stimulus for immunoprophylaxis in the center and in the children's family members. By the time most common-source outbreaks of hepatitis A are recognized, it is usually too late in the incubation period for IG to be effective; however, prophylaxis may limit the frequency of secondary cases. For travelers to tropical countries, developing countries, and other areas outside standard tourist routes, IG prophylaxis had been recommended before a vaccine became available. When such travel lasted <3 months, 0.02 mL/kg was given; for longer travel or residence in these areas, a dose of 0.06 mL/kg every 4–6 months was recommended. Administration of plasma-derived globulin is safe; all contemporary lots of IG are subjected to viral inactivation steps and must be free of HCV RNA as determined by PCR testing. Administration of IM lots of IG has not been associated with transmission of HBV, HCV, or HIV.

Formalin-inactivated vaccines made from strains of HAV attenuated in tissue culture have been shown to be safe, immunogenic, and effective in preventing hepatitis A. Hepatitis A vaccines are approved for use in persons who are at least 1 year old and appear to provide adequate protection beginning 4 weeks after a primary inoculation. If it can be given within 4 weeks of an expected exposure, such as by travel to an endemic area, hepatitis A vaccine is the preferred approach to *pre-exposure* immunoprophylaxis. If travel is more imminent, IG (0.02 mL/kg) should be administered at a different injection site, along with the first dose of vaccine. Because vaccination provides long-lasting protection (protective levels of anti-HAV should last 20 years after vaccination), persons whose risk will be sustained (e.g., frequent travelers or those remaining in endemic areas for prolonged periods) should be vaccinated, and vaccine should supplant the need for repeated IG injections. Shortly after its introduction, hepatitis A vaccine was recommended for children living in communities with a high incidence of HAV infection; in 1999, this recommendation was extended to include all children living in states, counties, and communities with high rates of HAV infection. As of 2006, the Advisory Committee on Immunization Practices of the U.S. Public Health Service recommended *routine hepatitis A vaccination of all children*. Other groups considered to be at increased risk for HAV infection and who are candidates for hepatitis A vaccination include military personnel, populations with cyclic outbreaks of hepatitis A (e.g., Alaskan natives), employees of day care centers, primate handlers, laboratory workers exposed to hepatitis A or fecal specimens, and patients with chronic liver disease. Because of an increased risk of fulminant hepatitis A—observed in some experiences but not confirmed in others—among patients with chronic hepatitis C, patients with chronic hepatitis C are candidates for hepatitis A vaccination, as are persons with chronic hepatitis B. Other populations whose recognized risk of hepatitis A is increased should be vaccinated, including men who have sex with men, injection drug users, persons with clotting disorders who require frequent administration of clotting-factor concentrates, persons traveling from the United States to countries with high or intermediate hepatitis A endemicity, postexposure prophylaxis for contacts of persons with hepatitis A, and household members and other close contacts of adopted children arriving from countries with high and moderate hepatitis A endemicity. Recommendations for dose and frequency differ for the two approved vaccine preparations (Table 360-7); all injections are IM. Hepatitis A vaccine has been reported to be effective in preventing secondary household and day care center–associated cases of acute hepatitis A. Because the vaccine provides long-lasting protection and is simpler to use, in 2006, the Immunization Practices Advisory Committee of the U.S. Public Health Service favored hepatitis A vaccine to IG for postexposure prophylaxis of healthy persons age 2–40 years; for younger or older persons, for immunosuppressed patients, and for patients with chronic liver disease, IG should continue to be used. In the United States, reported mortality resulting from hepatitis A declined in parallel with hepatitis A vaccine–associated reductions in the annual incidence of new infections.

TABLE 360-7 HEPATITIS A VACCINATION SCHEDULES

Age, years	No. of Doses	Dose	Schedule, months
HAVRIX (GlaxoSmithKline)[a]			
1–18	2	720 ELU[b] (0.5 mL)	0, 6–12
≥19	2	1440 ELU (1 mL)	0, 6–12
VAQTA (Merck)			
1–18	2	25 units (0.5 mL)	0, 6–18
≥19	2	50 units (1 mL)	0, 6–18

[a]A combination of this hepatitis A vaccine and hepatitis B vaccine, TWINRIX, is licensed for simultaneous protection against both of these viruses among adults (age ≥18 years). Each 1-mL dose contains 720 ELU of hepatitis A vaccine and 20 μg of hepatitis B vaccine. These doses are recommended at months 0, 1, and 6. [b]Enzyme-linked immunoassay units.

Abbreviation: ELU, enzyme-linked immunoassay unit.

Hepatitis B Until 1982, prevention of hepatitis B was based on *passive* immunoprophylaxis either with standard Ig, containing modest levels of anti-HBs, or hepatitis B immunoglobulin (HBIG), containing high titer anti-HBs. The efficacy of standard IG has never been established and remains questionable; even the efficacy of HBIG, demonstrated in several clinical trials, has been challenged, and its contribution appears to be in reducing the frequency of clinical *illness*, not in preventing *infection*. The first vaccine for *active* immunization, introduced in 1982, was prepared from purified, noninfectious 22-nm spherical HBsAg particles derived from the plasma of healthy HBsAg carriers. In 1987, the plasma-derived vaccine was supplanted by a genetically engineered vaccine derived from recombinant yeast. The latter vaccine consists of HBsAg particles that are nonglycosylated but are otherwise indistinguishable from natural HBsAg; two recombinant vaccines are licensed for use in the United States. Current recommendations can be divided into those for pre-exposure and postexposure prophylaxis.

For *pre-exposure* prophylaxis against hepatitis B in settings of frequent exposure (health workers exposed to blood; first-responder public safety workers; hemodialysis patients and staff; residents and staff of custodial institutions for the developmentally handicapped; injection drug users; inmates of long-term correctional facilities; persons with multiple sexual partners or who have had a sexually transmitted disease; men who have sex with men; persons such as hemophiliacs who require long-term, high-volume therapy with blood derivatives; household and sexual contacts of persons with chronic HBV infection; persons living in or traveling extensively in endemic areas; unvaccinated children under the age of 18; unvaccinated children who are Alaskan natives, Pacific Islanders, or residents in households of first-generation immigrants from endemic countries; persons born in countries with a prevalence of HBV infection ≥2%; patients with chronic liver disease; persons <age 60 with diabetes mellitus [those ≥60 at the discretion of their physicians]; persons with end-stage renal disease; persons with HIV infection), three IM (deltoid, not gluteal) injections of hepatitis B vaccine are recommended at 0, 1, and 6 months (other, optional schedules are summarized in Table 360-8). Pregnancy is *not* a contraindication to vaccination. In areas of low HBV endemicity such as the United States, despite the availability of safe and effective hepatitis B vaccines, a strategy of vaccinating persons in high-risk groups was not effective. The incidence of new hepatitis B cases continued to increase in the United States after the introduction of vaccines; <10% of all targeted persons in high-risk groups were actually vaccinated, and ~30% of persons with sporadic acute hepatitis B did not fall into any high-risk-group category. Therefore, to have an impact on the frequency of HBV infection in an area of low endemicity such as the United States, universal hepatitis B vaccination in childhood has been recommended. For unvaccinated children born after the implementation of universal infant vaccination, vaccination during early adolescence, at age 11–12 years, was recommended, and this recommendation has been extended to include all unvaccinated children age 0–19 years. In HBV-hyperendemic areas (e.g., Asia), universal vaccination of children has resulted in a marked 10- to 15-year decline in hepatitis B and its complications, including hepatocellular carcinoma.

The two available recombinant hepatitis B vaccines are comparable, one containing 10 μg of HBsAg (Recombivax-HB) and the other containing 20 μg of HBsAg (Engerix-B), and recommended doses for each injection vary for the two preparations (Table 360-8). Combinations of hepatitis B vaccine with other childhood vaccines are available as well (Table 360-8).

For unvaccinated persons sustaining an exposure to HBV, *post-exposure* prophylaxis with a combination of HBIG (for rapid

TABLE 360-8 PRE-EXPOSURE HEPATITIS B VACCINATION SCHEDULES

Target Group	No. of Doses	Dose	Schedule, months
RECOMBIVAX-HB (Merck)[a]			
Infants, children (<1–10 years)	3	5 µg (0.5 mL)	0, 1–2, 4–6
Adolescents (11–19 years)	3 or 4	5 µg (0.5 mL)	0–2, 1–4, 4–6 *or* 0, 12, 24 *or* 0, 1, 2, 12
	Or 2	10 µg (1 mL)	0, 4–6 (age 11–15)
Adults (≥20 years)	3	10 µg (1 mL)	0–2, 1–4, 4–6
Hemodialysis patients[b]			
<20 years	3	5 µg (0.5 mL)	0, 1, 6
≥20 years	3	40 µg (4 mL)	0, 1, 6
ENGERIX-B (GlaxoSmithKline)[c]			
Infants, children (<1–10 years)	3 or 4	10 µg (0.5 mL)	0, 1–2, 4–6 *or* 0, 1, 2, 12
Adolescents (10–19 years)	3 or 4	10 µg (0.5 mL)	0, 1–2, 4–6 *or* 0, 12, 24 *or* 0, 1, 2, 12
Adults (≥20 years)	3 or 4	20 µg (1 mL)	0–2, 1–4, 4–6 or 0, 1, 2, 12
Hemodialysis patients[b]			
<20 years	4	10 µg (0.5 mL)	0, 1, 2, 6
≥20 years	4	40 µg (2 mL)	0, 1, 2, 6

[a]This manufacturer produces a licensed combination of hepatitis B vaccine and vaccines against *Haemophilus influenzae* type b and *Neisseria meningitides*, Comvax, for use in infants and young children. Please consult product insert for dose and schedule. [b]This group also includes other immunocompromised persons. [c]This manufacturer produces two licensed combination hepatitis B vaccines: (1) Twinrix, recombinant hepatitis B vaccine plus inactivated hepatitis A vaccine, is licensed for simultaneous protection against both of these viruses among adults (age ≥18 years). Each 1-mL dose contains 720 ELU of hepatitis A vaccine and 20 µg of hepatitis B vaccine. These doses are recommended at months 0, 1, and 6. (2) Pediatrix, recombinant hepatitis B vaccine plus diphtheria and tetanus toxoid, pertussis, and inactivated poliovirus, is licensed for use in infants and young children. Please consult product insert for doses and schedules.

achievement of high-titer circulating anti-HBs) and hepatitis B vaccine (for achievement of long-lasting immunity as well as its apparent efficacy in attenuating clinical illness after exposure) is recommended. For *perinatal* exposure of infants born to HBsAg-positive mothers, a single dose of HBIG, 0.5 mL, should be administered IM in the thigh *immediately after birth*, followed by a complete course of three injections of recombinant hepatitis B vaccine (see doses above) to be started within the first 12 h of life. For those experiencing a direct percutaneous inoculation or transmucosal exposure to HBsAg-positive blood or body fluids (e.g., accidental *needle stick*, other mucosal penetration, or ingestion), a single IM dose of HBIG, 0.06 mL/kg, administered as soon after exposure as possible, is followed by a complete course of hepatitis B vaccine to begin within the first week. For those exposed by *sexual* contact to a patient with acute hepatitis B, a single IM dose of HBIG, 0.06 mL/kg, should be given within 14 days of exposure, to be followed by a complete course of hepatitis B vaccine. When both HBIG and hepatitis B vaccine are recommended, they may be given at the same time but at separate sites. Testing adults for anti-HBs after a course of vaccine is advisable to document the acquisition of immunity, but, because hepatitis B vaccine immunogenicity is nearly universal in infants, postvaccination anti-HBs testing of children is not recommended.

The precise duration of protection afforded by hepatitis B vaccine is unknown; however, ~80–90% of immunocompetent adult vaccinees retain protective levels of anti-HBs for at least 5 years, and 60–80% for 10 years, and protective antibody has been documented to last for at least two decades after vaccination in infancy. Thereafter and even after anti-HBs becomes undetectable, protection persists against clinical hepatitis B, hepatitis B surface antigenemia, and chronic HBV infection. Currently, *booster* immunizations are not recommended routinely, except in immunosuppressed persons who have lost detectable anti-HBs or immunocompetent persons who sustain percutaneous HBsAg-positive inoculations after losing detectable antibody. Specifically, for hemodialysis patients, annual anti-HBs testing is recommended after vaccination; booster doses are recommended when anti-HBs levels fall to <10 mIU/mL. As noted above, for persons at risk of both hepatitis A and B, a combined vaccine is available containing 720 enzyme-linked immunoassay units (ELUs) of inactivated HAV and 20 µg of recombinant HBsAg (at 0, 1, and 6 months).

Hepatitis D Infection with hepatitis D can be prevented by vaccinating susceptible persons with hepatitis B vaccine. No product is available for immunoprophylaxis to prevent HDV superinfection in HBsAg carriers; for them, avoidance of percutaneous exposures and limitation of intimate contact with persons who have HDV infection are recommended.

Hepatitis C IG is ineffective in preventing hepatitis C and is no longer recommended for postexposure prophylaxis in cases of perinatal, needle stick, or sexual exposure. Although prototype vaccines that induce antibodies to HCV envelope proteins have been developed, currently, hepatitis C vaccination is not feasible practically. Genotype and quasispecies viral heterogeneity as well as rapid evasion of neutralizing antibodies by this rapidly mutating virus, conspire to render HCV a difficult target for immunoprophylaxis with a vaccine. Prevention of transfusion-associated hepatitis C has been accomplished by the following successively introduced measures: exclusion of commercial blood donors and reliance on a volunteer blood supply; screening donor blood with surrogate markers such as ALT (no longer recommended) and anti-HBc, markers that identify segments of the blood donor population with an increased risk of bloodborne infections; exclusion of blood donors in high-risk groups for AIDS and the introduction of anti-HIV screening tests; and progressively sensitive serologic and virologic screening tests for HCV infection.

In the absence of active or passive immunization, prevention of hepatitis C includes behavior changes and precautions to limit exposures to infected persons. Recommendations designed to identify patients with clinically inapparent hepatitis as candidates for medical management have as a secondary benefit the identification of persons whose contacts could be at risk of becoming infected. A so-called look-back program has been recommended to identify persons who were transfused before 1992 with blood from a donor found subsequently to have hepatitis C. In addition, anti-HCV testing is recommended for persons born between 1945 and 1965, anyone who received a blood transfusion or a transplanted organ before the introduction of second-generation screening tests in 1992, those who ever used injection drugs (or took other illicit drugs by noninjection routes), chronically hemodialyzed patients, persons with clotting disorders who received clotting factors made before 1987 from pooled blood products, persons with elevated aminotransferase levels, health workers exposed to HCV-positive blood or contaminated needles, recipients of blood or organs from a donor found to be positive for hepatitis C, persons with HIV infection, health care and public safety personnel following a needle stick or other nonpercutaneous exposure to HCV-infected material, sexual partners of persons with hepatitis C, and children born to HCV-positive mothers (Table 360-4).

For stable, monogamous sexual partners, sexual transmission of hepatitis C is unlikely, and sexual barrier precautions are not recommended. For persons with multiple sexual partners or with sexually transmitted diseases, the risk of sexual transmission of hepatitis C is increased, and barrier precautions (latex condoms) are recommended. A person with hepatitis C should avoid sharing such items as razors, toothbrushes, and nail clippers with sexual partners and family members. No special precautions are recommended for babies born to mothers with hepatitis C, and breast-feeding does not have to be restricted.

Hepatitis E Whether IG prevents hepatitis E remains undetermined. Safe and effective recombinant genotype 1 vaccines, which protect against other genotypes as well, have been developed and are available in endemic areas but not in the United States.

361 Toxic and Drug-Induced Hepatitis

William M. Lee, Jules L. Dienstag

Liver injury is a possible consequence of ingestion of any xenobiotic, including industrial toxins, pharmacologic agents, and complementary and alternative medications (CAMs). Among patients with acute liver failure, drug-induced liver injury is the most common cause, and evidence for hepatotoxicity detected during clinical trials for drug development is the most common reason for failure of compounds to reach approval status. Drug-induced liver injury requires careful history taking to identify unrecognized exposure to chemicals used in work or at home, drugs taken by prescription or bought over the counter, and herbal or dietary supplement medicines. Hepatotoxic drugs can injure the hepatocyte directly, e.g., via a free-radical or metabolic intermediate that causes peroxidation of membrane lipids and that results in liver cell injury. Alternatively, a drug or its metabolite may activate components of the innate or adaptive immune system, stimulate apoptotic pathways, or initiate damage to bile excretory pathways (Fig. 361-1). Interference with bile canalicular pumps can allow endogenous bile acids, which can injure the liver, to accumulate. Such secondary injury, in turn, may lead to necrosis of hepatocytes; injure bile ducts, producing cholestasis; or block pathways of lipid movement, inhibit protein synthesis, or impair mitochondrial oxidation of fatty acids, resulting in lactic acidosis and intracellular triglyceride accumulation (expressed histologically as microvesicular steatosis). In other instances, drug metabolites sensitize hepatocytes to toxic cytokines. The differences observed between susceptible and nonsusceptible drug recipients may be attributable to HLA haplotypes that determine binding of drug-related haptens on the cell surface as well as to polymorphisms in elaboration of competing, protective cytokines, as has been suggested for acetaminophen hepatotoxicity (see below). Immune mechanisms may include cytotoxic lymphocytes or antibody-mediated cellular cytotoxicity. In addition, a role has been shown for activation of nuclear transporters, such as the constitutive androstane receptor (CAR) or, more recently, the pregnane X receptor (PXR), in the induction of drug hepatotoxicity.

DRUG METABOLISM

Most drugs, which are water-insoluble, undergo a series of metabolic steps, culminating in a water-soluble form appropriate for renal or biliary excretion. This process begins with oxidation or methylation mediated initially by the microsomal mixed-function oxygenases, cytochrome P450 (phase I reaction), followed by glucuronidation or sulfation (phase II reaction) or inactivation by glutathione. Most drug hepatotoxicity is mediated by a phase I toxic metabolite, but glutathione depletion, precluding inactivation of harmful compounds by glutathione S-transferase, can contribute as well.

LIVER INJURY CAUSED BY DRUGS

In general, two major types of chemical hepatotoxicity have been recognized: (1) direct toxic and (2) idiosyncratic. As shown in Table 361-1, direct toxic hepatitis occurs with predictable regularity in individuals exposed to the offending agent and is dose-dependent. The latent period between exposure and liver injury is usually short (often several hours), although clinical manifestations may be delayed for 24–48 h. Agents producing toxic hepatitis are generally systemic poisons or are converted in the liver to toxic metabolites. The direct hepatotoxins result in morphologic abnormalities that are reasonably characteristic and reproducible for each toxin. For example, carbon tetrachloride and trichloroethylene characteristically produce a centrilobular zonal necrosis, whereas yellow phosphorus poisoning typically results in periportal injury. The hepatotoxic octapeptides of *Amanita phalloides* usually produce massive hepatic necrosis; the lethal dose of the toxin is ~10 mg, the amount found in a single deathcap mushroom. Liver injury, which is often only one facet of the toxicity produced by the direct hepatotoxins, may go unrecognized until jaundice appears.

In idiosyncratic drug reactions, the occurrence of hepatitis is usually infrequent (1 in 10^3–10^5 patients) and unpredictable; the response is not as clearly dose-dependent as is injury associated with direct hepatotoxins, and liver injury may occur at any time during or shortly after exposure to the drug. That said, recent data suggest that most agents causing idiosyncratic toxicity are given at a daily dose exceeding 100 mg, suggesting a role for dose—drugs with low potency must be given in higher doses that engender greater chances for "off-target" effects. Adding to the difficulty of predicting or identifying idiosyncratic drug hepatotoxicity is the occurrence of mild, transient, nonprogressive serum aminotransferase elevations that resolve with continued drug use. Such "adaptation," the mechanism of which is unknown, is well recognized for drugs such as isoniazid, valproate, phenytoin, and HMG-CoA reductase inhibitors (statins). Extrahepatic manifestations of hypersensitivity, such as rash, arthralgias, fever, leukocytosis, and eosinophilia, occur in about one-quarter of patients with idiosyncratic hepatotoxic drug reactions but are characteristic for certain drugs and not others. Both primary immunologic injury and direct hepatotoxicity related to idiosyncratic differences in generation of toxic metabolites have been invoked to explain idiosyncratic drug reactions. The most current data appear to implicate the adaptive immune system responding to the formation of immune stimulatory compounds resulting from phase I metabolic activation of the offending drug. Differences in host susceptibility may result from varying kinetics of toxic metabolite generation and genetic polymorphisms in downstream drug-metabolizing pathways or cytokine activation; in addition, certain HLA haplotypes have been associated with hepatotoxicity of certain drugs such as amoxicillin-clavulanate and flucloxacillin. Occasionally, however, the clinical features of an allergic reaction (prominent tissue eosinophilia, autoantibodies, etc.) are difficult to ignore and suggest activation of IgE pathways. A few instances of drug hepatotoxicity are observed to be associated with autoantibodies, including a class of antibodies to liver-kidney microsomes, anti-LKM2, directed against a cytochrome P450 enzyme.

Idiosyncratic reactions lead to a morphologic pattern that is more variable than those produced by direct toxins; a single agent is often capable of causing a variety of lesions, although certain patterns tend to predominate. Depending on the agent involved, idiosyncratic hepatitis may result in a clinical and morphologic picture indistinguishable from that of viral hepatitis (e.g., isoniazid or ciprofloxacin). So-called hepatocellular injury is the most common form, featuring spotty necrosis in the liver lobule with a predominantly lymphocytic infiltrate resembling that observed in acute hepatitis A, B, or C. Drug-induced cholestasis ranges from mild to increasingly severe: (1) bland cholestasis with limited hepatocellular injury (e.g., estrogens, 17,α-substituted androgens); (2) inflammatory cholestasis (e.g., amoxicillin-clavulanic acid [the most frequently implicated antibiotic among cases of drug-induced liver injury], oxacillin, erythromycin estolate); (3) sclerosing cholangitis (e.g., after intrahepatic infusion of the chemotherapeutic agent floxuridine for hepatic metastases from a primary colonic carcinoma); and (4) disappearance of bile ducts, "ductopenic" cholestasis, similar to that observed in chronic rejection (Chap. 368) following liver transplantation (e.g., carbamazepine, levofloxacin). Cholestasis may result from binding of drugs to canalicular membrane transporters, accumulation of toxic bile acids resulting from canalicular pump failure, or genetic defects in canalicular transporter proteins. Clinically, the distinction between a hepatocellular and a cholestatic reaction is indicated by the R value, the ratio of alanine aminotransferase (ALT) to alkaline phosphatase values, both expressed as multiples of the upper limit of normal. An R value of >5.0 is associated with hepatocellular injury, R <2.0 with cholestatic injury, and R between 2.0 and 5.0 with mixed hepatocellular-cholestatic injury.

Morphologic alterations may also include bridging hepatic necrosis (e.g., methyldopa) or, infrequently, hepatic granulomas (e.g., sulfonamides). Some drugs result in macrovesicular or microvesicular steatosis or steatohepatitis, which, in some cases, has been linked to mitochondrial dysfunction and lipid peroxidation. Severe hepatotoxicity associated with steatohepatitis, most likely a result of mitochondrial toxicity, is being recognized with increasing frequency among patients receiving antiretroviral therapy with reverse transcriptase inhibitors for HIV infection (e.g., zidovudine, didanosine), although

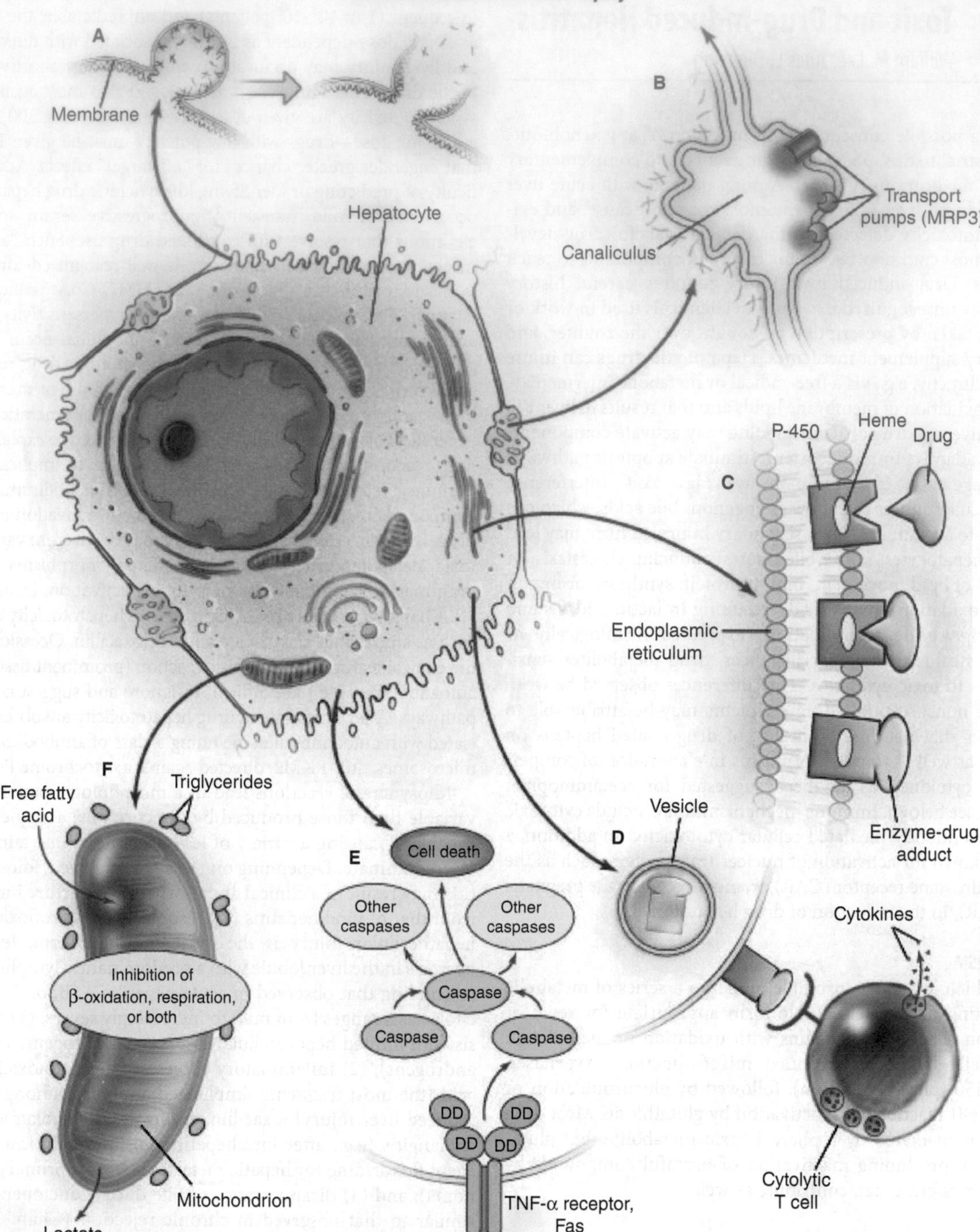

A. Rupture of cell membrane.
B. Injury of bile canaliculus (disruption of transport pumps).
C. P-450-drug covalent binding (drug adducts).
D. Drug adducts targeted by CTLs/cytokines.
E. Activation of apoptotic pathway by TNFα/Fas.
F. Inhibition of mitochondrial function.

FIGURE 361-1 Potential mechanisms of drug-induced liver injury. The normal hepatocyte may be affected adversely by drugs through (*A*) disruption of intracellular calcium homeostasis that leads to the disassembly of actin fibrils at the surface of the hepatocyte, resulting in blebbing of the cell membrane, rupture, and cell lysis; (*B*) disruption of actin filaments next to the canaliculus (the specialized portion of the cell responsible for bile excretion), leading to loss of villous processes and interruption of transport pumps such as multidrug resistance–associated protein 3 (MRP3), which, in turn, prevents the excretion of bilirubin and other organic compounds; (*C*) covalent binding of the heme-containing cytochrome P450 enzyme to the drug, thus creating nonfunctioning adducts; (*D*) migration of these enzyme-drug adducts to the cell surface in vesicles to serve as target immunogens for cytolytic attack by T cells, stimulating an immune response involving cytolytic T cells and cytokines; (*E*) activation of apoptotic pathways by tumor necrosis factor α (TNF-α) receptor or Fas (DD denotes death domain), triggering the cascade of intercellular caspases, resulting in programmed cell death; or (*F*) inhibition of mitochondrial function by a dual effect on both β-oxidation and the respiratory-chain enzymes, leading to failure of free fatty acid metabolism, a lack of aerobic respiration, and accumulation of lactate and reactive oxygen species (which may disrupt mitochondrial DNA). Toxic metabolites excreted in bile may damage bile-duct epithelium (not shown). CTLs, cytolytic T lymphocytes. *(Reproduced from WM Lee: Drug-induced hepatotoxicity. N Engl J Med 349:474, 2003, with permission.)*

TABLE 361-1 SOME FEATURES OF TOXIC AND DRUG-INDUCED HEPATIC INJURY

	Direct Toxic Effect[a]		Idiosyncratic[a]			Other[a]
Features	**Carbon Tetrachloride**	**Acetaminophen**	**Amoxicillin-Clavulanate**	**Isoniazid**	**Ciprofloxacin**	**Estrogens/Androgenic Steroids**
Predictable and dose-related toxicity	+	+	0	0	0	+
Latent period	Short	Short	Delayed onset	Variable	May be short	Variable
Arthralgia, fever, rash, eosinophilia	0	0	0	0	0	0
Liver morphology	Necrosis, fatty infiltration	Centrilobular necrosis	Mixed hepatocellular/cholestatic	Hepatocellular injury resembling viral hepatitis	Hepatocellular injury resembling viral hepatitis	Cholestasis *without* portal inflammation

[a]The drugs listed are typical examples.

many of these drugs have been withdrawn because of such hepatotoxicity (Chap. 226). Generally, such mitochondrial hepatotoxicity of these antiretroviral agents is reversible, but dramatic, nonreversible hepatotoxicity associated with mitochondrial injury (inhibition of DNA polymerase γ) was the cause of acute liver failure encountered during early clinical trials of now-abandoned fialuridine, a fluorinated pyrimidine analogue with potent antiviral activity against hepatitis B virus. Another potential target for idiosyncratic drug hepatotoxicity is sinusoidal lining cells; when these are injured, such as by high-dose chemotherapeutic agents (e.g., cyclophosphamide, melphalan, busulfan) administered prior to bone marrow transplantation, venoocclusive disease can result. Nodular regenerative hyperplasia, a subtle form of portal hypertension, may also result from vascular injury to portal venous endothelium following systemic chemotherapy, such as with oxaliplatin, as part of adjuvant treatment for colon cancer.

Not all adverse hepatic drug reactions can be classified as either toxic or idiosyncratic. For example, oral contraceptives, which combine estrogenic and progestational compounds, may result in impairment of hepatic tests and, occasionally, jaundice; however, they do not produce necrosis or fatty change, manifestations of hypersensitivity are generally absent, and susceptibility to the development of oral contraceptive–induced cholestasis appears to be genetically determined. Such estrogen-induced cholestasis is more common in women with cholestasis of pregnancy, a disorder linked to genetic defects in multidrug resistance–associated canalicular transporter proteins.

Any idiosyncratic reaction that occurs in <1:10,000 recipients will go unrecognized in most clinical trials, which involve only several thousand recipients. The U.S. Food and Drug Administration (FDA) and pharmaceutical companies have learned to look for even subtle indications of serious toxicity and monitor regularly the number of trial subjects in whom any aminotransferase elevations develop, as a possible surrogate for more serious toxicity. Even more valid as a predictor of severe hepatotoxicity is the occurrence of jaundice in patients enrolled in a clinical drug trial, so called "Hy's Law," named after Hyman Zimmerman, one of the pioneers of the field of drug hepatotoxicity. He recognized that, if jaundice occurred during a phase III trial, more serious liver injury was likely, with a 10:1 ratio between cases of jaundice and liver failure—10 patients with jaundice to 1 patient with acute liver failure. Thus, the finding of such Hy's Law cases during drug development often portends failure of approval, particularly if any of the subjects sustains a bad outcome. Troglitazone, a peroxisome proliferator-activated receptor γ agonist, was the first in its class of thiazolidinedione insulin-sensitizing agents. Although in retrospect, Hy's Law cases of jaundice had occurred during phase III trials, no instances of liver failure were recognized until well after the drug was introduced, underlining the importance of postmarketing surveillance in identifying toxic drugs and in leading to their withdrawal from use. Fortunately, such hepatotoxicity is not characteristic of the second-generation thiazolidinedione insulin-sensitizing agents rosiglitazone and pioglitazone; in clinical trials, the frequency of aminotransferase elevations in patients treated with these medications did not differ from that in placebo recipients, and isolated reports of liver injury among recipients are extremely rare.

Proving that an episode of liver injury is caused by a drug is difficult in many cases. Drug-induced liver injury is nearly always a presumptive diagnosis, and many other disorders produce a similar clinicopathologic picture. Thus, causality may be difficult to establish and requires several separate supportive assessment variables to lead to a high level of certainty, including temporal association (time of onset, time to resolution), clinical-biochemical features, type of injury (hepatocellular versus cholestatic), extrahepatic features, likelihood that a given agent is to blame based on its past record, and exclusion of other potential causes. Scoring systems such as the Roussel-Uclaf Causality Assessment Method (RUCAM) yield residual uncertainty and have not been adopted widely. Currently, the U.S. Drug-Induced Liver Injury Network (DILIN) relies on a structured expert opinion process requiring detailed data on each case and a comprehensive review by three experts who arrive at a consensus on a five-degree scale of likelihood (definite, highly likely, probable, possible, unlikely); however, this approach is not practical for routine clinical application.

Generally, drug hepatotoxicity is not more frequent in persons with underlying chronic liver disease, although the severity of the outcome may be amplified. Reported exceptions include hepatotoxicity of aspirin, methotrexate, isoniazid (only in certain experiences), antiretroviral therapy for HIV infection, and certain drugs such as conditioning regimens for bone marrow transplantation in the presence of hepatitis C.

TREATMENT TOXIC AND DRUG-INDUCED HEPATIC DISEASE

Treatment is largely supportive, except in acetaminophen hepatotoxicity (see below). In patients with fulminant hepatitis resulting from drug hepatotoxicity, liver transplantation may be lifesaving (Chap. 368). Withdrawal of the suspected agent is indicated at the first sign of an adverse reaction. A number of studies have suggested that lethal outcomes follow continued use of an agent in the face of symptoms and signs of liver injury. In the case of the direct toxins, liver involvement should not divert attention from renal or other organ involvement, which may also threaten survival. A number of agents are occasionally used but are of questionable value: glucocorticoids for drug hepatotoxicity with allergic features, silibinin for hepatotoxic mushroom poisoning, and ursodeoxycholic acid for cholestatic drug hepatotoxicity have never been shown to be effective and are not recommended.

In Table 361-2, several classes of chemical agents are listed together with examples of the pattern of liver injury produced by them. Certain drugs appear to be responsible for the development of chronic as well as acute hepatic injury. For example, nitrofurantoin, minocycline, hydralazine, and methyldopa have been associated with moderate to severe chronic hepatitis with autoimmune features. Methotrexate, tamoxifen, and amiodarone have been implicated in the development of cirrhosis. Portal hypertension in the absence of cirrhosis may result from alterations in hepatic architecture produced by vitamin A or arsenic intoxication, industrial exposure to vinyl chloride, or

TABLE 361-2 PRINCIPAL ALTERATIONS OF HEPATIC MORPHOLOGY PRODUCED BY SOME COMMONLY USED DRUGS AND CHEMICALS[a]

Principal Morphologic Change	Class of Agent	Example
Cholestasis	Anabolic steroid	Methyl testosterone, many other body-building supplements
	Antibiotic	Erythromycin estolate, nitrofurantoin, rifampin, amoxicillin-clavulanic acid, oxacillin
	Anticonvulsant	Carbamazepine
	Antidepressant	Duloxetine, mirtazapine, tricyclic antidepressants
	Anti-inflammatory	Sulindac
	Antiplatelet	Clopidogrel
	Antihypertensive	Irbesartan, fosinopril
	Antithyroid	Methimazole
	Calcium channel blocker	Nifedipine, verapamil
	Immunosuppressive	Cyclosporine
	Lipid-lowering	Ezetimibe
	Oncotherapeutic	Anabolic steroids, busulfan, tamoxifen, irinotecan, cytarabine, temozolomide
	Oral contraceptive	Norethynodrel with mestranol
	Oral hypoglycemic	Chlorpropamide
	Tranquilizer	Chlorpromazine[b]
Fatty liver	Antiarrhythmic	Amiodarone
	Antibiotic	Tetracycline (high-dose, IV)
	Anticonvulsant	Valproic acid
	Antiviral	Dideoxynucleosides (e.g., zidovudine), protease inhibitors (e.g., indinavir, ritonavir)
	Oncotherapeutic	Asparaginase, methotrexate, tamoxifen
Hepatitis	Anesthetic	Halothane, fluothane
	Antiandrogen	Flutamide
	Antibiotic	Isoniazid,[c] rifampicin, nitrofurantoin, telithromycin, minocycline,[d] pyrazinamide, trovafloxacin[e]
	Anticonvulsant	Phenytoin, carbamazepine, valproic acid, phenobarbital
	Antidepressant	Iproniazid, amitriptyline, trazodone, venlafaxine, fluoxetine, paroxetine, duloxetine, sertraline, nefazodone[e]
	Antifungal	Ketoconazole, fluconazole, itraconazole
	Antihypertensive	Methyldopa,[c] captopril, enalapril, lisinopril, losartan
	Anti-inflammatory	Ibuprofen, indomethacin, diclofenac, sulindac, bromfenac
	Antipsychotic	Risperidone
	Antiviral	Zidovudine, didanosine, stavudine, nevirapine, ritonavir, indinavir, tipranavir, zalcitabine
	Calcium channel blocker	Nifedipine, verapamil, diltiazem
	Cholinesterase inhibitor	Tacrine
	Diuretic	Chlorothiazide
	Laxative	Oxyphenisatin[c,e]
	Norepinephrine-reuptake inhibitor	Atomoxetine
	Oral hypoglycemic	Troglitazone,[e] acarbose
Mixed hepatitis/cholestatic	Antibiotic	Amoxicillin-clavulanic acid, trimethoprim-sulfamethoxazole
	Antibacterial	Clindamycin
	Antifungal	Terbinafine
	Antihistamine	Cyproheptadine
	Immunosuppressive	Azathioprine
	Lipid-lowering	Nicotinic acid, lovastatin, ezetimibe
Toxic (necrosis)	Analgesic	Acetaminophen
	Hydrocarbon	Carbon tetrachloride
	Metal	Yellow phosphorus
	Mushroom	*Amanita phalloides*
	Solvent	Dimethylformamide
Granulomas	Antiarrhythmic	Quinidine, diltiazem
	Antibiotic	Sulfonamides
	Anticonvulsant	Carbamazepine
	Anti-inflammatory	Phenylbutazone
	Xanthine oxidase inhibitor	Allopurinol
Vascular injury	Chemotherapeutic	Oxaliplatin, melphalan

[a]Several agents cause more than one type of liver lesion and appear under more than one category. [b]Rarely associated with primary biliary cirrhosis–like lesion. [c]Occasionally associated with chronic hepatitis or bridging hepatic necrosis or cirrhosis. [d]Associated with an autoimmune hepatitis–like syndrome. [e]Withdrawn from use because of severe hepatotoxicity.

administration of thorium dioxide. The latter three agents have also been associated with angiosarcoma of the liver. Oral contraceptives have been implicated in the development of hepatic adenoma and, rarely, hepatocellular carcinoma and hepatic vein occlusion (Budd-Chiari syndrome). Another unusual lesion, peliosis hepatis (blood cysts of the liver), has been observed in some patients treated with anabolic or contraceptive steroids. The existence of these hepatic disorders expands the spectrum of liver injury induced by chemical agents and emphasizes the need for a thorough drug history in all patients with liver dysfunction. A helpful LiverTox website that contains up-to-date information on drug-induced liver injury is available through the National Institute of Diabetes and Digestive and Kidney Diseases and the National Library of Medicine (*www.livertox.nih.gov*).

The following are patterns of adverse hepatic reactions for some prototypic agents.

ACETAMINOPHEN HEPATOTOXICITY (DIRECT TOXIN)

Acetaminophen represents the most prevalent cause of acute liver failure in the Western world; up to 72% of patients with acetaminophen hepatotoxicity in Scandinavia—somewhat lower frequencies in the United Kingdom and the United States—progress to encephalopathy and coagulopathy. Acetaminophen causes dose-related centrilobular hepatic necrosis after single-time-point ingestions, as intentional self-harm, or over extended periods, as unintentional overdoses, when multiple drug preparations or inappropriate drug amounts are used daily for several days, e.g., for relief of pain or fever. In these instances, 8 g/d, twice the daily recommended maximum dose, over several days can readily lead to liver failure. Use of opioid-acetaminophen combinations appears to be particularly harmful, because habituation to the opioid may occur with a gradual increase in opioid-acetaminophen combination dosing over days or weeks. A single dose of 10–15 g, occasionally less, may produce clinical evidence of liver injury. Fatal fulminant disease is usually (although not invariably) associated with ingestion of ≥25 g. Blood levels of acetaminophen correlate with severity of hepatic injury (levels >300 μg/mL 4 h after ingestion are predictive of the development of severe damage; levels <150 μg/mL suggest that hepatic injury is highly unlikely). Nausea, vomiting, diarrhea, abdominal pain, and shock are early manifestations occurring 4–12 h after ingestion. Then 24–48 h later, when these features are abating, hepatic injury becomes apparent. Maximal abnormalities and hepatic failure are evident 3–5 days after ingestion, and aminotransferase levels exceeding 10,000 IU/L are not uncommon (i.e., levels far exceeding those in patients with viral hepatitis). Renal failure and myocardial injury may be present. Whether or not a clear history of overdose can be elicited, clinical suspicion of acetaminophen hepatotoxicity should be raised by the presence of the extremely high aminotransferase levels in association with low bilirubin levels that are characteristic of this hyperacute injury. This biochemical signature should trigger further questioning of the subject if possible; however, denial or altered mentation may confound diagnostic efforts. In this setting, a presumptive diagnosis is reasonable, and the proven antidote, *N*-acetylcysteine—both safe and presumed to be effective even when injury has already begun to evolve—should be instituted.

Acetaminophen is metabolized predominantly by a phase II reaction to innocuous sulfate and glucuronide metabolites; however, a small proportion of acetaminophen is metabolized by a phase I reaction to a hepatotoxic metabolite formed from the parent compound by the cytochrome P450 CYP2E1. This metabolite, *N*-acetyl-p-benzoquinone-imine (NAPQI), is detoxified by binding to "hepatoprotective" glutathione to become harmless, water-soluble mercapturic acid, which undergoes renal excretion. When excessive amounts of NAPQI are formed, or when glutathione levels are low, glutathione levels are depleted and overwhelmed, permitting covalent binding to nucleophilic hepatocyte macromolecules forming acetaminophen-protein "adducts." These adducts, which can be measured in serum by high-performance liquid chromatography, hold promise as diagnostic markers of acetaminophen hepatotoxicity, and a point-of-care assay for acetaminophen-Cys adducts is under development. The binding of acetaminophen to hepatocyte macromolecules is believed to lead to hepatocyte necrosis; the precise sequence and mechanism are unknown. Hepatic injury may be potentiated by prior administration of alcohol, phenobarbital, isoniazid, or other drugs; by conditions that stimulate the mixed-function oxidase system; or by conditions such as starvation (including inability to maintain oral intake during severe febrile illnesses) that reduce hepatic glutathione levels. Alcohol induces cytochrome P450 CYP2E1; consequently, increased levels of the toxic metabolite NAPQI may be produced in chronic alcoholics after acetaminophen ingestion, but the role of alcohol in potentiating acute acetaminophen injury is still debated. Alcohol also suppresses hepatic glutathione production. Therefore, in chronic alcoholics, the toxic dose of acetaminophen may be as low as 2 g, and alcoholic patients should be warned specifically about the dangers of even standard doses of this commonly used drug. In a 2006 study, aminotransferase elevations were identified in 31–44% of normal subjects treated for 14 days with the maximal recommended dose of acetaminophen, 4 g daily (administered alone or as part of an acetaminophen-opioid combination); because these changes were transient and never associated with bilirubin elevation, the clinical relevance of these findings remains to be determined. Although underlying hepatitis C virus (HCV) infection was found to be associated with an increased risk of acute liver injury in patients hospitalized for acetaminophen overdose, generally, in patients with nonalcoholic liver disease, acetaminophen taken in recommended doses is well tolerated. Acetaminophen use in cirrhotic patients has not been associated with hepatic decompensation. On the other hand, because of the link between acetaminophen use and liver injury, and because of the limited safety margin between safe and toxic doses, the FDA has recommended that the daily dose of acetaminophen be reduced from 4 g to 3 g (even lower for persons with chronic alcohol use), that all acetaminophen-containing products be labeled prominently as containing acetaminophen, and that the potential for liver injury be prominent in the packaging of acetaminophen and acetaminophen-containing products. Within opioid combination products, the limit for the acetaminophen component has been lowered to 325 mg per tablet.

TREATMENT ACETAMINOPHEN OVERDOSAGE

Treatment includes gastric lavage, supportive measures, and oral administration of activated charcoal or cholestyramine to prevent absorption of residual drug. Neither charcoal nor cholestyramine appears to be effective if given >30 min after acetaminophen ingestion; if they are used, the stomach lavage should be done before other agents are administered orally. The chances of possible, probable, and high-risk hepatotoxicity can be derived from a nomogram plot (Fig. 361-2), readily available in emergency departments, as a function of measuring acetaminophen plasma levels 8 h after ingestion. In patients with high acetaminophen blood levels (>200 μg/mL measured at 4 h or >100 μg/mL at 8 h after ingestion), the administration of *N* acetylcysteine reduces the severity of hepatic necrosis. This agent provides sulfhydryl donor groups to replete glutathione, which is required to render harmless toxic metabolites that would otherwise bind covalently via sulfhydryl linkages to cell proteins, resulting in the formation of drug metabolite-protein adducts. Therapy should be begun within 8 h of ingestion but may be at least partially effective when given as late as 24–36 h after overdose. Later administration of sulfhydryl compounds is of uncertain value. Routine use of *N*-acetylcysteine has substantially reduced the occurrence of fatal acetaminophen hepatotoxicity. *N*-acetylcysteine may be given orally but is more commonly used as an IV solution, with a loading dose of 140 mg/kg over 1 h, followed by 70 mg/kg every 4 h for 15–20 doses. Whenever a patient with potential acetaminophen hepatotoxicity is encountered, a local poison control center should be contacted. Treatment can be stopped when plasma acetaminophen levels indicate that the risk of liver damage is low. If signs of hepatic failure (e.g., progressive jaundice, coagulopathy, confusion) occur despite *N*-acetylcysteine therapy for acetaminophen hepatotoxicity, liver transplantation may be the only option. Early arterial blood lactate levels among such patients with acute liver failure

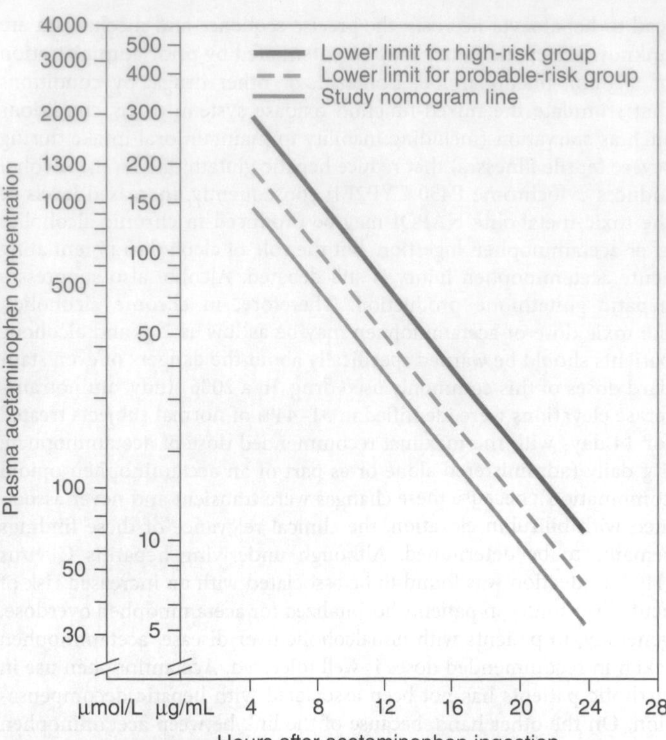

FIGURE 361-2 Nomogram to define risk of acetaminophen hepatotoxicity according to initial plasma acetaminophen concentration. *(After BH Rumack, H Matthew: Pediatrics 55:871, 1975.)*

may distinguish patients highly likely to require liver transplantation (lactate levels >3.5 mmol/L) from those likely to survive without liver replacement. Acute renal injury occurs in nearly 75% of patients with severe acetaminophen injury but is virtually always self-limited.

Survivors of acute acetaminophen overdose rarely, if ever, have ongoing liver injury or sequelae.

ISONIAZID HEPATOTOXICITY (TOXIC AND IDIOSYNCRATIC REACTION)

Isoniazid (INH) remains central to most antituberculous prophylactic and therapeutic regimens, despite its long-standing recognition as a hepatotoxin. In 10% of patients treated with INH, elevated serum aminotransferase levels develop during the first few weeks of therapy; however, these elevations in most cases are self-limited, mild (values for ALT <200 IU/L), and resolve despite continued drug use. This adaptive response allows continuation of the agent if symptoms and progressive enzyme elevations do not follow the initial elevations. Acute hepatocellular drug-induced liver injury secondary to INH is evident with a variable latency period up to 6 months and is more frequent in alcoholics and patients taking certain other medications, such as barbiturates, rifampin, and pyrazinamide. If the clinical threshold of encephalopathy is reached, severe hepatic injury is likely to be fatal or to require liver transplantation. Liver biopsy reveals morphologic changes similar to those of viral hepatitis or bridging hepatic necrosis. Substantial liver injury appears to be age-related, increasing substantially after age 35; the highest frequency is in patients over age 50, and the lowest is in patients under the age of 20. Even for patients >50 years of age monitored carefully during therapy, hepatotoxicity occurs in only ~2%, well below the risk estimate derived from earlier experiences. Fever, rash, eosinophilia, and other manifestations of drug allergy are distinctly unusual. Recently, antibodies to INH have been detected in INH recipients, but a link to causality of liver injury remains unclear. A clinical picture resembling chronic hepatitis has been observed in a few patients. Many public health programs that require INH prophylaxis for a positive tuberculin skin test or Quantiferon test include monthly monitoring of aminotransferase levels, although this practice has been called into question. Even more effective in limiting serious outcomes may be encouraging patients to be alert for symptoms such as nausea, fatigue, or jaundice, because most fatalities occur in the setting of continued INH use despite clinically apparent illness.

SODIUM VALPROATE HEPATOTOXICITY (TOXIC AND IDIOSYNCRATIC REACTION)

Sodium valproate, an anticonvulsant useful in the treatment of petit mal and other seizure disorders, has been associated with the development of severe hepatic toxicity and, rarely, fatalities, predominantly in children but also in adults. Among children listed as candidates for liver transplantation, valproate is the most common antiepileptic drug implicated. Asymptomatic elevations of serum aminotransferase levels have been recognized in as many as 45% of treated patients. These "adaptive" changes, however, appear to have no clinical importance, because major hepatotoxicity is not seen in the majority of patients despite continuation of drug therapy. In the rare patients in whom jaundice, encephalopathy, and evidence of hepatic failure are found, examination of liver tissue reveals microvesicular fat and bridging hepatic necrosis, predominantly in the centrilobular zone. Bile duct injury may also be apparent. Most likely, sodium valproate is not directly hepatotoxic, but its metabolite, 4-pentenoic acid, may be responsible for hepatic injury. Valproate hepatotoxicity is more common in persons with mitochondrial enzyme deficiencies and may be ameliorated by IV administration of carnitine, which valproate therapy can deplete. Recently, valproate toxicity has been linked to HLA haplotypes (*DR4* and *B*1502*) and to mutations in mitochondrial DNA polymerase gamma 1.

NITROFURANTOIN HEPATOTOXICITY (IDIOSYNCRATIC REACTION)

This commonly used antibiotic for urinary tract infections may cause an acute hepatitis leading to fatal outcome or, more frequently, chronic hepatitis of varying severity but indistinguishable from autoimmune chronic hepatitis. These two scenarios may reflect the frequent use and reuse of the drug for treatment of recurrent cystitis in women. Although most toxic agents manifest injury within 6 months of first ingestion, nitrofurantoin may have a longer latency period, in part perhaps because of its intermittent, recurrent use. Autoantibodies to nuclear components, smooth muscle, and mitochondria are seen and may subside after resolution of infection; however, glucocorticoid or other immunosuppressive medication may be necessary to resolve the autoimmune injury, and cirrhosis may be seen in cases that are not recognized quickly. Interstitial pulmonary fibrosis presenting as chronic cough and dyspnea may be present and resolve slowly with medication withdrawal. Histologic findings are identical to those of autoimmune hepatitis. A similar disease pattern can be observed with minocycline that is used repeatedly for the treatment of acne in teenagers as well as with hydralazine and alpha methyldopa.

AMOXICILLIN-CLAVULANATE HEPATOTOXICITY (IDIOSYNCRATIC MIXED REACTION)

Currently, the most common agent implicated as causing drug-induced liver injury in the United States and in Europe is amoxicillin-clavulanate (most frequent brand name: Augmentin). This medication causes a very specific syndrome of mixed or primarily cholestatic injury. Because hepatotoxicity may follow amoxicillin-clavulanate therapy after a relatively long latency period, the liver injury may begin to manifest at the time of drug withdrawal or after the drug has been withdrawn. The high prevalence of hepatotoxicity reflects in part the very frequent use of this drug for respiratory tract infections, including community-acquired pneumonia. The mechanism of hepatotoxicity is unclear, but the liver injury is thought to be caused by amoxicillin toxicity that is potentiated in some way by clavulanate, which itself appears not to be toxic. Symptoms include nausea, anorexia, fatigue, and jaundice—which may be prolonged—with pruritus. Rash is quite uncommon. On occasion, amoxicillin-clavulanate, like other cholestatic hepatotoxic drugs, causes permanent injury to small bile ducts, leading to the so-called "vanishing bile duct syndrome." In vanishing bile duct syndrome, initially, liver injury is minimal except for severe cholestasis; however, over time, histologic evidence of bile duct abnormalities is replaced by a paucity and eventual absence of discernible ducts on subsequent biopsies.

PHENYTOIN HEPATOTOXICITY (IDIOSYNCRATIC REACTION)

Phenytoin, formerly diphenylhydantoin, a mainstay in the treatment of seizure disorders, has been associated in rare instances with the development of severe hepatitis-like liver injury leading to fulminant hepatic failure. In many patients, the hepatitis is associated with striking fever, lymphadenopathy, rash (Stevens-Johnson syndrome or exfoliative dermatitis), leukocytosis, and eosinophilia, suggesting an immunologically mediated hypersensitivity mechanism. Despite these observations, evidence suggests that metabolic idiosyncrasy may be responsible for hepatic injury. In the liver, phenytoin is converted by cytochrome P450 to metabolites, including the highly reactive electrophilic arene oxides. These metabolites are normally metabolized further by epoxide hydrolases. A defect (genetic or acquired) in epoxide hydrolase activity could permit covalent binding of arene oxides to hepatic macromolecules, thereby leading to hepatic injury. Hepatic injury is usually manifest within the first 2 months after beginning phenytoin therapy. With the exception of an abundance of eosinophils in the liver, the clinical, biochemical, and histologic picture resembles that of viral hepatitis. In rare instances, bile duct injury may be the salient feature of phenytoin hepatotoxicity, with striking features of intrahepatic cholestasis. Asymptomatic elevations of aminotransferase and alkaline phosphatase levels have been observed in a sizable proportion of patients receiving long-term phenytoin therapy. These liver changes are believed by some authorities to represent the potent hepatic enzyme-inducing properties of phenytoin and are accompanied histologically by swelling of hepatocytes in the absence of necroinflammatory activity or evidence of chronic liver disease.

AMIODARONE HEPATOTOXICITY (TOXIC AND IDIOSYNCRATIC REACTION)

Therapy with this potent antiarrhythmic drug is accompanied in 15–50% of patients by modest elevations of serum aminotransferase levels that may remain stable or diminish despite continuation of the drug. Such abnormalities may appear days to many months after beginning therapy. A proportion of those with elevated aminotransferase levels have detectable hepatomegaly, and clinically important liver disease develops in <5% of patients. Features that represent a direct effect of the drug on the liver and that are common to the majority of long-term recipients are ultrastructural phospholipidosis, unaccompanied by clinical liver disease, and interference with hepatic mixed-function oxidase metabolism of other drugs. The cationic amphiphilic drug and its major metabolite desethylamiodarone accumulate in hepatocyte lysosomes and mitochondria and in bile duct epithelium. The relatively common elevations in aminotransferase levels are also considered a predictable, dose-dependent, direct hepatotoxic effect. On the other hand, in the rare patient with clinically apparent, symptomatic liver disease, liver injury resembling that seen in alcoholic liver disease is observed. The so-called pseudoalcoholic liver injury can range from steatosis to alcoholic hepatitis–like neutrophilic infiltration and Mallory's hyaline to cirrhosis. Electron-microscopic demonstration of phospholipid-laden lysosomal lamellar bodies can help to distinguish amiodarone hepatotoxicity from typical alcoholic hepatitis. This category of liver injury appears to be a metabolic idiosyncrasy that allows hepatotoxic metabolites to be generated. Rarely, an acute idiosyncratic hepatocellular injury resembling viral hepatitis or cholestatic hepatitis occurs. Hepatic granulomas have occasionally been observed. Because amiodarone has a long half-life, liver injury may persist for months after the drug is stopped.

ERYTHROMYCIN HEPATOTOXICITY (CHOLESTATIC IDIOSYNCRATIC REACTION)

The most important adverse effect associated with erythromycin, more common in children than adults, is the infrequent occurrence of a cholestatic reaction. Although most of these reactions have been associated with erythromycin estolate, other erythromycins may also be responsible. The reaction usually begins during the first 2 or 3 weeks of therapy and includes nausea, vomiting, fever, right upper quadrant abdominal pain, jaundice, leukocytosis, and moderately elevated aminotransferase and alkaline phosphatase levels. The clinical picture can resemble acute cholecystitis or bacterial cholangitis. Liver biopsy reveals variable cholestasis; portal inflammation comprising lymphocytes, polymorphonuclear leukocytes, and eosinophils; and scattered foci of hepatocyte necrosis. Symptoms and laboratory findings usually subside within a few days of drug withdrawal, and evidence of chronic liver disease has not been found on follow-up. The precise mechanism remains ill-defined.

ORAL CONTRACEPTIVE HEPATOTOXICITY (CHOLESTATIC REACTION)

The administration of oral contraceptive combinations of estrogenic and progestational steroids leads to intrahepatic cholestasis with pruritus and jaundice in a small number of patients weeks to months after taking these agents. Especially susceptible seem to be patients with recurrent idiopathic jaundice of pregnancy, severe pruritus of pregnancy, or a family history of these disorders. With the exception of liver biochemical tests, laboratory studies are normal, and extrahepatic manifestations of hypersensitivity are absent. Liver biopsy reveals cholestasis with bile plugs in dilated canaliculi and striking bilirubin staining of liver cells. In contrast to chlorpromazine-induced cholestasis, portal inflammation is absent. The lesion is reversible on withdrawal of the agent. The two steroid components appear to act synergistically on hepatic function, although the estrogen may be primarily responsible. Oral contraceptives are contraindicated in patients with a history of recurrent jaundice of pregnancy. Primarily benign, but rarely malignant, neoplasms of the liver, hepatic vein occlusion, and peripheral sinusoidal dilatation have also been associated with oral contraceptive therapy. Focal nodular hyperplasia of the liver is not more frequent among users of oral contraceptives.

ANABOLIC STEROIDS (CHOLESTATIC REACTION)

The most common form of liver injury caused by complementary and alternative medications is the profound cholestasis associated with anabolic steroids used by body builders. Unregulated agents sold in gyms and health food stores as diet supplements, which are taken by athletes to improve their performance, may contain anabolic steroids. Jaundice in a young male that is accompanied by a cholestatic, rather than a hepatitic, laboratory profile almost invariably will turn out to be caused by the use of one of a variety of androgen congeners. Such agents have the potential to injure bile transport pumps and to cause intense cholestasis; the time to onset is variable, and resolution, which is the rule, may require many weeks to months. Initially, anorexia, nausea, and malaise may occur, followed by pruritus in some but not all patients. Serum aminotransferase levels are usually <100 IU/L and serum alkaline phosphatase levels are generally moderately elevated with bilirubin levels frequently exceeding 342 μmol/L (20 mg/dL). Examination of liver tissue reveals cholestasis without substantial inflammation or necrosis. Anabolic steroids have also been used by prescription to treat bone marrow failure. In this setting, hepatic sinusoidal dilatation and peliosis hepatis have been reported in rare patients, as have hepatic adenomas and hepatocellular carcinoma.

TRIMETHOPRIM-SULFAMETHOXAZOLE HEPATOTOXICITY (IDIOSYNCRATIC REACTION)

This antibiotic combination is used routinely for urinary tract infections in immunocompetent persons and for prophylaxis against and therapy of *Pneumocystis carinii* pneumonia in immunosuppressed persons (transplant recipients, patients with AIDS). With its increasing use, its occasional hepatotoxicity is being recognized with growing frequency. Its likelihood is unpredictable, but when it occurs, trimethoprim-sulfamethoxazole hepatotoxicity follows a relatively uniform latency period of several weeks and is often accompanied by eosinophilia, rash, and other features of a hypersensitivity reaction. Biochemically and histologically, acute hepatocellular necrosis predominates, but cholestatic features are quite frequent. Occasionally, cholestasis without necrosis occurs, and, very rarely, a severe cholangiolytic pattern of liver injury is observed. In most cases, liver injury is self-limited, but rare fatalities have been recorded. The hepatotoxicity is attributable to the sulfamethoxazole component of the drug and is similar in features to that seen with other sulfonamides; tissue eosinophilia and granulomas may be seen. The risk of trimethoprim-sulfamethoxazole hepatotoxicity is increased in persons with HIV infection.

HMG-COA REDUCTASE INHIBITORS (STATINS) (IDIOSYNCRATIC MIXED HEPATOCELLULAR AND CHOLESTATIC REACTION)

Between 1 and 2% of patients taking lovastatin, simvastatin, pravastatin, fluvastatin, or one of the newer statin drugs for the treatment of hypercholesterolemia experience asymptomatic, reversible elevations (>threefold) of aminotransferase activity. Acute hepatitis-like histologic changes, centrilobular necrosis, and centrilobular cholestasis have been described in a very small number of cases. In a larger proportion, minor aminotransferase elevations appear during the first several weeks of therapy. Careful laboratory monitoring can distinguish between patients with minor, transitory changes, who may continue therapy and those with more profound and sustained abnormalities, who should discontinue therapy. Because clinically meaningful aminotransferase elevations are so rare after statin use and do not differ in meta-analyses from the frequency of such laboratory abnormalities in placebo recipients, a panel of liver experts recommended to the National Lipid Association's Safety Task Force that liver test monitoring was not necessary in patients treated with statins and that statin therapy need not be discontinued in patients found to have asymptomatic isolated aminotransferase elevations during therapy. Statin hepatotoxicity is not increased in patients with chronic hepatitis C, hepatic steatosis, or other underlying liver diseases, and statins can be used safely in these patients.

TOTAL PARENTERAL NUTRITION (STEATOSIS, CHOLESTASIS)

Total parenteral nutrition (TPN) is often complicated by cholestatic hepatitis attributable to steatosis, cholestasis, or gallstones (or gallbladder sludge). Steatosis or steatohepatitis may result from the excess carbohydrate calories in these nutritional supplements and is the predominant form of TPN-associated liver disorder in adults. The frequency of this complication has been reduced substantially by the introduction of balanced TPN formulas that rely on lipid as an alternative caloric source. Cholestasis and cholelithiasis, caused by the absence of stimulation of bile flow and secretion resulting from the lack of oral intake, is the predominant form of TPN-associated liver disease in infants, especially in premature neonates. Often, cholestasis in such neonates is multifactorial, contributed to by other factors such as sepsis, hypoxemia, and hypotension; occasionally, TPN-induced cholestasis in neonates culminates in chronic liver disease and liver failure. When TPN-associated liver test abnormalities occur in adults, balancing the TPN formula with more lipid is the intervention of first recourse. In infants with TPN-associated cholestasis, the addition of oral feeding may ameliorate the problem. Therapeutic interventions suggested, but not shown, to be of proven benefit, include cholecystokinin, ursodeoxycholic acid, *S* -adenosyl methionine, and taurine.

ALTERNATIVE AND COMPLEMENTARY MEDICINES (IDIOSYNCRATIC HEPATITIS, STEATOSIS)

Herbal medications that are of scientifically unproven efficacy and that lack prospective safety oversight by regulatory agencies currently account for more than 20% of drug-induced liver injury in the United States. Besides anabolic steroids, the most common category of dietary or herbal products is weight loss agents. Included among the herbal remedies associated with toxic hepatitis are Jin Bu Huan, xiao-chai-hu-tang, germander, chaparral, senna, mistletoe, skullcap, gentian, comfrey (containing pyrrolizidine alkaloids), ma huang, bee pollen, valerian root, pennyroyal oil, kava, celandine, Impila (*Callilepis laureola*), LipoKinetix, Hydroxycut, herbal nutritional supplements, and herbal teas containing *Camellia sinensis* (green tea extract). Well characterized are the acute hepatitis-like histologic lesions following Jin Bu Huan use: focal hepatocellular necrosis, mixed mononuclear portal tract infiltration, coagulative necrosis, apoptotic hepatocyte degeneration, tissue eosinophilia, and microvesicular steatosis. Megadoses of vitamin A can injure the liver, as can pyrrolizidine alkaloids, which often contaminate Chinese herbal preparations and can cause a venoocclusive injury leading to sinusoidal hepatic vein obstruction. Because some alternative medicines induce toxicity via active metabolites, alcohol and drugs that stimulate cytochrome P450 enzymes may enhance the toxicity of some of these products. Conversely, some alternative medicines also stimulate cytochrome P450 and may result in or amplify the toxicity of recognized drug hepatotoxins. Given the widespread use of such poorly defined herbal preparations, hepatotoxicity is likely to be encountered with increasing frequency; therefore, a drug history in patients with acute and chronic liver disease should include use of "alternative medicines" and other nonprescription preparations sold in so-called health food stores.

HIGHLY ACTIVE ANTIRETROVIRAL THERAPY (HAART) FOR HIV INFECTION (MITOCHONDRIAL TOXIC, IDIOSYNCRATIC, STEATOSIS; HEPATOCELLULAR, CHOLESTATIC, AND MIXED)

The recognition of drug hepatotoxicity in persons with HIV infection is complicated in this population by the many alternative causes of liver injury (chronic viral hepatitis, fatty infiltration, infiltrative disorders, mycobacterial infection, etc.), but drug hepatotoxicity associated with HAART is an emerging and common type of liver injury in HIV-infected persons (Chap. 226). Although no one antiviral agent is recognized as a potent hepatotoxin, combination regimens including reverse transcriptase and protease inhibitors cause hepatotoxicity in ~10% of treated patients. Implicated most frequently are combinations including nucleoside analogue reverse transcriptase inhibitors zidovudine, didanosine, and, to a lesser extent, stavudine; protease inhibitors ritonavir and indinavir (and amprenavir when used together with ritonavir), as well as tipranavir; and nonnucleoside reverse transcriptase inhibitors nevirapine and, to a lesser extent, efavirenz. These drugs cause predominantly hepatocellular injury but cholestatic injury as well, and prolonged (>6 months) use of reverse transcriptase inhibitors has been associated with mitochondrial injury, steatosis, and lactic acidosis. Indirect hyperbilirubinemia, resulting from direct inhibition of bilirubin-conjugating activity by UDP-glucuronosyltransferase, usually without elevation of aminotransferase or alkaline phosphatase activities, occurs in ~10% of patients treated with the protease inhibitor indinavir. Distinguishing the impact of HAART hepatotoxicity in patients with HIV and hepatitis virus co-infection is made challenging by the following: (1) both chronic hepatitis B and hepatitis C can affect the natural history of HIV infection and the response to HAART, and (2) HAART can have an impact on chronic viral hepatitis. For example, immunologic reconstitution with HAART can result in immunologically mediated liver-cell injury in patients with chronic hepatitis B co-infection if treatment with an antiviral agent for hepatitis B (e.g., the nucleoside analogue lamivudine) is withdrawn or if nucleoside analogue resistance emerges. Infection with HIV, especially with low CD4+ T cell counts, has been reported to increase the rate of hepatic fibrosis associated with chronic hepatitis C, and HAART therapy can increase levels of serum aminotransferases and HCV RNA in patients with hepatitis C co-infection. Didanosine or stavudine should not be used with ribavirin in patients with HIV/HCV co-infection because of an increased risk of severe mitochondrial toxicity and lactic acidosis.

Acknowledgment

Kurt J. Isselbacher, MD, contributed to this chapter in previous editions of Harrison's.

362 Chronic Hepatitis

Jules L. Dienstag

Chronic hepatitis represents a series of liver disorders of varying causes and severity in which hepatic inflammation and necrosis continue for at least 6 months. Milder forms are nonprogressive or only slowly progressive, while more severe forms may be associated with scarring and architectural reorganization, which, when advanced, lead ultimately to cirrhosis. Several categories of chronic hepatitis have been recognized. These include chronic viral hepatitis, drug-induced chronic hepatitis (Chap. 361), and autoimmune chronic hepatitis. In many cases, clinical and laboratory features are insufficient to allow assignment into one of these three categories; these "idiopathic" cases are also believed to represent autoimmune chronic hepatitis. Finally, clinical and laboratory features of chronic hepatitis are observed occasionally in patients with such hereditary/metabolic disorders as Wilson's disease (copper overload), α_1 antitrypsin deficiency (Chaps. 365 and 429), and nonalcoholic fatty liver disease (Chap. 367e) and even occasionally in patients with alcoholic liver injury (Chap. 363). Although all types of chronic hepatitis share certain clinical, laboratory, and histopathologic features, chronic viral and chronic autoimmune hepatitis are sufficiently distinct to merit separate discussions. For discussion of acute hepatitis, see Chap. 360.

CLASSIFICATION OF CHRONIC HEPATITIS

Common to all forms of chronic hepatitis are histopathologic distinctions based on localization and extent of liver injury. These vary from the milder forms, previously labeled *chronic persistent hepatitis* and *chronic lobular hepatitis*, to the more severe form, formerly called *chronic active hepatitis*. When first defined, these designations were believed to have prognostic implications, which were not corroborated by subsequent observations. Categorization of chronic hepatitis based primarily on histopathologic features has been replaced by a more informative classification based on a combination of clinical, serologic, and histologic variables. Classification of chronic hepatitis is based on (1) its *cause*; (2) its histologic activity, or *grade*; and (3) its degree of progression, or *stage*. Thus, neither clinical features alone nor histologic features—requiring liver biopsy—alone are sufficient to characterize and distinguish among the several categories of chronic hepatitis.

CLASSIFICATION BY CAUSE

Clinical and serologic features allow the establishment of a diagnosis of *chronic viral hepatitis*, caused by hepatitis B, hepatitis B plus D, or hepatitis C; *autoimmune hepatitis*, including several subcategories, I and II (perhaps III), based on serologic distinctions; *drug-associated chronic hepatitis*; and a category of unknown cause, or *cryptogenic chronic hepatitis* (Table 362-1). These are addressed in more detail below.

CLASSIFICATION BY GRADE

Grade, a histologic assessment of necroinflammatory activity, is based on examination of the liver biopsy. An assessment of important histologic features includes the degree of *periportal necrosis* and the disruption of the limiting plate of periportal hepatocytes by inflammatory cells (so-called *piecemeal necrosis* or *interface hepatitis*); the degree of confluent necrosis that links or forms bridges between vascular structures—between portal tract and portal tract or even more important bridges between portal tract and central vein—referred to as *bridging necrosis*; the degree of hepatocyte degeneration and focal necrosis within the lobule; and the degree of *portal inflammation*. Several scoring systems that take these histologic features into account have been devised, and the most popular are the histologic activity index (HAI), used commonly in the United States, and the METAVIR score, used in Europe (Table 362-2). Based on the presence and degree of these features of histologic activity, chronic hepatitis can be graded as mild, moderate, or severe.

TABLE 362-1 CLINICAL AND LABORATORY FEATURES OF CHRONIC HEPATITIS

Type of Hepatitis	Diagnostic Test(s)	Autoantibodies	Therapy
Chronic hepatitis B	HBsAg, IgG anti-HBc, HBeAg, HBV DNA	Uncommon	IFN-α, PEG IFN-α Oral agents: First-line: entecavir, tenofovir Second-line: lamivudine, adefovir, telbivudine
Chronic hepatitis C	Anti-HCV, HCV RNA	Anti-LKM1[a]	PEG IFN-α plus ribavirin Telaprevir[b] Boceprevir[b]
Chronic hepatitis D	Anti-HDV, HDV RNA, HBsAg, IgG anti-HBc	Anti-LKM3	IFN-α, PEG IFN-α[c]
Autoimmune hepatitis	ANA[d] (homogeneous), anti-LKM1 (±) Hyperglobulinemia	ANA, anti-LKM1 anti-SLA[e]	Prednisone, azathioprine
Drug-associated	—	Uncommon	Withdraw drug
Cryptogenic	All negative	None	Prednisone (?), azathioprine (?)

[a]Antibodies to liver-kidney microsomes type 1 (autoimmune hepatitis type II and some cases of hepatitis C). [b]Administered as a triple-drug combination with PEG IFN and ribavirin. Between the writing and publication of this chapter, two additional drugs were approved for hepatitis C, simeprevir and sofosbuvir (see *www.hcvguidelines.org*). [c]Early clinical trials suggested benefit of IFN-α therapy; PEG IFN-α is as effective, if not more so, and has supplanted standard IFN-α. [d]Antinuclear antibody (autoimmune hepatitis type I). [e]Antibodies to soluble liver antigen (autoimmune hepatitis type III).

Abbreviations: HBc, hepatitis B core; HBeAg, hepatitis B e antigen; HBsAg, hepatitis B surface antigen; HBV, hepatitis B virus; HCV, hepatitis C virus; HDV, hepatitis D virus; IFN-α, interferon α; IgG, immunoglobulin G; LKM, liver-kidney microsome; PEG IFN-α, pegylated interferon α; SLA, soluble liver antigen.

CLASSIFICATION BY STAGE

The stage of chronic hepatitis, which reflects the level of progression of the disease, is based on the degree of hepatic fibrosis. When fibrosis is so extensive that fibrous septa surround parenchymal nodules and alter the normal architecture of the liver lobule, the histologic lesion is defined as *cirrhosis*. Staging is based on the degree of fibrosis as categorized on a numerical scale from 0–6 (HAI) or 0–4 (METAVIR) (Table 362-2). Several noninvasive approaches have been introduced to provide approximations of hepatic histologic stage, including serum biomarkers of fibrosis and imaging determinations of liver elasticity.

CHRONIC VIRAL HEPATITIS

Both the enterically transmitted forms of viral hepatitis, hepatitis A and E, are self-limited and do not cause chronic hepatitis (rare reports notwithstanding in which acute hepatitis A serves as a trigger for the onset of autoimmune hepatitis in genetically susceptible patients or in which hepatitis E (Chap. 360) can cause chronic liver disease in immunosuppressed hosts, e.g., after liver transplantation). In contrast, the entire clinicopathologic spectrum of chronic hepatitis occurs in patients with chronic viral hepatitis B and C as well as in patients with chronic hepatitis D superimposed on chronic hepatitis B.

CHRONIC HEPATITIS B

The likelihood of chronicity after acute hepatitis B varies as a function of age. Infection at birth is associated with clinically silent acute infection but a 90% chance of chronic infection, whereas infection in young adulthood in immunocompetent persons is typically associated with clinically apparent acute hepatitis but a risk of chronicity of only approximately 1%. Most cases of chronic hepatitis B among adults, however, occur in patients who never had a recognized episode of clinically apparent acute viral hepatitis. The degree of liver injury (grade) in patients with chronic hepatitis B is variable, ranging from none in inactive carriers to mild to moderate to severe. Among adults

TABLE 362-2 HISTOLOGIC GRADING AND STAGING OF CHRONIC HEPATITIS

	Histologic Activity Index (HAI)[a]		METAVIR[b]	
Histologic Feature	**Severity**	**Score**	**Severity**	**Score**
Necroinflammatory Activity (grade)				
Periportal necrosis, including piecemeal necrosis and/or bridging necrosis (BN)	None	0	None	0
	Mild	1	Mild	1
	Mild/moderate	2	Moderate	2
	Moderate	3	Severe	3
	Severe	4		
			Bridging necrosis	Yes
				No
Intralobular necrosis — Confluent	—None	0	None or mild	0
	—Focal	1	Moderate	1
	—Zone 3 some	2	Severe	2
	—Zone 3 most	3		
	—Zone 3 + BN few	4		
	—Zone 3 + BN multiple	5		
	—Panacinar/multiacinar	6		
Focal	—None	0		
	—≤1 focus/10× field	1		
	—2–4 foci/10× field	2		
	—5–10 foci/10× field	3		
	—>10 foci/10× field	4		
Portal Inflammation	None	0		
	Mild	1		
	Moderate	2		
	Moderate/marked	3		
	Marked	4		
	Total	0–18		A0–A3[c]
Fibrosis (stage)				
None		0		F0
Portal fibrosis—some		1		F1
Portal fibrosis—most		2		F1
Bridging fibrosis—few		3		F2
Bridging fibrosis—many		4		F3
Incomplete cirrhosis		5		F4
Cirrhosis		6		F4
	Total	6		4

[a]Ishak K, Baptista A, Bianchi L, et al: Histologic grading and staging of chronic hepatitis. J Hepatol 22:696, 1995. [b]Bedossa P, Poynard T, French METAVIR Cooperative Study Group: An algorithm for grading activity in chronic hepatitis C. Hepatology 24:289, 1996. [c]Necroinflammatory grade: A0 = none; A1 = mild; A2 = moderate; A3 = severe.

with chronic hepatitis B, histologic features are of prognostic importance. In one long-term study of patients with chronic hepatitis B, investigators found a 5-year survival rate of 97% for patients with mild chronic hepatitis, 86% for patients with moderate to severe chronic hepatitis, and only 55% for patients with chronic hepatitis and postnecrotic cirrhosis. The 15-year survival in these cohorts was 77%, 66%, and 40%, respectively. On the other hand, more recent observations do not allow us to be so sanguine about the prognosis in patients with mild chronic hepatitis; among such patients followed for 1–13 years, progression to more severe chronic hepatitis and cirrhosis has been observed in more than a quarter of cases.

More important to consider than histology alone in patients with chronic hepatitis B is the degree of hepatitis B virus (HBV) replication. As reviewed in Chap. 360, chronic HBV infection can occur in the presence or absence of serum hepatitis B e antigen (HBeAg), and generally, for both HBeAg-reactive and HBeAg-negative chronic hepatitis B, the level of HBV DNA correlates with the level of liver injury and risk of progression. In *HBeAg-reactive chronic hepatitis B*, two phases have been recognized based on the relative level of HBV replication. The relatively *replicative phase* is characterized by the presence in the serum of HBeAg and HBV DNA levels well in excess of 10^3–10^4 IU/mL, sometimes exceeding 10^9 IU/mL; by the presence in the liver of detectable intrahepatocyte nucleocapsid antigens (primarily hepatitis B core antigen [HBcAg]); by high infectivity; and by accompanying liver injury. In contrast, the relatively *nonreplicative phase* is characterized by the absence of the conventional serum marker of HBV replication (HBeAg), the appearance of anti-HBe, levels of HBV DNA below a threshold of ~10^3 IU/mL, the absence of intrahepatocytic HBcAg, limited infectivity, and minimal liver injury. Patients in the replicative phase tend to have more severe chronic hepatitis, whereas those in the nonreplicative phase tend to have minimal or mild chronic hepatitis or to be inactive hepatitis B carriers. The likelihood in a patient with HBeAg-reactive chronic hepatitis B of converting spontaneously from relatively replicative to nonreplicative infection is approximately 10% per year. Distinctions in HBV replication and in histologic category, however, do not always coincide. In patients with HBeAg-reactive chronic HBV infection, especially when acquired at birth or in early childhood, as recognized commonly in Asian countries, a dichotomy is common between very high levels of HBV replication during the early decades of life (when the level of host tolerance of HBV is relatively high) and negligible levels of liver injury. Yet despite the relatively immediate, apparently benign nature of liver disease for many decades in this population, in the middle decades, activation of liver injury emerges as relative tolerance of the host to HBV declines, and these patients with childhood-acquired HBV infection are ultimately at increased risk later in life of cirrhosis, hepatocellular carcinoma (HCC) (Chap. 111), and liver-related death. **A discussion of the pathogenesis of liver injury in patients with chronic hepatitis B appears in Chap. 360.**

HBeAg-negative chronic hepatitis B (i.e., chronic HBV infection with active virus replication, readily detectable HBV DNA but without HBeAg [anti-HBe-reactive]), is more common than HBeAg-reactive chronic hepatitis B in Mediterranean and European countries and in Asia (and, correspondingly, in HBV genotypes other than A). Compared to patients with HBeAg-reactive chronic hepatitis B, patients with HBeAg-negative chronic hepatitis B have levels of HBV DNA that are several orders of magnitude lower (no more than 10^5–10^6 IU/mL) than those observed in the HBeAg-reactive subset. Most such cases represent precore or core-promoter mutations acquired late in the natural history of the disease (mostly early-life onset; age range 40–55 years, older than that for HBeAg-reactive chronic hepatitis B); these mutations prevent translation of HBeAg from the precore component of the HBV genome (precore mutants) or are characterized by downregulated transcription of precore mRNA (core-promoter mutants; Chap. 360). Although their levels of HBV DNA tend to be lower than among patients with HBeAg-reactive chronic hepatitis B, patients with HBeAg-negative chronic hepatitis B can have progressive liver injury (complicated by cirrhosis and HCC) and experience episodic reactivation of liver disease reflected in fluctuating levels of aminotransferase activity ("flares"). The biochemical and histologic activity of HBeAg-negative disease tends to correlate closely with levels of HBV replication, unlike the case mentioned above of Asian patients with HBeAg-reactive chronic hepatitis B during the early decades of their HBV infection. An important point worth reiterating is the observation that the level of HBV replication is the most important risk factor for the ultimate development of cirrhosis and HCC in both HBeAg-reactive and HBeAg-negative patients. Although levels of HBV DNA are lower and more readily suppressed by therapy to undetectable levels in HBeAg-negative (compared to HBeAg-reactive) chronic hepatitis B, achieving sustained responses that permit discontinuation of antiviral therapy is less likely in HBeAg-negative patients (see below). Inactive carriers are patients with circulating hepatitis B surface antigen (HBsAg), normal serum aminotransferase levels, undetectable HBeAg, and levels of HBV DNA that are either undetectable or present at a threshold of $\leq 10^3$ IU/mL. This serologic profile can occur not only in inactive carriers but also in patients with HBeAg-negative chronic hepatitis B during periods of relative inactivity; distinguishing between the two requires sequential biochemical and virologic monitoring over many months.

The spectrum of *clinical features* of chronic hepatitis B is broad, ranging from asymptomatic infection to debilitating disease or even end-stage, fatal hepatic failure. As noted above, the onset of the disease tends to be insidious in most patients, with the exception of the very few in whom chronic disease follows failure of resolution of clinically apparent acute hepatitis B. The clinical and laboratory features associated with progression from acute to chronic hepatitis B are discussed in Chap. 360.

Fatigue is a common symptom, and persistent or intermittent *jaundice* is a common feature in severe or advanced cases. Intermittent deepening of jaundice and recurrence of malaise and anorexia, as well as worsening fatigue, are reminiscent of acute hepatitis; such exacerbations may occur spontaneously, often coinciding with evidence of virologic reactivation; may lead to progressive liver injury; and, when superimposed on well-established cirrhosis, may cause hepatic decompensation. Complications of cirrhosis occur in end-stage chronic hepatitis and include ascites, edema, bleeding gastroesophageal varices, hepatic encephalopathy, coagulopathy, or hypersplenism. Occasionally, these complications bring the patient to initial clinical attention. Extrahepatic complications of chronic hepatitis B, similar to those seen during the prodromal phase of acute hepatitis B, are associated with deposition of circulating hepatitis B antigen–antibody immune complexes. These include arthralgias and arthritis, which are common, and the more rare purpuric cutaneous lesions (leukocytoclastic vasculitis), immune-complex glomerulonephritis, and generalized vasculitis (polyarteritis nodosa) (Chaps. 360 and 385).

Laboratory features of chronic hepatitis B do not distinguish adequately between histologically mild and severe hepatitis. Aminotransferase elevations tend to be modest for chronic hepatitis B but may fluctuate in the range of 100–1000 units. As is true for acute viral hepatitis B, alanine aminotransferase (ALT) tends to be more elevated than aspartate aminotransferase (AST); however, once cirrhosis is established, AST tends to exceed ALT. Levels of alkaline phosphatase activity tend to be normal or only marginally elevated. In severe cases, moderate elevations in serum bilirubin (51.3–171 μmol/L [3–10 mg/dL]) occur. Hypoalbuminemia and prolongation of the prothrombin time occur in severe or end-stage cases. Hyperglobulinemia and detectable circulating autoantibodies are distinctly absent in chronic hepatitis B (in contrast to autoimmune hepatitis). **Viral markers of chronic HBV infection are discussed in Chap. 360.**

TREATMENT CHRONIC HEPATITIS B

Although progression to cirrhosis is more likely in severe than in mild or moderate chronic hepatitis B, all forms of chronic hepatitis B can be progressive, and progression occurs primarily in patients with active HBV replication. Moreover, in populations of patients with chronic hepatitis B who are at risk for HCC (Chap. 111), the risk is highest for those with continued, high-level HBV replication and lower for persons in whom initially high-level HBV DNA falls spontaneously over time. Therefore, management of chronic hepatitis B is directed at suppressing the level of virus replication. Although clinical trials tend to focus on clinical endpoints achieved over 1–2 years (e.g., suppression of HBV DNA to undetectable levels, loss of HBeAg/HBsAg, improvement in histology, normalization of ALT), these short-term gains translate into reductions in the risk of clinical progression, hepatic decompensation, and death. To date, seven drugs have been approved for treatment of chronic hepatitis B: injectable interferon (IFN) α; pegylated interferon (long-acting IFN bound to polyethylene glycol, PEG [PEG IFN]); and the oral agents lamivudine, adefovir dipivoxil, entecavir, telbivudine, and tenofovir.

Antiviral therapy for hepatitis B has evolved rapidly since the mid-1990s, as has the sensitivity of tests for HBV DNA. When IFN and lamivudine were evaluated in clinical trials, HBV DNA was measured by insensitive hybridization assays with detection thresholds of 10^5–10^6 virions/mL; when adefovir, entecavir, telbivudine, tenofovir, and PEG IFN were studied in clinical trials, HBV DNA was measured by sensitive amplification assays (polymerase chain reaction [PCR]) with detection thresholds of 10^1–10^3 viral copies/mL or IU/mL. Recognition of these distinctions is helpful when comparing results of clinical trials that established the efficacy of these therapies (reviewed below in chronological order of publication of these efficacy trials).

INTERFERON

IFN-α was the first approved therapy for chronic hepatitis B. Although it is no longer used to treat hepatitis B, standard IFN is important historically, having provided important lessons about antiviral therapy in general. For immunocompetent adults with HBeAg-reactive chronic hepatitis B (who tend to have high-level HBV DNA [>10^5–10^6 virions/mL] and histologic evidence of chronic hepatitis on liver biopsy), a 16-week course of IFN given subcutaneously at a daily dose of 5 million units, or three times a week at a dose of 10 million units, results in a loss of HBeAg and hybridization-detectable HBV DNA (i.e., a reduction to levels below 10^5–10^6 virions/mL) in ~30% of patients, with a concomitant improvement in liver histology. Seroconversion from HBeAg to anti-HBe occurred in approximately 20%, and, in early trials, approximately 8% lost HBsAg. Successful IFN therapy and seroconversion are often accompanied by an acute hepatitis-like elevation in aminotransferase activity, which has been postulated to result from enhanced cytolytic T cell clearance of HBV-infected hepatocytes. Relapse after successful therapy is rare (1 or 2%). The likelihood of responding to IFN is higher in patients with lower levels of HBV DNA and substantial elevations of ALT. Although children can respond as well as adults, IFN therapy has not been effective in very young children infected at birth. Similarly, IFN therapy has not been effective in immunosuppressed persons, Asian patients with neonatal acquisition of infection and minimal-to-mild ALT elevations, or patients with decompensated chronic hepatitis B (in whom such therapy can actually be detrimental, sometimes precipitating decompensation, often associated with severe adverse effects). Among patients with HBeAg loss during therapy, long-term follow-up has demonstrated that 80% experience eventual loss of HBsAg (i.e., all serologic markers of infection, and normalization of ALT over a 9-year posttreatment period). In addition, improved long-term and complication-free survival as well as a reduction in the frequency of HCC have been documented among IFN responders, supporting the conclusion that successful antiviral therapy improves the natural history of chronic hepatitis B.

Initial trials of brief-duration IFN therapy in patients with *HBeAg-negative chronic hepatitis B* were disappointing, suppressing HBV replication transiently during therapy but almost never resulting in sustained antiviral responses. In subsequent IFN trials among patients with HBeAg-negative chronic hepatitis B, however, more protracted courses, lasting up to 1.5 years, have been reported to result in sustained remissions documented to last for several years, with suppressed HBV DNA and aminotransferase activity, in ~20%.

Complications of IFN therapy include systemic "flu-like" symptoms; marrow suppression; emotional lability (irritability, depression, anxiety); autoimmune reactions (especially autoimmune thyroiditis); and miscellaneous side effects such as alopecia, rashes, diarrhea, and numbness and tingling of the extremities. With the possible exception of autoimmune thyroiditis, all these side effects are reversible upon dose lowering or cessation of therapy.

Although no longer competitive with the newer generation of antivirals, IFN did represent the first successful antiviral approach and set a standard against which to measure subsequent drugs in the achievement of durable virologic, serologic, biochemical, and histologic responses; consolidation of virologic and biochemical benefit in the ensuing years after therapy; and improvement in the natural history of chronic hepatitis B. Standard IFN has been supplanted by long-acting PEG IFN (see below), and IFN nonresponders are now treated with one of the newer oral nucleoside analogues.

LAMIVUDINE

The first of the nucleoside analogues to be approved, the dideoxynucleoside lamivudine inhibits reverse transcriptase activity of both HIV and HBV and is a potent and effective agent for patients with chronic hepatitis B. Although generally superseded by newer, more potent agents, lamivudine is still used in regions of the world where newer agents are not yet approved are or not affordable. In clinical trials among patients with HBeAg-reactive chronic hepatitis B, lamivudine therapy at daily doses of 100 mg for 48–52 weeks suppressed HBV DNA by a median of approximately 5.5 $\log_{10}$ copies/mL and to undetectable levels, as measured by PCR amplification assays, in approximately 40% of patients. Therapy was associated with HBeAg loss in 32–33%; HBeAg seroconversion (i.e., conversion from HBeAg-reactive to anti-HBe-reactive) in 16–21%; normalization of ALT in 40–75%; improvement in histology in 50–60%; retardation in fibrosis in 20–30%; and prevention of progression to cirrhosis. HBeAg responses can occur even in subgroups who are resistant to IFN (e.g., those with high-level HBV DNA) or who failed in the past to respond to it. As is true for IFN therapy of chronic hepatitis B, patients with near-normal ALT activity tend not to experience HBeAg responses (despite suppression of HBV DNA), and those with ALT levels exceeding 5 × the upper limit of normal can expect 1-year HBeAg seroconversion rates of 50–60%. Generally, HBeAg seroconversions are confined to patients who achieve suppression of HBV DNA to $<10^4$ copies/mL (equivalent to $\sim10^3$ IU/mL). Lamivudine-associated HBeAg responses are accompanied by a posttreatment HBsAg seroconversion rate comparable to that seen after IFN-induced HBeAg responses. Among Western patients who undergo HBeAg responses during a year-long course of therapy and in whom the response is sustained for 4–6 months after cessation of therapy, the response is durable thereafter in the vast majority (>80%); therefore, the achievement of an HBeAg response represents a viable stopping point in therapy. Reduced durability has been reported in Asian patients; therefore, to support the durability of HBeAg responses, patients should receive a period of consolidation therapy of ≥6 months in Western patients and ≥1 year in Asian patients after HBeAg seroconversion. Close posttreatment monitoring is necessary to identify HBV reactivation promptly and to resume therapy. If HBeAg is unaffected by lamivudine therapy, the current approach is to continue therapy until an HBeAg response occurs, but long-term therapy may be required to suppress HBV replication and, in turn, limit liver injury; HBeAg seroconversions can increase to a level of 50% after 5 years of therapy. Histologic improvement continues to accrue with therapy beyond the first year; after a cumulative course of 3 years of lamivudine therapy, necroinflammatory activity is reduced in the majority of patients, and even cirrhosis has been shown to regress to precirrhotic stages in as many as three-quarters of patients.

Losses of HBsAg have been few during the first year of lamivudine therapy, and this observation had been cited as an advantage of IFN-based over lamivudine therapy; however, in head-to-head comparisons between standard IFN and lamivudine monotherapy, HBsAg losses were rare in both groups. Trials in which lamivudine and IFN were administered in combination failed to show a benefit of combination therapy over lamivudine monotherapy for either treatment-naïve patients or prior IFN nonresponders.

In patients with *HBeAg-negative chronic hepatitis B* (i.e., in those with precore and core-promoter HBV mutations), 1 year of lamivudine therapy results in HBV DNA suppression and normalization of ALT in three-quarters of patients and in histologic improvement in approximately two-thirds. Therapy has been shown to suppress HBV DNA by approximately 4.5 $\log_{10}$ copies/mL (baseline HBV DNA levels are lower than in patients with HBeAg-reactive hepatitis B) and to undetectable levels in approximately 70%, as measured by sensitive PCR amplification assays. Lacking HBeAg at the outset, patients with HBeAg-negative chronic hepatitis B cannot achieve an HBeAg response—a stopping point in HBeAg-reactive patients; almost invariably, when therapy is discontinued, reactivation is the rule. Therefore, these patients require long-term therapy; with successive years, the proportion with suppressed HBV DNA and normal ALT increases.

Clinical and laboratory side effects of lamivudine are negligible and indistinguishable from those observed in placebo recipients. Still, lamivudine doses should be reduced in patients with reduced creatinine clearance. During lamivudine therapy, transient ALT elevations, resembling those seen during IFN therapy and during spontaneous HBeAg-to-anti-HBe seroconversions, occur in one-fourth of patients. These ALT elevations may result from restored cytolytic T cell activation permitted by suppression of HBV replication. Similar ALT elevations, however, occur at an identical frequency in placebo recipients, but ALT elevations associated with HBeAg seroconversion are confined to lamivudine-treated patients. When therapy is stopped after a year of therapy, two- to threefold ALT elevations occur in 20–30% of lamivudine-treated patients, representing renewed liver-cell injury as HBV replication returns. Although these posttreatment flares are almost always transient and mild, rare severe exacerbations, especially in cirrhotic patients, have been observed, mandating close and careful clinical and virologic monitoring after discontinuation of treatment. Many authorities caution against discontinuing therapy in patients with cirrhosis, in whom posttreatment flares could precipitate decompensation.

Long-term monotherapy with lamivudine is associated with methionine-to-valine (M204V) or methionine-to-isoleucine (M204I) mutations, primarily at amino acid 204 in the tyrosine-methionine-aspartate-aspartate (YMDD) motif of HBV DNA polymerase, analogous to mutations that occur in HIV-infected patients treated with this drug. During a year of therapy, YMDD mutations occur in 15–30% of patients; the frequency increases with each year of therapy, reaching 70% at year 5. Ultimately, patients with YMDD mutants experience degradation of clinical, biochemical, and histologic responses; therefore, if treatment is begun with lamivudine monotherapy, the emergence of lamivudine resistance, reflected clinically by a breakthrough from suppressed levels of HBV DNA and ALT, is managed by adding another antiviral to which YMDD variants are sensitive (e.g., adefovir, tenofovir; see below).

Currently, although lamivudine is very safe and still used widely in other parts of the world, in the United States and Europe, lamivudine has been eclipsed by more potent antivirals that have superior resistance profiles (see below); it is no longer recommended as first-line therapy. Still, as the first successful oral antiviral agent for use in hepatitis B, lamivudine has provided proof of the concept that polymerase inhibitors can achieve virologic, serologic, biochemical, and histologic benefits. In addition, lamivudine has been shown to be effective in the treatment of patients with decompensated hepatitis B (for whom IFN is contraindicated), in some of whom decompensation can be reversed. Moreover, among patients with cirrhosis or advanced fibrosis, lamivudine has been shown to be effective in reducing the risk of progression to hepatic decompensation and, marginally, the risk of HCC. In the half decade following the introduction in the United States of lamivudine therapy for hepatitis B, referral of patients with HBV-associated end-stage liver disease for liver transplantation was reduced by ~30%, supporting further the beneficial impact of oral antiviral therapy on the natural history of chronic hepatitis B.

Because lamivudine monotherapy can result universally in the rapid emergence of YMDD variants in persons with HIV infection, patients with chronic hepatitis B should be tested for anti-HIV prior to therapy; if HIV infection is identified, lamivudine monotherapy at the HBV daily dose of 100 mg is contraindicated. These patients should be treated for both HIV and HBV with an HIV drug regimen that includes or is supplemented by at least two drugs active against HBV; antiretroviral therapy (ART) often contains two drugs with antiviral activity against HBV (e.g., tenofovir and emtricitabine), but if lamivudine is part of the regimen, the daily dose should be 300 mg (Chap. 226). The safety of lamivudine during pregnancy has not been established; however, the drug is not teratogenic in rodents and has been used safely in pregnant women with HIV infection and with HBV infection. Limited data even suggest that administration of lamivudine during the last months of pregnancy to mothers with high-level hepatitis B viremia (≥10^8 IU/mL) can reduce the likelihood of perinatal transmission of hepatitis B.

ADEFOVIR DIPIVOXIL

At an oral daily dose of 10 mg, the acyclic nucleotide analogue adefovir dipivoxil, the prodrug of adefovir, reduces HBV DNA by approximately 3.5–4 log_{10} copies/mL and is equally effective in treatment-naïve patients and IFN nonresponders. In HBeAg-reactive chronic hepatitis B, a 48-week course of adefovir dipivoxil was shown to achieve histologic improvement (and reduce the progression of fibrosis) and normalization of ALT in just over one-half of patients, HBeAg seroconversion in 12%, HBeAg loss in 23%, and suppression to an undetectable level of HBV DNA in 13–21%, as measured by PCR. Similar to IFN and lamivudine, adefovir dipivoxil is more likely to achieve an HBeAg response in patients with high baseline ALT (e.g., among adefovir-treated patients with ALT level >5 × the upper limit of normal), and HBeAg seroconversions occurred in 25%. The durability of adefovir-induced HBeAg responses is high (91% in one study); therefore, HBeAg response can be relied upon as a stopping point for adefovir therapy, after a period of consolidation therapy, as outlined above. Although data on the impact of additional therapy beyond 1 year are limited, biochemical, serologic, and virologic outcomes improve progressively as therapy is continued.

In patients with *HBeAg-negative chronic hepatitis B*, a 48-week course of 10 mg/d of adefovir dipivoxil resulted in histologic improvement in two-thirds, normalization of ALT in three-fourths, and suppression of HBV DNA to PCR-undetectable levels in one-half to two-thirds. As was true for lamivudine, because HBeAg responses—a potential stopping point—cannot be achieved in this group, reactivation is the rule when adefovir therapy is discontinued, and indefinite, long-term therapy is required. Treatment beyond the first year consolidates the gain of the first year; after 5 years of therapy, improvement in hepatic inflammation and regression of fibrosis were observed in three-fourths of patients, ALT was normal in 70%, and HBV DNA was undetectable in almost 70%. In one study, stopping adefovir after 5 years was followed by sustained suppression of HBV DNA and ALT, but most HBeAg-negative patients are treated indefinitely unless HBsAg loss, albeit very rare, is achieved.

Adefovir contains a flexible acyclic linker instead of the L-nucleoside ring of lamivudine, avoiding steric hindrance by mutated amino acids. In addition, the molecular structure of phosphorylated adefovir is very similar to that of its natural substrate; therefore, mutations to adefovir would also affect binding of the natural substrate, dATP. Hypothetically, these are among the reasons that resistance to adefovir dipivoxil is much less likely than resistance to lamivudine; no resistance was encountered in 1 year of clinical trial therapy. In subsequent years, however, adefovir resistance begins to emerge (asparagine to threonine at amino acid 236 [N236T] and alanine to valine or threonine at amino acid 181 [A181V/T], primarily), occurring in 2.5% after 2 years, but in 29% after 5 years of therapy (reported in HBeAg-negative patients). Among patients co-infected with HBV and HIV and who have normal CD4+ T cell counts, adefovir dipivoxil is effective in suppressing HBV dramatically (by 5 $logs_{10}$ in one study). Moreover, adefovir dipivoxil is effective in lamivudine-resistant, YMDD-mutant HBV and can be used when such lamivudine-induced variants emerge. When lamivudine resistance occurs, adding adefovir (i.e., maintaining lamivudine to preempt the emergence of adefovir resistance) is superior to switching to adefovir. Almost invariably, patients with adefovir-mutant HBV respond to lamivudine (or newer agents, such as entecavir, see below). When, in the past, adefovir had been evaluated as therapy for HIV infection, doses of 60–120 mg were required to suppress HIV, and, at these doses, the drug was nephrotoxic. Even at 30 mg/d, creatinine elevations of 44 μmol/L (0.5 mg/dL) occurred in 10% of patients; however, at the HBV-effective dose of 10 mg, such elevations of creatinine are rarely encountered. If any nephrotoxicity does occur, it rarely appears before 6–8 months of therapy. Although renal tubular injury is a rare potential side effect, and although creatinine monitoring is recommended during treatment, the therapeutic index of adefovir dipivoxil is high, and the nephrotoxicity observed in clinical trials at higher doses was reversible. For patients with underlying renal disease, frequency of administration of adefovir dipivoxil should be reduced to every 48 h for creatinine clearances of 30–49 mL/min; to every 72 h for creatinine clearances of 10–29 mL/min; and once a week, following dialysis, for patients undergoing hemodialysis. Adefovir dipivoxil is very well tolerated, and ALT elevations during and after withdrawal of therapy are similar to those observed and described above in clinical trials of lamivudine. An advantage of adefovir is its relatively favorable resistance profile; however, it is not as potent as the other approved oral agents, it does not suppress HBV DNA as rapidly or as uniformly as the others, it is the least likely of all agents to result in HBeAg seroconversion, and 20–50% of patients fail to suppress HBV DNA by 2 log_{10} ("primary nonresponders"). For these reasons, adefovir, which has been supplanted in both treatment-naïve and lamivudine-resistant patients by the more potent, less resistance-prone nucleotide analogue tenofovir (see below), is no longer recommended as first-line therapy.

PEGYLATED INTERFERON

After long-acting PEG IFN was shown to be effective in the treatment of hepatitis C (see below), this more convenient drug was evaluated in the treatment of chronic hepatitis B. Once-a-week PEG IFN is more effective than the more frequently administered, standard IFN, and several large-scale trials of PEG IFN versus oral nucleoside analogues have been conducted among patients with HBeAg-reactive and HBeAg-negative chronic hepatitis B.

In HBeAg-reactive chronic hepatitis B, two large-scale studies were done. One study evaluated PEG IFN-α 2b (100 μg weekly for 32 weeks, then 50 μg weekly for another 20 weeks for a total of 52 weeks, with a comparison arm of combination PEG IFN with oral lamivudine) in 307 subjects. The other study involved PEG IFN-α 2a (180 μg weekly for 48 weeks) in 814 primarily Asian patients, three-fourths of whom had ALT ≥2 × the upper limit of normal, with comparison arms of lamivudine monotherapy and combination PEG IFN plus lamivudine. At the end of therapy (48–52 weeks) in the PEG IFN monotherapy arms, HBeAg loss occurred in approximately 30%, HBeAg seroconversion in 22–27%, undetectable HBV DNA (<400 copies/mL by PCR) in 10–25%, normal ALT in 34–39%, and a mean reduction in HBV DNA of 2 log_{10} copies/mL (PEG IFN-α 2b) to 4.5 log_{10} copies/mL (PEG IFN-α 2a). Six months after completing PEG IFN monotherapy in these trials, HBeAg losses were present in approximately 35%, HBeAg seroconversion in approximately 30%, undetectable HBV DNA in 7–14%, normal ALT in 32–41%, and a mean reduction in HBV DNA of 2–2.4 log_{10} copies/mL. Although the combination of PEG IFN and lamivudine was superior at the end of therapy in one or more serologic, virologic, or biochemical outcomes, neither the combination arm (in both studies) nor the lamivudine monotherapy arm (in the PEG IFN-α 2a trial) demonstrated any benefit compared to the PEG IFN monotherapy arms 6 months after therapy. Moreover, HBsAg seroconversion occurred in 3–7% of PEG IFN recipients (with or without lamivudine); some of these seroconversions were identified by the end of therapy, but many were identified during the posttreatment follow-up period. The likelihood of HBeAg loss in PEG IFN–treated HBeAg-reactive patients is associated with HBV genotype A > B > C > D (shown for PEG IFN-α2b but not for α-2a).

Based on these results, some authorities concluded that PEG IFN monotherapy should be the first-line therapy of choice in HBeAg-reactive chronic hepatitis B; however, this conclusion has been challenged. Although a finite, 1-year course of PEG IFN results in a higher rate of sustained response (6 months after treatment) than is achieved with oral nucleoside/nucleotide analogue therapy, the comparison is confounded by the fact that oral agents are not discontinued at the end of 1 year. Instead, taken orally and free of side effects, therapy with oral agents is extended indefinitely or until after the occurrence of an HBeAg response. The rate of HBeAg responses after 2 years of oral-agent nucleoside analogue therapy is at least as high as, if not higher than, that achieved with PEG IFN after 1 year; favoring oral agents is the absence of injections, difficult-to-tolerate side effects, and laboratory monitoring as well as lower direct and indirect medical care costs and inconvenience. The association of HBsAg responses with PEG IFN therapy occurs in such a small proportion of patients that subjecting everyone to PEG IFN for the marginal gain of HBsAg responses during or immediately after therapy in such a very small minority is questionable. Moreover, HBsAg responses occur in a comparable proportion of patients treated with early-generation nucleoside/nucleotide analogues in the years after therapy, and, with the newer, more potent nucleoside analogues, the frequency of HBsAg loss during the first year of therapy equals that of PEG IFN and is exceeded during year 2 and beyond (see below). Of course, resistance is not an issue during PEG IFN therapy, but the risk of resistance is much lower with new agents (≤1% up to 3–6 years in previously treatment-naïve, entecavir-treated and tenofovir-treated patients; see below). Finally, the level of HBV DNA inhibition that can be achieved with the newer agents, and even with lamivudine, exceeds that which can be achieved with PEG IFN, in some cases by several orders of magnitude.

In HBeAg-negative chronic hepatitis B, a trial of PEG IFN-α 2a (180 μg weekly for 48 weeks versus comparison arms of lamivudine monotherapy and of combination therapy) in 564 patients showed that PEG IFN monotherapy resulted at the end of therapy in suppression of HBV DNA by a mean of 4.1 $\log_{10}$ copies/mL, undetectable HBV DNA (<400 copies/mL by PCR) in 63%, normal ALT in 38%, and loss of HBsAg in 4%. Although lamivudine monotherapy and combination lamivudine–PEG IFN therapy were both superior to PEG IFN at the end of therapy, no advantage of lamivudine monotherapy or combination therapy was apparent over PEG IFN monotherapy 6 months after therapy—suppression of HBV DNA by a mean of 2.3 $\log_{10}$ copies/mL, undetectable HBV DNA in 19%, and normal ALT in 59%. In subjects involved in this trial followed for up to 5 years, among the two-thirds followed who had been treated initially with PEG IFN, 17% maintained HBV DNA suppression to <400 copies/mL, but ALT remained normal in only 22%; HBsAg loss increased gradually to 12%. Among the half followed who had been treated initially with lamivudine monotherapy, HBV DNA remained <400 copies/mL in 7% and ALT normal in 16%; by year 5, 3.5% had lost HBsAg. As was the case for standard IFN therapy in HBeAg-negative patients, only a small proportion maintained responsiveness after completion of PEG IFN therapy, raising questions about the relative value of a finite period of PEG IFN, versus a longer course with a potent, low-resistance oral nucleoside analogue in these patients. Moreover, the value of PEG IFN for HBeAg-negative chronic hepatitis B has not been confirmed. In the only other controlled clinical trial of PEG IFN for HBeAg-negative chronic hepatitis B, the hepatitis C regimen of PEG IFN plus ribavirin was compared to PEG IFN monotherapy. In this trial, HBV DNA suppression (<400 copies/mL) occurred in only 7.5% of the two groups combined, and no study subject lost HBsAg.

In patients treated with PEG IFN, HBeAg and HBsAg responses have been associated with *IL28B* genotype CC, the favorable genotype identified in trials of PEG IFN for chronic hepatitis C. Also, reductions in quantitative HBsAg levels have been shown to correlate with and to be predictive of responsiveness to PEG IFN in chronic hepatitis B. If HBsAg levels fail to fall within the first 12–24 weeks or to reach <20,000 IU/mL by week 24, PEG IFN therapy is unlikely to be effective and should be discontinued.

ENTECAVIR

Entecavir, an oral cyclopentyl guanosine analogue polymerase inhibitor, appears to be the most potent of the HBV antivirals and is just as well tolerated as lamivudine. In a 709-subject clinical trial among HBeAg-reactive patients, oral entecavir, 0.5 mg daily, was compared to lamivudine, 100 mg daily. At 48 weeks, entecavir was superior to lamivudine in suppression of HBV DNA (mean 6.9 versus 5.5 $\log_{10}$ copies/mL), percentage with undetectable HBV DNA (<300 copies/mL by PCR; 67% versus 36%), histologic improvement (≥2-point improvement in necroinflammatory HAI score; 72% versus 62%), and normal ALT (68% versus 60%). The two treatments were indistinguishable in percentage with HBeAg loss (22% versus 20%) and seroconversion (21% versus 18%). Among patients treated with entecavir for 96 weeks, HBV DNA was undetectable cumulatively in 80% (versus 39% for lamivudine), and HBeAg seroconversions had occurred in 31% (versus 26% for lamivudine). After 3–6 years of entecavir, HBeAg seroconversions have been observed in 39–44% and HBsAg loss in 5–6%. Similarly, in a 638-subject clinical trial among HBeAg-negative patients, at week 48, oral entecavir, 0.5 mg daily, was superior to lamivudine, 100 mg daily, in suppression of HBV DNA (mean 5.0 versus 4.5 $\log_{10}$ copies/mL) and in percentage with undetectable HBV DNA (90% versus 72%), histologic improvement (70% versus 61%), and normal ALT (78% versus 71%). No resistance mutations were encountered in previously treatment-naïve, entecavir-treated patients during 96 weeks of therapy, and in a cohort of subjects treated for up to 6 years, resistance emerged in only 1.2%. Entecavir-induced HBeAg seroconversions are as durable as those achieved with other antivirals. Its high barrier to resistance coupled with its high potency renders entecavir a first-line drug for patients with chronic hepatitis B.

Entecavir is also effective against lamivudine-resistant HBV infection. In a trial of 286 lamivudine-resistant patients, entecavir, at a higher daily dose of 1 mg, was superior to lamivudine, as measured at week 48, in achieving suppression of HBV DNA (mean 5.1 versus 0.48 $\log_{10}$ copies/mL), undetectable HBV DNA (72% versus 19%), normal ALT (61% versus 15%), HBeAg loss (10% versus 3%), and HBeAg seroconversion (8% versus 3%). In this population of lamivudine-experienced patients, however, entecavir resistance emerged in 7% at 48 weeks. Although entecavir resistance requires both a YMDD mutation and a second mutation at one of several other sites (e.g., T184A, S202G/I, or M250V), resistance to entecavir in lamivudine-resistant chronic hepatitis B has been recorded to increase progressively to 43% at 4 years; therefore, entecavir is not as attractive a choice as adefovir or tenofovir for patients with lamivudine-resistant hepatitis B.

In clinical trials, entecavir has an excellent safety profile; in addition, on-treatment and posttreatment ALT flares are relatively uncommon and relatively mild in entecavir-treated patients. Doses should be reduced for patients with reduced creatinine clearance. Entecavir does have low-level antiviral activity against HIV and cannot be used as monotherapy to treat HBV infection in HIV/HBV co-infected persons.

TELBIVUDINE

Telbivudine, a cytosine analogue, is similar in efficacy to entecavir but slightly less potent in suppressing HBV DNA (a slightly less profound median 6.4 $\log_{10}$ reduction in HBeAg-reactive disease and a similar 5.2 $\log_{10}$ reduction in HBeAg-negative disease). In its registration trial, telbivudine at an oral daily dose of 600 mg suppressed HBV DNA to <300 copies/mL in 60% of HBeAg-positive and 88% of HBeAg-negative patients, reduced ALT to normal in 77% of HBeAg-positive and 74% of HBeAg-negative patients, and improved histology in 65% of HBeAg-positive and 67% of HBeAg-negative patients. Although resistance to telbivudine (M204I, not M204V, mutations) was less frequent than resistance to lamivudine at the end of 1 year, resistance mutations after 2 years of treatment occurred in up to 22%. Generally well tolerated, telbivudine has been associated with a low frequency of asymptomatic creatine kinase elevations and with a very low frequency of peripheral neuropathy; frequency of administration should be reduced for patients with impaired creatinine clearance. Its excellent potency notwithstanding, the inferior resistance profile of telbivudine has limited its appeal; telbivudine is neither recommended as first-line therapy nor widely used.

TENOFOVIR

Tenofovir disoproxil fumarate, an acyclic nucleotide analogue and potent antiretroviral agent used to treat HIV infection, is similar to adefovir but more potent in suppressing HBV DNA and inducing HBeAg responses; it is highly active against both wild-type and lamivudine-resistant HBV and active in patients whose response to adefovir is slow and/or limited. At an oral once-daily dose of 300 mg for 48 weeks, tenofovir suppressed HBV DNA by 6.2 $\log_{10}$ (to undetectable levels [<400 copies/mL] in 76%) in HBeAg-positive patients and by 4.6 $\log_{10}$ (to undetectable levels in 93%) in HBeAg-negative patients; reduced ALT to normal in 68% of HBeAg-positive and 76% of HBeAg-negative patients; and improved histology in 74% of HBeAg-positive and 72% of HBeAg-negative patients. In HBeAg-positive patients, HBeAg seroconversions occurred in 21% by the end of year 1, 27% by year 2, 34% by year 3, and 40% by year 5 of tenofovir treatment; HBsAg loss occurred in 3% by the end of year 1 and 6% at year 2, and 8% by year 5. After 5 years of tenofovir therapy, 87% of patients experienced histologic improvement, including reduction in fibrosis score (51%) and regression of cirrhosis (71%). The 5-year safety (negligible renal toxicity, in 1%, and mild reduction in bone density, in ~0.5%) and resistance profiles (none recorded through 5 years) of tenofovir are very favorable as well; therefore, tenofovir has supplanted adefovir both as first-line therapy for chronic hepatitis B and as add-on therapy for lamivudine-resistant chronic hepatitis B. Frequency of tenofovir administration should be reduced for patients with impaired creatinine clearance.

A comparison of the six antiviral therapies in current use appears in Table 362-3; their relative potencies in suppressing HBV DNA are shown in Fig. 362-1.

COMBINATION THERAPY

Although the combination of lamivudine and PEG IFN suppresses HBV DNA more profoundly during therapy than does monotherapy

TABLE 362-3 COMPARISON OF PEGYLATED INTERFERON (PEG IFN), LAMIVUDINE, ADEFOVIR, ENTECAVIR, TELBIVUDINE, AND TENOFOVIR THERAPY FOR CHRONIC HEPATITIS B[a]

Feature	PEG IFN[b]	Lamivudine	Adefovir	Entecavir	Telbivudine	Tenofovir
Route of administration	Subcutaneous injection	Oral	Oral	Oral	Oral	Oral
Duration of therapy[c]	48–52 weeks	≥52 weeks	≥48 weeks	≥48 weeks	≥52 weeks	≥48 weeks
Tolerability	Poorly tolerated	Well tolerated	Well tolerated; creatinine monitoring recommended	Well tolerated	Well tolerated	Well tolerated; creatinine monitoring recommended
HBeAg seroconversion						
1 yr Rx	18–20%	16–21%	12%	21%	22%	21%
>1 yr Rx	NA	up to 50% @ 5 yrs	43% @ 3 yrs[d]	31% @ 2 yrs 44% @ 6 yrs	30% @ 2 yrs	40% @ 5 yrs
Log_{10} HBV DNA reduction (mean copies/mL)						
HBeAg-reactive	4.5	5.5	median 3.5–5	6.9	6.4	6.2
HBeAg-negative	4.1	4.4–4.7	median 3.5–3.9	5.0	5.2	4.6
HBV DNA PCR negative (<300–400 copies/mL; <1000 copies/mL for adefovir) at end of yr 1						
HBeAg-reactive	10–25%	36–44%	13–21%	67% (91% @ 4 yrs)	60%	76%
HBeAg-negative	63%	60–73%	48–77%	90%	88%	93%
ALT normalization at end of yr 1						
HBeAg-reactive	39%	41–75%	48–61%	68%	77%	68%
HBeAg-negative	34–38%	62–79%	48–77%	78%	74%	76%
HBsAg loss yr 1	3–4%	≤1%	0%	2%	<1%	3%
>yr 1	12% 5 yr after 1 yr of Rx	No data	5% at yr 5	6% at yr 6	No data	8% at yr 5
Histologic improvement (≥2 point reduction in HAI) at yr 1						
HBeAg-reactive	38% 6 months after	49–62%	53–68%	72%	65%	74%
HBeAg-negative	48% 6 months after	61–66%	64%	70%	67%	72%
Viral resistance	None	15–30% @ 1 yr 70% @ 5 yrs	None @ 1 yr 29% @ 5 yrs	≤1% @ 1 yr[e] 1.2% @ 6 yrs[e]	Up to 5% @ yr 1 Up to 22% @ yr 2	0% @ yr 1 0% through yr 5
Pregnancy category	C	C[f]	C	C	B	B
Cost (US$) for 1 yr	~$18,000	~$2,500	~$6,500	~$8,700[g]	~$6,000	~$6,000

[a]Generally, these comparisons are based on data on each drug tested individually versus placebo in registration clinical trials; because, with rare exception, these comparisons are not based on head-to-head testing of these drugs, relative advantages and disadvantages should be interpreted cautiously. [b]Although standard interferon α administered daily or three times a week is approved as therapy for chronic hepatitis B, it has been supplanted by PEG IFN, which is administered once a week and is more effective. Standard interferon has no advantages over PEG IFN. [c]Duration of therapy in clinical efficacy trials; use in clinical practice may vary. [d]Because of a computer-generated randomization error that resulted in misallocation of drug versus placebo during the second year of clinical trial treatment, the frequency of HBeAg seroconversion beyond the first year is an estimate (Kaplan-Meier analysis) based on the small subset in whom adefovir was administered correctly. [e]7% during a year of therapy (43% at year 4) in lamivudine-resistant patients. [f]Despite its Class C designation, lamivudine has an extensive pregnancy safety record in women with HIV/AIDS. [g]Approximately $17,400 for lamivudine-refractory patients.

Abbreviations: ALT, alanine aminotransferase; HAI, histologic activity index; HBeAg, hepatitis B e antigen; HBsAg, hepatitis B surface antigen; HBV, hepatitis B virus; NA, not applicable; PEG IFN, pegylated interferon; PCR, polymerase chain reaction; Rx, therapy; yr, year.

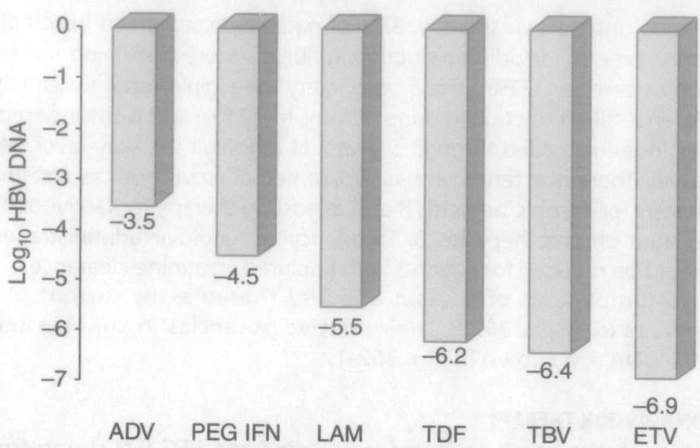

FIGURE 362-1 Relative potency of antiviral drugs for hepatitis B, as reflected by median $\log_{10}$ HBV DNA reduction in HBeAg-positive chronic hepatitis B. These data are from individual reports of large, randomized controlled registration trials that were the basis for approval of the drugs. In most instances, these data do not represent direct comparisons among the drugs, because study populations were different, baseline patient variables were not always uniform, and the sensitivity and dynamic range of the HBV DNA assays used in the trials varied. ADV, adefovir dipivoxil; ETV, entecavir; LAM, lamivudine; PEG IFN, pegylated interferon α2a; TBV, telbivudine; TDF, tenofovir disoproxil fumarate.

with either drug alone (and is much less likely to be associated with lamivudine resistance), this combination used for a year is no better than a year of PEG IFN in achieving sustained responses. To date, combinations of oral nucleoside/nucleotide agents have not achieved an enhancement in virologic, serologic, or biochemical efficacy over that achieved by the more potent of the combined drugs given individually. In a 2-year trial of combination entecavir and tenofovir versus entecavir monotherapy, for a small subgroup of patients with very high HBV DNA levels (≥10^8 IU/mL), a reduction in HBV DNA to <50 IU/mL was higher in the combination group (79% versus 62%); however, no differences in HBeAg responses or any other endpoint were observed between the combination-therapy and monotherapy groups, even in the high-HBV DNA subgroup. On the other hand, combining agents that are not cross-resistant (e.g., lamivudine and adefovir or tenofovir) has the potential to reduce the risk or perhaps even to preempt entirely the emergence of drug resistance. In the future, the treatment paradigm may shift from the current approach of sequential monotherapy to preemptive combination therapy, perhaps not for all patients but for subsets (e.g., patients with very high levels of HBV DNA, immunosuppressed patients); however, designing and executing clinical trials that demonstrate superior efficacy and resistance profile of combination therapy over monotherapy with entecavir or tenofovir will remain challenging.

NOVEL ANTIVIRALS AND STRATEGIES

In addition to the seven approved antiviral drugs for hepatitis B, emtricitabine, a fluorinated cytosine analogue very similar to lamivudine in structure, efficacy, and resistance profile, offers no advantage over lamivudine. A combination of emtricitabine and tenofovir is approved for the treatment of HIV infection and is an appealing combination therapy for hepatitis B, especially for lamivudine-resistant disease; however, neither emtricitabine nor the combination is approved yet for hepatitis B. Several initially promising antiviral agents have been abandoned because of toxicity (e.g., clevudine, which was linked to myopathy during its clinical development). Because direct-acting antivirals have been so successful in the management of chronic hepatitis B, more unconventional approaches—e.g., immunologic (e.g., toll receptor agonists) or genetic manipulation (e.g., RNA interference—gene silencing—to reduce HBV DNA transcription)—are not likely to be competitive, unless they can be shown to go beyond current antivirals in achieving recovery (HBsAg seroconversion) from HBV infection. Finally, initial emphasis in the development of antiviral therapy for hepatitis B was placed on monotherapy; whether combination regimens will yield additive or synergistic efficacy remains to be determined.

TREATMENT RECOMMENDATIONS

Several learned societies and groups of expert physicians have issued treatment recommendations for patients with chronic hepatitis B; the most authoritative and updated (and free of financial support by pharmaceutical companies) are those of the American Association for the Study of Liver Diseases (AASLD) and of the European Association for the Study of the Liver (EASL). Although the recommendations differ slightly, a consensus has emerged on most of the important points (Table 362-4). No treatment is recommended or available for inactive "nonreplicative" hepatitis B carriers (undetectable HBeAg with normal ALT and HBV DNA ≤10^3 IU/mL documented serially over time). In patients with detectable HBeAg and HBV DNA levels >2 × 10^4 IU/mL, treatment is recommended by the AASLD for those with ALT levels above 2 × the upper limit of normal. (The EASL recommends treatment in HBeAg-positive patients for HBV DNA levels >2 × 10^3 IU/mL and ALT above the upper limit of normal.) For HBeAg-positive patients with ALT ≤2 × the upper limit of normal, in whom sustained responses are not likely and who would require multiyear therapy, antiviral therapy is not recommended currently. This pattern is common during the early decades of life among Asian patients infected at birth; even in this group, therapy would be considered for those >40 years of age, ALT persistently at the high end of the twofold range, and/or with a family history of HCC, especially if the liver biopsy shows moderate to severe necroinflammatory activity or fibrosis. In this group, when, eventually, ALT becomes elevated later in life, antiviral therapy should be instituted. For patients with HBeAg-negative chronic hepatitis B, ALT >2 × the upper limit of normal (above the upper limit of normal according to EASL), and HBV DNA >2 × 10^3 IU/mL, antiviral therapy is recommended. If HBV DNA is >2 × 10^3 IU/mL and ALT is 1 to >2 × the upper limit of normal, liver biopsy should be considered to help in arriving at a decision to treat if substantial liver injury is present (treatment in this subset would be recommended according to EASL guidelines, because ALT is elevated).

For patients with compensated cirrhosis, because antiviral therapy has been shown to retard clinical progression, treatment is recommended regardless of HBeAg status and ALT as long as HBV DNA is detectable at >2 × 10^3 IU/mL (detectable at any level according to the EASL); monitoring without therapy is recommended for those with HBV DNA <2 × 10^3 IU/mL, unless ALT is elevated. For patients with decompensated cirrhosis, treatment is recommended regardless of serologic and biochemical status, as long as HBV DNA is detectable. Patients with decompensated cirrhosis should be evaluated as candidates for liver transplantation.

Among the seven available drugs for hepatitis B, PEG IFN has supplanted standard IFN, entecavir has supplanted lamivudine, and tenofovir has supplanted adefovir. PEG IFN, entecavir, or tenofovir is recommended as first-line therapy (Table 362-3). PEG IFN requires finite-duration therapy, achieves the highest rate of HBeAg responses after a year of therapy, and does not support viral mutations, but it requires subcutaneous injections and is associated with inconvenience, more intensive clinical and laboratory monitoring, and intolerability. Oral nucleoside analogues require long-term therapy in most patients, and when used alone, lamivudine and telbivudine foster the emergence of viral mutations, adefovir somewhat less so, and entecavir (except in lamivudine-experienced patients) and tenofovir rarely at all. Oral agents do not require injections or cumbersome laboratory monitoring, are very well tolerated, lead to improved histology in 50–90% of patients, suppress HBV DNA more profoundly than PEG IFN, and are effective even in patients who fail to respond to IFN-based therapy. Although oral agents are less likely to result in HBeAg responses during the first year of therapy, as compared to PEG IFN, treatment with oral agents tends to be extended beyond the first year and, by the end of the second year,

TABLE 362-4 RECOMMENDATIONS FOR TREATMENT OF CHRONIC HEPATITIS B[a]

HBeAg status	Clinical	HBV DNA (IU/mL)	ALT	Recommendation
HBeAg-reactive	[b]	$>2 \times 10^4$	$\leq 2 \times$ ULN[c,d]	No treatment; monitor. In patients >40, with family history of hepatocellular carcinoma, and/or ALT persistently at the high end of the twofold range, liver biopsy may help in decision to treat
	Chronic hepatitis	$>2 \times 10^4$[d]	$>2 \times$ ULN[d]	Treat[e]
	Cirrhosis compensated	$>2 \times 10^3$	< or > ULN	Treat[e] with oral agents, not PEG IFN
	Cirrhosis decompensated	$<2 \times 10^3$	>ULN	Consider treatment[f]
		Detectable	< or > ULN	Treat[e] with oral agents[g], not PEG IFN; refer for liver transplantation
		Undetectable	< or > ULN	Observe; refer for liver transplantation
HBeAg-negative	[b]	$\leq 2 \times 10^3$	≤ULN	Inactive carrier, treatment not necessary
	Chronic hepatitis	$>10^3$	1 to $>2 \times$ ULN[d]	Consider liver biopsy; treat[h] if biopsy shows moderate to severe inflammation or fibrosis
	Chronic hepatitis	$>10^4$	$>2 \times$ ULN[d]	Treat[h,i]
	Cirrhosis compensated	$>2 \times 10^3$	< or > ULN	Treate with oral agents, not PEG IFN
		$<2 \times 10^3$	>ULN	Consider treatment[f]
	Cirrhosis decompensated	Detectable	< or > ULN	Treat[h] with oral agents[g], not PEG IFN; refer for liver transplantation
		Undetectable	< or > ULN	Observe; refer for liver transplantation

[a]Based on practice guidelines of the American Association for the Study of Liver Diseases (AASLD). Except as indicated in footnotes, these guidelines are similar to those issued by the European Association for the Study of the Liver (EASL). [b]Liver disease tends to be mild or inactive clinically; most such patients do not undergo liver biopsy. [c]This pattern is common during early decades of life in Asian patients infected at birth. [d]According to the EASL guidelines, treat it HBV DNA is $>2 \times 10^3$ IU/mL and ALT >ULN. [e]One of the potent oral drugs with a high barrier to resistance (entecavir or tenofovir) or PEG IFN can be used as first-line therapy (see text). These oral agents, but not PEG IFN, should be used for interferon-refractory/intolerant and immunocompromised patients. PEG IFN is administered weekly by subcutaneous injection for a year; the oral agents are administered daily for at least a year and continued indefinitely or until at least 6 months after HBeAg seroconversion. [f]According to EASL guidelines, patients with compensated cirrhosis and detectable HBV DNA at any level, even with normal ALT, are candidates for therapy. Most authorities would treat indefinitely, even in HBeAg-positive disease after HBeAg seroconversion. [g]Because the emergence of resistance can lead to loss of antiviral benefit and further deterioration in decompensated cirrhosis, a low-resistance regimen is recommended—entecavir or tenofovir monotherapy or combination therapy with the more resistance-prone lamivudine (or telbivudine) plus adefovir. Therapy should be instituted urgently. [h]Because HBeAg seroconversion is not an option, the goal of therapy is to suppress HBV DNA and maintain a normal ALT. PEG IFN is administered by subcutaneous injection weekly for a year; caution is warranted in relying on a 6-month posttreatment interval to define a sustained response, because the majority of such responses are lost thereafter. Oral agents, entecavir or tenofovir, are administered daily, usually indefinitely or until, as very rarely occurs, virologic and biochemical responses are accompanied by HBsAg seroconversion. [i]For older patients and those with advanced fibrosis, consider lowering the HBV DNA threshold to $>2 \times 10^3$ IU/mL.

Abbreviations: AASLD, American Association for the Study of Liver Diseases; ALT, alanine aminotransferase; EASL, European Association for the Study of the Liver; HBeAg, hepatitis B e antigen; HBsAg, hepatitis B surface antigen; HBV, hepatitis B virus; PEG IFN, pegylated interferon; ULN, upper limit of normal.

yields HBeAg responses (and even HBsAg responses) comparable in frequency to those achieved after 1 year of PEG IFN (and without the associated side effects) (Table 362-5). Although adefovir and tenofovir are safe, creatinine monitoring is recommended. Substantial experience with lamivudine during pregnancy (see above) has identified no teratogenicity. Although interferons do not appear to cause congenital anomalies, interferons have antiproliferative properties and should be avoided during pregnancy. Adefovir during pregnancy has not been associated with birth defects; however, there may be an increased risk of spontaneous abortion. Data on the safety of entecavir during pregnancy have not been published. Sufficient data in animals and limited data in humans suggest that telbivudine and tenofovir can be used safely during pregnancy. In general, except perhaps for lamivudine, and until additional data become available, the other antivirals for hepatitis B should be avoided or used with extreme caution during pregnancy.

As noted above, some physicians prefer to begin with PEG IFN, while other physicians and patients prefer oral agents as first-line therapy. For patients with decompensated cirrhosis, the emergence of resistance can result in further deterioration and loss of antiviral effectiveness. Therefore, in this patient subset, the threshold for relying on therapy with a very favorable resistance profile (e.g., entecavir or tenofovir) or on combination therapy is low. PEG IFN should not be used in patients with compensated or decompensated cirrhosis.

For patients with end-stage chronic hepatitis B who undergo liver transplantation, reinfection of the new liver is almost universal in the absence of antiviral therapy. The majority of patients become high-level viremic carriers with minimal liver injury. Before the availability of antiviral therapy, an unpredictable proportion experienced severe hepatitis B–related liver injury, sometimes a fulminant-like hepatitis and sometimes a rapid recapitulation of the original severe chronic hepatitis B (Chap. 360). Currently, however, prevention of recurrent hepatitis B after liver transplantation has been achieved definitively by *combining* hepatitis B immune globulin with one of the oral nucleoside or nucleotide analogues (Chap. 368); preliminary data suggest that the newer, more potent, and less resistance-prone oral agents may be used instead of hepatitis B immune globulin for posttransplantation therapy.

Patients with HBV-HIV co-infection can have progressive HBV-associated liver disease and, occasionally, a severe exacerbation of hepatitis B resulting from immunologic reconstitution following ART. Lamivudine should never be used as monotherapy in patients with HBV-HIV infection because HIV resistance emerges rapidly to both viruses. Adefovir has been used successfully to treat chronic hepatitis B in HBV-HIV co-infected patients but is no longer considered a first-line agent for HBV. Entecavir has low-level activity against HIV and can result in selection of HIV resistance; therefore, it should be avoided in HBV-HIV co-infection. Tenofovir and the combination of tenofovir and emtricitabine in one pill are approved therapies for HIV and represent excellent choices for treating HBV infection in HBV-HIV co-infected patients. Generally, even for HBV-HIV co-infected patients who do not yet meet treatment criteria for HIV infection, treating for both HBV and HIV is recommended.

Patients with chronic hepatitis B who undergo cytotoxic chemotherapy for treatment of malignancies as well as patients treated with immunosuppressive, anticytokine, or antitumor necrosis factor therapies experience enhanced HBV replication and viral expression on hepatocyte membranes during chemotherapy coupled with suppression of cellular immunity. When chemotherapy is withdrawn, such patients are at risk for reactivation of hepatitis B, often severe and occasionally fatal. Such rebound reactivation represents restoration of cytolytic T cell function against a target organ enriched in HBV expression. Preemptive treatment with lamivudine prior to the initiation of chemotherapy has been shown to reduce the risk of such reactivation. The newer, more potent oral antiviral agents are

TABLE 362-5 PEGYLATED INTERFERON VERSUS ORAL NUCLEOSIDE ANALOGUES FOR THE TREATMENT OF CHRONIC HEPATITIS B

	PEG IFN	Nucleoside Analogues
Administration	Weekly injection	Daily, orally
Tolerability	Poorly tolerated, intensive monitoring	Well tolerated, limited monitoring
Duration of therapy	Finite 48 weeks	≥1 year, indefinite in most patients
Maximum mean HBV DNA suppression	4.5 $\log_{10}$	6.9 $\log_{10}$
Effective in high-level HBV DNA (≥10^9 IU/mL)	No	Yes
HBeAg seroconversion		
During 1 year of therapy	~30%	~20%
During >1 year of therapy	Not applicable	30% (year 2) to up to 50% (year 5)
HBeAg-negative posttreatment HBV DNA suppression	17% @ 5 years	7% @ 4 years (lamivudine)
HBsAg loss		
During 1 year of therapy	3–4%	0–3%
During >1 year of therapy	Not applicable	3–8% @ 5 years of therapy
After 1 year of therapy–HBeAg-negative	12% @ 5 years	3.5% @ 5 years
Antiviral resistance	None	Lamivudine: ~30% year 1, ~70% year 5
		Adefovir: 0% year 1, ~30% year 5
		Telbivudine: up to 4% year 1, 22% year 2
		Entecavir: ≤1.2% through year 6
		Tenofovir: 0% through year 5
Use in cirrhosis, transplantation, immunosuppressed	No	Yes
Cost, 1 year of therapy	++++	+ to ++

Abbreviations: HBV, hepatitis B virus; HBeAg, hepatitis B e antigen; HBsAg, hepatitis B surface antigen; PEG IFN, pegylated interferon.

even more effective in preventing hepatitis B reactivation and with a lower risk of antiviral drug resistance. The optimal duration of antiviral therapy after completion of chemotherapy is not known, but a suggested approach is 6 months for inactive hepatitis B carriers and longer-duration therapy in patients with baseline HBV DNA levels >2 × 10^3 IU/mL, until standard clinical endpoints are met (Table 362-4).

CHRONIC HEPATITIS D (DELTA HEPATITIS)

Chronic hepatitis D virus (HDV) may follow acute co-infection with HBV but at a rate no higher than the rate of chronicity of acute hepatitis B. That is, although HDV co-infection can increase the severity of acute hepatitis B, HDV does not increase the likelihood of progression to chronic hepatitis B. When, however, HDV superinfection occurs in a person who is already chronically infected with HBV, long-term HDV infection is the rule, and a worsening of the liver disease is the expected consequence. Except for severity, chronic hepatitis B plus D has similar clinical and laboratory features to those seen in chronic hepatitis B alone. Relatively severe and progressive chronic hepatitis, with or without cirrhosis, is the rule, and mild chronic hepatitis is the exception. Occasionally, however, mild hepatitis or even, rarely, inactive carriage occurs in patients with chronic hepatitis B plus D, and the disease may become indolent after several years of infection. A distinguishing serologic feature of chronic hepatitis D is the presence in the circulation of antibodies to liver-kidney microsomes (anti-LKM); however, the anti-LKM seen in hepatitis D, anti-LKM3, are directed against uridine diphosphate glucuronosyltransferase and are distinct from anti-LKM1 seen in patients with autoimmune hepatitis and in a subset of patients with chronic hepatitis C (see below). The clinical and laboratory features of chronic HDV infection are summarized in Chap. 360.

TREATMENT CHRONIC HEPATITIS D

Management is not well defined. Glucocorticoids are ineffective and are not used. Preliminary experimental trials of IFN-α suggested that conventional doses and durations of therapy lower levels of HDV RNA and aminotransferase activity only transiently during treatment but have no impact on the natural history of the disease. In contrast, high-dose IFN-α (9 million units three times a week) for 12 months may be associated with a sustained loss of HDV replication and clinical improvement in up to 50% of patients. Moreover, the beneficial impact of treatment has been observed to persist for 15 years and to be associated with a reduction in grade of hepatic necrosis and inflammation, reversion of advanced fibrosis (improved stage), and clearance of HDV RNA in some patients. A suggested approach to therapy has been high-dose, long-term IFN for at least a year and, in responders, extension of therapy until HDV RNA and HBsAg clearance. PEG IFN has also been shown to be effective in the treatment of chronic hepatitis D (e.g., after 48 weeks of therapy, associated with undetectable HDV RNA, durable for at least 24 posttreatment weeks, in a quarter of patients) and is a more convenient replacement for standard IFN. None of the nucleoside analogue antiviral agents for hepatitis B are effective in hepatitis D. In patients with end-stage liver disease secondary to chronic hepatitis D, liver transplantation has been effective. If hepatitis D recurs in the new liver without the expression of hepatitis B (an unusual serologic profile in immunocompetent persons but common in transplant patients), liver injury is limited. In fact, the outcome of transplantation for chronic hepatitis D is superior to that for chronic hepatitis B; in such patients, combination hepatitis B immune globulin and nucleoside analogue therapy for hepatitis B is indicated (Chap. 368).

CHRONIC HEPATITIS C

Regardless of the epidemiologic mode of acquisition of hepatitis C virus (HCV) infection, chronic hepatitis follows acute hepatitis C in 50–70% of cases; chronic infection is common even in those with a return to normal in aminotransferase levels after acute hepatitis C, adding up to an 85% likelihood of chronic HCV infection after acute hepatitis C. Few clues had emerged to explain host differences associated with chronic infection until recently, when variation in a single nucleotide polymorphism (SNP) on chromosome 19, *IL28B* (which codes for IFN-λ3), was identified that distinguished between responders and nonresponders to antiviral therapy (see below). The same variants correlated with spontaneous resolution after acute infection: 53% in genotype C/C, 30% in genotype C/T, but only 23% in genotype T/T. The association with HCV clearance after acute infection is even stronger when *IL28B* haplotype is combined with haplotype G/G of an SNP near HLA class II *DBQ1*03:01*.

In patients with chronic hepatitis C followed for 20 years, progression to cirrhosis occurs in about 20–25%. Such is the case even for patients with relatively clinically mild chronic hepatitis, including those without symptoms, with only modest elevations of aminotransferase activity, and with mild chronic hepatitis on liver biopsy. Even in cohorts of well-compensated patients with chronic hepatitis C referred for clinical research trials (no complications of chronic liver disease and with normal hepatic synthetic function), the prevalence of cirrhosis may be as high as 50%. Most cases of hepatitis C are identified initially in asymptomatic patients who have no history of acute hepatitis C (e.g., those discovered while attempting to donate blood, while undergoing lab testing as part of an application for life insurance, or as a result of routine laboratory tests). The source of HCV infection in many of these cases is not defined, although a long-forgotten percutaneous exposure (e.g., injection drug use) in the remote past can be elicited in a substantial proportion and probably accounts for most infections; most of these infections were acquired in the 1960s and 1970s, coming to clinical attention decades later.

Approximately one-third of patients with chronic hepatitis C have normal or near-normal aminotransferase activity; although one-third to one-half of these patients have chronic hepatitis on liver biopsy, the grade of liver injury and stage of fibrosis tend to be mild in the vast majority. In some cases, more severe liver injury has been reported—even, rarely, cirrhosis, most likely the result of previous histologic activity. Among patients with persistent normal aminotransferase activity sustained over ≥5–10 years, histologic progression has been shown to be rare; however, approximately one-fourth of patients with normal aminotransferase activity experience subsequent aminotransferase elevations, and histologic injury can be progressive once abnormal biochemical activity resumes. Therefore, continued clinical monitoring is indicated, even for patients with normal aminotransferase activity.

Despite this substantial rate of progression of chronic hepatitis C, and despite the fact that liver failure can result from end-stage chronic hepatitis C, the long-term prognosis for chronic hepatitis C in a majority of patients is relatively benign. Mortality over 10–20 years among patients with transfusion-associated chronic hepatitis C has been shown not to differ from mortality in a matched population of transfused patients in whom hepatitis C did not develop. Although death in the hepatitis group is more likely to result from liver failure, and although hepatic decompensation may occur in ~15% of such patients over the course of a decade, the majority (almost 60%) of patients remain asymptomatic and well compensated, with no clinical sequelae of chronic liver disease. Overall, chronic hepatitis C tends to be very slowly and insidiously progressive, if at all, in the vast majority of patients, whereas in approximately one-fourth of cases, chronic hepatitis C will progress eventually to end-stage cirrhosis. In fact, because HCV infection is so prevalent, and because a proportion of patients progress inexorably to end-stage liver disease, hepatitis C is the most frequent indication for liver transplantation (Chap. 368). In the United States, hepatitis C accounts for up to 40% of all chronic liver disease, and, as of 2007, mortality caused by hepatitis C surpassed that associated with HIV/AIDS. Moreover, because the prevalence of HCV infection is so much higher in the "baby boomer" cohort borne between 1945 and 1965, three-quarters of the mortality associated with hepatitis C occurs in this age cohort. Referral bias may account for the more severe outcomes described in cohorts of patients reported from tertiary care centers (20-year progression of >20%) versus the more benign outcomes in cohorts of patients monitored from initial blood-product-associated acute hepatitis or identified in community settings (20-year progression of only 4–7%). Still unexplained, however, are the wide ranges in reported progression to cirrhosis, from 2% over 17 years in a population of women with hepatitis C infection acquired from contaminated anti-D immune globulin to 30% over ≤11 years in recipients of contaminated intravenous immune globulin.

Progression of liver disease in patients with chronic hepatitis C has been reported to be more likely in patients with older age, longer duration of infection, advanced histologic stage and grade, more complex quasispecies diversity, increased hepatic iron, concomitant other liver disorders (alcoholic liver disease, chronic hepatitis B, hemochromatosis, α_1 antitrypsin deficiency, and steatohepatitis), HIV infection, and obesity. Among these variables, however, duration of infection appears to be one of the most important, and some of the others probably reflect disease duration to some extent (e.g., quasispecies diversity, hepatic iron accumulation). No other epidemiologic or clinical features of chronic hepatitis C (e.g., severity of acute hepatitis, level of aminotransferase activity, level of HCV RNA, presence or absence of jaundice during acute hepatitis) are predictive of eventual outcome. Despite the relatively benign nature of chronic hepatitis C over time in many patients, cirrhosis following chronic hepatitis C has been associated with the late development, after several decades, of HCC (Chap. 111); the annual rate of HCC in cirrhotic patients with hepatitis C is 1–4%, occurring primarily in patients who have had HCV infection for 30 years or more.

Perhaps the best prognostic indicator in chronic hepatitis C is liver histology; the rate of hepatic fibrosis may be slow, moderate, or rapid. Patients with mild necrosis and inflammation as well as those with limited fibrosis have an excellent prognosis and limited progression to cirrhosis. In contrast, among patients with moderate to severe necroinflammatory activity or fibrosis, including septal or bridging fibrosis, progression to cirrhosis is highly likely over the course of 10–20 years. The pace of fibrosis progression may be accelerated by such factors as concomitant HIV infection, other causes of liver disease, excessive alcohol use, and hepatic steatosis. Among patients with compensated cirrhosis associated with hepatitis C, the 10-year survival rate is close to 80%; mortality occurs at a rate of 2–6% per year; decompensation at a rate of 4–5% per year; and, as noted above, HCC at a rate of 1–4% per year. A discussion of the pathogenesis of liver injury in patients with chronic hepatitis C appears in Chap. 360.

Clinical features of chronic hepatitis C are similar to those described above for chronic hepatitis B. Generally, fatigue is the most common symptom; jaundice is rare. Immune complex–mediated extrahepatic complications of chronic hepatitis C are less common than in chronic hepatitis B (despite the fact that assays for immune complexes are often positive in patients with chronic hepatitis C), with the exception of essential mixed cryoglobulinemia (Chap. 360), which is linked to cutaneous vasculitis and membranoproliferative glomerulonephritis as well as lymphoproliferative disorders such as B-cell lymphoma and unexplained monoclonal gammopathy. In addition, chronic hepatitis C has been associated with extrahepatic complications unrelated to immune-complex injury. These include Sjögren's syndrome, lichen planus, porphyria cutanea tarda, type 2 diabetes mellitus, and the metabolic syndrome (including insulin resistance and steatohepatitis).

Laboratory features of chronic hepatitis C are similar to those in patients with chronic hepatitis B, but aminotransferase levels tend to fluctuate more (the characteristic episodic pattern of aminotransferase activity) and to be lower, especially in patients with long-standing disease. An interesting and occasionally confusing finding in patients with chronic hepatitis C is the presence of autoantibodies. Rarely, patients with autoimmune hepatitis (see below) and hyperglobulinemia have false-positive immunoassays for anti HCV. On the other hand, some patients with serologically confirmable chronic hepatitis C have circulating anti-LKM. These antibodies are anti-LKM1, as seen in patients with autoimmune hepatitis type 2 (see below), and are directed against a 33-amino-acid sequence of cytochrome P450 IID6. The occurrence of anti-LKM1 in some patients with chronic hepatitis C may result from the partial sequence homology between the epitope recognized by anti LKM1 and two segments of the HCV polyprotein. In addition, the presence of this autoantibody in some patients with chronic hepatitis C suggests that autoimmunity may be playing a role in the pathogenesis of chronic hepatitis C.

Histopathologic features of chronic hepatitis C, especially those that distinguish hepatitis C from hepatitis B, are described in Chap. 360.

TREATMENT CHRONIC HEPATITIS C

Therapy for chronic hepatitis C has evolved substantially in the two decades since IFN α was introduced for this indication. The therapeutic armamentarium has grown to include PEG IFN with ribavirin and, in 2011, the introduction of protease inhibitors telaprevir and boceprevir used in combination with PEG IFN and ribavirin in patients with HCV genotype 1. When first approved, IFN-α was administered via subcutaneous injection three times a week for 6 months but achieved a sustained virologic response (SVR) (Fig. 362-2) (a reduction of HCV RNA to undetectable levels by PCR when measured ≥6 months after completion of therapy) below 10%. Doubling the duration of therapy—but not increasing the dose or changing IFN preparations—increased the SVR rate to ~20%, and addition to the regimen of daily ribavirin, an oral guanosine nucleoside, increased the SVR rate to 40%. When used alone, ribavirin is ineffective and does not reduce HCV RNA levels appreciably, but ribavirin enhances the efficacy of IFN by reducing the likelihood of virologic relapse after the achievement of an end-treatment response (Fig. 362-2) (response measured during, and maintained to the end of, treatment). Proposed mechanisms to explain the role of ribavirin include subtle direct reduction of HCV replication, inhibition of host inosine monophosphate dehydrogenase activity (and associated depletion

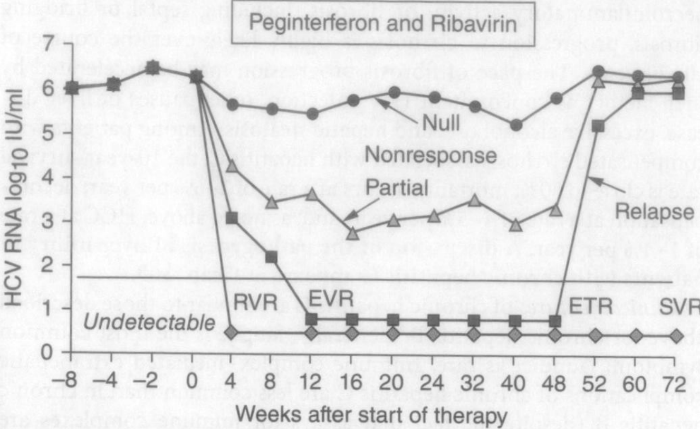

FIGURE 362-2 Classification of virologic responses based on outcomes during and after a 48-week course of pegylated interferon (PEG IFN) plus ribavirin antiviral therapy in patients with hepatitis C, genotype 1 or 4 (for genotype 2 or 3, the course would be 24 weeks). Nonresponders can be classified as null responders (hepatitis C virus [HCV] RNA reduction of <2 $\log_{10}$ IU/mL) or partial responders (HCV RNA reduction ≥2 $\log_{10}$ IU/mL but not suppressed to undetectable) by week 24 of therapy. In responders, HCV RNA can become undetectable, as shown with sensitive amplification assays, within 4 weeks (RVR, rapid virologic response); can be reduced by ≥2 $\log_{10}$ IU/mL within 12 weeks (early virologic response, EVR; if HCV RNA is undetectable at 12 weeks, the designation is "complete" EVR); or at the end of therapy, 48 weeks (ETR, end-treatment response). In responders, if HCV RNA remains undetectable for 24 weeks after ETR, week 72, the patient has a sustained virologic response (SVR), but if HCV RNA becomes detectable again, the patient is considered to have relapsed. In patients treated with protease inhibitor–based therapy, several additional milestones are monitored: (1) among boceprevir-treated patients, the level of HCV RNA reduction (>1 $\log_{10}$ or ≥1 $\log_{10}$ IU/mL) during the 4-week PEG IFN–ribavirin lead-in phase; (2) during boceprevir therapy, undetectable HCV RNA at week 8 (week 4 of triple-drug therapy; RVR); and (3) among telaprevir-treated patients, undetectable HCV RNA at week 4 and 12 (extended RVR). *(Reproduced with permission, courtesy of Marc G. Ghany, National Institute of Diabetes and Digestive and Kidney Diseases, National Institutes of Health and the American Association for the Study of Liver Diseases. Hepatology 49:1335, 2009.)*

of guanosine pools), immune modulation, induction of virologic mutational catastrophe, and enhancement of IFN-stimulated gene expression. IFN therapy results in activation of the JAK-STAT signal transduction pathway, which culminates in the intracellular elaboration of genes and their protein products that have antiviral properties. Hepatitis C proteins inhibit JAK-STAT signaling at several steps along the pathway, and exogenous IFN restores expression of IFN-stimulated genes and their antiviral effects.

Treatment with the combination of PEG IFN and ribavirin increased responsiveness (frequency of SVR) to as high as 55% overall, to >40% in genotypes 1 and 4, and to >80% in genotypes 2 and 3. Still, many important lessons about antiviral therapy for chronic hepatitis C were learned from the experience with IFN monotherapy and combination IFN-ribavirin therapy. Even in the absence of biochemical and virologic responses, histologic improvement occurs in approximately three-fourths of all treated patients. In chronic hepatitis C, unlike the case in hepatitis B, responses to therapy are not accompanied by transient, acute hepatitis-like aminotransferase elevations. Instead, ALT levels fall precipitously during therapy. Up to 90% of virologic responses are achieved within the first 12 weeks of therapy; responses thereafter are rare. Most relapses occur within the first 12 weeks after treatment; therefore, an SVR at week 12 posttreatment is roughly equivalent to a 24-week SVR. SVRs are very durable; normal ALT, improved histology, and absence of HCV RNA in serum and liver have been documented a decade after successful therapy, and "relapses" 2 years after sustained responses are almost unheard of. Thus, an SVR to antiviral therapy of chronic hepatitis C is tantamount to a cure.

Patient variables that tend to correlate with sustained virologic responsiveness to IFN-based therapy include favorable genotype (genotypes 2 and 3 as opposed to genotypes 1 and 4); low baseline HCV RNA level (<2 million copies/mL, which is equivalent to <800,000 IU/mL, the current convention of quantitation); histologically mild hepatitis and minimal fibrosis; age <40; female gender; and absence of obesity, insulin resistance, and type 2 diabetes mellitus. Patients with cirrhosis can respond, but they are less likely to do so. For patients treated with combination IFN-ribavirin, therapy for those with genotype 1 should last a full 48 weeks, whereas in those with genotypes 2 and 3, a 24-week course of therapy suffices (although refined tailoring of treatment duration may be indicated based on rapidity of response or associated cofactors, see below). The response rate in African Americans is disappointingly low for reasons that are not fully understood. Potentially contributing to, but not explaining entirely, low responsiveness in African Americans are a higher proportion with genotype 1, slower early viral kinetics during therapy, impaired HCV-specific immunity, and recently recognized host genetic differences in *IL28B* alleles, described below. The response rate in Latino patients is also low, despite the fact that the frequency of the favorable *IL28B* C allele is as common in Hispanic patients as in whites. Moreover, the likelihood of a sustained response is best if adherence to the treatment regimen is high (i.e., if patients receive ≥80% of the IFN and ribavirin doses and if they continue treatment for ≥80% of the anticipated duration of therapy). Other variables reported to correlate with increased responsiveness include brief duration of infection, low HCV quasispecies diversity, immunocompetence, absence of hepatic steatosis, and low liver iron levels. High levels of HCV RNA, more histologically advanced liver disease, and high quasispecies diversity all go hand in hand with advanced duration of infection, which is one of the most important clinical variables determining IFN responsiveness. The ironic fact, then, is that patients whose disease is least likely to progress are the ones *most* likely to respond to IFN and vice versa.

Genetic changes in the virus may explain differences in treatment responsiveness in some patients (e.g., among patients with genotype 1b, responsiveness to IFN is enhanced in those with amino-acid-substitution mutations in the nonstructural protein 5A gene). As described above in the discussion of spontaneous recovery from acute hepatitis C, IFN gene variants discovered recently in genome-wide association studies have been shown to have a substantial impact on responsiveness of patients with genotype 1 to antiviral therapy. In studies of patients treated with PEG IFN and ribavirin, variants of the *IL28B* SNP that code for IFN-λ3 (a type III IFN, the receptors for which are more discretely distributed than IFN-α receptors and more concentrated in hepatocytes) correlate significantly with responsiveness. Patients homozygous for the C allele at this locus have the highest frequency of achieving an SVR (~80%), those homozygous for the T allele at this locus are least likely to achieve an SVR (~25%), and those heterozygous at this locus (C/T) have an intermediate level of responsiveness (SVRs in ~35%). The fact that C/C is common in whites of European ancestry and even more so in Japanese persons but rare in African Americans helps explain the differences in observed responsiveness among these population groups.

Side effects of IFN therapy are described above in the section on treatment of chronic hepatitis B. The most pronounced side effect of ribavirin therapy is hemolysis; a reduction in hemoglobin of up to 2–3 g or in hematocrit of 5–10% can be anticipated. A small, unpredictable proportion of patients experience profound, brisk hemolysis, resulting in symptomatic anemia; therefore, close monitoring of blood counts is crucial, and ribavirin should be avoided in patients with anemia or hemoglobinopathies and in patients with coronary artery disease or cerebrovascular disease, in whom anemia can precipitate an ischemic event. When symptomatic anemia occurs, ribavirin dose reductions or addition of erythropoietin to boost red blood cell levels may be required; erythropoietin has been shown to improve patients' quality of life but not the likelihood of achieving an SVR. If ribavirin is stopped during therapy, SVR rates fall, but responsiveness can be maintained as long as ribavirin is not stopped and the total ribavirin dose exceeds 60% of the planned dose. In addition, ribavirin, which is excreted renally, should not be used in patients with renal insufficiency; the drug is teratogenic, precluding its use during pregnancy and mandating the scrupulous use of efficient contraception during therapy (IFNs, too, because of their antiproliferative properties, are contraindicated during pregnancy).

Ribavirin can also cause nasal and chest congestion, pruritus, and precipitation of gout. Combination IFN-ribavirin therapy is more difficult to tolerate than IFN monotherapy. In one large clinical trial of combination therapy versus monotherapy, among those in the 1-year treatment group, 21% of the combination group (but only 14% of the monotherapy group) had to discontinue treatment, whereas 26% of the combination group (but only 9% of the monotherapy group) required dose reductions.

Studies of viral kinetics have shown that despite a virion half-life in serum of only 2–3 h, the level of HCV is maintained by a high replication rate of 10^{12} hepatitis C virions per day. IFN-α blocks virion production or release with an efficacy that increases with increasing drug doses; moreover, the calculated death rate for infected cells during IFN therapy is inversely related to level of HCV RNA; patients with the most rapid death rate of infected hepatocytes are more likely to achieve undetectable HCV RNA at 3 months; in practice, failure to achieve an early virologic response (EVR), a ≥2-$\log_{10}$ reduction in HCV RNA by week 12, predicts failure to experience a subsequent SVR. Similarly, patients in whom HCV RNA becomes undetectable within 4 weeks (i.e., who achieve a rapid virologic response [RVR]) have a very high likelihood of achieving an SVR (Fig. 362-2). Therefore, to achieve rapid viral clearance from serum and the liver, *high-dose induction therapy* has been advocated. In practice, however, high-dose induction with IFN-based therapy has not yielded higher sustained response rates.

For the treatment of chronic hepatitis C, standard IFNs were supplanted by PEG IFNs. These have elimination times up to sevenfold longer than standard IFNs (i.e., a substantially longer half-life) and achieve prolonged concentrations, permitting administration once (rather than three times) a week. Instead of the frequent drug peaks (linked to side effects) and troughs (when drug is absent) associated with frequent administration of short-acting IFNs, administration of PEG IFNs results in drug concentrations that are more stable and sustained over time. Once-a-week PEG IFN monotherapy is twice as effective as monotherapy with its standard IFN counterpart, approaches the efficacy of combination standard IFN plus ribavirin, and is as well tolerated as standard IFNs, without more difficult-to-manage thrombocytopenia and leukopenia than standard IFNs. For most of the decade prior to 2011, when protease inhibitors were introduced for HCV genotype 1 (see below), the standard of care was a combination of PEG IFN plus ribavirin for all HCV genotypes.

Two PEG IFNs are available: PEG IFN-α2b and -α2a. PEG IFN-α2b consists of a 12-kD, linear PEG molecule bound to IFN-α2b, whereas PEG IFN-α2a consists of a larger, 40-kD, branched PEG molecule bound to IFN-α2a; because of its larger size and smaller volume of extravascular distribution, PEG IFN-α2a can be given at a uniform dose independent of weight, whereas the dose of the smaller PEG IFN-α2b, which has a much wider volume distribution, must be weight-based (Table 362-6). In the registration trial for PEG IFN-α2b plus ribavirin, the best regimen was 48 weeks of 1.5 μg/kg of PEG IFN once a week plus 800 mg of ribavirin daily. A post hoc analysis suggested that weight-based dosing of ribavirin would have been more effective than the fixed 800-mg dose used in the study (a broader dose/weight range was approved subsequently; see below). In the first registration trial for PEG IFN-α2a plus ribavirin, the best regimen was 48 weeks of 180 μg of PEG IFN plus 1000 mg (for patients <75 kg) to 1200 mg (for patients ≥75 kg) of ribavirin. SVRs of 54 and 56% were reported in these two studies, respectively. A subsequent study of PEG IFN-α2a plus ribavirin showed that, for patients with genotypes 2 and 3, a duration of 24 weeks and a ribavirin dose of 800 mg were sufficient. Among the three studies, for patients in the optimal treatment arm, SVR rates for patients with genotype 1 were 42–51%, and for patients with genotypes 2 and 3, rates were 76–82%. Between genotypes 2 and 3, genotype 3 is somewhat more refractory, and some authorities would extend therapy for a full 48 weeks in patients with genotype 3, especially if they have advanced hepatic fibrosis or cirrhosis and/or high-level HCV RNA.

TABLE 362-6 PEGYLATED INTERFERON (PEG IFN) α2a AND α2b FOR CHRONIC HEPATITIS C

	PEG IFN-α2b	PEG IFN-α2a
PEG size	12 kD linear	40 kD branched
Elimination half-life	54 h	65 h
Clearance	725 mL/h	60 mL/h
Dose	1.5 μg/kg (weight-based)	180 μg
Storage	Room temperature	Refrigerated
Ribavirin dose		
Genotype 1	800–1400 mg[a]	1000–1200 mg[b]
Genotype 2/3	800 mg	800 mg
Duration of therapy		
Genotype 1	48 weeks	48 weeks
Genotype 2/3	48 weeks[c]	24 weeks
Efficacy of combination therapy[d]	54%	56%
Genotype 1	40–42%	41–51%
Genotype 2/3	82%	76–78%

[a]In the registration trial for PEG IFN-α2b plus ribavirin, the optimal regimen was 1.5 μg of PEG IFN plus 800 mg of ribavirin; however, a post hoc analysis of this study suggested that higher ribavirin doses are better. In subsequent trials of PEG IFN-α2b with ribavirin in patients with genotype 1, the following daily ribavirin doses have been validated: 800 mg for patients weighing <65 kg, 1000 mg for patients weighing >65–85 kg, 1200 for patients weighing >85–105 kg, and 1400 mg for patients weighing >105 kg. [b]1000 mg for patients weighing <75 kg; 1200 mg for patients weighing ≥75 kg. [c]In the registration trial for PEG IFN-α2b plus ribavirin, all patients were treated for 48 weeks; however, data from other trials of standard interferons and the other PEG IFN demonstrated that 24 weeks suffices for patients with genotypes 2 and 3. For patients with genotype 3 who have advanced fibrosis/cirrhosis and/or high-level HCV RNA, a full 48 weeks is preferable. [d]Attempts to compare the two PEG IFN preparations based on the results of registration clinical trials are confounded by differences between trials of the two agents in methodologic details (different ribavirin doses, different methods for recording depression, and other side effects) and study-population composition (different proportion with bridging fibrosis/cirrhosis, proportion from the United States versus international, mean weight, proportion with genotype 1, and proportion with high-level HCV RNA). In the head-to-head comparison of the two PEG IFN preparations in the IDEAL trial reported in 2009, the two drugs were comparable in tolerability and efficacy. PEG IFN-α2b was administered at a weekly weight-based dose of 1.0 μg/kg or 1.5 μg/kg, and PEG IFN-α2a at a weekly fixed dose of 180 μg. For PEG IFN-α2b, daily ribavirin weight-based doses ranged between 800 and 1400 mg based on weight criteria (see footnote *a*, above), whereas for PEG IFN-α2a, daily ribavirin weight based doses ranged between 1000 and 1200 mg (see footnote *b*, above). For the two PEG IFN-α2b study arms, ribavirin dose reductions for ribavirin-associated adverse effects were done in 200- to 400-mg decrements; for PEG IFN-α2a, the ribavirin dose was reduced to 600 mg for intolerability. Sustained virologic responses occurred in 38.0% of the low-dose PEG IFN-α2b group, 39.8% of the standard, full-dose PEG IFN-α2b group, and 40.9% of the PEG IFN-α2a group.

Abbreviations: HCV RNA, hepatitis C virus RNA; PEG, polyethylene glycol.

In the initial registration trials for combination PEG IFN plus ribavirin, both combination PEG IFN regimens were compared to standard IFN-α2b plus ribavirin. Side effects of the combination PEG IFN-α2b regimen were comparable to those for the combination standard IFN regimen; however, when the combination PEG IFN-α2a regimen was compared with the combination standard IFN-α2b regimen, flu-like symptoms and depression were less common in the combination PEG IFN group. Although ascertainment of side effects differed between studies of the two drugs, when each was tested against standard IFN-α2b plus ribavirin, combination PEG IFN-α2a plus ribavirin appeared to be better tolerated. In a head-to-head trial of the two PEG IFNs (the IDEAL trial), the two PEG IFNs were found to be comparable in efficacy (achievement of SVR) and tolerability, although headache, nausea, fever, myalgia, depression, and drug discontinuation for any reason were less frequent in patients treated with PEG IFN-α2a than standard-dose PEG IFN-α2b. In contrast, neutropenia and rash were more frequent in patients treated with PEG IFN-α2a than standard-dose PEG IFN-α2b. In two subsequent head-to-head trials and a systematic review of randomized trials, PEG IFN-α2a was more effective than PEG IFN-α2b (SVR in genotypes 1–4: 48–55% versus 32–40%, respectively). In trials of PEG IFN-α2b among patients with HCV genotype 1, a broader range of weight-based daily ribavirin doses has been validated: 800 mg for weight <65 kg, 1000 mg for weight 65–85 kg, 1200 mg for weight >85–105 kg, and 1400 mg for weight >105 kg. Recommended doses for the two PEG IFNs plus ribavirin and other comparisons between the two therapies are shown in Table 362-6.

Until the 2011 introduction of protease inhibitors, unless ribavirin was contraindicated (see above), combination PEG IFN plus ribavirin was the recommended course of therapy—24 weeks for genotypes 2 and 3 and 48 weeks for genotype 1. For patients with genotypes 1 and 4, the standard of care now includes protease inhibitors or other direct-acting antiviral agents (see below); however, PEG IFN–ribavirin remained the standard of care for patients with genotypes 2 and 3 until late 2013. For patients treated with combination PEG IFN–ribavirin, measurement of quantitative HCV RNA levels at 12 weeks is helpful in guiding therapy; if a 2-$\log_{10}$ drop in HCV RNA has not been achieved by this time, chances for an SVR are negligible, and additional therapy is futile. If the 12-week HCV RNA has fallen by 2 $\log_{10}$ (EVR), the chances for an SVR at the end of therapy are approximately two-thirds; if the 12-week HCV RNA is undetectable ("complete" EVR), the chances for an SVR exceed 80% (Fig. 362-2). Because absence of an EVR is such a strong predictor of the absence of an ultimate SVR, therapy is discontinued for failure to achieve a 12-week 2-$\log_{10}$ drop in HCV RNA (EVR).

Studies have suggested that the frequency of an SVR to PEG IFN–ribavirin therapy can be increased in patients with baseline variables weighing against a response (e.g., HCV RNA $>8 \times 10^5$ IU/mL, weight >85 kg) by raising the dose of PEG IFN (e.g., to as high as 270 μg of PEG IFN-α2a) and/or the dose of ribavirin to as high as 1600 mg daily (if tolerated or supplemented by erythropoietin) or by tailoring treatment based on viral response to prolong the duration of viral clearance before discontinuing therapy, i.e., extending therapy from 48 to 72 weeks for patients with genotype 1 and a slow virologic response (i.e., those whose HCV RNA has not fallen rapidly to undetectable levels within 4 weeks [absence of RVR]). Tailoring therapy based on the kinetics of HCV RNA reduction has also been applied to abbreviating the duration of therapy in patients with genotype 1 (and 4). The results of several clinical trials suggest that, in patients with genotype 1 (and 4) who have a 4-week RVR (which occurs in ≤20%), especially in the subset with low baseline HCV RNA, 24 weeks of therapy with PEG IFN and weight-based ribavirin suffices, yielding SVR rates of ~90% and comparable to those achieved in this cohort with 48 weeks of therapy. Although initial reports suggested that, for patients with genotype 2 and (somewhat less so) genotype 3, in rapid virologic responders with undetectable HCV RNA at week 4, the total duration of therapy required to achieve an SVR could be as short as 12–16 weeks, a very sizable, definitive subsequent trial showed that relapse is increased if treatment duration is curtailed and that a full 24 weeks is superior for these genotypes (except for the minority with very low baseline levels of HCV RNA).

Persons with chronic HCV infection have been shown to suffer increased liver-related mortality. On the other hand, successful antiviral therapy of chronic hepatitis C resulting in an SVR has been shown to improve survival (and to reduce the need for liver transplantation), to lower the risk of liver failure and liver-related death and all-cause deaths, to slow the progression of chronic hepatitis C, and to reverse fibrosis and even cirrhosis. Although successful treatment reduces mortality in cirrhotic patients (and those with advanced fibrosis) and reduces the likelihood of HCC, the risk of liver-related death and HCC persists, albeit at a much reduced level, necessitating continued clinical monitoring and cancer surveillance after SVR in cirrhotics. On the other hand, in the absence of an SVR, routine-dose/duration IFN-based therapy does not reduce the risk of HCC. Similarly, for nonresponders to PEG IFN–ribavirin therapy, three trials of long-term maintenance therapy with PEG IFN have shown no benefit in reducing the risk of histologic progression or clinical decompensation, including the development of HCC. For PEG IFN–ribavirin nonresponders who have had a full, adequate course of therapy, the benefit of retreatment—with higher doses or a longer course of the original PEG IFN regimen or the alternative PEG IFN regimen or with a different type of IFN preparation (e.g., consensus IFN)—is marginal at best. Fortunately, such nonresponders can now be retreated with protease inhibitor-based therapy (see following).

FIRST-GENERATION PROTEASE INHIBITORS (2011–2013)

The HCV RNA genome encodes a single polyprotein, which is cleaved during and after translation by host and viral-encoded proteases. One protease involved in the cleavage of the viral polyprotein is an NS3-4A viral protein that has serine protease activity. Telaprevir and boceprevir are serine protease inhibitors that target NS3-4A. In 2011, telaprevir and boceprevir used in combination with PEG IFN and ribavirin were approved by the U.S. Food and Drug Administration (FDA) for the treatment of hepatitis C genotype 1 in adults with stable liver disease, both in patients who have not been treated before or who have failed previous treatment. Because the presently available HCV protease inhibitors have not been studied comprehensively in patients with genotypes other than 1, their use in these populations is not recommended.

Because resistance develops rapidly, both telaprevir and boceprevir must be used in combination with a PEG IFN and ribavirin-based regimen and should never be used alone. Ribavirin in particular appears to reduce relapse rates significantly in protease inhibitor–based regimens, such that those who cannot take or are intolerant to ribavirin are unlikely to benefit from the addition of these agents. All current telaprevir and boceprevir regimens consist of periods of triple therapy (protease inhibitor plus PEG IFN plus ribavirin) and periods of dual therapy (PEG IFN plus ribavirin). Telaprevir regimens begin with 12 weeks of triple therapy followed by dual therapy of a duration based on HCV RNA status at weeks 4 and 12 ("response-guided therapy") and prior treatment status. Boceprevir-based regimens consist of a 4-week lead-in period of dual (PEG IFN–ribavirin) therapy followed by triple therapy and, in some instances, a further extension of dual therapy, with duration of response-guided therapy based on HCV RNA status at weeks 4, 8, and 24 and prior treatment status (Table 362-7).

For patients with HCV genotype 1, protease inhibitors have significantly improved the frequency of RVRs and SVRs as compared to PEG IFN plus ribavirin alone. In treatment-naïve patients treated with telaprevir, an SVR was seen in up to 79% of patients who received 12 weeks of triple therapy followed by 12–36 weeks of dual therapy, and among those with EVRs (undetectable HCV RNA at weeks 4 and 12) and response-guided therapy stopped at week 24 (12 weeks of triple therapy, then 12 weeks of dual therapy), the rate of SVRs was 83–89% (92% in a subsequent study). In studies with boceprevir in treatment-naïve patients, SVRs were seen in 59–66% of patients, and among those with undetectable HCV RNA at 8 weeks, the SVR rate increased to 86–88%.

Protease inhibitors have also been studied in patients previously treated unsuccessfully with PEG IFN plus ribavirin. In studies with telaprevir, SVRs were seen in 83–88% of patients who had a previous relapse, 54–59% of partial responders (HCV RNA reduced by ≥2 $\log_{10}$ IU/mL but not to undetectable levels), and 29–33% of null responders (HCV RNA reduced by <2 $\log_{10}$ IU/mL). With boceprevir, SVRs occurred in 75% of prior relapsers and in 40–52% of previous partial responders; response rates in null responders are similar to those achieved with telaprevir-based therapy. In a substantial proportion of protease inhibitor nonresponders, resistance-associated variants can be identified, but these variants are not archived, and wild-type HCV reemerges in almost all cases within 1.5 to 2 years. SVRs to these protease inhibitors are highest in prior relapsers and

TABLE 362-7 INDICATIONS AND RECOMMENDATIONS FOR ANTIVIRAL THERAPY OF CHRONIC HEPATITIS C[a]

Standard Indications for Therapy

Detectable HCV RNA (with or without elevated ALT)

Portal/bridging fibrosis or moderate to severe hepatitis on liver biopsy (the necessity of a pretreatment biopsy is no longer embraced universally)

Indications for IFN/ribavirin-based therapy apply to adults as well as to children age 2–17, in whom treatment may be considered at reduced weight-based doses (see product inserts); protease inhibitors are not recommended for children age <18 years

Retreatment Recommended

Genotype 1

Relapsers, partial responders, or nonresponders after a previous course of standard IFN monotherapy or combination standard IFN/ribavirin therapy or PEG IFN/ribavirin

A course of PEG IFN/ribavirin plus protease inhibitor as below

Genotypes 2, 3, 4

Relapsers after a previous course of standard IFN monotherapy or combination standard IFN/ribavirin therapy

A course of PEG IFN plus ribavirin

Nonresponders to a previous course of standard IFN monotherapy or combination standard IFN/ribavirin therapy

A course of PEG IFN plus ribavirin—more likely to achieve a sustained virologic response in white patients without previous ribavirin therapy, with low baseline HCV RNA levels, with a ≥2-$\log_{10}$ reduction in HCV RNA during previous therapy, with genotypes 2 and 3, and without reduction in ribavirin dose

Antiviral Therapy Management Decisions Made on an Individual Basis

Children (age <18 years)—protease inhibitors not recommended.

Age >70 (in protease inhibitor trials, telaprevir trials included patients age 18–70; boceprevir trials included patients >18 years of age [no upper age cutoff])

Mild hepatitis on liver biopsy

Persons with severe renal insufficiency (require reduced doses of PEG IFN and ribavirin)

Long-Term Maintenance Therapy Recommended

Cutaneous vasculitis and glomerulonephritis associated with chronic hepatitis C

Long-Term Maintenance Therapy in Nonresponders Not Recommended

Antiviral Therapy Not Recommended

Decompensated cirrhosis (except, perhaps, in transplantation centers with experience in graded escalation, low-dose treatment to achieve undetectable HCV RNA prior to transplantation; results are mixed)

Pregnancy (teratogenicity of ribavirin)

Contraindications to use of antiviral medications

Therapeutic Regimens

HCV genotype 1

TREATMENT-NAÏVE (telaprevir and boceprevir) and PRIOR RELAPSERS (telaprevir)

PEG IFN-α2a 180 μg weekly plus weight-based ribavirin 1000 mg/d (<75 kg) to 1200 mg/d (≥75 kg) or

PEG IFN-α2b 1.5 μg/kg weekly plus weight-based ribavirin 800 mg/d (≤65 kg), 1000 mg/d (>65–85 kg), 1200 mg/d (>85–105 kg), or 1400 mg/d (>105 kg)

Plus response-guided therapy with a protease inhibitor consisting of either:

Boceprevir 800 mg three times daily with food started after a lead-in treatment of 4 weeks with PEG IFN–ribavirin

- Patients with undetectable HCV RNA at 8 and 24 weeks should receive triple-drug therapy (PEG IFN, ribavirin, boceprevir) through week 28 (4 weeks of PEG IFN–ribavirin then 24 weeks of triple-drug therapy). If HCV RNA is detectable at 4 weeks, continuing therapy through 48 weeks (4 weeks of PEG IFN–ribavirin then 44 weeks of triple drug therapy) may increase the sustained response rate.
- Patients with detectable HCV RNA at 8 weeks and undetectable at 24 weeks should receive triple-drug therapy (PEG IFN, ribavirin, boceprevir) through week 36 (4 weeks of PEG IFN–ribavirin then 32 weeks of triple-drug therapy) followed by a return to PEG IFN–ribavirin for 12 more weeks, for a total treatment duration of 48 weeks.
- Patients with cirrhosis who are treatment-naive and have undetectable HCV RNA at weeks 8 and 24 should continue triple-drug therapy (PEG IFN, ribavirin, boceprevir) through 48 weeks (4 weeks of PEG IFN–ribavirin then 44 weeks of triple-drug therapy).
- Stopping rules for futility: HCV RNA ≥100 IU/mL at week 12 or any detectable HCV RNA at week 24

or

Telaprevir 750 mg three times daily with fatty food started at the beginning of therapy without a PEG IFN–ribavirin lead-in

- Patients with undetectable HCV RNA at 4 and 12 weeks should receive triple-drug therapy (PEG IFN, ribavirin, telaprevir) for 12 weeks then PEG IFN and ribavirin for another 12 weeks, for a total of 24 weeks.
- Patients with detectable HCV RNA at 4 or 12 weeks and undetectable at 24 weeks should receive triple-drug therapy (PEG IFN, ribavirin, telaprevir) for 12 weeks, then PEG IFN–ribavirin for another 36 weeks, for a total treatment duration of 48 weeks.
- Patients with cirrhosis who are treatment-naïve and have undetectable HCV RNA at 4 and 12 weeks should receive triple-drug therapy for 12 weeks then PEG IFN–ribavirin for another 36 weeks, for a total treatment duration of 48 weeks.
- Stopping rules for futility: HCV RNA >1000 IU/mL at week 4 or 12 or any detectable HCV RNA at week 24

TREATMENT-EXPERIENCED

PEG IFN-α2a 180 μg weekly plus weight-based ribavirin 1000 mg/d (<75 kg) to 1200 mg/d (≥75 kg) or

PEG IFN-α2b 1.5 μg/kg weekly plus weight-based ribavirin 800 mg/d (≤65kg), 1000 mg/d (>65–85 kg), 1200 mg/d (>85–105 kg), or 1400 mg/d (>105 kg)

Plus a protease inhibitor consisting of either:

Response-guided therapy with boceprevir 800 mg three times daily with food started after a lead-in treatment of 4 weeks with PEG IFN–ribavirin

- For prior relapsers and partial responders (HCV RNA reduction of ≥2 $\log_{10}$ during previous therapy), follow the response-guided algorithm below; for prior null responders (HCV RNA reduction <2 $\log_{10}$ during previous therapy), a full 48-week course of therapy (4-week PEG IFN–ribavirin lead-in, followed by 44 weeks of triple-drug therapy [PEG IFN, ribavirin, boceprevir]) is recommended.

(Continued)

TABLE 362-7 INDICATIONS AND RECOMMENDATIONS FOR ANTIVIRAL THERAPY OF CHRONIC HEPATITIS C[a] (*CONTINUED*)

- Patients with undetectable HCV RNA at 8 and 24 weeks should receive triple-drug therapy (PEG IFN, ribavirin, boceprevir) through week 36 (4 weeks of PEG IFN–ribavirin then 32 weeks of triple-drug therapy). If HCV RNA is detectable at 4 weeks, continuing therapy through 48 weeks (4 weeks of PEG IFN–ribavirin then 44 weeks of triple therapy) may increase the sustained response rate.
- Patients with detectable HCV RNA at 8 weeks and undetectable at week 24 should receive triple-drug therapy (PEG IFN, ribavirin, boceprevir) through week 36 (4 weeks of PEG IFN–ribavirin then 32 weeks of triple-drug therapy), followed by a return to PEG IFN–ribavirin for 12 more weeks, for a total treatment duration of 48 weeks.
- Patients with cirrhosis who are treatment-experienced and have undetectable HCV RNA at weeks 8 and 24 should continue triple-drug therapy (PEG IFN, ribavirin, boceprevir) through 48 weeks (4 weeks of PEG IFN–ribavirin then 44 weeks of triple-drug therapy).
- Stopping rules for futility: HCV RNA ≥100 IU/mL at week 12 or any detectable HCV RNA at week 24

or

Telaprevir 750 mg three times daily with fatty food started at the beginning of therapy without a PEG IFN–ribavirin lead-in and without a response-guided approach, i.e., all patients receive a full 48-week course, independent of early responsiveness.

- For prior relapsers, follow guidelines for treatment-naïve patients above.
- Prior partial responders and null responders should receive triple-drug therapy (PEG IFN, ribavirin, telaprevir) for 12 weeks then PEG IFN and ribavirin for another 36 weeks, for a total of 48 weeks.
- Stopping rules for futility: HCV RNA >1000 IU/mL at week 4 or 12 or any detectable HCV RNA at week 24

HCV genotype 1 but protease inhibitors unavailable or contraindicated: 48 weeks of therapy

PEG IFN-α2a 180 μg weekly plus weight-based ribavirin 1000 mg/d (<75 kg) to 1200 mg/d (≥75 kg) or

PEG IFN-α2b 1.5 μg/kg weekly plus weight-based ribavirin 800 mg/d (≤65 kg), 1000 mg/d (>65–85 kg), 1200 mg/d (>85–105 kg), or 1400 mg/d (>105 kg)

HCV genotype 4: 48 weeks of PEG IFN–ribavirin therapy

PEG IFN-α2a 180 μg weekly plus weight-based ribavirin 1000 mg/d (<75 kg) to 1200 mg/d (≥75 kg) or

PEG IFN-α2b 1.5 μg/kg weekly plus weight-based ribavirin 800 mg/d (≤65 kg), 1000 mg/d (>65–85 kg), 1200 mg/d (>85–105 kg), or 1400 mg/d (>105 kg)

- Treatment should be discontinued in patients who do not achieve an early virologic response at week 12.
- Patients who do achieve an early virologic response should be retested at week 24, and treatment should be discontinued if HCV RNA remains detectable.

HCV genotypes 2 and 3: 24 weeks of therapy

PEG IFN-α2a 180 μg weekly plus ribavirin 800 mg/d or

PEG IFN-α2b 1.5 μg/kg weekly plus ribavirin 800 mg/d (for patients with genotype 3 who have advanced fibrosis and/or high-level HCV RNA, a full 48 weeks of therapy may be preferable)

For HCV/HIV co-infected patients: 48 weeks, regardless of genotype, of weekly PEG IFN-α2a (180 μg) or PEG IFN-α2b (1.5 μg/kg) plus a daily ribavirin dose of at least 600–800 mg, up to full weight-based 1000–1400 mg dosing if tolerated. Protease inhibitors may be used for genotype 1; however, because of potential drug-drug interactions between HCV protease inhibitors and HIV antiretroviral drugs, HCV protease inhibitors should be used cautiously in HCV/HIV co-infected patients. If protease inhibitors are used, a full 48-week course is recommended without response-guided therapy. For boceprevir, 4 weeks of PEG IFN–ribavirin lead-in, followed by 44 weeks of triple-drug therapy (PEG IFN, ribavirin, boceprevir). For telaprevir, 12 weeks of triple-drug therapy (PEG IFN, ribavirin, telaprevir), followed by 36 weeks of PEG IFN–ribavirin therapy. Stopping rules for futility are as noted above.

Features Associated with Reduced Responsiveness
Single nucleotide polymorphism (SNP) T allele (as opposed to C allele) at *IL28B* locus
Genotype 1a (compared to 1b)
High-level HCV RNA (>800,000 IU/mL)[b]
Advanced fibrosis (bridging fibrosis, cirrhosis)
Long-duration disease
Age >40[b]
High HCV quasispecies diversity
Immunosuppression
African-American ethnicity
Latino ethnicity
Obesity
Hepatic steatosis
Insulin resistance, type 2 diabetes mellitus[b]
Reduced adherence (lower drug doses and reduced duration of therapy)
For boceprevir, <1 $\log_{10}$ reduction in HCV RNA during 4-week PEG IFN–ribavirin lead-in
For protease inhibitor therapy, absence of extended rapid virologic response (eRVR), i.e., detectable HCV RNA, at weeks 4 and 12 for telaprevir; at weeks 8 and 24 for boceprevir

[a]As this chapter was going to press, two additional drugs were approved for hepatitis C, simeprevir and sofosbuvir. Rapidly evolving new recommendations are supplanting the recommendations in this table; for up-to-date treatment recommendations, please see *www.hcvguidelines.org*. [b]Less influential in patients treated with protease inhibitors.

Abbreviations: ALT, alanine aminotransferase; HCV, hepatitis C virus; IFN, interferon; PEG IFN, pegylated interferon; IU, international units (1 IU/mL is equivalent to ~2.5 copies/mL).

treatment-naïve patients (white > black ethnicity), lower in prior partial responders, lower still in prior null responders, and lowest in cirrhotic prior null responders (Fig. 362-3). Responses to protease inhibitor triple-drug regimens are higher in patients with *IL28B* C than non-C genotypes, HCV genotype 1b than genotype 1a, less advanced than more advanced fibrosis stage, whites than blacks, lower body mass index (BMI) than elevated BMI, and, for boceprevir, achievement of a >1 $\log_{10}$ HCV RNA reduction during 4 weeks of PEG IFN–ribavirin lead-in therapy. Age and HCV RNA level are less influential and insulin resistance is noninfluential on response to these antiviral agents.

Both protease inhibitors have potential toxicities. Telaprevir is associated with a severe, generalized (trunk and extremities), often confluent, maculopapular, pruritic rash in ~6% of treated patients. Other common side effects include pruritus, rectal burning, nausea, diarrhea, fatigue, and anemia, which may be relatively refractory,

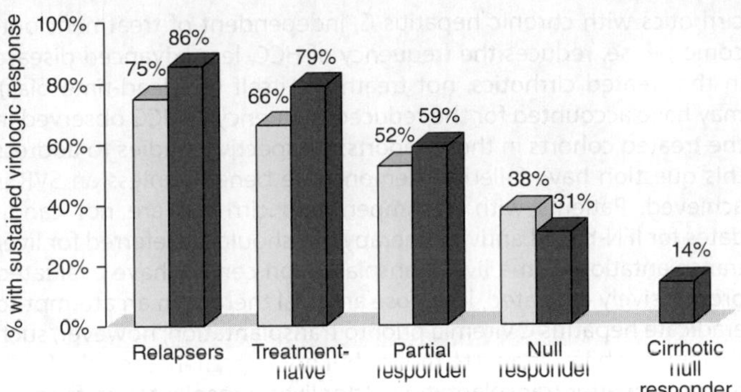

FIGURE 362-3 Maximal efficacy (sustained virologic responses, SVR) of telaprevir (*blue bars*) and boceprevir (*yellow bars*) reported in phase III clinical trials. *(Figure created using data from Bacon BR et al: N Engl J Med 364:1207, 2011; Jacobson IM et al: N Engl J Med 364:2405, 2011; Poordad F et al: N Engl J Med 364:1195, 2011; Zeuzem S et al: N Engl J Med 364:2417, 2011; Vierling JM et al: Hepatology 54 [Suppl 1]:796A-797A, 2011; Ghany MG et al: Hepatology 54:1433, 2011.)*

occasionally requiring transfusion. Complete blood counts should be obtained at baseline and then at 2, 4, 8, and 12 weeks after starting telaprevir. Anemia can occur in half of boceprevir-treated patients, as can neutropenia in up to 30% and thrombocytopenia in 3–4%. Complete blood counts should be obtained at baseline and then at 4, 8, and 12 weeks after starting boceprevir. Other side effects of boceprevir include fatigue, nausea, headache, dysgeusia (altered or unpleasant taste), dry mouth, vomiting, and diarrhea.

Use of protease inhibitors is further complicated by numerous drug-drug interactions. As telaprevir and boceprevir are both eliminated by and inhibit CYP3A4, these agents should not be administered with other medications that induce CYP3A4 or are dependent on CYP3A4 for elimination. Care should be taken to examine for any potential interactions between protease inhibitors and other medications the patient may be taking, because serious adverse events can occur. A convenient website is available to check for such drug-drug interactions (*www.hep-druginteractions.org*).

TREATMENT RECOMMENDATIONS*

Prior to therapy, HCV genotype should be determined, because the genotype dictates the duration of therapy and potentially the agents to be used. PEG IFN plus ribavirin represents the foundation of treatment for all HCV genotypes; patients infected with genotype 1 should also receive a protease inhibitor (telaprevir or boceprevir) when these are available and not contraindicated (Table 362-7). For chronic HCV genotype 1 infection, the AASLD and EASL published treatment guidelines in 2011 reflecting FDA-approved indications for the new protease inhibitors, and in 2012, United Kingdom and French consensus guidelines were published. For treatment-naïve patients and prior relapsers, response-guided therapy with telaprevir or boceprevir is recommended. For telaprevir, the regimen consists of 12 weeks of triple therapy, followed by 12 or 36 weeks of PEG IFN–ribavirin consolidation, depending on whether extended RVR milestones (HCV RNA undetectable at weeks 4 and 12) are met. For boceprevir, the regimen consists of a 4-week PEG IFN–ribavirin lead-in period, followed by 24–32 weeks of triple-drug therapy, depending on whether HCV RNA milestones (undetectable at weeks 8 and 24) are met; if HCV RNA is detectable at week 8 but undetectable at week 24, after 36 weeks of therapy (4-week PEG IFN–ribavirin lead-in plus 32 weeks of triple-drug therapy), an additional 12 weeks of PEG IFN–ribavirin consolidation is recommended. For prior partial and null responders, a full 48-week course of telaprevir (no lead-in period, no response-guided therapy) is recommended; for boceprevir, a 4-week PEG IFN–ribavirin lead-in period is followed by response-guided therapy (32 weeks of triple-drug therapy if HCV RNA is undetectable at weeks 8 and 24 or, if HCV RNA is still detectable at week 8 [but undetectable at week 24], 32 weeks of triple-drug therapy followed by 12 weeks of PEG IFN–ribavirin consolidation). For cirrhotic patients (and for any boceprevir-treated patient whose HCV RNA does not fall by >1 $\log_{10}$ by week 4), a full 48-week course without response-guided therapy should be considered.

Monitoring of HCV plasma RNA is crucial in assessing response to therapy. The goal of treatment is to eradicate HCV RNA, which is predicted by the absence of HCV RNA by PCR 6 months after stopping treatment (SVR). When therapy relied on PEG IFN and ribavirin, failure to achieve a 2-$\log_{10}$ drop in HCV RNA by week 12 of therapy (EVR) rendered it unlikely that further therapy would result in an SVR. When PEG IFN and ribavirin are part of a protease inhibitor regimen, HCV RNA should be measured at baseline and at weeks 4, 8 (for boceprevir), 12, and 24 to assess response to treatment and to aid in decisions regarding treatment duration (response-guided therapy), as well as 12 and 24 weeks after therapy. Stopping rules are important to prevent the emergence of resistance; if HCV RNA is > 1000 IU/mL at 4 or 12 weeks of telaprevir (or still detectable at week 24), or if HCV RNA is ≥100 IU/mL at week 12 of boceprevir (or detectable at week 24), all treatment should be stopped.

INDICATIONS FOR ANTIVIRAL THERAPY*

Patients with chronic hepatitis C who have detectable HCV RNA in serum, whether or not aminotransferase levels are increased, and chronic hepatitis of at least moderate grade and stage (portal or bridging fibrosis) are candidates for antiviral therapy with PEG IFN plus ribavirin. Most authorities recommend 800 mg of ribavirin for patients with genotypes 2 and 3 for both types of PEG IFN and weight-based 1000–1200 mg (when used with PEG IFN-α2a) or 800–1400 mg (when used with PEG IFN-α2b) ribavirin for patients with genotype 1 (and 4), unless ribavirin is contraindicated (Table 362-7). These PEG IFN and ribavirin doses are used with protease inhibitors for patients with genotype 1 (Table 362-7). Although patients with persistently normal ALT activity tend to progress histologically very slowly or not at all, they respond to antiviral therapy just as well as do patients with elevated ALT levels; therefore, although observation without therapy is an option, such patients are potential candidates for antiviral therapy. As noted above, therapy with IFN has been shown to improve survival and complication-free survival and to slow progression of (and to reverse) fibrosis.

HCV genotype determines the duration of PEG IFN and ribavirin therapy: 24 weeks for those with genotypes 2 and 3 and 48 weeks for patients with genotypes 4 and 1 (in patients for whom protease inhibitors are not available or contraindicated). For patients with genotype 4, treatment should be discontinued in patients who do not achieve an EVR at week 12. For patients with genotypes 2 and 3, a full, 24-week course is most effective, although the duration may be reduced to 12–16 weeks for patients with genotype 2, a low baseline level of viremia, and an RVR, especially to be considered for patients who tolerate therapy poorly. Also, consideration should be given to increasing the duration of therapy to 48 weeks for patients with genotype 3 who have advanced fibrosis and/or a high baseline level of viremia. As noted above, the absence of a 2-$\log_{10}$ drop in HCV RNA at week 12 (EVR) weighs heavily against the likelihood of an SVR; therefore, measuring HCV RNA at 12 weeks is recommended routinely (Fig. 362-2), and therapy can be discontinued if an EVR is not achieved. Among patients with genotype 4 who achieve an

*As this chapter was going to press, two additional antiviral drugs, a second-generation protease inhibitor simeprevir and nucleoside analogue polymerase inhibitor sofosbuvir were approved for the treatment of hepatitis C. Simerprevir, which is effective for genotype 1, must be administered, like first-generation protease inhibitors, for 12 weeks with PEG IFN and ribavirin, followed by another 12 weeks of PEG IFN and ribavirin (no response-guided therapy). Sofosbuvir, the more convenient and broadly applicable of the two new drugs, must be administered with PEG IFN and ribavirin but for only 12 weeks in patients with genotyes 1, 4-6; for patients with genotypes 2 and 3, PEG IFN is not required. Sofosbuvir plus ribavirin are administered for 12 weeks in genotype 2 and for 24 weeks in genotype 3. Antiviral therapy is evolving very rapidly; by the end of 2014, all-oral, interferon-free combinations (e.g., sofosbuvir plus the NS5a inhibitor ledipasvir) will supplant earlier treatment regimens. For updated treatment recommendations, please consult *www.hcvguidelines.org*.

EVR (≥2-$\log_{10}$ HCV RNA reduction) but in whom HCV RNA remains detectable at week 24, an SVR is unlikely, and therapy can be discontinued. Although response rates are lower in patients with certain pretreatment variables, selection for treatment should not be based on symptoms, genotype, HCV RNA level, mode of acquisition of hepatitis C, or advanced hepatic fibrosis. Patients with cirrhosis can respond and should not be excluded as candidates for therapy. For patients being treated with telaprevir and boceprevir, treating physicians should explain the negative impact of non-C *IL28B* genotype and advanced fibrosis on outcome.

Patients who have relapsed after, or failed to respond to (Fig. 362-2), a course of IFN monotherapy are potential candidates for retreatment with PEG IFN plus ribavirin (i.e., a more effective treatment regimen is required), and this approach remains current for patients with genotypes 2, 3, or 4; however, for patients with genotype 1, combination protease inhibitor/PEG IFN/ribavirin therapy is indicated. For patients with genotypes 2, 3, or 4 who were nonresponders to a prior course of IFN monotherapy, retreatment with IFN monotherapy or combination IFN plus ribavirin therapy is unlikely to achieve an SVR; however, a trial of combination PEG IFN plus ribavirin may be worthwhile, although an SVR is the outcome in <15–20% of patients. SVRs to retreatment of nonresponders are more frequent in those who had never received ribavirin in the past, those with genotypes 2 and 3, those with low pretreatment HCV RNA levels, and noncirrhotics, but less frequent in African Americans, those who failed to achieve a substantial reduction in HCV RNA during their previous course of therapy (null responders, Fig. 362-2), and those who required ribavirin dose reductions. Potential approaches to improving responsiveness to PEG IFN–ribavirin in prior nonresponders include longer duration of treatment; higher doses of PEG IFN, ribavirin, or both; and switching to a different IFN preparation; however, as noted above, none of these approaches achieves more than a marginal benefit. Treatment with a protease inhibitor–based regimen should be pursued in patients with genotype 1 who have relapsed after or not responded to prior treatment with IFN monotherapy or PEG IFN plus ribavirin, unless these protease inhibitors are not available or contraindicated (Table 362-7).

Early PEG IFN treatment is indicated for persons with acute hepatitis C; ribavirin, which is used frequently in such instances, has not been shown to improve efficacy over that of PEG IFN alone, and the new protease inhibitors have not been approved for acute hepatitis C **(Chap. 360)**. In patients with biochemically and histologically mild chronic hepatitis C, the rate of progression is slow, and monitoring without therapy is an option; however, such patients respond just as well to combination PEG IFN plus ribavirin therapy or triple-drug, protease-based therapy (for genotype 1) as those with elevated ALT and more histologically severe hepatitis. Therefore, therapy for these patients should be considered and the decision made based on such factors as patient motivation, genotype, stage of fibrosis, age, and comorbid conditions. A pretreatment liver biopsy to assess histologic grade and stage provides substantial information about progression of hepatitis C in the past, has prognostic value for future progression, and can identify such histologic factors as steatosis and stage of fibrosis, which can influence responsiveness to therapy. As therapy has improved for patients with a broad range of histologic severity, and as noninvasive laboratory markers and imaging correlates of fibrosis have gained popularity, some authorities, especially in Europe, place less value on, and do not recommend, pretreatment liver biopsies. On the other hand, serum markers of fibrosis are not considered sufficiently accurate, and histologic findings provide important prognostic information to physician and patient. Therefore, although the contemporary role of a pretreatment liver biopsy commands less of a consensus, a pretreatment liver biopsy still provides useful information and should be considered.

Patients with compensated cirrhosis can respond to therapy, although their likelihood of a sustained response is lower than in noncirrhotics; moreover, survival has been shown to improve after successful antiviral therapy in cirrhotics. Similarly, although several retrospective studies have suggested that antiviral therapy in cirrhotics with chronic hepatitis C, independent of treatment outcome per se, reduces the frequency of HCC, less advanced disease in the treated cirrhotics, not treatment itself (i.e., lead-time bias), may have accounted for the reduced frequency of HCC observed in the treated cohorts in these reports; prospective studies to address this question have failed to demonstrate benefit, unless an SVR is achieved. Patients with decompensated cirrhosis are not candidates for IFN-based antiviral therapy but should be referred for liver transplantation. Some liver transplantation centers have evaluated progressively escalated, low-dose antiviral therapy in an attempt to eradicate hepatitis C viremia prior to transplantation; however, such therapy has been shown to reduce but not to prevent the risk of HCV reinfection after transplantation. After liver transplantation for end-stage liver disease caused by hepatitis C, recurrent hepatitis C is the rule, and the pace of disease progression is more accelerated than in immunocompetent patients **(Chap. 368)**. Current therapy with PEG IFN and ribavirin after liver transplantation is unsatisfactory in most patients, but attempts to minimize immunosuppression are beneficial. Early experience with protease inhibitor–based therapy is encouraging, but inhibition of CYP3A4 by protease inhibitors can lead to markedly increased levels of immunosuppressive calcineurin inhibitors (especially tacrolimus), which requires intensive monitoring and can be very challenging. The cutaneous and renal vasculitis of HCV-associated essential mixed cryoglobulinemia **(Chap. 360)** may respond to antiviral therapy, but sustained responses are rare after discontinuation of therapy; therefore, prolonged, perhaps indefinite, therapy (as reported with IFN-based therapy) is recommended in this group (no indication for prolonged protease inhibitor therapy exists currently). Anecdotal reports suggest that antiviral therapy may be effective in porphyria cutanea tarda or lichen planus associated with hepatitis C.

In patients with HCV/HIV co-infection, hepatitis C is more progressive and severe than in HCV-monoinfected patients. Although patients with HCV/HIV co-infection respond to antiviral therapy for hepatitis C, they do not respond as well as patients with HCV infection alone. Four large national and international trials of antiviral therapy among patients with HCV/HIV co-infection have shown that PEG IFN (both α2a and α2b) plus ribavirin (daily doses ranging from flat-dosed 600–800 mg to weight-based 1000/1200 mg) is superior to standard IFN regimens; however, SVR rates were lower than in HCV-monoinfected patients, ranging from 14 to 38% for patients with genotypes 1 and 4 and from 44 to 73% for patients with genotypes 2 and 3. In the three largest trials, all patients, including those with genotypes 2 and 3, were treated for a full 48 weeks. In addition, tolerability of therapy was lower than in HCV-monoinfected patients; therapy was discontinued because of side effects in 12–39% of patients in these clinical trials. Based on these trials, weekly PEG IFN plus daily ribavirin at a daily dose of at least 600–800 mg, up to full weight-based doses, at doses recommended for HCV-monoinfected patients, if tolerated, is recommended for a full 48 weeks, regardless of genotype. An alternative recommendation for ribavirin doses was issued by a European Consensus Conference and consisted of standard, weight-based 1000–1200 mg for genotypes 1 and 4, but 800 mg for genotypes 2 and 3. A head-to-head trial of combination PEG IFN–ribavirin therapy in HCV/HIV co-infection demonstrated statistically indistinguishable efficacy of the two types of PEG IFN, despite a small advantage for PEG IFN-α2a: For PEG IFN-α2b and -α2a, SVRs occurred in 28% versus 32%, respectively, of patients with genotypes 1 and 4 and in 62% versus 71%, respectively, of patients with genotypes 2 and 3.

Although data are limited and recommendations pending, protease inhibitors may be used for genotype 1; however, because of potential drug-drug interactions between HCV protease inhibitors and HIV antiretroviral drugs (especially in ritonavir-boosted HIV protease inhibitors), HCV protease inhibitors should be used cautiously in HCV-HIV co-infected patients. If protease inhibitors are used, a full 48-week course is recommended without response-guided therapy: for boceprevir, 4 weeks of PEG IFN–ribavirin lead-in, followed by 44 weeks of triple-drug therapy (PEG IFN, ribavirin, boceprevir), and for telaprevir, 12 weeks of triple-drug therapy (PEG IFN, ribavirin, telaprevir), followed by 36 weeks of PEG IFN–ribavirin therapy. In preliminary trials among HIV-HCV co-infected patients, telaprevir-based triple-drug therapy (independent of whether they were receiving antiretroviral therapy [no antiretroviral drugs, efavirenz-tenofovir-emtricitabine, or ritonavir-boosted atazanavir-tenofovir-emtricitabine or lamivudine]) resulted in an SVR in 28 of 38 patients (74%), compared with 10 of 22 control patients (45%) treated with PEG IFN–ribavirin (60 study subjects); boceprevir-based triple-drug therapy (all were also receiving antiretroviral therapy) resulted in an SVR in 40 of 64 patients (63%), compared with 10 of 34 control patients (29%) treated with PEG IFN ribavirin (98 study subjects). Thus, for the prior standard of care, PEG IFN plus ribavirin, although the likelihood of an SVR is lower for HIV-HCV co-infected patients than for HCV-monoinfected patients, for protease inhibitor–based regimens, rates of SVR are comparable in HIV-HCV co-infected and HCV-monoinfected patients.

In HCV/HIV-infected patients, ribavirin can potentiate the toxicity of didanosine (e.g., lactic acidosis) and the lipoatrophy of stavudine, and zidovudine can exacerbate ribavirin-associated hemolytic anemia; therefore, these drug combinations should be avoided.

Patients with a history of injection drug use and alcoholism can be treated successfully for chronic hepatitis C, preferably in conjunction with drug and alcohol treatment programs. Because ribavirin is excreted renally, patients with end-stage renal disease, including those undergoing dialysis (which does not clear ribavirin), are not ideal candidates for ribavirin therapy. Rare reports suggest that reduced-dose ribavirin can be used, but the frequency of anemia is very high, and data on efficacy are limited. If patients with renal failure (glomerular filtration rate <60 mL/min) are treated, the PEG IFN-α2a dose should be reduced from 180 to 135 μg weekly and the PEG IFN-α2b dose reduced from 1.5 to 1 μg/kg weekly; similarly, the daily ribavirin dose in this population should be reduced to 200–800 mg (but not used or used cautiously at very low doses) if hemodialysis is required. Neither the optimal regimen nor the efficacy of therapy is well established in this population.

NOVEL ANTIVIRALS*

To date, attempts to develop better-tolerated ribavirin successors or improved types of IFN-α or longer acting IFNs than PEG IFN have not been successful. The demonstration that responsiveness to antiviral therapy is influenced by genetic variation in *IL28B*, which codes for IFN-λ (as noted above), raises the possibility that IFN-λ might be an effective or even more effective IFN for treating hepatitis C; early trials are in progress, but elevations of aminotransferase levels in treated subjects have raised concerns and delayed development. Beyond telaprevir and boceprevir, other direct antivirals that target HCV polymerase, protease, or NS5A (a membrane phosphoprotein component of the viral replication complex) are being investigated, as well as agents that can target host-encoded proteins. Among the novel antivirals are drugs with improved pharmacokinetic and resistance profiles, less treatment complexity, pangenotypic activity, fewer side effects, and fewer drug-drug interactions.* The pace of successful trials of all-oral regimens has accelerated. All-oral combinations of a second-generation protease inhibitor (asunaprevir) plus an NS5A inhibitor (daclatasvir); of a uridine nucleoside polymerase inhibitor (sofosbuvir)* plus ribavirin; of a polymerase inhibitor (sofosbuvir) plus an NS5A inhibitor (ledipasvir or daclatasvir) and ribavirin; and of combinations of a ritonavir-boosted protease inhibitor (ABT-450) plus a nonnucleoside polymerase inhibitor (ABT-333) plus an NS5A inhibitor (ABT-267) with or without ribavirin have been studied in clinical trials. Several of these drug combinations have achieved SVR rates exceeding 90%, even approaching 100%, for both treatment-naïve and treatment-experienced patients (including patients who failed to respond to first-generation protease inhibitors), across all HCV genotypes and independent of host *IL28B* genotype, and with treatment durations of 12–24 weeks or even shorter (8 weeks). Potentially, as early as 2014 or 2015, such combinations of direct antiviral agents will be used in drug cocktails that may replace IFN-based regimens entirely.

Less advanced is development of inhibitors of host proteins, such as oral, nonimmunosuppressive inhibitors of cyclophilin A (which interacts with NS5A during HCV replication) and subcutaneous antisense antagonists of host liver-expressed micro-RNA-122 (which promotes HCV replication). Given the accelerated progress of all-oral, short-treatment-duration, high-efficacy, direct-acting antivirals, these alternative approaches may not be practical or competitive.

AUTOIMMUNE HEPATITIS

DEFINITION

Autoimmune hepatitis is a chronic disorder characterized by continuing hepatocellular necrosis and inflammation, usually with fibrosis, which can progress to cirrhosis and liver failure. When fulfilling criteria of severity, this type of chronic hepatitis, when untreated, may have a 6-month mortality of as high as 40%. Based on contemporary estimates of the natural history of autoimmune hepatitis, the 10-year survival is 80–98% for treated and 67% for untreated patients. The prominence of extrahepatic features of autoimmunity and seroimmunologic abnormalities in this disorder supports an autoimmune process in its pathogenesis; this concept is reflected in the prior labels *lupoid* and *plasma cell hepatitis*. Autoantibodies and other typical features of autoimmunity, however, do not occur in all cases; among the broader categories of "idiopathic" or cryptogenic chronic hepatitis, many, perhaps the majority, are probably autoimmune in origin. Cases in which hepatotropic viruses, metabolic/genetic derangements (including nonalcoholic fatty liver disease), and hepatotoxic drugs have been excluded represent a spectrum of heterogeneous liver disorders of unknown cause, a proportion of which are most likely autoimmune hepatitis.

IMMUNOPATHOGENESIS

The weight of evidence suggests that the progressive liver injury in patients with autoimmune hepatitis is the result of a cell-mediated immunologic attack directed against liver cells. In all likelihood, predisposition to autoimmunity is inherited, whereas the liver specificity of this injury is triggered by environmental (e.g., chemical, drug [e.g., minocycline], or viral) factors. For example, patients have been described in whom apparently self-limited cases of acute hepatitis A, B, or C led to autoimmune hepatitis, presumably because of genetic susceptibility or predisposition. Evidence to support an autoimmune pathogenesis in this type of hepatitis includes the following: (1) In the liver, the histopathologic lesions are composed predominantly of cytotoxic T cells and plasma cells; (2) circulating autoantibodies (nuclear, smooth muscle, thyroid, etc.; see below), rheumatoid factor, and hyperglobulinemia are common; (3) other autoimmune disorders—such as thyroiditis, rheumatoid arthritis, autoimmune hemolytic anemia, ulcerative colitis, membranoproliferative glomerulonephritis, juvenile diabetes mellitus, celiac disease, and Sjögren's syndrome—occur with increased frequency in patients and in their relatives who have autoimmune hepatitis; (4) histocompatibility haplotypes associated with autoimmune diseases, such as HLA-B1, -B8, -DR3, and -DR4 as well as extended haplotype *DRB1*0301* and *DRB1*0401* alleles, are common in patients with autoimmune hepatitis; and (5) this type of chronic hepatitis is responsive to glucocorticoid/immunosuppressive therapy, effective in a variety of autoimmune disorders.

Cellular immune mechanisms appear to be important in the pathogenesis of autoimmune hepatitis. In vitro studies have suggested that in patients with this disorder, $CD4^+$ T lymphocytes are capable of becoming sensitized to hepatocyte membrane proteins and of destroying liver cells. Molecular mimicry by cross-reacting antigens that contain epitopes similar to liver antigens is postulated to activate these T cells, which infiltrate, and result in injury to, the liver. Abnormalities of immunoregulatory control over cytotoxic lymphocytes (impaired regulatory CD4+CD25+ T cell influences) may play a role as well. Studies of genetic predisposition to autoimmune hepatitis demonstrate that certain haplotypes are associated with the disorder, as enumerated above, as are polymorphisms in cytotoxic T lymphocyte antigens (*CTLA-4*) and tumor necrosis factor α (*TNFA*2*). The precise triggering factors, genetic influences, and cytotoxic and immunoregulatory mechanisms involved in this type of liver injury remain incompletely defined.

Intriguing clues into the pathogenesis of autoimmune hepatitis come from the observation that circulating autoantibodies are prevalent in patients with this disorder. Among the autoantibodies described in these patients are antibodies to nuclei (so-called antinuclear antibodies [ANAs], primarily in a homogeneous pattern) and smooth muscle (so-called anti-smooth-muscle antibodies, directed at actin, vimentin, and skeletin), antibodies to F-actin, antibodies to liver-kidney microsomes (anti-LKM, see below), antibodies to "soluble liver antigen" (directed against a uracil-guanine-adenine transfer RNA suppressor protein), antibodies to α-actinin, and antibodies to the liver-specific asialoglycoprotein receptor (or "hepatic lectin") and other hepatocyte membrane proteins. Although some of these provide helpful diagnostic markers, their involvement in the pathogenesis of autoimmune hepatitis has not been established.

Humoral immune mechanisms have been shown to play a role in the extrahepatic manifestations of autoimmune and idiopathic hepatitis. Arthralgias, arthritis, cutaneous vasculitis, and glomerulonephritis occurring in patients with autoimmune hepatitis appear to be mediated by the deposition of circulating immune complexes in affected tissue vessels, followed by complement activation, inflammation, and tissue injury. While specific viral antigen-antibody complexes can be identified in acute and chronic viral hepatitis, the nature of the immune complexes in autoimmune hepatitis has not been defined.

CLINICAL FEATURES

Many of the *clinical features* of autoimmune hepatitis are similar to those described for chronic viral hepatitis. The onset of disease may be insidious or abrupt; the disease may present initially like, and be confused with, acute viral hepatitis; a history of recurrent bouts of what had been labeled *acute hepatitis* is not uncommon. In approximately a quarter of patients, the diagnosis is made in the absence of symptoms, based on abnormal liver laboratory tests. A subset of patients with autoimmune hepatitis has distinct features. Such patients are predominantly young to middle-aged women with marked hyperglobulinemia and high-titer circulating ANAs. This is the group with positive lupus erythematosus (LE) preparations (initially labeled "*lupoid* " hepatitis) in whom other autoimmune features are common. Fatigue, malaise, anorexia, amenorrhea, acne, arthralgias, and jaundice are common. Occasionally, arthritis, maculopapular eruptions (including cutaneous vasculitis), erythema nodosum, colitis, pleurisy, pericarditis, anemia, azotemia, and sicca syndrome (keratoconjunctivitis, xerostomia) occur. In some patients, complications of cirrhosis, such as ascites and edema (associated with portal hypertension and hypoalbuminemia), encephalopathy, hypersplenism, coagulopathy, or variceal bleeding may bring the patient to initial medical attention.

The course of autoimmune hepatitis may be variable. In patients with mild disease or limited histologic lesions (e.g., piecemeal necrosis without bridging), progression to cirrhosis is limited, but, even in this subset, clinical monitoring is important to identify progression; up to half left untreated can progress to cirrhosis over the course of 15 years. In North America, cirrhosis at presentation is more common in African Americans than in whites. In those with severe symptomatic autoimmune hepatitis (aminotransferase levels >10 times normal, marked hyperglobulinemia, "aggressive" histologic lesions—bridging necrosis or multilobular collapse, cirrhosis), the 6-month mortality without therapy may be as high as 40%. Such severe disease accounts for only 20% of cases; the natural history of milder disease is variable, often accentuated by spontaneous remissions and exacerbations. Especially poor prognostic signs include the presence histologically of multilobular collapse at the time of initial presentation and failure of serum bilirubin to improve after 2 weeks of therapy. Death may result from hepatic failure, hepatic coma, other complications of cirrhosis (e.g., variceal hemorrhage), and intercurrent infection. In patients with established cirrhosis, HCC may be a late complication (Chap. 111) but occurs less frequently than in cirrhosis associated with viral hepatitis.

Laboratory features of autoimmune hepatitis are similar to those seen in chronic viral hepatitis. Liver biochemical tests are invariably abnormal but may not correlate with the clinical severity or histopathologic features in individual cases. Many patients with autoimmune hepatitis have normal serum bilirubin, alkaline phosphatase, and globulin levels with only minimal aminotransferase elevations. Serum AST and ALT levels are increased and fluctuate in the range of 100–1000 units. In severe cases, the serum bilirubin level is moderately elevated (51–171 μmol/L [3–10 mg/dL]). Hypoalbuminemia occurs in patients with very active or advanced disease. Serum alkaline phosphatase levels may be moderately elevated or near normal. In a small proportion of patients, marked elevations of alkaline phosphatase activity occur; in such patients, clinical and laboratory features overlap with those of primary biliary cirrhosis (Chap. 365). The prothrombin time is often prolonged, particularly late in the disease or during active phases.

Hypergammaglobulinemia (>2.5 g/dL) is common in autoimmune hepatitis, as is the presence of rheumatoid factor. As noted above, circulating autoantibodies are also prevalent, most characteristically ANAs in a homogeneous staining pattern. Smooth-muscle antibodies are less specific, seen just as frequently in chronic viral hepatitis. Because of the high levels of globulins achieved in the circulation of some patients with autoimmune hepatitis, occasionally the globulins may bind nonspecifically in solid-phase binding immunoassays for viral antibodies. This has been recognized most commonly in tests for antibodies to hepatitis C virus, as noted above. In fact, studies of autoantibodies in autoimmune hepatitis have led to the recognition of new categories of autoimmune hepatitis. *Type I autoimmune hepatitis* is the classic syndrome prevalent in North America and northern Europe occurring in young women, associated with marked hyperglobulinemia, lupoid features, circulating ANAs, and HLA- DR3 or HLA-DR4 (especially *B8-DRB1*03*). Also associated with type I autoimmune hepatitis are autoantibodies against actin and atypical perinuclear antineutrophilic cytoplasmic antibodies (pANCA).

Type II autoimmune hepatitis, often seen in children, more common in Mediterranean populations, and linked to HLA- DRB1 and HLA-DQB1 haplotypes, is associated not with ANA but with anti-LKM. Actually, anti-LKM represent a heterogeneous group of antibodies. In type II autoimmune hepatitis, the antibody is anti-LKM1, directed against cytochrome P450 2D6. This is the same anti-LKM seen in some patients with chronic hepatitis C. Anti-LKM2 is seen in drug-induced hepatitis, and anti-LKM3 (directed against uridine diphosphate glucuronyltransferases) is seen in patients with chronic hepatitis D. Another autoantibody observed in type II autoimmune hepatitis is directed against liver cytosol formiminotransferase cyclodeaminase (anti-liver cytosol 1). More controversial is whether or not a third category of autoimmune hepatitis exists, *type III autoimmune hepatitis*. These patients lack ANA and anti-LKM1 but have circulating antibodies to soluble liver antigen. Most of these patients are women and have clinical features similar to, perhaps more severe than, those of patients with type I autoimmune hepatitis. Type III autoimmune hepatitis does not appear to represent a distinct category but, instead, is part of the spectrum of type I autoimmune hepatitis; this subcategory has not been adopted by a consensus of international experts.

Liver biopsy abnormalities are similar to those described for chronic viral hepatitis. Expanding portal tracts and extending beyond the plate of periportal hepatocytes into the parenchyma (designated *interface hepatitis* or *piecemeal necrosis*) is a mononuclear cell infiltrate that, in autoimmune hepatitis, may include the presence of plasma cells. Necroinflammatory activity characterizes the lobular parenchyma, and evidence of hepatocellular regeneration is reflected by "rosette" formation, the occurrence of thickened liver cell plates, and regenerative "pseudolobules." Septal fibrosis, bridging fibrosis, and cirrhosis are frequent. In patients with early autoimmune hepatitis presenting as an acute-hepatitis-like illness, lobular and centrilobular (as opposed to the more common periportal) necrosis has been reported. Bile duct injury and granulomas are uncommon; however, a subgroup of patients with autoimmune hepatitis has histologic, biochemical, and serologic features overlapping those of primary biliary cirrhosis (Chap. 365).

DIAGNOSTIC CRITERIA

An international group has suggested a set of criteria for establishing a diagnosis of autoimmune hepatitis. Exclusion of liver disease caused by genetic disorders, viral hepatitis, drug hepatotoxicity, and alcohol are linked with such inclusive diagnostic criteria as hyperglobulinemia, autoantibodies, and characteristic histologic features. This international group has also suggested a comprehensive diagnostic scoring system that, rarely required for typical cases, may be helpful when typical features are not present. Factors that weigh in favor of the diagnosis include female gender; predominant aminotransferase elevation; presence and level of globulin elevation; presence of nuclear, smooth muscle, LKM1, and other autoantibodies; concurrent other autoimmune diseases; characteristic histologic features (interface hepatitis, plasma cells, rosettes); HLA-DR3 or -DR4 markers; and response to treatment (see below). A more simplified, more specific scoring system relies on four variables: autoantibodies, serum IgG level, typical or compatible histologic features, and absence of viral hepatitis markers. Weighing against the diagnosis are predominant alkaline phosphatase elevation, mitochondrial antibodies, markers of viral hepatitis, history of hepatotoxic drugs or excessive alcohol, histologic evidence of bile duct injury, or such atypical histologic features as fatty infiltration, iron overload, and viral inclusions.

DIFFERENTIAL DIAGNOSIS

Early during the course of chronic hepatitis, autoimmune hepatitis may resemble typical *acute viral hepatitis* (Chap. 360). Without histologic assessment, severe chronic hepatitis cannot be readily distinguished based on clinical or biochemical criteria from mild chronic hepatitis. In adolescence, *Wilson's disease* (Chaps. 365 and 429) may present with features of chronic hepatitis long before neurologic manifestations become apparent and before the formation of Kayser-Fleischer rings (copper deposition in Descemet's membrane in the periphery of the cornea). In this age group, serum ceruloplasmin and serum and urinary copper determinations plus measurement of liver copper levels establish the correct diagnosis. *Postnecrotic* or *cryptogenic cirrhosis* and *primary biliary cirrhosis* (Chap. 365) share clinical features with autoimmune hepatitis, and both alcoholic hepatitis (Chap. 363) and nonalcoholic steatohepatitis (Chap. 367e) may present with many features common to autoimmune hepatitis; historic, biochemical, serologic, and histologic assessments are usually sufficient to allow these entities to be distinguished from autoimmune hepatitis. Of course, the distinction between autoimmune and chronic viral hepatitis is not always straightforward, especially when viral antibodies occur in patients with autoimmune disease or when autoantibodies occur in patients with viral disease. Furthermore, the presence of extrahepatic features such as arthritis, cutaneous vasculitis, or pleuritis—not to mention the presence of circulating autoantibodies—may cause confusion with *rheumatologic disorders* such as rheumatoid arthritis and systemic lupus erythematosus. The existence of clinical and biochemical features of progressive necroinflammatory liver disease distinguishes chronic hepatitis from these other disorders, which are not associated with severe liver disease. Rarely, hepatic venous outflow obstruction (Budd-Chiari syndrome) may present with features suggestive of autoimmune hepatitis, but painful hepatomegaly, ascites, and vascular imaging provide distinguishing diagnostic clues. Other diagnostic considerations would include celiac disease and ischemic liver disease, which would be readily distinguishable by clinical and laboratory features from autoimmune hepatitis.

Finally, occasionally, features of autoimmune hepatitis overlap with features of autoimmune biliary disorders such as primary biliary cirrhosis, primary sclerosing cholangitis (Chaps. 365 and 369), or, even more rarely, mitochondrial antibody-negative autoimmune cholangitis. Such overlap syndromes are difficult to categorize, and often response to therapy may be the distinguishing factor that establishes the diagnosis.

TREATMENT AUTOIMMUNE HEPATITIS

The mainstay of management in autoimmune hepatitis is glucocorticoid therapy. Several controlled clinical trials have documented that such therapy leads to symptomatic, clinical, biochemical, and histologic improvement as well as increased survival. A therapeutic response can be expected in up to 80% of patients. Unfortunately, therapy has not been shown in clinical trials to prevent ultimate progression to cirrhosis; however, instances of reversal of fibrosis and cirrhosis have been reported in patients responding to treatment, and rapid treatment responses within 1 year do translate into a reduction in progression to cirrhosis. Although some advocate the use of prednisolone (the hepatic metabolite of prednisone), prednisone is just as effective and is favored by most authorities. Therapy may be initiated at 20 mg/d, but a popular regimen in the United States relies on an initiation dose of 60 mg/d. This high dose is tapered successively over the course of a month down to a maintenance level of 20 mg/d. An alternative, but equally effective, approach is to begin with half the prednisone dose (30 mg/d) along with azathioprine (50 mg/d). With azathioprine maintained at 50 mg/d, the prednisone dose is tapered over the course of a month down to a maintenance level of 10 mg/d. The advantage of the combination approach is a reduction, over the span of an 18-month course of therapy, in serious, life-threatening complications of steroid therapy (e.g., cushingoid features, hypertension, diabetes, osteoporosis) from 66% down to under 20%. Genetic analysis for thiopurine S-methyltransferase allelic variants does not correlate with azathioprine-associated cytopenias or efficacy and is not assessed routinely in patients with autoimmune hepatitis. In combination regimens, 6-mercaptopurine may be substituted for its prodrug azathioprine, but this is rarely required. Azathioprine alone, however, is not effective in achieving remission, nor is alternate-day glucocorticoid therapy. Limited experience with budesonide in noncirrhotic patients suggests that this steroid side effect–sparing drug may be effective. Although therapy has been shown to be effective for severe autoimmune hepatitis (AST ≥10 × the upper limit of normal or ≥5 × the upper limit of normal in conjunction with serum globulin greater than or equal to twice normal; bridging necrosis or multilobular necrosis on liver biopsy; presence of symptoms), therapy is not indicated for mild forms of chronic hepatitis, and the efficacy of therapy in mild or asymptomatic autoimmune hepatitis has not been established.

Improvement of fatigue, anorexia, malaise, and jaundice tends to occur within days to several weeks; biochemical improvement occurs over the course of several weeks to months, with a fall in serum bilirubin and globulin levels and an increase in serum albumin. Serum aminotransferase levels usually drop promptly, but improvements in AST and ALT alone do not appear to be reliable markers of recovery in individual patients; histologic improvement, characterized by a decrease in mononuclear infiltration and in hepatocellular necrosis, may be delayed for 6–24 months. Still, if interpreted cautiously, aminotransferase levels are valuable indicators of relative disease activity, and many authorities do *not* advocate for serial liver biopsies to assess therapeutic success or to guide decisions to alter or stop therapy. Rapidity of response is more common in older patients (≥69 years) and those with HLA *DBR1*04*; although rapid responders may progress less slowly to cirrhosis and liver transplantation, they are no less likely than slower responders to relapse after therapy. Therapy should continue for at least 12–18 months. After tapering and cessation of therapy, the likelihood of relapse is at least 50%, even if posttreatment histology has improved to show mild chronic hepatitis, and the majority of patients require therapy at maintenance doses indefinitely. Continuing azathioprine alone (2 mg/kg body weight daily) after cessation of prednisone therapy has been shown to reduce the frequency of relapse. Long-term maintenance with low-dose prednisone (≤10 mg daily) has also been shown to keep autoimmune hepatitis in check, but maintenance azathioprine is more effective in maintaining remission.

In medically refractory cases, an attempt should be made to intensify treatment with high-dose glucocorticoid monotherapy (60 mg daily) or combination glucocorticoid (30 mg daily) plus high-dose azathioprine (150 mg daily) therapy. After a month, doses of prednisone can be reduced by 10 mg a month, and doses of azathioprine can be reduced by 50 mg a month toward ultimate, conventional maintenance doses. Patients refractory to this regimen may be treated with cyclosporine, tacrolimus, or mycophenolate mofetil; however, to date, only limited anecdotal reports support these approaches. If medical therapy fails, or when chronic hepatitis progresses to cirrhosis and is associated with life-threatening complications of liver decompensation, liver transplantation is the only recourse (Chap. 368); failure of the bilirubin to improve after 2 weeks of therapy should prompt early consideration of the patient for liver transplantation. Recurrence of autoimmune hepatitis in the new liver occurs rarely in most experiences but in as many as 35–40% of cases in others.

Like all patients with chronic liver disease, patients with autoimmune hepatitis should be vaccinated against hepatitis A and B, ideally before immunosuppressive therapy is begun, if practical.

Acknowledgment

Kurt J. Isselbacher, MD, contributed to this chapter in previous editions of Harrison's.

363 Alcoholic Liver Disease

Mark E. Mailliard, Michael F. Sorrell

Chronic and excessive alcohol ingestion is one of the major causes of liver disease. The pathology of alcoholic liver disease consists of three major lesions, with the progressive injury rarely existing in a pure form: (1) fatty liver, (2) alcoholic hepatitis, and (3) cirrhosis. Fatty liver is present in >90% of daily as well as binge drinkers. A much smaller percentage of heavy drinkers will progress to alcoholic hepatitis, thought to be a precursor to cirrhosis. The prognosis of severe alcoholic liver disease is dismal; the mortality of patients with alcoholic hepatitis concurrent with cirrhosis is nearly 60% at 4 years. Although alcohol is considered a direct hepatotoxin, only between 10 and 20% of alcoholics will develop alcoholic hepatitis. The explanation for this apparent paradox is unclear but involves the complex interaction of facilitating factors, such as drinking patterns, diet, obesity, and gender. There are no diagnostic tools that can predict individual susceptibility to alcoholic liver disease.

GLOBAL CONSIDERATIONS

Alcohol is the world's third largest risk factor for disease burden. The harmful use of alcohol results in 2.5 million deaths each year. Most of the mortality attributed to alcohol is secondary to cirrhosis. Mortality from cirrhosis is declining in most Western countries, concurrent with a reduction in alcohol consumption, with the exceptions of the United Kingdom, Russia, Romania, and Hungary. These increases in cirrhosis and its complications are closely correlated with increased volume of alcohol consumed per capita population and are regardless of gender.

ETIOLOGY AND PATHOGENESIS

Quantity and duration of alcohol intake are the most important risk factors involved in the development of alcoholic liver disease (Table 363-1). The roles of beverage type(s), i.e. wine, beer, or spirits, and pattern of drinking (daily versus binge drinking) are less clear. Progress beyond the fatty liver stage seems to require additional risk factors that remain incompletely defined. Although there are genetic predispositions for alcoholism (Chap. 467), gender is a strong determinant for alcoholic liver disease. Women are more susceptible to alcoholic liver injury when compared to men. They develop advanced liver disease with substantially less alcohol intake. In general, the time it takes to develop liver disease is directly related to the amount of alcohol consumed. It is useful in estimating alcohol consumption to understand that one beer, four ounces of wine, or one ounce of 80% spirits all contain ~12 g of alcohol. The threshold for developing alcoholic liver disease is higher in men, while women are at increased risk for developing similar degrees of liver injury by consuming significantly less. Gender-dependent differences result from poorly understood effects of estrogen, proportion of body fat, and the gastric metabolism of alcohol. Obesity, a high-fat diet, and the protective effect of coffee have been postulated to play a part in the development of the pathogenic process.

TABLE 363-1 RISK FACTORS FOR ALCOHOLIC LIVER DISEASE

Risk Factor	Comment
Quantity	In men, 40–80 g/d of ethanol produces fatty liver; 160 g/d for 10–20 years causes hepatitis or cirrhosis. Only 15% of alcoholics develop alcoholic liver disease.
Gender	Women exhibit increased susceptibility to alcoholic liver disease at amounts >20 g/d; two drinks per day is probably safe.
Hepatitis C	HCV infection concurrent with alcoholic liver disease is associated with younger age for severity, more advanced histology, and decreased survival.
Genetics	Patatin-like phospholipase domain-containing protein 3 (PNPLA3) has been associated with alcoholic cirrhosis.
Fatty liver	Alcohol injury does not require malnutrition, but obesity and nonalcoholic fatty liver are risk factors. Patients should receive vigorous attention to nutritional support.

Chronic infection with hepatitis C virus (HCV) (Chap. 362) is an important comorbidity in the progression of alcoholic liver disease to cirrhosis in chronic and excessive drinkers. Even moderate alcohol intake of 20–50 g/d increases the risk of cirrhosis and hepatocellular cancer in HCV-infected individuals. Patients with both alcoholic liver injury and HCV infection develop decompensated liver disease at a younger age and have poorer overall survival. Increased liver iron stores and, rarely, porphyria cutanea tarda can occur as a consequence of the overlapping injurious processes secondary to alcohol abuse and HCV infection. In addition, alcohol intake of >50 g/d by HCV-infected patients decreases the efficacy of interferon-based antiviral therapy.

The pathogenesis of alcoholic liver injury is unclear. The present conceptual foundation is that alcohol acts as a direct hepatotoxin and that malnutrition does not have a major role. Ingestion of alcohol initiates an inflammatory cascade by its metabolism to acetaldehyde, resulting in a variety of metabolic responses. Steatosis from lipogenesis, fatty acid synthesis, and depression of fatty acid oxidation appears secondary to effects on sterol regulatory transcription factor and peroxisome proliferator-activated receptor α (PPAR-α). Intestinal-derived endotoxin initiates a pathogenic process through toll-like receptor 4 and tumor necrosis factor α (TNF-α) that facilitates hepatocyte apoptosis and necrosis. The cell injury and endotoxin release initiated by ethanol and its metabolites also activate innate and adaptive immunity pathways releasing proinflammatory cytokines (e.g., TNF-α), chemokines, and proliferation of T and B cells. The production of toxic protein-aldehyde adducts, generation of reducing equivalents, and oxidative stress also contribute to the liver injury. Hepatocyte injury and impaired regeneration following chronic alcohol ingestion are ultimately associated with stellate cell activation and collagen production, which are key events in fibrogenesis. The resulting fibrosis from continuing alcohol use determines the architectural derangement of the liver and associated pathophysiology.

PATHOLOGY

The liver has a limited repertoire in response to injury. Fatty liver is the initial and most common histologic response to hepatotoxic stimuli, including excessive alcohol ingestion. The accumulation of fat within the perivenular hepatocytes coincides with the location of alcohol dehydrogenase, the major enzyme responsible for alcohol metabolism. Continuing alcohol ingestion results in fat accumulation throughout the entire hepatic lobule. Despite extensive fatty change and distortion of the hepatocytes with macrovesicular fat, the cessation of drinking results in normalization of hepatic architecture and fat content. Alcoholic fatty liver has traditionally been regarded as entirely benign, but similar to the spectrum of nonalcoholic fatty liver disease (Chap. 367e), the appearance of steatohepatitis and certain pathologic features such as giant mitochondria, perivenular fibrosis, and macrovesicular fat may be associated with progressive liver injury.

The transition between fatty liver and the development of alcoholic hepatitis is blurred. The hallmark of alcoholic hepatitis is hepatocyte injury characterized by ballooning degeneration, spotty necrosis, polymorphonuclear infiltrate, and fibrosis in the perivenular and perisinusoidal space of Disse. Mallory-Denk bodies are often present in florid cases but are neither specific nor necessary to establish the diagnosis. Alcoholic hepatitis is thought to be a precursor to the development of cirrhosis. However, like fatty liver, it is potentially reversible with cessation of drinking. Cirrhosis is present in up to 50% of patients with biopsy-proven alcoholic hepatitis, and its regression is uncertain, even with abstention.

CLINICAL FEATURES

The clinical manifestations of alcoholic fatty liver are subtle and characteristically detected as a consequence of the patient's visit for a seemingly unrelated matter. Previously unsuspected hepatomegaly is often the only clinical finding. Occasionally, patients with fatty liver will present with right upper quadrant discomfort, nausea, and, rarely, jaundice. Differentiation of alcoholic fatty liver from nonalcoholic fatty liver is difficult unless an accurate drinking history is ascertained. In every instance where liver disease is present, a thoughtful and sensitive drinking history should be obtained. Standard, validated questions accurately detect alcohol-related problems (Chap. 467). Alcoholic hepatitis is associated with a wide gamut of clinical features. Fever, spider nevi, jaundice, and abdominal pain simulating an acute abdomen represent the extreme end of the spectrum, while many patients will be entirely asymptomatic. Portal hypertension, ascites, or variceal bleeding can occur in the absence of cirrhosis. Recognition of the clinical features of alcoholic hepatitis is central to the initiation of an effective and appropriate diagnostic and therapeutic strategy. It is important to recognize that patients with alcoholic cirrhosis often exhibit clinical features identical to other causes of cirrhosis.

LABORATORY FEATURES

Patients with alcoholic liver disease are often identified through routine screening tests. The typical laboratory abnormalities seen in fatty liver are nonspecific and include modest elevations of aspartate aminotransferase (AST), alanine aminotransferase (ALT), and γ-glutamyl transpeptidase (GGTP), often accompanied by hypertriglyceridemia and hyperbilirubinemia. In alcoholic hepatitis and in contrast to other causes of fatty liver, AST and ALT are usually elevated two- to sevenfold. They are rarely >400 IU, and the AST/ALT ratio is >1 (Table 363-2). Hyperbilirubinemia is accompanied by modest increases in the alkaline phosphatase level. Derangement in hepatocyte synthetic function indicates more serious disease. Hypoalbuminemia and coagulopathy are common in advanced liver injury. Ultrasonography is useful in detecting fatty infiltration of the liver and determining liver size. The demonstration by ultrasound of portal vein flow reversal, ascites, and intraabdominal venous collaterals indicates serious liver injury with less potential for complete reversal.

TABLE 363-2 LABORATORY DIAGNOSIS OF ALCOHOLIC FATTY LIVER AND ALCOHOLIC HEPATITIS

Test	Comment
AST	Increased two- to sevenfold, <400 IU/L, greater than ALT
ALT	Increased two- to sevenfold, <400 IU/L
AST/ALT	Usually >1
GGTP	Not specific to alcohol, easily inducible, elevated in all forms of fatty liver
Bilirubin	May be markedly increased in alcoholic hepatitis despite modest elevation in alkaline phosphatase

Abbreviations: ALT, alanine aminotransferase; AST, aspartate aminotransferase; GGTP, γ-glutamyl transpeptidase.

PROGNOSIS

Critically ill patients with alcoholic hepatitis have short-term (30-day) mortality rates >50%. Severe alcoholic hepatitis is heralded by coagulopathy (prothrombin time increased >5 s), anemia, serum albumin concentrations <25 g/L (2.5 mg/dL), serum bilirubin levels >137 μmol/L (8 mg/dL), renal failure, and ascites. A discriminant function calculated as 4.6 X (the prolongation of the prothrombin time above control [seconds]) + serum bilirubin (mg/dL) can identify patients with a poor prognosis (discriminant function >32). A Model for End-Stage Liver Disease (MELD) score (Chap. 368) ≥21 also is associated with significant mortality in alcoholic hepatitis. The presence of ascites, variceal hemorrhage, deep encephalopathy, or hepatorenal syndrome predicts a dismal prognosis. The pathologic stage of the injury can be helpful in predicting prognosis. Liver biopsy should be performed whenever possible to establish the diagnosis and to guide the therapeutic decisions.

TREATMENT ALCOHOLIC LIVER DISEASE

Complete abstinence from alcohol is the cornerstone in the treatment of alcoholic liver disease. Improved survival and the potential for reversal of histologic injury regardless of the initial clinical presentation are associated with total avoidance of alcohol ingestion. Referral of patients to experienced alcohol counselors and/or alcohol treatment programs should be routine in the management of patients with alcoholic liver disease. Attention should be directed to the nutritional and psychosocial states during the evaluation and treatment periods. Because of data suggesting that the pathogenic mechanisms in alcoholic hepatitis involve cytokine release and the perpetuation of injury by immunologic processes, glucocorticoids have been extensively evaluated in the treatment of alcoholic hepatitis. Patients with severe alcoholic hepatitis, defined as a discriminant function >32 or MELD >20, should be given prednisone, 40 mg/d, or prednisolone, 32 mg/d, for 4 weeks, followed by a steroid taper (Fig. 363-1). Exclusion criteria include active gastrointestinal bleeding, renal failure, or pancreatitis. Women with encephalopathy from severe alcoholic hepatitis may be particularly good candidates for glucocorticoids. A Lille score >0.45, at *http://www.lillemodel.com*, uses pretreatment variables plus the change in total bilirubin at day 7 of glucocorticoids to identify patients unresponsive to therapy.

The role of TNF-α expression and receptor activity in alcoholic liver injury has led to an examination of TNF inhibition as an alternative to glucocorticoids for severe alcoholic hepatitis. The nonspecific TNF inhibitor, pentoxifylline, demonstrated improved survival in the therapy of severe alcoholic hepatitis, primarily due to a decrease in hepatorenal syndrome (Fig. 363-2). Monoclonal antibodies that neutralize serum TNF-α should not be used in alcoholic hepatitis because of studies reporting increased deaths secondary to infection and renal failure.

Liver transplantation is an accepted indication for treatment in selected and motivated patients with end-stage cirrhosis. Outcomes are equal or superior to other indications for transplantation. In general, transplant candidacy should be reevaluated after a defined

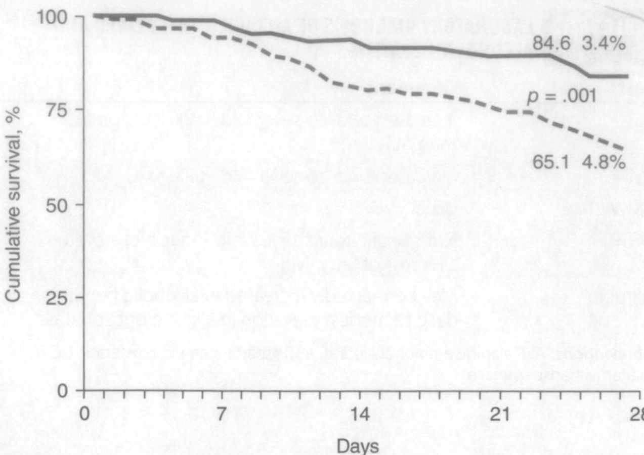

FIGURE 363-1 Effect of glucocorticoid therapy of severe alcoholic hepatitis on short-term survival: the result of a meta-analysis of individual data from three studies. Prednisolone, solid line; placebo, dotted line. *(Adapted from P Mathurin et al: J Hepatol 36:480, 2002, with permission from Elsevier Science.)*

period of sobriety. Patients presenting with alcoholic hepatitis have been largely excluded from transplant candidacy because of the perceived risk of increased surgical mortality and high rates of recidivism following transplantation. Recently, a European multidisciplinary group has reported excellent long-term transplant outcomes in highly selected patients with florid alcoholic hepatitis. General application of transplantation in such patients must await confirmatory outcomes by others.

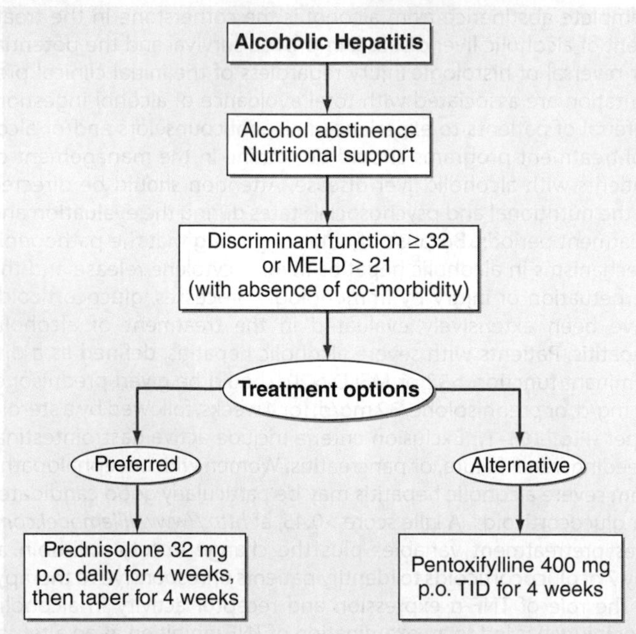

FIGURE 363-2 Treatment algorithm for alcoholic hepatitis. As identified by a calculated discriminant function >32 (see text), patients with severe alcoholic hepatitis, without the presence of gastrointestinal bleeding or infection, would be candidates for either glucocorticoids or pentoxifylline administration.

364 Nonalcoholic Fatty Liver Diseases and Nonalcoholic Steatohepatitis

Manal F. Abdelmalek, Anna Mae Diehl

INCIDENCE, PREVALENCE, AND NATURAL HISTORY

Nonalcoholic fatty liver disease (NAFLD) is the most common chronic liver disease in many parts of the world, including the United States. Population-based abdominal imaging studies have demonstrated fatty liver in at least 25% of American adults. Because the vast majority of these subjects deny hazardous levels of alcohol consumption (defined as greater than one drink per day in women or two drinks per day in men), they are considered to have NAFLD. NAFLD is strongly associated with overweight/obesity and insulin resistance. However, it can also occur in lean individuals and is particularly common in those with a paucity of adipose depots (i.e., lipodystrophy). Ethnic/racial factors also appear to influence liver fat accumulation; the documented prevalence of NAFLD is lowest in African Americans (~25%), highest in Americans of Hispanic ancestry (~50%), and intermediate in American whites (~33%).

NAFLD encompasses a spectrum of liver pathology with different clinical prognoses. The simple accumulation of triglyceride within hepatocytes (hepatic steatosis) is on the most clinically benign extreme of the spectrum. On the opposite, most clinically ominous extreme, are cirrhosis (Chap. 365) and primary liver cancer (Chap. 111). The risk of developing cirrhosis is extremely low in individuals with chronic hepatic steatosis, but increases as steatosis becomes complicated by histologically conspicuous hepatocyte death and inflammation (i.e., nonalcoholic steatohepatitis [NASH]). NASH itself is also a heterogeneous condition; sometimes it improves to steatosis or normal histology, sometimes it remains relatively stable for years, but sometimes it results in progressive accumulation of fibrous scar that eventuates in cirrhosis. Once NAFLD-related cirrhosis develops, the annual incidence of primary liver cancer is 1%.

Abdominal imaging is not able to determine which individuals with NAFLD have associated liver cell death and inflammation (i.e., NASH), and specific blood tests to diagnose NASH are not yet available. However, population-based studies that have used elevated serum ALT as a marker of liver injury indicate that about 6–8% of American adults have serum ALT elevations that cannot be explained by excessive alcohol consumption, other known causes of fatty liver disease (Table 364-1), viral hepatitis, or drug-induced or congenital liver diseases. Because the prevalence of such "cryptogenic" ALT elevations increases with body mass index, it is presumed that they are due to NASH. Hence, at any given point in time, NASH is present in about 25% of individuals who have NAFLD (i.e., about 6% of the general U.S. adult population has NASH). Smaller cross-sectional studies in which liver biopsies have been performed on NASH patients at tertiary referral centers consistently demonstrate advanced fibrosis or cirrhosis in about 25% of those cohorts. By extrapolation, therefore, cirrhosis develops in about 6% of individuals with NAFLD (i.e., in about 1.5–2% of the general U.S. population). The risk for advanced liver fibrosis is highest in individuals with NASH who are older than 45–50 years of age and overweight/obese or afflicted with type 2 diabetes.

To put these data in perspective, it is helpful to recall that the prevalence of hepatitis C–related cirrhosis in the United States is about 0.5%. Thus, NAFLD-related cirrhosis is about three to four times more common than cirrhosis caused by chronic hepatitis C infection. Consistent with these data, experts have predicted that NAFLD will surpass hepatitis C as the leading indication for liver transplantation in the United States within the next decade. Similar to cirrhosis caused by other liver diseases, cirrhosis caused by NAFLD increases the risk for primary liver cancer. Both hepatocellular carcinoma and intrahepatic cholangiocarcinoma (ICC) have also been reported to occur in NAFLD patients without cirrhosis, suggesting that NAFLD per se may be a premalignant condition. NAFLD, NASH, and NAFLD-related cirrhosis are not limited to adults. All have been well documented in children. As in adults, obesity and insulin resistance are the main risk

TABLE 364-1 ALTERNATIVE CAUSES OF HEPATIC STEATOSIS

- Alcoholic liver disease
- Hepatitis C (particularly genotype 3)
- Inborn errors of metabolism
  - Abetalipoproteinemia
  - Cholesterol ester storage disease
  - Galactosemia
  - Glycogen storage disease
  - Hereditary fructose intolerance
  - Homocystinuria
  - Systemic carnitine deficiency
  - Tyrosinemia
  - Weber-Christian syndrome
  - Wilson's disease
  - Wolman's disease
- Medications (see **Table 364–2**)
- Miscellaneous
  - Industrial exposure to petrochemical
  - Inflammatory bowel disease
  - Lipodystrophy
  - Bacterial overgrowth
  - Starvation
  - Parenteral nutrition
- Surgical procedures
  - Bilopancreatic diversion
  - Extensive small-bowel resection
  - Gastric bypass
  - Jejunoileal bypass
- Reye's syndrome
- Acute fatty liver of pregnancy
- HELLP syndrome (*h*emolytic anemia, *e*levated *l*iver enzymes, *l*ow *p*latelet count)

factors for pediatric NAFLD. Thus, the rising incidence and prevalence of childhood obesity suggests that NAFLD is likely to become an even greater contributor to society's burden of liver disease in the future.

PATHOGENESIS

The mechanisms underlying the pathogenesis and progression of NAFLD are not entirely clear. The best-understood mechanisms pertain to hepatic steatosis. This is proven to result when hepatocyte mechanisms for triglyceride synthesis (e.g., lipid uptake and de novo lipogenesis) overwhelm mechanisms for triglyceride disposal (e.g., degradative metabolism and lipoprotein export), leading to accumulation of fat (i.e., triglyceride) within hepatocytes. Obesity stimulates hepatocyte triglyceride accumulation by altering the intestinal microbiota to enhance both energy harvest from dietary sources and intestinal permeability. Reduced intestinal barrier function increases hepatic exposure to gut-derived products, which stimulate liver cells to generate inflammatory mediators that inhibit insulin actions. Obese adipose depots also produce excessive soluble factors (adipokines) that inhibit tissue insulin sensitivity. Insulin resistance promotes hyperglycemia. This drives the pancreas to produce more insulin to maintain glucose homeostasis. However, hyperinsulinemia also promotes lipid uptake, fat synthesis, and fat storage. The net result is hepatic triglyceride accumulation (i.e., steatosis).

Triglyceride per se is not hepatotoxic. However, its precursors (e.g., fatty acids and diacylglycerols) and metabolic by-products (e.g., reactive oxygen species) may damage hepatocytes, leading to hepatocyte lipotoxicity. Lipotoxicity also triggers the generation of other factors (e.g., inflammatory cytokines, hormonal mediators) that deregulate systems that normally maintain hepatocyte viability. The net result is increased hepatocyte death. Dying hepatocytes, in turn, release various factors that trigger wound healing responses that aim to replace (regenerate) lost hepatocytes. Such repair involves transient expansion of other cell types, such as myofibroblasts and progenitor cells, that make and degrade matrix, remodel the vasculature, and generate replacement hepatocytes, as well as the recruitment of immune cells that release factors that modulate liver injury and repair. NASH is the morphologic manifestation of lipotoxicity and resultant wound healing responses. Because the severity and duration of lipotoxic liver injury dictate the intensity and duration of repair, the histologic features and outcomes of NASH are variable. Cirrhosis and liver cancer are potential outcomes of chronic NASH. Cirrhosis results from futile repair, i.e., progressive accumulation of wound healing cells, fibrous matrix, and abnormal vasculature (scarring), rather than efficient reconstruction/regeneration of healthy hepatic parenchyma. Primary liver cancers develop when malignantly transformed liver cells escape mechanisms that normally control regenerative growth. The mechanisms responsible for futile repair (cirrhosis) and liver carcinogenesis are not well understood. Because normal liver regeneration is a very complex process, there are multiple opportunities for deregulation and, thus, pathogenic heterogeneity. To date, this heterogeneity has confounded development of both diagnostic tests and treatments for defective/deregulated liver repair (i.e., cirrhosis and cancer). Hence, current strategies focus on circumventing misrepair by preventing and/or reducing lipotoxic liver injury.

DIAGNOSIS

Diagnosing NAFLD requires demonstration of increased liver fat in the absence of hazardous levels of alcohol consumption. Thresholds for potentially dangerous alcohol ingestion have been set at more than one drink per day in women and two drinks per day in men based on epidemiologic evidence that the prevalence of serum aminotransferase elevations increases when alcohol consumption habitually exceeds these levels. In those studies, one drink was defined as having 10 g of ethanol and, thus, is equivalent to one can of beer, 4 ounces of wine, or 1.5 ounces (one shot) of distilled spirits. Other causes of liver fat accumulation (particularly exposure to certain drugs; Table 364-2) and liver injury (e.g., viral hepatitis, autoimmune liver disease, iron or copper overload, α_1 antitrypsin deficiency) must also be excluded. Thus, establishing the diagnosis of NAFLD does not require invasive testing: it can be accomplished by history and physical examination, liver imaging (ultrasound is an acceptable first-line test; computed tomography [CT] or magnetic resonance imaging [MRI] enhances sensitivity for liver fat detection but adds expense), and blood tests to exclude other liver diseases. It is important to emphasize that the liver may not be enlarged, and serum aminotransferases and liver function tests (e.g., bilirubin, albumin, prothrombin time) may be completely normal, in individuals with NAFLD. Because there is yet no one specific blood test for NAFLD, confidence in the diagnosis of NAFLD is increased by identification of NAFLD risk factors. The latter include increased body mass index, insulin resistance/type 2 diabetes mellitus, and other parameters indicative of the metabolic syndrome (e.g., systemic hypertension, dyslipidemia, hyperuricemia/gout, cardiovascular disease; Chap. 422) in the patient or family members.

Establishing the severity of NAFLD-related liver injury and related scarring (i.e., staging NAFLD) is more difficult than simply diagnosing NAFLD. Staging is critically important, however, because it is necessary to define prognosis and thereby determine treatment recommendations. The goal of staging is to distinguish patients with NASH from those with simple steatosis and to identify which of the NASH patients have advanced fibrosis. The 10-year probability of developing liver-related morbidity or mortality in steatosis is negligible, and hence, this subgroup of NAFLD patients tends to be managed conservatively (see below). In contrast, more intensive follow-up and therapy are justified in NASH patients, and the subgroup with advanced fibrosis merits the most intensive scrutiny and intervention because their 10-year risk of liver-related morbidity and mortality is clearly increased.

Staging approaches can be separated into noninvasive testing (i.e., blood testing, physical examination, and imaging) and invasive approaches (i.e., liver biopsy). Blood test evidence of hepatic dysfunction (e.g., hyperbilirubinemia, hypoalbuminemia, prothrombin time

TABLE 364-2 MEDICATIONS ASSOCIATED WITH HEPATIC STEATOSIS

- Cytotoxic and cytostatic drugs
  - L-Asparaginase
  - Azacitidine
  - Azaserine
  - Bleomycin
  - Methotrexate
  - Puromycin
  - Tetracycline
  - Doxycycline
- Metals
  - Antimony
  - Barium salts
  - Chromates
  - Phosphorus
  - Rare earths of low atomic number
  - Thallium compounds
  - Uranium compounds
- Other drugs and toxins
  - Amiodarone
  - 4,4′-Diethylaminoethoxyhexesterol
  - Ethionine
  - Ethyl bromide
  - Estrogens
  - Glucocorticoids
  - Highly active antiretroviral therapy
  - Hydralazine
  - Hypoglycin
  - Orotate
  - Perhexiline maleate
  - Safrole
  - Tamoxifen

prolongation) or portal hypertension (e.g., thrombocytopenia) and stigmata of portal hypertension on physical examination (e.g., spider angiomata, palmar erythema, splenomegaly, ascites, clubbing, encephalopathy) suggest a diagnosis of advanced NAFLD. Currently, however, liver biopsy is the gold standard for establishing the severity of liver injury and fibrosis because it is both more sensitive and specific than these other tests for establishing NAFLD severity. Although invasive, liver biopsy is seldom complicated by serious adverse sequelae such as significant bleeding, pain, or inadvertent puncture of other organs and thus is relatively safe. However, biopsy suffers from potential sampling error unless tissue cores of 2 cm or longer are acquired. Also, examination of tissue at a single point in time is not reliable for determining whether the pathologic processes are progressing or regressing. The risk of serial liver biopsies within short time intervals is generally deemed as unacceptable outside of research studies. These limitations of liver biopsy have stimulated efforts to develop noninvasive approaches to stage NAFLD. As is true for many other types of chronic liver disease, in NAFLD the levels of serum aminotransferases (aspartate aminotransferase [AST] and alanine aminotransferase [ALT]) do not reliably reflect the severity of liver cell injury, extent of liver cell death, or related liver inflammation and fibrosis. Thus, they are imperfect for determining which individuals with NAFLD have NASH. This has stimulated research to identify superior markers of liver injury. Serum levels of keratin 8 and keratin 18 appear to be promising surrogates. Keratins 8 and 18 (K8/18) are epithelial cytoskeletal proteins that undergo cleavage during programmed cell death (apoptosis). Both cleaved and full-length K8/18 are released into the blood as hepatocytes die, and studies suggest that serum levels of K8/18 differentiate individuals with NASH from those with simple steatosis or normal livers more reliably than do serum aminotransferase levels. Moreover, K8/18 levels appear to parallel the severity of liver fibrosis, with higher levels marking individuals who are likely to have worse scarring (i.e., advanced liver fibrosis or cirrhosis). While promising, testing for K8/18 has not yet become standard clinical practice. Other blood tests and imaging approaches that quantify liver fibrosis are also being developed. Recently, the U.S. Food and Drug Administration (FDA) approved an ultrasound-based test that measures liver stiffness as a surrogate marker of fibrosis (FibroScan®) (Chap. 358). This new tool will likely be used serially to monitor fibrosis progression and regression in NAFLD patients. Studies that compare the receiver operator characteristics of K8/18 plus FibroScan® versus liver biopsy for monitoring NAFLD evolution are forthcoming.

CLINICAL FEATURES OF NAFLD

Most subjects with NAFLD are asymptomatic. The diagnosis is often made when abnormal liver aminotransferases or features of fatty liver are noted during an evaluation performed for other reasons. NAFLD may also be diagnosed during the workup of vague right upper quadrant abdominal pain, hepatomegaly, or an abnormal-appearing liver at time of abdominal surgery. Obesity is present in 50–90% of subjects. Most patients with NAFLD also have other features of the metabolic syndrome (Chap. 422). Some have subtle stigmata of chronic liver disease, such as spider angiomata, palmer erythema, or splenomegaly. In a small minority of patients with advanced NAFLD, complications of end-stage liver disease (e.g., jaundice, features of portal hypertension such as ascites or variceal hemorrhage) may be the initial findings.

The association of NAFLD with obesity, diabetes, hypertriglyceridemia, hypertension, and cardiovascular disease is well known. Other associations include chronic fatigue, mood alterations, obstructive sleep apnea, thyroid dysfunction, and chronic pain syndrome. NAFLD is an independent risk factor for metabolic syndrome (Chap. 422). Longitudinal studies suggest that patients with NASH are at two- to threefold increased risk for the development of metabolic syndrome. Similarly, studies have shown that patients with NASH have a higher risk for the development of hypertension and diabetes mellitus. The presence of NAFLD is also independently associated with endothelial dysfunction, increased carotid intimal thickness, and the number of plaques in carotid and coronary arteries. Such data indicate that NAFLD has many deleterious effects on health in general.

TREATMENT OF NAFLD

Treatment of NAFLD can be divided into three components: (1) specific therapy of NAFLD-related liver disease; (2) treatment of NAFLD-associated comorbidities; and (3) treatment of the complications of advanced NAFLD. The subsequent discussion focuses on specific therapies for NAFLD, with some mention of their impact on major NAFLD comorbidities (insulin resistance/diabetes, obesity, and dyslipidemia). Treatment of the complications of advanced NAFLD involves management of the complications of cirrhosis and portal hypertension, including primary liver cancers. Approaches to accomplish these objectives are similar to those used in other chronic liver diseases and are covered elsewhere in the textbook (Chaps. 365 and 111).

At present, there are no FDA-approved therapies for the treatment of NAFLD. Thus, the current approach to NAFLD management focuses on treatment to improve the risk factors for NASH (i.e., obesity, insulin resistance, metabolic syndrome, dyslipidemia). Based on our understanding of the natural history of NAFLD, only patients with NASH or those with features of hepatic fibrosis on liver biopsy are considered currently for targeted pharmacologic therapies. This approach may change as our understanding of disease pathophysiology improves and potential targets of therapy evolve.

Diet and Exercise Lifestyle changes and dietary modification are the foundation for NAFLD treatment. Many studies indicate that lifestyle modification can improve serum aminotransferases and hepatic steatosis, with loss of at least 3–5% of body weight improving steatosis, but greater weight loss (up to 10%) necessary to improve steatohepatitis. The benefits of different dietary macronutrient contents (e.g., low-carbohydrate vs low-fat diets, saturated vs unsaturated fat diets) and different intensities of calorie restriction appear to be comparable. In adults with NAFLD, exercise regimens that improve fitness may be sufficient to reduce hepatic steatosis, but their impact on other aspects of liver histology remains unknown. Unfortunately, most NAFLD patients are unable to achieve sustained weight loss. Although pharmacologic therapies such as orlistat, topiramate, and phentermine to facilitate weight loss are available, their role in the treatment of NAFLD remains experimental.

Pharmacologic Therapies Several drug therapies have been tried in both research and clinical settings. No agent has yet been approved by the FDA for the treatment of NAFLD. Hence, this remains an area of active research. Because NAFLD is strongly associated with the metabolic syndrome and type 2 diabetes (Chaps. 417 and 418), the efficacy of various insulin-sensitizing agents has been examined. *Metformin*, an agent that mainly improves hepatic insulin sensitivity, has been evaluated in several small, open-label studies in adults and a recent larger, prospectively randomized trial in children (dubbed the TONIC study). Although several of the adult NASH studies suggested improvements in aminotransferases and/or liver histology, metformin did not improve liver histology in the TONIC study of children with NASH. Thus, it is not currently recommended as a treatment for NASH. Uncontrolled open-label studies have also investigated *thiazolidinediones (pioglitazone and rosiglitazone)* in adults with NASH. This class of drugs is known to improve systemic insulin resistance. Both pioglitazone and rosiglitazone reduced aminotransferases and improved some of the histologic features of NASH in small, uncontrolled studies. A large, National Institutes of Health–sponsored, randomized placebo-controlled clinical trial, the PIVENs Study (Pioglitazone vs Vitamin E vs Placebo for the Treatment of 247 Nondiabetic Adults with NASH), demonstrated that resolution of histologic NASH occurred more often in subjects treated with pioglitazone (30 mg/d) than with placebo for 18 months (47 vs 21%, p = .001). However, many subjects in the pioglitazone group gained weight, and liver fibrosis did not improve. Also, it should be noted that the long-term safety and efficacy of thiazolidinediones in patients with NASH has not been established. Five-year follow-up of subjects treated with rosiglitazone demonstrated no reduction in liver fibrosis, and rosiglitazone has been associated with increased long-term risk for cardiovascular mortality. Hence, it is not recommended as a treatment for NAFLD. Pioglitazone may be safer because in a recent large meta-analysis it was associated with reduced overall morality, myocardial infarction, and stroke. However, caution must be exercised when considering its use in patients with impaired myocardial function.

Antioxidants have also been evaluated for the treatment of NAFLD because oxidant stress is thought to contribute to the pathogenesis of NASH. *Vitamin E*, an inexpensive yet potent antioxidant, has been examined in several small pediatric and adult studies with varying results. In all of those studies, vitamin E was well tolerated, and most showed modest improvements in aminotransferase levels, radiographic features of hepatic steatosis, and/or histologic features of NASH. Vitamin E (800 IU/d) was also compared to placebo in the PIVENs and TONIC studies. In PIVENs, vitamin E was the only agent that achieved the predetermined primary endpoint (i.e., improvement in steatohepatitis, lobular inflammation, and steatosis score, without an increase in the fibrosis score). This endpoint was met in 43% of patients in the vitamin E group (p = .001 vs placebo), 34% in the pioglitazone group (p = .04 vs placebo), and 19% in the placebo group. Vitamin E also improved NASH histology in pediatric patients with NASH (TONIC trial). However, a recent population-based study suggested that chronic vitamin E therapy may increase the risk for cardiovascular mortality. Thus, vitamin E should only be considered as a first-line pharmacotherapy for nondiabetic NASH patients. Also, given its potentially negative effects on cardiovascular health, caution should be exercised until the risk-to-benefit ratio and long-term therapeutic efficacy of vitamin E are better defined. Ursodeoxycholic acid (a bile acid that improves certain cholestatic liver diseases) and *betaine* (metabolite of choline that raises SAM levels and decreases cellular oxidative damage) offer no histologic benefit over placebo in patients with NASH. Experimental evidence to support the use of *omega-3 fatty acids* in NAFLD exists; however, a recent large, multicenter, placebo-controlled study failed to demonstrate a histologic benefit. Other pharmacotherapies are also being evaluated in NAFLD (e.g., *probiotics, farnesoid X receptor agonists, anticytokine agents, glucagon-like peptide agonists, dipeptidyl IV antagonists*); however, sufficient data do not yet exist to justify their use as NASH treatments in standard clinical practice.

Statins are an important class of agents to treat dyslipidemia and decrease cardiovascular risk. There is no evidence to suggest that statins cause liver failure in patients with any chronic liver disease, including NAFLD. The incidence of liver enzyme elevations in NAFLD patients taking statins is also no different than that of healthy controls or patients with other chronic liver diseases. Moreover, several studies have suggested that statins may improve aminotransferases and histology in patients with NASH. Yet, there is continued reluctance to use statins in patients with NAFLD. The lack of evidence that statins harm the liver in NAFLD patients, combined with the increase risk for cardiovascular morbidity and mortality in NAFLD patients, warrants the use of statins to treat dyslipidemia in patients with NAFLD/NASH.

Bariatric Surgery Although interest in bariatric surgery as a treatment for NAFLD exists, a recently published Cochrane review concluded that lack of randomized clinical trials or adequate clinical studies prevents definitive assessment of benefits and harms of bariatric surgery as a treatment for NASH. Most studies of bariatric surgery have shown that bariatric surgery is generally safe in individuals with well-compensated chronic liver disease and improves hepatic steatosis and necroinflammation (i.e., features of NAFLD/NASH); however, effects on hepatic fibrosis have been variable. Concern lingers because some of the largest prospective studies suggest that hepatic fibrosis might progress after bariatric surgery. Thus, the Cochrane review deemed it premature to recommend bariatric surgery as a primary treatment for NASH. There is also general agreement that patients with NAFLD-related cirrhosis and portal hypertension should be excluded as candidates for bariatric surgery. However, given growing evidence for the benefits of bariatric surgery on metabolic syndrome complications in individuals with refractory obesity, it is not contraindicated in otherwise eligible patients with NAFLD or NASH.

Liver Transplantation Patients with NAFLD in whom end-stage liver disease develops should be evaluated for liver transplantation (Chap. 368). The outcomes of liver transplantation in well-selected patients with NAFLD are generally good, but comorbid medical conditions associated with NAFLD, such as diabetes mellitus, obesity, and cardiovascular disease, often limit transplant candidacy. NAFLD may recur after liver transplantation. The risk factors for recurrent or de novo NAFLD after liver transplantation are multifactorial and include hypertriglyceridemia, obesity, diabetes mellitus, and immunosuppressive therapies, particularly glucocorticoids.

GLOBAL HEALTH CONSIDERATIONS

The epidemic of obesity is now a global and accelerating phenomenon. Worldwide, there are over 1 billion overweight adults, of whom at least 300 million are obese. In the wake of the obesity epidemic follow numerous comorbidities, including NAFLD. NAFLD is the most common liver disease identified in Western countries and the fastest rising form of chronic liver disease worldwide. Present understanding of NAFLD natural history is based mainly on studies in whites who became overweight/obese and developed the metabolic syndrome in adulthood. The impact of the global childhood obesity epidemic on NAFLD pathogenesis/progression is unknown. Emerging evidence demonstrates that advanced NAFLD, including cirrhosis and primary liver cancer, can occur in children, prompting concerns that childhood-onset NAFLD might follow a more aggressive course than typical adult-acquired NAFLD. Some of the most populated parts of the world are in the midst of industrial revolutions, and certain environmental pollutants seem to exacerbate NAFLD. Some studies also suggest that the risk for NASH and NAFLD-related cirrhosis may be higher in certain ethnic groups such as Asians, certain Hispanics, and Native Americans and lower in others such as African Americans, compared with whites. Although all of these variables confound efforts to predict the net impact of this obesity-related liver disease on global health, it seems likely that NAFLD will remain a major cause of chronic liver disease worldwide for the foreseeable future.

365 Cirrhosis and Its Complications

Bruce R. Bacon

Cirrhosis is a condition that is defined histopathologically and has a variety of clinical manifestations and complications, some of which can be life-threatening. In the past, it has been thought that cirrhosis was never reversible; however, it has become apparent that when the underlying insult that has caused the cirrhosis has been removed, there can be reversal of fibrosis. This is most apparent with the successful treatment of chronic hepatitis C; however, reversal of fibrosis is also seen in patients with hemochromatosis who have been successfully treated and in patients with alcoholic liver disease who have discontinued alcohol use.

Regardless of the cause of cirrhosis, the pathologic features consist of the development of fibrosis to the point that there is architectural distortion with the formation of regenerative nodules. This results in a decrease in hepatocellular mass, and thus function, and an alteration of blood flow. The induction of fibrosis occurs with activation of hepatic stellate cells, resulting in the formation of increased amounts of collagen and other components of the extracellular matrix.

Clinical features of cirrhosis are the result of pathologic changes and mirror the severity of the liver disease. Most hepatic pathologists provide an assessment of grading and staging when evaluating liver biopsy samples. These grading and staging schemes vary between disease states and have been developed for most conditions, including chronic viral hepatitis, nonalcoholic fatty liver disease, and primary biliary cirrhosis. Advanced fibrosis usually includes bridging fibrosis with nodularity designated as stage 3 and cirrhosis designated as stage 4. Patients who have cirrhosis have varying degrees of compensated liver function, and clinicians need to differentiate between those who have stable, compensated cirrhosis and those who have decompensated cirrhosis. Patients who have developed complications of their liver disease and have become decompensated should be considered for liver transplantation. Many of the complications of cirrhosis will require specific therapy. *Portal hypertension* is a significant complicating feature of decompensated cirrhosis and is responsible for the development of ascites and bleeding from esophagogastric varices, two complications that signify decompensated cirrhosis. Loss of hepatocellular function results in jaundice, coagulation disorders, and hypoalbuminemia and contributes to the causes of portosystemic encephalopathy. The complications of cirrhosis are basically the same regardless of the etiology. Nonetheless, it is useful to classify patients by the cause of their liver disease (Table 365-1); patients can be divided into broad groups with alcoholic cirrhosis, cirrhosis due to chronic viral hepatitis, biliary cirrhosis, and other, less common causes such as cardiac cirrhosis, cryptogenic cirrhosis, and other miscellaneous causes.

ALCOHOLIC CIRRHOSIS

Excessive chronic alcohol use can cause several different types of chronic liver disease, including alcoholic fatty liver, alcoholic hepatitis, and alcoholic cirrhosis. Furthermore, use of excessive alcohol can contribute to liver damage in patients with other liver diseases, such as hepatitis C, hemochromatosis, and fatty liver disease related to obesity. Chronic alcohol use can produce fibrosis in the absence of accompanying inflammation and/or necrosis. Fibrosis can be centrilobular, pericellular, or periportal. When fibrosis reaches a certain degree, there is disruption of the normal liver architecture and replacement of liver cells by regenerative nodules. In alcoholic cirrhosis, the nodules are usually <3 mm in diameter; this form of cirrhosis is referred to as *micronodular*. With cessation of alcohol use, larger nodules may form, resulting in a mixed micronodular and macronodular cirrhosis.

TABLE 365-1 CAUSES OF CIRRHOSIS

Alcoholism	Cardiac cirrhosis
Chronic viral hepatitis	Inherited metabolic liver disease
Hepatitis B	Hemochromatosis
Hepatitis C	Wilson's disease
Autoimmune hepatitis	α_1 Antitrypsin deficiency
Nonalcoholic steatohepatitis	Cystic fibrosis
Biliary cirrhosis	Cryptogenic cirrhosis
Primary biliary cirrhosis	
Primary sclerosing cholangitis	
Autoimmune cholangiopathy	

Pathogenesis Alcohol is the most commonly used drug in the United States, and more than two-thirds of adults drink alcohol each year. Thirty percent have had a binge within the past month, and over 7% of adults regularly consume more than two drinks per day. Unfortunately, more than 14 million adults in the United States meet the diagnostic criteria for alcohol abuse or dependence. In the United States, chronic liver disease is the tenth most common cause of death in adults, and alcoholic cirrhosis accounts for approximately 40% of deaths due to cirrhosis.

Ethanol is mainly absorbed by the small intestine and, to a lesser degree, through the stomach. Gastric alcohol dehydrogenase (ADH) initiates alcohol metabolism. Three enzyme systems account for metabolism of alcohol in the liver. These include cytosolic ADH, the microsomal ethanol oxidizing system (MEOS), and peroxisomal catalase. The majority of ethanol oxidation occurs via ADH to form acetaldehyde, which is a highly reactive molecule that may have multiple effects. Ultimately, acetaldehyde is metabolized to acetate by aldehyde dehydrogenase (ALDH). Intake of ethanol increases intracellular accumulation of triglycerides by increasing fatty acid uptake and by reducing fatty acid oxidation and lipoprotein secretion. Protein synthesis, glycosylation, and secretion are impaired. Oxidative damage to hepatocyte membranes occurs due to the formation of reactive oxygen species; acetaldehyde is a highly reactive molecule that combines with proteins to form protein-acetaldehyde adducts. These adducts may interfere with specific enzyme activities, including microtubular formation and hepatic protein trafficking. With acetaldehyde-mediated hepatocyte damage, certain reactive oxygen species can result in Kupffer cell activation. As a result, profibrogenic cytokines are produced that initiate and perpetuate stellate cell activation, with the resultant production of excess collagen and extracellular matrix. Connective tissue appears in both periportal and pericentral zones and eventually connects portal triads with central veins forming regenerative nodules. Hepatocyte loss occurs, and with increased collagen production and deposition, together with continuing hepatocyte destruction, the liver contracts and shrinks in size. This process generally takes from years to decades to occur and requires repeated insults.

Clinical Features The diagnosis of alcoholic liver disease requires an accurate history regarding both amount and duration of alcohol consumption. Patients with alcoholic liver disease can present with nonspecific symptoms such as vague right upper quadrant abdominal pain, fever, nausea and vomiting, diarrhea, anorexia, and malaise. Alternatively, they may present with more specific complications of chronic liver disease, including ascites, edema, or upper gastrointestinal (GI) hemorrhage. Many cases present incidentally at the time of autopsy or elective surgery. Other clinical manifestations include the development of jaundice or encephalopathy. The abrupt onset of any of these complications may be the first event prompting the patient to seek medical attention. Other patients may be identified in the course of an evaluation of routine laboratory studies that are found to be abnormal. On physical examination, the liver and spleen may be enlarged, with the liver edge being firm and nodular. Other frequent findings include scleral icterus, palmar erythema (Fig. 365-1), spider angiomas (Fig. 365-2), parotid gland enlargement, digital clubbing, muscle wasting, or the development of edema and ascites. Men may have decreased body hair and gynecomastia as well as testicular atrophy, which may be a consequence of hormonal abnormalities or a direct toxic effect of alcohol on the testes. In women with advanced

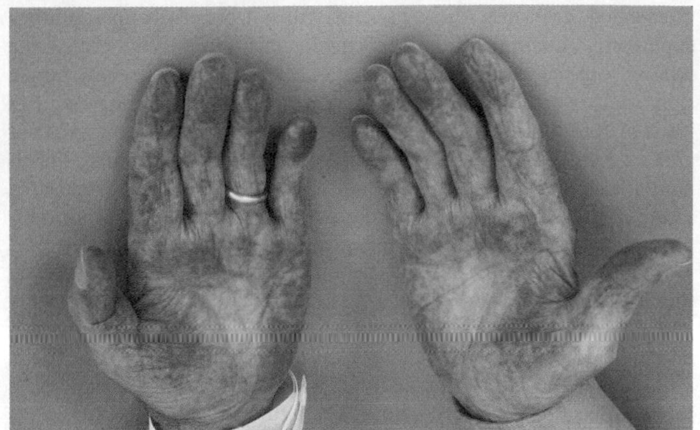

FIGURE 365-1 Palmar erythema. This figure shows palmar erythema in a patient with alcoholic cirrhosis. The erythema is peripheral over the palm with central pallor.

alcoholic cirrhosis, menstrual irregularities usually occur, and some women may be amenorrheic. These changes are often reversible following cessation of alcohol.

Laboratory tests may be completely normal in patients with early compensated alcoholic cirrhosis. Alternatively, in advanced liver disease, many abnormalities usually are present. Patients may be anemic either from chronic GI blood loss, nutritional deficiencies, or hypersplenism related to portal hypertension, or as a direct suppressive effect of alcohol on the bone marrow. A unique form of hemolytic anemia (with spur cells and acanthocytes) called *Zieve's syndrome* can occur in patients with severe alcoholic hepatitis. Platelet counts are often reduced early in the disease, reflective of portal hypertension with hypersplenism. Serum total bilirubin can be normal or elevated with advanced disease. Direct bilirubin is frequently mildly elevated in patients with a normal total bilirubin, but the abnormality typically progresses as the disease worsens. Prothrombin times are often prolonged and usually do not respond to administration of parenteral vitamin K. Serum sodium levels are usually normal unless patients have ascites and then can be depressed, largely due to ingestion of excess free water. Serum alanine and aspartate aminotransferases (ALT, AST) are typically elevated, particularly in patients who continue to drink, with AST levels being higher than ALT levels, usually by a 2:1 ratio.

Diagnosis Patients who have any of the above-mentioned clinical features, physical examination findings, or laboratory studies should be considered to have alcoholic liver disease. The diagnosis, however, requires accurate knowledge that the patient is continuing to use and abuse alcohol. Furthermore, other forms of chronic liver disease (e.g., chronic viral hepatitis or metabolic or autoimmune liver diseases) must be considered or ruled out, or if present, an estimate of relative causality along with the alcohol use should be determined. Liver biopsy can be helpful to confirm a diagnosis, but generally when patients present with alcoholic hepatitis and are still drinking, liver biopsy is withheld until abstinence has been maintained for at least 6 months to determine residual, nonreversible disease.

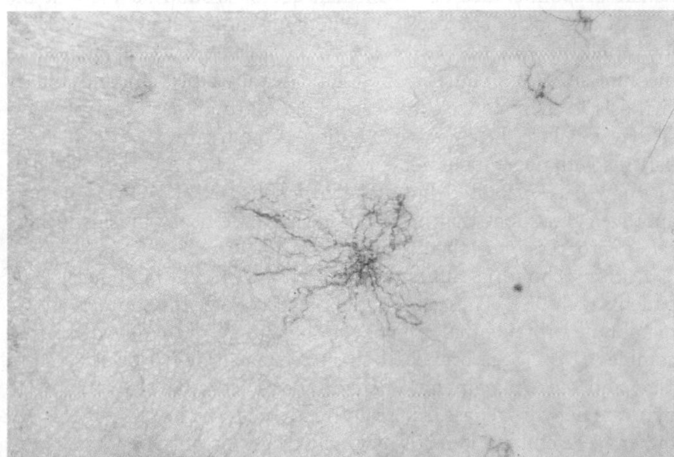

FIGURE 365-2 Spider angioma. This figure shows a spider angioma in a patient with hepatitis C cirrhosis. With release of central compression, the arteriole fills from the center and spreads out peripherally.

In patients who have had complications of cirrhosis and who continue to drink, there is a <50% 5-year survival. In contrast, in patients who are able to remain abstinent, the prognosis is significantly improved. In patients with advanced liver disease, the prognosis remains poor; however, in individuals who are able to remain abstinent, liver transplantation is a viable option.

TREATMENT ALCOHOLIC CIRRHOSIS

Abstinence is the cornerstone of therapy for patients with alcoholic liver disease. In addition, patients require good nutrition and long-term medical supervision to manage underlying complications that may develop. Complications such as the development of ascites and edema, variceal hemorrhage, or portosystemic encephalopathy all require specific management and treatment. Glucocorticoids are occasionally used in patients with severe alcoholic hepatitis in the absence of infection. Survival has been shown to improve in certain studies. Treatment is restricted to patients with a discriminant function (DF) value of >32. The DF is calculated as the serum total bilirubin plus the difference in the patient's prothrombin time compared to control (in seconds) multiplied by 4.6. In patients for whom this value is >32, there is improved survival at 28 days with the use of glucocorticoids.

Other therapies that have been used include oral pentoxifylline, which decreases the production of tumor necrosis factor α (TNF-α) and other proinflammatory cytokines. In contrast to glucocorticoids, with which complications can occur, pentoxifylline is relatively easy to administer and has few, if any, side effects. A variety of nutritional therapies have been tried with either parenteral or enteral feedings; however, it is unclear whether any of these modalities have significantly improved survival.

Recent studies have used parenterally administered inhibitors of TNF-α such as infliximab or etanercept. Early results have shown no adverse events; however, there was no clear-cut improvement in survival. Anabolic steroids, propylthiouracil, antioxidants, colchicine, and penicillamine have all been used but do not show clear-cut benefits and are not recommended.

As mentioned above, the cornerstone to treatment is cessation of alcohol use. Recent experience with medications that reduce craving for alcohol, such as acamprosate calcium, has been favorable. Patients may take other necessary medications even in the presence of cirrhosis. Acetaminophen use is often discouraged in patients with liver disease; however, if no more than 2 g of acetaminophen per day are consumed, there generally are no problems.

CIRRHOSIS DUE TO CHRONIC VIRAL HEPATITIS B OR C

Of patients exposed to the hepatitis C virus (HCV), approximately 80% develop chronic hepatitis C, and of those, about 20–30% will develop cirrhosis over 20–30 years. Many of these patients have had concomitant alcohol use, and the true incidence of cirrhosis due to hepatitis C alone is unknown. Nonetheless, this represents a significant number of patients. It is expected that an even higher percentage will go on to develop cirrhosis over longer periods of time. In the United States, approximately 5 to 6 million people have been exposed to HCV, with about 4 million who are chronically viremic. Worldwide, about 170 million individuals have hepatitis C, with some areas of the world (e.g., Egypt) having up to 15% of the population infected. HCV is a noncytopathic virus, and liver damage is probably immune-mediated. Progression of liver disease due to chronic hepatitis C is characterized by portal-based fibrosis with bridging fibrosis and nodularity developing, ultimately culminating in the development of cirrhosis. In cirrhosis due to chronic hepatitis C, the liver is small and shrunken with characteristic features of a mixed micro- and macronodular cirrhosis seen on liver biopsy. In addition to the increased fibrosis that is seen in cirrhosis due to hepatitis C, an inflammatory infiltrate is found in portal areas with interface hepatitis and occasionally some lobular hepatocellular injury and inflammation. In patients with HCV genotype 3, steatosis is often present.

Similar findings are seen in patients with cirrhosis due to chronic hepatitis B. Of adult patients exposed to hepatitis B, about 5% develop chronic hepatitis B, and about 20% of those patients will go on to develop cirrhosis. Special stains for hepatitis B core (HBc) and hepatitis B surface (HBs) antigen will be positive, and ground-glass hepatocytes signifying hepatitis B surface antigen (HBsAg) may be present. In the United States, there are about 2 million carriers of hepatitis B, whereas in other parts of the world where hepatitis B virus (HBV) is endemic (i.e., Asia, Southeast Asia, sub-Saharan Africa), up to 15% of the population may be infected, having acquired the infection vertically at the time of birth. Thus, over 300–400 million individuals are thought to have hepatitis B worldwide. Approximately 25% of these individuals may ultimately develop cirrhosis.

Clinical Features and Diagnosis Patients with cirrhosis due to either chronic hepatitis C or B can present with the usual symptoms and signs of chronic liver disease. Fatigue, malaise, vague right upper quadrant pain, and laboratory abnormalities are frequent presenting features. Diagnosis requires a thorough laboratory evaluation, including quantitative HCV RNA testing and analysis for HCV genotype, or hepatitis B serologies to include HBsAg, anti-HBs, HBeAg (hepatitis B e antigen), anti-HBe, and quantitative HBV DNA levels.

TREATMENT CIRRHOSIS DUE TO CHRONIC VIRAL HEPATITIS B OR C

Management of complications of cirrhosis revolves around specific therapy for treatment of whatever complications occur (e.g., esophageal variceal hemorrhage, development of ascites and edema, or encephalopathy). In patients with chronic hepatitis B, numerous studies have shown beneficial effects of antiviral therapy, which is effective at viral suppression, as evidenced by reducing aminotransferase levels and HBV DNA levels, and improving histology by reducing inflammation and fibrosis. Several clinical trials and case series have demonstrated that patients with decompensated liver disease can become compensated with the use of antiviral therapy directed against hepatitis B. Currently available therapy includes lamivudine, adefovir, telbivudine, entecavir, and tenofovir. Interferon α can also be used for treating hepatitis B, but it should not be used in cirrhotics.

Treatment of patients with cirrhosis due to hepatitis C is a little more difficult because the side effects of pegylated interferon and ribavirin therapy are often difficult to manage. Dose-limiting cytopenias (platelets, white blood cells, red blood cells) or severe side effects can result in discontinuation of treatment. Nonetheless, if patients can tolerate treatment, and if it is successful, the benefit is great and disease progression is reduced. Recent studies have shown that if platelets are <100,000, albumin is <3.5 g/dL, and Model for End-Stage Liver Disease (MELD) score is >10, the risk of severe complications of interferon-based antiviral therapy is significant. Recent approval of Direct Acting Antivirals (DAAs) has led to improved efficacy of treatment with regimens that are safe and well tolerated.

CIRRHOSIS FROM AUTOIMMUNE HEPATITIS AND NONALCOHOLIC FATTY LIVER DISEASE

Other causes of posthepatitic cirrhosis include autoimmune hepatitis and cirrhosis due to nonalcoholic steatohepatitis. Many patients with autoimmune hepatitis (AIH) present with cirrhosis that is already established. Typically, these patients will not benefit from immunosuppressive therapy with glucocorticoids or azathioprine because the AIH is "burned out." In this situation, liver biopsy does not show a significant inflammatory infiltrate. Diagnosis in this setting requires positive autoimmune markers such as antinuclear antibody (ANA) or anti-smooth-muscle antibody (ASMA). When patients with AIH present with cirrhosis and active inflammation accompanied by elevated liver enzymes, there can be considerable benefit from the use of immunosuppressive therapy.

Patients with nonalcoholic steatohepatitis are increasingly being found to have progressed to cirrhosis. With the epidemic of obesity that continues in Western countries, more and more patients are identified with nonalcoholic fatty liver disease (Chap. 364). Of these, a significant subset has nonalcoholic steatohepatitis and can progress to increased fibrosis and cirrhosis. Over the past several years, it has been increasingly recognized that many patients who were thought to have cryptogenic cirrhosis in fact have nonalcoholic steatohepatitis. As their cirrhosis progresses, they become catabolic and then lose the telltale signs of steatosis seen on biopsy. Management of complications of cirrhosis due to either AIH or nonalcoholic steatohepatitis is similar to that for other forms of cirrhosis.

BILIARY CIRRHOSIS

Biliary cirrhosis has pathologic features that are different from either alcoholic cirrhosis or posthepatitic cirrhosis, yet the manifestations of end-stage liver disease are the same. Cholestatic liver disease may result from necroinflammatory lesions, congenital or metabolic processes, or external bile duct compression. Thus, two broad categories reflect the anatomic sites of abnormal bile retention: *intrahepatic* and *extrahepatic*. The distinction is important for obvious therapeutic reasons. Extrahepatic obstruction may benefit from surgical or endoscopic biliary tract decompression, whereas intrahepatic cholestatic processes will not improve with such interventions and require a different approach.

The major causes of chronic cholestatic syndromes are primary biliary cirrhosis (PBC), autoimmune cholangitis (AIC), primary sclerosing cholangitis (PSC), and idiopathic adulthood ductopenia. These syndromes are usually clinically distinguished from each other by antibody testing, cholangiographic findings, and clinical presentation. However, they all share the histopathologic features of chronic cholestasis, such as cholate stasis; copper deposition; xanthomatous transformation of hepatocytes; and irregular, so-called biliary fibrosis. In addition, there may be chronic portal inflammation, interface activity, and chronic lobular inflammation. Ductopenia is a result of this progressive disease as patients develop cirrhosis.

PRIMARY BILIARY CIRRHOSIS

PBC is seen in about 100–200 individuals per million, with a strong female preponderance and a median age of around 50 years at the time of diagnosis. The cause of PBC is unknown; it is characterized by portal inflammation and necrosis of cholangiocytes in small- and medium-sized bile ducts. Cholestatic features prevail, and biliary cirrhosis is characterized by an elevated bilirubin level and progressive liver failure. Liver transplantation is the treatment of choice for patients with decompensated cirrhosis due to PBC. A variety of therapies have been proposed, but ursodeoxycholic acid (UDCA) is the only approved treatment that has some degree of efficacy by slowing the rate of progression of the disease.

Antimitochondrial antibodies (AMA) are present in about 90% of patients with PBC. These autoantibodies recognize intermitochondrial membrane proteins that are enzymes of the pyruvate dehydrogenase complex (PDC), the branched-chain 2-oxoacid dehydrogenase complex, and the 2-oxogluterate dehydrogenase complex. Most relate to pyruvate dehydrogenase. These autoantibodies are not pathogenic but rather are useful markers for making a diagnosis of PBC.

Pathology Histopathologic analyses of liver biopsies of patients with PBC have resulted in identifying four distinct stages of the disease as it progresses. The earliest lesion is termed *chronic nonsuppurative* *destructive cholangitis* and is a necrotizing inflammatory process of the portal tracts. Medium and small bile ducts are infiltrated with lymphocytes and undergo duct destruction. Mild fibrosis and sometimes bile stasis can occur. With progression, the inflammatory infiltrate becomes less prominent, but the number of bile ducts is reduced and there is proliferation of smaller bile ductules. Increased fibrosis ensues with the expansion of periportal fibrosis to bridging fibrosis. Finally, cirrhosis, which may be micronodular or macronodular, develops.

Clinical Features Currently, most patients with PBC are diagnosed well before the end-stage manifestations of the disease are present, and, as such, most patients are actually asymptomatic. When symptoms are present, they most prominently include a significant degree of fatigue out of proportion to what would be expected for either the severity of the liver disease or the age of the patient. Pruritus is seen in approximately 50% of patients at the time of diagnosis, and it can be debilitating. It might be intermittent and usually is most bothersome in the evening. In some patients, pruritus can develop toward the end of pregnancy, and there are examples of patients having been diagnosed with cholestasis of pregnancy rather than PBC. Pruritus that presents prior to the development of jaundice indicates severe disease and a poor prognosis.

Physical examination can show jaundice and other complications of chronic liver disease, including hepatomegaly, splenomegaly, ascites, and edema. Other features that are unique to PBC include hyperpigmentation, xanthelasma, and xanthomata, which are related to the altered cholesterol metabolism seen in this disease. Hyperpigmentation is evident on the trunk and the arms and is seen in areas of exfoliation and lichenification associated with progressive scratching related to the pruritus. Bone pain resulting from osteopenia or osteoporosis is occasionally seen at the time of diagnosis.

Laboratory Findings Laboratory findings in PBC show cholestatic liver enzyme abnormalities with an elevation in γ-glutamyl transpeptidase and alkaline phosphatase (ALP) along with mild elevations in aminotransferases (ALT and AST). Immunoglobulins, particularly IgM, are typically increased. Hyperbilirubinemia usually is seen once cirrhosis has developed. Thrombocytopenia, leukopenia, and anemia may be seen in patients with portal hypertension and hypersplenism. Liver biopsy shows characteristic features as described above and should be evident to any experienced hepatopathologist. Up to 10% of patients with characteristic PBC will have features of AIH as well and are defined as having "overlap" syndrome. These patients are usually treated as PBC patients and may progress to cirrhosis with the same frequency as typical PBC patients. Some patients require immunosuppressive medications as well.

Diagnosis PBC should be considered in patients with chronic cholestatic liver enzyme abnormalities. It is most often seen in middle-aged women. AMA testing may be negative, and it should be remembered that as many as 10% of patients with PBC may be AMA-negative. Liver biopsy is most important in this setting of AMA-negative PBC. In patients who are AMA-negative with cholestatic liver enzymes, PSC should be ruled out by way of cholangiography.

TREATMENT PRIMARY BILIARY CIRRHOSIS

Treatment of the typical manifestations of cirrhosis are no different for PBC than for other forms of cirrhosis. UDCA has been shown to improve both biochemical and histologic features of the disease. Improvement is greatest when therapy is initiated early; the likelihood of significant improvement with UDCA is low in patients with PBC who present with manifestations of cirrhosis. UDCA is given in doses of 13–15 mg/kg per day; the medication is usually well-tolerated, although some patients have worsening pruritus with initiation of therapy. A small proportion of patients may have diarrhea or headache as a side effect of the drug. UDCA has been shown to slow the rate of progression of PBC, but it does not reverse or cure the disease. Patients with PBC require long-term follow-up by a physician experienced with the disease. Certain patients may need to be considered for liver transplantation should their liver disease decompensate.

The main symptoms of PBC are fatigue and pruritus, and symptom management is important. Several therapies have been tried for treatment of fatigue, but none of them have been successful; frequent naps should be encouraged. Pruritus is treated with antihistamines, narcotic receptor antagonists (naltrexone), and rifampin. Cholestyramine, a bile salt–sequestering agent, has been helpful in some patients but is somewhat tedious and difficult to take. Plasmapheresis has been used rarely in patients with severe intractable pruritus. There is an increased incidence of osteopenia and osteoporosis in patients with cholestatic liver disease, and bone density testing should be performed. Treatment with a bisphosphonate should be instituted when bone disease is identified.

PRIMARY SCLEROSING CHOLANGITIS

As in PBC, the cause of PSC remains unknown. PSC is a chronic cholestatic syndrome that is characterized by diffuse inflammation and fibrosis involving the entire biliary tree, resulting in chronic cholestasis. This pathologic process ultimately results in obliteration of both the intra- and extrahepatic biliary tree, leading to biliary cirrhosis, portal hypertension, and liver failure. The cause of PSC remains unknown despite extensive investigation into various mechanisms related to bacterial and viral infections, toxins, genetic predisposition, and immunologic mechanisms, all of which have been postulated to contribute to the pathogenesis and progression of this syndrome.

Pathologic changes that can occur in PSC show bile duct proliferation as well as ductopenia and fibrous cholangitis (pericholangitis). Often, liver biopsy changes in PSC are not pathognomonic, and establishing the diagnosis of PSC must involve imaging of the biliary tree. Periductal fibrosis is occasionally seen on biopsy specimens and can be quite helpful in making the diagnosis. As the disease progresses, biliary cirrhosis is the final, end-stage manifestation of PSC.

Clinical Features The usual clinical features of PSC are those found in cholestatic liver disease, with fatigue, pruritus, steatorrhea, deficiencies of fat-soluble vitamins, and the associated consequences. As in PBC, the fatigue is profound and nonspecific. Pruritus can often be debilitating and is related to the cholestasis. The severity of pruritus does not correlate with the severity of the disease. Metabolic bone disease, as seen in PBC, can occur with PSC and should be treated (see above).

Laboratory Findings Patients with PSC typically are identified in the course of an evaluation of abnormal liver enzymes. Most patients have at least a twofold increase in ALP and may have elevated aminotransferases as well. Albumin levels may be decreased, and prothrombin times are prolonged in a substantial proportion of patients at the time of diagnosis. Some degree of correction of a prolonged prothrombin time may occur with parenteral vitamin K. A small subset of patients have aminotransferase elevations greater than five times the upper limit of normal and may have features of AIH on biopsy. These individuals are thought to have an overlap syndrome between PSC and AIH. Autoantibodies are frequently positive in patients with the overlap syndrome but are typically negative in patients who only have PSC. One autoantibody, the perinuclear antineutrophil cytoplasmic antibody (p-ANCA), is positive in about 65% of patients with PSC. Over 50% of patients with PSC also have ulcerative colitis (UC); accordingly, once a diagnosis of PSC is established, colonoscopy should be performed to look for evidence of UC.

Diagnosis The definitive diagnosis of PSC requires cholangiographic imaging. Over the last several years, magnetic resonance imaging (MRI) with magnetic resonance cholangiopancreatography (MRCP) has been used as the imaging technique of choice for initial evaluation. Once patients are screened in this manner, some investigators feel that endoscopic retrograde cholangiopancreatography (ERCP) should also be performed to be certain whether or not a dominant stricture is present. Typical cholangiographic findings in PSC are multifocal stricturing and beading involving both the intrahepatic and extrahepatic biliary tree. However, although involvement may be of the intrahepatic bile ducts alone or of the extrahepatic bile ducts alone, more commonly, both are involved. These strictures are typically short and with intervening segments of normal or slightly dilated bile ducts that are distributed diffusely, producing the classic beaded appearance. The gallbladder and cystic duct can be involved in up to 15% of cases. Patients with high-grade, diffuse stricturing of the intrahepatic bile ducts have an overall poor prognosis. Gradually, biliary cirrhosis develops, and patients will progress to decompensated liver disease with all the manifestations of ascites, esophageal variceal hemorrhage, and encephalopathy.

TREATMENT PRIMARY SCLEROSING CHOLANGITIS

There is no specific proven treatment for PSC. A recently completed study of high-dose (20 mg/kg per day) UDCA was found to be harmful. Some clinicians use UDCA at "PBC dosages" of 13–15 mg/kg per day with anecdotal improvement. Endoscopic dilatation of dominant strictures can be helpful, but the ultimate treatment is liver transplantation. A dreaded complication of PSC is the development of cholangiocarcinoma, which is a relative contraindication to liver transplantation. Symptoms of pruritus are common, and the approach is as mentioned previously for this problem in patients with PBC (see above).

CARDIAC CIRRHOSIS

Definition Patients with long-standing right-sided congestive heart failure may develop chronic liver injury and cardiac cirrhosis. This is an increasingly uncommon, if not rare, cause of chronic liver disease given the advances made in the care of patients with heart failure.

Etiology and Pathology In the case of long-term right-sided heart failure, there is an elevated venous pressure transmitted via the inferior vena cava and hepatic veins to the sinusoids of the liver, which become dilated and engorged with blood. The liver becomes enlarged and swollen, and with long-term passive congestion and relative ischemia due to poor circulation, centrilobular hepatocytes can become necrotic, leading to pericentral fibrosis. This fibrotic pattern can extend to the periphery of the lobule outward until a unique pattern of fibrosis causing cirrhosis can occur.

Clinical Features Patients typically have signs of congestive heart failure and will manifest an enlarged firm liver on physical examination. ALP levels are characteristically elevated, and aminotransferases may be normal or slightly increased with AST usually higher than ALT. It is unlikely that patients will develop variceal hemorrhage or encephalopathy.

Diagnosis The diagnosis is usually made in someone with clear-cut cardiac disease who has an elevated ALP and an enlarged liver. Liver biopsy shows a pattern of fibrosis that can be recognized by an experienced hepatopathologist. Differentiation from Budd-Chiari syndrome (BCS) can be made by seeing extravasation of red blood cells in BCS, but not in cardiac hepatopathy. Venoocclusive disease can also affect hepatic outflow and has characteristic features on liver biopsy. Venoocclusive disease can be seen under the circumstances of conditioning for bone marrow transplant with radiation and chemotherapy; it can also be seen with the ingestion of certain herbal teas as well as pyrrolizidine alkaloids. This is typically seen in Caribbean countries and rarely in the United States. Treatment is based on management of the underlying cardiac disease.

OTHER TYPES OF CIRRHOSIS

There are several other less common causes of chronic liver disease that can progress to cirrhosis. These include inherited metabolic liver diseases such as hemochromatosis, Wilson's disease, α_1 antitrypsin (α_1AT) deficiency, and cystic fibrosis. For all of these disorders, the manifestations of cirrhosis are similar, with some minor variations, to those seen in other patients with other causes of cirrhosis.

Hemochromatosis is an inherited disorder of iron metabolism that results in a progressive increase in hepatic iron deposition, which, over time, can lead to a portal-based fibrosis progressing to cirrhosis, liver failure, and hepatocellular cancer. While the frequency of hemochromatosis is relatively common, with genetic susceptibility occurring in 1 in 250 individuals, the frequency of end-stage manifestations due to the disease is relatively low, and fewer than 5% of those patients who are genotypically susceptible will go on to develop severe liver disease from hemochromatosis. Diagnosis is made with serum iron studies showing an elevated transferrin saturation and an elevated ferritin level, along with abnormalities identified by *HFE* mutation analysis. Treatment is straightforward, with regular therapeutic phlebotomy.

Wilson's disease is an inherited disorder of copper homeostasis with failure to excrete excess amounts of copper, leading to an accumulation in the liver. This disorder is relatively uncommon, affecting 1 in 30,000 individuals. Wilson's disease typically affects adolescents and young adults. Prompt diagnosis before end-stage manifestations become irreversible can lead to significant clinical improvement. Diagnosis requires determination of ceruloplasmin levels, which are low; 24-h urine copper levels, which are elevated; typical physical examination findings, including Kayser-Fleischer corneal rings; and characteristic liver biopsy findings. Treatment consists of copper-chelating medications.

α_1AT deficiency results from an inherited disorder that causes abnormal folding of the α_1AT protein, resulting in failure of secretion of that protein from the liver. It is unknown how the retained protein leads to liver disease. Patients with α_1AT deficiency at greatest risk for developing chronic liver disease have the ZZ phenotype, but only about 10–20% of such individuals will develop chronic liver disease. Diagnosis is made by determining α_1AT levels and phenotype. Characteristic periodic acid–Schiff (PAS)-positive, diastase-resistant globules are seen on liver biopsy. The only effective treatment is liver transplantation, which is curative.

Cystic fibrosis is an uncommon inherited disorder affecting whites of northern European descent. A biliary-type cirrhosis can occur, and some patients derive benefit from the chronic use of UDCA.

MAJOR COMPLICATIONS OF CIRRHOSIS

The clinical course of patients with advanced cirrhosis is often complicated by a number of important sequelae that can occur regardless of the underlying cause of the liver disease. These include portal hypertension and its consequences of gastroesophageal variceal hemorrhage, splenomegaly, ascites, hepatic encephalopathy, spontaneous bacterial peritonitis (SBP), hepatorenal syndrome, and hepatocellular carcinoma (Table 365-2).

PORTAL HYPERTENSION

Portal hypertension is defined as the elevation of the hepatic venous pressure gradient (HVPG) to >5 mmHg. Portal hypertension is caused by a combination of two simultaneously occurring hemodynamic processes: (1) increased intrahepatic resistance to the passage of blood

TABLE 365-2 COMPLICATIONS OF CIRRHOSIS

Portal hypertension	Coagulopathy
Gastroesophageal varices	Factor deficiency
Portal hypertensive gastropathy	Fibrinolysis
Splenomegaly, hypersplenism	Thrombocytopenia
Ascites	Bone disease
Spontaneous bacterial peritonitis	Osteopenia
Hepatorenal syndrome	Osteoporosis
Type 1	Osteomalacia
Type 2	Hematologic abnormalities
Hepatic encephalopathy	Anemia
Hepatopulmonary syndrome	Hemolysis
Portopulmonary hypertension	Thrombocytopenia
Malnutrition	Neutropenia

flow through the liver due to cirrhosis and regenerative nodules, and (2) increased splanchnic blood flow secondary to vasodilation within the splanchnic vascular bed. Portal hypertension is directly responsible for the two major complications of cirrhosis: variceal hemorrhage and ascites. *Variceal hemorrhage* is an immediate life-threatening problem with a 20–30% mortality rate associated with each episode of bleeding. The portal venous system normally drains blood from the stomach, intestines, spleen, pancreas, and gallbladder, and the portal vein is formed by the confluence of the superior mesenteric and splenic veins. Deoxygenated blood from the small bowel drains into the superior mesenteric vein along with blood from the head of the pancreas, the ascending colon, and part of the transverse colon. Conversely, the splenic vein drains the spleen and the pancreas and is joined by the inferior mesenteric vein, which brings blood from the transverse and descending colon as well as from the superior two-thirds of the rectum. Thus, the portal vein normally receives blood from almost the entire GI tract.

The causes of portal hypertension are usually subcategorized as prehepatic, intrahepatic, and posthepatic (Table 365-3). Prehepatic causes of portal hypertension are those affecting the portal venous system before it enters the liver; they include portal vein thrombosis and splenic vein thrombosis. Posthepatic causes encompass those affecting the hepatic veins and venous drainage to the heart; they include BCS, venoocclusive disease, and chronic right-sided cardiac congestion. Intrahepatic causes account for over 95% of cases of portal hypertension and are represented by the major forms of cirrhosis. Intrahepatic causes of portal hypertension can be further subdivided into presinusoidal, sinusoidal, and postsinusoidal causes. Postsinusoidal causes include venoocclusive disease, whereas presinusoidal causes include congenital hepatic fibrosis and schistosomiasis. Sinusoidal causes are related to cirrhosis from various causes.

Cirrhosis is the most common cause of portal hypertension in the United States, and clinically significant portal hypertension is present in >60% of patients with cirrhosis. Portal vein obstruction may be idiopathic or can occur in association with cirrhosis or with infection, pancreatitis, or abdominal trauma.

Coagulation disorders that can lead to the development of portal vein thrombosis include polycythemia vera; essential thrombocytosis; deficiencies in protein C, protein S, antithrombin 3, and factor V Leiden; and abnormalities in the gene regulating prothrombin production. Some patients may have a subclinical myeloproliferative disorder.

Clinical Features The three primary complications of portal hypertension are gastroesophageal varices with hemorrhage, ascites, and hypersplenism. Thus, patients may present with upper GI bleeding, which, on endoscopy, is found to be due to esophageal or gastric varices; with the development of ascites along with peripheral edema; or with an enlarged spleen with associated reduction in platelets and white blood cells on routine laboratory testing.

TABLE 365-3 CLASSIFICATION OF PORTAL HYPERTENSION

Prehepatic
Portal vein thrombosis
Splenic vein thrombosis
Massive splenomegaly (Banti's syndrome)
Hepatic
Presinusoidal
Schistosomiasis
Congenital hepatic fibrosis
Sinusoidal
Cirrhosis—many causes
Alcoholic hepatitis
Postsinusoidal
Hepatic sinusoidal obstruction (venoocclusive syndrome)
Posthepatic
Budd-Chiari syndrome
Inferior vena caval webs
Cardiac causes
Restrictive cardiomyopathy
Constrictive pericarditis
Severe congestive heart failure

ESOPHAGEAL VARICES Over the last decade, it has become common practice to screen known cirrhotics with endoscopy to look for esophageal varices. Such screening studies have shown that approximately one-third of patients with histologically confirmed cirrhosis have varices. Approximately 5–15% of cirrhotics per year develop varices, and it is estimated that the majority of patients with cirrhosis will develop varices over their lifetimes. Furthermore, it is anticipated that roughly one-third of patients with varices will develop bleeding. Several factors predict the risk of bleeding, including the severity of cirrhosis (Child's class, MELD score); the height of wedged-hepatic vein pressure; the size of the varix; the location of the varix; and certain endoscopic stigmata, including red wale signs, hematocystic spots, diffuse erythema, bluish color, cherry red spots, or white-nipple spots. Patients with tense ascites are also at increased risk for bleeding from varices.

Diagnosis In patients with cirrhosis who are being followed chronically, the development of portal hypertension is usually revealed by the presence of thrombocytopenia, the appearance of an enlarged spleen, or the development of ascites, encephalopathy, and/or esophageal varices with or without bleeding. In previously undiagnosed patients, any of these features should prompt further evaluation to determine the presence of portal hypertension and liver disease. Varices should be identified by endoscopy. Abdominal imaging, either by computed tomography (CT) or MRI, can be helpful in demonstrating a nodular liver and in finding changes of portal hypertension with intraabdominal collateral circulation. If necessary, interventional radiologic procedures can be performed to determine wedged and free hepatic vein pressures that will allow for the calculation of a wedged-to-free gradient, which is equivalent to the portal pressure. The average normal wedged-to-free gradient is 5 mmHg, and patients with a gradient >12 mmHg are at risk for variceal hemorrhage.

TREATMENT VARICEAL HEMORRHAGE

Treatment for variceal hemorrhage as a complication of portal hypertension is divided into two main categories: (1) primary prophylaxis and (2) prevention of rebleeding once there has been an initial variceal hemorrhage. Primary prophylaxis requires routine screening by endoscopy of all patients with cirrhosis. Once varices that are at increased risk for bleeding are identified, primary prophylaxis can be achieved either through nonselective beta blockade or by variceal band ligation. Numerous placebo-controlled clinical trials of either propranolol or nadolol have been reported in the literature. The most rigorous studies were those that only included patients with significantly enlarged varices or with hepatic vein pressure gradients >12 mmHg. Patients treated with beta blockers have a lower risk of variceal hemorrhage than those treated with placebo over 1 and 2 years of follow-up. There is also a decrease in mortality related to variceal hemorrhage. Unfortunately, overall survival was improved in only one study. Further studies have demonstrated that the degree of reduction of portal pressure is a significant feature to determine success of therapy. Therefore, it has been suggested that repeat measurements of hepatic vein pressure gradients may be used to guide pharmacologic therapy; however, this may be cost-prohibitive. Several studies have evaluated variceal band ligation and variceal sclerotherapy as methods for providing primary prophylaxis.

Endoscopic variceal ligation (EVL) has achieved a level of success and comfort with most gastroenterologists who see patients with these complications of portal hypertension. Thus, in patients with cirrhosis who are screened for portal hypertension and are found to have large varices, it is recommended that they receive either beta blockade or primary prophylaxis with EVL.

The approach to patients once they have had a variceal bleed is first to treat the acute bleed, which can be life-threatening, and then to prevent further bleeding. Prevention of further bleeding is usually accomplished with repeated variceal band ligation until varices are obliterated. Treatment of acute bleeding requires both fluid and blood-product replacement as well as prevention of subsequent bleeding with EVL.

The medical management of acute variceal hemorrhage includes the use of vasoconstricting agents, usually somatostatin or octreotide. Vasopressin was used in the past but is no longer commonly used. Balloon tamponade (Sengstaken-Blakemore tube or Minnesota tube) can be used in patients who cannot get endoscopic therapy immediately or who need stabilization prior to endoscopic therapy. Control of bleeding can be achieved in the vast majority of cases; however, bleeding recurs in the majority of patients if definitive endoscopic therapy has not been instituted. Octreotide, a direct splanchnic vasoconstrictor, is given at dosages of 50–100 μg/h by continuous infusion. Endoscopic intervention is used as first-line treatment to control bleeding acutely. Some endoscopists will use variceal injection therapy (sclerotherapy) as initial therapy, particularly when bleeding is vigorous. Variceal band ligation is used to control acute bleeding in over 90% of cases and should be repeated until obliteration of all varices is accomplished. When esophageal varices extend into the proximal stomach, band ligation is less successful. In these situations, when bleeding continues from gastric varices, consideration for a transjugular intrahepatic portosystemic shunt (TIPS) should be made. This technique creates a portosystemic shunt by a percutaneous approach using an expandable metal stent, which is advanced under angiographic guidance to the hepatic veins and then through the substance of the liver to create a direct portocaval shunt. This offers an alternative to surgery for acute decompression of portal hypertension. Encephalopathy can occur in as many as 20% of patients after TIPS and is particularly problematic in elderly patients and in patients with preexisting encephalopathy. TIPS should be reserved for individuals who fail endoscopic or medical management or who are poor surgical risks. TIPS can sometimes be used as a bridge to transplantation. Surgical esophageal transsection is a procedure that is rarely used and generally is associated with a poor outcome.

PREVENTION OF RECURRENT BLEEDING (FIG. 365-3)

Once patients have had an acute bleed and have been managed successfully, attention should be paid to preventing recurrent bleeding. This usually requires repeated variceal band ligation until varices are obliterated. Beta blockade may be of adjunctive benefit in patients who are having recurrent variceal band ligation; however, once varices have been obliterated, the need for beta blockade is lessened. Despite successful variceal obliteration, many patients will still have portal hypertensive gastropathy from which bleeding can occur. Nonselective beta blockade may be helpful to prevent further bleeding from portal hypertensive gastropathy once varices have been obliterated.

Portosystemic shunt surgery is less commonly performed with the advent of TIPS; nonetheless, this procedure should be considered for patients with good hepatic synthetic function who could benefit by having portal decompressive surgery.

SPLENOMEGALY AND HYPERSPLENISM

Congestive splenomegaly is common in patients with portal hypertension. Clinical features include the presence of an enlarged spleen on physical examination and the development of thrombocytopenia and leukopenia in patients who have cirrhosis. Some patients will have fairly significant left-sided and left upper quadrant abdominal pain related to an enlarged and engorged spleen. Splenomegaly itself usually requires no specific treatment, although splenectomy can be successfully performed under very special circumstances.

Hypersplenism with the development of thrombocytopenia is a common feature of patients with cirrhosis and is usually the first indication of portal hypertension.

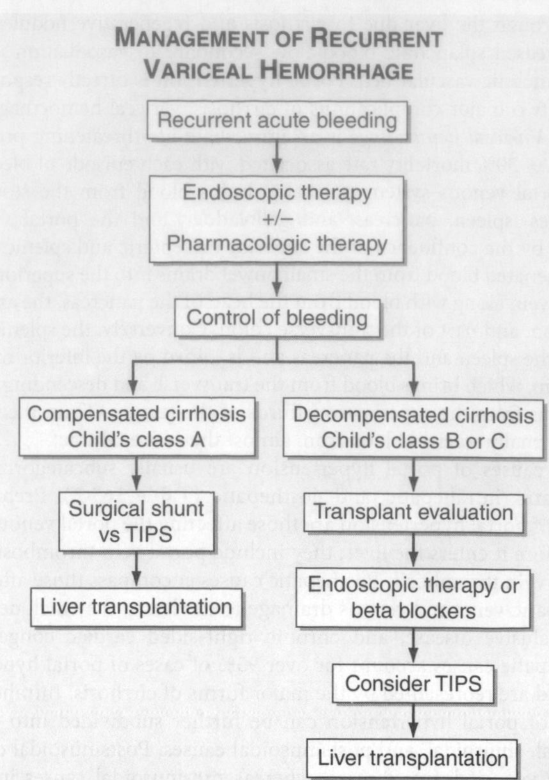

FIGURE 365-3 Management of recurrent variceal hemorrhage. This algorithm describes an approach to management of patients who have recurrent bleeding from esophageal varices. Initial therapy is generally with endoscopic therapy often supplemented by pharmacologic therapy. With control of bleeding, a decision needs to be made as to whether patients should go on to a surgical shunt or TIPS (if they are Child's class A) and be considered for transplant, or if they should have TIPS and be considered for transplant (if they are Child's class B or C). TIPS, transjugular intrahepatic portosystemic shunt.

ASCITES

Definition Ascites is the accumulation of fluid within the peritoneal cavity. Overwhelmingly, the most common cause of ascites is portal hypertension related to cirrhosis; however, clinicians should remember that malignant or infectious causes of ascites can be present as well, and careful differentiation of these other causes are obviously important for patient care.

Pathogenesis The presence of portal hypertension contributes to the development of ascites in patients who have cirrhosis (Fig. 365-4). There is an increase in intrahepatic resistance, causing increased portal pressure, but there is also vasodilation of the splanchnic arterial system, which, in turn, results in an increase in portal venous inflow. Both of these abnormalities result in increased production of splanchnic lymph. Vasodilating factors such as nitric oxide are responsible for the vasodilatory effect. These hemodynamic changes result in sodium retention by causing activation of the renin-angiotensin-aldosterone system with the development of hyperaldosteronism. The renal effects of increased aldosterone leading to sodium retention also contribute to the development of ascites. Sodium retention causes fluid accumulation and expansion of the extracellular fluid volume, which results in the formation of peripheral edema and ascites. Sodium retention is the consequence of a homeostatic response caused by underfilling of the arterial circulation secondary to arterial vasodilation in the splanchnic vascular bed. Because the retained fluid is constantly leaking out of the intravascular compartment into the peritoneal cavity, the sensation of vascular filling is not achieved, and the process continues. Hypoalbuminemia and reduced plasma oncotic pressure also contribute to the loss of fluid from the vascular compartment into the

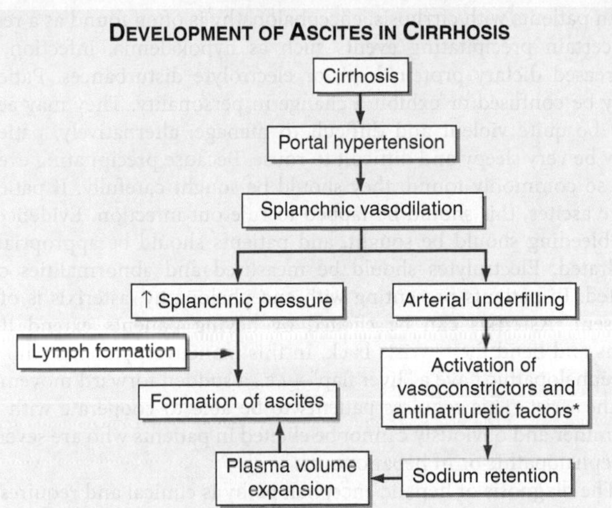

FIGURE 365-4 Development of ascites in cirrhosis. This flow diagram illustrates the importance of portal hypertension with splanchnic vasodilation in the development of ascites. *Antinatriuretic factors include the renin angiotensin aldosterone system and the sympathetic nervous system.

peritoneal cavity. Hypoalbuminemia is due to decreased synthetic function in a cirrhotic liver.

Clinical Features Patients typically note an increase in abdominal girth that is often accompanied by the development of peripheral edema. The development of ascites is often insidious, and it is surprising that some patients wait so long and become so distended before seeking medical attention. Patients usually have at least 1–2 L of fluid in the abdomen before they are aware that there is an increase. If ascitic fluid is massive, respiratory function can be compromised, and patients will complain of shortness of breath. Hepatic hydrothorax may also occur in this setting, contributing to respiratory symptoms. Patients with massive ascites are often malnourished and have muscle wasting and excessive fatigue and weakness.

Diagnosis Diagnosis of ascites is by physical examination and is often aided by abdominal imaging. Patients will have bulging flanks, may have a fluid wave, or may have the presence of shifting dullness. This is determined by taking patients from a supine position to lying on either their left or right side and noting the movement of the dullness to percussion. Subtle amounts of ascites can be detected by ultrasound or CT scanning. Hepatic hydrothorax is more common on the right side and implicates a rent in the diaphragm with free flow of ascitic fluid into the thoracic cavity.

When patients present with ascites for the first time, it is recommended that a diagnostic paracentesis be performed to characterize the fluid. This should include the determination of total protein and albumin content, blood cell counts with differential, and cultures. In the appropriate setting, amylase may be measured and cytology performed. In patients with cirrhosis, the protein concentration of the ascitic fluid is quite low, with the majority of patients having an ascitic fluid protein concentration <1 g/dL. The development of the serum ascites-to-albumin gradient (SAAG) has replaced the description of exudative or transudative fluid. When the gradient between the serum albumin level and the ascitic fluid albumin level is >1.1 g/dL, the cause of the ascites is most likely due to portal hypertension; this is usually in the setting of cirrhosis. When the gradient is <1.1 g/dL, infectious or malignant causes of ascites should be considered. When levels of ascitic fluid proteins are very low, patients are at increased risk for developing SBP. A high level of red blood cells in the ascitic fluid signifies a traumatic tap or perhaps a hepatocellular cancer or a ruptured omental varix. When the absolute level of polymorphonuclear leukocytes is >250/μL, the question of ascitic fluid infection should be strongly considered. Ascitic fluid cultures should be obtained using bedside inoculation of culture media.

TREATMENT ASCITES

Patients with small amounts of ascites can usually be managed with dietary sodium restriction alone. Most average diets in the United States contain 6–8 g of sodium per day, and if patients eat at restaurants or fast-food outlets, the amount of sodium in their diet can exceed this amount. Thus, it is often extremely difficult to get patients to change their dietary habits to ingest <2 g of sodium per day, which is the recommended amount. Patients are frequently surprised to realize how much sodium is in the standard U.S. diet; thus, it is important to make educational pamphlets available to the patient. Often, a simple recommendation is to eat fresh or frozen foods, avoiding canned or processed foods, which are usually preserved with sodium. When a moderate amount of ascites is present, diuretic therapy is usually necessary. Traditionally, spironolactone at 100–200 mg/d as a single dose is started, and furosemide may be added at 40–80 mg/d, particularly in patients who have peripheral edema. In patients who have never received diuretics before, the failure of the above-mentioned dosages suggests that they are not being compliant with a low-sodium diet. If compliance is confirmed and ascitic fluid is not being mobilized, spironolactone can be increased to 400–600 mg/d and furosemide increased to 120–160 mg/d. If ascites is still present with these dosages of diuretics in patients who are compliant with a low-sodium diet, then they are defined as having *refractory ascites*, and alternative treatment modalities including repeated large-volume paracentesis or a TIPS procedure should be considered (Fig. 365-5). Recent studies have shown that TIPS, while managing the ascites, does not improve survival in these patients. Unfortunately, TIPS is often associated with an increased frequency of hepatic encephalopathy and must be considered carefully on a case-by-case basis. The prognosis for patients with cirrhosis with ascites is poor, and some studies have shown that <50% of patients survive 2 years after the onset of ascites. Thus, there should be consideration for liver transplantation in patients with the onset of ascites.

SPONTANEOUS BACTERIAL PERITONITIS

SBP is a common and severe complication of ascites characterized by spontaneous infection of the ascitic fluid without an intraabdominal source. In patients with cirrhosis and ascites severe enough for hospitalization, SBP can occur in up to 30% of individuals and can have a 25% in-hospital mortality rate. Bacterial translocation is the presumed mechanism for development of SBP, with gut flora traversing the intestine

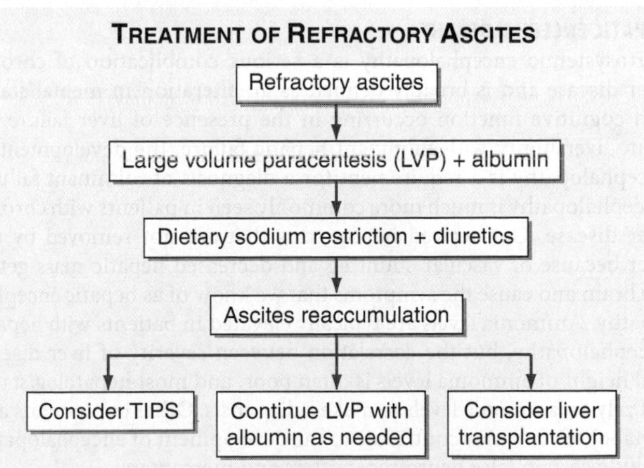

FIGURE 365-5 Treatment of refractory ascites. In patients who develop azotemia in the course of receiving diuretics in the management of their ascites, some will require repeated large-volume paracentesis (LVP), some may be considered for transjugular intrahepatic portosystemic shunt (TIPS), and some would be good candidates for liver transplantation. These decisions are all individualized.

into mesenteric lymph nodes, leading to bacteremia and seeding of the ascitic fluid. The most common organisms are *Escherichia coli* and other gut bacteria; however, gram-positive bacteria, including *Streptococcus viridans*, *Staphylococcus aureus*, and *Enterococcus* sp., can also be found. If more than two organisms are identified, secondary bacterial peritonitis due to a perforated viscus should be considered. The diagnosis of SBP is made when the fluid sample has an absolute neutrophil count >250/μL. Bedside cultures should be obtained when ascitic fluid is tapped. Patients with ascites may present with fever, altered mental status, elevated white blood cell count, and abdominal pain or discomfort, or they may present without any of these features. Therefore, it is necessary to have a high degree of clinical suspicion, and peritoneal taps are important for making the diagnosis. Treatment is with a second-generation cephalosporin, with cefotaxime being the most commonly used antibiotic. In patients with variceal hemorrhage, the frequency of SBP is significantly increased, and prophylaxis against SBP is recommended when a patient presents with upper GI bleeding. Furthermore, in patients who have had an episode(s) of SBP and recovered, once-weekly administration of antibiotics is used as prophylaxis for recurrent SBP.

HEPATORENAL SYNDROME

The hepatorenal syndrome (HRS) is a form of functional renal failure without renal pathology that occurs in about 10% of patients with advanced cirrhosis or acute liver failure. There are marked disturbances in the arterial renal circulation in patients with HRS; these include an increase in vascular resistance accompanied by a reduction in systemic vascular resistance. The reason for renal vasoconstriction is most likely multifactorial and is poorly understood. The diagnosis is made usually in the presence of a large amount of ascites in patients who have a stepwise progressive increase in creatinine. Type 1 HRS is characterized by a progressive impairment in renal function and a significant reduction in creatinine clearance within 1–2 weeks of presentation. Type 2 HRS is characterized by a reduction in glomerular filtration rate with an elevation of serum creatinine level, but it is fairly stable and is associated with a better outcome than that of type 1 HRS.

HRS is often seen in patients with refractory ascites and requires exclusion of other causes of acute renal failure. Treatment has, unfortunately, been difficult, and in the past, dopamine or prostaglandin analogues were used as renal vasodilating medications. Carefully performed studies have failed to show clear-cut benefit from these therapeutic approaches. Currently, patients are treated with midodrine, an α-agonist, along with octreotide and intravenous albumin. The best therapy for HRS is liver transplantation; recovery of renal function is typical in this setting. In patients with either type 1 or type 2 HRS, the prognosis is poor unless transplant can be achieved within a short period of time.

HEPATIC ENCEPHALOPATHY

Portosystemic encephalopathy is a serious complication of chronic liver disease and is broadly defined as an alteration in mental status and cognitive function occurring in the presence of liver failure. In acute liver injury with fulminant hepatic failure, the development of encephalopathy is a requirement for a diagnosis of fulminant failure. Encephalopathy is much more commonly seen in patients with chronic liver disease. Gut-derived neurotoxins that are not removed by the liver because of vascular shunting and decreased hepatic mass get to the brain and cause the symptoms that we know of as hepatic encephalopathy. Ammonia levels are typically elevated in patients with hepatic encephalopathy, but the correlation between severity of liver disease and height of ammonia levels is often poor, and most hepatologists do not rely on ammonia levels to make a diagnosis. Other compounds and metabolites that may contribute to the development of encephalopathy include certain false neurotransmitters and mercaptans.

Clinical Features In acute liver failure, changes in mental status can occur within weeks to months. Brain edema can be seen in these patients, with severe encephalopathy associated with swelling of the gray matter. Cerebral herniation is a feared complication of brain edema in acute liver failure, and treatment is meant to decrease edema with mannitol and judicious use of intravenous fluids.

In patients with cirrhosis, encephalopathy is often found as a result of certain precipitating events such as hypokalemia, infection, an increased dietary protein load, or electrolyte disturbances. Patients may be confused or exhibit a change in personality. They may actually be quite violent and difficult to manage; alternatively, patients may be very sleepy and difficult to rouse. Because precipitating events are so commonly found, they should be sought carefully. If patients have ascites, this should be tapped to rule out infection. Evidence of GI bleeding should be sought, and patients should be appropriately hydrated. Electrolytes should be measured and abnormalities corrected. In patients presenting with encephalopathy, asterixis is often present. Asterixis can be elicited by having patients extend their arms and bend their wrists back. In this maneuver, patients who are encephalopathic have a "liver flap"—i.e., a sudden forward movement of the wrist. This requires patients to be able to cooperate with the examiner and obviously cannot be elicited in patients who are severely encephalopathic or in hepatic coma.

The diagnosis of hepatic encephalopathy is clinical and requires an experienced clinician to recognize and put together all of the various features. Often when patients have encephalopathy for the first time, they are unaware of what is transpiring, but once they have been through the experience for the first time, they can identify when this is developing in subsequent situations and can often self-medicate to impair the development or worsening of encephalopathy.

TREATMENT HEPATIC ENCEPHALOPATHY

Treatment is multifactorial and includes management of the above-mentioned precipitating factors. Sometimes hydration and correction of electrolyte imbalance are all that is necessary. In the past, restriction of dietary protein was considered for patients with encephalopathy; however, the negative impact of that maneuver on overall nutrition is thought to outweigh the benefit when treating encephalopathy, and it is thus discouraged. There may be some benefit to replacing animal-based protein with vegetable-based protein in some patients with encephalopathy that is difficult to manage. The mainstay of treatment for encephalopathy, in addition to correcting precipitating factors, is to use lactulose, a nonabsorbable disaccharide, which results in colonic acidification. Catharsis ensues, contributing to the elimination of nitrogenous products in the gut that are responsible for the development of encephalopathy. The goal of lactulose therapy is to promote 2–3 soft stools per day. Patients are asked to titrate their amount of ingested lactulose to achieve the desired effect. Poorly absorbed antibiotics are often used as adjunctive therapies for patients who have had a difficult time with lactulose. The alternating administration of neomycin and metronidazole has commonly been used to reduce the individual side effects of each: neomycin for renal insufficiency and ototoxicity and metronidazole for peripheral neuropathy. More recently, rifaximin at 550 mg twice daily has been very effective in treating encephalopathy without the known side effects of neomycin or metronidazole. Zinc supplementation is sometimes helpful in patients with encephalopathy and is relatively harmless. The development of encephalopathy in patients with chronic liver disease is a poor prognostic sign, but this complication can be managed in the vast majority of patients.

MALNUTRITION IN CIRRHOSIS

Because the liver is principally involved in the regulation of protein and energy metabolism in the body, it is not surprising that patients with advanced liver disease are commonly malnourished. Once patients become cirrhotic, they are more catabolic, and muscle protein is metabolized. There are multiple factors that contribute to the malnutrition of cirrhosis, including poor dietary intake, alterations in gut nutrient absorption, and alterations in protein metabolism. Dietary supplementation for patients with cirrhosis is helpful in preventing patients from becoming catabolic.

ABNORMALITIES IN COAGULATION

Coagulopathy is almost universal in patients with cirrhosis. There is decreased synthesis of clotting factors and impaired clearance of anticoagulants. In addition, patients may have thrombocytopenia from hypersplenism due to portal hypertension. Vitamin K–dependent clotting factors are factors II, VII, IX, and X. Vitamin K requires biliary excretion for its subsequent absorption; thus, in patients with chronic cholestatic syndromes, vitamin K absorption is frequently diminished. Intravenous or intramuscular vitamin K can quickly correct this abnormality. More commonly, the synthesis of vitamin K–dependent clotting factors is diminished because of a decrease in hepatic mass, and, under these circumstances, administration of parenteral vitamin K does not improve the clotting factors or the prothrombin time. Platelet function is often abnormal in patients with chronic liver disease, in addition to decreases in platelet levels due to hypersplenism.

BONE DISEASE IN CIRRHOSIS

Osteoporosis is common in patients with chronic cholestatic liver disease because of malabsorption of vitamin D and decreased calcium ingestion. The rate of bone resorption exceeds that of new bone formation in patients with cirrhosis, resulting in bone loss. Dual x-ray absorptiometry (DEXA) is a useful method for determining osteoporosis or osteopenia in patients with chronic liver disease. When a DEXA scan shows decreased bone mass, treatment should be administered with bisphosphonates that are effective at inhibiting resorption of bone and efficacious in the treatment of osteoporosis.

HEMATOLOGIC ABNORMALITIES IN CIRRHOSIS

Numerous hematologic manifestations of cirrhosis are present, including anemia from a variety of causes including hypersplenism, hemolysis, iron deficiency, and perhaps folate deficiency from malnutrition. Macrocytosis is a common abnormality in red blood cell morphology seen in patients with chronic liver disease, and neutropenia may be seen as a result of hypersplenism.

366e Atlas of Liver Biopsies

Jules L. Dienstag, Atul K. Bhan

This is a digital-only chapter. It is available on the DVD that accompanies this book, as well as on Access Medicine/Harrison's Online, and the eBook and "app" editions of HPIM 19e.

Although clinical and laboratory features yield clues to the extent of inflammatory processes (disease grade), the degree of scarring and architectural distortion (disease stage), and the nature of the disease process, the liver biopsy is felt to represent the gold standard for assessing the degree of liver injury and fibrosis. Examination of liver histology provides not only a basis for quantitative scoring of disease activity and progression but also a wealth of qualitative information that can direct and inform diagnosis and management.

367e Genetic, Metabolic, and Infiltrative Diseases Affecting the Liver

Bruce R. Bacon

This is a digital-only chapter. It is available on the DVD that accompanies this book, as well as on Access Medicine/Harrison's Online, and the eBook and "app" editions of HPIM 19e.

There are a number of disorders of the liver that fit within the categories of genetic, metabolic, and infiltrative disorders. Inherited disorders include hemochromatosis, Wilson's disease, α_1 antitrypsin (α_1AT) deficiency, and cystic fibrosis (CF). Hemochromatosis is the most common inherited disorder affecting white populations, with the genetic susceptibility for the disease being identified in 1 in 250 individuals. Over the past 15 years, it has become increasingly apparent that nonalcoholic fatty liver disease (NAFLD) is the most common cause of elevated liver enzymes found in the U.S. population. This disorder is discussed in greater detail in Chap. 364. Infiltrative disorders of the liver are relatively rare.

368 Liver Transplantation

Raymond T. Chung, Jules L. Dienstag

Liver transplantation—the replacement of the native, diseased liver by a normal organ (allograft)—has matured from an experimental procedure reserved for desperately ill patients to an accepted, lifesaving operation applied more optimally in the natural history of end-stage liver disease. The preferred and technically most advanced approach is *orthotopic transplantation*, in which the native organ is removed and the donor organ is inserted in the same anatomic location. Pioneered in the 1960s by Thomas Starzl at the University of Colorado and, later, at the University of Pittsburgh and by Roy Calne in Cambridge, England, liver transplantation is now performed routinely worldwide. Success measured as 1-year survival has improved from ~30% in the 1970s to >90% today. These improved prospects for prolonged survival resulted from refinements in operative technique, improvements in organ procurement and preservation, advances in immunosuppressive therapy, and, perhaps most influentially, more enlightened patient selection and timing. Despite the perioperative morbidity and mortality, the technical and management challenges of the procedure, and its costs, liver transplantation has become the approach of choice for selected patients whose chronic or acute liver disease is progressive, life-threatening, and unresponsive to medical therapy. Based on the current level of success, the number of liver transplants has continued to grow each year; in 2012, 6256 patients received liver allografts in the United States. Still, the demand for new livers continues to outpace availability; as of mid-2013, 15,806 patients in the United States were on a waiting list for a donor liver. In response to this drastic shortage of donor organs, many transplantation centers supplement cadaver-organ liver transplantation with living-donor transplantation.

INDICATIONS

Potential candidates for liver transplantation are children and adults who, in the absence of contraindications (see below), suffer from severe, irreversible liver disease for which alternative medical or surgical treatments have been exhausted or are unavailable. *Timing of the operation is of critical importance.* Indeed, improved timing and better patient selection are felt to have contributed more to the increased success of liver transplantation in the 1980s and beyond than all the impressive technical and immunologic advances combined. Although the disease should be advanced, and although opportunities for spontaneous or medically induced stabilization or recovery should be allowed, the procedure should be done sufficiently early to give the surgical procedure a fair chance for success. Ideally, transplantation should be considered in patients with end-stage liver disease who are experiencing or have experienced a life-threatening complication of hepatic decompensation or whose quality of life has deteriorated to unacceptable levels. Although patients with well-compensated cirrhosis can survive for many years, many patients with quasi-stable chronic liver disease have much more advanced disease than may be apparent. As discussed below, the better the status of the patient prior to transplantation, the higher will be its anticipated success rate. The decision about *when* to transplant is complex and requires the combined judgment of an experienced team of hepatologists, transplant surgeons, anesthesiologists, and specialists in support services, not to mention the well-informed consent of the patient and the patient's family.

TRANSPLANTATION IN CHILDREN

Indications for transplantation in children are listed in Table 368-1. The most common is *biliary atresia. Inherited or genetic disorders of metabolism* associated with liver failure constitute another major indication for transplantation in children and adolescents. In Crigler-Najjar disease type I and in certain hereditary disorders of the urea cycle and of amino acid or lactate-pyruvate metabolism, transplantation may be the only way to prevent impending deterioration of central nervous system function, despite the fact that the native liver is structurally normal. Combined heart and liver transplantation has yielded dramatic improvement in cardiac function and in cholesterol levels in children with homozygous familial hypercholesterolemia; combined liver and kidney transplantation has been successful in patients with primary hyperoxaluria type I. In hemophiliacs with transfusion-associated hepatitis and liver failure, liver transplantation has been associated with recovery of normal factor VIII synthesis.

TRANSPLANTATION IN ADULTS

Liver transplantation is indicated for end-stage *cirrhosis* of all causes (Table 368-1). In *sclerosing cholangitis* and *Caroli's disease* (multiple cystic dilatations of the intrahepatic biliary tree), recurrent infections and sepsis associated with inflammatory and fibrotic obstruction of the biliary tree may be an indication for transplantation. Because prior biliary surgery complicates and is a relative contraindication for liver transplantation, surgical diversion of the biliary tree has been all but abandoned for patients with sclerosing cholangitis. In patients who undergo transplantation for *hepatic vein thrombosis* (*Budd-Chiari syndrome*), postoperative anticoagulation is essential; underlying myeloproliferative disorders may have to be treated but are not a contraindication to liver transplantation. If a donor organ can be located quickly, before life-threatening complications—including cerebral edema—set in, patients with acute liver failure are candidates for liver transplantation. Routine candidates for liver transplantation are patients with *alcoholic cirrhosis, chronic viral hepatitis*, and *primary hepatocellular malignancies*. Although all three of these categories are considered to be high risk, liver transplantation can be offered to carefully selected patients. Currently, chronic hepatitis C and alcoholic liver disease are the most common indications for liver transplantation, accounting for over 40% of all adult candidates who undergo the procedure. Patients with alcoholic cirrhosis can be considered as candidates for transplantation if they meet strict criteria for abstinence and reform; however, these criteria still do not prevent recidivism in up to a quarter of cases. In highly selected cases in a limited number of centers, transplantation for severe *acute* alcoholic hepatitis has been performed with success; however, because patients with acute alcoholic hepatitis are still actively using alcohol, and because continued alcohol abuse remains a concern, acute alcoholic hepatitis is not a routine indication for liver transplantation. Patients with chronic hepatitis C have early allograft and patient survival comparable to those of other subsets of patients after transplantation; however, reinfection in the donor organ is universal, recurrent hepatitis C is insidiously progressive, allograft cirrhosis develops in 20–30% at 5 years, and cirrhosis and late organ failure occur at a higher frequency beyond 5 years. With the introduction of highly effective direct acting antiviral agents targeting HCV, it is expected that allograft outcomes will improve significantly in the coming years. In patients with chronic hepatitis B, in the absence of measures to prevent recurrent hepatitis B, survival after transplantation is reduced by approximately 10–20%; however, prophylactic use of hepatitis B immune globulin (HBIg) during and after transplantation increases the success of transplantation to a level comparable to that seen in patients with nonviral causes of liver decompensation. Specific oral antiviral drugs (e.g., entecavir, tenofovir disoproxil fumarate) (Chap. 362) can be used both for prophylaxis against and for treatment of recurrent hepatitis B, facilitating further the management of patients undergoing liver transplantation for end-stage hepatitis B; most transplantation centers rely on antiviral drugs with or without HBIg to manage patients with hepatitis B. Issues of disease recurrence are discussed in more detail below. Patients with nonmetastatic primary hepatobiliary tumors—primary hepatocellular carcinoma (HCC), cholangiocarcinoma, hepatoblastoma, angiosarcoma, epithelioid hemangioendothelioma, and multiple or massive hepatic adenomata—have undergone liver transplantation; however, for some hepatobiliary malignancies, overall survival is significantly lower than that for other categories of liver disease. Most transplantation centers have reported 5-year recurrence-free survival rates in patients with unresectable HCC for single tumors <5 cm in diameter or for three or fewer lesions all <3 cm comparable to those seen in patients undergoing transplantation for nonmalignant indications. Consequently, liver transplantation is currently restricted to patients whose hepatic malignancies meet these criteria. Expanded criteria for patients with HCC continue to be evaluated. Because the likelihood of recurrent cholangiocarcinoma is very high, only highly selected patients with limited disease are being evaluated for transplantation after intensive chemotherapy and radiation.

TABLE 368-1 INDICATIONS FOR LIVER TRANSPLANTATION

Children	Adults
Biliary atresia	Primary biliary cirrhosis
Neonatal hepatitis	Secondary biliary cirrhosis
Congenital hepatic fibrosis	Primary sclerosing cholangitis
Alagille's syndrome[a]	Autoimmune hepatitis
Byler's disease[b]	Caroli's disease[c]
α_1-Antitrypsin deficiency	Cryptogenic cirrhosis
Inherited disorders of metabolism	Chronic hepatitis with cirrhosis
Wilson's disease	Hepatic vein thrombosis
Tyrosinemia	Fulminant hepatitis
Glycogen storage diseases	Alcoholic cirrhosis
Lysosomal storage diseases	Chronic viral hepatitis
Protoporphyria	Primary hepatocellular malignancies
Crigler-Najjar disease type I	Hepatic adenomas
Familial hypercholesterolemia	Nonalcoholic steatohepatitis
Primary hyperoxaluria type I	Familial amyloid polyneuropathy
Hemophilia	

[a]Arteriohepatic dysplasia, with paucity of bile ducts, and congenital malformations, including pulmonary stenosis. [b]Intrahepatic cholestasis, progressive liver failure, and mental and growth retardation. [c]Multiple cystic dilatations of the intrahepatic biliary tree.

CONTRAINDICATIONS

Absolute contraindications for transplantation include life-threatening systemic diseases, uncontrolled extrahepatic bacterial or fungal infections, preexisting advanced cardiovascular or pulmonary disease, multiple uncorrectable life-threatening congenital anomalies, metastatic malignancy, and active drug or alcohol abuse (Table 368-2). Because carefully selected patients in their sixties and even seventies have undergone transplantation successfully, advanced age per se is no longer considered an absolute contraindication; however, in older patients a more thorough preoperative evaluation should be undertaken to

TABLE 368-2 CONTRAINDICATIONS TO LIVER TRANSPLANTATION

Absolute	Relative
Uncontrolled extrahepatobiliary infection	Age >70
Active, untreated sepsis	Prior extensive hepatobiliary surgery
Uncorrectable, life-limiting congenital anomalies	Portal vein thrombosis
Active substance or alcohol abuse	Renal failure not attributable to liver disease
Advanced cardiopulmonary disease	Previous extrahepatic malignancy (not including nonmelanoma skin cancer)
Extrahepatobiliary malignancy (not including nonmelanoma malignancy skin cancer)	Severe obesity
Metastatic malignancy to the liver	Severe malnutrition/wasting
Cholangiocarcinoma	Medical noncompliance
AIDS	HIV seropositivity with failure to control HIV viremia or CD4 <100/μL
Life-threatening systemic diseases	Intrahepatic sepsis
	Severe hypoxemia secondary to right-to-left intrapulmonary shunts (Po_2 <50 mmHg)
	Severe pulmonary hypertension (mean pulmonary artery pressure >35 mmHg)
	Uncontrolled psychiatric disorder

exclude ischemic cardiac disease and other comorbid conditions. Advanced age (>70 years), however, should be considered a *relative contraindication*—that is, a factor to be taken into account with other relative contraindications. Other relative contraindications include portal vein thrombosis, HIV infection, preexisting renal disease not associated with liver disease (which may prompt consideration of combined liver and kidney transplantation), intrahepatic or biliary sepsis, severe hypoxemia (Po_2 <50 mmHg) resulting from right-to-left intrapulmonary shunts, portopulmonary hypertension with high mean pulmonary artery pressures (>35 mmHg), previous extensive hepatobiliary surgery, any uncontrolled serious psychiatric disorder, and lack of sufficient social supports. Any one of these relative contraindications is insufficient in and of itself to preclude transplantation. For example, the problem of portal vein thrombosis can be overcome by constructing a graft from the donor liver portal vein to the recipient's superior mesenteric vein. Now that highly active antiretroviral therapy has dramatically improved the survival of persons with HIV infection (Chap. 226), and because end-stage liver disease caused by chronic hepatitis C and B has emerged as a serious source of morbidity and mortality in the HIV infected population, liver transplantation has now been performed successfully in selected HIV-positive persons who have excellent control of HIV infection. Selected patients with CD4± T cell counts >100/μL and with pharmacologic suppression of HIV viremia have undergone transplantation for end-stage liver disease. HIV-infected persons who have received liver allografts for end-stage liver disease resulting from chronic hepatitis B have experienced survival rates compared to those of HIV-negative persons undergoing transplantation for the same indication. In contrast, recurrent hepatitis C virus (HCV) in the allograft has limited long-term success in persons with HCV-related end-stage liver disease. Again, it is expected that the availability of direct acting antiviral agents targeting HCV, will significantly improve allograft outcomes.

TECHNICAL CONSIDERATIONS

CADAVER DONOR SELECTION

Cadaver donor livers for transplantation are procured primarily from victims of head trauma. Organs from brain-dead donors up to age 60 are acceptable if the following criteria are met: hemodynamic stability, adequate oxygenation, absence of bacterial or fungal infection, absence of abdominal trauma, absence of hepatic dysfunction, and serologic exclusion of hepatitis B (HBV) and C viruses and HIV. Occasionally, organs from donors with hepatitis B and C are used (e.g., for recipients with prior hepatitis B and C, respectively). Organs from donors with antibodies to hepatitis B core antigen (anti-HBc) can also be used when the need is especially urgent, and recipients of these organs are treated prophylactically with antiviral drugs. Cardiovascular and respiratory functions are maintained artificially until the liver can be removed. Transplantation of organs procured from deceased donors who have succumbed to cardiac death can be performed successfully under selected circumstances, when ischemic time is minimized and liver histology preserved. Compatibility in ABO blood group and organ size between donor and recipient are important considerations in donor selection; however, ABO-incompatible, split liver, or reduced-donor-organ transplants can be performed in emergencies or marked donor scarcity. Tissue typing for human leukocyte antigen (HLA) matching is not required, and preformed cytotoxic HLA antibodies do not preclude liver transplantation. Following perfusion with cold electrolyte solution, the donor liver is removed and packed in ice. The use of University of Wisconsin (UW) solution, rich in lactobionate and raffinose, has permitted the extension of cold ischemic time up to 20 h; however, 12 h may be a more reasonable limit. Improved techniques for harvesting multiple organs from the same donor have increased the availability of donor livers, but the availability of donor livers is far outstripped by the demand. Currently in the United States, all donor livers are distributed through a nationwide organ-sharing network (United Network for Organ Sharing [UNOS]) designed to allocate available organs based on regional considerations and recipient acuity. Recipients who have the highest disease severity generally have the highest priority, but allocation strategies that balance highest urgency against best outcomes continue to evolve to distribute cadaver organs most effectively. Allocation based on the Child-Turcotte-Pugh (CTP) score, which uses five clinical variables (encephalopathy stage, ascites, bilirubin, albumin, and prothrombin time) and waiting time, has been replaced by allocation based on urgency alone, calculated by the Model for End-Stage Liver Disease (MELD) score. The MELD score is based on a mathematical model that includes bilirubin, creatinine, and prothrombin time expressed as international normalized ratio (INR) (Table 368-3). Neither waiting time (except as a tie breaker between two potential recipients with the same MELD scores) nor posttransplantation outcome is taken into account, but use of the MELD score

TABLE 368-3 UNITED NETWORK FOR ORGAN SHARING (UNOS) LIVER TRANSPLANTATION WAITING LIST CRITERIA

Status 1	Fulminant hepatic failure (including primary graft nonfunction and hepatic artery thrombosis within 7 days after transplantation as well as acute decompensated Wilson's disease)[a]
The Model for End-Stage Liver Disease (MELD) score, on a continuous scale,[b] determines allocation of the remainder of donor organs. This model is based on the following calculation:	
$3.78 \times \log_e$ bilirubin (mg/100 mL) ± $11.2 \times \log_e$ international normalized ratio (INR) ± $9.57 \times \log_e$ creatinine (mg/100 mL) ± 6.43 (v 0 for alcoholic and cholestatic liver disease, × 1 for all other types of liver disease).[c,d,e]	
Online calculators to determine MELD scores are available, such as the following: *http://optn.transplant.hrsa.gov/resources/professionalresources.asp?index=9.*	

[a]For children <18 years of age, status 1 includes acute or chronic liver failure plus hospitalization in an intensive care unit or inborn errors of metabolism. Status 1 is retained for those persons with fulminant hepatic failure and supersedes the MELD score. [b]The MELD scale is continuous, with 34 levels ranging between 6 and 40. Donor organs usually do not become available unless the MELD score exceeds 20. [c]Patients with stage T2 hepatocellular carcinoma receive 22 disease-specific points. [d]Creatinine is included because renal function is a validated predictor of survival in patients with liver disease. For adults undergoing dialysis twice a week, the creatinine in the equation is set to 4 mg/100 mL. [e]For children <18 years of age, the Pediatric End-Stage Liver Disease (PELD) scale is used. This scale is based on albumin, bilirubin, INR, growth failure, and age. Status 1 is retained.

has been shown to reduce waiting list mortality, to reduce waiting time prior to transplantation, to be the best predictor of pretransplantation mortality, to satisfy the prevailing view that medical need should be the decisive determinant, and to eliminate both the subjectivity inherent in the CTP scoring system (presence and degree of ascites and hepatic encephalopathy) and the differences in waiting times among different regions of the country. Recent data indicate that liver recipients with MELD scores <15 experienced higher posttransplantation mortality rates than similarly classified patients who remained on the wait list. This observation led to the modification of UNOS policy to allocate donor organs to candidates with MELD scores exceeding 15 within the local or regional procurement organization before offering the organ to local patients whose scores are <15. In addition, serum sodium, another important predictor of survival in liver transplantation candidates, is taken into consideration in allocating donor livers.

The highest priority (status 1) continues to be reserved for patients with fulminant hepatic failure or primary graft nonfunction. Because candidates for liver transplantation who have HCC may not be sufficiently decompensated to compete for donor organs based on urgency criteria alone, and because protracted waiting for cadaver donor organs often results in tumor growth beyond acceptable limits for transplantation, such patients are assigned disease-specific MELD points (Table 368–3). Other disease-specific MELD exceptions include portopulmonary hypertension, hepatopulmonary syndrome, familial amyloid polyneuropathy, primary hyperoxaluria (necessitating liver-kidney transplantation), cystic fibrosis liver disease, and highly selected cases of hilar cholangiocarcinoma.

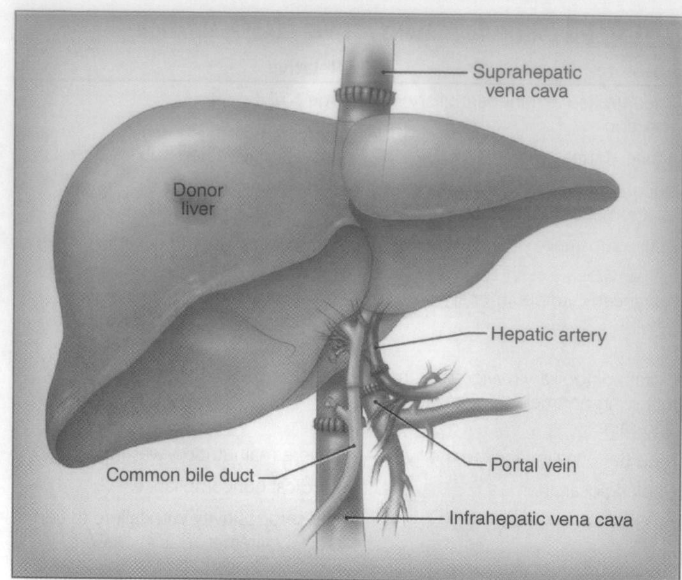

FIGURE 368-1 The anastomoses in orthotopic liver transplantation. The anastomoses are performed in the following sequence: (1) suprahepatic and infrahepatic vena cava, (2) portal vein, (3) hepatic artery, and (4) common bile duct-to-duct anastomosis. *(Adapted from JL Dienstag, AB Cosimi: N Engl J Med 367:1483, 2012.)*

LIVING DONOR TRANSPLANTATION

Occasionally, especially for liver transplantation in children, one cadaver organ can be split between two recipients (one adult and one child). A more viable alternative, transplantation of the right lobe of the liver from a healthy adult donor into an adult recipient, has gained increased popularity. Living donor transplantation of the left lobe (left lateral segment), introduced in the early 1990s to alleviate the extreme shortage of donor organs for small children, accounts currently for approximately one-third of all liver transplantation procedures in children. Driven by the shortage of cadaver organs, living donor transplantation involving the more sizable right lobe is being considered with increasing frequency in adults; however, living donor liver transplantation cannot be expected to solve the donor organ shortage; 246 such procedures were done in 2012, representing only about 4% of all liver transplant operations done in the United States.

Living donor transplantation can reduce waiting time and cold-ischemia time; is done under elective, rather than emergency, circumstances; and may be lifesaving in recipients who cannot afford to wait for a cadaver donor. The downside, of course, is the risk to the healthy donor (a mean of 10 weeks of medical disability; biliary complications in ~5%; postoperative complications such as wound infection, small-bowel obstruction, and incisional hernias in 9–19%; and even, in 0.2–0.4%, death) as well as the increased frequency of biliary (15–32%) and vascular (10%) complications in the recipient. Potential donors must participate voluntarily without coercion, and transplantation teams should go to great lengths to exclude subtle coercive or inappropriate psychological factors as well as outline carefully to both donor and recipient the potential benefits and risks of the procedure. Donors for the procedure should be 18–60 years old; have a compatible blood type with the recipient; have no chronic medical problems or history of major abdominal surgery; be related genetically or emotionally to the recipient; and pass an exhaustive series of clinical, biochemical, and serologic evaluations to unearth disqualifying medical disorders. The recipient should meet the same UNOS criteria for liver transplantation as recipients of a cadaver donor allograft. Comprehensive outcome data on adult-to-adult living donor liver transplantation are being collected (*www.nih-a2all.org*).

SURGICAL TECHNIQUE

Removal of the recipient's native liver is technically difficult, particularly in the presence of portal hypertension with its associated collateral circulation and extensive varices and especially in the presence of scarring from previous abdominal operations. The combination of portal hypertension and coagulopathy (elevated prothrombin time and thrombocytopenia) may translate into large blood product transfusion requirements. After the portal vein and infrahepatic and suprahepatic inferior vena cavae are dissected, the hepatic artery and common bile duct are dissected. Then the native liver is removed and the donor organ inserted. During the anhepatic phase, coagulopathy, hypoglycemia, hypocalcemia, and hypothermia are encountered and must be managed by the anesthesiology team. Caval, portal vein, hepatic artery, and bile duct anastomoses are performed in succession, the last by end-to-end suturing of the donor and recipient common bile ducts (Fig. 368-1) or by choledochojejunostomy to a Roux-en-Y loop if the recipient common bile duct cannot be used for reconstruction (e.g., in sclerosing cholangitis). A typical transplant operation lasts 8 h, with a range of 6–18 h. Because of excessive bleeding, large volumes of blood, blood products, and volume expanders may be required during surgery; however, blood requirements have fallen sharply with improvements in surgical technique, blood-salvage interventions, and experience.

As noted above, emerging alternatives to orthotopic liver transplantation include split-liver grafts, in which one donor organ is divided and inserted into two recipients; and living donor procedures, in which part of the left (for children), the left (for children or small adults), or the right (for adults) lobe of the liver is harvested from a living donor for transplantation into the recipient. In the adult procedure, once the right lobe is removed from the donor, the donor right hepatic vein is anastomosed to the recipient right hepatic vein remnant, followed by donor-to-recipient anastomoses of the portal vein and then the hepatic artery. Finally, the biliary anastomosis is performed, duct-to-duct if practical or via Roux-en-Y anastomosis. Heterotopic liver transplantation, in which the donor liver is inserted without removal of the native liver, has met with very limited success and acceptance, except in a very small number of centers. In attempts to support desperately ill patients until a suitable donor organ can be identified, several transplantation centers are studying extracorporeal perfusion with bioartificial liver cartridges constructed from hepatocytes bound to hollow fiber systems and used as temporary hepatic-assist devices, but their efficacy remains to be established. Areas of research with the potential to overcome the shortage of donor organs include hepatocyte transplantation and xenotransplantation with genetically modified organs of nonhuman origin (e.g., swine).

POSTOPERATIVE COURSE AND MANAGEMENT

IMMUNOSUPPRESSIVE THERAPY

The introduction in 1980 of cyclosporine as an immunosuppressive agent contributed substantially to the improvement in survival after liver transplantation. Cyclosporine, a calcineurin inhibitor, blocks early activation of T cells and is specific for T cell functions that result from the interaction of the T cell with its receptor and that involve the calcium-dependent signal transduction pathway. As a result, the activity of cyclosporine leads to inhibition of lymphokine gene activation, blocking interleukins 2, 3, and 4, tumor necrosis factor a, and other lymphokines. Cyclosporine also inhibits B cell functions. This process occurs without affecting rapidly dividing cells in the bone marrow, which may account for the reduced frequency of posttransplantation systemic infections. The most common and important side effect of cyclosporine therapy is nephrotoxicity. Cyclosporine causes dose-dependent renal tubular injury and direct renal artery vasospasm. Following renal function is therefore important in monitoring cyclosporine therapy, perhaps even a more reliable indicator than blood levels of the drug. Nephrotoxicity is reversible and can be managed by dose reduction. Other adverse effects of cyclosporine therapy include hypertension, hyperkalemia, tremor, hirsutism, glucose intolerance, and gingival hyperplasia.

Tacrolimus, a macrolide lactone antibiotic isolated from a Japanese soil fungus, *Streptomyces tsukubaensis*, has the same mechanism of action as cyclosporine but is 10–100 times more potent. Initially applied as "rescue" therapy for patients in whom rejection occurred despite the use of cyclosporine, tacrolimus was shown to be associated with a reduced frequency of acute, refractory, and chronic rejection. Although patient and graft survival are the same with these two drugs, the advantage of tacrolimus in minimizing episodes of rejection, reducing the need for additional glucocorticoid doses, and reducing the likelihood of bacterial and cytomegalovirus (CMV) infection has simplified the management of patients undergoing liver transplantation. In addition, the oral absorption of tacrolimus is more predictable than that of cyclosporine, especially during the early postoperative period when T-tube drainage interferes with the enterohepatic circulation of cyclosporine. As a result, in most transplantation centers, tacrolimus has now supplanted cyclosporine for primary immunosuppression, and many centers rely on oral rather than IV administration from the outset. For transplantation centers that prefer cyclosporine, a better-absorbed microemulsion preparation is available.

Although more potent than cyclosporine, tacrolimus is also more toxic and more likely to be discontinued for adverse events. The toxicity of tacrolimus is similar to that of cyclosporine; nephrotoxicity and neurotoxicity are the most commonly encountered adverse effects, and neurotoxicity (tremor, seizures, hallucinations, psychoses, coma) is more likely and more severe in tacrolimus-treated patients. Both drugs can cause diabetes mellitus, but tacrolimus does not cause hirsutism or gingival hyperplasia. Because of overlapping toxicity between cyclosporine and tacrolimus, especially nephrotoxicity, and because tacrolimus reduces cyclosporine clearance, these two drugs should not be used together. Because 99% of tacrolimus is metabolized by the liver, hepatic dysfunction reduces its clearance; in primary graft nonfunction (when, for technical reasons or because of ischemic damage prior to its insertion, the allograft is defective and does not function normally from the outset), tacrolimus doses have to be reduced substantially, especially in children. Both cyclosporine and tacrolimus are metabolized by the cytochrome P450 IIIA system, and, therefore, drugs that induce cytochrome P450 (e.g., phenytoin, phenobarbital, carbamazepine, rifampin) reduce available levels of cyclosporine and tacrolimus; and drugs that inhibit cytochrome P450 (e.g., erythromycin, fluconazole, ketoconazole, clotrimazole, itraconazole, verapamil, diltiazem, danazol, metoclopramide, the HIV protease inhibitor ritonavir, and the HCV protease inhibitors telaprevir and boceprevir) increase cyclosporine and tacrolimus blood levels. Indeed, itraconazole is used occasionally to help boost tacrolimus levels. Like azathioprine, cyclosporine and tacrolimus appear to be associated with a risk of lymphoproliferative malignancies (see below), which may occur earlier after cyclosporine or tacrolimus than after azathioprine therapy. Because of these side effects, combinations of cyclosporine or tacrolimus with prednisone and an antimetabolite (azathioprine or mycophenolic acid, see below)—all at reduced doses—are preferable regimens for immunosuppressive therapy.

Mycophenolic acid, a nonnucleoside purine metabolism inhibitor derived as a fermentation product from several *Penicillium* species, is another immunosuppressive drug being used for patients undergoing liver transplantation. Mycophenolate has been shown to be better than azathioprine, when used with other standard immunosuppressive drugs, in preventing rejection after renal transplantation and has been adopted widely as well for use in liver transplantation. The most common adverse effects of mycophenolate are bone marrow suppression and gastrointestinal complaints.

In patients with pretransplantation renal dysfunction or renal deterioration that occurs intraoperatively or immediately postoperatively, tacrolimus or cyclosporine therapy may not be practical; under these circumstances, induction or maintenance of immunosuppression with antithymocyte globulin (ATG, thymoglobulin) or monoclonal antibodies to T cells, OKT3, may be appropriate. Therapy with these agents has been especially effective in reversing acute rejection in the posttransplantation period and is the standard treatment for acute rejection that fails to respond to methylprednisolone boluses. Available data support the use of thymoglobulin induction to delay calcineurin inhibitor use and its attendant nephrotoxicity. IV infusions of thymoglobulin may be complicated by fever and chills, which can be ameliorated by premedication with antipyretics and a low dose of glucocorticoids. Infusions of OKT3 may be complicated by fever, chills, and diarrhea, or by pulmonary edema, which can be fatal. Because OKT3 is such a potent immunosuppressive agent, its use is also more likely to be complicated by opportunistic infection or lymphoproliferative disorders; therefore, because of the availability of alternative immunosuppressive drugs, OKT3 is now used sparingly.

Sirolimus, an inhibitor of the mammalian target of rapamycin (mTOR), blocks later events in T cell activation, is approved for use in kidney transplantation, but is not approved for use in liver transplant recipients because of the reported association with an increased frequency of hepatic artery thrombosis in the first month posttransplantation. In patients with calcineurin inhibitor–related nephrotoxicity, conversion to sirolimus has been demonstrated to be effective in preventing rejection with accompanying improvements in renal function. Because of its profound antiproliferative effects, sirolimus has also been suggested to be a useful immunosuppressive agent in patients with a prior or current history of malignancy, such as HCC. Side effects include hyperlipidemia, peripheral edema, oral ulcers, and interstitial pneumonitis. Everolimus is a hydroxyethyl derivative of sirolimus that, when used in conjunction with low-dose tacrolimus, also provides successful protection against acute rejection, with decreased renal impairment compared to that associated with standard tacrolimus dosing. Everolimus and sirolimus share a similar adverse events profile; therefore, neither of these agents is approved for routine use in liver allograft recipients.

The most important principle of immunosuppression is that the ideal approach strikes a balance between immunosuppression and immunologic competence. In general, given sufficient immunosuppression, acute liver allograft rejection is nearly always reversible. On one hand, incompletely treated acute rejection predisposes to the development of chronic rejection, which can threaten graft survival. On the other hand, if the cumulative dose of immunosuppressive therapy is too large, the patient may succumb to opportunistic infection. In hepatitis C, pulse glucocorticoids or OKT3 use accelerate recurrent allograft hepatitis. Further complicating matters, acute rejection can be difficult to distinguish histologically from recurrent hepatitis C. Therefore, immunosuppressive drugs must be used judiciously, with strict attention to the infectious consequences of such therapy and careful confirmation of the diagnosis of acute rejection. In this vein, efforts have been made to minimize the use of glucocorticoids, a mainstay of immunosuppressive regimens, and steroid-free immunosuppression can be achieved in some instances. Patients who undergo liver transplantation for autoimmune diseases such as primary biliary cirrhosis, autoimmune hepatitis, and primary sclerosing cholangitis are less likely to achieve freedom from glucocorticoids.

POSTOPERATIVE COMPLICATIONS

Complications of liver transplantation can be divided into nonhepatic and hepatic categories (Tables 368-4 and 368-5). In addition, both immediate postoperative and late complications are encountered. As a rule, patients who undergo liver transplantation have been chronically ill for protracted periods and may be malnourished and wasted. The impact of such chronic illness and the multisystem failure that accompanies liver failure continue to require attention in the postoperative period. Because of the massive fluid losses and fluid shifts that occur during the operation, patients may remain fluid-overloaded during the immediate postoperative period, straining cardiovascular reserve; this effect can be amplified in the face of transient renal dysfunction and pulmonary capillary vascular permeability. Continuous monitoring of cardiovascular and pulmonary function, measures to maintain the integrity of the intravascular compartment and to treat extravascular volume overload, and scrupulous attention to potential sources and sites of infection are of paramount importance. Cardiovascular instability may also result from the electrolyte imbalance that may accompany reperfusion of the donor liver as well as from restoration of systemic vascular resistance following implantation. Pulmonary function may be compromised further by paralysis of the right hemidiaphragm associated with phrenic nerve injury. The hyperdynamic state with increased cardiac output that is characteristic of patients with liver failure reverses rapidly after successful liver transplantation.

Other immediate management issues include renal dysfunction. Prerenal azotemia, acute kidney injury associated with hypoperfusion (acute tubular necrosis), and renal toxicity caused by antibiotics, tacrolimus, or cyclosporine are encountered frequently in the postoperative period, sometimes necessitating dialysis. Hemolytic-uremic syndrome can be associated with cyclosporine, tacrolimus, or OKT3. Occasionally, postoperative intraperitoneal bleeding may be sufficient to increase intraabdominal pressure, which, in turn, may reduce renal blood flow; this effect is rapidly reversible when abdominal distention is relieved by exploratory laparotomy to identify and ligate the bleeding site and to remove intraperitoneal clot.

Anemia may also result from acute upper gastrointestinal bleeding or from transient hemolytic anemia, which may be autoimmune, especially when blood group O livers are transplanted into blood group A or B recipients. This autoimmune hemolytic anemia is mediated by donor intrahepatic lymphocytes that recognize red blood cell A or B antigens on recipient erythrocytes. Transient in nature, this process resolves once the donor liver is repopulated by recipient bone marrow–derived lymphocytes; the hemolysis can be treated by transfusing blood group O red blood cells and/or by administering higher doses of glucocorticoids. Transient thrombocytopenia is also commonly encountered. Aplastic anemia, a late occurrence, is rare but has been reported in almost 30% of patients who underwent liver transplantation for acute, severe hepatitis of unknown cause.

Bacterial, fungal, or viral infections are common and may be life-threatening postoperatively. Early after transplant surgery, common postoperative infections predominate—pneumonia, wound infections, infected intraabdominal collections, urinary tract infections, and IV line infections—rather than opportunistic infections; these infections may involve the biliary tree and liver as well. Beyond the first postoperative month, the toll of immunosuppression becomes evident, and opportunistic infections—CMV, herpes viruses, fungal infections (*Aspergillus*, *Candida*, cryptococcal disease), mycobacterial infections, parasitic infections (*Pneumocystis*, *Toxoplasma*), bacterial infections (*Nocardia*, *Legionella*, *Listeria*)—predominate. Rarely, early infections represent those transmitted with the donor liver, either infections present in the donor or infections acquired during procurement processing. De novo viral hepatitis infections acquired from the donor organ or, almost unheard of now, from transfused blood products occur after typical incubation periods for these agents (well beyond the first month). Obviously, infections in an immunosuppressed host demand early recognition and prompt management; prophylactic antibiotic therapy is administered routinely in the immediate postoperative period. Use

TABLE 368-4 NONHEPATIC COMPLICATIONS OF LIVER TRANSPLANTATION

Fluid overload	
Cardiovascular instability	Arrhythmias
	Congestive heart failure
	Cardiomyopathy
Pulmonary compromise	Pneumonia
	Pulmonary capillary vascular permeability
	Fluid overload
Renal dysfunction	Prerenal azotemia
	Hypoperfusion injury (acute tubular necrosis)
	Drug nephrotoxicity
	↓ Renal blood flow secondary to ↑ intraabdominal pressure
Hematologic	Anemia secondary to gastrointestinal and/or intraabdominal bleeding
	Hemolytic anemia, aplastic anemia
	Thrombocytopenia
Infection	Bacterial: early, common postoperative infections
	Fungal/parasitic: late, opportunistic infections
	Viral: late, opportunistic infections, recurrent hepatitis
Neuropsychiatric	Seizures
	Metabolic encephalopathy
	Depression
	Difficult psychosocial adjustment
Diseases of donor	Infectious
	Malignant
Malignancy	B cell lymphoma (posttransplantation lymphoproliferative disorders)
	De novo neoplasms (particularly squamous cell skin carcinoma)

TABLE 368-5 HEPATIC COMPLICATIONS OF LIVER TRANSPLANTATION

Hepatic Dysfunction Common After Major Surgery	
Prehepatic	Pigment load
	Hemolysis
	Blood collections (hematomas, abdominal collections)
Intrahepatic	
Early	Hepatotoxic drugs and anesthesia
	Hypoperfusion (hypotension, shock, sepsis)
	Benign postoperative cholestasis
Late	Transfusion-associated hepatitis
	Exacerbation of primary hepatic disease
Posthepatic	Biliary obstruction
	↓ Renal clearance of conjugated bilirubin (renal dysfunction)
Hepatic Dysfunction Unique to Liver Transplantation	
Primary graft nonfunction	
Vascular compromise	Portal vein obstruction
	Hepatic artery thrombosis
	Anastomotic leak with intraabdominal bleeding
Bile duct disorder	Stenosis, obstruction, leak
Rejection	
Recurrent primary hepatic disease	

of sulfamethoxazole with trimethoprim reduces the incidence of postoperative *Pneumocystis carinii* pneumonia. Antiviral prophylaxis for CMV with ganciclovir should be administered in patients at high risk (e.g., when a CMV-seropositive donor organ is implanted into a CMV-seronegative recipient).

Neuropsychiatric complications include seizures (commonly associated with cyclosporine and tacrolimus toxicity), metabolic encephalopathy, depression, and difficult psychosocial adjustment. Rarely, diseases are transmitted by the allograft from the donor to the recipient. In addition to viral and bacterial infections, malignancies of donor origin have occurred. Posttransplantation lymphoproliferative disorders, especially B cell lymphoma, are a recognized complication associated with immunosuppressive drugs such as azathioprine, tacrolimus, and cyclosporine (see above). Epstein-Barr virus has been shown to play a contributory role in some of these tumors, which may regress when immunosuppressive therapy is reduced. De novo neoplasms appear at increased frequency after liver transplantation, particularly squamous cell carcinomas of the skin. Routine screening should be performed.

Long-term complications after liver transplantation attributable primarily to immunosuppressive medications include diabetes mellitus and osteoporosis (associated with glucocorticoids and calcineurin inhibitors) as well as hypertension, hyperlipidemia, and chronic renal insufficiency (associated with cyclosporine and tacrolimus). Monitoring and treating these disorders are routine components of posttransplantation care; in some cases, they respond to changes in immunosuppressive regimen, while in others, specific treatment of the disorder is introduced. Data from a large U.S. database showed that the prevalence of renal failure was 18% at year 5 and 25% at year 10 after liver transplantation. Similarly, the high frequency of diabetes, hypertension, hyperlipidemia, obesity, and the metabolic syndrome renders patients susceptible to cardiovascular disease after liver transplantation; although hepatic complications account for most of the mortality after liver transplantation, renal failure and cardiovascular disease are the other leading causes of late mortality after liver transplantation.

HEPATIC COMPLICATIONS

Hepatic dysfunction after liver transplantation is similar to the hepatic complications encountered after major abdominal and cardiothoracic surgery; however, in addition, hepatic complications include primary graft failure, vascular compromise, failure or stricture of the biliary anastomoses, and rejection. As in nontransplantation surgery, postoperative jaundice may result from prehepatic, intrahepatic, and posthepatic sources. *Prehepatic* sources represent the massive hemoglobin pigment load from transfusions, hemolysis, hematomas, ecchymoses, and other collections of blood. *Early intrahepatic* liver injury includes effects of hepatotoxic drugs and anesthesia; hypoperfusion injury associated with hypotension, sepsis, and shock; and benign postoperative cholestasis. *Late intrahepatic* sources of liver injury include exacerbation of primary disease. *Posthepatic* sources of hepatic dysfunction include biliary obstruction and reduced renal clearance of conjugated bilirubin. Hepatic complications unique to liver transplantation include primary graft failure associated with ischemic injury to the organ during harvesting; vascular compromise associated with thrombosis or stenosis of the portal vein or hepatic artery anastomoses; vascular anastomotic leak; stenosis, obstruction, or leakage of the anastomosed common bile duct; recurrence of primary hepatic disorder (see below); and rejection.

TRANSPLANT REJECTION

Despite the use of immunosuppressive drugs, rejection of the transplanted liver still occurs in a proportion of patients, beginning 1–2 weeks after surgery. Clinical signs suggesting rejection are fever, right upper quadrant pain, and reduced bile pigment and volume. Leukocytosis may occur, but the most reliable indicators are increases in serum bilirubin and aminotransferase levels. Because these tests lack specificity, distinguishing among rejection, biliary obstruction, primary graft nonfunction, vascular compromise, viral hepatitis, CMV infection, drug hepatotoxicity, and recurrent primary disease may be difficult. Radiographic visualization of the biliary tree and/or percutaneous liver biopsy often help to establish the correct diagnosis. Morphologic features of acute rejection include a mixed portal cellular infiltrate, bile duct injury, and/or endothelial inflammation ("endothelialitis"); some of these findings are reminiscent of graft-versus-host disease, primary biliary cirrhosis, or recurrent allograft hepatitis C. As soon as transplant rejection is suspected, treatment consists of IV methylprednisolone in repeated boluses; if this fails to abort rejection, many centers use thymoglobulin or OKT3. Caution should be exercised when managing acute rejection with pulse glucocorticoids or OKT3 in patients with HCV infection, because of the high risk of triggering recurrent allograft hepatitis C.

Chronic rejection is a relatively rare outcome that can follow repeated bouts of acute rejection or that occurs unrelated to preceding rejection episodes. Morphologically, chronic rejection is characterized by progressive cholestasis, focal parenchymal necrosis, mononuclear infiltration, vascular lesions (intimal fibrosis, subintimal foam cells, fibrinoid necrosis), and fibrosis. This process may be reflected as ductopenia—the vanishing bile duct syndrome, which is more common in patients undergoing liver transplantation for autoimmune liver disease. Reversibility of chronic rejection is limited; in patients with therapy-resistant chronic rejection, retransplantation has yielded encouraging results.

OUTCOME

SURVIVAL

The survival rate for patients undergoing liver transplantation has improved steadily since 1983. One-year survival rates have increased from ~70% in the early 1980s to 85–90% from 2003 to the present time. Currently, the 5-year survival rate exceeds 60%. An important observation is the relationship between clinical status before transplantation and outcome. For patients who undergo liver transplantation when their level of compensation is high (e.g., still working or only partially disabled), a 1-year survival rate of >85% is common. For those whose level of decompensation mandates continuous in-hospital care prior to transplantation, the 1-year survival rate is ~70%, whereas for those who are so decompensated that they require life support in an intensive care unit, the 1-year survival rate is ~50%. Since the adoption by UNOS in 2002 of the MELD system for organ allocation, posttransplantation survival has been found to be affected adversely for candidates with MELD scores >25, considered high disease severity. Thus, irrespective of allocation scheme, high disease severity before transplantation corresponds to diminished posttransplantation survival. Another important distinction in survival has been drawn between high- and low-risk patient categories. For patients who do not fit any "high-risk" designations, 1-year and 5-year survival rates of 85 and 80%, respectively, have been recorded. In contrast, among patients in high-risk categories—cancer, fulminant hepatitis, age >65, concurrent renal failure, respirator dependence, portal vein thrombosis, and history of a portacaval shunt or multiple right upper quadrant operations—survival statistics fall into the range of 60% at 1 year and 35% at 5 years. Survival after retransplantation for primary graft nonfunction is ~50%. Causes of failure of liver transplantation vary with time. Failures within the first 3 months result primarily from technical complications, postoperative infections, and hemorrhage. Transplant failures after the first 3 months are more likely to result from infection, rejection, or recurrent disease (such as malignancy or viral hepatitis).

RECURRENCE OF PRIMARY DISEASE

Features of autoimmune hepatitis, primary sclerosing cholangitis, and primary biliary cirrhosis overlap with those of rejection or posttransplantation bile duct injury. Whether autoimmune hepatitis and sclerosing cholangitis recur after liver transplantation is controversial; data supporting recurrent autoimmune hepatitis (in up to one-third of patients in some series) are more convincing than those supporting recurrent sclerosing cholangitis. Similarly, reports of recurrent primary biliary cirrhosis after liver transplantation have appeared; however, the histologic features of primary biliary cirrhosis and chronic rejection are virtually indistinguishable and occur as frequently in patients with primary biliary cirrhosis as in patients undergoing transplantation for other reasons. The presence of a florid inflammatory bile duct lesion is highly suggestive of the recurrence of primary biliary cirrhosis, but even this lesion can be observed in acute rejection. Hereditary disorders such as Wilson's disease and α_1-antitrypsin deficiency have not recurred after liver transplantation; however, recurrence of disordered iron metabolism has been observed in some patients with hemochromatosis. Hepatic vein thrombosis (Budd-Chiari syndrome) may recur; this can be minimized by treating underlying myeloproliferative disorders and by anticoagulation. Because cholangiocarcinoma recurs almost invariably, few centers now offer transplantation to such patients; however, a few highly selected patients with operatively confirmed stage I or II cholangiocarcinoma who undergo liver transplantation combined with neoadjuvant chemoradiation may experience excellent outcomes. In patients with intrahepatic HCC who meet criteria for transplantation, 1- and 5-year survivals are similar to those observed in patients undergoing liver transplantation for nonmalignant disease. Finally, metabolic disorders such as nonalcoholic steatohepatitis recur frequently, especially if the underlying metabolic predisposition is not altered. The metabolic syndrome occurs commonly after liver transplantation as a result of recurrent nonalcoholic fatty liver, immunosuppressive medications, and/or, in patients with hepatitis C related to the impact of HCV infection on insulin resistance, diabetes and fatty liver.

Hepatitis A can recur after transplantation for fulminant hepatitis A, but such acute reinfection has no serious clinical sequelae. In fulminant hepatitis B, recurrence is not the rule; however, in the absence of any prophylactic measures, hepatitis B usually recurs after transplantation for end-stage chronic hepatitis B. Before the introduction of prophylactic antiviral therapy, immunosuppressive therapy sufficient to prevent allograft rejection led inevitably to marked increases in hepatitis B viremia, regardless of pretransplantation levels. Overall graft and patient survival were poor, and some patients experienced a rapid recapitulation of severe injury—severe chronic hepatitis or even fulminant hepatitis—after transplantation. Also recognized in the era before availability of antiviral regimens was *fibrosing cholestatic hepatitis*, rapidly progressive liver injury associated with marked hyperbilirubinemia, substantial prolongation of the prothrombin time (both out of proportion to relatively modest elevations of aminotransferase activity), and rapidly progressive liver failure. This lesion has been suggested to represent a "choking off" of the hepatocyte by an overwhelming density of HBV proteins. Complications such as sepsis and pancreatitis were also observed more frequently in patients undergoing liver transplantation for hepatitis B prior to the introduction of antiviral therapy. The introduction of long-term prophylaxis with HBIg revolutionized liver transplantation for chronic hepatitis B. Preoperative hepatitis B vaccination, preoperative or postoperative interferon (IFN) therapy, or short-term (≤2 months) HBIg prophylaxis has not been shown to be effective, but a retrospective analysis of data from several hundred European patients followed for 3 years after transplantation has shown that long-term (≥6 months) prophylaxis with HBIg is associated with a lowering of the risk of HBV reinfection from ~75 to 35% and a reduction in mortality from ~50 to 20%.

As a result of long-term HBIg use following liver transplantation for chronic hepatitis B, similar improvements in outcome have been observed in the United States, with 1-year survival rates between 75% and 90%. Currently, with HBIg prophylaxis, the outcome of liver transplantation for chronic hepatitis B is indistinguishable from that for chronic liver disease unassociated with chronic hepatitis B; essentially, medical concerns regarding liver transplantation for chronic hepatitis B have been eliminated. Passive immunoprophylaxis with HBIg is begun during the anhepatic stage of surgery, repeated daily for the first 6 postoperative days, and then continued with infusions that are given either at regular intervals of 4–6 weeks or, alternatively, when anti-hepatitis B surface (HBs) levels fall below a threshold of 100 mIU/mL. The current approach in most centers is to continue HBIg indefinitely, which can add approximately $20,000 per year to the cost of care; some centers are evaluating regimens that shift to less frequent administration or to IM administration in the late posttransplantation period or, in low-risk patients, maintenance with antiviral therapy (see below) alone. Still, "breakthrough" HBV infection occasionally occurs.

Further improving the outcome of liver transplantation for chronic hepatitis B is the current availability of such antiviral drugs as lamivudine, adefovir, entecavir, and tenofovir disoproxil fumarate (Chap. 362). When these drugs are administered to patients with decompensated liver disease, a proportion improve sufficiently to postpone imminent liver transplantation. In addition, antiviral therapy can be used to prevent recurrence of HBV infection when administered *prior to* transplantation; to treat hepatitis B that recurs *after* transplantation, including in patients who break through HBIg prophylaxis; and to reverse the course of otherwise fatal fibrosing cholestatic hepatitis. Clinical trials have shown that lamivudine antiviral therapy reduces the level of HBV replication substantially, sometimes even resulting in clearance of hepatitis B surface antigen (HBsAg); reduces alanine aminotransferase (ALT) levels; and improves histologic features of necrosis and inflammation. Long-term use of lamivudine is safe and effective, but after several months, a proportion of patients become resistant to lamivudine, resulting from YMDD (tyrosine-methionine-aspartate-aspartate) mutations in the HBV polymerase motif (Chap. 362). In approximately one-half of such resistant patients, hepatic deterioration may ensue. Fortunately, adefovir and tenofovir disoproxil fumarate are available as well and can be used to treat lamivudine-associated YMDD variants, effectively "rescuing" patients experiencing hepatic decompensation after lamivudine breakthrough. Currently, most liver transplantation centers combine HBIg plus lamivudine, adefovir, entecavir, or tenofovir disoproxil fumarate. In low-risk patients with no detectable hepatitis B viremia at the time of transplantation, a number of clinical trials have suggested that antiviral prophylaxis can suffice, without HBIg or with a finite duration of HBIg, to prevent recurrent HBV infection of the allograft. Antiviral prophylactic approaches applied to patients undergoing liver transplantation for chronic hepatitis B are being used as well for patients without hepatitis B who receive organs from donors with antibody to hepatitis B core antigen (anti-HBc). Patients who undergo liver transplantation for chronic hepatitis B plus D are less likely to experience recurrent liver injury than patients undergoing liver transplantation for hepatitis B alone; still, such co-infected patients would also be offered standard posttransplantation prophylactic therapy for hepatitis B.

Accounting for up to 40% of all liver transplantation procedures, the most common indication for liver transplantation is end-stage liver disease resulting from chronic hepatitis C. Recurrence of HCV infection after liver transplantation can be documented in almost every patient. The clinical consequences of recurrent hepatitis C are limited during the first 5 years after transplantation. Nonetheless, despite the relative clinical benignity of recurrent hepatitis C in the early years after liver transplantation, and despite the negligible impact on patient survival during these early years, histologic studies have documented the presence of moderate to severe chronic hepatitis in more than one-half of all patients and cirrhosis in ~20% at 5 years. Allograft cirrhosis is even more common, occurring in up to two-thirds of patients at 5 years, if moderate hepatitis is detected in a 1-year liver biopsy. Not surprisingly, then, for patients undergoing liver transplantation for hepatitis C, allograft and patient survival are diminished substantially between 5 and 10 years after transplantation.

In a proportion of patients, even during the early posttransplantation period, recurrent hepatitis C may be sufficiently severe biochemically and histologically to merit antiviral therapy. Treatment with pegylated IFN can *suppress* HCV-associated liver injury but rarely leads to *sustained* benefit. Sustained virologic responses are the exception, and reduced tolerability is often dose-limiting. Preemptive combination antiviral therapy with pegylated IFN and the nucleoside analogue ribavirin immediately after transplantation does not appear to provide any advantage over therapy introduced after clinical hepatitis has occurred. Similarly, although IFN-based antiviral therapy is not recommended for patients with decompensated liver disease, some centers have experimented with pretransplantation antiviral therapy in an attempt to eradicate HCV replication prior to transplantation; preliminary results are promising, but IFN treatment of patients with end-stage liver disease can lead to worsening of hepatic decompensation, and HCV infection has recurred after transplantation in some of these recipients. Trials of hepatitis C immune globulin preparations to prevent recurrent hepatitis C after liver transplantation have not been successful. Similarly, a trial of a high-dose monoclonal antibody to the HCV E2 envelope glycoprotein delayed but did not prevent reappearance of viremia.

Although the current standard-of-care treatment of allograft hepatitis C is pegylated IFN and ribavirin, in a number of studies, the safety and efficacy of the addition of the approved HCV protease inhibitors telaprevir or boceprevir to pegylated IFN and ribavirin in genotype 1 infected patients with recurrent hepatitis C have been examined. Because of the profound inhibitory effects of the HCV protease inhibitors on the metabolism of the calcineurin inhibitors (increasing cyclosporine levels almost 5-fold and tacrolimus levels 70-fold), calcineurin inhibitor doses must be reduced to safe levels in these patients. In one multicenter study, treatment with a telaprevir- or boceprevir-based triple-drug regimen (with pegylated IFN and ribavirin) achieved rates of HCV clearance similar to those achieved in patients with chronic hepatitis C who had not undergone transplantation. Unfortunately, tolerability of these protease inhibitor–based regimens remains problematic in this population, particularly in persons with allograft cirrhosis, in whom the frequency of hepatic decompensation is increased. The approval of several new direct-acting antiviral (DAA) agents and of IFN-free DAA regimens against HCV will have a major impact on the management and outcome of both pretransplantation and posttransplantation HCV infection. Such therapeutic approaches (1) permit the clearance of viremia in a substantial proportion of decompensated cirrhotics, thereby preventing recurrent allograft infection and, possibly, even improving the clinical status of these patients, delaying or obviating the need for liver replacement; and (2) achieve sustained virologic responses in a much higher proportion of persons with allograft HCV infection, because of improvements in antiviral treatment efficacy and tolerability.

A small number of allograft recipients succumb to early HCV-associated liver injury, and a syndrome reminiscent of fibrosing cholestatic hepatitis (see above) has been observed rarely. Because patients with more episodes of rejection receive more immunosuppressive therapy, and because immunosuppressive therapy enhances HCV replication, patients with severe or multiple episodes of rejection are more likely to experience early recurrence of hepatitis C after transplantation. Both high viral levels and older donor age have been linked to recurrent HCV-induced liver disease and to earlier disease recurrence after transplantation.

Patients who undergo liver transplantation for end-stage alcoholic cirrhosis are at risk of resorting to drinking again after transplantation, a potential source of recurrent alcoholic liver injury. Currently, alcoholic liver disease is one of the more common indications for liver transplantation, accounting for 20–25% of all liver transplantation procedures, and most transplantation centers screen candidates carefully for predictors of continued abstinence. Recidivism is more likely in patients whose sobriety prior to transplantation was <6 months. For abstinent patients with alcoholic cirrhosis, liver transplantation can be undertaken successfully, with outcomes comparable to those for other categories of patients with chronic liver disease, when coordinated by a team approach that includes substance abuse counseling.

POSTTRANSPLANTATION QUALITY OF LIFE

Full rehabilitation is achieved in the majority of patients who survive the early postoperative months and escape chronic rejection or unmanageable infection. Psychosocial maladjustment interferes with medical compliance in a small number of patients, but most manage to adhere to immunosuppressive regimens, which must be continued indefinitely. In one study, 85% of patients who survived their transplant operations returned to gainful activities. In fact, some women have conceived and carried pregnancies to term after transplantation without demonstrable injury to their infants.

369 Diseases of the Gallbladder and Bile Ducts

Norton J. Greenberger, Gustav Paumgartner

PHYSIOLOGY OF BILE PRODUCTION AND FLOW

BILE SECRETION AND COMPOSITION

Bile formed in the hepatic lobules is secreted into a complex network of canaliculi, small bile ductules, and larger bile ducts that run with lymphatics and branches of the portal vein and hepatic artery in portal tracts situated between hepatic lobules. These interlobular bile ducts coalesce to form larger septal bile ducts that join to form the right and left hepatic ducts, which in turn, unite to form the common hepatic duct. The common hepatic duct is joined by the cystic duct of the gallbladder to form the common bile duct (CBD), which enters the duodenum (often after joining the main pancreatic duct) through the ampulla of Vater.

Hepatic bile is an isotonic fluid with an electrolyte composition resembling blood plasma. The electrolyte composition of gallbladder bile differs from that of hepatic bile because most of the inorganic anions, chloride and bicarbonate, have been removed by reabsorption across the gallbladder epithelium. As a result of water reabsorption, total solute concentration of bile increases from 3–4 g/dL in hepatic bile to 10–15 g/dL in gallbladder bile.

Major solute components of bile by moles percent include bile acids (80%), lecithin and traces of other phospholipids (16%), and unesterified cholesterol (4.0%). In the lithogenic state, the cholesterol value can be as high as 8–10%. Other constituents include conjugated bilirubin; proteins (all immunoglobulins, albumin, metabolites of hormones, and other proteins metabolized in the liver); electrolytes; mucus; and, often, drugs and their metabolites.

The total daily basal secretion of hepatic bile is ~500–600 mL. Many substances taken up or synthesized by the hepatocyte are secreted into the bile canaliculi. The canalicular membrane forms microvilli and is associated with microfilaments of actin, microtubules, and other contractile elements. Prior to their secretion into the bile, many substances are taken up into the hepatocyte, while others, such as phospholipids, a portion of primary bile acids, and some cholesterol, are synthesized de novo in the hepatocyte. Three mechanisms are important in regulating bile flow: (1) active transport of bile acids from hepatocytes into the bile canaliculi, (2) active transport of other organic anions, and (3) cholangiocellular secretion. The last is a secretin-mediated and cyclic AMP–dependent mechanism that results in the secretion of a sodium- and bicarbonate-rich fluid into the bile ducts.

Active vectorial secretion of biliary constituents from the portal blood into the bile canaliculi is driven by a set of polarized transport systems at the basolateral (sinusoidal) and the canalicular apical plasma membrane domains of the hepatocyte. Two sinusoidal bile salt uptake systems have been cloned in humans, the Na^+/taurocholate cotransporter (NTCP, SLC10A1) and the organic anion–transporting proteins (OATPs), which also transport a large variety of non-bile salt organic anions. Several ATP-dependent canalicular transport systems, "export pumps," (ATP-binding cassette transport proteins, also known as ABC transporters) have been identified, the most important of which are: the bile salt export pump (BSEP, ABCB11); the anionic conjugate export pump (MRP2, ABCC2), which mediates the canalicular excretion of various amphiphilic conjugates formed by phase II conjugation (e.g., bilirubin mono- and diglucuronides and drugs); the multidrug export pump (MDR1, ABCB1) for hydrophobic cationic compounds; and the phospholipid export pump (MDR3, ABCB4). Two hemitransporters ABCG5/G8, functioning as a couple, constitute the canalicular cholesterol and phytosterol transporter. F1C1 (ATP8B1) is an aminophospholipid transferase ("flippase") essential for maintaining the lipid asymmetry of the canalicular membrane. The canalicular membrane also contains ATP-independent transport systems such as the Cl/HCO_3 anion exchanger isoform 2 (AE2, SLC4A2) for canalicular bicarbonate secretion. For most of these transporters, genetic defects have been identified that are associated with various forms of cholestasis or defects of biliary excretion. F1C1 is defective in progressive familial intrahepatic cholestasis type 1 (PFIC1) and benign recurrent intrahepatic cholestasis type 1 (BRIC1) and results in ablation of all other ATP-dependent transporter functions. BSEP is defective in PFIC2 and BRIC2. Mutations of MRP2 (ABCC2) cause the Dubin-Johnson syndrome, an inherited form of conjugated hyperbilirubinemia (Chap. 359). A defective MDR3 (ABCB4) results in PFIC3. ABCG5/G8, the canalicular half transporters for cholesterol and other neutral sterols, are defective in sitosterolemia. The cystic fibrosis transmembrane regulator (CFTR, ABCC7) located on bile duct epithelial cells but not on canalicular membranes is defective in cystic fibrosis, which is associated with impaired cholangiocellular pH regulation during ductular bile formation and chronic cholestatic liver disease, occasionally resulting in biliary cirrhosis.

THE BILE ACIDS

The primary bile acids, cholic acid and chenodeoxycholic acid (CDCA), are synthesized from cholesterol in the liver, conjugated with glycine or taurine, and secreted into the bile. Secondary bile acids, including deoxycholate and lithocholate, are formed in the colon as bacterial metabolites of the primary bile acids. However, lithocholic acid is much less efficiently absorbed from the colon than deoxycholic acid. Another secondary bile acid, found in low concentration, is ursodeoxycholic acid (UDCA), a stereoisomer of CDCA. In healthy subjects, the ratio of glycine to taurine conjugates in bile is ~3:1.

Bile acids are detergent-like molecules that in aqueous solutions and above a critical concentration of about 2 m*M* form molecular aggregates called *micelles.* Cholesterol alone is sparingly soluble in aqueous environments, and its solubility in bile depends on both the total lipid concentration and the relative molar percentages of bile acids and lecithin. Normal ratios of these constituents favor the formation of solubilizing *mixed micelles,* while abnormal ratios promote the precipitation of cholesterol crystals in bile via an intermediate liquid crystal phase.

In addition to facilitating the biliary excretion of cholesterol, bile acids facilitate the normal intestinal absorption of dietary fats, mainly cholesterol and fat-soluble vitamins, via a micellar transport mechanism (Chap. 349). Bile acids also serve as a major physiologic driving force for hepatic bile flow and aid in water and electrolyte transport in the small bowel and colon.

ENTEROHEPATIC CIRCULATION

Bile acids are efficiently conserved under normal conditions. Unconjugated, and to a lesser degree also conjugated, bile acids are absorbed by *passive diffusion* along the entire gut. Quantitatively much more important for bile salt recirculation, however, is the *active transport* mechanism for conjugated bile acids in the distal ileum (Chap. 349). The reabsorbed bile acids enter the portal bloodstream and are taken up rapidly by hepatocytes, reconjugated, and resecreted into bile (enterohepatic circulation).

The normal bile acid pool size is approximately 2–4 g. During digestion of a meal, the bile acid pool undergoes at least one or more enterohepatic cycles, depending on the size and composition of the meal. Normally, the bile acid pool circulates ~5–10 times daily. Intestinal reabsorption of the pool is about 95% efficient; therefore, fecal loss of bile acids is in the range of 0.2–0.4 g/d. In the steady state, this fecal loss is compensated by an equal daily synthesis of bile acids by the liver, and, thus, the size of the bile acid pool is maintained. Bile acids in the intestine release fibroblast growth factor 19 (FGF19) into the circulation, which is transported to the liver where it suppresses synthesis of bile acids from cholesterol by inhibiting the rate-limiting enzyme cytochrome P450 7A1 (CYP7A1) and also promotes gallbladder relaxation. While the loss of bile salts in stool is usually matched by increased hepatic synthesis, the maximum rate of synthesis is ~5 g/d, which may be insufficient to replete the bile acid pool size when there is pronounced impairment of intestinal bile salt reabsorption.

The expression of ABC transporters in the enterohepatic circulation and of the rate-limiting enzymes of bile acid and cholesterol synthesis are regulated in a coordinated fashion by nuclear receptors, which are ligand-activated transcription factors. The hepatic BSEP (ABCB11) is upregulated by the farnesoid X receptor (FXR), a bile acid sensor that also represses bile acid synthesis. The expression of the cholesterol transporter, ABCG5/G8, is upregulated by the liver X receptor (LXR), which is an oxysterol sensor.

GALLBLADDER AND SPHINCTERIC FUNCTIONS

In the fasting state, the sphincter of Oddi offers a high-pressure zone of resistance to bile flow from the CBD into the duodenum. Its tonic contraction serves to (1) prevent reflux of duodenal contents into the pancreatic and bile ducts and (2) promote filling of the gallbladder. The major factor controlling the evacuation of the gallbladder is the peptide hormone cholecystokinin (CCK), which is released from the duodenal mucosa in response to the ingestion of fats and amino acids. CCK produces (1) powerful contraction of the gallbladder, (2) decreased resistance of the sphincter of Oddi, and (3) enhanced flow of biliary contents into the duodenum.

Hepatic bile is "concentrated" within the gallbladder by energy-dependent transmucosal absorption of water and electrolytes. Almost the entire bile acid pool may be sequestered in the gallbladder following an overnight fast for delivery into the duodenum with the first meal of the day. The normal capacity of the gallbladder is ~30 mL of bile.

DISEASES OF THE GALLBLADDER

CONGENITAL ANOMALIES

Anomalies of the biliary tract are not uncommon and include abnormalities in number, size, and shape (e.g., agenesis of the gallbladder, duplications, rudimentary or oversized "giant" gallbladders, and diverticula). *Phrygian cap* is a clinically innocuous entity in which a partial or complete septum (or fold) separates the fundus from the body. Anomalies of position or suspension are not uncommon and include left-sided gallbladder, intrahepatic gallbladder, retrodisplacement of the gallbladder, and "floating" gallbladder. The latter condition predisposes to acute torsion, volvulus, or herniation of the gallbladder.

GALLSTONES

Epidemiology and Pathogenesis Gallstones are quite prevalent in most Western countries. Gallstone formation increases after age 50. In the United States, the third National Health and Nutrition Examination Survey (NHANES III) has revealed an overall prevalence of gallstones of 7.9% in men and 16.6% in women. The prevalence was high in Mexican Americans (8.9% in men, 26.7% in women), intermediate for non-Hispanic whites (8.6% in men, 16.6% in women), and low for African Americans (5.3% in men, 13.9% in women).

Gallstones are formed because of abnormal bile composition. They are divided into two major types: cholesterol stones and pigment stones. Cholesterol stones account for more than 90% of all gallstones in Western industrialized countries. Cholesterol gallstones usually contain >50% cholesterol monohydrate plus an admixture of calcium salts, bile pigments, proteins, and fatty acids. Pigment stones are composed primarily of calcium bilirubinate; they contain <20% cholesterol and are classified into "black" and "brown" types, the latter forming secondary to chronic biliary infection.

CHOLESTEROL STONES AND BILIARY SLUDGE Cholesterol is essentially water insoluble and requires aqueous dispersion into either micelles or vesicles, both of which require the presence of a second lipid to solubilize the cholesterol. Cholesterol and phospholipids are secreted into bile as unilamellar bilayered vesicles, which are converted into mixed micelles consisting of bile acids, phospholipids, and cholesterol by the action of bile acids. If there is an excess of cholesterol in relation to phospholipids and bile acids, unstable, cholesterol-rich vesicles remain, which aggregate into large multilamellar vesicles from which cholesterol crystals precipitate (Fig. 369-1).

There are several important mechanisms in the formation of lithogenic (stone-forming) bile. The most important is increased biliary secretion of cholesterol. This may occur in association with obesity, the metabolic syndrome, high-caloric and cholesterol-rich diets,

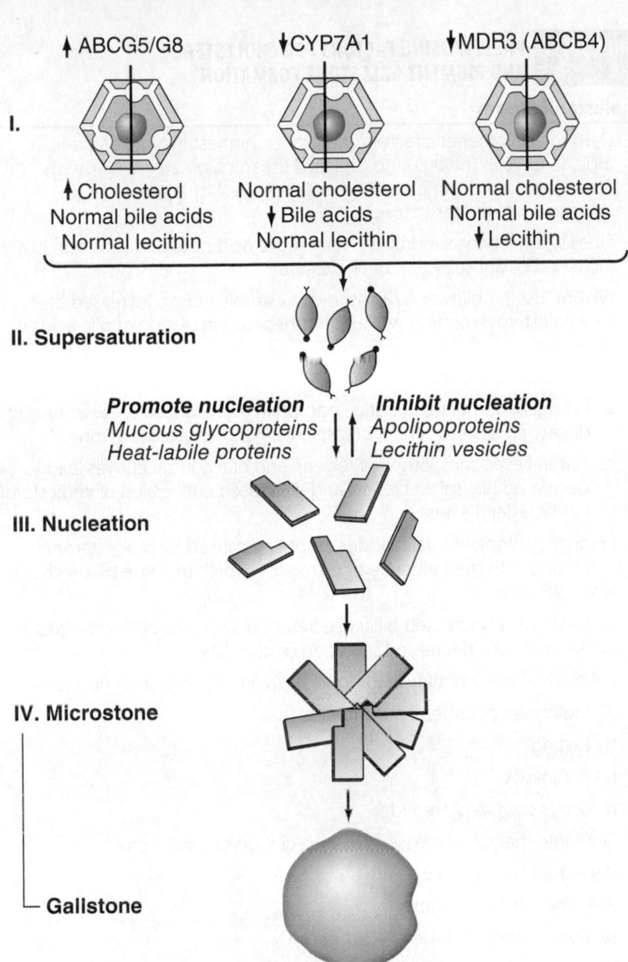

FIGURE 369-1 Scheme showing pathogenesis of cholesterol gallstone formation. Conditions or factors that increase the ratio of cholesterol to bile acids and phospholipids (lecithin) favor gallstone formation. ABCB4, ATP-binding cassette transporter; ABCG5/8, ATP-binding cassette (ABC) transporter G5/G8; CYP7A1, cytochrome P450 7A1; MDR3, multidrug resistance protein 3, also called phospholipid export pump.

or drugs (e.g., clofibrate) and may result from increased activity of hydroxymethylglutaryl-coenzyme A (HMG-CoA) reductase, the rate-limiting enzyme of hepatic cholesterol synthesis, and increased hepatic uptake of cholesterol from blood. In patients with gallstones, dietary cholesterol *increases* biliary cholesterol secretion. This does not occur in non-gallstone patients on high-cholesterol diets. In addition to environmental factors such as high-caloric and cholesterol-rich diets, genetic factors play an important role in gallstone disease. A large study of symptomatic gallstones in Swedish twins provided strong evidence for a role of genetic factors in gallstone pathogenesis. Genetic factors accounted for 25%, shared environmental factors for 13%, and individual environmental factors for 62% of the phenotypic variation among monozygotic twins. A single nucleotide polymorphism of the gene encoding the hepatic cholesterol transporter ABCG5/G8 has been found in 21% of patients with gallstones, but only in 9% of the general population. It is thought to cause a gain of function of the cholesterol transporter and to contribute to cholesterol hypersecretion. A high prevalence of gallstones is found among first-degree relatives of gallstone carriers and in certain ethnic populations such as American Indians, Chilean Indians, and Chilean Hispanics. A common genetic trait has been identified for some of these populations by mitochondrial DNA analysis. In some patients, impaired hepatic conversion of cholesterol to bile acids may also occur, resulting in an increase of the lithogenic cholesterol/bile acid ratio. Although most cholesterol stones have a polygenic basis, there are rare monogenic (Mendelian) causes. Recently, a mutation in the *CYP7A1* gene has been described that results in a deficiency of the enzyme cholesterol 7-hydroxylase, which catalyzes the initial step in cholesterol catabolism and bile acid synthesis. The homozygous state is associated with hypercholesterolemia and gallstones. Because the phenotype is expressed in the heterozygote state, mutations in the *CYP7A1* gene may contribute to the susceptibility to cholesterol gallstone disease in the population. Mutations in the *MDR3* (ABCB4) gene, which encodes the phospholipid export pump in the canalicular membrane of the hepatocyte, may cause defective phospholipid secretion into bile, resulting in cholesterol supersaturation of bile and formation of cholesterol gallstones in the gallbladder and in the bile ducts. Thus, an excess of biliary cholesterol in relation to bile acids and phospholipids is primarily due to hypersecretion of cholesterol, but hyposecretion of bile acids or phospholipids may contribute. An additional disturbance of bile acid metabolism that is likely to contribute to supersaturation of bile with cholesterol is enhanced conversion of cholic acid to deoxycholic acid, with replacement of the cholic acid pool by an expanded deoxycholic acid pool. It may result from enhanced dehydroxylation of cholic acid and increased absorption of newly formed deoxycholic acid. An increased deoxycholate secretion is associated with hypersecretion of cholesterol into bile.

While supersaturation of bile with cholesterol is an important prerequisite for gallstone formation, it is generally not sufficient by itself to produce cholesterol precipitation in vivo. Most individuals with supersaturated bile do not develop stones because the time required for cholesterol crystals to nucleate and grow is longer than the time bile remains in the gallbladder.

An important mechanism is *nucleation* of cholesterol monohydrate crystals, which is greatly accelerated in human lithogenic bile. Accelerated nucleation of cholesterol monohydrate in bile may be due to either an *excess of pronucleating factors* or a *deficiency of antinucleating factors*. Mucin and certain nonmucin glycoproteins, principally immunoglobulins, appear to be pronucleating factors, while apolipoproteins A-I and A-II and other glycoproteins appear to be antinucleating factors. Pigment particles may possibly play a role as nucleating factors. In a genome-wide analysis of serum bilirubin levels, the uridine diphosphate-glucuronyltransferase 1A1 (*UGT1A1*) Gilbert's syndrome gene variant was associated with the presence of gallstone disease. Because most gallstones associated with the *UGT1A1* variant were cholesterol stones, this finding points to the role of pigment particles in the pathogenesis of gallbladder stones. Cholesterol monohydrate crystal nucleation and crystal growth probably occur within the mucin gel layer. Vesicle fusion leads to liquid crystals, which, in turn, nucleate into solid cholesterol monohydrate crystals. Continued growth of the crystals occurs by direct nucleation of cholesterol molecules from supersaturated unilamellar or multilamellar biliary vesicles.

A third important mechanism in cholesterol gallstone formation is *gallbladder hypomotility*. If the gallbladder emptied all supersaturated or crystal-containing bile completely, stones would not be able to grow. A high percentage of patients with gallstones exhibit abnormalities of gallbladder emptying. Ultrasonographic studies show that gallstone patients display an increased gallbladder volume during fasting and also after a test meal (residual volume) and that fractional emptying after gallbladder stimulation is decreased. The incidence of gallstones is increased in conditions associated with infrequent or impaired gallbladder emptying such as fasting, parenteral nutrition, or pregnancy and in patients using drugs that inhibit gallbladder motility.

Biliary sludge is a thick, mucous material that, upon microscopic examination, reveals lecithin-cholesterol liquid crystals, cholesterol monohydrate crystals, calcium bilirubinate, and mucin gels. Biliary sludge typically forms a crescent-like layer in the most dependent portion of the gallbladder and is recognized by characteristic echoes on ultrasonography (see below). The presence of biliary sludge implies two abnormalities: (1) the normal balance between gallbladder mucin secretion and elimination has become deranged, and (2) nucleation of biliary solutes has occurred. That biliary sludge may be a precursor form of gallstone disease is evident from several observations. In one study, 96 patients with gallbladder sludge were followed prospectively by serial ultrasound studies. In 18%, biliary sludge disappeared and did not recur for at least 2 years. In 60%, biliary sludge disappeared and reappeared; in 14%, gallstones (8% asymptomatic, 6% symptomatic) developed; and in 6%, severe biliary pain with or without acute pancreatitis occurred. In 12 patients, cholecystectomies were performed, 6 for gallstone-associated biliary pain and 3 in symptomatic patients with sludge but without gallstones who had prior attacks of pancreatitis; the latter did not recur after cholecystectomy. It should be emphasized that biliary sludge can develop with disorders that cause gallbladder hypomotility; i.e., surgery, burns, total parenteral nutrition, pregnancy, and oral contraceptives—all of which are associated with gallstone formation. However, the presence of biliary sludge implies supersaturation of bile with either cholesterol or calcium bilirubinate.

Two other conditions are associated with cholesterol-stone or biliary-sludge formation: pregnancy and rapid weight reduction through a very-low-calorie diet. There appear to be two key changes during pregnancy that contribute to a "cholelithogenic state": (1) a marked increase in cholesterol saturation of bile during the third trimester and (2) sluggish gallbladder contraction in response to a standard meal, resulting in impaired gallbladder emptying. That these changes are related to pregnancy per se is supported by several studies that show reversal of these abnormalities quite rapidly after delivery. During pregnancy, gallbladder sludge develops in 20–30% of women and gallstones in 5–12%. Although biliary sludge is a common finding during pregnancy, it is usually asymptomatic and often resolves spontaneously after delivery. Gallstones, which are less common than sludge and frequently associated with biliary colic, may also disappear after delivery because of spontaneous dissolution related to bile becoming unsaturated with cholesterol postpartum.

Approximately 10–20% of persons with rapid weight reduction achieved through very-low-calorie dieting develop gallstones. In a study involving 600 patients who completed a 3-month, 520-kcal/d diet, UDCA in a dosage of 600 mg/d proved highly effective in preventing gallstone formation; gallstones developed in only 3% of UDCA recipients, compared to 28% of placebo-treated patients. In obese patients treated by gastric banding, 500 mg/d of UDCA reduced the risk of gallstone formation from 30% to 8% within a follow-up of 6 months.

To summarize, cholesterol gallstone disease occurs because of several defects, which include (1) bile supersaturation with cholesterol, (2) nucleation of cholesterol monohydrate with subsequent crystal retention and stone growth, and (3) abnormal gallbladder motor function with delayed emptying and stasis. Other important factors known to predispose to cholesterol-stone formation are summarized in Table 369-1.

PIGMENT STONES Black pigment stones are composed of either pure calcium bilirubinate or polymer-like complexes with calcium and mucin glycoproteins. They are more common in patients who have chronic hemolytic states (with increased conjugated bilirubin in bile), liver cirrhosis, Gilbert's syndrome, or cystic fibrosis. Gallbladder stones in patients with ileal diseases, ileal resection, or ileal bypass generally are also black pigment stones. Enterohepatic recycling of bilirubin in ileal disease states contributes to their pathogenesis. Brown pigment stones are composed of calcium salts of unconjugated bilirubin with varying amounts of cholesterol and protein. They are caused by the presence of increased amounts of unconjugated, insoluble bilirubin in bile that precipitates to form stones. Deconjugation of an excess of soluble bilirubin mono- and diglucuronides may be mediated by endogenous β-glucuronidase but may also occur by spontaneous hydrolysis. Sometimes, the enzyme is also produced when bile is chronically infected by bacteria, and such stones are brown. Pigment stone formation is frequent in Asia and is often associated with infections in the gallbladder and biliary tree (Table 369-1).

Diagnosis Procedures of potential use in the diagnosis of cholelithiasis and other diseases of the gallbladder are detailed in Table 369-2. Ultrasonography of the gallbladder is very accurate in the identification of cholelithiasis and has replaced oral cholecystography (Fig. 369-2A). Stones as small as 1.5 mm in diameter may be confidently identified provided that firm criteria are used (e.g., acoustic "shadowing" of opacities that are within the gallbladder lumen and that change with the patient's position [by gravity]). In major medical centers, the false-negative and false-positive rates for ultrasound in gallstone patients are ~2–4%. Biliary sludge is material of low echogenic activity that typically forms a layer in the most dependent position of the gallbladder. This layer shifts with postural changes but fails to produce acoustic shadowing; these two characteristics distinguish sludges from gallstones. Ultrasound can also be used to assess the emptying function of the gallbladder.

The plain abdominal film may detect gallstones containing sufficient calcium to be radiopaque (10–15% of cholesterol and ~50% of pigment stones). Plain radiography may also be of use in the diagnosis of emphysematous cholecystitis, porcelain gallbladder, limey bile, and gallstone ileus.

Oral cholecystography (OCG) has historically been a useful procedure for the diagnosis of gallstones but has been replaced by ultrasound and is regarded as obsolete. It may be used to assess the patency of the cystic duct and gallbladder emptying function. Further, OCG can also delineate the size and number of gallstones and determine whether they are calcified.

Radiopharmaceuticals such as ^{99m}Tc-labeled *N*-substituted iminodiacetic acids (HIDA, DIDA, DISIDA, etc.) are rapidly extracted from

TABLE 369-1 PREDISPOSING FACTORS FOR CHOLESTEROL AND PIGMENT GALLSTONE FORMATION

Cholesterol Stones

1. Demographic/genetic factors: Prevalence highest in North American Indians, Chilean Indians, and Chilean Hispanics, greater in Northern Europe and North America than in Asia, lowest in Japan; familial disposition; hereditary aspects
2. Obesity, metabolic syndrome: Normal bile acid pool and secretion but increased biliary secretion of cholesterol
3. Weight loss: Mobilization of tissue cholesterol leads to increased biliary cholesterol secretion while enterohepatic circulation of bile acids is decreased
4. Female sex hormones
   a. Estrogens stimulate hepatic lipoprotein receptors, increase uptake of dietary cholesterol, and increase biliary cholesterol secretion
   b. Natural estrogens, other estrogens, and oral contraceptives lead to decreased bile salt secretion and decreased conversion of cholesterol to cholesteryl esters
5. Pregnancy: Impaired gallbladder emptying caused by progesterone combined with the influence of estrogens, which increase biliary cholesterol secretion
6. Increasing age: Increased biliary secretion of cholesterol, decreased size of bile acid pool, decreased secretion of bile salts
7. Gallbladder hypomotility leading to stasis and formation of sludge
   a. Prolonged parenteral nutrition
   b. Fasting
   c. Pregnancy
   d. Drugs such as octreotide
8. Clofibrate therapy: Increased biliary secretion of cholesterol
9. Decreased bile acid secretion
   a. Primary biliary cirrhosis
   b. Genetic defect of the *CYP7A1* gene
10. Decreased phospholipid secretion: Genetic defect of the *MDR3* gene
11. Miscellaneous
    a. High-calorie, high-fat diet
    b. Spinal cord injury

Pigment Stones

1. Demographic/genetic factors: Asia, rural setting
2. Chronic hemolysis
3. Alcoholic liver cirrhosis
4. Pernicious anemia
5. Cystic fibrosis
6. Chronic biliary tract infection, parasite infections
7. Increasing age
8. Ileal disease, ileal resection or bypass

TABLE 369-2 DIAGNOSTIC EVALUATION OF THE GALLBLADDER

Diagnostic Advantages	Diagnostic Limitations	Comment
Gallbladder Ultrasound		
Rapid	Bowel gas	Procedure of choice for detection of stones
Accurate identification of gallstones (>95%)	Massive obesity	
Simultaneous scanning of GB, liver, bile ducts, pancreas	Ascites	
"Real-time" scanning allows assessment of GB volume, contractility		
Not limited by jaundice, pregnancy		
May detect very small stones		
Plain Abdominal X-Ray		
Low cost	Relatively low yield	Pathognomonic findings in: calcified gallstones
Readily available	? Contraindicated in pregnancy	Limey bile, porcelain GB
		Emphysematous cholecystitis
		Gallstone ileus
Radioisotope Scans (HIDA, DIDA, etc.)		
Accurate identification of cystic duct obstruction	? Contraindicated in pregnancy	Indicated for confirmation of suspected acute cholecystitis; less sensitive and less specific in chronic cholecystitis; useful in diagnosis of acalculous cholecystopathy, especially if given with CCK to assess gallbladder emptying
Simultaneous assessment of bile ducts	Serum bilirubin >103–205 μmol/L (6–12 mg/dL)	
	Cholecystogram of low resolution	

Abbreviations: CCK, cholecystokinin; GB, gallbladder.

the blood and are excreted into the biliary tree in high concentration even in the presence of mild to moderate serum bilirubin elevations. Failure to image the gallbladder in the presence of biliary ductal visualization may indicate cystic duct obstruction, acute or chronic cholecystitis, or surgical absence of the organ. Such scans have some application in the diagnosis of acute cholecystitis.

Symptoms of Gallstone Disease Gallstones usually produce symptoms by causing inflammation or obstruction following their migration into the cystic duct or CBD. The most specific and characteristic symptom of gallstone disease is biliary colic that is a constant and often long-lasting pain (see below). Obstruction of the cystic duct or CBD by a stone produces increased intraluminal pressure and distention of the viscus that cannot be relieved by repetitive biliary contractions. The resultant visceral pain is characteristically a severe, steady ache or fullness in the epigastrium or right upper quadrant (RUQ) of the abdomen with frequent radiation to the interscapular area, right scapula, or shoulder.

Biliary colic begins quite suddenly and may persist with severe intensity for 30 min to 5 h, subsiding gradually or rapidly. It is steady rather than intermittent, as would be suggested by the word *colic*, which must be regarded as a misnomer, although it is in widespread use. An episode of biliary pain persisting beyond 5 h should raise the suspicion of acute cholecystitis (see below). Nausea and vomiting frequently accompany episodes of biliary pain. An elevated level of serum bilirubin and/or alkaline phosphatase suggests a common duct stone. Fever or chills (rigors) with biliary pain usually imply a complication, i.e., cholecystitis, pancreatitis, or cholangitis. Complaints of short-lasting, vague epigastric fullness, dyspepsia, eructation, or flatulence, especially following a fatty meal, should not be confused with biliary pain. Such symptoms are frequently elicited from patients with or without gallstone disease

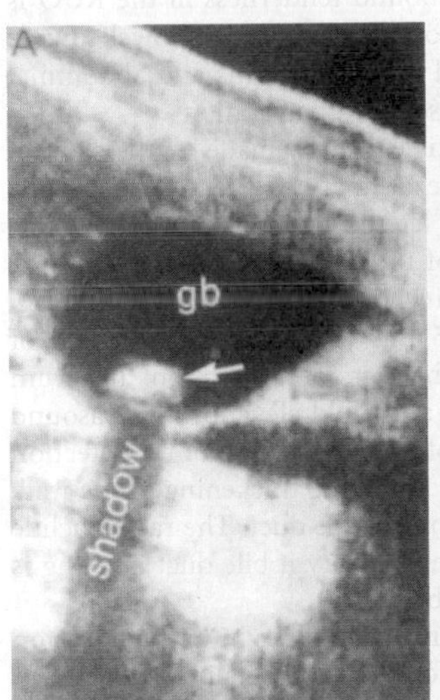

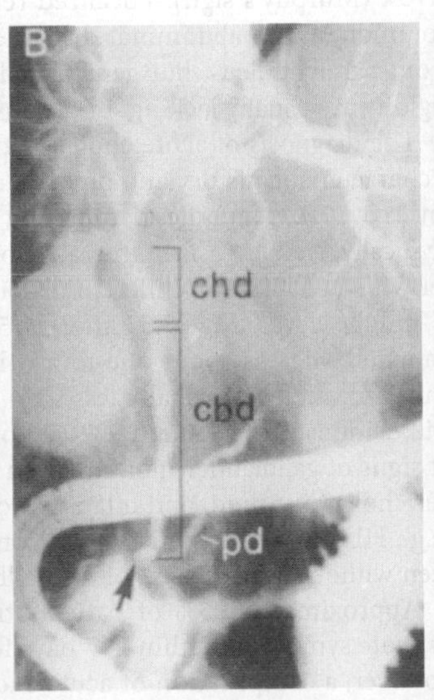

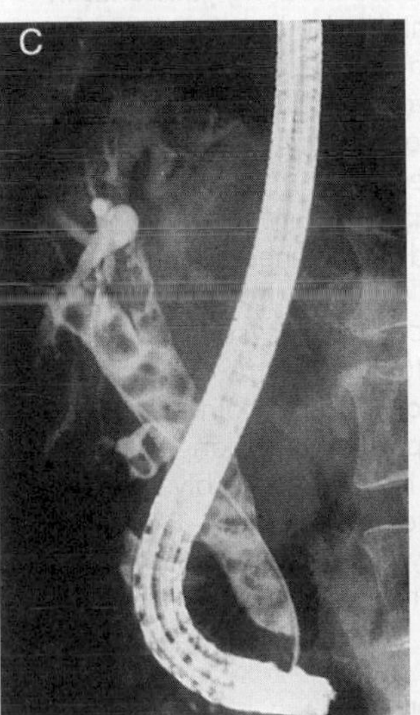

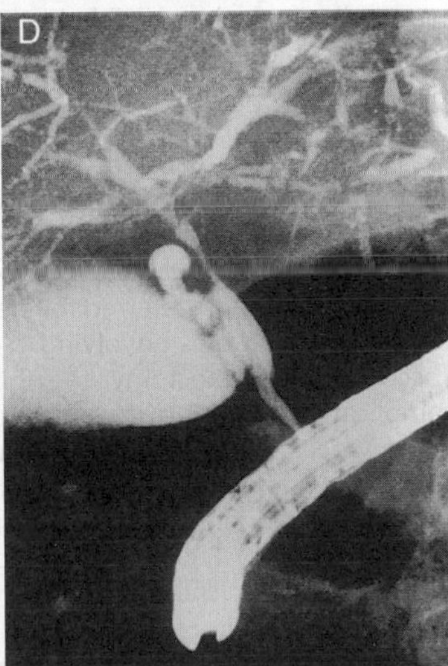

FIGURE 369-2 Examples of ultrasound and radiologic studies of the biliary tract. ***A.*** An ultrasound study showing a distended gallbladder (GB) containing a single large stone (*arrow*), which casts an acoustic shadow. ***B.*** Endoscopic retrograde cholangiopancreatogram (ERCP) showing normal biliary tract anatomy. In addition to the endoscope and large vertical gallbladder filled with contrast dye, the common hepatic duct (CHD), common bile duct (CBD), and pancreatic duct (PD) are shown. The *arrow* points to the ampulla of Vater. ***C.*** Endoscopic retrograde cholangiogram (ERC) showing choledocholithiasis. The biliary tract is dilated and contains multiple radiolucent calculi. ***D.*** ERCP showing sclerosing cholangitis. The common bile duct shows areas that are strictured and narrowed.

but are not specific for biliary calculi. Biliary colic may be precipitated by eating a fatty meal, by consumption of a large meal following a period of prolonged fasting, or by eating a normal meal; it is frequently nocturnal, occurring within a few hours of retiring.

Natural History Gallstone disease discovered in an asymptomatic patient or in a patient whose symptoms are not referable to cholelithiasis is a common clinical problem. Sixty to 80% of persons with asymptomatic gallstones remain asymptomatic over follow-up periods of up to 25 years. The probability of developing symptoms within 5 years after diagnosis is 2–4% per year and decreases in the years thereafter to 1–2%. The yearly incidence of complications is about 0.1–0.3%. Patients remaining asymptomatic for 15 years were found to be unlikely to develop symptoms during further follow-up, and most patients who did develop complications from their gallstones experienced *prior* warning symptoms. Similar conclusions apply to diabetic patients with silent gallstones. Decision analysis has suggested that (1) the cumulative risk of death due to gallstone disease while on expectant management is small, and (2) prophylactic cholecystectomy is not warranted.

Complications requiring cholecystectomy are much more common in gallstone patients who have developed symptoms of biliary pain. Patients found to have gallstones at a young age are more likely to develop symptoms from cholelithiasis than are patients >60 years at the time of initial diagnosis. Patients with diabetes mellitus and gallstones may be somewhat more susceptible to septic complications, but the magnitude of risk of septic biliary complications in diabetic patients is incompletely defined.

TREATMENT GALLSTONES

SURGICAL THERAPY

In asymptomatic gallstone patients, the risk of developing symptoms or complications requiring surgery is quite small (see above). Thus, a recommendation for cholecystectomy in a patient with gallstones should probably be based on assessment of three factors: (1) the presence of symptoms that are frequent enough or severe enough to interfere with the patient's general routine; (2) the presence of a prior complication of gallstone disease, i.e., history of acute cholecystitis, pancreatitis, gallstone fistula, etc.; or (3) the presence of an underlying condition predisposing the patient to increased risk of gallstone complications (e.g., calcified or porcelain gallbladder and/or a previous attack of acute cholecystitis regardless of current symptomatic status). Patients with very large gallstones (>3 cm in diameter) and patients harboring gallstones in a congenitally anomalous gallbladder might also be considered for prophylactic cholecystectomy. Although young age is a worrisome factor in asymptomatic gallstone patients, few authorities would now recommend routine cholecystectomy in all young patients with silent stones. Laparoscopic cholecystectomy is a minimal-access approach for the removal of the gallbladder together with its stones. Its advantages include a markedly shortened hospital stay, minimal disability, and decreased cost, and it is the procedure of choice for most patients referred for elective cholecystectomy.

From several studies involving >4000 patients undergoing laparoscopic cholecystectomy, the following key points emerge: (1) complications develop in ~4% of patients, (2) conversion to laparotomy occurs in 5%, (3) the death rate is remarkably low (i.e., <0.1%), and (4) the rate of bile duct injuries is low (i.e., 0.2–0.6%) and comparable with open cholecystectomy. These data indicate why laparoscopic cholecystectomy has become the "gold standard" for treating symptomatic cholelithiasis.

MEDICAL THERAPY—GALLSTONE DISSOLUTION

In carefully selected patients with a functioning gallbladder and with radiolucent stones <10 mm in diameter, complete dissolution can be achieved in ~50% of patients within 6 months to 2 years. For good results within a reasonable time period, this therapy should be limited to radiolucent stones smaller than 5 mm in diameter. The dose of UDCA should be 10–15 mg/kg per day. Stones larger than 10 mm in size rarely dissolve. Pigment stones are not responsive to UDCA therapy. Probably ≤10% of patients with *symptomatic* cholelithiasis are candidates for such treatment. However, in addition to the vexing problem of recurrent stones (30–50% over 3–5 years of follow-up), there is also the factor of taking an expensive drug for up to 2 years. The advantages and success of laparoscopic cholecystectomy have largely reduced the role of gallstone dissolution to patients who wish to avoid or are not candidates for elective cholecystectomy. However, patients with cholesterol gallstone disease who develop recurrent choledocholithiasis after cholecystectomy should be on long-term treatment with UDCA.

ACUTE AND CHRONIC CHOLECYSTITIS

Acute Cholecystitis Acute inflammation of the gallbladder wall usually follows obstruction of the cystic duct by a stone. Inflammatory response can be evoked by three factors: (1) *mechanical inflammation* produced by increased intraluminal pressure and distention with resulting ischemia of the gallbladder mucosa and wall, (2) *chemical inflammation* caused by the release of lysolecithin (due to the action of phospholipase on lecithin in bile) and other local tissue factors, and (3) *bacterial inflammation*, which may play a role in 50–85% of patients with acute cholecystitis. The organisms most frequently isolated by culture of gallbladder bile in these patients include *Escherichia coli*, *Klebsiella* spp., *Streptococcus* spp., and *Clostridium* spp.

Acute cholecystitis often begins as an attack of biliary pain that progressively worsens. Approximately 60–70% of patients report having experienced prior attacks that resolved spontaneously. As the episode progresses, however, the pain of acute cholecystitis becomes more generalized in the right upper abdomen. As with biliary colic, the pain of cholecystitis may radiate to the interscapular area, right scapula, or shoulder. Peritoneal signs of inflammation such as increased pain with jarring or on deep respiration may be apparent. The patient is anorectic and often nauseated. Vomiting is relatively common and may produce symptoms and signs of vascular and extracellular volume depletion. Jaundice is unusual early in the course of acute cholecystitis but may occur when edematous inflammatory changes involve the bile ducts and surrounding lymph nodes.

A low-grade fever is characteristically present, but shaking chills or rigors are not uncommon. The RUQ of the abdomen is almost invariably tender to palpation. An enlarged, tense gallbladder is palpable in 25–50% of patients. Deep inspiration or cough during subcostal palpation of the RUQ usually produces increased pain and inspiratory arrest (Murphy's sign). Localized rebound tenderness in the RUQ is common, as are abdominal distention and hypoactive bowel sounds from paralytic ileus, but generalized peritoneal signs and abdominal rigidity are usually lacking, in the absence of perforation.

The diagnosis of acute cholecystitis is usually made on the basis of a characteristic history and physical examination. The triad of sudden onset of RUQ tenderness, fever, and leukocytosis is highly suggestive. Typically, leukocytosis in the range of 10,000–15,000 cells per microliter with a left shift on differential count is found. The serum bilirubin is mildly elevated (<85.5 μmol/L [5 mg/dL]) in fewer than half of patients, whereas about one-fourth have modest elevations in serum aminotransferases (usually less than a fivefold elevation). Ultrasound will demonstrate calculi in 90–95% of cases and is useful for detection of signs of gallbladder inflammation including thickening of the wall, pericholecystic fluid, and dilatation of the bile duct. The radionuclide (e.g., HIDA) biliary scan may be confirmatory if bile duct imaging is seen without visualization of the gallbladder.

Approximately 75% of patients treated medically have remission of acute symptoms within 2–7 days following hospitalization. In 25%, however, a complication of acute cholecystitis will occur despite conservative treatment (see below). In this setting, prompt surgical intervention is required. Of the 75% of patients with acute cholecystitis who undergo remission of symptoms, ~25% will experience a recurrence of cholecystitis within 1 year, and 60% will have at least one recurrent bout within 6 years. In view of the natural history of the disease, acute cholecystitis is best treated by early surgery whenever possible.

Mirizzi's syndrome is a rare complication in which a gallstone becomes impacted in the cystic duct or neck of the gallbladder causing compression of the CBD, resulting in CBD obstruction and jaundice. Ultrasound shows gallstone(s) lying outside the hepatic duct. Endoscopic retrograde cholangiopancreatography (ERCP) (Fig. 369-2B), percutaneous transhepatic cholangiography (PTC), or magnetic resonance cholangiopancreatography (MRCP) will usually demonstrate the characteristic extrinsic compression of the CBD. Surgery consists of removing the cystic duct, diseased gallbladder, and the impacted stone. The preoperative diagnosis of Mirizzi's syndrome is important to avoid CBD injury.

ACALCULOUS CHOLECYSTITIS In 5–10% of patients with acute cholecystitis, calculi obstructing the cystic duct are not found at surgery. In >50% of such cases, an underlying explanation for acalculous inflammation is not found. An increased risk for the development of acalculous cholecystitis is especially associated with serious trauma or burns, with the postpartum period following prolonged labor, and with orthopedic and other nonbiliary major surgical operations in the postoperative period. It may possibly complicate periods of prolonged parenteral hyperalimentation. For some of these cases, biliary sludge in the cystic duct may be responsible. Other precipitating factors include vasculitis, obstructing adenocarcinoma of the gallbladder, diabetes mellitus, torsion of the gallbladder, "unusual" bacterial infections of the gallbladder (e.g., *Leptospira, Streptococcus, Salmonella*, or *Vibrio cholerae*), and parasitic infestation of the gallbladder. Acalculous cholecystitis may also be seen with a variety of other systemic disease processes (e.g., sarcoidosis, cardiovascular disease, tuberculosis, syphilis, actinomycosis).

Although the clinical manifestations of acalculous cholecystitis are indistinguishable from those of calculous cholecystitis, the setting of acute gallbladder inflammation complicating severe underlying illness is characteristic of acalculous disease. Ultrasound or computed tomography (CT) examinations demonstrating a large, tense, static gallbladder without stones and with evidence of poor emptying over a prolonged period may be diagnostically useful in some cases. The complication rate for acalculous cholecystitis exceeds that for calculous cholecystitis. Successful management of acute acalculous cholecystitis appears to depend primarily on early diagnosis and surgical intervention, with meticulous attention to postoperative care.

ACALCULOUS CHOLECYSTOPATHY Disordered motility of the gallbladder can produce recurrent biliary pain in patients without gallstones. Infusion of an octapeptide of CCK can be used to measure the gallbladder ejection fraction during cholescintigraphy. The surgical findings have included abnormalities such as chronic cholecystitis, gallbladder muscle hypertrophy, and/or a markedly narrowed cystic duct. Some of these patients may well have had antecedent gallbladder disease. The following criteria can be used to identify patients with acalculous cholecystopathy: (1) recurrent episodes of typical RUQ pain characteristic of biliary tract pain, (2) abnormal CCK cholescintigraphy demonstrating a gallbladder ejection fraction of <40%, and (3) infusion of CCK reproducing the patient's pain. An additional clue would be the identification of a large gallbladder on ultrasound examination. Finally, it should be noted that sphincter of Oddi dysfunction can also give rise to recurrent RUQ pain and CCK-scintigraphic abnormalities.

EMPHYSEMATOUS CHOLECYSTITIS So-called emphysematous cholecystitis is thought to begin with acute cholecystitis (calculous or acalculous) followed by ischemia or gangrene of the gallbladder wall and infection by gas-producing organisms. Bacteria most frequently cultured in this setting include anaerobes, such as *Clostridium welchii* or *Clostridium perfringens*, and aerobes, such as *E. coli*. This condition occurs most frequently in elderly men and in patients with diabetes mellitus. The clinical manifestations are essentially indistinguishable from those of nongaseous cholecystitis. The diagnosis is usually made on plain abdominal film by finding gas within the gallbladder lumen, dissecting within the gallbladder wall to form a gaseous ring, or in the pericholecystic tissues. The morbidity and mortality rates with emphysematous cholecystitis are considerable. Prompt surgical intervention coupled with appropriate antibiotics is mandatory.

Chronic Cholecystitis Chronic inflammation of the gallbladder wall is almost always associated with the presence of gallstones and is thought to result from repeated bouts of subacute or acute cholecystitis or from persistent mechanical irritation of the gallbladder wall by gallstones. The presence of bacteria in the bile occurs in >25% of patients with chronic cholecystitis. The presence of infected bile in a patient with *chronic* cholecystitis undergoing elective cholecystectomy probably adds little to the operative risk. Chronic cholecystitis may be asymptomatic for years, may progress to symptomatic gallbladder disease or to acute cholecystitis, or may present with complications (see below).

Complications of Cholecystitis • ***EMPYEMA AND HYDROPS*** Empyema of the gallbladder usually results from progression of acute cholecystitis with persistent cystic duct obstruction to superinfection of the stagnant bile with a pus-forming bacterial organism. The clinical picture resembles that of cholangitis with high fever; severe RUQ pain; marked leukocytosis; and often, prostration. Empyema of the gallbladder carries a high risk of gram-negative sepsis and/or perforation. Emergency surgical intervention with proper antibiotic coverage is required as soon as the diagnosis is suspected.

Hydrops or mucocele of the gallbladder may also result from prolonged obstruction of the cystic duct, usually by a large solitary calculus. In this instance, the obstructed gallbladder lumen is progressively distended, over a period of time, by mucus (mucocele) or by a clear transudate (hydrops) produced by mucosal epithelial cells. A visible, easily palpable, nontender mass sometimes extending from the RUQ into the right iliac fossa may be found on physical examination. The patient with hydrops of the gallbladder frequently remains asymptomatic, although chronic RUQ pain may also occur. Cholecystectomy is indicated, because empyema, perforation, or gangrene may complicate the condition.

GANGRENE AND PERFORATION Gangrene of the gallbladder results from ischemia of the wall and patchy or complete tissue necrosis. Underlying conditions often include marked distention of the gallbladder, vasculitis, diabetes mellitus, empyema, or torsion resulting in arterial occlusion. Gangrene usually predisposes to perforation of the gallbladder, but perforation may also occur in chronic cholecystitis without premonitory warning symptoms. *Localized perforations* are usually contained by the omentum or by adhesions produced by recurrent inflammation of the gallbladder. Bacterial superinfection of the walled-off gallbladder contents results in abscess formation. Most patients are best treated with cholecystectomy, but some seriously ill patients may be managed with cholecystostomy and drainage of the abscess. *Free perforation* is less common but is associated with a mortality rate of ~30%. Such patients may experience a sudden transient relief of RUQ pain as the distended gallbladder decompresses; this is followed by signs of generalized peritonitis.

FISTULA FORMATION AND GALLSTONE ILEUS Fistula formation into an adjacent organ adherent to the gallbladder wall may result from inflammation and adhesion formation. Fistulas into the duodenum are most common, followed in frequency by those involving the hepatic flexure of the colon, stomach or jejunum, abdominal wall, and renal pelvis. Clinically "silent" biliary-enteric fistulas occurring as a complication of acute cholecystitis have been found in up to 5% of patients undergoing cholecystectomy. Asymptomatic cholecystoenteric fistulas may sometimes be diagnosed by finding gas in the biliary tree on plain abdominal films. Barium contrast studies or endoscopy of the upper gastrointestinal tract or colon may demonstrate the fistula. Treatment in the symptomatic patient usually consists of cholecystectomy, CBD exploration, and closure of the fistulous tract.

Gallstone ileus refers to mechanical intestinal obstruction resulting from the passage of a large gallstone into the bowel lumen. The stone customarily enters the duodenum through a cholecystoenteric fistula at that level. The site of obstruction by the impacted gallstone is usually at the ileocecal valve, provided that the more proximal small bowel is of normal caliber. The majority of patients do not give a history of either prior biliary tract symptoms or complaints suggestive of acute cholecystitis or fistula formation. Large stones, >2.5 cm in diameter, are thought to predispose to fistula formation by gradual erosion through the gallbladder fundus. Diagnostic confirmation may occasionally be found on the plain abdominal film (e.g., small-intestinal obstruction with gas in the biliary tree and a calcified, ectopic gallstone) or following an upper gastrointestinal series (cholecystoduodenal fistula with small-bowel obstruction at the ileocecal valve). Laparotomy with stone extraction (or propulsion into the colon) remains the procedure of choice to relieve obstruction. Evacuation of large stones within the gallbladder should also be performed. In general, the gallbladder and its attachment to the intestines should be left alone.

LIMEY (MILK OF CALCIUM) BILE AND PORCELAIN GALLBLADDER Calcium salts in the lumen of the gallbladder in sufficient concentration may produce calcium precipitation and diffuse, hazy opacification of bile or a layering effect on plain abdominal roentgenography. This so-called limey bile, or milk of calcium bile, is usually clinically innocuous, but cholecystectomy is recommended, especially when it occurs in a hydropic gallbladder. In the entity called *porcelain gallbladder*, calcium salt deposition within the wall of a chronically inflamed gallbladder may be detected on the plain abdominal film. Cholecystectomy is advised in all patients with porcelain gallbladder because in a high percentage of cases this finding appears to be associated with the development of carcinoma of the gallbladder.

TREATMENT ACUTE CHOLECYSTITIS

MEDICAL THERAPY

Although surgical intervention remains the mainstay of therapy for acute cholecystitis and its complications, a period of in-hospital stabilization may be required before cholecystectomy. Oral intake is eliminated, nasogastric suction may be indicated, and extracellular volume depletion and electrolyte abnormalities are repaired. Meperidine or nonsteroidal anti-inflammatory drugs (NSAIDs) are usually employed for analgesia because they may produce less spasm of the sphincter of Oddi than drugs such as morphine. Intravenous antibiotic therapy is usually indicated in patients with severe acute cholecystitis, even though bacterial superinfection of bile may not have occurred in the early stages of the inflammatory process. Antibiotic therapy is guided by the most common organisms likely to be present, which are *E. coli*, *Klebsiella* spp., and *Streptococcus* spp. Effective antibiotics include ureidopenicillins such as piperacillin or mezlocillin, ampicillin sulbactam, ciprofloxacin, moxifloxacin, and third-generation cephalosporins. Anaerobic coverage by a drug such as metronidazole should be added if gangrenous or emphysematous cholecystitis is suspected. Imipenem and meropenem represent potent parenteral antibiotics that cover the whole spectrum of bacteria causing ascending cholangitis. They should, however, be reserved for the most severe, life-threatening infections when other regimens have failed (Chap. 186). Postoperative complications of wound infection, abscess formation, and sepsis are reduced in antibiotic-treated patients.

SURGICAL THERAPY

The optimal timing of surgical intervention in patients with acute cholecystitis depends on stabilization of the patient. The clear trend is toward earlier surgery, and this is due in part to requirements for shorter hospital stays. Urgent (emergency) cholecystectomy or cholecystostomy is probably appropriate in most patients in whom a complication of acute cholecystitis such as empyema, emphysematous cholecystitis, or perforation is suspected or confirmed. Patients with uncomplicated acute cholecystitis should undergo early elective laparoscopic cholecystectomy, ideally within 48–72 h after diagnosis. The complication rate is not increased in patients undergoing early as opposed to delayed (>6 weeks after diagnosis) cholecystectomy. Delayed surgical intervention is probably best reserved for (1) patients in whom the overall medical condition imposes an unacceptable risk for early surgery and (2) patients in whom the diagnosis of acute cholecystitis is in doubt. Thus, early cholecystectomy (within 72 h) is the treatment of choice for most patients with acute cholecystitis. Mortality figures for emergency cholecystectomy in most centers range from 1–3%, whereas the mortality risk for early elective cholecystectomy is ~0.5% in patients under age 60. Of course, the operative risks increase with age-related diseases of other organ systems and with the presence of long- or short-term complications of gallbladder disease. Seriously ill or debilitated patients with cholecystitis may be managed with cholecystostomy and tube drainage of the gallbladder. Elective cholecystectomy may then be done at a later date.

Postcholecystectomy Complications Early complications following cholecystectomy include atelectasis and other pulmonary disorders, abscess formation (often subphrenic), external or internal hemorrhage, biliary-enteric fistula, and bile leaks. Jaundice may indicate absorption of bile from an intraabdominal collection following a biliary leak or mechanical obstruction of the CBD by retained calculi, intraductal blood clots, or extrinsic compression.

Overall, cholecystectomy is a very successful operation that provides total or near-total relief of preoperative symptoms in 75–90% of patients. The most common cause of persistent postcholecystectomy symptoms is an overlooked symptomatic nonbiliary disorder (e.g., reflux esophagitis, peptic ulceration, pancreatitis, or—most often—irritable bowel syndrome). In a small percentage of patients, however, a disorder of the extrahepatic bile ducts may result in persistent symptomatology. These so-called postcholecystectomy syndromes may be due to (1) biliary strictures, (2) retained biliary calculi, (3) cystic duct stump syndrome, (4) stenosis or dyskinesia of the sphincter of Oddi, or (5) bile salt–induced diarrhea or gastritis.

CYSTIC DUCT STUMP SYNDROME In the absence of cholangiographically demonstrable retained stones, symptoms resembling biliary pain or cholecystitis in the postcholecystectomy patient have frequently been attributed to disease in a long (>1 cm) cystic duct remnant (cystic duct stump syndrome). Careful analysis, however, reveals that postcholecystectomy complaints are attributable to other causes in almost all patients in whom the symptom complex was originally thought to result from the existence of a long cystic duct stump. Accordingly, considerable care should be taken to investigate the possible role of other factors in the production of postcholecystectomy symptoms before attributing them to cystic duct stump syndrome.

PAPILLARY DYSFUNCTION, PAPILLARY STENOSIS, SPASM OF THE SPHINCTER OF ODDI, AND BILIARY DYSKINESIA Symptoms of biliary colic accompanied by signs of recurrent, intermittent biliary obstruction may be produced by acalculous cholecystopathy, papillary stenosis, papillary dysfunction, spasm of the sphincter of Oddi, and biliary dyskinesia. Papillary stenosis is thought to result from acute or chronic inflammation of the papilla of Vater or from glandular hyperplasia of the papillary segment. Five criteria have been used to define papillary stenosis: (1) upper abdominal pain, usually RUQ or epigastric; (2) abnormal liver tests; (3) dilatation of the CBD upon ERCP examination; (4) delayed (>45 min) drainage of contrast material from the duct; and (5) increased basal pressure of the sphincter of Oddi, a finding that may be of only minor significance. An alternative to ERCP is magnetic resonance cholangiography (MRC) if ERCP and/or biliary manometry are either unavailable or not feasible. After exclusion of acalculous cholecystopathy, treatment consists of endoscopic or surgical sphincteroplasty to ensure wide patency of the distal portions of both the bile and pancreatic ducts. The greater the number of the preceding criteria present, the greater is the likelihood that a patient does have a degree of papillary stenosis sufficient to justify correction. The factors usually considered as indications for sphincterotomy include (1) prolonged duration of symptoms, (2) lack of response to symptomatic treatment, (3) presence of severe disability, and (4) the patient's choice of sphincterotomy over surgery (given a clear understanding on his or her part of the risks involved in both procedures).

Criteria for diagnosing dyskinesia of the sphincter of Oddi are even more controversial than those for papillary stenosis. Proposed mechanisms include spasm of the sphincter, denervation sensitivity resulting in hypertonicity, and abnormalities of the sequencing or frequency rates of sphincteric-contraction waves. When thorough evaluation has failed to demonstrate another cause for the pain, and when cholangiographic and manometric criteria suggest a diagnosis of biliary dyskinesia, medical treatment with nitrites or anticholinergics to attempt pharmacologic relaxation of the sphincter has been proposed. Endoscopic biliary sphincterotomy (EBS) or surgical sphincteroplasty may be indicated in patients who fail to respond to a 2- to 3-month trial of medical therapy, especially if basal sphincter of Oddi pressures are elevated. EBS has become the procedure of choice for removing bile duct stones and for other biliary and pancreatic problems.

BILE SALT–INDUCED DIARRHEA AND GASTRITIS Postcholecystectomy patients may develop symptoms of dyspepsia, which have been attributed to duodenogastric reflux of bile. However, firm data linking these symptoms to bile gastritis after surgical removal of the gallbladder are lacking. Cholecystectomy induces persistent changes in gut transit, and these changes effect a noticeable modification of bowel habits. Cholecystectomy shortens gut transit time by accelerating passage of the fecal bolus through the colon with marked acceleration in the right colon, thus causing an increase in colonic bile acid output and a shift in bile acid composition toward the more diarrheagenic secondary bile acids, i.e. deoxycholic acid. Diarrhea that is severe enough, i.e., three or more watery movements per day, can be classified as postcholecystectomy diarrhea, and this occurs in 5–10% of patients undergoing elective cholecystectomy. Treatment with bile acid–sequestering agents such as cholestyramine or colestipol is often effective in ameliorating troublesome diarrhea.

THE HYPERPLASTIC CHOLECYSTOSES

The term *hyperplastic cholecystoses* is used to denote a group of disorders of the gallbladder characterized by excessive proliferation of normal tissue components.

Adenomyomatosis is characterized by a benign proliferation of gallbladder surface epithelium with glandlike formations, extramural sinuses, transverse strictures, and/or fundal nodule ("adenoma" or "adenomyoma") formation.

Cholesterolosis is characterized by abnormal deposition of lipid, especially cholesteryl esters, within macrophages in the lamina propria of the gallbladder wall. In its diffuse form ("strawberry gallbladder"), the gallbladder mucosa is brick red and speckled with bright yellow flecks of lipid. The localized form shows solitary or multiple "cholesterol polyps" studding the gallbladder wall. Cholesterol stones of the gallbladder are found in nearly half the cases. Cholecystectomy is indicated in both adenomyomatosis and cholesterolosis when symptomatic or when cholelithiasis is present.

The prevalence of gallbladder polyps in the adult population is ~5%, with a marked male predominance. Few significant changes have been found over a 5-year period in asymptomatic patients with gallbladder polyps <10 mm in diameter. Cholecystectomy is recommended in symptomatic patients, as well as in asymptomatic patients >50 years of age, or in those whose polyps are >10 mm in diameter or associated with gallstones or polyp growth on serial ultrasonography.

DISEASES OF THE BILE DUCTS

CONGENITAL ANOMALIES

Biliary Atresia and Hypoplasia Atretic and hypoplastic lesions of the extrahepatic and large intrahepatic bile ducts are the most common biliary anomalies of clinical relevance encountered in infancy. The clinical picture is one of severe obstructive jaundice during the first month of life, with pale stools. When biliary atresia is suspected on the basis of clinical, laboratory, and imaging findings, the diagnosis is confirmed by surgical exploration and operative cholangiography. Approximately 10% of cases of biliary atresia are treatable with Roux-en-Y choledochojejunostomy, with the Kasai procedure (hepatic portoenterostomy) being attempted in the remainder in an effort to restore some bile flow. Most patients, even those having successful biliary-enteric anastomoses, eventually develop chronic cholangitis, extensive hepatic fibrosis, and portal hypertension.

Choledochal Cysts Cystic dilatation may involve the free portion of the CBD, i.e., choledochal cyst, or may present as diverticulum formation in the intraduodenal segment. In the latter situation, chronic reflux of pancreatic juice into the biliary tree can produce inflammation and stenosis of the extrahepatic bile ducts leading to cholangitis or biliary obstruction. Because the process may be gradual, ~50% of patients present with onset of symptoms after age 10. The diagnosis may be made by ultrasound, abdominal CT, MRC, or cholangiography. Only one-third of patients show the classic triad of abdominal pain, jaundice, and an abdominal mass. Ultrasonographic detection of a cyst separate from the gallbladder should suggest the diagnosis of choledochal cyst, which can be confirmed by demonstrating the entrance of extrahepatic bile ducts into the cyst. Surgical treatment involves excision of the "cyst" and biliary-enteric anastomosis. Patients with choledochal cysts are at increased risk for the subsequent development of cholangiocarcinoma.

Congenital Biliary Ectasia Dilatation of intrahepatic bile ducts may involve either the major intrahepatic radicles (Caroli's disease), the inter- and intralobular ducts (congenital hepatic fibrosis), or both. In Caroli's disease, clinical manifestations include recurrent cholangitis, abscess formation in and around the affected ducts, and, often, brown pigment gallstone formation within portions of ectatic intrahepatic biliary radicles. Ultrasound, MRC, and CT are of great diagnostic value in demonstrating cystic dilatation of the intrahepatic bile ducts. Treatment with ongoing antibiotic therapy is usually undertaken in an effort to limit the frequency and severity of recurrent bouts of cholangitis. Progression to secondary biliary cirrhosis with portal hypertension, extrahepatic biliary obstruction, cholangiocarcinoma, or recurrent episodes of sepsis with hepatic abscess formation is common.

CHOLEDOCHOLITHIASIS

Pathophysiology and Clinical Manifestations Passage of gallstones into the CBD occurs in ~10–15% of patients with cholelithiasis. The incidence of common duct stones increases with increasing age of the patient, so that up to 25% of elderly patients may have calculi in the common duct at the time of cholecystectomy. Undetected duct stones are left behind in ~1–5% of cholecystectomy patients. The overwhelming majority of bile duct stones are cholesterol stones formed in the gallbladder, which then migrate into the extrahepatic biliary tree through the cystic duct. Primary calculi arising de novo in the ducts are usually brown pigment stones developing in patients with (1) hepatobiliary parasitism or chronic, recurrent cholangitis; (2) congenital anomalies of the bile ducts (especially Caroli's disease); (3) dilated, sclerosed, or strictured ducts; or (4) an *MDR3* (ABCB4) gene defect leading to impaired biliary phospholipids secretion (low phospholipid–associated cholesterol cholelithiasis). Common duct stones may remain asymptomatic for years, may pass spontaneously into the duodenum, or (most often) may present with biliary colic or a complication.

Complications • *CHOLANGITIS* Cholangitis may be acute or chronic, and symptoms result from inflammation, which usually is caused by at least partial obstruction to the flow of bile. Bacteria are present on bile culture in ~75% of patients with acute cholangitis early in the symptomatic course. The characteristic presentation of acute cholangitis involves biliary pain, jaundice, and spiking fevers with chills (Charcot's triad). Blood cultures are frequently positive, and leukocytosis is typical. *Nonsuppurative acute cholangitis* is most common and may respond relatively rapidly to supportive measures and to treatment with antibiotics. In *suppurative acute cholangitis*, however, the presence of pus under pressure in a completely obstructed ductal system leads to symptoms of severe toxicity—mental confusion, bacteremia, and septic shock. Response to antibiotics alone in this setting is relatively poor, multiple hepatic abscesses are often present, and the mortality rate approaches 100% unless prompt endoscopic or surgical relief of the obstruction and drainage of infected bile are carried out. Endoscopic management of bacterial cholangitis is as effective as surgical intervention. ERCP with endoscopic sphincterotomy is safe and the preferred initial procedure for both establishing a definitive diagnosis and providing effective therapy.

OBSTRUCTIVE JAUNDICE Gradual obstruction of the CBD over a period of weeks or months usually leads to initial manifestations of jaundice or pruritus without associated symptoms of biliary colic or cholangitis. Painless jaundice may occur in patients with choledocholithiasis, but is much more characteristic of biliary obstruction secondary to malignancy of the head of the pancreas, bile ducts, or ampulla of Vater.

In patients whose obstruction is secondary to choledocholithiasis, associated chronic calculous cholecystitis is very common, and the gallbladder in this setting may be unable to distend. The absence of a palpable gallbladder in most patients with biliary obstruction from duct stones is the basis for Courvoisier's law, i.e., that the presence of a palpably enlarged gallbladder suggests that the biliary obstruction is secondary to an underlying malignancy rather than to calculous disease. Biliary obstruction causes progressive dilatation of the intrahepatic bile ducts as intrabiliary pressures rise. Hepatic bile flow is suppressed, and reabsorption and regurgitation of conjugated bilirubin into the bloodstream lead to jaundice accompanied by dark urine (bilirubinuria) and light-colored (acholic) stools.

CBD stones should be suspected in any patient with cholecystitis whose serum bilirubin level is >85.5 μmol/L (5 mg/dL). The maximum bilirubin level is seldom >256.5 μmol/L (15.0 mg/dL) in patients with choledocholithiasis unless concomitant hepatic or renal disease or another factor leading to marked hyperbilirubinemia exists. Serum bilirubin levels ≥342.0 μmol/L (20 mg/dL) should suggest the possibility of neoplastic obstruction. The serum alkaline phosphatase level is almost always elevated in biliary obstruction. A rise in alkaline phosphatase often precedes clinical jaundice and may be the only abnormality in routine liver function tests. There may be a two- to tenfold elevation of serum aminotransferases, especially in association with acute obstruction. Following relief of the obstructing process, serum aminotransferase elevations usually return rapidly to normal, while the serum bilirubin level may take 1–2 weeks to return to normal. The alkaline phosphatase level usually falls slowly, lagging behind the decrease in serum bilirubin.

PANCREATITIS The most common associated entity discovered in patients with nonalcoholic acute pancreatitis is biliary tract disease. Biochemical evidence of pancreatic inflammation complicates acute cholecystitis in 15% of cases and choledocholithiasis in >30%, and the common factor appears to be the passage of gallstones through the common duct. Coexisting pancreatitis should be suspected in patients with symptoms of cholecystitis who develop (1) back pain or pain to the left of the abdominal midline, (2) prolonged vomiting with paralytic ileus, or (3) a pleural effusion, especially on the left side. Surgical treatment of gallstone disease is usually associated with resolution of the pancreatitis.

SECONDARY BILIARY CIRRHOSIS Secondary biliary cirrhosis may complicate prolonged or intermittent duct obstruction with or without recurrent cholangitis. Although this complication may be seen in patients with choledocholithiasis, it is more common in cases of prolonged obstruction from stricture or neoplasm. Once established, secondary biliary cirrhosis may be progressive even after correction of the obstructing process, and increasingly severe hepatic cirrhosis may lead to portal hypertension or to hepatic failure and death. Prolonged biliary obstruction may also be associated with clinically relevant deficiencies of the fat-soluble vitamins A, D, E, and K.

Diagnosis and Treatment The diagnosis of choledocholithiasis is usually made by cholangiography (Table 369-3), either preoperatively by endoscopic retrograde cholangiogram (ERC) (Fig. 369-2C) or MRCP or intraoperatively at the time of cholecystectomy. As many as 15% of patients undergoing cholecystectomy will prove to have CBD stones. When CBD stones are suspected prior to laparoscopic cholecystectomy, preoperative ERCP with endoscopic papillotomy and stone extraction is the preferred approach. It not only provides stone clearance but also defines the anatomy of the biliary tree in relationship to the cystic duct. CBD stones should be suspected in gallstone patients who have any of the following risk factors: (1) a history of jaundice or pancreatitis, (2) abnormal tests of liver function, and (3) ultrasonographic or MRCP evidence of a dilated CBD or stones in the duct. Alternatively, if intraoperative cholangiography reveals retained stones, postoperative ERCP can be carried out. The need for preoperative ERCP is expected to decrease further as laparoscopic techniques for bile duct exploration improve.

The widespread use of laparoscopic cholecystectomy and ERCP has decreased the incidence of complicated biliary tract disease and the need for choledocholithotomy and T-tube drainage of the bile ducts. EBS followed by spontaneous passage or stone extraction is the treatment of choice in the management of patients with common duct stones, especially in elderly or poor-risk patients.

TRAUMA, STRICTURES, AND HEMOBILIA

Most benign strictures of the extrahepatic bile ducts result from surgical trauma and occur in about 1 in 500 cholecystectomies. Strictures may present with bile leak or abscess formation in the immediate postoperative period or with biliary obstruction or cholangitis as long as 2 years or more following the inciting trauma. The diagnosis is established by percutaneous or endoscopic cholangiography. Endoscopic brushing of biliary strictures may be helpful in establishing the nature of the lesion and is more accurate than bile cytology alone. When positive exfoliative cytology is obtained, the diagnosis of a neoplastic stricture is established. This procedure is especially important in patients with primary sclerosing cholangitis (PSC) who are predisposed to the development of cholangiocarcinomas. Successful operative correction of non-PSC bile duct strictures by a skillful surgeon with duct-to-bowel anastomosis is usually possible, although mortality rates from surgical complications, recurrent cholangitis, or secondary biliary cirrhosis are high.

Hemobilia may follow traumatic or operative injury to the liver or bile ducts, intraductal rupture of a hepatic abscess or aneurysm of the hepatic artery, biliary or hepatic tumor hemorrhage, or mechanical complications of choledocholithiasis or hepatobiliary parasitism. Diagnostic procedures such as liver biopsy, PTC, and transhepatic biliary drainage catheter placement may also be complicated by hemobilia. Patients often present with a classic triad of biliary pain, obstructive jaundice, and melena or occult blood in the stools. The diagnosis is sometimes made by cholangiographic evidence of blood clot in the biliary tree, but selective angiographic verification may be required. Although minor episodes of hemobilia may resolve without operative intervention, surgical ligation of the bleeding vessel is frequently required.

EXTRINSIC COMPRESSION OF THE BILE DUCTS

Partial or complete biliary obstruction may be produced by extrinsic compression of the ducts. The most common cause of this form of obstructive jaundice is carcinoma of the head of the pancreas. Biliary obstruction may also occur as a complication of either acute or chronic pancreatitis or involvement of lymph nodes in the porta hepatis by lymphoma or metastatic carcinoma. The latter should be distinguished from cholestasis resulting from massive replacement of the liver by tumor.

HEPATOBILIARY PARASITISM

Infestation of the biliary tract by adult helminths or their ova may produce a chronic, recurrent pyogenic cholangitis with or without multiple hepatic abscesses, ductal stones, or biliary obstruction. This condition is relatively rare but does occur in inhabitants of southern China and elsewhere in Southeast Asia. The organisms most commonly involved are trematodes or flukes, including *Clonorchis sinensis, Opisthorchis viverrini* or *Opisthorchis felineus*, and *Fasciola hepatica*. The biliary tract also may be involved by intraductal migration of adult *Ascaris lumbricoides* from the duodenum or by intrabiliary rupture of hydatid cysts of the liver produced by *Echinococcus* spp. The diagnosis is made by cholangiography and the presence of characteristic ova on stool examination. When obstruction is present, the treatment of choice is laparotomy under antibiotic coverage, with common duct exploration and a biliary drainage procedure.

SCLEROSING CHOLANGITIS

Primary or idiopathic sclerosing cholangitis is characterized by a progressive, inflammatory, sclerosing, and obliterative process

TABLE 369-3 DIAGNOSTIC EVALUATION OF THE BILE DUCTS

Diagnostic Advantages	Diagnostic Limitations	Contraindications	Complications	Comment
Hepatobiliary Ultrasound				
Rapid Simultaneous scanning of GB, liver, bile ducts, pancreas Accurate identification of dilated bile ducts Not limited by jaundice, pregnancy Guidance for fine-needle biopsy	Bowel gas Massive obesity Ascites Barium Partial bile duct obstruction Poor visualization of distal CBD	None	None	Initial procedure of choice in investigating possible biliary tract obstruction
Computed Tomography				
Simultaneous scanning of GB, liver, bile ducts, pancreas Accurate identification of dilated bile ducts, masses Not limited by jaundice, gas, obesity, ascites High-resolution image Guidance for fine-needle biopsy	Extreme cachexia Movement artifact Ileus Partial bile duct obstruction	Pregnancy	Reaction to iodinated contrast, if used	Indicated for evaluation of hepatic or pancreatic masses Procedure of choice in investigating possible biliary obstruction if diagnostic limitations prevent HBUS
Magnetic Resonance Cholangiopancreatography				
Useful modality for visualizing pancreatic and biliary ducts Has excellent sensitivity for bile duct dilatation, biliary stricture, and intraductal abnormalities Can identify pancreatic duct dilatation or stricture, pancreatic duct stenosis, and pancreas divisum	Cannot offer therapeutic intervention High cost	Claustrophobia Certain metals (iron)	None	
Endoscopic Retrograde Cholangiopancreatography				
Simultaneous pancreatography Best visualization of distal biliary tract Bile or pancreatic cytology Endoscopic sphincterotomy and stone removal Biliary manometry	Gastroduodenal obstruction ? Roux-en-Y biliary-enteric anastomosis	Pregnancy ? Acute pancreatitis ? Severe cardiopulmonary disease	Pancreatitis Cholangitis, sepsis Infected pancreatic pseudocyst Perforation (rare) Hypoxemia, aspiration	Cholangiogram of choice in: Absence of dilated ducts ? Pancreatic, ampullary or gastroduodenal disease Prior biliary surgery Endoscopic sphincterotomy a treatment possibility
Percutaneous Transhepatic Cholangiogram				
Extremely successful when bile ducts dilated Best visualization of proximal biliary tract Bile cytology/culture Percutaneous transhepatic drainage	Nondilated or sclerosed ducts	Pregnancy Uncorrectable coagulopathy Massive ascites ? Hepatic abscess	Bleeding Hemobilia Bile peritonitis Bacteremia, sepsis	Indicated when ERCP is contraindicated or failed
Endoscopic Ultrasound				
Most sensitive method to detect ampullary stones				

Abbreviations: CBD, common bile duct; ERCP, endoscopic retrograde cholangiopancreatography; GB, gallbladder; HBUS, hepatobiliary ultrasound.

affecting the extrahepatic and/or the intrahepatic bile ducts. The disorder occurs up to 75% in association with inflammatory bowel disease, especially ulcerative colitis. It may also be associated with autoimmune pancreatitis; multifocal fibrosclerosis syndromes such as retroperitoneal, mediastinal, and/or periureteral fibrosis; Riedel's struma; or pseudotumor of the orbit.

Immunoglobulin G4 (IgG4)–associated cholangitis is a recently described biliary disease of unknown etiology that presents with biochemical and cholangiographic features indistinguishable from PSC, is often associated with autoimmune pancreatitis and other fibrosing conditions, and is characterized by elevated serum IgG4 and infiltration of IgG4-positive plasma cells in bile ducts and liver tissue. In contrast to PSC, it is not associated with inflammatory bowel disease and should be suspected if associated with increased serum IgG4 and unexplained pancreatic disease. Glucocorticoids are regarded as the initial treatment of choice. Relapse is common after steroid withdrawal, especially with proximal strictures. Long-term treatment with glucocorticoids and/or azathioprine may be needed after relapse or for inadequate response (Chap. 371).

Patients with primary sclerosing cholangitis often present with signs and symptoms of chronic or intermittent biliary obstruction: RUQ abdominal pain, pruritus, jaundice, or acute cholangitis. Late in the course, complete biliary obstruction, secondary biliary cirrhosis, hepatic failure, or portal hypertension with bleeding varices may occur. The diagnosis is usually established by finding multifocal, diffusely distributed strictures with intervening segments of normal or dilated ducts, producing a beaded appearance on cholangiography (Fig. 369-2D). The cholangiographic techniques of choice in suspected cases are MRCP and ERCP. When a diagnosis of sclerosing cholangitis has been established, a search for associated diseases, especially for chronic inflammatory bowel disease, should be carried out.

A recent study describes the natural history and outcome for 305 patients of Swedish descent with primary sclerosing cholangitis; 134 (44%) of the patients were asymptomatic at the time of diagnosis and, not surprisingly, had a significantly higher survival rate. The independent predictors of a bad prognosis were advanced age, serum bilirubin concentration, and liver histologic changes. Cholangiocarcinoma was found in 24 patients (8%). Inflammatory bowel disease was closely associated with primary sclerosing cholangitis and had a prevalence of 81% in this study population.

Small duct PSC is defined by the presence of chronic cholestasis and hepatic histology consistent with PSC but with normal findings on cholangiography. Small duct PSC is found in ~5% of patients with PSC and may represent an earlier stage of PSC associated with a significantly better long-term prognosis. However, such patients may progress to classic PSC and/or end-stage liver disease with consequent necessity of liver transplantation.

In patients with AIDS, cholangiopancreatography may demonstrate a broad range of biliary tract changes as well as pancreatic duct obstruction and occasionally pancreatitis (Chap. 226). Further, biliary tract lesions in AIDS include infection and cholangiopancreatographic changes similar to those of PSC. Changes noted include: (1) diffuse involvement of intrahepatic bile ducts alone, (2) involvement of both intra- and extrahepatic bile ducts, (3) ampullary stenosis, (4) stricture of the intrapancreatic portion of the CBD, and (5) pancreatic duct involvement. Associated infectious organisms include *Cryptosporidium*, *Mycobacterium avium-intracellulare*, cytomegalovirus, *Microsporidia*, and *Isospora*. In addition, acalculous cholecystitis occurs in up to 10% of patients. ERCP sphincterotomy, while not without risk, provides significant pain reduction in patients with AIDS-associated papillary stenosis. Secondary sclerosing cholangitis may occur as a long-term complication of choledocholithiasis, cholangiocarcinoma, operative or traumatic biliary injury, or contiguous inflammatory processes.

TREATMENT SCLEROSING CHOLANGITIS

Therapy with cholestyramine may help control symptoms of pruritus, and antibiotics are useful when cholangitis complicates the clinical picture. Vitamin D and calcium supplementation may help prevent the loss of bone mass frequently seen in patients with chronic cholestasis. Glucocorticoids, methotrexate, and cyclosporine have not been shown to be efficacious in PSC. UDCA in high dosage (20 mg/kg) improves serum liver tests, but an effect on survival has not been documented. In cases where high-grade biliary obstruction (dominant strictures) has occurred, balloon dilatation or stenting may be appropriate. Only rarely is surgical intervention indicated. Efforts at biliary-enteric anastomosis or stent placement may, however, be complicated by recurrent cholangitis and further progression of the stenosing process. The prognosis is unfavorable, with a median survival of 9–12 years following the diagnosis, regardless of therapy. Four variables (age, serum bilirubin level, histologic stage, and splenomegaly) predict survival in patients with PSC and serve as the basis for a risk score. PSC is one of the most common indications for liver transplantation.

SECTION 3 DISORDERS OF THE PANCREAS

370 Approach to the Patient with Pancreatic Disease

Darwin L. Conwell, Norton J. Greenberger, Peter A. Banks

GENERAL CONSIDERATIONS

As emphasized in Chap. 371, the etiologies as well as clinical manifestations of pancreatitis are quite varied. Although it is well-appreciated that pancreatitis is frequently secondary to biliary tract disease and alcohol abuse, it can also be caused by drugs, genetic mutations, trauma, and viral infections and is associated with metabolic and connective tissue disorders. In ~30% of patients with acute pancreatitis and 25–40% of patients with chronic pancreatitis, the etiology initially can be obscure.

The incidence of acute pancreatitis is about 5–35/100,000 new cases per year worldwide, with a mortality rate of about 3%. The incidence of chronic pancreatitis is about 4–8 new cases per 100,000 per year with a prevalence of 26–42 cases per 100,000. The number of patients admitted to the hospital who suffer with both acute and chronic pancreatitis in the United States is largely increasing and is now estimated to be 274,119 for acute pancreatitis and 19,724 for chronic pancreatitis. Acute pancreatitis is now the most common gastrointestinal diagnosis requiring hospitalization in the United States. Acute and chronic pancreatic disease costs an estimated 3 billion dollars annually in health care expenditures. These numbers may underestimate the true incidence and prevalence, because non–alcohol-induced pancreatitis has been largely ignored. At autopsy, the prevalence of chronic pancreatitis ranges from 0.04 to 5%.

The diagnosis of acute pancreatitis is generally clearly defined based on a combination of laboratory, imaging, and clinical symptoms. The diagnosis of chronic pancreatitis, especially in mild disease, is hampered by the relative inaccessibility of the pancreas to direct examination and the nonspecificity of the abdominal pain associated with chronic pancreatitis. Many patients with chronic pancreatitis do not have elevated blood amylase or lipase levels. Some patients with chronic pancreatitis develop signs and symptoms of pancreatic exocrine insufficiency, and thus, objective evidence for pancreatic disease can be demonstrated. However, there is a very large reservoir of pancreatic exocrine function. More than 90% of the pancreas must be damaged before maldigestion of fat and protein is manifested. Noninvasive, indirect tests of pancreatic exocrine function (fecal elastase) are much more likely to give abnormal results in patients with obvious advanced pancreatic disease (i.e., pancreatic calcification, steatorrhea, or diabetes mellitus) than in patients with occult disease. Invasive, direct tests of pancreatic secretory function (secretin tests) are the most sensitive and specific tests to detect early chronic pancreatic disease when imaging is equivocal or normal.

TESTS USEFUL IN THE DIAGNOSIS OF PANCREATIC DISEASE

Several tests have proved of value in the evaluation of pancreatic disease. Examples of specific tests and their usefulness in the diagnosis of acute and chronic pancreatitis are summarized in Table 370-1 and Fig. 370-1. At some institutions, pancreatic function tests are available and performed if the diagnosis of chronic pancreatic disease remains a possibility after noninvasive tests (ultrasound, computed tomography [CT], magnetic resonance cholangiopancreatography [MRCP]) or invasive tests (endoscopic retrograde cholangiopancreatography [ERCP], endoscopic ultrasonography [EUS]) have given normal or

TABLE 370-1 TESTS USEFUL IN THE DIAGNOSIS OF ACUTE AND CHRONIC PANCREATITIS AND PANCREATIC TUMORS

Test	Principle	Comment
Pancreatic Enzymes in Body Fluids		
Serum lipase	Pancreatic inflammation leads to increased serum enzyme levels	Enzyme measurement of choice for diagnosis of acute pancreatitis
Amylase		
1. Serum	Pancreatic inflammation leads to increased serum enzyme levels	Simple; reliable if test results are three times the upper limit of normal
2. Urine	Renal clearance of amylase is increased in acute pancreatitis	Infrequently used
3. Ascitic fluid	Disruption of gland or main pancreatic duct leads to increased amylase concentration	Can help establish source of ascites; false positives occur with intestinal obstruction and perforated ulcer; can also measure lipase
4. Pleural fluid	Exudative pleural effusion with pancreatitis	False positives occur with carcinoma of the lung and esophageal perforation
Studies Pertaining to Pancreatic Structure		
Radiologic and radionuclide tests		
1. Plain film of the abdomen	Can be abnormal in acute and chronic pancreatitis	Infrequently used
2. Upper gastrointestinal x-rays		Infrequently used
3. Ultrasonography (US)	Can provide information on edema, inflammation, calcification, pseudocysts, and mass lesions	Simple, noninvasive; sequential studies quite feasible; useful in diagnosis of gallstones; pancreas visualization limited by interference from overlying bowel gas
4. Computed tomography (CT) scan	Permits detailed visualization of pancreas and surrounding structures, pancreatic fluid collection, pseudocyst; assessment of necrosis or interstitial disease	Useful in the diagnosis of pancreatic calcification, dilated pancreatic ducts, and pancreatic tumors; may not be able to distinguish between inflammatory and neoplastic mass lesions
5. Magnetic resonance cholangiopancreatography (MRCP)	Three-dimensional imaging has been used to produce very good images of the pancreatic-biliary ductal system by a noninvasive technique	Has replaced ERCP as a diagnostic test; noninvasive
6. Endoscopic ultrasonography (EUS)	High frequency transducer used with EUS can produce very high-resolution images and depict changes in the pancreatic duct and parenchyma with great detail	Can be used to assess gallstones, chronic pancreatitis, and pancreatic carcinoma
7. Endoscopic retrograde cholangiopancreatography (ERCP)	Cannulation of pancreatic and common bile duct permits visualization of pancreatic-biliary ductal system	Primarily a therapeutic procedure; invasive
Pancreatic biopsy with US or CT guidance	Percutaneous aspiration biopsy of mass-forming lesions of the pancreas	High diagnostic yield; laparotomy avoided; can be done with EUS for the evaluation of chronic pancreatitis, autoimmune pancreatitis, and pancreatic carcinoma
Tests of Exocrine Pancreatic Function		
Direct stimulation of the pancreas with analysis of duodenal contents		
1. Secretin test	Secretin leads to increased output of pancreatic juice and HCO_3^-; pancreatic secretory response is related to the functional mass of pancreatic tissue	Sensitive enough to detect occult disease; involves duodenal intubation and fluoroscopic placement of gastroduodenal tube; poorly defined normal enzyme response; overlap in chronic pancreatitis; large secretory reserve capacity of the pancreas; currently done at only a few medical centers
2. Endoscopic secretin test	Replaces need for tube placement duodenum	Sensitive enough to detect occult disease; high negative predictive value; avoids intubation and fluoroscopy; requires sedation
Measurement of intraluminal digestion products		
1. Quantitative stool fat determination	Lack of lipolytic enzymes brings about impaired fat digestion	Reliable reference standard for defining severity of malabsorption; does not distinguish between maldigestion and malabsorption
Measurement of pancreatic enzymes in feces		
1. Elastase	Pancreatic secretion of proteolytic enzymes, not degraded in intestine	Diagnostic accuracy best if value is <100 μg/g performed on a solid stool

inconclusive results. In this regard, tests using *direct* stimulation of the pancreas with secretin are the most sensitive.

Pancreatic Enzymes in Body Fluids The serum amylase and lipase levels are widely used as screening tests for acute pancreatitis in the patient with acute abdominal pain or back pain. Values greater than three times the upper limit of normal in combination with epigastric pain strongly suggest the diagnosis if gut perforation or infarction is excluded. In acute pancreatitis, the serum amylase and lipase are usually elevated within 24 h of onset and remain so for 3–7 days. Levels usually return to normal within 7 days unless there is pancreatic ductal disruption, ductal obstruction, or pseudocyst formation. Approximately 85% of patients with acute pancreatitis have a threefold or greater elevated serum lipase and amylase levels. The values may be normal if (1) there is a delay (of 2–5 days) before blood samples are obtained, (2) the underlying disorder is chronic pancreatitis rather than acute pancreatitis, or (3) hypertriglyceridemia is present. Patients with hypertriglyceridemia and proven pancreatitis have been found to have spuriously low levels of amylase and perhaps lipase activity. In the absence of objective evidence of pancreatitis by abdominal ultrasound, CT scan, MRCP, or EUS, mild to moderate elevations of amylase and/or lipase are not helpful in making a diagnosis of chronic pancreatitis.

The serum amylase can be elevated in other conditions (Table 370-2), in part because the enzyme is found in many organs. In addition to the pancreas and salivary glands, small quantities of amylase are found in the tissues of the fallopian tubes, lung, thyroid, and tonsils and can be produced by various tumors (carcinomas of the lung, esophagus, breast, and ovary). Isoamylase determinations do not accurately

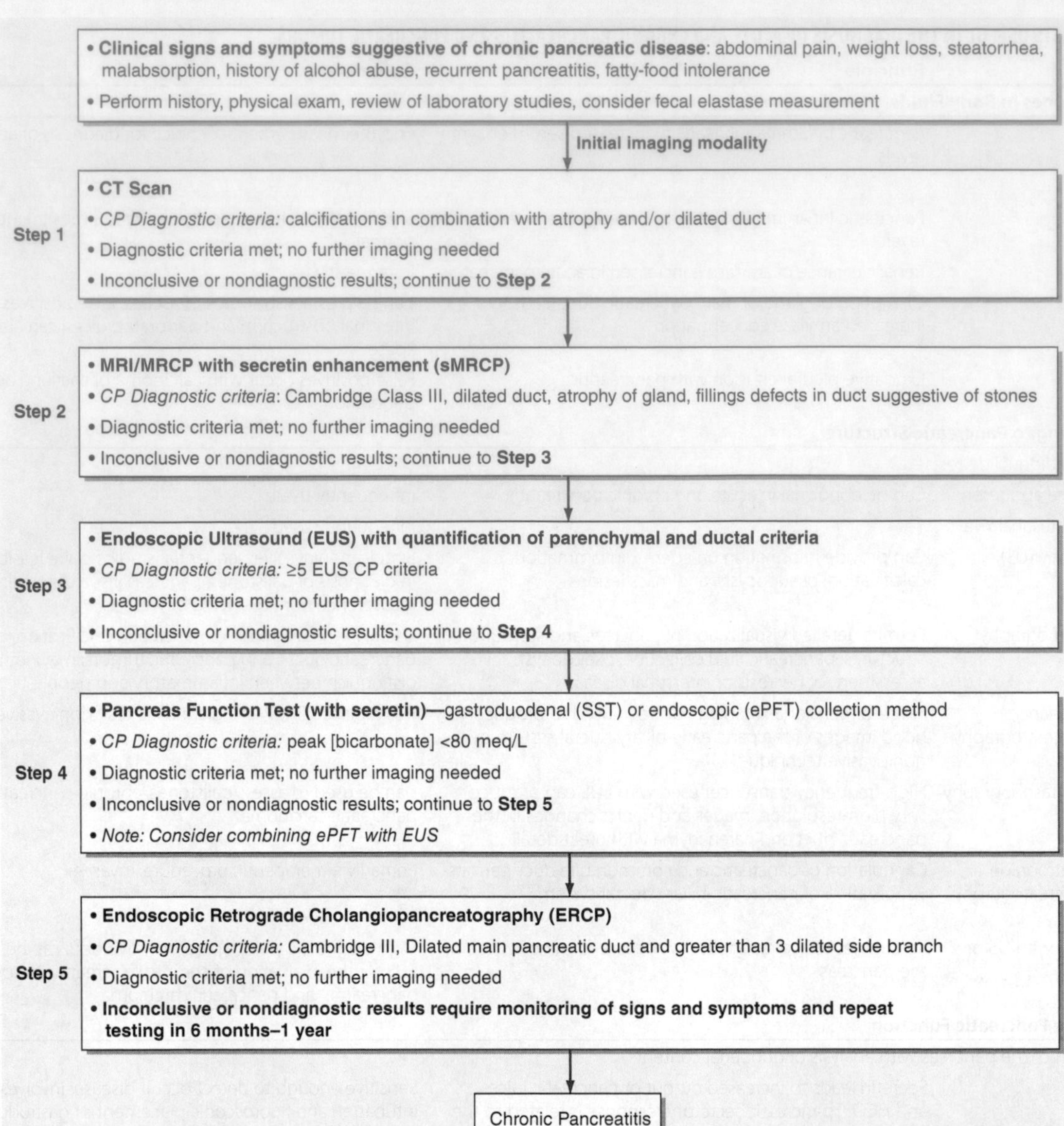

FIGURE 370-1 A stepwise diagnostic approach to the patient with suspected chronic pancreatitis (CP). Endoscopic ultrasonography (EUS) and magnetic resonance cholangiopancreatography (sMRCP/MRCP) are appropriate diagnostic alternatives to endoscopic retrograde cholangiopancreatography (ERCP). CT, computed tomography.

distinguish elevated blood amylase levels due to bona fide pancreatitis from elevated blood amylase levels due to a nonpancreatic source of amylase, especially when the blood amylase level is only moderately elevated. In patients with unexplained hyperamylasemia, measurement of macroamylase can avoid numerous tests in patients with this rare disorder.

Elevation of ascitic fluid amylase occurs in acute pancreatitis as well as in (1) ascites due to disruption of the main pancreatic duct or a leaking pseudocyst and (2) other abdominal disorders that simulate pancreatitis (e.g., intestinal obstruction, intestinal infarction, or perforated peptic ulcer). Elevation of pleural fluid amylase can occur in acute pancreatitis, chronic pancreatitis, carcinoma of the lung, and esophageal perforation. Lipase is the single best enzyme to measure for the diagnosis of acute pancreatitis. No single blood test is reliable for the diagnosis of acute pancreatitis in patients with renal failure. Pancreatic enzyme elevations are usually less than three times the upper limit of normal. Determining whether a patient with renal failure and abdominal pain has pancreatitis remains a difficult clinical problem. One study found that serum amylase levels were elevated in patients with renal dysfunction only when creatinine clearance was <0.8 mL/s (<50 mL/min). In such patients, the serum amylase level was invariably <500 IU/L in the absence of objective evidence of acute pancreatitis. In that study, serum lipase and trypsin levels paralleled serum amylase values. With these limitations in mind, the recommended screening test for acute pancreatitis in renal disease is serum lipase.

Studies Pertaining to Pancreatic Structure • ***RADIOLOGIC TESTS*** Plain films of the abdomen, which once provided useful information in patients with acute and chronic pancreatitis, have been superseded by other more detailed imaging procedures (ultrasound, EUS, CT, MRCP).

Ultrasonography (US) can provide important information in patients with acute pancreatitis, chronic pancreatitis, pseudocysts, and pancreatic carcinoma. Echographic appearances can indicate the presence of edema, inflammation, and calcification (not obvious on plain films of the abdomen), as well as pseudocysts, mass lesions, and gallstones. In acute pancreatitis, the pancreas is characteristically enlarged. In pancreatic pseudocyst, the usual appearance is primarily that of smooth, round fluid collection. Pancreatic carcinoma distorts the usual landmarks, and mass lesions >3.0 cm are usually detected as localized, solid lesions. US is often the initial investigation for most patients with suspected pancreatic disease. However, obesity and excess small- and large-bowel gas can interfere with pancreatic imaging by US studies.

Computed tomography (CT) is the best imaging study for initial evaluation of a suspected pancreatic disorder and for the assessment of

TABLE 370-2 CAUSES OF HYPERAMYLASEMIA AND HYPERAMYLASURIA

Pancreatic Disease

I. Pancreatitis
  A. Acute
  B. Chronic: ductal obstruction
  C. Complications of pancreatitis
    1. Pancreatic pseudocyst
    2. Ascites caused by pancreatic duct disruption
    3. Pancreatic necrosis
II. Pancreatic trauma
III. Pancreatic carcinoma

Nonpancreatic Disorders

I. Renal insufficiency
II. Salivary gland lesions
  A. Mumps
  B. Calculus
  C. Irradiation sialadenitis
  D. Maxillofacial surgery
III. "Tumor" hyperamylasemia
  A. Carcinoma of the lung, esophagus, breast, or ovary
IV. Macroamylasemia
V. Burns
VI. Diabetic ketoacidosis
VII. Pregnancy
VIII. Renal transplantation
IX. Cerebral trauma
X. Drugs: opiates

Other Abdominal Disorders

I. Biliary tract disease: cholecystitis, choledocholithiasis
II. Intraabdominal disease
  A. Perforated or penetrating peptic ulcer
  B. Intestinal obstruction or inflammation
  C. Ruptured ectopic pregnancy
  D. Peritonitis
  E. Aortic aneurysm
  F. Postoperative hyperamylasemia

complications of acute and chronic pancreatitis. It is especially useful in the detection of pancreatic and peripancreatic acute fluid collections, fluid-containing lesions such as pseudocysts, walled-off necrosis, calcium deposits **(see Chap. 371, Figs. 371-1, 371-2, and 371-4)**, and pancreatic neoplasms. Acute pancreatitis is characterized by (1) enlargement of the pancreatic outline, (2) distortion of the pancreatic contour, and/or (3) a pancreatic fluid that has a different attenuation coefficient than normal pancreas. Oral, water-soluble contrast agents are used to opacify the stomach and duodenum during CT scans; this strategy permits more precise delineation of various organs as well as mass lesions. Dynamic CT (using rapid IV administration of contrast) is useful in estimating the extent of pancreatic necrosis and in predicting morbidity and mortality. CT provides clear images much more rapidly and essentially negates artifact caused by patient movement. If acute pancreatitis is confirmed with serology and physical examination findings, CT scan in the first 3 days is not recommended to avoid overuse and minimize costs.

Endoscopic ultrasonography (EUS) produces high-resolution images of the pancreatic parenchyma and pancreatic duct with a transducer fixed to an endoscope that can be directed onto the surface of the pancreas through the stomach or duodenum. EUS and MRCP have largely replaced ERCP for diagnostic purposes in many centers. EUS allows one to obtain information about the pancreatic duct as well as the parenchyma and has few procedure-related complications associated with it, in contrast to the 5–10% of post-ERCP pancreatitis observed. EUS is also helpful in detecting common bile duct stones in acute

TABLE 370-3 ENDOSCOPIC ULTRASONOGRAPHIC CRITERIA FOR CHRONIC PANCREATITIS (TOTAL CRITERIA = 9)

Ductal	Parenchymal
Stones	Echogenic strands
Hyperechoic main duct margins	Echogenic foci
Main duct irregularity	Lobular contour
Main duct dilatation	Cyst
Visible side branches	

pancreatitis. Pancreatic masses can also be biopsied via EUS in cases with suspected pancreatic cancer, and one can deliver nerve-blocking agents through EUS fine-needle injection in patients suffering from pancreatic pain from chronic pancreatitis or cancer. EUS has been studied as a diagnostic modality for chronic pancreatitis. Criteria for abnormalities on EUS in severe chronic pancreatic disease have been developed. There is general agreement that the presence of five or more of the nine criteria listed in **Table 370-3** is highly predictive of chronic pancreatitis. Recent studies comparing EUS and ERCP to the secretin test in patients with unexplained abdominal pain suspected of having chronic pancreatitis show similar diagnostic accuracy in detecting early changes of chronic pancreatitis. The exact role of EUS versus CT, ERCP, or function testing in the early diagnosis of chronic pancreatitis has yet to be clearly defined.

Magnetic resonance imaging (MRI) and *magnetic resonance cholangiopancreatography* (MRCP) are now being used to view the bile ducts, pancreatic duct, and the pancreas parenchyma in both acute pancreatitis and chronic pancreatitis. For diagnostic imaging in chronic pancreatitis, non-breath-holding and three-dimensional turbo spin-echo techniques are being used to produce superb MRCP images. The main pancreatic duct and common bile duct can be seen well, but there is still a question as to whether changes can be detected consistently in the secondary ducts. The secondary ducts are not visualized in a normal pancreas. Secretin-enhanced MRCP is currently under investigation but is emerging as a method to better evaluate ductal changes. In anteroposterior imaging, T2 imaging of fluid collections can differentiate necrotic debris from fluid in suspected walled-off necrosis, and T1 imaging can diagnose hemorrhage in suspected pseudoaneurysm rupture.

Both EUS and MRCP have largely replaced ERCP in the diagnostic evaluation of pancreatic disease. As these techniques become more refined, especially with the administration of secretin, they may well be the diagnostic tests of choice to evaluate the pancreatic duct. ERCP is still needed for treatment of bile duct and pancreatic duct lesions. ERCP is primarily of therapeutic value after CT, EUS, or MRCP has detected abnormalities requiring invasive endoscopic treatment. ERCP can also be helpful at clarification of equivocal findings discovered with other imaging techniques **(see Chap. 371, Fig. 371-1)**. Pancreatic carcinoma is characterized by stenosis or obstruction of either the pancreatic duct or the common bile duct; both ductal systems are often abnormal (double-duct sign). In chronic pancreatitis, ERCP abnormalities in the main pancreatic duct and side branches have been outlined by the Cambridge classification. The presence of ductal stenosis and irregularity can make it difficult to distinguish chronic pancreatitis from carcinoma. It is important to be aware that ERCP changes interpreted as indicating chronic pancreatitis actually may be due to the effects of aging on the pancreatic duct or sequelae of a recent attack of acute pancreatitis. Although aging may cause impressive ductal alterations, it does not affect the results of pancreatic function tests (i.e., the secretin test). Elevated serum amylase levels after ERCP have been reported in the majority of patients, and clinical pancreatitis in 5–10% of patients. Recent data suggest that pancreatic duct stenting and rectal indomethacin can decrease the incidence of ERCP-induced pancreatitis. ERCP should rarely be done for diagnostic purposes and should especially be avoided in high-risk patients.

PANCREATIC BIOPSY WITH RADIOLOGIC GUIDANCE Percutaneous aspiration biopsy or a trucut biopsy of a pancreatic mass often distinguishes a pancreatic inflammatory mass from a pancreatic neoplasm.

TESTS OF EXOCRINE PANCREATIC FUNCTION

Pancreatic function tests (Table 370-1) can be divided into the following:

1. *Direct stimulation of the pancreas* by IV infusion of secretin followed by collection and measurement of duodenal contents

The secretin test, used to detect diffuse pancreatic disease, is based on the physiologic principle that the pancreatic secretory response is directly related to the functional mass of pancreatic tissue. In the standard assay, secretin is given IV in a dose of 0.2 μg/kg of synthetic human secretin as a bolus. Normal values for the standard secretin test are (1) volume output >2 mL/kg per hour, (2) bicarbonate (HCO_3^-) concentration >80 mmol/L, and (3) HCO_3^- output >10 mmol/L in 1 h. The most reproducible measurement, giving the highest level of discrimination between normal subjects and patients with chronic pancreatic exocrine insufficiency, appears to be the maximal bicarbonate concentration. A cutoff point below 80 mmol/L is considered abnormal and suggestive of abnormal secretory function that is most commonly observed in early chronic pancreatitis.

There may be a dissociation between the results of the secretin test and other tests of absorptive function. For example, patients with chronic pancreatitis often have abnormally low outputs of HCO_3^- after secretin but have normal fecal fat excretion. Thus the secretin test measures the secretory capacity of ductular epithelium, whereas fecal fat excretion indirectly reflects intraluminal lipolytic activity. Steatorrhea does not occur until intraluminal levels of lipase are markedly reduced, underscoring the fact that only small amounts of enzymes are necessary for intraluminal digestive activities. It must be emphasized that an abnormal secretin test result suggests only that chronic pancreatic damage is present.

2. *Measurement of fecal pancreatic enzymes* such as elastase

Measurement of *intraluminal digestion products* (i.e., undigested muscle fibers, stool fat, and fecal nitrogen) is discussed in Chap. 349. The amount of human elastase in stool reflects the pancreatic output of this proteolytic enzyme. Decreased elastase-1 activity (FE-1) in stool is an excellent test to detect severe pancreatic exocrine insufficiency (PEI) in patients with chronic pancreatitis and cystic fibrosis. FE-1 levels >200 μg/g are normal; levels of 100–200 μg/g are considered mild, and levels <100 μg/g are severe for PEI. Although the test is simple and noninvasive, it can give false-positive results and has a low sensitivity. Fecal levels <50 μg/g are definitive for PEI provided that the stool specimen is solid.

Tests useful in the diagnosis of exocrine pancreatic insufficiency and the differential diagnosis of malabsorption are also discussed in Chaps. 349 and 371.

371 Acute and Chronic Pancreatitis

Darwin L. Conwell, Peter Banks, Norton J. Greenberger

BIOCHEMISTRY AND PHYSIOLOGY OF PANCREATIC EXOCRINE SECRETION

GENERAL CONSIDERATIONS

The pancreas secretes 1500–3000 mL of isosmotic alkaline (pH >8) fluid per day containing about 20 enzymes. The pancreatic secretions provide the enzymes and bicarbonate needed to affect the major digestive activity of the gastrointestinal tract and provide an optimal pH for the function of these enzymes.

REGULATION OF PANCREATIC SECRETION

The exocrine pancreas is influenced by intimately interacting hormonal and neural systems. *Gastric acid* is the stimulus for the release of secretin from the duodenal mucosa (S cells), which stimulates the secretion of water and electrolytes from pancreatic ductal cells. Release of cholecystokinin (CCK) from the duodenal and proximal jejunal mucosa (Ito cells) is largely triggered by long-chain fatty acids, essential amino acids (tryptophan, phenylalanine, valine, methionine), and gastric acid itself. CCK evokes an enzyme-rich secretion from acinar cells in the pancreas. The *parasympathetic nervous system* (via the vagus nerve) exerts significant control over pancreatic secretion. Secretion evoked by secretin and CCK depends on permissive roles of vagal afferent and efferent pathways. This is particularly true for enzyme secretion, whereas water and bicarbonate secretions are heavily dependent on the hormonal effects of secretin and to a lesser extent CCK. Also, vagal stimulation affects the release of vasoactive intestinal peptide (VIP), a secretin agonist. Pancreatic exocrine secretion is also influenced by inhibitory neuropeptides such as somatostatin, pancreatic polypeptide, peptide YY, neuropeptide Y, enkephalin, pancreastatin, calcitonin gene–related peptides, glucagon, and galanin. Although pancreatic polypeptide and peptide YY may act primarily on nerves outside the pancreas, somatostatin acts at multiple sites. Nitric oxide (NO) is also an important neurotransmitter.

WATER AND ELECTROLYTE SECRETION

Bicarbonate is the ion of primary physiologic importance within pancreatic secretion. The ductal cells secrete bicarbonate predominantly derived from plasma (93%) more than from intracellular metabolism (7%). Bicarbonate enters the duct lumen through the sodium bicarbonate cotransporter with depolarization caused by chloride efflux through the cystic fibrosis transmembrane conductance regulator (CFTR). Secretin and VIP bind at the basolateral surface and cause an increase in secondary messenger intracellular cyclic AMP, and act on the apical surface of the ductal cells opening the CFTR in promoting secretion. CCK, acting as a neuromodulator, markedly potentiates the stimulatory effects of secretin. Acetylcholine also plays an important role in ductal cell secretion. Intraluminal bicarbonate secreted from the ductal cells helps neutralize gastric acid and creates the appropriate pH for the activity of pancreatic enzymes and bile salts on ingested food.

ENZYME SECRETION

The acinar cell is highly compartmentalized and is concerned with the secretion of pancreatic enzymes. Proteins synthesized by the rough endoplasmic reticulum are processed in the Golgi and then targeted to the appropriate site, whether that be zymogen granules, lysosomes, or other cell compartments. The zymogen granules migrate to the apical region of the acinar cell awaiting the appropriate neural or hormonal stimulatory response. The pancreas secretes amylolytic, lipolytic, and proteolytic enzymes into the duct lumen. *Amylolytic enzymes*, such as amylase, hydrolyze starch to oligosaccharides and to the disaccharide maltose. The *lipolytic enzymes* include lipase, phospholipase A_2, and cholesterol esterase. Bile salts inhibit lipase in isolation, but colipase, another constituent of pancreatic secretion, binds to lipase and prevents this inhibition. Bile salts activate phospholipase A and cholesterol esterase. *Proteolytic enzymes* include endopeptidases (trypsin, chymotrypsin), which act on internal peptide bonds of proteins and polypeptides; exopeptidases (carboxypeptidases, aminopeptidases), which act on the free carboxyl- and amino-terminal ends of peptides, respectively; and elastase. The proteolytic enzymes are secreted as inactive zymogen precursors. Ribonucleases (deoxyribonucleases, ribonuclease) are also secreted. *Enterokinase*, an enzyme found in the duodenal mucosa, cleaves the lysine-isoleucine bond of trypsinogen to form trypsin. Trypsin then activates the other proteolytic zymogens and phospholipase A_2 in a cascade phenomenon. All pancreatic enzymes have pH optima in the alkaline range. The nervous system initiates pancreatic enzyme secretion. The neurologic stimulation is cholinergic, involving extrinsic innervation by the vagus nerve and subsequent innervation by intrapancreatic cholinergic nerves. The stimulatory neurotransmitters are acetylcholine and gastrin-releasing peptides. These neurotransmitters activate calcium-dependent secondary messenger systems, resulting in the release of zymogens into the pancreas duct. VIP is present in intrapancreatic nerves and potentiates the effect of acetylcholine. In contrast to other species, there are no CCK receptors on acinar cells in humans. CCK in physiologic concentrations stimulates pancreatic secretion by stimulating afferent vagal and intrapancreatic nerves.

AUTOPROTECTION OF THE PANCREAS

Autodigestion of the pancreas is prevented by (1) the packaging of pancreatic proteases in precursor (proenzyme) form, (2) intracellular calcium homeostasis (low intracellular calcium in the cytosol of the acinar cell promotes the destruction of spontaneously activated trypsin), (3) acid-base balance, and (4) the synthesis of protective protease inhibitors (pancreatic secretory trypsin inhibitor [PSTI] or SPINK1), which can bind and inactivate about 20% of intracellular trypsin activity. Chymotrypsin C can also lyse and inactivate trypsin. These protease inhibitors are found in the acinar cell, the pancreatic secretions, and the α_1- and α_2-globulin fractions of plasma. Loss of any of these four protective mechanisms leads to premature enzyme activation, autodigestion, and acute pancreatitis.

ENTEROPANCREATIC AXIS AND FEEDBACK INHIBITION

Pancreatic enzyme secretion is controlled, at least in part, by a negative feedback mechanism induced by the presence of active serine proteases in the duodenum. To illustrate, perfusion of the duodenal lumen with phenylalanine (stimulates early digestion) causes a prompt increase in plasma CCK levels as well as increased secretion of chymotrypsin and other pancreatic enzymes. However, simultaneous perfusion with trypsin (stimulates late digestion) blunts both responses. Conversely, perfusion of the duodenal lumen with protease inhibitors actually leads to enzyme hypersecretion. The available evidence supports the concept that the duodenum contains a peptide called *CCK-releasing factor* (CCK-RF) that is involved in stimulating CCK release. It appears that serine proteases inhibit pancreatic secretion by inactivating a CCK-releasing peptide in the lumen of the small intestine. Thus, the integrative result of both bicarbonate and enzyme secretion depends on a feedback process for both bicarbonate and pancreatic enzymes. Acidification of the duodenum releases secretin, which stimulates vagal and other neural pathways to activate pancreatic duct cells, which secrete bicarbonate. This bicarbonate then neutralizes the duodenal acid, and the feedback loop is completed. Dietary proteins bind proteases, thereby leading to an increase in free CCK-RF. CCK is then released into the blood in physiologic concentrations, acting primarily through the neural pathways (vagal-vagal). This leads to acetylcholine-mediated pancreatic enzyme secretion. Proteases continue to be secreted from the pancreas until the protein within the duodenum is digested. At this point, pancreatic protease secretion is reduced to basic levels, thus completing this step in the feedback process.

ACUTE PANCREATITIS

GENERAL CONSIDERATIONS

Recent U.S. estimates from the National Inpatient Sample report that acute pancreatitis is the most common inpatient principal gastrointestinal diagnosis. The incidence of acute pancreatitis also varies in different countries and depends on cause (e.g., alcohol, gallstones, metabolic factors, drugs [Table 371-1]). The annual incidence ranges from 13–45/100,000 persons. Acute pancreatitis results in >250,000 hospitalizations per year. The median length of hospital stay is 4 days, with a median hospital cost of $6,096 and a mortality of 1%. The estimated cost annually approaches $2.6 billion. Hospitalization rates increase with age, are 88% higher among blacks, and are higher among males than females. The age-adjusted rate of hospital discharges with an acute pancreatitis diagnosis increased 62% between 1988 and 2004. From 2000 to 2009, the rate increased 30%. Thus, acute pancreatitis is increasing and is a significant burden on health care costs and resource utilization.

ETIOLOGY AND PATHOGENESIS

There are many causes of acute pancreatitis (Table 371-1), but the mechanisms by which these conditions trigger pancreatic inflammation have not been fully elucidated. Gallstones continue to be the leading cause of acute pancreatitis in most series (30–60%). The risk of acute pancreatitis in patients with at least one gallstone <5 mm in diameter is fourfold greater than that in patients with larger stones. Alcohol is the second most common cause, responsible for 15–30% of cases in the United States. The incidence of pancreatitis in alcoholics is surprisingly low (5/100,000), indicating that in addition to the amount of alcohol ingested, other factors affect a person's susceptibility to pancreatic injury such as cigarette smoking. Acute pancreatitis occurs in 5–10% of patients following endoscopic retrograde cholangiopancreatography (ERCP). Use of a prophylactic pancreatic duct stent and rectal nonsteroidal anti-inflammatory drugs (NSAIDs) has been shown to reduce pancreatitis after ERCP. Risk factors for post-ERCP pancreatitis include minor papilla sphincterotomy, sphincter of Oddi dysfunction, prior history of post-ERCP pancreatitis, age <60 years, >2 contrast injections into the pancreatic duct, and endoscopic trainee involvement.

Hypertriglyceridemia is the cause of acute pancreatitis in 1.3–3.8% of cases; serum triglyceride levels are usually >11.3 mmol/L (>1000 mg/dL). Most patients with hypertriglyceridemia, when subsequently examined, show evidence of an underlying derangement in lipid metabolism, probably unrelated to pancreatitis. Such patients are prone to recurrent episodes of pancreatitis. Any factor (e.g., drugs or alcohol) that causes an abrupt increase in serum triglycerides can precipitate a bout of acute pancreatitis. Patients with a deficiency of apolipoprotein CII have an increased incidence of pancreatitis; apolipoprotein CII

TABLE 371-1 CAUSES OF ACUTE PANCREATITIS

Common Causes
Gallstones (including microlithiasis)
Alcohol (acute and chronic alcoholism)
Hypertriglyceridemia
Endoscopic retrograde cholangiopancreatography (ERCP), especially after biliary manometry
Drugs (azathioprine, 6-mercaptopurine, sulfonamides, estrogens, tetracycline, valproic acid, anti-HIV medications, 5-aminosalicylic acid [5-ASA])
Trauma (especially blunt abdominal trauma)
Postoperative (abdominal and nonabdominal operations)
Uncommon Causes
Vascular causes and vasculitis (ischemic-hypoperfusion states after cardiac surgery)
Connective tissue disorders and thrombotic thrombocytopenic purpura (TTP)
Cancer of the pancreas
Hypercalcemia
Periampullary diverticulum
Pancreas divisum
Hereditary pancreatitis
Cystic fibrosis
Renal failure
Infections (mumps, coxsackievirus, cytomegalovirus, echovirus, parasites)
Autoimmune (e.g., type 1 and type 2)
Causes to Consider in Patients with Recurrent Bouts of Acute Pancreatitis Without an Obvious Etiology
Occult disease of the biliary tree or pancreatic ducts, especially microlithiasis, biliary sludge
Drugs
Alcohol abuse
Metabolic: Hypertriglyceridemia, hypercalcemia
Anatomic: Pancreas divisum
Pancreatic cancer
Intraductal papillary mucinous neoplasm (IPMN)
Hereditary pancreatitis
Cystic fibrosis
Autoimmune
Idiopathic

activates lipoprotein lipase, which is important in clearing chylomicrons from the bloodstream. Patients with diabetes mellitus who have developed ketoacidosis and patients who are on certain medications such as oral contraceptives may also develop high triglyceride levels. Approximately 0.1–2% of cases of acute pancreatitis are drug related. Drugs cause pancreatitis either by a hypersensitivity reaction or by the generation of a toxic metabolite, although in some cases, it is not clear which of these mechanisms is operative (Table 371-1).

Pathologically, acute pancreatitis varies from *interstitial pancreatitis* (pancreas blood supply maintained), which is generally self-limited to *necrotizing pancreatitis* (pancreas blood supply interrupted), in which the extent of necrosis may correlate with the severity of the attack and its systemic complications. Autodigestion is a currently accepted pathogenic theory; according to this theory, pancreatitis results when proteolytic enzymes (e.g., trypsinogen, chymotrypsinogen, proelastase, and lipolytic enzymes such as phospholipase A_2) are activated in the pancreas acinar cell rather than in the intestinal lumen. A number of factors (e.g., endotoxins, exotoxins, viral infections, ischemia, oxidative stress, lysosomal calcium, and direct trauma) are believed to facilitate premature activation of trypsin. Activated proteolytic enzymes, especially trypsin, not only digest pancreatic and peripancreatic tissues but also can activate other enzymes, such as elastase and phospholipase A_2. Spontaneous activation of trypsin also can occur.

ACTIVATION OF PANCREATIC ENZYMES IN THE PATHOGENESIS OF ACUTE PANCREATITIS

Several recent studies have suggested that pancreatitis is a disease that evolves in three phases. The *initial phase* is characterized by intrapancreatic digestive enzyme activation and acinar cell injury. Trypsin activation appears to be mediated by lysosomal hydrolases such as cathepsin B that become colocalized with digestive enzymes in intracellular organelles; it is currently believed that acinar cell injury is the consequence of trypsin activation. The *second phase* of pancreatitis involves the activation, chemoattraction, and sequestration of leukocytes and macrophages in the pancreas, resulting in an enhanced intrapancreatic inflammatory reaction. Neutrophil depletion induced by prior administration of an antineutrophil serum has been shown to reduce the severity of experimentally induced pancreatitis. There is also evidence to support the concept that neutrophils can activate trypsinogen. Thus, intrapancreatic acinar cell activation of trypsinogen could be a two-step process (i.e., an early neutrophil-independent and a later neutrophil-dependent phase). The *third phase* of pancreatitis is due to the effects of activated proteolytic enzymes and cytokines, released by the inflamed pancreas, on distant organs. Activated proteolytic enzymes, especially trypsin, not only digest pancreatic and peripancreatic tissues but also activate other enzymes such as elastase and phospholipase A_2. The active enzymes and cytokines then digest cellular membranes and cause proteolysis, edema, interstitial hemorrhage, vascular damage, coagulation necrosis, fat necrosis, and parenchymal cell necrosis. Cellular injury and death result in the liberation of bradykinin peptides, vasoactive substances, and histamine that can produce vasodilation, increased vascular permeability, and edema with profound effects on many organs. The systemic inflammatory response syndrome (SIRS) and acute respiratory distress syndrome (ARDS), as well as multiorgan failure, may occur as a result of this cascade of local and distant effects.

A number of genetic factors can increase the susceptibility and/or modify the severity of pancreatic injury in acute pancreatitis, recurrent pancreatitis, and chronic pancreatitis. All of the major genetic susceptibility factors center on the control of trypsin activity within the pancreatic acinar cell, in part because they were identified as candidate genes linked to intrapancreatic trypsin control. Five genetic variants have been identified as being associated with susceptibility to pancreatitis. The genes that have been identified include (1) cationic trypsinogen gene (*PRSS1*), (2) pancreatic secretory trypsin inhibitor (*SPINK1*), (3) the cystic fibrosis transmembrane conductance regulator gene (*CFTR*), (4) the chymotrypsin C gene (*CTRC*), and (5) the calcium-sensing receptor (*CASR*). Investigations of other genetic variants are currently under way, and new genes will be added to this list in the future. Multiple medical, ethical, and psychological issues arise when these genes are discovered, and referral to genetic counselors is recommended.

APPROACH TO THE PATIENT: Abdominal Pain

Abdominal pain is the major symptom of acute pancreatitis. Pain may vary from a mild discomfort to severe, constant, and incapacitating distress. Characteristically, the pain, which is steady and boring in character, is located in the epigastrium and periumbilical region, and may radiate to the back, chest, flanks, and lower abdomen. Nausea, vomiting, and abdominal distention due to gastric and intestinal hypomotility and chemical peritonitis are also frequent complaints.

Physical examination frequently reveals a distressed and anxious patient. Low-grade fever, tachycardia, and hypotension are fairly common. Shock is not unusual and may result from (1) hypovolemia secondary to exudation of blood and plasma proteins into the retroperitoneal space; (2) increased formation and release of kinin peptides, which cause vasodilation and increased vascular permeability; and (3) systemic effects of proteolytic and lipolytic enzymes released into the circulation. Jaundice occurs infrequently; when present, it usually is due to edema of the head of the pancreas with compression of the intrapancreatic portion of the common bile duct or passage of a biliary stone or sludge. Erythematous skin nodules due to subcutaneous fat necrosis may rarely occur. In 10–20% of patients, there are pulmonary findings, including basilar rales, atelectasis, and pleural effusion, the latter most frequently left sided. Abdominal tenderness and muscle rigidity are present to a variable degree, but compared with the intense pain, these signs may be less impressive. Bowel sounds are usually diminished or absent. An enlarged pancreas from acute fluid collection, walled off necrosis, or a pseudocyst may be palpable in the upper abdomen later in the course of the disease (i.e., 4–6 weeks). A faint blue discoloration around the umbilicus (Cullen's sign) may occur as the result of hemoperitoneum, and a blue-red-purple or green-brown discoloration of the flanks (Turner's sign) reflects tissue catabolism of hemoglobin from severe necrotizing pancreatitis with hemorrhage.

LABORATORY DATA

Serum amylase and lipase values threefold or more above normal virtually clinch the diagnosis if gut perforation, ischemia, and infarction are excluded. Serum lipase is the preferred test. However, it should be noted that there is no correlation between the severity of pancreatitis and the degree of serum lipase and amylase elevations. After 3–7 days, even with continuing evidence of pancreatitis, total serum amylase values tend to return toward normal. However, pancreatic isoamylase and lipase levels may remain elevated for 7–14 days. It should be recognized that amylase elevations in serum and urine occur in many conditions other than pancreatitis (see Chap. 370, Table 370-2). Importantly, patients with *acidemia* (arterial pH ≤7.32) may have spurious elevations in serum amylase. This finding explains why patients with diabetic ketoacidosis may have marked elevations in serum amylase without any other evidence of acute pancreatitis. Serum lipase activity increases in parallel with amylase activity and is more specific than amylase. A serum lipase measurement can be instrumental in differentiating a pancreatic or nonpancreatic cause for hyperamylasemia. *Leukocytosis* (15,000–20,000 leukocytes/μL) occurs frequently. Patients with more severe disease may show hemoconcentration with hematocrit values >44% and/or prerenal azotemia with a blood urea nitrogen (BUN) level >22 mg/dL resulting from loss of plasma into the retroperitoneal space and peritoneal cavity.

Hemoconcentration may be the harbinger of more severe disease (i.e., pancreatic necrosis), whereas azotemia is a significant risk factor for mortality. *Hyperglycemia* is common and is due to multiple factors, including decreased insulin release, increased glucagon release, and

TABLE 371-2 REVISED ATLANTA DEFINITIONS OF MORPHOLOGIC FEATURES OF ACUTE PANCREATITIS

Morphologic Feature	Definition	Computed Tomography Criteria
Interstitial pancreatitis	Acute inflammation of the pancreatic parenchyma and peripancreatic tissues, but without recognizable tissue necrosis	Pancreatic parenchyma enhancement by IV contrast agent No findings of peripancreatic necrosis
Necrotizing pancreatitis	Inflammation associated with pancreatic parenchymal necrosis and/or peripancreatic necrosis	Lack of pancreatic parenchymal enhancement by IV contrast agent and/or presence of findings of peripancreatic necrosis (see below—ANC and WON)
Acute pancreatic fluid collection	Peripancreatic fluid associated with interstitial edematous pancreatitis with no associated peripancreatic necrosis. This term applies only to areas of peripancreatic fluid seen within the first 4 weeks after onset of interstitial edematous pancreatitis and without the features of a pseudocyst.	Occurs in the setting of interstitial edematous pancreatitis Homogeneous collection with fluid density Confined by normal peripancreatic fascial planes No definable wall encapsulating the collection Adjacent to pancreas (no intrapancreatic extension)
Pancreatic pseudocyst	An encapsulated collection of fluid with a well-defined inflammatory wall usually outside the pancreas with minimal or no necrosis. This entity usually occurs >4 weeks after onset of interstitial edematous pancreatitis.	Well circumscribed, usually round or oval Homogeneous fluid density No nonliquid component Well-defined wall; that is, completely encapsulated Maturation usually requires >4 weeks after onset of acute pancreatitis; occurs after interstitial edematous pancreatitis
Acute necrotic collection (ANC)	A collection containing variable amounts of both fluid and necrosis associated with necrotizing pancreatitis; the necrosis can involve the pancreatic parenchyma and/or the peripancreatic tissues.	Occurs only in the setting of acute necrotizing pancreatitis Heterogeneous and nonliquid density of varying degrees in different locations (some appear homogeneous early in their course) No definable wall encapsulating the collection Location—intrapancreatic and/or extrapancreatic
Walled-off necrosis (WON)	A mature, encapsulated collection of pancreatic and/or peripancreatic necrosis that has developed a well-defined inflammatory wall. WON usually occurs >4 weeks after onset of necrotizing pancreatitis.	Heterogeneous with liquid and nonliquid density with varying degrees of loculations (some may appear homogeneous) Well-defined wall; that is, completely encapsulated Location—intrapancreatic and/or extrapancreatic Maturation usually requires 4 weeks after onset of acute necrotizing pancreatitis

Source: Modified from P Banks et al: Gut 62:102, 2013.

an increased output of adrenal glucocorticoids and catecholamines. *Hypocalcemia* occurs in ~25% of patients, and its pathogenesis is incompletely understood. Although earlier studies suggested that the response of the parathyroid gland to a decrease in serum calcium is impaired, subsequent observations have failed to confirm this phenomenon. Intraperitoneal saponification of calcium by fatty acids in areas of fat necrosis occurs occasionally, with large amounts (up to 6.0 g) dissolved or suspended in ascitic fluid. Such "soap formation" may also be significant in patients with pancreatitis, mild hypocalcemia, and little or no obvious ascites. *Hyperbilirubinemia* (serum bilirubin >68 mmoL or >4.0 mg/dL) occurs in ~10% of patients. However, jaundice is transient, and serum bilirubin levels return to normal in 4–7 days. Serum alkaline phosphatase and aspartate aminotransferase levels are also transiently elevated, and they parallel serum bilirubin values and may point to gallbladder-related disease or inflammation in the pancreatic head. *Hypertriglyceridemia* occurs in 5–10% of patients, and serum amylase levels in these individuals are often spuriously normal (Chap. 370). Approximately 5–10% of patients have *hypoxemia* (arterial PO_2 ≤60 mmHg), which may herald the onset of ARDS. Finally, the electrocardiogram is occasionally abnormal in acute pancreatitis with ST-segment and T-wave abnormalities simulating myocardial ischemia.

An abdominal ultrasound is recommended in the emergency ward as the initial diagnostic imaging modality and is most useful to evaluate for gallstone disease and the pancreatic head.

The revised Atlanta criteria have clearly outlined the morphologic features of acute pancreatitis on computed tomography (CT) scan as follows: (1) interstitial pancreatitis, (2) necrotizing pancreatitis, (3) acute pancreatic fluid collection, (4) pancreatic pseudocyst, (5) acute necrotic collection (ANC), and (6) walled-off pancreatic necrosis (WON) (Table 371-2 and Fig. 371-1). **Radiologic studies useful in the diagnosis of acute pancreatitis are discussed in Chap. 370 and listed in Table 370-1.**

DIAGNOSIS

Any severe acute pain in the abdomen or back should suggest the possibility of acute pancreatitis. The diagnosis is established by two of the following three criteria: (1) typical abdominal pain in the epigastrium that may radiate to the back, (2) threefold or greater elevation in serum lipase and/or amylase, and (3) confirmatory findings of acute pancreatitis on cross-sectional abdominal imaging. Patients also have associated nausea, emesis, fever, tachycardia, and abnormal findings on abdominal examination. Laboratory studies may reveal leukocytosis, hypocalcemia, and hyperglycemia. Although not required for diagnosis, markers of severity may include hemoconcentration (hematocrit >44%), admission azotemia (BUN >22 mg/dL), SIRS, and signs of organ failure (Table 371-3).

The *differential diagnosis* should include the following disorders: (1) perforated viscus, especially peptic ulcer; (2) acute cholecystitis and biliary colic; (3) acute intestinal obstruction; (4) mesenteric vascular occlusion; (5) renal colic; (6) inferior myocardial infarction; (7) dissecting aortic aneurysm; (8) connective tissue disorders with vasculitis; (9) pneumonia, and (10) diabetic ketoacidosis. It may be difficult to differentiate acute cholecystitis from acute pancreatitis, because an elevated serum amylase may be found in both disorders. Pain of biliary tract origin is more right sided or epigastric than periumbilical or left upper quadrant and can be more severe; ileus is usually absent. Ultrasound is helpful in establishing the diagnosis of cholelithiasis and cholecystitis. Intestinal obstruction due to mechanical factors can be differentiated from pancreatitis by the history of crescendo-decrescendo pain, findings on abdominal examination, and CT of the abdomen showing changes characteristic of mechanical obstruction. Acute mesenteric vascular occlusion is usually suspected in elderly debilitated patients with brisk leukocytosis, abdominal distention, and bloody diarrhea, confirmed by CT or magnetic resonance angiography. Vasculitides secondary to systemic lupus erythematosus and polyarteritis nodosa may be confused with pancreatitis, especially because pancreatitis may develop as a complication of these diseases. Diabetic ketoacidosis is often accompanied by abdominal pain and elevated total serum amylase levels, thus closely mimicking acute pancreatitis. However, the serum lipase level is not elevated in diabetic ketoacidosis.

CLINICAL COURSE, DEFINITIONS, AND CLASSIFICATIONS

The Revised Atlanta Classification (1) defines phases of acute pancreatitis, (2) defines severity of acute pancreatitis, and (3) clarifies imaging definitions as outlined below.

Phases of Acute Pancreatitis Two phases of acute pancreatitis have been defined, early (<2 weeks) and late (>2 weeks), which primarily

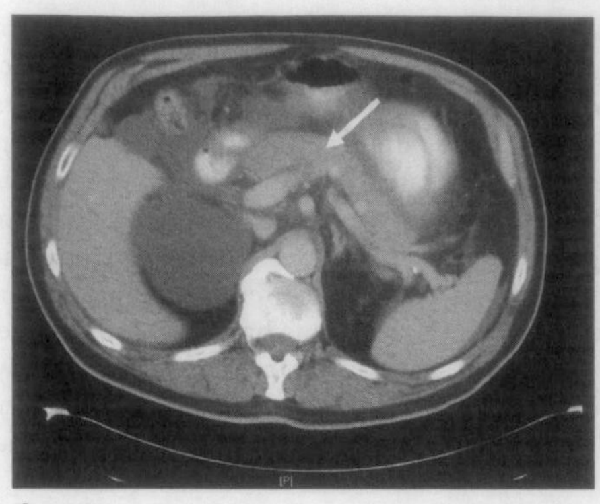

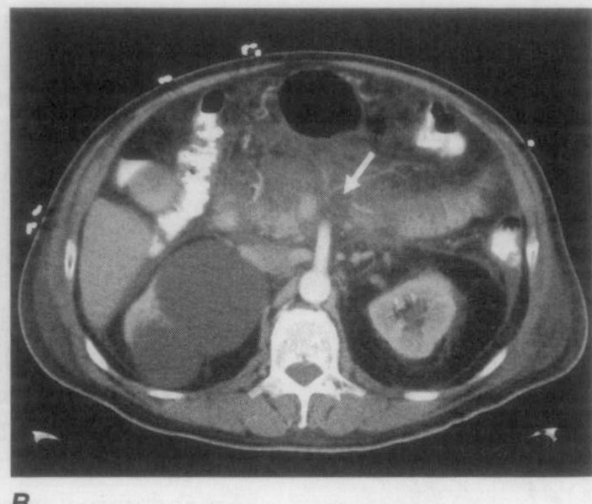

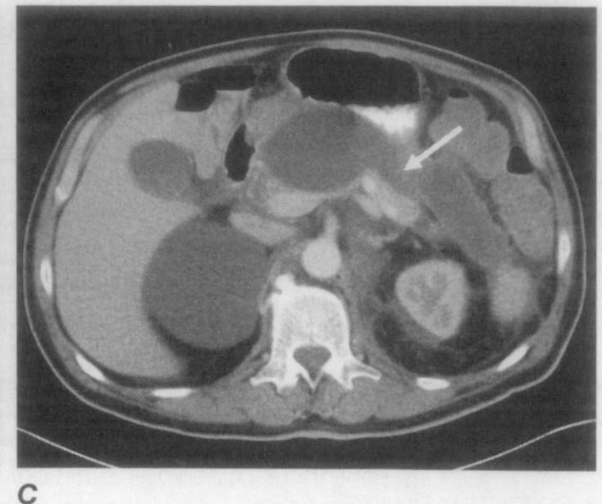

FIGURE 371-1 Acute pancreatitis: computed tomography (CT) evolution. ***A.*** Contrast-enhanced CT scan of the abdomen performed on admission for a patient with clinical and biochemical parameters suggestive of acute pancreatitis. Note the abnormal enhancement of the pancreatic parenchyma (*arrow*) suggestive of interstitial pancreatitis. ***B.*** Contrast-enhanced CT scan of the abdomen performed on the same patient 6 days later for persistent fever and systemic inflammatory response syndrome. The pancreas now demonstrates significant areas of nonenhancement consistent with development of necrosis, particularly in the body and neck region (*arrow*). Note that an early CT scan obtained within the first 48 h of hospitalization may underestimate or miss necrosis. ***C.*** Contrast-enhanced CT scan of the abdomen performed on the same patient 2 months after the initial episode of acute pancreatitis. CT now demonstrates evidence of a fluid collection consistent with walled-off pancreatic necrosis (*arrow*). *(Courtesy of Dr. KJ Mortele, Brigham and Women's Hospital; with permission.)*

describes the hospital course of the disease. In the *early phase* of acute pancreatitis, which lasts 1–2 weeks, severity is defined by clinical parameters rather than morphologic findings. Most patients exhibit SIRS, and if this persists, patients are predisposed to organ failure. Three organ systems should be assessed to define organ failure: respiratory, cardiovascular, and renal. Organ failure is defined as a score of 2 or more for one of these three organ systems using the modified Marshall scoring system. Persistent organ failure (>48 h) is the most important clinical finding in regard to severity of the acute pancreatitis episode. Organ failure that affects more than one organ is considered multisystem organ failure. CT imaging is usually not needed or recommended during the first 48 h of admission in acute pancreatitis.

The *late phase* is characterized by a protracted course of illness and may require imaging to evaluate for local complications. The important clinical parameter of severity, as in the early phase, is persistent organ failure. These patients may require supportive measures such as renal dialysis, ventilator support, or need for supplemental nutrition via the nasojejunal or parenteral route. The radiographic feature of greatest importance to recognize in this phase is the development of necrotizing pancreatitis on CT imaging. Necrosis generally prolongs hospitalization and, if infected, may require operative, endoscopic, or percutaneous intervention.

TABLE 371-3 SEVERE ACUTE PANCREATITIS

Risk Factors for Severity
• Age >60 years
• Obesity, BMI >30
• Comorbid disease (Charlson Comorbidity Index)
Markers of Severity at Admission or Within 24 h
• SIRS—defined by presence of 2 or more criteria:
• Core temperature <36° or >38°C
• Heart rate >90 beats/min
• Respirations >20/min or Pco_2 <32 mmHg
• White blood cell count >12,000/μL, <4000/μL, or 10% bands
• APACHE II
• Hemoconcentration (hematocrit >44%)
• Admission BUN (>22 mg/dL)
• BISAP Score
• (B) BUN >25 mg/dL
• (I) Impaired mental status
• (S) SIRS: ≥2 of 4 present
• (A) Age >60 years
• (P) Pleural effusion
• Organ failure (Modified Marshall Score)
• Cardiovascular: systolic BP <90 mmHg, heart rate >130 beats/min
• Pulmonary: Pao_2 <60 mmHg
• Renal: serum creatinine >2.0 mg%
Markers of Severity During Hospitalization
• Persistent organ failure
• Pancreatic necrosis

Abbreviations: APACHE II, Acute Physiology and Chronic Health Evaluation II; BMI, body mass index; BISAP, Bedside Index of Severity in Acute Pancreatitis; BP, blood pressure; BUN, blood urea nitrogen; SIRS, systemic inflammatory response syndrome.

Severity of Acute Pancreatitis Three severity classifications have also been defined: mild, moderately severe, and severe. *Mild acute pancreatitis* is without local complications or organ failure. Most patients with interstitial acute pancreatitis have mild pancreatitis. In mild acute pancreatitis, the disease is self-limited and subsides spontaneously, usually within 3–7 days after treatment is instituted. Oral intake can be resumed if the patient is hungry, has normal bowel function, and is without nausea and vomiting. Typically, a clear or full liquid diet has been recommended for the initial meal; however, a low-fat solid diet is a reasonable choice following recovery from mild acute pancreatitis.

Moderately severe acute pancreatitis is characterized by transient organ failure (resolves in <48 h) or local or systemic complications in the absence of persistent organ failure. These patients may or may not have necrosis, but may develop a local complication such as a fluid collection that requires a prolonged hospitalization greater than 1 week.

Severe acute pancreatitis is characterized by persistent organ failure (>48 h). Organ failure can be single or multiple. A CT scan or magnetic resonance imaging (MRI) should be obtained to assess for necrosis and/or complications. If a local complication is encountered, management is dictated by clinical symptoms, evidence of infection, maturity of fluid collection, and clinical stability of the patient. Prophylactic antibiotics are not recommended.

Imaging in Acute Pancreatitis Two types of pancreatitis are recognized on imaging as *interstitial* or *necrotizing* based on pancreatic perfusion. CT imaging is best evaluated 3–5 days into hospitalization when patients are not responding to supportive care to look for local complications such as necrosis. Recent studies report the overutilization of CT imaging in acute pancreatitis and its inability to be better than clinical judgment in the early days of acute pancreatitis management. The revised criteria also outline the terminology for local complications and fluid collections along with a CT imaging template to guide reporting of findings. Local morphologic features are summarized in Table 371-1. *Interstitial pancreatitis* occurs in 90–95% of admissions for acute pancreatitis and is characterized by diffuse gland enlargement, homogenous contrast enhancement, and mild inflammatory changes or peripancreatic stranding. Symptoms generally resolve with a week of hospitalization. *Necrotizing pancreatitis* occurs in 5–10% of acute pancreatitis admissions and does not evolve until several days of hospitalization. It is characterized by lack of pancreatic parenchymal enhancement by intravenous contrast agent and/or presence of findings of peripancreatic necrosis. According to the revised Atlanta criteria, the natural history of pancreatic and peripancreatic necrosis is variable because it may remain solid or liquefy, remain sterile or become infected, and persist or disappear over time. CT identification of local complications, particularly necrosis, is critical in patients who are not responding to therapy because patients with infected and sterile necrosis are at greatest risk of mortality (Figs. 371-1*B*, 371-2, and 371-3). The median prevalence of organ failure is 54% in necrotizing pancreatitis. The prevalence of organ failure is perhaps slightly higher in infected versus sterile necrosis. With single-organ system failure, the mortality is 3–10% but increases to 47% with multisystem organ failure.

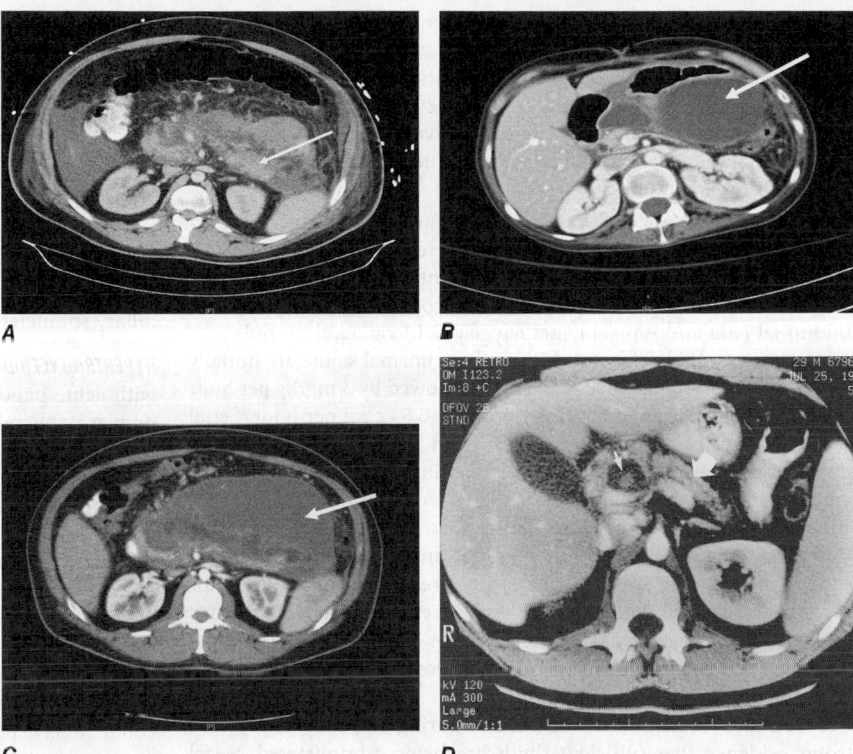

FIGURE 371-2 ***A.*** Acute necrotizing pancreatitis: computed tomography (CT) scan. Contrast-enhanced CT scan showing acute pancreatitis with necrosis. *Arrow* shows partially enhancing body/tail of pancreas surrounded by fluid with decreased enhancement in the neck/body of the pancreas. ***B.*** Acute fluid collection: CT scan. Contrast-enhanced CT scan showing fluid collection in the retroperitoneum (*arrow*) compressing the air-filled stomach arising from the pancreas in a patient with asparaginase-induced acute necrotizing pancreatitis. ***C.*** Walled off pancreatic necrosis: CT scan. CT scan showing marked walled-off necrosis of the pancreas and peripancreatic area (*arrow*) in a patient with necrotizing pancreatitis. Addendum: In past years, both of these CT findings (Figs. 371-2*B* and 371-2*C*) would have been misinterpreted as pseudocysts. ***D.*** Spiral CT showing a pseudocyst (*small arrow*) with a pseudoaneurysm (*light area in pseudocyst*). Note the demonstration of the main pancreatic duct (*big arrow*), even though this duct is minimally dilated by endoscopic retrograde cholangiopancreatography. *(A, B, C, courtesy of Dr. KJ Mortele, Brigham and Women's Hospital; D, courtesy of Dr. PR Ros, Brigham and Women's Hospital; with permission.)*

ACUTE PANCREATITIS MANAGEMENT

We will briefly describe the management of patients with acute pancreatitis from the time of diagnosis in the emergency ward to ongoing hospital admission and, finally, to time of discharge, highlighting salient features based on severity and complications. It is important to note that 85–90% of cases of acute pancreatitis are self-limited and subside spontaneously, usually within 3–7 days after initiation of treatment, and do not exhibit organ failure or local complications.

The management of acute pancreatitis begins in the emergency ward. After a diagnosis has been

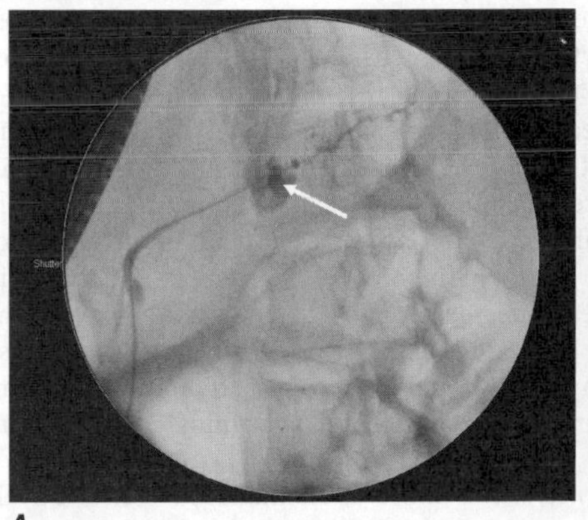

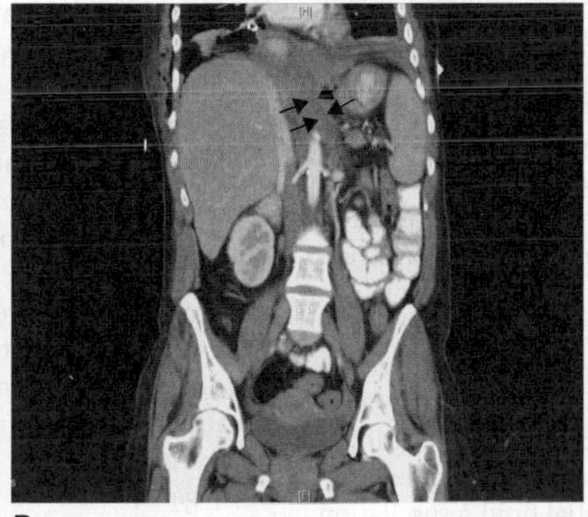

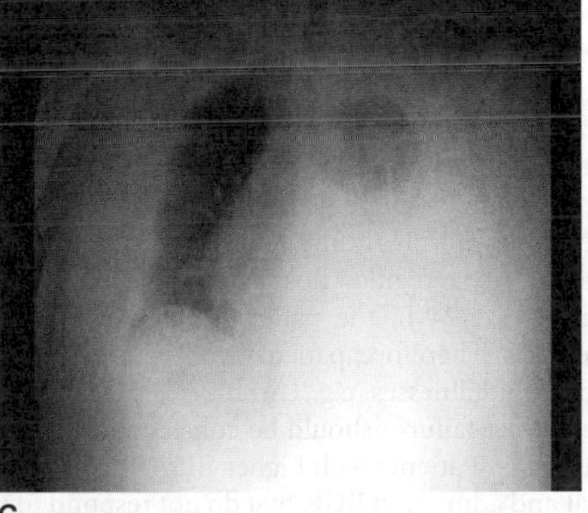

FIGURE 371-3 ***A.*** Pancreaticopleural fistula: pancreatic duct leak on endoscopic retrograde cholangiopancreatography. Pancreatic duct leak (*arrow*) demonstrated at the time of retrograde pancreatogram in a patient with acute exacerbation of alcohol-induced acute or chronic pancreatitis. ***B.*** Pancreaticopleural fistula: computed tomography (CT) scan. Contrast-enhanced CT scan (coronal view) with *arrows* showing fistula tract from pancreatic duct disruption in the pancreatic pleural fistula. ***C.*** Pancreaticopleural fistula: chest x-ray. Large pleural effusion in the left hemithorax from a disrupted pancreatic duct. Analysis of pleural fluid revealed elevated amylase concentration. *(Courtesy of Dr. KJ Mortele, Brigham and Women's Hospital; with permission.)*

confirmed, aggressive fluid resuscitation is initiated, intravenous analgesics are administered, severity is assessed, and a search for etiologies that may impact acute care is begun. Patients who do not respond to aggressive fluid resuscitation in the emergency ward should be considered for admission to a step-down or intensive care unit for aggressive fluid resuscitation, hemodynamic monitoring, and management of necrosis or organ failure.

Fluid Resuscitation and Monitoring Response to Therapy The most important treatment intervention for acute pancreatitis is safe, aggressive intravenous fluid resuscitation. The patient is made NPO to rest the pancreas and is given intravenous narcotic analgesics to control abdominal pain and supplemental oxygen (2 L) via nasal cannula.

Intravenous fluids of lactated Ringer's or normal saline are initially bolused at 15–20 cc/kg (1050–1400 mL), followed by 3 mg/kg per hour (200–250 mL/h), to maintain urine output >0.5 cc/kg per hour. Serial bedside evaluations are required every 6–8 h to assess vital signs, oxygen saturation, and change in physical examination. Lactated Ringer's solution has been shown to decrease systemic inflammation and may be a better crystalloid than normal saline. A *targeted resuscitation strategy* with measurement of hematocrit and BUN every 8–12 h is recommended to ensure adequacy of fluid resuscitation and monitor response to therapy, noting less aggressive resuscitation strategy may be needed in milder forms of pancreatitis. A rising BUN during hospitalization is not only associated with inadequate hydration but also higher in-hospital mortality.

A decrease in hematocrit and BUN during the first 12–24 h is strong evidence that sufficient fluids are being administered. Serial measurements and bedside assessment for fluid overload are continued, and fluid rates are maintained at the current rate. Adjustments in fluid resuscitation may be required in patients with cardiac, pulmonary, or renal disease. A rise in hematocrit or BUN during serial measurement should be treated with a repeat volume challenge with a 2-L crystalloid bolus followed by increasing the fluid rate by 1.5 mg/kg per hour. If the BUN or hematocrit fails to respond (i.e., remains elevated or does not decrease) to this bolus challenge and increase in fluid rate, consideration of transfer to an intensive care unit is strongly recommended for hemodynamic monitoring.

Assessment of Severity and Hospital Triage Severity of acute pancreatitis should be determined in the emergency ward to assist in patient triage to a regular hospital ward or step-down unit or direct admission to an intensive care unit. The Bedside Index of Severity in Acute Pancreatitis (BISAP) incorporates five clinical and laboratory parameters obtained within the first 24 h of hospitalization (Table 371-3)—BUN >25 mg/dL, impaired mental status (Glasgow coma score <15), SIRS, age >60 years, and pleural effusion on radiography—that can be useful in assessing severity. Presence of three or more of these factors was associated with substantially increased risk for in-hospital mortality among patients with acute pancreatitis. In addition, an elevated hematocrit >44% and admission BUN >22 mg/dL are also associated with more severe acute pancreatitis. Incorporating these indices with the overall patient response to initial fluid resuscitation in the emergency ward can be useful at triaging patients to the appropriate hospital acute care setting.

In general, patients with lower BISAP scores, hematocrits, and admission BUNs tend to respond to initial management and are triaged to a regular hospital ward for ongoing care. If SIRS is not present at 24 h, the patient is unlikely to develop organ failure or necrosis. Therefore, patients with persistent SIRS at 24 h or underlying comorbid illnesses (e.g., chronic obstructive pulmonary disease, congestive heart failure) should be considered for a step-down unit setting if available. Patients with higher BISAP scores and elevations in hematocrit and admission BUN that do not respond to initial fluid resuscitation and exhibit evidence of respiratory failure, hypotension, or organ failure should be considered for direct admission to an intensive care unit.

Special Considerations Based on Etiology A careful history, review of medications, selected laboratory studies (liver profile, serum triglycerides, serum calcium), and an abdominal ultrasound are recommended in the emergency ward to assess for etiologies that may impact acute management. An abdominal ultrasound is the initial imaging modality of choice and will evaluate the gallbladder and common duct and assess the pancreatic head.

GALLSTONE PANCREATITIS Patients with evidence of ascending cholangitis (rising white blood cell count, increasing liver enzymes) should undergo ERCP within 24–48 h of admission. Patients with gallstone pancreatitis are at increased risk of recurrence, and consideration should be given to performing a cholecystectomy during the same admission or within 4–6 weeks of discharge. An alternative for patients who are not surgical candidates would be to perform an endoscopic biliary sphincterotomy before discharge.

HYPERTRIGLYCERIDEMIA Serum triglycerides >1000 mg/dL are associated with acute pancreatitis. Initial therapy may include insulin, heparin, or plasmapheresis. Outpatient therapies include control of diabetes if present, administration of lipid-lowering agents, weight loss, and avoidance of drugs that elevate lipid levels.

Other potential etiologies that may impact acute hospital care include *hypercalcemia, autoimmune pancreatitis, post-ERCP pancreatitis*, and *drug-induced pancreatitis*. Treatment of hyperparathyroidism or malignancy is effective at reducing serum calcium. Autoimmune pancreatitis is responsive to glucocorticoid administration. Pancreatic duct stenting and rectal indomethacin administration are effective at decreasing pancreatitis after ERCP. Drugs that cause pancreatitis should be discontinued. Multiple drugs have been implicated, but only about 30 have been challenged (Class 1A) and found to be causative.

Nutritional Therapy A low-fat solid diet can be administered to subjects with mild acute pancreatitis after the abdominal pain has resolved. Enteral nutrition should be considered 2–3 days after admission in subjects with more severe pancreatitis instead of total parenteral nutrition (TPN). Enteral feeding maintains gut barrier integrity, limits bacterial translocation, is less expensive, and has fewer complications than TPN. The choice of gastric versus nasojejunal enteral feeding is currently under investigation.

Management of Local Complications (Table 371-4) Patients exhibiting signs of clinical deterioration despite aggressive fluid resuscitation and hemodynamic monitoring should be assessed for local complications, which may include necrosis, pseudocyst formation, pancreas duct disruption, peripancreatic vascular complications, and extrapancreatic infections. A multidisciplinary team approach is recommended including gastroenterology, surgery, interventional radiology, and intensive care specialists, and consideration should also be made for transfer to a pancreas center.

NECROSIS The management of necrosis requires a multidisciplinary team approach. Percutaneous aspiration of necrosis with Gram stain and culture should be performed if there are ongoing signs of possible pancreatic infection such as sustained leukocytosis, fever, or organ failure. There is currently no role for *prophylactic antibiotics* in necrotizing pancreatitis. It is reasonable to start broad-spectrum antibiotics in a patient who appears septic while awaiting the results of Gram stain and cultures. If cultures are negative, the antibiotics should be discontinued to minimize the risk of developing opportunistic or fungal superinfection. Repeated fine-needle aspiration and Gram stain with culture of pancreatic necrosis may be done every 5–7 days in the presence of persistent fever. Repeated CT or MRI imaging should also be considered with any change in clinical course to monitor for complications (e.g., thromboses, hemorrhage, abdominal compartment syndrome).

In general, *sterile necrosis* is most often managed conservatively unless complications arise. Once a diagnosis of *infected necrosis* is established and an organism identified, targeted antibiotics should be instituted. Pancreatic debridement (necrosectomy) should be considered for definitive management of *infected necrosis*, but clinical decisions are generally influenced by response to antibiotic treatment and overall clinical condition. Symptomatic local complications as outlined in the revised Atlanta criteria may require definitive therapy.

TABLE 371-4 COMPLICATIONS OF ACUTE PANCREATITIS

Local
Necrosis
Sterile
Infected
Walled-off necrosis
Pancreatic fluid collections
Pancreatic pseudocyst
Disruption of main pancreatic duct or secondary branches
Pancreatic ascites
Involvement of contiguous organs by necrotizing pancreatitis
Thrombosis of blood vessels (splenic vein, portal vein)
Pancreatic enteric fistula
Bowel infarction
Obstructive jaundice
Systemic
Pulmonary
Pleural effusion
Atelectasis
Mediastinal fluid
Pneumonitis
Acute respiratory distress syndrome
Hypoxemia (unrecognized)
Cardiovascular
Hypotension
Hypovolemia
Nonspecific ST-T changes in electrocardiogram simulating myocardial infarction
Pericardial effusion
Hematologic
Disseminated intravascular coagulation
Gastrointestinal hemorrhage
Peptic ulcer disease
Erosive gastritis
Hemorrhagic pancreatic necrosis with erosion into major blood vessels
Portal vein thrombosis, splenic vein thrombosis, variceal hemorrhage
Renal
Oliguria (<300 mL/d)
Azotemia
Renal artery and/or renal vein thrombosis
Acute tubular necrosis
Metabolic
Hyperglycemia
Hypertriglyceridemia
Hypocalcemia
Encephalopathy
Sudden blindness (Purtscher's retinopathy)
Central nervous system
Psychosis
Fat emboli
Fat necrosis
Subcutaneous tissues (erythematous nodules)
Bone
Miscellaneous (mediastinum, pleura, nervous system)

A step-up approach (percutaneous or endoscopic transgastric drainage followed, if necessary, by open necrosectomy) has been successfully reported by some pancreatic centers. One-third of the patients successfully treated with the step-up approach did not require major abdominal surgery. A recent randomized trial reported advantages to an initial endoscopic approach compared to an initial surgical necrosectomy approach in select patients requiring intervention for symptomatic WON. Taken together, a more conservative approach to the management of infected pancreatic necrosis has evolved over the years under the close supervision of a multidisciplinary team. If conservative therapy can be safely implemented for 4–6 weeks, to allow the pancreatic collections to resolve or "wall-off," surgical or endoscopic intervention is generally much safer and better tolerated by the patient.

PSEUDOCYST The incidence of pseudocyst is low, and most acute collections resolve over time. Less than 10% of patients have persistent fluid collections after 6 weeks that would meet the definition of a pseudocyst. Only symptomatic collections should be drained with surgery or endoscopy or by percutaneous route.

PANCREATIC DUCT DISRUPTION Pancreatic duct disruption may present with symptoms of increasing abdominal pain or shortness of breath in the setting of an enlarging fluid collection. Diagnosis can be confirmed on magnetic resonance cholangiopancreatography (MRCP) or ERCP. Placement of a bridging pancreatic stent for at least 6 weeks is >90% effective at resolving the leak. Nonbridging stents are less effective.

PERIVASCULAR COMPLICATIONS Perivascular complications may include *splenic vein thrombosis* with gastric varices and pseudoaneurysms. *Gastric varices* bleed less than 5% of the time. Life-threatening bleeding from a ruptured *pseudoaneurysm* can be diagnosed and treated with mesenteric angiography and embolization.

EXTRAPANCREATIC INFECTIONS Hospital-acquired infections occur in up to 20% of patients with acute pancreatitis. Patients should be continually monitored for the development pneumonia, urinary tract infection, and line infection. Continued culturing of urine, monitoring of chest x-rays, and routine changing of intravenous lines are important during hospitalization.

Follow-Up Care Hospitalizations for moderately severe and severe acute pancreatitis can last weeks to months and often involve a period of intensive care unit admission and outpatient rehabilitation or subacute nursing care. Follow-up evaluation should assess for development of diabetes, exocrine insufficiency, recurrent cholangitis, or development of infected fluid collections. As mentioned previously, cholecystectomy should be performed within 4–6 weeks of discharge if possible for patients with uncomplicated gallstone pancreatitis.

RECURRENT PANCREATITIS

Approximately 25% of patients who have had an attack of acute pancreatitis have a recurrence. The two most common etiologic factors are alcohol and cholelithiasis. In patients with recurrent pancreatitis without an obvious cause, the differential diagnosis should encompass occult biliary tract disease including microlithiasis, hypertriglyceridemia, drugs, pancreatic cancer, pancreas divisum, and cystic fibrosis (Table 371-1). In one series of 31 patients diagnosed initially as having idiopathic or recurrent acute pancreatitis, 23 were found to have occult gallstone disease. Thus, approximately two-thirds of patients with recurrent acute pancreatitis without an obvious cause actually have occult gallstone disease due to microlithiasis. Genetic defects as in hereditary pancreatitis and cystic fibrosis mutations can result in recurrent pancreatitis. Other diseases of the biliary tree and pancreatic ducts that can cause acute pancreatitis include choledochocele; ampullary tumors; pancreas divisum; and pancreatic duct stones, stricture, and tumor. Approximately 2–4% of patients with pancreatic carcinoma present with acute pancreatitis.

PANCREATITIS IN PATIENTS WITH AIDS

The incidence of acute pancreatitis is increased in patients with AIDS for two reasons: (1) the high incidence of infections involving the pancreas such as infections with cytomegalovirus, *Cryptosporidium*, and the *Mycobacterium avium* complex; and (2) the frequent use by patients with AIDS of medications such as didanosine, pentamidine, trimethoprim-sulfamethoxazole, and protease inhibitors. Incidence has been markedly reduced due to advances in therapy (Chap. 226).

CHRONIC PANCREATITIS AND PANCREATIC EXOCRINE INSUFFICIENCY

PATHOPHYSIOLOGY

Chronic pancreatitis is a disease process characterized by irreversible damage to the pancreas as distinct from the reversible changes noted in acute pancreatitis (Table 371-4). The events that initiate and then perpetuate the inflammatory process in the pancreas are becoming more clearly understood. Irrespective of the mechanism of injury, it is becoming apparent that stellate cell activation that results in cytokine expression and production of extracellular matrix proteins cause acute and chronic inflammation and collagen deposition in the pancreas. Thus, the condition is defined by the presence of histologic abnormalities, including chronic inflammation, fibrosis, and progressive destruction of both exocrine and eventually endocrine tissue (atrophy). A number of etiologies have been associated with chronic pancreatitis resulting in the cardinal manifestations of the disease such as abdominal pain, steatorrhea, weight loss, and diabetes mellitus (Table 371-5).

Although alcohol has been believed to be the primary cause of chronic pancreatitis, other factors contribute to the disease because not all heavy consumers of alcohol develop pancreatic disease. There is also a strong association between smoking and chronic pancreatitis. Cigarette smoke leads to an increased susceptibility to pancreatic autodigestion and predisposes to dysregulation of duct cell CFTR function.

TABLE 371-5 CHRONIC PANCREATITIS AND PANCREATIC EXOCRINE INSUFFICIENCY: TIGAR-O CLASSIFICATION SYSTEM

Toxic-metabolic
- Alcoholic
- Tobacco smoking
- Hypercalcemia
- Hyperlipidemia
- Chronic renal failure
- Medications—phenacetin abuse
- Toxins—organotin compounds (e.g., dibutylin dichloride, DBTC)

Idiopathic
- Early onset
- Late onset
- Tropical

Genetic
- Cationic trypsinogen (*PRSS1*)
- Cystic fibrosis transmembrane conductance regulator gene (*CFTR*)
- Calcium-sensing receptor (*CASR*)
- Chymotrypsin C gene (*CTRC*)
- Pancreatic secretory trypsin inhibitor gene (*SPINK1*)

Autoimmune
- Type 1 autoimmune chronic pancreatitis
- IgG4 systemic
- Type 2 autoimmune chronic pancreatitis

Recurrent and severe acute pancreatitis
- Postnecrotic (severe acute pancreatitis)
- Recurrent acute pancreatitis
- Vascular diseases/ischemia
- Radiation induced

Obstructive
- Pancreas divisum
- Duct obstruction (e.g., tumor)
- Preampullary duodenal wall cysts
- Posttraumatic pancreatic duct scars

Abbreviations: DBTC, dibutylin dichloride; TIGAR-O, toxic-metabolic, idiopathic, genetic, autoimmune, recurrent and severe acute pancreatitis, obstructive.

Smoking is an independent, dose-dependent risk factor for chronic pancreatitis and recurrent acute pancreatitis. Both continued alcohol and smoking exposure are associated with pancreatic fibrosis, calcifications, and progression of disease

Recent characterization of pancreatic stellate cells (PSCs) has added insight into the underlying cellular responses behind development of chronic pancreatitis. Specifically, PSCs are believed to play a role in maintaining normal pancreatic architecture that can shift toward fibrogenesis in the case of chronic pancreatitis. The sentinel acute pancreatitis event (SAPE) hypothesis uniformly describes the events in the pathogenesis of chronic pancreatitis. It is believed that alcohol or additional stimuli lead to matrix metalloproteinase–mediated destruction of normal collagen in pancreatic parenchyma, which later allows for pancreatic remodeling. Proinflammatory cytokines, tumor necrosis factor α (TNF-α), interleukin 1 (IL-1), and interleukin 6 (IL-6), as well as oxidant complexes, are able to induce PSC activity with subsequent new collagen synthesis. In addition to being stimulated by cytokines, oxidants, or growth factors, PSCs also possess transforming growth factor β (TGF-β)–mediated self-activating autocrine pathways that may explain disease progression in chronic pancreatitis even after removal of noxious stimuli.

ETIOLOGIC CONSIDERATIONS

Among adults in the United States, alcoholism is the most common cause of clinically apparent chronic pancreatitis, whereas cystic fibrosis is the most frequent cause in children. As many as 25% of adults in the United States with chronic pancreatitis have the *idiopathic* form. Recent investigations have indicated that up to 15% of patients with idiopathic pancreatitis may have pancreatitis due to genetic defects (Table 371-5).

Whitcomb and associates studied several large families with hereditary chronic pancreatitis and were able to identify a genetic defect that affects the gene encoding for trypsinogen. Several additional defects of this gene have also been described. The defect prevents the destruction of prematurely activated trypsin and allows it to be resistant to the intracellular protective effect of trypsin inhibitor. It is hypothesized that this continual activation of digestive enzymes within the gland leads to acute injury and, finally, chronic pancreatitis. Since the initial discovery of the *PRSS1* mutation defect, other genetic diseases have been detected (Table 371-5).

Several other groups of investigators have documented mutations of *CFTR*. This gene functions as a cyclic AMP–regulated chloride channel. In patients with cystic fibrosis, the high concentration of macromolecules can block the pancreatic ducts. It must be appreciated, however, that there is a great deal of heterogeneity in relationship to the *CFTR* gene defect. More than 1000 putative mutations of the *CFTR* gene have been identified. Attempts to elucidate the relationship between the genotype and pancreatic manifestations have been hampered by the number of mutations. The ability to detect *CFTR* mutations has led to the recognition that the clinical spectrum of the disease is broader than previously thought. Two studies have clarified the association between mutations of the *CFTR* gene and another monosymptomatic form of cystic fibrosis (i.e., chronic pancreatitis). It is estimated that in patients with idiopathic pancreatitis, the frequency of a single *CFTR* mutation is 11 times the expected frequency and the frequency of two mutant alleles is 80 times the expected frequency. In these studies, the patients were adults when the diagnosis of pancreatitis was made; none had any clinical evidence of pulmonary disease, and sweat test results were not diagnostic of cystic fibrosis. The prevalence of such mutations is unclear, and further studies are certainly needed. In addition, the therapeutic and prognostic implication of these findings with respect to managing pancreatitis remains to be determined. Long-term follow-up of affected patients is needed. *CFTR* mutations are common in the general population. It is unclear whether the *CFTR* mutation alone can lead to pancreatitis as an autosomal recessive disease. A study evaluated 39 patients with idiopathic chronic pancreatitis to assess the risk associated with these mutations. Patients with two *CFTR* mutations (compound heterozygotes) demonstrated *CFTR* function at a level between that seen in typical cystic fibrosis and cystic fibrosis carriers and had a 40-fold increased risk of pancreatitis. The presence of an *N34S SPINK1* mutation increased the risk 20-fold. A combination of two *CFTR* mutations and an *N34S SPINK1* mutation increased the risk of pancreatitis 900-fold. Knowledge of the genetic defects and downstream alterations in protein expression has led to the development of novel genetic therapy in cystic fibrosis children that potentiates the CFTR channel resulting in improvement in lung function, quality of life, and weight gain. Table 371-5 lists recognized causes of chronic pancreatitis and pancreatic exocrine insufficiency.

AUTOIMMUNE PANCREATITIS (TABLE 371-6)

Autoimmune pancreatitis (AIP) is an uncommon disorder of presumed autoimmune causation with characteristic laboratory, histologic, and morphologic findings. In type 1 AIP, the pancreas is involved as part of an IgG4 systemic disease (Chap. 391e) and meets HISORt criteria as defined below. The characteristic pancreatic histopathologic findings include lymphoplasmacytic infiltrate, storiform fibrosis, and abundant IgG4 cells. AIP type 2 is histologically confirmed idiopathic duct centric pancreatitis with granulocytic infiltration of the duct wall (termed GEL), but without IgG4 positive cells and systemic involvement. Although AIP was initially described as a primary pancreatic disorder, it is now recognized that it is associated with other disorders of presumed autoimmune etiology, and this has been termed IgG4 systemic disease (Chap. 391e). The clinical features include IgG4-associated cholangitis, rheumatoid arthritis, Sjögren's syndrome, ulcerative colitis, mediastinal fibrosis and adenopathy, autoimmune thyroiditis, tubulointerstitial nephritis, retroperitoneal fibrosis, chronic periaortitis, chronic sclerosing sialadenitis, and Mikulicz's disease. Mild symptoms, usually abdominal pain, and recurrent acute pancreatitis are unusual. Furthermore, AIP is not a common cause of idiopathic recurrent pancreatitis.

Weight loss and new onset of diabetes may also occur. An obstructive pattern on liver tests is common (i.e., disproportionately elevated serum alkaline phosphatase and minimally elevated serum aminotransferases). Elevated serum levels of IgG4 provide a marker for the disease, particularly in Western populations. Serum IgG4 normally accounts for only 5–6% of the total IgG4 in healthy patients but is elevated to values >280 mg/dL in those with AIP. CT scans reveal abnormalities in the majority of patients and include diffuse enlargement, focal enlargement, and a distinct enlargement at the head of the pancreas. ERCP or MRCP reveals strictures in the bile duct in more than one-third of patients with AIP; these may include common bile duct strictures, intrahepatic bile duct strictures, or proximal bile duct strictures, with accompanying narrowing of the pancreatic portion of the bile duct. This has been termed autoimmune IgG4 cholangitis. Characteristic histologic findings include extensive lymphoplasmacytic infiltrates with dense fibrosis around pancreatic ducts, as well as a lymphoplasmacytic infiltration, resulting in an obliterative phlebitis.

The Mayo Clinic HISORt criteria indicate that AIP can be diagnosed by the presence of at least two of the following: (1) *h*istology; (2) *i*maging; (3) *s*erology (elevated serum IgG4 levels); (4) *o*ther organ involvement; and (5) *r*esponse to glucocorticoid *t*herapy, with improvement in pancreatic and extrapancreatic manifestations.

Glucocorticoids have shown efficacy in alleviating symptoms, decreasing the size of the pancreas, and reversing histopathologic features in patients with AIP. Patients may respond dramatically to glucocorticoid therapy within a 2- to 4-week period. Prednisone is usually administered at an initial dose of 40 mg/d for 4 weeks followed by a taper of the daily dosage by 5 mg/wk based on monitoring of clinical parameters. Relief of symptoms, serial changes in abdominal imaging of the pancreas and bile ducts, decreased serum γ-globulin and IgG4 levels, and improvements in liver tests are parameters to follow. A poor response to glucocorticoids over a 2- to 4-week period should raise suspicion of pancreatic cancer or other forms of chronic pancreatitis. A recent multicenter international report reviewed 1064 patients with AIP. Clinical remission was achieved in 99% of type I and 92% of type II AIP patients with steroids. However, disease relapse occurred in 31% of type I and 9% of type II AIP patients. For treatment of disease relapse in type 1 AIP, glucocorticoids were successful in 201 of 295 (68%) patients, and azathioprine was successful in 52 of 58 patients (85%). A small number of patients responded favorably to 6-mercaptapurine, rituximab, cyclosporine, and cyclophosphamide. Types 1 and 2 AIP are highly responsive to initial glucocorticoid treatment. Relapse is common in type 1 patients, especially those with biliary tract strictures. Most relapses occur after glucocorticoids are discontinued. Patients with refractory symptoms and strictures generally require immunomodulator therapy as noted above. Appearance of interval cancers following a diagnosis of AIP is uncommon.

TABLE 371-6 CLINICAL FEATURES OF AUTOIMMUNE PANCREATITIS (AIP)

- Mild symptoms, usually abdominal pain, but without frequent attacks of acute pancreatitis
- Diffuse swelling and enlargement of the pancreas
- Two-thirds of patients present with either obstructive jaundice or a "mass" in the head of the pancreas mimicking carcinoma
- Diffuse irregular narrowing of the pancreatic duct (MRCP or ERCP)
- Increased levels of serum gamma globulins, especially IgG4
- Presence of other autoantibodies (ANA), rheumatoid factor (RF)
- Can occur with other autoimmune diseases: Sjögren's syndrome, primary sclerosing cholangitis, ulcerative colitis, rheumatoid arthritis
- Extrapancreatic bile duct changes such as stricture of the common bile duct and intrahepatic ducts
- Pancreatic calcifications (rare)
- Pancreatic biopsies reveal extensive fibrosis and lymphoplasmacytic infiltration
- Glucocorticoids are effective in alleviating symptoms, decreasing size of the pancreas, and reversing histopathologic changes

Abbreviations: ERCP, endoscopic retrograde cholangiopancreatography; MRCP, magnetic resonance cholangiopancreatography.

Clinical Features of Chronic Pancreatitis Patients with chronic pancreatitis seek medical attention predominantly because of two symptoms: abdominal pain or maldigestion and weight loss. The abdominal pain may be quite variable in location, severity, and frequency. The pain can be constant or intermittent with frequent pain-free intervals. Eating may exacerbate the pain, leading to a fear of eating with consequent weight loss. The spectrum of abdominal pain ranges from mild to quite severe, with narcotic dependence as a frequent consequence. Maldigestion is manifested as chronic diarrhea, steatorrhea, weight loss, and fatigue. Patients with chronic abdominal pain may or may not progress to maldigestion, and ~20% of patients will present with symptoms of maldigestion without a history of abdominal pain. Patients with chronic pancreatitis have significant morbidity and mortality and use appreciable amounts of societal resources. Despite steatorrhea, clinically apparent deficiencies of fat-soluble vitamins are surprisingly uncommon. Physical findings in these patients are usually unimpressive, so that there is a disparity between the severity of abdominal pain and the physical signs that usually consist of some mild tenderness.

The diagnosis of early or mild chronic pancreatitis can be challenging because there is no biomarker for the disease. In contrast to acute pancreatitis, the serum amylase and lipase levels are usually not strikingly elevated in chronic pancreatitis. Elevation of serum bilirubin and alkaline phosphatase may indicate cholestasis secondary to common bile duct stricture caused by chronic inflammation. Many patients have impaired glucose tolerance with elevated fasting blood glucose levels. The fecal elastase-1 and small-bowel biopsy are useful in the evaluation of patients with suspected pancreatic steatorrhea. The fecal elastase level will be abnormal and small-bowel histology will be normal in such patients. A decrease of fecal elastase level to <100 μg per gram of stool strongly suggests severe pancreatic exocrine insufficiency.

The radiographic evaluation of a patient with suspected chronic pancreatitis usually proceeds from a noninvasive to more invasive approach. Abdominal CT imaging (Fig. 371-4A,B) is the initial modality of choice, followed by MRI (Fig. 371-4C), endoscopic ultrasound, and pancreas function testing. In addition to excluding a

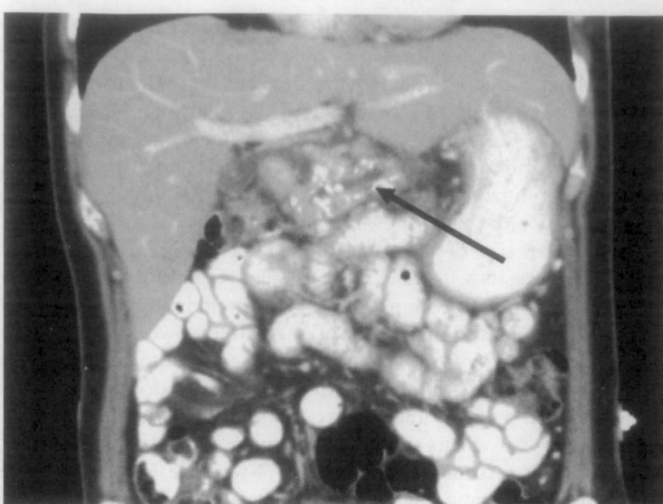

A

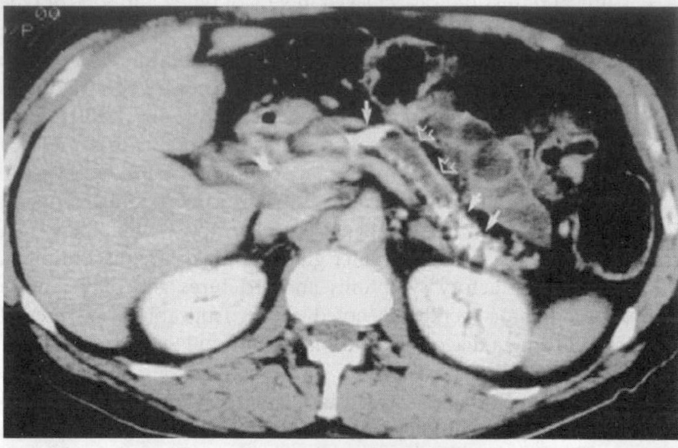

B

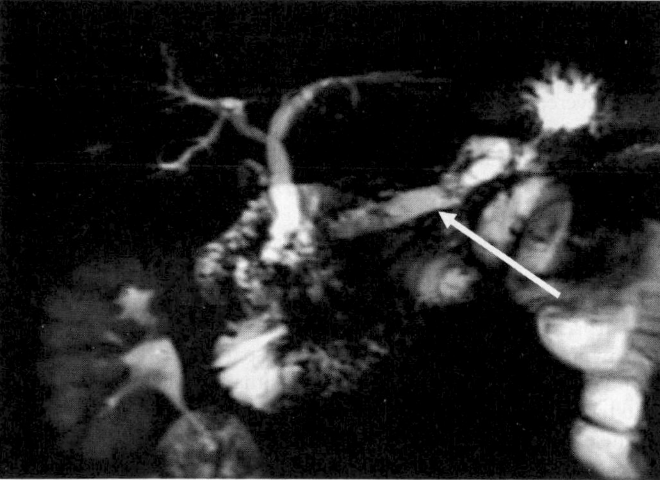

C

FIGURE 371-4 ***A.*** Chronic pancreatitis and pancreatic calculi: computed tomography (CT) scan. In this contrast-enhanced CT scan of the abdomen, there is evidence of an atrophic pancreas with multiple calcifications and stones in the parenchyma and dilated pancreatic duct (*arrow*). ***B.*** In this contrast-enhanced CT scan of the abdomen, there is evidence of an atrophic pancreas with multiple calcifications (*arrows*). Note the markedly dilated pancreatic duct seen in this section through the body and tail (*open arrows*). ***C.*** Chronic pancreatitis on magnetic resonance cholangiopancreatography (MRCP): dilated duct with filling defects. Gadolinium-enhanced magnetic resonance imaging/MRCP reveals a dilated pancreatic duct (*arrow*) in chronic pancreatitis with multiple filling defects suggestive of pancreatic duct calculi. *(A, C, courtesy of Dr. KJ Mortele, Brigham and Women's Hospital; with permission.)*

pseudocyst and pancreatic cancer, CT may show calcification, dilated ducts, or an atrophic pancreas. Although abdominal CT scanning and MRCP greatly aid in the diagnosis of pancreatic disease, the diagnostic test with the best sensitivity and specificity is the hormone stimulation test using secretin. The secretin test becomes abnormal when ≥60% of the pancreatic exocrine function has been lost. This usually correlates well with the onset of chronic abdominal pain. The role of endoscopic ultrasonography (EUS) in diagnosing early chronic pancreatitis is still being defined. A total of nine endosonographic features have been described in chronic pancreatitis. The presence of five or more features is considered diagnostic of chronic pancreatitis. EUS is not a sensitive enough test for detecting early chronic pancreatitis alone (Chap. 370) and may show positive features in patients who have dyspepsia or even normal aging individuals. Recent data suggest that EUS can be combined with endoscopic pancreatic function testing (EUS-ePFT) during a single endoscopy to screen for chronic pancreatitis in patients with chronic abdominal pain. Diffuse calcifications noted on plain film of the abdomen usually indicate significant damage to the pancreas and are pathognomic for chronic pancreatitis (Fig. 371-4*A*). Although alcohol is by far the most common cause of pancreatic calcification, such calcification may also be noted in hereditary pancreatitis, posttraumatic pancreatitis, hypercalcemic pancreatitis, idiopathic chronic pancreatitis, and tropical pancreatitis.

Complications of Chronic Pancreatitis The complications of chronic pancreatitis are protean and are listed in Table 371-7. Although most patients have impaired glucose tolerance, diabetic ketoacidosis and diabetic coma are uncommon. Likewise, end-organ damage (retinopathy, neuropathy, nephropathy) is also uncommon. A nondiabetic retinopathy may be due to either vitamin A and/or zinc deficiency. Gastrointestinal bleeding may occur from peptic ulceration, gastritis, a pseudocyst eroding into the duodenum, arterial bleeding into the pancreatic duct (hemosuccus pancreaticus), or ruptured varices secondary to splenic vein thrombosis due to chronic inflammation of the tail of the pancreas. Jaundice, cholestasis, and biliary cirrhosis may occur from the chronic inflammatory reaction around the intrapancreatic portion of the common bile duct. Twenty years after the diagnosis of calcific chronic pancreatitis, the cumulative risk of pancreatic carcinoma is 4%. Patients with hereditary pancreatitis are at a 10-fold higher risk for pancreatic cancer.

TREATMENT CHRONIC PANCREATITIS

STEATORRHEA

The treatment of steatorrhea with pancreatic enzymes is straightforward even though complete correction of steatorrhea is unusual. Enzyme therapy usually brings diarrhea under control and restores absorption of fat to an acceptable level and affects weight gain. Thus, pancreatic enzyme replacement has been the cornerstone of therapy. In treating steatorrhea, it is important to use a potent pancreatic formulation that will deliver sufficient lipase into the duodenum to correct maldigestion and decrease steatorrhea. In an attempt to standardize the enzyme activity, potency, and bioavailability, the U.S. Food and Drug Administration (FDA) required that all pancreas enzyme drugs in the United States obtain a New Drug Application (NDA) by April 2008. Table 371-8 lists frequently used formulations, but availability will be based on compliance with the FDA mandate. Recent data suggest that dosages up to

TABLE 371-7 COMPLICATIONS OF CHRONIC PANCREATITIS

Chronic abdominal pain	Jaundice
Narcotic addiction	Retinopathy
Diabetes mellitus/impaired glucose tolerance	Biliary stricture and/or biliary cirrhosis
Gastroparesis	Pseudocyst
Malabsorption/maldigestion	Metabolic bone disease
	Pancreatic cancer

TABLE 371-8 FDA-APPROVED PANCREATIC ENZYME (PANCRELIPASE) PREPARATIONS

	Enzyme Content/Unit Dose, U.S. Pharmacopeia Units		
Product	Lipase[a]	Amylase[a]	Protease[a]
Immediate-Release Capsule			
Non-enteric-coated			
Viokace 10,440	10,440	391,550	39,150
Viokace 20,880	20,880	78,300	78,300
Delayed-Release Capsules			
Enteric-coated mini-microspheres			
Creon 3000	3000	15,000	9500
Creon 6000	6000	30,000	19,000
Creon 12,000	12,000	60,000	38,000
Creon 24,000	24,000	120,000	76,000
Enteric-Coated Mini-Tablets			
Ultresa 13,800	13,800	27,600	27,600
Ultresa 20,700	20,700	41,400	41,400
Ultresa 23,000	23,000	46,000	46,000
Enteric-Coated Beads			
Zenpep 3000	3000	16,000	10,000
Zenpep 5000	5000	27,000	17,000
Zenpep 10,000	10,000	55,000	34,000
Zenpep 15,000	15,000	82,000	51,000
Zenpep 20,000	20,000	109,000	68,000
Zenpep 25,000	25,000	136,000	83,000
Enteric-Coated Micro-Tablets			
Pancreaze 4200	4200	17,500	10,000
Pancreaze 10,500	10,500	43,750	25,000
Pancreaze 16,800	16,800	70,000	40,000
Pancreaze 21,000	21,000	61,000	37,000
Bicarbonate-Buffered Enteric-Coated Microspheres			
Pertzye 8000	8000	30,250	28,750
Pertzye 16,000	16,000	60,500	57,500

[a]U.S. Pharmacopeia (USP) units per tablet or capsule

Note: The FDA has mandated all enzyme manufacturers to submit New Drug Applications (NDAs) for all pancreatic extract drug products after reviewing data that showed substantial variations among currently marketed products. Numerous manufacturers have investigations under way to seek FDA approval for the treatment of exocrine pancreatic insufficiency due to cystic fibrosis or other conditions under the new guidelines for this class of drugs (*www.fda.gov*).

80,000–100,000 units of lipase taken during the meal may be necessary to normalize nutritional parameters in malnourished chronic pancreatitis patients, and some may require acid suppression with proton pump inhibitors.

ABDOMINAL PAIN

The management of pain in patients with chronic pancreatitis is problematic.

Recent meta-analyses have shown no consistent benefit of *enzyme therapy* at reducing pain in chronic pancreatitis. In some patients with idiopathic chronic pancreatitis, conventional non-enteric-coated enzyme preparations containing high concentrations of serine proteases may relieve mild abdominal pain or discomfort. The pain relief experienced by these patients actually may be due to improvements in the dyspepsia from maldigestion.

Gastroparesis is also quite common in patients with chronic pancreatitis. It is important to recognize and treat with prokinetic drugs because treatment with enzymes may fail simply because gastric dysmotility is interfering with the delivery of enzymes into the upper intestine. A recent prospective study reported that pregabalin can improve pain in chronic pancreatitis and lower pain medication requirement.

Endoscopic treatment of chronic pancreatitis pain may involve sphincterotomy, stenting, stone extraction, and drainage of a pancreatic pseudocyst. Therapy directed to the pancreatic duct would seem to be most appropriate in the setting of a dominant stricture, especially if a ductal stone has led to obstruction. The use of endoscopic stenting for patients with chronic pain, but without a dominant stricture, has not been subjected to any controlled trials. It is now appreciated that significant complications can occur from stenting (i.e., bleeding, cholangitis, stent migration, pancreatitis, and stent clogging). In patients with large-duct disease usually from alcohol-induced chronic pancreatitis, ductal decompression with *surgical therapy* has been the therapy of choice. Among such patients, 80% seem to obtain immediate relief; however, at the end of 3 years, one-half of the patients have recurrence of pain. Two randomized prospective trials comparing endoscopic to surgical therapy for chronic pancreatitis demonstrated that surgical therapy was superior to endoscopy at decreasing pain and improving quality of life in selected patients with dilated ducts and abdominal pain. This would suggest that chronic pancreatitis patients with dilated ducts and pain should be considered for surgical intervention. The role of preoperative stenting prior to surgery as a predictor of response has yet to be proven.

A Whipple procedure, total pancreatectomy, and autologous islet cell transplantation have been used in selected patients with chronic pancreatitis and abdominal pain refractory to conventional therapy. The patients who have benefited the most from total pancreatectomy have chronic pancreatitis without prior pancreatic surgery or evidence of islet cell insufficiency. The role of this procedure remains to be fully defined but may be an option in lieu of ductal decompression surgery or pancreatic resection in patients with intractable, painful small-duct disease, particularly as the standard surgical procedures tend to decrease islet cell yield. Celiac plexus block has not resulted in long-lasting pain relief.

HEREDITARY PANCREATITIS

Hereditary pancreatitis is a rare disease that is similar to chronic pancreatitis except for an early age of onset and evidence of hereditary factors. A genomewide search using genetic linkage analysis identified the hereditary pancreatitis gene on chromosome 7. Mutations in ion codons 29 (exon 2) and 122 (exon 3) of the cationic trypsinogen gene cause autosomal dominant forms of hereditary pancreatitis. The codon 122 mutations lead to a substitution of the corresponding arginine with another amino acid, usually histidine. This substitution, when it occurs, eliminates a fail-safe trypsin self-destruction site necessary to eliminate trypsin that is prematurely activated within the acinar cell. These patients have recurring attacks of severe abdominal pain that may last from a few days to a few weeks. The serum amylase and lipase levels may be elevated during acute attacks but are usually normal. Patients frequently develop pancreatic calcification, diabetes mellitus, and steatorrhea; in addition, they have an increased incidence of pancreatic carcinoma, with the cumulative incidence being as high as 40% by age 70 years. A recent natural history study of hereditary pancreatitis in more than 200 patients from France reported that abdominal pain started in childhood at age 10 years, steatorrhea developed at age 29 years, diabetes at age 38 years, and pancreatic carcinoma at age 55 years. Such patients often require surgical ductal decompression for pain relief. Abdominal complaints in relatives of patients with hereditary pancreatitis should raise the question of pancreatic disease.

PSTI, or SPINK1, is a 56-amino-acid peptide that specifically inhibits trypsin by physically blocking its active site. SPINK1 acts as the first line of defense against prematurely activated trypsinogen in the acinar cell. Recently, it has been shown that the frequency of SPINK1 mutations in patients with idiopathic chronic pancreatitis is markedly increased, suggesting that these mutations may be associated with pancreatitis.

PANCREATIC ENDOCRINE TUMORS

Pancreatic endocrine tumors are discussed in Chap. 113.

ANNULAR PANCREAS

When the ventral pancreatic anlage fails to migrate correctly to make contact with the dorsal anlage, the result may be a ring of pancreatic tissue encircling the duodenum. Such an annular pancreas may cause intestinal obstruction in the neonate or the adult. Symptoms of postprandial fullness, epigastric pain, nausea, and vomiting may be present for years before the diagnosis is entertained. The radiographic findings are symmetric dilation of the proximal duodenum with bulging of the recesses on either side of the annular band, effacement but not destruction of the duodenal mucosa, accentuation of the findings in the right anterior oblique position, and lack of change on repeated examinations. The differential diagnosis should include duodenal webs, tumors of the pancreas or duodenum, postbulbar peptic ulcer, regional enteritis, and adhesions. Patients with annular pancreas have an increased incidence of pancreatitis and peptic ulcer. Because of these and other potential complications, the treatment is surgical even if the condition has been present for years. Retrocolic duodenojejeunostomy is the procedure of choice, although some surgeons advocate Billroth II gastrectomy, gastroenterostomy, and vagotomy.

PANCREAS DIVISUM

Pancreas divisum is present in 7–10% of the population and occurs when the embryologic ventral and dorsal pancreatic anlagen fail to fuse, so that pancreatic drainage is accomplished mainly through the accessory papilla. Pancreas divisum is the most common congenital anatomic variant of the human pancreas. Current evidence indicates that this anomaly does not predispose to the development of pancreatitis in the great majority of patients who harbor it. However, the combination of pancreas divisum and a small accessory orifice could result in dorsal duct obstruction. The challenge is to identify this subset of patients with dorsal duct pathology. Cannulation of the dorsal duct by ERCP is not as easily done as is cannulation of the ventral duct. Patients with pancreatitis and pancreas divisum demonstrated by MRCP or ERCP should be treated with conservative measures. In many of these patients, pancreatitis is idiopathic and unrelated to the pancreas divisum. Endoscopic or surgical intervention is indicated only if pancreatitis recurs and no other cause can be found. If marked dilation of the dorsal duct can be demonstrated, surgical ductal decompression should be performed. It should be stressed that the ERCP/MRCP appearance of pancreas divisum (i.e., a small-caliber ventral duct with an arborizing pattern) may be mistaken as representing an obstructed main pancreatic duct secondary to a mass lesion.

MACROAMYLASEMIA

In macroamylasemia, amylase circulates in the blood in a polymer form too large to be easily excreted by the kidney. Patients with this condition demonstrate an elevated serum amylase value and a low urinary amylase value. The presence of macroamylase can be documented by chromatography of the serum. The prevalence of macroamylasemia is 1.5% of the nonalcoholic general adult hospital population. Usually macroamylasemia is an incidental finding and is not related to disease of the pancreas or other organs. Macrolipasemia has now been documented in a few patients with cirrhosis or non-Hodgkin's lymphoma. In these patients, the pancreas appeared normal on ultrasound and CT examination. Lipase was shown to be complexed with immunoglobulin A. Thus, the possibility of *both* macroamylasemia and macrolipasemia should be considered in patients with elevated blood levels of these enzymes.

ACKNOWLEDGMENTS

This chapter represents a revised version of chapters by Drs. Norton J. Greenberger, Phillip P. Toskes, and Bechien Wu that were in previous editions of Harrison's.

SECTION 1 THE IMMUNE SYSTEM IN HEALTH AND DISEASE

372e Introduction to the Immune System

Barton F. Haynes, Kelly A. Soderberg, Anthony S. Fauci

This is a digital-only chapter. It is available on the DVD that accompanies this book, as well as on Access Medicine/Harrison's Online, and the eBook and "app" editions of HPIM 19e.

DEFINITIONS

- *Adaptive immune system*—recently evolved system of immune responses mediated by T and B lymphocytes. Immune responses by these cells are based on specific antigen recognition by clonotypic receptors that are products of genes that rearrange during development and throughout the life of the organism. Additional cells of the adaptive immune system include various types of antigen-presenting cells.
- *Antibody*—B cell–produced molecules encoded by genes that rearrange during B cell development consisting of immunoglobulin heavy and light chains that together form the central component of the B cell receptor for antigen. Antibody can exist as B cell–surface antigen-recognition molecules or as secreted molecules in plasma and other body fluids.

373e The Major Histocompatibility Complex

Gerald T. Nepom

This is a digital-only chapter. It is available on the DVD that accompanies this book, as well as on Access Medicine/Harrison's Online, and the eBook and "app" editions of HPIM 19e.

THE HLA COMPLEX AND ITS PRODUCTS

The human major histocompatibility complex (MHC), commonly called the human leukocyte antigen (HLA) complex, is a 4-megabase (Mb) region on chromosome 6 (6p21.3) that is densely packed with expressed genes. The best known of these genes are the HLA class I and class II genes, whose products are critical for immunologic specificity and transplantation histocompatibility, and they play a major role in susceptibility to a number of autoimmune diseases. Many other genes in the HLA region are also essential to the innate and antigen-specific functioning of the immune system. The HLA region shows extensive conservation with the MHC of other mammals in terms of genomic organization, gene sequence, and protein structure and function.

374 Primary Immune Deficiency Diseases

Alain Fischer

Immunity is intrinsic to life and an important tool in the fight for survival against pathogenic microorganisms. The human immune system can be divided into two major components: the innate immune system and the adaptive immune system (Chap. 372e). The innate immune system provides the rapid triggering of inflammatory responses based on the recognition (at the cell surface or within cells) of either molecules expressed by microorganisms or molecules that serve as "danger signals" released by cells under attack. These receptor/ligand interactions trigger signaling events that ultimately lead to inflammation. Virtually all cell lineages (not just immune cells) are involved in innate immune responses; however, myeloid cells (i.e., neutrophils and macrophages) play a major role because of their phagocytic capacity. The adaptive immune system operates by clonal recognition of antigens followed by a dramatic expansion of antigen-reactive cells and execution of an immune effector program. Most of the effector cells die off rapidly, whereas memory cells persist. Although both T and B lymphocytes recognize distinct chemical moieties and execute distinct adaptive immune responses, the latter is largely dependent on the former in generating long-lived humoral immunity. Adaptive responses utilize components of the innate immune system; for example, the antigen-presentation capabilities of dendritic cells help to determine the type of effector response. Not surprisingly, immune responses are controlled by a series of regulatory mechanisms.

Hundreds of gene products have been characterized as effectors or mediators of the immune system (Chap. 372e). Whenever the expression or function of one of these products is genetically impaired (provided the function is nonredundant), a primary immunodeficiency (PID) occurs.

PIDs are genetic diseases with primarily Mendelian inheritance. More than 250 conditions have now been described, and deleterious mutations in approximately 210 genes have been identified. The overall prevalence of PIDs has been estimated in various countries at 5 per 100,000 individuals; however, given the difficulty in diagnosing these rare and complex diseases, this figure is probably an underestimate. PIDs can involve all possible aspects of immune responses, from innate through adaptive, cell differentiation, and effector function and regulation. For the sake of clarity, PIDs should be classified according to (1) the arm of the immune system that is defective and (2) the mechanism of the defect (when known). Table 374-1 classifies the most prevalent PIDs according to this manner of classification; however, one should bear in mind that the classification of PIDs sometimes involves arbitrary decisions because of overlap and, in some cases, lack of data.

The consequences of PIDs vary widely as a function of the molecules that are defective. This concept translates into multiple levels of vulnerability to infection by pathogenic and opportunistic microorganisms, ranging from extremely broad (as in severe combined immunodeficiency [SCID]) to narrowly restricted to a single microorganism (as in Mendelian susceptibility to mycobacterial disease [MSMD]). The locations of the sites of infection and the causal microorganisms involved will thus help physicians arrive at proper diagnoses. PIDs can also lead to immunopathologic responses such as allergy (as in Wiskott-Aldrich syndrome), lymphoproliferation, and autoimmunity. A combination

TABLE 374-1 CLASSIFICATION OF PRIMARY IMMUNE DEFICIENCY DISEASES

Deficiencies of the Innate Immune System	
• Phagocytic cells:	
- Impaired production: severe congenital neutropenia (SCN)	
- Asplenia	
- Impaired adhesion: leukocyte adhesion deficiency (LAD)	
- Impaired killing: chronic granulomatous disease (CGD)	
• Innate immunity receptors and signal transduction:	
- Defects in Toll-like receptor signaling	
- Mendelian susceptibility to mycobacterial disease	
• Complement deficiencies:	
- Classical, alternative, and lectin pathways	
- Lytic phase	
Deficiencies of the Adaptive Immune System	
• T lymphocytes:	
- Impaired development	Severe combined immune deficiencies (SCIDs)
	DiGeorge syndrome
- Impaired survival, migration, function	Combined immunodeficiencies
	Hyper-IgE syndrome (autosomal dominant)
	DOCK8 deficiency
	CD40 ligand deficiency
	Wiskott-Aldrich syndrome
	Ataxia-telangiectasia and other DNA repair deficiencies
• B lymphocytes:	
- Impaired development	XL and AR agammaglobulinemia
- Impaired function	Hyper-IgM syndrome
	Common variable immunodeficiency (CVID)
	IgA deficiency
Regulatory Defects	
• Innate immunity	Autoinflammatory syndromes (outside the scope of this chapter)
	Severe colitis
• Adaptive immunity	Hemophagocytic lymphohistiocytosis (HLH)
	Autoimmune lymphoproliferation syndrome (ALPS)
	Autoimmunity and inflammatory diseases (IPEX, APECED)

Abbreviations: APECED, autoimmune polyendocrinopathy candidiasis ectodermal dysplasia; AR, autosomal recessive; IPEX, immunodysregulation polyendocrinopathy enteropathy X-linked syndrome; XL, X-linked.

of recurrent infections, inflammation, and autoimmunity can be observed in a number of PIDs, thus creating obvious therapeutic challenges. Finally, some PIDs increase the risk of cancer, notably but not exclusively lymphocytic cancers, e.g., lymphoma.

DIAGNOSIS OF PRIMARY IMMUNODEFICIENCIES

The most frequent symptom prompting the diagnosis of a PID is the presence of recurrent or unusually severe infections. As mentioned above, recurrent allergic or autoimmune manifestations may also alert the physician to a possible diagnosis of PID. In such cases, a detailed account of the subject's personal and family medical history should be obtained. It is of the utmost importance to gather as much medical information as possible on relatives and up to several generations of ancestors. In addition to the obvious focus on primary symptoms, the clinical examination should evaluate the size of lymphoid organs and, when appropriate, look for the characteristic signs of a number of complex syndromes that may be associated with a PID.

The performance of laboratory tests should be guided to some extent by the clinical findings. Infections of the respiratory tract (bronchi, sinuses) mostly suggest a defective antibody response. In general, invasive bacterial infections can result from complement deficiencies, signaling defects of innate immune responses, asplenia, or defective antibody responses. Viral infections, recurrent *Candida* infections, and opportunistic infections are generally suggestive of impaired T cell immunity. Skin infections and deep-seated abscesses primarily reflect innate immune defects (such as chronic granulomatous disease); however, they may also appear in the autosomal dominant hyper-IgE syndrome. Table 374-2 summarizes the laboratory tests that are most frequently used to diagnose a PID. More specific tests (notably genetic tests) are then used to make a definitive diagnosis.

The PIDs discussed below have been grouped together according to the affected cells and the mechanisms involved (Table 374-1, Fig. 374-1).

PRIMARY IMMUNODEFICIENCIES OF THE INNATE IMMUNE SYSTEM

PIDs of the innate immune system are relatively rare and account for approximately 10% of all PIDs.

SEVERE CONGENITAL NEUTROPENIA

Severe congenital neutropenia (SCN) consists of a group of inherited diseases that are characterized by severely impaired neutrophil counts (<500 polymorphonuclear leukocytes [PMN]/μL of blood). The condition is usually manifested from birth. SCN may also be cyclic (with a 3-week periodicity), and other neutropenia syndromes can also be intermittent. Although the most frequent inheritance pattern for SCN is autosomal dominant, autosomal recessive and X-linked recessive conditions also exist. Bacterial infections at the interface between the body and the external milieu (e.g., the orifices, wounds, and the respiratory tract) are common manifestations. Bacterial infections can rapidly progress through soft tissue and are followed by dissemination in the bloodstream. Severe visceral fungal infections can also ensue. The absence of pus is a hallmark of this condition.

Diagnosis of SCN requires examination of the bone marrow. Most SCNs are associated with a block in granulopoiesis at the promyelocytic stage (Fig. 374-1). SCN has multiple etiologies, and to date, mutations in 11 different genes have been identified. Most of these mutations result in isolated SCN, whereas others are syndromic (Chap. 80). The most frequent forms of SCN are caused by the premature cell death of granulocyte precursors, as observed in deficiencies of GFI1, HAX1, and elastase 2 (*ELANE*), with the latter accounting for 50% of SCN sufferers. Certain *ELANE* mutations cause cyclic neutropenia syndrome. A gain-of-function mutation in the *WASP* gene (see the section on "Wiskott-Aldrich syndrome" below) causes X-linked SCN, which is also associated with monocytopenia.

As mentioned above, SCN exposes the patient to life-threatening, disseminated bacterial and fungal infections. Treatment requires careful hygiene measures, notably in infants. Later in life, special oral and dental care is essential, along with the prevention of bacterial infection by prophylactic administration of trimethoprim/sulfamethoxazole. Subcutaneous injection of the cytokine granulocyte colony-stimulating factor (G-CSF) usually improves neutrophil development and thus prevents infection in most SCN diseases. However, there are two caveats: (1) a few cases of SCN with *ELANE* mutation are refractory to G-CSF and may require curative treatment via allogeneic hematopoietic stem cell transplantation (HSCT); and (2) a subset of G-CSF-treated patients carrying *ELANE* mutations are at a greater risk of developing acute myelogenous leukemia associated (in most cases) with somatic gain-of-function mutations of the G-CSF receptor gene.

ASPLENIA

Primary failure of the development of a spleen is an extremely rare disease that can be either syndromic (in Ivemark syndrome) or isolated with an autosomal dominant expression; in the latter case, mutations in the ribosomal protein SA gene were recently found. Due to the

TABLE 374-2 TESTS MOST FREQUENTLY USED TO DIAGNOSE A PRIMARY IMMUNE DEFICIENCY (PID)

Test	Information	PID Disease
• Blood cell counts and cell morphology	Neutrophil counts[a]	↓ Severe congenital neutropenia, ↑↑ LAD
	Lymphocyte counts[a]	T cell ID
	Eosinophilia	WAS, hyper-IgE syndrome
	Howell-Jolly bodies	Asplenia
• Chest x-ray	Thymic shadow	SCID, DiGeorge syndrome
	Costochondral junctions	Adenosine deaminase deficiency
• Bone x-ray	Metaphyseal ends	Cartilage hair hypoplasia
• Immunoglobulin serum levels	IgG, IgA, IgM	B cell ID
	IgE	Hyper-IgE syndrome, WAS, T cell ID
• Lymphocyte phenotype	T, B lymphocyte counts	T cell ID, agammaglobulinemia
• Dihydrorhodamine fluorescence (DHR) assay Nitroblue tetrazolium (NBT) assay	Reactive oxygen species production by PMNs	Chronic granulomatous disease
• CH50, AP50	Classic and alternative complement pathways	Complement deficiencies
• Ultrasonography of the abdomen	Spleen size	Asplenia

[a]Normal counts vary with age. For example, the lymphocyte count is between 3000 and 9000/μL of blood below the age of 3 months and between 1500 and 2500/μL in adults.

Abbreviations: ID, immunodeficiency; LAD, leukocyte adhesion deficiency; PMNs, polymorphonuclear leukocytes; SCID, severe combined immunodeficiency; WAS, Wiskott-Aldrich syndrome.

absence of natural filtration of microbes in the blood, asplenia predisposes affected individuals to fulminant infections by encapsulated bacteria. Although most infections occur in the first years of life, cases may also arise in adulthood. The diagnosis is confirmed by abdominal ultrasonography and the detection of Howell-Jolly bodies in red blood cells. Effective prophylactic measures (twice-daily oral penicillin and appropriate vaccination programs) usually prevent fatal outcomes.

GATA2 DEFICIENCY

Recently an immunodeficiency combining monocytopenia and dendritic and lymphoid (B and natural killer [NK]) cell deficiency (DCML), also called monocytopenia with nontuberculous mycobacterial infections (mono-MAC), has been described as a consequence of a dominant mutation in the gene *GATA2*, a transcription factor involved in hematopoiesis. This condition also predisposes to lymphedema,

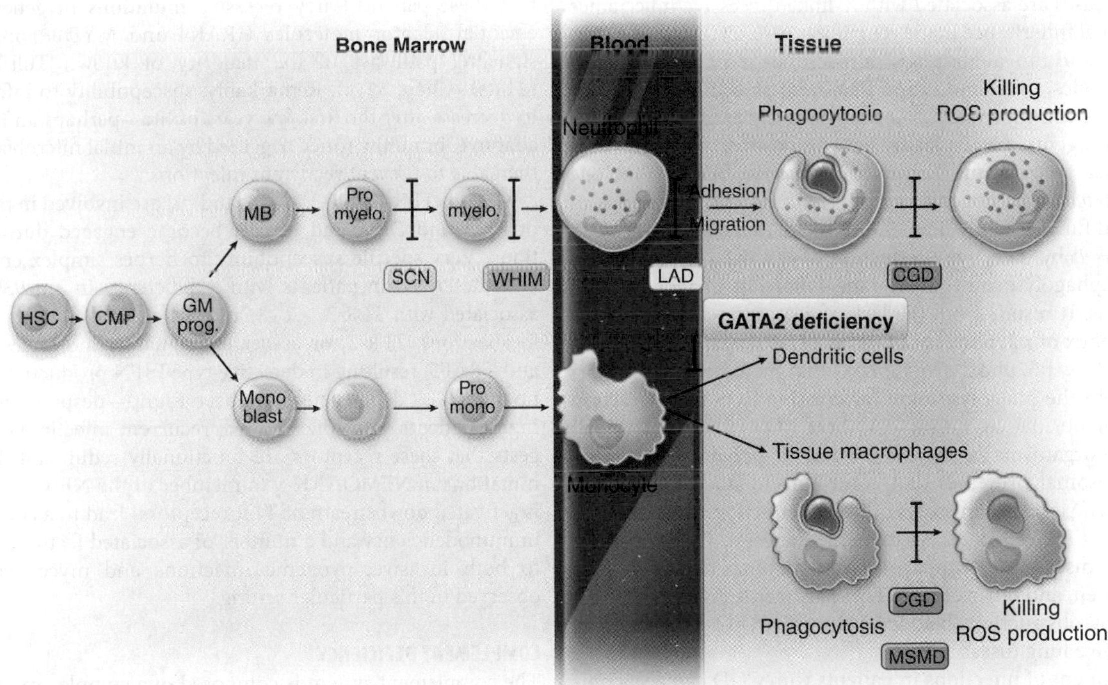

FIGURE 374-1 Differentiation of phagocytic cells and related primary immunodeficiencies (PIDs). Hematopoietic stem cells (HSCs) differentiate into common myeloid progenitors (CMPs) and then granulocyte-monocyte progenitors (GM-prog.), which, in turn, differentiate into neutrophils (MB: myeloblasts; Promyelo: promyelocytes; myelo: myelocytes) or monocytes (monoblasts and promonocytes). Upon activation, neutrophils adhere to the vascular endothelium, transmigrate, and phagocytose the targets. Reactive oxygen species (ROS) are delivered to the microorganism-containing phagosomes. Macrophages in tissues kill using the same mechanism. Following activation by interferon γ (not shown here), macrophages can be armed to kill intracellular pathogens such as mycobacteria. For sake of simplicity, not all cell differentiation stages are shown. The abbreviations for PIDs are contained in boxes placed at corresponding stages of the pathway. CGD, chronic granulomatous diseases; GATA2, zinc finger transcription factor; LAD, leukocyte adhesion deficiencies; MSMD, Mendelian susceptibility to mycobacterial disease; SCN, severe congenital neutropenia; WHIM, warts, hypogammaglobulinemia, infections, and myelokathexis.

myelodysplasia, and acute myeloid leukemia. Infections (bacterial and viral) are life-threatening, thus indicating, together with the malignant risk, HSCT.

LEUKOCYTE ADHESION DEFICIENCY (LAD)

Leukocyte adhesion deficiency (LAD) consists of three autosomal recessive conditions (LAD I, II, and III) (Chap. 80). The most frequent condition (LAD I) is caused by mutations in the β2 integrin gene; following leukocyte activation, β2 integrins mediate adhesion to inflamed endothelium expressing cognate ligands. LAD III results from a defect in a regulatory protein (kindlin, also known as Fermt 3) involved in activating the ligand affinity of β2 integrins. The extremely rare LAD II condition is the end result of a defect in selectin-mediated leukocyte rolling that occurs prior to β2 integrin binding. There is a primary defect in fucose transporter such that oligosaccharide selectin ligands are missing in this syndromic condition.

Given that neutrophils are not able to reach infected tissues, LAD renders the individual susceptible to bacterial and fungal infections in a way that is similar to that of patients with SCN. LAD also causes impaired wound healing and delayed loss of the umbilical cord. A diagnosis can be suspected in cases of pus-free skin/tissue infections and massive hyperleukocytosis (>30,000/μL) in the blood (mostly granulocytes). Patients with LAD III also develop bleeding because the β2 integrin in platelets is not functional. Use of immunofluorescence and functional assays to detect β2 integrin can help form a diagnosis. Severe forms of LAD may require HSCT, although gene therapy is also now being considered. Neutrophil-specific granule deficiency (a very rare condition caused by a mutation in the gene for transcription factor C/EBPα) results in a condition that is clinically similar to LAD.

CHRONIC GRANULOMATOUS DISEASES

Chronic granulomatous diseases (CGDs) are characterized by impaired phagocytic killing of microorganisms by neutrophils and macrophages (Chap. 80). The incidence is approximately 1 per 200,000 live births. About 70% of cases are associated with X-linked recessive inheritance versus autosomal inheritance in the remaining 30%. CGD causes deep-tissue bacterial and fungal abscesses in macrophage-rich organs such as the lymph nodes, liver, and lungs. Recurrent skin infections (such as folliculitis) are common and can prompt an early diagnosis of CGD. The infectious agents are typically catalase-positive bacteria (such as *Staphylococcus aureus* and *Serratia marcescens*) but also include *Burkholderia cepacia*, pathogenic mycobacteria (in certain regions of the world), and fungi (mainly filamentous molds, such as *Aspergillus*).

CGD is caused by defective production of reactive oxygen species (ROS) in the phagolysosome membrane following phagocytosis of microorganisms. It results from the lack of a component of NADPH oxidase (gp91phox or p22phox) or of the associated adapter/activating proteins (p47phox, p67phox, or p40phox) that mediate the transport of electrons into the phagolysosome for creating ROS by interaction with O_2. Under normal circumstances, these ROS either directly kill engulfed microorganisms or enable the rise in pH needed to activate the phagosomal proteases that contribute to microbial killing. Diagnosis of CGD is based on assays of ROS production in neutrophils and monocytes (Table 374-2). As its name suggests, CGD is also a granulomatous disease. Macrophage-rich granulomas can often arise in the liver, spleen, and other organs. These are sterile granulomas that cause disease by obstruction (bladder, pylorus, etc.) or inflammation (colitis, restrictive lung disease).

The management of infections in patients with CGD can be a complex process. The treatment of bacterial infections is generally based on combination therapy with antibiotics that are able to penetrate into cells. The treatment of fungal infections requires aggressive, long-term use of antifungals. Inflammatory/granulomatous lesions are usually steroid-sensitive; however, glucocorticoids often contribute to the spread of infections. Hence, there is strong need for new therapeutic options in what is still a poorly understood disease.

The treatment of CGD mostly relies on preventing infections. It has been unambiguously demonstrated that prophylactic usage of trimethoprim/sulfamethoxazole is both well tolerated and highly effective in reducing the risk of bacterial infection. Daily administration of azole derivatives (notably itraconazole) also reduces the frequency of fungal complications. It has long been suggested that interferon γ administration is helpful, although medical experts continue to disagree over this controversial issue. Patients may do reasonably well with prophylaxis and careful management. However, other patients develop severe and persistent fungal infections and/or chronic inflammatory complications that ultimately require HSCT. The latter is an established curative approach for CGD; however, the risk-versus-benefit ratio must be carefully assessed on a case-by-case basis. Gene therapy approaches are also being evaluated.

MENDELIAN SUSCEPTIBILITY TO MYCOBACTERIAL DISEASE (MSMD)

This group of diseases is characterized by a defect in the interleukin-12 (IL-12)–interferon (IFN) γ axis (including IL-12p40, IL-12 receptor [R] β_1, IFN-γ R_1 and R_2, STAT1, IRF8 and ISG515 deficiencies), which ultimately leads to impaired IFN-γ-dependent macrophage activation. Both recessive and dominant inheritance modes have been observed. The hallmark of this PID is a specific and narrow vulnerability to tuberculous and nontuberculous mycobacteria. The most severe phenotype (as observed in complete IFN-γ receptor deficiency) is characterized by disseminated infection that can be fatal even when aggressive and appropriate antimycobacterial therapy is applied. In addition to mycobacterial infections, MSMD patients (and particularly those with an IL-12/IL-12 R deficiency) are prone to developing *Salmonella* infections. Although MSMDs are very rare, they should be considered in any patient with persistent mycobacterial infection. Treatment with IFN-γ may efficiently bypass an IL-12/IL-12R deficiency.

TOLL-LIKE RECEPTOR (TLR) PATHWAY DEFICIENCIES

In a certain group of patients with early-onset, invasive *Streptococcus pneumoniae* infections or (less frequently) *Staphylococcus aureus* or other pyogenic infections, conventional screening for PIDs does not identify the cause of the defect in host defense. It has been established that these patients carry recessive mutations in genes that encode essential adaptor molecules (IRAK4 and MYD88) involved in the signaling pathways of the majority of known Toll-like receptors (TLRs) (Chap. 372e). Remarkably, susceptibility to infection appears to decrease after the first few years of life—perhaps an indication that adaptive immunity (once triggered by an initial microbial challenge) is then able to prevent recurrent infections.

Certain TLRs (TLR-3, -7, -8, and -9) are involved in the recognition of RNA and DNA and usually become engaged during viral infections. Very specific susceptibility to herpes simplex encephalitis has been described in patients with a deficiency in Unc93b (a molecule associated with TLR-3, -7, -8, and -9 required for correct subcellular localization), TLR-3, or associated signaling molecules TRIF, TBK1, and TRAF3, resulting in defective type I IFN production. The fact that no other TLR deficiencies have been found—despite extensive screening of patients with unexplained, recurrent infections—strongly suggests that these receptors are functionally redundant. Hypomorphic mutations in NEMO/IKK-γ (a member of the NF-κB complex, which is activated downstream of TLR receptors) lead to a complex, variable immunodeficiency and a number of associated features. Susceptibility to both invasive, pyogenic infections and mycobacteria may be observed in this particular setting.

COMPLEMENT DEFICIENCY

The complement system is composed of a complex cascade of plasma proteins (Chap. 372e) that leads to the deposition of C3b fragments on the surface of particles and the formation of immune complexes that can culminate in the activation of a lytic complex at the bacterial surface. C3 cleavage can be mediated via three pathways: the classic, alternate, and lectin pathways. C3b coats particles as part of the opsonization process that facilitates phagocytosis following binding to cognate receptors. A deficiency in any component of the classic pathway (C1q, C1r, C1s, C4, and C2) can predispose an individual to bacterial infections that are tissue-invasive or that occur in the respiratory tract. Likewise, a C3 deficiency or a deficiency in factor I (a protein that regulates C3 consumption, thus leading to a C3 deficiency due to its absence) also results in the same type of vulnerability to infection. It has recently been reported that a very rare deficiency in ficolin-3 predisposes affected individuals to bacterial infections. Deficiencies in the alternative pathway (factors D and properdin) are associated with the occurrence of invasive *Neisseria* infections.

Lastly, deficiencies of any complement component involved in the lytic phase (C5, C6, C7, C8, and, to a lesser extent, C9) predispose affected individuals to systemic infection by *Neisseria*. This is explained by the critical role of complement in the lysis of the thick cell wall possessed by this class of bacteria.

Diagnosis of a complement deficiency relies primarily on testing the status of the classic and alternate pathway via functional assays, i.e., the CH50 and AP50 tests, respectively. When either pathway is profoundly impaired, determination of the status of the relevant components in that pathway enables a precise diagnosis. Appropriate vaccinations and daily administration of oral penicillin are efficient means of preventing recurrent infections. It is noteworthy that several complement deficiencies (in the classic pathway and the lytic phase) may also predispose affected individuals to autoimmune diseases (notably systemic lupus erythematosus; Chap. 378).

PRIMARY IMMUNODEFICIENCIES OF THE ADAPTIVE IMMUNE SYSTEM

T LYMPHOCYTE DEFICIENCIES (TABLE 374-1, FIGS. 374-2 AND 374-3)

Given the central role of T lymphocytes in adaptive immune responses (Chap. 372e), PIDs involving T cells generally have severe pathologic consequences; this explains the poor overall prognosis and the need for early diagnosis and the early intervention with appropriate therapy. Several differentiation pathways of T cell effectors have been described, one or all of which may be affected by a given PID (Fig. 374-2). Follicular helper CD4+ T cells in germinal centers are required for T-dependent antibody production, including the generation of Ig class-switched, high-affinity antibodies. CD4+ T_H1 cells provide cytokine dependent (mostly IFN-γ-dependent) help to macrophages for intracellular killing of various microorganisms, including mycobacteria and *Salmonella*. CD4+ T_H2 cells produce IL-4, IL-5, and IL-13 and thus recruit and activate eosinophils and other cells required to fight helminth infections. CD4+ T_H17 cells produce IL-17 and IL-22 cytokines that recruit neutrophils to the skin and lungs to fight bacterial and fungal infections. Cytotoxic CD8+ T cells can kill infected cells, notably in the context of viral infections. In addition, certain T cell deficiencies predispose affected individuals to *Pneumocystis jiroveci* lung infections early in life and to chronic gut/biliary duct/liver infections by *Cryptosporidium* and related genera later on in life. Lastly, naturally occurring or induced regulatory T cells are essential for controlling inflammation (notably reactivity to commensal bacteria in the gut) and autoimmunity. The role of other T cell subsets with limited T cell receptor (TCR) diversity (such as γδTCR T cells or natural killer T [NKT] cells) in PIDs is less well known; however, these subsets can be defective in certain PIDs, and this finding can sometimes contribute to the diagnosis (e.g., NKT cell deficiency in X-linked proliferative syndrome). T cell deficiencies account for approximately 20% of all cases of PID.

Severe Combined Immunodeficiencies Severe combined immunodeficiencies (SCIDs) constitute a group of rare PIDs characterized by a profound block in T cell development and thus the complete absence of these cells. The developmental block is always the consequence of an intrinsic deficiency. The incidence of SCID is estimated to be 1 in 50,000 live births. Given the severity of the T cell deficiency, clinical consequences occur early in life (usually within 3 to 6 months of birth). The most frequent clinical manifestations are recurrent oral candidiasis, failure to thrive, and protracted diarrhea and/or acute interstitial pneumonitis caused by *Pneumocystis jiroveci* (although the latter can also be observed in the first year of life in children with B cell deficiencies). Severe viral infections or invasive bacterial infections can also occur. Patients may also experience complications related to infections caused by live vaccines (notably bacille Calmette-Guérin [BCG]) that may lead not only to local and regional infection but also to disseminated infection manifested by fever, splenomegaly, and skin and lytic bone lesions. A scaly skin eruption can be observed in a context of maternal T cell engraftment (see below). A diagnosis of SCID can be suspected based on the patient's clinical history and, possibly, a family history of deaths in very young children (suggestive of either X-linked or recessive inheritance). Lymphocytopenia is strongly suggestive of SCID in more than 90% of cases (Table 316-2). The absence of a thymic shadow on a chest x-ray can also be suggestive of SCID. An accurate diagnosis relies on precise determination of the number of circulating T, B, and NK lymphocytes and their subsets. T cell lymphopenia may be masked in some patients by the presence of maternal T cells

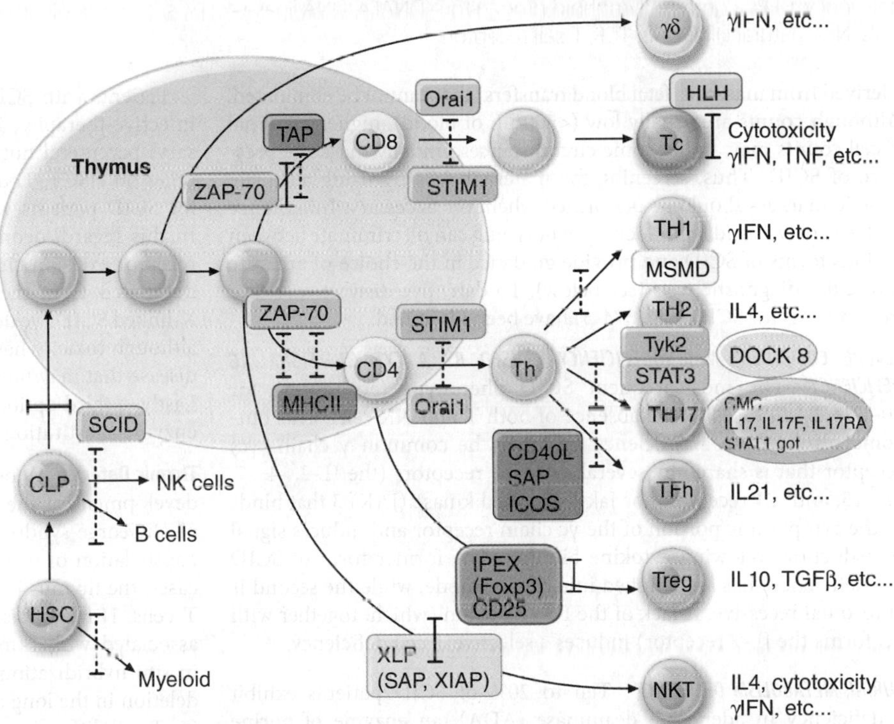

FIGURE 374-2 T cell differentiation, effector pathways, and related primary immunodeficiencies (PIDs). Hematopoietic stem cells (HSCs) differentiate into common lymphoid progenitors (CLPs), which, in turn, give rise to the T cell precursors that migrate to the thymus. The development of CD4+ and CD8+ T cells is shown. Known T cell effector pathways are indicated, i.e., γδ cells, cytotoxic T cells (Tc), T_H1, T_H2, T_H17, TFh (follicular helper) CD4 effector T cells, regulatory T cells (Treg), and natural killer T cells (NKTs); abbreviations for PIDs are contained in boxes. Vertical bars indicate a complete deficiency; broken bars a partial deficiency. SCID, severe combined immunodeficiency; ZAP-70, zeta-associated protein deficiency; MHCII, major histocompatibility complex class II deficiency; TAP, TAP1 and TAP2 deficiencies; Orai1, STIM1 deficiencies; HLH, hematopoietic lymphohistiocytosis; MSMD, Mendelian susceptibility to mycobacterial disease; Tyk2, DOCK8, autosomal recessive form of hyper-IgE syndrome; STAT3, autosomal dominant form of hyper-IgE syndrome; IL17F, IL17RA, STAT1 (gof: gain of function), CMC (chronic mucocutaneous candidiasis), CD40L, ICOS, SAP deficiencies; IPEX, immunodysregulation polyendocrinopathy enteropathy X-linked syndrome; XLP, X-linked proliferative syndromes.

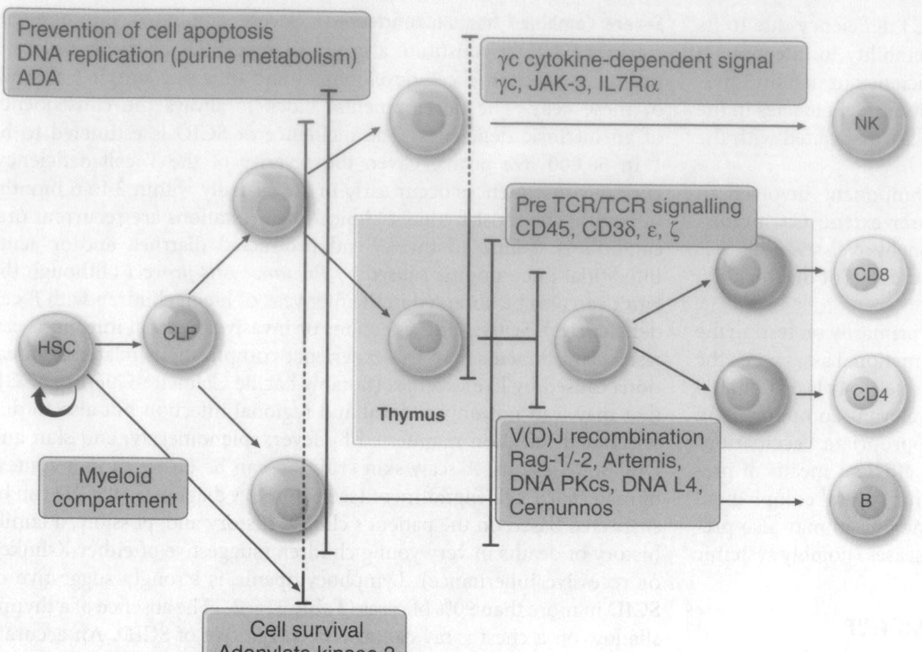

FIGURE 374-3 T cell differentiation and severe combined immunodeficiencies (SCIDs). The vertical bars indicate the five mechanisms currently known to lead to SCID. The names of deficient proteins are indicated in the boxes adjacent to the vertical bars. A broken line means that deficiency is partial or involves only some of the indicated immunodeficiencies. ADA, adenosine deaminase deficiency; CLPs, common lymphoid progenitors; DNAL4, DNA ligase 4; HSCs, hematopoietic stem cells; NKs, natural killer cells; TCR, T cell receptor.

(derived from maternal-fetal blood transfers) that cannot be eliminated. Although counts are usually low (<500/μL of blood), higher maternal T cell counts may, under some circumstances, initially mask the presence of SCID. Thus, screening for maternal cells by using adequate genetic markers should be performed whenever necessary. Inheritance pattern analysis and lymphocyte phenotyping can discriminate between various forms of SCID and provide guidance in the choice of accurate molecular diagnostic tests (see below). To date, five distinct causative mechanisms for SCID (Fig. 374-3) have been identified:

SEVERE COMBINED IMMUNODEFICIENCY CAUSED BY A CYTOKINE-SIGNALING DEFICIENCY The most frequent SCID phenotype (accounting for 40–50% of all cases) is the absence of both T and NK cells. This outcome results from a deficiency in either the common γ chain (γc) receptor that is shared by several cytokine receptors (the IL-2, -4, -7, -9, -15, and -21 receptors) or Jak-associated kinase (JAK) 3 that binds to the cytoplasmic portion of the γc chain receptor and induces signal transduction following cytokine binding. The former form of SCID (γc deficiency) has an X-linked inheritance mode, while the second is autosomal recessive. A lack of the IL-7Rα chain (which, together with γc, forms the IL-7 receptor) induces a selective T cell deficiency.

PURINE METABOLISM DEFICIENCY Ten to 20% of SCID patients exhibit a deficiency in adenosine deaminase (ADA), an enzyme of purine metabolism that deaminates adenosine (ado) and deoxyadenosine (dAdo). An ADA deficiency results in the accumulation of ado and dAdo metabolites that induce premature cell death of lymphocyte progenitors. The condition results in the absence of B and NK lymphocytes as well as T cells. The clinical expression of complete ADA deficiency typically occurs very early in life. Since ADA is a ubiquitous enzyme, its deficiency can also cause bone dysplasia with abnormal costochondral junctions and metaphyses (found in 50% of cases) and neurologic defects. The very rare purine nucleoside phosphorylase (PNP) deficiency causes a profound although incomplete T cell deficiency that is often associated with severe neurologic impairments.

DEFECTIVE REARRANGEMENTS OF T AND B CELL RECEPTORS A series of SCID conditions are characterized by a selective deficiency in T and B lymphocytes with autosomal recessive inheritance. These conditions account for 20–30% of SCID cases and result from mutations in genes encoding proteins that mediate the recombination of V(D)J gene elements in T and B cell antigen receptor genes (required for the generation of diversity in antigen recognition). The main deficiencies involve RAG-1, RAG-2, DNA-dependent protein kinase, and Artemis. A less severe (albeit variable) immunologic phenotype can result from other deficiencies in the same pathway, i.e., DNA ligase 4 and Cernunnos deficiencies. Given that these latter factors are involved in DNA repair, these deficiencies also cause developmental defects.

DEFECTIVE (PRE-)T CELL RECEPTOR SIGNALING IN THE THYMUS A selective T cell defect can be caused by a series of rare deficiencies in molecules involved in signaling via the pre-TCR or the TCR. These include deficiencies in CD3 subunits associated with the (pre-)TCR (i.e., CD3δ, ε, and ζ) and CD45.

RETICULAR DYSGENESIS Reticular dysgenesis is an extremely rare form of SCID that causes T and NK deficiencies with severe neutropenia and sensorineural deafness. It results from an adenylate kinase 2 deficiency.

Patients with SCID require appropriate care with aggressive anti-infective therapies, immunoglobulin replacement, and (when necessary) parenteral nutrition support. In most cases, curative treatment relies on HSCT. Today, HSCT provides a very high curative potential for SCID patients who are otherwise in reasonably good condition. In this regard, neonatal screening, based on quantification of T cell receptor excision circles (TRECs) on a Guthrie card sample, is being developed. Gene therapy has been found to be successful for cases of X-linked SCID (γc deficiency) and SCID caused by an ADA deficiency, although toxicity has become an issue in the treatment of the former disease that may now be overcome by use of newly generated vectors. Lastly, a third option for the treatment of ADA deficiency consists of enzyme substitution with a pegylated enzyme.

Thymic Defects A profound T cell defect can also result from faulty development of the thymus, as is most often observed in rare cases of DiGeorge syndrome—a relatively common condition leading to a constellation of developmental defects. In approximately 1% of such cases, the thymus is completely absent, leading to virtually no mature T cells. However, expansion of oligoclonal T cells can occur and is associated with skin lesions. Diagnosis (using immunofluorescence in situ hybridization) is based on the identification of a hemizygous deletion in the long arm of chromosome 22. To recover the capability for T cell differentiation, these cases require a thymic graft. CHARGE (coloboma of the eye, *h*eart anomaly, choanal *a*tresia, *r*etardation, genital and *e*ar anomalies) syndrome (CHD7 deficiency) is a less frequent cause of impaired thymus development. Lastly, the very rare "nude" defect is characterized by the absence of both hair and the thymus.

Omenn Syndrome *Omenn syndrome* consists of a subset of T cell deficiencies that present with a unique phenotype, including early-onset erythrodermia, alopecia, hepatosplenomegaly, and failure to thrive. These patients usually display T cell lymphocytosis, eosinophilia, and low B cell counts. It has been found that the T cells of these patients exhibit a low TCR heterogeneity. This peculiar syndrome is the consequence of hypomorphic mutations in genes usually associated with SCID, i.e., *RAG-1*, *RAG-2*, or (less frequently) *Artemis* or *IL-7Rα*. The impaired homeostasis of differentiating T cells thus causes this immune system–associated disease. These patients are very fragile, requiring simultaneous anti-infective therapy, nutritional support, and immunosuppression. HSCT provides a curative approach.

Functional T Cell Defects (Fig. 374-2) A subset of T cell PIDs with autosomal inheritance is characterized by partially preserved T cell differentiation but defective activation resulting in abnormal effector function. There are many causes of these defects, but all lead to susceptibility to viral and opportunistic infections, chronic diarrhea, and failure to thrive, with onset during childhood. Careful phenotyping and in vitro functional assays are required to identify these diseases, the best characterized of which are the following.

ZETA-ASSOCIATED PROTEIN 70 (ZAP70) DEFICIENCY Zeta associated protein 70 (ZAP70) is recruited to the TCR following antigen recognition. A ZAP70 deficiency leads typically to an almost complete absence of CD8+ T cells; CD4+ T cells are present but cannot be activated in vitro by TCR stimulation.

CALCIUM SIGNALING DEFECTS A small number of patients have been reported who exhibit a profound defect in in vitro T and B cell activation as a result of defective antigen receptor-mediated Ca^{2+} influx. This defect is caused by a mutation in the calcium channel gene (*ORAI-*) or its activator (*STIM-1*). It is noteworthy that these patients are also prone to autoimmune manifestations (blood cytopenias) and exhibit a nonprogressive muscle disease.

HUMAN LEUKOCYTE ANTIGEN (HLA) CLASS II DEFICIENCY Defective expression of HLA class II molecules is the hallmark of a group of four recessive genetic defects all of which affect molecules (RFX5, RFXAP, RFXANK, and CIITA) involved in the transactivation of the genes coding for HLA class II. As a result, low but variable CD4+ T cell counts are observed in addition to defective antigen-specific T and B cell responses. These patients are particularly susceptible to herpesvirus, adenovirus, and enterovirus infections and chronic gut/liver *Cryptosporidium* infections.

HLA CLASS I DEFICIENCY Defective expression of molecules involved in antigen presentation by HLA class I molecules (i.e., TAP-1, TAP-2, and Tapasin) leads to reduced CD8+ T cell counts, loss of HLA class I antigen expression, and a particular phenotype consisting of chronic obstructive pulmonary disease and severe vasculitis.

OTHER DEFECTS A variety of other T cell PIDs have been described, some of which are associated with a precise molecular defect (e.g., IL-2 inducible T cell kinase [ITK] deficiency, IL-21 receptor deficiency, CARD11 deficiency). These conditions are also characterized by profound vulnerability to infections, such as severe Epstein-Barr virus (EBV)–induced B cell proliferation and autoimmune disorders in ITK deficiency. Milder phenotypes are associated with CD8 and CD3γ deficiencies.

HSCT is indicated for most of these diseases, although the prognosis is worse than in SCID because many patients are chronically infected at the time of diagnosis. Fairly aggressive immunosuppression and myeloablation may be necessary to achieve engraftment of allogeneic stem cells.

T Cell Primary Immunodeficiencies with DNA Repair Defects This is a group of PIDs characterized by a combination of T and B cell defects of variable intensity, together with a number of nonimmunologic features resulting from DNA fragility. The autosomal recessive disorder *ataxia-telangiectasia* (AT) is the most frequently encountered condition in this group. It has an incidence of 1:40,000 live births and causes B cell defects (low IgA, IgG2 deficiency, and low antibody production), which often require immunoglobulin replacement. AT is associated with a progressive T cell immunodeficiency. As the name suggests, the hallmark features of AT are telangiectasia and cerebellar ataxia. The latter manifestations may not be detectable before the age of 3–4 years, so that AT should be considered in young children with IgA deficiency and recurrent and problematic infections. Diagnosis is based on a cytogenetic analysis showing excessive chromosomal rearrangements (mostly affecting chromosomes 7 and 14) in lymphocytes. AT is caused by a mutation in the gene encoding the ATM protein—a kinase that plays an important role in the detection and repair of DNA lesions (or cell death if the lesions are too numerous) by triggering several different pathways. Overall, AT is a progressive disease that carries a very high risk of lymphoma, leukemia, and (during adulthood) carcinomas. A variant of AT ("AT-like disease") is caused by mutation in the *MRE11* gene.

Nijmegen breakage syndrome (NBS) is a less common condition that also results from chromosome instability (with the same cytogenetic abnormalities as in AT). NBS is characterized by a severe T and B cell combined immune deficiency with autosomal recessive inheritance. Individuals with NBS exhibit microcephaly and a bird-like face, but have neither ataxia nor telangiectasia. The risk of malignancies is very high. NBS results from a deficiency in nibrin (NBSI, a protein associated with MRE11 and Rad50 that is involved in checking DNA lesions) caused by hypomorphic mutations.

Severe forms of *dyskeratosis congenita* (also known as Hoyeraal-Hreidarsson syndrome) combine a progressive immunodeficiency that can also include an absence of B and NK lymphocytes, progressive bone marrow failure, microcephaly, in utero growth retardation, and gastrointestinal disease. The disease can be X-linked or, more rarely, autosomal recessive. It is caused by the mutation of genes encoding telomere maintenance proteins, including dyskerin (DKC1).

Finally, *immunodeficiency with centromeric and facial anomalies* (ICF) is a complex syndrome of autosomal recessive inheritance that variably combines a mild T cell immune deficiency with a more severe B cell immune deficiency, coarse face, digestive disease, and mild mental retardation. A diagnostic feature is the detection by cytogenetic analysis of multiradial aspects in multiple chromosomes (most frequently 1, 9, and 16) corresponding to an abnormal DNA structure secondary to defective DNA methylation. It is the consequence of a deficiency in the DNA methyltransferase DNMT3B, or ZBTB24.

T Cell Primary Immunodeficiencies with Hyper-IgE Several T cell PIDs are associated with elevated serum IgE levels (as in Omenn syndrome). A condition sometimes referred to as *autosomal recessive hyper-IgE syndrome* is notably characterized by recurrent bacterial infections in the skin and respiratory tract and severe skin and mucosal infections by pox viruses and human papillomaviruses, together with severe allergic manifestations. T and B lymphocyte counts are low. Mutations in the *DOCK8* gene have been found in most of these patients. This condition is an indication for HSCT.

A very rare, related condition with autosomal recessive inheritance that causes a similar susceptibility to infection with various microbes (see above), including mycobacteria, reportedly results from a deficiency in Tyk-2, a JAK family kinase involved in the signaling of many different cytokine receptors.

Autosomal Dominant Hyper-IgE Syndrome This unique condition, the *autosomal dominant hyper-IgE syndrome*, is usually diagnosed by the combination of recurrent skin and lung infections that can be complicated by pneumatoceles. Infections are caused by pyogenic bacteria and fungi. Several other manifestations characterize hyper-IgE syndrome, including facial dysmorphy, defective loss of primary teeth, hyperextensibility, scoliosis, and osteoporosis. Elevated serum IgE levels are typical of this syndrome. Defective T_H17 effector responses have been shown to account at least in part for the specific patterns of susceptibility to particular microbes. This condition is caused by a heterozygous (dominant) mutation in the gene encoding the transcription factor STAT3 that is required in a number of signaling pathways following binding of cytokine to cytokine receptors (such as that of IL-6 and the IL-6 receptor). It also results in partially defective antibody production because of defective IL-21R signaling. Hence, immunoglobulin substitution can be considered as prophylaxis of bacterial infections.

Cartilage Hair Hypoplasia The autosomal recessive *cartilage hair hypoplasia* (CHH) disease is characterized by short-limb dwarfism, metaphyseal dysostosis, and sparse hair, together with a combined T and B cell PID of extremely variable intensity (ranging from quasi-SCID to no clinically significant immune defects). The condition can predispose to erythroblastopenia, autoimmunity, and tumors. It is caused by mutations in the *RMRP* gene for a noncoding ribosome-associated RNA.

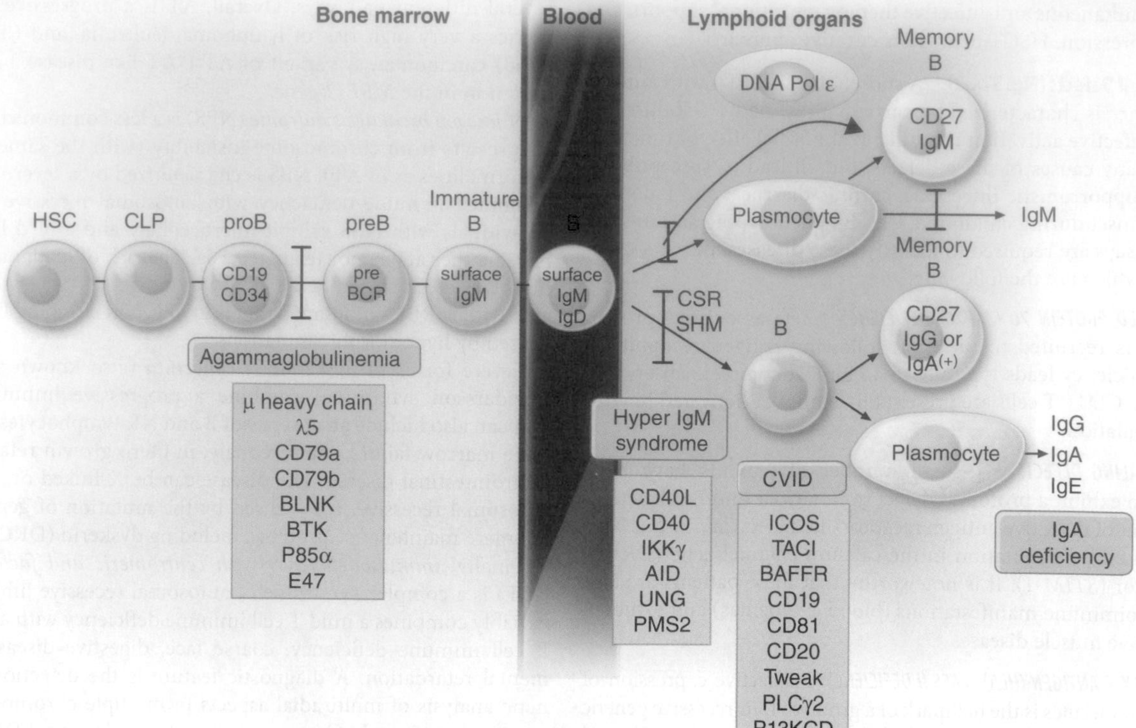

FIGURE 374-4 B cell differentiation and related primary immunodeficiencies (PIDs). Hematopoietic stem cells (HSCs) differentiate into common lymphoid progenitors (CLPs), which give rise to pre-B cells. The B cell differentiation pathway goes through the pre–B cell stage (expression of the μ heavy chain and surrogate light chain), the immature B cell stage (expression of surface IgM), and the mature B cell stage (expression of surface IgM and IgD). The main phenotypic characteristics of these cells are indicated. In lymphoid organs, B cells can differentiate into plasma cells and produce IgM or undergo (in germinal centers) Ig class switch recombination (CSR) and somatic mutation of the variable region of V genes (SHM) that enable selection of high-affinity antibodies. These B cells produce antibodies of various isotypes and generate memory B cells. PIDs are indicated in the purple boxes. CVID, common variable immunodeficiency.

CD40 Ligand and CD40 Deficiencies *Hyper-IgM syndrome* (HIGM) is a well-known PID that is usually classified as a B cell immune deficiency (see Fig. 374-4 and below). It results from defective immunoglobulin class switch recombination (CSR) in germinal centers and leads to profound deficiency in production of IgG, IgA, and IgE (although IgM production is maintained). Approximately half of HIGM sufferers are also prone to opportunistic infections, e.g., interstitial pneumonitis caused by *Pneumocystis jiroveci* (in young children), protracted diarrhea and cholangitis caused by *Cryptosporidium*, and infection of the brain with *Toxoplasma gondii*.

In the majority of cases, this condition has an X-linked inheritance and is caused by a deficiency in CD40 ligand (L). CD40L induces signaling events in B cells that are necessary for both CSR and adequate activation of other CD40-expressing cells that are involved in innate immune responses against the above-mentioned microorganisms. More rarely, the condition is caused by a deficiency in CD40 itself. The poorer prognosis of CD40L and CD40 deficiencies (relative to most other HIGM conditions) implies that (1) thorough investigations have to be performed in all cases of HIGM and (2) potentially curative HSCT should be discussed on a case-by-case basis for this group of patients.

Wiskott-Aldrich Syndrome *Wiskott-Aldrich syndrome* (WAS) is a complex, recessive, X-linked disease with an incidence of approximately 1 in 200,000 live births. It is caused by mutations in the *WASP* gene that affect not only T lymphocytes but also the other lymphocyte subsets, dendritic cells, and platelets. WAS is typically characterized by the following clinical manifestations: recurrent bacterial infections, eczema, and bleeding caused by thrombocytopenia. However, these manifestations are highly variable—mostly as a consequence of the many different *WASP* mutations that have been observed. Null mutations predispose affected individuals to invasive and bronchopulmonary infections, viral infections, severe eczema, and autoimmune manifestations. The latter include autoantibody-mediated blood cytopenia, glomerulonephritis, skin and visceral vasculitis (including brain vasculitis), erythema nodosum, and arthritis. Another possible consequence of WAS is lymphoma, which may be virally induced (e.g., by EBV or Kaposi's sarcoma–associated herpesvirus). Thrombocytopenia can be severe and compounded by the peripheral destruction of platelets associated with autoimmune disorders. Hypomorphic mutations usually lead to milder outcomes that are generally limited to thrombocytopenia. It is noteworthy that even patients with "isolated" X-linked thrombocytopenia can develop severe autoimmune disease or lymphoma later in life. The immunologic workup is not very informative; there can be a relative CD8+ T cell deficiency, frequently accompanied by low serum IgM levels and decreased antigen-specific antibody responses. A typical feature is reduced-sized platelets on a blood smear. Diagnosis is based on intracellular immunofluorescence analysis of WAS protein (WASp) expression in blood cells. WASp regulates the actin cytoskeleton and thus plays an important role in many lymphocyte functions, including cell adhesion and migration and the formation of synapses between antigen-presenting and target cells. Predisposition to autoimmune disorders is in part related to defective regulatory T cells. The treatment of WAS should match the severity of disease expression. Prophylactic antibiotics, immunoglobulin G (IgG) supplementation, and careful topical treatment of eczema are indicated. Although splenectomy improves platelet count in a majority of cases, this intervention is associated with a significant risk of infection (both before and after HSCT). Allogeneic HSCT is curative, with fairly good results overall. Gene therapy trials are also under way. A similar condition has been reported in a girl with a deficiency in the Wiskott-Aldrich interacting protein (WIP).

A few other complex PIDs are worth mentioning. *Sp110 deficiency* causes a T cell PID with liver venoocclusive disease and hypogammaglobulinemia. *Chronic mucocutaneous candidiasis* (CMC) is a heterogeneous disease, considering the different inheritance patterns that have been observed. In some cases, chronic candidiasis is associated with late-onset bronchopulmonary infections, bronchiectasis, and brain aneurysms. Moderate forms of CMC are related to autoimmunity and AIRE deficiency (see below). In this setting, predisposition to *Candida* infection is associated with the detection of autoantibodies to T_H17 cytokines. Recently, deficiencies in IL-17F and IL-17 receptor A and, above all, gain-of-function mutations in *STAT1* have been found to be associated with CMC. In all cases, CMC is related to defective T_H17 function. Innate immunodeficiency in CARD9 also predisposes to chronic invasive fungal infection.

B LYMPHOCYTE DEFICIENCIES (TABLE 374-1, FIG. 374-4)

Deficiencies that predominantly affect B lymphocytes are the most frequent PIDs and account for 60–70% of all cases. B lymphocytes make antibodies. Pentameric IgMs are found in the vascular compartment and are also secreted at mucosal surfaces. IgG antibodies diffuse freely into extravascular spaces, whereas IgA antibodies are produced and secreted predominantly from mucosa-associated lymphoid tissues. Although Ig isotypes have distinct effector functions, including Fc receptor–mediated and (indirectly) C_3 receptor–dependent phagocytosis of microorganisms, they share the ability to recognize and neutralize a given pathogen. Defective antibody production therefore allows the establishment of invasive, pyogenic bacterial infections as well as recurrent sinus and pulmonary infections (mostly caused by *Streptococcus pneumoniae*, *Haemophilus influenzae*, *Moraxella catarrhalis*, and, less frequently, gram-negative bacteria). If left untreated, recurrent bronchial infections lead to bronchiectasis and, ultimately, cor pulmonale and death. Parasitic infections such as caused by *Giardia lamblia* and bacterial infections caused by *Helicobacter* and *Campylobacter* of the gut are also observed. A complete lack of antibody production (namely agammaglobulinemia) can also predispose affected individuals to severe, chronic, disseminated enteroviral infections causing meningoencephalitis, hepatitis, and a dermatomyositis-like disease.

Even with the most profound of B cell deficiencies, infections rarely occur before the age of 6 months; this is because of transient protection provided by the transplacental passage of immunoglobulins during the last trimester of pregnancy. Conversely, a genetically nonimmunodeficient child born to a mother with hypogammaglobu linemia is, in the absence of maternal Ig substitution, usually prone to severe bacterial infections in utero and for several months after birth.

Diagnosis of B cell PIDs relies on the determination of serum Ig levels (Table 316-2). Determination of antibody production following immunization with tetanus toxoid vaccine or nonconjugated pneumococcal polysaccharide antigens can also help diagnose more subtle deficiencies. Another useful test is B cell phenotype determination in switched μ−δ− CD27+ and nonswitched memory B cells (μ+δ+ CD27+). In agammaglobulinemic patients, examination of bone marrow B cell precursors (Fig. 374-4) can help obtain a precise diagnosis and guide the choice of genetic tests.

Agammaglobulinemia Agammaglobulinemia is characterized by a profound defect in B cell development (<1% of the normal B cell blood count). In most patients, very low residual Ig isotypes can be detected in the serum. In 85% of cases, agammaglobulinemia is caused by a mutation in the *BTK* gene that is located on the X chromosome. The *BTK* gene product is a kinase that participates in (pre) B cell receptor signaling. When the kinase is defective, there is a block (albeit a leaky one) at the pre-B to B cell stage (Fig. 374-4). Detection of *BTK* by intracellular immunofluorescence of monocytes, and lack thereof in patients with X-linked agammaglobulinemia, is a useful diagnostic test. Not all of the mutations in *BTK* result in agammaglobulinemia, since some patients have a milder form of hypogammaglobulinemia and low but detectable B cell counts. These cases should not be confused with common variable immunodeficiency (CVID, see below). About 10% of agammaglobulinemia cases are caused by alterations in genes encoding elements of the pre-B cell receptor, i.e., the μ heavy chain, the λ5 surrogate light chain, Igα or Igβ, the scaffold protein BLNK, and the p85 α subunit of phosphatidylinositol 3 phosphate kinase (P13K). In 5% of cases, the defect is unknown. It is noteworthy that agammaglobulinemia can be observed in patients with ICF syndrome, despite the presence of normal peripheral B cell counts. Lastly, agammaglobulinemia can be a manifestation of a myelodysplastic syndrome (associated or not with neutropenia). Treatment of agammaglobulinemic patients is based on immunoglobulin replacement (see below). Profound hypogammaglobulinemia is also observed in adults, in association with thymoma.

Hyper-IgM (HIGM) Syndromes *HIGM* is a rare B cell PID characterized by defective Ig CSR. It results in very low serum levels of IgG and IgA and elevated or normal serum IgM levels. The clinical severity is similar to that seen in agammaglobulinemia, although chronic lung disease and sinusitis are less frequent and enteroviral infections are uncommon. As discussed above, a diagnosis of HIGM involves screening for an X-linked CD40L deficiency and an autosomal recessive CD40 deficiency, which affect both B and T cells. In 50% of cases affecting only B cells, these isolated HIGM syndromes result from mutations in the gene encoding activation-induced deaminase, the protein that induces CSR in B cell germinal centers. These patients usually have enlarged lymphoid organs. In the other 50% of cases, the etiology is unknown (except for rare UNG and PMS2 deficiencies). Furthermore, IgM-mediated autoimmunity and lymphomas can occur in HIGM syndrome. It is noteworthy that HIGM can result from fetal rubella syndrome or can be a predominant immunologic feature of other PIDs, such as the immunodeficiency associated with ectodermic anhydrotic hypoplasia X-linked NEMO deficiency and the combined T and B cell PIDs caused by DNA repair defects such as AT and Cernunnos deficiency.

Common Variable Immunodeficiency (CVID) CVID is an ill-defined condition characterized by low serum levels of one or more Ig isotypes. Its prevalence is estimated to be 1 in 20,000. The condition is recognized predominantly in adults, although clinical manifestations can occur earlier in life. Hypogammaglobulinemia is associated with at least partially defective antibody production in response to vaccine antigens. B lymphocyte counts are often normal but can be low. Besides infections, CVID patients may develop lymphoproliferation (splenomegaly), granulomatous lesions, colitis, antibody-mediated autoimmune disease, and lymphomas. A family history is found in 10% of cases. A clear-cut dominant inheritance pattern is found in some families, whereas recessive inheritance is observed more rarely. In most cases, no molecular cause can be identified. A small number of patients in Germany were found to carry mutations in the *ICOS* gene encoding a T cell-membrane protein that contributes to B cell activation and survival. In 10% of patients with CVID, monoallelic or biallelic mutations of the gene encoding TACI (a member of the tumor necrosis factor [TNF] receptor family that is expressed on B cells) have been found. In fact, heterozygous TACI mutations correspond to a genetic susceptibility factor, since similar heterozygous mutations are found in 1% of controls. The BAFF receptor was found to be defective in a kindred with CVID, although not all individuals carrying the mutation have CVID.

Recently a group of patients with hypogammaglobulinemia and lymphoproliferation were shown to exhibit dominant gain of function mutations in the *PIK3CD* gene encoding the p110δ form of P13 kinase. A diagnosis of CVID should be made after excluding the presence of hypomorphic mutations associated with agammaglobulinemia or more subtle T cell defects; this is particularly the case in children. It is possible that many cases of CVID result from a constellation of factors, rather than a single genetic defect. Recently, rare cases of hypogammaglobulinemia were found to be associated with CD19 and CD81 deficiencies. These patients have B cells that can be identified by typing for other B cell markers. Hypogammaglobulinemia can be associated with neutropenia and lymphopenia in the warts, hypogammaglobulinemia, infections, and myelokathexis syndrome (WHIM) caused by dominant gain-of-function mutation of *CXCR4*, resulting in cell retention in the bone marrow.

Selective Ig Isotype Deficiencies *IgA deficiency* and CVID represent polar ends of a clinical spectrum due to the same underlying gene defect(s) in a large subset of these patients. IgA deficiency is the most common PID; it can be found in 1 in every 600 individuals. It is asymptomatic in most cases; however, individuals may present with increased numbers of acute and chronic respiratory infections that may lead to bronchiectasis. In addition, over their lifetime, these patients experience an increased susceptibility to drug allergies, atopic disorders, and autoimmune diseases. Symptomatic IgA deficiency is probably related to CVID, since it can be found in relatives of patients with CVID. Furthermore, IgA deficiency may progress to CVID. It is thus important to assess serum Ig levels in IgA-deficient patients (especially when infections occur frequently) in order to detect changes that should prompt the initiation of immunoglobulin replacement. Selective IgG2 (+G4) deficiency (which in some cases may be associated with IgA deficiency) can also result in recurrent sinopulmonary infections and should thus be specifically sought in this clinical setting. These conditions are ill-defined and often transient during childhood. A pathophysiologic explanation has not been found.

Selective Antibody Deficiency to Polysaccharide Antigens Some patients with normal serum Ig levels are prone to *S. pneumoniae* and *H. influenzae* infections of the respiratory tract. Defective production of antibodies against polysaccharide antigens (such as those in the *S. pneumoniae* cell wall) can be observed and is probably causative. This condition may correspond to a defect in marginal zone B cells, a B cell subpopulation involved in T-independent antibody responses.

Immunoglobulin Replacement IgG antibodies have a half-life of 21–28 days. Thus, injection of plasma-derived polyclonal IgG containing a myriad of high-affinity antibodies can provide protection against disease-causing microorganisms in patients with defective IgG antibody production. This form of therapy should not be based on laboratory data alone (i.e., IgG and/or antibody deficiency) but should be guided by the occurrence or not of infections; otherwise, patients might be subjected to unjustified IgG infusions. Immunoglobulin replacement can be performed by IV or subcutaneous routes. In the former case, injections have to be repeated every 3–4 weeks, with a residual target level of 800 mg/mL in patients who had very low IgG levels prior to therapy. Subcutaneous injections are typically performed once a week, although the frequency can be adjusted on a case-by-case basis. A trough level of 800 mg/mL is desirable. Whatever the mode of administration, the main goal is to reduce the frequency of the respiratory tract infections and prevent chronic lung and sinus disease. The two routes appear to be equally safe and efficacious, and so the choice should be left to the preference of the patient.

In patients with chronic lung disease, chest physical therapy with good pulmonary toilet and the cyclic use of antibiotics are also needed. Immunoglobulin replacement is well tolerated by most patients, although the selection of the best-tolerated Ig preparation may be necessary in certain cases. Since IgG preparations contain a small proportion of IgAs, caution should be taken in patients with residual antibody production capacity and a complete IgA deficiency, as these subjects may develop anti-IgA antibodies that can trigger anaphylactic shock. These patients should be treated with IgA-free IgG preparations. Immunoglobulin replacement is a lifelong therapy; its rationale and procedures have to be fully understood and mastered by the patient and his or her family in order to guarantee the strict observance required for efficacy.

PRIMARY IMMUNODEFICIENCIES AFFECTING REGULATORY PATHWAYS (TABLE 374-1)

An increasing number of PIDs have been found to cause homeostatic dysregulation of the immune system, either alone or in association with increased vulnerability to infections. Defects of this type affecting the innate immune system and autoinflammatory syndromes will not be covered in this chapter. However, three specific entities (hemophagocytic lymphohistiocytosis, lymphoproliferation, and autoimmunity) will be described below.

HEMOPHAGOCYTIC LYMPHOHISTIOCYTOSIS

Hemophagocytic lymphohistiocytosis (HLH) is characterized by an unremitting activation of CD8+ T lymphocytes and macrophages that leads to organ damage (notably in the liver, bone marrow, and central nervous system). This syndrome results from a broad set of inherited diseases, all of which impair T and NK lymphocyte cytotoxicity. The manifestations of HLH are often induced by a viral infection. EBV is the most frequent trigger. In severe forms of HLH, disease onset may start during the first year of life or even (in rare cases) at birth.

Diagnosis relies on the identification of the characteristic symptoms of HLH (fever, hepatosplenomegaly, edema, neurologic diseases, blood cytopenia, increased liver enzymes, hypofibrinogenemia, high triglyceride levels, elevated markers of T cell activation, and hemophagocytic features in the bone marrow or cerebrospinal fluid). Functional assays of postactivation cytotoxic granule exocytosis (CD107 fluorescence at the cell membrane) can suggest genetically determined HLH. The conditions can be classified into three subsets:

1. Familial HLH with autosomal recessive inheritance, including perforin deficiency (30% of cases) that can be recognized by assessing intracellular perforin expression; Munc13-4 deficiency (30% of cases); syntaxin 11 deficiency (10% of cases); Munc18-2 deficiency (20% of cases); and a few residual cases that lack a known molecular defect.
2. HLH with partial albinism. Three conditions combine HLH and abnormal pigmentation, where hair examination can help in the diagnosis: Chédiak-Higashi syndrome, Griscelli syndrome, and Hermansky Pudlak syndrome type II. Chédiak-Higashi syndrome is also characterized by the presence of giant lysosomes within leukocytes (Chap. 80), in addition to a primary neurologic disorder with slow progression of symptoms over time.
3. X-linked proliferative syndrome (XLP) is characterized in most patients by the induction of HLH following EBV infection, while other patients develop progressive hypogammaglobulinemia similar to what is observed in CVID and/or certain lymphomas. XLP is caused by a mutation in the *SH2DIA* gene that encodes the adaptor protein SAP (associated with a SLAM family receptor). Several immunologic abnormalities have been described, including low 2B4-mediated NK cell cytotoxicity, impaired differentiation of NKT cells, defective antigen-induced T cell death, and defective T cell helper activity for B cells. A related disorder (XLP2) has recently been described. It is also X-linked and induces HLH (frequently after EBV infection), although the clinical manifestation may be less pronounced. The condition is associated with a deficiency of the antiapoptotic molecule XIAP. The pathophysiology of XLP2 and its relationship to XLP1 remain unclear.

HLH is a life-threatening complication. The treatment of this condition requires aggressive immunosuppression with either the cytotoxic agent etoposide or anti–T cell antibodies. Once remission has been achieved, HSCT should be performed, since it provides the only curative form of therapy.

AUTOIMMUNE LYMPHOPROLIFERATIVE SYNDROME

Autoimmune lymphoproliferative syndrome (ALPS) is characterized by nonmalignant T and B lymphoproliferation causing splenomegaly and enlarged lymph nodes; 70% of patients also display autoimmune manifestations such as autoimmune cytopenias, Guillain-Barré syndrome, uveitis, and hepatitis (Chaps. 79 and 372e). A hallmark of ALPS is the presence of CD4–CD8– TCRαβ+ T cells (2–50%) in the blood of affected individuals. Hypergammaglobulinemia involving IgG and IgA is also frequently observed. The syndrome is caused by a defect in Fas-mediated apoptosis of lymphocytes, which can thus accumulate and mediate autoimmunity. Furthermore, ALPS can lead to malignancies.

Most patients carry a heterozygous mutation in the gene encoding Fas that is characterized by dominant inheritance and variable penetrance, depending on the nature of the mutation. A rare and severe form of the disease with early onset can be observed in patients carrying a biallelic mutation of Fas, which profoundly impairs the protein's expression and/or function. Fas-ligand, caspase 10, caspase 8, and neuroblastoma RAS viral oncogene homologue (NRAS) mutations have also been reported in a few cases of ALPS. Many cases of ALPS have not been precisely delineated at the molecular level. A B cell–predominant ALPS has recently been found associated with a protein kinase Cδ gene mutation. Treatment of ALPS is essentially based on the use of proapoptotic drugs, which need to be carefully administered in order to avoid toxicity.

COLITIS, AUTOIMMUNITY, AND PRIMARY IMMUNODEFICIENCIES

Several PIDs (most of which are T cell–related) can cause severe gut inflammation. The prototypic example is *immunodysregulation polyendocrinopathy enteropathy X-linked syndrome* (IPEX), characterized by a widespread inflammatory enteropathy, food intolerance, skin rashes, autoimmune cytopenias, and diabetes. The syndrome is caused by loss-of-function mutations in the gene encoding the transcription factor FOXP3, which is required for the acquisition of effector function by regulatory T cells. In most cases of IPEX, CD4+CD25+ regulatory T cells are absent from the blood. This condition has a poor prognosis and requires aggressive immunosuppression. The only possible curative approach is allogeneic HSCT. IPEX-like syndromes that lack a FOXP3 mutation have also been described. In some cases, a CD25 deficiency has been found. Defective CD25 expression also impairs regulatory cell expansion/function. This functional T cell deficiency means that CD25-deficient patients are also at increased risk of opportunistic infections. It is noteworthy that abnormalities in regulatory T cells have been described in other PID settings, such as in Omenn syndrome, STAT5b deficiency, STIM1 (Ca flux) deficiency, and WAS; these abnormalities may account (at least in part) for the occurrence of inflammation and autoimmunity. The autoimmune features observed in a small fraction of patients with DiGeorge syndrome may have the same cause. Recently, severe inflammatory gut disease has been described in patients with a deficiency in the IL-10 receptor or IL-10.

A distinct autoimmune entity is observed in *autoimmune polyendocrinopathy candidiasis ectodermal dysplasia* (APECED) syndrome, which is characterized by autosomal recessive inheritance. It consists of multiple autoimmune manifestations that can affect solid organs in general and endocrine glands in particular. Mild, chronic *Candida* infection is often associated with this syndrome. The condition is due to mutations in the autoimmune regulator (*AIRE*) gene and results in impaired thymic expression of self-antigens by medullary epithelial cells and impaired negative selection of self-reactive T cells that leads to autoimmune manifestations.

A combination of hypogammaglobulinemia, autoantibody production, cold-induced urticaria or skin granulomas, or autoinflammation has been reported, and has been termed the *PLCγ2-associated antibody deficiency and immune dysregulation* (PLAID or APLAID).

CONCLUSION

The variety and complexity of the clinical manifestations of the many different PIDs strongly indicate that it is important to raise awareness of these diseases. Indeed, early diagnosis is essential for establishing an appropriate therapeutic regimen. Hence, patients with suspected PIDs must always be referred to experienced clinical centers that are able to perform appropriate molecular and genetic tests. A precise molecular diagnosis is not only necessary for initiating the most suitable treatment, but is also important for genetic counseling and prenatal diagnosis.

One pitfall that may hamper diagnosis is the high variability that is associated with many PIDs. Variable disease expression can result from the differing consequences of various mutations associated with a given condition, as exemplified by WAS and, to a lesser extent, X-linked agammaglobulinemia (XLA). There can also be effects of modifier genes (as also suspected in XLA) and environmental factors such as EBV infection that can be the main trigger of disease in XLP conditions. Furthermore, it has recently been established that somatic mutations in an affected gene can attenuate the phenotype of a number of T cell PIDs. This has been described for ADA deficiency, X-linked SCID, RAG deficiencies, NF-κB essential modulator (NEMO) deficiency, and, most frequently, WAS. In contrast, somatic mutations can create disease states analogous to PID, as reported for ALPS. Lastly, cytokine-neutralizing autoantibodies can mimic a PID, as shown for IFN-γ.

Many aspects of the pathophysiology of PIDs are still unknown, and the disease-causing gene mutations have not been identified in all cases (as illustrated by CVID and IgA deficiency). However, our medical understanding of PIDs has now reached the stage where scientifically based approaches to the diagnosis and treatment of these diseases can be implemented.

375e Primary Immunodeficiencies Associated with (or Secondary to) Other Diseases

Alain Fischer

This is a digital-only chapter. It is available on the DVD that accompanies this book, as well as on Access Medicine/Harrison's Online, and the eBook and "app" editions of HPIM 19e.

There are an increasing number of conditions in which a primary immunodeficiency (PID) has been described as one facet of a more complex disease setting. It is essential to consider associated diseases when a PID is identified as the primary manifestation and, conversely, not neglect the potentially harmful consequences of a PID that could be masked by other manifestations of a particular syndrome.

SECTION 2 DISORDERS OF IMMUNE-MEDIATED INJURY

376 Allergies, Anaphylaxis, and Systemic Mastocytosis

Joshua A. Boyce, K. Frank Austen

The term *atopy* implies a tendency to manifest asthma, rhinitis, urticaria, and atopic dermatitis alone or in combination, in association with the presence of allergen-specific IgE. However, individuals without an atopic background may also develop hypersensitivity reactions, particularly urticaria and anaphylaxis, associated with the presence of IgE. Inasmuch as the mast cell is a key effector cell in allergic rhinitis and asthma, and the dominant effector in urticaria, anaphylaxis, and systemic mastocytosis, its developmental biology, activation pathway, product profile, and target tissues will be considered in the introduction to these clinical disorders.

The binding of IgE to human mast cells and basophils, a process termed *sensitization*, prepares these cells for subsequent antigen-specific activation. The high-affinity Fc receptor for IgE, designated FcεRI, is composed of one α, one β, and two disulfide-linked γ chains, which together cross the plasma membrane seven times. The α chain is responsible for IgE binding, and the β and γ chains provide for signal transduction that follows the aggregation of the sensitized tetrameric receptors by polymeric antigen. The binding of IgE stabilizes the α chain at the plasma membrane, thus increasing the density of FcεRI receptors at the cell surface while sensitizing the cell for effector responses. This accounts for the correlation between serum IgE levels and the numbers of FcεRI receptors detected on circulating basophils.

Signal transduction is initiated through the action of a Src family–related tyrosine kinase termed Lyn that is constitutively associated with the β chain. Lyn transphosphorylates the canonical immunoreceptor tyrosine-based activation motifs (ITAMs) of the β and γ chains of the receptor, resulting in recruitment of more active Lyn to the β chain and of Syk tyrosine kinase. The phosphorylated tyrosines in the ITAMs function as binding sites for the tandem *src* homology two (SH2) domains within Syk. Syk activates not only phospholipase Cγ, which associates with the linker of activated T cells at the plasma membrane, but also phosphatidylinositol 3-kinase to provide phosphatidylinositol-3,4,5-trisphosphate, which allows membrane targeting of the Tec family kinase Btk and its activation by Lyn. In addition, the Src family tyrosine kinase Fyn becomes activated after aggregation of IgE receptors and phosphorylates the adapter protein Gab2 that enhances activation of phosphatidylinositol 3-kinase. Indeed, this additional input is essential for mast cell activation, but it can be partially inhibited by Lyn, indicating that the extent of mast cell activation is in part regulated by the interplay between these Src family kinases. Activated phospholipase Cγ cleaves phospholipid membrane substrates to provide inositol-1,4,5-trisphosphate (IP_3) and 1,2-diacylglycerols (1,2-DAGs) so as to mobilize intracellular calcium and activate protein kinase C, respectively. The subsequent opening of calcium-regulated activated channels provides the sustained elevations of intracellular calcium required to recruit the mitogen-activated protein kinases, ERK, JNK, and p38 (serine/threonine kinases), which provide cascades to augment arachidonic acid release and to mediate nuclear translocation of transcription factors for various cytokines. The calcium ion–dependent activation of phospholipases cleaves membrane phospholipids to generate lysophospholipids, which, like 1,2-DAG, may facilitate the fusion of the secretory granule perigranular membrane with the cell membrane, a step that releases the membrane-free granules containing the preformed mediators of mast cell effects.

The secretory granule of the human mast cell has a crystalline structure, unlike mast cells of lower species. IgE-dependent cell activation results in solubilization and swelling of the granule contents within the first minute of receptor perturbation; this reaction is followed by the ordering of intermediate filaments about the swollen granule, movement of the granule toward the cell surface, and fusion of the perigranular membrane with that of other granules and with the plasmalemma to form extracellular channels for mediator release while maintaining cell viability.

In addition to exocytosis, aggregation of FcεRI initiates two other pathways for generation of bioactive products, namely, lipid mediators and cytokines. The biochemical steps involved in expression of such cytokines as tumor necrosis factor α (TNF-α), interleukin (IL) 1, IL-6, IL-4, IL-5, IL-13, granulocyte-macrophage colony-stimulating factor (GM-CSF), and others, including an array of chemokines, have not been specifically defined for mast cells. Inhibition studies of cytokine production (IL-1β, TNF-α, and IL-6) in mouse mast cells with cyclosporine or FK506 reveal binding to the ligand-specific immunophilin and attenuation of the calcium ion- and calmodulin-dependent serine/threonine phosphatase, calcineurin.

Lipid mediator generation (Fig. 376-1) involves translocation of calcium ion–dependent cytosolic phospholipase A_2 to the outer nuclear membrane, with subsequent release of arachidonic acid for metabolic processing by the distinct prostanoid and leukotriene pathways. The constitutive prostaglandin endoperoxide synthase-1 (PGHS-1/cyclooxygenase-1) and the de novo inducible PGHS-2 (cyclooxygenase-2) convert released arachidonic acid to the sequential intermediates, prostaglandins G_2 and H_2. The glutathione-dependent hematopoietic prostaglandin D_2 (PGD_2) synthase then converts PGH_2 to PGD_2, the predominant mast cell prostanoid. The PGD_2 receptor DP_1 is expressed by platelets and epithelial cells, whereas DP_2 is expressed by T_H2 lymphocytes, eosinophils, and basophils. Mast cells also generate thromboxane A_2 (TXA_2), a short lived but powerful mediator that induces bronchoconstriction and platelet activation through the T prostanoid (TP) receptor.

For leukotriene biosynthesis, the released arachidonic acid is metabolized by 5-lipoxygenase (5-LO) in the presence of an integral nuclear membrane protein, 5-LO activating protein (FLAP). The calcium ion–dependent translocation of 5-LO to the nuclear membrane converts the arachidonic acid to the sequential intermediates, 5-hydroperoxyeicosatetraenoic acid (5-HPETE) and leukotriene (LT) A_4. LTA_4 is conjugated with reduced glutathione by LTC_4 synthase, an integral nuclear membrane protein homologous to FLAP. Intracellular LTC_4 is released by a carrier-specific export step for extracellular metabolism to the additional cysteinyl leukotrienes, LTD_4 and LTE_4, by the sequential removal of glutamic acid and glycine. Alternatively, cytosolic LTA_4 hydrolase converts some LTA_4 to the dihydroxy leukotriene LTB_4, which also undergoes specific export. Two receptors for LTB_4, BLT_1 and BLT_2, mediate chemotaxis of human neutrophils. Two receptors for the cysteinyl leukotrienes, $CysLT_1$ and $CysLT_2$, are present on smooth muscle of the airways and the microvasculature and on hematopoietic cells such as macrophages, eosinophils, and mast cells. Whereas the $CysLT_1$ receptor has a preference for LTD_4 and is blocked by the receptor antagonists in clinical use, the $CysLT_2$ receptor is equally responsive to LTD_4 and LTC_4, is unaffected by these antagonists, and is a negative regulator of the function of the $CysLT_1$ receptor. LTD_4, acting at $CysLT_1$ receptors, is the most potent known bronchoconstrictor, whereas LTE_4 induces a vascular leak and mediates the recruitment of eosinophils to the bronchial mucosa. Studies in gene-deleted mice indicate the existence of additional receptors for LTE_4. The lysophospholipid formed during the release of arachidonic acid from 1-*O*-alkyl-2-acyl-*sn*-glyceryl-3-phosphorylcholine can be acetylated in the second position to form platelet-activating factor (PAF). Serum levels of PAF correlated positively with the severity of anaphylaxis to peanut in a recent study, whereas the levels of PAF acetyl hydrolase (a PAF-degrading enzyme) were inversely related to the same outcome.

Unlike most other cells of bone marrow origin, mast cells circulate as committed progenitors lacking their characteristic secretory granules. These committed progenitors express *c-kit*, the receptor for stem cell factor (SCF). Unlike most other lineages, they retain and

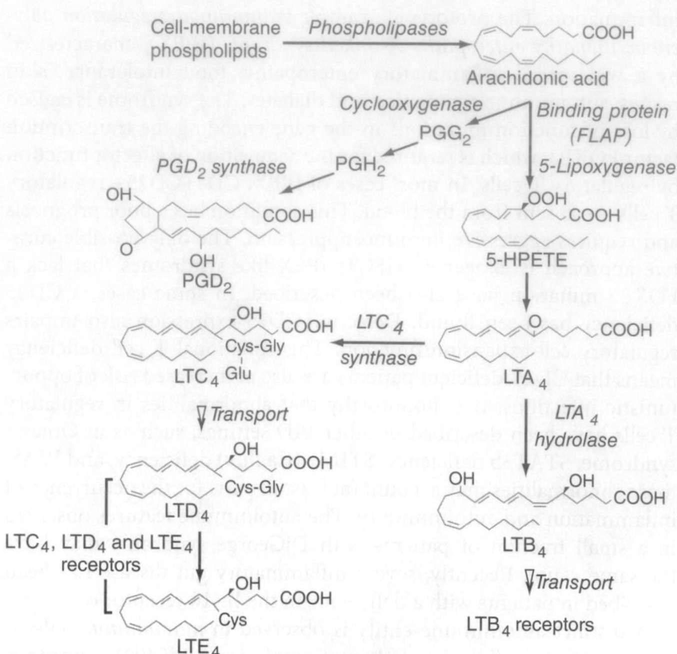

FIGURE 376-1 Pathways for biosynthesis and release of membrane-derived lipid mediators from mast cells. In the 5-lipoxygenase pathway, leukotriene A_4 (LTA_4) is the intermediate from which the terminal-pathway enzymes generate the distinct final products, leukotriene C_4 (LTC_4) and leukotriene B_4 (LTB_4), which leave the cell by separate saturable transport systems. Gamma glutamyl transpeptidase and a dipeptidase then cleave glutamic acid and glycine from LTC_4 to form LTD_4 and LTE_4, respectively. The major mast cell product of the cyclooxygenase system is PGD_2.

increase *c-kit* expression with maturation. The SCF interaction with *c-kit* is an absolute requirement for the development of constitutive tissue mast cells residing in skin and connective tissue sites and for the accumulation of mast cells at mucosal surfaces during T_H2-type immune responses. Several T cell-derived cytokines (IL-3, IL-4, IL-5, and IL-9) can potentiate SCF-dependent mast cell proliferation and/or survival in vitro in mice and humans. Indeed, mast cells are absent from the intestinal mucosa in clinical T cell deficiencies, but are present in the submucosa. Based on the immunodetection of secretory granule neutral proteases, mast cells in the lung parenchyma and intestinal mucosa selectively express tryptase, and those in the intestinal and airway submucosa, perivascular spaces, skin, lymph nodes, and breast parenchyma express tryptase, chymase, and carboxypeptidase A (CPA). In the mucosal epithelium of severe asthmatics, mast cells can express tryptase and CPA without chymase. The secretory granules of mast cells selectively positive for tryptase exhibit closed scrolls with a periodicity suggestive of a crystalline structure by electron microscopy, whereas the secretory granules of mast cells with multiple proteases are scroll-poor, with an amorphous or lattice-like appearance.

Mast cells are distributed at cutaneous and mucosal surfaces and in submucosal tissues about venules and could influence the entry of foreign substances by their rapid response capability (Fig. 376-2). Upon stimulus-specific activation and secretory granule exocytosis, histamine and acid hydrolases are solubilized, whereas the neutral proteases, which are cationic, remain largely bound to the anionic proteoglycans, heparin and chondroitin sulfate E, with which they function as a complex. Histamine and the various lipid mediators (PGD_2, $LTC_4/D_4/E_4$, PAF) alter venular permeability, thereby allowing influx of plasma proteins such as complement and immunoglobulins, whereas LTB_4 mediates leukocyte–endothelial cell adhesion and subsequent directed migration (chemotaxis). The accumulation of leukocytes and plasma opsonins facilitates defense of the microenvironment. The inflammatory response can also be detrimental, as in asthma, where the smooth-muscle constrictor activity of the cysteinyl leukotrienes is evident and much more potent than that of histamine.

The cellular component of the mast cell–mediated inflammatory response is augmented and sustained by cytokines and chemokines. IgE-dependent activation of human skin mast cells in situ elicits TNF-α production and release, which in turn induces endothelial cell responses favoring leukocyte adhesion. Similarly, activation of purified human lung mast cells or cord blood–derived cultured mast cells in vitro results in substantial production of proinflammatory (TNF-α) and immunomodulatory cytokines (IL-4, IL-5, IL-13) and chemokines. Bronchial biopsy specimens from patients with asthma reveal that mast cells are immunohistochemically positive for IL-4 and IL-5, but that the predominant localization of IL-4, IL-5, and GM-CSF is to T cells, defined as T_H2 by this profile. IL-4 modulates the T cell phenotype to the T_H2 subtype, determines the isotype switch to IgE (as does IL-13), and upregulates FcεRI-mediated expression of cytokines by mast cells based on in vitro studies.

An immediate and late cellular phase of allergic inflammation can be induced in the skin, nose, or lung of some allergic humans with local allergen challenge. The immediate phase in the nose involves pruritus and watery discharge; in the lung, it involves bronchospasm and mucus secretion; and in the skin, it involves a wheal-and-flare response with pruritus. The reduced nasal patency, reduced pulmonary function, or erythema with swelling at the skin site in a late-phase response at 6–8 h is associated with biopsy findings of infiltrating and activated T_H2 cells, eosinophils, basophils, and some neutrophils. The progression from early mast cell activation to late cellular infiltration has been used as an experimental surrogate of rhinitis or asthma. However, in asthma, there is an intrinsic hyperreactivity of the airways independent of the associated inflammation. Moreover, early- and late-phase responses (at least in the lung) are far more sensitive to blockade of IgE-dependent mast cell activation (or actions of histamine and cysteinyl leukotrienes) than are spontaneous or virally induced asthma exacerbations.

Consideration of the mechanism of immediate-type hypersensitivity diseases in the human has focused largely on the IgE-dependent recognition of otherwise innocuous substances. A region of chromosome 5 (5q23-31) contains genes implicated in the control of IgE levels including IL-4 and IL-13, as well as IL-3 and IL-9, which are involved in mucosal mast cell hyperplasia, and IL-5 and GM-CSF, which are central to eosinophil development and their enhanced tissue viability. Genes with linkage to the specific IgE response to particular allergens include those encoding the major histocompatibility complex (MHC) and certain chains of the T cell receptor (TCR-αδ). The complexity of atopy and the associated diseases includes susceptibility, severity, and therapeutic responses, each of which is among the separate variables modulated by both innate and adaptive immune stimuli.

The induction of allergic disease requires sensitization of a predisposed individual to a specific allergen. The greatest propensity for the development of atopic allergy occurs in childhood and early adolescence. The allergen is processed by antigen-presenting cells of the monocytic lineage (particularly dendritic cells) located throughout the body at surfaces that contact the outside environment, such as the nose, lungs, eyes, skin, and intestine. These antigen-presenting cells present the epitope-bearing peptides via their MHC to T helper cells and their subsets. The T cell response depends both on cognate recognition and on the cytokine microenvironment provided by the antigen-presenting dendritic cells, with IL-4 directing a T_H2 subset, interferon (IFN) γ a T_H1 profile, and IL-6 with transforming growth factor β (TGF-β) a T_H17 subset. Allergens not only present antigenic epitopes via dendritic cells but also contain pattern recognition ligands that facilitate the immune response by direct initiation of cytokine generation from innate cell types such as basophils, mast cells, eosinophils, and others. The T_H2 response is associated with activation of specific B cells that can also present allergens or that transform into plasma cells for antibody production. Synthesis and release into the plasma of allergen-specific IgE results in sensitization of FcεR1-bearing cells such as mast cells and basophils, which become activated on exposure to the specific allergen. In certain diseases, including those associated with atopy, the monocyte and eosinophil populations can express a trimeric FcεR1, which lacks the β chain, and yet respond to its aggregation. An additional recently recognized class of *c-kit*-expressing innate cells

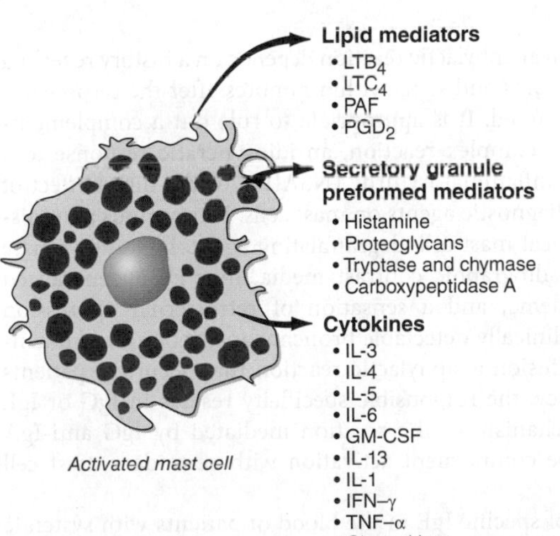

FIGURE 376-2 Bioactive mediators of three categories generated by IgE-dependent activation of murine mast cells can elicit common but sequential target cell effects leading to acute and sustained inflammatory responses. GM-CSF, granulocyte-macrophage colony-stimulating factor; IL, interleukin; IFN, interferon; LT, leukotriene; PAF, platelet-activating factor; PGD_2, prostaglandin D_2; TNF, tumor necrosis factor.

(termed nuocytes, natural helper cells, or group 2 innate lymphoid cells) can generate large quantities of IL-5 and IL-13 during antihelminth responses, are prominent in nasal polyps from humans, and could well contribute to inflammation in allergic diseases.

ANAPHYLAXIS

DEFINITION

Life-threatening anaphylactic responses of sensitized humans occur within minutes after systemic exposure to specific antigen. They are manifested by respiratory distress due to laryngeal edema and/or intense bronchospasm, often followed by vascular collapse, or by shock without antecedent respiratory difficulty. Cutaneous manifestations exemplified by pruritus and urticaria with or without angioedema are characteristic of such systemic anaphylactic reactions. Gastrointestinal manifestations include nausea, vomiting, crampy abdominal pain, and diarrhea.

PREDISPOSING FACTORS AND ETIOLOGY

There is no convincing evidence that age, sex, race, or geographic location predisposes a human to anaphylaxis except through exposure to specific immunogens. According to most studies, atopy does not predispose individuals to anaphylaxis from penicillin therapy or venom of a stinging insect but is a risk factor for allergens in food or latex. Risk factors for a poor outcome, however, include older age, use of beta blockers, and the presence of preexisting asthma. Severe hymenoptera anaphylaxis (generally with prominent hypotension) can be a presenting feature of underlying systemic mastocytosis. Additionally, some individuals suffering from recurrent episodes of idiopathic anaphylaxis possess morphologically aberrant mast cells in their bone marrow that express a mutant, constitutively active form of c-*kit*, even without evidence of frank mastocytosis.

The materials capable of eliciting the systemic anaphylactic reaction in humans include the following: heterologous proteins in the form of hormones (insulin, vasopressin, parathormone); enzymes (trypsin, chymotrypsin, penicillinase, streptokinase); pollen extracts (ragweed, grass, trees); nonpollen allergen extracts (dust mites, dander of cats, dogs, horses, and laboratory animals); food (peanuts, milk, eggs, seafood, nuts, grains, beans, gelatin in capsules); monoclonal antibodies; occupation-related products (latex rubber products); Hymenoptera venom (yellow jacket, yellow and white-faced hornets, paper wasp, honey bee, imported fire ants); polysaccharides such as dextran and thiomersal as a vaccine preservative; drugs such as protamine; antibiotics (penicillins, cephalosporins, amphotericin B, nitrofurantoin, quinolones); chemotherapy agents (carboplatin, paclitaxel, doxorubicin); local anesthetics (procaine, lidocaine); muscle relaxants (suxamethonium, gallamine, pancuronium); vitamins (thiamine, folic acid); diagnostic agents (sodium dehydrocholate, sulfobromophthalein); biologics (omalizumab, rituximab, etanercept); and occupation-related chemicals (ethylene oxide). Drugs function as haptens that form immunogenic conjugates with host proteins. The conjugating hapten may be the parent compound, a nonenzymatically derived storage product, or a metabolite formed in the host. Recombinant biologics can also induce the formation of IgE against the proteins or against glycosylated structures that serve as immunogens. Most recently, outbreaks of anaphylaxis to the anti-epidermal growth factor antibody cetuximab were reported in association with elevated titers of serum IgE to alpha-1,3-galactose, an oligosaccharide found on certain nonprimate proteins. Alpha-galactose antibodies also account for some episodes of delayed anaphylaxis to beef, lamb, and pork.

PATHOPHYSIOLOGY AND MANIFESTATIONS

Individuals differ in the time of appearance of symptoms and signs, but the hallmark of the anaphylactic reaction is the onset of some manifestation within seconds to minutes after introduction of the antigen (with the exception of alpha-galactose allergy), generally by injection or less commonly by ingestion. There may be upper or lower airway obstruction or both. Laryngeal edema may be experienced as a "lump" in the throat, hoarseness, or stridor, whereas bronchial obstruction is associated with a feeling of tightness in the chest and/or audible wheezing. Patients with asthma are predisposed to severe involvement of the lower airways and increased mortality. Flushing with diffuse erythema and a feeling of warmth may occur. A characteristic feature is the eruption of well-circumscribed, discrete cutaneous wheals with erythematous, raised, serpiginous borders and blanched centers. These urticarial eruptions are intensely pruritic and may be localized or disseminated. They may coalesce to form giant hives, and they seldom persist beyond 48 h. A localized, nonpitting, deeper edematous cutaneous process, angioedema, may also be present. It may be asymptomatic or cause a burning or stinging sensation. Angioedema of the bowel wall may cause sufficient intravascular volume depletion to precipitate cardiovascular collapse.

In fatal cases with clinical bronchial obstruction, the lungs show marked hyperinflation on gross and microscopic examination. The microscopic findings in the bronchi, however, are limited to luminal secretions, peribronchial congestion, submucosal edema, and eosinophilic infiltration, and the acute emphysema is attributed to intractable bronchospasm that subsides with death. The angioedema resulting in death by mechanical obstruction occurs in the epiglottis and larynx, but the process also is evident in the hypopharynx and to some extent in the trachea. On microscopic examination, there is wide separation of the collagen fibers and the glandular elements; vascular congestion and eosinophilic infiltration also are present. Patients dying of vascular collapse without antecedent hypoxia from respiratory insufficiency have visceral congestion with a presumptive loss of intravascular fluid volume. The associated electrocardiographic abnormalities, with or without infarction, in some patients may reflect a primary cardiac event mediated by mast cells (which are prominent near the coronary vessels) or may be secondary to a critical reduction in blood volume.

The angioedematous and urticarial manifestations of anaphylaxis have been attributed to the release of endogenous histamine. A role for the cysteinyl leukotrienes in causing marked bronchiolar constriction seems likely. Vascular collapse without respiratory distress in response to experimental challenge with the sting of a hymenopteran was associated with marked and prolonged elevations in blood histamine and intravascular coagulation and kinin generation. The finding that patients with systemic mastocytosis and episodic vascular collapse excrete large amounts of PGD_2 metabolites in addition to histamine suggests that PGD_2 is also of importance in the hypotensive anaphylactic reactions. As noted, serum PAF levels correlate with severity of anaphylaxis and are inversely proportional to the constitutive level of the acetylhydrolase involved in PAF inactivation. The actions of the array of mast cell–derived mediators are likely additive or synergistic at the target tissues.

DIAGNOSIS

The diagnosis of an anaphylactic reaction depends on a history revealing the onset of symptoms and signs within minutes after the responsible material is encountered. It is appropriate to rule out a complement-mediated immune complex reaction, an idiosyncratic response to a nonsteroidal anti-inflammatory drug (NSAID), or the direct effect of certain drugs or diagnostic agents on mast cells. Intravenous administration of a chemical mast cell–degranulating agent, including opiate derivatives and radiographic contrast media, may elicit generalized urticaria, angioedema, and a sensation of retrosternal oppression with or without clinically detectable bronchoconstriction or hypotension. In the transfusion anaphylactic reaction that occurs in patients with IgA deficiency, the responsible specificity resides in IgG or IgE anti-IgA; the mechanism of the reaction mediated by IgG anti-IgA is presumed to be complement activation with secondary mast cell participation.

The presence of specific IgE in the blood of patients with systemic anaphylaxis was demonstrated historically by passive transfer of the serum intradermally into a normal recipient, followed 24 h later by antigen challenge into the same site, with subsequent development of a wheal and flare (the *Prausnitz-Küstner reaction*). In current clinical practice, immunoassays using purified or recombinant antigens can demonstrate the presence of specific IgE in the serum of patients with anaphylactic reactions, and skin testing may be performed after the patient has recovered to elicit a local wheal and flare in response to the putative antigen. Elevations of tryptase levels in serum implicate mast cell activation in a systemic reaction and are particularly informative for anaphylaxis with episodes of hypotension during general anesthesia or when there has been a fatal outcome. However, because of the short half-life of tryptase, elevated levels are best detected within 4 h of a systemic reaction. Moreover, anaphylactic reactions to foods characteristically are not associated with elevations in serum tryptase.

TREATMENT ANAPHYLAXIS

Early recognition of an anaphylactic reaction is mandatory, since death can occur within minutes to hours after the first symptoms. Mild symptoms such as pruritus and urticaria can be controlled by administration of 0.3–0.5 mL of 1:1000 (1 mg/mL) epinephrine SC or IM, with repeated doses as required at 5- to 20-min intervals for a severe reaction. The failure to use epinephrine within the first 20 min of symptoms is a risk factor for poor outcome in studies of anaphylaxis to food. If the antigenic material was injected into an extremity, the rate of absorption may be reduced by prompt application of a tourniquet proximal to the reaction site, administration of 0.2 mL of 1:1000 epinephrine into the site, and removal without compression of an insect stinger, if present. An IV infusion should be initiated to provide a route for administration of 2.5 mL epinephrine, diluted 1:10,000, at 5- to 10-min intervals, volume expanders such as normal saline, and vasopressor agents such as dopamine if intractable hypotension occurs. Replacement of intravascular volume due to postcapillary venular leakage may require several liters of saline. Epinephrine provides both α- and β-adrenergic effects, resulting in vasoconstriction, bronchial smooth-muscle relaxation, and attenuation of enhanced venular permeability. Oxygen alone via a nasal catheter or with nebulized albuterol may be helpful, but either endotracheal intubation or a tracheostomy is mandatory for oxygen delivery if progressive hypoxia develops. Ancillary agents such as the antihistamine diphenhydramine, 50–100 mg IM or IV, and aminophylline, 0.25–0.5 g IV, are appropriate for urticaria-angioedema and bronchospasm, respectively. Intravenous glucocorticoids, 0.5–1 mg/kg of methylprednisolone, are not effective for the acute event but may alleviate later recurrence of bronchospasm, hypotension, or urticaria.

PREVENTION

Prevention of anaphylaxis must take into account the sensitivity of the individual, the dose and character of the diagnostic or therapeutic agent, and the effect of the route of administration on the rate of absorption. Beta blockers are relatively contraindicated in persons at risk for anaphylactic reactions, especially those sensitive to Hymenoptera venom or those undergoing immunotherapy for respiratory system allergy. If there is a definite history of a past anaphylactic reaction to a medication, it is advisable to select a structurally unrelated agent. A knowledge of cross-reactivity among agents is critical since, for example, cephalosporins have a cross-reactive ring structure with the penicillins. When skin testing, a prick or scratch skin test should precede an intradermal test, since the latter has a higher risk of causing anaphylaxis. These tests should be performed before the administration of certain materials that are likely to elicit anaphylactic reactions, such as allergenic extracts. Skin testing for antibiotics or chemotherapeutic agents should be performed only on patients with a positive clinical history consistent with an IgE-mediated reaction and in imminent need of the antibiotic in question; skin testing is of no value for non-IgE-mediated eruptions. With regard to penicillin, two-thirds of patients with a positive reaction history and positive skin tests to benzylpenicilloyl-polylysine (BPL) and/or the minor determinant mixture (MDM) of benzylpenicillin products experience allergic reactions with treatment, and these reactions are almost uniformly of the anaphylactic type in those patients with minor determinant reactivity. Even patients without a history of previous clinical reactions have a 2–6% incidence of positive skin tests to the two test materials, and about 3 per 1000 with a negative history experience anaphylaxis with therapy, with a mortality of about 1 per 100,000.

If an agent carrying a risk of eliciting an anaphylactic response is required because a non-cross-reactive alternative is not available, desensitization can be performed with most antibiotics and other classes of therapeutic agents by the IV, SC, or PO route. Typically, graded quantities of the drug are given by the selected route starting below the threshold dose for an adverse reaction and then doubling each dose until a therapeutic dosage is achieved. Due to the risk of systemic anaphylaxis during the course of desensitization, such a procedure should be performed under the supervision of a specialist and in a setting in which resuscitation equipment is at hand and an IV line is in place. Once a desensitized state is achieved, it is critical to continue administration of the therapeutic agent at regular intervals throughout the treatment period to prevent the reestablishment of a significant pool of sensitized cells.

A different form of protection involves the development of blocking antibody of the IgG class, which protects against Hymenoptera venom–induced anaphylaxis by interacting with antigen so that less reaches the sensitized tissue mast cells. The maximal risk for systemic anaphylactic reactions in persons with Hymenoptera sensitivity occurs in association with a currently positive skin test. Although there is little cross-reactivity between honey bee and yellow jacket venoms, there is a high degree of cross-reactivity between yellow jacket venom and the rest of the vespid venoms (yellow or white-faced hornets and wasps). Prevention involves modification of outdoor activities to exclude bare feet, wearing perfumed toiletries, eating in areas attractive to insects, clipping hedges or grass, and hauling away trash or fallen fruit. As with each anaphylactic sensitivity, the individual should wear an informational bracelet and have immediate access to an unexpired autoinjectable epinephrine kit. Venom immunotherapy for 5 years can induce a state of resistance to sting reactions that is independent of serum levels of specific IgG or IgE. For children under the age of 10 with a systemic reaction limited to skin, the likelihood of progression to more serious respiratory or vascular manifestations is low, and thus immunotherapy is not recommended.

URTICARIA AND ANGIOEDEMA

DEFINITION

Urticaria and angioedema may appear separately or together as cutaneous manifestations of localized nonpitting edema; a similar process may occur at mucosal surfaces of the upper respiratory or gastrointestinal tract. *Urticaria* involves only the superficial portion of the dermis, presenting as well-circumscribed wheals with erythematous raised serpiginous borders and blanched centers that may coalesce to become giant wheals. *Angioedema* is a well-demarcated localized edema involving the deeper layers of the skin, including the subcutaneous tissue, and can also involve the bowel wall. Recurrent episodes of urticaria and/or angioedema of less than 6 weeks' duration are considered acute, whereas attacks persisting beyond this period are designated chronic.

PREDISPOSING FACTORS AND ETIOLOGY

Urticaria and angioedema probably occur more frequently than reported because of the evanescent, self-limited nature of such eruptions, which seldom require medical attention when limited to the skin. Although persons in any age group may experience acute or chronic urticaria and/or angioedema, these lesions increase in frequency after adolescence, with the highest incidence occurring in persons in the third decade of life; indeed, one survey of college students indicated that 15–20% had experienced a pruritic wheal reaction.

The classification of urticaria-angioedema presented in Table 376-1 focuses on the different mechanisms for eliciting clinical disease and can be useful for differential diagnosis; nonetheless, most cases of chronic urticaria are idiopathic. Urticaria and/or angioedema occurring during the appropriate season in patients with seasonal respiratory allergy or as a result of exposure to animals or molds is attributed to inhalation or physical contact with pollens, animal dander, and mold spores, respectively. However, urticaria and angioedema secondary to inhalation are relatively uncommon compared to urticaria and

TABLE 376-1 CLASSIFICATION OF URTICARIA AND/OR ANGIOEDEMA

1. **IgE-dependent**
   a. Specific antigen sensitivity (pollens, foods, drugs, fungi, molds, Hymenoptera venom, helminths)
   b. Physical: dermographism, cold, solar, pressure, cholinergic
   c. Autoimmune
2. **Bradykinin-mediated**
   a. Hereditary angioedema: C1 inhibitor deficiency: null (type 1) and dysfunctional (type 2); mutated factor XII (type 3)
   b. Acquired angioedema: C1 inhibitor deficiency: anti-idiotype and anti-C1 inhibitor
   c. Angiotensin-converting enzyme inhibitors
3. **Complement-mediated**
   a. Necrotizing vasculitis
   b. Serum sickness
   c. Reactions to blood products
4. **Nonimmunologic**
   a. Direct mast cell–releasing agents (opiates, antibiotics, curare, D-tubocurarine, radiocontrast media)
   b. Agents that alter arachidonic acid metabolism (aspirin and nonsteroidal anti-inflammatory agents, azo dyes, and benzoates)
5. **Idiopathic**

angioedema elicited by ingestion of fresh fruits, shellfish, fish, milk products, chocolate, legumes including peanuts, and various drugs that may elicit not only the anaphylactic syndrome with prominent gastrointestinal complaints but also urticaria alone.

Additional etiologies include physical stimuli such as cold, heat, solar rays, exercise, and mechanical irritation. The physical urticarias can be distinguished by the precipitating event and other aspects of the clinical presentation. *Dermographism*, which occurs in 1–4% of the population, is defined by the appearance of a linear wheal at the site of a brisk stroke with a firm object or by any configuration appropriate to the eliciting event (Fig. 376-3). Dermographism has a prevalence that peaks in the second to third decades. It is not influenced by atopy and has a duration generally of <5 years. *Pressure urticaria*, which often accompanies chronic idiopathic urticaria, presents in response to a sustained stimulus such as a shoulder strap or belt, running (feet), or manual labor (hands). *Cholinergic urticaria* is distinctive in that the pruritic wheals are of small size (1–2 mm) and are surrounded by a large area of erythema; attacks are precipitated by fever, a hot bath or shower, or exercise and are presumptively attributed to a rise in core

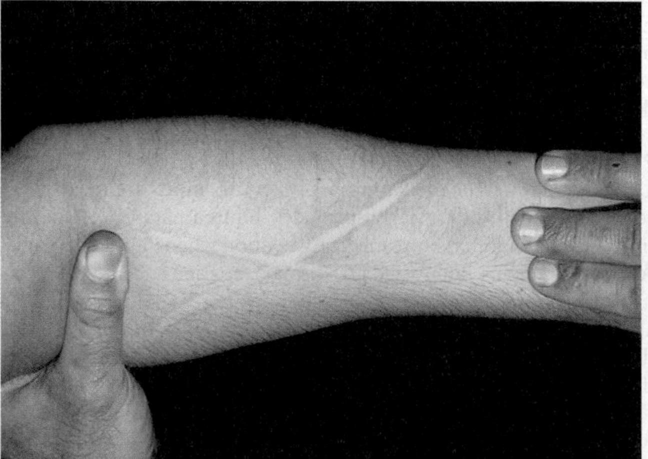

FIGURE 376-3 Dermographic urticarial lesion induced by stroking the forearm lightly with the edge of a tongue blade. The photograph, taken after 2 minutes, demonstrates a prominent wheal-and-flare reaction in the shape of an X. *(From LA Goldsmith et al [eds]: Fitzpatrick's Dermatology in General Medicine, 8th ed. New York, McGraw-Hill, 2012. Photograph provided by Allen P. Kaplan, MD, Medical University of South Carolina.)*

body temperature. *Exercise-induced anaphylaxis* can be precipitated by exertion alone or can be dependent on prior food ingestion. There is an association with the presence of IgE specific for α-5 gliadin, a component of wheat. The clinical presentation can be limited to flushing, erythema, and pruritic urticaria but may progress to angioedema of the face, oropharynx, larynx, or intestine or to vascular collapse; it is distinguished from cholinergic urticaria by presenting with wheals of conventional size and by not occurring with fever or a hot bath. *Cold urticaria* is local at body areas exposed to low ambient temperature or cold objects but can progress to vascular collapse with immersion in cold water (swimming). *Solar urticaria* is subdivided into six groups by the response to specific portions of the light spectrum. *Vibratory angioedema* may occur after years of occupational exposure or can be idiopathic; it may be accompanied by cholinergic urticaria. Other rare forms of physical allergy, always defined by stimulus-specific elicitation, include *local heat urticaria*, *aquagenic urticaria* from contact with water of any temperature (sometimes associated with polycythemia vera), and *contact urticaria* from direct interaction with some chemical substance.

Angioedema without urticaria due to the generation of bradykinin occurs with C1 inhibitor (C1INH) deficiency that may be inborn as an autosomal dominant characteristic or may be acquired through the appearance of an autoantibody. The angiotensin-converting enzyme (ACE) inhibitors can provoke a similar clinical presentation in 0.1–0.5% of hypertensive patients due to attenuated degradation of bradykinin. The urticaria and angioedema associated with classic serum sickness or with hypocomplementemic cutaneous necrotizing angiitis are believed to be immune-complex diseases. The drug reactions to mast cell granule–releasing agents and to NSAIDs may be systemic, resembling anaphylaxis, or limited to cutaneous sites.

PATHOPHYSIOLOGY AND MANIFESTATIONS

Urticarial eruptions are distinctly pruritic, may involve any area of the body from the scalp to the soles of the feet, and appear in crops of 12- to 36-h duration, with old lesions fading as new ones appear. Most of the physical urticarias (cold, cholinergic, dermatographism) are an exception, with individual lesions lasting less than 2 h. The most common sites for urticaria are the extremities and face, with angioedema often being periorbital and in the lips. Although self-limited in duration, angioedema of the upper respiratory tract may be life-threatening due to laryngeal obstruction, whereas gastrointestinal involvement may present with abdominal colic, with or without nausea and vomiting, and may result in unnecessary surgical intervention. No residual discoloration occurs with either urticaria or angioedema unless there is an underlying vasculitic process leading to superimposed extravasation of erythrocytes.

The pathology is characterized by edema of the superficial dermis in urticaria and of the subcutaneous tissue and deep dermis in angioedema. Collagen bundles in affected areas are widely separated, and the venules are sometimes dilated. Any perivenular infiltrate consists of lymphocytes, monocytes, eosinophils, and neutrophils that are present in varying combination and numbers.

Perhaps the best-studied example of IgE- and mast cell–mediated urticaria and angioedema is *cold urticaria*. Cryoglobulins or cold agglutinins are present in up to 5% of these patients. Immersion of an extremity in an ice bath precipitates angioedema of the distal portion with urticaria at the air interface within minutes of the challenge. Histologic studies reveal marked mast cell degranulation with associated edema of the dermis and subcutaneous tissues. The histamine level in the plasma of venous effluent of the cold-challenged and angioedematous extremity is markedly increased, but no such increase appears in the plasma of effluent of the contralateral normal extremity. Elevated levels of histamine have been found in the plasma of venous effluent and in the fluid of suction blisters at experimentally induced lesional sites in patients with dermographism, pressure urticaria, vibratory angioedema, light urticaria, and heat urticaria. By ultrastructural analysis, the pattern of mast cell degranulation in cold urticaria resembles an IgE-mediated response with solubilization of granule contents, fusion of the perigranular and cell membranes, and discharge of granule contents, whereas in a dermographic lesion, there is additional superimposed zonal (piecemeal) degranulation. There are several reports of resolution of cold urticaria by treatment with monoclonal anti-human IgE (omalizumab). Elevations of plasma histamine levels with biopsy-proven mast cell degranulation have also been demonstrated with generalized attacks of *cholinergic urticaria* and *exercise-related anaphylaxis* precipitated experimentally in subjects exercising on a treadmill while wearing a wet suit; however, only subjects with cholinergic urticaria have a concomitant decrease in pulmonary function.

Up to 40% of patients with chronic urticaria have an autoimmune cause for their disease including autoantibodies to IgE (5–10%) or, more commonly, to the α chain of FcεRI (35–45%). In these patients, autologous serum injected into their own skin can induce a wheal-and-flare reaction involving mast cell activation. The presence of these antibodies can also be recognized by their capacity to release histamine or induce activation markers such as CD63 or CD203 on basophils. An association with antibodies to microsomal peroxidase and/or thyroglobulin has been observed often with clinically significant Hashimoto's thyroiditis. In vitro studies reveal that these autoantibodies can mediate basophil degranulation with enhancement by serum as a source of the anaphylatoxic fragment, C5a.

Hereditary angioedema is an autosomal dominant disease due to a deficiency of C1INH (type 1) in about 85% of patients and to a dysfunctional protein (type 2) in the remainder. A third type of hereditary angioedema has been described in which C1INH function is normal, and the causal lesion is a mutant form of factor XII, which leads to generation of excessive bradykinin. In the acquired form of C1INH deficiency, there is excessive consumption due either to immune complexes formed between anti-idiotypic antibody and monoclonal IgG presented by B cell lymphomas or to an autoantibody directed to C1INH. C1INH blocks the catalytic function of activated factor XII (Hageman factor) and of kallikrein, as well as the C1r/C1s components of C1. During clinical attacks of angioedema, C1INH-deficient patients have elevated plasma levels of bradykinin, particularly in the venous effluent of an involved extremity, and reduced levels of prekallikrein and high-molecular-weight kininogen, from which bradykinin is cleaved. The parallel decline in the complement substrates C4 and C2 reflects the action of activated C1 during such attacks. Mice with targeted disruption of the gene for C1INH exhibit a chronic increase in vascular permeability. The pathobiology is aggravated by administration of an ACE inhibitor (captopril) and is attenuated by breeding the C1INH null strain to a bradykinin 2 receptor (Bk2R) null strain. As ACE is also described as kininase II, the use of blockers results in impaired bradykinin degradation and explains the angioedema that occurs idiosyncratically in hypertensive patients with a normal C1INH. Bradykinin mediated angioedema, whether caused by ACE inhibitors or by C1INH deficiency, is noteworthy for the conspicuous absence of concomitant urticaria.

DIAGNOSIS

The rapid onset and self-limited nature of urticarial and angioedematous eruptions are distinguishing features. Additional characteristics are the occurrence of the urticarial crops in various stages of evolution and the asymmetric distribution of the angioedema. Urticaria and/or angioedema involving IgE-dependent mechanisms are often appreciated by historic considerations implicating specific allergens or physical stimuli, by seasonal incidence, and by exposure to certain environments. Direct reproduction of the lesion with physical stimuli is particularly valuable because it so often establishes the cause of the lesion. The diagnosis of an environmental allergen based on the clinical history can be confirmed by skin testing or assay for allergen-specific IgE in serum. IgE-mediated urticaria and/or angioedema may or may not be associated with an elevation of total IgE or with peripheral eosinophilia. Fever, leukocytosis, and an elevated sedimentation rate are absent.

The classification of urticarial and angioedematous states presented in Table 376-1 in terms of possible mechanisms necessarily includes some differential diagnostic points. Hypocomplementemia is not observed in IgE-mediated mast cell disease and may reflect either an acquired abnormality generally attributed to the formation of immune complexes or a genetic or acquired deficiency of C1INH. Chronic recurrent urticaria, generally in females, associated with arthralgias, an elevated sedimentation rate, and normo- or hypocomplementemia suggests an underlying cutaneous necrotizing angiitis. Vasculitic urticaria typically persists longer than 72 h, whereas conventional urticaria often has a duration of 12–36 h. Confirmation depends on a biopsy that reveals cellular infiltration, nuclear debris, and fibrinoid necrosis of the venules. The same pathobiologic process accounts for the urticaria in association with such diseases as systemic lupus erythematosus or viral hepatitis with or without associated arteritis. Serum sickness per se or a similar clinical entity due to drugs includes not only urticaria but also pyrexia, lymphadenopathy, myalgia, and arthralgia or arthritis. Urticarial reactions to blood products or intravenous administration of immunoglobulin are defined by the event and generally are not progressive unless the recipient is IgA-deficient in the former case or the reagent is aggregated in the latter.

The diagnosis of hereditary angioedema is suggested not only by family history but also by the lack of pruritus and of urticarial lesions, the prominence of recurrent gastrointestinal attacks of colic, and episodes of laryngeal edema. Laboratory diagnosis depends on demonstrating a deficiency of C1INH antigen (type 1) or a nonfunctional protein (type 2) by a catalytic inhibition assay. While levels of C1 are normal, its substrates, C4 and C2, are chronically depleted and fall further during attacks due to the activation of additional C1. Patients with the acquired forms of C1INH deficiency have the same clinical manifestations but differ in the lack of a familial element. Furthermore, their sera exhibit a reduction of C1 function and C1q protein as well as C1INH, C4, and C2. Inborn C1INH deficiency and ACE inhibitor–elicited angioedema are associated with elevated levels of bradykinin. Lastly, type 3 hereditary angioedema is associated with normal levels of complement proteins.

Urticaria and angioedema are distinct from contact sensitivity, a vesicular eruption that progresses to chronic thickening of the skin with continued allergenic exposure. They also differ from atopic dermatitis, a condition that may present as erythema, edema, papules, vesiculation, and oozing proceeding to a subacute and chronic stage in which vesiculation is less marked or absent and scaling, fissuring, and lichenification predominate in a distribution that characteristically involves the flexor surfaces. In cutaneous mastocytosis, the reddish brown macules and papules, characteristic of urticaria pigmentosa, urticate with pruritus upon trauma; and in systemic mastocytosis, without or with urticaria pigmentosa, there is episodic systemic flushing with or without urtication but no angioedema.

TREATMENT URTICARIA AND ANGIOEDEMA

Identification and subsequent elimination of the etiologic factor(s) provide the most satisfactory therapeutic program; this approach is feasible to varying degrees with IgE-mediated reactions to allergens or physical stimuli. For most forms of urticaria, H_1 antihistamines such as chlorpheniramine or diphenhydramine effectively attenuate both urtication and pruritus, but because of their side effects, nonsedating agents such as loratadine, desloratadine, and fexofenadine, or low-sedating agents such as cetirizine or levocetirizine generally are used first. Cyproheptadine in dosages beginning at 8 mg and ranging up to 32 mg daily and especially hydroxyzine in dosages beginning at 40 mg and ranging up to 200 mg daily have proven effective when H_1 antihistamines fail. The addition of an H_2 antagonist such as cimetidine, ranitidine, or famotidine in conventional dosages may add benefit when H_1 antihistamines are inadequate. Doxepin, a dibenzoxepin tricyclic compound with both H_1 and H_2 receptor antagonist activity, is yet another alternative. A $CysLT_1$ receptor antagonist such as montelukast, 10 mg/d, or zafirlukast, 20 mg twice a day, can be important add-on therapy.

Topical glucocorticoids are of no value, and systemic glucocorticoids are generally avoided in idiopathic, allergen-induced, or physical urticarias due to their long-term toxicity. Systemic glucocorticoids are useful in the management of patients with pressure urticaria, vasculitic urticaria (especially with eosinophil prominence), idiopathic angioedema with or without urticaria, or chronic urticaria that responds poorly to conventional treatment. With persistent vasculitic urticaria, hydroxychloroquine, dapsone, or colchicine may be added to the regimen after hydroxyzine and before or along with systemic glucocorticoids. Cyclosporine can be efficacious for patients with chronic idiopathic or chronic autoimmune urticaria that is severe and poorly responsive to other modalities and/or where a glucocorticoid requirement is excessive. For chronic urticaria induced by autoantibody activation of mast cells and basophils or cold urticaria, monoclonal anti-IgE antibodies such as omalizumab may be considered.

The therapy of inborn C1INH deficiency has been simplified by the finding that attenuated androgens correct the biochemical defect and afford prophylactic protection; their efficacy is attributed to production by the normal gene of an amount of functional C1INH sufficient to control the spontaneous activation of C1. The antifibrinolytic agent ε-aminocaproic acid may be used for preoperative prophylaxis but is contraindicated in patients with thrombotic tendencies or ischemia due to arterial atherosclerosis. Infusion of isolated C1INH protein may be used for prophylaxis or treatment of an acute attack; a bradykinin 2 receptor antagonist and ecallantide, a kallikrein inhibitor, which are administered SC, are each being assessed for amelioration of attacks. Treatment of the underlying hematologic malignancy is indicated for acquired C1INH deficiency.

SYSTEMIC MASTOCYTOSIS

DEFINITION

Systemic mastocytosis is defined by a clonal expansion of mast cells that in most instances is indolent and nonmalignant. The mast cell expansion is generally recognized only in bone marrow and in the normal peripheral distribution sites of the cells, such as skin, gastrointestinal mucosa, liver, and spleen. Mastocytosis occurs at any age and has a slight preponderance in males. The prevalence of systemic mastocytosis is not known, a familial occurrence is rare, and atopy is not increased.

CLASSIFICATION AND PATHOPHYSIOLOGY

A consensus classification for mastocytosis recognizes cutaneous mastocytosis with variants and four systemic forms (Table 376-2). Cutaneous mastocytosis is the most common diagnosis in children, whereas the form designated as *indolent systemic mastocytosis* (ISM) accounts for the majority of adult patients; it implies that there is no evidence of an associated hematologic disorder, liver disease, or lymphadenopathy and is not known to alter life expectancy. In *systemic mastocytosis associated with clonal hematologic non–mast cell lineage disease* (SM-AHNMD), the prognosis is determined by the nature of the associated disorder, which can range from dysmyelopoiesis to leukemia. In *aggressive systemic mastocytosis* (ASM), mast cell infiltration/proliferation in multiple organs such as liver, spleen, gut, and/or bone results in a poor prognosis; a subset of patients with this form has prominent eosinophilia with hepatosplenomegaly and lymphadenopathy. *Mast cell leukemia* (MCL) is the rarest form of the disease and is invariably fatal at present; the peripheral blood contains circulating, metachromatically staining, atypical mast cells. An aleukemic form of MCL is recognized without circulating mast cells when the percentage of high-grade immature mast cells in bone marrow smears exceeds 20% in a nonspicular area. Mast cell sarcoma and extracutaneous mastocytomas are rare solid mast cell tumors with malignant and benign features, respectively.

TABLE 376-2 CLASSIFICATION OF MASTOCYTOSIS

Cutaneous mastocytosis (CM)
- Urticaria pigmentosa (UP)/maculopapular cutaneous mastocytosis (MPCM)
- Variants: plaque form, nodular form; telangiectasia macularis eruptiva perstans (TMEP)
- Solitary mastocytoma of skin
- Diffuse cutaneous mastocytosis

Indolent systemic mastocytosis (ISM)

Systemic mastocytosis with an associated clonal hematologic non–mast cell lineage disease (SM-AHNMD)

Aggressive systemic mastocytosis (ASM)

Mast cell leukemia (MCL)

Mast cell sarcoma (MCS)

Extracutaneous mastocytoma

Source: Modified from SH Swerdlow et al (eds): *World Health Organization Classification of Tumors: Pathology and Genetics in Tumors of Hematopoietic and Lymphoid Tissues.* Lyon, IARC Press, 2008.

A point mutation of A to T at codon 816 of *c-kit* that causes an aspartic acid to valine substitution is found in multiple cell lineages in patients with mastocytosis, resulting in a somatic gain-in-function mutation. This substitution, as well as other rare mutations of *c-kit*, is characteristic of patients with all forms of systemic mastocytosis but is also present in some children with cutaneous mastocytosis, as might be anticipated because mast cells are of bone marrow lineage. The prognosis for patients with cutaneous mastocytosis and for almost all with ISM is a normal life expectancy, whereas that for patients with SM-AHNMD is determined by a non–mast cell component. ASM and MCL carry a poorer prognosis. In infants and children with cutaneous manifestations, namely, urticaria pigmentosa or bullous lesions, visceral involvement is usually lacking, and resolution is common.

CLINICAL MANIFESTATIONS

The clinical manifestations of systemic mastocytosis, distinct from a leukemic complication, are due to tissue occupancy by the mast cell mass, the tissue response to that mass, and the release of bioactive substances acting at both local and distal sites. The pharmacologically induced manifestations are pruritus, flushing, palpitations and vascular collapse, gastric distress, lower abdominal crampy pain, and recurrent headache. The increase in local cell burden is evidenced by the lesions of urticaria pigmentosa at skin sites and may be a direct local cause of bone pain and/or malabsorption. Mast cell–mediated fibrotic changes occur in liver, spleen, and bone marrow but not in gastrointestinal tissue or skin. Immunofluorescent analysis of bone marrow and skin lesions in ISM and of spleen, lymph node, and skin in ASM has revealed only one mast cell phenotype, namely, scroll-poor cells expressing tryptase, chymase, and CPA.

The cutaneous lesions of urticaria pigmentosa are reddish-brown macules or papules that respond to trauma with urtication and erythema (Darier's sign). The apparent incidence of these lesions is ≥80% in patients with ISM and <50% in those with SM-AHNMD or ASM. Approximately 1% of patients with ISM have skin lesions that appear as tan-brown macules with striking patchy erythema and associated telangiectasia (telangiectasia macularis eruptiva perstans). In the upper gastrointestinal tract, gastritis and peptic ulcer are significant problems. In the lower intestinal tract, the occurrence of diarrhea and abdominal pain is attributed to increased motility due to mast cell mediators; this problem can be aggravated by malabsorption, which can also cause secondary nutritional insufficiency and osteomalacia. The periportal fibrosis associated with mast cell infiltration and a prominence of eosinophils may lead to portal hypertension and ascites. In some patients, flushing and recurrent vascular collapse are markedly aggravated by an idiosyncratic response to a minimal dosage of NSAIDs. The neuropsychiatric disturbances are clinically most evident as impaired recent memory, decreased attention span, and "migraine-like" headaches. Patients may experience exacerbation of a specific clinical sign or symptom with alcohol ingestion, temperature changes, stress, use of mast cell–interactive narcotics, or ingestion of NSAIDs.

DIAGNOSIS

Although the diagnosis of mastocytosis is generally suspected on the basis of the clinical history and physical findings, and can be supported by laboratory procedures, it can be established only by a tissue diagnosis. By convention, the diagnosis of systemic mastocytosis depends heavily on bone marrow biopsy to meet the criteria of one major plus one minor or three minor findings (Table 376-3). The bone marrow provides the major criterion by revealing aggregates of mast cells, often in paratrabecular and perivascular locations with lymphocytes and eosinophils, as well as the minor criteria of an abnormal mast cell morphology, an aberrant mast cell membrane immunophenotype, or a codon 816 mutation in any cell type. A serum total tryptase level

TABLE 376-3 DIAGNOSTIC CRITERIA FOR SYSTEMIC MASTOCYTOSIS[a]

Major: Multifocal dense infiltrates of mast cells in bone marrow or other extracutaneous tissues with confirmation by immunodetection of tryptase or metachromasia
Minor: Abnormal mast cell morphology with a spindle shape and/or multilobed or eccentric nucleus
Aberrant mast cell surface phenotype with expression of CD25 (IL-2 receptor) and CD2 in addition to C117 (c-*kit*)
Detection of codon 816 mutation in peripheral blood cells, bone marrow cells, or lesional tissue
Total serum tryptase >20 ng/mL

[a]Diagnosis requires either the major criterion and one minor criterion or three minor criteria.

and/or a 24-h urine collection for measurement of histamine, histamine metabolites, or metabolites of PGD_2 are noninvasive approaches to consider before bone marrow biopsy. The pro-β and α forms of tryptase are elevated in more than one-half of patients with systemic mastocytosis and provide a minor criterion; the fully processed ("mature") β form is increased in patients undergoing an anaphylactic reaction. Additional studies directed by the presentation include a bone densitometry, bone scan, or skeletal survey; contrast studies of the upper gastrointestinal tract with small-bowel follow-through, computed tomography scan, or endoscopy; and a neuropsychiatric evaluation. Osteoporosis is increased in mastocytosis and may lead to pathologic fractures.

The differential diagnosis requires the exclusion of other flushing disorders. The 24-h urine assessment of 5-hydroxy-indoleacetic acid and metanephrines should exclude a carcinoid tumor or a pheochromocytoma. Some patients presenting with recurrent mast cell activation symptoms without an obvious increase in mast cell burden in skin or bone marrow have been shown to carry aberrant mast cells with clonality markers of D816C c-*kit* mutation or surface CD25 expression. Most patients with recurrent anaphylaxis, including the idiopathic group, present with angioedema and/or wheezing, which are not manifestations of systemic mastocytosis.

TREATMENT SYSTEMIC MASTOCYTOSIS

The management of systemic mastocytosis uses a stepwise and symptom/sign–directed approach that includes an H_1 antihistamine for flushing and pruritus, an H_2 antihistamine or proton pump inhibitor for gastric acid hypersecretion, oral cromolyn sodium for diarrhea and abdominal pain, and aspirin for severe flushing with or without associated vascular collapse, despite use of H_1 and H_2 antihistamines, to block biosynthesis of PGD_2. Systemic glucocorticoids appear to alleviate the malabsorption. Mast cell cytoreductive therapy consisting of IFN-α or cladribine is generally reserved for advanced, nonindolent variants of systemic mastocytosis. Their efficacy in ASM is variable, perhaps because of dosage limitations due to side effects. Chemotherapy is appropriate for the frank leukemias. A self-injectable epinephrine prescription is recommended for most patients due to increased incidence of anaphylaxis. Although c-*kit* is a receptor tyrosine kinase, the gain-in-function mutation of codon 816 is not susceptible to inhibition by imatinib mesylate.

ALLERGIC RHINITIS

DEFINITION

Allergic rhinitis is characterized by sneezing; rhinorrhea; obstruction of the nasal passages; conjunctival, nasal, and pharyngeal itching; and lacrimation, all occurring in a temporal relationship to allergen exposure. Although commonly seasonal due to elicitation by airborne pollens, it can be perennial in an environment of chronic exposure to house dust mites, animal danders, or insect products. In North America, the incidence of allergic rhinitis is about 7%. The overall prevalence in North America is nearly 20%, with the peak prevalence of nearly 40% occurring in childhood and adolescence.

PREDISPOSING FACTORS AND ETIOLOGY

Allergic rhinitis generally occurs in atopic individuals, often in association with atopic dermatitis, food allergy, urticaria, and/or asthma (Chap. 309). Up to 40% of patients with rhinitis manifest asthma, whereas ~70% of individuals with asthma experience rhinitis. Symptoms generally appear before the fourth decade of life and tend to diminish gradually with aging, although complete spontaneous remissions are uncommon. A relatively small number of weeds that depend on wind rather than insects for pollination, as well as grasses and some trees, produce sufficient quantities of pollen suitable for wide distribution by air currents to elicit seasonal allergic rhinitis. The dates of pollination of these species generally vary little from year to year in a particular locale but may be quite different in another climate. In the temperate areas of North America, trees typically pollinate from March through May, grasses in June and early July, and ragweed from mid-August to early October. Molds, which are widespread in nature because they occur in soil or decaying organic matter, propagate spores in a pattern that depends on climatic conditions. Perennial allergic rhinitis occurs in response to allergens that are present throughout the year, including animal dander, cockroach-derived proteins, mold spores, or dust mites such as *Dermatophagoides farinae* and *Dermatophagoides pteronyssinus*. Dust mites are scavengers of human skin and excrete cysteine protease allergens in their feces. In up to one-half of patients with perennial rhinitis, no clear-cut allergen can be demonstrated as causative. The ability of many allergens to cause rhinitis rather than lower respiratory tract symptoms (particularly pollens) may be attributed to their large size, 10–100 μm, and retention within the nose.

PATHOPHYSIOLOGY AND MANIFESTATIONS

Episodic rhinorrhea, sneezing, obstruction of the nasal passages with lacrimation, and pruritus of the conjunctiva, nasal mucosa, and oropharynx are the hallmarks of allergic rhinitis. The nasal mucosa is pale and boggy, the conjunctiva congested and edematous, and the pharynx generally unremarkable. Swelling of the turbinates and mucous membranes with obstruction of the sinus ostia and eustachian tubes precipitates secondary infections of the sinuses and middle ear, respectively. Nasal polyps, representing mucosal protrusions containing edema fluid with variable numbers of eosinophils and degranulated mast cells, can increase obstructive symptoms and can concurrently arise within the nasopharynx or sinuses. However, atopy is not a risk factor for nasal polyps, which instead may occur in the setting of the aspirin-intolerant triad of rhinosinusitis and asthma and in patients with chronic staphylococcal colonization, which produces superantigens leading to an intense T_H2 inflammatory response.

The nose presents a large mucosal surface area through the folds of the turbinates and serves to adjust the temperature and moisture content of inhaled air and to filter out particulate materials >10 μm in size by impingement in a mucous blanket; ciliary action moves the entrapped particles toward the pharynx. Entrapment of pollen and digestion of the outer coat by mucosal enzymes such as lysozymes release protein allergens generally of 10,000–40,000 molecular weight. The initial interaction occurs between the allergen and intraepithelial mast cells and then proceeds to involve deeper perivenular mast cells, both of which are sensitized with specific IgE. During the symptomatic season when the mucosae are already swollen and hyperemic, there is enhanced adverse reactivity to the seasonal pollen. Biopsy specimens of nasal mucosa during seasonal rhinitis show submucosal edema with infiltration by eosinophils, along with some basophils and neutrophils.

The mucosal surface fluid contains IgA that is present because of its secretory piece and also IgE, which apparently arrives by diffusion from plasma cells in proximity to mucosal surfaces. IgE fixes to mucosal and submucosal mast cells, and the intensity of the clinical response to inhaled allergens is quantitatively related to the naturally occurring pollen dose. In sensitive individuals, the introduction of allergen into the nose is associated with sneezing, "stuffiness," and discharge, and the fluid contains histamine, PGD_2, and leukotrienes. Thus the mast cells of the nasal mucosa and submucosa generate and release mediators through IgE-dependent reactions that are capable of producing tissue edema and eosinophilic infiltration.

DIAGNOSIS

The diagnosis of seasonal allergic rhinitis depends largely on an accurate history of occurrence coincident with the pollination of the offending weeds, grasses, or trees. The continuous character of perennial allergic rhinitis due to contamination of the home or place of work makes historic analysis difficult, but there may be variability in symptoms that can be related to exposure to animal dander, dust mite and/or cockroach allergens, fungal spores, or work-related allergens such as latex. Patients with perennial rhinitis commonly develop the problem in adult life, and manifest nasal congestion and a postnasal discharge, often associated with thickening of the sinus membranes demonstrated by radiography. Perennial nonallergic rhinitis with eosinophilia syndrome (NARES) occurs in the middle decades of life and is characterized by nasal obstruction, anosmia, chronic sinusitis, and frequent aspirin intolerance. The term *vasomotor rhinitis* or *perennial nonallergic rhinitis* designates a condition of enhanced reactivity of the nasopharynx in which a symptom complex resembling perennial allergic rhinitis occurs with nonspecific stimuli, including chemical odors, temperature and humidity variations, and position changes but occurs without tissue eosinophilia or an allergic etiology. Other entities to be excluded are structural abnormalities of the nasopharynx; exposure to irritants; gustatory rhinitis associated with cholinergic activation that occurs while eating or ingesting alcohol; hypothyroidism; upper respiratory tract infection; pregnancy with prominent nasal mucosal edema; prolonged topical use of α-adrenergic agents in the form of nose drops (rhinitis medicamentosa); and the use of certain therapeutic agents such as rauwolfia, β-adrenergic antagonists, estrogens, progesterone, ACE inhibitors, aspirin and other NSAIDS, and drugs for erectile dysfunction (phosphodiesterase-5 inhibitors).

The nasal secretions of allergic patients are rich in eosinophils, and a modest peripheral eosinophilia is a common feature. Local or systemic neutrophilia implies infection. Total serum IgE is frequently elevated, but the demonstration of immunologic specificity for IgE is critical to an etiologic diagnosis. A skin test by the intracutaneous route (puncture or prick) with the allergens of interest provides a rapid and reliable approach to identifying allergen-specific IgE that has sensitized cutaneous mast cells. A positive intracutaneous skin test with 1:10–1:20 weight/volume of extract has a high predictive value for the presence of allergy. An intradermal test with a 1:500–1:1000 dilution of 0.05 mL may follow if indicated by history when the intracutaneous test is negative, but while more sensitive, it is less reliable due to the reactivity of some asymptomatic individuals at the test dose. Skin testing by the intracutaneous route for food allergens can be supportive of the clinical history. A double-blind, placebo-controlled challenge may document a food allergy, but such a procedure does bear the risk of an anaphylactic reaction. An elimination diet is safer but is tedious and less definitive. Food allergy is uncommon as a cause of allergic rhinitis.

Newer methodology for detecting total IgE, including the development of enzyme-linked immunosorbent assays (ELISA) employing anti-IgE bound to either a solid-phase or a liquid-phase particle, provides rapid and cost-effective determinations. Measurements of specific anti-IgE in serum are obtained by its binding to an allergen and quantitation by subsequent uptake of labeled anti-IgE. As compared to the skin test, the assay of specific IgE in serum is less sensitive but has high specificity.

PREVENTION

Avoidance of exposure to the offending allergen is the most effective means of controlling allergic diseases; removal of pets from the home to avoid animal danders, utilization of air-filtration devices to minimize the concentrations of airborne pollens, elimination of cockroach-derived proteins by chemical destruction of the pest and careful food storage, travel to areas where the allergen is not being generated, and even a change of domicile to eliminate a mold spore problem may be necessary. Control of dust mites by allergen avoidance includes use of plastic-lined covers for mattresses, pillows, and comforters; using a filter-equipped vacuum cleaner; washing bedding and clothes at temperatures >54.5°C (above 130°F); and elimination of carpets and drapes.

TREATMENT ALLERGIC RHINITIS

Although allergen avoidance is the most cost-effective means of managing allergic rhinitis, treatment with pharmacologic agents represents the standard approach to seasonal or perennial allergic rhinitis. Oral H_1 antihistamines are effective for nasopharyngeal itching, sneezing, and watery rhinorrhea and for such ocular manifestations as itching, tearing, and erythema, but they are less efficacious for the nasal congestion. The older antihistamines are sedating, and they induce psychomotor impairment, including reduced eye-hand coordination and impaired automobile driving skills. Their anticholinergic (muscarinic) effects include visual disturbance, urinary retention, and constipation. Because the newer H_1 antihistamines such as fexofenadine, loratadine, desloratadine, cetirizine, levocetirizine, olopatadine, bilastine, and azelastine are less lipophilic and more H_1 selective, their ability to cross the blood-brain barrier is reduced, and thus their sedating and anticholinergic side effects are minimized. These newer antihistamines do not differ appreciably in efficacy for relief of rhinitis and/or sneezing. Azelastine nasal spray may benefit individuals with nonallergic vasomotor rhinitis, but it has an adverse effect of dysgeusia (taste perversion) in some patients. Because antihistamines have little effect on congestion, α-adrenergic agents such as phenylephrine or oxymetazoline are generally used topically to alleviate nasal congestion and obstruction. However, the duration of their efficacy is limited because of rebound rhinitis (i.e., 7- to 14-day use can lead to rhinitis medicamentosa) and such systemic responses as hypertension. Oral α-adrenergic agonist decongestants containing pseudoephedrine are standard for the management of nasal congestion, generally in combination with an antihistamine. While oral antihistamines typically reduce nasal and ocular symptoms by about one-third, pseudoephedrine must be added to achieve a similar reduction in nasal congestion. These pseudoephedrine combination products can cause insomnia and are precluded from use in patients with narrow angle glaucoma, urinary retention, severe hypertension, marked coronary artery disease, or a first-trimester pregnancy. The $CysLT_1$ blocker montelukast is approved for treatment of both seasonal and perennial rhinitis, and it reduces both nasal and ocular symptoms by about 20%. Cromolyn sodium, a nasal spray, is essentially without side effects and is used prophylactically on a continuous basis during the season. Intranasal high-potency glucocorticoids are the most potent drugs available for the relief of established rhinitis, seasonal or perennial, and are effective in relieving nasal congestion. They provide efficacy with substantially reduced side effects as compared with this same class of agent administered orally. Their most frequent side effect is local irritation, with *Candida* overgrowth being a rare occurrence. The currently available intranasal glucocorticoids—beclomethasone, flunisolide, triamcinolone, budesonide, fluticasone propionate, fluticasone furoate, ciclesonide, and mometasone furoate—are equally effective for nasal symptom relief, including nasal congestion; these agents all achieve up to 70% overall symptom relief with some variation in the time period for onset of benefit. Topical ipratropium is an anticholinergic agent effective in reducing rhinorrhea, including that in patients with perennial symptoms, and it can be additionally efficacious when combined with intranasal glucocorticoids. Local treatment with cromolyn sodium is effective in treating mild allergic conjunctivitis. Topical antihistamines such as olopatadine, azelastine, ketotifen, or epinastine administered to the eye provide rapid relief of itching and redness and are more effective than oral antihistamines.

Immunotherapy, often termed *hyposensitization*, consists of repeated subcutaneous injections of gradually increasing concentrations of the allergen(s) considered to be specifically responsible for the symptom complex. Controlled studies of ragweed, grass, dust mite, and cat dander allergens administered for treatment of allergic rhinitis have demonstrated at least partial relief of symptoms and

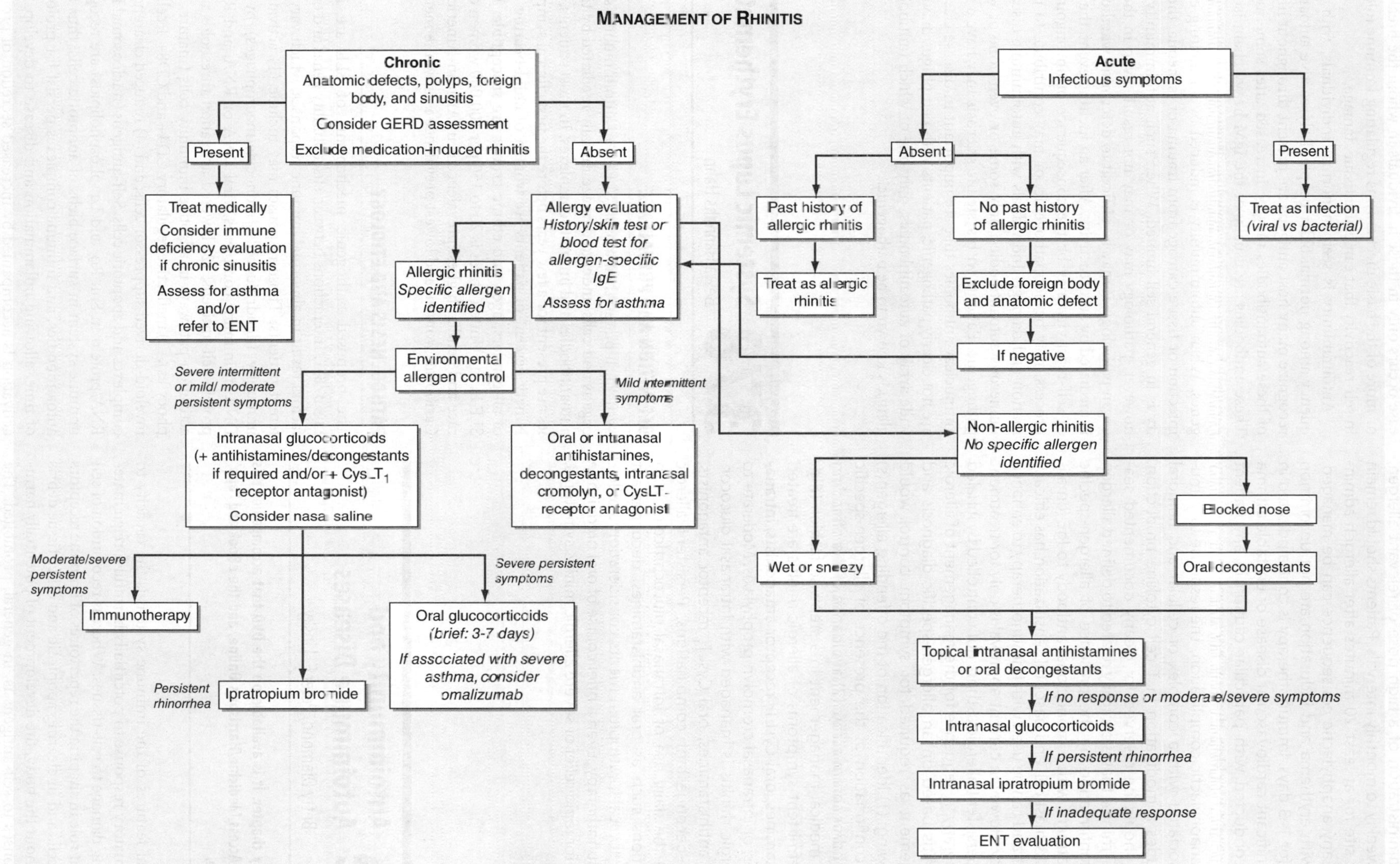

FIGURE 376-4 Algorithm for the diagnosis and management of rhinitis. ENT, ear, nose, and throat; GERD, gastroesophageal reflux disease.

signs. The duration of such immunotherapy is 3–5 years, with discontinuation being based on minimal symptoms over two consecutive seasons of exposure to the allergen. Clinical benefit appears related to the administration of a high dose of relevant allergen, advancing from weekly to monthly intervals. Patients should remain at the treatment site for at least 20 minutes after allergen administration so that any anaphylactic consequence can be managed. Local reactions with erythema and induration are not uncommon and may persist for 1–3 days. Immunotherapy is contraindicated in patients with significant cardiovascular disease or unstable asthma and should be conducted with particular caution in any patient requiring β-adrenergic blocking therapy because of the difficulty in managing an anaphylactic complication. The response to immunotherapy is associated with a complex of cellular and humoral effects that includes a modulation in T cell cytokine production. Immunotherapy should be reserved for clearly documented seasonal or perennial rhinitis that is clinically related to defined allergen exposure with confirmation by the presence of allergen-specific IgE. Systemic treatment with a monoclonal antibody to IgE (omalizumab) that blocks mast cell and basophil sensitization has efficacy for allergic rhinitis and can be used with immunotherapy to enhance safety and efficacy. However, current approval is only for treatment of patients with persistent allergic asthma not controlled by inhaled glucocorticoid therapy. A sequence for the management of allergic or perennial rhinitis based on an allergen-specific diagnosis and stepwise management as required for symptom control would include the following: (1) identification of the offending allergen(s) by history with confirmation of the presence of allergen-specific IgE by skin test and/or serum assay; (2) avoidance of the offending allergen; and (3) medical management in a stepwise fashion (Fig. 376-4). Mild intermittent symptoms of allergic rhinitis are treated with oral antihistamines, oral $CysLT_1$ receptor antagonists, intranasal antihistamines, or intranasal cromolyn prophylaxis. Moderate to more severe allergic rhinitis is managed with intranasal glucocorticoids plus oral antihistamines, oral $CysLT_1$ receptor antagonists, or antihistamine-decongestant combinations. Persistent allergic rhinitis requiring the daily use of intranasal glucocorticoids with add-on interventions such as oral antihistamines, decongestant combinations, or topical ipratropium merits consideration of allergen-specific immunotherapy. Even a brief course of oral prednisone can be indicated for rapid relief of severe allergic rhinitis symptoms.

377e Autoimmunity and Autoimmune Diseases

Betty Diamond, Peter E. Lipsky

This is a digital-only chapter. It is available on the DVD that accompanies this book, as well as on Access Medicine/Harrison's Online, and the eBook and "app" editions of HPIM 19e.

One of the central features of the immune system is the capacity to mount an inflammatory response to potentially harmful foreign materials while avoiding damage to self-tissues. Whereas recognition of self plays an important role in shaping the repertoires of immune receptors on both T and B cells and in clearing apoptotic and other tissue debris from sites throughout the body, the development of potentially harmful immune responses to self-antigens is, in general, prohibited. The essential feature of an *autoimmune disease* is that tissue injury is caused by the immunologic reaction of the organism against its own tissues. *Autoimmunity*, on the other hand, refers merely to the presence of antibodies or T lymphocytes that react with self-antigens and does not necessarily imply that the self-reactivity has pathogenic consequences. Autoimmunity is present in all individuals; however, autoimmune disease occurs only in those individuals in whom the breakdown of one or more of the basic mechanisms regulating immune tolerance results in self-reactivity that can cause tissue damage.

Autoimmunity is seen in normal individuals, with a higher frequency among normal older people. Polyreactive autoantibodies that recognize many host antigens are present throughout life. Expression of these autoantibodies may be increased after some inciting events. These antibodies are usually of the IgM heavy chain isotype and are encoded by nonmutated germline immunoglobulin variable region genes. When autoimmunity is induced by an inciting event, such as infection or tissue damage from trauma or ischemia, the autoreactivity is in general self-limited. When such autoimmunity does persist, however, pathology may or may not result. Even in the presence of organ pathology, it may be difficult to determine whether the damage is mediated by autoreactivity. After an inciting event, the development of self-reactivity may be the consequence of an ongoing pathologic process, may be nonpathogenic, or may contribute to tissue inflammation and damage. Individuals with autoimmune disease may have numerous autoantibodies, only some or even none of which may be pathogenic. Patients with systemic sclerosis may have a wide array of antinuclear antibodies that are important in disease classification but are not clearly pathogenic; patients with pemphigus may also exhibit a wide array of autoantibodies, only one of which (antibody to desmoglein) is known to be pathogenic.

378 Systemic Lupus Erythematosus

Bevra Hannahs Hahn

DEFINITION AND PREVALENCE

Systemic lupus erythematosus (SLE) is an autoimmune disease in which organs and cells undergo damage initially mediated by tissue-binding autoantibodies and immune complexes. In most patients, autoantibodies are present for a few years before the first clinical symptom appears. Ninety percent of patients are women of child-bearing years; people of all genders, ages, and ethnic groups are susceptible. Prevalence of SLE in the United States is 20 to 150 per 100,000 women depending on race and gender; highest prevalence is in African-American and Afro-Caribbean women, and lowest prevalence is in white men.

PATHOGENESIS AND ETIOLOGY

The proposed pathogenic mechanisms of SLE are illustrated in Fig. 378-1. Interactions between susceptibility genes and environmental factors result in abnormal immune responses, which vary between different patients. Those responses may include (1) activation of innate immunity (dendritic cells, monocyte/macrophages) by CpG DNA, DNA in immune complexes, viral DNA or RNA, and RNA in RNA/protein self-antigens; (2) lowered activation thresholds and abnormal activation pathways in adaptive immunity cells (mature T and B lymphocytes); (3) ineffective regulatory CD4+ and CD8+ T cells, B cells, and myeloid-derived suppressor cells; and (4) reduced clearance of immune complexes and apoptotic cells. Self-antigens (nucleosomal DNA/protein; RNA/protein in Sm, Ro, and La; phospholipids) are recognized by the immune system in surface blebs of apoptotic cells; thus autoantigens, autoantibodies, and immune complexes persist for prolonged periods of time, allowing inflammation and disease to develop. Immune cell activation is accompanied by increased secretion of proinflammatory type 1 and 2 interferons (IFNs), tumor necrosis factor α (TNF-α), interleukin (IL) 17 and B cell-maturation/survival cytokines B lymphocyte stimulator (BLyS/BAFF), and IL-10. Upregulation of genes induced by

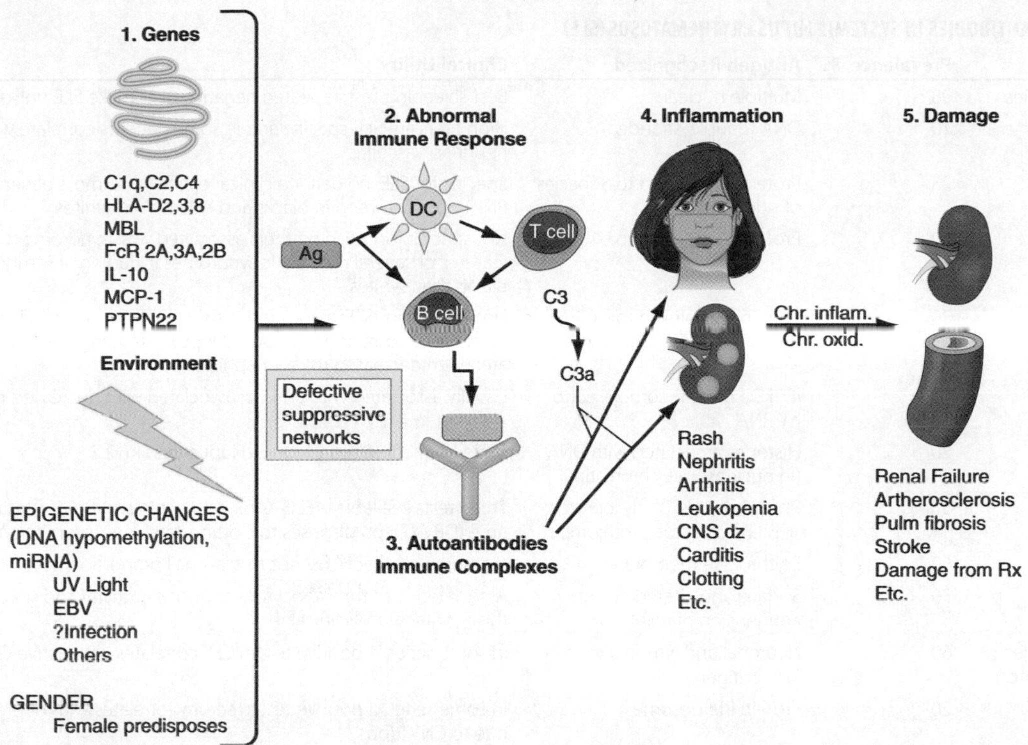

FIGURE 378-1 Pathogenesis of systemic lupus erythematosus (SLE). Genes confirmed in more than one genome-wide association analysis in northern European whites (several confirmed in Asians as well) as increasing susceptibility to SLE or lupus nephritis are listed (reviewed in SG Guerra et al: Arthritis Res Ther 14:211, 2012). Gene-environment interactions (reviewed in KH Costenbader et al: Autoimmune Rev 11:604, 2012) result in abnormal immune responses that generate pathogenic autoantibodies and immune complexes that deposit in tissue, activate complement, cause inflammation, and over time lead to irreversible organ damage (reviewed in GC Tsokos: N Engl J Med 365:2110, 2011; and BH Hahn, in DJ Wallace, BH Hahn [eds]: *Dubois' Lupus Erythematosus and Related Syndromes*, 8th ed. New York, Elsevier, 2013). Ag, antigen; C1q, complement system; C3, complement component; CNS, central nervous system; DC, dendritic cell; EBV, Epstein Barr virus; HLA, human leukocyte antigen; FcR, immunoglobulin Fc-binding receptor; IL, interleukin; MCP, monocyte chemotactic protein; PTPN, phosphotyrosine phosphatase; UV, ultraviolet.

IFNs is a genetic "signature" in peripheral blood cells of 50–60% of SLE patients. Decreased production of other cytokines also contributes to SLE: lupus T and natural killer (NK) cells fail to produce enough IL-2 and transforming growth factor beta (TGF-β) to induce and sustain regulatory CD4+ and CD8+ T cells. The result of these abnormalities is sustained production of autoantibodies (referred to in Fig. 378-1 and described in Table 378-1) and immune complexes; pathogenic subsets bind target tissues, with activation of complement, leading to release of cytokines, chemokines, vasoactive peptides, oxidants, and proteolytic enzymes. This results in activation of multiple tissue cells (endothelial cells, tissue-fixed macrophages, mesangial cells, podocytes, renal tubular epithelial cells) and influx into target tissues of T and B cells, monocyte/macrophages, and dendritic cells. In the setting of chronic inflammation, accumulation of growth factors and products of chronic oxidation contribute to irreversible tissue damage, including fibrosis/sclerosis in glomeruli, arteries, lungs, and other tissues.

SLE is a multigenic disease. Rare single-gene defects confer high hazard ratios (HRs) for SLE (5 to 25), including homozygous deficiencies of early components of complement (C1q,r,s; C2; C4) and a mutation in *TREX1* on the X chromosome. In most genetically susceptible individuals, normal alleles of multiple genes each contribute a small amount to abnormal immune/inflammation/tissue damage responses; if enough predisposing variations are present, disease results. Approximately 45 predisposing genes (examples listed in Fig. 378-1) have been identified in recent genome-wide association studies in different racial groups. Individually, they confer an HR for SLE of 1.5–3 and account for approximately 18% of disease susceptibility, suggesting that environmental exposures and epigenetics play major roles. Predisposing, antigen-presenting human leukocyte antigen (HLA) molecules are most commonly found, in multiple ethnic groups (HLA DRB1 *0301 and *1501, as well as multiple genes across the major histocompatibility complex (MHC) 120-gene region). Other genetic factors in whites include innate immunity pathway gene polymorphisms, especially associated with IFN-α (*STAT4, IRF5, IRAK1, TNFAIP3, PTPN22*), genes in lymphocyte signaling pathways (*PTPN22, PDCD-1, Ox40L, BANK-1, LYN, BLK*), genes that affect clearance of apoptotic cells or immune complexes (*C1q, FCRGIIA, FCRGIIIA, CRP, ITGAM*), genes that influence neutrophil adherence (*ITGAM*), and genes that influence DNA repair (*TREX-1*). Some polymorphisms influence clinical manifestations; such as single nucleotide polymorphisms (SNPs) of *STAT4* that associate with severe disease, anti-DNA, nephritis, and antiphospholipid syndrome, and an allele of *FCGRIIA* encoding a receptor that binds immune complexes poorly and predisposes to nephritis. Some gene effects are in promoter regions (e.g., IL-10), and others are conferred by copy numbers (e.g., C4A). In addition to genome-encoded susceptibility and protective genes, the influence of certain microRNAs (miRNAs) on gene transcription, as well as post-transcriptional epigenetic modification of DNA (which is hypomethylated in T cells of SLE patients), probably play major roles in disease susceptibility.

Some gene polymorphisms contribute to several autoimmune diseases, such as *STAT4* and *CTLA4*. All of these gene polymorphisms/transcription/epigenetic combinations influence immune responses to the external and internal environment; when such responses are too high and/or too prolonged and/or inadequately regulated, autoimmune disease results.

Female sex is permissive for SLE with evidence for hormone effects, genes on the X chromosome, and epigenetic differences between genders playing a role. Females of many mammalian species make higher antibody responses than males. Women exposed to

TABLE 378-1 AUTOANTIBODIES IN SYSTEMIC LUPUS ERYTHEMATOSUS (SLE)

Antibody	Prevalence, %	Antigen Recognized	Clinical Utility
Antinuclear antibodies	98	Multiple nuclear	Best screening test; repeated negative tests make SLE unlikely
Anti-dsDNA	70	DNA (double-stranded)	High titers are SLE-specific and in some patients correlate with disease activity, nephritis, vasculitis
Anti-Sm	25	Protein complexed to 6 species of nuclear U1 RNA	Specific for SLE; no definite clinical correlations; most patients also have anti-RNP; more common in blacks and Asians than whites
Anti-RNP	40	Protein complexed to U1 RNA	Not specific for SLE; high titers associated with syndromes that have overlap features of several rheumatic syndromes including SLE; more common in blacks than whites
Anti-Ro (SS-A)	30	Protein complexed to hY RNA, primarily 60 kDa and 52 kDa	Not specific for SLE; associated with sicca syndrome, predisposes to subacute cutaneous lupus, and to neonatal lupus with congenital heart block; associated with decreased risk for nephritis
Anti-La (SS-B)	10	47-kDa protein complexed to hY RNA	Usually associated with anti-Ro; associated with decreased risk for nephritis
Antihistone	70	Histones associated with DNA (in nucleosome, chromatin)	More frequent in drug-induced lupus than in SLE
Antiphospholipid	50	Phospholipids, β_2 glycoprotein 1 (β_2G1) cofactor, prothrombin	Three tests available—ELISAs for cardiolipin and β_2G1, sensitive prothrombin time (DRVVT); predisposes to clotting, fetal loss, thrombocytopenia
Antierythrocyte	60	Erythrocyte membrane	Measured as direct Coombs test; a small proportion develops overt hemolysis
Antiplatelet	30	Surface and altered cytoplasmic antigens on platelets	Associated with thrombocytopenia, but sensitivity and specificity are not good; this is not a useful clinical test
Antineuronal (includes antiglutamate receptor)	60	Neuronal and lymphocyte surface antigens	In some series, a positive test in CSF correlates with active CNS lupus
Antiribosomal P	20	Protein in ribosomes	In some series, a positive test in serum correlates with depression or psychosis due to CNS lupus

Abbreviations: CNS, central nervous system; CSF, cerebrospinal fluid; DRVVT, dilute Russell viper venom time; ELISA, enzyme-linked immunosorbent assay.

estrogen-containing oral contraceptives or hormone replacement have an increased risk of developing SLE (1.2- to 2-fold). Estradiol binds to receptors on T and B lymphocytes, increasing activation and survival of those cells, thus favoring prolonged immune responses. Genes on the X chromosome that influence SLE, such as *TREX-1*, may play a role in gender predisposition, possibly because some genes on the second X in females are not silent. People with XXY karyotype (Klinefelter's syndrome) have a significantly increased risk for SLE.

Several environmental stimuli may influence SLE (Fig. 378-1). Exposure to ultraviolet light causes flares of SLE in approximately 70% of patients, possibly by increasing apoptosis in skin cells or by altering DNA and intracellular proteins to make them antigenic. Some infections induce normal immune responses that involve certain T and B cells that recognize self-antigens; such cells are not appropriately regulated, and autoantibody production occurs. Most SLE patients have autoantibodies for 3 years or more before the first symptoms of disease, suggesting that regulation controls the degree of autoimmunity for years before quantities and qualities of autoantibodies and pathogenic B and T cells cause clinical disease. Epstein-Barr virus (EBV) may be one infectious agent that can trigger SLE in susceptible individuals. Children and adults with SLE are more likely to be infected by EBV than age-, sex-, and ethnicity-matched controls. EBV contains amino acid sequences that mimic sequences on human spliceosomes (RNA/protein antigens) often recognized by autoantibodies in people with SLE. Current tobacco smoking increases risk for SLE (odds ratio [OR] 1.5). Prolonged occupational exposure to silica (e.g., inhalation of soap powder dust or soil in farming activities) increases risk (OR 4.3) in African-American women. Thus, interplay between genetic susceptibility, environment, gender, and abnormal immune responses results in autoimmunity (Chap. 377e).

PATHOLOGY

In SLE, biopsies of affected skin show deposition of Ig at the dermal-epidermal junction (DEJ), injury to basal keratinocytes, and inflammation dominated by T lymphocytes in the DEJ and around blood vessels and dermal appendages. Clinically unaffected skin may also show Ig deposition at the DEJ.

In renal biopsies, the pattern and severity of injury are important in diagnosis and in selecting the best therapy. Most recent clinical studies of lupus nephritis have used the International Society of Nephrology (ISN) and the Renal Pathology Society (RPS) classification (Table 378-2). In the ISN/RPS classification, the addition of "a" for active and "c" for chronic changes gives physicians information regarding the potential reversibility of disease. The system focuses on glomerular disease, although the presence of tubular interstitial and vascular disease is important to clinical outcomes. In general, class III and IV disease, as well as class V accompanied by III or IV disease, should be treated with aggressive immunosuppression if possible, because there is a high risk for end-stage renal disease (ESRD) if patients are untreated or undertreated. In contrast, treatment for lupus nephritis is not recommended in patients with class I or II disease or with extensive irreversible changes. In the recent Systemic Lupus International Collaborating Clinic (SLICC) criteria for classification of SLE, a diagnosis can be established on the basis of renal histology without meeting additional criteria (Table 378-3).

Histologic abnormalities in blood vessels may also determine therapy. Patterns of vasculitis are not specific for SLE but may indicate active disease: leukocytoclastic vasculitis is most common (Chap. 385).

Lymph node biopsies are usually performed to rule out infection or malignancies. In SLE, they show nonspecific diffuse chronic inflammation.

DIAGNOSIS

The diagnosis of SLE is based on characteristic clinical features and autoantibodies. Current criteria for classification are listed in Table 378-3, and an algorithm for diagnosis and initial therapy is shown in Fig. 378-2. The criteria are intended for confirming the diagnosis of SLE in patients included in studies; the author uses them in individual patients for estimating the probability that a disease is SLE. Any combination of four or more criteria, with at least one in the clinical and one in the immunologic category, well documented at any time during an individual's history, makes it likely that the patient has SLE. (Specificity and sensitivity are ~93% and ~92%, respectively.) In many patients, criteria accrue over time. Antinuclear antibodies (ANA) are positive in >98% of patients during the course of disease; repeated negative tests by immunofluorescent methods suggest that the diagnosis is not SLE, unless other autoantibodies are present (Fig. 378-2). High-titer IgG antibodies to double-stranded DNA and antibodies to the Sm antigen are both specific for SLE and, therefore, favor the diagnosis in the presence of compatible clinical manifestations. The

TABLE 378-2 CLASSIFICATION OF LUPUS NEPHRITIS (INTERNATIONAL SOCIETY OF NEPHROLOGY AND RENAL PATHOLOGY SOCIETY)

Class I: Minimal Mesangial Lupus Nephritis
Normal glomeruli by light microscopy, but mesangial immune deposits by immunofluorescence.
Class II: Mesangial Proliferative Lupus Nephritis
Purely mesangial hypercellularity of any degree or mesangial matrix expansion by light microscopy, with mesangial immune deposits. A few isolated subepithelial or subendothelial deposits may be visible by immunofluorescence or electron microscopy, but not by light microscopy.
Class III: Focal Lupus Nephritis
Active or inactive focal, segmental or global endo- or extracapillary glomerulonephritis involving ≤50% of all glomeruli, typically with focal subendothelial immune deposits, with or without mesangial alterations.
Class III (A): Active lesions—focal proliferative lupus nephritis
Class III (A/C): Active and chronic lesions—focal proliferative and sclerosing lupus nephritis
Class III (C): Chronic inactive lesions with glomerular scars—focal sclerosing lupus nephritis
Class IV: Diffuse Lupus Nephritis
Active or inactive diffuse, segmental or global endo- or extracapillary glomerulonephritis involving ≥50% of all glomeruli, typically with diffuse subendothelial immune deposits, with or without mesangial alterations. This class is divided into diffuse segmental (IV-S) lupus nephritis when ≥50% of the involved glomeruli have segmental lesions, and diffuse global (IV-G) lupus nephritis when ≥50% of the involved glomeruli have global lesions. Segmental is defined as a glomerular lesion that involves less than one-half of the glomerular tuft. This class includes cases with diffuse wire loop deposits but with little or no glomerular proliferation.
Class IV-S (A): Active lesions—diffuse segmental proliferative lupus nephritis
Class IV-G (A): Active lesions—diffuse global proliferative lupus nephritis
Class IV-S (A/C): Active and chronic lesions—diffuse segmental proliferative and sclerosing lupus nephritis
Class IV-G (A/C): Active and chronic lesions—diffuse global proliferative and sclerosing lupus nephritis
Class IV-S (C): Chronic inactive lesions with scars—diffuse segmental sclerosing lupus nephritis
Class IV-G (C): Chronic inactive lesions with scars—diffuse global sclerosing lupus nephritis
Class V: Membranous Lupus Nephritis
Global or segmental subepithelial immune deposits or their morphologic sequelae by light microscopy and by immunofluorescence or electron microscopy, with or without mesangial alterations. Class V lupus nephritis may occur in combination with class III or IV, in which case both will be diagnosed. Class V lupus nephritis may show advanced sclerosis.
Class VI: Advanced Sclerotic Lupus Nephritis
≥90% of glomeruli globally sclerosed without residual activity.

Note: Indicate and grade (mild, moderate, severe) tubular atrophy, interstitial inflammation and fibrosis, and severity of arteriosclerosis or other vascular lesions.

Source: JJ Weening et al: Kidney Int 65:521, 2004. Reprinted by permission from Macmillan Publishers Ltd, Copyright 2004.

TABLE 378-3 SYSTEMIC LUPUS INTERNATIONAL COLLABORATING CLINIC CRITERIA FOR CLASSIFICATION OF SYSTEMIC LUPUS ERYTHEMATOSUS

Clinical Manifestations	Immunologic Manifestations
Skin	ANA > reference negative value
Acute, subacute cutaneous LE	Anti-dsDNA
Chronic cutaneous LE	Anti-Sm
Oral ulcers	Antiphospholipid
Alopecia	Low serum complement
Synovitis	Positive direct Coombs test
Renal	
Prot/Cr ≥0.5	
RBC casts	
Biopsy[a]	
Neurologic	
Seizures, psychosis, mononeuritis, myelitis, peripheral or cranial neuropathies, acute confusional state	
Hemolytic anemia	
Leukopenia (<4000) or	
Lymphopenia (<1000)	
Thrombocytopenia (<100,000)	

[a]Renal biopsy read as systemic lupus qualifies for classification as SLE even if none of the other above features are present.

Interpretation: Presence of any 4 criteria (must have at least 1 in each category) qualifies patient to be classified as having SLE with 93% specificity and 92% sensitivity.

Abbreviations: ANA, antinuclear antibody; Cr, creatinine; LE, lupus erythematosus; Prot, protein.

Source: M Petri et al: Arthritis Rheum 64:2677, 2012. Because these criteria are new, currently ongoing clinical studies use prior American College of Rheumatology Criteria; see EM Tan et al: Arthritis Rheum 25:1271, 1982; update MC Hochberg: Arthritis Rheum 40:1725, 1997.

presence in an individual of multiple autoantibodies without clinical symptoms should not be considered diagnostic for SLE, although such persons are at increased risk.

INTERPRETATION OF CLINICAL MANIFESTATIONS

When a diagnosis of SLE is made, it is important to establish the severity and potential reversibility of the illness and to estimate the possible consequences of various therapeutic interventions. In the following paragraphs, descriptions of some disease manifestations begin with relatively mild problems and progress to those more life-threatening.

OVERVIEW AND SYSTEMIC MANIFESTATIONS

At its onset, SLE may involve one or several organ systems; over time, additional manifestations may occur (Tables 378-3 and 378-4). Most of the autoantibodies characteristic of each person are present at the time clinical manifestations appear (Tables 378-1 and 378-3). Severity of SLE varies from mild and intermittent to severe and fulminant. Approximately 85% of patients have either continuing active disease (while being treated) or one or more flares of active disease annually. Permanent complete remissions (absence of symptoms with no treatment) are rare. Systemic symptoms, particularly fatigue and myalgias/arthralgias, are present most of the time. Severe systemic illness requiring glucocorticoid therapy can occur with fever, prostration, weight loss, and anemia with or without other organ-targeted manifestations.

MUSCULOSKELETAL MANIFESTATIONS

Most people with SLE have intermittent polyarthritis, varying from mild to disabling, characterized by soft tissue swelling and tenderness in joints and/or tendons, most commonly in hands, wrists, and knees. Joint deformities (hands and feet) develop in only 10%. Erosions on joint x-rays are rare but can be identified by ultrasound in almost half of patients. Some individuals have rheumatoid-like arthritis with erosions and fulfill criteria for both RA and SLE ("rhupus"); they may be coded as having both diseases. If pain persists in a single joint, such as knee, shoulder, or hip, a diagnosis of ischemic necrosis of bone should be considered, particularly if there are no other manifestations of active SLE because its prevalence is increased in SLE, especially in patients treated with systemic glucocorticoids. Myositis with clinical muscle weakness, elevated creatine kinase levels, positive magnetic resonance imaging (MRI) scan, and muscle necrosis and inflammation on biopsy can occur, although most patients have myalgias without frank myositis. Glucocorticoid therapies (commonly) and antimalarial therapies (rarely) can cause muscle weakness; these adverse effects must be distinguished from active inflammatory disease.

CUTANEOUS MANIFESTATIONS

Lupus dermatitis can be classified as acute, subacute, or chronic, and there are many different types of lesions encompassed within these groups. Discoid lupus erythematosus (DLE) is the most common

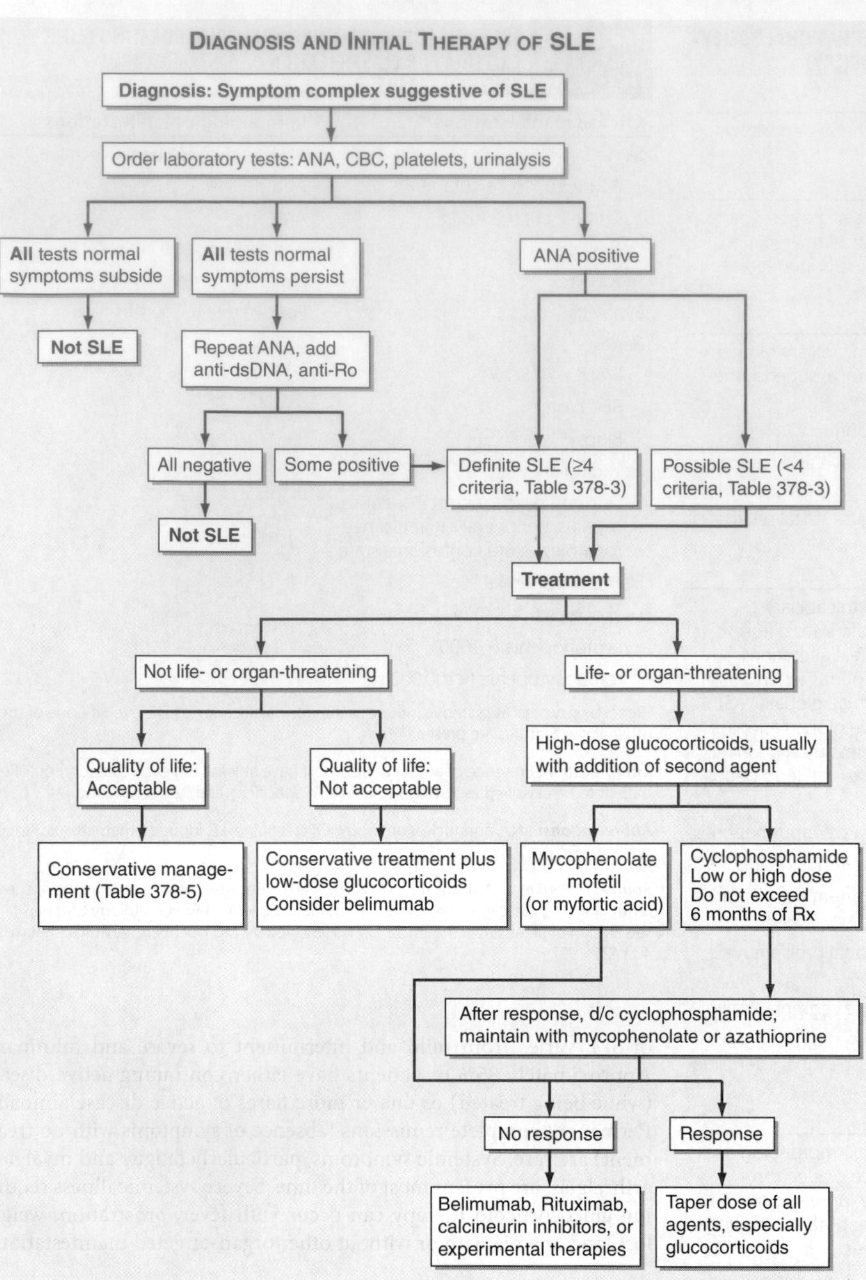

FIGURE 378-2 Algorithm for diagnosis and initial therapy of systemic lupus erythematosus (SLE). For guidelines on management of lupus and lupus nephritis, see BH Hahn et al: Arthritis Care Res (Hoboken) 64:797, 2012; GK Bertsias et al: Ann Rheum Dis 71:1771, 2012; and G Bertsias et al: Ann Rheum Dis 67:195, 2008. For details on mycophenolate and cyclophosphamide induction and maintenance therapies, see L Henderson et al: Cochrane Database Syst Rev 12:CD002922, 2012; Z Touma et al: J Rheumatol 38:69, 2011; EM Ginzler et al: Arthritis Rheum 62:211, 2010; FA Houssiau et al: Ann Rheum Dis 69:61, 2010; and MA Dooley et al: N Engl J Med 365:1886, 2011. For belimumab in treatment, see BH Hahn: N Eng J Med 368:1528, 2013. For rituximab, see L Lightstone: Lupus 22:390, 2013; and BH Rovin et al: Arthritis Rheum 64:1215, 2012. ANA, antinuclear antibodies; CBC, complete blood count.

chronic dermatitis in lupus; lesions are roughly circular with slightly raised, scaly hyperpigmented erythematous rims and depigmented, atrophic centers in which all dermal appendages are permanently destroyed. Lesions can be disfiguring, particularly on the face and scalp. Treatment consists primarily of topical or locally injected glucocorticoids and systemic antimalarials. Only 5% of people with DLE have SLE (although half have positive ANA); however, among individuals with SLE, as many as 20% have DLE. The most common acute SLE rash is a photosensitive, slightly raised erythema, occasionally scaly, on the face (particularly the cheeks and nose—the "butterfly" rash), ears, chin, V region of the neck and chest, upper back, and extensor surfaces of the arms. Worsening of this rash often accompanies flare of systemic disease. Subacute cutaneous lupus erythematosus (SCLE) consists of scaly red patches similar to psoriasis, or circular flat red-rimmed lesions. Patients with these manifestations are exquisitely photosensitive; most have antibodies to Ro (SS-A). Other SLE rashes include recurring urticaria, lichen planus-like dermatitis, bullae, and panniculitis ("lupus profundus"). Rashes can be minor or severe; they may be the major disease manifestation. Small ulcerations on the oral or nasal mucosa are common in SLE; the lesions resemble aphthous ulcers.

RENAL MANIFESTATIONS

Nephritis is usually the most serious manifestation of SLE, particularly because nephritis and infection are the leading causes of mortality in the first decade of disease. Because nephritis is asymptomatic in most lupus patients, urinalysis should be ordered in any person suspected of having SLE. The classification of lupus nephritis is primarily histologic (see "Pathology," above, and Table 378-2). Renal biopsy is recommended for every SLE patient with any clinical evidence of nephritis; results are used to plan current and near-future therapies. Patients with dangerous proliferative forms of glomerular damage (ISN III and IV) usually have microscopic hematuria and proteinuria (>500 mg per 24 h); approximately one-half develop nephrotic syndrome, and most develop hypertension. If diffuse proliferative glomerulonephritis (DPGN) is inadequately treated, virtually all patients develop ESRD within 2 years of diagnosis. Therefore, aggressive immunosuppression is indicated (usually systemic glucocorticoids plus a cytotoxic drug), unless damage is irreversible (Fig. 378-2, Table 378-5). African Americans are more likely to develop ESRD than are whites, even with the most current therapies. Overall in the United States, ~20% of individuals with lupus DPGN die or develop ESRD within 10 years of diagnosis. Such individuals require aggressive control of SLE and of the complications of renal disease and of therapy. Approximately 20% of SLE patients with proteinuria (usually nephrotic) have membranous glomerular changes without proliferative changes on renal biopsy. Their outcome is better than for those with DPGN, but patients with class V and nephrotic range proteinuria should be treated in the same way as those with classes III or IV proliferative disease. Lupus nephritis tends to be an ongoing disease, with flares requiring re-treatment or increased treatment over many years. For most people with lupus nephritis, accelerated atherosclerosis becomes important after several years of disease; attention must be given to control of systemic inflammation, blood pressure, hyperlipidemia, and hyperglycemia.

NERVOUS SYSTEM MANIFESTATIONS

There are many central nervous system (CNS) and peripheral nervous system manifestations of SLE; in some patients, these are the major cause of morbidity and mortality. It is useful to approach this diagnostically by asking first whether the symptoms result from SLE or another condition (such as infection in immunosuppressed

TABLE 378-4 CLINICAL MANIFESTATIONS OF SLE AND PREVALENCE OVER THE ENTIRE COURSE OF DISEASE[a]

Manifestation	Prevalence, %
Systemic: Fatigue, malaise, fever, anorexia, weight loss	95
Musculoskeletal	95
Arthralgias/myalgias	95
Nonerosive polyarthritis	60
Hand deformities	10
Myopathy/myositis	25/5
Ischemic necrosis of bone	15
Cutaneous	80
Photosensitivity	70
Malar rash	50
Oral ulcers	40
Alopecia	40
Discoid rash	20
Vasculitis rash	20
Other (e.g., urticaria, subacute cutaneous lupus)	15
Hematologic	85
Anemia (chronic disease)	70
Leukopenia (<4000/μL)	65
Lymphopenia (<1500/μL)	50
Thrombocytopenia (<100,000/μL)	15
Lymphadenopathy	15
Splenomegaly	15
Hemolytic anemia	10
Neurologic	60
Cognitive disorder	50
Mood disorder	40
Headache	25
Seizures	20
Mono-, polyneuropathy	15
Stroke, TIA	10
Acute confusional state or movement disorder	2–5
Aseptic meningitis, myelopathy	<1
Cardiopulmonary	60
Pleurisy, pericarditis, effusions	30–50
Myocarditis, endocarditis	10
Lupus pneumonitis	10
Coronary artery disease	10
Interstitial fibrosis	5
Pulmonary hypertension, ARDS, hemorrhage	<5
Shrinking lung syndrome	<5
Renal	30–50
Proteinuria ≥500 mg/24 h, cellular casts	30–50
Nephrotic syndrome	25
End-stage renal disease	5–10
Gastrointestinal	40
Nonspecific (nausea, mild pain, diarrhea)	30
Abnormal liver enzymes	40
Vasculitis	5
Thrombosis	15
Venous	10
Arterial	5
Ocular	15
Sicca syndrome	15
Conjunctivitis, episcleritis	10
Vasculitis	5

[a]Numbers indicate percentage of patients who have the manifestation at some time during the course of illness.

Abbreviations: ARDS, acute respiratory distress syndrome; TIA, transient ischemic attack.

individuals or side effects of therapies). If symptoms are related to SLE, it should be determined whether they are caused by a diffuse process (requiring immunosuppression) or vascular occlusive disease (requiring anticoagulation). The most common manifestation of diffuse CNS lupus is cognitive dysfunction, including difficulties with memory and reasoning. Headaches are also common. When excruciating, they often indicate SLE flare; when milder, they are difficult to distinguish from migraine or tension headaches. Seizures of any type may be caused by lupus; treatment often requires both antiseizure and immunosuppressive therapies. Psychosis can be the dominant manifestation of SLE; it must be distinguished from glucocorticoid-induced psychosis. The latter usually occurs in the first weeks of glucocorticoid therapy, at daily doses of ≥40 mg of prednisone or equivalent; psychosis resolves over several days after glucocorticoids are decreased or stopped. Myelopathy is not rare and is often disabling; rapid initiation of immunosuppressive therapy starting with high-dose glucocorticoids is standard of care.

VASCULAR OCCLUSIONS

The prevalence of transient ischemic attacks, strokes, and myocardial infarctions is increased in patients with SLE. These vascular events are increased in, but not exclusive to, SLE patients with antibodies to phospholipids (antiphospholipid antibodies), which are associated with hypercoagulability and acute thrombotic events (Chap. 379). Chronic SLE with or without antiphospholipid antibodies is associated with accelerated atherosclerosis. Ischemia in the brain can be caused by focal occlusion (either noninflammatory or associated with vasculitis) or by embolization from carotid artery plaque or from fibrinous vegetations of Libman-Sacks endocarditis. Appropriate tests for antiphospholipid antibodies (see below) and for sources of emboli should be ordered in such patients to estimate the need for, intensity of, and duration of anti-inflammatory and/or anticoagulant therapies. In SLE, myocardial infarctions are primarily manifestations of accelerated atherosclerosis. The increased risk for vascular events is three- to tenfold overall, and is highest in women <49 years old. Characteristics associated with increased risk for atherosclerosis include older age, hypertension, dyslipidemia, dysfunctional proinflammatory high-density lipoproteins, repeated high scores for disease activity, high cumulative or daily doses of glucocorticoids, and high levels of homocysteine. When it is most likely that an event results from clotting, long-term anticoagulation is the therapy of choice. Two processes can occur at once—vasculitis plus bland vascular occlusions—in which case it is appropriate to treat with anticoagulation plus immunosuppression. Statin therapies reduce levels of low-density lipoproteins (LDL) in SLE patients; reduction of cardiac events by statins has been shown in SLE patients with renal transplants but not in other SLE cohorts to date.

PULMONARY MANIFESTATIONS

The most common pulmonary manifestation of SLE is pleuritis with or without pleural effusion. This manifestation, when mild, may respond to treatment with nonsteroidal anti-inflammatory drugs (NSAIDs); when more severe, patients require a brief course of glucocorticoid therapy. Pulmonary infiltrates also occur as a manifestation of active SLE and are difficult to distinguish from infection on imaging studies. Life-threatening pulmonary manifestations include interstitial inflammation leading to fibrosis, shrinking lung syndrome, and intraalveolar hemorrhage; all of these probably require early aggressive immunosuppressive therapy as well as supportive care.

CARDIAC MANIFESTATIONS

Pericarditis is the most frequent cardiac manifestation; it usually responds to anti-inflammatory therapy and infrequently leads to tamponade. More serious cardiac manifestations are myocarditis and fibrinous endocarditis of Libman-Sacks. The endocardial involvement can lead to valvular insufficiencies, most commonly of the mitral or aortic valves, or to embolic events. It has not been proven that glucocorticoid or other immunosuppressive therapies lead to improvement of lupus myocarditis or endocarditis, but it is usual practice to administer a trial of high-dose steroids along with appropriate supportive therapy for

TABLE 378-5 MEDICATIONS FOR THE MANAGEMENT OF SLE

Medication	Dose Range	Drug Interactions	Serious or Common Adverse Effects
NSAIDs, salicylates (Ecotrin[a] and St. Joseph's aspirin[a] approved by FDA for use in SLE)	Doses toward upper limit of recommended range usually required	A2R/ACE inhibitors, glucocorticoids, fluconazole, methotrexate, thiazides	NSAIDs: Higher incidence of aseptic meningitis, elevated liver enzymes, decreased renal function, vasculitis of skin; entire class, especially COX-2-specific inhibitors, may increase risk for myocardial infarction Salicylates: ototoxicity, tinnitus Both: GI events and symptoms, allergic reactions, dermatitis, dizziness, acute renal failure, edema, hypertension
Topical glucocorticoids	Mid potency for face; mid to high potency for other areas	None known	Atrophy of skin, contact dermatitis, folliculitis, hypopigmentation, infection
Topical sunscreens	SPF 15 at least; 30+ preferred	None known	Contact dermatitis
Hydroxychloroquine[a] (quinacrine can be added or substituted)	200–400 mg qd (100 mg qd)	None known	Retinal damage, agranulocytosis, aplastic anemia, ataxia, cardiomyopathy, dizziness, myopathy, ototoxicity, peripheral neuropathy, pigmentation of skin, seizures, thrombocytopenia. Quinacrine usually causes diffuse yellow skin coloration.
DHEA (dehydroepiandrosterone)	200 mg qd	Unclear	Acne, menstrual irregularities, high serum levels of testosterone
Methotrexate (for dermatitis, arthritis)	10–25 mg once a week, PO or SC, with folic acid; decrease dose if CrCl <60 mL/min	Acitretin, leflunomide, NSAIDs and salicylates, penicillins, probenecid, sulfonamides, trimethoprim	Anemia, bone marrow suppression, leukopenia, thrombocytopenia, hepatotoxicity, nephrotoxicity, infections, neurotoxicity, pulmonary fibrosis, pneumonitis, severe dermatitis, seizures.
Glucocorticoids, oral[a] (several specific brands are approved by FDA for use in SLE)	Prednisone, prednisolone: 0.5–1 mg/kg per day for severe SLE 0.07–0.3 mg/kg per day or qod for milder disease	A2R/ACE antagonists, antiarrhythmics class III, cyclosporine, NSAIDs and salicylates, phenothiazines, phenytoins, quinolones, rifampin, risperidone, thiazides, sulfonylureas, warfarin	Infection, VZV infection, hypertension, hyperglycemia, hypokalemia, acne, allergic reactions, anxiety, aseptic necrosis of bone, cushingoid changes, CHF, fragile skin, insomnia, menstrual irregularities, mood swings, osteoporosis, psychosis
Methylprednisolone sodium succinate, IV[a] (FDA approved for lupus nephritis)	For severe disease, 1 g IV qd × 3 days	As for oral glucocorticoids	As for oral glucocorticoids (if used repeatedly); anaphylaxis
Cyclophosphamide[b] IV	Low dose (for whites of northern European backgrounds): 500 mg every 2 weeks for 6 doses, then begin maintenance with MMF or AZA. High dose: 7–25 mg/kg q month × 6; consider mesna administration with dose	Allopurinol, bone marrow suppressants, colony-stimulating factors, doxorubicin, rituximab, succinylcholine, zidovudine	Infection, VZV infection, bone marrow suppression, leukopenia, anemia, thrombocytopenia, hemorrhagic cystitis (less with IV), carcinoma of the bladder, alopecia, nausea, diarrhea, malaise, malignancy, ovarian and testicular failure. Ovarian failure is probably not a problem with low dose.
Oral	1.5–3 mg/kg per day; decrease dose for CrCl <25 mL/min		
Mycophenolate mofetil (MMF)[b] or mycophenolic acid (MPA)	MMF: 2–3 g/d PO for induction therapy, 1–2 g/d for maintenance therapy; max 1 g bid if CrCl <25 mL/min MPA: 360–1080 mg bid; caution if CrCl <25 mL/min	Acyclovir, antacids, azathioprine, bile acid-binding resins, ganciclovir, iron, salts, probenecid, oral contraceptives	Infection, leukopenia, anemia, thrombocytopenia, lymphoma, lymphoproliferative disorders, malignancy, alopecia, cough, diarrhea, fever, GI symptoms, headache, hypertension, hypercholesterolemia, hypokalemia, insomnia, peripheral edema, elevated liver enzymes, tremor, rash
Azathioprine (AZA)[b]	2–3 mg/kg per day PO for induction; 1–2 mg/kg per day for maintenance; decrease frequency of dose if CrCl <50 mL/min	ACE inhibitors, allopurinol, bone marrow suppressants, interferons, mycophenolate mofetil, rituximab, warfarin, zidovudine	Infection, VZV infection, bone marrow suppression, leukopenia, anemia, thrombocytopenia, pancreatitis, hepatotoxicity, malignancy, alopecia, fever, flulike illness, GI symptoms
Belimumab	10 mg/kg IV wks 0, 2, and 4, then monthly	IVIg	Infusion reactions, allergy, infections probable
Rituximab (for patients resistant to above therapies)	375 mg/m² q wk × 4 or 1 g q 2 wks × 2	IVIg	Infection (including PML), infusion reactions, headache, arrhythmias, allergic responses

[a]Indicates medication is approved for use in SLE by the U.S. Food and Drug Administration. [b]Indicates the medication has been used with glucocorticoids in the trials showing efficacy.

Abbreviations: A2R, angiotensin II receptor; ACE, angiotensin-converting enzyme; CHF, congestive heart failure; CrCl, creatinine clearance; FDA, U.S. Food and Drug Administration; GI, gastrointestinal; IVIg, intravenous immunoglobulin; NSAIDs, nonsteroidal anti-inflammatory drugs; PML, progressive multifocal leukoencephalopathy; SLE, systemic lupus erythematosus; SPF, sun protection factor; VZV, varicella-zoster virus.

heart failure, arrhythmia, or embolic events. As discussed above, patients with SLE are at increased risk for myocardial infarction, usually due to accelerated atherosclerosis, which probably results from immune attack, chronic inflammation, and/or chronic oxidative damage to arteries.

HEMATOLOGIC MANIFESTATIONS

The most frequent hematologic manifestation of SLE is anemia, usually normochromic normocytic, reflecting chronic illness. Hemolysis can be rapid in onset and severe, requiring high-dose glucocorticoid therapy, which is effective in most patients. Leukopenia is also common and almost always consists of lymphopenia, not granulocytopenia; lymphopenia rarely predisposes to infections and by itself usually does not require therapy. Thrombocytopenia may be a recurring problem. If platelet counts are >40,000/μL and abnormal bleeding is absent, therapy may not be required. High-dose glucocorticoid therapy (e.g., 1 mg/kg per day of prednisone or equivalent) is usually effective for the first few episodes of severe thrombocytopenia. Recurring or prolonged hemolytic anemia or thrombocytopenia, or disease requiring an unacceptably high dose of daily glucocorticoids, should be treated with an additional strategy (see "Management of Systemic Lupus Erythematosus" below).

GASTROINTESTINAL MANIFESTATIONS

Nausea, sometimes with vomiting, and diarrhea can be manifestations of an SLE flare, as can diffuse abdominal pain probably caused by autoimmune peritonitis and/or intestinal vasculitis. Increases in serum aspartate aminotransferase (AST) and alanine aminotransferase (ALT) are common when SLE is active. These manifestations usually improve promptly during systemic glucocorticoid therapy. Vasculitis involving the intestine may be life-threatening; perforations, ischemia, bleeding, and sepsis are frequent complications. Aggressive immunosuppressive therapy with high-dose glucocorticoids is recommended for short-term control; evidence of recurrence is an indication for additional therapies.

OCULAR MANIFESTATIONS

Sicca syndrome (Sjögren's syndrome; Chap. 383) and nonspecific conjunctivitis are common in SLE and rarely threaten vision. In contrast, retinal vasculitis and optic neuritis are serious manifestations: blindness can develop over days to weeks. Aggressive immunosuppression is recommended, although there are no controlled trials to prove effectiveness. Complications of systemic and intraorbital glucocorticoid therapy include cataracts (common) and glaucoma.

LABORATORY TESTS

Laboratory tests serve (1) to establish or rule out the diagnosis; (2) to follow the course of disease, particularly to suggest that a flare is occurring or organ damage is developing; and (3) to identify adverse effects of therapies.

TESTS FOR AUTOANTIBODIES (TABLES 378-1 AND 378-3)

Diagnostically, the most important autoantibodies to detect are ANA because the test is positive in >95% of patients, usually at the onset of symptoms. A few patients develop ANA within 1 year of symptom onset; repeated testing may thus be useful. ANA tests using immunofluorescent methods are more reliable than enzyme-linked immunosorbent assays (ELISAs) and/or bead assays, which have less specificity. ANA-negative lupus exists but is rare in adults and is usually associated with other autoantibodies (anti-Ro or anti-DNA). High-titer IgG antibodies to double-stranded DNA (dsDNA) (but not to single-stranded DNA) are specific for SLE. ELISA and immunofluorescent reactions of sera with the dsDNA in the flagellate *Crithidia luciliae* have ~60% sensitivity for SLE; identification of high-avidity anti-dsDNA in the Farr assay is not as sensitive but may correlate better with risk for nephritis. Titers of anti-dsDNA vary over time. In some patients, increases in quantities of anti-dsDNA herald a flare, particularly of nephritis or vasculitis, especially when associated with declining levels of C3 or C4 complement. Antibodies to Sm are also specific for SLE and assist in diagnosis; anti-Sm antibodies do not usually correlate with disease activity or clinical manifestations. Antiphospholipid antibodies are not specific for SLE, but their presence fulfills one classification criterion, and they identify patients at increased risk for venous or arterial clotting, thrombocytopenia, and fetal loss. There are three widely accepted tests that measure different antibodies (anticardiolipin, anti-β_2-glycoprotein, and the lupus anticoagulant). ELISA is used for anticardiolipin and anti-β_2-glycoprotein (both internationally standardized with good reproducibility); a sensitive phospholipid-based activated prothrombin time such as the dilute Russell venom viper test is used to identify the lupus anticoagulant. The higher the titers of IgG anticardiolipin (>40 IU is considered high), and the greater the number of different antiphospholipid antibodies that are detected, the greater is the risk for a clinical episode of clotting. Quantities of antiphospholipid antibodies may vary markedly over time; repeated testing is justified if clinical manifestations of the antiphospholipid syndrome (APS) appear (Chap. 379). To classify a patient as having APS, with or without SLE, by international criteria requires the presence of one or more clotting episodes and/or repeated fetal losses plus at least two positive tests for antiphospholipid antibodies, at least 12 weeks apart; however, many patients with APS do not meet these stringent criteria, which are intended for inclusion of patients into studies.

An additional autoantibody test with predictive value (not used for diagnosis) detects anti-Ro/SS-A, which indicates increased risk for neonatal lupus, sicca syndrome, and SCLE. Women with child-bearing potential and SLE should be screened for antiphospholipid antibodies and anti-Ro, because both antibodies have the potential to cause fetal harm.

STANDARD TESTS FOR DIAGNOSIS

Screening tests for complete blood count, platelet count, and urinalysis may detect abnormalities that contribute to the diagnosis and influence management decisions.

TESTS FOR FOLLOWING DISEASE COURSE

It is useful to follow tests that indicate the status of organ involvement known to be present during SLE flares. These might include urinalysis for hematuria and proteinuria, hemoglobin levels, platelet counts, and serum levels of creatinine or albumin. There is great interest in identification of additional markers of disease activity. Candidates include levels of anti-DNA and anti-C1q antibodies, several components of complement (C3 is most widely available), activated complement products (including those that bind to the C4d receptor on erythrocytes), IFN-inducible gene expression in peripheral blood cells, serum levels of BLyS (B lymphocyte stimulator, also called BAFF), and urinary levels of TNF-like weak inducer of apoptosis (TWEAK), neutrophil gelatinase-associated lipocalin (NGAL), or monocyte chemotactic protein 1 (MCP-1). None is uniformly agreed upon as a reliable indicator of flare or of response to therapeutic interventions. It is likely that a panel of multiple proteins will be developed to predict both impending flare and response to recently instituted therapies. For now, the physician should determine for each patient whether certain laboratory test changes predict flare. If so, altering therapy in response to these changes may be advisable (30 mg of prednisone daily for 2 weeks has been shown to prevent flares in patients with rising anti-DNA plus falling complement). In addition, given the increased prevalence of atherosclerosis in SLE, it is advisable to follow the recommendations of the National Cholesterol Education Program for testing and treatment, including scoring of SLE as an independent risk factor, similar to diabetes mellitus.

MANAGEMENT OF SYSTEMIC LUPUS ERYTHEMATOSUS

There is no cure for SLE, and complete sustained remissions are rare. Therefore, the physician should plan to induce remissions of acute flares and then maintain improvements with strategies that suppress symptoms to an acceptable level and prevent organ damage. Usually patients will endure some adverse effects of medications. Therapeutic choices depend on (1) whether disease manifestations are life-threatening or likely to cause organ damage, justifying aggressive therapies; (2) whether manifestations are potentially reversible; and (3) the best approaches to preventing complications of disease and its treatments. Therapies, doses, and adverse effects are listed in Table 378-5.

CONSERVATIVE THERAPIES FOR MANAGEMENT OF NON-LIFE-THREATENING DISEASE

Among patients with fatigue, pain, and autoantibodies indicative of SLE, but without major organ involvement, management can be directed to suppression of symptoms. Analgesics and antimalarials are mainstays. NSAIDs are useful analgesics/anti-inflammatories, particularly for arthritis/arthralgias. However, two major issues indicate caution in using NSAIDs. First, SLE patients compared with the general population are at increased risk for NSAID-induced aseptic meningitis, elevated serum transaminases, hypertension, and renal dysfunction. Second, all NSAIDs, particularly those that inhibit cyclooxygenase-2 specifically, may increase risk for myocardial infarction. Acetaminophen to control pain may be a good strategy, but NSAIDs are more effective in some patients. The relative hazards of NSAIDs compared with low-dose glucocorticoid therapy have not been established. Antimalarials (hydroxychloroquine, chloroquine, and quinacrine) often reduce dermatitis, arthritis, and fatigue. A randomized, placebo-controlled, prospective trial has shown that withdrawal of hydroxychloroquine results in increased numbers of disease flares; hydroxychloroquine also reduces accrual of tissue damage, including renal damage, over time. Because of potential retinal toxicity, patients receiving antimalarials should undergo ophthalmologic examinations annually. A placebo-controlled prospective trial suggests that administration of dehydroepiandrosterone may reduce disease activity. If quality of life is inadequate despite these conservative measures, treatment with low doses of systemic glucocorticoids may be necessary. The clinician may also consider treatment with belimumab (anti-BLyS) in these patients, although published clinical trials enrolled patients who had failed to respond to conservative therapies. Lupus dermatitis should be managed with topical sunscreens, antimalarials, topical glucocorticoids, and/or tacrolimus, and if severe or unresponsive, systemic glucocorticoids with or without mycophenolate mofetil.

LIFE-THREATENING SLE: PROLIFERATIVE FORMS OF LUPUS NEPHRITIS

Guidelines for management of lupus nephritis have been published recently by the American College of Rheumatology and the European League Against Rheumatism (encompassed and referenced in Fig. 378-2 and Table 378-5). The mainstay of treatment for any inflammatory life-threatening or organ-threatening manifestations of SLE is systemic glucocorticoids (0.5–1 mg/kg per day PO or 500–1000 mg of methylprednisolone sodium succinate IV daily for 3 days followed by 0.5–1 mg/kg of daily prednisone or equivalent). Evidence that glucocorticoid therapy is life-saving comes from retrospective studies from the pre-dialysis era; survival was significantly better in people with DPGN treated with high-dose daily glucocorticoids (40–60 mg of prednisone daily for 4–6 months) versus lower doses. Currently, high doses are recommended for much shorter periods; recent trials of interventions for severe SLE use 4–6 weeks of 0.5–1 mg/kg per day of prednisone or equivalent. Thereafter, doses are tapered as rapidly as the clinical situation permits, usually to a maintenance dose ranging from 5 to 10 mg of prednisone or equivalent per day. Most patients with an episode of severe SLE require many years of maintenance therapy with low-dose glucocorticoids, which can be increased to prevent or treat disease flares. Frequent attempts to gradually reduce the glucocorticoid requirement are recommended because virtually everyone develops important adverse effects (Table 378-5). High-quality clinical studies regarding initiating therapy for severe, active SLE with IV pulses of high-dose glucocorticoids are not available. Most recent clinical trials in lupus nephritis have initiated therapy with high-dose IV glucocorticoid pulses (500–1000 mg daily for 3–5 days). This approach must be tempered by safety considerations, such as the presence of conditions adversely affected by glucocorticoids (e.g., infection, hyperglycemia, hypertension, osteoporosis).

Cytotoxic/immunosuppressive agents added to glucocorticoids are recommended to treat serious SLE. Almost all prospective controlled trials in SLE involving cytotoxic agents have been conducted in combination with glucocorticoids in patients with lupus nephritis. Therefore, the following recommendations apply to treatment of nephritis. Either cyclophosphamide (an alkylating agent) or mycophenolate mofetil (a relatively lymphocyte-specific inhibitor of inosine monophosphatase and therefore of purine synthesis) is an acceptable choice for induction of improvement in severely ill patients; azathioprine (a purine analogue and cycle-specific antimetabolite) may be effective but is slower to influence response and associated with more flares. In patients whose renal biopsies show ISN grade III or IV disease, early treatment with combinations of glucocorticoids and cyclophosphamide reduces progression to ESRD and death. Shorter-term studies with glucocorticoids plus mycophenolate mofetil (prospective randomized trials of 6 months, follow-up studies of 36 months) show that this regimen is similar to cyclophosphamide in achieving improvement. Comparisons are complicated by effects of race, since higher proportions of African Americans (and other non-Asian, nonwhite races) respond to mycophenolate than to cyclophosphamide, whereas similar proportions of whites and Asians respond to each drug. Regarding toxicity, diarrhea is more common with mycophenolate mofetil; amenorrhea, leukopenia, and nausea are more common with cyclophosphamide. Importantly, rates of severe infections and death are similar in meta-analyses. Two different regimens of IV cyclophosphamide are available. For white patients with northern European backgrounds, low doses of cyclophosphamide (500 mg every 2 weeks for six total doses, followed by azathioprine or mycophenolate maintenance) are as effective as standard high doses, with less toxicity. Ten-year follow-up has shown no differences between the high-dose and low-dose groups (death or ESRD in 9–20% of patients in each group). The majority of the European patients were white; it is not clear whether the data apply to U.S. populations. High-dose cyclophosphamide (500–1000 mg/m^2 body surface area given monthly IV for 6 months, followed by azathioprine or mycophenolate maintenance) is an acceptable approach for patients with severe nephritis (e.g., multiple cellular crescents and/or fibrinoid necrosis on renal biopsy, or rapidly progressive glomerulonephritis). Cyclophosphamide and mycophenolate responses begin 3–16 weeks after treatment is initiated, whereas glucocorticoid responses may begin within 24 h.

For maintenance therapy, mycophenolate and azathioprine probably are similar in efficacy and toxicity; both are safer than cyclophosphamide. In a recently published multicenter study, mycophenolate was superior to azathioprine in maintaining renal function and survival in patients who responded to induction therapy with either cyclophosphamide or mycophenolate. The incidence of ovarian failure, a common effect of high-dose cyclophosphamide therapy (but probably not of low-dose therapy), can be reduced by treatment with a gonadotropin-releasing hormone agonist (e.g., leuprolide 3.75 mg intramuscularly) prior to each monthly cyclophosphamide dose. Patients with high serum creatinine levels (e.g., ≥265 μmol/L [≥3.0 mg/dL]) many months in duration and high chronicity scores on renal biopsy are not likely to respond to any of these therapies. In general, it may be better to induce improvement in an African-American or Hispanic patient with proliferative glomerulonephritis with mycophenolate mofetil (2–3 g daily) rather than cyclophosphamide, with the option to switch if no evidence of response is detectable after 3–6 months of treatment. For whites and Asians, induction with either mycophenolate mofetil or cyclophosphamide is acceptable. Cyclophosphamide may be discontinued when it is clear that a patient is improving. The number of SLE flares is reduced by maintenance therapy with mycophenolate mofetil (1.5–2 g daily) or azathioprine (1–2.5 mg/kg per day). Both cyclophosphamide and mycophenolate mofetil are potentially teratogenic; patients should be off either medication for at least 3 months before attempting to conceive. Azathioprine can be used if necessary to control active SLE in patients who are pregnant. If azathioprine is used either for induction or maintenance therapy, patients may be prescreened for homozygous deficiency of the TMPT enzyme (which is required to metabolize the 6-mercaptopurine product of azathioprine) because they are at higher risk for bone marrow suppression.

Good improvement occurs in ~80% of lupus nephritis patients receiving either cyclophosphamide or mycophenolate at 1–2 years of follow-up. However, in some studies, at least 50% of these individuals have flares of nephritis over the next 5 years, and re-treatment is required; such individuals are more likely to progress to ESRD. Long-term outcome of lupus nephritis to most interventions is better in whites than in African Americans. Methotrexate (a folinic acid antagonist) may have a role in the treatment of arthritis and dermatitis but probably not in nephritis or other life-threatening disease. Small controlled trials (in Asia) of leflunomide, a relatively lymphocyte-specific pyrimidine antagonist licensed for use in rheumatoid arthritis, have suggested it can suppress disease activity in some SLE patients. Cyclosporine and tacrolimus, which inhibit production of IL-2 and T lymphocyte functions, have not been studied in prospective controlled trials in SLE in the United States; several studies in Asia have shown they are effective in lupus nephritis. Because they have potential nephrotoxicity but little bone marrow toxicity, the author uses them for periods of a few months in patients with steroid-resistant cytopenias of SLE or in steroid-resistant patients who have developed bone marrow suppression from standard cytotoxic agents.

Use of biologics directed against B cells for active SLE is under intense study. Use of anti-CD20 (rituximab), particularly in patients with SLE who are resistant to the more standard combination therapies discussed above, is controversial. Several open trials have shown efficacy in a majority of such patients, both for nephritis and for extrarenal lupus. However, recent prospective placebo-controlled randomized trials, one in renal and one in nonrenal SLE, did not show a difference between anti-CD20 and placebo when added to standard combination therapies. In contrast, recent trials of standard therapy plus belimumab (anti-BLyS, which binds soluble BLyS/BAFF, which is required for maturation of naïve and transitional B cells to plasma cells and memory B cells) showed improvement in 51% of SLE patients compared to 36% of those on placebo; these differences were statistically significant. The U.S. Food and Drug Administration (FDA) has approved belimumab for treatment of seropositive patients with SLE who have failed standard treatments. The belimumab trial did not include patients with active nephritis or CNS disease. Post hoc analyses have shown that the SLE patient most likely to respond to belimumab has fairly robust clinical activity (a Systemic Lupus Erythematosus Disease Activity Index [SLEDAI] score of ≥10), positive anti-DNA, and low serum complement. SLEDAI is a widely used measure of SLE disease activity; scores >3 reflect clinically active disease. At this time, it is useful to add belimumab to the therapeutic armamentarium in SLE, and it is clear that some patients benefit. However, its role in management of lupus nephritis is not yet known.

SPECIAL CONDITIONS IN SLE THAT MAY REQUIRE ADDITIONAL OR DIFFERENT THERAPIES

Crescentic Lupus Nephritis The presence of cellular or fibrotic crescents in glomeruli with proliferative glomerulonephritis indicates a worse prognosis than in patients without this feature. There are no large prospective multinational controlled trials showing efficacy of cyclophosphamide, mycophenolate, cyclosporine, or tacrolimus in such cases. Most authorities currently recommend that high-dose cyclophosphamide is the induction therapy of choice, in addition to high-dose glucocorticoids. One prospective trial from China showed superiority of mycophenolate to cyclophosphamide.

Membranous Lupus Nephritis Most SLE patients with membranous (INS-V) nephritis also have proliferative changes and should be treated for proliferative disease. However, some have pure membranous changes. Treatment for this group is less well defined. Some authorities do not recommend immunosuppression unless proteinuria is in the nephrotic range (although treatment with angiotensin-converting enzyme inhibitors or angiotensin II receptor blockers is recommended). In those patients, recent prospective controlled trials suggest that alternate-day glucocorticoids plus cyclophosphamide or mycophenolate mofetil or cyclosporine are all effective in the majority of patients in reducing proteinuria. It is more controversial whether they preserve renal function over the long term.

Pregnancy and Lupus Fertility rates for men and women with SLE are probably normal. However, rate of fetal loss is increased (approximately two- to threefold) in women with SLE. Fetal demise is higher in mothers with high disease activity, antiphospholipid antibodies, and/or active nephritis. Suppression of disease activity can be achieved by administration of systemic glucocorticoids. A placental enzyme, 11-β-dehydrogenase 2, deactivates glucocorticoids; it is more effective in deactivating prednisone and prednisolone than the fluorinated glucocorticoids dexamethasone and betamethasone. Glucocorticoids are listed by the FDA as pregnancy category A (no evidence of teratogenicity in human studies); cyclosporine, tacrolimus, and rituximab are listed as category C (may be teratogenic in animals but no good evidence in humans); azathioprine, hydroxychloroquine, mycophenolate mofetil, and cyclophosphamide are category D (there is evidence of teratogenicity in humans, but benefits might outweigh risks in certain situations); and methotrexate is category X (risks outweigh benefits). Therefore, active SLE in pregnant women should be controlled with hydroxychloroquine and, if necessary, prednisone/prednisolone at the lowest effective doses for the shortest time required. Azathioprine may be added if these treatments do not suppress disease activity. Adverse effects of prenatal glucocorticoid exposure (primarily betamethasone) on offspring may include low birth weight, developmental abnormalities in the CNS, and predilection toward adult metabolic syndrome. It is likely that each of these glucocorticoids and immunosuppressive medications gets into breast milk, at least in low levels; patients should consider not breastfeeding if they need therapy for SLE. In SLE patients with antiphospholipid antibodies (on at least two occasions) and prior fetal losses, treatment with heparin (usually low-molecular-weight) plus low-dose aspirin has been shown in prospective controlled trials to increase significantly the proportion of live births; however, a recent prospective trial showed no differences in fetal outcomes in women taking aspirin compared to those taking aspirin plus low-molecular-weight heparin. An additional potential problem for the fetus is the presence of antibodies to Ro, sometimes associated with neonatal lupus consisting of rash and congenital heart block with or without cardiomyopathy. The cardiac manifestations can be life-threatening; therefore the presence of anti-Ro requires vigilant monitoring of fetal heart rates with prompt intervention (delivery if possible) if distress occurs. Recent evidence shows that hydroxychloroquine treatment of an anti-Ro-positive mother whose infant develops congenital heart block significantly reduces the chance that subsequent fetuses will develop heart block. There is some evidence that dexamethasone treatment of a mother in whom first- or second-degree heart block is detected in utero may sometimes prevent progression of heart block. Women with SLE usually tolerate pregnancy without disease flares. However, a small proportion develops severe flares requiring aggressive glucocorticoid therapy or early delivery. Poor maternal outcomes are highest in women with active nephritis or irreversible organ damage in kidneys, brain, or heart.

Lupus and Antiphospholipid Syndrome (APS) Patients with SLE who have venous or arterial clotting and/or repeated fetal losses and at least two positive tests for antiphospholipid antibodies have APS and should be managed with long-term anticoagulation (Chap. 379). A target international normalized ratio (INR) of 2.0–2.5 is recommended for patients with one episode of venous clotting; an INR of 3.0–3.5 is recommended for patients with recurring clots or arterial clotting, particularly in the CNS. Recommendations are based on both retrospective and prospective studies of posttreatment clotting events and adverse effects from anticoagulation.

Microvascular Thrombotic Crisis (Thrombotic Thrombocytopenic Purpura, Hemolytic-Uremic Syndrome) This syndrome of hemolysis, thrombocytopenia, and microvascular thrombosis in kidneys, brain, and other tissues carries a high mortality rate and occurs most commonly in young individuals with lupus nephritis. The most useful laboratory tests are identification of schistocytes on peripheral blood smears, elevated serum levels of lactate dehydrogenase, and antibodies to

ADAMS13. Plasma exchange or extensive plasmapheresis is usually life-saving; most authorities recommend concomitant glucocorticoid therapy; there is no evidence that cytotoxic drugs are effective.

Lupus Dermatitis Patients with any form of lupus dermatitis should minimize exposure to ultraviolet light, using appropriate clothing and sunscreens with a sun protection factor of at least 30. Topical glucocorticoids and antimalarials (such as hydroxychloroquine) are effective in reducing lesion severity in most patients and are relatively safe. Systemic treatment with retinoic acid is a useful strategy in patients with inadequate improvement on topical glucocorticoids and antimalarials; adverse effects are potentially severe (particularly fetal abnormalities), and there are stringent reporting requirements for its use in the United States. Extensive, pruritic, bullous, or ulcerating dermatitides usually improve promptly after institution of systemic glucocorticoids; tapering may be accompanied by flare of lesions, thus necessitating use of a second medication such as hydroxychloroquine, retinoids, or cytotoxic medications such as methotrexate, azathioprine, or mycophenolate mofetil. In therapy-resistant lupus dermatitis there are reports of success with topical tacrolimus (caution must be exerted because of the possible increased risk for malignancies) or with systemic dapsone or thalidomide (the extreme danger of fetal deformities from thalidomide requires permission from and supervision by the supplier).

PREVENTIVE THERAPIES

Prevention of complications of SLE and its therapy include providing appropriate vaccinations (the administration of influenza and pneumococcal vaccines has been studied in patients with SLE; flare rates are similar to those receiving placebo) and suppressing recurrent urinary tract infections. Vaccination with attenuated live viruses is generally discouraged in patients who are immunosuppressed. Strategies to prevent osteoporosis should be initiated in most patients likely to require long-term glucocorticoid therapy and/or with other predisposing factors. Postmenopausal women can be protected from steroid-induced osteoporosis with either bisphosphonates or denosumab. Safety of long-term use of these strategies in premenopausal women is not well established. Control of hypertension and appropriate prevention strategies for atherosclerosis, including monitoring and treatment of dyslipidemias, management of hyperglycemia, and management of obesity, are recommended.

EXPERIMENTAL THERAPIES

Studies of highly targeted experimental therapies for SLE are in progress. They include targeting (1) activated B lymphocytes with anti-CD22 or TACI-Ig, (2) inhibition of IFN-α, (3) inhibition of B/T cell second signal coactivation with CTLA-Ig, (4) inhibition of innate immune activation via TLR7 or TLR7 and 9, (5) induction of regulatory T cells with peptides from immunoglobulins or autoantigens; (6) suppression of T cells, B cells, and monocyte/macrophages with laquinimod; and (7) inhibition of lymphocyte activation by blockade of Jak/Stat. A few studies have used vigorous untargeted immunosuppression with high-dose cyclophosphamide plus anti-T cell strategies, with rescue by transplantation of autologous hematopoietic stem cells for the treatment of severe and refractory SLE. One U.S. report showed an estimated mortality rate over 5 years of 15% and sustained remission in 50%. It is hoped that in the next edition of this text, we will be able to recommend more effective and less toxic approaches to treatment of SLE based on some of these strategies.

PATIENT OUTCOMES, PROGNOSIS, AND SURVIVAL

Survival in patients with SLE in the United States, Canada, Europe, and China is approximately 95% at 5 years, 90% at 10 years, and 78% at 20 years. In the United States, African Americans and Hispanic Americans with a mestizo heritage have a worse prognosis than whites, whereas Africans in Africa and Hispanic Americans with a Puerto Rican origin do not. The relative importance of gene mixtures and environmental differences accounting for ethnic differences is not known. Poor prognosis (~50% mortality in 10 years) in most series is associated with (at the time of diagnosis) high serum creatinine levels (>124 μmol/L [>1.4 mg/dL]), hypertension, nephrotic syndrome (24-h urine protein excretion >2.6 g), anemia (hemoglobin <124 g/L [<12.4 g/dL]), hypoalbuminemia, hypocomplementemia, antiphospholipid antibodies, male sex, ethnicity (African American, Hispanic with mestizo heritage), and low socioeconomic status. Data regarding outcomes in SLE patients with renal transplants show mixed results: some series show a twofold increase in graft rejection compared to patients with other causes of ESRD, whereas others show no differences. Overall patient survival is comparable (85% at 2 years). Lupus nephritis occurs in approximately 10% of transplanted kidneys. Disability in patients with SLE is common due primarily to chronic fatigue, arthritis, and pain, as well as renal disease. As many as 25% of patients may experience remissions, sometimes for a few years, but these are rarely permanent. The leading causes of death in the first decade of disease are systemic disease activity, renal failure, and infections; subsequently, thromboembolic events become increasingly frequent causes of mortality.

DRUG-INDUCED LUPUS

This is a syndrome of positive ANA associated with symptoms such as fever, malaise, arthritis or intense arthralgias/myalgias, serositis, and/or rash. The syndrome appears during therapy with certain medications and biologic agents, is predominant in whites, has less female predilection than SLE, rarely involves kidneys or brain, is rarely associated with anti-dsDNA, is commonly associated with antibodies to histones, and usually resolves over several weeks after discontinuation of the offending medication. The list of substances that can induce lupus-like disease is long. Among the most frequent are the antiarrhythmics procainamide, disopyramide, and propafenone; the antihypertensive hydralazine; several angiotensin-converting enzyme inhibitors and beta blockers; the antithyroid propylthiouracil; the antipsychotics chlorpromazine and lithium; the anticonvulsants carbamazepine and phenytoin; the antibiotics isoniazid, minocycline, and nitrofurantoin (Macrodantin); the antirheumatic sulfasalazine; the diuretic hydrochlorothiazide; the antihyperlipidemics lovastatin and simvastatin; and IFNs and TNF inhibitors. ANA usually appears before symptoms; however, many of the medications mentioned above induce ANA in patients who never develop symptoms of drug-induced lupus. It is appropriate to test for ANA at the first hint of relevant symptoms and to use test results to help decide whether to withdraw the suspect agent.

379 Antiphospholipid Syndrome

Haralampos M. Moutsopoulos, Panayiotis G. Vlachoyiannopoulos

DEFINITIONS

Antiphospholipid syndrome (APS) is an autoantibody-mediated acquired thrombophilia characterized by recurrent arterial or venous thrombosis and/or pregnancy morbidity. The major autoantibodies detected in the patient's sera are directed against phospholipid (PL)-binding plasma proteins, mainly against a 43-kDa plasma apolipoprotein known as β2 glycoprotein I (β2GPI) and prothrombin. The plasma concentration of β2GPI is 50–200 μg/mL. β2GPI consists of 326 amino acids arranged in five domains (I through V). Domain V forms a positively charged patch, suitable to interact with negatively charged PL. In plasma, β2GPI has a circular conformation with domain V binding to and concealing the B cell epitopes lying on domain I. Another group of antibodies termed *lupus anticoagulant* (LA) elongate clotting times in vitro; this elongation is not corrected by adding normal plasma to the detection system (Table 379-1). Patients with APS often possess antibodies recognizing *Treponema pallidum* PL/cholesterol complexes, which are detected as biologic false-positive serologic tests for syphilis

TABLE 379-1 CLASSIFICATION AND NOMENCLATURE OF ANTIPHOSPHOLIPID ANTIBODIES

Name	Assay for their Detection	Comments
Antibodies against cardiolipin (aCL)	Enzyme-linked immunosorbent assay (ELISA) using as antigen cardiolipin (CL), a negatively charged phospholipid	aCL from patients with APS recognize β2GPI existing in the human serum as well as in bovine serum, which is used to block the nonspecific bindings sites on the ELISA plate. CL simply stabilizes β2GPI at high concentration on the polystyrene surface.
Antibodies against β2GPI (anti-β2GPI)	ELISA using as antigen affinity purified or recombinant β2GPI in the absence of PL	Antibodies recognize β2GPI bound in the absence of CL to an oxidized polystyrene surface, where oxygen atoms in the moieties C-O or C=O were introduced by γ-irradiation.
Lupus anticoagulant (LA)	Activated partial thromboplastin time (aPTT) Kaolin clotting time (KCT) Dilute Russel viper venom test (DRVVT)	Antibodies recognize β2GPI or prothrombin (PT) and elongate aPTT, implying that they interfere with the generation of thrombin by prothrombin. Prolongation of the clotting times is an in vitro phenomenon, and LA induces thromboses in vivo.

Abbreviations: APL, antiphospholipid syndrome; β2GPI, β2 glycoprotein I; PL, phospholipid.

(BFP-STS) and Venereal Disease Research Laboratory (VDRL) tests. APS may occur alone (primary) or in association with any other autoimmune disease (secondary). Catastrophic APS (CAPS) is defined as a rapidly progressive thromboembolic disease involving simultaneously three or more organs, organ systems, or tissues leading to corresponding functional defects.

EPIDEMIOLOGY

Anti-PL (aPL)-binding plasma protein antibodies occur in 1–5% of the general population. Their prevalence increases with age; however, it is questionable whether they induce thrombotic events in elderly individuals. One-third of patients with systemic lupus erythematosus (SLE) (Chap. 378) possess these antibodies, whereas their prevalence in other autoimmune connective tissue disorders, such as systemic sclerosis (scleroderma), Sjögren's syndrome, dermatomyositis, rheumatoid arthritis, and early undifferentiated connective tissue disease, ranges from 6 to 15%. One-third of aPL-positive individuals experience thrombotic events or pregnancy morbidity.

PATHOGENESIS

The trigger for the induction of antibodies to PL-binding proteins is not known. However infections, oxidative stress, major physical stresses such as surgery, and discontinuation of anticoagulant treatment may induce the exacerbation of the disease. Experimental data have shown that these phenomena are induced via (1) conformational changes of β2GPI either complexed with microbial antigens or dimerization through interaction with endothelial cell surface receptor annexin 2/TLR4, the platelet receptors apolipoprotein E receptor 2′ (apoER2′) and/or GPIb/IX/V receptor, and/or the chemokine platelet factor 4 (PF4); or (2) impaired defensive mechanisms such as reduced generation of endothelial nitric oxide synthase. Adherence of β2GPI to apoER2′, GPIb/IX/V receptor, and/or PF4 induces activation of endothelial cells, platelets, and monocytes. This process activates downstream pathways such as p38 mitogen-activated protein (p38 MAP) kinase and nuclear factor (NF)-κB, leading to the following events: secretion of proinflammatory cytokines, such as interleukin (IL) 1, IL-6, and IL-8; the expression of adhesion molecules; inhibition of cell-surface plasminogen activation; and expression of tissue factor. The above events change the phenotype of these cells to a prothrombotic form. In addition, anti-β2GPI antibodies induce fetal injury in mice through complement activation, as shown by the evidence that C4-deficient mice were protected from fetal injury.

CLINICAL MANIFESTATIONS AND LABORATORY FINDINGS

Clinical manifestations represent mainly a direct or indirect expression of venous or arterial thrombosis and/or pregnancy morbidity (Table 379-2). Clinical features associated with venous thrombosis are superficial and deep vein thrombosis, cerebral venous thrombosis, signs and symptoms of intracranial hypertension, retinal vein thrombosis, pulmonary emboli, pulmonary arterial hypertension, and Budd-Chiari syndrome. Livedo reticularis consists of a mottled reticular vascular pattern that appears as a lace-like, purplish discoloration of the skin. It is probably caused by swelling of the venules owing to obstruction of capillaries by thrombi. This clinical manifestation correlates with vascular lesions such as those in the central nervous system as well as aseptic bone necrosis. Arterial thrombosis is manifested as migraines, cognitive dysfunction, transient ischemic attacks, stroke, myocardial infarction, arterial thrombosis of upper and lower

TABLE 379-2 CLINICAL FEATURES OF ANTIPHOSPHOLIPID SYNDROME

Manifestation	%
Venous Thrombosis and Related Consequences	
Deep vein thrombosis	39
Livedo reticularis	24
Pulmonary embolism	14
Superficial thrombophlebitis	12
Thrombosis in various other sites	11
Arterial Thrombosis and Related Consequences	
Stroke	20
Cardiac valve thickening/dysfunction and/or Libman-Sacks vegetations	14
Transient ischemic attack	11
Myocardial ischemia (infarction or angina) and coronary bypass thrombosis	10
Leg ulcers and/or digital gangrene	9
Arterial thrombosis in the extremities	7
Retinal artery thrombosis/amaurosis fugax	7
Ischemia of visceral organs or avascular necrosis of bone	6
Multi-infarct dementia	3
Neurologic Manifestations of Uncertain Etiology	
Migraine	20
Epilepsy	7
Chorea	1
Cerebellar ataxia	1
Transverse myelopathy	0.5
Renal Manifestations Due to Various Reasons (Renal Artery/Renal Vein/Glomerular Thrombosis, Fibrous Intima Hyperplasia)	3
Osteoarticular Manifestations	
Arthralgia	39
Arthritis	27
Obstetric Manifestations (Referred to the Number of Pregnancies)	
Preeclampsia	10
Eclampsia	4
Fetal Manifestations (Referred to the Number of Pregnancies)	
Early fetal loss (<10 weeks)	35
Late fetal loss (≥10 weeks)	17
Premature birth among the live births	11
Hematologic Manifestations	
Thrombocytopenia	30
Autoimmune hemolytic anemia	10

Source: Adapted from R Cervera et al: Arthritis Rheum 46:1019, 2002.

extremities, ischemic leg ulcers, digital gangrene, avascular necrosis of bone, retinal artery occlusion leading to painless transient vision loss, renal artery stenosis, and glomerular lesions, as well as infarcts of spleen, pancreas, and adrenals. Libman-Sacks endocarditis consists of very small vegetations, histologically characterized by organized platelet-fibrin microthrombi surrounded by growing fibroblasts and macrophages. Glomerular lesions are manifested with hypertension, mildly elevated serum creatinine levels, proteinuria, and mild hematuria. Histologically, these lesions are characterized in an acute phase by thrombotic microangiopathy involving glomerular capillaries, and in a chronic phase with fibrous intima hyperplasia, fibrous and/or fibrocellular occlusions of arterioles, and focal cortical atrophy (Table 379-2). Premature atherosclerosis has been recognized as a rare feature of APS. Coombs-positive hemolytic anemia and thrombocytopenia are laboratory findings associated with APS. Discontinuation of therapy, major surgery, infection, and trauma may trigger CAPS.

DIAGNOSIS AND DIFFERENTIAL DIAGNOSIS

The diagnosis of APS should be seriously considered in cases of thrombosis, cerebral vascular accidents in individuals younger than 55 years of age, or pregnancy morbidity in the presence of livedo reticularis or thrombocytopenia. In these cases, aPL antibodies should be measured. The presence of at least one clinical and one laboratory criterion ensures the diagnosis even in the presence of other causes of thrombophilia. Clinical criteria include: (1) vascular thrombosis defined as one or more clinical episodes of arterial, venous, or small vessel thrombosis in any tissue or organ; and (2) pregnancy morbidity, defined as (a) one or more unexplained deaths of a morphologically normal fetus at or beyond the tenth week of gestation; (b) one or more premature births of a morphologically normal neonate before the thirty-fourth week of gestation because of eclampsia, severe preeclampsia, or placental insufficiency; or (c) three or more unexplained consecutive spontaneous abortions before the tenth week of gestation. Laboratory criteria include (1) LA, (2) anticardiolipin (aCL), and/or (3) anti-β2GPI antibodies, at intermediate or high titers on two occasions, 12 weeks apart.

Differential diagnosis is based on the exclusion of other inherited or acquired causes of thrombophilia (Chap. 141), Coombs-positive hemolytic anemia (Chap. 129), and thrombocytopenia (Chap. 140). Livedo reticularis with or without a painful ulceration on the lower extremities also may be a manifestation of disorders affecting (1) the vascular wall, such as polyarteritis nodosa, SLE, cryoglobulinemia, and lymphomas; or (2) the vascular lumen, such as myeloproliferative disorders, atherosclerosis, hypercholesterolemia, or other causes of thrombophilia.

TREATMENT ANTIPHOSPHOLIPID SYNDROME

After the first thrombotic event, APS patients should be placed on warfarin for life, aiming to achieve an international normalized ratio (INR) ranging from 2.5 to 3.5, alone or in combination with 80 mg of aspirin daily. Pregnancy morbidity is prevented by a combination of heparin with aspirin 80 mg daily. IV immunoglobulin (IVIg) 400 mg/kg every day for 5 days may also prevent abortions, whereas glucocorticoids are ineffective. Patients with aPL in the absence of any clinical event who are simultaneously positive for aCL, anti-β2GPI, and LA or have SLE are at risk to develop thrombotic events and can be protected by aspirin 80 mg daily.

Some patients with APS and patients with CAPS have recurrent thrombotic events despite appropriate anticoagulation. In these cases, IVIg 400 mg/kg every day for 5 days may be of benefit. Patients with CAPS, who are treated in the intensive care unit, are unable to receive warfarin; in this situation, therapeutic doses of low-molecular-weight heparin should be administered. In cases of heparin-induced thrombocytopenia and thrombosis syndrome, inhibitors of phospholipid-bound activated factor X (FXa), such as fondaparinux 7.5 mg SC daily or rivaroxaban 10 mg PO daily, are effective. The above drugs are administered by fixed doses and do not require close monitoring; their safety during the first trimester of pregnancy has not been clearly established.

380 Rheumatoid Arthritis

Ankoor Shah, E. William St. Clair

INTRODUCTION

Rheumatoid arthritis (RA) is a chronic inflammatory disease of unknown etiology marked by a symmetric, peripheral polyarthritis. It is the most common form of chronic inflammatory arthritis and often results in joint damage and physical disability. Because it is a systemic disease, RA may result in a variety of extraarticular manifestations, including fatigue, subcutaneous nodules, lung involvement, pericarditis, peripheral neuropathy, vasculitis, and hematologic abnormalities.

Insights gained by a wealth of basic and clinical research over the past two decades have revolutionized the contemporary paradigms for the diagnosis and management of RA. Serum antibodies to cyclic citrullinated peptides (anti-CCPs) are routinely used along with rheumatoid factor as a biomarker of diagnostic and prognostic significance. Advances in imaging modalities have improved our ability to detect joint inflammation and destruction in RA. The science of RA has taken a major leap forward with the identification of new disease-related genes and further deciphering of the molecular pathways of disease pathogenesis. The relative importance of these different mechanisms has been highlighted by the observed benefits of the new class of highly targeted biologic and small-molecule therapies. Despite these gains, incomplete understanding of the initiating pathogenic pathways of RA remains a sizable barrier to its cure and prevention.

The last two decades have witnessed a remarkable improvement in the outcomes of RA. The historic descriptions of crippling arthritis are currently encountered much less frequently. Much of this progress can be traced to the expanded therapeutic armamentarium and the adoption of early treatment intervention. The shift in treatment strategy dictates a new mind-set for primary care practitioners—namely, one that demands early referral of patients with inflammatory arthritis to a rheumatologist for prompt diagnosis and initiation of therapy. Only then will patients achieve their best outcomes.

CLINICAL FEATURES

The incidence of RA increases between 25 and 55 years of age, after which it plateaus until the age of 75 and then decreases. The presenting symptoms of RA typically result from inflammation of the joints, tendons, and bursae. Patients often complain of early morning joint stiffness lasting more than 1 h that eases with physical activity. The earliest involved joints are typically the small joints of the hands and feet. The initial pattern of joint involvement may be monoarticular, oligoarticular (≤4 joints), or polyarticular (>5 joints), usually in a symmetric distribution. Some patients with inflammatory arthritis will present with too few affected joints to be classified as having RA—so-called undifferentiated inflammatory arthritis. Those with an undifferentiated arthritis who are most likely to be diagnosed later with RA have a higher number of tender and swollen joints, test positive for serum rheumatoid factor (RF) or anti-CCP antibodies, and have higher scores for physical disability.

Once the disease process of RA is established, the wrists, metacarpophalangeal (MCP), and proximal interphalangeal (PIP) joints stand out as the most frequently involved joints (Fig. 380-1). Distal interphalangeal (DIP) joint involvement may occur in RA, but it usually is a manifestation of coexistent osteoarthritis. Flexor tendon tenosynovitis is a frequent hallmark of RA and leads to decreased range of motion, reduced grip strength, and "trigger" fingers. Progressive destruction of the joints and soft tissues may lead to chronic, irreversible deformities. Ulnar deviation results from subluxation of the MCP joints, with subluxation of the proximal phalanx to the volar side of the hand. Hyperextension of the PIP joint with flexion of the DIP joint ("swan-neck deformity"), flexion of the PIP joint with hyperextension of the DIP joint ("boutonnière deformity"), and subluxation of the first MCP joint with hyperextension of the first interphalangeal (IP) joint ("Z-line

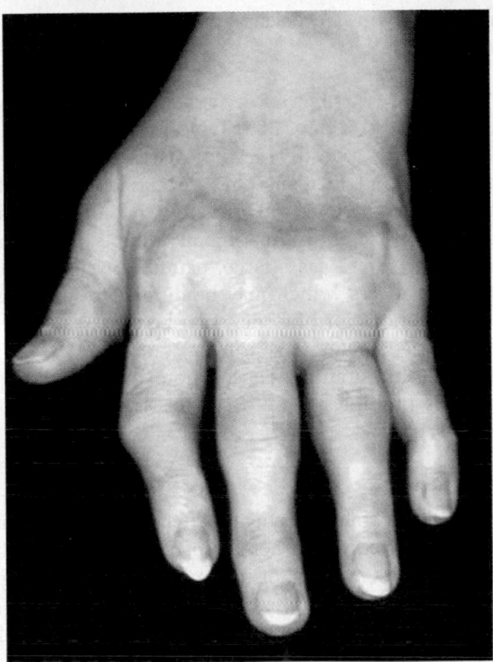

FIGURE 380-1 Metacarpophalangeal and proximal interphalangeal joint swelling in rheumatoid arthritis. *(Courtesy of the American College of Rheumatology Image Bank.)*

deformity") also may result from damage to the tendons, joint capsule, and other soft tissues in these small joints. Inflammation about the ulnar styloid and tenosynovitis of the extensor carpi ulnaris may cause subluxation of the distal ulna, resulting in a "piano-key movement" of the ulnar styloid. Although metatarsophalangeal (MTP) joint involvement in the feet is an early feature of disease, chronic inflammation of the ankle and midtarsal regions usually comes later and may lead to pes planovalgus ("flat feet"). Large joints, including the knees and shoulders, are often affected in established disease, although these joints may remain asymptomatic for many years after onset.

Atlantoaxial involvement of the cervical spine is clinically noteworthy because of its potential to cause compressive myelopathy and neurologic dysfunction. Neurologic manifestations are rarely a presenting sign or symptom of atlantoaxial disease, but they may evolve over time with progressive instability of C1 on C2. The prevalence of atlantoaxial subluxation has been declining in recent years, and occurs now in less than 10% of patients. Unlike the spondyloarthritides (Chap. 384), RA rarely affects the thoracic and lumbar spine. Radiographic abnormalities of the temporomandibular joint occur commonly in patients with RA, but they are generally not associated with significant symptoms or functional impairment.

Extraarticular manifestations may develop during the clinical course of RA, even prior to the onset of arthritis (Fig. 380-2). Patients most likely to develop extraarticular disease have a history of smoking, have early onset of significant physical disability, and test positive for serum RF. Subcutaneous nodules, secondary Sjögren's syndrome, pulmonary nodules, and anemia are among the most frequently observed

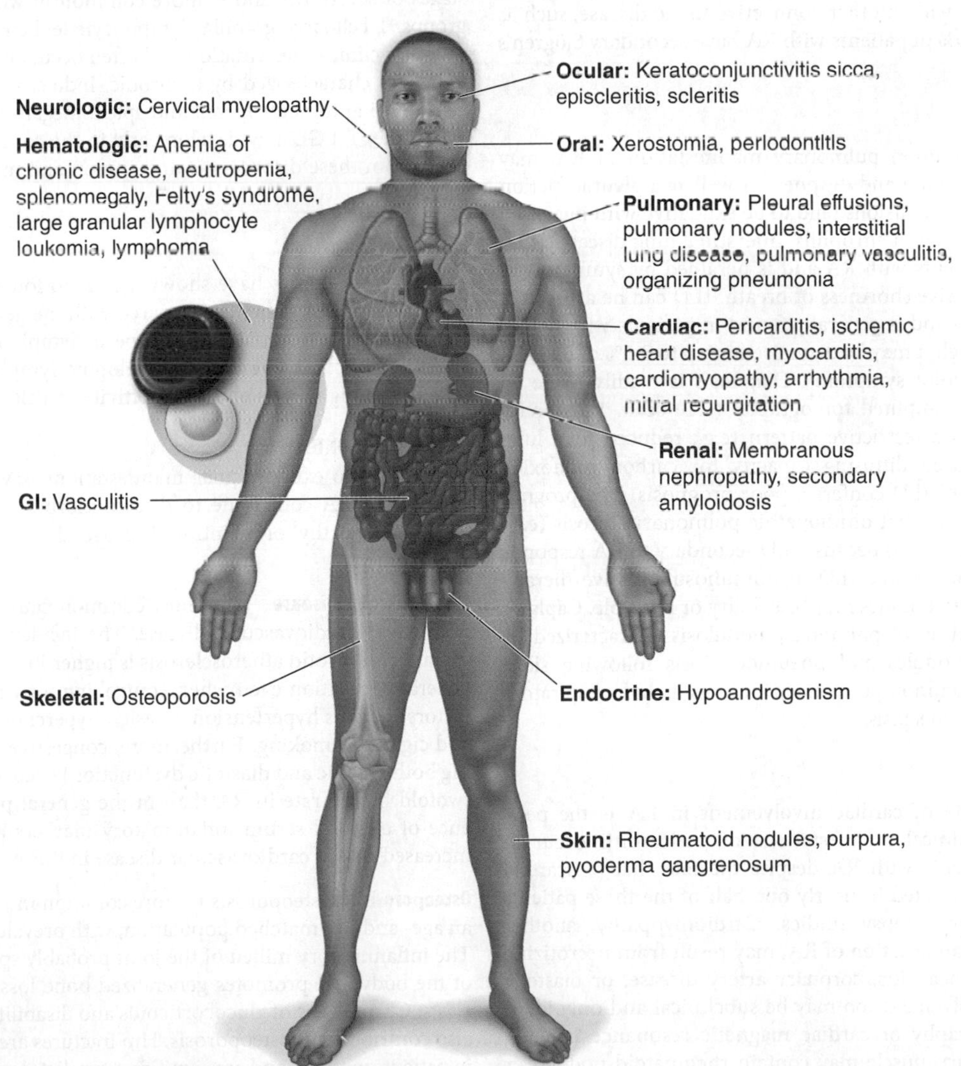

FIGURE 380-2 Extraarticular manifestations of rheumatoid arthritis.

extraarticular manifestations. Recent studies have shown a decrease in the incidence and severity of at least some extraarticular manifestations, particularly Felty's syndrome and vasculitis.

The most common systemic and extraarticular features of RA are described in more detail in the sections below.

CONSTITUTIONAL

These signs and symptoms include weight loss, fever, fatigue, malaise, depression, and in the most severe cases, cachexia; they generally reflect a high degree of inflammation and may even precede the onset of joint symptoms. In general, the presence of a fever of >38.3°C (101°F) at any time during the clinical course should raise suspicion of systemic vasculitis (see below) or infection.

NODULES

Subcutaneous nodules occur in 30–40% of patients and more commonly in those with the highest levels of disease activity, the disease-related shared epitope (see below), a positive test for serum RF, and radiographic evidence of joint erosions. When palpated, the nodules are generally firm; nontender; and adherent to periosteum, tendons, or bursae; developing in areas of the skeleton subject to repeated trauma or irritation such as the forearm, sacral prominences, and Achilles tendon. They may also occur in the lungs, pleura, pericardium, and peritoneum. Nodules are typically benign, although they can be associated with infection, ulceration, and gangrene.

SJÖGREN'S SYNDROME

Secondary Sjögren's syndrome (Chap. 383) is defined by the presence of either keratoconjunctivitis sicca (dry eyes) or xerostomia (dry mouth) in association with another connective tissue disease, such as RA. Approximately 10% of patients with RA have secondary Sjögren's syndrome.

PULMONARY

Pleuritis, the most common pulmonary manifestation of RA, may produce pleuritic chest pain and dyspnea, as well as a pleural friction rub and effusion. Pleural effusions tend to be exudative with increased numbers of monocytes and neutrophils. Interstitial lung disease (ILD) may also occur in patients with RA and is heralded by symptoms of dry cough and progressive shortness of breath. ILD can be associated with cigarette smoking and is generally found in patients with higher disease activity, although it may be diagnosed in up to 3.5% of patients prior to the onset of joint symptoms. Diagnosis is readily made by high-resolution chest computed tomography (CT) scan. Pulmonary function testing shows a restrictive pattern (e.g., reduced total lung capacity) with a reduced diffusing capacity for carbon monoxide (DL_{CO}). The presence of ILD confers a poor prognosis. The prognosis is not quite as poor as that of idiopathic pulmonary fibrosis (e.g., usual interstitial pneumonitis) because ILD secondary to RA responds more favorably than idiopathic ILD to immunosuppressive therapy (Chap. 315). Pulmonary nodules may be solitary or multiple. Caplan's syndrome is a rare subset of pulmonary nodulosis characterized by the development of nodules and pneumoconiosis following silica exposure. Other less common pulmonary findings include respiratory bronchiolitis and bronchiectasis.

CARDIAC

The most frequent site of cardiac involvement in RA is the pericardium. However, clinical manifestations of pericarditis occur in less than 10% of patients with RA despite the fact that pericardial involvement may be detected in nearly one-half of the these patients by echocardiogram or autopsy studies. Cardiomyopathy, another clinically important manifestation of RA, may result from necrotizing or granulomatous myocarditis, coronary artery disease, or diastolic dysfunction. This involvement too may be subclinical and only identified by echocardiography or cardiac magnetic resonance imaging (MRI). Rarely, the heart muscle may contain rheumatoid nodules or be infiltrated with amyloid. Mitral regurgitation is the most common valvular abnormality in RA, occurring at a higher frequency than the general population.

VASCULITIS

Rheumatoid vasculitis (Chap. 385) typically occurs in patients with long-standing disease, a positive test for serum RF, and hypocomplementemia. The overall incidence has decreased significantly in the last decade to be less than 1% of patients. The cutaneous signs vary and include petechiae, purpura, digital infarcts, gangrene, livedo reticularis, and in severe cases large, painful lower extremity ulcerations. Vasculitic ulcers, which may be difficult to distinguish from those caused by venous insufficiency, may be treated successfully with immunosuppressive agents (requiring cytotoxic treatment in severe cases) as well as skin grafting. Sensorimotor polyneuropathies, such as mononeuritis multiplex, may occur in association with systemic rheumatoid vasculitis.

HEMATOLOGIC

A normochromic, normocytic anemia often develops in patients with RA and is the most common hematologic abnormality. The degree of anemia parallels the degree of inflammation, correlating with the levels of serum C-reactive protein (CRP) and erythrocyte sedimentation rate (ESR). Platelet counts may also be elevated in RA as an acute-phase reactant. Immune-mediated thrombocytopenia is rare in this disease.

Felty's syndrome is defined by the clinical triad of neutropenia, splenomegaly, and nodular RA and is seen in less than 1% of patients, although its incidence appears to be declining in the face of more aggressive treatment of the joint disease. It typically occurs in the late stages of severe RA and is more common in whites than other racial groups. T cell large granular lymphocyte leukemia (T-LGL) may have a similar clinical presentation and often occurs in association with RA. T-LGL is characterized by a chronic, indolent clonal growth of LGL cells, leading to neutropenia and splenomegaly. As opposed to Felty's syndrome, T-LGL may develop early in the course of RA. Leukopenia apart from these disorders is uncommon and most often due to drug therapy.

LYMPHOMA

Large cohort studies have shown a two- to fourfold increased risk of lymphoma in RA patients compared with the general population. The most common histopathologic type of lymphoma is a diffuse large B cell lymphoma. The risk of developing lymphoma increases if the patient has high levels of disease activity or Felty's syndrome.

ASSOCIATED CONDITIONS

In addition to extraarticular manifestations, several conditions associated with RA contribute to disease morbidity and mortality rates. They are worthy of mention because they affect chronic disease management.

Cardiovascular Disease The most common cause of death in patients with RA is cardiovascular disease. The incidence of coronary artery disease and carotid atherosclerosis is higher in RA patients than in the general population even when controlling for traditional cardiac risk factors, such as hypertension, obesity, hypercholesterolemia, diabetes, and cigarette smoking. Furthermore, congestive heart failure (including both systolic and diastolic dysfunction) occurs at an approximately twofold higher rate in RA than in the general population. The presence of elevated serum inflammatory markers appears to confer an increased risk of cardiovascular disease in this population.

Osteoporosis Osteoporosis is more common in patients with RA than an age- and sex-matched population, with prevalence rates of 20–30%. The inflammatory milieu of the joint probably spills over into the rest of the body and promotes generalized bone loss by activating osteoclasts. Chronic use of glucocorticoids and disability-related immobility also contributes to osteoporosis. Hip fractures are more likely to occur in patients with RA and are significant predictors of increased disability and mortality rate in this disease.

Hypoandrogenism Men and postmenopausal women with RA have lower mean serum testosterone, luteinizing hormone (LH), and dehydroepiandrosterone (DHEA) levels than control populations. It has thus been hypothesized that hypoandrogenism may play a role in the pathogenesis of RA or arise as a consequence of the chronic inflammatory response. It is also important to realize that patients receiving chronic glucocorticoid therapy may develop hypoandrogenism owing to inhibition of LH and follicle-stimulating hormone (FSH) secretion from the pituitary gland. Because low testosterone levels may lead to osteoporosis, men with hypoandrogenism should be considered for androgen replacement therapy.

EPIDEMIOLOGY

RA affects approximately 0.5–1% of the adult population worldwide. There is evidence that the overall incidence of RA has been decreasing in recent decades, whereas the prevalence has remained the same because individuals with RA are living longer. The incidence and prevalence of RA varies based on geographic location, both globally and among certain ethnic groups within a country (Fig. 380-3). For example, the Native American Yakima, Pima, and Chippewa tribes of North America have reported prevalence rates in some studies of nearly 7%. In contrast, many population studies from Africa and Asia show lower prevalence rates for RA in the range of 0.2–0.4%.

Like many other autoimmune diseases, RA occurs more commonly in females than in males, with a 2–3:1 ratio. Interestingly, studies of RA from some of the Latin American and African countries show an even greater predominance of disease in females compared to males, with ratios of 6–8:1. Given this preponderance of females, various theories have been proposed to explain the possible rôle of estrogen in disease pathogenesis. Most of the theories center on the role of estrogens in enhancing the immune response. For example, some experimental studies have shown that estrogen can stimulate production of tumor necrosis factor a (TNF-α), a major cytokine in the pathogenesis of RA.

GENETIC CONSIDERATIONS

It has been recognized for over 30 years that genetic factors contribute to the occurrence of RA as well as to its severity. The likelihood that a first-degree relative of a patient will share the diagnosis of RA is 2–10 times greater than in the general population. There remains, however, some uncertainty in the extent to which genetics plays a role in the causative mechanisms of RA. Although twin studies imply that genetic factors may explain up to 60% of the occurrence of RA, the more commonly stated estimate falls in the range of 10–25%. The estimate of genetic influence may vary across studies due to gene–environment interactions.

The alleles known to confer the greatest risk of RA are located within the major histocompatibility complex (MHC). It has been estimated that one-third of the genetic risk for RA resides within this locus. Most, but probably not all, of this risk is associated with allelic variation in the HLA-DRB1 gene, which encodes the MHC II β-chain molecule. The disease-associated HLA-DRB1 alleles share an amino acid sequence at positions 70–74 in the third hypervariable regions of the HLA-DR β-chain, termed the *shared epitope (SE).* Carriership of the SE alleles is associated with production of anti-CCP antibodies and worse disease outcomes. Some of these HLA-DRB1 alleles bestow a high risk of disease (*0401), whereas others confer a more moderate risk (*0101, *0404, *1001, and *0901). Additionally, there is regional variation. In Greece, for example, where RA tends to be milder than in western European countries, RA susceptibility has been associated with the *0101 SE allele. By comparison, the *0401 or *0404 alleles are found in approximately 50–70% of northern Europeans and are the predominant risk alleles in this group. The most common disease susceptibility SE alleles in Asians, namely the Japanese, Koreans, and Chinese, are *0405 and *0901. Lastly, disease susceptibility of Native American populations such as the Pima and Tlingit Indians, where the prevalence of RA can be as high as 7%, is associated with the SE allele *1042. The risk of RA conferred by these SE alleles is less in African and Hispanic Americans than in individuals of European ancestry.

Genome-wide association studies (GWAS) have made possible the identification of several non-MHC-related genes that contribute to RA susceptibility. GWAS are based on the detection of single-nucleotide polymorphisms (SNPs), which allow for examination of the genetic architecture of complex diseases such as RA. There are approximately 10 million common SNPs within a human genome consisting of 3 billion base pairs. As a rule, GWAS identify only common variants, namely, those with a frequency of more than 5% in the general population.

Overall, several themes have emerged from GWAS in RA. First, the non-MHC loci identified as risk alleles for RA have only a modest

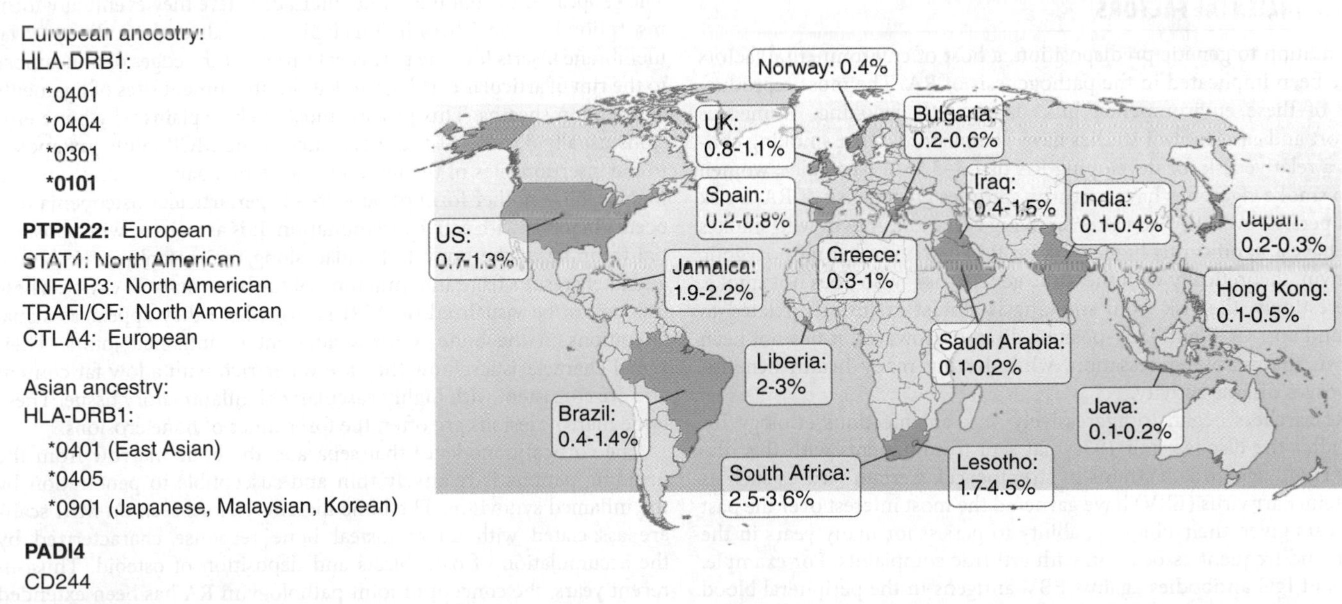

FIGURE 380-3 Global prevalence rates of rheumatoid arthritis (RA) with genetic associations. Listed are the major genetic alleles associated with RA. Although human leukocyte antigen (HLA)-DRB1 mutations are found globally, some alleles have been associated with RA in only certain ethnic groups.

effect on risk; they also contribute to the risk for developing other autoimmune diseases, such as type 1 diabetes mellitus, systemic lupus erythematosus, and multiple sclerosis. Second, although most of the non-HLA associations are described in patients with anti-CCP antibody-positive disease, there are several risk loci that are unique to anti-CCP antibody-negative disease. Third, risk alleles vary among ethnic groups. And fourth, the risk loci mostly reside in genes encoding proteins involved in the regulation of the immune response. However, the risk alleles identified by GWAS only account at present for approximately 5% of the genetic risk, suggesting that rare variants or other classes of DNA variants, such as variants in copy number, may be yet found that significantly contribute to the overall risk model.

Recently, imputation of SNP data from a GWAS meta-analysis shows amino acid substitutions in the MHC locus independently associated with the risk for RA are at position 11, 71, and 74 in HLA-DRβ1, position 9 of HLA-B, and position 9 of HLA-DPβ1. The amino acids at position 11, 71, and 74 are located in the antigen-binding grove of the HLA-DRβ1 molecule, highlighting positions 71 and 74 that form part of the original shared epitope.

Among the best examples of the non-MHC genes contributing to the risk of RA is the gene encoding protein tyrosine phosphatase non-receptor 22 (*PTPN22*). This gene varies in frequency among patients from different parts of Europe (e.g., 3–10%), but is absent in patients of East Asian ancestry. *PTPN22* encodes lymphoid tyrosine phosphatase, a protein that regulates T and B cell function. Inheritance of the risk allele for *PTPN22* produces a gain-of-function in the protein that is hypothesized to result in the abnormal thymic selection of autoreactive T and B cells and appears to be associated exclusively with anti-CCP-positive disease. The peptidyl arginine deiminase type IV (*PADI4*) gene is another risk allele that encodes an enzyme involved in the conversion of arginine to citrulline and is postulated to play a role in the development of antibodies to citrullinated antigens. A polymorphism in *PADI4* has been associated with RA only in Asian populations.

Epigenetics is the study of heritable traits that affect gene expression but do not modify DNA sequence. It may provide a link between environmental exposure and predisposition to disease. The best-studied mechanisms include posttranslational histone modifications and DNA methylation. Although studies of epigenetic phenomena are limited, DNA methylation patterns have been shown to differ between RA patients and healthy controls, as well as patients with osteoarthritis.

ENVIRONMENTAL FACTORS

In addition to genetic predisposition, a host of environmental factors have been implicated in the pathogenesis of RA. The most reproducible of these environmental links is cigarette smoking. Numerous cohort and case control studies have demonstrated that smoking confers a relative risk for developing RA of 1.5–3.5. In particular, women who smoke cigarettes have a nearly 2.5 times greater risk of RA, a risk that persists even 15 years after smoking cessation. A twin who smokes will have a significantly higher risk for RA than his or her monozygotic co-twin, theoretically with the same genetic risk, who does not smoke. Interestingly, the risk from smoking is almost exclusively related to RF and anti-CCP antibody-positive disease. However, it has not been shown that smoking cessation, while having many health benefits, improves disease activity.

Researchers began to aggressively seek an infectious etiology for RA after the discovery in 1931 that sera from patients with this disease could agglutinate strains of streptococci. Certain viruses such as Epstein-Barr virus (EBV) have garnered the most interest over the past 30 years given their ubiquity, ability to persist for many years in the host, and frequent association with arthritic complaints. For example, titers of IgG antibodies against EBV antigens in the peripheral blood and saliva are significantly higher in patients with RA than the general population. EBV DNA has also been found in synovial fluid and synovial cells of RA patients. Because the evidence for these links is largely circumstantial, it has not been possible to directly implicate infection as a causative factor in RA.

PATHOLOGY

RA affects the synovial tissue and underlying cartilage and bone. The synovial membrane, which covers most articular surfaces, tendon sheaths, and bursae, normally is a thin layer of connective tissue. In joints, it faces the bone and cartilage, bridging the opposing bony surfaces and inserting at periosteal regions close to the articular cartilage. It consists primarily of two cell types—type A synoviocytes (macrophage-derived) and type B synoviocytes (fibroblast-derived). The synovial fibroblasts are the most abundant and produce the structural components of joints, including collagen, fibronectin, and laminin, as well as other extracellular constituents of the synovial matrix. The sublining layer consists of blood vessels and a sparse population of mononuclear cells within a loose network of connective tissue. Synovial fluid, an ultrafiltrate of blood, diffuses through the subsynovial lining tissue across the synovial membrane and into the joint cavity. Its main constituents are hyaluronan and lubricin. Hyaluronan is a glycosaminoglycan that contributes to the viscous nature of synovial fluid, which along with lubricin, lubricates the surface of the articular cartilage.

The pathologic hallmarks of RA are synovial inflammation and proliferation, focal bone erosions, and thinning of articular cartilage. Chronic inflammation leads to synovial lining hyperplasia and the formation of pannus, a thickened cellular membrane containing fibroblast-like synoviocytes and granulation-reactive fibrovascular tissue that invades the underlying cartilage and bone. The inflammatory infiltrate is made up of no less than six cell types: T cells, B cells, plasma cells, dendritic cells, mast cells, and, to a lesser extent, granulocytes. The T cells comprise 30–50% of the infiltrate, with the other cells accounting for the remainder. The topographical organization of these cells is complex and may vary among individuals with RA. Most often, the lymphocytes are diffusely organized among the tissue resident cells; however, in some cases, the B cells, T cells, and dendritic cells may form higher levels of organization, such as lymphoid follicles and germinal center–like structures. Growth factors secreted by synovial fibroblasts and macrophages promote the formation of new blood vessels in the synovial sublining that supply the increasing demands for oxygenation and nutrition required by the infiltrating leukocytes and expanding synovial tissue.

The structural damage to the mineralized cartilage and subchondral bone is mediated by the osteoclast. Osteoclasts are multinucleated giant cells that can be identified by their expression of CD68, tartrate-resistant acid phosphatase, cathepsin K, and the calcitonin receptor. They appear at the pannus-bone interface where they eventually form resorption lacunae. These lesions typically localize where the synovial membrane inserts into the periosteal surface at the edges of bones close to the rim of articular cartilage and at the attachment sites of ligaments and tendon sheaths. This process most likely explains why bone erosions usually develop at the radial sites of the MCP joints juxtaposed to the insertion sites of the tendons, collateral ligaments, and synovial membrane. Another form of bone loss is periarticular osteopenia that occurs in joints with active inflammation. It is associated with substantial thinning of the bony trabeculae along the metaphyses of bones, and likely results from inflammation of the bone marrow cavity. These lesions can be visualized on MRI scans, where they appear as signal alterations in the bone marrow adjacent to inflamed joints. Their signal characteristics show they are water-rich with a low fat content and are consistent with highly vascularized inflammatory tissue. These bone marrow lesions are often the forerunner of bone erosions.

The cortical bone layer that separates the bone marrow from the invading pannus is relatively thin and susceptible to penetration by the inflamed synovium. The bone marrow lesions seen on MRI scans are associated with an endosteal bone response characterized by the accumulation of osteoblasts and deposition of osteoid. Thus, in recent years, the concept of joint pathology in RA has been extended to include the bone marrow cavity. Finally, generalized osteoporosis, which results in the thinning of trabecular bone throughout the body, is a third form of bone loss found in patients with RA.

Articular cartilage is an avascular tissue comprised of a specialized matrix of collagens, proteoglycans, and other proteins. It is organized in four distinct regions (superficial, middle, deep, and calcified cartilage zones)—chondrocytes constitute the unique cellular component in these layers. Originally, cartilage was considered to be an inert tissue, but it is now known to be a highly responsive tissue that reacts to inflammatory mediators and mechanical factors, which in turn, alter the balance between cartilage anabolism and catabolism. In RA, the initial areas of cartilage degradation are juxtaposed to the synovial pannus. The cartilage matrix is characterized by a generalized loss of proteoglycan, most evident in the superficial zones adjacent to the synovial fluid. Degradation of cartilage may also take place in the perichondrocytic zone and in regions adjacent to the subchondral bone.

PATHOGENESIS

The pathogenic mechanisms of synovial inflammation are likely to result from a complex interplay of genetic, environmental, and immunologic factors that produces dysregulation of the immune system and a breakdown in self-tolerance (Fig. 380-4). Precisely what triggers these initiating events and what genetic and environmental factors disrupt the immune system remains a mystery. However, a detailed molecular picture is emerging of the mechanisms underlying the chronic inflammatory response and the destruction of the articular cartilage and bone.

In RA, the preclinical stage appears to be characterized by a breakdown in self-tolerance. This idea is supported by the finding that autoantibodies, such as RF and anti-CCP antibodies, may be found in sera from patients many years before clinical disease can be detected. However, the antigenic targets of anti-CCP antibodies and RF are not restricted to the joint, and their role in disease pathogenesis remains speculative. Anti-CCP antibodies are directed against deaminated peptides, which result from posttranslational modification by the enzyme PADI4. They recognize citrulline-containing regions of several different matrix proteins, including filaggrin, keratin, fibrinogen, and vimentin, and are present at higher levels in the joint fluid compared to the serum. Other autoantibodies have been found in a minority of patients with RA, but they also occur in the setting of other types of arthritis. They bind to a diverse array of autoantigens, including type II collagen, human cartilage gp-39, aggrecan, calpastatin, BiP (immunoglobulin binding protein), and glucose-6-phosphate isomerase.

In theory, environmental stimulants may synergize with other factors to bring about inflammation in RA. People who smoke display higher citrullination of proteins in bronchoalveolar fluid than those who do not smoke. Thus, it has been speculated that long-term exposure to tobacco smoke might induce citrullination of cellular proteins in the lung and stimulate the expression of a neoepitope capable of inducing self-reactivity, which in turns, leads to formation of immune complexes and joint inflammation. Exposure to silicone dust and mineral oil, which has adjuvant effects, has also been linked to an increased risk for anti-CCP antibody-positive RA.

How might microbes or their products be involved in the initiating events of RA? The immune system is alerted to the presence of microbial infections through Toll-like receptors (TLRs). There are 10 TLRs in humans that recognize a variety of microbial products, including bacterial cell-surface lipopolysaccharides and heat-shock proteins (TLR4), lipoproteins (TLR2), double-strand RNA viruses (TLR3), and unmethylated CpG DNA from bacteria (TLR9). TLR2, -3, and -4 are abundantly expressed by synovial fibroblasts in early RA and, when bound by their ligands, upregulate production of proinflammatory cytokines. Although such events could amplify inflammatory pathways in RA, a specific role for TLRs in disease pathogenesis has not been elucidated.

The pathogenesis of RA is built upon the concept that self-reactive T cells drive the chronic inflammatory response. In theory, self-reactive T cells might arise in RA from abnormal central (thymic) selection due to defects in DNA repair leading to an imbalance of T cell death and life, or defects in the cell signaling apparatus lowering the threshold for T cell activation. Similarly, abnormal selection of the T cell repertoire in the periphery might lead to a breakdown in T cell tolerance. The support for these theories comes mainly from studies of arthritis in mouse models. It has not been shown that patients with RA have abnormal thymic selection of T cells or defective apoptotic pathways regulating cell death. At least some antigen stimulation inside the joint seems likely, owing to the fact that T cells in the synovium express a cell-surface phenotype indicating prior antigen exposure and show evidence of clonal expansion. Of interest, peripheral blood T cells from patients with RA have been shown to display a fingerprint of premature aging that mostly affects inexperienced naïve T cells. In these studies, the most glaring findings have been the loss of telomeric sequences and a decrease in the thymic output of new T cells. Although intriguing, it is not clear how generalized T cell abnormalities might provoke a systemic disease dominated by synovitis.

There is substantial evidence supporting a role for CD4+ T cells in the pathogenesis of RA. First, the co-receptor CD4 on the surface of T cells binds to invariant sites on MHC class II molecules, stabilizing the MHC-peptide–T cell receptor complex during T cell activation. Because the SE on MHC class II molecules is a risk factor for RA, it follows that CD4+ T cell activation may play a role in the pathogenesis of this disease. Second, CD4+ memory T cells are enriched in the synovial tissue from patients with RA and can be implicated through "guilt by association." Third, CD4+ T cells have been shown to be important in the initiation of arthritis in animal models. Fourth, some, but not all, T cell–directed therapies have shown clinical efficacy in this disease. Taken together, these lines of evidence suggest that CD4+ T cells play an important role in orchestrating the chronic inflammatory response in RA. However, other cell types, such as CD8+ T cells, natural killer (NK) cells, and B cells are present in synovial tissue and may also influence pathogenic responses.

In the rheumatoid joint, by mechanisms of cell-cell contact and release of soluble mediators, activated T cells stimulate macrophages and fibroblast-like synoviocytes to generate proinflammatory mediators and proteases that drive the synovial inflammatory response and destroy the cartilage and bone. CD4+ T cell activation is dependent on two signals: (1) T cell receptor binding to peptide-MHC on antigen-presenting cells; and (2) CD28 binding to CD80/86 on antigen-presenting cells. CD4+ T cells also provide help to B cells, which in turn, produce antibodies that may promote further inflammation in the joint. The previous T cell–centric model for the pathogenesis of RA was based on a T_H1-driven paradigm, which came from studies indicating that CD4+ T helper (T_H) cells differentiated into T_H1 and T_H2 subsets, each with their distinctive cytokine profiles. T_H1 cells were found to mainly produce interferon γ (IFN-γ), lymphotoxin β, and TNF-α, whereas T_H2 cells predominately secreted interleukin (IL)-4, IL-5, IL-6, IL-10, and IL-13. The recent discovery of another subset of T_H cells, namely the T_H17 lineage, has revolutionized our concepts concerning the pathogenesis of RA. In humans, naïve T cells are induced to differentiate into T_H17 cells by exposure to transforming growth factor β (TGF-β), IL-1, IL-6, and IL-23. Upon activation, T_H17 cells secrete a variety of proinflammatory mediators such as IL-17, IL-21, IL-22, TNF-α, IL-26, IL-6, and granulocyte-macrophage colony-stimulating factor (GM-CSF). Substantial evidence now exists from both animal models and humans that IL-17 plays an important role not only in promoting joint inflammation, but also in destroying cartilage and subchondral bone

The immune system has evolved mechanisms to counterbalance the potential harmful immune-mediated inflammatory responses provoked by infectious agents and other triggers. Among these negative regulators are regulatory T (T_{reg}) cells, which are produced in the thymus and induced in the periphery to suppress immune-mediated inflammation. They are characterized by the surface expression of CD25 and the transcription factor forkhead box P3 (FOXP3) and orchestrate dominant tolerance through contact with other immune cells and secretion of inhibitory cytokines, such as TGF-β, IL-10, and IL-35. T_{reg} cells appear to be heterogeneous and capable of suppressing distinct classes (T_H1, T_H2, T_H17) of the immune response. In RA, the data that T_{reg} numbers are deficient compared to normal healthy controls are contradictory and inconclusive. Although some experimental evidence suggests that T_{reg} suppressive activity is lost due to dysfunctional expression of cytotoxic T lymphocyte antigen 4

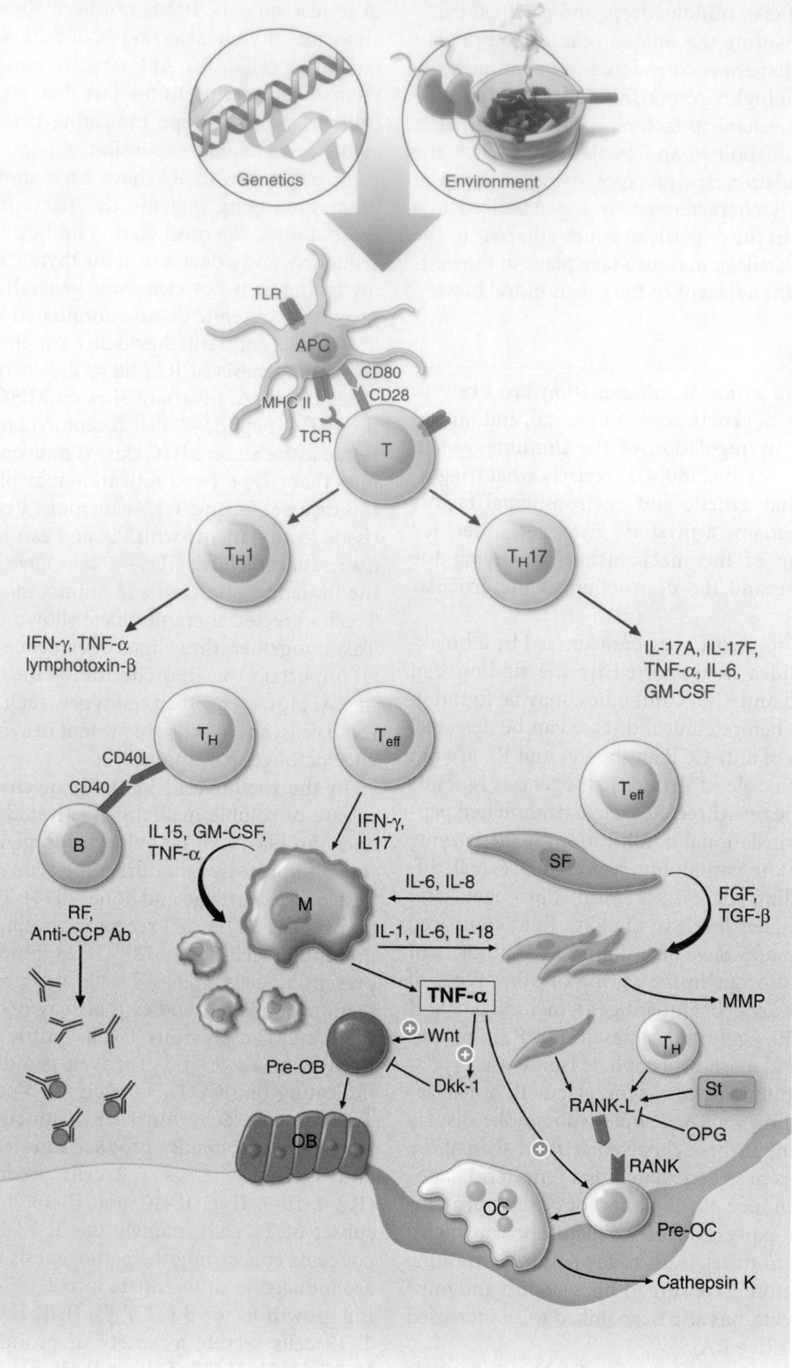

FIGURE 380-4 Pathophysiologic mechanisms of inflammation and joint destruction. Genetic predisposition along with environmental factors may trigger the development of rheumatoid arthritis (RA), with subsequent synovial T cell activation. CD4+ T cells become activated by antigen-presenting cells (APCs) through interactions between the T cell receptor and class II major histocompatibility complex (MHC)-peptide antigen (signal 1) with co-stimulation through the CD28-CD80/86 pathway, as well as other pathways (signal 2). In theory, ligands binding Toll-like receptors (TLRs) may further stimulate activation of APCs inside the joint. Synovial CD4+ T cells differentiate into T_H1 and T_H17 cells, each with their distinctive cytokine profile. CD4+ T_H cells in turn activate B cells, some of which are destined to differentiate into autoantibody-producing plasma cells. Immune complexes, possibly comprised of rheumatoid factors (RFs) and anti–cyclic citrullinated peptides (CCP) antibodies, may form inside the joint, activating the complement pathway and amplifying inflammation. T effector cells stimulate synovial macrophages (M) and fibroblasts (SF) to secrete proinflammatory mediators, among which is tumor necrosis factor α (TNF-α). TNF-α upregulates adhesion molecules on endothelial cells, promoting leukocyte influx into the joint. It also stimulates the production of other inflammatory mediators, such as interleukin 1 (IL-1), IL-6, and granulocyte-macrophage colony-stimulating factor (GM-CSF). TNF-α has a critically important function in regulating the balance between bone destruction and formation. It upregulates the expression of dickkopf-1 (DKK-1), which can then internalize Wnt receptors on osteoblast precursors. Wnt is a soluble mediator that promotes osteoblastogenesis and bone formation. In RA, bone formation is inhibited through the Wnt pathway, presumably due to the action of elevated levels of DKK-1. In addition to inhibiting bone formation, TNF-α stimulates osteoclastogenesis. However, it is not sufficient by itself to induce the differentiation of osteoclast precursors (Pre-OC) into activated osteoclasts capable of eroding bone. Osteoclast differentiation requires the presence of macrophage colony-stimulating factor (M-CSF) and receptor activator of nuclear factor-kB (RANK) ligand (RANKL), which binds to RANK on the surface of Pre-OC. Inside the joint, RANKL is mainly derived from stromal cells, synovial fibroblasts, and T cells. Osteoprotegerin (OPG) acts as a decoy receptor for RANKL, thereby inhibiting osteoclastogenesis and bone loss. FGF, fibroblast growth factor; IFN, interferon; TGF, transforming growth factor.

(CTLA-4), the nature of T_{reg} defects in RA, if they exist, remains unclear.

Cytokines, chemokines, antibodies, and endogenous danger signals bind to receptors on the surface of immune cells and stimulate a cascade of intracellular signaling events that can amplify the inflammatory response. Signaling molecules and their binding partners in these pathways are the target of small-molecule drugs designed to interfere with signal transduction and block these reinforcing inflammatory loops. Examples of signal molecules in these critical inflammatory pathways include Janus kinase (JAK)/signal transducers and activators of transcription (STAT), spleen tyrosine kinase (Syk), mitogen-activated protein kinases (MAPKs), and nuclear factor-κB (NF-κB). These pathways exhibit significant cross-talk and are found in many cell types. Some signal transducers, such as JAK3, are primarily expressed in hematopoietic cells and play an important role in the inflammatory response in RA.

Activated B cells are also important players in the chronic inflammatory response. B cells give rise to plasma cells, which in turn, produce antibodies, including RF and anti-CCP antibodies. RFs may form large immune complexes inside the joint that contribute to the pathogenic process by fixing complement and promoting the release of proinflammatory chemokines and chemoattractants. In mouse models of arthritis, RF-containing immune complexes and anti-CCP-containing immune complexes synergize with other mechanisms to exacerbate the synovial inflammatory response.

RA is often considered to be a macrophage-driven disease because this cell type is the predominant source of proinflammatory cytokines inside the joint. Key proinflammatory cytokines released by synovial macrophages include TNF-α, IL-1, IL-6, IL-12, IL-15, IL-18, and IL-23. Synovial fibroblasts, the other major cell type in this microenvironment, produce the cytokines IL-1 and IL-6 as well as TNF-α. TNF-α is a pivotal cytokine in the pathobiology of synovial inflammation. It upregulates adhesion molecules on endothelial cells, promoting the influx of leukocytes into the synovial microenvironment; activates synovial fibroblasts; stimulates angiogenesis; promotes pain receptor sensitizing pathways; and drives osteoclastogenesis. Fibroblasts secrete matrix metalloproteinases (MMPs) as well as other proteases that are chiefly responsible for the breakdown of articular cartilage.

Osteoclast activation at the site of the pannus is closely tied to the presence of focal bone erosion. Receptor activator of nuclear factor-κB ligand (RANKL) is expressed by stromal cells, synovial fibroblasts, and T cells. Upon binding to its receptor RANK on osteoclast progenitors, RANKL stimulates osteoclast differentiation and bone resorption. RANKL activity is regulated by osteoprotegerin (OPG), a decoy receptor of RANKL that blocks osteoclast formation. Monocytic cells in the synovium serve as the precursors of osteoclasts and, when exposed to macrophage colony-stimulating factor (M-CSF) and RANKL, fuse to form polykaryons termed *preosteoclasts*. These precursor cells undergo further differentiation into osteoclasts with the characteristic ruffled membrane. Cytokines such as TNF-α, IL-1, IL-6, and IL-17 increase the expression of RANKL in the joint and thus promote osteoclastogenesis. Osteoclasts also secrete cathepsin K, which is a cysteine protease that degrades the bone matrix by cleaving collagen. Stimulation of osteoclasts also contributes to generalized bone loss and osteoporosis.

Increased bone loss is only part of the story in RA, as decreased bone formation plays a crucial role in bone remodeling at sites of inflammation. Recent evidence shows that inflammation suppresses bone formation. The proinflammatory cytokine TNF-α plays a key role in actively suppressing bone formation by enhancing the expression of dickkopf-1 (DKK-1). DKK-1 is an important inhibitor of the Wnt pathway, which acts to promote osteoblast differentiation and bone formation. The Wnt system is a family of soluble glycoproteins that bind to cell-surface receptors known as frizzled (fz) and low-density lipoprotein (LDL) receptor–related proteins (LRPs) and promote cell growth. In animal models, increased levels of DKK-1 are associated with decreased bone formation, whereas inhibition of DKK-1 protects against structural damage in the joint. Wnt proteins also induce the formation of OPG and thereby shut down bone resorption, emphasizing their key role in tightly regulating the balance between bone resorption and formation.

DIAGNOSIS

The clinical diagnosis of RA is largely based on signs and symptoms of a chronic inflammatory arthritis, with laboratory and radiographic results providing important supplemental information. In 2010, a collaborative effort between the American College of Rheumatology (ACR) and the European League Against Rheumatism (EULAR) revised the 1987 ACR classification criteria for RA in an effort to improve early diagnosis with the goal of identifying patients who would benefit from early introduction of disease-modifying therapy (Table 380-1). Application of the newly revised criteria yields a score of 0–10, with a score of ≥ 6 fulfilling the requirements for definite RA. The new classification criteria differ in several ways from the older criteria set. The new criteria include a positive test for serum anti-CCP antibodies (also termed ACPA, anti-citrullinated peptide antibodies) as an item, which carries greater specificity for the diagnosis of RA than a positive test for RF. The newer classification criteria also do not take into account whether the patient has rheumatoid nodules or radiographic joint damage because these findings occur rarely in early RA. It is important to emphasize that the new 2010 ACR-EULAR criteria are "classification criteria" as opposed to "diagnostic criteria" and serve to distinguish patients at the onset of disease who have a high likelihood of evolution to chronic disease with persistent synovitis and joint damage. The presence of radiographic joint erosions or subcutaneous nodules may inform the diagnosis in the later stages of the disease.

LABORATORY FEATURES

Patients with systemic inflammatory diseases such as RA will often present with elevated nonspecific inflammatory markers such as an ESR or CRP. Detection of serum RF and anti-CCP antibodies is important in differentiating RA from other polyarticular diseases, although RF lacks diagnostic specificity and may be found in association with other chronic inflammatory diseases in which arthritis figures in the clinical manifestations.

IgM, IgG, and IgA isotypes of RF occur in sera from patients with RA, although the IgM isotype is the one most frequently measured by commercial laboratories. Serum IgM RF has been found in 75–80% of patients with RA; therefore, a negative result does not exclude the presence of this disease. It is also found in other connective tissue diseases, such as primary Sjögren's syndrome, systemic lupus erythematosus, and type II mixed essential cryoglobulinemia, as well as chronic infections such as subacute bacterial endocarditis and hepatitis B and C. Serum RF may also be detected in 1–5% of the healthy population.

TABLE 380-1 CLASSIFICATION CRITERIA FOR RHEUMATOID ARTHRITIS

		Score
Joint involvement	1 large joint (shoulder, elbow, hip, knee, ankle)	0
	2–10 large joints	1
	1–3 small joints (MCP, PIP, thumb IP, MTP, wrists)	2
	4–10 small joints	3
	>10 joints (at least 1 small joint)	5
Serology	Negative RF and negative ACPA	0
	Low-positive RF or low-positive anti-CCP antibodies (≤3 times ULN)	2
	High-positive RF or high-positive anti-CCP antibodies (>3 times ULN)	3
Acute-phase reactants	Normal CRP and normal ESR	0
	Abnormal CRP or abnormal ESR	1
Duration of symptoms	<6 weeks	0
	≥6 weeks	1

Note: These criteria are aimed at classification of newly presenting patients who have at least one joint with definite clinical synovitis that is not better explained by another disease. A score of ≥6 fulfills requirements for definite RA.

Abbreviations: ACPA, anti-citrullinated peptide antibodies; CCP, cyclic citrullinated peptides; CRP, C-reactive protein; ESR, erythrocyte sedimentation rate; IP, interphalangeal joint; MCP, metacarpophalangeal joint; MTP, metatarsophalangeal joint; PIP, proximal interphalangeal joint; RF, rheumatoid factor; ULN, upper limit of normal.

Source: D Aletaha et al: Arthritis Rheum 62:2569, 2010.

The presence of serum anti-CCP antibodies has about the same sensitivity as serum RF for the diagnosis of RA. However, its diagnostic specificity approaches 95%, so a positive test for anti-CCP antibodies in the setting of an early inflammatory arthritis is useful for distinguishing RA from other forms of arthritis. There is some incremental value in testing for the presence of both RF and anti-CCP, as some patients with RA are positive for RF but negative for anti-CCP and visa versa. The presence of RF or anti-CCP antibodies also has prognostic significance, with anti-CCP antibodies showing the most value for predicting worse outcomes.

SYNOVIAL FLUID ANALYSIS

Typically, synovial fluid from patients with RA reflects an inflammatory state. Synovial fluid white blood cell (WBC) counts can vary widely, but generally range between 5000 and 50,000 WBC/μL compared to <2000 WBC/μL for a noninflammatory condition such as osteoarthritis. In contrast to the synovial tissue, the overwhelming cell type in the synovial fluid is the neutrophil. Clinically, the analysis of synovial fluid is most useful for confirming an inflammatory arthritis (as opposed to osteoarthritis), while at the same time excluding infection or a crystal-induced arthritis such as gout or pseudogout (Chap. 395).

JOINT IMAGING

Joint imaging is a valuable tool not only for diagnosing RA, but also for tracking progression of any joint damage. Plain x-ray is the most common imaging modality, but it is limited to visualization of the bony structures and inferences about the state of the articular cartilage based on the amount of narrowing of the joint space. MRI and ultrasound techniques offer the added value of detecting changes in the soft tissues such as synovitis, tenosynovitis, and effusions as well as greater sensitivity for identifying bony abnormalities. Plain radiographs are usually relied upon in clinical practice for the purpose of diagnosis and monitoring of affected joints. However, in selected cases, MRI and ultrasound can provide additional diagnostic information that may guide clinical decision making. Musculoskeletal ultrasound with power Doppler is increasingly used in rheumatology clinical practice for detecting synovitis and bone erosion.

Plain Radiography Classically in RA, the initial radiographic finding is periarticular osteopenia. Practically speaking, however, this finding is difficult to appreciate on plain films and, in particular, on the newer digitalized x-rays. Other findings on plain radiographs include soft tissue swelling, symmetric joint space loss, and subchondral erosions, most frequently in the wrists and hands (MCPs and PIPs) and the feet (MTPs). In the feet, the lateral aspect of the fifth MTP is often targeted first, but other MTP joints may be involved at the same time. X-ray imaging of advanced RA may reveal signs of severe destruction, including joint subluxation and collapse (Fig. 380-5).

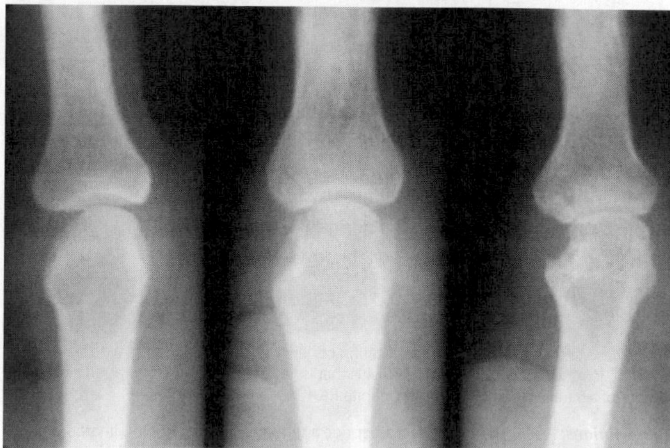

FIGURE 380-5 X-ray demonstrating progression of erosions on the proximal interphalangeal joint. *(Courtesy of the American College of Rheumatology.)*

MRI MRI offers the greatest sensitivity for detecting synovitis and joint effusions, as well as early bone and bone marrow changes. These soft tissue abnormalities often occur before osseous changes are noted on x-ray. Presence of bone marrow edema has been recognized to be an early sign of inflammatory joint disease and can predict the subsequent development of erosions on plain radiographs as well as MRI scans. Cost and availability of MRI are the main factors limiting its routine clinical use.

Ultrasound Ultrasound, including power color Doppler, has the ability to detect more erosions than plain radiography, especially in easily accessible joints. It can also reliably detect synovitis, including increased joint vascularity indicative of inflammation. The usefulness of ultrasound is dependent on the experience of the sonographer; however, it does offer the advantages of portability, lack of radiation, and low expense relative to MRI, factors that make it attractive as a clinical tool.

CLINICAL COURSE

The natural history of RA is complex and affected by a number of factors including age of onset, gender, genotype, phenotype (i.e., extraarticular manifestations or variants of RA), and comorbid conditions, which make for a truly heterogeneous disease. There is no simple way to predict the clinical course. It is important to realize that as many as 10% of patients with inflammatory arthritis fulfilling ACR classification criteria for RA will undergo a spontaneous remission within 6 months (particularly seronegative patients). However, the vast majority of patients will exhibit a pattern of persistent and progressive disease activity that waxes and wanes in intensity over time. A minority of patients will show intermittent and recurrent explosive attacks of inflammatory arthritis interspersed with periods of disease quiescence. Finally, an aggressive form of RA may occur in an unfortunate few with inexorable progression of severe erosive joint disease, although this highly destructive course is less common in the modern treatment era of biologics.

Disability, as measured by the Health Assessment Questionnaire (HAQ), shows gradual worsening of disability over time in the face of poorly controlled disease activity and disease progression. Disability may result from both a disease activity–related component that is potentially reversible with therapy and a joint damage–related component owing to the cumulative and largely irreversible effects of cartilage and bone breakdown. Early in the course of disease, the extent of joint inflammation is the primary determinant of disability, while in the later stages of disease, the amount of joint damage is the dominant contributing factor. Previous studies have shown that more than one-half of patients with RA are unable to work 10 years after the onset of their disease; however, increased employability and less work absenteeism has been reported recently with the use of newer therapies and earlier treatment intervention.

The overall mortality rate in RA is two times greater than the general population, with ischemic heart disease being the most common cause of death followed by infection. Median life expectancy is shortened by an average of 7 years for men and 3 years for women compared to control populations. Patients at higher risk for shortened survival are those with systemic extraarticular involvement, low functional capacity, low socioeconomic status, low education, and chronic prednisone use.

TREATMENT RHEUMATOID ARTHRITIS

The amount of clinical disease activity in patients with RA reflects the overall burden of inflammation and is the variable most influencing treatment decisions. Joint inflammation is the main driver of joint damage and is the most important cause of functional disability in the early stages of disease. Several composite indices have been developed to assess clinical disease activity. The ACR 20, 50, and 70 improvement criteria (which corresponds to a 20%, 50%, and 70% improvement, respectively, in joint counts, physician/patient assessment of disease severity, pain scale, serum levels of acute-phase reactants [ESR or CRP], and a functional assessment of disability using a self-administered patient questionnaire) are a composite index with a dichotomous response variable. The ACR improvement criteria are commonly used in clinical trials as an endpoint for comparing the proportion of responders between treatment groups. In contrast, the Disease Activity Score (DAS), Simplified Disease Activity Index (SDAI), and the Clinical Disease Activity Index (CDAI) are continuous measures of disease activity. These scales are increasingly used in clinical practice for tracking disease status and, in particular, for documenting treatment response.

Several developments during the past two decades have changed the therapeutic landscape in RA. They include (1) the emergence of methotrexate as the disease-modifying antirheumatic drug (DMARD) of first choice for the treatment of early RA; (2) the development of novel highly efficacious biologicals that can be used alone or in combination with methotrexate; and (3) the proven superiority of combination DMARD regimens over methotrexate alone. The medications used for the treatment of RA may be divided into broad categories: nonsteroidal anti-inflammatory drugs (NSAIDs); glucocorticoids, such as prednisone and methylprednisolone; conventional DMARDs; and biologic DMARDs (Table 380-2). Although disease for some patients with RA is managed adequately with a single DMARD, such as methotrexate, the situation in most cases demands the use of a combination DMARD regimen that may vary in its components over the treatment course depending on fluctuations in disease activity and emergence of drug-related toxicities and comorbidities.

NSAIDs

NSAIDs were formerly viewed as the core of all other RA therapy, but they are now considered to be adjunctive therapy for management of symptoms uncontrolled by other measures. NSAIDs exhibit both analgesic and anti-inflammatory properties. The anti-inflammatory effects of NSAIDs derive from their ability to nonselectively inhibit cyclooxygenase (COX)-1 and COX-2. Although the results of clinical trials suggest NSAIDs are roughly equivalent in their efficacy, experience suggests that some individuals may preferentially respond to a particular NSAID. Chronic use should be minimized due to the possibility of side effects, including gastritis and peptic ulcer disease as well as impairment of renal function.

GLUCOCORTICOIDS

Glucocorticoids may serve in several ways to control disease activity in RA. First, they may be administered in low to moderate doses to achieve rapid disease control before the onset of fully effective DMARD therapy, which often takes several weeks or even months. Second, a 1- to 2-week burst of glucocorticoids may be prescribed for the management of acute disease flares, with dose and duration guided by the severity of the exacerbation. Chronic administration of low doses (5–10 mg/d) of prednisone (or its equivalent) may also be warranted to control disease activity in patients with an inadequate response to DMARD therapy. Low-dose prednisone therapy has been shown in prospective studies to retard radiographic progression of joint disease; however, the benefits of this approach must be carefully weighed against the risks. Best practices minimize chronic use of low-dose prednisone therapy owing to the risk of osteoporosis and other long-term complications; however, the use of chronic prednisone therapy is unavoidable in many cases. High-dose glucocorticoids may be necessary for treatment of severe extraarticular manifestations of RA, such as ILD. Finally, if a patient exhibits one or a few actively inflamed joints, the clinician may consider intraarticular injection of an intermediate-acting glucocorticoid such as triamcinolone acetonide. This approach may allow for rapid control of inflammation in the setting of a limited number of affected joints. Caution must be exercised to appropriately exclude joint infection, as it often mimics an RA flare.

Osteoporosis ranks as an important long-term complication of chronic prednisone use. The ACR recommends primary prevention of glucocorticoid-induced osteoporosis with a bisphosphonate in any patient receiving 5 mg/d or more of prednisone for greater than 3 months. Although prednisone use is known to increase the risk of peptic ulcer disease, especially with concomitant NSAID use, no evidence-based guidelines have been published regarding the use of gastrointestinal ulcer prophylaxis in this situation.

DMARDs

DMARDs are so named because of their ability to slow or prevent structural progression of RA. The conventional DMARDs include hydroxychloroquine, sulfasalazine, methotrexate, and leflunomide; they exhibit a delayed onset of action of approximately 6–12 weeks. Methotrexate is the DMARD of choice for the treatment of RA and is the anchor drug for most combination therapies. It was approved for the treatment of RA in 1986 and remains the benchmark for the efficacy and safety of new disease-modifying therapies. At the dosages used for the treatment of RA, methotrexate has been shown to stimulate adenosine release from cells, producing an anti-inflammatory effect. The clinical efficacy of leflunomide, an inhibitor of pyrimidine synthesis, appears similar to that of methotrexate; it has been shown in well-designed trials to be effective for the treatment of RA as monotherapy or in combination with methotrexate and other DMARDs.

Although similar to the other DMARDs in its slow onset of action, hydroxychloroquine has not been shown to delay radiographic progression of disease and thus is not considered to be a true DMARD. In clinical practice, hydroxychloroquine is generally used for treatment of early, mild disease or as adjunctive therapy in combination with other DMARDs. Sulfasalazine is used in a similar manner and has been shown in randomized, controlled trials to reduce radiographic progression of disease. Minocycline, gold salts, penicillamine, azathioprine, and cyclosporine have all been used for the treatment of RA with varying degrees of success; however, they are used sparingly now due to their inconsistent clinical efficacy or unfavorable toxicity profile.

BIOLOGICALS

Biologic DMARDs have revolutionized the treatment of RA over the past decade (Table 380-2). They are protein therapeutics designed mostly to target cytokines and cell-surface molecules. The TNF inhibitors were the first biologicals approved for the treatment of RA. Anakinra, an IL-1 receptor antagonist, was approved shortly thereafter; however, its benefits have proved to be relatively modest compared with the other biologicals and is rarely used for the treatment of RA with the availability of other more effective agents. Abatacept, rituximab, and tocilizumab are the newest members of this class.

Anti-TNF Agents The development of TNF inhibitors was originally spurred by the experimental finding that TNF is a critical upstream mediator of joint inflammation. Currently, five agents that inhibit TNF-α are approved for the treatment of RA. There are three different anti-TNF monoclonal antibodies. Infliximab is a chimeric (part mouse and human) monoclonal antibody, whereas adalimumab and golimumab are humanized monoclonal antibodies. Certolizumab pegol is a pegylated Fc-free fragment of a humanized monoclonal antibody with binding specificity for TNF-α. Lastly, etanercept is a soluble fusion protein comprising the TNF receptor 2 in covalent linkage with the Fc portion of IgG1. All of the TNF inhibitors have been shown in randomized controlled clinical trials to reduce the signs and symptoms of RA, slow radiographic progression of joint damage, and improve physical function and quality of life. Anti-TNF drugs are typically used in combination with background methotrexate therapy. This combination regimen, which affords maximal benefit in many cases, is often the next step for treatment of patients with an inadequate response to methotrexate therapy. Etanercept, adalimumab, certolizumab pegol, and golimumab have also been approved for use as monotherapy.

Anti-TNF agents should be avoided in patients with active infection or a history of hypersensitivity to these agents and are contraindicated in patients with chronic hepatitis B infection or class III/IV congestive

TABLE 380-2 DMARDs USED FOR THE TREATMENT OF RHEUMATOID ARTHRITIS

Drug	Dosage	Serious Toxicities	Other Common Side Effects	Initial Evaluation	Monitoring
Hydroxychloroquine	200–400 mg/d orally (≤6.5 mg/kg)	Irreversible retinal damage Cardiotoxicity Blood dyscrasia	Nausea Diarrhea Headache Rash	Eye examination if >40 years old or prior ocular disease	Funduscopic and visual field testing every 12 months
Sulfasalazine	Initial: 500 mg orally twice daily Maintenance: 1000–1500 mg twice daily	Granulocytopenia Hemolytic anemia (with G6PD deficiency)	Nausea Diarrhea Headache	CBC, LFTs G6PD level	CBC every 2–4 weeks for first 3 months, then every 3 months
Methotrexate	10–25 mg/week orally or SQ Folic acid 1 mg/d to reduce toxicities	Hepatotoxicity Myelosuppression Infection Interstitial pneumonitis Pregnancy category X	Nausea Diarrhea Stomatitis/mouth ulcers Alopecia Fatigue	CBC, LFTs Viral hepatitis panel[a] Chest x-ray	CBC, creatinine, LFTs every 2–3 months
Leflunomide	10–20 mg/d	Hepatotoxicity Myelosuppression Infection Pregnancy category X	Alopecia Diarrhea	CBC, LFTs Viral hepatitis panel[a]	CBC, creatinine, LFTs every 2–3 months
TNF-α Inhibitors	Infliximab: 3 mg/kg IV at weeks 0, 2, 6, then every 8 weeks. May increase dose up to 10 mg/kg every 4 weeks	↑ Risk bacterial, fungal infections Reactivation of latent TB ↑ Lymphoma risk (controversial) Drug-induced lupus Neurologic deficits	Infusion reaction ↑ LFTs	PPD skin test	LFTs periodically
	Etanercept: 50 mg SQ weekly, or 25 mg SQ biweekly	As above	Injection site reaction	PPD skin test	Monitor for injection site reactions
	Adalimumab: 40 mg SQ every other week	As above	Injection site reaction	PPD skin test	Monitor for injection site reactions
	Golimumab: 50 mg SQ monthly	As above	Injection site reaction	PPD skin test	Monitor for injection site reactions
	Certolizumab: 400 mg SQ weeks 0, 2, 4, then 200 mg every other week	As above	Injection site reaction	PPD skin test	Monitor for injection site reactions
Abatacept	Weight based: <60 kg: 500 mg 60–100 kg: 750 mg >100 kg: 1000 mg IV dose at weeks 0, 2, and 4, and then every 4 weeks OR 125 mg SQ weekly	↑ Risk bacterial, viral infections	Headache Nausea	PPD skin test	Monitor for infusion reactions
Anakinra	100 mg SQ daily	↑ Risk bacterial, viral infections Reactivation of latent TB Neutropenia	Injection site reaction Headache	PPD skin test CBC with differential	CBC every month for 3 months, then every 4 months for 1 year Monitor for injection site reactions
Rituximab	1000 mg IV × 2, days 0 and 14 May repeat course every 24 weeks or more Premedicate with methyl-prednisolone 100 mg to decrease infusion reaction	↑ Risk bacterial, viral infections Infusion reaction Cytopenia Hepatitis B reactivation	Rash Fever	CBC Viral hepatitis panel[a]	CBC at regular intervals

(Continued)

TABLE 380-2 DMARDs USED FOR THE TREATMENT OF RHEUMATOID ARTHRITIS (*CONTINUED*)

Drug	Dosage	Serious Toxicities	Other Common Side Effects	Initial Evaluation	Monitoring
Tocilizumab	4–8 mg/kg 4–8 mg/kg IV monthly OR 162 mg SQ every other week (<100 kg weight) 162 mg SQ every week (≥100 kg weight)	Risk of infection Infusion reaction LFT elevation Dyslipidemia Cytopenias		PPD skin test	CBC and LFTs at regular intervals
Tofacitinib	5 mg orally BID	Risk of infection LFT elevation Dyslipidemia Neutropenia	Upper respiratory tract infections Diarrhea Headache Nasopharyngitis	PPD skin test	CBC, LFTs, and lipids at regular intervals

[a]Viral hepatitis panel: hepatitis B surface antigen, hepatitis C viral antibody.

Abbreviations: CBC, complete blood count; DMARDs, disease-modifying antirheumatic drugs; G6PD, glucose-6-phosphate dehydrogenase; IV, intravenous; LFTs, liver function tests; PPD, purified protein derivative; SQ, subcutaneous; TB, tuberculosis.

heart failure. The major concern is the increased risk for infection, including serious bacterial infections, opportunistic fungal infection, and reactivation of latent tuberculosis. For this reason, all patients are screened for latent tuberculosis according to national guidelines prior to starting anti-TNF therapy (Chap. 202). In the United States, patients are skin tested using an intradermal injection of purified protein derivative (PPD); individuals with skin reactions of more than 5 mm are presumed to have had previous exposure to tuberculosis and are evaluated for active disease and treated accordingly. The QuantiFERON IFN-γ release assay may also be used in selected circumstances to screen for previous exposure to tuberculosis.

Anakinra Anakinra, the recombinant form of the naturally occurring IL-1 receptor antagonist. Although anakinra has seen limited use for the treatment of RA, it has enjoyed a resurgence of late as an effective therapy of some rare inherited syndromes dependent on IL-1 production, including neonatal-onset inflammatory disease, Muckle-Wells syndrome, and familial cold urticaria, as well as systemic juvenile-onset inflammatory arthritis and adult-onset Still's disease. Anakinra should not be combined with an anti-TNF drug due to the high rate of serious infections as observed with this regimen in a clinical trial.

Abatacept Abatacept is a soluble fusion protein consisting of the extracellular domain of human CTLA-4 linked to the modified portion of human IgG. It inhibits the co-stimulation of T cells by blocking CD28-CD80/86 interactions and may also inhibit the function of antigen-presenting cells by reverse signaling through CD80 and CD86. Abatacept has been shown in clinical trials to reduce disease activity, slow radiographic progression of damage, and improve functional disability. Many patients receive abatacept in combination with methotrexate or another DMARD such as leflunomide. Abatacept therapy has been associated with an increased risk of infection.

Rituximab Rituximab is a chimeric monoclonal antibody directed against CD20, a cell-surface molecule expressed by most mature B lymphocytes. It works by depleting B cells, which in turn, leads to a reduction in the inflammatory response by unknown mechanisms. These mechanisms may include a reduction in autoantibodies, inhibition of T cell activation, and alteration of cytokine production. Rituximab has been approved for the treatment of refractory RA in combination with methotrexate and has been shown to be more effective for patients with seropositive than seronegative disease. Rituximab therapy has been associated with mild to moderate infusion reactions as well as an increased risk of infection. Notably, there have been isolated reports of a potentially lethal brain disorder, progressive multifocal leukoencephalopathy (PML), in association with rituximab therapy, although the absolute risk of this complication appears to be very low in patients with RA. Most of these cases have occurred on a background of previous or current exposure to other potent immunosuppressive drugs.

Tocilizumab Tocilizumab is a humanized monoclonal antibody directed against the membrane and soluble forms of the IL-6 receptor. IL-6 is a proinflammatory cytokine implicated in the pathogenesis of RA, with detrimental effects on both joint inflammation and damage. IL-6 binding to its receptor activates intracellular signaling pathways that affect the acute-phase response, cytokine production, and osteoclast activation. Clinical trials attest to the clinical efficacy of tocilizumab therapy for RA, both as monotherapy and in combination with methotrexate and other DMARDs. Tocilizumab has been associated with an increased risk of infection, neutropenia, and thrombocytopenia; however, the hematologic abnormalities appear to be reversible upon stopping the drug. In addition, this agent has been shown to increase LDL cholesterol; however, it is not known as yet if this effect on lipid levels increases the risk for development of atherosclerotic disease.

SMALL-MOLECULE INHIBITORS

Because some patients do not adequately respond to conventional DMARDS or biologic therapy, other therapeutic targets have been investigated to fill this gap. Recently, drug development in RA has focused attention on the intracellular signaling pathways that transduce the positive signals of cytokines and other inflammatory mediators that create the positive feedback loops in the immune response. These synthetic DMARDs aim to provide the same efficacy as biological therapies in an oral formulation.

Tofacitinib Tofacitinib is a small-molecule inhibitor that primarily inhibits JAK1 and JAK3, which mediate signaling of the receptors for the common γ-chain-related cytokines IL-2, -4, -7, -9, -15, and -21 as well as IFN-γ and IL-6. These cytokines all play roles in promoting T and B cell activation as well as inflammation. Tofacitinib, an oral agent, has been shown in randomized, placebo-controlled clinical trials to improve the signs and symptoms of RA significantly over placebo. Major adverse events include elevated serum transaminases indicative of liver injury, neutropenia, increased cholesterol levels, and elevation in serum creatinine. Its use is also associated with an increased risk of infections. Tofacitinib can be used as monotherapy or in combination with methotrexate.

APPROACH TO THE PATIENT: Rheumatoid Arthritis

The original treatment pyramid for RA is now considered to be obsolete and has evolved into a new strategy that focuses on several goals: (1) early, aggressive therapy to prevent joint damage and disability; (2) frequent modification of therapy with utilization of combination therapy where appropriate; (3) individualization of therapy in an attempt to maximize response and minimize side effects; and (4) achieving, whenever possible, remission of clinical disease activity. A considerable amount of evidence supports this intensive treatment approach.

As mentioned earlier, methotrexate is the DMARD of first choice for initial treatment of moderate to severe RA. Failure to achieve adequate improvement with methotrexate therapy calls for a change in DMARD therapy, usually transition to an effective combination regimen. Effective combinations include: methotrexate, sulfasalazine, and hydroxychloroquine (oral triple therapy); methotrexate and leflunomide; and methotrexate plus a biological. The combination of methotrexate and an anti-TNF agent, for example, has been shown in randomized, controlled trials to be superior to methotrexate alone not only for reducing signs and symptoms of disease, but also for retarding the progression of structural joint damage. Predicting which patients will ultimately show radiologic joint damage is imprecise at best, although some factors such as an elevated serum level of acute-phase reactants, high burden of joint inflammation, and the presence of erosive disease are associated with increased likelihood of developing structural injury.

In 2012 a joint task force of the ACR and EULAR updated the treatment guidelines for RA. They do make a distinction between patients with early RA (<6 months of disease duration) and patients with established RA. These guidelines highlight the need to switch or add DMARD therapy after 3 months of worsening or persistent moderate/high disease activity. If disease still persists after 3 months of intense DMARD therapy, addition of a biologic agent is warranted. Treatment with a biologic agent or aggressive combination DMARD therapy was also recommended as initial therapy in certain patients with high disease activity and poor prognosis. However, it has not been clearly established that this more intensive initial approach is superior to starting with methotrexate alone and, in the absence of an inadequate therapeutic response, moving rapidly to combination therapy.

Some patients may not respond to an anti-TNF drug or may be intolerant of its side effects. Initial responders to an anti-TNF agent that later worsen may benefit from switching to another anti-TNF agent. The 2012 guidelines recommend that with loss or lack of effectiveness of anti-TNF after 3 months, one should switch to another anti-TNF or non-TNF biologic agent. In patients with high disease activity and a serious adverse event from an anti-TNF agent, a non-TNF drug should be used.

Studies have also shown that oral triple therapy (hydroxychloroquine, methotrexate, and sulfasalazine) is a reasonable first step for the treatment of early RA, including its use as a step-up strategy where treatment is initiated with methotrexate alone and then combined at 6 months with hydroxychloroquine and sulfasalazine if the disease is not adequately controlled.

A clinical state defined as low disease activity or remission is the optimal goal of therapy, although most patients never achieve remission despite every effort to achieve it. Composite indices, such as the Disease Activity Score-28 (DAS-28), are useful for classifying states of low disease activity and remission; however, they are imperfect tools due to the limitations of the clinical joint examination in which low-grade synovitis may escape detection. Complete remission has been stringently defined as the total absence of all articular and extraarticular inflammation and immunologic activity related to RA. However, evidence for this state can be difficult to demonstrate in clinical practice. In an effort to standardize and simplify the definition of remission for clinical trials, the ACR and EULAR developed two provisional operational definitions of remission in RA (Table 380-3). A patient may be considered in remission if he or she (1) meets all of the clinical and laboratory criteria listed in Table 380-3 or (2) has a composite SDAI score of <3.3. The SDAI is calculated by taking the sum of a tender joint and swollen joint count (using 28 joints), patient global assessment (0–10 scale), physician global assessment (0–10 scale), and CRP (in mg/dL). This definition of remission does not take into account the possibility of subclinical synovitis or that damage alone may produce a tender or swollen joint. Ignoring the semantics of these definitions, the aforementioned remission criteria are nonetheless useful for setting a level of disease control that will likely result in minimal or no progression of structural damage and disability.

TABLE 380-3 ACR/EULAR PROVISIONAL DEFINITION OF REMISSION IN RHEUMATOID ARTHRITIS

At any time point, patient must satisfy all of the following:

- Tender joint count ≤1
- Swollen joint count ≤1
- C-reactive protein ≤1 mg/dL
- Patient global assessment ≤1 (on a 0–10 scale)

OR

At any time point, patient must have a Simplified Disease Activity Index score of ≤3.3

Source: Adapted from DT Felson et al: Arthritis Rheum 63:573, 2011.

PHYSICAL THERAPY AND ASSISTIVE DEVICES

All patients should receive a prescription for exercise and physical activity. Dynamic strength training, community-based comprehensive physical therapy, and physical-activity coaching (emphasizing 30 min of moderately intensive activity most days a week) have all been shown to improve muscle strength and perceived health status. Foot orthotics for painful valgus deformity decrease foot pain and resulting disability and functional limitations. Judicious use of wrist splints can also decrease pain; however, their benefits may be offset by decreased dexterity and a variable effect on grip strength.

SURGERY

Surgical procedures may improve pain and disability in RA—most notably the hands, wrists, and feet, typically after the failure of medical therapy with varying degrees of reported long-term success. For large joints, such as the knee, hip, shoulder, or elbow, total joint arthroplasty is an option for advanced joint disease. A few surgical options exist for dealing with the smaller hand joints. Silicone implants are the most common prosthetic for MCP arthroplasty and are generally implanted in patients with severe decreased arc of motion, marked flexion contractures, MCP joint pain with radiographic abnormalities, and severe ulnar drift. Arthrodesis and total wrist arthroplasty are reserved for patients with severe disease who have substantial pain and functional impairment. These two procedures appear to have equal efficacy in terms of pain control and patient satisfaction. Numerous surgical options exist for correction of hallux valgus in the forefoot, including arthrodesis and arthroplasty, as well as primarily arthrodesis for refractory hindfoot pain.

OTHER MANAGEMENT CONSIDERATIONS

Pregnancy Up to 75% of female RA patients will note overall improvement in symptoms during pregnancy, but often will flare after delivery. Flares during pregnancy are generally treated with low doses of prednisone; hydroxychloroquine and sulfasalazine are probably the safest DMARDs to use during pregnancy. Methotrexate and leflunomide therapy are contraindicated during pregnancy due to their teratogenicity in animals and humans. The experience with biologic agents has been insufficient to make specific recommendations for their use during pregnancy. Most rheumatologists avoid their use in this setting; however, exceptions are considered depending on the circumstances.

Elderly Patients RA presents in up to one-third of patients after the age of 60; however, older individuals may receive less aggressive treatment due to concerns about increased risks of drug toxicity. Studies suggest that conventional DMARDs and biologic agents are equally effective and safe in younger and older patients. Due to comorbidities, many elderly patients have an increased risk of infection. Aging also leads to a gradual decline in renal function that may raise the risk for side effects from NSAIDs and some DMARDS, such as methotrexate. Renal function must be taken into consideration before prescribing methotrexate, which is mostly cleared by the kidneys. To reduce the risks of side effects, methotrexate doses may need to be adjusted downward for the drop in renal function that usually comes with the seventh and eighth decades of life. Methotrexate is usually not prescribed for patients with a serum creatinine greater than 2 mg/dL.

GLOBAL CHALLENGES

Developing countries are finding an increase in the incidence of noncommunicable, chronic diseases such as diabetes, cardiovascular disease, and RA in the face of ongoing poverty, rampant infectious disease, and poor access to modern health care facilities. In these areas, patients tend to have a greater delay in diagnosis and limited access to specialists, and thus greater disease activity and disability at presentation. In addition, infection risk remains a significant issue for the treatment of RA in developing countries because of the immunosuppression associated with the use of glucocorticoids and most DMARDs. For example, in some developing countries, patients undergoing treatment for RA have a substantial increase in the incidence of tuberculosis, which demands the implementation of far more comprehensive screening practices and liberal use of isoniazid prophylaxis than in developed countries. The increased prevalence of hepatitis B and C, as well as human immunodeficiency virus (HIV), in these developing countries also poses challenges. Reactivation of viral hepatitis has been observed in association with some of the DMARDs, such as rituximab. Also, reduced access to antiretroviral therapy may limit the control of HIV infection and therefore the choice of DMARD therapies.

Despite these challenges, one should attempt to initiate early treatment of RA in the developing countries with the resources at hand. Sulfasalazine and methotrexate are all reasonably accessible throughout the world where they can be used as both monotherapy and in combination with other drugs. The use of biologic agents is increasing in the developed countries as well as in other areas around the world, although their use is limited by high cost; national protocols restrict their use, and concerns remain about the risk for opportunistic infections.

SUMMARY

Improved understanding of the pathogenesis of RA and its treatment has dramatically revolutionized the management of this disease. The outcomes of patients with RA are vastly superior to those of the prebiologic modifier era; more patients than in years past are able to avoid significant disability and continue working, albeit with some job modifications in many cases. The need for early and aggressive treatment of RA as well as frequent follow-up visits for monitoring of drug therapy has implications for our health care system. Primary care physicians and rheumatologists must be prepared to work together as a team to reach the ambitious goals of best practice. In many settings, rheumatologists have reengineered their practice in a way that places high priority on consultations for any new patient with early inflammatory arthritis.

The therapeutic regimens for RA are becoming increasingly complex with the rapidly expanding therapeutic armamentarium. Patients receiving these therapies must be carefully monitored by both the primary care physician and the rheumatologist to minimize the risk of side effects and identify quickly any complications of chronic immunosuppression. Also, prevention and treatment of RA-associated conditions such as ischemic heart disease and osteoporosis will likely benefit from a team approach owing to the value of multidisciplinary care.

Research will continue to search for new therapies with superior efficacy and safety profiles and investigate treatment strategies that can bring the disease under control more rapidly and nearer to remission. However, prevention and cure of RA will likely require new breakthroughs in our understanding of disease pathogenesis. These insights may come from genetic studies illuminating critical pathways in the mechanisms of joint inflammation. Equally ambitious is the lofty goal of biomarker discovery that will open the door to personalized medicine for the care of patients with RA.

381 Acute Rheumatic Fever

Jonathan R. Carapetis

Acute rheumatic fever (ARF) is a multisystem disease resulting from an autoimmune reaction to infection with group A streptococcus. Although many parts of the body may be affected, almost all of the manifestations resolve completely. The major exception is cardiac valvular damage (rheumatic heart disease [RHD]), which may persist after the other features have disappeared.

GLOBAL CONSIDERATIONS

ARF and RHD are diseases of poverty. They were common in all countries until the early twentieth century, when their incidence began to decline in industrialized nations. This decline was largely attributable to improved living conditions—particularly less crowded housing and better hygiene—which resulted in reduced transmission of group A streptococci. The introduction of antibiotics and improved systems of medical care had a supplemental effect.

The virtual disappearance of ARF and reduction in the incidence of RHD in industrialized countries during the twentieth century unfortunately was not replicated in developing countries, where these diseases continue unabated. RHD is the most common cause of heart disease in children in developing countries and is a major cause of mortality and morbidity in adults as well. It has been estimated that between 15 and 19 million people worldwide are affected by RHD, with approximately one-quarter of a million deaths occurring each year. Some 95% of ARF cases and RHD deaths now occur in developing countries, with particularly high rates in sub-Saharan Africa, Pacific nations, Australasia, and South and Central Asia. The pathogenetic pathway from exposure to group A streptococcus followed by pharyngeal infection and subsequent development of ARF, ARF recurrences, and development of RHD and its complications is associated with a range of risk factors and, therefore, potential interventions at each point (Fig. 381-1). In affluent countries, many of these risk factors are well controlled, and where needed, interventions are in place. Unfortunately, the greatest burden of disease is found in developing countries, most of which do not have the resources, capacity, and/or interest to tackle this multifaceted disease. In particular, almost none of the developing countries has a coordinated, register-based RHD control program, which is proven to be cost effective in reducing the burden of RHD. Enhancing awareness of RHD and mobilizing resources for its control in developing countries are issues requiring international attention.

EPIDEMIOLOGY

ARF is mainly a disease of children age 5–14 years. Initial episodes become less common in older adolescents and young adults and are rare in persons age >30 years. By contrast, recurrent episodes of ARF remain relatively common in adolescents and young adults. This pattern contrasts with the prevalence of RHD, which peaks between 25 and 40 years. There is no clear gender association for ARF, but RHD more commonly affects females, sometimes up to twice as frequently as males.

PATHOGENESIS

ORGANISM FACTORS

Based on currently available evidence, ARF is exclusively caused by infection of the upper respiratory tract with group A streptococci (Chap. 173). Although classically, certain M-serotypes (particularly types 1, 3, 5, 6, 14, 18, 19, 24, 27, and 29) were associated with ARF, in high-incidence regions, it is now thought that any strain of group A streptococcus has the potential to cause ARF. The potential role of skin infection and of groups C and G streptococci is currently being investigated.

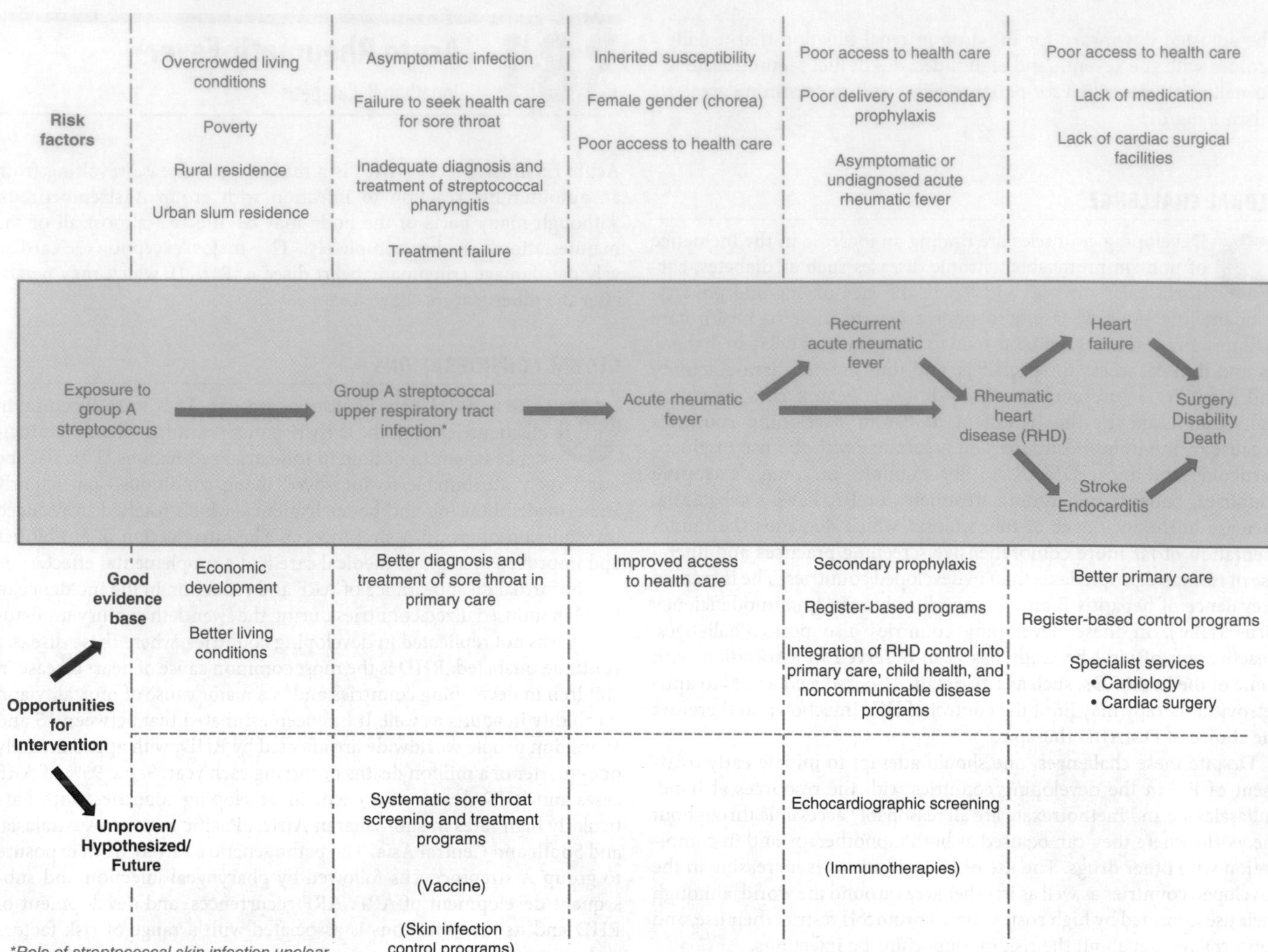

FIGURE 381-1 Pathogenetic pathway for acute rheumatic fever and rheumatic heart disease, with associated risk factors and opportunities for intervention at each step. Interventions in *parentheses* are either unproven or currently unavailable.

HOST FACTORS

Approximately 3–6% of any population may be susceptible to ARF, and this proportion does not vary dramatically between populations. Findings of familial clustering of cases and concordance in monozygotic twins—particularly for chorea—confirm that susceptibility to ARF is an inherited characteristic, with 44% concordance in monozygotic twins compared to 12% in dizygotic twins, and heritability more recently estimated at 60%. Most evidence for host factors focuses on immunologic determinants. Some human leukocyte antigen (HLA) class II alleles, particularly HLA-DR7 and HLA-DR4, appear to be associated with susceptibility, whereas other class II alleles have been associated with protection (HLA-DR5, HLA-DR6, HLA-DR51, HLA-DR52, and HLA-DQ). Associations have also been described with polymorphisms at the tumor necrosis factor α locus (TNF-α-308 and TNF-α-238), high levels of circulating mannose-binding lectin, and Toll-like receptors.

THE IMMUNE RESPONSE

The most widely accepted theory of rheumatic fever pathogenesis is based on the concept of molecular mimicry, whereby an immune response targeted at streptococcal antigens (mainly thought to be on the M protein and the *N*-acetylglucosamine of group A streptococcal carbohydrate) also recognizes human tissues. In this model, cross-reactive antibodies bind to endothelial cells on the heart valve, leading to activation of the adhesion molecule VCAM-1, with resulting recruitment of activated lymphocytes and lysis of endothelial cells in the presence of complement. The latter leads to release of peptides including laminin, keratin, and tropomyosin, which, in turn, activates cross-reactive T cells that invade the heart, amplifying the damage and causing epitope spreading. An alternative hypothesis proposes that the initial damage is due to streptococcal invasion of epithelial surfaces, with binding of M protein to type IV collagen RHD allowing it to become immunogenic, but not through the mechanism of molecular mimicry.

CLINICAL FEATURES

There is a latent period of ~3 weeks (1–5 weeks) between the precipitating group A streptococcal infection and the appearance of the clinical features of ARF. The exceptions are chorea and indolent carditis, which may follow prolonged latent periods lasting up to 6 months. Although many patients report a prior sore throat, the preceding group A streptococcal infection is commonly subclinical; in these cases, it can only be confirmed using streptococcal antibody testing. The most common clinical features are polyarthritis (present in 60–75% of cases) and carditis (50–60%). The prevalence of chorea in ARF varies substantially between populations, ranging from <2 to 30%. Erythema marginatum and subcutaneous nodules are now rare, being found in <5% of cases.

HEART INVOLVEMENT

Up to 60% of patients with ARF progress to RHD. The endocardium, pericardium, or myocardium may be affected. Valvular damage is the hallmark of rheumatic carditis. The mitral valve is almost always

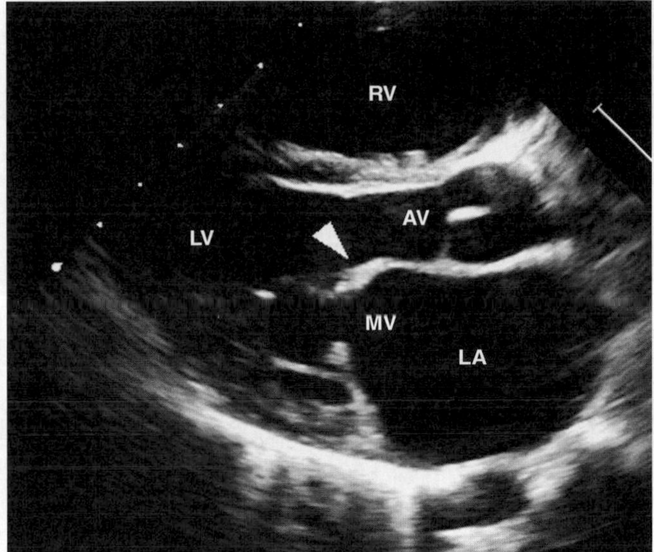

FIGURE 381-2 Transthoracic echocardiographic image from a 5-year-old boy with chronic rheumatic heart disease. This diastolic image demonstrates leaflet thickening, restriction of the anterior mitral valve leaflet tip and doming of the body of the leaflet toward the interventricular septum. This appearance (marked by the *arrowhead*) is commonly described as a "hockey stick" or an "elbow" deformity. AV, aortic valve; LA, left atrium; LV, left ventricle; MV, mitral valve; RV, right ventricle. *(Courtesy of Dr. Bo Remenyi, Department of Paediatric and Congenital Cardiac Services, Starship Children's Hospital, Auckland, New Zealand.)*

affected, sometimes together with the aortic valve; isolated aortic valve involvement is rare. Damage to the pulmonary or tricuspid valves is usually secondary to increased pulmonary pressures resulting from left-sided valvular disease. Early valvular damage leads to regurgitation. Over ensuing years, usually as a result of recurrent episodes, leaflet thickening, scarring, calcification, and valvular stenosis may develop (Fig. 381-2). See Videos 381-1 and 381-2 on the DVD. Therefore, the characteristic manifestation of carditis in previously unaffected individuals is mitral regurgitation, sometimes accompanied by aortic regurgitation. Myocardial inflammation may affect electrical conduction pathways, leading to P-R interval prolongation (first-degree atrioventricular block or rarely higher level block) and softening of the first heart sound.

People with RHD are often asymptomatic for many years before their valvular disease progresses to cause cardiac failure. Moreover, particularly in resource-poor settings, the diagnosis of ARF is often not made, so children, adolescents, and young adults may have RHD but not know it. These cases can be diagnosed using echocardiography; auscultation is poorly sensitive and specific for RHD diagnosis in asymptomatic patients. Echocardiographic screening of school-aged children in populations with high rates of RHD is becoming more widespread and has been facilitated by improving technologies in portable echocardiography and the availability of consensus guidelines for the diagnosis of RHD on echocardiography (Table 381-1). Although a diagnosis of definite RHD on screening echocardiography should lead to commencement of secondary prophylaxis, the clinical significance of borderline RHD has yet to be determined.

JOINT INVOLVEMENT

The most common form of joint involvement in ARF is arthritis, i.e., objective evidence of inflammation, with hot, swollen, red, and/or tender joints, and involvement of more than one joint (i.e., polyarthritis). Polyarthritis is typically migratory, moving from one joint to another over a period of hours. ARF almost always affects the large joints—most commonly the knees, ankles, hips, and elbows—and is asymmetric. The pain is severe and usually disabling until anti-inflammatory medication is commenced.

TABLE 381-1 WORLD HEART FEDERATION CRITERIA FOR ECHOCARDIOGRAPHIC DIAGNOSIS OF RHEUMATIC HEART DISEASE (RHD) IN INDIVIDUALS <20 YEARS OF AGE[a]

Definite RHD (either A, B, C, or D):
(A) Pathologic MR and at least two morphologic features of RHD of the mitral valve
(B) MS mean gradient ≥4 mmHg (note: congenital MV anomalies must be excluded)
(C) Pathologic AR and at least two morphologic features of RHD of the AV (note: bicuspid AV and dilated aortic root must be excluded)
(D) Borderline disease of both the MV and AV
Borderline RHD (either A, B, or C):
(A) At least two morphologic features of RHD of the MV without pathologic MR or MS
(B) Pathologic MR
(C) Pathologic AR
Normal Echocardiographic Findings (all of A, B, C, and D):
(A) MR that does not meet all four Doppler criteria (physiologic MR)
(B) AR that does not meet all four Doppler criteria (physiologic AR)
(C) An isolated morphologic feature of RHD of the MV (e.g., valvular thickening), without any associated pathologic stenosis or regurgitation
(D) Morphologic feature of RHD of the AV (e.g., valvular thickening), without any associated pathologic stenosis or regurgitation
Definitions of Pathologic Regurgitation and Morphologic Features of RHD:
Pathologic MR: All of the following: seen in two views; in at least one view, jet length ≥2 cm; peak velocity ≥3 m/s; pansystolic jet in at least one envelope
Pathologic AR: All of the following: seen in two views; in at least one view, jet length ≥1 cm; peak velocity ≥3 m/s; pandiastolic jet in at least one envelope
Morphologic features of RHD in MV: anterior MV leaflet thickening ≥3 mm (age specific); chordal thickening; restricted leaflet motion; excessive leaflet tip motion during systole
Morphologic features of RHD in AV: irregular or focal thickening; coaptation defect; restricted leaflet motion; prolapse

[a]For criteria in individuals >20 years of age, see source document.

Abbreviations: AR, aortic regurgitation; AV, aortic valve; MR, mitral regurgitation; MS, mitral stenosis; MV, mitral valve.

Source: Adapted from Remenyi B et al: World Heart Federation criteria for echocardiographic diagnosis of rheumatic heart disease-an evidence-based guideline. Nat Rev Cardiol 9:297–309, 2012.

Less severe joint involvement is also relatively common and has been recognized as a potential major manifestation in high-risk populations in diagnostic guidelines from Australia, but at the time of writing, this was not reflected in the Jones criteria. Arthralgia without objective joint inflammation usually affects large joints in the same migratory pattern as polyarthritis. In some populations, aseptic monoarthritis may be a presenting feature of ARF, which may, in turn, result from early commencement of anti-inflammatory medication before the typical migratory pattern is established.

The joint manifestations of ARF are highly responsive to salicylates and other nonsteroidal anti-inflammatory drugs (NSAIDs). Indeed, joint involvement that persists for more than 1 or 2 days after starting salicylates is unlikely to be due to ARF.

CHOREA

Sydenham's chorea commonly occurs in the absence of other manifestations, follows a prolonged latent period after group A streptococcal infection, and is found mainly in females. The choreiform movements affect particularly the head (causing characteristic darting movements of the tongue) and the upper limbs (Chap. 448). They may be generalized or restricted to one side of the body (hemi-chorea). In mild cases, chorea may be evident only on careful examination, whereas in the most severe cases, the affected individuals are unable to perform activities of daily living. There is often associated emotional lability or obsessive-compulsive traits, which may last longer than the choreiform movements (which usually resolve within 6 weeks but sometimes may take up to 6 months).

SKIN MANIFESTATIONS

The classic rash of ARF is *erythema marginatum* (Chap. 24), which begins as pink macules that clear centrally, leaving a serpiginous, spreading edge. The rash is evanescent, appearing and disappearing before the examiner's eyes. It occurs usually on the trunk, sometimes on the limbs, but almost never on the face.

Subcutaneous nodules occur as painless, small (0.5–2 cm), mobile lumps beneath the skin overlying bony prominences, particularly of the hands, feet, elbows, occiput, and occasionally the vertebrae. They are a delayed manifestation, appearing 2–3 weeks after the onset of disease, last for just a few days up to 3 weeks, and are commonly associated with carditis.

OTHER FEATURES

Fever occurs in most cases of ARF, although rarely in cases of pure chorea. Although high-grade fever (≥39°C) is the rule, lower grade temperature elevations are not uncommon. Elevated acute-phase reactants are also present in most cases.

EVIDENCE OF A PRECEDING GROUP A STREPTOCOCCAL INFECTION

With the exception of chorea and low-grade carditis, both of which may become manifest many months later, evidence of a preceding group A streptococcal infection is essential in making the diagnosis of ARF. Because most cases do not have a positive throat swab culture or rapid antigen test, serologic evidence is usually needed. The most common serologic tests are the anti-streptolysin O (ASO) and anti-DNase B (ADB) titers. Where possible, age-specific reference ranges should be determined in a local population of healthy people without a recent group A streptococcal infection.

CONFIRMING THE DIAGNOSIS

Because there is no definitive test, the diagnosis of ARF relies on the presence of a combination of typical clinical features together with evidence of the precipitating group A streptococcal infection, and the exclusion of other diagnoses. This uncertainty led Dr. T. Duckett Jones in 1944 to develop a set of criteria (subsequently known as the *Jones criteria*) to aid in the diagnosis. At the time of writing, the Jones criteria were undergoing revision but had not yet been released. The existing diagnostic guideline is a World Health Organization update of the 1992 Jones Criteria (Table 381-2), though it should be noted that other guidelines, including those from Australia and New Zealand, suggest more sensitive criteria for making the diagnosis in patients from settings or populations at high risk of ARF.

TABLE 381-2 2002–2003 WORLD HEALTH ORGANIZATION CRITERIA FOR THE DIAGNOSIS OF RHEUMATIC FEVER AND RHEUMATIC HEART DISEASE (BASED ON THE 1992 REVISED JONES CRITERIA)

Diagnostic Categories	Criteria
Primary episode of rheumatic fever[a]	Two major or one major and two minor manifestations plus evidence of preceding group A streptococcal infection
Recurrent attack of rheumatic fever in a patient without established rheumatic heart disease	Two major or one major and two minor manifestations plus evidence of preceding group A streptococcal infection
Recurrent attack of rheumatic fever in a patient with established rheumatic heart disease[b]	Two minor manifestations plus evidence of preceding group A streptococcal infection[c]
Rheumatic chorea Insidious onset rheumatic carditis[b]	Other major manifestations or evidence of group A streptococcal infection not required
Chronic valve lesions of rheumatic heart disease (patients presenting for the first time with pure mitral stenosis or mixed mitral valve disease and/or aortic valve disease)[d]	Do not require any other criteria to be diagnosed as having rheumatic heart disease
Major manifestations	Carditis Polyarthritis Chorea Erythema marginatum Subcutaneous nodules
Minor manifestations	Clinical: fever, polyarthralgia Laboratory: elevated erythrocyte sedimentation rate or leukocyte count[e] Electrocardiogram: prolonged P-R interval
Supporting evidence of a preceding streptococcal infection within the last 45 days	Elevated or rising anti-streptolysin O or other streptococcal antibody, *or* A positive throat culture, *or* Rapid antigen test for group A streptococcus, *or* Recent scarlet fever[e]

[a]Patients may present with polyarthritis (or with only polyarthralgia or monoarthritis) and with several (three or more) other minor manifestations, together with evidence of recent group A streptococcal infection. Some of these cases may later turn out to be rheumatic fever. It is prudent to consider them as cases of "probable rheumatic fever" (once other diagnoses are excluded) and advise regular secondary prophylaxis. Such patients require close follow-up and regular examination of the heart. This cautious approach is particularly suitable for patients in vulnerable age groups in high-incidence settings. [b]Infective endocarditis should be excluded. [c]Some patients with recurrent attacks may not fulfill these criteria. [d]Congenital heart disease should be excluded. [e]1992 Revised Jones criteria do not include elevated leukocyte count as a laboratory minor manifestation (but do include elevated C-reactive protein), and do not include recent scarlet fever as supporting evidence of a recent streptococcal infection.

Source: Reprinted with permission from WHO Expert Consultation on Rheumatic Fever and Rheumatic Heart Disease (2001: Geneva, Switzerland): *Rheumatic Fever and Rheumatic Heart Disease: Report of a WHO Expert Consultation* (WHO Tech Rep Ser, 923). Geneva, World Health Organization, 2004.

TREATMENT ACUTE RHEUMATIC FEVER

Patients with possible ARF should be followed closely to ensure that the diagnosis is confirmed, treatment of heart failure and other symptoms is undertaken, and preventive measures including commencement of secondary prophylaxis, inclusion on an ARF registry, and health education are commenced. Echocardiography should be performed on all possible cases to aid in making the diagnosis and to determine the severity at baseline of any carditis. Other tests that should be performed are listed in Table 381-3.

There is no treatment for ARF that has been proven to alter the likelihood of developing, or the severity of, RHD. With the exception of treatment of heart failure, which may be life-saving in cases of severe carditis, the treatment of ARF is symptomatic.

ANTIBIOTICS

All patients with ARF should receive antibiotics sufficient to treat the precipitating group A streptococcal infection (Chap. 173). Penicillin is the drug of choice and can be given orally (as phenoxymethyl penicillin, 500 mg [250 mg for children ≤27 kg] PO twice daily, or amoxicillin, 50 mg/kg [maximum, 1 g] daily, for 10 days) or as a single dose of 1.2 million units (600,000 units for children ≤27 kg) IM benzathine penicillin G.

SALICYLATES AND NSAIDS

These may be used for the treatment of arthritis, arthralgia, and fever, once the diagnosis is confirmed. They are of no proven value in the treatment of carditis or chorea. Aspirin is the drug of choice, delivered at a dose of 50–60 mg/kg per day, up to a maximum of 80–100 mg/kg per day (4–8 g/d in adults) in four to five divided doses. At higher doses, the patient should be monitored for symptoms of salicylate toxicity such as nausea, vomiting, or tinnitus; if symptoms appear, lower doses should be used. When the acute

TABLE 381-3 RECOMMENDED TESTS IN CASES OF POSSIBLE ACUTE RHEUMATIC FEVER

Recommended for All Cases
White blood cell count
Erythrocyte sedimentation rate
C-reactive protein
Blood cultures if febrile
Electrocardiogram (if prolonged P-R interval or other rhythm abnormality, repeat in 2 weeks and again at 2 months if still abnormal)
Chest x-ray if clinical or echocardiographic evidence of carditis
Echocardiogram (consider repeating after 1 month if negative)
Throat swab (preferably before giving antibiotics)—culture for group A streptococcus
Antistreptococcal serology: both anti-streptolysin O and anti-DNase B titers, if available (repeat 10–14 days later if first test not confirmatory)
Tests for Alternative Diagnoses, Depending on Clinical Features
Repeated blood cultures if possible endocarditis
Joint aspirate (microscopy and culture) for possible septic arthritis
Copper, ceruloplasmin, antinuclear antibody, drug screen for choreiform movements
Serology and autoimmune markers for arboviral, autoimmune, or reactive arthritis

Source: Reprinted with permission from Menzies School of Health Research.

symptoms are substantially resolved, usually within the first 2 weeks, patients on higher doses can have the dose reduced to 50–60 mg/kg per day for a further 2–4 weeks. Fever, joint manifestations, and elevated acute-phase reactants sometimes recur up to 3 weeks after the medication is discontinued. This does not indicate a recurrence and can be managed by recommencing salicylates for a brief period. Naproxen at a dose of 10–20 mg/kg per day is a suitable alternative to aspirin and has the advantage of twice-daily dosing.

CONGESTIVE HEART FAILURE

Glucocorticoids The use of glucocorticoids in ARF remains controversial. Two meta-analyses have failed to demonstrate a benefit of glucocorticoids compared to placebo or salicylates in improving the short- or longer term outcome of carditis. However, the studies included in these meta-analyses all took place >40 years ago and did not use medications in common usage today. Many clinicians treat cases of severe carditis (causing heart failure) with glucocorticoids in the belief that they may reduce the acute inflammation and result in more rapid resolution of failure. However, the potential benefits of this treatment should be balanced against the possible adverse effects. If used, prednisone or prednisolone is recommended at a dose of 1–2 mg/kg per day (maximum, 80 mg), usually for a few days or up to a maximum of 3 weeks.

MANAGEMENT OF HEART FAILURE

See Chap. 280.

BED REST

Traditional recommendations for long-term bed rest, once the cornerstone of management, are no longer widely practiced. Instead, bed rest should be prescribed as needed while arthritis and arthralgia are present and for patients with heart failure. Once symptoms are well controlled, gradual mobilization can commence as tolerated.

CHOREA

Medications to control the abnormal movements do not alter the duration or outcome of chorea. Milder cases can usually be managed by providing a calm environment. In patients with severe chorea, carbamazepine or sodium valproate is preferred to haloperidol. A response may not be seen for 1–2 weeks, and medication should be continued for 1–2 weeks after symptoms subside. There is recent evidence that corticosteroids are effective and lead to more rapid symptom reduction in chorea. They should be considered in severe or refractory cases. Prednisone or prednisolone may be commenced at 0.5 mg/kg daily, with weaning as early as possible, preferably after 1 week if symptoms are reduced, although slower weaning or temporary dose escalation may be required if symptoms worsen.

INTRAVENOUS IMMUNOGLOBULIN (IVIG)

Small studies have suggested that IVIg may lead to more rapid resolution of chorea but have shown no benefit on the short- or long-term outcome of carditis in ARF without chorea. In the absence of better data, IVIg is *not* recommended except in cases of severe chorea refractory to other treatments.

PROGNOSIS

Untreated, ARF lasts on average 12 weeks. With treatment, patients are usually discharged from hospital within 1–2 weeks. Inflammatory markers should be monitored every 1–2 weeks until they have normalized (usually within 4–6 weeks), and an echocardiogram should be performed after 1 month to determine if there has been progression of carditis. Cases with more severe carditis need close clinical and echocardiographic monitoring in the longer term.

Once the acute episode has resolved, the priority in management is to ensure long-term clinical follow-up and adherence to a regimen of secondary prophylaxis. Patients should be entered onto the local ARF registry (if present) and contact made with primary care practitioners to ensure a plan for follow-up and administration of secondary prophylaxis before the patient is discharged. Patients and their families should also be educated about their disease, emphasizing the importance of adherence to secondary prophylaxis.

PREVENTION

PRIMARY PREVENTION

Ideally, primary prevention would entail elimination of the major risk factors for streptococcal infection, particularly overcrowded housing. This is difficult to achieve in most places where ARF is common.

Therefore, the mainstay of primary prevention for ARF remains primary prophylaxis (i.e., the timely and complete treatment of group A streptococcal sore throat with antibiotics). If commenced within 9 days of sore throat onset, a course of penicillin (as outlined above for treatment of ARF) will prevent almost all cases of ARF that would otherwise have developed. In settings where ARF and RHD are common but microbiologic diagnosis of group A streptococcal pharyngitis is not available, such as in resource-poor countries, primary care guidelines often recommend that all patients with sore throat be treated with penicillin or, alternatively, that a clinical algorithm be used to identify patients with a higher likelihood of group A streptococcal pharyngitis. Although imperfect, such approaches recognize the importance of ARF prevention at the expense of overtreating many cases of sore throat that are not caused by group A streptococcus.

SECONDARY PREVENTION

The mainstay of controlling ARF and RHD is secondary prevention. Because patients with ARF are at dramatically higher risk than the general population of developing a further episode of ARF after a group A streptococcal infection, they should receive long-term penicillin prophylaxis to prevent recurrences. The best antibiotic for secondary prophylaxis is benzathine penicillin G (1.2 million units, or 600,000 units if ≤27 kg) delivered every 4 weeks. It can be given every 3 weeks, or even every 2 weeks, to persons considered to be at particularly high risk, although in settings where good compliance with an every-4-week dosing schedule can be achieved, more frequent dosing is rarely needed. Oral penicillin V (250 mg) can be given twice daily instead but is less effective than benzathine penicillin G. Penicillin-allergic patients can receive erythromycin (250 mg) twice daily.

The duration of secondary prophylaxis is determined by many factors, in particular the duration since the last episode of ARF

TABLE 381-4 AMERICAN HEART ASSOCIATION RECOMMENDATIONS FOR DURATION OF SECONDARY PROPHYLAXIS[a]

Category of Patient	Duration of Prophylaxis
Rheumatic fever without carditis	For 5 years after the last attack or 21 years of age (whichever is longer)
Rheumatic fever with carditis but no residual valvular disease	For 10 years after the last attack, or 21 years of age (whichever is longer)
Rheumatic fever with persistent valvular disease, evident clinically or on echocardiography	For 10 years after the last attack, or 40 years of age (whichever is longer); sometimes lifelong prophylaxis

[a]These are only recommendations and must be modified by individual circumstances as warranted. Note that some organizations recommend a minimum of 10 years of prophylaxis after the most recent episode, or until 21 years of age (whichever is longer), regardless of the presence of carditis with the initial episode.

Source: Adapted from AHA Scientific Statement Prevention of Rheumatic Fever and Diagnosis and Treatment of Acute Streptococcal Pharyngitis. Circulation 119:1541, 2009.

(recurrences become less likely with increasing time), age (recurrences are less likely with increasing age), and the severity of RHD (if severe, it may be prudent to avoid even a very small risk of recurrence because of the potentially serious consequences) (Table 381-4). Secondary prophylaxis is best delivered as part of a coordinated RHD control program, based around a registry of patients. Registries improve the ability to follow patients and identify those who default from prophylaxis and to institute strategies to improve adherence.

VIDEO 381-1A Transthoracic echocardiographic images of a 9-year-old girl with first episode of acute rheumatic fever. Images demonstrate the typical echocardiographic findings of acute rheumatic carditis. The valve leaflets are relatively thin and highly mobile. The failure of coaptation of the mitral valve leaflets is the result of chordal elongation and annular dilatation. The mitral valve regurgitation is moderate with a typical posterolaterally directed regurgitant jet of rheumatic carditis. ***A.*** Acute rheumatic carditis (apical four-chamber view echocardiogram).

VIDEO 381-1B Transthoracic echocardiographic images of a 9-year-old girl with first episode of acute rheumatic fever. Images demonstrate the typical echocardiographic findings of acute rheumatic carditis. The valve leaflets are relatively thin and highly mobile. The failure of coaptation of the mitral valve leaflets is the result of chordal elongation and annular dilatation. The mitral valve regurgitation is moderate with a typical posterolaterally directed regurgitant jet of rheumatic carditis. ***B.*** Acute rheumatic carditis (apical four-chamber view color Doppler echocardiogram).

VIDEO 381-1C Transthoracic echocardiographic images of a 9-year-old girl with first episode of acute rheumatic fever. Images demonstrate the typical echocardiographic findings of acute rheumatic carditis. The valve leaflets are relatively thin and highly mobile. The failure of coaptation of the mitral valve leaflets is the result of chordal elongation and annular dilatation. The mitral valve regurgitation is moderate with a typical posterolaterally directed regurgitant jet of rheumatic carditis. ***C.*** Acute rheumatic carditis (parasternal long-axis view echocardiogram).

VIDEO 381-1D Transthoracic echocardiographic images of a 9-year-old girl with first episode of acute rheumatic fever. Images demonstrate the typical echocardiographic findings of acute rheumatic carditis. The valve leaflets are relatively thin and highly mobile. The failure of coaptation of the mitral valve leaflets is the result of chordal elongation and annular dilatation. The mitral valve regurgitation is moderate with a typical posterolaterally directed regurgitant jet of rheumatic carditis. ***D.*** Acute rheumatic carditis (parasternal long-axis view color Doppler echocardiogram).

VIDEO 381-2A Transthoracic echocardiographic images are from a 5-year-old boy with chronic rheumatic heart disease with severe mitral valve regurgitation and moderate mitral valve stenosis. Images demonstrate the typical echocardiographic findings in advanced chronic rheumatic heart disease. Both the anterior and posterior mitral valve leaflets are markedly thickened. During diastole, the motion of the anterior mitral valve leaflet tip is restricted with doming of the body of the leaflet toward the interventricular septum. This appearance is commonly described as a "hockey stick" or an "elbow" deformity. ***A.*** Chronic rheumatic heart disease (parasternal long-axis view).

VIDEO 381-2B Transthoracic echocardiographic images are from a 5-year-old boy with chronic rheumatic heart disease with severe mitral valve regurgitation and moderate mitral valve stenosis. Images demonstrate the typical echocardiographic findings in advanced chronic rheumatic heart disease. Both the anterior and posterior mitral valve leaflets are markedly thickened. During diastole, the motion of the anterior mitral valve leaflet tip is restricted with doming of the body of the leaflet toward the interventricular septum. This appearance is commonly described as a "hockey stick" or an "elbow" deformity. ***B.*** Chronic rheumatic heart disease (apical two-chamber view echocardiogram).

382 Systemic Sclerosis (Scleroderma) and Related Disorders

John Varga

DEFINITION

Systemic sclerosis (SSc) is an uncommon connective tissue disorder characterized by multisystem involvement, heterogeneous clinical manifestations, a chronic and often progressive course, and significant disability and mortality. Multiple genes contribute to disease susceptibility; however, environmental exposures are likely to play a major role in causing SSc. The early stage of the disease is associated with prominent inflammatory features. Over time, functional and structural alterations in multiple vascular beds and progressive visceral organ dysfunction due to fibrosis dominate the clinical picture. Although thickened skin (scleroderma) is the distinguishing hallmark of SSc, skin induration can occur in localized forms of scleroderma and other disorders (Table 382-1). Patients with SSc can be broadly

TABLE 382-1 CONDITIONS ASSOCIATED WITH SKIN INDURATION

- Systemic sclerosis (SSc)
  - Limited cutaneous SSc
  - Diffuse cutaneous SSc
- Localized scleroderma
  - Guttate (plaque) morphea, diffuse (pansclerotic) morphea, bullous morphea
  - Linear scleroderma, coup de sabre, hemifacial atrophy
- Pansclerotic morphea
- Overlap syndromes
  - Mixed connective tissue disease
  - SSc/polymyositis
- Stiff skin syndrome
- Diabetic scleredema and scleredema of Buschke
- Scleromyxedema (papular mucinosis)
- Chronic graft-versus-host disease
- Diffuse fasciitis with eosinophilia (Shulman's disease, eosinophilic fasciitis)
- Chemically induced and drug-associated scleroderma-like conditions
  - Vinyl chloride–induced disease
  - Eosinophilia-myalgia syndrome (associated with L-tryptophan)
  - Nephrogenic systemic fibrosis (associated with gadolinium)
- Paraneoplastic syndrome

TABLE 382-2 SUBSETS OF SYSTEMIC SCLEROSIS (SSC): FEATURES OF LIMITED CUTANEOUS SSC VERSUS DIFFUSE CUTANEOUS SSC

Characteristic Feature	Limited Cutaneous SSc	Diffuse Cutaneous SSc
Skin involvement	Indolent onset. Limited to fingers, distal to elbows, face; slow progression	Rapid onset. Diffuse: fingers, extremities, face, trunk; rapid progression
Raynaud's phenomenon	Antedates skin involvement, sometimes by years; may be associated with critical ischemia in the digits	Onset coincident with skin involvement; critical ischemia less common
Musculoskeletal	Mild arthralgia	Severe arthralgia, carpal tunnel syndrome, tendon friction rubs
Interstitial lung disease	Slowly progressive, generally mild	Frequent, early onset and progression, can be severe
Pulmonary arterial hypertension	Frequent, late, may occur as an isolated complication	Often occurs in association with interstitial lung disease
Scleroderma renal crisis	Very rare	Occurs in 15%; generally early (<4 years from disease onset)
Calcinosis cutis	Frequent, prominent	Less common, mild
Characteristic autoantibodies	Anticentromere	Anti–topoisomerase I (Scl-70), anti-RNA polymerase III

grouped into diffuse cutaneous and limited cutaneous subsets defined by the pattern of skin involvement, as well as clinical and laboratory features (Table 382-2). Diffuse cutaneous SSc (dcSSc) is associated with extensive skin induration, starting in the fingers and ascending from distal to proximal limbs and the trunk. These patients often have early interstitial lung disease and acute renal involvement. In contrast, in patients with limited cutaneous SSc (lcSSc), Raynaud's phenomenon may precede other manifestations of SSc by years. In these patients, skin involvement remains limited to the fingers (sclerodactyly), distal limbs, and face, and the trunk is not affected. The constellation of calcinosis cutis, Raynaud's phenomenon, esophageal dysmotility, sclerodactyly, and telangiectasia, seen in some lcSSc patients, is termed the *CREST syndrome*. Visceral organ involvement in lcSSc tends to show insidious progression, and pulmonary arterial hypertension (PAH), interstitial lung disease, hypothyroidism, and primary biliary cirrhosis may occur as late complications. In some patients, Raynaud's phenomenon and other characteristic features of SSc occur in the absence of skin thickening. This syndrome has been termed *SSc sine scleroderma*.

EPIDEMIOLOGY

SSc is an acquired sporadic disease with a worldwide distribution and affecting all races. In the United States, the incidence is estimated at 9–19 cases per million per year. The only community-based survey of SSc yielded a prevalence of 286 cases per million. There are an estimated 100,000 cases in the United States, although this number may be significantly higher if patients who do not meet strict classification criteria are also included. Rates of SSc in England, Australia, and Japan appear to be lower. Age, gender, and ethnicity are important in disease susceptibility. In common with other connective tissue diseases, SSc shows a strong female predominance (4.6:1), which is most pronounced in the childbearing years and declines after menopause. Although SSc can present at any age, the peak age of onset for both limited and diffuse cutaneous forms is 30–50 years. The incidence is higher in blacks than whites, and disease onset occurs at an earlier age. Furthermore, blacks with SSc are more likely to have diffuse cutaneous disease associated with interstitial lung involvement and a worse prognosis.

GENETIC CONSIDERATIONS

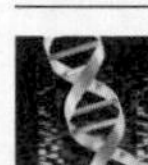

In general, SSc shows modest heritability, and the genetic associations identified to date make only a small contribution to disease susceptibility. Concordance rates for SSc are low (4.7%) in monozygotic twins, although concordance for antinuclear antibody (ANA) positivity is significantly higher. On the other hand, evidence for genetic contribution to disease susceptibility is provided by the observation that 1.6% of SSc patients have a first-degree relative with SSc, a prevalence rate markedly increased compared to the general population. The risk of Raynaud's phenomenon, interstitial lung disease, and other autoimmune diseases, including systemic lupus erythematosus (SLE) (Chap. 378), rheumatoid arthritis (Chap. 380), and autoimmune thyroiditis (Chap. 405), is also increased. Approaches to study the role of genetics in SSc use candidate gene single nucleotide polymorphism (SNP) analysis and genome-wide association studies (GWASs). Candidate gene studies in SSc have shown associations with multiple gene variants, many related to B and T lymphocyte activation and signaling (*BANK1, BLK, CD247, CSK, IRAK1, IL2RA, PTPN22,* and *TNIP1*). *IRAK1*, which codes for a gene involved in both innate and adaptive immunity, is the first X-linked gene associated with SSc and may contribute to female predominance. Other gene variants associated with SSc are involved in innate immunity and the interferon pathways (*IRF5, IRF7, STAT4, TNFAIP3,* and *TLR2*). In addition, candidate gene studies and GWAS both identified association with genes in the major histocompatibility complex (MHC), including *NOTCH4* and *PSORSC1*. In addition to disease susceptibility, some of these genetic loci are associated with particular SSc disease manifestations or serologic subsets, including interstitial lung disease (ILD) (*CTGF, CD226*), PAH (*TNIP1*), and scleroderma renal crisis (*HLA-DRB1**). Although the functional consequences of these gene variants are currently not well understood, they may result in altered immune function, leading to increased susceptibility to autoimmunity and inflammation. Of note, many of the genetic variants associated with SSc are also seen in other autoimmune disorders, including SLE, rheumatoid arthritis, and psoriasis, suggesting common pathways shared among these conditions. The genetic associations identified to date only explain a fraction of the heritability of SSc, and GWASs, fine mapping, and resequencing of DNA regions of interest to identify additional genetic susceptibility factors in SSc, particularly rare variants, are currently ongoing.

ENVIRONMENTAL AND OCCUPATIONAL RISK FACTORS

Given the relatively modest genetic contribution to disease susceptibility, environmental factors, such as infectious agents, intestinal microbiota, and occupational, dietary, and drug exposures, are likely to play a major role in causing SSc. Patients with SSc show evidence of chronic infection of lesional tissue with Epstein-Barr virus (EBV). They also have increased antibodies to human cytomegalovirus (hCMV), and anti–topoisomerase I (Scl-70) autoantibodies recognize hCMV-associated antigenic epitopes, suggesting molecular mimicry as a possible mechanistic link between hCMV infection and SSc. An epidemic of a novel syndrome with features suggestive of SSc occurred in Spain in the 1980s. The outbreak, termed *toxic oil syndrome*, was linked to contaminated rapeseed oils used for cooking. Another epidemic outbreak, termed *eosinophilia-myalgia syndrome* (EMS), occurred a decade later and was linked to the consumption of L-tryptophan-containing dietary supplements. Although both of these novel toxic-epidemic syndromes were characterized by scleroderma-like chronic skin changes and variable visceral organ involvement, they were associated with clinical, pathologic, and laboratory features distinguishing them from SSc. Occupational exposures tentatively linked with SSc include silica dust in miners, polyvinyl chloride, epoxy resins, and aromatic hydrocarbons including toluene and trichloroethylene. Drugs implicated in SSc-like illnesses include bleomycin, pentazocine, and cocaine, and appetite suppressants linked with pulmonary hypertension. Although case reports and series describing SSc in women with silicone breast implants had raised concern regarding a possible causal role of silicone in SSc, large-scale epidemiologic investigations found no evidence of increased prevalence of SSc.

PATHOGENESIS

The following three cardinal pathophysiologic processes account for the protean clinical manifestations of SSc: (1) diffuse microangiopathy, (2) inflammation and autoimmunity, and (3) visceral and vascular fibrosis in multiple organs (Fig. 382-1). Autoimmunity and altered vascular reactivity are early manifestations. Complex and dynamic interplay between these processes initiates and then amplifies the fibrotic process.

ANIMAL MODELS OF DISEASE

No single animal model of SSc fully reproduces the three cardinal processes that underlie the pathogenesis, but some recapitulate selected aspects of the human disease, including fibrosis, microvascular involvement, and autoimmunity. Tight-skin mice (Tsk1) develop spontaneous skin thickening due to a mutation in the fibrillin-1 gene. The mutant fibrillin-1 protein disrupts extracellular matrix assembly and causes aberrant activation of transforming growth factor β (TGF-β). Fibrillin-1 mutations are associated with Marfan's disease as well as the stiff skin syndrome but not SSc. Skin and lung fibrosis can be induced in mice by injection of bleomycin, HOCl, or double-stranded RNA or by transplantation of human leukocyte antigen (HLA)–mismatched bone marrow or spleen cells. Targeted genetic modifications in mice give rise to new disease models for dissecting the pathogenetic roles of individual molecules, cell types, and networks. For example, mice lacking Smad3, an intracellular TGF-β signal transducer, adiponectin, or the nuclear receptor peroxisome proliferator-activated receptor (PPAR) γ or overexpressing Wnt10b or adiponectin were either resistant or hypersensitive to chemically induced experimental scleroderma. These mouse models have potential utility in preclinical evaluation of potential therapies.

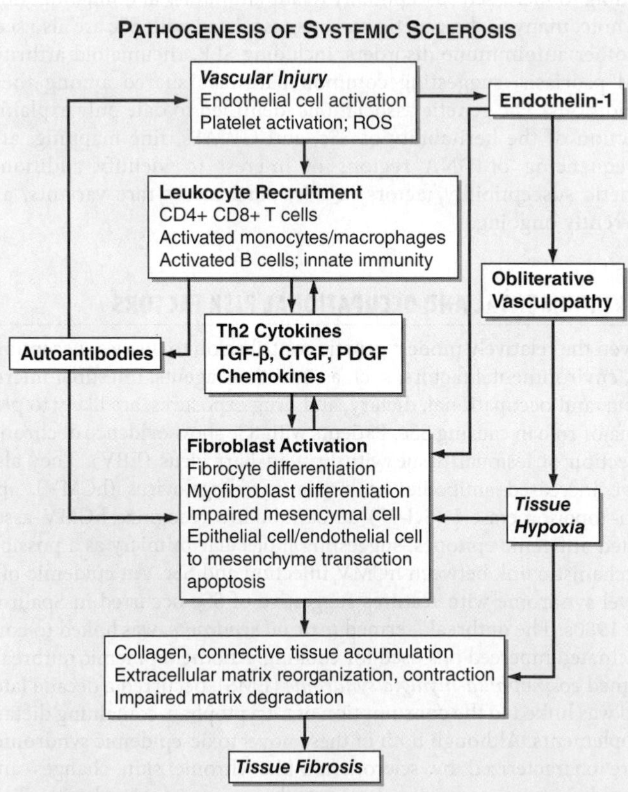

FIGURE 382-1 Initial vascular injury in a genetically susceptible individual leads to functional and structural vascular alterations, inflammation, and autoimmunity. The inflammatory and immune responses initiate and sustain fibroblast activation and differentiation, resulting in pathologic fibrogenesis and irreversible tissue damage. Vascular damage results in tissue ischemia that further contributes to progressive fibrosis and atrophy. CTGF, connective tissue growth factor; PDGF, platelet-derived growth factor; TGF-β, transforming growth factor β.

MICROANGIOPATHY

Involvement of small blood vessels in SSc affects multiple vascular beds and has important clinical sequelae including Raynaud's phenomenon, ischemic digital ulcers, scleroderma renal crisis, and PAH. Raynaud's phenomenon, an early disease manifestation, is characterized by an altered blood-flow response to cold challenge. This initially reversible functional abnormality is associated with autonomic and peripheral nervous system alterations, including impaired production of the neuropeptide calcitonin gene-related peptide from sensory afferent nerves and heightened sensitivity of α_2-adrenergic receptors on vascular smooth-muscle cells. Isolated (primary) Raynaud's phenomenon is extremely common and generally benign and nonprogressive. In contrast, SSc-associated Raynaud's phenomenon is often progressive and complicated by irreversible structural changes, culminating in ischemic digital ulcers and loss of digits. Viruses, vascular cytotoxic factors, thrombogenic microparticles, complement and autoantibodies to phospholipids, β2 glycoprotein I (β2GPI), and endothelial cells are suspected triggers of endothelial cell injury in SSc. Endothelial injury results in dysregulated production of endothelium-derived vasodilatory (nitric oxide and prostacyclin) and vasoconstricting (endothelin-1) substances, as well as increased expression of intercellular adhesion molecule 1 (ICAM-1) and other surface adhesion molecules. Microvessels show enhanced permeability and transendothelial leukocyte diapedesis, abnormal activation of coagulation cascades, elevated thrombin production, and impaired fibrinolysis. Spontaneous platelet aggregation causes release of serotonin, platelet-derived growth factor (PDGF), and platelet alpha granules including thromboxane, a potent vasoconstrictor. Smooth-muscle cell–like myointimal cells proliferate, the basement membrane is thickened and reduplicated, and fibrosis of the adventitial layers develops. The vasculopathic process affects capillaries, as well as arterioles, and even large vessels in many organs, resulting in reduced blood flow and tissue ischemia. Progressive luminal occlusion due to intimal and medial hypertrophy, combined with persistent endothelial cell damage and adventitial fibrosis, establish a vicious cycle that culminates in the striking absence of blood vessels (rarefaction) in late-stage disease. Recurrent ischemia-reperfusion generates reactive oxygen species (ROS) that further damage the endothelium through peroxidation of membrane lipids. Paradoxically, the process of revascularization that normally reestablishes blood flow to ischemic tissue is defective in SSc despite elevated levels of vascular endothelial growth factor (VEGF) and other angiogenic factors. Moreover, the number of bone marrow–derived circulating endothelial progenitor cells is reduced. Thus, widespread capillary loss, obliterative vasculopathy of small and medium-sized arteries, and failure to repair damaged vessels are hallmarks of SSc.

IMMUNE DYSREGULATION

Cellular Immunity The following observations highlight the autoimmune nature of SSc: presence of circulating autoantibodies; familial clustering of SSc with other autoimmune diseases; detection of immune cells, including T cells with oligoclonal antigen receptors, in target organs; elevated circulating levels and spontaneous secretion from blood mononuclear cells of inflammatory cytokines and chemokines such as interleukin (IL) 1, IL-4, IL-10, IL-17, IL-33, CCL2, and CXCL4; and the association with variants in genes functionally implicated in immune responses. Genetic studies in SSc reveal strong and consistent associations with major histocompatibility locus alleles, as well as non-HLA-linked genes encoding mediators of both adaptive and innate immune responses (*CD247*, *STAT4*, *IRF5*, *CD226*, and *TNFSF4*). In early SSc, mononuclear inflammatory cell infiltrates comprised of activated T cells, monocytes/macrophages, and dendritic cells can be seen in skin, lungs, and other affected organs prior to appearance of fibrosis or vascular damage. Dendritic cells and T cells can often be found in close proximity to activated fibroblasts and myofibroblasts. Tissue-infiltrating T cells express CD45 and HLA-DR activation markers and display restricted T cell receptor signatures indicative of oligoclonal expansion in response to (unknown) antigen.

TABLE 382-3 AUTOANTIBODIES AND ASSOCIATED FEATURES IN SYSTEMIC SCLEROSIS (SSC)

Target Antigen	SSc Subset	Characteristic Clinical Association
Topoisomerase I	dcSSc	Tendon friction rubs, early ILD, cardiac involvement, scleroderma renal crisis
Centromere proteins	lcSSc	Digital ischemic ulcers, calcinosis cutis, isolated PAH, overlap syndromes; renal crisis rare
RNA polymerase III	dcSSc	Rapidly progressive skin involvement, tendon friction rubs, joint contractures, GAVE, renal crisis, contemporaneous cancers
U3-RNP (fibrillarin)	dcSSc	PAH, ILD, scleroderma renal crisis, myositis
Th/TO	lcSSc	ILD, PAH
PM/Scl	lcSSc	Calcinosis cutis, ILD, myositis overlap
Ku	Overlap	SLE, myositis
U1-RNP	MCTD	PAH, arthritis, myositis

Abbreviations: dcSSc, diffuse cutaneous SSc; GAVE, gastric antral vascular ectasia, ILD, interstitial lung disease; lcSSc, limited cutaneous SSc; MCTD, mixed connective tissue disease; PAH, pulmonary arterial hypertension; SLE, systemic lupus erythematosus.

Circulating T cells have elevated levels of chemokine receptors and α_1 integrin adhesion molecules, accounting for their enhanced binding to endothelium and to fibroblasts. Endothelial cells express ICAM-1 and other adhesion molecules that facilitate leukocyte diapedesis. Activated macrophages and T cells show a T_H2-polarized type 2 immune response driven by dendritic cells and thymic stromal lymphopoietin. T_H2 cytokines such as IL-4 and IL-13 induce fibroblast activation and alternate M2 macrophage polarization, whereas the T_H1 cytokine interferon γ (IFN-γ) blocks cytokine-mediated fibroblast activation. Alternately activated M2 macrophages produce TGF-β and promote fibrosis. Although the frequency of circulating regulatory T cells that enforce immune tolerance is elevated in SSc, their immunosuppressive function is defective. Molecular characterization of SSc skin biopsies using DNA microarrays identifies a subset showing markedly elevated expression of inflammation-associated genes, particularly chemokines and their receptors, interferon response genes, and mediators of innate immunity. Evidence of activated innate immunity and toll-like receptor signaling, indicative of activation by type 1 interferon produced by plasmacytoid dendritic cells, is prominent in peripheral blood cells.

Humoral Autoimmunity Circulating ANAs can be detected in virtually all patients with SSc. In addition, a number of SSc-specific autoantibodies have been described. These SSc-specific antibodies show strong association with distinct disease endophenotypes (Table 382-3). While most are directed against intracellular proteins associated with cell proliferation, such as topoisomerase I and RNA polymerases I, II, and III, others are directed against cell-surface antigens, receptors, or secreted proteins. Autoantibodies have clinical utility as diagnostic and prognostic biomarkers in SSc, and some, such as antibodies directed against the angiotensin II receptor or the PDGF receptor, may have a direct pathogenic role.

A variety of mechanisms have been proposed for the development of autoantibodies in SSc. Proteolytic cleavage, increased expression, or altered subcellular localization of certain cellular proteins in SSc could lead to their recognition as neoepitopes by the immune system, resulting in breakdown of immune tolerance. B cells are implicated in both the autoimmune and fibrotic process in SSc. In addition to antibody production, B cells also present antigen, secrete IL-6 and TGF-β, and modulate T cell and dendritic cell function.

FIBROSIS

Fibrosis affecting multiple organs, a distinguishing feature of SSc, is characterized by progressive replacement of normal tissue architecture with dense, stiff, and acellular connective tissue. Fibrosis characteristically follows, and is thought to be a consequence of, inflammation, autoimmunity, and microvascular damage. Fibroblasts are mesenchymal cells responsible for maintaining the functional and structural integrity of connective tissue. Upon activation by TGF-β and other extracellular cues, fibroblasts proliferate; migrate; secrete collagens, growth factors, chemokines, and cytokines; and transdifferentiate into contractile myofibroblasts. Under normal conditions, these fibrotic responses constitute self-limited physiologic remodeling necessary for tissue repair and regeneration. When these responses become sustained and amplified, pathologic fibrosis results. Autocrine stimulatory signaling by endogenously produced TGF-β and fibrotic mediators such as hypoxia, ROS, thrombin, Wnt ligands, connective tissue growth factor (CTGF), PDGF, lysophosphatidic acid, endothelin-1, mechanical forces, and endogenous ligands for toll-like receptors are responsible for maintaining sustained fibroblast activation underlying progressive fibrosis in SSc.

In addition to tissue-resident fibroblasts and transformation of epithelial cells into fibroblasts, bone marrow–derived circulating mesenchymal progenitor cells also contribute to fibrosis. The factors that regulate the differentiation of mesenchymal progenitor cells and their trafficking from the circulation into lesional tissue are unknown. Epithelial and endothelial cells, mesenchymal progenitor cells, and tissue fibroblasts can differentiate into smooth-muscle-like myofibroblasts. Although myofibroblasts can be detected transiently during normal wound healing, they persist in fibrotic tissue, possibly due to resistance to apoptosis, and contribute to scar formation via production of collagen and TGF-β and contraction of the surrounding extracellular matrix.

Explanted SSc fibroblasts may display an abnormally activated phenotype ex vivo, with variably increased rates of collagen gene transcription, spontaneous ROS generation, and constitutive expression of alpha smooth muscle actin stress fibers. The persistence of the "scleroderma phenotype" of these cells during their serial passage in vitro may reflect autocrine TGF-β stimulatory loops, deregulated microRNA expressions, histone acetylation, and other epigenetic modifications.

PATHOLOGY

The distinguishing pathologic hallmark of SSc is the combination of widespread capillary loss and obliterative microangiopathy, together with fibrosis in the skin and internal organs. In early disease, perivascular inflammatory cell infiltrates composed of T lymphocytes, monocytes/macrophages, plasma cells, mast cells, and occasionally B cells may be detected in multiple organs. A bland noninflammatory obliterative vasculopathy as a late finding is prominent in the heart, lungs, kidneys, and intestinal tract. Fibrosis is found in the skin, lungs, gastrointestinal tract, heart, tendon sheaths, perifascicular tissue surrounding skeletal muscle, and some endocrine organs. In these tissues, accumulation of collagens, fibronectin, proteoglycans, tenascin, cartilage oligomeric matrix protein (COMP), and other structural macromolecules progressively disrupts normal architecture, resulting in impaired function of affected organs.

SKIN

In the skin, fibrosis causes dermal expansion and obliteration of the hair follicles, eccrine glands, and other appendages (Fig. 382-2A). Collagen fiber accumulation is most prominent in the reticular dermis, and the fibrotic process invades the subjacent adipose layer with entrapment of adipocytes. With disease progression, the intradermal adipose layer is diminished and may completely disappear. The epidermis is atrophic, and the rete pegs are effaced.

LUNGS

Patchy infiltration of the alveolar walls with T lymphocytes, macrophages, and eosinophils occurs in early disease. With progression, interstitial fibrosis and vascular damage dominate the pathologic picture, often coexisting within the same lesions in patients with dcSSc. Pulmonary fibrosis is characterized by expansion of the alveolar interstitium, with accumulation of collagen and other matrix proteins. The most common histologic pattern in SSc-associated ILD is nonspecific interstitial pneumonia (NSIP), distinct from the usual interstitial pneumonia (UIP) pattern characteristically seen in patients with

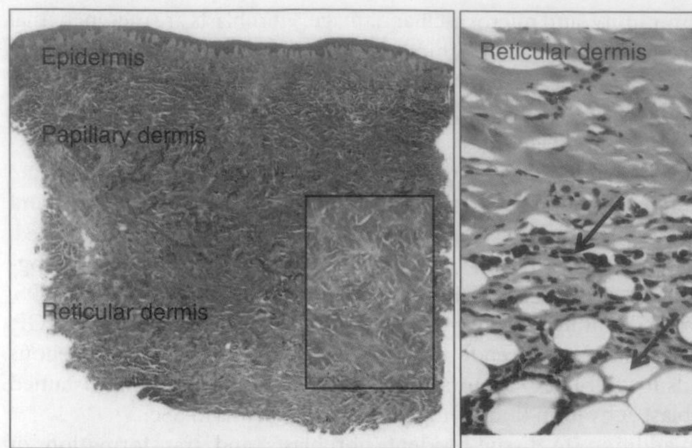

A

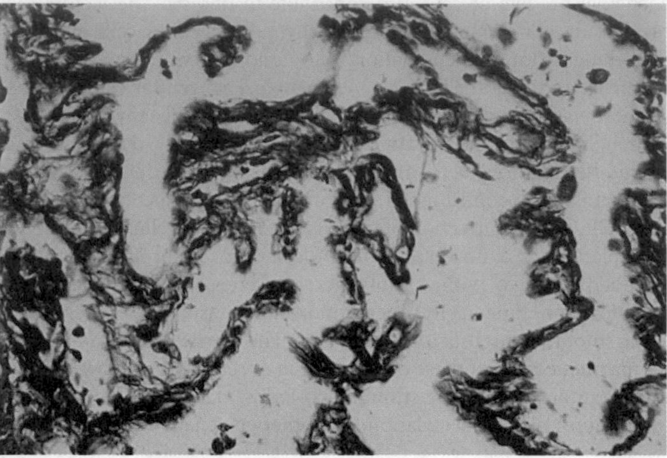

B

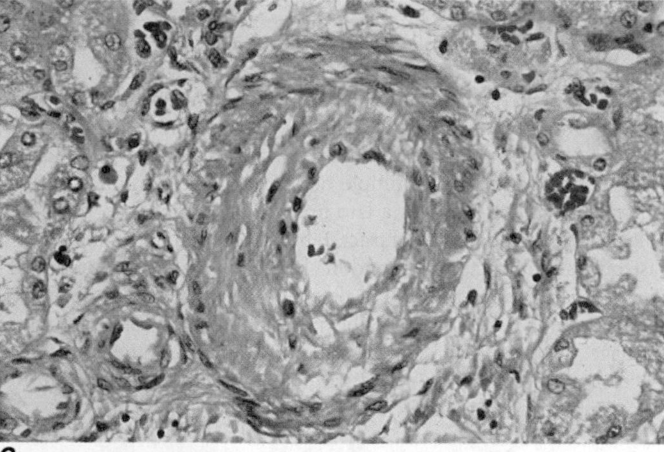

C

FIGURE 382-2 Pathologic findings in systemic sclerosis (SSc). ***A. Left panel:*** The skin is thickened due the marked expansion of the dermis. Inset, higher magnification showing thick hyalinized collagen bundles replace skin appendages. ***Right panel:*** Inflammation in the reticular dermis. Mononuclear inflammatory cells infiltrating the dermis and intradermal adipose tissue. ***B.*** Early interstitial lung disease. Diffuse fibrosis of the alveolar septae and a chronic inflammatory cell infiltrate. Trichrome stain. ***C.*** Pulmonary arterial obliterative vasculopathy. Striking intimal hyperplasia and narrowing of the lumen of a small pulmonary artery, with minimal interstitial fibrosis, in a patient with limited cutaneous SSc.

idiopathic pulmonary fibrosis (Fig. 382-2*B*). Progressive thickening of the alveolar septae results in obliteration of the airspaces and loss of pulmonary blood vessels. This process impairs gas exchange and contributes to pulmonary hypertension. Intimal thickening of the pulmonary arteries, best seen with elastin stain, underlies pulmonary hypertension (Fig. 382-2*C*) and, at autopsy, is often associated with multiple pulmonary emboli and evidence of myocardial fibrosis.

GASTROINTESTINAL TRACT

Pathologic changes can be found at any level from the mouth to the rectum. The lower esophagus shows prominent atrophy of the muscular layers and characteristic vascular lesions; striated muscle in the upper third of the esophagus is generally spared. Replacement of the normal intestinal tract architecture results in diminished peristaltic activity, with gastroesophageal reflux, dysmotility, and small-bowel obstruction. Chronic reflux is associated with esophageal inflammation, ulcerations, and stricture formation and may lead to Barrett's metaplasia.

KIDNEYS

In the kidneys, vascular lesions affecting the interlobular and arcuate arteries predominate. Chronic renal ischemia is associated with shrunken glomeruli. Acute scleroderma renal crisis is associated with a classic thrombotic microangiopathic pathology: reduplication of elastic lamina, marked intimal proliferation, and narrowing of the lumen in small renal arteries, commonly accompanied by thrombosis and hemolysis.

HEART

The heart is frequently affected, with prominent involvement of the myocardium and pericardium. The characteristic arteriolar lesions are concentric intimal hypertrophy and luminal narrowing, accompanied by contraction band necrosis reflecting ischemia-reperfusion injury and myocardial fibrosis. Fibrosis of the conduction system is common, especially at the sinoatrial node. Despite the prominent role of ischemia in SSc, the frequency of atherosclerotic coronary artery disease is comparable to the general population.

OTHER ORGANS

Synovitis may be found in early SSc; however, with disease progression, the synovium becomes fibrotic. Fibrosis of tendon sheaths and fascia produces palpable and sometimes audible tendon friction rubs. Inflammation and, in later stages, atrophy and fibrosis of the muscles are common findings. Fibrosis of the thyroid gland and of the minor salivary glands may be seen.

CLINICAL FEATURES

OVERVIEW

Virtually every organ can be clinically affected (Table 382-4). Most patients with SSc can be classified as lcSSc or dcSSc (Table 382-2). Although stratification of SSc patients into diffuse and limited cutaneous subsets is useful, disease expression is far more complex, and several distinct endophenotypes exist within each subset. For example, 10–15% of patients with lcSSc develop PAH without significant ILD. Other patients have systemic features of SSc without appreciable skin involvement (SSc sine scleroderma). Unique clinical phenotypes of SSc associate with specific autoantibodies (Table 382-3). Patients with "overlap" have typical SSc features coexisting with clinical and laboratory evidence of another autoimmune disease such as polymyositis, Sjögren's syndrome, polyarthritis, autoimmune liver disease, or SLE.

TABLE 382-4 FREQUENCY OF CLINICAL ORGAN INVOLVEMENT: LIMITED CUTANEOUS AND DIFFUSE CUTANEOUS FORMS OF SYSTEMIC SCLEROSIS (SSC)

Features	Limited Cutaneous SSc (%)	Diffuse Cutaneous SSc (%)
Skin involvement	90[a]	100
Raynaud's phenomenon	99	98
Esophageal involvement	90	80
Pulmonary fibrosis	35	65
Pulmonary arterial hypertension	15	15
Myopathy	11	23
Cardiac involvement	9	12
Scleroderma renal crisis	2	15

[a]Approximately 10% of limited cutaneous SSc patients have SSc sine scleroderma.

INITIAL CLINICAL PRESENTATION

The initial presentation is quite different in the diffuse and the limited cutaneous forms of the disease. In dcSSc, the interval between Raynaud's phenomenon and onset of other disease manifestations is typically brief (weeks to months). Soft tissue swelling and intense pruritus are signs of the early inflammatory "edematous" phase. The fingers, hands, distal limbs, and face are usually affected first. Diffuse skin hyperpigmentation and carpal tunnel syndrome can occur. Arthralgias, muscle weakness, fatigue, and decreased joint mobility are common. During the ensuing weeks to months, the inflammatory edematous phase evolves into the "fibrotic" phase, with skin induration associated with hair loss, reduced production of skin oils, and a decline in sweating capacity. Progressive flexion contractures of the fingers ensue. The wrists, elbows, shoulders, hip girdles, knees, and ankles become stiff due to fibrosis of the supporting joint structures. While advancing skin involvement is the most visible manifestation of early dcSSc, important and frequently clinically silent internal organ involvement develops during this stage. The initial 4 years from disease onset is the period of rapidly evolving pulmonary and renal damage. If organ failure does not occur during this period, the systemic process may stabilize.

Compared to dcSSc, the course of lcSSc is characteristically more indolent. In these patients, the interval between Raynaud's phenomenon and onset of manifestations such as gastroesophageal reflux, cutaneous telangiectasia, or soft tissue calcifications can be several years. On the other hand, scleroderma renal crisis and severe pulmonary fibrosis are uncommon in lcSSc. Clinically evident cardiac involvement and PAH develop in more than 15%. Overlap with keratoconjunctivitis sicca, polyarthritis, cutaneous vasculitis, and biliary cirrhosis is seen in some patients with lcSSc.

ORGAN INVOLVEMENT

RAYNAUD'S PHENOMENON

Raynaud's phenomenon, the most frequent extracutaneous complication of SSc, is characterized by episodes of reversible vasoconstriction in the fingers and toes. Vasoconstriction may also affect the tip of the nose and earlobes. Attacks are triggered by a decrease in temperature, as well as emotional stress and vibration. Typical attacks start with pallor, followed by cyanosis of variable duration. Hyperemia ensues spontaneously or with rewarming of the digit. The progression of the three color phases reflects the underlying vasoconstriction, ischemia, and reperfusion.

As much as 3–5% of the general population has Raynaud's phenomenon. In the absence of signs or symptoms of an underlying condition, Raynaud's phenomenon is classified as primary and represents an exaggerated physiologic response to cold. Secondary Raynaud's phenomenon can occur as a complication of SSc and other connective tissue diseases, hematologic and endocrine conditions, and occupational disorders, and can complicate the use of beta blockers and anticancer drugs such as cisplatin and bleomycin. Distinguishing primary versus secondary Raynaud's phenomenon presents a diagnostic challenge. Primary Raynaud's phenomenon is supported by the following: absence of an underlying cause; a family history of Raynaud's phenomenon; absence of digital tissue necrosis, ulceration, or gangrene; and a negative ANA test. Secondary Raynaud's phenomenon tends to develop at an older age (>30 years), is clinically more severe (episodes more frequent, prolonged, and painful), and is frequently associated with ischemic digital ulcers and loss of digits (Fig. 382-3). Nailfold capillaroscopy, where the cutaneous capillaries at the nail bed are viewed under a drop of grade B immersion oil using a low-power stereoscopic microscope, can be helpful in the evaluation of Raynaud's phenomenon. Primary Raynaud's phenomenon is associated with normal capillaries that appear as regularly spaced parallel vascular loops, whereas in patients with Raynaud's associated with SSc and other connective tissue diseases, nailfold capillaries are distorted with widened and irregular loops, dilated lumen, and areas of vascular "dropout." In addition to digits, cold-induced episodic Raynaud's-like vasospasm has been documented in the pulmonary, renal, gastrointestinal, and coronary circulations in SSc.

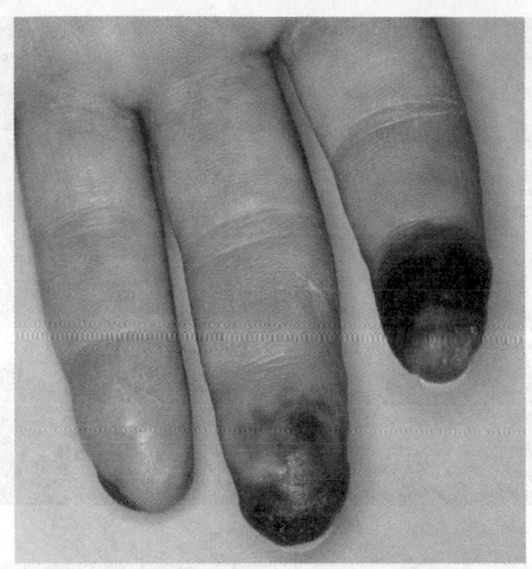

FIGURE 382-3 Digital necrosis. Sharply demarcated necrosis of the fingertip in a patient with limited cutaneous systemic sclerosis (SSc) associated with severe Raynaud's phenomenon.

SKIN FEATURES

While early-stage SSc is associated with edematous skin changes, skin thickening is the hallmark that distinguishes SSc from other connective tissue diseases. The distribution of skin thickening is invariably symmetric and bilateral. It typically starts in the fingers and then characteristically advances from distal to proximal extremities in an ascending fashion. The involved skin is firm, coarse, and thickened, and the extremities and trunk may be darkly pigmented. In some patients, diffuse tanning in the absence of sun exposure is a very early manifestation of skin involvement. In dark-skinned patients, vitiligo-like hypopigmentation may occur. Because pigment loss spares the perifollicular areas, the skin may have a "salt-and-pepper" appearance, most prominently on the scalp, upper back, and chest. Dermal sclerosis due to collagen accumulation obliterates hair follicles, sweat glands, and eccrine and sebaceous glands, resulting in hair loss, decreased sweating, and dry skin. Transverse creases on the dorsum of the fingers disappear (Fig. 382-4). Fixed flexion contractures of the fingers cause reduced hand mobility and lead to muscle atrophy. Skin thickening in combination with fibrosis of the subjacent tendons accounts for contractures of the wrists, elbows, and knees. Thick ridges at the neck due

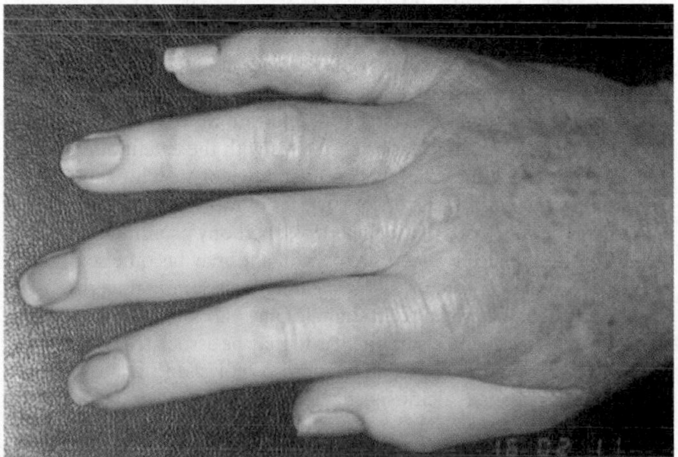

FIGURE 382-4 Sclerodactyly. Note skin induration on the fingers, and fixed flexion contractures at the proximal interphalangeal joints in a patient with limited cutaneous systemic sclerosis (SSc).

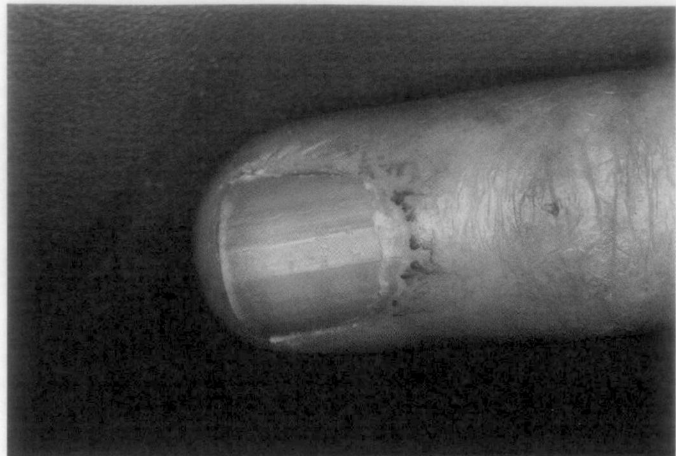

A

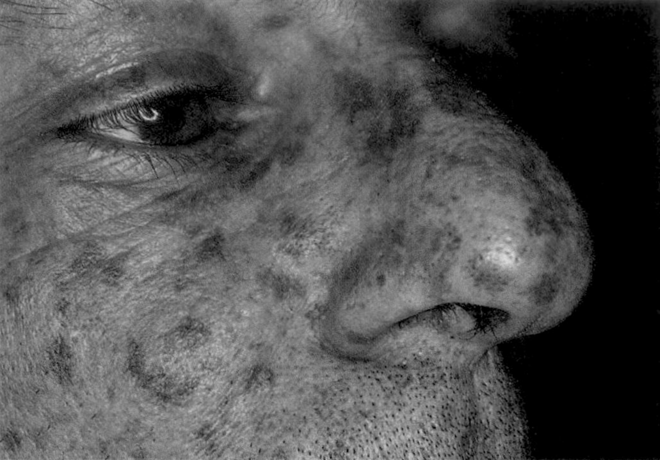

B

FIGURE 382-5 Cutaneous vascular changes. ***A.*** Capillary changes at the nailfold in a patient with limited cutaneous systemic sclerosis (lcSSc). ***B.*** Telangiectasia on the face.

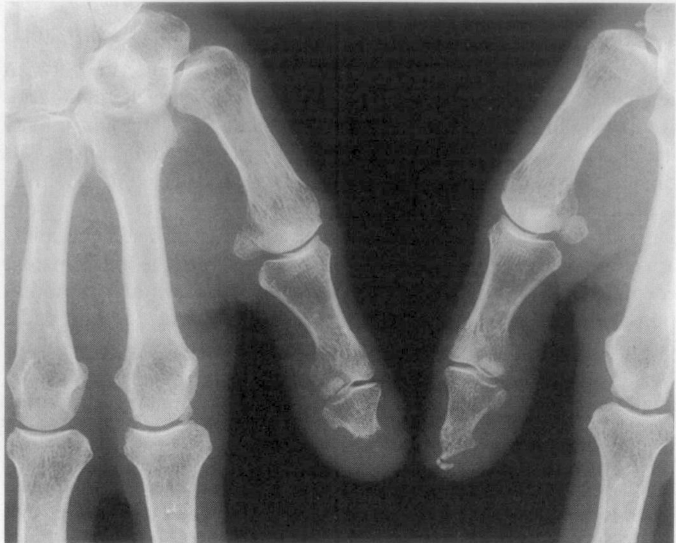

FIGURE 382-6 Acro-osteolysis. Note dissolution of terminal phalanges in a patient with long-standing limited cutaneous systemic sclerosis (lcSSc) and Raynaud's phenomenon.

to firm adherence of skin to the underlying platysma muscle interfere with neck extension. The face assumes a characteristic "mauskopf" appearance with taut and shiny skin, loss of wrinkles, and occasionally an expressionless facies due to reduced mobility of the eyelids, cheeks, and mouth. Thinning of the lips with accentuation of the central incisor teeth and fine wrinkles (radial furrowing) around the mouth complete the picture. Reduced oral aperture (microstomia) interferes with eating and oral hygiene. The nose assumes a pinched, beak-like appearance.

In established SSc, the skin is firmly bound to the subcutaneous fat (tethering) and undergoes thinning and atrophy. Telangiectasias are dilated skin capillaries 2–20 mm in diameter frequently seen in lcSSc. These lesions, reminiscent of hereditary hemorrhagic telangiectasia, are prominent on the face, hands, lips, and oral mucosa (Fig. 382-5). A greater number of telangiectasias correlates with the extent of microvascular complications, including PAH. Breakdown of atrophic skin leads to chronic ulcerations at the extensor surfaces of the proximal interphalangeal joints, the volar pads of the fingertips, and bony prominences such as the elbows and malleoli. Ulcers are painful and may become secondarily infected, resulting in osteomyelitis. Healing of ischemic fingertip ulcerations leaves characteristic fixed digital "pits." Loss of soft tissue at the fingertips due to ischemia is frequent and may be associated with striking resorption of the terminal phalanges (acro-osteolysis) (Fig. 382-6).

Calcium deposits (calcinosis) in the skin and soft tissues occur in patients with lcSSc who are positive for anticentromere antibodies. The deposits, varying in size from tiny punctate lesions to large conglomerate masses, are composed of calcium hydroxyapatite crystals and can be readily visualized on plain x-rays. Frequent locations include the finger pads, palms, extensor surfaces of the forearms, and the olecranon and prepatellar bursae (Fig. 382-7). They may occasionally ulcerate through the overlying skin, producing drainage of chalky white material, pain, and local inflammation. Paraspinal soft tissue calcifications may cause neurologic complications.

PULMONARY FEATURES

Pulmonary involvement is frequent in SSc and is the leading cause of death. The two principal forms are ILD and pulmonary vascular disease. Patients with SSc frequently develop some degree of both complications. Less frequent pulmonary manifestations include aspiration pneumonitis complicating chronic gastroesophageal reflux, pulmonary hemorrhage due to endobronchial telangiectasia, obliterative bronchiolitis, pleural reactions, restrictive ventilatory defect due to chest wall fibrosis, spontaneous pneumothorax, and drug-induced lung toxicity. The incidence of lung cancer is increased.

Interstitial Lung Disease (ILD) Evidence of ILD can be found in up to 90% of patients with SSc at autopsy and 85% by thin-section high-resolution computed tomography (HRCT). In contrast, clinically significant ILD develops in 16–43%; the frequency varies depending on the detection method used. Risk factors include male gender, African-American race, diffuse skin involvement, severe gastroesophageal reflux, and the presence of topoisomerase I autoantibodies, as well as a low forced vital capacity (FVC) or single-breath diffusing capacity of the lung for carbon monoxide (DLco) at initial presentation. In these patients, the most rapid progression in lung disease occurs early in

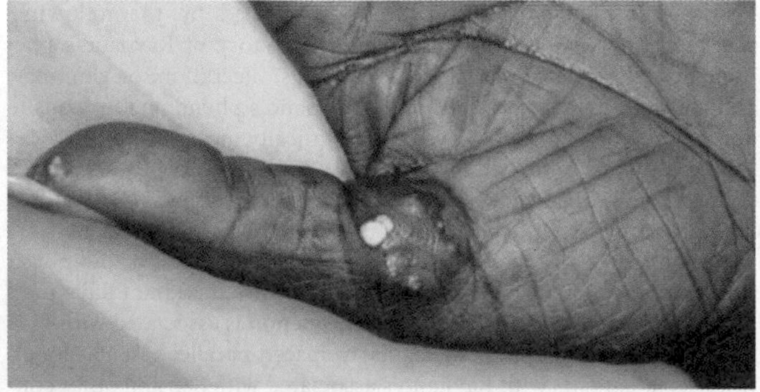

FIGURE 382-7 Calcinosis cutis. Note large calcific deposit breaking through the skin in a patient with limited cutaneous systemic sclerosis (lcSSc).

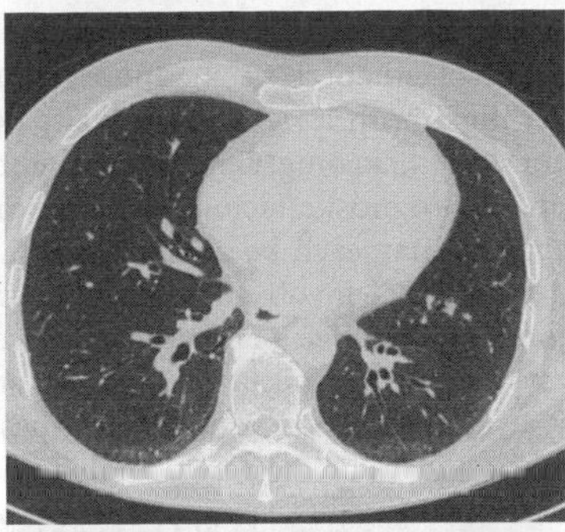

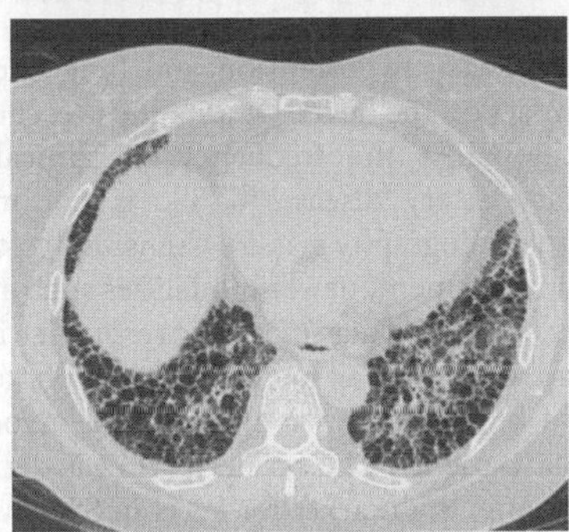

FIGURE 382-8 HRCT images of the chest from patients with systemic sclerosis. *Top panel:* Early interstitial lung disease. Mild changes with sub pleural reticulations and ground glass opacities in the lower lobes of the lung. Patient in supine position. ***Bottom panel:*** Extensive lung fibrosis with ground glass opacities, coarse reticular honeycombing, and traction bronchiectasis. *(Courtesy of Rishi Agrawal, MD.)*

the course of the disease (within the first 3 years), when the FVC can decline by 30% per year.

Pulmonary involvement can remain asymptomatic until it is advanced. The most common presenting respiratory symptoms—exertional dyspnea, fatigue, and reduced exercise tolerance—are subtle and slowly progressive. A chronic dry cough may be present. Physical examination may reveal "Velcro" crackles at the lung bases. Pulmonary function testing (PFT) is a sensitive method for detecting early pulmonary involvement. The most common abnormalities are reductions in FVC, total lung capacity (TLC), and DLco. A reduction in DLco that is significantly out of proportion to the reduction in lung volumes should raise suspicion for pulmonary vascular disease, but may also be due to anemia. Oxygen desaturation with exercise is common.

Chest radiography can rule out infection and other causes of pulmonary involvement, but compared to HRCT, it is relatively insensitive for detection of early ILD. HRCT shows subpleural reticular linear opacities and ground-glass opacifications, predominantly in the lower lobes, even in asymptomatic patients (Fig. 382-8). Additional HRCT findings include mediastinal lymphadenopathy, pulmonary nodules, traction bronchiectasis, and uncommonly, honeycomb changes. The extent of pulmonary interstitial changes on HRCT is a predictor of mortality in SSc. Bronchoalveolar lavage (BAL) can demonstrate inflammation in the lower respiratory tract and may be useful for ruling out infection. Although an elevated proportion of neutrophils (>2%) and/or eosinophils (>3%) in the BAL fluid is correlated with more extensive lung disease on HRCT and is associated with more rapid decline in FVC and reduced survival, BAL is not useful for identifying reversible alveolitis. Lung biopsy is indicated only in patients with atypical findings on chest radiographs and should be thoracoscopically guided. The histologic pattern on lung biopsy may predict the risk of progression of ILD. The most common pattern in SSc, NSIP, carries a better prognosis than UIP.

Pulmonary Arterial Hypertension (PAH) PAH, defined as a mean pulmonary arterial pressure ≥25 mmHg with a pulmonary capillary wedge pressure ≤15 mmHg, develops in approximately 15% of patients with SSc and can occur in association with ILD or as an isolated abnormality. The natural history of SSc-associated PAH is variable, but in many patients, it follows a downhill course with development of right heart failure. The median survival of SSc patients with untreated PAH is 1 year following diagnosis. Risk factors for PAH include limited cutaneous disease, older age at disease onset, severe Raynaud's phenomenon, and the presence of antibodies to centromere, U1-RNP, U3-RNP (fibrillarin), and B23.

The initial symptom of PAH is typically exertional dyspnea and reduced exercise capacity. With disease progression, angina, exertional near-syncope, and symptoms and signs of right-sided heart failure appear. Physical examination may show tachypnea, a prominent split S_2 heart sound, palpable right ventricular heave, elevated jugular venous pressure, and dependent edema. Doppler echocardiography provides a noninvasive method for estimating the pulmonary arterial pressure. In light of the poor prognosis of untreated PAH, all SSc patients should be screened for its presence at initial evaluation. Echocardiographic estimates of pulmonary arterial systolic pressures >40 mmHg at rest suggest PAH. Pulmonary function testing may show a reduced DLco in isolation or out of proportion with the severity of restriction. Right heart catheterization is the gold standard for diagnosing PAH. Because echocardiography can result in over- or underestimation of pulmonary arterial pressures in SSc, cardiac catheterization is always required to confirm the presence of PAH; accurately assess its severity, including the degree of right heart dysfunction; and rule out venoocclusive disease and other cardiac causes of pulmonary hypertension. Yearly echocardiographic screening for PAH is recommended in most patients with SSc; an isolated decline in DLco may also be indicative of developing PAH. Serum levels of brain natriuretic peptide (BNP) and N-terminal pro-BNP correlate with the presence and severity of PAH in SSc, as well as survival. While BNP measurements can be useful in screening for PAH and in monitoring the response to treatment, elevated BNP levels are not specific for PAH and also occur in other forms of right and left heart disease. The prognosis of SSc-associated PAH is worse, and treatment response poorer, than in idiopathic PAH

GASTROINTESTINAL INVOLVEMENT

The gastrointestinal tract is affected in up to 90% of SSc patients with both limited and diffuse cutaneous forms of the disease. The pathologic features of atrophy of smooth muscle, intact mucosa, and obliterative small-vessel vasculopathy are similar throughout the length of the gastrointestinal tract.

Upper Gastrointestinal Tract Involvement Oropharyngeal manifestations due to a combination of xerostomia, reduced oral aperture, periodontal disease, and resorption of the mandibular condyles are frequent and cause much distress. The frenulum of the tongue may be shortened. Most patients have symptoms of gastroesophageal reflux disease (GERD): heartburn, regurgitation, and dysphagia. A combination of reduced lower esophageal sphincter pressure resulting in gastroesophageal reflux, impaired esophageal clearance of refluxed gastric contents due to diminished motility in the distal two-thirds of the esophagus, and delayed gastric emptying accounts for GERD. Manometry shows abnormal upper intestinal motility in most patients with SSc. Extraesophageal manifestations of GERD include hoarseness, chronic cough, and aspiration pneumonitis, which may aggravate underlying ILD. Chest computed tomography (CT) scan characteristically shows a dilated esophagus with intraluminal air. Endoscopy may be necessary to rule out opportunistic infections with *Candida*, herpes virus, and cytomegalovirus. Severe erosive esophagitis may be found on endoscopy in patients with minimal symptoms. Esophageal strictures and Barrett's esophagus may complicate chronic GERD. Because Barrett's esophagus is associated with an increased risk of adenocarcinoma, SSc patients with Barrett's esophagus need periodic endoscopy and esophageal biopsy.

Gastroparesis with early satiety, abdominal distention, and aggravated reflux symptoms is common. The presence and severity of gastroparesis can be assessed by radionuclide gastric emptying studies. Gastric antral vascular ectasia (GAVE) in the antrum may occur. These subepithelial lesions, reflecting the diffuse small-vessel vasculopathy of SSc, are described as "watermelon stomach" due to their endoscopic appearance. Patients with GAVE can have recurrent episodes of gastrointestinal bleeding, resulting in chronic unexplained anemia.

Lower Gastrointestinal Tract Involvement Impaired intestinal motility may result in malabsorption and chronic diarrhea secondary to bacterial overgrowth. Fat and protein malabsorption and vitamin B_{12} and vitamin D deficiency ensue, sometimes culminating in severe malnutrition. Disturbed intestinal motor function can also cause intestinal pseudo-obstruction, with symptoms of nausea and abdominal distension that are indistinguishable from those of delayed gastric emptying. Patients present with recurrent episodes of acute abdominal pain, nausea, and vomiting. Radiographic studies show acute intestinal obstruction, and the major diagnostic challenge is to differentiate pseudoobstruction, which responds to supportive care and intravenous nutritional supplementation, from mechanical obstruction.

Colonic involvement may cause severe constipation, fecal incontinence, gastrointestinal bleeding from telangiectasia, and rectal prolapse. In late-stage SSc, wide-mouth sacculations or diverticula occur in the colon, occasionally causing perforation and bleeding. An occasional radiologic finding is pneumatosis cystoides intestinalis due to air trapping in the bowel wall that may rarely rupture and cause benign pneumoperitoneum. Although the liver is rarely affected, primary biliary cirrhosis may coexist with SSc.

RENAL INVOLVEMENT: SCLERODERMA RENAL CRISIS

Scleroderma renal crisis occurs in 10–15% of patients and generally within 4 years of the onset of the disease. Prior to the advent of angiotensin-converting enzyme (ACE) inhibitors, short-term survival in scleroderma renal crisis was <10%. The pathogenesis involves obliterative vasculopathy and luminal narrowing of the renal arcuate and interlobular arteries. Progressive reduction in renal blood flow, aggravated by vasospasm, leads to juxtaglomerular hyperplasia, increased renin secretion, and activation of angiotensin, with further renal vasoconstriction resulting in a vicious cycle that culminates in accelerated hypertension. Risk factors for scleroderma renal crisis include African-American race, male gender, and dcSSc with extensive and progressive skin involvement. Up to 50% of patients with scleroderma renal crisis have anti-RNA polymerase III antibodies. Palpable tendon friction rubs, pericardial effusion, new unexplained anemia, and thrombocytopenia may be harbingers of impending scleroderma renal crisis. High-risk patients with early SSc should be counseled to check their blood pressure daily. Patients with lcSSc or anticentromere antibodies rarely develop scleroderma renal crisis. Because there is an association between glucocorticoid use and scleroderma renal crisis, prednisone should be used in high-risk SSc patients only when absolutely required and at low doses (<10 mg/d).

Patients characteristically present with accelerated hypertension and progressive oliguric renal insufficiency. However, approximately 10% of patients with scleroderma renal crisis present with normal blood pressure. Normotensive renal crisis is generally associated with a poor outcome. Headache, blurred vision, and congestive heart failure may accompany elevation of blood pressure. Urinalysis typically shows mild proteinuria, granular casts, and microscopic hematuria; thrombocytopenia and microangiopathic hemolysis with fragmented red blood cells can be seen. Progressive oliguric renal failure over several days generally follows. In some cases, scleroderma renal crisis is misdiagnosed as thrombotic thrombocytopenic purpura or other forms of thrombotic microangiopathy. In these cases, a renal biopsy may be of some benefit. In addition, biopsy findings of vascular thrombosis and glomerular ischemic collapse predict poor renal outcomes. Oliguria or a creatinine >3 mg/dL at presentation predicts poor outcome, with permanent hemodialysis and high mortality. Rarely, crescentic glomerulonephritis occurs in the setting of SSc and may be associated with myeloperoxidase-specific antineutrophil cytoplasmic antibodies. Membranous glomerulonephritis may occur in patients treated with D-penicillamine. Asymptomatic renal function impairment occurs in up to half of SSc patients. Such subclinical renal involvement is associated with other vascular manifestations of SSc and rarely progresses.

CARDIAC INVOLVEMENT

Although it is often silent, cardiac involvement in SSc is frequently detected when patients are screened with sensitive diagnostic tools. Clinically evident cardiac involvement is associated with poor outcomes. Cardiac disease in SSc may be primary or secondary to PAH, ILD, or renal involvement. It occurs more frequently in patients with dcSSc than in those with lcSSc and generally develops within 3 years of the onset of skin thickening. Clinically evident cardiac involvement in SSc is a poor prognostic factor. The endocardium, myocardium, and pericardium may each be affected separately or together. Manifestations of pericardial involvement include acute pericarditis, pericardial effusions, constrictive pericarditis, and cardiac tamponade. Conduction system fibrosis occurs commonly and may be silent or manifested by atrial and ventricular tachycardias or heart block. Recurrent vasospasm and ischemia-reperfusion injury contribute to myocardial fibrosis, resulting in asymptomatic systolic or diastolic left ventricular dysfunction that may progress to overt heart failure. Systemic and pulmonary hypertension and lung and renal involvement may also impact on the heart. Despite the presence of widespread obliterative vasculopathy, the frequency of clinical or pathologic epicardial coronary artery disease in SSc is not increased. While conventional echocardiography has low sensitivity for detecting SSc preclinical heart involvement, newer modalities such as tissue Doppler echocardiography (TDE), cardiac magnetic resonance imaging (cMRI), thallium perfusion, and nuclear imaging (single photon emission CT [SPECT]) reveal a high prevalence of abnormal myocardial function or perfusion in SSc patients. The serum level of N-terminal pro-BNP, a ventricular hormone, is a marker for PAH in SSc, but may also have utility as a marker of primary cardiac involvement.

MUSCULOSKELETAL COMPLICATIONS

Carpal tunnel syndrome occurs frequently and may be a presenting manifestation. Generalized arthralgia and stiffness are prominent in early disease. Mobility of small and large joints is progressively impaired, especially in dcSSc. Most commonly affected are the hands. Contractures develop at the proximal interphalangeal joints and wrists. Large joint contractures can be accompanied by tendon friction rubs, characterized by leathery crepitation that can be heard or palpated upon passive movement, that are due to extensive fibrosis and adhesion of the tendon sheaths and fascial planes at the affected joint. Presence of tendon friction rubs is associated with increased risk for renal and cardiac complications and reduced survival. True joint inflammation is uncommon; however, occasional patients develop erosive polyarthritis in the hands. Muscle weakness is common and may indicate deconditioning, disuse atrophy, and malnutrition. Less commonly, inflammatory myositis indistinguishable from idiopathic polymyositis may occur. A chronic noninflammatory myopathy characterized by atrophy and fibrosis in the absence of elevated muscle enzyme levels can be seen in late-stage SSc. Bone resorption occurs most commonly in the terminal phalanges, where it causes loss of the distal tufts (acro-osteolysis) (Fig. 382-5). Resorption of the mandibular condyles can lead to bite difficulties. Osteolysis can also affect the ribs and distal clavicles.

OTHER DISEASE MANIFESTATIONS

Many SSc patients develop dry eyes and dry mouth (sicca complex). Biopsy of the minor salivary glands shows fibrosis rather than focal lymphocytic infiltration characteristic of primary Sjögren's syndrome (Chap. 383). Hypothyroidism is common and generally due to fibrosis of the thyroid gland. The frequency of macrovascular involvement, including peripheral vascular and coronary artery disease, may be increased. Whereas the central nervous system is generally spared, sensory trigeminal neuropathy due to fibrosis or vasculopathy can occur, presenting with gradual onset of pain and numbness. Pregnancy in women with SSc may be associated with an increased rate of adverse fetal outcomes. Furthermore, cardiopulmonary involvement may worsen during pregnancy, and new onset of scleroderma renal crisis has been described. Erectile dysfunction is frequent in men with SSc and may be the initial disease manifestation. Inability to attain or maintain penile erection is due to vascular insufficiency and fibrosis.

Malignancy in SSc Epidemiologic studies indicate an increased risk of cancer in SSc. Lung cancer and esophageal adenocarcinoma typically occur in the setting of long-standing ILD or gastroesophageal reflux disease and may be caused by chronic inflammation and repair. In contrast, breast, lung, and ovarian carcinomas and lymphomas tend to occur in close temporal association with the clinical onset of SSc, particularly in patients who have autoantibodies to RNA polymerase III. In these cases, SSc may represent a paraneoplastic syndrome triggered by the antitumor immune response.

LABORATORY EVALUATION AND BIOMARKERS

A mild normocytic or microcytic anemia is frequent in patients with SSc and may indicate gastrointestinal bleeding caused by GAVE or chronic esophagitis. Macrocytic anemia may be caused by folate and vitamin B_{12} deficiency due to small-bowel bacterial overgrowth and malabsorption or by drugs such as methotrexate or alkylating agents. Microangiopathic hemolytic anemia caused by mechanical fragmentation of red blood cells during their passage through microvessels coated with fibrin or platelet thrombi is a hallmark of the thrombotic microangiopathy associated with scleroderma renal crisis. Thrombocytopenia and leukopenia may indicate drug toxicity. In contrast to other connective tissue diseases, the erythrocyte sedimentation rate (ESR) is generally normal; an elevation may signal coexisting myositis or malignancy.

Antinuclear autoantibodies are present in almost all patients with SSc and can be detected at disease onset. Autoantibodies against topoisomerase I (Scl-70) and centromere are mutually exclusive and quite specific for SSc (Table 382-3). Topoisomerase I antibodies are detected in 31% of patients with dcSSc, but in only 13% of patients with lcSSc. They are associated with increased risk of ILD and poor outcomes. Anticentromere antibodies are detected in 38% of patients with lcSSc, but in only 2% of patients with dcSSc and rarely in patients with Raynaud's phenomenon and Sjögren's syndrome. Anticentromere antibodies in SSc are associated with PAH, but only infrequently with significant cardiac or renal involvement or ILD. Nucleolar immunofluorescence pattern on serologic testing reflects antibodies to U3-RNP (fibrillarin), Th/To, or PM/Scl, whereas a speckled immunofluorescence pattern indicates antibodies to RNA polymerase III. Although antibodies to β2GPI occur in antiphospholipid antibody syndrome and are not specific for SSc, their presence in SSc is associated with an increased risk of ischemic lesions in the fingers.

DIAGNOSIS, STAGING, AND MONITORING

The diagnosis of SSc is made primarily on clinical grounds and is generally straightforward in patients with established disease. The presence of skin induration, with a characteristic symmetric distribution pattern associated with typical visceral organ manifestations, establishes the diagnosis with a high degree of certainty. Although the conditions listed in Table 382-1 can be associated with skin induration, the distribution pattern of skin lesions, together with the absence of Raynaud's phenomenon or typical visceral organ manifestations or SSc-specific autoantibodies, differentiates these conditions from SSc. Occasionally, full-thickness biopsy of the skin is required for establishing the diagnosis of scleredema, scleromyxedema, or nephrogenic systemic fibrosis. In lcSSc, a history of antecedent Raynaud's phenomenon and gastroesophageal reflux symptoms, coupled with the presence of sclerodactyly and capillary changes on nailfold capillaroscopy, often in combinations with cutaneous telangiectasia and calcinosis, helps to establish the diagnosis. The finding of digital tip pitting scars and radiologic evidence of pulmonary fibrosis in the lower lobes are particularly helpful diagnostically. Primary Raynaud's phenomenon is a common benign condition that must be differentiated from early or limited SSc. Nailfold microscopy is particularly helpful in this situation, because in primary Raynaud's phenomenon, the nailfold capillaries are normal, whereas in SSc, capillary abnormalities, as well as serum autoantibodies, can be detected even before other disease manifestations.

Establishing the diagnosis of SSc at an early stage of the disease may be a challenge. In dcSSc, initial symptoms are often nonspecific and relate to inflammation. Patients complain of fatigue, swelling, aching, and stiffness, and Raynaud's phenomenon may initially be absent. Physical examination may reveal diffuse upper extremity edema and puffy fingers. Patients at this stage are sometimes diagnosed as early rheumatoid arthritis, SLE, myositis, or, most commonly, undifferentiated connective tissue disease. Within weeks to months, Raynaud's phenomenon and characteristic clinical features appear accompanied by advancing induration of the skin. The presence of antinuclear and SSc-specific autoantibodies provides a high degree of diagnostic specificity. Raynaud's phenomenon with fingertip ulcerations or other evidence of digital ischemia, coupled with telangiectasia, distal esophageal dysmotility, unexplained ILD or PAH, or accelerated hypertension with renal failure in the absence of clinically evident skin induration, suggests the diagnosis of SSc sine scleroderma. These patients may have anticentromere antibodies.

TREATMENT SYSTEMIC SCLEROSIS

OVERVIEW: MANAGEMENT PRINCIPLES To date, no therapy has been shown to significantly alter the natural history of SSc. In contrast, multiple interventions are highly effective in alleviating the symptoms, slowing the progression of the cumulative organ damage, and reducing disability. A significant reduction in disease-related mortality has been noted during the past 25 years. In light of the marked heterogeneity in disease manifestations, organ complications, and natural history, treatment must be tailored to each individual patient's unique needs.

A thorough investigation should be undertaken at baseline. Optimal management incorporates the following principles (Table 382-5): prompt and accurate diagnosis; classification and risk stratification based on clinical and laboratory evaluation; early recognition of organ-based complications and assessment of their extent, severity, and likelihood of deterioration; regular monitoring for disease progression, activity, new complications, and response to therapy; adjusting therapy; and continuing patient education. In order to minimize irreversible organ damage, the management of life-threatening complications must be proactive, with regular screening and initiation of appropriate intervention at the earliest possible opportunity. In light of the complex and multisystemic nature of the SSc, a team-based management approach integrating multiple specialists should be pursued whenever possible. Most patients are treated with combinations of drugs that impact different aspects of the disease. We encourage patients to become familiar with the spectrum of potential complications and understand therapeutic options and natural history, and empower them to partner with their treating physicians. This requires a long term relationship between patient and physician, with ongoing counseling and encouragement.

DISEASE-MODIFYING THERAPY: IMMUNOSUPPRESSIVE AGENTS Immunosuppressive agents used in the treatment of other autoimmune or connective tissue diseases have generally shown modest or no benefit in SSc. Glucocorticoids may alleviate stiffness and aching in early-stage dcSSc but do not influence the progression of skin or internal organ involvement, and their use is associated with an increased risk of scleroderma renal crisis. Therefore, glucocorticoids should be given only when absolutely necessary, at the lowest dose possible, and for brief periods only. The use of cyclophosphamide has been extensively studied in light of its efficacy in the treatment of vasculitis (Chap. 385), SLE (Chap. 378), and other autoimmune diseases (Chap. 377e).

Both oral and intermittent IV cyclophosphamide were shown to reduce the progression of SSc-associated ILD, with stabilization and, rarely, modest improvement of pulmonary function and HRCT findings after 1 year of treatment. Improvement in respiratory symptoms and skin induration was also noted. These beneficial effects wane upon discontinuation of therapy. The benefits of cyclophosphamide need to be balanced against its potential toxicity, including bone marrow suppression, opportunistic infections, hemorrhagic cystitis and bladder cancer, premature ovarian failure, and late secondary malignancies.

TABLE 382-5 KEY PRINCIPLES IN MANAGEMENT

- Establish early and accurate diagnosis.
- Evaluate internal organ involvement.
- Define clinical disease stage and activity.
- Tailor individualized therapy to each patient's unique needs.
- Assess treatment response, and adjust therapy as needed; monitor for disease progression and new complications.

Methotrexate was associated with a modest skin improvement in small studies. Mycophenolate mofetil treatment was associated with improved skin induration in uncontrolled studies and was generally well tolerated. Small studies support the use of rituximab in SSc patients with skin involvement and ILD. The use of cyclosporine, azathioprine, extracorporeal photopheresis, thalidomide, rapamycin, imatinib, and IV immunoglobulin is currently not well supported by the literature. Intensive immune ablation using a conditioning regimen of high-dose chemotherapy with or without irradiation, followed by autologous stem cell reconstitution, has resulted in durable disease remission in some cases and is undergoing evaluation in randomized clinical trials. In light of its potential morbidity and mortality, as well as significant cost, autologous stem cell transplantation in SSc is still considered experimental.

Antifibrotic Therapy Because widespread tissue fibrosis in SSc causes progressive organ damage, drugs that interfere with the fibrotic process represent a rational therapeutic approach. D-Penicillamine has been extensively used as an antifibrotic agent. In retrospective studies, D-penicillamine stabilized and improved skin induration, prevented new internal organ involvement, and improved survival. However, a randomized controlled clinical trial in early active SSc found no difference in the extent of skin involvement between patients treated with standard-dose (750 mg/d) or very low-dose (125 mg every other day) D-penicillamine. Recent clinical trials show benefit of pirfenidone and of nintedanib in patients with idiopathic pulmonary fibrosis, with significant slowing of the loss of lung function. Whether these two new drugs will have comparable efficacy in the treatment of SSc-associated lung disease is still under investigation.

Vascular Therapy The goal of therapy is to control Raynaud's phenomenon, prevent the development and enhance the healing of ischemic complications, and slow the progression of obliterative vasculopathy. Patients should dress warmly, minimize cold exposure or stress, and avoid drugs that precipitate or exacerbate vasospastic episodes. Some patients with Raynaud's may respond to biofeedback therapy. Extended-release dihydropyridine calcium channel blockers such as nifedipine, amlodipine, or diltiazem can ameliorate Raynaud's phenomenon, but their use is often limited by side effects (palpitations, dependent edema, worsening gastroesophageal reflux). While ACE inhibitors do not reduce the frequency or severity of episodes, angiotensin II receptor blockers such as losartan are effective and generally well tolerated. Patients with Raynaud's phenomenon unresponsive to these therapies may require the addition of α_1-adrenergic receptor blockers (e.g., prazosin), 5-phosphodiesterase inhibitors (e.g., sildenafil), serotonin reuptake inhibitors (e.g., fluoxetine), topical nitroglycerine, and intermittent infusions of IV prostaglandins. Low-dose aspirin and dipyridamole prevent platelet aggregation and may have a role as adjunctive agents. In patients with ischemic ulcers, the endothelin-1 receptor antagonist bosentan reduces the risk of new ulcers. Digital sympathectomy and local injections of botulinum type A (Botox) into the digits are options in patients with severe ischemia and impending loss of the digits. Empirical long-term therapy with statins and antioxidants may retard the progression of vascular damage and obliteration. Vasodilators such as ACE inhibitors, calcium channel blockers, and endothelin receptor blockers may also improve myocardial perfusion and left ventricular function.

TREATMENT OF GASTROINTESTINAL COMPLICATIONS Because oral problems including decreased oral aperture, decreased saliva production, gum recession and periodontal disease leading to teeth loss are common, regular dental care is recommended. Gastroesophageal reflux is very common and may occur in the absence of symptoms; therefore all patients with SSc should be treated. Patients should be instructed to elevate the head of the bed, eat frequent small meals, and avoid oral intake before bedtime. Proton pump inhibitors reduce acid reflux and may need to be given in relatively high doses. Prokinetic agents such as domperidone may be helpful, especially if delayed gastric emptying is present. Episodic gastrointestinal bleeding from gastric antral vascular ectasia (watermelon stomach) may be amenable to treatment with endoscopic laser photocoagulation, although recurrence can occur. Bacterial overgrowth due to small-bowel dysmotility causes abdominal bloating and diarrhea and may lead to malabsorption and severe malnutrition. Treatment with short courses of rotating broad-spectrum antibiotics such as metronidazole, erythromycin, and tetracycline can eradicate bacterial overgrowth. Parenteral hyperalimentation is indicated if malnutrition develops. Chronic hypomotility of the small bowel may respond to octreotide, but pseudo-obstruction is difficult to treat. Fecal incontinence, a frequently underreported complication of SSc, may respond to anti-diarrheal medication and biofeedback therapy.

TREATMENT OF PULMONARY ARTERIAL HYPERTENSION (PAH) In patients with SSc, PAH carries an extremely poor prognosis and accounts for 30% of deaths. Because PAH is asymptomatic until advanced, patients with SSc should be screened for its presence at initial evaluation, and on a yearly basis thereafter. Treatment is generally started with an oral endothelin-1 receptor antagonist such as bosentan or a phosphodiesterase type 5 inhibitor such as sildenafil. Patients may also require diuretics and digoxin when appropriate. If hypoxemia is documented, supplemental oxygen should be prescribed in order to avoid hypoxia-induced secondary pulmonary vasoconstriction. Prostacyclin analogues such as epoprostenol or treprostinil can be given by continuous IV or SC infusion, or via intermittent nebulized inhalations. Combination therapy with different classes of agents, such as an endothelin-1 antagonist and a phosphodiesterase inhibitor, is often necessary. Lung transplantation remains an option for selected patients who fail medical therapy.

TREATMENT OF RENAL CRISIS Scleroderma renal crisis is a medical emergency. Since the outcome is largely determined by the extent of renal damage present at the time that aggressive therapy is initiated, prompt recognition of impending or early scleroderma renal crisis is essential, and efforts should be made to avoid its occurrence. High-risk SSc patients with early disease, extensive and progressive skin involvement, tendon friction rubs, and anti-RNA polymerase III antibodies should be instructed to monitor their blood pressure daily and report significant alterations immediately. Potentially nephrotoxic drugs should be avoided, and glucocorticoids should be used only when absolutely necessary and at low doses. Patients presenting with scleroderma renal crisis should be immediately hospitalized. Once other causes of renal disease are excluded, treatment should be started promptly with titration of short-acting ACE inhibitors, with the goal of achieving rapid normalization of the blood pressure. In patients with hypertension persisting despite ACE inhibitor therapy, addition of angiotensin II receptor blockers, calcium channel blockers, and direct renin inhibitors should be considered. Anecdotal evidence indicates responses to endothelin-1 receptor blockers and prostacyclins. Up to two-thirds of patients with scleroderma renal crisis go on to dialysis. The outcome of scleroderma renal crisis is worse in patients with antibodies to topoisomerase I compared to those with antibodies to RNA polymerase III. Substantial renal recovery can occur following scleroderma renal crisis, and dialysis can be discontinued, in 30–50% of the patients. Kidney transplantation is appropriate for those unable to discontinue dialysis after 2 years. Survival of transplanted SSc patients is comparable to that of patients with other connective tissue diseases, and recurrence of renal crisis is rare.

SKIN CARE Because skin involvement in SSc is never life-threatening and because it stabilizes and may even regress spontaneously, over time, the management of SSc should not be dictated by its cutaneous manifestations. The inflammatory symptoms of early skin involvement can be controlled with antihistamines and cautious short-term use of low-dose glucocorticoids (<5 mg/d of prednisone). Retrospective studies have shown that D-penicillamine reduced the extent and progression of skin induration; however, these benefits could not be substantiated in a controlled prospective trial. Cyclophosphamide and methotrexate have modest effects on skin induration. Because the skin is dry, the use of hydrophilic ointments and bath oils is encouraged. Regular skin massage is helpful. Telangiectasia may present a cosmetic problem, especially on the face. Treatment with pulsed dye laser may have short-term benefit. Ischemic digital ulcers should be protected by occlusive dressing to promote healing and prevent infection. Infected skin ulcers are treated with topical antibiotics. Surgical debridement may be indicated. No therapy has been shown to be effective in preventing the formation of calcific soft tissue deposits or promoting their dissolution.

TREATMENT OF MUSCULOSKELETAL COMPLICATIONS Arthralgia and joint stiffness are common and distressing manifestations most prominent in early-stage disease. Short courses of nonsteroidal anti-inflammatory agents, weekly methotrexate, and cautious use of low-dose corticosteroids may alleviate these symptoms. Physical and occupational therapy can be effective for maintaining musculoskeletal function and improving long-term outcomes.

COURSE

The natural history of SSc is highly variable and difficult to predict, especially in early stages of the disease, when the specific subset—diffuse or limited cutaneous form—is not clear. Patient with dcSSc tend to have a more rapidly progressive course and worse prognosis than those with lcSSc.

In dcSSc, inflammatory symptoms such as fatigue, edema, arthralgia, and pruritus tend to subside, and the extent of skin thickening reaches a plateau at 2–4 years after disease onset, followed by slow regression. It is during the early edematous/inflammatory stage, generally lasting <3 years, that important visceral organ involvement occurs. While existing visceral organ involvement, such as pulmonary fibrosis, may progress even after skin involvement peaks, new organ involvement is rare. Scleroderma renal crisis almost invariably occurs within the first 4 years of disease. In late-stage disease (>6 years), the skin is usually soft and atrophic. Skin regression characteristically occurs in an order that is the reverse of initial involvement, with softening on the trunks followed by proximal and finally distal extremities; however, sclerodactyly and finger contractures generally persist. Relapse or recurrence of skin thickening after the peak of skin involvement has been reached is uncommon. Patients with lcSSc follow a clinical course that is markedly different than that of dcSSc. Raynaud's phenomenon typically precedes other disease manifestations by years or even decades. Visceral organ complications such as PAH and ILD generally develop late and progress slowly.

PROGNOSIS

SSc confers a substantial increase in the risk of premature death. Age- and gender-adjusted mortality rates are fivefold to eightfold higher compared to the general population, and more than half of all patients with SSc die from their disease. In one population-based study of SSc, the median survival was 11 years. In patients with dcSSc, 5- and 10-year survival rates are 70% and 55%, respectively, whereas in patients with lcSSc, 5- and 10-year survival rates are 90% and 75%, respectively. The prognosis correlates with the extent of skin involvement, which itself is a surrogate for visceral organ involvement. Major causes of death are PAH, pulmonary fibrosis, gastrointestinal involvement, and cardiac disease. Scleroderma renal crisis is associated with a 30% 3-year mortality. Lung cancer and excess cardiovascular deaths also contribute to increased mortality. Markers of poor prognosis include male gender, African-American race, older age at disease onset, extensive skin thickening with truncal involvement, palpable tendon friction rubs, and evidence of significant or progressive visceral organ involvement. Laboratory predictors of increased mortality at initial evaluation include an elevated ESR, anemia, proteinuria and anti–topoisomerase I antibodies. In one study, SSc patients with extensive skin involvement, lung vital capacity <55% predicted, significant gastrointestinal involvement (pseudoobstruction or malabsorption), evidence of cardiac involvement (arrhythmias or congestive heart failure), or scleroderma renal crisis had a cumulative 9-year survival <40%. The severity of PAH is strongly associated with mortality, and SSc patients who had a mean pulmonary arterial pressure ≥45 mmHg had a 33% 3-year survival. The advent of ACE inhibitors in scleroderma renal crisis had a dramatic impact on survival, increasing from <10% at 1 year in the pre–ACE inhibitor era to >70% 3-year survival at the present time. Moreover, 10-year survival in SSc has improved from <60% in the 1970s to >66–78% in the 1990s, a trend that reflects both earlier detection and better management of complications.

LOCALIZED SCLERODERMA

The term *scleroderma* is commonly used to describe a group of localized skin disorders (Table 382-1). These occur more commonly in children than in adults. In contrast to SSc, localized scleroderma is rarely complicated by Raynaud's phenomenon or significant internal organ involvement. Morphea presents as solitary or multiple circular patches of thickened skin or, rarely, as widespread induration (generalized or pansclerotic morphea); the fingers are spared. Linear scleroderma—streaks of thickened skin, typically in one or both lower extremities—may affect the subcutaneous tissues, leading to fibrosis and atrophy of supporting structures, muscle, and bone. In children, the growth of affected long bones can be retarded. When linear scleroderma lesions cross joints, significant contractures can develop.

MIXED CONNECTIVE TISSUE DISEASE

Patients who have lcSSc coexisting with features of SLE, polymyositis, and rheumatoid arthritis may have mixed connective tissue disease (MCTD). This overlap syndrome is generally associated with the presence of high titers of autoantibodies to U1-RNP. The characteristic initial presentation is Raynaud's phenomenon associated with puffy fingers and myalgia. Gradually, lcSSc features of sclerodactyly, calcinosis, and cutaneous telangiectasia develop. Skin rashes suggestive of SLE (malar rash, photosensitivity) or of dermatomyositis (heliotrope rash on the eyelids, erythematous rash on the knuckles) occur. Arthralgia is common, and some patients develop erosive polyarthritis. Pulmonary fibrosis and isolated or secondary PAH may develop. Other manifestations include esophageal dysmotility, pericarditis, Sjögren's syndrome, and renal disease, especially membranous glomerulonephritis. Laboratory evaluation indicates features of inflammation with elevated ESR and hypergammaglobulinemia. While anti-U1RNP antibodies are detected in the serum in high titers, SSc-specific autoantibodies are not found. In contrast to SSc, patients with MCTD often show a good response to treatment with glucocorticoids, and the long-term prognosis is better than that of SSc. Whether MCTD is a truly distinct entity or is, rather, a subset of SLE or SSc remains controversial.

EOSINOPHILIC FASCIITIS

Eosinophilic fasciitis is a rare idiopathic disorder associated with induration of the skin that generally develops rapidly. Adults are primarily affected. The skin has a coarse cobblestone "peau d'orange" appearance. In contrast to SSc, internal organ involvement is rare, and Raynaud's phenomenon and SSc-associated autoantibodies are absent. Furthermore, skin involvement spares the fingers. Full-thickness excisional biopsy of the lesional skin reveals fibrosis of the subcutaneous fascia and is generally required for diagnosis. Inflammation and eosinophil infiltration in the fascia are variably present. In the acute phase of the illness, peripheral blood eosinophilia may be prominent. MRI appears to be a sensitive tool for the diagnosis of eosinophilic fasciitis. In some patients, eosinophilic fasciitis occurs in association with, or preceding, myelodysplastic syndromes or multiple myeloma. Treatment with glucocorticoids leads to prompt resolution of the eosinophilia. In contrast, skin changes generally show slow and variable improvement. The prognosis of patients with eosinophilic fasciitis is good.

383 Sjögren's Syndrome

Haralampos M. Moutsopoulos, Athanasios G. Tzioufas

DEFINITION, INCIDENCE, AND PREVALENCE

Sjögren's syndrome is a chronic, slowly progressive autoimmune disease characterized by lymphocytic infiltration of the exocrine glands resulting in xerostomia and dry eyes. Approximately one-third of patients present with systemic manifestations; a small but significant number of patients develop malignant lymphoma. The disease presents alone (primary Sjögren's syndrome) or in association with other autoimmune rheumatic diseases (secondary Sjögren's syndrome) (Table 383-1).

Middle-aged women (female-to-male ratio, 9:1) are primarily affected, although Sjögren's syndrome may occur at any age, including childhood. The prevalence of primary Sjögren's syndrome is ~0.5–1%, while 30% of patients with autoimmune rheumatic diseases suffer from secondary Sjögren's syndrome.

PATHOGENESIS

Sjögren's syndrome is characterized by both lymphocytic infiltration of the exocrine glands and B lymphocyte hyperreactivity. An oligomonoclonal B cell process, which is characterized by cryoprecipitable monoclonal immunoglobulins (IgMκ) with rheumatoid factor activity, is evident in up to 25% of patients.

Sera from patients with Sjögren's syndrome often contain autoantibodies to non-organ-specific antigens such as immunoglobulins (rheumatoid factors) and extractable nuclear and cytoplasmic antigens (Ro/SS-A, La/SS-B). Ro/SS-A autoantigen consists of two polypeptides (52 and 60 kDa, respectively) in conjunction with cytoplasmic RNAs, whereas the 48-kDa La/SS-B protein is bound to RNA III polymerase transcripts. Autoantibodies to Ro/SS-A and La/SS-B antigens are usually detected at the time of diagnosis and are associated with earlier disease onset, longer disease duration, salivary gland enlargement, and more intense lymphocytic infiltration of minor salivary glands.

The major infiltrating cells in the affected exocrine glands are activated T and B lymphocytes. T cells predominate in mild lesions, whereas B cells are dominant in more severe lesions. Macrophages and dendritic cells also are found. The number of macrophages positive for interleukin (IL) 18 has been shown to correlate with parotid gland enlargement and low levels of the C4 component of complement, both of which are adverse predictors for lymphoma development.

Ductal and acinar epithelial cells appear to play a significant role in the initiation and perpetuation of autoimmune injury. These cells (1) express class II major histocompatibility complex (MHC) molecules, costimulatory molecules, and abberant expression of intracellular autoantigens on cell membranes and thus are able to provide signals essential for lymphocytic activation; (2) inappropriately produce proinflammatory cytokines and lymphoattractant chemokines necessary for sustaining the autoimmune lesion and allowing progression to more sophisticated ectopic germinal center formation, which occurs in one-fifth of patients; and (3) express functional receptors of innate immunity, particularly Toll-like receptors (TLRs) 3, 7, and 9, that may account for the perpetuation of the autoimmune response.

TABLE 383-1 ASSOCIATION OF SJÖGREN'S SYNDROME WITH OTHER AUTOIMMUNE DISEASES

Rheumatoid arthritis
Systemic lupus erythematosus
Scleroderma
Mixed connective tissue disease
Primary biliary cirrhosis
Vasculitis
Chronic active hepatitis

Both infiltrating T and B cells have a tendency to be resistant to apoptosis. Levels of B cell–activating factor (BAFF) have been found to be elevated in patients with Sjögren's syndrome, especially those with hypergammaglobulinemia, and probably accounts for this antiapoptotic effect. Glandular epithelial cells seem to have an active role in the production of BAFF, which may be expressed and secreted after stimulation with type I interferon as well as with viral or synthetic double-stranded RNA. The triggering factor for epithelial activation appears to be a persistent enteroviral infection (possibly with coxsackievirus strains). Type I and type II interferon signatures have been described in ductal epithelial cells and T cells, respectively; their detection implies that interferons exert direct and cross-regulating effects on the pathogenic process.

A defect in cholinergic activity mediated through the M3 receptor and redistribution of the water-channel protein aquaporin 5, both leading to neuroepithelial dysfunction and diminished glandular secretions, have been proposed.

Molecular analysis of human leukocyte antigen (HLA) class II genes has revealed that Sjögren's syndrome, regardless of the patient's ethnic origin, is highly associated with the HLA DQA1*0501 allele. Genome-wide association studies have disclosed an increased prevalence of single-nucleotide polymorphisms in genes of IRF-5 and STAT-4, which participate in the activation of the type I interferon pathway.

CLINICAL MANIFESTATIONS

The majority of patients with Sjögren's syndrome have symptoms related to diminished lacrimal and salivary gland function. In most patients, the primary syndrome runs a slow and benign course. The initial manifestations can be mucosal or nonspecific dryness, and 8–10 years may elapse from the initial symptoms to full-blown development of the disease.

The principal oral symptom of Sjögren's syndrome is dryness (xerostomia). Patients report difficulty in swallowing dry food, an inability to speak continuously, a burning sensation, an increase in dental caries, and problems in wearing complete dentures. Physical examination shows a dry, erythematous, sticky oral mucosa. There is atrophy of the filiform papillae on the dorsum of the tongue, and saliva from the major glands is either not expressible or cloudy. Enlargement of the parotid or other major salivary glands occurs in two-thirds of patients with primary Sjögren's syndrome but is uncommon in those with the secondary syndrome. Diagnostic tests include sialometry, sialography, and scintigraphy. Newer imaging techniques, including ultrasound, MRI, and magnetic resonance sialography of the major salivary glands, are also being used. Biopsy of the labial minor salivary gland permits histopathologic confirmation of focal lymphocytic infiltrates.

Ocular involvement is the other major manifestation of Sjögren's syndrome. Patients usually describe a sandy or gritty feeling under the eyelids. Other symptoms include burning, accumulation of secretions in thick strands at the inner canthi, decreased tearing, redness, itching, eye fatigue, and increased photosensitivity. These symptoms, which define *keratoconjunctivitis sicca*, are attributed to the destruction of corneal and bulbar conjunctival epithelium. Diagnostic evaluation of keratoconjunctivitis sicca includes measurement of tear flow by Schirmer I test and determination of tear composition, with assessment of tear breakup time or tear lysozyme content. Slit-lamp examination of the cornea and conjunctiva after rose bengal staining reveals punctuate corneal ulcerations and attached filaments of corneal epithelium.

Involvement of other exocrine glands, which occurs less frequently, includes a decrease in mucous gland secretions of the upper and lower respiratory tree, resulting in dry nose, throat, and trachea (xerotrachea). In addition, diminished secretion of the exocrine glands of the gastrointestinal tract leads to esophageal mucosal atrophy, atrophic gastritis, and subclinical pancreatitis. Dyspareunia due to dryness of the external genitalia and dry skin also may occur.

Extraglandular (systemic) manifestations are seen in one-third of patients with Sjögren's syndrome (Table 383-2) but are very rare in patients whose Sjögren's syndrome is associated with rheumatoid

TABLE 383-2 PREVALENCE OF EXTRAGLANDULAR MANIFESTATIONS IN PRIMARY SJÖGREN'S SYNDROME

Clinical Manifestation	Percent	Remarks
Arthralgias/arthritis	60	Usually non-erosive, leading to Jaccoud's arthropathy.
Raynaud's phenomenon	37	In one-third of patients, precedes sicca manifestations.
Lymphadenopathy	14	Lymphoma should be excluded.
Lung involvement	14	Small airway disease is the predominant pathology.
Vasculitis	11	The most common clinical manifestation is cutaneous palpable purpura.
Kidney involvement	9	Interstitial kidney disease is usually asymptomatic. Glomerulonephritis is associated with cryoglobulinemia.
Liver involvement	6	Primary biliary cirrhosis stage I.
Lymphoma	6	Glandular MALT[a] lymphoma is most common.
Peripheral neuropathy	2	Polyneuropathy, either sensory or sensorimotor.
Myositis	1	Sporadic causes of myositis and inclusion body myositis have been reported.

[a]Mucosa-associated lymphoid tissue.

TABLE 383-3 DIFFERENTIAL DIAGNOSIS OF SICCA SYMPTOMS

Xerostomia	Dry Eye	Bilateral Parotid Gland Enlargement
Viral infections	Inflammation	Viral infections
Drugs	Stevens-Johnson syndrome	Mumps
Psychotherapeutic	Pemphigoid	Influenza
Parasympatholytic	Chronic conjunctivitis	Epstein-Barr virus
Antihypertensive	Chronic blepharitis	Coxsackievirus A
Psychogenic origin	Sjögren's syndrome	Cytomegalovirus
Irradiation	Toxicity	HIV, HCV
Diabetes mellitus	Burns	Sarcoidosis
Trauma	Drugs	IgG4 syndrome
Sjögren's syndrome	Neurologic conditions	Sjögren's syndrome
Amyloidosis	Impaired lacrimal gland function	Metabolic disorders
	Impaired eyelid function	Diabetes mellitus
	Miscellaneous	Hyperlipoproteinemias
	Trauma	Chronic pancreatitis
	Hypovitaminosis A	Hepatic cirrhosis
	Blink abnormality	Endocrine
	Anesthetic cornea	Acromegaly
	Lid scarring	Gonadal hypofunction
	Epithelial irregularity	

arthritis. Patients with primary Sjögren's syndrome more often report easy fatigability, low-grade fever, Raynaud's phenomenon, myalgias, and arthralgias. Most patients with primary Sjögren's syndrome experience at least one episode of non-erosive arthritis during the course of their disease. Manifestations of pulmonary involvement are frequently evident histologically but are rarely important clinically. Dry cough is the major manifestation that is attributed to small airway disease. Renal involvement includes interstitial nephritis, clinically manifested by hyposthenuria and renal tubular dysfunction with or without acidosis. Untreated acidosis may lead to nephrocalcinosis. Glomerulonephritis is a rare finding that occurs in patients with mixed cryoglobulinemia or with systemic lupus erythematosus overlapping with Sjögren's syndrome. Vasculitis affects small and medium-sized vessels. The most common clinical features are purpura, recurrent urticaria, skin ulcerations, glomerulonephritis, and mononeuritis multiplex.

Different autoantibodies may determine the clinical expression of the disease. Patients positive for anticentromere autoantibody present with a clinical picture similar to that of limited scleroderma (Chap. 382). Antimitochondrial antibodies may connote liver involvement in the form of primary biliary cirrhosis (Chap. 369). Autoantibodies to 21-hydroxylate have recently been described in almost 20% of patients; their presence is associated with a blunted adrenal response.

Central nervous system involvement is rarely recognized. A few cases of myelitis associated with antibody to aquaporin 4 have been described.

Lymphoma is a well-known manifestation of Sjögren's syndrome that usually presents later in the illness. Persistent parotid gland enlargement, purpura, leukopenia, cryoglobulinemia, low C4 complement levels, and ectopic germinal centers in minor salivary gland biopsy samples are manifestations suggesting the development of lymphoma. It is interesting that the same risk factors account for glomerulonephritis and lymphoma and that these risk factors are the ones that confer increased mortality risk. Most lymphomas are extranodal, low-grade marginal-zone B cell lymphomas and are usually detected incidentally during evaluation of the labial biopsy. The affected lymph nodes are usually peripheral. Survival rates are decreased in patients with B symptoms, lymph node mass >7 cm in diameter, and high or intermediate histologic grade.

Routine laboratory tests in Sjögren's syndrome reveal mild normochromic, normocytic anemia. An elevated erythrocyte sedimentation rate is found in ~70% of patients.

DIAGNOSIS AND DIFFERENTIAL DIAGNOSIS

Primary Sjögren's syndrome is diagnosed if (1) the patient presents with eye and/or mouth dryness, (2) eye tests disclose keratoconjunctivitis sicca, (3) mouth evaluation reveals the classic manifestations of the syndrome, and/or (4) the patient's serum reacts with Ro/SS-A and/or La/SS-B autoantigens. Labial biopsy is needed when the diagnosis is uncertain or to rule out other conditions that may cause dry mouth or eyes or parotid gland enlargement (Tables 383-3 and 383-4). Validated diagnostic criteria have been established by a European study and have now been further improved by a European-American study group (Table 383-5). Hepatitis C virus infection should be ruled out since, apart from serologic tests, the clinicopathologic picture is almost identical to that of Sjögren's syndrome. Enlargement of major salivary glands, particularly in seronegative patients, should raise the suspicion of IgG4-related syndrome, which may present also as chronic pancreatitis, interstitial nephritis, retroperitoneal fibrosis, and aortitis.

TREATMENT SJÖGREN'S SYNDROME

Treatment of Sjögren's syndrome is aimed at symptom relief and limitation of the damaging local effects of chronic xerostomia and keratoconjunctivitis sicca through substitution for or stimulation of the missing secretions (Fig. 383-1).

TABLE 383-4 DIFFERENTIAL DIAGNOSIS OF SJÖGREN'S SYNDROME

HIV Infection and Sicca Syndrome	Sjögren's Syndrome	Sarcoidosis
Predominant in young males	Predominant in middle-aged women	No age or sex preference
Lack of autoantibodies to Ro/SS-A and/or La/SS-B	Presence of autoantibodies	Lack of autoantibodies to Ro/SS-A and/or La/SS-B
Lymphoid infiltrates of salivary glands by CD8+ T lymphocytes	Lymphoid infiltrates of salivary glands by CD4+ T lymphocytes	Granulomas in salivary glands
Association with HLA-DR5	Association with HLA-DR3 and DRw52	Unknown
Positive serologic tests for HIV	Negative serologic tests for HIV	Negative serologic tests for HIV

TABLE 383-5 REVISED INTERNATIONAL CLASSIFICATION CRITERIA FOR SJÖGREN'S SYNDROME[a,b,c]

I. Ocular symptoms: a positive response to at least one of three validated questions.
  1. Have you had daily, persistent, troublesome dry eyes for more than 3 months?
  2. Do you have a recurrent sensation of sand or gravel in the eyes?
  3. Do you use tear substitutes more than three times a day?

II. Oral symptoms: a positive response to at least one of three validated questions.
  1. Have you had a daily feeling of dry mouth for more than 3 months?
  2. Have you had recurrent or persistently swollen salivary glands as an adult?
  3. Do you frequently drink liquids to aid in swallowing dry foods?

III. Ocular signs: objective evidence of ocular involvement defined as a positive result to at least one of the following two tests:
  1. Shirmer's I test, performed without anesthesia (≤5 mm in 5 min)
  2. Rose Bengal score or other ocular dye score (≥4 according to van Bijsterveld's scoring system)

IV. Histopathology: In minor salivary glands focal lymphocytic sialoadenitis, with a focus score ≥1.

V. Salivary gland involvement: objective evidence of salivary gland involvement defined by a positive result to at least one of the following diagnostic tests:
  1. Unstimulated whole salivary flow (≤1.5 mL in 15 min)
  2. Parotid sialography
  3. Salivary scintigraphy

VI. Antibodies in the serum to Ro/SS-A or La/SS-B antigens, or both.

[a]Exclusion criteria: past head and neck radiation treatment, hepatitis C infection, AIDS, preexisting lymphoma, sarcoidosis, graft-versus-host disease, use of anticholinergic drugs. [b]Primary Sjögren's syndrome: any four of the six items, as long as item IV (histopathology) or VI (serology) is positive; or any three of the four objective-criteria items (III, IV, V, VI). [c]In patients with a potentially associated disease (e.g., another well-defined connective tissue disease), the presence of item I or item II plus any two from among items III, IV, and V may be considered indicative of secondary Sjögren's syndrome.

Source: From C Vitali et al: Ann Rheum Dis 61:554, 2002. ©2002 with permission from BMJ Publishing Group Ltd.

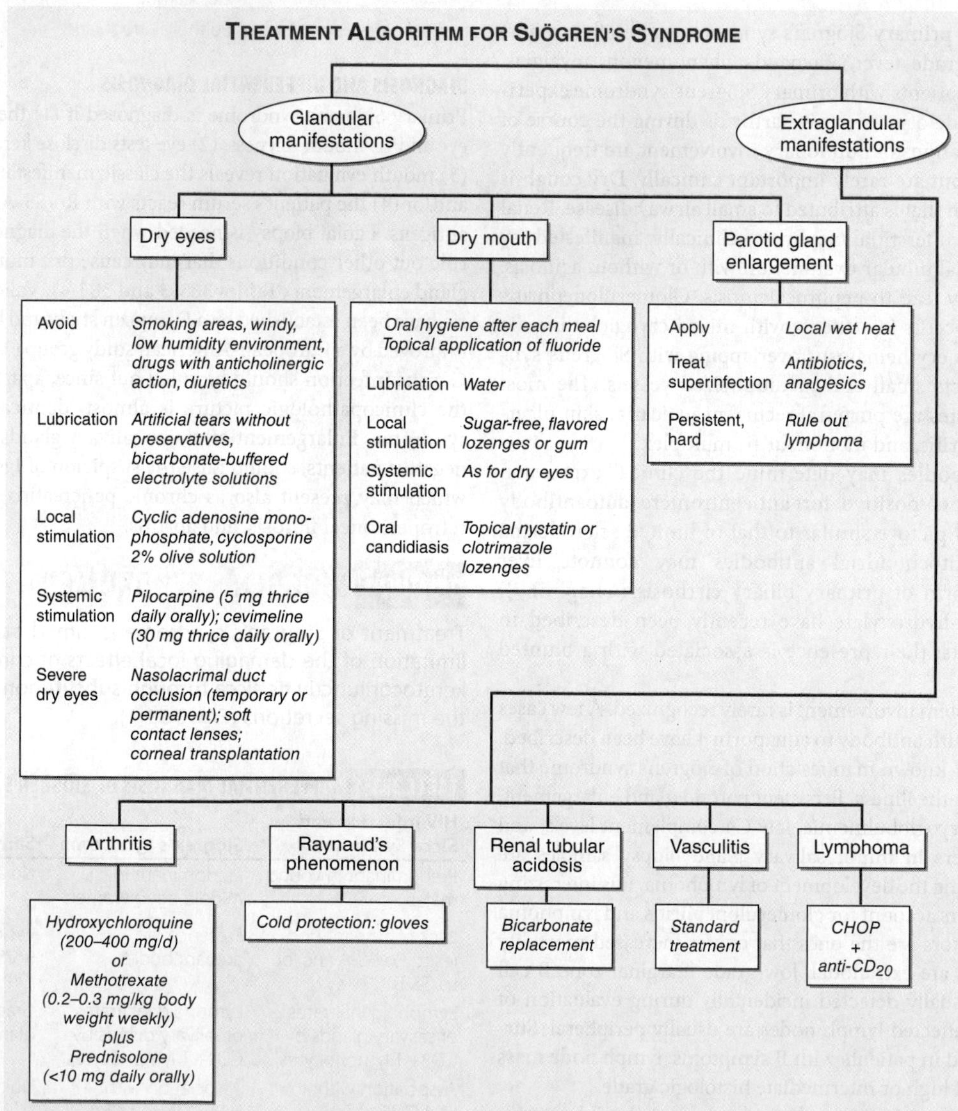

FIGURE 383-1 Treatment algorithm for Sjögren's syndrome. CHOP, cyclophosphamide, adriamycin (hydroxydaunorubicin), vincristine (oncovin), and prednisone.

To replace deficient tears, several ophthalmic preparations are readily available (hydroxypropyl methylcellulose; polyvinyl alcohol; 0.5% methylcellulose; Hypo Tears). If corneal ulcerations are present, eye patching and boric acid ointments are recommended. Certain drugs that may decrease lacrimal and salivary secretions, such as diuretics, antihypertensive drugs, anticholinergics, and antidepressants, should be avoided.

For xerostomia, the best replacement is water. Propionic acid gels may be used to treat vaginal dryness. To stimulate secretions, orally administered pilocarpine (5 mg thrice daily) or cevimeline (30 mg thrice daily) appears to improve sicca manifestations, and both are well tolerated. Hydroxychloroquine (200 mg) is helpful for arthralgias and mild arthritis.

Patients with renal tubular acidosis should receive sodium bicarbonate by mouth (0.5–2 mmol/kg in four divided doses). Glucocorticoids (1 mg/kg per day) and/or immunosuppressive agents (e.g., cyclophosphamide) are indicated only for the treatment of systemic vasculitis. Anti–tumor necrosis factor agents are ineffective. Monoclonal antibody to CD20 appears to be effective in patients with systemic disease, particularly in those with vasculitis, arthritis, and fatigability. Combination of anti-CD-20 with a classic CHOP regimen (cyclosporine, adriamycin [hydroxydaunorubicin], vincristine [oncovin], and prednisone) leads to increased survival rates among patients with high-grade lymphomas.

384 The Spondyloarthritides

Joel D. Taurog, John D. Carter

The spondyloarthritides are a group of overlapping disorders that share certain clinical features and genetic associations. These disorders include ankylosing spondylitis (AS), reactive arthritis, psoriatic arthritis and spondylitis, enteropathic arthritis and spondylitis, juvenile-onset spondyloarthritis (SpA), and undifferentiated SpA. The similarities in clinical manifestations and genetic predisposition suggest that these disorders share pathogenic mechanisms.

ANKYLOSING SPONDYLITIS

AS is an inflammatory disorder of unknown cause that primarily affects the axial skeleton; peripheral joints and extraarticular structures are also frequently involved. The disease usually begins in the second or third decade; male-to-female prevalence is between 2:1 and 3:1. The term *axial spondyloarthritis* is coming into common use, supported by criteria formulated in 2009 (Table 384-1). This classification includes both definite AS and early stages that do not yet meet classical criteria for AS, but it probably also includes other conditions with a different natural history.

EPIDEMIOLOGY

AS shows a striking correlation with the histocompatibility antigen HLA-B27 and occurs worldwide roughly in proportion to the prevalence of B27 (Chap. 373e). In North American whites, the prevalence of B27 is 7%, whereas it is 90% in patients with AS, independent of disease severity.

In population surveys, AS is present in 1–6% of adults inheriting B27, whereas the prevalence is 10–30% among B27+ adult first-degree relatives of AS probands. Concordance rate in identical twins is about 65%. Susceptibility to AS is determined largely by genetic factors, with B27 comprising less than one-half of the genetic component. Genome-wide single-nucleotide polymorphism (SNP) analysis has identified over 30 additional susceptibility alleles.

TABLE 384-1 ASAS CRITERIA FOR CLASSIFICATION OF AXIAL SPONDYLOARTHRITIS (TO BE APPLIED FOR PATIENTS WITH BACK PAIN ≥3 MONTHS AND AGE OF ONSET <45 YEARS)[a]

Sacroiliitis on Imaging Plus ≥1 SpA Feature	or	HLA-B27 Plus ≥2 Other SpA Features
Sacroiliitis on imaging		SpA features
• Active (acute) inflammation on MRI highly suggestive of SpA-associated sacroiliitis[b]		• Inflammatory back pain[d]
		• Arthritis[e]
and/or		• Enthesitis (heel)[f]
• Definite radiographic sacroiliitis according to modified New York criteria[c]		• Anterior uveitis[g]
		• Dactylitis[e]
		• Psoriasis[e]
		• Crohn's disease or ulcerative colitis[e]
		• Good response to NSAIDs[h]
		• Family history of SpA[i]
		• HLA-B27
		• Elevated CRP[j]

[a]Sensitivity 83%, specificity 84%. The imaging arm (sacroiliitis) alone has a sensitivity of 66% and a specificity of 97%. [b]Bone marrow edema and/or osteitis on short tau inversion recovery (STIR) or gadolinium-enhanced T1 image. [c]Bilateral grade ≥2 or unilateral grade 3 or 4. [d]See text for criteria. [e]Past or present, diagnosed by a physician. [f]Past or present pain or tenderness on examination at calcaneus insertion of Achilles tendon or plantar fascia. [g]Past or present, confirmed by an ophthalmologist. [h]Substantial relief of back pain at 24–48 h after a full dose of NSAID. [i]First- or second-degree relatives with ankylosing spondylitis (AS), psoriasis, uveitis, reactive arthritis (ReA), or inflammatory bowel disease (IBD). [j]After exclusion of other causes of elevated CRP.

Abbreviations: ASAS, Assessment of Spondyloarthritis International Society; CRP, C-reactive protein; MRI, magnetic resonance imaging; NSAIDs, nonsteroidal anti-inflammatory drugs; SpA, spondyloarthritis.

Source: From M Rudwaleit et al: Ann Rheum Dis 68:777, 2009. Copyright 2009, with permission from BMJ Publishing Group Ltd.

PATHOLOGY

Sacroiliitis is often the earliest manifestation of AS. Knowledge of its pathology comes from both biopsy and autopsy studies that cover a range of disease durations. Synovitis and myxoid marrow represent the earliest changes, followed by pannus and subchondral granulation tissue. Marrow edema, enthesitis, and chondroid differentiation are also found. Macrophages, T cells, plasma cells, and osteoclasts are prevalent. Eventually the eroded joint margins are gradually replaced by fibrocartilage regeneration and then by ossification. The joint may become totally obliterated.

In the spine, the specimens studied have either been surgically resected in advanced disease or taken from autopsies. There is inflammatory granulation tissue in the paravertebral connective tissue at the junction of annulus fibrosus and vertebral bone, and in some cases along the entire outer annulus. The outer annular fibers are eroded and eventually replaced by bone, forming the beginning of a syndesmophyte, which then grows by continued endochondral ossification, ultimately bridging the adjacent vertebral bodies. Ascending progression of this process leads to the "bamboo spine." Other lesions in the spine include diffuse osteoporosis (loss of trabecular bone despite accretion of periosteal bone), erosion of vertebral bodies at the disk margin, "squaring" or "barreling" of vertebrae, and inflammation and destruction of the disk-bone border. Inflammatory arthritis of the apophyseal (facet) joints is common, with synovitis, inflammation at the bony attachment of the joint capsule, and subchondral bone marrow granulation tissue. Erosion of joint cartilage by pannus is often followed by bony ankylosis. This may precede formation of syndesmophytes bridging the adjacent disks. Bone mineral density is diminished in the spine and proximal femur early in the course of the disease.

Peripheral synovitis in AS shows marked vascularity, which is also evident as tortuous macrovascularity seen during arthroscopy. Lining layer hyperplasia, lymphoid infiltration, and pannus formation are also found. Central cartilaginous erosions caused by proliferation of subchondral granulation tissue are common. It should be emphasized that the characteristics of peripheral arthritis in AS and other forms of SpA are similar, and distinct from those of rheumatoid arthritis.

Inflammation in the fibrocartilaginous enthesis, the region where a tendon, ligament, or joint capsule attaches to bone, is a characteristic lesion in AS and other SpAs, both at axial and peripheral sites. Enthesitis is associated with prominent edema of the adjacent bone marrow and is often characterized by erosive lesions that eventually undergo ossification.

Subclinical intestinal inflammation has been found in the colon or distal ileum in a majority of patients with SpA. The histology is described below under "Enteropathic Arthritis."

PATHOGENESIS

The pathogenesis of AS is immune-mediated, but there is little direct evidence for antigen-specific autoimmunity, and there is evidence to suggest more of an autoinflammatory pathogenesis. Uncertainty remains regarding the primary site of disease initiation. The dramatic response of the disease to therapeutic blockade of tumor necrosis factor α (TNF-α) indicates that this cytokine plays a central role in the immunopathogenesis of AS. Other genes related to TNF pathways show association with AS, including *TNFRSF1A*, *LTBR*, and *TBKBP1*. More recent evidence strongly implicates the interleukin (IL) 23/IL-17 cytokine pathway in AS pathogenesis. At least five genes in this pathway show association with AS, including *IL23R*, *PTER4*, *IL12B*, *CARD9*, and *TYK2*. All of these genes are also associated with inflammatory bowel disease (IBD), and three of them are associated with psoriasis. Serum levels of IL-23 and IL-17 are elevated in AS patients. Mice expressing high levels of IL-23 show spontaneous infiltration in the entheses of CD3+CD4–CD8– cells bearing IL-23 receptors and producing IL-17 and IL-22. This finding suggests the possibility that site-specific innate immune cells may play a critical role in the anatomic specificity of the lesions. Mast cells and, to a lesser extent, neutrophils appear to be the major IL-17-producing cells in peripheral arthritis, whereas neutrophils producing IL-17 are prominent in apophyseal joints. High levels of circulating γδ T cells expressing IL-23 receptors and producing IL-17 have been found in AS patients.

Other associated genes encode other cytokines or cytokine receptors (*IL6R*, *IL1R1*, *IL1R2*, *IL7R*, *IL27*), transcription factors involved in the differentiation of immune cells (*RUNX3*, *EOMES*, *BACH2*, *NKX2-3*, *TBX21*), or other molecules involved in activation or regulation of immune or inflammatory responses (*FCGR2A*, *ZMIZ1*, *NOS2*, *ICOSLG*).

The inflamed sacroiliac joint is infiltrated with CD4+ and CD8+ T cells and macrophages and shows high levels of TNF-α, particularly early in the disease. Abundant transforming growth factor β (TGF-β) has been found in more advanced lesions. Peripheral synovitis in AS and the other spondyloarthritides is characterized by neutrophils, macrophages expressing CD68 and CD163, CD4+ and CD8+ T cells, and B cells. There is prominent staining for intercellular adhesion molecule 1 (ICAM-1), vascular cell adhesion molecule 1 (VCAM-1), matrix metalloproteinase 3 (MMP-3), and myeloid-related proteins 8 and 14 (MRP-8 and MRP-14). Unlike rheumatoid arthritis (RA) synovium, citrullinated proteins and cartilage gp39 peptide–major histocompatibility complexes (MHCs) are absent. However, citrullinated proteins can be seen in the circulation.

No specific event or exogenous agent that triggers the onset of disease has been identified, although overlapping features with reactive arthritis and IBD and the involvement of the IL-23/IL-17 pathway suggest that enteric bacteria may play a role, and microdamage from mechanical stress at enthesial sites has also been implicated.

It is firmly established that HLA-B27 plays a direct role in AS pathogenesis, but its precise role at the molecular level remains unresolved. Rats transgenic for HLA-B27 develop arthritis and spondylitis, and this is unaffected by the absence of CD8. It thus appears that classical peptide antigen presentation to CD8+ T cells may not be the primary disease mechanism. However, the association of AS with ERAP1, which strongly influences the MHC class I peptide repertoire, is only found in B27+ patients, and this suggests that peptide binding to B27 is nonetheless important. The pairs of ERAP1 alleles found in AS patients show diminished peptidase activity, compared with those found in healthy controls. The B27 heavy chain has an unusual tendency to misfold, a process that may be proinflammatory. Genetic and functional studies in humans have suggested a role for natural killer (NK) cells in AS, possibly through interaction with B27 heavy chain homodimers. SpA-prone B27 rats show defective dendritic cell function and share with AS patients a characteristic "reverse interferon" gene expression signature in antigen-presenting cells.

New bone formation in AS appears to be largely based on enchondral bone formation and occurs only in the periosteal compartment. It correlates with lack of regulation of the Wnt signaling pathway, which controls the differentiation of mesenchymal cells into osteophytes, by the inhibitors DKK-1 and sclerostin. Indirect evidence and data from animal models also implicate bone morphogenic proteins, hedgehog proteins, and prostaglandin E_2. There is sharp controversy as to whether vertebral new bone formation in AS is a sequela of inflammation or whether it arises independently of inflammation. The second hypothesis is based on the observation that syndesmophyte formation is not suppressed by anti-TNF-α therapy that potently suppresses inflammation. TNF-α is also a known inducer of DKK-1, which inhibits bone formation. Recent magnetic resonance imaging (MRI) studies suggest that it is vertebral inflammatory lesions that undergo metaplasia to fat (increased T1-weighted signal) that are the predominant site of subsequent syndesmophytes despite anti-TNF-α therapy, whereas early acute inflammatory lesions resolve. A recent study suggested that the rate of syndesmophyte formation decreases after >4 years of anti-TNF-α therapy.

CLINICAL MANIFESTATIONS

The symptoms of the disease are usually first noticed in late adolescence or early adulthood; the median age in Western countries is approximately 23 years. In 5% of patients, symptoms begin after age 40. The initial symptom is usually dull pain, insidious in onset, felt deep in the lower lumbar or gluteal region, accompanied by low-back morning stiffness of up to a few hours' duration that improves with activity and returns following inactivity. Within a few months, the pain has usually become persistent and bilateral. Nocturnal exacerbation of pain often forces the patient to rise and move around.

In some patients, bony tenderness (presumably reflecting enthesitis or osteitis) may accompany back pain or stiffness, whereas in others it may be the predominant complaint. Common sites include the costosternal junctions, spinous processes, iliac crests, greater trochanters, ischial tuberosities, tibial tubercles, and heels. Hip and shoulder ("root" joint) arthritis is considered part of the axial disease. Hip arthritis occurs in 25–35% of patients. Shoulder arthritis is much less common. Severe isolated hip arthritis or bony chest pain may be the presenting complaint, and symptomatic hip disease can dominate the clinical picture. Arthritis of peripheral joints other than the hips and shoulders, usually asymmetric, occurs in up to 30% of patients. Neck pain and stiffness from involvement of the cervical spine are usually relatively late manifestations but are occasionally dominant symptoms. Rare patients, particularly in the older age group, present with predominantly constitutional symptoms.

AS often has a juvenile onset in developing countries. Peripheral arthritis and enthesitis usually predominate, with axial symptoms supervening in late adolescence.

Initially, physical findings mirror the inflammatory process. The most specific findings involve loss of spinal mobility, with limitation of anterior and lateral flexion and extension of the lumbar spine and of chest expansion. Limitation of motion is usually out of proportion to the degree of bony ankylosis and is thought to possibly reflect muscle spasm secondary to pain and inflammation. Pain in the sacroiliac joints may be elicited either with direct pressure or with stress on the joints. In addition, there is commonly tenderness upon palpation of the posterior spinous processes and other sites of symptomatic bony tenderness.

The modified Schober test is a useful measure of lumbar spine flexion. The patient stands erect, with heels together, and marks are made on the spine at the lumbosacral junction (identified by a horizontal line between the posterosuperior iliac spines) and 10 cm above. The patient then bends forward maximally with knees fully extended, and the distance between the two marks is measured. This distance increases by ≥5 cm in the case of normal mobility and by <4 cm in the case of decreased mobility. Chest expansion is measured as the difference between maximal inspiration and maximal forced expiration in the fourth intercostal space in males or just below the breasts in females, with the patient's hands resting on or just behind the head. Normal chest expansion is ≥5 cm. Lateral bending measures the distance the patient's middle finger travels down the leg with maximal lateral bending. Normal is >10 cm.

Limitation or pain with motion of the hips or shoulders is usually present if these joints are involved. It should be emphasized that early in the course of mild cases, symptoms may be subtle and nonspecific, and the physical examination may be unrevealing.

The course of the disease is extremely variable, ranging from the individual with mild stiffness and normal radiographs to the patient with a totally fused spine and severe bilateral hip arthritis, accompanied by severe peripheral arthritis and extraarticular manifestations. Pain tends to be persistent early in the disease and intermittent later, with alternating exacerbations and quiescent periods. In a typical severe untreated case with progression of the spondylitis to syndesmophyte formation, the patient's posture undergoes characteristic changes, with obliterated lumbar lordosis, buttock atrophy, and accentuated thoracic kyphosis. There may be a forward stoop of the neck or flexion contractures at the hips, compensated by flexion at the knees. Disease progression can be estimated clinically from loss of height, limitation of chest expansion and spinal flexion, and occiput-to-wall distance. Occasional individuals are encountered with advanced deformities who report having never had significant symptoms.

The factors most predictive of radiographic progression (see below) are the presence of existing syndesmophytes, high inflammatory makers, and smoking. In some but not all studies, onset of AS in adolescence and early hip involvement correlate with a worse prognosis. In women, AS tends to progress less frequently to total spinal ankylosis, although there may be an increased prevalence of isolated cervical ankylosis and peripheral arthritis. In industrialized countries, peripheral arthritis (distal to hips and shoulders) occurs in less than one-half of patients with AS, usually as a late manifestation, whereas in developing countries, the prevalence is much higher, with onset typically early in the disease course. Pregnancy has no consistent effect on AS, with symptoms improving, remaining the same, or deteriorating in one-third of pregnant patients, respectively.

The most serious complication of the spinal disease is spinal fracture, which can occur with even minor trauma to the rigid, osteoporotic spine. The lower cervical spine is most commonly involved. These fractures are often displaced and cause spinal cord injury. A recent survey suggested a >10% lifetime risk of fracture. Occasionally, fracture through a diskovertebral junction and adjacent neural arch, termed *pseudoarthrosis*, most common in the thoracolumbar spine, can be an unrecognized source of persistent localized pain and/or neurologic dysfunction. Wedging of thoracic vertebrae is common and correlates with accentuated kyphosis.

The most common extraarticular manifestation is acute anterior uveitis, which occurs in up to 40% of patients and can antedate the spondylitis. Attacks are typically unilateral, causing pain, photophobia, and increased lacrimation. These tend to recur, often in the opposite eye. Cataracts and secondary glaucoma are not uncommon sequelae. Up to 60% of patients with AS have inflammation in the colon or ileum. This is usually asymptomatic, but frank IBD occurs in 5–10% of patients with AS (see "Enteropathic Arthritis," below). About 10% of patients meeting criteria for AS have psoriasis (see "Psoriatic Arthritis," below). Aortic insufficiency, sometimes leading to congestive heart failure, occurs in a small percentage of patients, occasionally early. Third-degree heart block may occur alone or together with aortic insufficiency. Subclinical pulmonary lesions and cardiac dysfunction may be relatively common. Cauda equina syndrome and upper pulmonary lobe fibrosis are rare late complications. Retroperitoneal fibrosis is a rare associated condition. Prostatitis has been reported to have an increased prevalence. Amyloidosis is rare (Chap. 137).

Several validated measures of disease activity and functional outcome are in widespread use in the study and management of AS, particularly the Bath Ankylosing Spondylitis Disease Activity Index (BASDAI) and the Ankylosing Spondylitis Disease Activity Score (ASDAS), both measures of disease activity; the Bath Ankylosing Spondylitis Functional Index (BASFI), a measure of limitation in activities of daily living; and several measures of radiographic changes. The Harris hip score, although not specific for AS, can be helpful. Despite persistence of the disease, most patients remain gainfully employed. Some but not all studies of survival in AS have suggested that AS shortens life span, compared with the general population. Mortality attributable to AS is largely the result of spinal trauma, aortic insufficiency, respiratory failure, amyloid nephropathy, or complications of therapy such as upper gastrointestinal hemorrhage. The impact of anti-TNF therapy on outcome and mortality is not yet known, except for significantly improved work productivity.

LABORATORY FINDINGS

No laboratory test is diagnostic of AS. In most ethnic groups, HLA-B27 is present in 80–90% of patients. Erythrocyte sedimentation rate (ESR) and C-reactive protein (CRP) are often, but not always, elevated. Mild anemia may be present. Patients with severe disease may show an elevated alkaline phosphatase level. Elevated serum IgA levels are common. Rheumatoid factor, anti-cyclic citrullinated peptide (CCP), and antinuclear antibodies (ANAs) are largely absent unless caused by a coexistent disease, although ANAs may appear with anti-TNF therapy. Circulating levels of CD8+ T cells tend to be low, and serum matrix metalloproteinase 3 levels correlate with disease activity. Synovial fluid from peripheral joints in AS is nonspecifically inflammatory. In cases with restriction of chest wall motion, decreased vital capacity and increased functional residual capacity are common, but airflow is normal and ventilatory function is usually well maintained.

RADIOGRAPHIC FINDINGS

Radiographically demonstrable sacroiliitis, usually symmetric, is eventually present in AS. The earliest changes by standard radiography are blurring of the cortical margins of the subchondral bone, followed by erosions and sclerosis. Progression of the erosions leads to "pseudowidening" of the joint space; as fibrous and then bony ankylosis supervene, the joints may become obliterated.

In the lumbar spine, progression of the disease leads to straightening, caused by loss of lordosis, and reactive sclerosis, caused by osteitis of the anterior corners of the vertebral bodies with subsequent erosion, leading to "squaring" or even "barreling" of one or more vertebral bodies. Progressive ossification leads to eventual formation of marginal syndesmophytes, visible on plain films as bony bridges connecting successive vertebral bodies anteriorly and laterally.

Years may elapse before unequivocal sacroiliac abnormalities are evident on plain radiographs, and consequently, MRI is being increasingly used in diagnosing AS. Active sacroiliitis is best visualized by dynamic MRI with fat saturation, either T2-weighed turbo spin-echo sequence or short tau inversion recovery (STIR) with high resolution, or T1-weighted images with contrast enhancement. These techniques sensitively identify early intraarticular inflammation, cartilage changes, and underlying bone marrow edema in sacroiliitis (Fig. 384-1). They are also highly sensitive for evaluation of acute and chronic spinal changes (Fig. 384-2).

Reduced bone mineral density can be detected by dual-energy x-ray absorptiometry of the femoral neck and the lumbar spine. Use of a lateral projection of the L3 vertebral body can prevent falsely elevated readings related to spinal ossification.

DIAGNOSIS

It is important to establish the diagnosis of early AS before the development of irreversible deformity. This goal presents a challenge for several reasons: (1) Back pain is very common, but AS is much less common; (2) an early presumptive diagnosis often relies on clinical grounds requiring considerable expertise; and (3) young individuals with symptoms of AS often do not seek medical care. The widely used modified New York criteria (1984) are based on the presence of definite radiographic sacroiliitis and are too insensitive in early

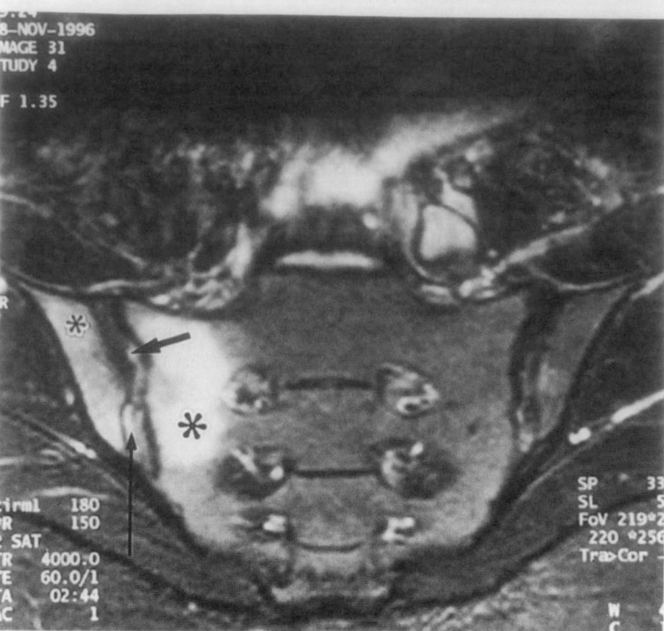

FIGURE 384-1 Early sacroiliitis in a patient with ankylosing spondylitis, indicated by prominent edema in the juxtaarticular bone marrow (*asterisks*), synovium and joint capsule (*thin arrow*), and interosseous ligaments (*thick arrow*) on a short tau inversion recovery (STIR) magnetic resonance image. *(From M Bollow et al: Zeitschrift für Rheumatologie 58:61, 1999. Reproduced with permission.)*

or mild cases. In 2009, new criteria for axial SpA were proposed by the Assessment of Spondyloarthritis International Society (ASAS) (Table 384-1). They are applicable to individuals with ≥3 months of back pain with age of onset <45 years old. Active inflammation of the sacroiliac joints as determined by dynamic MRI is considered equivalent to definite radiographic sacroiliitis (see below).

AS must be differentiated from numerous other causes of low-back pain, some far more common than AS. To qualify as the criterion for inflammatory back pain of axial SpA (Table 384-1), the chronic (≥3 months) back pain should have four or more of the following characteristic features: (1) age of onset <40 years old; (2) insidious onset; (3) improvement with exercise; (4) no improvement with rest; and (5) pain at night with improvement upon getting up. Other common features of inflammatory back pain include morning stiffness >30 min, awakening from back pain during only the second half of the night, and alternating buttock pain. In clinical decision-making, all of these features are additive. The most common causes of back pain other than AS are primarily mechanical or degenerative rather than primarily inflammatory and tend not to show clustering of these features.

Less-common metabolic, infectious, and malignant causes of back pain must also be differentiated from AS, including infectious spondylitis, spondylodiskitis, and sacroiliitis, and primary or metastatic tumor. Ochronosis can produce a phenotype that is clinically and radiographically similar to AS. Calcification and ossification of paraspinous ligaments occur in *diffuse idiopathic skeletal hyperostosis* (DISH), which occurs in the middle-aged and elderly and is usually not symptomatic. Ligamentous calcification gives the appearance of "flowing wax" on the anterior bodies of the vertebrae. Intervertebral disk spaces are preserved, and sacroiliac and apophyseal joints appear normal, helping to differentiate DISH from spondylosis and from AS, respectively.

TREATMENT ANKYLOSING SPONDYLITIS

All management of AS should include an exercise program designed to maintain posture and range of motion. Nonsteroidal anti-inflammatory drugs (NSAIDs) are the first line of pharmacologic therapy for AS. These agents reduce pain and tenderness and increase mobility in many patients with AS. There is mounting evidence that continuous high-dose NSAID therapy slows radiographic progression, particularly in patients who are at higher risk for progression. However, many patients with AS have continued symptoms despite NSAID therapy and are likely to benefit from anti-TNF-α therapy. Patients with AS treated with infliximab (chimeric human/mouse anti-TNF-α monoclonal antibody), etanercept (soluble p75 TNF-α receptor–IgG fusion protein), adalimumab, or golimumab (human anti-TNF-α monoclonal antibodies, or certolizumab pegol [humanized mouse anti-TNF-α monoclonal antibody]) have shown rapid, profound, and sustained reductions in all clinical and laboratory measures of disease activity. In a good response, there is significant improvement in both objective and subjective indicators of disease activity and function, including morning stiffness, pain, spinal mobility, peripheral joint swelling, CRP, and ESR. MRI studies indicate substantial resolution of bone marrow edema, enthesitis, and joint effusions in the sacroiliac joints, spine, and peripheral joints (Fig. 384-2). Similar results have been obtained in large randomized controlled trials of all four agents and

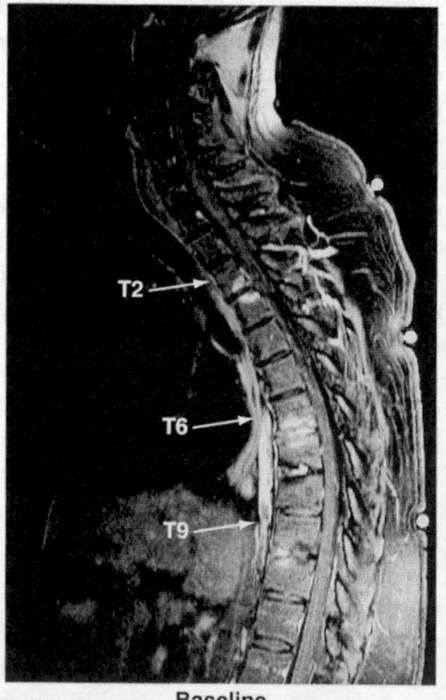

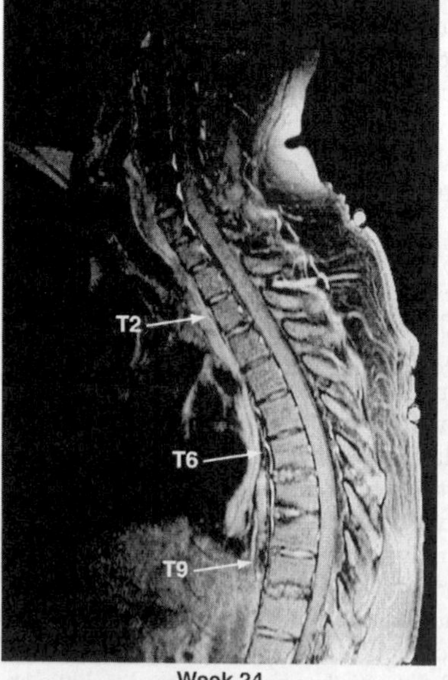

FIGURE 384-2 Spinal inflammation (spondylodiskitis) in a patient with ankylosing spondylitis and its dramatic response to treatment with infliximab. Gadolinium-enhanced T1-weighted magnetic resonance images, with fat saturation, at baseline and after 24 weeks of infliximab therapy. *(From J Braun et al: Arthritis Rheum 54:1646, 2006.)*

many open-label studies. About one-half of the patients achieve a ≥50% reduction in the BASDAI. The response tends to be stable over time, and partial or full remissions are common. Predictors of the best responses include younger age, shorter disease duration, higher baseline inflammatory markers, and lower baseline functional disability. Nonetheless, some patients with long-standing disease and even spinal ankylosis can obtain significant benefit. Increased bone mineral density is found as early as 24 weeks after onset of therapy. There is evidence that anti-TNF therapy does not prevent syndesmophyte formation, although this may apply mainly during the early years of therapy. A mechanism for this has been proposed based on the observation that TNF-α inhibits new bone formation by upregulating DKK-1, a negative regulator of the wingless (Wnt) signaling pathway that promotes osteoblast activity. Serum DKK-1 levels are inappropriately low in AS patients and are also suppressed by anti-TNF therapy.

Infliximab is given intravenously, 3–5 mg/kg body weight, and then repeated 2 weeks later, again 6 weeks later, and then at 8-week intervals. Etanercept is given by subcutaneous injection, 50 mg once weekly. Adalimumab is given by subcutaneous injection, 40 mg biweekly. Golimumab is given by subcutaneous injection, 50 or 100 mg every 4 weeks. Certolizumab pegol is given by subcutaneous injection, 400 mg every 4 weeks.

Although these potent immunosuppressive agents have thus far been relatively safe, patients are at increased risk for serious infections, including disseminated tuberculosis. Hypersensitivity infusion or injection site reactions are not uncommon. Cases of anti-TNF-induced psoriasis have been increasingly recognized. Rare cases of systemic lupus erythematosus–related disease have been reported, as have hematologic disorders such as pancytopenia, demyelinating disorders, exacerbation of congestive heart failure, and severe liver disease. The overall incidence of malignancy does not appear to be increased in AS patients treated with anti-TNF therapy, but isolated cases of hematologic malignancy have occurred shortly after the start of treatment.

Because of the expense, potentially serious side effects, and unknown long-term effects of these agents, their use should be restricted to patients with a definite diagnosis and active disease (BASDAI ≥4 out of 10 and expert opinion) that is inadequately responsive to therapy with at least two different NSAIDs. Before initiation of anti-TNF therapy, all patients should be tested for tuberculin (TB) reactivity, and reactors (≥5 mm on PPD testing or a positive quantiferon test) should be treated with anti-TB agents. Contraindications include active infection or high risk of infection; malignancy or premalignancy; and history of systemic lupus erythematosus, multiple sclerosis, or related autoimmunity. Pregnancy and breast-feeding are relative contraindications. Continuation beyond 12 weeks of therapy requires either a 50% reduction in BASDAI or absolute reduction of ≥2 out of 10, and favorable expert opinion. Switching to a second anti-TNF agent may be effective, especially if there was a response to the first that was lost rather than primary failure. Sulfasalazine, in doses of 2–3 g/d, has been shown to be of modest benefit, primarily for peripheral arthritis. A therapeutic trial of this agent should precede any use of anti-TNF agents in patients with predominantly peripheral arthritis. Methotrexate, although widely used, has not been shown to be of benefit in AS, nor has any therapeutic role for gold or oral glucocorticoids been documented. Potential benefit in AS has been reported for thalidomide, 200 mg/d, perhaps acting through inhibition of TNF-α.

Ustekinumab (anti-IL-12/23) and secukinumab (anti-IL-17) monoclonal antibodies have shown promising efficacy in clinical trials, but have not yet been approved for use in AS.

The most common indication for surgery in patients with AS is severe hip joint arthritis, the pain and stiffness of which are usually dramatically relieved by total hip arthroplasty. Rare patients may benefit from surgical correction of extreme flexion deformities of the spine or of atlantoaxial subluxation.

Attacks of uveitis are usually managed effectively with local glucocorticoid administration in conjunction with mydriatic agents, although systemic glucocorticoids, immunosuppressive drugs, or anti-TNF therapy may be required. TNF inhibitors reduce the frequency of attacks of uveitis in patients with AS, although cases of new or recurrent uveitis after use of a TNF inhibitor have been observed, especially with etanercept.

Coexistent cardiac disease may require pacemaker implantation and/or aortic valve replacement. Management of axial osteoporosis is at present similar to that used for primary osteoporosis, since data specific for AS are not available.

REACTIVE ARTHRITIS

Reactive arthritis (ReA) refers to acute nonpurulent arthritis complicating an infection elsewhere in the body. In recent years, the term has been used primarily to refer to SpA following enteric or urogenital infections.

Other forms of reactive and infection-related arthritis not associated with B27 and showing a spectrum of clinical features different from SpA, such as Lyme disease and rheumatic fever, are discussed in Chaps. 210 and 381.

HISTORIC BACKGROUND

The association of acute arthritis with episodes of diarrhea or urethritis has been recognized for centuries. A large number of cases during World Wars I and II focused attention on the triad of arthritis, urethritis, and conjunctivitis, often with additional mucocutaneous lesions, which became widely known by eponyms that are now of historic interest only.

The identification of bacterial species capable of triggering the clinical syndrome and the finding that many patients possess the B27 antigen led to the unifying concept of ReA as a clinical syndrome triggered by specific etiologic agents in a genetically susceptible host. A similar spectrum of clinical manifestations can be triggered by enteric infection with any of several *Shigella*, *Salmonella*, *Yersinia*, and *Campylobacter* species; by genital infection with *Chlamydia trachomatis*; and by other agents as well. The triad of arthritis, urethritis, and conjunctivitis represents a small part of the spectrum of the clinical manifestations of ReA and only a minority of patients present with this "classic triad" of symptoms. Although emerging data suggest that asymptomatic *Chlamydia trachomatis* infections might trigger ReA, for the purposes of this chapter, the use of the term *ReA* will be restricted to those cases of SpA in which there is at least presumptive evidence for a related symptomatic antecedent infection. Patients with clinical features of ReA who lack evidence of an antecedent infection will be considered to have *undifferentiated spondyloarthritis*, discussed below.

EPIDEMIOLOGY

Initial reports may have overestimated the association of ReA with HLA-B27, since 60–85% of patients who developed ReA triggered by *Shigella*, *Yersinia*, or *Chlamydia* were B27-positive. However, other studies demonstrated a lower prevalence of B27 in ReA triggered by *Salmonella*, with one study suggesting no association in *Campylobacter*-induced ReA. Several more recent community-based or common-source epidemic studies demonstrated that the prevalence of B27 in ReA was below 50%. The most common age range is 18–40 years, but ReA can occur rarely in children and occasionally in older adults.

The attack rate of postenteric ReA generally ranges from 1% to about 30% depending on the study and causative organism, whereas the attack rate of postchlamydial ReA is about 4–8%. The gender ratio in ReA following enteric infection is nearly 1:1, whereas venereally acquired ReA occurs mainly in men. The overall prevalence and incidence of ReA are difficult to assess because of the lack of validated diagnostic criteria, variable prevalence and arthritogenic potential of the triggering infectious agents, and inconstant genetic susceptibility factors in different populations. In Scandinavia, an annual incidence of 10–28:100,000 has been reported. The spondyloarthritides were formerly almost unknown in sub-Saharan Africa. However, ReA and other peripheral SpAs have now become the most common rheumatic diseases in Africans in the wake of the AIDS epidemic, without association to B27, which is very rare in these populations. ReA is often the first manifestation of HIV infection and often remits with disease progression. In contrast,

Western white patients with HIV and SpA are usually B27-positive, and the arthritis flares as AIDS advances.

PATHOLOGY

Synovial histology is similar to that of other SpAs. Enthesitis shows increased vascularity and macrophage infiltration of fibrocartilage. Microscopic histopathologic evidence of inflammation mimicking IBD has routinely been demonstrated in the colon and ileum of patients with postenteric ReA and less commonly in postvenereal ReA. The skin lesions of keratoderma blennorrhagica, associated mainly with venereally acquired ReA, are histologically indistinguishable from pustular psoriatic lesions.

ETIOLOGY AND PATHOGENESIS

The bacteria identified as definitive triggers of ReA include several *Salmonella* spp., *Shigella* spp., *Yersinia enterocolitica, Yersinia pseudotuberculosis, Campylobacter jejuni,* and *Chlamydia trachomatis.* These triggering microbes are gram-negative bacteria with a lipopolysaccharide component to their cell walls. All four *Shigella* species (*Shigella sonnei, Shigella boydii, Shigella flexneri,* and *Shigella dysenteriae*) have been implicated in cases of ReA, with *S. flexneri* and *S. sonnei* being the most common. After *Salmonella* infection, individuals of Caucasian descent may be more likely than those of Asian descent to develop ReA. Children may be less susceptible to ReA caused by *Salmonella* and *Campylobacter. Yersinia* species in Europe and Scandinavia may have greater arthritogenic potential than in other parts of the world, and *C. trachomatis* appears to be a common cause worldwide. The ocular serovars of *C. trachomatis* appear to be particularly, perhaps uniquely, arthritogenic.

There is also evidence implicating *Clostridium difficile, Campylobacter coli,* certain toxigenic *Escherichia coli,* and possibly *Ureaplasma urealyticum* and *Mycoplasma genitalium* as potential triggers of ReA. *Chlamydia pneumoniae* is another trigger of ReA, albeit far less common than *C. trachomatis.* There have also been numerous isolated reports of acute arthritis preceded by other bacterial, viral, or parasitic infections, and even following intravesicular bacillus Calmette-Guérin (BCG) treatment for bladder cancer.

It has not been determined whether ReA occurs by the same pathogenic mechanism following infection with each of these microorganisms, nor has the mechanism been elucidated in the case of any one of the known bacterial triggers. Most, if not all, of the organisms well established to be triggers share a capacity to attack mucosal surfaces, to invade host cells, and to survive intracellularly. Antigens from *Chlamydia, Yersinia, Salmonella,* and *Shigella* have been shown to be present in the synovium and/or synovial fluid leukocytes of patients with ReA for long periods following the acute attack. In ReA triggered by *Y. enterocolitica,* bacterial lipopolysaccharide (LPS) and heat-shock protein antigens have been found in peripheral blood cells years after the triggering infection. *Yersinia* DNA and *C. trachomatis* DNA and RNA have been detected in synovial tissue from ReA patients, suggesting the presence of viable organisms despite uniform failure to culture the organism from these specimens. In *C. trachomatis*–induced ReA specifically, the bacterial load in synovial tissue of patients with remitting disease is lower than that of active disease, but mRNAs encoding proinflammatory proteins are equal to or higher than those of active disease. The specificity of these findings is unclear, however, since chromosomal bacterial DNA and 16S rRNA from a very wide variety of bacteria have also been found in synovium in other rheumatic diseases, albeit less frequently. In several older studies, synovial T cells that specifically responded to antigens of the inciting organism were reported and characterized as predominantly CD4+ with a T_H2 or T regulatory phenotype. More recent work has documented high levels of IL-17 in ReA synovial fluid, but the source has not been identified. HLA-B27 seems to be associated with more severe and chronic forms of the "classic triad" of ReA, but its pathogenic role remains to be determined. HLA-B27 significantly prolongs the intracellular survival of *Y. enterocolitica* and *Salmonella enteritidis* in human and mouse cell lines. Prolonged intracellular bacterial survival, promoted by B27, other factors, or both, may permit trafficking of infected leukocytes from the site of primary infection to joints, where an innate and/or adaptive immune response to persistent bacterial antigens may then promote arthritis.

CLINICAL FEATURES

The clinical manifestations of ReA constitute a spectrum that ranges from an isolated, transient monoarthritis or enthesitis to severe multisystem disease. A careful history will usually elicit evidence of an antecedent infection 1–4 weeks before onset of symptoms of the reactive disease, particularly in postenteric ReA. However, in a sizable minority, no clinical or laboratory evidence of an antecedent infection can be found, particularly in the case of postchlamydial ReA. In cases of presumed venereally acquired reactive disease, there is often a history of a recent new sexual partner, even without laboratory evidence of infection.

Constitutional symptoms are common, including fatigue, malaise, fever, and weight loss. The musculoskeletal symptoms are usually acute in onset. Arthritis is usually asymmetric and additive, with involvement of new joints occurring over a few days to 1–2 weeks. The joints of the lower extremities, especially the knee, ankle, and subtalar, metatarsophalangeal, and toe interphalangeal joints, are most commonly involved, but the wrist and fingers can be involved as well. The arthritis is usually quite painful, and tense joint effusions are not uncommon, especially in the knee. Dactylitis, or "sausage digit," a diffuse swelling of a solitary finger or toe, is a distinctive feature of ReA and other peripheral spondyloarthritides but can be seen in polyarticular gout and sarcoidosis. Tendinitis and fasciitis are particularly characteristic lesions, producing pain at multiple insertion sites (entheses), especially the Achilles insertion, the plantar fascia, and sites along the axial skeleton. Spinal, low-back, and buttock pain are quite common and may be caused by insertional inflammation, muscle spasm, acute sacroiliitis, or, presumably, arthritis in intervertebral joints.

Urogenital lesions may occur throughout the course of the disease. In males, urethritis may be marked or relatively asymptomatic and may be either an accompaniment of the triggering infection or a result of the reactive phase of the disease; interestingly, it occurs in both postvenereal and postenteric ReA. Prostatitis is also common. Similarly, in females, cervicitis or salpingitis may be caused either by the infectious trigger or by the sterile reactive process.

Ocular disease is common, ranging from transient, asymptomatic conjunctivitis to an aggressive anterior uveitis that occasionally proves refractory to treatment and may result in blindness.

Mucocutaneous lesions are frequent. Oral ulcers tend to be superficial, transient, and often asymptomatic. The characteristic skin lesions, *keratoderma blennorrhagica,* consist of vesicles and/or pustules that become hyperkeratotic, ultimately forming a crust before disappearing. They are most common on the palms and soles but may occur elsewhere as well. In patients with HIV infection, these lesions are often extremely severe and extensive, sometimes dominating the clinical picture (Chap. 226). Lesions may occur on the glans penis, termed *circinate balanitis;* these consist of vesicles that quickly rupture to form painless superficial erosions, which in circumcised individuals can form crusts similar to those of keratoderma blennorrhagica. Nail changes are common and consist of onycholysis, distal yellowish discoloration, and/or heaped-up hyperkeratosis.

Less-frequent or rare manifestations of ReA include cardiac conduction defects, aortic insufficiency, central or peripheral nervous system lesions, and pleuropulmonary infiltrates.

Arthritis typically persists for 3–5 months, but more chronic courses do occur. Chronic joint symptoms persist in about 15% of patients and in up to 60% of patients in hospital-based series, but these tend to be less severe than in the acute stage. Recurrences of the acute syndrome are also common. Work disability or forced change in occupation is common in those with persistent joint symptoms. Chronic heel pain is often particularly distressing. Low-back pain, sacroiliitis, and frank AS are also common sequelae. In most studies, HLA-B27–positive patients have shown a worse outcome than B27-negative patients. Patients with *Yersinia-* or *Salmonella*-induced arthritis have less chronic disease than those whose initial episode follows epidemic shigellosis.

LABORATORY AND RADIOGRAPHIC FINDINGS

The ESR and acute-phase reactants are usually elevated during the acute phase of the disease, often markedly so. Mild anemia may be present. Synovial fluid is nonspecifically inflammatory. In most ethnic groups, 30–50% of the patients are B27-positive. The triggering infection usually does not persist at the site of primary mucosal infection through the time of onset of the reactive disease, but it may be possible to culture the organism, e.g., in the case of *Yersinia*- or *Chlamydia*-induced disease. Serologic evidence of exposure to one of the causative organisms with elevation of antibodies is nonspecific and is of questionable utility. Polymerase chain reaction (PCR) for chlamydial DNA in first-voided urine specimens may have high sensitivity in the acute stage but is less useful with chronic disease.

In early or mild disease, radiographic changes may be absent or confined to juxtaarticular osteoporosis. With long-standing persistent disease, radiographic features share those of psoriatic arthritis; marginal erosions and loss of joint space can be seen in affected joints. Periostitis with reactive new bone formation is characteristic, as in all the SpAs. Spurs at the insertion of the plantar fascia are common.

Sacroiliitis and spondylitis may be seen as late sequelae. Sacroiliitis is more commonly asymmetric than in AS, and spondylitis, rather than ascending symmetrically, can begin anywhere along the lumbar spine. The syndesmophytes are described as nonmarginal; they are coarse, asymmetric, and "comma"-shaped, arising from the middle of a vertebral body, a pattern less commonly seen in primary AS. Progression to spinal fusion is uncommon.

DIAGNOSIS

ReA is a clinical diagnosis with no definitively diagnostic laboratory test or radiographic finding. The diagnosis should be entertained in any patient with an acute inflammatory, asymmetric, additive arthritis or tendinitis. The evaluation should include questioning regarding possible triggering events such as an episode of diarrhea or dysuria. On physical examination, attention must be paid to the distribution of the joint and tendon involvement and to possible sites of extraarticular involvement, such as the eyes, mucous membranes, skin, nails, and genitalia. Synovial fluid analysis may be helpful in excluding septic or crystal-induced arthritis. Culture, serology, or molecular methods may help to identify a triggering infection, but they cannot be relied upon.

Although typing for B27 has low negative predictive value in ReA, it may have prognostic significance in terms of severity, chronicity, and the propensity for spondylitis and uveitis. Furthermore, if positive, it can be helpful diagnostically in atypical cases. HIV testing is often indicated and may be necessary in order to select appropriate therapy.

It is important to differentiate ReA from disseminated gonococcal disease (Chap. 181), both of which can be venereally acquired and associated with urethritis. Unlike ReA, gonococcal arthritis and tenosynovitis tend to involve both upper and lower extremities equally, spare the axial skeleton, and be associated with characteristic vesicular skin lesions. A positive gonococcal culture from the urethra or cervix does not exclude a diagnosis of ReA; however, culturing gonococci from blood, skin lesion, or synovium establishes the diagnosis of disseminated gonococcal disease. PCR assay for *Neisseria gonorrhoeae* and *C. trachomatis* may be helpful. Occasionally, only a therapeutic trial of antibiotics can distinguish the two.

ReA shares many features in common with psoriatic arthropathy. However, psoriatic arthritis is usually gradual in onset; the arthritis tends to affect primarily the upper extremities; there is less associated periarthritis; and there are usually no associated mouth ulcers, urethritis, or bowel symptoms.

TREATMENT REACTIVE ARTHRITIS

Most patients with ReA benefit to some degree from high-dose NSAIDs, although acute symptoms are rarely completely ameliorated, and some patients fail to respond at all. Indomethacin, 75–150 mg/d in divided doses, is the initial treatment of choice, but other NSAIDs may be tried.

Prompt, appropriate antibiotic treatment of acute chlamydial urethritis or enteric infection may prevent the emergence of ReA, but is not universally successful. Data regarding the potential benefit of antibiotic therapy that is initiated after onset of arthritis are conflicting, but several trials suggest no benefit. One long-term follow-up study suggested that although antibiotic therapy had no effect on the acute episode of ReA, it helped prevent subsequent chronic SpA. Another such study failed to demonstrate any long-term benefit. A promising recent double-blind placebo-controlled study assessing combination antibiotics showed that a majority of patients with chronic ReA due to *Chlamydia* benefited significantly from a 6-month course of rifampin 300 mg daily plus azithromycin 500 mg daily for 5 days, then twice weekly, or 6 months of rifampin 300 mg daily plus doxycycline 100 mg twice daily. The possibility remains that acute *Chlamydia*-induced ReA might respond more favorably to antibiotic therapy than the postenteric variety.

Multicenter trials have suggested that sulfasalazine, up to 3 g/d in divided doses, may be beneficial to patients with persistent ReA.[1] Patients with persistent disease may respond to azathioprine, 1–2 mg/kg per day, or to methotrexate, up to 20 mg per week; however, these therapeutic regimens have never formally been studied. Although no controlled trials of anti-TNF-α in ReA have been reported, anecdotal evidence supports the use of these agents in severe chronic cases, although lack of response has also been observed.[1]

Tendinitis and other enthesitic lesions may benefit from intralesional glucocorticoids. Uveitis may require aggressive treatment to prevent serious sequelae (see above). Skin lesions ordinarily require only symptomatic topical treatment. In patients with HIV infection and ReA, many of whom have severe skin lesions, the skin lesions in particular respond to antiretroviral therapy. Cardiac complications are managed conventionally; management of neurologic complications is symptomatic.

Comprehensive management includes counseling of patients in the avoidance of sexually transmitted disease and exposure to enteropathogens, as well as appropriate use of physical therapy, vocational counseling, and continued surveillance for long-term complications such as AS. Patients with a history of ReA are at increased risk for recurrent attacks following repeated exposures.

PSORIATIC ARTHRITIS

Psoriatic arthritis (PsA) refers to an inflammatory musculoskeletal disease that has both autoimmune and autoinflammatory features characteristically occurring in individuals with psoriasis.

HISTORIC BACKGROUND

The association between arthritis and psoriasis was noted in the nineteenth century. In the 1960s, on the basis of epidemiologic and clinical studies, it became clear that unlike RA, the arthritis associated with psoriasis was usually seronegative, often involved the distal interphalangeal (DIP) joints of the fingers and the spine and sacroiliac joints, had distinctive radiographic features, and showed considerable familial aggregation. In the 1970s, PsA was included in the broader category of the spondyloarthritides because of features similar to those of AS and ReA.

EPIDEMIOLOGY

Estimates of the prevalence of PsA among individuals with psoriasis range from 5 to 42%. The prevalence of PsA appears to be increasing in parallel with disease awareness; recent data using screening tools suggest that 20% or more of patients with psoriasis have undiagnosed PsA. The duration and severity of psoriasis increase one's likelihood of developing PsA. In white populations, psoriasis is estimated to have a prevalence of

[1]Azathioprine, methotrexate, sulfasalazine, pamidronate, and thalidomide have not been approved for this purpose by the U.S. Food and Drug Administration at the time of publication.

1–3%. Psoriasis and PsA are less common in other races in the absence of HIV infection, and the prevalence of PsA in individuals with psoriasis may be less common. First-degree relatives of PsA patients have an elevated risk for psoriasis, for PsA itself, and for other forms of SpA. Of patients with psoriasis, up to 30% have an affected first-degree relative. In monozygotic twins, the reported concordance for psoriasis varies from 35 to 72%, and for PsA from 10 to 30%. A variety of HLA associations have been found. The *HLA-Cw*0602* gene is directly associated with psoriasis, particularly familial juvenile-onset (type I) psoriasis. HLA-B27 is associated with psoriatic spondylitis (see below). HLA-DR7, -DQ3, and -B57 are associated with PsA because of linkage disequilibrium with Cw6. Other associations with PsA include HLA-B13, -B37, -B38, -B39, -C12, and -DR4. A recent genome-wide scan found association of both psoriasis and PsA with a polymorphism at the HCP5 locus closely linked to HLA-B, and also to IL-23R, IL-12B (chromosome 5q31), IL-13, and several other chromosomal regions. Certain genetic loci are associated with PsA but not psoriasis, e.g., RUNX3 and IL-13.

PATHOLOGY

The inflamed synovium in PsA resembles that of RA, although with somewhat less hyperplasia and cellularity than in RA. As noted with AS above, the synovial vascular pattern in PsA is generally greater and more tortuous than in RA, independent of disease duration. Some studies have indicated a higher tendency to synovial fibrosis in PsA. Unlike RA, PsA shows prominent enthesitis, with histology similar to that of the other spondyloarthritides.

PATHOGENESIS

PsA is almost certainly immune-mediated and probably shares pathogenic mechanisms with psoriasis. PsA synovium is characterized by lining layer hyperplasia; diffuse infiltration with T cells, B cells, macrophages, and NK receptor–expressing cells, with upregulation of leukocyte homing receptors; and neutrophil proliferation with angiogenesis. Clonally expanded T cell subpopulations are frequent and have been demonstrated both in the synovium and the skin. Plasmacytoid dendritic cells are thought to play a key role in psoriasis, and there is some evidence for their participation in PsA. There is abundant synovial overexpression of proinflammatory cytokines, and synovial tissue staining has identified an overexpression of monocyte-derived cytokines, such as myeloid-related protein (S100A8/A9). Interferon γ, TNF-α, and IL-1β, -2, -6, -8, -10, -12, -13, and -15 are found in PsA synovium or synovial fluid. T_H17-derived cytokines are important in PsA, given the genetic association with genes in the IL-12/IL-23 axis and the therapeutic response to an antibody to the shared IL-12/23 p40 subunit (see below). T_H17 cells have been identified from the dermal extracts of psoriatic lesions and the synovial fluid of PsA patients. The majority of these CD4+ IL-17+ T cells are of memory phenotype (CD4RO[+]CD45RA[–]CD11a[+]). Consistent with the extensive bone remodeling in PsA, patients with PsA have been found to have a marked increase in osteoclastic precursors in peripheral blood and upregulation of receptor activator of nuclear factor κβ ligand (RANKL) in the synovial lining layer. Increased serum levels of TNF-α, RANKL, leptin, and omentin positively correlate with these osteoclastic precursors.

CLINICAL FEATURES

In 60–70% of cases, psoriasis precedes joint disease. In 15–20% of cases, the two manifestations appear within 1 year of each other. In about 15–20% of cases, the arthritis precedes the onset of psoriasis and can present a diagnostic challenge. The frequency in men and women is almost equal, although the frequency of disease patterns differs somewhat in the two sexes. The disease can begin in childhood or late in life but typically begins in the fourth or fifth decade, at an average age of 37 years.

The spectrum of arthropathy associated with psoriasis is quite broad. Many classification schemes have been proposed. In the original scheme of Wright and Moll, five patterns are described: (1) arthritis of the DIP joints; (2) asymmetric oligoarthritis; (3) symmetric polyarthritis similar to RA; (4) axial involvement (spine and sacroiliac joints); and (5) arthritis mutilans, a highly destructive form of disease. These patterns frequently coexist, and the pattern that persists chronically often differs from that of the initial presentation. A simpler scheme in recent use contains three patterns: oligoarthritis, polyarthritis, and axial arthritis.

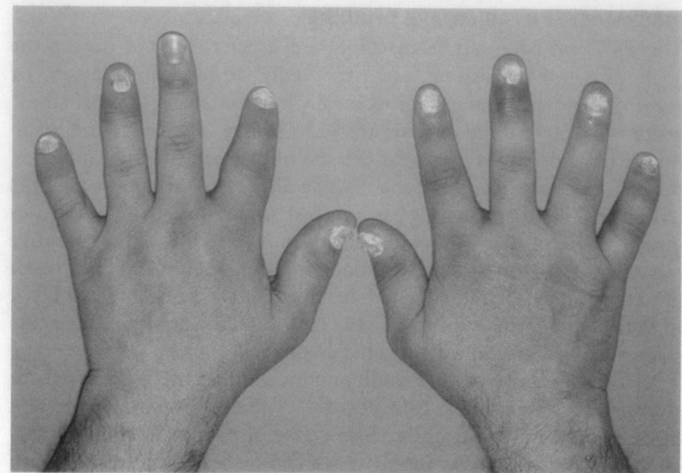

FIGURE 384-3 Characteristic lesions of psoriatic arthritis. Inflammation is prominent in the distal interphalangeal joints (left 5th, 4th, 2nd; right 2nd, 3rd, and 5th) and proximal interphalangeal joints (left 2nd, right 2nd, 4th, and 5th). There is dactylitis in the left 2nd finger and thumb, with pronounced telescoping of the left 2nd finger. Nail dystrophy (hyperkeratosis and onycholysis) affects each of the fingers except the left 3rd finger, the only finger without arthritis. *(Courtesy of Donald Raddatz, MD; with permission.)*

Nail changes in the fingers or toes occur in up to 90% of patients with PsA, compared with 40% of psoriatic patients without arthritis, and pustular psoriasis is said to be associated with more severe arthritis. Several articular features distinguish PsA from other joint disorders; such hallmark features include dactylitis and enthesitis. Dactylitis occurs in >30%; enthesitis and tenosynovitis are also common and are probably present in most patients, although often not appreciated on physical examination. Shortening of digits because of underlying osteolysis is particularly characteristic of PsA (Fig. 384-3), and there is a much greater tendency than in RA for both fibrous and bony ankylosis of small joints. Rapid ankylosis of one or more proximal interphalangeal (PIP) joints early in the course of disease is not uncommon. Back and neck pain and stiffness are also common in PsA.

Arthropathy confined to the DIP joints occurs in about 5% of cases. Accompanying nail changes in the affected digits are almost always present. These joints are also often affected in the other patterns of PsA. Approximately 30% of patients have asymmetric oligoarthritis. This pattern commonly involves a knee or another large joint with a few small joints in the fingers or toes, often with dactylitis. Symmetric polyarthritis occurs in about 40% of PsA patients at presentation. It may be indistinguishable from RA in terms of the joints involved, but other features characteristic of PsA are usually also present. Almost any peripheral joint can be involved. Axial arthropathy without peripheral involvement is found in about 5% of PsA patients. It may be clinically indistinguishable from idiopathic AS, although more neck involvement and less thoracolumbar spinal involvement are characteristic, and nail changes are not found in idiopathic AS. A small percentage of PsA patients have arthritis mutilans, in which there can be widespread shortening of digits ("telescoping"), sometimes coexisting with ankylosis and contractures in other digits.

Six patterns of nail involvement are identified: pitting, horizontal ridging, onycholysis, yellowish discoloration of the nail margins, dystrophic hyperkeratosis, and combinations of these findings. Other extraarticular manifestations of the spondyloarthritides are common. Eye involvement, either conjunctivitis or uveitis, is reported in 7–33% of PsA patients. Unlike the uveitis associated with AS, the uveitis in PsA is more often bilateral, chronic, and/or posterior. Aortic valve insufficiency has been found in <4% of patients, usually after longstanding disease.

Widely varying estimates of clinical outcome have been reported in PsA. At its worst, severe PsA with arthritis mutilans is potentially at least as crippling and ultimately fatal as severe RA. Unlike RA, however, many patients with PsA experience temporary remissions. Overall, erosive disease develops in the majority of patients, progressive disease with deformity and disability is common, and in some large published series, mortality was found to be significantly increased compared with the general population. There appears to be a greater incidence of cardiovascular death in psoriatic disease.

The psoriasis and associated arthropathy seen with HIV infection both tend to be severe and can occur in populations with very little psoriasis in noninfected individuals. Severe enthesopathy, dactylitis, and rapidly progressive joint destruction are seen, but axial involvement is very rare. This condition is prevented by or responds well to antiretroviral therapy.

LABORATORY AND RADIOGRAPHIC FINDINGS

There are no laboratory tests diagnostic of PsA. ESR and CRP are often elevated. A small percentage of patients may have low titers of rheumatoid factor or antinuclear antibodies. About 10% of patients have anti-CCP antibodies. Uric acid may be elevated in the presence of extensive psoriasis. HLA-B27 is found in 50–70% of patients with axial disease, but in ≤20% of patients with only peripheral joint involvement.

The peripheral and axial arthropathies in PsA show a number of radiographic features that distinguish them from RA and AS, respectively. Characteristics of peripheral PsA include DIP involvement, including the classic "pencil-in-cup" deformity; marginal erosions with adjacent bony proliferation ("whiskering"); small-joint ankylosis; osteolysis of phalangeal and metacarpal bone, with telescoping of digits; and periostitis and proliferative new bone at sites of enthesitis. Characteristics of axial PsA include asymmetric sacroiliitis. When compared with idiopathic AS, axial PsA manifests less zygapophyseal joint arthritis; nonmarginal, bulky, "comma"-shaped syndesmophytes that tend to be fewer and less symmetric and delicate than the marginal syndesmophytes of AS; fluffy hyperperiostosis on anterior vertebral bodies; severe cervical spine involvement, with a tendency to atlantoaxial subluxation but relative sparing of the thoracolumbar spine; and paravertebral ossification. Ultrasound and MRI both readily demonstrate enthesitis and tendon sheath effusions that can be difficult to assess on physical examination. A recent MRI study of 68 PsA patients found sacroiliitis in 35%, unrelated to B27 but correlated with restricted spinal movement.

DIAGNOSIS

Classification criteria for PsA were published in 2006 (Classification of Psoriatic Arthritis [CASPAR] criteria) that have been widely accepted (Table 384-2). The sensitivity and specificity of these criteria exceed 90%, and they are useful for early diagnosis. The criteria are based on the history, presence of psoriasis, characteristic peripheral or spinal joint symptoms, signs, and imaging. Diagnosis can be challenging when the arthritis precedes psoriasis, the psoriasis is undiagnosed or obscure, or the joint involvement closely resembles another form of arthritis. A high index of suspicion is needed in any patient with an undiagnosed inflammatory arthropathy. The history should include inquiry about psoriasis in the patient and family members. Patients should be asked to disrobe for the physical examination, and psoriasiform lesions should be sought in the scalp, ears, umbilicus, and gluteal folds in addition to more accessible sites; the finger and toe nails should also be carefully examined. Axial symptoms or signs, dactylitis, enthesitis, ankylosis, the pattern of joint involvement, and characteristic radiographic changes can be helpful clues. The differential diagnosis includes all other forms of arthritis, which can occur coincidentally in individuals with psoriasis. The differential diagnosis of isolated DIP involvement is short. Osteoarthritis (Heberden's nodes) is usually not inflammatory; gout involving more than one DIP joint often involves other sites and may be accompanied by tophi; the very rare entity multicentric reticulohistiocytosis involves other joints and has characteristic small pearly periungual skin nodules; and the uncommon entity inflammatory osteoarthritis, like the others, lacks the nail changes of PsA. Radiography can be helpful in all of these cases and in distinguishing between psoriatic spondylitis and idiopathic AS. A history of trauma to an affected joint preceding the onset of arthritis is said to occur more frequently in PsA than in other types of arthritis, perhaps reflecting the Koebner phenomenon in which psoriatic skin lesions can arise at sites of the skin trauma.

TABLE 384-2 THE CASPAR (*CLASSIFICATION CRITERIA FOR PSORIATIC ARTHRITIS*) CRITERIA[a]

To meet the CASPAR criteria, a patient must have inflammatory articular disease (joint, spine, or entheseal) with ≥3 points from any of the following five categories:

1. Evidence of current psoriasis,[b,c] a personal history of psoriasis, or a family history of psoriasis[d]
2. Typical psoriatic nail dystrophy[e] observed on current physical examination
3. A negative test result for rheumatoid factor
4. Either current dactylitis[f] or a history of dactylitis recorded by a rheumatologist
5. Radiographic evidence of juxtaarticular new bone formation[g] in the hand or foot

[a]Specificity of 99% and sensitivity of 91%. [b]Current psoriasis is assigned 2 points; all other features are assigned 1 point. [c]Psoriatic skin or scalp disease present at the time of examination, as judged by a rheumatologist or dermatologist. [d]History of psoriasis in a first- or second-degree relative. [e]Onycholysis, pitting, or hyperkeratosis. [f]Swelling of an entire digit. [g]Ill-defined ossification near joint margins, excluding osteophyte formation.

Source: From W Taylor et al: Arthritis Rheum, 54:2665, 2006.

TREATMENT PSORIATIC ARTHRITIS

Ideally, coordinated therapy is directed at both the skin and joints in PsA. As described above for AS, use of the anti-TNF-α agents has revolutionized the treatment of PsA. Prompt and dramatic resolution of both arthritis and skin lesions has been observed in large, randomized controlled trials of etanercept, infliximab, adalimumab, and golimumab. Many of the responding patients had long-standing disease that was resistant to all previous therapy, as well as extensive skin disease. The clinical response is often more dramatic than in RA, and delay of disease progression has been demonstrated radiographically. The potential additive effect of methotrexate to anti-TNF-α agents in PsA remains uncertain. As noted above, anti-TNF therapy, paradoxically, has been reported to trigger exacerbation or de novo appearance of psoriasis, typically the palmoplantar pustular variety. In some cases, the therapy can nevertheless be continued.

Ustekinumab, a monoclonal antibody to the shared IL-23/IL-12p40 subunit, is an efficacious treatment for psoriasis and has shown promise in PsA in clinical trials. Other newer drugs that have shown efficacy for both psoriasis and PsA include the anti-IL-17 pathway agents, such as secukinumab and brodalumab, and an oral phosphodiesterase-4 inhibitor, apremilast. Data on the oral Jak inhibitor, tofacitinib, has been very limited but promising.

Other treatment for PsA has been based on drugs that have efficacy in RA and/or in psoriasis. Until recently, controlled clinical trial data on methotrexate in doses of 15–25 mg/week and sulfasalazine (usually given in doses of 2–3 g/d) suggesting clinical efficacy have been somewhat limited, but neither regimen effectively halts progression of erosive joint disease. A recent double-blind trial assessing methotrexate 15 mg weekly in PsA demonstrated no benefit to the joint-based inflammation, but improvement was seen in patient and assessor global scores and skin scores. Other agents with efficacy in psoriasis reported to benefit PsA are cyclosporine, retinoic acid derivatives, and psoralens plus ultraviolet A light (PUVA). There is controversy regarding the efficacy in PsA of gold and antimalarials, which have been widely used in RA. The pyrimidine synthetase inhibitor leflunomide has been shown in a randomized controlled trial to be beneficial in both psoriasis and PsA.

All of these treatments require careful monitoring. Immunosuppressive therapy may be used cautiously in HIV-associated PsA if the HIV infection is well controlled.

UNDIFFERENTIATED AND JUVENILE-ONSET SPONDYLOARTHRITIS

Many patients, usually young adults, present with some features of one or more of the spondyloarthritides discussed above. Until recently, these patients were said to have *undifferentiated spondyloarthritis*, or simply *spondyloarthritis*, as defined by the 1991 European Spondyloarthropathy Study Group criteria. For example, a patient may present with inflammatory synovitis of one knee, Achilles tendinitis, and dactylitis of one digit. Some of these patients may have ReA in which the triggering infection remains clinically silent. In some other cases, the patient subsequently develops IBD or psoriasis, or the process eventually meets criteria for AS. This diagnosis of undifferentiated SpA was also commonly applied to patients with inflammatory back pain, who did meet modified New York criteria for AS. Most of these would now be classified under the new category of axial SpA (Table 384-1).

Comparable to the classification criteria for axial symptoms, the ASAS has recently formulated criteria for peripheral SpA. This is intended to exclude patients with axial symptoms and thus to divide the universe of patients with SpA into axial and exclusively peripheral subsets. These criteria are shown in Table 384-3.

Approximately one-half of the patients with undifferentiated SpA are HLA-B27-positive, and thus the absence of B27 is not useful in establishing or excluding the diagnosis. In familial cases, which are much more frequently B27-positive, there is often eventual progression to classical AS.

In juvenile-onset SpA, which begins between ages 7 and 16, most commonly in boys (60–80%), an asymmetric, predominantly lower-extremity oligoarthritis and enthesitis without extraarticular features is the typical mode of presentation. The prevalence of B27 in this condition, which has been termed the *seronegative enthesopathy and arthropathy (SEA) syndrome*, is approximately 80%. Many, but not all, of these patients go on to develop AS in late adolescence or adulthood.

Management of undifferentiated SpA is similar to that of the other spondyloarthritides. Response to anti-TNF-α therapy has been documented, and this therapy is indicated in severe, persistent cases not responsive to other treatment.

Current pediatric textbooks and journals should be consulted for information on management of juvenile-onset SpA.

ENTEROPATHIC ARTHRITIS

HISTORIC BACKGROUND

A relationship between arthritis and IBD was observed in the 1930s. The relationship was further defined by the epidemiologic studies in the 1950s and 1960s and included in the concept of the spondyloarthritides in the 1970s.

TABLE 384-3 ASAS CRITERIA FOR PERIPHERAL SPONDYLOARTHRITIS[a]

Arthritis[b]	*or*	Enthesitis
	plus	
One or more of the following:		
• Uveitis		
• Psoriasis		
• Crohn's disease or ulcerative colitis		
OR two or more of the following:		
• Arthritis		
• Enthesitis		
• Dactylitis		
• Inflammatory back pain ever		
• Family history for SpA		

[a]Sensitivity 79.5%, specificity 83.3% [b]Peripheral arthritis, usually predominantly lower limb and/or asymmetric.

Source: M Rudawaleit et al: Ann Rheum Dis 70:25, 2011.

EPIDEMIOLOGY

Both of the common forms of IBD, ulcerative colitis (UC) and Crohn's disease (CD) (Chap. 351), are associated with SpA. UC and CD both have an estimated prevalence of 0.05–0.1%, and the incidence of each is thought to have increased in recent decades. AS and peripheral arthritis are both associated with UC and CD. Wide variations have been reported in the estimated frequencies of these associations. In recent series, AS was diagnosed in 1–10%, and peripheral arthritis in 10–50% of patients with IBD. Inflammatory back pain and enthesopathy are common, and many patients have sacroiliitis on imaging studies.

The prevalence of UC or CD in patients with AS is thought to be 5–10%. However, investigation of unselected SpA patients by ileocolonoscopy has revealed that from one-third to two-thirds of patients with AS have subclinical intestinal inflammation that is evident either macroscopically or histologically. These lesions have also been found in patients with undifferentiated SpA or ReA (both enterically and urogenitally acquired).

Both UC and CD have a tendency to familial aggregation, more so for CD. HLA associations have been weak and inconsistent. HLA-B27 is found in up to 70% of patients with IBD and AS, but in ≤15% of patients with IBD and peripheral arthritis or IBD alone. Three alleles of the *NOD2/CARD15* gene on chromosome 16 have been found in approximately one-half of patients with CD. These alleles are not associated with the spondyloarthritides per se. However, they are found significantly more often in (1) CD patients with sacroiliitis than in those without sacroiliitis, and (2) SpA patients with chronic inflammatory gut lesions than in those with normal gut histology. These associations are independent of HLA-B27. In addition to *NOD2*, over 100 other genes have been found to be associated with CD, UC, or both. Around 20 of these are also associated with AS.

PATHOLOGY

Available data for IBD-associated peripheral arthritis suggest a synovial histology similar to other spondyloarthritides. Association with arthropathy does not affect the gut histology of UC or CD (Chap. 351). The subclinical inflammatory lesions in the colon and distal ileum associated with SpA have been classified as either acute or chronic. The former resemble acute bacterial enteritis, with largely intact architecture and neutrophilic infiltration in the lamina propria. The latter resemble the lesions of CD, with distortion of villi and crypts, aphthoid ulceration, and mononuclear cell infiltration in the lamina propria.

PATHOGENESIS

Both IBD and SpA are immune-mediated, but the specific pathogenic mechanisms are poorly understood, and the connection between the two is obscure. The shared genetics evidently reflects shared pathogenic mechanisms. A number of rodent models showing various immune perturbations manifest both IBD and arthritis. Several lines of evidence indicate trafficking of leukocytes between the gut and the joint. Mucosal leukocytes from IBD patients have been shown to bind avidly to synovial vasculature through several different adhesion molecules. Macrophages expressing CD163 are prominent in the inflammatory lesions of both gut and synovium in the spondyloarthritides.

CLINICAL FEATURES

AS associated with IBD is clinically indistinguishable from idiopathic AS. It runs a course independent of the bowel disease, and in some patients, it precedes the onset of IBD, sometimes by many years. Peripheral arthritis may also begin before onset of overt bowel disease. The spectrum of peripheral arthritis includes acute self-limited attacks of oligoarthritis that often coincide with relapses of IBD, and more chronic and symmetric polyarticular arthritis that runs a course independent of IBD activity. The patterns of joint involvement are similar in UC and CD. In general, erosions and deformities are infrequent in IBD-associated peripheral arthritis, and joint surgery is infrequently required. Isolated destructive hip arthritis is a rare complication of CD, apparently distinct from osteonecrosis and septic arthritis. Dactylitis and enthesopathy are occasionally found. In addition to the ~20% of IBD patients with SpA, a comparable percentage have arthralgias or fibromyalgia symptoms.

Other extraintestinal manifestations of IBD are seen in addition to arthropathy, including uveitis, pyoderma gangrenosum, erythema nodosum, and finger clubbing, all somewhat more commonly in CD than UC. The uveitis shares the features described above for PsA-associated uveitis.

LABORATORY AND RADIOGRAPHIC FINDINGS

Laboratory findings reflect the inflammatory and metabolic manifestations of IBD. Joint fluid is usually at least mildly inflammatory. Of patients with AS and IBD, 30–70% carry the HLA-B27 gene, compared with >85% of patients with AS alone and 50–70% of those with AS and psoriasis. Hence, definite or probable AS in a B27-negative individual in the absence of psoriasis should prompt a search for occult IBD. Radiographic changes in the axial skeleton are the same as in uncomplicated AS. Erosions are uncommon in peripheral arthritis but may occur, particularly in the metatarsophalangeal joints. Isolated destructive hip disease has been described.

DIAGNOSIS

Diarrhea and arthritis are both common conditions that can coexist for a variety of reasons. When etiopathogenically related, ReA and IBD-associated arthritis are the most common causes. Rare causes include celiac disease, blind loop syndromes, and Whipple's disease. In most cases, diagnosis depends on investigation of the bowel disease.

TREATMENT ENTEROPATHIC ARTHRITIS

Treatment of CD has been improved by therapy with anti-TNF agents. Infliximab, adalimumab, and certolizumab pegol are effective for induction and maintenance of clinical remission in CD, and infliximab has been shown to be effective in fistulizing CD. IBD-associated arthritis also responds to these agents. Other treatment for IBD, including sulfasalazine and related drugs, systemic glucocorticoids, and immunosuppressive drugs, is also usually of benefit for associated peripheral arthritis. NSAIDs are generally helpful and well tolerated, but they can precipitate flares of IBD. As noted above for psoriasis, rare cases of IBD, either CD or UC, have apparently been precipitated by anti-TNF therapy, usually etanercept, given for any of several rheumatic diseases.

SAPHO SYNDROME

The syndrome of synovitis, acne, pustulosis, hyperostosis, and osteitis (SAPHO) is characterized by a variety of skin and musculoskeletal manifestations. Dermatologic manifestations include palmoplantar pustulosis, acne conglobata, acne fulminans, and hidradenitis suppurativa. The main musculoskeletal findings are sternoclavicular and spinal hyperostosis, chronic recurrent foci of sterile osteomyelitis, and axial or peripheral arthritis. Cases with one or a few manifestations are probably the rule. The ESR is usually elevated, sometimes dramatically. In some cases, bacteria, most often *Propionibacterium acnes*, have been cultured from bone biopsy specimens and occasionally other sites. IBD was coexistent in 8% of patients in one large series. B27 is not associated. Either bone scan or computed tomography scan is helpful diagnostically. An MRI report described characteristic vertebral body corner cortical erosions in 12 of 12 patients. High-dose NSAIDs may provide relief from bone pain. A number of uncontrolled series and case reports describe successful therapy with pamidronate or other bisphosphonates. Response to anti-TNF-α therapy has also been observed, although in a few cases this has been associated with a flare of skin manifestations. Successful prolonged antibiotic therapy has also been reported. Recent reports suggest a possible autoinflammatory pathogenesis and successful treatment with the IL-1 receptor antagonist anakinra.

385 The Vasculitis Syndromes

Carol A. Langford, Anthony S. Fauci

DEFINITION

Vasculitis is a clinicopathologic process characterized by inflammation of and damage to blood vessels. The vessel lumen is usually compromised, and this is associated with ischemia of the tissues supplied by the involved vessel. A broad and heterogeneous group of syndromes may result from this process, since any type, size, and location of blood vessel may be involved. Vasculitis and its consequences may be the primary or sole manifestation of a disease; alternatively, vasculitis may be a secondary component of another disease. Vasculitis may be confined to a single organ, such as the skin, or it may simultaneously involve several organ systems.

CLASSIFICATION

A major feature of the vasculitic syndromes as a group is the fact that there is a great deal of heterogeneity at the same time as there is considerable overlap among them. This heterogeneity and overlap in addition to a lack of understanding of the pathogenesis of these syndromes have been major impediments to the development of a coherent classification system for these diseases. Table 385-1 lists the major vasculitis syndromes. The distinguishing and overlapping features of these syndromes are discussed below.

PATHOPHYSIOLOGY AND PATHOGENESIS

Generally, most of the vasculitic syndromes are assumed to be mediated at least in part by immunopathogenic mechanisms that occur in response to certain antigenic stimuli. However, evidence supporting this hypothesis is for the most part indirect and may reflect epiphenomena as opposed to true causality. Furthermore, it is unknown why some individuals might develop vasculitis in response to certain antigenic stimuli, whereas others do not. It is likely that a number of factors are involved in the ultimate expression of a vasculitic syndrome. These include the genetic predisposition, environmental exposures, and the regulatory mechanisms associated with immune response to certain antigens. Although immune complex formation, antineutrophil cytoplasmic antibodies (ANCA), and pathogenic T lymphocyte responses (Table 385-2) have been among the prominent hypothesized

TABLE 385-1 VASCULITIS SYNDROMES

Primary Vasculitis Syndromes	Secondary Vasculitis Syndromes
Granulomatosis with polyangiitis (Wegener's)	Vasculitis associated with probable etiology
Microscopic polyangiitis	Drug-induced vasculitis
Eosinophilic granulomatosis with polyangiitis (Churg-Strauss)	Hepatitis C virus–associated cryoglobulinemic vasculitis
IgA vasculitis (Henoch-Schönlein)	Hepatitis B virus–associated vasculitis
Cryoglobulinemic vasculitis	Cancer-associated vasculitis
Polyarteritis nodosa	Vasculitis associated with systemic disease
Kawasaki disease	Lupus vasculitis
Giant cell arteritis	Rheumatoid vasculitis
Takayasu arteritis	Sarcoid vasculitis
Behçet's disease	
Cogan's syndrome	
Single-organ vasculitis	
Cutaneous leukocytoclastic angiitis	
Cutaneous arteritis	
Primary central nervous system vasculitis	
Isolated aortitis	

Source: Adapted from JC Jennette et al: Arthritis Rheum 65:1, 2013.

TABLE 385-2 POTENTIAL MECHANISMS OF VESSEL DAMAGE IN VASCULITIS SYNDROMES

Pathogenic immune-complex formation and/or deposition
IgA vasculitis (Henoch-Schönlein)
Lupus vasculitis
Serum sickness and cutaneous vasculitis syndromes
Hepatitis C virus–associated cryoglobulinemic vasculitis
Hepatitis B virus–associated vasculitis
Production of antineutrophilic cytoplasmic antibodies
Granulomatosis with polyangiitis (Wegener's)
Microscopic polyangiitis
Eosinophilic granulomatosis with polyangiitis (Churg-Strauss)
Pathogenic T lymphocyte responses and granuloma formation
Giant cell arteritis
Takayasu arteritis
Granulomatosis with polyangiitis (Wegener's)
Eosinophilic granulomatosis with polyangiitis (Churg-Strauss)

Source: Adapted from MC Sneller, AS Fauci: Med Clin North Am 81:221, 1997.

mechanisms, it is likely that the pathogenesis of individual forms of vasculitis is complex and varied.

PATHOGENIC IMMUNE-COMPLEX FORMATION

Deposition of immune complexes was the first and most widely accepted pathogenic mechanism of vasculitis. However, the causal role of immune complexes has not been clearly established in most of the vasculitic syndromes. Circulating immune complexes need not result in deposition of the complexes in blood vessels with ensuing vasculitis, and many patients with active vasculitis do not have demonstrable circulating or deposited immune complexes. The actual antigen contained in the immune complex has only rarely been identified in vasculitic syndromes. In this regard, hepatitis B antigen has been identified in both the circulating and deposited immune complexes in a subset of patients who have features of a systemic vasculitis, most notably in polyarteritis nodosa (see "Polyarteritis Nodosa"). Cryoglobulinemic vasculitis is strongly associated with hepatitis C virus infection; hepatitis C virions and hepatitis C virus antigen-antibody complexes have been identified in the cryoprecipitates of these patients (see "Cryoglobulinemic Vasculitis").

The mechanisms of tissue damage in immune complex–mediated vasculitis resemble those described for serum sickness. In this model, antigen-antibody complexes are formed in antigen excess and are deposited in vessel walls whose permeability has been increased by vasoactive amines such as histamine, bradykinin, and leukotrienes released from platelets or from mast cells as a result of IgE-triggered mechanisms. The deposition of complexes results in activation of complement components, particularly C5a, which is strongly chemotactic for neutrophils. These cells then infiltrate the vessel wall, phagocytose the immune complexes, and release their intracytoplasmic enzymes, which damage the vessel wall. As the process becomes subacute or chronic, mononuclear cells infiltrate the vessel wall. The common denominator of the resulting syndrome is compromise of the vessel lumen with ischemic changes in the tissues supplied by the involved vessel. Several variables may explain why only certain types of immune complexes cause vasculitis and why only certain vessels are affected in individual patients. These include the ability of the reticuloendothelial system to clear circulating complexes from the blood, the size and physicochemical properties of immune complexes, the relative degree of turbulence of blood flow, the intravascular hydrostatic pressure in different vessels, and the preexisting integrity of the vessel endothelium.

ANTINEUTROPHIL CYTOPLASMIC ANTIBODIES (ANCA)

ANCA are antibodies directed against certain proteins in the cytoplasmic granules of neutrophils and monocytes. These autoantibodies are present in a high percentage of patients with active granulomatosis with polyangiitis (Wegener's) and microscopic polyangiitis, and in a lower percentage of patients with eosinophilic granulomatosis with polyangiitis (Churg-Strauss). Because these diseases share the presence of ANCA and small-vessel vasculitis, some investigators have come to refer to them collectively as "ANCA-associated vasculitis." However, as these diseases possess unique clinical phenotypes in which ANCA may be absent, it remains our opinion that granulomatosis with polyangiitis (Wegener's), microscopic polyangiitis, and eosinophilic granulomatosis with polyangiitis (Churg-Strauss) should continue to be viewed as separate entities.

There are two major categories of ANCA based on different targets for the antibodies. The terminology of *cytoplasmic ANCA* (cANCA) refers to the diffuse, granular cytoplasmic staining pattern observed by immunofluorescence microscopy when serum antibodies bind to indicator neutrophils. Proteinase-3, a 29-kDa neutral serine proteinase present in neutrophil azurophilic granules, is the major cANCA antigen. More than 90% of patients with typical active granulomatosis with polyangiitis (Wegener's) have detectable antibodies to proteinase-3 (see below). The terminology of *perinuclear ANCA* (pANCA) refers to the more localized perinuclear or nuclear staining pattern of the indicator neutrophils. The major target for pANCA is the enzyme myeloperoxidase; other targets that can produce a pANCA pattern of staining include elastase, cathepsin G, lactoferrin, lysozyme, and bactericidal/permeability-increasing protein. However, only antibodies to myeloperoxidase have been convincingly associated with vasculitis. Antimyeloperoxidase antibodies have been reported to occur in variable percentages of patients with microscopic polyangiitis, eosinophilic granulomatosis with polyangiitis (Churg-Strauss), isolated necrotizing crescentic glomerulonephritis, and granulomatosis with polyangiitis (Wegener's) (see below). A pANCA pattern of staining that is not due to antimyeloperoxidase antibodies has been associated with nonvasculitic entities such as rheumatic and nonrheumatic autoimmune diseases, inflammatory bowel disease, certain drugs, and infections such as endocarditis and bacterial airway infections in patients with cystic fibrosis.

It is unclear why patients with these vasculitis syndromes develop antibodies to myeloperoxidase or proteinase-3 or what role these antibodies play in disease pathogenesis. There are a number of in vitro observations that suggest possible mechanisms whereby these antibodies can contribute to the pathogenesis of the vasculitis syndromes. Proteinase-3 and myeloperoxidase reside in the azurophilic granules and lysosomes of resting neutrophils and monocytes, where they are apparently inaccessible to serum antibodies. However, when neutrophils or monocytes are primed by tumor necrosis factor α (TNF-α) or interleukin 1 (IL-1), proteinase-3 and myeloperoxidase translocate to the cell membrane, where they can interact with extracellular ANCA. The neutrophils then degranulate and produce reactive oxygen species that can cause tissue damage. Furthermore, ANCA-activated neutrophils can adhere to and kill endothelial cells in vitro. Activation of neutrophils and monocytes by ANCA also induces the release of proinflammatory cytokines such as IL-1 and IL-8. Adoptive transfer experiments in genetically engineered mice provide further evidence for a direct pathogenic role of ANCA in vivo. In contradiction, however, a number of clinical and laboratory observations argue against a primary pathogenic role for ANCA. Patients may have active granulomatosis with polyangiitis (Wegener's) in the absence of ANCA; the absolute height of the antibody titers does not correlate well with disease activity; and patients with granulomatosis with polyangiitis (Wegener's) in remission may continue to have high antiproteinase-3 (cANCA) titers for years (see below).

PATHOGENIC T LYMPHOCYTE RESPONSES AND GRANULOMA FORMATION

The histopathologic feature of granulomatous vasculitis has provided evidence to support a role of pathogenic T lymphocyte responses and cell-mediated immune injury. Vascular endothelial cells can express HLA class II molecules following activation by cytokines such as interferon (IFN) γ. This allows these cells to participate in immunologic reactions such as interaction with CD4+ T lymphocytes in a manner similar to antigen-presenting macrophages. Endothelial cells can secrete IL-1, which may activate T lymphocytes and initiate or propagate in situ immunologic processes within the blood vessel. In addition, IL-1 and TNF-α are potent inducers of endothelial-leukocyte adhesion molecule 1 (ELAM-1) and vascular cell adhesion molecule 1 (VCAM-1), which may enhance the adhesion of leukocytes to endothelial cells in the blood vessel wall.

APPROACH TO THE PATIENT: General Principles of Diagnosis

The diagnosis of vasculitis is often considered in any patient with an unexplained systemic illness. However, there are certain clinical abnormalities that when present alone or in combination should suggest a diagnosis of vasculitis. These include palpable purpura, pulmonary infiltrates and microscopic hematuria, chronic inflammatory sinusitis, mononeuritis multiplex, unexplained ischemic events, and glomerulonephritis with evidence of multisystem disease. A number of nonvasculitic diseases may also produce some or all of these abnormalities. Thus, the first step in the workup of a patient with suspected vasculitis is to exclude other diseases that produce clinical manifestations that can mimic vasculitis (Table 385-3). It is particularly important to exclude infectious diseases with features that overlap those of vasculitis, especially if the patient's clinical condition is deteriorating rapidly and empirical immunosuppressive treatment is being contemplated.

Once diseases that mimic vasculitis have been excluded, the workup should follow a series of progressive steps that establish the diagnosis of vasculitis and determine, where possible, the category of the vasculitis syndrome (Fig. 385-1). This approach is of considerable importance since several of the vasculitis syndromes require aggressive therapy with glucocorticoids and other immunosuppressive agents, whereas other syndromes usually resolve spontaneously and require symptomatic treatment only. The definitive diagnosis of vasculitis is usually made based on biopsy of involved tissue. The yield of "blind" biopsies of organs with no subjective or objective evidence of involvement is very low and should be avoided. When syndromes such as polyarteritis nodosa, Takayasu arteritis, or primary central nervous system (CNS) vasculitis are suspected, arteriogram of organs with suspected involvement should be performed.

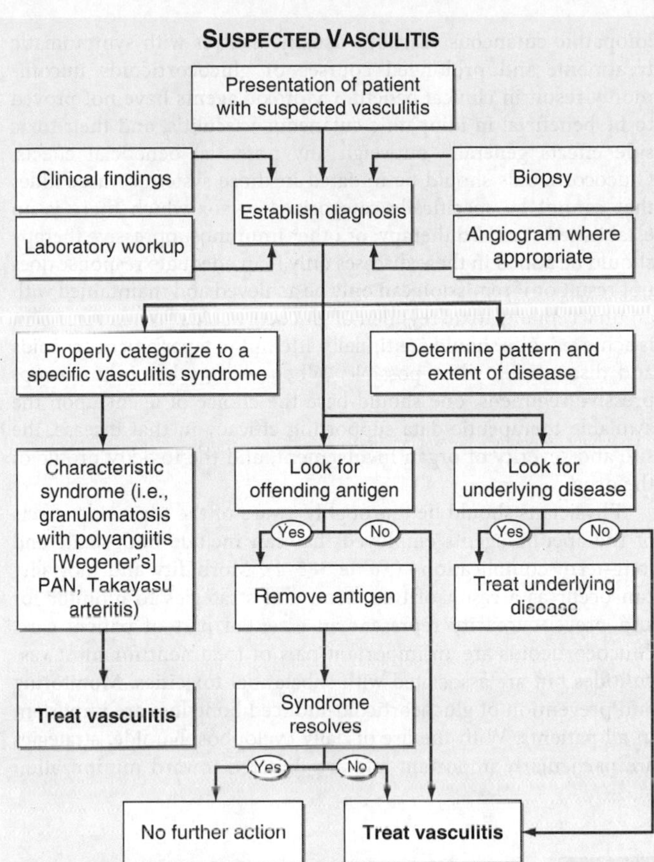

FIGURE 385-1 Algorithm for the approach to a patient with suspected diagnosis of vasculitis. PAN, polyarteritis nodosa.

GENERAL PRINCIPLES OF TREATMENT Once a diagnosis of vasculitis has been established, a decision regarding therapeutic strategy must be made (Fig. 385-1). If an offending antigen that precipitates the vasculitis is recognized, the antigen should be removed where possible. If the vasculitis is associated with an underlying disease such as an infection, neoplasm, or connective tissue disease, the underlying disease should be treated. If the syndrome represents a primary vasculitic disease, treatment should be initiated according to the category of the vasculitis syndrome. Specific therapeutic regimens are discussed below for the individual vasculitis syndromes; however, certain general principles regarding therapy should be considered. Decisions regarding treatment should be based on the use of regimens for which there has been published literature supporting efficacy for that particular vasculitic disease. Since the potential toxic side effects of certain therapeutic regimens may be substantial, the risk-versus-benefit ratio of any therapeutic approach should be weighed carefully. On the one hand, glucocorticoids and/or other immunosuppressive agents should be instituted immediately in diseases where irreversible organ system dysfunction and high morbidity and mortality rates have been clearly established. Granulomatosis with polyangiitis (Wegener's) is the prototype of a severe systemic vasculitis requiring such a therapeutic approach (see below). On the other hand, when feasible, aggressive therapy should be avoided for vasculitic manifestations that rarely result in irreversible organ system dysfunction and that usually do not respond to such therapy. For example, isolated

TABLE 385-3 CONDITIONS THAT CAN MIMIC VASCULITIS

Infectious diseases
Bacterial endocarditis
Disseminated gonococcal infection
Pulmonary histoplasmosis
Coccidioidomycosis
Syphilis
Lyme disease
Rocky Mountain spotted fever
Whipple's disease
Coagulopathies/thrombotic microangiopathies
Antiphospholipid syndrome
Thrombotic thrombocytopenic purpura
Neoplasms
Atrial myxoma
Lymphoma
Carcinomatosis
Drug toxicity
Cocaine
Levamisole
Amphetamines
Ergot alkaloids
Methysergide
Arsenic
Sarcoidosis
Atheroembolic disease
Antiglomerular basement membrane disease (Goodpasture's syndrome)
Amyloidosis
Migraine
Reversible cerebral vasoconstrictive syndrome

idiopathic cutaneous vasculitis usually resolves with symptomatic treatment, and prolonged courses of glucocorticoids uncommonly result in clinical benefit. Cytotoxic agents have not proved to be beneficial in idiopathic cutaneous vasculitis, and their toxic side effects generally outweigh any potential beneficial effects. Glucocorticoids should be initiated in those systemic vasculitides that cannot be specifically categorized or for which there is no established standard therapy; or other immunosuppressive therapy should be added in these diseases only if an adequate response does not result or if remission can only be achieved and maintained with an unacceptably toxic regimen of glucocorticoids. When remission is achieved, one should continually attempt to taper glucocorticoids and discontinue when possible. When using other immunosuppressive regimens, one should base the choice of agent upon the available therapeutic data supporting efficacy in that disease, the site and severity of organ involvement, and the toxicity profile of the drug.

Physicians should be thoroughly aware of the toxic side effects of therapeutic agents employed that can include both acute and long-term complications (Table 385-4). Morbidity and mortality can occur as a result of treatment, and strategies to monitor for and prevent toxicity represent an essential part of patient care. Glucocorticoids are an important part of treatment for most vasculitides but are associated with substantial toxicities. Monitoring and prevention of glucocorticoid-induced bone loss are important in all patients. With the use of daily cyclophosphamide, strategies are particularly important and are directed toward minimization of bladder toxicity and prevention of leukopenia. Instructing the patient to take cyclophosphamide all at once in the morning with a large amount of fluid throughout the day in order to maintain a dilute urine can reduce the risk of bladder injury. Bladder cancer can occur several years after discontinuation of cyclophosphamide therapy; therefore, monitoring for bladder cancer should continue indefinitely in patients who have received cyclophosphamide. Bone marrow suppression is an important toxicity of cyclophosphamide and can be observed during glucocorticoid tapering or over time, even after periods of stable measurements. Monitoring of the complete blood count every 1–2 weeks for as long as the patient receives cyclophosphamide can effectively prevent cytopenias. Maintaining the white blood cell (WBC) count at >3000/μL and the neutrophil count at >1500/μL is essential to reduce the risk of life-threatening infections.

Methotrexate and azathioprine are also associated with bone marrow suppression, and complete blood counts should be obtained every 1–2 weeks for the first 1–2 months after their initiation and once a month thereafter. To lessen toxicity, methotrexate is often given together with folic acid, 1 mg daily, or folinic acid, 5–10 mg once a week 24 h following methotrexate. Prior to initiation of azathioprine, thiopurine methyltransferase (TPMT), an enzyme involved in the metabolism of azathioprine, should be assayed because inadequate levels may result in severe cytopenia.

Infection represents a significant toxicity for all vasculitis patients treated with immunosuppressive therapy. Infections with *Pneumocystis jiroveci* and certain fungi can be seen even in the face of WBCs that are within normal limits, particularly in patients receiving glucocorticoids. All vasculitis patients who are receiving daily glucocorticoids in combination with another immunosuppressive agent should receive trimethoprim-sulfamethoxazole (TMP-SMX) or another prophylactic therapy to prevent *P. jiroveci* infection.

Finally, it should be emphasized that each patient is unique and requires individual decision-making. The above outline should serve as a framework to guide therapeutic approaches; however, flexibility should be practiced in order to provide maximal therapeutic efficacy with minimal toxic side effects in each patient.

TABLE 385-4 MAJOR TOXIC SIDE EFFECTS OF DRUGS USED IN THE TREATMENT OF SYSTEMIC VASCULITIS

Glucocorticoids	
Osteoporosis	Growth suppression in children
Cataracts	Hypertension
Glaucoma	Avascular necrosis of bone
Diabetes mellitus	Myopathy
Electrolyte abnormalities	Alterations in mood
Metabolic abnormalities	Psychosis
Suppression of inflammatory and immune responses leading to opportunistic infections	Pseudotumor cerebri Peptic ulcer diathesis Pancreatitis
Cushingoid features	
Cyclophosphamide	
Bone marrow suppression	Hypogammaglobulinemia
Cystitis	Pulmonary fibrosis
Bladder carcinoma	Myelodysplasia
Gonadal suppression	Oncogenesis
Gastrointestinal intolerance	Teratogenicity
	Opportunistic infections
Methotrexate	
Gastrointestinal intolerance	Pneumonitis
Stomatitis	Teratogenicity
Bone marrow suppression	Opportunistic infections
Hepatotoxicity (may lead to fibrosis or cirrhosis)	
Azathioprine	
Gastrointestinal intolerance	Opportunistic infections
Bone marrow suppression	Hypersensitivity
Hepatotoxicity	
Rituximab	
Infusion reactions	Opportunistic infections
Progressive multifocal leukoencephalopathy	Hepatitis B reactivation Tumor lysis syndrome
Mucocutaneous reactions	

GRANULOMATOSIS WITH POLYANGIITIS (WEGENER'S)

DEFINITION

Granulomatosis with polyangiitis (Wegener's) is a distinct clinicopathologic entity characterized by granulomatous vasculitis of the upper and lower respiratory tracts together with glomerulonephritis. In addition, variable degrees of disseminated vasculitis involving both small arteries and veins may occur.

INCIDENCE AND PREVALENCE

Granulomatosis with polyangiitis (Wegener's) is an uncommon disease with an estimated prevalence of 3 per 100,000. It is extremely rare in blacks compared with whites; the male-to-female ratio is 1:1. The disease can be seen at any age; ~15% of patients are <19 years of age, but only rarely does the disease occur before adolescence; the mean age of onset is ~40 years.

PATHOLOGY AND PATHOGENESIS

The histopathologic hallmarks of granulomatosis with polyangiitis (Wegener's) are necrotizing vasculitis of small arteries and veins together with granuloma formation, which may be either intravascular or extravascular (Fig. 385-2). Lung involvement typically appears as multiple, bilateral, nodular cavitary infiltrates (Fig. 385-3), which on biopsy almost invariably reveal the typical necrotizing granulomatous vasculitis. Upper airway lesions, particularly those in the sinuses and nasopharynx, typically reveal inflammation, necrosis, and granuloma formation, with or without vasculitis.

In its earliest form, renal involvement is characterized by a focal and segmental glomerulitis that may evolve into a rapidly progressive

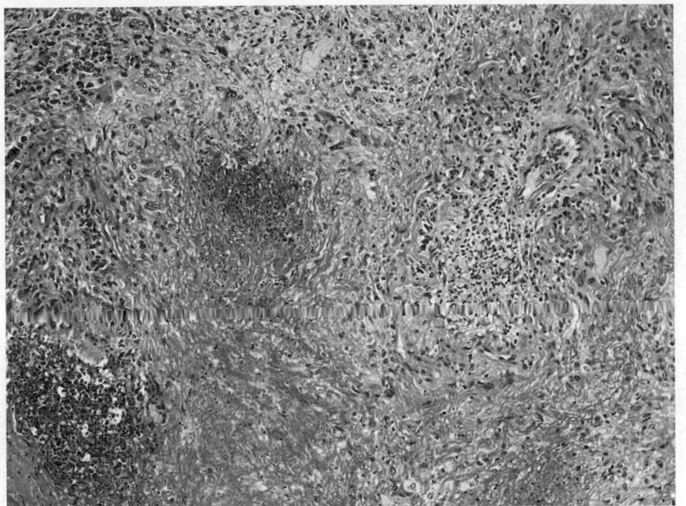

FIGURE 385-2 Lung histology in granulomatosis with polyangiitis (Wegener's). This area of geographic necrosis has a serpiginous border of histiocytes and giant cells surrounding a central necrotic zone. Vasculitis is also present with neutrophils and lymphocytes infiltrating the wall of a small arteriole (*upper right*). *(Courtesy of William D. Travis, MD; with permission.)*

crescentic glomerulonephritis. Granuloma formation is only rarely seen on renal biopsy. In contrast to other forms of glomerulonephritis, evidence of immune complex deposition is not found in the renal lesion of granulomatosis with polyangiitis (Wegener's). In addition to the classic triad of disease of the upper and lower respiratory tracts and kidney, virtually any organ can be involved with vasculitis, granuloma, or both.

The immunopathogenesis of this disease is unclear, although the involvement of upper airways and lungs with granulomatous vasculitis suggests an aberrant cell-mediated immune response to an exogenous or even endogenous antigen that enters through or resides in the upper airway. Chronic nasal carriage of *Staphylococcus aureus* has been reported to be associated with a higher relapse rate of granulomatosis with polyangiitis (Wegener's); however, there is no evidence for a role of this organism in the pathogenesis of the disease.

Peripheral blood mononuclear cells obtained from patients with granulomatosis with polyangiitis (Wegener's) manifest increased secretion of IFN-γ but not of IL-4, IL-5, or IL-10 compared to normal controls. In addition, TNF-α production from peripheral blood mononuclear cells and CD4+ T cells is elevated. Furthermore, monocytes from patients with granulomatosis with polyangiitis (Wegener's) produce increased amounts of IL-12. These findings indicate an unbalanced T_H1-type T cell cytokine pattern in this disease that may have pathogenic and perhaps ultimately therapeutic implications.

A high percentage of patients with granulomatosis with polyangiitis (Wegener's) develop ANCA, and these autoantibodies may play a role in the pathogenesis of this disease (see above).

CLINICAL AND LABORATORY MANIFESTATIONS

Involvement of the upper airways occurs in 95% of patients with granulomatosis with polyangiitis (Wegener's). Patients often present with severe upper respiratory tract findings such as paranasal sinus pain and drainage and purulent or bloody nasal discharge, with or without nasal mucosal ulceration (Table 385-5). Nasal septal perforation may follow, leading to saddle nose deformity. Serous otitis media may occur as a result of eustachian tube blockage. Subglottic tracheal stenosis resulting from active disease or scarring occurs in ~16% of patients and may result in severe airway obstruction.

TABLE 385-5 GRANULOMATOSIS WITH POLYANGIITIS (WEGENER'S): FREQUENCY OF CLINICAL MANIFESTATIONS IN 158 PATIENTS STUDIED AT THE NATIONAL INSTITUTES OF HEALTH

Manifestation	Percentage at Disease Onset	Percentage Throughout Course of Disease
Kidney		
Glomerulonephritis	18	77
Ear/Nose/Throat	73	92
Sinusitis	51	85
Nasal disease	36	68
Otitis media	25	44
Hearing loss	14	42
Subglottic stenosis	1	16
Ear pain	9	14
Oral lesions	3	10
Lung	45	85
Pulmonary infiltrates	25	66
Pulmonary nodules	24	58
Hemoptysis	12	30
Pleuritis	10	28
Eyes		
Conjunctivitis	5	18
Dacryocystitis	1	18
Scleritis	6	16
Proptosis	2	15
Eye pain	3	11
Visual loss	0	8
Retinal lesions	0	4
Corneal lesions	0	1
Iritis	0	2
Other[a]		
Arthralgias/arthritis	32	67
Fever	23	50
Cough	19	46
Skin abnormalities	13	46
Weight loss (>10% body weight)	15	35
Peripheral neuropathy	1	15
Central nervous system disease	1	8
Pericarditis	2	6
Hyperthyroidism	1	3

[a]Fewer than 1% had parotid, pulmonary artery, breast, or lower genitourinary (urethra, cervix, vagina, testicular) involvement.

Source: GS Hoffman et al: Ann Intern Med 116:488, 1992.

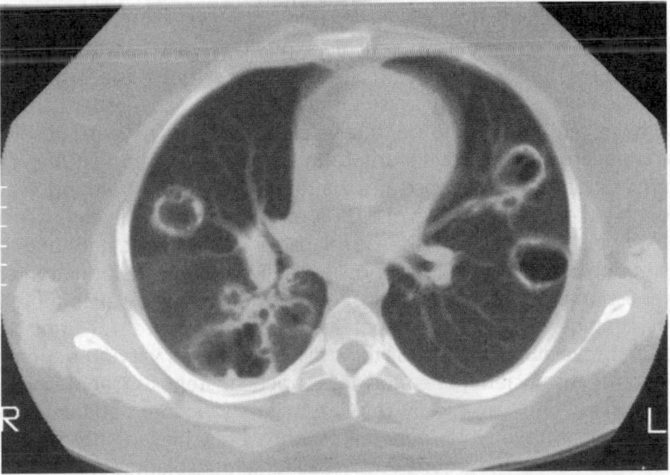

FIGURE 385-3 Computed tomography scan of a patient with granulomatosis with polyangiitis (Wegener's). The patient developed multiple, bilateral, and cavitary infiltrates.

Pulmonary involvement may be manifested as asymptomatic infiltrates or may be clinically expressed as cough, hemoptysis, dyspnea, and chest discomfort. It is present in 85–90% of patients. Endobronchial disease, either in its active form or as a result of fibrous scarring, may lead to obstruction with atelectasis.

Eye involvement (52% of patients) may range from a mild conjunctivitis to dacryocystitis, episcleritis, scleritis, granulomatous sclerouveitis, ciliary vessel vasculitis, and retroorbital mass lesions leading to proptosis.

Skin lesions (46% of patients) appear as papules, vesicles, palpable purpura, ulcers, or subcutaneous nodules; biopsy reveals vasculitis, granuloma, or both. Cardiac involvement (8% of patients) manifests as pericarditis, coronary vasculitis, or, rarely, cardiomyopathy. Nervous system manifestations (23% of patients) include cranial neuritis, mononeuritis multiplex, or, rarely, cerebral vasculitis and/or granuloma.

Renal disease (77% of patients) generally dominates the clinical picture and, if left untreated, accounts directly or indirectly for most of the mortality rate in this disease. Although it may smolder in some cases as a mild glomerulitis with proteinuria, hematuria, and red blood cell casts, it is clear that once clinically detectable renal functional impairment occurs, rapidly progressive renal failure usually ensues unless appropriate treatment is instituted.

While the disease is active, most patients have nonspecific symptoms and signs such as malaise, weakness, arthralgias, anorexia, and weight loss. Fever may indicate activity of the underlying disease but more often reflects secondary infection, usually of the upper airway.

Characteristic laboratory findings include a markedly elevated erythrocyte sedimentation rate (ESR), mild anemia and leukocytosis, mild hypergammaglobulinemia (particularly of the IgA class), and mildly elevated rheumatoid factor. Thrombocytosis may be seen as an acute-phase reactant. Approximately 90% of patients with active granulomatosis with polyangiitis (Wegener's) have a positive antiproteinase-3 ANCA. However, in the absence of active disease, the sensitivity drops to ~60–70%. A small percentage of patients with granulomatosis with polyangiitis (Wegener's) may have antimyeloperoxidase rather than antiproteinase-3 antibodies, and up to 20% may lack ANCA.

Patients with granulomatosis with polyangiitis (Wegener's) have been found to have an increased incidence of venous thrombotic events. Although routine anticoagulation for all patients is not recommended, a heightened awareness for any clinical features suggestive of deep venous thrombosis or pulmonary emboli is warranted.

DIAGNOSIS

The diagnosis of granulomatosis with polyangiitis (Wegener's) is made by the demonstration of necrotizing granulomatous vasculitis on tissue biopsy in a patient with compatible clinical features. Pulmonary tissue offers the highest diagnostic yield, almost invariably revealing granulomatous vasculitis. Biopsy of upper airway tissue usually reveals granulomatous inflammation with necrosis but may not show vasculitis. Renal biopsy can confirm the presence of pauci-immune glomerulonephritis.

The specificity of a positive antiproteinase-3 ANCA for granulomatosis with polyangiitis (Wegener's) is very high, especially if active glomerulonephritis is present. However, the presence of ANCA should be adjunctive and, with rare exceptions, should not substitute for a tissue diagnosis. False-positive ANCA titers have been reported in certain infectious and neoplastic diseases.

In its typical presentation, the clinicopathologic complex of granulomatosis with polyangiitis (Wegener's) usually provides ready differentiation from other disorders. However, if all the typical features are not present at once, it needs to be differentiated from the other vasculitides, antiglomerular basement membrane disease (Goodpasture's syndrome) (Chap. 338), relapsing polychondritis (Chap. 389), tumors of the upper airway or lung, and infectious diseases such as histoplasmosis (Chap. 236), mucocutaneous leishmaniasis (Chap. 251), and rhinoscleroma (Chap. 44) as well as noninfectious granulomatous diseases.

Of particular note is the differentiation from other *midline destructive diseases*. These diseases lead to extreme tissue destruction and mutilation localized to the midline upper airway structures including the sinuses; erosion through the skin of the face commonly occurs, a feature that is extremely rare in granulomatosis with polyangiitis (Wegener's). Although blood vessels may be involved in the intense inflammatory reaction and necrosis, primary vasculitis is not seen. *Upper airway neoplasms* and specifically *extranodal natural killer (NK)/T cell lymphoma (nasal type)* are important causes of midline destructive disease. These lesions are diagnosed based on histology, which reveals polymorphous atypical lymphoid cells with an NK cell immunophenotype, typically Epstein-Barr virus (Chap. 134). Such cases are treated based on their degree of dissemination, and localized lesions have responded to irradiation. Upper airway lesions should never be irradiated in granulomatosis with polyangiitis (Wegener's). Cocaine-induced tissue injury can be another important mimic of granulomatosis with polyangiitis (Wegener's) in patients who present with isolated midline destructive disease. ANCA that target human neutrophil elastase can be found in patients with cocaine-induced midline destructive lesions and can complicate the differentiation from granulomatosis with polyangiitis (Wegener's). This has been further confounded by the high frequency of levamisole adulteration of cocaine, which can result in cutaneous infarction and serologic changes that may mimic vasculitis. Granulocytopenia is a common finding in levamisole-induced disease that would not be associated with granulomatosis with polyangiitis (Wegener's).

Granulomatosis with polyangiitis (Wegener's) must also be differentiated from *lymphomatoid granulomatosis*, which is an Epstein-Barr virus–positive B cell proliferation that is associated with an exuberant T cell reaction. Lymphomatoid granulomatosis is characterized by lung, skin, CNS, and kidney involvement in which atypical lymphocytoid and plasmacytoid cells infiltrate nonlymphoid tissue in an angioinvasive manner. In this regard, it clearly differs from granulomatosis with polyangiitis (Wegener's) in that it is not an inflammatory vasculitis in the classic sense but an angiocentric perivascular infiltration of atypical mononuclear cells. Up to 50% of patients may develop a true malignant lymphoma.

TREATMENT GRANULOMATOSIS WITH POLYANGIITIS (WEGENER'S)

Prior to the introduction of effective therapy, granulomatosis with polyangiitis (Wegener's) was universally fatal within a few months of diagnosis. Glucocorticoids alone led to some symptomatic improvement, with little effect on the ultimate course of the disease. The development of treatment with cyclophosphamide dramatically changed patient outcome such that marked improvement was seen in >90% of patients, complete remission in 75% of patients, and 5-year patient survival was seen in over 80%.

Despite the ability to successfully induce remission, 50–70% of remissions are later associated with one or more relapses. The determination of relapse should be based on objective evidence of disease activity, taking care to rule out other features that may have a similar appearance such as infection, medication toxicity, or chronic disease sequelae. The ANCA titer can be misleading and should not be used to assess disease activity. Many patients who achieve remission continue to have elevated titers for years. Results from a large prospective study found that increases in ANCA were not associated with relapse and that only 43% relapsed within 1 year of an increase in ANCA levels. Thus, a rise in ANCA by itself is not a harbinger of immediate disease relapse and should not lead to reinstitution or increase in immunosuppressive therapy. Reinduction of remission after relapse is almost always achieved; however, a high percentage of patients ultimately have some degree of damage from irreversible features of their disease, such as varying degrees of renal insufficiency, hearing loss, tracheal stenosis, saddle nose deformity, and chronically impaired sinus function. Patients who developed irreversible renal failure but who achieved subsequent remission have undergone successful renal transplantation.

Because long-term cyclophosphamide is associated with substantial toxicity, approaches have been developed that seek to minimize the duration of exposure to cyclophosphamide while still taking advantage of its efficacy for severe disease. Treatment of granulomatosis with polyangiitis (Wegener's) is currently viewed as having two phases: *induction*, where active disease is put into remission, followed by *maintenance*. The decision regarding which agents to use for induction and maintenance is based on disease severity together with individual patient factors that include contraindication, relapse history, and comorbidities.

CYCLOPHOSPHAMIDE INDUCTION FOR SEVERE DISEASE

For patients with severe disease, daily cyclophosphamide combined with glucocorticoids has been repeatedly proved to effectively induce remission and prolong survival. At the initiation of therapy, glucocorticoids are usually given as prednisone, 1 mg/kg per day for the first month, followed by gradual tapering on an alternate-day or daily schedule with discontinuation after ~6–9 months.

Cyclophosphamide is given in doses of 2 mg/kg per day orally, but as it is renally eliminated, dosage reduction should be considered in patients with renal insufficiency. Some reports have indicated therapeutic success with less frequent and severe toxic side effects using IV cyclophosphamide. In a recent randomized trial, IV cyclophosphamide 15 mg/kg, three infusions given every 2 weeks, then every 3 weeks thereafter, was compared to cyclophosphamide 2 mg/kg daily given for 3 months followed by 1.5 mg/kg daily. Although IV cyclophosphamide was found to have a comparable rate of remission with a lower cumulative cyclophosphamide dose and occurrence of leukopenia, the use of a consolidation phase and an insufficient frequency of blood count monitoring may have negatively influenced the results in those who received daily cyclophosphamide. Of note in this study was that relapse occurred in 19% of those who received IV cyclophosphamide as compared to 9% who received daily oral administration. We continue to strongly favor daily cyclophosphamide with utilization of blood count monitoring every 1–2 weeks (as discussed above) and limiting the duration of induction exposure to 3–6 months.

In patients with imminently life-threatening disease, such as rapidly progressive glomerulonephritis with a creatinine greater than 4.0 mg/dL or pulmonary hemorrhage requiring mechanical ventilation, a regimen of daily cyclophosphamide and glucocorticoids is the treatment of choice to induce remission. Adjunctive plasmapheresis was found to further improve renal recovery in a study of patients with rapidly progressive glomerulonephritis who had a creatinine of greater than 5.8 mg/dL.

REMISSION MAINTENANCE AFTER CYCLOPHOSPHAMIDE

After 3–6 months of induction treatment, cyclophosphamide should be stopped and switched to another agent for remission maintenance. The agents with which there has been the greatest published experience are methotrexate and azathioprine. Methotrexate is administered orally or subcutaneously starting at a dosage of 0.3 mg/kg as a single weekly dose, not to exceed 15 mg/week. If the treatment is well tolerated after 1–2 weeks, the dosage should be increased by 2.5 mg weekly up to a dosage of 20–25 mg/week and maintained at that level. Azathioprine, 2 mg/kg per day, has also proved effective in maintaining remission following induction with daily cyclophosphamide. In a randomized trial comparing methotrexate to azathioprine for remission maintenance, comparable rates of toxicity and relapse were seen. Therefore, the choice of agent is often based on toxicity profile, because methotrexate cannot be given to patients with renal insufficiency or chronic liver disease, as well as on other individual patient factors. In patients who are unable to receive methotrexate or azathioprine or who have relapsed through such treatment, mycophenolate mofetil, 1000 mg twice a day, may also sustain remission following cyclophosphamide induction.

The optimal duration of maintenance therapy is uncertain. In the absence of toxicity, maintenance therapy is usually given for a minimum of 2 years past remission, after which time consideration can be given for tapering over a 6–12 month period until discontinuation. Patients with significant organ damage or a history of relapse may benefit from longer-term continuation of a maintenance agent.

RITUXIMAB INDUCTION FOR SEVERE DISEASE

Rituximab is a chimeric monoclonal antibody directed against CD20 present on normal and malignant B lymphocytes that is U.S. Food and Drug Administration (FDA) approved for the treatment of granulomatosis with polyangiitis (Wegener's) and microscopic polyangiitis. In two randomized trials that enrolled ANCA-positive patients with severe active granulomatosis with polyangiitis (Wegener's) or microscopic polyangiitis, rituximab 375 mg/m^2 once a week for 4 weeks in combination with glucocorticoids was found to be as effective as cyclophosphamide with glucocorticoids for inducing disease remission. In the trial, which also enrolled patients with relapsing disease, rituximab was found to be statistically superior to cyclophosphamide.

Although the data support that rituximab is effective for remission induction of severe active granulomatosis with polyangiitis (Wegener's) or microscopic polyangiitis, there remain a number of ongoing questions regarding rituximab that must be considered in weighing its use in the individual patient. The optimal approach to remission maintenance after treatment with rituximab remains unclear, as does whether this should include conventional maintenance agents such as methotrexate or azathioprine versus scheduled retreatment with rituximab. In addition, there are no long-term safety data with rituximab in granulomatosis with polyangiitis (Wegener's) or microscopic polyangiitis.

Although rituximab does not have the bladder toxicity or infertility concerns, as can occur with cyclophosphamide, in both of the randomized trials, the rate of adverse events was similar in the rituximab and cyclophosphamide arms. Serious side effects of rituximab include infusion reactions, severe mucocutaneous reactions, and rare reports of progressive multifocal leukoencephalopathy. Because rituximab can bring about reactivation of hepatitis B, all patients should undergo hepatitis screening prior to treatment with rituximab.

OTHER BIOLOGIC THERAPIES

Etanercept, a dimeric fusion protein containing the 75-kDa TNF receptor bound to human IgG1, was not found to sustain remission when used adjunctively to standard therapy and should not be used in the treatment of granulomatosis with polyangiitis (Wegener's).

METHOTREXATE INDUCTION FOR NONSEVERE DISEASE

For selected patients whose disease is not immediately life threatening, methotrexate together with glucocorticoids given at the dosages described above may be considered as an alternative for induction therapy, which is then continued for maintenance.

TRIMETHOPRIM-SULFAMETHOXAZOLE

Although certain reports have indicated that TMP-SMX may be of benefit in the treatment of granulomatosis with polyangiitis (Wegener's) isolated to the sinonasal tissues, it should never be used alone to treat active granulomatosis with polyangiitis (Wegener's) outside of the upper airway such as in patients with renal or pulmonary disease. In a study examining the effect of TMP-SMX on relapse, decreased relapses were shown only with regard to upper airway disease, and no differences in major organ relapses were observed.

ORGAN-SPECIFIC TREATMENT

Not all manifestations of granulomatosis with polyangiitis (Wegener's) require or respond to immunosuppressive therapy. In managing non–major organ disease, such as that isolated to the sinus, joints, or skin, the risks of treatment should be carefully weighed against the benefits. Treatment with cyclophosphamide is rarely if ever justified for the treatment of isolated sinus disease in granulomatosis with polyangiitis (Wegener's). Although patients with non–major organ disease may be effectively treated without immunosuppressive therapy, these individuals must be monitored closely for the development of disease activity affecting the lungs, kidneys, or other major organs. Subglottic stenosis and endobronchial stenosis are examples of disease manifestations that do not typically respond to systemic immunosuppressive treatment.

MICROSCOPIC POLYANGIITIS

DEFINITION

The term *microscopic polyarteritis* was introduced into the literature by Davson in 1948 in recognition of the presence of glomerulonephritis in patients with polyarteritis nodosa. In 1992, the Chapel Hill Consensus Conference on the Nomenclature of Systemic Vasculitis adopted the term *microscopic polyangiitis* to connote a necrotizing vasculitis with few or no immune complexes affecting small vessels (capillaries, venules, or arterioles). Glomerulonephritis is very common in microscopic polyangiitis, and pulmonary capillaritis often occurs. The absence of granulomatous inflammation in microscopic polyangiitis is said to differentiate it from granulomatosis with polyangiitis (Wegener's).

INCIDENCE AND PREVALENCE

The incidence of microscopic polyangiitis has not yet been reliably established due to its previous inclusion as part of polyarteritis nodosa. The mean age of onset is ~57 years of age, and males are slightly more frequently affected than females.

PATHOLOGY AND PATHOGENESIS

The vasculitis seen in microscopic polyangiitis has a predilection to involve capillaries and venules in addition to small and medium-sized arteries. Immunohistochemical staining reveals a paucity of immunoglobulin deposition in the vascular lesion of microscopic polyangiitis, suggesting that immune-complex formation does not play a role in the pathogenesis of this syndrome. The renal lesion seen in microscopic polyangiitis is identical to that of granulomatosis with polyangiitis (Wegener's). Like granulomatosis with polyangiitis (Wegener's), microscopic polyangiitis is highly associated with the presence of ANCA, which may play a role in pathogenesis of this syndrome (see above).

CLINICAL AND LABORATORY MANIFESTATIONS

Because of its predilection to involve the small vessels, microscopic polyangiitis and granulomatosis with polyangiitis (Wegener's) share similar clinical features. Disease onset may be gradual, with initial symptoms of fever, weight loss, and musculoskeletal pain; however, it is often acute. Glomerulonephritis occurs in at least 79% of patients and can be rapidly progressive, leading to renal failure. Hemoptysis may be the first symptom of alveolar hemorrhage, which occurs in 12% of patients. Other manifestations include mononeuritis multiplex and gastrointestinal tract and cutaneous vasculitis. Upper airway disease and pulmonary nodules are not typically found in microscopic polyangiitis and, if present, suggest granulomatosis with polyangiitis (Wegener's).

Features of inflammation may be seen, including an elevated ESR, anemia, leukocytosis, and thrombocytosis. ANCA are present in 75% of patients with microscopic polyangiitis, with antimyeloperoxidase antibodies being the predominant ANCA associated with this disease.

DIAGNOSIS

The diagnosis is based on histologic evidence of vasculitis or pauci-immune glomerulonephritis in a patient with compatible clinical features of multisystem disease. Although microscopic polyangiitis is strongly ANCA-associated, no studies have as yet established the sensitivity and specificity of ANCA in this disease.

TREATMENT MICROSCOPIC POLYANGIITIS

The 5-year survival rate for patients with treated microscopic polyangiitis is 74%, with disease-related mortality occurring from alveolar hemorrhage or gastrointestinal, cardiac, or renal disease. Studies on treatment have come from trials that have included patients with granulomatosis with polyangiitis (Wegener's) or microscopic polyangiitis. Currently, the treatment approach for microscopic polyangiitis is the same as is used for granulomatosis with polyangiitis (Wegener's) (see "Granulomatosis with Polyangiitis [Wegener's]" for a detailed description of this therapeutic regimen), and patients with immediately life-threatening disease should be treated with the combination of prednisone and daily cyclophosphamide or rituximab. Disease relapse has been observed in at least 34% of patients. Treatment for such relapses would be similar to that used at the time of initial presentation and based on site and severity of disease.

EOSINOPHILIC GRANULOMATOSIS WITH POLYANGIITIS (CHURG-STRAUSS)

DEFINITION

Eosinophilic granulomatosis with polyangiitis (Churg-Strauss) was described in 1951 by Churg and Strauss and is characterized by asthma, peripheral and tissue eosinophilia, extravascular granuloma formation, and vasculitis of multiple organ systems.

INCIDENCE AND PREVALENCE

Eosinophilic granulomatosis with polyangiitis (Churg-Strauss) is an uncommon disease with an estimated annual incidence of 1–3 per million. The disease can occur at any age with the possible exception of infants. The mean age of onset is 48 years, with a female-to-male ratio of 1.2:1.

PATHOLOGY AND PATHOGENESIS

The necrotizing vasculitis of eosinophilic granulomatosis with polyangiitis (Churg-Strauss) involves small and medium-sized muscular arteries, capillaries, veins, and venules. A characteristic histopathologic feature of eosinophilic granulomatosis with polyangiitis (Churg-Strauss) is granulomatous reactions that may be present in the tissues or even within the walls of the vessels themselves. These are usually associated with infiltration of the tissues with eosinophils. This process can occur in any organ in the body; lung involvement is predominant, with skin, cardiovascular system, kidney, peripheral nervous system, and gastrointestinal tract also commonly involved. Although the precise pathogenesis of this disease is uncertain, its strong association with asthma and its clinicopathologic manifestations, including eosinophilia, granuloma, and vasculitis, point to aberrant immunologic phenomena.

CLINICAL AND LABORATORY MANIFESTATIONS

Patients with eosinophilic granulomatosis with polyangiitis (Churg-Strauss) often exhibit nonspecific manifestations such as fever, malaise, anorexia, and weight loss, which are characteristic of a multisystem disease. The pulmonary findings in eosinophilic granulomatosis with polyangiitis (Churg-Strauss) clearly dominate the clinical picture with severe asthmatic attacks and the presence of pulmonary infiltrates. Mononeuritis multiplex is the second most common manifestation and occurs in up to 72% of patients. Allergic rhinitis and sinusitis develop in up to 61% of patients and are often observed early in the course of disease. Clinically recognizable heart disease occurs in ~14% of patients and is an important cause of mortality. Skin lesions occur in ~51% of patients and include purpura in addition to cutaneous and subcutaneous nodules. The renal disease in eosinophilic granulomatosis with polyangiitis (Churg-Strauss) is less common and generally less severe than that of granulomatosis with polyangiitis and microscopic polyangiitis.

The characteristic laboratory finding in virtually all patients with eosinophilic granulomatosis with polyangiitis (Churg-Strauss) is a striking eosinophilia, which reaches levels >1000 cells/μL in >80% of patients. Evidence of inflammation as evidenced by elevated ESR, fibrinogen, or α_2-globulins can be found in 81% of patients. The other laboratory findings reflect the organ systems involved. Approximately 48% of patients with eosinophilic granulomatosis with polyangiitis (Churg-Strauss) have circulating ANCA that is usually antimyeloperoxidase.

DIAGNOSIS

Although the diagnosis of eosinophilic granulomatosis with polyangiitis (Churg-Strauss) is optimally made by biopsy in a patient with the characteristic clinical manifestations (see above), histologic confirmation can be challenging because the pathognomonic features often do not occur simultaneously. In order to be diagnosed with eosinophilic granulomatosis with polyangiitis (Churg-Strauss), a patient should have evidence of asthma, peripheral blood eosinophilia, and clinical features consistent with vasculitis.

TREATMENT EOSINOPHILIC GRANULOMATOSIS WITH POLYANGIITIS (CHURG-STRAUSS)

The prognosis of untreated eosinophilic granulomatosis with polyangiitis (Churg-Strauss) is poor, with a reported 5-year survival of 25%. With treatment, prognosis is favorable, with one study finding a 78-month actuarial survival rate of 72%. Myocardial involvement is the most frequent cause of death and is responsible for 39% of patient mortality. Echocardiography should be performed in all newly diagnosed patients because this may influence therapeutic decisions.

Glucocorticoids alone appear to be effective in many patients. Dosage tapering is often limited by asthma, and many patients require low-dose prednisone for persistent asthma many years after clinical recovery from vasculitis. In glucocorticoid failure or in patients who present with fulminant multisystem disease, particularly cardiac involvement, the treatment of choice is a combined regimen of daily cyclophosphamide and prednisone (see "Granulomatosis with Polyangiitis [Wegener's]" for a detailed description of this therapeutic regimen). Recent studies of mepolizumab (anti-IL-5 antibody) in eosinophilic granulomatosis with polyangiitis (Churg-Strauss) have been encouraging, but this treatment requires further investigation.

POLYARTERITIS NODOSA

DEFINITION

Polyarteritis nodosa was described in 1866 by Kussmaul and Maier. It is a multisystem, necrotizing vasculitis of small and medium-sized muscular arteries in which involvement of the renal and visceral arteries is characteristic. Polyarteritis nodosa does not involve pulmonary arteries, although bronchial vessels may be involved; granulomas, significant eosinophilia, and an allergic diathesis are not observed.

INCIDENCE AND PREVALENCE

It is difficult to establish an accurate incidence of polyarteritis nodosa because previous reports have included polyarteritis nodosa and microscopic polyangiitis as well as other related vasculitides. Polyarteritis nodosa, as currently defined, is felt to be a very uncommon disease.

PATHOLOGY AND PATHOGENESIS

The vascular lesion in polyarteritis nodosa is a necrotizing inflammation of small and medium-sized muscular arteries. The lesions are segmental and tend to involve bifurcations and branchings of arteries. They may spread circumferentially to involve adjacent veins. However, involvement of venules is not seen in polyarteritis nodosa and, if present, suggests microscopic polyangiitis (see below). In the acute stages of disease, polymorphonuclear neutrophils infiltrate all layers of the vessel wall and perivascular areas, which results in intimal proliferation and degeneration of the vessel wall. Mononuclear cells infiltrate the area as the lesions progress to the subacute and chronic stages. Fibrinoid necrosis of the vessels ensues with compromise of the lumen, thrombosis, infarction of the tissues supplied by the involved vessel, and, in some cases, hemorrhage. As the lesions heal, there is collagen deposition, which may lead to further occlusion of the vessel lumen. Aneurysmal dilations up to 1 cm in size along the involved arteries are characteristic of polyarteritis nodosa. Granulomas and substantial eosinophilia with eosinophilic tissue infiltrations are not characteristically found and suggest eosinophilic granulomatosis with polyangiitis (Churg-Strauss) (see above).

Multiple organ systems are involved, and the clinicopathologic findings reflect the degree and location of vessel involvement and the resulting ischemic changes. As mentioned above, pulmonary arteries are not involved in polyarteritis nodosa, and bronchial artery involvement is uncommon. The pathology in the kidney in classic polyarteritis nodosa is that of arteritis without glomerulonephritis. In patients with significant hypertension, typical pathologic features of glomerulosclerosis may be seen. In addition, pathologic sequelae of hypertension may be found elsewhere in the body.

The presence of a polyarteritis nodosa–like vasculitis in patients with hepatitis B together with the isolation of circulating immune complexes composed of hepatitis B antigen and immunoglobulin, and the demonstration by immunofluorescence of hepatitis B antigen, IgM, and complement in the blood vessel walls, strongly suggest the role of immunologic phenomena in the pathogenesis of this disease. A polyarteritis nodosa–like vasculitis has also been reported in patients with hepatitis C. Hairy cell leukemia can be associated with polyarteritis nodosa; the pathogenic mechanisms of this association are unclear.

CLINICAL AND LABORATORY MANIFESTATIONS

Nonspecific signs and symptoms are the hallmarks of polyarteritis nodosa. Fever, weight loss, and malaise are present in over one-half of cases. Patients usually present with vague symptoms such as weakness, malaise, headache, abdominal pain, and myalgias that can rapidly progress to a fulminant illness. Specific complaints related to the vascular involvement within a particular organ system may also dominate the presenting clinical picture as well as the entire course of the illness (Table 385-6). In polyarteritis nodosa, renal involvement most commonly manifests as hypertension, renal insufficiency, or hemorrhage due to microaneurysms.

There are no diagnostic serologic tests for polyarteritis nodosa. In >75% of patients, the leukocyte count is elevated with a predominance of neutrophils. Eosinophilia is seen only rarely and, when present at high levels, suggests the diagnosis of eosinophilic granulomatosis with polyangiitis (Churg-Strauss). The anemia of chronic disease may be seen, and an elevated ESR is almost always present. Other common laboratory findings reflect the particular organ involved. Hypergammaglobulinemia may be present, and all patients should be screened for hepatitis B and C. Antibodies against myeloperoxidase or proteinase-3 (ANCA) are rarely found in patients with polyarteritis nodosa.

DIAGNOSIS

The diagnosis of polyarteritis nodosa is based on the demonstration of characteristic findings of vasculitis on biopsy material of involved

TABLE 385-6 CLINICAL MANIFESTATIONS RELATED TO ORGAN SYSTEM INVOLVEMENT IN POLYARTERITIS NODOSA

Organ System	Percent Incidence	Clinical Manifestations
Renal	60	Renal failure, hypertension
Musculoskeletal	64	Arthritis, arthralgia, myalgia
Peripheral nervous system	51	Peripheral neuropathy, mononeuritis multiplex
Gastrointestinal tract	44	Abdominal pain, nausea and vomiting, bleeding, bowel infarction and perforation, cholecystitis, hepatic infarction, pancreatic infarction
Skin	43	Rash, purpura, nodules, cutaneous infarcts, livedo reticularis, Raynaud's phenomenon
Cardiac	36	Congestive heart failure, myocardial infarction, pericarditis
Genitourinary	25	Testicular, ovarian, or epididymal pain
Central nervous system	23	Cerebral vascular accident, altered mental status, seizure

Source: From TR Cupps, AS Fauci: *The Vasculitides*. Philadelphia, Saunders, 1981.

organs. In the absence of easily accessible tissue for biopsy, the arteriographic demonstration of involved vessels, particularly in the form of aneurysms of small and medium-sized arteries in the renal, hepatic, and visceral vasculature, is sufficient to make the diagnosis. This should consist of a catheter-directed dye arteriogram because magnetic resonance and computed tomography arteriograms do not have sufficient resolution at the current time to visualize the vessels affected in polyarteritis nodosa. Aneurysms of vessels are not pathognomonic of polyarteritis nodosa; furthermore, aneurysms need not always be present, and arteriographic findings may be limited to stenotic segments and obliteration of vessels. Biopsy of symptomatic organs such as nodular skin lesions, painful testes, and nerve/muscle provides the highest diagnostic yields.

TREATMENT POLYARTERITIS NODOSA

The prognosis of untreated polyarteritis nodosa is extremely poor, with a reported 5-year survival rate between 10 and 20%. Death usually results from gastrointestinal complications, particularly bowel infarcts and perforation, and cardiovascular causes. Intractable hypertension often compounds dysfunction in other organ systems, such as the kidneys, heart, and CNS, leading to additional late morbidity and mortality in polyarteritis nodosa. With the introduction of treatment, survival rate has increased substantially. Favorable therapeutic results have been reported in polyarteritis nodosa with the combination of prednisone and cyclophosphamide (see "Granulomatosis with Polyangiitis [Wegener's]" for a detailed description of this therapeutic regimen). In less severe cases of polyarteritis nodosa, glucocorticoids alone have resulted in disease remission. In patients with hepatitis B who have a polyarteritis nodosa–like vasculitis, antiviral therapy represents an important part of therapy and has been used in combination with glucocorticoids and plasma exchange. Careful attention to the treatment of hypertension can lessen the acute and late morbidity and mortality rates associated with renal, cardiac, and CNS complications of polyarteritis nodosa. Following successful treatment, relapse of polyarteritis nodosa has been estimated to occur in 10–20% of patients.

GIANT CELL ARTERITIS AND POLYMYALGIA RHEUMATICA

DEFINITION

Giant cell arteritis, historically referred to as *temporal arteritis*, is an inflammation of medium- and large-sized arteries. It characteristically involves one or more branches of the carotid artery, particularly the temporal artery. However, it is a systemic disease that can involve arteries in multiple locations, particularly the aorta and its main branches.

Giant cell arteritis is closely associated with *polymyalgia rheumatica*, which is characterized by stiffness, aching, and pain in the muscles of the neck, shoulders, lower back, hips, and thighs. Most commonly, polymyalgia rheumatica occurs in isolation, but it may be seen in 40–50% of patients with giant cell arteritis. In addition, ~10–20% of patients who initially present with features of isolated polymyalgia rheumatica later go on to develop giant cell arteritis. This strong clinical association together with data from pathophysiologic studies has increasingly supported that giant cell arteritis and polymyalgia rheumatica represent differing clinical spectrums of a single disease process.

INCIDENCE AND PREVALENCE

Giant cell arteritis occurs almost exclusively in individuals >50 years. It is more common in women than in men and is rare in blacks. The incidence of giant cell arteritis varies widely in different studies and in different geographic regions. A high incidence has been found in Scandinavia and in regions of the United States with large Scandinavian populations, compared to a lower incidence in southern Europe. The annual incidence rates in individuals ≥50 years range from 6.9 to 32.8 per 100,000 population. Familial aggregation has been reported, as has an association with HLA-DR4. In addition, genetic linkage studies have demonstrated an association of giant cell arteritis with alleles at the HLA-DRB1 locus, particularly HLA-DRB1*04 variants. In Olmsted County, Minnesota, the annual incidence of polymyalgia rheumatica in individuals ≥50 years is 58.7 per 100,000 population.

PATHOLOGY AND PATHOGENESIS

Although the temporal artery is most frequently involved in giant cell arteritis, patients often have a systemic vasculitis of multiple medium- and large-sized arteries, which may go undetected. Histopathologically, the disease is a panarteritis with inflammatory mononuclear cell infiltrates within the vessel wall with frequent giant cell formation. There is proliferation of the intima and fragmentation of the internal elastic lamina. Pathophysiologic findings in organs result from the ischemia related to the involved vessels.

Experimental data support that giant cell arteritis is an antigen-driven disease in which activated T lymphocytes, macrophages, and dendritic cells play a critical role in the disease pathogenesis. Sequence analysis of the T cell receptor of tissue-infiltrating T cells in lesions of giant cell arteritis indicates restricted clonal expansion, suggesting the presence of an antigen residing in the arterial wall. Giant cell arteritis is believed to be initiated in the adventitia where CD4+ T cells enter through the vasa vasorum, become activated, and orchestrate macrophage differentiation. T cells recruited to vasculitic lesions in patients with giant cell arteritis produce predominantly IL-2 and IFN-γ, and the latter has been suggested to be involved in the progression to overt arteritis. Recent data demonstrate that at least two separate lineages of CD4 T cells--IFN-γ-producing T_H1 cells and IL-17-producing T_H17 cells—participate in vascular inflammation and may have differing levels of responsiveness to glucocorticoids.

CLINICAL AND LABORATORY MANIFESTATIONS

Giant cell arteritis is most commonly characterized clinically by the complex of fever, anemia, high ESR, and headaches in a patient over the age of 50 years. Other phenotypic manifestations include features of systemic inflammation including malaise, fatigue, anorexia, weight loss, sweats, arthralgias, polymyalgia rheumatica, or large-vessel disease.

In patients with involvement of the cranial arteries, headache is the predominant symptom and may be associated with a tender, thickened, or nodular artery, which may pulsate early in the disease but may become occluded later. Scalp pain and claudication of the jaw and tongue may occur. A well-recognized and dreaded complication of giant cell arteritis, particularly in untreated patients, is ischemic optic neuropathy, which may lead to serious visual symptoms, even sudden blindness in some patients. However, most patients have complaints relating to the head or eyes before visual loss. Attention to such symptoms with institution of appropriate therapy (see below) will usually avoid this complication. Other cranial ischemic complications include strokes and scalp or tongue infarction.

Up to one-third of patients can have large-vessel disease that can be the primary presentation of giant cell arteritis or can emerge at a later point in patients who have had previous cranial arteritis features or polymyalgia rheumatica. Manifestations of large-vessel disease can include subclavian artery stenosis that can present as arm claudication or aortic aneurysms involving the thoracic and to a lesser degree the abdominal aorta, which carry risks of rupture or dissection.

Characteristic laboratory findings in addition to the elevated ESR include a normochromic or slightly hypochromic anemia. Liver function abnormalities are common, particularly increased alkaline phosphatase levels. Increased levels of IgG and complement have been reported. Levels of enzymes indicative of muscle damage such as serum creatine kinase are not elevated.

DIAGNOSIS

The diagnosis of giant cell arteritis and its associated clinicopathologic syndrome can often be suggested clinically by the demonstration of the complex of fever, anemia, and high ESR with or without symptoms of polymyalgia rheumatica in a patient >50 years. The diagnosis is confirmed by biopsy of the temporal artery. Since involvement of the vessel may be segmental, positive yield is increased by obtaining a biopsy segment of 3–5 cm together with serial sectioning of biopsy specimens. Ultrasonography of the temporal artery has been reported to be helpful in diagnosis. A temporal artery biopsy should be obtained as quickly as possible in the setting of ocular signs and symptoms, and under these circumstances, therapy should not be delayed pending a biopsy. In this regard, it has been reported that temporal artery biopsies may show vasculitis even after ~14 days of glucocorticoid therapy. A dramatic clinical response to a trial of glucocorticoid therapy can further support the diagnosis.

Large-vessel disease may be suggested by symptoms and findings on physical examination such as diminished pulses or bruits. It is confirmed by vascular imaging, most commonly through magnetic resonance or computed tomography.

Isolated polymyalgia rheumatica is a clinical diagnosis made by the presence of typical symptoms of stiffness, aching, and pain in the muscles of the hip and shoulder girdle, an increased ESR, the absence of clinical features suggestive of giant cell arteritis, and a prompt therapeutic response to low-dose prednisone.

TREATMENT GIANT CELL ARTERITIS AND POLYMYALGIA RHEUMATICA

Acute disease-related mortality directly from giant cell arteritis is very uncommon, with fatalities occurring from cerebrovascular events or myocardial infarction. However, patients are at risk of late mortality from aortic aneurysm rupture or dissection as patients with giant cell arteritis are 18 times more likely to develop thoracic aortic aneurysms than the general population.

The goals of treatment in giant cell arteritis are to reduce symptoms and, most importantly, to prevent visual loss. The treatment approach for cranial and large-vessel disease in giant cell arteritis is currently the same. Giant cell arteritis and its associated symptoms are exquisitely sensitive to glucocorticoid therapy. Treatment should begin with prednisone, 40–60 mg/d for ~1 month, followed by a gradual tapering. When ocular signs and symptoms occur, consideration should be given for the use of methylprednisolone 1000 mg daily for 3 days to protect remaining vision. Although the optimal duration of glucocorticoid therapy has not been established, most series have found that patients require treatment for ≥2 years. Symptom recurrence during prednisone tapering develops in 60–85% of patients with giant cell arteritis, requiring a dosage increase. The ESR can serve as a useful indicator of inflammatory disease activity in monitoring and tapering therapy and can be used to judge the pace of the tapering schedule. However, minor increases in the ESR can occur as glucocorticoids are being tapered and do not necessarily reflect an exacerbation of arteritis, particularly if the patient remains symptom-free. Under these circumstances, the tapering should continue with caution. Glucocorticoid toxicity occurs in 35–65% of patients and represents an important cause of patient morbidity. Aspirin 81 mg daily has been found to reduce the occurrence of cranial ischemic complications in giant cell arteritis and should be given in addition to glucocorticoids in patients who do not have contraindications. The use of weekly methotrexate as a glucocorticoid-sparing agent has been examined in two randomized placebo-controlled trials that reached conflicting conclusions. Infliximab, a monoclonal antibody to TNF, was studied in a randomized trial and was not found to provide benefit. Recent reports have shown favorable response of giant cell arteritis to tocilizumab (anti-IL-6 receptor), but this treatment requires further study before use in clinical practice.

Patients with isolated polymyalgia rheumatica respond promptly to prednisone, which can be started at a lower dose of 10–20 mg/d. Similar to giant cell arteritis, the ESR can serve as a useful indicator in monitoring and prednisone reduction. Recurrent polymyalgia symptoms develop in the majority of patients during prednisone tapering. One study of weekly methotrexate found that the use of this drug reduced the prednisone dose on average by only 1 mg and did not decrease prednisone-related side effects. A randomized trial in polymyalgia rheumatica did not find infliximab to lessen relapse or glucocorticoid requirements.

TAKAYASU ARTERITIS

DEFINITION

Takayasu arteritis is an inflammatory and stenotic disease of medium- and large-sized arteries characterized by a strong predilection for the aortic arch and its branches.

INCIDENCE AND PREVALENCE

Takayasu arteritis is an uncommon disease with an estimated annual incidence rate of 1.2–2.6 cases per million. It is most prevalent in adolescent girls and young women. Although it is more common in Asia, it is neither racially nor geographically restricted.

PATHOLOGY AND PATHOGENESIS

The disease involves medium- and large sized arteries, with a strong predilection for the aortic arch and its branches; the pulmonary artery may also be involved. The most commonly affected arteries seen by arteriography are listed in Table 385-7. The involvement of the major branches of the aorta is much more marked at their origin than distally. The disease is a panarteritis with inflammatory mononuclear cell infiltrates and occasionally giant cells. There are marked intimal proliferation and fibrosis, scarring and vascularization of the media, and disruption and degeneration of the elastic lamina. Narrowing of the lumen occurs with or without thrombosis. The vasa vasorum are frequently involved. Pathologic changes in various organs reflect the compromise of blood flow through the involved vessels.

Immunopathogenic mechanisms, the precise nature of which is uncertain, are suspected in this disease. As with several of the vasculitis syndromes, circulating immune complexes have been demonstrated, but their pathogenic significance is unclear.

CLINICAL AND LABORATORY MANIFESTATIONS

Takayasu arteritis is a systemic disease with generalized as well as vascular symptoms. The generalized symptoms include malaise, fever, night sweats, arthralgias, anorexia, and weight loss, which may occur months before vessel involvement is apparent. These symptoms may merge into those related to vascular compromise and organ ischemia. Pulses are commonly absent in the involved vessels, particularly the subclavian artery. The frequency of arteriographic abnormalities and the potentially associated clinical

TABLE 385-7 FREQUENCY OF ARTERIOGRAPHIC ABNORMALITIES AND POTENTIAL CLINICAL MANIFESTATIONS OF ARTERIAL INVOLVEMENT IN TAKAYASU ARTERITIS

Artery	Percentage of Arteriographic Abnormalities	Potential Clinical Manifestations
Subclavian	93	Arm claudication, Raynaud's phenomenon
Common carotid	58	Visual changes, syncope, transient ischemic attacks, stroke
Abdominal aorta[a]	47	Abdominal pain, nausea, vomiting
Renal	38	Hypertension, renal failure
Aortic arch or root	35	Aortic insufficiency, congestive heart failure
Vertebral	35	Visual changes, dizziness
Coeliac axis[a]	18	Abdominal pain, nausea, vomiting
Superior mesenteric[a]	18	Abdominal pain, nausea, vomiting
Iliac	17	Leg claudication
Pulmonary	10–40	Atypical chest pain, dyspnea
Coronary	<10	Chest pain, myocardial infarction

[a]Arteriographic lesions at these locations are usually asymptomatic but may potentially cause these symptoms.

Source: G Kerr et al: Ann Intern Med 120:919, 1994.

manifestations are listed in Table 385-7. Hypertension occurs in 32–93% of patients and contributes to renal, cardiac, and cerebral injury.

Characteristic laboratory findings include an elevated ESR, mild anemia, and elevated immunoglobulin levels.

DIAGNOSIS

The diagnosis of Takayasu arteritis should be suspected strongly in a young woman who develops a decrease or absence of peripheral pulses, discrepancies in blood pressure, and arterial bruits. The diagnosis is confirmed by the characteristic pattern on arteriography, which includes irregular vessel walls, stenosis, poststenotic dilation, aneurysm formation, occlusion, and evidence of increased collateral circulation. Complete aortic arteriography by catheter-directed dye arteriography or magnetic resonance arteriography should be obtained in order to fully delineate the distribution and degree of arterial disease. Histopathologic demonstration of vessel wall inflammation that is predominantly lymphocytic with granuloma formation and giant cells involving the media and adventitia adds confirmatory data; however, tissue is rarely readily available for examination. IgG4-related disease is a potential cause of aortitis and periaortitis that is histologically differentiated from Takayasu arteritis by a dense lymphoplasmacytic infiltrate rich in IgG4-positive plasma cells, a storiform pattern of fibrosis, and obliterative phlebitis.

TREATMENT TAKAYASU ARTERITIS

The long-term outcome of patients with Takayasu arteritis has varied widely between studies. Although two North American reports found overall survival to be ≥94%, the 5-year mortality rate from other studies has ranged from 0 to 35%. Disease-related mortality most often occurs from congestive heart failure, cerebrovascular events, myocardial infarction, aneurysm rupture, or renal failure. Even in the absence of life-threatening disease, Takayasu arteritis can be associated with significant morbidity. The course of the disease is variable, and although spontaneous remissions may occur, Takayasu arteritis is most often chronic and relapsing. Although glucocorticoid therapy in doses of 40–60 mg prednisone per day alleviates symptoms, there are no convincing studies that indicate that it increases survival. The combination of glucocorticoid therapy for acute signs and symptoms and an aggressive surgical and/or arterioplastic approach to stenosed vessels has markedly improved outcome and decreased morbidity by lessening the risk of stroke, correcting hypertension due to renal artery stenosis, and improving blood flow to ischemic viscera and limbs. Unless it is urgently required, surgical correction of stenosed arteries should be undertaken only when the vascular inflammatory process is well controlled with medical therapy. In individuals who are refractory to or unable to taper glucocorticoids, methotrexate in doses up to 25 mg per week has yielded encouraging results. Preliminary results with anti-TNF therapies have been encouraging, but will require further study through randomized trials to determine efficacy.

IgA VASCULITIS (HENOCH-SCHÖNLEIN)

DEFINITION

IgA vasculitis (Henoch-Schönlein) is a small-vessel vasculitis characterized by palpable purpura (most commonly distributed over the buttocks and lower extremities), arthralgias, gastrointestinal signs and symptoms, and glomerulonephritis.

INCIDENCE AND PREVALENCE

IgA vasculitis (Henoch-Schönlein) is usually seen in children; most patients range in age from 4 to 7 years; however, the disease may also be seen in infants and adults. It is not a rare disease; in one series it accounted for between 5 and 24 admissions per year at a pediatric hospital. The male-to-female ratio is 1.5:1. A seasonal variation with a peak incidence in spring has been noted.

PATHOLOGY AND PATHOGENESIS

The presumptive pathogenic mechanism for IgA (Henoch-Schönlein) vasculitis is immune-complex deposition. A number of inciting antigens have been suggested including upper respiratory tract infections, various drugs, foods, insect bites, and immunizations. IgA is the antibody class most often seen in the immune complexes and has been demonstrated in the renal biopsies of these patients.

CLINICAL AND LABORATORY MANIFESTATIONS

In pediatric patients, palpable purpura is seen in virtually all patients; most patients develop polyarthralgias in the absence of frank arthritis. Gastrointestinal involvement, which is seen in almost 70% of pediatric patients, is characterized by colicky abdominal pain usually associated with nausea, vomiting, diarrhea, or constipation and is frequently accompanied by the passage of blood and mucus per rectum; bowel intussusception may occur. Renal involvement occurs in 10–50% of patients and is usually characterized by mild glomerulonephritis leading to proteinuria and microscopic hematuria, with red blood cell casts in the majority of patients (Chap. 338); it usually resolves spontaneously without therapy. Rarely, a progressive glomerulonephritis will develop. In adults, presenting symptoms are most frequently related to the skin and joints, while initial complaints related to the gut are less common. Although certain studies have found that renal disease is more frequent and more severe in adults, this has not been a consistent finding. However, the course of renal disease in adults may be more insidious and thus requires close follow-up. Myocardial involvement can occur in adults but is rare in children.

Laboratory studies generally show a mild leukocytosis, a normal platelet count, and occasionally eosinophilia. Serum complement components are normal, and IgA levels are elevated in about one-half of patients.

DIAGNOSIS

The diagnosis of IgA vasculitis (Henoch-Schönlein) is based on clinical signs and symptoms. Skin biopsy specimen can be useful in confirming leukocytoclastic vasculitis with IgA and C3 deposition by immunofluorescence. Renal biopsy is rarely needed for diagnosis but may provide prognostic information in some patients.

TREATMENT IgA VASCULITIS (HENOCH-SCHÖNLEIN)

The prognosis of IgA vasculitis (Henoch-Schönlein) is excellent. Mortality is exceedingly rare, and 1–5% of children progress to end-stage renal disease. Most patients recover completely, and some do not require therapy. Treatment is similar for adults and children. When glucocorticoid therapy is required, prednisone, in doses of 1 mg/kg per day and tapered according to clinical response, has been shown to be useful in decreasing tissue edema, arthralgias, and abdominal discomfort; however, it has not proved beneficial in the treatment of skin or renal disease and does not appear to shorten the duration of active disease or lessen the chance of recurrence. Patients with rapidly progressive glomerulonephritis have been anecdotally reported to benefit from intensive plasma exchange combined with cytotoxic drugs. Disease recurrences have been reported in 10–40% of patients.

CRYOGLOBULINEMIC VASCULITIS

DEFINITION

Cryoglobulins are cold-precipitable monoclonal or polyclonal immunoglobulins. Cryoglobulinemia may be associated with a systemic vasculitis characterized by palpable purpura, arthralgias, weakness, neuropathy, and glomerulonephritis. Although this can be observed in association with a variety of underlying disorders including multiple myeloma, lymphoproliferative disorders, connective tissue diseases, infection, and liver disease, in many instances it appears to be idiopathic. Because of the apparent absence of an underlying disease and the presence of cryoprecipitate containing oligoclonal/polyclonal immunoglobulins, this entity was referred to as *essential mixed cryoglobulinemia*. Since the discovery of hepatitis C, it has been established that the vast majority of patients who were considered to have essential mixed cryoglobulinemia have cryoglobulinemic vasculitis related to hepatitis C infection.

INCIDENCE AND PREVALENCE

The incidence of cryoglobulinemic vasculitis has not been established. It has been estimated, however, that 5% of patients with chronic hepatitis C will develop cryoglobulinemic vasculitis.

PATHOLOGY AND PATHOGENESIS

Skin biopsies in cryoglobulinemic vasculitis reveal an inflammatory infiltrate surrounding and involving blood vessel walls, with fibrinoid necrosis, endothelial cell hyperplasia, and hemorrhage. Deposition of immunoglobulin and complement is common. Abnormalities of uninvolved skin including basement membrane alterations and deposits in vessel walls may be found. Membranoproliferative glomerulonephritis is responsible for 80% of all renal lesions in cryoglobulinemic vasculitis.

The association between hepatitis C and cryoglobulinemic vasculitis has been supported by the high frequency of documented hepatitis C infection, the presence of hepatitis C RNA and anti–hepatitis C antibodies in serum cryoprecipitates, evidence of hepatitis C antigens in vasculitic skin lesions, and the effectiveness of antiviral therapy (see below). Current evidence suggests that in the majority of cases, cryoglobulinemic vasculitis occurs when an aberrant immune response to hepatitis C infection leads to the formation of immune complexes consisting of hepatitis C antigens, polyclonal hepatitis C–specific IgG, and monoclonal IgM rheumatoid factor. The deposition of these immune complexes in blood vessel walls triggers an inflammatory cascade that results in cryoglobulinemic vasculitis.

CLINICAL AND LABORATORY MANIFESTATIONS

The most common clinical manifestations of cryoglobulinemic vasculitis are cutaneous vasculitis, arthritis, peripheral neuropathy, and glomerulonephritis. Renal disease develops in 10–30% of patients. Life-threatening rapidly progressive glomerulonephritis or vasculitis of the CNS, gastrointestinal tract, or heart occurs infrequently.

The presence of circulating cryoprecipitates is the fundamental finding in cryoglobulinemic vasculitis. Rheumatoid factor is almost always found and may be a useful clue to the disease when cryoglobulins are not detected. Hypocomplementemia occurs in 90% of patients. An elevated ESR and anemia occur frequently. Evidence for hepatitis C infection must be sought in all patients by testing for hepatitis C antibodies and hepatitis C RNA.

TREATMENT CRYOGLOBULINEMIC VASCULITIS

Acute mortality directly from cryoglobulinemic vasculitis is uncommon, but the presence of glomerulonephritis is a poor prognostic sign for overall outcome. In such patients, 15% progress to end-stage renal disease, with 40% later experiencing fatal cardiovascular disease, infection, or liver failure. As indicated above, the majority of cases are associated with hepatitis C infection. In such patients, treatment with antiviral therapy (Chap. 360) can prove beneficial and should be considered first-line therapy for hepatitis C–associated cryoglobulinemic vasculitis. Clinical improvement with antiviral therapy is dependent on the virologic response. Patients who clear hepatitis C from the blood have objective improvement in their vasculitis along with significant reductions in levels of circulating cryoglobulins, IgM, and rheumatoid factor. However, substantial portions of patients with hepatitis C do not have a sustained virologic response to such therapy, and the vasculitis typically relapses with the return of viremia. While transient improvement can be observed with glucocorticoids, a complete response is seen in only 7% of patients. Plasmapheresis and cytotoxic agents have been used in anecdotal reports. These observations have not been confirmed, and such therapies carry significant risks. Randomized trials with rituximab (anti-CD20) in hepatitis C–associated cryoglobulinemic vasculitis have provided evidence of benefit such that this agent should be considered in patients with active vasculitis either in combination with antiviral therapy or alone in patients who have relapsed through, are intolerant to, or have contraindications to antiviral agents.

SINGLE-ORGAN VASCULITIS

The potential for vasculitis to affect single organs has become increasingly recognized. This has been defined as vasculitis in arteries or veins of any size in a single organ that has no features that indicate that it is a limited expression of a systemic vasculitis. Examples include isolated aortitis, testicular vasculitis, vasculitis of the breast, isolated cutaneous vasculitis, and primary CNS vasculitis. In some instances, this may be discovered at the time of surgery such as orchiectomy for a testicular mass where there is concern for neoplasm that is found instead to be vasculitis. Some patients originally diagnosed with single-organ vasculitis may later develop additional manifestations of a more systemic disease. In instances where there is no evidence of systemic vasculitis and the affected organ has been removed in its entirety, the patient may be followed closely without immunosuppressive therapy. In other instances, such as primary CNS vasculitis or some patients with isolated cutaneous vasculitis, medical intervention is warranted.

IDIOPATHIC CUTANEOUS VASCULITIS

DEFINITION

The term *cutaneous vasculitis* is defined broadly as inflammation of the blood vessels of the dermis. Due to its heterogeneity, cutaneous vasculitis has been described by a variety of terms including *hypersensitivity vasculitis* and *cutaneous leukocytoclastic angiitis*. However, cutaneous vasculitis is not one specific disease but a manifestation that can be seen in a variety of settings. In >70% of cases, cutaneous vasculitis occurs either as part of a primary systemic vasculitis or as a secondary vasculitis related to an inciting agent or an underlying disease (see "Secondary Vasculitis," below). In the remaining 30% of cases, cutaneous vasculitis occurs idiopathically.

INCIDENCE AND PREVALENCE

Cutaneous vasculitis represents the most commonly encountered vasculitis in clinical practice. The exact incidence of idiopathic cutaneous vasculitis has not been determined due to the predilection for cutaneous vasculitis to be associated with an underlying process and the variability of its clinical course.

PATHOLOGY AND PATHOGENESIS

The typical histopathologic feature of cutaneous vasculitis is the presence of vasculitis of small vessels. Postcapillary venules are the most commonly involved vessels; capillaries and arterioles may be involved less frequently. This vasculitis is characterized by a *leukocytoclasis*, a term that refers to the nuclear debris remaining from the neutrophils that have infiltrated in and around the vessels during the acute stages. In the subacute or chronic stages, mononuclear cells predominate; in certain subgroups, eosinophilic infiltration is seen. Erythrocytes often extravasate from the involved vessels, leading to palpable purpura. *Cutaneous arteritis* can also occur, which involves slightly larger-sized vessels within the dermis.

CLINICAL AND LABORATORY MANIFESTATIONS

The hallmark of idiopathic cutaneous vasculitis is the predominance of skin involvement. Skin lesions may appear typically as palpable purpura; however, other cutaneous manifestations of the vasculitis may occur, including macules, papules, vesicles, bullae, subcutaneous nodules, ulcers, and recurrent or chronic urticaria. The skin lesions may be pruritic or even quite painful, with a burning or stinging sensation. Lesions most commonly occur in the lower extremities in ambulatory patients or in the sacral area in bedridden patients due to the effects of hydrostatic forces on the postcapillary venules. Edema may accompany certain lesions, and hyperpigmentation often occurs in areas of recurrent or chronic lesions.

There are no specific laboratory tests diagnostic of idiopathic cutaneous vasculitis. A mild leukocytosis with or without eosinophilia is characteristic, as is an elevated ESR. Laboratory studies should be aimed toward ruling out features to suggest an underlying disease or a systemic vasculitis.

DIAGNOSIS

The diagnosis of cutaneous vasculitis is made by the demonstration of vasculitis on biopsy. An important diagnostic principle in patients with cutaneous vasculitis is to search for an etiology of the vasculitis—be it an exogenous agent, such as a drug or an infection, or an endogenous condition, such as an underlying disease (Fig. 385-1). In addition, a careful physical and laboratory examination should be performed to rule out the possibility of systemic vasculitis. This should start with the least invasive diagnostic approach and proceed to the more invasive only if clinically indicated.

TREATMENT IDIOPATHIC CUTANEOUS VASCULITIS

When an antigenic stimulus is recognized as the precipitating factor in the cutaneous vasculitis, it should be removed; if this is a microbe, appropriate antimicrobial therapy should be instituted. If the vasculitis is associated with another underlying disease, treatment of the latter often results in resolution of the former. In situations where disease is apparently self-limited, no therapy, except possibly symptomatic therapy, is indicated. When cutaneous vasculitis persists and when there is no evidence of an inciting agent, an associated disease, or an underlying systemic vasculitis, the decision to treat should be based on weighing the balance between the degree of symptoms and the risk of treatment. Some cases of idiopathic cutaneous vasculitis resolve spontaneously, whereas others remit and relapse. In patients with persistent vasculitis, a variety of therapeutic regimens have been tried with variable results. In general, the treatment of idiopathic cutaneous vasculitis has not been satisfactory. Fortunately, since the disease is generally limited to the skin, this lack of consistent response to therapy usually does not lead to a life-threatening situation. Agents with which there have been anecdotal reports of success include dapsone, colchicine, hydroxychloroquine, and nonsteroidal anti-inflammatory agents. Glucocorticoids are often used in the treatment of idiopathic cutaneous vasculitis. Therapy is usually instituted as prednisone, 1 mg/kg per day, with rapid tapering where possible, either directly to discontinuation or by conversion to an alternate-day regimen followed by ultimate discontinuation. In cases that prove refractory to glucocorticoids, a trial of a cytotoxic agent may be indicated. Patients with chronic vasculitis isolated to cutaneous venules rarely respond dramatically to any therapeutic regimen, and cytotoxic agents should be used only as a last resort in these patients. Methotrexate and azathioprine have been used in such situations in anecdotal reports. Although cyclophosphamide is the most effective therapy for the systemic vasculitides, it should almost never be used for idiopathic cutaneous vasculitis because of the potential toxicity.

PRIMARY CENTRAL NERVOUS SYSTEM (CNS) VASCULITIS

Primary CNS vasculitis is an uncommon clinicopathologic entity characterized by vasculitis restricted to the vessels of the CNS without other apparent systemic vasculitis. The inflammatory process is usually composed of mononuclear cell infiltrates with or without granuloma formation.

Patients may present with headaches, altered mental function, and focal neurologic defects. Systemic symptoms are generally absent. Devastating neurologic abnormalities may occur depending on the extent of vessel involvement. The diagnosis can be suggested by abnormal magnetic resonance imaging of the brain, an abnormal lumbar puncture, and/or demonstration of characteristic vessel abnormalities on arteriography (Fig. 385-4), but it is confirmed by biopsy of the brain parenchyma and leptomeninges. In the absence of a brain biopsy, care should be taken not to misinterpret as true primary vasculitis arteriographic abnormalities that might actually be related to another

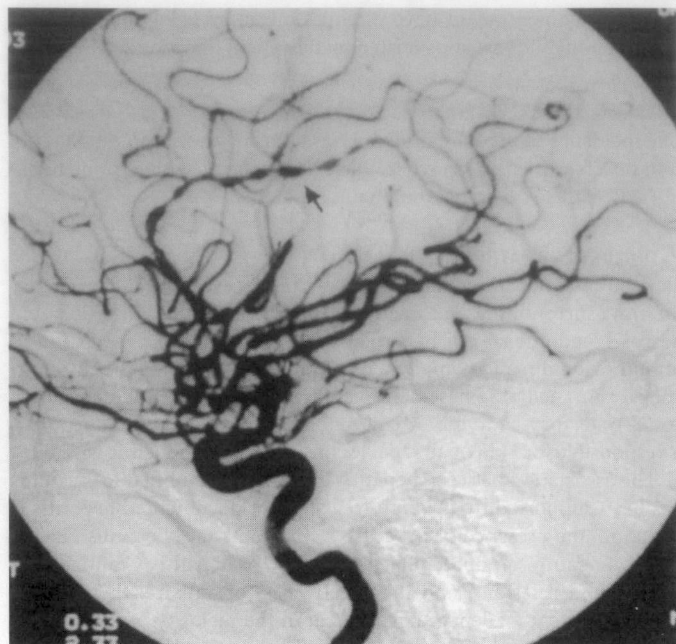

FIGURE 385-4 Cerebral arteriogram from a 32-year-old male with primary central nervous system vasculitis. Dramatic beading (*arrow*) typical of vasculitis is seen.

cause. An important entity in the differential diagnosis is reversible cerebral vasoconstrictive syndrome, which typically presents with "thunderclap" headache and is associated with arteriographic abnormalities that mimic primary CNS vasculitis that are reversible. Other diagnostic considerations include infection, atherosclerosis, emboli, connective tissue disease, sarcoidosis, malignancy, and drug-associated causes. The prognosis of granulomatous primary CNS vasculitis is poor; however, some reports indicate that glucocorticoid therapy, alone or together with cyclophosphamide administered as described above, has induced clinical remissions.

BEHÇET'S DISEASE

Behçet's disease is a clinicopathologic entity characterized by recurrent episodes of oral and genital ulcers, iritis, and cutaneous lesions. The underlying pathologic process is a leukocytoclastic venulitis, although vessels of any size and in any organ can be involved. This disorder is described in detail in Chap. 387.

COGAN'S SYNDROME

Cogan's syndrome is characterized by interstitial keratitis together with vestibuloauditory symptoms. It may be associated with a systemic vasculitis, particularly aortitis with involvement of the aortic valve. Glucocorticoids are the mainstay of treatment. Initiation of treatment as early as possible after the onset of hearing loss improves the likelihood of a favorable outcome.

KAWASAKI DISEASE

Kawasaki disease is an acute, febrile, multisystem disease of children. Some 80% of cases occur prior to the age of 5, with the peak incidence occurring at ≤2 years. It is characterized by nonsuppurative cervical adenitis and changes in the skin and mucous membranes such as edema; congested conjunctivae; erythema of the oral cavity, lips, and palms; and desquamation of the skin of the fingertips. Although the disease is generally benign and self-limited, it is associated with coronary artery aneurysms in ~25% of cases, with an overall case fatality rate of 0.5–2.8%. These complications usually occur between the third and fourth weeks of illness during the convalescent stage. Vasculitis of the coronary arteries is seen in almost all the fatal cases that have been autopsied. There is typical intimal proliferation and infiltration of the vessel wall with mononuclear cells. Beadlike aneurysms and thromboses may be seen along the artery. Other manifestations include pericarditis, myocarditis, myocardial ischemia and infarction, and cardiomegaly.

Apart from the up to 2.8% of patients who develop fatal complications, the prognosis of this disease for uneventful recovery is excellent. High-dose IV γ-globulin (2 g/kg as a single infusion over 10 h) together with aspirin (100 mg/kg per day for 14 days followed by 3–5 mg/kg per day for several weeks) have been shown to be effective in reducing the prevalence of coronary artery abnormalities when administered early in the course of the disease. Surgery may be necessary for Kawasaki disease patients who have giant coronary artery aneurysms or other coronary complications. Surgical treatment most commonly includes thromboendarterectomy, thrombus clearing, aneurysmal reconstruction, and coronary artery bypass grafting.

POLYANGIITIS OVERLAP SYNDROMES

Some patients with systemic vasculitis manifest clinicopathologic characteristics that do not fit precisely into any specific disease but have overlapping features of different vasculitides. Active systemic vasculitis in such settings has the same potential for causing irreversible organ system damage as when it occurs in one of the defined syndromes listed in Table 385-1. The diagnostic and therapeutic considerations as well as the prognosis for these patients depend on the sites and severity of active vasculitis. Patients with vasculitis that could potentially cause irreversible damage to a major organ system should be treated as described under "Granulomatosis with Polyangiitis (Wegener's)."

SECONDARY VASCULITIS

DRUG-INDUCED VASCULITIS

Vasculitis associated with drug reactions usually presents as palpable purpura that may be generalized or limited to the lower extremities or other dependent areas; however, urticarial lesions, ulcers, and hemorrhagic blisters may also occur (Chap. 74). Signs and symptoms may be limited to the skin, although systemic manifestations such as fever, malaise, and polyarthralgias may occur. Although the skin is the predominant organ involved, systemic vasculitis may result from drug reactions. Drugs that have been implicated in vasculitis include allopurinol, thiazides, gold, sulfonamides, phenytoin, and penicillin (Chap. 74).

An increasing number of drugs have been reported to cause vasculitis associated with antimyeloperoxidase ANCA. Of these, the best evidence of causality exists for hydralazine and propylthiouracil. The clinical manifestations in ANCA-positive drug-induced vasculitis can range from cutaneous lesions to glomerulonephritis and pulmonary hemorrhage. Outside of drug discontinuation, treatment should be based on the severity of the vasculitis. Patients with immediately life-threatening small-vessel vasculitis should initially be treated with glucocorticoids and cyclophosphamide as described for granulomatosis with polyangiitis (Wegener's). Following clinical improvement, consideration may be given for tapering such agents along a more rapid schedule.

SERUM SICKNESS AND SERUM SICKNESS–LIKE REACTIONS

These reactions are characterized by the occurrence of fever, urticaria, polyarthralgias, and lymphadenopathy 7–10 days after primary exposure and 2–4 days after secondary exposure to a heterologous protein (classic serum sickness) or a nonprotein drug such as penicillin or sulfa (serum sickness–like reaction). Most of the manifestations are not due to a vasculitis; however, occasional patients will have typical cutaneous venulitis that may progress rarely to a systemic vasculitis.

VASCULITIS ASSOCIATED WITH OTHER UNDERLYING DISEASES

Certain *infections* may directly trigger an inflammatory vasculitic process. For example, rickettsias can invade and proliferate in the endothelial cells of small blood vessels causing a vasculitis (Chap. 211). In addition, the inflammatory response around blood vessels associated with certain systemic fungal diseases such as histoplasmosis (Chap. 236) may mimic a primary vasculitic process. A leukocytoclastic vasculitis predominantly involving the skin with occasional involvement of other organ systems may be a minor component of many other infections. These include *subacute bacterial endocarditis, Epstein-Barr virus infection, HIV infection*, and a number of other infections.

Vasculitis can be associated with certain *malignancies*, particularly lymphoid or reticuloendothelial neoplasms. Leukocytoclastic venulitis confined to the skin is the most common finding; however, widespread systemic vasculitis may occur. Of particular note is the association of *hairy cell leukemia* (Chap. 134) with polyarteritis nodosa.

A number of *connective tissue diseases* have vasculitis as a secondary manifestation of the underlying primary process. Foremost among these are *systemic lupus erythematosus* (Chap. 378), *rheumatoid arthritis* (Chap. 380), *inflammatory myositis* (Chap. 388), *relapsing polychondritis* (Chap. 389), and *Sjögren's syndrome* (Chap. 383). The most common form of vasculitis in these conditions is the small-vessel venulitis isolated to the skin. However, certain patients may develop a fulminant systemic necrotizing vasculitis.

Secondary vasculitis has also been observed in association with *ulcerative colitis, congenital deficiencies of various complement components, sarcoidosis, primary biliary cirrhosis, α_1-antitrypsin deficiency*, and *intestinal bypass surgery*.

386e Atlas of the Vasculitic Syndromes

Carol A. Langford, Anthony S. Fauci

This is a digital-only chapter. It is available on the DVD that accompanies this book, as well as on Access Medicine/Harrison's Online, and the eBook and "app" editions of HPIM 19e.

Diagnosis of the vasculitic syndromes is usually based on characteristic histologic or arteriographic findings in a patient who has clinically compatible features. The images provided in this atlas highlight some of the characteristic histologic and radiographic findings that may be seen in the vasculitic diseases. These images demonstrate the importance that tissue histology may have in securing the diagnosis of vasculitis, the utility of diagnostic imaging in the vasculitic diseases, and the improvements in the care of vasculitis patients that have resulted from radiologic innovations.

Tissue biopsies represent vital information in many patients with a suspected vasculitic syndrome, not only in confirming the presence of vasculitis and other characteristic histologic features, but also in ruling out other diseases that can have similar clinical presentations. The determination of where biopsies should be performed is based on the presence of clinical disease in an affected organ, the likelihood of a positive diagnostic yield from data contained in the published literature, and the risk of performing a biopsy in an affected site. Common sites where biopsies may be performed include the lung, kidney, and skin. Other sites such as sural nerve, brain, testicle, and gastrointestinal tissues may also demonstrate features of vasculitis and be appropriate locations for biopsy when clinically affected.

387 Behçet's Syndrome

Haralampos M. Moutsopoulos

DEFINITION, INCIDENCE, AND PREVALENCE

Behçet's syndrome is a multisystem disorder presenting with recurrent oral and genital ulcerations as well as ocular involvement. The diagnosis is clinical and based on internationally agreed diagnostic criteria (Table 387-1).

The syndrome affects young males and females from the Mediterranean region, the Middle East, and the Far East, suggesting a link with the ancient Silk Route. Males and females are affected equally, but males often have more severe disease. Blacks are very infrequently affected.

PATHOGENESIS

The etiology and pathogenesis of this syndrome remain obscure. The disease appears to be in the crossroads of autoinflammatory and autoimmune disorders. The main pathologic lesion is systemic perivasculitis with early neutrophil infiltration and endothelial swelling. In some patients, diffuse inflammatory disease, involving all layers of large vessels and resulting to formation of pseudoaneurysms, suggests vasculitis of vasa vasorum. Apart from activated neutrophils, increased numbers of infiltrating T_H1, T_H17, cytotoxic CD8+, and γδ T cells are observed, suggesting a link between innate and adaptive autoreactive immune response. Circulating autoantibodies against α-enolase of endothelial cells, selenium binding protein, and anti-*Saccharomyces cerevisiae* antibodies have been observed, but their pathogenic role remains unclear. A recent genome-wide association study confirmed the known association of Behçet's syndrome with HLA-B*51 and identified a second, independent association within the major histocompatibility complex (MHC) class I region. In addition, an association with interleukin (IL) 10 and the IL-23R–IL-12RB2 locus was also observed. Interestingly, the disease-associated IL-10 variant was correlated with diminished mRNA expression and low protein production.

CLINICAL FEATURES

The recurrent aphthous ulcerations are a sine qua non for the diagnosis. The ulcers are usually painful, are shallow or deep with a central yellowish necrotic base, appear singly or in crops, and are located anywhere in the oral cavity. Small ulcers, less than 10 mm in diameter, are seen in 85% of patients, whereas large or herpetiform lesions are less frequent. The ulcers persist for 1–2 weeks and subside without leaving scars. The genital ulcers are less common but more specific, are painful, do not affect the glans penis or urethra, and produce scrotal scars.

Skin involvement is observed in 80% of patients and includes folliculitis, erythema nodosum, an acne-like exanthem, and, infrequently, vasculitis, Sweet syndrome, and pyoderma gangrenosum. Nonspecific skin inflammatory reactivity to any scratches or intradermal saline injection (pathergy test) is a common and specific manifestation.

Eye involvement with scarring and bilateral panuveitis is the most dreaded complication, since it occasionally progresses rapidly to blindness. The eye disease, occurring in 50% of patients, is usually present at the onset but may also develop within the first few years. In addition to iritis, posterior uveitis, retinal vessel occlusions, and optic neuritis can be seen in some patients with the syndrome.

Nondeforming arthritis or arthralgias are seen in 50% of patients and affect the knees and ankles.

TABLE 387-1 DIAGNOSTIC CRITERIA OF BEHÇET'S SYNDROME

Recurrent oral ulceration plus two of the following:

- Recurrent genital ulceration
- Eye lesions
- Skin lesions
- Pathergy test

Superficial or deep peripheral vein thrombosis is seen in 30% of patients. Pulmonary emboli are a rare complication. The superior vena cava is obstructed occasionally, producing a dramatic clinical picture. Arterial involvement occurs in less than 5% of patients and presents with aortitis or peripheral arterial aneurysm and arterial thrombosis. Pulmonary artery vasculitis presenting with dyspnea, cough, chest pain, hemoptysis, and infiltrates on chest roentgenograms has been reported in 5% of patients and should be differentiated from thromboembolic disease since it warrants anti-inflammatory and not thrombolytic therapy.

Neurologic involvement (5–10%) appears mainly in the parenchymal form (80%); it is associated with brainstem involvement and has a serious prognosis (*central nervous system [CNS]-Behçet's syndrome*). IL-6 is persistently raised in cerebrospinal fluid of these patients. Cerebral venous thrombosis is most frequently observed in the superior sagittal and transverse sinuses and is associated with headache and increased intracranial pressure. Magnetic resonance imaging (MRI) and/or proton magnetic resonance spectroscopy (MRS) are very sensitive and should be employed if CNS-Behçet's syndrome is suspected.

Gastrointestinal involvement is seen more frequently in patients from Japan and consists of mucosal ulcerations of the gut, resembling Crohn's disease.

Epididymitis is seen in 5% of patients, whereas amyloidosis of AA type and glomerulonephritis are uncommon.

Laboratory findings are mainly nonspecific indices of inflammation, such as leukocytosis and elevated erythrocyte sedimentation rate, as well as C-reactive protein levels.

TREATMENT BEHÇET'S SYNDROME

The severity of the syndrome usually abates with time. Apart from the patients with CNS-Behçet's syndrome and major vessel disease, the life expectancy seems to be normal and the only serious complication is blindness.

Mucous membrane involvement may respond to topical glucocorticoids in the form of mouthwash or paste. In more serious cases, thalidomide (100 mg/d) is effective. Thrombophlebitis is treated with aspirin, 325 mg/d. Colchicine can be beneficial for the mucocutaneous manifestations and arthritis. Uveitis and CNS-Behçet's syndrome require systemic glucocorticoid therapy (prednisone, 1 mg/kg per day) and azathioprine (2–3 mg/kg per day). Cyclosporine (5 mg/kg) has been used for sight-threatening uveitis, alone or in combination with azathioprine. Pulse doses of cyclophosphamide are useful early in the course of the disease for pulmonary or peripheral arterial aneurysms. Anti–tumor necrosis factor therapy is recommended in panuveitis refractory to immunosuppressives. Administration of this therapy improves visual acuity in more than two-thirds of patients.

388 Polymyositis, Dermatomyositis, and Inclusion Body Myositis

Marinos C. Dalakas

The inflammatory myopathies represent the largest group of acquired and potentially treatable causes of skeletal muscle weakness. They are classified into three major groups: polymyositis (PM), dermatomyositis (DM), and inclusion body myositis (IBM).

CLINICAL FEATURES

The prevalence of the inflammatory myopathies is estimated at 1 in 100,000. PM as a stand-alone entity is a rare disease. DM affects both children and adults and women more often than men. IBM is three times more frequent in men than in women, more common in whites than blacks, and is most likely to affect persons age >50 years.

These disorders present as progressive and symmetric muscle weakness except for IBM, which can have an asymmetric pattern. Patients usually report increasing difficulty with everyday tasks requiring the use of proximal muscles, such as getting up from a chair, climbing steps, stepping onto a curb, lifting objects, or combing hair. Fine-motor movements that depend on the strength of distal muscles, such as buttoning a shirt, sewing, knitting, or writing, are affected only late in the course of PM and DM, but fairly early in IBM. Falling is common in IBM because of early involvement of the quadriceps muscle, with buckling of the knees. Ocular muscles are spared, even in advanced, untreated cases; if these muscles are affected, the diagnosis of inflammatory myopathy should be questioned. Facial muscles are unaffected in PM and DM, but mild facial muscle weakness is common in patients with IBM. In all forms of inflammatory myopathy, pharyngeal and neck-flexor muscles are often involved, causing dysphagia or difficulty in holding up the head (*head drop*). In advanced and rarely in acute cases, respiratory muscles may also be affected. Severe weakness, if untreated, is almost always associated with muscle wasting. Sensation remains normal. The tendon reflexes are preserved but may be absent in severely weakened or atrophied muscles, especially in IBM, where atrophy of the quadriceps and the distal muscles is common. Myalgia and muscle tenderness may occur in a small number of patients, usually early in the disease, and particularly in DM associated with connective tissue disorders. Weakness in PM and DM progresses subacutely over a period of weeks or months and rarely acutely; by contrast, IBM progresses very slowly, over years, simulating a late-life muscular dystrophy (Chap. 462e) or slowly progressive motor neuron disorder (Chap. 452).

SPECIFIC FEATURES

(Table 388-1)

TABLE 388-1 FEATURES ASSOCIATED WITH INFLAMMATORY MYOPATHIES

Characteristic	Polymyositis	Dermatomyositis	Inclusion Body Myositis
Age at onset	>18 years	Adulthood and childhood	>50 years
Familial association	No	No	Yes, in some rare cases
Extramuscular manifestations	Yes	Yes	Yes
Associated conditions			
Connective tissue diseases	Yes[a]	Scleroderma and mixed connective tissue disease (overlap syndromes)	Yes, in up to 20% of cases[a]
Systemic autoimmune diseases[b]	Frequent	Infrequent	Infrequent
Malignancy	No	Yes, in up to 15% of cases	No
Viruses	Yes[c]	Unproven	Yes[c]
Drugs[d]	Yes	Yes, rarely	No
Parasites and bacteria[e]	Yes	No	No

[a]Systemic lupus erythematosus, rheumatoid arthritis, Sjögren's syndrome, systemic sclerosis, mixed connective tissue disease. [b]Crohn's disease, vasculitis, sarcoidosis, primary biliary cirrhosis, adult celiac disease, chronic graft-versus-host disease, discoid lupus, ankylosing spondylitis, Behçet's syndrome, myasthenia gravis, acne fulminans, dermatitis herpetiformis, psoriasis, Hashimoto's disease, granulomatous diseases, agammaglobulinemia, monoclonal gammopathy, hypereosinophilic syndrome, Lyme disease, Kawasaki disease, autoimmune thrombocytopenia, hypergammaglobulinemic purpura, hereditary complement deficiency, IgA deficiency. [c]HIV (human immunodeficiency virus) and HTLV-1 (human T cell lymphotropic virus type 1). [d]Drugs include penicillamine (dermatomyositis and polymyositis), zidovudine (polymyositis), statins (necrotizing, toxic, or autoimmune myositis), and contaminated tryptophan (dermatomyositis-like illness). Other myotoxic drugs may cause myopathy but not an inflammatory myopathy (see text for details). [e]Parasites (protozoa, cestodes, nematodes), tropical and bacterial myositis (pyomyositis).

Polymyositis The actual onset of PM is often not easily determined, and patients typically delay seeking medical advice for several weeks or even months. This is in contrast to DM, in which the rash facilitates early recognition (see below). PM mimics many other myopathies and is a diagnosis of exclusion. It is a subacute inflammatory myopathy affecting adults, and rarely children, who *do not have* any of the following: rash, involvement of the extraocular and facial muscles, family history of a neuromuscular disease, history of exposure to myotoxic drugs or toxins, endocrinopathy, neurogenic disease, muscular dystrophy, biochemical muscle disorder (deficiency of a muscle enzyme), or IBM as excluded by muscle biopsy analysis (see below). As an isolated entity, PM is a rare (and overdiagnosed) disorder; more commonly, PM occurs in association with a systemic autoimmune or connective tissue disease or with a known viral or bacterial infection. Drugs, especially D-penicillamine, statins, or zidovudine (AZT), may also trigger an inflammatory myopathy similar to PM.

Dermatomyositis DM is a distinctive entity identified by a characteristic rash accompanying, or more often preceding, muscle weakness. The rash may consist of a blue-purple discoloration on the upper eyelids with edema (heliotrope rash; see Fig. 73-3), a flat red rash on the face and upper trunk, and erythema of the knuckles with a raised violaceous scaly eruption (*Gottron's sign*; see Fig. 73-4). The erythematous rash can also occur on other body surfaces, including the knees, elbows, malleoli, neck and anterior chest (often in a *V sign*), or back and shoulders (*shawl sign*), and may worsen after sun exposure. In some patients, the rash is pruritic, especially on the scalp, chest, and back. Dilated capillary loops at the base of the fingernails are also characteristic. The cuticles may be irregular, thickened, and distorted, and the lateral and palmar areas of the fingers may become rough and cracked, with irregular, "dirty" horizontal lines, resembling *mechanic's hands*. The weakness can be mild, moderate, or severe enough to lead to quadriparesis. At times, the muscle strength appears normal, hence the term *dermatomyositis sine myositis*. When muscle biopsy is performed in such cases, however, significant perivascular and perimysial inflammation is often seen.

DM usually occurs alone but may overlap with scleroderma and mixed connective tissue disease. Fasciitis and thickening of the skin, similar to that seen in chronic cases of DM, have occurred in patients with the *eosinophilia-myalgia syndrome* associated with the ingestion of contaminated L-tryptophan.

Inclusion Body Myositis In patients ≥50 years of age, IBM is the most common of the inflammatory myopathies. It is often misdiagnosed as PM and is suspected only later when a patient with presumed PM does not respond to therapy. Weakness and atrophy of the distal muscles, especially foot extensors and deep finger flexors, occur in almost all cases of IBM and may be a clue to early diagnosis. Some patients present with falls because their knees collapse due to early quadriceps weakness. Others present with weakness in the small muscles of the hands, especially finger flexors, and complain of inability to hold objects such as golf clubs or perform tasks such as turning keys or tying knots. On occasion, the weakness and accompanying atrophy can be asymmetric and selectively involve the quadriceps, iliopsoas, triceps, biceps, and finger flexors, resembling a lower motor neuron disease. Dysphagia is common, occurring in up to 60% of IBM patients, and may lead to episodes of choking. Sensory examination is generally normal; some patients have mildly diminished vibratory sensation at the ankles that presumably is age-related. The pattern of distal weakness, which superficially resembles motor neuron or peripheral nerve disease, results from the myopathic process affecting distal muscles selectively. Disease progression is slow but steady, and most patients require an assistive device such as cane, walker, or wheelchair within several years of onset.

In at least 20% of cases, IBM is associated with systemic autoimmune or connective tissue diseases. Familial aggregation of typical IBM may occur; such cases have been designated as *familial inflammatory IBM*. This disorder is distinct from *hereditary inclusion body myopathy* (h-IBM), which describes a heterogeneous group of recessive, and less frequently dominant, inherited syndromes; the h-IBMs are noninflammatory myopathies. A subset of h-IBM that spares the quadriceps muscles has emerged as a distinct entity. This disorder, originally described in Iranian Jews and now seen in many ethnic groups, is linked to chromosome 9p1 and results from mutations in the UDP-*N*-acetylglucosamine 2-epimerase/*N*-acetylmannosamine kinase (*GNE*) gene.

ASSOCIATED CLINICAL FINDINGS

Extramuscular Manifestations These may be present to a varying degree in patients with PM or DM, and include:

1. *Systemic symptoms*, such as fever, malaise, weight loss, arthralgia, and Raynaud's phenomenon, especially when inflammatory myopathy is associated with a connective tissue disorder.
2. *Joint contractures*, mostly in DM and especially in children.
3. *Dysphagia and gastrointestinal symptoms*, due to involvement of oropharyngeal striated muscles and upper esophagus, especially in DM and IBM.
4. *Cardiac disturbances*, including atrioventricular conduction defects, tachyarrhythmias, dilated cardiomyopathy, a low ejection fraction, and congestive heart failure, which may rarely occur either from the disease itself or from hypertension associated with long-term use of glucocorticoids.
5. *Pulmonary dysfunction*, due to weakness of the thoracic muscles, interstitial lung disease, or drug-induced pneumonitis (e.g., from methotrexate), which may cause dyspnea, nonproductive cough, and aspiration pneumonia. Interstitial lung disease may precede myopathy or occur early in the disease and develops in up to 10% of patients with PM or DM, most of whom have antibodies to t-RNA synthetases, as described below.
6. *Subcutaneous calcifications*, in DM, sometimes extruding on the skin and causing ulcerations and infections.
7. *Arthralgias*, synovitis, or deforming arthropathy with subluxation in the interphalangeal joints, which can occur in some patients with DM and PM who have Jo-1 antibodies (see below).

Association with Malignancies Although all the inflammatory myopathies can have a chance association with malignant lesions, especially in older age groups, the incidence of malignant conditions appears to be specifically increased only in patients with DM and not in those with PM or IBM. The most common tumors associated with DM are ovarian cancer, breast cancer, melanoma, colon cancer, and non-Hodgkin's lymphoma. The extent of the search that should be conducted for an occult neoplasm in adults with DM depends on the clinical circumstances. Tumors in these patients are usually uncovered by abnormal findings in the medical history and physical examination and not through an extensive blind search. The weight of evidence argues against performing expensive, invasive, and nondirected tumor searches. A complete annual physical examination with pelvic, breast (mammogram, if indicated), and rectal examinations (with colonoscopy according to age and family history); urinalysis; complete blood count; blood chemistry tests; and a chest film should suffice in most cases. In Asians, nasopharyngeal cancer is common, and a careful examination of ears, nose, and throat is indicated. If malignancy is clinically suspected, screening with a whole-body positron emission tomography (PET) scan should be considered.

Overlap Syndromes These describe the association of inflammatory myopathies with connective tissue diseases. A well-characterized overlap syndrome occurs in patients with DM who also have manifestations of systemic sclerosis or mixed connective tissue disease, such as sclerotic thickening of the dermis, contractures, esophageal hypomotility, microangiopathy, and calcium deposits (Table 388-1). By contrast, signs of rheumatoid arthritis, systemic lupus erythematosus, or Sjögren's syndrome are very rare in patients with DM. Patients with the overlap syndrome of DM and systemic sclerosis may have a specific antinuclear antibody, the anti-PM/Scl, directed against a nucleolar-protein complex.

PATHOGENESIS

An autoimmune etiology of the inflammatory myopathies is indirectly supported by an association with other autoimmune or connective tissue diseases; the presence of various autoantibodies; an association with specific major histocompatibility complex (MHC) genes; demonstration of T cell–mediated myocytotoxicity or complement-mediated microangiopathy; and a response to immunotherapy.

Autoantibodies and Immunogenetics Various autoantibodies against nuclear antigens (antinuclear antibodies) and cytoplasmic antigens are found in up to 30% of patients with inflammatory myopathies. The antibodies to cytoplasmic antigens are directed against ribonucleoproteins involved in protein synthesis (antisynthetases) or translational transport (anti-signal-recognition particles). The antibody directed against the histidyl-transfer RNA synthetase, called *anti-Jo-1*, accounts for 75% of all the antisynthetases and is clinically useful because up to 80% of patients with anti-Jo-1 antibodies have interstitial lung disease. Some patients with the anti-Jo-1 antibody also have Raynaud's phenomenon, nonerosive arthritis, and the MHC molecules DR3 and DRw52. DR3 haplotypes (molecular designation DRB1*0301, DQB1*0201) occur in up to 75% of patients with PM and IBM, whereas in juvenile DM, there is an increased frequency of DQA1*0501 (Chap. 373e). Antibodies against the cytosolic 5′-nucleotidase 1A, an enzyme abundantly expressed in muscle and thought to be involved in DNA degradation and repair, have been detected in one-third of IBM patients. Although the pathogenic significance of these antibodies is still unknown, they highlight the presence of an immune response, as discussed below.

Immunopathologic Mechanisms In DM, humoral immune mechanisms are implicated, resulting in a microangiopathy and muscle ischemia (Fig. 388-1). Endomysial inflammatory infiltrates are composed of B cells located in proximity to CD4 T cells, plasmacytoid dendritic cells, and macrophages; there is a relative absence of lymphocytic invasion of nonnecrotic muscle fibers. Activation of the complement C5b-9 membranolytic attack complex is thought to be a critical early event that triggers release of proinflammatory cytokines and chemokines, induces expression of vascular cell adhesion molecule (VCAM) 1 and intercellular adhesion molecule (ICAM) 1 on endothelial cells, and facilitates migration of activated lymphoid cells to the perimysial and endomysial spaces. Necrosis of the endothelial cells, reduced numbers of endomysial capillaries, ischemia, and muscle-fiber destruction resembling microinfarcts occur. The remaining capillaries often have dilated lumens in response to the ischemic process. Larger intramuscular blood vessels may also be affected in the same pattern. Residual perifascicular atrophy reflects the endofascicular hypoperfusion that is prominent in the periphery of muscle fascicles. Increased expression of type I interferon–inducible proteins is also noted in these regions.

By contrast, in PM and IBM, a mechanism of T cell–mediated cytotoxicity is likely. CD8 T cells, along with macrophages, initially surround and eventually invade and destroy healthy, nonnecrotic muscle fibers that aberrantly express class I MHC molecules. MHC-I expression, absent from the sarcolemma of normal muscle fibers, is probably induced by cytokines secreted by activated T cells and macrophages. The CD8/MHC-I complex is characteristic of PM and IBM; its detection can aid in confirming the histologic diagnosis of PM, as discussed below. The cytotoxic CD8 T cells contain perforin and granzyme granules directed toward the surface of the muscle fibers and capable of inducing myonecrosis. Analysis of T cell receptor molecules expressed by the infiltrating CD8 cells has revealed clonal expansion and conserved sequences in the antigen-binding region, both suggesting an antigen-driven T cell response. Whether the putative antigens are endogenous (e.g., muscle) or exogenous (e.g., viral) sequences is unknown. Viruses have not been identified within the muscle fibers. Co-stimulatory molecules and their counterreceptors, which are fundamental for T cell activation and antigen recognition, are strongly upregulated in PM and IBM. As noted above, the possibility that B cells and the humoral immune system might also play a role in IBM is suggested by the identification of anti-cytosolic 5′-nucleotidase

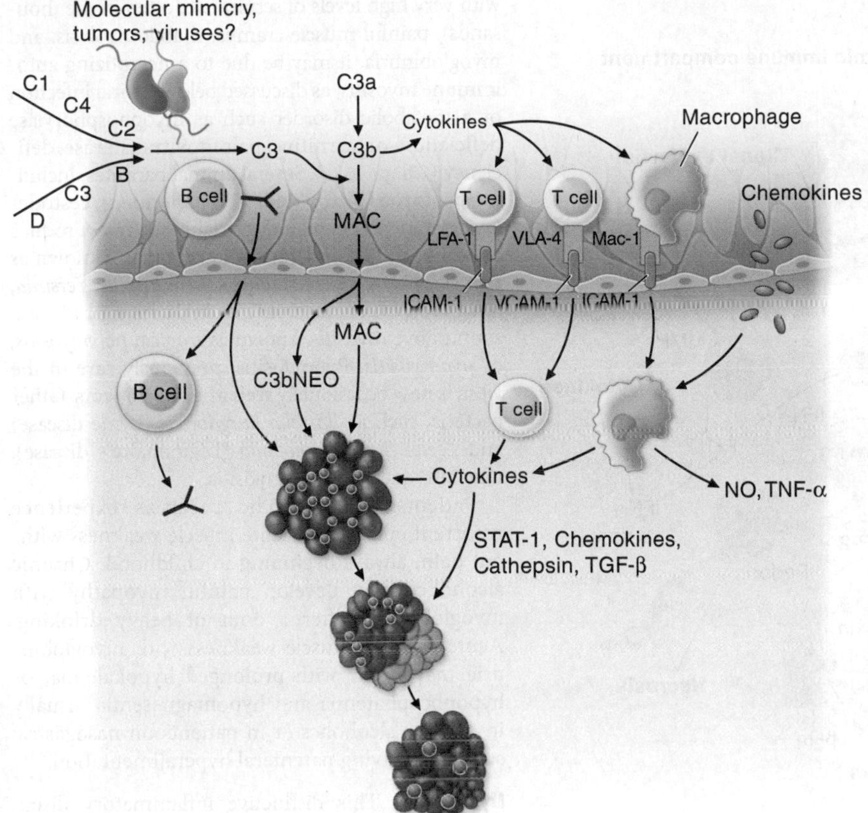

FIGURE 388-1 Immunopathogenesis of dermatomyositis. Activation of complement, possibly by autoantibodies (Y), against endothelial cells and formation of C3 via the classic or alternative pathway. Activated C3 leads to formation of C3b, C3bNEO, and membrane attack complexes (MAC), which are deposited in and around the endothelial cell wall of the endomysial capillaries. Deposition of MAC leads to destruction of capillaries, ischemia, or microinfarcts, most prominent in the periphery of the fascicles, and perifascicular atrophy. B cells, plasmacytoid dendritic cells, CD4 T cells, and macrophages traffic from the circulation to the muscle. Endothelial expression of vascular cell adhesion molecule (VCAM) and intercellular adhesion molecule (ICAM) is induced by cytokines released by the mononuclear cells. Integrins, specifically very late activation antigen (VLA)-4 and lymphocyte function–associated antigen (LFA)-1, bind VCAM and ICAM and promote T cell and macrophage infiltration of muscle through the endothelial cell wall.

1A antibodies in some patients. Key molecules involved in T cell–mediated cytotoxicity are depicted in Fig. 388-2.

The Role of Nonimmune Factors in IBM In IBM, the presence of Congo red–positive amyloid deposits within some vacuolated muscle fibers and abnormal mitochondria with cytochrome oxidase–negative fibers suggest that, in addition to the autoimmune component, there is also a degenerative process. Similar to Alzheimer's disease, the intracellular amyloid deposits in IBM are immunoreactive against amyloid precursor protein (APP), β-amyloid, chymotrypsin, apolipoprotein E, presenilin, ubiquitin, and phosphorylated tau, but it is unclear whether these deposits, which are also seen in other vacuolar myopathies, are directly pathogenic or represent secondary phenomena. The same is true for the mitochondrial abnormalities, which may also be secondary to the effects of aging or a bystander effect of upregulated cytokines. Expression of cytokines and upregulation of MHC class I by the muscle fibers may cause an endoplasmic reticulum stress response resulting in intracellular accumulation of stressor molecules or misfolded glycoproteins and activation of nuclear factor κB (NF-κB), leading to further cytokine activation.

Association with Viral Infections and the Role of Retroviruses Several viruses, including coxsackieviruses, influenza, paramyxoviruses, mumps, cytomegalovirus, and Epstein-Barr virus, have been indirectly associated with myositis. For the coxsackieviruses, an autoimmune myositis triggered by molecular mimicry has been proposed because of structural homology between histidyl-transfer RNA synthetase that is the target of the Jo-1 antibody (see above) and genomic RNA of an animal picornavirus, the encephalomyocarditis virus. Sensitive polymerase chain reaction (PCR) studies, however, have repeatedly failed to confirm the presence of such viruses in muscle biopsies.

The best evidence of a viral connection in PM and IBM is with the retroviruses. Some individuals infected with HIV or with human T cell lymphotropic virus 1 (HTLV-1) develop PM or IBM; a similar disorder has been described in nonhuman primates infected with the simian immunodeficiency virus. The inflammatory myopathy may occur as the initial manifestation of a retroviral infection, or myositis may develop later in the disease course. Retroviral antigens have been detected only in occasional endomysial macrophages and not within the muscle fibers themselves, suggesting that persistent infection and viral replication within the muscle does not occur. Histologic findings are identical to retroviral-negative PM or IBM. The infiltrating T cells in the muscle have a clonal bias and a number of them are retroviral-specific. This disorder should be distinguished from a toxic myopathy related to long-term therapy with AZT, characterized by fatigue, myalgia, mild muscle weakness, and mild elevation of creatine kinase (CK). AZT-induced myopathy, which generally improves when the drug is discontinued, is a mitochondrial disorder characterized histologically by "ragged-red" fibers. AZT inhibits γ-DNA polymerase, an enzyme found solely in the mitochondrial matrix.

GLOBAL ISSUES

Inadequate data exist with respect to possible differences in the prevalence of the inflammatory myopathies in various parts of the world. PM appears to be reported more often in Asia and southern Europe, whereas IBM seems to be more frequently recognized in North America, northern Europe, and Australia. Whether this represents differences in diagnostic methods and disease awareness or true disease prevalence remains unclear. Pyomyositis and parasitic myositis are clearly more common in the tropics, whereas HIV-associated PM and IBM are more commonly encountered in areas endemic for HIV. In patients from Asia, nasopharyngeal cancer appears to be a malignancy more commonly associated with DM, necessitating the need to specifically search for these tumors in this population.

DIFFERENTIAL DIAGNOSIS

The clinical picture of the typical skin rash and proximal or diffuse muscle weakness has few causes other than DM. However, proximal muscle weakness without skin involvement can be due to many conditions other than PM or IBM.

Subacute or Chronic Progressive Muscle Weakness This may be due to denervating conditions such as the spinal muscular atrophies or amyotrophic lateral sclerosis (Chap. 452). In addition to the muscle weakness, upper motor neuron signs in the latter and signs of denervation detected by electromyography (EMG) aid in the diagnosis. The muscular dystrophies (Chap. 462e) may be additional considerations; however, these disorders usually develop over years rather than weeks or months and rarely present after the age of 30 years. It may be difficult, even with a muscle biopsy, to distinguish chronic PM from a rapidly advancing muscular dystrophy. This is particularly true of facioscapulohumeral muscular dystrophy, dysferlin myopathy, and

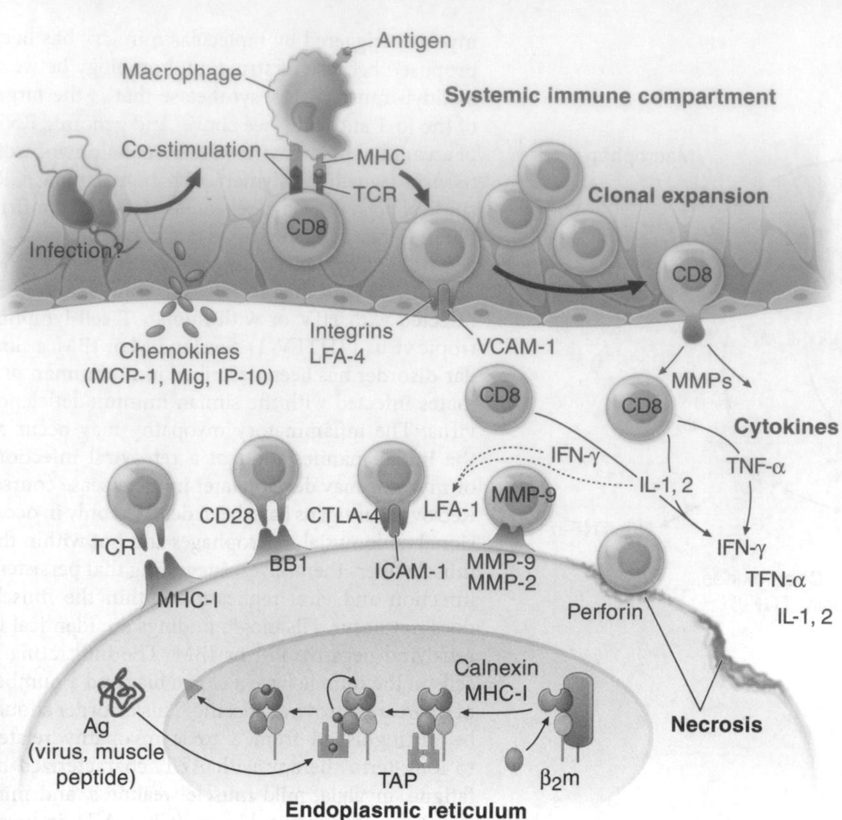

FIGURE 388-2 Cell-mediated mechanisms of muscle damage in polymyositis (PM) and inclusion body myositis (IBM). Antigen-specific CD8 cells are expanded in the periphery, cross the endothelial barrier, and bind directly to muscle fibers via T cell receptor (TCR) molecules that recognize aberrantly expressed major histocompatibility complex (MHC)-I. Engagement of co-stimulatory molecules (BB1 and ICOSL) with their ligands (CD28, CTLA-4, and ICOS), along with ICAM-1/LFA-1, stabilize the CD8–muscle fiber interaction. Metalloproteinases (MMPs) facilitate the migration of T cells and their attachment to the muscle surface. Muscle fiber necrosis occurs via perforin granules released by the autoaggressive T cells. A direct myocytotoxic effect exerted by the cytokines interferon (IFN) γ, interleukin (IL) 1, or tumor necrosis factor (TNF) α may also play a role. Death of the muscle fiber is mediated by necrosis. MHC class I molecules consist of a heavy chain and a light chain (β_2 microglobulin [β_2m]) complexed with an antigenic peptide that is transported into the endoplasmic reticulum by TAP proteins (Chap. 373e).

the dystrophinopathies where inflammatory cell infiltration is often found early in the disease. Such doubtful cases should always be given an adequate trial of glucocorticoid therapy and undergo genetic testing to exclude muscular dystrophy. Identification of the MHC/CD8 lesion by muscle biopsy is helpful to identify cases of PM. Some metabolic myopathies, including glycogen storage disease due to myophosphorylase or acid maltase deficiency, lipid storage myopathies due to carnitine deficiency, and mitochondrial diseases produce weakness that is often associated with other characteristic clinical signs; diagnosis rests upon histochemical and biochemical studies of the muscle biopsy. The endocrine myopathies such as those due to hypercorticosteroidism, hyper- and hypothyroidism, and hyper- and hypoparathyroidism require the appropriate laboratory investigations for diagnosis. Muscle wasting in patients with an underlying neoplasm may be due to disuse, cachexia, or rarely a paraneoplastic neuromyopathy (Chap. 122).

Diseases of the neuromuscular junction, including myasthenia gravis or the Lambert-Eaton myasthenic syndrome, cause fatiguing weakness that also affects ocular and other cranial muscles (Chap. 461). Repetitive nerve stimulation and single-fiber EMG studies aid in diagnosis.

Acute Muscle Weakness This may be caused by an acute neuropathy such as Guillain-Barré syndrome (Chap. 460), transverse myelitis (Chap. 456), a neurotoxin (Chap. 462e), or a neurotropic viral infection such as poliomyelitis or West Nile virus (Chap. 164). When acute weakness is associated with very high levels of serum CK (often in the thousands), painful muscle cramps, rhabdomyolysis, and myoglobinuria, it may be due to a necrotizing autoimmune myositis, as discussed below, a viral infection or a metabolic disorder such as myophosphorylase deficiency, or carnitine palmitoyltransferase deficiency (Chap. 462e). Several animal parasites, including protozoa (*Toxoplasma*, *Trypanosoma*), cestodes (cysticerci), and nematodes (trichinae), may produce a focal or diffuse inflammatory myopathy known as *parasitic polymyositis*. *Staphylococcus aureus*, *Yersinia*, *Streptococcus*, or anaerobic bacteria may produce a suppurative myositis, known as *tropical polymyositis*, or *pyomyositis*. Pyomyositis, previously rare in the west, is now occasionally seen in AIDS patients. Other bacteria, such as *Borrelia burgdorferi* (Lyme disease) and *Legionella pneumophila* (Legionnaire's disease), may infrequently cause myositis.

Patients with periodic paralysis experience recurrent episodes of acute muscle weakness without pain, always beginning in childhood. Chronic alcoholics may develop painful myopathy with myoglobinuria after a bout of heavy drinking. Acute painless muscle weakness with myoglobinuria may occur with prolonged hypokalemia, or hypophosphatemia and hypomagnesemia, usually in chronic alcoholics or in patients on nasogastric suction receiving parenteral hyperalimentation.

Myofasciitis This distinctive inflammatory disorder affecting muscle and fascia presents as diffuse myalgias, skin induration, fatigue, and mild muscle weakness; mild elevations of serum CK are usually present. The most common form is eosinophilic myofasciitis characterized by peripheral blood eosinophilia and eosinophilic infiltrates in the endomysial tissue. In some patients, the eosinophilic myositis/fasciitis occurs in the context of parasitic infections, vasculitis, mixed connective tissue disease, hypereosinophilic syndrome, or toxic exposures (e.g., toxic oil syndrome, contaminated L-tryptophan) or with mutations in the calpain gene. A distinct subset of myofasciitis is characterized by pronounced infiltration of the connective tissue around the muscle by sheets of periodic acid–Schiff-positive macrophages and occasional CD8 T cells (macrophagic myofasciitis or inflammatory myositis with abundant macrophages [IMAM]). A focal form of this disorder, limited to sites of previous vaccinations, administered months or years earlier, has been linked to an aluminum-containing substrate in vaccines. This disorder, which to date has not been observed outside of France, responds to glucocorticoid therapy, and the overall prognosis seems favorable.

Necrotizing Autoimmune Myositis This is an increasingly recognized entity that has distinct features, even though it is often labeled as PM. It presents as an acute or subacute onset of symmetric muscle weakness; CK is typically extremely high. The weakness can be severe. Coexisting interstitial lung disease and cardiomyopathy may be present. The disorder may develop after a viral infection, in association with cancer, or in patients taking statins when the myopathy continues to worsen after statin withdrawal. Some patients have antibodies against signal recognition particle (SRP) or against the 3-hydroxy-3-methylglutaryl-coenzyme A reductase (HMGCR), a 100-kDa protein considered the pharmacologic target of statins. The muscle biopsy demonstrates necrotic fibers infiltrated by macrophages but only rare, if any, T cell infiltrates. Muscle MHC-I expression is only slightly and focally upregulated. The capillaries may be swollen with hyalinization, thickening of the capillary wall, and deposition of complement. Most patients respond to immunotherapy, but some are resistant.

Hyperacute Necrotizing Fasciitis/Myositis (Flesh-Eating Disease) This a fulminant infectious disease, seen most often in the tropics or in conditions with poor hygiene, characterized by widespread necrosis of the superficial fascia and muscle of a limb; if the scrotum, perineum, and abdominal wall are affected, the condition is referred to as Fournier's gangrene. It may be caused by group A β-hemolytic *Streptococcus*, methicillin-sensitive *S. aureus*, *Pseudomonas aeruginosa*, *Vibrio vulnificus*, clostridial species (gas gangrene; Chap. 179), or polymicrobial infection with anaerobes and facultative bacteria (Chap. 201); toxins from these bacteria may act as superantigens (Chap. 372e). The port of bacterial entry is usually a trivial cut or skin abrasion, and the source is contact with carriers of the organism. Individuals with diabetes mellitus, immunodeficiency states, or systemic illnesses such as liver failure are most susceptible. Systemic varicella is a predisposing factor in children.

The disease presents with swelling, pain, and redness in the involved area followed by a rapid tissue necrosis of fascia and muscle that progresses at an estimated rate of 3 cm/h. Emergency debridement, antibiotics, IV immunoglobulin (IVIg), and even hyperbaric oxygen have been recommended. In progressive or advanced cases, amputation of the affected limb may be necessary to avoid a fatal outcome.

Drug-Induced Myopathies D-Penicillamine, procainamide, and statins may produce a true myositis resembling PM or necrotizing myositis. A DM-like illness has been associated with the contaminated preparations of L-tryptophan. As noted above, AZT causes a mitochondrial myopathy. Other drugs may elicit a toxic noninflammatory myopathy that is histologically different from DM, PM, or IBM. These include cholesterol-lowering agents such as clofibrate, lovastatin, simvastatin, or pravastatin, especially when combined with cyclosporine, amiodarone, or gemfibrozil. Mild statin-induced myopathic symptoms (such as myalgia, fatigue, or asymptomatic elevations of CK) are self-limited and usually improve after discontinuation of the drug. In rare patients, however, muscle weakness continues to progress even after the statin is withdrawn; in these cases, a diagnostic muscle biopsy is indicated and search for antibodies to HMGCR is suggested; if histologic evidence of PM or necrotizing myositis is present, immunotherapy should be initiated. Rhabdomyolysis and myoglobinuria have been rarely associated with amphotericin B, ε-aminocaproic acid, fenfluramine, heroin, and phencyclidine. The use of amiodarone, chloroquine, colchicine, carbimazole, emetine, etretinate, and ipecac syrup; chronic laxative or licorice use resulting in hypokalemia; and glucocorticoid or growth hormone administration have also been associated with myopathic muscle weakness. Some neuromuscular blocking agents such as pancuronium, in combination with glucocorticoids, may cause an acute critical illness myopathy. A careful drug history is essential for diagnosis of these drug-induced myopathies, which do not require immunosuppressive therapy except when an autoimmune myopathy has been triggered, as noted above.

"Weakness" due to Muscle Pain and Muscle Tenderness A number of conditions including *polymyalgia rheumatica* (Chap. 385) and arthritic disorders of adjacent joints may enter into the differential diagnosis of inflammatory myopathy, even though they do not cause myositis. The muscle biopsy is either normal or discloses type II muscle fiber atrophy. Patients with *fibrositis* and *fibromyalgia* (Chap. 396) complain of focal or diffuse muscle tenderness, fatigue, and aching, which is sometimes poorly differentiated from joint pain. Some patients, however, have muscle tenderness, painful muscles on movement, and signs suggestive of a collagen vascular disorder, such as an increased erythrocyte sedimentation rate, C-reactive protein, antinuclear antibody, or rheumatoid factor, along with modest elevation of the serum CK and aldolase. They demonstrate a "break-away" pattern of weakness with difficulty sustaining effort but not true muscle weakness. The muscle biopsy is usually normal or nonspecific. Many such patients show some response to nonsteroidal anti-inflammatory agents or glucocorticoids, although most continue to have indolent complaints. An indolent fasciitis in the setting of an ill-defined connective tissue disorder may be at times present, and these patients should not be labeled as having a psychosomatic disorder. *Chronic fatigue syndrome*, which may follow a viral infection, can present with debilitating fatigue, sore throat, painful lymphadenopathy, myalgia, arthralgia, sleep disorder, and headache (Chap. 464e). These patients do not have muscle weakness, and the muscle biopsy is normal.

DIAGNOSIS

The clinically suspected diagnosis of PM, DM, IBM, or necrotizing myositis is confirmed by analysis of serum muscle enzymes, EMG findings, and muscle biopsy (Table 388-2).

The most sensitive enzyme is CK, which in active disease can be elevated as much as 50-fold. Although the CK level usually parallels disease activity, it can be normal in some patients with active IBM or DM, especially when associated with a connective tissue disease. The CK is always elevated in patients with active PM. Along with the CK, the serum glutamic-oxaloacetic and glutamate pyruvate transaminases, lactate dehydrogenase, and aldolase may be elevated.

Needle EMG shows myopathic potentials characterized by short-duration, low-amplitude polyphasic units on voluntary activation and increased spontaneous activity with fibrillations, complex repetitive discharges, and positive sharp waves. Mixed potentials (polyphasic units of short and long duration) indicating a chronic process and muscle fiber regeneration are often present in IBM. These EMG findings are not diagnostic of an inflammatory myopathy but are useful

TABLE 388-2 CRITERIA FOR DIAGNOSIS OF INFLAMMATORY MYOPATHIES

	Polymyositis			
Criterion	Definite	Probable	Dermatomyositis	Inclusion Body Myositis
Myopathic muscle weakness[a]	Yes	Yes	Yes[b]	Yes; slow onset, early involvement of distal muscles, frequent falls
Electromyographic findings	Myopathic	Myopathic	Myopathic	Myopathic with mixed potentials
Muscle enzymes	Elevated (up to 50-fold)	Elevated (up to 50-fold)	Elevated (up to 50-fold) or normal	Elevated (up to 10-fold) or normal
Muscle biopsy findings[c]	"Primary" inflammation with the CD8/MHC-I complex and no vacuoles	Ubiquitous MHC-I expression but minimal inflammation and no vacuoles[d]	Perifascicular, perimysial, or perivascular infiltrates, perifascicular atrophy	Primary inflammation with CD8/MHC-I complex; vacuolated fibers with β-amyloid deposits; cytochrome oxygenase–negative fibers; signs of chronic myopathy[e]
Rash or calcinosis	Absent	Absent	Present[f]	Absent

[a]Myopathic muscle weakness, affecting proximal muscles more than distal ones and sparing eye and facial muscles, is characterized by a subacute onset (weeks to months) and rapid progression in patients who have no family history of neuromuscular disease, no endocrinopathy, no exposure to myotoxic drugs or toxins, and no biochemical muscle disease (excluded on the basis of muscle biopsy findings). [b]In some cases with the typical rash, the muscle strength is seemingly normal (dermatomyositis sine myositis); these patients often have new onset of easy fatigue and reduced endurance. Careful muscle testing may reveal mild muscle weakness. [c]See text for details. [d]An adequate trial of prednisone or other immunosuppressive drugs is warranted in probable cases. If, in retrospect, the disease is unresponsive to therapy, another muscle biopsy should be considered to exclude other diseases or possible evolution in inclusion body myositis. [e]If the muscle biopsy does not contain vacuolated fibers but shows chronic myopathy with hypertrophic fibers, primary inflammation with the CD8/MHC-I complex, and cytochrome oxygenase–negative fibers, the diagnosis is probable inclusion body myositis. [f]If rash is absent but muscle biopsy findings are characteristic of dermatomyositis, the diagnosis is probable dermatomyositis.

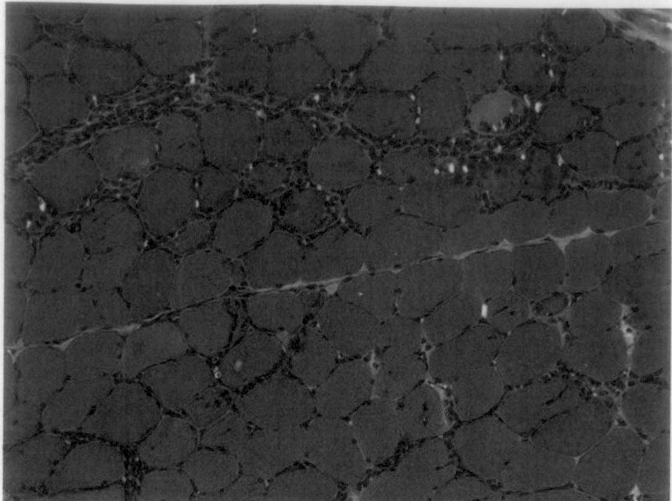

FIGURE 388-3 Cross-section of a muscle biopsy from a patient with polymyositis demonstrates scattered inflammatory foci with lymphocytes invading or surrounding muscle fibers. Note lack of chronic myopathic features (increased connective tissue, atrophic or hypertrophic fibers) as seen in inclusion body myositis.

to identify the presence of active or chronic myopathy and to exclude neurogenic disorders.

Magnetic resonance imaging (MRI) is not routinely used for the diagnosis of PM, DM, or IBM. However, it may provide information or guide the location of the muscle biopsy in certain clinical settings.

Muscle biopsy—despite occasional variability in demonstrating all of the typical pathologic findings—is the most sensitive and specific test for establishing the diagnosis of inflammatory myopathy and for excluding other neuromuscular diseases. Inflammation is the histologic hallmark for these diseases; however, additional features are characteristic of each subtype (Figs. 388-3, 388-4, and 388-5).

In PM the inflammation is *primary*, a term used to indicate that the inflammation is not reactive and the T cell infiltrates, located primarily within the muscle fascicles (endomysially), surround individual, healthy muscle fibers and result in phagocytosis and necrosis (Fig. 388-3). The MHC-I molecule is ubiquitously expressed on the sarcolemma, even in fibers not invaded by CD8+ cells. The CD8/MHC-I lesion is characteristic and useful to confirm or establish the diagnosis and to exclude disorders with secondary, nonspecific, inflammation, such as in some muscular dystrophies. When the disease is chronic, connective tissue is increased and may react positively with alkaline phosphatase. In necrotizing myositis, there are abundant necrotic fibers invaded or

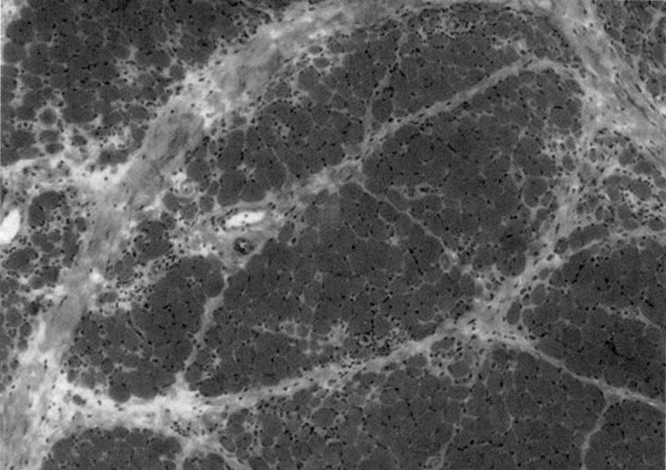

FIGURE 388-4 Cross-section of a muscle biopsy from a patient with dermatomyositis demonstrates atrophy of the fibers at the periphery of the fascicle (perifascicular atrophy).

surrounded by macrophages, but no lymphocytic infiltrates or MHC-I expression beyond the necrotic fibers.

In DM the endomysial inflammation is predominantly perivascular or in the interfascicular septae and around—rather than within—the muscle fascicles (Fig. 388-4). The intramuscular blood vessels show endothelial hyperplasia with tubuloreticular profiles, fibrin thrombi, and obliteration of capillaries. The muscle fibers undergo necrosis, degeneration, and phagocytosis, often in groups involving a portion of a muscle fasciculus in a wedge-like shape or at the periphery of the fascicle, due to microinfarcts within the muscle. This results in perifascicular atrophy, characterized by 2–10 layers of atrophic fibers at the periphery of the fascicles. The presence of perifascicular atrophy is diagnostic of DM, *even in the absence of inflammation*.

In IBM (Fig. 388-5), there is endomysial inflammation with T cells invading MHC-I-expressing nonvacuolated muscle fibers; basophilic granular deposits distributed around the edge of slit-like vacuoles (rimmed vacuoles); loss of fibers, replaced by fat and connective tissue, hypertrophic fibers, and angulated or round fibers; rare eosinophilic cytoplasmic inclusions; abnormal mitochondria characterized by the presence of ragged-red fibers or cytochrome oxidase–negative fibers; and amyloid deposits within or next to the vacuoles best visualized with crystal violet or Congo-red staining viewed with fluorescent optics. Electron microscopy demonstrates filamentous inclusions in the vicinity of the rimmed vacuoles. In at least 15% of patients with the typical clinical phenotype of IBM, there is brisk inflammation in the muscle biopsy but no vacuoles or amyloid deposits, leading to an erroneous diagnosis of PM. Such patients are often referred to as having "clinical IBM." Close clinicopathologic correlations are therefore essential; if uncertain, a repeat muscle biopsy from another site is often helpful.

TREATMENT THERAPY OF INFLAMMATORY MYOPATHIES

The goal of therapy is to improve muscle strength, thereby improving function in activities of daily living, and ameliorate the extramuscular manifestations (rash, dysphagia, dyspnea, fever). When strength improves, the serum CK falls concurrently; however, the reverse is not always true. Unfortunately, there is a common tendency to "chase" or treat the CK level instead of the muscle weakness, a practice that has led to prolonged and unnecessary use of immunosuppressive drugs and erroneous assessment of their efficacy. It is prudent to discontinue these drugs if, after an adequate trial, there is no objective improvement in muscle strength whether or not CK levels are reduced. Agents used in the treatment of PM and DM include the following:

1. *Glucocorticoids*. Oral prednisone is the initial treatment of choice; the effectiveness and side effects of this therapy determine the future need for stronger immunosuppressive drugs. High-dose prednisone, at least 1 mg/kg per day, is initiated as early in the disease as possible. After 3–4 weeks, prednisone is tapered slowly over a period of 10 weeks to 1 mg/kg every other day. If there is evidence of efficacy and no serious side effects, the dosage is then further reduced by 5 or 10 mg every 3–4 weeks until the lowest possible dose that controls the disease is reached. The efficacy of prednisone is determined by an objective increase in muscle strength and activities of daily living, which almost always occurs by the third month of therapy. A feeling of increased energy or a reduction of the CK level without a concomitant increase in muscle strength is not a reliable sign of improvement. If prednisone provides no objective benefit after ~3 months of high-dose therapy, the disease is probably unresponsive to the drug and tapering should be accelerated while the next-in-line immunosuppressive drug is started. Although controlled trials have not been performed, almost all patients with true PM or DM respond to glucocorticoids to *some degree and for some period of time*; in general, DM responds better than PM.

The long-term use of prednisone may cause increased weakness associated with a normal or unchanged CK level; this effect is referred to as *steroid myopathy*. In a patient who previously

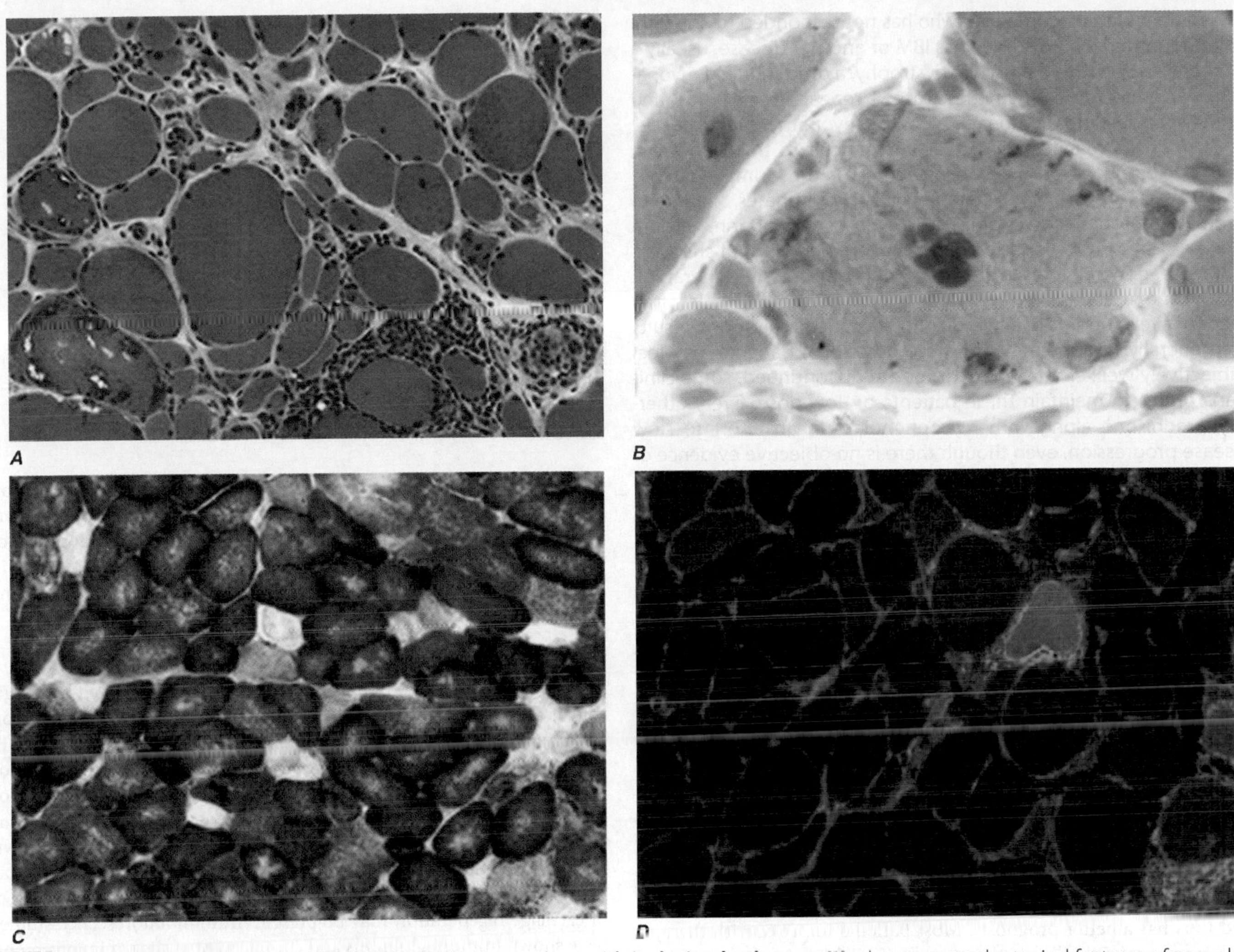

FIGURE 388-5 Cross-sections of a muscle biopsy from a patient with inclusion body myositis demonstrate the typical features of vacuoles with lymphocytic infiltrates surrounding nonvacuolated or necrotic fibers (***A***), tiny endomysial deposits of amyloid visualized with crystal violet (***B***), cytochrome oxidase–negative fibers, indicative of mitochondrial dysfunction (***C***), and ubiquitous major histocompatibility complex class I expression at the periphery of all fibers (***D***).

responded to high doses of prednisone, the development of new weakness may be related to steroid myopathy or to disease activity that either will respond to a higher dose of glucocorticoids or has become glucocorticoid-resistant. In uncertain cases, the prednisone dosage can be steadily increased or decreased as desired: the cause of the weakness is usually evident in 2–8 weeks.

2. *Other immunosuppressive drugs*. Approximately 75% of patients ultimately require additional treatment. This occurs when a patient fails to respond adequately to glucocorticoids after a 3-month trial, the patient becomes glucocorticoid-resistant, glucocorticoid-related side effects appear, attempts to lower the prednisone dose repeatedly result in a new relapse, or rapidly progressive disease with evolving severe weakness and respiratory failure develops.

   The following drugs are commonly used but have never been tested in controlled studies: (1) *Azathioprine* is well tolerated, has few side effects, and appears to be as effective for long-term therapy as other drugs. The dose is up to 3 mg/kg daily. (2) *Methotrexate* has a faster onset of action than azathioprine. It is given orally starting at 7.5 mg weekly for the first 3 weeks (2.5 mg every 12 h for 3 doses), with gradual dose escalation by 2.5 mg per week to a total of 25 mg weekly. A rare side effect is methotrexate pneumonitis, which can be difficult to distinguish from the interstitial lung disease of the primary myopathy associated with Jo-1 antibodies (described above). (3) *Mycophenolate mofetil* also has a faster onset of action than azathioprine. At doses up to 2.5 or 3 g/d in two divided doses, it is well tolerated for long-term use. (4) Monoclonal anti-CD20 antibody (rituximab) has been shown in a small uncontrolled series to benefit patients with DM and PM, but a controlled study did not show differences between patients randomized 8 weeks apart. (5) *Cyclosporine* has inconsistent and mild benefit. (6) *Cyclophosphamide* (0.5–1 g/m^2 IV monthly for 6 months) has limited success and significant toxicity. (7) Tacrolimus (formerly known as Fk506) has been effective in some difficult cases of PM especially with interstitial lung disease.

3. *Immunomodulation*. In a controlled trial of patients with refractory DM, IVIg improved not only strength and rash but also the underlying immunopathology. The benefit is often short-lived (≤8 weeks), and repeated infusions every 6–8 weeks are generally required to maintain improvement. A dose of 2 g/kg divided over 2–5 days per course is recommended. Uncontrolled observations suggest that IVIg may also be beneficial for patients with PM. Neither plasmapheresis nor leukapheresis appears to be effective in PM and DM.

The following sequential empirical approach to the treatment of PM and DM is suggested: *Step 1*: high-dose prednisone; *Step 2*: azathioprine, mycophenolate, or methotrexate for steroid-sparing effect; *Step 3*: IVIg; *Step 4*: a trial, with guarded optimism, of one of the following agents, chosen according to the patient's age, degree of disability, tolerance, experience with the drug, and general health: rituximab, cyclosporine, cyclophosphamide, or tacrolimus. Patients with interstitial lung disease may benefit from aggressive treatment with cyclophosphamide or tacrolimus.

A patient with presumed PM who has not responded to any form of immunotherapy most likely has IBM or another disease, usually a metabolic myopathy, a muscular dystrophy, a drug-induced myopathy, or an endocrinopathy. In these cases, a repeat muscle biopsy and a renewed search for another cause of the myopathy is indicated.

Calcinosis, a manifestation of DM, is difficult to treat; however, new calcium deposits may be prevented if the primary disease responds to the available therapies. Bisphosphonates, aluminum hydroxide, probenecid, colchicine, low doses of warfarin, calcium blockers, and surgical excision have all been tried without success.

IBM is generally resistant to immunosuppressive therapies. Prednisone together with azathioprine or methotrexate is often tried for a few months in newly diagnosed patients, although results are generally disappointing. Because occasional patients may feel subjectively weaker after these drugs are discontinued, some clinicians prefer to maintain these patients on low-dose, every-other-day prednisone along with mycophenolate in an effort to slow disease progression, even though there is no objective evidence or controlled study to support this practice. In two controlled studies of IVIg in IBM, minimal benefit in up to 30% of patients was found; the strength gains, however, were not of sufficient magnitude to justify its routine use. Another trial of IVIg combined with prednisone was ineffective. Nonetheless, some experts believe that a 2- to 3-month trial with IVIg may be reasonable for selected patients with IBM who experience rapid progression of muscle weakness or choking episodes due to worsening dysphagia.

PROGNOSIS

The 5-year survival rate for treated patients with PM and DM is ~95%, and the 10-year survival rate is 84%; death is usually due to pulmonary, cardiac, or other systemic complications. The prognosis is worse for patients who are severely affected at presentation, when initial treatment is delayed, and in cases with severe dysphagia or respiratory difficulties. Older patients and those with associated cancer also have a worse prognosis. DM responds more favorably to therapy than PM and thus has a better prognosis. Most patients improve with therapy, and many make a full functional recovery, which is often sustained with maintenance therapy. Up to 30% may be left with some residual muscle weakness. Relapses may occur at any time.

IBM has the least favorable prognosis of the inflammatory myopathies. Most patients will require the use of an assistive device such as a cane, walker, or wheelchair within 5–10 years of onset. In general, the older the age of onset in IBM, the more rapidly progressive is the course.

389 Relapsing Polychondritis

Carol A. Langford

Relapsing polychondritis is an uncommon disorder of unknown cause characterized by inflammation of cartilage predominantly affecting the ears, nose, and laryngotracheobronchial tree. Other manifestations include scleritis, neurosensory hearing loss, polyarthritis, cardiac abnormalities, skin lesions, and glomerulonephritis. Relapsing polychondritis has been estimated to have an incidence of 3.5 per million population per year. The peak age of onset is between the ages of 40 and 50 years, but relapsing polychondritis may affect children and the elderly. It is found in all races, and both sexes are equally affected. No familial tendency is apparent. A significantly higher frequency of HLA-DR4 has been found in patients with relapsing polychondritis than in healthy individuals. A predominant subtype allele(s) of HLA-DR4 was not found. Approximately 30% of patients with relapsing polychondritis will have another rheumatologic disorder, the most frequent being systemic vasculitis, followed by rheumatoid arthritis, and systemic lupus erythematosus (SLE). Nonrheumatic disorders associated with relapsing polychondritis include Hashimoto's thyroiditis, primary biliary cirrhosis, and myelodysplastic syndrome (Table 389-1). In most cases, these disorders antedate the appearance of relapsing polychondritis, usually by months or years; however, in other instances, the onset of relapsing polychondritis can accompany disease presentation.

TABLE 389-1 DISORDERS ASSOCIATED WITH RELAPSING POLYCHONDRITIS[a]

Systemic vasculitis
Rheumatoid arthritis
Systemic lupus erythematosus
Overlapping connective tissue disease
Spondyloarthritides
Behçet's disease
Polymyalgia rheumatica
Primary biliary cirrhosis
Pulmonary fibrosis
Hashimoto's thyroiditis
Myelodysplastic syndrome

[a]Systemic vasculitis is the most common association, followed by rheumatoid arthritis and systemic lupus erythematosus.

Source: Modified from CJ Michet et al: Ann Intern Med 104:74, 1986.

PATHOLOGY AND PATHOPHYSIOLOGY

The earliest abnormality of hyaline and elastic cartilage noted histologically is a focal or diffuse loss of basophilic staining indicating depletion of proteoglycan from the cartilage matrix. Inflammatory infiltrates are found adjacent to involved cartilage and consist predominantly of mononuclear cells and occasional plasma cells. In acute disease, polymorphonuclear white cells may also be present. Destruction of cartilage begins at the outer edges and advances centrally. There is lacunar breakdown and loss of chondrocytes. Degenerating cartilage is replaced by granulation tissue and later by fibrosis and focal areas of calcification. Small loci of cartilage regeneration may be present. Immunofluorescence studies have shown immunoglobulins and complement at sites of involvement. Extracellular granular material observed in the degenerating cartilage matrix by electron microscopy has been interpreted to be enzymes, immunoglobulins, or proteoglycans.

Immunologic mechanisms play a role in the pathogenesis of relapsing polychondritis. The accumulating data strongly suggest that both humoral and cell-mediated immunity play an important role in the pathogenesis of relapsing polychondritis. Immunoglobulin and complement deposits are found at sites of inflammation. In addition, antibodies to type II collagen and to matrilin-1 and immune complexes are detected in the sera of some patients. The possibility that an immune response to type II collagen may be important in the pathogenesis is supported experimentally by the occurrence of auricular chondritis in rats immunized with type II collagen. Antibodies to type II collagen are found in the sera of these animals, and immune deposits are detected at sites of ear inflammation. Humoral immune responses to type IX and type XI collagen, matrilin-1, and cartilage oligomeric matrix protein have been demonstrated in some patients. In a study, rats immunized with matrilin-1 were found to develop severe inspiratory stridor and swelling of the nasal septum. The rats had severe inflammation with erosions of the involved cartilage, which was characterized by increased numbers of CD4+ and CD8+ T cells in the lesions. The cartilage of the joints and ear pinna was not involved. All had IgG antibodies to matrilin-1. Matrilin-1 is a noncollagenous protein present in the extracellular matrix in cartilage. It is present in high concentrations in the trachea and is also present in the nasal septum but not in articular cartilage. A subsequent study demonstrated serum anti-matrilin-1 antibodies in approximately 13% of patients with relapsing polychondritis; approximately 70% of these patients had respiratory symptoms. Cell-mediated immunity may also be operative in causing tissue injury, since lymphocyte transformation can be demonstrated when lymphocytes of patients are exposed to cartilage extracts. T cells specific for type II collagen have been found in some

TABLE 389-2 CLINICAL MANIFESTATIONS OF RELAPSING POLYCHONDRITIS

Clinical Feature	Presenting	Cumulative
	Frequency, %	
Auricular chondritis	43	89
Arthritis	32	72
Nasal chondritis	21	61
Ocular inflammation	18	59
Laryngotracheal symptoms	23	55
Reduced hearing	7	40
Saddle nose deformity	11	25
Cutaneous	4	25
Laryngotracheal stricture	15	23
Vasculitis	2	14
Elevated creatinine	7	13
Aortic or mitral regurgitation	0	12

Source: Modified from PD Kent et al: Curr Opin Rheumatol 16:56, 2004.

patients, and CD4+ T cells have been observed at sites of cartilage inflammation.

CLINICAL MANIFESTATIONS

The onset of relapsing polychondritis is frequently abrupt, with the appearance of one or two sites of cartilaginous inflammation. The pattern of cartilaginous involvement and the frequency of episodes vary widely among patients. Noncartilaginous presentations may also occur. Systemic inflammatory features such as fever, fatigue, and weight loss occur and may precede the clinical signs of relapsing polychondritis by several weeks. Relapsing polychondritis may go unrecognized for several months or even years in patients who only initially manifest intermittent joint pain and/or swelling, or who have unexplained eye inflammation, hearing loss, valvular heart disease, or pulmonary symptoms.

Auricular chondritis is the most frequent presenting manifestation of relapsing polychondritis, occurring in 40% of patients and eventually affecting about 85% of patients (Table 389-2). One or both ears are involved, either sequentially or simultaneously. Patients experience the sudden onset of pain, tenderness, and swelling of the cartilaginous portion of the ear (Fig. 389-1). This typically involves the pinna of the ears, sparing the earlobes because they do not contain cartilage. The overlying skin has a beefy red or violaceous color. Prolonged or recurrent episodes lead to cartilage destruction and result in a flabby or

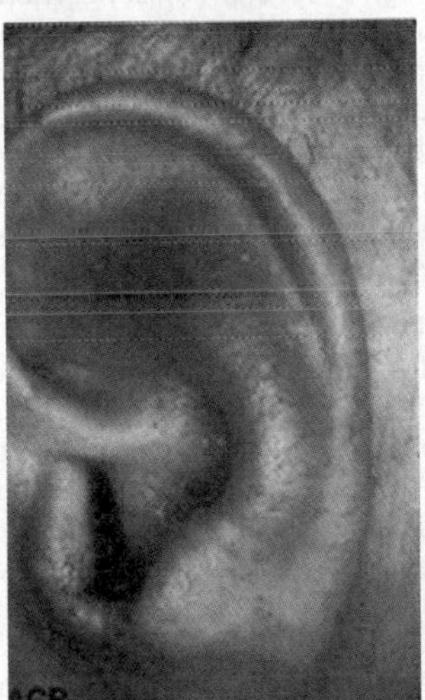

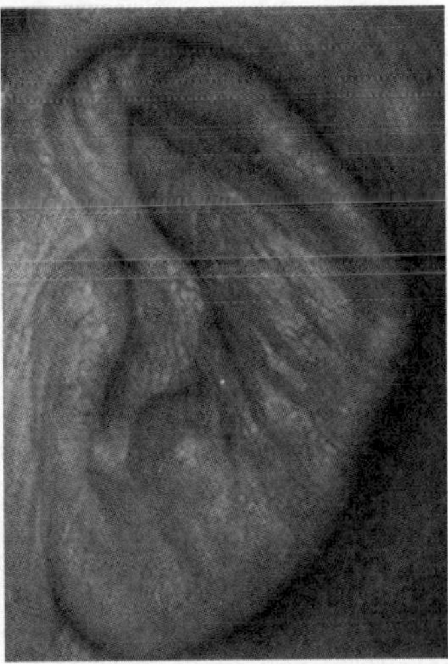

FIGURE 389-1 ***Left.*** The pinna is erythematous, swollen, and tender. Not shown is the ear lobule that is spared as there is no underlying cartilage. ***Right.*** The pinna is thickened and deformed. The destruction of the underlying cartilage results in a floppy ear. *(Reprinted from the Clinical Slide Collection on the Rheumatic Diseases, ©1991, 1995, 1997, 1998, 1999. Used by permission of the American College of Rheumatology.)*

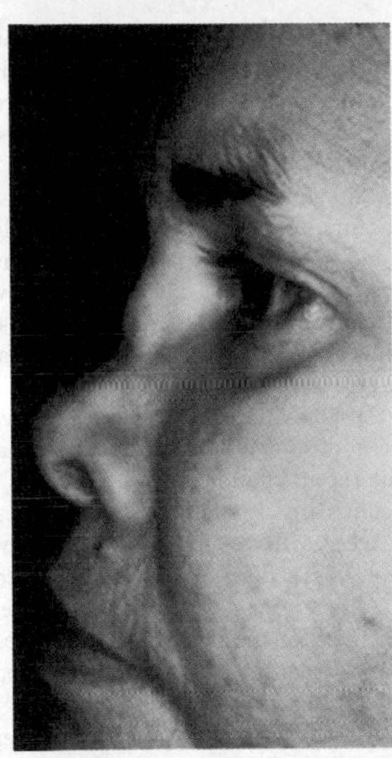

FIGURE 389-2 Saddle nose results from destruction and collapse of the nasal cartilage. *(Reprinted from the Clinical Slide Collection on the Rheumatic Diseases, ©1991, 1995, 1997, 1998, 1999. Used by permission of the American College of Rheumatology.)*

droopy ear. Swelling may close off the eustachian tube or the external auditory meatus, either of which can impair hearing. Inflammation of the internal auditory artery or its cochlear branch produces hearing loss, vertigo, ataxia, nausea, and vomiting. Vertigo is almost always accompanied by hearing loss.

Approximately 61% of patients will develop nasal involvement, with 21% having this at the time of presentation. Patients may experience nasal stuffiness, rhinorrhea, and epistaxis. The bridge of the nose and surrounding tissue become red, swollen, and tender and may collapse, producing a saddle nose deformity (Fig. 389-2). In some patients, nasal deformity develops insidiously without overt inflammation. Saddle nose is observed more frequently in younger patients, especially in women.

Joint involvement is the presenting manifestation in relapsing polychondritis in approximately one-third of patients and may be present for several months before other features appear. Eventually, more than one-half of the patients will have arthralgias or arthritis. The arthritis is usually asymmetric and oligo- or polyarticular, and it involves both large and small peripheral joints. An episode of arthritis lasts from a few days to several weeks and resolves spontaneously without joint erosion or deformity. Attacks of arthritis may not be temporally related to other manifestations of relapsing polychondritis. Joint fluid has been reported to be noninflammatory. In addition to peripheral joints, inflammation may involve the costochondral, sternomanubrial, and sternoclavicular cartilages. Destruction of these cartilages may result in a pectus excavatum deformity or even a flail anterior chest wall.

Eye manifestations occur in more than one-half of patients and include conjunctivitis, episcleritis, scleritis, iritis, uveitis, and keratitis. Ocular inflammation can be severe and visually threatening. Other manifestations include eyelid and periorbital edema, proptosis, optic neuritis, extraocular muscle palsies, retinal vasculitis, and renal vein occlusion.

Laryngotracheobronchial involvement occurs in ~50% of patients and is among the most serious manifestations of relapsing polychondritis. Symptoms include hoarseness, a nonproductive cough, and tenderness over the larynx and proximal trachea. Mucosal edema, strictures, and/or collapse of laryngeal or tracheal cartilage may cause stridor and life-threatening airway obstruction necessitating tracheostomy. Involvement can extend into the lower airways resulting in tracheobronchomalacia. Collapse of cartilage in bronchi leads to pneumonia and, when extensive, to respiratory insufficiency.

Cardiac valvular regurgitation occurs in about 5–10% of patients and is due to progressive dilation of the valvular ring or to destruction of the valve cusps. Aortic regurgitation occurs in about 7% of patients, with the mitral and other heart valves being affected less often. Other cardiac manifestations include pericarditis, myocarditis, coronary vasculitis, and conduction abnormalities. Aneurysms of the proximal, thoracic, or abdominal aorta may occur even in the absence of active chondritis and occasionally rupture.

Renal disease occurs in about 10% of patients. The most common renal lesions include mesangial expansion or segmental necrotizing glomerulonephritis, which have been reported to have small amounts of electron-dense deposits in the mesangium where there is also faint deposition of C3 and/or IgG or IgM. Tubulointerstitial disease and IgA nephropathy have also been reported.

Approximately 25% of patients have skin lesions, which can include purpura, erythema nodosum, erythema multiforme, angioedema/urticaria, livedo reticularis, and panniculitis.

Features of vasculitis are seen in up to 25% of patients and can affect any size vessel. Large vessel vasculitis may present with aortic aneurysms, and medium vessel disease may affect the coronary, hepatic, mesenteric, or renal arteries or vessel supplying nerves. Skin vessel disease and involvement of the postcapillary venules can also occur. A variety of primary vasculitides have also been reported to occur in association with relapsing polychondritis (Chap. 385). One specific overlap is the "MAGIC" syndrome (*m*outh *a*nd *g*enital ulcers with *i*nflamed *c*artilage) in which patients present with features of both relapsing polychondritis and Behçet's disease (Chap. 387).

LABORATORY FINDINGS AND DIAGNOSTIC IMAGING

There are no laboratory features that are diagnostic for relapsing polychondritis. Mild leukocytosis and normocytic, normochromic anemia are often present. Eosinophilia is observed in 10% of patients. The erythrocyte sedimentation rate and C-reactive protein are usually elevated. Rheumatoid factor and antinuclear antibody tests are occasionally positive in low titers, and complement levels are normal. Antibodies to type II collagen are present in fewer than one-half of the patients and are not specific. Circulating immune complexes may be detected, especially in patients with early active disease. Elevated levels of γ globulin may be present. Antineutrophil cytoplasmic antibodies (ANCA), either cytoplasmic (cANCA) or perinuclear (pANCA), are found in some patients with active disease. However, on target antigen–specific testing, there are only occasional reports of positive myeloperoxidase-ANCA, and proteinase 3-ANCA are very rarely found in relapsing polychondritis.

The upper and lower airways can be evaluated by imaging techniques such as computed tomography and magnetic resonance imaging (MRI). Bronchoscopy provides direct visualization of the airways but can be a high-risk procedure in patients with airway compromise. Pulmonary function testing with flow-volume loops can show inspiratory and/or expiratory obstruction. Imaging can also be useful to detect extracartilaginous disease. The chest film may show widening of the ascending or descending aorta due to an aneurysm, and cardiomegaly when aortic insufficiency is present. MRI can assess aortic aneurysmal dilatation. Electrocardiography and echocardiography can be useful in further evaluating for cardiac features of disease.

DIAGNOSIS

Diagnosis is based on recognition of the typical clinical features. Biopsies of the involved cartilage from the ear, nose, or respiratory tract will confirm the diagnosis but are only necessary when clinical features are not typical. Diagnostic criteria were suggested in 1976 by McAdam et al and modified by Damiani and Levine in 1979. These criteria continue to be generally used in clinical practice. McAdam et al proposed the following: (1) recurrent chondritis of both auricles; (2) nonerosive inflammatory arthritis; (3) chondritis of nasal cartilage; (4) inflammation of ocular structures, including conjunctivitis, keratitis, scleritis/episcleritis, and/or uveitis; (5) chondritis of the laryngeal and/or tracheal cartilages; and (6) cochlear and/or vestibular damage manifested by neurosensory hearing loss, tinnitus, and/or vertigo. The diagnosis is certain when three or more of these features are present along with a positive biopsy from the ear, nasal, or respiratory cartilage. Damiani and Levine later suggested that the diagnosis could be made when one or more of the above features and a positive biopsy were present, when two or more separate sites of cartilage inflammation were present that responded to glucocorticoids or dapsone, or when three or more of the above features were present.

The differential diagnosis of relapsing polychondritis is centered around its sites of clinical involvement. Patients with granulomatosis with polyangiitis (Wegener's) may have a saddle nose and tracheal involvement but can be distinguished by the primary inflammation occurring in the mucosa at these sites, the absence of auricular involvement, and the presence of pulmonary parenchymal disease. Patients with Cogan's syndrome have interstitial keratitis and vestibular and auditory abnormalities, but this syndrome does not involve the respiratory tract or ears. Reactive arthritis may initially resemble relapsing polychondritis because of oligoarticular arthritis and eye involvement, but it is distinguished in time by the appearance of urethritis and typical mucocutaneous lesions and the absence of nose or ear cartilage involvement. Rheumatoid arthritis may initially suggest relapsing polychondritis because of arthritis and eye inflammation. The arthritis in rheumatoid arthritis, however, is erosive and symmetric. In addition, rheumatoid factor titers are usually high compared with those in relapsing polychondritis, and anti-cyclic citrullinated peptide is usually not seen. Bacterial infection of the pinna may be mistaken for relapsing polychondritis but differs by usually involving only one ear, including the earlobe. Auricular cartilage may also be damaged by trauma or frostbite. Nasal destructive disease and auricular abnormalities can also be seen in patients using cocaine adulterated with levamisole. Ear involvement in this setting differs from relapsing polychondritis by typically manifesting as purpuric plaques with necrosis extending to the pinna, which does not contain cartilage.

TREATMENT RELAPSING POLYCHONDRITIS

In patients with active chondritis, prednisone, 40–60 mg/d, is often effective in suppressing disease activity; it is tapered gradually once disease is controlled. In some patients, prednisone can be stopped, whereas in others, low doses in the range of 5–10 mg/d are required for continued suppression of disease. Dapsone 50–100 mg/d has been effective for cartilage inflammation and joint features in some patients. Other immunosuppressive drugs such as cyclophosphamide, methotrexate, azathioprine, or cyclosporine should be reserved for patients who have severe organ-threatening disease, fail to respond to prednisone, or require high doses to control disease activity. Patients with significant ocular inflammation often require intraocular glucocorticoids as well as high doses of prednisone. There are a small number of reports on the use of tumor necrosis factor antagonists, rituximab (anti-CD20), and tocilizumab (anti-interleukin 6 receptor), which are too few in number to assess efficacy. Heart valve replacement or repair of an aortic aneurysm may be necessary. When airway obstruction is severe, tracheostomy is required. Stents may be necessary in patients with tracheobronchial collapse.

PATIENT OUTCOME, PROGNOSIS, AND SURVIVAL

The course of relapsing polychondritis is highly variable. Some patients experience inflammatory episodes lasting from a few days to several weeks that then subside spontaneously or with treatment. Attacks may recur at intervals varying from weeks to months. In other patients, the disease has a chronic, smoldering course that may be severe. In one study, the 5-year estimated survival rate was 74% and the 10-year survival rate was 55%. In contrast to earlier series, only about one-half of the deaths could be attributed to relapsing polychondritis or complications of treatment. Airway complications accounted for only 10% of all fatalities. In general, patients with more widespread disease have a worse prognosis.

Acknowledgment

This chapter represents a revised version of the text authored by Dr. Bruce C. Gilliland that appeared in previous editions of Harrison's Principles of Internal Medicine. Dr. Gilliland passed away on February 17, 2007, and had been a contributor to Harrison's since the 11th edition.

390 Sarcoidosis

Robert P. Baughman, Elyse E. Lower

DEFINITION

Sarcoidosis is an inflammatory disease characterized by the presence of noncaseating granulomas. The disease is often multisystem and requires the presence of involvement in two or more organs for a specific diagnosis. The finding of granulomas is not specific for sarcoidosis, and other conditions known to cause granulomas must be ruled out. These conditions include mycobacterial and fungal infections, malignancy, and environmental agents such as beryllium. Although sarcoidosis can affect virtually every organ of the body, the lung is most commonly affected. Other organs commonly affected are the liver, skin, and eye. The clinical outcome of sarcoidosis varies, with remission occurring in over one-half of patients within a few years of diagnosis; however, the remaining patients may develop a chronic disease that lasts for decades.

ETIOLOGY

Despite multiple investigations, the cause of sarcoidosis remains unknown. Currently, the most likely etiology is an infectious or noninfectious environmental agent that triggers an inflammatory response in a genetically susceptible host. Among the possible infectious agents, careful studies have shown a much higher incidence of *Propionibacter acnes* in the lymph nodes of sarcoidosis patients compared to controls. An animal model has shown that *P. acnes* can induce a granulomatous response in mice similar to sarcoidosis. Others have demonstrated the presence of a mycobacterial protein (*Mycobacterium tuberculosis* catalase-peroxidase [mKatG]) in the granulomas of some sarcoidosis patients. This protein is very resistant to degradation and may represent the persistent antigen in sarcoidosis. Immune response to this and other mycobacterial proteins has been documented by another laboratory. These studies suggest that a mycobacterium similar to *M. tuberculosis* could be responsible for sarcoidosis. The mechanism exposure/infection with such agents has been the focus of other studies. Environmental exposures to insecticides and mold have been associated with an increased risk for disease. In addition, health care workers appear to have an increased risk. Also, sarcoidosis in a donor organ has occurred after transplantation into a sarcoidosis patient. Some authors have suggested that sarcoidosis is not due to a single agent but represents a particular host response to multiple agents. Some studies have been able to correlate the environmental exposures to genetic markers. These studies have supported the hypothesis that a genetically susceptible host is a key factor in the disease.

INCIDENCE, PREVALENCE, AND GLOBAL IMPACT

Sarcoidosis is seen worldwide, with the highest prevalence reported in the Nordic population. In the United States, the disease has been reported more commonly in African Americans than whites, with the ratio of African Americans to whites ranging from 3:1 to 17:0. Women appear to be slightly more susceptible than men. The higher incidence in African Americans may have been influenced by the fact that African Americans seem to develop more extensive and chronic pulmonary disease. Because most sarcoidosis clinics are run by pulmonologists, a selection bias may have occurred. Worldwide, the prevalence of the disease varies from 20–60 per 100,000 for many groups such as Japanese, Italians, and American whites. Higher rates occur in Ireland and Nordic countries. In one closely observed community in Sweden, the lifetime risk for developing sarcoidosis was 3%.

Sarcoidosis often occurs in young, otherwise healthy adults. It is uncommon to diagnose the disease in someone under age 18. However, it has become clear that a second peak in incidence develops around age 60. In a study of >700 newly diagnosed sarcoidosis patients in the United States, one-half of the patients were ≥40 years at the time of diagnosis.

Although most cases of sarcoidosis are sporadic, a familial form of the disease exists. At least 5% of patients with sarcoidosis will have a family member with sarcoidosis. Sarcoidosis patients who are Irish or African American seem to have a two to three times higher rate of familial disease.

PATHOPHYSIOLOGY AND IMMUNOPATHOGENESIS

The granuloma is the pathologic hallmark of sarcoidosis. A distinct feature of sarcoidosis is the local accumulation of inflammatory cells. Extensive studies in the lung using bronchoalveolar lavage (BAL) have demonstrated that the initial inflammatory response is an influx of T helper cells. In addition, there is an accumulation of activated monocytes. Figure 390-1 is a proposed model for sarcoidosis. Using the HLA-CD4 complex, antigen-presenting cells present an unknown antigen to the helper T cell. Studies have clarified that specific HLA haplotypes such as HLA-DRB1*1101 are associated with an increased risk for developing sarcoidosis. In addition, different HLA haplotypes are associated with different clinical outcomes.

The macrophage/helper T cell cluster leads to activation with the increased release of several cytokines. These include interleukin (IL)-2 released from the T cell and interferon γ and tumor necrosis factor (TNF) released by the macrophage. The T cell is a necessary part of the initial inflammatory response. In advanced, untreated HIV infection, patients who lack helper T cells rarely develop sarcoidosis. In contrast, several reports confirm that sarcoidosis becomes unmasked as HIV-infected individuals receive antiretroviral therapy, with subsequent restoration of their immune system. In contrast, treatment of established pulmonary sarcoidosis with cyclosporine, a drug that downregulates helper T cell responses, seems to have little impact on sarcoidosis.

The granulomatous response of sarcoidosis can resolve with or without therapy. However, in at least 20% of patients with sarcoidosis, a chronic form of the disease develops. This persistent form of the disease is associated with the secretion of high levels of IL-8. Also, studies have reported that patients with this chronic form of disease release excessive amounts of TNF in areas of inflammation. Specific

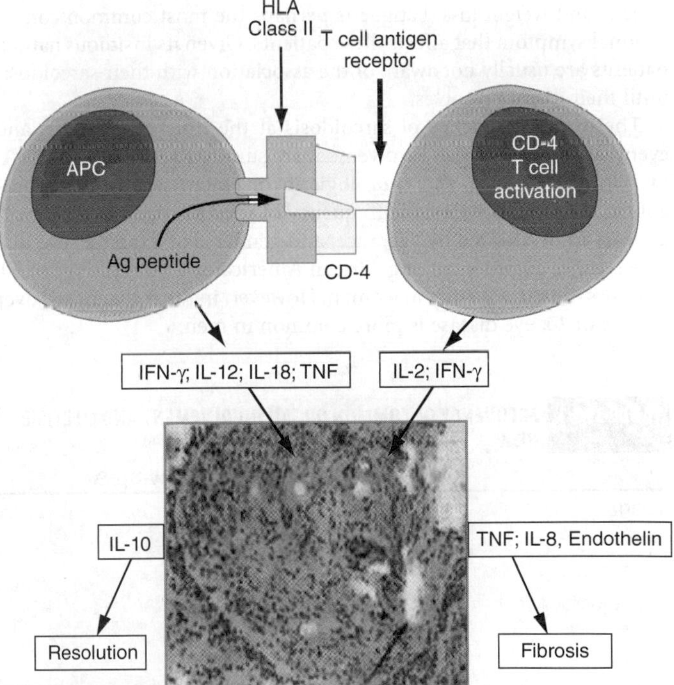

FIGURE 390-1 Schematic representation of initial events of sarcoidosis. The antigen-presenting cell and helper T cell complex leads to the release of multiple cytokines. This forms a granuloma. Over time, the granuloma may resolve or lead to chronic disease, including fibrosis. APC, antigen-presenting cell; HLA, human leukocyte antigen; IFN, interferon; IL, interleukin; TNF, tumor necrosis factor.

gene signatures have been associated with more severe disease, such as cardiac, neurologic, and fibrotic pulmonary disease.

At diagnosis the natural history of the disease may be difficult to predict. One form of the disease, *Löfgren's syndrome*, consists of erythema nodosum and hilar adenopathy on chest roentgenogram. In some cases, periarticular arthritis may be identified without erythema nodosum. Löfgren's syndrome is associated with a good prognosis, with >90% of patients experiencing disease resolution within 2 years. Recent studies have demonstrated that the HLA-DRB1*03 was found in two-thirds of Scandinavian patients with Löfgren's syndrome. More than 95% of those patients who were HLA-DRB1*03 positive had resolution of their disease within 2 years, whereas nearly one-half of the remaining patients had disease for more than 2 years. It remains to be determined whether these observations can be applied to a non-Scandinavian population.

CLINICAL MANIFESTATIONS

The presentation of sarcoidosis ranges from patients who are asymptomatic to those with organ failure. It is unclear how often sarcoidosis is asymptomatic. In countries where routine chest roentgenogram screening is performed, 20–30% of pulmonary cases are detected in asymptomatic individuals. The inability to screen for other asymptomatic forms of the disease would suggest that as many as one-third of sarcoidosis patients are asymptomatic.

Respiratory complaints including cough and dyspnea are the most common presenting symptoms. In many cases, the patient presents with a 2- to 4-week history of these symptoms. Unfortunately, due to the nonspecific nature of pulmonary symptoms, the patient may see physicians for up to a year before a diagnosis is confirmed. For these patients, the diagnosis of sarcoidosis is usually only suggested when a chest roentgenogram is performed.

Symptoms related to cutaneous and ocular disease are the next two most common complaints. Skin lesions are often nonspecific. However, because these lesions are readily observed, the patient and treating physician are often led to a diagnosis. In contrast to patients with pulmonary disease, patients with cutaneous lesions are more likely to be diagnosed within 6 months of symptoms.

Nonspecific constitutional symptoms include fatigue, fever, night sweats, and weight loss. Fatigue is perhaps the most common constitutional symptom that affects these patients. Given its insidious nature, patients are usually not aware of the association with their sarcoidosis until their disease resolves.

The overall incidence of sarcoidosis at the time of diagnosis and eventual common organ involvement are summarized in Table 390-1. Over time, skin, eye, and neurologic involvement seem more apparent. In the United States, the frequency of specific organ involvement appears to be affected by age, race, and gender. For example, eye disease is more common among African Americans. Under the age of 40, it occurs more frequently in women. However, in those diagnosed over the age of 40, eye disease is more common in men.

TABLE 390-1 FREQUENCY OF COMMON ORGAN INVOLVEMENT AND LIFETIME RISK[a]

	Presentation, %[b]	Follow-Up, %[c]
Lung	95	94
Skin	24	43
Eye	12	29
Extrathoracic lymph node	15	16
Liver	12	14
Spleen	7	8
Neurologic	5	16
Cardiac	2	3

[a]Patients could have more than one organ involved. [b]From ACCESS study of 736 patients evaluated within 6 months of diagnosis. [c]From follow-up of 1024 sarcoidosis patients seen at the University of Cincinnati Interstitial Lung Disease and Sarcoidosis Clinic from 2002–2006.

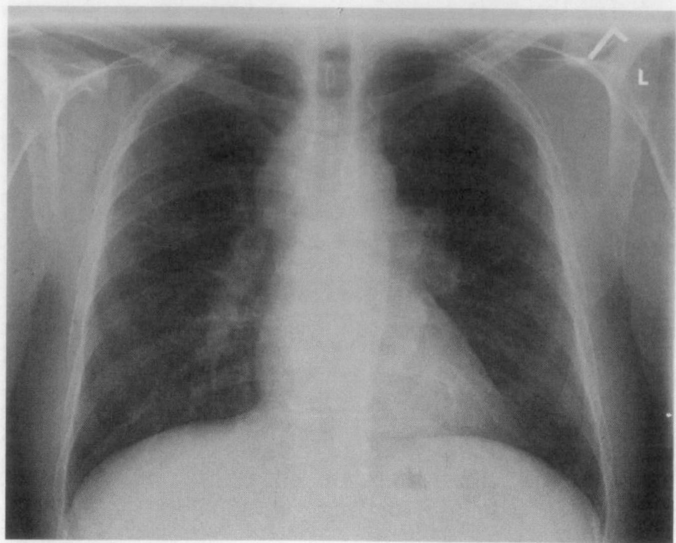

FIGURE 390-2 Posterior-anterior chest roentgenogram demonstrating bilateral hilar adenopathy, stage 1 disease.

LUNG

Lung involvement occurs in >90% of sarcoidosis patients. The most commonly used method for detecting lung disease is still the chest roentgenogram. Figure 390-2 illustrates the chest roentgenogram from a sarcoidosis patient with bilateral hilar adenopathy. Although the computed tomography (CT) scan has changed the diagnostic approach to interstitial lung disease, the CT scan is not usually considered a monitoring tool for patients with sarcoidosis. Figure 390-3 demonstrates some of the characteristic CT features, including peribronchial thickening and reticular nodular changes, which are predominantly subpleural. The peribronchial thickening seen on CT scan seems to explain the high yield of granulomas from bronchial biopsies performed for diagnosis.

Although the CT scan is more sensitive, the standard scoring system described by Scadding in 1961 for chest roentgenograms remains the preferred method of characterizing the chest involvement. Stage 1 is hilar adenopathy alone (Fig. 390-2), often with right paratracheal involvement. Stage 2 is a combination of adenopathy plus infiltrates, whereas stage 3 reveals infiltrates alone. Stage 4 consists of fibrosis. Usually the infiltrates in sarcoidosis are predominantly an upper lobe process. Only in a few noninfectious diseases is an upper lobe

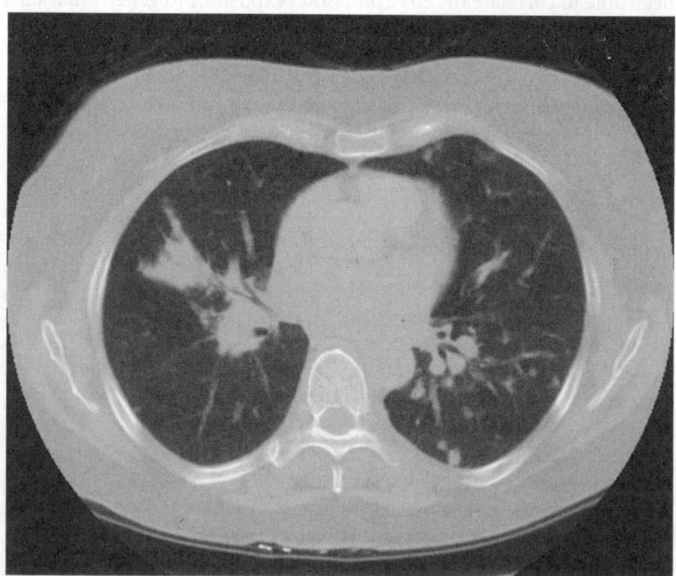

FIGURE 390-3 High-resolution computed tomography scan of chest demonstrating patchy reticular nodularity, including areas of confluence.

predominance noted. In addition to sarcoidosis, the differential diagnosis of upper lobe disease includes hypersensitivity pneumonitis, silicosis, and Langerhans cell histiocytosis. For infectious diseases, tuberculosis and *Pneumocystis* pneumonia can often present as upper lobe diseases.

Lung volumes, mechanics, and diffusion are all useful in evaluating interstitial lung diseases such as sarcoidosis. The diffusion of carbon monoxide (DL_{CO}) is the most sensitive test for an interstitial lung disease. Reduced lung volumes are a reflection of the restrictive lung disease seen in sarcoidosis. However, a third of the patients presenting with sarcoidosis still have lung volumes within the normal range, despite abnormal chest roentgenograms and dyspnea.

Approximately one-half of sarcoidosis patients present with obstructive disease, reflected by a reduced ratio of forced vital capacity expired in 1 second (FEV_1/FVC). Cough is a very common symptom. Airway involvement causing varying degrees of obstruction underlies the cough in most sarcoidosis patients. Airway hyperreactivity, as determined by methacholine challenge, will be positive in some of these patients. A few patients with cough will respond to traditional bronchodilators as the only form of treatment. In some cases, high-dose inhaled glucocorticoids alone are useful. Airway obstruction can be due to large airway stenosis, which can become fibrotic and unresponsive to anti-inflammatory therapy.

Pulmonary arterial hypertension is reported in at least 5% of sarcoidosis patients. Either direct vascular involvement or the consequence of fibrotic changes in the lung can lead to pulmonary arterial hypertension. In sarcoidosis patients with end-stage fibrosis awaiting lung transplant, 70% will have pulmonary arterial hypertension. This is a much higher incidence than that reported for other fibrotic lung diseases. In less advanced, but still symptomatic, patients, pulmonary arterial hypertension has been noted in up to 50% of the cases. Because sarcoidosis-associated pulmonary arterial hypertension may respond to therapy, evaluation for this should be considered in persistently dyspneic patients.

SKIN

Skin involvement is eventually identified in over a third of patients with sarcoidosis. The classic cutaneous lesions include erythema nodosum, maculopapular lesions, hyper- and hypopigmentation, keloid formation, and subcutaneous nodules. A specific complex of involvement of the bridge of the nose, the area beneath the eyes, and the cheeks is referred to as *lupus pernio* (Fig. 390-4) and is diagnostic for a chronic form of sarcoidosis.

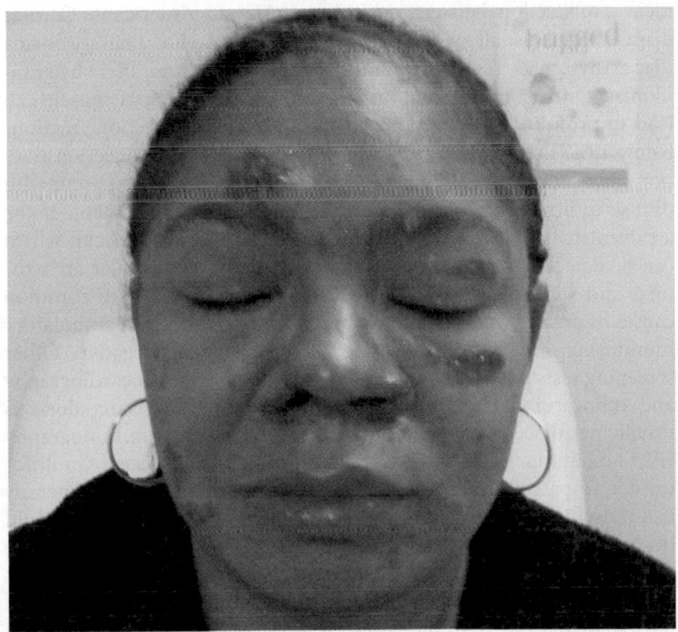

FIGURE 390-4 Chronic inflammatory lesions around nose, eyes, and cheeks, referred to as lupus pernio.

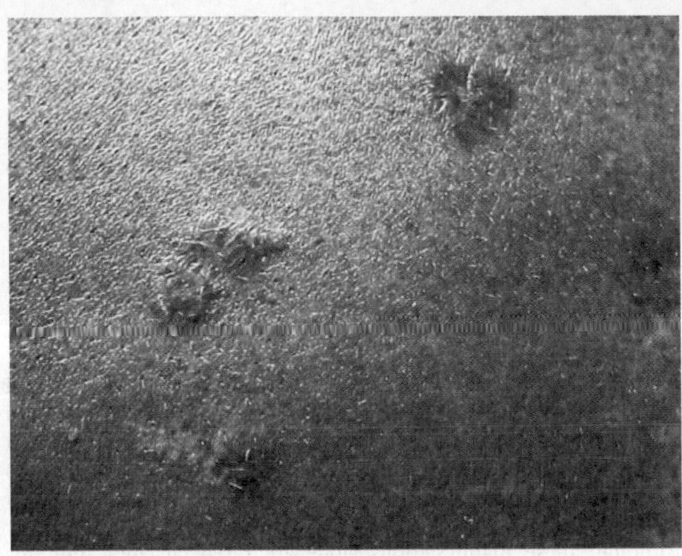

FIGURE 390-5 Maculopapular lesions on the trunk of a sarcoidosis patient.

In contrast, erythema nodosum is a transient rash that can be seen in association with hilar adenopathy and uveitis (Löfgren's syndrome). Erythema nodosum is more common in women and in certain self-described demographic groups including whites and Puerto Ricans. In the United States, the other manifestations of skin sarcoidosis, especially lupus pernio, are more common in African Americans than whites.

The maculopapular lesions from sarcoidosis are the most common chronic form of the disease (Fig. 390-5). These are often overlooked by the patient and physician, because they are chronic and not painful. Initially, these lesions are usually purplish papules and are often indurated. They can become confluent and infiltrate large areas of the skin. With treatment, the color and induration may fade. Because these lesions are caused by noncaseating granulomas, the diagnosis of sarcoidosis can be readily made by a skin biopsy.

EYE

The frequency of ocular manifestations for sarcoidosis varies depending on race. In Japan, >70% of sarcoidosis patients develop ocular disease, whereas in the United States only 30% have eye disease, with problems more common in African Americans than whites. Although the most common manifestation is an anterior uveitis, over a quarter of patients will have inflammation at the posterior of the eye, including retinitis and pars planitis. Although symptoms such as photophobia, blurred vision, and increased tearing can occur, some asymptomatic patients still have active inflammation. Initially asymptomatic patients with ocular sarcoidosis can eventually develop blindness. Therefore, it is recommended that all patients with sarcoidosis receive a dedicated ophthalmologic examination. Sicca is seen in over one-half of the chronic sarcoidosis patients. Dry eyes appear to be a reflection of prior lacrimal gland disease. Although the patient may no longer have active inflammation, the dry eyes may require natural tears or other lubricants.

LIVER

Using biopsies to detect granulomatous disease, liver involvement can be identified in over one-half of sarcoidosis patients. However, using liver function studies, only 20–30% of patients will have evidence of liver involvement. The most common abnormality of liver function is an elevation of the alkaline phosphatase level, consistent with an obstructive pattern. In addition, elevated transaminase levels can occur. An elevated bilirubin level is a marker for more advanced liver disease. Overall, only 5% of sarcoidosis patients have sufficient symptoms from their liver disease to require specific therapy. Although symptoms can be due to hepatomegaly, more frequently symptoms result from extensive intrahepatic cholestasis leading to portal hypertension. In this case, ascites and esophageal varices can occur. It is rare that a sarcoidosis patient will require a liver transplant, because even the patient with cirrhosis due to sarcoidosis can respond to systemic therapy. On a cautionary note, patients with both sarcoidosis and hepatitis C should avoid therapy with interferon a because of its association with the development or worsening of granulomatous disease.

BONE MARROW AND SPLEEN

One or more bone marrow manifestations can be identified in many sarcoidosis patients. The most common hematologic problem is lymphopenia, which is a reflection of sequestration of the lymphocytes into the areas of inflammation. Anemia occurs in 20% of patients, and leukopenia is less common. Bone marrow examination will reveal granulomas in about a third of patients. Although splenomegaly can be detected in 5–10% of patients, splenic biopsy reveals granulomas in 60% of patients. The CT scan can be relatively specific for sarcoidosis involvement of the spleen (Fig. 390-6). Both bone marrow and spleen involvement are more common in African Americans than whites. Although these manifestations alone are rarely an indication for therapy, on rare occasion, splenectomy may be indicated for massive symptomatic splenomegaly or profound pancytopenia. Nonthoracic lymphadenopathy can occur in up to 20% of patients.

CALCIUM METABOLISM

Hypercalcemia and/or hypercalciuria occurs in about 10% of sarcoidosis patients. It is more common in whites than African Americans and in men. The mechanism of abnormal calcium metabolism is increased production of 1,25-dihydroxyvitamin D by the granuloma itself. The 1,25-dihydroxyvitamin D causes increased intestinal absorption of calcium, leading to hypercalcemia with a suppressed parathyroid hormone (PTH) level (Chap. 424). Increased exogenous vitamin D from diet or sunlight exposure may exacerbate this problem. Serum calcium should be determined as part of the initial evaluation of all sarcoidosis patients, and a repeat determination may be useful during the summer months with increased sun exposure. In patients with a history of renal calculi, a 24-h urine calcium measurement should be obtained. If a sarcoidosis patient with a history of renal calculi is to be placed on calcium supplements, a follow-up 24-h urine calcium level should be measured.

RENAL DISEASE

Direct kidney involvement occurs in <5% of sarcoidosis patients. It is associated with granulomas in the kidney itself and can lead to nephritis.

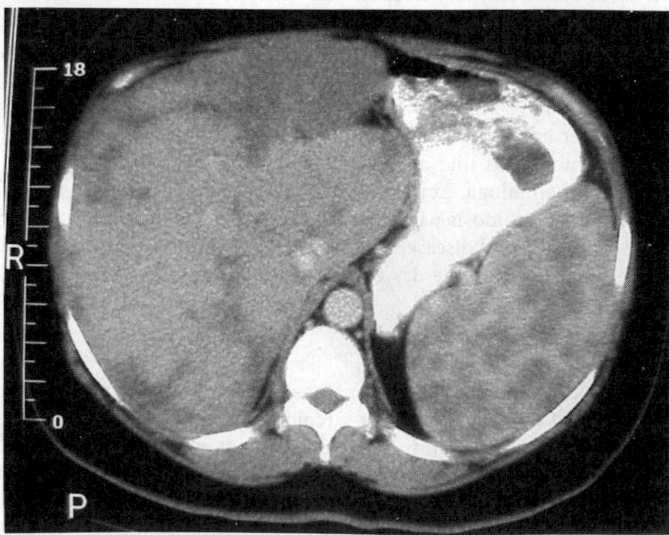

FIGURE 390-6 Computed tomography scan of the abdomen after oral and intravenous contrast. The stomach is compressed by the enlarged spleen. Within the spleen, areas of hypo- and hyperdensity are identified.

However, hypercalcemia is the most likely cause of sarcoidosis-associated renal disease. In 1–2% of sarcoidosis patients, acute renal failure may develop as a result of hypercalcemia. Successful treatment of hypercalcemia with glucocorticoids and other therapies often improves but usually does not totally resolve the renal dysfunction.

NERVOUS SYSTEM

Neurologic disease is reported in 5–10% of sarcoidosis patients and appears to be of equal frequency across all ethnic groups. Any part of the central or peripheral nervous system can be affected. The presence of granulomatous inflammation is often visible on magnetic resonance imaging (MRI) studies. The MRI with gadolinium enhancement may demonstrate space-occupying lesions, but the MRI can be negative due to small lesions or the effect of systemic therapy in reducing the inflammation. The cerebral spinal fluid (CSF) findings include lymphocytic meningitis with a mild increase in protein. The CSF glucose is usually normal but can be low. Certain areas of the nervous system are more commonly affected in neurosarcoidosis. These include cranial nerve involvement, basilar meningitis, myelopathy, and anterior hypothalamic disease with associated diabetes insipidus (Chap. 404). Seizures and cognitive changes also occur. Of the cranial nerves, seventh nerve paralysis can be transient and mistaken for Bell's palsy (idiopathic seventh nerve paralysis). Because this form of neurosarcoidosis often resolves within weeks and may not recur, it may have occurred prior to a definitive diagnosis of sarcoidosis. Optic neuritis is another cranial nerve manifestation of sarcoidosis. This manifestation is more chronic and usually requires long-term systemic therapy. It can be associated with both anterior and posterior uveitis. Differentiating between neurosarcoidosis and multiple sclerosis can be difficult at times. Optic neuritis can occur in both diseases. In some patients with sarcoidosis, multiple enhancing white matter abnormalities may be detected by MRI, suggesting multiple sclerosis. In such cases, the presence of meningeal enhancement or hypothalamic involvement suggests neurosarcoidosis, as does evidence of extraneurologic disease such as pulmonary or skin involvement, which also suggests sarcoidosis. Because the response of neurosarcoidosis to glucocorticoids and cytotoxic therapy is different from that of multiple sclerosis, differentiating between these disease entities is important.

CARDIAC

The presence of cardiac involvement is influenced by race. Although over a quarter of Japanese sarcoidosis patients develop cardiac disease, only 5% of sarcoidosis patients in the United States and Europe develop symptomatic cardiac disease. However, there is no apparent racial predilection between whites and African Americans. Cardiac disease, which usually presents as either congestive heart failure or cardiac arrhythmias, results from infiltration of the heart muscle by granulomas. Diffuse granulomatous involvement of the heart muscle can lead to profound dysfunction with left ventricular ejection fractions below 10%. Even in this situation, improvement in the ejection fraction can occur with systemic therapy. Arrhythmias can also occur with diffuse infiltration or with more patchy cardiac involvement. If the atrioventricular (AV) node is infiltrated, heart block can occur, which can be detected by routine electrocardiography. Ventricular arrhythmias and sudden death due to ventricular tachycardia are common causes of death. Arrhythmias are best detected using 24-h ambulatory monitoring, and electrophysiology studies may be negative. Other screening tests for cardiac disease include routine electrocardiography and echocardiography. The confirmation of cardiac sarcoidosis is usually performed with either MRI or positron emission tomography (PET) scanning. Because ventricular arrhythmias are usually multifocal due to patchy multiple granulomas in the heart, ablation therapy is not useful. Patients with significant ventricular arrhythmias should be considered for an implanted defibrillator, which appears to have reduced the rate of death in cardiac sarcoidosis. Although systemic therapy can be useful in treating the arrhythmias, patients may still have malignant arrhythmias up to 6 months after starting successful treatment, and the risk for recurrent arrhythmias occurs whenever medications are tapered.

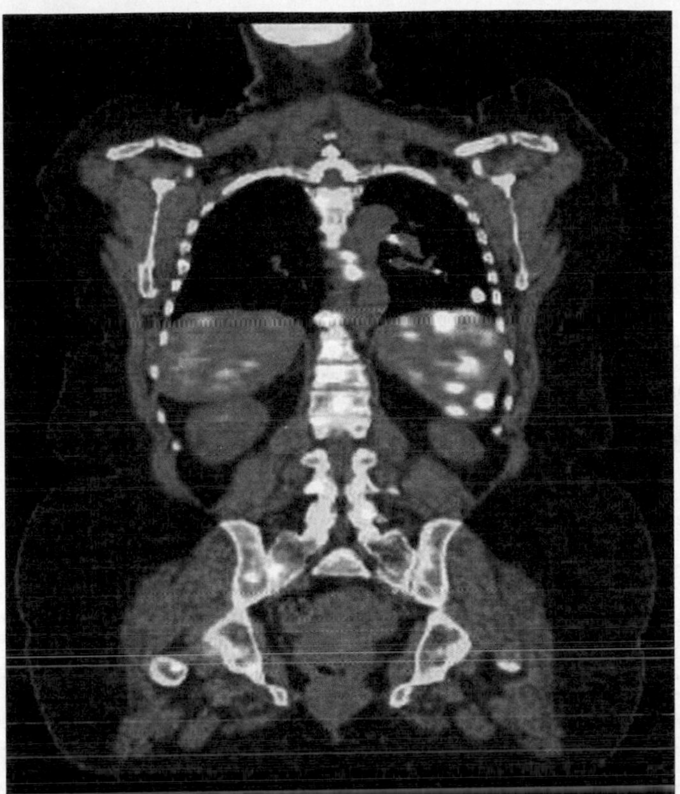

FIGURE 390-7 Positron emission tomography and computed tomography scan merged demonstrating increased activity in spleen, ribs, and spine of patient with sarcoidosis.

MUSCULOSKELETAL SYSTEM

Direct granulomatous involvement of bone and muscle can be documented by radiography (x-ray, MRI, PET scan [Fig. 390-7], or gallium scan) or confirmed by biopsy in about 10% of sarcoidosis patients. However, a larger percentage of sarcoidosis patients complain of myalgias and arthralgias. These complaints are similar to those reported by patients with other inflammatory diseases, including chronic infections such as mononucleosis. Fatigue associated with sarcoidosis may be overwhelming for many patients. Recent studies have demonstrated a link between fatigue and small peripheral nerve fiber disease in sarcoidosis.

OTHER ORGAN INVOLVEMENT

Although sarcoidosis can affect any organ of the body, rarely does it involve the breast, testes, ovary, or stomach. Because of the rarity of involvement, a mass in one of these areas requires a biopsy to rule out other diseases including cancer. For example, in a study of breast problems in female sarcoidosis patients, a breast lesion was more likely to be a granuloma from sarcoidosis than from breast cancer. However, findings on the physical examination or mammogram cannot reliably differentiate between these lesions. More importantly, as women with sarcoidosis age, breast cancer becomes more common. Therefore, it is recommended that routine screening including mammography be performed along with other imaging studies (ultrasound, MRI) or biopsy as clinically indicated.

COMPLICATIONS

Sarcoidosis is usually a self-limited, non-life-threatening disease. However, organ-threatening disease can occur. These complications can include blindness, paraplegia, or renal failure. Death from sarcoidosis occurs in about 5% of patients seen in sarcoidosis referral clinics. The usual causes of death related to sarcoidosis are from lung, cardiac, neurologic, or liver involvement. In respiratory failure, an elevation of the right atrial pressure is a poor prognostic finding. Lung complications can also include infections such as mycetoma, which can subsequently lead to massive bleeding. In addition, the use of immunosuppressive agents can increase the incidence of serious infections.

LABORATORY FINDINGS

The chest roentgenogram remains the most commonly used tool to assess lung involvement in sarcoidosis. As noted above, the chest roentgenogram classifies involvement into four stages, with stages 1 and 2 having hilar and paratracheal adenopathy. The CT scan has been used increasingly in evaluating interstitial lung disease. In sarcoidosis, the presence of adenopathy and a nodular infiltrate is not specific for sarcoidosis. Adenopathy up to 2 cm can be seen in other inflammatory lung diseases such as idiopathic pulmonary fibrosis. However, adenopathy >2 cm in the short axis supports the diagnosis of sarcoidosis over other interstitial lung diseases.

The PET scan has increasingly replaced gallium-67 scanning to identify areas of granulomatous disease in the chest and other parts of the body (Fig. 390-7). Both tests can be used to identify potential areas for biopsy. Cardiac PET scanning has also proved useful in assessing cardiac sarcoidosis. The identification of hypermetabolic activity may be due to the granulomas from sarcoidosis and not to disseminated malignancy.

MRI has also proved useful in the assessment of extrapulmonary sarcoidosis. Gadolinium enhancement has been demonstrated in areas of inflammation in the brain, heart, and bone. MRI scans may detect asymptomatic lesions. Like PET scan, MRI changes appear similar to those seen with malignancy and infection. In some cases, biopsy may be necessary to determine the cause of the radiologic abnormality.

Serum levels of angiotensin-converting enzyme (ACE) can be helpful in the diagnosis of sarcoidosis. However, the test has somewhat low sensitivity and specificity. Elevated levels of ACE are reported in 60% of patients with acute disease and only 20% of patients with chronic disease. Although there are several causes for mild elevation of ACE, including diabetes, elevations of >50% of the upper limit of normal are seen in only a few conditions including sarcoidosis, leprosy, Gaucher's disease, hyperthyroidism, and disseminated granulomatous infections such as miliary tuberculosis. Because the ACE level is determined by a biologic assay, the concurrent use of an ACE inhibitor such as lisinopril will lead to a very low ACE level.

DIAGNOSIS

The diagnosis of sarcoidosis requires both compatible clinical features and pathologic findings. Because the cause of sarcoidosis remains elusive, the diagnosis cannot be made with 100% certainty. Nevertheless, the diagnosis can be made with reasonable certainty based on history and physical features along with laboratory and pathologic findings.

Patients are usually evaluated for possible sarcoidosis based on two scenarios (Fig. 390-8). In the first scenario, a patient may undergo a biopsy revealing a noncaseating granuloma in either a pulmonary or an extrapulmonary organ. If the clinical presentation is consistent with sarcoidosis and there is no alternative cause for the granulomas identified, then the patient is felt to have sarcoidosis.

In the second scenario, signs or symptoms suggesting sarcoidosis such as the presence of bilateral adenopathy may be present in an otherwise asymptomatic patient or a patient with uveitis or a rash consistent with sarcoidosis. At this point, a diagnostic procedure should be performed. For the patient with a compatible skin lesion, a skin biopsy should be considered. Other biopsies to consider could include liver, extrathoracic lymph node, or muscle. In some cases, a biopsy of the affected organ may not be easy to perform (such as a brain or spinal cord lesion). In other cases, such as an endomyocardial biopsy, the likelihood of a positive biopsy is low. Because of the high rate of pulmonary involvement in these cases, the lung may be easier to approach by bronchoscopy. During the bronchoscopy, a transbronchial biopsy, bronchial biopsy, or transbronchial needle aspirate can be performed. The endobronchial ultrasonography-guided (EBUS) transbronchial needle aspirate can assist in diagnosing sarcoidosis in patients with mediastinal adenopathy (stage 1 or 2 radiographic pulmonary disease), whereas transbronchial biopsy has a higher diagnostic yield for those

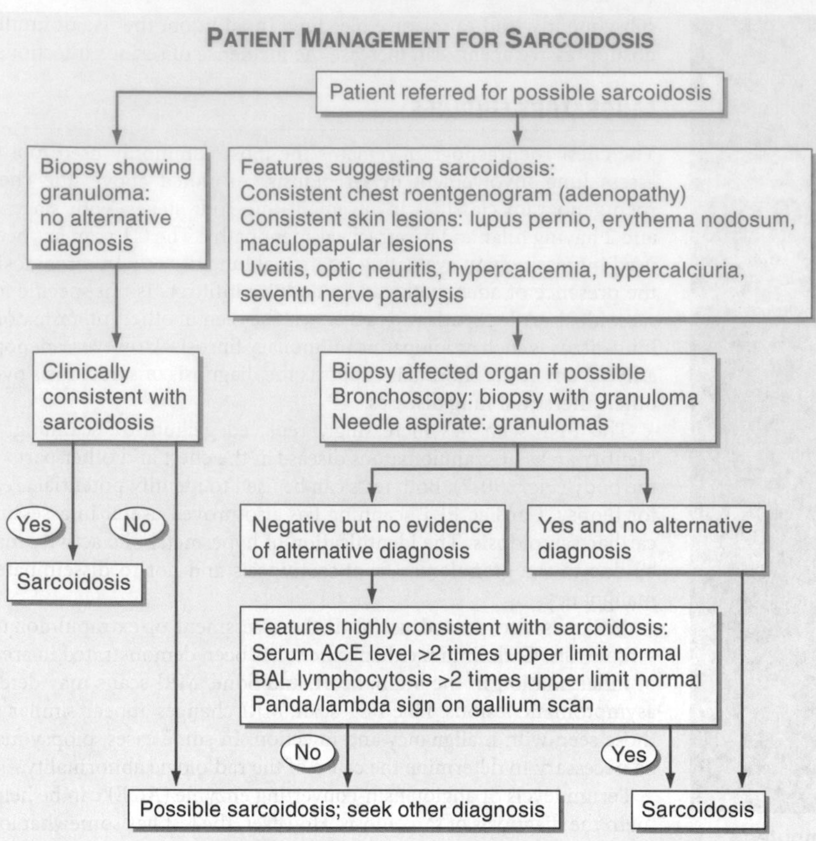

FIGURE 390-8 Proposed approach to management of patient with possible sarcoidosis. Presence of one or more of these features supports the diagnosis of sarcoidosis: uveitis, optic neuritis, hypercalcemia, hypercalciuria, seventh cranial nerve paralysis, diabetes insipidus. ACE, angiotensin-converting enzyme; BAL, bronchoalveolar lavage.

with only parenchymal lung disease (stage 3). These tests are complementary and may be performed together.

If the biopsy reveals granulomas, an alternative diagnosis such as infection or malignancy must be excluded. Bronchoscopic washings can be sent for cultures for fungi and tuberculosis. For the pathologist, the more tissue that is provided, the more comfortable is the diagnosis of sarcoidosis. A needle aspirate may be adequate in an otherwise classic case of sarcoidosis, but may be insufficient in a patient in whom lymphoma or fungal infection is a likely alternative diagnosis. Because granulomas can be seen on the edge of a lymphoma, the presence of a few granulomas from a needle aspirate may not be sufficient to clarify the diagnosis. Mediastinoscopy provides a larger sample to confirm the presence or absence of lymphoma in the mediastinum. Alternatively, for most patients, evidence of extrathoracic disease (e.g., eye involvement) may further support the diagnosis of sarcoidosis.

For patients with negative pathology, positive supportive tests may increase the likelihood of the diagnosis of sarcoidosis. These tests include an elevated ACE level, which can also be elevated in other granulomatous diseases but not in malignancy. A positive PET scan can support the diagnosis if multiple organs are affected. A BAL is often performed during the bronchoscopy. An increase in the percentage of lymphocytes supports the diagnosis of sarcoidosis. The use of the lymphocyte markers CD4 and CD8 can be used to determine the CD4/CD8 ratio of these increased lymphocytes in the BAL fluid. A ratio of >3.5 is strongly supportive of sarcoidosis but is less sensitive than an increase in lymphocytes alone. Although in general, an increase in BAL lymphocytes is supportive of the diagnosis, other conditions must be considered.

Supportive findings, when combined with commonly associated but nondiagnostic clinical features of the disease, improve the diagnostic probability of sarcoidosis. These clinical features include uveitis, renal stones, hypercalcemia, seventh cranial nerve paralysis, or erythema nodosum. The presence of one or more of these features in a patient suspected of having sarcoidosis increases the probability of sarcoidosis.

The *Kviem-Siltzbach procedure* is a specific diagnostic test for sarcoidosis. An intradermal injection of specially prepared tissue derived from the spleen of a known sarcoidosis patient is biopsied 4–6 weeks after injection. If noncaseating granulomas are seen, this is highly specific for the diagnosis of sarcoidosis. Unfortunately, there is no commercially available Kviem-Siltzbach reagent, and some locally prepared batches have lower specificity. Thus, this test is of historic interest and is rarely used in current clinical practice.

Because the diagnosis of sarcoidosis can never be certain, over time other features may arise that lead to an alternative diagnosis. Conversely, evidence for new organ involvement may eventually confirm the diagnosis of sarcoidosis.

PROGNOSIS

The risk of death or loss of organ function remains low in sarcoidosis. Poor outcomes usually occur in patients who present with advanced disease in whom treatment seems to have little impact. In these cases, irreversible fibrotic changes have frequently occurred. Over the past 20 years, the reported mortality from sarcoidosis has increased in the United States and England. Whether this is due to heightened awareness of the chronic nature of this disease or to other factors such as more widespread immunosuppressive therapy usage remains unclear.

For the majority of patients, initial presentation occurs during the granulomatous phase of the disease as depicted in Fig. 390-1. It is clear that many patients resolve their disease within 2–5 years. These patients are felt to have acute, self-limiting sarcoidosis. However, there is a form of the disease that does not resolve within the first 2–5 years. These chronic patients can be identified at presentation by certain risk factors at presentation such as fibrosis on chest roentgenogram, presence of lupus pernio, bone cysts, cardiac or neurologic disease (except isolated seventh nerve paralysis), and presence of renal calculi due to hypercalciuria. Recent studies also indicate that patients who require glucocorticoids for any manifestation of their disease in the first 6 months of presentation have a >50% chance of having chronic disease. In contrast, <10% of patients who require no systemic therapy in the first 6 months will require chronic therapy.

TREATMENT SARCOIDOSIS

Indications for therapy should be based on symptoms or presence of organ- or life-threatening disease, including disease involving the eye, heart, or nervous system. The patient with asymptomatic elevated liver function tests or an abnormal chest roentgenogram probably does not benefit from treatment. However, these patients should be monitored for evidence of progressive, symptomatic disease.

One approach to therapy is summarized in **Figs. 390-9 and 390-10**. We have divided the approach into treating acute versus chronic disease. For acute disease, no therapy remains a viable option for patients with no or mild symptoms. For symptoms confined to only one organ, topical therapy is preferable. For multiorgan disease or disease too extensive for topical therapy, an approach to systemic therapy is outlined. Glucocorticoids remain the drugs of choice for this disease. However, the decision to continue to treat with glucocorticoids or to add steroid-sparing agents depends on the tolerability, duration, and dosage of glucocorticoids.

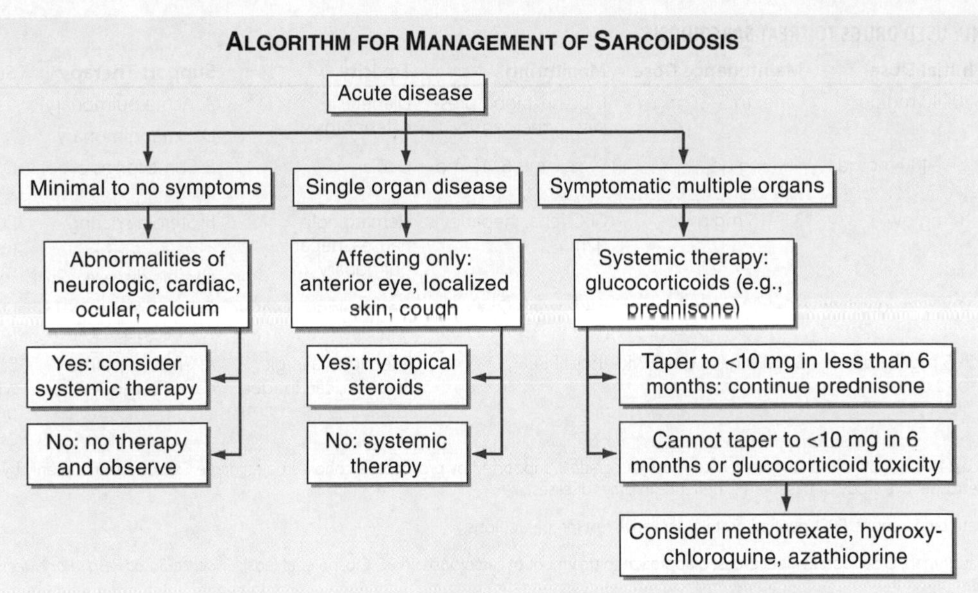

FIGURE 390-9 The management of acute sarcoidosis is based on level of symptoms and extent of organ involvement. In patients with mild symptoms, no therapy may be needed unless specified manifestations are noted.

Table 390-2 summarizes the dosage and monitoring of several commonly used drugs. According to the available trials, evidence-based recommendations are made. Most of these recommendations are for pulmonary disease because most of the trials were performed only in pulmonary disease. Treatment recommendations for extrapulmonary disease are usually similar with a few modifications. For example, the dosage of glucocorticoids is usually higher for neurosarcoidosis and lower for cutaneous disease. There was some suggestion that higher doses would be beneficial for cardiac sarcoidosis, but one study found that initial prednisone doses >40 mg/d were associated with a worse outcome because of toxicity.

Systemic therapies for sarcoidosis are usually immunosuppressive including glucocorticoids, cytotoxics, or biologics. Although most patients receive glucocorticoids as their initial systemic therapy, toxicity associated with prolonged therapy often leads to steroid-sparing alternatives. The antimalarial drugs such as hydroxychloroquine are more effective for skin than pulmonary disease. Minocycline may also be useful for cutaneous sarcoidosis. For pulmonary and other extrapulmonary disease, cytotoxic agents are often used. These include methotrexate, azathioprine, leflunomide, mycophenolate, and cyclophosphamide. The most widely studied cytotoxic agent has been methotrexate. This agent works in approximately two-thirds of sarcoidosis patients, regardless of the disease manifestation. In one retrospective study comparing methotrexate to azathioprine, both drugs were equally effective. However, methotrexate was associated with significantly less toxicity. As noted in Table 390-2, specific guidelines for monitoring therapy have been recommended. Cytokine modulators such as thalidomide and pentoxifylline have also been used in a limited number of cases.

The biologic anti-TNF agents have recently been studied in sarcoidosis, with prospective randomized trials completed for both etanercept and infliximab. Etanercept has a limited role as a steroid-sparing agent. Conversely, infliximab significantly improved lung function when administered to glucocorticoid and cytotoxic pretreated patients with chronic disease The difference in response between these two agents is similar to that observed in

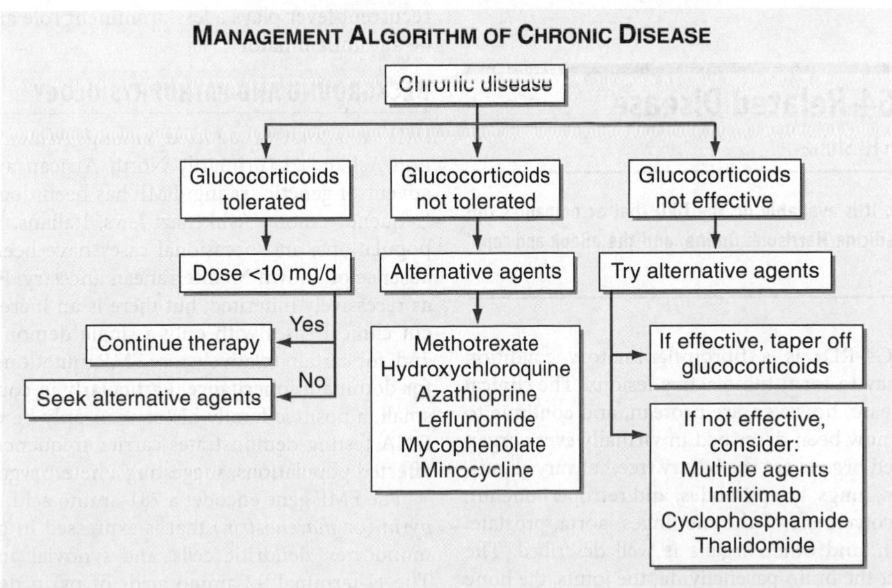

FIGURE 390-10 Approach to chronic disease is based on whether glucocorticoid therapy is tolerated or not.

TABLE 390-2 COMMONLY USED DRUGS TO TREAT SARCOIDOSIS

Drug	Initial Dose	Maintenance Dose	Monitoring	Toxicity	Support Therapy[a]	Support Monitoring[a]
Prednisone	20–40 mg qd	Taper to 5–10 mg	Glucose, blood pressure, bone density	Diabetes, osteoporosis	A: Acute pulmonary D: Extrapulmonary	
Hydroxychloroquine	200–400 mg qd	400 mg qd	Eye exam q6–12 mo	Ocular	B: Some forms of disease	D: Routine eye exam
Methotrexate	10 mg qwk	2.5–15 mg qwk	CBC, renal, hepatic q2mo	Hematologic, nausea, hepatic, pulmonary	B: Steroid sparing C: Some forms chronic disease	D: Routine hematologic, renal, and hepatic monitoring
Azathioprine	50–150 mg qd	50–200 mg qd	CBC, renal q2mo	Hematologic, nausea	C: Some forms chronic disease	D: Routine hematologic monitoring
Infliximab	3–5 mg/kg q2wk for 2 doses	3–10 mg/kg q4–8 wk	Initial PPD	Infections, allergic reaction, carcinogen	A: Chronic pulmonary disease	B: Caution in patients with latent tuberculosis or advanced congestive heart failure

[a]Grade A: supported by at least two double-blind randomized control trials; grade B: supported by prospective cohort studies; grade C: supported primarily by two or more retrospective studies; grade D: only one retrospective study or based on experience in other diseases.

Abbreviations: CBC, complete blood count; PPD, purified protein derivative test for tuberculosis.

Source: Adapted from RP Baughman, O Selroos: Evidence-based approach to treatment of sarcoidosis, in PG Gibson et al (eds): *Evidence-Based Respiratory Medicine.* Oxford, BMJ Books Blackwell, 2005, pp 491–508.

Crohn's disease, where infliximab is effective and etanercept is not. However, there is a higher risk for reactivation of tuberculosis with infliximab compared to etanercept. The differential response rate could be explained by differences in mechanism of action because etanercept is a TNF receptor antagonist and infliximab is a monoclonal antibody against TNF. In contrast to etanercept, infliximab also binds to TNF on the surface of some cells that release TNF, which leads to cell lysis. This effect has been documented in Crohn's disease. Adalimumab is a humanized monoclonal anti-TNF antibody that also appears effective for sarcoidosis when dosed at higher strengths, as recommended for the treatment of Crohn's disease. The role of the newer therapeutic agents for sarcoidosis is still evolving. However, these targeted therapies confirm that TNF may be an important target, especially in the treatment of chronic disease. However, these agents are not a panacea, because sarcoidosis-like disease has occurred in patients treated with anti-TNF agents for nonsarcoidosis indications.

391e IgG4-Related Disease

John H. Stone

This is a digital-only chapter. It is available on the DVD that accompanies this book, as well as on Access Medicine/Harrison's Online, and the eBook and "app" editions of HPIM 19e.

IgG4-related disease (IgG4-RD) is a fibroinflammatory condition characterized by a tendency to form tumefactive lesions. The clinical manifestations of this disease, however, are protean, and continue to be defined. IgG4-RD has now been described in virtually every organ system. Commonly affected organs are the biliary tree, salivary glands, periorbital tissues, kidneys, lungs, lymph nodes, and retroperitoneum. In addition, IgG4-RD involvement of the meninges, aorta, prostate, thyroid, pericardium, skin, and other organs is well described. The disease is believed to affect the brain parenchyma, the joints, the bone marrow, and the bowel mucosa only rarely (if ever).

392 Familial Mediterranean Fever and Other Hereditary Autoinflammatory Diseases

Daniel L. Kastner

Familial Mediterranean fever (FMF) is the prototype of a group of inherited diseases (Table 392-1) that are characterized by recurrent episodes of fever with serosal, synovial, or cutaneous inflammation and, in some individuals, the eventual development of systemic AA amyloidosis (Chap. 137). Because of the relative infrequency of high-titer autoantibodies or antigen-specific T cells, the term *autoinflammatory* has been proposed to describe these disorders, rather than autoimmune. The innate immune system, with its myeloid effector cells and germline receptors for pathogen-associated molecular patterns and endogenous danger signals, plays a predominant role in the pathogenesis of the autoinflammatory diseases. Although the hereditary recurrent fevers comprise a major category of the autoinflammatory diseases, other inherited disorders of inflammation in which recurrent fever plays a less prominent role are now also considered to be autoinflammatory.

BACKGROUND AND PATHOPHYSIOLOGY

FMF was first recognized among Armenians, Arabs, Turks, and non-Ashkenazi (primarily North African and Iraqi) Jews. With the advent of genetic testing, FMF has been documented with increasing frequency among Ashkenazi Jews, Italians, and other Mediterranean populations, and occasional cases have been confirmed even in the absence of known Mediterranean ancestry. FMF is generally regarded as recessively inherited, but there is an increasing awareness of clear-cut clinical cases with only a single demonstrable genetic mutation, and, for certain relatively rare FMF mutations, there is strong evidence for dominant inheritance. Particularly in countries where families are small, a positive family history can only be elicited in ~50% of cases. DNA testing demonstrates carrier frequencies as high as 1:3 among affected populations, suggesting a heterozygote advantage.

The FMF gene encodes a 781-amino acid, ~95 kDa protein denoted *pyrin* (or *marenostrin*) that is expressed in granulocytes, eosinophils, monocytes, dendritic cells, and synovial and peritoneal fibroblasts. The N-terminal 92 amino acids of pyrin define a motif, the PYRIN domain, that is similar in structure to death domains, death effector

TABLE 392-1 THE HEREDITARY RECURRENT FEVER SYNDROMES

	FMF	TRAPS	HIDS	MWS	FCAS	NOMID
Ethnicity	Jewish, Arab, Turkish, Armenian, Italian	Any ethnic group	Predominantly Dutch, northern European	Any ethnic group	Any ethnic group	Any ethnic group
Inheritance	Recessive[a]	Dominant	Recessive	Dominant	Dominant	Most commonly de novo mutations; somatic mosaicism in a significant minority
Gene/chromosome	*MEFV*/16p13.3	*TNFRSF1A*/12p13	*MVK*/12q24	*NLRP3*/1q44	*NLRP3*/1q44	*NLRP3*/1q44
Protein	Pyrin	p55 TNF receptor	Mevalonate kinase	Cryopyrin (NLRP3)	Cryopyrin (NLRP3)	Cryopyrin (NLRP3)
Attack length	1–3 days	Often >7 days	3–7 days	1–2 days	Minutes–3 days	Continuous, with flares
Serosa	Pleurisy, peritonitis; asymptomatic pericardial effusions	Pleurisy, peritonitis, pericarditis	Abdominal pain, but seldom peritonitis; pleurisy, pericarditis uncommon	Abdominal pain; pleurisy, pericarditis rare	Rare	Rare
Skin	Erysipeloid erythema	Centrifugally migrating erythema	Diffuse maculopapular rash; oral ulcers	Diffuse urticaria-like rash	Cold-induced urticaria-like rash	Diffuse urticaria-like rash
Joints	Acute monoarthritis; chronic hip arthritis (rare)	Acute monoarthritis, arthralgia	Arthralgia, oligoarthritis	Arthralgia, large joint oligoarthritis	Polyarthralgia	Epiphyseal, patellar overgrowth, clubbing
Muscle	Exercise-induced myalgia common; protracted febrile myalgia rare	Migratory myalgia	Uncommon	Myalgia common	Sometimes myalgia	Sometimes myalgia
Eyes, ears	Uncommon	Periorbital edema, conjunctivitis, rarely uveitis	Uncommon	Conjunctivitis, episcleritis, optic disc edema; sensorineural hearing loss	Conjunctivitis	Conjunctivitis, uveitis, optic disc edema, blindness, sensorineural hearing loss
CNS	Aseptic meningitis rare	Headache	Headache	Headache	Headache	Aseptic meningitis, seizures
Amyloidosis	Most common in M694V homozygotes	~15% of cases, most often cysteine mutations, T50M	Uncommon	~25% of cases	Uncommon	Late complication
Treatment	Oral colchicine prophylaxis, IL-1 inhibitors for refractory cases	Glucocorticoids, etanercept, IL-1 inhibitors	NSAIDs for fever; IL-1 and TNF inhibitors	Anakinra, rilonacept, canakinumab	Anakinra, rilonacept, canakinumab	Anakinra

[a]A substantial percentage of patients with clinical FMF have only a single demonstrable MEFV mutation on DNA sequencing.

Abbreviations: FCAS, familial cold autoinflammatory syndrome; FMF, familial Mediterranean fever; HIDS, hyperimmunoglobulinemia D with periodic fever syndrome; IL, interleukin; MWS, Muckle-Wells syndrome; NOMID, neonatal-onset multisystem inflammatory disease; NSAIDs, nonsteroidal anti-inflammatories; TNF, tumor necrosis factor; TRAPS, TNF receptor-associated periodic syndrome.

domains, and caspase recruitment domains. PYRIN domains mediate homotypic protein-protein interactions and have been found in several other proteins, including cryopyrin (NLRP3), which is mutated in three other recurrent fever syndromes. Through a number of mechanisms, including the interaction of the PYRIN domain with an intermediary adaptor protein, pyrin regulates caspase-1 (interleukin [IL] 1β-converting enzyme), and thereby IL-1β secretion. Mice bearing FMF-associated pyrin mutations exhibit inflammation and excessive IL-1 production.

ACUTE ATTACKS

Febrile episodes in FMF may begin even in early infancy; 90% of patients have had their first attack by age 20. Typical FMF episodes generally last 24–72 h, with arthritic attacks tending to last somewhat longer. In some patients, the episodes occur with great regularity, but more often, the frequency of attacks varies over time, ranging from as often as once every few days to remissions lasting several years. Attacks are often unpredictable, although some patients relate them to physical exertion, emotional stress, or menses; pregnancy may be associated with remission.

If measured, fever is nearly always present throughout FMF attacks. Severe hyperpyrexia and even febrile seizures may be seen in infants, and fever is sometimes the only manifestation of FMF in young children.

Over 90% of FMF patients experience abdominal attacks at some time. Episodes range in severity from dull, aching pain and distention with mild tenderness on direct palpation to severe generalized pain with absent bowel sounds, rigidity, rebound tenderness, and air-fluid levels on upright radiographs. Computed tomography (CT) scanning may demonstrate a small amount of fluid in the abdominal cavity. If such patients undergo exploratory laparotomy, a sterile, neutrophil-rich peritoneal exudate is present, sometimes with adhesions from previous episodes. Ascites is rare.

Pleural attacks are usually manifested by unilateral, sharp, stabbing chest pain. Radiographs may show atelectasis and sometimes an effusion. If performed, thoracentesis demonstrates an exudative fluid rich in neutrophils. After repeated attacks, pleural thickening may develop.

FMF arthritis is most frequent among individuals homozygous for the M694V mutation, which is especially common in the non-Ashkenazi Jewish population. Acute arthritis in FMF is usually monoarticular, affecting the knee, ankle, or hip, although other patterns can be seen, particularly in children. Large sterile effusions rich in neutrophils are frequent, without commensurate erythema or warmth. Even after repeated arthritic attacks, radiographic changes are rare. Before the advent of colchicine prophylaxis, chronic arthritis of the knee or hip was seen in ~5% of FMF patients with arthritis. Chronic sacroiliitis can occur in FMF irrespective of the HLA-B27 antigen, even in the face of colchicine therapy. In the United States, FMF patients are much more likely to have arthralgia than arthritis.

The most characteristic cutaneous manifestation of FMF is erysipelas-like erythema, a raised erythematous rash that most commonly occurs on the dorsum of the foot, ankle, or lower leg alone or in combination with abdominal pain, pleurisy, or arthritis. Biopsy demonstrates perivascular infiltrates of granulocytes and monocytes. This rash is seen most often in M694V homozygotes and is relatively rare in the United States.

Exercise-induced (nonfebrile) myalgia is common in FMF, and a small percentage of patients develop a protracted febrile myalgia that can last several weeks. Symptomatic pericardial disease is rare, although some patients have small pericardial effusions as an incidental echocardiographic finding. Unilateral acute scrotal inflammation may occur in prepubertal boys. Aseptic meningitis has been reported in FMF, but the causal connection is controversial. Vasculitis, including Henoch-Schönlein purpura and polyarteritis nodosa (Chap. 385), may be seen at increased frequency in FMF. The M694V FMF mutation has recently been shown to be a risk factor for Behçet's disease.

Laboratory features of FMF attacks are consistent with acute inflammation and include an elevated erythrocyte sedimentation rate, leukocytosis, thrombocytosis (in children), and elevations in C-reactive protein, fibrinogen, haptoglobin, and serum immunoglobulins. Transient albuminuria and hematuria may also be seen.

AMYLOIDOSIS

Before the advent of colchicine prophylaxis, systemic amyloidosis was a common complication of FMF. It is caused by deposition of a fragment of serum amyloid A, an acute-phase reactant, in the kidneys, adrenals, intestine, spleen, lung, and testes (Chap. 137). Amyloidosis should be suspected in patients who have proteinuria between attacks; renal or rectal biopsy is used most often to establish the diagnosis. Risk factors include the M694V homozygous genotype, positive family history (independent of FMF mutational status), the SAA 1 genotype, male gender, noncompliance with colchicine therapy, and having grown up in the Middle East.

DIAGNOSIS

For typical cases, physicians experienced with FMF can often make the diagnosis on clinical grounds alone. Clinical criteria sets for FMF have been shown to have high sensitivity and specificity in parts of the world where the pretest probability of FMF is high. Genetic testing can provide a useful adjunct in ambiguous cases or for physicians not experienced in FMF. Most of the more severe disease-associated FMF mutations are in exon 10 of the gene, with a smaller group of milder variants in exon 2. An updated list of mutations for FMF and other hereditary recurrent fevers can be found online at *http://fmf.igh.cnrs.fr/infevers/*.

Genetic testing has permitted a broadening of the clinical spectrum and geographic distribution of FMF and may be of prognostic value. Most studies indicate that M694V homozygotes have an earlier age of onset and a higher frequency of arthritis, rash, and amyloidosis. In contrast, the E148Q variant is quite common in certain populations and is more likely to affect overall levels of inflammation than to cause clinical FMF. E148Q is sometimes found in *cis* with exon 10 mutations, which may complicate the interpretation of genetic test results. Only ~70% of patients with clinically typical FMF have two identifiable mutations in *trans*. The inability to identify a second mutation even after intensive molecular analysis suggests that one FMF mutation may be sufficient to cause disease under some circumstances. In these cases clinical judgment is very important, and sometimes a therapeutic trial of colchicine may help to confirm the diagnosis. Genetic testing of unaffected individuals is usually inadvisable, because of the possibility of nonpenetrance and the potential impact of a positive test on future insurability.

If a patient is seen during his or her first attack, the differential diagnosis may be broad, although delimited by the specific organ involvement. After several attacks the differential diagnosis may include the other hereditary recurrent fever syndromes (Table 392-1); the syndrome of periodic fever with aphthous ulcers, pharyngitis, and cervical adenopathy (PFAPA); systemic-onset juvenile rheumatoid arthritis or adult Still's disease; porphyria; hereditary angioedema; inflammatory bowel disease; and, in women, gynecologic disorders.

TREATMENT FAMILIAL MEDITERRANEAN FEVER

The treatment of choice for FMF is daily oral colchicine, which decreases the frequency and intensity of attacks and prevents the development of amyloidosis in compliant patients. Intermittent dosing at the onset of attacks is not as effective as daily prophylaxis and is of unproven value in preventing amyloidosis. The usual adult dose of colchicine is 1.2–1.8 mg/d, which causes substantial reduction in symptoms in two-thirds of patients and some improvement in >90%. Children may require lower doses, although not proportionately to body weight.

Common side effects of colchicine include bloating, abdominal cramps, lactose intolerance, and diarrhea. They can be minimized by starting at a low dose and gradually advancing as tolerated, splitting the dose, use of simethicone for flatulence, and avoidance of dairy products. If taken by either parent at the time of conception, colchicine may cause a small increase in the risk of trisomy 21 (Down's syndrome). In elderly patients with renal insufficiency, colchicine can cause a myoneuropathy characterized by proximal muscle weakness and elevation of the creatine kinase. Cyclosporine inhibits hepatic excretion of colchicine by its effects on the MDR-1 transport system, sometimes leading to colchicine toxicity in patients who have undergone renal transplantation for amyloidosis. Intravenous colchicine should generally not be administered to patients already taking oral colchicine, because severe, sometimes fatal, toxicity can occur in this setting.

For FMF patients who do not respond to colchicine or cannot tolerate therapeutic doses, injectable IL-1 inhibitors appear to be effective in preventing the acute attacks. In a small randomized placebo-controlled trial, weekly subcutaneous rilonacept, a recombinant IL-1 receptor fusion protein, significantly reduced the frequency of attacks. There is also substantial anecdotal experience with daily subcutaneous anakinra, a recombinant IL-1 receptor antagonist, in preventing the acute attacks of FMF, and in some cases reducing established amyloid deposits. Canakinumab, a monoclonal antibody to IL-1β, and tumor necrosis factor (TNF) inhibitors may also have a role in the treatment of colchicine-unresponsive or intolerant patients. Bone marrow transplantation has been suggested for refractory FMF, but the risk-benefit ratio is currently regarded as unacceptable.

OTHER HEREDITARY RECURRENT FEVERS

Within 5 years of the discovery of the FMF gene, three additional genes causing five other hereditary recurrent fever syndromes were identified, catalyzing a paradigm shift in diagnosis and treatment of these disorders.

TNF RECEPTOR-ASSOCIATED PERIODIC SYNDROME (TRAPS)

TRAPS is caused by dominantly inherited mutations in the extracellular domains of the 55-kDa TNF receptor (TNFR1, p55). Although originally described in a large Irish family (and hence the name *familial Hibernian fever*), TRAPS has a broad ethnic distribution. TRAPS episodes often begin in childhood. The duration of attacks ranges from 1–2 days to as long as several weeks, and in severe cases symptoms may be nearly continuous. In addition to peritoneal, pleural, and synovial attacks similar to FMF, TRAPS patients frequently have ocular inflammation (most often conjunctivitis and/or periorbital edema), and a distinctive migratory myalgia with overlying painful erythema may be present. TRAPS patients generally respond better to glucocorticoids than to prophylactic colchicine. Untreated, about 15% develop amyloidosis. The diagnosis of TRAPS is based on the demonstration of *TNFRSF1A* mutations in the presence of characteristic symptoms. Two particular variants, R92Q and P46L, are common in certain populations and may act more as functional polymorphisms than as disease-causing mutations. In contrast, pathogenic *TNFRSF1A* mutations, including a number of substitutions at highly conserved cysteine residues, are associated with intracellular TNFR1 misfolding, aggregation, and retention, with consequent ligand independent kinase activation, mitochondrial reactive oxygen species production, and proinflammatory cytokine release. Etanercept, a TNF inhibitor, ameliorates TRAPS attacks, but the long-term experience with this agent has been less favorable. Perhaps because of the ligand-independent signaling abnormalities in TRAPS, IL-1 inhibition has been beneficial in a large percentage of the patients in whom it has been used. Monoclonal anti-TNF antibodies should be avoided, because they may exacerbate TRAPS attacks.

HYPERIMMUNOGLOBULINEMIA D WITH PERIODIC FEVER SYNDROME (HIDS)

HIDS is a recessively inherited recurrent fever syndrome found primarily in individuals of northern European ancestry. It is caused by mutations in mevalonate kinase (*MVK*), encoding an enzyme involved in the synthesis of cholesterol and nonsterol isoprenoids. Attacks usually begin in infancy and last 3–5 days. Clinically distinctive features include painful cervical adenopathy, a diffuse maculopapular rash sometimes affecting the palms and soles, and aphthous ulcers; pleurisy is rare, as is amyloidosis. Although originally defined by the persistent elevation of serum IgD, disease activity is not related to IgD levels, and some patients with FMF or TRAPS may have modestly increased serum IgD. Moreover, occasional patients with *MVK* mutations and recurrent fever have normal IgD levels. For these reasons, some have proposed renaming this disorder *mevalonate kinase deficiency (MKD)*. All patients with mutations have markedly elevated urinary mevalonate levels during their febrile attacks, although the inflammatory manifestations are likely to be due to a deficiency of isoprenoids rather than an excess of mevalonate. There is currently no established treatment for HIDS/MKD, although intermittent or continuous IL-1 inhibition and TNF inhibitors have been effective in small series.

THE CRYOPYRINOPATHIES, OR CRYOPYRIN-ASSOCIATED PERIODIC SYNDROMES (CAPS)

Three hereditary febrile syndromes, familial cold autoinflammatory syndrome (FCAS), Muckle-Wells syndrome (MWS), and neonatal-onset multisystem inflammatory disease (NOMID), are all caused by mutations in *NLRP3* (formerly known as *CIAS1*), the gene encoding cryopyrin (or NLRP3), and represent a clinical spectrum of disease. FCAS patients develop chills, fever, headache, arthralgia, conjunctivitis, and an urticaria-like rash in response to generalized cold exposure. In MWS, an urticarial rash is noted, but it is not usually induced by cold; MWS patients also develop fevers, abdominal pain, limb pain, arthritis, conjunctivitis, and, over time, sensorineural hearing loss. NOMID is the most severe of the three disorders, with chronic aseptic meningitis, a characteristic arthropathy, and rash. Like the FMF protein, pyrin, cryopyrin has an N-terminal PYRIN domain. Cryopyrin regulates IL-1β production through the formation of a macromolecular complex termed the *inflammasome*. Peripheral blood leukocytes from patients with FCAS, MWS, and NOMID release increased amounts of IL-1β upon in vitro stimulation, relative to healthy controls. Macrophages from cryopyrin-deficient mice exhibit decreased IL-1β production in response to certain gram-positive bacteria, bacterial RNA, and monosodium urate crystals. Patients with all three cryopyrinopathies show a dramatic response to injections of IL-1 inhibitors. Approximately one-third of patients with clinical manifestations of NOMID do not have germline mutations in *NLRP3*, but have been found to be mosaic for somatic *NLRP3* mutations. Such patients also respond dramatically to IL-1 inhibition. Similarly, somatic mosaicism in *NLRP3* has been found in Schnitzler's syndrome, which presents in middle age with recurrent fever, urticarial rash, elevated acute phase reactants, monoclonal IgM gammopathy, and abnormal bone remodeling. IL-1 inhibition is the treatment of choice for Schnitzler's syndrome.

OTHER INHERITED AUTOINFLAMMATORY DISEASES

There are a number of other Mendelian autoinflammatory diseases in which recurrent fevers are not a prominent clinical sign but that involve abnormalities of innate immunity. The syndrome of pyogenic arthritis with pyoderma gangrenosum and acne (PAPA) is a dominantly inherited disorder that presents with episodes of sterile pyogenic monoarthritis often induced by trauma, severe pyoderma gangrenosum, and severe cystic acne, usually beginning in puberty. It is caused by mutations in *PSTPIP1*, which encodes a pyrin-binding protein, and the arthritic manifestations often respond to IL-1 inhibition. Patients with the recessively inherited deficiency of the IL-1 receptor antagonist (DIRA) present with a generalized pustular rash and multifocal sterile osteomyelitis, and show dramatic clinical responses to anakinra, the recombinant form of the protein they lack. IL-36 is another member of the IL-1 family of cytokines that is regulated by an endogenous receptor antagonist. The recessively inherited deficiency of the IL-36 receptor antagonist (DITRA) presents with episodes of generalized pustular psoriasis and dramatic systemic inflammation.

Whereas PAPA, DIRA, and DITRA all involve mutations in IL-1-related molecules, other autoinflammatory diseases are caused by mutations in other components of innate immunity. *Blau's syndrome* is caused by mutations in *CARD15* (also known as *NOD2*), which regulates nuclear factor-κB activation. Blau's syndrome is characterized by granulomatous dermatitis, uveitis, and arthritis; distinct *CARD15* variants predispose to Crohn's disease. Recessive mutations in one or more components of the proteasome lead to excessive interferon signaling and the syndrome of chronic atypical neutrophilic dermatosis with lipodystrophy and elevated temperature (CANDLE), a severe form of generalized panniculitis. De novo gain-of-function mutations in TMEM173, encoding the stimulator of interferon genes (STING), cause severe vasculopathy and pulmonary fibrosis. Recessive loss-of-function mutations in CERCR1, encoding adenosine deaminase 2 (ADA2), cause a vasculopathy that can manifest as livedoid rash, early-onset lacunar strokes, or polyarteritis nodosa.

Finally, it should be noted that a number of common, genetically complex disorders are now sometimes considered autoinflammatory, because of evidence that components of the innate immune system, such as the inflammasome, may play a role in the pathogenesis. Two prominent examples are gout and atherosclerosis. Large clinical trials of IL-1 inhibitors have been initiated in both conditions.

393 Approach to Articular and Musculoskeletal Disorders

John J. Cush

Musculoskeletal complaints account for >315 million outpatient visits per year and over 20% of all outpatient visits in the United States. The Centers for Disease Control and Prevention estimate that 22.7% (52.5 million) of the U.S. population has physician-diagnosed arthritis and 22 million have significant functional limitation. While many patients will have self-limited conditions requiring minimal evaluation and only symptomatic therapy and reassurance, specific musculoskeletal presentations or their persistence may herald a more serious condition that requires further evaluation or laboratory testing to establish a diagnosis. The goal of the musculoskeletal evaluation is to formulate a differential diagnosis that leads to an accurate diagnosis and timely therapy, while avoiding excessive diagnostic testing and unnecessary treatment (Table 393-1). There are several urgent conditions that must be diagnosed promptly to avoid significant morbid or mortal sequelae. These "red flag" diagnoses include septic arthritis, acute crystal-induced arthritis (e.g., gout), and fracture. Each may be suspected by its acute onset and monarticular or focal musculoskeletal pain (see below).

Despite well-known links between certain disorders and laboratory testing, the majority of individuals with musculoskeletal complaints can be diagnosed with a thorough history and a comprehensive physical and musculoskeletal examination. The initial encounter should determine whether the musculoskeletal complaint signals a red flag condition (septic arthritis, gout, or fracture) or not. The evaluation should proceed to ascertain if the complaint is (1) *articular* or *nonarticular* in origin, (2) *inflammatory* or *noninflammatory* in nature, (3) *acute* or *chronic* in duration, and (4) *localized (monarticular)* or *widespread* (*polyarticular*) in distribution.

With such an approach and an understanding of the pathophysiologic processes, the musculoskeletal complaint or presentation can be characterized (e.g., acute inflammatory monarthritis or a chronic noninflammatory, nonarticular widespread pain) to narrow the diagnostic possibilities. A diagnosis can be made in the vast majority of individuals. However, some patients will not fit immediately into an established diagnostic category. Many musculoskeletal disorders resemble each other at the outset, and some may take weeks or months (but not years) to evolve into a recognizable diagnostic entity. This consideration should temper the desire to establish a definitive diagnosis at the first encounter.

TABLE 393-1 EVALUATION OF PATIENTS WITH MUSCULOSKELETAL COMPLAINTS

Goals
- Accurate diagnosis
- Timely provision of therapy
- Avoidance of unnecessary diagnostic testing
- Identification of acute, focal/monarticular "red flag" conditions

Approach
- Determination of chronology (acute vs chronic)
- Determination of the nature of the pathologic process (inflammatory vs noninflammatory)
- Determination of the extent of involvement (monarticular, polyarticular, focal, widespread)
- Anatomic localization of complaint (articular vs nonarticular)
- Consider the most common disorders first
- Formulate a differential diagnosis

ARTICULAR VERSUS NONARTICULAR

The musculoskeletal evaluation must discriminate the anatomic origin(s) of the patient's complaint. For example, ankle pain can result from a variety of pathologic conditions involving disparate anatomic structures, including gonococcal arthritis, calcaneal fracture, Achilles tendinitis, plantar fasciitis, cellulitis, and peripheral or entrapment neuropathy. Distinguishing between articular and nonarticular conditions requires a careful and detailed examination. Articular structures include the synovium, synovial fluid, articular cartilage, intraarticular ligaments, joint capsule, and juxtaarticular bone. Nonarticular (or periarticular) structures, such as supportive extraarticular ligaments, tendons, bursae, muscle, fascia, bone, nerve, and overlying skin, may be involved in the pathologic process. Although musculoskeletal complaints are often ascribed to the joints, nonarticular disorders more frequently underlie such complaints. Distinguishing between these potential sources of pain may be challenging to the unskilled examiner. Articular disorders may be characterized by deep or diffuse pain, pain or limited range of motion on active and passive movement, and swelling (caused by synovial proliferation, effusion, or bony enlargement), crepitation, instability, "locking," or deformity. By contrast, nonarticular disorders tend to be painful on active, but not passive (or assisted), range of motion. Periarticular conditions often demonstrate point or focal tenderness in regions adjacent to articular structures, are elicited with a specific movement or position, and have physical findings remote from the joint capsule. Moreover, nonarticular disorders seldom demonstrate swelling, crepitus, instability, or deformity of the joint itself.

INFLAMMATORY VERSUS NONINFLAMMATORY DISORDERS

In the course of a musculoskeletal evaluation, the examiner should determine the nature of the underlying pathologic process and whether inflammatory or noninflammatory findings exist. Inflammatory disorders may be infectious (*Neisseria gonorrhoeae* or *Mycobacterium tuberculosis*), crystal-induced (gout, pseudogout), immune-related (rheumatoid arthritis [RA], systemic lupus erythematosus [SLE]), reactive (rheumatic fever, reactive arthritis), or idiopathic. Inflammatory disorders may be identified by any of the four cardinal signs of inflammation (erythema, warmth, pain, or swelling), systemic symptoms (fatigue, fever, rash, weight loss), or laboratory evidence of inflammation (elevated erythrocyte sedimentation rate [ESR] or C-reactive protein [CRP], thrombocytosis, anemia of chronic disease, or hypoalbuminemia). Articular stiffness commonly accompanies chronic musculoskeletal disorders. The duration of stiffness may be prolonged (hours) with inflammatory disorders (such as RA or polymyalgia rheumatica) and may improve with activity. By contrast, intermittent stiffness (also known as gel phenomenon) is typical of noninflammatory conditions (such as osteoarthritis [OA]), shorter in duration (<60 min), and exacerbated by activity. Fatigue may accompany inflammation (as seen in RA and polymyalgia rheumatica) but may also be a consequence of fibromyalgia (a noninflammatory disorder), chronic pain, poor sleep, depression, anemia, cardiac failure, endocrinopathy, or malnutrition. Noninflammatory disorders may be related to trauma (rotator cuff tear), repetitive use (bursitis, tendinitis), degeneration or ineffective repair (OA), neoplasm (pigmented villonodular synovitis), or pain amplification (fibromyalgia). Noninflammatory disorders are often characterized by pain without synovial swelling or warmth, absence of inflammatory or systemic features, daytime gel phenomena rather than morning stiffness, and normal (for age) or negative laboratory investigations.

Identification of the nature of the underlying process and the site of the complaint will enable the examiner to characterize the musculoskeletal presentation (e.g., acute inflammatory monarthritis, chronic noninflammatory, nonarticular widespread pain), narrow the diagnostic considerations, and assess the need for immediate diagnostic or

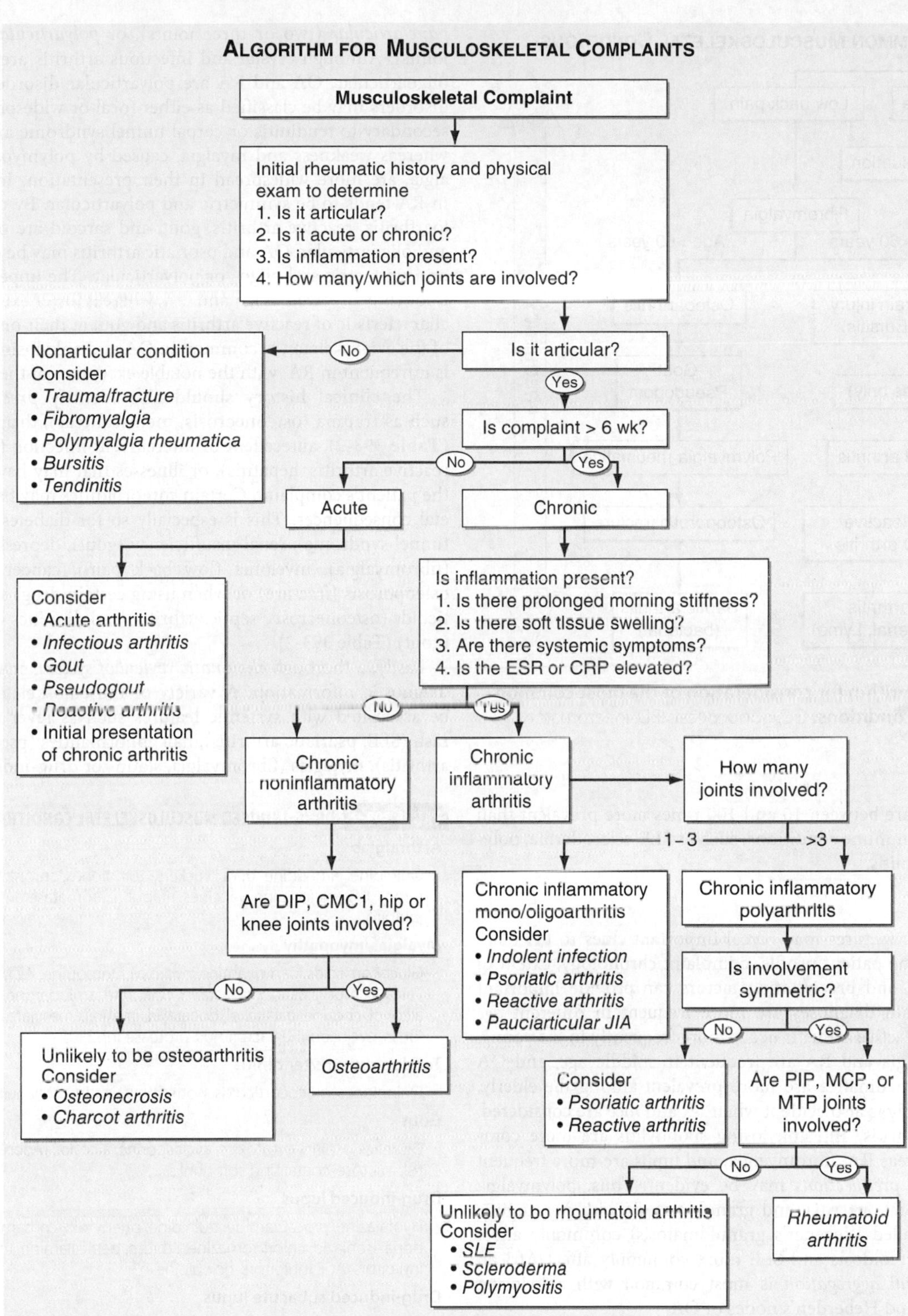

FIGURE 393-1 Algorithm for the diagnosis of musculoskeletal complaints. An approach to formulating a differential diagnosis (shown in italics). CMC, carpometacarpal; CRP, C-reactive protein; DIP, distal interphalangeal; ESR, erythrocyte sedimentation rate; JIA, juvenile idiopathic arthritis; MCP, metacarpophalangeal; MTP, metatarsophalangeal; PIP, proximal interphalangeal; PMR, polymyalgia rheumatica; SLE, systemic lupus erythematosus.

therapeutic intervention or for continued observation. Figure 393-1 presents an algorithmic approach to the evaluation of patients with musculoskeletal complaints. This approach relies on clinical and historic features, rather than laboratory testing, to diagnose many common rheumatic disorders.

A simpler, alternative approach would consider the most commonly encountered complaints first, based on frequency in younger versus older populations. The most prevalent causes of musculoskeletal complaints are shown in Fig. 393-2. Because trauma, fracture, overuse syndromes, and fibromyalgia are among the most common causes of joint pain, these should be considered during the initial encounter. If these possibilities are excluded, other frequently occurring disorders should be considered according to the patient's age. Hence, those younger than 60 years are commonly affected by repetitive use/strain disorders, gout (men only), RA, spondyloarthritis, and uncommonly, infectious arthritis. Patients over age 60 years are frequently affected by OA, crystal (gout and pseudogout) arthritis, polymyalgia rheumatica, osteoporotic fracture, and uncommonly, septic arthritis.

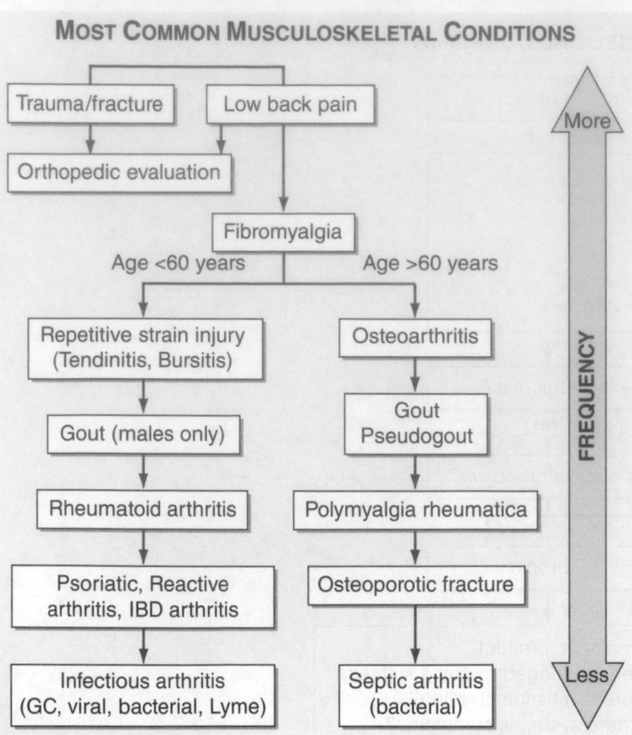

FIGURE 393-2 Algorithm for consideration of the most common musculoskeletal conditions. GC, gonococcal; IBD, inflammatory bowel disease.

These conditions are between 10 and 100 times more prevalent than other serious autoimmune conditions, such as SLE, scleroderma, polymyositis, and vasculitis.

CLINICAL HISTORY

Additional historic features may reveal important clues to the diagnosis. Aspects of the patient profile, complaint chronology, extent of joint involvement, and precipitating factors can provide important information. Certain diagnoses are more frequent in different *age* groups. SLE and reactive arthritis occur more frequently in the young, whereas fibromyalgia and RA are frequent in middle age, and OA and polymyalgia rheumatica are more prevalent among the elderly. Diagnostic clustering is also evident when *sex* and *race* are considered. Gout, spondyloarthritis, and ankylosing spondylitis are more common in men, whereas RA, fibromyalgia, and lupus are more frequent in women. *Racial predilections* may be evident. Thus, polymyalgia rheumatica, giant cell arteritis, and granulomatosis with polyangiitis (GPA; formerly called Wegener's granulomatosis) commonly affect whites, whereas sarcoidosis and SLE more commonly affect African Americans. *Familial aggregation* is most common with ankylosing spondylitis, gout, and Heberden's nodes of OA.

The chronology of the complaint is an important diagnostic feature and can be divided into the *onset, evolution*, and *duration*. The onset of disorders such as septic arthritis or gout tends to be abrupt, whereas OA, RA, and fibromyalgia may have more indolent presentations. The patients' complaints may evolve differently and be classified as chronic (OA), intermittent (crystal or Lyme arthritis), migratory (rheumatic fever, gonococcal or viral arthritis), or additive (RA, psoriatic arthritis). Musculoskeletal disorders are typically classified as acute or chronic based on a symptom duration that is either less than or greater than 6 weeks, respectively. Acute arthropathies tend to be infectious, crystal-induced, or reactive. Chronic conditions include noninflammatory or immunologic arthritides (e.g., OA, RA) and nonarticular disorders (e.g., fibromyalgia).

The *extent* or *distribution* of articular involvement is often informative. Articular disorders are classified based on the number of joints involved, as either *monarticular* (one joint), *oligoarticular* or *pauciarticular* (two or three joints), or *polyarticular* (four or more joints). Although crystal and infectious arthritis are often mono- or oligoarticular, OA and RA are polyarticular disorders. Nonarticular disorders may be classified as either focal or widespread. Complaints secondary to tendinitis or carpal tunnel syndrome are typically focal, whereas weakness and myalgia, caused by polymyositis or fibromyalgia, are more widespread in their presentation. Joint involvement in RA tends to be symmetric and polyarticular. By contrast, spondyloarthritis, reactive arthritis, gout, and sarcoid are often asymmetric and oligoarticular. OA and psoriatic arthritis may be either symmetric or asymmetric and oligo- or polyarticular. The upper extremities are frequently involved in RA and OA, whereas lower extremity arthritis is characteristic of reactive arthritis and gout at their onset. Involvement of the axial skeleton is common in OA and ankylosing spondylitis but is infrequent in RA, with the notable exception of the cervical spine.

The clinical history should also identify *precipitating events*, such as trauma (osteonecrosis, meniscal tear), drug administration (Table 393-2), antecedent or intercurrent infection (rheumatic fever, reactive arthritis, hepatitis), or illnesses that may have contributed to the patient's complaint. Certain comorbidities may have musculoskeletal consequences. This is especially so for diabetes mellitus (carpal tunnel syndrome), renal insufficiency (gout), depression or insomnia (fibromyalgia), myeloma (low back pain), cancer (myositis), and osteoporosis (fracture) or when using certain drugs such as glucocorticoids (osteonecrosis, septic arthritis) and diuretics or chemotherapy (gout) (Table 393-2).

Lastly, a thorough *rheumatic review of systems* may disclose useful diagnostic information. A variety of musculoskeletal disorders may be associated with systemic features such as fever (SLE, infection), rash (SLE, psoriatic arthritis), nail abnormalities (psoriatic or reactive arthritis), myalgias (fibromyalgia, statin- or drug-induced myopathy),

TABLE 393-2 DRUG-INDUCED MUSCULOSKELETAL CONDITIONS

Arthralgias
Quinidine, cimetidine, beta blockers, quinolones, chronic acyclovir, interferons, IL-2, nicardipine, vaccines, rifabutin, aromatase and HIV protease inhibitors
Myalgias/myopathy
Glucocorticoids, penicillamine, hydroxychloroquine, AZT, lovastatin, simvastatin, atorvastatin, pravastatin, clofibrate, amiodarone, interferon, IL-2, alcohol, cocaine, paclitaxel, docetaxel, imatinib mesylate, colchicine, quinolones, cyclosporine, tacrolimus, protease inhibitors
Tendon rupture/tendinitis
Quinolones, glucocorticoids, isotretinoin, statins, collagenase injections
Gout
Diuretics, aspirin, cytotoxics, cyclosporine, alcohol, moonshine, ethambutol, fructose-containing soft drinks
Drug-induced lupus
Hydralazine, procainamide, quinidine, phenytoin, carbamazepine, methyldopa, isoniazid, chlorpromazine, lithium, penicillamine, tetracyclines, TNF inhibitors, ACE inhibitors, ticlopidine
Drug-induced subacute lupus
Proton pump inhibitors, calcium channel blockers (diltiazem), ACE inhibitors, TNF inhibitors, terbinafine, interferons (α and β-1a), paclitaxel, docetaxel, HCTZ
Osteonecrosis
Glucocorticoids, alcohol, radiation, bisphosphonates
Osteopenia
Glucocorticoids, chronic heparin, phenytoin
Scleroderma
Vinyl chloride, bleomycin, baricitinib, pentazocine, organic solvents, carbidopa, tryptophan, rapeseed oil
Vasculitis
Allopurinol, amphetamines, cocaine (often levamisole adulterated), thiazides, penicillamine, propylthiouracil, montelukast, TNF inhibitors, hepatitis B vaccine, trimethoprim/sulfamethoxazole, minocycline, hydralazine

Abbreviations: ACE, angiotensin-converting enzyme; AZT, zidovudine; HCTZ, hydrochlorothiazide; IL-2, interleukin 2; TNF, tumor necrosis factor.

or weakness (polymyositis, neuropathy). In addition, some conditions are associated with involvement of other organ systems including the eyes (Behçet's disease, sarcoidosis, spondyloarthritis), gastrointestinal tract (scleroderma, inflammatory bowel disease), genitourinary tract (reactive arthritis, gonococcemia), or nervous system (Lyme disease, vasculitis).

RHEUMATOLOGIC EVALUATION OF THE ELDERLY

The incidence of rheumatic diseases rises with age, such that 58% of those >65 years will have joint complaints. Musculoskeletal disorders in elderly patients are often not diagnosed because the signs and symptoms may be insidious, overlooked, or overshadowed by comorbidities. These difficulties are compounded by the diminished reliability of laboratory testing in the elderly, who often manifest nonpathologic abnormal results. For example, the ESR may be misleadingly elevated, and low-titer positive tests for rheumatoid factor and antinuclear antibodies (ANAs) may be seen in up to 15% of elderly patients. Although nearly all rheumatic disorders afflict the elderly, geriatric patients are particularly prone to OA, osteoporosis, osteoporotic fractures, gout, pseudogout, polymyalgia rheumatica, vasculitis, and drug-induced disorders (Table 393-2). The elderly should be approached in the same manner as other patients with musculoskeletal complaints, but with an emphasis on identifying the potential rheumatic consequences of medical comorbidities and therapies. The physical examination should identify the nature of the musculoskeletal complaint as well as coexisting diseases that may influence diagnosis and choice of treatment.

RHEUMATOLOGIC EVALUATION OF THE HOSPITALIZED PATIENT

Evaluation of a hospitalized patient with rheumatic complaints differs from that of an outpatient, owing to greater symptom severity, more acute presentations, and greater interplay of comorbidities. Patients with rheumatic disorders tend to be admitted for one of several reasons: (1) acute onset of inflammatory arthritis; (2) undiagnosed systemic or febrile illness; (3) musculoskeletal trauma; (4) exacerbation or deterioration of an existing autoimmune disorder (e.g., SLE); or (5) new medical comorbidities (e.g., thrombotic event, lymphoma, infection) arising in patients with an established rheumatic disorder. Notably, rheumatic patients are seldom if ever admitted because of widespread pain or serologic abnormalities or for the initiation of new therapies.

Acute monarticular inflammatory arthritis may be a "red flag" condition (e.g., septic arthritis, gout, pseudogout) that will require arthrocentesis and, on occasion, hospitalization if infection is suspected. However, new-onset inflammatory polyarthritis will have a wider differential diagnosis (e.g., RA, hepatitis-related arthritis, serum sickness, drug-induced lupus, polyarticular septic arthritis) and may require targeted laboratory investigations rather than synovial fluid analyses. Patients with febrile, multisystem disorders will require exclusion of crystal, infectious, or neoplastic etiologies and an evaluation driven by the dominant symptom/finding with the greatest specificity. Conditions worthy of consideration may include gout or pseudogout, vasculitis (giant cell arteritis in the elderly or polyarteritis nodosa in younger patients), adult-onset Still's disease, SLE, antiphospholipid antibody syndrome, and sarcoidosis. Because the misdiagnosis of connective tissue disorders is common, patients who present with a reported preexisting rheumatic condition (e.g., SLE, RA, ankylosing spondylitis) should have their diagnosis confirmed by careful history, physical and musculoskeletal examination, and review of their medical records. It is important to note that when established rheumatic disease patients are admitted to the hospital, it is usually not for a medical problem related to their autoimmune disease, but rather because of either a comorbid condition or complication of drug therapy. Patients with chronic inflammatory disorders (e.g., RA, SLE, psoriasis) have an augmented risk of infection, cardiovascular events, and neoplasia.

Certain conditions, such as acute gout, can be precipitated in hospitalized patients by surgery, dehydration, or other events and should be considered when hospitalized patients are evaluated for the acute onset of a musculoskeletal condition. Lastly, overly aggressive and unfocused laboratory testing will often yield abnormal findings that are better explained by the patient's preexisting condition(s) rather than a new inflammatory or autoimmune disorder.

PHYSICAL EXAMINATION

The goal of the physical examination is to ascertain the structures involved, the nature of the underlying pathology, the functional consequences of the process, and the presence of systemic or extraarticular manifestations. A knowledge of topographic anatomy is necessary to identify the primary site(s) of involvement and differentiate articular from nonarticular disorders. The musculoskeletal examination depends largely on careful inspection, palpation, and a variety of specific physical maneuvers to elicit diagnostic signs (Table 393-3). Although most articulations of the appendicular skeleton can be examined in this manner, adequate inspection and palpation are not possible for many axial (e.g., zygapophyseal) and inaccessible (e.g., sacroiliac or hip) joints. For such joints, there is a greater reliance on specific maneuvers and imaging for assessment.

Examination of involved and uninvolved joints will determine whether *pain*, *warmth*, *erythema*, or *swelling* is present. The locale and level of pain elicited by palpation or movement should be quantified. One standard would be to count the number of tender joints on palpation of 28 easily examined joints (proximal interphalangeals, metacarpophalangeals, wrists, elbows, shoulders, and knees). Similarly, the number of swollen joints (0–28) can be counted and recorded. Careful examination should distinguish between true articular swelling (caused by bony hypertrophy, synovial effusion or proliferation) and nonarticular (or periarticular) involvement, which usually extends beyond the normal joint margins. Synovial effusion can be distinguished from synovial hypertrophy or bony hypertrophy by palpation or specific maneuvers. For example, small to moderate knee effusions may be identified by the "bulge sign" or "ballottement of the patellae." Bursal effusions (e.g., effusions of the olecranon or prepatellar bursa) are often focal, periarticular, overlie bony prominences, and are fluctuant with sharply defined borders. Joint *stability* can be assessed by stabilizing the proximal joint, by palpation, and by the application of manual stress to the distal appendage. *Subluxation* or *dislocation*, which may be secondary to traumatic, mechanical, or inflammatory

TABLE 393-3 GLOSSARY OF MUSCULOSKELETAL TERMS

Crepitus
A palpable (less commonly audible) vibratory or crackling sensation elicited with joint motion; fine joint crepitus is common and often insignificant in large joints; coarse joint crepitus indicates advanced cartilaginous and degenerative changes (as in osteoarthritis)

Subluxation
Alteration of joint alignment such that articulating surfaces incompletely approximate each other

Dislocation
Abnormal displacement of articulating surfaces such that the surfaces are not in contact

Range of motion
For diarthrodial joints, the arc of measurable movement through which the joint moves in a single plane

Contracture
Loss of full movement resulting from a fixed resistance caused either by tonic spasm of muscle (reversible) or by fibrosis of periarticular structures (permanent)

Deformity
Abnormal shape or size resulting from bony hypertrophy, malalignment of articulating structures, or damage to periarticular supportive structures

Enthesitis
Inflammation of the entheses (tendinous or ligamentous insertions on bone)

Epicondylitis
Infection or inflammation involving an epicondyle

causes, can be assessed by inspection and palpation. Joint *swelling* or *volume* can be assessed by palpation. Distention of the articular capsule usually causes pain and evident enlargement or fluctuance. The patient will attempt to minimize the pain by maintaining the joint in the position of least intraarticular pressure and greatest volume, usually partial flexion. For this reason, inflammatory effusions may give rise to flexion contractures. Clinically, this may be detected as fluctuant or "squishy" swelling in larger joints and grape-like compressibility in smaller joints. Inflammation may result in fixed flexion deformities or diminished range of motion—especially on extension, when intraarticular pressure is increased. Active and passive *range of motion* should be assessed in all planes, with contralateral comparison. A goniometer may be used to quantify the arc of movement. Each joint should be passively manipulated through its full range of motion (including, as appropriate, flexion, extension, rotation, abduction, adduction, lateral bending, inversion, eversion, supination, pronation, medial/lateral deviation, and plantar- or dorsiflexion). Extreme range of motion may be seen with hypermobility syndrome, with joint pain and connective tissue laxity, often associated with Ehlers-Danlos or Marfan's syndrome. Limitation of motion is frequently caused by inflammation, effusion, pain, deformity, contracture, or restriction from neuromyopathic causes. If passive motion exceeds active motion, a periarticular process (e.g., tendinitis, tendon rupture, or myopathy) should be considered. *Contractures* may reflect antecedent synovial inflammation or trauma. Minor joint *crepitus* is common during joint palpation and maneuvers but only indicates significant cartilage degeneration as it becomes coarser (e.g., OA). Joint *deformity* usually indicates a long-standing or aggressive pathologic process. Deformities may result from ligamentous destruction, soft tissue contracture, bony enlargement, ankylosis, erosive disease, subluxation, trauma, or loss of proprioception. Examination of the musculature will document strength, atrophy, pain, or spasm. Appendicular muscle weakness should be characterized as proximal or distal. Muscle strength should be assessed by observing the patient's performance (e.g., walking, rising from a chair, grasping, writing). Strength may also be graded on a 5-point scale: 0 for no movement; 1 for trace movement or twitch; 2 for movement with gravity eliminated; 3 for movement against gravity only; 4 for movement against gravity and resistance; and 5 for normal strength. The examiner should assess for often-overlooked nonarticular or periarticular involvement, especially when articular complaints are not supported by objective findings referable to the joint capsule. The identification of soft tissue/nonarticular pain will prevent unwarranted and often expensive additional evaluations. Specific maneuvers may reveal common nonarticular abnormalities, such as a carpal tunnel syndrome (which can be identified by Tinel's or Phalen's sign). Other examples of soft tissue abnormalities include olecranon bursitis, epicondylitis (e.g., tennis elbow), enthesitis (e.g., Achilles tendinitis), and tender trigger points associated with fibromyalgia.

APPROACH TO REGIONAL RHEUMATIC COMPLAINTS

Although all patients should be evaluated in a logical and thorough manner, many cases with focal musculoskeletal complaints are caused by commonly encountered disorders that exhibit a predictable pattern of onset, evolution, and localization; they can often be diagnosed immediately on the basis of limited historic information and selected maneuvers or tests. Although nearly every joint could be approached in this manner, the evaluation of four common involved anatomic regions—the hand, shoulder, hip, and knee—are reviewed here.

HAND PAIN

Focal or unilateral hand pain may result from trauma, overuse, infection, or a reactive or crystal-induced arthritis. By contrast, bilateral hand complaints commonly suggest a degenerative (e.g., OA), systemic, or inflammatory/immune (e.g., RA) etiology. The distribution or pattern of joint involvement is highly suggestive of certain disorders (Fig. 393-3). Thus, OA (or degenerative arthritis) may manifest as distal interphalangeal (DIP) and proximal interphalangeal (PIP) joint pain with bony hypertrophy sufficient to produce Heberden's and Bouchard's nodes, respectively. Pain, with or without bony swelling, involving the base of the thumb (first carpometacarpal joint) is also highly suggestive of OA. By contrast, RA tends to cause symmetric, polyarticular involvement of the PIP, metacarpophalangeal (MCP), intercarpal, and carpometacarpal joints (wrist) with pain and palpable synovial tissue hypertrophy. Psoriatic arthritis may mimic the pattern of joint involvement seen in OA (DIP and PIP joints), but can be distinguished by the presence of inflammatory signs (erythema, warmth, synovial swelling), with or without carpal involvement, nail pitting, or onycholysis. Whereas lateral or medial subluxations at the PIP or DIP joints are most likely due to inflammatory OA or psoriatic arthritis, dorsal or ventral deformities (swan neck or boutonnière deformities) are typical of RA. Hemochromatosis should be considered when degenerative changes (bony hypertrophy) are seen at the second and third MCP joints with associated radiographic chondrocalcinosis or episodic, inflammatory wrist arthritis.

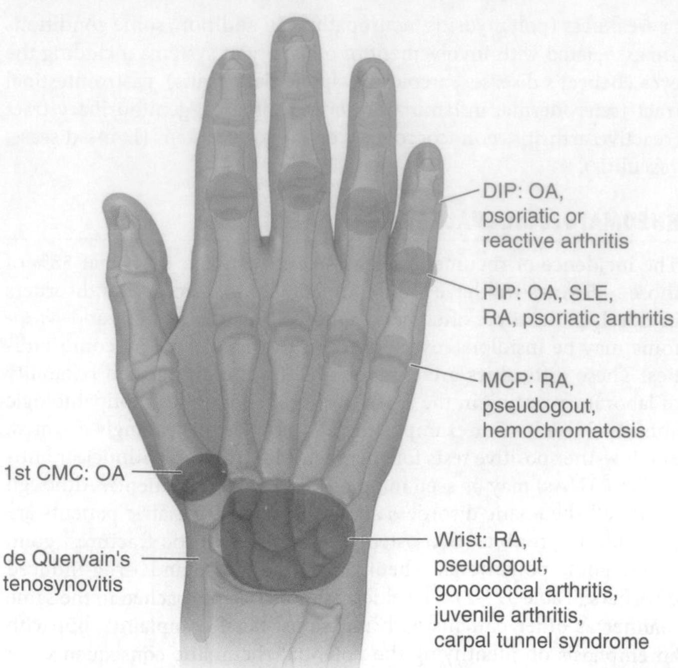

FIGURE 393-3 Sites of hand or wrist involvement and their potential disease associations. CMC, carpometacarpal; DIP, distal interphalangeal; MCP, metacarpophalangeal; OA, osteoarthritis; PIP, proximal interphalangeal; RA, rheumatoid arthritis; SLE, systemic lupus erythematosus. *(From JJ Cush et al: Evaluation of musculoskeletal complaints, in Rheumatology: Diagnosis and Therapeutics, 2nd ed, JJ Cush et al [eds]. Philadelphia, Lippincott Williams & Wilkins, 2005, pp 3–20. Used with permission from Dr. John J. Cush.)*

Dactylitis manifests as soft tissue swelling of the whole digit and may have a sausage-like appearance. Common causes of dactylitis include psoriatic arthritis, spondyloarthritis, juvenile spondylitis, mixed connective tissue disease, scleroderma, sarcoidosis, and sickle cell disease. Soft tissue swelling over the dorsum of the hand and wrist may suggest an inflammatory extensor tendon tenosynovitis possibly caused by gonococcal infection, gout, or inflammatory arthritis (e.g., RA). Tenosynovitis is suggested by localized warmth, swelling, or pitting edema and may be confirmed when the soft tissue swelling tracks with tendon movement, such as flexion and extension of fingers, or when pain is induced while stretching the extensor tendon sheaths (flexing the digits distal to the MCP joints and maintaining the wrist in a fixed, neutral position).

Focal wrist pain localized to the radial aspect may be caused by de Quervain's tenosynovitis resulting from inflammation of the tendon sheath(s) involving the abductor pollicis longus or extensor pollicis brevis (Fig. 393-3). This commonly results from overuse or follows pregnancy and may be diagnosed with Finkelstein's test. A positive result is present when radial wrist pain is induced after the thumb is flexed and placed inside a clenched fist and the patient actively deviates the hand downward with ulnar deviation at the wrist. Carpal tunnel syndrome is another common disorder of the upper extremity and results from compression of the median nerve within the carpal tunnel. Manifestations include pain in the wrist that may radiate with paresthesia to the thumb, second and third fingers, and radial half of the fourth finger and, at times, atrophy of thenar musculature. Carpal tunnel syndrome is commonly associated with pregnancy, edema, trauma, OA, inflammatory arthritis, and infiltrative disorders (e.g., amyloidosis). The diagnosis may be suggested by a positive Tinel's or Phalen's sign. With each test, paresthesia in a median nerve distribution is induced or increased by either "thumping" the volar aspect of the wrist (Tinel's sign) or pressing the extensor surfaces of both flexed wrists against each other (Phalen's sign). The low sensitivity and moderate specificity of these tests may require nerve conduction velocity testing to confirm a suspected diagnosis.

SHOULDER PAIN

During the evaluation of shoulder disorders, the examiner should carefully note any history of trauma, fibromyalgia, infection, inflammatory disease, occupational hazards, or previous cervical disease. In addition, the patient should be questioned as to the activities or movement(s) that elicit shoulder pain. While arthritis is suggested by pain on movement in all planes, pain with specific active motion suggests a periarticular (nonarticular) process. Shoulder pain may originate in the glenohumeral or acromioclavicular joints, subacromial (subdeltoid) bursa, periarticular soft tissues (e.g., fibromyalgia, rotator cuff tear/tendinitis), or cervical spine (Fig. 393-4). Shoulder pain is referred frequently from the cervical spine but may also be referred from intrathoracic lesions (e.g., a Pancoast tumor) or from gallbladder, hepatic, or diaphragmatic disease. These same visceral causes may also manifest as focal scapular pain. Fibromyalgia should be suspected

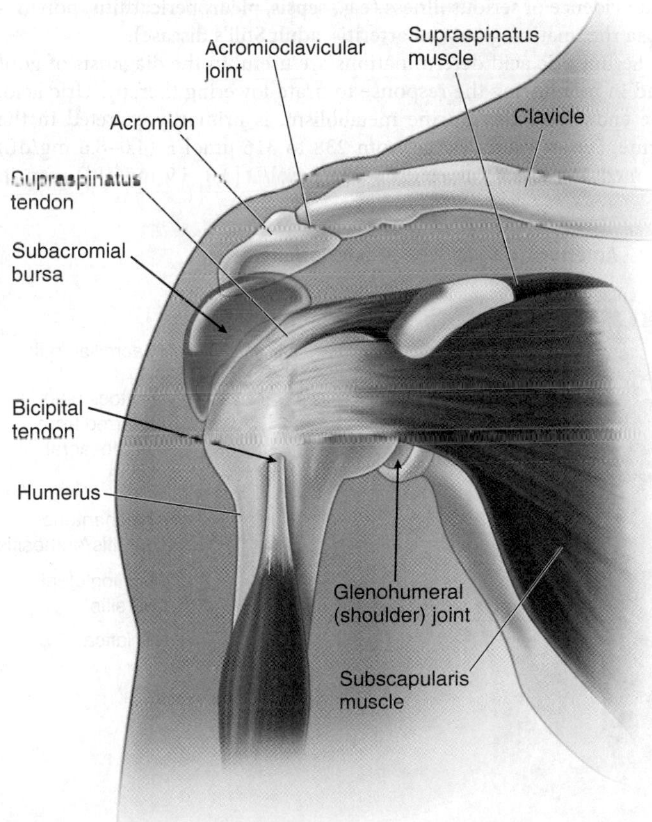

FIGURE 393-4 Origins of shoulder pain. The schematic diagram of the shoulder indicates with arrows the anatomic origins of shoulder pain.

when glenohumeral pain is accompanied by diffuse periarticular (i.e., subacromial, bicipital) pain and tender points (i.e., trapezius or supraspinatus). The shoulder should be put through its full range of motion both actively and passively (with examiner assistance): forward flexion, extension, abduction, adduction, and internal and external rotation. Manual inspection of the periarticular structures will often provide important diagnostic information. Glenohumeral involvement is best detected by placing the thumb over the glenohumeral joint just medial and inferior to the coracoid process and applying pressure anteriorly while internally and externally rotating the humeral head. Pain localized to this region is indicative of glenohumeral pathology. Synovial effusion or tissue is seldom palpable but, if present, may suggest infection, RA, amyloidosis, or an acute tear of the rotator cuff. The examiner should apply direct manual pressure over the subacromial bursa that lies lateral to and immediately beneath the acromion (Fig. 393-4). Subacromial bursitis is a frequent cause of shoulder pain. Anterior to the subacromial bursa, the bicipital tendon traverses the bicipital groove. This tendon is best identified by palpating it in its groove as the patient rotates the humerus internally and externally. Direct pressure over the tendon may reveal pain indicative of bicipital tendinitis. Palpation of the acromioclavicular joint may disclose local pain, bony hypertrophy, or, uncommonly, synovial swelling. Whereas OA and RA commonly affect the acromioclavicular joint, OA seldom involves the glenohumeral joint, unless there is a traumatic or occupational cause.

Rotator cuff tendinitis or tear is a very common cause of shoulder pain. Nearly 30 percent of the elderly will have shoulder pain, with rotator cuff tendinitis or tear as the primary cause. The rotator cuff is formed by four tendons that attach the scapula to the proximal humerus (supraspinatus, infraspinatus, teres minor, and subscapularis tendons). Of these, the supraspinatus muscle is the most commonly damaged. Rotator cuff tendinitis is suggested by pain on active abduction (but not passive abduction), pain over the lateral deltoid muscle, night pain, and evidence of the impingement signs (pain with overhead arm activities). The Neer test for impingement is performed by the examiner raising the patient's arm into forced flexion while stabilizing and preventing rotation of the scapula. A positive sign is present if pain develops before 180° of forward flexion. Tear of the rotator cuff is common in the elderly and often results from trauma; it may manifest in the same manner as tendinitis. The drop arm test is abnormal with supraspinatus pathology and is demonstrated by passive abduction of the arm to 90° by the examiner. If the patient is unable to hold the arm up actively or unable to lower the arm slowly without dropping, the test is positive. Tendinitis or tear of the rotator cuff is best confirmed by magnetic resonance imaging (MRI) or ultrasound.

KNEE PAIN

Knee pain may result from intraarticular (OA, RA) or periarticular (anserine bursitis, collateral ligament strain) processes or be referred from hip pathology. A careful history should delineate the chronology of the knee complaint and whether there are predisposing conditions, trauma, or medications that might underlie the complaint. For example, patellofemoral disease (e.g., OA) may cause anterior knee pain that worsens with climbing stairs. Observation of the patient's gait is also important. The knee should be carefully inspected in the upright (weight-bearing) and supine positions for swelling, erythema, malalignment, visible trauma, muscle wasting, and leg length discrepancy. The most common malalignment in the knee is *genu varum* (bowlegs) or *genu valgum* (knock-knees) resulting from asymmetric cartilage loss medially or laterally. Bony swelling of the knee joint commonly results from hypertrophic osseous changes seen with disorders such as OA and neuropathic arthropathy. Swelling caused by hypertrophy of the synovium or synovial effusion may manifest as a fluctuant, ballotable, or soft tissue enlargement in the suprapatellar pouch (suprapatellar reflection of the synovial cavity) or regions lateral and medial to the patella. Synovial effusions may also be detected by balloting the patella downward toward the femoral groove or by eliciting a "bulge sign." With the knee extended, the examiner should manually compress, or "milk," synovial fluid down from the suprapatellar pouch and lateral to the patellae. The application of manual pressure lateral to the patella may cause an observable shift in synovial fluid (bulge) to the medial aspect. The examiner should note that this maneuver is only effective in detecting small to moderate effusions (<100 mL). Inflammatory disorders such as RA, gout, pseudogout, and psoriatic arthritis may involve the knee joint and produce significant pain, stiffness, swelling, or warmth. A popliteal or *Baker's cyst* may be palpated with the knee partially flexed and is best viewed posteriorly with the patient standing and knees fully extended to visualize isolated or unilateral popliteal swelling or fullness.

Anserine bursitis is an often missed periarticular cause of knee pain in adults. The pes anserine bursa underlies the insertion of the conjoined tendons (sartorius, gracilis, semitendinosus) on the anteromedial proximal tibia and may be painful following trauma, overuse, or inflammation. It is often tender in patients with fibromyalgia, obesity, and knee OA. Other forms of bursitis may also present as knee pain. The prepatellar bursa is superficial and is located over the inferior portion of the patella. The infrapatellar bursa is deeper and lies beneath the patellar ligament before its insertion on the tibial tubercle.

Internal derangement of the knee may result from trauma or degenerative processes. Damage to the meniscal cartilage (medial or lateral) frequently presents as chronic or intermittent knee pain. Such an injury should be suspected when there is a history of trauma, athletic activity, or chronic knee arthritis, and when the patient relates symptoms of "locking" or "giving way" of the knee. With the knee flexed 90° and the patient's foot on the table, pain elicited during palpation over the joint line or when the knee is stressed laterally or medially may suggest a meniscal tear. A positive McMurray test may also indicate a meniscal tear. To perform this test, the knee is first flexed at 90°, and the leg is then extended while the lower extremity is simultaneously torqued medially or laterally. A painful click during inward rotation may indicate a lateral meniscus tear, and pain during outward rotation may indicate a tear in the medial meniscus. Lastly, damage to the cruciate ligaments should be suspected with acute onset of pain, possibly with swelling, a history of trauma, or a synovial fluid aspirate that is grossly bloody. Examination of the cruciate ligaments is best accomplished by eliciting a drawer sign. With the patient recumbent, the knee should be partially flexed and the foot stabilized on the examining surface. The examiner should manually attempt to displace the tibia anteriorly or posteriorly with respect to the femur. If anterior movement is detected, then anterior cruciate ligament damage is likely. Conversely, significant posterior movement may indicate posterior cruciate damage. Contralateral comparison will assist the examiner in detecting significant anterior or posterior movement.

HIP PAIN

The hip is best evaluated by observing the patient's gait and assessing range of motion. The vast majority of patients reporting "hip pain" localize their pain unilaterally to the posterior gluteal musculature (Fig. 393-5). Such pain tends to radiate down the posterolateral aspect of the thigh and may or may not be associated with complaints of low back pain. This presentation frequently results from degenerative arthritis of the lumbosacral spine or disks and commonly follows a dermatomal distribution with involvement of nerve roots between L4 and S1. Sciatica is caused by impingement of the L4, L5, or S1 nerve (i.e., from a herniated disk) and manifests as unilateral neuropathic pain extending from the gluteal region down the posterolateral leg to the foot. Some individuals instead localize their "hip pain" laterally to the area overlying the trochanteric bursa. Because of the depth of this bursa, swelling and warmth are usually absent. Diagnosis of trochanteric bursitis or enthesitis can be confirmed by inducing point tenderness over the trochanteric bursa. Gluteal and trochanteric pain are common findings in fibromyalgia. Range of movement may be limited by pain. Pain in the hip joint is less common and tends to be located anteriorly, over the inguinal ligament; it may radiate medially to the groin. Uncommonly, iliopsoas bursitis may mimic true hip joint pain. Diagnosis of iliopsoas bursitis may be suggested by a history of trauma or inflammatory arthritis. Pain associated with iliopsoas bursitis is localized to the groin or anterior thigh and tends to worsen with hyperextension of the hip; many patients prefer to flex and externally rotate the hip to reduce the pain from a distended bursa.

LABORATORY INVESTIGATIONS

The vast majority of musculoskeletal disorders can be easily diagnosed by a complete history and physical examination. An additional objective of the initial encounter is to determine whether additional investigations or immediate therapy is required. Additional evaluation is indicated with: (1) monarticular conditions; (2) traumatic or inflammatory conditions; (3) the presence of neurologic findings; (4) systemic manifestations; or (5) chronic symptoms (>6 weeks) and a lack of response to symptomatic measures. The extent and nature of the additional investigation should be dictated by the clinical features and suspected pathologic process. Laboratory tests should be used to confirm a specific clinical diagnosis and not be used to screen or evaluate patients with vague rheumatic complaints. Indiscriminate use of broad batteries of diagnostic tests and radiographic procedures is rarely a useful or cost-effective means to establish a diagnosis.

Besides a complete blood count, including a white blood cell (WBC) and differential count, the routine evaluation should include a determination of an acute-phase reactant such as the ESR or CRP, which can be useful in discriminating inflammatory from noninflammatory disorders. Both are inexpensive, easily obtained, and may be elevated with infection, inflammation, autoimmune disorders, neoplasia, pregnancy, renal insufficiency, advanced age, or hyperlipidemia. Extreme elevation of the acute-phase reactants (CRP, ESR) is seldom seen without evidence of serious illness (e.g., sepsis, pleuropericarditis, polymyalgia rheumatica, giant cell arteritis, adult Still's disease).

Serum uric acid determinations are useful in the diagnosis of gout and in monitoring the response to urate-lowering therapy. Uric acid, the end product of purine metabolism, is primarily excreted in the urine. Serum values range from 238 to 516 μmol/L (4.0–8.6 mg/dL) in men; the lower values (178–351 μmol/L [3.0–5.9 mg/dL]) seen in

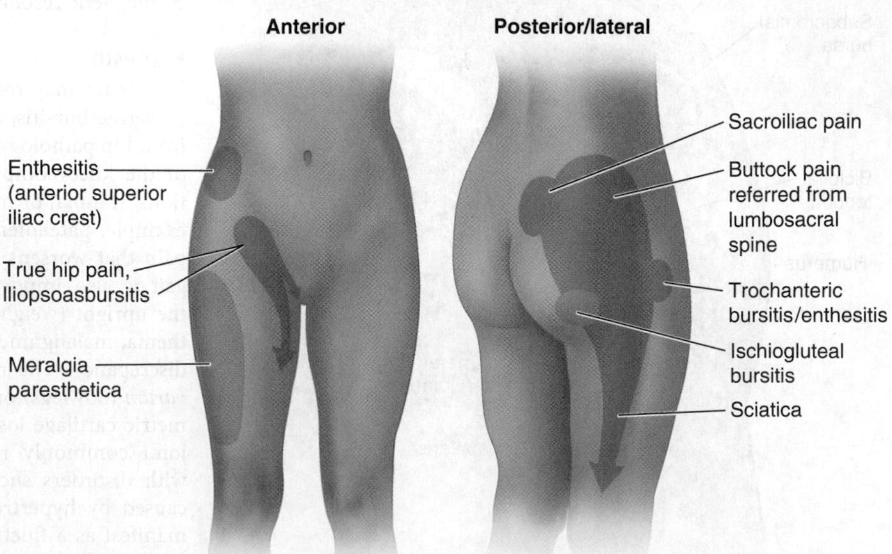

FIGURE 393-5 Origins of hip pain and dysesthesias. *(From JJ Cush et al: Evaluation of musculoskeletal complaints, in Rheumatology: Diagnosis and Therapeutics, 2nd ed, JJ Cush et al [eds]. Philadelphia, Lippincott Williams & Wilkins, 2005, pp 3–20. Used with permission from Dr. John J. Cush.)*

women are caused by the uricosuric effects of estrogen. Urinary uric acid levels are normally <750 mg per 24 h. Although hyperuricemia (especially levels >535 μmol/L [9 mg/dL]) is associated with an increased incidence of gout and nephrolithiasis, levels may not correlate with the severity of articular disease. Uric acid levels (and the risk of gout) may be increased by inborn errors of metabolism (Lesch-Nyhan syndrome), disease states (renal insufficiency, myeloproliferative disease, psoriasis), or drugs (alcohol, cytotoxic therapy, thiazides). Although nearly all patients with gout will demonstrate hyperuricemia at some time during their illness, up to 50% of patients with an acute gouty attack will have normal serum uric acid levels. Monitoring serum uric acid may be useful in assessing the response to urate-lowering therapy or chemotherapy, with the target goal being a serum urate <6 mg/dL.

Serologic tests for rheumatoid factor (RF), cyclic anticitrullinated peptide (CCP or ACPA) antibodies, ANAs, complement levels, Lyme and antineutrophil cytoplasmic antibodies (ANCA), or antistreptolysin O (ASO) titer should be carried out only when there is clinical evidence to specifically suggest an associated diagnosis, because these have poor predictive value when used for screening, especially when the pretest probability is low. For most of these, there is no value to repeated or serial serologic testing. Although 4–5% of a healthy population will have positive tests for RF and ANAs, only 1% and <0.4% of the population will have RA or SLE, respectively. IgM RF (autoantibodies against the Fc portion of IgG) is found in 80% of patients with RA and may also be seen in low titers in patients with chronic infections (tuberculosis, leprosy, hepatitis); other autoimmune diseases (SLE, Sjögren's syndrome); and chronic pulmonary, hepatic, or renal diseases. When considering RA, both serum RF and anti-CCP antibodies should be obtained as these are complementary. Both are comparably sensitive, but CCP antibodies are more specific than RF. In RA, the presence of anti-CCP and RF antibodies may indicate a greater risk for more severe, erosive polyarthritis. ANAs are found in nearly all patients with SLE and may also be seen in patients with other autoimmune diseases (polymyositis, scleroderma, antiphospholipid syndrome, Sjögren's syndrome), drug-induced lupus (Table 393-2), chronic liver or renal disorders, and advanced age. Positive ANAs are found in 5% of adults and in up to 14% of elderly or chronically ill individuals. The ANA test is very sensitive but poorly specific for lupus, as only 1–2% of all positive results will be caused by lupus alone. The interpretation of a positive ANA test may depend on the magnitude of the titer and the pattern observed by immunofluorescence microscopy (Table 393-4). Diffuse and speckled patterns are least specific, whereas a peripheral, or rim, pattern (related to autoantibodies against double-strand [native] DNA) is highly specific and suggestive of lupus. Centromeric patterns are seen in patients with limited scleroderma (calcinosis, Raynaud's phenomenon, esophageal involvement, sclerodactyly, telangiectasia [CREST] syndrome) or primary biliary sclerosis, and nucleolar patterns may be seen in patients with diffuse systemic sclerosis or inflammatory myositis.

TABLE 393-4 ANTINUCLEAR ANTIBODY (ANA) PATTERNS AND CLINICAL ASSOCIATIONS

ANA Pattern	Antigen Identified	Clinical Correlate
Diffuse	Deoxyribonucleoprotein	Nonspecific
	Histones	Drug-induced lupus, lupus
Peripheral (rim)	ds-DNA	50% of SLE (specific)
Speckled	U1-RNP	>90% of MCTD
	Sm	30% of SLE (specific)
	Ro (SS-A)	Sjögren's 60%, SCLE, neonatal lupus, ANA(−) lupus
	La (SS-B)	50% of Sjögren's, 15% lupus
	Scl-70	40% of diffuse scleroderma
	PM-1	Polymyositis (PM), dermatomyositis
	Jo-1	PM w/pneumonitis + arthritis
Nucleolar	RNA polymerase I, others	40% of PSS
Centromere	Kinetochore	75% CREST (limited scleroderma)

Abbreviations: ANA, antinuclear antibody; CREST, calcinosis, *R*aynaud phenomenon, esophageal involvement, sclerodactyly, and *t*elangiectasia; MCTD, mixed connective tissue disease; PSS, progressive systemic sclerosis; SCLE, subacute cutaneous lupus erythematosus; SLE, systemic lupus erythematosus.

Aspiration and analysis of synovial fluid are always indicated in acute monarthritis or when an infectious or crystal-induced arthropathy is suspected. Synovial fluid may distinguish between noninflammatory and inflammatory processes by analysis of the appearance, viscosity, and cell count. Tests for synovial fluid glucose, protein, lactate dehydrogenase, lactic acid, or autoantibodies are not recommended because they have no diagnostic value. Normal synovial fluid is clear or a pale straw color and is viscous, primarily because of the high levels of hyaluronate. Noninflammatory synovial fluid is clear, viscous, and amber-colored, with a WBC count of <2000/μL and a predominance of mononuclear cells. The viscosity of synovial fluid is assessed by expressing fluid from the syringe one drop at a time. Normally, there is a stringing effect, with a long tail behind each synovial drop. Effusions caused by OA or trauma will have normal viscosity. Inflammatory fluid is turbid and yellow, with an increased WBC count (2000–50,000/μL) and a polymorphonuclear leukocyte predominance. Inflammatory fluid has reduced viscosity, diminished hyaluronate, and little or no tail following each drop of synovial fluid. Such effusions are found in RA, gout, and other inflammatory arthritides. Septic fluid is opaque and purulent, with a WBC count usually >50,000/μL, a predominance of polymorphonuclear leukocytes (>75%), and low viscosity. Such effusions are typical of septic arthritis but may also occur with RA or gout. In addition, hemorrhagic synovial fluid may be seen with trauma, hemarthrosis, or neuropathic arthritis. An algorithm for synovial fluid aspiration and analysis is shown in Fig. 393-6. Synovial fluid should be analyzed immediately for appearance, viscosity, and cell count. Monosodium urate crystals (observed in gout) are seen by polarized microscopy and are long, needle-shaped, negatively birefringent, and usually intracellular. In chondrocalcinosis and pseudogout, calcium pyrophosphate dihydrate crystals are usually short, rhomboid-shaped, and positively birefringent. Whenever infection is suspected, synovial fluid should be Gram stained and cultured appropriately. If gonococcal arthritis is suspected, nucleic acid amplification tests should be used to detect either *Chlamydia trachomatis* or *N. gonorrhoeae* infection. Synovial fluid from patients with chronic monarthritis should also be cultured for *M. tuberculosis* and fungi. Last, it should be noted that crystal-induced arthritis and septic arthritis occasionally occur together in the same joint.

DIAGNOSTIC IMAGING IN JOINT DISEASES

Conventional radiography has been a valuable tool in the diagnosis and staging of articular disorders. Plain x-rays are most appropriate and cost effective when there is a history of trauma, suspected chronic infection, progressive disability, or monarticular involvement; when therapeutic alterations are considered; or when a baseline assessment is desired for what appears to be a chronic process. However, in acute inflammatory arthritis, early radiography is rarely helpful in establishing a diagnosis and may only reveal soft tissue swelling or juxtaarticular demineralization. As the disease progresses, calcification (of soft tissues, cartilage, or bone), joint space narrowing, erosions, bony ankylosis, new bone formation (sclerosis, osteophytes, or periostitis), or subchondral cysts may develop and suggest specific clinical entities. Consultation with a radiologist will help define the optimal imaging modality, technique, or positioning and prevent the need for further studies.

Additional imaging techniques may possess greater diagnostic sensitivity and facilitate early diagnosis in a limited number of articular disorders and in selected circumstances and are indicated when conventional radiography is inadequate or nondiagnostic (Table 393-5). *Ultrasonography* is useful in the detection of soft tissue abnormalities, such as tendinitis, tenosynovitis, enthesitis, bursitis, and entrapment neuropathies. Wider use, lower cost, better technology, and enhanced site-specific transducers now allow for routine use in outpatient care. Owing to low cost, portability, and wider use, ultrasound use has grown and is the preferred method for the evaluation of synovial (Baker's) cysts, rotator cuff tears, tendinitis and tendon injury, and

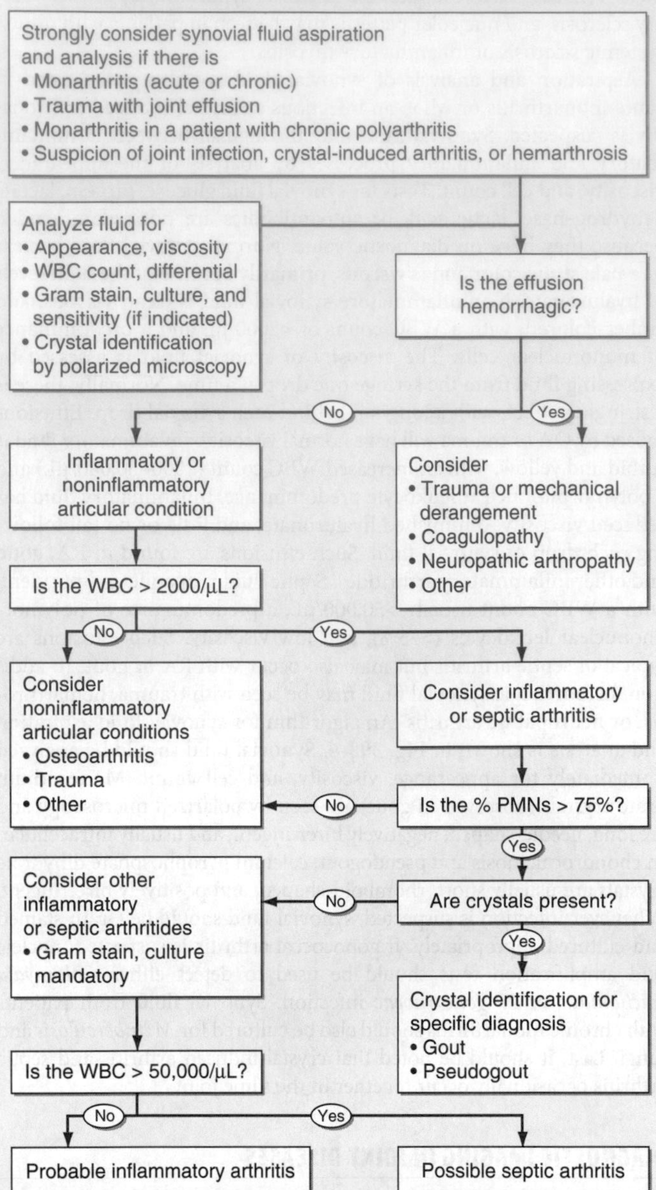

FIGURE 393-6 Algorithmic approach to the use and interpretation of synovial fluid aspiration and analysis. PMNs, polymorphonuclear (leukocytes); WBC, white blood cell (count).

crystal deposition on cartilage. Use of power Doppler allows for early detection of synovitis and bony erosions. *Radionuclide scintigraphy* is a very sensitive, but poorly specific, means of detecting inflammatory or metabolic alterations in bone or periarticular soft tissue structures. Scintigraphy is best suited for total-body assessment (extent and distribution) of skeletal involvement (neoplasia, Paget's disease) and the assessment of patients with undiagnosed polyarthralgias, looking for occult arthritis. The use of scintigraphy has declined with greater use and declining cost of ultrasound and MRI. The limited tissue contrast resolution of scintigraphy may obscure the distinction between a bony or periarticular process and may necessitate the additional use of MRI. Scintigraphy using ^{99m}Tc, ^{67}Ga, or ^{111}In-labeled WBCs has been applied to a variety of articular disorders with variable success (Table 393-5). Although [^{99m}Tc] diphosphate scintigraphy may be useful in identifying osseous infection, neoplasia, inflammation, increased blood flow, bone remodeling, heterotopic bone formation, or avascular necrosis, MRI is preferred in most instances. Gallium scanning uses ^{67}Ga, which binds serum and cellular transferrin and lactoferrin and is preferentially taken up by neutrophils, macrophages,

TABLE 393-5 DIAGNOSTIC IMAGING TECHNIQUES FOR MUSCULOSKELETAL DISORDERS

Method	Imaging Time, h	Cost[a]	Current Indications
Ultrasound	<1	++	Synovial (Baker's) cysts
			Rotator cuff tears
			Bursitis, tendinitis, tendon injury
			Enthesitis
			Carpal tunnel syndrome
			Urate or calcium pyrophosphate deposition on cartilage
			Early detection of synovial inflammation or erosions
			Ultrasound-guided injection/arthrocentesis
Radionuclide scintigraphy			
^{99m}Tc	1–4	++	Metastatic bone survey
			Evaluation of Paget's disease
			Identifying occult arthritis in patients with undiagnosed polyarthralgia
^{111}In-WBC	24	+++	Acute infection
			Prosthetic infection
			Acute osteomyelitis
^{67}Ga	24–48	++++	Acute and chronic infection
			Acute osteomyelitis
Computed tomography (CT)	<1	+++	Herniated intervertebral disk
			Sacroiliitis
			Spinal stenosis
			Spinal trauma
			Osteoid osteoma
			Stress fracture
Dual-energy CT	<1	NA	Uric acid deposition
			Tophus localization
Magnetic resonance imaging	1/2–2	++++	Avascular necrosis
			Osteomyelitis
			Septic arthritis, infected prosthetic joints
			Early sacroiliitis
			Intraarticular derangement and soft tissue injury
			Derangements of axial skeleton and spinal cord
			Herniated intervertebral disk
			Pigmented villonodular synovitis
			Inflammatory and metabolic muscle pathology

[a]Relative cost for imaging study.

Abbreviations: NA, not commercially available; WBC, white blood cell.

bacteria, and tumor tissue (e.g., lymphoma). As such, it is primarily used in the identification of occult infection or malignancy. Scanning with ^{111}In-labeled WBCs has been used to detect osteomyelitis and infectious or inflammatory arthritis. Despite their utility, ^{111}In-labeled WBC or ^{67}Ga scanning has largely been replaced by MRI, except when there is a suspicion of septic joint or prosthetic joint infections.

Computed tomography (CT) provides detailed visualization of the axial skeleton. Articulations previously considered difficult to visualize by radiography (e.g., zygapophyseal, sacroiliac, sternoclavicular, hip joints) can be effectively evaluated using CT. CT has been demonstrated to be useful in the diagnosis of low back pain syndromes (e.g., spinal stenosis vs herniated disk), sacroiliitis, osteoid osteoma, and stress fractures. Helical or spiral CT (with or without contrast angiography) is a novel technique that is rapid, cost effective, and sensitive

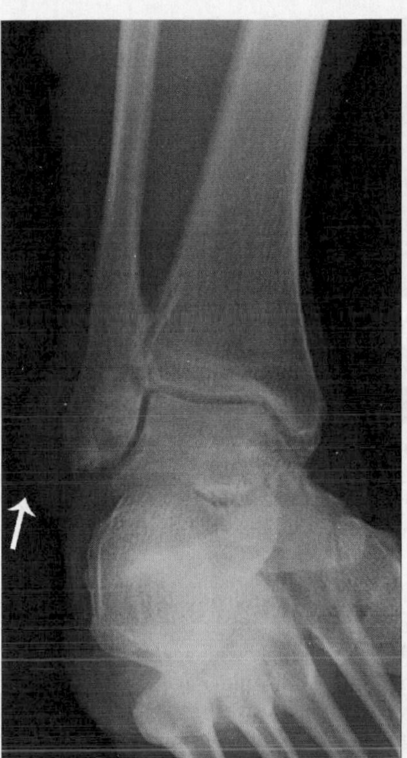

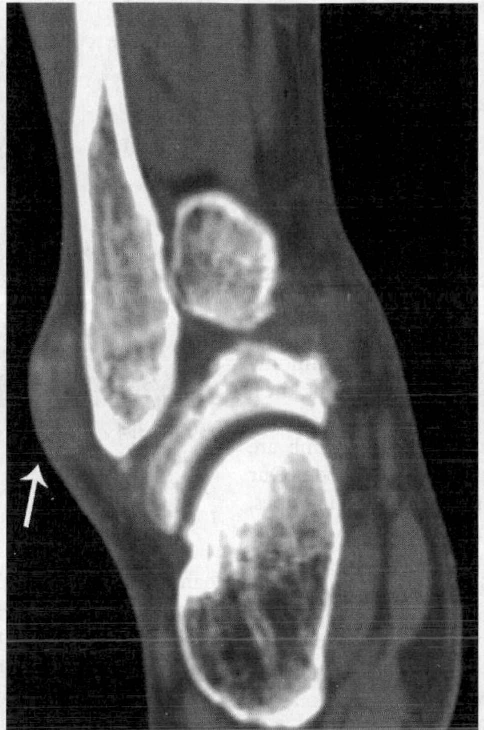

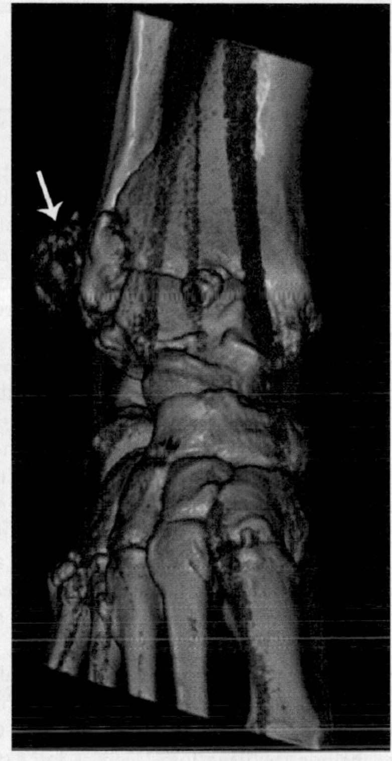

FIGURE 393-7 Dual-energy computed tomography (DECT) scan from a 45-year-old woman with right ankle swelling around the lateral malleolus. Three-dimensional volume-rendered coronal reformatted DECT image shows that the mass is composed of monosodium urate (*red*) in keeping with tophus (*arrow*). *(Used with permission from S Nicolaou et al: AJR 194:1072, 2010.)*

in diagnosing pulmonary embolism or obscure fractures, often in the setting of initially equivocal findings. High-resolution CT can be advocated in the evaluation of suspected or established infiltrative lung disease (e.g., scleroderma or rheumatoid lung). The recent use of hybrid (positron emission tomography [PET] or single-photon emission CT [SPECT]) CT scans in metastatic evaluations has incorporated CT to provide better anatomic localization of scintigraphic abnormalities.

^{18}F-Fluorodeoxyglucose (FDG) is the most commonly used radiopharmaceutical in PET scanning. FDG-PET/CT scans have been seldom used in the evaluation of septic or inflammatory arthritis. Dual-energy CT (DECT) scanning, developed in urology to identify urinary calculi, has been a highly sensitive and specific method used to identify and quantify uric acid deposition in tissues (Fig. 393-7).

MRI has significantly advanced the ability to image musculoskeletal structures. MRI has the advantages of providing multiplanar images with fine anatomic detail and contrast resolution (Fig. 393-8) that allows for the superior ability to visualize bone marrow and soft tissue periarticular structures. Although more costly with a longer procedural time than CT, the MRI has become the preferred technique when evaluating complex musculoskeletal disorders.

MRI can image fascia, vessels, nerve, muscle, cartilage, ligaments, tendons, pannus, synovial effusions, and bone marrow. Visualization of particular structures can be enhanced by altering the pulse sequence to produce either T1- or T2-weighted spin echo, gradient echo, or inversion recovery (including short tau inversion recovery [STIR]) images. Because of its sensitivity to changes in marrow fat, MRI is a sensitive but nonspecific means of detecting osteonecrosis, osteomyelitis, and marrow inflammation indicating overlying synovitis or osteitis (Fig. 393-8). Because of its enhanced soft tissue resolution, MRI is more sensitive than arthrography or CT in the diagnosis of soft tissue injuries (e.g., meniscal and rotator cuff tears); intraarticular derangements; marrow abnormalities (osteonecrosis, myeloma); and spinal cord or nerve root damage, synovitis, or cartilage damage or loss.

Acknowledgment

The author acknowledges the contributions of Dr. Peter E. Lipsky to this chapter in previous editions.

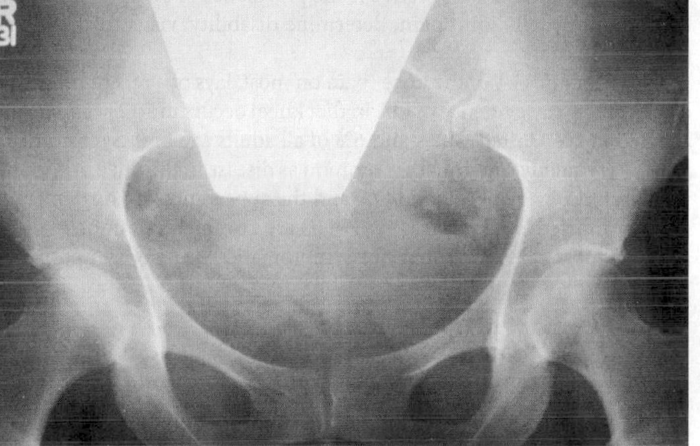

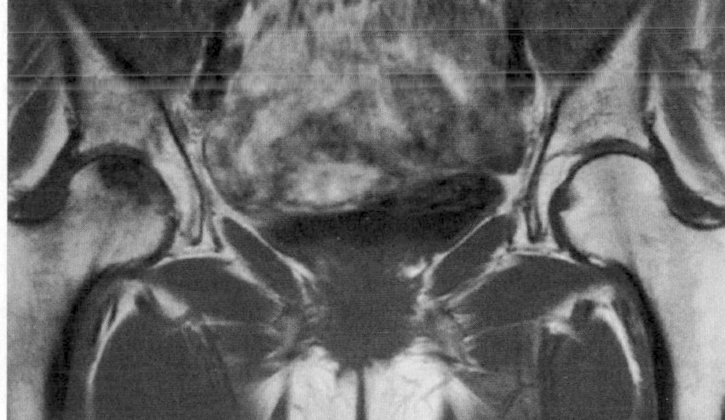

FIGURE 393-8 Superior sensitivity of magnetic resonance imaging (MRI) in the diagnosis of osteonecrosis of the femoral head. A 45-year-old woman receiving high-dose glucocorticoids developed right hip pain. Conventional x-rays (*top*) demonstrated only mild sclerosis of the right femoral head. T1-weighted MRI (*bottom*) demonstrated low-density signal in the right femoral head, diagnostic of osteonecrosis.

394 Osteoarthritis

David T. Felson

Osteoarthritis (OA) is the most common type of arthritis. Its high prevalence, especially in the elderly, and the high rate of disability related to disease make it a leading cause of disability in the elderly. Because of the aging of Western populations and because obesity, a major risk factor, is increasing in prevalence, the occurrence of OA is on the rise. In the United States, OA prevalence will increase by 66–100% by 2020.

OA affects certain joints, yet spares others (Fig. 394-1). Commonly affected joints include the cervical and lumbosacral spine, hip, knee, and first metatarsal phalangeal joint (MTP). In the hands, the distal and proximal interphalangeal joints and the base of the thumb are often affected. Usually spared are the wrist, elbow, and ankle. Our joints were designed, in an evolutionary sense, for brachiating apes, animals that still walked on four limbs. We thus develop OA in joints that were ill designed for human tasks such as pincer grip (OA in the thumb base) and walking upright (OA in knees and hips). Some joints, like the ankles, may be spared because their articular cartilage may be uniquely resistant to loading stresses.

OA can be diagnosed based on structural abnormalities or on the symptoms these abnormalities evoke. According to cadaveric studies, by elderly years, structural changes of OA are nearly universal. These include cartilage loss (seen as joint space loss on x-rays) and osteophytes. Many persons with x-ray evidence of OA have no joint symptoms, and although the prevalence of structural abnormalities is of interest in understanding disease pathogenesis, what matters more from a clinical perspective is the prevalence of symptomatic OA. Symptoms, usually joint pain, determine disability, visits to clinicians, and disease costs.

Symptomatic OA of the knee (pain on most days of a recent month in a knee plus x-ray evidence of OA in that knee) occurs in ~12% of persons age ≥60 in the United States and 6% of all adults age ≥30. Symptomatic hip OA is roughly one-third as common as disease in the knee. Although radiographically evident hand OA and the appearance of bony enlargement in affected hand joints (Fig. 394-2) are extremely common in older persons, most cases are often not symptomatic. Even so, symptomatic hand OA occurs in ~10% of elderly individuals and often produces measurable limitation in function.

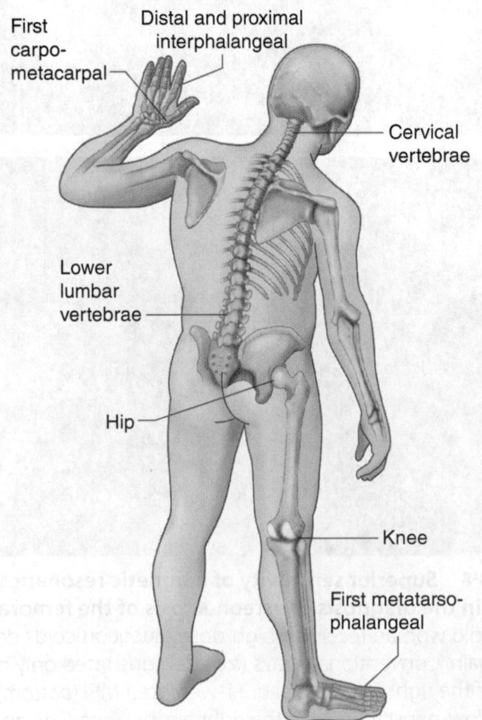

FIGURE 394-1 Joints commonly affected by osteoarthritis.

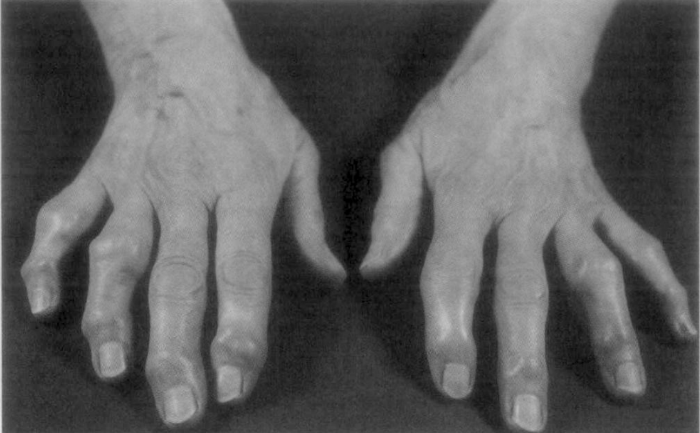

FIGURE 394-2 Severe osteoarthritis of the hands affecting the distal interphalangeal joints (Heberden's nodes) and the proximal interphalangeal joints (Bouchard's nodes). There is no clear bony enlargement of the other common site in the hands, the thumb base.

The prevalence of OA rises strikingly with age. Regardless of how it is defined, OA is uncommon in adults under age 40 and highly prevalent in those over age 60. It is also a disease that, at least in middle-aged and elderly persons, is much more common in women than in men, and sex differences in prevalence increase with age.

X-ray evidence of OA is common in the lower back and neck, but back pain and neck pain have not been tied to findings of OA on x-ray. Thus, back pain and neck pain are treated separately (Chap. 22).

DEFINITION

OA is joint failure, a disease in which all structures of the joint have undergone pathologic change, often in concert. The pathologic sine qua non of disease is hyaline articular cartilage loss, present in a focal and, initially, nonuniform manner. This is accompanied by increasing thickness and sclerosis of the subchondral bony plate, by outgrowth of osteophytes at the joint margin, by stretching of the articular capsule, by mild synovitis in many affected joints, and by weakness of muscles bridging the joint. In knees, meniscal degeneration is part of the disease. There are numerous pathways that lead to joint failure, but the initial step is often joint injury in the setting of a failure of protective mechanisms.

JOINT PROTECTIVE MECHANISMS AND THEIR FAILURE

Joint protectors include joint capsule and ligaments, muscle, sensory afferents, and underlying bone. Joint capsule and ligaments serve as joint protectors by providing a limit to excursion, thereby fixing the range of joint motion.

Synovial fluid reduces friction between articulating cartilage surfaces, thereby serving as a protector against friction-induced cartilage wear. This lubrication function depends on *hyaluronic acid* and on *lubricin*, a mucinous glycoprotein secreted by synovial fibroblasts whose concentration diminishes after joint injury and in the face of synovial inflammation.

The ligaments, along with overlying skin and tendons, contain mechanoreceptor sensory afferent nerves. These mechanoreceptors fire at different frequencies throughout a joint's range of motion, providing feedback by way of the spinal cord to muscles and tendons. As a consequence, these muscles and tendons can assume the right tension at appropriate points in joint excursion to act as optimal joint protectors, anticipating joint loading.

Muscles and tendons that bridge the joint are key joint protectors. Their coordinated contractions at the appropriate time in joint movement provide the appropriate power and acceleration for the limb to accomplish its tasks. Focal stress across the joint is minimized by muscle contraction that decelerates the joint before impact and assures that when joint impact arrives, it is distributed broadly across the joint surface.

Failure of these joint protectors increases the risk of joint injury and OA. For example, in animals, OA develops rapidly when a sensory nerve to the joint is sectioned and joint injury induced. Similarly, in humans, Charcot's arthropathy, a severe and rapidly progressive OA, develops when minor joint injury occurs in the presence of posterior column peripheral neuropathy. Another example of joint protector failure is rupture of ligaments, a well-known cause of the early development of OA.

CARTILAGE AND ITS ROLE IN JOINT FAILURE

In addition to being a primary target tissue for disease, cartilage also functions as a joint protector. A thin rim of tissue at the ends of two opposing bones, cartilage is lubricated by synovial fluid to provide an almost frictionless surface across which these two bones move. The compressible stiffness of cartilage compared to bone provides the joint with impact-absorbing capacity.

The earliest changes of OA may occur in cartilage, and abnormalities there can accelerate disease development. The two major macromolecules in cartilage are type 2 collagen, which provides cartilage its tensile strength, and aggrecan, a proteoglycan macromolecule linked with hyaluronic acid, which consists of highly negatively charged glycosaminoglycans. In normal cartilage, type 2 collagen is woven tightly, constraining the aggrecan molecules in the interstices between collagen strands, forcing these highly negatively charged molecules into close proximity with one another. The aggrecan molecule, through electrostatic repulsion of its negative charges, gives cartilage its compressive stiffness. Chondrocytes, the cells within this avascular tissue, synthesize all elements of the matrix and produce enzymes that break down the matrix. Synovium and chondrocytes synthesize and release cytokines and growth factors, which provide feedback that modulates synthesis of matrix molecules (Fig. 394-3). Cartilage matrix synthesis and catabolism are in a dynamic equilibrium influenced by the cytokine and growth factor environment. Mechanical and osmotic stress on chondrocytes induces these cells to alter gene expression and increase production of inflammatory cytokines and matrix-degrading enzymes. While chondrocytes synthesize numerous enzymes, matrix metalloproteinases (MMP) (especially collagenases and ADAMTS-5) are critical enzymes in the breakdown of cartilage matrix. Both collagenase and aggrecanases act primarily in the territorial matrix surrounding chondrocytes; however, as the osteoarthritic process develops, their activities and effects spread throughout the matrix, especially in the superficial layers of cartilage.

The synovium, cartilage, and bone all influence disease development through cytokines, chemokines, and even complement activation (Fig. 394-3). These act on chondrocyte cell surface receptors and ultimately have transcriptional effects. Matrix fragments released from cartilage stimulate synovitis. Among the most important cytokines are interleukin (IL) 1β, which exerts transcriptional effects on chondrocytes, stimulating production of proteinases and suppressing cartilage matrix synthesis. Tumor necrosis factor (TNF) α may play a similar role to that of IL-1. These cytokines also induce chondrocytes to synthesize prostaglandin E_2 and nitric oxide, which have complex effects on matrix synthesis and degradation. At early stages in the matrix response to injury and in the healthy response to loading, the net effect of cytokine stimulation may be matrix synthesis, but ultimately, the combination of effects on chondrocytes triggers matrix degradation. Enzymes in the matrix are held in check by activation inhibitors, including tissue inhibitor of metalloproteinase (TIMP). Growth factors are also part of this complex network, with BMP-2 and transforming growth factor β playing prominent roles in stimulating the development of osteophytes. Whereas healthy articular cartilage is avascular in part due to angiogenesis inhibitors present in cartilage, disease is characterized by the invasion of blood vessels into cartilage from underlying bone and proliferation of vessels within synovium. This is influenced by vascular endothelial growth factor (VEGF) synthesis in the cartilage and bone. With these blood vessels come nerves that may bring nociceptive innervation.

Probably as a result of chronic oxidative damage, articular chondrocytes exhibit an age-related decline in synthetic capacity while maintaining the ability to produce proinflammatory mediators and matrix-degrading enzymes, findings characteristic of a senescent secretory phenotype. These chondrocytes are unable to maintain tissue homeostasis (such as after insults of a mechanical or inflammatory nature). Thus, with age, cartilage is easily damaged by minor sometimes unnoticed injuries, including those that are part of daily activities.

OA cartilage is characterized by gradual depletion of aggrecan, an unfurling of the tightly woven collagen matrix, and loss of type 2 collagen. With these changes comes increasing vulnerability of cartilage, which loses its compressive stiffness.

RISK FACTORS

Joint vulnerability and joint loading are the two major factors contributing to the development of OA. On the one hand, a vulnerable joint whose protectors are dysfunctional can develop OA with minimal

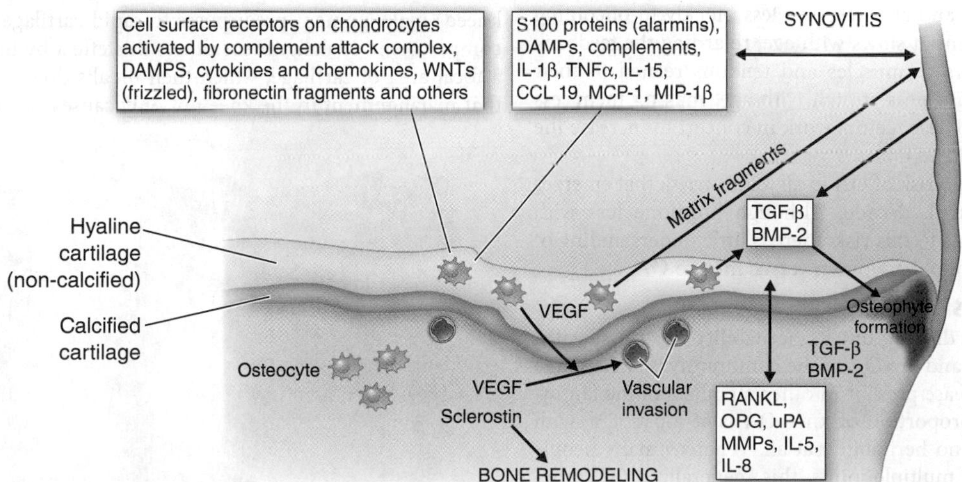

FIGURE 394-3 Selected factors involved in the osteoarthritic process including chondrocytes, bone, and synovium. Synovitis causes release of cytokines, alarmins, damage-associated molecular pattern (DAMP) molecules, and complement, which activate chondrocytes through cell surface receptors. Chondrocytes produce matrix molecules (collagen type 2, aggrecan) and the enzymes responsible for the degradation of the matrix (e.g., ADAMTS-5 and matrix metalloproteinases [MMPs]). Bone invasion occurs through the calcified cartilage, triggered by vascular endothelial growth factor (VEGF) and other molecules. IL, interleukin; TGF, transforming growth factor; TNF, tumor necrosis factor. *(From RF Loeser et al: Arthritis Rheum 64:1697, 2012.)*

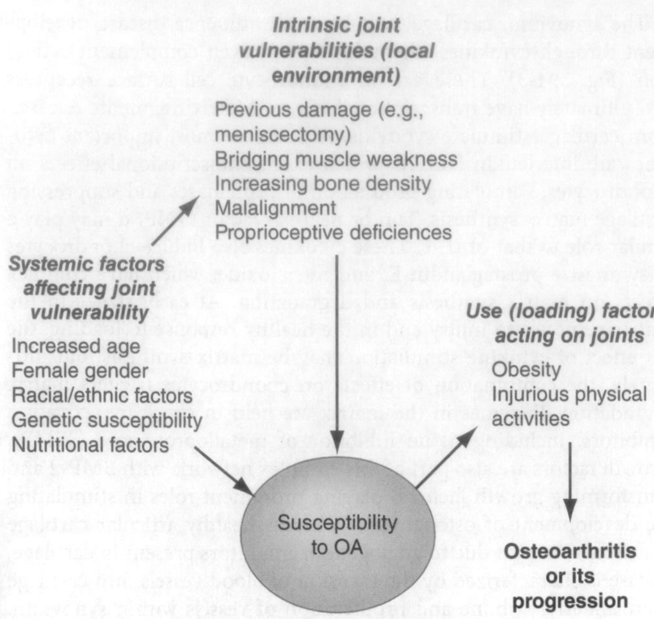

FIGURE 394-4 Risk factors for osteoarthritis (OA) either contribute to the susceptibility of the joint (systemic factors or factors in the local joint environment) or increase risk by the load they put on the joint. Usually a combination of loading and susceptibility factors is required to cause disease or its progression.

levels of loading, perhaps even levels encountered during everyday activities. On the other hand, in a young joint with competent protectors, a major acute injury or long-term overloading is necessary to precipitate disease. Risk factors for OA can be understood in terms of their effect either on joint vulnerability or on loading (Fig. 394-4).

SYSTEMIC RISK FACTORS

Age is the most potent risk factor for OA. Radiographic evidence of OA is rare in individuals under age 40; however, in some joints, such as the hands, OA occurs in >50% of persons over age 70. Aging increases joint vulnerability through several mechanisms. Whereas dynamic loading of joints stimulates cartilage matrix synthesis by chondrocytes in young cartilage, aged cartilage is less responsive to these stimuli. Partly because of this failure to synthesize matrix with loading, cartilage thins with age, and thinner cartilage experiences higher shear stress at basal layers and is at greater risk of cartilage damage. Also, joint protectors fail more often with age. Muscles that bridge the joint become weaker with age and also respond less quickly to oncoming impulses. Sensory nerve input slows with age, retarding the feedback loop of mechanoreceptors to muscles and tendons related to their tension and position. Ligaments stretch with age, making them less able to absorb impulses. These factors work in concert to increase the vulnerability of older joints to OA.

Older women are at high risk of OA in all joints, a risk that emerges as women reach their sixth decade. Although hormone loss with menopause may contribute to this risk, there is little understanding of the unique vulnerability of older women versus men to OA.

HERITABILITY AND GENETICS

OA is a highly heritable disease, but its heritability is joint specific. Fifty percent of the hand and hip OA in the community is attributable to inheritance, i.e., to disease present in other members of the family. However, the heritable proportion of knee OA is at most 30%, with some studies suggesting no heritability at all. Whereas many people with OA have disease in multiple joints, this "generalized OA" phenotype is rarely inherited and is more often a consequence of aging.

Emerging evidence has identified genetic mutations that confer a high risk of OA, the best replicated is a polymorphism within the growth differentiation factor 5 gene. This polymorphism diminishes the quantity of GDF5; GDF5 has its main influence on joint shape, and genes predisposing to OA are likely to increase risk of disease based on their effects on joint development and shape.

GLOBAL CONSIDERATIONS

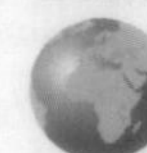

Hip OA is rare in China and in immigrants from China to the United States. However, OA in the knees is at least as common, if not more so, in Chinese than in whites from the United States, and knee OA represents a major cause of disability in China, especially in rural areas. Anatomic differences between Chinese and white hips may account for much of the difference in hip OA prevalence, with white hips having a higher prevalence of anatomic predispositions to the development of OA. Persons from Africa, but not African Americans, may also have a very low rate of hip OA.

RISK FACTORS IN THE JOINT ENVIRONMENT

Some risk factors increase vulnerability of the joint through local effects on the joint environment. With changes in joint anatomy, for example, load across the joint is no longer distributed evenly across the joint surface, but rather shows an increase in focal stress. In the hip, three uncommon developmental abnormalities occurring in utero or in childhood, congenital dysplasia, Legg-Perthes disease, and slipped capital femoral epiphysis, leave a child with distortions of hip joint anatomy that often lead to OA later in life. Girls are predominantly affected by acetabular dysplasia, a mild form of congenital dislocation, whereas the other abnormalities more often affect boys. Depending on the severity of the anatomic abnormalities, hip OA occurs either in young adulthood (severe abnormalities) or middle age (mild abnormalities).

Major injuries to a joint also can produce anatomic abnormalities that leave the joint susceptible to OA. For example, a fracture through the joint surface often causes OA in joints in which the disease is otherwise rare such as the ankle and the wrist. Avascular necrosis can lead to collapse of dead bone at the articular surface, producing anatomic irregularities and subsequent OA.

Tears of ligamentous and fibrocartilaginous structures that protect the joints, such as the anterior cruciate ligament and the meniscus in the knee and the labrum in the hip, can lead to premature OA. Meniscal tears increase with age and when chronic are often asymptomatic but lead to adjacent cartilage damage and accelerated OA. Even injuries in which the affected person never received a diagnosis may increase risk of OA. For example, in the Framingham Study subjects, men with a history of major knee injury, but no surgery, had a 3.5-fold increased risk for subsequent knee OA.

Another source of anatomic abnormality is malalignment across the joint (Fig. 394-5). This factor has been best studied in the knee, which is the fulcrum of the longest lever arm in the body. Varus (bowlegged) knees with OA are at exceedingly high risk of cartilage loss in the medial or inner compartment of the knee, whereas valgus (knockkneed) malalignment predisposes to rapid cartilage loss in the lateral compartment. Malalignment causes this effect by increasing stress on a focal area of cartilage, which then breaks down. There is evidence that malalignment in the knee not only causes cartilage loss but leads

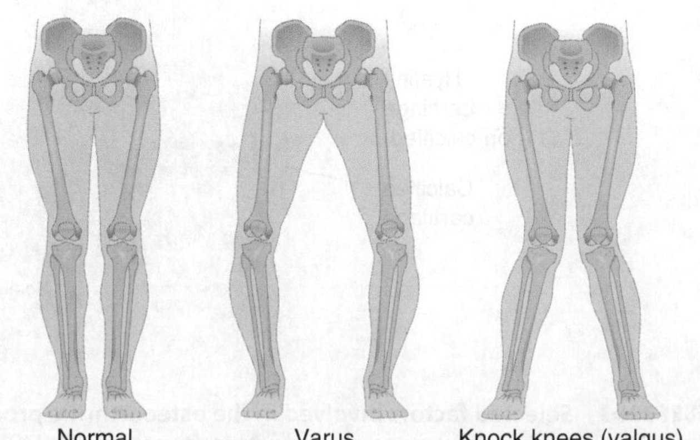

FIGURE 394-5 The two types of limb malalignment in the frontal plane: varus, in which the stress is placed across the medial compartment of the knee joint, and valgus, which places excess stress across the lateral compartment of the knee.

to underlying bone damage, producing bone marrow lesions seen on magnetic resonance imaging (MRI). Malalignment in the knee often produces such a substantial increase in focal stress within the knee (as evidenced by its destructive effects on subchondral bone) that severely malaligned knees may be destined to progress regardless of the status of other risk factors.

Weakness in the quadriceps muscles bridging the knee increases the risk of the development of painful OA in the knee.

Patients with knee OA have impaired proprioception across their knees, and this may predispose them to further disease progression. The role of bone in serving as a shock absorber for impact load is not well understood, but persons with increased bone density are at high risk of OA, suggesting that the resistance of bone to impact during joint use may play a role in disease development.

LOADING FACTORS

Obesity Three to six times body weight is transmitted across the knee during single-leg stance. Any increase in weight may be multiplied by this factor to reveal the excess force across the knee in overweight persons during walking. Obesity is a well-recognized and potent risk factor for the development of knee OA and, less so, for hip OA. Obesity precedes the development of disease and is not just a consequence of the inactivity present in those with disease. It is a stronger risk factor for disease in women than in men, and in women, the relationship of weight to the risk of disease is linear, so that with each increase in weight, there is a commensurate increase in risk. Weight loss in women lowers the risk of developing symptomatic disease. Not only is obesity a risk factor for OA in weight-bearing joints, but obese persons have more severe symptoms from the disease.

Obesity's effect on the development and progression of disease is mediated mostly through the increased loading in weight-bearing joints that occurs in overweight persons. However, a modest association of obesity with an increased risk of hand OA suggests that there may be a systemic metabolic factor circulating in obese persons that affects disease risk also.

Repeated Use of Joint and Exercise There are two categories of repetitive joint use, occupational use and leisure time physical activities. Workers performing repetitive tasks as part of their occupations for many years are at high risk of developing OA in the joints they use repeatedly. For example, farmers are at high risk for hip OA, and miners have high rates of OA in knees and spine. Workers whose jobs require regular knee bending or lifting or carrying heavy loads have a high rate of knee OA. One reason why workers may get disease is that during long days at work, their muscles may gradually become exhausted, no longer serving as effective joint protectors.

It is widely recommended for people to adopt an exercise-filled lifestyle, and long-term studies of exercise suggest no consistent association of exercise with OA risk in the majority of persons. However, persons who already have injured joints may put themselves at greater risk by engaging in certain types of exercise. For example, persons who have already sustained major knee injuries are at increased risk of progressive knee OA as a consequence of running. In addition, compared to nonrunners, elite runners (professional runners and those on Olympic teams) have high risks of both knee and hip OA. Lastly, although recreational runners are not at increased risk of knee OA, studies suggest that they have a modest increased risk of disease in the hip.

PATHOLOGY

The pathology of OA provides evidence of the involvement of many joint structures in disease. Cartilage initially shows surface fibrillation and irregularity. As disease progresses, focal erosions develop there, and these eventually extend down to the subjacent bone. With further progression, cartilage erosion down to bone expands to involve a larger proportion of the joint surface, even though OA remains a focal disease with nonuniform loss of cartilage (Fig. 394-6).

After an injury to cartilage, chondrocytes undergo mitosis and clustering. Although the metabolic activity of these chondrocyte clusters is high, the net effect of this activity is to promote proteoglycan depletion in the matrix surrounding the chondrocytes. This is because the catabolic is greater than the synthetic activity. As disease develops, collagen matrix becomes damaged, the negative charges of proteoglycans get exposed, and cartilage swells from ionic attraction to water molecules. Because in damaged cartilage proteoglycans are no longer forced into close proximity, cartilage does not bounce back after loading as it did when healthy, and cartilage becomes vulnerable to further injury. Chondrocytes at the basal level of cartilage undergo apoptosis.

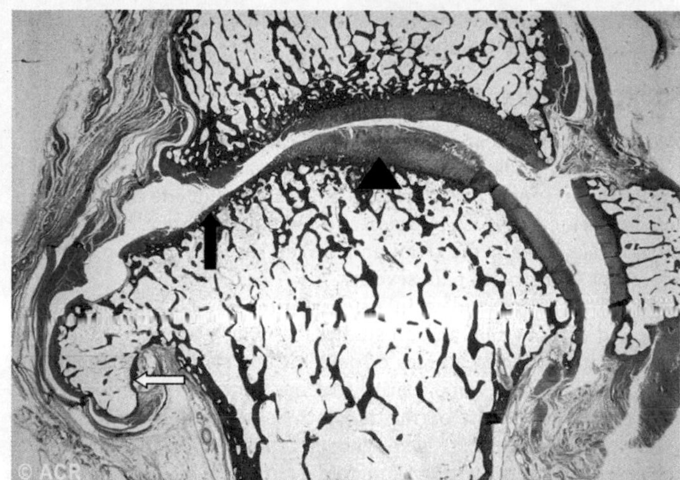

FIGURE 394-6 Pathologic changes of osteoarthritis in a toe joint. Note the nonuniform loss of cartilage (*arrowhead vs solid arrow*), the increased thickness of the subchondral bone envelope (*solid arrow*), and the osteophyte (*open arrow*). *(From the American College of Rheumatology slide collection.)*

With loss of cartilage come alterations in subchondral bone. Stimulated by growth factors and cytokines, osteoclasts and osteoblasts in the subchondral bony plate, just underneath cartilage, become activated. Bone formation produces a thickening and stiffness of the subchondral plate that occurs even before cartilage ulcerates. Trauma to bone during joint loading may be the primary factor driving this bone response, with healing from injury (including microcracks) producing stiffness. Small areas of osteonecrosis usually exist in joints with advanced disease. Bone death may also be caused by bone trauma with shearing of microvasculature, leading to a cutoff of vascular supply to some bone areas.

At the margin of the joint, near areas of cartilage loss, osteophytes form. These start as outgrowths of new cartilage, and with neurovascular invasion from the bone, this cartilage ossifies. Osteophytes are an important radiographic hallmark of OA. In malaligned joints, osteophytes grow larger on the side of the joint subject to most loading stress (e.g., in varus knees, osteophytes grow larger on the medial side).

The synovium produces lubricating fluids that minimize shear stress during motion. In healthy joints, the synovium consists of a single discontinuous layer filled with fat and containing two types of cells, macrophages and fibroblasts, but in OA, it can sometimes become edematous and inflamed. There is a migration of macrophages from the periphery into the tissue, and cells lining the synovium proliferate. Enzymes secreted by the synovium digest cartilage matrix that has been released from the surface of the cartilage.

Additional pathologic changes occur in the capsule, which stretches, becomes edematous, and can become fibrotic.

The pathology of OA is not identical across joints. In hand joints with severe OA, for example, there are often cartilage erosions in the center of the joint probably produced by bony pressure from the opposite side of the joint.

Basic calcium phosphate and calcium pyrophosphate dihydrate crystals are present microscopically in most joints with end-stage OA. Their role in osteoarthritic cartilage is unclear, but their release from cartilage into the joint space and joint fluid likely triggers synovial inflammation, which can, in turn, produce release of enzymes and trigger nociceptive stimulation.

SOURCES OF PAIN

Because cartilage is aneural, cartilage loss in a joint is not accompanied by pain. Thus, pain in OA likely arises from structures outside the cartilage. Innervated structures in the joint include the synovium, ligaments, joint capsule, muscles, and subchondral bone. Most of these are not visualized by the x-ray, and the severity of x-ray changes in OA correlates poorly with pain severity.

Based on MRI studies in osteoarthritic knees comparing those with and without pain and on studies mapping tenderness in unanesthetized joints, likely sources of pain include synovial inflammation, joint effusions, and bone marrow edema. Modest synovitis develops in many but not all osteoarthritic joints. Some diseased joints have no synovitis, whereas others have synovial inflammation that approaches the severity of joints with rheumatoid arthritis (Chap. 380). The presence of synovitis on MRI is correlated with the presence and severity of knee pain. Capsular stretching from fluid in the joint stimulates nociceptive fibers there, inducing pain. Increased focal loading as part of the disease not only damages cartilage but probably also injures the underlying bone. As a consequence, bone marrow edema appears on the MRI; histologically, this edema signals the presence of microcracks and scar, which are the consequences of trauma. These lesions may stimulate bone nociceptive fibers. Also, hemostatic pressure within bone rises in OA, and the increased pressure itself may stimulate nociceptive fibers, causing pain.

Pain may arise from outside the joint also, including bursae near the joints. Common sources of pain near the knee are anserine bursitis and iliotibial band syndrome.

Persons with chronic OA pain may develop nervous system alterations as a consequence of disease, changes which decrease inhibitory controls on nociception and its distribution. This may produce allodynia and hyperalgesia in some patients with OA.

CLINICAL FEATURES

Joint pain from OA is activity-related. Pain comes on either during or just after joint use and then gradually resolves. Examples include knee or hip pain with going up or down stairs, pain in weight-bearing joints when walking, and, for hand OA, pain when cooking. Early in disease, pain is episodic, triggered often by a day or two of overactive use of a diseased joint, such as a person with knee OA taking a long run and noticing a few days of pain thereafter. As disease progresses, the pain becomes continuous and even begins to be bothersome at night. Stiffness of the affected joint may be prominent, but morning stiffness is usually brief (<30 min).

In knees, buckling may occur, in part, due to weakness of muscles crossing the joint. Mechanical symptoms, such as buckling, catching, or locking, could also signify internal derangement, such as meniscal tears, and need to be evaluated. In the knee, pain with activities requiring knee flexion, such as stair climbing and arising from a chair, often emanates from the patellofemoral compartment of the knee, which does not actively articulate until the knee is bent ~35°.

OA is the most common cause of chronic knee pain in persons over age 45, but the differential diagnosis is long. Inflammatory arthritis is likely if there is prolonged morning stiffness and many other joints are affected. Bursitis occurs commonly around knees and hips. A physical examination should focus on whether tenderness is over the joint line (at the junction of the two bones around which the joint is articulating) or is outside of it. Anserine bursitis, medial and distal to the knee, is an extremely common cause of chronic knee pain that may respond to a glucocorticoid injection. Prominent nocturnal pain in the absence of end-stage OA merits a distinct workup. For hip pain, OA can be detected by loss of internal rotation on passive movement, and pain isolated to an area lateral to the hip joint usually reflects the presence of trochanteric bursitis.

No blood tests are routinely indicated for workup of patients with OA unless symptoms and signs suggest inflammatory arthritis.

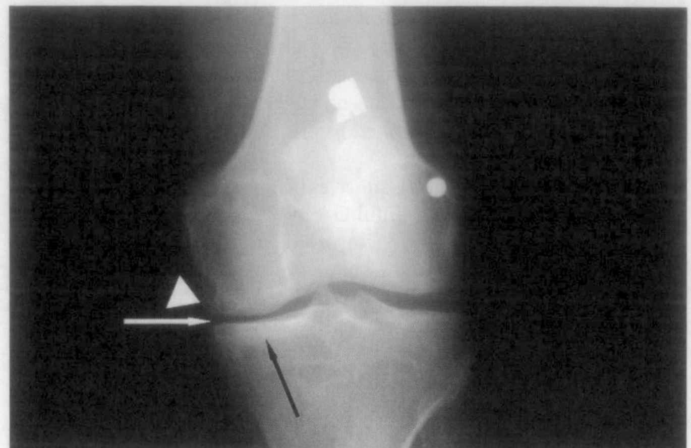

FIGURE 394-7 X-ray of knee with medial osteoarthritis. Note the narrowed joint space on medial side of the joint only (*white arrow*), the sclerosis of the bone in the medial compartment providing evidence of cortical thickening (*black arrow*), and the osteophytes in the medial femur (*white wedge*).

Examination of the synovial fluid is often more helpful diagnostically than an x-ray. If the synovial fluid white count is >1000/μL, inflammatory arthritis or gout or pseudogout is likely, the latter two being also identified by the presence of crystals.

X-rays are indicated to evaluate chronic hand pain and hip pain thought to be due to OA, as the diagnosis is often unclear without confirming radiographs. For knee pain, x-rays should be obtained if symptoms or signs are not typical of OA or if knee pain persists after inauguration of effective treatment. In OA, radiographic findings (Fig. 394-7) correlate poorly with the presence and severity of pain. Further, radiographs may be normal in early disease as they are insensitive to cartilage loss and other early findings.

Although MRI may reveal the extent of pathology in an osteoarthritic joint, it is not indicated as part of the diagnostic workup. Findings such as meniscal tears and cartilage and bone lesions occur in most patients with OA in the knee, but almost never warrant a change in therapy.

TREATMENT OSTEOARTHRITIS

The goals of the treatment of OA are to alleviate pain and minimize loss of physical function. To the extent that pain and loss of function are consequences of inflammation, of weakness across the joint, and of laxity and instability, the treatment of OA involves addressing each of these impairments. Comprehensive therapy consists of a multimodality approach including nonpharmacologic and pharmacologic elements.

Patients with mild and intermittent symptoms may need only reassurance or nonpharmacologic treatments. Patients with ongoing, disabling pain are likely to need both nonpharmacotherapy and pharmacotherapy.

Treatments for knee OA have been more completely evaluated than those for hip and hand OA or for disease in other joints. Thus, although the principles of treatment are identical for OA in all joints, we shall focus below on the treatment of knee OA, noting specific recommendations for disease in other joints, especially when they differ from those for the knee.

NONPHARMACOTHERAPY

Because OA is a mechanically driven disease, the mainstay of treatment involves altering loading across the painful joint and improving the function of joint protectors, so they can better distribute load across the joint. Ways of lessening focal load across the joint include:

1. avoiding activities that overload the joint, as evidenced by their causing pain;
2. improving the strength and conditioning of muscles that bridge the joint, so as to optimize their function; and
3. unloading the joint, either by redistributing load within the joint with a brace or a splint or by unloading the joint during weight bearing with a cane or a crutch.

The simplest effective treatment for many patients is to avoid activities that precipitate pain. For example, for the middle-aged patient whose long-distance running brings on symptoms of knee OA, a less demanding form of weight-bearing activity may alleviate all symptoms. For an older person whose daily constitutionals up and down hills bring on knee pain, routing the constitutional away from hills might eliminate symptoms.

Each pound of weight increases the loading across the knee three- to sixfold. Weight loss may have a commensurate multiplier effect, unloading both knees and hips and probably relieving pain in those joints.

In hand joints affected by OA, splinting, by limiting motion, often minimizes pain for patients with involvement especially in the base of the thumb. Weight-bearing joints such as knees and hips can be unloaded by using a cane in the hand opposite to the affected joint for partial weight bearing. A physical therapist can help teach the patient how to use the cane optimally, including ensuring that its height is optimal for unloading. Crutches or walkers can serve a similar beneficial function.

Exercise Osteoarthritic pain in knees or hips during weight bearing results in lack of activity and poor mobility, and because OA is so common, the inactivity that results represents a public health concern, increasing the risk of cardiovascular disease and obesity. Aerobic capacity is poor in most elders with symptomatic knee OA, worse than others of the same age.

Weakness in muscles that bridge osteoarthritic joints is multifactorial in etiology. First, there is a decline in strength with age. Second, with limited mobility comes disuse muscle atrophy. Third, patients with painful knee or hip OA alter their gait so as to lessen loading across the affected joint, and this further diminishes muscle use. Fourth, "arthrogenous inhibition" may occur, whereby contraction of muscles bridging the joint is inhibited by a nerve afferent feedback loop emanating in a swollen and stretched joint capsule; this prevents maximal attainment of voluntary maximal strength. Because adequate muscle strength and conditioning are critical to joint protection, weakness in a muscle that bridges a diseased joint makes the joint more susceptible to further damage and pain. The degree of weakness correlates strongly with the severity of joint pain and the degree of physical limitation. One of the cardinal elements of the treatment of OA is to improve the functioning of muscles surrounding the joint.

For knee and hip OA, trials have shown that exercise lessens pain and improves physical function. Most effective exercise regimens consist of aerobic and/or resistance training, the latter of which focuses on strengthening muscles across the joint. Exercises are likely to be effective, especially if they train muscles for the activities a person performs daily. Activities that increase pain in the joint should be avoided, and the exercise regimen needs to be individualized to optimize effectiveness. Range-of-motion exercises, which do not strengthen muscles, and isometric exercises that strengthen muscles, but not through range of motion, are unlikely to be effective by themselves. Low-impact exercises, including water aerobics and water resistance training, are often better tolerated by patients than exercises involving impact loading, such as running or treadmill exercises. A patient should be referred to an exercise class or to a therapist who can create an individualized regimen, and then an individualized home-based regimen can be crafted. In addition to conventional exercise regimens, tai chi may be effective for knee OA. However, there is no strong evidence that patients with hand OA benefit from therapeutic exercise.

Adherence over the long term is the major challenge to an exercise prescription. In trials involving patients with knee OA, who are engaged in exercise treatment, from a third to over half of patients stopped exercising by 6 months. Less than 50% continued regular exercise at 1 year. The strongest predictor of a patient's continued exercise is a previous personal history of successful exercise. Physicians should reinforce the exercise prescription at each clinic visit, help the patient recognize barriers to ongoing exercise, and identify convenient times for exercise to be done routinely. The combination of exercise with calorie restriction and weight loss is especially effective in lessening pain.

Correction of Malalignment Malalignment in the frontal plane (varus-valgus) markedly increases the stress across the joint, which can lead to progression of disease and to pain and disability (Fig. 394-5). Correcting malalignment, either surgically or with bracing, may relieve pain in persons whose knees are malaligned. Malalignment develops over years as a consequence of gradual anatomic alterations of the joint and bone, and correcting it is often very challenging. One way is with a fitted brace, which takes an often varus osteoarthritic knee and straightens it by putting valgus stress across the knee. Unfortunately, many patients are unwilling to wear a realigning knee brace; in addition, in patients with obese legs, braces may slip with usage and lose their realigning effect. They are indicated for willing patients who can learn to put them on correctly and on whom they do not slip.

Other ways of correcting malalignment across the knee include the use of orthotics in footwear. Unfortunately, although they may have modest effects on knee alignment, trials have heretofore not demonstrated efficacy of a lateral wedge orthotic versus placebo wedges.

Pain from the patellofemoral compartment of the knee can be caused by tilting of the patella or patellar malalignment with the patella riding laterally or medially in the femoral trochlear groove. Using a brace to realign the patella, or tape to pull the patella back into the trochlear sulcus or reduce its tilt, has been shown, when compared to placebo taping in clinical trials, to lessen patellofemoral pain. However, patients may find it difficult to apply tape, and skin irritation from the tape is common. Commercial patellar braces may be a solution, but there is insufficient evidence on their efficacy to recommend them.

Although their effect on malalignment is questionable, neoprene sleeves pulled to cover the knee lessen pain and are easy to use and popular among patients. The explanation for their therapeutic effect on pain is unclear.

In patients with knee OA, acupuncture produces modest pain relief compared to placebo needles and may be an adjunctive treatment.

PHARMACOTHERAPY

Although nonpharmacologic approaches to therapy constitute its mainstay, pharmacotherapy serves an important adjunctive role in OA treatment. Available drugs are administered using oral, topical, and intraarticular routes.

Acetaminophen, Nonsteroidal Anti-Inflammatory Drugs (NSAIDs), and Cyclooxygenase-2 (COX-2) Inhibitors Acetaminophen (paracetamol) is the initial analgesic of choice for patients with OA in knees, hips, or hands. For some patients, it is adequate to control symptoms, in which case more toxic drugs such as NSAIDs can be avoided. Doses up to 1 g three times daily can be used (Table 394-1).

NSAIDs are the most popular drugs to treat osteoarthritic pain. They can be administered either topically or orally. In clinical trials, oral NSAIDs produce ~30% greater improvement in pain than high-dose acetaminophen. Occasional patients treated with NSAIDs experience dramatic pain relief, whereas others experience little improvement. Initially, NSAIDs should be administered topically or taken orally on an "as needed" basis because side effects are less frequent with low intermittent doses. If occasional medication use is insufficiently effective, then daily treatment may be indicated, with

TABLE 394-1 PHARMACOLOGIC TREATMENT FOR OSTEOARTHRITIS

Treatment	Dosage	Comments
Acetaminophen	Up to 1 g tid	Prolongs half-life of warfarin. Make sure patient is not taking other treatments containing acetaminophen to avoid hepatic toxicity.
Oral NSAIDs and COX-2 inhibitors		Take with food. Increased risk of myocardial infarction and stroke for some NSAIDs and especially COX-2 inhibitors. High rates of gastrointestinal side effects, including ulcers and bleeding, occur. Patients at high risk for gastrointestinal side effects should also take either a proton pump inhibitor or misoprostol.[a] There is an increase in gastrointestinal side effects or bleeding when taken with acetylsalicylic acid. Can also cause edema and renal insufficiency.
Naproxen	375–500 mg bid	
Salsalate	1500 mg bid	
Ibuprofen	600–800 mg 3–4 times a day	
Topical NSAIDs		Rub onto joint. Few systemic side effects. Skin irritation common.
Diclofenac Na 1% gel	4 g qid (for knees, hands)	
Opiates	Various	Common side effects include dizziness, sedation, nausea or vomiting, dry mouth, constipation, urinary retention, and pruritus. Respiratory and central nervous system depression can occur.
Capsaicin	0.025–0.075% cream 3–4 times a day	Can irritate mucous membranes.
Intraarticular injections		
Steroids		
Hyaluronans	Varies from 3–5 weekly injections depending on preparation	Mild to moderate pain at injection site. Controversy exists regarding efficacy.

[a]Patients at high risk include those with previous gastrointestinal events, persons ≥60 years, and persons taking glucocorticoids. Trials have shown the efficacy of proton pump inhibitors and misoprostol in the prevention of ulcers and bleeding. Misoprostol is associated with a high rate of diarrhea and cramping; therefore, proton pump inhibitors are more widely used to reduce NSAID-related gastrointestinal symptoms.

Abbreviations: COX-2, cyclooxygenase-2; NSAIDs, nonsteroidal anti-inflammatory drugs.

Source: Adapted from DT Felson: N Engl J Med 354:841, 2006.

an anti-inflammatory dose selected (Table 394-1). Patients should be reminded to take low-dose aspirin and ibuprofen at different times to eliminate a drug interaction.

NSAIDs taken orally have substantial and frequent side effects, the most common of which is upper gastrointestinal toxicity, including dyspepsia, nausea, bloating, gastrointestinal bleeding, and ulcer disease. Some 30–40% of patients experience upper gastrointestinal (GI) side effects so severe as to require discontinuation of medication. To minimize the risk of nonsteroidal-related GI side effects, patients should not take two NSAIDs and should take medications after food; if risk is high, patients should take a gastroprotective agent, such as a proton pump inhibitor. Certain oral agents are safer to the stomach than others, including nonacetylated salicylates and nabumetone. Major NSAID-related GI side effects can occur in patients who do not complain of upper GI symptoms. In one study of patients hospitalized for GI bleeding, 81% had no premonitory symptoms.

Because of the increased rates of cardiovascular events associated with COX-2 inhibitors and with some conventional NSAIDs such as diclofenac, many of these drugs are not appropriate long-term treatment choices for older persons with OA, especially those at high risk of heart disease or stroke. The American Heart Association has identified rofecoxib and all other COX-2 inhibitors as putting patients at high risk, although low doses of celecoxib (≤200 mg/d) may not be associated with an elevation of risk. The only conventional NSAID that appears safe from a cardiovascular perspective is naproxen, but it does have GI toxicity.

There are other common side effects of NSAIDs, including the tendency to develop edema because of prostaglandin inhibition of afferent blood supply to glomeruli in the kidneys and, for similar reasons, a predilection toward reversible renal insufficiency. Blood pressure may increase modestly in some NSAID-treated patients. Oral NSAIDs should not be used in patients with stage IV or V renal disease and should be used with caution in those with stage III disease.

NSAIDs can be placed into a gel or topical solution with another chemical modality that enhances penetration of the skin barrier creating a topical NSAID. When absorbed through the skin, plasma concentrations are an order of magnitude lower than with the same amount of drug administered orally or parenterally. However, when these drugs are administered topically in proximity to a superficial joint (knees, hands, but not hips), the drug can be found in joint tissues such as the synovium and cartilage. Trial results have varied but generally have found that topical NSAIDs are slightly less efficacious than oral agents, but have far fewer GI and systemic side effects. Unfortunately, topical NSAIDs often cause local skin irritation where the medication is applied, inducing redness, burning, or itching in up to 40% of patients (see Table 394-1).

Intraarticular Injections: Glucocorticoids and Hyaluronic Acid Because synovial inflammation is likely to be a major cause of pain in patients with OA, local anti-inflammatory treatments administered intraarticularly may be effective in ameliorating pain, at least temporarily. Glucocorticoid injections provide such efficacy, but response is variable, with some patients having little relief of pain whereas others experience pain relief lasting several months. Glucocorticoid injections are useful to get patients over acute flares of pain and may be especially indicated if the patient has coexistent OA and crystal deposition disease, especially from calcium pyrophosphate dihydrate crystals (Chap. 395). There is no evidence that repeated glucocorticoid injections into the joint are dangerous.

Hyaluronic acid injections can be given for treatment of symptoms in knee and hip OA, but there is controversy as to whether they have efficacy versus placebo (Table 394-1).

Other Classes of Drugs and Nutraceuticals For patients with symptomatic knee or hip OA who have not had an adequate response to the treatments above and are either unwilling to undergo or are not candidates for total joint arthroplasty, opioid analgesics have shown modest efficacy and can be tried. Opioid management plans and patient selection are critical. Another option is the use of duloxetine, which has demonstrated modest efficacy in OA.

Recent guidelines recommend against the use of glucosamine or chondroitin for OA. Large publicly supported trials have failed to show that, compared with placebo, these compounds relieve pain in persons with disease.

Optimal nonsurgical therapy for OA is often achieved by trial and error, with each patient having idiosyncratic responses to specific treatments. When medical therapies have failed and the patient has an unacceptable reduction in their quality of life and ongoing pain and disability, then at least for knee and hip OA, total joint arthroplasty is indicated.

SURGERY

For knee OA, several operations are available. Arthroscopic debridement and lavage have diminished in popularity after randomized trials evaluating this operation have showed that its efficacy is no greater than that of sham surgery or no treatment for relief of pain or disability. Even mechanical symptoms such as buckling, which are extremely common in patients with knee OA, do not respond to arthroscopic debridement. Although arthroscopic meniscectomy is indicated for acute meniscal tears in which symptoms such as locking and acute pain are clearly related temporally to a knee injury that produced the tear, recent trials show that doing a partial meniscectomy in persons with OA and a symptomatic meniscal tear does not relieve knee pain or improve function.

For patients with knee OA isolated to the medial compartment, operations to realign the knee to lessen medial loading can relieve pain. These include a high tibial osteotomy, in which the tibia is broken just below the tibial plateau and realigned so as to load the lateral, nondiseased compartment, or a unicompartmental replacement with realignment. Each surgery may provide the patient with years of pain relief before a total knee replacement is required.

Ultimately, when the patient with knee or hip OA has failed medical treatment modalities and remains in pain, with limitations of physical function that compromise the quality of life, the patient should be referred for total knee or hip arthroplasty. These are highly efficacious operations that relieve pain and improve function in the vast majority of patients, although rates of success are higher for hip than knee replacement. Currently failure rates for both are ~1% per year, although these rates are higher in obese patients. The chance of surgical success is greater in centers where at least 25 such operations are performed yearly or with surgeons who perform multiple operations annually. The timing of knee or hip replacement is critical. If the patient suffers for many years until their functional status has declined substantially, with considerable muscle weakness, postoperative functional status may not improve to a level achieved by others who underwent operation earlier in their disease course.

Cartilage Regeneration Chondrocyte transplantation has not been found to be efficacious in OA, perhaps because OA includes pathology of joint mechanics, which is not corrected by chondrocyte transplants. Similarly, abrasion arthroplasty (chondroplasty) has not been well studied for efficacy in OA, but it produces fibrocartilage in place of damaged hyaline cartilage. Both of these surgical attempts to regenerate and reconstitute articular cartilage may be more likely to be efficacious early in disease when joint malalignment and many of the other noncartilage abnormalities that characterize OA have not yet developed.

395 Gout and Other Crystal-Associated Arthropathies

H. Ralph Schumacher, Lan X. Chen

The use of polarizing light microscopy during synovial fluid analysis in 1961 by McCarty and Hollander and the subsequent application of other crystallographic techniques, such as electron microscopy, energy-dispersive elemental analysis, and x-ray diffraction, have allowed investigators to identify the roles of different microcrystals, including monosodium urate (MSU), calcium pyrophosphate (CPP), calcium apatite (apatite), and calcium oxalate (CaOx), in inducing acute or chronic arthritis or periarthritis. The clinical events that result from deposition of MSU, CPP, apatite, and CaOx have many similarities but also have important differences. Because of often similar clinical presentations, the need to perform synovial fluid analysis to distinguish the type of crystal involved must be emphasized. Polarized light microscopy alone can identify most typical crystals; apatite, however, is an exception. Aspiration and analysis of effusions are also important to assess the possibility of infection. Apart from the identification of specific microcrystalline materials or organisms, synovial fluid characteristics in crystal-associated diseases are nonspecific, and synovial fluid can be inflammatory or noninflammatory. Without crystal identification, these diseases can be confused with rheumatoid or other types of arthritis. A list of possible musculoskeletal manifestations of crystal-associated arthritis is shown in Table 395-1.

TABLE 395-1 MUSCULOSKELETAL MANIFESTATIONS OF CRYSTAL-INDUCED ARTHRITIS

Acute mono- or polyarthritis	Destructive arthropathies
Bursitis	Chronic inflammatory arthritis
Tendinitis	Spinal arthritis
Enthesitis	Peculiar type of osteoarthritis
Tophaceous deposits	Carpal tunnel syndrome

GOUT

Gout is a metabolic disease that most often affects middle-aged to elderly men and postmenopausal women. It results from an increased body pool of urate with hyperuricemia. It typically is characterized by episodic acute arthritis or chronic arthritis caused by deposition of MSU crystals in joints and connective tissue tophi and the risk for deposition in kidney interstitium or uric acid nephrolithiasis (Chap. 431e).

ACUTE AND CHRONIC ARTHRITIS

Acute arthritis is the most common early clinical manifestation of gout. Usually, only one joint is affected initially, but polyarticular acute gout can occur in subsequent episodes. The metatarsophalangeal joint of the first toe often is involved, but tarsal joints, ankles, and knees also are affected commonly. Especially in elderly patients or in advanced disease, finger joints may be involved. Inflamed Heberden's or Bouchard's nodes may be a first manifestation of gouty arthritis. The first episode of acute gouty arthritis frequently begins at night with dramatic joint pain and swelling. Joints rapidly become warm, red, and tender, with a clinical appearance that often mimics that of cellulitis. Early attacks tend to subside spontaneously within 3–10 days, and most patients have intervals of varying length with no residual symptoms until the next episode. Several events may precipitate acute gouty arthritis: dietary excess, trauma, surgery, excessive ethanol ingestion, hypouricemic therapy, and serious medical illnesses such as myocardial infarction and stroke.

After many acute mono- or oligoarticular attacks, a proportion of gouty patients may present with a chronic nonsymmetric synovitis, causing potential confusion with rheumatoid arthritis (Chap. 380). Less commonly, chronic gouty arthritis will be the only manifestation, and, more rarely, the disease will manifest only as periarticular tophaceous deposits in the absence of synovitis. Women represent only 5–20% of all patients with gout. Most women with gouty arthritis are postmenopausal and elderly, have osteoarthritis and arterial hypertension that causes mild renal insufficiency, and usually are receiving diuretics. Premenopausal gout is rare. Kindreds of precocious gout in young females caused by decreased renal urate clearance and renal insufficiency have been described.

Laboratory Diagnosis Even if the clinical appearance strongly suggests gout, the presumptive diagnosis ideally should be confirmed by needle aspiration of acutely or chronically involved joints or tophaceous deposits. Acute septic arthritis, several of the other crystalline-associated arthropathies, palindromic rheumatism, and psoriatic arthritis may present with similar clinical features. During acute gouty

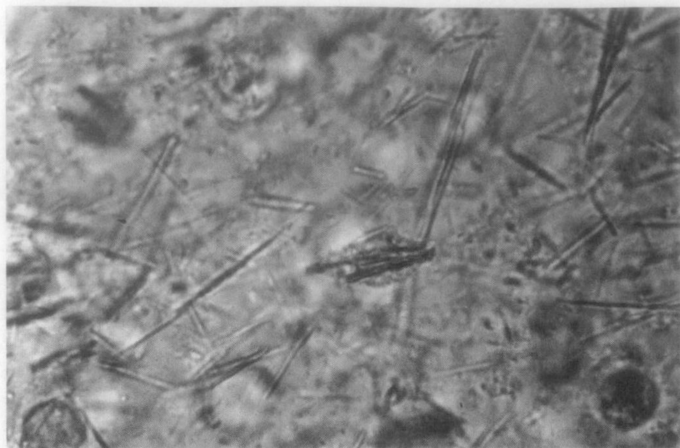

FIGURE 395-1 Extracellular and intracellular monosodium urate crystals, as seen in a fresh preparation of synovial fluid, illustrate needle- and rod-shaped crystals. These crystals are strongly negative birefringent crystals under compensated polarized light microscopy; 400×.

attacks, needle-shaped MSU crystals typically are seen both intracellularly and extracellularly (Fig. 395-1). With compensated polarized light, these crystals are brightly birefringent with negative elongation. Synovial fluid leukocyte counts are elevated from 2000 to 60,000/μL. Effusions appear cloudy due to the increased numbers of leukocytes. Large amounts of crystals occasionally produce a thick pasty or chalky joint fluid. Bacterial infection can coexist with urate crystals in synovial fluid; if there is any suspicion of septic arthritis, joint fluid must be cultured.

MSU crystals also can often be demonstrated in the first metatarsophalangeal joint and in knees not acutely involved with gout. Arthrocentesis of these joints is a useful technique to establish the diagnosis of gout between attacks.

Serum uric acid levels can be normal or low at the time of an acute attack, as inflammatory cytokines can be uricosuric and effective initiation of hypouricemic therapy can precipitate attacks. This limits the value of serum uric acid determinations for the diagnosis of gout. Nevertheless, serum urate levels are almost always elevated at some time and are important to use to follow the course of hypouricemic therapy. A 24-h urine collection for uric acid can, in some cases, be useful in assessing the risk of stones, elucidating overproduction or underexcretion of uric acid, and deciding whether it may be appropriate to use a uricosuric therapy (Chap. 431e). Excretion of >800 mg of uric acid per 24 h on a regular diet suggests that causes of overproduction of purine should be considered. Urinalysis, serum creatinine, hemoglobin, white blood cell (WBC) count, liver function tests, and serum lipids should be obtained because of possible pathologic sequelae of gout and other associated diseases requiring treatment and as baselines because of possible adverse effects of gout treatment.

Radiographic Features Cystic changes, well-defined erosions with sclerotic margins (often with overhanging bony edges), and soft tissue masses are characteristic radiographic features of advanced chronic tophaceous gout. Ultrasound may aid earlier diagnosis by showing a double contour sign overlying the articular cartilage. Dual-energy computed tomography (CT) can show specific features establishing the presence of urate crystals.

TREATMENT GOUT

ACUTE GOUTY ARTHRITIS

The mainstay of treatment during an acute attack is the administration of anti-inflammatory drugs such as nonsteroidal anti-inflammatory drugs (NSAIDs), colchicine, or glucocorticoids. NSAIDs are used most often in individuals without complicating comorbid conditions. Both colchicine and NSAIDs may be poorly tolerated and dangerous in the elderly and in the presence of renal insufficiency and gastrointestinal disorders. Ice pack applications and rest of the involved joints can be helpful. Colchicine given orally is a traditional and effective treatment if used early in an attack. Useful regimens are one 0.6-mg tablet given every 8 h with subsequent tapering or 1.2 mg followed by 0.6 mg in 1 h with subsequent day dosing depending on response. This is generally better tolerated than the formerly advised higher dose regimens. The drug must be at least temporarily discontinued promptly at the first sign of loose stools, and symptomatic treatment must be given for the diarrhea. Intravenous colchicine has been taken off the market. NSAIDs given in full anti-inflammatory doses are effective in ~90% of patients, and the resolution of signs and symptoms usually occurs in 5–8 days. The most effective drugs are any of those with a short half-life and include indomethacin, 25–50 mg tid; naproxen, 500 mg bid; ibuprofen, 800 mg tid; diclofenac, 50 mg tid; and celecoxib 800 mg followed by 400 mg 12 h later, then 400 mg bid.

Glucocorticoids given IM or orally, for example, prednisone, 30–50 mg/d as the initial dose and gradually tapered with the resolution of the attack, can be effective in polyarticular gout. For a single joint or a few involved joints, intraarticular triamcinolone acetonide, 20–40 mg, or methylprednisolone, 25–50 mg, have been effective and well tolerated. Based on recent evidence on the essential role of the inflammasome and interleukin 1β (IL-1β) in acute gout, anakinra has been used, and other inhibitors of IL-1β, including canakinumab and rilonacept, are under investigation.

HYPOURICEMIC THERAPY

Ultimate control of gout requires correction of the basic underlying defect: the hyperuricemia. Attempts to normalize serum uric acid to <300–360 μmol/L (5.0–6.0 mg/dL) to prevent recurrent gouty attacks and eliminate tophaceous deposits are critical and entail a commitment to hypouricemic regimens and medications that generally are required for life. Hypouricemic drug therapy should be considered when, as in most patients, the hyperuricemia cannot be corrected by simple means (control of body weight, low-purine diet, increase in liquid intake, limitation of ethanol use, decreased use of fructose-containing foods and beverages, and avoidance of diuretics). The decision to initiate hypouricemic therapy usually is made taking into consideration the number of acute attacks (urate lowering may be cost-effective after two attacks), serum uric acid levels (progression is more rapid in patients with serum uric acid >535 μmol/L [>9.0 mg/dL]), the patient's willingness to commit to lifelong therapy, or the presence of uric acid stones. Urate-lowering therapy should be initiated in any patient who already has tophi or chronic gouty arthritis. Uricosuric agents such as probenecid can be used in patients with good renal function who underexcrete uric acid, with <600 mg in a 24-h urine sample. Urine volume should be maintained by ingestion of 1500 mL of water every day. Probenecid can be started at a dose of 250 mg twice daily and increased gradually as needed up to 3 g per day to achieve and maintain a serum uric acid level of less than 6 mg/dL. Probenecid is generally not effective in patients with serum creatinine levels >177 μmol/L (2 mg/dL). These patients may require allopurinol or benzbromarone (not available in the United States). Benzbromarone is another uricosuric drug that is more effective in patients with chronic kidney disease. Some agents used to treat common comorbidities, including losartan, fenofibrate, and amlodipine, have some mild uricosuric effects.

The xanthine oxidase inhibitor allopurinol is by far the most commonly used hypouricemic agent and is the best drug to lower serum urate in overproducers, urate stone formers, and patients with renal disease. It can be given in a single morning dose, usually 100 mg initially and increasing up to 800 mg if needed. In patients with chronic renal disease, the initial allopurinol dose should be lower and adjusted depending on the serum creatinine concentration; for example, with a creatinine clearance of 10 mL/min, one generally would use 100 mg every other day. Doses can be increased gradually to reach the target urate level of less than 6 mg/dL. Toxicity of allopurinol has been recognized increasingly in patients who use thiazide diuretics, in patients allergic to penicillin and ampicillin, and in Asians expressing HLA-B*5801. The most serious side effects include life-threatening toxic epidermal necrolysis, systemic vasculitis, bone marrow suppression, granulomatous hepatitis, and renal failure. Patients with mild cutaneous reactions to allopurinol can reconsider the use of a uricosuric agent, undergo an attempt at desensitization to allopurinol, or take febuxostat, a new, chemically unrelated specific xanthine oxidase inhibitor. Febuxostat is approved in the United States at 40 or 80 mg once a day and does not require dose adjustment in mild to moderate renal disease. Pegloticase is a pegylated uricase, now available for patients who do not tolerate or fail full doses of other treatments. It is given intravenously usually at 8 mg every 2 weeks and can dramatically lower serum uric acid in up to 50% of such patients. New uricosurics are also undergoing investigation.

Urate-lowering drugs are generally not initiated during acute attacks but after the patient is stable and low-dose colchicine has been initiated to decrease the risk of the flares that often occur with urate lowering. Colchicine anti-inflammatory prophylaxis in doses of 0.6 mg one to two times daily should be given along with the hypouricemic therapy until the patient is normouricemic and without gouty attacks for 6 months or as long as tophi are present. Colchicine should not be used in dialysis patients and is given in lower doses in patients with renal disease or with P glycoprotein or CYP3A4 inhibitors such as clarithromycin that can increase toxicity of colchicine.

CALCIUM PYROPHOSPHATE DEPOSITION (CPPD) DISEASE

PATHOGENESIS

The deposition of CPP crystals in articular tissues is most common in the elderly, occurring in 10–15% of persons age 65–75 years and 30–50% of those >85 years. In most cases, this process is asymptomatic and the cause of CPPD is uncertain. Because >80% of patients are >60 years and 70% have preexisting joint damage from other conditions, it is likely that biochemical changes in aging or diseased cartilage favor crystal nucleation. In patients with CPPD arthritis, there is increased production of inorganic pyrophosphate and decreased levels of pyrophosphatases in cartilage extracts. Mutations in the *ANKH* gene, as described in both familial and sporadic cases, can increase elaboration and extracellular transport of pyrophosphate. The increase in pyrophosphate production appears to be related to enhanced activity of ATP pyrophosphohydrolase and 5′-nucleotidase, which catalyze the reaction of ATP to adenosine and pyrophosphate. This pyrophosphate could combine with calcium to form CPP crystals in matrix vesicles or on collagen fibers. There are decreased levels of cartilage glycosaminoglycans that normally inhibit and regulate crystal nucleation. High activities of transglutaminase enzymes also may contribute to the deposition of CPP crystals.

Release of CPP crystals into the joint space is followed by the phagocytosis of those crystals by monocyte macrophages and neutrophils, which respond by releasing chemotactic and inflammatory substances and, as with MSU crystals, activating the inflammasome.

A minority of patients with CPPD arthropathy have metabolic abnormalities or hereditary CPP disease (Table 395-2). These associations suggest that a variety of different metabolic products may enhance CPP crystal deposition either by directly altering cartilage or by inhibiting inorganic pyrophosphatases. Included among these conditions are hyperparathyroidism, hemochromatosis, hypophosphatasia, hypomagnesemia, and possibly myxedema. The presence of CPPD arthritis in individuals <50 years old should lead to consideration of these metabolic disorders (Table 395-2) and inherited forms of disease, including those identified in a variety of ethnic groups. Genomic DNA studies performed on different kindreds have shown a possible location of genetic defects on chromosome 8q or on chromosome 5p in a region that expresses the gene of the membrane pyrophosphate channel (*ANKH* gene). As noted above, mutations described in the *ANKH* gene in kindreds with CPPD arthritis can increase extracellular

TABLE 395-2 CONDITIONS ASSOCIATED WITH CALCIUM PYROPHOSPHATE CRYSTAL DEPOSITION DISEASE

Aging
Disease-associated
Primary hyperparathyroidism
Hemochromatosis
Hypophosphatasia
Hypomagnesemia
Chronic gout
Postmeniscectomy
Gitelman's syndrome
Epiphyseal dysplasias

pyrophosphate and induce CPP crystal formation. Investigation of younger patients with CPPD should include inquiry for evidence of familial aggregation and evaluation of serum calcium, phosphorus, alkaline phosphatase, magnesium, iron, and transferrin.

CLINICAL MANIFESTATIONS

CPPD arthropathy may be asymptomatic, acute, subacute, or chronic or may cause acute synovitis superimposed on chronically involved joints. Acute CPPD arthritis originally was termed *pseudogout* by McCarty and co-workers because of its striking similarity to gout. Other clinical manifestations of CPPD include (1) association with or enhancement of peculiar forms of osteoarthritis; (2) induction of severe destructive disease that may radiographically mimic neuropathic arthritis; (3) production of chronic symmetric synovitis that is clinically similar to rheumatoid arthritis; (4) intervertebral disk and ligament calcification with restriction of spine mobility, the crowned dens syndrome, or spinal stenosis (most commonly seen in the elderly); and (5) rarely periarticular tophus-like nodules.

The knee is the joint most frequently affected in CPPD arthropathy. Other sites include the wrist, shoulder, ankle, elbow, and hands. The temporomandibular joint may be involved. Clinical and radiographic evidence indicates that CPPD deposition is polyarticular in at least two-thirds of patients. When the clinical picture resembles that of slowly progressive osteoarthritis, diagnosis may be difficult. Joint distribution may provide important clues suggesting CPPD disease. For example, primary osteoarthritis less often involves metacarpophalangeal, wrist, elbow, shoulder, or ankle joints. If radiographs or ultrasound reveal punctate and/or linear radiodense deposits within fibrocartilaginous joint menisci or articular hyaline cartilage (*chondrocalcinosis*), the diagnostic likelihood of CPPD disease is further increased. *Definitive diagnosis* requires demonstration of typical rhomboid or rodlike crystals (generally weakly positively birefringent or nonbirefringent with polarized light) in synovial fluid or articular tissue (Fig. 395-2). In the absence of joint effusion or indications to obtain a synovial biopsy, chondrocalcinosis is presumptive of CPPD. One exception is chondrocalcinosis due to CaOx in some patients with chronic renal failure.

Acute attacks of CPPD arthritis may be precipitated by trauma. Rapid diminution of serum calcium concentration, as may occur in severe medical illness or after surgery (especially parathyroidectomy), can also lead to attacks.

In as many as 50% of cases, episodes of CPPD-induced inflammation are associated with low-grade fever and, on occasion, temperatures as high as 40°C (104°F). In such cases, synovial fluid analysis with microbial cultures is essential to rule out the possibility of infection. In fact, infection in a joint with any microcrystalline deposition process can lead to crystal shedding and subsequent synovitis from both crystals and microorganisms. The leukocyte count in synovial fluid in acute CPPD can range from several thousand cells to 100,000 cells/μL, with the mean being about 24,000 cells/μL and the predominant cell being the neutrophil. CPP crystals may be seen inside tissue fragments and fibrin clots and in neutrophils (Fig. 395-2). CPP crystals may coexist with MSU and apatite in some cases.

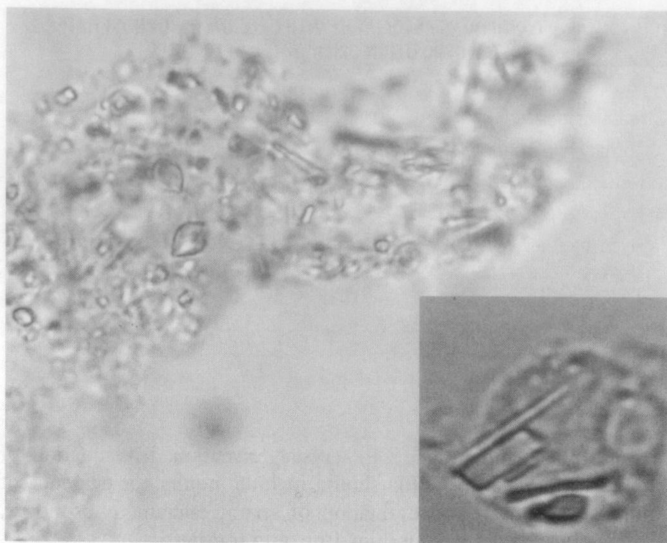

FIGURE 395-2 Intracellular and extracellular calcium pyrophosphate (CPP) crystals, as seen in a fresh preparation of synovial fluid, illustrate rectangular, rod-shaped, and rhomboid crystals that are weakly positively or nonbirefringent crystals (compensated polarized light microscopy; 400×).

TREATMENT CPPD DISEASE

Untreated acute attacks may last a few days to as long as a month. Treatment by rest, joint aspiration, and NSAIDs or by intraarticular glucocorticoid injection may result in more rapid return to prior status. For patients with frequent recurrent attacks, daily prophylactic treatment with low doses of colchicine may be helpful in decreasing the frequency of the attacks. Severe polyarticular attacks usually require short courses of glucocorticoids or, as recently reported, an IL-1β antagonist, anakinra. Unfortunately, there is no effective way to remove CPP deposits from cartilage and synovium. Uncontrolled studies suggest that the administration of NSAIDS (with a gastric protective agent if required), hydroxychloroquine, or even methotrexate may be helpful in controlling persistent synovitis. Patients with progressive destructive large-joint arthropathy may require joint replacement.

CALCIUM APATITE DEPOSITION DISEASE

PATHOGENESIS

Apatite is the primary mineral of normal bone and teeth. Abnormal accumulation of basic calcium phosphates, largely carbonate substituted apatite, can occur in areas of tissue damage (dystrophic calcification), hypercalcemic or hyperparathyroid states (metastatic calcification), and certain conditions of unknown cause (Table 395-3). In chronic renal failure, hyperphosphatemia can contribute to extensive apatite deposition both in and around joints. Familial aggregation is rarely seen; no association with *ANKH* mutations has been described thus far. Apatite crystals are deposited primarily on matrix vessels. Incompletely understood alterations in matrix proteoglycans, phosphatases, hormones, and cytokines probably can influence crystal formation.

Apatite aggregates are commonly present in synovial fluid in an extremely destructive chronic arthropathy of the elderly that occurs most often in the shoulders (Milwaukee shoulder) and in a similar process in hips, knees, and erosive osteoarthritis of fingers. Joint destruction is associated with damage to cartilage and supporting structures, leading to instability and deformity. Progression tends to be indolent. Symptoms range from minimal to severe pain and disability that may lead to joint replacement surgery. Whether severely affected patients represent an extreme synovial tissue response to the apatite crystals that are so common in osteoarthritis is uncertain. Synovial lining cell or fibroblast cultures exposed to apatite (or CPP) crystals can undergo mitosis and markedly increase the release of prostaglandin E_2, various cytokines, and also collagenases and neutral proteases, underscoring the destructive potential of abnormally stimulated synovial lining cells.

TABLE 395-3 CONDITIONS ASSOCIATED WITH APATITE DEPOSITION DISEASE

Aging
Osteoarthritis
Hemorrhagic shoulder effusions in the elderly (Milwaukee shoulder)
Destructive arthropathy
Tendinitis, bursitis
Tumoral calcinosis (sporadic cases)
Disease-associated
Hyperparathyroidism
Milk-alkali syndrome
Renal failure/long-term dialysis
Connective tissue diseases (e.g., systemic sclerosis, dermatomyositis, SLE)
Heterotopic calcification after neurologic catastrophes (e.g., stroke, spinal cord injury)
Heredity
Bursitis, arthritis
Tumoral calcinosis
Fibrodysplasia ossificans progressiva

Abbreviation: SLE, systemic lupus erythematosus.

CLINICAL MANIFESTATIONS

Periarticular or articular deposits may occur and may be associated with acute reversible inflammation and/or chronic damage to the joint capsule, tendons, bursa, or articular surfaces. The most common sites of apatite deposition include bursae and tendons in and/or around the knees, shoulders, hips, and fingers. Clinical manifestations include asymptomatic radiographic abnormalities, acute synovitis, bursitis, tendinitis, and chronic destructive arthropathy. Although the true incidence of apatite arthritis is not known, 30–50% of patients with osteoarthritis have apatite microcrystals in their synovial fluid. Such crystals frequently can be identified in clinically stable osteoarthritic joints, but they are more likely to come to attention in persons experiencing acute or subacute worsening of joint pain and swelling. The synovial fluid leukocyte count in apatite arthritis is usually low (<2000/μL) despite dramatic symptoms, with predominance of mononuclear cells.

DIAGNOSIS

Intra- and/or periarticular calcifications with or without erosive, destructive, or hypertrophic changes may be seen on radiographs (Fig. 395-3). They should be distinguished from the linear calcifications typical of CPPD.

Definitive diagnosis of apatite arthropathy, also called basic calcium phosphate disease, depends on identification of crystals from synovial fluid or tissue (Fig. 395-3). Individual crystals are very small and can be seen only by electron microscopy. Clumps of crystals may appear as 1- to 20-μm shiny intra- or extracellular nonbirefringent globules or aggregates that stain purplish with Wright's stain and bright red with alizarin red S. Tetracycline binding and other investigative techniques are under consideration as labeling alternatives. Absolute identification depends on electron microscopy with energy-dispersive elemental analysis, x-ray diffraction, infrared spectroscopy, or Raman microspectroscopy, but these techniques usually are not required in clinical diagnosis.

TREATMENT CALCIUM APATITE DEPOSITION DISEASE

Treatment of apatite arthritis or periarthritis is nonspecific. Acute attacks of bursitis or synovitis may be self-limiting, resolving in days to several weeks. Aspiration of effusions and the use of either NSAIDs or oral colchicine for 2 weeks or intra- or periarticular injection of a depot glucocorticoid appear to shorten the duration and

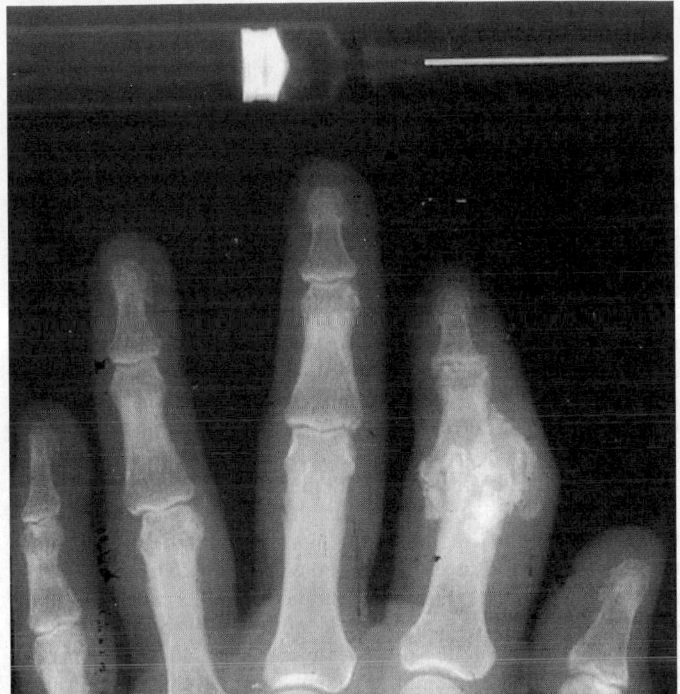

A

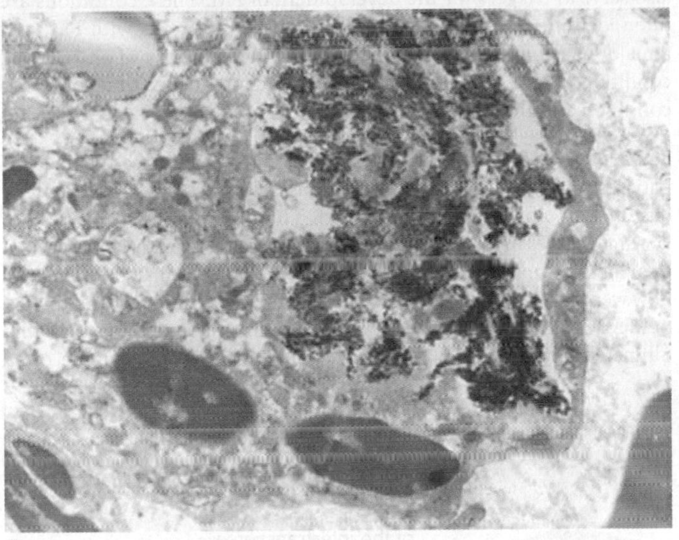

B

FIGURE 395-3 ***A.*** Radiograph showing calcification due to apatite crystals surrounding an eroded joint. ***B.*** An electron micrograph demonstrates dark needle-shaped apatite crystals within a vacuole of a synovial fluid mononuclear cell (30,000×).

intensity of symptoms. Local injection of disodium ethylenediaminetetraacetic acid (EDTA) and SC anakinra have been suggested as effective in single studies of acute calcific tendinitis at the shoulder. Other reports have described that IV gamma globulin, rituximab, calcium channel blockers, or bisphosphonates may help diffuse calcinosis. Periarticular apatite deposits may be resorbed with resolution of attacks. Agents to lower serum phosphate levels may lead to resorption of deposits in renal failure patients receiving hemodialysis. In patients with underlying severe destructive articular changes, response to medical therapy is usually less rewarding.

CAOX DEPOSITION DISEASE

PATHOGENESIS

Primary oxalosis is a rare hereditary metabolic disorder (Chap. 434e). Enhanced production of oxalic acid may result from at least two

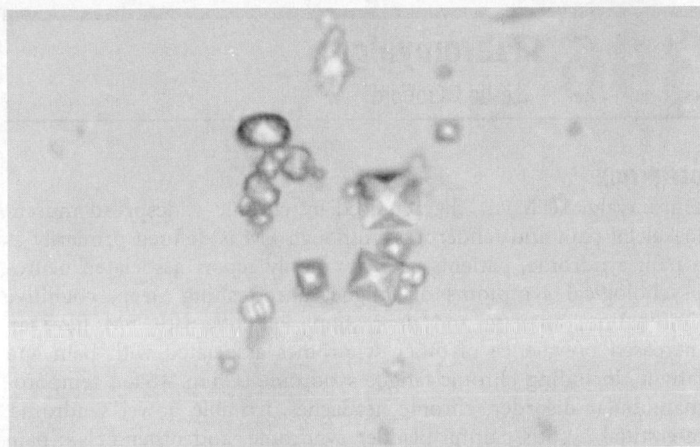

FIGURE 395-4 Bipyramidal and small polymorphic calcium oxalate crystals from synovial fluid are a classic finding in calcium oxalate arthropathy (ordinary light microscopy; 400×).

different enzyme defects, leading to hyperoxalemia and deposition of CaOx crystals in tissues. Nephrocalcinosis and renal failure are typical results. Acute and/or chronic CaOx arthritis, periarthritis, and bone disease may complicate primary oxalosis during later years of illness.

Secondary oxalosis is more common than the primary disorder. In chronic renal disease, calcium oxalate deposits have long been recognized in visceral organs, blood vessels, bones, and cartilage and are now known to be one of the causes of arthritis in chronic renal failure. Thus far, reported patients have been dependent on long-term hemodialysis or peritoneal dialysis (Chap. 336), and many had received ascorbic acid supplements. Ascorbic acid is metabolized to oxalate, which is inadequately cleared in uremia and by dialysis. Such supplements and foods high in oxalate content usually are avoided in dialysis programs because of the risk of enhancing hyperoxalosis and its sequelae.

CLINICAL MANIFESTATIONS AND DIAGNOSIS

CaOx aggregates can be found in bone, articular cartilage, synovium, and periarticular tissues. From these sites, crystals may be shed, causing acute synovitis. Persistent aggregates of CaOx can, like apatite and CPP, stimulate synovial cell proliferation and enzyme release, resulting in progressive articular destruction. Deposits have been documented in fingers, wrists, elbows, knees, ankles, and feet.

Clinical features of acute CaOx arthritis may not be distinguishable from those due to urate, CPP, or apatite. Radiographs may reveal chondrocalcinosis or soft tissue calcifications. CaOx-induced synovial effusions are usually noninflammatory, with <2000 leukocytes/μL, or mildly inflammatory. Neutrophils or mononuclear cells can predominate. CaOx crystals have a variable shape and variable birefringence to polarized light. The most easily recognized forms are bipyramidal, have strong birefringence (Fig. 395-4), and stain with alizarin red S.

TREATMENT CALCIUM OXALATE DEPOSITION DISEASE

Treatment of CaOx arthropathy with NSAIDs, colchicine, intraarticular glucocorticoids, and/or an increased frequency of dialysis has produced only slight improvement. In primary oxalosis, liver transplantation has induced a significant reduction in crystal deposits (Chap. 434e).

ACKNOWLEDGMENT

This chapter has been revised for this and the previous two editions from an original version written by Antonio Reginato, MD, in earlier editions of Harrison's Principles of Internal Medicine.

396 Fibromyalgia

Leslie J. Crofford

DEFINITION

Fibromyalgia (FM) is characterized by chronic widespread musculoskeletal pain and tenderness. Although FM is defined primarily as a pain syndrome, patients also commonly report associated neuropsychological symptoms of fatigue, unrefreshing sleep, cognitive dysfunction, anxiety, and depression. Patients with FM have an increased prevalence of other syndromes associated with pain and fatigue, including chronic fatigue syndrome (Chap. 464e), temporomandibular disorder, chronic headaches, irritable bowel syndrome, interstitial cystitis/painful bladder syndrome, and other pelvic pain syndromes. Available evidence implicates the central nervous system as key to maintaining pain and other core symptoms of FM and related conditions. The presence of FM is associated with substantial negative consequences for physical and social functioning.

EPIDEMIOLOGY

In clinical settings, a diagnosis of FM is made in ~2% of the population and is far more common in women than in men, with a ratio of ~9:1. However, in population-based survey studies worldwide, the prevalence rate is ~2–5%, with a female-to-male ratio of only 2–3:1 and with some variability depending on the method of ascertainment. The prevalence data are similar across socioeconomic classes. Cultural factors may play a role in determining whether patients with FM symptoms seek medical attention; however, even in cultures in which secondary gain is not expected to play a significant role, the prevalence of FM remains in this range.

CLINICAL MANIFESTATIONS

Pain and Tenderness At presentation, patients with FM most commonly report "pain all over." These patients have pain that is typically both above and below the waist on both sides of the body and involves the axial skeleton (neck, back, or chest). The pain attributable to FM is poorly localized, difficult to ignore, severe in its intensity, and associated with a reduced functional capacity. For a diagnosis of FM, pain should have been present most of the day on most days for at least 3 months.

The clinical pain of FM is associated with increased evoked pain sensitivity. In clinical practice, this elevated sensitivity may be determined by a tender-point examination in which the examiner uses the thumbnail to exert pressure of ~4 kg/m^2 (or the amount of pressure leading to blanching of the tip of the thumbnail) on well-defined musculotendinous sites (Fig. 396-1). Previously, the classification criteria of the American College of Rheumatology required that 11 of 18 sites be perceived as painful for a diagnosis of FM. In practice, tenderness is a continuous variable, and strict application of a categorical threshold for diagnostic specifics is not necessary. Newer criteria eliminate the need for tender points and focus instead on clinical symptoms of widespread pain and neuropsychological symptoms. The newer criteria perform well in a clinical setting in comparison to the older, tender-point criteria. However, it appears that when the new criteria are applied to populations, the result is an increase in prevalence of FM and a change in the sex ratio (see "Epidemiology," earlier).

Patients with FM often have peripheral pain generators that are thought to serve as triggers for the more widespread pain attributed to central nervous system factors. Potential pain generators such as arthritis, bursitis, tendinitis, neuropathies, and other inflammatory or degenerative conditions should be identified by history and physical examination. More subtle pain generators may include joint hypermobility and scoliosis. In addition, patients may have chronic myalgias triggered by infectious, metabolic, or psychiatric conditions that can also serve as triggers for the development of FM. These conditions are often identified in the differential diagnosis of patients with FM, and a major challenge is to distinguish the ongoing activity of a triggering condition from FM that is occurring as a consequence of a comorbid condition and that should itself be treated.

Neuropsychological Symptoms In addition to widespread pain, FM patients typically report fatigue, stiffness, sleep disturbance, cognitive dysfunction, anxiety, and depression. These symptoms are present to varying degrees in most FM patients but are not present in every patient or at all times in a given patient. Relative to pain, such symptoms may, however, have an equal or even greater impact on function and quality of life. Fatigue is highly prevalent in patients under primary care who ultimately are diagnosed with FM. Pain, stiffness, and fatigue often

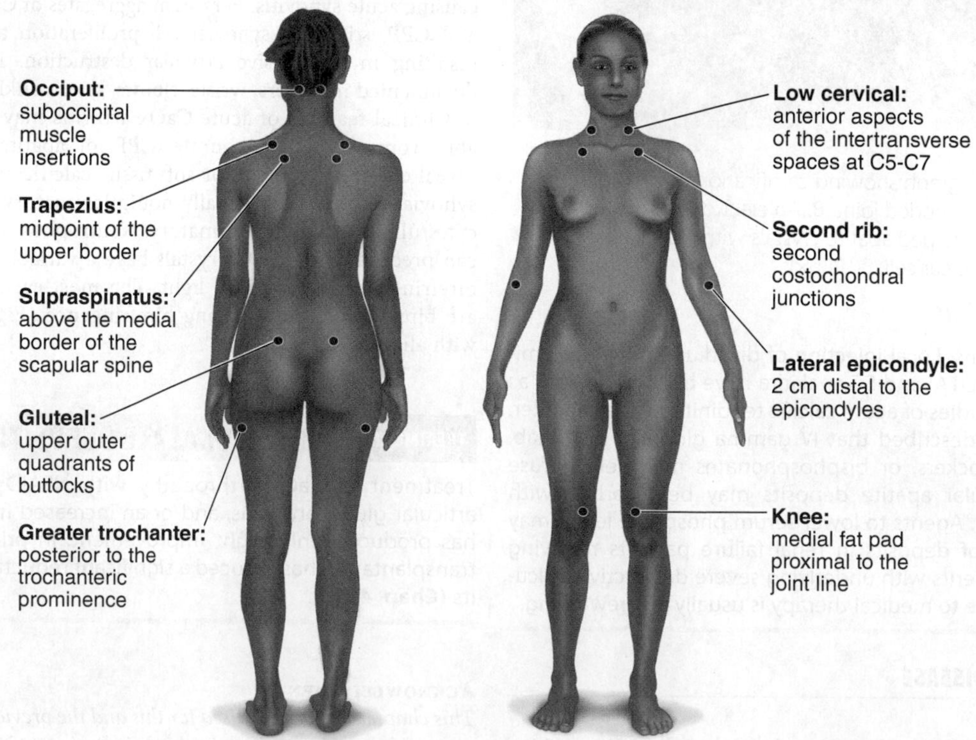

FIGURE 396-1 Tender-point assessment in patients with fibromyalgia. *(Figure created using data from F Wolfe et al: Arthritis Care Res 62:600, 2010.)*

are worsened by exercise or unaccustomed activity (postexertional malaise). The sleep complaints include difficulty falling asleep, difficulty staying asleep, and early-morning awakening. Regardless of the specific complaint, patients awake feeling unrefreshed. Patients with FM may meet criteria for restless legs syndrome and sleep-disordered breathing; frank sleep apnea can also be documented. Cognitive issues are characterized as slowness in processing, difficulties with attention or concentration, problems with word retrieval, and short-term memory loss. Studies have demonstrated altered cognitive function in these domains in patients with FM, though speed of processing is age-appropriate. Symptoms of anxiety and depression are common, and the lifetime prevalence of mood disorders in patients with FM approaches 80%. Although depression is neither necessary nor sufficient for the diagnosis of FM, it is important to screen for major depressive disorders by querying for depressed mood and anhedonia. Analysis of genetic factors that are likely to predispose to FM reveals shared neurobiologic pathways with mood disorders, providing the basis for comorbidity (see later in this chapter).

Overlapping Syndromes Because FM can overlap in presentation with other chronic pain conditions, review of systems often reveals headaches, facial/jaw pain, regional myofascial pain particularly involving the neck or back, and arthritis. Visceral pain involving the gastrointestinal tract, bladder, and pelvic or perineal region is often present as well. Patients may or may not meet defined criteria for specific syndromes. It is important for patients to understand that shared pathways may mediate symptoms and that treatment strategies effective for one condition may help with global symptom management.

Comorbid Conditions FM is often comorbid with chronic musculoskeletal, infectious, metabolic, or psychiatric conditions. Whereas FM affects only 2–5% of the general population, it occurs in 20% or more of patients with degenerative or inflammatory rheumatic disorders, likely because these conditions serve as peripheral pain generators to alter central pain-processing pathways. Similarly, chronic infectious, metabolic, or psychiatric diseases associated with musculoskeletal pain can mimic FM and/or serve as a trigger for the development of FM. It is particularly important for clinicians to be sensitive to pain management of these comorbid conditions so that when FM emerges—characterized by pain outside the boundaries of what could reasonably be explained by the triggering condition, development of neuropsychological symptoms, or tenderness on physical examination—treatment of central pain processes will be undertaken as opposed to a continued focus on treatment of peripheral or inflammatory causes of pain.

Psychosocial Considerations Symptoms of FM often have their onset and are exacerbated during periods of high-level real or perceived stress. This pattern may reflect an interaction among central stress physiology, vigilance or anxiety, and central pain-processing pathways. An understanding of current psychosocial stressors will aid in patient management, as many factors that exacerbate symptoms cannot be addressed by pharmacologic approaches. Furthermore, there is a high prevalence of exposure to previous interpersonal and other forms of violence in patients with FM and related conditions. If posttraumatic stress disorder is an issue, the clinician should be aware of it and consider treatment options.

Functional Impairment It is crucial to evaluate the impact of FM symptoms on function and role fulfillment. In defining the success of a management strategy, improved function is a key measure. Functional assessment should include physical, mental, and social domains. A recognition of the ways in which role functioning falls short will be helpful in the establishment of treatment goals.

DIFFERENTIAL DIAGNOSIS

Because musculoskeletal pain is such a common complaint, the differential diagnosis of FM is broad. Table 396-1 lists some of the more common conditions that should be considered. Patients with inflammatory causes for widespread pain should be identifiable on the basis of specific history, physical findings, and laboratory or radiographic tests.

TABLE 396-1 COMMON CONDITIONS IN THE DIFFERENTIAL DIAGNOSIS OF FIBROMYALGIA

Inflammatory
Polymyalgia rheumatica
Inflammatory arthritis: rheumatoid arthritis, spondyloarthritides
Connective tissue diseases: systemic lupus erythematosus, Sjögren's syndrome
Infectious
Hepatitis C
HIV infection
Lyme disease
Parvovirus B19 infection
Epstein-Barr virus infection
Noninflammatory
Degenerative joint/spine/disk disease
Myofascial pain syndromes
Bursitis, tendinitis, repetitive strain injuries
Endocrine
Hypo- or hyperthyroidism
Hyperparathyroidism
Neurologic Diseases
Multiple sclerosis
Neuropathic pain syndromes
Psychiatric Disease
Major depressive disorder
Drugs
Statins
Aromatase inhibitors

LABORATORY OR RADIOGRAPHIC TESTING

Routine laboratory and radiographic tests yield normal results in FM. Thus diagnostic testing is focused on exclusion of other diagnoses and evaluation for pain generators or comorbid conditions (Table 396-2). Most patients with new chronic widespread pain should be assessed for the most common entities in the differential diagnosis. Radiographic testing should be used sparingly and only for diagnosis of inflammatory arthritis. After the patient has been evaluated thoroughly, repeat testing is discouraged unless the symptom complex changes. Particularly to be discouraged is advanced imaging (MRI) of the spine unless there are features suggesting inflammatory spine disease or neurologic symptoms.

GENETICS AND PHYSIOLOGY

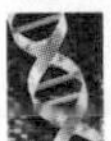

As in most complex diseases, it is likely that a number of genes contribute to vulnerability to the development of FM. To date, these genes appear to be in pathways controlling pain and stress

TABLE 396-2 LABORATORY AND RADIOGRAPHIC TESTING IN PATIENTS WITH FIBROMYALGIA SYMPTOMS

Routine
Erythrocyte sedimentation rate (ESR) or C-reactive protein (CRP)
Complete blood count (CBC)
Thyroid-stimulating hormone (TSH)
Guided by History and Physical Examination
Complete metabolic panel
Antinuclear antibody (ANA)
Anti-SSA (anti–Sjögren's syndrome A) and anti-SSB
Rheumatoid factor and anti–cyclic citrullinated peptide (anti-CCP)
Creatine phosphokinase (CPK)
Viral and bacterial serologies
Spine and joint radiographs

Source: LM Arnold et al: J Women's Health 21:231, 2012; MA Fitzcharles et al: J Rheumatol 40:1388, 2013.

responses. Some of the genetic underpinnings of FM are shared across other chronic pain conditions. Genes associated with metabolism, transport, and receptors of serotonin and other monoamines have been implicated in FM and overlapping conditions. Genes associated with other pathways involved in pain transmission have also been described as vulnerability factors for FM. Taken together, the pathways in which polymorphisms have been identified in FM patients further implicate central factors in mediation of the physiology that leads to the clinical manifestations of FM.

Psychophysical testing of patients with FM has demonstrated altered sensory afferent pain processing and impaired descending noxious inhibitory control leading to hyperalgesia and allodynia. Functional MRI and other research imaging procedures clearly demonstrate activation of the brain regions involved in the experience of pain in response to stimuli that are innocuous in study participants without FM. Pain perception in FM patients is influenced by the emotional and cognitive dimensions, such as catastrophizing and perceptions of control, providing a solid basis for recommendations for cognitive and behavioral treatment strategies.

APPROACH TO THE PATIENT: Fibromyalgia

FM is common and has an extraordinary impact on the patient's function and health-related quality of life. However, its symptoms and impact can be managed effectively by physicians and other health professionals. Developing a partnership with patients is essential for improving the outcome of FM, with a goal of understanding the factors involved, implementing a treatment strategy, and choosing appropriate nonpharmacologic and pharmacologic treatments.

TREATMENT FIBROMYALGIA

NONPHARMACOLOGIC TREATMENT

Patients with chronic pain, fatigue, and other neuropsychological symptoms require a framework for understanding the symptoms that have such an important impact on their function and quality of life. Explaining the genetics, triggers, and physiology of FM can be an important adjunct in relieving associated anxiety and in reducing the overall cost of health care resources. In addition, patients must be educated regarding expectations for treatment. The physician should focus on improved function and quality of life rather than elimination of pain. Illness behaviors, such as frequent physician visits, should be discouraged and behaviors that focus on improved function strongly encouraged.

Treatment strategies should include physical conditioning, with encouragement to begin at low levels of aerobic exercise and to proceed with slow but consistent advancement. Patients who have been physically inactive or who report postexertional malaise may do best in supervised or water-based programs at the start. Activities that promote improved physical function with relaxation, such as yoga and Tai Chi, may also be helpful. Strength training may be recommended after patients reach their aerobic goals. Exercise programs are helpful in reducing tenderness and enhancing self-efficacy. Cognitive-behavioral strategies to improve sleep hygiene and reduce illness behaviors can also be helpful in management.

PHARMACOLOGIC APPROACHES

It is essential for the clinician to treat any comorbid triggering condition and to clearly delineate for the patient the treatment goals for each medication. For example, glucocorticoids or nonsteroidal anti-inflammatory drugs may be useful for management of inflammatory triggers but are not effective against FM-related symptoms. At present, the treatment approaches that have proved most successful in FM patients target afferent or descending pain pathways. Table 396-3 lists the drugs with demonstrated effectiveness. It should be emphasized strongly that opioid analgesics are to be avoided in patients with FM. These agents have no demonstrated efficacy in FM and are associated with opioid-induced hyperalgesia that can worsen both symptoms and function. Use of single agents to treat multiple symptom domains is strongly encouraged. For example, if a patient's symptom complex is dominated by pain and sleep disturbance, use of an agent that exerts both analgesic and sleep-promoting effects is desirable. These agents include sedating antidepressants such as amitriptyline and alpha-2-delta ligands such as gabapentin and pregabalin. For patients whose pain is associated with fatigue, anxiety, or depression, drugs that have both analgesic and antidepressant/anxiolytic effects, such as duloxetine or milnacipran, may be the best first choice.

TABLE 396-3 PHARMACOLOGIC AGENTS EFFECTIVE FOR TREATMENT OF FIBROMYALGIA

Antidepressants: balanced serotonin–norepinephrine reuptake inhibitors
Amitriptyline[a]
Duloxetine[b,c]
Milnacipran[b,c]
Anticonvulsants: ligands of the alpha-2-delta subunit of voltage-gated calcium channels
Gabapentin
Pregabalin[b]

[a]RA Moore et al: Cochrane Database Syst Rev 12:CD008242, 2012. [b]Approved by the U.S. Food and Drug Administration. [c]W Hauser et al: Cochrane Database Syst Rev 1: CD010292, 2013.

Source: LM Arnold: Arthritis Rheum 56:1336, 2007.

397 Arthritis Associated with Systemic Disease, and Other Arthritides

Carol A. Langford, Brian F. Mandell

ARTHRITIS ASSOCIATED WITH SYSTEMIC DISEASE

ARTHROPATHY OF ACROMEGALY

Acromegaly is the result of excessive production of growth hormone by an adenoma in the anterior pituitary gland (Chap. 403). The excessive secretion of growth hormone along with insulin-like growth factor I stimulates proliferation of cartilage, periarticular connective tissue, and bone, resulting in several musculoskeletal problems, including osteoarthritis, back pain, muscle weakness, and carpal tunnel syndrome.

Osteoarthritis is a common feature, most often affecting the knees, shoulders, hips, and hands. Single or multiple joints may be affected. Hypertrophy of cartilage initially produces radiographic widening of the joint space. The newly synthesized cartilage is abnormally susceptible to fissuring, ulceration, and destruction. Ligamental laxity of joints further contributes to the development of osteoarthritis. Cartilage degrades, the joint space narrows, and subchondral sclerosis and osteophytes develop. Joint examination reveals crepitus and laxity. Joint fluid is noninflammatory. Calcium pyrophosphate dihydrate crystals are found in the cartilage in some cases of acromegaly arthropathy and, when shed into the joint, can elicit attacks of pseudogout. Chondrocalcinosis may be observed on radiographs. Back pain is extremely common, perhaps as a result of spine hypermobility. Spine radiographs show normal or widened intervertebral disk spaces, hypertrophic anterior osteophytes, and ligamental calcification. The latter changes are similar to those observed in patients with diffuse idiopathic skeletal hyperostosis. Dorsal kyphosis in conjunction with elongation of the ribs contributes to the development of the barrel chest seen in acromegalic patients. The hands and feet become enlarged as a result of soft tissue proliferation. The fingers are thickened and have spadelike distal tufts. One-third of patients have a thickened heel pad. Approximately 25% of patients exhibit Raynaud's phenomenon. Carpal tunnel syndrome occurs in about half of patients. The median nerve is compressed by excess connective tissue in the carpal tunnel. Patients with acromegaly may develop proximal muscle weakness, which is thought to be caused by the effect of growth hormone on muscle. Serum muscle enzyme levels and electromyographic findings are normal. Muscle biopsy specimens contain muscle fibers of varying size without inflammation.

ARTHROPATHY OF HEMOCHROMATOSIS

Hemochromatosis is a disorder of iron storage. Absorption of excessive amounts of iron from the intestine leads to iron deposition in parenchymal cells, which results in impairment of organ function (Chap. 428). Symptoms of hemochromatosis usually begin between the ages of 40 and 60 but can appear earlier. Arthropathy, which occurs in 20–40% of patients, usually begins after the age of 50 and may be the first clinical feature of hemochromatosis. The arthropathy is an osteoarthritis-like disorder affecting the small joints of the hands and later the larger joints, such as knees, ankles, shoulders, and hips. The second and third metacarpophalangeal joints of both hands are often the first and most prominent joints affected; this clinical picture may provide an important clue to the possibility of hemochromatosis because these joints are not predominantly affected by "routine" osteoarthritis. Patients experience some morning stiffness and pain with use of involved joints. The affected joints are enlarged and mildly tender. Radiographs show narrowing of the joint space, subchondral sclerosis, subchondral cysts, and juxtaarticular proliferation of bone. Hooklike osteophytes are seen in up to 20% of patients; although they are regarded as a characteristic feature of hemochromatosis, they can also occur in osteoarthritis and are not disease specific. The synovial fluid is noninflammatory. The synovium shows mild to moderate proliferation of iron-containing lining cells, fibrosis, and some mononuclear cell infiltration. In approximately half of patients, there is evidence of calcium pyrophosphate deposition disease, and some patients late in the course of disease experience episodes of acute pseudogout (Chap. 395). An early diagnosis is suggested by high serum transferrin saturation, which is more sensitive than ferritin elevation.

Iron may damage the articular cartilage in several ways. Iron catalyzes superoxide-dependent lipid peroxidation, which may play a role in joint damage. In animal models, ferric iron has been shown to interfere with collagen formation and increase the release of lysosomal enzymes from cells in the synovial membrane. Iron inhibits synovial tissue pyrophosphatase in vitro and therefore may inhibit pyrophosphatase in vivo, resulting in chondrocalcinosis.

TREATMENT ARTHROPATHY OF HEMOCHROMATOSIS

The treatment of hemochromatosis is repeated phlebotomy. Unfortunately, this treatment has little effect on established arthritis, which, along with chondrocalcinosis, may progress. Symptom-based treatment of the arthritis consists of administration of acetaminophen and nonsteroidal anti-inflammatory drugs (NSAIDs), as tolerated. Acute pseudogout attacks are treated with high doses of an NSAID or a short course of glucocorticoids. Hip or knee total joint replacement has been successful in advanced disease.

HEMOPHILIC ARTHROPATHY

Hemophilia is a sex-linked recessive genetic disorder characterized by the absence or deficiency of factor VIII (hemophilia A, or classic hemophilia) or factor IX (hemophilia B, or Christmas disease) (Chap. 141). Hemophilia A constitutes 85% of cases. Spontaneous hemarthrosis is a common problem with both types of hemophilia and can lead to a deforming arthritis. The frequency and severity of hemarthrosis are related to the degree of clotting factor deficiency. Hemarthrosis is not common in other disorders of coagulation such as von Willebrand disease, factor V deficiency, warfarin therapy, or thrombocytopenia.

Hemarthrosis occurs after 1 year of age, when a child begins to walk and run. In order of frequency, the joints most commonly affected are the knees, ankles, elbows, shoulders, and hips. Small joints of the hands and feet are occasionally involved.

In the initial stage of arthropathy, hemarthrosis produces a warm, tensely swollen, and painful joint. The patient holds the affected joint in flexion and guards against any movement. Blood in the joint remains liquid because of the absence of intrinsic clotting factors and the absence of tissue thromboplastin in the synovium. The synovial blood is resorbed over a period of ≥1 week, with the precise interval depending on the size of the hemarthrosis. Joint function usually returns to normal or baseline in ~2 weeks. Low-grade temperature elevation may accompany hemarthrosis, but a fever >101°F (38.3°C) warrants concern about infection.

Recurrent hemarthrosis may result in chronic arthritis. The involved joints remain swollen, and flexion deformities develop. Joint motion may be restricted and function severely limited. Restricted joint motion or laxity with subluxation is a feature of end-stage disease.

Bleeding into muscle and soft tissue also causes musculoskeletal dysfunction. When bleeding into the iliopsoas muscle occurs, the hip is held in flexion because of the pain, resulting in a hip flexion contracture. Rotation of the hip is preserved, which distinguishes this problem from hemarthrosis or other causes of hip synovitis. Expansion of the hematoma may place pressure on the femoral nerve, resulting in femoral neuropathy. Hemorrhage into a closed compartment space, such as the calf or the volar compartment in the forearm, can result in muscle necrosis, neuropathy, and flexion deformities of the ankles, wrists, and fingers. When bleeding involves periosteum or bone, a painful pseudotumor forms. These pseudotumors occur distal to the elbows or knees in children and improve with treatment of hemophilia. Surgical removal is indicated if the pseudotumor continues to enlarge. In adults, pseudotumors develop in the femur and pelvis and are usually refractory to treatment. When bleeding occurs in muscle, cysts may develop within the muscle. Needle aspiration of a cyst is contraindicated because this procedure can induce further bleeding; however, if the cyst becomes secondarily infected, drainage may be necessary (after factor repletion).

Septic arthritis is rare in hemophilia and is difficult to distinguish from acute hemarthrosis on physical examination. If there is serious suspicion of an infected joint, the joint should be aspirated immediately, the fluid cultured, and treatment with broad-spectrum antibiotics administered, with coverage for microorganisms including *Staphylococcus*, until culture results become available. Clotting-factor deficiency should be corrected before arthrocentesis to minimize the risk of traumatic bleeding.

Radiographs of joints reflect the stage of disease. In early stages, there is only capsule distention; later, juxtaarticular osteopenia, marginal erosions, and subchondral cysts develop. Late in the disease, the joint space is narrowed and there is bony overgrowth similar to that in osteoarthritis.

TREATMENT HEMARTHROSIS

The treatment of musculoskeletal bleeding is initiated with the immediate infusion of factor VIII or IX at the first sign of joint or muscle hemorrhage. Patients who have developed factor inhibitors are at elevated risk for joint damage and may benefit from receiving recombinant activated factor VII or activated prothrombin complex concentrate. The joint should be rested in a position of forced extension, as tolerated, to avoid contracture. Analgesia should be provided; nonselective NSAIDs, which can diminish platelet function, should be avoided if possible. Selective cyclooxygenase-2 inhibitors do not interfere with platelet function, although cardiovascular and gastrointestinal risks must still be weighed. Synovectomy—open or arthroscopic—may be attempted in patients with chronic symptomatic synovial proliferation and recurrent hemarthrosis, although hypertrophied synovium is highly vascular and subject to bleeding. Both types of synovectomy reduce the number of hemarthroses. Open surgical synovectomy, however, is associated with some loss of range of motion. Both require aggressive prophylaxis against bleeding. Radiosynovectomy with either yttrium 90 silicate or phosphorus 31 colloid has been effective and may be attempted when surgical synovectomy is not practical. Total joint replacement is indicated for severe joint destruction and incapacitating pain.

ARTHROPATHIES ASSOCIATED WITH HEMOGLOBINOPATHIES

Sickle Cell Disease Sickle cell disease (Chap. 127) is associated with several musculoskeletal abnormalities (Table 397-1). Children under the age of 5 years may develop diffuse swelling, tenderness, and warmth of the hands and feet lasting 1–3 weeks. This condition, referred to as *sickle cell dactylitis* or *hand-foot syndrome*, has also been observed in sickle cell thalassemia. Dactylitis is believed to result from infarction of the bone marrow and cortical bone leading to periostitis and soft tissue swelling. Radiographs show periosteal elevation, subperiosteal new-bone formation, and areas of radiolucency and increased density involving the metacarpals, metatarsals, and proximal phalanges. These bone changes disappear after several months. The syndrome leaves little or no residual damage. Because hematopoiesis ceases in the small bones of the hands and feet with age, the syndrome is rarely seen after age 5.

Sickle cell crisis is associated with periarticular pain and occasionally with joint effusions. The joint and periarticular area are warm and tender. Knees and elbows are most often affected, but other joints can be involved. Joint effusions are usually noninflammatory. Acute synovial infarction can cause a sterile effusion with high neutrophil counts in synovial fluid. Synovial biopsies have shown mild lining-cell proliferation and microvascular thrombosis with infarctions. Scintigraphic studies have shown decreased marrow uptake adjacent to the involved joint. The treatment for sickle cell crisis is detailed in Chap. 127.

Patients with sickle cell disease seem predisposed to osteomyelitis, which commonly involves the long tubular bones (Chap. 158); *Salmonella* is a particularly common cause (Chap. 190). Radiographs of the involved site initially show periosteal elevation, with subsequent disruption of the cortex. Treatment of the infection results in healing of the bone lesion. In addition, sickle cell disease is associated with bone infarction resulting from vaso-occlusion secondary to the sickling of red cells. Bone infarction also occurs in hemoglobin sickle cell disease and sickle cell thalassemia (Chap. 127). The bone pain in sickle cell crisis is due to infarction of bone and bone marrow. In children, infarction of the epiphyseal growth plate interferes with normal growth of the affected extremity. Radiographically, infarction of the bone cortex results in periosteal elevation and irregular thickening of the bone cortex. Infarction in the bone marrow leads to lysis, fibrosis, and new bone formation. Clinical distinction between osteomyelitis and bone infarctions can be difficult; imaging can be helpful.

Avascular necrosis of the head of the femur occurs in ~5% of patients. It also occurs in the humeral head and less commonly in the distal femur, tibial condyles, distal radius, vertebral bodies, and other juxtaarticular sites. Irregularity of the femoral head and other articular surfaces often results in degenerative joint disease. Radiography of the affected joint may show patchy radiolucency and density followed by flattening of the bone. MRI is a sensitive technique for detecting early avascular necrosis as well as bone infarction elsewhere. Total hip replacement and placement of prostheses in other joints may improve function and relieve joint pain in these patients.

Septic arthritis is occasionally encountered in sickle cell disease (Chap. 157). Multiple joints may be infected. Joint infection may result from bacteremia due to splenic dysfunction or from contiguous osteomyelitis. The more common microorganisms include *Staphylococcus aureus*, *Streptococcus*, and *Salmonella*. *Salmonella* does not cause septic arthritis as frequently as it causes osteomyelitis. Acute gouty arthritis is uncommon in sickle cell disease, even though 40% of patients are hyperuricemic. However, it may occur in patients generally not expected to get gout (young patients, female patients). Hyperuricemia is due to overproduction of uric acid secondary to increased red cell turnover as well as suboptimal renal excretion. Attacks may be polyarticular, and diagnostic arthrocentesis should be performed to distinguish infection from gout or synovial infarction.

The bone marrow hyperplasia in sickle cell disease results in widening of the medullary cavities, thinning of the cortices, and coarse trabeculations and central cupping of the vertebral bodies. These changes are also seen to a lesser degree in hemoglobin sickle cell disease and sickle cell thalassemia. In normal individuals red marrow is located mostly in the axial skeleton, but in sickle cell disease red marrow is found in the bones of the extremities and even in the tarsal and carpal bones. Vertebral compression may lead to dorsal kyphosis, and softening of the bone in the acetabulum may result in protrusio acetabuli.

TABLE 397-1 MUSCULOSKELETAL ABNORMALITIES IN SICKLE CELL DISEASE

Sickle Cell Dactylitis	Avascular Necrosis
Joint effusions in sickle cell crises	Bone changes secondary to marrow hyperplasia
Osteomyelitis	Septic arthritis
Infarction of bone	Gouty arthritis
Infarction of bone marrow	

Thalassemia A congenital disorder of hemoglobin synthesis, β thalassemia is characterized by impaired production of β chains (Chap. 127). Bone and joint abnormalities occur in β thalassemia, being most common in the major and intermedia groups. In one study, ~50% of patients with β thalassemia had evidence of symmetric ankle arthropathy characterized by a dull aching pain that was aggravated by weight bearing. The onset came most often in the second or third decade of life. The degree of ankle pain in these patients varied. Some patients experienced self-limited ankle pain that occurred only after strenuous physical activity and lasted several days or weeks. Other patients had chronic ankle pain that became worse with walking. Symptoms eventually abated in a few patients. Compression of the ankle, calcaneus, or forefoot was painful in some patients. Synovial fluid from two patients was noninflammatory. Radiographs of the ankle showed osteopenia, widened medullary spaces, thin cortices, and coarse trabeculations—findings that are largely the result of bone marrow expansion. The joint space was preserved. Specimens of bone from three patients revealed osteomalacia, osteopenia, and microfractures. Increased numbers of osteoblasts as well as increased foci of bone resorption were present on the bone surface. Iron staining was found in the bone trabeculae, in osteoid, and in the cement line. Synovium showed hyperplasia of lining cells, which contained deposits of hemosiderin. This arthropathy was considered to be related to the underlying bone pathology. The role of iron overload or abnormal bone metabolism in the pathogenesis of this arthropathy is not known. The arthropathy was treated with analgesics and splints. Patients also received transfusions to decrease hematopoiesis and bone marrow expansion.

In patients with β-thalassemia major and β-thalassemia intermedia, other joints are also involved, including the knees, hips, and shoulders. Acquired hemochromatosis with arthropathy has been described in a patient with thalassemia. Gouty arthritis and septic arthritis can occur. Avascular necrosis is not a feature of thalassemia because there is no sickling of red cells leading to thrombosis and infarction.

β-Thalassemia minor (also known as *β-thalassemia trait*) is likewise associated with joint manifestations. Chronic seronegative oligoarthritis affecting predominantly ankles, wrists, and elbows has been described; the affected patients had mild persistent synovitis without large effusions or joint erosions. Recurrent episodes of acute asymmetric arthritis have also been reported; episodes last <1 week and may affect the knees, ankles, shoulders, elbows, wrists, and metacarpal phalangeal joints. The mechanism underlying this arthropathy is unknown. Treatment with NSAIDs is not particularly effective.

MUSCULOSKELETAL DISORDERS ASSOCIATED WITH HYPERLIPIDEMIA

(See also Chap. 421) Musculoskeletal or cutaneous manifestations may be the first clinical indication of a specific hereditary disorder of lipoprotein metabolism. Patients with familial hypercholesterolemia (previously referred to as *type II hyperlipoproteinemia*) may have recurrent migratory polyarthritis involving the knees and other large peripheral joints and, to a lesser degree, peripheral small joints. Pain ranges from moderate to incapacitating. The involved joints can be warm, erythematous, swollen, and tender. Arthritis usually has a sudden onset, lasts from a few days to 2 weeks, and does not cause joint damage. Episodes may suggest acute gout attacks. Several attacks occur per year. Synovial fluid from involved joints is not inflammatory and contains few white cells and no crystals. Joint involvement may actually represent inflammatory periarthritis or peritendinitis and not true arthritis. The recurrent, transient nature of the arthritis may suggest rheumatic fever, especially because patients with hyperlipoproteinemia may have an elevated erythrocyte sedimentation rate and elevated antistreptolysin O titers (the latter being quite common). Attacks of tendinitis, including the large Achilles and patellar tendons, may come on gradually and last only a few days or may be acute as described above. Patients may be asymptomatic between attacks. Achilles tendinitis and other joint manifestations often precede the appearance of xanthomas and may be the first clinical indication of hyperlipoproteinemia. Attacks of tendinitis may follow treatment with a lipid-lowering drug. Over time, patients may develop tendinous xanthomas in the Achilles, patellar, and extensor tendons of the hands and feet. Xanthomas have also been reported in the peroneal tendon, the plantar aponeurosis, and the periosteum overlying the distal tibia. These xanthomas are located within tendon fibers. Tuberous xanthomas are soft subcutaneous masses located over the extensor surfaces of the elbows, knees, and hands as well as on the buttocks. They appear during childhood in homozygous patients and after the age of 30 in heterozygous patients. Patients with elevated plasma levels of very-low-density lipoprotein (VLDL) and triglycerides (previously referred to as *type IV hyperlipoproteinemia*) may also have a mild inflammatory arthritis affecting large and small peripheral joints, usually in an asymmetric pattern, with only a few joints involved at a time. The onset of arthritis usually comes in middle age. Arthritis may be persistent or recurrent, with episodes lasting a few days or weeks. Some patients may experience severe joint pain or morning stiffness. Joint tenderness and periarticular hyperesthesia may also be present, as may synovial thickening. Joint fluid is usually noninflammatory and without crystals but may have increased white blood cell counts with predominantly mononuclear cells. Radiographs may show juxtaarticular osteopenia and cystic lesions. Large bone cysts have been noted in a few patients. Xanthoma and bone cysts are also observed in other lipoprotein disorders. The pathogenesis of arthritis in patients with familial hypercholesterolemia or with elevated levels of VLDL and triglycerides is not well understood. NSAIDs or analgesics usually provide adequate relief of symptoms when used on an as-needed basis.

Patients may improve clinically as they are treated with lipid-lowering agents; however, patients treated with an HMG-CoA reductase inhibitor may experience myalgias, and a few patients develop myopathy, myositis, or even rhabdomyolysis. Patients who develop myositis during statin therapy may be susceptible to this adverse effect because of an underlying muscle disorder and should be reevaluated after discontinuation of the drug. Myositis has also been reported with the use of niacin (Chap. 388) but is less common than myalgias.

Musculoskeletal syndromes have not clearly been associated with the more common mixed hyperlipidemias seen in general practice.

OTHER ARTHRITIDES

NEUROPATHIC JOINT DISEASE

Neuropathic joint disease (Charcot joint) is a progressive destructive arthritis associated with loss of pain sensation, proprioception, or both. Normal muscular reflexes that modulate joint movement are impaired. Without these protective mechanisms, joints are subjected to repeated trauma, resulting in progressive cartilage and bone damage. Today, diabetes mellitus is the most frequent cause of neuropathic joint disease (Fig. 397-1). A variety of other disorders are associated with neuropathic arthritis, including tabes dorsalis, leprosy, yaws, syringomyelia, meningomyelocele, congenital indifference to pain, peroneal muscular atrophy (Charcot-Marie-Tooth disease), and amyloidosis. An arthritis resembling neuropathic joint disease has been reported in patients who have received intraarticular glucocorticoid injections, but this is a rare complication and was not observed in one series of patients with knee osteoarthritis who received intraarticular glucocorticoid injections every 3 months for 2 years. The distribution of joint involvement depends on the underlying neurologic disorder (Table 397-2). In tabes dorsalis, the knees, hips, and ankles are most commonly affected; in syringomyelia, the glenohumeral joint, elbow, and wrist; and in diabetes mellitus, the tarsal and tarsometatarsal joints.

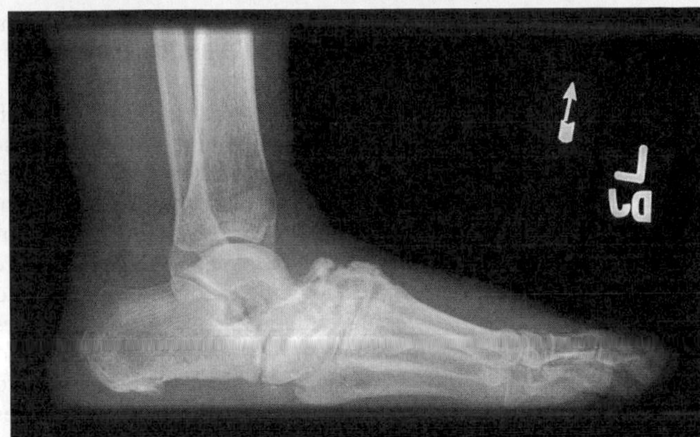

FIGURE 397-1 Charcot arthropathy associated with diabetes mellitus. Lateral foot radiograph demonstrating complete loss of the arch due to bony fragmentation and dislocation in the midfoot. *(Courtesy of Andrew Neckers, MD, and Jean Schils, MD; with permission.)*

PATHOLOGY AND PATHOPHYSIOLOGY

The pathologic changes in the neuropathic joint are similar to those found in the severe osteoarthritic joint. There is fragmentation and eventual loss of articular cartilage with eburnation of the underlying bone. Osteophytes are found at the joint margins. With more advanced disease, erosions are present on the joint surface. Fractures, devitalized bone, intraarticular loose bodies, and microscopic fragments of cartilage and bone may be present.

At least two underlying mechanisms are believed to be involved in the pathogenesis of neuropathic arthritis. An abnormal autonomic nervous system is thought to be responsible for the dysregulated blood flow to the joint with subsequent resorption of bone. Loss of bone, particularly in the diabetic foot, may be the initial finding. With the loss of deep pain, proprioception, and protective neuromuscular reflexes, the joint is subjected to repeated microtrauma, resulting in ligamental tears and bone fractures. The injury that follows frequent intraarticular glucocorticoid injections is thought to be due to the analgesic effect of glucocorticoids, leading to overuse of an already damaged joint; the result is accelerated cartilage damage, although steroid-induced cartilage damage be more common in some other animal species than in humans. It is not understood why only a few patients with neuropathy develop clinically evident neuropathic arthritis.

CLINICAL MANIFESTATIONS

Neuropathic joint disease usually begins in a single joint and then becomes apparent in other joints, depending on the underlying neurologic disorder. The involved joint becomes progressively enlarged as a result of bony overgrowth and synovial effusion. Loose bodies may be palpated in the joint cavity. Joint instability, subluxation, and crepitus occur as the disease progresses. Neuropathic joints may develop rapidly, and a totally disorganized joint with multiple bony fragments may evolve within weeks or months. The amount of pain experienced

TABLE 397-2 DISORDERS ASSOCIATED WITH NEUROPATHIC JOINT DISEASE

Diabetes mellitus	Amyloidosis
Tabes dorsalis	Leprosy
Meningomyelocele	Congenital indifference to pain
Syringomyelia	Peroneal muscular atrophy

by the patient is less than would be anticipated from the degree of joint damage. Patients may experience sudden joint pain from intraarticular fractures of osteophytes or condyles.

Neuropathic arthritis is encountered most often in patients with diabetes mellitus, with an incidence of ~0.5%. The onset of disease usually comes at an age of ≥50 years in a patient who has had diabetes for several years, but exceptions occur. The tarsal and tarsometatarsal joints are most often affected, with the metatarsophalangeal and talotibial joints next most commonly involved. The knees and spine are occasionally involved. Patients often attribute the onset of foot pain to antecedent trauma such as twisting of the foot. Neuropathic changes may develop rapidly after a foot fracture or dislocation. The foot and ankle are often swollen. Downward collapse of the tarsal bones leads to convexity of the sole, referred to as a "rocker foot." Large osteophytes may protrude from the top of the foot. Calluses frequently form over the metatarsal heads and may lead to infected ulcers and osteomyelitis. The value of protective inserts and orthotics, as well as regular foot examination, cannot be overstated. Radiographs may show resorption and tapering of the distal metatarsal bones. The term *Lisfranc fracture-dislocation* is sometimes used to describe the destructive changes at the tarsometatarsal joints.

DIAGNOSIS

The diagnosis of neuropathic arthritis is based on the clinical features and characteristic radiographic findings in a patient with underlying sensory neuropathy. The differential diagnosis of neuropathic arthritis depends upon the severity of the process and includes osteomyelitis, avascular necrosis, advanced osteoarthritis, stress fractures, and calcium pyrophosphate deposition disease. Radiographs in neuropathic arthritis initially show changes of osteoarthritis with joint space narrowing, subchondral bone sclerosis, osteophytes, and joint effusions; marked destructive and hypertrophic changes follow later. The radiographic findings of neuropathic arthritis may be difficult to differentiate from those of osteomyelitis, especially in the diabetic foot. The joint margins in a neuropathic joint tend to be distinct, while in osteomyelitis they are blurred. Imaging studies may be helpful, but cultures of tissue from the joint are often required to exclude osteomyelitis. MRI and bone scans using indium 111–labeled white blood cells or indium 111–labeled immunoglobulin G, which will show increased uptake in osteomyelitis but not in a neuropathic joint, may be useful. A technetium bone scan will not distinguish osteomyelitis from neuropathic arthritis, as increased uptake is observed in both. The joint fluid in neuropathic arthritis is noninflammatory; may be xanthochromic or even bloody; and may contain fragments of synovium, cartilage, and bone. The finding of calcium pyrophosphate dihydrate crystals supports the diagnosis of crystal-associated arthropathy. In the absence of such crystals, an increased number of leukocytes may indicate osteomyelitis.

TREATMENT NEUROPATHIC JOINT DISEASE

The primary focus of treatment is to stabilize the joint. Treatment of the underlying disorder, even if successful, does not usually affect established joint disease. Braces and splints are helpful. Their use requires close surveillance, because patients may be unable to appreciate pressure from a poorly adjusted brace. In the diabetic patient, early recognition of Charcot foot and its treatment—prohibition of weight bearing by the foot for at least 8 weeks—may possibly prevent severe disease from developing. Fusion of an unstable joint may improve function and reduce pain, but nonunion is frequent, especially when immobilization of the joint is inadequate.

HYPERTROPHIC OSTEOARTHROPATHY AND CLUBBING

Hypertrophic osteoarthropathy (HOA) is characterized by clubbing of digits and, in more advanced stages, by periosteal new-bone formation and synovial effusions. HOA may be primary or familial and may begin in childhood. Secondary HOA is associated with intrathoracic malignancies, suppurative and some hypoxemic lung diseases, congenital heart disease, and a variety of other disorders. Clubbing is almost always a feature of HOA but can occur as an isolated manifestation (Fig. 397-2). The presence of clubbing in isolation may be congenital or represent either an early stage or one element in the spectrum of HOA. Isolated acquired clubbing has the same clinical significance as clubbing associated with periostitis.

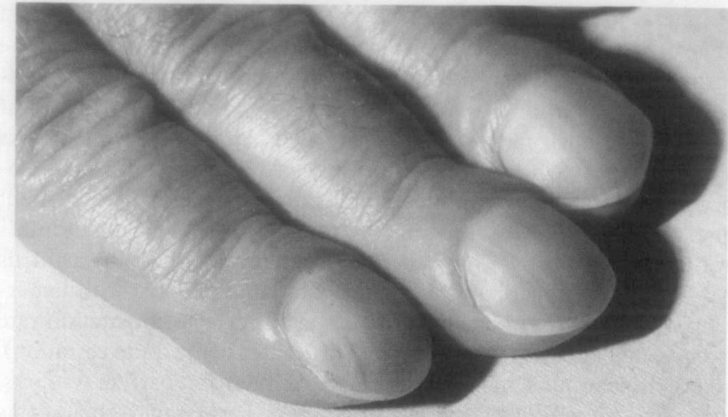

FIGURE 397-2 Clubbing of the fingers. *(Reprinted from the Clinical Slide Collection on the Rheumatic Diseases, © 1991, 1995. Used by permission of the American College of Rheumatology.)*

Pathology and Pathophysiology of Acquired HOA In HOA, bone changes in the distal extremities begin as periostitis followed by new bone formation. At this stage, a radiolucent area may be observed between the new periosteal bone and the subjacent cortex. As the process progresses, multiple layers of new bone are deposited and become contiguous with the cortex, with consequent cortical thickening. The outer portion of the bone is laminated in appearance, with an irregular surface. Initially, the process of periosteal new-bone formation involves the proximal and distal diaphyses of the tibia, fibula, radius, and ulna and, less frequently, the femur, humerus, metacarpals, metatarsals, and phalanges. Occasionally, scapulae, clavicles, ribs, and pelvic bones are also affected. The adjacent interosseous membranes may become ossified. The distribution of bone manifestations is usually bilateral and symmetric. The soft tissue overlying the distal third of the arms and legs may be thickened. Proliferation of connective tissue occurs in the nail bed and volar pad of digits, giving the distal phalanges a clubbed appearance. Small blood vessels in the clubbed digits are dilated and have thickened walls. In addition, the number of arteriovenous anastomoses is increased.

Several theories have been suggested for the pathogenesis of HOA, but many have been disproved or have not explained the condition's development in all clinical disorders with which it is associated. Previously proposed neurogenic and humoral theories are no longer considered likely explanations for HOA. Studies have suggested a role for platelets in the development of HOA. It has been observed that megakaryocytes and large platelet particles present in the venous circulation are fragmented in their passage through normal lung. In patients with cyanotic congenital heart disease and in other disorders associated with right-to-left shunts, these large platelet particles bypass the lung and reach the distal extremities, where they can interact with endothelial cells. Platelet–endothelial cell activation in the distal portion of the extremities may result in the release of platelet-derived growth factor (PDGF) and other factors leading to the proliferation of connective tissue and periosteum. Stimulation of fibroblasts by PDGF and transforming growth factor β results in cell growth and collagen synthesis. Elevated plasma levels of von Willebrand factor antigen have been found in patients with both primary and secondary forms of HOA, indicating endothelial activation or damage. Abnormalities of collagen synthesis have been demonstrated in the involved skin of patients with primary HOA. Other factors are undoubtedly involved in the pathogenesis of HOA, and further studies are needed to elucidate this disorder.

Clinical Manifestations Primary or familial HOA, also referred to as *pachydermoperiostitis* or *Touraine-Solente-Golé syndrome*, usually begins insidiously at puberty. In a smaller proportion of patients, the onset comes in the first year of life. The disorder is inherited as an autosomal dominant trait with variable expression and is nine times more common among boys than among girls. Approximately one-third of patients have a family history of primary HOA.

Primary HOA is characterized by clubbing, periostitis, and unusual skin features. A small number of patients with this syndrome do not express clubbing. The skin changes and periostitis are prominent features of this syndrome. The skin becomes thickened and coarse. Deep nasolabial folds develop, and the forehead may become furrowed. Patients may have heavy-appearing eyelids and ptosis. The skin is often greasy, and there may be excessive sweating of the hands and feet. Patients may also experience acne vulgaris, seborrhea, and folliculitis. In a few patients, the skin over the scalp becomes very thick and corrugated, a feature that has been descriptively termed *cutis verticis gyrata*. The distal extremities, particularly the legs, become thickened as a consequence of the proliferation of new bone and soft tissue; when the process is extensive, the distal lower extremities resemble those of an elephant. The periostitis usually is not painful, which it can be in secondary HOA. Clubbing of the fingers may be extensive, producing large, bulbous deformities and clumsiness. Clubbing also affects the toes. Patients may experience articular and periarticular pain, especially in the ankles and knees, and joint motion may be mildly restricted by periarticular bone overgrowth. Noninflammatory effusions occur in the wrists, knees, and ankles. Synovial hypertrophy is not found. Associated abnormalities observed in patients with primary HOA include hypertrophic gastropathy, bone marrow failure, female escutcheon, gynecomastia, and cranial suture defects. In patients with primary HOA, the symptoms disappear when adulthood is reached.

HOA secondary to an underlying disease occurs more frequently than primary HOA. It accompanies a variety of disorders and may precede clinical features of the associated disorder by months. Clubbing is more frequent than the full syndrome of HOA in patients with associated illnesses. Because clubbing evolves over months and is usually asymptomatic, it is often recognized first by the physician and not the patient. Patients may experience a burning sensation in their fingertips. Clubbing is characterized by widening of the fingertips, enlargement of the distal volar pad, convexity of the nail contour, and the loss of the normal 15° angle between the proximal nail and cuticle. The thickness of the digit at the base of the nail is greater than the thickness at the distal interphalangeal joint. An objective measurement of finger clubbing can be made by determining the diameter at the base of the nail and at the distal interphalangeal joint of all 10 digits. Clubbing is present when the sum of the individual digit ratios is >10. At the bedside, clubbing can be appreciated by having the patient place the dorsal surface of the distal phalanges of the fourth fingers together with the nails opposing each other. Normally, an open area is visible between the bases of the opposing fingernails; when clubbing is present, this open space is no longer visible. The base of the nail feels spongy when compressed, and the nail can be easily rocked on its bed. When clubbing is advanced, the finger may have a drumstick appearance, and the distal interphalangeal joint can be hyperextended. Periosteal involvement in the distal extremities may produce a burning or deep-seated aching pain. The pain, which can be quite incapacitating, is aggravated by dependency and relieved by elevation of the affected limbs. Pressure applied over the distal forearms and legs or gentle percussion of distal long bones like the tibia may be quite painful.

Patients may experience joint pain, most often in the ankles, wrists, and knees. Joint effusions may be present; usually, they are small and noninflammatory. The small joints of the hands are rarely affected. Severe joint or long bone pain may be the presenting symptom of an underlying lung malignancy and may precede the appearance of clubbing. In addition, the progression of HOA tends to be more rapid when associated with malignancies, most notably bronchogenic carcinoma. Noninflammatory but variably painful knee effusions may occur prior to the appearance of clubbing and symptoms of distal periostitis. Unlike primary HOA, secondary HOA does not commonly include excessive sweating and oiliness of the skin or thickening of the facial skin.

TABLE 397-3 DISORDERS ASSOCIATED WITH HYPERTROPHIC OSTEOARTHROPATHY

Pulmonary
Bronchogenic carcinoma and other neoplasms
Lung abscesses, empyema, bronchiectasis
Chronic interstitial pneumonitis
Cystic fibrosis
Sarcoidosis
Gastrointestinal
Inflammatory bowel disease
Sprue
Neoplasms: esophagus, liver, bowel
Cardiovascular
Cyanotic congenital heart disease
Subacute bacterial endocarditis
Infected arterial grafts[a]
Aortic aneurysm[b]
Aneurysm of major extremity artery[a]
Patent ductus arteriosus[b]
Arteriovenous fistula of major extremity vessel[a]
Thyroid (thyroid acropachy)
Hyperthyroidism (Graves' disease)

[a]Unilateral involvement. [b]Bilateral lower-extremity involvement.

HOA occurs in 5–10% of patients with intrathoracic malignancies, the most common being bronchogenic carcinoma and pleural tumors (Table 397-3). Lung metastases infrequently cause HOA. HOA is also seen in patients with intrathoracic infections, including lung abscesses, empyema, and bronchiectasis, but is uncommon in pulmonary tuberculosis. HOA may accompany chronic interstitial pneumonitis, sarcoidosis, and cystic fibrosis. In cystic fibrosis, clubbing is more common than the full syndrome of HOA. Other causes of clubbing include congenital heart disease with right-to-left shunts, bacterial endocarditis, Crohn's disease, ulcerative colitis, sprue, and neoplasms of the esophagus, liver, and small and large bowel. In patients who have congenital heart disease with right-to-left shunts, clubbing alone occurs more often than the full syndrome of HOA.

Unilateral clubbing has been found in association with aneurysms of major extremity arteries, with infected arterial grafts, and with arteriovenous fistulas of brachial vessels. Clubbing of the toes but not the fingers has been associated with an infected abdominal aortic aneurysm and patent ductus arteriosus. Clubbing of a single digit may follow trauma and has been reported in tophaceous gout and sarcoidosis. While clubbing occurs more commonly than the full syndrome in most diseases, periostitis in the absence of clubbing has been observed in the affected limb of patients with infected arterial grafts.

Hyperthyroidism (Graves' disease), treated or untreated, is occasionally associated with clubbing and periostitis of the bones of the hands and feet. This condition is referred to as *thyroid acropachy*. Periostitis may be asymptomatic and occurs in the midshaft and diaphyseal portion of the metacarpal and phalangeal bones. Significant hand-joint pain may occur; this pain may respond to successful therapy for thyroid dysfunction. The long bones of the extremities are seldom affected. Elevated levels of long-acting thyroid stimulator are found in the sera of these patients.

Laboratory Findings The laboratory abnormalities reflect the underlying disorder. The synovial fluid of involved joints has <500 white cells/μL, and the cells are predominantly mononuclear. Radiographs show a faint radiolucent line beneath the new periosteal bone along the shaft of long bones at their distal end. These changes are observed most frequently at the ankles, wrists, and knees. The ends of the distal phalanges may show osseous resorption. Radionuclide studies show pericortical linear uptake along the cortical margins of long bones that may precede any radiographic changes.

TREATMENT HYPERTROPHIC OSTEOARTHROPATHY

The treatment of HOA aims to identify the associated disorder and treat it appropriately. The symptoms and signs of HOA may disappear completely with removal of or effective chemotherapy for a tumor or with antibiotic therapy for a chronic pulmonary infection and drainage of the infected site. Vagotomy or percutaneous block of the vagus nerve leads to symptomatic relief in some patients. NSAIDs or analgesics may help control symptoms of HOA.

REFLEX SYMPATHETIC DYSTROPHY SYNDROME

The reflex sympathetic dystrophy syndrome is now referred to as *complex regional pain syndrome, type 1*, according to the new classification system of the International Association for the Study of Pain. This syndrome is characterized by pain and swelling, usually of a distal extremity, accompanied by vasomotor instability, trophic skin changes, and the rapid development of bony demineralization. Reflex sympathetic dystrophy syndrome, including its treatment, is covered in greater detail in Chap. 454.

TIETZE SYNDROME AND COSTOCHONDRITIS

Tietze syndrome is manifested by painful swelling of one or more costochondral articulations. The age of onset is usually before 40, and both sexes are affected equally. In most patients, only one joint is involved, usually the second or third costochondral joint. The onset of anterior chest pain may be sudden or gradual. The pain may radiate to the arms or shoulders and is aggravated by sneezing, coughing, deep inspirations, or twisting motions of the chest. The term *costochondritis* is often used interchangeably with *Tietze syndrome*, but some workers restrict the former term to pain of the costochondral articulations without swelling. Costochondritis is observed in patients over age 40; tends to affect the third, fourth, and fifth costochondral joints; and occurs more often in women. Both syndromes may mimic cardiac or upper abdominal causes of pain. Rheumatoid arthritis, ankylosing spondylitis, and reactive arthritis may involve costochondral joints but are distinguished easily by their other clinical features. Other skeletal causes of anterior chest wall pain are xiphoidalgia and the slipping rib syndrome, which usually involves the tenth rib. Malignancies such as breast cancer, prostate cancer, plasma cell cytoma, and sarcoma can invade the ribs, thoracic spine, or chest wall and produce symptoms suggesting Tietze syndrome. Patients with osteomalacia may have significant rib pain, with or without documented microfractures. These conditions should be distinguishable by radiography, bone scanning, vitamin D measurement, or biopsy. Analgesics, anti-inflammatory drugs, and local glucocorticoid injections usually relieve symptoms of costochondritis/Tietze syndrome. Care should be taken to avoid overdiagnosing these syndromes in patients with acute chest pain syndromes; many patients will be tender to overly vigorous palpation of the costochondral joints.

MYOFASCIAL PAIN SYNDROME

Myofascial pain syndrome is characterized by multiple areas of localized musculoskeletal pain and tenderness in association with tender points. The pain is deep and aching and may be accompanied by a burning sensation. Myofascial pain may be regional and follow trauma, overuse, or prolonged static contraction of a muscle or muscle group, which may occur when an individual is reading or writing at a desk or working at a computer. In addition, this syndrome may be associated with underlying osteoarthritis of the neck or low back. Pain may be referred from tender points to defined areas distant from the area of original tenderness. Palpation of the tender point reproduces or accentuates the pain. The tender points are usually located in the center of a muscle belly, but they can occur at other sites such as costosternal junctions, the xiphoid process, ligamentous and tendinous insertions, fascia, and fatty areas. Tender point sites in muscle have been described as feeling indurated and taut, and palpation may cause the muscle to twitch. These findings, however, have been shown not to be unique to myofascial pain syndrome: in a controlled study, they were also present in some "normal" subjects. Myofascial pain most often involves the posterior neck, low back, shoulders, and chest. Chronic pain in the muscles of the posterior neck may involve referral of pain from a tender point in the erector neck muscle or upper trapezius to the head, leading to persistent headaches that may last for days. Tender points in the paraspinal muscles of the low back may refer pain to the buttock. Pain may be referred down the leg from a tender point in the gluteus medius and can mimic sciatica. A tender point in the infraspinatus muscle may produce local and referred pain over the lateral deltoid and down the outside of the arm into the hand. Injection of a local anesthetic such as 1% lidocaine into the tender point site often results in at least transient pain relief. Another useful technique is first to spray an agent such as ethyl chloride from the tender point toward the area of referred pain and then to stretch the muscle. This maneuver may need to be repeated several times. Massage and application of ultrasound to the affected area also may be beneficial. Patients should be instructed in methods to prevent muscle stresses related to work and recreation. Posture and resting positions are important in preventing muscle tension. The prognosis in most patients is good. In some patients, regionally localized myofascial pain syndrome may seem to evolve into more generalized fibromyalgia (Chap. 396). Abnormal or nonrestorative sleep is a common accompaniment in these patients and may need to be specifically addressed.

NEOPLASIAS AND ARTHRITIS

Primary tumors and tumor-like disorders of synovium are uncommon but should be considered in the differential diagnosis of monarticular joint disease. In addition, metastases to bone and primary bone tumors adjacent to a joint may produce joint symptoms.

Pigmented villonodular synovitis (PVNS) is characterized by the slowly progressive, exuberant, benign proliferation of synovial tissue, usually involving a single joint. The most common age of onset is in the third decade, and women are affected slightly more often than men. The cause of this disorder is unknown.

The synovium has a brownish color and numerous large, finger-like villi that fuse to form pedunculated nodules. There is marked hyperplasia of synovial cells in the stroma of the villi. Hemosiderin granules and lipids are found in the cytoplasm of macrophages and in the interstitial tissue. Multinucleated giant cells may be present. The proliferative synovium grows into the subsynovial tissue and invades adjacent cartilage and bone.

The clinical picture of PVNS is characterized by the insidious onset of persistent swelling and pain in affected joints, most commonly the knee. Other joints affected include the hips, ankles, calcaneocuboid joints, elbows, and small joints of the fingers or toes. The disease may also involve the common flexor sheath of the hands or fingers. Less often, tendon sheaths in the wrist, ankle, or foot may be involved. Symptoms of pain, a catching sensation, or stiffness may initially be mild and intermittent and may be present for years before the patient seeks medical attention. Radiographs may show joint space narrowing, erosions, and subchondral cysts. The diagnosis of PVNS is strongly suggested by gradient echo MRI, which reveals a synovial mass lesion of low signal intensity typical of tissue containing hemosiderin (Fig. 397-3). The joint fluid contains blood and is dark red or almost black in color. Lipid-containing macrophages may be present in the fluid. The joint fluid may be clear if hemorrhage has not occurred. Some patients have polyarticular involvement.

The treatment for PVNS is complete synovectomy. With incomplete synovectomy, the villonodular synovitis recurs, and the rate of tissue growth may be faster than it was originally. Irradiation of the involved joint has been successful in some patients.

Synovial chondromatosis is a disorder characterized by multiple focal metaplastic growths of normal-appearing cartilage in the synovium or tendon sheath. Segments of cartilage break loose and continue to grow as loose bodies. When calcification and ossification of loose bodies occur, the disorder is referred to as *synovial osteochondromatosis*. The disorder is usually monarticular and affects young to middle-aged individuals. The knee is most often involved, followed by hip, elbow, and shoulder. Symptoms are pain, swelling, and decreased

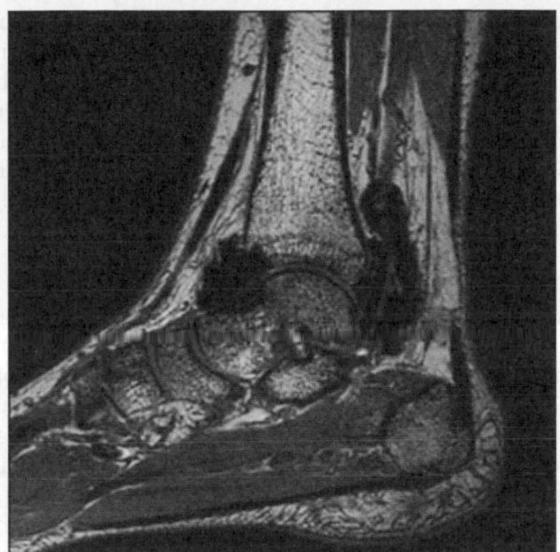

FIGURE 397-3 Pigmented villonodular synovitis. MRI gradient echo sagittal image showing a mass that abuts the neck of the talus with marked low signal typical of tissue containing hemosiderin. *(Courtesy of Donald Flemming, MD; with permission.)*

motion of the joint. Radiographs may show several rounded calcifications within the joint cavity. Treatment is synovectomy; however, as in PVNS, the tumor may recur.

Synovial sarcoma is a malignant neoplasm often found near a large joint of both upper and lower extremities, being more common in the lower extremity. It seldom arises within the joint itself. Synovial sarcomas constitute 10% of soft tissue sarcomas. The tumor is believed to arise from primitive mesenchymal tissue that differentiates into epithelial cells and/or spindle cells. Small foci of calcification may be present in the tumor mass. Synovial sarcoma occurs most often in young adults and is more common in men. The tumor presents as a slowly growing deep-seated mass near a joint, without much pain. The area of the knee is the most common site, followed by the foot, ankle, elbow, and shoulder. Other primary sites include the buttocks, abdominal wall, retroperitoneum, and mediastinum. The tumor spreads along tissue planes. The most common site of visceral metastasis is the lung. The diagnosis is made by biopsy. Treatment consists of wide resection of the tumor, including adjacent muscle and regional lymph nodes, followed by chemotherapy and radiation therapy. Amputation of the involved distal extremity may be required. Chemotherapy may be beneficial in some patients with metastatic disease. Isolated sites of pulmonary metastasis can be surgically removed. The 5-year survival rate with treatment is variable and depends on the staging of the tumor, ranging from ~25% to >60%. Synovial sarcomas tend to recur locally and metastasize to regional lymph nodes, lungs, and skeleton.

In addition to the rare direct metastases of solid cell tumors to the highly vascular synovium, neoplasia arising from nonarticular organ sites can affect joints in other ways. Acute leukemias in children can mimic juvenile inflammatory arthritis with severe joint pain and fever. In adults, chronic and acute myeloid leukemia can infiltrate the synovium in rare instances. The rarely occurring hairy cell leukemia has a peculiar tendency to cause episodic inflammatory oligoarthritis and tenosynovitis; these episodes are dramatic and mimic acute gout attacks. They respond to potent anti-inflammatory therapy with glucocorticoids; with remission of the leukemia, they may abate. Carcinomas can be associated with several paraneoplastic articular syndromes, including HOA (discussed above). Acute palmar fasciitis with polyarthritis is a well-described but rare condition associated with certain cancers, mainly adenocarcinomas. Clinically, this syndrome is fairly abrupt in onset, with pain in the metacarpophalangeal and proximal interphalangeal joints of the hands and rapidly evolving contractures of the fingers due to thickening of the palmar (flexor) tendons. A similar syndrome can be seen in diabetics. Paraneoplastic arthritis has been described and may occur in several patterns: asymmetric disease predominantly affecting the lower extremity joints and symmetric polyarthritis with hand joint involvement. Tumors are often found after the onset of the arthritis, and many patients have a preceding period of malaise or weight loss. The onset is often acute, and patients tend to be older men. These features should raise the specter of an underlying malignancy (or a viral infection such as hepatitis C) as the cause of the arthritis. In one series, the symptoms resolved with successful therapy for the malignancy and did not recur with relapse of the malignancy. Dermatomyositis has a well-described association with neoplasms and may include joint pain and arthritis. Malignancy-associated arthritis may be responsive to NSAIDs and to treatment of the primary neoplasm.

ACKNOWLEDGMENT

This chapter represents a revised version of the chapter authored by Dr. Bruce C. Gilliland that appeared in previous editions of Harrison's. Dr. Gilliland passed away on February 17, 2007. He had been a contributor to Harrison's Principles of Internal Medicine since the 11th edition.

398 Periarticular Disorders of the Extremities

Carol A. Langford

A number of periarticular disorders have become increasingly common, due in part to greater participation in recreational sports by individuals of a wide range of ages. Periarticular disorders most commonly affect the knee or shoulder. With the exception of bursitis, hip pain is most often articular or is being referred from disease affecting another structure (Chap 393). This chapter discusses some of the more common periarticular disorders.

BURSITIS

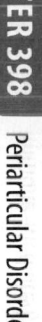

Bursitis is inflammation of a bursa, which is a thin-walled sac lined with synovial tissue. The function of the bursa is to facilitate movement of tendons and muscles over bony prominences. Excessive frictional forces from overuse, trauma, systemic disease (e.g., rheumatoid arthritis, gout), or infection may cause bursitis. *Subacromial bursitis* (subdeltoid bursitis) is the most common form of bursitis. The subacromial bursa, which is contiguous with the subdeltoid bursa, is located between the undersurface of the acromion and the humeral head and is covered by the deltoid muscle. Bursitis is caused by repetitive overhead motion and often accompanies rotator cuff tendinitis. Another frequently encountered form is *trochanteric bursitis*, which involves the bursa around the insertion of the gluteus medius onto the greater trochanter of the femur. Patients experience pain over the lateral aspect of the hip and upper thigh and have tenderness over the posterior aspect of the greater trochanter. External rotation and resisted abduction of the hip elicit pain. *Olecranon bursitis* occurs over the posterior elbow, and when the area is acutely inflamed, infection or gout should be excluded by aspirating the bursa and performing a Gram stain and culture on the fluid as well as examining the fluid for urate crystals. *Achilles bursitis* involves the bursa located above the insertion of the tendon to the calcaneus and results from overuse and wearing tight shoes. *Retrocalcaneal bursitis* involves the bursa that is located between the calcaneus and posterior surface of the Achilles tendon. The pain is experienced at the back of the heel, and swelling appears on the medial and/or lateral side of the tendon. It occurs in association with spondyloarthritides, rheumatoid arthritis, gout, or trauma. *Ischial bursitis* affects the bursa separating the gluteus medius from the ischial tuberosity and develops from prolonged sitting and pivoting on hard surfaces. *Iliopsoas bursitis* affects the bursa that lies between the iliopsoas muscle and hip joint and is lateral to the femoral vessels. Pain is experienced over this area and is made worse by hip extension and flexion. *Anserine bursitis* is an inflammation of the sartorius bursa located over the medial side of the tibia just below the knee and under the conjoint tendon and is manifested by pain on climbing stairs. Tenderness is present over the insertion of the conjoint tendon of the sartorius, gracilis, and semitendinosus. *Prepatellar bursitis* occurs in the bursa situated between the patella and overlying skin and is caused by kneeling on hard surfaces. Gout or infection may also occur at this site. Bursitis is typically diagnosed by history and physical examination, but visualization by ultrasound may play a useful role in selected instances for diagnosis and directed guidance of glucocorticoid injection. Treatment of bursitis consists of prevention of the aggravating situation, rest of the involved part, administration of a nonsteroidal anti-inflammatory drug (NSAID) where appropriate for an individual patient, or local glucocorticoid injection.

ROTATOR CUFF TENDINITIS AND IMPINGEMENT SYNDROME

Tendinitis of the rotator cuff is the major cause of a painful shoulder and is currently thought to be caused by inflammation of the tendon(s). The rotator cuff consists of the tendons of the supraspinatus, infraspinatus, subscapularis, and teres minor muscles, and inserts on the humeral tuberosities. Of the tendons forming the rotator cuff, the supraspinatus tendon is the most often affected, probably because of its repeated impingement (*impingement syndrome*) between the humeral head and the undersurface of the anterior third of the acromion and coracoacromial ligament above as well as the reduction in its blood supply that occurs with abduction of the arm (Fig. 398-1). The tendon of the infraspinatus and that of the long head of the biceps are less commonly involved. The process begins with edema and hemorrhage of the rotator cuff, which evolves to fibrotic thickening and eventually to rotator cuff degeneration with tendon tears and bone spurs. Subacromial bursitis also accompanies this syndrome. Symptoms usually appear after injury or overuse, especially with activities involving elevation of the arm with some degree of forward flexion. Impingement syndrome occurs in persons participating in baseball, tennis, swimming, or occupations that require repeated elevation of the arm. Those over age 40 are particularly susceptible. Patients complain of a dull aching in the shoulder, which may interfere with sleep. Severe pain is experienced when the arm is actively abducted into an overhead position. The arc between 60° and 120° is especially painful. Tenderness is present over the lateral aspect of the humeral head just below the acromion. NSAIDs, local glucocorticoid injection, and physical therapy may relieve symptoms. Surgical decompression of the subacromial space may be necessary in patients refractory to conservative treatment.

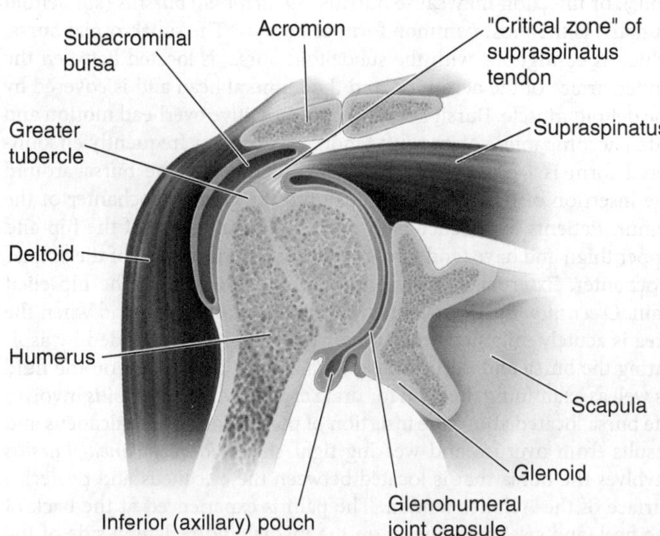

FIGURE 398-1 Coronal section of the shoulder illustrating the relationships of the glenohumeral joint, the joint capsule, the subacromial bursa, and the rotator cuff (supraspinatus tendon). *(From F Kozin, in Arthritis and Allied Conditions, 13th ed, WJ Koopman [ed]. Baltimore, Williams & Wilkins, 1997, with permission.)*

Patients may tear the supraspinatus tendon acutely by falling on an outstretched arm or lifting a heavy object. Symptoms are pain along with weakness of abduction and external rotation of the shoulder. Atrophy of the supraspinatus muscles develops. The diagnosis is established by arthrogram, ultrasound, or magnetic resonance imaging (MRI). Surgical repair may be necessary in patients who fail to respond to conservative measures. In patients with moderate-to-severe tears and functional loss, surgery is indicated.

CALCIFIC TENDINITIS

This condition is characterized by deposition of calcium salts, primarily hydroxyapatite, within a tendon. The exact mechanism of calcification is not known but may be initiated by ischemia or degeneration of the tendon. The supraspinatus tendon is most often affected because it is frequently impinged on and has a reduced blood supply when the arm is abducted. The condition usually develops after age 40. Calcification within the tendon may evoke acute inflammation, producing sudden and severe pain in the shoulder. However, it may be asymptomatic or not related to the patient's symptoms. Diagnosis of calcific tendonitis can be made by ultrasound or radiograph. Most cases are self-limited and respond to conservative therapy with physical therapy and/or NSAIDs. A subset of patients is refractory and requires ultrasound-guided percutaneous needle aspiration and lavage or surgery.

BICIPITAL TENDINITIS AND RUPTURE

Bicipital tendinitis, or tenosynovitis, is produced by friction on the tendon of the long head of the biceps as it passes through the bicipital groove. When the inflammation is acute, patients experience anterior shoulder pain that radiates down the biceps into the forearm. Abduction and external rotation of the arm are painful and limited. The bicipital groove is very tender to palpation. Pain may be elicited along the course of the tendon by resisting supination of the forearm with the elbow at 90° (Yergason's supination sign). Acute rupture of the tendon may occur with vigorous exercise of the arm and is often painful. In a young patient, it should be repaired surgically. Rupture of the tendon in an older person may be associated with little or no pain and is recognized by the presence of persistent swelling of the biceps produced by the retraction of the long head of the biceps. Surgery is usually not necessary in this setting.

DE QUERVAIN'S TENOSYNOVITIS

In this condition, inflammation involves the abductor pollicis longus and the extensor pollicis brevis as these tendons pass through a fibrous sheath at the radial styloid process. The usual cause is repetitive twisting of the wrist. It may occur in pregnancy, and it also occurs in mothers who hold their babies with the thumb outstretched. Patients experience pain on grasping with their thumb, such as with pinching. Swelling and tenderness are often present over the radial styloid process. The Finkelstein sign is positive, which is elicited by having the patient place the thumb in the palm and close the fingers over it. The wrist is then ulnarly deviated, resulting in pain over the involved tendon sheath in the area of the radial styloid. Treatment consists initially of splinting the wrist and an NSAID. When severe or refractory to conservative treatment, glucocorticoid injections can be very effective.

PATELLAR TENDINITIS (JUMPER'S KNEE)

Tendinitis involves the patellar tendon at its attachment to the lower pole of the patella. Patients may experience pain when jumping during basketball or volleyball, going up stairs, or doing deep knee squats. Tenderness is noted on examination over the lower pole of the patella. Treatment consists of rest, icing, and NSAIDs, followed by strengthening and increasing flexibility.

ILIOTIBIAL BAND SYNDROME

The iliotibial band is a thick connective tissue that runs from the ilium to the fibula. Patients with iliotibial band syndrome most commonly present with aching or burning pain at the site where the band courses over the lateral femoral condyle of the knee; pain may also radiate up the thigh, toward the hip. Predisposing factors for iliotibial band syndrome include a varus alignment of the knee, excessive running distance, poorly fitted shoes, or continuous running on uneven terrain. Treatment consists of rest, NSAIDs, physical therapy, and addressing risk factors such as shoes and running surface. Glucocorticoid injection into the area of tenderness can provide relief, but running must be avoided for at least 2 weeks after the injection. Surgical release of the iliotibial band has been helpful in rare patients for whom conservative treatment has failed.

ADHESIVE CAPSULITIS

Often referred to as "frozen shoulder," adhesive capsulitis is characterized by pain and restricted movement of the shoulder, usually in the absence of intrinsic shoulder disease. Adhesive capsulitis may follow bursitis or tendinitis of the shoulder or be associated with systemic disorders such as chronic pulmonary disease, myocardial infarction, and diabetes mellitus. Prolonged immobility of the arm contributes to the development of adhesive capsulitis. Pathologically, the capsule of the shoulder is thickened, and a mild chronic inflammatory infiltrate and fibrosis may be present.

Adhesive capsulitis occurs more commonly in women after age 50. Pain and stiffness usually develop gradually but progress rapidly in some patients. Night pain is often present in the affected shoulder, and pain may interfere with sleep. The shoulder is tender to palpation, and both active and passive movement are restricted. Radiographs of the shoulder show osteopenia. The diagnosis is typically made by physical examination but can be confirmed if necessary by arthrography, in that only a limited amount of contrast material, usually <15 mL, can be injected under pressure into the shoulder joint.

In most patients, the condition improves spontaneously 1–3 years after onset. While pain usually improves, many patients are left with some limitation of shoulder motion. Early mobilization of the arm following an injury to the shoulder may prevent the development of this disease. Physical therapy provides the foundation of treatment for adhesive capsulitis. Local injections of glucocorticoids and NSAIDs may also provide relief of symptoms. Slow but forceful injection of contrast material into the joint may lyse adhesions and stretch the capsule, resulting in improvement of shoulder motion. Manipulation under anesthesia may be helpful in some patients.

LATERAL EPICONDYLITIS (TENNIS ELBOW)

Lateral epicondylitis, or tennis elbow, is a painful condition involving the soft tissue over the lateral aspect of the elbow. The pain originates at or near the site of attachment of the common extensors to the lateral epicondyle and may radiate into the forearm and dorsum of the wrist. The pain usually appears after work or recreational activities involving repeated motions of wrist extension and supination against resistance. Most patients with this disorder injure themselves in activities other than tennis, such as pulling weeds, carrying suitcases or briefcases, or using a screwdriver. The injury in tennis usually occurs when hitting a backhand with the elbow flexed. Shaking hands and opening doors can reproduce the pain. Striking the lateral elbow against a solid object may also induce pain.

The treatment is usually rest along with administration of an NSAID. Ultrasound, icing, and friction massage may also help relieve pain. When pain is severe, the elbow is placed in a sling or splinted at 90° of flexion. When the pain is acute and well localized, injection of a glucocorticoid using a small-gauge needle may be effective. Following injection, the patient should be advised to rest the arm for at least 1 month and avoid activities that would aggravate the elbow. Once symptoms have subsided, the patient should begin rehabilitation to strengthen and increase flexibility of the extensor muscles before resuming physical activity involving the arm. A forearm band placed 2.5–5.0 cm (1–2 in.) below the elbow may help to reduce tension on the extensor muscles at their attachment to the lateral epicondyle. The patient should be advised to restrict activities requiring forcible extension and supination of the wrist. Improvement may take several months. The patient may continue to experience mild pain but, with care, can usually avoid the return of debilitating pain. Occasionally, surgical release of the extensor aponeurosis may be necessary.

MEDIAL EPICONDYLITIS

Medial epicondylitis is an overuse syndrome resulting in pain over the medial side of the elbow with radiation into the forearm. The cause of this syndrome is considered to be repetitive resisted motions of wrist flexion and pronation, which lead to microtears and granulation tissue at the origin of the pronator teres and forearm flexors, particularly the flexor carpi radialis. This overuse syndrome is usually seen in patients >35 years and is much less common than lateral epicondylitis. It occurs most often in work-related repetitive activities but also occurs with recreational activities such as swinging a golf club or throwing a baseball. On physical examination, there is tenderness just distal to the medial epicondyle over the origin of the forearm flexors. Pain can be reproduced by resisting wrist flexion and pronation with the elbow extended. Radiographs are usually normal. The differential diagnosis of patients with medial elbow symptoms includes tears of the pronator teres, acute medial collateral ligament tear, and medial collateral ligament instability. Ulnar neuritis has been found in 25–50% of patients with medial epicondylitis and is associated with tenderness over the ulnar nerve at the elbow as well as hypesthesia and paresthesia on the ulnar side of the hand.

The initial treatment of medial epicondylitis is conservative, involving rest, NSAIDs, friction massage, ultrasound, and icing. Some patients may require splinting. Injections of glucocorticoids at the painful site may also be effective. Patients should be instructed to rest for at least 1 month. Also, patients should start physical therapy once the pain has subsided. In patients with chronic debilitating medial epicondylitis that remains unresponsive after at least a year of treatment, surgical release of the flexor muscle at its origin may be necessary and is often successful.

PLANTAR FASCIITIS

Plantar fasciitis is a common cause of foot pain in adults, with the peak incidence occurring in people between the ages of 40 and 60 years. The pain originates at or near the site of the plantar fascia attachment to the medial tuberosity of the calcaneus. Several factors that increase the risk of developing plantar fasciitis include obesity, pes planus (flat foot or absence of the foot arch when standing), pes cavus (high-arched foot), limited dorsiflexion of the ankle, prolonged standing, walking on hard surfaces, and faulty shoes. In runners, excessive running and a change to a harder running surface may precipitate plantar fasciitis.

The diagnosis of plantar fasciitis can usually be made on the basis of history and physical examination alone. Patients experience severe pain with the first steps on arising in the morning or following inactivity during the day. The pain usually lessens with weight-bearing activity during the day, only to worsen with continued activity. Pain is made worse on walking barefoot or up stairs. On examination, maximal tenderness is elicited on palpation over the inferior heel corresponding to the site of attachment of the plantar fascia.

Imaging studies may be indicated when the diagnosis is not clear. Plain radiographs may show heel spurs, which are of little diagnostic significance. Ultrasonography in plantar fasciitis can demonstrate thickening of the fascia and diffuse hypoechogenicity, indicating edema at the attachment of the plantar fascia to the calcaneus. MRI is a sensitive method for detecting plantar fasciitis, but it is usually not required for establishing the diagnosis.

The differential diagnosis of inferior heel pain includes calcaneal stress fractures, the spondyloarthritides, rheumatoid arthritis, gout, neoplastic or infiltrative bone processes, and nerve compression/entrapment syndromes.

Resolution of symptoms occurs within 12 months in more than 80% of patients with plantar fasciitis. The patient is advised to reduce or discontinue activities that can exacerbate plantar fasciitis. Initial treatment consists of ice, heat, massage, and stretching. Orthotics provide medial arch support and can be effective. Foot strapping or taping are commonly performed, and some patients may benefit by wearing a night splint designed to keep the ankle in a neutral position. A short course of NSAIDs can be given to patients when the benefits outweigh the risks. Local glucocorticoid injections have also been shown to be efficacious but may carry an increased risk for plantar fascia rupture. Plantar fasciotomy is reserved for those patients who have failed to improve after at least 6–12 months of conservative treatment.

ACKNOWLEDGMENT

This chapter represents a revised version of the chapter authored by Dr. Bruce C. Gilliland that was in the previous editions of Harrison's. Dr. Gilliland passed away on February 17, 2007, and had been a contributor to Harrison's Principles of Internal Medicine since the 11th edition.

SECTION 1 ENDOCRINOLOGY

399 Approach to the Patient with Endocrine Disorders

J. Larry Jameson

The management of endocrine disorders requires a broad understanding of intermediary metabolism, reproductive physiology, bone metabolism, and growth. Accordingly, the practice of endocrinology is intimately linked to a conceptual framework for understanding hormone secretion, hormone action, and principles of feedback control (Chap. 400e). The endocrine system is evaluated primarily by measuring hormone concentrations, arming the clinician with valuable diagnostic information. Most disorders of the endocrine system are amenable to effective treatment once the correct diagnosis is determined. Endocrine deficiency disorders are treated with physiologic hormone replacement; hormone excess conditions, which usually are caused by benign glandular adenomas, are managed by removing tumors surgically or reducing hormone levels medically.

SCOPE OF ENDOCRINOLOGY

The specialty of endocrinology encompasses the study of glands and the hormones they produce. The term *endocrine* was coined by Starling to contrast the actions of hormones secreted internally (*endocrine*) with those secreted externally (*exocrine*) or into a lumen, such as the gastrointestinal tract. The term *hormone,* derived from a Greek phrase meaning "to set in motion," aptly describes the dynamic actions of hormones as they elicit cellular responses and regulate physiologic processes through feedback mechanisms.

Unlike many other specialties in medicine, it is not possible to define endocrinology strictly along anatomic lines. The classic endocrine glands—pituitary, thyroid, parathyroid, pancreatic islets, adrenals, and gonads—communicate broadly with other organs through the nervous system, hormones, cytokines, and growth factors. In addition to its traditional synaptic functions, the brain produces a vast array of peptide hormones, and this has led to the discipline of neuroendocrinology. Through the production of hypothalamic releasing factors, the central nervous system (CNS) exerts a major regulatory influence over pituitary hormone secretion (Chap. 401e). The peripheral nervous system stimulates the adrenal medulla. The immune and endocrine systems are also intimately intertwined. The adrenal hormone cortisol is a powerful immunosuppressant. Cytokines and interleukins (ILs) have profound effects on the functions of the pituitary, adrenal, thyroid, and gonads. Common endocrine diseases such as autoimmune thyroid disease and type 1 diabetes mellitus are caused by dysregulation of immune surveillance and tolerance. Less common diseases such as polyglandular failure, Addison's disease, and lymphocytic hypophysitis also have an immunologic basis.

The interdigitation of endocrinology with physiologic processes in other specialties sometimes blurs the role of hormones. For example, hormones play an important role in maintenance of blood pressure, intravascular volume, and peripheral resistance in the cardiovascular system. Vasoactive substances such as catecholamines, angiotensin II, endothelin, and nitric oxide are involved in dynamic changes of vascular tone in addition to their multiple roles in other tissues. The heart is the principal source of atrial natriuretic peptide, which acts in classic endocrine fashion to induce natriuresis at a distant target organ (the kidney). Erythropoietin, a traditional circulating hormone, is made in the kidney and stimulates erythropoiesis in bone marrow (Chap. 77). The kidney is also integrally involved in the renin-angiotensin axis (Chap. 406) and is a primary target of several hormones, including parathyroid hormone (PTH), mineralocorticoids, and vasopressin. The gastrointestinal tract produces a surprising number of peptide hormones, such as cholecystokinin, ghrelin, gastrin, secretin, and vasoactive intestinal peptide, among many others. Carcinoid and islet tumors can secrete excessive amounts of these hormones, leading to specific clinical syndromes (Chap. 113). Many of these gastrointestinal hormones are also produced in the CNS, where their functions are poorly understood. Adipose tissue produces leptin, which acts centrally to control appetite, along with adiponectin, resistin, and other hormones that regulate metabolism. As hormones such as inhibin, ghrelin, and leptin are discovered, they become integrated into the science and practice of medicine on the basis of their functional roles rather than their tissues of origin.

Characterization of hormone receptors frequently reveals unexpected relationships to factors in nonendocrine disciplines. The growth hormone (GH) and leptin receptors, for example, are members of the cytokine receptor family. The G protein–coupled receptors (GPCRs), which mediate the actions of many peptide hormones, are used in numerous physiologic processes, including vision, smell, and neurotransmission.

PATHOLOGIC MECHANISMS OF ENDOCRINE DISEASE

Endocrine diseases can be divided into three major types of conditions: (1) hormone excess, (2) hormone deficiency, and (3) hormone resistance (Table 399-1).

CAUSES OF HORMONE EXCESS

Syndromes of hormone excess can be caused by neoplastic growth of endocrine cells, autoimmune disorders, and excess hormone administration. Benign endocrine tumors, including parathyroid, pituitary, and adrenal adenomas, often retain the capacity to produce hormones, perhaps reflecting the fact that these tumors are relatively well differentiated. Many endocrine tumors exhibit subtle defects in their "set points" for feedback regulation. For example, in Cushing's disease, impaired feedback inhibition of adrenocorticotropic hormone (ACTH) secretion is associated with autonomous function. However, the tumor cells are not completely resistant to feedback, as evidenced by ACTH suppression by higher doses of dexamethasone (e.g., high-dose dexamethasone test) (Chap. 406). Similar set point defects are also typical of parathyroid adenomas and autonomously functioning thyroid nodules.

The molecular basis of some endocrine tumors, such as the multiple endocrine neoplasia (MEN) syndromes (MEN 1, 2A, 2B), have provided important insights into tumorigenesis (Chap. 408). MEN 1 is characterized primarily by the triad of parathyroid, pancreatic islet, and pituitary tumors. MEN 2 predisposes to medullary thyroid carcinoma, pheochromocytoma, and hyperparathyroidism. The *MEN1* gene, located on chromosome 11q13, encodes a putative tumor-suppressor gene, menin. Analogous to the paradigm first described for retinoblastoma, the affected individual inherits a mutant copy of the *MEN1* gene, and tumorigenesis ensues after a somatic "second hit"

TABLE 399-1 CAUSES OF ENDOCRINE DYSFUNCTION

Type of Endocrine Disorder	Examples
Hyperfunction	
Neoplastic	
Benign	Pituitary adenomas, hyperparathyroidism, autonomous thyroid or adrenal nodules, pheochromocytoma
Malignant	Adrenal cancer, medullary thyroid cancer, carcinoid
Ectopic	Ectopic ACTH, SIADH secretion
Multiple endocrine neoplasia (MEN)	MEN 1, MEN 2
Autoimmune	Graves' disease
Iatrogenic	Cushing's syndrome, hypoglycemia
Infectious/inflammatory	Subacute thyroiditis
Activating receptor mutations	LH, TSH, Ca^{2+}, PTH receptors, $G_s\alpha$
Hypofunction	
Autoimmune	Hashimoto's thyroiditis, type 1 diabetes mellitus, Addison's disease, polyglandular failure
Iatrogenic	Radiation-induced hypopituitarism, hypothyroidism, surgical
Infectious/inflammatory	Adrenal insufficiency, hypothalamic sarcoidosis
Hormone mutations	GH, LHβ, FSHβ, vasopressin
Enzyme defects	21-Hydroxylase deficiency
Developmental defects	Kallmann syndrome, Turner's syndrome, transcription factors
Nutritional/vitamin deficiency	Vitamin D deficiency, iodine deficiency
Hemorrhage/infarction	Sheehan's syndrome, adrenal insufficiency
Hormone Resistance	
Receptor mutations	
Membrane	GH, vasopressin, LH, FSH, ACTH, GnRH, GHRH, PTH, leptin, Ca^{2+}
Nuclear	AR, TR, VDR, ER, GR, PPARγ
Signaling pathway mutations	Albright's hereditary osteodystrophy
Postreceptor	Type 2 diabetes mellitus, leptin resistance

Abbreviations: ACTH, adrenocorticotropic hormone; AR, androgen receptor; ER, estrogen receptor; FSH, follicle-stimulating hormone; GHRH, growth hormone–releasing hormone; GnRH, gonadotropin-releasing hormone; GR, glucocorticoid receptor; LH, luteinizing hormone; PPAR, peroxisome proliferator activated receptor; PTH, parathyroid hormone; SIADH, syndrome of inappropriate antidiuretic hormone; TR, thyroid hormone receptor; TSH, thyroid-stimulating hormone; VDR, vitamin D receptor.

leads to loss of function of the normal *MEN1* gene (through deletion or point mutations).

In contrast to inactivation of a tumor-suppressor gene, as occurs in MEN 1 and most other inherited cancer syndromes, MEN 2 is caused by activating mutations in a single allele. In this case, activating mutations of the *RET* protooncogene, which encodes a receptor tyrosine kinase, leads to thyroid C cell hyperplasia in childhood before the development of medullary thyroid carcinoma. Elucidation of this pathogenic mechanism has allowed early genetic screening for *RET* mutations in individuals at risk for MEN 2, permitting identification of those who may benefit from prophylactic thyroidectomy and biochemical screening for pheochromocytoma and hyperparathyroidism.

Mutations that activate hormone receptor signaling have been identified in several GPCRs. For example, activating mutations of the luteinizing hormone (LH) receptor cause a dominantly transmitted form of male-limited precocious puberty, reflecting premature stimulation of testosterone synthesis in Leydig cells (Chap. 411). Activating mutations in these GPCRs are located predominantly in the transmembrane domains and induce receptor coupling to $G_s\alpha$ even in the absence of hormone. Consequently, adenylate cyclase is activated, and cyclic adenosine monophosphate (AMP) levels increase in a manner that mimics hormone action. A similar phenomenon results from activating mutations in $G_s\alpha$. When these mutations occur early in development, they cause McCune-Albright syndrome. When they occur only in somatotropes, the activating $G_s\alpha$ mutations cause GH-secreting tumors and acromegaly (Chap. 403).

In autoimmune Graves' disease, antibody interactions with the thyroid-stimulating hormone (TSH) receptor mimic TSH action, leading to hormone overproduction (Chap. 405). Analogous to the effects of activating mutations of the TSH receptor, these stimulating autoantibodies induce conformational changes that release the receptor from a constrained state, thereby triggering receptor coupling to G proteins.

CAUSES OF HORMONE DEFICIENCY

Most examples of hormone deficiency states can be attributed to glandular destruction caused by autoimmunity, surgery, infection, inflammation, infarction, hemorrhage, or tumor infiltration (Table 399-1). Autoimmune damage to the thyroid gland (Hashimoto's thyroiditis) and pancreatic islet β cells (type 1 diabetes mellitus) is a prevalent cause of endocrine disease. Mutations in a number of hormones, hormone receptors, transcription factors, enzymes, and channels can also lead to hormone deficiencies.

HORMONE RESISTANCE

Most severe hormone resistance syndromes are due to inherited defects in membrane receptors, nuclear receptors, or the pathways that transduce receptor signals. These disorders are characterized by defective hormone action despite the presence of increased hormone levels. In complete androgen resistance, for example, mutations in the androgen receptor result in a female phenotypic appearance in genetic (XY) males, even though LH and testosterone levels are increased (Chap. 408). In addition to these relatively rare genetic disorders, more common acquired forms of functional hormone resistance include insulin resistance in type 2 diabetes mellitus, leptin resistance in obesity, and GH resistance in catabolic states. The pathogenesis of functional resistance involves receptor downregulation and postreceptor desensitization of signaling pathways; functional forms of resistance are generally reversible.

CLINICAL EVALUATION OF ENDOCRINE DISORDERS

Because most glands are relatively inaccessible, the physical examination usually focuses on the manifestations of hormone excess or deficiency as well as direct examination of palpable glands, such as the thyroid and gonads. For these reasons, it is important to evaluate patients in the context of their presenting symptoms, review of systems, family and social history, and exposure to medications that may affect the endocrine system. Astute clinical skills are required to detect subtle symptoms and signs suggestive of underlying endocrine disease. For example, a patient with Cushing's syndrome may manifest specific findings, such as central fat redistribution, striae, and proximal muscle weakness, in addition to features seen commonly in the general population, such as obesity, plethora, hypertension, and glucose intolerance. Similarly, the insidious onset of hypothyroidism—with mental slowing, fatigue, dry skin, and other features—can be difficult to distinguish from similar, nonspecific findings in the general population. Clinical judgment that is based on knowledge of disease prevalence and pathophysiology is required to decide when to embark on more extensive evaluation of these disorders. Laboratory testing plays an essential role in endocrinology by allowing quantitative assessment of hormone levels and dynamics. Radiologic imaging tests such as computed tomography (CT) scan, magnetic resonance imaging (MRI), thyroid scan, and ultrasound are also used for the diagnosis of endocrine disorders. However, these tests generally are employed only after a hormonal abnormality has been established by biochemical testing.

HORMONE MEASUREMENTS AND ENDOCRINE TESTING

Immunoassays are the most important diagnostic tool in endocrinology, as they allow sensitive, specific, and quantitative determination of steady-state and dynamic changes in hormone concentrations. Immunoassays use antibodies to detect specific hormones. For many peptide hormones, these measurements are now configured to use two different antibodies to increase binding affinity and specificity. There are many variations of these assays; a common format involves using one antibody to capture the antigen (hormone) onto an immobilized surface and a second antibody, coupled to a chemiluminescent (immunochemiluminescent assay [ICMA]) or radioactive (immunoradiometric assay [IRMA]) signal, to detect the antigen. These assays are sensitive enough to detect plasma hormone concentrations in the picomolar to nanomolar range, and they can readily distinguish structurally related proteins, such as PTH from PTH-related peptide (PTHrP). A variety of other techniques are used to measure specific hormones, including mass spectroscopy, various forms of chromatography, and enzymatic methods; bioassays are now rarely used.

Most hormone measurements are based on plasma or serum samples. However, urinary hormone determinations remain useful for the evaluation of some conditions. Urinary collections over 24 h provide an integrated assessment of the production of a hormone or metabolite, many of which vary during the day. It is important to assure complete collections of 24-h urine samples; simultaneous measurement of creatinine provides an internal control for the adequacy of collection and can be used to normalize some hormone measurements. A 24-h urine free cortisol measurement largely reflects the amount of unbound cortisol, thus providing a reasonable index of biologically available hormone. Other commonly used urine determinations include 17-hydroxycorticosteroids, 17-ketosteroids, vanillylmandelic acid, metanephrine, catecholamines, 5-hydroxyindoleacetic acid, and calcium.

The value of quantitative hormone measurements lies in their correct interpretation in a clinical context. The normal range for most hormones is relatively broad, often varying by a factor of two- to tenfold. The normal ranges for many hormones are sex- and age-specific. Thus, using the correct normative database is an essential part of interpreting hormone tests. The pulsatile nature of hormones and factors that can affect their secretion, such as sleep, meals, and medications, must also be considered. Cortisol values increase fivefold between midnight and dawn; reproductive hormone levels vary dramatically during the female menstrual cycle.

For many endocrine systems, much information can be gained from basal hormone testing, particularly when different components of an endocrine axis are assessed simultaneously. For example, low testosterone and elevated LH levels suggest a primary gonadal problem, whereas a hypothalamic-pituitary disorder is likely if both LH and testosterone are low. Because TSH is a sensitive indicator of thyroid function, it is generally recommended as a first-line test for thyroid disorders. An elevated TSH level is almost always the result of primary hypothyroidism, whereas a low TSH is most often caused by thyrotoxicosis. These predictions can be confirmed by determining the free thyroxine level. In the less common circumstance when free thyroxine and TSH are both low, it is important to consider secondary hypopituitarism caused by hypothalamic-pituitary disease. Elevated calcium and PTH levels suggest hyperparathyroidism, whereas PTH is suppressed in hypercalcemia caused by malignancy or granulomatous diseases. A suppressed ACTH in the setting of hypercortisolemia, or increased urine free cortisol, is seen with hyperfunctioning adrenal adenomas.

It is not uncommon, however, for baseline hormone levels associated with pathologic endocrine conditions to overlap with the normal range. In this circumstance, dynamic testing is useful to separate the two groups further. There are a multitude of dynamic endocrine tests, but all are based on principles of feedback regulation, and most responses can be rationalized based on principles that govern the regulation of endocrine axes. *Suppression tests* are used in the setting of suspected endocrine hyperfunction. An example is the dexamethasone suppression test used to evaluate Cushing's syndrome (Chaps. 403 and 406). *Stimulation tests* generally are used to assess endocrine hypofunction. The ACTH stimulation test, for example, is used to assess the adrenal gland response in patients with suspected adrenal insufficiency. Other stimulation tests use hypothalamic-releasing factors such as corticotropin releasing hormone (CRH) and growth hormone–releasing hormone (GHRH) to evaluate pituitary hormone reserve (Chap. 403). Insulin-induced hypoglycemia also evokes pituitary ACTH and GH responses. Stimulation tests based on reduction or inhibition of endogenous hormones are now used infrequently. Examples include metyrapone inhibition of cortisol synthesis and clomiphene inhibition of estrogen feedback.

SCREENING AND ASSESSMENT OF COMMON ENDOCRINE DISORDERS

Many endocrine disorders are prevalent in the adult population (Table 399-2) and can be diagnosed and managed by general internists, family practitioners, or other primary health care providers. The high prevalence and clinical impact of certain endocrine diseases justifies vigilance for features of these disorders during routine physical examinations; laboratory screening is indicated in selected high-risk populations.

TABLE 399-2 EXAMPLES OF PREVALENT ENDOCRINE AND METABOLIC DISORDERS IN THE ADULT

Disorder	Approx. Prevalence in Adults[a]	Screening/Testing Recommendations[b]	Chapter(s)
Obesity	34% BMI ≥30 68% BMI ≥25	Calculate BMI Measure waist circumference Exclude secondary causes Consider comorbid complications	416
Type 2 diabetes mellitus	>7%	Beginning at age 45, screen every 3 years, or earlier in high-risk groups: Fasting plasma glucose (FPG) >126 mg/dL Random plasma glucose >200 mg/dL An elevated HbA1c Consider comorbid complications	417
Hyperlipidemia	20–25%	Cholesterol screening at least every 5 years; more often in high-risk groups Lipoprotein analysis (LDL, HDL) for increased cholesterol, CAD, diabetes Consider secondary causes	421
Metabolic syndrome	35%	Measure waist circumference, FPG, BP, lipids	422
Hypothyroidism	5–10%, women 0.5–2%, men	TSH; confirm with free T_4 Screen women after age 35 and every 5 years thereafter	405
Graves' disease	1–3%, women 0.1%, men	TSH, free T_4	405
Thyroid nodules and neoplasia	2–5% palpable >25% by ultrasound	Physical examination of thyroid Fine-needle aspiration biopsy	405
Osteoporosis	5–10%, women 2–5%, men	Bone mineral density measurements in women >65 years or in postmenopausal women or men at risk Exclude secondary causes	425
Hyperparathyroidism	0.1–0.5%, women > men	Serum calcium PTH, if calcium is elevated Assess comorbid conditions	424
Infertility	10%, couples	Investigate both members of couple Semen analysis in male Assess ovulatory cycles in female Specific tests as indicated	411, 412
Polycystic ovarian syndrome	5–10%, women	Free testosterone, DHEAS Consider comorbid conditions	412
Hirsutism	5–10%	Free testosterone, DHEAS Exclude secondary causes Additional tests as indicated	68
Menopause	Median age, 51	FSH	413
Hyperprolactinemia	15% in women with amenorrhea or galactorrhea	PRL level MRI, if not medication-related	403
Erectile dysfunction	10–25%	Careful history, PRL, testosterone Consider secondary causes (e.g., diabetes)	67
Hypogonadism, male	1–2%	Testosterone, LH	411
Gynecomastia	15%	Often, no tests are indicated Consider Klinefelter's syndrome Consider medications, hypogonadism, liver disease	411
Klinefelter's syndrome	0.2%, men	Karyotype Testosterone	410
Vitamin D deficiency	10%	Measure serum 25-OH vitamin D Consider secondary causes	423
Turner's syndrome	0.03%, women	Karyotype Consider comorbid conditions	410

[a]The prevalence of most disorders varies among ethnic groups and with aging. Data based primarily on U.S. population. [b]See individual chapters for additional information on eva and treatment. Early testing is indicated in patients with signs and symptoms of disease and in those at increased risk.

Abbreviations: BMI, body mass index; BP, blood pressure; CAD, coronary artery disease; DHEAS, dehydroepiandrosterone; FSH, follicle-stimulating hormone; HDL, high-density lip tein; LDL, low-density lipoprotein; LH, luteinizing hormone; MRI, magnetic resonance imaging; PRL, prolactin; PTH, parathyroid hormone; TSH, thyroid-stimulating hormone.

400e Mechanisms of Hormone Action

J. Larry Jameson

This is a digital-only chapter. It is available on the DVD that accompanies this book, as well as on Access Medicine/Harrison's Online, and the eBook and "app" editions of HPIM 19e.

CLASSES OF HORMONES

Hormones can be divided into five major types: (1) *amino acid derivatives* such as dopamine, catecholamine, and thyroid hormone; (2) *small neuropeptides* such as gonadotropin-releasing hormone (GnRH), thyrotropin-releasing hormone (TRH), somatostatin, and vasopressin; (3) *large proteins* such as insulin, luteinizing hormone (LH), and parathyroid hormone (PTH); (4) *steroid hormones* such as cortisol and estrogen that are synthesized from cholesterol-based precursors; and (5) *vitamin derivatives* such as retinoids (vitamin A) and vitamin D. A variety of *peptide growth factors*, most of which act locally, share actions with hormones. As a rule, amino acid derivatives and peptide hormones interact with cell-surface membrane receptors. Steroids, thyroid hormones, vitamin D, and retinoids are lipid-soluble and interact with intracellular nuclear receptors, although many also interact with membrane receptors or intracellular signaling proteins as well.

401e Anterior Pituitary: Physiology of Pituitary Hormones

Shlomo Melmed, J. Larry Jameson

This is a digital-only chapter. It is available on the DVD that accompanies this book, as well as on Access Medicine/Harrison's Online, and the eBook and "app" editions of HPIM 19e.

The anterior pituitary often is referred to as the "master gland" because, together with the hypothalamus, it orchestrates the complex regulatory functions of many other endocrine glands. The anterior pituitary gland produces six major hormones: (1) prolactin (PRL), (2) growth hormone (GH), (3) adrenocorticotropic hormone (ACTH), (4) luteinizing hormone (LH), (5) follicle-stimulating hormone (FSH), and (6) thyroid-stimulating hormone (TSH). Pituitary hormones are secreted in a pulsatile manner, reflecting stimulation by an array of specific hypothalamic releasing factors. Each of these pituitary hormones elicits specific responses in peripheral target tissues. The hormonal products of those peripheral glands, in turn, exert feedback control at the level of the hypothalamus and pituitary to modulate pituitary function. Pituitary tumors cause characteristic hormone excess syndromes. Hormone deficiency may be inherited or acquired. Fortunately, there are efficacious treatments for many pituitary hormone excess and deficiency syndromes. Nonetheless, these diagnoses are often elusive; this emphasizes the importance of recognizing subtle clinical manifestations and performing the correct laboratory diagnostic tests. **For discussion of disorders of the posterior pituitary, or neurohypophysis, see Chap. 404.**

402 Hypopituitarism

Shlomo Melmed, J. Larry Jameson

Inadequate production of anterior pituitary hormones leads to features of hypopituitarism. Impaired production of one or more of the anterior pituitary trophic hormones can result from inherited disorders; more commonly, adult hypopituitarism is acquired and reflects the compressive mass effects of tumors or the consequences of local pituitary or hypothalamic traumatic, inflammatory, or vascular damage. These processes also may impair synthesis or secretion of hypothalamic hormones, with resultant pituitary failure (Table 402-1).

DEVELOPMENTAL AND GENETIC CAUSES OF HYPOPITUITARISM

Pituitary Dysplasia Pituitary dysplasia may result in aplastic, hypoplastic, or ectopic pituitary gland development. Because pituitary development follows midline cell migration from the nasopharyngeal Rathke's pouch, midline craniofacial disorders may be associated with

TABLE 402-1 ETIOLOGY OF HYPOPITUITARISM[a]

Development/structural
Transcription factor defect
Pituitary dysplasia/aplasia
Congenital central nervous system mass, encephalocele
Primary empty sella
Congenital hypothalamic disorders (septo-optic dysplasia, Prader-Willi syndrome, Laurence-Moon-Biedl syndrome, Kallmann syndrome)
Traumatic
Surgical resection
Radiation damage
Head injuries
Neoplastic
Pituitary adenoma
Parasellar mass (germinoma, ependymoma, glioma)
Rathke's cyst
Craniopharyngioma
Hypothalamic hamartoma, gangliocytoma
Pituitary metastases (breast, lung, colon carcinoma)
Lymphoma and leukemia
Meningioma
Infiltrative/inflammatory
Lymphocytic hypophysitis
Hemochromatosis
Sarcoidosis
Histiocytosis X
Granulomatous hypophysitis
Transcription factor antibodies
Vascular
Pituitary apoplexy
Pregnancy-related (infarction with diabetes; postpartum necrosis)
Sickle cell disease
Arteritis
Infections
Fungal (histoplasmosis)
Parasitic (toxoplasmosis)
Tuberculosis
Pneumocystis carinii

[a]Trophic hormone failure associated with pituitary compression or destruction usually occurs sequentially: growth hormone > follicle-stimulating hormone > luteinizing hormone > thyroid-stimulating hormone > adrenocorticotropic hormone. During childhood, growth retardation is often the presenting feature, and in adults, hypogonadism is the earliest symptom.

pituitary dysplasia. Acquired pituitary failure in the newborn also can be caused by birth trauma, including cranial hemorrhage, asphyxia, and breech delivery.

SEPTO-OPTIC DYSPLASIA Hypothalamic dysfunction and hypopituitarism may result from dysgenesis of the septum pellucidum or corpus callosum. Affected children have mutations in the *HESX1* gene, which is involved in early development of the ventral prosencephalon. These children exhibit variable combinations of cleft palate, syndactyly, ear deformities, hypertelorism, optic nerve hypoplasia, micropenis, and anosmia. Pituitary dysfunction leads to diabetes insipidus, growth hormone (GH) deficiency and short stature, and, occasionally, thyroid-stimulating hormone (TSH) deficiency.

Tissue-Specific Factor Mutations Several pituitary cell–specific transcription factors, such as Pit-1 and Prop-1, are critical for determining the development and committed function of differentiated anterior pituitary cell lineages. Autosomal dominant or recessive Pit-1 mutations cause combined GH, prolactin (PRL), and TSH deficiencies. These patients usually present with growth failure and varying degrees of hypothyroidism. The pituitary may appear hypoplastic on magnetic resonance imaging (MRI).

Prop-1 is expressed early in pituitary development and appears to be required for Pit-1 function. Familial and sporadic *PROP1* mutations result in combined GH, PRL, TSH, and gonadotropin deficiency. Over 80% of these patients have growth retardation; by adulthood, all are deficient in TSH and gonadotropins, and a small minority later develop adrenocorticotropic hormone (ACTH) deficiency. Because of gonadotropin deficiency, these individuals do not enter puberty spontaneously. In some cases, the pituitary gland appears enlarged on MRI. *TPIT* mutations result in ACTH deficiency associated with hypocortisolism.

Developmental Hypothalamic Dysfunction • ***KALLMANN SYNDROME*** Kallmann syndrome results from defective hypothalamic gonadotropin-releasing hormone (GnRH) synthesis and is associated with anosmia or hyposmia due to olfactory bulb agenesis or hypoplasia (Chap. 411). Classically, the syndrome may also be associated with color blindness, optic atrophy, nerve deafness, cleft palate, renal abnormalities, cryptorchidism, and neurologic abnormalities such as mirror movements. The initial genetic cause was identified in the X-linked *KAL* gene, mutations of which impair embryonic migration of GnRH neurons from the hypothalamic olfactory placode to the hypothalamus. Based on further studies, at least a dozen other genetic abnormalities, in addition to KAL mutations, have been found to cause isolated GnRH deficiency. Autosomal recessive (i.e., *GPR54*, *KISS1*) and dominant (i.e., *FGFR1*) modes of transmission have been described, and there is a growing list of genes associated with GnRH deficiency (*GNRH1, PROK2, PROKR2, CH7, PCSK1, FGF8, NELF, WDR11, TAC3, TACR3*). A fraction of patients have digenic mutations. Associated clinical features, in addition to GnRH deficiency, vary depending on the genetic cause. GnRH deficiency prevents progression through puberty. Males present with delayed puberty and pronounced hypogonadal features, including micropenis, probably the result of low testosterone levels during infancy. Females present with primary amenorrhea and failure of secondary sexual development.

Kallmann syndrome and other causes of congenital GnRH deficiency are characterized by low luteinizing hormone (LH) and follicle-stimulating hormone (FSH) levels and low concentrations of sex steroids (testosterone or estradiol). In sporadic cases of isolated gonadotropin deficiency, the diagnosis is often one of exclusion after other known causes of hypothalamic-pituitary dysfunction have been eliminated. Repetitive GnRH administration restores normal pituitary gonadotropin responses, pointing to a hypothalamic defect in these patients.

Long-term treatment of males with human chorionic gonadotropin (hCG) or testosterone restores pubertal development and secondary sex characteristics; women can be treated with cyclic estrogen and progestin. Fertility also may be restored by the administration of gonadotropins or by using a portable infusion pump to deliver subcutaneous, pulsatile GnRH.

BARDET-BIEDL SYNDROME This very rare genetically heterogeneous disorder is characterized by mental retardation, renal abnormalities, obesity, and hexadactyly, brachydactyly, or syndactyly. Central diabetes insipidus may or may not be associated. GnRH deficiency occurs in 75% of males and half of affected females. Retinal degeneration begins in early childhood, and most patients are blind by age 30. Numerous subtypes of Bardet-Biedl syndrome (BBS) have been identified, with genetic linkage to at least nine different loci. Several of the loci encode genes involved in basal body cilia function, and this may account for the diverse clinical manifestations.

LEPTIN AND LEPTIN RECEPTOR MUTATIONS Deficiencies of leptin or its receptor cause a broad spectrum of hypothalamic abnormalities, including hyperphagia, obesity, and central hypogonadism (Chap. 415e). Decreased GnRH production in these patients results in attenuated pituitary FSH and LH synthesis and release.

PRADER-WILLI SYNDROME This is a contiguous gene syndrome that results from deletion of the paternal copies of the imprinted *SNRPN* gene, the *NECDIN* gene, and possibly other genes on chromosome 15q. Prader-Willi syndrome is associated with hypogonadotropic hypogonadism, hyperphagia-obesity, chronic muscle hypotonia, mental retardation, and adult-onset diabetes mellitus (Chap. 83e). Multiple somatic defects also involve the skull, eyes, ears, hands, and feet. Diminished hypothalamic oxytocin- and vasopressin-producing nuclei have been reported. Deficient GnRH synthesis is suggested by the observation that chronic GnRH treatment restores pituitary LH and FSH release.

ACQUIRED HYPOPITUITARISM

Hypopituitarism may be caused by accidental or neurosurgical trauma; vascular events such as apoplexy; pituitary or hypothalamic neoplasms, craniopharyngioma, lymphoma, or metastatic tumors; inflammatory disease such as lymphocytic hypophysitis; infiltrative disorders such as sarcoidosis, hemochromatosis (Chap. 428), and tuberculosis; or irradiation.

Increasing evidence suggests that patients with brain injury, including contact sports trauma, subarachnoid hemorrhage, and irradiation, have transient hypopituitarism and require intermittent long-term endocrine follow-up, because permanent hypothalamic or pituitary dysfunction will develop in 25–40% of these patients.

Hypothalamic Infiltration Disorders These disorders—including sarcoidosis, histiocytosis X, amyloidosis, and hemochromatosis—frequently involve both hypothalamic and pituitary neuronal and neurochemical tracts. Consequently, diabetes insipidus occurs in half of patients with these disorders. Growth retardation is seen if attenuated GH secretion occurs before puberty. Hypogonadotropic hypogonadism and hyperprolactinemia are also common.

Inflammatory Lesions Pituitary damage and subsequent secretory dysfunction can be seen with chronic site infections such as tuberculosis, with opportunistic fungal infections associated with AIDS, and in tertiary syphilis. Other inflammatory processes, such as granulomas and sarcoidosis, may mimic the features of a pituitary adenoma. These lesions may cause extensive hypothalamic and pituitary damage, leading to trophic hormone deficiencies.

Cranial Irradiation Cranial irradiation may result in long-term hypothalamic and pituitary dysfunction, especially in children and adolescents, as they are more susceptible to damage after whole-brain or head and neck therapeutic irradiation. The development of hormonal abnormalities correlates strongly with irradiation dosage and the time interval after completion of radiotherapy. Up to two-thirds of patients ultimately develop hormone insufficiency after a median dose of 50 Gy (5000 rad) directed at the skull base. The development of hypopituitarism occurs over 5–15 years and usually reflects hypothalamic damage rather than primary destruction of pituitary cells. Although the pattern of hormone loss is variable, GH deficiency is most common, followed by gonadotropin and ACTH deficiency. When deficiency of one or more hormones is documented, the possibility of diminished reserve of other hormones is likely. Accordingly, anterior pituitary function should be continually evaluated over the long term in previously irradiated patients, and replacement therapy instituted when appropriate (see below).

Lymphocytic Hypophysitis This occurs most often in postpartum women; it usually presents with hyperprolactinemia and MRI evidence of a prominent pituitary mass that often resembles an adenoma, with mildly elevated PRL levels. Pituitary failure caused by diffuse lymphocytic infiltration may be transient or permanent but requires immediate evaluation and treatment. Rarely, isolated pituitary hormone deficiencies have been described, suggesting a selective autoimmune process targeted to specific cell types. Most patients manifest symptoms of progressive mass effects with headache and visual disturbance. The erythrocyte sedimentation rate often is elevated. Because the MRI image may be indistinguishable from that of a pituitary adenoma, hypophysitis should be considered in a postpartum woman with a newly diagnosed pituitary mass before an unnecessary surgical intervention is undertaken. The inflammatory process often resolves after several months of glucocorticoid treatment, and pituitary function may be restored, depending on the extent of damage.

Pituitary Apoplexy Acute intrapituitary hemorrhagic vascular events can cause substantial damage to the pituitary and surrounding sellar structures. Pituitary apoplexy may occur spontaneously in a preexisting adenoma; postpartum (Sheehan's syndrome); or in association with diabetes, hypertension, sickle cell anemia, or acute shock. The hyperplastic enlargement of the pituitary, which occurs normally during pregnancy, increases the risk for hemorrhage and infarction. Apoplexy is an endocrine emergency that may result in severe hypoglycemia, hypotension and shock, central nervous system (CNS) hemorrhage, and death. Acute symptoms may include severe headache with signs of meningeal irritation, bilateral visual changes, ophthalmoplegia, and, in severe cases, cardiovascular collapse and loss of consciousness. Pituitary computed tomography (CT) or MRI may reveal signs of intratumoral or sellar hemorrhage, with pituitary stalk deviation and compression of pituitary tissue.

Patients with no evident visual loss or impaired consciousness can be observed and managed conservatively with high-dose glucocorticoids. Those with significant or progressive visual loss, cranial nerve palsy, or loss of consciousness require urgent surgical decompression. Visual recovery after sellar surgery is inversely correlated with the length of time after the acute event. Therefore, severe ophthalmoplegia or visual deficits are indications for early surgery. Hypopituitarism is common after apoplexy.

Empty Sella A partial or apparently totally empty sella is often an incidental MRI finding, and may be associated with intracranial hypertension. These patients usually have normal pituitary function, implying that the surrounding rim of pituitary tissue is fully functional. Hypopituitarism, however, may develop insidiously. Pituitary masses also may undergo clinically silent infarction and involution with development of a partial or totally empty sella by cerebrospinal fluid (CSF) filling the dural herniation. Rarely, small but functional pituitary adenomas may arise within the rim of normal pituitary tissue, and they are not always visible on MRI.

PRESENTATION AND DIAGNOSIS

The clinical manifestations of hypopituitarism depend on which hormones are lost and the extent of the hormone deficiency. GH deficiency causes growth disorders in children and leads to abnormal body composition in adults (see below). Gonadotropin deficiency causes menstrual disorders and infertility in women and decreased sexual function, infertility, and loss of secondary sexual characteristics in men. TSH and ACTH deficiency usually develop later in the course of pituitary failure. TSH deficiency causes growth retardation in children and features of hypothyroidism in children and adults. The secondary form of adrenal insufficiency caused by ACTH deficiency leads to hypocortisolism with relative preservation of mineralocorticoid production. PRL deficiency causes failure of lactation. When lesions involve the posterior pituitary, polyuria and polydipsia reflect loss of vasopressin secretion. In patients with long-standing pituitary damage, epidemiologic studies document an increased mortality rate, primarily from increased cardiovascular and cerebrovascular disease. Previous head or neck irradiation is also a determinant of increased mortality rates in patients with hypopituitarism, especially from cerebrovascular disease.

LABORATORY INVESTIGATION

Biochemical diagnosis of pituitary insufficiency is made by demonstrating low levels of respective pituitary trophic hormones in the setting of low levels of target hormones. For example, low free thyroxine in the setting of a low or inappropriately normal TSH level suggests secondary hypothyroidism. Similarly, a low testosterone level without elevation of gonadotropins suggests hypogonadotropic hypogonadism. Provocative tests may be required to assess pituitary reserve (Table 402-2). GH responses to insulin-induced hypoglycemia, arginine, L-dopa, growth hormone–releasing hormone (GHRH), or growth hormone–releasing peptides (GHRPs) can be used to assess GH reserve. Corticotropin-releasing hormone (CRH) administration induces ACTH release, and administration of synthetic ACTH (cosyntropin) evokes adrenal cortisol release as an indirect indicator of pituitary ACTH reserve (Chap. 406). ACTH reserve is most reliably assessed by measuring ACTH and cortisol levels during insulin-induced hypoglycemia. However, this test should be performed cautiously in patients with suspected adrenal insufficiency because of enhanced susceptibility to hypoglycemia and hypotension. Administering insulin to induce hypoglycemia is contraindicated in patients with active coronary artery disease or known seizure disorders.

TREATMENT HYPOPITUITARISM

Hormone replacement therapy, including glucocorticoids, thyroid hormone, sex steroids, growth hormone, and vasopressin, is usually safe and free of complications. Treatment regimens that mimic physiologic hormone production allow for maintenance of satisfactory clinical homeostasis. Effective dosage schedules are outlined in Table 402-3. Patients in need of glucocorticoid replacement require careful dose adjustments during stressful events such as acute illness, dental procedures, trauma, and acute hospitalization.

DISORDERS OF GROWTH AND DEVELOPMENT

Skeletal Maturation and Somatic Growth The growth plate is dependent on a variety of hormonal stimuli, including GH, insulin-like growth factor (IGF) I, sex steroids, thyroid hormones, paracrine growth factors, and cytokines. The growth-promoting process also requires caloric energy, amino acids, vitamins, and trace metals and consumes about 10% of normal energy production. Malnutrition impairs chondrocyte activity, increases GH resistance, and reduces circulating IGF-I and IGFBP3 levels.

Linear bone growth rates are very high in infancy and are pituitary-dependent. Mean growth velocity is ~6 cm/year in later childhood and usually is maintained within a given range on a standardized percentile chart. Peak growth rates occur during midpuberty when bone age is 12 (girls) or 13 (boys). Secondary sexual development is associated with elevated sex steroids that cause progressive epiphyseal growth plate closure. *Bone age* is delayed in patients with all forms of true GH deficiency or GH receptor defects that result in attenuated GH action.

Short stature may occur as a result of constitutive intrinsic growth defects or because of acquired extrinsic factors that impair growth. In general, delayed bone age in a child with short stature is suggestive of a hormonal or systemic disorder, whereas normal bone age in a short child is more likely to be caused by a genetic cartilage dysplasia or growth plate disorder (Chap. 427).

GH Deficiency in Children • ***GH DEFICIENCY*** Isolated GH deficiency is characterized by short stature, micropenis, increased fat, high-pitched voice, and a propensity to hypoglycemia due to relatively unopposed insulin action. Familial modes of inheritance are seen in at least one-third of these individuals and may be autosomal dominant, recessive,

TABLE 402-2 TESTS OF PITUITARY SUFFICIENCY

Hormone	Test	Blood Samples	Interpretation
Growth hormone (GH)	Insulin tolerance test: Regular insulin (0.05–0.15 U/kg IV)	−30, 0, 30, 60, 120 min for glucose and GH	Glucose <40 mg/dL; GH should be >3 μg/L
	GHRH test: 1 μg/kg IV	0, 15, 30, 45, 60, 120 min for GH	Normal response is GH >3 μg/L
	L-Arginine test: 30 g IV over 30 min	0, 30, 60, 120 min for GH	Normal response is GH >3 μg/L
	L-Dopa test: 500 mg PO	0, 30, 60, 120 min for GH	Normal response is GH >3 μg/L
Prolactin	TRH test: 200–500 μg IV	0, 20, and 60 min for TSH and PRL	Normal prolactin is >2 μg/L and increase >200% of baseline
ACTH	Insulin tolerance test: regular insulin (0.05–0.15 U/kg IV)	−30, 0, 30, 60, 90 min for glucose and cortisol	Glucose <40 mg/dL Cortisol should increase by >7 μg/dL or to >20 μg/dL
	CRH test: 1 μg/kg ovine CRH IV at 8 A.M.	0, 15, 30, 60, 90, 120 min for ACTH and cortisol	Basal ACTH increases 2- to 4-fold and peaks at 20–100 pg/mL Cortisol levels >20–25 μg/dL
	Metyrapone test: Metyrapone (30 mg/kg) at midnight	Plasma 11-deoxycortisol and cortisol at 8 A.M.; ACTH can also be measured	Plasma cortisol should be <4 g/dL to assure an adequate response Normal response is 11-deoxycortisol >7.5 μg/dL or ACTH >75 pg/mL
	Standard ACTH stimulation test: ACTH 1-24 (cosyntropin), 0.25 mg IM or IV	0, 30, 60 min for cortisol and aldosterone	Normal response is cortisol >21 g/dL and aldosterone response of >4 ng/dL above baseline
	Low-dose ACTH test: ACTH 1-24 (cosyntropin), 1 μg IV	0, 30, 60 min for cortisol	Cortisol should be >21 g/dL
	3-day ACTH stimulation test consists of 0.25 mg ACTH 1-24 given IV over 8 h each day		Cortisol >21 g/dL
TSH	Basal thyroid function tests: T_4, T_3, TSH	Basal measurements	Low free thyroid hormone levels in the setting of TSH levels that are not appropriately increased indicate pituitary insufficiency
	TRH test: 200–500 μg IV	0, 20, 60 min for TSH and PRL[a]	TSH should increase by >5 mU/L unless thyroid hormone levels are increased
LH, FSH	LH, FSH, testosterone, estrogen	Basal measurements	Basal LH and FSH should be increased in postmenopausal women Low testosterone levels in the setting of low LH and FSH indicate pituitary insufficiency
	GnRH test: GnRH (100 μg) IV	0, 30, 60 min for LH and FSH	In most adults, LH should increase by 10 IU/L and FSH by 2 IU/L Normal responses are variable
Multiple hormones	Combined anterior pituitary test: GHRH (1 g/kg), CRH (1 μg/kg), GnRH (100 g), TRH (200 μg) are given IV	−30, 0, 15, 30, 60, 90, 120 min for GH, ACTH, cortisol, LH, FSH, and TSH	Combined or individual releasing hormone responses must be elevated in the context of basal target gland hormone values and may not be uniformly diagnostic (see text)

[a]Evoked PRL response indicates lactotrope integrity.

Abbreviations: T_3, triiodothyronine; T_4, thyroxine; TRH, thyrotropin-releasing hormone. For other abbreviations, see text.

or X-linked. About 10% of children with GH deficiency have mutations in the *GH-N* gene, including gene deletions and a wide range of point mutations. Mutations in transcription factors Pit-1 and Prop-1, which control somatotrope development, result in GH deficiency in combination with other pituitary hormone deficiencies, which may become manifest only in adulthood. The diagnosis of *idiopathic GH deficiency* (IGHD) should be made only after known molecular defects have been rigorously excluded.

GHRH RECEPTOR MUTATIONS Recessive mutations of the GHRH receptor gene in subjects with severe proportionate dwarfism are associated with low basal GH levels that cannot be stimulated by exogenous GHRH, GHRP, or insulin-induced hypoglycemia, as well as anterior pituitary hypoplasia The syndrome exemplifies the importance of the GHRH receptor for somatotrope cell proliferation and hormonal responsiveness.

GH INSENSITIVITY This is caused by defects of GH receptor structure or signaling. Homozygous or heterozygous mutations of the GH receptor are associated with partial or complete GH insensitivity and growth failure (*Laron's syndrome*). The diagnosis is based on normal or high GH levels, with decreased circulating GH-binding protein (GHBP), and low IGF-I levels. Very rarely, defective IGF-I, IGF-I receptor, or IGF-I signaling defects are also encountered. *STAT5B* mutations result in both immunodeficiency as well as abrogated GH signaling, leading to short stature with normal or elevated GH levels and low IGF-I levels. Circulating GH receptor antibodies may rarely cause peripheral GH insensitivity.

NUTRITIONAL SHORT STATURE Caloric deprivation and malnutrition, uncontrolled diabetes, and chronic renal failure represent secondary causes of abrogated GH receptor function. These conditions also stimulate production of proinflammatory cytokines, which act to exacerbate the block of GH-mediated signal transduction. Children with these conditions typically exhibit features of acquired short stature with normal or elevated GH and low IGF-I levels.

PSYCHOSOCIAL SHORT STATURE Emotional and social deprivation lead to growth retardation accompanied by delayed speech, discordant hyperphagia, and an attenuated response to administered GH. A nurturing environment restores growth rates.

PRESENTATION AND DIAGNOSIS

Short stature is commonly encountered in clinical practice, and the decision to evaluate these children requires clinical judgment in association with auxologic data and family history. Short stature should be evaluated comprehensively if a patient's height is >3 standard deviations (SD) below the mean for age or if the growth rate has decelerated. Skeletal maturation is best evaluated by measuring a radiologic bone age, which is based mainly on the degree of wrist bone growth plate fusion. Final height can be predicted using standardized scales (Bayley-Pinneau or Tanner-Whitehouse) or

TABLE 402-3 HORMONE REPLACEMENT THERAPY FOR ADULT HYPOPITUITARISM[a]

Trophic Hormone Deficit	Hormone Replacement
ACTH	Hydrocortisone (10–20 mg A.M.; 5–10 mg P.M.)
	Cortisone acetate (25 mg A.M.; 12.5 mg P.M.)
	Prednisone (5 mg A.M.)
TSH	L-Thyroxine (0.075–0.15 mg daily)
FSH/LH	Males
	Testosterone gel (5–10 g/d)
	Testosterone skin patch (5 mg/d)
	Testosterone enanthate (200 mg IM every 2 weeks)
	Females
	Conjugated estrogen (0.65–1.25 mg qd for 25 days)
	Progesterone (5–10 mg qd) on days 16–25
	Estradiol skin patch (0.025–0.1 mg every week), adding progesterone on days 16–25 if uterus intact
	For fertility: menopausal gonadotropins, human chorionic gonadotropins
GH	Adults: Somatotropin (0.1–1.25 mg SC qd)
	Children: Somatotropin (0.02–0.05 mg/kg per day)
Vasopressin	Intranasal desmopressin (5–20 g twice daily)
	Oral 300–600 μg qd

[a]All doses shown should be individualized for specific patients and should be reassessed during stress, surgery, or pregnancy. Male and female fertility requirements should be managed as discussed in **Chaps. 411 and 412**.

Note: For abbreviations, see text.

estimated by adding 6.5 cm (boys) or subtracting 6.5 cm (girls) from the midparental height.

LABORATORY INVESTIGATION

Because GH secretion is pulsatile, GH deficiency is best assessed by examining the response to provocative stimuli, including exercise, insulin-induced hypoglycemia, and other pharmacologic tests that normally increase GH to >7 μg/L in children. Random GH measurements do not distinguish normal children from those with true GH deficiency. Adequate adrenal and thyroid hormone replacement should be assured before testing. Age- and sex-matched IGF-I levels are not sufficiently sensitive or specific to make the diagnosis but can be useful to confirm GH deficiency. Pituitary MRI may reveal pituitary mass lesions or structural defects. Molecular analyses for known mutations should be undertaken when the cause of short stature remains cryptic, or when additional clinical features suggest a genetic cause.

TREATMENT DISORDERS OF GROWTH AND DEVELOPMENT

Replacement therapy with recombinant GH (0.02–0.05 mg/kg per day SC) restores growth velocity in GH-deficient children to ~10 cm/year. If pituitary insufficiency is documented, other associated hormone deficits should be corrected, especially adrenal steroids. GH treatment is also moderately effective for accelerating growth rates in children with Turner's syndrome and chronic renal failure.

In patients with GH insensitivity and growth retardation due to mutations of the GH receptor, treatment with IGF-I bypasses the dysfunctional GH receptor.

ADULT GH DEFICIENCY (AGHD)

This disorder usually is caused by acquired hypothalamic or pituitary somatotrope damage. Acquired pituitary hormone deficiency follows a typical pattern in which loss of adequate GH reserve foreshadows subsequent hormone deficits. The sequential order of hormone loss is usually GH → FSH/LH → TSH → ACTH. Patients previously diagnosed with childhood-onset GH deficiency should be retested as adults to affirm the diagnosis.

TABLE 402-4 FEATURES OF ADULT GROWTH HORMONE DEFICIENCY

Clinical

- Impaired quality of life
  - Decreased energy and drive
  - Poor concentration
  - Low self-esteem
  - Social isolation
- Body composition changes
  - Increased body fat mass
  - Central fat deposition
  - Increased waist-to-hip ratio
  - Decreased lean body mass
- Reduced exercise capacity
  - Reduced maximum O_2 uptake
  - Impaired cardiac function
  - Reduced muscle mass
- Cardiovascular risk factors
  - Impaired cardiac structure and function
  - Abnormal lipid profile
  - Decreased fibrinolytic activity
  - Atherosclerosis
  - Omental obesity

Imaging

- Pituitary: mass or structural damage
- Bone: reduced bone mineral density
- Abdomen: excess omental adiposity

Laboratory

- Evoked GH <3 ng/mL
- IGF-I and IGFBP3 low or normal
- Increased LDL cholesterol
- Concomitant gonadotropin, TSH, and/or ACTH reserve deficits may be present

Abbreviation: LDL, low-density lipoprotein. For other abbreviations, see text.

PRESENTATION AND DIAGNOSIS

The clinical features of AGHD include changes in body composition, lipid metabolism, and quality of life and cardiovascular dysfunction (Table 402-4). Body composition changes are common and include reduced lean body mass, increased fat mass with selective deposition of intraabdominal visceral fat, and increased waist-to-hip ratio. Hyperlipidemia, left ventricular dysfunction, hypertension, and increased plasma fibrinogen levels also may be present. Bone mineral content is reduced, with resultant increased fracture rates. Patients may experience social isolation, depression, and difficulty maintaining gainful employment. Adult hypopituitarism is associated with a threefold increase in cardiovascular mortality rates in comparison to age- and sex-matched controls, and this may be due to GH deficiency, as patients in these studies were replaced with other deficient pituitary hormones.

LABORATORY INVESTIGATION

AGHD is rare, and in light of the nonspecific nature of associated clinical symptoms, patients appropriate for testing should be selected carefully on the basis of well-defined criteria. With few exceptions, testing should be restricted to patients with the following predisposing factors: (1) pituitary surgery, (2) pituitary or hypothalamic tumor or granulomas, (3) history of cranial irradiation, (4) radiologic evidence of a pituitary lesion, (5) childhood requirement for GH replacement therapy, and rarely (6) unexplained low age- and sex-matched IGF-I levels. The transition of a GH-deficient adolescent to adulthood requires retesting to document subsequent adult GH deficiency. Up to 20% of patients previously treated for childhood-onset GH deficiency are found to be GH-sufficient on repeat testing as adults.

A significant proportion (~25%) of truly GH-deficient adults have low-normal IGF-I levels. Thus, as in the evaluation of GH deficiency in children, valid age- and sex-matched IGF-I measurements provide a useful index of therapeutic responses but are not sufficiently sensitive for diagnostic purposes. The most validated test to distinguish pituitary-sufficient patients from those with AGHD is insulin-induced (0.05–0.1 U/kg) hypoglycemia. After glucose reduction to ~40 mg/dL, most individuals experience neuroglycopenic symptoms (Chap. 420), and peak GH release occurs at 60 min and remains elevated for up to 2 h. About 90% of healthy adults exhibit GH responses >5 μg/L; AGHD is defined by a peak GH response to hypoglycemia of <3 μg/L. Although insulin-induced hypoglycemia is safe when performed under appropriate supervision, it is contraindicated in patients with diabetes, ischemic heart disease, cerebrovascular disease, or epilepsy and in elderly patients. Alternative stimulatory tests include intravenous arginine (30 g), GHRH (1 μg/kg), GHRP-6 (90 μg), and glucagon (1 mg). Combinations of these tests may evoke GH secretion in subjects who are not responsive to a single test.

TREATMENT ADULT GH DEFICIENCY

Once the diagnosis of AGHD is unequivocally established, replacement of GH may be indicated. Contraindications to therapy include the presence of an active neoplasm, intracranial hypertension, and uncontrolled diabetes and retinopathy. The starting dose of 0.1–0.2 mg/d should be titrated (up to a maximum of 1.25 mg/d) to maintain IGF-I levels in the mid-normal range for age- and sex-matched controls (Fig. 402-1). Women require higher doses than men, and elderly patients require less GH. Long-term GH maintenance sustains normal IGF-I levels and is associated with persistent body composition changes (e.g., enhanced lean body mass and lower body fat). High-density lipoprotein cholesterol increases, but total cholesterol and insulin levels may not change significantly. Lumbar spine bone mineral density increases, but this response is gradual (>1 year). Many patients note significant improvement in quality of life when evaluated by standardized questionnaires. The effect of GH replacement on mortality rates in GH-deficient patients is currently the subject of long-term prospective investigation.

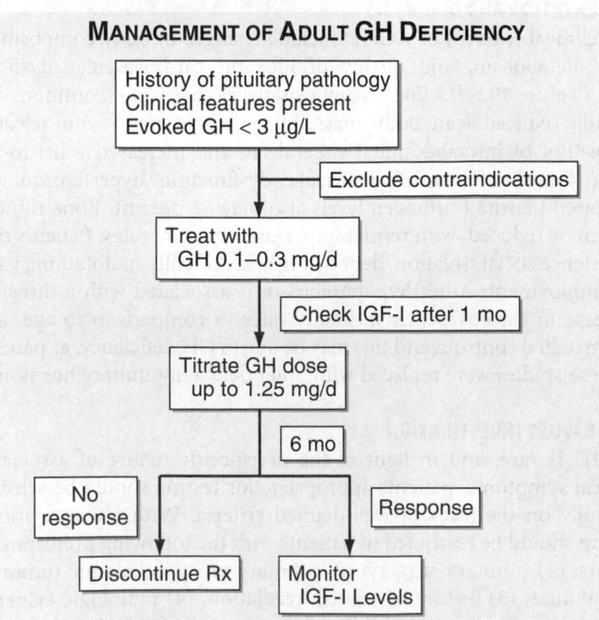

FIGURE 402-1 Management of adult growth hormone (GH) deficiency. IGF, insulin-like growth factor; Rx, Treatment.

About 30% of patients exhibit reversible dose-related fluid retention, joint pain, and carpal tunnel syndrome, and up to 40% exhibit myalgias and paresthesia. Patients receiving insulin require careful monitoring for dosing adjustments, as GH is a potent counterregulatory hormone for insulin action. Patients with type 2 diabetes mellitus initially develop further insulin resistance. However, glycemic control usually improves with the sustained loss of abdominal fat associated with long-term GH replacement. Headache, increased intracranial pressure, hypertension, and tinnitus occur rarely. Pituitary tumor regrowth and progression of skin lesions or other tumors are being assessed in long-term surveillance programs. To date, development of these potential side effects does not appear significant.

ACTH DEFICIENCY

PRESENTATION AND DIAGNOSIS

Secondary adrenal insufficiency occurs as a result of pituitary ACTH deficiency. It is characterized by fatigue, weakness, anorexia, nausea, vomiting, and, occasionally, hypoglycemia. In contrast to primary adrenal failure, hypocortisolism associated with pituitary failure usually is not accompanied by hyperpigmentation or mineralocorticoid deficiency.

ACTH deficiency is commonly due to glucocorticoid withdrawal after treatment-associated suppression of the hypothalamic-pituitary-adrenal (HPA) axis. Isolated ACTH deficiency may occur after surgical resection of an ACTH-secreting pituitary adenoma that has suppressed the HPA axis; this phenomenon is in fact suggestive of a surgical cure. The mass effects of other pituitary adenomas or sellar lesions may lead to ACTH deficiency, but usually in combination with other pituitary hormone deficiencies. Partial ACTH deficiency may be unmasked in the presence of an acute medical or surgical illness, when clinically significant hypocortisolism reflects diminished ACTH reserve. Rarely, *TPIT* or *POMC* mutations result in primary ACTH deficiency.

LABORATORY DIAGNOSIS

Inappropriately low ACTH levels in the setting of low cortisol levels are characteristic of diminished ACTH reserve. Low basal serum cortisol levels are associated with blunted cortisol responses to ACTH stimulation and impaired cortisol response to insulin-induced hypoglycemia, or testing with metyrapone or CRH. For a description of provocative ACTH tests, see Chap. 406.

TREATMENT ACTH DEFICIENCY

Glucocorticoid replacement therapy improves most features of ACTH deficiency. The total daily dose of hydrocortisone replacement preferably should not exceed 25 mg daily, divided into two or three doses. Prednisone (5 mg each morning) is longer acting and has fewer mineralocorticoid effects than hydrocortisone. Some authorities advocate lower maintenance doses in an effort to avoid cushingoid side effects. Doses should be increased severalfold during periods of acute illness or stress.

GONADOTROPIN DEFICIENCY

Hypogonadism is the most common presenting feature of adult hypopituitarism even when other pituitary hormones are also deficient. It is often a harbinger of hypothalamic or pituitary lesions that impair GnRH production or delivery through the pituitary stalk. As noted below, hypogonadotropic hypogonadism is a common presenting feature of hyperprolactinemia.

A variety of inherited and acquired disorders are associated with *isolated hypogonadotropic hypogonadism* (IHH) (Chap. 411). Hypothalamic defects associated with GnRH deficiency include Kallmann syndrome and mutations in more than a dozen genes that regulate GnRH neuron migration, development, and function (see above). Mutations in GPR54, DAX1, kisspeptin, the GnRH receptor, and the LHβ or FSHβ subunit genes also cause pituitary gonadotropin deficiency. Acquired forms of GnRH deficiency leading to hypogonadotropism are seen in association with anorexia nervosa, stress, starvation, and extreme exercise but also may be idiopathic. Hypogonadotropic hypogonadism in these disorders is reversed by removal of the stressful stimulus or by caloric replenishment.

PRESENTATION AND DIAGNOSIS

In premenopausal women, hypogonadotropic hypogonadism presents as diminished ovarian function leading to oligomenorrhea or amenorrhea, infertility, decreased vaginal secretions, decreased libido, and breast atrophy. In hypogonadal adult men, secondary testicular failure is associated with decreased libido and potency, infertility, decreased muscle mass with weakness, reduced beard and body hair growth, soft testes, and characteristic fine facial wrinkles. Osteoporosis occurs in both untreated hypogonadal women and men.

LABORATORY INVESTIGATION

Central hypogonadism is associated with low or inappropriately normal serum gonadotropin levels in the setting of low sex hormone concentrations (testosterone in men, estradiol in women). Because gonadotropin secretion is pulsatile, valid assessments may require repeated measurements or the use of pooled serum samples. Men have reduced sperm counts.

Intravenous GnRH (100 μg) stimulates gonadotropes to secrete LH (which peaks within 30 min) and FSH (which plateaus during the ensuing 60 min). Normal responses vary according to menstrual cycle stage, age, and sex of the patient. Generally, LH levels increase about threefold, whereas FSH responses are less pronounced. In the setting of gonadotropin deficiency, a normal gonadotropin response to GnRH indicates intact pituitary gonadotrope function and suggests a hypothalamic abnormality. An absent response, however, does not reliably distinguish pituitary from hypothalamic causes of hypogonadism. For this reason, GnRH testing usually adds little to the information gained from baseline evaluation of the hypothalamic-pituitary-gonadotrope axis except in cases of isolated GnRH deficiency (e.g., Kallmann syndrome).

MRI examination of the sellar region and assessment of other pituitary functions usually are indicated in patients with documented central hypogonadism.

TREATMENT GONADOTROPIN DEFICIENCY

In males, testosterone replacement is necessary to achieve and maintain normal growth and development of the external genitalia, secondary sex characteristics, male sexual behavior, and androgenic anabolic effects, including maintenance of muscle function and bone mass. Testosterone may be administered by intramuscular injections every 1–4 weeks or by using skin patches that are replaced daily (Chap. 411). Testosterone gels are also available. Gonadotropin injections (hCG or human menopausal gonadotropin [hMG]) over 12–18 months are used to restore fertility. Pulsatile GnRH therapy (25–150 ng/kg every 2 h), administered by a subcutaneous infusion pump, is also effective for treatment of hypothalamic hypogonadism when fertility is desired.

In premenopausal women, cyclical replacement of estrogen and progesterone maintains secondary sexual characteristics and integrity of genitourinary tract mucosa and prevents premature osteoporosis (Chap. 412). Gonadotropin therapy is used for ovulation induction. Follicular growth and maturation are initiated using hMG or recombinant FSH; hCG or human luteinizing hormone (hLH) is subsequently injected to induce ovulation. As in men, pulsatile GnRH therapy can be used to treat hypothalamic causes of gonadotropin deficiency.

DIABETES INSIPIDUS

See Chap. 404 for diagnosis and treatment of diabetes insipidus.

403 Anterior Pituitary Tumor Syndromes

Shlomo Melmed, J. Larry Jameson

HYPOTHALAMIC, PITUITARY, AND OTHER SELLAR MASSES

EVALUATION OF SELLAR MASSES

Local Mass Effects Clinical manifestations of sellar lesions vary, depending on the anatomic location of the mass and the direction of its extension (Table 403-1). The dorsal sellar diaphragm presents the least resistance to soft tissue expansion from the sella; consequently, pituitary adenomas frequently extend in a suprasellar direction. Bony invasion may occur as well.

Headaches are common features of small intrasellar tumors, even with no demonstrable suprasellar extension. Because of the confined nature of the pituitary, small changes in intrasellar pressure stretch the dural plate; however, headache severity correlates poorly with adenoma size or extension.

Suprasellar extension can lead to visual loss by several mechanisms, the most common being compression of the optic chiasm, but rarely, direct invasion of the optic nerves or obstruction of cerebrospinal fluid (CSF) flow leading to secondary visual disturbances can occur. Pituitary stalk compression by a hormonally active or inactive intrasellar mass may compress the portal vessels, disrupting pituitary access to hypothalamic hormones and dopamine; this results in early hyperprolactinemia and later concurrent loss of other pituitary hormones. This "stalk section" phenomenon may also be caused by trauma, whiplash injury with posterior clinoid stalk compression, or skull base fractures. Lateral mass invasion may impinge on the cavernous sinus and compress its neural contents, leading to cranial nerve III,

TABLE 403-1 FEATURES OF SELLAR MASS LESIONS[a]

Impacted Structure	Clinical Impact
Pituitary	Hypogonadism
	Hypothyroidism
	Growth failure and adult hyposomatotropism
	Hypoadrenalism
Optic chiasm	Loss of red perception
	Bitemporal hemianopia
	Superior or bitemporal field defect
	Scotoma
	Blindness
Hypothalamus	Temperature dysregulation
	Appetite and thirst disorders
	Obesity
	Diabetes insipidus
	Sleep disorders
	Behavioral dysfunction
	Autonomic dysfunction
Cavernous sinus	Ophthalmoplegia with or without ptosis or diplopia
	Facial numbness
Frontal lobe	Personality disorder
	Anosmia
Brain	Headache
	Hydrocephalus
	Psychosis
	Dementia
	Laughing seizures

[a]As the intrasellar mass expands, it first compresses intrasellar pituitary tissue, then usually invades dorsally through the dura to lift the optic chiasm or laterally to the cavernous sinuses. Bony erosion is rare, as is direct brain compression. Microadenomas may present with headache.

IV, and VI palsies as well as effects on the ophthalmic and maxillary branches of the fifth cranial nerve (Chap. 455). Patients may present with diplopia, ptosis, ophthalmoplegia, and decreased facial sensation, depending on the extent of neural damage. Extension into the sphenoid sinus indicates that the pituitary mass has eroded through the sellar floor. Aggressive tumors rarely invade the palate roof and cause nasopharyngeal obstruction, infection, and CSF leakage. Temporal and frontal lobe involvement may rarely lead to uncinate seizures, personality disorders, and anosmia. Direct hypothalamic encroachment by an invasive pituitary mass may cause important metabolic sequelae, including precocious puberty or hypogonadism, diabetes insipidus, sleep disturbances, dysthermia, and appetite disorders.

Magnetic Resonance Imaging Sagittal and coronal T1-weighted magnetic resonance imaging (MRI) before and after administration of gadolinium allows precise visualization of the pituitary gland with clear delineation of the hypothalamus, pituitary stalk, pituitary tissue and surrounding suprasellar cisterns, cavernous sinuses, sphenoid sinus, and optic chiasm. Pituitary gland height ranges from 6 mm in children to 8 mm in adults; during pregnancy and puberty, the height may reach 10–12 mm. The upper aspect of the adult pituitary is flat or slightly concave, but in adolescent and pregnant individuals, this surface may be convex, reflecting physiologic pituitary enlargement. The stalk should be midline and vertical. Computed tomography (CT) scan is reserved to define the extent of bony erosion or the presence of calcification.

Anterior pituitary gland soft tissue consistency is slightly heterogeneous on MRI, and signal intensity resembles that of brain matter on T1-weighted imaging (Fig. 403-1). Adenoma density is usually lower than that of surrounding normal tissue on T1-weighted imaging, and the signal intensity increases with T2-weighted images. The high phospholipid content of the posterior pituitary results in a "pituitary bright spot."

Sellar masses are encountered commonly as incidental findings on MRI, and most of them are pituitary adenomas (incidentalomas). In the absence of hormone hypersecretion, these small intrasellar lesions can be monitored safely with MRI, which is performed annually and then less often if there is no evidence of further growth. Resection should be considered for incidentally discovered larger macroadenomas, because about one-third become invasive or cause local pressure effects. If hormone hypersecretion is evident, specific therapies are indicated as described below. When larger masses (>1 cm) are encountered, they should also be distinguished from nonadenomatous lesions. Meningiomas often are associated with bony hyperostosis; craniopharyngiomas may be calcified and are usually hypodense, whereas gliomas are hyperdense on T2-weighted images.

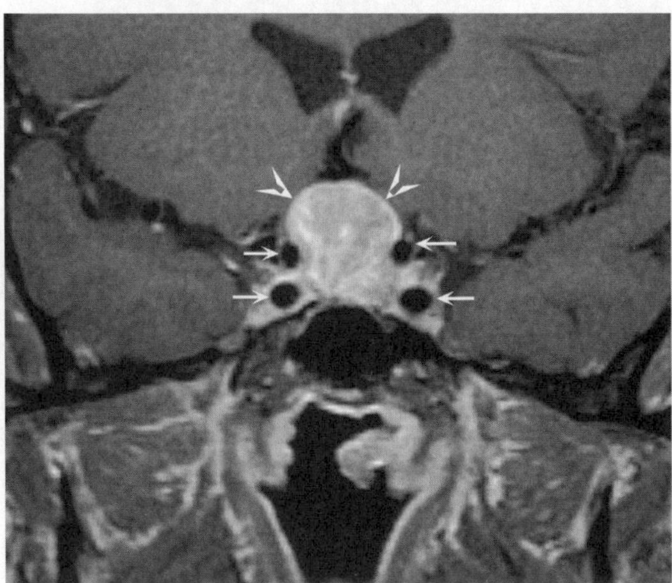

FIGURE 403-1 Pituitary adenoma. Coronal T1-weighted postcontrast magnetic resonance image shows a homogeneously enhancing mass (*arrowheads*) in the sella turcica and suprasellar region compatible with a pituitary adenoma; the *small arrows* outline the carotid arteries.

TABLE 403-2 SCREENING TESTS FOR FUNCTIONAL PITUITARY ADENOMAS

	Test	Comments
Acromegaly	Serum IGF-I	Interpret IGF-I relative to age- and sex-matched controls
	Oral glucose tolerance test with GH obtained at 0, 30, and 60 min	Normal subjects should suppress growth hormone to <1 g/L
Prolactinoma	Serum PRL	Exclude medications
		MRI of the sella should be ordered if PRL is elevated
Cushing's disease	24-h urinary free cortisol	Ensure urine collection is total and accurate
	Dexamethasone (1 mg) at 11 P.M. and fasting plasma cortisol measured at 8 A.M.	Normal subjects suppress to <5 g/dL
	ACTH assay	Distinguishes adrenal adenoma (ACTH suppressed) from ectopic ACTH or Cushing's disease (ACTH normal or elevated)

Abbreviations: ACTH, adrenocorticotropin hormone; GH, growth hormone; IGF-I, insulin-like growth factor I; MRI, magnetic resonance imaging; PRL, prolactin.

Ophthalmologic Evaluation Because optic tracts may be contiguous to an expanding pituitary mass, reproducible visual field assessment using perimetry techniques should be performed on all patients with sellar mass lesions that impinge the optic chiasm (Chap. 39). Bitemporal hemianopia, often more pronounced superiorly, is observed classically. It occurs because nasal ganglion cell fibers, which cross in the optic chiasm, are especially vulnerable to compression of the ventral optic chiasm. Occasionally, homonymous hemianopia occurs from postchiasmal compression or monocular temporal field loss from prechiasmal compression. Invasion of the cavernous sinus can produce diplopia from ocular motor nerve palsy. Early diagnosis reduces the risk of optic atrophy, vision loss, or eye misalignment.

Laboratory Investigation The presenting clinical features of functional pituitary adenomas (e.g., acromegaly, prolactinomas, or Cushing's syndrome) should guide the laboratory studies (Table 403-2). However, for a sellar mass with no obvious clinical features of hormone excess, laboratory studies are geared toward determining the nature of the tumor and assessing the possible presence of hypopituitarism. When a pituitary adenoma is suspected based on MRI, initial hormonal evaluation usually includes (1) basal prolactin (PRL); (2) insulin-like growth factor (IGF) I; (3) 24-h urinary free cortisol (UFC) and/or overnight oral dexamethasone (1 mg) suppression test; (4) α subunit, follicle-stimulating hormone (FSH), and luteinizing hormone (LH); and (5) thyroid function tests. Additional hormonal evaluation may be indicated based on the results of these tests. Pending more detailed assessment of hypopituitarism, a menstrual history, measurement of testosterone and 8 A.M. cortisol levels, and thyroid function tests usually identify patients with pituitary hormone deficiencies that require hormone replacement before further testing or surgery.

Histologic Evaluation Immunohistochemical staining of pituitary tumor specimens obtained at transsphenoidal surgery confirms clinical and laboratory studies and provides a histologic diagnosis when hormone studies are equivocal and in cases of clinically nonfunctioning tumors. Occasionally, ultrastructural assessment by electron microscopy is required for diagnosis.

TREATMENT HYPOTHALAMIC, PITUITARY, AND OTHER SELLAR MASSES

OVERVIEW Successful management of sellar masses requires accurate diagnosis as well as selection of optimal therapeutic modalities. Most pituitary tumors are benign and slow-growing. Clinical features result from local mass effects and hormonal hyper- or hyposecretion syndromes caused directly by the adenoma or occurring as a consequence of treatment. Thus, lifelong management and follow-up are necessary for these patients.

MRI with gadolinium enhancement for pituitary visualization, new advances in transsphenoidal surgery and in stereotactic radiotherapy (including gamma-knife radiotherapy), and novel therapeutic agents have improved pituitary tumor management. The goals of pituitary tumor treatment include normalization of excess pituitary secretion, amelioration of symptoms and signs of hormonal hypersecretion syndromes, and shrinkage or ablation of large tumor masses with relief of adjacent structure compression. Residual anterior pituitary function should be preserved during treatment and sometimes can be restored by removing the tumor mass. Ideally, adenoma recurrence should be prevented.

TRANSSPHENOIDAL SURGERY Transsphenoidal rather than transfrontal resection is the desired surgical approach for pituitary tumors, except for the rare invasive suprasellar mass surrounding the frontal or middle fossa or the optic nerves or invading posteriorly behind the clivus. Intraoperative microscopy facilitates visual distinction between adenomatous and normal pituitary tissue as well as microdissection of small tumors that may not be visible by MRI (**Fig. 403-2**). Transsphenoidal surgery also avoids the cranial invasion and manipulation of brain tissue required by subfrontal surgical approaches. Endoscopic techniques with three-dimensional intraoperative localization have also improved visualization and access to tumor tissue. Individual surgical experience is a major determinant of outcome efficacy with these techniques.

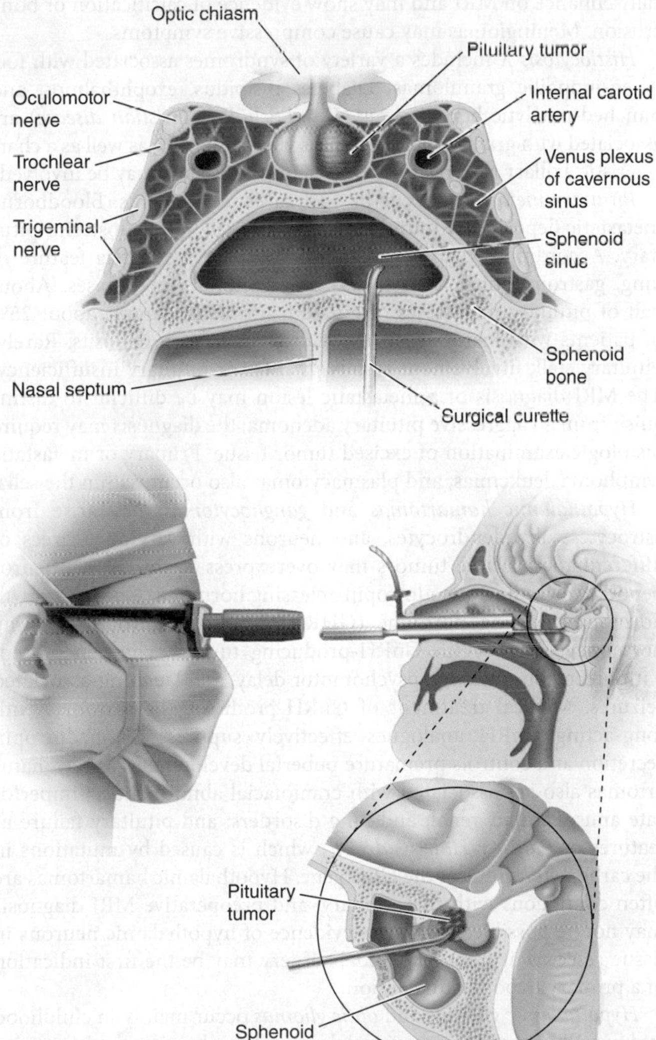

FIGURE 403-2 **Transsphenoidal resection of pituitary mass via the endonasal approach.** *(Adapted from R Fahlbusch: Endocrinol Metab Clin 21:669, 1992.)*

In addition to correction of hormonal hypersecretion, pituitary surgery is indicated for mass lesions that impinge on surrounding structures. Surgical decompression and resection are required for an expanding pituitary mass accompanied by persistent headache, progressive visual field defects, cranial nerve palsies, hydrocephalus, and, occasionally, intrapituitary hemorrhage and apoplexy. Transsphenoidal surgery sometimes is used for pituitary tissue biopsy to establish a histologic diagnosis.Whenever possible, the pituitary mass lesion should be selectively excised; normal pituitary tissue should be manipulated or resected only when critical for effective mass dissection. Nonselective hemihypophysectomy or total hypophysectomy may be indicated if no hypersecreting mass lesion is clearly discernible, multifocal lesions are present, or the remaining nontumorous pituitary tissue is obviously necrotic. This strategy, however, increases the likelihood of hypopituitarism and the need for lifelong hormone replacement.

Preoperative mass effects, including visual field defects and compromised pituitary function, may be reversed by surgery, particularly when the deficits are not long-standing. For large and invasive tumors, it is necessary to determine the optimal balance between maximal tumor resection and preservation of anterior pituitary function, especially for preserving growth and reproductive function in younger patients. Similarly, tumor invasion outside the sella is rarely amenable to surgical cure; the surgeon must judge the risk-versus-benefit ratio of extensive tumor resection.

Side Effects Tumor size, the degree of invasiveness, and experience of the surgeon largely determine the incidence of surgical complications. Operative mortality rate is about 1%. Transient diabetes insipidus and hypopituitarism occur in up to 20% of patients. Permanent diabetes insipidus, cranial nerve damage, nasal septal perforation, or visual disturbances may be encountered in up to 10% of patients. CSF leaks occur in 4% of patients. Less common complications include carotid artery injury, loss of vision, hypothalamic damage, and meningitis. Permanent side effects are rare after surgery for microadenomas.

RADIATION

Radiation is used either as a primary therapy for pituitary or parasellar masses or, more commonly, as an adjunct to surgery or medical therapy. Focused megavoltage irradiation is achieved by precise MRI localization, using a high-voltage linear accelerator and accurate isocentric rotational arcing. A major determinant of accurate irradiation is reproduction of the patient's head position during multiple visits and maintenance of absolute head immobility. A total of <50 Gy (5000 rad) is given as 180-cGy (180-rad) fractions divided over about 6 weeks. Stereotactic radiosurgery delivers a large single high-energy dose from a cobalt-60 source (gamma knife), linear accelerator, or cyclotron. Long-term effects of gamma-knife surgery are unclear but appear to be similar to those encountered with conventional radiation. Proton beam therapy is available in some centers and provides concentrated radiation doses within a localized region.

The role of radiation therapy in pituitary tumor management depends on multiple factors, including the nature of the tumor, the age of the patient, and the availability of surgical and radiation expertise. Because of its relatively slow onset of action, radiation therapy is usually reserved for postsurgical management. As an adjuvant to surgery, radiation is used to treat residual tumor and in an attempt to prevent regrowth. Irradiation offers the only means for potentially ablating significant postoperative residual nonfunctioning tumor tissue. In contrast, PRL- and growth hormone (GH)-secreting tumor tissues are amenable to medical therapy.

Side Effects In the short term, radiation may cause transient nausea and weakness. Alopecia and loss of taste and smell may be more long-lasting. Failure of pituitary hormone synthesis is common in patients who have undergone head and neck or pituitary-directed irradiation. More than 50% of patients develop loss of GH, adrenocorticotropin hormone (ACTH), thyroid-stimulating hormone (TSH), and/or gonadotropin secretion within 10 years, usually due to hypothalamic damage. Lifelong follow-up with testing of anterior pituitary hormone reserve is therefore required after radiation treatment. Optic nerve damage with impaired vision due to optic neuritis is reported in about 2% of patients who undergo pituitary irradiation. Cranial nerve damage is uncommon now that radiation doses are ≤2 Gy (200 rad) at any one treatment session and the maximum dose is <50 Gy (5000 rad). The use of stereotactic radiotherapy may reduce damage to adjacent structures. Radiotherapy for pituitary tumors has been associated with adverse mortality rates, mainly from cerebrovascular disease. The cumulative risk of developing a secondary tumor after conventional radiation is 1.3% after 10 years and 1.9% after 20 years.

MEDICAL

Medical therapy for pituitary tumors is highly specific and depends on tumor type. For prolactinomas, dopamine agonists are the treatment of choice. For acromegaly, somatostatin analogues and GH receptor antagonists are indicated. For TSH-secreting tumors, somatostatin analogues and occasionally dopamine agonists are indicated. ACTH-secreting tumors and nonfunctioning tumors are generally not responsive to medications and require surgery and/or irradiation.

SELLAR MASSES

Sellar masses other than pituitary adenomas may arise from brain, hypothalamic, or pituitary tissues. Each exhibit features related to the lesion location but also unique to the specific etiology.

Hypothalamic Lesions Lesions involving the anterior and preoptic hypothalamic regions cause paradoxical vasoconstriction, tachycardia, and hyperthermia. Acute hyperthermia usually is due to a hemorrhagic insult, but poikilothermia may also occur. Central disorders of thermoregulation result from posterior hypothalamic damage. The *periodic hypothermia syndrome* is characterized by episodic attacks of rectal temperatures <30°C (86°F), sweating, vasodilation, vomiting, and bradycardia (Chap. 478e). Damage to the ventromedial hypothalamic nuclei by craniopharyngiomas, hypothalamic trauma, or inflammatory disorders may be associated with *hyperphagia* and *obesity*. This region appears to contain an energy-satiety center where melanocortin receptors are influenced by leptin, insulin, pro-opiomelanocortin (POMC) products, and gastrointestinal peptides (Chap. 415e). Polydipsia and hypodipsia are associated with damage to central osmoreceptors located in preoptic nuclei (Chap. 404). Slow-growing hypothalamic lesions can cause increased somnolence and disturbed sleep cycles as well as obesity, hypothermia, and emotional outbursts. Lesions of the central hypothalamus may stimulate sympathetic neurons, leading to elevated serum catecholamine and cortisol levels. These patients are predisposed to cardiac arrhythmias, hypertension, and gastric erosions.

Craniopharyngiomas are benign, suprasellar cystic masses that present with headaches, visual field deficits, and variable degrees of hypopituitarism. They are derived from Rathke's pouch and arise near the pituitary stalk, commonly extending into the suprasellar cistern. Craniopharyngiomas are often large, cystic, and locally invasive. Many are partially calcified, exhibiting a characteristic appearance on skull x-ray and CT images. More than half of all patients present before age 20, usually with signs of increased intracranial pressure, including headache, vomiting, papilledema, and hydrocephalus. Associated symptoms include visual field abnormalities, personality changes and cognitive deterioration, cranial nerve damage, sleep difficulties, and weight gain. Hypopituitarism can be documented in about 90%, and diabetes insipidus occurs in about 10% of patients. About half of affected children present with growth retardation. MRI is generally superior to CT for evaluating cystic structure and tissue components of craniopharyngiomas. CT is useful to define calcifications and evaluate invasion into surrounding bony structures and sinuses.

Treatment usually involves transcranial or transsphenoidal surgical resection followed by postoperative radiation of residual tumor. Surgery alone is curative in less than half of patients because of recurrences due to adherence to vital structures or because of small tumor deposits in the hypothalamus or brain parenchyma. The goal of surgery is to remove as much tumor as possible without risking complications associated with efforts to remove firmly adherent or inaccessible tissue. In the absence of radiotherapy, about 75% of craniopharyngiomas recur, and 10-year survival is less than 50%. In patients with incomplete resection, radiotherapy improves 10-year survival to 70–90% but is associated with increased risk of secondary malignancies. Most patients require lifelong pituitary hormone replacement.

Developmental failure of Rathke's pouch obliteration may lead to *Rathke's cysts*, which are small (<5 mm) cysts entrapped by squamous epithelium and are found in about 20% of individuals at autopsy. Although Rathke's cleft cysts do not usually grow and are often diagnosed incidentally, about a third present in adulthood with compressive symptoms, diabetes insipidus, and hyperprolactinemia due to stalk compression. Rarely, hydrocephalus develops. The diagnosis is suggested preoperatively by visualizing the cyst wall on MRI, which distinguishes these lesions from craniopharyngiomas. Cyst contents range from CSF-like fluid to mucoid material. *Arachnoid cysts* are rare and generate an MRI image that is isointense with CSF.

Sella chordomas usually present with bony clival erosion, local invasiveness, and, on occasion, calcification. Normal pituitary tissue may be visible on MRI, distinguishing chordomas from aggressive pituitary adenomas. Mucinous material may be obtained by fine-needle aspiration.

Meningiomas arising in the sellar region may be difficult to distinguish from nonfunctioning pituitary adenomas. Meningiomas typically enhance on MRI and may show evidence of calcification or bony erosion. Meningiomas may cause compressive symptoms.

Histiocytosis X includes a variety of syndromes associated with foci of eosinophilic granulomas. Diabetes insipidus, exophthalmos, and punched-out lytic bone lesions (*Hand-Schüller-Christian disease*) are associated with granulomatous lesions visible on MRI, as well as a characteristic axillary skin rash. Rarely, the pituitary stalk may be involved.

Pituitary metastases occur in ~3% of cancer patients. Bloodborne metastatic deposits are found almost exclusively in the posterior pituitary. Accordingly, diabetes insipidus can be a presenting feature of lung, gastrointestinal, breast, and other pituitary metastases. About half of pituitary metastases originate from breast cancer; about 25% of patients with metastatic breast cancer have such deposits. Rarely, pituitary stalk involvement results in anterior pituitary insufficiency. The MRI diagnosis of a metastatic lesion may be difficult to distinguish from an aggressive pituitary adenoma; the diagnosis may require histologic examination of excised tumor tissue. Primary or metastatic lymphoma, leukemias, and plasmacytomas also occur within the sella.

Hypothalamic hamartomas and *gangliocytomas* may arise from astrocytes, oligodendrocytes, and neurons with varying degrees of differentiation. These tumors may overexpress hypothalamic neuropeptides, including gonadotropin-releasing hormone (GnRH), growth hormone–releasing hormone (GHRH), and corticotropin-releasing hormone (CRH). With GnRH-producing tumors, children present with precocious puberty, psychomotor delay, and laughing-associated seizures. Medical treatment of GnRH-producing hamartomas with long-acting GnRH analogues effectively suppresses gonadotropin secretion and controls premature pubertal development. Rarely, hamartomas also are associated with craniofacial abnormalities; imperforate anus; cardiac, renal, and lung disorders; and pituitary failure as features of *Pallister-Hall syndrome*, which is caused by mutations in the carboxy terminus of the *GLI3* gene. Hypothalamic hamartomas are often contiguous with the pituitary, and preoperative MRI diagnosis may not be possible. Histologic evidence of hypothalamic neurons in tissue resected at transsphenoidal surgery may be the first indication of a primary hypothalamic lesion.

Hypothalamic gliomas and *optic gliomas* occur mainly in childhood and usually present with visual loss. Adults have more aggressive tumors; about a third are associated with neurofibromatosis.

Brain germ cell tumors may arise within the sellar region. They include *dysgerminomas*, which frequently are associated with diabetes insipidus and visual loss. They rarely metastasize. *Germinomas, embryonal carcinomas, teratomas,* and *choriocarcinomas* may arise in the parasellar region and produce hCG. These germ cell tumors present with precocious puberty, diabetes insipidus, visual field defects, and thirst disorders. Many patients are GH-deficient with short stature.

PITUITARY ADENOMAS AND HYPERSECRETION SYNDROMES

Pituitary adenomas are the most common cause of pituitary hormone hypersecretion and hyposecretion syndromes in adults. They account for ~15% of all intracranial neoplasms and have been identified with a population prevalence of ~80/100,000. At autopsy, up to one-quarter of all pituitary glands harbor an unsuspected microadenoma (<10 mm diameter). Similarly, pituitary imaging detects small clinically inapparent pituitary lesions in at least 10% of individuals.

Pathogenesis Pituitary adenomas are benign neoplasms that arise from one of the five anterior pituitary cell types. The clinical and biochemical phenotypes of pituitary adenomas depend on the cell type from which they are derived. Thus, tumors arising from lactotrope (PRL), somatotrope (GH), corticotrope (ACTH), thyrotrope (TSH), or gonadotrope (LH, FSH) cells hypersecrete their respective hormones (Table 403-3). Plurihormonal tumors express various combinations of GH, PRL, TSH, ACTH, or the glycoprotein hormone α or β subunits. They may be diagnosed by careful immunocytochemistry or may manifest as clinical syndromes that combine features of these hormonal hypersecretory syndromes. Morphologically, these tumors may arise from a single polysecreting cell type or include cells with mixed function within the same tumor.

Hormonally active tumors are characterized by autonomous hormone secretion with diminished feedback responsiveness to physiologic inhibitory pathways. Hormone production does not always correlate with tumor size. Small hormone-secreting adenomas may cause significant clinical perturbations, whereas larger adenomas that produce less hormone may be clinically silent and remain undiagnosed (if no central compressive effects occur). About one-third of all adenomas are clinically nonfunctioning and produce no distinct clinical hypersecretory syndrome. Most of them arise from gonadotrope cells and may secrete small amounts of α- and β-glycoprotein hormone subunits or, very rarely, intact circulating gonadotropins. True pituitary carcinomas with documented extracranial metastases are exceedingly rare.

Almost all pituitary adenomas are monoclonal in origin, implying the acquisition of one or more somatic mutations that confer a selective growth advantage. Consistent with their clonal origin, complete surgical resection of small pituitary adenomas usually cures hormone hypersecretion. Nevertheless, hypothalamic hormones such as GHRH and CRH also enhance mitotic activity of their respective pituitary target cells in addition to their role in pituitary hormone regulation. Thus, patients who harbor rare abdominal or chest tumors that elaborate ectopic GHRH or CRH may present with somatotrope or corticotrope hyperplasia with GH or ACTH hypersecretion.

Several etiologic genetic events have been implicated in the development of pituitary tumors. The pathogenesis of sporadic forms of acromegaly has been particularly informative as a model of tumorigenesis. GHRH, after binding to its G protein–coupled somatotrope receptor, uses cyclic adenosine monophosphate (AMP) as a second messenger to stimulate GH secretion and somatotrope proliferation. A subset (~35%) of GH-secreting pituitary tumors contains sporadic mutations in Gsα (Arg 201 → Cys or His; Gln 227 → Arg). These mutations attenuate intrinsic GTPase activity, resulting in constitutive elevation of cyclic AMP, Pit-1 induction, and activation of cyclic AMP response element binding protein (CREB), thereby promoting somatotrope cell proliferation and GH secretion.

Characteristic loss of heterozygosity (LOH) in various chromosomes has been documented in large or invasive macroadenomas, suggesting the presence of putative tumor suppressor genes at these loci in up to 20% of sporadic pituitary tumors, including GH-, PRL-, and ACTH-producing adenomas and some nonfunctioning tumors. Lineage-specific cell cycle disruptions with elevated levels of CDK inhibitors are present in most of these adenomas.

Compelling evidence also favors growth factor promotion of pituitary tumor proliferation. Basic fibroblast growth factor (bFGF) is abundant in the pituitary and stimulates pituitary cell mitogenesis, whereas epithelial growth factor (EGF) receptor signaling induces both hormone synthesis and cell proliferation. Other factors involved in initiation and promotion of pituitary tumors include loss of negative-feedback inhibition (as seen with primary hypothyroidism or hypogonadism) and estrogen-mediated or paracrine angiogenesis. Growth characteristics and neoplastic behavior also may be influenced by several activated oncogenes, including *RAS* and pituitary tumor transforming gene (*PTTG*), or inactivation of growth suppressor genes, including *MEG3*.

Genetic Syndromes Associated with Pituitary Tumors Several familial syndromes are associated with pituitary tumors, and the genetic mechanisms for some of them have been unraveled (Table 403-4).

Multiple endocrine neoplasia (MEN) 1 is an autosomal dominant syndrome characterized primarily by a genetic predisposition to parathyroid, pancreatic islet, and pituitary adenomas (Chap. 408). MEN1 is caused by inactivating germline mutations in *MENIN*, a constitutively expressed tumor-suppressor gene located on chromosome 11q13.

TABLE 403-3 CLASSIFICATION OF PITUITARY ADENOMAS[a]

Adenoma Cell Origin	Hormone Product	Clinical Syndrome
Lactotrope	PRL	Hypogonadism, galactorrhea
Gonadotrope	FSH, LH, subunits	Silent or hypogonadism
Somatotrope	GH	Acromegaly/gigantism
Corticotrope	ACTH	Cushing's disease
Mixed growth hormone and prolactin cell	GH, PRL	Acromegaly, hypogonadism, galactorrhea
Other plurihormonal cell	Any	Mixed
Acidophil stem cell	PRL, GH	Hypogonadism, galactorrhea, acromegaly
Mammosomatotrope	PRL, GH	Hypogonadism, galactorrhea, acromegaly
Thyrotrope	TSH	Thyrotoxicosis
Null cell	None	Pituitary failure
Oncocytoma	None	Pituitary failure

[a]Hormone-secreting tumors are listed in decreasing order of frequency. All tumors may cause local pressure effects, including visual disturbances, cranial nerve palsy, and headache.

Note: For abbreviations, see text.

Source: Adapted from S Melmed, in JL Jameson (ed): *Principles of Molecular Medicine.* Totowa, NJ, Humana Press, 1998.

TABLE 403-4 FAMILIAL PITUITARY TUMOR SYNDROMES

	Gene Mutated	Clinical Features
Multiple endocrine neoplasia 1 (MEN 1)	*MEN1* (11q13)	Hyperparathyroidism Pancreatic neuroendocrine tumors Foregut carcinoids Adrenal adenomas Skin lesions Pituitary adenomas (40%)
Multiple endocrine neoplasia 4 (MEN 4)	*CDKNIB* (12p13)	Hyperparathyroidism Pituitary adenomas Other tumors
Carney complex	*PRKAR1A* (17q23-24)	Pituitary hyperplasia and adenomas (10%) Atrial myxomas Schwannomas Adrenal hyperplasia Lentigines
Familial pituitary adenomas	*AIP* (11q13.3)	Acromegaly/gigantism (~15% of afflicted families)

Loss of heterozygosity or a somatic mutation of the remaining normal *MENIN* allele leads to tumorigenesis. About half of affected patients develop prolactinomas; acromegaly and Cushing's syndrome are less commonly encountered.

Carney's syndrome is characterized by spotty skin pigmentation, myxomas, and endocrine tumors, including testicular, adrenal, and pituitary adenomas. Acromegaly occurs in about 20% of these patients. A subset of patients have mutations in the R1α regulatory subunit of protein kinase A (*PRKAR1A*).

McCune-Albright syndrome consists of polyostotic fibrous dysplasia, pigmented skin patches, and a variety of endocrine disorders, including acromegaly, adrenal adenomas, and autonomous ovarian function (Chap. 426e). Hormonal hypersecretion results from constitutive cyclic AMP production caused by inactivation of the GTPase activity of Gsα. The Gsα mutations occur postzygotically, leading to a mosaic pattern of mutant expression.

Familial acromegaly is a rare disorder in which family members may manifest either acromegaly or gigantism. A subset of families with a predisposition for familial pituitary tumors, especially acromegaly, have been found to harbor germline mutations in the *AIP* gene, which encodes the aryl hydrocarbon receptor interacting protein.

HYPERPROLACTINEMIA

Etiology Hyperprolactinemia is the most common pituitary hormone hypersecretion syndrome in both men and women. PRL-secreting pituitary adenomas (prolactinomas) are the most common cause of PRL levels >200 μg/L (see below). Less pronounced PRL elevation can also be seen with microprolactinomas but is more commonly caused by drugs, pituitary stalk compression, hypothyroidism, or renal failure (Table 403-5).

Pregnancy and lactation are the important physiologic causes of hyperprolactinemia. Sleep-associated hyperprolactinemia reverts to normal within an hour of awakening. Nipple stimulation and sexual orgasm also may increase PRL. Chest wall stimulation or trauma (including chest surgery and herpes zoster) invoke the reflex suckling arc with resultant hyperprolactinemia. Chronic renal failure elevates PRL by decreasing peripheral clearance. Primary hypothyroidism is associated with mild hyperprolactinemia, probably because of compensatory TRH secretion.

Lesions of the hypothalamic-pituitary region that disrupt hypothalamic dopamine synthesis, portal vessel delivery, or lactotrope responses are associated with hyperprolactinemia. Thus, hypothalamic tumors, cysts, infiltrative disorders, and radiation-induced damage cause elevated PRL levels, usually in the range of 30–100 μg/L. Plurihormonal adenomas (including GH and ACTH tumors) may hypersecrete PRL directly. Pituitary masses, including clinically nonfunctioning pituitary tumors, may compress the pituitary stalk to cause hyperprolactinemia.

Drug-induced inhibition or disruption of dopaminergic receptor function is a common cause of hyperprolactinemia (Table 403-5). Thus, antipsychotics and antidepressants are a relatively common cause of mild hyperprolactinemia. Most patients receiving risperidone have elevated prolactin levels, sometimes exceeding 200 μg/L. Methyldopa inhibits dopamine synthesis, and verapamil blocks dopamine release, also leading to hyperprolactinemia. Hormonal agents that induce PRL include estrogens and thyrotropin-releasing hormone (TRH).

Presentation and Diagnosis Amenorrhea, galactorrhea, and infertility are the hallmarks of hyperprolactinemia in women. If hyperprolactinemia develops before menarche, primary amenorrhea results. More commonly, hyperprolactinemia develops later in life and leads to oligomenorrhea and ultimately to amenorrhea. If hyperprolactinemia is sustained, vertebral bone mineral density can be reduced compared with age-matched controls, particularly when it is associated with pronounced hypoestrogenemia. Galactorrhea is present in up to 80% of hyperprolactinemic women. Although usually bilateral and spontaneous, it may be unilateral or expressed only manually. Patients also may complain of decreased libido, weight gain, and mild hirsutism.

In men with hyperprolactinemia, diminished libido, infertility, and visual loss (from optic nerve compression) are the usual presenting symptoms. Gonadotropin suppression leads to reduced testosterone,

TABLE 403-5 ETIOLOGY OF HYPERPROLACTINEMIA

I. **Physiologic hypersecretion**
- Pregnancy
- Lactation
- Chest wall stimulation
- Sleep
- Stress

II. **Hypothalamic–pituitary stalk damage**
- Tumors
  - Craniopharyngioma
  - Suprasellar pituitary mass
  - Meningioma
  - Dysgerminoma
  - Metastases
- Empty sella
- Lymphocytic hypophysitis
- Adenoma with stalk
- Compression
- Granulomas
- Rathke's cyst
- Irradiation
- Trauma
  - Pituitary stalk section
  - Suprasellar surgery

III. **Pituitary hypersecretion**
- Prolactinoma
- Acromegaly

IV. **Systemic disorders**
- Chronic renal failure
- Hypothyroidism
- Cirrhosis
- Pseudocyesis
- Epileptic seizures

V. **Drug-induced hypersecretion**
- Dopamine receptor blockers
  - Atypical antipsychotics: risperidone
  - Phenothiazines: chlorpromazine, perphenazine
  - Butyrophenones: haloperidol
  - Thioxanthenes
  - Metoclopramide
- Dopamine synthesis inhibitors
  - α-Methyldopa
- Catecholamine depletors
  - Reserpine
- Opiates
- H_2 antagonists
  - Cimetidine, ranitidine
- Imipramines
  - Amitriptyline, amoxapine
- Serotonin reuptake inhibitors
  - Fluoxetine
- Calcium channel blockers
  - Verapamil
  - Estrogens
  - Thyrotropin-releasing hormone

Note: Hyperprolactinemia >200 μg/L almost invariably is indicative of a prolactin-secreting pituitary adenoma. Physiologic causes, hypothyroidism, and drug-induced hyperprolactinemia should be excluded before extensive evaluation.

impotence, and oligospermia. True galactorrhea is uncommon in men with hyperprolactinemia. If the disorder is long-standing, secondary effects of hypogonadism are evident, including osteopenia, reduced muscle mass, and decreased beard growth.

The diagnosis of idiopathic hyperprolactinemia is made by exclusion of known causes of hyperprolactinemia in the setting of a normal pituitary MRI. Some of these patients may harbor small microadenomas below visible MRI sensitivity (~2 mm).

GALACTORRHEA

Galactorrhea, the inappropriate discharge of milk-containing fluid from the breast, is considered abnormal if it persists longer than 6 months after childbirth or discontinuation of breast-feeding. Postpartum galactorrhea associated with amenorrhea is a self limiting disorder usually associated with moderately elevated PRL levels. Galactorrhea may occur spontaneously, or it may be elicited by nipple pressure. In both men and women, galactorrhea may vary in color and consistency (transparent, milky, or bloody) and arise either unilaterally or bilaterally. Mammography or ultrasound is indicated for bloody discharges (particularly from a single nipple), which may be caused by breast cancer. Galactorrhea is commonly associated with hyperprolactinemia caused by any of the conditions listed in Table 403-5. Acromegaly is associated with galactorrhea in about one-third of patients. Treatment of galactorrhea usually involves managing the underlying disorder (e.g., replacing T_4 for hypothyroidism, discontinuing a medication, treating prolactinoma).

Laboratory Investigation Basal, fasting morning PRL levels (normally <20 μg/L) should be measured to assess hypersecretion. Both false-positive and false-negative results may be encountered. In patients with markedly elevated PRL levels (>1000 μg/L), reported results may be falsely lowered because of assay artifacts; sample dilution is required to measure these high values accurately. Falsely elevated values may be caused by aggregated forms of circulating PRL, which are usually biologically inactive (macroprolactinemia). Hypothyroidism should be excluded by measuring TSH and T_4 levels.

TREATMENT HYPERPROLACTINEMIA

Treatment of hyperprolactinemia depends on the cause of elevated PRL levels. Regardless of the etiology, however, treatment should be aimed at normalizing PRL levels to alleviate suppressive effects on gonadal function, halt galactorrhea, and preserve bone mineral density. Dopamine agonists are effective for most causes of hyperprolactinemia (see the treatment section for prolactinoma, below) regardless of the underlying cause.

If the patient is taking a medication known to cause hyperprolactinemia, the drug should be withdrawn, if possible. For psychiatric patients who require neuroleptic agents, supervised dose titration or the addition of a dopamine agonist can help restore normoprolactinemia and alleviate reproductive symptoms. However, dopamine agonists may worsen the underlying psychiatric condition, especially at high doses. Hyperprolactinemia usually resolves after adequate thyroid hormone replacement in hypothyroid patients or after renal transplantation in patients undergoing dialysis. Resection of hypothalamic or sellar mass lesions can reverse hyperprolactinemia caused by stalk compression and reduced dopamine tone. Granulomatous infiltrates occasionally respond to glucocorticoid administration. In patients with irreversible hypothalamic damage, no treatment may be warranted. In up to 30% of patients with hyperprolactinemia—usually without a visible pituitary microadenoma—the condition may resolve spontaneously.

PROLACTINOMA

Etiology and Prevalence Tumors arising from lactotrope cells account for about half of all functioning pituitary tumors, with a population prevalence of ~10/100,000 in men and ~30/100,000 in women. Mixed tumors that secrete combinations of GH and PRL, ACTH and PRL, and rarely TSH and PRL are also seen. These plurihormonal tumors are usually recognized by immunohistochemistry, sometimes without apparent clinical manifestations from the production of additional hormones. Microadenomas are classified as <1 cm in diameter and usually do not invade the parasellar region. Macroadenomas are >1 cm in diameter and may be locally invasive and impinge on adjacent structures. The female-to-male ratio for microprolactinomas is 20:1, whereas the sex ratio is near 1:1 for macroadenomas. Tumor size generally correlates directly with PRL concentrations; values >250 μg/L usually are associated with macroadenomas. Men tend to present with larger tumors than women, possibly because the features of male hypogonadism are less readily evident. PRL levels remain stable in most patients, reflecting the slow growth of these tumors. About 5% of microadenomas progress in the long term to macroadenomas.

Presentation and Diagnosis Women usually present with amenorrhea, infertility, and galactorrhea. If the tumor extends outside the sella, visual field defects or other mass effects may be seen. Men often present with impotence, loss of libido, infertility, or signs of central nervous system (CNS) compression, including headaches and visual defects. Assuming that physiologic and medication-induced causes of hyperprolactinemia are excluded (Table 403-5), the diagnosis of prolactinoma is likely with a PRL level >200 μg/L. PRL levels <100 μg/L may be caused by microadenomas, other sellar lesions that decrease dopamine inhibition, or nonneoplastic causes of hyperprolactinemia. For this reason, an MRI should be performed in all patients with hyperprolactinemia. It is important to remember that hyperprolactinemia caused secondarily by the mass effects of nonlactotrope lesions is also corrected by treatment with dopamine agonists despite failure to shrink the underlying mass. Consequently, PRL suppression by dopamine agonists does not necessarily indicate that the underlying lesion is a prolactinoma.

TREATMENT PROLACTINOMA

Because microadenomas rarely progress to become macroadenomas, no treatment may be needed if patients are asymptomatic and fertility is not desired; these patients should be monitored by regular serial PRL measurements and MRI scans.For symptomatic microadenomas, therapeutic goals include control of hyperprolactinemia, reduction of tumor size, restoration of menses and fertility, and resolution of galactorrhea. Dopamine agonist doses should be titrated to achieve maximal PRL suppression and restoration of reproductive function (Fig. 403-3). A normalized PRL level does not ensure reduced tumor size. However, tumor shrinkage usually is not seen in those who do not respond with lowered PRL levels. For macroadenomas, formal visual field testing should be performed before initiating dopamine agonists. MRI and visual fields should be assessed at 6- to 12-month intervals until the mass shrinks and annually thereafter until maximum size reduction has occurred.

MEDICAL

Oral dopamine agonists (cabergoline and bromocriptine) are the mainstay of therapy for patients with micro- or macroprolactinomas. Dopamine agonists suppress PRL secretion and synthesis as well as lactotrope cell proliferation. In patients with microadenomas who have achieved normoprolactinemia and significant reduction of tumor mass, the dopamine agonist may be withdrawn after 2 years. These patients should be monitored carefully for evidence of prolactinoma recurrence. About 20% of patients (especially males) are resistant to dopaminergic treatment; these adenomas may exhibit decreased D_2 dopamine receptor numbers or a postreceptor defect. D_2 receptor gene mutations in the pituitary have not been reported.

Cabergoline An ergoline derivative, cabergoline is a long-acting dopamine agonist with high D_2 receptor affinity. The drug effectively suppresses PRL for >14 days after a single oral dose and induces prolactinoma shrinkage in most patients. Cabergoline (0.5–1.0 mg twice weekly) achieves normoprolactinemia and resumption of normal gonadal function in ~80% of patients with microadenomas; galactorrhea improves or resolves in 90% of patients. Cabergoline normalizes PRL and shrinks ~70% of macroprolactinomas. Mass

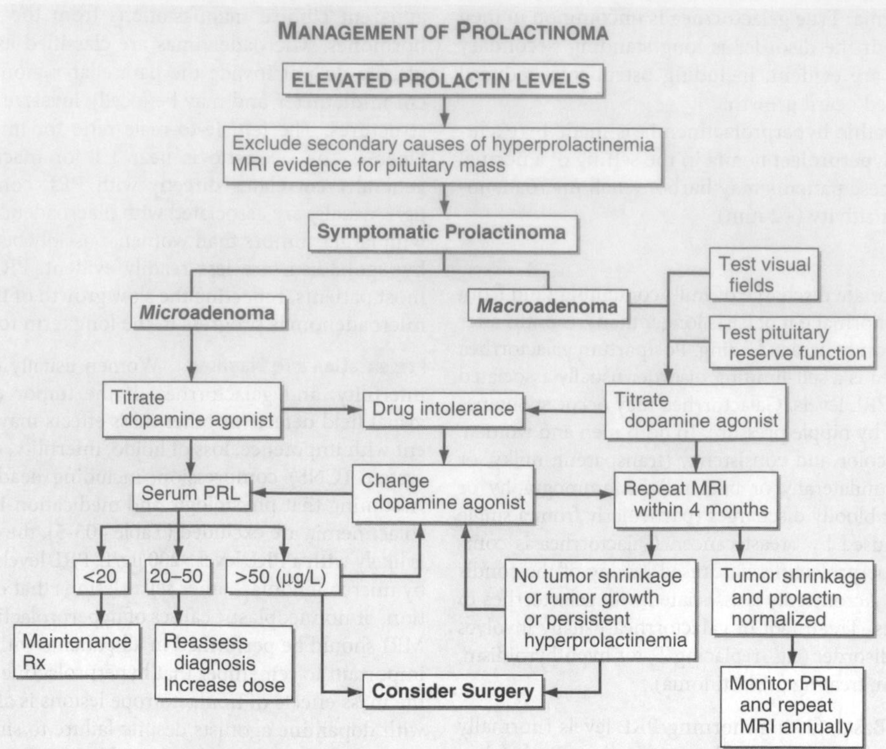

FIGURE 403-3 Management of prolactinoma. MRI, magnetic resonance imaging; PRL, prolactin.

effect symptoms, including headaches and visual disorders, usually improve dramatically within days after cabergoline initiation; improvement of sexual function requires several weeks of treatment but may occur before complete normalization of prolactin levels. After initial control of PRL levels has been achieved, cabergoline should be reduced to the lowest effective maintenance dose. In ~5% of treated patients harboring a microadenoma, hyperprolactinemia may resolve and not recur when dopamine agonists are discontinued after long-term treatment. Cabergoline also may be effective in patients resistant to bromocriptine. Adverse effects and drug intolerance are encountered less commonly than with bromocriptine.

BROMOCRIPTINE

The ergot alkaloid bromocriptine mesylate is a dopamine receptor agonist that suppresses prolactin secretion. Because it is short-acting, the drug is preferred when pregnancy is desired. In microadenomas, bromocriptine rapidly lowers serum prolactin levels to normal in up to 70% of patients, decreases tumor size, and restores gonadal function. In patients with macroadenomas, prolactin levels are also normalized in 70% of patients, and tumor mass shrinkage (≥50%) is achieved in most patients.

Therapy is initiated by administering a low bromocriptine dose (0.625–1.25 mg) at bedtime with a snack, followed by gradually increasing the dose. Most patients are controlled with a daily dose of ≤7.5 mg (2.5 mg tid).

SIDE EFFECTS

Side effects of dopamine agonists include constipation, nasal stuffiness, dry mouth, nightmares, insomnia, and vertigo; decreasing the dose usually alleviates these problems. Nausea, vomiting, and postural hypotension with faintness may occur in ~25% of patients after the initial dose. These symptoms may persist in some patients. In general, fewer side effects are reported with cabergoline. For the approximately 15% of patients who are intolerant of oral bromocriptine, cabergoline may be better tolerated. Intravaginal administration of bromocriptine is often efficacious in patients with intractable gastrointestinal side effects. Auditory hallucinations, delusions, and mood swings have been reported in up to 5% of patients and may be due to the dopamine agonist properties or to the lysergic acid derivative of the compounds. Rare reports of leukopenia, thrombocytopenia, pleural fibrosis, cardiac arrhythmias, and hepatitis have been described. Patients with Parkinson's disease who receive at least 3 mg of cabergoline daily have been reported to be at risk for development of cardiac valve regurgitation. Studies analyzing over 500 prolactinoma patients receiving recommended doses of cabergoline (up to 2 mg weekly) have shown no evidence for an increased incidence of valvular disorders. Nevertheless, because no controlled prospective studies in pituitary tumor patients are available, it is prudent to perform echocardiograms before initiating standard-dose cabergoline therapy.

Surgery Indications for surgical adenoma debulking include dopamine resistance or intolerance and the presence of an invasive macroadenoma with compromised vision that fails to improve after drug treatment. Initial PRL normalization is achieved in about 70% of microprolactinomas after surgical resection, but only 30% of macroadenomas can be resected successfully. Follow-up studies have shown that hyperprolactinemia recurs in up to 20% of patients within the first year after surgery; long-term recurrence rates exceed 50% for macroadenomas. Radiotherapy for prolactinomas is reserved for patients with aggressive tumors that do not respond to maximally tolerated dopamine agonists and/or surgery.

PREGNANCY

The pituitary increases in size during pregnancy, reflecting the stimulatory effects of estrogen and perhaps other growth factors on pituitary vascularity and lactotrope cell hyperplasia. About 5% of microadenomas significantly increase in size, but 15–30% of macroadenomas grow during pregnancy. Bromocriptine has been used for more than 30 years to restore fertility in women with hyperprolactinemia, without evidence of teratogenic effects. Nonetheless, most authorities recommend strategies to minimize fetal exposure to the drug. For women taking bromocriptine who desire pregnancy, mechanical contraception should be used through three regular menstrual cycles to allow for conception timing. When pregnancy is confirmed, bromocriptine should be discontinued and PRL levels followed serially, especially if headaches or visual symptoms occur. For women harboring macroadenomas, regular visual field testing is recommended, and the drug should be reinstituted if tumor growth is apparent. Although pituitary MRI may be safe during pregnancy, this procedure should be reserved for symptomatic patients with severe headache and/or visual field defects. Surgical decompression may be indicated if vision is threatened. Although comprehensive data support the efficacy and relative safety of bromocriptine-facilitated fertility, patients should be advised of potential unknown deleterious effects and the risk of tumor growth during pregnancy. Because cabergoline is long-acting with a high D_2-receptor affinity, it is not recommended for use in women when fertility is desired.

ACROMEGALY

Etiology GH hypersecretion is usually the result of a somatotrope adenoma but may rarely be caused by extrapituitary lesions (Table 403-6). In addition to the more common GH-secreting somatotrope adenomas, mixed mammosomatotrope tumors and acidophilic stem-cell adenomas secrete both GH and PRL. In patients with acidophilic stem-cell adenomas, features of hyperprolactinemia (hypogonadism and galactorrhea) predominate over the less clinically evident signs of acromegaly. Occasionally, mixed plurihormonal tumors are encountered that also secrete ACTH, the glycoprotein hormone α subunit, or TSH in addition to GH. Patients with partially empty sellas may present with GH hypersecretion due to a small GH-secreting adenoma within the compressed rim of pituitary tissue; some of these may reflect the spontaneous necrosis of tumors that were previously larger. GH-secreting tumors rarely arise from ectopic pituitary tissue remnants in the nasopharynx or midline sinuses.

There are case reports of ectopic GH secretion by tumors of pancreatic, ovarian, lung, or hematopoietic origin. Rarely, excess GHRH production may cause acromegaly because of chronic stimulation of somatotropes. These patients present with classic features of acromegaly, elevated GH levels, pituitary enlargement on MRI, and pathologic characteristics of pituitary hyperplasia. The most common cause of GHRH-mediated acromegaly is a chest or abdominal carcinoid tumor. Although these tumors usually express positive GHRH immunoreactivity, clinical features of acromegaly are evident in only a minority of patients with carcinoid disease. Excessive GHRH also may be elaborated by hypothalamic tumors, usually choristomas or neuromas.

TABLE 403-6 CAUSES OF ACROMEGALY

	Prevalence, %
Excess Growth Hormone Secretion	
Pituitary	98
Densely or sparsely granulated GH cell adenoma	60
Mixed GH cell and PRL cell adenoma	25
Mammosomatotrope cell adenoma	10
Plurihormonal adenoma	
GH cell carcinoma or metastases	
Multiple endocrine neoplasia 1 (GH cell adenoma)	
McCune-Albright syndrome	
Ectopic sphenoid or parapharyngeal sinus pituitary adenoma	
Extrapituitary tumor	
Pancreatic islet cell tumor	<1
Lymphoma	
Excess Growth Hormone–Releasing Hormone Secretion	
Central	<1
Hypothalamic hamartoma, choristoma, ganglioneuroma	<1
Peripheral	<1
Bronchial carcinoid, pancreatic islet cell tumor, small cell lung cancer, adrenal adenoma, medullary thyroid carcinoma, pheochromocytoma	

Abbreviations: GH, growth hormone; PRL, prolactin.

Source: Adapted from S Melmed: N Engl J Med 355:2558–2573, 2006.

Presentation and Diagnosis Protean manifestations of GH and IGF-I hypersecretion are indolent and often are not clinically diagnosed for 10 years or more. Acral bony overgrowth results in frontal bossing, increased hand and foot size, mandibular enlargement with prognathism, and widened space between the lower incisor teeth. In children and adolescents, initiation of GH hypersecretion before epiphyseal long bone closure is associated with development of pituitary gigantism (Fig. 403-4). Soft tissue swelling results in increased heel pad thickness, increased shoe or glove size, ring tightening, characteristic coarse facial features, and a large fleshy nose. Other commonly encountered clinical features include hyperhidrosis, a deep and hollow-sounding voice, oily skin, arthropathy, kyphosis, carpal tunnel syndrome, proximal muscle weakness and fatigue, acanthosis nigricans, and skin tags. Generalized visceromegaly occurs, including cardiomegaly, macroglossia, and thyroid gland enlargement.

The most significant clinical impact of GH excess occurs with respect to the cardiovascular system. Coronary heart disease, cardiomyopathy with arrhythmias, left ventricular hypertrophy, decreased diastolic function, and hypertension ultimately occur in most patients if untreated. Upper airway obstruction with sleep apnea occurs in more than 60% of patients and is associated with both soft tissue laryngeal airway obstruction and central sleep dysfunction. Diabetes mellitus develops in 25% of patients with acromegaly, and most patients are intolerant of a glucose load (as GH counteracts the action of insulin). Acromegaly is associated with an increased risk of colon polyps and mortality from colonic malignancy; polyps are diagnosed in up to one-third of patients. Overall mortality is increased about threefold and is due primarily to cardiovascular and cerebrovascular disorders and respiratory disease. Unless GH levels are controlled, survival is reduced by an average of 10 years compared with an age-matched control population.

Laboratory Investigation Age-matched serum IGF-I levels are elevated in acromegaly. Consequently, an IGF-I level provides a useful laboratory screening measure when clinical features raise the possibility of acromegaly. Due to the pulsatility of GH secretion, measurement of a single random GH level is not useful for the diagnosis or exclusion of acromegaly and does not correlate with disease severity. The diagnosis of acromegaly is confirmed by demonstrating the failure of GH suppression to <0.4 μg/L within 1–2 h of an oral glucose load (75 g). When newer ultrasensitive GH assays are used, normal nadir GH levels are even lower (<0.05 μg/L). About 20% of patients exhibit a paradoxical GH rise after glucose. PRL should be measured, as it is elevated in ~25% of patients with acromegaly. Thyroid function, gonadotropins, and sex steroids may be attenuated because of tumor mass effects. Because most patients will undergo surgery with glucocorticoid coverage, tests of ACTH reserve in asymptomatic patients are more efficiently deferred until after surgery.

TREATMENT ACROMEGALY

The goal of treatment is to control GH and IGF-I hypersecretion, ablate or arrest tumor growth, ameliorate comorbidities, restore mortality rates to normal, and preserve pituitary function.

Surgical resection of GH-secreting adenomas is the initial treatment for most patients (Fig. 403-5). Somatostatin analogues are used as adjuvant treatment for preoperative shrinkage of large invasive macroadenomas, immediate relief of debilitating symptoms, and reduction of GH hypersecretion; in frail patients experiencing morbidity; and in patients who decline surgery or, when surgery fails, to achieve biochemical control. Irradiation or repeat surgery may be required for patients who cannot tolerate or do not respond to adjunctive medical therapy. The high rate of late hypopituitarism and the slow rate (5–15 years) of biochemical response are the

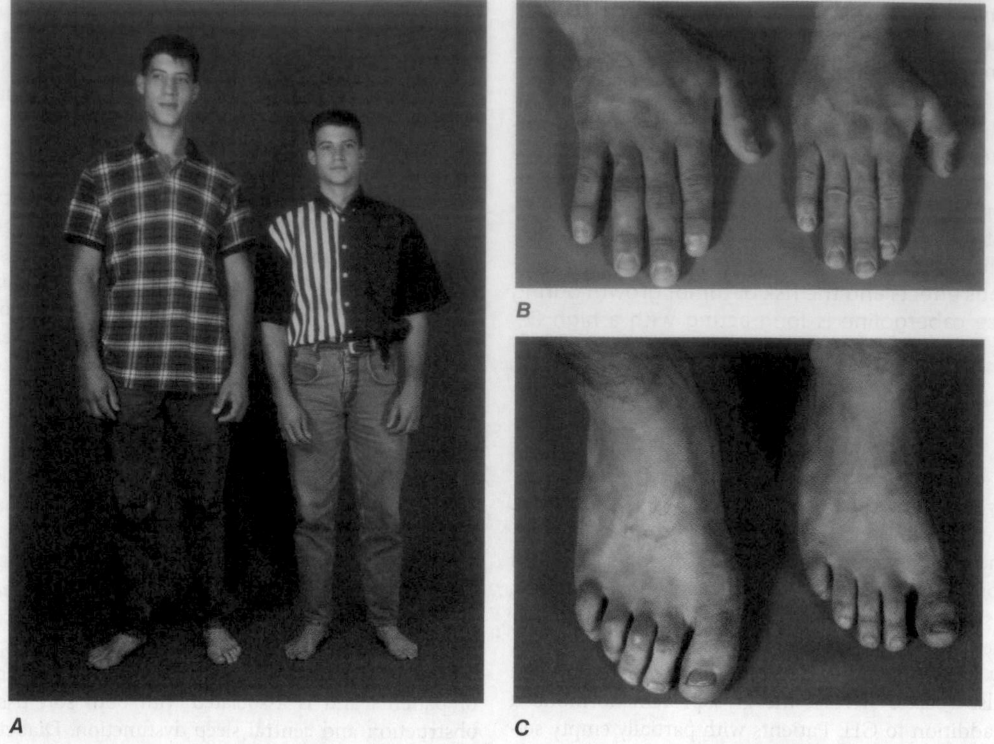

FIGURE 403-4 Features of acromegaly/gigantism. A 22-year-old man with gigantism due to excess growth hormone is shown to the left of his identical twin. The increased height and prognathism (***A***) and enlarged hand (***B***) and foot (***C***) of the affected twin are apparent. Their clinical features began to diverge at the age of approximately 13 years. *(Reproduced from R Gagel, IE McCutcheon: N Engl J Med 324:524, 1999; with permission.)*

main disadvantages of radiotherapy. Irradiation is also relatively ineffective in normalizing IGF-I levels. Stereotactic ablation of GH-secreting adenomas by gamma-knife radiotherapy is promising, but initial reports suggest that long-term results and side effects are similar to those observed with conventional radiation. Somatostatin analogues may be required while awaiting the full benefits of radiotherapy. Systemic co-morbid sequelae of acromegaly, including cardiovascular disease, diabetes, and arthritis, should be managed aggressively. Mandibular surgical repair may be indicated.

SURGERY

Transsphenoidal surgical resection by an experienced surgeon is the preferred primary treatment for both microadenomas (remission rate ~70%) and macroadenomas (<50% in remission). Soft tissue swelling improves immediately after tumor resection. GH levels return to normal within an hour, and IGF-I levels are normalized within 3–4 days. In ~10% of patients, acromegaly may recur several years after apparently successful surgery; hypopituitarism develops in up to 15% of patients after surgery.

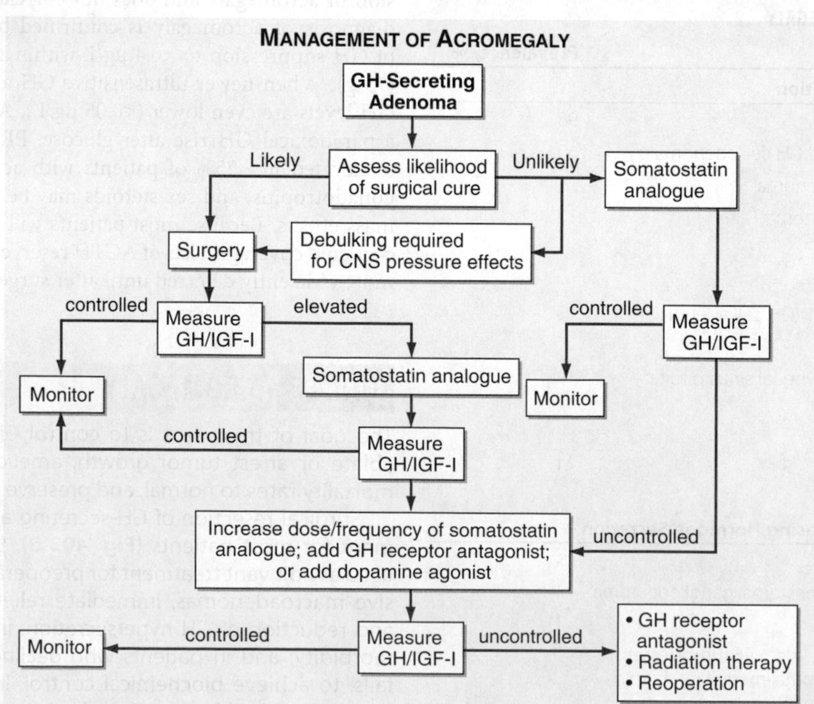

FIGURE 403-5 Management of acromegaly. GH, growth hormone; CNS, central nervous system; IGF, insulin-like growth factor. *(Adapted from S Melmed et al: J Clin Endocrinol Metab 94:1509–1517, 2009; © The Endocrine Society.)*

SOMATOSTATIN ANALOGUES

Somatostatin analogues exert their therapeutic effects through SSTR2 and SSTR5 receptors, both of which are expressed by GH-secreting tumors. Octreotide acetate is an eight-amino-acid synthetic somatostatin analogue. In contrast to native somatostatin, the analogue is relatively resistant to plasma degradation. It has a 2-h serum half-life and possesses fortyfold greater potency than native somatostatin to suppress GH. Octreotide is administered by subcutaneous injection, beginning with 50 μg tid; the dose can be increased gradually up to 1500 μg/d. Fewer than 10% of patients do not respond to the analogue. Octreotide suppresses integrated GH levels and normalizes IGF-I levels in ~60% of treated patients.

The long acting somatostatin depot formulations, octreotide and lanreotide, are the preferred medical treatment for patients with acromegaly. *Sandostatin-LAR* is a sustained-release, long-acting formulation of octreotide incorporated into microspheres that sustain drug levels for several weeks after intramuscular injection. GH suppression occurs for as long as 6 weeks after a 30-mg intramuscular injection; long-term monthly treatment sustains GH and IGF-I suppression and also reduces pituitary tumor size in ~50% of patients. *Lanreotide* autogel, a slow-release depot somatostatin preparation, is a cyclic somatostatin octapeptide analogue that suppresses GH and IGF-I hypersecretion after a 60-mg subcutaneous injection. Long-term (4–6 weeks) administration controls GH hypersecretion in about two-thirds of treated patients and improves patient compliance because of the long interval required between drug injections. Rapid relief of headache and soft tissue swelling occurs in ~75% of patients within days to weeks of somatostatin analogue initiation. Most patients report symptomatic improvement, including amelioration of headache, perspiration, obstructive apnea, and cardiac failure.

Side Effects Somatostatin analogues are well tolerated in most patients. Adverse effects are short-lived and mostly relate to drug-induced suppression of gastrointestinal motility and secretion. Transient nausea, abdominal discomfort, fat malabsorption, diarrhea, and flatulence occur in one-third of patients, and these symptoms usually remit within 2 weeks. Octreotide suppresses postprandial gallbladder contractility and delays gallbladder emptying; up to 30% of patients develop long-term echogenic sludge or asymptomatic cholesterol gallstones. Other side effects include mild glucose intolerance due to transient insulin suppression, asymptomatic bradycardia, hypothyroxinemia, and local injection site discomfort.

GH RECEPTOR ANTAGONIST

Pegvisomant antagonizes endogenous GH action by blocking peripheral GH binding to its receptor. Consequently, serum IGF-I levels are suppressed, reducing the deleterious effects of excess endogenous GH. Pegvisomant is administered by daily subcutaneous injection (10–20 mg) and normalizes IGF-I in ~70% of patients. GH levels, however, remain elevated as the drug does not target the pituitary adenoma. Side effects include reversible liver enzyme elevation, lipodystrophy, and injection site pain. Tumor size should be monitored by MRI.

Combined treatment with monthly somatostatin analogues and weekly or biweekly pegvisomant injections has been used effectively in resistant patients.

DOPAMINE AGONISTS

Bromocriptine and cabergoline may modestly suppress GH secretion in some patients. Very high doses of bromocriptine (≥20 mg/d) or cabergoline (0.5 mg/d) are usually required to achieve modest GH therapeutic efficacy. Combined treatment with octreotide and cabergoline may induce additive biochemical control compared with either drug alone.

RADIATION

External radiation therapy or high-energy stereotactic techniques are used as adjuvant therapy for acromegaly. An advantage of radiation is that patient compliance with long-term treatment is not required. Tumor mass is reduced, and GH levels are attenuated over time. However, 50% of patients require at least 8 years for GH levels to be suppressed to <5 μg/L; this level of GH reduction is achieved in about 90% of patients after 18 years but represents suboptimal GH suppression. Patients may require interim medical therapy for several years before attaining maximal radiation benefits. Most patients also experience hypothalamic-pituitary damage, leading to gonadotropin, ACTH, and/or TSH deficiency within 10 years of therapy.

In summary, surgery is the preferred primary treatment for GH-secreting microadenomas (Fig. 403-5). The high frequency of GH hypersecretion after macroadenoma resection usually necessitates adjuvant or primary medical therapy for these larger tumors. Patients unable to receive or respond to unimodal medical treatment may benefit from combined treatments, or can be offered radiation.

CUSHING'S SYNDROME (ACTH-PRODUCING ADENOMA)

(See also Chap. 406)

Etiology and Prevalence Pituitary corticotrope adenomas account for 70% of patients with endogenous causes of Cushing's syndrome. However, it should be emphasized that iatrogenic hypercortisolism is the most common cause of cushingoid features. Ectopic tumor ACTH production, cortisol-producing adrenal adenomas, adrenal carcinoma, and adrenal hyperplasia account for the other causes; rarely, ectopic tumor CRH production is encountered.

ACTH-producing adenomas account for about 10–15% of all pituitary tumors. Because the clinical features of Cushing's syndrome often lead to early diagnosis, most ACTH-producing pituitary tumors are relatively small microadenomas. However, macroadenomas also are seen and some ACTH-expressing adenomas are clinically silent. Cushing's disease is 5–10 times more common in women than in men. These pituitary adenomas exhibit unrestrained ACTH secretion, with resultant hypercortisolemia. However, they retain partial suppressibility in the presence of high doses of administered glucocorticoids, providing the basis for dynamic testing to distinguish pituitary from nonpituitary causes of Cushing's syndrome.

Presentation and Diagnosis The diagnosis of Cushing's syndrome presents two great challenges: (1) to distinguish patients with pathologic cortisol excess from those with physiologic or other disturbances of cortisol production and (2) to determine the etiology of pathologic cortisol excess.

Typical features of chronic cortisol excess include thin skin, central obesity, hypertension, plethoric moon facies, purple striae and easy bruisability, glucose intolerance or diabetes mellitus, gonadal dysfunction, osteoporosis, proximal muscle weakness, signs of hyperandrogenism (acne, hirsutism), and psychological disturbances (depression, mania, and psychoses) (Table 403-7). Hematopoietic features of hypercortisolism include leukocytosis, lymphopenia, and eosinopenia. Immune suppression includes delayed hypersensitivity and infection propensity. These protean yet commonly encountered manifestations of hypercortisolism make it challenging to decide which patients mandate formal laboratory evaluation. Certain features make pathologic causes of hypercortisolism more likely; they include characteristic central redistribution of fat, thin skin with striae and bruising, and proximal muscle weakness. In children and young females, early osteoporosis may be particularly prominent. The primary cause of death is cardiovascular disease, but life-threatening infections and risk of suicide are also increased.

Rapid development of features of hypercortisolism associated with skin hyperpigmentation and severe myopathy suggests an ectopic tumor source of ACTH. Hypertension, hypokalemic alkalosis, glucose intolerance, and edema are also more pronounced in these patients. Serum potassium levels <3.3 mmol/L are evident in ~70% of patients with ectopic ACTH secretion but are seen in <10% of patients with pituitary-dependent Cushing's syndrome.

Laboratory Investigation The diagnosis of Cushing's syndrome is based on laboratory documentation of endogenous hypercortisolism. Measurement of 24-h urine free cortisol (UFC) is a precise and cost-effective screening test. Alternatively, the failure to suppress plasma cortisol after an overnight 1-mg dexamethasone suppression test can

TABLE 403-7 CLINICAL FEATURES OF CUSHING'S SYNDROME (ALL AGES)

Symptoms/Signs	Frequency, %
Obesity or weight gain (>115% ideal body weight)	80
Thin skin	80
Moon facies	75
Hypertension	75
Purple skin striae	65
Hirsutism	65
Menstrual disorders (usually amenorrhea)	60
Plethora	60
Abnormal glucose tolerance	55
Impotence	55
Proximal muscle weakness	50
Truncal obesity	50
Acne	45
Bruising	45
Mental changes	45
Osteoporosis	40
Edema of lower extremities	30
Hyperpigmentation	20
Hypokalemic alkalosis	15
Diabetes mellitus	15

Source: Adapted from MA Magiokou et al, in ME Wierman (ed): *Diseases of the Pituitary*. Totowa, NJ, Humana, 1997.

be used to identify patients with hypercortisolism. As nadir levels of cortisol occur at night, elevated midnight serum or salivary samples of cortisol are suggestive of Cushing's syndrome. Basal plasma ACTH levels often distinguish patients with ACTH-independent (adrenal or exogenous glucocorticoid) from those with ACTH-dependent (pituitary, ectopic ACTH) Cushing's syndrome. Mean basal ACTH levels are about eightfold higher in patients with ectopic ACTH secretion than in those with pituitary ACTH-secreting adenomas. However, extensive overlap of ACTH levels in these two disorders precludes using ACTH measurements to make the distinction. Preferably, dynamic testing based on differential sensitivity to glucocorticoid feedback or ACTH stimulation in response to CRH or cortisol reduction is used to distinguish ectopic from pituitary sources of excess ACTH (Table 403-8). Very rarely, circulating CRH levels are elevated, reflecting ectopic tumor-derived secretion of CRH and often ACTH. For further discussion of dynamic testing for Cushing's syndrome, see Chap. 406.

Most ACTH-secreting pituitary tumors are <5 mm in diameter, and about half are undetectable by sensitive MRI. The high prevalence of incidental pituitary microadenomas diminishes the ability to distinguish ACTH-secreting pituitary tumors accurately from nonsecreting incidentalomas.

Inferior Petrosal Venous Sampling Because pituitary MRI with gadolinium enhancement is insufficiently sensitive to detect small (<2 mm) pituitary ACTH-secreting adenomas, bilateral inferior petrosal sinus ACTH sampling before and after CRH administration may be required to distinguish these lesions from ectopic ACTH-secreting tumors that may have similar clinical and biochemical characteristics. Simultaneous assessment of ACTH in each inferior petrosal vein and in the diagnosis of peripheral circulation provides a strategy for confirming and localizing pituitary ACTH production. Sampling is performed at baseline and 2, 5, and 10 min after intravenous bovine CRH (1 μg/kg) injection. An increased ratio (>2) of inferior petrosal:peripheral vein ACTH confirms pituitary Cushing's syndrome. After CRH injection, peak petrosal:peripheral ACTH ratios ≥3 confirm the presence of a pituitary ACTH-secreting tumor. The sensitivity of this test is >95%, with very rare false-positive results. False-negative results may be encountered in patients with aberrant venous drainage. Petrosal sinus catheterizations are technically difficult, and about 0.05% of patients develop neurovascular complications. The procedure should not be performed in patients with hypertension, in patients with known cerebrovascular disease, or in the presence of a well-visualized pituitary adenoma on MRI.

TABLE 403-8 DIFFERENTIAL DIAGNOSIS OF ACTH-DEPENDENT CUSHING'S SYNDROME[a]

	ACTH-Secreting Pituitary Tumor	Ectopic ACTH Secretion
Etiology	Pituitary corticotrope adenoma	Bronchial, abdominal carcinoid
	Plurihormonal adenoma	Small cell lung cancer
		Thymoma
Sex	F > M	M > F
Clinical features	Slow onset	Rapid onset
		Pigmentation
		Severe myopathy
Serum potassium <3.3μg/L	<10%	75%
24-h urinary free cortisol (UFC)	High	High
Basal ACTH level	Inappropriately high	Very high
Dexamethasone suppression		
1 mg overnight		
Low-dose (0.5 mg q6h)	Cortisol >5 μg/dL	Cortisol >5 μg/dL
High-dose (2 mg q6h)	Cortisol <5 μg/dL	Cortisol >5 μg/dL
UFC >80% suppressed	Microadenomas: 90%	10%
	Macroadenomas: 50%	
Inferior petrosal sinus sampling (IPSS)		
Basal		
IPSS: peripheral	>2	<2
CRH-induced		
IPSS: peripheral	>3	<3

[a]ACTH-independent causes of Cushing's syndrome are diagnosed by suppressed ACTH levels and an adrenal mass in the setting of hypercortisolism. Iatrogenic Cushing's syndrome is excluded by history.

Abbreviations: ACTH, adrenocorticotropic hormone; CRH, corticotropin-releasing hormone; F, female; M, male.

TREATMENT CUSHING'S SYNDROME

Selective transsphenoidal resection is the treatment of choice for Cushing's disease (Fig. 403-6). The remission rate for this procedure is ~80% for microadenomas but <50% for macroadenomas. However, surgery is rarely successful when the adenoma is not visible on MRI. After successful tumor resection, most patients experience a postoperative period of symptomatic ACTH deficiency that may last up to 12 months. This usually requires low-dose cortisol replacement, as patients experience both steroid withdrawal symptoms and have a suppressed hypothalamic-pituitary-adrenal axis. Biochemical recurrence occurs in approximately 5% of patients in whom surgery was initially successful.

When initial surgery is unsuccessful, repeat surgery is sometimes indicated, particularly when a pituitary source for ACTH is well documented. In older patients, in whom issues of growth and fertility are less important, hemi- or total hypophysectomy may be necessary if a discrete pituitary adenoma is not recognized. Pituitary irradiation may be used after unsuccessful surgery, but it cures only about 15% of patients. Because the effects of radiation are slow and only partially effective in adults, steroidogenic inhibitors are used in combination with pituitary irradiation to block adrenal effects of persistently high ACTH levels.

Pasireotide (600 or 900 ug/day subcutaneously), a somatostatin analog with high affinity for SST5 > SST2 receptors, has been approved for treating patients with ACTH-secreting pituitary tumors when surgery is not an option or has been unsuccessful. In clinical trials, the drug lowered plasma ACTH levels, normalized 24-h urinary free cortisol levels in about 25% of patients, and resulted in up to 40% mean pituitary tumor shrinkage. Side effects include development of

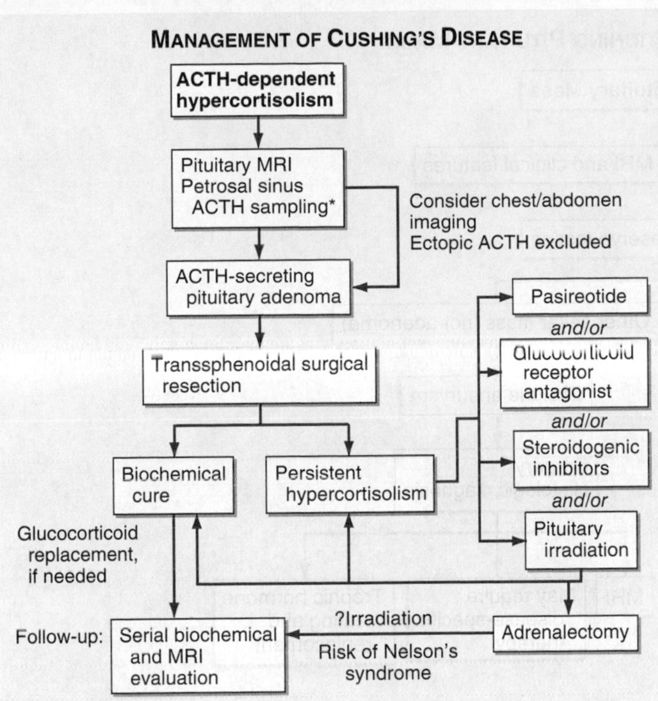

FIGURE 403-6 Management of Cushing's syndrome. ACTH, adrenocorticotropin hormone; MRI, magnetic resonance imaging. *, Not usually required.

hyperglycemia and diabetes in about 70% of patients, likely due to suppressed pancreatic secretion of insulin and incretins. Because patients with hypercortisolism are insulin-resistant, hyperglycemia should be rigorously managed. Other side effects are similar to those encountered for somatostatin analogs and include transient abdominal discomfort, diarrhea, nausea, and gallstones (20% of patients). The drug requires consistent long-term administration.

Ketoconazole, an imidazole derivative antimycotic agent, inhibits several P450 enzymes and effectively lowers cortisol in most patients with Cushing's disease when administered twice daily (600–1200 mg/d). Elevated hepatic transaminases, gynecomastia, impotence, gastrointestinal upset, and edema are common side effects.

Mifepristone (300–1200 mg/d), a glucocorticoid receptor antagonist, blocks peripheral cortisol action and is approved to treat hyperglycemia in Cushing's disease. Because the drug does not target the pituitary tumor, both ACTH and cortisol levels remain elevated, thus obviating a reliable circulating biomarker. Side effects are largely due to general antagonism of other steroid hormones and include hypokalemia, endometrial hyperplasia, hypoadrenalism, and hypertension.

Metyrapone (2–4 g/d) inhibits 11β-hydroxylase activity and normalizes plasma cortisol in up to 75% of patients. Side effects include nausea and vomiting, rash, and exacerbation of acne or hirsutism. *Mitotane* (o,p′-DDD; 3–6 g/d orally in four divided doses) suppresses cortisol hypersecretion by inhibiting 11β-hydroxylase and cholesterol side-chain cleavage enzymes and by destroying adrenocortical cells. Side effects of mitotane include gastrointestinal symptoms, dizziness, gynecomastia, hyperlipidemia, skin rash, and hepatic enzyme elevation. It also may lead to hypoaldosteronism. Other agents include *aminoglutethimide* (250 mg tid), *trilostane* (200–1000 mg/d), *cyproheptadine* (24 mg/d), and IV *etomidate* (0.3 mg/kg per hour). Glucocorticoid insufficiency is a potential side effect of agents used to block steroidogenesis.

The use of steroidogenic inhibitors has decreased the need for bilateral adrenalectomy. Surgical removal of both adrenal glands corrects hypercortisolism but may be associated with significant morbidity rates and necessitates permanent glucocorticoid and mineralocorticoid replacement. Adrenalectomy in the setting of residual corticotrope adenoma tissue predisposes to the development of *Nelson's syndrome*, a disorder characterized by rapid pituitary tumor enlargement and increased pigmentation secondary to high ACTH levels. Prophylactic radiation therapy may be indicated to prevent the development of Nelson's syndrome after adrenalectomy.

NONFUNCTIONING AND GONADOTROPIN-PRODUCING PITUITARY ADENOMAS

Etiology and Prevalence Nonfunctioning pituitary adenomas include those that secrete little or no pituitary hormones as well as tumors that produce too little hormone to result in recognizable clinical features. They are the most common type of pituitary adenoma and are usually macroadenomas at the time of diagnosis because clinical features are not apparent until tumor mass effects occur. Based on immunohistochemistry, most clinically nonfunctioning adenomas can be shown to originate from gonadotrope cells. These tumors typically produce small amounts of intact gonadotropins (usually FSH) as well as uncombined α, LH β, and FSH β subunits. Tumor secretion may lead to elevated α and FSH β subunits and, rarely, to increased LH β subunit levels. Some adenomas express α subunits without FSH or LH. TRH administration often induces an atypical increase of tumor-derived gonadotropins or subunits.

Presentation and Diagnosis Clinically nonfunctioning tumors often present with optic chiasm pressure and other symptoms of local expansion or may be incidentally discovered on an MRI performed for another indication (incidentaloma). Rarely, menstruwal disturbances or ovarian hyperstimulation occur in women with large tumors that produce FSH and LH. More commonly, adenoma compression of the pituitary stalk or surrounding pituitary tissue leads to attenuated LH and features of hypogonadism. PRL levels are usually slightly increased, also because of stalk compression. It is important to distinguish this circumstance from true prolactinomas, as nonfunctioning tumors do not shrink in response to treatment with dopamine agonists.

Laboratory Investigation The goal of laboratory testing in clinically nonfunctioning tumors is to classify the type of the tumor, identify hormonal markers of tumor activity, and detect possible hypopituitarism. Free α subunit levels may be elevated in 10–15% of patients with nonfunctioning tumors. In female patients, peri- or postmenopausal basal FSH concentrations are difficult to distinguish from tumor-derived FSH elevation. Premenopausal women have cycling FSH levels, also preventing clear-cut diagnostic distinction from tumor-derived FSH. In men, gonadotropin-secreting tumors may be diagnosed because of slightly increased gonadotropins (FSH > LH) in the setting of a pituitary mass. Testosterone levels are usually low despite the normal or increased LH level, perhaps reflecting reduced LH bioactivity or the loss of normal LH pulsatility. Because this pattern of hormone test results is also seen in primary gonadal failure and, to some extent, with aging (Chap. 411), the finding of increased gonadotropins alone is insufficient for the diagnosis of a gonadotropin-secreting tumor. In the majority of patients with gonadotrope adenomas, TRH administration stimulates LH β subunit secretion; this response is not seen in normal individuals. GnRH testing, however, is not helpful for making the diagnosis. For nonfunctioning and gonadotropin-secreting tumors, the diagnosis usually rests on immunohistochemical analyses of surgically resected tumor tissue, as the mass effects of these tumors usually necessitate resection.

Although acromegaly or Cushing's syndrome usually presents with unique clinical features, clinically inapparent (silent) somatotrope or corticotrope adenomas may only be diagnosed by immunostaining of resected tumor tissue. If PRL levels are <100 μg/L in a patient harboring a pituitary mass, a nonfunctioning adenoma causing pituitary stalk compression should be considered.

TREATMENT NONFUNCTIONING AND GONADOTROPIN-PRODUCING PITUITARY ADENOMAS

Asymptomatic small nonfunctioning microadenomas adenomas with no threat to vision may be followed with regular MRI and visual field testing without immediate intervention. However, for macroadenomas, transsphenoidal surgery is indicated to reduce tumor size and relieve mass effects (Fig. 403-7). Although it is not usually

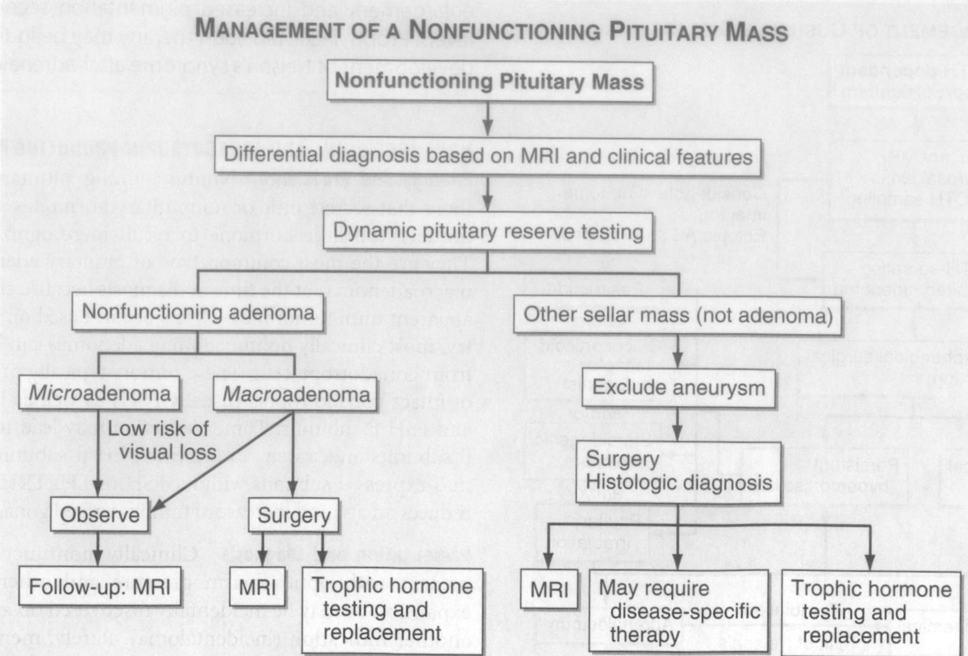

FIGURE 403-7 Management of a nonfunctioning pituitary mass. MRI, magnetic resonance imaging.

possible to remove all adenoma tissue surgically, vision improves in 70% of patients with preoperative visual field defects. Preexisting hypopituitarism that results from tumor mass effects may improve or resolve completely. Beginning about 6 months postoperatively, MRI scans should be performed yearly to detect tumor regrowth. Within 5–6 years after successful surgical resection, ~15% of nonfunctioning tumors recur. When substantial tumor remains after transsphenoidal surgery, adjuvant radiotherapy may be indicated to prevent tumor regrowth. Radiotherapy may be deferred if no postoperative residual mass is evident. Nonfunctioning pituitary tumors respond poorly to dopamine agonist treatment and somatostatin analogues are largely ineffective for shrinking these tumors. The selective GnRH antagonist Nal-Glu GnRH suppresses FSH hypersecretion but has no effect on adenoma size.

TSH-SECRETING ADENOMAS

TSH-producing macroadenomas are very rare but are often large and locally invasive when they occur. Patients usually present with thyroid goiter and hyperthyroidism, reflecting overproduction of TSH. Diagnosis is based on demonstrating elevated serum free T_4 levels, inappropriately normal or high TSH secretion, and MRI evidence of a pituitary adenoma. Elevated uncombined α subunits are seen in many patients.

It is important to exclude other causes of inappropriate TSH secretion, such as resistance to thyroid hormone, an autosomal dominant disorder caused by mutations in the thyroid hormone β receptor (Chap. 405). The presence of a pituitary mass and elevated β subunit levels are suggestive of a TSH-secreting tumor. Dysalbuminemic hyperthyroxinemia syndromes, caused by mutations in serum thyroid hormone binding proteins, are also characterized by elevated thyroid hormone levels, but with normal rather than suppressed TSH levels. Moreover, free thyroid hormone levels are normal in these disorders, most of which are familial.

TREATMENT TSH-SECRETING ADENOMAS

The initial therapeutic approach is to remove or debulk the tumor mass surgically, usually using a transsphenoidal approach. Total resection is not often achieved as most of these adenomas are large and locally invasive. Normal circulating thyroid hormone levels are achieved in about two-thirds of patients after surgery. Thyroid ablation or antithyroid drugs (methimazole and propylthiouracil) can be used to reduce thyroid hormone levels. Somatostatin analogue treatment effectively normalizes TSH and α subunit hypersecretion, shrinks the tumor mass in 50% of patients, and improves visual fields in 75% of patients; euthyroidism is restored in most patients. Because somatostatin analogues markedly suppress TSH, biochemical hypothyroidism often requires concomitant thyroid hormone replacement, which may also further control tumor growth.

404 Disorders of the Neurohypophysis

Gary L. Robertson

The neurohypophysis, or posterior pituitary, is formed by axons that originate in large cell bodies in the supraoptic and paraventricular nuclei of the hypothalamus. It produces two hormones: (1) arginine vasopressin (AVP), also known as antidiuretic hormone, and (2) oxytocin. AVP acts on the renal tubules to reduce water loss by concentrating the urine. Oxytocin stimulates postpartum milk letdown in response to suckling. A deficiency of AVP secretion or action causes diabetes insipidus (DI), a syndrome characterized by the production of large amounts of dilute urine. Excessive or inappropriate AVP production impairs urinary water excretion and predisposes to hyponatremia if water intake is not reduced in parallel with urine output.

VASOPRESSIN

SYNTHESIS AND SECRETION

AVP is a nonapeptide composed of a six-member disulfide ring and a tripeptide tail (Fig. 404-1). It is synthesized via a polypeptide precursor that includes AVP, neurophysin, and copeptin, all encoded by a single gene on chromosome 20. After preliminary processing and folding, the precursor is packaged in neurosecretory vesicles, where it is transported down the axon; further processed to AVP, neurophysin, and copeptin; and stored in neurosecretory vesicles until released by exocytosis into peripheral blood.

AVP secretion is regulated primarily by the "effective" osmotic pressure of body fluids. This control is mediated by specialized hypothalamic cells known as *osmoreceptors*, which are extremely sensitive

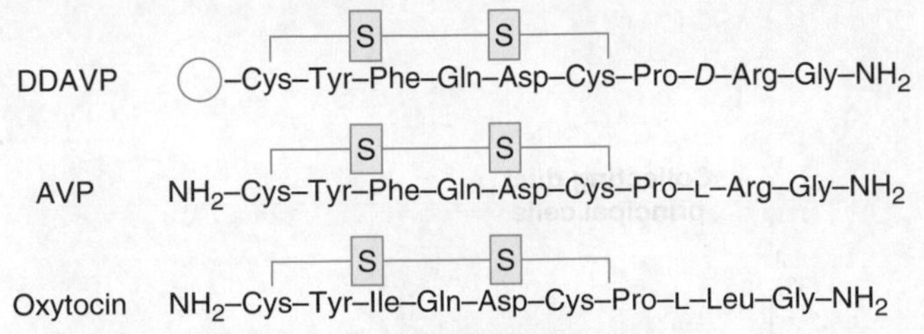

DDAVP ○–Cys–Tyr–Phe–Gln–Asp–Cys–Pro–*D*–Arg–Gly–NH_2 (S–S bridge between Cys residues)

AVP NH_2–Cys–Tyr–Phe–Gln–Asp–Cys–Pro–L–Arg–Gly–NH_2 (S–S bridge between Cys residues)

Oxytocin NH_2–Cys–Tyr–Ile–Gln–Asp–Cys–Pro–L–Leu–Gly–NH_2 (S–S bridge between Cys residues)

FIGURE 404-1 Primary structures of arginine vasopressin (AVP), oxytocin, and desmopressin (DDAVP).

to small changes in the plasma concentration of sodium and its anions but normally are insensitive to other solutes such as urea and glucose. The osmoreceptors appear to include inhibitory as well as stimulatory components that function in concert to form a threshold, or set point, control system. Below this threshold, plasma AVP is suppressed to levels that permit the development of a maximum water diuresis. Above it, plasma AVP rises steeply in direct proportion to plasma osmolarity, quickly reaching levels sufficient to effect a maximum antidiuresis. The absolute levels of plasma osmolarity/sodium at which minimally and maximally effective levels of plasma AVP occur, vary appreciably from person to person, apparently due to genetic influences on the set and sensitivity of the system. However, the average threshold, or set point, for AVP release corresponds to a plasma osmolarity or sodium of about 280 mosmol/L or 135 meq/L, respectively; levels only 2–4% higher normally result in maximum antidiuresis.

Although it is relatively stable in a healthy adult, the set point of the osmoregulatory system can be lowered by pregnancy, the menstrual cycle, estrogen, and relatively large, acute reductions in blood pressure or volume. Those reductions are mediated largely by neuronal afferents that originate in transmural pressure receptors of the heart and large arteries and project via the vagus and glossopharyngeal nerves to the brainstem, from which postsynaptic projections ascend to the hypothalamus. These pathways maintain a tonic inhibitory tone that decreases when blood volume or pressure falls by >10–20%. This baroregulatory system is probably of minor importance in the physiology of AVP secretion because the hemodynamic changes required to affect it usually do not occur during normal activities. However, the baroregulatory system undoubtedly plays an important role in AVP secretion in patients with disorders that produce large, acute disturbances of hemodynamic function. However, the baroregulatory system undoubtedly plays an important role in AVP secretion in patients with disorders that produce large, acute disturbances of hemodynamic function.

AVP secretion also can be stimulated by nausea, acute hypoglycemia, glucocorticoid deficiency, smoking, and, possibly, hyperangiotensinemia. The emetic stimuli are extremely potent since they typically elicit immediate, 50- to 100-fold increases in plasma AVP even when the nausea is transient and is not associated with vomiting or other symptoms. They appear to act via the emetic center in the medulla and can be blocked completely by treatment with antiemetics such as fluphenazine. There is no evidence that pain or other noxious stresses have any effect on AVP unless they elicit a vasovagal reaction with its associated nausea and hypotension.

ACTION

The most important, if not the only, physiologic action of AVP is to reduce water excretion by promoting concentration of urine. This antidiuretic effect is achieved by increasing the hydroosmotic permeability of cells that line the distal tubule and medullary collecting ducts of the kidney (Fig. 404-2). In the absence of AVP, these cells are impermeable to water and reabsorb little, if any, of the relatively large volume of dilute filtrate that enters from the proximal nephron. The lack of reabsorption results in the excretion of very large volumes (as much as 0.2 mL/kg per min) of maximally dilute urine (specific gravity and osmolarity ~1.000 and 50 mosmol/L, respectively), a condition known as *water diuresis.* In the presence of AVP, these cells become selectively permeable to water, allowing the water to diffuse back down the osmotic gradient created by the hypertonic renal medulla. As a result, the dilute fluid passing through the tubules is concentrated and the rate of urine flow decreases. The magnitude of this effect varies in direct proportion to the plasma AVP concentration and the rate of solute excretion. At maximum levels of AVP and normal rates of solute excretion, it approximates a urine flow rate as low as 0.35 mL/min and a urine osmolarity as high as 1200 mosmol/L. This effect is reduced by a solute diuresis such as glucosuria in diabetes mellitus. Antidiuresis is mediated via binding to G protein–coupled V_2 receptors on the serosal surface of the cell, activation of adenyl cyclase, and insertion into the luminal surface of water channels composed of a protein known as *aquaporin 2* (AQP2). The V_2 receptors and aquaporin 2 are encoded by genes on chromosomes Xq28 and 12q13, respectively.

At high concentrations, AVP also causes contraction of smooth muscle in blood vessels in the skin and gastrointestinal tract, induces glycogenolysis in the liver, and potentiates adrenocorticotropic hormone (ACTH) release by corticotropin-releasing factor. These effects are mediated by V_{1a} or V_{1b} receptors that are coupled to phospholipase C. Their role, if any, in human physiology/pathophysiology is uncertain.

METABOLISM

AVP distributes rapidly into a space roughly equal to the extracellular fluid volume. It is cleared irreversibly with a half-life ($t_{1/2}$) of 10–30 min. Most AVP clearance is due to degradation in the liver and kidneys. During pregnancy, the metabolic clearance of AVP is increased three- to fourfold due to placental production of an N terminal peptidase.

THIRST

Because AVP cannot reduce water loss below a certain minimum level obligated by urinary solute load and evaporation from skin and lungs, a mechanism for ensuring adequate intake is essential for preventing dehydration. This vital function is performed by the thirst mechanism. Like AVP, thirst is regulated primarily by an osmostat that is situated in the anteromedial hypothalamus and is able to detect very small changes in the plasma concentration of sodium and its anions. The thirst osmostat appears to be "set" about 3% higher than the AVP osmostat. This arrangement ensures that thirst, polydipsia, and dilution of body fluids do not occur until plasma osmolarity/sodium starts to exceed the defensive capacity of the antidiuretic mechanism.

OXYTOCIN

Oxytocin is also a nonapeptide that differs from AVP only at positions 3 and 8 (Fig. 404-1). However, it has relatively little antidiuretic effect and seems to act mainly on mammary ducts to facilitate milk letdown during nursing. It also may help initiate or facilitate labor by stimulating contraction of uterine smooth muscle, but it is not clear if this action is physiologic or necessary for normal delivery.

DEFICIENCIES OF AVP SECRETION AND ACTION

DIABETES INSIPIDUS

Clinical Characteristics A decrease of 75% or more in the secretion or action of AVP usually results in DI, a syndrome characterized by the production of abnormally large volumes of dilute urine. The 24-h urine volume exceeds 50 mL/kg body weight, and the osmolarity is less than 300 mosmol/L. The polyuria produces symptoms of urinary frequency, enuresis, and/or nocturia, which may disturb sleep and cause mild daytime fatigue or somnolence. It also results in a slight rise in plasma osmolarity that stimulates thirst and a commensurate increase in fluid intake (polydipsia). Overt clinical signs of dehydration are uncommon unless thirst and/or the compensatory increase of fluid intake are also impaired.

Etiology A primary deficiency of AVP secretion usually results from agenesis or irreversible destruction of the neurohypophysis. It is referred to variously as *neurohypophyseal DI, neurogenic DI, pituitary DI, cranial DI,* or *central DI.* It can be caused by a variety of congenital, acquired, or genetic disorders, but in about one-half of all adult patients, it is idiopathic (Table 404-1). Pituitary DI caused by surgery in or around the neurohypophysis usually appears within 24 h. After a few days, it may transition to a 2- to 3-week period of inappropriate antidiuresis, after which the DI may or may not recur permanently.

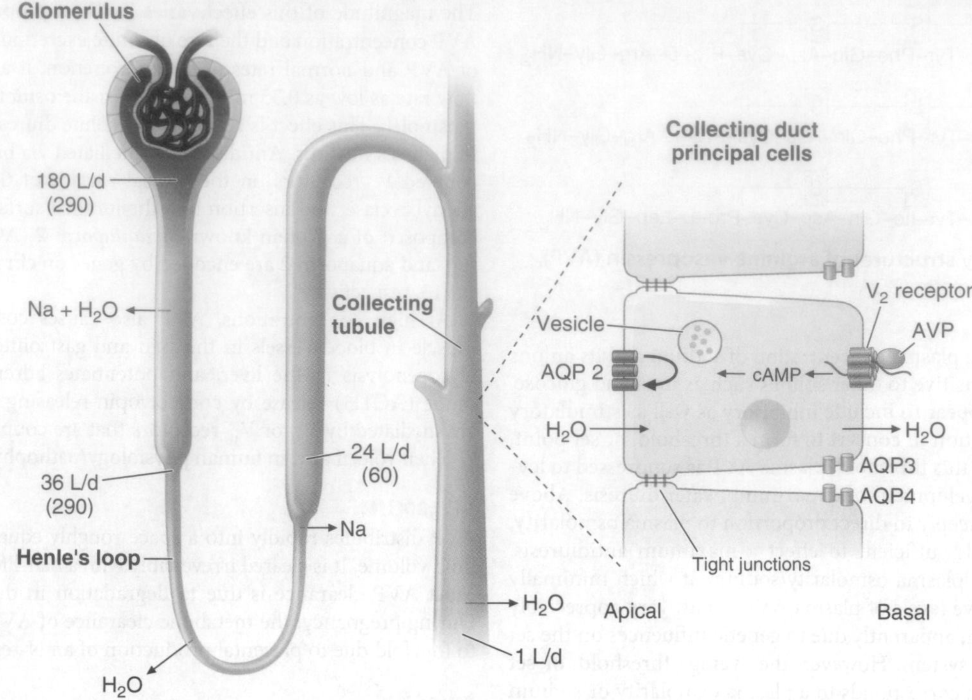

FIGURE 404-2 Antidiuretic effect of arginine vasopressin (AVP) in the regulation of urine volume. In a typical 70-kg adult, the kidney filters ~180 L/d of plasma. Of this, ~144 L (80%) is reabsorbed isosmotically in the proximal tubule and another 8 L (4–5%) is reabsorbed without solute in the descending limb of Henle's loop. The remainder is diluted to an osmolarity of ~60 mmol/kg by selective reabsorption of sodium and chloride in the ascending limb. In the absence of AVP, the urine issuing from the loop passes largely unmodified through the distal tubules and collecting ducts, resulting in a maximum water diuresis. In the presence of AVP, solute-free water is reabsorbed osmotically through the principal cells of the collecting ducts, resulting in the excretion of a much smaller volume of concentrated urine. This antidiuretic effect is mediated via a G protein–coupled V_2 receptor that increases intracellular cyclic AMP, thereby inducing translocation of aquaporin 2 (AQP 2) water channels into the apical membrane. The resultant increase in permeability permits an influx of water that diffuses out of the cell through AQP 3 and AQP 4 water channels on the basal-lateral surface. The net rate of flux across the cell is determined by the number of AQP 2 water channels in the apical membrane and the strength of the osmotic gradient between tubular fluid and the renal medulla. Tight junctions on the lateral surface of the cells serve to prevent unregulated water flow.

Five genetic forms of pituitary DI are now known. By far, the most common is transmitted in an autosomal dominant mode and is caused by diverse mutations in the coding region of one allele of the AVP–neurophysin II (or *AVP-NPII*) gene. All the mutations alter one or more amino acids known to be critical for correct processing and/or folding of the prohormone, thus interfering with its trafficking through the endoplasmic reticulum. The misfolded mutant precursor accumulates and interferes with production of AVP by the normal allele, eventually destroying the magnocellular neurons in which it is produced. The AVP deficiency and DI are usually not present at birth but develop gradually over a period of several months to years, progressing from partial to severe at different rates depending on the mutation. Once established, the deficiency of AVP is permanent, but for unknown reasons, the DI occasionally improves or remits spontaneously in late middle age. The parvocellular neurons that make AVP and the magnocellular neurons that make oxytocin appear to be unaffected. There are also rare autosomal recessive forms of pituitary DI. One is due to an inactivating mutation in the AVP portion of the gene; another is due to a large deletion involving the majority of the AVP gene and regulatory sequences in the intergenic region. A third form is caused by mutations of the *WFS 1* gene responsible for Wolfram's syndrome (DI, diabetes mellitus, optic atrophy, and neural deafness [DIDMOAD]). An X-linked recessive form linked to a region on Xq28 has also been described.

A primary deficiency of plasma AVP also can result from increased metabolism by an N-terminal aminopeptidase produced by the placenta. It is referred to as *gestational DI* because the signs and symptoms manifest during pregnancy and usually remit several weeks after delivery.

Secondary deficiencies of AVP secretion result from inhibition by excessive intake of fluids. They are referred to as *primary polydipsia* and can be divided into three subcategories. One of them, *dipsogenic DI*, is characterized by inappropriate thirst caused by a reduction in the set of the osmoregulatory mechanism. It sometimes occurs in association with multifocal diseases of the brain such as neurosarcoid, tuberculous meningitis, and multiple sclerosis but is often idiopathic. The second subtype, *psychogenic polydipsia*, is not associated with thirst, and the polydipsia seems to be a feature of psychosis or obsessive compulsive disorder. The third subtype, *iatrogenic polydipsia*, results from recommendations to increase fluid intake for its presumed health benefits.

Primary deficiencies in the antidiuretic action of AVP result in *nephrogenic DI*. The causes can be genetic, acquired, or drug induced (Table 404-1). The most common genetic form is transmitted in a semirecessive X-linked manner. It is caused by mutations in the coding region of the V_2 receptor gene that impair trafficking and/or ligand binding of the mutant receptor. There are also autosomal recessive or dominant forms of nephrogenic DI. They are caused by *AQP2* gene mutations that result in complete or partial defects in trafficking and function of the water channels that mediate antidiuresis in the distal and collecting tubules of the kidney.

Secondary deficiencies in the antidiuretic response to AVP result from polyuria per se. They are caused by washout of the medullary concentration gradient and/or suppression of aquaporin function. They usually resolve 24–48 h after the polyuria is corrected but can complicate interpretation of some acute tests used for differential diagnosis.

Pathophysiology In pituitary, gestational, or nephrogenic DI, the polyuria results in a small (1–2%) decrease in body water and a commensurate increase in plasma osmolarity and sodium that stimulates thirst and a compensatory increase in water intake. As a result, *hypernatremia and other overt physical or laboratory signs of dehydration do not develop unless the patient also has a defect in thirst or fails to increase fluid intake for some other reason.*

TABLE 404-1 CAUSES OF DIABETES INSIPIDUS

Pituitary diabetes insipidus

Acquired

- Head trauma (closed and penetrating) including pituitary surgery
- Neoplasms
  - Primary
    - Craniopharyngioma
    - Pituitary adenoma (suprasellar)
    - Dysgerminoma
    - Meningioma
  - Metastatic (lung, breast)
  - Hematologic (lymphoma, leukemia)
- Granulomas
  - Sarcoidosis
  - Histiocytosis
  - Xanthoma disseminatum
- Infectious
  - Chronic meningitis
  - Viral encephalitis
  - Toxoplasmosis
- Inflammatory
  - Lymphocytic infundibuloneurohypophysitis
  - Granulomatosis with polyangiitis (Wegener's)
  - Lupus erythematosus
  - Scleroderma
- Chemical toxins
  - Tetrodotoxin
  - Snake venom
- Vascular
  - Sheehan's syndrome
  - Aneurysm (internal carotid)
  - Aortocoronary bypass
  - Hypoxic encephalopathy
- Idiopathic

Congenital malformations

- Septo-optic dysplasia
- Midline craniofacial defects
- Holoprosencephaly
- Hypogenesis, ectopia of pituitary

Genetic

- Autosomal dominant (*AVP-neurophysin gene*)
- Autosomal recessive
- Type A (*AVP neurophysin gene*)
- Type B (*AVP-neurophysin gene*)
- Type C (*Wolfram's [4p-WFS 1] gene*)
- X-linked recessive (Xq28)

Gestational diabetes insipidus

Pregnancy (second and third trimesters)

Nephrogenic diabetes insipidus

Acquired

- Drugs
  - Lithium
  - Demeclocycline
  - Methoxyflurane
  - Amphotericin B
  - Aminoglycosides
  - Cisplatin
  - Rifampin
  - Foscarnet
- Metabolic
  - Hypercalcemia, hypercalciuria
  - Hypokalemia
- Obstruction (ureter or urethra)
- Vascular
  - Sickle cell disease and trait
  - Ischemia (acute tubular necrosis)
- Granulomas
  - Sarcoidosis
- Neoplasms
  - Sarcoma
- Infiltration
  - Amyloidosis
- Idiopathic

Genetic

- X-linked recessive (*AVP receptor-2 gene*)
- Autosomal recessive (*AQP2 gene*)
- Autosomal dominant (*AQP2 gene*)

Primary polydipsia

Acquired

- Psychogenic
  - Schizophrenia
  - Obsessive compulsive disorder
- Dipsogenic (abnormal thirst)
  - Granulomas (sarcoidosis)
  - Infectious (tuberculous meningitis)
  - Head trauma (closed and penetrating)
  - Demyelination (multiple sclerosis)
  - Drugs
  - Idiopathic
  - Iatrogenic

In pituitary and nephrogenic DI, the severity of the defect in AVP secretion or action varies significantly from patient to patient. In some, the defect is so severe that it cannot be overcome by even an intense stimulus such as nausea or severe dehydration. In others, the defect in AVP secretion or action is incomplete, and a modest stimulus such as a few hours of fluid deprivation, smoking, or a vasovagal reaction can raise urine osmolarity as high as 800 mosmol/L. However, even when the defects are partial, the relation of urine osmolarity to plasma AVP in patients with nephrogenic DI (Fig. 404-3A) or of plasma AVP to plasma osmolarity and sodium in patients with pituitary DI (Fig. 404-3B) is subnormal.

In primary polydipsia, the pathogenesis of the polydipsia and polyuria is the reverse of that in pituitary, nephrogenic, and gestational DI. In primary polydipsia, an abnormality in cognition or thirst causes excessive intake of fluids and an increase in body water that reduces plasma osmolarity/sodium, AVP secretion, and urinary concentration. Dilution of the urine, in turn, results in a compensatory increase in urinary free-water excretion that usually offsets the increase in intake and stabilizes plasma osmolarity/sodium at a level only 1–2% below basal. Thus, hyponatremia or clinically appreciable overhydration is uncommon unless the polydipsia is very severe or the compensatory water diuresis is impaired by a drug or disease that stimulates or mimics the antidiuretic effect of endogenous AVP. A rise in plasma osmolarity and sodium produced by fluid deprivation or hypertonic saline infusion increases plasma AVP normally. However, the resultant increase in urine concentration is often subnormal because polyuria per se temporarily reduces the capacity of the kidney to concentrate the urine. Thus, the maximum level of urine osmolarity achieved during fluid deprivation is often indistinguishable from that in patients with partial pituitary or partial nephrogenic DI.

Differential Diagnosis When symptoms of urinary frequency, enuresis, nocturia, and/or persistent thirst are present in the absence of glucosuria, the possibility of DI should be evaluated by collecting a 24-h urine on ad libitum fluid intake. If the volume exceeds 50 mL/kg per day (3500 mL in a 70-kg male) and the osmolarity is below 300 mosmol/L, DI is confirmed and the patient should be evaluated further to determine the type in order to select the appropriate therapy.

The type of DI can sometimes be inferred from the clinical setting or medical history. Often, however, such information is lacking, ambiguous, or misleading, and other approaches to differential diagnosis are needed. If basal plasma osmolarity and sodium are within normal limits, the traditional approach is to determine the effect of fluid deprivation and injection of antidiuretic hormone on urine osmolarity. This approach suffices for differential diagnosis *if* fluid deprivation raises plasma osmolarity and sodium above the normal range *without* inducing concentration of the urine. In that event, primary polydipsia and partial defects in AVP secretion and action are excluded, and the effect on urine osmolarity of injecting 2 μg of the AVP analogue, desmopressin, indicates whether the patient has severe pituitary DI or severe nephrogenic DI. However, this approach is of little or no diagnostic value if fluid deprivation results in concentration of the urine because the increases in urine osmolarity achieved both before and after the injection of desmopressin are similar in patients with *partial* pituitary DI, *partial* nephrogenic DI, and primary polydipsia. These disorders can be differentiated by measuring plasma AVP during fluid deprivation and relating it to the concurrent level of plasma and urine osmolarity (Fig. 404-3). However, this approach does not always differentiate clearly between partial pituitary DI and primary polydipsia unless the measurement is made when plasma osmolarity and sodium are at or above the normal range. This level is difficult to achieve by fluid deprivation alone once urinary concentration occurs. Therefore it is usually necessary to give a short infusion of 3% saline condition (0.1 mL/kg body weight per minute for 60 to 90 minutes) and repeat the measurement of plasma AVP.

A simpler but equally reliable way to differentiate between pituitary DI, nephrogenic DI, and primary polydipsia is to measure basal plasma

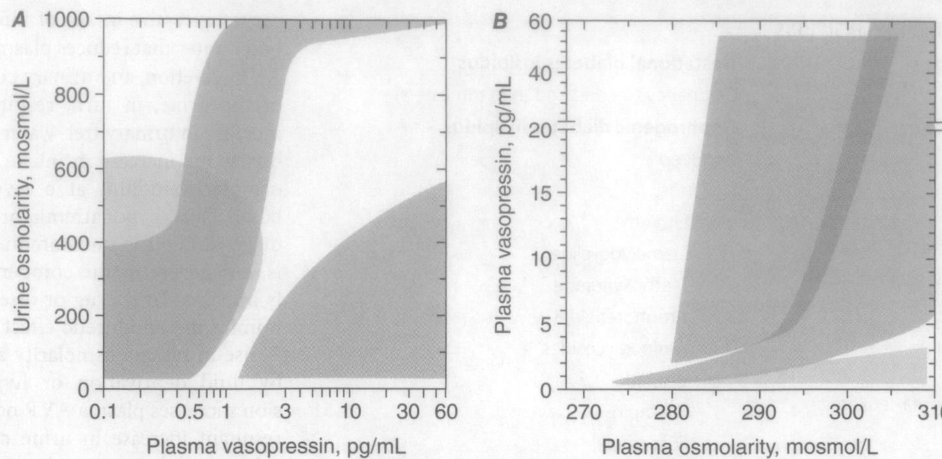

FIGURE 404-3 Relationship of plasma AVP to urine osmolarity (*A*) and plasma osmolarity (*B*) before and during fluid deprivation–hypertonic saline infusion test in patients who are normal or have primary polydipsia (blue zones), pituitary diabetes insipidus (green zones), or nephrogenic diabetes insipidus (pink zones).

AVP to determine if a brain magnetic resonance imaging (MRI) is needed and sufficient for diagnosis (Fig. 404-4). If plasma AVP *on ad libitum fluid intake* is normal or elevated (>1 pg/mL) when measured by a sensitive and specific assay, both primary polydipsia and pituitary DI are excluded and the diagnosis of nephrogenic DI can be confirmed, if desired, by a 1- to 2-day outpatient trial of desmopressin

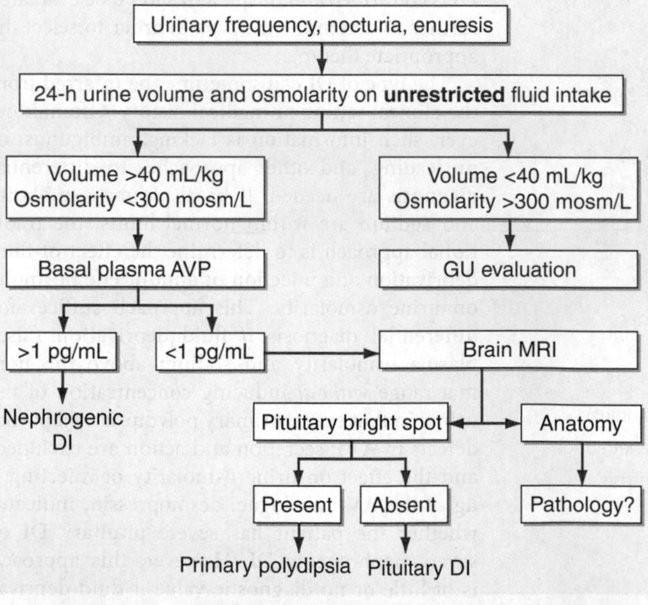

Urinary frequency, nocturia, enuresis

24-h urine volume and osmolarity on **unrestricted** fluid intake

Volume >40 mL/kg
Osmolarity <300 mosm/L

Volume <40 mL/kg
Osmolarity >300 mosm/L

Basal plasma AVP

GU evaluation

>1 pg/mL

<1 pg/mL

Brain MRI

Nephrogenic DI

Pituitary bright spot

Anatomy

Present

Absent

Pathology?

Primary polydipsia

Pituitary DI

FIGURE 404-4 Simplified approach to the differential diagnosis of diabetes insipidus. When symptoms suggest diabetes insipidus (DI), the syndrome should be differentiated from a genitourinary (GU) abnormality by measuring the 24-h urine volume and osmolarity on unrestricted fluid intake. If DI is confirmed, basal plasma arginine vasopressin (AVP) should be measured on unrestricted fluid intake. If AVP is normal or elevated (>1 pg/mL), the patient probably has nephrogenic DI. However, if plasma AVP is low or undetectable, the patient has either pituitary DI or primary polydipsia. In that case, magnetic resonance imaging (MRI) of the brain can be performed to differentiate between these two conditions by determining whether or not the normal posterior pituitary bright spot is visible on T1-weighted midsagittal images. In addition, the MRI anatomy of the pituitary hypothalamic area can be examined to look for evidence of pathology that sometimes causes pituitary DI or the dipsogenic form of primary polydipsia. MRI is not reliable for differential diagnosis unless nephrogenic DI has been excluded because the bright spot is also absent, small, or faint in this condition.

therapy. If, however, basal plasma AVP is low or undetectable (<1 pg/mL), nephrogenic DI is very unlikely and MRI of the brain can be used to differentiate pituitary DI from primary polydipsia. In most healthy adults and children, the posterior pituitary emits a hyperintense signal visible in T1-weighted midsagittal images. This "bright spot" is almost always present in patients with primary polydipsia but is always absent or abnormally small in patients with pituitary DI, even if their AVP deficiency is partial. The MRI is also useful in searching for pathology responsible for pituitary DI or the dipsogenic form of primary polydipsia (Fig. 404-2). The principal caveat is that MRI is not reliable for differential diagnosis of DI in patients with empty sella because they typically lack a bright spot even when their AVP secretion and action are normal. MRI also cannot be used to differentiate pituitary from nephrogenic DI because many patients with nephrogenic DI also lack a posterior pituitary bright spot, probably because they have an abnormally high rate of AVP secretion and turnover.

If MRI and/or AVP assays with the requisite sensitivity and specificity are unavailable and a fluid deprivation test is impractical or undesirable, a third way to differentiate between pituitary DI, nephrogenic DI, and primary polydipsia is a trial of desmopressin therapy. Such a trial should be conducted with very close monitoring of serum sodium as well as urine output, preferably in hospital, because desmopressin will produce hyponatremia in 8–24 h if the patient has primary polydipsia.

TREATMENT DIABETES INSIPIDUS

The signs and symptoms of uncomplicated pituitary DI can be eliminated by treatment with desmopressin (DDAVP), a synthetic analogue of AVP (Fig. 404-1). DDAVP acts selectively at V2 receptors to increase urine concentration and decrease urine flow in a dose-dependent manner. It is also more resistant to degradation than is AVP and has a three- to fourfold longer duration of action. DDAVP can be given by IV or SC injection, nasal inhalation, or orally by means of a tablet of melt. The doses required to control pituitary DI completely vary widely, depending on the patient and the route of administration. However, among adults, they usually range from 1–2 μg qd or bid by injection, 10–20 μg bid or tid by nasal spray, or 100–400 μg bid or tid orally. The onset of antidiuresis is rapid, ranging from as little as 15 min after injection to 60 min after oral administration. When given in a dose that normalizes 24-h urinary osmolarity (400–800 mosmol/L) and volume (15–30 mL/kg body weight), DDAVP produces a slight (1–3%) increase in total body water and a decrease in plasma osmolarity/sodium that rapidly eliminates thirst and polydipsia (Fig. 404-5). Consequently, water balance is maintained within the normal range. Hyponatremia does not develop unless urine volume is reduced too far (to less than 10 mL/kg per day) or fluid intake is excessive due to an associated

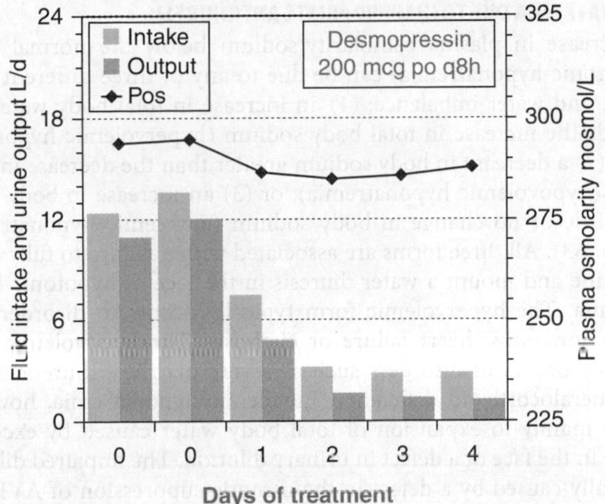

FIGURE 404-5 Effect of desmopressin therapy on fluid intake (*blue bars*), urine output (*orange bars*), and plasma osmolarity (*red line*) in a patient with uncomplicated pituitary diabetes insipidus. Note that treatment rapidly reduces fluid intake and urine output to normal, with only a slight increase in body water as evidenced by the slight decrease in plasma osmolarity.

abnormality in thirst or cognition. Fortunately, thirst abnormalities are rare, and if the patient is taught to drink only when truly thirsty, DDAVP can be given safely in doses sufficient to normalize urine output (~15–30 mL/kg per day) without the need for allowing intermittent escape to prevent water intoxication.

Primary polydipsia cannot be treated safely with DDAVP or any other antidiuretic drug because eliminating the polyuria does not eliminate the urge to drink. Therefore, it invariably produces hyponatremia and/or other signs of water intoxication, usually within 8–24 h if urine output is normalized completely. There is no consistently effective way to correct dipsogenic or psychogenic polydipsia, but the iatrogenic form may respond to patient education. To minimize the risk of water intoxication, all patients should be warned about the use of other drugs such as thiazide diuretics or carbamazepine (Tegretol) that can impair urinary free-water excretion directly or indirectly.

The polyuria and polydipsia of nephrogenic DI are not affected by treatment with standard doses of DDAVP. If resistance is partial, it may be overcome by tenfold higher doses, but this treatment is too expensive and inconvenient for long-term use. However, treatment with conventional doses of a thiazide diuretic and/or amiloride in conjunction with a low-sodium diet and a prostaglandin synthesis inhibitor (e.g., indomethacin) usually reduces the polyuria and polydipsia by 30–70% and may eliminate them completely in some patients. Side effects such as hypokalemia and gastric irritation can be minimized by the use of amiloride or potassium supplements and by taking medications with meals.

HYPODIPSIC HYPERNATREMIA

An increase in plasma osmolarity/sodium above the normal range (hypertonic hypernatremia) can be caused by either a decrease in total body water or an increase in total body sodium. The former results from a failure to drink enough to replace normal or increased urinary and insensible water loss. The deficient intake can be due either to water deprivation or a lack of thirst (hypodipsia). The most common cause of an increase in total body sodium is primary hyperaldosteronism (Chap. 406). Rarely, it can also result from ingestion of hypertonic saline in the form of sea water or incorrectly prepared infant formula. However, even in these forms of hypernatremia, inadequate intake of water also contributes. This chapter focuses on hypodipsic hypernatremia, the form of hypernatremia due to a primary defect in the thirst mechanism.

Clinical Characteristics Hypodipsic hypernatremia is a syndrome characterized by chronic or recurrent hypertonic dehydration. The hypernatremia varies widely in severity and usually is associated with signs of hypovolemia such as tachycardia, postural hypotension, azotemia, hyperuricemia, and hypokalemia due to secondary hyperaldosteronism. Muscle weakness, pain, rhabdomyolysis, hyperglycemia, hyperlipidemia, and acute renal failure may also occur. Obtundation or coma may be present but are often absent. Despite inappropriately low levels of plasma AVP, DI usually is not evident at presentation but may develop during rehydration as blood volume, blood pressure, and plasma osmolarity/sodium return toward normal, further reducing plasma AVP.

Etiology Hypodipsia is usually due to hypogenesis or destruction of the osmoreceptors in the anterior hypothalamus that regulate thirst. These defects can result from various congenital malformations of midline brain structures or may be acquired due to diseases such as occlusions of the anterior communicating artery, primary or metastatic tumors in the hypothalamus, head trauma, surgery, granulomatous diseases such as sarcoidosis and histiocytosis, AIDS, and cytomegalovirus encephalitis. Because of their proximity, the osmoreceptors that regulate AVP secretion also are usually impaired. Thus, AVP secretion responds poorly or not at all to hyperosmotic stimulation (Fig. 404-6) but, in most cases, increases normally to nonosmotic

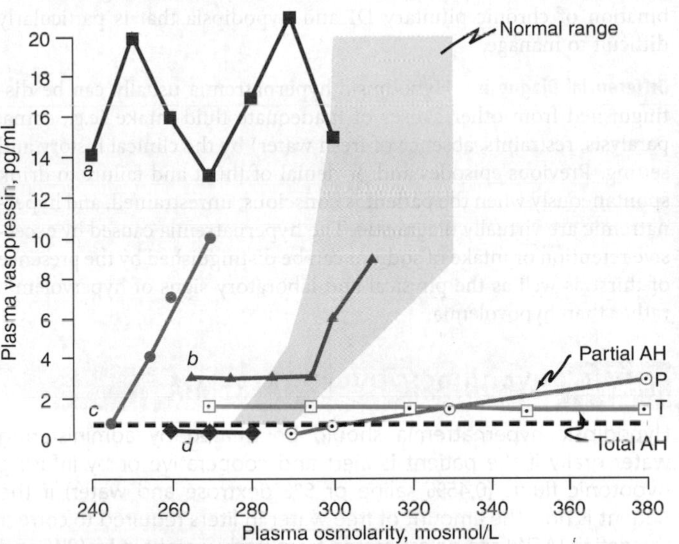

FIGURE 404-6 Heterogeneity of osmoregulatory dysfunction in adipsic hypernatremia (AH) and the syndrome of inappropriate antidiuresis (SIAD). Each line depicts schematically the relationship of plasma arginine vasopressin (AVP) to plasma osmolarity during water loading and/or infusion of 3% saline in a patient with either AH (*open symbols*) or SIAD (*closed symbols*). The shaded area indicates the normal range of the relationship. The horizontal broken line indicates the plasma AVP level below which the hormone is undetectable and urinary concentration usually does not occur. Lines P and T represent patients with a selective deficiency in the osmoregulation of thirst and AVP that is either partial (○) or total (□). In the latter, plasma AVP does not change in response to increases or decreases in plasma osmolarity but remains within a range sufficient to concentrate the urine even if overhydration produces hypotonic hyponatremia. In contrast, if the osmoregulatory deficiency is partial (○), rehydration of the patient suppresses plasma AVP to levels that result in urinary dilution and polyuria before plasma osmolarity and sodium are reduced to normal. Lines *a*–*d* represent different defects in the osmoregulation of plasma AVP observed in patients with SIADH or SIAD. In *a* (■), plasma AVP is markedly elevated and fluctuates widely without relation to changes in plasma osmolarity, indicating complete loss of osmoregulation. In *b* (▲), plasma AVP remains fixed at a slightly elevated level until plasma osmolarity reaches the normal range, at which point it begins to rise appropriately, indicating a selective defect in the inhibitory component of the osmoregulatory mechanism. In *c* (●), plasma AVP rises in close correlation with plasma osmolarity before the latter reaches the normal range, indicating downward resetting of the osmostat. In *d* (◆), plasma AVP appears to be osmoregulated normally, suggesting that the inappropriate antidiuresis is caused by some other abnormality.

stimuli such as nausea or large reductions in blood volume or blood pressure, indicating that the neurohypophysis is intact.

Pathophysiology Hypodipsia results in a failure to drink enough water to replenish obligatory renal and extrarenal losses. Consequently, plasma osmolarity and sodium rise often to extremely high levels before the disorder is recognized. In most cases, urinary loss of water contributes little, if any, to the dehydration because AVP continues to be secreted in the small amounts necessary to concentrate the urine. In some patients this appears to be due to hypovolemic stimulation and/or incomplete destruction of AVP osmoreceptors because plasma AVP declines and DI develops during rehydration (Fig. 404-6). In others, however, plasma AVP does not decline during rehydration even if they are overhydrated. Consequently, they develop a hyponatremic syndrome indistinguishable from inappropriate antidiuresis. This suggests that the AVP osmoreceptors normally provide inhibitory and stimulatory input to the neurohypophysis and the patients can no longer osmotically stimulate or suppress tonic secretion of the hormone because both inputs have been totally eliminated by the same pathology that destroyed the osmoregulation of thirst. In a few patients, the neurohypophysis is also destroyed, resulting in a combination of chronic pituitary DI and hypodipsia that is particularly difficult to manage.

Differential Diagnosis Hypodipsic hypernatremia usually can be distinguished from other causes of inadequate fluid intake (e.g., coma, paralysis, restraints, absence of fresh water) by the clinical history and setting. Previous episodes and/or denial of thirst and failure to drink spontaneously when the patient is conscious, unrestrained, and hypernatremic are virtually diagnostic. The hypernatremia caused by excessive retention or intake of sodium can be distinguished by the presence of thirst as well as the physical and laboratory signs of hypervolemia rather than hypovolemia.

TREATMENT HYPODIPSIC HYPERNATREMIA

Hypodipsic hypernatremia should be treated by administering water orally if the patient is alert and cooperative or by infusing hypotonic fluids (0.45% saline or 5% dextrose and water) if the patient is not. The amount of free water in liters required to correct the deficit (ΔFW) can be estimated from body weight in kg (BW) and the serum sodium concentration in mmol/L (S_{Na}) by the formula $\Delta FW = 0.5BW \times ([S_{Na} - 140]/140)$. If serum glucose ($S_{Glu}$) is elevated, the measured S_{Na} should be corrected (S_{Na}^*) by the formula $S_{Na}^* = S_{Na} + ([S_{Glu} - 90]/36)$. This amount plus an allowance for continuing insensible and urinary losses should be given over a 24- to 48-h period. Close monitoring of serum sodium as well as fluid intake and urinary output is essential because, depending on the extent of osmoreceptor deficiency, some patients will develop AVP-deficient DI, requiring DDAVP therapy to complete rehydration; others will develop hyponatremia and a syndrome of inappropriate antidiuresis (SIAD)-like picture if overhydrated. If hyperglycemia and/or hypokalemia are present, insulin and/or potassium supplements should be given with the expectation that both can be discontinued soon after rehydration is complete. Plasma urea/creatinine should be monitored closely for signs of acute renal failure caused by rhabdomyolysis, hypovolemia, and hypotension.

Once the patient has been rehydrated, an MRI of the brain and tests of anterior pituitary function should be performed to look for the cause and collateral defects in other hypothalamic functions. A long-term management plan to prevent or minimize recurrence of the fluid and electrolyte imbalance also should be developed. This should include a practical method to regulate fluid intake in accordance with variations in water balance as indicated by changes in body weight or serum sodium determined by home monitoring analyzers. Prescribing a constant fluid intake is ineffective and potentially dangerous because it does not take into account the large, uncontrolled variations in insensible loss that inevitably result from changes in ambient temperature and physical activity.

HYPONATREMIA DUE TO INAPPROPRIATE ANTIDIURESIS

A decrease in plasma osmolarity/sodium below the normal range (hypotonic hyponatremia) can be due to any of three different types of salt and water imbalance: (1) an increase in total body water that exceeds the increase in total body sodium (hypervolemic hyponatremia); (2) a decrease in body sodium greater than the decrease in body water (hypovolemic hyponatremia); or (3) an increase in body water with little or no change in body sodium (euvolemic hyponatremia) (Chap. 63). All three forms are associated with a failure to fully dilute the urine and mount a water diuresis in the face of hypotonic hyponatremia. The hypervolemic form typically occurs in disorders like severe congestive heart failure or cirrhosis. The hypovolemic form typically occurs in disorders such as severe diarrhea, diuretic abuse, or mineralocorticoid deficiency. Euvolemic hyponatremia, however, is due mainly to expansion of total body water caused by excessive intake in the face of a defect in urinary dilution. The impaired dilution is usually caused by a defect in the osmotic suppression of AVP that can have either of two causes. One is a nonhemodynamic stimulus such as nausea or a cortisol deficiency, which can be corrected quickly by treatment with antiemetics or cortisol. The other is a primary defect in osmoregulation caused by another disorder such as malignancy, stroke, or pneumonia that cannot be easily or quickly corrected. The latter is commonly known as the syndrome of inappropriate antidiuretic hormone (SIADH). Much less often, euvolemic hyponatremia can also result from AVP-independent activation of renal V_2 receptors, a variant known as nephrogenic inappropriate antidiuresis or NSIAD. Both of the latter will be discussed in this chapter.

Clinical Characteristics Antidiuresis of any cause decreases the volume and increases the concentration of urine. If not accompanied by a commensurate reduction in fluid intake or an increase in insensible loss, the reduction in urine output results in excess water retention which expands and dilutes body fluids. If the hyponatremia develops gradually or has been present for more than a few days, it may be largely asymptomatic. However, if it develops acutely, it is usually accompanied by symptoms and signs of water intoxication that may include mild headache, confusion, anorexia, nausea, vomiting, coma, and convulsions. Severe acute hyponatremia may be lethal. Other clinical signs and symptoms vary greatly, depending on the type of hyponatremia. The hypervolemic form is characterized by generalized edema and other signs of marked volume expansion. The opposite is evident in the hypovolemic form. However, overt signs of volume expansion or contraction are absent in SIADH, SIAD, and other forms of euvolemic hyponatremia.

Etiology In SIADH, the inappropriate secretion of AVP can have many different causes. They include ectopic production of AVP by lung cancer or other neoplasms; eutopic release induced by various diseases or drugs; and exogenous administration of AVP, DDAVP, or large doses of oxytocin (Table 404-2). The ectopic forms result from abnormal expression of the *AVP-NPII* gene by primary or metastatic malignancies. The eutopic forms occur most often in patients with acute infections or strokes but have also been associated with many other neurologic diseases and injuries. The mechanisms by which these diseases interfere with osmotic suppression of AVP are not known. The defect in osmoregulation can take any of four distinct forms (Fig. 404-6). In one of the most common (reset osmostat), AVP secretion remains fully responsive to changes in plasma osmolarity/sodium, but the threshold, or set point, of the osmoregulatory system is abnormally low. These patients differ from those with the other types of SIADH in that they are able to maximally suppress plasma AVP and dilute their urine if their fluid intake is high enough to reduce their plasma osmolarity and/or sodium to the new set point. In most patients, SIADH is self-limited and remits spontaneously within 2–3 weeks, but about 10% of cases are chronic. Another, smaller subgroup (~10% of the total) has inappropriate antidiuresis without a demonstrable defect in the osmoregulation of plasma AVP (Fig. 404-6). In some of them, all young boys, the inappropriate antidiuresis has been traced to a constitutively activating mutation of the V_2 receptor gene. This unusual variant may be referred to as familial nephrogenic SIAD (NSIAD) to distinguish it from

TABLE 404-2 CAUSES OF SYNDROME OF INAPPROPRIATE ANTIDIURETIC HORMONE (SIADH)

Neoplasms	Neurologic
Carcinomas	Guillain-Barré syndrome
Lung	Multiple sclerosis
Duodenum	Delirium tremens
Pancreas	Amyotrophic lateral sclerosis
Ovary	Hydrocephalus
Bladder, ureter	Psychosis
Other neoplasms	Peripheral neuropathy
Thymoma	Congenital malformations
Mesothelioma	Agenesis corpus callosum
Bronchial adenoma	Cleft lip/palate
Carcinoid	Other midline defects
Gangliocytoma	Metabolic
Ewing's sarcoma	Acute intermittent porphyria
Head trauma (closed and penetrating)	Pulmonary
	Asthma
Infections	Pneumothorax
Pneumonia, bacterial or viral	Positive-pressure respiration
Abscess, lung or brain	Drugs
Cavitation (aspergillosis)	Vasopressin or desmopressin
Tuberculosis, lung or brain	Serotonin reuptake inhibitors
Meningitis, bacterial or viral	Oxytocin, high dose
Encephalitis	Vincristine
AIDS	Carbamazepine
Vascular	Nicotine
Cerebrovascular occlusions, hemorrhage	Phenothiazines
	Cyclophosphamide
Cavernous sinus thrombosis	Tricyclic antidepressants
	Monoamine oxidase inhibitors

other possible causes of the syndrome. The inappropriate antidiuresis in these patients appears to be permanent, although the hyponatremia is variable owing presumably to individual differences in fluid intake.

Pathophysiology Impaired osmotic suppression of antidiuresis results in excessive retention of water and dilution of body fluids only if water intake exceeds insensible and urinary losses. The excess intake is sometimes due to an associated defect in the osmoregulation of thirst (dipsogenic) but can also be psychogenic or iatrogenic, including excessive IV administration of hypotonic fluids. In SIADH and other forms of euvolemic hyponatremia, the decrease in plasma osmolarity/sodium and the increase in extracellular and intracellular volume are proportional to the amount of water retained. Thus, an increase in body water of 10% (~4 L in a 70-kg adult) reduces plasma osmolarity and sodium by approximately 10% (~28 mosmol/L or 14 meq/L). An increase in body water of this magnitude is rarely detectable on physical examination but will be reflected in a weight gain of about 4 kg. It also increases glomerular filtration and atrial natriuretic hormone and suppresses plasma renin activity, thereby increasing urinary sodium excretion. The resultant reduction in total body sodium decreases the expansion of extracellular volume but aggravates the hyponatremia and further expands intracellular volume. The latter further increases brain swelling and intracranial pressure, which probably produces most of the symptoms of acute water intoxication. Within a few days, this swelling may be counteracted by inactivation or elimination of intracellular solutes, resulting in the remission of symptoms even though the hyponatremia persists.

In type I (hypervolemic) or type II (hypovolemic) hyponatremia, osmotic suppression of AVP secretion appears to be counteracted by a hemodynamic stimulus resulting from a large reduction in cardiac output and/or effective blood volume. The resultant antidiuresis is enhanced by decreased distal delivery of glomerular filtrate that results from increased reabsorption of sodium in proximal nephron. If the reduction in urine output is not associated with a commensurate reduction in water intake or an increase in insensible loss, body fluids are expanded and diluted, resulting in hyponatremia despite an increase in body sodium. Unlike SIADH and other forms of euvolemic hyponatremia, however, glomerular filtration is reduced and plasma renin activity and aldosterone are elevated. Thus, the rate of urinary sodium excretion is low (unless sodium reabsorption is impaired by a diuretic), and the hyponatremia is usually accompanied by edema, hypokalemia, azotemia, and hyperuricemia. In type II (hypovolemic) hyponatremia, sodium and water are also retained as an appropriate compensatory response to the severe depletion.

Differential Diagnosis SIADH is a diagnosis of exclusion that usually can be made from the history, physical examination, and basic laboratory data. If hyperglycemia is present, its contribution to the reduction in plasma sodium can be estimated either by measuring plasma osmolarity for a more accurate estimate of the true "effective" tonicity of body fluids or by correcting the measured plasma sodium for the reduction caused by the hyperglycemia using the simplified formula

$$\text{corrected } P_{na} = \text{measured } P_{na} + (P_{glu} - 90)/36$$

where P_{na} = plasma sodium in meq/L and P_{glu} = plasma glucose in mg/dL.

If the plasma osmolarity and/or corrected plasma sodium are below normal limits, hypotonic hyponatremia is present and further evaluation to determine the type should be undertaken in order to administer safe and effective treatment. This differentiation is usually possible by evaluating standard clinical indicators of the extracellular fluid volume (Table 404-3). If these findings are ambiguous or contradictory, measuring plasma renin activity or the *rate* of urinary sodium excretion may be helpful *provided* that the hyponatremia is not in the recovery phase or is due to a primary defect in renal conservation of sodium, diuretic abuse, or hyporeninemic hypoaldosteronism. The latter may be suspected if serum potassium is elevated instead of low, as it usually is in types I and II hyponatremia. Measurements of plasma AVP are currently of no value in differentiating SIADH from the other types of hyponatremia since the plasma levels are elevated similarly in all. In patients who fulfill the clinical criteria for type III (euvolemic) hyponatremia, morning plasma cortisol should also be measured to exclude secondary adrenal insufficiency. If it is normal and there is no history of nausea/vomiting, the diagnosis of SIADH is confirmed, and a careful search for occult lung cancer or other common causes of the syndrome (Table 404-2) should be undertaken.

SIAD due to an activating mutation of the V_2 receptor gene should be suspected if the hyponatremia occurs in a child or several members of the family or is refractory to treatment with a vaptan (see below). In that case, plasma AVP should be measured to confirm that it is appropriately suppressed while the hyponatremia and antidiuresis are present, and the V_2 receptor gene should be sequenced, if possible.

TREATMENT HYPONATREMIA

The management of hyponatremia differs depending on the type and the severity and duration of symptoms. In acute symptomatic SIADH, the aim should be to raise plasma osmolarity and/or plasma sodium at a rate approximating 1% an hour until they reach levels of about 270 mosmol/L or 130 meq/L, respectively. This can be accomplished in either of two ways. One is to infuse hypertonic (3%) saline at a rate of about 0.05 mL/kg body weight per minute. This treatment also has the advantage of correcting the sodium deficiency that is partly responsible for the hyponatremia and often produces a solute diuresis that serves to remove some of the excess water. The other treatment is to reduce body water by giving an AVP receptor-2 antagonist (vaptan) to block the antidiuretic effect of AVP and increase urine output (Fig. 404-7). One of the vaptans, a combined V_2/V_{1a} antagonist (Conivaptan), has been approved for short-term, in-hospital IV treatment of SIADH, and others are in various stages of development. With either approach, fluid intake should be restricted to less than urine

TABLE 404-3 DIFFERENTIAL DIAGNOSIS OF HYPONATREMIA BASED ON CLINICAL ASSESSMENT OF EXTRACELLULAR FLUID VOLUME (ECFV)

Clinical Findings	Type I, Hypervolemic	Type II, Hypovolemic	Type III, Euvolemic	SIADH and SIAD Euvolemic
History				
CHF, cirrhosis, or nephrosis	Yes	No	No	No
Salt and water loss	No	Yes	No	No
ACTH–cortisol deficiency and/or nausea and vomiting	No	No	Yes	No
Physical examination				
Generalized edema, ascites	Yes	No	No	No
Postural hypotension	Maybe	Maybe	Maybe[a]	No
Laboratory				
BUN, creatinine	High-normal	High-normal	Low-normal	Low-normal
Uric acid	High-normal	High-normal	Low-normal	Low-normal
Serum potassium	Low-normal	Low-normal[b]	Normal[c]	Normal
Serum urate	High	High	Low	Low
Serum albumin	Low-normal	High-normal	Normal	Normal
Serum cortisol	Normal-high	Normal-high[d]	Low[e]	Normal
Plasma renin activity	High	High	Low[f]	Low
Urinary sodium (meq per unit of time)[g]	Low	Low[h]	High[i]	High[i]

[a]Postural hypotension may occur in secondary (ACTH-dependent) adrenal insufficiency even though extracellular fluid volume and aldosterone are usually normal. [b]Serum potassium may be high if hypovolemia is due to aldosterone deficiency. [c]Serum potassium may be low if vomiting causes alkalosis. [d]Serum cortisol is low if hypovolemia is due to primary adrenal insufficiency (Addison's disease). [e]Serum cortisol will be normal or high if the cause is nausea and vomiting rather than secondary (ACTH-dependent) adrenal insufficiency. [f]Plasma renin activity may be high if the cause is secondary (ACTH) adrenal insufficiency. [g]Urinary sodium should be expressed as the *rate of excretion* rather than the concentration. In a hyponatremic adult, an excretion rate >25 meq/d (or 25 μeq/mg of creatinine) could be considered high. [h]The rate of urinary sodium excretion may be high if the hypovolemia is due to diuretic abuse, primary adrenal insufficiency, or other causes of renal sodium wasting. [i]The rate of urinary sodium excretion may be low if intake is curtailed by symptoms or treatment.

Abbreviations: ACTH, adrenocorticotropic hormone; BUN, blood urea nitrogen; CHF, congestive heart failure; SIAD, syndrome of inappropriate antidiuresis.

output, and serum sodium should be checked at least once every 2h to ensure it is not raised too fast or too far. Doing so may result in central pontine myelinolysis, an acute, potentially fatal neurologic syndrome characterized by quadriparesis, ataxia, and abnormal extraocular movements.

In chronic and/or minimally symptomatic SIADH, the hyponatremia can and should be corrected more gradually. This can be achieved by restricting total fluid intake to less than the sum of urinary and insensible losses. Because the water derived from food

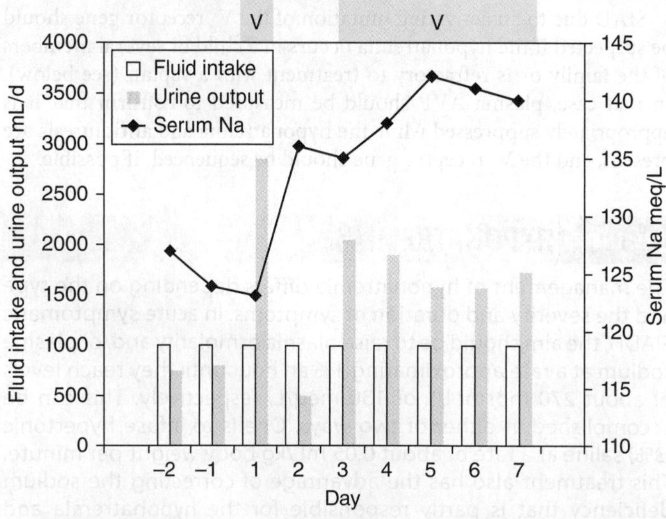

FIGURE 404-7 The effect of vaptan therapy on water balance in a patient with chronic syndrome of inappropriate antidiuretic hormone (SIADH). The periods of vaptan (V) therapy are indicated by the green shaded boxes at the top. Urine output is indicated by orange bars. Fluid intake is shown by the open bars. Intake was restricted to 1 L/d throughout. Serum sodium is indicated by the black line. Note that sodium increased progressively when vaptan increased urine output to levels that clearly exceeded fluid intake.

(300–700 mL/d) usually approximates basal insensible losses in adults, the aim should be to reduce total discretionary intake (all liquids) to approximately 500 mL less than urinary output. Adherence to this regimen is often problematic and, even if achieved, usually reduces body water and increases serum sodium by only about 1–2% per day. Hence, additional approaches are usually desirable if not necessary. The best approach for treatment of chronic SIADH is the administration of an oral vaptan, tolvaptan, a selective V_2 antagonist that also increases urinary water excretion by blocking the antidiuretic effect of AVP. Some restriction of fluid intake may also be necessary to achieve satisfactory control of the hyponatremia. It is approved for treatment of nonemergent SIADH with initial in-hospital dosing. Other approaches include demeclocycline, 150–300 mg PO tid or qid, or fludrocortisone, 0.05–0.2 mg PO bid. The effect of the demeclocycline manifests in 7–14 days and is due to induction of a reversible form of nephrogenic DI. Potential side effects include phototoxicity and azotemia. The effect of fludrocortisone also requires 1–2 weeks and is partly due to increased retention of sodium and possibly inhibition of thirst. It also increases urinary potassium excretion, which may require replacement through dietary adjustments or supplements and may induce hypertension, occasionally necessitating discontinuation of the treatment.

In euvolemic hyponatremia caused by protracted nausea and vomiting or isolated glucocorticoid deficiency (type III), all abnormalities can be corrected quickly and completely by giving an antiemetic or stress doses of hydrocortisone (for glucocorticoid deficiency). As with other treatments, care must be taken to ensure that serum sodium does not rise too quickly or too far.

In SIAD due to an activating mutation of the V_2 receptor, the V_2 antagonists usually do not block the antidiuresis or raise plasma osmolarity/sodium. In that condition, use of an osmotic diuretic such as urea is reported to be effective in preventing or correcting hyponatremia. However, some vaptans may be effective in patients with a different type of activating mutation so the response to this therapy may be neither predictable nor diagnostic.

In hypervolemic hyponatremia, fluid restriction is also appropriate and somewhat effective if it can be maintained. However, infusion of hypertonic saline is contraindicated because it further increases total body sodium and edema and may precipitate cardiovascular decompensation. However, as in SIADH, the V_2 receptor antagonists are also safe and effective in the treatment of hypervolemic hyponatremia caused by congestive heart failure. Tolvaptan is approved by the Food and Drug Administration for this indication with the caveat that treatment should be initiated or reinitiated in hospital. Its use should also be limited to 30 days at a time because of reports that longer periods may be associated with abnormal liver chemistries.

In hypovolemic hyponatremia, the defect in AVP secretion and water balance usually can be corrected easily and quickly by stopping the loss of sodium and water and/or replacing the deficits by mouth or IV infusion of normal or hypertonic saline. As with the treatment of other forms of hyponatremia, care must be taken to ensure that plasma sodium does not increase too rapidly or too far. Fluid restriction and administration of AVP antagonists are contraindicated in type II hyponatremia because they would only aggravate the underlying volume depletion and could result in hemodynamic collapse.

GLOBAL PERSPECTIVES

The incidence, clinical characteristics, etiology, pathophysiology, differential diagnosis, and treatments of fluid and electrolyte disorders in tropical and nonindustrialized countries differ in some respects from those in the United States and other industrialized parts of the world. Hyponatremia, for example, appears to be more common and is more likely to be due to infectious diseases such as cholera, shigellosis, and other diarrheal disorders. In these circumstances, hyponatremia is probably due to gastrointestinal losses of salt and water (hypovolemia type II), but other abnormalities, including undefined infectious toxins, also may contribute. The causes of DI are similar worldwide except that malaria and venoms from snake or insect bites are much more common.

405 Disorders of the Thyroid Gland

J. Larry Jameson, Susan J. Mandel, Anthony P. Weetman

The thyroid gland produces two related hormones, thyroxine (T_4) and triiodothyronine (T_3) (Fig. 405-1). Acting through thyroid hormone receptors α and β, these hormones play a critical role in cell differentiation during development and help maintain thermogenic and metabolic homeostasis in the adult. Autoimmune disorders of the thyroid gland can stimulate overproduction of thyroid hormones (*thyrotoxicosis*) or cause glandular destruction and hormone deficiency (*hypothyroidism*). In addition, benign nodules and various forms of thyroid cancer are relatively common and amenable to detection by physical examination.

ANATOMY AND DEVELOPMENT

The thyroid (Greek *thyreos*, shield, plus *eidos*, form) consists of two lobes connected by an isthmus. It is located anterior to the trachea between the cricoid cartilage and the suprasternal notch. The normal thyroid is 12–20 g in size, highly vascular, and soft in consistency. Four parathyroid glands, which produce parathyroid hormone (Chap. 424), are located posterior to each pole of the thyroid. The recurrent laryngeal nerves traverse the lateral borders of the thyroid gland and must be identified during thyroid surgery to avoid injury and vocal cord paralysis.

The thyroid gland develops from the floor of the primitive pharynx during the third week of gestation. The developing gland migrates along the thyroglossal duct to reach its final location in the neck. This feature accounts for the rare ectopic location of thyroid tissue at the base of the tongue (lingual thyroid) as well as the occurrence of thyroglossal duct cysts along this developmental tract. Thyroid hormone synthesis normally begins at about 11 weeks' gestation.

Neural crest derivatives from the ultimobranchial body give rise to thyroid medullary C cells that produce calcitonin, a calcium-lowering hormone. The C cells are interspersed throughout the thyroid gland, although their density is greatest in the juncture of the upper one-third and lower two-thirds of the gland. Calcitonin plays a minimal role in calcium homeostasis in humans but the C-cells are important because of their involvement in medullary thyroid cancer.

Thyroid gland development is orchestrated by the coordinated expression of several developmental transcription factors. Thyroid transcription factor (TTF)-1, TTF-2, and paired homeobox 8 (PAX-8) are expressed selectively, but not exclusively, in the thyroid gland. In combination, they dictate thyroid cell development and the induction of thyroid-specific genes such as thyroglobulin (Tg), thyroid peroxidase (TPO), the sodium iodide symporter (Na^+/I^-, NIS), and the thyroid-stimulating hormone receptor (TSH-R). Mutations in these developmental transcription factors or their downstream target genes are rare causes of thyroid agenesis or dyshormonogenesis, although the causes of most forms of congenital hypothyroidism remain unknown (Table 405-1). Because congenital hypothyroidism occurs in approximately 1 in 4000 newborns, neonatal screening is now performed in most industrialized countries (see below). Transplacental passage of maternal thyroid hormone occurs before the fetal thyroid gland begins to function and provides partial hormone support to a fetus with congenital hypothyroidism. Early thyroid hormone replacement in newborns with congenital hypothyroidism prevents potentially severe developmental abnormalities.

The thyroid gland consists of numerous spherical follicles composed of thyroid follicular cells that surround secreted colloid, a proteinaceous fluid containing large amounts of thyroglobulin, the protein precursor of thyroid hormones (Fig. 405-2). The thyroid follicular cells are polarized—the basolateral surface is apposed to the bloodstream and an apical surface faces the follicular lumen. Increased demand for thyroid hormone is regulated by thyroid-stimulating hormone (TSH), which binds to its receptor on the basolateral surface of the follicular cells. This binding leads to Tg reabsorption from the follicular lumen and proteolysis within the cytoplasm, yielding thyroid hormones for secretion into the bloodstream.

REGULATION OF THE THYROID AXIS

TSH, secreted by the thyrotrope cells of the anterior pituitary, plays a pivotal role in control of the thyroid axis and serves as the most useful

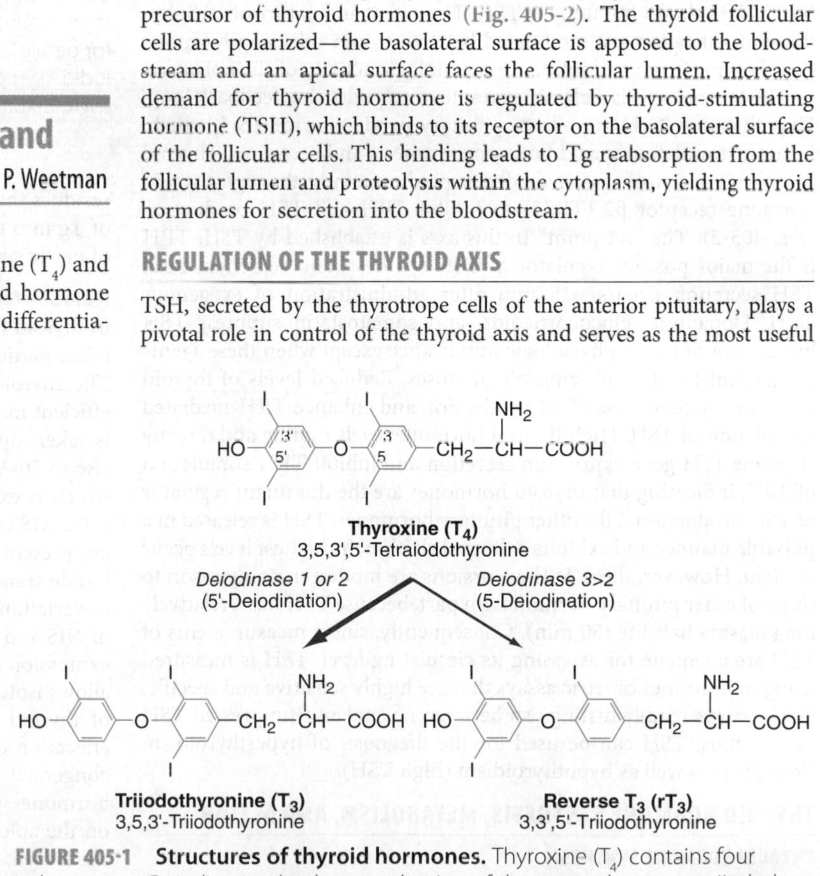

Thyroxine (T_4)
3,5,3',5'-Tetraiodothyronine

Deiodinase 1 or 2
(5'-Deiodination)

Deiodinase 3>2
(5-Deiodination)

Triiodothyronine (T_3)
3,5,3'-Triiodothyronine

Reverse T_3 (rT_3)
3,3',5'-Triiodothyronine

FIGURE 405-1 Structures of thyroid hormones. Thyroxine (T_4) contains four iodine atoms. Deiodination leads to production of the potent hormone triiodothyronine (T_3) or the inactive hormone reverse T_3.

TABLE 405-1 GENETIC CAUSES OF CONGENITAL HYPOTHYROIDISM

Defective Gene Protein	Inheritance	Consequences
PROP-1	Autosomal recessive	Combined pituitary hormone deficiencies with preservation of adrenocorticotropic hormone
PIT-1	Autosomal recessive Autosomal dominant	Combined deficiencies of growth hormone, prolactin, thyroid-stimulating hormone (TSH)
TSHβ	Autosomal recessive	TSH deficiency
TTF-1 (TITF-1)	Autosomal dominant	Variable thyroid hypoplasia, choreoathetosis, pulmonary problems
TTF-2 (FOXE-1)	Autosomal recessive	Thyroid agenesis, choanal atresia, spiky hair
PAX-8	Autosomal dominant	Thyroid dysgenesis
TSH-receptor	Autosomal recessive	Resistance to TSH
$G_{s\alpha}$ (Albright hereditary osteodystrophy)	Autosomal dominant	Resistance to TSH
Na^+/I^- symporter	Autosomal recessive	Inability to transport iodide
DUOX2 (THOX2)	Autosomal dominant	Organification defect
DUOXA2	Autosomal recessive	Organification defect
Thyroid peroxidase	Autosomal recessive	Defective organification of iodide
Thyroglobulin	Autosomal recessive	Defective synthesis of thyroid hormone
Pendrin	Autosomal recessive	Pendred syndrome: sensorineural deafness and partial organification defect in thyroid
Dehalogenase 1	Autosomal recessive	Loss of iodide reutilization

physiologic marker of thyroid hormone action. TSH is a 31-kDa hormone composed of α and β subunits; the α subunit is common to the other glycoprotein hormones (luteinizing hormone, follicle-stimulating hormone, human chorionic gonadotropin [hCG]), whereas the TSH β subunit is unique to TSH. The extent and nature of carbohydrate modification are modulated by thyrotropin-releasing hormone (TRH) stimulation and influence the biologic activity of the hormone.

The thyroid axis is a classic example of an endocrine feedback loop. Hypothalamic TRH stimulates pituitary production of TSH, which, in turn, stimulates thyroid hormone synthesis and secretion. Thyroid hormones act via negative feedback predominantly through thyroid hormone receptor β2 (TRβ2) to inhibit TRH and TSH production (Fig. 405-2). The "set-point" in this axis is established by TSH. TRH is the major positive regulator of TSH synthesis and secretion. Peak TSH secretion occurs ~15 min after administration of exogenous TRH. Dopamine, glucocorticoids, and somatostatin suppress TSH but are not of major physiologic importance except when these agents are administered in pharmacologic doses. Reduced levels of thyroid hormone increase basal TSH production and enhance TRH-mediated stimulation of TSH. High thyroid hormone levels rapidly and directly suppress TSH gene expression secretion and inhibit TRH stimulation of TSH, indicating that thyroid hormones are the dominant regulator of TSH production. Like other pituitary hormones, TSH is released in a pulsatile manner and exhibits a diurnal rhythm; its highest levels occur at night. However, these TSH excursions are modest in comparison to those of other pituitary hormones, in part, because TSH has a relatively long plasma half-life (50 min). Consequently, single measurements of TSH are adequate for assessing its circulating level. TSH is measured using immunoradiometric assays that are highly sensitive and specific. These assays readily distinguish between normal and suppressed TSH values; thus, TSH can be used for the diagnosis of hyperthyroidism (low TSH) as well as hypothyroidism (high TSH).

THYROID HORMONE SYNTHESIS, METABOLISM, AND ACTION

THYROID HORMONE SYNTHESIS

Thyroid hormones are derived from Tg, a large iodinated glycoprotein. After secretion into the thyroid follicle, Tg is iodinated on tyrosine residues that are subsequently coupled via an ether linkage. Reuptake of Tg into the thyroid follicular cell allows proteolysis and the release of newly synthesized T_4 and T_3.

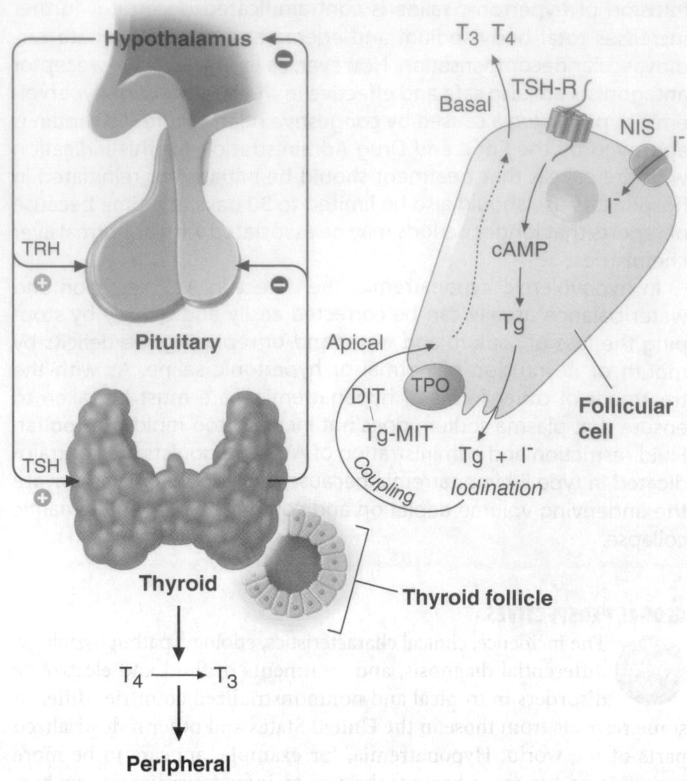

FIGURE 405-2 Regulation of thyroid hormone synthesis. ***Left.*** Thyroid hormones T_4 and T_3 feed back to inhibit hypothalamic production of thyrotropin-releasing hormone (TRH) and pituitary production of thyroid-stimulating hormone (TSH). TSH stimulates thyroid gland production of T_4 and T_3. ***Right.*** Thyroid follicles are formed by thyroid epithelial cells surrounding proteinaceous colloid, which contains thyroglobulin. Follicular cells, which are polarized, synthesize thyroglobulin and carry out thyroid hormone biosynthesis (see text for details). DIT, diiodotyrosine; MIT, monoiodotyrosine; NIS, sodium iodide symporter; Tg, thyroglobulin; TPO, thyroid peroxidase; TSH-R, thyroid-stimulating hormone receptor.

Iodine Metabolism and Transport Iodide uptake is a critical first step in thyroid hormone synthesis. Ingested iodine is bound to serum proteins, particularly albumin. Unbound iodine is excreted in the urine. The thyroid gland extracts iodine from the circulation in a highly efficient manner. For example, 10–25% of radioactive tracer (e.g., ^{123}I) is taken up by the normal thyroid gland over 24 h; this value can rise to 70–90% in Graves' disease. Iodide uptake is mediated by NIS, which is expressed at the basolateral membrane of thyroid follicular cells. NIS is most highly expressed in the thyroid gland, but low levels are present in the salivary glands, lactating breast, and placenta. The iodide transport mechanism is highly regulated, allowing adaptation to variations in dietary supply. Low iodine levels increase the amount of NIS and stimulate uptake, whereas high iodine levels suppress NIS expression and uptake. The selective expression of NIS in the thyroid allows isotopic scanning, treatment of hyperthyroidism, and ablation of thyroid cancer with radioisotopes of iodine, without significant effects on other organs. Mutation of the *NIS* gene is a rare cause of congenital hypothyroidism, underscoring its importance in thyroid hormone synthesis. Another iodine transporter, pendrin, is located on the apical surface of thyroid cells and mediates iodine efflux into the lumen. Mutation of the *pendrin* gene causes *Pendred syndrome*, a disorder characterized by defective organification of iodine, goiter, and sensorineural deafness.

Iodine deficiency is prevalent in many mountainous regions and in central Africa, central South America, and northern Asia (Fig. 405-3). Europe remains mildly iodine-deficient, and health surveys indicate that iodine intake has been falling in the United States and Australia. The World Health Organization (WHO) estimates that about 2 billion people are iodine-deficient, based on urinary excretion data. In areas of relative iodine deficiency, there is an increased prevalence of goiter and, when deficiency is severe, hypothyroidism and cretinism. *Cretinism* is characterized by mental and growth retardation and occurs when children who live in iodine-deficient regions are not treated with iodine or thyroid hormone to restore normal thyroid hormone levels during early life. These children are often born to mothers with iodine deficiency, and it is likely that maternal thyroid hormone deficiency worsens the condition. Concomitant selenium deficiency may also contribute to the neurologic manifestations of cretinism. Iodine supplementation of salt, bread, and other food substances has markedly reduced the prevalence of cretinism. Unfortunately, however, iodine deficiency remains the most common cause of preventable mental deficiency, often because of societal resistance to food additives or the cost of supplementation. In addition to overt cretinism, mild iodine deficiency can lead to subtle reduction of IQ. Oversupply of iodine, through supplements or foods enriched in iodine (e.g., shellfish, kelp), is associated with an increased incidence of autoimmune thyroid disease. The recommended average daily intake of iodine is 150–250 μg/d for adults, 90–120 μg/d for children, and 250 μg/d for pregnant and lactating women. Urinary iodine is >10 μg/dL in iodine-sufficient populations.

Organification, Coupling, Storage, and Release After iodide enters the thyroid, it is trapped and transported to the apical membrane of thyroid follicular cells, where it is oxidized in an organification reaction that involves TPO and hydrogen peroxide produced by dual oxidase (DUOX) and DUOX maturation factor (DUOXA). The reactive iodine atom is added to selected tyrosyl residues within Tg, a large (660 kDa) dimeric protein that consists of 2769 amino acids. The iodotyrosines in Tg are then coupled via an ether linkage in a reaction that is also catalyzed by TPO. Either T_4 or T_3 can be produced by this reaction, depending on the number of iodine atoms present in the iodotyrosines. After coupling, Tg is taken back into the thyroid cell, where it is processed in lysosomes to release T_4 and T_3. Uncoupled mono- and diiodotyrosines (MIT, DIT) are deiodinated by the enzyme dehalogenase, thereby recycling any iodide that is not converted into thyroid hormones.

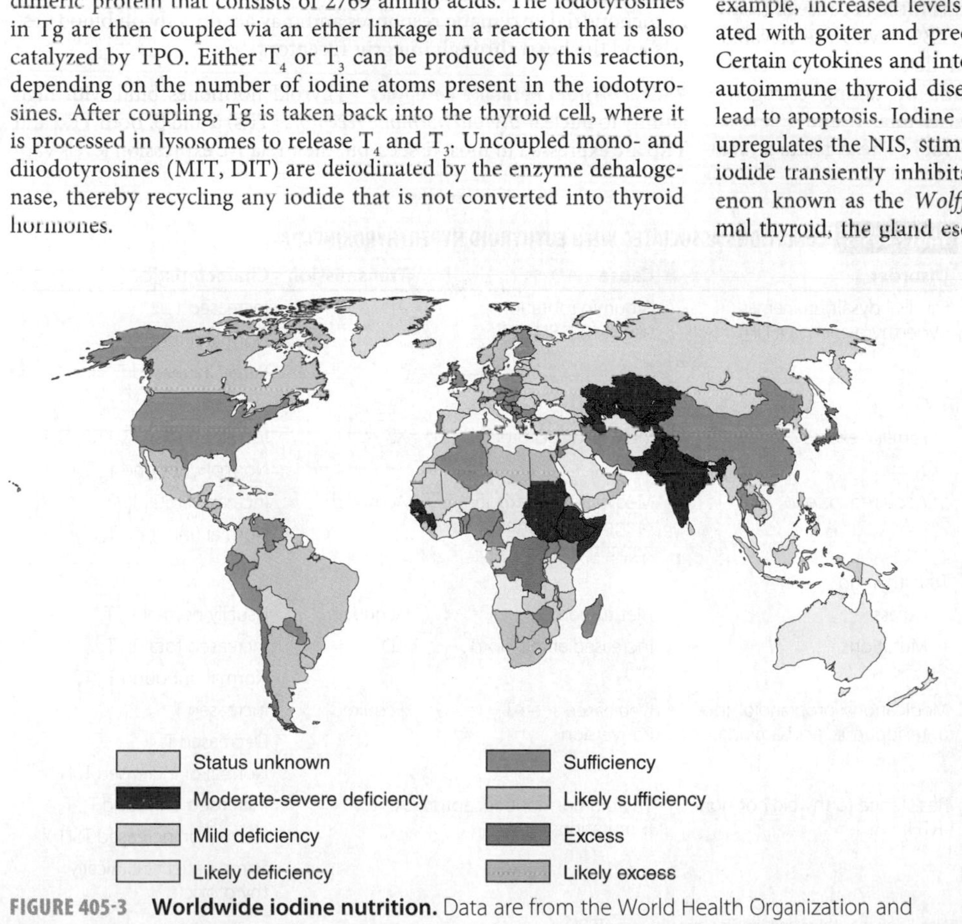

Disorders of thyroid hormone synthesis are rare causes of congenital hypothyroidism. The vast majority of these disorders are due to recessive mutations in TPO or Tg, but defects have also been identified in the TSH-R, NIS, pendrin, hydrogen peroxide generation, and dehalogenase. Because of the biosynthetic defect, the gland is incapable of synthesizing adequate amounts of hormone, leading to increased TSH and a large goiter.

TSH Action TSH regulates thyroid gland function through the TSH-R, a seven-transmembrane G protein–coupled receptor (GPCR). The TSH-R is coupled to the α subunit of stimulatory G protein ($G_{s\alpha}$), which activates adenylyl cyclase, leading to increased production of cyclic adenosine monophosphate (AMP). TSH also stimulates phosphatidylinositol turnover by activating phospholipase C. The functional role of the TSH-R is exemplified by the consequences of naturally occurring mutations. Recessive loss-of-function mutations cause thyroid hypoplasia and congenital hypothyroidism. Dominant gain-of-function mutations cause sporadic or familial hyperthyroidism that is characterized by goiter, thyroid cell hyperplasia, and autonomous function. Most of these activating mutations occur in the transmembrane domain of the receptor. They mimic the conformational changes induced by TSH binding or the interactions of thyroid-stimulating immunoglobulins (TSI) in Graves' disease. Activating TSH-R mutations also occur as somatic events, leading to clonal selection and expansion of the affected thyroid follicular cell and autonomously functioning thyroid nodules (see below).

Other Factors That Influence Hormone Synthesis and Release Although TSH is the dominant hormonal regulator of thyroid gland growth and function, a variety of growth factors, most produced locally in the thyroid gland, also influence thyroid hormone synthesis. These include insulin-like growth factor I (IGF-I), epidermal growth factor, transforming growth factor β (TGF-β), endothelins, and various cytokines. The quantitative roles of these factors are not well understood, but they are important in selected disease states. In acromegaly, for example, increased levels of growth hormone and IGF-I are associated with goiter and predisposition to multinodular goiter (MNG). Certain cytokines and interleukins (ILs) produced in association with autoimmune thyroid disease induce thyroid growth, whereas others lead to apoptosis. Iodine deficiency increases thyroid blood flow and upregulates the NIS, stimulating more efficient iodine uptake. Excess iodide transiently inhibits thyroid iodide organification, a phenomenon known as the *Wolff-Chaikoff effect*. In individuals with a normal thyroid, the gland escapes from this inhibitory effect and iodide organification resumes; the suppressive action of high iodide may persist, however, in patients with underlying autoimmune thyroid disease.

Status unknown
Moderate-severe deficiency
Mild deficiency
Likely deficiency
Sufficiency
Likely sufficiency
Excess
Likely excess

FIGURE 405-3 Worldwide iodine nutrition. Data are from the World Health Organization and the International Council for the Control of Iodine Deficiency Disorders (*http://indorgs.virginia.edu/iccidd/mi/cidds.html*).

THYROID HORMONE TRANSPORT AND METABOLISM

Serum Binding Proteins T_4 is secreted from the thyroid gland in about twentyfold excess over T_3 (Table 405-2). Both hormones are bound to plasma proteins, including thyroxine-binding globulin (TBG), transthyretin (TTR, formerly known as thyroxine-binding prealbumin, or TBPA), and albumin. The plasma-binding proteins increase the pool of circulating hormone, delay hormone clearance, and may modulate hormone delivery to selected tissue sites. The concentration of TBG is relatively low (1–2 mg/dL), but because of its high affinity for thyroid hormones ($T_4 > T_3$), it carries about 80% of the bound hormones. Albumin has relatively low affinity for thyroid hormones but has a high plasma concentration (~3.5 g/dL), and it binds up to 10% of T_4 and 30% of T_3. TTR carries about 10% of T_4 but little T_3.

TABLE 405-2 CHARACTERISTICS OF CIRCULATING T_4 AND T_3

Hormone Property	T_4	T_3
Serum concentrations		
Total hormone	8 μg/dL	0.14 μg/dL
Fraction of total hormone in the unbound form	0.02%	0.3%
Unbound (free) hormone	$21 \times 10^{-12} M$	$6 \times 10^{-12} M$
Serum half-life	7 d	2 d
Fraction directly from the thyroid	100%	20%
Production rate, including peripheral conversion	90 μg/d	32 μg/d
Intracellular hormone fraction	~20%	~70%
Relative metabolic potency	0.3	1
Receptor binding	$10^{-10} M$	$10^{-11} M$

When the effects of the various binding proteins are combined, approximately 99.98% of T_4 and 99.7% of T_3 are protein-bound. Because T_3 is less tightly bound than T_4, the fraction of unbound T_3 is greater than unbound T_4, but there is less unbound T_3 in the circulation because it is produced in smaller amounts and cleared more rapidly than T_4. The unbound or "free" concentrations of the hormones are $\sim 2 \times 10^{-11} M$ for T_4 and $\sim 6 \times 10^{-12} M$ for T_3, which roughly correspond to the thyroid hormone receptor binding constants for these hormones (see below). The unbound hormone is thought to be biologically available to tissues. Nonetheless, the homeostatic mechanisms that regulate the thyroid axis are directed toward maintenance of normal concentrations of unbound hormones.

Abnormalities of Thyroid Hormone Binding Proteins A number of inherited and acquired abnormalities affect thyroid hormone binding proteins. X-linked TBG deficiency is associated with very low levels of total T_4 and T_3. However, because unbound hormone levels are normal, patients are euthyroid and TSH levels are normal. It is important to recognize this disorder to avoid efforts to normalize total T_4 levels, because this leads to thyrotoxicosis and is futile because of rapid hormone clearance in the absence of TBG. TBG levels are elevated by estrogen, which increases sialylation and delays TBG clearance. Consequently, in women who are pregnant or taking estrogen-containing contraceptives, elevated TBG increases total T_4 and T_3 levels; however, unbound T_4 and T_3 levels are normal. These features are part of the explanation for why women with hypothyroidism require increased amounts of L-thyroxine replacement as TBG levels are increased by pregnancy or estrogen treatment. Mutations in TBG, TTR, and albumin may increase the binding affinity for T_4 and/or T_3 and cause disorders known as *euthyroid hyperthyroxinemia* or *familial dysalbuminemic hyperthyroxinemia* (FDH) (Table 405-3). These disorders result in increased total T_4 and/or T_3, but unbound hormone levels are normal. The familial nature of the disorders, and the fact that TSH levels are normal rather than suppressed, should suggest this diagnosis. Unbound hormone levels (ideally measured by dialysis) are normal in FDH. The diagnosis can be confirmed by using tests that measure the affinities of radiolabeled hormone binding to specific transport proteins or by performing DNA sequence analyses of the abnormal transport protein genes.

Certain medications, such as salicylates and salsalate, can displace thyroid hormones from circulating binding proteins. Although these drugs transiently perturb the thyroid axis by increasing free thyroid hormone levels, TSH is suppressed until a new steady state is reached, thereby restoring euthyroidism. Circulating factors associated with acute illness may also displace thyroid hormone from binding proteins (see "Sick Euthyroid Syndrome," below).

Deiodinases T_4 may be thought of as a precursor for the more potent T_3. T_4 is converted to T_3 by the deiodinase enzymes (Fig. 405-1). Type I deiodinase, which is located primarily in thyroid, liver, and kidneys, has a relatively low affinity for T_4. Type II deiodinase has a higher affinity for T_4 and is found primarily in the pituitary gland, brain, brown fat, and thyroid gland. Expression of type II deiodinase allows it to regulate T_3 concentrations locally, a property that may be important in the context of levothyroxine (T_4) replacement. Type II deiodinase is also regulated by thyroid hormone; hypothyroidism induces the enzyme, resulting in enhanced $T_4 \rightarrow T_3$ conversion in tissues such as brain and pituitary. $T_4 \rightarrow T_3$ conversion is impaired by fasting, systemic illness or acute trauma, oral contrast agents, and a variety of medications (e.g., propylthiouracil, propranolol, amiodarone, glucocorticoids). Type III deiodinase inactivates T_4 and T_3 and is the most important source of reverse T_3 (rT_3), including in the sick euthyroid syndrome. This enzyme is expressed in the human placenta but is not active in healthy individuals. In the sick euthyroid syndrome, especially with hypoperfusion, the type III deiodinase is activated in muscle and liver. Massive hemangiomas that express type III deiodinase are a rare cause of hypothyroidism in infants.

THYROID HORMONE ACTION

Thyroid Hormone Transport Circulating thyroid hormones enter cells by passive diffusion and via specific transporters such as the monocarboxylate 8 transporter (MCT8), MCT10, and organic anion-transporting polypeptide 1C1. Mutations in the *MCT8* gene have been identified in patients with X-linked psychomotor retardation and thyroid function abnormalities (low T_4, high T_3, and high TSH). After entering cells, thyroid hormones act primarily through nuclear receptors, although they also have nongenomic actions through stimulating mitochondrial enzymatic responses and may act directly on blood vessels and the heart through integrin receptors.

Nuclear Thyroid Hormone Receptors Thyroid hormones bind with high affinity to nuclear *thyroid hormone receptors* (TRs) α and β. Both TRα and TRβ are expressed in most tissues, but their relative expression levels vary

TABLE 405-3 CONDITIONS ASSOCIATED WITH EUTHYROID HYPERTHYROXINEMIA

Disorder	Cause	Transmission	Characteristics
Familial dysalbuminemic hyperthyroxinemia (FDH)	Albumin mutations, usually R218H	AD	Increased T_4 Normal unbound T_4 Rarely increased T_3
TBG			
Familial excess	Increased TBG production	XL	Increased total T_4, T_3 Normal unbound T_4, T_3
Acquired excess	Medications (estrogen), pregnancy, cirrhosis, hepatitis	Acquired	Increased total T_4, T_3 Normal unbound T_4, T_3
Transthyretin[a]			
Excess	Islet tumors	Acquired	Usually normal T_4, T_3
Mutations	Increased affinity for T_4 or T_3	AD	Increased total T_4, T_3 Normal unbound T_4, T_3
Medications: propranolol, ipodate, iopanoic acid, amiodarone	Decreased $T_4 \rightarrow T_3$ conversion	Acquired	Increased T_4 Decreased T_3 Normal or increased TSH
Resistance to thyroid hormone (RTH)	Thyroid hormone receptor β mutations	AD	Increased unbound T_4, T_3 Normal or increased TSH Some patients clinically thyrotoxic

[a]Also known as thyroxine-binding prealbumin (TBPA).

Abbreviations: AD, autosomal dominant; TBG, thyroxine-binding globulin; TSH, thyroid-stimulating hormone; XL, X-linked.

among organs; TRα is particularly abundant in brain, kidneys, gonads, muscle, and heart, whereas TRβ expression is relatively high in the pituitary and liver. Both receptors are variably spliced to form unique isoforms. The TRβ2 isoform, which has a unique amino terminus, is selectively expressed in the hypothalamus and pituitary, where it plays a role in feedback control of the thyroid axis (see above). The TRα2 isoform contains a unique carboxy terminus that precludes thyroid hormone binding; it may function to block the action of other TR isoforms.

The TRs contain a central DNA-binding domain and a C-terminal ligand-binding domain. They bind to specific DNA sequences, termed *thyroid response elements* (TREs), in the promoter regions of target genes (Fig. 405-4). The receptors bind as homodimers or, more commonly, as heterodimers with retinoic acid X receptors (RXRs) (Chap. 400e). The activated receptor can either stimulate gene transcription (e.g., myosin heavy chain α) or inhibit transcription (e.g., TSH β-subunit gene), depending on the nature of the regulatory elements in the target gene.

Thyroid hormones (T_3 and T_4) bind with similar affinities to TRα and TRβ. However, structural differences in the ligand binding domains provide the potential for developing receptor-selective agonists or antagonists, and these are under investigation. T_3 is bound with 10–15 times greater affinity than T_4, which explains its increased hormonal potency. Although T_4 is produced in excess of T_3, receptors are occupied mainly by T_3, reflecting $T_4 \rightarrow T_3$ conversion by peripheral tissues, greater T_3 bioavailability in the plasma, and the greater affinity of receptors for T_3. After binding to TRs, thyroid hormone induces conformational changes in the receptors that modify its interactions with accessory transcription factors. Importantly, in the absence of thyroid hormone binding, the aporeceptors bind to co-repressor proteins that inhibit gene transcription. Hormone binding dissociates the co-repressors and allows the recruitment of co-activators that enhance transcription. The discovery of TR interactions with co-repressors explains the fact that TR silences gene expression in the absence of hormone binding. Consequently, hormone deficiency has a profound effect on gene expression because it causes gene repression as well as loss of hormone-induced stimulation. This concept has been corroborated by the finding that targeted deletion of the TR genes in mice has a less pronounced phenotypic effect than hormone deficiency.

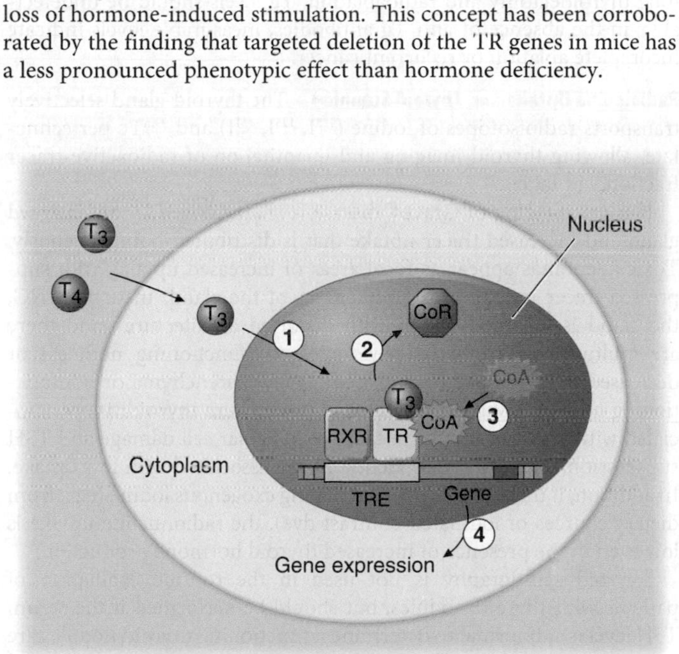

FIGURE 405-4 Mechanism of thyroid hormone receptor action. The thyroid hormone receptor (TR) and retinoid X receptor (RXR) form heterodimers that bind specifically to thyroid hormone response elements (TRE) in the promoter regions of target genes. In the absence of hormone, TR binds co-repressor (CoR) proteins that silence gene expression. The numbers refer to a series of ordered reactions that occur in response to thyroid hormone: (1) T_4 or T_3 enters the nucleus; (2) T_3 binding dissociates CoR from TR; (3) co-activators (CoA) are recruited to the T_3-bound receptor; and (4) gene expression is altered.

Thyroid Hormone Resistance Resistance to thyroid hormone (RTH) is an autosomal dominant disorder characterized by elevated thyroid hormone levels and inappropriately normal or elevated TSH. Individuals with RTH do not, in general, exhibit signs and symptoms that are typical of hypothyroidism because hormone resistance is partial and is compensated by increased levels of thyroid hormone. The clinical features of RTH can include goiter, attention deficit disorder, mild reduction in IQ, delayed skeletal maturation, tachycardia, and impaired metabolic responses to thyroid hormone.

Classical forms of RTH are caused by mutations in the TRβ gene. These mutations, located in restricted regions of the ligand-binding domain, cause loss of receptor function. However, because the mutant receptors retain the capacity to dimerize with RXRs, bind to DNA, and recruit co-repressor proteins, they function as antagonists of the remaining normal TRβ and TRα receptors. This property, referred to as "dominant negative" activity, explains the autosomal dominant mode of transmission. The diagnosis is suspected when unbound thyroid hormone levels are increased without suppression of TSH. Similar hormonal abnormalities are found in other affected family members, although the TRβ mutation arises de novo in about 20% of patients. DNA sequence analysis of the TRβ gene provides a definitive diagnosis. RTH must be distinguished from other causes of euthyroid hyperthyroxinemia (e.g., FDH) and inappropriate secretion of TSH by TSH-secreting pituitary adenomas (Chap. 403). In most patients, no treatment is indicated; the importance of making the diagnosis is to avoid inappropriate treatment of mistaken hyperthyroidism and to provide genetic counseling.

A distinct form of RTH is caused by mutations in the TRα gene. Affected patients have many clinical features of congenital hypothyroidism including growth retardation, skeletal dysplasia, and severe constipation. In contrast to RTH caused by mutations in TRβ, thyroid function tests include normal TSH, low or normal T_4, and normal or elevated T_3 levels. These distinct clinical and laboratory features underscore the different tissue distribution and functional roles of TRβ and TRα. Optimal treatment of patients with RTH caused by TRα mutations has not been established.

PHYSICAL EXAMINATION

In addition to the examination of the thyroid itself, the physical examination should include a search for signs of abnormal thyroid function and the extrathyroidal features of ophthalmopathy and dermopathy (see below). Examination of the neck begins by inspecting the seated patient from the front and side and noting any surgical scars, obvious masses, or distended veins. The thyroid can be palpated with both hands from behind or while facing the patient, using the thumbs to palpate each lobe. It is best to use a combination of these methods, especially when nodules are small. The patient's neck should be slightly flexed to relax the neck muscles. After locating the cricoid cartilage, the isthmus, which is attached to the lower one-third of the thyroid lobes, can be identified and then followed laterally to locate either lobe (normally, the right lobe is slightly larger than the left). By asking the patient to swallow sips of water, thyroid consistency can be better appreciated as the gland moves beneath the examiner's fingers.

Features to be noted include thyroid size, consistency, nodularity, and any tenderness or fixation. An estimate of thyroid size (normally 12–20 g) should be made, and a drawing is often the best way to record findings. However, ultrasound is the method of choice when it is important to determine thyroid size accurately. The size, location, and consistency of any nodules should also be defined. A bruit or thrill over the gland, located over the insertion of the superior and inferior thyroid arteries (supero- or inferolaterally), indicates increased vascularity, as occurs in hyperthyroidism. If the lower borders of the thyroid lobes are not clearly felt, a goiter may be retrosternal. Large retrosternal goiters can cause venous distention over the neck and difficulty breathing, especially when the arms are raised (Pemberton's sign). With any central mass above the thyroid, the tongue should be extended, as thyroglossal cysts then move upward. The thyroid examination is not complete without assessment for lymphadenopathy in the supraclavicular and cervical regions of the neck.

Measurement of Thyroid Hormones The enhanced sensitivity and specificity of *TSH assays* have greatly improved laboratory assessment of thyroid function. Because TSH levels change dynamically in response to alterations of T_4 and T_3, a logical approach to thyroid testing is to first determine whether TSH is suppressed, normal, or elevated. With rare exceptions (see below), a normal TSH level excludes a primary abnormality of thyroid function. This strategy depends on the use of immunochemiluminometric assays (ICMAs) for TSH that are sensitive enough to discriminate between the lower limit of the reference range and the suppressed values that occur with thyrotoxicosis. Extremely sensitive (fourth-generation) assays can detect TSH levels ≤0.004 mIU/L, but, for practical purposes, assays sensitive to ≤0.1 mIU/L are sufficient. The widespread availability of the TSH ICMA has rendered the TRH stimulation test obsolete, because the failure of TSH to rise after an intravenous bolus of 200–400 μg TRH has the same implications as a suppressed basal TSH measured by ICMA.

The finding of an abnormal TSH level must be followed by measurements of circulating thyroid hormone levels to confirm the diagnosis of hyperthyroidism (suppressed TSH) or hypothyroidism (elevated TSH). Radioimmunoassays are widely available for serum *total* T_4 and *total* T_3. T_4 and T_3 are highly protein-bound, and numerous factors (illness, medications, genetic factors) can influence protein binding. It is useful, therefore, to measure the free, or unbound, hormone levels, which correspond to the biologically available hormone pool. Two direct methods are used to measure *unbound thyroid hormones*: (1) unbound thyroid hormone competition with radiolabeled T_4 (or an analogue) for binding to a solid-phase antibody, and (2) physical separation of the unbound hormone fraction by ultracentrifugation or equilibrium dialysis. Although early unbound hormone immunoassays suffered from artifacts, newer assays correlate well with the results of the more technically demanding and expensive physical separation methods. An indirect method that is now less commonly used to estimate unbound thyroid hormone levels is to calculate the free T_3 or free T_4 index from the total T_4 or T_3 concentration and the *thyroid hormone binding ratio* (THBR). The latter is derived from the *T_3-resin uptake test*, which determines the distribution of radiolabeled T_3 between an absorbent resin and the unoccupied thyroid hormone binding proteins in the sample. The binding of the labeled T_3 to the resin is increased when there is reduced unoccupied protein binding sites (e.g., TBG deficiency) or increased total thyroid hormone in the sample; it is decreased under the opposite circumstances. The product of THBR and total T_3 or T_4 provides the *free T_3 or T_4 index*. In effect, the index corrects for anomalous total hormone values caused by abnormalities in hormone-protein binding.

Total thyroid hormone levels are *elevated* when TBG is increased due to estrogens (pregnancy, oral contraceptives, hormone therapy, tamoxifen, selective estrogen receptor modulators, inflammatory liver disease) and *decreased* when TBG binding is reduced (androgens, nephrotic syndrome). Genetic disorders and acute illness can also cause abnormalities in thyroid hormone binding proteins, and various drugs (phenytoin, carbamazepine, salicylates, and nonsteroidal anti-inflammatory drugs [NSAIDs]) can interfere with thyroid hormone binding. Because unbound thyroid hormone levels are normal and the patient is euthyroid in all of these circumstances, assays that measure unbound hormone are preferable to those for total thyroid hormones.

For most purposes, the unbound T_4 level is sufficient to confirm thyrotoxicosis, but 2–5% of patients have only an elevated T_3 level (T_3 toxicosis). Thus, unbound T_3 levels should be measured in patients with a suppressed TSH but normal unbound T_4 levels.

There are several clinical conditions in which the use of TSH as a screening test may be misleading, particularly without simultaneous unbound T_4 determinations. Any severe nonthyroidal illness can cause abnormal TSH levels (see below). Although hypothyroidism is the most common cause of an elevated TSH level, rare causes include a TSH-secreting pituitary tumor (Chap. 403), thyroid hormone resistance, and assay artifact. Conversely, a suppressed TSH level, particularly <0.01 mIU/L, usually indicates thyrotoxicosis. However, subnormal TSH levels between 0.01 and 0.1 mIU/L may be seen during the first trimester of pregnancy (due to hCG secretion), after treatment of hyperthyroidism (because TSH can remain suppressed for several months), and in response to certain medications (e.g., high doses of glucocorticoids or dopamine). Importantly, secondary hypothyroidism, caused by hypothalamic-pituitary disease, is associated with a variable (low to high-normal) TSH level, which is inappropriate for the low T_4 level. Thus, *TSH should not be used as an isolated laboratory test to assess thyroid function in patients with suspected or known pituitary disease.*

Tests for the end-organ effects of thyroid hormone excess or depletion, such as estimation of basal metabolic rate, tendon reflex relaxation rates, or serum cholesterol, are not useful as clinical determinants of thyroid function.

Tests to Determine the Etiology of Thyroid Dysfunction Autoimmune thyroid disease is detected most easily by measuring circulating antibodies against TPO and Tg. Because antibodies to Tg alone are uncommon, it is reasonable to measure only TPO antibodies. About 5–15% of euthyroid women and up to 2% of euthyroid men have thyroid antibodies; such individuals are at increased risk of developing thyroid dysfunction. Almost all patients with autoimmune hypothyroidism, and up to 80% of those with Graves' disease, have TPO antibodies, usually at high levels.

TSIs are antibodies that stimulate the TSH-R in Graves' disease. They are most commonly measured by commercially available tracer displacement assays called TRAb (TSH receptor antibody) with the assumption that elevated levels in the setting of clinical hyperthyroidism reflect stimulatory effects on the TSH receptor. A bioassay is less commonly used. The main use of these assays is to predict neonatal thyrotoxicosis caused by high maternal levels of TRAb or TSI (>3× upper limit of normal) in the last trimester of pregnancy.

Serum Tg levels are increased in all types of thyrotoxicosis except *thyrotoxicosis factitia* caused by self-administration of thyroid hormone. Tg levels are particularly increased in thyroiditis, reflecting thyroid tissue destruction and release of Tg. The main role for Tg measurement, however, is in the follow-up of thyroid cancer patients. After total thyroidectomy and radioablation, Tg levels should be undetectable; in the absence of anti-Tg antibodies, measurable levels indicate incomplete ablation or recurrent cancer.

Radioiodine Uptake and Thyroid Scanning The thyroid gland selectively transports radioisotopes of iodine (^{123}I, ^{125}I, ^{131}I) and ^{99m}Tc pertechnetate, allowing thyroid imaging and quantitation of radioactive tracer fractional uptake.

Nuclear imaging of Graves' disease is characterized by an enlarged gland and increased tracer uptake that is distributed homogeneously. Toxic adenomas appear as focal areas of increased uptake, with suppressed tracer uptake in the remainder of the gland. In toxic MNG, the gland is enlarged—often with distorted architecture—and there are multiple areas of relatively increased (functioning nodules) or decreased tracer uptake (suppressed thyroid parenchyma or nonfunctioning nodules). Subacute, viral, and postpartum thyroiditis are associated with very low uptake because of follicular cell damage and TSH suppression. Thyrotoxicosis factitia is also associated with low uptake. In addition, if there is excessive circulating exogenous iodine (e.g., from dietary sources of iodinated contrast dye), the radionuclide uptake is low even in the presence of increased thyroid hormone production.

Thyroid scintigraphy is not used in the routine evaluation of patients with thyroid nodules, but should be performed if the serum TSH level is subnormal to determine if functioning thyroid nodules are present. Functioning or "hot" nodules are almost never malignant, and fine-needle aspiration (FNA) biopsy is not indicated. The vast majority of thyroid nodules do not produce thyroid hormone ("cold" nodules), and these are more likely to be malignant (~5–10%). Whole-body and thyroid scanning is also used in the treatment and surveillance of thyroid cancer. After thyroidectomy for thyroid cancer, the TSH level is raised by either using a thyroid hormone withdrawal protocol or recombinant human TSH injection (see below). Administration of ^{131}I allows whole-body scanning (WBS) to confirm remnant ablation and to detect any functioning metastases. In addition, WBS may be helpful in surveillance of patients at risk for recurrence.

TABLE 405-4 GRAYSCALE SONOGRAPHIC FEATURES ASSOCIATED WITH THYROID CANCER

	Median Sensitivity [range]	Median Specificity [range]
Hypoechoic compared with surrounding thyroid	81% [48–90%]	53% [36–92%]
Marked hypoechogenicity	41% [27–59%]	94% [92–94%]
Microcalcifications	44% [26–73%]	89% [69–98%]
Irregular, microlobulated margins	55% [17–84%]	79% [62–85%]
Solid consistency	86% [78–91%]	48% [30–58%]
Taller than wide shape on transverse view	48% [33–84%]	92% [82–93%]

Thyroid Ultrasound Ultrasonography is valuable for the diagnosis and evaluation of patients with nodular thyroid disease (Table 405-4). Evidence-based guidelines recommend thyroid ultrasonography for all patients suspected of having thyroid nodules by either physical examination or another imaging study. Using 10- to 12-MHz linear transducers, resolution and image quality are excellent, allowing the characterization of nodules and cysts >3 mm. Certain sonographic patterns are highly suggestive of malignancy (e.g., hypoechoic solid nodules with infiltrative borders and microcalcifications), whereas other features correlate with benignity (e.g., spongiform nodules defined as those with multiple small internal cystic areas) (Fig. 405-5). In addition to evaluating thyroid nodules, ultrasound is useful for monitoring nodule size and for the aspiration of nodules or cystic lesions. Ultrasound-guided FNA biopsy of thyroid lesions lowers the rate of inadequate sampling and decreases sample error, thereby reducing the false-negative rate of FNA cytology. Ultrasonography of the central and lateral cervical lymph node compartments is indispensable in the evaluation thyroid cancer patients, preoperatively and during follow-up.

HYPOTHYROIDISM

Iodine deficiency remains a common cause of hypothyroidism worldwide. In areas of iodine sufficiency, autoimmune disease (Hashimoto's thyroiditis) and iatrogenic causes (treatment of hyperthyroidism) are most common (Table 405-5).

TABLE 405-5 CAUSES OF HYPOTHYROIDISM

Primary
Autoimmune hypothyroidism: Hashimoto's thyroiditis, atrophic thyroiditis
Iatrogenic: ^{131}I treatment, subtotal or total thyroidectomy, external irradiation of neck for lymphoma or cancer
Drugs: iodine excess (including iodine-containing contrast media and amiodarone), lithium, antithyroid drugs, *p*-aminosalicylic acid, interferon α and other cytokines, aminoglutethimide, tyrosine kinase inhibitors (e.g., sunitinib)
Congenital hypothyroidism: absent or ectopic thyroid gland, dyshormonogenesis, TSH-R mutation
Iodine deficiency
Infiltrative disorders: amyloidosis, sarcoidosis, hemochromatosis, scleroderma, cystinosis, Riedel's thyroiditis
Overexpression of type 3 deiodinase in infantile hemangioma and other tumors
Transient
Silent thyroiditis, including postpartum thyroiditis
Subacute thyroiditis
Withdrawal of supraphysiologic thyroxine treatment in individuals with an intact thyroid
After ^{131}I treatment or subtotal thyroidectomy for Graves' disease
Secondary
Hypopituitarism: tumors, pituitary surgery or irradiation, infiltrative disorders, Sheehan's syndrome, trauma, genetic forms of combined pituitary hormone deficiencies
Isolated TSH deficiency or inactivity
Bexarotene treatment
Hypothalamic disease: tumors, trauma, infiltrative disorders, idiopathic

Abbreviations: TSH, thyroid-stimulating hormone; TSH-R, TSH receptor.

CONGENITAL HYPOTHYROIDISM

Prevalence Hypothyroidism occurs in about 1 in 4000 newborns. It may be transient, especially if the mother has TSH-R blocking antibodies or has received antithyroid drugs, but permanent hypothyroidism occurs in the majority. Neonatal hypothyroidism is due to thyroid gland dysgenesis in 80–85%, to inborn errors of thyroid hormone synthesis in 10–15%, and is TSH-R antibody-mediated in 5% of affected newborns. The developmental abnormalities are twice as common in girls. Mutations that cause congenital hypothyroidism are being increasingly identified, but most remain idiopathic (Table 405-1).

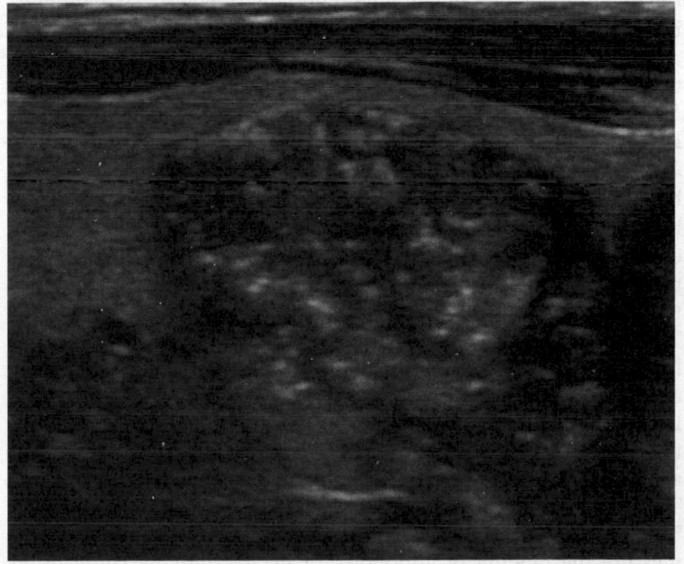

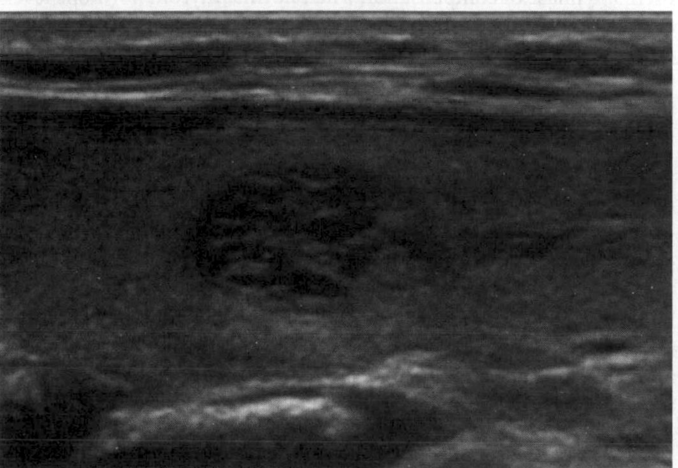

A B

FIGURE 405-5 Sonographic patterns of thyroid nodules. ***A.*** High suspicion ultrasound pattern for thyroid malignancy (hypoechoic solid nodule with irregular borders and microcalcifications). ***B.*** Very low suspicion ultrasound pattern for thyroid malignancy (spongiform nodule with microcystic areas comprises over >50% of nodule volume).

TABLE 405-6 SIGNS AND SYMPTOMS OF HYPOTHYROIDISM (DESCENDING ORDER OF FREQUENCY)

Symptoms	Signs
Tiredness, weakness	Dry coarse skin; cool peripheral extremities
Dry skin	Puffy face, hands, and feet (myxedema)
Feeling cold	Diffuse alopecia
Hair loss	Bradycardia
Difficulty concentrating and poor memory	Peripheral edema
Constipation	Delayed tendon reflex relaxation
Weight gain with poor appetite	Carpal tunnel syndrome
Dyspnea	Serous cavity effusions
Hoarse voice	
Menorrhagia (later oligomenorrhea or amenorrhea)	
Paresthesia	
Impaired hearing	

Clinical Manifestations The majority of infants appear normal at birth, and <10% are diagnosed based on clinical features, which include prolonged jaundice, feeding problems, hypotonia, enlarged tongue, delayed bone maturation, and umbilical hernia. Importantly, permanent neurologic damage results if treatment is delayed. Typical features of adult hypothyroidism may also be present (Table 405-6). Other congenital malformations, especially cardiac, are four times more common in congenital hypothyroidism.

Diagnosis and Treatment Because of the severe neurologic consequences of untreated congenital hypothyroidism, neonatal screening programs have been established. These are generally based on measurement of TSH or T_4 levels in heel-prick blood specimens. When the diagnosis is confirmed, T_4 is instituted at a dose of 10–15 μg/kg per day, and the dose is adjusted by close monitoring of TSH levels. T_4 requirements are relatively great during the first year of life, and a high circulating T_4 level is usually needed to normalize TSH. Early treatment with T_4 results in normal IQ levels, but subtle neurodevelopmental abnormalities may occur in those with the most severe hypothyroidism at diagnosis or when treatment is delayed or suboptimal.

AUTOIMMUNE HYPOTHYROIDISM

Classification Autoimmune hypothyroidism may be associated with a goiter (Hashimoto's, or *goitrous thyroiditis*) or, at the later stages of the disease, minimal residual thyroid tissue (*atrophic thyroiditis*). Because the autoimmune process gradually reduces thyroid function, there is a phase of compensation when normal thyroid hormone levels are maintained by a rise in TSH. Although some patients may have minor symptoms, this state is called *subclinical hypothyroidism*. Later, unbound T_4 levels fall and TSH levels rise further; symptoms become more readily apparent at this stage (usually TSH >10 mIU/L), which is referred to as *clinical hypothyroidism* or *overt hypothyroidism*.

Prevalence The mean annual incidence rate of autoimmune hypothyroidism is up to 4 per 1000 women and 1 per 1000 men. It is more common in certain populations, such as the Japanese, probably because of genetic factors and chronic exposure to a high-iodine diet. The mean age at diagnosis is 60 years, and the prevalence of overt hypothyroidism increases with age. Subclinical hypothyroidism is found in 6–8% of women (10% over the age of 60) and 3% of men. The annual risk of developing clinical hypothyroidism is about 4% when subclinical hypothyroidism is associated with positive TPO antibodies.

Pathogenesis In Hashimoto's thyroiditis, there is a marked lymphocytic infiltration of the thyroid with germinal center formation, atrophy of the thyroid follicles accompanied by oxyphil metaplasia, absence of colloid, and mild to moderate fibrosis. In atrophic thyroiditis, the fibrosis is much more extensive, lymphocyte infiltration is less pronounced, and thyroid follicles are almost completely absent. Atrophic thyroiditis likely represents the end stage of Hashimoto's thyroiditis rather than a distinct disorder.

As with most autoimmune disorders, susceptibility to autoimmune hypothyroidism is determined by a combination of genetic and environmental factors, and the risk of either autoimmune hypothyroidism or Graves' disease is increased among siblings. HLA-DR polymorphisms are the best documented genetic risk factors for autoimmune hypothyroidism, especially HLA-DR3, -DR4, and -DR5 in Caucasians. A weak association also exists between polymorphisms in *CTLA-4*, a T cell–regulatory gene, and autoimmune hypothyroidism. Both of these genetic associations are shared by other autoimmune diseases, which may explain the relationship between autoimmune hypothyroidism and other autoimmune diseases, especially type 1 diabetes mellitus, Addison's disease, pernicious anemia, and vitiligo. HLA-DR and *CTLA-4* polymorphisms account for approximately half of the genetic susceptibility to autoimmune hypothyroidism. Other contributory loci remain to be identified. A gene on chromosome 21 may be responsible for the association between autoimmune hypothyroidism and Down's syndrome. The female preponderance of thyroid autoimmunity is most likely due to sex steroid effects on the immune response, but an X chromosome–related genetic factor is also possible and may account for the high frequency of autoimmune hypothyroidism in Turner's syndrome. Environmental susceptibility factors are poorly defined at present. A high iodine intake and decreased exposure to microorganisms in childhood increase the risk of autoimmune hypothyroidism. These factors may account for the increase in prevalence over the last two to three decades.

The thyroid lymphocytic infiltrate in autoimmune hypothyroidism is composed of activated CD4+ and CD8+ T cells as well as B cells. Thyroid cell destruction is primarily mediated by the CD8+ cytotoxic T cells, which destroy their targets by either perforin-induced cell necrosis or granzyme B–induced apoptosis. In addition, local T cell production of cytokines, such as tumor necrosis factor (TNF), IL-1, and interferon γ (IFN-γ), may render thyroid cells more susceptible to apoptosis mediated by death receptors, such as Fas, which are activated by their respective ligands on T cells. These cytokines also impair thyroid cell function directly and induce the expression of other proinflammatory molecules by the thyroid cells themselves, such as cytokines, HLA class I and class II molecules, adhesion molecules, CD40, and nitric oxide. Administration of high concentrations of cytokines for therapeutic purposes (especially IFN-α) is associated with increased autoimmune thyroid disease, possibly through mechanisms similar to those in sporadic disease.

Antibodies to TPO and Tg are clinically useful markers of thyroid autoimmunity, but any pathogenic effect is restricted to a secondary role in amplifying an ongoing autoimmune response. TPO antibodies fix complement, and complement membrane-attack complexes are present in the thyroid in autoimmune hypothyroidism. However, transplacental passage of Tg or TPO antibodies has no effect on the fetal thyroid, which suggests that T cell–mediated injury is required to initiate autoimmune damage to the thyroid.

Up to 20% of patients with autoimmune hypothyroidism have antibodies against the TSH-R, which, in contrast to TSI, do not stimulate the receptor but prevent the binding of TSH. These TSH-R-blocking antibodies, therefore, cause hypothyroidism and, especially in Asian patients, thyroid atrophy. Their transplacental passage may induce transient neonatal hypothyroidism. Rarely, patients have a mixture of TSI and TSH-R-blocking antibodies, and thyroid function can oscillate between hyperthyroidism and hypothyroidism as one or the other antibody becomes dominant. Predicting the course of disease in such individuals is difficult, and they require close monitoring of thyroid function. Bioassays can be used to document that TSH-R-blocking antibodies reduce the cyclic AMP–inducing effect of TSH on cultured TSH-R-expressing cells, but these assays are difficult to perform. Thyrotropin-binding inhibitory immunoglobulin (TBII) assays that measure the binding of antibodies to the receptor by competition with radiolabeled TSH do not distinguish between TSI- and TSH-R-blocking antibodies, but a positive result in a patient with spontaneous hypothyroidism is strong evidence for the presence of blocking antibodies. The use of these assays does not generally alter clinical management, although it may be useful to confirm the cause of transient neonatal hypothyroidism.

Clinical Manifestations The main clinical features of hypothyroidism are summarized in Table 405-6. The onset is usually insidious, and the patient may become aware of symptoms only when euthyroidism is restored. Patients with Hashimoto's thyroiditis may present because of goiter rather than symptoms of hypothyroidism. The goiter may not be large, but it is usually irregular and firm in consistency. It is often possible to palpate a pyramidal lobe, normally a vestigial remnant of the thyroglossal duct. Rarely is uncomplicated Hashimoto's thyroiditis associated with pain.

Patients with atrophic thyroiditis or the late stage of Hashimoto's thyroiditis present with symptoms and signs of hypothyroidism. The skin is dry, and there is decreased sweating, thinning of the epidermis, and hyperkeratosis of the stratum corneum. Increased dermal glycosaminoglycan content traps water, giving rise to skin thickening without pitting (*myxedema*). Typical features include a puffy face with edematous eyelids and nonpitting pretibial edema (Fig. 405-6). There is pallor, often with a yellow tinge to the skin due to carotene accumulation. Nail growth is retarded, and hair is dry, brittle, difficult to manage, and falls out easily. In addition to diffuse alopecia, there is thinning of the outer third of the eyebrows, although this is not a specific sign of hypothyroidism.

Other common features include constipation and weight gain (despite a poor appetite). In contrast to popular perception, the weight gain is usually modest and due mainly to fluid retention in the myxedematous tissues. Libido is decreased in both sexes, and there may be oligomenorrhea or amenorrhea in long-standing disease, but menorrhagia is also common. Fertility is reduced, and the incidence of miscarriage is increased. Prolactin levels are often modestly increased (Chap. 403) and may contribute to alterations in libido and fertility and cause galactorrhea.

Myocardial contractility and pulse rate are reduced, leading to a reduced stroke volume and bradycardia. Increased peripheral resistance may be accompanied by hypertension, particularly diastolic. Blood flow is diverted from the skin, producing cool extremities. Pericardial effusions occur in up to 30% of patients but rarely compromise cardiac function. Although alterations in myosin heavy chain isoform expression have been documented, cardiomyopathy is unusual. Fluid may also accumulate in other serous cavities and in the middle ear, giving rise to conductive deafness. Pulmonary function is generally normal, but dyspnea may be caused by pleural effusion, impaired respiratory muscle function, diminished ventilatory drive, or sleep apnea.

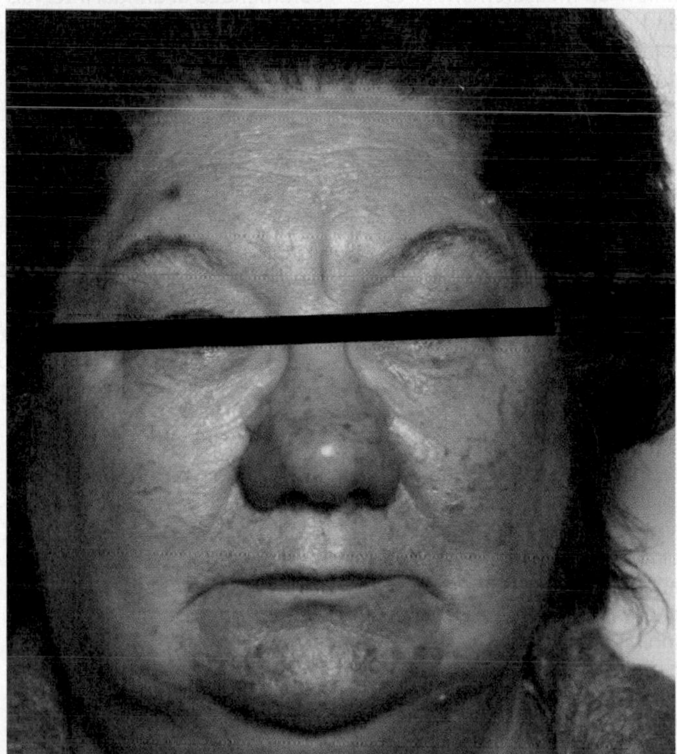

FIGURE 405-6 Facial appearance in hypothyroidism. Note puffy eyes and thickened skin.

Carpal tunnel and other entrapment syndromes are common, as is impairment of muscle function with stiffness, cramps, and pain. On examination, there may be slow relaxation of tendon reflexes and pseudomyotonia. Memory and concentration are impaired. Experimentally, positron emission tomography (PET) scans examining glucose metabolism in hypothyroid subjects show lower regional activity in the amygdala, hippocampus, and perigenual anterior cingulated cortex, among other regions, and this activity corrects after thyroxine replacement. Rare neurologic problems include reversible cerebellar ataxia, dementia, psychosis, and myxedema coma. *Hashimoto's encephalopathy* has been defined as a steroid-responsive syndrome associated with TPO antibodies, myoclonus, and slow-wave activity on electroencephalography, but the relationship with thyroid autoimmunity or hypothyroidism is not established. The hoarse voice and occasionally clumsy speech of hypothyroidism reflect fluid accumulation in the vocal cords and tongue.

The features described above are the consequence of thyroid hormone deficiency. However, autoimmune hypothyroidism may be associated with signs or symptoms of other autoimmune diseases, particularly vitiligo, pernicious anemia, Addison's disease, alopecia areata, and type 1 diabetes mellitus. Less common associations include celiac disease, dermatitis herpetiformis, chronic active hepatitis, rheumatoid arthritis, systemic lupus erythematosus (SLE), myasthenia gravis, and Sjögren's syndrome. Thyroid-associated ophthalmopathy, which usually occurs in Graves' disease (see below), occurs in about 5% of patients with autoimmune hypothyroidism.

Autoimmune hypothyroidism is uncommon in children and usually presents with slow growth and delayed facial maturation. The appearance of permanent teeth is also delayed. Myopathy, with muscle swelling, is more common in children than in adults. In most cases, puberty is delayed, but precocious puberty sometimes occurs. There may be intellectual impairment if the onset is before 3 years and the hormone deficiency is severe.

Laboratory Evaluation A summary of the investigations used to determine the existence and cause of hypothyroidism is provided in Fig. 405-7. A normal TSH level excludes primary (but not secondary) hypothyroidism. If the TSH is elevated, an unbound T_4 level is needed to confirm the presence of clinical hypothyroidism, but T_4 is inferior to TSH when used as a screening test, because it will not detect subclinical hypothyroidism. Circulating unbound T_3 levels are normal in about 25% of patients, reflecting adaptive deiodinase responses to hypothyroidism. T_3 measurements are, therefore, not indicated.

Once clinical or subclinical hypothyroidism is confirmed, the etiology is usually easily established by demonstrating the presence of TPO antibodies, which are present in >90% of patients with autoimmune hypothyroidism. TBII can be found in 10–20% of patients, but measurement is not needed routinely. If there is any doubt about the cause of a goiter associated with hypothyroidism, FNA biopsy can be used to confirm the presence of autoimmune thyroiditis. Other abnormal laboratory findings in hypothyroidism may include increased creatine phosphokinase, elevated cholesterol and triglycerides, and anemia (usually normocytic or macrocytic). Except when accompanied by iron deficiency, the anemia and other abnormalities gradually resolve with thyroxine replacement.

Differential Diagnosis An asymmetric goiter in Hashimoto's thyroiditis may be confused with a MNG or thyroid carcinoma, in which thyroid antibodies may also be present. Ultrasound can be used to show the presence of a solitary lesion or an MNG rather than the heterogeneous thyroid enlargement typical of Hashimoto's thyroiditis. FNA biopsy is useful in the investigation of focal nodules. Other causes of hypothyroidism are discussed below and in Table 405-5 but rarely cause diagnostic confusion.

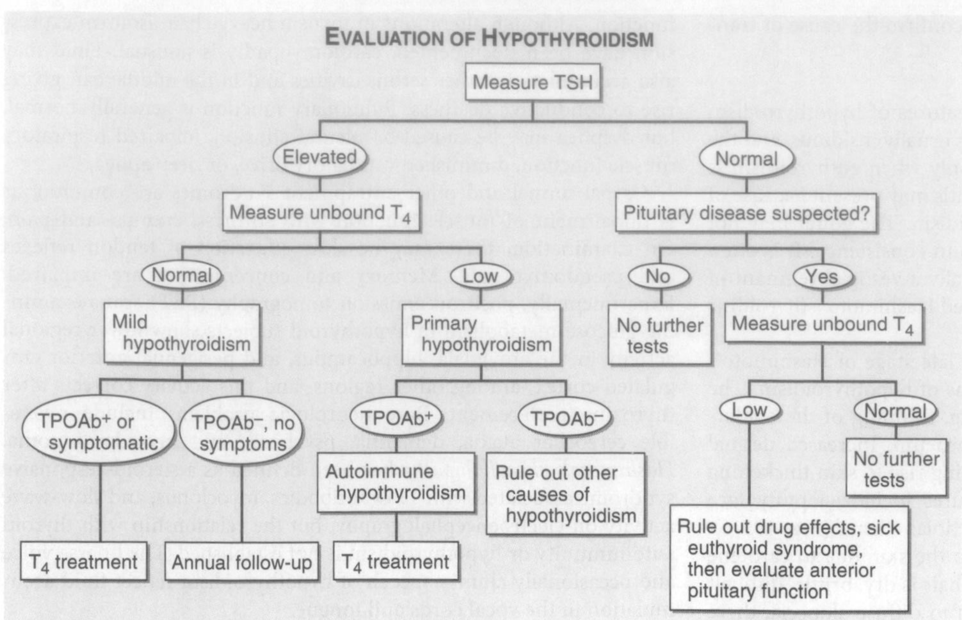

FIGURE 405-7 Evaluation of hypothyroidism. TPOAb+, thyroid peroxidase antibodies present; TPOAb−, thyroid peroxidase antibodies not present; TSH, thyroid-stimulating hormone.

OTHER CAUSES OF HYPOTHYROIDISM

Iatrogenic hypothyroidism is a common cause of hypothyroidism and can often be detected by screening before symptoms develop. In the first 3–4 months after radioiodine treatment, transient hypothyroidism may occur due to reversible radiation damage. Low-dose thyroxine treatment can be withdrawn if recovery occurs. Because TSH levels are suppressed by hyperthyroidism, unbound T_4 levels are a better measure of thyroid function than TSH in the months following radioiodine treatment. Mild hypothyroidism after subtotal thyroidectomy may also resolve after several months, as the gland remnant is stimulated by increased TSH levels.

Iodine deficiency is responsible for endemic goiter and cretinism but is an uncommon cause of adult hypothyroidism unless the iodine intake is very low or there are complicating factors, such as the consumption of thiocyanates in cassava or selenium deficiency. Although hypothyroidism due to iodine deficiency can be treated with thyroxine, public health measures to improve iodine intake should be advocated to eliminate this problem. Iodized salt or bread or a single bolus of oral or intramuscular iodized oil have all been used successfully.

Paradoxically, chronic iodine excess can also induce goiter and hypothyroidism. The intracellular events that account for this effect are unclear, but individuals with autoimmune thyroiditis are especially susceptible. Iodine excess is responsible for the hypothyroidism that occurs in up to 13% of patients treated with amiodarone (see below). Other drugs, particularly lithium, may also cause hypothyroidism. Transient hypothyroidism caused by thyroiditis is discussed below.

Secondary hypothyroidism is usually diagnosed in the context of other anterior pituitary hormone deficiencies; isolated TSH deficiency is very rare (Chap. 402). TSH levels may be low, normal, or even slightly increased in secondary hypothyroidism; the latter is due to secretion of immunoactive but bioinactive forms of TSH. The diagnosis is confirmed by detecting a low unbound T_4 level. The goal of treatment is to maintain T_4 levels in the upper half of the reference range, because TSH levels cannot be used to monitor therapy.

TREATMENT HYPOTHYROIDISM

CLINICAL HYPOTHYROIDISM

If there is no residual thyroid function, the daily replacement dose of levothyroxine is usually 1.6 μg/kg body weight (typically 100–150 μg), ideally taken at least 30 min before breakfast. In many patients, however, lower doses suffice until residual thyroid tissue is destroyed. In patients who develop hypothyroidism after the treatment of Graves' disease, there is often underlying autonomous function, necessitating lower replacement doses (typically 75–125 μg/d).

Adult patients under 60 years old without evidence of heart disease may be started on 50–100 μg levothyroxine (T_4) daily. The dose is adjusted on the basis of TSH levels, with the goal of treatment being a normal TSH, ideally in the lower half of the reference range. TSH responses are gradual and should be measured about 2 months after instituting treatment or after any subsequent change in levothyroxine dosage. The clinical effects of levothyroxine replacement are slow to appear. Patients may not experience full relief from symptoms until 3–6 months after normal TSH levels are restored. Adjustment of levothyroxine dosage is made in 12.5- or 25-μg increments if the TSH is high; decrements of the same magnitude should be made if the TSH is suppressed. Patients with a suppressed TSH of any cause, including T_4 overtreatment, have an increased risk of atrial fibrillation and reduced bone density.

Although desiccated animal thyroid preparations (thyroid extract USP) are available, they are not recommended because the ratio of T_3 to T_4 is nonphysiologic. The use of levothyroxine combined with liothyronine (triiodothyronine, T_3) has been investigated, but benefit has not been confirmed in prospective studies. There is no place for liothyronine alone as long-term replacement, because the short half-life necessitates three or four daily doses and is associated with fluctuating T_3 levels.

Once full replacement is achieved and TSH levels are stable, follow-up measurement of TSH is recommended at annual intervals and may be extended to every 2–3 years if a normal TSH is maintained over several years. It is important to ensure ongoing adherence, however, as patients do not feel any symptomatic difference after missing a few doses of levothyroxine, and this sometimes leads to self-discontinuation.

In patients of normal body weight who are taking ≥200 μg of levothyroxine per day, an elevated TSH level is often a sign of poor adherence to treatment. This is also the likely explanation for fluctuating TSH levels, despite a constant levothyroxine dosage. Such patients often have normal or high unbound T_4 levels, despite an elevated TSH, because they remember to take medication for a few days before testing; this is sufficient to normalize T_4, but not TSH levels. It is important to consider variable adherence, because this pattern of thyroid function tests is otherwise suggestive of disorders associated with inappropriate TSH secretion (Table 405-3). Because T_4 has a long half-life (7 days), patients who miss a dose can be advised to take two doses of the skipped tablets at once. Other causes of increased levothyroxine requirements must be excluded, particularly malabsorption (e.g., celiac disease, small-bowel surgery), estrogen or selective estrogen receptor modulator therapy, ingestion with a meal, and drugs that interfere with T_4 absorption or metabolism such as cholestyramine, ferrous sulfate, calcium supplements, proton pump inhibitors, lovastatin, aluminum hydroxide, rifampicin, amiodarone, carbamazepine, phenytoin, and tyrosine kinase inhibitors.

SUBCLINICAL HYPOTHYROIDISM

By definition, subclinical hypothyroidism refers to biochemical evidence of thyroid hormone deficiency in patients who have few or no apparent clinical features of hypothyroidism. There are no universally accepted recommendations for the management of subclinical hypothyroidism, but levothyroxine is recommended if the patient is a woman who wishes to conceive or is pregnant, or when TSH levels are above 10 mIU/L. When TSH levels are below 10 mIU/L, treatment should be considered when patients have suggestive symptoms of hypothyroidism, positive TPO antibodies, or any evidence of heart disease. It is important to confirm that any elevation of TSH is sustained over a 3-month period before treatment is given. As long as excessive treatment is avoided, there is no risk in correcting a slightly increased TSH. Treatment is administered by starting with a low dose of levothyroxine (25–50 μg/d) with the goal of normalizing TSH. If levothyroxine is not given, thyroid function should be evaluated annually.

SPECIAL TREATMENT CONSIDERATIONS

Rarely, levothyroxine replacement is associated with pseudotumor cerebri in children. Presentation appears to be idiosyncratic and occurs months after treatment has begun.

Women with a history or high risk of hypothyroidism should ensure that they are euthyroid prior to conception and during early pregnancy because maternal hypothyroidism may adversely affect fetal neural development and cause preterm delivery. The presence of thyroid autoantibodies alone, in a euthyroid patient, is also associated with miscarriage and preterm delivery; it is unclear if levothyroxine therapy improves outcomes. Thyroid function should be evaluated immediately after pregnancy is confirmed and every 4 weeks during the first half of the pregnancy, with less frequent testing after 20 weeks' gestation (every 6–8 weeks depending on whether levothyroxine dose adjustment is ongoing). The levothyroxine dose may need to be increased by up to 50% during pregnancy, with a goal TSH of less than 2.5 mIU/L during the first trimester and less than 3.0 mIU/L during the second and third trimesters. After delivery, thyroxine doses typically return to prepregnancy levels. Pregnant women should be counseled to separate ingestion of prenatal vitamins and iron supplements from levothyroxine by at least 4 h.

Elderly patients may require 20% less thyroxine than younger patients. In the elderly, especially patients with known coronary artery disease, the starting dose of levothyroxine is 12.5–25 μg/d with similar increments every 2–3 months until TSH is normalized. In some patients, it may be impossible to achieve full replacement despite optimal antianginal treatment. *Emergency surgery* is generally safe in patients with untreated hypothyroidism, although routine surgery in a hypothyroid patient should be deferred until euthyroidism is achieved.

Myxedema coma still has a 20–40% mortality rate, despite intensive treatment, and outcomes are independent of the T_4 and TSH levels. Clinical manifestations include reduced level of consciousness, sometimes associated with seizures, as well as the other features of hypothyroidism (Table 405-6). Hypothermia can reach 23°C (74°F). There may be a history of treated hypothyroidism with poor compliance, or the patient may be previously undiagnosed. Myxedema coma almost always occurs in the elderly and is usually precipitated by factors that impair respiration, such as drugs (especially sedatives, anesthetics, and antidepressants), pneumonia, congestive heart failure, myocardial infarction, gastrointestinal bleeding, or cerebrovascular accidents. Sepsis should also be suspected. Exposure to cold may also be a risk factor. Hypoventilation, leading to hypoxia and hypercapnia, plays a major role in pathogenesis; hypoglycemia and dilutional hyponatremia also contribute to the development of myxedema coma.

Levothyroxine can initially be administered as a single IV bolus of 500 μg, which serves as a loading dose. Although further levothyroxine is not strictly necessary for several days, it is usually continued at a dose of 50–100 μg/d. If suitable IV preparation is not available, the same initial dose of levothyroxine can be given by nasogastric tube (although absorption may be impaired in myxedema). An alternative is to give liothyronine (T_3) intravenously or via nasogastric tube, in doses ranging from 10 to 25 μg every 8–12 h. This treatment has been advocated because $T_4 \rightarrow T_3$ conversion is impaired in myxedema coma. However, excess liothyronine has the potential to provoke arrhythmias. Another option is to combine levothyroxine (200 μg) and liothyronine (25 μg) as a single, initial IV bolus followed by daily treatment with levothyroxine (50–100 μg/d) and liothyronine (10 μg every 8 h).

Supportive therapy should be provided to correct any associated metabolic disturbances. External warming is indicated only if the temperature is <30°C, as it can result in cardiovascular collapse (Chap. 478e). Space blankets should be used to prevent further heat loss. Parenteral hydrocortisone (50 mg every 6 h) should be administered, because there is impaired adrenal reserve in profound hypothyroidism. Any precipitating factors should be treated, including the early use of broad-spectrum antibiotics, pending the exclusion of infection. Ventilatory support with regular blood gas analysis is usually needed during the first 48 h. Hypertonic saline or IV glucose may be needed if there is severe hyponatremia or hypoglycemia; hypotonic IV fluids should be avoided because they may exacerbate water retention secondary to reduced renal perfusion and inappropriate vasopressin secretion. The metabolism of most medications is impaired, and sedatives should be avoided if possible or used in reduced doses. Medication blood levels should be monitored, when available, to guide dosage.

THYROTOXICOSIS

Thyrotoxicosis is defined as the state of thyroid hormone excess and is not synonymous with *hyperthyroidism*, which is the result of excessive thyroid function. However, the major etiologies of thyrotoxicosis are hyperthyroidism caused by Graves' disease, toxic MNG, and toxic adenomas. Other causes are listed in Table 405-7.

GRAVES' DISEASE

Epidemiology Graves' disease accounts for 60–80% of thyrotoxicosis. The prevalence varies among populations, reflecting genetic factors and iodine intake (high iodine intake is associated with an increased prevalence of Graves' disease). Graves' disease occurs in up to 2% of women but is one-tenth as frequent in men. The disorder rarely begins before adolescence and typically occurs between 20 and 50 years of age; it also occurs in the elderly.

TABLE 405-7 CAUSES OF THYROTOXICOSIS

Primary Hyperthyroidism
Graves' disease
Toxic multinodular goiter
Toxic adenoma
Functioning thyroid carcinoma metastases
Activating mutation of the TSH receptor
Activating mutation of $G_{s\alpha}$ (McCune-Albright syndrome)
Struma ovarii
Drugs: iodine excess (Jod-Basedow phenomenon)
Thyrotoxicosis Without Hyperthyroidism
Subacute thyroiditis
Silent thyroiditis
Other causes of thyroid destruction: amiodarone, radiation, infarction of adenoma
Ingestion of excess thyroid hormone (thyrotoxicosis factitia) or thyroid tissue
Secondary Hyperthyroidism
TSH-secreting pituitary adenoma
Thyroid hormone resistance syndrome: occasional patients may have features of thyrotoxicosis
Chorionic gonadotropin-secreting tumors[a]
Gestational thyrotoxicosis[a]

[a]Circulating TSH levels are low in these forms of secondary hyperthyroidism.

Abbreviations: TSH, thyroid-stimulating hormone.

Pathogenesis As in autoimmune hypothyroidism, a combination of environmental and genetic factors, including polymorphisms in HLA-DR, the immunoregulatory genes *CTLA-4*, *CD25*, *PTPN22*, *FCRL3*, and *CD226*, as well as the TSH-R, contribute to Graves' disease susceptibility. The concordance for Graves' disease in monozygotic twins is 20–30%, compared to <5% in dizygotic twins. Indirect evidence suggests that stress is an important environmental factor, presumably operating through neuroendocrine effects on the immune system. Smoking is a minor risk factor for Graves' disease and a major risk factor for the development of ophthalmopathy. Sudden increases in iodine intake may precipitate Graves' disease, and there is a threefold increase in the occurrence of Graves' disease in the postpartum period. Graves' disease may occur during the immune reconstitution phase after highly active antiretroviral therapy (HAART) or alemtuzumab treatment.

The hyperthyroidism of Graves' disease is caused by TSI that are synthesized in the thyroid gland as well as in bone marrow and lymph nodes. Such antibodies can be detected by bioassays or by using the more widely available TBII assays. The presence of TBII in a patient with thyrotoxicosis implies the existence of TSI, and these assays are useful in monitoring pregnant Graves' patients in whom high levels of TSI can cross the placenta and cause neonatal thyrotoxicosis. Other thyroid autoimmune responses, similar to those in autoimmune hypothyroidism (see above), occur concurrently in patients with Graves' disease. In particular, TPO antibodies occur in up to 80% of cases and serve as a readily measurable marker of autoimmunity. Because the coexisting thyroiditis can also affect thyroid function, there is no direct correlation between the level of TSI and thyroid hormone levels in Graves' disease. In the long term, spontaneous autoimmune hypothyroidism may develop in up to 15% of patients with Graves' disease.

Cytokines appear to play a major role in thyroid-associated ophthalmopathy. There is infiltration of the extraocular muscles by activated T cells; the release of cytokines such as IFN-γ, TNF, and IL-1 results in fibroblast activation and increased synthesis of glycosaminoglycans that trap water, thereby leading to characteristic muscle swelling. Late in the disease, there is irreversible fibrosis of the muscles. Orbital fibroblasts may be particularly sensitive to cytokines, perhaps explaining the anatomic localization of the immune response. Though the pathogenesis of thyroid-associated ophthalmopathy remains unclear, there is mounting evidence that the TSH-R may be a shared autoantigen that is expressed in the orbit; this would explain the close association with autoimmune thyroid disease. Increased fat is an additional cause of retrobulbar tissue expansion. The increase in intraorbital pressure can lead to proptosis, diplopia, and optic neuropathy.

Clinical Manifestations Signs and symptoms include features that are common to any cause of thyrotoxicosis (Table 405-8) as well as those specific for Graves' disease. The clinical presentation depends on the severity of thyrotoxicosis, the duration of disease, individual susceptibility to excess thyroid hormone, and the patient's age. In the elderly, features of thyrotoxicosis may be subtle or masked, and patients may present mainly with fatigue and weight loss, a condition known as *apathetic thyrotoxicosis*.

TABLE 405-8 SIGNS AND SYMPTOMS OF THYROTOXICOSIS (DESCENDING ORDER OF FREQUENCY)

Symptoms	Signs[a]
Hyperactivity, irritability, dysphoria	Tachycardia; atrial fibrillation in the elderly
Heat intolerance and sweating	Tremor
Palpitations	Goiter
Fatigue and weakness	Warm, moist skin
Weight loss with increased appetite	Muscle weakness, proximal myopathy
Diarrhea	Lid retraction or lag
Polyuria	Gynecomastia
Oligomenorrhea, loss of libido	

[a]Excludes the signs of ophthalmopathy and dermopathy specific for Graves' disease.

Thyrotoxicosis may cause unexplained weight loss, despite an enhanced appetite, due to the increased metabolic rate. Weight gain occurs in 5% of patients, however, because of increased food intake. Other prominent features include hyperactivity, nervousness, and irritability, ultimately leading to a sense of easy fatigability in some patients. Insomnia and impaired concentration are common; apathetic thyrotoxicosis may be mistaken for depression in the elderly. Fine tremor is a frequent finding, best elicited by having patients stretch out their fingers while feeling the fingertips with the palm. Common neurologic manifestations include hyperreflexia, muscle wasting, and proximal myopathy without fasciculation. Chorea is rare. Thyrotoxicosis is sometimes associated with a form of hypokalemic periodic paralysis; this disorder is particularly common in Asian males with thyrotoxicosis, but it occurs in other ethnic groups as well.

The most common cardiovascular manifestation is sinus tachycardia, often associated with palpitations, occasionally caused by supraventricular tachycardia. The high cardiac output produces a bounding pulse, widened pulse pressure, and an aortic systolic murmur and can lead to worsening of angina or heart failure in the elderly or those with preexisting heart disease. Atrial fibrillation is more common in patients >50 years of age. Treatment of the thyrotoxic state alone converts atrial fibrillation to normal sinus rhythm in about half of patients, suggesting the existence of an underlying cardiac problem in the remainder.

The skin is usually warm and moist, and the patient may complain of sweating and heat intolerance, particularly during warm weather. Palmar erythema, onycholysis, and, less commonly, pruritus, urticaria, and diffuse hyperpigmentation may be evident. Hair texture may become fine, and a diffuse alopecia occurs in up to 40% of patients, persisting for months after restoration of euthyroidism. Gastrointestinal transit time is decreased, leading to increased stool frequency, often with diarrhea and occasionally mild steatorrhea. Women frequently experience oligomenorrhea or amenorrhea; in men, there may be impaired sexual function and, rarely, gynecomastia. The direct effect of thyroid hormones on bone resorption leads to osteopenia in long-standing thyrotoxicosis; mild hypercalcemia occurs in up to 20% of patients, but hypercalciuria is more common. There is a small increase in fracture rate in patients with a previous history of thyrotoxicosis.

In Graves' disease, the thyroid is usually diffusely enlarged to two to three times its normal size. The consistency is firm, but not nodular. There may be a thrill or bruit, best detected at the inferolateral margins of the thyroid lobes, due to the increased vascularity of the gland and the hyperdynamic circulation.

Lid retraction, causing a staring appearance, can occur in any form of thyrotoxicosis and is the result of sympathetic overactivity. However, Graves' disease is associated with specific eye signs that comprise *Graves' ophthalmopathy* (Fig. 405-8A). This condition is also called *thyroid-associated ophthalmopathy*, because it occurs in the absence of hyperthyroidism in 10% of patients. Most of these individuals have autoimmune hypothyroidism or thyroid antibodies. The onset of Graves' ophthalmopathy occurs within the year before or after the diagnosis of thyrotoxicosis in 75% of patients but can sometimes precede or follow thyrotoxicosis by several years, accounting for some cases of euthyroid ophthalmopathy.

Some patients with Graves' disease have little clinical evidence of ophthalmopathy. However, the enlarged extraocular muscles typical of the disease, and other subtle features, can be detected in almost all patients when investigated by ultrasound or computed tomography (CT) imaging of the orbits. Unilateral signs are found in up to 10% of patients. The earliest manifestations of ophthalmopathy are usually a sensation of grittiness, eye discomfort, and excess tearing. About one-third of patients have proptosis, best detected by visualization of the sclera between the lower border of the iris and the lower eyelid, with the eyes in the primary position. Proptosis can be measured using an exophthalmometer. In severe cases, proptosis may cause corneal exposure and damage, especially if the lids fail to close during sleep. Periorbital edema, scleral injection, and chemosis are also frequent. In 5–10% of patients, the muscle swelling is so severe that diplopia results, typically, but not exclusively, when the patient looks up and laterally. The most serious manifestation is compression of the optic nerve at

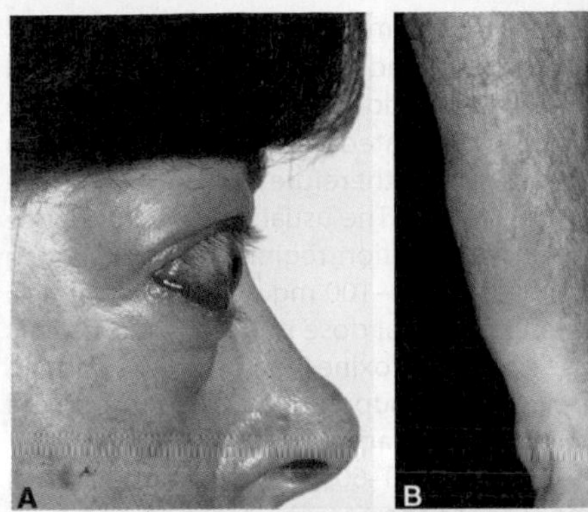

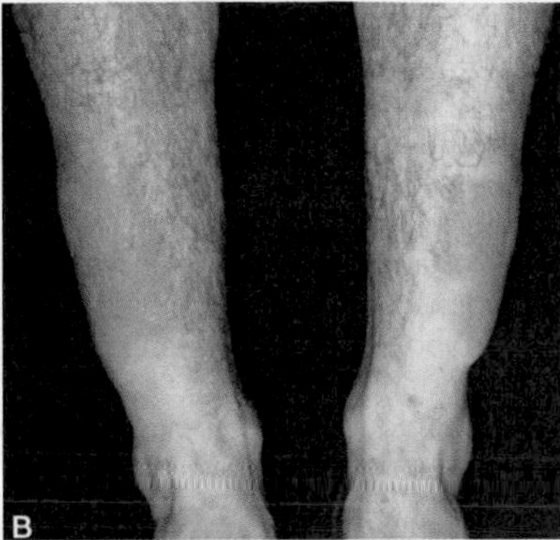

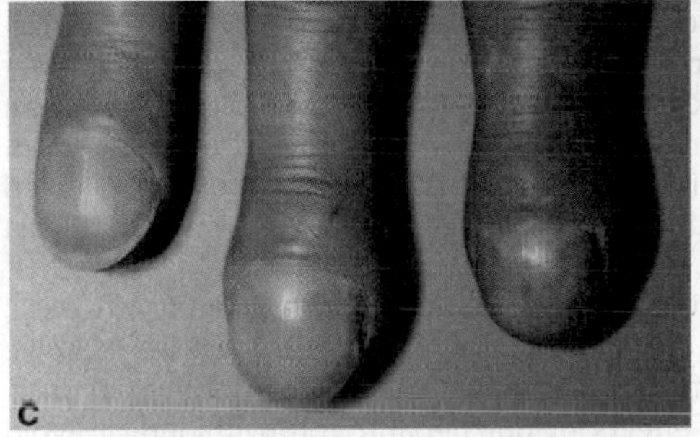

FIGURE 405-8 Features of Graves' disease. ***A.*** Ophthalmopathy in Graves' disease; lid retraction, periorbital edema, conjunctival injection, and proptosis are marked. ***B.*** Thyroid dermopathy over the lateral aspects of the shins. ***C.*** Thyroid acropachy.

the apex of the orbit, leading to papilledema; peripheral field defects; and, if left untreated, permanent loss of vision.

The "NO SPECS" scoring system to evaluate ophthalmopathy is an acronym derived from the following changes:

0 – **N**o signs or symptoms
1 = **O**nly signs (lid retraction or lag), no symptoms
2 – **S**oft tissue involvement (periorbital edema)
3 = **P**roptosis (>22 mm)
4 = **E**xtraocular muscle involvement (diplopia)
5 = **C**orneal involvement
6 = **S**ight loss

Although useful as a mnemonic, the NO SPECS scheme is inadequate to describe the eye disease fully, and patients do not necessarily progress from one class to another; alternative scoring systems that assess disease activity are preferable for monitoring purposes. When Graves' eye disease is active and severe, referral to an ophthalmologist is indicated and objective measurements are needed, such as lid-fissure width; corneal staining with fluorescein; and evaluation of extraocular muscle function (e.g., Hess chart), intraocular pressure and visual fields, acuity, and color vision.

Thyroid dermopathy occurs in <5% of patients with Graves' disease (Fig. 405-8*B*), almost always in the presence of moderate or severe ophthalmopathy. Although most frequent over the anterior and lateral aspects of the lower leg (hence the term *pretibial myxedema*), skin changes can occur at other sites, particularly after trauma. The typical lesion is a noninflamed, indurated plaque with a deep pink or purple color and an "orange skin" appearance. Nodular involvement can occur, and the condition can rarely extend over the whole lower leg and foot, mimicking elephantiasis. *Thyroid acropachy* refers to a form of clubbing found in <1% of patients with Graves' disease (Fig. 405-8*C*). It is so strongly associated with thyroid dermopathy that an alternative cause of clubbing should be sought in a Graves' patient without coincident skin and orbital involvement.

Laboratory Evaluation Investigations used to determine the existence and cause of thyrotoxicosis are summarized in Fig. 405-9. In Graves' disease, the TSH level is suppressed, and total and unbound thyroid hormone levels are increased. In 2–5% of patients (and more in areas of borderline iodine intake), only T_3 is increased (T_3 toxicosis). The converse state of T_4 toxicosis, with elevated total and unbound T_4 and normal T_3 levels, is occasionally seen when hyperthyroidism is induced by excess iodine, providing surplus substrate for thyroid hormone synthesis. Measurement of TPO antibodies or TRAb may be useful if the diagnosis is unclear clinically but is not needed routinely. Associated abnormalities that may cause diagnostic confusion in thyrotoxicosis include elevation of bilirubin, liver enzymes, and ferritin. Microcytic anemia and thrombocytopenia may occur.

Differential Diagnosis Diagnosis of Graves' disease is straightforward in a patient with biochemically confirmed thyrotoxicosis, diffuse goiter on palpation, ophthalmopathy, and often a personal or family history of autoimmune disorders. For patients with thyrotoxicosis who lack these features, the diagnosis is generally established by a radionuclide (^{99m}Tc, ^{123}I, or ^{131}I) scan and uptake of the thyroid, which will distinguish the diffuse, high uptake of Graves' disease from destructive thyroiditis, ectopic thyroid tissue, and factitious thyrotoxicosis. Scintigraphy is the preferred diagnostic test; however, TRAb measurement can be used to assess autoimmune activity. In secondary hyperthyroidism due to a

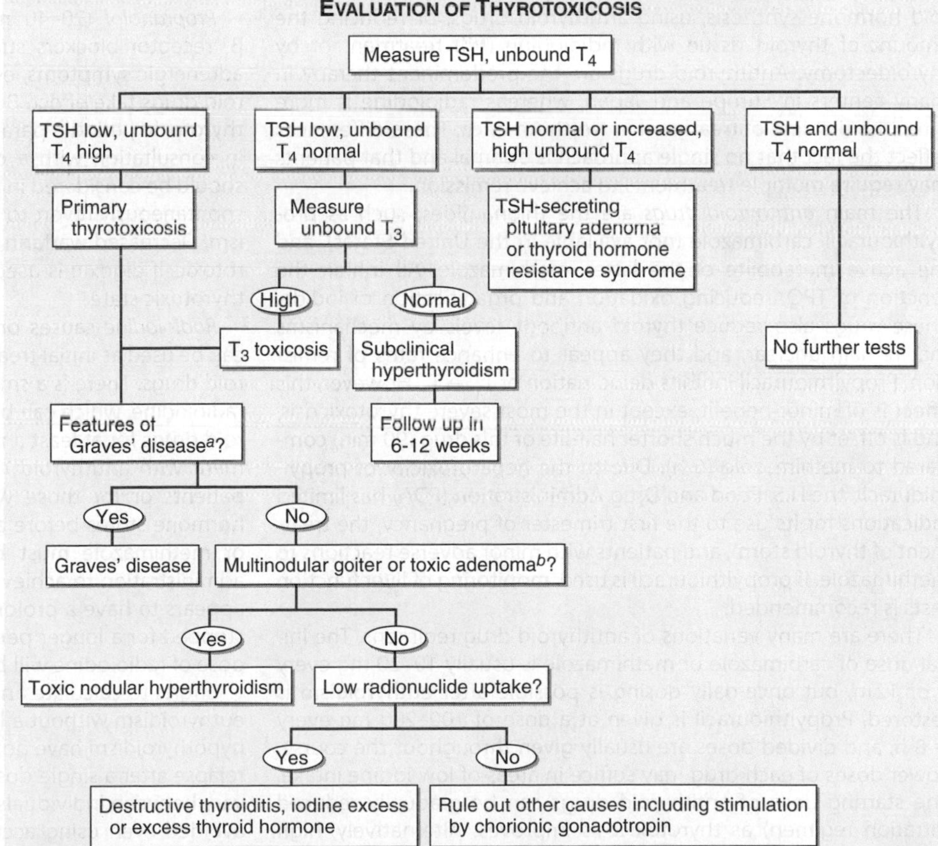

FIGURE 405-9 Evaluation of thyrotoxicosis. [a]Diffuse goiter, positive TPO antibodies or TRAb, ophthalmopathy, dermopathy. [b]Can be confirmed by radionuclide scan. TSH, thyroid-stimulating hormone.

TSH-secreting pituitary tumor, there is also a diffuse goiter. The presence of a nonsuppressed TSH level and the finding of a pituitary tumor on CT or magnetic resonance scan (MRI) scan suggest this diagnosis.

Clinical features of thyrotoxicosis can mimic certain aspects of other disorders, including panic attacks, mania, pheochromocytoma, and weight loss associated with malignancy. The diagnosis of thyrotoxicosis can be easily excluded if the TSH and unbound T_4 and T_3 levels are normal. A normal TSH also excludes Graves' disease as a cause of diffuse goiter.

Clinical Course Clinical features generally worsen without treatment; mortality was 10–30% before the introduction of satisfactory therapy. Some patients with mild Graves' disease experience spontaneous relapses and remissions. Rarely, there may be fluctuation between hypo- and hyperthyroidism due to changes in the functional activity of TSH-R antibodies. About 15% of patients who enter remission after treatment develop hypothyroidism 10–15 years later as a result of the destructive autoimmune process.

The clinical course of ophthalmopathy does not follow that of the thyroid disease. Ophthalmopathy typically worsens over the initial 3–6 months, followed by a plateau phase over the next 12–18 months, with spontaneous improvement, particularly in the soft tissue changes. However, the course is more fulminant in up to 5% of patients, requiring intervention in the acute phase if there is optic nerve compression or corneal ulceration. Diplopia may appear late in the disease due to fibrosis of the extraocular muscles. Radioiodine treatment for hyperthyroidism worsens the eye disease in a small proportion of patients (especially smokers). Antithyroid drugs or surgery have no adverse effects on the clinical course of ophthalmopathy. Thyroid dermopathy, when it occurs, usually appears 1–2 years after the development of Graves' hyperthyroidism; it may improve spontaneously.

TREATMENT GRAVES' DISEASE

The *hyperthyroidism* of Graves' disease is treated by reducing thyroid hormone synthesis, using antithyroid drugs, or reducing the amount of thyroid tissue with radioiodine (^{131}I) treatment or by thyroidectomy. Antithyroid drugs are the predominant therapy in many centers in Europe and Japan, whereas radioiodine is more often the first line of treatment in North America. These differences reflect the fact that no single approach is optimal and that patients may require multiple treatments to achieve remission.

The main *antithyroid drugs* are the thionamides, such as propylthiouracil, carbimazole (not available in the United States), and the active metabolite of the latter, methimazole. All inhibit the function of TPO, reducing oxidation and organification of iodide. These drugs also reduce thyroid antibody levels by mechanisms that remain unclear, and they appear to enhance rates of remission. Propylthiouracil inhibits deiodination of $T_4 \rightarrow T_3$. However, this effect is of minor benefit, except in the most severe thyrotoxicosis, and is offset by the much shorter half-life of this drug (90 min) compared to methimazole (6 h). Due to the hepatotoxicity of propylthiouracil, the U.S. Food and Drug Administration (FDA) has limited indications for its use to the first trimester of pregnancy, the treatment of thyroid storm, and patients with minor adverse reactions to methimazole. If propylthiouracil is used, monitoring of liver function tests is recommended.

There are many variations of antithyroid drug regimens. The initial dose of carbimazole or methimazole is usually 10–20 mg every 8 or 12 h, but once-daily dosing is possible after euthyroidism is restored. Propylthiouracil is given at a dose of 100–200 mg every 6–8 h, and divided doses are usually given throughout the course. Lower doses of each drug may suffice in areas of low iodine intake. The starting dose of antithyroid drugs can be gradually reduced (titration regimen) as thyrotoxicosis improves. Alternatively, high doses may be given combined with levothyroxine supplementation (block-replace regimen) to avoid drug-induced hypothyroidism. The titration regimen is preferred to minimize the dose of antithyroid drug and provide an index of treatment response.

Thyroid function tests and clinical manifestations are reviewed 4–6 weeks after starting treatment, and the dose is titrated based on unbound T_4 levels. Most patients do not achieve euthyroidism until 6–8 weeks after treatment is initiated. TSH levels often remain suppressed for several months and therefore do not provide a sensitive index of treatment response. The usual daily maintenance doses of antithyroid drugs in the titration regimen are 2.5–10 mg of carbimazole or methimazole and 50–100 mg of propylthiouracil. In the block-replace regimen, the initial dose of antithyroid drug is held constant, and the dose of levothyroxine is adjusted to maintain normal unbound T_4 levels. When TSH suppression is alleviated, TSH levels can also be used to monitor therapy.

Maximum remission rates (up to 30–60% in some populations) are achieved by 12–18 months for the titration regimen and by 6 months for the block-replace regimen. For unclear reasons, remission rates appear to vary in different geographic regions. Younger patients, males, smokers, and patients with severe hyperthyroidism and large goiters are most likely to relapse when treatment stops, but outcomes are difficult to predict. All patients should be followed closely for relapse during the first year after treatment and at least annually thereafter.

The common minor side effects of antithyroid drugs are rash, urticaria, fever, and arthralgia (1–5% of patients). These may resolve spontaneously or after substituting an alternative antithyroid drug. Rare but major side effects include hepatitis (propylthiouracil; avoid use in children) and cholestasis (methimazole and carbimazole); an SLE-like syndrome; and, most important, agranulocytosis (<1%). It is essential that antithyroid drugs are stopped and not restarted if a patient develops major side effects. Written instructions should be provided regarding the symptoms of possible agranulocytosis (e.g., sore throat, fever, mouth ulcers) and the need to stop treatment pending an urgent complete blood count to confirm that agranulocytosis is not present. Management of agranulocytosis is described in Chap. 130. It is not useful to monitor blood counts prospectively, because the onset of agranulocytosis is idiosyncratic and abrupt.

Propranolol (20–40 mg every 6 h) or longer-acting selective β_1 receptor blockers such as atenolol may be helpful to control adrenergic symptoms, especially in the early stages before antithyroid drugs take effect. Beta blockers are also useful in patients with thyrotoxic periodic paralysis, pending correction of thyrotoxicosis. In consultation with a cardiologist, anticoagulation with warfarin should be considered in all patients with atrial fibrillation who often spontaneously revert to sinus rhythm with control of hyperthyroidism. Decreased warfarin doses are required when patients are thyrotoxic. If digoxin is used, increased doses are often needed in the thyrotoxic state.

Radioiodine causes progressive destruction of thyroid cells and can be used as initial treatment or for relapses after a trial of antithyroid drugs. There is a small risk of thyrotoxic crisis (see below) after radioiodine, which can be minimized by pretreatment with antithyroid drugs for at least a month before treatment. Antecedent treatment with antithyroid drugs should be considered for all elderly patients or for those with cardiac problems to deplete thyroid hormone stores before administration of radioiodine. Carbimazole or methimazole must be stopped 3–5 days before radioiodine administration to achieve optimum iodine uptake. Propylthiouracil appears to have a prolonged radioprotective effect and should be stopped for a longer period before radioiodine is given, or a larger dose of radioiodine will be necessary.

Efforts to calculate an optimal dose of radioiodine that achieves euthyroidism without a high incidence of relapse or progression to hypothyroidism have not been successful. Some patients inevitably relapse after a single dose because the biologic effects of radiation vary between individuals, and hypothyroidism cannot be uniformly avoided even using accurate dosimetry. A practical strategy is to give a fixed dose based on clinical features, such as the severity of thyrotoxicosis, the size of the goiter (increases the dose needed), and the level of radioiodine uptake (decreases the dose needed). ^{131}I dosage generally ranges between 370 MBq (10 mCi) and 555 MBq

(15 mCi). Most authorities favor an approach aimed at thyroid ablation (as opposed to euthyroidism), given that levothyroxine replacement is straightforward and most patients ultimately progress to hypothyroidism over 5–10 years, frequently with some delay in the diagnosis of hypothyroidism.

Certain radiation safety precautions are necessary in the first few days after radioiodine treatment, but the exact guidelines vary depending on local protocols. In general, patients need to avoid close, prolonged contact with children and pregnant women for 5–7 days because of possible transmission of residual isotope and exposure to radiation emanating from the gland. Rarely, there may be mild pain due to radiation thyroiditis 1–2 weeks after treatment. Hyperthyroidism can persist for 2–3 months before radioiodine takes full effect. For this reason, β-adrenergic blockers or antithyroid drugs can be used to control symptoms during this interval. Persistent hyperthyroidism can be treated with a second dose of radioiodine, usually 6 months after the first dose. The risk of hypothyroidism after radioiodine depends on the dosage but is at least 10–20% in the first year and 5% per year thereafter. Patients should be informed of this possibility before treatment and require close follow-up during the first year followed by annual thyroid function testing.

Pregnancy and breast-feeding are absolute contraindications to radioiodine treatment, but patients can conceive safely 6 months after treatment. The presence of severe ophthalmopathy requires caution, and some authorities advocate the use of prednisone, 40 mg/d, at the time of radioiodine treatment, tapered over 6–12 weeks to prevent exacerbation of ophthalmopathy. The overall risk of cancer after radioiodine treatment in adults is not increased. Although many physicians avoid radioiodine in children and adolescents because of the theoretical risks of malignancy, emerging evidence suggests that radioiodine can be used safely in older children.

Subtotal or near-total thyroidectomy is an option for patients who relapse after antithyroid drugs and prefer this treatment to radioiodine. Some experts recommend surgery in young individuals, particularly when the goiter is very large. Careful control of thyrotoxicosis with antithyroid drugs, followed by potassium iodide (3 drops SSKI orally tid), is needed prior to surgery to avoid thyrotoxic crisis and to reduce the vascularity of the gland. The major complications of surgery—bleeding, laryngeal edema, hypoparathyroidism, and damage to the recurrent laryngeal nerves—are unusual when the procedure is performed by highly experienced surgeons. Recurrence rates in the best series are <2%, but the rate of hypothyroidism is only slightly less than that following radioiodine treatment.

The titration regimen of antithyroid drugs should be used to manage Graves' disease in *pregnancy* because transplacental passage of these drugs may produce fetal hypothyroidism and goiter if the maternal dose is excessive. If available, propylthiouracil should be used in early gestation because of the association of rare cases of fetal *aplasia cutis* and other defects, such as choanal atresia with carbimazole and methimazole. As noted above, because of its rare association with hepatotoxicity, propylthiouracil should be limited to the first trimester and then maternal therapy should be converted to methimazole (or carbimazole) at a ratio of 15–20 mg of propylthiouracil to 1 mg of methimazole The lowest effective antithyroid drug dose should be used throughout gestation to maintain the maternal serum free T_4 level at the upper limit of the nonpregnant normal reference range. It is often possible to stop treatment in the last trimester because TSIs tend to decline in pregnancy. Nonetheless, the transplacental transfer of these antibodies rarely causes *fetal* or *neonatal thyrotoxicosis*. Poor intrauterine growth, a fetal heart rate of >160 beats/min, and high levels of maternal TSI in the last trimester may herald this complication. Antithyroid drugs given to the mother can be used to treat the fetus and may be needed for 1–3 months after delivery, until the maternal antibodies disappear from the baby's circulation. The postpartum period is a time of major risk for relapse of Graves' disease. Breast-feeding is safe with low doses of antithyroid drugs. Graves' disease in *children* is usually managed with methimazole or carbimazole (avoid propylthiouracil), often given as a prolonged course of the titration regimen. Surgery or radioiodine may be indicated for severe disease.

Thyrotoxic crisis, or *thyroid storm*, is rare and presents as a life-threatening exacerbation of hyperthyroidism, accompanied by fever, delirium, seizures, coma, vomiting, diarrhea, and jaundice. The mortality rate due to cardiac failure, arrhythmia, or hyperthermia is as high as 30%, even with treatment. Thyrotoxic crisis is usually precipitated by acute illness (e.g., stroke, infection, trauma, diabetic ketoacidosis), surgery (especially on the thyroid), or radioiodine treatment of a patient with partially treated or untreated hyperthyroidism. Management requires intensive monitoring and supportive care, identification and treatment of the precipitating cause, and measures that reduce thyroid hormone synthesis. Large doses of propylthiouracil (500–1000 mg loading dose and 250 mg every 4 h) should be given orally or by nasogastric tube or per rectum; the drug's inhibitory action on $T_4 \rightarrow T_3$ conversion makes it the antithyroid drug of choice. If not available, methimazole can be used in doses up to 30 mg every 12 h. One hour after the first dose of propylthiouracil, stable iodide is given to block thyroid hormone synthesis via the Wolff-Chaikoff effect (the delay allows the antithyroid drug to prevent the excess iodine from being incorporated into new hormone). A saturated solution of potassium iodide (5 drops SSKI every 6 h) or, where available, ipodate or iopanoic acid (500 mg per 12 h) may be given orally. Sodium iodide, 0.25 g IV every 6 h, is an alternative but is not generally available. Propranolol should also be given to reduce tachycardia and other adrenergic manifestations (60–80 mg PO every 4 h; or 2 mg IV every 4 h). Although other β-adrenergic blockers can be used, high doses of propranolol decrease $T_4 \rightarrow T_3$ conversion, and the doses can be easily adjusted. Caution is needed to avoid acute negative inotropic effects, but controlling the heart rate is important, as some patients develop a form of high-output heart failure. Short-acting IV esmolol can be used to decrease heart rate while monitoring for signs of heart failure. Additional therapeutic measures include glucocorticoids (e.g., hydrocortisone 300 mg IV bolus, then 100 mg every 8 h), antibiotics if infection is present, cooling, oxygen, and IV fluids.

Ophthalmopathy requires no active treatment when it is mild or moderate, because there is usually spontaneous improvement. General measures include meticulous control of thyroid hormone levels, cessation of smoking, and an explanation of the natural history of ophthalmopathy. Discomfort can be relieved with artificial tears (e.g., 1% methylcellulose), eye ointment, and the use of dark glasses with side frames. Periorbital edema may respond to a more upright sleeping position or a diuretic. Corneal exposure during sleep can be avoided by using patches or taping the eyelids shut. Minor degrees of diplopia improve with prisms fitted to spectacles. Severe ophthalmopathy, with optic nerve involvement or chemosis resulting in corneal damage, is an emergency requiring joint management with an ophthalmologist. Pulse therapy with IV methylprednisolone (e.g., 500 mg of methylprednisolone once weekly for 6 weeks, then 250 mg once weekly for 6 weeks) is preferable to oral glucocorticoids, which are used for moderately active disease. When glucocorticoids are ineffective, orbital decompression can be achieved by removing bone from any wall of the orbit, thereby allowing displacement of fat and swollen extraocular muscles. The transantral route is used most often because it requires no external incision. Proptosis recedes an average of 5 mm, but there may be residual or even worsened diplopia. Once the eye disease has stabilized, surgery may be indicated for relief of diplopia and correction of the appearance. External beam radiotherapy of the orbits has been used for many years, but the efficacy of this therapy remains unclear, and it is best reserved for those with moderately active disease who have failed or are not candidates for glucocorticoid therapy. Other immunosuppressive agents such as rituximab have shown some benefit, but their role is yet to be established.

Thyroid dermopathy does not usually require treatment, but it can cause cosmetic problems or interfere with the fit of shoes. Surgical removal is not indicated. If necessary, treatment consists of topical, high-potency glucocorticoid ointment under an occlusive dressing. Octreotide may be beneficial in some cases.

OTHER CAUSES OF THYROTOXICOSIS

Destructive thyroiditis (subacute or silent thyroiditis) typically presents with a short thyrotoxic phase due to the release of preformed thyroid hormones and catabolism of Tg (see "Subacute Thyroiditis," below). True hyperthyroidism is absent, as demonstrated by a low radionuclide uptake. Circulating Tg levels are usually increased. Other causes of thyrotoxicosis with low or absent thyroid radionuclide uptake include *thyrotoxicosis factitia*, iodine excess, and, rarely, ectopic thyroid tissue, particularly teratomas of the ovary (*struma ovarii*) and functional metastatic follicular carcinoma. Whole-body radionuclide studies can demonstrate ectopic thyroid tissue, and thyrotoxicosis factitia can be distinguished from destructive thyroiditis by the clinical features and low levels of Tg. Amiodarone treatment is associated with thyrotoxicosis in up to 10% of patients, particularly in areas of low iodine intake (see below).

TSH-secreting pituitary adenoma is a rare cause of thyrotoxicosis. It is characterized by the presence of an inappropriately normal or increased TSH level in a patient with hyperthyroidism, diffuse goiter, and elevated T_4 and T_3 levels (**Chap. 403**). Elevated levels of the α-subunit of TSH, released by the TSH-secreting adenoma, support this diagnosis, which can be confirmed by demonstrating the pituitary tumor on MRI or CT scan. A combination of transsphenoidal surgery, sella irradiation, and octreotide may be required to normalize TSH, because many of these tumors are large and locally invasive at the time of diagnosis. Radioiodine or antithyroid drugs can be used to control thyrotoxicosis.

Thyrotoxicosis caused by *toxic MNG* and *hyperfunctioning solitary nodules* is discussed below.

THYROIDITIS

A clinically useful classification of thyroiditis is based on the onset and duration of disease (**Table 405-9**).

ACUTE THYROIDITIS

Acute thyroiditis is rare and due to suppurative infection of the thyroid. In children and young adults, the most common cause is the presence of a piriform sinus, a remnant of the fourth branchial pouch that connects the oropharynx with the thyroid. Such sinuses are predominantly left-sided. A long-standing goiter and degeneration in a thyroid malignancy are risk factors in the elderly. The patient presents with thyroid pain, often referred to the throat or ears, and a small, tender goiter that may be asymmetric. Fever, dysphagia, and erythema over the thyroid are common, as are systemic symptoms of a febrile illness and lymphadenopathy.

TABLE 405-9 CAUSES OF THYROIDITIS

Acute
Bacterial infection: especially *Staphylococcus, Streptococcus,* and *Enterobacter*
Fungal infection: *Aspergillus, Candida, Coccidioides, Histoplasma,* and *Pneumocystis*
Radiation thyroiditis after ^{131}I treatment
Amiodarone (may also be subacute or chronic)
Subacute
Viral (or granulomatous) thyroiditis
Silent thyroiditis (including postpartum thyroiditis)
Mycobacterial infection
Drug induced (interferon, amiodarone)
Chronic
Autoimmunity: focal thyroiditis, Hashimoto's thyroiditis, atrophic thyroiditis
Riedel's thyroiditis
Parasitic thyroiditis: echinococcosis, strongyloidiasis, cysticercosis
Traumatic: after palpation

The differential diagnosis of *thyroid pain* includes subacute or, rarely, chronic thyroiditis; hemorrhage into a cyst; malignancy including lymphoma; and, rarely, amiodarone-induced thyroiditis or amyloidosis. However, the abrupt presentation and clinical features of acute thyroiditis rarely cause confusion. The erythrocyte sedimentation rate (ESR) and white cell count are usually increased, but thyroid function is normal. FNA biopsy shows infiltration by polymorphonuclear leukocytes; culture of the sample can identify the organism. Caution is needed in immunocompromised patients as fungal, mycobacterial, or *Pneumocystis* thyroiditis can occur in this setting. Antibiotic treatment is guided initially by Gram stain and, subsequently, by cultures of the FNA biopsy. Surgery may be needed to drain an abscess, which can be localized by CT scan or ultrasound. Tracheal obstruction, septicemia, retropharyngeal abscess, mediastinitis, and jugular venous thrombosis may complicate acute thyroiditis but are uncommon with prompt use of antibiotics.

SUBACUTE THYROIDITIS

This is also termed *de Quervain's thyroiditis, granulomatous thyroiditis,* or *viral thyroiditis.* Many viruses have been implicated, including mumps, coxsackie, influenza, adenoviruses, and echoviruses, but attempts to identify the virus in an individual patient are often unsuccessful and do not influence management. The diagnosis of subacute thyroiditis is often overlooked because the symptoms can mimic pharyngitis. The peak incidence occurs at 30–50 years, and women are affected three times more frequently than men.

Pathophysiology The thyroid shows a characteristic patchy inflammatory infiltrate with disruption of the thyroid follicles and multinucleated giant cells within some follicles. The follicular changes progress to granulomas accompanied by fibrosis. Finally, the thyroid returns to normal, usually several months after onset. During the initial phase of follicular destruction, there is release of Tg and thyroid hormones, leading to increased circulating T_4 and T_3 and suppression of TSH (**Fig. 405-10**). During this destructive phase, radioactive iodine uptake is low or undetectable. After several weeks, the thyroid is depleted of stored thyroid hormone and a phase of hypothyroidism typically occurs, with low unbound T_4 (and sometimes T_3) and moderately increased TSH levels. Radioactive iodine uptake returns to normal or is even increased as a result of the rise in TSH. Finally, thyroid hormone and TSH levels return to normal as the disease subsides.

Clinical Manifestations The patient usually presents with a painful and enlarged thyroid, sometimes accompanied by fever. There may be

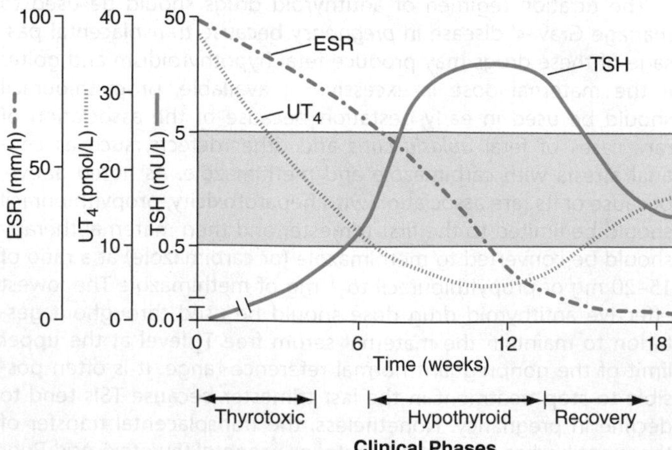

FIGURE 405-10 Clinical course of subacute thyroiditis. The release of thyroid hormones is initially associated with a thyrotoxic phase and suppressed thyroid-stimulating hormone (TSH). A hypothyroid phase then ensues, with low T_4 and TSH levels that are initially low but gradually increase. During the recovery phase, increased TSH levels combined with resolution of thyroid follicular injury lead to normalization of thyroid function, often several months after the beginning of the illness. ESR, erythrocyte sedimentation rate; UT_4, free or unbound T_4.

features of thyrotoxicosis or hypothyroidism, depending on the phase of the illness. Malaise and symptoms of an upper respiratory tract infection may precede the thyroid-related features by several weeks. In other patients, the onset is acute, severe, and without obvious antecedent. The patient typically complains of a sore throat, and examination reveals a small goiter that is exquisitely tender. Pain is often referred to the jaw or ear. Complete resolution is the usual outcome, but late-onset permanent hypothyroidism occurs in 15% of cases, particularly in those with coincidental thyroid autoimmunity. A prolonged course over many months, with one or more relapses, occurs in a small percentage of patients.

Laboratory Evaluation As depicted in Fig. 405-10, thyroid function tests characteristically evolve through three distinct phases over about 6 months: (1) thyrotoxic phase, (2) hypothyroid phase, and (3) recovery phase. In the thyrotoxic phase, T_4 and T_3 levels are increased, reflecting their discharge from the damaged thyroid cells, and TSH is suppressed. The T_4/T_3 ratio is greater than in Graves' disease or thyroid autonomy, in which T_3 is often disproportionately increased. The diagnosis is confirmed by a high ESR and low uptake of radioiodine (<5%) or ^{99m}Tc pertechnetate (as compared to salivary gland pertechnetate concentration). The white blood cell count may be increased, and thyroid antibodies are negative. If the diagnosis is in doubt, FNA biopsy may be useful, particularly to distinguish unilateral involvement from bleeding into a cyst or neoplasm.

TREATMENT SUBACUTE THYROIDITIS

Relatively large doses of aspirin (e.g., 600 mg every 4–6 h) or NSAIDs are sufficient to control symptoms in many cases. If this treatment is inadequate, or if the patient has marked local or systemic symptoms, glucocorticoids should be given. The usual starting dose is 40–60 mg of prednisone, depending on severity. The dose is gradually tapered over 6–8 weeks, in response to improvement in symptoms and the ESR. If a relapse occurs during glucocorticoid withdrawal, treatment should be started again and withdrawn more gradually. In these patients, it is useful to wait until the radioactive iodine uptake normalizes before stopping treatment. Thyroid function should be monitored every 2–4 weeks using TSH and unbound T_4 levels. Symptoms of thyrotoxicosis improve spontaneously but may be ameliorated by β-adrenergic blockers; antithyroid drugs play no role in treatment of the thyrotoxic phase. Levothyroxine replacement may be needed if the hypothyroid phase is prolonged, but doses should be low enough (50–100 μg daily) to allow TSH-mediated recovery.

SILENT THYROIDITIS

Painless thyroiditis, or *"silent" thyroiditis*, occurs in patients with underlying autoimmune thyroid disease and has a clinical course similar to that of subacute thyroiditis. The condition occurs in up to 5% of women 3–6 months after pregnancy and is then termed *postpartum thyroiditis*. Typically, patients have a brief phase of thyrotoxicosis lasting 2–4 weeks, followed by hypothyroidism for 4–12 weeks, and then resolution; often, however, only one phase is apparent. The condition is associated with the presence of TPO antibodies antepartum, and it is three times more common in women with type 1 diabetes mellitus. As in subacute thyroiditis, the uptake of ^{99m}Tc pertechnetate or radioactive iodine is initially suppressed. In addition to the painless goiter, silent thyroiditis can be distinguished from subacute thyroiditis by a normal ESR and the presence of TPO antibodies. Glucocorticoid treatment is not indicated for silent thyroiditis. Severe thyrotoxic symptoms can be managed with a brief course of propranolol, 20–40 mg three or four times daily. Thyroxine replacement may be needed for the hypothyroid phase but should be withdrawn after 6–9 months, as recovery is the rule. Annual follow-up thereafter is recommended, because a proportion of these individuals develop permanent hypothyroidism. The condition may recur in subsequent pregnancies.

DRUG-INDUCED THYROIDITIS

Patients receiving cytokines such as IFN-α or IL-2 may develop painless thyroiditis. IFN-α, which is used to treat chronic hepatitis B or C and hematologic and skin malignancies, causes thyroid dysfunction in up to 5% of treated patients. It has been associated with painless thyroiditis, hypothyroidism, and Graves' disease, and is most common in women with TPO antibodies prior to treatment. For discussion of amiodarone, see "Amiodarone Effects on Thyroid Function," below.

CHRONIC THYROIDITIS

Focal thyroiditis is present in 20–40% of euthyroid autopsy cases and is associated with serologic evidence of autoimmunity, particularly the presence of TPO antibodies. The most common clinically apparent cause of chronic thyroiditis is *Hashimoto's thyroiditis*, an autoimmune disorder that often presents as a firm or hard goiter of variable size (see above). *Riedel's thyroiditis* is a rare disorder that typically occurs in middle-aged women. It presents with an insidious, painless goiter with local symptoms due to compression of the esophagus, trachea, neck veins, or recurrent laryngeal nerves. Dense fibrosis disrupts normal gland architecture and can extend outside the thyroid capsule. Despite these extensive histologic changes, thyroid dysfunction is uncommon. The goiter is hard, nontender, often asymmetric, and fixed, leading to suspicion of a malignancy. Diagnosis requires open biopsy as FNA biopsy is usually inadequate. Treatment is directed to surgical relief of compressive symptoms. Tamoxifen may also be beneficial. There is an association between Riedel's thyroiditis and IgG4-related systemic disease causing idiopathic fibrosis at other sites (retroperitoneum, mediastinum, biliary tree, lung, and orbit).

SICK EUTHYROID SYNDROME (NONTHYROIDAL ILLNESS)

Any acute, severe illness can cause abnormalities of circulating TSH or thyroid hormone levels in the absence of underlying thyroid disease, making these measurements potentially misleading. The major cause of these hormonal changes is the release of cytokines such as IL-6. Unless a thyroid disorder is strongly suspected, the routine testing of thyroid function should be avoided in acutely ill patients.

The most common hormone pattern in sick euthyroid syndrome (SES) is a decrease in total and unbound T_3 levels (low T_3 syndrome) with normal levels of T_4 and TSH. The magnitude of the fall in T_3 correlates with the severity of the illness. T_4 conversion to T_3 via peripheral 5′ (outer ring) deiodination is impaired, leading to increased reverse T_3 (rT_3). Since rT_3 is metabolized by 5′ deiodination, its clearance is also reduced. Thus, decreased clearance rather than increased production is the major basis for increased rT_3. Also, T_4 is alternately metabolized to the hormonally inactive T_3 sulfate. It is generally assumed that this low T_3 state is adaptive, because it can be induced in normal individuals by fasting. Teleologically, the fall in T_3 may limit catabolism in starved or ill patients.

Very sick patients may exhibit a dramatic fall in total T_4 and T_3 levels (low T_4 syndrome). With decreased tissue perfusion, muscle and liver expression of the type 3 deiodinase leads to accelerated T_4 and T_3 metabolism. This state has a poor prognosis. Another key factor in the fall in T_4 levels is altered binding to TBG. The commonly used free T_4 assays are subject to artifact when serum binding proteins are low and underestimate the true free T_4 level. Fluctuation in TSH levels also creates challenges in the interpretation of thyroid function in sick patients. TSH levels may range from <0.1 mIU/L in very ill patients, especially with dopamine or glucocorticoid therapy, to >20 mIU/L during the recovery phase of SES. The exact mechanisms underlying the subnormal TSH seen in 10% of sick patients and the increased TSH seen in 5% remain unclear but may be mediated by cytokines including IL-12 and IL-18.

Any severe illness can induce changes in thyroid hormone levels, but certain disorders exhibit a distinctive pattern of abnormalities. Acute liver disease is associated with an initial rise in total (but not unbound) T_3 and T_4 levels due to TBG release; these levels become subnormal with progression to liver failure. A transient increase in total and unbound T_4 levels, usually with a normal T_3 level, is seen in 5–30% of acutely ill psychiatric patients. TSH values may be transiently low, normal, or high in these patients. In the early stage of HIV infection, T_3 and T_4 levels rise, even if there is weight loss. T_3 levels fall with progression to AIDS, but TSH usually remains normal. Renal disease is often accompanied by low T_3 concentrations, but with normal rather than increased rT_3 levels, due to an unknown factor that increases uptake of rT_3 into the liver.

The diagnosis of SES is challenging. Historic information may be limited, and patients often have multiple metabolic derangements. Useful features to consider include previous history of thyroid disease and thyroid function tests, evaluation of the severity and time course of the patient's acute illness, documentation of medications that may affect thyroid function or thyroid hormone levels, and measurements of rT_3 together with unbound thyroid hormones and TSH. The diagnosis of SES is frequently presumptive, given the clinical context and pattern of laboratory values; only resolution of the test results with clinical recovery can clearly establish this disorder. Treatment of SES with thyroid hormone (T_4 and/or T_3) is controversial, but most authorities recommend monitoring the patient's thyroid function tests during recovery, without administering thyroid hormone, unless there is historic or clinical evidence suggestive of hypothyroidism. Sufficiently large randomized controlled trials using thyroid hormone are unlikely to resolve this therapeutic controversy in the near future, because clinical presentations and outcomes are highly variable.

AMIODARONE EFFECTS ON THYROID FUNCTION

Amiodarone is a commonly used type III antiarrhythmic agent (Chap. 277). It is structurally related to thyroid hormone and contains 39% iodine by weight. Thus, typical doses of amiodarone (200 mg/d) are associated with very high iodine intake, leading to greater than forty-fold increases in plasma and urinary iodine levels. Moreover, because amiodarone is stored in adipose tissue, high iodine levels persist for >6 months after discontinuation of the drug. Amiodarone inhibits deiodinase activity, and its metabolites function as weak antagonists of thyroid hormone action. Amiodarone has the following effects on thyroid function: (1) acute, transient suppression of thyroid function; (2) hypothyroidism in patients susceptible to the inhibitory effects of a high iodine load; and (3) thyrotoxicosis that may be caused by either a Jod-Basedow effect from the iodine load, in the setting of MNG or incipient Graves' disease, or a thyroiditis-like condition.

The initiation of amiodarone treatment is associated with a transient decrease of T_4 levels, reflecting the inhibitory effect of iodine on T_4 release. Soon thereafter, most individuals escape from iodide-dependent suppression of the thyroid (Wolff-Chaikoff effect), and the inhibitory effects on deiodinase activity and thyroid hormone receptor action become predominant. These events lead to the following pattern of thyroid function tests: increased T_4, decreased T_3, increased rT_3, and a transient TSH increase (up to 20 mIU/L). TSH levels normalize or are slightly suppressed within 1–3 months.

The incidence of hypothyroidism from amiodarone varies geographically, apparently correlating with iodine intake. Hypothyroidism occurs in up to 13% of amiodarone-treated patients in iodine-replete countries, such as the United States, but is less common (<6% incidence) in areas of lower iodine intake, such as Italy or Spain. The pathogenesis appears to involve an inability of the thyroid gland to escape from the Wolff-Chaikoff effect in autoimmune thyroiditis. Consequently, amiodarone-associated hypothyroidism is more common in women and individuals with positive TPO antibodies. It is usually unnecessary to discontinue amiodarone for this side effect, because levothyroxine can be used to normalize thyroid function. TSH levels should be monitored, because T_4 levels are often increased for the reasons described above.

The management of amiodarone-induced thyrotoxicosis (AIT) is complicated by the fact that there are different causes of thyrotoxicosis and because the increased thyroid hormone levels exacerbate underlying arrhythmias and coronary artery disease. Amiodarone treatment causes thyrotoxicosis in 10% of patients living in areas of low iodine intake and in 2% of patients in regions of high iodine intake. There are two major forms of AIT, although some patients have features of both. Type 1 AIT is associated with an underlying thyroid abnormality (preclinical Graves' disease or nodular goiter). Thyroid hormone synthesis becomes excessive as a result of increased iodine exposure (Jod-Basedow phenomenon). Type 2 AIT occurs in individuals with no intrinsic thyroid abnormalities and is the result of drug-induced lysosomal activation leading to destructive thyroiditis with histiocyte accumulation in the thyroid; the incidence rises as cumulative amiodarone dosage increases. Mild forms of type 2 AIT can resolve spontaneously or can occasionally lead to hypothyroidism. Color-flow Doppler thyroid scanning shows increased vascularity in type 1 AIT but decreased vascularity in type 2 AIT. Thyroid scintiscans are difficult to interpret in this setting because the high endogenous iodine levels diminish tracer uptake. However, the presence of normal or rarely increased uptake favors type 1 AIT.

In AIT, the drug should be stopped, if possible, although this is often impractical because of the underlying cardiac disorder. Discontinuation of amiodarone will not have an acute effect because of its storage and prolonged half-life. High doses of antithyroid drugs can be used in type 1 AIT but are often ineffective. In type 2 AIT, oral contrast agents, such as sodium ipodate (500 mg/d) or sodium tyropanoate (500 mg, 1–2 doses/d), rapidly reduce T_4 and T_3 levels, decrease $T_4 \rightarrow T_3$ conversion, and may block tissue uptake of thyroid hormones. Potassium perchlorate, 200 mg every 6 h, has been used to reduce thyroidal iodide content. Perchlorate treatment has been associated with agranulocytosis, although the risk appears relatively low with short-term use. Glucocorticoids, as administered for subacute thyroiditis, have modest benefit in type 2 AIT. Lithium blocks thyroid hormone release and can also provide some benefit. Near-total thyroidectomy rapidly decreases thyroid hormone levels and may be the most effective long-term solution if the patient can undergo the procedure safely.

THYROID FUNCTION IN PREGNANCY

Five factors alter thyroid function in pregnancy: (1) the transient increase in hCG during the first trimester, which stimulates the TSH-R; (2) the estrogen-induced rise in TBG during the first trimester, which is sustained during pregnancy; (3) alterations in the immune system, leading to the onset, exacerbation, or amelioration of an underlying autoimmune thyroid disease (see above); (4) increased thyroid hormone metabolism by the placenta; and (5) increased urinary iodide excretion, which can cause impaired thyroid hormone production in areas of marginal iodine sufficiency. Women with a precarious iodine intake (<50 μg/d) are most at risk of developing a goiter during pregnancy or giving birth to an infant with a goiter and hypothyroidism. The World Health Organization recommends a daily iodine intake of 250 μg during pregnancy and prenatal vitamins should contain 150 μg per tablet.

The rise in circulating hCG levels during the first trimester is accompanied by a reciprocal fall in TSH that persists into the middle of pregnancy. This reflects the weak binding of hCG, which is present at very high levels, to the TSH-R. Rare individuals have been described with variant TSH-R sequences that enhance hCG binding and TSH-R activation. hCG-induced changes in thyroid function can result in transient gestational hyperthyroidism that may be associated with *hyperemesis gravidarum*, a condition characterized by severe nausea and vomiting and risk of volume depletion. However, since the hyperthyroidism is not causal, antithyroid drugs are not indicated unless concomitant Graves' disease is suspected. Parenteral fluid replacement usually suffices until the condition resolves.

During pregnancy, subclinical hypothyroidism occurs in 2% of women, but overt hypothyroidism is present in only 1 in 500. Prospective randomized controlled trials have not shown a benefit for universal thyroid disease screening in pregnancy. Targeted TSH testing for hypothyroidism is recommended for women planning a pregnancy if they have a strong family history of autoimmune thyroid disease, other autoimmune disorders (e.g., type 1 diabetes), prior preterm delivery or recurrent miscarriage, or signs or symptoms of thyroid disease. Thyroid hormone requirements are increased by up to 50% during pregnancy in levothyroxine-treated hypothyroid women (see above section on treatment of hypothyroidism).

GOITER AND NODULAR THYROID DISEASE

Goiter refers to an enlarged thyroid gland. Biosynthetic defects, iodine deficiency, autoimmune disease, and nodular diseases can each lead to goiter, although by different mechanisms. Biosynthetic defects and iodine deficiency are associated with reduced efficiency of thyroid hormone synthesis, leading to increased TSH, which stimulates thyroid growth as a compensatory mechanism to overcome the block in hormone synthesis. Graves' disease and Hashimoto's thyroiditis are also associated with goiter. In Graves' disease, the goiter results mainly from the TSH-R–mediated effects of TSI. The goitrous form of Hashimoto's thyroiditis occurs because of acquired defects in hormone synthesis, leading to elevated levels of TSH and its consequent growth effects. Lymphocytic infiltration and immune system–induced growth factors also contribute to thyroid enlargement in Hashimoto's thyroiditis. Nodular disease is characterized by the disordered growth of thyroid cells, often combined with the gradual development of fibrosis. Because the management of goiter depends on the etiology, the detection of thyroid enlargement on physical examination should prompt further evaluation to identify its cause.

Nodular thyroid disease is common, occurring in about 3–7% of adults when assessed by physical examination. Using ultrasound, nodules are present in up to 50% of adults, with the majority being <1 cm in diameter. Thyroid nodules may be solitary or multiple, and they may be functional or nonfunctional.

DIFFUSE NONTOXIC (SIMPLE) GOITER

Etiology and Pathogenesis When diffuse enlargement of the thyroid occurs in the absence of nodules and hyperthyroidism, it is referred to as a *diffuse nontoxic goiter*. This is sometimes called *simple goiter*, because of the absence of nodules, or *colloid goiter*, because of the presence of uniform follicles that are filled with colloid. Worldwide, diffuse goiter is most commonly caused by iodine deficiency and is termed *endemic goiter* when it affects >5% of the population. In nonendemic regions, *sporadic goiter* occurs, and the cause is usually unknown. Thyroid enlargement in teenagers is sometimes referred to as *juvenile goiter*. In general, goiter is more common in women than men, probably because of the greater prevalence of underlying autoimmune disease and the increased iodine demands associated with pregnancy.

In *iodine-deficient areas*, thyroid enlargement reflects a compensatory effort to trap iodide and produce sufficient hormone under conditions in which hormone synthesis is relatively inefficient. Somewhat surprisingly, TSH levels are usually normal or only slightly increased, suggesting increased sensitivity to TSH or activation of other pathways that lead to thyroid growth. Iodide appears to have direct actions on thyroid vasculature and may indirectly affect growth through vasoactive substances such as endothelins and nitric oxide. Endemic goiter is also caused by exposure to environmental *goitrogens* such as cassava root, which contains a thiocyanate; vegetables of the Cruciferae family (known as cruciferous vegetables) (e.g., Brussels sprouts, cabbage, and cauliflower); and milk from regions where goitrogens are present in grass. Although relatively rare, inherited defects in thyroid hormone synthesis lead to a diffuse nontoxic goiter. Abnormalities at each step in hormone synthesis, including iodide transport (NIS), Tg synthesis, organification and coupling (TPO), and the regeneration of iodide (dehalogenase), have been described.

CLINICAL MANIFESTATIONS AND DIAGNOSIS

If thyroid function is preserved, most goiters are asymptomatic. Examination of a diffuse goiter reveals a symmetrically enlarged, nontender, generally soft gland without palpable nodules. Goiter is defined, somewhat arbitrarily, as a lateral lobe with a volume greater than the thumb of the individual being examined. If the thyroid is markedly enlarged, it can cause tracheal or esophageal compression. These features are unusual, however, in the absence of nodular disease and fibrosis. *Substernal goiter* may obstruct the thoracic inlet. *Pemberton's sign* refers to symptoms of faintness with evidence of facial congestion and external jugular venous obstruction when the arms are raised above the head, a maneuver that draws the thyroid into the thoracic inlet. Respiratory flow measurements and CT or MRI should be used to evaluate substernal goiter in patients with obstructive signs or symptoms.

Thyroid function tests should be performed in all patients with goiter to exclude thyrotoxicosis or hypothyroidism. It is not unusual, particularly in iodine deficiency, to find a low total T_4, with normal T_3 and TSH, reflecting enhanced $T_4 \rightarrow T_3$ conversion. A low TSH with a normal free T_3 and free T_4, particularly in older patients, suggests the possibility of thyroid autonomy or undiagnosed Graves' disease, and is termed *subclinical thyrotoxicosis*. The benefit of treatment (typically with radioiodine) in subclinical thyrotoxicosis, versus follow-up and implementing treatment if free T_3 or free T_4 levels become abnormal, is unclear, but treatment is increasingly recommended in the elderly to reduce the risk of atrial fibrillation and bone loss. TPO antibodies may be useful to identify patients at increased risk of autoimmune thyroid disease. Low urinary iodine levels (<50 μg/L) support a diagnosis of iodine deficiency. Thyroid scanning is not generally necessary but will reveal increased uptake in iodine deficiency and most cases of dyshormonogenesis. Ultrasound is not generally indicated in the evaluation of diffuse goiter unless a nodule is palpable on physical examination.

TREATMENT DIFFUSE NONTOXIC (SIMPLE) GOITER

Iodine replacement induces variable regression of goiter in iodine deficiency, depending on how long it has been present and the degree of fibrosis that has developed. Surgery is rarely indicated for diffuse goiter. Exceptions include documented evidence of tracheal compression or obstruction of the thoracic inlet, which are more likely to be associated with substernal MNGs (see below). Subtotal or near-total thyroidectomy for these or cosmetic reasons should be performed by an experienced surgeon to minimize complication rates. Surgery should be followed by replacement with levothyroxine, with the aim of keeping the TSH level at the lower end of the reference range to prevent regrowth of the goiter.

NONTOXIC MULTINODULAR GOITER

Etiology and Pathogenesis Depending on the population studied, MNG or nodular enlargement of the thyroid occurs in up to 12% of adults. MNG is more common in women than men and increases in prevalence with age. It is more common in iodine-deficient regions but also occurs in regions of iodine sufficiency, reflecting multiple genetic, autoimmune, and environmental influences on the pathogenesis.

There is typically wide variation in nodule size. Histology reveals a spectrum of morphologies ranging from hypercellular regions to cystic areas filled with colloid. Fibrosis is often extensive, and areas of hemorrhage or lymphocytic infiltration may be seen. Using molecular techniques, most nodules within an MNG are polyclonal in origin, suggesting a hyperplastic response to locally produced growth factors and cytokines. TSH, which is usually not elevated, may play a permissive or contributory role. Monoclonal lesions also occur within an MNG, reflecting mutations in genes that confer a selective growth advantage to the progenitor cell.

Clinical Manifestations Most patients with nontoxic MNG are asymptomatic and euthyroid. MNG typically develops over many years and is detected on routine physical examination, when an individual notices an enlargement in the neck, or as an incidental finding on imaging. If the goiter is large enough, it can ultimately lead to compressive symptoms including difficulty swallowing, respiratory distress (tracheal compression), or plethora (venous congestion), but these symptoms are uncommon. Symptomatic MNGs are usually extraordinarily large and/or develop fibrotic areas that cause compression. Sudden pain in an MNG is usually caused by hemorrhage into a nodule but should raise the possibility of invasive malignancy. Hoarseness, reflecting laryngeal nerve involvement, also suggests malignancy.

Diagnosis On examination, thyroid architecture is distorted, and multiple nodules of varying size can be appreciated. Because many nodules are deeply embedded in thyroid tissue or reside in posterior or substernal locations, it is not possible to palpate all nodules. Pemberton's sign, characterized by facial suffusion when the patient's arms are elevated above the head, suggests that the goiter has increased pressure in the thoracic inlet. A TSH level should be measured to exclude subclinical hyper- or hypothyroidism, but thyroid function is usually normal. Tracheal deviation is common, but compression must usually exceed 70% of the tracheal diameter before there is significant airway compromise. Pulmonary function testing can be used to assess the functional effects of compression, which characteristically causes inspiratory stridor. CT or MRI can be used to evaluate the anatomy of the goiter and the extent of substernal extension or tracheal narrowing. A barium swallow may reveal the extent of esophageal compression. The risk of malignancy in MNG is similar to that in solitary nodules. Ultrasonography can be used to identify which nodules should be biopsied based on sonographic features (see section above on ultrasound) and size. For nodules with more suspicious imaging characteristics (e.g., hypoechogenicity, microcalcifications, irregular margins), biopsy is recommended when ≥1 cm.

TREATMENT NONTOXIC MULTINODULAR GOITER

Most nontoxic MNGs can be managed conservatively. T_4 suppression is rarely effective for reducing goiter size and introduces the risk of subclinical or overt thyrotoxicosis, particularly if there is underlying autonomy or if it develops during treatment. If levothyroxine is used, it should be started at low doses (50 μg daily) and advanced gradually while monitoring the TSH level to avoid excessive suppression. Contrast agents and other iodine-containing substances should be avoided because of the risk of inducing the *Jod-Basedow effect*, characterized by enhanced thyroid hormone production by autonomous nodules. Radioiodine is used with increasing frequency in areas where large goiters are more prevalent because it can decrease goiter size and may selectively ablate regions of autonomy. Dosage of ^{131}I depends on the size of the goiter and radioiodine uptake but is usually about 3.7 MBq (0.1 mCi) per gram of tissue, corrected for uptake (typical dose 370–1070 MBq [10 to 29 mCi]). Repeat treatment may be needed and effectiveness may be increased by concurrent administration of low-dose recombinant TSH (0.1 mg IM). It is possible to achieve a 40–50% reduction in goiter size in most patients. Earlier concerns about radiation-induced thyroid swelling and tracheal compression have diminished, as studies have shown this complication to be rare. When acute compression occurs, glucocorticoid treatment or surgery may be needed. Radiation-induced hypothyroidism is less common than after treatment for Graves' disease. However, posttreatment autoimmune thyrotoxicosis may occur in up to 5% of patients treated for nontoxic MNG. Surgery remains highly effective but is not without risk, particularly in older patients with underlying cardiopulmonary disease.

TOXIC MULTINODULAR GOITER

The pathogenesis of toxic MNG appears to be similar to that of nontoxic MNG; the major difference is the presence of functional autonomy in toxic MNG. The molecular basis for autonomy in toxic MNG remains unknown. As in nontoxic goiters, many nodules are polyclonal, whereas others are monoclonal and vary in their clonal origins. Genetic abnormalities known to confer functional autonomy, such as activating TSH-R or $G_s\alpha$ mutations (see below), are not usually found in the autonomous regions of toxic MNG goiter.

In addition to features of goiter, the clinical presentation of toxic MNG includes subclinical hyperthyroidism or mild thyrotoxicosis. The patient is usually elderly and may present with atrial fibrillation or palpitations, tachycardia, nervousness, tremor, or weight loss. Recent exposure to iodine, from contrast dyes or other sources, may precipitate or exacerbate thyrotoxicosis. The TSH level is low. The uncombined T_4 level may be normal or minimally increased; T_3 is often elevated to a greater degree than T_4. Thyroid scan shows heterogeneous uptake with multiple regions of increased and decreased uptake; 24-h uptake of radioiodine may not be increased but is usually in the upper normal range.

Prior to definitive treatment of the hyperthyroidism, ultrasound imaging should be performed to assess the presence of discrete nodules corresponding to areas of decreased uptake ("cold" nodules). If present, FNA may be indicated based on sonographic features and size cutoffs. The cytology results, if indeterminate or suspicious, may direct the therapy to surgery.

TREATMENT TOXIC MULTINODULAR GOITER

Antithyroid drugs normalize thyroid function and are particularly useful in the elderly or ill patients with limited lifespan. In contrast to Graves' disease, spontaneous remission does not occur and so treatment is long-term. Radioiodine is generally the treatment of choice; it treats areas of autonomy as well as decreasing the mass of the goiter. Sometimes, however, a degree of autonomy remains, presumably because multiple autonomous regions emerge as soon as others are treated, and further radioiodine treatment may be necessary. Surgery provides definitive treatment of underlying thyrotoxicosis as well as goiter. Patients should be rendered euthyroid using an antithyroid drug before operation.

HYPERFUNCTIONING SOLITARY NODULE

A solitary, autonomously functioning thyroid nodule is referred to as *toxic adenoma*. The pathogenesis of this disorder has been unraveled by demonstrating the functional effects of mutations that stimulate the TSH-R signaling pathway. Most patients with solitary hyperfunctioning nodules have acquired somatic, activating mutations in the TSH-R (Fig. 405-11). These mutations, located primarily in the receptor transmembrane domain, induce constitutive receptor coupling to $G_{S\alpha}$, increasing cyclic AMP levels and leading to enhanced thyroid follicular cell proliferation and function. Less commonly, somatic mutations are identified in $G_{S\alpha}$. These mutations, which are similar to those seen in

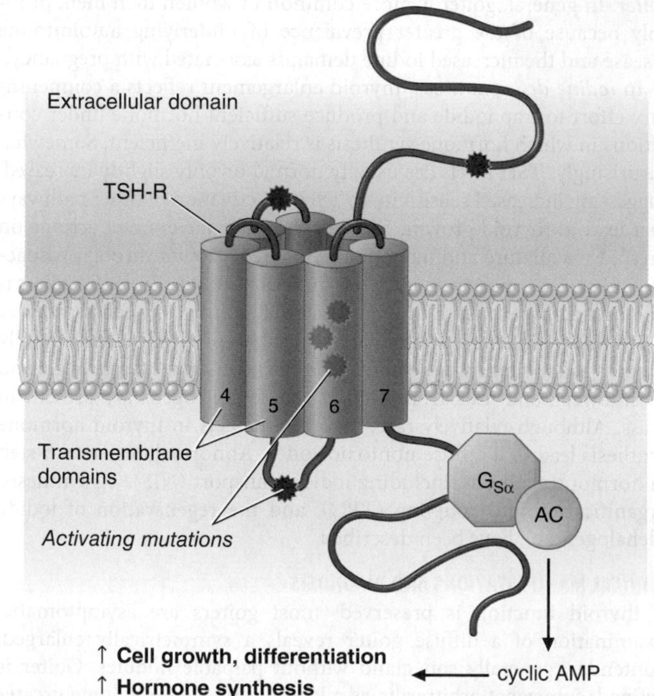

FIGURE 405-11 Activating mutations of the thyroid-stimulating hormone receptor (TSH-R). Mutations (*) that activate TSH-R reside mainly in transmembrane 5 and intracellular loop 3, although mutations have occurred in a variety of different locations. The effect of these mutations is to induce conformational changes that mimic TSH binding, thereby leading to coupling to stimulatory G protein ($G_{S\alpha}$) and activation of adenylate cyclase (AC), an enzyme that generates cyclic AMP.

McCune-Albright syndrome (Chap. 412) or in a subset of somatotrope adenomas (Chap. 403), impair guanosine triphosphate (GTP) hydrolysis, causing constitutive activation of the cyclic AMP signaling pathway. In most series, activating mutations in either the TSH-R or the $G_{s\alpha}$ subunit genes are identified in >90% of patients with solitary hyperfunctioning nodules.

Thyrotoxicosis is usually mild. The disorder is suggested by a subnormal TSH level; the presence of the thyroid nodule, which is generally large enough to be palpable; and the absence of clinical features suggestive of Graves' disease or other causes of thyrotoxicosis. A thyroid scan provides a definitive diagnostic test, demonstrating focal uptake in the hyperfunctioning nodule and diminished uptake in the remainder of the gland, as activity of the normal thyroid is suppressed.

TREATMENT HYPERFUNCTIONING SOLITARY NODULE

Radioiodine ablation is usually the treatment of choice. Because normal thyroid function is suppressed, ^{131}I is concentrated in the hyperfunctioning nodule with minimal uptake and damage to normal thyroid tissue. Relatively large radioiodine doses (e.g., 370–1110 MBq [10–29.9 mCi] ^{131}I) have been shown to correct thyrotoxicosis in about 75% of patients within 3 months. Hypothyroidism occurs in <10% of those patients over the next 5 years. Surgical resection is also effective and is usually limited to enucleation of the adenoma or lobectomy, thereby preserving thyroid function and minimizing risk of hypoparathyroidism or damage to the recurrent laryngeal nerves. Medical therapy using antithyroid drugs and beta blockers can normalize thyroid function but is not an optimal long-term treatment. Using ultrasound guidance, repeated ethanol injections and percutaneous radiofrequency thermal ablation have been used successfully in some centers to ablate hyperfunctioning nodules, and these techniques have also been used to reduce the size of nonfunctioning thyroid nodules.

BENIGN NEOPLASMS

The various types of benign thyroid nodules are listed in Table 405-10. These lesions are common (5–10% adults), particularly when assessed by sensitive techniques such as ultrasound. The risk of malignancy is very low for *macrofollicular adenomas* and *normofollicular adenomas. Microfollicular, trabecular, and Hürthle cell variants* raise greater concern, and the histology is more difficult to interpret. Many are mixed cystic/solid lesions on ultrasound and may appear spongiform reflecting the pathology of macrofollicular structure. However, the majority of solid nodules (whether hypo-, iso-, or hyperechoic) are also benign. FNA, usually performed with ultrasound guidance, is the diagnostic procedure of choice to evaluate thyroid nodules (see the "Approach to the Patient" section on thyroid nodules). Pure thyroid cysts, <2% of all thyroid growths, consist of colloid and are benign as well. Cysts frequently recur, even after repeated aspiration, and may require surgical excision if they are large. Ethanol ablation to sclerose the cyst has been used successfully for patients who are symptomatic.

TSH suppression with levothyroxine therapy does not decrease thyroid nodule size in iodine-sufficient populations. However, if there is relative iodine deficiency, both iodine and levothyroxine therapy may decrease nodule volume. If levothyroxine is administered in this situation and the nodule has not decreased in size after 6–12 months of suppressive therapy, treatment should be discontinued because little benefit is likely to accrue from long-term treatment; the risk of iatrogenic subclinical thyrotoxicosis should also be considered.

THYROID CANCER

Thyroid carcinoma is the most common malignancy of the endocrine system. Malignant tumors derived from the follicular epithelium are classified according to histologic features. Differentiated tumors, such as papillary thyroid cancer (PTC) or follicular thyroid cancer (FTC), are often curable, and the prognosis is good for patients identified with early-stage disease. In contrast, anaplastic thyroid cancer (ATC) is aggressive, responds poorly to treatment, and is associated with a bleak prognosis.

The incidence of thyroid cancer is ~12/100,000 per year in the United States and increases with age. Prognosis is worse in older persons (>65 years). Thyroid cancer is twice as common in women as men, but male gender is associated with a worse prognosis. Additional important risk factors include a history of childhood head or neck irradiation, large nodule size (≥4 cm), evidence for local tumor fixation or invasion into lymph nodes, and the presence of metastases (Table 405-11). Several unique features of thyroid cancer facilitate its management: (1) thyroid nodules are amenable to biopsy by FNA; (2) iodine radioisotopes can be used to diagnose (^{123}I) and treat (^{131}I) differentiated thyroid cancer, reflecting the unique uptake of this anion by the thyroid gland; and (3) serum markers allow the detection of

TABLE 405-10 CLASSIFICATION OF THYROID NEOPLASMS

Benign	
Follicular epithelial cell adenomas	
Macrofollicular (colloid)	
Normofollicular (simple)	
Microfollicular (fetal)	
Trabecular (embryonal)	
Hürthle cell variant (oncocytic)	
Malignant	**Approximate Prevalence, %**
Follicular epithelial cell	
Well-differentiated carcinomas	
Papillary carcinomas	80–90
Pure papillary	
Follicular variant	
Diffuse sclerosing variant	
Tall cell, columnar cell variants	
Follicular carcinomas	5–10
Minimally invasive	
Widely invasive	
Hürthle cell carcinoma (oncocytic)	
Insular carcinoma	
Undifferentiated (anaplastic) carcinomas	
C cell (calcitonin-producing)	
Medullary thyroid cancer	<10
Sporadic	
Familial	
MEN 2	
Other malignancies	
Lymphomas	1–2
Sarcomas	
Metastases	
Others	

Abbreviation: MEN, multiple endocrine neoplasia.

TABLE 405-11 RISK FACTORS FOR THYROID CARCINOMA IN PATIENTS WITH THYROID NODULE

History of head and neck irradiation, including total-body irradiation for bone marrow transplant and brain radiation for childhood leukemia	Family history of thyroid cancer, MEN 2, or other genetic syndromes associated with thyroid malignancy (e.g., Cowden's syndrome, familial polyposis, Carney complex)
Exposure to ionizing radiation from fallout in childhood or adolescence	Vocal cord paralysis, hoarse voice
Age <20 or >65 years	Nodule fixed to adjacent structures
Increased nodule size (>4 cm)	Extrathyroidal extension
New or enlarging neck mass	Lateral cervical lymphadenopathy
Male gender	

Abbreviation: MEN, multiple endocrine neoplasia.

residual or recurrent disease, including the use of Tg levels for PTC and FTC, and calcitonin for medullary thyroid cancer (MTC).

CLASSIFICATION

Thyroid neoplasms can arise in each of the cell types that populate the gland, including thyroid follicular cells, calcitonin-producing C cells, lymphocytes, and stromal and vascular elements, as well as metastases from other sites (Table 405-10). The American Joint Committee on Cancer (AJCC) has designated a staging system using the tumor, node, metastasis (TNM) classification (Table 405-12). Several other classification and staging systems are also widely used, some of which place greater emphasis on histologic features or risk factors such as age or gender.

PATHOGENESIS AND GENETIC BASIS

Radiation Early studies of the pathogenesis of thyroid cancer focused on the role of external radiation, which predisposes to chromosomal breaks, leading to genetic rearrangements and loss of tumor-suppressor genes. External radiation of the mediastinum, face, head, and neck region was administered in the past to treat an array of conditions, including acne and enlargement of the thymus, tonsils, and adenoids. Radiation exposure increases the risk of benign and malignant thyroid nodules, is associated with multicentric cancers, and shifts the incidence of thyroid cancer to an earlier age group. Radiation from nuclear fallout also increases the risk of thyroid cancer. Children seem more predisposed to the effects of radiation than adults. Of note, radiation derived from ^{131}I therapy appears to contribute minimal increased risk of thyroid cancer.

TSH and Growth Factors Many differentiated thyroid cancers express TSH receptors and, therefore, remain responsive to TSH. Higher serum TSH levels, even within normal range, are associated with increased thyroid cancer risk in patients with thyroid nodules. These observations provide the rationale for T_4 suppression of TSH in patients with thyroid cancer. Residual expression of TSH receptors also allows TSH-stimulated uptake of ^{131}I therapy (see below).

TABLE 405-12 THYROID CANCER CLASSIFICATION[a]

Papillary or Follicular Thyroid Cancers		
	<45 years	>45 years
Stage I	Any T, any N, M0	T1, N0, M0
Stage II	Any T, any N, M1	T2, N0, M0
Stage III	—	T3, N0, M0 T1–T3, N1a, M0
Stage IVA	—	T4a, any N, M0 T1–T3, N1b, M0
Stage IVB		T4b, any N, M0
Stage IVC		Any T, any N, M1
Anaplastic Thyroid Cancer		
Stage IV	All cases are stage IV	
Medullary Thyroid Cancer		
Stage I	T1, N0, M0	
Stage II	T2 or T3, N0, M0	
Stage III	T1–T3, N1a, M0	
Stage IVA	T4a, any N, M0 T1–T3, N1b, M0	
Stage IVB	T4b, any N, M0	
Stage IVC	Any T, any N, M1	

[a]Criteria include: T, the size and extent of the primary tumor (T1a ≤1 cm; T1b >1 cm but ≤2 cm; T2 >2 cm but ≤4 cm; T3 >4 cm or any tumor with extension into perithyroidal soft tissue or sternothyroid muscle; T4a invasion into subcutaneous soft tissues, larynx, trachea, esophagus, or recurrent laryngeal nerve; T4b invasion into prevertebral fascia or encasement of carotid artery or mediastinal vessels); N, the absence (N0) or presence (N1a level IV central compartment; N1b levels II–V lateral compartment, upper mediastinal or retro/parapharyngeal) of regional node involvement; M, the absence (M0) or presence (M1) of distant metastases.

Source: American Joint Committee on Cancer staging system for thyroid cancers using the TNM classification, 7th edition.

Oncogenes and Tumor-Suppressor Genes Thyroid cancers are monoclonal in origin, consistent with the idea that they originate as a consequence of mutations that confer a growth advantage to a single cell. In addition to increased rates of proliferation, some thyroid cancers exhibit impaired apoptosis and features that enhance invasion, angiogenesis, and metastasis. Thyroid neoplasms have been analyzed for a variety of genetic alterations, but without clear evidence of an ordered acquisition of somatic mutations as they progress from the benign to the malignant state. On the other hand, certain mutations are relatively specific for thyroid neoplasia, some of which correlate with histologic classification (Table 405-13).

As described above, activating mutations of the TSH-R and the $G_{S\alpha}$ subunit are associated with autonomously functioning nodules. Although these mutations induce thyroid cell growth, this type of nodule is almost always benign.

Activation of the RET-RAS-BRAF signaling pathway is seen in up to 70% of PTCs, although the types of mutations are heterogeneous. A variety of rearrangements involving the *RET* gene on chromosome 10 bring this receptor tyrosine kinase under the control of other promoters, leading to receptor overexpression. *RET* rearrangements occur in 20–40% of PTCs in different series and were observed with increased frequency in tumors developing after the Chernobyl radiation accident. Rearrangements in PTC have also been observed for another tyrosine kinase gene, *TRK1*, which is located on chromosome 1. To date, the identification of PTC with *RET* or *TRK1* rearrangements has not proven useful for predicting prognosis or treatment responses. *BRAF V600E* mutations appear to be the most common genetic alteration in PTC. These mutations activate the kinase, which stimulates the mitogen-activated protein MAP kinase (MAPK) cascade. *RAS* mutations, which also stimulate the MAPK cascade, are found in about 20–30% of thyroid neoplasms (*NRAS* > *HRAS* > *KRAS*), including both PTC and FTC. Of note, simultaneous *RET*, *BRAF*, and *RAS* mutations rarely occur in the same tumor, suggesting that activation of the MAPK cascade is critical for tumor development, independent of the step that initiates the cascade.

RAS mutations also occur in FTCs. In addition, a rearrangement of the thyroid developmental transcription factor PAX8 with the nuclear receptor PPARγ is identified in a significant fraction of FTCs. Overall, about 70% of follicular cancers have mutations or genetic rearrangements. Loss of heterozygosity of 3p or 11q, consistent with deletions of tumor-suppressor genes, is also common in FTCs.

Most of the mutations seen in differentiated thyroid cancers have also been detected in ATCs. *BRAF* mutations are seen in up to 50% of ATCs. Mutations in *CTNNB1*, which encodes β-catenin, occur in about two-thirds of ATCs, but not in PTC or FTC. Mutations of the tumor-suppressor *P53* also play an important role in the development of ATC. Because *P53* plays a role in cell cycle surveillance, DNA repair, and apoptosis, its loss may contribute to the rapid acquisition of genetic instability as well as poor treatment responses (Chap. 102e) (Table 405-13).

The role of molecular diagnostics in the clinical management of thyroid cancer is under investigation. In principle, analyses of specific mutations might aid in classification, prognosis, or choice of treatment. Although *BRAF V600E* mutations are associated with loss of iodine uptake by tumor cells, there is no clear evidence to date that this information alters clinical decision making. Higher recurrence rates have been variably reported in patients with *BRAF*-positive PTC, but the impact on survival rates is unclear. Sequencing of thyroid cancers as part of the Cancer Genome Atlas (TCGA) is likely to lead to new classification schemes based on molecular abnormalities in tumors.

MTC, when associated with multiple endocrine neoplasia (MEN) type 2, harbors an inherited mutation of the *RET* gene. Unlike the rearrangements of *RET* seen in PTC, the mutations in MEN 2 are

TABLE 405-13 GENETIC ALTERATIONS IN THYROID NEOPLASIA

Gene/Protein	Type of Gene	Chromosomal Location	Genetic Abnormality	Tumor
TSH receptor	GPCR receptor	14q31	Point mutations	Toxic adenoma, differentiated carcinomas
$G_{s\alpha}$	G protein	20q13.2	Point mutations	Toxic adenoma, differentiated carcinomas
RET/PTC	Receptor tyrosine kinase	10q11.2	Rearrangements	PTC (more common in radiation-induced tumors)
			PTC1: inv(10)(q11.2q21)	
			PTC2: t(10;17)(q11.2;q23)	
			PTC3: ELE1/TK	
RET	Receptor tyrosine kinase	10q11.2	Point mutations	MEN 2, medullary thyroid cancer
BRAF	MEK kinase	7q24	Point mutations, rearrangements	PTC, ATC
TRK	Receptor tyrosine kinase	1q23-24	Rearrangements	Multinodular goiter, papillary thyroid cancer
RAS	Signal transducing p21	NRAS 1p13.2 (most common); HRAS 11p15.5; KRAS 12p12.1	Point mutations	Follicular thyroid cancer, PTC follicular variant, adenomas
p53	Tumor suppressor, cell cycle control, apoptosis	17p13	Point mutations Deletion, insertion	Anaplastic cancer
APC	Tumor suppressor, adenomatous polyposis coli gene	5q21-q22	Point mutations	Anaplastic cancer, also associated with familial polyposis coli
p16 (MTS1, CDKN2A)	Tumor suppressor, cell cycle control	9p21	Deletions	Differentiated carcinomas
p21/WAF	Tumor suppressor, cell cycle control	6p21.2	Overexpression	Anaplastic cancer
MET	Receptor tyrosine kinase	7q31	Overexpression	Follicular thyroid cancer
c-MYC	Receptor tyrosine kinase	8q24.12-13	Overexpression	Differentiated carcinoma
PTEN	Phosphatase	10q23	Point mutations	PTC in Cowden's syndrome (multiple hamartomas, breast tumors, gastrointestinal polyps, thyroid tumors)
CTNNB1	β-Catenin	3p22	Point mutations	Anaplastic cancer
Loss of heterozygosity (LOH)	? Tumor suppressors	3p; 11q13, other loci	Deletions	Differentiated thyroid carcinomas, anaplastic cancer
PAX8-PPARγ1	Transcription factor nuclear receptor fusion	t(2;3)(q13;p25)	Translocation	Follicular adenoma or carcinoma, rare PTC follicular variant

Abbreviations: APC, adenomatous polyposis coli; ATC, anaplastic thyroid cancer; BRAF, v-raf homologue, B1; CDKN2A, cyclin-dependent kinase inhibitor 2A; c-MYC, cellular homologue of myelocytomatosis virus protooncogene; ELE1/TK, RET-activating gene ele1/tyrosine kinase; GPCR, G protein–coupled receptor; $G_{s\alpha}$, G-protein stimulating α-subunit; MEK, mitogen extracellular signal-regulated kinase; MEN 2, multiple endocrine neoplasia-2; MET, met protooncogene (hepatocyte growth factor receptor); MTS, multiple tumor suppressor; p53, p53 tumor suppressor gene; PTC, papillary thyroid cancer; PTEN, phosphatase and tensin homologue; RAS, rat sarcoma protooncogene; RET, rearranged during transfection protooncogene; p21, p21 tumor suppressor; PAX8, paired domain transcription factor; PPARγ1, peroxisome-proliferator activated receptor γ1; TRK, tyrosine kinase receptor; TSH, thyroid-stimulating hormone; WAF, wild-type p53 activated fragment.

Source: Adapted with permission from P Kopp, JL Jameson, in JL Jameson (ed): *Principles of Molecular Medicine*. Totowa, NJ, Humana Press, 1998.

point mutations that induce constitutive activity of the tyrosine kinase (Chap. 408). MTC is preceded by hyperplasia of the C cells, raising the likelihood that as-yet-unidentified "second hits" lead to cellular transformation. A subset of sporadic MTC contains somatic mutations that activate *RET*.

WELL-DIFFERENTIATED THYROID CANCER

Papillary PTC is the most common type of thyroid cancer, accounting for 70–90% of well-differentiated thyroid malignancies. Microscopic PTC is present in up to 25% of thyroid glands at autopsy, but most of these lesions are very small (several millimeters) and are not clinically significant. Characteristic cytologic features of PTC help make the diagnosis by FNA or after surgical resection; these include psammoma bodies, cleaved nuclei with an "orphan-Annie" appearance caused by large nucleoli, and the formation of papillary structures.

PTC tends to be multifocal and to invade locally within the thyroid gland as well as through the thyroid capsule and into adjacent structures in the neck. It has a propensity to spread via the lymphatic system but can metastasize hematogenously as well, particularly to bone and lung. Because of the relatively slow growth of the tumor, a significant burden of pulmonary metastases may accumulate, sometimes with remarkably few symptoms. The prognostic implication of lymph node spread is debated. Lymph node involvement by thyroid cancer can be well tolerated but appears to increase the risk of recurrence and mortality, particularly in older patients. The staging of PTC by the TNM system is outlined in Table 405-12. Most papillary cancers are identified in the early stages (>80% stages I or II) and have an excellent prognosis, with survival curves similar to expected survival (Fig. 405-12). Mortality is markedly increased in stage IV disease, especially in the presence of distant metastases (stage IVC), but this group comprises only about 1% of patients. The treatment of PTC is described below.

Follicular The incidence of FTC varies widely in different parts of the world; it is more common in iodine-deficient regions. Currently, FTC accounts for only about 5% of all thyroid cancers diagnosed in the United States. FTC is difficult to diagnose by FNA because the distinction between benign and malignant follicular neoplasms rests largely on evidence of invasion into vessels, nerves, or adjacent structures. FTC tends to spread by hematogenous routes leading to bone, lung, and central nervous system metastases. Mortality rates associated with FTC are less favorable than for PTC, in part because a larger proportion of patients present with stage IV disease. Poor prognostic features include distant metastases, age >50 years, primary tumor size >4 cm, Hürthle cell histology, and the presence of marked vascular invasion.

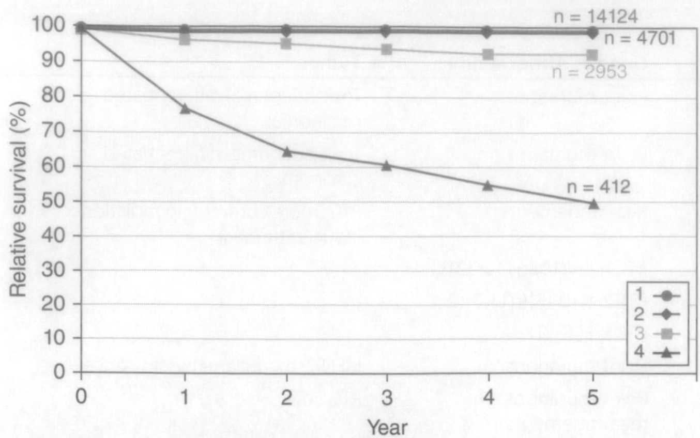

FIGURE 405-12 Survival rates of patients with different stages of papillary cancer. *(Adapted with permission from Edge SB, Byrd DR: Thyroid, in Compton CC, Fritz AB, Greene FL, Trotti A [eds]: AJCC Cancer Staging Manual, 7th ed. New York, Springer, 2010, pp 87–92.)*

TREATMENT WELL-DIFFERENTIATED THYROID CANCER

SURGERY

All well-differentiated thyroid cancers should be surgically excised. In addition to removing the primary lesion, surgery allows accurate histologic diagnosis and staging, and multicentric disease is commonly found in the contralateral thyroid lobe. Preoperative sonography should be performed in all patients to assess the central and lateral cervical lymph node compartments for suspicious adenopathy, which if present, can undergo FNA and then be removed at surgery. Bilateral, near-total thyroidectomy has been shown to reduce recurrence rates in all patients except those with T1a tumors (≤1 cm). If cytology is diagnostic for thyroid cancer, bilateral surgery should be done. If malignancy is identified pathologically after lobectomy, completion surgery is recommended unless the tumor is T1a or is a minimally invasive follicular cancer. Bilateral surgery for patients at higher risk allows monitoring of serum Tg levels and administration of radioiodine for remnant ablation and potential treatment of iodine-avid metastases, if indicated. Therefore, near-total thyroidectomy is preferable in almost all patients; complication rates are acceptably low if the surgeon is highly experienced in the procedure.

TSH SUPPRESSION THERAPY

Because most tumors are still TSH-responsive, levothyroxine suppression of TSH is a mainstay of thyroid cancer treatment. Although TSH suppression clearly provides therapeutic benefit, there are no prospective studies that define the optimal level of TSH suppression. The degree of TSH suppression should be individualized based on a patient's risk of recurrence. It should be adjusted over time as surveillance blood tests and imaging confirm absence of disease or, alternatively, indicate possible residual/recurrent cancer. For patients at low risk of recurrence, TSH should be suppressed into the low but detectable range (0.1–0.5 mIU/L). If subsequent surveillance testing indicates no evidence of disease, the TSH target may rise to the lower half of the normal range. For patients at high risk of recurrence or with known metastatic disease, TSH levels should be kept to <0.1 mIU/L if there are no strong contraindications to mild thyrotoxicosis. In this instance, unbound T_4 must also be monitored to avoid excessive treatment.

RADIOIODINE TREATMENT

After near-total thyroidectomy, substantial thyroid tissue often remains, particularly in the thyroid bed and surrounding the parathyroid glands. Postsurgical radioablation of the remnant thyroid eliminates residual normal thyroid, facilitating the use of Tg determinations and radioiodine scanning for long-term follow-up. In addition, well-differentiated thyroid cancer often incorporates radioiodine, although less efficiently than normal thyroid follicular cells. Radioiodine uptake is determined primarily by expression of the NIS and is stimulated by TSH, requiring expression of the TSH-R. The retention time for radioactivity is influenced by the extent to which the tumor retains differentiated functions such as iodide trapping and organification. Consequently, for patients at risk of recurrence and for those with known distant metastatic disease, ^{131}I ablation may also potentially treat residual tumor cells.

Indications Not all patients benefit from radioiodine therapy. Neither recurrence nor survival rates are improved in stage I patients with T1 tumors (≤2 cm) confined to the thyroid. However, in higher risk patients (larger tumors, more aggressive variants of papillary cancer, tumor vascular invasion, presence of large-volume lymph node metastases), radioiodine reduces recurrence and may increase survival.

^{131}I Thyroid Ablation and Treatment As noted above, the decision to use ^{131}I for thyroid ablation should be coordinated with the surgical approach, because radioablation is much more effective when there is minimal remaining normal thyroid tissue. Radioiodine is administered after iodine depletion (patient follows a low-iodine diet for 1≤2 weeks) and in the presence of elevated serum TSH levels to stimulate uptake of the isotope into both the remnant and potentially any residual tumor. To achieve high serum TSH levels, there are two approaches. A patient may be withdrawn from thyroid hormone so that endogenous TSH is secreted and, ideally, the serum TSH level is >25 mIU/L at the time of ^{131}I therapy. A typical strategy is to treat the patient for several weeks postoperatively with liothyronine (25 μg qd or bid), followed by thyroid hormone withdrawal for 2 weeks. Alternatively, recombinant human TSH (rhTSH) is administered as two daily consecutive injections (0.9 mg) with administration of ^{131}I 24 h after the second injection. The patient can continue to take levothyroxine and remains euthyroid. Both approaches have equal success in achieving remnant ablation.

A pretreatment scanning dose of ^{131}I (usually 111–185 MBq [3–5 mCi]) or ^{123}I (74 MBq [2 mCi]) can reveal the amount of residual tissue and provides guidance about the dose needed to accomplish ablation. However, because of concerns about radioactive "stunning" that impairs subsequent treatment, there is a trend to avoid pretreatment scanning with ^{131}I and use either ^{123}I or proceed directly to ablation, unless there is suspicion that the amount of residual tissue will alter therapy or that there is distant metastatic disease. In the United States, outpatient doses of up to 6475 MBq (175 mCi) can be given at most centers. The administered dose depends on the indication for therapy with lower doses of 1850–2775 MBq (50–75 mCi) given for remnant ablation but higher doses of 3700–5500 MBq (100–150 mCi) used as adjuvant therapy when residual disease may be present. A WBS following radioiodine treatment is used to confirm the ^{131}I uptake in the remnant and to identify possible metastatic disease.

Follow-Up Whole-Body Thyroid Scanning and Thyroglobulin Determinations Serum thyroglobulin is a sensitive marker of residual/recurrent thyroid cancer after ablation of the residual postsurgical thyroid tissue. However, newer Tg assays have functional sensitivities as low as 0.1 ng/mL, as opposed to older assays with functional sensitivities of 1 ng/mL, reducing the number of patients with truly undetectable serum Tg levels. Because the vast majority of papillary thyroid cancer recurrences are in cervical lymph nodes, a neck ultrasound should be performed about 6 months after thyroid ablation; ultrasound has been shown to be more sensitive than WBS in this scenario.

In low-risk patients who have no clinical evidence of residual disease after ablation and a basal Tg <1 ng/mL on levothyroxine, an rhTSH-stimulated Tg level should be obtained 6–12 months after ablation, without WBS. If stimulated Tg levels are low (<1 ng/mL) and, ideally, undetectable, the risk of recurrence is <5% at 5 years. Newer data indicate that rhTSH stimulation may not be required for patients with undetectable basal Tg levels in sensitive assays, if there is documented absence of Tg antibodies. These patients can be followed with unstimulated Tg every 6–12 months and neck ultrasound as indicated. Levothyroxine dosing may then be titrated to a higher TSH level of 0.5–1.5 mIU/L.

The use of WBS is reserved for patients with known iodine-avid metastases or those with elevated serum thyroglobulin levels and negative imaging with ultrasound, chest CT, and neck cross-sectional imaging who may require additional ^{131}I therapy.

In addition, most authorities advocate radioiodine treatment for scan-negative, Tg-positive (Tg >5–10 ng/mL) patients, as many derive therapeutic benefit from a large dose of ^{131}I. For such patients, rhTSH preparation is not FDA approved for the treatment of metastatic disease, and the traditional approach of thyroid hormone withdrawal should be followed. This involves switching patients from levothyroxine (T_4) to the more rapidly cleared hormone liothyronine (T_3), thereby allowing TSH to increase more quickly. Whenever ^{131}I is administered, posttherapy WBS is the gold standard to assess iodine-avid metastases.

In addition to radioiodine, external beam radiotherapy is also used to treat specific metastatic lesions, particularly when they cause bone pain or threaten neurologic injury (e.g., vertebral metastases).

New Potential Therapies Kinase inhibitors are being explored as a means to target pathways known to be active in thyroid cancer, including the RAS, BRAF, EGFR, VEGFR, and angiogenesis pathways. A multicenter randomized controlled trial of the multikinase inhibitor sorafenib in 417 patients with progressive metastatic thyroid cancer reported a doubling of progression-free survival to 10.8 months in the treatment group compared with the placebo group. Ongoing trials are exploring whether differentiation protocols with kinase inhibitors or other approaches might enhance radioiodine uptake and efficacy.

ANAPLASTIC AND OTHER FORMS OF THYROID CANCER

Anaplastic Thyroid Cancer As noted above, ATC is a poorly differentiated and aggressive cancer. The prognosis is poor, and most patients die within 6 months of diagnosis. Because of the undifferentiated state of these tumors, the uptake of radioiodine is usually negligible, but it can be used therapeutically if there is residual uptake. Chemotherapy has been attempted with multiple agents, including anthracyclines and paclitaxel, but it is usually ineffective. External beam radiation therapy can be attempted and continued if tumors are responsive.

Thyroid Lymphoma Lymphoma in the thyroid gland often arises in the background of Hashimoto's thyroiditis. A rapidly expanding thyroid mass suggests the possibility of this diagnosis. Diffuse large-cell lymphoma is the most common type in the thyroid. Biopsies reveal sheets of lymphoid cells that can be difficult to distinguish from small-cell lung cancer or ATC. These tumors are often highly sensitive to external radiation. Surgical resection should be avoided as initial therapy because it may spread disease that is otherwise localized to the thyroid. If staging indicates disease outside of the thyroid, treatment should follow guidelines used for other forms of lymphoma (Chap. 134).

MEDULLARY THYROID CARCINOMA

MTC can be sporadic or familial and accounts for about 5% of thyroid cancers. There are three familial forms of MTC: MEN 2A, MEN 2B, and familial MTC without other features of MEN (Chap. 408). In general, MTC is more aggressive in MEN 2B than in MEN 2A, and familial MTC is more aggressive than sporadic MTC. Elevated serum calcitonin provides a marker of residual or recurrent disease. All patients with MTC should be tested for *RET* mutations, because genetic counseling and testing of family members can be offered to those individuals who test positive for mutations.

The management of MTC is primarily surgical. Unlike tumors derived from thyroid follicular cells, these tumors do not take up radioiodine. External radiation treatment and chemotherapy may provide palliation in patients with advanced disease (Chap. 408).

APPROACH TO THE PATIENT: Thyroid Nodules

Palpable thyroid nodules are found in about 5% of adults, but the prevalence varies considerably worldwide. Given this high prevalence rate, practitioners commonly identify thyroid nodules either on physical examination or as incidental findings on imaging performed for another indication (e.g., carotid ultrasound, cervical spine MRI). The main goal of this evaluation is to identify, in a cost-effective manner, the small subgroup of individuals with malignant lesions.

Nodules are more common in iodine-deficient areas, in women, and with aging. Most palpable nodules are >1 cm in diameter, but the ability to feel a nodule is influenced by its location within the gland (superficial versus deeply embedded), the anatomy of the patient's neck, and the experience of the examiner. More sensitive methods of detection, such as CT, thyroid ultrasound, and pathologic studies, reveal thyroid nodules in up to 50% of glands in individuals over the age of 50. The presence of these thyroid incidentalomas has led to much debate about how to detect nodules and which nodules to investigate further.

An approach to the evaluation of a solitary nodule is outlined in Fig. 405-13. Most patients with thyroid nodules have normal thyroid function tests. Nonetheless, thyroid function should be assessed by measuring a TSH level, which may be suppressed by one or more autonomously functioning nodules. If the TSH is suppressed, a radionuclide scan is indicated to determine if the identified nodule is "hot," as lesions with increased uptake are almost never malignant and FNA is unnecessary. Otherwise, the next step in evaluation is performance of a thyroid ultrasound for three reasons: (1) Ultrasound will confirm if the palpable nodule is indeed a nodule. About 15% of "palpable" nodules are not confirmed on imaging, and therefore, no further evaluation is required. (2) Ultrasound will assess if there are additional nonpalpable nodules for which FNA may be recommended based on imaging features and size. (3) Ultrasound will characterize the imaging features of the nodule, which, combined with the nodule's size, facilitate decision making about FNA.

Evidence-based guidelines from both the American Thyroid Association and the American Association of Clinical Endocrinologists provide recommendations for nodule FNA based on sonographic imaging features and size cut offs, with lower size cut offs for nodules with more suspicious ultrasound characteristics. FNA biopsy, ideally performed with ultrasound guidance, has good sensitivity and specificity when performed by physicians familiar with the procedure and when the results are interpreted by experienced cytopathologists. The technique is particularly useful for detecting PTC. However, the distinction between benign and malignant follicular lesions is often not possible using cytology alone.

In several large studies, FNA biopsies yielded the following findings: 65% benign, 5% malignant or suspicious for malignancy, 10% nondiagnostic or yielding insufficient material for diagnosis, and 20% indeterminate. The Bethesda System is now widely used to provide more uniform terminology for reporting thyroid nodule FNA cytology results. This six-tiered classification system with the respective estimated malignancy rates is shown in Table 405-14. Specifically, the Bethesda System subcategorized cytology specimens previously labeled as indeterminate into three categories: atypia or follicular lesion of undetermined significance (AUS/FLUS), follicular neoplasm, and suspicious for malignancy.

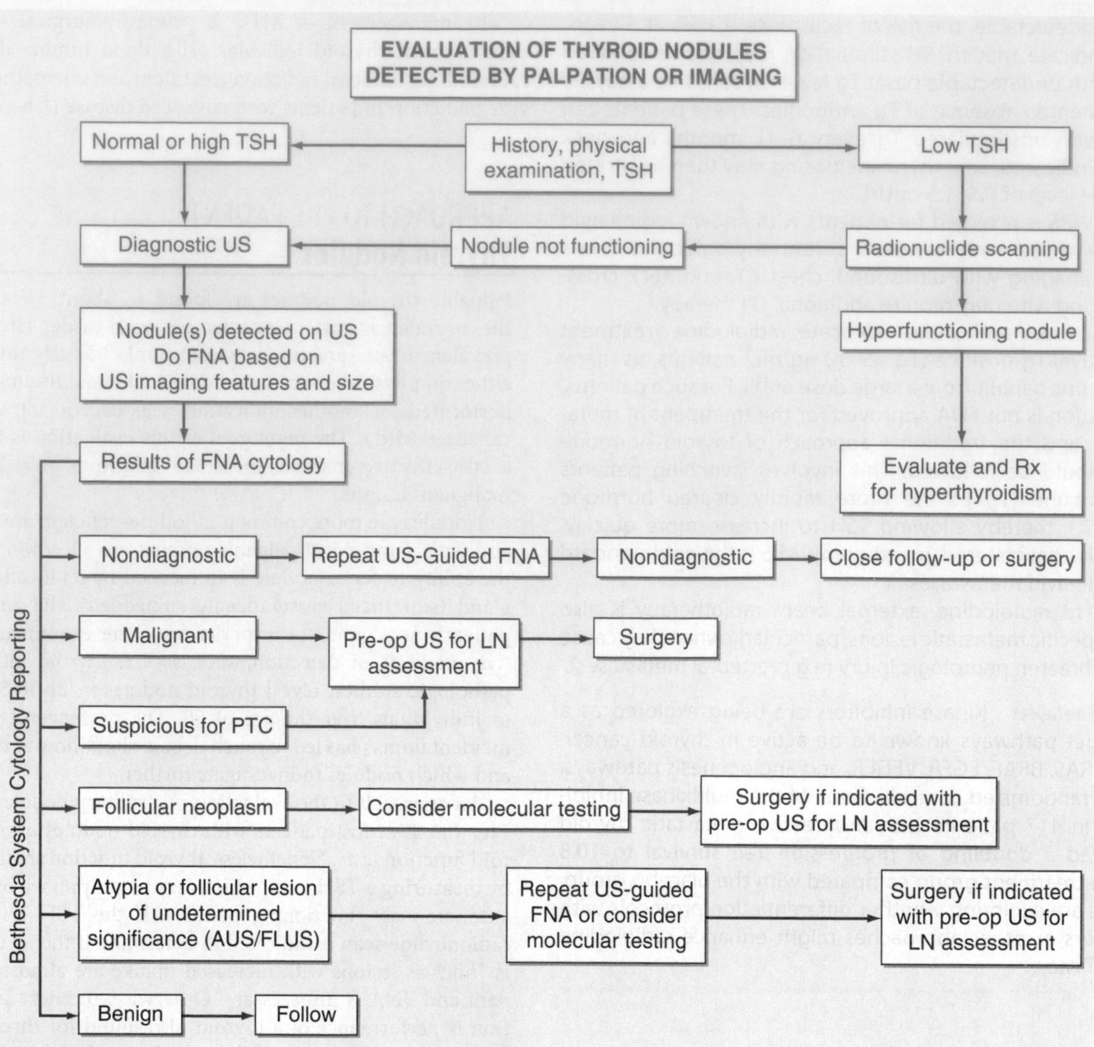

FIGURE 405-13 Approach to the patient with a thyroid nodule. See text and references for details. FNA, fine-needle aspiration; LN, lymph node; PTC, papillary thyroid cancer; TSH, thyroid-stimulating hormone; US, ultrasound.

Cytology results indicative of malignancy mandate surgery, after performing preoperative sonography to evaluate the cervical lymph nodes. Nondiagnostic cytology specimens generally result from cystic lesions but may also occur in fibrous long-standing nodules. Ultrasound-guided FNA is indicated when a repeat FNA is necessary. Repeat FNA will yield a diagnostic cytology in about 50% of cases. Benign nodules should be monitored by ultrasound for growth, and repeat FNA should be considered if the nodule enlarges. The use of levothyroxine to suppress serum TSH is not effective in shrinking nodules in iodine-replete populations, and therefore, levothyroxine should not be used.

The three new cytology classifications introduced by the Bethesda System are associated with different risks of malignancy (Table 405-14).

TABLE 405-14 BETHESDA CLASSIFICATION FOR THYROID CYTOLOGY

Diagnostic Category	Risk of Malignancy
Nondiagnostic or unsatisfactory	1–5%
Benign	2–4%
Atypia or follicular lesion of unknown significance (AUS/FLUS)	15–20%
Follicular neoplasm	20–30%
Suspicious for malignancy	60–75%
Malignant	97–100%

For nodules with suspicious for malignancy cytology, surgery is recommended after ultrasound assessment of cervical lymph nodes. Options to be discussed with the patient include: (1) lobectomy with intraoperative frozen section; (2) near-total thyroidectomy; and (3) mutational analysis mainly for *BRAF V600E*, which is virtually diagnostic of PTC, and bilateral rather than unilateral thyroid surgery is required.

On the other hand, the majority of nodules with AUS/FLUS and follicular neoplasm cytology results are benign; only 10–30% are malignant. The traditional approach for these patients is diagnostic lobectomy for histopathologic diagnosis. Therefore, up to 85% of patients undergo surgery for benign nodules. A high-sensitivity (~90%) novel molecular test using gene expression profiling technology may reduce the need for unnecessary surgery in these two groups. In a multicenter trial of over 265 such nodules, a negative gene expression classifier test reduced the risk of malignancy to about 6%, leading to clinical recommendations for follow-up rather than surgery.

The evaluation of a thyroid nodule is stressful for most patients. They are concerned about the possibility of thyroid cancer, whether verbalized or not. It is constructive, therefore, to review the diagnostic approach and to reassure patients when no malignancy is found. When a suspicious lesion or thyroid cancer is identified, the generally favorable prognosis and available treatment options can be reassuring.

406 Disorders of the Adrenal Cortex

Wiebke Arlt

The adrenal cortex produces three classes of corticosteroid hormones: glucocorticoids (e.g., cortisol), mineralocorticoids (e.g., aldosterone), and adrenal androgen precursors (e.g., dehydroepiandrosterone [DHEA]) (Fig. 406-1). Glucocorticoids and mineralocorticoids act through specific nuclear receptors, regulating aspects of the physiologic stress response as well as blood pressure and electrolyte homeostasis. Adrenal androgen precursors are converted in the gonads and peripheral target cells to sex steroids that act via nuclear androgen and estrogen receptors.

Disorders of the adrenal cortex are characterized by deficiency or excess of one or several of the three major corticosteroid classes. Hormone deficiency can be caused by inherited glandular or enzymatic disorders or by destruction of the pituitary or adrenal gland by autoimmune disorders, infection, infarction, or iatrogenic events such as surgery or hormonal suppression. Hormone excess is usually the result of neoplasia, leading to increased production of adrenocorticotropic hormone (ACTH) by the pituitary or neuroendocrine cells (ectopic ACTH) or increased production of glucocorticoids, mineralocorticoids, or adrenal androgen precursors by adrenal nodules. Adrenal nodules are increasingly identified incidentally during abdominal imaging performed for other reasons.

ADRENAL ANATOMY AND DEVELOPMENT

The normal adrenal glands weigh 6–11 g each. They are located above the kidneys and have their own blood supply. Arterial blood flows initially to the subcapsular region and then meanders from the outer cortical zona glomerulosa through the intermediate zona fasciculata to the inner zona reticularis and eventually to the adrenal medulla. The right suprarenal vein drains directly into the vena cava, while the left suprarenal vein drains into the left renal vein.

During early embryonic development, the adrenals originate from the urogenital ridge and then separate from gonads and kidneys at about the sixth week of gestation. Concordant with the time of sexual differentiation (seventh to ninth week of gestation, Chap. 410), the adrenal cortex starts to produce cortisol and the adrenal sex steroid

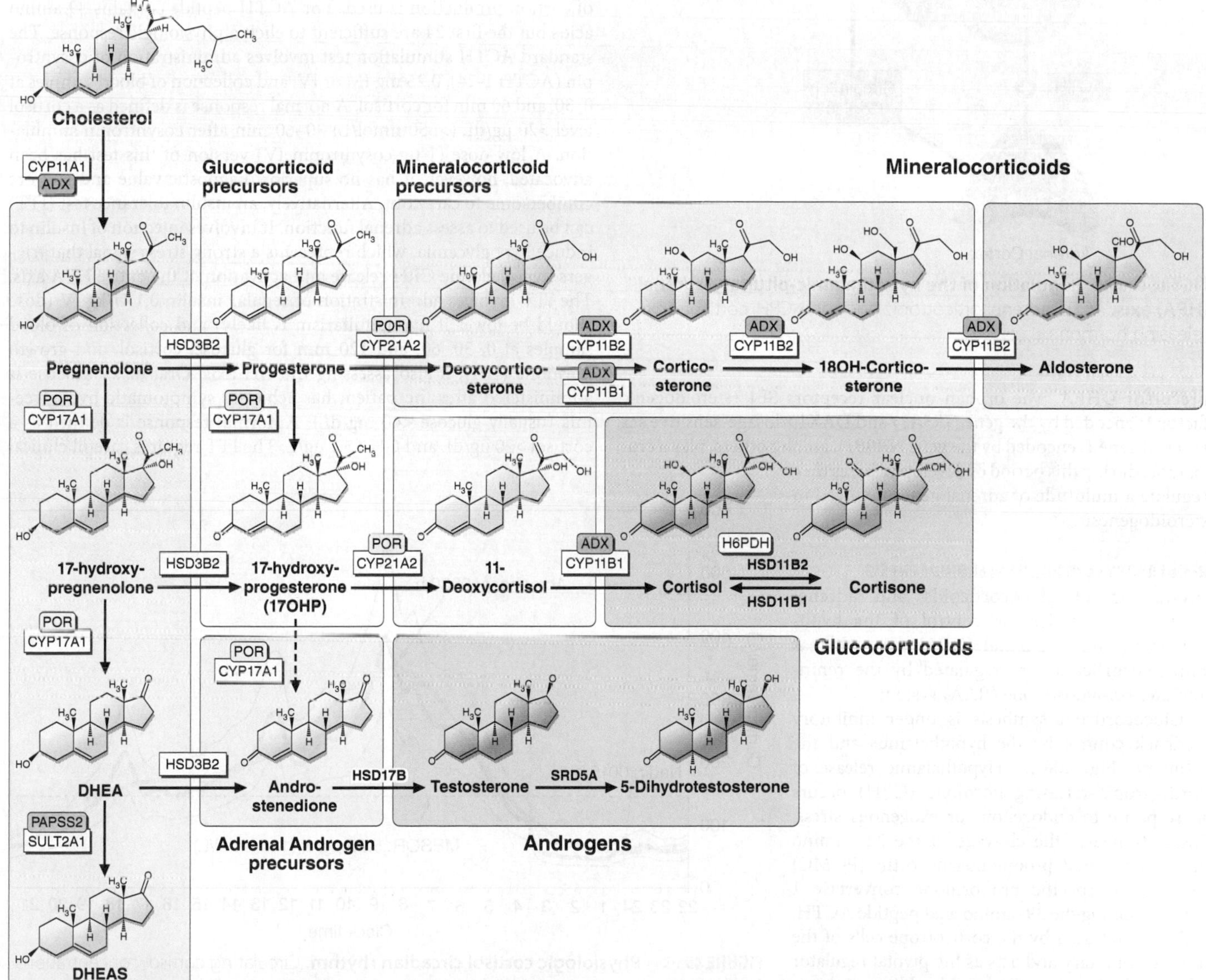

FIGURE 406-1 Adrenal steroidogenesis. ADX, adrenodoxin; CYP11A1, side chain cleavage enzyme; CYP11B1, 11β-hydroxylase; CYP11B2, aldosterone synthase; CYP17A1, 17α-hydroxylase/17,20 lyase; CYP21A2, 21-hydroxylase; DHEA, dehydroepiandrosterone; DHEAS, dehydroepiandrosterone sulfate; H6PDH, hexose-6-phosphate dehydrogenase; HSD11B1, 11β-hydroxysteroid dehydrogenase type 1; HSD11B2, 11β-hydroxysteroid dehydrogenase type 2; HSD17B, 17β-hydroxysteroid dehydrogenase; HSD3B2, 3β-hydroxysteroid dehydrogenase type 2; PAPSS2, PAPS synthase type 2; POR, P450 oxidoreductase; SRD5A, 5α-reductase; SULT2A1, DHEA sulfotransferase.

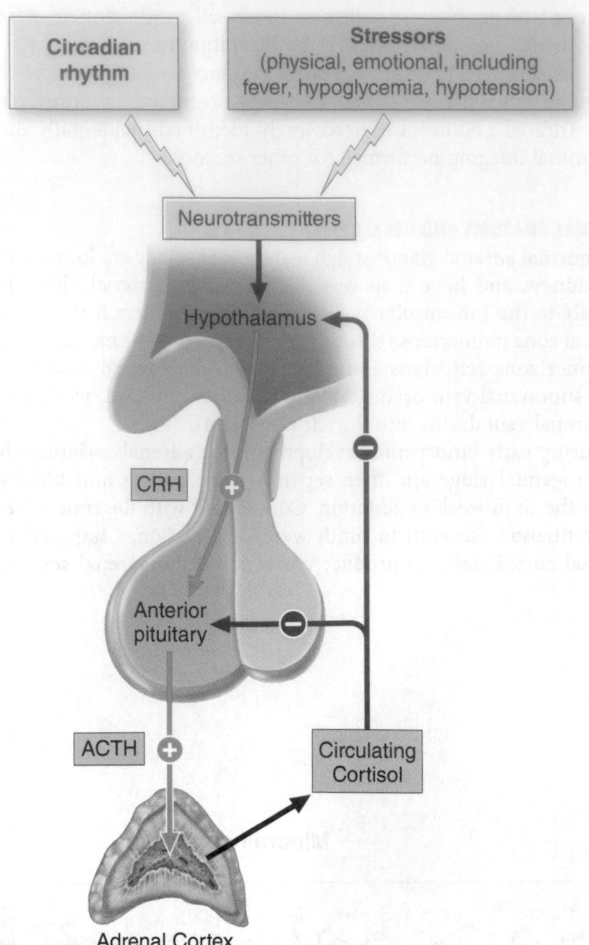

FIGURE 406-2 Regulation of the hypothalamic-pituitary-adrenal (HPA) axis. ACTH, adrenocorticotropic hormone; CRH, corticotropin-releasing hormone.

precursor DHEA. The orphan nuclear receptors SF1 (steroidogenic factor 1; encoded by the gene *NR5A1*) and DAX1 (dosage-sensitive sex reversal gene 1; encoded by the gene *NR0B1*), among others, play a crucial role during this period of development, as they regulate a multitude of adrenal genes involved in steroidogenesis.

REGULATORY CONTROL OF STEROIDOGENESIS

Production of glucocorticoids and adrenal androgens is under the control of the hypothalamic-pituitary-adrenal (HPA) axis, whereas mineralocorticoids are regulated by the renin-angiotensin-aldosterone (RAA) system.

Glucocorticoid synthesis is under inhibitory feedback control by the hypothalamus and the pituitary (Fig. 406-2). Hypothalamic release of corticotropin-releasing hormone (CRH) occurs in response to endogenous or exogenous stress. CRH stimulates the cleavage of the 241–amino acid polypeptide proopiomelanocortin (POMC) by pituitary-specific prohormone convertase 1 (PC1), yielding the 39–amino acid peptide ACTH. ACTH is released by the corticotrope cells of the anterior pituitary and acts as the pivotal regulator of adrenal cortisol synthesis, with additional short-term effects on mineralocorticoid and adrenal androgen synthesis. The release of CRH, and subsequently ACTH, occurs in a pulsatile fashion that follows a circadian rhythm under the control of the hypothalamus, specifically its suprachiasmatic nucleus (SCN), with additional regulation by a complex network of cell-specific clock genes. Reflecting the pattern of ACTH secretion, adrenal cortisol secretion exhibits a distinct circadian rhythm, starting to rise in the early morning hours prior to awakening, with peak levels in the morning and low levels in the evening (Fig. 406-3).

Diagnostic tests assessing the HPA axis make use of the fact that it is regulated by negative feedback. Glucocorticoid excess is diagnosed by employing a dexamethasone suppression test. Dexamethasone, a potent synthetic glucocorticoid, suppresses CRH/ACTH by binding hypothalamic-pituitary glucocorticoid receptors and, therefore, results in downregulation of endogenous cortisol synthesis. Various versions of the dexamethasone suppression test are described in detail in Chap. 403. If cortisol production is autonomous (e.g., adrenal nodule), ACTH is already suppressed and dexamethasone has little additional effect. If cortisol production is driven by an ACTH-producing pituitary adenoma, dexamethasone suppression is ineffective at low doses but usually induces suppression at high doses. If cortisol production is driven by an ectopic source of ACTH, the tumors are usually resistant to dexamethasone suppression. Thus, the dexamethasone suppression test is useful to establish the diagnosis of Cushing's syndrome and to assist with the differential diagnosis of cortisol excess.

Conversely, to assess glucocorticoid deficiency, ACTH stimulation of cortisol production is used. The ACTH peptide contains 39 amino acids but the first 24 are sufficient to elicit a physiologic response. The standard ACTH stimulation test involves administration of cosyntropin (ACTH 1-24), 0.25 mg IM or IV, and collection of blood samples at 0, 30, and 60 min for cortisol. A normal response is defined as a cortisol level >20 μg/dL (>550 nmol/L) 30–60 min after cosyntropin stimulation. A low-dose (1 μg cosyntropin IV) version of this test has been advocated; however, it has no superior diagnostic value and is more cumbersome to carry out. Alternatively, an insulin tolerance test (ITT) can be used to assess adrenal function. It involves injection of insulin to induce hypoglycemia, which represents a strong stress signal that triggers hypothalamic CRH release and activation of the entire HPA axis. The ITT involves administration of regular insulin 0.1 U/kg IV (dose should be lower if hypopituitarism is likely) and collection of blood samples at 0, 30, 60, and 120 min for glucose, cortisol, and growth hormone (GH), if also assessing the GH axis. Oral or IV glucose is administered after the patient has achieved symptomatic hypoglycemia (usually glucose <40 mg/dL). A normal response is defined as a cortisol >20 μg/dL and GH >5.1 μg/L. The ITT requires careful clinical

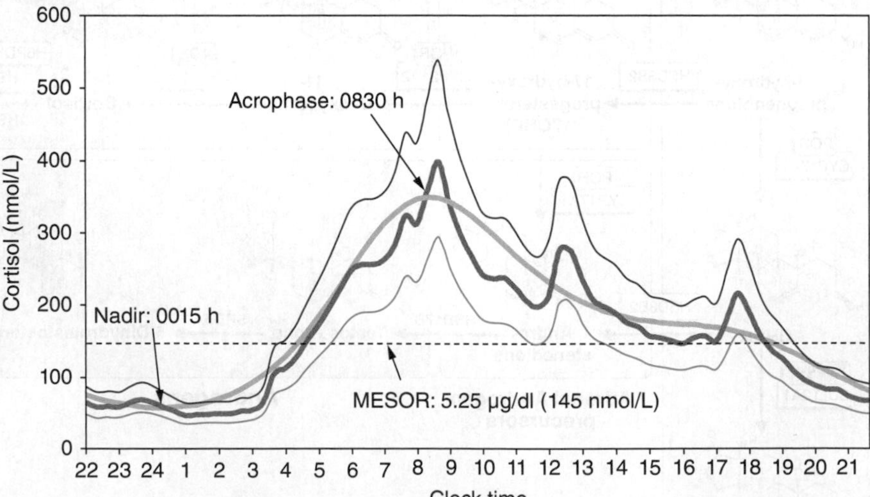

FIGURE 406-3 Physiologic cortisol circadian rhythm. Circulating cortisol concentrations (geometrical mean ± standard deviation values and fitted cosinor) drop under the rhythm-adjusted mean (MESOR) in the early evening hours, with nadir levels around midnight and a rise in the early morning hours; peak levels are observed ~8:30 AM (acrophase). *(Modified after M Debono et al: Modified-release hydrocortisone to provide circadian cortisol profiles. J Clin Endocrinol Metab 94:1548, 2009.)*

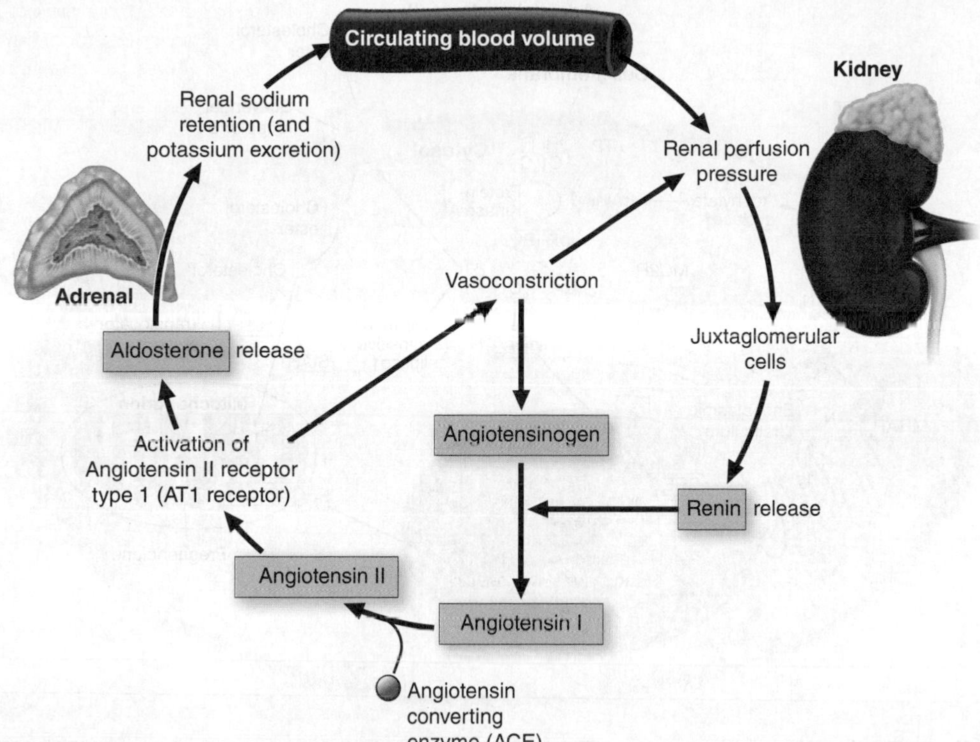

FIGURE 406-4 Regulation of the renin-angiotensin-aldosterone (RAA) system.

monitoring and sequential measurements of glucose. It is contraindicated in patients with coronary disease, cerebrovascular disease, or seizure disorders, which has made the short cosyntropin test the commonly accepted first-line test.

Mineralocorticoid production is controlled by the RAA regulatory cycle, which is initiated by the release of renin from the juxtaglomerular cells in the kidney, resulting in cleavage of angiotensinogen to angiotensin I in the liver (Fig. 406-4). Angiotensin-converting enzyme (ACE) cleaves angiotensin I to angiotensin II, which binds and activates the angiotensin II receptor type 1 (AT1 receptor [AT1R]), resulting in increased adrenal aldosterone production and vasoconstriction. Aldosterone enhances sodium retention and potassium excretion, and increases the arterial perfusion pressure, which in turn regulates renin release. Because mineralocorticoid synthesis is primarily under the control of the RAA system, hypothalamic-pituitary damage does not significantly impact the capacity of the adrenal to synthesize aldosterone.

Similar to the HPA axis, the assessment of the RAA system can be used for diagnostic purposes. If mineralocorticoid excess is present, there is a counter-regulatory downregulation of plasma renin (see below for testing). Conversely, in mineralocorticoid deficiency, plasma renin is markedly increased. Physiologically, oral or IV sodium loading results in suppression of aldosterone, a response that is attenuated or absent in patients with autonomous mineralocorticoid excess.

STEROID HORMONE SYNTHESIS, METABOLISM, AND ACTION

ACTH stimulation is required for the initiation of steroidogenesis. The ACTH receptor MC2R (melanocortin 2 receptor) interacts with the MC2R-accessory protein MRAP, and the complex is transported to the adrenocortical cell membrane, where it binds to ACTH (Fig. 406-5). ACTH stimulation generates cyclic AMP (cAMP), which upregulates the protein kinase A (PKA) signaling pathway. Inactive PKA is a tetramer of two regulatory and two catalytic subunits that is dissociated by cAMP into a dimer of two regulatory subunits bound to cAMP and two free and active catalytic subunits. PKA activation impacts steroidogenesis in three distinct ways: (1) increases the import of cholesterol esters; (2) increases the activity of hormone-sensitive lipase, which cleaves cholesterol esters to cholesterol for import into the mitochondrion; and (3) increases the availability and phosphorylation of CREB (cAMP response element binding), a transcription factor that enhances transcription of CYP11A1 and other enzymes required for glucocorticoid synthesis.

Adrenal steroidogenesis occurs in a zone-specific fashion, with mineralocorticoid synthesis occurring in the outer zona glomerulosa, glucocorticoid synthesis in the zona fasciculata, and adrenal androgen synthesis in the inner zona reticularis (Fig. 406-1). All steroidogenic pathways require cholesterol import into the mitochondrion, a process initiated by the action of the steroidogenic acute regulatory (StAR) protein, which shuttles cholesterol from the outer to the inner mitochondrial membrane. The majority of steroidogenic enzymes are cytochrome P450 (CYP) enzymes, which are either located in the mitochondrion (side chain cleavage enzyme, CYP11A1; 11β-hydroxylase, CYP11B1; aldosterone synthase, CYP11B2) or in the endoplasmic reticulum membrane (17α-hydroxylase, CYP17A1; 21-hydroxylase, CYP21A2; aromatase, CYP19A1). These enzymes require electron donation via specific redox cofactor enzymes, P450 oxidoreductase (POR), and adrenodoxin/adrenodoxin reductase (ADX/ADR) for the microsomal and mitochondrial CYP enzymes, respectively. In addition, the short-chain dehydrogenase 3β-hydroxysteroid dehydrogenase type 2 (3β-HSD2), also termed Δ4,Δ5 isomerase, plays a major role in adrenal steroidogenesis.

The cholesterol side chain cleavage enzyme CYP11A1 generates pregnenolone. Glucocorticoid synthesis requires conversion of pregnenolone to progesterone by 3β-HSD2, followed by conversion to 17-hydroxyprogesterone by CYP17A1, further hydroxylation at carbon 21 by CYP21A2, and eventually, 11β-hydroxylation by CYP11B1 to generate active cortisol (Fig. 406-1). Mineralocorticoid synthesis also requires progesterone, which is first converted to deoxycorticosterone by CYP21A2 and then converted via corticosterone and 18-hydroxycorticosterone to aldosterone in three steps catalyzed by CYP11B2. For adrenal androgen synthesis, pregnenolone undergoes conversion by CYP17A1, which uniquely catalyzes two enzymatic reactions. Via its 17α-hydroxylase activity, CYP17A1 converts pregnenolone to 17-hydroxypregnenolone, followed by generation of the universal sex steroid precursor DHEA via CYP17A1 17,20 lyase activity. The majority of DHEA is secreted by the adrenal in the form of its sulfate ester, DHEAS, generated by DHEA sulfotransferase (SULT2A1).

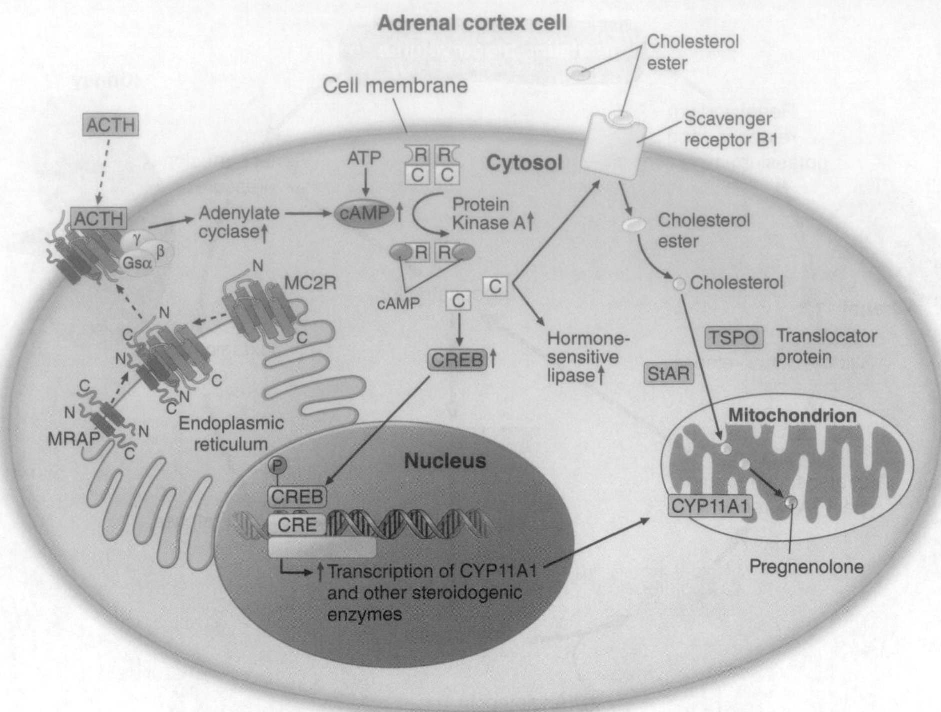

FIGURE 406-5 ACTH effects on adrenal steroidogenesis. ACTH, adrenocorticotropic hormone; binding protein; MRAP, MC2R-accessory protein; protein kinase A catalytic subunit (C; *PRKACA*), PKA regulatory subunit (R; *PRKAR1A*); StAR, steroidogenic acute regulatory (protein); TSPO, translocator protein.

Following its release from the adrenal, cortisol circulates in the bloodstream mainly bound to cortisol-binding globulin (CBG) and to a lesser extent to albumin, with only a minor fraction circulating as free, unbound hormone. Free cortisol is thought to enter cells directly, not requiring active transport. In addition, in a multitude of peripheral target tissues of glucocorticoid action, including adipose, liver, muscle, and brain, cortisol is generated from inactive cortisone within the cell by the enzyme 11β-hydroxysteroid dehydrogenase type 1 (11β-HSD1) (Fig. 406-6). Thereby, 11β-HSD1 functions as a tissue-specific prereceptor regulator of glucocorticoid action. For the conversion of inactive cortisone to active cortisol, 11β-HSD1 requires nicotinamide adenine dinucleotide phosphate (NADPH [reduced form]), which is provided by the enzyme hexose-6-phosphate dehydrogenase (H6PDH). Like the catalytic domain of 11β-HSD1, H6PDH is located in the lumen of the endoplasmic reticulum, and converts glucose-6-phosphate (G6P) to 6-phosphogluconate (6PGL), thereby regenerating NADP+ to NADPH, which drives the activation of cortisol from cortisone by 11β-HSD1.

In the cytosol of target cells, cortisol binds and activates the glucocorticoid receptor (GR), which results in dissociation of heat shock

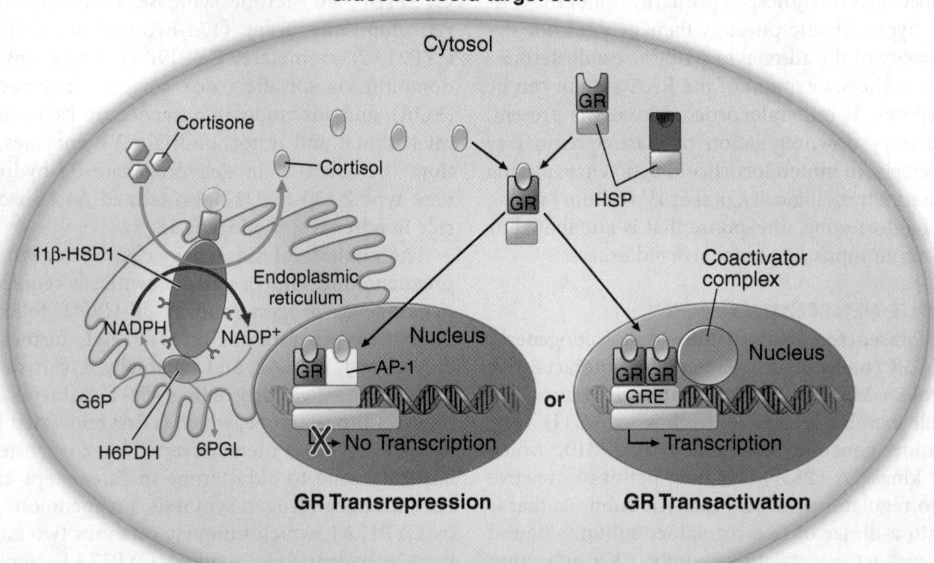

FIGURE 406-6 Prereceptor activation of cortisol and glucocorticoid receptor (GR) action. AP-1 activator protein-1; G6P, glucose-6-phosphate; GRE, glucocorticoid response elements; HSP, heat shock proteins; NADPH, nicotinamide adenine dinucleotide phosphate (reduced form); 6PGL, 6-phosphogluconate.

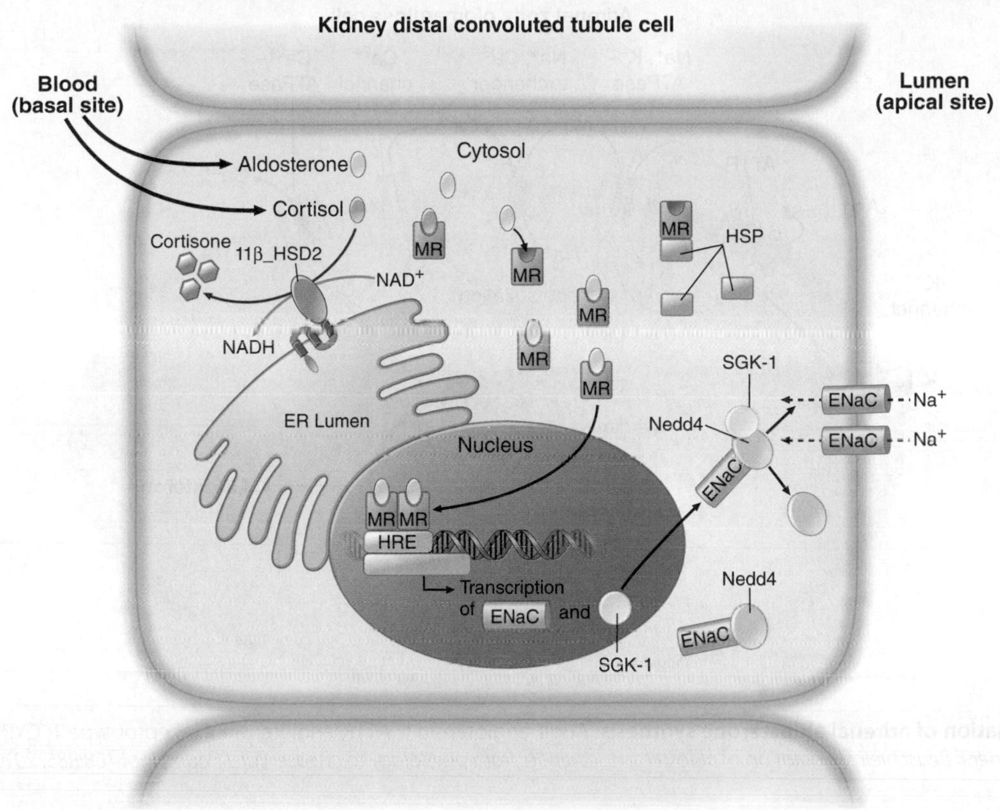

FIGURE 406-7 Prereceptor inactivation of cortisol and mineralocorticoid receptor action. ENaC, epithelial sodium channel; HRE, hormone response element; NADH, nicotinamide adenine dinucleotide; SGK-1, serum glucocorticoid-inducible kinase-1.

proteins (HSP) from the receptor and subsequent dimerization (Fig. 406-6). Cortisol-bound GR dimers translocate to the nucleus and activate glucocorticoid response elements (GRE) in the DNA sequence, thereby enhancing transcription of glucocorticoid-regulated genes (GR transactivation). However, cortisol-bound GR can also form heterodimers with transcription factors such as AP-1 or NF-κB, resulting in transrepression of proinflammatory genes, a mechanism of major importance for the anti-inflammatory action of glucocorticoids. It is important to note that corticosterone also exerts glucocorticoid activity, albeit much weaker than cortisol itself. However, in rodents, corticosterone is the major glucocorticoid, and in patients with 17-hydroxylase deficiency, lack of cortisol can be compensated for by higher concentrations of corticosterone that accumulates as a consequence of the enzymatic block.

Cortisol is inactivated to cortisone by the microsomal enzyme 11β-hydroxysteroid dehydrogenase type 2 (11β-HSD2) (Fig. 406-7), mainly in the kidney, but also in the colon, salivary glands, and other target tissues. Cortisol and aldosterone bind the mineralocorticoid receptor (MR) with equal affinity; however, cortisol circulates in the bloodstream at about a thousandfold higher concentration. Thus, only rapid inactivation of cortisol to cortisone by 11β-HSD2 prevents MR activation by excess cortisol, thereby acting as a tissue-specific modulator of the MR pathway. In addition to cortisol and aldosterone, deoxycorticosterone (DOC) (Fig. 406-1) also exerts mineralocorticoid activity. DOC accumulation due to 11β-hydroxylase deficiency or due to tumor-related excess production can result in mineralocorticoid excess.

Aldosterone synthesis in the adrenal zona glomerulosa cells is driven by the enzyme aldosterone synthase (CYP11B2). The binding of angiotensin II to the AT1 receptor causes glomerulosa cell membrane depolarization by increasing intracellular sodium through inhibition of sodium potassium (Na^+/K^+) ATPase enzymes as well as potassium channels. This drives an increase in intracellular calcium by opening of voltage-dependent calcium channels or inhibition of calcium (Ca^{2+}) ATPase enzymes. Consequently, the calcium signaling pathway is triggered, resulting in upregulation of CYP11B2 transcription (Fig. 406-8).

Analogous to cortisol action via the GR, aldosterone (or cortisol) binding to the MR in the kidney tubule cell dissociates the HSP–receptor complex, allowing homodimerization of the MR, and translocation of the hormone-bound MR dimer to the nucleus (Fig. 406-7). The activated MR enhances transcription of the epithelial sodium channel (ENaC) and serum glucocorticoid-inducible kinase 1 (SGK-1). In the cytosol, interaction of ENaC with Nedd4 prevents cell surface expression of ENaC. However, SGK-1 phosphorylates serine residues within the Nedd4 protein, reduces the interaction between Nedd4 and ENaC, and consequently, enhances the trafficking of ENaC to the cell surface, where it mediates sodium retention.

CUSHING'S SYNDROME

(See also Chap. 403) Cushing's syndrome reflects a constellation of clinical features that result from chronic exposure to excess glucocorticoids of any etiology. The disorder can be ACTH-dependent (e.g., pituitary corticotrope adenoma, ectopic secretion of ACTH by nonpituitary tumor) or ACTH-independent (e.g., adrenocortical adenoma, adrenocortical carcinoma, nodular adrenal hyperplasia), as well as iatrogenic (e.g., administration of exogenous glucocorticoids to treat various inflammatory conditions). The term *Cushing's disease* refers specifically to Cushing's syndrome caused by a pituitary corticotrope adenoma.

Epidemiology Cushing's syndrome is generally considered a rare disease. It occurs with an incidence of 1–2 per 100,000 population per year. However, it is debated whether mild cortisol excess may be more prevalent among patients with several features of Cushing's such as centripetal obesity, type 2 diabetes, and osteoporotic vertebral fractures, recognizing that these are relatively nonspecific and common in the population.

In the overwhelming majority of patients, Cushing's syndrome is caused by an ACTH-producing corticotrope adenoma of the pituitary (Table 406-1), as initially described by Harvey Cushing in 1912. Cushing's disease more frequently affects women, with the exception of prepubertal cases, where it is more common in boys. By contrast,

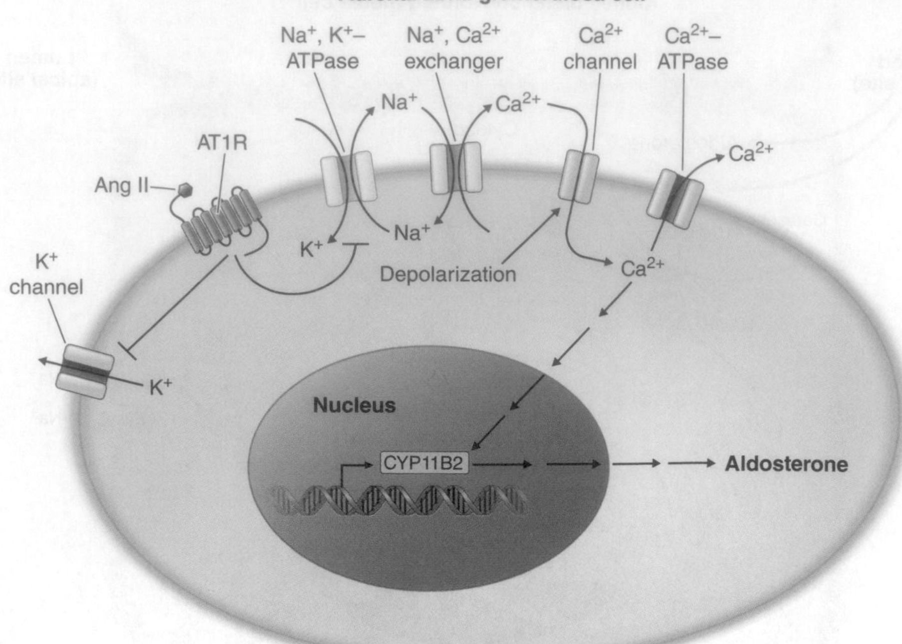

FIGURE 406-8 Regulation of adrenal aldosterone synthesis. AngII, angiotensin II; AT1R, angiotensin II receptor type 1; CYP11B2, aldosterone synthase. *(Modified after F Beuschlein: Regulation of aldosterone secretion: from physiology to disease. Eur J Endocrinol 168:R85, 2013.)*

ectopic ACTH syndrome is more frequently identified in men. Only 10% of patients with Cushing's syndrome have a primary, adrenal cause of their disease (e.g., autonomous cortisol excess independent of ACTH), and most of these patients are women. Overall, the medical use of glucocorticoids for immunosuppression, or for the treatment of inflammatory disorders, is the most common cause of Cushing's syndrome.

Etiology In at least 90% of patients with Cushing's disease, ACTH excess is caused by a corticotrope pituitary microadenoma, often only a few millimeters in diameter. Pituitary macroadenomas (i.e., tumors >1 cm in size) are found in only 5–10% of patients. Pituitary corticotrope adenomas usually occur sporadically but very rarely can be found in the context of multiple endocrine neoplasia type 1 (MEN 1) (Chap. 408).

Ectopic ACTH production is predominantly caused by occult carcinoid tumors, most frequently in the lung, but also in thymus or pancreas. Because of their small size, these tumors are often difficult to locate. Advanced small-cell lung cancer can cause ectopic ACTH production. In rare cases, ectopic CRH and/or ACTH production has been found to originate from medullary thyroid carcinoma or pheochromocytoma, the latter co-secreting catecholamines and ACTH.

TABLE 406-1 CAUSES OF CUSHING'S SYNDROME

Causes of Cushing's Syndrome	Female:Male Ratio	%
ACTH-Dependent Cushing's		90
Cushing's disease (= ACTH-producing pituitary adenoma)	4:1	75
Ectopic ACTH syndrome (due to ACTH secretion by bronchial or pancreatic carcinoid tumors, small-cell lung cancer, medullary thyroid carcinoma, pheochromocytoma and others)	1:1	15
ACTH-Independent Cushing's	4:1	10
Adrenocortical adenoma		5–10
Adrenocortical carcinoma		1
Rare causes: macronodular adrenal hyperplasia; primary pigmented nodular adrenal disease (micro- and/or macronodular); McCune-Albright syndrome		<1

Abbreviation: ACTH, adrenocorticotropic hormone.

The majority of patients with ACTH-independent cortisol excess harbor a cortisol-producing adrenal adenoma; intratumor mutations, i.e., somatic mutations in the PKA catalytic subunit PRKACA, have been identified as cause of disease in 40% of these tumors. Adrenocortical carcinomas may also cause ACTH-independent disease and are often large, with excess production of several corticosteroid classes.

A rare but notable cause of adrenal cortisol excess is macronodular adrenal hyperplasia with low circulating ACTH, but with evidence for autocrine stimulation of cortisol production via intraadrenal ACTH production. These hyperplastic nodules are often also characterized by ectopic expression of G protein–coupled receptors not usually found in the adrenal, including receptors for luteinizing hormone, vasopressin, serotonin, interleukin 1, catecholamines, or gastric inhibitory peptide (GIP), the cause of food-dependent Cushing's. Activation of these receptors results in upregulation of PKA signaling, as physiologically occurs with ACTH, with a subsequent increase in cortisol production. A combination of germline and somatic mutations in the tumor-suppressor gene *ARMC5* have been identified as a prevalent cause of Cushing's due to macronodular adrenal hyperplasia. Germline mutations in the PKA catalytic subunit PRKACA can represent a rare cause of macronodular adrenal hyperplasia associated with cortisol excess.

Mutations in one of the regulatory subunits of PKA, PRKAR1A, are found in patients with primary pigmented nodular adrenal disease (PPNAD) as part of *Carney's complex*, an autosomal dominant multiple neoplasia condition associated with cardiac myxomas, hyperlentiginosis, Sertoli cell tumors, and PPNAD. PPNAD can present as micronodular or macronodular hyperplasia, or both. Phosphodiesterases can influence intracellular cAMP and can thereby impact PKA activation. Mutations in PDE11A and PDE8B have been identified in patients with bilateral adrenal hyperplasia and Cushing's, with and without evidence of PPNAD.

Another rare cause of ACTH-independent Cushing's is *McCune-Albright syndrome*, also associated with polyostotic fibrous dysplasia, unilateral café-au-lait spots, and precocious puberty. McCune-Albright syndrome is caused by activating mutations in the stimulatory

TABLE 406-2 SIGNS AND SYMPTOMS OF CUSHING'S SYNDROME

Body Compartment/ System	Signs and Symptoms
Body fat	Weight gain, central obesity, rounded face, fat pad on back of neck ("buffalo hump")
Skin	Facial plethora, thin and brittle skin, easy bruising, broad and purple stretch marks, acne, hirsutism
Bone	Osteopenia, osteoporosis (vertebral fractures), decreased linear growth in children
Muscle	Weakness, proximal myopathy (prominent atrophy of gluteal and upper leg muscles with difficulty climbing stairs or getting up from a chair)
Cardiovascular system	Hypertension, hypokalemia, edema, atherosclerosis
Metabolism	Glucose intolerance/diabetes, dyslipidemia
Reproductive system	Decreased libido, in women amenorrhea (due to cortisol-mediated inhibition of gonadotropin release)
Central nervous system	Irritability, emotional lability, depression, sometimes cognitive defects; in severe cases, paranoid psychosis
Blood and immune system	Increased susceptibility to infections, increased white blood cell count, eosinopenia, hypercoagulation with increased risk of deep vein thrombosis and pulmonary embolism

G protein alpha subunit 1, GNAS-1 (guanine nucleotide binding protein alpha stimulating activity polypeptide 1), and such mutations have also been found in bilateral macronodular hyperplasia without other McCune-Albright features and, in rare instances, also in isolated cortisol-producing adrenal adenomas (Table 406-1; Chap. 426e).

Clinical Manifestations Glucocorticoids affect almost all cells of the body, and thus signs of cortisol excess impact multiple physiologic systems (Table 406-2), with upregulation of gluconeogenesis, lipolysis, and protein catabolism causing the most prominent features. In addition, excess glucocorticoid secretion overcomes the ability of 11β-HSD2 to rapidly inactivate cortisol to cortisone in the kidney, thereby exerting mineralocorticoid actions, manifest as diastolic hypertension, hypokalemia, and edema. Excess glucocorticoids also interfere with central regulatory systems, leading to suppression of gonadotropins with subsequent hypogonadism and amenorrhea, and suppression of the hypothalamic-pituitary-thyroid axis, resulting in decreased thyroid-stimulating hormone (TSH) secretion.

The majority of clinical signs and symptoms observed in Cushing's syndrome are relatively nonspecific and include features such as obesity, diabetes, diastolic hypertension, hirsutism, and depression that are commonly found in patients who do not have Cushing's. Therefore, careful clinical assessment is an important aspect of evaluating suspected cases. A diagnosis of Cushing's should be considered when several clinical features are found in the same patient, in particular when more specific features are found. These include fragility of the skin, with easy bruising and broad (>1 cm), purplish striae (Fig. 406-9), and signs of proximal myopathy, which becomes most obvious when trying to stand up from a chair without the use of hands or when climbing stairs. Clinical manifestations of Cushing's do not differ substantially among the different causes of Cushing's. In ectopic ACTH syndrome, hyperpigmentation of the knuckles, scars, or skin areas exposed to increased friction can be observed (Fig. 406-9) and is caused by stimulatory effects of excess ACTH and other POMC cleavage products on melanocyte pigment production. Furthermore, patients with ectopic ACTH syndrome, and some with adrenocortical carcinoma as the cause of Cushing's, may have a more brisk onset and rapid progression of clinical signs and symptoms.

Patients with Cushing's syndrome can be acutely endangered by deep vein thrombosis, with subsequent pulmonary embolism due to a hypercoagulable state associated with Cushing's. The majority of patients also experience psychiatric symptoms, mostly in the form of anxiety or depression, but acute paranoid or depressive psychosis

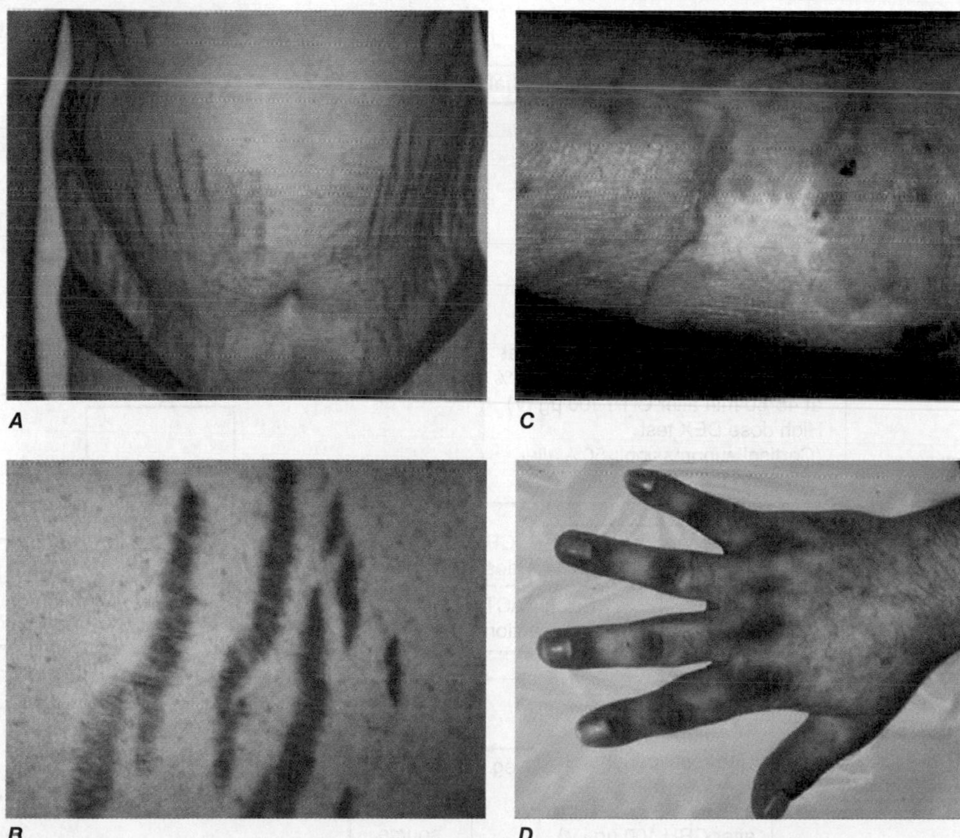

FIGURE 406-9 Clinical features of Cushing's syndrome. ***A.*** Note central obesity and broad, purple stretch marks (***B.*** close-up). ***C.*** Note thin and brittle skin in an elderly patient with Cushing's syndrome. ***D.*** Hyperpigmentation of the knuckles in a patient with ectopic adrenocorticotropic hormone (ACTH) excess.

may also occur. Even after cure, long-term health may be affected by persistently impaired health-related quality of life and increased risk of cardiovascular disease and osteoporosis with vertebral fractures, depending on the duration and degree of exposure to significant cortisol excess.

Diagnosis The most important first step in the management of patients with suspected Cushing's syndrome is to establish the correct diagnosis. Most mistakes in clinical management, leading to unnecessary imaging or surgery, are made because the diagnostic protocol is not followed (Fig. 406-10). This protocol requires establishing the diagnosis of Cushing's beyond doubt prior to employing any tests used for the differential diagnosis of the condition. In principle, after excluding exogenous glucocorticoid use as the cause of clinical signs and symptoms, suspected cases should be tested if there are multiple and progressive features of Cushing's, particularly features with a potentially higher discriminatory value. Exclusion of Cushing's is also indicated in patients with incidentally discovered adrenal masses.

A diagnosis of Cushing's can be considered as established if the results of several tests are consistently suggestive of Cushing's. These tests may include increased 24-h urinary free cortisol excretion in three separate collections, failure to appropriately suppress morning cortisol after overnight exposure to dexamethasone, and evidence of loss of diurnal cortisol secretion with high levels at midnight, the time of the physiologically lowest secretion (Fig. 406-10). Factors potentially affecting the outcome of these diagnostic tests have to be excluded such as incomplete 24-h urine collection or rapid inactivation of dexamethasone due to concurrent intake of CYP3A4-inducing drugs (e.g., antiepileptics, rifampicin). Concurrent intake of oral contraceptives that raise CBG and thus total cortisol can cause failure to suppress after dexamethasone. If in doubt, testing should be repeated after 4–6 weeks off estrogens. Patients with pseudo-Cushing states, i.e., alcohol-related, and those with cyclic Cushing's may require further testing to safely confirm or exclude the diagnosis of Cushing's. In addition, the biochemical assays employed can affect the test results, with specificity representing a common problem with antibody-based

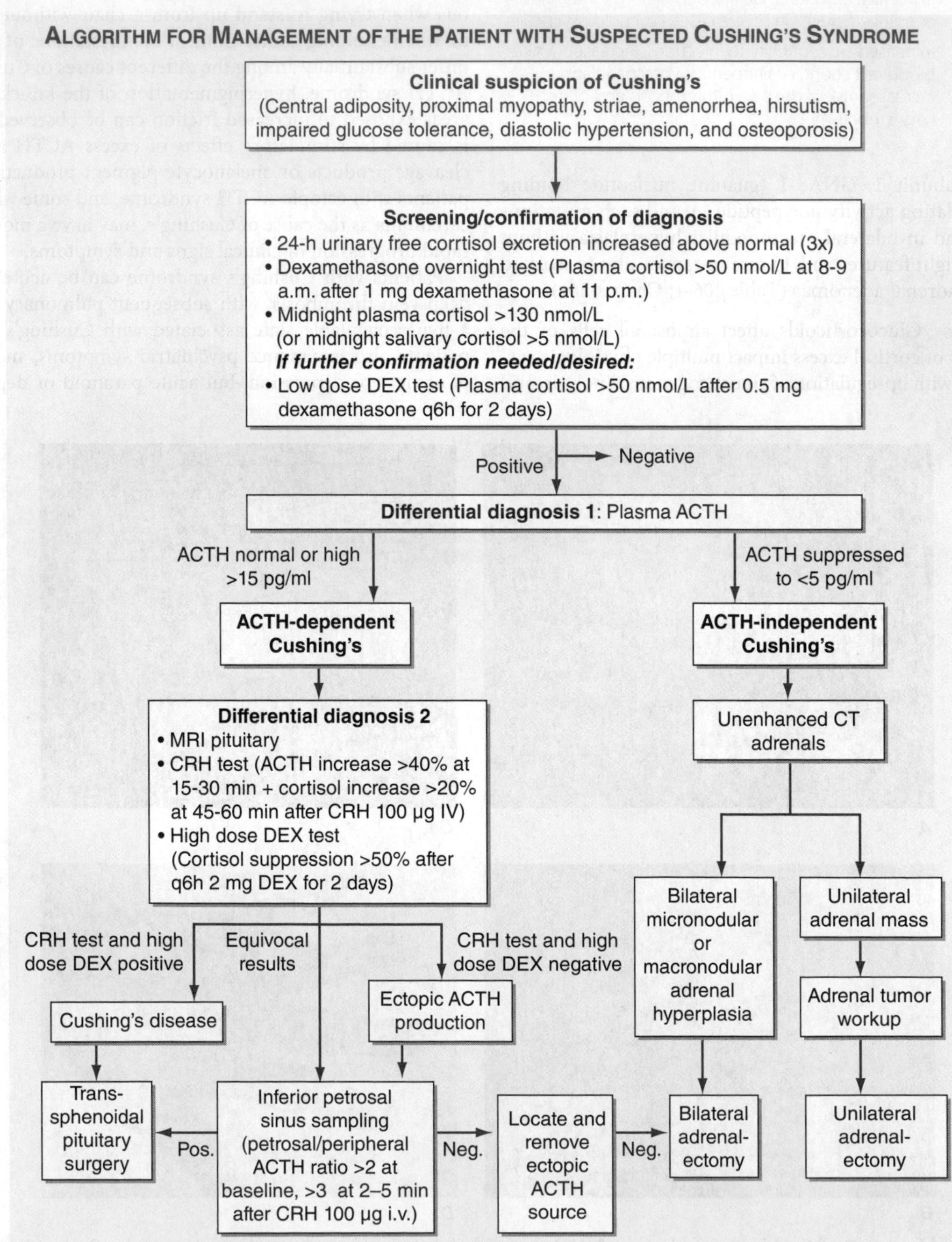

FIGURE 406-10 **Management of the patient with suspected Cushing's syndrome.** ACTH, adrenocorticotropic hormone; CRH, corticotropin-releasing hormone; CT, computed tomography; DEX, dexamethasone; MRI, magnetic resonance imaging.

assays for the measurement of urinary free cortisol. These assays have been greatly improved by the introduction of highly specific tandem mass spectrometry.

Differential Diagnosis The evaluation of patients with confirmed Cushing's should be carried out by an endocrinologist and begins with the differential diagnosis of ACTH-dependent and ACTH-independent cortisol excess (Fig. 406-10). Generally, plasma ACTH levels are suppressed in cases of autonomous adrenal cortisol excess, as a consequence of enhanced negative feedback to the hypothalamus and pituitary. By contrast, patients with ACTH-dependent Cushing's have normal or increased plasma ACTH, with very high levels being found in some patients with ectopic ACTH syndrome. Importantly, imaging should only be used after it is established whether the cortisol excess is ACTH-dependent or ACTH-independent, because nodules in the pituitary or the adrenal are a common finding in the general population. In patients with confirmed ACTH-independent excess, adrenal imaging is indicated (Fig. 406-11), preferably using an unenhanced computed tomography (CT) scan. This allows assessment of adrenal morphology and determination of precontrast tumor density in Hounsfield units (HU), which helps to distinguish between benign and malignant adrenal lesions.

For ACTH-dependent cortisol excess (Chap. 403), a magnetic resonance image (MRI) of the pituitary is the investigation of choice, but it may not show an abnormality in up to 40% of cases because of small tumors below the sensitivity of detection. Characteristically, pituitary corticotrope adenomas fail to enhance following gadolinium administration on T1-weighted MRI images. In all cases of confirmed ACTH-dependent Cushing's, further tests are required for the differential diagnosis of pituitary Cushing's disease and ectopic ACTH syndrome. These tests exploit the fact that most pituitary corticotrope adenomas still display regulatory features, including residual ACTH suppression by high-dose glucocorticoids and CRH responsiveness. In contrast, ectopic sources of ACTH are typically resistant to dexamethasone suppression and unresponsive to CRH (Fig. 406-10). However, it should be noted that a small minority of ectopic ACTH-producing tumors exhibit dynamic responses similar to pituitary corticotrope tumors. If the two tests show discordant results, or if there is any other reason for doubt, the differential diagnosis can be further clarified by performing bilateral inferior petrosal sinus sampling (IPSS) with concurrent blood sampling for ACTH in the right and left inferior petrosal sinus and a peripheral vein. An increased central/peripheral plasma ACTH ratio >2 at baseline and >3 at 2–5 min after CRH injection is indicative of Cushing's disease (Fig. 406-10), with very high sensitivity and specificity. Of note, the results of the IPSS cannot be reliably used for lateralization (i.e., prediction of the location of the tumor within the pituitary), because there is broad interindividual variability in the venous drainage of the pituitary region. Importantly, no cortisol-lowering agents should be used prior to IPSS.

If the differential diagnostic testing indicates ectopic ACTH syndrome, then further imaging should include high-resolution, fine-cut CT scanning of the chest and abdomen for scrutiny of the lung, thymus, and pancreas. If no lesions are identified, an MRI of the chest can be considered because carcinoid tumors usually show high signal intensity on T2-weighted images. Furthermore, octreotide scintigraphy can be helpful in some cases because ectopic ACTH-producing tumors often express somatostatin receptors. Depending on the suspected cause, patients with ectopic ACTH syndrome should also undergo blood sampling for fasting gut hormones, chromogranin A, calcitonin, and biochemical exclusion of pheochromocytoma.

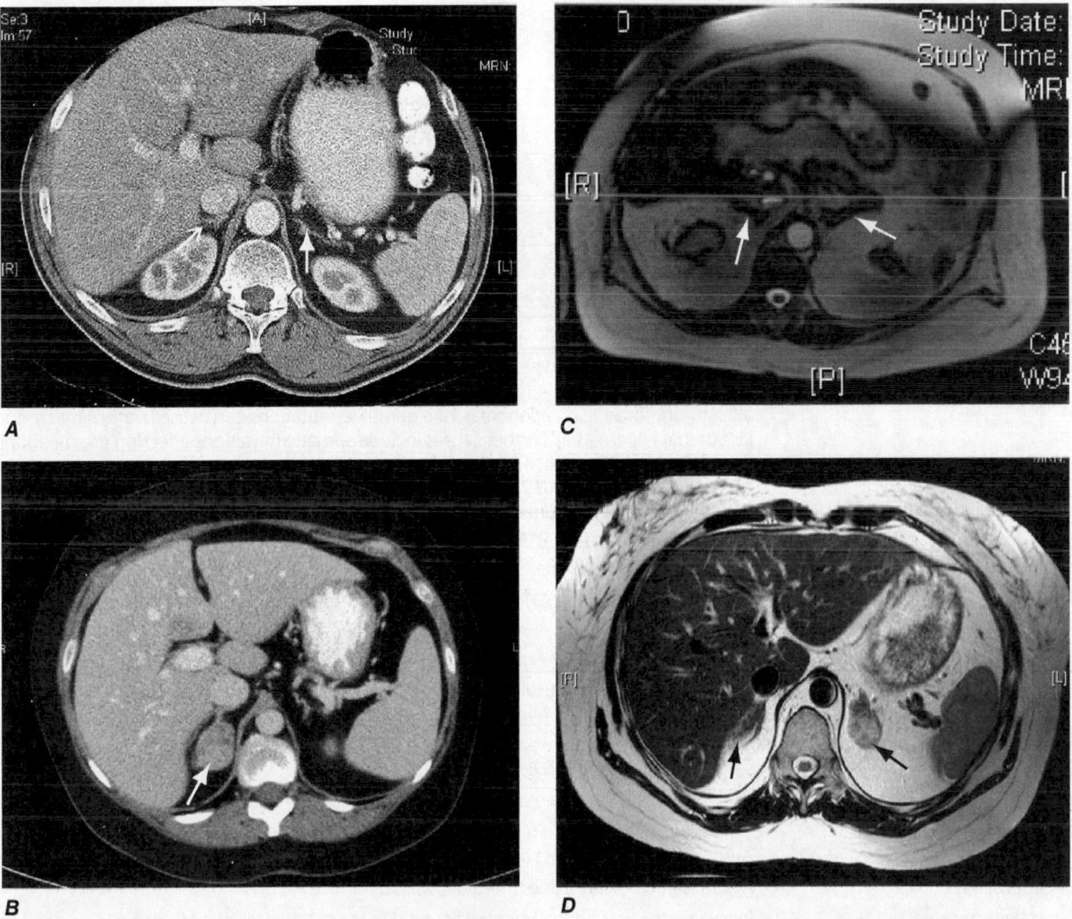

FIGURE 406-11 **Adrenal imaging in Cushing's syndrome.** ***A.*** Adrenal computed tomography (CT) showing normal bilateral adrenal morphology (*arrows*). ***B.*** CT scan depicting a right adrenocortical adenoma (*arrow*) causing Cushing's syndrome. ***C.*** Magnetic resonance imaging (MRI) showing bilateral adrenal hyperplasia due to excess adrenocorticotropic hormone stimulation in Cushing's disease. ***D.*** MRI showing bilateral macronodular hyperplasia causing Cushing's syndrome.

TREATMENT CUSHING'S SYNDROME

Overt Cushing's is associated with a poor prognosis if left untreated. In ACTH-independent disease, treatment consists of surgical removal of the adrenal tumor. For smaller tumors, a minimally invasive approach can be used, whereas for larger tumors and those suspected of malignancy, an open approach is preferred.

In Cushing's disease, the treatment of choice is selective removal of the pituitary corticotrope tumor, usually via an endoscopic transsphenoidal approach. This results in an initial cure rate of 70–80% when performed by a highly experienced surgeon. However, even after initial remission following surgery, long-term follow-up is important because late relapse occurs in a significant number of patients. If pituitary disease recurs, there are several options, including second surgery, radiotherapy, stereotactic radiosurgery, and bilateral adrenalectomy. These options need to be applied in a highly individualized fashion.

In some patients with very severe, overt Cushing's (e.g., difficult to control hypokalemic hypertension or acute psychosis), it may be necessary to introduce medical therapy to rapidly control the cortisol excess during the period leading up to surgery. Similarly, patients with metastasized, glucocorticoid-producing carcinomas may require long-term antiglucocorticoid drug treatment. In case of ectopic ACTH syndrome, in which the tumor cannot be located, one must carefully weigh whether drug treatment or bilateral adrenalectomy is the most appropriate choice, with the latter facilitating immediate cure but requiring life-long corticosteroid replacement. In this instance, it is paramount to ensure regular imaging follow-up for identification of the ectopic ACTH source.

Oral agents with established efficacy in Cushing's syndrome are metyrapone and ketoconazole. Metyrapone inhibits cortisol synthesis at the level of 11β-hydroxylase (Fig. 406-1), whereas the antimycotic drug ketoconazole inhibits the early steps of steroidogenesis. Typical starting doses are 500 mg tid for metyrapone (maximum dose, 6 g) and 200 mg tid for ketoconazole (maximum dose, 1200 mg). Mitotane, a derivative of the insecticide o,p'DDD, is an adrenolytic agent that is also effective for reducing cortisol. Because of its side effect profile, it is most commonly used in the context of adrenocortical carcinoma, but low-dose treatment (500–1000 mg/d) has also been used in benign Cushing's. In severe cases of cortisol excess, etomidate can be used to lower cortisol. It is administered by continuous IV infusion in low, nonanesthetic doses.

After the successful removal of an ACTH- or cortisol-producing tumor, the HPA axis will remain suppressed. Thus, hydrocortisone replacement needs to be initiated at the time of surgery and slowly tapered following recovery, to allow physiologic adaptation to normal cortisol levels. Depending on degree and duration of cortisol excess, the HPA axis may require many months or even years to resume normal function.

MINERALOCORTICOID EXCESS

Epidemiology Following the first description of a patient with an aldosterone-producing adrenal adenoma (*Conn's syndrome*), mineralocorticoid excess was thought to represent a rare cause of hypertension. However, in studies systematically screening all patients with hypertension, a much higher prevalence is now recognized, ranging from 5 to 12%. The prevalence is higher when patients are preselected for hypokalemic hypertension.

Etiology The most common cause of mineralocorticoid excess is primary aldosteronism, reflecting excess production of aldosterone by the adrenal zona glomerulosa. Bilateral micronodular hyperplasia is somewhat more common than unilateral adrenal adenomas (Table 406-3). Somatic mutations in channels and enzymes responsible for increasing sodium and calcium influx in adrenal zona glomerulosa cells have been identified as prevalent causes of aldosterone-producing adrenal adenomas (Table 406-3) and, in the case of germline mutations, also of primary aldosteronism due to bilateral macronodular adrenal hyperplasia. However, bilateral adrenal hyperplasia as a cause of mineralocorticoid excess is usually micronodular but can also contain larger nodules that might be mistaken for a unilateral adenoma. In rare instances, primary aldosteronism is caused by an adrenocortical carcinoma. Carcinomas should be considered in younger patients and in those with larger tumors, because benign aldosterone-producing adenomas usually measure <2 cm in diameter.

A rare cause of aldosterone excess is glucocorticoid-remediable aldosteronism (GRA), which is caused by a chimeric gene resulting

TABLE 406-3 CAUSES OF MINERALOCORTICOID EXCESS

Causes of Mineralocorticoid Excess	Mechanism	%
Primary Aldosteronism		
Adrenal (Conn's) adenoma	Autonomous aldosterone excess can be caused by somatic (intratumor) mutations in the potassium channel GIRK4 (encoded by *KCNJ5*; identified as cause of disease in 40% of aldosterone-producing adenomas; rare germline mutations can cause bilateral macronodular adrenal hyperplasia). Further causes include somatic mutations affecting the α-subunit of the Na^+/K^+-ATPase (encoded by *ATP1A1*), the plasma membrane calcium-transporting ATPase 3 (encoded by *ATP2B3*), and somatic or germline mutations in *CACNA1D* encoding the voltage-gated calcium channel Cav1.3. All mutations result in upregulation of CYP11B2 and hence aldosterone synthesis.	60
Bilateral (micronodular) adrenal hyperplasia	Autonomous aldosterone excess	60
Glucocorticoid-remediable hyperaldosteronism (dexamethasone-suppressible hyperaldosteronism)	Crossover between the *CYP11B1* and *CYP11B2* genes results in ACTH-driven aldosterone production	<1
Other Causes (Rare)		<1
Syndrome of apparent mineralocorticoid excess (SAME)	Mutations in *HSD11B2* result in lack of renal inactivation of cortisol to cortisone, leading to excess activation of the MR by cortisol	
Cushing's syndrome	Cortisol excess overcomes the capacity of HSD11B2 to inactivate cortisol to cortisone, consequently flooding the MR	
Glucocorticoid resistance	Upregulation of cortisol production due to GR mutations results in flooding of the MR by cortisol	
Adrenocortical carcinoma	Autonomous aldosterone and/or DOC excess	
Congenital adrenal hyperplasia	Accumulation of DOC due to mutations in *CYP11B1* or *CYP17A1*	
Progesterone-induced hypertension	Progesterone acts as an abnormal ligand due to mutations in the MR gene	
Liddle's syndrome	Mutant ENaC β or γ subunits resulting in reduced degradation of ENaC keeping the membrane channel in open conformation for longer, enhancing mineralocorticoid action	

Abbreviations: ACTH, adrenocorticotropic hormone; DOC, deoxycorticosterone; ENaC, epithelial sodium channel; GR, glucocorticoid receptor; HSD11B2, 11β-hydroxysteroid dehydrogenase type 2; MR, mineralocorticoid receptor.

from cross-over of promoter sequences between the *CYP11B1* and *CYP11B2* genes that are involved in glucocorticoid and mineralocorticoid synthesis, respectively (Fig. 406-1). This rearrangement brings *CYP11B2* transcription under the control of ACTH receptor signaling; consequently, aldosterone production is regulated by ACTH rather than by renin. The family history can be helpful because there may be evidence for dominant transmission of hypertension. Recognition of the disorder is important because it can be associated with early-onset hypertension and strokes. In addition, glucocorticoid suppression can reduce aldosterone production.

Other rare causes of mineralocorticoid excess are listed in Table 406-3. An important cause is excess binding and activation of the mineralocorticoid receptor by a steroid other than aldosterone. Cortisol acts as a potent mineralocorticoid if it escapes efficient inactivation to cortisone by 11β-HSD2 in the kidney (Fig. 406-7). This can be caused by inactivating mutations in the *HSD11B2* gene resulting in the syndrome of apparent mineralocorticoid excess (SAME) that characteristically manifests with severe hypokalemic hypertension in childhood. However, milder mutations may cause normokalemic hypertension manifesting in adulthood (type II SAME). Inhibition of 11β-HSD2 by excess licorice ingestion also results in hypokalemic hypertension, as does overwhelming of 11β-HSD2 conversion capacity by cortisol excess in Cushing's syndrome. Deoxycorticosterone (DOC) also binds and activates the mineralocorticoid receptor and can cause hypertension if its circulating concentrations are increased. This can arise through autonomous DOC secretion by an adrenocortical carcinoma, but also when DOC accumulates as a consequence of an adrenal enzymatic block, as seen in congenital adrenal hyperplasia due to CYP11B1 (11β hydroxylase) or CYP17A1 (17α-hydroxylase) deficiency (Fig. 406-1). Progesterone can cause hypokalemic hypertension in rare individuals who harbor a mineralocorticoid receptor mutation that enhances binding and activation by progesterone; physiologically, progesterone normally exerts antimineralocorticoid activity. Finally, excess mineralocorticoid activity can be caused by mutations in the β or γ subunits of the ENaC, disrupting its interaction with Nedd4 (Fig. 406-7), and thereby decreasing receptor internalization and degradation. The constitutively active ENAC drives hypokalemic hypertension, resulting in an autosomal dominant disorder termed *Liddle's syndrome.*

Clinical Manifestations Excess activation of the mineralocorticoid receptor leads to potassium depletion and increased sodium retention, with the latter causing an expansion of extracellular and plasma volume. Increased ENaC activity also results in hydrogen depletion that can cause metabolic alkalosis. Aldosterone also has direct effects on the vascular system, where it increases cardiac remodeling and decreases compliance. Aldosterone excess may cause direct damage to the myocardium and the kidney glomeruli, in addition to secondary damage due to systemic hypertension.

The clinical hallmark of mineralocorticoid excess is hypokalemic hypertension; serum sodium tends to be normal due to the concurrent fluid retention, which in some cases can lead to peripheral edema. Hypokalemia can be exacerbated by thiazide drug treatment, which leads to increased delivery of sodium to the distal renal tubule, thereby driving potassium excretion. Severe hypokalemia can be associated with muscle weakness, overt proximal myopathy, or even hypokalemic paralysis. Severe alkalosis contributes to muscle cramps and, in severe cases, can cause tetany.

Diagnosis Diagnostic screening for mineralocorticoid excess is not currently recommended for all patients with hypertension, but should be restricted to those who exhibit hypertension associated with drug resistance, hypokalemia, an adrenal mass, or onset of disease before the age of 40 years (Fig. 406-12). The accepted screening test is concurrent measurement of plasma renin and aldosterone with subsequent calculation of the aldosterone-renin ratio (ARR) (Fig. 406-12); serum potassium needs to be normalized prior to testing. Stopping antihypertensive medication can be cumbersome, particularly in patients with severe hypertension. Thus, for practical purposes, in the first instance the patient can remain on the usual antihypertensive medications, with the exception that mineralocorticoid receptor antagonists need to be ceased at least 4 weeks prior to ARR measurement. The remaining antihypertensive drugs usually do not affect the outcome of ARR testing, except that beta blocker treatment can cause false-positive results and ACE/AT1R inhibitors can cause false-negative results in milder cases (Table 406-4).

ARR screening is positive if the ratio is >750 pmol/L per ng/mL per hour, with a concurrently high normal or increased aldosterone (Fig. 406-12). If one relies on the ARR only, the likelihood of a false-positive ARR becomes greater when renin levels are very low. The characteristics of the biochemical assays are also important. Some labs measure plasma renin activity, whereas others measure plasma renin concentrations. Antibody-based assays for the measurement of serum aldosterone lack the reliability of tandem mass spectrometry assays, but these are not yet ubiquitously available.

Diagnostic confirmation of mineralocorticoid excess in a patient with positive ARR screening result should be undertaken by an endocrinologist as the tests lack optimized validation. The most straightforward is the saline infusion test, which involves the IV administration of 2 L of physiologic saline over a 4-h period. Failure of aldosterone to suppress below 140 pmol/L (5 ng/dL) is indicative of autonomous mineralocorticoid excess. Alternative tests are the oral sodium loading test (300 mmol NaCl/d for 3 days) or the fludrocortisone suppression test (0.1 mg q6h with 30 mmol NaCl q8h for 4 days); the latter can be difficult because of the risk of profound hypokalemia and increased hypertension. In patients with overt hypokalemic hypertension, strongly positive ARR, and concurrently increased aldosterone levels, confirmatory testing is usually not necessary.

Differential Diagnosis and Treatment After the diagnosis of hyperaldosteronism is established, the next step is to use adrenal imaging to further assess the cause. Fine-cut CT scanning of the adrenal region is the method of choice because it provides excellent visualization of adrenal morphology. CT will readily identify larger tumors suspicious of malignancy but may miss lesions smaller than 5 mm. The differentiation between bilateral micronodular hyperplasia and a unilateral adenoma is only required if a surgical approach is feasible and desired. Consequently, selective adrenal vein sampling (AVS) should only be carried out in surgical candidates with either no obvious lesion on CT or evidence of a unilateral lesion in patients older than 40 years, because the latter patients have a high likelihood of harboring a coincidental, endocrine-inactive adrenal adenoma (Fig. 406-12). AVS is used to compare aldosterone levels in the inferior vena cava and between the right and left adrenal veins. AVS requires concurrent measurement of cortisol to document correct placement of the catheter in the adrenal veins and should demonstrate a cortisol gradient >3 between the vena cava and each adrenal vein. Lateralization is confirmed by an aldosterone/cortisol ratio that is at least twofold higher on one side than the other. AVS is a complex procedure that requires a highly skilled interventional radiologist. Even then, the right adrenal vein can be difficult to cannulate correctly, which, if not achieved, invalidates the procedure. There is also no agreement as to whether the two adrenal veins should be cannulated simultaneously or successively and whether ACTH stimulation enhances the diagnostic value of AVS.

Patients younger than 40 years with confirmed mineralocorticoid excess and a unilateral lesion on CT can go straight to surgery, which is also indicated in patients with confirmed lateralization documented by a valid AVS procedure. Laparoscopic adrenalectomy is the preferred approach. Patients who are not surgical candidates, or with evidence of bilateral hyperplasia based on CT or AVS, should be treated medically (Fig. 406-12). Medical treatment, which can also be considered prior to surgery to avoid postsurgical hypoaldosteronism, consists primarily of the mineralocorticoid receptor antagonist spironolactone. It can be started at 12.5–50 mg bid and titrated up to a maximum of 400 mg/d to control blood pressure and normalize potassium. Side effects include menstrual irregularity, decreased libido, and gynecomastia. The more selective MR antagonist eplerenone can also be used. Doses start at 25 mg bid, and it can be titrated up to 200 mg/d. Another useful drug is the sodium channel blocker amiloride (5–10 mg bid).

In patients with normal adrenal morphology and family history of early-onset, severe hypertension, a diagnosis of GRA should be

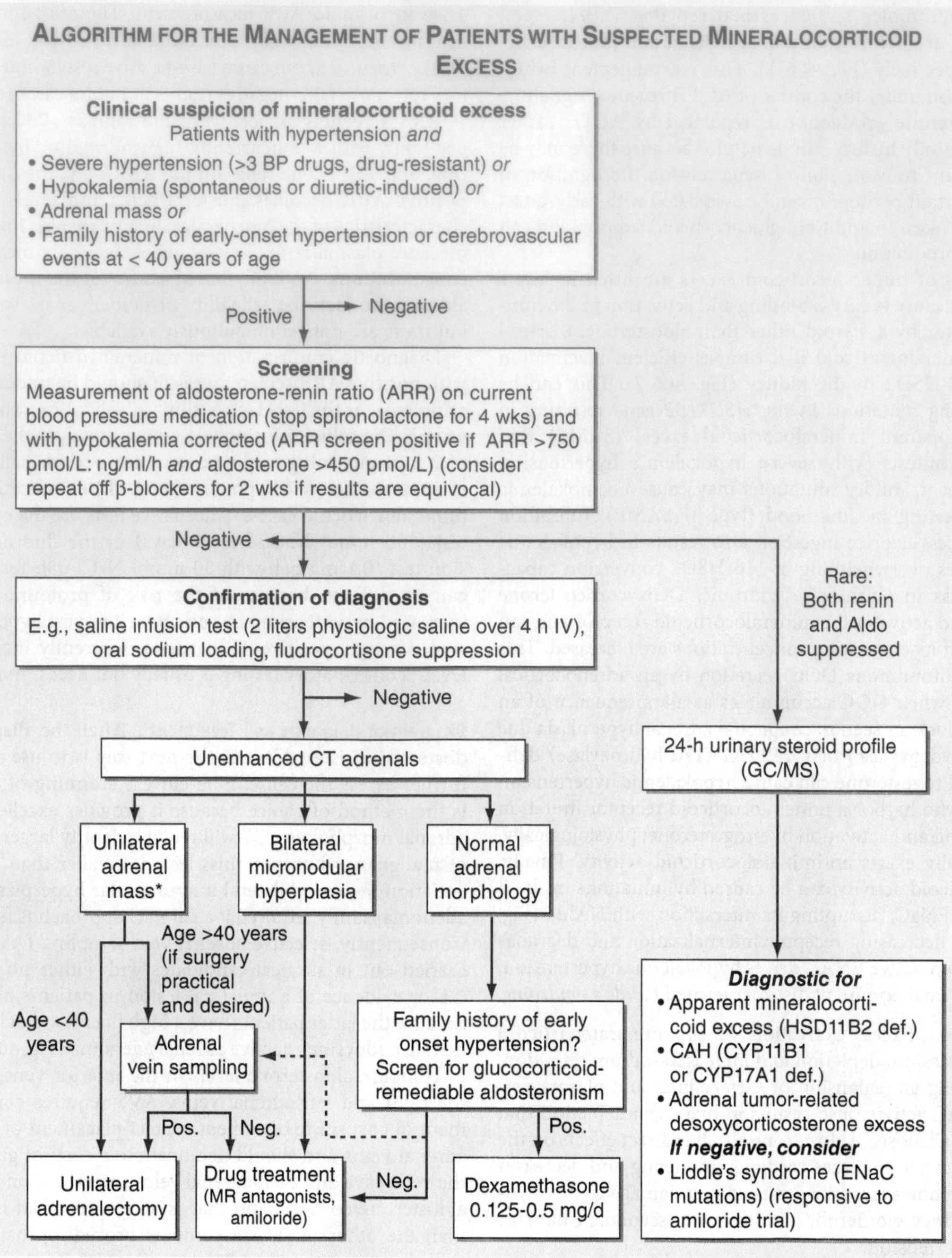

ALGORITHM FOR THE MANAGEMENT OF PATIENTS WITH SUSPECTED MINERALOCORTICOID EXCESS

Clinical suspicion of mineralocorticoid excess
Patients with hypertension *and*
- Severe hypertension (>3 BP drugs, drug-resistant) *or*
- Hypokalemia (spontaneous or diuretic-induced) *or*
- Adrenal mass *or*
- Family history of early-onset hypertension or cerebrovascular events at < 40 years of age

Positive → Negative

Screening
Measurement of aldosterone-renin ratio (ARR) on current blood pressure medication (stop spironolactone for 4 wks) and with hypokalemia corrected (ARR screen positive if ARR >750 pmol/L: ng/ml/h *and* aldosterone >450 pmol/L) (consider repeat off β-blockers for 2 wks if results are equivocal)

Negative

Confirmation of diagnosis
E.g., saline infusion test (2 liters physiologic saline over 4 h IV), oral sodium loading, fludrocortisone suppression

Rare: Both renin and Aldo suppressed

Negative

Unenhanced CT adrenals

24-h urinary steroid profile (GC/MS)

Unilateral adrenal mass*

Bilateral micronodular hyperplasia

Normal adrenal morphology

Age >40 years (if surgery practical and desired)

Age <40 years

Adrenal vein sampling

Family history of early onset hypertension? Screen for glucocorticoid-remediable aldosteronism

Diagnostic for
- Apparent mineralocorticoid excess (HSD11B2 def.)
- CAH (CYP11B1 or CYP17A1 def.)
- Adrenal tumor-related desoxycorticosterone excess

If negative, consider
- Liddle's syndrome (ENaC mutations) (responsive to amiloride trial)

Pos. Neg.

Pos.

Neg.

Unilateral adrenalectomy

Drug treatment (MR antagonists, amiloride)

Dexamethasone 0.125-0.5 mg/d

FIGURE 406-12 Management of patients with suspected mineralocorticoid excess. *Perform adrenal tumor workup (see Fig. 406-13). BP, blood pressure; CAH, congenital adrenal hyperplasia; CT, computed tomography; GC/MS, gas chromatography/mass spectrometry; PRA, plasma renin activity.

TABLE 406-4 EFFECTS OF ANTIHYPERTENSIVE DRUGS ON THE ALDOSTERONE-RENIN-RATIO (ARR)

Drug	Effect on Renin	Effect on Aldosterone	Net Effect on ARR
β Blockers	↓	↑	↑
α_1 Blockers	→	→	→
α_2 Sympathomimetics	→	→	→
ACE inhibitors	↑	↓	↓
AT1R blockers	↑	↓	↓
Calcium antagonists	→	→	→
Diuretics	(↑)	(↑)	→/(↓)

Abbreviations: ACE, angiotensin-converting enzyme; AT1R, angiotensin II receptor type 1.

considered and can be evaluated using genetic testing. Treatment of GRA consists of administering dexamethasone, using the lowest dose possible to control blood pressure. Some patients also require additional MR antagonist treatment.

The diagnosis of nonaldosterone-related mineralocorticoid excess is based on documentation of suppressed renin and suppressed aldosterone in the presence of hypokalemic hypertension. This testing is best carried out by employing urinary steroid metabolite profiling by gas chromatography/mass spectrometry (GC/MS). An increased free cortisol over free cortisone ratio is suggestive of SAME and can be treated with dexamethasone. Steroid profiling by GC/MS also detects the steroids associated with CYP11B1 and CYP17A1 deficiency or the irregular steroid secretion pattern in a DOC-producing adrenocortical carcinoma (Fig. 406-12). If the GC/MS profile is normal, then Liddle's syndrome should be considered. It is very sensitive to amiloride treatment but will not respond to MR antagonist treatment, because the defect is due to a constitutively active ENaC.

APPROACH TO THE PATIENT: INCIDENTALLY DISCOVERED ADRENAL MASS

Epidemiology Incidentally discovered adrenal masses, commonly termed adrenal "incidentalomas," are common, with a prevalence of at least 2% in the general population as documented in CT and autopsy series. The prevalence increases with age, with 1% of 40-year-olds and 7% of 70-year-olds harboring an adrenal mass.

Etiology Most solitary adrenal tumors are monoclonal neoplasms. Several genetic syndromes, including MEN 1 (*MEN1*), MEN 2 (*RET*), Carney's complex (*PRKAR1A*), and McCune-Albright (*GNAS1*), can have adrenal tumors as one of their features. Somatic mutations in *MEN1*, *GNAS1*, and *PRKAR1A* have been identified in a small proportion of sporadic adrenocortical adenomas. Aberrant expression of membrane receptors (gastric inhibitory peptide, α- and β-adrenergic, luteinizing hormone, vasopressin V1, and interleukin 1 receptors) have been identified in some sporadic cases of macronodular adrenocortical hyperplasia.

The majority of adrenal nodules are endocrine-inactive adrenocortical adenomas. However, larger series suggest that up to 25% of adrenal nodules are hormonally active, due to a cortisol- or aldosterone-producing adrenocortical adenoma or a pheochromocytoma associated with catecholamine excess (Table 406-5). Adrenocortical carcinoma is rare but is the cause of an adrenal mass in 5% of patients. However, the most common cause of a malignant adrenal mass is metastasis originating from another solid tissue tumor (Table 406-5).

Differential Diagnosis and Treatment Patients with an adrenal mass >1 cm require a diagnostic evaluation. Two key questions need to be addressed: (1) Does the tumor autonomously secrete hormones that could have a detrimental effect on health? (2) Is the adrenal mass benign or malignant?

Hormone secretion by an adrenal mass occurs along a continuum, with a gradual increase in clinical manifestations in parallel with hormone levels. Exclusion of catecholamine excess from a pheochromocytoma arising from the adrenal medulla is a mandatory part of the diagnostic workup (Fig. 406-13). Furthermore, autonomous cortisol and aldosterone secretion resulting in Cushing's syndrome or primary aldosteronism, respectively, require exclusion. Adrenal incidentalomas can be associated with lower levels of autonomous cortisol secretion, and patients may lack overt clinical features of Cushing's syndrome. Nonetheless, they may exhibit one or more components of the metabolic syndrome (e.g., obesity, type 2 diabetes, or hypertension). There is ongoing debate about the optimal treatment for these patients with mild or subclinical Cushing's syndrome. Overproduction of adrenal androgen precursors, DHEA and its sulfate, is rare and most frequently seen in the context of adrenocortical carcinoma, as are increased levels of steroid precursors such as 17-hydroxyprogesterone.

For the differentiation of benign from malignant adrenal masses, imaging is relatively sensitive, although specificity is suboptimal. CT is the procedure of choice for imaging the adrenal glands (Fig. 406-11). The risk of adrenocortical carcinoma, pheochromocytoma, and benign adrenal myelolipoma increases with the diameter of the adrenal mass. However, size alone is of poor predictive value, with only 80% sensitivity and 60% specificity for the differentiation of benign from malignant masses when using a 4-cm cut-off. Metastases are found with similar frequency in adrenal masses of all sizes. Tumor density on unenhanced CT is of additional diagnostic value, with most adrenocortical adenomas being lipid rich and thus presenting with low attenuation values (i.e., densities of <10 HU). By contrast, adrenocortical carcinomas, but also pheochromocytomas, usually have high attenuation values (i.e., densities >20 HU on precontrast scans). Generally, benign lesions are rounded and homogenous, whereas most malignant lesions appear lobulated and inhomogeneous. Pheochromocytoma and adrenomyelolipoma may also exhibit lobulated and inhomogeneous features. Additional information can be obtained from CT by assessment of contrast wash-out after 15 min, which is >50% in benign lesions but <40% in malignant lesions, which usually have a more extensive vascularization. MRI also allows for the visualization of the adrenal glands with somewhat lower resolution than CT. However, because it does not involve exposure to ionizing radiation, it is preferred in children, young adults, and during pregnancy. MRI has a valuable role in the characterization of indeterminate adrenal lesions using chemical shift analysis, with malignant tumors rarely showing loss of signal on opposed-phase MRI.

Fine-needle aspiration (FNA) or CT-guided biopsy of an adrenal mass is almost never indicated. FNA of a pheochromocytoma can cause a life-threatening hypertensive crisis. FNA of an adrenocortical carcinoma violates the tumor capsule and can cause needle track metastasis. FNA should only be considered in a patient with a history of nonadrenal malignancy and a newly detected adrenal mass, after careful exclusion of pheochromocytoma, and if the outcome will influence therapeutic management. It is important to recognize that in 25% of patients with a previous history of nonadrenal malignancy, a newly detected mass on CT is not a metastasis.

Adrenal masses associated with confirmed hormone excess or suspected malignancy are usually treated surgically (Fig. 406-13) or, if adrenalectomy is not feasible or desired, with medication. Preoperative exclusion of glucocorticoid excess is particularly important for the prediction of postoperative suppression of the contralateral adrenal gland, which requires glucocorticoid replacement peri- and postoperatively. If the initial decision is for observation, imaging and biochemical testing should be repeated about a year after the first assessment. However, this may be performed earlier in patients with borderline imaging or hormonal findings. There is no agreement with regard to the required long-term follow-up beyond 1 year in patients with normal biochemistry and no evidence of increased tumor size at follow-up.

TABLE 406-5 CLASSIFICATION OF UNILATERAL ADRENAL MASSES

Mass	Approximate Prevalence (%)
Benign	
Adrenocortical adenoma	
Endocrine-inactive	60–85
Cortisol-producing	5–10
Aldosterone-producing	2–5
Pheochromocytoma	5–10
Adrenal myelolipoma	<1
Adrenal ganglioneuroma	<0.1
Adrenal hemangioma	<0.1
Adrenal cyst	<1
Adrenal hematoma/hemorrhagic infarction	<1
Indeterminate	
Adrenocortical oncocytoma	<1
Malignant	
Adrenocortical carcinoma	2–5
Malignant pheochromocytoma	<1
Adrenal neuroblastoma	<0.1
Lymphomas (including primary adrenal lymphoma)	<1
Metastases (most frequent: breast, lung)	15

Note: Bilateral adrenal enlargement/masses may be caused by congenital adrenal hyperplasia, bilateral macronodular hyperplasia, bilateral hemorrhage (due to antiphospholipid syndrome or sepsis-associated Waterhouse-Friderichsen syndrome), granuloma, amyloidosis, or infiltrative disease including tuberculosis.

ADRENOCORTICAL CARCINOMA

Adrenocortical carcinoma (ACC) is a rare malignancy with an annual incidence of 1–2 per million population. ACC is generally considered a highly malignant tumor; however, it presents with broad interindividual variability with regard to biologic characteristics and clinical behavior. Somatic mutations in the tumor-suppressor gene *TP53* are found in 25% of apparently sporadic ACC. Germline *TP53* mutations are the cause of the Li-Fraumeni syndrome associated with multiple solid organ cancers including ACC and are found in 25% of pediatric

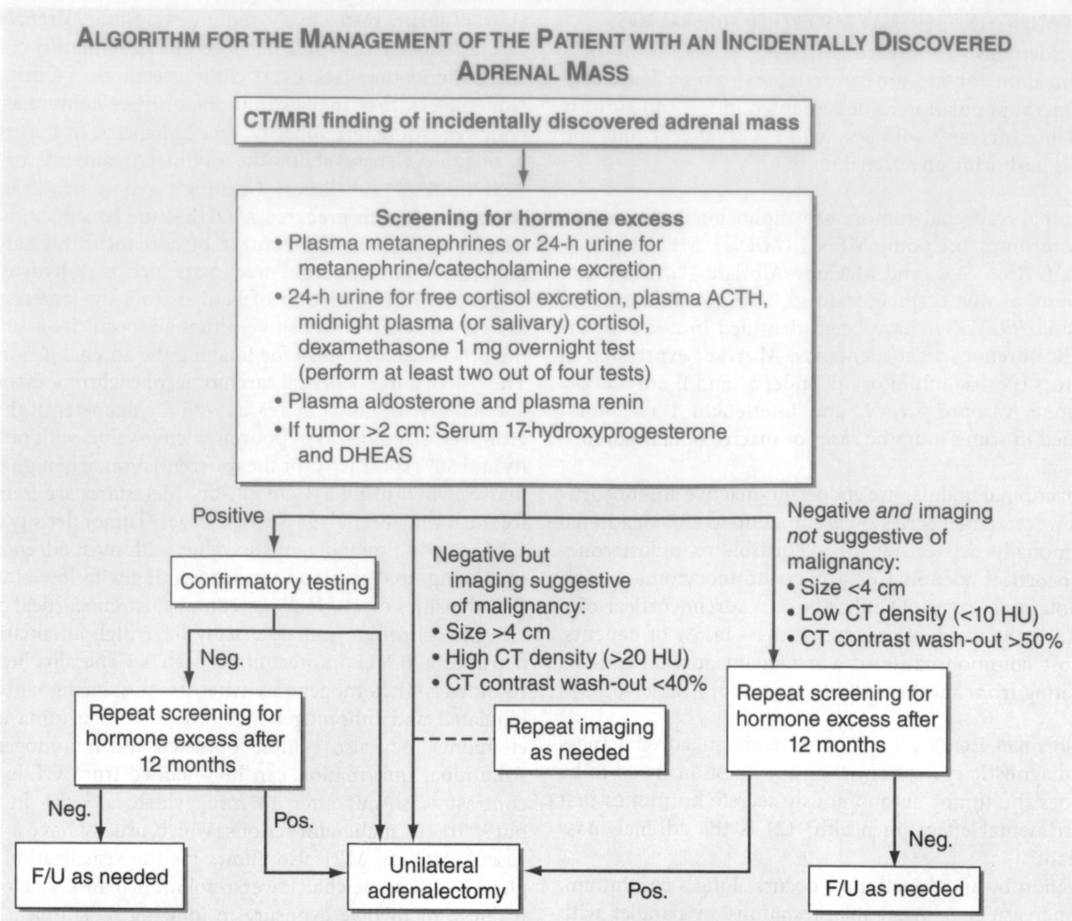

FIGURE 406-13 Management of the patient with an incidentally discovered adrenal mass. CT, computed tomography; F/U, follow-up; MRI, magnetic resonance imaging.

ACC cases; the *TP53* mutation R337H is found in almost all pediatric ACC in Brazil. Other genetic changes identified in ACC include alterations in the Wnt/β-catenin pathway and in the insulin-like growth factor 2 (IGF2) cluster; IGF2 overexpression is found in 90% of ACC.

Patients with large adrenal tumors suspicious of malignancy should be managed by a multidisciplinary specialist team, including an endocrinologist, an oncologist, a surgeon, a radiologist, and a histopathologist. FNA is not indicated in suspected ACC: first, cytology and also histopathology of a core biopsy cannot differentiate between benign and malignant primary adrenal masses; second, FNA violates the tumor capsule and may even cause needle canal metastasis. Even when the entire tumor specimen is available, the histopathologic differentiation between benign and malignant lesions is a diagnostic challenge. The most common histopathologic classification is the Weiss score, taking into account high nuclear grade; mitotic rate (>5/HPF); atypical mitosis; <25% clear cells; diffuse architecture; and presence of necrosis, venous invasion, and invasion of sinusoidal structures and tumor capsule. The presence of three or more elements suggests ACC.

Although 60–70% of ACCs show biochemical evidence of steroid overproduction, in many patients, this is not clinically apparent due to the relatively inefficient steroid production by the adrenocortical cancer cells. Excess production of glucocorticoids and adrenal androgen precursors are most common. Mixed excess production of several corticosteroid classes by an adrenal tumor is generally indicative of malignancy.

Tumor staging at diagnosis (Table 406-6) has important prognostic implications and requires scanning of the chest and abdomen for local organ invasion, lymphadenopathy, and metastases. Intravenous contrast medium is necessary for maximum sensitivity for hepatic metastases. An adrenal origin may be difficult to determine on standard axial CT imaging if the tumors are large and invasive, but CT reconstructions and MRI are more informative (Fig. 406-14) using multiple planes and different sequences. Vascular and adjacent organ invasion is diagnostic of malignancy. 18-Fluoro-2-deoxy-D-glucose positron emission tomography (18-FDG PET) is highly sensitive for the detection of malignancy and can be used to detect small metastases or local recurrence that may not be obvious on CT (Fig. 406-14). However, FDG PET is not specific and therefore cannot be used for differentiating benign from malignant adrenal lesions. Metastasis in ACC most frequently occurs to liver and lung.

There is no established grading system for ACC, and the Weiss score carries no prognostic value; the most important prognostic histopathologic parameter is the Ki67 proliferation index, with Ki67 <10% indicative of slow to moderate growth velocity, whereas a Ki67 ≥10% is associated with poor prognosis including high risk of recurrence and rapid progression.

Cure of ACC can only be achieved by early detection and complete surgical removal. Capsule violation during primary surgery, metastasis at diagnosis, and primary treatment in a nonspecialist center are major determinants of poor survival. If the primary tumor invades adjacent organs, en bloc removal of kidney and spleen should be considered to reduce the risk of recurrence. Surgery can also be considered in a patient with metastases if there is severe tumor-related hormone excess. This indication needs to be carefully weighed against surgical risk, including thromboembolic complications, and the resulting delay in the introduction of other therapeutic options. Patients with confirmed ACC and successful removal of the primary tumor should receive adjuvant treatment with mitotane (o,p'DDD), particularly in patients with a high risk of recurrence as determined by tumor size >8 cm, histopathologic signs of vascular invasion, capsule invasion or violation, and a Ki67 proliferation index ≥10%. Adjuvant mitotane should be continued for at least 2 years, if the patient can tolerate side effects. Regular monitoring of plasma mitotane levels is mandatory (therapeutic range 14–20 mg/L; neurotoxic complications more frequent at >20 mg/L). Mitotane is usually started at 500 mg tid, with stepwise increases to a maximum dose of 2000 mg tid

TABLE 406-6 CLASSIFICATION SYSTEM FOR STAGING OF ADRENOCORTICAL CARCINOMA

ENSAT Stage	TNM Stage	TNM Definitions
I	T1,N0,M0	T1, tumor ≤5 cm N0, no positive lymph node M0, no distant metastases
II	T2,N0,M0	T2, tumor >5 cm N0, no positive lymph node M0, no distant metastases
III	T1–T2,N1,M0 T3–T4,N0–N1,M0	N1, positive lymph node(s) M0, no distant metastases T3, tumor infiltration into surrounding tissue T4, tumor invasion into adjacent organs *or* venous tumor thrombus in vena cava or renal vein
IV	T1–T4,N0–N1,M1	M1, presence of distant metastases

Abbreviations: ENSAT, European Network for the Study of Adrenal Tumors; TNM, tumor, node, metastasis.

in days (high-dose saturation) or weeks (low-dose saturation) as tolerated. Once therapeutic range plasma mitotane levels are achieved, the dose can be tapered to maintenance doses mostly ranging from 1000 to 1500 mg tid. Mitotane treatment results in disruption of cortisol synthesis and thus requires glucocorticoid replacement; glucocorticoid replacement dose should be at least double of that usually used in adrenal insufficiency (i.e., 20 mg tid) because mitotane induces hepatic CYP3A4 activity resulting in rapid inactivation of glucocorticoids. Mitotane also increases circulating CBG, thereby decreasing the available free cortisol fraction. Single metastases can be addressed surgically or with radiofrequency ablation as appropriate. If the tumor recurs or progresses during mitotane treatment, chemotherapy should be considered; the established first-line chemotherapy regimen is the combination of cisplatin, etoposide, and doxorubicin plus continuing mitotane. Painful bone metastasis responds to irradiation. Overall survival in ACC is still poor, with 5-year survival rates of 30–40% and a median survival of 15 months in metastatic ACC.

ADRENAL INSUFFICIENCY

Epidemiology The prevalence of well-documented, permanent adrenal insufficiency is 5 in 10,000 in the general population. Hypothalamic-pituitary origin of disease is most frequent, with a prevalence of 3 in 10,000, whereas primary adrenal insufficiency has a prevalence of 2 in 10,000. Approximately one-half of the latter cases are acquired, mostly caused by autoimmune destruction of the adrenal glands; the other one-half are genetic, most commonly caused by distinct enzymatic blocks in adrenal steroidogenesis affecting glucocorticoid synthesis (i.e., congenital adrenal hyperplasia.)

Adrenal insufficiency arising from suppression of the HPA axis as a consequence of exogenous glucocorticoid treatment is much more common, occurring in 0.5–2% of the population in developed countries.

Etiology *Primary adrenal insufficiency* is most commonly caused by autoimmune adrenalitis. Isolated autoimmune adrenalitis accounts for 30–40%, whereas 60–70% develop adrenal insufficiency as part of autoimmune polyglandular syndromes (APS) (Chap. 408) (Table 406-7). APS1, also termed APECED (autoimmune polyendocrinopathy-candidiasis-ectodermal dystrophy), is the underlying cause in 10% of patients affected by APS. APS1 is transmitted in an autosomal recessive manner and is caused by mutations in the autoimmune regulator gene *AIRE*. Associated autoimmune conditions overlap with those seen in APS2, but may also include total alopecia, primary hypoparathyroidism, and, in rare cases, lymphoma. APS1 patients invariably develop chronic mucocutaneous candidiasis, usually manifest in childhood, and preceding adrenal insufficiency by years or decades. The much more prevalent APS2 is of polygenic inheritance, with confirmed associations with the *HLA DR3* gene region in the major histocompatibility complex and distinct gene regions involved in immune regulation (*CTLA-4, PTPN22, CLEC16A*). Coincident autoimmune disease most frequently includes thyroid autoimmune disease, vitiligo, and premature ovarian failure. Less commonly, additional features may include type 1 diabetes and pernicious anemia caused by vitamin B_{12} deficiency.

X-linked adrenoleukodystrophy has an incidence of 1:20,000 males and is caused by mutations in the *X-ALD* gene encoding the peroxisomal membrane transporter protein ABCD1; its disruption results in accumulation of very long chain (>24 carbon atoms) fatty acids. Approximately 50% of cases manifest in early childhood with rapidly progressive white matter disease (cerebral ALD); 35% present during adolescence or in early adulthood with neurologic features indicative of myelin and peripheral nervous system involvement (adrenomyeloneuropathy [AMN]). In the remaining 15%, adrenal insufficiency is the sole manifestation of disease. Of note, distinct mutations manifest with variable penetrance and phenotypes within affected families.

Rarer causes of adrenal insufficiency involve destruction of the adrenal glands as a consequence of infection, hemorrhage, or infiltration

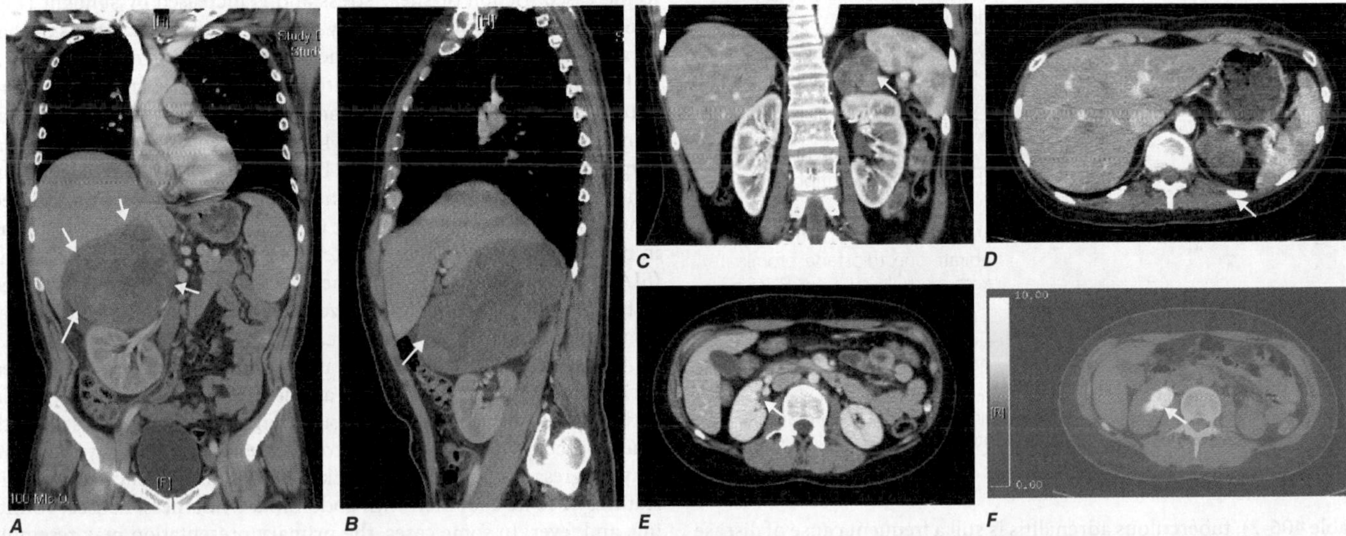

FIGURE 406-14 Imaging in adrenocortical carcinoma. Magnetic resonance imaging scan with (*A*) frontal and (*B*) lateral views of a right adrenocortical carcinoma that was detected incidentally. Computed tomography (CT) scan with (*C*) coronal and (*D*) transverse views depicting a right-sided adrenocortical carcinoma. Note the irregular border and inhomogeneous structure. CT scan (*E*) and positron emission tomography/CT (*F*) visualizing a peritoneal metastasis of an adrenocortical carcinoma in close proximity to the right kidney (*arrow*).

TABLE 406-7 CAUSES OF PRIMARY ADRENAL INSUFFICIENCY

Diagnosis	Gene	Associated Features
Autoimmune polyglandular syndrome 1 (APS1)	*AIRE*	Hypoparathyroidism, chronic mucocutaneous candidiasis, other autoimmune disorders, rarely lymphomas
Autoimmune polyglandular syndrome 2 (APS2)	Associations with HLA-DR3, CTLA-4	Hypothyroidism, hyperthyroidism, premature ovarian failure, vitiligo, type 1 diabetes mellitus, pernicious anemia
Isolated autoimmune adrenalitis	Associations with HLA-DR3, CTLA-4	
Congenital adrenal hyperplasia (CAH)	*CYP21A2, CYP11B1, CYP17A1, HSD3B2, POR*	See Table 406-10 (see also Chap. 410)
Congenital lipoid adrenal hyperplasia (CLAH)	*STAR, CYP11A1*	46,XY DSD, gonadal failure (see also Chap. 410)
Adrenal hypoplasia congenita (AHC)	*NR0B1 (DAX-1), NR5A1 (SF-1)*	46,XY DSD, gonadal failure (see also Chap. 410)
Adrenoleukodystrophy (ALD), adrenomyeloneuropathy (AMN)	*X-ALD*	Demyelination of central nervous system (ALD) or spinal cord and peripheral nerves (AMN)
Familial glucocorticoid deficiency	*MC2R*	Tall stature
	MRAP	None
	STAR	None
	NNT	None
	MCM4	Growth retardation, natural killer cell deficiency
Triple A syndrome	*AAAS*	Alacrima, achalasia, neurologic impairment
Smith-Lemli-Opitz syndrome	*SLOS*	Cholesterol synthesis disorder associated with mental retardation, craniofacial malformations, growth failure
Kearns-Sayre syndrome	Mitochondrial DNA deletions	Progressive external ophthalmoplegia, pigmentary retinal degeneration, cardiac conduction defects, gonadal failure, hypoparathyroidism, type 1 diabetes,
IMAGe syndrome	*CDKN1C*	Intrauterine growth retardation, metaphyseal dysplasia, genital anomalies
Adrenal infections		Tuberculosis, HIV, CMV, cryptococcosis, histoplasmosis, coccidioidomycosis
Adrenal infiltration		Metastases, lymphomas, sarcoidosis, amyloidosis, hemochromatosis
Adrenal hemorrhage		Meningococcal sepsis (Waterhouse-Friderichsen syndrome), primary antiphospholipid syndrome
Drug-induced		Mitotane, aminoglutethimide, abiraterone, trilostane, etomidate, ketoconazole, suramin, RU486
Bilateral adrenalectomy		E.g., in the management of Cushing's or after bilateral nephrectomy

Abbreviations: AIRE, autoimmune regulator; CMV, cytomegalovirus; DSD, disordered sex development; MC2R, ACTH receptor; MCM4, mini chromosome maintenance-deficient 4 homologue; MRAP, MC2R-accessory protein; NNT, nicotinamide nucleotide transhydrogenase.

(Table 406-7); tuberculous adrenalitis is still a frequent cause of disease in developing countries. Adrenal metastases rarely cause adrenal insufficiency, and this occurs only with bilateral, bulky metastases.

Inborn causes of primary adrenal insufficiency other than congenital adrenal hyperplasia are rare, causing less than 1% of cases. However, their elucidation provides important insights into adrenal gland development and physiology. Mutations causing primary adrenal insufficiency (Table 406-7) include factors regulating adrenal development and steroidogenesis (DAX-1, SF-1), cholesterol synthesis, import and cleavage (DHCR7, StAR, CYP11A1), and elements of the adrenal ACTH response pathway (MC2R, MRAP) (Fig. 406-5), and factors involved in redox regulation (NNT) and DNA repair (MCM4, CDKN1C).

Secondary adrenal insufficiency is the consequence of dysfunction of the hypothalamic-pituitary component of the HPA axis (Table 406-8). Excluding iatrogenic suppression, the overwhelming majority of cases are caused by pituitary or hypothalamic tumors or their treatment by surgery or irradiation (Chap. 403). Rarer causes include pituitary apoplexy, either as a consequence of an infarcted pituitary adenoma or transient reduction in the blood supply of the pituitary during surgery or after rapid blood loss associated with parturition, also termed Sheehan's syndrome. Isolated ACTH deficiency is rarely caused by autoimmune disease or pituitary infiltration (Table 406-8). Mutations in the ACTH precursor POMC or in factors regulating pituitary development are genetic causes of ACTH deficiency (Table 406-8).

Clinical Manifestations In principle, the clinical features of primary adrenal insufficiency (Addison's disease) are characterized by the loss of both glucocorticoid and mineralocorticoid secretion (Table 406-9). In secondary adrenal insufficiency, only glucocorticoid deficiency is present, as the adrenal itself is intact and thus still amenable to regulation by the RAA system. Adrenal androgen secretion is disrupted in both primary and secondary adrenal insufficiency (Table 406-9). Hypothalamic-pituitary disease can lead to additional clinical manifestations due to involvement of other endocrine axes (thyroid, gonads, growth hormone, prolactin) or visual impairment with bitemporal hemianopia caused by chiasmal compression. It is important to recognize that iatrogenic adrenal insufficiency caused by exogenous glucocorticoid suppression of the HPA axis may result in all symptoms associated with glucocorticoid deficiency (Table 406-9), if exogenous glucocorticoids are stopped abruptly. However, patients will appear clinically cushingoid as a result of the preceding overexposure to glucocorticoids.

Chronic adrenal insufficiency manifests with relatively nonspecific signs and symptoms such as fatigue and loss of energy, often resulting in delayed or missed diagnoses (e.g., as depression or anorexia). A distinguishing feature of primary adrenal insufficiency is hyperpigmentation, which is caused by excess ACTH stimulation of melanocytes. Hyperpigmentation is most pronounced in skin areas exposed to increased friction or shear stress and is increased by sunlight (Fig. 406-15). Conversely, in secondary adrenal insufficiency, the skin has an alabaster-like paleness due to lack of ACTH secretion.

Hyponatremia is a characteristic biochemical feature in primary adrenal insufficiency and is found in 80% of patients at presentation. Hyperkalemia is present in 40% of patients at initial diagnosis. Hyponatremia is primarily caused by mineralocorticoid deficiency but can also occur in secondary adrenal insufficiency due to diminished inhibition of antidiuretic hormone (ADH) release by cortisol, resulting in mild syndrome of inappropriate secretion of antidiuretic hormone (SIADH). Glucocorticoid deficiency also results in slightly increased TSH concentrations that normalize within days to weeks after initiation of glucocorticoid replacement.

Acute adrenal insufficiency usually occurs after a prolonged period of nonspecific complaints and is more frequently observed in patients with primary adrenal insufficiency, due to the loss of both glucocorticoid and mineralocorticoid secretion. Postural hypotension may progress to hypovolemic shock. Adrenal insufficiency may mimic features of acute abdomen with abdominal tenderness, nausea, vomiting, and fever. In some cases, the primary presentation may resemble neurologic disease, with decreased responsiveness, progressing to stupor and coma. An adrenal crisis can be triggered by an intercurrent illness, surgical or other stress, or increased glucocorticoid inactivation (e.g., hyperthyroidism).

TABLE 406-8 CAUSES OF SECONDARY ADRENAL INSUFFICIENCY

Diagnosis	Gene	Associated Features
Pituitary tumors (endocrine active and inactive adenomas, very rare: carcinoma)		Depending on tumor size and location: visual field impairment (bilateral hemianopia), hyperprolactinemia, secondary hypothyroidism, hypogonadism, growth hormone deficiency
Other mass lesions affecting the hypothalamic-pituitary region		Craniopharyngioma, meningioma, ependymoma, metastases
Pituitary irradiation		Radiotherapy administered for pituitary tumors, brain tumors, or craniospinal irradiation in leukemia
Autoimmune hypophysitis		Often associated with pregnancy; may present with panhypopituitarism or isolated ACTH deficiency; can be associated with autoimmune thyroid disease, more rarely with vitiligo, premature ovarian failure, type 1 diabetes, pernicious anemia
Pituitary apoplexy/hemorrhage		Hemorrhagic infarction of large pituitary adenomas or pituitary infarction consequent to traumatic major blood loss (e.g., surgery or pregnancy: Sheehan's syndrome)
Pituitary infiltration		Tuberculosis, actinomycosis, sarcoidosis, histiocytosis X, granulomatosis with polyangiitis (Wegener's), metastases
Drug-induced		Chronic glucocorticoid excess (endogenous or exogenous)
Congenital isolated ACTH deficiency	*TBX19* (Tpit)	
Combined pituitary hormone deficiency (CPHD)	*PROP-1*	Progressive development of CPHD in the order GH, PRL, TSH, LH/FSH, ACTH
	HESX1	CPHD and septo-optic dysplasia
	LHX3	CPHD and limited neck rotation, sensorineural deafness
	LHX4	CPHD and cerebellar abnormalities
	SOX3	CPHD and variable mental retardation
Proopiomelanocortin (POMC) deficiency	*POMC*	Early-onset obesity, red hair pigmentation

Abbreviations: ACTH, adrenocorticotropic hormone; GH, growth hormone; LH/FSH, luteinizing hormone/follicle-stimulating hormone; PRL, prolactin; TSH, thyroid-stimulating hormone.

Diagnosis The diagnosis of adrenal insufficiency is established by the short cosyntropin test, a safe and reliable tool with excellent predictive diagnostic value (Fig. 406-16). The cut-off for failure is usually defined at cortisol levels of <500–550 nmol/L (18–20 μg/dL) sampled 30–60 min after ACTH stimulation; the exact cut-off is dependent on the locally available assay. During the early phase of HPA disruption (e.g., within 4 weeks of pituitary insufficiency), patients may still respond to exogenous ACTH stimulation. In this circumstance, the ITT is an alternative choice but is more invasive and should be carried out only under a specialist's supervision (see above). Induction of hypoglycemia is contraindicated in individuals with diabetes mellitus, cardiovascular disease, or history of seizures. Random serum cortisol measurements are of limited diagnostic value, because baseline cortisol levels may be coincidentally low due to the physiologic diurnal rhythm of cortisol secretion (Fig. 406-3). Similarly, many patients with secondary adrenal insufficiency have relatively normal baseline cortisol levels but fail to mount an appropriate cortisol response to ACTH, which can only be revealed by stimulation testing. Importantly, tests to establish the diagnosis of adrenal insufficiency should never delay treatment. Thus, in a patient with suspected adrenal crisis, it is reasonable to draw baseline cortisol levels, provide replacement therapy, and defer formal stimulation testing until a later time.

TABLE 406-9 SIGNS AND SYMPTOMS OF ADRENAL INSUFFICIENCY

Signs and Symptoms Caused by Glucocorticoid Deficiency
TB>Fatigue, lack of energy
Weight loss, anorexia
Myalgia, joint pain
Fever
Normochromic anemia, lymphocytosis, eosinophilia
Slightly increased TSH (due to loss of feedback inhibition of TSH release)
Hypoglycemia (more frequent in children)
Low blood pressure, postural hypotension
Hyponatremia (due to loss of feedback inhibition of AVP release)
Signs and Symptoms Caused by Mineralocorticoid Deficiency (Primary Adrenal Insufficiency Only)
Abdominal pain, nausea, vomiting
Dizziness, postural hypotension
Salt craving
Low blood pressure, postural hypotension
Increased serum creatinine (due to volume depletion)
Hyponatremia
Hyperkalemia
Signs and Symptoms Caused by Adrenal Androgen Deficiency
Lack of energy
Dry and itchy skin (in women)
Loss of libido (in women)
Loss of axillary and pubic hair (in women)
Other Signs and Symptoms
Hyperpigmentation (primary adrenal insufficiency only) (due to excess of proopiomelanocortin [POMC]-derived peptides)
Alabaster-colored pale skin (secondary adrenal insufficiency only) (due to deficiency of POMC-derived peptides)

Abbreviations: AVP, arginine vasopressin; TSH, thyroid-stimulating hormone.

Once adrenal insufficiency is confirmed, measurement of plasma ACTH is the next step, with increased or inappropriately low levels defining primary and secondary origin of disease, respectively (Fig. 406-16). In primary adrenal insufficiency, increased plasma renin will confirm the presence of mineralocorticoid deficiency. At initial presentation, patients with primary adrenal insufficiency should undergo screening for steroid autoantibodies as a marker of autoimmune adrenalitis. If these tests are negative, adrenal imaging by CT is indicated to investigate possible hemorrhage, infiltration, or masses. In male patients with negative autoantibodies in the plasma, very-long-chain fatty acids should be measured to exclude X-ALD. Patients with inappropriately low ACTH, in the presence of confirmed cortisol deficiency, should undergo hypothalamic-pituitary imaging by MRI. Features suggestive of preceding pituitary apoplexy, such as sudden-onset severe headache or history of previous head trauma, should be carefully explored, particularly in patients with no obvious MRI lesion.

TREATMENT ACUTE ADRENAL INSUFFICIENCY

Acute adrenal insufficiency requires immediate initiation of rehydration, usually carried out by saline infusion at initial rates of 1 L/h with continuous cardiac monitoring. Glucocorticoid replacement should be initiated by bolus injection of 100 mg hydrocortisone, followed by the administration of 100–200 mg hydrocortisone over 24 h, either by continuous infusion or by bolus IV or IM injections. Mineralocorticoid replacement can be initiated once the daily hydrocortisone dose has been reduced to <50 mg because at higher doses hydrocortisone provides sufficient stimulation of mineralocorticoid receptors.

Glucocorticoid replacement for the treatment of chronic adrenal insufficiency should be administered at a dose that replaces the physiologic daily cortisol production, which is usually achieved by

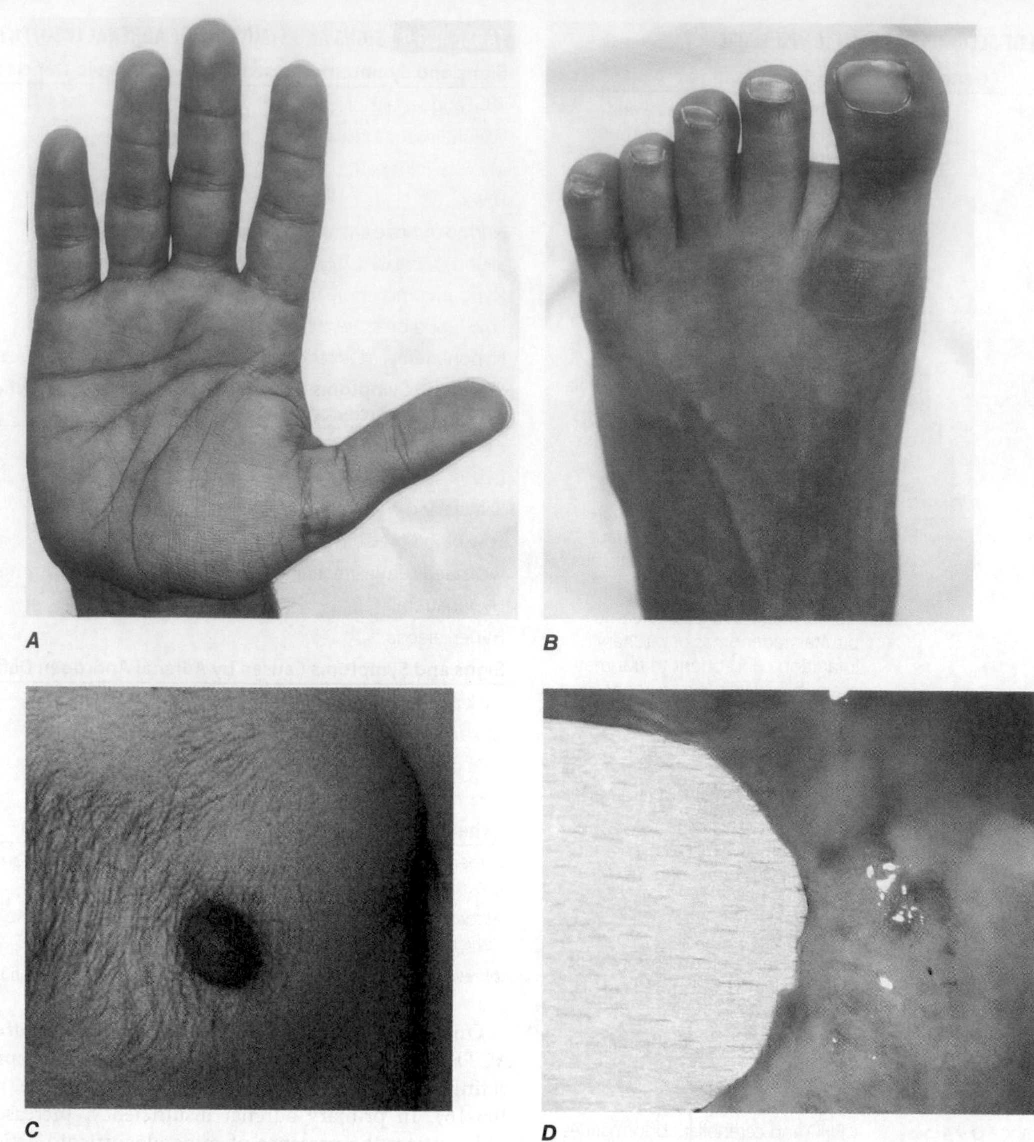

FIGURE 406-15 Clinical features of Addison's disease. Note the hyperpigmentation in areas of increased friction including (***A***) palmar creases, (***B***) dorsal foot, (***C***) nipples and axillary region, and (***D***) patchy hyperpigmentation of the oral mucosa.

the oral administration of 15–25 mg hydrocortisone in two to three divided doses. Pregnancy may require an increase in hydrocortisone dose by 50% during the last trimester. In all patients, at least one-half of the daily dose should be administered in the morning. Currently available glucocorticoid preparations fail to mimic the physiologic cortisol secretion rhythm (Fig. 406-3). Long-acting glucocorticoids such as prednisolone or dexamethasone are not preferred because they result in increased glucocorticoid exposure due to extended glucocorticoid receptor activation at times of physiologically low cortisol secretion. There are no well-established dose equivalencies, but as a guide, equipotency can be assumed for 1 mg hydrocortisone, 1.6 mg cortisone acetate, 0.2 mg prednisolone, 0.25 mg prednisone, and 0.025 mg dexamethasone.

Monitoring of glucocorticoid replacement is mainly based on the history and examination for signs and symptoms suggestive of glucocorticoid over- or underreplacement, including assessment of body weight and blood pressure. Plasma ACTH, 24-h urinary free cortisol, or serum cortisol day curves reflect whether hydrocortisone has been taken or not, but do not convey reliable information about replacement quality. In patients with isolated primary adrenal insufficiency, monitoring should include screening for autoimmune thyroid disease, and female patients should be made aware of the possibility of premature ovarian failure. Supraphysiologic glucocorticoid treatment with doses equivalent to 30 mg hydrocortisone or more will affect bone metabolism, and these patients should undergo regular bone mineral density evaluation. All patients with adrenal insufficiency need to be instructed about the requirement for stress-related glucocorticoid dose adjustments. These generally consist of doubling the routine oral glucocorticoid dose in the case of intercurrent illness with fever and bed rest and the need for IV hydrocortisone injection at a daily dose of 100 mg in cases of prolonged vomiting, surgery, or trauma. Patients living or traveling in regions with delayed access to acute health care should carry a hydrocortisone self-injection emergency kit, in addition to their usual steroid emergency cards and bracelets.

Mineralocorticoid replacement in primary adrenal insufficiency should be initiated at a dose of 100–150 μg fludrocortisone. The adequacy of treatment can be evaluated by measuring blood pressure, sitting and standing, to detect a postural drop indicative of hypovolemia. In addition, serum sodium, potassium, and plasma renin should be measured regularly. Renin levels should be kept in the upper normal reference range. Changes in glucocorticoid dose may also impact on mineralocorticoid replacement as cortisol also binds the mineralocorticoid receptor; 40 mg hydrocortisone is equivalent to 100 μg fludrocortisone. In patients living or traveling in areas with hot or tropical weather conditions, the fludrocortisone dose should be increased by 50–100 μg during the summer. Mineralocorticoid dose may also need to be adjusted during pregnancy, due to the antimineralocorticoid activity of progesterone, but this is less often required than hydrocortisone dose adjustment.

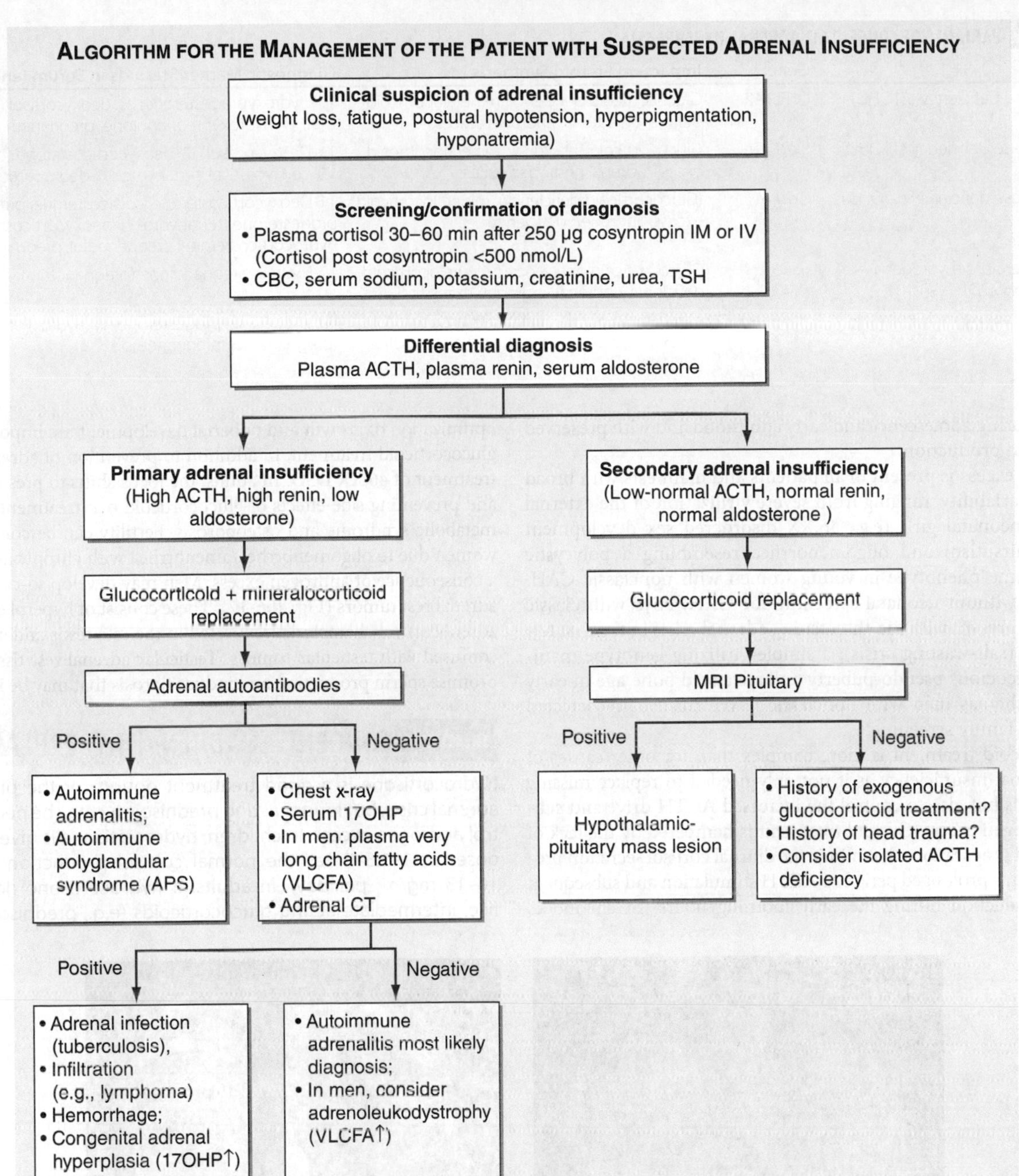

FIGURE 406-16 Management of the patient with suspected adrenal insufficiency. ACTH, adrenocorticotropic hormone; CBC, complete blood count; MRI, magnetic resonance imaging; PRA, plasma renin activity; TSH, thyroid-stimulating hormone.

Plasma renin cannot serve as a monitoring tool during pregnancy, because renin rises physiologically during gestation.

Adrenal androgen replacement is an option in patients with lack of energy, despite optimized glucocorticoid and mineralocorticoid replacement. It may also be indicated in women with features of androgen deficiency, including loss of libido. Adrenal androgen replacement can be achieved by once-daily administration of 25–50 mg DHEA. Treatment is monitored by measurement of DHEAS, androstenedione, testosterone, and sex hormone–binding globulin (SHBG) 24 h after the last DHEA dose.

CONGENITAL ADRENAL HYPERPLASIA

(See also Chap. 410) Congenital adrenal hyperplasia (CAH) is caused by mutations in genes encoding steroidogenic enzymes involved in glucocorticoid synthesis (*CYP21A2, CYP17A1, HSD3B2, CYP11B1*) or in the cofactor enzyme P450 oxidoreductase that serves as an electron donor to CYP21A2 and CYP17A1 (Fig. 406-1). Invariably, patients affected by CAH exhibit glucocorticoid deficiency. Depending on the exact step of enzymatic block, they may also have excess production of mineralocorticoids or deficient production of sex steroids (Table 406-10). The diagnosis of CAH is readily established by measurement of the steroids accumulating before the distinct enzymatic block, either in serum or in urine, preferably by the use of mass spectrometry–based assays (Table 406-10).

Mutations in *CYP21A2* are the most prevalent cause of CAH, responsible for 90–95% of cases. 21-Hydroxylase deficiency disrupts glucocorticoid and mineralocorticoid synthesis (Fig. 406-1), resulting in diminished negative feedback via the HPA axis. This leads to increased pituitary ACTH release, which drives increased synthesis of adrenal androgen precursors and subsequent androgen excess. The degree of impairment of glucocorticoid and mineralocorticoid secretion depends on the severity of mutations. Major loss-of-function mutations result in combined glucocorticoid and mineralocorticoid deficiency (classic CAH, neonatal presentation), whereas less severe mutations affect glucocorticoid synthesis only (simple virilizing CAH, neonatal or early childhood presentation). The mildest mutations result in the least severe clinical phenotype, nonclassic CAH, usually

TABLE 406-10 VARIANTS OF CONGENITAL ADRENAL HYPERPLASIA

Variant	Gene	Impact on Steroid Synthesis	Diagnostic Marker Steroids in Serum (and Urine)
21-Hydroxylase deficiency (21OHD)	*CYP21A2*	Glucocorticoid deficiency, mineralocorticoid deficiency, adrenal androgen excess	17-Hydroxyprogesterone, 21-deoxycortisol (pregnanetriol, 17-hydroxypregnanolone, pregnanetriolone)
11β-Hydroxylase deficiency (11OHD)	*CYP11B1*	Glucocorticoid deficiency, mineralocorticoid excess, adrenal androgen excess	11-Deoxycortisol, 11-deoxycorticosterone (tetrahydro-11-deoxycortisol, tetrahydro-11-deoxycorticosterone)
17α-Hydroxylase deficiency (17OHD)	*CYP17A1*	(Glucocorticoid deficiency), mineralocorticoid excess, androgen deficiency	11-Deoxycorticosterone, corticosterone, pregnenolone, progesterone (tetrahydro-11-deoxycorticosterone, tetrahydrocorticosterone, pregnenediol, pregnanediol)
3β-Hydroxysteroid dehydrogenase deficiency (3bHSDD)	*HSD3B2*	Glucocorticoid deficiency, (mineralocorticoid deficiency), adrenal androgen excess	17-Hydroxypregnanolone (pregnanetriol)
P450 oxidoreductase deficiency (ORD)	*POR*	Glucocorticoid deficiency, (mineralocorticoid excess), androgen deficiency, skeletal malformations	Pregnenolone, progesterone, 17-hydroxyprogesterone (pregnanediol, pregnanetriol)

presenting during adolescence and early adulthood and with preserved glucocorticoid production.

Androgen excess is present in all patients and manifests with broad phenotypic variability, ranging from severe virilization of the external genitalia in neonatal girls (e.g., 46,XX disordered sex development [DSD]) to hirsutism and oligomenorrhea resembling a polycystic ovary syndrome phenotype in young women with nonclassic CAH. In countries without neonatal screening for CAH, boys with classic CAH usually present with life-threatening adrenal crisis in the first few weeks of life (salt-wasting crisis); a simple-virilizing genotype manifests with precocious pseudo-puberty and advanced bone age in early childhood, whereas men with nonclassic CAH are usually detected only through family screening.

Glucocorticoid treatment is more complex than for other causes of primary adrenal insufficiency as it not only needed to replace missing glucocorticoids but also to control the increased ACTH drive and subsequent androgen excess. Current treatment is hampered by the lack of glucocorticoid preparations that mimic the diurnal cortisol secretion profile, resulting in a prolonged period of ACTH stimulation and subsequent androgen production during the early morning hours. In childhood, optimization of growth and pubertal development are important goals of glucocorticoid treatment, in addition to prevention of adrenal crisis and treatment of 46,XX DSD. In adults, the focus shifts to preserving fertility and preventing side effects of glucocorticoid overtreatment, namely, the metabolic syndrome and osteoporosis. Fertility can be compromised in women due to oligomenorrhea/amenorrhea with chronic anovulation as a consequence of androgen excess. Men may develop so-called testicular adrenal rest tumors (Fig. 406-17). These consist of hyperplastic cells with adrenocortical characteristics located in the rete testis and should not be confused with testicular tumors. Testicular adrenal rest tissue can compromise sperm production and induce fibrosis that may be irreversible.

TREATMENT CONGENITAL ADRENAL HYPERPLASIA

Hydrocortisone is a good treatment option for the prevention of adrenal crisis, but longer acting prednisolone may be needed to control androgen excess. In children, hydrocortisone is given in divided doses at 1–1.5 times the normal cortisol production rate (about 10–13 mg/m^2 per day). In adults, if hydrocortisone does not suffice, intermediate-acting glucocorticoids (e.g., prednisone) may be

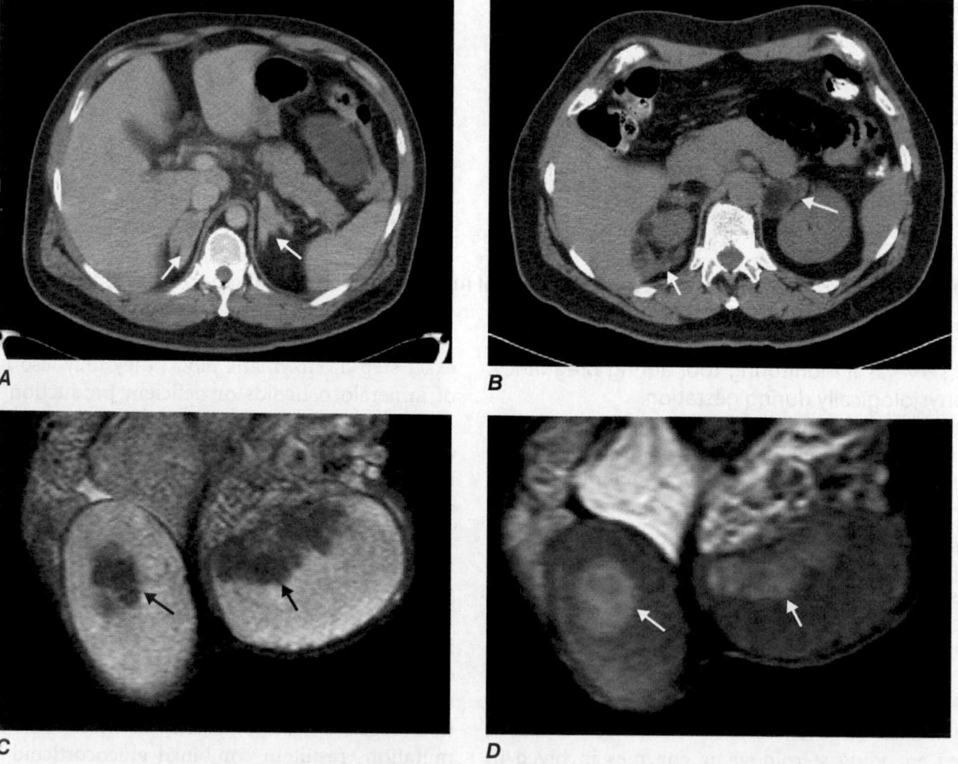

FIGURE 406-17 Imaging in congenital adrenal hyperplasia (CAH). Adrenal computed tomography scans showing homogenous bilateral hyperplasia in a young patient with classic CAH (***A***) and macronodular bilateral hyperplasia (***B***) in a middle-aged patient with classic CAH with longstanding poor disease control. Magnetic resonance imaging scan with T1-weighted (***C***) and T2-weighted (***D***) images showing bilateral testicular adrenal rest tumors (*arrows*) in a young patient with salt-wasting congenital adrenal hyperplasia. *(Courtesy of N. Reisch.)*

given, using the lowest dose necessary to suppress excess androgen production. For achieving fertility, dexamethasone treatment may be required, but should be only given for the shortest possible time period to limit adverse metabolic side effects. Biochemical monitoring should include androstenedione and testosterone, aiming for the normal sex-specific reference range. 17-Hydroxyprogesterone (17OHP) is a useful marker of overtreatment, indicated by 17OHP levels within the normal range of healthy controls. Glucocorticoid overtreatment may suppress the hypothalamic-pituitary-gonadal axis. Thus, treatment needs to be carefully titrated against clinical features of disease control. Stress dose glucocorticoids should be given at double or triple the daily dose for surgery, acute illness, or severe trauma. Poorly controlled CAH can result in adrenocortical hyperplasia, which gave the disease its name, and may present as macronodular hyperplasia subsequent to long-standing ACTH excess (Fig. 406-17). The nodular areas can develop autonomous adrenal androgen production and may be unresponsive to glucocorticoid treatment.

Mineralocorticoid requirements change during life and are higher in children, explained by relative mineralocorticoid resistance that diminishes with ongoing maturation of the kidney. Children with CAH usually receive mineralocorticoid and salt replacement. However, young adults with CAH should undergo reassessment of their mineralocorticoid reserve. Plasma renin should be regularly monitored and kept within the upper half of the normal reference range.

407 Pheochromocytoma

Hartmut P. H. Neumann

Pheochromocytomas and paragangliomas are catecholamine-producing tumors derived from the sympathetic or parasympathetic nervous system. These tumors may arise sporadically or be inherited as features of multiple endocrine neoplasia type 2, von Hippel–Lindau disease, or several other pheochromocytoma-associated syndromes. The diagnosis of pheochromocytomas identifies a potentially correctable cause of hypertension, and their removal can prevent hypertensive crises that can be lethal. The clinical presentation is variable, ranging from an adrenal incidentaloma to a hypertensive crisis with associated cerebrovascular or cardiac complications.

EPIDEMIOLOGY

Pheochromocytoma is estimated to occur in 2–8 of 1 million persons per year, and ~0.1% of hypertensive patients harbor a pheochromocytoma. The mean age at diagnosis is ~40 years, although the tumors can occur from early childhood until late in life. The classic "rule of tens" for pheochromocytomas states that ~10% are bilateral, 10% are extra-adrenal, and 10% are malignant.

ETIOLOGY AND PATHOGENESIS

Pheochromocytomas and paragangliomas are well-vascularized tumors that arise from cells derived from the sympathetic (e.g., adrenal medulla) or parasympathetic (e.g., carotid body, glomus vagale) paraganglia (Fig. 407-1). The name *pheochromocytoma* reflects the black-colored staining caused by chromaffin oxidation of catecholamines; although a variety of terms have been used to describe these tumors, most clinicians use this designation to describe symptomatic catecholamine-producing tumors, including those in extra-adrenal retroperitoneal, pelvic, and thoracic sites. The term *paraganglioma* is used to describe catecholamine-producing tumors in the skull base and neck; these tumors may secrete little or no catecholamine. In contrast to common clinical parlance, the World Health Organization (WHO) restricts the term *pheochromocytoma* to adrenal tumors and applies the term *paraganglioma* to tumors at all other sites.

The etiology of sporadic pheochromocytomas and paragangliomas is unknown. However, 25–33% of patients have an inherited condition, including germ-line mutations in the classically recognized *RET, VHL, NF1, SDHB, SDHC,* and *SDHD* genes or in the more recently recognized *SDHA, SDHAF2, TMEM127,* and *MAX* genes. Biallelic gene inactivation has been demonstrated for the *VHL, NF1,* and *SDH* genes, whereas *RET* mutations activate receptor tyrosine kinase activity. SDH is an enzyme of the Krebs cycle and the mitochondrial respiratory chain. The VHL protein is a component of a ubiquitin E3 ligase. *VHL* mutations reduce protein degradation, resulting in upregulation of components involved in cell cycle progression, glucose metabolism, and oxygen sensing.

CLINICAL FEATURES

Its clinical presentation is so variable that pheochromocytoma has been termed "the great masquerader" (Table 407-1). Among the presenting manifestations, episodes of palpitation, headache, and profuse sweating are typical, and these manifestations constitute a classic triad. The presence of all three manifestations in association with hypertension makes pheochromocytoma a likely diagnosis. However, a pheochromocytoma can be asymptomatic for years, and some tumors grow to a considerable size before patients note symptoms.

The dominant sign is hypertension. Classically, patients have episodic hypertension, but sustained hypertension is also common. Catecholamine crises can lead to heart failure, pulmonary edema, arrhythmias, and intracranial hemorrhage. During episodes of hormone release, which can occur at widely divergent intervals, patients are anxious and pale, and they experience tachycardia and palpitations. These paroxysms generally last <1 h and may be precipitated by surgery, positional changes, exercise, pregnancy, urination (particularly with bladder pheochromocytomas), and various medications (e.g., tricyclic antidepressants, opiates, metoclopramide).

DIAGNOSIS

The diagnosis is based on documentation of catecholamine excess by biochemical testing and localization of the tumor by imaging. These two criteria are of equal importance, although measurement of catecholamines or metanephrines (their methylated metabolites) is traditionally the first step in diagnosis.

Biochemical testing Pheochromocytomas and paragangliomas synthesize and store catecholamines, which include norepinephrine (noradrenaline), epinephrine (adrenaline), and dopamine. Elevated plasma and urinary levels of catecholamines and metanephrines form the cornerstone of diagnosis. The characteristic fluctuations in the hormonal activity of tumors results in considerable variation in serial catecholamine measurements. However, most tumors continuously leak O-methylated metabolites, which are detected by measurement of metanephrines.

Catecholamines and metanephrines can be measured by different methods, including high-performance liquid chromatography, enzyme-linked immunosorbent assay, and liquid chromatography/mass spectrometry. When pheochromocytoma is suspected on clinical grounds (i.e., when values are three times the upper limit of normal), this diagnosis is highly likely regardless of the assay used. However, as summarized in Table 407-2, the sensitivity and specificity of available biochemical tests vary greatly, and these differences are important in assessing patients with borderline elevations of different compounds. Urinary tests for metanephrines (total or fractionated) and catecholamines are widely available and are used commonly for initial evaluation. Among these tests, those for the fractionated metanephrines and catecholamines are the most sensitive. Plasma tests are more convenient and include measurements of catecholamines and metanephrines. Measurements of plasma metanephrine are the most sensitive and are less susceptible to false-positive elevations from stress, including venipuncture. Although the incidence of false-positive test results has been reduced by the introduction of newer assays, physiologic stress responses and medications that increase catecholamine levels still can confound testing. Because the tumors are relatively rare, borderline elevations are likely to represent false-positive results. In

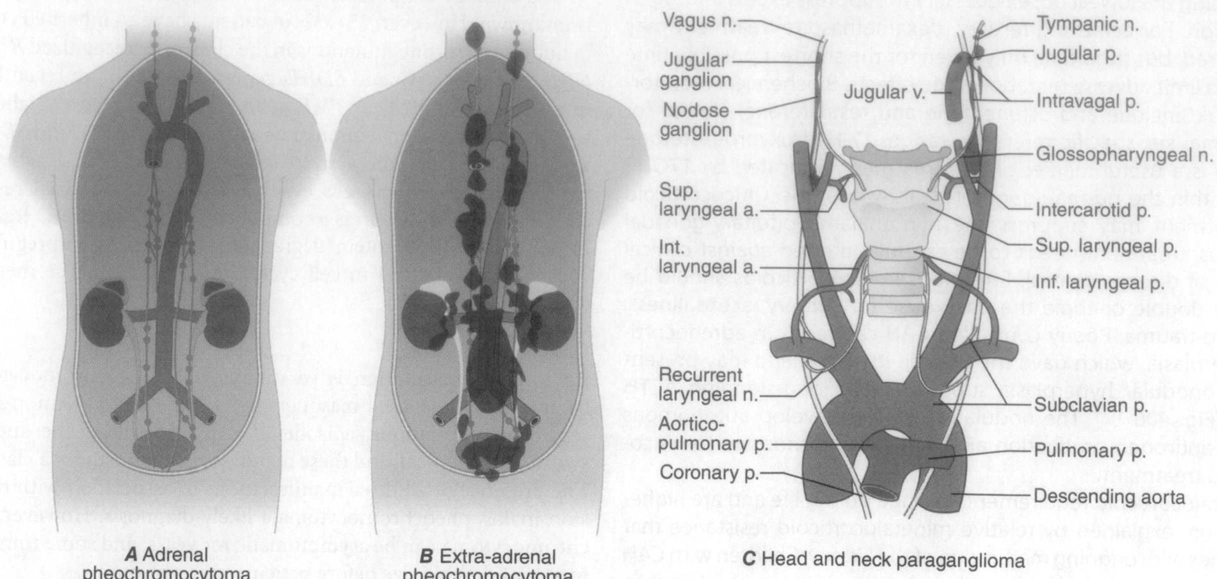

FIGURE 407-1 The paraganglial system and topographic sites (in red) of pheochromocytomas and paragangliomas. *(Parts A and B from WM Manger, RW Gifford: Clinical and experimental pheochromocytoma. Cambridge, Blackwell Science, 1996; Part C from GG Glenner, PM Grimley: Tumors of the Extra-adrenal Paraganglion System [Including Chemoreceptors], Atlas of Tumor Pathology, 2nd Series, Fascicle 9. Washington, DC, AFIP, 1974.)*

TABLE 407-1 CLINICAL FEATURES ASSOCIATED WITH PHEOCHROMOCYTOMA, LISTED BY FREEQUENCY OF OCCURRENCE

1. Headaches	10. Weight loss
2. Profuse sweating	11. Paradoxical response to antihypertensive drugs
3. Palpitations and tachycardia	12. Polyuria and polydipsia
4. Hypertension, sustained or paroxysmal	13. Constipation
5. Anxiety and panic attacks	14. Orthostatic hypotension
6. Pallor	15. Dilated cardiomyopathy
7. Nausea	16. Erythrocytosis
8. Abdominal pain	17. Elevated blood sugar
9. Weakness	18. Hypercalcemia

TABLE 407-2 BIOCHEMICAL AND IMAGING METHODS USED FOR DIAGNOSIS OF PHEOCHROMOCYTOMA AND PARAGANGLIOMA

Diagnostic Method	Sensitivity	Specificity
24-h urinary tests		
Catecholamines	+++	+++
Fractionated metanephrines	++++	++
Total metanephrines	+++	++++
Plasma tests		
Catecholamines	+++	++
Free metanephrines	++++	+++
Imaging		
CT	++++	+++
MRI	++++	+++
MIBG scintigraphy	+++	++++
Somatostatin receptor scintigraphy[a]	++	++
^{18}Fluoro-DOPA PET/CT	+++	++++

[a]Values are particularly high in head and neck paragangliomas.

Abbreviations: MIBG, metaiodobenzylguanidine; PET/CT, positron emission tomography plus CT. For the biochemical tests, the ratings correspond globally to sensitivity and specificity rates as follows: ++, <85%; +++, 85–95%; and ++++, >95%.

this circumstance, it is important to exclude dietary or drug-related factors (withdrawal of levodopa or use of sympathomimetics, diuretics, tricyclic antidepressants, alpha and beta blockers) that might cause false-positive results and then to repeat testing or perform a clonidine suppression test (i.e., the measurement of plasma normetanephrine 3 h after oral administration of 300 μg of clonidine). Other pharmacologic tests, such as the phentolamine test and the glucagon provocation test, are of relatively low sensitivity and are not recommended.

Diagnostic Imaging A variety of methods have been used to localize pheochromocytomas and paragangliomas (Table 407-2). CT and MRI are similar in sensitivity and should be performed with contrast. T2-weighted MRI with gadolinium contrast is optimal for detecting pheochromocytomas and is somewhat better than CT for imaging extraadrenal pheochromocytomas and paragangliomas. About 5% of adrenal incidentalomas, which usually are detected by CT or MRI, prove to be pheochromocytomas upon endocrinologic evaluation.

Tumors also can be localized by procedures using radioactive tracers, including ^{131}I- or ^{123}I-metaiodobenzylguanidine (MIBG) scintigraphy, ^{111}In-somatostatin analogue scintigraphy, ^{18}F-DOPA positron emission tomography (PET), or ^{18}F-fluorodeoxyglucose (FDG) PET. Because these agents exhibit selective uptake in paragangliomas, nuclear imaging is particularly useful in the hereditary syndromes.

Differential Diagnosis When the possibility of a pheochromocytoma is being entertained, other disorders to consider include essential hypertension, anxiety attacks, use of cocaine or amphetamines, mastocytosis or carcinoid syndrome (usually without hypertension), intracranial lesions, clonidine withdrawal, autonomic epilepsy, and factitious crises (usually from use of sympathomimetic amines). When an asymptomatic adrenal mass is identified, likely diagnoses other than pheochromocytoma include a nonfunctioning adrenal adenoma, an aldosteronoma, and a cortisol-producing adenoma (Cushing's syndrome).

TREATMENT PHEOCHROMOCYTOMA

Complete tumor removal, the ultimate therapeutic goal, can be achieved by partial or total adrenalectomy. It is important to preserve the normal adrenal cortex, particularly in hereditary disorders in which bilateral pheochromocytomas are most likely. Preoperative preparation of the patient is important. Before surgery, blood pressure should be consistently below 160/90 mmHg. Classically, blood pressure has been controlled by α-adrenergic blockers (oral phenoxybenzamine, 0.5–4 mg/kg of body weight). Because patients are volume-constricted, liberal salt intake and hydration are necessary to avoid severe orthostasis. Oral prazosin or intravenous phentolamine can be used to manage paroxysms while adequate alpha blockade is awaited. Beta blockers (e.g., 10 mg of propranolol three or four times per day) can then be added. Other antihypertensives, such as calcium channel blockers or angiotensin-converting enzyme inhibitors, have also been used effectively.

Surgery should be performed by teams of surgeons and anesthesiologists with experience in the management of pheochromocytomas. Blood pressure can be labile during surgery, particularly at the outset of intubation or when the tumor is manipulated. Nitroprusside infusion is useful for intraoperative hypertensive crises, and hypotension usually responds to volume infusion.

Minimally invasive techniques (laparoscopy or retroperitoneoscopy) have become the standard approaches in pheochromocytoma surgery. They are associated with fewer complications, a faster recovery, and optimal cosmetic results. Extra-adrenal abdominal and most thoracic pheochromocytomas also can also be removed endoscopically. Postoperatively, catecholamine normalization should be documented. An adrenocorticotropic hormone test should be used to exclude cortisol deficiency when bilateral adrenal cortex–sparing surgery has been performed.

MALIGNANT PHEOCHROMOCYTOMA

About 5–10% of pheochromocytomas and paragangliomas are malignant. The diagnosis of malignant pheochromocytoma is problematic. The typical histologic criteria of cellular atypia, presence of mitoses, and invasion of vessels or adjacent tissues are insufficient for the diagnosis of malignancy in pheochromocytoma. Thus, the term *malignant pheochromocytoma* is restricted to tumors with distant metastases, most commonly found by nuclear medicine imaging in lungs, bone, or liver—locations suggesting a vascular pathway of spread. Because hereditary syndromes are associated with multifocal tumor sites, these features should be anticipated in patients with germ-line mutations of *RET, VHL, SDHD*, or *SDHB*. However, distant metastases also occur in these syndromes, especially in carriers of *SDHB* mutations.

Treatment of malignant pheochromocytoma or paraganglioma is challenging. Options include tumor mass reduction, alpha blockers for symptoms, chemotherapy, and nuclear medicine radiotherapy. The first-line choice is nuclear medicine therapy for scintigraphically documented metastases, preferably with ^{131}I-MIBG in 200-mCi doses at monthly intervals over three to six cycles. Averbuch's chemotherapy protocol includes dacarbazine (600 mg/m^2 on days 1 and 2), cyclophosphamide (750 mg/m^2 on day 1), and vincristine (1.4 mg/m^2 on day 1), all repeated every 21 days for three to six cycles. Palliation (stable disease to shrinkage) is achieved in about one-half of patients. Other chemotherapeutic options are sunitinib and temozolomide/thalidomide. The prognosis of metastatic pheochromocytoma or paraganglioma is variable, with 5-year survival rates of 30–60%.

PHEOCHROMOCYTOMA IN PREGNANCY

Pheochromocytomas occasionally are diagnosed in pregnancy. Endoscopic removal, preferably in the fourth to sixth month of gestation, is possible and can be followed by uneventful childbirth. Regular screening in families with inherited pheochromocytomas provides an opportunity to identify and remove asymptomatic tumors in women of reproductive age.

PHEOCHROMOCYTOMA-ASSOCIATED SYNDROMES

About 25–33% of patients with a pheochromocytoma or paraganglioma have an inherited syndrome. At diagnosis, patients with inherited syndromes are a mean of ~15 years younger than patients with sporadic tumors.

Neurofibromatosis type 1 (NF1) was the first described pheochromocytoma-associated syndrome (Chap. 118). The *NF1* gene functions as a tumor suppressor by regulating the Ras signaling cascade. Classic features of neurofibromatosis include multiple neurofibromas, café au lait spots, axillary freckling of the skin, and Lisch nodules of the iris (Fig. 407-2). Pheochromocytomas occur in only ~1% of these patients

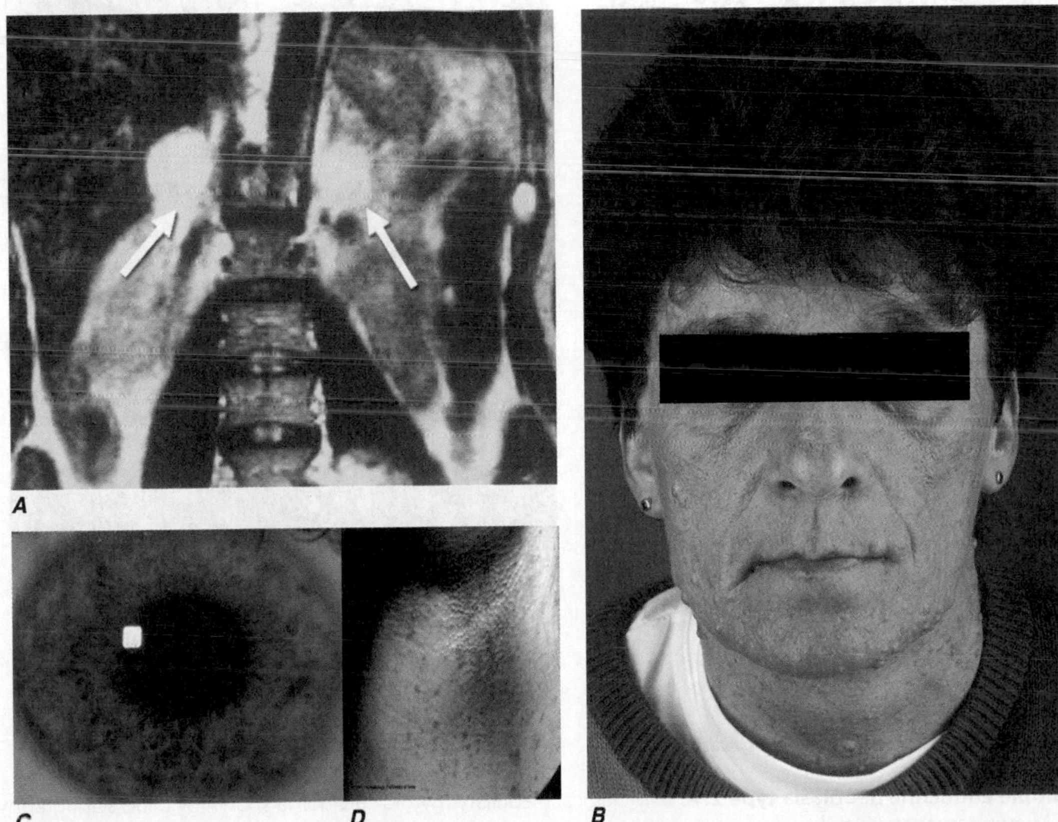

FIGURE 407-2 Neurofibromatosis. *A.* MRI of bilateral adrenal pheochromocytoma. ***B.*** Cutaneous neurofibromas. ***C.*** Lisch nodules of the iris. ***D.*** Axillary freckling. *(Part A from HPH Neumann et al: Keio J Med 54:15, 2005; with permission.)*

and are located predominantly in the adrenals. Malignant pheochromocytoma is not uncommon.

The best-known pheochromocytoma-associated syndrome is the autosomal dominant disorder *multiple endocrine neoplasia type 2* (MEN2) (Chap. 408). Both types of MEN2 (2A and 2B) are caused by mutations in *RET* (*re*arranged during *t*ransfection), which encodes a tyrosine kinase. The locations of RET mutations correlate with the severity of disease and the type of MEN2 (Chap. 408). MEN2A is characterized by medullary thyroid carcinoma (MTC), pheochromocytoma, and hyperparathyroidism; MEN2B also includes MTC and pheochromocytoma as well as multiple mucosal neuromas, marfanoid habitus, and other developmental disorders, though it typically lacks hyperparathyroidism. MTC is found in virtually all patients with MEN2, but pheochromocytoma occurs in only ~50% of these patients. Nearly all pheochromocytomas in MEN2 are benign and located in the adrenals, often bilaterally (Fig. 407-3). Pheochromocytoma may be symptomatic before MTC. Prophylactic thyroidectomy is being performed in many carriers of *RET* mutations; pheochromocytomas should be excluded before any surgery in these patients.

Von Hippel–Lindau syndrome (VHL) is an autosomal dominant disorder that predisposes to retinal and cerebellar hemangioblastomas, which also occur in the brainstem and spinal cord (Fig. 407-4). Other important features of VHL are clear cell renal carcinomas, pancreatic neuroendocrine tumors, endolymphatic sac tumors of the inner ear, cystadenomas of the epididymis and broad ligament, and multiple pancreatic or renal cysts.

The *VHL* gene (among other genes) encodes an E3 ubiquitin ligase that regulates expression of hypoxia-inducible factor 1. Loss of *VHL* is associated with increased expression of vascular endothelial growth factor (VEGF), which induces angiogenesis. Although the *VHL* gene can be inactivated by all types of mutations, patients with pheochromocytoma predominantly have missense mutations. About 20–30% of patients with VHL have pheochromocytomas, but in some families the incidence can reach 90%. The recognition of pheochromocytoma as a VHL-associated feature provides an opportunity to diagnose retinal, central nervous system, renal, and pancreatic tumors at a stage when effective treatment may still be possible.

The *paraganglioma syndromes (PGLs)* have been classified by genetic analyses of families with head and neck paragangliomas. The susceptibility genes encode subunits of the enzyme succinate dehydrogenase (SDH), a component in the Krebs cycle and the mitochondrial electron transport chain. SDH is formed by four subunits (A–D). Mutations of *SDHB* (PGL4), *SDHC* (PGL3), *SDHD* (PGL1), and *SDHAF2* (PGL2) predispose to the PGLs. The transmission of the disease in carriers of *SDHB* and *SDHC* germ-line mutations is autosomal dominant. In contrast, in *SDHD* and *SDHAF2* families, only the progeny of affected fathers develop tumors if they inherit the mutation. PGL1 is most common, followed by PGL4; PGL2 and PGL3 are rare. Adrenal, extra-adrenal abdominal, and thoracic pheochromocytomas, which are components of PGL1 and PGL4, are rare in PGL3 and absent in PGL2 (Fig. 407-5). About one-third of patients with PGL4 develop metastases.

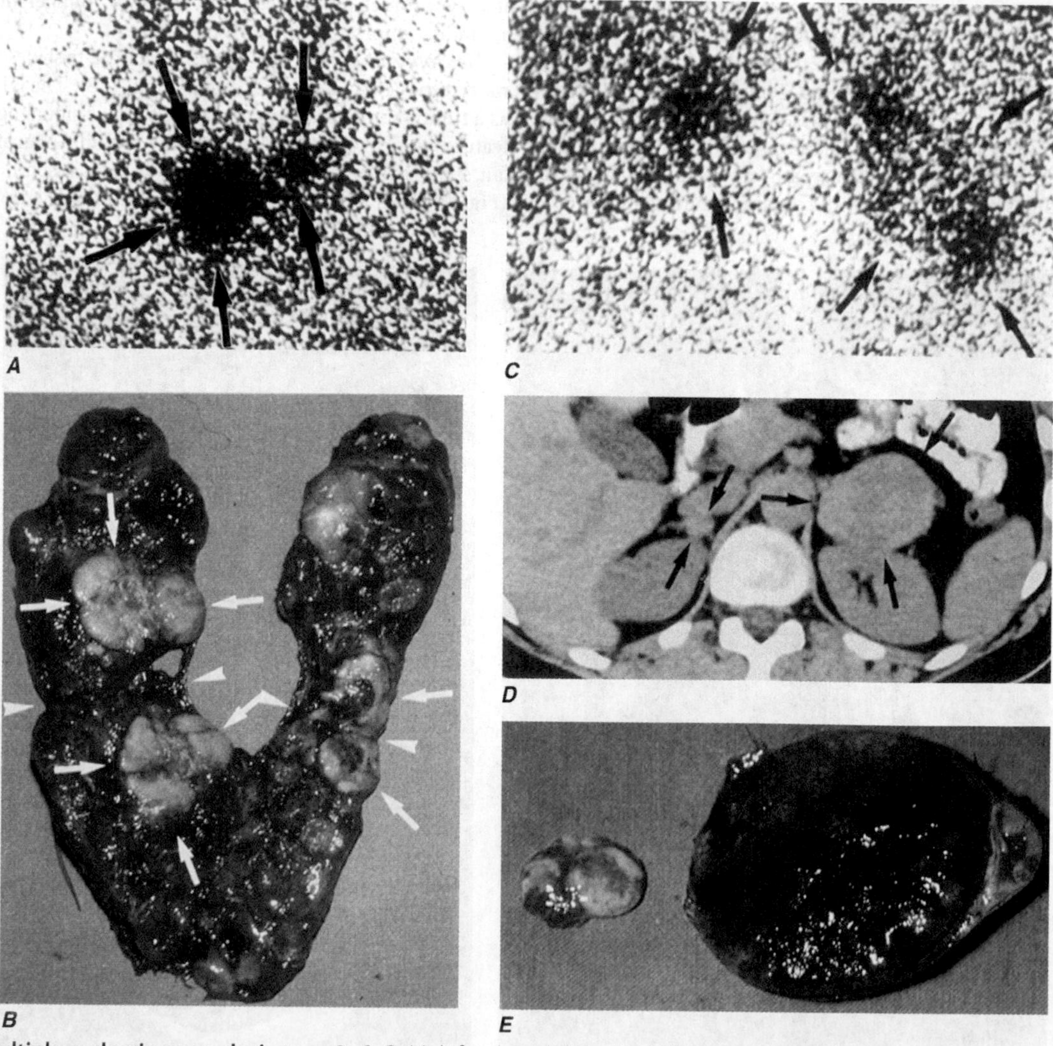

FIGURE 407-3 Multiple endocrine neoplasia type 2. *A, B.* Multifocal medullary thyroid carcinoma shown by MIBG scintigraphy (*A*) and operative specimen (*B*). Arrows demonstrate the tumors; arrowheads show the tissue bridge of the cut specimen. ***C–E.*** Bilateral adrenal pheochromocytoma shown by MIBG scintigraphy (*C*), CT imaging (*D*), and operative specimens (*E*). *(From HPH Neumann et al: Keio J Med 54:15, 2005; with permission.)*

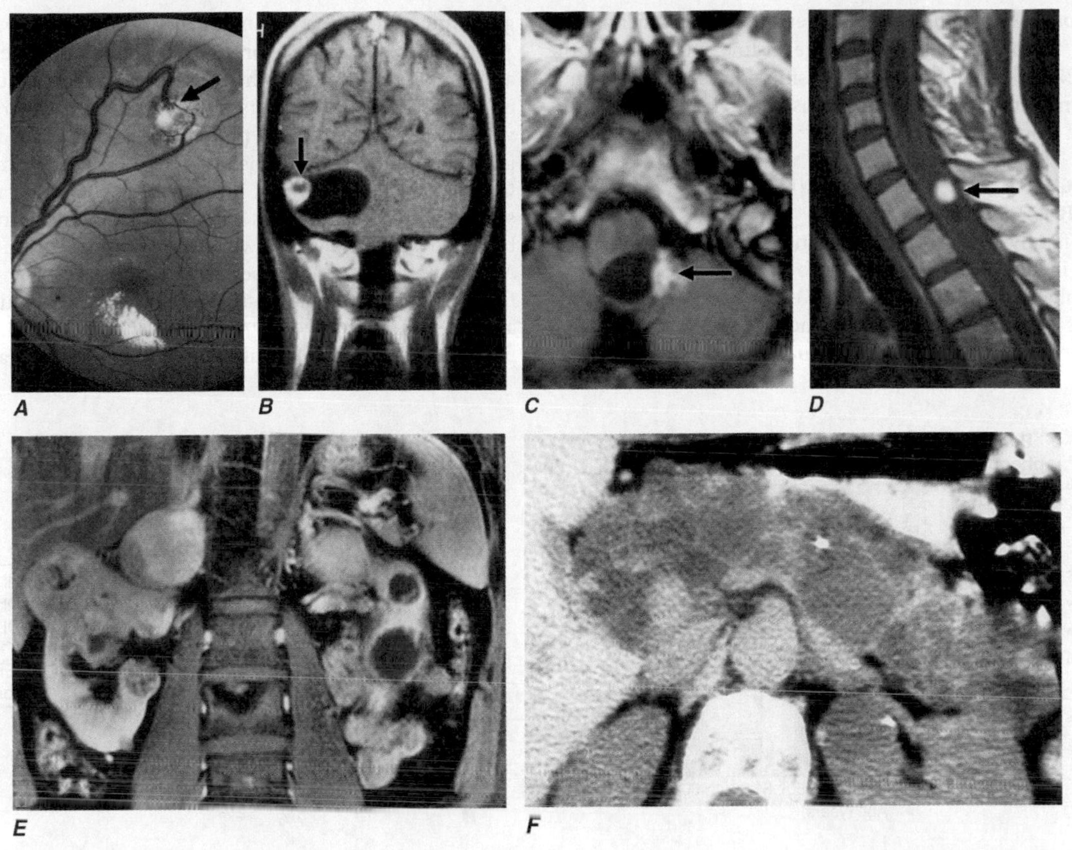

FIGURE 407-4 Von Hippel–Lindau disease. ***A.*** Retinal angioma. All subsequent panels show findings on MRI: ***B–D.*** Hemangioblastomas of the cerebellum (***B***) in brainstem (***C***) and spinal cord (***D***). ***E.*** Bilateral pheochromocytomas and bilateral renal clear cell carcinomas ***F.*** Multiple pancreatic cysts. *(Parts A and D from HPH Neumann et al: Adv Nephrol Necker Hosp 27:361, 1997. © Elsevier. Part B from SH Morgan, J-P Grunfeld [eds]: Inherited Disorders of the Kidney. Oxford, UK, Oxford University Press, 1998. Part F from HPH Neumann et al: Contrib Nephrol 136:193, 2001. © S. Karger AG, Basel.)*

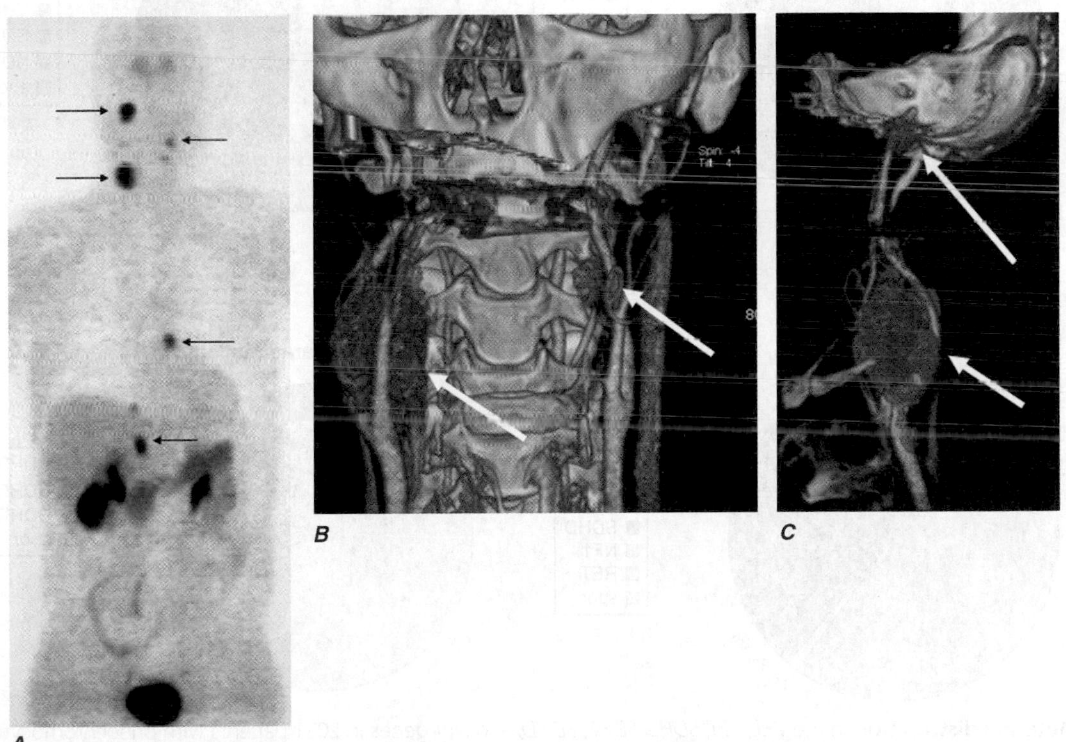

FIGURE 407-5 Paraganglioma syndrome. A patient with the SDHD W5X mutation and PGL1 underwent incomplete resection of a left carotid body tumor. ***A.*** ^{18}F-DOPA positron emission tomography demonstrating tumor uptake in the right jugular glomus, the right carotid body, the left carotid body, the left coronary glomus, and the right adrenal gland. Note the physiologic accumulation of the radiopharmaceutical agent in the kidneys, liver, gallbladder, renal pelvis, and urinary bladder. ***B*** and ***C.*** CT angiography with three-dimensional reconstruction. Arrows point to the paraganglial tumors. *(From S Hoegerle et al: Eur J Nucl Med Mol Imaging 30:689, 2003; with permission.)*

Familial pheochromocytoma (FP) has been attributed to hereditary, mainly adrenal tumors in patients with germ-line mutations in the genes *TMEM127, MAX,* and *SDHA*. Transmission is also autosomal dominant, and mutations of *MAX*, like those of *SDHD*, cause tumors only if inherited from the father.

GUIDELINES FOR GENETIC SCREENING OF PATIENTS WITH PHEOCHROMOCYTOMA OR PARAGANGLIOMA

In addition to family history, general features suggesting an inherited syndrome include young age, multifocal tumors, extra-adrenal tumors, and malignant tumors (Fig. 407-6). Because of the relatively high prevalence of familial syndromes among patients who present with pheochromocytoma or paraganglioma, it is useful to identify germ-line mutations even in patients without a known family history. A first step is to search for clinical features of inherited syndromes and to obtain an in-depth, multigenerational family history. Each of these syndromes exhibits autosomal dominant transmission with variable penetrance, but a proband with a mother affected by paraganglial tumors is not predisposed to PLG1 (*SDHD* mutation carrier). Cutaneous neurofibromas, café au lait spots, and axillary freckling suggest neurofibromatosis. Germ-line mutations in *NF1* have not been reported in patients with sporadic pheochromocytomas. Thus, *NF1* testing need not be performed in the absence of other clinical features of neurofibromatosis. A personal or family history of MTC or an elevation of serum calcitonin strongly suggests MEN 2 and should prompt testing for *RET* mutations. A history of visual impairment or

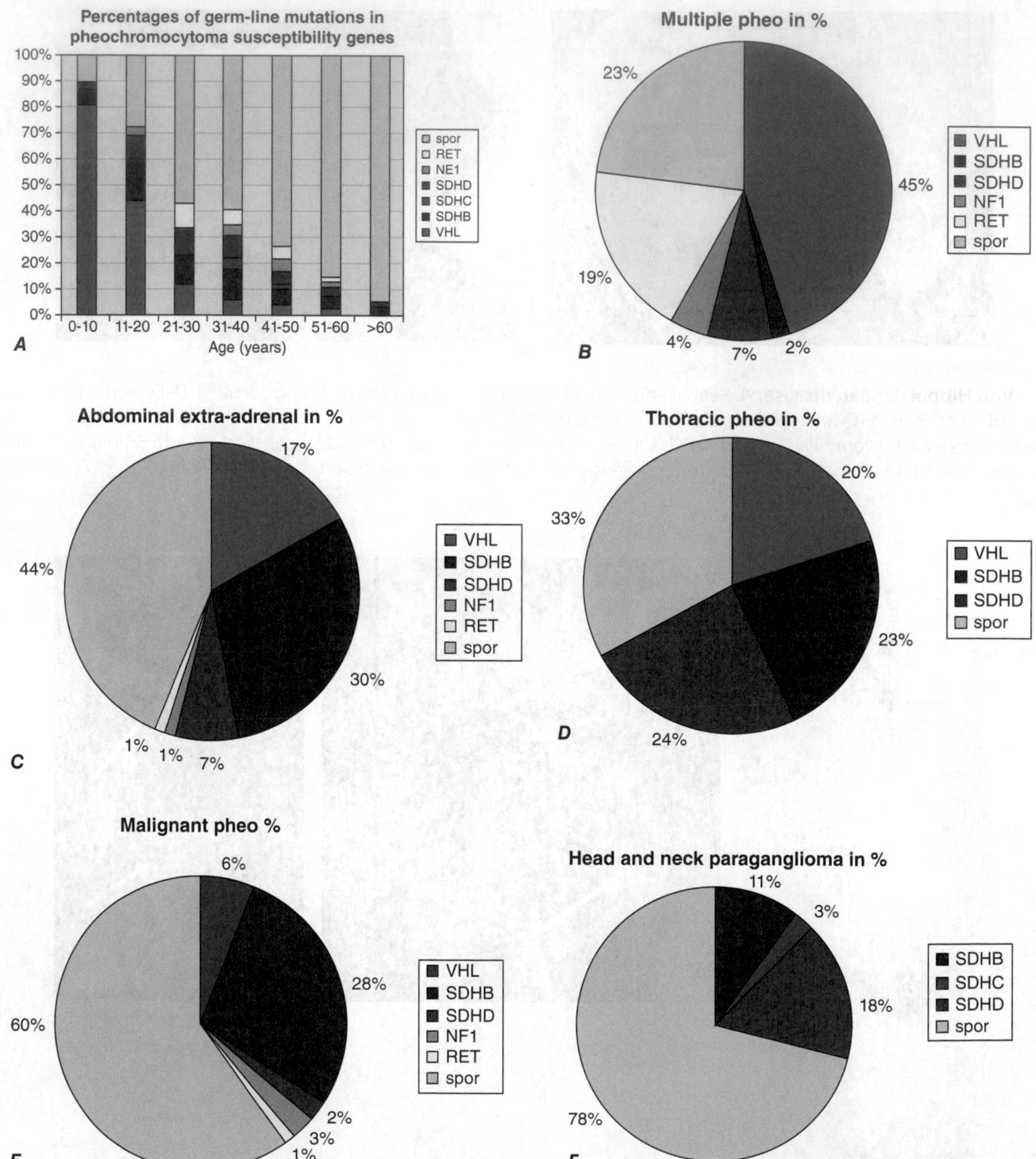

FIGURE 407-6 Mutation distribution in the *VHL, RET, SDHB, SDHC, SDHD,* and *NF1* genes in 2021 patients with pheochromocytomas and paragangliomas from the European-American Pheochromocytoma-Paraganglioma Registry based in Freiburg, Germany, as updated on March 1, 2014. ***A.*** Correlation with age. The bars depict the frequency of sporadic (spor) or various inherited forms of pheochromocytoma in different age groups. The inherited disorders are much more common among younger individuals presenting with pheochromocytoma. Patients with mutations in the *TMEM127, MAX,* and *SDHA* genes are not included, since they contribute <1% in decades 4–7 only. ***B–F.*** Germ-line mutations according to multiple (*B*), extra-adrenal retroperitoneal (*C*), thoracic (*D*), and malignant (*E*) pheochromocytomas and head and neck paragangliomas (*F*). *(Data from the Freiburg International Pheochromocytoma and Paraganglioma Registry, 2014.)*

tumors of the cerebellum, kidney, brainstem, or spinal cord suggests the possibility of VHL. A personal and/or family history of head and neck paraganglioma suggests PGL1 or PGL4.

A single adrenal pheochromocytoma in a patient with an otherwise unremarkable history may still be associated with mutations of *VHL, RET, SDHB*, or *SDHD* (in decreasing order of frequency). Two-thirds of extra-adrenal tumors are associated with one of these syndromes, and multifocal tumors occur with decreasing frequency in carriers of *RET, SDHD, VHL*, and *SDHB* mutations. About 30% of head and neck paragangliomas are associated with germ-line mutations of one of the SDH subunit genes (most often *SDHD*) and are rare in carriers of *VHL, RET*, and *TMEM127* mutations (Fig. 407-6F).

Immunohistochemistry is helpful in the preselection of hereditary pheochromocytoma. Negative immunostaining with antibodies to SDHB, TMEM127, and MAX may predict mutations of the *SDH, TMEM127*, and *MAX* genes, respectively.

Once the underlying syndrome is diagnosed, the benefit of genetic testing can be extended to relatives. For this purpose, it is necessary to identify the germ-line mutation in the proband and, after genetic counseling, to perform DNA sequence analyses of the responsible gene in relatives to determine whether they are affected (Chap. 84). Other family members may benefit when individuals who carry a germ-line mutation are biochemically screened for paraganglial tumors.

Asymptomatic paraganglial tumors, now often detected in patients with hereditary tumors and their relatives, are challenging to manage. Watchful waiting strategies have been introduced. Head and neck paragangliomas—mainly carotid body, jugular, and vagal tumors—are increasingly treated by radiation, since surgery is frequently associated with permanent palsy of cranial nerves II, VII, IX, X, XI, and XII. Nevertheless, tympanic paragangliomas are symptomatic early, and most of these tumors can easily be resected, with subsequent improvement of hearing and alleviation of tinnitus.

408 Multiple Endocrine Neoplasia

Rajesh V. Thakker

Multiple endocrine neoplasia (MEN) is characterized by a predilection for tumors involving two or more endocrine glands. Four major forms of MEN are recognized and referred to as MEN types 1–4 (MEN 1–4) (Table 408-1). Each type of MEN is inherited as an autosomal dominant syndrome or may occur sporadically; that is, without a family history. However, this distinction between familial and sporadic forms is often difficult because family members with the disease may have died before symptoms developed. In addition to MEN 1–4, at least six other syndromes are associated with multiple endocrine and other organ neoplasias (MEONs) (Table 408-2). These MEONs include the hyperparathyroidism-jaw tumor syndrome, Carney complex, von Hippel-Lindau disease (Chap. 407), neurofibromatosis type 1 (Chap. 118), Cowden's syndrome, and McCune-Albright syndrome (Chap. 426e); all of these are inherited as autosomal dominant disorders, except for McCune-Albright syndrome, which is caused by mosaic expression of a postzygotic somatic cell mutation (Table 408-2).

A diagnosis of a MEN or MEON syndrome may be established in an individual by one of three criteria: (1) clinical features (two or more of the associated tumors [or lesions] in an individual); (2) familial pattern (one of the associated tumors [or lesions] in a first-degree relative of a patient with a clinical diagnosis of the syndrome); and (3) genetic analysis (a germline mutation in the associated gene in an individual, who may be clinically affected or asymptomatic). Mutational analysis in MEN and MEON syndromes is helpful in clinical practice to: (1) confirm the clinical diagnosis; (2) identify family members who harbor the mutation and require screening for relevant tumor detection and early/appropriate treatment; and (3) identify the ~50% of family members who do not harbor the germline mutation and can, therefore, be alleviated of the anxiety of developing associated tumors. This latter aspect also helps to reduce health care costs by reducing the need for unnecessary biochemical and radiologic investigations.

MULTIPLE ENDOCRINE NEOPLASIA TYPE 1

Clinical Manifestations MEN type 1 (MEN 1), which is also referred to as Wermer's syndrome, is characterized by the triad of tumors involving the parathyroids, pancreatic islets, and anterior pituitary. In addition, adrenal cortical tumors, carcinoid tumors usually of the foregut, meningiomas, facial angiofibromas, collagenomas, and lipomas may also occur in some patients with MEN 1. Combinations of the affected glands and their pathologic features (e.g., hyperplastic adenomas of the parathyroid glands) may differ in members of the same family and even between identical twins. In addition, a nonfamilial (e.g., sporadic) form occurs in 8–14% of patients with MEN 1, and molecular genetic studies have confirmed the occurrence of de novo mutations of the *MEN1* gene in approximately 10% of patients with MEN 1. The prevalence of MEN 1 is approximately 0.25% based on randomly chosen postmortem studies but is 1–18% among patients with primary hyperparathyroidism, 16–38% among patients with pancreatic islet tumors, and <3% among patients with pituitary tumors. The disorder affects all age groups, with a reported age range of 5 to 81 years, with clinical and biochemical manifestations developing in the vast majority by the fifth decade. The clinical manifestations of MEN 1 are related to the sites of tumors and their hormonal products. In the absence of treatment, endocrine tumors are associated with an earlier mortality in patients with MEN 1, with a 50% probability of death by the age of 50 years. The cause of death is usually a malignant tumor, often from a pancreatic neuroendocrine tumor (NET) or foregut carcinoid. In addition, the treatment outcomes of patients with MEN 1–associated tumors are not as successful as those in patients with non–MEN 1 tumors. This is because MEN 1–associated tumors, with the exception of pituitary NETs, are usually multiple, making it difficult to achieve a successful surgical cure. Occult metastatic disease is also more prevalent in MEN 1, and the tumors may be larger, more aggressive, and resistant to treatment.

Parathyroid Tumors (See also Chap. 424) Primary hyperparathyroidism occurs in approximately 90% of patients and is the most common feature of MEN 1. Patients may have asymptomatic hypercalcemia or vague symptoms associated with hypercalcemia (e.g., polyuria, polydipsia, constipation, malaise, or dyspepsia). Nephrolithiasis and osteitis fibrosa cystica (less commonly) may also occur. Biochemical investigations reveal hypercalcemia, usually in association with elevated circulating parathyroid hormone (PTH) (Table 408-3). The hypercalcemia is usually mild, and severe hypercalcemia or parathyroid cancer is a rare occurrence. Additional differences in the primary hyperparathyroidism of patients with MEN 1, as opposed to those without MEN 1, include an earlier age at onset (20–25 years vs 55 years) and an equal male-to-female ratio (1:1 vs 1:3). Preoperative imaging (e.g., neck ultrasound with ^{99m}Tc-sestamibi parathyroid scintigraphy) is of limited benefit because all parathyroid glands may be affected, and neck exploration may be required irrespective of preoperative localization studies.

TREATMENT PARATHYROID TUMORS

Surgical removal of the abnormally overactive parathyroids in patients with MEN 1 is the definitive treatment. However, it is controversial whether to perform subtotal (e.g., removal of 3.5 glands) or total parathyroidectomy with or without autotransplantation of parathyroid tissue in the forearm, and whether surgery should be performed at an early or late stage. Minimally invasive parathyroidectomy is not recommended because all four parathyroid glands are usually affected with multiple adenomas or hyperplasia. Surgical experience should be taken into account given the variability in pathology in MEN 1. Calcimimetics (e.g., cinacalcet), which act via

TABLE 408-1 MULTIPLE ENDOCRINE NEOPLASIA (MEN) SYNDROMES

Type (Chromosomal Location)	Tumors (Estimated Penetrance)	Gene and Most Frequently Mutated Codons
MEN 1 (11q13)	Parathyroid adenoma (90%)	*MEN1*
	Enteropancreatic tumor (30–70%)	83/84, 4-bp del (≈4%)
	• Gastrinoma (>50%)	119, 3-bp del (≈3%)
	• Insulinoma (10–30%)	209-211, 4-bp del (≈8%)
	• Nonfunctioning and PPoma (20–55%)	418, 3-bp del (≈4%)
	• Glucagonoma (<3%)	514-516, del or ins (≈7%)
	• VIPoma (<1%)	Intron 4 ss (≈10%)
	Pituitary adenoma (15–50%)	
	• Prolactinoma (60%)	
	• Somatotrophinoma (25%)	
	• Corticotropinoma (<5%)	
	• Nonfunctioning (<5%)	
	Associated tumors	
	• Adrenal cortical tumor (20–70%)	
	• Pheochromocytoma (<1%)	
	• Bronchopulmonary NET (2%)	
	• Thymic NET (2%)	
	• Gastric NET (10%)	
	• Lipomas (>33%)	
	• Angiofibromas (85%)	
	• Collagenomas (70%)	
	• Meningiomas (8%)	
MEN 2 (10 cen-10q11.2)		
MEN 2A	MTC (90%)	*RET*
	Pheochromocytoma (>50%)	634, e.g., Cys → Arg (~85%)
	Parathyroid adenoma (10–25%)	
MTC only	MTC (100%)	*RET* 618, missense (>50%)
MEN 2B (also known as MEN 3)	MTC (>90%)	*RET* 918, Met → Thr (>95%)
	Pheochromocytoma (>50%)	
	Associated abnormalities (40–50%)	
	• Mucosal neuromas	
	• Marfanoid habitus	
	• Medullated corneal nerve fibers	
	• Megacolon	
MEN 4 (12p13)	Parathyroid adenoma[a]	*CDKN1B*; no common mutations identified to date
	Pituitary adenoma[a]	
	Reproductive organ tumors[a] (e.g., testicular cancer, neuroendocrine cervical carcinoma)	
	?Adrenal + renal tumors[a]	

[a]Insufficient numbers reported to provide prevalence information.

Note: Autosomal dominant inheritance of the MEN syndromes has been established.

Abbreviations: del, deletion; ins, insertion; MTC, medullary thyroid cancer; NET, neuroendocrine tumor; PPoma, pancreatic polypeptide–secreting tumor; VIPoma, vasoactive intestinal polypeptide–secreting tumor.

Source: Reproduced from RV Thakker et al: J Clin Endocrinol Metab 97:2990, 2012.

the calcium-sensing receptor, have been used to treat primary hyperparathyroidism in some patients when surgery is unsuccessful or contraindicated.

Pancreatic Tumors (See also Chap. 113) The incidence of pancreatic islet cell tumors, which are NETs, in patients with MEN 1 ranges from 30 to 80% in different series. Most of these tumors (Table 408-1) produce excessive amounts of hormone (e.g., gastrin, insulin, glucagon, vasoactive intestinal polypeptide [VIP]) and are associated with distinct clinical syndromes, although some are nonfunctioning or nonsecretory. These pancreatic islet cell tumors have an earlier age at onset in patients with MEN 1 than in patients without MEN 1.

Gastrinoma Gastrin-secreting tumors (gastrinomas) are associated with marked gastric acid production and recurrent peptic ulcerations, a combination referred to as the Zollinger-Ellison syndrome. Gastrinomas occur more often in patients with MEN 1 who are older than age 30 years. Recurrent severe multiple peptic ulcers, which may perforate, and cachexia are major contributors to the high mortality. Patients with Zollinger-Ellison syndrome may also suffer from diarrhea and steatorrhea. The diagnosis is established by demonstration of an elevated fasting serum gastrin concentration in association with increased basal gastric acid secretion (Table 408-3). However, the diagnosis of Zollinger-Ellison syndrome may be difficult in hypercalcemic MEN 1 patients, because hypercalcemia can also cause hypergastrinemia.

TABLE 408-2 MULTIPLE ENDOCRINE AND OTHER ORGAN NEOPLASIA SYNDROMES (MEONs)

Disease[a]	Gene Product	Chromosomal Location
Hyperparathyroidism-jaw tumor (HPT-JT)	Parafibromin	1q31.2
Carney complex		
CNC1	PPKAR1A	17q24.2
CNC2	?[b]	2p16
von Hippel-Lindau disease (VHL)	pVHL (elongin)	3p25
Neurofibromatosis type 1 (NF1)	Neurofibromin	17q11.2
Cowden's syndrome (CWD)		
CWD1	PTEN	10q23.31
CWD2	SDHB	1p36.13
CWD3	SDHD	11q23.1
CWD4	KLLN	10q23.31
CWD5	PIK3CA	3q26.32
CWD6	AKT1	14q32.33
McCune-Albright syndrome (MAS)	Gsα	20q13.32

[a]The inheritance for these disorders is autosomal dominant, except MAS, which is due to mosaicism that results from the postzygotic somatic cell mutation of the *GNAS1* gene, encoding Gsα. [b]?, unknown.

Ultrasonography, endoscopic ultrasonography, computed tomography (CT), nuclear magnetic resonance imaging (MRI), selective abdominal angiography, venous sampling, and somatostatin receptor scintigraphy are helpful in localizing the tumor prior to surgery. Gastrinomas represent more than 50% of all pancreatic NETs in patients with MEN 1, and approximately 20% of patients with gastrinomas will be found to have MEN 1. Gastrinomas, which may also occur in the duodenal mucosa, are the major cause of morbidity and mortality in patients with MEN 1. Most MEN 1 gastrinomas are malignant and metastasize before a diagnosis is established.

TREATMENT GASTRINOMA

Medical treatment of patients with MEN 1 and Zollinger-Ellison syndrome is directed toward reducing basal acid output to <10 mmol/L. Parietal cell H^+-K^+-adenosine triphosphatase (ATPase) inhibitors (e.g., omeprazole or lansoprazole) reduce acid output and are the drugs of choice for gastrinomas. Some patients may also require additional treatment with the histamine H_2 receptor antagonists, cimetidine or ranitidine. The role of surgery in the treatment of gastrinomas in patients with MEN 1 is controversial. The goal of surgery is to reduce the risk of distant metastatic disease and improve survival. For a nonmetastatic gastrinoma situated in the pancreas, surgical excision is often effective. However, the risk of hepatic metastases increases with tumor size, such that 25–40% of patients with pancreatic NETs >4 cm develop hepatic metastases, and 50–70% of patients with tumors 2–3 cm in size have lymph node metastases. Survival in MEN 1 patients with gastrinomas <2.5 cm in size is 100% at 15 years, but 52% at 15 years, if metastatic disease is present. The presence of lymph node metastases does not appear to adversely affect survival. Surgery for gastrinomas that are >2–2.5 cm has been recommended, because the disease-related survival in these patients is improved following surgery. In addition, duodenal gastrinomas, which occur more frequently in patients with MEN 1, have been treated successfully with surgery. However, in most patients with MEN 1, gastrinomas are multiple or extrapancreatic, and with the exception of duodenal gastrinomas, surgery is rarely successful. For example, the results of one study revealed that only ~15% of patients with MEN 1 were free of disease immediately after surgery, and at 5 years, this number had decreased to ~5%; the respective outcomes in patients without MEN 1 were better, at 45% and 40%. Given these findings, most specialists recommend a nonsurgical management for gastrinomas in MEN 1, except as noted earlier for smaller, isolated lesions. Treatment of disseminated gastrinomas is difficult. Chemotherapy with streptozotocin and 5-fluorouracil; hormonal therapy with octreotide or lanreotide, which are human somatostatin analogues; hepatic artery embolization; administration of human leukocyte interferon; and removal of all resectable tumor have been successful in some patients.

Insulinoma These β islet cell insulin-secreting tumors represent 10–30% of all pancreatic tumors in patients with MEN 1. Patients with an insulinoma present with hypoglycemic symptoms (e.g., weakness, headaches, sweating, faintness, seizures, altered behavior, weight gain) that typically develop after fasting or exertion and improve after glucose intake. The most reliable test is a supervised 72-h fast. Biochemical investigations reveal increased plasma insulin concentrations in association with hypoglycemia (Table 408-3). Circulating concentrations of C peptide and proinsulin, which are also increased, are useful in establishing the diagnosis. It also is important to demonstrate the absence of sulfonylureas in plasma and urine samples obtained during the investigation of hypoglycemia (Table 408-3). Surgical success is greatly enhanced by preoperative localization by endoscopic ultrasonography, CT scanning, or celiac axis angiography. Additional localization methods may include preoperative and perioperative percutaneous transhepatic portal venous sampling, selective intraarterial stimulation with hepatic venous sampling, and intraoperative direct pancreatic ultrasonography. Insulinomas occur in association with gastrinomas in 10% of patients with MEN 1, and the two tumors may arise at different times. Insulinomas occur more often in patients with MEN 1 who are younger than 40 years, and some arise in individuals younger than 20 years. In contrast, in patients without MEN 1, insulinomas generally occur in those older than 40 years. Insulinomas may be the first manifestation of MEN 1 in 10% of patients, and approximately 4% of patients with insulinomas will have MEN 1.

TABLE 408-3 BIOCHEMICAL AND RADIOLOGICAL SCREENING IN MULTIPLE ENDOCRINE NEOPLASIA TYPE 1

Tumor	Age to Begin (Years)	Biochemical Test (Plasma or Serum) Annually	Imaging Test (Time Interval)
Parathyroid	8	Calcium, PTH	None
Pancreatic NETs			
Gastrinoma	20	Gastrin (± gastric pH)	None
Insulinoma	5	Fasting glucose, insulin	None
Other pancreatic NET	<10	Chromogranin A; pancreatic polypeptide, glucagon, vasoactive intestinal peptide	MRI, CT, or EUS (annually)
Anterior pituitary	5	Prolactin, IGF-I	MRI (every 3 years)
Adrenal	<10	None unless symptoms or signs of functioning tumor and/or tumor >1 cm identified on imaging	MRI or CT (annually with pancreatic imaging)
Thymic and bronchial carcinoid	15	None	CT or MRI (every 1–2 years)

Abbreviations: CT, computed tomography; EUS, endoscopic ultrasound; IGF-I, insulin-like growth factor I; MRI, magnetic resonance imaging; PTH, parathyroid hormone.

Source: Reproduced from RV Thakker et al: J Clin Endocrinol Metab 97:2990, 2012.

TREATMENT INSULINOMA

Medical treatment, which consists of frequent carbohydrate meals and diazoxide or octreotide, is not always successful, and surgery is the optimal treatment. Surgical treatment, which ranges from enucleation of a single tumor to a distal pancreatectomy or partial pancreatectomy, has been curative in many patients. Chemotherapy may include streptozotocin, 5-fluorouracil, and doxorubicin. Hepatic artery embolization has been used for metastatic disease.

Glucagonoma These glucagon-secreting pancreatic NETs occur in <3% of patients with MEN 1. The characteristic clinical manifestations of a skin rash (necrolytic migratory erythema), weight loss, anemia, and stomatitis may be absent. The tumor may have been detected in an asymptomatic patient with MEN 1 undergoing pancreatic imaging or by the finding of glucose intolerence and hyperglucagonemia.

TREATMENT GLUCAGONOMA

Surgical removal of the glucagonoma is the treatment of choice. However, treatment may be difficult because approximately 50–80% of patients have metastases at the time of diagnosis. Medical treatment with somatostatin analogues (e.g., octreotide or lanreotide) or chemotherapy with streptozotocin and 5-fluorouracil has been successful in some patients, and hepatic artery embolization has been used to treat metastatic disease.

Vasoactive Intestinal Peptide (VIP) Tumors (VIPomas) VIPomas have been reported in only a few patients with MEN 1. This clinical syndrome is characterized by watery diarrhea, hypokalemia, and achlorhydria and is also referred to as the Verner-Morrison syndrome, the WDHA (watery diarrhea, hypokalemia, and achlorhydria) syndrome, or the VIPoma syndrome. The diagnosis is established by excluding laxative and diuretic abuse, by confirming a stool volume in excess of 0.5–1.0 L/d during a fast, and by documenting a markedly increased plasma VIP concentration.

TREATMENT VIPOMAS

Surgical management of VIPomas, which are mostly located in the tail of the pancreas, can be curative. However, in patients with unresectable tumor, somatostatin analogues, such as octreotide and lanreotide, may be effective. Streptozotocin with 5-fluorouracil may be beneficial, along with hepatic artery embolization for the treatment of metastases.

Pancreatic Polypeptide-Secreting Tumors (Ppomas) and Nonfunctioning Pancreatic NETs PPomas are found in a large number of patients with MEN 1. No pathologic sequelae of excessive polypeptide (PP) secretion are apparent, and the clinical significance of PP is unknown. Many PPomas may have been unrecognized or classified as nonfunctioning pancreatic NETs, which likely represent the most common enteropancreatic NET associated with MEN 1 (Fig. 408-1). The absence of both a clinical syndrome and specific biochemical abnormalities may result in a delayed diagnosis of nonfunctioning pancreatic NETs, which are associated with a worse prognosis than other functioning tumors, including insulinoma and gastrinoma. The optimum screening method and its timing interval for nonfunctioning pancreatic NETs remain to be established. At present, endoscopic ultrasound likely represents the most sensitive method of detecting small pancreatic tumors, but somatostatin receptor scintography is the most reliable method for detecting metastatic disease (Table 408-3).

TREATMENT PPOMAS AND NONFUNCTIONING PANCREATIC NETS

The management of nonfunctioning pancreatic NETs in the asymptomatic patient is controversial. One recommendation is to undertake surgery irrespective of tumor size after biochemical assessment is complete. Alternatively, other experts recommend surgery based on tumor size, using either >1 cm or >3 cm at different centers. Pancreatoduodenal surgery is successful in removing the tumors in 80% of patients, but more than 40% of patients develop complications, including diabetes mellitus, frequent steatorrhea, early and late dumping syndromes, and other gastrointestinal symptoms. However, ~50–60% of patients treated surgically survive >5 years. When considering these recommendations, it is important to consider that occult metastatic disease (e.g., tumors not detected by imaging investigations) is likely to be present in a substantial proportion of these patients at the time of presentation. Inhibitors of tyrosine kinase receptors (TKRs) and of the mammalian

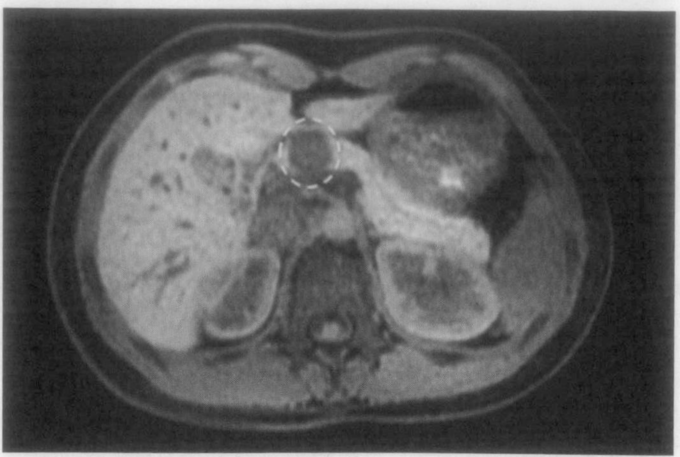

A

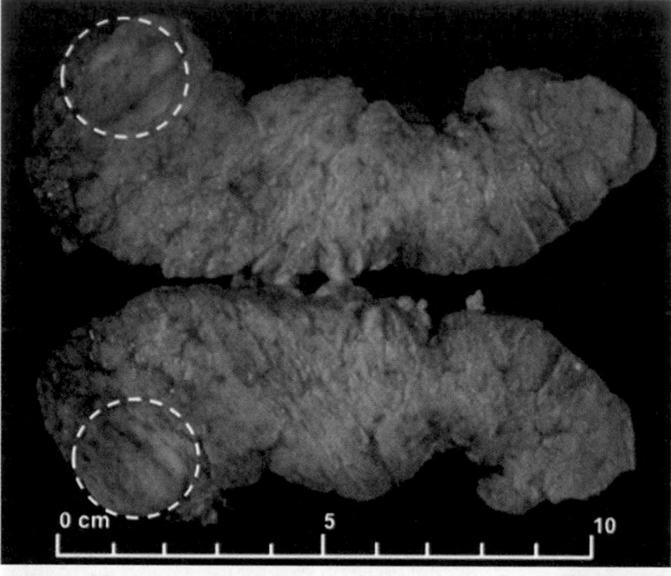

B

FIGURE 408-1 Pancreatic nonfunctioning neuroendocrine tumor (NET) in a 14-year-old patient with multiple endocrine neoplasia type 1 (MEN 1). ***A.*** An abdominal magnetic resonance imaging scan revealed a low-intensity >2.0 cm (anteroposterior maximal diameter) tumor within the neck of pancreas. There was no evidence of invasion of adjacent structures or metastases. The tumor is indicated by *white dashed circle*. ***B.*** The pancreatic NET was removed by surgery, and macroscopic examination confirmed the location of the tumor (*white dashed circles*) in the neck of the pancreas. Immunohistochemistry showed the tumor to immunostain for chromogranin A, but not gastrointestinal peptides or menin, thereby confirming that it was a nonsecreting NET due to loss of menin expression. *(Part A adapted with permission from PJ Newey et al: J Clin Endocrinol Metab 10:3640, 2009.)*

target of rapamycin (mTOR) signaling pathway have been reported to be effective in treating pancreatic NETs and in doubling the progression-free survival time.

Other Pancreatic NETs NETs secreting growth hormone–releasing hormone (GHRH), GHRHomas, have been reported rarely in patients with MEN 1. It is estimated that ~33% of patients with GHRHomas have other MEN 1–related tumors. GHRHomas may be diagnosed by demonstrating elevated serum concentrations of growth hormone and GHRH. More than 50% of GHRHomas occur in the lung, 30% occur in the pancreas, and 10% are found in the small intestine. Somatostatinomas secrete somatostatin, a peptide that inhibits the secretion of a variety of hormones, resulting in hyperglycemia, cholelithiasis, low acid output, steatorrhea, diarrhea, abdominal pain, anemia, and weight loss. Although 7% of pancreatic NETs secrete somatostatin, the clinical features of somatostatinoma syndrome are unusual in patients with MEN 1.

Pituitary Tumors (See also Chap. 403) Pituitary tumors occur in 15–50% of patients with MEN 1 (Table 408-1). These occur as early as 5 years of age or as late as the ninth decade. MEN 1 pituitary adenomas are more frequent in women than men and significantly are macroadenomas (i.e., diameter >1 cm). Moreover, about one-third of these pituitary tumors show invasive features such as infiltration of tumor cells into surrounding normal juxtatumoral pituitary tissue. However, no specific histologic parameters differentiate between MEN 1 and non–MEN 1 pituitary tumors. Approximately 60% of MEN 1 associated pituitary tumors secrete prolactin, <25% secrete growth hormone, 5% secrete adrenocorticotropic hormone (ACTH), and the remainder appear to be nonfunctioning, with some secreting glycoprotein subunits (Table 408-1). However, pituitary tumors derived from MEN 1 patients may exhibit immunoreactivity to several hormones. In particular, there is a greater frequency of somatolactotrope tumors. Prolactinomas are the first manifestation of MEN 1 in ~15% of patients, whereas somatotrope tumors occur more often in patients older than 40 years of age. Fewer than 3% of patients with anterior pituitary tumors will have MEN 1. Clinical manifestations are similar to those in patients with sporadic pituitary tumors without MEN 1 and depend on the hormone secreted and the size of the pituitary tumor. Thus, patients may have symptoms of hyperprolactinemia (e.g., amenorrhea, infertility, and galactorrhea in women, or impotence and infertility in men) or have features of acromegaly or Cushing's disease. In addition, enlarging pituitary tumors may compress adjacent structures such as the optic chiasm or normal pituitary tissue, causing visual disturbances and/or hypopituitarism. In asymptomatic patients with MEN 1, periodic biochemical monitoring of serum prolactin and insulin-like growth factor I (IGF-I) levels, as well as MRI of the pituitary, can lead to early identification of pituitary tumors (Table 408-3). In patients with abnormal results, hypothalamic-pituitary testing should characterize the nature of the pituitary lesion and its effects on the secretion of other pituitary hormones.

TREATMENT PITUITARY TUMORS

Treatment of pituitary tumors in patients with MEN 1 consists of therapies similar to those used in patients without MEN 1 and includes appropriate medical therapy (e.g., bromocriptine or cabergoline for prolactinoma; or octreotide or lanreotide for somatotrope tumors) or selective transsphenoidal adenomectomy, if feasible, with radiotherapy reserved for residual unresectable tumor tissue. Pituitary tumors in MEN 1 patients may be more aggressive and less responsive to medical or surgical treatments.

Associated Tumors Patients with MEN 1 may also develop carcinoid tumors, adrenal cortical tumors, facial angiofibromas, collagenomas, thyroid tumors, and lipomatous tumors.

Carcinoid Tumors (See also Chap. 113) Carcinoid tumors occur in more than 3% of patients with MEN 1 (Table 408-1). The carcinoid tumor may be located in the bronchi, gastrointestinal tract, pancreas, or thymus. At the time of diagnosis, most patients are asymptomatic and do not have clinical features of the carcinoid syndrome. Importantly, no hormonal or biochemical abnormality (e.g., plasma chromogranin A) is consistently observed in individuals with thymic or bronchial carcinoid tumors. Thus, screening for these tumors is dependent on radiologic imaging. The optimum method for screening has not been established. CT and MRI are sensitive for detecting thymic and bronchial tumors (Table 408-3), although repeated CT scanning raises concern about exposure to repeated doses of ionizing radiation. Octreotide scintigraphy may also reveal some thymic and bronchial carcinoids, although there is insufficient evidence to recommend its routine use. Gastric carcinoids, of which the type II gastric enterochromaffin-like (ECL) cell carcinoids (ECLomas) are associated with MEN 1 and Zollinger-Ellison syndrome, may be detected incidentally at the time of gastric endoscopy for dyspeptic symptoms in MEN 1 patients. These tumors, which may be found in >10% of MEN 1 patients, are usually multiple and smaller than 1.5 cm. Bronchial carcinoids in patients with MEN 1 occur predominantly in women (male-to-female ratio, 1:4). In contrast, thymic carcinoids in European patients with MEN 1 occur predominantly in men (male-to-female ratio, 20:1), with cigarette smokers having a higher risk for these tumors; thymic carcinoids in Japanese patients with MEN 1 have a less marked sex difference (male-to-female ratio 2:1). The course of thymic carcinoids in MEN 1 appears to be particularly aggressive. The presence of thymic tumors in patients with MEN 1 is associated with a median survival after diagnosis of approximately 9.5 years, with 70% of patients dying as a direct result of the tumor.

TREATMENT CARCINOID TUMORS

If resectable, surgical removal of carcinoid tumors is the treatment of choice. For unresectable tumors and those with metastatic disease, treatment with radiotherapy or chemotherapeutic agents (e.g., cisplatin, etoposide) may be used. In addition, somatostatin analogues, such as octreotide or lanreotide, have resulted in symptom improvement and regression of some tumors. Little is known about the malignant potential of gastric type II ECLomas, but treatment with somatostatin analogues, such as octreotide or lanreotide, has resulted in regression of these ECLomas.

Adrenocortical Tumors (See also Chap. 406) Asymptomatic adrenocortical tumors occur in 20–70% of patients with MEN 1 depending on the radiologic screening methods used (Table 408-1). Most of these tumors, which include cortical adenomas, hyperplasia, multiple adenomas, nodular hyperplasia, cysts, and carcinomas, are nonfunctioning. Indeed, <10% of patients with enlarged adrenal glands have hormonal hypersecretion, with primary hyperaldosteronism and ACTH-independent Cushing's syndrome being encountered most commonly. Occasionally, hyperandrogenemia may occur in association with adrenocortical carcinoma. Pheochromocytoma in association with MEN 1 is rare. Biochemical investigation (e.g., plasma renin and aldosterone concentrations, low-dose dexamethasone suppression test, urinary catecholamines, and/or metanephrines) should be undertaken in those with symptoms or signs suggestive of functioning adrenal tumors or in those with tumors >1 cm. Adrenocortical carcinoma occurs in approximately 1% of MEN 1 patients but increases to >10% for adrenal tumors larger than 1 cm.

TREATMENT ADRENOCORTICAL TUMORS

Consensus has not been reached about the management of MEN 1–associated nonfunctioning adrenal tumors, because the majority are benign. However, the risk of malignancy increases with size, particularly for tumors with a diameter >4 cm. Indications for surgery for adrenal tumors include: size >4 cm in diameter; atypical or suspicious radiologic features (e.g., increased Hounsfield unit on unenhanced CT scan) and size of 1–4 cm in diameter; or significant measurable growth over a 6-month period. The treatment of functioning (e.g., hormone-secreting) adrenal tumors is similar to that for tumors occurring in non–MEN 1 patients.

Meningioma Central nervous system (CNS) tumors, including ependymomas, schwannomas, and meningiomas, have been reported in MEN 1 patients (Table 408-1). Meningiomas are found in <10% of patients with other clinical manifestations of MEN 1 (e.g., primary hyperparathyroidism) for >15 years. The majority of meningiomas are not associated with symptoms, and 60% do not enlarge. The treatment of MEN 1–associated meningiomas is similar to that in non–MEN 1 patients.

Lipomas Subcutaneous lipomas occur in >33% of patients with MEN 1 (Table 408-1) and are frequently multiple. In addition, visceral, pleural, or retroperitoneal lipomas may occur in patients with MEN 1. Management is conservative. However, when surgically removed for cosmetic reasons, they typically do not recur.

Facial Angiofibromas and Collagenomas The occurrence of multiple facial angiofibromas in patients with MEN 1 may range from >20 to >90%, and occurrence of collagenomas may range from 0 to >70% (Table 408-1). These cutaneous findings may allow presymptomatic diagnosis of MEN 1 in the relatives of a patient with MEN 1. Treatment for these cutaneous lesions is usually not required.

Thyroid Tumors Thyroid tumors, including adenomas, colloid goiters, and carcinomas, have been reported to occur in >25% of patients with MEN 1. However, the prevalence of thyroid disorders in the general population is high, and it has been suggested that the association of thyroid abnormalities in patients with MEN 1 may be incidental. The treatment of thyroid tumors in MEN 1 patients is similar to that for non–MEN 1 patients.

Genetics and Screening The *MEN1* gene is located on chromosome 11q13 and consists of 10 exons, which encode a 610–amino acid protein, menin, that regulates transcription, genome stability, cell division, and proliferation. The pathophysiology of MEN 1 follows the Knudson two-hit hypothesis with a tumor-suppressor role for menin. Inheritance of a germline *MEN1* mutation predisposes an individual to developing a tumor that arises following a somatic mutation, which may be a point mutation or more commonly a deletion, leading to loss of heterozygosity (LOH) in the tumor DNA. The germline mutations of the *MEN1* gene are scattered throughout the entire 1830-bp coding region and splice sites, and there is no apparent correlation between the location of *MEN1* mutations and clinical manifestations of the disorder, in contrast with the situation in patients with MEN 2 (Table 408-1). More than 10% of *MEN1* germline mutations arise de novo and may be transmitted to subsequent generations. Some families with MEN 1 mutations develop parathyroid tumors as the sole endocrinopathy, and this condition is referred to as familial isolated hyperparathyroidism (FIHP). However, between 5 and 25% of patients with MEN 1 do not harbor germline mutations or deletions of the *MEN1* gene. Such patients with MEN 1–associated tumors but without *MEN1* mutations may represent phenocopies or have mutations involving other genes. Other genes associated with MEN 1–like features include: *CDC73*, which encodes parafibromin, whose mutations result in the hyperparathyroid-jaw tumor syndrome; the calcium-sensing receptor gene (*CaSR*), whose mutations result in familial benign hypocalciuric hypercalcemia (FBHH); and the aryl hydrocarbon receptor interacting protein gene (*AIP*), a tumor suppressor located on chromosome 11q13 whose mutations are associated with familial isolated pituitary adenomas (FIPA). Genetic testing to determine the *MEN1* mutation status in symptomatic family members within a MEN 1 kindred, as well as to all index cases (e.g., patients) with two or more endocrine tumors, is advisable. If an *MEN1* mutation is not identified in the index case with two or more endocrine tumors, then clinical and genetic tests for other disorders such as hyperparathyroid-jaw tumor syndrome, FBHH, FIPA, MEN 2, or MEN 4 should be considered, because these patients may represent phenocopies for MEN 1.

The current guidelines recommend that *MEN1* mutational analysis should be undertaken in: (1) an index case with two or more MEN 1–associated endocrine tumors (e.g., parathyroid, pancreatic, or pituitary tumors); (2) asymptomatic first-degree relatives of a known *MEN1* mutation carrier; and (3) first-degree relatives of a *MEN1* mutation carrier with symptoms, signs, or biochemical or radiologic evidence for one or more MEN 1–associated tumors. In addition, *MEN1* mutational analysis should be considered in patients with suspicious or atypical MEN 1. This would include individuals with parathyroid adenomas before the age of 30 years or multigland parathyroid disease; individuals with gastrinoma or multiple pancreatic NETs at any age; or individuals who have two or more MEN 1–associated tumors that are not part of the classical triad of parathyroid, pancreatic islet, and anterior pituitary tumors (e.g., parathyroid tumor plus adrenal tumor). Family members, including asymptomatic individuals who have been identified to harbor a *MEN1* mutation, will require biochemical and radiologic screening (Table 408-3). In contrast, relatives who do not harbor the *MEN1* mutation have a risk of developing MEN 1–associated endocrine tumors that is similar to that of the general population; thus, relatives without the *MEN1* mutation do not require repeated screening.

Mutational analysis in asymptomatic individuals should be undertaken at the earliest opportunity and, if possible, in the first decade of life because tumors have developed in some children by the age of 5 years. Appropriate biochemical and radiologic investigations (Table 408-3) aimed at detecting the development of tumors should then be undertaken in affected individuals. Mutant gene carriers should undergo biochemical screening at least once per annum and also have baseline pituitary and abdominal imaging (e.g., MRI or CT), which should then be repeated at 1- to 3-year intervals (Table 408-3). Screening should commence after 5 years of age and should continue for life because the disease may develop as late as the eighth decade. The screening history and physical examination elicit the symptoms and signs of hypercalcemia, nephrolithiasis, peptic ulcer disease, neuroglycopenia, hypopituitarism, galactorrhea and amenorrhea in women, acromegaly, Cushing's disease, and visual field loss and the presence of subcutaneous lipomas, angiofibromas, and collagenomas. Biochemical screening should include measurements of serum calcium, PTH, gastrointestinal hormones (e.g., gastrin, insulin with a fasting glucose, glucagon, VIP, PP), chromogranin A, prolactin, and IGF-I in all individuals. More specific endocrine function tests should be undertaken in individuals who have symptoms or signs suggestive of a specific clinical syndrome. Biochemical screening for the development of MEN 1 tumors in asymptomatic members of families with MEN 1 is of great importance to reduce morbidity and mortality from the associated tumors.

MULTIPLE ENDOCRINE NEOPLASIA TYPE 2 AND TYPE 3

Clinical Manifestations MEN type 2 (MEN 2), which is also called Sipple's syndrome, is characterized by the association of medullary thyroid carcinoma (MTC), pheochromocytomas, and parathyroid tumors (Table 408-1). Three clinical variants of MEN 2 are recognized: MEN 2A, MEN 2B, and MTC only. MEN 2A, which is often referred to as MEN 2, is the most common variant. In MEN 2A, MTC is associated with pheochromocytomas in 50% of patients (may be bilateral) and with parathyroid tumors in 20% of patients. MEN 2A may rarely occur in association with Hirschsprung's disease, caused by the absence of autonomic ganglion cells in the terminal hindgut, resulting in colonic dilatation, severe constipation, and obstruction. MEN 2A may also be associated with cutaneous lichen amyloidosis, which is a pruritic lichenoid lesion that is usually located on the upper back. MEN 2B, which is also referred to as MEN 3, represents 5% of all cases of MEN 2 and is characterized by the occurrence of MTC and pheochromocytoma in association with a Marfanoid habitus; mucosal neuromas of the lips, tongue, and eyelids; medullated corneal fibers; and intestinal autonomic ganglion dysfunction leading to multiple diverticulae and megacolon. Parathyroid tumors do not usually occur in MEN 2B. MTC only (FMTC) is a variant in which MTC is the sole manifestation of the syndrome. However, the distinction between

TABLE 408-4 RECOMMENDATIONS FOR TESTS AND SURGERY IN MEN 2 AND MEN 3[a]

RET Mutation, Exon (Ex) Location, and Codon Involved	Risk[b]	Recommended Age (years) for Test/Intervention				
		RET Mutational Analysis	First Serum Calcitonin and Neck Ultrasound	Prophylactic Thyroidectomy	Screening for Pheochromocytoma	Screening for PHPT
Ex13 (768, 790)[c]; Ex14 (804)[c]; Ex15 (891)[c]	+	<3–5	<3–5	5[d]	20	20
Ex10 (609, 611, 618, 620)[c]; Ex11 (630)[c]	++	<3–5	<3–5	<5[e]	20	20
Ex11 (634)[c]	+++	<3–5	<3–5	<5	8	20
Ex15 (883)[f]; Ex16 (918)[f]	++++	ASAP and by <1	ASAP and by <0.5–1	ASAP and by <1	8	—[g]

[a]Adapted from American Thyroid Association Guidelines, RT Kloos et al: Thyroid 6:565, 2009. [b]Risk for early development of metastasis and aggressive growth of medullary thyroid cancer: ++++, highest; +++, high; ++, intermediate; and +, lowest. [c]Mutations associated with MEN 2A (or medullary thyroid carcinoma only). [d]Consider surgery at 5 years or later if serum calcitonin is normal, neck ultrasound is normal, and there is a less aggressive family history and family preference. [e]Consider surgery before 5 years or later if serum calcitonin is normal, neck ultrasound is normal, and there is a less aggressive family history and family preference. [f]Mutations associated with MEN 2B (MEN 3). [g]Not required because PHPT is not a feature of MEN 2B (MEN 3).

Abbreviations: ASAP, as soon as possible; MEN, multiple endocrine neoplasia; PHPT, primary hyperparathyroidism.

FMTC and MEN 2A is difficult and should only be considered if there are at least four family members above the age of 50 years who are affected by MTC but not pheochromocytomas or primary hyperparathyroidism. All of the MEN 2 variants are due to mutations of the rearranged during transfection (*RET*) protooncogene, which encodes a TKR. Moreover, there is a correlation between the locations of *RET* mutations and MEN 2 variants. Thus, ~95% of MEN 2A patients have mutations involving the cysteine-rich extracellular domain, with mutations of codon 634 accounting for ~85% of MEN 2A mutations; FMTC patients also have mutations of the cysteine-rich extracellular domain, with most mutations occurring in codon 618. In contrast, ~95% of MEN 2B/MEN 3 patients have mutations of codon 918 of the intracellular tyrosine kinase domain (Table 408-1 and Table 408-4).

Medullary Thyroid Carcinoma MTC is the most common feature of MEN 2A and MEN 2B and occurs in almost all affected individuals. MTC represents 5–10% of all thyroid gland carcinomas, and 20% of MTC patients have a family history of the disorder. The use of *RET* mutational analysis to identify family members at risk for hereditary forms of MTC has altered the presentation of MTC from that of symptomatic tumors to a preclinical disease for which prophylactic thyroidectomy (Table 408-4) is undertaken to improve the prognosis and ideally result in cure. However, in patients who do not have a known family history of MEN 2A, FMTC, or MEN 2B, and therefore have not had *RET* mutational analysis, MTC may present as a palpable mass in the neck, which may be asymptomatic or associated with symptoms of pressure or dysphagia in >15% of patients. Diarrhea occurs in 30% of patients and is associated either with elevated circulating concentrations of calcitonin or tumor-related secretion of serotonin and prostaglandins. Some patients may also experience flushing. In addition, ectopic ACTH production by MTC may cause Cushing's syndrome. The diagnosis of MTC relies on the demonstration of hypercalcitoninemia (>90 pg/mL in the basal state); stimulation tests using IV pentagastrin (0.5 mg/kg) and or calcium infusion (2 mg/kg) are rarely used now, reflecting improvements in the assay for calcitonin. Neck ultrasonography with fine-needle aspiration of the nodules can confirm the diagnosis. Radionucleotide thyroid scans may reveal MTC tumors as "cold" nodules. Radiography may reveal dense irregular calcification within the involved portions of the thyroid gland and in lymph nodes involved with metastases. Positron emission tomography (PET) may help to identify the MTC and metastases (Fig. 408-2). Metastases of MTC usually occur to the cervical lymph nodes in the early stages and to the mediastinal nodes, lung, liver, trachea, adrenal, esophagus, and bone in later stages. Elevations in serum calcitonin concentrations are often the first sign of recurrence or persistent disease, and the serum calcitonin doubling time is useful for determining prognosis. MTC can have an aggressive clinical course, with early metastases and death in approximately 10% of patients. A family history of aggressive MTC or MEN 2B may be elicited.

TREATMENT MEDULLARY THYROID CARCINOMA

Individuals with *RET* mutations who do not have clinical manifestations of MTC should be offered prophylactic surgery between the ages of <1 and 5 years. The timing of surgery will depend on the type of *RET* mutation and its associated risk for early development, metastasis, and aggressive growth of MTC (Table 408-4). Such patients should have a total thyroidectomy with a systematic central neck dissection to remove occult nodal metastasis, although

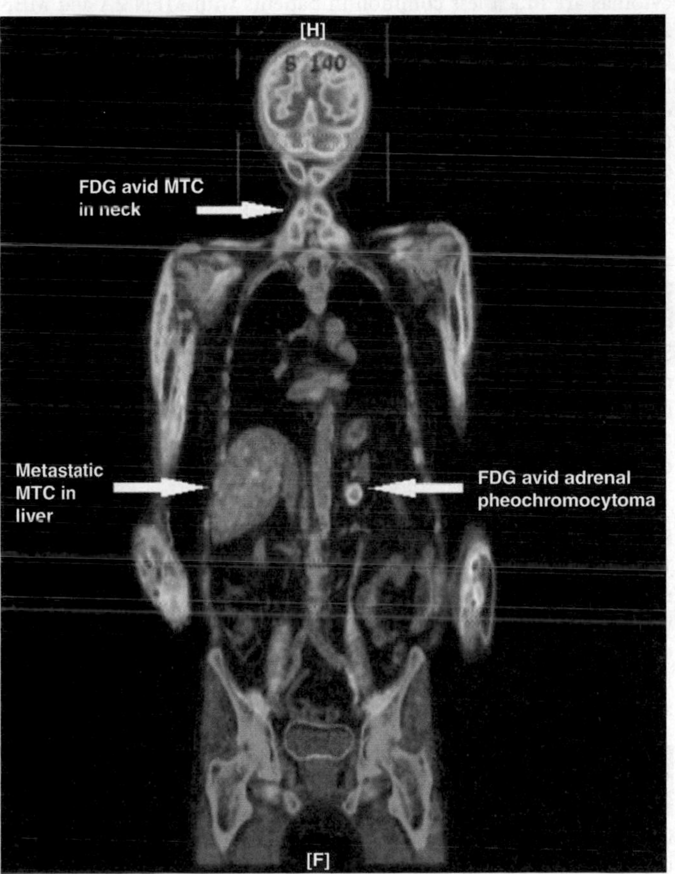

FIGURE 408-2 Fluorodeoxyglucose (FDG) positron emission tomography scan in a patient with multiple endocrine neoplasia type 2A, showing medullary thyroid cancer (MTC) with hepatic and skeletal (left arm) metastasis and a left adrenal pheochromocytoma. Note the presence of excreted FDG compound in the bladder. *(Reproduced with permission from A Naziat et al: Clin Endocrinol [Oxf] 78:966, 2013.)*

the value of undertaking a central neck dissection has been subject to debate. Prophylactic thyroidectomy, with life-long thyroxine replacement, has dramatically improved outcomes in patients with MEN 2 and MEN 3, such that ~90% of young patients with *RET* mutations who had a prophylactic thyroidectomy have no evidence of persistent or recurrent MTC at 7 years after surgery. In patients with clinically evident MTC, a total thyroidectomy with bilateral central resection is recommended, and an ipsilateral lateral neck dissection should be undertaken if the primary tumor is >1 cm in size or there is evidence of nodal metastasis in the central neck. Surgery is the only curative therapy for MTC. The 10-year survival in patients with metastatic MTC is ~20%. For inoperable MTC or metastatic disease, the tyrosine kinase inhibitors, vandetanib and cabozantinib, have improved the progression-free survival times. Other types of chemotherapy are of limited efficacy, but radiotherapy may help to palliate local disease.

Pheochromocytoma (See also Chap. 407) These noradrenaline- and adrenaline-secreting tumors occur in >50% of patients with MEN 2A and MEN 2B and are a major cause of morbidity and mortality. Patients may have symptoms and signs of catecholamine secretion (e.g., headaches, palpitations, sweating, poorly controlled hypertension), or they may be asymptomatic with detection through biochemical screening based on a history of familial MEN 2A, MEN 2B, or MTC. Pheochromocytomas in patients with MEN 2A and MEN 2B differ significantly in distribution when compared with patients without MEN 2A and MEN 2B. Extra-adrenal pheochromocytomas, which occur in 10% of patients without MEN 2A and MEN 2B, are observed rarely in patients with MEN 2A and MEN 2B. Malignant pheochromocytomas are much less common in patients with MEN 2A and MEN 2B. The biochemical and radiologic investigation of pheochromocytoma in patients with MEN 2A and MEN 2B is similar to that in non–MEN 2 patients and includes the measurement of plasma (obtained from supine patients) and urinary free fractionated metanephrines (e.g., normetanephrine and metanephrines measured separately), CT or MRI scanning, radionuclide scanning with meta-iodo-(^{123}I or ^{131}I)-benzyl guanidine (MIBG), and PET using (^{18}F)-fluorodopamine or (^{18}F)-fluoro-2-dexoxy-D-glucose (Fig. 408-2).

TREATMENT PHEOCHROMOCYTOMA

Surgical removal of pheochromocytoma, using α and β adrenoreceptor blockade before and during the operation, is the recommended treatment. Endoscopic adrenal-sparing surgery, which decreases postoperative morbidity, hospital stay, and expense, as opposed to open surgery, has become the method of choice.

Parathyroid Tumors (See also Chap. 424) Parathyroid tumors occur in 10–25% of patients with MEN 2A. However, >50% of these patients do not have hypercalcemia. The presence of abnormally enlarged parathyroids, which are unusually hyperplastic, is often seen in the normocalcemic patient undergoing thyroidectomy for MTC. The biochemical investigation and treatment of hypercalcemic patients with MEN 2A is similar to that of patients with MEN 1.

Genetics and Screening To date, approximately 50 different *RET* mutations have been reported, and these are located in exons 5, 8, 10, 11, 13, 14, 15, and 16. *RET* germline mutations are detected in >95% of MEN 2A, FMTC, and MEN 2B families, with Cys634Arg being most common in MEN 2A, Cys618Arg being most common in FMTC, and Met918Thr being most common in MEN 2B (Tables 408-1 and 408-4). Between 5 and 10% of patients with MTC or MEN 2A–associated tumors have de novo *RET* germline mutations, and ~50% of patients with MEN 2B have de novo *RET* germline mutations. These de novo *RET* germline mutations always occur on the paternal allele. Approximately 5% of patients with sporadic pheochromocytoma have a germline *RET* mutation, but such germline *RET* mutations do not appear to be associated with sporadic primary hyperparathyroidism. Thus, *RET* mutational analysis should be performed in: (1) all patients with MTC who have a family history of tumors associated with MEN 2, FMTC, or MEN 3, such that the diagnosis can be confirmed and genetic testing offered to asymptomatic relatives; (2) all patients with MTC and pheochromocytoma without a known family history of MEN 2 or MEN 3; (3) all patients with MTC, but without a family history of MEN 2, FMTC, or MEN 3, because these patients may have a de novo germline *RET* mutations; (4) all patients with bilateral pheochromocytoma; and (5) patients with unilateral pheochromocytoma, particularly if this occurs with increased calcitonin levels.

Screening for MEN 2/MEN 3–associated tumors in patients with *RET* germline mutations should be undertaken annually and include serum calcitonin measurements, a neck ultrasound for MTC, plasma and 24-h urinary fractionated metanephrines for pheochromocytoma, and albumin-corrected serum calcium or ionized calcium with PTH for primary hyperparathyroidism. In patients with MEN 2–associated *RET* mutations, screening for MTC should begin by 3 to 5 years; for pheochromocytoma by 20 years; and for primary hyperparathyroidism by 20 years of age (Table 408-4).

MULTIPLE ENDOCRINE NEOPLASIA TYPE 4

Clinical Manifestations Patients with MEN 1–associated tumors, such as parathyroid adenomas, pituitary adenomas, and pancreatic NETs, occurring in association with gonadal, adrenal, renal, and thyroid tumors have been reported to have mutations of the gene encoding the 196–amino acid cyclin-dependent kinase inhibitor (CK1) p27 kip1 (*CDNKIB*). Such families with MEN 1–associated tumors and *CDNKIB* mutations are designated to have MEN 4 (Table 408-1). The investigations and treatments for the MEN 4–associated tumors are similar to those for MEN 1 and non–MEN 1 tumors.

Genetics and Screening To date, eight different MEN 4–associated mutations of *CDNKIB*, which is located on chromosome 12p13, have been reported, and all of these are associated with a loss of function. These MEN 4 patients may represent ~3% of the 5–10% of patients with MEN 1 who do not have mutations of the *MEN1* gene. Germline *CDNKIB* mutations may rarely be found in patients with sporadic (i.e., nonfamilial) forms of primary hyperparathyroidism.

HYPERPARATHYROIDISM-JAW TUMOR SYNDROME (SEE ALSO CHAP. 424)

Clinical Manifestations Hyperparathyroidism-jaw tumor (HPT-JT) syndrome is an autosomal dominant disorder characterized by the development of parathyroid tumors (15% are carcinomas) and fibro-osseous jaw tumors. In addition, some patients may also develop Wilms' tumors, renal cysts, renal hematomas, renal cortical adenomas, papillary renal cell carcinomas, pancreatic adenocarcinomas, uterine tumors, testicular mixed germ cell tumors with a major seminoma component, and Hürthle cell thyroid adenomas. The parathyroid tumors may occur in isolation and without any evidence of jaw tumors, and this may cause confusion with other hereditary hypercalcemic disorders, such as MEN 1. However, genetic testing to identify the causative mutation will help to establish the correct diagnosis. The investigation and treatment for HPT-JT-associated tumors are similar to those in non-HPT-JT patients, except that early parathyroidectomy is advisable because of the increased frequency of parathyroid carcinoma.

Genetics and Screening The gene that causes HPT-JT is located on chromosome 1q31.2 and encodes a 531–amino acid protein, parafibromin (Table 408-2). Parafibromin is also referred to as cell division cycle protein 73 (CDC73) and has a role in transcription. Genetic testing in families helps to identify mutation carriers who should be periodically screened for the development of tumors (Table 408-5).

VON HIPPEL-LINDAU DISEASE (SEE ALSO CHAP. 407)

Clinical Manifestations von Hippel-Lindau (VHL) disease is an autosomal dominant disorder characterized by hemangioblastomas of the retina and CNS; cysts involving the kidneys, pancreas, and epididymis; renal cell carcinomas; pheochromocytomas; and pancreatic islet cell tumors. The retinal and CNS hemangioblastomas are benign vascular tumors that may be multiple; those in the CNS may cause symptoms

TABLE 408-5 HPT-JT SCREENING GUIDELINES

Tumor[a]	Test	Frequency[b]
Parathyroid	Serum Ca, PTH	6–12 months
Ossifying jaw fibroma	Panoramic jaw x-ray with neck shielding[c]	5 years
Renal	Abdominal MRI[c,d]	5 years
Uterine	Ultrasound (transvaginal or transabdominal) and additional imaging ± D&C if indicated[e]	Annual

[a]Screening for most common HPT-JT–associated tumors is considered. Assessment for other reported tumor types may be indicated (e.g., pancreatic, thyroid, testicular tumors). [b]Frequency of repeating test after baseline tests performed. [c]X rays and imaging involving ionizing radiation should ideally be avoided to minimize risk of generating subsequent mutations. [d]Ultrasound scan recommended if MRI unavailable. [e]Such selective pelvic imaging should be considered after obtaining a detailed menstrual history.

Abbreviations: Ca, calcium; D&C, dilatation and curettage; HPT-JT, hyperparathyroidism-jaw tumor syndrome; MRI, magnetic resonance imaging; PTH, parathyroid hormone.

Source: Reproduced from PJ Newey et al: Hum Mutat 31:295, 2010.

by compressing adjacent structures and/or increasing intracranial pressure. In the CNS, the cerebellum and spinal cord are the most frequently involved sites. The renal abnormalities consist of cysts and carcinomas, and the lifetime risk of a renal cell carcinoma (RCC) in VHL is 70%. The endocrine tumors in VHL consist of pheochromocytomas and pancreatic islet cell tumors. The clinical presentation of pheochromocytoma in VHL disease is similar to that in sporadic cases, except there is a higher frequency of bilateral or multiple tumors, which may involve extra-adrenal sites in VHL disease. The most frequent pancreatic lesions in VHL are multiple cyst-adenomas, which rarely cause clinical disease. However, nonsecreting pancreatic islet cell tumors occur in <10% of VHL patients, who are usually asymptomatic. The pancreatic tumors in these patients are often detected by regular screening using abdominal imaging. Pheochromocytomas should be investigated and treated as described earlier for MEN 2. The pancreatic islet cell tumors frequently become malignant, and early surgery is recommended.

Genetics and Screening The *VHL* gene, which is located on chromosome 3p26-p25, is widely expressed in human tissues and encodes a 213–amino acid protein (pVHL) (Table 408-2). A wide variety of germline *VHL* mutations have been identified. *VHL* acts as a tumor-suppressor gene. A correlation appears to exist between the type of mutation and the clinical phenotype; large deletions and protein-truncating mutations are associated with a low incidence of pheochromocytomas, whereas some missense mutations in VHL patients are associated with pheochromocytoma (referred to as VHL type 2C). Other missense mutations may be associated with hemangioblastomas and RCC but not pheochromocytoma (referred to as VHL type 1), whereas distinct missense mutations are associated with hemangioblastomas, RCC, and pheochromocytoma (VHL type 2B). VHL type 2A, which refers to the occurrence of hemangioblastomas and pheochromocytoma without RCC, is associated with rare missense mutations. The basis for these complex genotype-phenotype relationships remains to be elucidated. One major function of pVHL, which is also referred to as elongin, is to downregulate the expression of vascular endothelial growth factor (VEGF) and other hypoxia-inducible mRNAs. Thus, pVHL, in complex with other proteins, regulates the expression of hypoxia-inducible factors (HIF-1 and HIF-2) such that loss of functional pVHL leads to a stabilization of the HIF protein complexes, resulting in VEGF overexpression and tumor angiogenesis. Screening for the development of pheochromocytomas and pancreatic islet cell tumors is as described earlier for MEN 2 and MEN 1, respectively (Tables 408-3 and 408-4).

NEUROFIBROMATOSIS

Clinical Manifestations Neurofibromatosis type 1 (NF1), which is also referred to as von Recklinghausen's disease, is an autosomal dominant disorder characterized by the following manifestations: neurologic (e.g., peripheral and spinal neurofibromas); ophthalmologic (e.g., optic gliomas and iris hamartomas such as Lisch nodules); dermatologic (e.g., café au lait macules); skeletal (e.g., scoliosis, macrocephaly, short stature, and pseudoarthrosis); vascular (e.g., stenoses of renal and intracranial arteries); and endocrine (e.g., pheochromocytoma, carcinoid tumors, and precocious puberty). Neurofibromatosis type 2 (NF2) is also an autosomal dominant disorder but is characterized by the development of bilateral vestibular schwannomas (acoustic neuromas) that lead to deafness, tinnitus, or vertigo. Some patients with NF2 also develop meningiomas, spinal schwannomas, peripheral nerve neurofibromas, and café au lait macules. Endocrine abnormalities are not found in NF2 and are associated solely with NF1. Pheochromocytomas, carcinoid tumors, and precocious puberty occur in about 1% of patients with NF1, and growth hormone deficiency has been also reported. The features of pheochromocytomas in NF1 are similar to those in non-NF1 patients, with 90% of tumors being located within the adrenal medulla and the remaining 10% at an extra-adrenal location, which often involves the para-aortic region. Primary carcinoid tumors are often periampullary and may also occur in the ileum but rarely in the pancreas, thyroid, or lungs. Hepatic metastases are associated with symptoms of the carcinoid syndrome, which include flushing, diarrhea, bronchoconstriction, and tricuspid valve disease. Precocious puberty is usually associated with the extension of an optic glioma into the hypothalamus with resultant early activation of gonadotropin-releasing hormone secretion. Growth hormone deficiency has also been observed in some NF1 patients, who may or may not have optic chiasmal gliomas, but it is important to note that short stature is frequent in the absence of growth hormone deficiency in patients with NF1. The investigation and treatment for tumors are similar to those undertaken for each respective tumor type in non-NF1 patients.

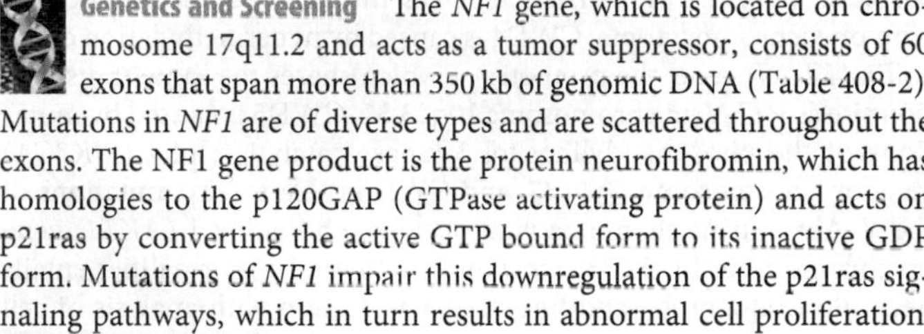

Genetics and Screening The *NF1* gene, which is located on chromosome 17q11.2 and acts as a tumor suppressor, consists of 60 exons that span more than 350 kb of genomic DNA (Table 408-2). Mutations in *NF1* are of diverse types and are scattered throughout the exons. The NF1 gene product is the protein neurofibromin, which has homologies to the p120GAP (GTPase activating protein) and acts on p21ras by converting the active GTP bound form to its inactive GDP form. Mutations of *NF1* impair this downregulation of the p21ras signaling pathways, which in turn results in abnormal cell proliferation. Screening for the development of pheochromocytomas and carcinoid tumors is as described earlier for MEN 2 and MEN 1, respectively (Tables 408-3 and 408-4).

CARNEY COMPLEX

Clinical Manifestations Carney complex (CNC) is an autosomal dominant disorder characterized by spotty skin pigmentation (usually of the face, labia, and conjunctiva), myxomas (usually of the eyelids and heart, but also the tongue, palate, breast, and skin), psammomatous melanotic schwannomas (usually of the sympathetic nerve chain and upper gastrointestinal tract), and endocrine tumors that involve the adrenals, Sertoli cells, somatotropes, thyroid, and ovary. Cushing's syndrome, the result of primary pigmented nodular adrenal disease (PPNAD), is the most common endocrine manifestation of CNC and may occur in one-third of patients. Patients with CNC and Cushing's syndrome often have an atypical appearance by being thin (as opposed to having truncal obesity). In addition, they may have short stature, muscle and skin wasting, and osteoporosis. These patients often have levels of urinary free cortisol that are normal or increased only marginally. Cortisol production may fluctuate periodically with days or weeks of hypercortisolism; this pattern is referred to as "periodic Cushing's syndrome." Patients with Cushing's syndrome usually have loss of the circadian rhythm of cortisol production. Acromegaly, the result of a somatotrope tumor, affects ~10% of patients with CNC. Testicular tumors may also occur in one-third of patients with CNC. These may either be large-cell calcifying Sertoli cell tumors, adrenocortical rests, or Leydig cell tumors. The Sertoli cell tumors occasionally may be estrogen-secreting and lead to precocious puberty or gynecomastia. Some patients with CNC have been reported to develop thyroid follicular tumors, ovarian cysts, or breast duct adenomas.

Genetics and Screening CNC type 1 (CNC1) is due to mutations of the protein kinase A (PKA) regulatory subunit 1 α (R1α) (*PPKAR1A*), a tumor suppressor, whose gene is located on chromosome 17q.24.2 (Table 408-2). The gene causing CNC type 2 (CNC2) is located on chromosome 2p16 and has not yet been identified. It is interesting to note, however, that some tumors do not show LOH of 2p16 but instead show genomic instability, suggesting that this CNC gene may not be a tumor suppressor. Screening and treatment of these endocrine tumors are similar to those described earlier for patients with MEN 1 and MEN 2 (Tables 408-3 and 408-4).

COWDEN'S SYNDROME

Clinical Manifestations Multiple hamartomatous lesions, especially of the skin, mucous membranes (e.g., buccal, intestinal, and colonic), breast, and thyroid are characteristic of Cowden's (CWD) syndrome, which is an autosomal dominant disorder. Thyroid abnormalities occur in two-thirds of patients with CWD syndrome, and these usually consist of multinodular goiters or benign adenomas, although <10% of patients may have a follicular thyroid carcinoma. Breast abnormalities occur in >75% of patients and consist of either fibrocystic disease or adenocarcinomas. The investigation and treatment for CWD tumors are similar to those undertaken for non-CWD patients.

Genetics and Screening CWD syndrome is genetically heterogenous, and six types (CWD1–6) are recognized (Table 408-2). CWD is due to mutations of the phosphate and tensin homologue deleted on chromosome 10 (*PTEN*) gene, located on chromosome 10q23.31. CWD2 is caused by mutations of the succinate dehydrogenase subunit B (*SDHB*) gene, located on chromosome 1p36.13; and CWD3 is caused by mutations of the *SDHD* gene, located on chromosome 11q13.1. *SDHB* and *SDHD* mutations are also associated with pheochromocytoma. CWD4 is caused by hypermethylation of the Killin (*KLLN*) gene, the promoter of which shares the same transcription site as *PTEN* on chromosome 10q23.31. CWD5 is caused by mutations of the phosphatidylinositol 3-kinase catalytic alpha (*PIK3CA*) gene on chromosome 3q26.32, and CWD6 is caused by mutations of the V-Akt murine thymoma viral oncogene homolog 1 (*AKT1*) gene on chromosome 14q32.33. Screening for thyroid abnormalities entails neck ultrasonography and fine-needle aspiration with analysis of cell cytology.

MCCUNE-ALBRIGHT SYNDROME (SEE ALSO CHAP. 426e)

Clinical Manifestations McCune-Albright syndrome (MAS) is characterized by the triad of polyostotic fibrous dysplasia, which may be associated with hypophosphatemic rickets; café au lait skin pigmentation; and peripheral precocious puberty; other endocrine abnormalities include thyrotoxicosis, which may be associated with a multinodular goiter, somatotrope tumors, and Cushing's syndrome (due to adrenal tumors). Investigation and treatment for each endocrinopathy are similar to those used in patients without MAS.

Genetics and Screening MAS is a disorder of mosaicism that results from postzygotic somatic cell mutations of the G protein α stimulating subunit (Gsα), encoded by the *GNAS1* gene, located on chromosome 20q13.32 (Table 408-2). The Gsα mutations, which include Arg201Cys, Arg201His, Glu227Arg, or Glu227His, are activating and are found only in cells of the abnormal tissues. Screening for hyperfunction of relevant endocrine glands and development of hypophosphatemia, which may be associated with elevated serum fibroblast growth factor 23 (FGF23) concentrations, is undertaken in MAS patients.

ACKNOWLEDGMENTS

The author is grateful to the Medical Research Council (UK) for support and to Mrs. Tracey Walker for typing the manuscript.

409 Autoimmune Polyendocrine Syndromes

Peter A. Gottlieb

Polyglandular deficiency syndromes have been given many different names, reflecting the wide spectrum of disorders that have been associated with these syndromes and the heterogeneity of their clinical presentations. The name used in this chapter for this group of disorders is *autoimmune polyendocrine syndrome* (APS). In general, these disorders are divided into two major categories, APS type 1 (APS-1) and APS type 2 (APS-2). Some groups have further subdivided APS-2 into APS type 3 (APS-3) and APS type 4 (APS-4) depending on the type of autoimmunity involved. For the most part, this additional classification does not clarify our understanding of disease pathogenesis or prevention of complications in individual patients. Importantly, there are many nonendocrine disease associations included in these syndromes, suggesting that although the underlying autoimmune disorder predominantly involves endocrine targets, it does not exclude other tissues. The disease associations found in APS-1 and APS-2 are summarized in Table 409-1. Understanding these syndromes and their disease manifestations can lead to early diagnosis and treatment of additional disorders in patients and their family members.

TABLE 409-1 DISEASE ASSOCIATIONS WITH AUTOIMMUNE POLYENDOCRINE SYNDROMES

Autoimmune Polyendocrine Syndrome Type 1	Autoimmune Polyendocrine Syndrome Type 2	Other Autoimmune Polyendocrine Disorders
Endocrine	**Endocrine**	IPEX (immune dysfunction polyendocrinopathy X-linked)
Addison's disease	Addison's disease	Thymic tumors
Hypoparathyroidism	Type 1 diabetes	Anti-insulin receptor antibodies
Hypogonadism	*Graves' disease or autoimmune thyroiditis*	POEMS syndrome
Graves' disease or autoimmune thyroiditis	*Hypogonadism*	Insulin autoimmune syndrome (Hirata's syndrome)
Type 1 diabetes		Adult combined pituitary hormone deficiency (CPHD) with anti-Pit1 autoantibodies
		Kearns-Sayre syndrome
		DIDMOAD syndrome
Nonendocrine	**Nonendocrine**	Congenital rubella associated with thyroiditis and/or diabetes
Mucocutaneous candidiasis	Celiac disease, dermatitis herpetiformis	
Chronic active hepatitis	Pernicious anemia	
Pernicious anemia	Vitiligo	
Vitiligo	*Alopecia*	
Asplenism	*Myasthenia gravis*	
Ectodermal dysplasia	*IgA deficiency*	
Alopecia	*Parkinson's disease*	
Malabsorption syndromes	*Idiopathic thrombocytopenia*	
IgA deficiency		

Abbreviations: DIDMOAD, diabetes insipidus, diabetes mellitus, progressive bilateral optic atrophy, and sensorineural deafness; POEMS, polyneuropathy, organomegaly, endocrinopathy, M-protein, and skin changes.

Note: Italics denote less common disorders.

APS-1

APS-1 (Online Mendelian Inheritance in Man [OMIM] 240300) has also been called autoimmune polyendocrinopathy–candidiasis–ectodermal dystrophy (APECED). Mucocutaneous candidiasis, hypoparathyroidism, and Addison's disease form the three major components of this disorder. However, as summarized in Table 409-1, many other organ systems can be involved over time. APS-1 is rare, with fewer than 500 cases reported in the literature. It is an autosomal recessive disorder caused by mutations in the *AIRE* gene (autoimmune regulator gene) found on chromosome 21. This gene is most highly expressed in thymic medullary epithelial cells (mTECs) where it appears to control the expression of tissue-specific self-antigens (e.g., insulin). Deletion of this regulator leads to decreased expression of tissue-specific self-antigens and is hypothesized to allow autoreactive T cells to avoid clonal deletion, which normally occurs during T cell maturation in the thymus. The *AIRE* gene is also expressed in epithelial cells found in peripheral lymphoid organs, but its role in these extrathymic cells remains controversial. A number of mutations have been described in this gene, and there is a higher frequency within certain ethnic groups including Iranian Jews, Sardinians, Finns, Norwegians, and Irish.

Clinical Manifestations APS-1 develops very early in life, often in infancy (Table 409-2). Chronic mucocutaneous candidiasis without signs of systemic disease is often the first manifestation. It affects the mouth and nails more frequently than the skin and esophagus. Chronic oral candidiasis can result in atrophic disease with areas suggestive of leukoplakia, which can pose a risk for future carcinoma. The etiology is associated with anticytokine autoantibodies (anti-IL-17A, -IL-17F, and -IL-22) related to T helper (T_H) 17 T cells and depressed production of these cytokines by peripheral blood mononuclear cells. Hypoparathyroidism usually develops next, followed by adrenal insufficiency. The time from development of one component of the disorder to the next can be many years, and the order of disease appearance is variable.

Chronic candidiasis is nearly always present and is not very responsive to treatment. Hypoparathyroidism is found in >85% of cases, and Addison's disease is found in nearly 80%. Gonadal failure appears to affect women more than men (70% vs 25%, respectively), and hypoplasia of the dental enamel also occurs frequently (77% of patients). Other endocrine disorders that occur less frequently include type 1 diabetes (23%) and autoimmune thyroid disease (18%). Nonendocrine manifestations that present less frequently include alopecia (40%), vitiligo (26%), intestinal malabsorption (18%), pernicious anemia (31%), chronic active hepatitis (17%), and nail dystrophy. An unusual and debilitating manifestation of the disorder is the development of refractory diarrhea/obstipation that may be related to autoantibody-mediated destruction of enterochromaffin or enterochromaffin-like cells.

TABLE 409-2 COMPARISON OF APS-1 AND APS-2

APS-1	APS-2
Early onset: infancy	Later onset
Siblings often affected and at risk	Multigenerational
Equivalent sex distribution	Females > males affected
Monogenic: *AIRE* gene, chromosome 21, autosomal recessive	Polygenic: *HLA, MICA, PTPN22, CTLA4*
Not HLA associated for entire syndrome, some specific component risk	DR3/DR4 associated; other HLA class III gene associations noted
Autoantibodies to type 1 interferons and IL-17 and IL-22	No autoantibodies to cytokines
Autoantibodies to specific target organs	Autoantibodies to specific target organs
Asplenism	No defined immunodeficiency
Mucocutaneous candidiasis	Association with other nonendocrine immunologic disorders like myasthenia gravis and idiopathic thrombocytopenic purpura

Abbreviations: APS, autoimmune polyendocrine syndrome; IL, interleukin.

The incidence rates for many of these disorders peak in the first or second decade of life, but the individual disease components continue to emerge over time. Therefore, prevalence rates may be higher than originally reported.

Diagnosis The diagnosis of APS-1 is usually made clinically when two of the three major component disorders are found in an individual patient. Siblings of individuals with APS-1 should be considered affected even if only one component disorder has been detected due to the known inheritance of the syndrome. Genetic analysis of the *AIRE* gene should be undertaken to identify mutations. Initial sequencing may detect the common mutations, but rare mutations are continually being noted, and an initial negative genetic analysis should not dissuade one from the clinical diagnosis until more extensive DNA sequencing can be performed. Detection of anti-interferon α and anti-interferon o antibodies can identify nearly 100% of cases with APS-1. The autoantibody arises independent of the type of *AIRE* gene mutation and is not found in other autoimmune disorders.

Diagnosis of each underlying disorder should be done based on their typical clinical presentations (Table 409-3). Mucocutaneous candidiasis may present throughout the gastrointestinal tract, and it may be detected in the oral mucosa or from stool samples. Evaluation by a gastroenterologist to examine the esophagus for candidiasis or secondary stricture may be merited based on symptoms. Other gastrointestinal manifestations of APS-1, including malabsorption and obstipation, may also bring these young patients to the attention of gastroenterologists for first evaluation. Specific physical examination findings of hyperpigmentation, vitiligo, alopecia, tetany, and signs of hyper- or hypothyroidism should be considered as signs of development of component disorders.

The development of disease-specific autoantibody assays can help confirm disease and also detect risk for future disease. For example, where possible, detection of anticytokine antibodies to interleukin (IL) 17 and IL-22 would confirm the diagnosis of mucocutaneous candidiasis due to APS-1. The presence of anti-21-hydroxylase antibody or anti-17-hydroxylase antibody (which may be found more commonly in adrenal insufficiency associated with APS-1) would confirm the presence or risk for Addison's disease. Other autoantibodies found in type 1 diabetes (e.g., anti-GAD65), pernicious anemia, and other component conditions should be screened for on a regular basis (6- to 12-month intervals depending on the age of the subject).

Laboratory tests, including a complete metabolic panel, phosphorous and magnesium, thyroid-stimulating hormone (TSH), adrenocorticotropic hormone (ACTH; morning), hemoglobin A_{1c}, plasma vitamin B_{12} level, and complete blood count with peripheral smear looking for Howell-Jolly bodies (asplenism), should also be performed at these time points. Detection of abnormal physical findings or test results should prompt subsequent examinations of the relevant organ system (e.g., presence of Howell-Jolly bodies indicates need for ultrasound of spleen).

TREATMENT APS-1

Therapy of individual disease components is carried out as outlined in other relevant chapters. Replacement of deficient hormones (e.g., adrenal, pancreas, ovaries/testes) will treat most of the endocrinopathies noted. Several unique issues merit special emphasis. Adrenal insufficiency can be masked by primary hypothyroidism by prolonging the half-life of cortisol. The caveat therefore is that replacement therapy with thyroid hormone can precipitate an adrenal crisis in an undiagnosed individual. Hence, all patients with hypothyroidism and the possibility of APS should be screened for adrenal insufficiency to allow treatment with glucocorticoids prior to the initiation of thyroid hormone replacement. Treatment of mucocutaneous candidiasis with ketoconazole in an individual with subclinical adrenal insufficiency may also precipitate adrenal crisis. Furthermore, mucocutaneous candidiasis may be difficult to eradicate entirely. Severe cases of disease involvement may require systemic immunomodulatory therapy, but this is not commonly needed.

TABLE 409-3 CLINICAL FEATURES AND RECOMMENDED FOLLOW-UP FOR APS-1 AND APS-2

Component Disease	Recommended Evaluation
APS-1	
Addison's disease	Sodium, potassium, ACTH, cortisol, 21- and 17-hydroxylase autoantibodies
Diarrhea	History
Ectodermal dysplasia	Physical examination
Hypoparathyroidism	Serum calcium, phosphate, PTH
Hepatitis	Liver function tests
Hypothyroidism/ Graves' disease	TSH; thyroid peroxidase and/or thyroglobulin autoantibodies and anti-TSH receptor Ab
Male hypogonadism	FSH/LH, testosterone
Malabsorption	Physical examination, anti-IL-17 and anti-IL-22 autoantibodies
Mucocutaneous candidiasis	Physical examination, mucosal swab, stool samples
Obstipation	History
Ovarian failure	FSH/LH, estradiol
Pernicious anemia	CBC, vitamin B_{12} levels
Splenic atrophy	Blood smear for Howell-Jolly bodies; platelet count; ultrasound if positive
Type 1 diabetes	Glucose, hemoglobin A_{1c}, diabetes-associated autoantibodies (insulin, GAD65, IA-2, ZnT8)
APS-2	
Addison's disease	21-Hydroxylase autoantibodies, ACTH stimulation testing if positive
Alopecia	Physical examination
Autoimmune hyper- or hypothyroidism	TSH; thyroid peroxidase and/or thyroglobulin autoantibodies, anti-TSH receptor Ab
Celiac disease	Transglutaminase autoantibodies; small intestine biopsy if positive
Cerebellar ataxia	Dictated by signs and symptoms of disease
Chronic inflammatory demyelinating polyneuropathy	Dictated by signs and symptoms of disease
Hypophysitis	Dictated by signs and symptoms of disease, anti-Pit1 autoantibody
Idiopathic heart block	Dictated by signs and symptoms of disease
IgA deficiency	IgA level
Myasthenia gravis	Dictated by signs and symptoms of disease, antiacetylcholinesterase Ab
Myocarditis	Dictated by signs and symptoms of disease
Pernicious anemia	Anti–parietal cell autoantibodies
	CBC, vitamin B_{12} levels if positive
Serositis	Dictated by signs and symptoms of disease
Stiff man syndrome	Dictated by signs and symptoms of disease
Vitiligo	Physical examination, NALP-1 polymorphism

Abbreviations: Ab, antibody; ACTH, adrenocorticotropic hormone; APS, autoimmune polyendocrine syndrome; CBC, complete blood count; FSH, follicle-stimulating hormone; IL, interleukin; LH, luteinizing hormone; PTH, parathyroid hormone; TSH, thyroid-stimulating hormone.

APS-2

APS-2 (OMIM 269200) is more common than APS-1 with a prevalence of 1 in 100,000. It has a gender bias and occurs more often in female patients with a ratio of at least 3:1 compared to male patients. In contrast to APS-1, APS-2 often has its onset in adulthood with a peak incidence between 20 and 60 years of age. It shows a familial, multigenerational heritage (Table 409-2). The presence of two or more of the following endocrine deficiencies in the same patient defines the presence of APS-2: primary adrenal insufficiency (Addison's disease; 50–70%), Graves' disease or autoimmune thyroiditis (15–69%), type 1 diabetes mellitus (T1D; 40–50%), and primary hypogonadism. Frequently associated autoimmune conditions include celiac disease (3–15%), myasthenia gravis, vitiligo, alopecia, serositis, and pernicious anemia. These conditions occur with increased frequency in affected patients but are also are found in their family members (Table 409-3).

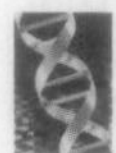

Genetic Considerations The overwhelming risk factor for APS-2 has been localized to the genes in the human lymphocyte antigen complex on chromosome 6. Primary adrenal insufficiency in APS-2, but not APS-1, is strongly associated with both HLA-DR3 and HLA-DR4. Other class I and class II genes and alleles, such as HLA-B8, HLA-DQ2 and HLA-DQ8, and HLA-DR subtype such as DRB1*0404, appear to contribute to organ-specific disease susceptibility (Table 409-4). HLA-B8- and HLA-DR3-associated illnesses include selective IgA deficiency, juvenile dermatomyositis, dermatitis herpetiformis, alopecia, scleroderma, autoimmune thrombocytopenia purpura, hypophysitis, metaphyseal osteopenia, and serositis.

Several other immune genes have been proposed to be associated with Addison's disease and therefore with APS-2 (Table 409-3). The "5.1" allele of a major histocompatibility complex (MHC) gene is an atypical class I HLA molecule MIC-A. The MIC-A5.1 allele has a very strong association with Addison's disease that is not accounted for by linkage disequilibrium with DR3 or DR4. Its role is complicated because certain HLA class I genes can offset this effect. PTPN22 codes for a polymorphism in a protein tyrosine phosphatase, which acts on intracellular signaling pathways in both T and B lymphocytes. It has been implicated in T1D, Addison's disease, and other autoimmune conditions. CTLA4 is a receptor on the T cell surface that modulates the activation state of the cell as part of the signal 2 pathway. Polymorphisms of this gene appear to cause downregulation of the cell surface expression of the receptor, leading to decreased T cell activation and proliferation. This appears to contribute to disease in Addison's disease and potentially other components of APS-2. Allelic variants of the IL-2Rα are linked to development of T1D and autoimmune thyroid disease and could contribute to the phenotype of APS-2 in certain individuals.

Diagnosis When one of the component disorders is present, a second associated disorder occurs more commonly than in the general population (Table 409-3). There is controversy as to which tests to use and how often to screen individuals for disease. A strong family history of autoimmunity should raise suspicion in an individual with an initial component diagnosis. The development of a rarer form of autoimmunity, such as Addison's disease, should prompt more extensive screening for other linked disorders compared to the diagnosis of autoimmune thyroid disease, which is relatively common.

Circulating autoantibodies, as previously discussed, can precede the development of disease by many years but would allow the clinician to follow the patient and identify the disease onset at its earliest time point (Tables 409-3 and 409-4). For each of the endocrine components of the disorder, appropriate autoantibody assays are listed and, if positive, should prompt physiologic testing to diagnose clinical or subclinical disease. For Addison's disease, antibodies to 21-hydroxylase antibodies are highly diagnostic for risk of adrenal insufficiency. However, individuals may take many years to develop overt hypoadrenalism. Screening of 21-hydroxylase antibody–positive patients can be performed measuring morning ACTH and cortisol on a yearly basis. Rising ACTH values over time or low morning cortisol in association with signs or symptoms of adrenal insufficiency should prompt testing via the cosyntropin stimulation test (Chap. 406). T1D can be screened for by measuring autoantibodies including anti-insulin, anti-GAD65, anti-IA-2, and anti-ZnT8. Risk for progression to disease can be based on the number of antibodies, and in some cases the titer (insulin autoantibody), as well as other metabolic factors (impaired oral glucose tolerance test). National Institutes of Health–sponsored trial groups such as Type 1 Diabetes TrialNet are screening first- and second-degree family members for these autoantibodies and identifying prediabetic individuals who may qualify for intervention trials to change the course of the disease prior to onset.

TABLE 409-4 APS-2 AND OTHER POLYENDOCRINE DISORDER ASSOCIATIONS

Disease	HLA Association	Initiating Factor	Mechanism	Autoantigen
Graves' Disease	DR3	Iodine Anti-CD52	Antibody	TSH receptor
Myasthenia gravis	DR3, DR7	Thymoma Penicillamine	Antibody	Acetylcholine receptor
Anti-insulin receptor	?	SLE or other autoimmune disease	Antibody	Insulin receptor
Hypoparathyroidism	?	?	Antibody	Cell surface inhibitor
Insulin autoimmune syndrome	DR4, DRB1*0406	Methimazole Sulfhydryl-containing drugs	Antibody	Insulin
Celiac disease	DQ2/DQ8	Gluten diet	T cell	Transglutaminase
Type 1 diabetes	DR3/DR4 DQ2/DQ8	? Congenital rubella	T cell	Insulin, GAD65, IA-2, ZnT8, IGRP
Addison's disease	DR3/DR4 DRB1*0404	Unknown	T cell	21-Hydroxylase P450-5cc
Thyroiditis	DR3/DQB1*0201 DQA1*0301	Iodine Interferon α	T cell	Thyroglobulin Thyroid peroxidase
Pernicious anemia	?	?	T cell	Intrinsic factor H+/K+ ATPase
Vitiligo	?	Melanoma Antigen Immunization	?	Melanocyte
Chromosome dysgenesis–trisomy 21 and Turner's syndrome	DQA1*0301	?	?	Thyroid, islet, transglutaminase
Hypophysitis	?	Pit-1, TDRD6	?	Pituitary, Pit-1

Abbreviations: APS, autoimmune polyendocrine syndrome; SLE, systemic lupus erythematosus; TSH, thyroid-stimulating hormone.

Screening tests for thyroid disease can include anti–thyroid peroxidase (TPO) or anti-thyroglobulin autoantibodies or anti-TSH receptor antibodies for Graves' disease. Yearly measurements of TSH can then be used to follow these individuals. Celiac disease can be screened for using the anti–tissue transglutaminase (tTg) antibody test. For those <20 years of age, testing every 1–2 years should be performed, whereas less frequent testing is indicated after the age of 20 because the majority of individuals who develop celiac disease have the antibody earlier in life. Positive tTg antibody test results should be confirmed on repeat testing, followed by small-bowel biopsy to document pathologic changes of celiac disease. Many patients have asymptomatic celiac disease that is nevertheless associated with osteopenia and impaired growth. If left untreated, symptomatic celiac disease has been reported to be associated with an increased risk of gastrointestinal malignancy, especially lymphoma.

The knowledge of the particular disease associations should guide other autoantibody or laboratory testing. A complete history and physical examination should be performed every 1–3 years including CBC, metabolic panel, TSH, and vitamin B_{12} levels to screen for most of the possible abnormalities. More specific tests should be based on specific findings from the history and physical.

TREATMENT APS-2

With the exception of Graves' disease, the management of each of the endocrine components of APS-2 involves hormone replacement and is covered in detail in the chapters on adrenal (Chap. 406), thyroid (Chap. 405), gonadal (Chaps. 411 and 412), and parathyroid disease (Chap. 424). As noted for APS-1, adrenal insufficiency can be masked by primary hypothyroidism and should be considered and treated as discussed above. In patients with T1D, decreasing insulin requirements or hypoglycemia, without obvious secondary causes, may indicate the emergence of adrenal insufficiency. Hypocalcemia in APS-2 patients is more likely due to malabsorption than hypoparathyroidism.

Immunotherapy for autoimmune endocrine disease has been reserved for T1D, for the most part, reflecting the lifetime burden of the disease for the individual patient and society. Although several immunotherapies (e.g., modified anti-CD3, rituximab, abatacept) can prolong the honeymoon phase of T1D, none has achieved long-term success. Active research using new approaches and combination therapy may change the treatment of this disease or other autoimmune conditions that share similar pathways. Furthermore, treatment of subclinical disease diagnosed by the presence of autoantibodies may provide a mechanism to preempt the development of overt disease and is the subject of active basic and clinical research.

IPEX

*I*mmune dysregulation, *p*olyendocrinopathy, *e*nteropathy, and *X*-linked disease (IPEX; OMIM 304790) is a rare X-linked recessive disorder. The disease onset is in infancy and is characterized by severe enteropathy, T1D, and skin disease, as well as variable association with several other autoimmune disorders. Many infants die within the first days of life, but the course is variable, with some children surviving for 12–15 years. Early onset of T1D, often at birth, is highly suggestive of the diagnosis because nearly 80% of IPEX patients develop T1D. Although treatment of the individual disorders can temporarily improve the situation, treatment of the underlying immune deficiency is required and includes immunosuppressive therapy generally followed by hematopoietic stem cell transplantation. Transplantation is the only life-saving form of therapy and can be fully curative by normalizing the imbalanced immune system found in this disorder.

IPEX is caused by mutations in the *FOXP3* gene, which is also mutated in the Scurfy mouse, an animal model that shares much of the phenotype of IPEX patients. The FOXP3 transcription factor is expressed in regulatory T cells designated CD4+CD25+FOXP3+ (Treg). Lack of this factor causes a profound deficiency of this Treg population and results in rampant autoimmunity due to the lack of peripheral tolerance normally provided by these cells. Certain mutations may lead to varying forms of expression of the full syndrome, and there are rare cases where the *FOXP3* gene is intact but other genes involved in this pathway (e.g., CD25, IL-2Rα) may be causative.

THYMIC TUMORS

Thymomas and thymic hyperplasia are associated with several autoimmune diseases, with the most common being myasthenia gravis (44%) and red cell aplasia (20%). Graves' disease, T1D, and Addison's disease may also be associated with thymic tumors. Patients with myasthenia gravis and thymoma may have unique anti–acetylcholine receptor autoantibodies. Many thymomas lack AIRE expression within the thymoma, and this could be a potential factor in the development of autoimmunity. In support of this concept, thymoma is the one other disease with "frequent" development of anticytokine antibodies and mucocutaneous candidiasis in adults. The majority of tumors are malignant, and temporary remissions of the autoimmune condition can occur with resection of the tumor.

ANTI-INSULIN RECEPTOR ANTIBODIES

This is a very rare disorder where severe insulin resistance (type B) is caused by the presence of anti-insulin receptor antibodies. It is associated with acanthosis nigricans, which can also be associated with other forms of less severe insulin resistance. About one-third of patients have an associated autoimmune illness such as systemic lupus erythematosus or Sjögren's syndrome. Therefore, the presence of antinuclear antibodies, elevated erythrocyte sedimentation rate, hyperglobulinemia, leukopenia, and hypocomplementemia may accompany the presentation. The presence of anti-insulin receptor autoantibodies leads to marked insulin resistance, requiring more than 100,000 units of insulin to be given daily with only partial control of hyperglycemia. Patients can also have severe hypoglycemia due to partial activation of the insulin receptor by the antibody. The course of the disease is variable, and several patients have had spontaneous remissions. Therapy targeting B lymphocytes including rituximab, cyclophosphamide, and pulse steroids can induce remission of the disease.

INSULIN AUTOIMMUNE SYNDROME (HIRATA'S SYNDROME)

The insulin autoimmune syndrome, associated with Graves' disease and methimazole therapy (or other sulfhydryl-containing medications), is of particular interest due to a remarkably strong association with a specific HLA haplotype. Such patients with elevated titers of anti-insulin autoantibodies frequently present with hypoglycemia. In Japan, the disease is restricted to HLA-DR4-positive individuals with DRB1*0406. Curiously, a recent report demonstrated that five out of six Caucasian patients taking lipoic acid (sulfhydryl group) who developed insulin autoimmune syndrome were primarily DRB1*0403 (which is related to DRB1*0406); the sixth was DRB1*0406. In Hirata's syndrome the anti-insulin autoantibodies are often polyclonal. Discontinuation of the medication generally leads to resolution of the syndrome over time.

POEMS SYNDROME

POEMS (*p*olyneuropathy, *o*rganomegaly, *e*ndocrinopathy, *M*-protein, and *s*kin changes; also known as Crow-Fukase syndrome; OMIM 192240) patients usually present with a progressive sensorimotor polyneuropathy, diabetes mellitus (50%), primary gonadal failure (70%), and a plasma cell dyscrasia with sclerotic bony lesions. Associated findings can be hepatosplenomegaly, lymphadenopathy, and hyperpigmentation. Patients often present in the fifth to sixth decade of life and have a median survival after diagnosis of less than 3 years. The syndrome is assumed to be secondary to circulating immunoglobulins, but patients have excess vascular endothelial growth factor as well as elevated levels of other inflammatory cytokines such as IL1-β, IL-6, and tumor necrosis factor α. A small series of patients have been treated with thalidomide, leading to a decrease in vascular endothelial growth factor. Hyperglycemia responds to small, subcutaneous doses of insulin. The hypogonadism is due to primary gonadal disease with elevated plasma levels of follicle-stimulating hormone and luteinizing hormone. Temporary resolution of the features of POEMS, including normalization of blood glucose, may occur after radiotherapy for localized plasma cell lesions of bone or after chemotherapy, thalidomide, plasmapheresis, autologous stem cell transplantation, or treatment with all-*trans*-retinoic acid.

OTHER DISORDERS

Other diseases can exhibit polyendocrine deficiencies, including Kearns-Sayre syndrome, DIDMOAD syndrome (*d*iabetes *i*nsipidus, *d*iabetes *m*ellitus, progressive bilateral *o*ptic *a*trophy, and sensorineural *d*eafness; also termed Wolfram's syndrome), Down's syndrome or trisomy 21 (OMIM 190685), Turner's syndrome (monosomy X, 45,X), and congenital rubella.

Kearns-Sayre syndrome (OMIM 530000) is a rare mitochondrial DNA disorder characterized by myopathic abnormalities leading to ophthalmoplegia and progressive weakness in association with several endocrine abnormalities, including hypoparathyroidism, primary gonadal failure, diabetes mellitus, and hypopituitarism. Crystalline mitochondrial inclusions are found in muscle biopsy specimens, and such inclusions have also been observed in the cerebellum. Antiparathyroid antibodies have not been described; however, antibodies to the anterior pituitary gland and striated muscle have been identified, and the disease may have autoimmune components. These mitochondrial DNA mutations occur sporadically and do not appear to be associated with a familial syndrome.

Wolfram's syndrome (OMIM 222300, chromosome 4; OMIM 598500, mitochondrial) is a rare autosomal recessive disease that is also called DIDMOAD. Neurologic and psychiatric disturbances are prominent in most patients and can cause severe disability. The disease is caused by defects in wolframin, a 100-kDa transmembrane protein that has been localized to the endoplasmic reticulum and is found in neuronal and neuroendocrine tissue. Its expression induces ion channel activity with a resultant increase in intracellular calcium and may play an important role in intracellular calcium homeostasis. Wolfram's syndrome appears to be a slowly progressive neurodegenerative process, and there is nonautoimmune selective destruction of the pancreatic beta cells. Diabetes mellitus with an onset in childhood is usually the first manifestation. Diabetes mellitus and optic atrophy are present in all reported cases, but expression of the other features is variable.

Down's syndrome, or trisomy 21 (OMIM 190685), is associated with the development of T1D, thyroiditis, and celiac disease. Patients with Turner's syndrome also appear to be at increased risk for the development of thyroid disease and celiac disease. It is recommended to screen patients with trisomy 21 and Turner's syndrome for associated autoimmune diseases on a regular basis.

SECTION 2 REPRODUCTIVE ENDOCRINOLOGY

410 Disorders of Sex Development

John C. Achermann, J. Larry Jameson

Sex development begins in utero but continues into young adulthood with the achievement of sexual maturity and reproductive capability. The major determinants of sex development can be divided into three components: chromosomal sex, gonadal sex (sex determination), and phenotypic sex (sex differentiation) (Fig. 410-1). Variations at each of these stages can result in disorders (or differences) of sex development (DSDs) (Table 410-1). In the newborn period, approximately 1 in 4000 babies require investigation because of ambiguous (atypical) genitalia. Urgent assessment is required, because some causes such as congenital adrenal hyperplasia (CAH) can be associated with life-threatening adrenal crises. Support for the parents and clear communication about the diagnosis and management options are essential. The involvement of an experienced multidisciplinary team is important for counseling, planning appropriate investigations, and discussing long-term well-being. DSDs can also present at other ages and to a range of health professionals. Subtler forms of gonadal dysfunction (e.g., Klinefelter's syndrome [KS], Turner's syndrome [TS]) often are diagnosed later in life by internists. Because these conditions are associated with a variety of psychological, reproductive, and potential medical consequences, an open dialogue must be established between the patient and health care providers to ensure continuity and attention to these issues.

SEX DEVELOPMENT

Chromosomal sex, defined by a karyotype, describes the X and/or Y chromosome complement (46,XY; 46,XX) that is established at the time of fertilization. The presence of a normal Y chromosome determines that testis development will occur even in the presence of multiple X chromosomes (e.g., 47,XXY or 48,XXXY). The loss of an X chromosome impairs gonad development (45,X or 45,X/46,XY mosaicism). Fetuses with no X chromosome (45,Y) are not viable.

Gonadal sex refers to the histologic and functional characteristics of gonadal tissue as testis or ovary. The embryonic gonad is bipotential and can develop (from ~42 days after conception) into either a testis or an ovary, depending on which genes are expressed (Fig. 410-2). Testis development is initiated by expression of the Y chromosome gene *SRY*

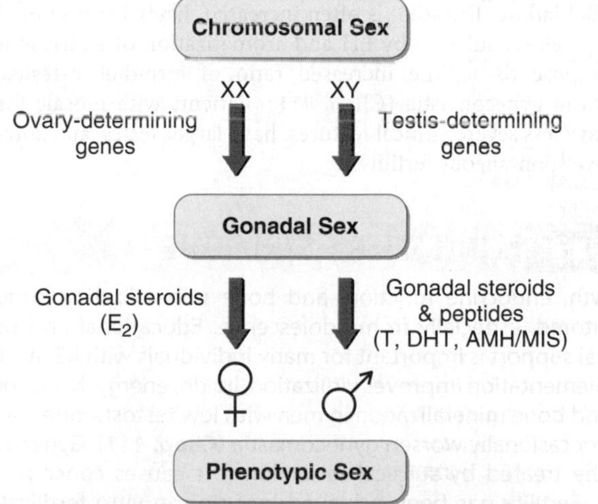

FIGURE 410-1 Sex development can be divided into three major components: chromosomal sex, gonadal sex, and phenotypic sex. DHT, dihydrotestosterone; MIS, müllerian-inhibiting substance also known as anti-müllerian hormone, AMH; T, testosterone.

(sex-determining region on the Y chromosome) that encodes an HMG box transcription factor. *SRY* is expressed transiently in cells destined to become Sertoli cells and serves as a pivotal switch to establish the testis lineage. Mutation of *SRY* prevents testis development in 46,XY individuals, whereas translocation of *SRY* in 46,XX individuals is sufficient to induce testis development and a male phenotype. Other genes are necessary to continue testis development. *SOX9* (*SRY*-related HMG-box gene 9) is upregulated by *SRY* in the developing testis but is suppressed in the ovary. *WT1* (Wilms' tumor–related gene 1) acts early in the genetic pathway and regulates the transcription of several genes, including *SF1* (*NR5A1*), *DAX1* (*NR0B1*), and *AMH* (encoding müllerian-inhibiting substance [MIS]). *SF1* encodes steroidogenic factor 1, a nuclear receptor that functions in cooperation with other transcription factors to regulate a large array of adrenal and gonadal genes, including *SOX9* and many genes involved in steroidogenesis. *SF1* mutations causing loss of function are found in ~10% of XY patients with gonadal dysgenesis and impaired androgenization. In contrast, duplication of a related gene *DAX1* also impairs testis development, revealing the exquisite sensitivity of the testis-determining pathway to gene dosage effects. *DAX1* loss-of-function mutations cause adrenal hypoplasia, hypogonadotropic hypogonadism, and testicular dysgenesis. In addition to the genes mentioned above, studies of humans and mice indicate that at least 30 other genes are also involved in gonad development (Fig. 410-2). These genes encode an array of signaling molecules and paracrine growth factors in addition to transcription factors.

Although ovarian development once was considered a "default" process, it is now clear that specific genes are expressed during the earliest stages of ovary development. Some of these factors may repress testis development (e.g., WNT4, R-spondin-1) (Fig. 410-2). Once the ovary has formed, additional factors are required for normal follicular development (e.g., follicle-stimulating hormone [FSH] receptor, *GDF9*). Steroidogenesis in the ovary requires the development of follicles that contain granulosa cells and theca cells surrounding the oocytes (Chap. 412). Thus, there is relatively limited ovarian steroidogenesis until puberty.

Germ cells also develop in a sex dimorphic manner. In the developing ovary, primordial germ cells (PGCs) proliferate and enter meiosis, whereas they proliferate and then undergo mitotic arrest in the developing testis. PGC entry into meiosis is initiated by retinoic acid that activates *STRA8* (stimulated by retinoic acid 8) and other genes involved in meiosis. The developing testis produces high levels of CYP26B1, an enzyme that degrades retinoic acid, preventing PGC entry into meiosis. Approximately 7 million germ cells are present in the fetal ovary in the second trimester, and 1 million remain at birth. Only 400 are ovulated during a woman's reproductive life span (Chap. 412).

Phenotypic sex refers to the structures of the external and internal genitalia and secondary sex characteristics. The developing testis releases anti-müllerian hormone (AMH; also known as müllerian-inhibiting substance [MIS]) from Sertoli cells and testosterone from Leydig cells. AMH is a member of the transforming growth factor (TGF) β family and acts through specific receptors to cause regression of the müllerian structures from 60–80 days after conception. At ~60–140 days after conception, testosterone supports the development of wolffian structures, including the epididymides, vasa deferentia, and seminal vesicles. Testosterone is the precursor for dihydrotestosterone (DHT), a potent androgen that promotes development of the external genitalia, including the penis and scrotum (65–100 days, and thereafter) (Fig. 410-3). The urogenital sinus develops into the prostate and prostatic urethra in the male and into the urethra and lower portion of the vagina in the female. The genital tubercle becomes the glans penis in the male and the clitoris in the female. The urogenital swellings form the scrotum or the labia majora, and the urethral folds fuse to form the shaft of the penis and the male urethra or the labia minora. In the female, wolffian ducts regress and the müllerian ducts form the

TABLE 410-1 CLASSIFICATION OF DISORDERS OF SEX DEVELOPMENT (DSDS)

Sex Chromosome DSD	46,XY DSD (see Table 410-3)	46,XX DSD (see Table 410-4)
47,XXY (Klinefelter's syndrome and variants)	**Disorders of gonadal (testis) development**	**Disorders of gonadal (ovary) development**
45,X (Turner's syndrome and variants)	Complete or partial gonadal dysgenesis (e.g., SRY, SOX9, SF1, WT1, DHH, MAP3K1)	Gonadal dysgenesis
45,X/46,XY mosaicism (mixed gonadal dysgenesis)	Impaired fetal Leydig cell function (e.g., *SF1/NR5A1, CXorf6/MAMLD1*)	Ovotesticular DSD
46,XX/46,XY (chimerism/mosaicism)	Ovotesticular DSD	Testicular DSD (e.g., *SRY*+, dup *SOX9, RSPO1*)
	Testis regression	**Androgen excess**
	Disorders in androgen synthesis or action	Fetal
	Disorders of androgen biosynthesis	3β-Hydroxysteroid dehydrogenase II (*HSD3β2*)
	LH receptor (*LHCGR*)	21-Hydroxylase (*CYP21A2*)
	Smith-Lemli-Opitz syndrome	P450 oxidoreductase (*POR*)
	Steroidogenic acute regulatory (*StAR*) protein	11β-Hydroxylase (*CYP11B1*)
	Cholesterol side-chain cleavage (*CYP11A1*)	Glucocorticoid receptor mutations
	3β-Hydroxysteroid dehydrogenase II (*HSD3B2*)	Fetoplacental
	17α-Hydroxylase/17,20-lyase (*CYP17A1*)	Aromatase deficiency (*CYP19*)
	P450 oxidoreductase (*POR*)	Oxidoreductase deficiency (*POR*)
	Cytochrome b5 (*CYB5A*)	Maternal
	17β-Hydroxysteroid dehydrogenase III (*HSD17B3*)	Maternal virilizing tumors (e.g., luteomas)
	5α-Reductase II (*SRD5A2*)	Androgenic drugs
	Aldo-keto reductase 1C2 (*AKR1C2*)	**Other**
	Disorders of androgen action	Syndromic associations (e.g., cloacal anomalies)
	Androgen insensitivity syndrome	Müllerian agenesis/hypoplasia (e.g., MRKH)
	Drugs and environmental modulators	Uterine abnormalities (e.g., MODY5)
	Other	Vaginal atresia (e.g., McKusick-Kaufman)
	Syndromic associations of male genital development	Labial adhesions
	Persistent müllerian duct syndrome	
	Vanishing testis syndrome	
	Isolated hypospadias	
	Congenital hypogonadotropic hypogonadism	
	Cryptorchidism	
	Environmental influences	

Source: Modified from IA Hughes: Arch Dis Child 91:554, 2006.

fallopian tubes, uterus, and upper segment of the vagina. A female phenotype will develop in the absence of the gonad, but estrogen is needed for maturation of the uterus and breast at puberty.

DISORDERS OF CHROMOSOMAL SEX

Variations in sex chromosome number and structure can present as DSDs (e.g., 45,X/46,XY). KS (47,XXY) and TS (45,X) do not usually present with genital ambiguity but are associated with gonadal dysfunction (Table 410-2).

KLINEFELTER'S SYNDROME (47,XXY)

Pathophysiology The classic form of KS (47,XXY) occurs after meiotic nondisjunction of the sex chromosomes during gametogenesis (40% during spermatogenesis, 60% during oogenesis) (Chap. 83e). Mosaic forms of KS (46,XY/47,XXY) are thought to result from chromosomal mitotic nondisjunction within the zygote and occur in at least 10% of individuals with this condition. Other chromosomal variants of KS (e.g., 48,XXYY, 48,XXXY) have been reported but are less common.

Clinical Features KS is characterized by small testes, infertility, gynecomastia, tall stature/increased leg length, and hypogonadism in phenotypic males. It has an incidence of at least 1 in 1000 men, but approximately 75% of cases are not diagnosed. Of those who are diagnosed, only 10% are identified prepubertally, usually because of small genitalia or cryptorchidism. Others are diagnosed after puberty, usually based on impaired androgenization and/or gynecomastia. Developmental delay, speech difficulties, and poor motor skills may be features but are variable, especially in adolescence. Later in life, body habitus or infertility leads to the diagnosis. Testes are small and firm (median length 2.5 cm [4 mL volume]; almost always <3.5 cm [12 mL]) and typically seem inappropriately small for the degree of androgenization. Biopsies are not usually necessary but typically reveal seminiferous tubule hyalinization and azoospermia. Other clinical features of KS are listed in Table 410-2. Plasma concentrations of FSH and luteinizing hormone (LH) are increased in most adults with 47,XXY, and plasma testosterone is decreased (50–75%), reflecting primary gonadal failure. Estradiol is often increased, likely because of chronic Leydig cell stimulation by LH and aromatization of androstenedione by adipose tissue; the increased ratio of estradiol-to-testosterone results in gynecomastia (Chap. 411). Patients with mosaic forms of KS have less severe clinical features, have larger testes, and sometimes achieve spontaneous fertility.

TREATMENT KLINEFELTER'S SYNDROME

Growth, endocrine function, and bone mineralization should be monitored, especially from adolescence. Educational and psychological support is important for many individuals with KS. Androgen supplementation improves virilization, libido, energy, hypofibrinolysis, and bone mineralization in men with low testosterone levels but may occasionally worsen gynecomastia (Chap. 411). Gynecomastia can be treated by surgical reduction if it causes concern (Chap. 411). Fertility has been achieved by using in vitro fertilization in men with oligospermia or with intracytoplasmic sperm injection (ICSI) after retrieval of spermatozoa by testicular sperm extraction techniques. In specialized centers, successful spermatozoa retrieval using this technique is possible in >50% of men with nonmosaic

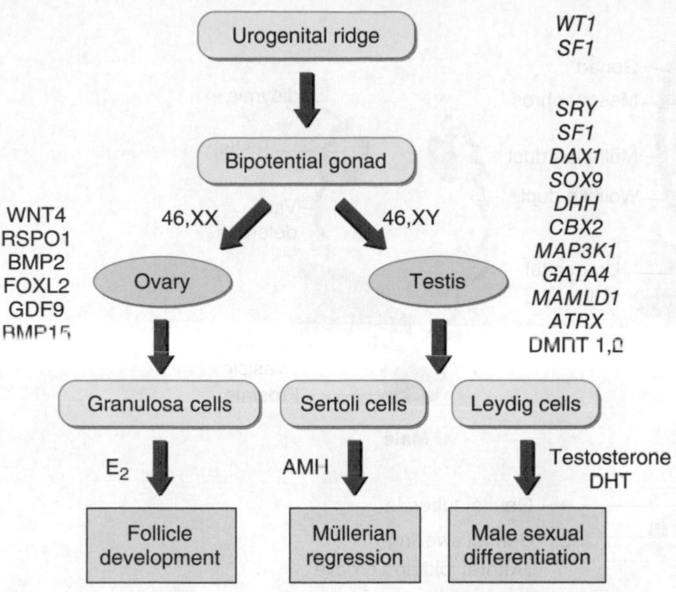

FIGURE 410-2 The genetic regulation of gonadal development. AMH, anti müllerian hormone (müllerian-inhibiting substance); *ATRX*, α-thalassemia, mental retardation on the X; BMP2 and 15, bone morphogenic factors 2 and 15; *CBX2*, chromobox homologue 2; *DAX1*, dosage sensitive sex-reversal, adrenal hypoplasia congenita on the X chromosome, gene 1; *DHH*, desert hedgehog; DHT, dihydrotestosterone; *DMRT 1,2*, doublesex MAB3-related transcription factor 1,2; *FOXL2*, forkhead transcription factor L2; *GATA4*, GATA binding protein 4; GDF9, growth differentiation factor 9; *MAMLD1*, mastermind-like domain containing 1; *MAP3K1*, mitogen-activated protein kinase kinase kinase 1; RSPO1, R-spondin 1; *SF1*, steroidogenic factor 1 (also known as NR5A1); *SOX9*, *SRY*-related HMG-box gene 9; *SRY*, sex-determining region on the Y chromosome; *WNT4*, wingless-type MMTV integration site 4; *WT1*, Wilms' tumor–related gene 1.

KS. Results may be better in younger men. After ICSI and embryo transfer, successful pregnancies can be achieved in ~50% of these cases. The risk of transmission of this chromosomal abnormality needs to be considered, and preimplantation screening may be desired, although this outcome is much less common than originally predicted. Long-term monitoring of men with KS is important given the increased risk of breast cancer, cardiovascular disease, metabolic syndrome, and autoimmune disorders. Because most men with KS are never diagnosed, it is important that all internists consider this diagnosis in men with these features who might be seeking medical advice for other conditions.

TURNER'S SYNDROME (GONADAL DYSGENESIS; 45,X)

Pathophysiology Approximately one-half of women with TS have a 45,X karyotype, about 20% have 45,X/46,XX mosaicism, and the remainder have structural abnormalities of the X chromosome such as X fragments, isochromosomes, or rings. The clinical features of TS result from haploinsufficiency of multiple X chromosomal genes (e.g., short stature homeobox, *SHOX*). However, imprinted genes also may be affected when the inherited X has different parental origins.

Clinical Features TS is characterized by bilateral streak gonads, primary amenorrhea, short stature, and multiple congenital anomalies in phenotypic females. It affects ~1 in 2500 women and is diagnosed at different ages depending on the dominant clinical features (Table 410-2). Prenatally, a diagnosis of TS usually is made incidentally after chorionic villus sampling or amniocentesis for unrelated reasons such as advanced maternal age. Prenatal ultrasound findings include increased nuchal translucency. The postnatal diagnosis of TS should be considered in female neonates or infants with lymphedema, nuchal folds, low hairline, or left-sided cardiac defects and in girls with unexplained growth failure or pubertal delay. Although limited spontaneous pubertal development occurs in up to 30% of girls with TS (10%, 45,X; 30–40%, 45,X/46,XX) and ~2% reach menarche, the vast majority of women with TS develop complete ovarian insufficiency. Therefore, this diagnosis should be considered in all women who present with primary or secondary amenorrhea and elevated gonadotropin levels.

TREATMENT TURNER'S SYNDROME

The management of girls and women with TS requires a multidisciplinary approach because of the number of potentially involved organ systems. Detailed cardiac and renal evaluation should be performed at the time of diagnosis. Individuals with congenital heart

TABLE 410-2 CLINICAL FEATURES OF CHROMOSOMAL DISORDERS OF SEX DEVELOPMENT (DSD)

Disorder	Common Chromosomal Complement	Gonad	Genitalia: External	Genitalia: Internal	Breast Development
Klinefelter's syndrome	47,XXY or 46,XY/47,XXY	Hyalinized testes	Male	Male	Gynecomastia
	Clinical Features: Small testes, azoospermia, decreased facial and axillary hair, decreased libido, tall stature and increased leg length, decreased penile length, increased risk of breast tumors, thromboembolic disease, learning difficulties, speech delay and decreased verbal IQ, obesity, diabetes mellitus, metabolic syndrome, varicose veins, hypothyroidism, systemic lupus erythematosus, epilepsy				
Turner's syndrome	45,X or 45,X/46,XX	Streak gonad or immature ovary	Female	Hypoplastic female	Immature female
	Clinical Features: Infancy: lymphedema, web neck, shield chest, low-set hairline, cardiac defects and coarctation of the aorta, urinary tract malformations, and horseshoe kidney Childhood: short stature, cubitus valgus, short neck, short fourth metacarpals, hypoplastic nails, micrognathia, scoliosis, otitis media and sensorineural hearing loss, ptosis and amblyopia, multiple nevi and keloid formation, autoimmune thyroid disease, visuospatial learning difficulties Adulthood: pubertal failure and primary amenorrhea, hypertension, obesity, dyslipidemia, impaired glucose tolerance and insulin resistance, autoimmune thyroid disease, cardiovascular disease, aortic root dilation, osteoporosis, inflammatory bowel disease, chronic hepatic dysfunction, increased risk of colon cancer, hearing loss				
45,X/46,XY mosaicism	45,X/46,XY	Testis or streak gonad	Variable	Variable	Usually male
	Clinical Features: Short stature, increased risk of gonadal tumors, some Turner's syndrome features				
Ovotesticular DSD (true hermaphroditism)	46,XX/46,XY	Testis and ovary or ovotestis	Variable	Variable	Gynecomastia
	Clinical Features: Possible increased risk of gonadal tumors				

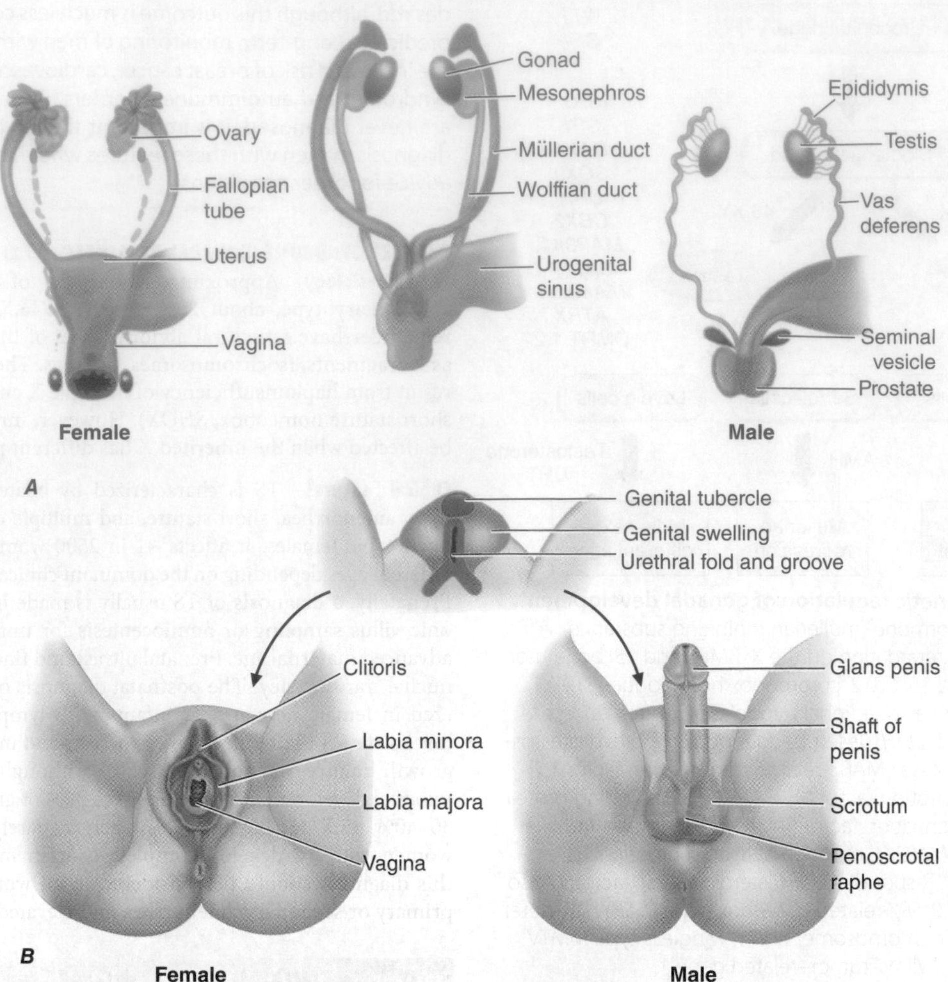

FIGURE 410-3 Sex development. ***A.*** Internal urogenital tract. ***B.*** External genitalia. *(After E Braunwald et al [eds]: Harrison's Principles of Internal Medicine, 15th ed. New York, McGraw-Hill, 2001.)*

defects (CHDs) (30%) (bicuspid aortic valve, 30–50%; coarctation of the aorta, 30%; aortic root dilation, 5%) require long-term follow-up by an experienced cardiologist, antibiotic prophylaxis for dental or surgical procedures, and serial magnetic resonance imaging (MRI) of aortic root dimensions, because progressive aortic root dilation is associated with increased risk of aortic dissection. Individuals found to have congenital renal and urinary tract malformations (30%) are at risk for urinary tract infections, hypertension, and nephrocalcinosis. Hypertension can occur independently of cardiac and renal malformations and should be monitored and treated as in other patients with essential hypertension. Clitoral enlargement or other evidence of virilization suggests the presence of covert, translocated Y chromosomal material and is associated with increased risk of gonadoblastoma. Regular assessment of thyroid function, weight, dentition, hearing, speech, vision, and educational issues should be performed during childhood. Otitis media and middle-ear disease are prevalent in childhood (50–85%), and sensorineural hearing loss becomes progressively common with age (70–90%). Autoimmune hypothyroidism (15–30%) can occur in childhood but has a mean age of onset in the third decade. Counseling about long-term growth and fertility issues should be provided. Patient support groups are active throughout the world and can play an invaluable role.

Short stature can be an issue for some girls because untreated final height rarely exceeds 150 cm in nonmosaic 45,X TS. High-dose recombinant growth hormone stimulates growth rate in children with TS and is occasionally combined with low doses of the nonaromatizable anabolic steroid oxandrolone (up to 0.05 mg/kg per day) in an older child (>9 years). However, final height increments are often about 5–10 cm, and individualization of treatment response to regimens may be beneficial. Girls with evidence of ovarian insufficiency require estrogen replacement to induce breast and uterine development, support growth, and maintain bone mineralization. Most physicians now initiate low-dose estrogen therapy (one-tenth to one-eighth of the adult replacement dose) to induce puberty at an age-appropriate time (~12 years). Doses of estrogen are increased gradually to allow development over a 2- to 4-year period. Progestins are added later to regulate withdrawal bleeds. Some women with TS have achieved successful pregnancy after ovum donation and in vitro fertilization but are high risk, and cardiac assessment is required. Long-term follow-up of women with TS involves careful surveillance of sex hormone replacement and reproductive function, bone mineralization, cardiac function and aortic root dimensions, blood pressure, weight and glucose tolerance, hepatic and lipid profiles, thyroid function, and hearing. This service is provided by a dedicated TS clinic in some centers.

45,X/46,XY MOSAICISM (MIXED GONADAL DYSGENESIS)

The phenotype of individuals with 45,X/46,XY mosaicism (sometimes called *mixed gonadal dysgenesis*) can vary considerably. Some have a predominantly female phenotype with somatic features of TS, streak gonads, and müllerian structures, and are managed as TS with a Y chromosome. Most 45,X/46,XY individuals have a male phenotype and testes, and the diagnosis is made incidentally after amniocentesis or during investigation of infertility. In practice, most newborns referred for assessment have atypical genitalia and variable somatic features. Management is complex and needs to be individualized. A female sex-of-rearing is often assigned if uterine structures are present, gonads are intraabdominal, and phallic development is incomplete. In such situations, gonadectomy usually is considered to prevent further androgen secretion at puberty and prevent risk of gonadoblastoma (up to 25%). Individuals raised as males usually require reconstructive surgery for hypospadias and removal of dysgenetic or streak gonads if the gonads cannot be brought down into the scrotum. Scrotal testes can be preserved but require regular examination for tumor development and sonography at the time of puberty. Biopsy for carcinoma in situ is recommended in adolescence, and testosterone supplementation may be required to support androgenization in puberty or if low testosterone is detected in adulthood. Height potential is usually attenuated; some children receive recombinant growth hormone using TS protocols. Screening for cardiac, renal, and other TS features should be considered, and psychological support offered for the family and young person.

OVOTESTICULAR DSD

Ovotesticular DSD (formerly called *true hermaphroditism*) occurs when both an ovary and a testis—or when an ovotestis—are found in one individual. Most individuals with this diagnosis have a 46,XX karyotype, especially in sub-Saharan Africa, and present with ambiguous genitalia at birth or with breast development and phallic development at puberty. A 46,XX/46,XY chimeric karyotype is less common and has a variable phenotype.

DISORDERS OF GONADAL AND PHENOTYPIC SEX

Disorders of gonadal and phenotypic sex can result in underandrogenization of individuals with a 46,XY karyotype (46,XY DSD) and the excess androgenization of individuals with a 46,XX karyotype (46,XX DSD) (Table 410-1). These disorders cover a spectrum of phenotypes ranging from "46,XY phenotypic females" or "46,XX phenotypic males" to individuals with atypical genitalia.

46,XY DSD

Underandrogenization of the 46,XY fetus (formerly called *male pseudohermaphroditism*) reflects defects in androgen production or action. It can result from disorders of testis development, defects of androgen synthesis, or resistance to testosterone and DHT (Table 410-1).

Disorders of Testis Development • *TESTICULAR DYSGENESIS* *Pure* (or *complete*) *gonadal dysgenesis* (*Swyer's syndrome*) is associated with streak gonads, müllerian structures (due to insufficient AMH/MIS secretion), and a complete absence of androgenization. Phenotypic females with this condition often present because of absent pubertal development and are found to have a 46,XY karyotype. Serum sex steroids, AMH/MIS, and inhibin B are low, and LH and FSH are elevated. Patients with *partial gonadal dysgenesis* (*dysgenetic testes*) may produce enough MIS to regress the uterus and sufficient testosterone for partial androgenization, and therefore usually present in the newborn period with atypical genitalia. Gonadal dysgenesis can result from mutations or deletions of testis-promoting genes (*WT1*, *CBX2*, *SF1*, *SRY*, *SOX9*, *MAP3K1*, *DHH*, *GATA4*, *ATRX*, *ARX*, *DMRT*) or duplication of chromosomal loci containing "antitestis" genes (e.g., *WNT4/RSPO1*, *DAX1*) (Table 410-3). Among these, deletions or mutations of *SRY* and heterozygous mutations of *SF1* (*NR5A1*) appear to be most common but still account collectively for <25% of cases. Associated clinical features may be present, reflecting additional functional roles for these genes. For example, renal dysfunction occurs in patients with specific *WT1* mutations (Denys-Drash and Frasier's syndromes), primary adrenal failure occurs in some patients with *SF1* mutations, and severe cartilage abnormalities (campomelic dysplasia) are the predominant clinical feature of *SOX9* mutations. A family history of DSD, infertility, or early menopause is important because mutations in *SF1/NR5A1* can be inherited from a mother in a sex-limited dominant manner (which can mimic X-linked inheritance). In some cases, a woman may later develop primary ovarian insufficiency because of the effect of *SF1* on the ovary. Intraabdominal dysgenetic testes should be removed to prevent malignancy, and estrogens can be used to induce secondary sex characteristics and uterine development in 46,XY individuals raised as females, if it is felt that a female gender identity is established. *Absent (vanishing) testis syndrome* (*bilateral anorchia*) reflects regression of the testis during development. The etiology is unknown, but the absence of müllerian structures indicates adequate secretion of AMH early in utero. In most cases, androgenization of the external genitalia is either normal or slightly impaired (e.g., small penis, hypospadias). These individuals can be offered testicular prostheses and should receive androgen replacement in adolescence.

Disorders of Androgen Synthesis Defects in the pathway that regulates androgen synthesis (Fig. 410-4) cause underandrogenization of the 46,XY fetus (Table 410-1). Müllerian regression is unaffected because Sertoli cell function is preserved. Most of these conditions can present with a spectrum of genital phenotypes, ranging from female-typical external genitalia or clitoromegaly in the more severe situations to penoscrotal hypospadias or a small phallus in others.

LH RECEPTOR Mutations in the LH receptor (LHCGR) cause Leydig cell hypoplasia and androgen deficiency, due to impaired actions of human chorionic gonadotropin in utero and LH late in gestation and during the neonatal period. As a result, testosterone and DHT synthesis are insufficient for complete androgenization.

STEROIDOGENIC ENZYME PATHWAYS Mutations in *steroidogenic acute regulatory protein* (*StAR*) and *CYP11A1* affect both adrenal and gonadal steroidogenesis (Fig. 410-4) (Chap. 406). Affected individuals (46,XY) usually have severe early-onset salt-losing adrenal failure and a female phenotype, although later-onset milder variants have been reported. Defects in *3β-hydroxysteroid dehydrogenase type 2* (*HSD3β2*) also cause adrenal insufficiency in severe cases, but the accumulation of dehydroepiandrosterone (DHEA) has a mild androgenizing effect, resulting in ambiguous genitalia or hypospadias. Salt loss occurs in many but not all cases. Patients with CAH due to *17α-hydroxylase* (*CYP17*) *deficiency* have variable underandrogenization and develop hypertension and hypokalemia due to the potent salt-retaining effects of corticosterone and 11-deoxycorticosterone. Patients with complete loss of 17α-hydroxylase function often present as phenotypic females who fail to enter puberty and are found to have inguinal testes and hypertension in adolescence. Some mutations in *CYP17* selectively impair 17,20-lyase activity without altering 17α-hydroxylase activity, leading to underandrogenization without mineralocorticoid excess and hypertension. Disruption of the coenzyme, *cytochrome b5* (*CYB5A*), can present similarly, and methemoglobinemia is usually present. Mutations in *P450 oxidoreductase* (*POR*) affect multiple steroidogenic enzymes, leading to impaired androgenization and a biochemical pattern of apparent combined 21-hydroxylase and 17α-hydroxylase deficiency, sometimes with skeletal abnormalities (Antley-Bixler craniosynostosis). Defects in *17β-hydroxysteroid dehydrogenase type 3* (*HSD17β3*) and *5α-reductase type 2* (*SRD5A2*) interfere with the synthesis of testosterone and DHT, respectively. These conditions are characterized by minimal or absent androgenization in utero, but some phallic development can occur during adolescence due to the action of other enzyme isoforms. Individuals with 5α-reductase type 2 deficiency have normal wolffian structures and usually do not develop breast tissue. At puberty, the increase in testosterone induces muscle mass and other virilizing features despite DHT deficiency. Some individuals change gender from female to male at puberty. Thus, the management of this disorder is challenging. DHT cream can improve prepubertal phallic growth in patients raised as male. Gonadectomy before adolescence and estrogen replacement at puberty can be considered in individuals raised as females who have a female gender identity. Disruption of alternative pathways to fetal DHT production might also present with 46,XY DSD (*AKR1C2/AKR1C4*).

Disorders of Androgen Action • *ANDROGEN INSENSITIVITY SYNDROME* Mutations in the androgen receptor cause resistance to androgen (testosterone, DHT) action or the *androgen insensitivity syndrome* (*AIS*). AIS is a spectrum of disorders that affects at least 1 in 100,000 46,XY individuals. Because the androgen receptor is X-linked, only 46,XY offspring are affected if the mother is a carrier of a mutation. XY individuals with *complete AIS* (formerly called *testicular feminization syndrome*) have a female phenotype, normal breast development

TABLE 410-3 SELECTED GENETIC CAUSES OF 46,XY DISORDERS OF SEX DEVELOPMENT (DSDs)

Gene	Inheritance	Gonad	Uterus	External Genitalia	Associated Features
Disorders of Testis Development					
WT1	AD	Dysgenetic testis	+/–	Female or ambiguous	Wilms' tumor, renal abnormalities, gonadal tumors (WAGR, Denys-Drash and Frasier's syndromes)
CBX2	AD	Ovary	+	Female	
SF1	AR/AD (SL)	Dysgenetic testis/Leydig dysfunction	+/–	Female or ambiguous	Primary adrenal failure; primary ovarian insufficiency in female (46,XX) relatives
SRY	Y	Dysgenetic testis or ovotestis	+/–	Female or ambiguous	
SOX9	AD	Dysgenetic testis or ovotestis	+/–	Female or ambiguous	Campomelic dysplasia
MAP3K1	AD (SL)	Dysgenetic testis	+/–	Female or ambiguous	
DHH	AR	Dysgenetic testis	+	Female	Minifascicular neuropathy
GATA4	AD	Dysgenetic testis	–	Ambiguous or male	Congenital heart disease
ATRX	X	Dysgenetic testis	–	Female or ambiguous	α Thalassemia, developmental delay
ARX	X	Dysgenetic testis	–	Male or ambiguous	Developmental delay; X-linked lissencephaly
MAMLD1	X	Dysgenetic testis/Leydig dysfunction	–	Hypospadias	
DAX1	dupXp21	Dysgenetic testis	+/–	Female or ambiguous	
WNT4/RSPO1	dup1p35	Dysgenetic testis	+	Ambiguous	
Disorders of Androgen Synthesis					
LHR	AR	Testis	–	Female, ambiguous or micropenis	Leydig cell hypoplasia
DHCR7	AR	Testis	–	Variable	Smith-Lemli-Opitz syndrome: coarse facies, second-third toe syndactyly, failure to thrive, developmental delay, cardiac and visceral abnormalities
StAR	AR	Testis	–	Female or ambiguous	Congenital lipoid adrenal hyperplasia (primary adrenal failure)
CYP11A1	AR	Testis	–	Ambiguous	Primary adrenal failure
HSD3B2	AR	Testis	–	Ambiguous	CAH, primary adrenal failure ± salt loss, partial androgenization due to ↑ DHEA
CYP17	AR	Testis	–	Female or ambiguous	CAH, hypertension due to ↑ corticosterone and 11-deoxycorticosterone, except in isolated 17,20-lyase deficiency
CYB5A	AR	Testis	–	Ambiguous	Apparent isolated 17,20-lyase deficiency; methemoglobinemia
POR	AR	Testis	–	Ambiguous or male	Mixed features of 21-hydroxylase deficiency and 17α-hydroxylase/17,20-lyase deficiency, sometimes associated with Antley-Bixler craniosynostosis
HSD17B3	AR	Testis	–	Female or ambiguous	Partial androgenization at puberty, ↑ androstenedione-to-testosterone ratio
SRD5A2	AR	Testis	–	Ambiguous or micropenis	Partial androgenization at puberty, ↑ testosterone-to-dihydrotestosterone ratio
AKR1C2 (AKR1C4)	AR	Testis	–	Female or ambiguous	Decreased fetal DHT production
Disorders of Androgen Action					
Androgen receptor	X	Testis	–	Female, ambiguous, micropenis or normal male	Phenotypic spectrum from complete androgen insensitivity syndrome (female external genitalia) and partial androgen insensitivity (ambiguous) to normal male genitalia and infertility

Abbreviations: AD, autosomal dominant; *AKR1C2*, aldo-keto reductase family 1 member 2; AR, autosomal recessive; *ARX*, aristaless related homeobox, X-linked; *ATRX*, α-thalassemia, mental retardation on the X; CAH, congenital adrenal hyperplasia; *CBX2*, chromobox homologue 2; *CYB5A*, cytochrome b5 POR, P450 oxidoreductase; *CYP11A1*, P450 cholesterol side-chain cleavage; *CYP17*, 17α-hydroxylase and 17,20-lyase; *DAX1*, dosage sensitive sex-reversal, adrenal hypoplasia congenita on the X chromosome, gene 1; DHEA, dehydroepiandrosterone; *DHCR7*, sterol 7 δ reductase; *DHH*, desert hedgehog; *GATA4*, GATA binding protein 4; *HSD17B3*, 17β-hydroxysteroid dehydrogenase type 3; *HSD3B2*, 3β-hydroxysteroid dehydrogenase type 2; *LHR*, LH receptor; *MAP3K1*, mitogen-activated protein kinase kinase kinase 1; *SF1*, steroidogenic factor 1; SL, sex-limited; *SOX9*, *SRY*-related HMG-box gene 9; *SRD5A2*, 5α-reductase type 2; *SRY*, sex-related gene on the Y chromosome; *StAR*, steroidogenic acute regulatory protein; WAGR, Wilms' tumor, aniridia, genitourinary anomalies, and mental retardation; *WNT4*, wingless-type mouse mammary tumor virus integration site, 4; *WT1*, Wilms' tumor–related gene 1.

(due to aromatization of testosterone), a short vagina but no uterus (because MIS production is normal), scanty pubic and axillary hair, and a female gender identity and sex role behavior. Gonadotropins and testosterone levels can be low, normal, or elevated, depending on the degree of androgen resistance and the contribution of estradiol to feedback inhibition of the hypothalamic-pituitary-gonadal axis. AMH/MIS levels in childhood are normal or high. Most patients present with inguinal hernias (containing testes) in childhood or with primary amenorrhea in late adolescence. Gonadectomy sometimes is offered for girls diagnosed in childhood, because there is a low risk of malignancy, and estrogen replacement is prescribed. Alternatively, the gonads can be left in situ until breast development is complete and removed because of tumor risk. Some adults with complete AIS decline gonadectomy, but should be counseled about the risk of malignancy, especially because early detection of premalignant changes by imaging or biomarkers is currently not possible. The use of graded dilators in adolescence is usually sufficient to dilate the vagina for sexual intercourse.

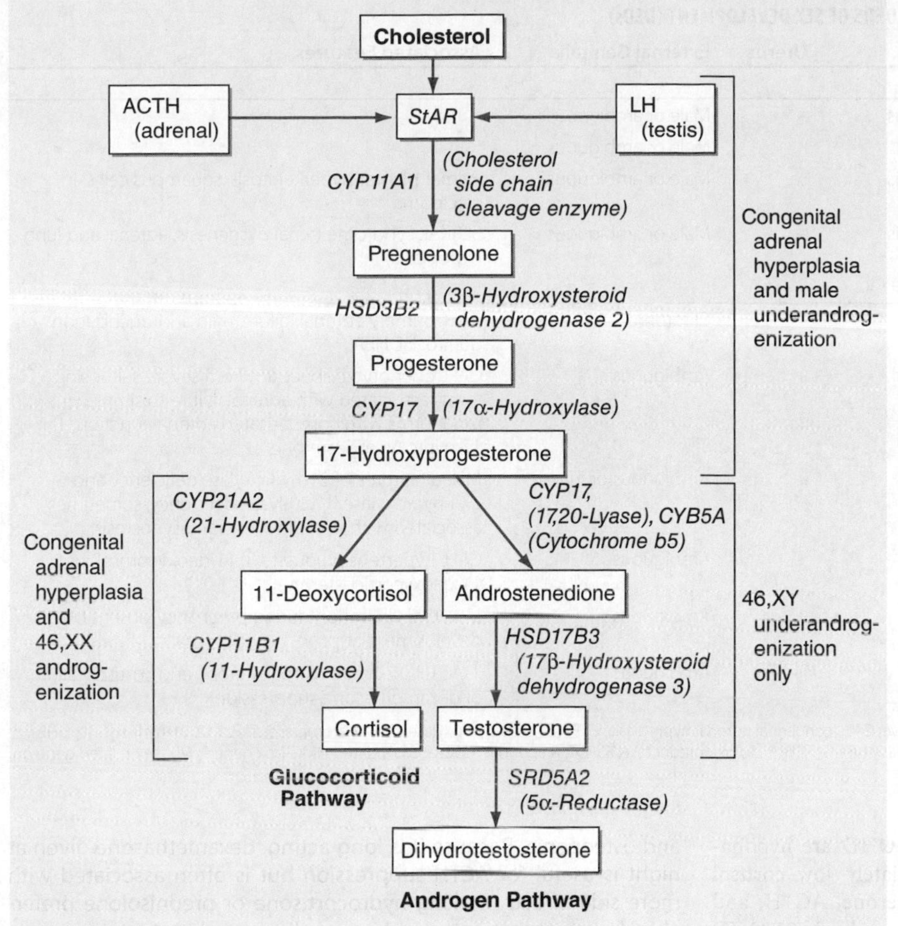

FIGURE 410-4 Simplified overview of glucocorticoid and androgen synthesis pathways. Defects in *CYP21A2* and *CYP11B1* shunt steroid precursors into the androgen pathway and cause androgenization of the 46,XX fetus. Testosterone is synthesized in the testicular Leydig cells and converted to dihydrotestosterone peripherally. Defects in enzymes involved in androgen synthesis result in underandrogenization of the 46,XY fetus. *StAR*, steroidogenic acute regulatory protein. *(After E Braunwald et al [eds]: Harrison's Principles of Internal Medicine, 15th ed. New York, McGraw-Hill, 2001.)*

Partial AIS (Reifenstein's syndrome) results from androgen receptor mutations that maintain residual function. Patients often present in infancy with penoscrotal hypospadias and small undescended testes and with gynecomastia at the time of puberty. Those individuals raised as males usually require hypospadias repair in childhood and may need breast reduction in adolescence. Some boys enter puberty spontaneously. High-dose testosterone has been given to support development if puberty does not progress, but long-term data are limited. More severely underandrogenized patients present with clitoral enlargement and labial fusion and may be raised as females. The surgical and psychosexual management of these patients is complex and requires active involvement of the parents and the patient during the appropriate stages of development. *Azoospermia* and male-factor infertility also have been described in association with mild loss-of-function mutations in the androgen receptor.

OTHER DISORDERS AFFECTING 46,XY MALES

Persistent müllerian duct syndrome is the presence of a uterus in an otherwise phenotypic male. This condition can result from mutations in AMH or its receptor (AMHR2). The uterus may be removed, but only if damage to the vasa deferentia and blood supply can be avoided. *Isolated hypospadias* occurs in ~1 in 250 males and is usually repaired surgically. Most cases are idiopathic, although evidence of penoscrotal hypospadias, poor phallic development, and/or bilateral cryptorchidism requires investigation for an underlying DSD (e.g., partial gonadal dysgenesis, mild defect in testosterone action, or even severe forms of 46,XX CAH). Unilateral undescended testes (cryptorchidism) affect more than 3% of boys at birth. Orchidopexy should be considered if the testis has not descended by 6–9 months of age. Bilateral cryptorchidism occurs less frequently and should raise suspicion of gonadotropin deficiency or DSD. A small subset of patients with cryptorchidism may have mutations in the insulin-like 3 (*INSL3*) gene or its receptor LGR8 (also known as *GREAT*), which mediates normal testicular descent. *Syndromic associations* and *intrauterine growth retardation* also occur relatively frequently in association with impaired testicular function or target tissue responsiveness, but the underlying etiology of many of these conditions is unknown.

46,XX DSD

Inappropriate androgenization of the 46,XX fetus (formerly called *female pseudohermaphroditism*) occurs when the gonad (ovary) contains androgen-secreting testicular material or after increased androgen exposure, which is usually adrenal in origin (Table 410-1).

46,XX Testicular/Ovotesticular DSD Testicular tissue can develop in 46,XX testicular DSD (46,XX males) after translocation of *SRY*, duplication of *SOX9*, or defects in *RSPO1* (Table 410-4).

Increased Androgen Exposure • ***21-HYDROXYLASE DEFICIENCY (CONGENITAL ADRENAL HYPERPLASIA)*** The *classic form* of 21-hydroxylase deficiency (21-OHD) is the most common cause of CAH (Chap. 406). It has an incidence between 1 in 10,000 and 1 in 15,000 and is the most common cause of androgenization in chromosomal 46,XX females (Table 410-4). Affected individuals are homozygous or compound heterozygous for severe mutations in the enzyme 21-hydroxylase (*CYP21A2*). This mutation causes a block in adrenal glucocorticoid and mineralocorticoid synthesis, increasing 17-hydroxyprogesterone and shunting steroid precursors into the androgen synthesis pathway (Fig. 410-4). Glucocorticoid insufficiency causes a compensatory elevation of adrenocorticotropin (ACTH), resulting in adrenal hyperplasia and additional synthesis of steroid precursors proximal to the enzymatic block. Increased androgen synthesis in utero causes androgenization of the 46,XX fetus in the first trimester. Ambiguous genitalia are seen at birth, with varying degrees of clitoral enlargement and labial fusion. Excess androgen production causes gonadotropin-independent precocious puberty in males with 21 OHD.

The *salt-wasting* form of 21-OHD results from severe combined glucocorticoid and mineralocorticoid deficiency. A salt-wasting crisis usually manifests between 5 and 21 days of life and is a potentially life-threatening event that requires urgent fluid resuscitation and steroid treatment. Thus, a diagnosis of 21-OHD should be considered in any baby with atypical genitalia with bilateral nonpalpable gonads. Males (46,XY) with 21-OHD have no genital abnormalities at birth but are equally susceptible to adrenal insufficiency and salt-losing crises.

Females with the *classic simple virilizing* form of 21-OHD also present with genital ambiguity. They have impaired cortisol biosynthesis but do not develop salt loss. Patients with *nonclassic 21-OHD* produce normal amounts of cortisol and aldosterone but at the expense of producing excess androgens. Hirsutism (60%), oligomenorrhea (50%), and acne (30%) are the most common presenting features. This is one of the most common recessive disorders in humans, with an incidence as high as 1 in 100 to 500 in many populations and 1 in 27 in Ashkenazi Jews of Eastern European origin.

TABLE 410-4 SELECTED GENETIC CAUSES OF 46,XX DISORDERS OF SEX DEVELOPMENT (DSDs)

Gene	Inheritance	Gonad	Uterus	External Genitalia	Associated Features
Testicular/Ovotesticular DSD					
SRY	Translocation	Testis or ovotestis	–	Male or ambiguous	
SOX9	dup17q24	Unknown	–	Male or ambiguous	
RSPO1	AR	Testis or ovotestis	±	Male or ambiguous	Palmar plantar hyperkeratosis, squamous cell skin carcinoma
WNT4	AR	Testis or ovotestis	–	Male or ambiguous	SERKAL syndrome (renal dysgenesis, adrenal and lung hypoplasia)
Increased Androgen Synthesis					
HSD3B2	AR	Ovary	+	Clitoromegaly	CAH, primary adrenal failure, mild androgenization due to ↑ DHEA
CYP21A2	AR	Ovary	+	Ambiguous	CAH, phenotypic spectrum from severe salt-losing forms associated with adrenal failure to simple virilizing forms with compensated adrenal function, ↑ 17-hydroxyprogesterone
POR	AR	Ovary	+	Ambiguous or female	Mixed features of 21-hydroxylase deficiency and 17α-hydroxylase/17,20-lyase deficiency, sometimes associated with Antley-Bixler craniosynostosis
CYP11B1	AR	Ovary	+	Ambiguous	CAH, hypertension due to ↑ 11-deoxycortisol and 11-deoxycorticosterone
CYP19	AR	Ovary	+	Ambiguous	Maternal virilization during pregnancy, absent breast development at puberty
Glucocorticoid receptor	AR	Ovary	+	Ambiguous	↑ ACTH, 17-hydroxyprogesterone and cortisol; failure of dexamethasone suppression

Abbreviations: ACTH, adrenocorticotropin; AR, autosomal recessive; CAH, congenital adrenal hyperplasia; *CYP11B1*, 11β-hydroxylase; *CYP19*, aromatase; *CYP21A2*, 21-hydroxylase; DHEA, dehydroepiandrosterone; *HSD3B2*, 3β-hydroxysteroid dehydrogenase type 2; *POR*, P450 oxidoreductase; *RSPO1*, R-spondin 1; *SOX9*, *SRY*-related HMG-box gene 9; *SRY*, sex-related gene on the Y chromosome.

Biochemical features of acute salt-wasting 21-OHD are hyponatremia, hyperkalemia, hypoglycemia, inappropriately low cortisol and aldosterone, and elevated 17-hydroxyprogesterone, ACTH, and plasma renin activity. Presymptomatic diagnosis of classic 21-OHD is now made by neonatal screening tests for increased 17-hydroxyprogesterone in many centers. In most cases, 17-hydroxyprogesterone is markedly increased. In adults, ACTH stimulation (0.25 mg of cosyntropin IV) with assays for 17-hydroxyprogesterone at 0 and 30 min can be useful for detecting nonclassic 21-OHD and heterozygotes (Chap. 406).

TREATMENT CONGENITAL ADRENAL HYPERPLASIA

Acute salt-wasting crises require fluid resuscitation, IV hydrocortisone, and correction of hypoglycemia. Once the patient is stabilized, glucocorticoids must be given to correct the cortisol insufficiency and suppress ACTH stimulation, thereby preventing further virilization, rapid skeletal maturation, and the development of polycystic ovaries. Typically, hydrocortisone (10–15 mg/m^2 per day in three divided doses) is used in childhood with a goal of partially suppressing 17-hydroxyprogesterone (100 to <1000 ng/dL). The aim of treatment is to use the lowest glucocorticoid dose that adequately suppresses adrenal androgen production without causing signs of glucocorticoid excess such as impaired growth and obesity. Salt-wasting conditions are treated with mineralocorticoid replacement. Infants usually need salt supplements up to the first year of life. Plasma renin activity and electrolytes are used to monitor mineralocorticoid replacement. Some patients with simple virilizing 21-OHD also benefit from mineralocorticoid supplements. Parents and patients should be educated about the need for increased doses of steroids during sickness, and patients should carry medic alert systems.

Steroid treatment for older adolescents and adults varies depending on lifestyle, age, and factors such as a desire to optimize fertility. Hydrocortisone remains a useful approach, but treatment with prednisolone at night may provide more complete ACTH suppression. Steroid doses should be adjusted to individual requirements because overtreatment can result in iatrogenic Cushing's-like features, including weight gain, insulin resistance, hypertension, and osteopenia. Because it is long acting, dexamethasone given at night is useful for ACTH suppression but is often associated with more side effects, making hydrocortisone or prednisolone preferable for most patients. Androstenedione and testosterone may be useful measurements of long-term control, with less fluctuation than 17-hydroxyprogesterone. Mineralocorticoid requirements often decrease in adulthood, and doses should be reassessed and reduced to avoid hypertension in adults. In very severe cases, adrenalectomy has been advocated but incurs the risks of surgery and total adrenal insufficiency.

Girls with significant genital androgenization due to classic 21-OHD usually undergo vaginal reconstruction and sometimes clitoral reduction (maintaining the glans and nerve supply), but the optimal timing of these procedures is debated, as is the need for the individual to be able to consent. There is a higher threshold for undertaking clitoral surgery in some centers because long-term sensation and ability to achieve orgasm can be affected, but the long-term results of newer techniques are not yet known. Full information about all options should be provided. If surgery is performed in infancy, surgical revision or regular vaginal dilatation may be needed in adolescence or adulthood, and long-term psychological support and psychosexual counseling may be appropriate. Women with 21-OHD frequently develop polycystic ovaries and have reduced fertility, especially when control is poor. Fecundity is achieved in 60–90% of women with good metabolic control, but ovulation induction (or even adrenalectomy) may be required. Dexamethasone should be avoided in pregnancy. Men with poorly controlled 21-OHD may develop testicular adrenal rests and are at risk for reduced fertility. Prenatal treatment of 21-OHD by the administration of dexamethasone to mothers is still under evaluation. However, pending methods to diagnose the disorder early in pregnancy, both affected and nonaffected fetuses will be exposed because treatment is started ideally before 6 to 7 weeks. The long-term effects of prenatal dexamethasone exposure on fetal development are still under evaluation, and current guidelines recommend full informed consent before treatment, ideally in a protocol that allows long-term follow-up of all children treated. Newer techniques such as cell-free fetal DNA testing may potentially reduce treatment of nonaffected fetuses.

The treatment of other forms of CAH includes mineralocorticoid and glucocorticoid replacement for salt-losing conditions (e.g., *StAR, CYP11A1, HSD3β2*), suppression of ACTH drive with glucocorticoids in disorders associated with hypertension (e.g., *CYP17, CYP11B1*), and appropriate sex hormone replacement in adolescence and adulthood, when necessary.

OTHER CAUSES Increased androgen synthesis can also occur in CAH due to defects in *POR, 11β-hydroxylase (CYP11B1)*, and *3β-hydroxysteroid dehydrogenase type 2 (HSD3B2)* and with mutations in the genes encoding *aromatase (CYP19)* and the glucocorticoid receptor. Increased androgen exposure in utero can occur with maternal virilizing tumors and with ingestion of androgenic compounds.

OTHER DISORDERS AFFECTING 46,XX FEMALES

Congenital absence of the vagina occurs in association with *müllerian agenesis* or *hypoplasia* as part of the Mayer-Rokitansky-Kuster-Hauser (MRKH) syndrome (rarely caused by *WNT4* mutations). This diagnosis should be considered in otherwise phenotypically normal females with primary amenorrhea. Associated features include renal (agenesis) and cervical spinal abnormalities.

GLOBAL CONSIDERATIONS

The approach to a child or adolescent with ambiguous genitalia or another DSD requires cultural sensitivity, as the concepts of sex and gender vary widely. Rare genetic DSDs can occur more frequently in specific populations (e.g., *5α-reductase type 2* in the Dominican Republic). Different forms of CAH also show ethnic and geographic variability. In many countries, appropriate biochemical tests may not be readily available, and access to appropriate forms of treatment and support may be limited.

411 Disorders of the Testes and Male Reproductive System

Shalender Bhasin, J. Larry Jameson

The male reproductive system regulates sex differentiation, virilization, and the hormonal changes that accompany puberty, ultimately leading to spermatogenesis and fertility. Under the control of the pituitary hormones—luteinizing hormone (LH) and follicle-stimulating hormone (FSH)—the Leydig cells of the testes produce testosterone and germ cells are nurtured by Sertoli cells to divide, differentiate, and mature into sperm. During embryonic development, testosterone and dihydrotestosterone (DHT) induce the wolffian duct and virilization of the external genitalia. During puberty, testosterone promotes somatic growth and the development of secondary sex characteristics. In the adult, testosterone is necessary for spermatogenesis, stimulation of libido and normal sexual function, and maintenance of muscle and bone mass. This chapter focuses on the physiology of the testes and disorders associated with decreased androgen production, which may be caused by gonadotropin deficiency or by primary testis dysfunction. A variety of testosterone formulations now allow more physiologic androgen replacement. Infertility occurs in ~5% of men and is increasingly amenable to treatment by hormone replacement or by using sperm transfer techniques. For further discussion of sexual dysfunction, disorders of the prostate, and testicular cancer, see Chaps. 67, 115, and 116, respectively.

DEVELOPMENT AND STRUCTURE OF THE TESTIS

The fetal testis develops from the undifferentiated gonad after expression of a genetic cascade that is initiated by the *SRY* (sex-related gene on the Y chromosome) (Chap. 410). SRY induces differentiation of Sertoli cells, which surround germ cells and, together with peritubular myoid cells, form testis cords that will later develop into seminiferous tubules. Fetal Leydig cells and endothelial cells migrate into the gonad from the adjacent mesonephros but may also arise from interstitial cells that reside between testis cords. Leydig cells produce testosterone, which supports the growth and differentiation of wolffian duct structures that develop into the epididymis, vas deferens, and seminal vesicles. Testosterone is also converted to DHT (see below), which induces formation of the prostate and the external male genitalia, including the penis, urethra, and scrotum. Testicular descent through the inguinal canal is controlled in part by Leydig cell production of insulin-like factor 3 (INSL3), which acts via a receptor termed *Great* (*G protein–coupled receptor affecting testis descent*). Sertoli cells produce müllerian-inhibiting substance (MIS), which causes regression of the müllerian structures, including the fallopian tube, uterus, and upper segment of the vagina.

NORMAL MALE PUBERTAL DEVELOPMENT

Although *puberty* commonly refers to the maturation of the reproductive axis and the development of secondary sex characteristics, it involves a coordinated response of multiple hormonal systems including the adrenal gland and the growth hormone (GH) axis (Fig. 411-1). The development of secondary sex characteristics is initiated by *adrenarche*, which usually occurs between 6 and 8 years of age when the adrenal gland begins to produce greater amounts of androgens from the zona reticularis, the principal site of dehydroepiandrosterone (DHEA) production. The sex maturation process is greatly accelerated by the activation of the hypothalamic-pituitary axis and the production of gonadotropin-releasing hormone (GnRH). The GnRH pulse generator in the hypothalamus is active during fetal life and early infancy but is restrained until the early stages of puberty by a neuroendocrine brake imposed by the inhibitory actions of glutamate, γ-aminobutyric acid (GABA), and neuropeptide Y. Although the pathways that initiate reactivation of the GnRH pulse generator at the onset of puberty have been elusive, mounting evidence supports involvement of GPR54, a G protein–coupled receptor that binds an endogenous ligand, kisspeptin. Individuals with mutations of GPR54 fail to enter puberty, and experiments in primates demonstrate that infusion of the ligand is sufficient to induce premature puberty. Kisspeptin signaling plays an important role in mediating the feedback action of sex steroids on gonadotropin secretion and in regulating the tempo of sexual maturation at puberty. Leptin, a hormone produced by adipose cells, plays a permissive role in the resurgence of GnRH secretion at the onset of puberty, as leptin-deficient individuals also fail to enter puberty (Chap. 415e). The adipocyte hormone leptin, gut hormone ghrelin, neuropeptide Y, and kisspeptin integrate the signals

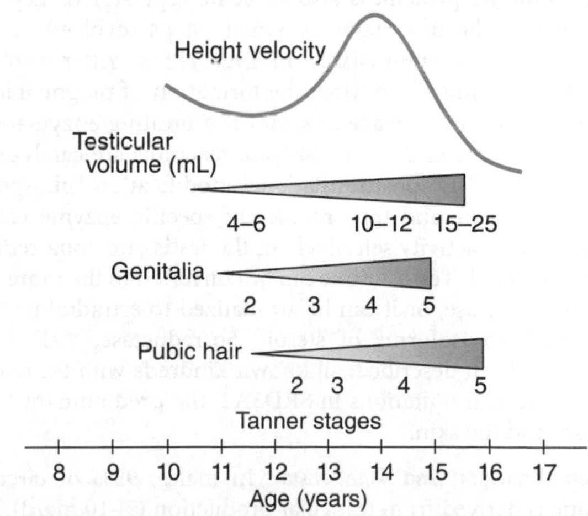

FIGURE 411-1 Pubertal events in males. Sexual maturity ratings for genitalia and pubic hair and divided into five stages. *(From WA Marshall, JM Tanner: Variations in the pattern of pubertal changes in boys. Arch Dis Child 45:13, 1970.)*

originating in energy stores and metabolic tissues with mechanisms that control onset of puberty through regulation of GnRH secretion. Energy deficit and excess and metabolic stress are associated with disturbed reproductive maturation and timing of pubertal onset.

The early stages of puberty are characterized by nocturnal surges of LH and FSH. Growth of the testes is usually the first sign of puberty, reflecting an increase in seminiferous tubule volume. Increasing levels of testosterone deepen the voice and increase muscle growth. Conversion of testosterone to DHT leads to growth of the external genitalia and pubic hair. DHT also stimulates prostate and facial hair growth and initiates recession of the temporal hairline. The growth spurt occurs at a testicular volume of about 10–12 mL. GH increases early in puberty and is stimulated in part by the rise in gonadal steroids. GH increases the level of insulin-like growth factor I (IGF-I), which enhances linear bone growth. The prolonged pubertal exposure to gonadal steroids (mainly estradiol) ultimately causes epiphyseal closure and limits further bone growth.

REGULATION OF TESTICULAR FUNCTION

REGULATION OF THE HYPOTHALAMIC-PITUITARY-TESTIS AXIS IN ADULT MAN

Hypothalamic GnRH regulates the production of the pituitary gonadotropins LH and FSH (Fig. 411-2). GnRH is released in discrete pulses approximately every 2 h, resulting in corresponding pulses of LH and FSH. These dynamic hormone pulses account in part for the wide variations in LH and testosterone, even within the same individual. LH acts primarily on the Leydig cell to stimulate testosterone synthesis. The regulatory control of androgen synthesis is mediated by testosterone and estrogen feedback on both the hypothalamus and the pituitary. FSH acts on the Sertoli cell to regulate spermatogenesis and the production of Sertoli products such as inhibin B, which acts to selectively suppress pituitary FSH. Despite these somewhat distinct Leydig and Sertoli cell–regulated pathways, testis function is integrated at several levels: GnRH regulates both gonadotropins; spermatogenesis requires high levels of testosterone; and numerous paracrine interactions between Leydig and Sertoli cells are necessary for normal testis function.

THE LEYDIG CELL: ANDROGEN SYNTHESIS

LH binds to its seven-transmembrane, G protein–coupled receptor to activate the cyclic AMP pathway. Stimulation of the LH receptor induces *st*eroid *a*cute *r*egulatory (StAR) protein, along with several steroidogenic enzymes involved in androgen synthesis. LH receptor mutations cause Leydig cell hypoplasia or agenesis, underscoring the importance of this pathway for Leydig cell development and function. The rate-limiting process in testosterone synthesis is the delivery of cholesterol by the StAR protein to the inner mitochondrial membrane. Peripheral benzodiazepine receptor, a mitochondrial cholesterol-binding protein, is also an acute regulator of Leydig cell steroidogenesis. The five major enzymatic steps involved in testosterone synthesis are summarized in Fig. 411-3. After cholesterol transport into the mitochondrion, the formation of pregnenolone by CYP11A1 (side chain cleavage enzyme) is a limiting enzymatic step. The 17α-hydroxylase and the 17,20-lyase reactions are catalyzed by a single enzyme, CYP17; posttranslational modification (phosphorylation) of this enzyme and the presence of specific enzyme cofactors confer 17,20-lyase activity selectively in the testis and zona reticularis of the adrenal gland. Testosterone can be converted to the more potent DHT by 5α-reductase, or it can be aromatized to estradiol by CYP19 (aromatase). Two isoforms of steroid 5α-reductase, SRD5A1 and SRD5A2, have been described; all known kindreds with 5α-reductase deficiency have had mutations in SRD5A2, the predominant form in the prostate and the skin.

Testosterone Transport and Metabolism In males, 95% of circulating testosterone is derived from testicular production (3–10 mg/d). Direct secretion of testosterone by the adrenal and the peripheral conversion of androstenedione to testosterone collectively account for another 0.5 mg/d of testosterone. Only a small amount of DHT (70 μg/d) is secreted directly by the testis; most circulating DHT is derived from peripheral conversion of testosterone. Most of the daily production of estradiol (~45 μg/d) in men is derived from aromatase-mediated peripheral conversion of testosterone and androstenedione.

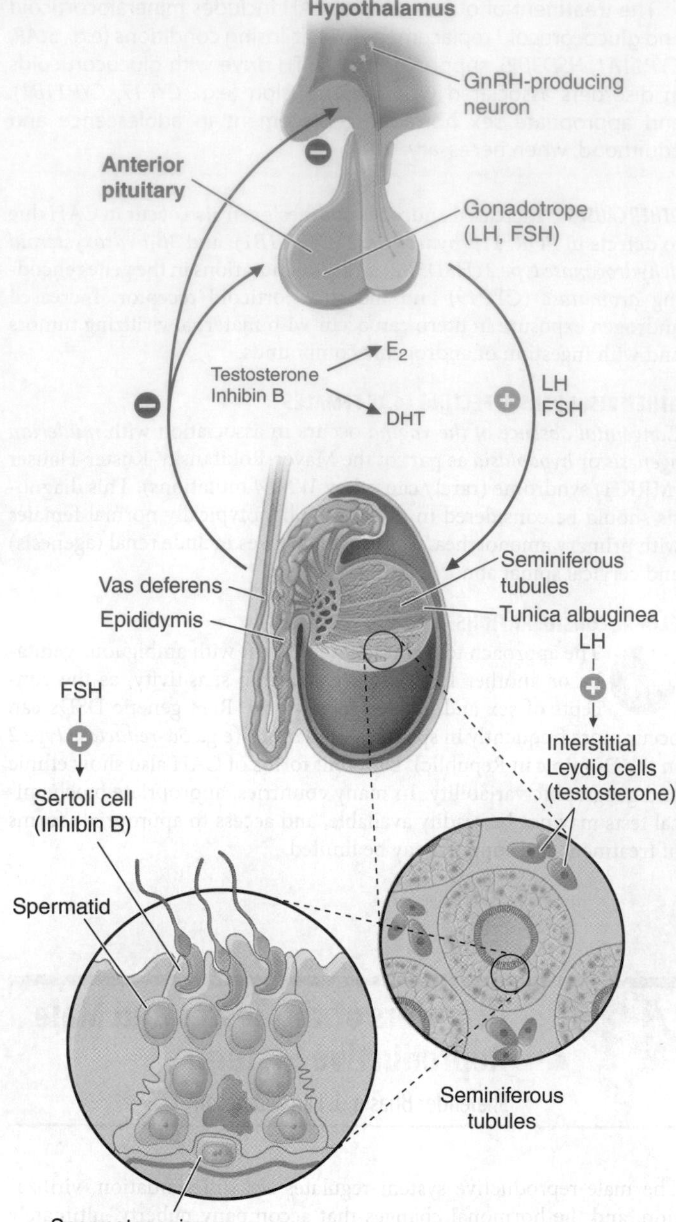

FIGURE 411-2 Human pituitary gonadotropin axis, structure of testis, and seminiferous tubule. E_2, 17β-estradiol; DHT, dihydrotestosterone; FSH, follicle-stimulating hormones; GnRH, gonadotropin-releasing; LH, luteinizing hormone.

Circulating testosterone is bound to two plasma proteins: sex hormone–binding globulin (SHBG) and albumin (Fig. 411-4). SHBG binds testosterone with much greater affinity than albumin. Only 0.5–3% of testosterone is unbound. According to the "free hormone" hypothesis, only the unbound fraction is biologically active; however, albumin-bound hormone dissociates readily in the capillaries and may be bioavailable. SHBG-bound testosterone also may be internalized through endocytic pits by binding to a protein called megalin. SHBG concentrations are decreased by androgens, obesity, diabetes mellitus, insulin, and nephrotic syndrome. Conversely, estrogen administration, hyperthyroidism, many chronic inflammatory illnesses, infections such as HIV or hepatitis B and C, and aging are associated with high SHBG concentrations.

Testosterone is metabolized predominantly in the liver, although some degradation occurs in peripheral tissues, particularly the

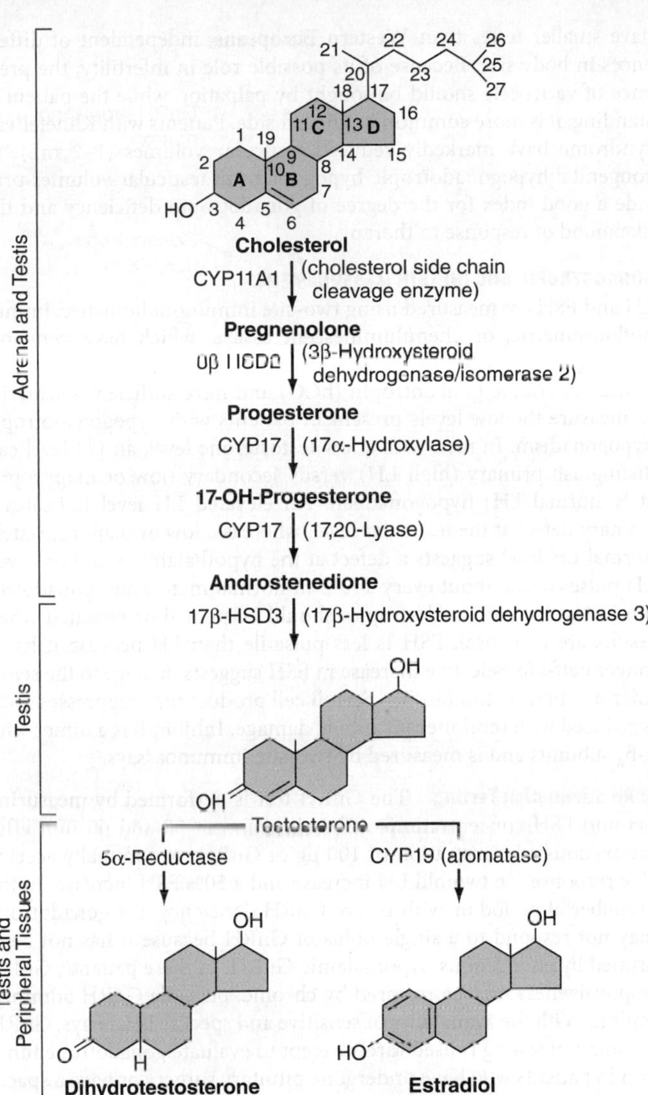

FIGURE 411-3 The biochemical pathway in the conversion of 27-carbon sterol cholesterol to androgens and estrogens.

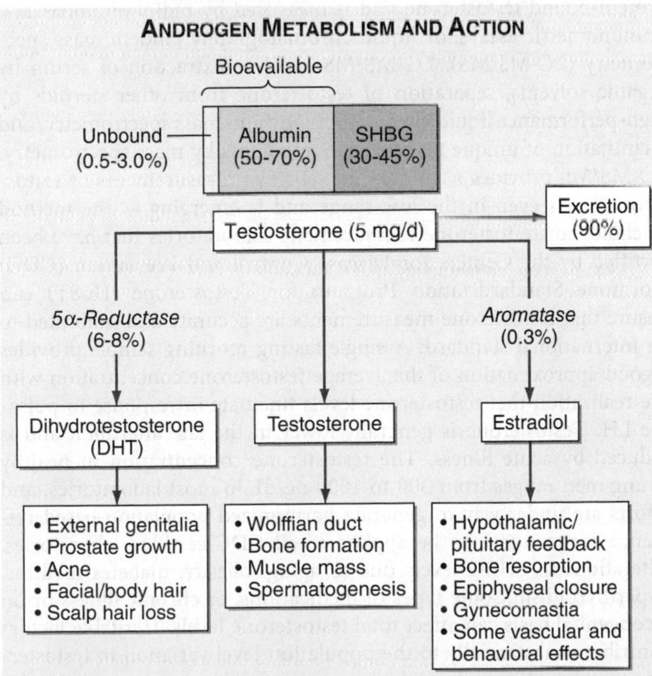

FIGURE 411-4 Androgen metabolism and actions. SHBG, sex hormone–binding globulin.

prostate and the skin. In the liver, testosterone is converted by a series of enzymatic steps that involve 5α- and 5β-reductases, 3α- and 3β-hydroxysteroid dehydrogenases, and 17β-hydroxysteroid dehydrogenase into androsterone, etiocholanolone, DHT, and 3-α-androstanediol. These compounds undergo glucuronidation or sulfation before being excreted by the kidneys.

Mechanism of Androgen Action Testosterone exerts some of its biologic effects by binding to androgen receptor, either directly or after its conversion to DHT by the steroid 5-α reductase. Testosterone's effects on the skeletal muscle, erythropoiesis, and bone in men do not require its obligatory conversion to DHT. However, the conversion of testosterone to DHT is necessary for the masculinization of the urogenital sinus and genital tubercle. Aromatization of testosterone to estradiol mediates additional effects of testosterone on the bone resorption, epiphyseal closure, sexual desire, vascular endothelium, and fat. DHT can also be converted in some tissues by 3-keto reductase/3β-hydroxysteroid dehydrogenase enzymes to 5α-androstane-3β,17β-diol, which is a high-affinity ligand and agonist of estrogen receptor β.

The androgen receptor (AR) is structurally related to the nuclear receptors for estrogen, glucocorticoids, and progesterone (Chap. 400e). The AR is encoded by a gene on the long arm of the X chromosome and has a molecular mass of about 110 kDa. A polymorphic region in the amino terminus of the receptor, which contains a variable number of glutamine repeats, modifies the transcriptional activity of the receptor. The AR protein is distributed in both the cytoplasm and the nucleus. The ligand binding to the AR induces conformational changes that allow the recruitment and assembly of tissue-specific cofactors and causes it to translocate into the nucleus, where it binds to DNA or other transcription factors already bound to DNA. Thus, the AR is a ligand-regulated transcription factor that regulates the expression of androgen-dependent genes in a tissue-specific manner. Some androgen effects may be mediated by nongenomic AR signal transduction pathways. Testosterone binds to AR with half the affinity of DHT. The DHT-AR complex also has greater thermostability and a slower dissociation rate than the testosterone-AR complex. However, the molecular basis for selective testosterone versus DHT actions remains incompletely explained.

THE SEMINIFEROUS TUBULES: SPERMATOGENESIS

The seminiferous tubules are convoluted, closed loops with both ends emptying into the rete testis, a network of progressively larger efferent ducts that ultimately form the epididymis (Fig. 411-2). The seminiferous tubules total about 600 m in length and comprise about two-thirds of testis volume. The walls of the tubules are formed by polarized Sertoli cells that are apposed to peritubular myoid cells. Tight junctions between Sertoli cells create a blood-testis barrier. Germ cells compose the majority of the seminiferous epithelium (~60%) and are intimately embedded within the cytoplasmic extensions of the Sertoli cells, which function as "nurse cells." Germ cells progress through characteristic stages of mitotic and meiotic divisions. A pool of type A spermatogonia serve as stem cells capable of self-renewal. Primary spermatocytes are derived from type B spermatogonia and undergo meiosis before progressing to spermatids that undergo spermiogenesis (a differentiation process involving chromatin condensation, acquisition of an acrosome, elongation of cytoplasm, and formation of a tail) and are released from Sertoli cells as mature spermatozoa. The complete differentiation process into mature sperm requires 74 days. Peristaltic-type action by peritubular myoid cells transports sperm into the efferent ducts. The spermatozoa spend an additional 21 days in the epididymis, where they undergo further maturation and capacitation. The normal adult testes produce >100 million sperm per day.

Naturally occurring mutations in the *FSHβ* gene and in the FSH receptor confirm an important, but not essential, role for this pathway in spermatogenesis. Females with these mutations are hypogonadal and infertile because ovarian follicles do not mature; males exhibit variable degrees of reduced spermatogenesis, presumably because of impaired Sertoli cell function. Because Sertoli cells produce inhibin B, an inhibitor of FSH, seminiferous tubule damage (e.g., by radiation) causes a selective increase of FSH. Testosterone reaches very high concentrations locally in the testis and is essential for spermatogenesis. The cooperative actions of FSH and testosterone are important in the progression of meiosis and spermiation. FSH and testosterone regulate germ cell survival via the intrinsic and the extrinsic apoptotic mechanisms. FSH may also play an important role in supporting spermatogonia. Gonadotropin-regulated testicular RNA helicase (GRTH/DDX25), a testis-specific gonadotropin/androgen-regulated RNA helicase, is present in germ cells and Leydig cells and may be an important factor in the paracrine regulation of germ cell development. Several cytokines and growth factors are also involved in the regulation of spermatogenesis by paracrine and autocrine mechanisms. A number of knockout mouse models exhibit impaired germ cell development or spermatogenesis, presaging possible mutations associated with male infertility. The human Y chromosome contains a small pseudoautosomal region that can recombine with homologous regions of the X chromosome. Most of the Y chromosome does not recombine with the X chromosome and is referred to as the male-specific region of the Y (MSY). The MSY contains 156 transcription units that encode for 26 proteins, including nine families of Y-specific multicopy genes; many of these Y-specific genes are also testis-specific and necessary for spermatogenesis. Microdeletions of several Y chromosome azoospermia factor (*AZF*) genes (e.g., RNA-binding motif, *RBM*; deleted in azoospermia, *DAZ*) are associated with oligospermia or azoospermia.

TREATMENT MALE FACTOR INFERTILITY

Treatment options for male factor infertility have expanded greatly in recent years. Secondary hypogonadism is highly amenable to treatment with pulsatile GnRH or gonadotropins (see below). Assisted reproductive technologies such as the in vitro fertilization (IVF) and intracytoplasmic sperm injection (ICSI) have provided new opportunities for patients with primary testicular failure and disorders of sperm transport. Choice of initial treatment options depends on sperm concentration and motility. Expectant management should be attempted initially in men with mild male factor infertility (sperm count of 15–20 × 10^6/mL and normal motility). Moderate male factor infertility (10–15 × 10^6/mL and 20–40% motility) should begin with intrauterine insemination alone or in combination with treatment of the female partner with clomiphene or gonadotropins, but it may require IVF with or without ICSI. For men with a severe defect (sperm count of <10 × 10^6/mL, 10% motility), IVF with ICSI or donor sperm should be used.

CLINICAL AND LABORATORY EVALUATION OF MALE REPRODUCTIVE FUNCTION

HISTORY AND PHYSICAL EXAMINATION

The history should focus on developmental stages such as puberty and growth spurts, as well as androgen-dependent events such as early morning erections, frequency and intensity of sexual thoughts, and frequency of masturbation or intercourse. Although libido and the overall frequency of sexual acts are decreased in androgen-deficient men, young hypogonadal men may achieve erections in response to visual erotic stimuli. Men with acquired androgen deficiency often report decreased energy and increased irritability.

The physical examination should focus on secondary sex characteristics such as hair growth, gynecomastia, testicular volume, prostate, and height and body proportions. *Eunuchoid proportions* are defined as an arm span >2 cm greater than height and suggest that androgen deficiency occurred before epiphyseal fusion. Hair growth in the face, axilla, chest, and pubic regions is androgen-dependent; however, changes may not be noticeable unless androgen deficiency is severe and prolonged. Ethnicity also influences the intensity of hair growth (Chap. 68). Testicular volume is best assessed by using a Prader orchidometer. Testes range from 3.5 to 5.5 cm in length, which corresponds to a volume of 12–25 mL. Advanced age does not influence testicular size, although the consistency becomes less firm. Asian men generally have smaller testes than Western Europeans, independent of differences in body size. Because of its possible role in infertility, the presence of varicocele should be sought by palpation while the patient is standing; it is more common on the left side. Patients with Klinefelter's syndrome have markedly reduced testicular volumes (1–2 mL). In congenital hypogonadotropic hypogonadism, testicular volumes provide a good index for the degree of gonadotropin deficiency and the likelihood of response to therapy.

GONADOTROPIN AND INHIBIN MEASUREMENTS

LH and FSH are measured using two-site immunoradiometric, immunofluorometric, or chemiluminescent assays, which have very low cross-reactivity with other pituitary glycoprotein hormones and human chorionic gonadotropin (hCG) and have sufficient sensitivity to measure the low levels present in patients with hypogonadotropic hypogonadism. In men with a low testosterone level, an LH level can distinguish primary (high LH) versus secondary (low or inappropriately normal LH) hypogonadism. An elevated LH level indicates a primary defect at the testicular level, whereas a low or inappropriately normal LH level suggests a defect at the hypothalamic-pituitary level. LH pulses occur about every 1–3 h in normal men. Thus, gonadotropin levels fluctuate, and samples should be pooled or repeated when results are equivocal. FSH is less pulsatile than LH because it has a longer half-life. Selective increase in FSH suggests damage to the seminiferous tubules. Inhibin B, a Sertoli cell product that suppresses FSH, is reduced with seminiferous tubule damage. Inhibin B is a dimer with α-β_B subunits and is measured by two-site immunoassays.

GnRH Stimulation Testing The GnRH test is performed by measuring LH and FSH concentrations at baseline and at 30 and 60 min after intravenous administration of 100 μg of GnRH. A minimally acceptable response is a twofold LH increase and a 50% FSH increase. In the prepubertal period or with severe GnRH deficiency, the gonadotrope may not respond to a single bolus of GnRH because it has not been primed by endogenous hypothalamic GnRH; in these patients, GnRH responsiveness may be restored by chronic, pulsatile GnRH administration. With the availability of sensitive and specific LH assays, GnRH stimulation testing is used rarely except to evaluate gonadotrope function in patients who have undergone pituitary surgery or have a space-occupying lesion in the hypothalamic-pituitary region.

TESTOSTERONE ASSAYS

Total Testosterone Total testosterone includes both unbound and protein-bound testosterone and is measured by radioimmunoassays, immunometric assays, or liquid chromatography tandem mass spectrometry (LC-MS/MS). LC-MS/MS involves extraction of serum by organic solvents, separation of testosterone from other steroids by high-performance liquid chromatography and mass spectrometry, and quantitation of unique testosterone fragments by mass spectrometry. LC-MS/MS provides accurate and sensitive measurements of testosterone levels even in the low range and is emerging as the method of choice for testosterone measurement. Laboratories that have been certified by the Centers for Disease Control and Prevention (CDC) Hormone Standardization Program for Testosterone (HoST) can ensure that testosterone measurements are accurate and calibrated to an international standard. A single fasting morning sample provides a good approximation of the average testosterone concentration with the realization that testosterone levels fluctuate in response to pulsatile LH. Testosterone is generally lower in the late afternoon and is reduced by acute illness. The testosterone concentration in healthy young men ranges from 300 to 1000 ng/dL in most laboratories, and efforts are under way to generate harmonized population-based reference ranges that can be applied to all CDC-certified laboratories. Alterations in SHBG levels due to aging, obesity, diabetes mellitus, hyperthyroidism, some types of medications, or chronic illness or on a congenital basis can affect total testosterone levels. Heritable factors contribute substantially to the population-level variation in testosterone levels, and genome-wide association studies have revealed polymorphisms in the *SHBG* gene as important contributors to variation in testosterone levels.

Measurement of Unbound Testosterone Levels Most circulating testosterone is bound to SHBG and to albumin; only 0.5–3% of circulating testosterone is unbound, or "free." The unbound testosterone concentration can be measured by equilibrium dialysis or calculated from total testosterone, SHBG, and albumin concentrations. Recent research has shown that testosterone binding to SHBG is a multistep process that involves complex homoallostery within the SHBG dimer; a novel allosteric model of testosterone binding to SHBG dimers provides good estimates of free testosterone concentrations. The previous law of mass action equations based on linear models of testosterone binding to SHBG have been shown to be erroneous. Tracer analogue methods are relatively inexpensive and convenient, but they are inaccurate. *Bioavailable testosterone* refers to unbound testosterone plus testosterone that is loosely bound to albumin; it can be determined by the ammonium sulfate precipitation method.

hCG Stimulation Test The hCG stimulation test is performed by administering a single injection of 1500–4000 IU of hCG intramuscularly and measuring testosterone levels at baseline and 24, 48, 72, and 120 h after hCG injection. An alternative regimen involves three injections of 1500 units of hCG on successive days and measuring testosterone levels 24 h after the last dose. An acceptable response to hCG is a doubling of the testosterone concentration in adult men. In prepubertal boys, an increase in testosterone to >150 ng/dL indicates the presence of testicular tissue. No response may indicate an absence of testicular tissue or marked impairment of Leydig cell function. Measurement of MIS, a Sertoli cell product, is also used to detect the presence of testes in prepubertal boys with cryptorchidism.

SEMEN ANALYSIS

Semen analysis is the most important step in the evaluation of male infertility. Samples are collected by masturbation following a period of abstinence for 2–3 days. Semen volumes and sperm concentrations vary considerably among fertile men, and several samples may be needed before concluding that the results are abnormal. Analysis should be performed within an hour of collection. Using semen samples from over 4500 men in 14 countries, whose partners had a time-to-pregnancy of less than 12 months, the World Health Organization (WHO) has generated the following one-sided reference limits for semen parameters: semen volume, 1.5 mL; total sperm number, 39 million per ejaculate; sperm concentration, 15 million/mL; vitality, 58% live; progressive motility, 32%; total (progressive + nonprogressive) motility, 40%; morphologically normal forms, 4.0%. Some men with low sperm counts are nevertheless fertile. A variety of tests for sperm function can be performed in specialized laboratories, but these add relatively little to the treatment options.

TESTICULAR BIOPSY

Testicular biopsy is useful in some patients with oligospermia or azoospermia as an aid in diagnosis and indication for the feasibility of treatment. Using local anesthesia, fine-needle aspiration biopsy is performed to aspirate tissue for histology. Alternatively, open biopsies can be performed under local or general anesthesia when more tissue is required. A normal biopsy in an azoospermic man with a normal FSH level suggests obstruction of the vas deferens, which may be correctable surgically. Biopsies are also used to harvest sperm for ICSI and to classify disorders such as hypospermatogenesis (all stages present but in reduced numbers), germ cell arrest (usually at primary spermatocyte stage), and Sertoli cell–only syndrome (absent germ cells) or hyalinization (sclerosis with absent cellular elements).

DISORDERS OF SEXUAL DIFFERENTIATION

See Chap. 410.

DISORDERS OF PUBERTY

The onset and tempo of puberty varies greatly in the general population and is affected by genetic and environmental factors. Although some of the variance in the timing of puberty is explained by heritable factors, the genes involved remain unknown.

PRECOCIOUS PUBERTY

Puberty in boys before age 9 is considered precocious. *Isosexual precocity* refers to premature sexual development consistent with phenotypic sex and includes features such as the development of facial hair and phallic growth. Isosexual precocity is divided into gonadotropin-dependent and gonadotropin-independent causes of androgen excess (Table 411-1). *Heterosexual precocity* refers to the premature development of estrogenic features in boys, such as breast development.

Gonadotropin-Dependent Precocious Puberty This disorder, called *central precocious puberty* (CPP), is less common in boys than in girls. It is caused by premature activation of the GnRH pulse generator, sometimes because of central nervous system (CNS) lesions such as hypothalamic hamartomas, but it is often idiopathic. CPP is characterized by gonadotropin levels that are inappropriately elevated for age. Because pituitary priming has occurred, GnRH elicits LH and FSH responses typical of those seen in puberty or in adults. Magnetic resonance imaging (MRI) should be performed to exclude a mass, structural defect, infection, or inflammatory process. Mutations in *MKRN3*, an imprinted gene encoding makorin ring-finger protein 3, which is expressed only from the paternally inherited allele, have been associated with CPP.

Gonadotropin-Independent Precocious Puberty In gonadotropin-independent precocious puberty, androgens from the testis or the adrenal are increased, but gonadotropins are low. This group of disorders includes hCG-secreting tumors; congenital adrenal hyperplasia; sex steroid–producing tumors of the testis, adrenal, and ovary; accidental or deliberate exogenous sex steroid administration; hypothyroidism; and activating mutations of the LH receptor or $G_s\alpha$ subunit.

TABLE 411-1 CAUSES OF PRECOCIOUS OR DELAYED PUBERTY IN BOYS

I. Precocious puberty
   A. Gonadotropin-dependent
      1. Idiopathic
      2. Hypothalamic hamartoma or other lesions
      3. CNS tumor or inflammatory state
   B. Gonadotropin-independent
      1. Congenital adrenal hyperplasia
      2. hCG-secreting tumor
      3. McCune-Albright syndrome
      4. Activating LH receptor mutation
      5. Exogenous androgens
II. Delayed puberty
   A. Constitutional delay of growth and puberty
   B. Systemic disorders
      1. Chronic disease
      2. Malnutrition
      3. Anorexia nervosa
   C. CNS tumors and their treatment (radiotherapy and surgery)
   D. Hypothalamic-pituitary causes of pubertal failure (low gonadotropins)
      1. Congenital disorders (see Table 411-2)
      2. Acquired disorders
         a. Pituitary tumors
         b. Hyperprolactinemia
   E. Gonadal causes of pubertal failure (elevated gonadotropins)
      1. Klinefelter's syndrome
      2. Bilateral undescended testes
      3. Orchitis
      4. Chemotherapy or radiotherapy
      5. Anorchia
   F. Androgen insensitivity

Abbreviations: CNS, central nervous system; GnRH, gonadotropin-releasing hormone; hCG, human chronic gonadotropin; LH, luteinizing hormone.

FAMILIAL MALE-LIMITED PRECOCIOUS PUBERTY Also called *testotoxicosis*, familial male-limited precocious puberty is an autosomal dominant disorder caused by activating mutations in the LH receptor, leading to constitutive stimulation of the cyclic AMP pathway and testosterone production. Clinical features include premature androgenization in boys, growth acceleration in early childhood, and advanced bone age followed by premature epiphyseal fusion. Testosterone is elevated, and LH is suppressed. Treatment options include inhibitors of testosterone synthesis (e.g., ketoconazole), AR antagonists (e.g., flutamide and bicalutamide), and aromatase inhibitors (e.g., anastrazole).

MCCUNE-ALBRIGHT SYNDROME This is a sporadic disorder caused by somatic (postzygotic) activating mutations in the $G_s\alpha$ subunit that links G protein–coupled receptors to intracellular signaling pathways (Chap. 426e). The mutations impair the guanosine triphosphatase activity of the $G_s\alpha$ protein, leading to constitutive activation of adenylyl cyclase. Like activating LH receptor mutations, this stimulates testosterone production and causes gonadotropin-independent precocious puberty. In addition to sexual precocity, affected individuals may have autonomy in the adrenals, pituitary, and thyroid glands. Café au lait spots are characteristic skin lesions that reflect the onset of the somatic mutations in melanocytes during embryonic development. Polyostotic fibrous dysplasia is caused by activation of the parathyroid hormone receptor pathway in bone. Treatment is similar to that in patients with activating LH receptor mutations. Bisphosphonates have been used to treat bone lesions.

CONGENITAL ADRENAL HYPERPLASIA Boys with congenital adrenal hyperplasia (CAH) who are not well controlled with glucocorticoid suppression of adrenocorticotropic hormone (ACTH) can develop premature virilization because of excessive androgen production by the adrenal gland (Chaps. 406 and 410). LH is low, and the testes are small. Adrenal rests may develop within the testis of poorly controlled patients with CAH because of chronic ACTH stimulation; adrenal rests do not require surgical removal and regress with effective glucocorticoid therapy. Some children with CAH may develop gonadotropin-dependent precocious puberty with early maturation of the hypothalamic-pituitary-gonadal axis, elevated gonadotropins, and testicular growth.

Heterosexual Sexual Precocity Breast enlargement in prepubertal boys can result from familial aromatase excess, estrogen-producing tumors in the adrenal gland, Sertoli cell tumors in the testis, marijuana smoking, or exogenous estrogens or androgens. Occasionally, germ cell tumors that secrete hCG can be associated with breast enlargement due to excessive stimulation of estrogen production (see "Gynecomastia," below).

APPROACH TO THE PATIENT: Precocious Puberty

After verification of precocious development, serum LH and FSH levels should be measured to determine whether gonadotropins are increased in relation to chronologic age (gonadotropin-dependent) or whether sex steroid secretion is occurring independent of LH and FSH (gonadotropin-independent). In children with gonadotropin-dependent precocious puberty, CNS lesions should be excluded by history, neurologic examination, and MRI scan of the head. If organic causes are not found, one is left with the diagnosis of idiopathic central precocity. Patients with high testosterone but suppressed LH concentrations have gonadotropin-independent sexual precocity; in these patients, DHEA sulfate (DHEAS) and 17α-hydroxyprogesterone should be measured. High levels of testosterone and 17α-hydroxyprogesterone suggest the possibility of CAH due to 21α-hydroxylase or 11β-hydroxylase deficiency. If testosterone and DHEAS are elevated, adrenal tumors should be excluded by obtaining a computed tomography (CT) scan of the adrenal glands. Patients with elevated testosterone but without increased 17α-hydroxyprogesterone or DHEAS should undergo careful evaluation of the testis by palpation and ultrasound to exclude a Leydig cell neoplasm. Activating mutations of the LH receptor should be considered in children with gonadotropin-independent precocious puberty in whom CAH, androgen abuse, and adrenal and testicular neoplasms have been excluded.

TREATMENT PRECOCIOUS PUBERTY

In patients with a known cause (e.g., a CNS lesion or a testicular tumor), therapy should be directed toward the underlying disorder. In patients with idiopathic CPP, long-acting GnRH analogues can be used to suppress gonadotropins and decrease testosterone, halt early pubertal development, delay accelerated bone maturation, prevent early epiphyseal closure, promote final height gain, and mitigate the psychosocial consequences of early pubertal development without causing osteoporosis. The treatment is most effective for increasing final adult height if it is initiated before age 6. Puberty resumes after discontinuation of the GnRH analogue. Counseling is an important aspect of the overall treatment strategy.

In children with gonadotropin-independent precocious puberty, inhibitors of steroidogenesis, such as ketoconazole, and AR antagonists have been used empirically. Long-term treatment with spironolactone (a weak androgen antagonist) and ketoconazole has been reported to normalize growth rate and bone maturation and to improve predicted height in small, nonrandomized trials in boys with familial male-limited precocious puberty. Aromatase inhibitors, such as testolactone and letrozole, have been used as an adjunct to antiandrogen and GnRH analogue therapy for children with familial male-limited precocious puberty, CAH, and McCune-Albright syndrome.

DELAYED PUBERTY

Puberty is delayed in boys if it has not ensued by age 14, an age that is 2–2.5 standard deviations above the mean for healthy children. Delayed puberty is more common in boys than in girls. There are four main categories of delayed puberty: (1) constitutional delay of growth and puberty (~60% of cases); (2) functional hypogonadotropic hypogonadism caused by systemic illness or malnutrition (~20% of cases); (3) hypogonadotropic hypogonadism caused by genetic or acquired defects in the hypothalamic-pituitary region (~10% of cases); and (4) hypergonadotropic hypogonadism secondary to primary gonadal failure (~15% of cases) (Table 411-1). Functional hypogonadotropic hypogonadism is more common in girls than in boys. Permanent causes of hypogonadotropic or hypergonadotropic hypogonadism are identified in >25% of boys with delayed puberty.

APPROACH TO THE PATIENT: Delayed Puberty

Any history of systemic illness, eating disorders, excessive exercise, social and psychological problems, and abnormal patterns of linear growth during childhood should be verified. Boys with pubertal delay may have accompanying emotional and physical immaturity relative to their peers, which can be a source of anxiety. Physical examination should focus on height; arm span; weight; visual fields; and secondary sex characteristics, including hair growth, testicular volume, phallic size, and scrotal reddening and thinning. Testicular size >2.5 cm generally indicates that the child has entered puberty.

The main diagnostic challenge is to distinguish those with constitutional delay, who will progress through puberty at a later age, from those with an underlying pathologic process. Constitutional delay should be suspected when there is a family history and when there are delayed bone age and short stature. Pituitary priming by pulsatile GnRH is required before LH and FSH are synthesized and secreted normally. Thus, blunted responses to exogenous GnRH can be seen in patients with constitutional delay, GnRH deficiency, or pituitary disorders (see "GnRH Stimulation Testing," above). On the other hand, low-normal basal gonadotropin levels or a normal response to exogenous GnRH is consistent with an early stage of puberty, which is often heralded by nocturnal GnRH secretion. Thus, constitutional delay is a diagnosis of exclusion that requires ongoing evaluation until the onset of puberty and the growth spurt.

TREATMENT DELAYED PUBERTY

If therapy is considered appropriate, it can begin with 25–50 mg testosterone enanthate or testosterone cypionate every 2 weeks, or by using a 2.5-mg testosterone patch or 25-mg testosterone gel. Because aromatization of testosterone to estrogen is obligatory for mediating androgen effects on epiphyseal fusion, concomitant treatment with aromatase inhibitors may allow attainment of greater final adult height. Testosterone treatment should be interrupted after 6 months to determine if endogenous LH and FSH secretion have ensued. Other causes of delayed puberty should be considered when there are associated clinical features or when boys do not enter puberty spontaneously after a year of observation or treatment.

Reassurance without hormonal treatment is appropriate for many individuals with presumed constitutional delay of puberty. However, the impact of delayed growth and pubertal progression on a child's social relationships and school performance should be weighed. Also, boys with constitutional delay of puberty are less likely to achieve their full genetic height potential and have reduced total-body bone mass as adults, mainly due to narrow limb bones and vertebrae as a result of impaired periosteal expansion during puberty. Administration of androgen therapy to boys with constitutional delay does not affect final height, and when administered with an aromatase inhibitor, it may improve final height.

DISORDERS OF THE MALE REPRODUCTIVE AXIS DURING ADULTHOOD

HYPOGONADOTROPIC HYPOGONADISM

Because LH and FSH are trophic hormones for the testes, impaired secretion of these pituitary gonadotropins results in secondary hypogonadism, which is characterized by low testosterone in the setting of low LH and FSH. Those with the most severe deficiency have complete absence of pubertal development, sexual infantilism, and, in some cases, hypospadias and undescended testes. Patients with partial gonadotropin deficiency have delayed or arrested sex development. The 24-h LH secretory profiles are heterogeneous in patients with hypogonadotropic hypogonadism, reflecting variable abnormalities of LH pulse frequency or amplitude. In severe cases, basal LH is low and there are no LH pulses. A smaller subset of patients has low-amplitude LH pulses or markedly reduced pulse frequency. Occasionally, only sleep-entrained LH pulses occur, reminiscent of the pattern seen in the early stages of puberty. Hypogonadotropic hypogonadism can be classified into congenital and acquired disorders. Congenital disorders most commonly involve GnRH deficiency, which leads to gonadotropin deficiency. Acquired disorders are much more common than congenital disorders and may result from a variety of sellar mass lesions or infiltrative diseases of the hypothalamus or pituitary.

Congenital Disorders Associated with Gonadotropin Deficiency Congenital hypogonadotropic hypogonadism is a heterogeneous group of disorders characterized by decreased gonadotropin secretion and testicular dysfunction either due to impaired function of the GnRH pulse generator or the gonadotrope. The disorders characterized by GnRH deficiency represent a family of oligogenic disorders whose phenotype spans a wide spectrum. Some individuals with GnRH deficiency may suffer from complete absence of pubertal development, while others may manifest varying degrees of gonadotropin deficiency and pubertal delay, and a subset that carries the same mutations as their affected family members may even have normal reproductive function. In approximately 10% of men with idiopathic hypogonadotropic hypogonadism, reversal of gonadotropin deficiency may occur in adult life after sex steroid therapy. Also, a small fraction of men with idiopathic hypogonadotropic hypogonadism may present with androgen deficiency and infertility in adult life after having gone through apparently normal pubertal development. Nutritional, emotional, or metabolic stress may unmask gonadotropin deficiency and reproductive dysfunction (analogous to hypothalamic amenorrhea) in some patients who harbor mutations in the candidate genes but who previously had normal reproductive function. The clinical phenotype may include isolated anosmia or hyposmia. These striking variations in phenotypic presentation of GnRH deficiency have highlighted the important role of oligogenicity and gene-gene and gene-environment interactions in shaping the clinical phenotype.

Mutations in a number of genes involved in the development and migration of GnRH neurons or in the regulation of GnRH secretion have been linked to GnRH deficiency, although the genetic defect remains elusive in nearly two-thirds of cases. Familial hypogonadotropic hypogonadism can be transmitted as an X-linked (20%), autosomal recessive (30%), or autosomal dominant (50%) trait. Some individuals with idiopathic hypogonadotropic hypogonadism (IHH) have sporadic mutations in the same genes that cause inherited forms of the disorder. The genetic defects associated with GnRH deficiency can be conveniently classified as anosmic (Kallmann's syndrome) or normosmic (Table 411-2), although the occurrence of both anosmic and normosmic forms of GnRH deficiency in the same families suggests commonality of pathophysiologic mechanisms. *Kallmann's syndrome*, the anosmic form of GnRH deficiency, can result from mutations in one or more genes associated with olfactory bulb morphogenesis and the migration of GnRH neurons from their origin in the region of the olfactory placode, along the scaffold established by the olfactory nerves, through the cribriform plate into their final location into the preoptic region of the hypothalamus. Thus, mutations in *KAL1*, *FGF8*, *FGFR1*, *NELF*, *PROK2*, *PROK2R*, and *CHD7* have been described in patients with Kallmann's syndrome. An X-linked form of IHH is caused by mutations in the *KAL1* gene, which encodes anosmin, a protein that mediates the migration of neural progenitors of the olfactory bulb and GnRH-producing neurons. These individuals have GnRH deficiency and variable combinations of anosmia or hyposmia, renal defects, and neurologic abnormalities including mirror movements. Mutations in the *FGFR1* gene cause an autosomal dominant form of hypogonadotropic hypogonadism that clinically resembles Kallmann's syndrome; mutations in its putative ligand, *FGF8* gene product, have also been associated with IHH. Prokineticin 2 (*PROK2*) also encodes a protein involved in migration and development of olfactory and GnRH neurons. Recessive mutations in *PROK2* or in its receptor, *PROKR2*, have been associated with both anosmic and normosmic forms of hypogonadotropic hypogonadism.

Normosmic GnRH deficiency results from defects in pulsatile GnRH secretion, its regulation, or its action on the gonadotrope and has been associated with mutations in *GnRHR*, *GNRH1*, *KISS1R*, *TAC3*, *TACR3*, and *NROB1* (*DAX1*). Some mutations, such as those in *PROK2*, *PROKR2*, and *CHD7*, have been associated with both the anosmic and normosmic forms of IHH. *GnRHR* mutations, the most frequent identifiable cause of normosmic IHH, account for ~40% of autosomal recessive and 10% of sporadic cases of hypogonadotropic hypogonadism. These patients have decreased LH response to exogenous GnRH. Some receptor mutations alter GnRH binding affinity, allowing apparently normal responses to pharmacologic doses of exogenous GnRH, whereas other mutations may alter signal transduction downstream of hormone binding. Mutations of the *GnRH1* gene have also been reported in patients with hypogonadotropic hypogonadism, although they are rare. G protein–coupled receptor *KISS1R* (*GPR54*) and its cognate ligand, kisspeptin (*KISS1*), are important regulators of sexual maturation in primates. Recessive mutations in *GPR54* cause gonadotropin deficiency without anosmia. Patients retain responsiveness to exogenous GnRH, suggesting an abnormality in the neural pathways controlling GnRH release. The genes encoding neurokinin B (*TAC3*), which is involved in preferential activation of GnRH release in early development, and its receptor (*TAC3R*) have been implicated

TABLE 411-2 CAUSES OF CONGENITAL HYPOGONADOTROPIC HYPOGONADISM

Gene	Locus	Inheritance	Associated Features
A. Hypogonadotropic Hypogonadism due to GnRH Deficiency			
A1. GnRH Deficiency Associated with Hyposmia or Anosmia			
KAL1	Xp22	X-linked	Anosmia, renal agenesis, synkinesia, cleft lip/palate, oculomotor/visuospatial defects, gut malformations
NELF	9q34.3	AR	Anosmia, hypogonadotropic hypogonadism
FGFR1	8p11-p12	AD	Anosmia, cleft lip/palate, synkinesia, syndactyly
PROK2	3p21	AR	Anosmia/sleep dysregulation
PROK2R	20p12.3	AR	Variable
CHD7	8q12.1		Anosmia, other features of CHARGE syndrome
A2. GnRH Deficiency with Normal Sense of Smell			
GNRHR	4q21	AR	None
GnRH1	8p21	AR	None
KISS1R	19p13	AR	None
TAC3	12q13	AR	Microphallus, cryptorchidism, reversal of GnRH deficiency
TAC3R	4q25	AR	Microphallus, cryptorchidism, reversal of GnRH deficiency
LEPR	1p31	AR	Obesity
LEP	7q31	AR	Obesity
FGF8	10q24	AR	Skeletal abnormalities
B. Hypogonadotropic Hypogonadism not due to GnRH Deficiency			
PC1	5q15-21	AR	Obesity, diabetes mellitus, ACTH deficiency
HESX1	3p21	AR	Septo-optic dysplasia, CPHD
		AD	Isolated GH insufficiency
LHX3	9q34	AR	CPHD (ACTH spared), cervical spine rigidity
PROP1	5q35	AR	CPHD (ACTH usually spared)
FSHβ	11p13	AR	↑ LH
LHβ	19q13	AR	↑ FSH
SF1 (NR5A1)	9p33	AD/AR	Primary adrenal failure, XY sex reversal

Abbreviations: ACTH, adrenocorticotropic hormone; AD, autosomal dominant; AR, autosomal recessive; CHARGE, eye coloboma, choanal atresia, growth and developmental retardation, genitourinary anomalies, ear anomalies; CPHD, combined pituitary hormone deficiency; *DAX1*, dosage-sensitive sex-reversal, adrenal hypoplasia congenita, X-chromosome; *FGFR1*, fibroblast growth factor receptor 1; FSH, follicle-stimulating hormone; *FSHβ*, follicle-stimulating hormone β-subunit; GH, growth hormone; GnRH, gonadotropin-releasing hormone; *GNRHR*, gonadotropin-releasing hormone receptor; *GPR54*, G protein–coupled receptor 54; *HESX1*, homeo box gene expressed in embryonic stem cells 1; *KAL1*, interval-1 gene; *LEP*, leptin; *LEPR*, leptin receptor; LH, luteinizing hormone; *LHβ*, luteinizing hormone β-subunit; *LHX3*, LIM homeobox gene 3; *NELF*, nasal embryonic LHRH factor; *PC1*, prohormone convertase 1; *PROK2*, prokineticin 2; *PROP1*, Prophet of Pit 1; *SF1*, steroidogenic factor 1; *TAC3*, tachykinin 3; *TAC3R*, tachykinin 3 receptor.

in some families with normosmic IHH. Mutations in more than one gene (digenicity or oligogenicity) may contribute to clinical heterogeneity in IHH patients. X-linked hypogonadotropic hypogonadism also occurs in *adrenal hypoplasia congenita*, a disorder caused by mutations in the *DAX1* gene, which encodes a nuclear receptor in the adrenal gland and reproductive axis. Adrenal hypoplasia congenita is characterized by absent development of the adult zone of the adrenal cortex, leading to neonatal adrenal insufficiency. Puberty usually does not occur or is arrested, reflecting variable degrees of gonadotropin deficiency. Although sexual differentiation is normal, **most** patients have testicular dysgenesis and impaired spermatogenesis despite gonadotropin replacement. Less commonly, adrenal hypoplasia congenita, sex reversal, and hypogonadotropic hypogonadism can be caused by mutations of steroidogenic factor 1 (SF1). Rarely, recessive mutations in the *LHβ* or *FSHβ* gene have been described in patients with selective deficiencies of these gonadotropins. In approximately 10% of men with IHH, reversal of gonadotropin deficiency may occur in adult life. Also, a small fraction of men with IHH may present with androgen deficiency and infertility in adult life after having gone through apparently normal pubertal development.

A number of homeodomain transcription factors are involved in the development and differentiation of the specialized hormone-producing cells within the pituitary gland (Table 411-2). Patients with mutations of *PROP1* have combined pituitary hormone deficiency that includes GH, prolactin (PRL), thyroid-stimulating hormone (TSH), LH, and FSH, but not ACTH. *LHX3* mutations cause combined pituitary hormone deficiency in association with cervical spine rigidity. *HESX1* mutations cause septo-optic dysplasia and combined pituitary hormone deficiency.

Prader-Willi syndrome is characterized by obesity, hypotonic musculature, mental retardation, hypogonadism, short stature, and small hands and feet. Prader-Willi syndrome is a genomic imprinting disorder caused by deletions of the proximal portion of the paternally derived chromosome 15q11-15q13 region, which contains a bipartite imprinting center, uniparental disomy of the maternal alleles, or mutations of the genes/loci involved in imprinting (Chap. 83e). *Laurence-Moon syndrome* is an autosomal recessive disorder characterized by obesity, hypogonadism, mental retardation, polydactyly, and retinitis pigmentosa. Recessive mutations of leptin, or its receptor, cause severe obesity and pubertal arrest, apparently because of hypothalamic GnRH deficiency (Chap. 415e).

Acquired Hypogonadotropic Disorders • ***SEVERE ILLNESS, STRESS, MALNUTRITION, AND EXERCISE*** These factors may cause reversible gonadotropin deficiency. Although gonadotropin deficiency and reproductive dysfunction are well documented in these conditions in women, men exhibit similar but less pronounced responses. Unlike women, most male runners and other endurance athletes have normal gonadotropin and sex steroid levels, despite low body fat and frequent intensive exercise. Testosterone levels fall at the onset of illness and recover during recuperation. The magnitude of gonadotropin suppression generally correlates with the severity of illness. Although hypogonadotropic hypogonadism is the most common cause of androgen deficiency in patients with acute illness, some have elevated levels of LH and FSH, which suggest primary gonadal dysfunction. The pathophysiology of reproductive dysfunction during acute illness is unknown but likely involves a combination of cytokine and/or glucocorticoid effects. There is a high frequency of low testosterone levels in patients with chronic illnesses such as HIV infection, end-stage renal disease, chronic obstructive lung disease, and many types of cancer and in patients receiving glucocorticoids. About 20% of HIV-infected men with low testosterone levels have elevated LH and FSH levels; these patients presumably have primary testicular dysfunction. The remaining 80% have either normal or low LH and FSH levels; these men have a central hypothalamic-pituitary defect or a dual defect involving both the testis and the hypothalamic-pituitary centers. Muscle wasting is common in chronic diseases associated with hypogonadism, which also leads to debility, poor quality of life, and adverse outcome of disease. There is great interest in exploring strategies that can reverse androgen deficiency or attenuate the sarcopenia associated with chronic illness.

Men using opioids for relief of cancer or noncancerous pain or because of addiction often have suppressed testosterone and LH levels and high prevalence of sexual dysfunction and osteoporosis; the degree of suppression is dose-related and particularly severe with long-acting opioids such as methadone. Opioids suppress GnRH secretion and alter the sensitivity to feedback inhibition by gonadal steroids. Men who are heavy users of marijuana have decreased testosterone secretion and sperm production. The mechanism of marijuana-induced hypogonadism is decreased GnRH secretion. Gynecomastia observed in marijuana users can also be caused by plant estrogens in crude preparations. Androgen deprivation therapy in men with prostate cancer has been associated with increased risk of bone fractures, diabetes mellitus, cardiovascular events, fatigue, sexual dysfunction, and poor quality of life.

OBESITY In men with mild to moderate obesity, SHBG levels decrease in proportion to the degree of obesity, resulting in lower total testosterone levels. However, free testosterone levels usually remain within the normal range. The decrease in SHBG levels is caused by increased circulating insulin, which inhibits SHBG production. Estradiol levels are higher in obese men compared to healthy, nonobese controls, because of aromatization of testosterone to estradiol in adipose tissue. Weight loss is associated with reversal of these abnormalities including an increase in total and free testosterone levels and a decrease in estradiol levels. A subset of obese men with moderate to severe obesity may have a defect in the hypothalamic-pituitary axis as suggested by low free testosterone in the absence of elevated gonadotropins. Weight gain in adult men can accelerate the rate of age-related decline in testosterone levels.

HYPERPROLACTINEMIA (See also Chap. 403) Elevated PRL levels are associated with hypogonadotropic hypogonadism. PRL inhibits hypothalamic GnRH secretion either directly or through modulation of tuberoinfundibular dopaminergic pathways. A PRL-secreting tumor may also destroy the surrounding gonadotropes by invasion or compression of the pituitary stalk. Treatment with dopamine agonists reverses gonadotropin deficiency, although there may be a delay relative to PRL suppression.

SELLAR MASS LESIONS Neoplastic and nonneoplastic lesions in the hypothalamus or pituitary can directly or indirectly affect gonadotrope function. In adults, pituitary adenomas constitute the largest category of space-occupying lesions affecting gonadotropin and other pituitary hormone production. Pituitary adenomas that extend into the suprasellar region can impair GnRH secretion and mildly increase PRL secretion (usually <50 μg/L) because of impaired tonic inhibition by dopaminergic pathways. These tumors should be distinguished from prolactinomas, which typically secrete higher PRL levels. The presence of diabetes insipidus suggests the possibility of a craniopharyngioma, infiltrative disorder, or other hypothalamic lesions (Chap. 404).

HEMOCHROMATOSIS (See also Chap. 428) Both the pituitary and testis can be affected by excessive iron deposition. However, the pituitary defect is the predominant lesion in most patients with hemochromatosis and hypogonadism. The diagnosis of hemochromatosis is suggested by the association of characteristic skin discoloration, hepatic enlargement or dysfunction, diabetes mellitus, arthritis, cardiac conduction defects, and hypogonadism.

PRIMARY TESTICULAR CAUSES OF HYPOGONADISM

Common causes of primary testicular dysfunction include Klinefelter's syndrome, uncorrected cryptorchidism, cancer chemotherapy, radiation to the testes, trauma, torsion, infectious orchitis, HIV infection, anorchia syndrome, and myotonic dystrophy. Primary testicular disorders may be associated with impaired spermatogenesis, decreased androgen production, or both. See Chap. 410 for disorders of testis development, androgen synthesis, and androgen action.

Klinefelter's Syndrome (See also Chap. 410) Klinefelter's syndrome is the most common chromosomal disorder associated with testicular dysfunction and male infertility. It occurs in about 1 in 600 live-born males. Azoospermia is the rule in men with Klinefelter's syndrome who have the 47,XXY karyotype; however, men with mosaicism may have germ cells, especially at a younger age. The clinical phenotype of Klinefelter's syndrome can be heterogeneous possibly because of mosaicism, polymorphisms in AR gene, variable testosterone levels, or other genetic factors. Testicular histology shows hyalinization of seminiferous tubules and absence of spermatogenesis. Although their function is impaired, the number of Leydig cells appears to increase. Testosterone is decreased and estradiol is increased, leading to clinical features of undervirilization and gynecomastia. Men with Klinefelter's syndrome are at increased risk of systemic lupus erythematosus, Sjögren's syndrome, breast cancer, diabetes mellitus, osteoporosis, non-Hodgkin's lymphoma, and lung cancer, and reduced risk of prostate cancer. Periodic mammography for breast cancer surveillance is recommended for men with Klinefelter's syndrome. Fertility has been achieved by intracytoplasmic injection of sperm retrieved surgically from testicular biopsies of men with Klinefelter's syndrome, including some men with the nonmosaic form of Klinefelter's syndrome. The karyotypes 48,XXXY and 49,XXXXY are associated with a more severe phenotype, increased risk of congenital malformations, and lower intelligence than 47,XXY individuals.

Cryptorchidism Cryptorchidism occurs when there is incomplete descent of the testis from the abdominal cavity into the scrotum. About 3% of full-term and 30% of premature male infants have at least one undescended testis at birth, but descent is usually complete by the first few weeks of life. The incidence of cryptorchidism is <1% by 9 months of age. Androgens regulate predominantly the inguinoscrotal descent of the testes through degeneration of the craniosuspensory ligament and a shortening of the gubernaculums, respectively. Mutations in *INSL3* and leucine-rich repeat family of G protein–coupled receptor 8 (*LGR8*), which regulate the transabdominal portion of testicular descent, have been found in some patients with cryptorchidism.

Cryptorchidism is associated with increased risk of malignancy, infertility, inguinal hernia, and torsion. Unilateral cryptorchidism, even when corrected before puberty, is associated with decreased sperm count, possibly reflecting unrecognized damage to the fully descended testis or other genetic factors. Epidemiologic, clinical, and molecular evidence supports the idea that cryptorchidism, hypospadias, impaired spermatogenesis, and testicular cancer may be causally related to common genetic and environment perturbations and are components of the testicular dysgenesis syndrome.

Acquired Testicular Defects *Viral orchitis* may be caused by the mumps virus, echovirus, lymphocytic choriomeningitis virus, and group B arboviruses. Orchitis occurs in as many as one-fourth of adult men with mumps; the orchitis is unilateral in about two-thirds and bilateral in the remainder. Orchitis usually develops a few days after the onset of parotitis but may precede it. The testis may return to normal size and function or undergo atrophy. Semen analysis returns to normal for three-fourths of men with unilateral involvement but for only one-third of men with bilateral orchitis. *Trauma*, including testicular torsion, can also cause secondary atrophy of the testes. The exposed position of the testes in the scrotum renders them susceptible to both thermal and physical trauma, particularly in men with hazardous occupations.

The testes are sensitive to *radiation damage*. Doses >200 mGy (20 rad) are associated with increased FSH and LH levels and damage to the spermatogonia. After ~800 mGy (80 rad), oligospermia or azoospermia develops, and higher doses may obliterate the germinal epithelium. Permanent androgen deficiency in adult men is uncommon after therapeutic radiation; however, most boys given direct testicular radiation therapy for acute lymphoblastic leukemia have permanently low testosterone levels. Sperm banking should be considered before patients undergo radiation treatment or chemotherapy.

Drugs interfere with testicular function by several mechanisms, including inhibition of testosterone synthesis (e.g., ketoconazole), blockade of androgen action (e.g., spironolactone), increased estrogen (e.g., marijuana), or direct inhibition of spermatogenesis (e.g., chemo therapy).

Combination chemotherapy for acute leukemia, Hodgkin's disease, and testicular and other cancers may impair Leydig cell function and cause infertility. The degree of gonadal dysfunction depends on the type of chemotherapeutic agent and the dose and duration of therapy. Because of high response rates and the young age of these men, infertility and androgen deficiency have emerged as important long-term complications of cancer chemotherapy. Cyclophosphamide and combination regimens containing procarbazine are particularly toxic to germ cells. Thus, 90% of men with Hodgkin's lymphoma receiving MOPP (mechlorethamine, vincristine, procarbazine, prednisone) therapy develop azoospermia or extreme oligozoospermia; newer regimens that do not include procarbazine, such as ABVD (doxorubicin, bleomycin, vinblastine, dacarbazine), are less toxic to germ cells.

Alcohol, when consumed in excess for prolonged periods, decreases testosterone, independent of liver disease or malnutrition. Elevated estradiol and decreased testosterone levels may occur in men taking digitalis.

The occupational and recreational history should be carefully evaluated in all men with infertility because of the toxic effects of many *chemical agents* on spermatogenesis. Known environmental hazards include pesticides (e.g., vinclozolin, dicofol, atrazine), sewage contaminants (e.g., ethinyl estradiol in birth control pills, surfactants such as octylphenol, nonyphenol), plasticizers (e.g., pthalates), flame retardants (e.g., polychlorinated biphenyls, polybrominated diphenol ethers), industrial pollutants (e.g., heavy metals cadmium and lead, dioxins, polycyclic aromatic hydrocarbons), microwaves, and ultrasound. In some populations, sperm density is said to have declined by as much as 40% in the past 50 years. Environmental estrogens or antiandrogens may be partly responsible.

Testicular failure also occurs as a part of *polyglandular autoimmune insufficiency* (Chap. 408). Sperm antibodies can cause isolated male infertility. In some instances, these antibodies are secondary phenomena resulting from duct obstruction or vasectomy. Granulomatous diseases can affect the testes, and testicular atrophy occurs in 10–20% of men with lepromatous leprosy because of direct tissue invasion by the mycobacteria. The tubules are involved initially, followed by endarteritis and destruction of Leydig cells.

Systemic disease can cause primary testis dysfunction in addition to suppressing gonadotropin production. In cirrhosis, a combined testicular and pituitary abnormality leads to decreased testosterone production independent of the direct toxic effects of ethanol. Impaired hepatic extraction of adrenal androstenedione leads to extraglandular conversion to estrone and estradiol, which partially suppresses LH. Testicular atrophy and gynecomastia are present in approximately one-half of men with cirrhosis. In chronic renal failure, androgen synthesis and sperm production decrease despite elevated gonadotropins. The elevated LH level is due to reduced clearance, but it does not restore normal testosterone production. About one-fourth of men with renal failure have hyperprolactinemia. Improvement in testosterone production with hemodialysis is incomplete, but successful renal transplantation may return testicular function to normal. Testicular atrophy is present in one-third of men with sickle cell anemia. The defect may be at either the testicular or the hypothalamic-pituitary level. Sperm density can decrease temporarily after acute febrile illness in the absence of a change in testosterone production. Infertility in men with celiac disease is associated with a hormonal pattern typical of androgen resistance, namely elevated testosterone and LH levels.

Neurologic diseases associated with altered testicular function include myotonic dystrophy, spinobulbar muscular atrophy, and paraplegia. In myotonic dystrophy, small testes may be associated with impairment of both spermatogenesis and Leydig cell function. Spinobulbar muscular atrophy is caused by an expansion of the glutamine repeat sequences in the amino-terminal region of the AR; this expansion impairs function of the AR, but it is unclear how the alteration is related to the neurologic manifestations. Men with spinobulbar muscular atrophy often have undervirilization and infertility as a late manifestation. Spinal cord lesions that cause paraplegia can lead to a temporary decrease in testosterone levels and may cause persistent defects in spermatogenesis; some patients retain the capacity for penile erection and ejaculation.

ANDROGEN INSENSITIVITY SYNDROMES

Mutations in the AR cause resistance to the action of testosterone and DHT. These X-linked mutations are associated with variable degrees of defective male phenotypic development and undervirilization (Chap. 410). Although not technically hormone-insensitivity syndromes, two genetic disorders impair testosterone conversion to active sex steroids. Mutations in the *SRD5A2* gene, which encodes 5α-reductase type 2, prevent the conversion of testosterone to DHT, which is necessary for the normal development of the male external genitalia. Mutations in the *CYP19* gene, which encodes aromatase, prevent testosterone conversion to estradiol. Males with *CYP19* mutations have delayed epiphyseal fusion, tall stature, eunuchoid proportions, and osteoporosis, consistent with evidence from an estrogen receptor–deficient individual that these testosterone actions are mediated indirectly via estrogen.

GYNECOMASTIA

Gynecomastia refers to enlargement of the male breast. It is caused by excess estrogen action and is usually the result of an increased estrogen-to-androgen ratio. True gynecomastia is associated with glandular breast tissue that is >4 cm in diameter and often tender. Glandular tissue enlargement should be distinguished from excess adipose tissue: glandular tissue is firmer and contains fibrous-like cords. Gynecomastia occurs as a normal physiologic phenomenon in the newborn (due to transplacental transfer of maternal and placental estrogens), during puberty (high estrogen-to-androgen ratio in early stages of puberty), and with aging (increased fat tissue and increased aromatase activity), but it can also result from pathologic conditions associated with androgen deficiency or estrogen excess. The prevalence of gynecomastia increases with age and body mass index (BMI), likely because of increased aromatase activity in adipose tissue. Medications that alter androgen metabolism or action may also cause gynecomastia. The relative risk of breast cancer is increased in men with gynecomastia, although the absolute risk is relatively small.

PATHOLOGIC GYNECOMASTIA

Any cause of *androgen deficiency* can lead to gynecomastia, reflecting an increased estrogen-to-androgen ratio, because estrogen synthesis still occurs by aromatization of residual adrenal and gonadal androgens. Gynecomastia is a characteristic feature of Klinefelter's syndrome (Chap. 410). *Androgen insensitivity* disorders also cause gynecomastia. *Excess estrogen production* may be caused by tumors, including Sertoli cell tumors in isolation or in association with Peutz-Jeghers syndrome or Carney complex. Tumors that produce hCG, including some testicular tumors, stimulate Leydig cell estrogen synthesis. *Increased conversion of androgens to estrogens* can be a result of increased availability of substrate (androstenedione) for extraglandular estrogen formation (CAH, hyperthyroidism, and most feminizing adrenal tumors) or of diminished catabolism of androstenedione (liver disease) so that estrogen precursors are shunted to aromatase in peripheral sites. Obesity is associated with increased aromatization of androgen precursors to estrogens. Extraglandular aromatase activity can also be increased in tumors of the liver or adrenal gland or rarely as an inherited disorder. Several families with *increased peripheral aromatase activity* inherited as an autosomal dominant or as an X-linked disorder have been described. In some families with this disorder, an inversion in chromosome 15q21.2-3 causes the CYP19 gene to be activated by the regulatory elements of contiguous genes, resulting in excessive estrogen production in the fat and other extragonadal tissues. *Drugs* can cause gynecomastia by acting directly as estrogenic substances (e.g., oral contraceptives, phytoestrogens, digitalis) or by inhibiting androgen synthesis (e.g., ketoconazole) or action (e.g., spironolactone).

Because up to two-thirds of pubertal boys and half of hospitalized men have palpable glandular tissue that is benign, detailed investigation or intervention is not indicated in all men presenting with gynecomastia (Fig. 411-5). In addition to the extent of gynecomastia, recent onset, rapid growth, tender tissue, and occurrence in a lean subject should prompt more extensive evaluation. This should include a careful drug history, measurement and examination of the testes, assessment of virilization, evaluation of liver function, and hormonal measurements including testosterone, estradiol, and androstenedione, LH, and hCG. A karyotype should be obtained in men with very small testes to exclude Klinefelter's syndrome. Despite extensive evaluation, the etiology is established in fewer than one-half of patients.

TREATMENT GYNECOMASTIA

When the primary cause can be identified and corrected, breast enlargement usually subsides over several months. However, if gynecomastia is of long duration, surgery is the most effective therapy. Indications for surgery include severe psychological and/or cosmetic problems, continued growth or tenderness, or suspected malignancy. In patients who have painful gynecomastia and in

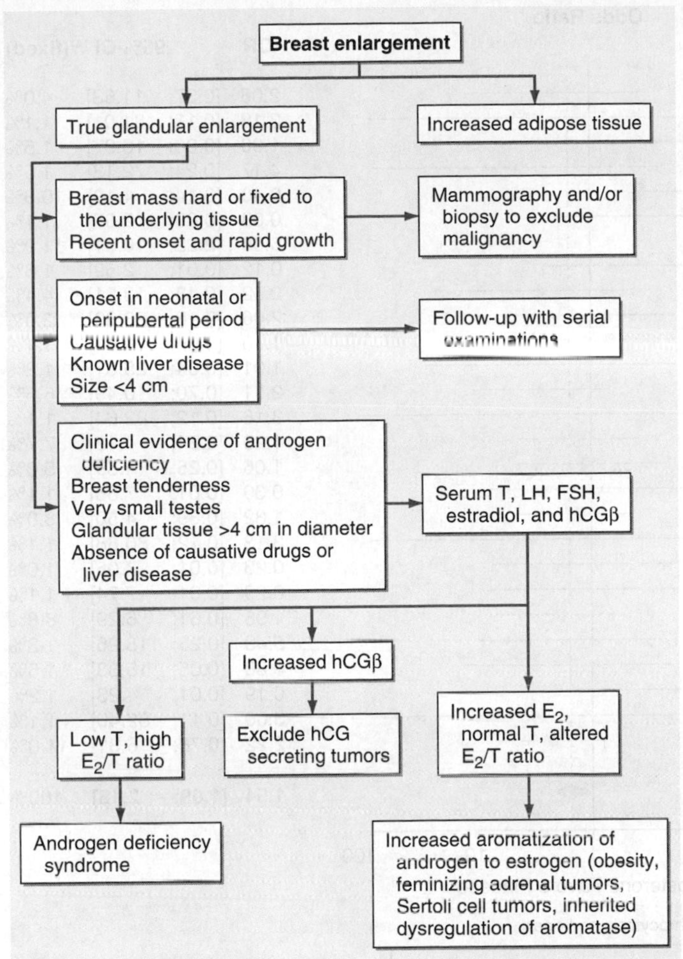

FIGURE 411-5 Evaluation of gynecomastia. E_2, 17β-estradiol; hCGβ, human chorionic gonadotropin β; T, testosterone.

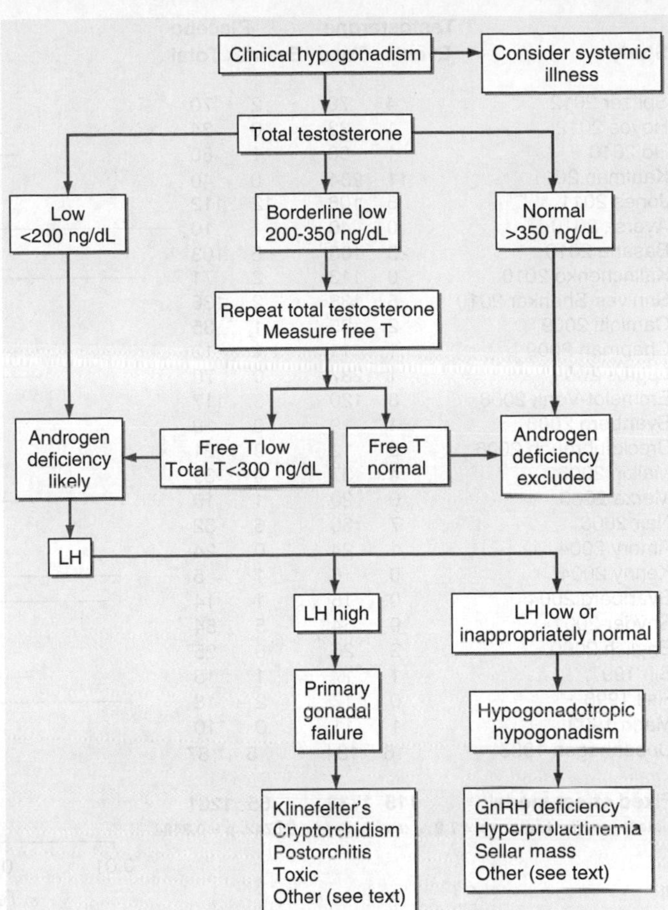

FIGURE 411-6 Evaluation of hypogonadism. GnRH, gonadotropin-releasing hormone; LH, luteinizing hormone; T, testosterone.

whom surgery cannot be performed, treatment with antiestrogens such as tamoxifen (20 mg/d) can reduce pain and breast tissue size in over half the patients. Estrogen receptor antagonists, tamoxifen and raloxifene, have been reported in small trials to reduce breast size in men with pubertal gynecomastia, although complete regression of breast enlargement is unusual with the use of estrogen receptor antagonists. Aromatase inhibitors can be effective in the early proliferative phase of the disorder. However, in a randomized trial in men with established gynecomastia, anastrozole proved no more effective than placebo in reducing breast size. Tamoxifen is effective in the prevention and treatment of breast enlargement and breast pain in men with prostate cancer who are receiving antiandrogen therapy.

AGING-RELATED CHANGES IN MALE REPRODUCTIVE FUNCTION

A number of cross-sectional and longitudinal studies (e.g., The Baltimore Longitudinal Study of Aging, the Framingham Heart Study, the Massachusetts Male Aging Study, and the European Male Aging Study) have established that testosterone concentrations decrease with advancing age. This age-related decline starts in the third decade of life and progresses slowly; the rate of decline in testosterone concentrations is greater in obese men, men with chronic illness, and those taking medications than in healthy older men. Because SHBG concentrations are higher in older men than in younger men, free or bioavailable testosterone concentrations decline with aging to a greater extent than total testosterone concentrations. The age-related decline in testosterone is due to defects at all levels of the hypothalamic-pituitary-testicular axis: pulsatile GnRH secretion is attenuated, LH response to GnRH is reduced, and testicular response to LH is impaired. However, the gradual rise of LH with aging suggests that testis dysfunction is the main cause of declining androgen levels. The term *andropause* has been used to denote age-related decline in testosterone concentrations; this term is a misnomer because there is no discrete time when testosterone concentrations decline abruptly. The approach to evaluating hypogonadism is summarized in Fig. 411-6.

In epidemiologic surveys, low total and bioavailable testosterone concentrations have been associated with decreased appendicular skeletal muscle mass and strength, decreased self-reported physical function, higher visceral fat mass, insulin resistance, and increased risk of coronary artery disease and mortality, although the associations are weak. An analysis of signs and symptoms in older men in the European Male Aging Study revealed a syndromic association of sexual symptoms with total testosterone levels below 320 ng/dL and free testosterone levels below 64 pg/mL in community-dwelling older men. In systematic reviews of randomized controlled trials, testosterone therapy of healthy older men with low or low-normal testosterone levels was associated with greater increments in lean body mass, grip strength, and self-reported physical function compared with placebo. Testosterone therapy also induced greater improvement in vertebral but not femoral bone mineral density. Testosterone therapy of older men with sexual dysfunction and unequivocally low testosterone levels improves libido, but testosterone effects on erectile function and response to selective phosphodiesterase inhibitors have been inconsistent. Testosterone therapy has not been shown to improve depression scores, fracture risk, cognitive function, response to phosphodiesterase inhibitors, or clinical outcomes in older men. Furthermore, neither the long-term risks nor clinical benefits of testosterone therapy in older men have been demonstrated in adequately powered trials. Although there is no evidence that testosterone causes prostate cancer, there is concern that testosterone therapy might cause subclinical prostate cancers to grow. Testosterone therapy is associated with increased risk of detection of prostate events (Fig. 411-7).

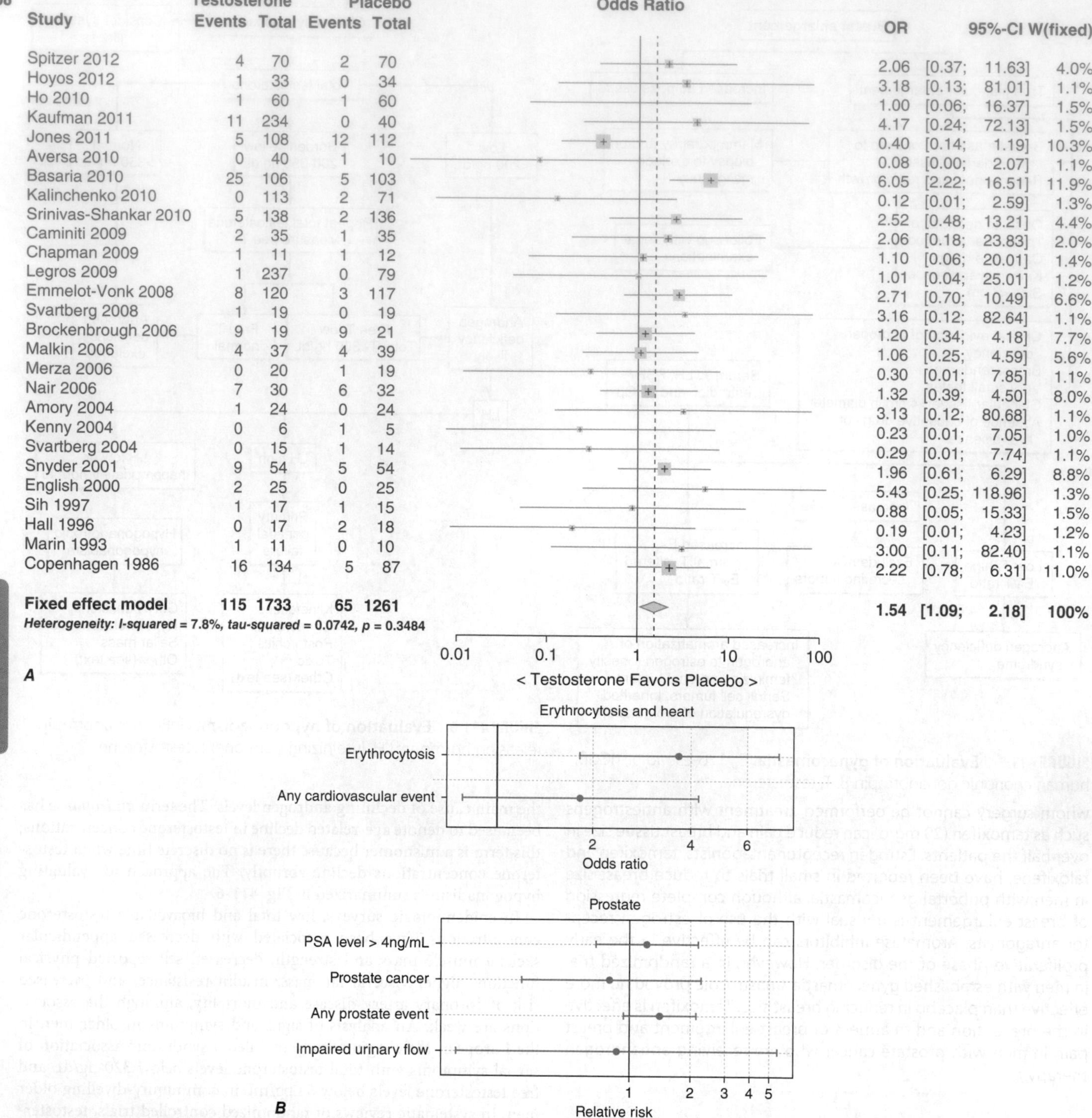

Study
Testosterone Events Total
Placebo Events Total
Odds Ratio
OR 95%-CI W(fixed)
Spitzer 2012 4 70 2 70 2.06 [0.37; 11.63] 4.0%
Hoyos 2012 1 33 0 34 3.18 [0.13; 81.01] 1.1%
Ho 2010 1 60 1 60 1.00 [0.06; 16.37] 1.5%
Kaufman 2011 11 234 0 40 4.17 [0.24; 72.13] 1.5%
Jones 2011 5 108 12 112 0.40 [0.14; 1.19] 10.3%
Aversa 2010 0 40 1 10 0.08 [0.00; 2.07] 1.1%
Basaria 2010 25 106 5 103 6.05 [2.22; 16.51] 11.9%
Kalinchenko 2010 0 113 2 71 0.12 [0.01; 2.59] 1.3%
Srinivas-Shankar 2010 5 138 2 136 2.52 [0.48; 13.21] 4.4%
Caminiti 2009 2 35 1 35 2.06 [0.18; 23.83] 2.0%
Chapman 2009 1 11 1 12 1.10 [0.06; 20.01] 1.4%
Legros 2009 1 237 0 79 1.01 [0.04; 25.01] 1.2%
Emmelot-Vonk 2008 8 120 3 117 2.71 [0.70; 10.49] 6.6%
Svartberg 2008 1 19 0 19 3.16 [0.12; 82.64] 1.1%
Brockenbrough 2006 9 19 9 21 1.20 [0.34; 4.18] 7.7%
Malkin 2006 4 37 4 39 1.06 [0.25; 4.59] 5.6%
Merza 2006 0 20 1 19 0.30 [0.01; 7.85] 1.1%
Nair 2006 7 30 6 32 1.32 [0.39; 4.50] 8.0%
Amory 2004 1 24 0 24 3.13 [0.12; 80.68] 1.1%
Kenny 2004 0 6 1 5 0.23 [0.01; 7.05] 1.0%
Svartberg 2004 0 15 1 14 0.29 [0.01; 7.74] 1.1%
Snyder 2001 9 54 5 54 1.96 [0.61; 6.29] 8.8%
English 2000 2 25 0 25 5.43 [0.25; 118.96] 1.3%
Sih 1997 1 17 1 15 0.88 [0.05; 15.33] 1.5%
Hall 1996 0 17 2 18 0.19 [0.01; 4.23] 1.2%
Marin 1993 1 11 0 10 3.00 [0.11; 82.40] 1.1%
Copenhagen 1986 16 134 5 87 2.22 [0.78; 6.31] 11.0%
Fixed effect model 115 1733 65 1261 1.54 [1.09; 2.18] 100%
Heterogeneity: I-squared = 7.8%, tau-squared = 0.0742, p = 0.3484
0.01 0.1 1 10 100
< Testosterone Favors Placebo >
A
Erythrocytosis and heart
Erythrocytosis
Any cardiovascular event
2 4 6
Odds ratio
Prostate
PSA level > 4ng/mL
Prostate cancer
Any prostate event
Impaired urinary flow
1 2 3 4 5
Relative risk
B

FIGURE 411-7 Meta-analyses of cardiovascular and prostate adverse events associated with testosterone therapy. ***A.*** A meta-analysis of cardiovascular-related events in randomized testosterone trials of 12 weeks or longer in duration. Randomization to testosterone was associated with a significantly increased risk of cardiovascular-related event (odds ratio [OR] 1.54). *(Modified with permission from L Xu et al: Testosterone therapy and cardiovascular events among men: a systematic review and meta-analysis of placebo-controlled randomized trials BMC Med 11:108, 2013.)* ***B.*** The relative risk of prostate events and the associated 95% confidence intervals (CIs) in a meta-analysis of randomized testosterone trials. PSA, prostate-specific antigen. *(Data were derived from a meta-analysis by MM Fernández-Balsells et al: J Clin Endocrinol Metab 95:2560, 2010, and the figure was reproduced with permission from M Spitzer et al: Nat Rev Endocrinol 9:414, 2013.)*

One randomized testosterone trial in older men with mobility limitation and high burden of chronic conditions, such as diabetes, heart disease, hypertension, and hyperlipidemia, reported a greater number of cardiovascular events in men randomized to the testosterone arm of the study than in those randomized to the placebo arm. Since then, two large retrospective analyses of patient databases have reported higher frequency of cardiovascular events, including myocardial infarction, in older men with preexisting heart disease (Fig. 411-7).

Population screening of all older men for low testosterone levels is not recommended, and testing should be restricted to men who have symptoms or physical features attributable to androgen deficiency. Testosterone therapy is not recommended for all older men with low testosterone levels. In older men with significant symptoms of androgen deficiency who have testosterone levels below 200 ng/dL, testosterone therapy may be considered on an individualized basis and should be instituted after careful discussion of the risks and benefits (see "Testosterone Replacement," below).

Testicular morphology, semen production, and fertility are maintained up to a very old age in men. Although concern has been expressed about age-related increases in germ cell mutations and impairment of DNA repair mechanisms, there is no clear evidence that the frequency of chromosomal aneuploidy is increased in the sperm of older men. However, the incidence of autosomal dominant diseases, such as achondroplasia, polyposis coli, Marfan's syndrome, and Apert's syndrome, increases in the offspring of men who are advanced in age, consistent with transmission of sporadic missense mutations. Advanced paternal age may be associated with increased rates of de novo mutations, which may contribute to an increased risk of neurodevelopmental diseases such as schizophrenia and autism. The somatic mutations in male germ cells that enhance the proliferation of germ cells could lead to within-testis expansion of mutant clonal lines, thus favoring the propagation of germ cells carrying these pathogenic mutations and increasing the risk of mutations in the offspring of older fathers (the "selfish spermatogonial selection" hypothesis).

APPROACH TO THE PATIENT: Androgen Deficiency

Hypogonadism is often characterized by decreased sex drive, reduced frequency of sexual activity, inability to maintain erections, reduced beard growth, loss of muscle mass, decreased testicular size, and gynecomastia. Erectile dysfunction and androgen deficiency are two distinct clinical disorders that can coexist in middle-aged and older men. Less than 10% of patients with erectile dysfunction have testosterone deficiency. Thus, it is useful to evaluate men presenting with erectile dysfunction for androgen deficiency. Except when extreme, these clinical features of androgen deficiency may be difficult to distinguish from changes that occur with normal aging. Moreover, androgen deficiency may develop gradually. Several epidemiologic studies, such as the Framingham Heart Study, the Massachusetts Male Aging Study, the Baltimore Longitudinal Study of Aging, and the Study of Osteoporotic Fractures in Men, have reported a high prevalence of low testosterone levels in middle-aged and older men. The age-related decline in testosterone should be distinguished from classical hypogonadism due to diseases of the testes, the pituitary, and the hypothalamus.

When symptoms or clinical features suggest possible androgen deficiency, the laboratory evaluation is initiated by the measurement of total testosterone, preferably in the morning using a reliable assay, such as LC-MS/MS that has been calibrated to an international testosterone standard (Fig. 411-6). A consistently low total testosterone level <300 ng/dL measured by a reliable assay, in association with symptoms, is evidence of testosterone deficiency. An early-morning testosterone level >400 ng/dL makes the diagnosis of androgen deficiency unlikely. In men with testosterone levels between 200 and 400 ng/dL, the total testosterone level should be repeated and a free testosterone level should be measured. In older men and in patients with other clinical states that are associated with alterations in SHBG levels, a direct measurement of free testosterone level by equilibrium dialysis can be useful in unmasking testosterone deficiency.

When androgen deficiency has been confirmed by the consistently low testosterone concentrations, LH should be measured to classify the patient as having primary (high LH) or secondary (low or inappropriately normal LH) hypogonadism. An elevated LH level indicates that the defect is at the testicular level. Common causes of primary testicular failure include Klinefelter's syndrome, HIV infection, uncorrected cryptorchidism, cancer chemotherapeutic agents, radiation, surgical orchiectomy, or prior infectious orchitis. Unless causes of primary testicular failure are known, a karyotype should be performed in men with low testosterone and elevated LH to exclude Klinefelter's syndrome. Men who have low testosterone levels but "inappropriately normal" or low LH levels have secondary hypogonadism; their defect resides at the hypothalamic-pituitary level. Common causes of acquired secondary hypogonadism include space-occupying lesions of the sella, hyperprolactinemia, chronic illness, hemochromatosis, excessive exercise, and the use of anabolic-androgenic steroids, opiates, marijuana, glucocorticoids, and alcohol. Measurement of PRL and MRI scan of the hypothalamic-pituitary region can help exclude the presence of a space-occupying lesion. Patients in whom known causes of hypogonadotropic hypogonadism have been excluded are classified as having IHH. It is not unusual for congenital causes of hypogonadotropic hypogonadism, such as Kallmann's syndrome, to be diagnosed in young adults.

TREATMENT ANDROGEN DEFICIENCY

GONADOTROPINS

Gonadotropin therapy is used to establish or restore fertility in patients with gonadotropin deficiency of any cause. Several gonadotropin preparations are available. Human menopausal gonadotropin (hMG; purified from the urine of postmenopausal women) contains 75 IU FSH and 75 IU LH per vial. hCG (purified from the urine of pregnant women) has little FSH activity and resembles LH in its ability to stimulate testosterone production by Leydig cells. Recombinant LH is now available. Because of the expense of hMG, treatment is usually begun with hCG alone, and hMG is added later to promote the FSH-dependent stages of spermatid development. Recombinant human FSH (hFSH) is now available and is indistinguishable from purified urinary hFSH in its biologic activity and pharmacokinetics in vitro and in vivo, although the mature β subunit of recombinant hFSH has seven fewer amino acids. Recombinant hFSH is available in ampoules containing 75 IU (~7.5 μg FSH), which accounts for >99% of protein content. Once spermatogenesis is restored using combined FSH and LH therapy, hCG alone is often sufficient to maintain spermatogenesis.

Although a variety of treatment regimens are used, 1000–2000 IU of hCG or recombinant human LH (rhLH) administered intramuscularly three times weekly is a reasonable starting dose. Testosterone levels should be measured 6–8 weeks later and 48–72 h after the hCG or rhLH injection; the hCG/rhLH dose should be adjusted to achieve testosterone levels in the mid-normal range. Sperm counts should be monitored on a monthly basis. It may take several months for spermatogenesis to be restored; therefore, it is important to forewarn patients about the potential length and expense of the treatment and to provide conservative estimates of success rates. If testosterone levels are in the mid-normal range but the sperm concentrations are low after 6 months of therapy with hCG alone, FSH should be added. This can be done by using hMG, highly purified urinary hFSH, or recombinant hFSH. The selection of FSH dose is empirical. A common practice is to start with the addition of 75 IU FSH three times each week in conjunction with the hCG/rhLH injections. If sperm densities are still low after 3 months of combined treatment, the FSH dose should be increased to 150 IU. Occasionally, it may take ≥18–24 months for spermatogenesis to be restored.

The two best predictors of success using gonadotropin therapy in hypogonadotropic men are testicular volume at presentation and time of onset. In general, men with testicular volumes >8 mL have better response rates than those who have testicular volumes >4 mL. Patients who became hypogonadotropic after puberty experience higher success rates than those who have never undergone pubertal changes. Spermatogenesis can usually be reinitiated by hCG alone, with high rates of success for men with postpubertal onset of hypogonadotropism. The presence of a primary testicular abnormality, such as cryptorchidism, will attenuate testicular response to gonadotropin therapy. Prior androgen therapy does not preclude subsequent response to gonadotropin therapy, although some studies suggest that it may attenuate response to subsequent gonadotropin therapy.

Androgen therapy is indicated to restore testosterone levels to normal to correct features of androgen deficiency. Testosterone replacement improves libido and overall sexual activity; increases energy, lean muscle mass, and bone density; and decreases fat mass. The benefits of testosterone replacement therapy have only been proven in men who have documented androgen deficiency, as demonstrated by testosterone levels that are well below the lower limit of normal.

Testosterone is available in a variety of formulations with distinct pharmacokinetics (Table 411-3). Testosterone serves as a prohormone and is converted to 17β-estradiol by aromatase and to 5α-dihydrotestosterone by steroid 5α-reductase. Therefore, when evaluating testosterone formulations, it is important to consider whether the formulation being used can achieve physiologic estradiol and DHT concentrations, in addition to normal testosterone concentrations. Although testosterone concentrations at the lower end of the normal male range can restore sexual function, it is not

TABLE 411-3 CLINICAL PHARMACOLOGY OF SOME TESTOSTERONE FORMULATIONS

Formulation	Regimen	Pharmacokinetic Profile	DHT and E_2	Advantages	Disadvantages
Testosterone enanthate or cypionate	150–200 mg IM q2wk or 75–100 mg/wk	After a single IM injection, serum T levels rise into the supraphysiologic range, then decline gradually into the hypogonadal range by the end of the dosing interval	DHT and E_2 levels rise in proportion to the increase in T levels; T:DHT and T:E_2 ratios do not change	Corrects symptoms of androgen deficiency; relatively inexpensive, if self-administered; flexibility of dosing	Requires IM injection; peaks and valleys in serum T levels
Topical testosterone gels and axillary testosterone solution	Available in sachets, tubes, and pumps	When used in appropriate doses, these topical formulations restore serum T and E_2 levels to the physiologic male range	Serum DHT levels are higher and T:DHT ratios are lower in hypogonadal men treated with the transdermal gels than in healthy eugonadal men	Corrects symptoms of androgen deficiency, provides flexibility of dosing, ease of application, good skin tolerability	Potential of transfer to a female partner or child by direct skin-to-skin contact; skin irritation in a small proportion of treated men; moderately high DHT levels; considerable interindividual and intraindivudal variation in on-treatment T levels
Transdermal testosterone patch	1 or 2 patches, designed to nominally deliver 5–10 mg T over 24 h applied every day on nonpressure areas	Restores serum T, DHT, and E_2 levels to the physiologic male range	T:DHT and T:E_2 levels are in the physiologic male range	Ease of application, corrects symptoms of androgen deficiency	Serum T levels in some androgen-deficient men may be in the low-normal range; these men may need application of 2 patches daily; skin irritation at the application site occurs frequently in many patients
Buccal, bioadhesive, testosterone tablets	30-mg controlled-release, bioadhesive tablets bid	Absorbed from the buccal mucosa	Normalizes serum T and DHT levels in hypogonadal men	Corrects symptoms of androgen deficiency in healthy, hypogonadal men	Gum-related adverse events in 16% of treated men
Testosterone pellets	2–6 pellets implanted SC; dose and regimen vary with formulation	Serum T peaks at 1 month and then is sustained in normal range for 3–6 months, depending on formulation	T:DHT and T:E_2 ratios do not change	Corrects symptoms of androgen deficiency	Requires surgical incision for insertions; pellets may extrude spontaneously
17-α-Methyl testosterone	This 17-α-alkylated compound should *not* be used because of potential for liver toxicity	Orally active			Clinical responses are variable; potential for liver toxicity; should *not* be used for treatment of androgen deficiency
Oral testosterone undecanoate[a]	40–80 mg PO bid or tid with meals	When administered in oleic acid, T undecanoate is absorbed through the lymphatics, bypassing the portal system; considerable variability in the same individual on different days and among individuals	High DHT:T ratio	Convenience of oral administration	Not approved in the United States; variable clinical responses, variable serum T levels, high DHT:T ratio
Injectable long-acting testosterone undecanoate in oil[a]	European regimen 1000 mg IM, followed by 1000 mg at 6 weeks, and 1000 mg every 10–14 weeks	When administered at a dose of 750–1000 mg IM, serum T levels are maintained in the normal range in a majority of treated men	DHT and E_2 levels rise in proportion to the increase in T levels; T:DHT and T:E_2 ratios do not change	Corrects symptoms of androgen deficiency; requires infrequent administration	Requires IM injection of a large volume (4 mL); cough reported immediately after injection in a very small number of men
Testosterone-in-adhesive matrix patch[a]	2 × 60 cm^2 patches delivering approximately 4.8 mg of T/d	Restores serum T, DHT, and E_2 to the physiologic range	T:DHT and T:E_2 are in the physiologic range	Lasts 2 d	Some skin irritation

[a]These formulations are not approved for clinical use in the United States, but are available outside the United States in many countries. Physicians in those countries where these formulations are available should follow the approved drug regimens.

Abbreviations: DHT, dihydrotestosterone; E_2, estradiol; T, testosterone.

clear whether low-normal testosterone levels can maintain bone mineral density and muscle mass. The current recommendation is to restore testosterone levels to the mid-normal range.

Oral Derivatives of Testosterone Testosterone is well-absorbed after oral administration but is quickly degraded during the first pass through the liver. Therefore, it is difficult to achieve sustained blood levels of testosterone after oral administration of crystalline testosterone. 17α-Alkylated derivatives of testosterone (e.g., 17α-methyl testosterone, oxandrolone, fluoxymesterone) are relatively resistant to hepatic degradation and can be administered orally; however, because of the potential for hepatotoxicity, including cholestatic jaundice, peliosis, and hepatoma, these formulations should not be used for testosterone replacement. Hereditary angioedema due to C1 esterase deficiency is the only exception to this general recommendation; in this condition, oral 17α-alkylated androgens are useful because they stimulate hepatic synthesis of the C1 esterase inhibitor.

Injectable Forms of Testosterone The esterification of testosterone at the 17β-hydroxy position makes the molecule hydrophobic and extends its duration of action. The slow release of testosterone ester from an oily depot in the muscle accounts for its extended duration of action. The longer the side chain, the greater is the hydrophobicity of the ester and the longer is the duration of action. Thus, testosterone enanthate, cypionate, and undecanoate with longer side chains have longer duration of action than testosterone propionate. Within 24 h after intramuscular administration of 200 mg testosterone enanthate or cypionate, testosterone levels rise into the high-normal or supraphysiologic range and then gradually decline into the hypogonadal range over the next 2 weeks. A bimonthly regimen of testosterone enanthate or cypionate therefore results in peaks and troughs in testosterone levels that are accompanied by changes in a patient's mood, sexual desire, and energy level. The kinetics of testosterone enanthate and cypionate are similar. Estradiol and DHT levels are normal if testosterone replacement is physiologic.

Transdermal Testosterone Patch The nongenital testosterone patch, when applied in an appropriate dose, can normalize testosterone, DHT, and estradiol levels 4–12 h after application. Sexual function and well-being are restored in androgen-deficient men treated with the nongenital patch. One 5-mg patch may not be sufficient to increase testosterone into the mid-normal male range in all hypogonadal men; some patients may need two 5-mg patches daily to achieve the targeted testosterone concentrations. The use of testosterone patches may be associated with skin irritation in some individuals.

Testosterone Gel Several transdermal testosterone gels (e.g., Androgel, Testim, Fortesta, and Axiron), when applied topically to the skin in appropriate doses (Table 411-3), can maintain total and free testosterone concentrations in the normal range in hypogonadal men. The current recommendations are to begin with an initial U.S. Food and Drug Administration–approved dose and adjust the dose based on testosterone levels. The advantages of the testosterone gel include the ease of application and its flexibility of dosing. A major concern is the potential for inadvertent transfer of the gel to a sexual partner or to children who may come in close contact with the patient. The ratio of DHT to testosterone concentrations is higher in men treated with the testosterone gel than in healthy men. Also, there is considerable intra- and interindividual variation in serum testosterone levels in men treated with the transdermal gel due to variations in transdermal absorption and plasma clearance of testosterone. Therefore, monitoring of serum testosterone levels and multiple dose adjustments may be required to achieve and maintain testosterone levels in the target range.

Buccal Adhesive Testosterone A buccal testosterone tablet, which adheres to the buccal mucosa and releases testosterone as it is slowly dissolved, has been approved. After twice-daily application of 30-mg tablets, serum testosterone levels are maintained within the normal male range in a majority of treated hypogonadal men. The adverse effects include buccal ulceration and gum problems in a few subjects. The effects of food and brushing on absorption have not been studied in detail.

Implants of crystalline testosterone can be inserted in the subcutaneous tissue by means of a trocar through a small skin incision. Testosterone is released by surface erosion of the implant and absorbed into the systemic circulation. Two to six 200-mg implants can maintain testosterone in the mid- to high-normal range for up to 6 months. Potential drawbacks include incising the skin for insertion and removal and spontaneous extrusions and fibrosis at the site of the implant.

Testosterone Formulations Not Available in the United States Testosterone undecanoate, when administered orally in oleic acid, is absorbed preferentially through the lymphatics into the systemic circulation and is spared the first-pass degradation in the liver. Doses of 40–80 mg orally, two or three times daily, are typically used. However, the clinical responses are variable and suboptimal. DHT-to-testosterone ratios are higher in hypogonadal men treated with oral testosterone undecanoate, as compared to eugonadal men.

After initial priming, long-acting testosterone undecanoate in oil, when administered intramuscularly every 12 weeks, maintains serum testosterone, estradiol, and DHT in the normal male range and corrects symptoms of androgen deficiency in a majority of treated men. However, large injection volume (4 mL) is its relative drawback.

Novel Androgen Formulations A number of androgen formulations with better pharmacokinetics or more selective activity profiles are under development. A long-acting ester, testosterone undecanoate, when injected intramuscularly, can maintain circulating testosterone concentrations in the male range for 7–12 weeks. Initial clinical trials have demonstrated the feasibility of administering testosterone by the sublingual or buccal routes. 7α-Methyl-19-nortestosterone is an androgen that cannot be 5α-reduced; therefore, compared to testosterone, it has relatively greater agonist activity in muscle and gonadotropin suppression but lesser activity on the prostate.

Selective AR modulators (SARMs) are a class of AR ligands that bind the AR and display tissue-selective actions. A number of nonsteroidal SARMs that act as full agonists on the muscle and bone and that spare the prostate to varying degrees have advanced to phase 3 human trials. Nonsteroidal SARMs do not serve as substrates for either the steroid 5α-reductase or the CYP19 aromatase. SARM binding to AR induces specific conformational changes in the AR protein, which then modulates protein-protein interactions between AR and its coregulators, resulting in tissue-specific regulation of gene expression.

Pharmacologic Uses of Androgens Androgens and SARMs are being evaluated as anabolic therapies for functional limitations associated with aging and chronic illness. Testosterone supplementation increases skeletal muscle mass, maximal voluntary strength, and muscle power in healthy men, hypogonadal men, older men with low testosterone levels, HIV-infected men with weight loss, and men receiving glucocorticoids. These anabolic effects of testosterone are related to testosterone dose and circulating concentrations. Systematic reviews have confirmed that testosterone therapy of HIV-infected men with weight loss promotes improvements in body weight, lean body mass, muscle strength, and depression indices, leading to the recommendation that testosterone be considered as an adjunctive therapy in HIV-infected men who are experiencing unexplained weight loss and who have low testosterone levels. Similarly, in glucocorticoid-treated men, testosterone therapy should be considered to maintain muscle mass and strength and vertebral bone mineral density. It is unknown whether testosterone therapy of older men with functional limitations is safe and effective in improving physical function, vitality, and health-related quality of life and reducing disability. Concerns about potential adverse effects of testosterone on prostate and cardiovascular event rates have encouraged the development of SARMs that are preferentially anabolic and spare the prostate.

Testosterone administration induces hypertrophy of both type 1 and 2 fibers and increases satellite cell (muscle progenitor cells) and myonuclear number. Androgens promote the differentiation of mesenchymal, multipotent progenitor cells into the myogenic lineage and inhibit their differentiation into the adipogenic lineage. Testosterone may have additional effects on satellite cell replication and muscle protein synthesis, which may contribute to an increase in skeletal muscle mass.

Other indications for androgen therapy are in selected patients with anemia due to bone marrow failure (an indication largely supplanted by erythropoietin) or for hereditary angioedema.

Male Hormonal Contraception Based on Combined Administration of Testosterone and Gonadotropin Inhibitors Supraphysiologic doses of testosterone (200 mg testosterone enanthate weekly) suppress LH and FSH secretion and induce azoospermia in 50% of Caucasian men and >95% of Chinese men. The WHO-supported multicenter efficacy trials have demonstrated that suppression of spermatogenesis to azoospermia or severe oligozoospermia (<3 million/mL) by administration of testosterone enanthate to men results in highly effective contraception. Because of concern about long-term adverse effects of supraphysiologic testosterone doses, regimens that combine other gonadotropin inhibitors, such as GnRH antagonists and progestins with replacement doses of testosterone, are being investigated. Oral etonogestrel daily in combination with intramuscular testosterone decanoate every 4–6 weeks induced azoospermia or severe oligozoospermia (sperm density <1 million/mL) in 99% of treated men over a 1-year period. This regimen was associated with weight gain, deceased testicular volume, and decreased plasma high-density lipoprotein (HDL) cholesterol, and its long-term safety has not been demonstrated. SARMs that are more potent inhibitors of gonadotropins than testosterone and spare the prostate hold promise for their contraceptive potential.

Recommended Regimens for Androgen Replacement Testosterone esters are administered typically at doses of 75–100 mg intramuscularly every week, or 150–200 mg every 2 weeks. One or two 5-mg nongenital testosterone patches can be applied daily over the skin of the back, thigh, or upper arm away from pressure areas. Testosterone gels are typically applied over a covered area of skin at initial doses that vary with the formulation; patients should wash their hands after gel application. Bioadhesive buccal testosterone tablets at a dose of 30 mg are typically applied twice daily on the buccal mucosa.

Establishing Efficacy of Testosterone Replacement Therapy Because a clinically useful marker of androgen action is not available, restoration of testosterone levels to the mid-normal range remains the goal of therapy. Measurements of LH and FSH are not useful in assessing the adequacy of testosterone replacement. Testosterone should be measured 3 months after initiating therapy to assess adequacy of therapy. There is substantial interindividual variability in serum testosterone levels, especially with transdermal gels, presumably due to genetic differences in testosterone clearance and transdermal absorption. In patients who are treated with testosterone enanthate or cypionate, testosterone levels should be 350–600 ng/dL 1 week after the injection. If testosterone levels are outside this range, adjustments should be made either in the dose or in the interval between injections. In men on transdermal patch, gel, or buccal testosterone therapy, testosterone levels should be in the mid-normal range (500–700 ng/dL) 4–12 h after application. If testosterone levels are outside this range, the dose should be adjusted. Multiple dose adjustments are often necessary to achieve testosterone levels in the desired therapeutic range.

Restoration of sexual function, secondary sex characteristics, energy, and well-being and maintenance of muscle and bone health are important objectives of testosterone replacement therapy. The patient should be asked about sexual desire and activity, the presence of early morning erections, and the ability to achieve and maintain erections adequate for sexual intercourse. Some hypogonadal men continue to complain about sexual dysfunction even after testosterone replacement has been instituted; these patients may benefit from counseling. The hair growth in response to androgen replacement is variable and depends on ethnicity. Hypogonadal men with prepubertal onset of androgen deficiency who begin testosterone therapy in their late twenties or thirties may find it difficult to adjust to their newly found sexuality and may benefit from counseling. If the patient has a sexual partner, the partner should be included in counseling because of the dramatic physical and sexual changes that occur with androgen treatment.

Contraindications for Androgen Administration Testosterone administration is contraindicated in men with a history of prostate or breast cancer (Table 411-4). Testosterone therapy should not be administered without further urologic evaluation to men with a palpable prostate nodule or induration; to men with prostate-specific antigen levels >4 ng/mL or >3 ng/mL in men at high risk for prostate cancer such as African Americans or men with first-degree relatives with prostate cancer; or to men with severe lower urinary tract symptoms (American Urological Association lower urinary tract symptom score >19). Testosterone replacement should not be administered to men with baseline hematocrit ≥50%, severe untreated obstructive sleep apnea, uncontrolled or poorly controlled congestive heart failure, or myocardial infarction, stroke, or acute coronary syndrome in the preceding 6 months.

Monitoring Potential Adverse Experiences The clinical effectiveness and safety of testosterone replacement therapy should be assessed 3 to 6 months after initiating testosterone therapy and annually thereafter (Table 411-5). Potential adverse effects include acne, oiliness of skin, erythrocytosis, breast tenderness and enlargement, leg edema, induction and exacerbation of obstructive sleep apnea, and increased risk of detection of prostate events. In addition, there may be formulation-specific adverse effects such as skin irritation with transdermal patch, risk of gel transfer to a sexual partner with testosterone gels, buccal ulceration and gum problems with buccal testosterone, and pain and mood fluctuation with injectable testosterone esters. Older men with preexisting heart disease may be at increased risk of cardiovascular events after initiation of testosterone therapy.

HEMOGLOBIN LEVELS Administration of testosterone to androgen-deficient men is typically associated with a ~3% increase in hemoglobin

TABLE 411-4 CONDITIONS IN WHICH TESTOSTERONE ADMINISTRATION IS ASSOCIATED WITH A RISK OF ADVERSE OUTCOME

Conditions in which testosterone administration is associated with very high risk of serious adverse outcomes:
Metastatic prostate cancer
Breast cancer
Conditions in which testosterone administration is associated with moderate to high risk of adverse outcomes:
Undiagnosed prostate nodule or induration
PSA >4 ng/mL (>3 ng/mL in individuals at high risk for prostate cancer, such as African Americans or men with first-degree relatives who have prostate cancer)
Erythrocytosis (hematocrit >50%)
Severe lower urinary tract symptoms associated with benign prostatic hypertrophy as indicated by American Urological Association/International Prostate Symptom Score >19
Uncontrolled or poorly controlled congestive heart failure
Myocardial infarction, stroke, or acute coronary syndrome in the preceding 6 months

Abbreviation: PSA, prostate-specific antigen.

Source: Reproduced from the Endocrine Society Guideline for Testosterone Therapy of Androgen Deficiency Syndromes in Men (S Bhasin et al: J Clin Endocrinol Metab 95:2536, 2010).

TABLE 411-5 MONITORING MEN RECEIVING TESTOSTERONE THERAPY

1. Evaluate the patient 3–6 months after treatment initiation and then annually to assess whether symptoms have responded to treatment and whether the patient is suffering from any adverse effects.
2. Monitor testosterone level 3–6 months after initiation of testosterone therapy:
   - Therapy should aim to raise serum testosterone level into the mid-normal range.
   - Injectable testosterone enanthate or cypionate: Measure serum testosterone level midway between injections. If testosterone is >700 ng/dL (24.5 nmol/L) or >400 ng/dL (14.1 nmol/L), adjust dose or frequency.
   - Transdermal patches: Assess testosterone level 3–12 h after application of the patch; adjust dose to achieve testosterone level in the mid-normal range.
   - Buccal testosterone bioadhesive tablet: Assess level immediately before or after application of fresh system.
   - Transdermal gels and solution: Assess testosterone level 2–8 h after patient has been on treatment for at least 2 weeks; adjust dose to achieve serum testosterone level in the mid-normal range.
   - Testosterone pellets: Measure testosterone levels at the end of the dosing interval. Adjust the number of pellets and/or the dosing interval to achieve serum testosterone levels in the normal range.
   - Oral testosterone undecanoate[a]: Monitor serum testosterone level 3–5 h after ingestion.
   - Injectable testosterone undecanoate: Measure serum testosterone level just prior to each subsequent injection and adjust the dosing interval to maintain serum testosterone in mid-normal range.
3. Check hematocrit at baseline, at 3–6 months, and then annually. If hematocrit is >54%, stop therapy until hematocrit decreases to a safe level; evaluate the patient for hypoxia and sleep apnea; reinitiate therapy with a reduced dose.
4. Measure bone mineral density of lumbar spine and/or femoral neck after 1–2 years of testosterone therapy in hypogonadal men with osteoporosis or low trauma fracture, consistent with regional standard of care.
5. In men 40 years of age or older with baseline PSA >0.6 ng/mL, perform digital rectal examination and check PSA level before initiating treatment, at 3–6 months, and then in accordance with guidelines for prostate cancer screening depending on the age and race of the patient.
6. Obtain urologic consultation if there is:
   - An increase in serum PSA concentration >1.4 ng/mL within any 12-month period of testosterone treatment.
   - A PSA velocity of >0.4 ng/mL per year using the PSA level after 6 months of testosterone administration as the reference (only applicable if PSA data are available for a period exceeding 2 years).
   - Detection of a prostatic abnormality on digital rectal examination.
   - An AUA/IPSS prostate symptom score of >19.
7. Evaluate formulation-specific adverse effects at each visit:
   - Buccal testosterone tablets: Inquire about alterations in taste and examine the gums and oral mucosa for irritation.
   - Injectable testosterone esters (enanthate, cypionate, and undecanoate): Ask about fluctuations in mood or libido and, rarely, cough after injections.
   - Testosterone patches: Look for skin reaction at the application site.
   - Testosterone gels: Advise patients to cover the application sites with a shirt and to wash the skin with soap and water before having skin-to-skin contact, because testosterone gels leave a testosterone residue on the skin that can be transferred to a woman or child who might come in close contact. Serum testosterone levels are maintained when the application site is washed 4–6 h after application of the testosterone gel.
   - Testosterone pellets: Look for signs of infection, fibrosis, or pellet extrusion.

[a]Not approved for clinical use in the United States.

Abbreviations: AUA/IPSS, American Urological Association/International Prostate Symptom Score; PSA, prostate-specific antigen.

Source: Reproduced with permission from the Endocrine Society Guideline for Testosterone Therapy of Androgen Deficiency Syndromes in Adult Men (S Bhasin et al: J Clin Endocrinol Metab 95:2536, 2010).

levels, due to increased erythropoiesis, suppression of hepcidin, and increased iron availability for erythropoiesis. The magnitude of hemoglobin increase during testosterone therapy is greater in older men than younger men and in men who have sleep apnea, a significant smoking history, or chronic obstructive lung disease. The frequency of erythrocytosis is higher in hypogonadal men treated with injectable testosterone esters than in those treated with transdermal formulations, presumably due to the higher testosterone dose delivered by the typical regimens of testosterone esters. Erythrocytosis is the most frequent adverse event reported in testosterone trials in middle-aged and older men and is also the most frequent cause of treatment discontinuation in these trials. If hematocrit rises above 54%, testosterone therapy should be stopped until hematocrit has fallen to <50%. After evaluation of the patient for hypoxia and sleep apnea, testosterone therapy may be reinitiated at a lower dose.

PROSTATE AND SERUM PROSTATE-SPECIFIC ANTIGEN LEVELS Testosterone replacement therapy increases prostate volume to the size seen in age-matched controls but does not increase prostate volume beyond that expected for age. There is no evidence that testosterone therapy causes prostate cancer. However, androgen administration can exacerbate preexisting metastatic prostate cancer. Many older men harbor microscopic foci of cancer in their prostates. It is not known whether long-term testosterone administration will induce these microscopic foci to grow into clinically significant cancers.

Prostate-specific antigen (PSA) levels are lower in testosterone-deficient men and are restored to normal after testosterone replacement. There is considerable test-retest variability in PSA measurements. Increments in PSA levels after testosterone supplementation in androgen-deficient men are generally <0.5 ng/mL, and increments >1.0 ng/mL over a 3- to 6-month period are unusual. The 90% confidence interval for the change in PSA values in men with benign prostatic hypertrophy, measured 3–6 months apart, is 1.4 ng/mL. Therefore, the Endocrine Society expert panel suggested that an increase in PSA >1.4 ng/mL in any 1 year after starting testosterone therapy, if confirmed, should lead to urologic evaluation. PSA velocity criterion can be used for patients who have sequential PSA measurements for >2 years; a change of >0.40 ng/mL per year merits closer urologic follow-up.

CARDIOVASCULAR RISK In epidemiologic studies, testosterone concentrations are negatively related to the risk of diabetes mellitus, heart disease, and all-cause and cardiovascular mortality. A recent testosterone trial in older men with mobility limitation was stopped early because of the higher rates of cardiovascular events in the testosterone arm than in the placebo arm of this trial. Meta-analyses of testosterone trials have found a significant increase in cardiovascular event rates in older men receiving testosterone therapy. Inferences about adverse events from previous trials included in these meta-analyses are limited by poor ascertainment, small numbers of events, heterogeneity of study populations, and small numbers of participants. Two retrospective analyses also found a higher frequency of cardiovascular events in association with testosterone therapy in older men with preexisting heart disease. Retrospective database analyses are limited by their inherent inability to verify the indication for treatment, diagnoses, or other relevant quantitative information and are susceptible to confounding by many other factors. Adequately powered prospective studies are needed to determine the effect on testosterone replacement on cardiovascular risk.

Androgen Abuse by Athletes and Recreational Bodybuilders The illicit use of androgenic-anabolic steroids (AAS) to enhance athletic performance first surfaced in the 1950s among power lifters and spread rapidly to other sports, professional as well as high school athletes, and recreational bodybuilders. In the early 1980s, the use of AAS spread beyond the athletic community into the general population, and now as many as 3 million Americans, most of them men, have likely used these compounds. Most AAS users are not athletes, but rather recreational weightlifters, who use these drugs to look lean and more muscular. The most commonly used AAS include testosterone esters, nandrolone, stanozolol, methandienone, and methenolol. AAS users generally use increasing doses of multiple steroids in a practice known as stacking.

The adverse effects of long-term AAS abuse remain poorly understood. Most of the information about the adverse effects of AAS has emerged from case reports, uncontrolled studies, or clinical trials that used replacement doses of testosterone. The adverse event data from clinical trials using physiologic replacement doses of testosterone have been extrapolated unjustifiably to AAS users who may administer 10–100 times the replacement doses of testosterone over many years and to support the claim that AAS use is safe. A substantial fraction of androgenic steroid users also use other drugs that are perceived to be muscle building or performance enhancing, such as GH; erythropoiesis-stimulating agents; insulin; and stimulants such as amphetamine, clenbuterol, cocaine, ephedrine, and thyroxine; and drugs perceived to reduce adverse effects such as hCG, aromatase inhibitors, or estrogen antagonists. The men who abuse androgenic steroids are more likely to engage in other high-risk behaviors than nonusers. The adverse events associated with AAS use may be due to AAS themselves, concomitant use of other drugs, high-risk behaviors, and host characteristics that may render these individuals more susceptible to AAS use or to other high-risk behaviors.

The high rates of mortality and morbidities observed in AAS users are alarming. One Finnish study reported 4.6 times the risk of death among elite power lifters than in age-matched men from the general population. The causes of death among power lifters included suicides, myocardial infarction, hepatic coma, and non-Hodgkin's lymphoma. A retrospective review of patient records in Sweden also reported higher standardized mortality ratios for AAS users than for nonusers. Thiblin and colleagues found that 32% of deaths among AAS users were suicidal, 26% homicidal, and 35% accidental. The median age of death among AAS users (24 years) is even lower than that for heroin or amphetamine users.

Numerous reports of cardiac death among young AAS users raise concerns about the adverse cardiovascular effects of AAS. High doses of AAS may induce proatherogenic dyslipidemia, increase thrombosis risk via effects on clotting factors and platelets, and induce vasospasm through their effects on vascular nitric oxide.

Replacement doses of testosterone, when administered parenterally, are associated with only a small decrease in HDL cholesterol and little or no effect on total cholesterol, low-density lipoprotein (LDL) cholesterol, and triglyceride levels. In contrast, supraphysiologic doses of testosterone and orally administered, 17α-alkylated, nonaromatizable AAS are associated with marked reductions in HDL cholesterol and increases in LDL cholesterol.

Recent studies of AAS users using tissue Doppler and strain imaging and MRI have reported diastolic and systolic dysfunction, including significantly lower early and late diastolic tissue velocities, reduced E/A ratio, and reduced peak systolic strain in AAS users than in nonusers. Power athletes using AAS often have short QT intervals but increased QT dispersion, which may predispose them to ventricular arrhythmias. Long-term AAS use may be associated with myocardial hypertrophy and fibrosis. Myocardial tissue of power lifters using AAS has been shown to be infiltrated with fibrous tissue and fat droplets. The finding of ARs on myocardial cells suggests that AAS might be directly toxic to myocardial cells.

Long-term AAS use suppresses LH and FSH secretion and inhibits endogenous testosterone production and spermatogenesis. Men who have used AAS for more than a few months experience marked suppression of the hypothalamic-pituitary-testicular (HPT) axis after stopping AAS that may be associated with sexual dysfunction, fatigue, infertility, and depression; in some AAS users, HPT suppression may last more than a year, and in a few individuals, complete recovery may never occur. The symptoms of androgen deficiency caused by androgen withdrawal may cause some men to revert back to using AAS, leading to continued use and AAS dependence. As many as 30% of AAS users develop a syndrome of AAS dependence, characterized by long-term AAS use despite adverse medical and psychiatric effects.

Supraphysiologic doses of testosterone may also impair insulin sensitivity. Orally administered androgens also have been associated with insulin resistance and diabetes.

Unsafe injection practices, high-risk behaviors, and increased rates of incarceration render AAS users at increased risk of HIV and hepatitis B and C. In one survey, nearly 1 in 10 gay men had injected AAS or other substances, and AAS users were more likely to report high-risk unprotected anal sex than other men.

Some AAS users develop hypomanic or manic symptoms during AAS exposure (irritability, aggressiveness, reckless behavior, and occasional psychotic symptoms, sometimes associated with violence) and major depression (sometimes associated with suicidality) during AAS withdrawal. Users may also develop other forms of illicit drug use, which may be potentiated or exacerbated by AAS.

Elevated liver enzymes, cholestatic jaundice, hepatic neoplasms, and peliosis hepatis have been reported with oral, 17α-alkylated AAS. AAS use may cause muscle hypertrophy without compensatory adaptations in tendons, ligaments, and joints, thus increasing the risk of tendon and joint injuries. AAS use is associated with acne, baldness, and increased body hair.

The suspicion of AAS use may be raised by the increased hemoglobin and hematocrit, suppressed LH and FSH and testosterone levels, low high-density lipoproteins cholesterol, and low testicular volume and sperm density in a person who looks highly muscular. Accredited laboratories use gas chromatography–mass spectrometry or liquid chromatography–mass spectrometry to detect anabolic steroid abuse. In recent years, the availability of high-resolution mass spectrometry and tandem mass spectrometry has further improved the sensitivity of detecting androgen abuse. Illicit testosterone use is detected generally by the application of the measurement of the urinary testosterone-to-epitestosterone ratio and further confirmed by the use of the ^{13}C:^{12}C ratio in testosterone by the use of isotope ratio combustion mass spectrometry. Exogenous testosterone administration increases urinary testosterone glucuronide excretion and consequently the testosterone-to-epitestosterone ratio. Ratios >4 suggest exogenous testosterone use but can also reflect genetic variation. Genetic variations in the uridine diphosphoglucuronyl transferase 2B17 (*UGT2B17*), the major enzyme for testosterone glucuronidation, affect the testosterone-to-epitestosterone ratio. Synthetic testosterone has a lower ^{13}C:^{12}C ratio than endogenously produced testosterone, and these differences in ^{13}C:^{12}C ratio can be detected by isotope ratio combustion mass spectrometry, which is used to confirm exogenous testosterone use in individuals with a high testosterone-to-epitestosterone ratio.

412 Disorders of the Female Reproductive System

Janet E. Hall

The female reproductive system regulates the hormonal changes responsible for puberty and adult reproductive function. Normal reproductive function in women requires the dynamic integration of hormonal signals from the hypothalamus, pituitary, and ovary, resulting in repetitive cycles of follicle development, ovulation, and preparation of the endometrial lining of the uterus for implantation should conception occur. It is critical to understand pubertal development in normal girls (and boys) as a yardstick for identifying precocious and delayed puberty.

For further discussion of related topics, see the following chapters: amenorrhea and pelvic pain (Chap. 69), infertility and contraception (Chap. 414), menopause (Chap. 413), disorders of sex development (Chap. 410), and disorders of the male reproductive system (Chap. 411).

DEVELOPMENT OF THE OVARY AND EARLY FOLLICULAR GROWTH

The ovary orchestrates the development and release of a mature oocyte and also elaborates hormones (e.g., estrogen, progesterone, inhibin, relaxin) that are critical for pubertal development and preparation of the uterus for conception, implantation, and the early stages of pregnancy. To achieve these functions in repeated monthly cycles, the ovary undergoes some of the most dynamic changes of any organ in the body. Primordial germ cells can be identified by the third week of gestation, and their migration to the genital ridge is complete by 6 weeks of gestation. Germ cells persist within the genital ridge, are then referred to as *oogonia*, and are essential for induction of ovarian development. Although one X chromosome undergoes X inactivation in somatic cells, it is reactivated in oogonia and genes on both X chromosomes are required for normal ovarian development. A streak ovary containing only stromal cells is found in patients with 45,X Turner's syndrome (Chap. 410).

The germ cell population expands, and starting at ~8 weeks of gestation, oogonia begin to enter prophase of the first meiotic division and become primary oocytes. This allows the oocyte to be surrounded by a single layer of flattened granulosa cells to form a primordial follicle (Fig. 412-1). Granulosa cells are derived from mesonephric cells that invade the ovary early in its development, pushing the germ cells to the periphery. The weight of evidence supports the concept that for the most part, the ovary contains a nonrenewable pool of germ cells. Through the combined processes of mitosis, meiosis, and atresia, the population of oogonia reaches its maximum of 6–7 million by 20 weeks of gestation, after which there is a progressive loss of both oogonia and primordial follicles through the process of atresia. At birth, oogonia are no longer present in the ovary, and only 1–2 million germ cells remain in the form of primordial follicles (Fig. 412-2). The oocyte persists in prophase of the first meiotic division until just before ovulation, when meiosis resumes.

The quiescent primordial follicles are recruited to further growth and differentiation through a highly regulated process that limits the size of the developing cohort to ensure that folliculogenesis can continue throughout the reproductive life span. This initial recruitment of primordial follicles to form primary follicles (Fig. 412-1) is characterized by growth of the oocyte and the transition from squamous to cuboidal granulosa cells. The theca interna cells that surround the developing follicle begin to form as the primary follicle grows. Acquisition of a zona pellucida by the oocyte and the presence of several layers of surrounding cuboidal granulosa cells mark the development of secondary follicles. It is at this stage that granulosa cells develop follicle-stimulating hormone (FSH), estradiol, and androgen receptors and communicate with one another through the development of gap junctions.

Bidirectional signaling between the germ cells and the somatic cells in the ovary is a necessary component underlying the maturation

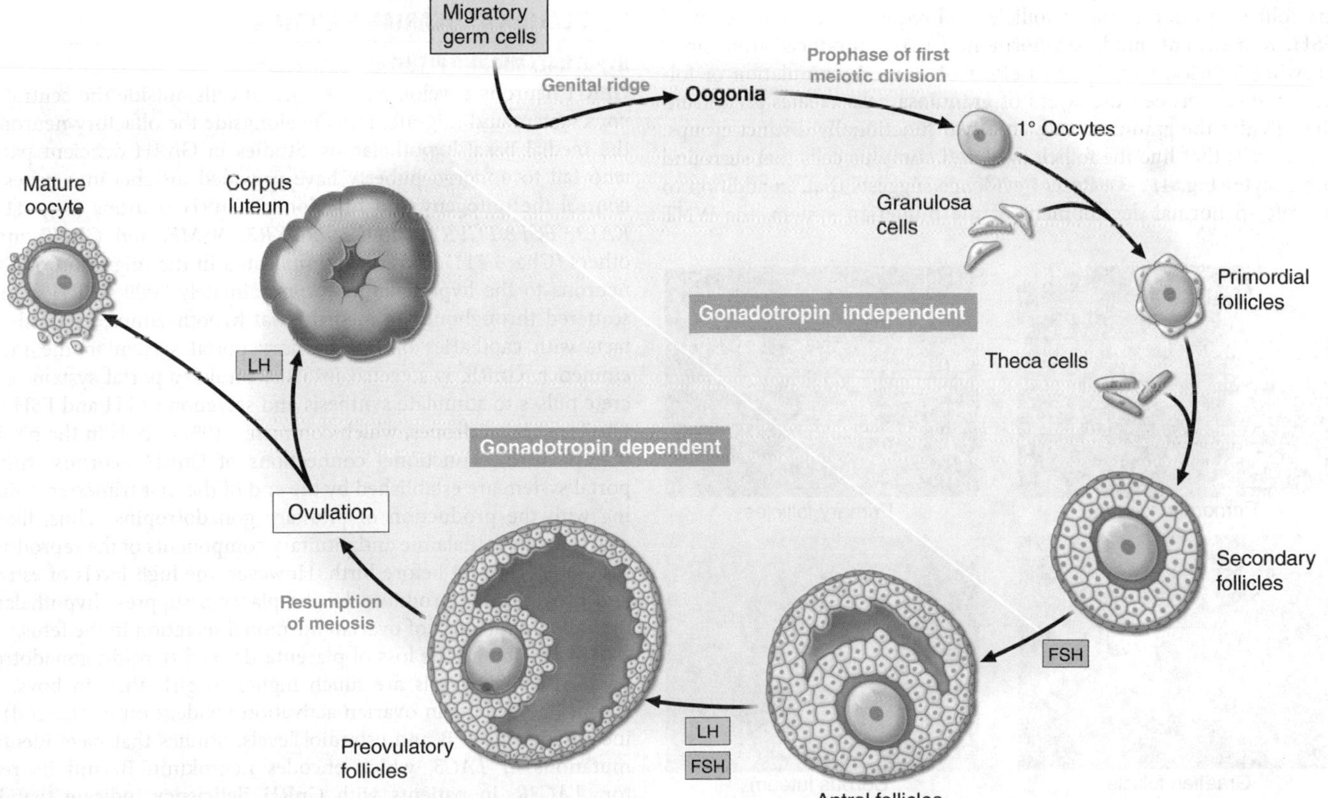

FIGURE 412-1 Stages of ovarian development from the arrival of the migratory germ cells at the genital ridge through gonadotropin-independent and gonadotropin-dependent phases that ultimately result in ovulation of a mature oocyte. FSH, follicle-stimulating hormone; LH, luteinizing hormone.

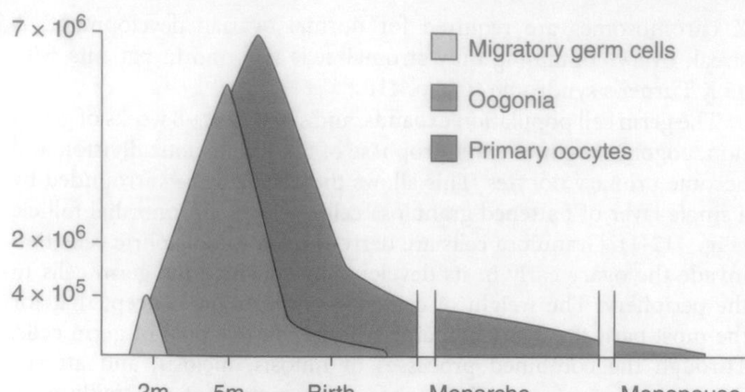

FIGURE 412-2 Ovarian germ cell number is maximal at midgestation and then decreases precipitously.

of the oocyte and the capacity for hormone secretion. For example, oocyte-derived growth differentiation factor 9 (GDF-9) and bone morphogenic protein-15 (BMP-15), also known as GDF-9b, are required for migration of pregranulosa and pretheca cells to the outer surface of the developing follicle and, hence, initial follicle formation. GDF-9 is also required for formation of secondary follicles, as are granulosa cell–derived KIT ligand (KITL) and the forkhead transcription factor (FOXL2). All of these genes are potential candidates for premature ovarian failure in women, and mutations in the human *FOXL2* gene have been shown to cause the syndrome of blepharophimosis/ptosis/epicanthus inversus, which is associated with ovarian failure.

DEVELOPMENT OF A MATURE FOLLICLE

The early stages of follicle growth are primarily driven by intraovarian factors and may take up to a year from development of the primary follicle to the dominant follicle stage. Further maturation to the preovulatory state, including the resumption of meiosis in the oocyte, requires the combined stimulus of FSH and luteinizing hormone (LH) (Fig. 412-1) and can be accomplished within weeks. Recruitment of secondary follicles from the resting follicle pool requires the direct action of FSH, whereas anti-müllerian hormone (AMH) produced from small growing follicles, restrains this effect of FSH. Accumulation of follicular fluid between the layers of granulosa cells creates an antrum that divides the granulosa cells into two functionally distinct groups: mural cells that line the follicle wall and cumulus cells that surround the oocyte (Fig. 412-3). Recent evidence suggests that, in addition to its role in normal development of the müllerian system, the WNT signaling pathway is required for normal antral follicle development and may also play a role in ovarian steroidogenesis. A single dominant follicle emerges from the growing follicle pool within the first 5–7 days after the onset of menses, and the majority of follicles fall off their growth trajectory and become atretic. Autocrine actions of activin and BMP-6, derived from the granulosa cells, and paracrine actions of GDF-9, BMP-15, BMP-6, and Gpr149, derived from the oocyte, are involved in granulosa cell proliferation and modulation of FSH responsiveness. Differential exposure to these factors may explain the mechanism whereby a given follicle is selected for continued growth to the preovulatory stage. The dominant follicle can be distinguished by its size, evidence of granulosa cell proliferation, large number of FSH receptors, high aromatase activity, and elevated concentrations of estradiol and inhibin A in follicular fluid.

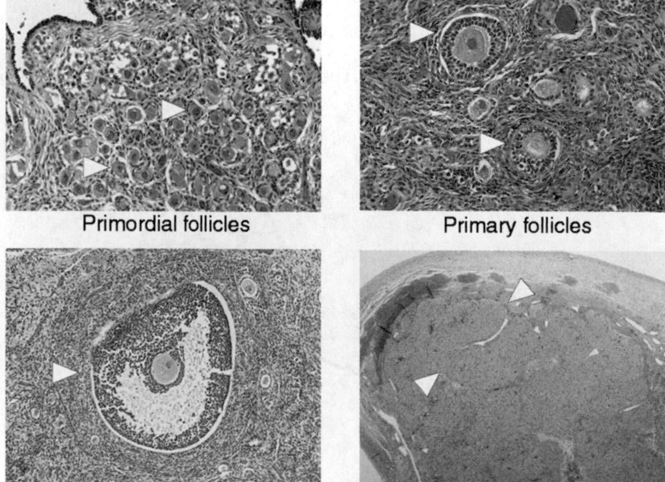

FIGURE 412-3 Development of ovarian follicles. The Graafian follicle is also known as a tertiary or preovulatory follicle. *(Courtesy of JH Eichhorn and D. Roberts, Massachusetts General Hospital; with permission.)*

The dominant follicle undergoes rapid expansion during the 5–6 days prior to ovulation, reflecting granulosa cell proliferation and accumulation of follicular fluid. FSH induces LH receptors on the granulosa cells, and the preovulatory, or Graafian, follicle moves to the outer ovarian surface in preparation for ovulation. The LH surge triggers the resumption of meiosis, the suppression of granulosa cell proliferation, and the induction of cyclooxygenase 2 (COX-2), prostaglandins, the progesterone receptor, and the epidermal growth factor (EGF)-like growth factors amphiregulin, epiregulin, betacellulin, and neuroregulin 1, all of which are required for ovulation. EGF-like factors are thought to mediate these follicular responses to LH. Ovulation also involves production of extracellular matrix leading to expansion of the cumulus cell population that surrounds the oocyte and the controlled expulsion of the egg and follicular fluid. Both progesterone and prostaglandins (induced by the ovulatory stimulus) are essential for this process. After ovulation, luteinization is induced by LH in conjunction with the acquisition of a rich vascular network in response to vascular endothelial growth factor (VEGF) and basic fibroblast growth factor (FGF). Traditional regulators of central reproductive control, gonadotropin-releasing hormone (GnRH) and its receptor (GnRHR), are also produced in the ovary and may be involved in corpus luteum function.

REGULATION OF OVARIAN FUNCTION

HYPOTHALAMIC AND PITUITARY SECRETION

GnRH neurons develop from epithelial cells outside the central nervous system and migrate, initially alongside the olfactory neurons, to the medial basal hypothalamus. Studies in GnRH-deficient patients who fail to undergo puberty have provided insights into genes that control the ontogeny and function of GnRH neurons (Fig. 412-4). *KAL1*, *FGF8/FGFR1*, *PROK2/PROKR2*, *NSMF*, and *CDH7*, among others (Chap. 411), have been implicated in the migration of GnRH neurons to the hypothalamus. Approximately 7000 GnRH neurons, scattered throughout the medial basal hypothalamus, establish contacts with capillaries of the pituitary portal system in the median eminence. GnRH is secreted into the pituitary portal system in discrete pulses to stimulate synthesis and secretion of LH and FSH from pituitary gonadotropes, which comprise ~10% of cells in the pituitary (Chap. 401e). Functional connections of GnRH neurons with the portal system are established by the end of the first trimester, coinciding with the production of pituitary gonadotropins. Thus, like the ovary, the hypothalamic and pituitary components of the reproductive system are present before birth. However, the high levels of estradiol and progesterone produced by the placenta suppress hypothalamic-pituitary stimulation of ovarian hormonal secretion in the fetus.

After birth and the loss of placenta-derived steroids, gonadotropin levels rise. FSH levels are much higher in girls than in boys. This rise in FSH results in ovarian activation (evident on ultrasound) and increased inhibin B and estradiol levels. Studies that have identified mutations in *TAC3*, which encodes neurokinin B, and its receptor, *TAC3R*, in patients with GnRH deficiency indicate that both are involved in control of GnRH secretion and may be particularly important at this early stage of development. By 12–20 months of age, the reproductive axis is again suppressed, and a period of relative quiescence persists until puberty (Fig. 412-5). At the onset of puberty,

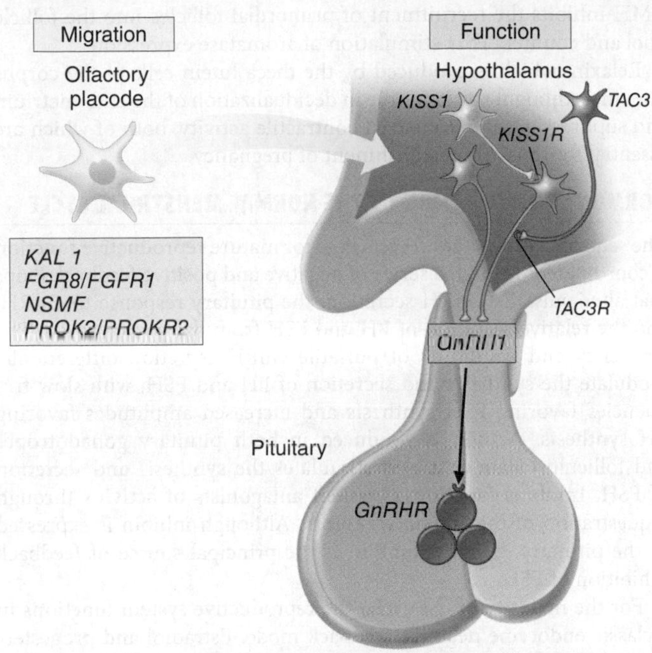

FIGURE 412-4 Establishment of a functional gonadotropin-releasing hormone (GnRH) system requires the participation of a number of genes that are essential for development and migration of GnRH neurons from the olfactory placode to the hypothalamus in addition to genes involved in the functional control of GnRH secretion and action.

pulsatile GnRH secretion induces pituitary gonadotropin production. In the early stages of puberty, LH and FSH secretion are apparent only during sleep, but as puberty develops, pulsatile gonadotropin secretion occurs throughout the day and night.

The mechanisms responsible for the childhood quiescence and pubertal reactivation of the reproductive axis remain incompletely understood. GnRH neurons in the hypothalamus respond to both excitatory and inhibitory factors. Increased sensitivity to the inhibitory influence of gonadal steroids has long been implicated in the inhibition of GnRH secretion during childhood but has not been definitively established in the human. Metabolic signals, such as adipocyte-derived leptin, play a permissive role in reproductive function (Chap. 415e). Studies of patients with isolated GnRH deficiency reveal that mutations in the G protein–coupled receptor 54 (*GPR54*) gene (now known as *KISS1R*) preclude the onset of puberty. The ligand for this receptor, metastin, is derived from the parent peptide, kisspeptin-1 (*KISS1*), and is a powerful stimulant for GnRH release. A potential role for kisspeptin in the onset of puberty has been suggested by upregulation of *KISS1* and *KISS1R* transcripts in the hypothalamus at the time of puberty. *TAC3* and dynorphin (*Dyn*), which appear to play an inhibitory rather than stimulatory role in GnRH control, are co-expressed with *KISS1* in KNDy neurons that project to GnRH neurons. This system is intimately involved with estrogen negative feedback regulation of GnRH secretion.

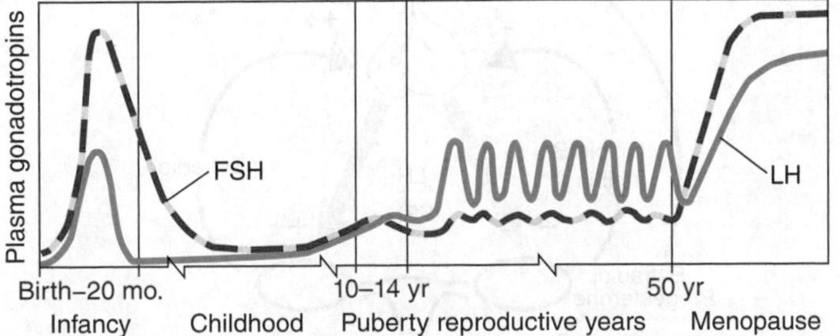

FIGURE 412-5 Follicle-stimulating hormone (FSH) and luteinizing hormone (LH) are increased during the neonatal years but go through a period of childhood quiescence before increasing again during puberty. Gonadotropin levels are cyclic during the reproductive years and increase dramatically with the loss of negative feedback that accompanies menopause.

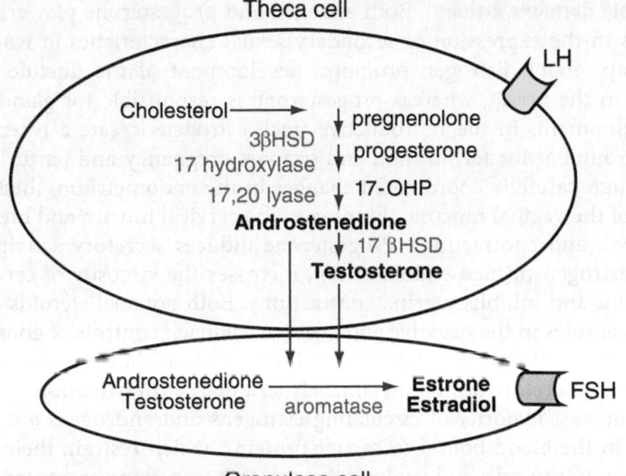

FIGURE 412-6 Estrogen production in the ovary requires the cooperative function of the theca and granulosa cells under the control of luteinizing hormone (LH) and follicle-stimulating hormone (FSH). HSD, hydroxysteroid dehydrogenase; OHP, hydroxyprogesterone.

OVARIAN STEROIDS

Ovarian steroid-producing cells do not store hormones but produce them in response to LH and FSH during the normal menstrual cycle. The sequence of steps and the enzymes involved in the synthesis of steroid hormones are similar in the ovary, adrenal, and testis. However, the enzymes required to catalyze specific steps are compartmentalized and may not be abundant or even present in all cell types. Within the developing ovarian follicle, estrogen synthesis from cholesterol requires close integration between theca and granulosa cells—sometimes called the *two-cell model for steroidogenesis* (Fig. 412-6). FSH receptors are confined to the granulosa cells, whereas LH receptors are restricted to the theca cells until the late stages of follicular development, when they are also found on granulosa cells. The theca cells surrounding the follicle are highly vascularized and use cholesterol, derived primarily from circulating lipoproteins, as the starting point for the synthesis of androstenedione and testosterone under the control of LH. Androstenedione and testosterone are transferred across the basal lamina to the granulosa cells, which receive no direct blood supply. The mural granulosa cells are particularly rich in aromatase and, under the control of FSH, produce estradiol, the primary steroid secreted from the follicular phase ovary and the most potent estrogen. Theca cell–produced androstenedione and, to a lesser extent, testosterone are also secreted into peripheral blood, where they can be converted to dihydrotestosterone in skin and to estrogens in adipose tissue. The hilar interstitial cells of the ovary are functionally similar to Leydig cells and are also capable of secreting androgens. Although stromal cells proliferate in response to androgens (as in polycystic ovarian syndrome [PCOS]), they do not secrete androgens.

Development of the rich capillary network following rupture of the follicle at the time of ovulation makes it possible for large molecules such as low-density lipoprotein (LDL) to reach the luteinized granulosa and theca lutein cells. As in the follicle, both cell types are required for steroidogenesis in the corpus luteum. The large luteinized granulosa cells are the main source of progesterone production, whereas the smaller theca lutein cells produce 17-hydroxyprogesterone, a substrate for aromatization to estradiol by the luteinized granulosa cells. LH is critical for normal structure and function of the corpus luteum. Because LH and human chorionic gonadotropin (hCG) bind to a common receptor, the role of LH in support of the corpus luteum can be replaced by hCG in the first 10 weeks after conception, and hCG is commonly used for luteal phase support in the treatment of infertility.

Steroid Hormone Actions Both estrogen and progesterone play critical roles in the expression of secondary sexual characteristics in women (Chap. 400e). Estrogen promotes development of the ductule system in the breast, whereas progesterone is responsible for glandular development. In the reproductive tract, estrogens create a receptive environment for fertilization and support pregnancy and parturition through carefully coordinated changes in the endometrium, thickening of the vaginal mucosa, thinning of the cervical mucus, and uterine growth and contractions. Progesterone induces secretory activity in the estrogen-primed endometrium, increases the viscosity of cervical mucus, and inhibits uterine contractions. Both gonadal steroids play critical roles in the negative and positive feedback controls of gonadotropin secretion. Progesterone also increases basal body temperature and has therefore been used clinically as a marker of ovulation.

The vast majority of circulating estrogens and androgens are carried in the blood bound to carrier proteins, which restrain their free diffusion into cells and prolong their clearance, serving as a reservoir. High-affinity binding proteins include sex hormone–binding globulin (SHBG), which binds androgens with somewhat greater affinity than estrogens, and corticosteroid-binding globulin (CBG), which also binds progesterone. Modulations in binding protein levels by insulin, androgens, and estrogens contribute to high bioavailable testosterone levels in PCOS and to high circulating estrogen and progesterone levels during pregnancy.

Estrogens act primarily through binding to the nuclear receptors, estrogen receptor (ER) α and β. Transcriptional coactivators and corepressors modulate ER action (Chap. 400e). Both ER subtypes are present in the hypothalamus, pituitary, ovary, and reproductive tract. Although ERα and -β exhibit some functional redundancy, there is also a high degree of specificity, particularly in expression within cell types. For example, ERα functions in the ovarian theca cells, whereas ERβ is critical for granulosa cell function. There is also evidence for membrane-initiated signaling by estrogen. Similar signaling mechanisms pertain for progesterone with evidence of transcriptional regulation through progesterone receptor (PR) A and B protein isoforms, as well as rapid membrane signaling.

OVARIAN PEPTIDES

Inhibin was initially isolated from gonadal fluids based on its ability to selectively inhibit FSH secretion from pituitary cells. Inhibin is a heterodimer composed of an α subunit and a βA or βB subunit to form inhibin A or inhibin B, both of which are secreted from the ovary. Activin is a homodimer of inhibin β subunits with the capacity to stimulate the synthesis and secretion of FSH. Inhibins and activins are members of the transforming growth factor β (TGF-β) superfamily of growth and differentiation factors. During the purification of inhibin, follistatin, an unrelated monomeric protein that inhibits FSH secretion, was discovered. Within the pituitary, follistatin inhibits FSH secretion indirectly through binding and neutralizing activin.

Inhibin B is secreted from the granulosa cells of small antral follicles, whereas inhibin A is present in both granulosa and theca cells and is secreted by dominant follicles. Inhibin A is also present in luteinized granulosa cells and is a major secretory product of the corpus luteum. Inhibin B is constitutively secreted by granulosa cells and increases in serum in conjunction with recruitment of secondary follicles to the pool of actively growing follicles under the control of FSH. Inhibin B has been used clinically as a marker of ovarian reserve. Inhibin B is an important inhibitor of FSH, independent of estradiol, during the menstrual cycle. Although activin is also secreted from the ovary, the excess of follistatin in serum, combined with its nearly irreversible binding of activin, make it unlikely that ovarian activin plays an endocrine role in FSH regulation. However, there is evidence that activin plays an autocrine/paracrine role in the ovary, in addition to its intrapituitary role in modulation of FSH production.

AMH (also known as müllerian-inhibiting substance) is important in ovarian biology in addition to the function from which it derived its name (i.e., promotion of the degeneration of the müllerian system during embryogenesis in the male). AMH is produced by granulosa cells from small follicles and, like inhibin B, is a marker of ovarian reserve. AMH inhibits the recruitment of primordial follicles into the follicle pool and counters FSH stimulation of aromatase expression.

Relaxin, which is produced by the theca lutein cells of the corpus luteum, is thought to play a role in decidualization of the endometrium and suppression of myometrial contractile activity, both of which are essential for the early establishment of pregnancy.

HORMONAL INTEGRATION OF THE NORMAL MENSTRUAL CYCLE

The sequence of changes responsible for mature reproductive function is coordinated through a series of negative and positive feedback loops that alter pulsatile GnRH secretion, the pituitary response to GnRH, and the relative secretion of LH and FSH from the gonadotrope. The frequency and amplitude of pulsatile GnRH secretion differentially modulate the synthesis and secretion of LH and FSH, with slow frequencies favoring FSH synthesis and increased amplitudes favoring LH synthesis. Activin is produced in both pituitary gonadotropes and folliculostellate cells and stimulates the synthesis and secretion of FSH. Inhibins function as potent antagonists of activins through sequestration of the activin receptors. Although inhibin is expressed in the pituitary, gonadal inhibin is the principal source of feedback inhibition of FSH.

For the majority of the cycle, the reproductive system functions in a classic endocrine negative feedback mode. Estradiol and progesterone inhibit GnRH secretion, and the inhibins act at the pituitary to selectively inhibit FSH synthesis and secretion (Fig. 412-7). This negative feedback control of FSH is critical for development of the single mature oocyte that characterizes normal reproductive function in women. In addition to these negative feedback controls, the menstrual cycle is uniquely dependent on estrogen-induced positive feedback to produce an LH surge that is essential for ovulation of a mature follicle. Estrogen negative feedback in women occurs primarily at the hypothalamus with a small pituitary contribution, whereas estrogen positive feedback occurs at the pituitary with hypothalamic GnRH secretion playing a permissive role.

THE FOLLICULAR PHASE

The follicular phase is characterized by recruitment of a cohort of secondary follicles and the ultimate selection of a dominant preovulatory follicle (Fig. 412-8). The follicular phase begins, by convention, on the first day of menses. However, follicle recruitment is initiated by the rise in FSH that begins in the late luteal phase of the previous cycle in conjunction with the loss of negative feedback of gonadal steroids and likely inhibin A. The fact that a 20–30% increase in FSH is adequate for follicular recruitment speaks to the marked sensitivity of the resting follicle pool to FSH. The resultant granulosa cell proliferation is responsible for increasing early follicular phase levels of inhibin B. Inhibin B in conjunction with rising levels of estradiol, and

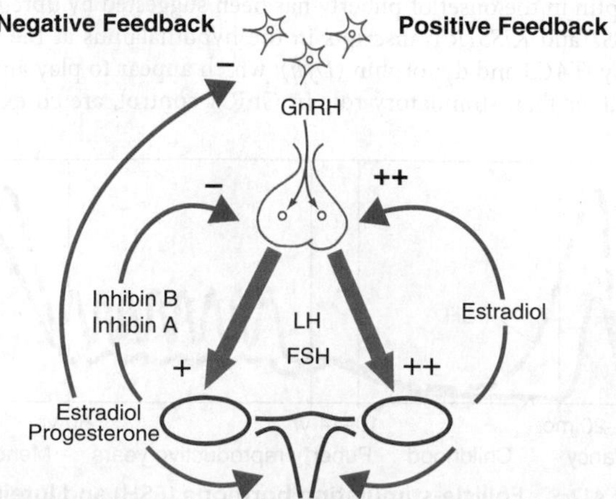

FIGURE 412-7 The reproductive system in women is critically dependent on both negative feedback of gonadal steroids and inhibin to modulate follicle-stimulating hormone (FSH) secretion and on estrogen positive feedback to generate the preovulatory luteinizing hormone (LH) surge. GnRH, gonadotropin-releasing hormone.

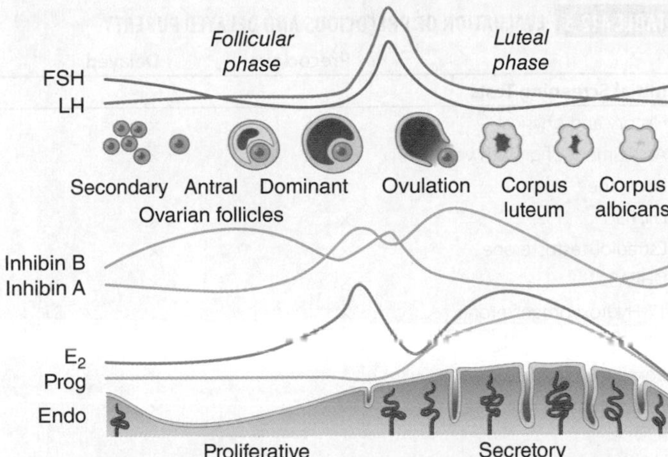

FIGURE 412-8 Relationship between gonadotropins, follicle development, gonadal secretion, and endometrial changes during the normal menstrual cycle. E_2, estradiol; Endo, endometrium; FSH, follicle-stimulating hormone; LH, luteinizing hormone; Prog, progesterone.

probably inhibin A, restrain FSH secretion during this critical period such that only a single follicle matures in the vast majority of cycles. The increased risk of multiple gestation associated with the increased levels of FSH characteristic of advanced maternal age, or with exogenous gonadotropin administration in the treatment of infertility, attests to the importance of negative feedback regulation of FSH. With further growth of the dominant follicle, estradiol and inhibin A increase exponentially and the follicle acquires LH receptors. Increasing levels of estradiol are responsible for proliferative changes in the endometrium. The exponential rise in estradiol results in positive feedback on the pituitary, leading to the generation of an LH surge (and a smaller FSH surge), thereby triggering ovulation and luteinization of the granulosa cells.

THE LUTEAL PHASE

The luteal phase begins with the formation of the corpus luteum from the ruptured follicle (Fig. 412-8). Progesterone and inhibin A are produced from the luteinized granulosa cells, which continue to aromatize theca-derived androgen precursors, producing estradiol. The combined actions of estrogen and progesterone are responsible for the secretory changes in the endometrium that are necessary for implantation. The corpus luteum is supported by LH but has a finite life span because of diminished sensitivity to LH. The demise of the corpus luteum results in a progressive decline in hormonal support of the endometrium. Inflammation or local hypoxia and ischemia result in vascular changes in the endometrium, leading to the release of cytokines, cell death, and shedding of the endometrium.

If conception occurs, hCG produced by the trophoblast binds to LH receptors on the corpus luteum, maintaining steroid hormone production and preventing involution of the corpus luteum. The corpus luteum is essential for the hormonal maintenance of the endometrium during the first 6–10 weeks of pregnancy until this function is taken over by the placenta.

CLINICAL ASSESSMENT OF OVARIAN FUNCTION

Menstrual bleeding should become regular within 2–4 years of menarche, although anovulatory and irregular cycles are common before that. For the remainder of adult reproductive life, the cycle length counted from the first day of menses to the first day of subsequent menses is ~28 days, with a range of 25–35 days. However, cycle-to-cycle variability for an individual woman is ±2 days. Luteal phase length is relatively constant between 12 and 14 days in normal cycles; thus, the major variability in cycle length is due to variations in the follicular phase. The duration of menstrual bleeding in ovulatory cycles varies between 4 and 6 days. There is a gradual shortening of cycle length with age such that women over the age of 35 have cycles that are shorter than during their younger reproductive years. Anovulatory cycles increase as women approach menopause, and bleeding patterns may be erratic.

Women who report regular monthly bleeding with cycles that do not vary by >4 days generally have ovulatory cycles, but several other clinical signs can be used to assess the likelihood of ovulation. Some women experience *mittelschmerz*, described as midcycle pelvic discomfort that is thought to be caused by the rapid expansion of the dominant follicle at the time of ovulation. A constellation of premenstrual moliminal symptoms such as bloating, breast tenderness, and food cravings often occur several days before menses in ovulatory cycles, but their absence cannot be used as evidence of anovulation. Methods that can be used to determine whether ovulation is likely include a serum progesterone level >5 ng/mL ~7 days before expected menses, an increase in basal body temperature of 0.24°C (>0.5°F) in the second half of the cycle due to the thermoregulatory effect of progesterone, or the detection of the urinary LH surge using ovulation predictor kits. Because ovulation occurs ~36 h after the LH surge, urinary LH can be helpful in timing intercourse to coincide with ovulation.

Ultrasound can be used to detect the growth of the fluid-filled antrum of the developing follicle and to assess endometrial proliferation in response to increasing estradiol levels in the follicular phase, as well as the characteristic echogenicity of the secretory endometrium of the luteal phase.

PUBERTY

NORMAL PUBERTAL DEVELOPMENT IN GIRLS

The first menstrual period (*menarche*) occurs relatively late in the series of developmental milestones that characterize normal pubertal development (Table 412-1). Menarche is preceded by the appearance of pubic and then axillary hair (*adrenarche*) as a result of maturation of the zona reticularis in the adrenal gland and increased adrenal androgen secretion, particularly dehydroepiandrosterone (DHEA). The triggers for adrenarche remain unknown but may involve increases in body mass index, as well as in utero and neonatal factors. Menarche is also preceded by breast development (*thelarche*). The breast is exquisitely sensitive to the very low levels of estrogen that result from peripheral conversion of adrenal androgens and the low levels of estrogen secreted from the ovary early in pubertal maturation. Breast development precedes the appearance of pubic and axillary hair in ~60% of girls. The interval between the onset of breast development and menarche is ~2 years. There has been a gradual decline in the age of menarche over the past century, attributed in large part to improvement in nutrition, and there is a relationship between adiposity and earlier sexual maturation in girls. In the United States, menarche occurs at an average age of 12.5 years (Table 412-1). Much of the variation in the timing of puberty is due to genetic factors, with heritability estimates of 50–80%. Both adrenarche and thelarche occur ~1 year earlier in black compared with white girls, although the timing of menarche differs by only 6 months between these ethnic groups.

Other important hormonal changes also occur in conjunction with puberty. Growth hormone (GH) levels increase early in puberty, stimulated in part by the pubertal increases in estrogen secretion. GH increases insulin-like growth factor-I (IGF-I), which enhances linear growth. The growth spurt is generally less pronounced in girls than in boys, with a peak growth velocity of ~7 cm/year. Linear growth is ultimately limited by closure of epiphyses in the long bones as a result of prolonged exposure to estrogen. Puberty is also associated with mild insulin resistance.

TABLE 412-1 MEAN AGE (YEARS) OF PUBERTAL MILESTONES IN GIRLS

	Onset of Breast/ Pubic Hair Development	Age of Peak Height Velocity	Menarche	Final Breast/ Pubic Hair Development	Adult Height
White	10.2	11.9	12.6	14.3	17.1
Black	9.6	11.5	12	13.6	16.5

Source: From FM Biro et al: J Pediatr 148:234, 2006.

TABLE 412-2 DIFFERENTIAL DIAGNOSIS OF PRECOCIOUS PUBERTY

Central (GnRH Dependent)	Peripheral (GnRH Independent)
Idiopathic	Congenital adrenal hyperplasia
CNS tumors	Estrogen-producing tumors
Hamartomas	Adrenal tumors
Astrocytomas	Ovarian tumors
Adenomyomas	Gonadotropin/hCG-producing tumors
Gliomas	Exogenous exposure to estrogen or androgen
Germinomas	McCune-Albright syndrome
CNS infection	Aromatase excess syndrome
Head trauma	
Iatrogenic	
Radiation	
Chemotherapy	
Surgical	
CNS malformation	
Arachnoid or suprasellar cysts	
Septo-optic dysplasia	
Hydrocephalus	

Abbreviations: CNS, central nervous system; GnRH, gonadotropin-releasing hormone; hCG, human chorionic gonadotropin.

TABLE 412-3 EVALUATION OF PRECOCIOUS AND DELAYED PUBERTY

	Precocious	Delayed
Initial Screening Tests		
History and physical	×	×
Assessment of growth velocity	×	×
Bone age	×	×
LH, FSH	×	×
Estradiol, testosterone	×	×
DHEAS	×	×
17-Hydroxyprogesterone	×	
TSH, T_4	×	×
Complete blood count		×
Sedimentation rate, C-reactive protein		×
Electrolytes, renal function		×
Liver enzymes		×
IGF-I, IGFBP-3		×
Urinalysis		×
Secondary Tests		
Pelvic ultrasound	×	×
Cranial MRI	×	×
β-hCG	×	
GnRH/agonist stimulation test	×	×
ACTH stimulation test	×	
Inflammatory bowel disease panel	×	×
Celiac disease panel		×
Prolactin		×
Karyotype		×

Abbreviations: ACTH, adrenocorticotropic hormone; DHEAS, dehydroepiandrosterone sulfate; FSH, follicle-stimulating hormone; hCG, human chorionic gonadotropin; IGF-I, insulin-like growth factor-I; IGFBP-3, IGF-binding protein 3; LH, luteinizing hormone; MRI, magnetic resonance imaging; TSH, thyroid-stimulating hormone; T_4, thyroxine.

DISORDERS OF PUBERTY

The differential diagnosis of precocious and delayed puberty is similar in boys (Chap. 411) and girls. However, there are differences in the timing of normal puberty and differences in the relative frequency of specific disorders in girls compared with boys.

Precocious Puberty Traditionally, precocious puberty has been defined as the development of secondary sexual characteristics before the age of 8 in girls based on data from Marshall and Tanner in British girls studied in the 1960s. More recent studies led to recommendations that girls be evaluated for precocious puberty if breast development or pubic hair is present at <7 years of age for white girls or <6 years for black girls.

Precocious puberty in girls is most often centrally mediated (Table 412-2), resulting from early activation of the hypothalamic-pituitary-ovarian axis. It is characterized by pulsatile LH secretion (which is initially associated with deep sleep) and an enhanced LH and FSH response to exogenous GnRH (two- to threefold stimulation) (Table 412-3). True precocity is marked by advancement in bone age of >2 standard deviations, a recent history of growth acceleration, and progression of secondary sexual characteristics. In girls, centrally mediated precocious puberty is idiopathic in ~85% of cases; however, neurogenic causes must be considered. Mutations in genes associated with GnRH deficiency have been reported in small numbers of patients with idiopathic precocious puberty (*KISS, KISS1R, TAC3, TAC3R*, and *DAX-1*), but their frequency is insufficient to warrant their use in clinical testing. GnRH agonists that induce pituitary desensitization are the mainstay of treatment to prevent premature epiphyseal closure and preserve adult height, as well as to manage psychosocial repercussions of precocious puberty.

Peripherally mediated precocious puberty does not involve activation of the hypothalamic-pituitary-ovarian axis and is characterized by suppressed gonadotropins in the presence of elevated estradiol. Management of peripheral precocious puberty involves treating the underlying disorder (Table 412-2) and limiting the effects of gonadal steroids using aromatase inhibitors, inhibitors of steroidogenesis, and ER blockers. It is important to be aware that central precocious puberty can also develop in girls whose precocity was initially peripherally mediated, as in McCune-Albright syndrome and congenital adrenal hyperplasia.

Incomplete and intermittent forms of precocious puberty may also occur. For example, premature breast development may occur in girls before the age of 2 years, with no further progression and without significant advancement in bone age, estrogen production, or compromised height. Premature adrenarche can also occur in the absence of progressive pubertal development, but it must be distinguished from late-onset congenital adrenal hyperplasia and androgen-secreting tumors, in which case it may be termed *heterosexual precocity*. Premature adrenarche may be associated with obesity, hyperinsulinemia, and the subsequent predisposition to PCOS.

Delayed Puberty Delayed puberty (Table 412-4) is defined as the absence of secondary sexual characteristics by age 13 in girls. The diagnostic considerations are very similar to those for primary amenorrhea (Chap. 69). Between 25 and 40% of delayed puberty in girls is of ovarian origin, with Turner's syndrome accounting for the majority of such patients. Functional hypogonadotropic hypogonadism encompasses diverse etiologies such as systemic illnesses, including celiac disease and chronic renal disease, and endocrinopathies such as diabetes and hypothyroidism. In addition, girls appear to be particularly susceptible to the adverse effects of decreased energy balance resulting from exercise, dieting, and/or eating disorders. Together these reversible conditions account for ~25% of delayed puberty in girls. Congenital hypogonadotropic hypogonadism in girls or boys can be caused by mutations in several different genes or combinations of genes (Fig. 412-4, Chap. 411, Table 411-2). Approximately 50% of girls with congenital hypogonadotropic hypogonadism, with or without anosmia, have a history of some degree of breast development, and 10% report one to two episodes of vaginal bleeding. Family studies suggest that genes identified in association with absent puberty may also cause delayed puberty, and recent reports have further suggested that a genetic susceptibility to environmental stresses such as diet and exercise may account for at least some cases of functional hypothalamic amenorrhea. Although neuroanatomic causes of delayed puberty are considerably less common in girls than in boys, it is always important to rule these out in the setting of hypogonadotropic hypogonadism.

TABLE 412-4 DIFFERENTIAL DIAGNOSIS OF DELAYED PUBERTY

Hypergonadotropic
Ovarian
Turner's syndrome
Gonadal dysgenesis
Chemotherapy/radiation therapy
Galactosemia
Autoimmune oophoritis
Congenital lipoid hyperplasia
Steroidogenic enzyme abnormalities
17α-Hydroxylase deficiency
Aromatase deficiency
Gonadotropin/receptor mutations
FSHβ, LHR, FSHR
Androgen resistance syndrome
Hypogonadotropic
Genetic
Hypothalamic syndromes
Leptin/leptin receptor
HESX1 (septo-optic dysplasia)
PC1 (prohormone convertase)
IHH and Kallmann's syndrome
KAL1, FGF8, FGFR1, NSMF, PROK2, PROKR2,
KISS1, KISS1R, TAC3, TAC3R, GnRH1, GnRHR, SEM3A, HS6ST1, WDR11, CHD7
Abnormalities of pituitary development/function
PROP1
CNS tumors/infiltrative disorders
Craniopharyngioma
Astrocytoma, germinoma, glioma
Prolactinomas, other pituitary tumors
Histiocytosis X
Chemotherapy/radiation
Functional
Chronic diseases
Malnutrition
Excessive exercise
Eating disorders

Abbreviations: *CHD7*, chromodomain-helicase-DNA-binding protein 7; CNS, central nervous system; *FGF8*, fibroblast growth factor 8; *FGFR1*, fibroblast growth factor 1 receptor; *FSHβ*, follicle-stimulating hormone β chain; *FSHR*, FSH receptor; *GNRHR*, gonadotropin-releasing hormone receptor; *HESX1*, homeobox, embryonic stem cell expressed 1; *HS6ST1*, heparin sulfate 6-O sulfotransferase 1; IHH, idiopathic hypogonadotropic hypogonadism; KAL, Kallmann; *KISS1*, kisspeptin 1; *KISSR1*, KISS1 receptor; *LHR*, luteinizing hormone receptor; *NSMF*, NMDA receptor synaptonuclear signaling and neuronal migration factor; *PROK2*, prokineticin 2; *PROKR2* prokineticin receptor 2; *PROP1*, prophet of Pit1, paired-like homeodomain transcription factor *SEMA3A*, semaphorin-3A; *WDR11*, WD repeat-containing protein 11.

413 Menopause and Postmenopausal Hormone Therapy

JoAnn E. Manson, Shari S. Bassuk

Menopause is the permanent cessation of menstruation due to loss of ovarian follicular function. It is diagnosed retrospectively after 12 months of amenorrhea. The average age at menopause is 51 years among U.S. women. *Perimenopause* refers to the time period preceding menopause, when fertility wanes and menstrual cycle irregularity increases, until the first year after cessation of menses. The onset of perimenopause precedes the final menses by 2–8 years, with a mean duration of 4 years. Smoking accelerates the menopausal transition by 2 years.

Although the peri- and postmenopausal transitions share many symptoms, the physiology and clinical management of the two differ. Low-dose oral contraceptives have become a therapeutic mainstay in perimenopause, whereas postmenopausal hormone therapy (HT) has been a common method of symptom alleviation after menstruation ceases.

PERIMENOPAUSE

PHYSIOLOGY

Ovarian mass and fertility decline sharply after age 35 and even more precipitously during perimenopause; depletion of primary follicles, a process that begins before birth, occurs steadily until menopause (Chap. 412). In perimenopause, intermenstrual intervals shorten significantly (typically by 3 days) as a result of an accelerated follicular phase. Follicle-stimulating hormone (FSH) levels rise because of altered folliculogenesis and reduced inhibin secretion. In contrast to the consistently high FSH and low estradiol levels seen in menopause, perimenopause is characterized by "irregularly irregular" hormone levels. The propensity for anovulatory cycles can produce a hyperestrogenic, hypoprogestagenic environment that may account for the increased incidence of endometrial hyperplasia or carcinoma, uterine polyps, and leiomyoma observed among women of perimenopausal age. Mean serum levels of selected ovarian and pituitary hormones during the menopausal transition are shown in Fig. 413-1. With transition into menopause, estradiol levels fall markedly, whereas estrone levels are relatively preserved, a pattern reflecting peripheral aromatization of adrenal and ovarian androgens. Levels of FSH increase more than those of luteinizing hormone, presumably because of the loss of inhibin as well as estrogen feedback.

DIAGNOSTIC TESTS

The Stages of Reproductive Aging Workshop +10 (STRAW+10) classification provides a comprehensive framework for the clinical assessment of ovarian aging. As shown in Fig. 413-2, menstrual cycle characteristics are the principal criteria for characterizing the menopausal transition, with biomarker measures as supportive criteria. Because of their extreme intraindividual variability, FSH and estradiol levels are imperfect diagnostic indicators of perimenopause in menstruating women. However, a consistently low FSH level in the early follicular phase (days 2–5) of the menstrual cycle does not support a diagnosis of perimenopause, while levels >25 IU/L in a random blood sample are characteristic of the late menopause transition. FSH measurement can also aid in assessing fertility; levels of <20 IU/L, 20 to <30 IU/L, and ≥30 IU/L measured on day 3 of the cycle indicate a good, fair, and poor likelihood of achieving pregnancy, respectively. Antimüllerian hormone and inhibin B may also be useful for assessing reproductive aging.

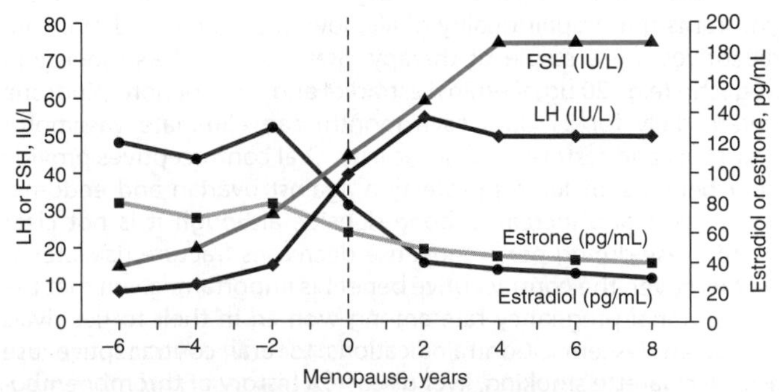

FIGURE 413-1 Mean serum levels of ovarian and pituitary hormones during the menopausal transition. FSH, follicle-stimulating hormone; LH, luteinizing hormone. *(From JL Shifren, I Schiff: J Womens Health Gend Based Med 9 Suppl 1:S3, 2000.)*

Stage	−5	−4	−3b	−3a	−2	−1	+1a	+1b	+1c	+2
Terminology	Reproductive				Menopausal transition		Postmenopause			
	Early	Peak	Late		Early	Late	Early			Late
					Perimenopause					
Duration	*Variable*				*Variable*	1–3 years	2 years (1+1)		3–6 years	*Remaining lifespan*
Principal criteria										
Menstrual cycle	Variable to regular	Regular	Regular	Subtle changes in flow/length	*Variable Length* Persistent ≥7-day difference in length of consecutive cycles	Interval of amenorrhea of ≥60 days				
Supportive criteria										
Endocrine										
FSH				Variable*	↑ Variable*	↑ >25 IU/L**	↑ Variable		Stabilizes	
AMH			Low	Low	Low	Low	Low		Very low	
Inhibin B			Low	Low	Low	Low	Low		Very low	
Antral follicle count			Low	Low	Low	Low	Very low		Very low	
Descriptive characteristics										
Symptoms						Vasomotor symptoms *Likely*	Vasomotor symptoms *Most likely*			*Increasing symptoms of urogenital atrophy*

*Blood draw on cycle days 2–5 ↑ = elevated.
**Approximate expected level based on assays using current international pituitary standard.

FIGURE 413-2 The Stages of Reproductive Aging Workshop +10 (STRAW +10) staging system for reproductive aging in women. AMH, antimüllerian hormone; FSH, follicle-stimulating hormone. *(From SD Harlow et al: Menopause 14:387, 2012. Reproduced with permission.)*

SYMPTOMS

Determining whether symptoms that develop in midlife are due to ovarian senescence or to other age-related changes is difficult. There is strong evidence that the menopausal transition can cause hot flashes, night sweats, irregular bleeding, and vaginal dryness, and there is moderate evidence that it can cause sleep disturbances in some women. There is inconclusive or insufficient evidence that ovarian aging is a major cause of mood swings, depression, impaired memory or concentration, somatic symptoms, urinary incontinence, or sexual dysfunction. In one U.S. study, nearly 60% of women reported hot flashes in the 2 years before their final menses. Symptom intensity, duration, frequency, and effects on quality of life are highly variable.

TREATMENT PERIMENOPAUSE

PERIMENOPAUSAL THERAPY

For women with irregular or heavy menses or hormone-related symptoms that impair quality of life, low-dose combined oral contraceptives are a staple of therapy. Static doses of estrogen and progestin (e.g., 20 μg of ethinyl estradiol and 1 mg of norethindrone acetate daily for 21 days each month) can eliminate vasomotor symptoms and restore regular cyclicity. Oral contraceptives provide other benefits, including protection against ovarian and endometrial cancers and increased bone density, although it is not clear whether use during perimenopause decreases fracture risk later in life. Moreover, the contraceptive benefit is important, given that the unintentional pregnancy rate among women in their forties rivals that of adolescents. Contraindications to oral contraceptive use include cigarette smoking, liver disease, a history of thromboembolism or cardiovascular disease, breast cancer, or unexplained vaginal bleeding. Progestin-only formulations (e.g., 0.35 mg of norethindrone daily) or medroxyprogesterone (Depo-Provera) injections (e.g., 150 mg IM every 3 months) may provide an alternative for the treatment of perimenopausal menorrhagia in women who smoke or have cardiovascular risk factors. Although progestins neither regularize cycles nor reduce the number of bleeding days, they reduce the volume of menstrual flow.

Nonhormonal strategies to reduce menstrual flow include the use of nonsteroidal anti-inflammatory agents such as mefenamic acid (an initial dose of 500 mg at the start of menses, then 250 mg qid for 2–3 days) or, when medical approaches fail, endometrial ablation. It should be noted that menorrhagia requires an evaluation to rule out uterine disorders. Transvaginal ultrasound with saline enhancement is useful for detecting leiomyomata or polyps, and endometrial aspiration can identify hyperplastic changes.

TRANSITION TO MENOPAUSE

For sexually active women using contraceptive hormones to alleviate perimenopausal symptoms, the question of when and if to switch to HT must be individualized. Doses of estrogen and progestogen (either synthetic progestins or natural forms of progesterone) in HT are lower than those in oral contraceptives and have not been documented to prevent pregnancy. Although a 1-year absence of spontaneous menses reliably indicates ovulation cessation, it is not possible to assess the natural menstrual pattern while a woman is taking an oral contraceptive. Women willing to switch to a barrier method of contraception should do so; if menses occur spontaneously, oral contraceptive use can be resumed. The average age of final menses among relatives can serve as a guide for when to initiate this process, which can be repeated yearly until menopause has occurred.

MENOPAUSE AND POSTMENOPAUSAL HORMONE THERAPY

One of the most complex health care decisions facing women is whether to use postmenopausal HT. Once prescribed primarily to relieve vasomotor symptoms, HT has been promoted as a strategy to forestall various disorders that accelerate after menopause, including osteoporosis and cardiovascular disease. In 2000, nearly 40% of postmenopausal women age 50–74 in the United States had used HT. This widespread use occurred despite the paucity of conclusive data, until recently, on the health consequences of such therapy. Although many women rely on their health care providers for a definitive answer to the question of whether to use postmenopausal hormones, balancing the benefits and risks for an individual patient is challenging.

Although observational studies suggest that HT prevents cardiovascular and other chronic diseases, the apparent benefits may result at least in part from differences between women who opt to take postmenopausal hormones and women who do not. Those choosing HT tend to be healthier, have greater access to medical care, are more compliant with prescribed treatments, and maintain a more health-promoting lifestyle. Randomized trials, which eliminate these confounding factors, have not consistently confirmed the benefits found in observational studies. Indeed, the largest HT trial to date, the Women's Health Initiative (WHI), which examined more than 27, 000 postmenopausal women age 50–79 (mean age, 63) for an average of 5–7 years, was stopped early because of an overall unfavorable benefit-risk ratio in the estrogen-progestin arm and an excess risk of stroke that was not offset by a reduced risk of coronary heart disease (CHD) in the estrogen-only arm.

The following summary offers a decision-making guide based on a synthesis of currently available evidence. Prevention of cardiovascular disease is eliminated from the equation due to lack of evidence for such benefits in recent randomized clinical trials.

BENEFITS AND RISKS OF POSTMENOPAUSAL HORMONE THERAPY

See Table 413-1.

Definite Benefits • ***SYMPTOMS OF MENOPAUSE*** Compelling evidence, including data from randomized clinical trials, indicates that estrogen therapy is highly effective for controlling vasomotor and genitourinary symptoms. Alternative approaches, including the use of antidepressants (such as paroxetine, 7.5 mg/d; or venlafaxine, 75–150 mg/d), gabapentin (300–900 mg/d), clonidine (0.1–0.2 mg/d), or vitamin E (400–800 IU/d), or the consumption of soy-based products or other phytoestrogens, may also alleviate vasomotor symptoms, although they are less effective than HT. Paroxetine is the only nonhormonal drug approved by the U.S. Food and Drug Administration for treatment of vasomotor symptoms. Bazedoxifene, an estrogen agonist/antagonist, in combination with conjugated estrogens has also received approval for vasomotor symptom management. For genitourinary symptoms, the efficacy of vaginal estrogen is similar to that of oral or transdermal estrogen; oral ospemifene is an additional option.

OSTEOPOROSIS (See also Chap. 425)

Bone density By reducing bone turnover and resorption rates, estrogen slows the aging-related bone loss experienced by most postmenopausal women. More than 50 randomized trials have demonstrated that postmenopausal estrogen therapy, with or without a progestogen, rapidly increases bone mineral density at the spine by 4–6% and at the hip by 2–3% and that those increases are maintained during treatment.

Fractures Data from observational studies indicate a 50–80% lower risk of vertebral fracture and a 25–30% lower risk of hip, wrist, and other peripheral fractures among current estrogen users; addition of a progestogen does not appear to modify this benefit. In the WHI, 5–7 years of either combined estrogen-progestin or estrogen-only therapy was associated with a 33% reduction in hip fractures and 25–30% fewer total fractures among a population unselected for osteoporosis. Bisphosphonates (such as alendronate, 10 mg/d or 70 mg once per week; risedronate, 5 mg/d or 35 mg once per week; or ibandronate, 2.5 mg/d or 150 mg once per month or 3 mg every 3 months IV) and raloxifene (60 mg/d), a selective estrogen receptor modulator (SERM), have been shown in randomized trials to increase bone mass density and decrease fracture rates. Other options for treatment of osteoporosis are bazedoxifene in combination with conjugated estrogens and parathyroid hormone (teriparatide, 20 μg/d SC). These agents, unlike estrogen, do not appear to have adverse effects on the endometrium or breast. Increased physical activity, adequate calcium intake (1000–1200 mg/d through diet or supplements in two or three divided doses), and adequate vitamin D intake (600–1000 IU/d) may also reduce the risk of osteoporosis-related fractures. According to the Institute of Medicine's 2011 report, 25-hydroxyvitamin D blood levels of ≥50 nmol/L are sufficient for bone-density maintenance and fracture prevention. The Fracture Risk Assessment (FRAX®) score, an algorithm that combines an individual's bone-density score with age and other risk factors to predict her 10-year risk of hip and major osteoporotic fracture, may be of use in guiding decisions about pharmacologic treatment (see *www.shef.ac.uk/FRAX/*).

Definite Risks • ***ENDOMETRIAL CANCER (WITH ESTROGEN ALONE)*** A combined analysis of 30 observational studies found a tripling of endometrial cancer risk among short-term users (1–5 years) of unopposed estrogen and a nearly tenfold increased risk among long-term users (≥10 years). These findings are supported by results from the randomized Postmenopausal Estrogen/Progestin Interventions (PEPI) trial, in which 24% of women assigned to unopposed estrogen for 3 years developed atypical endometrial hyperplasia—a premalignant lesion—as opposed to only 1% of women assigned to placebo. Use of a progestogen, which opposes the effects of estrogen on the endometrium, eliminates these risks and may even reduce risk (see later).

VENOUS THROMBOEMBOLISM A meta-analysis of observational studies found that current oral estrogen use was associated with a 2.5-fold increase in risk of venous thromboembolism in postmenopausal women. A meta-analysis of randomized trials, including the WHI, found a 2.1-fold increase in risk. Results from the WHI indicate a nearly twofold increase in risk of pulmonary embolism and deep vein thrombosis with estrogen-progestin and a 35–50% increase in these risks with estrogen-only therapy. Transdermal estrogen, taken alone or with certain progestogens (micronized progesterone or pregnane derivatives), appears to be a safer alternative with respect to thrombotic risk.

BREAST CANCER (WITH ESTROGEN-PROGESTIN) An increased risk of breast cancer has been found among current or recent estrogen users in observational studies; this risk is directly related to duration of use. In a meta-analysis of 51 case-control and cohort studies, short-term use (<5 years) of postmenopausal HT did not appreciably elevate breast cancer incidence, whereas long-term use (≥5 years) was associated with a 35% increase in risk. In contrast to findings for endometrial cancer, combined estrogen-progestin regimens appear to increase breast cancer risk more than estrogen alone. Data from randomized trials also indicate that estrogen-progestin raises breast cancer risk. In the WHI, women assigned to receive combination hormones for an average of 5.6 years were 24% more likely to develop breast cancer than women assigned to placebo, but 7.1 years of estrogen-only therapy did not increase risk. Indeed, the WHI showed a trend toward a reduction in breast cancer risk with estrogen alone, although it is unclear whether this finding would pertain to formulations of estrogen other than conjugated equine estrogens or to treatment durations of >7 years. In the Heart and Estrogen/Progestin Replacement Study (HERS), 4 years of combination therapy was associated with a 27% increase in breast cancer risk. Although the latter finding was not statistically significant, the totality of evidence strongly implicates estrogen-progestin therapy in breast carcinogenesis.

Some observational data suggest that the length of the interval between menopause onset and HT initiation may influence the association between such therapy and breast cancer risk, with a "gap time" of <3–5 years conferring a higher HT-associated breast cancer risk. (This pattern of findings contrasts with that for CHD, as discussed later in this Chapter.) However, this association remains inconclusive and may be a spurious finding attributable to higher rates of screening mammography and thus earlier cancer detection in HT users than in nonusers, especially in early menopause. Indeed, in the WHI trial, hazard ratios for HT and breast cancer risk did not differ among women

TABLE 413-1 BENEFITS AND RISKS OF POSTMENOPAUSAL HORMONE THERAPY IN THE OVERALL STUDY POPULATION OF WOMEN 50–79 YEARS OF AGE IN THE INTERVENTION PHASE OF THE WOMEN'S HEALTH INITIATIVE (WHI) ESTROGEN-PROGESTIN AND ESTROGEN-ALONE TRIALS[a]

		Estrogen-Progestin		Estrogen Alone	
Outcome	**Effect**	**Relative Benefit or Risk**	**Absolute Benefit or Risk[b]**	**Relative Benefit or Risk**	**Absolute Benefit or Risk[b]**
Definite Benefits					
Symptoms of menopause	Definite improvement	↓65–90% decreased risk[c]		↓65–90% decreased risk[c]	
Osteoporosis	Definite increase in bone mineral density and decrease in fracture risk	↓33% decreased risk for hip fracture	6 fewer cases (11 vs. 17) of hip fracture	↓33% decreased risk for hip fracture	6 fewer cases (13 vs. 19) of hip fracture
Definite Risks[h]					
Endometrial cancer	Definite increase in risk with estrogen alone (see below for estrogen-progestin)	See below	See below		4.6 excess cases (observational studies)
Pulmonary embolism	Definite increase in risk	↑98% increased risk	9 excess cases (18 vs. 9)	↑35% increased risk (n.s.)	4 excess cases (14 vs. 10)
Deep vein thrombosis	Definite increase in risk	↑87% increased risk	11.5 excess cases (25 vs. 14)	↑48% increased risk	7.5 excess cases (23 vs. 15)
Breast cancer	Definite increase in risk with long-term use (≥5 years) of estrogen-progestin	↑24% increased risk	8.5 excess cases (43 vs. 35)	↓21% decreased risk (n.s.)	7 fewer cases (28 vs. 35)
Gallbladder disease	Definite increase in risk	↑57% increased risk	47 excess cases (131 vs. 84)	↑55% increased risk	58 excess cases (164 vs. 106)
Probable or Uncertain Risks and Benefits[h]					
Coronary heart disease[d]	Probable increase in risk among older women and women many years past menopause; possible decrease in risk or no effect in younger or recently menopausal women[e]	↑18% increased risk (n.s.)	6 excess cases (41 vs. 35)	No increase in risk	No difference in risk
Myocardial infarction	Significant interaction by age group for estrogen alone, with reduced risk in younger—but not older—women (p for trend by age = .02)	↑24% increased risk (n.s.)	6 excess cases (35 vs. 29)	No increase in risk[e]	No difference in risk[e]
Stroke	Probable increase in risk	↑37% increased risk	9 excess cases (33 vs. 24)	↑35% increased risk	11 excess cases (45 vs. 34)
Ovarian cancer	Probable increase in risk with long-term use (≥5 years)	↑41% increased risk (n.s.)	1 excess cases (5 vs. 4)	Not available	Not available
Endometrial cancer	Probable decrease in risk with estrogen-progestin during long-term follow-up (see above for estrogen alone)	↓33% decreased risk[f]	3 fewer cases (7 vs. 10)	See above	See above
Urinary incontinence	Probable increase in risk	↑49% increased risk	549 excess cases (1661 vs. 1112)	↑61% increased risk	852 excess cases (2255 vs. 1403)
Colorectal cancer	Probable decrease in risk with estrogen-progestin; possible increase in risk in older women with estrogen alone (p for trend by age = .02 for estrogen alone)	↓38% decreased risk	6.5 fewer cases (10 vs. 17)	No increase or decrease in risk[e]	No difference in risk[e]
Type 2 diabetes	Probable decrease in risk	↓19% decreased risk	16 fewer cases (72 vs. 88)	↓14% decreased risk	21 fewer cases (134 vs. 155)
Dementia (age ≥65)	Increase in risk in older women (but inconsistent data from observational studies and randomized trials)	↑101% increased risk	23 excess cases (46 vs. 23)	↑47% increased risk (n.s.)	15 excess cases (44 vs. 29)
Total mortality	Possible increase in risk among older women and women many years past menopause; possible decrease in risk or no effect in younger or recently menopausal women (p for trend by age <.05 for both trials combined)	No increase in risk	No difference in risk	No increase in risk[e]	No difference in risk[e]
Global index[g]	Probable increase in risk or no effect among older women and women many years past menopause; possible decrease in risk or no effect in younger or recently menopausal women (p for trend by age = 0.02 for estrogen alone)	↑12% increased risk	20.5 excess cases (189 vs. 168)	No increase in risk[e]	No difference in risk[e]

[a]The estrogen-progestin arm of the WHI assessed 5.6 years of conjugated equine estrogen (0.625 mg/d) plus medroxyprogesterone acetate (2.5 mg/d) versus placebo. The estrogen-alone arm of the WHI assessed 7.1 years of conjugated equine estrogen (0.625 mg/d) versus placebo. [b]Number of cases per 10, 000 women per year. [c]The WHI was not designed to assess the effect of HT on menopausal symptoms. Data from other randomized trials suggest that HT reduces risk for menopausal symptoms by 65–90%. [d]*Coronary heart disease* is defined as nonfatal myocardial infarction or coronary death. [e]There was a significant interaction by age; that is, the association between HT and the specified outcome was different in younger women and older women. [f]This is the risk reduction that was observed during a cumulative 12-year follow-up period (5.6 years of treatment plus 6.8 years of postintervention observation). [g]The *global index* is a composite outcome representing the first event for each participant from among the following: coronary heart disease, stroke, pulmonary embolism, breast cancer, colorectal cancer, endometrial cancer (estrogen-progestin arm only), hip fracture, and death. Because participants can experience more than one type of event, the global index cannot be derived by a simple summing of the component events. [h]Includes some outcomes where results were divergent between the estrogen-progestin arm and the estrogen-alone arm.

Abbreviation: n.s., not statistically significant.

Source: Data from JE Manson et al: JAMA 310:1353, 2013.

50–59, those 60–69, and those 70–79 years of age at trial entry. (There was insufficient power to examine finer age categories.) Additional research is needed to clarify the issue.

GALLBLADDER DISEASE Large observational studies report a two- to threefold increased risk of gallstones or cholecystectomy among postmenopausal women taking oral estrogen. In the WHI, women randomized to estrogen-progestin or estrogen alone were ~55% more likely to develop gallbladder disease than those assigned to placebo. Risks were also increased in HERS. Transdermal HT might be a safer alternative, but further research is needed.

Probable or Uncertain Risks and Benefits • ***CORONARY HEART DISEASE/STROKE*** Until recently, HT had been enthusiastically recommended as a possible cardioprotective agent. In the past three decades, multiple observational studies suggested, in the aggregate, that estrogen use leads to a 35–50% reduction in CHD incidence among postmenopausal women. The biologic plausibility of such an association is supported by data from randomized trials demonstrating that exogenous estrogen lowers plasma low-density lipoprotein (LDL) cholesterol levels and raises high-density lipoprotein (HDL) cholesterol levels by 10–15%. Administration of estrogen also favorably affects lipoprotein(a) levels, LDL oxidation, endothelial vascular function, fibrinogen, and plasminogen activator inhibitor 1. However, estrogen therapy has unfavorable effects on other biomarkers of cardiovascular risk: it boosts triglyceride levels; promotes coagulation via factor VII, prothrombin fragments 1 and 2, and fibrinopeptide A elevations; and raises levels of the inflammatory marker C-reactive protein.

Randomized trials of estrogen or combined estrogen-progestin in women with preexisting cardiovascular disease have not confirmed the benefits reported in observational studies. In HERS (a secondary-prevention trial designed to test the efficacy and safety of estrogen-progestin therapy with regard to clinical cardiovascular outcomes), the 4-year incidence of coronary death and nonfatal myocardial infarction was similar in the active-treatment and placebo groups, and a 50% increase in risk of coronary events was noted during the first year among participants assigned to the active-treatment group. Although it is possible that progestin may mitigate estrogen's benefits, the Estrogen Replacement and Atherosclerosis (ERA) trial indicated that angiographically determined progression of coronary atherosclerosis was unaffected by either opposed or unopposed estrogen treatment. Moreover, no cardiovascular benefit was found in the Papworth Hormone Replacement Therapy Atherosclerosis Study, a trial of transdermal estradiol with and without norethindrone; the Women's Estrogen for Stroke Trial (WEST), a trial of oral 17β-estradiol; or the Estrogen in the Prevention of Reinfarction Trial (ESPRIT), a trial of oral estradiol valerate. Thus, in clinical trials, HT has not proved effective for the secondary prevention of cardiovascular disease in postmenopausal women.

Primary-prevention trials also suggest an early increase in cardiovascular risk and an absence of cardioprotection with postmenopausal HT. In the WHI, women assigned to 5.6 years of estrogen-progestin therapy were 18% more likely to develop CHD (defined in primary analyses as nonfatal myocardial infarction or coronary death) than those assigned to placebo, although this risk elevation was not statistically significant. However, during the trial's first year, there was a significant 80% increase in risk, which diminished in subsequent years (p for trend by time = .03). In the estrogen-only arm of the WHI, no overall effect on CHD was observed during the 7.1 years of the trial or in any specific year of follow-up. This pattern of results was similar to that for the outcome of total myocardial infarction.

However, a closer look at available data suggests that timing of initiation of HT may critically influence the association between such therapy and CHD. Estrogen may slow early stages of atherosclerosis but have adverse effects on advanced atherosclerotic lesions. It has been hypothesized that the prothrombotic and proinflammatory effects of estrogen manifest themselves predominantly among women with subclinical lesions who initiate HT well after the menopausal transition, whereas women with less arterial damage who start HT early in menopause may derive cardiovascular benefit because they have not yet developed advanced lesions. Nonhuman primate data support this concept. Conjugated estrogens had no effect on the extent of coronary artery plaque in cynomolgus monkeys assigned to receive estrogen alone or combined with progestin starting 2 years (~6 years in human terms) after oophorectomy and well after the establishment of atherosclerosis. However, administration of exogenous hormones immediately after oophorectomy, during the early stages of atherosclerosis, reduced the extent of plaque by 70%.

Lending further credence to this hypothesis are results of subgroup analyses of observational and clinical trial data. For example, among women who entered the WHI trial with a relatively favorable cholesterol profile, estrogen with or without progestin led to a 40% lower risk of incident CHD. Among women who entered with a worse cholesterol profile, therapy resulted in a 73% higher risk (p for interaction = .02). The presence or absence of the metabolic syndrome (Chap. 422) also strongly influenced the relation between HT and incident CHD. Among women with the metabolic syndrome, HT more than doubled CHD risk, whereas no association was observed among women without the syndrome. Moreover, although there was no association between estrogen-only therapy and CHD in the WHI trial cohort as a whole, such therapy was associated with a CHD risk reduction of 40% among participants age 50–59; in contrast, a risk reduction of only 5% was observed among those age 60–69, and a risk increase of 9% was found among those age 70–79 (p for trend by age = .08). For the outcome of total myocardial infarction, estrogen alone was associated with a borderline-significant 45% reduction and a nonsignificant 24% increase in risk among the youngest and oldest women, respectively (p for trend by age = .02). Estrogen was also associated with lower levels of coronary artery calcified plaque in the younger age group. Although age did not have a similar effect in the estrogen-progestin arm of the WHI, CHD risks increased with years since menopause (p for trend = .08), with a significantly elevated risk among women who were ≥20 years past menopause. For the outcome of total myocardial infarction, estrogen-progestin was associated with a 9% risk reduction among women <10 years past menopause as opposed to a 16% increase in risk among women 10–19 years past menopause and a twofold increase in risk among women >20 years past menopause (p for trend = .01). In the large observational Nurses' Health Study, women who chose to start HT within 4 years of menopause experienced a lower risk of CHD than did nonusers, whereas those who began therapy ≥10 years after menopause appeared to receive little coronary benefit. Observational studies include a high proportion of women who begin HT within 3–4 years of menopause, whereas clinical trials include a high proportion of women ≥12 years past menopause; this difference helps to reconcile some of the apparent discrepancies between the two types of studies.

For the outcome of stroke, WHI participants assigned to estrogen-progestin or estrogen alone were ~35% more likely to suffer a stroke than those assigned to placebo. Whether or not age at initiation of HT influences stroke risk is not well understood. In the WHI and the Nurses' Health Study, HT was associated with an excess risk of stroke in all age groups. Further research is needed on age, time since menopause, and other individual characteristics (including biomarkers) that predict increases or decreases in cardiovascular risk associated with exogenous HT. Furthermore, it remains uncertain whether different doses, formulations, or routes of administration of HT will produce different cardiovascular effects.

COLORECTAL CANCER Observational studies have suggested that HT reduces risks of colon and rectal cancer, although the estimated magnitudes of the relative benefits have ranged from 8% to 34% in various meta-analyses. In the WHI (the sole trial to examine the issue), estrogen-progestin was associated with a significant 38% reduction in colorectal cancer over a 5.6-year period, although no benefit was seen with 7 years of estrogen-only therapy. However, a modifying effect of age was observed, with a doubling of risk with HT in women age 70–79 but no risk elevation in younger women (p for trend by age = .02).

COGNITIVE DECLINE AND DEMENTIA A meta-analysis of 10 case-control and two cohort studies suggested that postmenopausal HT is associated with a 34% decreased risk of dementia. Subsequent randomized trials (including the WHI), however, have failed to demonstrate any benefit of estrogen or estrogen-progestin therapy on the progression of mild to moderate Alzheimer's disease and/or have indicated a potential adverse effect of HT on the incidence of dementia, at least in women ≥65 years of age. Among women randomized to HT (as opposed to placebo) at age 50–55 in the WHI, no effect on cognition was observed during the postintervention phase. Determining whether timing of initiation of HT influences cognitive outcomes will require further study.

OVARIAN CANCER AND OTHER DISORDERS On the basis of limited observational and randomized data, it has been hypothesized that HT increases the risk of ovarian cancer and reduces the risk of type 2 diabetes mellitus. Results from the WHI support these hypotheses. The WHI also found that HT use was associated with an increased risk of urinary incontinence and that estrogen-progestin was associated with increased rates of lung cancer mortality.

ENDOMETRIAL CANCER (WITH ESTROGEN-PROGESTIN) In the WHI, use of estrogen-progestin was associated with a nonsignificant 17% reduction in risk of endometrial cancer. A significant reduction in risk emerged during the postintervention period (see later).

ALL-CAUSE MORTALITY In the overall WHI cohort, estrogen with or without progestin was not associated with all-cause mortality. However, there was a trend toward reduced mortality in younger women, particularly with estrogen alone. For women 50–59, 60–69, and 70–79 years of age, relative risks (RRs) associated with estrogen-only therapy were 0.70, 1.01, and 1.21, respectively (p for trend = .04).

OVERALL BENEFIT-RISK PROFILE Estrogen-progestin was associated with an unfavorable benefit-risk profile (excluding relief from menopausal symptoms) as measured by a "global index"—a composite outcome including CHD, stroke, pulmonary embolism, breast cancer, colorectal cancer, endometrial cancer, hip fracture, and death (Table 413-1)—in the WHI cohort as a whole, and this association did not vary by 10-year age group. Estrogen-only therapy was associated with a neutral benefit-risk profile in the WHI cohort as a whole. However, there was a significant trend toward a more favorable benefit-risk profile among younger women and a less favorable profile among older women, with RRs of 0.84, 0.99, and 1.17 for women 50–59, 60–69, and 70–79 years of age, respectively (p for trend by age = .02).

CHANGES IN HEALTH STATUS AFTER DISCONTINUATION OF HORMONE THERAPY In the WHI, many but not all risks and benefits associated with active use of HT dissipated within 5–7 years after discontinuation of therapy. For estrogen-progestin, an elevated risk of breast cancer persisted (RR = 1.28 [95% confidence interval, 1.11–1.48]) during a cumulative 12-year follow-up period (5.6 years of treatment plus 6.8 years of postintervention observation), but most cardiovascular disease risks became neutral. A reduction in hip fracture risk persisted (RR = 0.81 [0.68–0.97]), and a significant reduction in endometrial cancer risk emerged (RR = 0.67 [0.49–0.91]). For estrogen alone, the reduction in breast cancer risk became statistically significant (RR = 0.79 [0.65–0.97]) during a cumulative 12-year follow-up period (6.8 years of treatment plus 5.1 years of postintervention observation), and significant differences by age group persisted for total myocardial infarction and the global index, with more favorable results for younger women.

APPROACH TO THE PATIENT: Postmenopausal Hormone Therapy

The rational use of postmenopausal HT requires balancing the potential benefits and risks. Figure 413-3 provides one approach to decision making. The clinician should first determine whether the patient has moderate to severe menopausal symptoms—the primary indication for initiation of systemic HT. Systemic HT may also be used to prevent osteoporosis in women at high risk of fracture who cannot tolerate alternative osteoporosis therapies. (Vaginal estrogen or other medications may be used to treat urogenital symptoms in the absence of vasomotor symptoms.) The benefits and risks of such therapy should be reviewed with the patient, giving more emphasis to absolute than to relative measures of effect and pointing out uncertainties in clinical knowledge where relevant. Because chronic disease rates generally increase with age, absolute risks tend to be greater in older women, even when relative risks remain similar. Potential side effects—especially vaginal bleeding that may result from use of the combined estrogen-progestogen formulations recommended for women with an intact uterus—should be noted. The patient's own preference regarding therapy should be elicited and factored into the decision. Contraindications to HT should be assessed routinely and include unexplained vaginal bleeding, active liver disease, venous thromboembolism, history of endometrial cancer (except stage 1 without deep invasion) or breast cancer, and history of CHD, stroke, transient ischemic attack, or diabetes. Relative contraindications include hypertriglyceridemia (>400 mg/dL) and active gallbladder disease; in such cases, transdermal estrogen may be an option. Primary prevention of heart disease should not be viewed as an expected benefit of HT, and an increase in the risk of stroke as well as a small early increase in the risk of coronary artery disease should be considered. Nevertheless, such therapy may be appropriate if the noncoronary benefits of treatment clearly outweigh the risks. A woman who suffers an acute coronary event or stroke while taking HT should discontinue therapy immediately.

Short-term use (<5 years for estrogen-progestogen and <7 years for estrogen alone) is appropriate for relief of menopausal symptoms among women without contraindications to such use. However, such therapy should be avoided by women with an elevated baseline risk of future cardiovascular events. Women who have contraindications for or are opposed to HT may derive benefit from the use of certain antidepressants (including venlafaxine, fluoxetine, or paroxetine), gabapentin, clonidine, soy, or black cohosh and, for genitourinary symptoms, intravaginal estrogen creams or devices, or ospemifene.

Long-term use (≥5 years for estrogen-progestogen and ≥7 years for estrogen alone) is more problematic because a heightened risk of breast cancer must be factored into the decision, especially for estrogen-progestogen. Reasonable candidates for such use include the small percentage of postmenopausal women who have persistent severe vasomotor symptoms along with an increased risk of osteoporosis (e.g., those with osteopenia, a personal or family history of nontraumatic fracture, or a weight below 125 lbs), who also have no personal or family history of breast cancer in a first-degree relative or other contraindications, and who have a strong personal preference for therapy. Poor candidates are women with elevated cardiovascular risk, those at increased risk of breast cancer (e.g., women who have a first-degree relative with breast cancer, susceptibility genes such as *BRCA1* or *BRCA2*, or a personal history of cellular atypia detected by breast biopsy), and those at low risk of osteoporosis. Even for reasonable candidates, strategies to minimize dose and duration of use should be employed. For example, women using HT to relieve intense vasomotor symptoms in early postmenopause should consider discontinuing therapy within 5 years, resuming it only if such symptoms persist. Because of the role of progestogens in increasing breast cancer risk, regimens that employ cyclic rather than continuous progestogen exposure as well as formulations other than medroxyprogesterone acetate should be considered if treatment is extended. For prevention of osteoporosis, alternative therapies such as bisphosphonates or SERMs should be considered. Research on alternative progestogens and androgen-containing preparations has been limited, particularly with respect to long-term safety. Additional research on the effects of these agents on cardiovascular disease, glucose tolerance, and breast cancer will be of particular interest.

In addition to HT, lifestyle choices such as smoking abstention, adequate physical activity, and a healthy diet can play a role in controlling symptoms and preventing chronic disease. An expanding array of pharmacologic options (e.g., bisphosphonates, SERMs, and other agents for osteoporosis; cholesterol-lowering or antihypertensive agents for cardiovascular disease) should also reduce the widespread reliance on hormone use. However, short-term HT may still benefit some women.

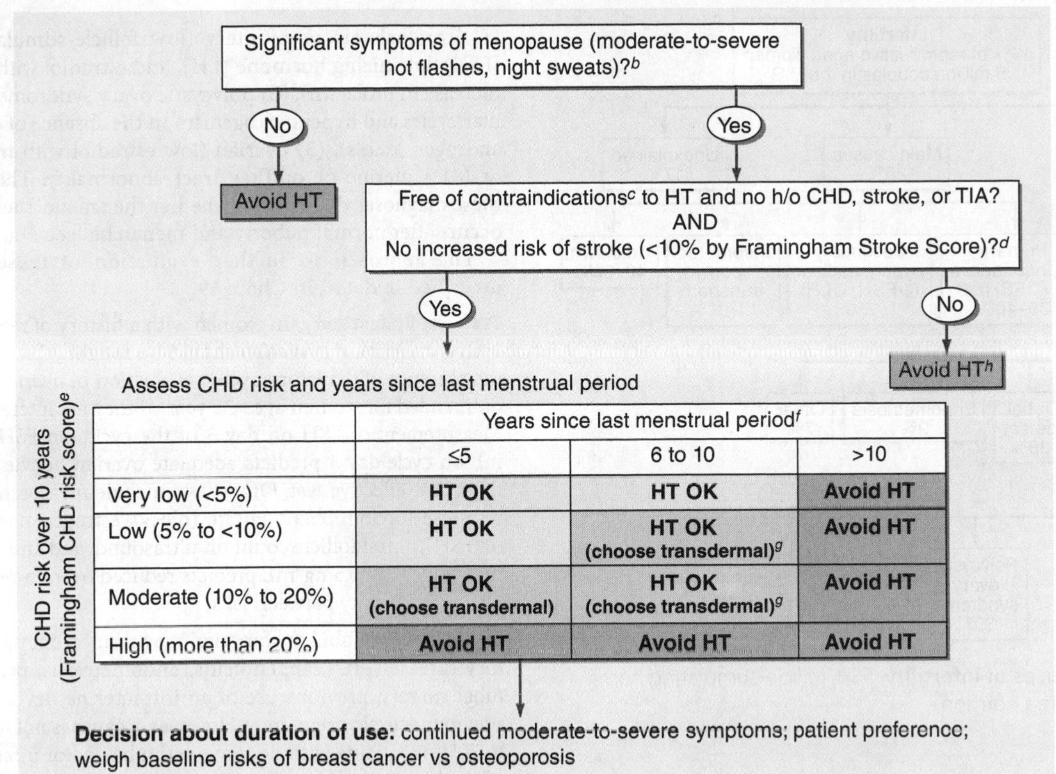

FIGURE 413-3 Chart for identifying appropriate candidates for postmenopausal hormone therapy (HT).[a]
[a]Reassess each step at least once every 6–12 months (assuming the patient's continued preference for HT). [b]Women who are at high risk of osteoporotic fracture but are unable to tolerate alternative preventive medications may also be reasonable candidates for systemic HT even if they do not have moderate to severe vasomotor symptoms. Women who have vaginal dryness without moderate to severe vasomotor symptoms may be candidates for vaginal estrogen. [c]Traditional contraindications are unexplained vaginal bleeding; active liver disease; history of venous thromboembolism due to pregnancy, oral contraceptive use, or an unknown etiology; blood-clotting disorder; history of breast or endometrial cancer; and diabetes. Oral HT should be avoided but transdermal HT may be an option (see *g* below) for other contraindications, including high triglyceride levels (>400 mg/dL); active gallbladder disease; and history of venous thromboembolism due to past immobility, surgery, or bone fracture. [d]Ten-year risk of stroke, based on Framingham Stroke Risk Score (RB D'Agostino et al: Stroke risk profile: Adjustment for antihypertensive medication. The Framingham Study. Stroke 25:40, 1994), as modified by JE Manson, SS Bassuk: *Hot Flashes, Hormones & Your Health*. New York, McGraw-Hill, 2007. [e]Ten-year risk of CHD, based on Framingham Coronary Heart Disease Risk Score (Expert Panel on Detection, Evaluation, and Treatment of High Blood Cholesterol in Adults: JAMA 285:2486, 2001), as modified by JE Manson, SS Bassuk: Hot Flashes, Hormones & Your Health. New York, McGraw-Hill, 2007. [f]Women >10 years past menopause are not good candidates for initiation (first use) of HT. [g]Avoid oral HT. Transdermal HT may be an option because it has a less adverse effect on clotting factors, triglyceride levels, and inflammation factors than oral HT. [h]Consider selective serotonin or serotonin–norepinephrine reuptake inhibitor, gabapentin, clonidine, soy, or another alternative.
Abbreviations: CHD, coronary heart disease; h/o, history of; TIA, transient ischemic attack. *(Adapted from JE Manson, SS Bassuk: Hot Flashes, Hormones & Your Health. New York, McGraw-Hill, 2007.*

414 Infertility and Contraception

Janet E. Hall

INFERTILITY

DEFINITION AND PREVALENCE

Infertility has traditionally been defined as the inability to conceive after 12 months of unprotected sexual intercourse. In women who ultimately conceived, pregnancy occurred in ~50% within 3 months, 75–82% within 6 months, and 85–92% within 12 months. The World Health Organization (WHO) considers infertility as a disability (an impairment of function) and thus access to health care falls under the Convention on the Rights of Persons with Disability. Thirty-four million women, predominantly from developing countries, have infertility resulting from maternal sepsis and unsafe abortion. In populations <60 years old, infertility is ranked the fifth highest serious global disability. In the United States, the rate of infertility in married women age 15–44 is 6% based on the National Survey of Family Growth, although prospective studies suggest that it may be as high as 12–15%. The infertility rate has remained relatively stable over the past 30 years in most countries. However, the proportion of couples without children has risen, reflecting both higher numbers of couples in childbearing years and a trend to delay childbearing. This trend has important implications because of an age-related decrease in fecundability: the incidence of primary infertility increases from ~8% between the ages of 18 and 38 to 25% and 30% between the ages of 35 and 39 and 40 and 44, respectively. It is estimated that 14% of couples in the United States have received medical assistance for infertility; of these, two-thirds received counseling, ~12% underwent infertility testing of the female and/or male partner, and 17% received drugs to induce ovulation.

CAUSES OF INFERTILITY

The spectrum of infertility ranges from reduced conception rates or the need for medical intervention to irreversible causes of infertility. Infertility can be attributed primarily to male factors in 25% of couples and female factors in 58% of couples and is unexplained in about 17% of couples (Fig. 414-1). Not uncommonly, both male and female factors contribute to infertility. Decreases in the ability to conceive as a

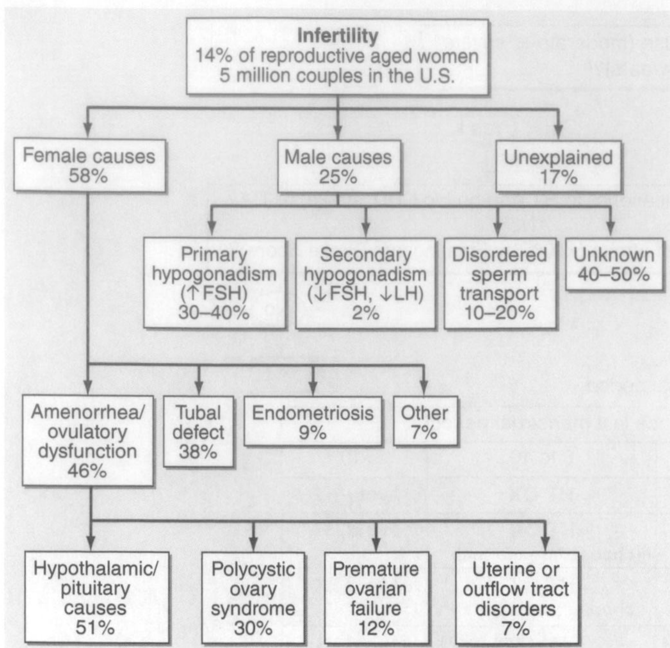

FIGURE 414-1 Causes of infertility. FSH, follicle-stimulating hormone; LH, luteinizing hormone.

function of age in women has led to recommendations that women >34 years old who are not at increased risk of infertility seek attention after 6 months, rather than 12 months as suggested for younger women, and receive an expedited work-up and approach to treatment.

APPROACH TO THE PATIENT: Infertility

INITIAL EVALUATION

In all couples presenting with infertility, the initial evaluation includes discussion of the appropriate timing of intercourse and discussion of modifiable risk factors such as smoking, alcohol, caffeine, and obesity. The range of required investigations should be reviewed as well as a brief description of infertility treatment options, including adoption. Initial investigations are focused on determining whether the primary cause of the infertility is male, female, or both. These investigations include a semen analysis in the male, confirmation of ovulation in the female, and, in the majority of situations, documentation of tubal patency in the female. In some cases, after an extensive workup excluding all male and female factors, a specific cause cannot be identified, and infertility may ultimately be classified as unexplained.

PSYCHOLOGICAL ASPECTS OF INFERTILITY

Infertility is invariably associated with psychological stress related not only to the diagnostic and therapeutic procedures themselves but also to repeated cycles of hope and loss associated with each new procedure or cycle of treatment that does not result in the birth of a child. These feelings are often combined with a sense of isolation from friends and family. Counseling and stress-management techniques should be introduced early in the evaluation of infertility. Importantly, infertility and its treatment do not appear to be associated with long-term psychological sequelae.

FEMALE CAUSES

Abnormalities in menstrual function constitute the most common cause of female infertility. These disorders, which include ovulatory dysfunction and abnormalities of the uterus or outflow tract, may present as amenorrhea or as irregular or short menstrual cycles. A careful history and physical examination and a limited number of laboratory tests will help to determine whether the abnormality is (1) hypothalamic or pituitary (low follicle-stimulating hormone [FSH], luteinizing hormone [LH], and estradiol with or without an increase in prolactin), (2) polycystic ovary syndrome (PCOS; irregular cycles and hyperandrogenism in the absence of other causes of androgen excess), (3) ovarian (low estradiol with increased FSH), or (4) a uterine or outflow tract abnormality. The frequency of these diagnoses depends on whether the amenorrhea is primary or occurs after normal puberty and menarche (see Fig. 69-2).

The approach to further evaluation of these disorders is described in detail in Chap. 69.

Ovulatory Dysfunction In women with a history of regular menstrual cycles, *evidence of ovulation* should be sought (Chap. 412). Even in the presence of ovulatory cycles, evaluation of *ovarian reserve* is recommended for women age >35 years if they are interested in fertility. Measurement of FSH on day 3 of the cycle (an FSH level <10 IU/mL on cycle day 3 predicts adequate ovarian oocyte reserve) is the most cost-effective test. Other tests include measurement of FSH in response to clomiphene citrate (blocks estrogen negative feedback on FSH), antral follicle count on ultrasound, and anti-müllerian hormone (AMH; <0.5 ng/mL predicts reduced ovarian reserve although there is variability between labs).

Tubal Disease Tubal dysfunction may result from pelvic inflammatory disease (PID), appendicitis, endometriosis, pelvic adhesions, tubal surgery, previous use of an intrauterine device (IUD), and a previous ectopic pregnancy. However, a cause is not identified in up to 50% of patients with documented tubal factor infertility. Because of the high prevalence of tubal disease, evaluation of tubal patency by hysterosalpingogram (HSG) or laparoscopy should occur early in the majority of couples with infertility. Subclinical infections with *Chlamydia trachomatis* may be an underdiagnosed cause of tubal infertility and requires the treatment of both partners.

Endometriosis *Endometriosis* is defined as the presence of endometrial glands or stroma outside the endometrial cavity and uterine musculature and accounts for 40% of infertility not due to ovulatory disorders, tubal obstruction, or male factor. Its presence is suggested by a history of dyspareunia (painful intercourse), worsening dysmenorrhea that often begins before menses, or a thickened rectovaginal septum or deviation of the cervix on pelvic examination. Mild endometriosis does not appear to impair fertility; the pathogenesis of the infertility associated with moderate and severe endometriosis may be multifactorial with impairments of folliculogenesis, fertilization, and implantation, as well as adhesions. Endometriosis is often clinically silent, however, and can only be excluded definitively by laparoscopy.

MALE CAUSES (SEE ALSO CHAP. 411)

Known causes of male infertility include primary testicular disease, genetic disorders (particularly Y chromosome microdeletions), disorders of sperm transport, and hypothalamic-pituitary disease resulting in secondary hypogonadism. However, the etiology is not ascertained in up to one-half of men with suspected male factor infertility. The key initial diagnostic test is a *semen analysis*. Testosterone levels should be measured if the sperm count is low on repeated examination or if there is clinical evidence of hypogonadism. Gonadotropin levels will help to determine a gonadal versus a central cause of hypogonadism.

TREATMENT INFERTILITY

In addition to addressing the negative impact of smoking on fertility and pregnancy outcome, counseling about nutrition and weight is a fundamental component of infertility and pregnancy management. Both low and increased body mass index (BMI) are associated with infertility in women and with increased morbidity during pregnancy. Obesity has also been associated with infertility in men. The treatment of infertility should be tailored to the problems unique to each couple. In many situations, including unexplained infertility, mild-to-moderate endometriosis, and/or borderline semen parameters, a stepwise approach to infertility is optimal, beginning with low-risk interventions and moving to more invasive, higher risk interventions only if necessary. After determination of all infertility factors and their correction, if possible, this approach might include, in increasing order of complexity: (1) expectant management, (2) clomiphene citrate or an aromatase inhibitor (see below) with or without intrauterine insemination (IUI), (3) gonadotropins with or without IUI, and (4) in vitro fertilization (IVF). The time used for evaluation, correction of problems identified, and expectant management can be longer in women age <30 years, but this process should be advanced rapidly in women age >35 years. In some situations, expectant management will not be appropriate.

OVULATORY DYSFUNCTION

Treatment of ovulatory dysfunction should first be directed at identification of the etiology of the disorder to allow specific management when possible. Dopamine agonists, for example, may be indicated in patients with hyperprolactinemia (Chap. 403); lifestyle modification may be successful in women with obesity, low body weight, or a history of intensive exercise.

Medications used for ovulation induction include agents that increase FSH through alteration of negative feedback, gonadotropins, and pulsatile GnRH. *Clomiphene citrate* is a nonsteroidal estrogen antagonist that increases FSH and LH levels by blocking estrogen negative feedback at the hypothalamus. The efficacy of clomiphene for ovulation induction is highly dependent on patient selection. In appropriate patients, it induces ovulation in ~60% of women with PCOS and has traditionally been the initial treatment of choice. Combination with agents that modify insulin levels such as metformin does not appear to improve outcome. Clomiphene citrate is less successful in patients with hypogonadotropic hypogonadism. *Aromatase inhibitors* have also been investigated for the treatment of infertility. Studies suggest they may have advantages over clomiphene, but these medications have not been approved for this indication.

Gonadotropins are highly effective for ovulation induction in women with hypogonadotropic hypogonadism and PCOS and are used to induce the development of multiple follicles in unexplained infertility and in older reproductive-age women. Disadvantages include a significant risk of multiple gestation and the risk of ovarian hyperstimulation, particularly in women with polycystic ovaries, with or without other features of PCOS. Careful monitoring and a conservative approach to ovarian stimulation reduce these risks. Currently available gonadotropins include urinary preparations of LH and FSH, highly purified FSH, and recombinant FSH. Although FSH is the key component, LH is essential for steroidogenesis in hypogonadotropic patients, and LH or human chorionic gonadotropin (hCG) may improve results through effects on terminal differentiation of the oocyte. These methods are commonly combined with IUI.

None of these methods are effective in women with premature ovarian failure, in whom donor oocyte or adoption is the method of choice.

TUBAL DISEASE

If hysterosalpingography suggests a tubal or uterine cavity abnormality or if a patient is age ≥35 at the time of initial evaluation, laparoscopy with tubal lavage is recommended, often with a hysteroscopy. Although tubal reconstruction may be attempted if tubal disease is identified, it is generally being replaced by the use of IVF. These patients are at increased risk of developing an ectopic pregnancy.

ENDOMETRIOSIS

Although 60% of women with minimal or mild endometriosis may conceive within 1 year without treatment, laparoscopic resection or ablation appears to improve conception rates. Medical management of advanced stages of endometriosis is widely used for symptom control but has not been shown to enhance fertility. In moderate and severe endometriosis, conservative surgery is associated with pregnancy rates of 50 and 39%, respectively, compared with rates of 25 and 5% with expectant management alone. In some patients, IVF may be the treatment of choice.

MALE FACTOR INFERTILITY

The treatment options for male factor infertility have expanded greatly in recent years (Chap. 411). Secondary hypogonadism is highly amenable to treatment with gonadotropins or pulsatile gonadotropin-releasing hormone (GnRH) where available. In vitro techniques have provided new opportunities for patients with primary testicular failure and disorders of sperm transport. Choice of initial treatment options depends on sperm concentration and motility. Expectant management should be attempted initially in men with mild male factor infertility (sperm count of 15 to 20 × 10^6/mL and normal motility). Moderate male factor infertility (10 to 15 × 10^6/mL and 20–40% motility) should begin with IUI alone or in combination with treatment of the female partner with ovulation induction, but it may require IVF with or without intracytoplasmic sperm injection (ICSI). For men with a severe defect (sperm count of <10 × 10^6/mL, 10% motility), IVF with ICSI or donor sperm should be used. If ICSI is performed because of azoospermia due to congenital bilateral absence of the vas deferens, genetic testing and counseling should be provided because of the risk of cystic fibrosis.

ASSISTED REPRODUCTIVE TECHNOLOGIES

The development of assisted reproductive technologies (ARTs) has dramatically altered the treatment of male and female infertility. IVF is indicated for patients with many causes of infertility that have not been successfully managed with more conservative approaches. IVF or ICSI is often the treatment of choice in couples with a significant male factor or tubal disease, whereas IVF using donor oocytes is used in patients with premature ovarian failure and in women of advanced reproductive age. Success rates are influenced by cause of infertility and age, varying between 15 and 40%. Success rates are highest in anovulatory women and lowest in women with decreased ovarian reserve. In the United States, success rates are higher in white than in black, Asian, or Hispanic women. Although often effective, IVF is expensive and requires careful monitoring of ovulation induction and invasive techniques, including the aspiration of multiple follicles. IVF is associated with a significant risk of multiple gestation, particularly in women age <35, in whom the rate can be as high as 30%, which has led to specific recommendations for numbers of embryos or blastocysts to transfer based on age and specific prognostic factors.

CONTRACEPTION

Although use of contraception worldwide has increased in the last two decades, as of 2010, 146 million women worldwide age 15–49 years who were married or in a union had an unmet need for family planning. The absolute number of married women who use contraception or have an unmet need for family planning is projected to grow from 900 million (876–922 million) in 2010 to 962 million (927–992 million) in 2015.

Only 15% of couples in the United States report having unprotected sexual intercourse in the past 3 months. However, despite the wide availability and widespread use of a variety of effective methods of contraception, approximately one-half of all births in the United States are the result of unintended pregnancy. Teenage pregnancies continue to represent a serious public health problem in the United States, with >1 million unintended pregnancies each year—a significantly greater incidence than in other industrialized nations.

Of the contraceptive methods available (Table 414-1), a reversible form of contraception is used by >50% of couples, whereas sterilization (male or female) has been used as a permanent form of contraception by over one-third of couples. Pregnancy termination is relatively safe when directed by health care professionals but is rarely the option of choice.

TABLE 414-1 EFFECTIVENESS OF DIFFERENT FORMS OF CONTRACEPTION

Method of Contraception	Theoretical[a] Effectiveness, %	Actual[a] Effectiveness, %	Percent Continuing Use at 1 Year[b]	Contraceptive Methods Used by U.S. Women[c]
Barrier methods				
Condoms	98	88	63	18
Diaphragm	94	82	58	2
Cervical cap	94	82	50	<1
Spermicides	97	79	43	1
Sterilization				
Male	99.9	99.9	100	9
Female	99.8	99.6	100	27
Intrauterine device				1
Copper T380	99	97	78	
Progestasert	98	97	81	
Mirena	99.9	99.8		
Hormonal contraceptives	99.7	92	72	31
Combination pill				
Progestin only pill				
Transdermal patch				
Vaginal ring				
Monthly injection				
Long-acting progestins				

[a]Adapted from J Trussel et al: Obstet Gynecol 76:558, 1990. [b]Adapted from Contraceptive Technology Update. Contraceptive Technology, Feb. 1996, Vol 17, No 1, pp 13–24. [c]Adapted from LJ Piccinino, WD Mosher: Fam Plan Perspective 30:4, 1998.

No single contraceptive method is ideal, although all are safer than carrying a pregnancy to term. The effectiveness of a given method of contraception does not just depend on the efficacy of the method itself. Discrepancies between theoretical and actual effectiveness emphasize the importance of patient education and compliance when considering various forms of contraception (Table 414-1). Knowledge of the advantages and disadvantages of each contraceptive is essential for counseling an individual about the methods that are safest and most consistent with his or her lifestyle. The WHO has extensive family planning resources for the physician and patient that can be accessed online. Similar resources for determining medical eligibility are available through the Centers for Disease Control and Prevention (CDC). Considerations for contraceptive use in obese patients and after bariatric surgery are discussed below.

BARRIER METHODS

Barrier contraceptives (such as condoms, diaphragms, and cervical caps) and spermicides are easily available, reversible, and have fewer side effects than hormonal methods. However, their effectiveness is highly dependent on adherence and proper use (Table 414-1). A major advantage of barrier contraceptives is the protection provided against sexually transmitted infections (STIs) (Chap. 163). Consistent use is associated with a decreased risk of HIV, gonorrhea, nongonococcal urethritis, and genital herpes, probably due in part to the concomitant use of spermicides. Natural membrane condoms may be less effective than latex condoms, and petroleum-based lubricants can degrade condoms and decrease their efficacy for preventing HIV infection. Barrier methods used by women include the diaphragm, cervical cap, and contraceptive sponge. The cervical cap and sponge are less effective than the diaphragm, and there have been rare reports of toxic shock syndrome with the diaphragm and contraceptive sponge.

STERILIZATION

Sterilization is the method of birth control most frequently chosen by fertile men and multiparous women >30 years old (Table 414-1). Sterilization refers to a procedure that prevents fertilization by surgical interruption of the fallopian tubes in women or the vas deferens in men. Although tubal ligation and vasectomy are potentially reversible, these procedures should be considered permanent and should not be undertaken without patient counseling.

Several methods of *tubal ligation* have been developed, all of which are highly effective with a 10-year cumulative pregnancy rate of 1.85 per 100 women. However, when pregnancy does occur, the risk of ectopic pregnancy may be as high as 30%. The success rate of tubal reanastomosis depends on the method of ligation used, but even after successful reversal, the risk of ectopic pregnancy remains high. In addition to prevention of pregnancy, tubal ligation reduces the risk of ovarian cancer, possibly by limiting the upward migration of potential carcinogens.

Vasectomy is a highly effective outpatient surgical procedure that has little risk. The development of azoospermia may be delayed for 2–6 months, and other forms of contraception must be used until two sperm-free ejaculations provide proof of sterility. Reanastomosis may restore fertility in 30–50% of men, but the success rate declines with time after vasectomy and may be influenced by factors such as the development of antisperm antibodies.

INTRAUTERINE DEVICES

IUDs inhibit pregnancy through several mechanisms, primarily via a spermicidal effect caused by a sterile inflammatory reaction induced by the presence of a foreign body in the uterine cavity (copper IUDs) or by the release of progestins (Progestasert, Mirena). IUDs provide a high level of efficacy in the absence of systemic metabolic effects, and ongoing motivation is not required to ensure efficacy once the device has been placed. However, only 1% of women in the United States use this method compared to a utilization rate of 15–30% in much of Europe and Canada, despite evidence that the newer devices are not associated with increased rates of pelvic infection and infertility, as occurred with earlier devices. An IUD should not be used in women at high risk for development of STI or in women at high risk for bacterial endocarditis. The IUD may not be effective in women with uterine leiomyomas because they alter the size or shape of the uterine cavity. IUD use is associated with increased menstrual blood flow, although this is less pronounced with the progestin-releasing IUD, which is associated with a more frequent occurrence of spotting or amenorrhea.

HORMONAL METHODS

Oral Contraceptive Pills Because of their ease of use and efficacy, oral contraceptive pills are the most widely used form of hormonal contraception. They act by suppressing ovulation, changing cervical mucus, and altering the endometrium. The current formulations are made from synthetic estrogens and progestins. The estrogen component of the pill consists of ethinyl estradiol or mestranol, which is metabolized to ethinyl estradiol. Multiple synthetic progestins are used. Norethindrone and its derivatives are used in many formulations. Low-dose norgestimate and the more recently developed (third-generation) progestins (desogestrel, gestodene, drospirenone) have a less androgenic profile; levonorgestrel appears to be the most androgenic of the progestins and should be avoided in patients with hyperandrogenism. The three major formulations of oral contraceptives are (1) fixed-dose estrogen-progestin combination, (2) phasic estrogen-progestin combination, and (3) progestin only. Each of these formulations is administered daily for 3 weeks followed by a week of

TABLE 414-2 ORAL CONTRACEPTIVES: CONTRAINDICATIONS AND DISEASE RISK

Contraindications
Absolute
Previous thromboembolic event or stroke
History of an estrogen-dependent tumor
Active liver disease
Pregnancy
Undiagnosed abnormal uterine bleeding
Hypertriglyceridemia
Women age >35 years who smoke heavily
Relative
Hypertension
Women receiving anticonvulsant drug therapy
Women following bariatric surgery (malabsorptive procedure)
Disease Risks
Increased
Coronary heart disease—increased in smokers >35; no relation to progestin type
Hypertension—relative risk 1.8 (current users) and 1.2 (previous users)
Venous thrombosis—relative risk ~4; may be higher with third-generation progestin, drospirenone, and patch; compounded by obesity (tenfold increased risk compared with nonobese, no OCP); markedly increased with factor V Leiden or prothrombin gene mutations
Stroke—slight increase; unclear relation to migraine headache
Cerebral vein thrombosis—relative risk ~13–15; synergistic with prothrombin gene mutation
Cervical cancer—relative risk 2–4
Breast cancer—may increase risk in carriers of *BRCA1* and possibly *BRCA2*
Decreased
Ovarian cancer—50% reduction in risk
Endometrial cancer—40% reduction in risk

Abbreviation: OCP, oral contraceptive pill.

no medication during which menstrual bleeding generally occurs. Two extended oral contraceptives are approved for use in the United States; Seasonale is a 3-month preparation with 84 days of active drug and 7 days of placebo, whereas Lybrel is a continuous preparation. Current doses of ethinyl estradiol range from 10 to 50 μg. However, indications for the 50-μg dose are rare, and the majority of formulations contain 30–35 μg of ethinyl estradiol. The reduced estrogen and progestin content in the second- and third-generation pills has decreased both side effects and risks associated with oral contraceptive use (Table 414-2). At the currently used doses, patients must be cautioned not to miss pills due to the potential for ovulation. Side effects, including breakthrough bleeding, amenorrhea, breast tenderness, and weight gain, often respond to a change in formulation. Even the lower dose oral contraceptives have been associated with an increased risk of cardiovascular disease (myocardial infarction, stroke, venous thromboembolism [VTE]), but the absolute excess risk is extremely low. VTE risk is higher with the third-generation than the second-generation progestins, and the risk of stroke and VTE is also higher with drospirenone (although not cyproterone), but the absolute excess risk is small and may be outweighed by contraceptive benefits and reduction in ovarian and endometrial cancer risk.

The microdose progestin-only minipill is less effective as a contraceptive, having a pregnancy rate of 2–7 per 100 women-years. However, it may be appropriate for women at increased risk for cardiovascular disease or for women who cannot tolerate synthetic estrogens.

Alternative Methods A *weekly contraceptive patch* (Ortho Evra) is available and has similar efficacy to oral contraceptives. Approximately 2% of patches fail to adhere, and a similar percentage of women have skin reactions. Efficacy is lower in women weighing >90 kg. The amount of estrogen delivered may be comparable to that of a 40-μg ethinyl estradiol oral contraceptive, raising the possibility of increased risk of VTE, which must be balanced against potential benefits for women not able to successfully use other methods. A *monthly contraceptive estrogen/progestin injection* (Lunelle) is highly effective, with a first-year failure rate of <0.2%, but it may be less effective in obese women. Its use is associated with bleeding irregularities that diminish over time. Fertility returns rapidly after discontinuation. A *monthly vaginal ring* (NuvaRing) that is intended to be left in place during intercourse is also available for contraceptive use. It is highly effective, with a 12-month failure rate of 0.7%. Ovulation returns within the first recovery cycle after discontinuation.

Long-Term Contraceptives Long-term progestin administration acts primarily by inhibiting ovulation and causing changes in the endometrium and cervical mucus that result in decreased implantation and sperm transport. Depot medroxyprogesterone acetate (Depo-Provera, DMPA), the only injectable form available in the United States, is effective for 3 months, but return of fertility after discontinuation may be delayed for up to 12–18 months. DMPA is now available for both SC and IM injection. Irregular bleeding, amenorrhea, and weight gain are the most common side effects. This form of contraception may be particularly good for women in whom an estrogen-containing contraceptive is contraindicated (e.g., migraine exacerbation, sickle cell anemia, fibroids).

POSTCOITAL CONTRACEPTION

The probability of pregnancy without relation to time of the month is 8%, but the probability varies significantly in relation to proximity to ovulation and may be as high has 30%. In order of efficacy, methods of postcoital contraception include the following:

1. Copper IUD insertion within a maximum of 5 days has a reported efficacy of 99–100% and prevents pregnancy by its spermicidal effect; insertion is frequently available through family planning clinics.
2. Oral antiprogestins (ulipristal acetate, 30 mg single dose, available worldwide, or mifepristone, 600 mg single dose, not available for this indication in the United States) prevent pregnancy by delaying or preventing ovulation; when administered, ideally within 72 h but up to 120 h after intercourse, they have an efficacy of 98–99%; require a prescription.
3. Levonorgestrel (1.5 mg as a single dose) delays or prevents ovulation and is not effective after ovulation; should be taken within 72 h of unprotected intercourse, and has an efficacy that varies between 60 and 94%; it is available over the counter.

Combined estrogen and progestin regimens have lower efficacy and are no longer recommended. A pregnancy test is not necessary before the use of oral methods, but pregnancy should be excluded before IUD insertion. Risk factors for failure of oral regimens include close proximity to ovulation and unprotected intercourse after use. In addition, there is an increased risk of pregnancy in obese and overweight women using levonorgestrel for postcoital contraception and an increased risk in obese women using an antiprogestin.

IMPACT OF OBESITY ON CONTRACEPTIVE CHOICE

Approximately one-third of adults in the United States are obese. Although obesity is associated with some reduction in fertility, the vast majority of obese women can conceive. The risk of pregnancy-associated complications is higher in obese women. Intrauterine contraception may be more effective than oral or transdermal methods for obese women. The WHO guidelines provide no restrictions (class 1) for the use of intrauterine contraception, DMPA, and progestin-only pills for obese women (BMI ≥30) in the absence of coexistent medical problems, whereas methods that include estrogen (pill, patch, ring) are considered class 2 (advantages generally outweigh theoretical or proven risks) due to the increased risk of thromboembolic disease. There are no restrictions to the use of any contraceptive methods following restrictive bariatric surgery procedures, but both combined and progestin-only pills are relatively less effective following procedures associated with malabsorption.

415e Biology of Obesity

Jeffrey S. Flier, Eleftheria Maratos-Flier

This is a digital-only chapter. It is available on the DVD that accompanies this book, as well as on Access Medicine/Harrison's Online, and the eBook and "app" editions of HPIM 19e.

In a world where food supplies are intermittent, the ability to store energy in excess of what is required for immediate use is essential for survival. Fat cells, residing within widely distributed adipose tissue depots, are adapted to store excess energy efficiently as triglyceride and, when needed, to release stored energy as free fatty acids for use at other sites. This physiologic system, orchestrated through endocrine and neural pathways, permits humans to survive starvation for as long as several months. However, in the presence of nutritional abundance and a sedentary lifestyle, and influenced importantly by genetic endowment, this system increases adipose energy stores and produces adverse health consequences.

DEFINITION AND MEASUREMENT

Obesity is a state of excess adipose tissue mass. Although often viewed as equivalent to increased body weight, this need not be the case—lean but very muscular individuals may be overweight by numerical standards without having increased adiposity. Body weights are distributed continuously in populations, so that choice of a medically meaningful distinction between lean and obese is somewhat arbitrary. Obesity is therefore defined by assessing its linkage to morbidity or mortality.

416 Evaluation and Management of Obesity

Robert F. Kushner

More than 66% of U.S. adults are categorized as overweight or obese, and the prevalence of obesity is increasing rapidly in most of the industrialized world. Children and adolescents also are becoming more obese, indicating that the current trends will accelerate over time. Obesity is associated with an increased risk of multiple health problems, including hypertension, type 2 diabetes, dyslipidemia, obstructive sleep apnea, nonalcoholic fatty liver disease, degenerative joint disease, and some malignancies. Thus, it is important for physicians to identify, evaluate, and treat patients for obesity and associated comorbid conditions.

EVALUATION

Physicians should screen all adult patients for obesity and offer intensive counseling and behavioral interventions to promote sustained weight loss. The five main steps in the evaluation of obesity, as described below, are (1) a focused obesity-related history, (2) a physical examination to determine the degree and type of obesity, (3) assessment of comorbid conditions, (4) determination of fitness level, and (5) assessment of the patient's readiness to adopt lifestyle changes.

The Obesity-Focused History Information from the history should address the following seven questions:

- What factors contribute to the patient's obesity?
- How is the obesity affecting the patient's health?
- What is the patient's level of risk from obesity?
- What does the patient find difficult about managing weight?
- What are the patient's goals and expectations?
- Is the patient motivated to begin a weight management program?
- What kind of help does the patient need?

Although the vast majority of cases of obesity can be attributed to behavioral factors that affect diet and physical activity patterns, the history may suggest secondary causes that merit further evaluation. Disorders to consider include polycystic ovarian syndrome, hypothyroidism, Cushing's syndrome, and hypothalamic disease. Drug-induced weight gain also should be considered. Common causes include medications for diabetes (insulin, sulfonylureas, thiazolidinediones); steroid hormones; psychotropic agents; mood stabilizers (lithium); antidepressants (tricyclics, monoamine oxidase inhibitors, paroxetine, mirtazapine); and antiepileptic drugs (valproate, gabapentin, carbamazepine). Other medications, such as nonsteroidal anti-inflammatory drugs and calcium channel blockers, may cause peripheral edema but do not increase body fat.

The patient's current diet and physical activity patterns may reveal factors that contribute to the development of obesity and may identify behaviors to target for treatment. This type of historic information is best obtained by the combination of a questionnaire and an interview.

Body Mass Index (BMI) and Waist Circumference Three key anthropometric measurements are important in evaluating the degree of obesity: weight, height, and waist circumference. The BMI, calculated as weight (kg)/height $(m)^2$ or as weight (lbs)/height $(inches)^2 \times 703$, is used to classify weight status and risk of disease (Tables 416-1 and 416-2). BMI provides an estimate of body fat and is related to disease risk. Lower BMI thresholds for overweight and obesity have been proposed for the Asia-Pacific region since this population appears to be at risk for glucose and lipid abnormalities at lower body weights.

Excess abdominal fat, assessed by measurement of waist circumference or waist-to-hip ratio, is independently associated with a higher risk for diabetes mellitus and cardiovascular disease. Measurement of the waist circumference is a surrogate for visceral adipose tissue and should be performed in the horizontal plane above the iliac crest (Table 416-3).

Physical Fitness Several prospective studies have demonstrated that physical fitness, reported by questionnaire or measured by a maximal treadmill exercise test, is an important predictor of all-cause mortality rate independent of BMI and body composition. These observations highlight the importance of taking a physical activity and exercise history during examination as well as emphasizing physical activity as a treatment approach.

Obesity-Associated Comorbid Conditions The evaluation of comorbid conditions should be based on presentation of symptoms, risk factors, and index of suspicion. For all patients, a fasting lipid panel should be performed (total, low-density lipoprotein, and high-density lipoprotein cholesterol and triglyceride levels) and a fasting blood glucose level and blood pressure determined. Symptoms and diseases that are directly or indirectly related to obesity are listed in Table 416-4. Although individuals vary, the number and severity of organ-specific comorbid conditions usually rise with increasing levels of obesity. Patients at very high absolute risk include those with the following: established coronary heart disease; presence of other atherosclerotic diseases, such as peripheral arterial disease, abdominal aortic aneurysm, and symptomatic carotid artery disease; type 2 diabetes; and sleep apnea.

Assessing the Patient's Readiness to Change An attempt to initiate lifestyle changes when the patient is not ready usually leads to frustration and may hamper future weight-loss efforts. Assessment includes

TABLE 416-1 BODY MASS INDEX (BMI)

BMI	19	20	21	22	23	24	25	26	27	28	29	30	31	32	33	34	35
Height (Inches)								Body Weight (Pounds)									
58	91	96	100	105	110	115	119	124	129	134	138	143	148	153	158	162	167
59	94	99	104	109	114	119	124	128	133	138	143	148	153	158	163	168	173
60	97	102	107	112	118	123	128	133	138	143	148	153	158	163	168	174	179
61	100	106	111	116	122	127	132	137	143	148	153	158	164	169	174	180	185
62	104	109	115	120	126	131	136	142	147	153	158	164	169	175	180	186	191
63	107	113	118	124	130	135	141	146	152	158	163	169	175	180	186	191	197
64	110	116	122	128	134	140	145	151	157	163	169	174	180	186	192	197	204
65	114	120	126	132	138	144	150	156	162	168	174	180	186	192	198	204	210
66	118	124	130	136	142	148	155	161	167	173	179	186	192	198	204	210	216
67	121	127	134	140	146	153	159	166	172	178	185	191	198	204	211	217	223
68	125	131	138	144	151	158	164	171	177	184	190	197	203	210	216	223	230
69	128	135	142	149	155	162	169	176	182	189	196	203	209	216	223	230	236
70	132	139	146	153	160	167	174	181	188	195	202	209	216	222	229	236	243
71	136	143	150	157	165	172	179	186	193	200	208	215	222	229	236	243	250
72	140	147	154	162	169	177	184	191	199	206	213	221	228	235	242	250	258
73	144	151	159	166	174	182	189	197	204	212	219	227	235	242	250	257	265
74	148	155	163	171	179	186	194	202	210	218	225	233	241	249	256	264	272
75	152	160	168	176	184	192	200	208	216	224	232	240	248	256	264	272	279
76	156	164	172	180	189	197	205	213	221	230	238	246	254	263	271	279	287

BMI	36	37	38	39	40	41	42	43	44	45	46	47	48	49	50	51	52	53	54
58	172	177	181	186	191	196	201	205	210	215	220	224	229	234	239	244	248	253	258
59	178	183	188	193	198	203	208	212	217	222	227	232	237	242	247	252	257	262	267
60	184	189	194	199	204	209	215	220	225	230	235	240	245	250	255	261	266	271	276
61	190	195	201	206	211	217	222	227	232	238	243	248	254	259	264	269	275	280	285
62	196	202	207	213	218	224	229	235	240	246	251	256	262	267	273	278	284	289	295
63	203	208	214	220	225	231	237	242	248	254	259	265	270	278	282	287	293	299	304
64	209	215	221	227	232	238	244	250	256	262	267	273	279	285	291	296	302	308	314
65	216	222	228	234	240	246	252	258	264	270	276	282	288	294	300	306	312	318	324
66	223	229	235	241	247	253	260	266	272	278	284	291	297	303	309	315	322	328	334
67	230	236	242	249	255	261	268	274	280	287	293	299	306	312	319	325	331	338	344
68	236	243	249	256	262	269	276	282	289	295	302	308	315	322	328	335	341	348	354
69	243	250	257	263	270	277	284	291	297	304	311	318	324	331	338	345	351	358	365
70	250	257	264	271	278	285	292	299	306	313	320	327	334	341	348	355	362	369	376
71	257	265	272	279	286	293	301	308	315	322	329	338	343	351	358	365	372	379	386
72	265	272	279	287	294	302	309	316	324	331	338	346	353	361	368	375	383	390	397
73	272	280	288	295	302	310	318	325	333	340	348	355	363	371	378	386	393	401	408
74	280	287	295	303	311	319	326	334	342	350	358	365	373	381	389	396	404	412	420
75	287	295	303	311	319	327	335	343	351	359	367	375	383	391	399	407	415	423	431
76	295	304	312	320	328	336	344	353	361	369	377	385	394	402	410	418	426	435	443

patient motivation and support, stressful life events, psychiatric status, time availability and constraints, and appropriateness of goals and expectations. Readiness can be viewed as the balance of two opposing forces: (1) motivation, or the patient's desire to change; and (2) resistance, or the patient's resistance to change.

TABLE 416-2 CLASSIFICATION OF WEIGHT STATUS AND DISEASE RISK

Classification	Body Mass Index (kg/m²)	Obesity Class	Disease Risk
Underweight	<18.5	—	—
Healthy weight	18.5–24.9	—	—
Overweight	25.0–29.9	—	Increased
Obesity	30.0–34.9	I	High
Obesity	35.0–39.9	II	Very high
Extreme obesity	≥40	III	Extremely high

Source: Adapted from the National Institutes of Health, National Heart, Lung, and Blood Institute: *Clinical Guidelines on the Identification, Evaluation, and Treatment of Overweight and Obesity in Adults.* U.S. Department of Health and Human Services, U.S. Public Health Service, 1998.

A helpful method to begin a readiness assessment is to use the motivational interviewing technique of "anchoring" the patient's interest and confidence to change on a numerical scale. With this technique, the patient is asked to rate—on a scale from 0 to 10, with 0 being not so important (or confident) and 10 being very important (or confident)—his or her level of interest in and confidence about losing weight at this time. This exercise helps establish readiness to change and also serves as a basis for further dialogue.

TREATMENT OBESITY

THE GOAL OF THERAPY

The primary goals of treatment are to improve obesity-related comorbid conditions and to reduce the risk of developing future comorbidities. Information obtained from the history, physical examination, and diagnostic tests is used to determine risk and develop a treatment plan (**Fig. 416-1**). The decision of how aggressively to treat the patient and which modalities to use is determined by the patient's risk status, expectations, and available resources.

TABLE 416-3 ETHNIC-SPECIFIC CUTPOINT VALUES FOR WAIST CIRCUMFERENCE

Ethnic Group	Waist Circumference
Europeans	
Men	>94 cm (>37 in)
Women	>80 cm (>31.5 in)
South Asians and Chinese	
Men	>90 cm (>35 in)
Women	>80 cm (>31.5 in)
Japanese	
Men	>85 cm (>33.5 in)
Women	>90 cm (>35 in)
Ethnic South and Central Americans	Use South Asian recommendations until more specific data are available.
Sub-Saharan Africans	Use European data until more specific data are available.
Eastern Mediterranean and Middle Eastern (Arab) populations	Use European data until more specific data are available.

Source: From KGMM Alberti et al for the IDF Epidemiology Task Force Consensus Group: Lancet 366:1059, 2005.

Not all patients who are deemed obese by BMI alone need to be treated, as exemplified by the concepts of obesity paradox or the metabolically healthy obese. However, patients who present with obesity-related comorbidities and who would benefit from weight loss intervention should be managed proactively. Therapy for obesity always begins with lifestyle management and may include pharmacotherapy or surgery, depending on BMI risk category (Table 416-5). Setting an initial weight-loss goal of 8–10% over 6 months is a realistic target.

TABLE 416-4 OBESITY-RELATED ORGAN SYSTEMS REVIEW

Cardiovascular	**Respiratory**
Hypertension	Dyspnea
Congestive heart failure	Obstructive sleep apnea
Cor pulmonale	Hypoventilation syndrome
Varicose veins	Pickwickian syndrome
Pulmonary embolism	Asthma
Coronary artery disease	**Gastrointestinal**
Endocrine	Gastroesophageal reflux disease
Metabolic syndrome	Nonalcoholic fatty-liver disease
Type 2 diabetes	Cholelithiasis
Dyslipidemia	Hernias
Polycystic ovarian syndrome	Colon cancer
Musculoskeletal	**Genitourinary**
Hyperuricemia and gout	Urinary stress incontinence
Immobility	Obesity-related glomerulopathy
Osteoarthritis (knees and hips)	Hypogonadism (male)
Low back pain	Breast and uterine cancer
Carpal tunnel syndrome	Pregnancy complications
Psychological	**Neurologic**
Depression/low self-esteem	Stroke
Body image disturbance	Idiopathic intracranial hypertension
Social stigmatization	Meralgia paresthetica
Integument	Dementia
Striae distensae	
Stasis pigmentation of legs	
Lymphedema	
Cellulitis	
Intertrigo, carbuncles	
Acanthosis nigricans	
Acrochordons (skin tags)	
Hidradenitis suppurativa	

LIFESTYLE MANAGEMENT

Obesity care involves attention to three essential elements of lifestyle: dietary habits, physical activity, and behavior modification. Because obesity is fundamentally a disease of energy imbalance, all patients must learn how and when energy is consumed (diet), how and when energy is expended (physical activity), and how to incorporate this information into their daily lives (behavioral therapy). Lifestyle management has been shown to result in a modest (typically 3–5 kg) weight loss when compared with no treatment or usual care.

Diet Therapy The primary focus of diet therapy is to reduce overall calorie consumption. Guidelines from the National Heart, Lung, and Blood Institute recommend initiating treatment with a calorie deficit of 500–1000 kcal/d compared with the patient's habitual diet. This reduction is consistent with a goal of losing ~1–2 lbs per week. The calorie deficit can be instituted through dietary substitutions or alternatives. Examples include choosing smaller portion sizes, eating more fruits and vegetables, consuming more whole-grain cereals, selecting leaner cuts of meat and skimmed dairy products, reducing consumption of fried foods and other foods with added fats and oils, and drinking water instead of sugar-sweetened beverages. It is important that dietary counseling remain patient centered and that the goals set be practical, realistic, and achievable.

The macronutrient composition of the diet will vary with the patient's preference and medical condition. The 2010 U.S. Department of Agriculture Dietary Guidelines for Americans (Chap. 95e), which focus on health promotion and risk reduction, can be applied to treatment of overweight or obese patients. The recommendations include maintaining a diet rich in whole grains, fruits, vegetables, and dietary fiber; consuming two servings (8 oz) of fish high in omega 3 fatty acids per week; decreasing sodium intake to <2300 mg/d; consuming 3 cups of milk (or equivalent low-fat or fat-free dairy products) per day; limiting cholesterol intake to <300 mg/d; and keeping total fat intake at 20–35% of daily calories and saturated fat intake at <10% of daily calories. Application of these guidelines to specific calorie goals can be found on the website *www.choosemyplate.gov*. The revised Dietary Reference Intakes for Macronutrients released by the Institute of Medicine recommends that 45–65% of calories come from carbohydrates, 20–35% from fat, and 10–35% from protein. The guidelines also recommend daily fiber intake of 38 g (men) and 25 g (women) for persons over 50 years of age and 30 g (men) and 21 g (women) for those under age 50.

Since portion control is one of the most difficult strategies for patients to manage, the use of pre-prepared products such as meal replacements is a simple and convenient suggestion. Examples include frozen entrees, canned beverages, and bars. Use of meal replacements in the diet has been shown to result in a 7–8% weight loss.

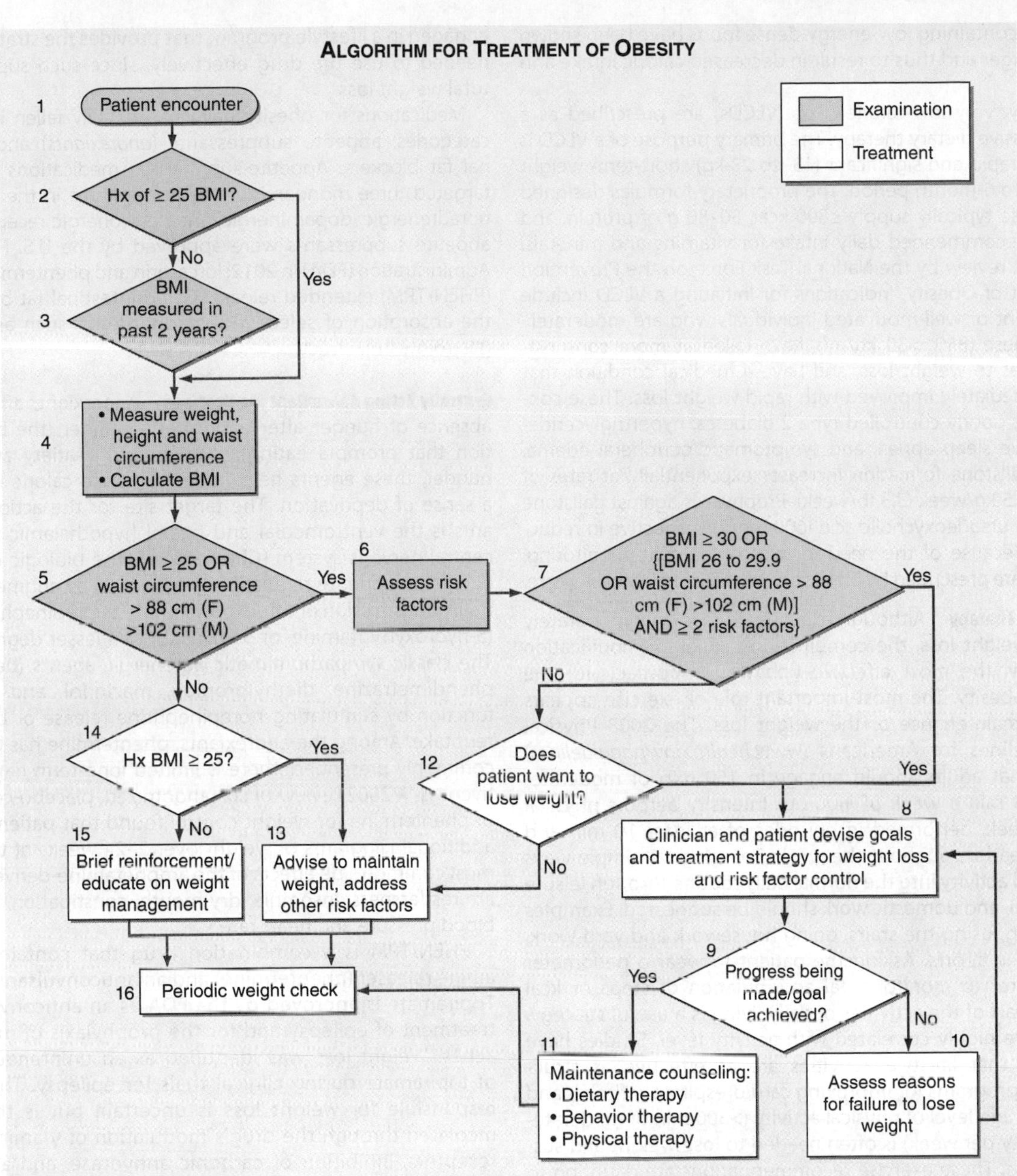

FIGURE 416-1 Algorithm for the treatment of obesity. This algorithm applies only to assessment for overweight and obesity and subsequent decisions based on that assessment. It does not reflect initial overall assessment for other conditions that the physician may wish to perform. BMI, body mass index; Hx, history. *(From the National, Heart, Lung, and Blood Institute: Clinical guidelines on the identification, evaluation, and treatment of overweight and obesity in adults: The evidence report. Washington, DC, US Department of Health and Human Services, 1998.)*

Numerous randomized trials comparing diets of different macronutrient composition (e.g., low-carbohydrate, low-fat, Mediterranean) have shown that weight loss depends primarily on reduction of total caloric intake and adherence to the prescribed diet, not the specific proportions of carbohydrate, fat, and protein in the diet. The macronutrient composition will ultimately be determined by the patient's taste preferences, cooking style, and culture. However, the patient's underlying medical problems are also important in guiding the recommended dietary composition. The dietary prescription will vary according to the patient's metabolic profile and risk factors. A consultation with a registered dietitian for medical nutrition therapy is particularly useful in considering patient preference and treatment of comorbid diseases.

TABLE 416-5 A GUIDE TO OPTING FOR TREATMENT FOR OBESITY

	BMI Category (kg/m²)				
Treatment	**25–26.9**	**27–29.9**	**30–34.9**	**35–39.9**	**≥40**
Diet, exercise, behavioral therapy	With comorbidities	With comorbidities	+	+	+
Pharmacotherapy	—	With comorbidities	+	+	+
Surgery	—	—	—	With comorbidities	+

Source: From the National Heart, Lung, and Blood Institute, North American Association for the Study of Obesity (2000).

Another dietary approach to consider is based on the concept of *energy density*, which refers to the number of calories (i.e., amount of energy) a food contains per unit of weight. People tend to ingest a constant volume of food regardless of caloric or macronutrient content. Adding water or fiber to a food decreases its energy density by increasing weight without affecting caloric content. Examples of foods with low-energy density include soups, fruits, vegetables, oatmeal, and lean meats. Dry foods and high-fat foods such as pretzels, cheese, egg yolks, potato chips, and red meat have a high-energy density. Diets containing low-energy-dense foods have been shown to control hunger and thus to result in decreased caloric intake and weight loss.

Occasionally, very low-calorie diets (VLCDs) are prescribed as a form of aggressive dietary therapy. The primary purpose of a VLCD is to promote a rapid and significant (13- to 23-kg) short-term weight loss over a 3- to 6-month period. The proprietary formulas designed for this purpose typically supply ≤800 kcal, 50–80 g of protein, and 100% of the recommended daily intake for vitamins and minerals. According to a review by the National Task Force on the Prevention and Treatment of Obesity, indications for initiating a VLCD include the involvement of well-motivated individuals who are moderately to severely obese (BMI, >30 kg/m^2), have failed at more conservative approaches to weight loss, and have a medical condition that would be immediately improved with rapid weight loss. These conditions include poorly controlled type 2 diabetes, hypertriglyceridemia, obstructive sleep apnea, and symptomatic peripheral edema. The risk for gallstone formation increases exponentially at rates of weight loss >1.5 kg/week (3.3 lb/week). Prophylaxis against gallstone formation with ursodeoxycholic acid (600 mg/d) is effective in reducing this risk. Because of the need for close metabolic monitoring, VLCDs usually are prescribed by physicians specializing in obesity care.

Physical Activity Therapy Although exercise alone is only moderately effective for weight loss, the combination of dietary modification and exercise is the most effective behavioral approach for the treatment of obesity. The most important role of exercise appears to be in the maintenance of the weight loss. The 2008 Physical Activity Guidelines for Americans (*www.health.gov/paguidelines*) recommend that adults should engage in 150 min of moderate-intensity or 75 min a week of vigorous-intensity aerobic physical activity per week, performed in episodes of at least 10 min and preferably spread throughout the week. Focusing on simple ways to add physical activity into the normal daily routine through leisure activities, travel, and domestic work should be suggested. Examples include walking, using the stairs, doing housework and yard work, and engaging in sports. Asking the patient to wear a pedometer or accelerometer to monitor total accumulation of steps or kcal expended as part of the activities of daily living is a useful strategy. Step counts are highly correlated with activity level. Studies have demonstrated that lifestyle activities are as effective as structured exercise programs for improving cardiorespiratory fitness and weight loss. A high level of physical activity (>300 min of moderate-intensity activity per week) is often needed to lose weight and sustain weight loss. These exercise recommendations are daunting to most patients and need to be implemented gradually. Consultation with an exercise physiologist or personal trainer may be helpful.

Behavioral Therapy Cognitive behavioral therapy is used to help change and reinforce new dietary and physical activity behaviors. Strategies include self-monitoring techniques (e.g., journaling, weighing, and measuring food and activity); stress management; stimulus control (e.g., using smaller plates, not eating in front of the television or in the car); social support; problem solving; and cognitive restructuring to help patients develop more positive and realistic thoughts about themselves. When recommending any behavioral lifestyle change, the patient should be asked to identify what, when, where, and how the behavioral change will be performed. The patient should keep a record of the anticipated behavioral change so that progress can be reviewed at the next office visit. Because these techniques are time-consuming to implement, their supervision is often undertaken by ancillary office staff, such as a nurse-clinician or registered dietitian.

PHARMACOTHERAPY

Adjuvant pharmacologic treatments should be considered for patients with a BMI ≥30 kg/m^2 or—for patients who have concomitant obesity-related diseases and for whom dietary and physical activity therapy has not been successful—a BMI ≥27 kg/m^2. When an antiobesity medication is prescribed, patients should be actively engaged in a lifestyle program that provides the strategies and skills needed to use the drug effectively, since such support increases total weight loss.

Medications for obesity have traditionally fallen into two major categories: appetite suppressants (*anorexiants*) and gastrointestinal fat blockers. Appetite-suppressing medications have primarily targeted three monoamine receptor systems in the hypothalamus: noradrenergic, dopaminergic, and serotonergic receptors. Two new appetite suppressants were approved by the U.S. Food and Drug Administration (FDA) in 2012: lorcaserin and phentermine/topiramate (PHEN/TPM) extended release. Gastrointestinal fat blockers reduce the absorption of selective macronutrients, such as fat, from the gastrointestinal tract.

Centrally Acting Anorexiant Medications Anorexiants affect *satiety* (the absence of hunger after eating) and hunger (the biologic sensation that prompts eating). By increasing satiety and decreasing hunger, these agents help patients reduce caloric intake without a sense of deprivation. The target site for the actions of anorexiants is the ventromedial and lateral hypothalamic regions in the central nervous system (**Chap. 415e**). The biologic effect of these agents on appetite regulation is produced by augmentation of the neurotransmission of three monoamines: norepinephrine; serotonin (5-hydroxytryptamine, or 5-HT); and, to a lesser degree, dopamine. The classic sympathomimetic adrenergic agents (benzphetamine, phendimetrazine, diethylpropion, mazindol, and phentermine) function by stimulating norepinephrine release or by blocking its reuptake. Among the anorexiants, phentermine has been the most commonly prescribed; there is limited long-term data on its effectiveness. A 2002 review of six randomized, placebo-controlled trials of phentermine for weight control found that patients lost 0.6–6.0 additional kilograms of weight over 2–24 weeks of treatment. The most common side effects of the amphetamine-derived anorexiants are restlessness, insomnia, dry mouth, constipation, and increased blood pressure and heart rate.

PHEN/TPM is a combination drug that contains a catecholamine releaser (phentermine) and an anticonvulsant (topiramate). Topiramate is approved by the FDA as an anticonvulsant for the treatment of epilepsy and for the prophylaxis of migraine headaches. Weight loss was identified as an unintended side effect of topiramate during clinical trials for epilepsy. The mechanism responsible for weight loss is uncertain but is thought to be mediated through the drug's modulation of γ-aminobutyric acid receptors, inhibition of carbonic anhydrase, and antagonism of glutamate. PHEN/TPM has undergone two 1-year pivotal randomized, placebo-controlled, double-blind trials of efficacy and safety: EQUIP and CONQUER. In a third study, SEQUEL, 78% of CONQUER participants continued to receive their blinded treatment for an additional year. All participants received diet and exercise counseling. Participant numbers, eligibility, characteristics, and weight loss outcomes are displayed in **Table 416-6**. Intention-to-treat 1-year placebo-subtracted weight loss for the PHEN/TPM 15-mg/92-mg dose was 9.3% and 8.6%, respectively, in the EQUIP and CONQUER trials. Clinical and statistical dose-dependent improvements were seen in selected cardiovascular and metabolic outcome measurements that were related to the weight loss. The most common adverse events experienced by the drug-randomized group were paresthesias, dry mouth, constipation, dysgeusia, and insomnia. Because of an increased risk of congenital fetal oral-cleft formation from topiramate, the FDA approval of PHEN/TPM stipulated a Risk Evaluation and Mitigation Strategies requirement to educate prescribers about the need for active birth control among women of childbearing age and a contraindication for use during pregnancy.

Lorcaserin is a selective 5-HT2C receptor agonist with a functional selectivity ~15 times that of 5-HT2A receptors and 100 times that of 5-HT2B receptors. This selectivity is important, since the drug-induced valvulopathy documented with two other serotonergic agents that were removed from the market—fenfluramine

TABLE 416-6 CLINICAL TRIALS FOR WEIGHT LOSS MEDICATIONS[a]

	Lorcaserin		PHEN/TPM[d]	
	BLOOM[b]	BLOSSOM[c]	EQUIP	CONQUER
No. of participants (ITT-LOCF)	3182	4008	1230	2448
Age (years)	18–65	18–65	≥35	27–45
BMI (kg/m²)	27–45	27–45	18–70	18–70
Comorbid conditions (cardiovascular and metabolic)	≥1	≥1	≥1	≥2
Mean weight loss (%) with treatment vs. placebo	5.8 vs. 2.2	4.8 vs. 2.8	11 vs. 1.6	10.4 vs. 1.8
Placebo subtracted weight loss (%)	3.6	3.0	9.3	8.6
Categorical change in 5% weight loss with treatment vs. placebo	47.5 vs. 20.3	47.2 vs. 25	67 vs. 17	70 vs. 21
Completion rate (%)	Lorcaserin, 55.4; placebo, 45.1	55.5	59.9	62

[a]Table shows a comparison of two 1-year prospective, randomized, double-blind trials of lorcaserin (BLOOM and BLOSSOM) and phentermine-topiramate extended release (EQUIP and CONQUER). [b]Lorcaserin dose: 10 mg bid. [c]Lorcaserin dose: 10 mg bid or qd. [d]Phentermine-topiramate extended release dose: 15 mg/92 mg.

Abbreviations: BMI, body mass index (see Table 416-1); ITT-LOCF, intention to treat, last observation carried forward; PHEN/TPM, phentermine-topiramate extended release.

and dexfenfluramine—was due to activation of the 5-HT2B receptors expressed on cardiac valvular interstitial cells. By activating the 5-HT2C receptor, lorcaserin is thought to decrease food intake through the pro-opiomelanocortin system of neurons.

Lorcaserin has undergone two randomized, placebo-controlled, double-blind trials for efficacy and safety. Participants were randomized to receive lorcaserin (10 mg bid) or placebo in the BLOOM study and to receive lorcaserin (10 mg bid or qd) or placebo in the BLOSSOM study. All participants received diet and exercise counseling. Participant numbers, eligibility, characteristics, and weight loss outcomes are displayed in Table 416-6. Overweight or obese subjects had at least one coexisting condition (hypertension, dyslipidemia, cardiovascular disease, impaired glucose tolerance, or sleep apnea)—medical conditions that are commonly seen in the office setting. Intention-to-treat 1-year placebo-subtracted weight loss was 3.6% and 3.0%, respectively, in the BLOOM and BLOSSOM trials. Echocardiography was performed at the screening visit and at scheduled time points over the course of the studies. There was no difference in the development of FDA-defined valvulopathy between drug-treated and placebo-treated participants at 1 year or 2 years. Modest statistical improvements consistent with the weight loss were seen in selected cardiovascular and metabolic outcome measurements. The most common adverse events experienced by the drug group were headache, dizziness, and nausea.

In approving both PHEN/TPM and lorcaserin, the FDA introduced a new provision with important clinical relevance: a prescription trial period to assess effectiveness. Response to both medications should be assessed after 3 months of treatment. For lorcaserin, the medication should be discontinued if the patient has not lost at least 5% of body weight by that point. For PHEN/TPM, if the patient has not lost at least 3% of body weight at 3 months, the clinician can either escalate the dose and reassess progress at 6 months or discontinue treatment entirely.

Peripherally Acting Medications Orlistat (Xenical™) is a synthetic hydrogenated derivative of a naturally occurring lipase inhibitor, lipostatin, that is produced by the mold *Streptomyces toxytricini*. This drug is a potent, slowly reversible inhibitor of pancreatic, gastric, and carboxylester lipases and phospholipase A_2, which are required for the hydrolysis of dietary fat into fatty acids and monoacylglycerols. Orlistat acts in the lumen of the stomach and small intestine by forming a covalent bond with the active site of these lipases. Taken at a therapeutic dose of 120 mg tid, orlistat blocks the digestion and absorption of ~30% of dietary fat. After discontinuation of the drug, fecal fat content usually returns to normal within 48–72 h.

Multiple randomized, double-blind, placebo-controlled studies have shown that, after 1 year, orlistat produces a weight loss of ~9–10%, whereas placebo recipients have a 4–6% weight loss. Because orlistat is minimally (<1%) absorbed from the gastrointestinal tract, it has no systemic side effects. The drug's tolerability is related to the malabsorption of dietary fat and the subsequent passage of fat in the feces. Adverse gastrointestinal effects, including flatus with discharge, fecal urgency, fatty/oily stool, and increased defecation, are reported in at least 10% of orlistat-treated patients. These side effects generally are experienced early, diminish as patients control their dietary fat intake, and only infrequently cause patients to withdraw from clinical trials. When taken concomitantly, psyllium mucilloid is helpful in controlling orlistat-induced gastrointestinal side effects. Because serum concentrations of the fat-soluble vitamins D and E and β-carotene may be reduced by orlistat treatment, vitamin supplements are recommended to prevent potential deficiencies. Orlistat was approved for over-the-counter use in 2007.

Antiobesity Drugs in Development Two additional medications are currently in development. Bupropion and naltrexone (Contrave™)—a dopamine and norepinephrine reuptake inhibitor and an opioid receptor antagonist, respectively—are theoretically combined to dampen the motivation/reinforcement that food brings (dopamine effect) and the pleasure/palatability of eating (opioid effect). In the COR-1 randomized, double-blind, placebo-controlled trial, 1742 enrolled participants, who were 18–65 years of age and had BMIs of 30–45 kg/m², were randomized to receive naltrexone (16 mg/d) plus bupropion (360 mg/d), naltrexone (32 mg/d) plus bupropion (360 mg/d), or placebo. Mean change in body weight for the three groups was 5.0%, 6.1%, and 1.3%, respectively. The most common adverse events were nausea, headache, constipation, dizziness, vomiting, and dry mouth. However, the FDA rejected the drug in 2011 because of cardiovascular concerns and concluded that a large-scale study of the long-term cardiovascular effects of naltrexone would be needed before approval could be considered.

Liraglutide, a glucagon-like peptide 1 receptor agonist currently approved for the treatment of type 2 diabetes, has independent weight loss effects via hypothalamic neural activation causing appetite suppression. In a double-blind, placebo-controlled trial, 564 adults with BMIs of 30–40 kg/m² were randomized to receive once-daily SC liraglutide (1.2, 1.8, 2.4, or 3.0 mg), placebo, or open-label orlistat (120 mg tid) for 1 year. The liraglutide and placebo recipients were switched to 2.4 mg of liraglutide during the second year and then to 3.0 mg for an additional year. One-year placebo-subtracted mean weight loss was 5.8 kg for liraglutide and 3.8 kg more than those on orlistat. The most common side effects were nausea, vomiting, and change in bowel habits.

Bariatric surgery (Fig. 416-2) can be considered for patients with severe obesity (BMI, ≥40 kg/m^2) or for those with moderate obesity (BMI, ≥35 kg/m^2) associated with a serious medical condition. Weight loss surgeries have traditionally been classified into three categories on the basis of anatomic changes: restrictive, restrictive malabsorptive, and malabsorptive. More recently, however, the clinical benefits of bariatric surgery in achieving weight loss and alleviating metabolic comorbidities have been attributed largely to changes in the physiologic responses of gut hormones and in adipose tissue metabolism. Metabolic effects resulting from bypassing the foregut include altered responses of ghrelin, glucagon-like peptide 1, peptide YY3-36, and oxyntonodulin. Additional effects on food intake and body weight control may be attributed to changes in vagal signaling. The loss of fat mass, particularly visceral fat, is associated with multiple metabolic, adipokine, and inflammatory changes that include improved insulin sensitivity and glucose disposal; reduced free fatty acid flux; increased adiponectin levels; and decreased interleukin 6, tumor necrosis factor α, and high-sensitivity C-reactive protein levels.

Restrictive surgeries limit the amount of food the stomach can hold and slow the rate of gastric emptying. *Laparoscopic adjustable gastric banding* is the prototype of this category. The first banding device, the LAP-BAND, was approved for use in the United States in 2001 and the second, the REALIZE band, in 2007. In contrast to previous devices, these bands have diameters that are adjustable by way of their connection to a reservoir that is implanted under the skin. Injection of saline into the reservoir and removal of saline from the reservoir tighten and loosen the band's internal diameter, respectively, thus changing the size of the gastric opening. The mean percentage of total body weight lost at 5 years is estimated at 20–25%. In *laparoscopic sleeve gastrectomy*, the stomach is restricted by stapling and dividing it vertically, removing ~80% of the greater curvature, and leaving a slim banana-shaped remnant stomach along the lesser curvature. Weight loss after this procedure is superior to that after laparoscopic adjustable gastric banding.

The three restrictive-malabsorptive bypass procedures combine the elements of gastric restriction and selective malabsorption. These procedures are Roux-en-Y gastric bypass, biliopancreatic diversion, and biliopancreatic diversion with duodenal switch (Fig. 416-2). Roux-en-Y is the most commonly undertaken and most accepted bypass procedure. It may be performed with an open incision or by laparoscopy.

These procedures generally produce a 30–35% average total body weight loss that is maintained in nearly 60% of patients at 5 years. In general, mean weight loss is greater after the combined restrictive-malabsorptive procedures than after the restrictive procedures. Significant improvement in multiple obesity-related comorbid conditions, including type 2 diabetes, hypertension, dyslipidemia, obstructive sleep apnea, quality of life, and long-term cardiovascular events, has been reported. A meta-analysis of controlled clinical trials comparing bariatric surgery versus no surgery showed that surgery was associated with a reduced odds ratio (OR) risk of global mortality (OR = 0.55), cardiovascular death (OR = 0.58), and all-cause mortality (OR = 0.70).

Among the observed improvements in comorbidities, the prevention and treatment of type 2 diabetes resulting from bariatric surgery has garnered the most attention. Fifteen-year data from the Swedish Obese Subjects study demonstrated a marked reduction (i.e., by 78%) in the incidence of type 2 diabetes development among obese patients who underwent bariatric surgery. Several randomized controlled studies have shown greater weight loss and more improved glycemic control at 1 and 2 years among surgical patients than among patients receiving conventional medical therapy. A retrospective cohort study of more than 4000 adults with diabetes found that, overall, 68.2% of patients experienced an initial complete type 2 diabetes remission within 5 years after surgery. However, among these patients, one-third redeveloped type 2 diabetes within 5 years. The rapid improvement seen in diabetes after restrictive-malabsorptive procedures is thought to be due to surgery-specific, weight-independent effects on glucose homeostasis brought about by alteration of gut hormones.

The mortality rate from bariatric surgery is generally <1% but varies with the procedure, the patient's age and comorbid conditions, and the experience of the surgical team. The most common surgical complications include stomal stenosis or marginal ulcers (occurring in 5–15% of patients) that present as prolonged nausea and vomiting after eating or inability to advance the diet to solid foods. These complications typically are treated by endoscopic balloon dilation and acid suppression therapy, respectively. For patients who undergo laparoscopic adjustable gastric banding, there are no intestinal absorptive abnormalities other than mechanical reduction in gastric size and outflow. Therefore, selective deficiencies are uncommon unless eating habits become unbalanced. In contrast, the restrictive-malabsorptive procedures carry an increased risk for micronutrient deficiencies of vitamin B_{12}, iron, folate, calcium, and vitamin D. Patients with restrictive-malabsorptive procedures require lifelong supplementation with these micronutrients.

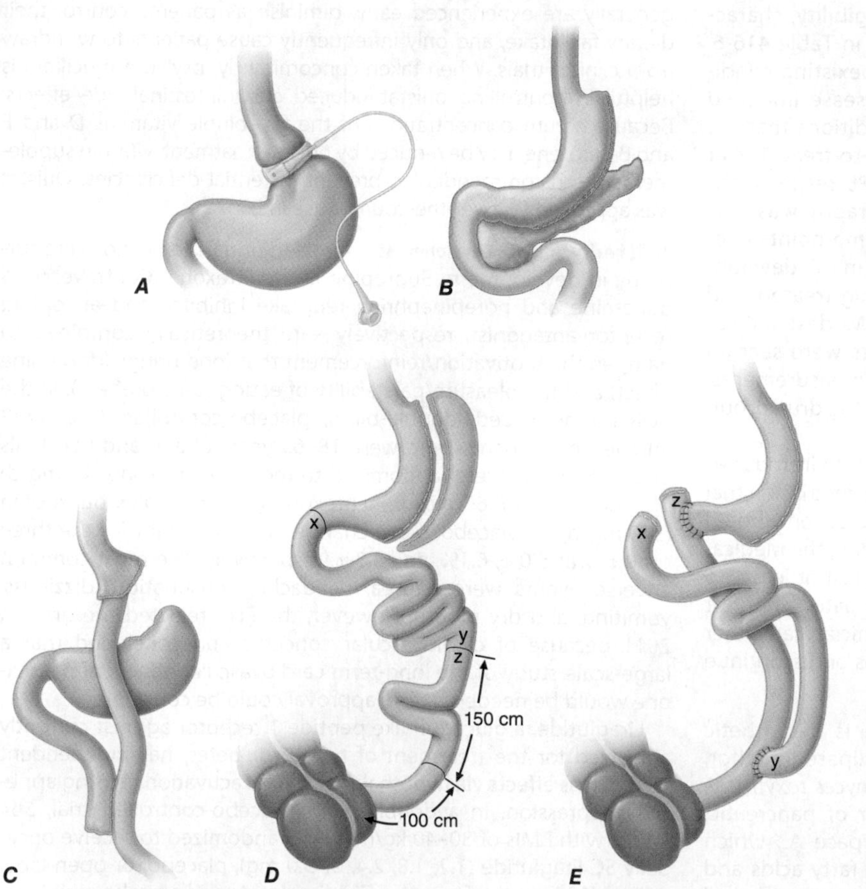

FIGURE 416-2 Bariatric surgical procedures. Examples of operative interventions used for surgical manipulation of the gastrointestinal tract. ***A.*** Laparoscopic adjustable gastric banding. ***B.*** Laparoscopic sleeve gastrectomy. ***C.*** The Roux-en-Y gastric bypass. ***D.*** Biliopancreatic diversion with duodenal switch. ***E.*** Biliopancreatic diversion. *(From ML Kendrick, GF Dakin: Mayo Clin Proc 815:518, 2006; with permission.)*

417 Diabetes Mellitus: Diagnosis, Classification, and Pathophysiology

Alvin C. Powers

Diabetes mellitus (DM) refers to a group of common metabolic disorders that share the phenotype of hyperglycemia. Several distinct types of DM are caused by a complex interaction of genetics and environmental factors. Depending on the etiology of the DM, factors contributing to hyperglycemia include reduced insulin secretion, decreased glucose utilization, and increased glucose production. The metabolic dysregulation associated with DM causes secondary pathophysiologic changes in multiple organ systems that impose a tremendous burden on the individual with diabetes and on the health care system. In the United States, DM is the leading cause of end-stage renal disease (ESRD), nontraumatic lower extremity amputations, and adult blindness. It also predisposes to cardiovascular diseases. With an increasing incidence worldwide, DM will be likely a leading cause of morbidity and mortality in the future.

CLASSIFICATION

DM is classified on the basis of the pathogenic process that leads to hyperglycemia, as opposed to earlier criteria such as age of onset or type of therapy (Fig. 417-1). There are two broad categories of DM, designated type 1 and type 2 (Table 417-1). However, there is increasing recognition of other forms of diabetes in which the pathogenesis is better understood. These other forms of diabetes may share features of type 1 and/or type 2 DM. Both type 1 and type 2 DM are preceded by a phase of abnormal glucose homeostasis as the pathogenic processes progress. Type 1 DM is the result of complete or near-total insulin deficiency. Type 2 DM is a heterogeneous group of disorders characterized by variable degrees of insulin resistance, impaired insulin secretion, and increased glucose production. Distinct genetic and metabolic defects in insulin action and/or secretion give rise to the common phenotype of hyperglycemia in type 2 DM and have important potential therapeutic implications now that pharmacologic agents are available to target specific metabolic derangements. Type 2 DM is preceded by a period of abnormal glucose homeostasis classified as impaired fasting glucose (IFG) or impaired glucose tolerance (IGT).

Two features of the current classification of DM merit emphasis from previous classifications. First, the terms *insulin-dependent diabetes mellitus* (IDDM) and *non-insulin-dependent diabetes mellitus* (NIDDM) are obsolete. Because many individuals with type 2 DM eventually require insulin treatment for control of

		Hyperglycemia			
		Pre-diabetes*	Diabetes Mellitus		
Type of Diabetes	Normal glucose tolerance	Impaired fasting glucose or impaired glucose tolerance	Not insulin requiring	Insulin required for control	Insulin required for survival
Type 1					
Type 2					
Other specific types					
Gestational Diabetes					
Time (years)					
FPG	<5.6 mmol/L (100 mg/dL)	5.6–6.9 mmol/L (100–125 mg/dL)	≥7.0 mmol/L (126 mg/dL)		
2-h PG	<7.8 mmol/L (140 mg/dL)	7.8–11.0 mmol/L (140–199 mg/dL)	≥11.1 mmol/L (200 mg/dL)		
HbA1C	<5.6%	5.7–6.4%	≥6.5%		

FIGURE 417-1 Spectrum of glucose homeostasis and diabetes mellitus (DM). The spectrum from normal glucose tolerance to diabetes in type 1 DM, type 2 DM, other specific types of diabetes, and gestational DM is shown from left to right. In most types of DM, the individual traverses from normal glucose tolerance to impaired glucose tolerance to overt diabetes (these should be viewed not as abrupt categories but as a spectrum). *Arrows* indicate that changes in glucose tolerance may be bidirectional in some types of diabetes. For example, individuals with type 2 DM may return to the impaired glucose tolerance category with weight loss; in gestational DM, diabetes may revert to impaired glucose tolerance or even normal glucose tolerance after delivery. The fasting plasma glucose (FPG), the 2-h plasma glucose (PG) after a glucose challenge, and the hemoglobin A_{1c} (HbA_{1c}) for the different categories of glucose tolerance are shown at the lower part of the figure. These values do not apply to the diagnosis of gestational DM. Some types of DM may or may not require insulin for survival. *Some use the term *increased risk for diabetes* or *intermediate hyperglycemia* (World Health Organization) rather than *prediabetes*. (*Adapted from the American Diabetes Association, 2014.*)

TABLE 417-1 ETIOLOGIC CLASSIFICATION OF DIABETES MELLITUS

I. Type 1 diabetes (beta cell destruction, usually leading to absolute insulin deficiency)
   - A. Immune-mediated
   - B. Idiopathic

II. Type 2 diabetes (may range from predominantly insulin resistance with relative insulin deficiency to a predominantly insulin secretory defect with insulin resistance)

III. Other specific types of diabetes
   - A. Genetic defects of beta cell development or function characterized by mutations in:
     1. Hepatocyte nuclear transcription factor (HNF) 4α (MODY 1)
     2. Glucokinase (MODY 2)
     3. HNF-1α (MODY 3)
     4. Insulin promoter factor-1 (IPF-1; MODY 4)
     5. HNF-1β (MODY 5)
     6. NeuroD1 (MODY 6)
     7. Mitochondrial DNA
     8. Subunits of ATP-sensitive potassium channel
     9. Proinsulin or insulin
     10. Other pancreatic islet regulators/proteins such as *KLF11, PAX4, BLK, GATA4, GATA6, SLC2A2* (GLUT2), *RFX6, GLIS3*
   - B. Genetic defects in insulin action
     1. Type A insulin resistance
     2. Leprechaunism
     3. Rabson-Mendenhall syndrome
     4. Lipodystrophy syndromes
   - C. Diseases of the exocrine pancreas—pancreatitis, pancreatectomy, neoplasia, cystic fibrosis, hemochromatosis, fibrocalculous pancreatopathy, mutations in carboxyl ester lipase
   - D. Endocrinopathies—acromegaly, Cushing's syndrome, glucagonoma, pheochromocytoma, hyperthyroidism, somatostatinoma, aldosteronoma
   - E. Drug- or chemical-induced—glucocorticoids, vacor (a rodenticide), pentamidine, nicotinic acid, diazoxide, β-adrenergic agonists, thiazides, calcineurin and mTOR inhibitors, hydantoins, asparaginase, α-interferon, protease inhibitors, antipsychotics (atypicals and others), epinephrine
   - F. Infections—congenital rubella, cytomegalovirus, coxsackievirus
   - G. Uncommon forms of immune-mediated diabetes—"stiff-person" syndrome, anti-insulin receptor antibodies
   - H. Other genetic syndromes sometimes associated with diabetes—Wolfram's syndrome, Down's syndrome, Klinefelter's syndrome, Turner's syndrome, Friedreich's ataxia, Huntington's chorea, Laurence-Moon-Biedl syndrome, myotonic dystrophy, porphyria, Prader-Willi syndrome

IV. Gestational diabetes mellitus (GDM)

Abbreviation: MODY, maturity-onset diabetes of the young.

Source: Adapted from American Diabetes Association: Diabetes Care 37(Suppl 1):S14, 2014.

glycemia, the use of the term NIDDM generated considerable confusion. A second difference is that age or treatment modality is not a criterion. Although type 1 DM most commonly develops before the age of 30, an autoimmune beta cell destructive process can develop at any age. It is estimated that between 5 and 10% of individuals who develop DM after age 30 years have type 1 DM. Although type 2 DM more typically develops with increasing age, it is now being diagnosed more frequently in children and young adults, particularly in obese adolescents.

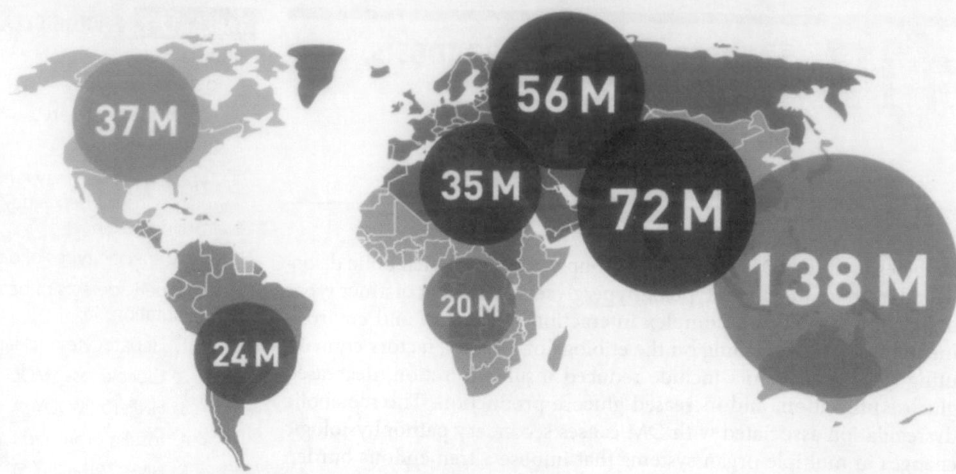

FIGURE 417-2 Worldwide prevalence of diabetes mellitus. Global estimate is 382 million individuals with diabetes. Regional estimates of the number of individuals with diabetes (20–79 years of age) are shown (2013). *(Used with permission from the IDF Diabetes Atlas, the International Diabetes Federation, 2013.)*

OTHER TYPES OF DM

Other etiologies for DM include specific genetic defects in insulin secretion or action, metabolic abnormalities that impair insulin secretion, mitochondrial abnormalities, and a host of conditions that impair glucose tolerance (Table 417-1). *Maturity-onset diabetes of the young* (MODY) and *monogenic diabetes* are subtypes of DM characterized by autosomal dominant inheritance, early onset of hyperglycemia (usually <25 years; sometimes in neonatal period), and impaired insulin secretion (discussed below). Mutations in the insulin receptor cause a group of rare disorders characterized by severe insulin resistance.

DM can result from pancreatic exocrine disease when the majority of pancreatic islets are destroyed. Cystic fibrosis–related DM is an important consideration in that patient population. Hormones that antagonize insulin action can also lead to DM. Thus, DM is often a feature of endocrinopathies such as acromegaly and Cushing's disease. Viral infections have been implicated in pancreatic islet destruction but are an extremely rare cause of DM. A form of acute onset of type 1 diabetes, termed *fulminant diabetes*, has been noted in Japan and may be related to viral infection of islets.

GESTATIONAL DIABETES MELLITUS

Glucose intolerance developing during pregnancy is classified as gestational diabetes mellitus (GDM). Insulin resistance is related to the metabolic changes of late pregnancy, and the increased insulin requirements may lead to IGT or diabetes. GDM occurs in ~7% (range 1–14%) of pregnancies in the United States; most women revert to normal glucose tolerance postpartum but have a substantial risk (35–60%) of developing DM in the next 10–20 years. The International Association of the Diabetes and Pregnancy Study Groups and the American Diabetes Association (ADA) recommend that diabetes diagnosed at the initial prenatal visit should be classified as "overt" diabetes rather than GDM. With the rising rates of obesity, the number of women being diagnosed with GDM or overt diabetes is rising worldwide.

EPIDEMIOLOGY AND GLOBAL CONSIDERATIONS

The worldwide prevalence of DM has risen dramatically over the past two decades, from an estimated 30 million cases in 1985 to 382 million in 2013 (Fig. 417-2). Based on current trends, the International Diabetes Federation projects that 592 million individuals will have diabetes by the year 2035 (see *http://www.idf.org/*). Although the prevalence of both type 1 and type 2 DM is increasing worldwide, the prevalence of type 2 DM is rising much more rapidly, presumably because of increasing obesity, reduced activity levels as countries become more industrialized, and the aging of the population. In 2013, the prevalence of diabetes in individuals from age 20–79 ranged from 23 to 37% in the 10 countries with the highest prevalence (Tuvalu, Federated States of Micronesia, Marshall Islands, Kiribati, Vanuatu, Cook Islands, Saudi Arabia, Nauru, Kuwait, and Qatar, in descending order of prevalence). The countries with the greatest number of individuals with diabetes in 2013 are China (98.4 million), India (65.1 million), United States (24.4 million), Brazil (11.9 million), and the Russian Federation (10.9 million). Up to 80% of individuals with diabetes live in low-income or medium-income countries. In the most recent estimate for the United States (2012), the Centers for Disease Control and Prevention (CDC) estimated that 9.3% of the population had diabetes (~28% of the individuals with diabetes were undiagnosed; globally, it is estimated that 50% of individuals may be undiagnosed). The CDC estimated that the incidence and prevalence of diabetes doubled from 1990–2008, but appears to have plateaued from 2008–2012. DM increases with age. In 2012, the prevalence of DM in the United Sates was estimated to be 0.2% in individuals age <20 years and 12% in individuals age >20 years. In individuals age >65 years, the prevalence of DM was 26.9%. The prevalence is similar in men and women throughout most age ranges (14% and 11%, respectively, in individuals age >20 years). Worldwide, most individuals with diabetes are between the ages of 40 and 59 years.

There is considerable geographic variation in the incidence of both type 1 and type 2 DM. Scandinavia has the highest incidence of type 1 DM; the lowest incidence is in the Pacific Rim where it is 20- to 30-fold lower. Northern Europe and the United States have an intermediate rate. Much of the increased risk of type 1 DM is believed to reflect the frequency of high-risk human leukocyte antigen (HLA) alleles among ethnic groups in different geographic locations. The prevalence of type 2 DM and its harbinger, IGT, is highest in certain Pacific islands and the Middle East and intermediate in countries such as India and the United States. This variability is likely due to genetic, behavioral, and environmental factors. DM prevalence also varies among different ethnic populations within a given country, with indigenous populations usually having a greater incidence of diabetes than the general population of the country. For example, the CDC estimated that the age-adjusted prevalence of DM in the United States (age >20 years; 2010–2012) was 8% in non-Hispanic whites, 9% in Asian Americans, 13% in Hispanics, 13% in non-Hispanic blacks, and 16% in American-Indian and Alaskan native populations. The onset of type 2 DM occurs, on average, at an earlier age in ethnic groups other than non-Hispanic whites. In Asia, the prevalence of diabetes is increasing rapidly, and the diabetes phenotype appears to be somewhat different from that in the United States and Europe, with an onset at a lower body mass index (BMI) and younger age, greater visceral adiposity, and reduced insulin secretory capacity.

Diabetes is a major cause of mortality, but several studies indicate that diabetes is likely underreported as a cause of death. In the United States, diabetes was listed as the seventh leading cause of death in 2010. A recent estimate suggested that diabetes was responsible for almost 5.1 million deaths or 8% of deaths worldwide in 2013. In 2013, it was estimated that $548 billion or 11% of health care expenditures worldwide were spent on individuals with diabetes.

TABLE 417-2 CRITERIA FOR THE DIAGNOSIS OF DIABETES MELLITUS

- Symptoms of diabetes plus random blood glucose concentration ≥11.1 mmol/L (200 mg/dL)[a] *or*
- Fasting plasma glucose ≥7.0 mmol/L (126 mg/dL)[b] *or*
- Hemoglobin A_{1c} ≥ 6.5%[c] *or*
- 2-h plasma glucose ≥11.1 mmol/L (200 mg/dL) during an oral glucose tolerance test[d]

[a]Random is defined as without regard to time since the last meal. [b]Fasting is defined as no caloric intake for at least 8 h. [c]Hemoglobin A_{1c} test should be performed in a laboratory using a method approved by the National Glycohemoglobin Standardization Program and correlated to the reference assay of the Diabetes Control and Complications Trial. Point-of-care hemoglobin A_{1c} should not be used for diagnostic purposes. [d]The test should be performed using a glucose load containing the equivalent of 75 g anhydrous glucose dissolved in water, not recommended for routine clinical use.

Note: In the absence of unequivocal hyperglycemia and acute metabolic decompensation, these criteria should be confirmed by repeat testing on a different day.

Source: Adapted from American Diabetes Association: Diabetes Care 37(Suppl 1):S14, 2014.

DIAGNOSIS

Glucose tolerance is classified into three broad categories: normal glucose homeostasis, DM, or impaired glucose homeostasis. Glucose tolerance can be assessed using the fasting plasma glucose (FPG), the response to oral glucose challenge, or the hemoglobin A_{1c} (HbA_{1c}). An FPG <5.6 mmol/L (100 mg/dL), a plasma glucose <140 mg/dL (11.1 mmol/L) following an oral glucose challenge, and an HbA_{1c} <5.7% are considered to define normal glucose tolerance. The International Expert Committee with members appointed by the ADA, the European Association for the Study of Diabetes, and the International Diabetes Federation have issued diagnostic criteria for DM (Table 417-2) based on the following premises: (1) the FPG, the response to an oral glucose challenge (oral glucose tolerance test [OGTT]), and HbA_{1c} differ among individuals, and (2) DM is defined as the level of glycemia at which diabetes-specific complications occur rather than on deviations from a population-based mean. For example, the prevalence of retinopathy in Native Americans (Pima Indian population) begins to increase at an FPG >6.4 mmol/L (116 mg/dL) (Fig. 417-3).

An FPG ≥7.0 mmol/L (126 mg/dL), a glucose ≥11.1 mmol/L (200 mg/dL) 2 h after an oral glucose challenge, or an HbA_{1c} ≥6.5% warrants the diagnosis of DM (Table 417-2). A random plasma glucose concentration ≥11.1 mmol/L (200 mg/dL) accompanied by classic symptoms of DM (polyuria, polydipsia, weight loss) is also sufficient for the diagnosis of DM (Table 417-2).

Abnormal glucose homeostasis (Fig. 417-1) is defined as (1) FPG = 5.6–6.9 mmol/L (100–125 mg/dL), which is defined as *impaired fasting glucose* (IFG); (2) plasma glucose levels between 7.8 and 11 mmol/L (140 and 199 mg/dL) following an oral glucose challenge, which is termed *impaired glucose tolerance* (IGT); or (3) HbA_{1c} of 5.7–6.4%. An HbA_{1c} of 5.7–6.4%, IFG, and IGT do not identify the same individuals, but individuals in all three groups are at greater risk of progressing to type 2 DM, have an increased risk of cardiovascular disease, and should be counseled about ways to decrease these risks (see below). Some use the terms *prediabetes*, *increased risk of diabetes*, or *intermediate hyperglycemia* (World Health Organization) for this category. These values for the fasting plasma glucose, the glucose following an oral glucose challenge, and HbA_{1c} are continuous variables and not discrete categories. The current criteria for the diagnosis of DM emphasize the HbA_{1c} or the FPG as the most reliable and convenient tests for identifying DM in asymptomatic individuals (however, some individuals may meet criteria for one test but not the other). OGTT, although still a valid means for diagnosing DM, is not often used in routine clinical care.

The diagnosis of DM has profound implications for an individual from both a medical and a financial standpoint. Thus, abnormalities on screening tests for diabetes should be repeated before making a definitive diagnosis of DM, unless acute metabolic derangements or a markedly elevated plasma glucose are present (Table 417-2). These criteria also allow for the diagnosis of DM to be withdrawn in situations when the glucose intolerance reverts to normal.

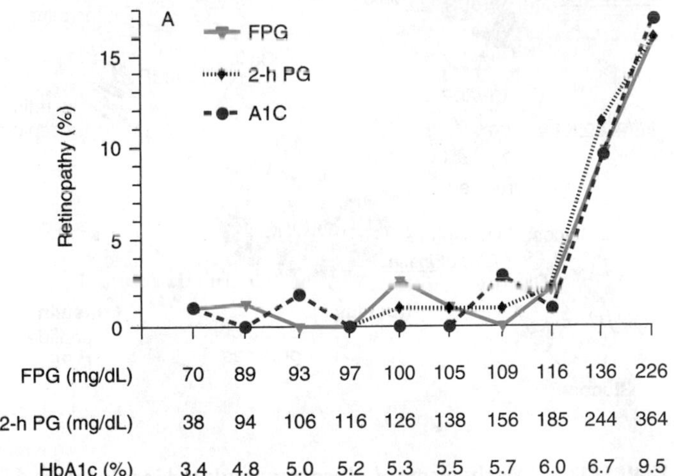

FIGURE 417-3 Relationship of diabetes-specific complication and glucose tolerance. This figure shows the incidence of retinopathy in Pima Indians as a function of the fasting plasma glucose (FPG), the 2-h plasma glucose after a 75-g oral glucose challenge (2-h PG), or the hemoglobin A_{1c} (HbA_{1c}). Note that the incidence of retinopathy greatly increases at a fasting plasma glucose >116 mg/dL, a 2-h plasma glucose of 185 mg/dL, or an HbA_{1c} >6.5%. (Blood glucose values are shown in mg/dL; to convert to mmol/L, divide value by 18.) *(Copyright 2002, American Diabetes Association. From Diabetes Care 25[Suppl 1]: S5–S20, 2002.)*

SCREENING

Widespread use of the FPG or the HbA_{1c} as a screening test for type 2 DM is recommended because (1) a large number of individuals who meet the current criteria for DM are asymptomatic and unaware that they have the disorder, (2) epidemiologic studies suggest that type 2 DM may be present for up to a decade before diagnosis, (3) some individuals with type 2 DM have one or more diabetes-specific complications at the time of their diagnosis, (4) treatment of type 2 DM may favorably alter the natural history of DM, diagnosis of prediabetes should spur efforts for diabetes prevention. The ADA recommends screening all individuals >45 years every 3 years and screening individuals at an earlier age if they are overweight (BMI >25 kg/m^2 or ethnically relevant definition for overweight) and have one additional risk factor for diabetes (Table 417-3). In contrast to type 2 DM, a long asymptomatic period of hyperglycemia is rare prior to the diagnosis of type 1 DM. A number of immunologic markers for type 1 DM are becoming available (discussed below), but their routine use outside a clinical trial is discouraged, pending the identification of clinically beneficial interventions for individuals at high risk for developing type 1 DM.

TABLE 417-3 RISK FACTORS FOR TYPE 2 DIABETES MELLITUS

Family history of diabetes (i.e., parent or sibling with type 2 diabetes)
Obesity (BMI ≥25 kg/m^2 or ethnically relevant definition for overweight)
Physical inactivity
Race/ethnicity (e.g., African American, Latino, Native American, Asian American, Pacific Islander)
Previously identified with IFG, IGT, or an hemoglobin A_{1c} of 5.7–6.4%
History of GDM or delivery of baby >4 kg (9 lb)
Hypertension (blood pressure ≥140/90 mmHg)
HDL cholesterol level <35 mg/dL (0.90 mmol/L) and/or a triglyceride level >250 mg/dL (2.82 mmol/L)
Polycystic ovary syndrome or acanthosis nigricans
History of cardiovascular disease

Abbreviations: BMI, body mass index; GDM, gestational diabetes mellitus; HDL, high-density lipoprotein; IFG, impaired fasting glucose; IGT, impaired glucose tolerance.

Source: Adapted from American Diabetes Association: Diabetes Care 37(Suppl 1):S14, 2014.

OVERALL REGULATION OF GLUCOSE HOMEOSTASIS

Glucose homeostasis reflects a balance between hepatic glucose production and peripheral glucose uptake and utilization. Insulin is the most important regulator of this metabolic equilibrium, but neural input, metabolic signals, and other hormones (e.g., glucagon) result in integrated control of glucose supply and utilization (Fig. 417-4). The organs that regulate glucose and lipids communicate by neural and humoral mechanisms with fat and muscle producing adipokines, myokines, and metabolites that influence liver function. In the fasting state, low insulin levels increase glucose production by promoting hepatic gluconeogenesis and glycogenolysis and reduce glucose uptake in insulin-sensitive tissues (skeletal muscle and fat), thereby promoting mobilization of stored precursors such as amino acids and free fatty acids (lipolysis). Glucagon, secreted by pancreatic alpha cells when blood glucose or insulin levels are low, stimulates glycogenolysis and gluconeogenesis by the liver and renal medulla (Chap. 420). Postprandially, the glucose load elicits a rise in insulin and fall in glucagon, leading to a reversal of these processes. Insulin, an anabolic hormone, promotes the storage of carbohydrate and fat and protein synthesis. The major portion of postprandial glucose is used by skeletal muscle, an effect of insulin-stimulated glucose uptake. Other tissues, most notably the brain, use glucose in an insulin-independent fashion. Factors secreted by skeletal myocytes (irisin), adipocytes (leptin, resistin, adiponectin, etc.), and bone also influence glucose homeostasis.

INSULIN BIOSYNTHESIS

Insulin is produced in the beta cells of the pancreatic islets. It is initially synthesized as a single-chain 86-amino-acid precursor polypeptide, preproinsulin. Subsequent proteolytic processing removes the amino-terminal signal peptide, giving rise to proinsulin. Proinsulin is structurally related to insulin-like growth factors I and II, which bind weakly to the insulin receptor. Cleavage of an internal 31-residue fragment from proinsulin generates the C peptide and the A (21 amino acids) and B (30 amino acids) chains of insulin, which are connected by disulfide bonds. The mature insulin molecule and C peptide are stored together and co-secreted from secretory granules in the beta cells. Because C peptide is cleared more slowly than insulin, it is a useful marker of insulin secretion and allows discrimination of endogenous and exogenous sources of insulin in the evaluation of hypoglycemia (Chaps. 420 and 113). Pancreatic beta cells co-secrete islet amyloid polypeptide (IAPP) or amylin, a 37-amino-acid peptide, along with insulin. The role of IAPP in normal physiology is incompletely defined, but it is the major component of the amyloid fibrils found in the islets of patients with type 2 diabetes, and an analogue is sometimes used in treating type 1 and type 2 DM. Human insulin is produced by recombinant DNA technology; structural alterations at one or more amino acid residues modify its physical and pharmacologic characteristics (Chap. 418).

INSULIN SECRETION

Glucose is the key regulator of insulin secretion by the pancreatic beta cell, although amino acids, ketones, various nutrients, gastrointestinal peptides, and neurotransmitters also influence insulin secretion. Glucose levels >3.9 mmol/L (70 mg/dL) stimulate insulin synthesis, primarily by enhancing protein translation and processing. Glucose stimulation of insulin secretion begins with its transport into the beta cell by a facilitative glucose transporter (Fig. 417-5). Glucose phosphorylation by glucokinase is the rate-limiting step that controls glucose-regulated insulin secretion. Further metabolism of glucose-6-phosphate via glycolysis generates ATP, which inhibits the activity of an ATP-sensitive K^+ channel. This channel consists of two separate proteins: one is the binding site for certain oral hypoglycemics (e.g., sulfonylureas, meglitinides); the other is an inwardly rectifying K^+ channel protein (Kir6.2). Inhibition of this K^+ channel induces beta cell membrane depolarization, which opens voltage-dependent calcium channels (leading to an influx of calcium) and stimulates insulin secretion. Insulin secretory profiles reveal a pulsatile pattern of hormone release, with small secretory bursts occurring about every 10 min, superimposed upon greater amplitude oscillations of about 80–150 min. Incretins are released from neuroendocrine cells of the gastrointestinal tract following food ingestion and amplify glucose-stimulated insulin secretion and suppress glucagon secretion. Glucagon-like peptide 1 (GLP-1), the most potent incretin, is released from L cells in the small intestine and stimulates insulin secretion only when the blood glucose is above the fasting level. Incretin analogues or pharmacologic agents that prolong the activity of endogenous GLP-1 enhance insulin secretion.

INSULIN ACTION

Once insulin is secreted into the portal venous system, ~50% is removed and degraded by the liver. Unextracted insulin enters the

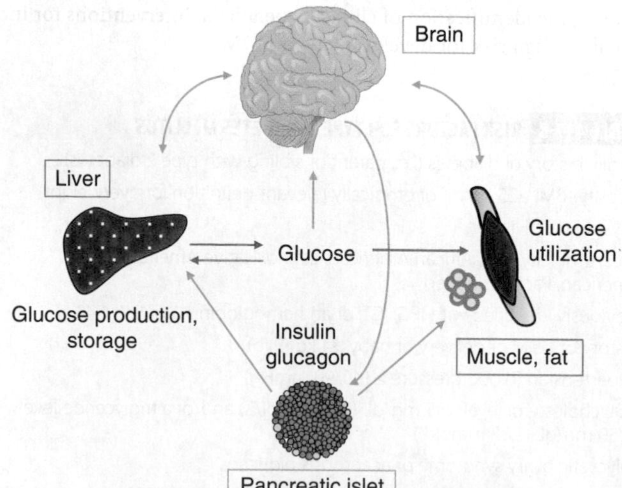

FIGURE 417-4 Regulation of glucose homeostasis. The organs shown contribute to glucose utilization, production, or storage. See text for a description of the communications (*arrows*), which can be neural or humoral.

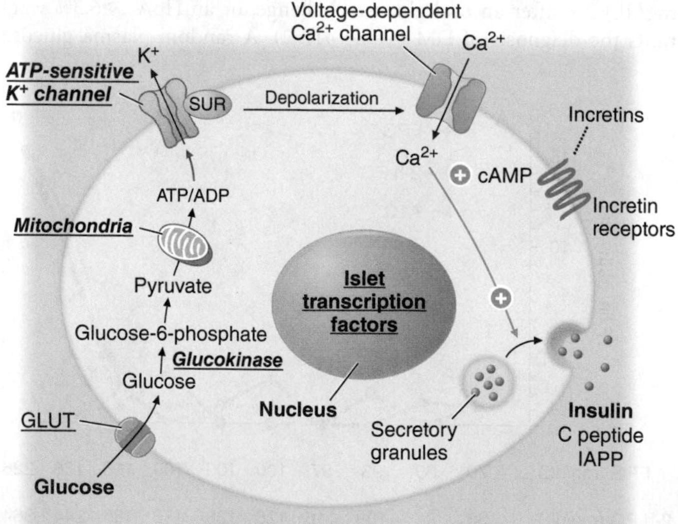

FIGURE 417-5 Mechanisms of glucose-stimulated insulin secretion and abnormalities in diabetes. Glucose and other nutrients regulate insulin secretion by the pancreatic beta cell. Glucose is transported by a glucose transporter (GLUT1 and/or GLUT2 in humans, GLUT2 in rodents); subsequent glucose metabolism by the beta cell alters ion channel activity, leading to insulin secretion. The SUR receptor is the binding site for some drugs that act as insulin secretagogues. Mutations in the events or proteins underlined are a cause of monogenic forms of diabetes. ADP, adenosine diphosphate; ATP, adenosine triphosphate; cAMP, cyclic adenosine monophosphate; IAPP, islet amyloid polypeptide or amylin; SUR, sulfonylurea receptor.

systemic circulation where it binds to receptors in target sites. Insulin binding to its receptor stimulates intrinsic tyrosine kinase activity, leading to receptor autophosphorylation and the recruitment of intracellular signaling molecules, such as insulin receptor substrates (IRS). IRS and other adaptor proteins initiate a complex cascade of phosphorylation and dephosphorylation reactions, resulting in the widespread metabolic and mitogenic effects of insulin. As an example, activation of the phosphatidylinositol-3′-kinase (PI-3-kinase) pathway stimulates translocation of a facilitative glucose transporter (e.g., GLUT4) to the cell surface, an event that is crucial for glucose uptake by skeletal muscle and fat. Activation of other insulin receptor signaling pathways induces glycogen synthesis, protein synthesis, lipogenesis, and regulation of various genes in insulin-responsive cells.

PATHOGENESIS

TYPE 1 DM

Type 1 DM is the result of interactions of genetic, environmental, and immunologic factors that ultimately lead to the destruction of the pancreatic beta cells and insulin deficiency. Type 1 DM, which can develop at any age, develops most commonly before 20 years of age. Worldwide, the incidence of type 1 DM is increasing at the rate of 3–4% per year for uncertain reasons. Type 1 DM results from autoimmune beta cell destruction, and most, but not all, individuals have evidence of islet-directed autoimmunity. Some individuals who have the clinical phenotype of type 1 DM lack immunologic markers indicative of an autoimmune process involving the beta cells and the genetic markers of type 1 DM. These individuals are thought to develop insulin deficiency by unknown, nonimmune mechanisms and may be ketosis prone; many are African American or Asian in heritage. The temporal development of type 1 DM is shown schematically as a function of beta cell mass in Fig. 417-6. Individuals with a genetic susceptibility are thought to have normal beta cell mass at birth but begin to lose beta cells secondary to autoimmune destruction that occurs over months to years. This autoimmune process is thought to be triggered by an infectious or environmental stimulus and to be sustained by a beta cell–specific molecule. In the majority of patients, immunologic markers appear after the triggering event but before diabetes becomes clinically overt. Beta cell mass then begins to decrease, and insulin secretion progressively declines, although normal glucose tolerance is maintained. The rate of decline in beta cell mass varies widely among individuals, with some patients progressing rapidly to clinical diabetes and others evolving more slowly. Features of diabetes do not become evident until a majority of beta cells are destroyed (70–80%). At this point, residual functional beta cells exist but are insufficient in number to maintain glucose tolerance. The events that trigger the transition from glucose intolerance to frank diabetes are often associated with increased insulin requirements, as might occur during infections or puberty. After the initial clinical presentation of type 1 DM, a "honeymoon" phase may ensue during which time glycemic control is achieved with modest doses of insulin or, rarely, insulin is not needed. However, this fleeting phase of endogenous insulin production from residual beta cells disappears and the individual becomes insulin deficient. Many individuals with long-standing type 1 DM produce a small amount of insulin (as reflected by C-peptide production), and some individuals with more than 50 years of type 1 DM have insulin-positive cells in the pancreas at autopsy.

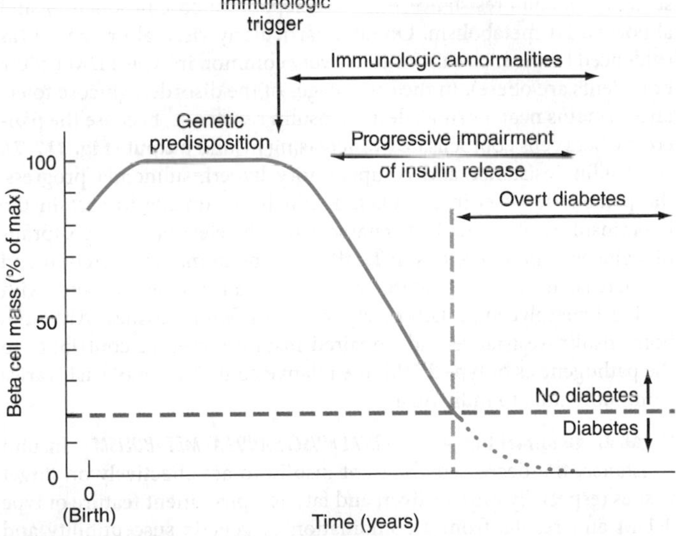

FIGURE 417-6 Temporal model for development of type 1 diabetes. Individuals with a genetic predisposition are exposed to a trigger that initiates an autoimmune process, resulting in a gradual decline in beta cell mass. The downward slope of the beta cell mass varies among individuals and may not be continuous. This progressive impairment in insulin release results in diabetes when ~80% of the beta cell mass is destroyed. A "honeymoon" phase may be seen in the first 1 or 2 years after the onset of diabetes and is associated with reduced insulin requirements. *(Adapted from ER Kaufman: Medical Management of Type 1 Diabetes, 6th ed. American Diabetes Association, Alexandria, VA, 2012.)*

GENETIC CONSIDERATIONS

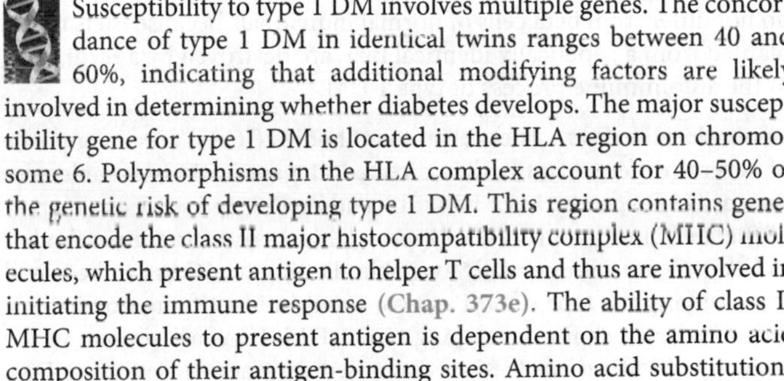

Susceptibility to type 1 DM involves multiple genes. The concordance of type 1 DM in identical twins ranges between 40 and 60%, indicating that additional modifying factors are likely involved in determining whether diabetes develops. The major susceptibility gene for type 1 DM is located in the HLA region on chromosome 6. Polymorphisms in the HLA complex account for 40–50% of the genetic risk of developing type 1 DM. This region contains genes that encode the class II major histocompatibility complex (MHC) molecules, which present antigen to helper T cells and thus are involved in initiating the immune response (Chap. 373e). The ability of class II MHC molecules to present antigen is dependent on the amino acid composition of their antigen-binding sites. Amino acid substitutions may influence the specificity of the immune response by altering the binding affinity of different antigens for class II molecules.

Most individuals with type 1 DM have the HLA DR3 and/or DR4 haplotype. Refinements in genotyping of HLA loci have shown that the haplotypes DQA1*0301, DQB1*0302, and DQB1*0201 are most strongly associated with type 1 DM. These haplotypes are present in 40% of children with type 1 DM as compared to 2% of the normal U.S. population. However, most individuals with predisposing haplotypes do not develop diabetes.

In addition to MHC class II associations, genome association studies have identified at least 20 different genetic loci that contribute susceptibility to type 1 DM (polymorphisms in the promoter region of the insulin gene, the CTLA-4 gene, interleukin 2 receptor, *CTLA4*, and PTPN22, etc.). Genes that confer protection against the development of the disease also exist. The haplotype DQA1*0102, DQB1*0602 is extremely rare in individuals with type 1 DM (<1%) and appears to provide protection from type 1 DM.

Although the risk of developing type 1 DM is increased tenfold in relatives of individuals with the disease, the risk is relatively low: 3–4% if the parent has type 1 DM and 5–15% in a sibling (depending on which HLA haplotypes are shared). Hence, most individuals with type 1 DM do not have a first-degree relative with this disorder.

Pathophysiology Although other islet cell types (alpha cells [glucagon-producing], delta cells [somatostatin-producing], or PP cells [pancreatic polypeptide-producing]) are functionally and embryologically similar to beta cells and express most of the same proteins as beta cells, they are spared from the autoimmune destruction. Pathologically, the pancreatic islets have a modest infiltration of lymphocytes (a process termed *insulitis*). After beta cells are destroyed, it is thought that the inflammatory process abates and the islets become atrophic. Studies of the autoimmune process in humans and in animal models of type 1 DM (NOD mouse and BB rat) have identified the following abnormalities in the humoral and cellular arms of the immune system: (1) islet cell autoantibodies; (2) activated lymphocytes in the islets, peripancreatic lymph nodes, and systemic circulation; (3) T lymphocytes that proliferate when stimulated with islet proteins; and (4) release of cytokines within the insulitis. Beta cells seem to be particularly susceptible to the toxic effect of some cytokines (tumor necrosis factor α [TNF-α], interferon γ, and interleukin 1 [IL-1]). The precise mechanisms of beta cell death are not known but may involve formation of nitric oxide metabolites, apoptosis, and direct CD8+ T cell cytotoxicity. The islet destruction is mediated by T lymphocytes rather than islet autoantibodies, as these antibodies do not generally react with the cell surface of islet cells and are not capable of transferring DM to animals. Efforts to suppress the autoimmune process at the time of diagnosis of diabetes have largely been ineffective or only temporarily effective in slowing beta cell destruction.

Pancreatic islet molecules targeted by the autoimmune process include insulin, glutamic acid decarboxylase (GAD; the biosynthetic enzyme for the neurotransmitter GABA), ICA-512/IA-2 (homology with tyrosine phosphatases), and a beta cell–specific zinc transporter (ZnT-8). Most of the autoantigens are not beta cell–specific, which raises the question of how the beta cells are selectively destroyed. Current theories favor initiation of an autoimmune process directed at one beta cell molecule, which then spreads to other islet molecules as the immune process destroys beta cells and creates a series of secondary autoantigens. The beta cells of individuals who develop type 1 DM do not differ from beta cells of normal individuals because islets transplanted from a genetically identical twin are destroyed by a recurrence of the autoimmune process of type 1 DM.

Immunologic Markers Islet cell autoantibodies (ICAs) are a composite of several different antibodies directed at pancreatic islet molecules such as GAD, insulin, IA-2/ICA-512, and ZnT-8, and serve as a marker of the autoimmune process of type 1 DM. Assays for autoantibodies to GAD-65 are commercially available. Testing for ICAs can be useful in classifying the type of DM as type 1 and in identifying nondiabetic individuals at risk for developing type 1 DM. ICAs are present in the majority of individuals (>85%) diagnosed with new-onset type 1 DM, in a significant minority of individuals with newly diagnosed type 2 DM (5–10%), and occasionally in individuals with GDM (<5%). ICAs are present in 3–4% of first-degree relatives of individuals with type 1 DM. In combination with impaired insulin secretion after IV glucose tolerance testing, they predict a >50% risk of developing type 1 DM within 5 years. At present, the measurement of ICAs in nondiabetic individuals is a research tool because no treatments have been demonstrated to prevent the occurrence or progression to type 1 DM.

Environmental Factors Numerous environmental events have been proposed to trigger the autoimmune process in genetically susceptible individuals; however, none have been conclusively linked to diabetes. Identification of an environmental trigger has been difficult because the event may precede the onset of DM by several years (Fig. 417-6). Putative environmental triggers include viruses (coxsackie, rubella, enteroviruses most prominently), bovine milk proteins, and nitrosourea compounds. There is increasing interest in the microbiome and type 1 diabetes (Chap. 86e).

Prevention of Type 1 DM A number of interventions have prevented diabetes in animal models. None of these interventions have been successful in preventing type 1 DM in humans. For example, the Diabetes Prevention Trial–Type 1 concluded that administering insulin (IV or PO) to individuals at high risk for developing type 1 DM did not prevent type 1 DM. This is an area of active clinical investigation.

TYPE 2 DM

Insulin resistance and abnormal insulin secretion are central to the development of type 2 DM. Although the primary defect is controversial, most studies support the view that insulin resistance precedes an insulin secretory defect but that diabetes develops only when insulin secretion becomes inadequate. Type 2 DM likely encompasses a range of disorders with common phenotype of hyperglycemia. Most of our current understanding (and the discussion below) of the pathophysiology and genetics is based on studies of individuals of European descent. It is becoming increasing apparent that DM in other ethnic groups (Asian, African, and Latin American) has a somewhat different, but yet undefined, pathophysiology. In general, Latinos have greater insulin resistance and East Asians and South Asians have more beta cell dysfunction, but both defects are present in both populations. East and South Asians appear to develop type 2 DM at a younger age and a lower BMI. In some groups, DM that is ketosis prone (often obese) or ketosis-resistant (often lean) is seen.

GENETIC CONSIDERATIONS

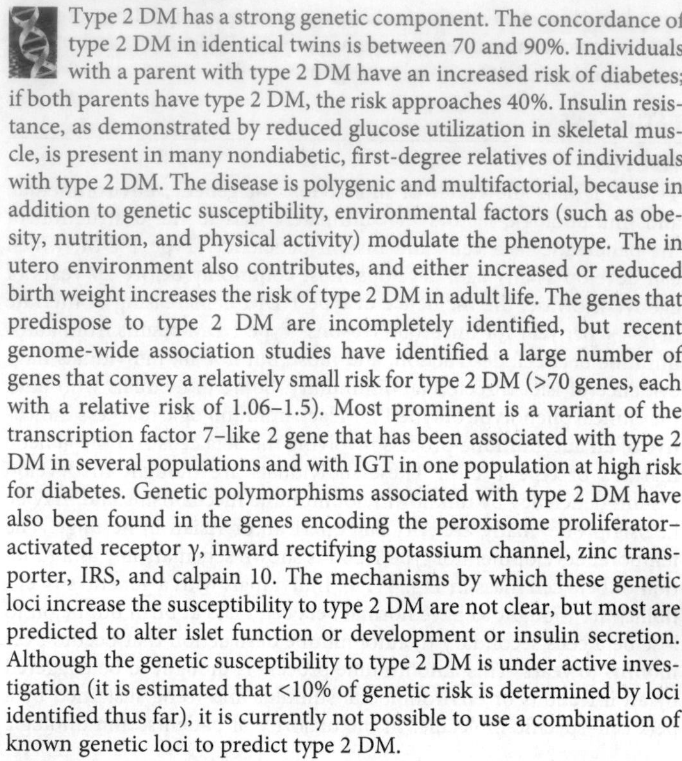

Type 2 DM has a strong genetic component. The concordance of type 2 DM in identical twins is between 70 and 90%. Individuals with a parent with type 2 DM have an increased risk of diabetes; if both parents have type 2 DM, the risk approaches 40%. Insulin resistance, as demonstrated by reduced glucose utilization in skeletal muscle, is present in many nondiabetic, first-degree relatives of individuals with type 2 DM. The disease is polygenic and multifactorial, because in addition to genetic susceptibility, environmental factors (such as obesity, nutrition, and physical activity) modulate the phenotype. The in utero environment also contributes, and either increased or reduced birth weight increases the risk of type 2 DM in adult life. The genes that predispose to type 2 DM are incompletely identified, but recent genome-wide association studies have identified a large number of genes that convey a relatively small risk for type 2 DM (>70 genes, each with a relative risk of 1.06–1.5). Most prominent is a variant of the transcription factor 7–like 2 gene that has been associated with type 2 DM in several populations and with IGT in one population at high risk for diabetes. Genetic polymorphisms associated with type 2 DM have also been found in the genes encoding the peroxisome proliferator–activated receptor γ, inward rectifying potassium channel, zinc transporter, IRS, and calpain 10. The mechanisms by which these genetic loci increase the susceptibility to type 2 DM are not clear, but most are predicted to alter islet function or development or insulin secretion. Although the genetic susceptibility to type 2 DM is under active investigation (it is estimated that <10% of genetic risk is determined by loci identified thus far), it is currently not possible to use a combination of known genetic loci to predict type 2 DM.

Pathophysiology Type 2 DM is characterized by impaired insulin secretion, insulin resistance, excessive hepatic glucose production, and abnormal fat metabolism. Obesity, particularly visceral or central (as evidenced by the hip-waist ratio), is very common in type 2 DM (≥80% of patients are obese). In the early stages of the disorder, glucose tolerance remains near-normal, despite insulin resistance, because the pancreatic beta cells compensate by increasing insulin output (Fig. 417-7). As insulin resistance and compensatory hyperinsulinemia progress, the pancreatic islets in certain individuals are unable to sustain the hyperinsulinemic state. IGT, characterized by elevations in postprandial glucose, then develops. A further decline in insulin secretion and an increase in hepatic glucose production lead to overt diabetes with fasting hyperglycemia. Ultimately, beta cell failure ensues. Although both insulin resistance and impaired insulin secretion contribute to the pathogenesis of type 2 DM, the relative contribution of each varies from individual to individual.

Metabolic Abnormalities • ***ABNORMAL MUSCLE AND FAT METABOLISM*** Insulin resistance, the decreased ability of insulin to act effectively on target tissues (especially muscle, liver, and fat), is a prominent feature of type 2 DM and results from a combination of genetic susceptibility and obesity. Insulin resistance is relative, however, because supranormal levels of circulating insulin will normalize the plasma glucose. Insulin dose-response curves exhibit a rightward shift, indicating reduced sensitivity, and a reduced maximal response, indicating an overall decrease in maximum glucose utilization (30–60% lower than in normal individuals). Insulin resistance impairs glucose utilization by insulin-sensitive tissues and increases hepatic glucose output; both effects contribute to the hyperglycemia. Increased hepatic glucose output predominantly accounts for increased FPG levels, whereas decreased peripheral glucose usage results in postprandial hyperglycemia. In skeletal muscle, there is a greater impairment in nonoxidative

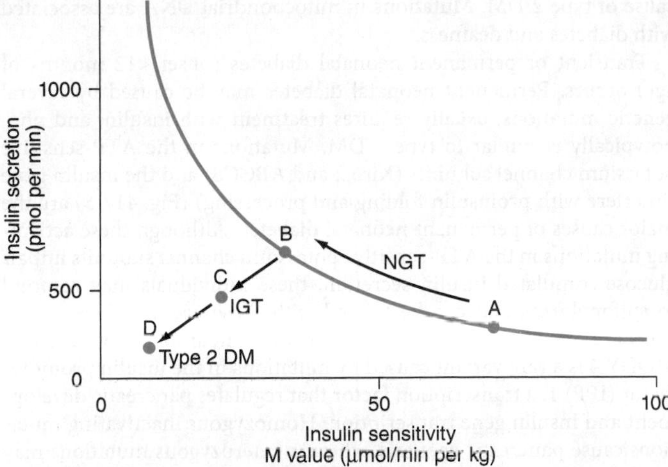

FIGURE 417-7 Metabolic changes during the development of type 2 diabetes mellitus (DM). Insulin secretion and insulin sensitivity are related, and as an individual becomes more insulin resistant (by moving from point A to point B), insulin secretion increases. A failure to compensate by increasing the insulin secretion results initially in impaired glucose tolerance (IGT; point C) and ultimately in type 2 DM (point D). NGT, normal glucose tolerance. *(Adapted from SE Kahn: J Clin Endocrinol Metab 86:4047, 2001; RN Bergman, M Ader: Trends Endocrinol Metab 11:351, 2000.)*

glucose usage (glycogen formation) than in oxidative glucose metabolism through glycolysis. Glucose metabolism in insulin-independent tissues is not altered in type 2 DM.

The precise molecular mechanism leading to insulin resistance in type 2 DM has not been elucidated. Insulin receptor levels and tyrosine kinase activity in skeletal muscle are reduced, but these alterations are most likely secondary to hyperinsulinemia and are not a primary defect. Therefore, "postreceptor" defects in insulin-regulated phosphorylation/dephosphorylation appear to play the predominant role in insulin resistance. Abnormalities include the accumulation of lipid within skeletal myocytes, which may impair mitochondrial oxidative phosphorylation and reduce insulin-stimulated mitochondrial ATP production. Impaired fatty acid oxidation and lipid accumulation within skeletal myocytes also may generate reactive oxygen species such as lipid peroxides. Of note, not all insulin signal transduction pathways are resistant to the effects of insulin (e.g., those controlling cell growth and differentiation using the mitogenic-activated protein kinase pathway). Consequently, hyperinsulinemia may increase the insulin action through these pathways, potentially accelerating diabetes-related conditions such as atherosclerosis.

The obesity accompanying type 2 DM, particularly in a central or visceral location, is thought to be part of the pathogenic process (Chap. 415e). In addition to these white fat depots, humans now are recognized to have brown fat, which has much greater thermogenic capacity. Efforts are under way to increase the activity or quantity of brown fat (e.g., a myokine, irisin, may convert white to brown fat). The increased adipocyte mass leads to increased levels of circulating free fatty acids and other fat cell products. For example, adipocytes secrete a number of biologic products (nonesterified free fatty acids, retinol-binding protein 4, leptin, TNF-α, resistin, IL-6, and adiponectin). In addition to regulating body weight, appetite, and energy expenditure, adipokines also modulate insulin sensitivity. The increased production of free fatty acids and some adipokines may cause insulin resistance in skeletal muscle and liver. For example, free fatty acids impair glucose utilization in skeletal muscle, promote glucose production by the liver, and impair beta cell function. In contrast, the production by adipocytes of adiponectin, an insulin-sensitizing peptide, is reduced in obesity, and this may contribute to hepatic insulin resistance. Adipocyte products and adipokines also produce an inflammatory state and may explain why markers of inflammation such as IL-6 and C-reactive protein are often elevated in type 2 DM. In addition, inflammatory cells have been found infiltrating adipose tissue. Inhibition of inflammatory signaling pathways such as the nuclear factor-κB (NF-κB) pathway appears to reduce insulin resistance and improve hyperglycemia in animal models and is being tested in humans.

IMPAIRED INSULIN SECRETION Insulin secretion and sensitivity are interrelated (Fig. 417-7). In type 2 DM, insulin secretion initially increases in response to insulin resistance to maintain normal glucose tolerance. Initially, the insulin secretory defect is mild and selectively involves glucose-stimulated insulin secretion, including a greatly reduced first secretory phase. The response to other nonglucose secretagogues, such as arginine, is preserved, but overall beta function is reduced by as much as 50% at the onset of type 2 DM. Abnormalities in proinsulin processing are reflected by increased secretion of proinsulin in type 2 DM. Eventually, the insulin secretory defect is progressive.

The reason(s) for the decline in insulin secretory capacity in type 2 DM is unclear. The assumption is that a second genetic defect—superimposed upon insulin resistance—leads to beta cell failure. Beta cell mass is decreased by approximately 50% in individuals with long-standing type 2 DM. Islet amyloid polypeptide or amylin, co-secreted by the beta cell, forms the amyloid fibrillar deposit found in the islets of individuals with long-standing type 2 DM. Whether such islet amyloid deposits are a primary or secondary event is not known. The metabolic environment of diabetes may also negatively impact islet function. For example, chronic hyperglycemia paradoxically impairs islet function ("glucose toxicity") and leads to a worsening of hyperglycemia. Improvement in glycemic control is often associated with improved islet function. In addition, elevation of free fatty acid levels ("lipotoxicity") and dietary fat may also worsen islet function. Reduced GLP-1 action may contribute to the reduced insulin secretion.

INCREASED HEPATIC GLUCOSE AND LIPID PRODUCTION In type 2 DM, insulin resistance in the liver reflects the failure of hyperinsulinemia to suppress gluconeogenesis, which results in fasting hyperglycemia and decreased glycogen storage by the liver in the postprandial state. Increased hepatic glucose production occurs early in the course of diabetes, although likely after the onset of insulin secretory abnormalities and insulin resistance in skeletal muscle. As a result of insulin resistance in adipose tissue, lipolysis and free fatty acid flux from adipocytes are increased, leading to increased lipid (very-low-density lipoprotein [VLDL] and triglyceride) synthesis in hepatocytes. This lipid storage or steatosis in the liver may lead to nonalcoholic fatty liver disease (Chap. 367e) and abnormal liver function tests. This is also responsible for the dyslipidemia found in type 2 DM (elevated triglycerides, reduced high-density lipoprotein [HDL], and increased small dense low-density lipoprotein [LDL] particles).

Insulin Resistance Syndromes The insulin resistance condition comprises a spectrum of disorders, with hyperglycemia representing one of the most readily diagnosed features. The *metabolic syndrome*, the *insulin resistance syndrome*, and *syndrome X* are terms used to describe a constellation of metabolic derangements that includes insulin resistance, hypertension, dyslipidemia (decreased HDL and elevated triglycerides), central or visceral obesity, type 2 DM or IGT/IFG, and accelerated cardiovascular disease. This syndrome is discussed in Chap. 422.

A number of relatively rare forms of severe insulin resistance include features of type 2 DM or IGT (Table 417-1). Mutations in the insulin receptor that interfere with binding or signal transduction are a rare cause of insulin resistance. Acanthosis nigricans and signs of hyperandrogenism (hirsutism, acne, and oligomenorrhea in women) are also common physical features. Two distinct syndromes of severe insulin resistance have been described in adults: (1) type A, which affects young women and is characterized by severe hyperinsulinemia, obesity, and features of hyperandrogenism; and (2) type B, which affects middle-aged women and is characterized by severe hyperinsulinemia, features of hyperandrogenism, and autoimmune disorders. Individuals with the type A insulin resistance syndrome have an undefined defect in the insulin-signaling pathway; individuals with the type B insulin resistance syndrome have autoantibodies directed at the insulin receptor. These receptor autoantibodies may block insulin binding or may stimulate the insulin receptor, leading to intermittent hypoglycemia.

Polycystic ovary syndrome (PCOS) is a common disorder that affects premenopausal women and is characterized by chronic anovulation and hyperandrogenism (Chap. 412). Insulin resistance is seen in a significant subset of women with PCOS, and the disorder substantially increases the risk for type 2 DM, independent of the effects of obesity.

Prevention Type 2 DM is preceded by a period of IGT or IFG, and a number of lifestyle modifications and pharmacologic agents prevent or delay the onset of DM. Individuals with prediabetes or increased risk of diabetes should be referred to a structured program to reduce body weight and increase physical activity as well as being screened for cardiovascular disease. The Diabetes Prevention Program (DPP) demonstrated that intensive changes in lifestyle (diet and exercise for 30 min/d five times/week) in individuals with IGT prevented or delayed the development of type 2 DM by 58% compared to placebo. This effect was seen in individuals regardless of age, sex, or ethnic group. In the same study, metformin prevented or delayed diabetes by 31% compared to placebo. The lifestyle intervention group lost 5–7% of their body weight during the 3 years of the study. Studies in Finnish and Chinese populations noted similar efficacy of diet and exercise in preventing or delaying type 2 DM. A number of agents, including α-glucosidase inhibitors, metformin, thiazolidinediones, GLP-1 receptor pathway modifiers, and orlistat, prevent or delay type 2 DM but are not approved for this purpose. Individuals with a strong family history of type 2 DM and individuals with IFG or IGT should be strongly encouraged to maintain a normal BMI and engage in regular physical activity. Pharmacologic therapy for individuals with prediabetes is currently controversial because its cost-effectiveness and safety profile are not known. The ADA has suggested that metformin be considered in individuals with both IFG and IGT who are at very high risk for progression to diabetes (age <60 years, BMI ≥35 kg/m^2, family history of diabetes in first-degree relative, and women with a history of GDM). Individuals with IFG, IGT, or an HbA_{1c} of 5.7–6.4% should be monitored annually to determine if diagnostic criteria for diabetes are present.

GENETICALLY DEFINED, MONOGENIC FORMS OF DIABETES MELLITUS RELATED TO REDUCED INSULIN SECRETION

Several monogenic forms of DM have been identified. More than 10 different variants of MODY, caused by mutations in genes encoding islet-enriched transcription factors or glucokinase (Fig. 417-5; Table 417-1), are transmitted as autosomal dominant disorders. MODY 1, MODY 3, and MODY 5 are caused by mutations in hepatocyte nuclear transcription factor (HNF) 4α, HNF-1α, and HNF-1β, respectively. As their names imply, these transcription factors are expressed in the liver but also in other tissues, including the pancreatic islets and kidney. These factors most likely affect islet development or the expression of genes important in glucose-stimulated insulin secretion or the maintenance of beta cell mass. For example, individuals with an HNF-1α mutation (MODY 3) have a progressive decline in glycemic control but may respond to sulfonylureas. In fact, some of these patients were initially thought to have type 1 DM but were later shown to respond to a sulfonylurea, and insulin was discontinued. Individuals with a HNF-1β mutation have progressive impairment of insulin secretion and hepatic insulin resistance, and require insulin treatment (minimal response to sulfonylureas). These individuals often have other abnormalities such as renal cysts, mild pancreatic exocrine insufficiency, and abnormal liver function tests. Individuals with MODY 2, the result of mutations in the glucokinase gene, have mild-to-moderate, stable hyperglycemia that does not respond to oral hypoglycemic agents. Glucokinase catalyzes the formation of glucose-6-phosphate from glucose, a reaction that is important for glucose sensing by the beta cells (Fig. 417-5) and for glucose utilization by the liver. As a result of glucokinase mutations, higher glucose levels are required to elicit insulin secretory responses, thus altering the set point for insulin secretion. Studies of populations with type 2 DM suggest that mutations in MODY-associated genes are an uncommon (<5%) cause of type 2 DM. Mutations in mitochondrial DNA are associated with diabetes and deafness.

Transient or permanent neonatal diabetes (onset <12 months of age) occurs. Permanent neonatal diabetes may be caused by several genetic mutations, usually requires treatment with insulin, and phenotypically is similar to type 1 DM. Mutations in the ATP-sensitive potassium channel subunits (Kir6.2 and ABCC8) and the insulin gene (interfere with proinsulin folding and processing) (Fig. 417-5) are the major causes of permanent neonatal diabetes. Although these activating mutations in the ATP-sensitive potassium channel subunits impair glucose-stimulated insulin secretion, these individuals may respond to sulfonylureas and can be treated with these agents. These mutations are often associated with a spectrum of neurologic dysfunction. MODY 4 is a rare variant caused by mutations in the insulin promoter factor (IPF) 1, a transcription factor that regulates pancreatic development and insulin gene transcription. Homozygous inactivating mutations cause pancreatic agenesis, whereas heterozygous mutations may result in DM. Mutations in the transcription factor of *GATA6* are the most common cause of pancreatic agenesis. Homozygous glucokinase mutations cause a severe form of neonatal diabetes.

APPROACH TO THE PATIENT: Diabetes Mellitus

Once the diagnosis of DM is made, attention should be directed to symptoms related to diabetes (acute and chronic) and classifying the type of diabetes. DM and its complications produce a wide range of symptoms and signs; those secondary to acute hyperglycemia may occur at any stage of the disease, whereas those related to chronic hyperglycemia begin to appear during the second decade of hyperglycemia (Chap. 419). Individuals with previously undetected type 2 DM may present with chronic complications of DM at the time of diagnosis. The history and physical examination should assess for symptoms or signs of acute hyperglycemia and should screen for the chronic complications and conditions associated with DM.

HISTORY

A complete medical history should be obtained with special emphasis on DM-relevant aspects such as weight, family history of DM and its complications, risk factors for cardiovascular disease, exercise, smoking, and ethanol use. Symptoms of hyperglycemia include polyuria, polydipsia, weight loss, fatigue, weakness, blurry vision, frequent superficial infections (vaginitis, fungal skin infections), and slow healing of skin lesions after minor trauma. Metabolic derangements relate mostly to hyperglycemia (osmotic diuresis) and to the catabolic state of the patient (urinary loss of glucose and calories, muscle breakdown due to protein degradation and decreased protein synthesis). Blurred vision results from changes in the water content of the lens and resolves as the hyperglycemia is controlled.

In a patient with established DM, the initial assessment should also include special emphasis on prior diabetes care, including the type of therapy, prior HbA_{1c} levels, self-monitoring blood glucose results, frequency of hypoglycemia, presence of DM-specific complications, and assessment of the patient's knowledge about diabetes, exercise, and nutrition. Diabetes-related complications may afflict several organ systems, and an individual patient may exhibit some, all, or none of the symptoms related to the complications of DM (Chap. 419). In addition, the presence of DM-related comorbidities should be sought (cardiovascular disease, hypertension, dyslipidemia). Pregnancy plans should be ascertained in women of childbearing age.

PHYSICAL EXAMINATION

In addition to a complete physical examination, special attention should be given to DM-relevant aspects such as weight or BMI, retinal examination, orthostatic blood pressure, foot examination, peripheral pulses, and insulin injection sites. Blood pressure >140/80 mmHg is considered hypertension in individuals with diabetes. Because periodontal disease is more frequent in DM, the teeth and gums should also be examined.

An annual foot examination should (1) assess blood flow, sensation (vibratory sensation [128-MHz tuning fork at the base of the great toe], the ability to sense touch with a monofilament [5.07, 10-g monofilament], pinprick sensation, testing for ankle reflexes, and vibration perception threshold using a biothesiometer), ankle reflexes, and nail care; (2) look for the presence of foot deformities such as hammer or claw toes and Charcot foot; and (3) identify sites of potential ulceration. The ADA recommends annual screening for distal symmetric neuropathy beginning with the initial diagnosis of diabetes and annual screening for autonomic neuropathy 5 years after diagnosis of type 1 DM and at the time of diagnosis of type 2 DM. This includes testing for loss of protective sensation (LOPS) using monofilament testing plus one of the following tests: vibration, pinprick, ankle reflexes, or vibration perception threshold (using a biothesiometer). If the monofilament test or one of the other tests is abnormal, the patient is diagnosed with LOPS and counseled accordingly (Chap. 419).

CLASSIFICATION OF DM IN AN INDIVIDUAL PATIENT

The etiology of diabetes in an individual with new-onset disease can usually be assigned on the basis of clinical criteria. Individuals with type 1 DM tend to have the following characteristics: (1) onset of disease prior to age 30 years; (2) lean body habitus; (3) requirement of insulin as the initial therapy; (4) propensity to develop ketoacidosis; and (5) an increased risk of other autoimmune disorders such as autoimmune thyroid disease, adrenal insufficiency, pernicious anemia, celiac disease, and vitiligo. In contrast, individuals with type 2 DM often exhibit the following features: (1) develop diabetes after the age of 30 years; (2) are usually obese (80% are obese, but elderly individuals may be lean); (3) may not require insulin therapy initially; and (4) may have associated conditions such as insulin resistance, hypertension, cardiovascular disease, dyslipidemia, or PCOS. In type 2 DM, insulin resistance is often associated with abdominal obesity (as opposed to hip and thigh obesity) and hypertriglyceridemia. Although most individuals diagnosed with type 2 DM are older, the age of diagnosis is declining, and there is a marked increase among overweight children and adolescents. Some individuals with phenotypic type 2 DM present with diabetic ketoacidosis but lack autoimmune markers and may be later treated with oral glucose-lowering agents rather than insulin (this clinical picture is sometimes referred to as *ketosis-prone type 2 DM*). On the other hand, some individuals (5–10%) with the phenotypic appearance of type 2 DM do not have absolute insulin deficiency but have autoimmune markers (GAD and other ICA autoantibodies) suggestive of type 1 DM (termed *latent autoimmune diabetes of the adult*). Such individuals are more likely to be <50 years of age, thinner, and have a personal or family history of other autoimmune disease than individuals with type 2 DM. They are much more likely to require insulin treatment within 5 years. Monogenic forms of diabetes (discussed above) should be considered in those with diabetes onset at <30 years of age, an autosomal pattern of diabetes inheritance, and the lack of nearly complete insulin deficiency. Despite recent advances in the understanding of the pathogenesis of diabetes, it remains difficult to categorize some patients unequivocally. Individuals who deviate from the clinical profile of type 1 and type 2 DM, or who have other associated defects such as deafness, pancreatic exocrine disease, and other endocrine disorders, should be classified accordingly (Table 417-1).

LABORATORY ASSESSMENT

The laboratory assessment should first determine whether the patient meets the diagnostic criteria for DM (Table 417-2) and then assess the degree of glycemic control (Chap. 418). In addition to the standard laboratory evaluation, the patient should be screened for DM-associated conditions (e.g., albuminuria, dyslipidemia, thyroid dysfunction).

The classification of the type of DM may be facilitated by laboratory assessments. Serum insulin or C-peptide measurements often do not distinguish type 1 from type 2 DM, but a low C-peptide level confirms a patient's need for insulin. Many individuals with new-onset type 1 DM retain some C-peptide production. Measurement of islet cell antibodies at the time of diabetes onset may be useful if the type of DM is not clear based on the characteristics described above.

418 Diabetes Mellitus: Management and Therapies

Alvin C. Powers

OVERALL GOALS

The goals of therapy for type 1 or type 2 diabetes mellitus (DM) are to (1) eliminate symptoms related to hyperglycemia, (2) reduce or eliminate the long-term microvascular and macrovascular complications of DM (Chap. 419), and (3) allow the patient to achieve as normal a lifestyle as possible. To reach these goals, the physician should identify a target level of glycemic control for each patient, provide the patient with the educational and pharmacologic resources necessary to reach this level, and monitor/treat DM-related complications. Symptoms of diabetes usually resolve when the plasma glucose is <11.1 mmol/L (200 mg/dL), and thus most DM treatment focuses on achieving the second and third goals. This chapter first reviews the ongoing treatment of diabetes in the outpatient setting and then discusses the treatment of severe hyperglycemia, as well as the treatment of diabetes in hospitalized patients.

The care of an individual with either type 1 or type 2 DM requires a multidisciplinary team. Central to the success of this team are the patient's participation, input, and enthusiasm, all of which are essential for optimal diabetes management. Members of the health care team include the primary care provider and/or the endocrinologist or diabetologist, a certified diabetes educator, a nutritionist, and a psychologist. In addition, when the complications of DM arise, subspecialists (including neurologists, nephrologists, vascular surgeons, cardiologists, ophthalmologists, and podiatrists) with experience in DM-related complications are essential.

ONGOING ASPECTS OF COMPREHENSIVE DIABETES CARE

A number of names are sometimes applied to different approaches to diabetes care, such as intensive insulin therapy, intensive glycemic control, and "tight control." The current chapter, and other sources, uses the term *comprehensive diabetes care* to emphasize the fact that optimal diabetes therapy involves more than plasma glucose management and medications. Although glycemic control is central to optimal diabetes therapy, comprehensive diabetes care of both type 1 and type 2 DM should also detect and manage DM-specific complications (Chap. 419) and modify risk factors for DM-associated diseases. The key elements of comprehensive diabetes care are summarized in Table 418-1. In addition to the physical aspects of DM, social, family, financial, cultural, and employment-related issues may impact diabetes care. The International Diabetes Federation (IDF), recognizing that resources available for diabetes care vary widely throughout the world, has issued guidelines for "recommended care" (a well-developed service base and with health care funding systems consuming a significant part of their national wealth), "limited care" (health care settings with very limited resources), and "comprehensive care" (health care settings with considerable resources). This chapter provides guidance

TABLE 418-1 GUIDELINES FOR ONGOING, COMPREHENSIVE MEDICAL CARE FOR PATIENTS WITH DIABETES

- Optimal and individualized glycemic control
- Self-monitoring of blood glucose (individualized frequency)
- HbA_{1c} testing (2–4 times/year)
- Patient education in diabetes management (annual); diabetes-self management education and support
- Medical nutrition therapy and education (annual)
- Eye examination (annual or biannual; **Chap. 419**)
- Foot examination (1–2 times/year by physician; daily by patient; **Chap. 419**)
- Screening for diabetic nephropathy (annual; **Chap. 419**)
- Blood pressure measurement (quarterly)
- Lipid profile and serum creatinine (estimate GFR) (annual; **Chap. 419**)
- Influenza/pneumococcal/hepatitis B immunizations
- Consider antiplatelet therapy (**Chap. 419**)

Abbreviations: GFR, glomerular filtration rate; HbA_{1c}, hemoglobin A_{1c}.

for this comprehensive level of diabetes care. The treatment goals for patients with diabetes are summarized in Table 418-2 and should be individualized.

DETECTION AND PREVENTION OF COMPLICATIONS RELATED TO DIABETES

The morbidity and mortality rates of DM-related complications (Chap. 419) can be greatly reduced by timely and consistent surveillance procedures (Table 418-1). These screening procedures are indicated for all individuals with DM, but many individuals with diabetes do not receive comprehensive diabetes care. A comprehensive eye examination should be performed by a qualified optometrist or ophthalmologist. Because many individuals with type 2 DM have had asymptomatic diabetes for several years before diagnosis, the American Diabetes Association (ADA) recommends the following ophthalmologic examination schedule: (1) individuals with type 1 DM should have an initial eye examination within 5 years of diagnosis, (2) individuals with type 2 DM should have an initial eye examination at the time of diabetes diagnosis, (3) women with DM who are pregnant or contemplating pregnancy should have an eye examination prior to conception and during the first trimester, and (4) if eye exam is normal, repeat examination in 2–3 years is appropriate.

TABLE 418-2 TREATMENT GOALS FOR ADULTS WITH DIABETES[a]

Index	Goal
Glycemic control[b]	
HbA_{1c}	<7.0%[c]
Preprandial capillary plasma glucose	4.4–7.2 mmol/L (80–130 mg/dL)
Peak postprandial capillary plasma glucose[d]	<10.0 mmol/L (<180 mg/dL)
Blood pressure	<140/90 mmHg[e]
Lipids[f]	
Low-density lipoprotein	<2.6 mmol/L (100 mg/dL)[g]
High-density lipoprotein	>1 mmol/L (40 mg/dL) in men
	>1.3 mmol/L (50 mg/dL) in women
Triglycerides	<1.7 mmol/L (150 mg/dL)

[a]As recommended by the American Diabetes Association; goals should be individualized for each patient (see text). Goals may be different for certain patient populations. [b]HbA_{1c} is primary goal. [c]Diabetes Control and Complications Trial–based assay. [d]1–2 h after beginning of a meal. [e]Goal of <130/80 mmHg may be appropriate for younger individuals [f]In decreasing order of priority. Recent guidelines from the American College of Cardiology and American Heart Association no longer advocate specific LDL and HDL goals (**see Chaps. 291e and 419**). [g]Goal of <1.8 mmol/L (70 mg/dL) may be appropriate for individuals with cardiovascular disease.

Abbreviation: HbA_{1c}, hemoglobin A_{1c}.

Source: Adapted from American Diabetes Association: Diabetes Care 38(Suppl 1):S1, 2015.

PATIENT EDUCATION ABOUT DM, NUTRITION, AND EXERCISE

The patient with type 1 or type 2 DM should receive education about nutrition, exercise, care of diabetes during illness, and medications to lower the plasma glucose. Along with improved compliance, patient education allows individuals with DM to assume greater responsibility for their care. Patient education should be viewed as a continuing process with regular visits for reinforcement; it should not be a process that is completed after one or two visits to a nurse educator or nutritionist. The ADA refers to education about the individualized management plan for the patient as diabetes self-management education (DSME) and diabetes self-management support (DSMS). DSME and DSMS are ways to improve the patient's knowledge, skills, and abilities necessary for diabetes self-care and should also emphasize psychosocial issues and emotional well-being. More frequent contact between the patient and the diabetes management team (e.g., electronic, telephone) improves glycemic control.

Diabetes Education The diabetes educator is a health care professional (nurse, dietician, or pharmacist) with specialized patient education skills who is certified in diabetes education (e.g., American Association of Diabetes Educators). Education topics important for optimal diabetes care include self-monitoring of blood glucose; urine ketone monitoring (type 1 DM); insulin administration; guidelines for diabetes management during illnesses; prevention and management of hypoglycemia (Chap. 420); foot and skin care; diabetes management before, during, and after exercise; and risk factor–modifying activities.

Psychosocial Aspects Because the individual with DM can face challenges that affect many aspects of daily life, psychosocial assessment and treatment are a critical part of providing comprehensive diabetes care. The individual with DM must accept that he or she may develop complications related to DM. Even with considerable effort, normoglycemia can be an elusive goal, and solutions to worsening glycemic control may not be easily identifiable. The patient should view him- or herself as an essential member of the diabetes care team and not as someone who is cared for by the diabetes management team. Emotional stress may provoke a change in behavior so that individuals no longer adhere to a dietary, exercise, or therapeutic regimen. This can lead to the appearance of either hyper- or hypoglycemia. Eating disorders, including binge eating disorders, bulimia, and anorexia nervosa, appear to occur more frequently in individuals with type 1 or type 2 DM.

Nutrition *Medical nutrition therapy* (MNT) is a term used by the ADA to describe the optimal coordination of caloric intake with other aspects of diabetes therapy (insulin, exercise, weight loss). Primary prevention measures of MNT are directed at preventing or delaying the onset of type 2 DM in high-risk individuals (obese or with prediabetes) by promoting weight reduction. Medical treatment of obesity is a rapidly evolving area and is discussed in Chap. 416. Secondary prevention measures of MNT are directed at preventing or delaying diabetes-related complications in diabetic individuals by improving glycemic control. Tertiary prevention measures of MNT are directed at managing diabetes-related complications (cardiovascular disease, nephropathy) in diabetic individuals. MNT in patients with diabetes and cardiovascular disease should incorporate dietary principles used in nondiabetic patients with cardiovascular disease. Although the recommendations for all three types of MNT overlap, this chapter emphasizes secondary prevention measures of MNT. Pharmacologic approaches that facilitate weight loss and bariatric surgery should be considered in selected patients (Chaps. 415e and 416).

In general, the components of optimal MNT are similar for individuals with type 1 or type 2 DM and similar to those for the general population (fruits, vegetables, fiber-containing foods, and low fat; Table 418-3). MNT education is an important component of comprehensive diabetes care and should be reinforced by regular patient education. Historically, nutrition education imposed restrictive, complicated regimens on the patient. Current practices have greatly changed, although many patients and health care providers still view the diabetic diet as monolithic and static. For example, MNT now includes foods

TABLE 418-3 NUTRITIONAL RECOMMENDATIONS FOR ADULTS WITH DIABETES OR PREDIABETES[a]

Weight loss diet (in prediabetes and type 2 DM)
- Hypocaloric diet that is low-carbohydrate

Fat in diet (optimal % of diet is not known; should be individualized)
- Minimal *trans* fat consumption
- Mediterranean-style diet rich in monounsaturated fatty acids may be better

Carbohydrate in diet (optimal % of diet is not known; should be individualized)
- Monitor carbohydrate intake in regard to calories
- Sucrose containing foods may be consumed with adjustments in insulin dose, but minimize intake
- Amount of carbohydrate determined by estimating grams of carbohydrate in diet (type 1 DM)
- Use glycemic index to predict how consumption of a particular food may affect blood glucose
- Fructose preferred over sucrose or starch

Protein in diet (optimal % of diet is not known; should be individualized)

Other components
- Dietary fiber, vegetable, fruits, whole grains, dairy products, and sodium intake as advised for general population
- Nonnutrient sweeteners
- Routine supplements of vitamins, antioxidants, or trace elements not advised

[a]See text for differences for patients with type 1 or type 2 diabetes.

Source: Adapted from American Diabetes Association: Diabetes Care 37(Suppl 1):S14, 2014.

with sucrose and seeks to modify other risk factors such as hyperlipidemia and hypertension rather than focusing exclusively on weight loss in individuals with type 2 DM. The *glycemic index* is an estimate of the postprandial rise in the blood glucose when a certain amount of that food is consumed. Consumption of foods with a low glycemic index appears to reduce postprandial glucose excursions and improve glycemic control. Reduced-calorie and nonnutritive sweeteners are useful. Currently, evidence does not support supplementation of the diet with vitamins, antioxidants (vitamin C and E), or micronutrients (chromium) in patients with diabetes.

The goal of MNT in the individual with type 1 DM is to coordinate and match the caloric intake, both temporally and quantitatively, with the appropriate amount of insulin. MNT in type 1 DM and self-monitoring of blood glucose must be integrated to define the optimal insulin regimen. The ADA encourages patients and providers to use carbohydrate counting or exchange systems to estimate the nutrient content of a meal or snack. Based on the patient's estimate of the carbohydrate content of a meal, an insulin-to-carbohydrate ratio determines the bolus insulin dose for a meal or snack. MNT must be flexible enough to allow for exercise, and the insulin regimen must allow for deviations in caloric intake. An important component of MNT in type 1 DM is to minimize the weight gain often associated with intensive diabetes management.

The goals of MNT in type 2 DM should focus on weight loss and address the greatly increased prevalence of cardiovascular risk factors (hypertension, dyslipidemia, obesity) and disease in this population. The majority of these individuals are obese, and weight loss is strongly encouraged and should remain an important goal. Hypocaloric diets and modest weight loss (5–7%) often result in rapid and dramatic glucose lowering in individuals with new-onset type 2 DM. Nevertheless, numerous studies document that long-term weight loss is uncommon. MNT for type 2 DM should emphasize modest caloric reduction (low-carbohydrate) and increased physical activity. Increased consumption of soluble, dietary fiber may improve glycemic control in individuals with type 2 DM. Weight loss and exercise improve insulin resistance.

Exercise Exercise has multiple positive benefits including cardiovascular risk reduction, reduced blood pressure, maintenance of muscle mass, reduction in body fat, and weight loss. For individuals with type 1 or type 2 DM, exercise is also useful for lowering plasma glucose (during and following exercise) and increasing insulin sensitivity. In patients with diabetes, the ADA recommends 150 min/week (distributed over at least 3 days) of moderate aerobic physical activity with no gaps longer than 2 days. The exercise regimen should also include resistance training.

Despite its benefits, exercise presents challenges for individuals with DM because they lack the normal glucoregulatory mechanisms (normally, insulin falls and glucagon rises during exercise). Skeletal muscle is a major site for metabolic fuel consumption in the resting state, and the increased muscle activity during vigorous, aerobic exercise greatly increases fuel requirements. Individuals with type 1 DM are prone to either hyperglycemia or hypoglycemia during exercise, depending on the preexercise plasma glucose, the circulating insulin level, and the level of exercise-induced catecholamines. If the insulin level is too low, the rise in catecholamines may increase the plasma glucose excessively, promote ketone body formation, and possibly lead to ketoacidosis. Conversely, if the circulating insulin level is excessive, this relative hyperinsulinemia may reduce hepatic glucose production (decreased glycogenolysis, decreased gluconeogenesis) and increase glucose entry into muscle, leading to hypoglycemia.

To avoid exercise-related hyper- or hypoglycemia, individuals with type 1 DM should (1) monitor blood glucose before, during, and after exercise; (2) delay exercise if blood glucose is >14 mmol/L (250 mg/dL) and ketones are present; (3) if the blood glucose is <5.6 mmol/L (100 mg/dL), ingest carbohydrate before exercising; (4) monitor glucose during exercise and ingest carbohydrate to prevent hypoglycemia; (5) decrease insulin doses (based on previous experience) before exercise and inject insulin into a nonexercising area; and (6) learn individual glucose responses to different types of exercise and increase food intake for up to 24 h after exercise, depending on intensity and duration of exercise. In individuals with type 2 DM, exercise-related hypoglycemia is less common but can occur in individuals taking either insulin or insulin secretagogues.

Despite asymptomatic cardiovascular disease appearing at a younger age in both type 1 and type 2 DM, routine screening for coronary artery disease has not been shown to be effective and is not recommended (Chap. 419). Untreated proliferative retinopathy is a relative contraindication to vigorous exercise, because this may lead to vitreous hemorrhage or retinal detachment.

MONITORING THE LEVEL OF GLYCEMIC CONTROL

Optimal monitoring of glycemic control involves plasma glucose measurements by the patient and an assessment of long-term control by the physician (measurement of hemoglobin A_{1c} [HbA_{1c}] and review of the patient's self-measurements of plasma glucose). These measurements are complementary: the patient's measurements provide a picture of short-term glycemic control, whereas the HbA_{1c} reflects average glycemic control over the previous 2–3 months.

Self-Monitoring of Blood Glucose Self-monitoring of blood glucose (SMBG) is the standard of care in diabetes management and allows the patient to monitor his or her blood glucose at any time. In SMBG, a small drop of blood and an easily detectable enzymatic reaction allow measurement of the capillary plasma glucose. Many glucose monitors can rapidly and accurately measure glucose (calibrated to provide plasma glucose value even though blood glucose is measured) in small amounts of blood (3–10 μL) obtained from the fingertip; alternative testing sites (e.g., forearm) are less reliable, especially when the blood glucose is changing rapidly (postprandially). A large number of blood glucose monitors are available, and the certified diabetes educator is critical in helping the patient select the optimal device and learn to use it properly. By combining glucose measurements with diet history, medication changes, and exercise history, the diabetes management team and patient can improve the treatment program.

The frequency of SMBG measurements must be individualized and adapted to address the goals of diabetes care. Individuals with type 1

DM or individuals with type 2 DM taking multiple insulin injections each day should routinely measure their plasma glucose three or more times per day to estimate and select mealtime boluses of short-acting insulin and to modify long-acting insulin doses. Most individuals with type 2 DM require less frequent monitoring, although the optimal frequency of SMBG has not been clearly defined. Individuals with type 2 DM who are taking insulin should use SMBG more frequently than those on oral agents. Individuals with type 2 DM who are on oral medications should use SMBG as a means of assessing the efficacy of their medication and the impact of diet. Because plasma glucose levels fluctuate less in these individuals, one to two SMBG measurements per day (or fewer in patients who are on oral agents or are diet-controlled) may be sufficient. Most measurements in individuals with type 1 or type 2 DM should be performed prior to a meal and supplemented with postprandial measurements to assist in reaching postprandial glucose targets (Table 418-2).

Devices for continuous glucose monitoring (CGM) have been approved by the U.S. Food and Drug Administration (FDA), and others are in various stages of development. These devices do not replace the need for traditional glucose measurements and require calibration with SMBG. This rapidly evolving technology requires substantial expertise on the part of the diabetes management team and the patient. Current CGM systems measure the glucose in interstitial fluid, which is in equilibrium with the blood glucose. These devices provide useful short-term information about the patterns of glucose changes as well as an enhanced ability to detect hypoglycemic episodes. Alarms notify the patient if the blood glucose falls into the hypoglycemic range. Clinical experience with these devices is rapidly growing, and they are most useful in individuals with hypoglycemia unawareness, individuals with frequent hypoglycemia, or those who have not achieved glycemic targets despite major efforts. The utility of CGM in the intensive care unit (ICU) setting remains to be determined.

Assessment of Long-Term Glycemic Control Measurement of glycated hemoglobin (HbA_{1c}) is the standard method for assessing long-term glycemic control. When plasma glucose is consistently elevated, there is an increase in nonenzymatic glycation of hemoglobin; this alteration reflects the glycemic history over the previous 2–3 months, because erythrocytes have an average life span of 120 days (glycemic level in the preceding month contributes about 50% to the HbA_{1c} value). Measurement of HbA_{1c} at the "point of care" allows for more rapid feedback and may therefore assist in adjustment of therapy.

HbA_{1c} should be measured in all individuals with DM during their initial evaluation and as part of their comprehensive diabetes care. As the primary predictor of long-term complications of DM, the HbA_{1c} should mirror, to a certain extent, the short-term measurements of SMBG. These two measurements are complementary in that recent intercurrent illnesses may impact the SMBG measurements but not the HbA_{1c}. Likewise, postprandial and nocturnal hyperglycemia may not be detected by the SMBG of fasting and preprandial capillary plasma glucose but will be reflected in the HbA_{1c}. In standardized assays, the HbA_{1c} approximates the following mean plasma glucose values: an HbA_{1c} of 6% = 7.0 mmol/L (126 mg/dL), 7% = 8.6 mmol/L (154 mg/dL), 8% = 10.2 mmol/L (183 mg/dL), 9% = 11.8 mmol/L (212 mg/dL), 10% = 13.4 mmol/L (240 mg/dL), 11% = 14.9 mmol/L (269 mg/dL), and 12% = 16.5 mmol/L (298 mg/dL). In patients achieving their glycemic goal, the ADA recommends measurement of the HbA_{1c} at least twice per year. More frequent testing (every 3 months) is warranted when glycemic control is inadequate or when therapy has changed. Laboratory standards for the HbA_{1c} test have been established and should be correlated to the reference assay of the Diabetes Control and Complications Trial (DCCT). Clinical conditions such hemoglobinopathies, anemias, reticulocytosis, transfusions, and uremia may interfere with the HbA_{1c} result. The degree of glycation of other proteins, such as albumin, can be used as an alternative indicator of glycemic control when the HbA_{1c} is inaccurate. The fructosamine assay (measuring glycated albumin) reflects the glycemic status over the prior 2 weeks.

PHARMACOLOGIC TREATMENT OF DIABETES

Comprehensive care of type 1 and type 2 DM requires an emphasis on nutrition, exercise, and monitoring of glycemic control but also usually involves glucose-lowering medication(s). This chapter discusses classes of such medications but does not describe every glucose-lowering agent available worldwide. The initial step is to select an individualized, glycemic goal for the patient.

ESTABLISHMENT OF TARGET LEVEL OF GLYCEMIC CONTROL

Because the complications of DM are related to glycemic control, normoglycemia or near-normoglycemia is the desired, but often elusive, goal for most patients. Normalization or near-normalization of the plasma glucose for long periods of time is extremely difficult, as demonstrated by the DCCT and United Kingdom Prospective Diabetes Study (UKPDS). Regardless of the level of hyperglycemia, improvement in glycemic control will lower the risk of diabetes-specific complications (Chap. 419).

The target for glycemic control (as reflected by the HbA_{1c}) must be individualized, and the goals of therapy should be developed in consultation with the patient after considering a number of medical, social, and lifestyle issues. The ADA calls this a *patient-centered approach*, and other organizations such as the IDF and American Association of Clinical Endocrinologists (AACE) also suggest an individualized glycemic goal. Important factors to consider include the patient's age and ability to understand and implement a complex treatment regimen, presence and severity of complications of diabetes, known cardiovascular disease (CVD), ability to recognize hypoglycemic symptoms, presence of other medical conditions or treatments that might affect survival or the response to therapy, lifestyle and occupation (e.g., possible consequences of experiencing hypoglycemia on the job), and level of support available from family and friends.

In general, the ADA suggests that the goal is to achieve an HbA_{1c} as close to normal as possible without significant hypoglycemia. In most individuals, the target HbA_{1c} should be <7% (Table 418-2) with a more stringent target for some patients. For instance, the HbA_{1c} goal in a young adult with type 1 DM may be 6.5%. A higher HbA_{1c} goal may be appropriate for the very young or old or in individuals with limited life span or comorbid conditions. For example, an appropriate HbA_{1c} goal in elderly individuals with multiple, chronic illnesses and impaired activities of daily living might be 8.0 or 8.5%. A major consideration is the frequency and severity of hypoglycemia, because this becomes more common with a more stringent HbA_{1c} goal.

More stringent glycemic control (HbA_{1c} of ≤6%) is not beneficial, and may be detrimental, in patients with type 2 DM and a high risk of CVD. Large clinical trials (UKPDS, Action to Control Cardiovascular Risk in Diabetes [ACCORD], Action in Diabetes and Vascular Disease: Preterax and Diamicron MR Controlled Evaluation [ADVANCE], Veterans Affairs Diabetes Trial [VADT]; Chap. 419) have examined glycemic control in type 2 DM in individuals with low risk of CVD, with high risk of CVD, or with established CVD and have found that more intense glycemic control is not beneficial and, in some patient populations, may have a negative impact on some outcomes. These divergent outcomes stress the need for individualized glycemic goals based on the following general guidelines: (1) early in the course of type 2 diabetes when the CVD risk is lower, improved glycemic control likely leads to improved cardiovascular outcome, but this benefit occurs more than a decade after the period of improved glycemic control; (2) intense glycemic control in individuals with established CVD or at high risk for CVD is not advantageous, and may be deleterious, over a follow-up of 3–5 years; an HbA_{1c} goal <7.0% is not appropriate in this population; (3) hypoglycemia in such high-risk populations (elderly, CVD) should be avoided; and (4) improved glycemic control reduces microvascular complications of diabetes (Chap. 419) even if it does not improve macrovascular complications like CVD.

TYPE 1 DIABETES MELLITUS

General Aspects The ADA recommendations for fasting and bedtime glycemic goals and HbA_{1c} targets are summarized in Table 418-2.

The goal is to design and implement insulin regimens that mimic physiologic insulin secretion. Because individuals with type 1 DM partially or completely lack endogenous insulin production, administration of basal insulin is essential for regulating glycogen breakdown, gluconeogenesis, lipolysis, and ketogenesis. Likewise, insulin replacement for meals should be appropriate for the carbohydrate intake and promote normal glucose utilization and storage.

Intensive Management Intensive diabetes management has the goal of achieving euglycemia or near-normal glycemia. This approach requires multiple resources, including thorough and continuing patient education, comprehensive recording of plasma glucose measurements and nutrition intake by the patient, and a variable insulin regimen that matches glucose intake and insulin dose. Insulin regimens usually include multiple-component insulin regimens, multiple daily injections (MDIs), or insulin infusion devices (each discussed below).

The benefits of intensive diabetes management and improved glycemic control include a reduction in the microvascular complications of DM and a reduction in diabetes-related complications. From a psychological standpoint, the patient experiences greater control over his or her diabetes and often notes an improved sense of well-being, greater flexibility in the timing and content of meals, and the capability to alter insulin dosing with exercise. In addition, intensive diabetes management prior to and during pregnancy reduces the risk of fetal malformations and morbidity. Intensive diabetes management is encouraged in newly diagnosed patients with type 1 DM because it may prolong the period of C-peptide production, which may result in better glycemic control and a reduced risk of serious hypoglycemia. Although intensive management confers impressive benefits, it is also accompanied by significant personal and financial costs and is therefore not appropriate for all individuals.

Insulin Preparations Current insulin preparations are generated by recombinant DNA technology and consist of the amino acid sequence of human insulin or variations thereof. In the United States, most insulin is formulated as U-100 (100 units/mL). Regular insulin formulated as U-500 (500 units/mL) is available and sometimes useful in patients with severe insulin resistance. Human insulin has been formulated with distinctive pharmacokinetics or genetically modified to more closely mimic physiologic insulin secretion. Insulins can be classified as short-acting or long-acting (Table 418-4). For example, one short-acting insulin formulation, insulin lispro, is an insulin analogue in which the 28th and 29th amino acids (lysine and proline) on the insulin B chain have been reversed by recombinant DNA technology. Insulin aspart and insulin glulisine are genetically modified insulin analogues with properties similar to lispro. All three of the insulin analogues have full biologic activity but less tendency for self-aggregation, resulting in more rapid absorption and onset of action and a shorter duration of action. These characteristics are particularly advantageous for allowing entrainment of insulin injection and action to rising plasma glucose levels following meals. The shorter duration of action also appears to be associated with a decreased number of hypoglycemic episodes, primarily because the decay of insulin action corresponds to the decline in plasma glucose after a meal. Thus, insulin aspart, lispro, or glulisine is preferred over regular insulin for prandial coverage. Insulin glargine is a long-acting biosynthetic human insulin that differs from normal insulin in that asparagine is replaced by glycine at amino acid 21, and two arginine residues are added to the C terminus of the B chain. Compared to neutral protamine Hagedorn (NPH) insulin, the onset of insulin glargine action is later, the duration of action is longer (~24 h), and there is a less pronounced peak. A lower incidence of hypoglycemia, especially at night, has been reported with insulin glargine when compared to NPH insulin. The most recent evidence does not support an association between glargine and increased cancer risk. Insulin detemir has a fatty acid side chain that prolongs its action by slowing absorption and catabolism. Twice-daily injections of glargine or detemir are sometimes required to provide 24-h coverage. Regular and NPH insulin have the native insulin amino acid sequence.

Basal insulin requirements are provided by long-acting (NPH insulin, insulin glargine, or insulin detemir) insulin formulations. These are usually prescribed with short-acting insulin in an attempt to mimic physiologic insulin release with meals. Although mixing of NPH and short-acting insulin formulations is common practice, this mixing may alter the insulin absorption profile (especially the short-acting insulins). For example, lispro absorption is delayed by mixing with NPH. The alteration in insulin absorption when the patient mixes different insulin formulations should not prevent mixing insulins. However, the following guidelines should be followed: (1) mix the different insulin formulations in the syringe immediately before injection (inject within 2 min after mixing); (2) do not store insulin as a mixture; (3) follow the same routine in terms of insulin mixing and administration to standardize the physiologic response to injected insulin; and (4) do not mix insulin glargine or detemir with other insulins. The miscibility of some insulins allows for the production of combination insulins that contain 70% NPH and 30% regular (70/30), or equal mixtures of NPH and regular (50/50). By including the insulin analogue mixed with protamine, several combinations have a short-acting and long-acting profile (Table 418-4). Although more convenient for the patient (only two injections/day), combination insulin formulations do not allow independent adjustment of short-acting and long-acting activity. Several insulin formulations are available as insulin "pens," which may be more convenient for some patients. Insulin delivery by inhalation has recently been approved but is not yet available. Other insulins, such as one with a duration of action of several days, are under development but are not currently available in the United States.

TABLE 418-4 PROPERTIES OF INSULIN PREPARATIONS[a]

Preparation	Time of Action: Onset, h	Peak, h	Effective Duration, h
Short-acting			
Aspart	<0.25	0.5–1.5	2–4
Glulisine	<0.25	0.5–1.5	2–4
Lispro	<0.25	0.5–1.5	2–4
Regular	0.5–1.0	2–3	3–6
Long-acting			
Detemir	1–4	—[b]	12-24[c]
Glargine	2–4	—[b]	20-24
NPH	2–4	4–10	10–16
Insulin combinations[d]			
75/25–75% protamine lispro, 25% lispro	<0.25	Dual[e]	10–16
70/30–70% protamine aspart, 30% aspart	<0.25	Dual[e]	15-18
50/50–50% protamine lispro, 50% lispro	<0.25	Dual[e]	10–16
70/30–70% NPH, 30% regular	0.5–1	Dual[e]	10–16

[a]Insulin preparations available in the United States; others are available in the United Kingdom and Europe. [b]Glargine and detemir have minimal peak activity. [c]Duration is dose-dependent (shorter at lower doses). [d]Other insulin combinations are available [e]Dual: two peaks—one at 2–3 h and the second one several hours later.

Source: Adapted from FR Kaufman: *Medical Management of Type 1 Diabetes*, 6th edition. Alexandria, VA. American Diabetes Association, 2012.

Insulin Regimens Representations of the various insulin regimens that may be used in type 1 DM are illustrated in Fig. 418-1. Although the insulin profiles are depicted as "smooth," symmetric curves, there is considerable patient-to-patient variation in the peak and duration. In all regimens, long-acting insulins (NPH, glargine, or detemir) supply basal insulin, whereas regular, insulin aspart, glulisine, or lispro insulin provides prandial insulin. Short-acting insulin analogues should be injected just before (<10 min) or just after a meal; regular insulin is given 30–45 min prior to a meal. Sometimes short-acting insulin analogues are injected just after a meal (gastroparesis, unpredictable food intake).

A shortcoming of current insulin regimens is that injected insulin immediately enters the systemic circulation, whereas endogenous

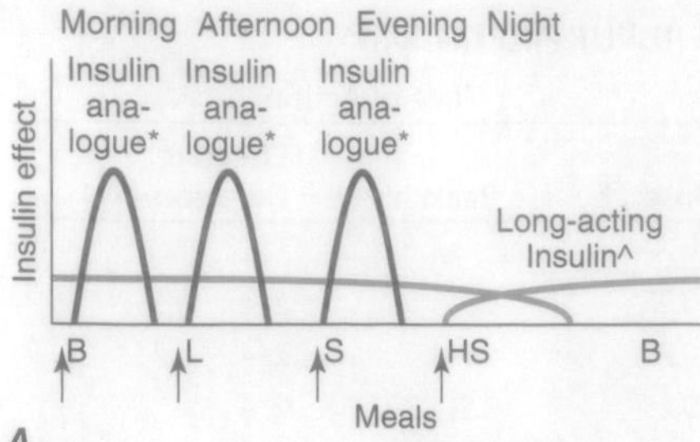

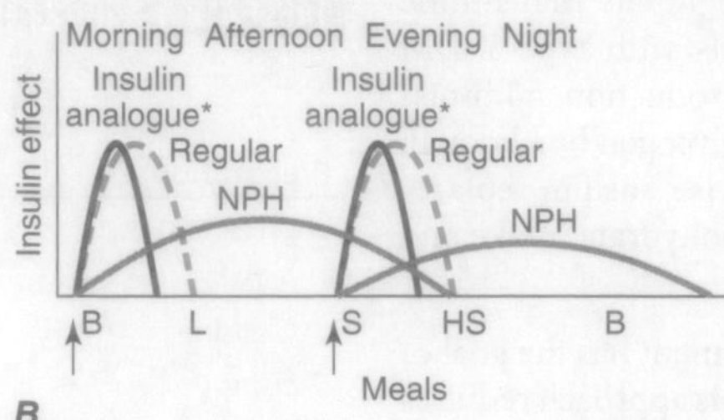

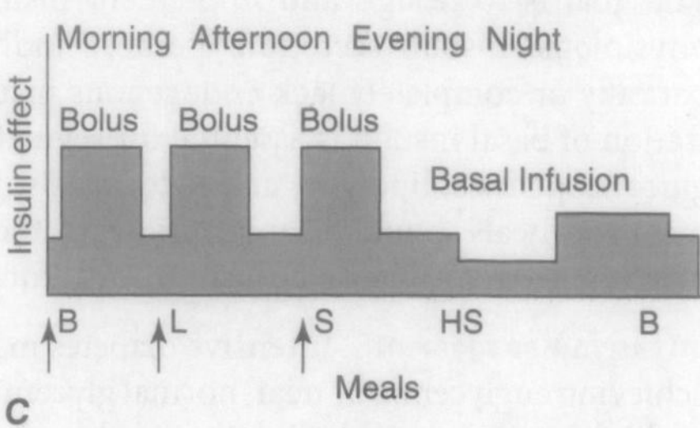

FIGURE 418-1 Representative insulin regimens for the treatment of diabetes. For each panel, the *y*-axis shows the amount of insulin effect and the *x*-axis shows the time of day. B, breakfast; HS, bedtime; L, lunch; S, supper. *Lispro, glulisine, or insulin aspart can be used. The time of insulin injection is shown with a *vertical arrow*. The type of insulin is noted above each insulin curve. ***A.*** Multiple-component insulin regimen consisting of long-acting insulin (^glargine or detemir) to provide basal insulin coverage and three shots of glulisine, lispro, or insulin aspart to provide glycemic coverage for each meal. ***B.*** Injection of two shots of long-acting insulin (NPH) and short-acting insulin analogue (glulisine, lispro, insulin aspart [*solid red line*], or regular insulin [*green dashed line*]). Only one formulation of short-acting insulin is used. ***C.*** Insulin administration by insulin infusion device is shown with the basal insulin and a bolus injection at each meal. The basal insulin rate is decreased during the evening and increased slightly prior to the patient awakening in the morning. Glulisine, lispro, or insulin aspart is used in the insulin pump. *(Adapted from H Lebovitz [ed]: Therapy for Diabetes Mellitus. American Diabetes Association, Alexandria, VA, 2004.)*

insulin is secreted into the portal venous system. Thus, exogenous insulin administration exposes the liver to subphysiologic insulin levels. No insulin regimen reproduces the precise insulin secretory pattern of the pancreatic islet. However, the most physiologic regimens entail more frequent insulin injections, greater reliance on short-acting insulin, and more frequent capillary plasma glucose measurements. In general, individuals with type 1 DM require 0.5–1 U/kg per day of insulin divided into multiple doses, with ~50% of the insulin given as basal insulin.

Multiple-component insulin regimens refer to the combination of basal insulin and bolus insulin (preprandial short-acting insulin). The timing and dose of short-acting, preprandial insulin are altered to accommodate the SMBG results, anticipated food intake, and physical activity. Such regimens offer the patient with type 1 diabetes more flexibility in terms of lifestyle and the best chance for achieving near normoglycemia. One such regimen, shown in Fig. 418-1*B*, consists of basal insulin with glargine or detemir and preprandial lispro, glulisine, or insulin aspart. The insulin aspart, glulisine, or lispro dose is based on individualized algorithms that integrate the preprandial glucose and the anticipated carbohydrate intake. To determine the meal component of the preprandial insulin dose, the patient uses an insulin-to-carbohydrate ratio (a common ratio for type 1 DM is 1–1.5 units/10 g of carbohydrate, but this must be determined for each individual). To this insulin dose is added the supplemental or correcting insulin based on the preprandial blood glucose (one formula uses 1 unit of insulin for every 2.7 mmol/L [50 mg/dL] over the preprandial glucose target; another formula uses [body weight in kg] × [blood glucose – desired glucose in mg/dL]/1500). An alternative multiple-component insulin regimen consists of bedtime NPH insulin, a small dose of NPH insulin at breakfast (20–30% of bedtime dose), and preprandial short-acting insulin. Other variations of this regimen are in use but have the disadvantage that NPH has a significant peak, making hypoglycemia more common. Frequent SMBG (more than three times per day) is absolutely essential for these types of insulin regimens.

In the past, one commonly used regimen consisted of twice-daily injections of NPH mixed with a short-acting insulin before the morning and evening meals (Fig. 418-1*B*). Such regimens usually prescribe two-thirds of the total daily insulin dose in the morning (with about two-thirds given as long-acting insulin and one-third as short-acting) and one-third before the evening meal (with approximately one-half given as long-acting insulin and one-half as short-acting). The drawback to such a regimen is that it forces a rigid schedule on the patient, in terms of daily activity and the content and timing of meals. Although it is simple and effective at avoiding severe hyperglycemia, it does not generate near-normal glycemic control in individuals with type 1 DM. Moreover, if the patient's meal pattern or content varies or if physical activity is increased, hyperglycemia or hypoglycemia may result. Moving the long-acting insulin from before the evening meal to bedtime may avoid nocturnal hypoglycemia and provide more insulin as glucose levels rise in the early morning (so-called dawn phenomenon). The insulin dose in such regimens should be adjusted based on SMBG results with the following general assumptions: (1) the fasting glucose is primarily determined by the prior evening long-acting insulin; (2) the pre-lunch glucose is a function of the morning short-acting insulin; (3) the pre-supper glucose is a function of the morning long-acting insulin; and (4) the bedtime glucose is a function of the pre-supper, short-acting insulin. This is not an optimal regimen for the patient with type 1 DM, but is sometimes used for patients with type 2 DM.

Continuous SC insulin infusion (CSII) is a very effective insulin regimen for the patient with type 1 DM (Fig. 418-1*C*). To the basal insulin infusion, a preprandial insulin ("bolus") is delivered by the insulin infusion device based on instructions from the patient, who uses an individualized algorithm incorporating the preprandial plasma glucose and anticipated carbohydrate intake. These sophisticated insulin infusion devices can accurately deliver small doses of insulin (microliters per hour) and have several advantages: (1) multiple basal infusion rates can be programmed to accommodate nocturnal versus daytime basal insulin requirement; (2) basal infusion rates can be altered during periods of exercise; (3) different waveforms of insulin infusion with meal-related bolus allow better matching of insulin depending on meal composition; and (4) programmed algorithms consider prior insulin administration and blood glucose values in calculating the insulin dose. These devices require instruction by a health professional with considerable experience with insulin-infusion devices and very frequent patient interactions with the diabetes management team. Insulin-infusion devices present unique challenges, such as infection at the infusion site, unexplained hyperglycemia because the infusion set becomes obstructed, or diabetic ketoacidosis if the pump becomes disconnected. Because most physicians use lispro, glulisine, or insulin aspart in CSII, the extremely short half-life of these insulins quickly leads to insulin deficiency if the delivery system is interrupted. Essential to the safe use of infusion devices is thorough patient education about pump function and frequent SMBG. Efforts to create a closed-loop system in which data from continuous glucose measurement regulate the insulin infusion rate are under way.

Other Agents That Improve Glucose Control The role of amylin, a 37-amino-acid peptide co-secreted with insulin from pancreatic beta cells, in normal glucose homeostasis is uncertain. However, based on the rationale that patients who are insulin deficient are also amylin deficient, an analogue of amylin (pramlintide) was created and found to reduce postprandial glycemic excursions in type 1 and type 2 diabetic patients taking insulin. Pramlintide injected just before a meal slows gastric emptying and suppresses glucagon but does not alter insulin levels. Pramlintide is approved for insulin-treated patients with type 1 and type 2 DM. Addition of pramlintide produces a modest reduction in the HbA_{1c} and seems to dampen meal-related glucose excursions. In type 1 DM, pramlintide is started as a 15-μg SC injection before each meal and titrated up to a maximum of 30–60 μg as tolerated. In type 2 DM, pramlintide is started as a 60-μg SC injection before each meal and may be titrated up to a maximum of 120 μg. The major side effects are nausea and vomiting, and dose escalations should be slow to limit these side effects. Because pramlintide slows gastric emptying, it may influence absorption of other medications and should not be used in combination with other drugs that slow GI motility. The short-acting insulin given before the meal should initially be reduced to avoid hypoglycemia and then titrated as the effects of the pramlintide become evident. α-Glucosidase inhibitors are sometimes used with insulin in type 1 DM.

TYPE 2 DIABETES MELLITUS

General Aspects The goals of glycemia-controlling therapy for type 2 DM are similar to those in type 1 DM. Whereas glycemic control tends to dominate the management of type 1 DM, the care of individuals with type 2 DM must also include attention to the treatment of conditions associated with type 2 DM (e.g., obesity, hypertension, dyslipidemia, CVD) and detection/management of DM-related complications (Fig. 418-2). Reduction in cardiovascular risk is of paramount importance because this is the leading cause of mortality in these individuals.

Type 2 DM management should begin with MNT (discussed above). An exercise regimen to increase insulin sensitivity and promote weight loss should also be instituted. Pharmacologic approaches to the management of type 2 DM include oral glucose-lowering agents, insulin, and other agents that improve glucose control; most physicians and patients prefer oral glucose-lowering agents as the initial choice. Any therapy that improves glycemic control reduces "glucose toxicity" to beta cells and improves endogenous insulin secretion. However, type 2 DM is a progressive disorder and ultimately requires multiple therapeutic agents and often insulin in most patients.

Glucose-Lowering Agents Advances in the therapy of type 2 DM have generated oral glucose-lowering agents that target different pathophysiologic processes in type 2 DM. Based on their mechanisms of action, glucose-lowering agents are subdivided into agents that increase insulin secretion, reduce glucose production, increase insulin sensitivity, enhance GLP-1 action, or promote urinary excretion of glucose (Table 418-5). Glucose-lowering agents other than insulin (with the exception of amylin analogue and α-glucosidase inhibitors) are ineffective in type 1 DM and should not be used for glucose management of severely ill individuals with type 2 DM. Insulin is sometimes the initial glucose-lowering agent in type 2 DM.

BIGUANIDES Metformin, representative of this class of agents, reduces hepatic glucose production and improves peripheral glucose utilization slightly (Table 418-5). Metformin activates AMP-dependent protein kinase and enters cells through organic cation transporters (polymorphisms of these may influence the response to metformin). Recent evidence indicates that metformin's mechanism for reducing hepatic glucose production is to antagonize glucagon's ability to generate cAMP in hepatocytes. Metformin reduces fasting plasma glucose (FPG) and insulin levels, improves the lipid profile, and promotes modest weight loss. An extended-release form is available and may have fewer gastrointestinal side effects (diarrhea, anorexia, nausea, metallic taste). Because of its relatively slow onset of action and gastrointestinal symptoms with higher doses, the initial dose should be low and then escalated every 2–3 weeks based on SMBG measurements. Metformin is effective as monotherapy and can be used in combination with other oral agents or with insulin. The major toxicity of metformin, lactic acidosis, is very rare and can be prevented by careful patient selection. Vitamin B_{12} levels are ~30% lower during metformin treatment. Metformin should not be used in patients with renal insufficiency (glomerular filtration rate [GFR] <60 mL/min), any form of acidosis, unstable congestive heart failure (CHF), liver disease, or severe hypoxemia. Some feel that that these guidelines are too restrictive and prevent individuals with mild to moderate renal impairment from being safely treated with metformin. The National Institute for Health and Clinical Excellence in the United Kingdom suggests that metformin be used at a GFR >30 mL/min, with a reduced dose when the GFR is <45 mL/min. Metformin should be discontinued in hospitalized patients, in patients who can take nothing orally, and in those receiving radiographic contrast material. Insulin should be used until metformin can be restarted.

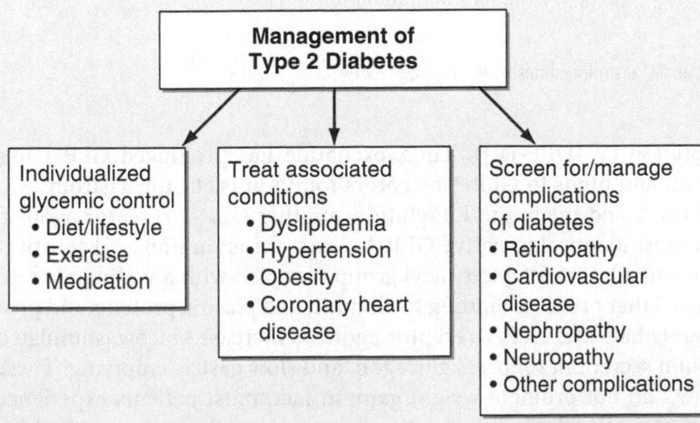

FIGURE 418-2 Essential elements in comprehensive care of type 2 diabetes.

INSULIN SECRETAGOGUES—AGENTS THAT AFFECT THE ATP-SENSITIVE K^+ CHANNEL Insulin secretagogues stimulate insulin secretion by interacting with the ATP-sensitive potassium channel on the beta cell (Chap. 417). These drugs are most effective in individuals with type 2 DM of relatively recent onset (<5 years) who have residual endogenous insulin production. First-generation sulfonylureas (chlorpropamide, tolazamide, tolbutamide) have a longer half-life, a greater incidence of hypoglycemia, and more frequent drug interactions, and are no longer used. Second-generation sulfonylureas have a more rapid onset of action and better coverage of the postprandial glucose rise, but the shorter half-life of some agents may require more than once-a-day dosing. Sulfonylureas reduce both fasting and postprandial glucose and should be initiated at low doses and increased at 1- to 2-week intervals based on SMBG. In general, sulfonylureas increase insulin acutely and thus should be taken shortly before a meal; with chronic therapy, though, the insulin release is more sustained. Glimepiride and glipizide can be given in a single daily dose and are preferred over glyburide, especially in the elderly. Repaglinide, nateglinide, and mitiglinide are not sulfonylureas but also interact with the ATP-sensitive potassium channel. Because of their short half-life, these agents are given with each meal or immediately before to reduce meal-related glucose excursions.

Insulin secretagogues, especially the longer acting ones, have the potential to cause hypoglycemia, especially in elderly individuals. Hypoglycemia is usually related to delayed meals, increased physical activity, alcohol intake, or renal insufficiency. Individuals who ingest an overdose of some agents develop prolonged and serious hypoglycemia and should be monitored closely in the hospital (Chap. 420). Most sulfonylureas are metabolized in the liver to compounds (some of which are active) that are cleared by the kidney. Thus, their use in individuals with significant hepatic or renal dysfunction is not advisable. Weight gain, a common side effect of sulfonylurea therapy, results from the increased insulin levels and improvement in glycemic control. Some sulfonylureas have significant drug interactions with alcohol and some medications including warfarin, aspirin, ketoconazole, α-glucosidase inhibitors, and fluconazole. A related isoform of ATP-sensitive potassium channels is present in the myocardium and the brain. All of these agents except glyburide have a low affinity for this isoform. Despite concerns that this agent might affect the myocardial response to ischemia and observational studies suggesting that sulfonylureas increase cardiovascular risk, studies have not shown an increased cardiac mortality with glyburide or other agents in this class.

TABLE 418-5 AGENTS USED FOR TREATMENT OF TYPE 1 OR TYPE 2 DIABETES

	Mechanism of Action	Examples[a]	HbA_{1c} Reduction (%)[b]	Agent-Specific Advantages	Agent-Specific Disadvantages	Contraindications
Oral						
Biguanides[c*]	↓ Hepatic glucose production	Metformin	1–2	Weight neutral, do not cause hypoglycemia, inexpensive, extensive experience, ↓ CV events	Diarrhea, nausea, lactic acidosis	Serum creatinine >1.5 mg/dL (men) >1.4 mg/dL (women) (see text), CHF, radiographic contrast studies, hospitalized patients, acidosis
α-Glucosidase inhibitors[c**]	↓ GI glucose absorption	Acarbose, miglitol, voglibose	0.5–0.8	Reduce postprandial glycemia	GI flatulence, liver function tests	Renal/liver disease
Dipeptidyl peptidase IV inhibitors[c***]	Prolong endogenous GLP-1 action	Alogliptin, Anagliptin, Gemigliptin, linagliptin, saxagliptin, sitagliptin, teneligliptin, vildagliptin	0.5–0.8	Well tolerated, do not cause hypoglycemia		Reduced dose with renal disease; one associated with increase heart failure risk; possible association with ACE inhibitor–induced angioedema
Insulin secretagogues: Sulfonylureas[c*]	↑ Insulin secretion	Glibornuride, gliclazide, glimepiride, glipizide, gliquidone, glyburide, glyclopyramide	1–2	Short onset of action, lower postprandial glucose, inexpensive	Hypoglycemia, weight gain	Renal/liver disease
Insulin secretagogues: Nonsulfonylureas[c***]	↑ Insulin secretion	Nateglinide, repaglinide, mitiglinide	0.5–1.0	Short onset of action, lower postprandial glucose	Hypoglycemia	Renal/liver disease
Sodium-glucose co-transporter 2 inhibitors[***]	↑ Urinary glucose excretion	Canagliflozin, dapagliflozin, empagliflozin	0.5–1.0	Insulin secretion and action independent	Urinary and vaginal infections, dehydration, exacerbate tendency to hyperkalemia	Limited clinical experience; moderate renal insufficiency
Thiazolidinediones[c***]	↓ Insulin resistance, ↑ glucose utilization	Rosiglitazone, pioglitazone	0.5–1.4	Lower insulin requirements	Peripheral edema, CHF, weight gain, fractures, macular edema	CHF, liver disease
Parenteral						
Amylin agonists[c,d***]	Slow gastric emptying, ↓ glucagon	Pramlintide	0.25–0.5	Reduce postprandial glycemia, weight loss	Injection, nausea, ↑ risk of hypoglycemia with insulin	Agents that also slow GI motility
GLP-1 receptor agonists[c***]	↑ Insulin, ↓ glucagon, slow gastric emptying, satiety	Exenatide, liraglutide, dulaglutide	0.5–1.0	Weight loss, do not cause hypoglycemia	Injection, nausea, ↑ risk of hypoglycemia with insulin secretagogues	Renal disease, agents that also slow GI motility; medullary carcinoma of thyroid
Insulin[c,d****]	↑ Glucose utilization, ↓ hepatic glucose production, and other anabolic actions	See text and Table 418-4	Not limited	Known safety profile	Injection, weight gain, hypoglycemia	
Medical nutrition therapy and physical activity[c]	↓ Insulin resistance, ↑ insulin secretion	Low-calorie, low-fat diet, exercise	1–3	Other health benefits	Compliance difficult, long-term success low	

[a]Examples are approved for use in at least one country, but may not be available in the United States or all countries. Examples may not include all agents in the class. [b]HbA1c reduction (absolute) depends partly on starting HbA_{1c}. [c]Used for treatment of type 2 diabetes. [d]Used in conjunction with insulin for treatment of type 1 diabetes. Cost of agent: *low, **moderate, ***high, ****variable.

Note: Some agents used to treat type 2 DM are not included in table (see text).

Abbreviations: ACE, angiotensin-converting enzyme; CHF, congestive heart failure; CV, cardiovascular; GI, gastrointestinal; HbA_{1c}, hemoglobin A_{1c}.

INSULIN SECRETAGOGUES—AGENTS THAT ENHANCE GLP-1 RECEPTOR SIGNALING "Incretins" amplify glucose-stimulated insulin secretion (Chap. 417). Agents that either act as a GLP-1 receptor agonist or enhance endogenous GLP-1 activity are approved for the treatment of type 2 DM (Table 418-5). Agents in this class do not cause hypoglycemia because of the glucose-dependent nature of incretin-stimulated insulin secretion (unless there is concomitant use of an agent that can lead to hypoglycemia—sulfonylureas, etc.). Exenatide, a synthetic version of a peptide initially identified in the saliva of the Gila monster (exendin-4), is an analogue of GLP-1. Unlike native GLP-1, which has a half-life of >5 min, differences in the exenatide amino acid sequence render it resistant to the enzyme that degrades GLP-1 (dipeptidyl peptidase IV [DPP-IV]). Thus, exenatide has prolonged GLP-1-like action and binds to GLP-1 receptors found in islets, the gastrointestinal tract, and the brain. Liraglutide, another GLP-1 receptor agonist, is almost identical to native GLP-1 except for an amino acid substitution and addition of a fatty acyl group (coupled with a γ-glutamic acid spacer) that promote binding to albumin and plasma proteins and prolong its half-life. GLP-1 receptor agonists increase glucose-stimulated insulin secretion, suppress glucagon, and slow gastric emptying. These agents do not promote weight gain; in fact, most patients experience modest weight loss and appetite suppression. Treatment with these agents should start at a low dose to minimize initial side effects (nausea being the limiting one). GLP-1 receptor agonists, available in twice daily, daily, and weekly injectable formulations, can be used as combination therapy with metformin, sulfonylureas, and thiazolidinediones. Some patients taking insulin secretagogues may require a reduction in those agents to prevent hypoglycemia. The major side effects are nausea, vomiting, and diarrhea. Some formulations carry a black box warning from the FDA because of an increased risk of thyroid C-cell tumors in rodents and are contraindicated in individuals with medullary carcinoma of the thyroid or multiple endocrine neoplasia. Because GLP-1 receptor agonists slow gastric emptying, they may influence the absorption of other drugs. Whether GLP-1 receptor agonists enhance beta cell survival, promote beta cell proliferation, or alter the natural history of type 2 DM is not known. Other GLP-1 receptor agonists and formulations are under development.

DPP-IV inhibitors inhibit degradation of native GLP-1 and thus enhance the incretin effect. DPP-IV, which is widely expressed on the cell surface of endothelial cells and some lymphocytes, degrades a wide range of peptides (not GLP-1 specific). DPP-IV inhibitors promote insulin secretion in the absence of hypoglycemia or weight gain and appear to have a preferential effect on postprandial blood glucose. The levels of GLP-1 action in the patient are greater with the GLP-1 receptor agonists than with DPP-IV inhibitors. DPP-IV inhibitors are used either alone or in combination with other oral agents in type 2 DM. Reduced doses should be given to patients with renal insufficiency. Initial concerns about the pancreatic side effects of GLP-1 receptor agonists and DPP-IV inhibitors (pancreatitis, possible premalignant lesions) appear to be unfounded.

α-GLUCOSIDASE INHIBITORS α-Glucosidase inhibitors reduce postprandial hyperglycemia by delaying glucose absorption; they do not affect glucose utilization or insulin secretion (Table 418-5). Postprandial hyperglycemia, secondary to impaired hepatic and peripheral glucose disposal, contributes significantly to the hyperglycemic state in type 2 DM. These drugs, taken just before each meal, reduce glucose absorption by inhibiting the enzyme that cleaves oligosaccharides into simple sugars in the intestinal lumen. Therapy should be initiated at a low dose with the evening meal and increased to a maximal dose over weeks to months. The major side effects (diarrhea, flatulence, abdominal distention) are related to increased delivery of oligosaccharides to the large bowel and can be reduced somewhat by gradual upward dose titration. α-Glucosidase inhibitors may increase levels of sulfonylureas and increase the incidence of hypoglycemia. Simultaneous treatment with bile acid resins and antacids should be avoided. These agents should not be used in individuals with inflammatory bowel disease, gastroparesis, or a serum creatinine >177 μmol/L (2 mg/dL). This class of agents is not as potent as other oral agents in lowering the HbA_{1c} but is unique because it reduces the postprandial glucose rise even in individuals with type 1 DM. If hypoglycemia from other diabetes treatments occurs while taking these agents, the patient should consume glucose because the degradation and absorption of complex carbohydrates will be retarded.

THIAZOLIDINEDIONES Thiazolidinediones (Table 418-5) reduce insulin resistance by binding to the PPAR γ (peroxisome proliferator–activated receptor γ) nuclear receptor (which forms a heterodimer with the retinoid X receptor). The PPAR-γ receptor is found at highest levels in adipocytes but is expressed at lower levels in many other tissues. Agonists of this receptor regulate a large number of genes, promote adipocyte differentiation, reduce hepatic fat accumulation, and promote fatty acid storage. Thiazolidinediones promote a redistribution of fat from central to peripheral locations. Circulating insulin levels decrease with use of the thiazolidinediones, indicating a reduction in insulin resistance. Although direct comparisons are not available, the two currently available thiazolidinediones appear to have similar efficacy. The prototype of this class of drugs, troglitazone, was withdrawn from the U.S. market after reports of hepatotoxicity and an association with an idiosyncratic liver reaction that sometimes led to hepatic failure. Although rosiglitazone and pioglitazone do not appear to induce the liver abnormalities seen with troglitazone, the FDA recommends measurement of liver function tests prior to initiating therapy.

Rosiglitazone raises low-density lipoprotein (LDL), high-density lipoprotein (HDL), and triglycerides slightly. Pioglitazone raises HDL to a greater degree and LDL a lesser degree but lowers triglycerides. The clinical significance of the lipid changes with these agents is not known and may be difficult to ascertain because most patients with type 2 DM are also treated with a statin.

Thiazolidinediones are associated with weight gain (2–3 kg), a small reduction in the hematocrit, and a mild increase in plasma volume. Peripheral edema and CHF are more common in individuals treated with these agents. These agents are contraindicated in patients with liver disease or CHF (class III or IV). The FDA has issued an alert that rare patients taking these agents may experience a worsening of diabetic macular edema. An increased risk of fractures has been noted in women taking these agents. Thiazolidinediones have been shown to induce ovulation in premenopausal women with polycystic ovary syndrome. Women should be warned about the risk of pregnancy because the safety of thiazolidinediones in pregnancy is not established.

Concerns about increased cardiovascular risk associated with rosiglitazone led to considerable restrictions on its use and to the FDA issuing a "black box" warning in 2007. However, based on new information, the FDA has revised its guidelines and categorizes rosiglitazone similar to other drugs for type 2 DM. Because of a possible increased risk of bladder cancer, pioglitazone is part of an ongoing FDA safety review.

Sodium-Glucose Co-Transporter 2 Inhibitors (SLGT2) These agents (Table 418-5) lower the blood glucose by selectively inhibiting this co-transporter, which is expressed almost exclusively in the proximal, convoluted tubule in the kidney. This inhibits glucose reabsorption, lowers the renal threshold for glucose, and leads to increased urinary glucose excretion. Thus, the glucose-lowering effect is insulin independent and not related to changes in insulin sensitivity or secretion. Because these agents are the newest class to treat type 2 DM (Table 418-5), clinical experience is limited. Due to the increased urinary glucose, urinary or vaginal infections are more common, and the diuretic effect can lead to reduced intravascular volume. As part of the FDA approval of canagliflozin in 2013, postmarketing studies for cardiovascular outcomes and for monitoring bladder and urinary cancer risk are under way.

OTHER THERAPIES FOR TYPE 2 DM

Bile acid–binding resins Evidence indicates that bile acids, by signaling through nuclear receptors, may have a role in metabolism. Bile acid metabolism is abnormal in type 2 DM. The bile acid–binding resin colesevelam has been approved for the treatment of type 2 DM (already approved for treatment of hypercholesterolemia). Because bile acid–binding resins are minimally absorbed into the systemic circulation, how bile acid–binding resins lower blood glucose is not known. The most common side effects are gastrointestinal (constipation, abdominal pain, and nausea). Bile acid–binding resins can increase plasma triglycerides and should be used cautiously in patients with a tendency for hypertriglyceridemia. The role of this class of drugs in the treatment of type 2 DM is not yet defined.

Bromocriptine A formulation of the dopamine receptor agonist bromocriptine (Cycloset) has been approved by the FDA for the treatment of type 2 DM. However, its role in the treatment of type 2 DM is uncertain.

INSULIN THERAPY IN TYPE 2 DM Insulin should be considered as the initial therapy in type 2 DM, particularly in lean individuals or those with severe weight loss, in individuals with underlying renal or hepatic disease that precludes oral glucose-lowering agents, or in individuals who are hospitalized or acutely ill. Insulin therapy is ultimately required by a substantial number of individuals with type 2 DM because of the progressive nature of the disorder and the relative insulin deficiency that develops in patients with long-standing diabetes. Both physician and patient reluctance often delay the initiation of insulin therapy, but glucose control and patient well-being are improved by insulin therapy in patients who have not reached the glycemic target.

Because endogenous insulin secretion continues and is capable of providing some coverage of mealtime caloric intake, insulin is usually initiated in a single dose of long-acting insulin (0.3–0.4 U/kg per day), given in the evening (NPH) or just before bedtime (NPH, glargine, detemir). Because fasting hyperglycemia and increased hepatic glucose production are prominent features of type 2 DM, bedtime insulin is more effective in clinical trials than a single dose of morning insulin. Glargine given at bedtime has less nocturnal hypoglycemia than NPH insulin. Some physicians prefer a relatively low, fixed starting dose of long-acting insulin (5–15 units) or a weight-based dose (0.2 units/kg). The insulin dose may then be adjusted in 10% increments as dictated by SMBG results. Both morning and bedtime long-acting insulin may be used in combination with oral glucose-lowering agents. Initially, basal insulin may be sufficient, but often prandial insulin coverage with multiple insulin injections is needed as diabetes progresses (see insulin regimens used for type 1 DM). Other insulin formulations that have a combination of short-acting and long-acting insulin (Table 418-4) are sometimes used in patients with type 2 DM because of convenience but do not allow independent adjustment of short-acting and long-acting insulin dose and often do not achieve the same degree of glycemic control as basal/bolus regimens. In selected patients with type 2 DM, insulin-infusion devices may be considered.

CHOICE OF INITIAL GLUCOSE-LOWERING AGENT The level of hyperglycemia and the patient's individualized goal (see "Establishment of Target Level of Glycemic Control") should influence the initial choice of therapy. Assuming that maximal benefit of MNT and increased physical activity has been realized, patients with mild to moderate hyperglycemia (FPG <11.1–13.9 mmol/L [200–250 mg/dL]) often respond well to a single, oral glucose-lowering agent. Patients with more severe hyperglycemia (FPG >13.9 mmol/L [250 mg/dL]) may respond partially but are unlikely to achieve normoglycemia with oral monotherapy. A stepwise approach that starts with a single agent and adds a second agent to achieve the glycemic target can be used (see "Combination therapy with glucose-lowering agents," below). Insulin can be used as initial therapy in individuals with severe hyperglycemia (FPG <13.9–16.7 mmol/L [250–300 mg/dL]) or in those who are symptomatic from the hyperglycemia. This approach is based on the rationale that more rapid glycemic control will reduce "glucose toxicity" to the islet cells, improve endogenous insulin secretion, and possibly allow oral glucose-lowering agents to be more effective. If this occurs, the insulin may be discontinued.

Insulin secretagogues, biguanides, α-glucosidase inhibitors, thiazolidinediones, GLP-1 receptor agonists, DPP-IV inhibitors, SLGT2 inhibitors, and insulin are approved for monotherapy of type 2 DM. Although each class of oral glucose-lowering agents has advantages and disadvantages (Table 418-5), certain generalizations apply: (1) insulin secretagogues, biguanides, GLP-1 receptor agonists, and thiazolidinediones improve glycemic control to a similar degree (1–2% reduction in HbA_{1c}) and are more effective than α-glucosidase inhibitors, DPP-IV inhibitors, and SLGT2 inhibitors; (2) assuming a similar degree of glycemic improvement, no clinical advantage to one class of drugs has been demonstrated; any therapy that improves glycemic control is likely beneficial; (3) insulin secretagogues, GLP-1 receptor agonists, DPP-IV inhibitors, α-glucosidase inhibitors, and SLGT2 inhibitors begin to lower the plasma glucose immediately, whereas the glucose-lowering effects of the biguanides and thiazolidinediones are delayed by weeks; (4) not all agents are effective in all individuals with type 2 DM; (5) biguanides, α-glucosidase inhibitors, GLP-1 receptor agonists, DPP-IV inhibitors, thiazolidinediones, and SLGT2 inhibitors do not directly cause hypoglycemia; (6) most individuals will eventually require treatment with more than one class of oral glucose-lowering agents or insulin, reflecting the progressive nature of type 2 DM; and (7) durability of glycemic control is slightly less for glyburide compared to metformin or rosiglitazone.

Considerable clinical experience exists with metformin and sulfonylureas because they have been available for several decades. It is assumed that the α-glucosidase inhibitors, GLP-1 agonists, DPP-IV inhibitors, thiazolidinediones, and SLGT2 inhibitors will reduce

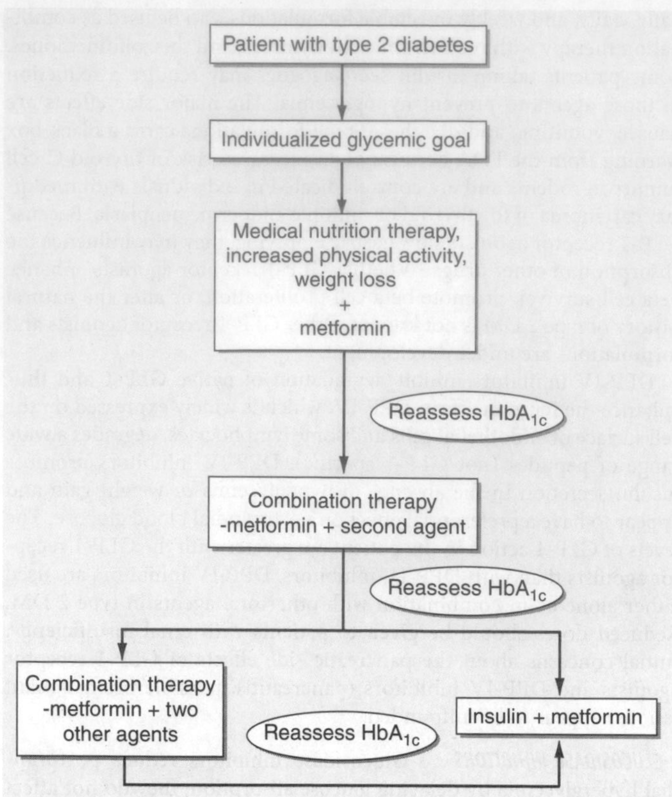

FIGURE 418-3 Glycemic management of type 2 diabetes. See text for discussion of treatment of severe hyperglycemia or symptomatic hyperglycemia. Agents that can be combined with metformin include insulin secretagogues, thiazolidinediones, α-glucosidase inhibitors, DPP-IV inhibitors, GLP-1 receptor agonists, SLGT2 inhibitors, and insulin. HbA_{1c}, hemoglobin HbA_{1c}.

DM-related complications by improving glycemic control, but long-term data are not yet available. The thiazolidinediones are theoretically attractive because they target a fundamental abnormality in type 2 DM, namely insulin resistance. However, all of these agents are currently more costly than metformin and sulfonylureas.

Treatment algorithms by several professional societies (ADA/European Association for the Study of Diabetes [EASD], IDF, AACE) suggest metformin as initial therapy because of its efficacy, known side effect profile, and low cost (Fig. 418-3). Metformin's advantages are that it promotes mild weight loss, lowers insulin levels, and improves the lipid profile slightly. Based on SMBG results and the HbA_{1c}, the dose of metformin should be increased until the glycemic target is achieved or maximum dose is reached. If metformin is not tolerated, then initial therapy with an insulin secretagogue or DPP-IV inhibitor is reasonable.

COMBINATION THERAPY WITH GLUCOSE-LOWERING AGENTS A number of combinations of therapeutic agents are successful in type 2 DM (metformin + second oral agent, metformin + GLP-1 receptor agonist, or metformin + insulin), and the dosing of agents in combination is the same as when the agents are used alone. Because mechanisms of action of the first and second agents should be different, the effect on glycemic control is usually additive. There are little data to support the choice of one combination over another combination. Medication costs vary considerably (Table 418-5), and this often factors into medication choice. Several fixed-dose combinations of oral agents are available, but evidence that they are superior to titration of single agent to a maximum dose and then addition of a second agent is lacking. If adequate control is not achieved with the combination of two agents (based on reassessment of the HbA_{1c} every 3 months), a third oral agent or basal insulin should be added (Fig. 418-3). Treatment approaches vary considerably from country to country. For example, α-glucosidase inhibitors are used commonly in South Asian patients

(Indian), but infrequently in the United States or Europe. Whether this reflects an underlying difference in the disease or physician preference is not clear.

Treatment with insulin becomes necessary as type 2 DM enters the phase of relative insulin deficiency (as seen in long-standing DM) and is signaled by inadequate glycemic control with one or two oral glucose-lowering agents. Insulin alone or in combination should be used in patients who fail to reach the glycemic target. For example, a single dose of long-acting insulin at bedtime is often effective in combination with metformin. In contrast, insulin secretagogues have little utility once insulin therapy is started. Experience using incretin therapies and insulin is limited. As endogenous insulin production falls further, multiple injections of long-acting and short-acting insulin regimens are necessary to control postprandial glucose excursions. These insulin regimens are identical to the long-acting and short-acting combination regimens discussed above for type 1 DM. Because the hyperglycemia of type 2 DM tends to be more "stable," these regimens can be increased in 10% increments every 2–3 days using the fasting blood glucose results. Weight gain and hypoglycemia are the major adverse effects of insulin therapy. The daily insulin dose required can become quite large (1–2 units/kg per day) as endogenous insulin production falls and insulin resistance persists. Individuals who require >1 unit/kg per day of long-acting insulin should be considered for combination therapy with metformin or a thiazolidinedione. The addition of metformin or a thiazolidinedione can reduce insulin requirements in some individuals with type 2 DM, while maintaining or even improving glycemic control. Insulin plus a thiazolidinedione promotes weight gain and is associated with peripheral edema. Addition of a thiazolidinedione to a patient's insulin regimen may necessitate a reduction in the insulin dose to avoid hypoglycemia. Patients requiring large doses of insulin (>200 units/day) can be treated with a more concentrated form of insulin, U-500.

EMERGING THERAPIES

Whole pancreas transplantation (performed concomitantly with a renal transplant) may normalize glucose tolerance and is an important therapeutic option in type 1 DM with end-stage renal disease, although it requires substantial expertise and is associated with the side effects of immunosuppression. Pancreatic islet transplantation has been plagued by limitations in pancreatic islet supply and graft survival and remains an area of clinical investigation. Many individuals with long-standing type 1 DM still produce very small amounts of insulin or have insulin-positive cells within the pancreas. This suggests that beta cells may slowly regenerate but are quickly destroyed by the autoimmune process. Thus, efforts to suppress the autoimmune process and to stimulate beta cell regeneration are being tested both at the time of diagnosis and in years after the diagnosis of type 1 DM. Closed-loop pumps that infuse the appropriate amount of insulin in response to changing glucose levels are potentially feasible now that CGM technology has been developed. Bi-hormonal pumps that deliver both insulin and glucagon are under development. New therapies under development for type 2 DM include activators of glucokinase, inhibitors of 11 β-hydroxysteroid dehydrogenase-1, GPR40 agonists, monoclonal antibodies to reduce inflammation, and salsalate.

Bariatric surgery for obese individuals with type 2 DM has shown considerable promise, sometimes with dramatic resolution of the diabetes or major reductions in the needed dose of glucose-lowering therapies (Chap. 416). Several large, unblinded clinical trials have demonstrated a much greater efficacy of bariatric surgery compared to medical management in the treatment of type 2 DM; the durability of the diabetes reversal or improvement is uncertain. The ADA clinical guidelines state that bariatric surgery should be considered in individuals with DM and a body mass index >35 kg/m^2.

ADVERSE EFFECTS OF THERAPY FOR DIABETES MELLITUS

As with any therapy, the benefits of efforts directed toward glycemic control must be balanced against the risks of treatment (Table 418-5). Side effects of intensive treatment include an increased frequency of serious hypoglycemia, weight gain, increased economic costs, and greater demands on the patient. In the DCCT, quality of life was very similar in the intensive and standard therapy groups. The most serious complication of therapy for DM is hypoglycemia, and its treatment with oral glucose or glucagon injection is discussed in Chap. 420. Severe, recurrent hypoglycemia warrants examination of treatment regimen and glycemic goal for the individual patient. Weight gain occurs with most (insulin, insulin secretagogues, thiazolidinediones) but not all (metformin, α-glucosidase inhibitors, GLP-1 receptor agonists, DPP-IV inhibitors) therapies. The weight gain is partially due to the anabolic effects of insulin and the reduction in glucosuria. As a result of recent controversies about the optimal glycemic goal and concerns about safety, the FDA now requires information about the cardiovascular safety profile as part of its evaluation of new treatments for type 2 DM.

ACUTE DISORDERS RELATED TO SEVERE HYPERGLYCEMIA

Individuals with type 1 or type 2 DM and severe hyperglycemia (>16.7 mmol/L [300 mg/dL]) should be assessed for clinical stability, including mentation and hydration. Depending on the patient and the rapidity and duration of the severe hyperglycemia, an individual may require more intense and rapid therapy to lower the blood glucose. However, many patients with poorly controlled diabetes and hyperglycemia have few symptoms. The physician should assess if the patient is stable or if diabetic ketoacidosis or a hyperglycemic hyperosmolar state should be considered. Ketones, an indicator of diabetic ketoacidosis, should be measured in individuals with type 1 DM when the plasma glucose is >16.7 mmol/L (300 mg/dL), during a concurrent illness, or with symptoms such as nausea, vomiting, or abdominal pain. Blood measurement of β-hydroxybutyrate is preferred over urine testing with nitroprusside-based assays that measure only acetoacetate and acetone.

Diabetic ketoacidosis (DKA) and hyperglycemic hyperosmolar state (HHS) are acute, severe disorders directly related to diabetes. DKA was formerly considered a hallmark of type 1 DM, but also occurs in individuals who lack immunologic features of type 1 DM and who can sometimes subsequently be treated with oral glucose-lowering agents (these obese individuals with type 2 DM are often of Hispanic or African-American descent). HHS is primarily seen in individuals with type 2 DM. Both disorders are associated with absolute or relative insulin deficiency, volume depletion, and acid-base abnormalities. DKA and HHS exist along a continuum of hyperglycemia, with or without ketosis. The metabolic similarities and differences in DKA and HHS are highlighted in Table 418-6. Both

TABLE 418-6 LABORATORY VALUES IN DIABETIC KETOACIDOSIS (DKA) AND HYPERGLYCEMIC HYPEROSMOLAR STATE (HHS) (REPRESENTATIVE RANGES AT PRESENTATION)

	DKA	HHS
Glucose,[a] mmol/L (mg/dL)	13.9–33.3 (250–600)	33.3–66.6 (600–1200)
Sodium, meq/L	125–135	135–145
Potassium[a,b]	Normal to ↑	Normal
Magnesium[a]	Normal	Normal
Chloride[a]	Normal	Normal
Phosphate[a,b]	Normal	Normal
Creatinine	Slightly ↑	Moderately ↑
Osmolality (mOsm/mL)	300–320	330–380
Plasma ketones[a]	++++	+/–
Serum bicarbonate,[a] meq/L	<15	Normal to slightly ↓
Arterial pH	6.8–7.3	>7.3
Arterial P_{CO_2},[a] mmHg	20–30	Normal
Anion gap[a](Na – [Cl + HCO_3])	↑	Normal to slightly ↑

[a]Large changes occur during treatment of DKA. [b]Although plasma levels may be normal or high at presentation, total-body stores are usually depleted.

disorders are associated with potentially serious complications if not promptly diagnosed and treated.

DIABETIC KETOACIDOSIS

Clinical Features The symptoms and physical signs of DKA are listed in Table 418-7 and usually develop over 24 h. DKA may be the initial symptom complex that leads to a diagnosis of type 1 DM, but more frequently, it occurs in individuals with established diabetes. Nausea and vomiting are often prominent, and their presence in an individual with diabetes warrants laboratory evaluation for DKA. Abdominal pain may be severe and can resemble acute pancreatitis or ruptured viscus. Hyperglycemia leads to glucosuria, volume depletion, and tachycardia. Hypotension can occur because of volume depletion in combination with peripheral vasodilatation. Kussmaul respirations and a fruity odor on the patient's breath (secondary to metabolic acidosis and increased acetone) are classic signs of the disorder. Lethargy and central nervous system depression may evolve into coma with severe DKA but should also prompt evaluation for other reasons for altered mental status (e.g., infection, hypoxemia). Cerebral edema, an extremely serious complication of DKA, is seen most frequently in children. Signs of infection, which may precipitate DKA, should be sought on physical examination, even in the absence of fever. Tissue ischemia (heart, brain) can also be a precipitating factor. Omission of insulin because of an eating disorder, mental health disorders, or an unstable psychosocial environment may sometimes be a factor precipitating DKA.

Pathophysiology DKA results from relative or absolute insulin deficiency combined with counterregulatory hormone excess (glucagon, catecholamines, cortisol, and growth hormone). Both insulin deficiency and glucagon excess, in particular, are necessary for DKA to develop. The decreased ratio of insulin to glucagon promotes gluconeogenesis, glycogenolysis, and ketone body formation in the liver, as well as increases in substrate delivery from fat and muscle (free fatty acids, amino acids) to the liver. Markers of inflammation (cytokines, C-reactive protein) are elevated in both DKA and HHS

The combination of insulin deficiency and hyperglycemia reduces the hepatic level of fructose-2,6-bisphosphate, which alters the activity of phosphofructokinase and fructose-1,6-bisphosphatase. Glucagon excess decreases the activity of pyruvate kinase, whereas insulin deficiency increases the activity of phosphoenolpyruvate carboxykinase. These changes shift the handling of pyruvate toward glucose synthesis and away from glycolysis. The increased levels of glucagon and catecholamines in the face of low insulin levels promote glycogenolysis. Insulin deficiency also reduces levels of the GLUT4 glucose transporter, which impairs glucose uptake into skeletal muscle and fat and reduces intracellular glucose metabolism.

Ketosis results from a marked increase in free fatty acid release from adipocytes, with a resulting shift toward ketone body synthesis in the liver. Reduced insulin levels, in combination with elevations in catecholamines and growth hormone, increase lipolysis and the release of free fatty acids. Normally, these free fatty acids are converted to triglycerides or very-low-density lipoprotein (VLDL) in the liver. However, in DKA, hyperglucagonemia alters hepatic metabolism to favor ketone body formation, through activation of the enzyme carnitine palmitoyltransferase I. This enzyme is crucial for regulating fatty acid transport into the mitochondria, where beta oxidation and conversion to ketone bodies occur. At physiologic pH, ketone bodies exist as ketoacids, which are neutralized by bicarbonate. As bicarbonate stores are depleted, metabolic acidosis ensues. Increased lactic acid production also contributes to the acidosis. The increased free fatty acids increase triglyceride and VLDL production. VLDL clearance is also reduced because the activity of insulin-sensitive lipoprotein lipase in muscle and fat is decreased. Hypertriglyceridemia may be severe enough to cause pancreatitis.

DKA is often precipitated by increased insulin requirements, as occurs during a concurrent illness (Table 418-7). Failure to augment insulin therapy often compounds the problem. Complete omission or inadequate administration of insulin by the patient or health care team (in a hospitalized patient with type 1 DM) may precipitate DKA. Patients using insulin-infusion devices with short-acting insulin may develop DKA, because even a brief interruption in insulin delivery (e.g., mechanical malfunction) quickly leads to insulin deficiency.

Laboratory Abnormalities and Diagnosis The timely diagnosis of DKA is crucial and allows for prompt initiation of therapy. DKA is characterized by hyperglycemia, ketosis, and metabolic acidosis (increased anion gap) along with a number of secondary metabolic derangements (Table 418-6). Occasionally, the serum glucose is only minimally elevated. Serum bicarbonate is frequently <10 mmol/L, and arterial pH ranges between 6.8 and 7.3, depending on the severity of the acidosis. Despite a total-body potassium deficit, the serum potassium at presentation may be mildly elevated, secondary to the acidosis. Total-body stores of sodium, chloride, phosphorus, and magnesium are reduced in DKA but are not accurately reflected by their levels in the serum because of hypovolemia and hyperglycemia. Elevated blood urea nitrogen (BUN) and serum creatinine levels reflect intravascular volume depletion. Interference from acetoacetate may falsely elevate the serum creatinine measurement. Leukocytosis, hypertriglyceridemia, and hyperlipoproteinemia are commonly found as well. Hyperamylasemia may suggest a diagnosis of pancreatitis, especially when accompanied by abdominal pain. However, in DKA the amylase is usually of salivary origin and thus is not diagnostic of pancreatitis. Serum lipase should be obtained if pancreatitis is suspected.

The measured serum sodium is reduced as a consequence of the hyperglycemia (1.6-mmol/L [1.6-meq] reduction in serum sodium for each 5.6-mmol/L [100-mg/dL] rise in the serum glucose). A normal serum sodium in the setting of DKA indicates a more profound water deficit. In "conventional" units, the calculated serum osmolality (2 × [serum sodium + serum potassium] + plasma glucose [mg/dL]/18 + BUN/2.8) is mildly to moderately elevated, although to a lesser degree than that found in HHS (see below).

In DKA, the ketone body, β-hydroxybutyrate, is synthesized at a threefold greater rate than acetoacetate; however, acetoacetate is preferentially detected by a commonly used ketosis detection reagent (nitroprusside). Serum ketones are present at significant levels (usually positive at serum dilution of ≥1:8). The nitroprusside tablet, or stick, is often used to detect urine ketones; certain medications such as captopril or penicillamine may cause false-positive reactions. Serum or plasma assays for β-hydroxybutyrate are preferred because they more accurately reflect the true ketone body level.

The metabolic derangements of DKA exist along a spectrum, beginning with mild acidosis with moderate hyperglycemia evolving into more severe findings. The degree of acidosis and hyperglycemia do not necessarily correlate closely because a variety of factors determine the level of hyperglycemia (oral intake, urinary glucose loss). Ketonemia is a consistent finding in DKA and distinguishes it from simple hyperglycemia. The differential diagnosis of DKA includes starvation ketosis, alcoholic ketoacidosis (bicarbonate usually >15 meq/L), and other forms of increased anion-gap acidosis (Chap. 66).

TABLE 418-7 MANIFESTATIONS OF DIABETIC KETOACIDOSIS

Symptoms	Physical Findings
Nausea/vomiting	Tachycardia
Thirst/polyuria	Dehydration/hypotension
Abdominal pain	Tachypnea/Kussmaul respirations/respiratory distress
Shortness of breath	Abdominal tenderness (may resemble acute pancreatitis or surgical abdomen)
Precipitating events	Lethargy/obtundation/cerebral edema/possibly coma
Inadequate insulin administration	
Infection (pneumonia/UTI/gastroenteritis/sepsis)	
Infarction (cerebral, coronary, mesenteric, peripheral)	
Drugs (cocaine)	
Pregnancy	

Abbreviation: UTI, urinary tract infection.

TREATMENT DIABETIC KETOACIDOSIS

The management of DKA is outlined in Table 418-8. After initiating IV fluid replacement and insulin therapy, the agent or event that precipitated the episode of DKA should be sought and aggressively treated. If the patient is vomiting or has altered mental status, a nasogastric tube should be inserted to prevent aspiration of gastric contents. Central to successful treatment of DKA is careful monitoring and frequent reassessment to ensure that the patient and the metabolic derangements are improving. A comprehensive flow sheet should record chronologic changes in vital signs, fluid intake and output, and laboratory values as a function of insulin administered.

After the initial bolus of normal saline, replacement of the sodium and free water deficit is carried out over the next 24 h (fluid deficit is often 3–5 L). When hemodynamic stability and adequate urine output are achieved, IV fluids should be switched to 0.45% saline depending on the calculated volume deficit. The change to 0.45% saline helps to reduce the trend toward hyperchloremia later in the course of DKA. Alternatively, initial use of lactated Ringer's IV solution may reduce the hyperchloremia that commonly occurs with normal saline.

A bolus of IV (0.1 units/kg) short-acting insulin should be administered immediately (Table 418-8), and subsequent treatment should provide continuous and adequate levels of circulating insulin. IV administration is preferred (0.1 units/kg of regular insulin per hour) because it ensures rapid distribution and allows adjustment of the infusion rate as the patient responds to therapy. In mild episodes of DKA, short-acting insulin can be used SC. IV insulin should be continued until the acidosis resolves and the patient is metabolically stable. As the acidosis and insulin resistance associated with DKA resolve, the insulin infusion rate can be decreased (to 0.05–0.1 units/kg per hour). Long-acting insulin, in combination with SC short-acting insulin, should be administered as soon as the patient resumes eating, because this facilitates transition to an outpatient insulin regimen and reduces length of hospital stay. It is crucial to continue the insulin infusion until adequate insulin levels are achieved by administering long-acting insulin by the SC route. Even relatively brief periods of inadequate insulin administration in this transition phase may result in DKA relapse.

Hyperglycemia usually improves at a rate of 4.2–5.6 mmol/L (75–100 mg/dL) per hour as a result of insulin-mediated glucose disposal, reduced hepatic glucose release, and rehydration. The latter reduces catecholamines, increases urinary glucose loss, and expands the intravascular volume. The decline in the plasma glucose within the first 1–2 h may be more rapid and is mostly related to volume expansion. When the plasma glucose reaches 13.9 mmol/L (250 mg/dL), glucose should be added to the 0.45% saline infusion to maintain the plasma glucose in the 8.3–13.9 mmol/L (150–250 mg/dL) range, and the insulin infusion should be continued. Ketoacidosis begins to resolve as insulin reduces lipolysis, increases peripheral ketone body use, suppresses hepatic ketone body formation, and promotes bicarbonate regeneration. However, the acidosis and ketosis resolve more slowly than hyperglycemia. As ketoacidosis improves, β-hydroxybutyrate is converted to acetoacetate. Ketone body levels may appear to increase if measured by laboratory assays that use the nitroprusside reaction, which only detects acetoacetate and acetone. The improvement in acidosis and anion gap, a result of bicarbonate regeneration and decline in ketone bodies, is reflected by a rise in the serum bicarbonate level and the arterial pH. Depending on the rise of serum chloride, the anion gap (but not bicarbonate) will normalize. A hyperchloremic acidosis (serum bicarbonate of 15–18 mmol/L [15–18 meq/L]) often follows successful treatment and gradually resolves as the kidneys regenerate bicarbonate and excrete chloride.

Potassium stores are depleted in DKA (estimated deficit 3–5 mmol/kg [3–5 meq/kg]). During treatment with insulin and fluids, various factors contribute to the development of hypokalemia. These include insulin-mediated potassium transport into cells, resolution of the acidosis (which also promotes potassium entry into cells), and urinary loss of potassium salts of organic acids. Thus, potassium repletion should commence as soon as adequate urine output and a normal serum potassium are documented. If the initial serum potassium level is elevated, then potassium repletion should be delayed until the potassium falls into the normal range. Inclusion of 20–40 meq of potassium in each liter of IV fluid is reasonable, but additional potassium supplements may also be required. To reduce the amount of chloride administered, potassium phosphate or acetate can be substituted for the chloride salt. The goal is to maintain the serum potassium at >3.5 mmol/L (3.5 meq/L).

Despite a bicarbonate deficit, bicarbonate replacement is not usually necessary. In fact, theoretical arguments suggest that bicarbonate administration and rapid reversal of acidosis may impair cardiac function, reduce tissue oxygenation, and promote hypokalemia. The results of most clinical trials do not support the routine use of bicarbonate replacement, and one study in children found that bicarbonate use was associated with an increased risk of cerebral edema. However, in the presence of severe acidosis (arterial pH <7.0), the ADA advises bicarbonate (50 mmol/L [meq/L] of sodium bicarbonate in 200 mL of sterile water with 10 meq/L KCl per hour for 2 h until the pH is >7.0). Hypophosphatemia may result from increased glucose usage, but randomized clinical trials have not demonstrated that phosphate replacement is beneficial in DKA. If the serum phosphate is <0.32 mmol/L (1 mg/dL), then phosphate supplement should be considered and the serum calcium monitored. Hypomagnesemia may develop during DKA therapy and may also require supplementation.

TABLE 418-8 MANAGEMENT OF DIABETIC KETOACIDOSIS

1. Confirm diagnosis (↑ plasma glucose, positive serum ketones, metabolic acidosis).
2. Admit to hospital; intensive care setting may be necessary for frequent monitoring or if pH <7.00 or unconscious.
3. Assess:
   Serum electrolytes (K^+, Na^+, Mg^{2+}, Cl^-, bicarbonate, phosphate)
   Acid-base status—pH, HCO_3^-, P_{CO_2}, β-hydroxybutyrate
   Renal function (creatinine, urine output)
4. Replace fluids: 2–3 L of 0.9% saline over first 1–3 h (10–20 mL/kg per hour); subsequently, 0.45% saline at 250–500 mL/h; change to 5% glucose and 0.45% saline at 150–250 mL/h when plasma glucose reaches 250 mg/dL (13.9 mmol/L).
5. Administer short-acting insulin: IV (0.1 units/kg), then 0.1 units/kg per hour by continuous IV infusion; increase two- to threefold if no response by 2–4 h. If the initial serum potassium is <3.3 mmol/L (3.3 meq/L), do not administer insulin until the potassium is corrected.
6. Assess patient: What precipitated the episode (noncompliance, infection, trauma, pregnancy, infarction, cocaine)? Initiate appropriate workup for precipitating event (cultures, CXR, ECG).
7. Measure capillary glucose every 1–2 h; measure electrolytes (especially K^+, bicarbonate, phosphate) and anion gap every 4 h for first 24 h.
8. Monitor blood pressure, pulse, respirations, mental status, fluid intake and output every 1–4 h.
9. Replace K^+: 10 meq/h when plasma K^+ <5.0–5.2 meq/L (or 20–30 meq/L of infusion fluid), ECG normal, urine flow and normal creatinine documented; administer 40–80 meq/h when plasma K^+ <3.5 meq/L or if bicarbonate is given. If initial serum potassium is >5.2 mmol/L (5.2 meq/L), do not supplement K^+ until the potassium is corrected.
10. See text about bicarbonate or phosphate supplementation.
11. Continue above until patient is stable, glucose goal is 8.3–13.9 mmol/L (150–250 mg/dL), and acidosis is resolved. Insulin infusion may be decreased to 0.05–0.1 units/kg per hour.
12. Administer long-acting insulin as soon as patient is eating. Allow for a 2–4 hour overlap in insulin infusion and SC insulin injection.

Abbreviations: CXR, chest x-ray; ECG, electrocardiogram.

Source: Adapted from M Sperling, in *Therapy for Diabetes Mellitus and Related Disorders*, American Diabetes Association, Alexandria, VA, 1998; and AE Kitabchi et al: Diabetes Care 32:1335, 2009.

With appropriate therapy, the mortality rate of DKA is low (<1%) and is related more to the underlying or precipitating event, such as infection or myocardial infarction. Venous thrombosis, upper gastrointestinal bleeding, and acute respiratory distress syndrome occasionally complicate DKA. The major nonmetabolic complication of DKA therapy is cerebral edema, which most often develops in children as DKA is resolving. The etiology of and optimal therapy for cerebral edema are not well established, but overreplacement of free water should be avoided.

Following treatment, the physician and patient should review the sequence of events that led to DKA to prevent future recurrences. Foremost is patient education about the symptoms of DKA, its precipitating factors, and the management of diabetes during a concurrent illness. During illness or when oral intake is compromised, patients should (1) frequently measure the capillary blood glucose; (2) measure urinary ketones when the serum glucose is >16.5 mmol/L (300 mg/dL); (3) drink fluids to maintain hydration; (4) continue or increase insulin; and (5) seek medical attention if dehydration, persistent vomiting, or uncontrolled hyperglycemia develop. Using these strategies, early DKA can be prevented or detected and treated appropriately on an outpatient basis.

HYPERGLYCEMIC HYPEROSMOLAR STATE

Clinical Features The prototypical patient with HHS is an elderly individual with type 2 DM, with a several-week history of polyuria, weight loss, and diminished oral intake that culminates in mental confusion, lethargy, or coma. The physical examination reflects profound dehydration and hyperosmolality and reveals hypotension, tachycardia, and altered mental status. Notably absent are symptoms of nausea, vomiting, and abdominal pain and the Kussmaul respirations characteristic of DKA. HHS is often precipitated by a serious, concurrent illness such as myocardial infarction or stroke. Sepsis, pneumonia, and other serious infections are frequent precipitants and should be sought. In addition, a debilitating condition (prior stroke or dementia) or social situation that compromises water intake usually contributes to the development of the disorder.

Pathophysiology Relative insulin deficiency and inadequate fluid intake are the underlying causes of HHS. Insulin deficiency increases hepatic glucose production (through glycogenolysis and gluconeogenesis) and impairs glucose utilization in skeletal muscle (see above discussion of DKA). Hyperglycemia induces an osmotic diuresis that leads to intravascular volume depletion, which is exacerbated by inadequate fluid replacement. The absence of ketosis in HHS is not understood. Presumably, the insulin deficiency is only relative and less severe than in DKA. Lower levels of counterregulatory hormones and free fatty acids have been found in HHS than in DKA in some studies. It is also possible that the liver is less capable of ketone body synthesis or that the insulin/glucagon ratio does not favor ketogenesis.

Laboratory Abnormalities and Diagnosis The laboratory features in HHS are summarized in Table 418-6. Most notable are the marked hyperglycemia (plasma glucose may be >55.5 mmol/L [1000 mg/dL]), hyperosmolality (>350 mosmol/L), and prerenal azotemia. The measured serum sodium may be normal or slightly low despite the marked hyperglycemia. The corrected serum sodium is usually increased (add 1.6 meq to measured sodium for each 5.6-mmol/L [100-mg/dL] rise in the serum glucose). In contrast to DKA, acidosis and ketonemia are absent or mild. A small anion-gap metabolic acidosis may be present secondary to increased lactic acid. Moderate ketonuria, if present, is secondary to starvation.

TREATMENT HYPERGLYCEMIC HYPEROSMOLAR STATE

Volume depletion and hyperglycemia are prominent features of both HHS and DKA. Consequently, therapy of these disorders shares several elements (Table 418-8). In both disorders, careful monitoring of the patient's fluid status, laboratory values, and insulin infusion rate is crucial. Underlying or precipitating problems should be aggressively sought and treated. In HHS, fluid losses and dehydration are usually more pronounced than in DKA due to the longer duration of the illness. The patient with HHS is usually older, more likely to have mental status changes, and more likely to have a life-threatening precipitating event with accompanying comorbidities. Even with proper treatment, HHS has a substantially higher mortality rate than DKA (up to 15% in some clinical series).

Fluid replacement should initially stabilize the hemodynamic status of the patient (1–3 L of 0.9% normal saline over the first 2–3 h). Because the fluid deficit in HHS is accumulated over a period of days to weeks, the rapidity of reversal of the hyperosmolar state must balance the need for free water repletion with the risk that too rapid a reversal may worsen neurologic function. If the serum sodium is >150 mmol/L (150 meq/L), 0.45% saline should be used. After hemodynamic stability is achieved, the IV fluid administration is directed at reversing the free water deficit using hypotonic fluids (0.45% saline initially, then 5% dextrose in water [D_5W]). The calculated free water deficit (which averages 9–10 L) should be reversed over the next 1–2 days (infusion rates of 200–300 mL/h of hypotonic solution). Potassium repletion is usually necessary and should be dictated by repeated measurements of the serum potassium. In patients taking diuretics, the potassium deficit can be quite large and may be accompanied by magnesium deficiency. Hypophosphatemia may occur during therapy and can be improved by using KPO_4 and beginning nutrition.

As in DKA, rehydration and volume expansion lower the plasma glucose initially, but insulin is also required. A reasonable regimen for HHS begins with an IV insulin bolus of 0.1 unit/kg followed by IV insulin at a constant infusion rate of 0.1 unit/kg per hour. If the serum glucose does not fall, increase the insulin infusion rate by twofold. As in DKA, glucose should be added to IV fluid when the plasma glucose falls to 13.9 mmol/L (250 mg/dL), and the insulin infusion rate should be decreased to 0.05–0.1 unit/kg per hour. The insulin infusion should be continued until the patient has resumed eating and can be transferred to a SC insulin regimen. The patient should be discharged from the hospital on insulin, although some patients can later switch to oral glucose-lowering agents.

MANAGEMENT OF DIABETES IN A HOSPITALIZED PATIENT

Virtually all medical and surgical subspecialties are involved in the care of hospitalized patients with diabetes. Hyperglycemia, whether in a patient with known diabetes or in someone without known diabetes, appears to be a predictor of poor outcome in hospitalized patients. General anesthesia, surgery, infection, or concurrent illness raises the levels of counterregulatory hormones (cortisol, growth hormone, catecholamines, and glucagon) and cytokines that may lead to transient insulin resistance and hyperglycemia. These factors increase insulin requirements by increasing glucose production and impairing glucose utilization and thus may worsen glycemic control. The concurrent illness or surgical procedure may lead to variable insulin absorption and also prevent the patient with DM from eating normally and, thus, may promote hypoglycemia. Glycemic control should be assessed on admission using the HbA_{1c}. Electrolytes, renal function, and intravascular volume status should be assessed as well. The high prevalence of CVD in individuals with DM (especially in type 2 DM) may necessitate preoperative cardiovascular evaluation (Chap. 419).

The goals of diabetes management during hospitalization are near-normoglycemia, avoidance of hypoglycemia, and transition back to the outpatient diabetes treatment regimen. Upon hospital admission, frequent glycemic monitoring should begin, as should planning for diabetes management after discharge. Glycemic control appears to improve the clinical outcomes in a variety of settings, but optimal glycemic goals for the hospitalized patient are incompletely defined.

In a number of cross-sectional studies of patients with diabetes, a greater degree of hyperglycemia was associated with worse cardiac, neurologic, and infectious outcomes. In some studies, patients who do not have preexisting diabetes but who develop modest blood glucose elevations during their hospitalization appear to benefit from achieving near-normoglycemia using insulin treatment. However, a large randomized clinical trial (Normoglycemia in Intensive Care Evaluation Survival Using Glucose Algorithm Regulation [NICE-SUGAR]) of individuals in the ICU (most of whom were receiving mechanical ventilation) found an increased mortality rate and a greater number of episodes of severe hypoglycemia with very strict glycemic control (target blood glucose of 4.5–6 mmol/L or 81–108 mg/dL) compared to individuals with a more moderate glycemic goal (mean blood glucose of 8 mmol/L or 144 mg/dL). Currently, most data suggest that very strict blood glucose control in acutely ill patients likely worsens outcomes and increases the frequency of hypoglycemia. The ADA suggests the following glycemic goals for hospitalized patients: (1) in critically ill patients: glucose of 7.8–10.0 mmol/L or 140–180 mg/dL; (2) in non–critically ill patients: premeal glucose <7.8 mmol/L (140 mg/dL) and at other times blood glucose <10 mmol/L (180 mg/dL).

Critical aspects for optimal diabetes care in the hospital include the following. (1) A hospital system approach to treatment of hyperglycemia and prevention of hypoglycemia is needed. Inpatient diabetes management teams consisting of nurse practitioners and physicians are increasingly common. (2) Diabetes treatment plans should focus on the transition from the ICU and the transition from the inpatient to outpatient setting. (3) Adjustment of the discharge treatment regimen of patients whose diabetes was poorly controlled on admission (as reflected by the HbA_{1c}) is necessary.

The physician caring for an individual with diabetes in the perioperative period, during times of infection or serious physical illness, or simply when the patient is fasting for a diagnostic procedure must monitor the plasma glucose vigilantly, adjust the diabetes treatment regimen, and provide glucose infusion as needed. Hypoglycemia is frequent in hospitalized patients, and many of these episodes are avoidable. Hospital systems should have a diabetes management protocol to avoid inpatient hypoglycemia. Measures to reduce or prevent hypoglycemia include frequent glucose monitoring and anticipating potential modifications of insulin/glucose administration because of changes in the clinical situation or treatment (e.g., tapering of glucocorticoids) or interruption of enteral or parenteral infusions or PO intake.

Depending on the severity of the patient's illness and the hospital setting, the physician can use either an insulin infusion or SC insulin. Insulin infusions are preferred in the ICU or in a clinically unstable setting. The absorption of SC insulin may be variable in such situations. Insulin infusions can also effectively control plasma glucose in the perioperative period and when the patient is unable to take anything by mouth. Regular insulin is used rather than insulin analogues for IV insulin infusion because it is less expensive and equally effective. The physician must consider carefully the clinical setting in which an insulin infusion will be used, including whether adequate ancillary personnel are available to monitor the plasma glucose frequently and whether they can adjust the insulin infusion rate to maintain the plasma glucose within the optimal range. Insulin-infusion algorithms should integrate the insulin sensitivity of the patient, frequent blood glucose monitoring, and the trend of changes in the blood glucose to determine the insulin-infusion rate. Insulin-infusion algorithms jointly developed and implemented by nursing and physician staff are advised. Because of the short half-life of IV regular insulin, it is necessary to administer long-acting insulin prior to discontinuation of the insulin infusion (2–4 h before the infusion is stopped) to avoid a period of insulin deficiency.

In patients who are not critically ill or not in the ICU, basal or "scheduled" insulin is provided by SC, long-acting insulin supplemented by prandial and/or "corrective" insulin using a short-acting insulin (insulin analogues preferred). The use of "sliding scale," short-acting insulin alone, where no insulin is given unless the blood glucose is elevated, is inadequate for inpatient glucose management and should not be used. The short-acting, preprandial insulin dose should include coverage for food consumption (based on anticipated carbohydrate intake) plus a corrective or supplemental insulin based on the patient's insulin sensitivity and the blood glucose. For example, if the patient is thin (and likely insulin-sensitive), a corrective insulin supplement might be 1 unit for each 2.7 mmol/L (50 mg/dL) over the glucose target. If the patient is obese and insulin-resistant, then the insulin supplement might be 2 units for each 2.7 mmol/L (50 mg/dL) over the glucose target. It is critical to individualize the regimen and adjust the basal or "scheduled" insulin dose frequently, based on the corrective insulin required. A consistent carbohydrate diabetes meal plan for hospitalized patients provides a predictable amount of carbohydrate for a particular meal each day (but not necessarily the same amount for breakfast, lunch, and supper). The hospital diet should be determined by a nutritionist; terms such as *ADA diet* or *low-sugar diet* are no longer used.

Individuals with type 1 DM who are undergoing general anesthesia and surgery or who are seriously ill should receive continuous insulin, either through an IV insulin infusion or by SC administration of a reduced dose of long-acting insulin. Short-acting insulin alone is insufficient. Prolongation of a surgical procedure or delay in the recovery room is not uncommon and may result in periods of insulin deficiency leading to DKA. Insulin infusion is the preferred method for managing patients with type 1 DM in the perioperative period or when serious concurrent illness is present (0.5–1.0 units/h of regular insulin). If the diagnostic or surgical procedure is brief and performed under local or regional anesthesia, a reduced dose of SC, long-acting insulin may suffice (30–50% reduction, with short-acting insulin withheld or reduced). This approach facilitates the transition back to long-acting insulin after the procedure. Glucose may be infused to prevent hypoglycemia. The blood glucose should be monitored frequently during the illness or in the perioperative period.

Individuals with type 2 DM can be managed with either an insulin infusion or SC long-acting insulin (25–50% reduction depending on clinical setting) plus preprandial, short-acting insulin. Oral glucose-lowering agents should be discontinued upon admission and are not useful in regulating the plasma glucose in clinical situations where the insulin requirements and glucose intake are changing rapidly. Moreover, these oral agents may be dangerous if the patient is fasting (e.g., hypoglycemia with sulfonylureas). Metformin should be withheld when radiographic contrast media will be given or if unstable CHF, acidosis, or declining renal function is present.

SPECIAL CONSIDERATIONS IN DIABETES MELLITUS

TOTAL PARENTERAL NUTRITION

(See also Chap. 98e) Total parenteral nutrition (TPN) greatly increases insulin requirements. In addition, individuals not previously known to have DM may become hyperglycemic during TPN and require insulin treatment. IV insulin infusion is the preferred treatment for hyperglycemia, and rapid titration to the required insulin dose is done most efficiently using a separate insulin infusion. After the total insulin dose has been determined, insulin may be added directly to the TPN solution or, preferably, given as a separate infusion or subcutaneously. Often, individuals receiving either TPN or enteral nutrition receive their caloric loads continuously and not at "meal times"; consequently, SC insulin regimens must be adjusted.

GLUCOCORTICOIDS

Glucocorticoids increase insulin resistance, decrease glucose utilization, increase hepatic glucose production, and impair insulin secretion. These changes lead to a worsening of glycemic control in individuals with DM and may precipitate diabetes in other individuals ("steroid-induced diabetes"). The effects of glucocorticoids on glucose homeostasis are dose-related, usually reversible, and most pronounced in the postprandial period. If the FPG is near the normal range, oral diabetes agents (e.g., sulfonylureas, metformin) may be sufficient to reduce hyperglycemia. If the FPG is >11.1 mmol/L (200 mg/dL), oral agents are usually not efficacious and insulin therapy is required. Short-acting insulin may be required to supplement long-acting insulin in order to control postprandial glucose excursions.

REPRODUCTIVE ISSUES

Reproductive capacity in either men or women with DM appears to be normal. Menstrual cycles may be associated with alterations in glycemic control in women with DM. Pregnancy is associated with marked insulin resistance; the increased insulin requirements often precipitate DM and lead to the diagnosis of gestational diabetes mellitus (GDM). Glucose, which at high levels is a teratogen to the developing fetus, readily crosses the placenta, but insulin does not. Thus, hyperglycemia from the maternal circulation may stimulate insulin secretion in the fetus. The anabolic and growth effects of insulin may result in macrosomia. GDM complicates ~7% (range 1–14%) of pregnancies. The incidence of GDM is greatly increased in certain ethnic groups, including African Americans and Latinas, consistent with a similar increased risk of type 2 DM. Current recommendations advise screening for glucose intolerance between weeks 24 and 28 of pregnancy in women with increased risk for GDM (≥25 years; obesity; family history of DM; member of an ethnic group such as Latina, Native American, Asian American, African American, or Pacific Islander). Therapy for GDM is similar to that for individuals with pregnancy-associated diabetes and involves MNT and insulin, if hyperglycemia persists. Oral glucose-lowering agents are not approved for use during pregnancy, but studies using metformin or glyburide have shown efficacy and have not found toxicity. However, many physicians use insulin to treat GDM. With current practices, the morbidity and mortality rates of the mother with GDM and the fetus are not different from those in the nondiabetic population. Individuals who develop GDM are at marked increased risk for developing type 2 DM in the future and should be screened periodically for DM. Most individuals with GDM revert to normal glucose tolerance after delivery, but some will continue to have overt diabetes or impairment of glucose tolerance after delivery. In addition, children of women with GDM appear to be at risk for obesity and glucose intolerance and have an increased risk of diabetes beginning in the later stages of adolescence.

Pregnancy in individuals with known DM requires meticulous planning and adherence to strict treatment regimens. Intensive diabetes management and normalization of the HbA_{1c} are essential for individuals with existing DM who are planning pregnancy. The most crucial period of glycemic control is soon after fertilization. The risk of fetal malformations is increased 4–10 times in individuals with uncontrolled DM at the time of conception, and normal plasma glucose during the preconception period and throughout the periods of organ development in the fetus should be the goal.

LIPODYSTROPHIC DM

Lipodystrophy, or the loss of subcutaneous fat tissue, may be generalized in certain genetic conditions such as leprechaunism. Generalized lipodystrophy is associated with severe insulin resistance and is often accompanied by acanthosis nigricans and dyslipidemia. Localized lipodystrophy associated with insulin injections has been reduced considerably by the use of human insulin.

Protease Inhibitors and Lipodystrophy Protease inhibitors used in the treatment of HIV disease (Chap. 226) have been associated with a centripetal accumulation of fat (visceral and abdominal area), accumulation of fat in the dorsocervical region, loss of extremity fat, decreased insulin sensitivity (elevations of the fasting insulin level and reduced glucose tolerance on IV glucose tolerance testing), and dyslipidemia. Although many aspects of the physical appearance of these individuals resemble Cushing's syndrome, increased cortisol levels do not account for this appearance. The possibility remains that this is related to HIV infection by some undefined mechanism, because some features of the syndrome were observed before the introduction of protease inhibitors. Therapy for HIV-related lipodystrophy is not well established.

419 Diabetes Mellitus: Complications

Alvin C. Powers

Diabetes-related complications affect many organ systems and are responsible for the majority of morbidity and mortality associated with the disease. Strikingly, in the United States, diabetes is the leading cause of new blindness in adults, renal failure, and nontraumatic lower extremity amputation. Diabetes-related complications usually do not appear until the second decade of hyperglycemia. Because type 2 diabetes mellitus (DM) often has a long asymptomatic period of hyperglycemia before diagnosis, many individuals with type 2 DM have complications at the time of diagnosis. Fortunately, many of the diabetes-related complications can be prevented or delayed with early detection, aggressive glycemic control, and efforts to minimize the risks of complications.

Diabetes-related complications can be divided into vascular and nonvascular complications and are similar for type 1 and type 2 DM (Table 419-1). The vascular complications of DM are further subdivided into microvascular (retinopathy, neuropathy, nephropathy) and macrovascular complications (coronary heart disease [CHD], peripheral arterial disease [PAD], cerebrovascular disease). Microvascular complications are diabetes-specific, whereas macrovascular complications are similar to those in nondiabetics but occur at greater frequency in individuals with diabetes. Nonvascular complications include gastroparesis, infections, skin changes, and hearing loss. Whether type 2 DM increases the risk of dementia or impaired cognitive function is not clear.

GLYCEMIC CONTROL AND COMPLICATIONS

The microvascular complications of both type 1 and type 2 DM result from chronic hyperglycemia (Fig. 419-1). Evidence implicating a causative role for chronic hyperglycemia in the development of macrovascular complications is less conclusive. CHD events and mortality rate are two to four times greater in patients with type 2 DM and correlate with fasting and postprandial plasma glucose levels as well the

TABLE 419-1 DIABETES-RELATED COMPLICATIONS

Microvascular
- Eye disease
  - Retinopathy (nonproliferative/proliferative)
  - Macular edema
- Neuropathy
  - Sensory and motor (mono- and polyneuropathy)
  - Autonomic
- Nephropathy (albuminuria and declining renal function)

Macrovascular
- Coronary heart disease
- Peripheral arterial disease
- Cerebrovascular disease

Other
- Gastrointestinal (gastroparesis, diarrhea)
- Genitourinary (uropathy/sexual dysfunction)
- Dermatologic
- Infectious
- Cataracts
- Glaucoma
- Cheiroarthropathy[a]
- Periodontal disease
- Hearing loss

Other comorbid conditions associated with diabetes (relationship to hyperglycemia is uncertain): depression, obstructive sleep apnea, fatty liver disease, hip fracture, osteoporosis (in type 1 diabetes), cognitive impairment or dementia, low testosterone in men

[a]Thickened skin and reduced joint mobility.

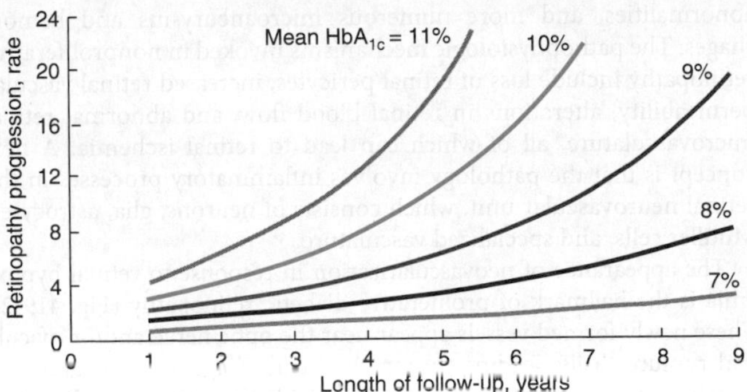

FIGURE 419-1 Relationship of glycemic control and diabetes duration to diabetic retinopathy. The progression of retinopathy in individuals in the Diabetes Control and Complications Trial is graphed as a function of the length of follow-up with different curves for different hemoglobin A_{1c} (HbA_{1c}) values. *(Adapted from The Diabetes Control and Complications Trial Research Group: Diabetes 44:968, 1995.)*

hemoglobin A_{1c} (HbA_{1c}). Other factors such as dyslipidemia and hypertension also play important roles in macrovascular complications.

The Diabetes Control and Complications Trial (DCCT) provided definitive proof that reduction in chronic hyperglycemia can prevent many complications of type 1 DM (Fig. 419-1). This large multicenter clinical trial randomized more than 1400 individuals with type 1 DM to either intensive or conventional diabetes management and prospectively evaluated the development of diabetes-related complications during a mean follow-up of 6.5 years. Individuals in the intensive diabetes management group received multiple administrations of insulin each day (injection or pump) along with extensive educational, psychological, and medical support. Individuals in the conventional diabetes management group received twice-daily insulin injections and quarterly nutritional, educational, and clinical evaluation. The goal in the former group was normoglycemia; the goal in the latter group was prevention of symptoms of diabetes. Individuals in the intensive diabetes management group achieved a substantially lower HbA_{1c} (7.3%) than individuals in the conventional diabetes management group (9.1%). After the DCCT results were reported in 1993, study participants continue to be followed in the Epidemiology of Diabetes Intervention and Complications (EDIC) trial, which recently completed 30 years of follow-up (DCCT + EDIC). At the end of the DCCT phase, study participants in both intensive and conventional arms were offered intensive therapy. However, during the subsequent follow-up of more than 18 years, the initial separation in glycemic control disappeared with both arms maintaining a mean HbA_{1c} of 8.0%.

The DCCT phase demonstrated that improvement of glycemic control reduced nonproliferative and proliferative retinopathy (47% reduction), microalbuminuria (39% reduction), clinical nephropathy (54% reduction), and neuropathy (60% reduction). Improved glycemic control also slowed the progression of early diabetic complications. During the DCCT phase, weight gain (4.6 kg) and severe hypoglycemia (requiring assistance of another person to treat) were more common in the intensive therapy group. The benefits of an improvement in glycemic control occurred over the entire range of HbA_{1c} values (Fig. 419-1), indicating that at any HbA_{1c} level, an improvement in glycemic control is beneficial. The results of the DCCT predicted that individuals in the intensive diabetes management group would gain 7.7 additional years of vision, 5.8 additional years free from end-stage renal disease (ESRD), and 5.6 years free from lower extremity amputations. If all complications of DM were combined, individuals in the intensive diabetes management group would experience 15.3 more years of life without significant microvascular or neurologic complications of DM, compared to individuals who received standard therapy. This translates into an additional 5.1 years of life expectancy for individuals in the intensive diabetes management group. The 30-year follow-up data in the intensively treated group show a continued reduction in retinopathy, nephropathy, and cardiovascular disease. For example, individuals in the intensive therapy group had a 42–57% reduction in cardiovascular events (nonfatal myocardial infarction [MI], stroke, or death from a cardiovascular event) at a mean follow-up of 17 years, even though their subsequent glycemic control was the same as those in the conventional diabetes management group from years 6.5–17. During the EDIC phase, less than 1% of the cohort had become blind, lost a limb to amputation, or required dialysis.

The United Kingdom Prospective Diabetes Study (UKPDS) studied the course of >5000 individuals with type 2 DM for >10 years. This study used multiple treatment regimens and monitored the effect of intensive glycemic control and risk factor treatment on the development of diabetic complications. Newly diagnosed individuals with type 2 DM were randomized to (1) intensive management using various combinations of insulin, a sulfonylurea, or metformin or (2) conventional therapy using dietary modification and pharmacotherapy with the goal of symptom prevention. In addition, individuals were randomly assigned to different antihypertensive regimens. Individuals in the intensive treatment arm achieved an HbA_{1c} of 7%, compared to a 7.9% HbA_{1c} in the standard treatment group. The UKPDS demonstrated that each percentage point reduction in HbA_{1c} was associated with a 35% reduction in microvascular complications. As in the DCCT, there was a continuous relationship between glycemic control and development of complications. Improved glycemic control also reduced the cardiovascular event rate in the follow-up period of >10 years.

One of the major findings of the UKPDS was that strict blood pressure control significantly reduced both macro- and microvascular complications. In fact, the beneficial effects of blood pressure control were greater than the beneficial effects of glycemic control. Lowering blood pressure to moderate goals (144/82 mmHg) reduced the risk of DM-related death, stroke, microvascular endpoints, retinopathy, and heart failure (risk reductions between 32 and 56%).

Similar reductions in the risks of retinopathy and nephropathy were also seen in a small trial of lean Japanese individuals with type 2 DM randomized to either intensive glycemic control or standard therapy with insulin (Kumamoto study). These results demonstrate the effectiveness of improved glycemic control in individuals of different ethnicity and, presumably, a different etiology of DM (i.e., phenotypically different from those in the DCCT and UKPDS). The Action to Control Cardiovascular Risk in Diabetes (ACCORD) and Action in Diabetes and Vascular Disease: Preterax and Diamicron MR Controlled Evaluation (ADVANCE) trials also found that improved glycemic control reduced microvascular complications.

Thus, these large clinical trials in type 1 and type 2 DM indicate that chronic hyperglycemia plays a causative role in the pathogenesis of diabetic microvascular complications. In both the DCCT and the UKPDS, cardiovascular events were reduced at follow-up of >10 years, even though the improved glycemic control was not maintained. The positive impact of a period of improved glycemic control on later disease has been termed a *legacy effect* or *metabolic memory*.

A summary of the features of diabetes-related complications includes the following. (1) Duration and degree of hyperglycemia correlate with complications. (2) Intensive glycemic control is beneficial in all forms of DM. (3) Blood pressure control is critical, especially in type 2 DM. (4) Survival in patients with type 1 DM is improving, and diabetes-related complications are declining. (5) Not all individuals with diabetes develop diabetes-related complications. Other incompletely defined factors appear to modulate the development of complications. For example, despite long-standing DM, some individuals never develop nephropathy or retinopathy. Many of these patients have glycemic control that is indistinguishable from those who develop microvascular complications, suggesting a genetic susceptibility for developing particular complications.

MECHANISMS OF COMPLICATIONS

Although chronic hyperglycemia is an important etiologic factor leading to complications of DM, the mechanism(s) by which it leads to such diverse cellular and organ dysfunction is unknown. An emerging hypothesis is that hyperglycemia leads to epigenetic changes (Chap. 82) that influence gene expression in affected cells. For example, this may explain the legacy effect or metabolic memory mentioned above.

Four theories, which are not mutually exclusive, on how hyperglycemia might lead to the chronic complications of DM include the following pathways. (1) Increased intracellular glucose leads to the formation of advanced glycosylation end products, which bind to a cell surface receptor, via the nonenzymatic glycosylation of intra- and extracellular proteins, leading to cross-linking of proteins, accelerated atherosclerosis, glomerular dysfunction, endothelial dysfunction, and altered extracellular matrix composition. (2) Hyperglycemia increases glucose metabolism via the sorbitol pathway related to the enzyme aldose reductase. However, testing of this theory in humans, using aldose reductase inhibitors, has not demonstrated beneficial effects. (3) Hyperglycemia increases the formation of diacylglycerol, leading to activation of protein kinase C, which alters the transcription of genes for fibronectin, type IV collagen, contractile proteins, and extracellular matrix proteins in endothelial cells and neurons. (4) Hyperglycemia increases the flux through the hexosamine pathway, which generates fructose-6-phosphate, a substrate for O-linked glycosylation and proteoglycan production, leading to altered function by glycosylation of proteins such as endothelial nitric oxide synthase or by changes in gene expression of transforming growth factor β (TGF-β) or plasminogen activator inhibitor-1.

Growth factors may play an important role in some diabetes-related complications, and their production is increased by most of these proposed pathways. Vascular endothelial growth factor A (VEGF-A) is increased locally in diabetic proliferative retinopathy and decreases after laser photocoagulation. TGF-β is increased in diabetic nephropathy and stimulates basement membrane production of collagen and fibronectin by mesangial cells. A possible unifying mechanism is that hyperglycemia leads to increased production of reactive oxygen species or superoxide in the mitochondria; these compounds may activate all four of the pathways described above. Although hyperglycemia serves as the initial trigger for complications of diabetes, it is still unknown whether the same pathophysiologic processes are operative in all complications or whether some pathways predominate in certain organs.

OPHTHALMOLOGIC COMPLICATIONS OF DIABETES MELLITUS

DM is the leading cause of blindness between the ages of 20 and 74 in the United States. The gravity of this problem is highlighted by the finding that individuals with DM are 25 times more likely to become legally blind than individuals without DM. Severe vision loss is primarily the result of progressive diabetic retinopathy and clinically significant macular edema. Diabetic retinopathy is classified into two stages: nonproliferative and proliferative. Nonproliferative diabetic retinopathy usually appears late in the first decade or early in the second decade of the disease and is marked by retinal vascular microaneurysms, blot hemorrhages, and cotton-wool spots (Fig. 419-2). Mild nonproliferative retinopathy may progress to more extensive disease, characterized by changes in venous vessel caliber, intraretinal microvascular abnormalities, and more numerous microaneurysms and hemorrhages. The pathophysiologic mechanisms invoked in nonproliferative retinopathy include loss of retinal pericytes, increased retinal vascular permeability, alterations in retinal blood flow, and abnormal retinal microvasculature, all of which can lead to retinal ischemia. A new concept is that the pathology involves inflammatory processes in the retinal neurovascular unit, which consists of neurons, glia, astrocytes, Muüller cells, and specialized vasculature.

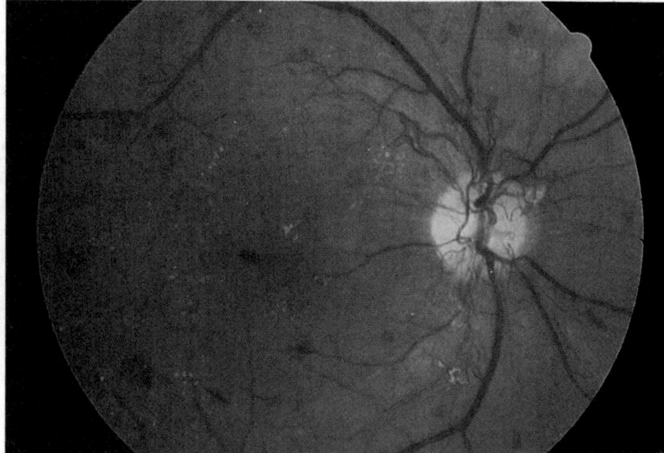

FIGURE 419-2 Diabetic retinopathy results in scattered hemorrhages, yellow exudates, and neovascularization. This patient has neovascular vessels proliferating from the optic disc, requiring urgent panretinal laser photocoagulation.

The appearance of neovascularization in response to retinal hypoxemia is the hallmark of proliferative diabetic retinopathy (Fig. 419-2). These newly formed vessels appear near the optic nerve and/or macula and rupture easily, leading to vitreous hemorrhage, fibrosis, and ultimately retinal detachment. Not all individuals with nonproliferative retinopathy go on to develop proliferative retinopathy, but the more severe the nonproliferative disease, the greater the chance of evolution to proliferative retinopathy within 5 years. This creates an important opportunity for early detection and treatment of diabetic retinopathy. Clinically significant macular edema can occur in the context of nonproliferative or proliferative retinopathy. Fluorescein angiography and optical coherence tomography are useful to detect macular edema, which is associated with a 25% chance of moderate visual loss over the next 3 years. Duration of DM and degree of glycemic control are the best predictors of the development of retinopathy; hypertension and nephropathy are also risk factors. Nonproliferative retinopathy is found in many individuals who have had DM for >20 years. Although there is genetic susceptibility for retinopathy, it confers less influence than either the duration of DM or the degree of glycemic control.

TREATMENT DIABETIC RETINOPATHY

The most effective therapy for diabetic retinopathy is prevention. Intensive glycemic and blood pressure control will delay the development or slow the progression of retinopathy in individuals with either type 1 or type 2 DM. Paradoxically, during the first 6–12 months of improved glycemic control, established diabetic retinopathy may transiently worsen. Fortunately, this progression is temporary, and in the long term, improved glycemic control is associated with less diabetic retinopathy. Individuals with known retinopathy may be candidates for prophylactic laser photocoagulation when initiating intensive therapy. Once advanced retinopathy is present, improved glycemic control imparts less benefit, although adequate ophthalmologic care can prevent most blindness.

Regular, comprehensive eye examinations are essential for all individuals with DM (see Table 418-1). Most diabetic eye disease can be successfully treated if detected early. Routine, nondilated eye examinations by the primary care provider or diabetes specialist are inadequate to detect diabetic eye disease, which requires an ophthalmologist for optimal care of these disorders. Laser photocoagulation is very successful in preserving vision. Proliferative retinopathy is usually treated with panretinal laser photocoagulation, whereas macular edema is treated with focal laser photocoagulation and anti–vascular endothelial growth factor therapy (ocular injection). Aspirin therapy (650 mg/d) does not appear to influence the natural history of diabetic retinopathy.

RENAL COMPLICATIONS OF DIABETES MELLITUS

Diabetic nephropathy is the leading cause of chronic kidney disease (CKD), ESRD, and CKD requiring renal replacement therapy. Furthermore, the prognosis of diabetic patients on dialysis is poor, with survival comparable to many forms of cancer. Albuminuria in individuals with DM is associated with an increased risk of cardiovascular disease. Individuals with diabetic nephropathy commonly have diabetic retinopathy.

Like other microvascular complications, the pathogenesis of diabetic nephropathy is related to chronic hyperglycemia. The mechanisms by which chronic hyperglycemia leads to diabetic nephropathy, although incompletely defined, involve the effects of soluble factors (growth factors, angiotensin II, endothelin, advanced glycation end products [AGEs]), hemodynamic alterations in the renal microcirculation (glomerular hyperfiltration or hyperperfusion, increased glomerular capillary pressure), and structural changes in the glomerulus (increased extracellular matrix, basement membrane thickening, mesangial expansion, fibrosis). Some of these effects may be mediated through angiotensin II receptors. Smoking accelerates the decline in renal function. Because only 20–40% of patients with diabetes develop diabetic nephropathy, additional genetic or environmental susceptibility factors remain unidentified. Known risk factors include race and a family history of diabetic nephropathy. Diabetic nephropathy and ESRD secondary to DM develop more commonly in African Americans, Native Americans, and Hispanic individuals with diabetes.

The natural history of diabetic nephropathy is characterized by a fairly predictable sequence of events that was initially defined for individuals with type 1 DM but appears to be similar in type 2 DM (Fig. 419-3). Glomerular hyperperfusion and renal hypertrophy occur in the first years after the onset of DM and are associated with an increase of the glomerular filtration rate (GFR). During the first 5 years of DM, thickening of the glomerular basement membrane, glomerular hypertrophy, and mesangial volume expansion occur as the GFR returns to normal. After 5–10 years of type 1 DM, many individuals begin to excrete small amounts of albumin in the urine. The American Diabetes Association (ADA) recently suggested that the terms previously used to refer to increased urinary protein (microalbuminuria as defined as 30–299 mg/d in a 24-h collection or 30–299 μg/mg creatinine in a spot collection or macroalbuminuria as defined as >300 mg/24 h) be replaced by the phrases "persistent albuminuria (30–299 mg/24 h)" and "persistent albuminuria (≥300 mg/24 h)" to better reflect the continuous nature of albumin excretion in the urine as risk factor for nephropathy and cardiovascular disease (CVD). This chapter uses the terms *microalbuminuria* and *macroalbuminuria*. Although the appearance of microalbuminuria in type 1 DM is an important risk factor for progression to macroalbuminuria, only ~50% of individuals progress to macroalbuminuria over the next 10 years. In some individuals with type 1 diabetes and microalbuminuria of short duration, the microalbuminuria regresses. Microalbuminuria is also a risk factor for CVD. Once macroalbuminuria is present, there is a steady decline in GFR, and ~50% of individuals reach ESRD in 7–10 years. Once macroalbuminuria develops, blood pressure rises slightly and the pathologic changes are likely irreversible.

The nephropathy that develops in type 2 DM differs from that of type 1 DM in the following respects: (1) microalbuminuria or macroalbuminuria may be present when type 2 DM is diagnosed, reflecting its long asymptomatic period; (2) hypertension more commonly accompanies microalbuminuria or macroalbuminuria in type 2 DM; and (3) microalbuminuria may be less predictive of diabetic nephropathy and likelihood of progression to macroalbuminuria in type 2 DM, in large part due to increased CV mortality in this population. Finally, it should be noted that albuminuria in type 2 DM may be secondary to factors unrelated to DM, such as hypertension, congestive heart failure (CHF), prostate disease, or infection.

As part of comprehensive diabetes care (Chap. 418), albuminuria should be detected at an early stage when effective therapies can be instituted. Because some individuals with type 1 or type 2 DM have a decline in GFR in the absence of albuminuria, annual measurement of the serum creatinine to estimate GFR should also be performed.

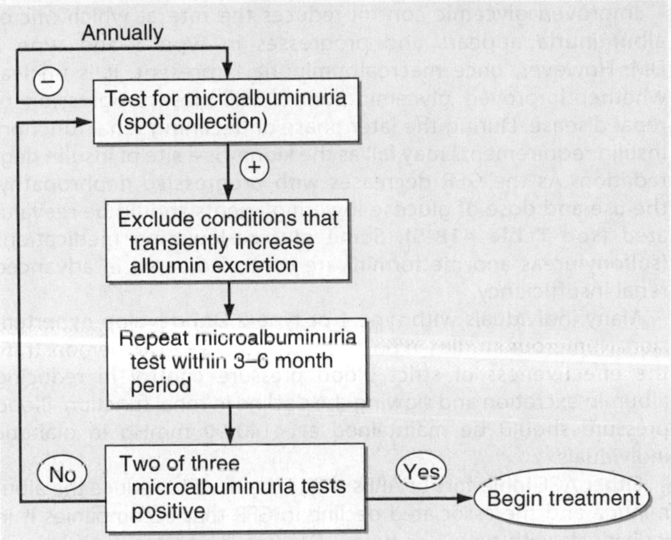

FIGURE 419-4 Screening for microalbuminuria should be performed in patients with type 1 diabetes for ≥5 years, in patients with type 2 diabetes, and during pregnancy. Non-diabetes-related conditions that might increase microalbuminuria are urinary tract infection, hematuria, heart failure, febrile illness, severe hyperglycemia, severe hypertension, and vigorous exercise. *(Adapted from RA DeFranzo, in Therapy for Diabetes Mellitus and Related Disorders, 3rd ed. American Diabetes Association, Alexandria, VA, 1998.)*

An annual microalbuminuria measurement (albumin-to-creatinine ratio in spot urine) is advised in individuals with type 1 or type 2 DM (Fig. 419-4). The urine protein measurement in a routine urinalysis does not detect these low levels of albumin excretion. Screening for albuminuria should commence 5 years after the onset of type 1 DM and at the time of diagnosis of type 2 DM.

Type IV renal tubular acidosis (hyporeninemic hypoaldosteronism) may occur in type 1 or 2 DM. These individuals develop a propensity to hyperkalemia and acidemia, which may be exacerbated by medications (especially angiotensin-converting enzyme [ACE] inhibitors, angiotensin receptor blockers [ARBs], and spironolactone). Patients with DM are predisposed to radiocontrast-induced nephrotoxicity. Risk factors for radiocontrast-induced nephrotoxicity are preexisting nephropathy and volume depletion. Individuals with DM undergoing radiographic procedures with contrast dye should be well hydrated before and after dye exposure, and the serum creatinine should be monitored for 24–48 h following the procedure. Metformin should be held if indicated.

TREATMENT DIABETIC NEPHROPATHY

The optimal therapy for diabetic nephropathy is prevention by control of glycemia **(Chap. 418 outlines glycemic goals and approaches)**. Interventions effective in slowing progression of albuminuria include (1) improved glycemic control, (2) strict blood pressure control, and (3) administration of an ACE inhibitor or ARB. Dyslipidemia should also be treated.

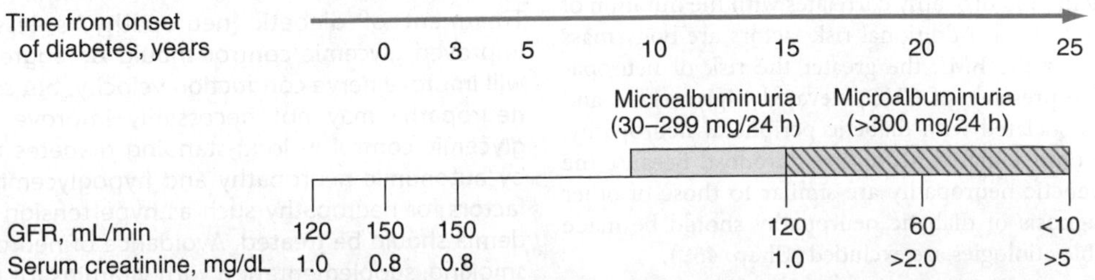

FIGURE 419-3 Time course of development of diabetic nephropathy. The relationship of time from onset of diabetes, the glomerular filtration rate (GFR), and the serum creatinine are shown. *(Adapted from RA DeFranzo, in Therapy for Diabetes Mellitus and Related Disorders, 3rd ed. American Diabetes Association, Alexandria, VA, 1998.)*

Improved glycemic control reduces the rate at which microalbuminuria appears and progresses in type 1 and type 2 DM. However, once macroalbuminuria is present, it is unclear whether improved glycemic control will slow progression of renal disease. During the later phase of declining renal function, insulin requirements may fall as the kidney is a site of insulin degradation. As the GFR decreases with progressive nephropathy, the use and dose of glucose-lowering agents should be reevaluated (see Table 418-5). Some glucose-lowering medications (sulfonylureas and metformin) are contraindicated in advanced renal insufficiency.

Many individuals with type 1 or type 2 DM develop hypertension. Numerous studies in both type 1 and type 2 DM demonstrate the effectiveness of strict blood pressure control in reducing albumin excretion and slowing the decline in renal function. Blood pressure should be maintained at <140/90 mmHg in diabetic individuals.

Either ACE inhibitors or ARBs should be used to reduce the albuminuria and the associated decline in GFR that accompanies it in individuals with type 1 or type 2 DM (see "Hypertension," below). Although direct comparisons of ACE inhibitors and ARBs are lacking, most experts believe that the two classes of drugs are equivalent in patient with diabetes. ARBs can be used as an alternative in patients who develop ACE inhibitor–associated cough or angioedema. After 2–3 months of therapy in patients with microalbuminuria, the drug dose is increased until the maximum tolerated dose is reached. Recent studies do not show benefit of intervention prior to onset of microalbuminuria. The combination of an ACE inhibitor and an ARB is not recommended and appears to be detrimental. If use of either ACE inhibitors or ARBs is not possible or the blood pressure is not controlled, then, diuretics, calcium channel blockers (nondihydropyridine class), or beta blockers should be used. These salutary effects are mediated by reducing intraglomerular pressure and inhibition of angiotensin-driven sclerosing pathways, in part through inhibition of TGF-β-mediated pathways.

The ADA does not suggest restriction of protein intake in diabetic individuals with albuminuria because studies have failed to show benefit.

Nephrology consultation should be considered when albuminuria appears and again when the estimated GFR is <60 mL/min per 1.743 m². As compared with nondiabetic individuals, hemodialysis in patients with DM is associated with more frequent complications, such as hypotension (due to autonomic neuropathy or loss of reflex tachycardia), more difficult vascular access, and accelerated progression of retinopathy. Complications of atherosclerosis are the leading cause of death in diabetic individuals with nephropathy and hyperlipidemia should be treated aggressively. Renal transplantation from a living related donor is the preferred therapy but requires chronic immunosuppression. Combined pancreas-kidney transplant offers the promise of normoglycemia and freedom from dialysis.

NEUROPATHY AND DIABETES MELLITUS

Diabetic neuropathy occurs in ~50% of individuals with long-standing type 1 and type 2 DM. It may manifest as polyneuropathy, mononeuropathy, and/or autonomic neuropathy. As with other complications of DM, the development of neuropathy correlates with the duration of diabetes and glycemic control. Additional risk factors are body mass index (BMI) (the greater the BMI, the greater the risk of neuropathy) and smoking. The presence of CVD, elevated triglycerides, and hypertension is also associated with diabetic peripheral neuropathy. Both myelinated and unmyelinated nerve fibers are lost. Because the clinical features of diabetic neuropathy are similar to those of other neuropathies, the diagnosis of diabetic neuropathy should be made only after other possible etiologies are excluded (Chap. 459).

Polyneuropathy/Mononeuropathy The most common form of diabetic neuropathy is distal symmetric polyneuropathy. It most frequently presents with distal sensory loss and pain, but up to 50% of patients do not have symptoms of neuropathy. Hyperesthesia, paresthesia, and dysesthesia also may occur. Any combination of these symptoms may develop as neuropathy progresses. Symptoms may include a sensation of numbness, tingling, sharpness, or burning that begins in the feet and spreads proximally. Neuropathic pain develops in some of these individuals, occasionally preceded by improvement in their glycemic control. Pain typically involves the lower extremities, is usually present at rest, and worsens at night. Both an acute (lasting <12 months) and a chronic form of painful diabetic neuropathy have been described. The acute form is sometimes treatment-related, occurring in the context of improved glycemic control. As diabetic neuropathy progresses, the pain subsides and eventually disappears, but a sensory deficit in the lower extremities persists. Physical examination reveals sensory loss, loss of ankle deep-tendon reflexes, and abnormal position sense.

Diabetic polyradiculopathy is a syndrome characterized by severe disabling pain in the distribution of one or more nerve roots. It may be accompanied by motor weakness. Intercostal or truncal radiculopathy causes pain over the thorax or abdomen. Involvement of the lumbar plexus or femoral nerve may cause severe pain in the thigh or hip and may be associated with muscle weakness in the hip flexors or extensors (diabetic amyotrophy). Fortunately, diabetic polyradiculopathies are usually self-limited and resolve over 6–12 months.

Mononeuropathy (dysfunction of isolated cranial or peripheral nerves) is less common than polyneuropathy in DM and presents with pain and motor weakness in the distribution of a single nerve. Mononeuropathies can occur at entrapment sites such as carpal tunnel or be noncompressive. A vascular etiology for noncompressive mononeuropathies has been suggested, but the pathogenesis is unknown. Involvement of the third cranial nerve is most common and is heralded by diplopia. Physical examination reveals ptosis and ophthalmoplegia with normal pupillary constriction to light. Sometimes other cranial nerves, such as IV, VI, or VII (Bell's palsy), are affected. Peripheral mononeuropathies or simultaneous involvement of more than one nerve (mononeuropathy multiplex) may also occur.

Autonomic Neuropathy Individuals with long-standing type 1 or 2 DM may develop signs of autonomic dysfunction involving the cholinergic, noradrenergic, and peptidergic (peptides such as pancreatic polypeptide, substance P, etc.) systems. DM-related autonomic neuropathy can involve multiple systems, including the cardiovascular, gastrointestinal, genitourinary, sudomotor, and metabolic systems. Autonomic neuropathies affecting the cardiovascular system cause a resting tachycardia and orthostatic hypotension. Reports of sudden death have also been attributed to autonomic neuropathy. Gastroparesis and bladder-emptying abnormalities are often caused by the autonomic neuropathy seen in DM (discussed below). Hyperhidrosis of the upper extremities and anhidrosis of the lower extremities result from sympathetic nervous system dysfunction. Anhidrosis of the feet can promote dry skin with cracking, which increases the risk of foot ulcers. Autonomic neuropathy may reduce counterregulatory hormone release (especially catecholamines), leading to an inability to sense hypoglycemia appropriately (hypoglycemia unawareness; Chap. 420), thereby subjecting the patient to the risk of severe hypoglycemia and complicating efforts to improve glycemic control.

TREATMENT DIABETIC NEUROPATHY

Treatment of diabetic neuropathy is less than satisfactory. Improved glycemic control should be aggressively pursued and will improve nerve conduction velocity, but symptoms of diabetic neuropathy may not necessarily improve. Efforts to improve glycemic control in long-standing diabetes may be confounded by autonomic neuropathy and hypoglycemia unawareness. Risk factors for neuropathy such as hypertension and hypertriglyceridemia should be treated. Avoidance of neurotoxins (alcohol) and smoking, supplementation with vitamins for possible deficiencies (B_{12}, folate; Chap. 96e), and symptomatic treatment are the mainstays of therapy. Loss of sensation in the foot places the patient at risk for ulceration and its sequelae; consequently, prevention of such problems is of paramount importance. Patients with symptoms or signs of neuropathy should check their feet daily and take precautions (footwear) aimed at preventing calluses or ulcerations. If foot deformities are present, a podiatrist should be involved.

Chronic, painful diabetic neuropathy is difficult to treat but may respond to duloxetine, amitriptyline, gabapentin, valproate, pregabalin, or opioids. Two agents, duloxetine and pregabalin, have been approved by the U.S. Food and Drug Administration (FDA) for pain associated with diabetic neuropathy, but no treatments are satisfactory. No direct comparisons of agents are available, and it is reasonable to switch agents if there is no response or if side effects develop. Referral to a pain management center may be necessary. Because the pain of acute diabetic neuropathy may resolve over time, medications may be discontinued as progressive neuronal damage from DM occurs.

Therapy of orthostatic hypotension secondary to autonomic neuropathy is also challenging. A variety of agents have limited success (fludrocortisone, midodrine, clonidine, octreotide, and yohimbine), but each has significant side effects. Nonpharmacologic maneuvers (adequate salt intake, avoidance of dehydration and diuretics, and lower extremity support hose) may offer some benefit.

GASTROINTESTINAL/GENITOURINARY DYSFUNCTION

Long-standing type 1 and 2 DM may affect the motility and function of the gastrointestinal (GI) and genitourinary systems. The most prominent GI symptoms are delayed gastric emptying (gastroparesis) and altered small- and large-bowel motility (constipation or diarrhea). Gastroparesis may present with symptoms of anorexia, nausea, vomiting, early satiety, and abdominal bloating. Microvascular complications (retinopathy and neuropathy) are usually present. Nuclear medicine scintigraphy after ingestion of a radiolabeled meal may document delayed gastric emptying, but may not correlate well with the patient's symptoms. Noninvasive "breath tests" following ingestion of a radiolabeled meal have been developed, but are not yet validated. Although parasympathetic dysfunction secondary to chronic hyperglycemia is important in the development of gastroparesis, hyperglycemia itself also impairs gastric emptying. Nocturnal diarrhea, alternating with constipation, is a feature of DM related GI autonomic neuropathy. In type 1 DM, these symptoms should also prompt evaluation for celiac sprue because of its increased frequency. Esophageal dysfunction in long-standing DM may occur but is usually asymptomatic.

Diabetic autonomic neuropathy may lead to genitourinary dysfunction including cystopathy and female sexual dysfunction (reduced sexual desire, dyspareunia, reduced vaginal lubrication). Symptoms of diabetic cystopathy begin with an inability to sense a full bladder and a failure to void completely. As bladder contractility worsens, bladder capacity and the postvoid residual increase, leading to symptoms of urinary hesitancy, decreased voiding frequency, incontinence, and recurrent urinary tract infections. Diagnostic evaluation includes cystometry and urodynamic studies.

Erectile dysfunction and retrograde ejaculation are very common in DM and may be one of the earliest signs of diabetic neuropathy (Chap. 67). Erectile dysfunction, which increases in frequency with the age of the patient and the duration of diabetes, may occur in the absence of other signs of diabetic autonomic neuropathy.

TREATMENT GASTROINTESTINAL/GENITOURINARY DYSFUNCTION

Current treatments for these complications of DM are inadequate. Improved glycemic control should be a primary goal, because some aspects (neuropathy, gastric function) may improve. Smaller, more frequent meals that are easier to digest (liquid) and low in fat and fiber may minimize symptoms of gastroparesis. Metoclopramide has been used but is now restricted in both the United States and Europe and not advised for long-term use. Gastric electrical stimulatory devices are available but not approved. Diabetic diarrhea in the absence of bacterial overgrowth is treated symptomatically (Chap. 349).

Diabetic cystopathy should be treated with scheduled voiding or self-catheterization. Drugs that inhibit type 5 phosphodiesterase are effective for erectile dysfunction, but their efficacy in individuals with DM is slightly lower than in the nondiabetic population (Chap. 67). Sexual dysfunction in women may be improved with use of vaginal lubricants, treatment of vaginal infections, and systemic or local estrogen replacement.

CARDIOVASCULAR MORBIDITY AND MORTALITY

CVD is increased in individuals with type 1 or type 2 DM. The Framingham Heart Study revealed a marked increase in PAD, coronary artery disease, MI, and CHF (risk increase from one- to fivefold) in DM. In addition, the prognosis for individuals with diabetes who have coronary artery disease or MI is worse than for nondiabetics. CHD is more likely to involve multiple vessels in individuals with DM. In addition to CHD, cerebrovascular disease is increased in individuals with DM (threefold increase in stroke). Thus, after controlling for all known cardiovascular risk factors, type 2 DM increases the cardiovascular death rate twofold in men and fourfold in women.

The American Heart Association has designated DM as a "CHD risk equivalent," and type 2 DM patients without a prior MI have a similar risk for coronary artery–related events as nondiabetic individuals who have had a prior MI. However, the cardiovascular risk assessment in type 2 DM should encompass a more nuanced approach. Cardiovascular risk is lower and not equivalent in a younger individual with a brief duration of type 2 DM compared to an older individual with long-standing type 2DM. Because of the extremely high prevalence of underlying CVD in individuals with diabetes (especially in type 2 DM), evidence of atherosclerotic vascular disease (e.g., cardiac stress test) should be sought in an individual with diabetes who has symptoms suggestive of cardiac ischemia or peripheral or carotid arterial disease. The screening of asymptomatic individuals with diabetes for CHD, even with a risk-factor scale, is not recommended because recent studies have not shown a clinical benefit. The absence of chest pain ("silent ischemia") is common in individuals with diabetes, and a thorough cardiac evaluation should be considered prior to major surgical procedures.

The increase in cardiovascular morbidity and mortality rates in diabetes appears to relate to the synergism of hyperglycemia with other cardiovascular risk factors. Risk factors for macrovascular disease in diabetic individuals include dyslipidemia, hypertension, obesity, reduced physical activity, and cigarette smoking. Additional risk factors more prevalent in the diabetic population include microalbuminuria, macroalbuminuria, an elevation of serum creatinine, abnormal platelet function and endothelial dysfunction The possibility of atherogenic potential of insulin is suggested by the data in nondiabetic individuals showing higher serum insulin levels (indicative of insulin resistance) in association with greater risk of cardiovascular morbidity and mortality. However, treatment with insulin and the sulfonylureas did not increase the risk of CVD in individuals with type 2 DM.

TREATMENT CARDIOVASCULAR DISEASE

In general, the treatment of coronary disease is not different in the diabetic individual (Chap. 293). Revascularization procedures for CHD, including percutaneous coronary interventions (PCI) and coronary artery bypass grafting (CABG), may be less efficacious in the diabetic individual. Initial success rates of PCI in diabetic individuals are similar to those in the nondiabetic population, but diabetic patients have higher rates of restenosis and lower long-term patency and survival rates in older studies.

Aggressive cardiovascular risk modification in all individuals with DM and glycemic control should be individualized, as discussed in Chap. 418. In patients with known CHD and type 2 DM, an ACE inhibitor (or ARB), a statin, and acetylsalicylic acid (ASA; aspirin) should be considered. Past trepidation about using beta blockers in individuals who have diabetes should not prevent use of these agents because they clearly benefit diabetic patients after MI. In patients with CHF, thiazolidinediones should not be used (Chap. 418). However, metformin can be used in patients with stable CHF if the renal function is normal.

Antiplatelet therapy reduces cardiovascular events in individuals with DM who have CHD and is recommended. Current recommendations by the ADA include the use of aspirin for primary prevention of coronary events in diabetic individuals with an increased 10-year cardiovascular risk >10% (at least one risk factor such as hypertension, smoking, family history, albuminuria, or dyslipidemia in men >50 years or women >60 years of age). ASA is not recommended for primary prevention in those with a 10-year cardiovascular risk <10%. The aspirin dose is the same as in nondiabetic individuals.

Cardiovascular Risk Factors • ***DYSLIPIDEMIA*** Individuals with DM may have several forms of dyslipidemia (Chap. 421). Because of the additive cardiovascular risk of hyperglycemia and hyperlipidemia, lipid abnormalities should be assessed aggressively and treated as part of comprehensive diabetes care (Chap. 418). The most common pattern of dyslipidemia is hypertriglyceridemia and reduced high-density lipoprotein (HDL) cholesterol levels. DM itself does not increase levels of low-density lipoprotein (LDL), but the small dense LDL particles found in type 2 DM are more atherogenic because they are more easily glycated and susceptible to oxidation.

Almost all treatment studies of diabetic dyslipidemia have been performed in individuals with type 2 DM because of the greater frequency of dyslipidemia in this form of diabetes. Interventional studies have shown that the beneficial effects of LDL reduction with statins are similar in the diabetic and nondiabetic populations. Large prospective trials of primary and secondary intervention for CHD have included some individuals with type 2 DM, and subset analyses have consistently found that reductions in LDL reduce cardiovascular events and morbidity in individuals with DM. No prospective studies have addressed similar questions in individuals with type 1 DM. Because the frequency of CVD is low in children and young adults with diabetes, assessment of cardiovascular risk should be incorporated into the guidelines discussed below.

Based on the guidelines provided by the ADA, priorities in the treatment of dyslipidemia are as follows: (1) lower the LDL cholesterol, (2) raise the HDL cholesterol, and (3) decrease the triglycerides. A treatment strategy depends on the pattern of lipoprotein abnormalities. Initial therapy for all forms of dyslipidemia should include dietary changes, as well as the same lifestyle modifications recommended in the nondiabetic population (smoking cessation, blood pressure control, weight loss, increased physical activity). The dietary recommendations for individuals with DM include increased monounsaturated fat and carbohydrates and reduced saturated fats and cholesterol (Chap. 421). According to guidelines of the ADA, the target lipid values in diabetic individuals (age >40 years) without CVD should be as follows: LDL <2.6 mmol/L (100 mg/dL); HDL >1 mmol/L (40 mg/dL) in men and >13 mmol/L (50 mg/dL) in women; and triglycerides <1.7 mmol/L (150 mg/dL). In patients >40 years, the ADA recommends addition of a statin, regardless of the LDL level, in patients with CHD and those without CHD who have CHD risk factors. Recently released guidelines by the American College of Cardiology (ACC) and American Heart Association (AHA) differ slightly and recommend that diabetic individuals aged 40–75 without CHD and a LDL of 70–189 mg/dl receive "moderate" intensity statin therapy (Chap. 291e). Improvement in glycemic control will lower triglycerides and have a modest beneficial effect by raising HDL.

If the patient is known to have CHD, the ADA recommends an LDL goal of <18 mmol/L (70 mg/dL) as an "option" (in keeping with evidence that such a goal is beneficial in nondiabetic individuals with CHD [Chap. 421]). The ACC/AHA guidelines do not advocate a specific LDL for statin therapy. HMG-CoA reductase inhibitors are the agents of choice for lowering LDL. Combination therapy with an HMG-CoA reductase inhibitor and a fibrate or another lipid-lowering agent (ezetimibe, niacin) may be considered but increases the possibility of side effects such as myositis and has not been shown to be beneficial. Nicotinic acid effectively raises HDL and can be used in patients with diabetes, but may worsen glycemic control and increase insulin resistance and has not been shown to provide additional benefit beyond statin therapy alone. Bile acid–binding resins should not be used if hypertriglyceridemia is present. In large clinical trials, statin usage is associated with a mild increase in the risk of developing type 2 DM. This risk is greatest in individuals with other risk factors for type 2 DM (Chap. 417). However, the cardiovascular benefits of statin use outweigh the mildly increased risk of diabetes.

HYPERTENSION Hypertension can accelerate other complications of DM, particularly CVD, nephropathy, and retinopathy. In targeting a goal of blood pressure of <140/80 mmHg, therapy should first emphasize lifestyle modifications such as weight loss, exercise, stress management, and sodium restriction. The BP goal should be individualized. In some younger individuals, the provider may target a blood pressure of <130/80 mmHg. Realizing that more than one agent is usually required to reach the blood pressure goal, the ADA recommends that all patients with diabetes and hypertension be treated with an ACE inhibitor or an ARB. Subsequently, agents that reduce cardiovascular risk (beta blockers, thiazide diuretics, and calcium channel blockers) should be incorporated into the regimen. ACE inhibitors and ARBs are likely equivalent in most patients with diabetes and renal disease. Serum potassium and renal function should be monitored.

Because of the high prevalence of atherosclerotic disease in individuals with type 2 DM, the possibility of renovascular hypertension should be considered when the blood pressure is not readily controlled.

LOWER EXTREMITY COMPLICATIONS

DM is the leading cause of nontraumatic lower extremity amputation in the United States. Foot ulcers and infections are also a major source of morbidity in individuals with DM. The reasons for the increased incidence of these disorders in DM involve the interaction of several pathogenic factors: neuropathy, abnormal foot biomechanics, PAD, and poor wound healing. The peripheral sensory neuropathy interferes with normal protective mechanisms and allows the patient to sustain major or repeated minor trauma to the foot, often without knowledge of the injury. Disordered proprioception causes abnormal weight bearing while walking and subsequent formation of callus or ulceration. Motor and sensory neuropathy lead to abnormal foot muscle mechanics and to structural changes in the foot (hammer toe, claw toe deformity, prominent metatarsal heads, Charcot joint). Autonomic neuropathy results in anhidrosis and altered superficial blood flow in the foot, which promote drying of the skin and fissure formation. PAD and poor wound healing impede resolution of minor breaks in the skin, allowing them to enlarge and to become infected.

Many individuals with type 2 DM develop a foot ulcer (great toe or metatarsophalangeal areas are most common), and a significant subset who develop an ulceration will ultimately undergo amputation (14–24% risk with that ulcer or subsequent ulceration). Risk factors for foot ulcers or amputation include male sex, diabetes for >10 years, peripheral neuropathy, abnormal structure of foot (bony abnormalities, callus, thickened nails), PAD, smoking, history of previous ulcer or amputation, visual impairment, and poor glycemic control. Large calluses are often precursors to or overlie ulcerations.

TREATMENT LOWER EXTREMITY COMPLICATIONS

The optimal therapy for foot ulcers and amputations is prevention through identification of high-risk patients, education of the patient, and institution of measures to prevent ulceration. High-risk patients should be identified during the routine, annual foot examination performed on all patients with DM (see "Ongoing Aspects of Comprehensive Diabetes Care" in Chap. 418). If the monofilament test or one of the other tests is abnormal, the patient is diagnosed with loss of protective sensation (LOPS; Chap. 417). Providers should consider screening for asymptomatic PAD in individuals >50 years of age who have diabetes and other risk factors using ankle-brachial index testing in high-risk individuals (Chap. 302). Patient education should emphasize (1) careful selection of footwear, (2) daily inspection of the feet to detect early signs of poor-fitting footwear or minor trauma, (3) daily foot hygiene to keep the skin clean and moist, (4) avoidance of self-treatment of foot abnormalities and high-risk behavior (e.g., walking barefoot), and (5) prompt consultation with a health care provider if an abnormality arises. Patients at high risk for ulceration or amputation may benefit from evaluation by a foot care specialist. Calluses and nail deformities should be treated by a podiatrist. Interventions directed at risk factor modification include orthotic shoes and devices, callus management, nail care, and prophylactic measures to reduce increased skin pressure from abnormal bony architecture. Attention to other risk factors for vascular disease (smoking, dyslipidemia, hypertension) and improved glycemic control are also important.

Despite preventive measures, foot ulceration and infection are common and represent a serious problem. Due to the multifactorial pathogenesis of lower extremity ulcers, management of these lesions is multidisciplinary and often demands expertise in orthopedics, vascular surgery, endocrinology, podiatry, and infectious diseases. The plantar surface of the foot is the most common site of ulceration. Ulcers may be primarily neuropathic (no accompanying infection) or may have surrounding cellulitis or osteomyelitis. Cellulitis without ulceration is also frequent and should be treated with antibiotics that provide broad-spectrum coverage, including anaerobes (see below).

An infected ulcer is a clinical diagnosis, because superficial culture of any ulceration will likely find multiple possible bacterial species. The infection surrounding the foot ulcer is often the result of multiple organisms, with aerobic gram-positive cocci (staphylococci including MRSA, Group A and B streptococci) being most common and with aerobic gram-negative bacilli and/or obligate anaerobes as co-pathogens.

Gas gangrene may develop in the absence of clostridial infection. Cultures taken from the surface of the ulcer are not helpful; a culture from the debrided ulcer base or from purulent drainage or aspiration of the wound is the most helpful. Wound depth should be determined by inspection and probing with a blunt-tipped sterile instrument. Plain radiographs of the foot should be performed to assess the possibility of osteomyelitis in chronic ulcers that have not responded to therapy. Magnetic resonance imaging (MRI) is the most specific modality, with nuclear medicine scans and labeled white cell studies as alternatives. Surgical debridement is often necessary.

Osteomyelitis is best treated by a combination of prolonged antibiotics (IV, then oral) and/or possibly debridement of infected bone. The possible contribution of vascular insufficiency should be considered in all patients. Peripheral arterial bypass procedures are often effective in promoting wound healing and in decreasing the need for amputation of the ischemic limb (Chap. 302).

A consensus statement from the ADA identified six interventions with demonstrated efficacy in diabetic foot wounds: (1) off-loading, (2) debridement, (3) wound dressings, (4) appropriate use of antibiotics, (5) revascularization, and (6) limited amputation. Off-loading is the complete avoidance of weight bearing on the ulcer, which removes the mechanical trauma that retards wound healing. Bed rest and a variety of orthotic devices or contact casting limit weight bearing on wounds or pressure points. Surgical debridement is important and effective, but clear efficacy of other modalities for wound cleaning (enzymes, soaking, whirlpools) is lacking. Dressings such as hydrocolloid dressings promote wound healing by creating a moist environment and protecting the wound. Antiseptic agents should be avoided. Topical antibiotics are of limited value. Referral for physical therapy, orthotic evaluation, and rehabilitation should occur once the infection is controlled.

Mild or non-limb-threatening infections can be treated with oral antibiotics directed predominantly at methicillin-susceptible staphylococci and streptococci (e.g., dicloxacillin, cephalosporin, amoxicillin/clavulanate). However the increasing prevalence of MRSA often requires the use of clindamycin, doxycycline, or trimethoprim-sulfamethoxazole. Trimethoprim-sulfamethoxazole exhibits less reliable coverage of streptococci than the β-lactams, and diabetic patients may develop adverse effects including acute kidney injury and hyperkalemia. Surgical debridement of necrotic tissue, local wound care (avoidance of weight bearing over the ulcer), and close surveillance for progression of infection are crucial. More severe infections require IV antibiotics as well as bed rest and local wound care. Urgent surgical debridement may be required. Optimization of glycemic control should be a goal. IV antibiotics should provide broad-spectrum coverage directed toward *Staphylococcus aureus*, including MRSA, streptococci, gram-negative aerobes, and anaerobic bacteria. Initial antimicrobial regimens include vancomycin plus a β-lactam/β-lactamase inhibitor or carbapenem or vancomycin plus a combination of quinolone plus metronidazole. Daptomycin, ceftaroline, or linezolid may be substituted for vancomycin. If the infection surrounding the ulcer is not improving with IV antibiotics, reassessment of antibiotic coverage and reconsideration of the need for surgical debridement or revascularization are indicated. With clinical improvement, oral antibiotics and local wound care can be continued on an outpatient basis with close follow-up.

INFECTIONS

Individuals with DM have a greater frequency and severity of infection. The reasons for this include incompletely defined abnormalities in cell-mediated immunity and phagocyte function associated with hyperglycemia, as well as diminished vascularization. Hyperglycemia aids the colonization and growth of a variety of organisms (*Candida* and other fungal species). Many common infections are more frequent and severe in the diabetic population, whereas several rare infections are seen almost exclusively in the diabetic population. Examples of this latter category include rhinocerebral mucormycosis, emphysematous infections of the gallbladder and urinary tract, and "malignant" or invasive otitis externa. Invasive otitis externa is usually secondary to *P. aeruginosa* infection in the soft tissue surrounding the external auditory canal, usually begins with pain and discharge, and may rapidly progress to osteomyelitis and meningitis. These infections should be sought, in particular, in patients presenting with severe hyperglycemia (Chap. 418).

Pneumonia, urinary tract infections, and skin and soft tissue infections are all more common in the diabetic population. In general, the organisms that cause pulmonary infections are similar to those found in the nondiabetic population; however, gram-negative organisms, *S. aureus*, and *Mycobacterium tuberculosis* are more frequent pathogens. Urinary tract infections (either lower tract or pyelonephritis) are the result of common bacterial agents such as *Escherichia coli*, although several yeast species (*Candida* and *Torulopsis glabrata*) are commonly observed. Complications of urinary tract infections include emphysematous pyelonephritis and emphysematous cystitis. Bacteriuria occurs frequently in individuals with diabetic cystopathy. Susceptibility to furunculosis, superficial candidal infections, and vulvovaginitis are increased. Poor glycemic control is a common denominator in individuals with these infections. Diabetic individuals have an increased rate of colonization of *S. aureus* in the skinfolds and nares. Diabetic patients also have a greater risk of postoperative wound infections.

DERMATOLOGIC MANIFESTATIONS

The most common skin manifestations of DM are xerosis and pruritus and are usually relieved by skin moisturizers. Protracted wound healing and skin ulcerations are also frequent complications. Diabetic dermopathy, sometimes termed *pigmented pretibial papules*, or "diabetic skin spots," begins as an erythematous macule or papule that evolves into an area of circular hyperpigmentation. These lesions result from minor mechanical trauma in the pretibial region and are more common in elderly men with DM. Bullous diseases, such as bullosa diabeticorum (shallow ulcerations or erosions in the pretibial region), are also seen. *Necrobiosis lipoidica diabeticorum* is an uncommon disorder, accompanying diabetes in predominantly young women. This usually begins in the pretibial region as an erythematous plaque or papules that gradually enlarge, darken, and develop irregular margins, with atrophic centers and central ulceration. They are often painful. Vitiligo occurs at increased frequency in individuals with type 1 DM. *Acanthosis nigricans* (hyperpigmented velvety plaques seen on the neck, axilla, or extensor surfaces) is sometimes a feature of severe insulin resistance and accompanying diabetes. Generalized or localized *granuloma annulare* (erythematous plaques on the extremities or trunk) and *scleredema* (areas of skin thickening on the back or neck at the site of previous superficial infections) are more common in the diabetic population. *Lipoatrophy* and *lipohypertrophy* can occur at insulin injection sites but are now unusual with the use of human insulin.

420 Hypoglycemia

Philip E. Cryer, Stephen N. Davis

Hypoglycemia is most commonly caused by drugs used to treat diabetes mellitus or by exposure to other drugs, including alcohol. However, a number of other disorders, including critical organ failure, sepsis and inanition, hormone deficiencies, non-β-cell tumors, insulinoma, and prior gastric surgery, can cause hypoglycemia (Table 420-1). Hypoglycemia is most convincingly documented by *Whipple's triad:* (1) symptoms consistent with hypoglycemia, (2) a low plasma glucose concentration measured with a precise method (not a glucose monitor), and (3) relief of symptoms after the plasma glucose level is raised. The lower limit of the fasting plasma glucose concentration is normally ~70 mg/dL (~3.9 mmol/L), but lower venous glucose levels occur normally, late after a meal, during pregnancy, and during prolonged fasting (>24 h). Hypoglycemia can cause serious morbidity; if severe and prolonged, it can be fatal. It should be considered in any patient with episodes of confusion, an altered level of consciousness, or a seizure.

TABLE 420-1 CAUSES OF HYPOGLYCEMIA IN ADULTS

Ill or medicated individual

1. Drugs
   - Insulin or insulin secretagogue
   - Alcohol
   - Others
2. Critical illness
   - Hepatic, renal or cardiac failure
   - Sepsis
   - Inanition
3. Hormone deficiency
   - Cortisol
   - Glucagon and epinephrine (in insulin-deficient diabetes)
4. Non–islet cell tumor

Seemingly well individual

5. Endogenous hyperinsulinism
   - Insulinoma
   - Functional β-cell disorders (nesidioblastosis)
     - Noninsulinoma pancreatogenous hypoglycemia
     - Post–gastric bypass hypoglycemia
   - Insulin autoimmune hypoglycemia
     - Antibody to insulin
     - Antibody to insulin receptor
   - Insulin secretagogue
   - Other
6. Accidental, surreptitious, or malicious hypoglycemia

Source: From PE Cryer et al: J Clin Endocrinol Metab 94:709, 2009. ©The Endocrine Society, 2009.

SYSTEMIC GLUCOSE BALANCE AND GLUCOSE COUNTERREGULATION

Glucose is an obligate metabolic fuel for the brain under physiologic conditions. The brain cannot synthesize glucose or store more than a few minutes' supply as glycogen and therefore requires a continuous supply of glucose from the arterial circulation. As the arterial plasma glucose concentration falls below the physiologic range, blood-to-brain glucose transport becomes insufficient to support brain energy metabolism and function. However, redundant glucose counterregulatory mechanisms normally prevent or rapidly correct hypoglycemia.

Plasma glucose concentrations are normally maintained within a relatively narrow range—roughly 70–110 mg/dL (3.9–6.1 mmol/L) in the fasting state, with transient higher excursions after a meal—despite wide variations in exogenous glucose delivery from meals and in endogenous glucose utilization by, for example, exercising muscle. Between meals and during fasting, plasma glucose levels are maintained by endogenous glucose production, hepatic glycogenolysis, and hepatic (and renal) gluconeogenesis (Fig. 420-1). Although hepatic glycogen stores are usually sufficient to maintain plasma glucose levels for ~8 h, this period can be shorter if glucose demand is increased by exercise or if glycogen stores are depleted by illness or starvation.

Gluconeogenesis normally requires low insulin levels and the presence of anti-insulin (counterregulatory) hormones together with a coordinated supply of precursors from muscle and adipose tissue to the liver (and kidneys). Muscle provides lactate, pyruvate, alanine, glutamine, and other amino acids. Triglycerides in adipose tissue are broken down into fatty acids and glycerol, which is a gluconeogenic precursor. Fatty acids provide an alternative oxidative fuel to tissues other than the brain (which requires glucose).

Systemic glucose balance—maintenance of the normal plasma glucose concentration—is accomplished by a network of hormones, neural signals, and substrate effects that regulate endogenous glucose production and glucose utilization by tissues other than the brain (Chap. 417). Among the regulatory factors, insulin plays a dominant role (Table 420-2; Fig. 420-1). As plasma glucose levels decline within the physiologic range in the fasting state, pancreatic β-cell insulin secretion decreases, thereby increasing hepatic glycogenolysis and hepatic (and renal) gluconeogenesis. Low insulin levels also reduce glucose utilization in peripheral tissues, inducing lipolysis and proteolysis and consequently releasing gluconeogenic precursors. Thus, a decrease in insulin secretion is the first defense against hypoglycemia.

As plasma glucose levels decline just below the physiologic range, glucose counterregulatory (plasma glucose–raising) hormones are released (Table 420-2; Fig. 420-1). Among these, pancreatic α-cell glucagon, which stimulates hepatic glycogenolysis, plays a primary role. Glucagon is the second defense against hypoglycemia. Adrenomedullary epinephrine, which stimulates hepatic glycogenolysis and gluconeogenesis (and renal gluconeogenesis), is not normally critical. However, it becomes critical when glucagon is deficient. Epinephrine is the third defense against hypoglycemia. When hypoglycemia is prolonged beyond ~4 h, cortisol and growth hormone also support glucose production and restrict glucose utilization to a limited amount (~20% compared to epinephrine). Thus cortisol and growth hormone play no role in defense against acute hypoglycemia.

As plasma glucose levels fall further, symptoms prompt behavioral defense against hypoglycemia, including the ingestion of food (Table 420-2; Fig. 420-1). The normal glycemic thresholds for these responses to decreasing plasma glucose concentrations are shown in Table 420-2. However, these thresholds are dynamic. They shift to higher-than-normal glucose levels in people with poorly controlled diabetes, who can experience symptoms of hypoglycemia when their glucose levels decline toward the normal range (*pseudohypoglycemia*). On the other hand, thresholds shift to lower-than-normal glucose levels in people with recurrent hypoglycemia; e.g., patients with aggressively treated diabetes or an insulinoma have symptoms at glucose levels lower than those that cause symptoms in healthy individuals.

Clinical Manifestations Neuroglycopenic manifestations of hypoglycemia are the direct result of central nervous system glucose deprivation. These features include behavioral changes, confusion, fatigue, seizure, loss of consciousness, and, if hypoglycemia is severe and prolonged,

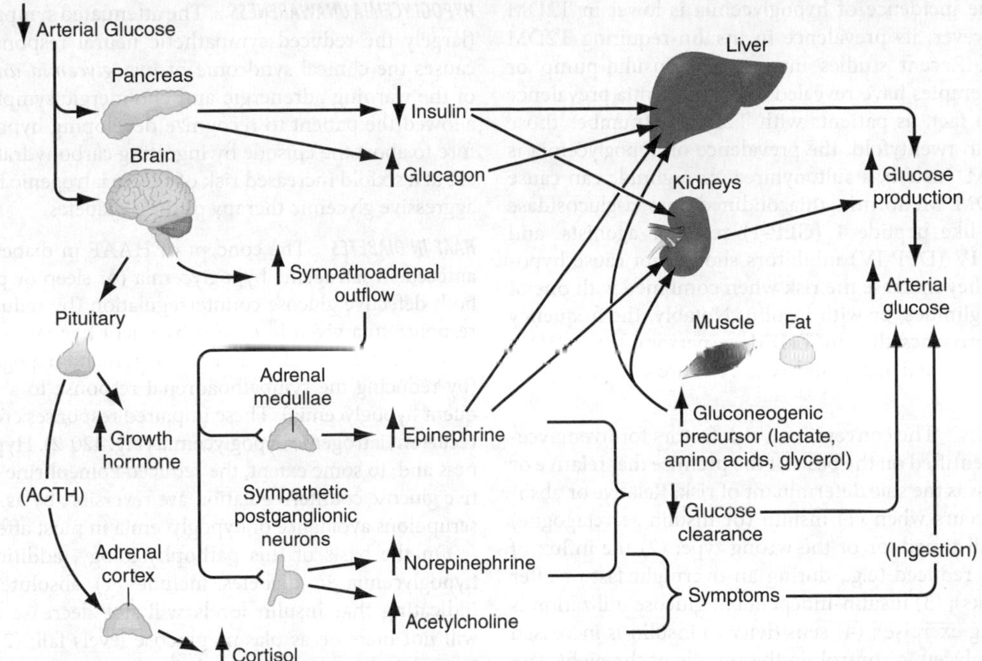

FIGURE 420-1 Physiology of glucose counterregulation: mechanisms that normally prevent or rapidly correct hypoglycemia. In insulin-deficient diabetes, the key counterregulatory responses—suppression of insulin and increases in glucagon—are lost, and stimulation of sympathoadrenal outflow is attenuated. ACTH, adrenocorticotropic hormone.

death. Neurogenic (or autonomic) manifestations of hypoglycemia result from the perception of physiologic changes caused by the central nervous system–mediated sympathoadrenal discharge that is triggered by hypoglycemia. They include *adrenergic* symptoms (mediated largely by norepinephrine released from sympathetic postganglionic neurons but perhaps also by epinephrine released from the adrenal medullae), such as palpitations, tremor, and anxiety, as well as *cholinergic* symptoms (mediated by acetylcholine released from sympathetic postganglionic neurons), such as sweating, hunger, and paresthesias. Clearly, these are nonspecific symptoms. Their attribution to hypoglycemia requires that the corresponding plasma glucose concentration be low and that the symptoms resolve after the glucose level is raised (as delineated by Whipple's triad).

Common signs of hypoglycemia include diaphoresis and pallor. Heart rate and systolic blood pressure are typically increased but may not be raised in an individual who has experienced repeated, recent episodes of hypoglycemia. Neuroglycopenic manifestations are often observable. Transient focal neurologic deficits occur occasionally. Permanent neurologic deficits are rare.

Etiology and Pathophysiology Hypoglycemia is most commonly a result of the treatment of diabetes. This topic is therefore addressed before other causes of hypoglycemia are considered.

HYPOGLYCEMIA IN DIABETES

Impact and Frequency Hypoglycemia is the limiting factor in the glycemic management of diabetes mellitus. First, it causes recurrent morbidity in most people with type 1 diabetes (T1DM) and in many with advanced type 2 diabetes (T2DM), and it is sometimes fatal. Second, it precludes maintenance of euglycemia over a lifetime of diabetes and thus full realization of the well-established microvascular benefits of glycemic control. Third, it causes a vicious cycle of recurrent hypoglycemia by producing hypoglycemia-associated autonomic failure—i.e., the clinical syndromes of defective glucose counterregulation and of hypoglycemia unawareness (see later).

Hypoglycemia is a fact of life for people with T1DM. They suffer an average of two episodes of symptomatic hypoglycemia per week and at least one episode of severe, at least temporarily disabling hypoglycemia each year. An estimated 6–10% of people with T1DM die as a result

TABLE 420-2 PHYSIOLOGIC RESPONSES TO DECREASING PLASMA GLUCOSE CONCENTRATIONS

Response	Glycemic Threshold, mmol/L (mg/dL)	Physiologic Effects	Role in Prevention or Correction of Hypoglycemia (Glucose Counterregulation)
↓ Insulin	4.4–4.7 (80–85)	↑ R_a (↓ R_d)	Primary glucose regulatory factor/first defense against hypoglycemia
↑ Glucagon	3.6–3.9 (65–70)	↑ R_a	Primary glucose counterregulatory factor/second defense against hypoglycemia
↑ Epinephrine	3.6–3.9 (65–70)	↑ R_a, ↓ R_c	Third defense against hypoglycemia, critical when glucagon is deficient
↑ Cortisol and growth hormone	3.6–3.9 (65–70)	↑ R_a, ↓ R_c	Involved in defense against prolonged hypoglycemia; not critical
Symptoms	2.8–3.1 (50–55)	Recognition of hypoglycemia	Prompt behavioral defense against hypoglycemia (food ingestion)
↓ Cognition	<2.8 (<50)	—	Compromises behavioral defense against hypoglycemia

Note: R_a, rate of glucose appearance, glucose production by the liver and kidneys; R_c, rate of glucose clearance, glucose utilization relative to the ambient plasma glucose by insulin-sensitive tissues; R_d, rate of glucose disappearance, glucose utilization by insulin-sensitive tissues such as skeletal muscle. R_d by the brain is not altered by insulin, glucagon, epinephrine, cortisol, or growth hormone.

Source: From PE Cryer, in S Melmed et al (eds): *Williams Textbook of Endocrinology*, 12th ed. New York, Elsevier, 2012.

of hypoglycemia. The incidence of hypoglycemia is lower in T2DM than in T1DM. However, its prevalence in insulin-requiring T2DM is surprisingly high. Recent studies investigating insulin-pump or multiple-injection therapies have revealed a hypoglycemia prevalence approaching 70%. In fact, as patients with T2DM outnumber those with T1DM by ten- to twentyfold, the prevalence of hypoglycemia is now greater in T2DM. Insulin, a sulfonylurea, or a glinide can cause hypoglycemia in T2DM. Metformin, thiazolidinediones, α-glucosidase inhibitors, glucagon-like peptide 1 (GLP-1) receptor agonists, and dipeptidyl peptidase IV (DPP-IV) inhibitors should not cause hypoglycemia. However, they increase the risk when combined with one of the sulfonylureas or glinides, or with insulin. Notably, the frequency of hypoglycemia approaches that in T1DM as persons with T2DM develop absolute insulin deficiency and require more complex treatment with insulin.

Conventional Risk Factors The conventional risk factors for hypoglycemia in diabetes are identified on the basis of the premise that relative or absolute insulin excess is the sole determinant of risk. Relative or absolute insulin excess occurs when (1) insulin (or insulin secretagogue) doses are excessive, ill-timed, or of the wrong type; (2) the influx of exogenous glucose is reduced (e.g., during an overnight fast or after missed meals or snacks); (3) insulin-independent glucose utilization is increased (e.g., during exercise); (4) sensitivity to insulin is increased (e.g., with improved glycemic control, in the middle of the night, late after exercise, or with increased fitness or weight loss); (5) endogenous glucose production is reduced (e.g., after alcohol ingestion); and (6) insulin clearance is reduced (e.g., in renal failure). However, these conventional risk factors alone explain a minority of episodes; other factors are typically involved.

Hypoglycemia-Associated Autonomic Failure (HAAF) While marked insulin excess alone can cause hypoglycemia, iatrogenic hypoglycemia in diabetes is typically the result of the interplay of relative or absolute therapeutic insulin excess and compromised physiologic and behavioral defenses against falling plasma glucose concentrations (Table 420-2; Fig. 420-2). Defective glucose counterregulation compromises physiologic defense (particularly decrements in insulin and increments in glucagon and epinephrine), and hypoglycemia unawareness compromises behavioral defense (ingestion of carbohydrate).

DEFECTIVE GLUCOSE COUNTERREGULATION In the setting of absolute endogenous insulin deficiency, insulin levels do not decrease as plasma glucose levels fall; the first defense against hypoglycemia is lost. Furthermore, probably because the decrement in intraislet insulin is normally a signal to stimulate glucagon secretion, glucagon levels do not increase as plasma glucose levels fall further; a second defense against hypoglycemia is lost. Finally, the increase in epinephrine levels, a third defense against hypoglycemia, in response to a given level of hypoglycemia is typically attenuated. The glycemic threshold for the sympathoadrenal (adrenomedullary epinephrine and sympathetic neural norepinephrine) response is shifted to lower plasma glucose concentrations. That shift is typically the result of recent antecedent iatrogenic hypoglycemia. In the setting of absent decrements in insulin and of absent increments in glucagon, the attenuated increment in epinephrine causes the clinical syndrome of defective glucose counterregulation. Affected patients are at ≥25-fold greater risk of severe iatrogenic hypoglycemia during aggressive glycemic therapy for their diabetes than are patients with normal epinephrine responses. This functional—and potentially reversible—disorder is distinct from classic diabetic autonomic neuropathy—a structural and irreversible disorder.

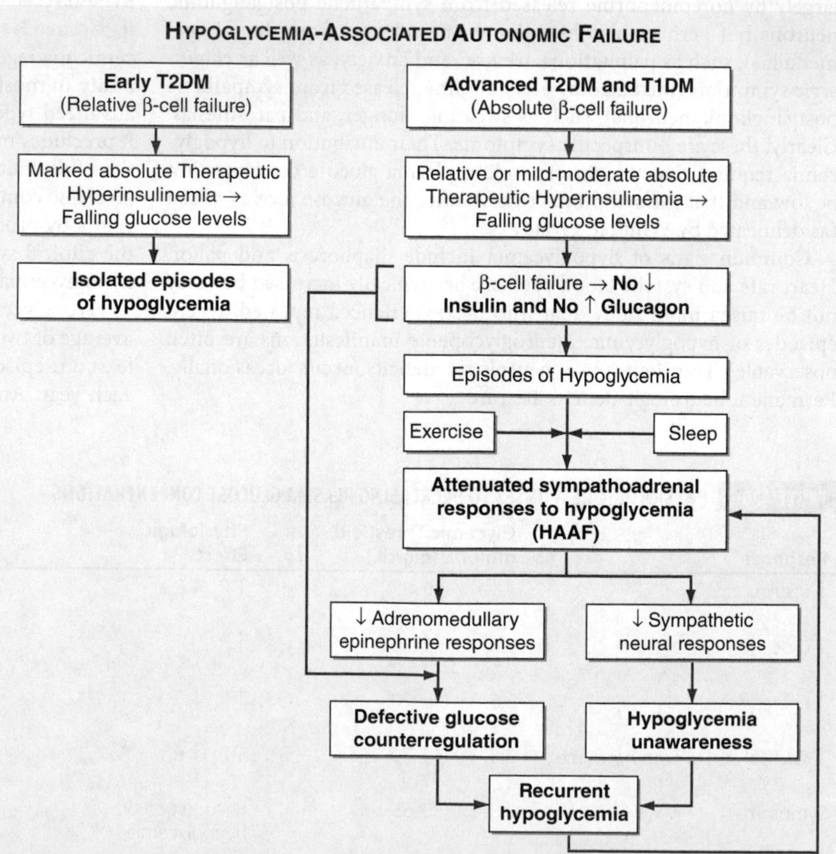

FIGURE 420-2 Hypoglycemia-associated autonomic failure (HAAF) in insulin-deficient diabetes. T1DM, type 1 diabetes mellitus; T2DM, type 2 diabetes mellitus. *(Modified from PE Cryer: Hypoglycemia in Diabetes. Pathophysiology, Prevalence, and Prevention, 2nd ed. © American Diabetes Association, 2012.)*

HYPOGLYCEMIA UNAWARENESS The attenuated sympathoadrenal response (largely the reduced sympathetic neural response) to hypoglycemia causes the clinical syndrome of *hypoglycemia unawareness*—i.e., loss of the warning adrenergic and cholinergic symptoms that previously allowed the patient to recognize developing hypoglycemia and therefore to abort the episode by ingesting carbohydrates. Affected patients are at a sixfold increased risk of severe iatrogenic hypoglycemia during aggressive glycemic therapy of their diabetes.

HAAF IN DIABETES The concept of HAAF in diabetes posits that recent antecedent iatrogenic hypoglycemia (or sleep or prior exercise) causes both defective glucose counterregulation (by reducing the epinephrine response to a given level of subsequent hypoglycemia in the setting of absent insulin and glucagon responses) and hypoglycemia unawareness (by reducing the sympathoadrenal response to a given level of subsequent hypoglycemia). These impaired responses create a vicious cycle of recurrent iatrogenic hypoglycemia (Fig. 420-2). Hypoglycemia unawareness and, to some extent, the reduced epinephrine component of defective glucose counterregulation are reversible by as little as 2–3 weeks of scrupulous avoidance of hypoglycemia in most affected patients.

On the basis of this pathophysiology, additional risk factors for hypoglycemia in diabetes include (1) absolute insulin deficiency, indicating that insulin levels will not decrease and glucagon levels will not increase as plasma glucose levels fall; (2) a history of severe hypoglycemia or of hypoglycemia unawareness, implying recent antecedent hypoglycemia, as well as prior exercise or sleep, indicating that the sympathoadrenal response will be attenuated; and (3) lower hemoglobin A_{1c} (HbA_{1c}) levels or lower glycemic goals that, all other factors being equal, increase the probability of recent antecedent hypoglycemia.

Hypoglycemia Risk Factor Reduction Several recent multicenter, randomized, controlled trials investigating the potential benefits of tight glucose control in either inpatient or outpatient settings have reported a high prevalence of severe hypoglycemia. In the NICE-SUGAR study, attempts to control in-hospital plasma glucose values towards physiologic levels resulted in increased mortality risk. The ADVANCE and ACCORD studies and the Veterans Affairs Diabetes Trial (VADT) also found a significant incidence of severe hypoglycemia among T2DM patients. Severe hypoglycemia with accompanying serious cardiovascular morbidity and mortality also occurred in the standard (e.g., not receiving intensified treatment) control group in both the ACCORD study and the VADT. Thus, severe hypoglycemia can and does occur at HbA_{1c} values of 8–9% in both T1DM and T2DM. Somewhat surprisingly, all three studies found little or no benefit of intensive glucose control to reduce macrovascular events in T2DM. In fact, the ACCORD study was ended early because of the increased mortality rate in the intensive glucose control arm. Whether iatrogenic hypoglycemia was the cause of the increased mortality risk is not known. In light of these findings, some new recommendations and paradigms have been formulated. Whereas there is little debate regarding the need to reduce hyperglycemia in the hospital, the glycemic maintenance goals have been modified to lie between 140 and 180 mg/dL. Accordingly, the benefits of insulin therapy and reduced hyperglycemia can be obtained while the prevalence of hypoglycemia is reduced.

Similarly, evidence exists that intensive glucose control can reduce the prevalence of microvascular disease in both T1DM and T2DM. These benefits need to be weighed against the increased prevalence of hypoglycemia. Certainly, the level of glucose control (i.e., the HbA_{1c} level) should be evaluated for each patient. Multicenter trials have demonstrated that individuals with recently diagnosed T1DM or T2DM can have better glycemic control with less hypoglycemia. In addition, there is still long-term benefit in reducing HbA_{1c} values from higher to lower, albeit still above recommended levels. Perhaps a reasonable therapeutic goal is the lowest HbA_{1c} level that does not cause severe hypoglycemia and that preserves awareness of hypoglycemia.

Pancreatic transplantation (both whole-organ and islet-cell) has been used in part as a treatment for severe hypoglycemia. Generally, rates of hypoglycemia are reduced after transplantation. This decrease appears to be due to increased physiologic insulin and glucagon responses during hypoglycemia.

The use of continuous glucose monitors offers some promise as a method of reducing hypoglycemia while improving HbA_{1c}. Other interventions to stimulate counterregulatory responses, such as selective serotonin-reuptake inhibitors, β-adrenergic receptor antagonists, opiate receptor antagonists, and fructose, remain experimental and have not been assessed in large-scale clinical trials.

Thus, intensive glycemic therapy (Chap. 418) needs to be applied along with the patient's education and empowerment, frequent self-monitoring of blood glucose, flexible insulin (and other drug) regimens (including the use of insulin analogues, both short- and longer-acting), individualized glycemic goals, and ongoing professional guidance, support, and consideration of both the conventional risk factors and those indicative of compromised glucose counterregulation. Given a history of hypoglycemia unawareness, a 2- to 3-week period of scrupulous avoidance of hypoglycemia is indicated.

HYPOGLYCEMIA WITHOUT DIABETES

There are many causes of hypoglycemia (Table 420-1). Because hypoglycemia is common in insulin- or insulin secretagogue–treated diabetes, it is often reasonable to assume that a clinically suspicious episode is the result of hypoglycemia. On the other hand, because hypoglycemia is rare in the absence of relevant drug-treated diabetes, it is reasonable to conclude that a hypoglycemic disorder is present only in patients in whom Whipple's triad can be demonstrated.

Particularly when patients are ill or medicated, the initial diagnostic focus should be on the possibility of drug involvement and then on critical illnesses, hormone deficiency, or non–islet cell tumor hypoglycemia. In the absence of any of these etiologic factors and in a seemingly well individual, the focus should shift to possible endogenous hyperinsulinism or accidental, surreptitious, or even malicious hypoglycemia.

Drugs Insulin and insulin secretagogues suppress glucose production and stimulate glucose utilization. Ethanol blocks gluconeogenesis but not glycogenolysis. Thus, alcohol-induced hypoglycemia typically occurs after a several-day ethanol binge during which the person eats little food, with consequent glycogen depletion. Ethanol is usually measurable in blood at the time of presentation, but its levels correlate poorly with plasma glucose concentrations. Because gluconeogenesis becomes the predominant route of glucose production during prolonged hypoglycemia, alcohol can contribute to the progression of hypoglycemia in patients with insulin-treated diabetes.

Many other drugs have been associated with hypoglycemia. These include commonly used drugs such as angiotensin-converting enzyme inhibitors and angiotensin receptor antagonists, β-adrenergic receptor antagonists, quinolone antibiotics, indomethacin, quinine, and sulfonamides.

Critical Illness Among hospitalized patients, serious illnesses such as renal, hepatic, or cardiac failure; sepsis; and inanition are second only to drugs as causes of hypoglycemia.

Rapid and extensive hepatic destruction (e.g., toxic hepatitis) causes fasting hypoglycemia because the liver is the major site of endogenous glucose production. The mechanism of hypoglycemia in patients with cardiac failure is unknown. Hepatic congestion and hypoxia may be involved. Although the kidneys are a source of glucose production, hypoglycemia in patients with renal failure is also caused by the reduced clearance of insulin and the reduced mobilization of gluconeogenic precursors in renal failure.

Sepsis is a relatively common cause of hypoglycemia. Increased glucose utilization is induced by cytokine production in macrophage-rich tissues such as the liver, spleen, and lung. Hypoglycemia develops if glucose production fails to keep pace. Cytokine-induced inhibition of gluconeogenesis in the setting of nutritional glycogen depletion, in combination with hepatic and renal hypoperfusion, may also contribute to hypoglycemia.

Hypoglycemia can be seen with starvation, perhaps because of loss of whole-body fat stores and subsequent depletion of gluconeogenic precursors (e.g., amino acids), necessitating increased glucose utilization.

Hormone Deficiencies Neither cortisol nor growth hormone is critical to the prevention of hypoglycemia, at least in adults. Nonetheless, hypoglycemia can occur with prolonged fasting in patients with primary adrenocortical failure (Addison's disease) or hypopituitarism. Anorexia and weight loss are typical features of chronic cortisol deficiency and likely result in glycogen depletion. Cortisol deficiency is associated with impaired gluconeogenesis and low levels of gluconeogenic precursors; these associations suggest that substrate-limited gluconeogenesis, in the setting of glycogen depletion, is the cause of hypoglycemia. Growth hormone deficiency can cause hypoglycemia in young children. In addition to extended fasting, high rates of glucose utilization (e.g., during exercise or in pregnancy) or low rates of glucose production (e.g., after alcohol ingestion) can precipitate hypoglycemia in adults with previously unrecognized hypopituitarism.

Hypoglycemia is not a feature of the epinephrine-deficient state that results from bilateral adrenalectomy when glucocorticoid replacement is adequate, nor does it occur during pharmacologic adrenergic blockade when other glucoregulatory systems are intact. Combined deficiencies of glucagon and epinephrine play a key role in the pathogenesis of iatrogenic hypoglycemia in people with insulin-deficient diabetes, as discussed earlier. Otherwise, deficiencies of these hormones are not usually considered in the differential diagnosis of a hypoglycemic disorder.

Non-β-Cell Tumors Fasting hypoglycemia, often termed *non–islet cell tumor hypoglycemia*, occurs occasionally in patients with large mesenchymal or epithelial tumors (e.g., hepatomas, adrenocortical carcinomas, carcinoids). The glucose kinetic patterns resemble those of hyperinsulinism (see next), but insulin secretion is suppressed appropriately during hypoglycemia. In most instances, hypoglycemia is due to overproduction of an incompletely processed form of insulin-like growth factor II ("big IGF-II") that does not complex normally with circulating binding proteins and thus more readily gains access to target tissues. The tumors are usually apparent clinically, plasma ratios of IGF-II to IGF-I are high, and free IGF-II levels (and levels of pro-IGF-II [1–21]) are elevated. Curative surgery is seldom possible, but reduction of tumor bulk may ameliorate hypoglycemia. Therapy with a glucocorticoid, a growth hormone, or both has also been reported to alleviate hypoglycemia. Hypoglycemia attributed to ectopic IGF-I production has been reported but is rare.

Endogenous Hyperinsulinism Hypoglycemia due to endogenous hyperinsulinism can be caused by (1) a primary β-cell disorder—typically a β-cell tumor (*insulinoma*), sometimes multiple insulinomas, or a functional β-cell disorder with β-cell hypertrophy or hyperplasia; (2) an antibody to insulin or to the insulin receptor; (3) a β-cell secretagogue such as a sulfonylurea; or perhaps (4) ectopic insulin secretion, among other very rare mechanisms. None of these causes is common.

The fundamental pathophysiologic feature of endogenous hyperinsulinism caused by a primary β-cell disorder or an insulin secretagogue is the failure of insulin secretion to fall to very low levels during hypoglycemia. This feature is assessed by measurement of plasma insulin, C-peptide (the connecting peptide that is cleaved from proinsulin to produce insulin), proinsulin, and glucose concentrations during hypoglycemia. Insulin, C-peptide, and proinsulin levels need not be high relative to normal, euglycemic values; rather, they are inappropriately high in the setting of a low plasma glucose concentration. Critical diagnostic findings are a plasma insulin concentration ≥3 μU/mL (≥18 pmol/L), a plasma C-peptide concentration ≥0.6 ng/mL (≥0.2 nmol/L), and a plasma proinsulin concentration ≥5.0 pmol/L when the plasma glucose concentration is <55 mg/dL (<3.0 mmol/L) with symptoms of hypoglycemia. A low plasma β-hydroxybutyrate concentration (≤2.7 mmol/L) and an increment in plasma glucose level of >25 mg/dL (>1.4 mmol/L) after IV administration of glucagon (1.0 mg) indicate increased insulin (or IGF) actions.

The diagnostic strategy is (1) to measure plasma glucose, insulin, C-peptide, proinsulin, and β-hydroxybutyrate concentrations and to screen for circulating oral hypoglycemic agents during an episode of hypoglycemia and (2) to assess symptoms during the episode and seek their resolution following correction of hypoglycemia by IV injection of glucagon (i.e., to document Whipple's triad). This is straightforward if the patient is hypoglycemic when seen. Since endogenous hyperinsulinemic disorders usually, but not invariably, cause fasting hypoglycemia, a diagnostic episode may develop after a relatively short outpatient fast. Serial sampling during an inpatient diagnostic fast of up to 72 h or after a mixed meal is more problematic. An alternative is to give patients a detailed list of the required measurements and ask them to present to an emergency room, with the list, during a symptomatic episode. Obviously, a normal plasma glucose concentration during a symptomatic episode indicates that the symptoms are not the result of hypoglycemia.

An *insulinoma*—an insulin-secreting pancreatic islet β-cell tumor—is the prototypical cause of endogenous hyperinsulinism and therefore should be sought in patients with a compatible clinical syndrome. However, insulinoma is not the only cause of endogenous hyperinsulinism. Some patients with fasting endogenous hyperinsulinemic hypoglycemia have diffuse islet involvement with β-cell hypertrophy and sometimes hyperplasia. This pattern is commonly referred to as *nesidioblastosis*, although β-cells budding from ducts are not invariably found. Other patients have a similar islet pattern but with postprandial hypoglycemia, a disorder termed *noninsulinoma pancreatogenous hypoglycemia*. Postgastric bypass postprandial hypoglycemia, which most often follows Roux-en-Y gastric bypass, is also characterized by diffuse islet involvement and endogenous hyperinsulinism. Some have suggested that exaggerated GLP-1 responses to meals cause hyperinsulinemia and hypoglycemia, but the relevant pathogenesis has not been clearly established. If medical treatments with agents such as an α-glucosidase inhibitor, diazoxide, or octreotide fail, partial pancreatectomy may be required. Autoimmune hypoglycemias include those caused by an antibody to insulin that binds post-meal insulin and then gradually disassociates, with consequent late postprandial hypoglycemia. Alternatively, an insulin receptor antibody can function as an agonist. The presence of an insulin secretagogue, such as a sulfonylurea or a glinide, results in a clinical and biochemical pattern similar to that of an insulinoma but can be distinguished by the presence of the circulating secretagogue. Finally, there are reports of very rare phenomena such as ectopic insulin secretion, a gain-of-function insulin receptor mutation, and exercise-induced hyperinsulinemia.

Insulinomas are uncommon, with an estimated yearly incidence of 1 in 250, 000. Because more than 90% of insulinomas are benign, they are a treatable cause of potentially fatal hypoglycemia. The median age at presentation is 50 years in sporadic cases, but the tumor usually presents in the third decade when it is a component of multiple endocrine neoplasia type 1 (Chap. 408). More than 99% of insulinomas are within the substance of the pancreas, and the tumors are usually small (<2.0 cm in diameter in 90% of cases). Therefore, they come to clinical attention because of hypoglycemia rather than mass effects. CT or MRI detects ~70–80% of insulinomas. These methods detect metastases in the roughly 10% of patients with a malignant insulinoma. Transabdominal ultrasound often identifies insulinomas, and endoscopic ultrasound has a sensitivity of ~90%. Somatostatin receptor scintigraphy is thought to detect insulinomas in about half of patients. Selective pancreatic arterial calcium injections, with the endpoint of a sharp increase in hepatic venous insulin levels, regionalize insulinomas with high sensitivity, but this invasive procedure is seldom necessary except to confirm endogenous hyperinsulinism in the diffuse islet disorders. Intraoperative pancreatic ultrasonography almost invariably localizes insulinomas that are not readily palpable by the surgeon. Surgical resection of a solitary insulinoma is generally curative. Diazoxide, which inhibits insulin secretion, or the somatostatin analogue octreotide can be used to treat hypoglycemia in patients with unresectable tumors; everolimus, an mTOR (mammalian target of rapamycin) inhibitor, is promising.

ACCIDENTAL, SURREPTITIOUS, OR MALICIOUS HYPOGLYCEMIA

Accidental ingestion of an insulin secretagogue (e.g., as the result of a pharmacy or other medical error) or even accidental administration of insulin can occur. Factitious hypoglycemia, caused by surreptitious or even malicious administration of insulin or an insulin secretagogue, shares many clinical and laboratory features with insulinoma. It is most common among health care workers, patients with diabetes or their relatives, and people with a history of other factitious illnesses. However, it should be considered in all patients being evaluated for hypoglycemia of obscure cause. Ingestion of an insulin secretagogue causes hypoglycemia with increased C-peptide levels, whereas exogenous insulin causes hypoglycemia with low C-peptide levels reflecting suppression of insulin secretion.

Analytical error in the measurement of plasma glucose concentrations is rare. On the other hand, glucose monitors used to guide treatment of diabetes are not quantitative instruments, particularly at low glucose levels, and should not be used for the definitive diagnosis of hypoglycemia. Even with a quantitative method, low measured glucose concentrations can be artifactual—e.g., the result of continued glucose metabolism by the formed elements of the blood ex vivo, particularly in the presence of leukocytosis, erythrocytosis, or thrombocytosis or with delayed separation of the serum from the formed elements (pseudohypoglycemia).

INBORN ERRORS OF METABOLISM CAUSING HYPOGLYCEMIA

Nondiabetic hypoglycemia also results from inborn errors of metabolism. Such hypoglycemia most commonly occurs in infancy but can also occur in adulthood. Cases in adults can be classified into those resulting in fasting hypoglycemia, postprandial hypoglycemia, and exercise-induced hypoglycemia.

Fasting Hypoglycemia Although rare, disorders of glycogenolysis can result in fasting hypoglycemia. These disorders include glycogen storage disease (GSD) of types 0, I, III, and IV and Fanconi-Bickel syndrome (Chap. 433e). Patients with GSD types I and III characteristically have high blood lactate levels before and after meals, respectively. Both groups have hypertriglyceridemia, but ketones are high in GSD type III. Defects in fatty acid oxidation also result in fasting hypoglycemia. These defects can include (1) defects in the carnitine cycle; (2) fatty-acid β-oxidation disorders; (3) electron transfer disturbances; and (4) ketogenesis disorders. Finally, defects in gluconeogenesis (fructose-1, 6-biphosphatase) have been reported to result in recurrent hypoglycemia and lactic acidosis.

Postprandial Hypoglycemia Inborn errors of metabolism resulting in postprandial hypoglycemia are also rare. These errors include (1) glucokinase, SUR1, and Kir6.2 potassium channel mutations; (2) congenital disorders of glycosylation; and (3) inherited fructose intolerance.

Exercise-Induced Hypoglycemia Exercise-induced hypoglycemia, by definition, follows exercise. It results in hyperinsulinemia caused by increased activity of monocarboxylate transporter 1 in β cells.

APPROACH TO THE PATIENT: Hypoglycemia

In addition to the recognition and documentation of hypoglycemia as well as its treatment (often on an urgent basis), diagnosis of the hypoglycemic mechanism is critical for the selection of therapy that prevents, or at least minimizes, recurrent hypoglycemia.

RECOGNITION AND DOCUMENTATION

Hypoglycemia is suspected in patients with typical symptoms; in the presence of confusion, an altered level of consciousness, or a seizure; or in a clinical setting in which hypoglycemia is known to occur. Blood should be drawn, whenever possible, before the administration of glucose to allow documentation of a low plasma glucose concentration. Convincing documentation of hypoglycemia requires the fulfillment of Whipple's triad. Thus, the ideal time to measure the plasma glucose level is during a symptomatic episode. A normal glucose level excludes hypoglycemia as the cause of the symptoms. A low glucose level confirms that hypoglycemia is the cause of the symptoms, provided the latter resolve after the glucose level is raised. When the cause of the hypoglycemic episode is obscure, additional measurements—made while the glucose level is low and before treatment—should include plasma insulin, C-peptide, proinsulin, and β-hydroxybutyrate levels; also critical are screening for circulating oral hypoglycemic agents and assessment of symptoms before and after the plasma glucose concentration is raised.

When the history suggests prior hypoglycemia and no potential mechanism is apparent, the diagnostic strategy is to evaluate the patient as just described and assess for Whipple's triad during and after an episode of hypoglycemia. On the other hand, while it cannot be ignored, a distinctly low plasma glucose concentration measured in a patient without corresponding symptoms raises the possibility of an artifact (pseudohypoglycemia).

DIAGNOSIS OF THE HYPOGLYCEMIC MECHANISM

In a patient with documented hypoglycemia, a plausible hypoglycemic mechanism can often be deduced from the history, physical examination, and available laboratory data (Table 420-1). Drugs, particularly alcohol or agents used to treat diabetes, should be the first consideration—even in the absence of known use of a relevant drug—given the possibility of surreptitious, accidental, or malicious drug administration. Other considerations include evidence of a relevant critical illness, hormone deficiencies (less commonly), and a non-β-cell tumor that can be pursued diagnostically (rarely). Absent one of these mechanisms in an otherwise seemingly well individual, the physician should consider endogenous hyperinsulinism and proceed with measurements and assessment of symptoms during spontaneous hypoglycemia or under conditions that might elicit hypoglycemia.

URGENT TREATMENT

If the patient is able and willing, oral treatment with glucose tablets or glucose-containing fluids, candy, or food is appropriate. A reasonable initial dose is 20 g of glucose. If the patient is unable or unwilling (because of neuroglycopenia) to take carbohydrates orally, parenteral therapy is necessary. IV administration of glucose (25 g) should be followed by a glucose infusion guided by serial plasma glucose measurements. If IV therapy is not practical, SC or IM glucagon (1.0 mg in adults) can be used, particularly in patients with T1DM. Because it acts by stimulating glycogenolysis, glucagon is ineffective in glycogen-depleted individuals (e.g., those with alcohol-induced hypoglycemia). Glucagon also stimulates insulin secretion and is therefore less useful in T2DM. The somatostatin analogue octreotide can be used to suppress insulin secretion in sulfonylurea-induced hypoglycemia. These treatments raise plasma glucose concentrations only transiently, and patients should therefore be urged to eat as soon as is practical to replete glycogen stores.

PREVENTION OF RECURRENT HYPOGLYCEMIA

Prevention of recurrent hypoglycemia requires an understanding of the hypoglycemic mechanism. Offending drugs can be discontinued or their doses reduced. Hypoglycemia caused by a sulfonylurea can persist for hours or even days. Underlying critical illnesses can often be treated. Cortisol and growth hormone can be replaced if levels are deficient. Surgical, radiotherapeutic, or chemotherapeutic reduction of a non–islet cell tumor can alleviate hypoglycemia even if the tumor cannot be cured; glucocorticoid or growth hormone administration also may reduce hypoglycemic episodes in such patients. Surgical resection of an insulinoma is curative; medical therapy with diazoxide or octreotide can be used if resection is not possible and in patients with a nontumor β-cell disorder. Partial pancreatectomy may be necessary in the latter patients. The treatment of autoimmune hypoglycemia (e.g., with glucocorticoid or immunosuppressive drugs) is problematic, but these disorders are sometimes self-limited. Failing these treatments, frequent feedings and avoidance of fasting may be required. Administration of uncooked cornstarch at bedtime or even an overnight intragastric infusion of glucose may be necessary for some patients.

421 Disorders of Lipoprotein Metabolism

Daniel J. Rader, Helen H. Hobbs

Lipoproteins are complexes of lipids and proteins that are essential for transport of cholesterol, triglycerides, and fat-soluble vitamins. Previously, lipoprotein disorders were the purview of specialized lipidologists, but the demonstration that lipid-lowering therapy significantly reduces the clinical complications of atherosclerotic cardiovascular disease (ASCVD) has brought the diagnosis and treatment of these disorders into the domain of the internist. The number of individuals who are candidates for lipid-lowering therapy continues to increase. Therefore, the appropriate diagnosis and management of lipoprotein disorders is of critical importance in the practice of medicine. This chapter reviews normal lipoprotein physiology, the pathophysiology of disorders of lipoprotein metabolism, the effects of diet and other environmental factors that influence lipoprotein metabolism, and the practical approaches to the diagnosis and management of lipoprotein disorders.

LIPOPROTEIN METABOLISM

LIPOPROTEIN CLASSIFICATION AND COMPOSITION

Lipoproteins are large macromolecular complexes composed of lipids and proteins that transport poorly soluble lipids (primarily triglycerides, cholesterol, and fat-soluble vitamins) through body fluids

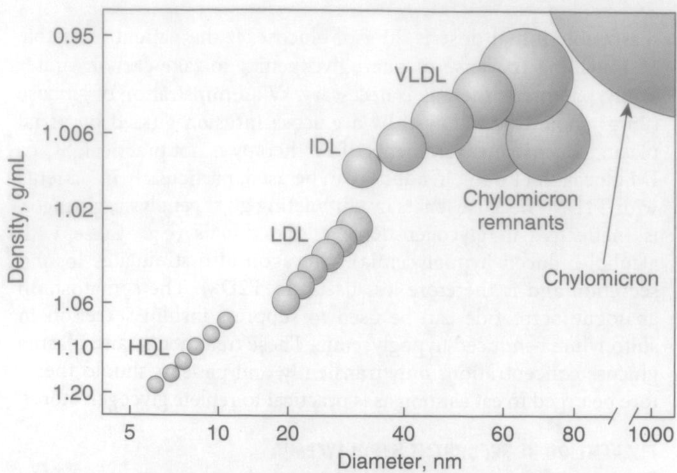

FIGURE 421-1 The density and size distribution of the major classes of lipoprotein particles. Lipoproteins are classified by density and size, which are inversely related. HDL, high-density lipoprotein; IDL, intermediate-density lipoprotein; LDL, low-density lipoprotein; VLDL, very-low-density lipoprotein.

(plasma, interstitial fluid, and lymph) to and from tissues. Lipoproteins play an essential role in the absorption of dietary cholesterol, long-chain fatty acids, and fat-soluble vitamins; the transport of triglycerides, cholesterol, and fat-soluble vitamins from the liver to peripheral tissues; and the transport of cholesterol from peripheral tissues to the liver and intestine.

Lipoproteins contain a core of hydrophobic lipids (triglycerides and cholesteryl esters) surrounded by a shell of hydrophilic lipids (phospholipids, unesterified cholesterol) and proteins (called apolipoproteins) that interact with body fluids. The plasma lipoproteins are divided into five major classes based on their relative density (**Fig. 421-1 and Table 421-1**): chylomicrons, very-low-density lipoproteins (VLDLs), intermediate-density lipoproteins (IDLs), low-density lipoproteins (LDLs), and high-density lipoproteins (HDLs). Each lipoprotein class comprises a family of particles that vary in density, size, and protein composition. Because lipid is less dense than water, the density of a lipoprotein particle is primarily determined by the amount of lipid per particle. Chylomicrons are the most lipid-rich and therefore least dense lipoprotein particles, whereas HDLs have the least lipid and are therefore the most dense lipoproteins. In addition to their density, lipoprotein particles can be classified according to their size, determined either by nondenaturing gel electrophoresis or by nuclear magnetic resonance profiling. There is a strong inverse relationship between density and size, with the largest particles being the most buoyant (chylomicrons) and the smallest particles being the most dense (HDL).

The proteins associated with lipoproteins, called *apolipoproteins* (**Table 421-2**), are required for the assembly, structure, function, and metabolism of lipoproteins. Apolipoproteins activate enzymes important in lipoprotein metabolism and act as ligands for cell surface receptors. ApoB is a very large protein and is the major structural protein of chylomicrons, VLDLs, IDLs, and LDLs; one molecule

TABLE 421-2 MAJOR APOLIPOPROTEINS

Apolipoprotein	Primary Source	Lipoprotein Association	Function
ApoA-I	Intestine, liver	HDL, chylomicrons	Structural protein for HDL Activates LCAT
ApoA-II	Liver	HDL, chylomicrons	Structural protein for HDL
ApoA-IV	Intestine, liver	HDL, chylomicrons	Unknown
ApoA-V	Liver	VLDL, chylomicrons	Promotes LPL-mediated triglyceride lipolysis
Apo(a)	Liver	Lp(a)	Unknown
ApoB-48	Intestine	Chylomicrons, chylomicron remnants	Structural protein for chylomicrons
ApoB-100	Liver	VLDL, IDL, LDL, Lp(a)	Structural protein for VLDL, LDL, IDL, Lp(a) Ligand for binding to LDL receptor
ApoC-I	Liver	Chylomicrons, VLDL, HDL	Unknown
ApoC-II	Liver	Chylomicrons, VLDL, HDL	Cofactor for LPL
ApoC-III	Liver, intestine	Chylomicrons, VLDL, HDL	Inhibits LPL activity and lipoprotein binding to receptors
ApoE	Liver	Chylomicron remnants, IDL, HDL	Ligand for binding to LDL receptor and other receptors

Abbreviations: HDL, high-density lipoprotein; IDL, intermediate-density lipoprotein; LCAT, lecithin-cholesterol acyltransferase; LDL, low-density lipoprotein; Lp(a), lipoprotein A; LPL, lipoprotein lipase; VLDL, very-low-density lipoprotein.

TABLE 421-1 MAJOR LIPOPROTEIN CLASSES

				Apolipoproteins		
Lipoprotein	**Density, g/mL**[a]	**Size, nm**[b]	**Electrophoretic Mobility**[c]	**Major**	**Other**	**Other Constituents**
Chylomicrons	0.930	75–1200	Origin	ApoB-48	A-I, A-V, C-I, C-II, C-III, E	Retinyl esters
Chylomicron remnants	0.930–1.006	30–80	Slow pre-β	ApoB-48	A-I, A-V, C-I, C-II, C-III, E	Retinyl esters
VLDL	0.930–1.006	30–80	Pre-β	ApoB-100	A-I, A-II, A-V, C-I, C-II, C-III, E	Vitamin E
IDL	1.006–1.019	25–35	Slow pre-β	ApoB-100	C-I, C-II, C-III, E	Vitamin E
LDL	1.019–1.063	18–25	β	ApoB-100		Vitamin E
HDL	1.063–1.210	5–12	α	ApoA-I	A-II, A-IV, A-V, C-III, E	LCAT, CETP, paroxonase
Lp(a)	1.050–1.120	25	Pre-β	ApoB-100	Apo(a)	Oxidized phospholipids

[a]The density of the particle is determined by ultracentrifugation. [b]The size of the particle is measured using gel electrophoresis. [c]The electrophoretic mobility of the particle on agarose gel electrophores reflects the size and surface charge of the particle, with β being the position of LDL and α being the position of HDL.

Note: All of the lipoprotein classes contain phospholipids, esterified and unesterified cholesterol, and triglycerides to varying degrees.

Abbreviations: CETP, cholesteryl ester transfer protein; HDL, high-density lipoprotein; IDL, intermediate-density lipoprotein; LCAT, lecithin-cholesterol acyltransferase; LDL, low-density lipoprotein; Lp(a), lipoprotein A; VLDL, very-low-density lipoprotein.

of apoB, either apoB-48 (chylomicron) or apoB-100 (VLDL, IDL, or LDL), is present on each lipoprotein particle. The human liver synthesizes apoB-100, and the intestine makes apoB-48, which is derived from the same gene by mRNA editing. HDLs have different apolipoproteins that define this lipoprotein class, most importantly apoA-I, which is synthesized in the liver and intestine and is found on virtually all HDL particles. ApoA-II is the second most abundant HDL apolipoprotein and is on approximately two-thirds of the HDL particles. ApoC-I, apoC-II, and apoC-III participate in the metabolism of triglyceride-rich lipoproteins. ApoE also plays a critical role in the metabolism and clearance of triglyceride-rich particles. Most apolipoproteins, other than apoB, exchange actively among lipoprotein particles in the blood. Apolipoprotein(a) [apo(a)] is a distinctive apolipoprotein and is discussed more below.

TRANSPORT OF INTESTINALLY DERIVED DIETARY LIPIDS BY CHYLOMICRONS

One critical role of lipoproteins is the efficient transport of dietary lipids from the intestine to tissues that require fatty acids for energy or store and metabolize lipids (Fig. 421-2). Dietary triglycerides are hydrolyzed by lipases within the intestinal lumen and emulsified with bile acids to form micelles. Dietary cholesterol, fatty acids, and fat-soluble vitamins are absorbed in the proximal small intestine. Cholesterol and retinol are esterified (by the addition of a fatty acid) in the enterocyte to form cholesteryl esters and retinyl esters, respectively. Longer-chain fatty acids (>12 carbons) are incorporated into triglycerides and packaged with apoB-48, cholesteryl esters, retinyl esters, phospholipids, and cholesterol to form chylomicrons. Nascent chylomicrons are secreted into the intestinal lymph and delivered via the thoracic duct directly to the systemic circulation, where they are extensively processed by peripheral tissues before reaching the liver. The particles encounter lipoprotein lipase (LPL), which is anchored to a glycosylphosphatidylinositol-anchored protein, GPIHBP1, that is attached to the endothelial surfaces of capillaries in adipose tissue, heart, and skeletal muscle (Fig. 421-2). The triglycerides of chylomicrons are hydrolyzed by LPL, and free fatty acids are released. ApoC-II, which is transferred to circulating chylomicrons from HDL, acts as a required cofactor for LPL in this reaction. The released free fatty acids are taken up by adjacent myocytes or adipocytes and either oxidized to generate energy or reesterified and stored as triglyceride. Some of the released free fatty acids bind albumin before entering cells and are transported to other tissues, especially the liver. The chylomicron particle progressively shrinks in size as the hydrophobic core is hydrolyzed and the hydrophilic lipids (cholesterol and phospholipids) and apolipoproteins on the particle surface are transferred to HDL, creating chylomicron remnants.

Chylomicron remnants are rapidly removed from the circulation by the liver through a process that requires apoE as a ligand for receptors in the liver. Consequently, few, if any, chylomicrons or chylomicron remnants are generally present in the blood after a 12-h fast, except in patients with certain disorders of lipoprotein metabolism.

TRANSPORT OF HEPATICALLY DERIVED LIPIDS BY VLDL AND LDL

Another key role of lipoproteins is the transport of hepatic lipids from the liver to the periphery (Fig. 421-2). VLDL particles resemble chylomicrons in protein composition but contain apoB-100 rather than apoB-48 and have a higher ratio of cholesterol to triglyceride (~1 mg of cholesterol for every 5 mg of triglyceride). The triglycerides of VLDL are derived predominantly from the esterification of long-chain fatty acids in the liver. The packaging of hepatic triglycerides with the other major components of the nascent VLDL particle (apoB-100, cholesteryl esters, phospholipids, and vitamin E) requires the action of the enzyme microsomal triglyceride transfer protein (MTP). After secretion into the plasma, VLDL acquires multiple copies of apoE and apolipoproteins of the C series by transfer from HDL. As with chylomicrons, the triglycerides of VLDL are hydrolyzed by LPL, especially in muscle, heart, and adipose tissue. After the VLDL remnants dissociate from LPL, they are referred to as IDLs, which contain roughly similar amounts of cholesterol and triglyceride. The liver removes approximately 40–60% of IDL by LDL receptor–mediated endocytosis via binding to apoE. The remainder of IDL is remodeled by hepatic lipase (HL) to form LDL. During this process, phospholipids and triglyceride in the particle are hydrolyzed, and all apolipoproteins except apoB-100 are transferred to other lipoproteins. Approximately 70% of LDL is removed from the circulation by the liver in a similar manner as IDL; however, in this case, apoB, rather than apoE, binds the LDL receptor.

Lp(a) is a lipoprotein similar to LDL in lipid and protein composition, but it contains an additional protein called apolipoprotein(a) [apo(a)]. Apo(a) is synthesized in the liver and attached to apoB-100 by a disulfide linkage. The major site of clearance of Lp(a) is the liver, but the uptake pathway is not known.

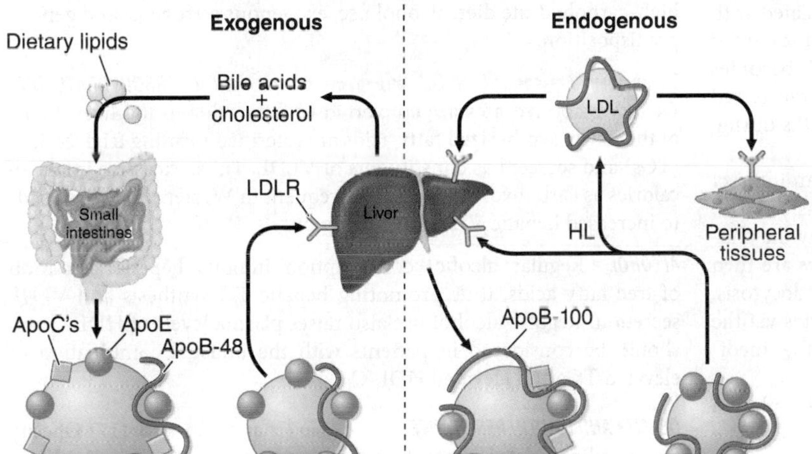

HDL METABOLISM AND REVERSE CHOLESTEROL TRANSPORT

All nucleated cells synthesize cholesterol, but only hepatocytes and enterocytes can effectively excrete cholesterol from the body, into either the bile or the gut lumen. In the liver, cholesterol is secreted into the bile, either directly or after conversion to bile acids. Cholesterol in peripheral cells is transported from the plasma membranes of peripheral cells to the liver and intestine by a process termed "reverse cholesterol transport" that is facilitated by HDL (Fig. 421-3).

Nascent HDL particles are synthesized by the intestine and the liver. Newly secreted apoA-I rapidly acquires phospholipids and unesterified cholesterol from its site

FIGURE 421-2 The exogenous and endogenous lipoprotein metabolic pathways. The exogenous pathway transports dietary lipids to the periphery and the liver. The endogenous pathway transports hepatic lipids to the periphery. FFA, free fatty acid; HL, hepatic lipase; IDL, intermediate-density lipoprotein; LDL, low-density lipoprotein; LDLR, low-density lipoprotein receptor; LPL, lipoprotein lipase; VLDL, very-low-density lipoprotein.

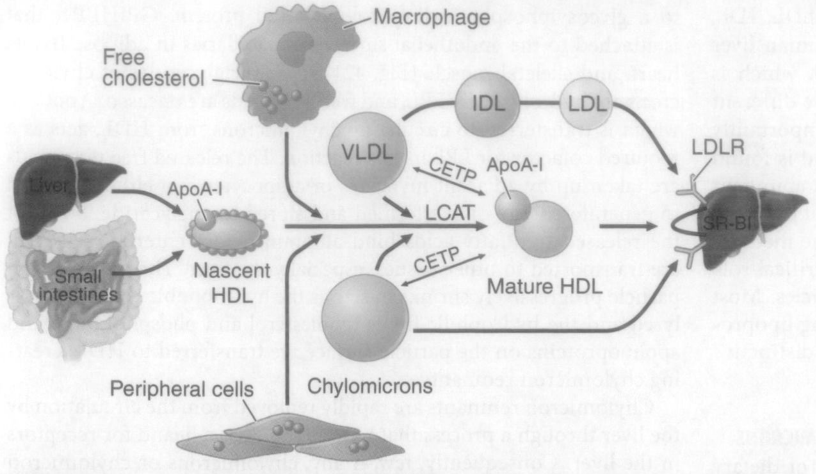

FIGURE 421-3 High-density lipoprotein (HDL) metabolism and reverse cholesterol transport. This pathway transports excess cholesterol from the periphery back to the liver for excretion in the bile. The liver and the intestine produce nascent HDLs. Free cholesterol is acquired from macrophages and other peripheral cells and esterified by lecithin-cholesterol acyltransferase (LCAT), forming mature HDLs. HDL cholesterol can be selectively taken up by the liver via SR-BI (scavenger receptor class BI). Alternatively, HDL cholesteryl ester can be transferred by cholesteryl ester transfer protein (CETP) from HDLs to very-low-density lipoproteins (VLDLs) and chylomicrons, which can then be taken up by the liver. IDL, intermediate-density lipoprotein; LDL, low-density lipoprotein; LDLR, low-density lipoprotein receptor.

of synthesis (intestine or liver) via efflux promoted by the membrane protein ATP-binding cassette protein A1 (ABCA1). This process results in the formation of discoidal HDL particles, which then recruit additional unesterified cholesterol from cells or circulating lipoproteins. Within the HDL particle, the cholesterol is esterified by lecithin-cholesterol acyltransferase (LCAT), a plasma enzyme associated with HDL, and the more hydrophobic cholesteryl ester moves to the core of the HDL particle. As HDL acquires more cholesteryl ester, it becomes spherical, and additional apolipoproteins and lipids are transferred to the particles from the surfaces of chylomicrons and VLDLs during lipolysis.

HDL cholesterol is transported to hepatocytes by both an indirect and a direct pathway. HDL cholesteryl esters can be transferred to apoB-containing lipoproteins in exchange for triglyceride by the cholesteryl ester transfer protein (CETP). The cholesteryl esters are then removed from the circulation by LDL receptor–mediated endocytosis. HDL cholesterol can also be taken up directly by hepatocytes via the scavenger receptor class B1 (SR-B1), a cell surface receptor that mediates the selective transfer of lipids to cells.

HDL particles undergo extensive remodeling within the plasma compartment by a variety of lipid transfer proteins and lipases. The phospholipid transfer protein (PLTP) transfers phospholipids from other lipoproteins to HDL or among different classes of HDL particles. After CETP- and PLTP-mediated lipid exchange, the triglyceride-enriched HDL becomes a much better substrate for HL, which hydrolyzes the triglycerides and phospholipids to generate smaller HDL particles. A related enzyme called *endothelial lipase* hydrolyzes HDL phospholipids, generating smaller HDL particles that are catabolized faster. Remodeling of HDL influences the metabolism, function, and plasma concentrations of HDL.

DISORDERS OF ELEVATED CHOLESTEROL AND TRIGLYCERIDES

Disorders of lipoprotein metabolism are collectively referred to as "dyslipidemias." Dyslipidemias are generally characterized clinically by increased plasma levels of cholesterol, triglycerides, or both, variably accompanied by reduced levels of HDL cholesterol. Because plasma lipids are commonly screened (see below), dyslipidemia is frequently seen in clinical practice. The majority of patients with dyslipidemia have some combination of genetic predisposition (often polygenic) and environmental contribution (lifestyle, medical condition, or drug). Many, but not all, patients with dyslipidemia are at increased risk for ASCVD, the primary reason for making the diagnosis, as intervention may reduce this risk. In addition, patients with substantially elevated levels of triglycerides may be at risk for acute pancreatitis and require intervention to reduce this risk.

Although literally hundreds of proteins influence lipoprotein metabolism and may interact to produce dyslipidemia in an individual patient, there are a limited number of discrete "nodes" that regulate lipoprotein metabolism. These include: (1) assembly and secretion of triglyceride-rich VLDLs by the liver; (2) lipolysis of triglyceride-rich lipoproteins by LPL; (3) receptor-mediated uptake of apoB-containing lipoproteins by the liver; (4) cellular cholesterol metabolism in the hepatocyte and the enterocyte; and (5) neutral lipid transfer and phospholipid hydrolysis in the plasma. The following discussion will focus on these regulatory nodes, recognizing that in many cases these nodes interact with and influence each other.

DYSLIPIDEMIA CAUSED BY EXCESSIVE HEPATIC SECRETION OF VLDL

Excessive production of VLDL by the liver is one of the most common causes of dyslipidemia. Individuals with excessive hepatic VLDL production usually have elevated fasting triglycerides and low levels of HDL cholesterol (HDL-C), with variable elevations in LDL cholesterol (LDL-C) but usually elevated plasma levels of apoB. A cluster of other metabolic risk factors are often found in association with VLDL overproduction, including obesity, glucose intolerance, insulin resistance, and hypertension (the so-called metabolic syndrome, Chap. 422). Some of the major factors that drive hepatic VLDL secretion include obesity, insulin resistance, a high-carbohydrate diet, alcohol use, exogenous estrogens, and genetic predisposition.

Secondary Causes of VLDL Overproduction • ***HIGH-CARBOHYDRATE DIET*** Dietary carbohydrates are converted to fatty acids in the liver. Some of the newly synthesized fatty acids are esterified forming triglycerides (TGs) and secreted as constituents of VLDL. Thus, excessive intake of calories as carbohydrates, which is frequent in Western societies, leads to increased hepatic VLDL-TG secretion.

ALCOHOL Regular alcohol consumption inhibits hepatic oxidation of free fatty acids, thus promoting hepatic TG synthesis and VLDL secretion. Regular alcohol use also raises plasma levels of HDL-C and should be considered in patients with the unusual combination of elevated TGs and elevated HDL-C.

OBESITY AND INSULIN RESISTANCE **(See also Chaps. 416 and 417)** Obesity and insulin resistance are frequently accompanied by dyslipidemia characterized by elevated plasma levels of TG, low HDL-C, variable levels of LDL-C, and increased levels of small dense LDL. The increase in adipocyte mass and accompanying decreased insulin sensitivity associated with obesity have multiple effects on lipid metabolism, with one of the major effects being excessive hepatic VLDL production. More free fatty acids are delivered from the expanded and insulin-resistant adipose tissue to the liver, where they are reesterified in hepatocytes to form TGs, which are packaged into VLDLs for secretion into the circulation. In addition, the increased insulin levels promote increased fatty acid synthesis in the liver. In insulin-resistant patients who progress to type 2 diabetes mellitus, dyslipidemia remains common, even when the patient is under relatively good glycemic control. In addition to increased VLDL production, insulin resistance can also result in decreased LPL activity, resulting in reduced catabolism of chylomicrons and VLDLs and more severe hypertriglyceridemia (see below).

NEPHROTIC SYNDROME **(See also Chap. 335)** Nephrotic syndrome is a classic cause of excessive VLDL production. The molecular mechanism of VLDL overproduction remains poorly understood but has been attributed to the effects of hypoalbuminemia leading to increased hepatic protein synthesis. Effective treatment of the underlying renal disease often normalizes the lipid profile, but most patients with chronic nephrotic syndrome require lipid-lowering drug therapy.

CUSHING'S SYNDROME (See also Chap. 406) Endogenous or exogenous glucocorticoid excess is associated with increased VLDL synthesis and secretion and hypertriglyceridemia. Patients with Cushing's syndrome frequently have dyslipidemia especially characterized by hypertriglyceridemia and low HDL-C, although elevations in plasma levels of LDL-C can also be seen.

Primary (Genetic) Causes of VLDL Overproduction Genetic variation influences hepatic VLDL production. A number of genes have been identified in which common and low-frequency variants likely contribute to increased VLDL production, likely involving interactions with diet and other environmental factors. The best recognized inherited condition associated with VLDL overproduction is familial combined hyperlipidemia.

FAMILIAL COMBINED HYPERLIPIDEMIA (FCHL) FCHL is generally characterized by elevations in plasma levels of TGs (VLDL) and LDL-C (including small dense LDL) and reduced plasma levels of HDL-C. It is estimated to occur in approximately 1 in 100–200 individuals and is an important cause of premature coronary heart disease (CHD); approximately 20% of patients who develop CHD under age 60 have FCHL. FCHL can manifest in childhood but is usually not fully expressed until adulthood. The disease clusters in families, with affected family members typically have one of three possible phenotypes: (1) elevated plasma levels of LDL-C, (2) elevated plasma levels of TGs due to elevation in VLDL, or (3) elevated plasma levels of both LDL-C and TG. The lipoprotein profile can switch among these three phenotypes in the same individual over time and may depend on factors such as diet, exercise, weight, and insulin sensitivity. Patients with FCHL almost always have significantly elevated plasma levels of apoB. The levels of apoB are disproportionately high relative to the plasma LDL-C concentration, indicating the presence of small, dense LDL particles, which are characteristic of this syndrome.

Individuals with this phenotype generally share the same metabolic defect, namely overproduction of VLDL by the liver. The molecular etiology of this condition remains poorly understood, and no single gene has been identified in which mutations cause this disorder. It is likely that defects in a combination of genes can cause the condition, suggesting that a more appropriate term for the disorder might be *polygenic combined hyperlipidemia.*

The presence of a mixed dyslipidemia (plasma TG levels between 200 and 600 mg/dL and total cholesterol levels between 200 and 400 mg/dL, usually with HDL-C levels <40 mg/dL in men and <50 mg/dL in women) and a family history of mixed dyslipidemia and/or premature CHD strongly suggests the diagnosis. Individuals with this phenotype should be treated aggressively due to significantly increased risk of premature CHD. Decreased dietary intake of simple carbohydrates, aerobic exercise, and weight loss can all have beneficial effects on the lipid profile. Patients with diabetes should be aggressively treated to maintain good glucose control. Most patients with FCHL require lipid-lowering drug therapy, starting with statins, to reduce lipoprotein levels and lower the risk of cardiovascular disease.

LIPODYSTROPHY Lipodystrophy is a condition in which the generation of adipose tissue generally or in certain fat depots is impaired. Lipodystrophies are often associated with insulin resistance and elevated plasma levels of VLDL and chylomicrons due to increased fatty acid synthesis and VLDL production, as well as reduced clearance of TG-rich particles. This disorder can be especially difficult to control. Patients with congenital generalized lipodystrophy are very rare and have nearly complete absence of subcutaneous fat, accompanied by profound insulin resistance and leptin deficiency, and accumulation of TGs in multiple tissues including the liver. Some patients with generalized lipodystrophy have been treated successfully with leptin administration. Partial lipodystrophy is somewhat more common and can be caused by mutations in several different genes, most notably lamin A. Partial lipodystrophy is usually characterized by increased truncal fat accompanied by markedly reduced or absent subcutaneous fat in the extremities and buttocks. These patients generally have insulin resistance, often quite severe, accompanied by type 2 diabetes, hepatosteatosis, and dyslipidemia. The dyslipidemia is usually characterized by elevated TGs and cholesterol and can be difficult to manage clinically. Patients with partial lipodystrophy are at substantially increased risk of atherosclerotic vascular disease and should therefore be treated aggressively for their dyslipidemia with statins and, if necessary, additional lipid-lowering therapies.

DYSLIPIDEMIA CAUSED BY IMPAIRED LIPOLYSIS OF TRIGLYCERIDE-RICH LIPOPROTEINS

Impaired lipolysis of the TGs in TG-rich lipoproteins (TRLs) also commonly contributes to dyslipidemia. As noted above, LPL is the key enzyme responsible for hydrolyzing the TGs in chylomicrons and VLDL. LPL is synthesized and secreted into the extracellular space from adipocytes, myocytes, and cardiomyocytes. It is then transported from the subendothelial to the vascular endothelial surfaces by GPIHPB1. LPL is also synthesized in macrophages. Individuals with impaired LPL activity, whether secondary or due to a primary genetic disorder, have elevated fasting TGs and low levels of HDL-C, usually without elevation in LDL-C or apoB. Insulin resistance, in addition to causing excessive VLDL production, can also cause impaired LPL activity and lipolysis. A number of common and low-frequency genetic variants have been described that influence LPL activity, and single-gene Mendelian disorders that reduce LPL activity have also been described (Table 421-3).

Secondary Causes of Impaired Lipolysis of TRLs • *OBESITY AND INSULIN RESISTANCE* (See also Chaps. 415e, 416, and 417) In addition to hepatic overproduction of VLDL, as discussed above, obesity, insulin resistance, and type 2 diabetes have been reported to be associated with variably reduced LPL activity. This may be due in part to the effects of tissue insulin resistance leading to reduced transcription of LPL in skeletal muscle and adipose, as well as to increased production of the LPL inhibitor apoC III by the liver. This reduction in LPL activity often contributes to the dyslipidemia seen in these patients.

Primary (Genetic) Causes and Genetic Predisposition to Impaired Lipolysis of TRLs • *FAMILIAL CHYLOMICRONEMIA SYNDROME* As noted above, LPL is required for the hydrolysis of TGs in chylomicrons and VLDLs, and apoC-II is a cofactor for LPL. Genetic deficiency or inactivity of either protein results in impaired lipolysis and profound elevations in plasma chylomicrons. These patients can also have elevated plasma levels of VLDL, but chylomicronemia predominates. The fasting plasma is turbid, and if left at 4°C (39.2°F) for a few hours, the chylomicrons float to the top and form a creamy supernatant. In these disorders, collectively called the *familial chylomicronemia syndrome*, fasting TG levels are almost invariably >1000 mg/dL. Fasting cholesterol levels are also elevated but to a lesser degree.

LPL deficiency has autosomal recessive inheritance and has a frequency of approximately 1 in 1 million in the population. *ApoC-II deficiency* is also recessive in inheritance pattern and is even less common than LPL deficiency. Multiple different mutations in the LPL and *APOC2* genes cause these diseases. Obligate LPL heterozygotes often have mild-to-moderate elevations in plasma TG levels, whereas individuals heterozygous for mutation in apoC-II do not have hypertriglyceridemia.

Both LPL and apoC-II deficiency usually present in childhood with recurrent episodes of severe abdominal pain due to acute pancreatitis. On funduscopic examination, the retinal blood vessels are opalescent (lipemia retinalis). Eruptive xanthomas, which are small, yellowish-white papules, often appear in clusters on the back, buttocks, and extensor surfaces of the arms and legs. These typically painless skin lesions may become pruritic. Hepatosplenomegaly results from the uptake of circulating chylomicrons by reticuloendothelial cells in the liver and spleen. For unknown reasons, some patients with persistent

TABLE 421-3 PRIMARY HYPERLIPOPROTEINEMIAS CAUSED BY KNOWN SINGLE-GENE MUTATIONS

Genetic Disorder	Protein (Gene) Defect	Lipoproteins Elevated	Clinical Findings	Genetic Transmission	Estimated Incidence
Hypertriglyceridemia					
Lipoprotein lipase deficiency	LPL (*LPL*)	Chylomicrons, VLDL	Eruptive xanthomas, hepatosplenomegaly, pancreatitis	AR	~1/1,000,000
Familial apoC-II deficiency	ApoC-II (*APOC2*)	Chylomicrons, VLDL	Eruptive xanthomas, hepatosplenomegaly, pancreatitis	AR	<1/1,000,000
ApoA-V deficiency	ApoA-V (*APOA5*)	Chylomicrons, VLDL	Eruptive xanthomas, hepatosplenomegaly, pancreatitis	AR	<1/1,000,000
GPIHBP1 deficiency	*GPIHBP1*	Chylomicrons	Eruptive xanthomas, pancreatitis	AR	<1/1,000,000
Combined Hyperlipidemia					
Familial hepatic lipase deficiency	Hepatic lipase (*LIPC*)	VLDL remnants, HDL	Pancreatitis, CHD	AR	<1/1,000,000
Familial dysbetalipoproteinemia	ApoE (*APOE*)	Chylomicron remnants, VLDL remnants	Palmar and tuberoeruptive xanthomas, CHD, PVD	AR	~1/10,000
Hypercholesterolemia					
Familial hypercholesterolemia	LDL receptor (*LDLR*)	LDL	Tendon xanthomas, CHD	AD	~1/250 to 1/500
Familial defective apoB-100	ApoB-100 (*APOB*)	LDL	Tendon xanthomas, CHD	AD	<~1/1500
Autosomal dominant hypercholesterolemia, type 3	PCSK9 (*PCSK9*)	LDL	Tendon xanthomas, CHD	AD	<1/1,000,000
Autosomal recessive hypercholesterolemia	ARH (*LDLRAP*)	LDL	Tendon xanthomas, CHD	AR	<1/1,000,000
Sitosterolemia	*ABCG5* or *ABCG8*	LDL	Tendon xanthomas, CHD	AR	<1/1,000,000

Abbreviations: AD, autosomal dominant; apo, apolipoprotein; AR, autosomal recessive; ARH, autosomal recessive hypercholesterolemia; CHD, coronary heart disease; LDL, low-density lipoprotein; LPL, lipoprotein lipase; PVD, peripheral vascular disease; VLDL, very-low density lipoprotein.

and pronounced chylomicronemia never develop pancreatitis, eruptive xanthomas, or hepatosplenomegaly. Premature CHD is not generally a feature of familial chylomicronemia syndromes.

The diagnoses of LPL and apoC-II deficiency are established enzymatically in specialized laboratories by assaying TG lipolytic activity in postheparin plasma. Blood is sampled after an IV heparin injection to release the endothelial-bound LPL. LPL activity is profoundly reduced in both LPL and apoC-II deficiency; in patients with apoC-II deficiency, it normalizes after the addition of normal plasma (providing a source of apoC-II). Molecular sequencing of the genes can be used to confirm the diagnosis.

The major therapeutic intervention in familial chylomicronemia syndrome is dietary fat restriction (to as little as 15 g/d) with fat-soluble vitamin supplementation. Consultation with a registered dietician familiar with this disorder is essential. Caloric supplementation with medium-chain TGs, which are absorbed directly into the portal circulation, can be useful, but there is uncertainty about their hepatic safety with prolonged use. If dietary fat restriction alone is not successful in resolving the chylomicronemia, fish oils have been effective in some patients. In patients with apoC-II deficiency, apoC-II can be provided by infusing fresh-frozen plasma to resolve the chylomicronemia in the acute setting. Management of patients with familial chylomicronemia syndrome is particularly challenging during pregnancy when VLDL production is increased. A gene therapy approach, called alipogene tiparvovec, is approved for LPL deficiency in Europe; it involves multiple intramuscular injections of an adeno-associated viral vector encoding a gain-of-function LPL variant, leading to skeletal myocyte expression of LPL.

APOA-V DEFICIENCY Another apolipoprotein, ApoA-V, facilitates the association of VLDL and chylomicrons with LPL and promotes their hydrolysis. Individuals harboring loss-of-function mutations in both *APOA5* alleles develop hyperchylomicronemia. Heterozygosity for variants in *APOA5* that reduce its function contributes to the polygenic basis of hypertriglyceridemia.

GPIHBP1 DEFICIENCY Homozygosity for mutations that interfere with GPIHBP1 synthesis or folding cause severe hypertriglyceridemia by compromising the transport of LPL to the vascular endothelium. The frequency of chylomicronemia due to mutations in GHIHBP1 has not been established but appears to be very rare.

FAMILIAL HYPERTRIGLYCERIDEMIA (FHTG) FHTG is characterized by elevated fasting TGs without a clear secondary cause, average to below average LDL-C levels, low HDL-C levels, and a family history of hypertriglyceridemia. Plasma LDL-C levels are often reduced due to defective conversion of TG-rich particles to LDL. In contrast to FCHL, apoB levels are not elevated. The identification of other first-degree relatives with hypertriglyceridemia is useful in making the diagnosis. Unlike in FCHL, this condition is not generally associated with a significantly increased risk of CHD. However, if the hypertriglyceridemia is exacerbated by environmental factors, medical conditions, or drugs, the TGs can rise to a level at which acute pancreatitis is a risk. Indeed, management of patients with this condition is mostly geared toward reduction of TGs to prevent pancreatitis.

Individuals with this phenotype generally have reduced lipolysis of TRLs, although overproduction of VLDL by the liver can also contribute. No single gene has been identified in which mutations cause this disorder, whereas combinations of gene variants have been shown to cause this phenotype. A more appropriate term for this condition might be *polygenic hypertriglyceridemia.*

It is important to consider and rule out secondary causes of the hypertriglyceridemia as discussed above. Increased intake of simple carbohydrates, obesity, insulin resistance, alcohol use, estrogen treatment, and certain medications can exacerbate this phenotype. Patients who are at high risk for CHD due to other risk factors should be treated with statin therapy. In patients who are otherwise not at high risk for CHD, lipid-lowering drug therapy can frequently be avoided with appropriate dietary and lifestyle changes. Patients with plasma TG levels >500 mg/dL after a trial of diet and exercise should be considered for drug therapy with a fibrate or fish oil to reduce TGs in order to prevent pancreatitis.

DYSLIPIDEMIA CAUSED BY IMPAIRED HEPATIC UPTAKE OF APOB-CONTAINING LIPOPROTEINS

Impaired uptake of LDL and remnant lipoproteins by the liver is another common cause of dyslipidemia. As discussed above, the LDL receptor is the major receptor responsible for uptake of LDL and remnant particles by the liver. Downregulation of LDL receptor activity or genetic variation that reduces the activity of the LDL receptor pathway leads to elevations in LDL-C. One major factor that reduces LDL receptor activity is a diet high in saturated and *trans* fats. Other medical conditions that reduce LDL receptor activity include hypothyroidism and estrogen deficiency. In addition, genetic variation in a number of genes influences LDL clearance, and mutations in some of these genes cause several discrete Mendelian disorders of elevated LDL-C (Table 421-3).

Secondary Causes of Impaired Hepatic Uptake of Lipoproteins • ***HYPOTHYROIDISM*** (See also Chap. 405) Hypothyroidism is associated with elevated plasma LDL-C levels due primarily to a reduction in hepatic LDL receptor function and delayed clearance of LDL. Thyroid hormone increases hepatic expression of the LDL receptor. Hypothyroid patients also frequently have increased levels of circulating IDL, and some patients with hypothyroidism also have mild hypertriglyceridemia. Because hypothyroidism is often subtle and therefore easily overlooked, all patients presenting with elevated plasma levels of LDL-C, especially if there has been an unexplained increase in LDL-C, should be screened for hypothyroidism. Thyroid replacement therapy usually ameliorates the hypercholesterolemia; if not, the patient probably has a primary lipoprotein disorder and may require lipid-lowering drug therapy with a statin.

CHRONIC KIDNEY DISEASE (See also Chap. 335) Chronic kidney disease (CKD) is often associated with mild hypertriglyceridemia (<300 mg/dL) due to the accumulation of VLDLs and remnant lipoproteins in the circulation. TG lipolysis and remnant clearance are both reduced in patients with renal failure. Because the risk of ASCVD is increased in end-stage renal disease, subjects with hyperlipidemia, they should usually be aggressively treated with lipid-lowering agents, even though there is inadequate data at present to indicate that this population benefits from LDL-lowering therapy.

Patients with solid organ transplants often have increased lipid levels due to the effect of the drugs required for immunosuppression. These patients can present a difficult clinical management problem, since statins should be used cautiously in these patients due to untoward muscle-related side effects.

Primary (Genetic) Causes of Impaired Hepatic Uptake of Lipoproteins Genetic variation contributes substantially to elevated LDL-C levels in the general population. It has been estimated that at least 50% of variation in LDL-C is genetically determined. Many patients with elevated LDL-C have *polygenic hypercholesterolemia* characterized by hypercholesterolemia in the absence of secondary causes of hypercholesterolemia (other than dietary factors) or a primary Mendelian disorder. In patients who are genetically predisposed to higher LDL-C levels, diet plays a key role; indeed increased saturated and *trans* fats in the diet shifts the entire distribution of LDL levels in the population to the right. Inheritance of several variants that together elevate LDL-C, coupled with diet, is generally the cause of this condition; <10% of first-degree relatives themselves have hypercholesterolemia. However, single-gene (Mendelian) causes of elevated LDL-C are relatively common and should be considered in the differential diagnosis of elevated LDL-C.

FAMILIAL HYPERCHOLESTEROLEMIA (FH) FH, also known as autosomal dominant hypercholesterolemia (ADH) type 1, is an autosomal co-dominant disorder characterized by elevated plasma levels of LDL-C in the absence of hypertriglyceridemia. FH is caused by loss-of-function mutations in the gene encoding the LDL receptor. The reduction in LDL receptor activity in the liver results in a reduced rate of clearance of LDL from the circulation. The plasma level of LDL increases to a level such that the rate of LDL production equals the rate of LDL clearance by residual LDL receptor as well as non-LDL receptor mechanisms. More than 1600 different mutations have been reported in association with FH. The elevated levels of LDL-C in FH are primarily due to delayed removal of LDL from the blood; in addition, because the removal of IDL is also delayed, the production of LDL from IDL is also increased. Individuals with two mutated LDL receptor alleles (FH homozygotes, or compound heterozygotes) have much higher LDL-C levels than those with one mutant allele (FH heterozygotes).

Heterozygous FH is caused by the inheritance of one mutant LDL receptor allele. The population frequency of heterozygous FH due to LDL receptor mutations was originally estimated to be 1 in 500 individuals, but recent data suggest it may be as high as approximately 1 in 250 individuals, making it one of the most common single-gene disorders in humans. FH has a higher prevalence in certain founder populations, such as South African Afrikaners, Christian Lebanese, and French Canadians. Heterozygous FH is characterized by elevated plasma levels of LDL-C (usually 200–400 mg/dL) and normal levels of TGs. Patients with heterozygous FH have hypercholesterolemia from birth, and disease recognition is usually based on detection of hypercholesterolemia on routine screening, the appearance of tendon xanthomas, or the development of symptomatic cardiovascular disease. Inheritance is dominant, meaning that the condition was inherited from one parent and ~50% of the patient's siblings can be expected to have hypercholesterolemia. The family history is frequently positive for premature CHD on the side of the family from which the mutation was inherited. Physical findings in many, but not all, patients with heterozygous FH include corneal arcus and tendon xanthomas particularly involving the dorsum of the hands and the Achilles tendons. Untreated heterozygous FH is associated with a markedly increased risk of cardiovascular disease. Untreated men with heterozygous FH have an ~50% chance of having a myocardial infarction before age 60 years, and women with heterozygous FH are at substantially increased risk as well. The age of onset of cardiovascular disease is highly variable and depends on the specific molecular defect, the level of LDL-C, and coexisting cardiovascular risk factors. FH heterozygotes with elevated plasma levels of Lp(a) (see below) appear to be at greater risk for cardiovascular disease.

No definitive diagnostic test for heterozygous FH is available, except in certain founder populations where selected mutations predominate. Most LDL receptor mutations are private and require sequencing of the LDL receptor gene for identification. Sequencing for clinical diagnosis is available but not standard of care and is rarely performed in the United States, because the clinical utility of identifying the specific mutation has not been demonstrated. A family history of hypercholesterolemia and/or premature coronary disease is supportive of the diagnosis. Secondary causes of significant hypercholesterolemia such as hypothyroidism, nephrotic syndrome, and obstructive liver disease should be excluded.

Heterozygous FH patients should be aggressively treated to lower plasma levels of LDL-C, starting in childhood. Initiation of a diet low in saturated and *trans* fats is recommended, but heterozygous FH patients virtually always require lipid-lowering drug therapy for effective control of their LDL-C levels. Statins are effective in heterozygous FH and are clearly the drug class of choice, and usually a more potent member of the class. However, some heterozygous FH patients cannot achieve adequate control of their LDL-C levels even with high-dose statin therapy and require additional drugs; a cholesterol absorption inhibitor and/or a bile acid sequestrant are the next-line classes of drugs. Currently, heterozygous FH patients whose LDL-C levels remain markedly elevated (>200 mg/dL with cardiovascular disease [CVD] or >300 mg/dL without CVD) on maximally tolerated drug therapy are candidates for LDL apheresis, a physical method of purging the blood of LDL in which the LDL particles are selectively removed from the circulation; LDL apheresis is usually performed every 2 weeks. A new class of drugs known as PCSK9 inhibitors is under clinical development and has the potential to effectively control LDL-C levels in the vast majority of patients with heterozygous FH who are inadequately controlled on a statin alone or who are statin intolerant.

Homozygous FH is caused by mutations in both alleles of the LDL receptor and therefore much rarer than heterozygous FH. Patients with homozygous FH have been classified into those patients with virtually no detectable LDL receptor activity (*receptor negative*) and those patients with markedly reduced but detectable LDL receptor activity (*receptor defective*). LDL-C levels in patients with homozygous FH range from about 400 to >1000 mg/dL, with receptor-defective patients at the lower end and receptor-negative patients at the higher end of the range. TGs are usually normal. Many patients with homozygous FH, particularly receptor-negative patients, present in childhood with cutaneous xanthomas on the hands, wrists, elbows, knees, heels, or buttocks. The devastating consequence of homozygous FH is accelerated ASCVD, which often presents in childhood or early adulthood. Atherosclerosis often develops first in the aortic root, where it can cause aortic valvular or supravalvular stenosis, and typically extends into the coronary ostia, which become stenotic. Symptoms can be atypical, and sudden death is not uncommon. Untreated, receptor-negative patients with homozygous FH rarely survive beyond the second decade; patients with receptor-defective LDL receptor defects have a better prognosis but almost invariably develop clinically apparent atherosclerotic vascular disease by age 30, and often much sooner. Carotid and femoral disease develops later in life and is usually not clinically significant.

Homozygous FH should be suspected in a child or young adult with LDL >400 mg/dL without secondary cause. Cutaneous xanthomas, evidence of CVD, and hypercholesterolemia in both parents all are supportive of the diagnosis. Although the specific mutations in the LDL receptor can usually be identified by DNA sequencing, this is not generally performed, and the diagnosis is usually made on clinical grounds.

Patients with homozygous FH must be treated aggressively to delay the onset and progression of CVD. Receptor defective patients sometimes respond to statins and other LDL-lowering drug classes such as a cholesterol absorption inhibitor or a bile acid sequestrant, which upregulate the LDL receptor activity. Two drugs that reduce the hepatic production of VLDL and thus LDL, a small-molecule inhibitor of the microsomal TG transfer protein (MTP) and an antisense oligonucleotide to apoB, are approved in the United States for the treatment of adults with homozygous FH and can be considered. PCSK9 inhibitors, which work through increasing LDL receptor availability, appear to have some benefit in receptor-defective patients and are under clinical development. LDL apheresis is used to lower plasma LDL levels in these patients and can promote regression of xanthomas as well as slow the progression of atherosclerosis. Because the liver is quantitatively the most important tissue for removing circulating LDLs via the LDL receptor, liver transplantation is effective in decreasing plasma LDL-C levels in this disorder but is infrequently used because of the associated problems with immunosuppression.

FAMILIAL DEFECTIVE APOB-100 (FDB) FDB, also known as autosomal dominant hypercholesterolemia (ADH) type 2, is a dominantly inherited disorder that clinically resembles heterozygous FH with elevated LDL-C levels and normal TGs. FDB is caused by mutations in the gene encoding apoB-100, specifically in LDL receptor–binding domain of apoB-100. Several different mutations have been identified, but a single mutation predominates: substitution of glutamine for arginine at position 3500. The mutation results in a reduction in the affinity of LDL binding to the LDL receptor, so LDL is removed from the circulation at a reduced rate. FDB is less common than FH but is more prevalent in individuals of central European descent; the Lancaster County (United States) Amish are a founder population in which the prevalence of FDB is as high as 1 in 10 individuals. FDB is characterized by elevated plasma LDL-C levels with normal TGs; tendon xanthomas can be seen, although not as frequently as in FH, and there is an associated increase in risk of CHD. Patients with FDB cannot be clinically distinguished from patients with heterozygous FH, although patients with FDB tend to have somewhat lower plasma levels of LDL-C than FH heterozygotes, presumably due to the fact that IDL clearance is not impaired in this disorder. Homozygotes for FDB mutations have higher LDL-C levels than FDB heterozygotes but are not as severely affected as homozygous FH patients. The apoB-100 gene mutations can be detected directly through sequencing of the receptor-binding region of the apoB gene or genotyping for the most common mutation, but genetic diagnosis is not generally performed because there is no direct implication for clinical management. As with FH, patients are treated with statins first and, if necessary, with additional classes of LDL-lowering drugs.

AUTOSOMAL DOMINANT HYPERCHOLESTEROLEMIA DUE TO MUTATIONS IN PCSK9 (ADH-PCSK9 OR ADH3) ADH-PCSK9, also known as autosomal dominant hypercholesterolemia (ADH) type 3, is a very rare autosomal dominant disorder caused by gain-of-function mutations in proprotein convertase subtilisin/kexin type 9 (PCSK9). PCSK9 is a secreted protein that binds to the LDL receptor, targeting it for degradation. Normally, after LDL binds to the LDL receptor, it is internalized along with the receptor, and in the low pH of the endosome, the LDL receptor dissociates from the LDL and recycles to the cell surface. When PCSK9 binds the receptor, the complex is internalized and the receptor is directed to the lysosome, rather than to the cell surface. The missense mutations in PCSK9 that cause hypercholesterolemia enhance the activity of PCSK9. As a consequence, the number of hepatic LDL receptors is reduced. Patients with ADH-PCSK9 are similar clinically to patients with FH. They may be particularly responsive to PCSK9 inhibitors in clinical development. Loss-of-function mutations in PCSK9 cause low LDL-C levels (see below).

AUTOSOMAL RECESSIVE HYPERCHOLESTEROLEMIA (ARH) ARH is a very rare disorder that is mostly seen in individuals of Sardinian descent. The disease is caused by mutations in a protein, ARH (also called LDLR adaptor protein, LDLRAP), which is required for LDL receptor–mediated endocytosis in the liver. ARH binds to the cytoplasmic domain of the LDL receptor and links the receptor to the endocytic machinery. In the absence of LDLRAP, LDL binds to the extracellular domain of the LDL receptor, but the lipoprotein-receptor complex fails to be internalized. ARH, like homozygous FH, is characterized by hypercholesterolemia, tendon xanthomas, and premature coronary artery disease (CAD). The levels of plasma LDL-C tend to be intermediate between the levels present in FH homozygotes and FH heterozygotes, and CAD is not usually symptomatic until the third decade. LDL receptor function in cultured fibroblasts is normal or only modestly reduced in ARH, whereas LDL receptor function in lymphocytes and the liver is negligible. Unlike FH homozygotes, the hyperlipidemia responds to treatment with statins, but these patients usually require additional therapy to lower plasma LDL-C to acceptable levels.

SITOSTEROLEMIA Sitosterolemia is a rare autosomal recessive disease that can result in severe hypercholesterolemia, tendon xanthomas, and premature ASCVD. Sitosterolemia is caused by loss-of-function mutations in either of two members of the ATP-binding cassette (ABC) half transporter family, *ABCG5* and *ABCG8*. These genes are expressed in enterocytes and hepatocytes. The proteins heterodimerize to form a functional complex that transports plant sterols such as sitosterol and campesterol, and animal sterols, predominantly cholesterol, across the biliary membrane of hepatocytes into the bile and across the intestinal luminal surface of enterocytes into the gut lumen. In normal individuals, <5% of dietary plant sterols are absorbed by the proximal small intestine. The small amounts of plant sterols that enter the circulation are preferentially excreted into the bile. Thus, levels of plant sterols are kept very low in tissues. In sitosterolemia, the intestinal absorption of sterols is increased and biliary and fecal excretion of the sterols is reduced, resulting in increased plasma and tissue levels of both plant sterols and cholesterol. The increase in hepatic sterol levels results in transcriptional suppression of the expression of the LDL receptor, resulting in reduced uptake of LDL and substantially increased LDL-C levels. In addition to the usual clinical picture of hypercholesterolemia (i.e., tendon xanthomas and premature ASCVD), these patients also have anisocytosis and poikilocytosis of erythrocytes and megathrombocytes due to the incorporation of plant sterols into cell membranes. Episodes of hemolysis and splenomegaly are a distinctive clinical feature of this disease compared to other genetic forms of hypercholesterolemia and can be a clue to the diagnosis.

Sitosterolemia should be suspected in a patient with severe hypercholesterolemia without a family history of such or who responds dramatically to dietary therapy and/or ezetimibe but not statins. Sitosterolemia can be diagnosed by a laboratory finding of a substantial increase in the plasma level of sitosterol and/or other plant sterols. It is important to make the diagnosis, because bile acid sequestrants and cholesterol-absorption inhibitors are the most effective agents to reduce LDL-C and plasma plant sterol levels in these patients.

CHOLESTERYL ESTER STORAGE DISEASE (CESD) CESD, also known as *lysosomal acid lipase deficiency*, is an autosomal recessive disorder characterized by elevated LDL-C, usually in association with low HDL-C, together with progressive fatty liver ultimately leading to hepatic fibrosis. Plasma TG levels can also be mild to moderately increased in this disorder. The most severe form of this disorder, Wolman's disease, presents in infancy and is rapidly fatal. Both Wolman's disease and CESD are caused by loss-of-function variants in both alleles of the gene encoding lysosomal acid lipase (LAL; gene name *LIPA*). LAL is responsible for hydrolyzing neutral lipids, particularly TGs and cholesteryl esters, after delivery to the lysosome by cell-surface receptors such as the LDL receptor. It is particularly important in the liver, which clears large amounts of lipoproteins from the circulation. Genetic deficiency of LAL results in accumulation of neutral lipid in the hepatocytes, leading to hepatosplenomegaly, microvesicular steatosis, and ultimately fibrosis and end-stage liver disease. The etiology of the elevated LDL-C levels is uncertain; one study suggested that VLDL production is increased, but impaired LDL receptor–mediated clearance of LDL is also likely.

CESD should be particularly suspected in nonobese patients with elevated LDL-C, low HDL-C, and evidence of fatty liver in the absence of overt insulin resistance. The diagnosis can be made with a dried blood spot assay of LAL activity and confirmed by DNA genotyping for the most common mutation, followed if necessary by sequencing of the gene to find the second mutation. Liver biopsy is required to assess the degree of inflammation and fibrosis. It is important to make the diagnosis because it has implications for liver monitoring and potentially for therapeutic approaches under development.

FAMILIAL DYSBETALIPOPROTEINEMIA (FDBL) FDBL (also known as *type III hyperlipoproteinemia*) is usually a recessive disorder characterized by a mixed hyperlipidemia (elevated cholesterol and TGs) due to the accumulation of remnant lipoprotein particles (chylomicron remnants and VLDL remnants, or IDL). ApoE is present in multiple copies on chylomicron remnants and IDL, and mediates their removal via hepatic lipoprotein receptors (Fig. 421-2). FDBL is due to genetic variants of apoE, most commonly apoE2, that result in an apoE protein with reduced ability to bind lipoprotein receptors. The *APOE* gene is polymorphic in sequence, resulting in the expression of three common isoforms: apoE3, which is the most common; and apoE2 and apoE4, which both differ from apoE3 by a single amino acid. Although associated with slightly higher LDL-C levels and increased CHD risk, the apoE4 allele is not associated with FDBL. Individuals who carry one or two apoE4 alleles have an increased risk of Alzheimer's disease. ApoE2 has a lower affinity for the LDL receptor; therefore, chylomicron remnants and IDL containing apoE2 are removed from plasma at a slower rate. Individuals who are homozygous for the E2 allele (the E2/E2 genotype) comprise the most common subset of patients with FDBL.

Approximately 0.5% of the general population are apoE2/E2 homozygotes, but only a small minority of these individuals actually develop hyperlipidemia characteristic of FDBL. In most cases, an additional, sometimes identifiable, factor precipitates the development of hyperlipoproteinemia. The most common precipitating factors are a high-fat diet, diabetes mellitus, obesity, hypothyroidism, renal disease, HIV infection, estrogen deficiency, alcohol use, or certain drugs. The disease seldom presents in women before menopause. Other mutations in apoE can cause a dominant form of FDBL where the hyperlipidemia is fully manifest in the heterozygous state, but these mutations are very rare.

Patients with FDBL usually present in adulthood with hyperlipidemia, xanthomas, or premature coronary or peripheral vascular disease. In FDBL, in contrast to other disorders of elevated TGs, the plasma levels of cholesterol and TG are often elevated to a similar degree, and the level of HDL-C is usually normal or reduced. Two distinctive types of xanthomas, tuberoeruptive and palmar, are seen in FDBL patients. Tuberoeruptive xanthomas begin as clusters of small papules on the elbows, knees, or buttocks and can grow to the size of small grapes. Palmar xanthomas (alternatively called *xanthomata striata palmaris*) are orange-yellow discolorations of the creases in the palms and wrists. Both of these xanthoma types are virtually pathognomonic for FDBL. Subjects with FDBL have premature ASCVD and tend to have more peripheral vascular disease than is typically seen in FH.

The definitive diagnosis of FDBL can be made either by the documentation of very high levels of remnant lipoproteins or by identification of the apoE2/E2 genotype. A variety of methods are used to identify remnant lipoproteins in the plasma, including "β-quantification" by ultracentrifugation (ratio of directly measured VLDL-C to total plasma TG >0.30), lipoprotein electrophoresis (broad β band), or nuclear magnetic resonance lipoprotein profiling. The Friedewald formula for calculation of LDL-C is not valid in FDBL because the VLDL particles are depleted in TG and enriched in cholesterol. The plasma levels of LDL-C are actually low in this disorder due to defective metabolism of VLDL to LDL. DNA-based methods (apoE genotyping) can be performed to confirm homozygosity for apoE2. However, absence of the apoE2/E2 genotype does not strictly rule out the diagnosis of FDBL, because other mutations in apoE can (rarely) cause this condition.

Because FDBL is associated with increased risk of premature ASCVD, it should be treated aggressively. Other metabolic conditions that can worsen the hyperlipidemia (see above) should be managed. Patients with FDBL are typically diet-responsive and can respond favorably to weight reduction and to low-cholesterol, low-fat diets. Alcohol intake should be curtailed. Pharmacologic therapy is often required, and statins are the first line in management. In the event of statin intolerance or insufficient control of hyperlipidemia, cholesterol absorption inhibitors, fibrates, and niacin are also effective in the treatment of FDBL.

HEPATIC LIPASE DEFICIENCY Hepatic lipase (HL; gene name *LIPC*) is a member of the same gene family as LPL and hydrolyzes TGs and phospholipids in remnant lipoproteins and HDL. Hydrolysis of lipids in remnant particles by HL contributes to their hepatic uptake via an apoE-mediated process. HL deficiency is a very rare autosomal recessive disorder characterized by elevated plasma levels of cholesterol and TGs (mixed hyperlipidemia) due to the accumulation of lipoprotein remnants, accompanied by elevated plasma level of HDL-C. The diagnosis is confirmed by measuring HL activity in postheparin plasma and/or confirmation of loss-of-function mutations in both alleles of HL/*LIPC*. Due to the small number of patients with HL deficiency, the association of this genetic defect with ASCVD is not entirely clear, although anecdotally patients with HL deficiency who have premature CVD have been described. As with FDBL, statin therapy is recommended to reduce remnant lipoproteins and cardiovascular risk.

Additional Secondary Causes of Dyslipidemia

Many of the secondary causes of dyslipidemia (Table 421-4) have been described above. Additional considerations are discussed here.

LIVER DISORDERS (See also Chap. 357) Because the liver is the principal site of formation and clearance of lipoproteins, liver disorders can affect plasma lipid levels in a variety of ways. Hepatitis due to infection, drugs, or alcohol is often associated with increased VLDL synthesis and mild to moderate hypertriglyceridemia. Severe hepatitis and liver failure are associated with dramatic reductions in plasma cholesterol and TGs due to reduced lipoprotein biosynthetic capacity.

Cholestasis is associated with hypercholesterolemia, which can be very severe. A major pathway by which cholesterol is excreted from the body is via secretion into bile, either directly or after conversion to bile acids, and cholestasis blocks this critical excretory pathway. In cholestasis, free cholesterol, coupled with phospholipids, is secreted into the plasma as a constituent of a lamellar particle called *LP-X*. The particles can deposit in skinfolds, producing lesions resembling those seen in patients with FDBL (xanthomata strata palmaris). Planar and eruptive xanthomas can also be seen in patients with cholestasis.

DRUGS Many drugs have an impact on lipid metabolism and can result in significant alterations in the lipoprotein profile (Table 421-4). Estrogen administration is associated with increased VLDL and HDL synthesis, resulting in elevated plasma levels of both TGs and HDL-C. This lipoprotein pattern is distinctive because the levels of plasma TG and HDL-C are typically inversely related. Plasma TG levels should be monitored when birth control pills or postmenopausal estrogen

TABLE 421-4 SECONDARY CAUSES OF DYSLIPIDEMIA

LDL		HDL					
Elevated	**Reduced**	**Elevated**	**Reduced**	**VLDL Elevated**	**IDL Elevated**	**Chylomicrons Elevated**	**Lp(a) Elevated**
Hypothyroidism	Severe liver disease	Alcohol	Smoking	Obesity	Multiple myeloma	Autoimmune disease	Chronic kidney disease Nephrotic syndrome
Nephrotic syndrome Cholestasis	Malabsorption Malnutrition Gaucher's disease	Exercise Exposure to chlorinated hydrocarbons	DM type 2 Obesity Malnutrition	DM type 2 Glycogen storage disease	Monoclonal gammopathy	DM type 2	Inflammation Menopause
Acute intermittent porphyria	Chronic infectious disease	Drugs: estrogen	Gaucher's disease	Nephrotic syndrome Hepatitis Alcohol	Autoimmune disease		Orchidectomy
Anorexia nervosa Hepatoma Drugs: thiazides, cyclosporin, carbamazepine	Hyperthyroidism Drugs: niacin toxicity		Cholesteryl ester storage disease Drugs: anabolic steroids, beta blockers	Renal failure Sepsis Stress Cushing's syndrome Pregnancy Acromegaly Lipodystrophy Drugs: estrogen, beta blockers, glucocorticoids, bile acid binding resins, retinoic acid	Hypothyroidism		Hypothyroidism Acromegaly Drugs: growth hormone, isotretinoin

Abbreviations: DM, diabetes mellitus; HDL, high-density lipoprotein; IDL, intermediate-density lipoprotein; LDL, low-density lipoprotein; Lp(a), lipoprotein A; VLDL, very-low-density lipoprotein.

therapy is initiated to ensure that the increase in VLDL production does not lead to severe hypertriglyceridemia. Use of low-dose preparations of estrogen or the estrogen patch can minimize the effect of exogenous estrogen on lipids.

INHERITED CAUSES OF LOW LEVELS OF ApoB-CONTAINING LIPOPROTEINS

Plasma concentrations of LDL-C <60 mg/dL are unusual. Although in some cases LDL-C levels in this range may be reflective of malnutrition or serious chronic illness, LDL-C <60 mg/dL in an otherwise healthy individual suggests an inherited condition. The major inherited causes of low LDL-C are reviewed here.

Abetalipoproteinemia The synthesis and secretion of apoB-containing lipoproteins in the enterocytes of the proximal small bowel and in the hepatocytes of the liver involve a complex series of events that coordinate the coupling of various lipids with apoB-48 and apoB-100, respectively. Abetalipoproteinemia is a rare autosomal recessive disease caused by loss-of-function mutations in the gene encoding microsomal TG transfer protein (MTP; gene name *MTTP*), a protein that transfers lipids to nascent chylomicrons and VLDLs in the intestine and liver, respectively. Plasma levels of cholesterol and TG are extremely low in this disorder, and chylomicrons, VLDLs, LDLs, and apoB are undetectable in plasma. The parents of patients with abetalipoproteinemia (obligate heterozygotes) have normal plasma lipid and apoB levels. Abetalipoproteinemia usually presents in early childhood with diarrhea and failure to thrive due to fat malabsorption. The initial neurologic manifestations are loss of deep tendon reflexes, followed by decreased distal lower extremity vibratory and proprioceptive sense, dysmetria, ataxia, and the development of a spastic gait, often by the third or fourth decade. Patients with abetalipoproteinemia also develop a progressive pigmented retinopathy presenting with decreased night and color vision, followed by reductions in daytime visual acuity and ultimately progressing to near-blindness. The presence of spinocerebellar degeneration and pigmented retinopathy in this disease has resulted in some patients with abetalipoproteinemia being misdiagnosed as having Friedreich's ataxia.

Most of the clinical manifestations of abetalipoproteinemia result from defects in the absorption and transport of fat-soluble vitamins. Vitamin E and retinyl esters are normally transported from enterocytes to the liver by chylomicrons, and vitamin E is dependent on VLDL for transport out of the liver and into the circulation. As a consequence of the inability of these patients to secrete apoB-containing particles, patients with abetalipoproteinemia are markedly deficient in vitamin E and are also mildly to moderately deficient in vitamins A and K. Patients with abetalipoproteinemia should be referred to specialized centers for confirmation of the diagnosis and appropriate therapy. Treatment consists of a low-fat, high-caloric, vitamin-enriched diet accompanied by large supplemental doses of vitamin E. It is imperative that treatment be initiated as soon as possible to prevent development of neurologic sequelae, which can progress even with appropriate therapy. New therapies for this serious disease are needed.

Familial Hypobetalipoproteinemia (FHBL) FHBL generally refers to a condition of low total cholesterol, LDL-C, and apoB due to mutations in apoB. Most of the mutations causing FHBL result in a truncated apoB protein, resulting in impaired assembly and secretion of chylomicrons from enterocytes and VLDL from the liver. Mutations that result in VLDL particles containing a truncated apoB protein are cleared from the circulation at an accelerated rate, which also contributes to patients with this disorder having low levels of LDL-C and apoB. Individuals heterozygous for these mutations usually have LDL-C levels <60–80 mg/dL and also tend to have lower levels of plasma TG. Many FHBL patients have elevated levels of hepatic fat (due to reduced VLDL export) and sometimes have increased levels of liver transaminases, although it appears that these patients infrequently develop associated inflammation and fibrosis.

Mutations in both apoB alleles cause homozygous FHBL, an extremely rare disorder resembling abetalipoproteinemia with nearly undetectable LDL-C and apoB. The neurologic defects in this form of hypobetalipoproteinemia tend to be less severe than is typically seen in abetalipoproteinemia. Homozygous hypobetalipoproteinemia can be distinguished from abetalipoproteinemia by examining the inheritance pattern of the plasma LDL-C level. The levels of LDL-C and apoB are normal in the parents of patients with abetalipoproteinemia and low in those of patients with homozygous hypobetalipoproteinemia.

PCSK9 Deficiency Another inherited cause of low LDL-C results from loss-of-function mutations in PCSK9. PCSK9 is a secreted protein that binds to the extracellular domain of the LDL receptor in the liver and promotes the degradation of the receptor. Heterozygosity for nonsense mutations in PCSK9 that interfere with the synthesis of the protein are associated with increased hepatic LDL receptor activity and reduced plasma levels of LDL-C. Such mutations are particularly frequent in individuals of African descent. Individuals who are heterozygous for a loss-of-function mutation in PCSK9 have an ~30–40% reduction in plasma levels of LDL-C and have a substantial protection from CHD relative to those without a PCSK9 mutation, presumably due to having lower plasma cholesterol levels since birth. This observation led to the development of PCSK9 inhibitors as a new strategy for reducing LDL-C levels and cardiovascular risk. Homozygotes for these nonsense mutations have been reported and have extremely low LDL-C levels (<20 mg/dL) but appear otherwise healthy. A sequence variation of somewhat higher frequency (R46L) is found predominantly in individuals of European descent. This mutation impairs, but does not completely destroy, PCSK9 function. As a consequence, the plasma levels of LDL-C in individuals carrying this mutation are more modestly reduced (~15–20%); individuals with these mutations have a 45% reduction in ASCVD risk.

DISORDERS OF REDUCED HDL CHOLESTEROL

Low levels of HDL-C are very commonly encountered in clinical practice. Low HDL-C is an important independent predictor of increased cardiovascular risk and has been used regularly in standardized risk calculators, including the most recent one from the American Heart Association (AHA)/American College of Cardiology (ACC). However, it remains very uncertain whether low HDL-C is directly causal for the development of ASCVD. HDL metabolism is strongly influenced by TRLs, insulin resistance, and inflammation, among other environmental and medical factors. Thus the HDL-C measurement integrates a number of cardiovascular risk factors, potentially explaining its strong inverse association with ASCVD.

The majority of patients with low HDL-C have some combination of genetic predisposition and secondary factors. Variants in dozens of genes have been shown to influence HDL-C levels. Even more important quantitatively, obesity and insulin resistance have strong suppressive effects on HDL-C, and low HDL-C in these conditions is widely observed. Furthermore, the vast majority of patients with elevated TGs have reduced levels of HDL-C. Most patients with low HDL-C who have been studied in detail have accelerated catabolism of HDL and its associated apoA-I as the physiologic basis for the low HDL-C. Importantly, although HDL-C remains an important biomarker for assessing cardiovascular risk, it is not currently a direct target of intervention for raising the level in order to reduce cardiovascular risk. Certain therapeutic approaches in clinical development, such as inhibitors of CETP (see below), have the potential to change this paradigm.

INHERITED CAUSES OF VERY LOW LEVELS OF HDL-C

Mutations in genes encoding proteins that play critical roles in HDL synthesis and catabolism can result in reductions in plasma levels of HDL-C. Unlike the genetic forms of hypercholesterolemia, which are invariably associated with premature coronary atherosclerosis, genetic forms of hypoalphalipoproteinemia (low HDL-C) are often not associated with clearly increased risk of ASCVD.

Gene Deletions in the *APOA5-A1-C3-A4* Locus and Coding Mutations in *APOA1* Complete genetic deficiency of apoA-I due to a complete deletion of the *APOA1* gene results in the virtual absence of circulating HDL and appears to increase the risk of premature ASCVD. The genes encoding *APOA5*, *APOA1*, *APOC3*, and *APOA4* are clustered together on chromosome 11. Some patients with no apoA-I have genomic deletions that include other genes in the cluster. ApoA-I is required for LCAT activity. In the absence of LCAT, free cholesterol levels increase in both plasma (not HDL) and in tissues. The free cholesterol can form deposits in the cornea and in the skin, resulting in corneal opacities and planar xanthomas. Premature CHD is associated with apoA-I deficiency.

Missense and nonsense mutations in the apoA-I gene are present in some patients with low plasma levels of HDL-C (usually 15–30 mg/dL), but are a rare cause of low plasma HDL-C levels. Most individuals with low plasma HDL-C levels due to missense mutations in apoA-I do not appear to have premature CHD. Patients who are heterozygous for an Arg173Cys substitution in apoA-I (so-called apoA-I_{Milano}) have very low plasma levels of HDL-C due to impaired LCAT activation and accelerated clearance of the HDL particles containing the abnormal apoA-I. Despite having very low plasma levels of HDL-C, these individuals do not have an increased risk of premature CHD.

A few selected missense mutations in apoA-I and apoA-II promote the formation of amyloid fibrils, which can cause systemic amyloidosis.

Tangier Disease (*ABCA1* Deficiency) Tangier disease is a rare autosomal co-dominant form of extremely low plasma HDL-C levels that is caused by mutations in the gene encoding ABCA1, a cellular transporter that facilitates efflux of unesterified cholesterol and phospholipids from cells to apoA-I (Fig. 421-3). ABCA1 in the liver and intestine rapidly lipidates the apoA-I secreted from the basolateral membranes of these tissues. In the absence of ABCA1, the nascent, poorly lipidated apoA-I is immediately cleared from the circulation. Thus, patients with Tangier disease have extremely low circulating plasma levels of HDL-C (<5 mg/dL) and apoA-I (<5 mg/dL). Cholesterol accumulates in the reticuloendothelial system of these patients, resulting in hepatosplenomegaly and pathognomonic enlarged, grayish yellow or orange tonsils. An intermittent peripheral neuropathy (mononeuritis multiplex) or a sphingomyelia-like neurologic disorder can also be seen in this disorder. Tangier disease is probably associated with some increased risk of premature atherosclerotic disease, although the association is not as robust as might be anticipated, given the very low levels of HDL-C and apoA-I in these patients. Patients with Tangier disease also have low plasma levels of LDL-C, which may attenuate the atherosclerotic risk. Obligate heterozygotes for ABCA1 mutations have moderately reduced plasma HDL-C levels (15–30 mg/dL), and their risk of premature CHD remains uncertain.

Familial LCAT Deficiency This rare autosomal recessive disorder is caused by mutations in LCAT, an enzyme synthesized in the liver and secreted into the plasma, where it circulates associated with lipoproteins (Fig. 421-3). As reviewed above, the enzyme is activated by apoA-I and mediates the esterification of cholesterol to form cholesteryl esters. Consequently, in familial LCAT deficiency, the proportion of free cholesterol in circulating lipoproteins is greatly increased (from ~25% to >70% of total plasma cholesterol). Deficiency in this enzyme interferes with the maturation of HDL particles and results in rapid catabolism of circulating apoA-I.

Two genetic forms of familial LCAT deficiency have been described in humans: complete deficiency (also called *classic LCAT deficiency*) and partial deficiency (also called *fish-eye disease*). Progressive corneal opacification due to the deposition of free cholesterol in the cornea, very low plasma levels of HDL-C (usually <10 mg/dL), and variable hypertriglyceridemia are characteristic of both disorders. In partial LCAT deficiency, there are no other known clinical sequelae. In contrast, patients with complete LCAT deficiency have hemolytic anemia and progressive renal insufficiency that eventually leads to end-stage renal disease. Remarkably, despite the extremely low plasma levels of HDL-C and apoA-I, premature ASCVD is not a consistent feature of either LCAT deficiency or fish eye disease. The diagnosis can be confirmed in a specialized laboratory by assaying plasma LCAT activity or by sequencing the *LCAT* gene.

Primary Hypoalphalipoproteinemia The condition of low plasma levels of HDL-C (the "alpha lipoprotein") is referred to as *hypoalphalipoproteinemia*. Primary hypoalphalipoproteinemia is defined as a plasma HDL-C level below the tenth percentile in the setting of relatively normal cholesterol and TG levels, no apparent secondary causes of low plasma HDL-C, and no clinical signs of LCAT deficiency or Tangier disease. This syndrome is often referred to as *isolated low HDL*. A family history of low HDL-C facilitates the diagnosis of an inherited condition, which may follow an autosomal dominant pattern. The metabolic etiology of this disease appears to be primarily accelerated catabolism of HDL and its apolipoproteins. Some of these patients may have ABCA1 mutations and therefore technically have heterozygous Tangier disease. Several kindreds with primary hypoalphalipoproteinemia and an increased incidence of premature CHD have been described, although it is not clear if the low HDL-C level is the cause of the accelerated atherosclerosis in these families. Association of hypoalphalipoproteinemia with premature CHD may depend on the specific nature of the gene defect or the underlying metabolic defect that either directly or indirectly causes the low plasma HDL-C level.

INHERITED CAUSES OF VERY HIGH LEVELS OF HDL-C

CETP Deficiency Loss-of-function mutations in both alleles of the gene encoding CETP cause substantially elevated HDL-C levels (usually >150 mg/dL). As noted above, CETP transfers cholesteryl esters from HDL to apoB-containing lipoproteins (Fig. 421-3). Absence of this transfer activity results in an increase in the cholesteryl ester content of HDL and a reduction in plasma levels of LDL-C. The large, cholesterol-rich HDL particles circulating in these patients are cleared at a reduced rate. CETP deficiency was first diagnosed in Japanese persons and is rare outside of Japan. The relationship of CETP deficiency to ASCVD remains unresolved. Heterozygotes for CETP deficiency have only modestly elevated HDL-C levels. Based on the phenotype of high HDL-C in CETP deficiency, pharmacologic inhibition of CETP is under development as a new therapeutic approach to both raise HDL-C levels and lower LDL-C levels, but whether it will reduce risk of ASCVD remains to be determined.

SCREENING, DIAGNOSIS, AND MANAGEMENT OF DISORDERS OF LIPOPROTEIN METABOLISM

SCREENING

Plasma lipid and lipoprotein levels should be measured in all adults, preferably after a 12-h overnight fast. In most clinical laboratories, the total cholesterol and TGs in the plasma are measured enzymatically, and then the cholesterol in the supernatant is measured after precipitation of apoB-containing lipoproteins to determine the HDL-C. The LDL-C is then estimated using the following equation:

$$\text{LDL-C} = \text{total cholesterol} - (\text{TG}/5) - \text{HDL-C}$$

(The VLDL cholesterol content is estimated by dividing the plasma TG by 5, reflecting the ratio of TG to cholesterol in VLDL particles.) This formula (the Friedewald formula) is reasonably accurate if test results are obtained on fasting plasma and if the TG level does not exceed ~200 mg/dL; by convention it cannot be used if the TG level is >400 mg/dL. LDL-C can be directly measured by a number of methods. Further evaluation and treatment are based primarily on the clinical assessment of absolute cardiovascular risk using risk calculators such as the AHA/ACC risk calculator based on a large amount of observational data.

DIAGNOSIS

A critical first step in managing a lipoprotein disorder is to attempt to determine the class or classes of lipoproteins that are increased or decreased in the patient. Once the hyperlipidemia is accurately classified, efforts should be directed to rule out any possible secondary causes of the hyperlipidemia (Table 421-4). Although many patients with hyperlipidemia have a primary (i.e., genetic) cause of their lipid disorder, secondary factors frequently contribute to the hyperlipidemia. A careful social, medical, and family history should be obtained. A fasting glucose should be obtained in the initial workup of all subjects with an elevated TG level. Nephrotic syndrome and chronic renal insufficiency should be excluded by obtaining urine protein and serum creatinine. Liver function tests should be performed to rule out hepatitis and cholestasis. Hypothyroidism should be ruled out by measuring serum thyroid-stimulating hormone.

Once secondary causes have been ruled out, attempts should be made to diagnose the primary lipid disorder because the underlying genetic defect can provide important prognostic information regarding the risk of developing CHD, the response to drug therapy, and the management of other family members. Obtaining the correct diagnosis often requires a detailed family medical history, lipid analyses in family members, and sometimes specialized testing.

Severe Hypertriglyceridemia If the fasting plasma TG level is >1000 mg/dL, the patient has chylomicronemia. If the cholesterol-to-TG ratio is >10, familial chylomicronemia syndrome must be considered, and LPL activity measured in postheparin plasma can help with making that diagnosis. Most adults with chylomicronemia also have elevated VLDL levels. These individuals usually do not have a Mendelian disorder but instead are genetically predisposed and have secondary factors (diet, obesity, glucose intolerance, alcohol ingestion, estrogen therapy) that contribute to the hyperlipidemia. Such patients are a risk of acute pancreatitis and should be treated to reduce their TG levels and thus their risk of pancreatitis.

Severe Hypercholesterolemia If the levels of LDL-C are very high (greater than a ninety-fifth percentile for age and sex), it is likely that the patient has a genetic cause of hypercholesterolemia. At present, there is no compelling reason to perform molecular studies to further refine the molecular diagnosis because the clinical management is not affected. Recessive forms of severe hypercholesterolemia are rare, but if a patient with severe hypercholesterolemia has parents with normal cholesterol levels, ARH, sitosterolemia, and CESD should be considered. Patients with more moderate hypercholesterolemia that does not segregate in families as a monogenic trait are likely to have polygenic hypercholesterolemia.

Combined Hyperlipidemia The most common errors in the diagnosis of lipid disorders involve patients with combined hyperlipidemia. Elevations in the plasma levels of both cholesterol and TGs are seen in patients with increased plasma levels of VLDL and LDL or of remnant lipoproteins. A β-quantification to determine the VLDL cholesterol/TG ratio in plasma (see discussion of FDBL) or a direct measurement of the plasma LDL-C should be performed at least once prior to initiation of lipid-lowering therapy to determine if the hyperlipidemia is due to the accumulation of remnants or to an increase in both LDL and VLDL. Measurement of plasma apoB levels can help identify patients with FCHL who may require more aggressive treatment.

APPROACH TO THE PATIENT: Lipoprotein Disorders

The major goals in the clinical management of lipoprotein disorders are: (1) prevention of acute pancreatitis in patients with severe hypertriglyceridemia; and (2) prevention of CVD and related cardiovascular events.

MANAGEMENT OF SEVERE HYPERTRIGLYCERIDEMIA TO PREVENT PANCREATITIS

Although the observational relationship between severe hypertriglyceridemia, particularly chylomicronemia, and acute pancreatitis is well-established, there has never been a clinical trial designed or powered to prove that intervention to reduce TGs reduces the risk of pancreatitis. Nevertheless, it is generally considered appropriate medical practice to intervene in patients with TGs >500 mg/dL in order to reduce the risk of pancreatitis. It remains controversial whether individuals with severe hypertriglyceridemia are at increased risk for ASCVD.

Lifestyle Modifying the lifestyle of the patient with severe hypertriglyceridemia often is associated with a significant reduction in plasma TG level. Patients who drink alcohol should be encouraged to decrease or preferably eliminate their intake. Patients with severe hypertriglyceridemia often benefit from a formal dietary consultation with a dietician intimately familiar with counseling patients on the dietary management of high TGs. Dietary fat intake should be restricted to reduce the formation of chylomicrons in the intestine. The excessive intake of simple carbohydrates should be discouraged because insulin drives TG production in the liver. Aerobic exercise and even increase in regular physical activity can have a positive effect in reducing TG levels and should be strongly encouraged. For patients who are overweight, weight loss can help to reduce TG levels. In extreme cases, bariatric surgery has been shown to not only produce effective weight loss but also substantially reduce plasma TG levels.

Pharmacologic Therapy for Severe Hypertriglyceridemia Despite the above interventions, however, many patients with severe hypertriglyceridemia require pharmacologic therapy (Table 421-5). Patients who persist in having fasting TG >500 mg/dL despite active lifestyle management are candidates for pharmacologic therapy. There are three classes of drugs that are used for management of these patients: fibrates, omega-3 fatty acids (fish oils), and niacin. In addition, statins can reduce plasma TG levels and also reduce ASCVD risk.

FIBRATES Fibric acid derivatives, or fibrates, are agonists of PPARα, a nuclear receptor involved in the regulation of lipid metabolism. Fibrates stimulate LPL activity (enhancing TG hydrolysis), reduce apoC-III synthesis (enhancing lipoprotein remnant clearance), promote β-oxidation of fatty acids, and may reduce VLDL TG production. Fibrates are a first-line therapy for severe hypertriglyceridemia (>500 mg/dL). This class of therapeutic agents sometimes lowers but more often raises the plasma level of LDL-C in individuals with severe hypertriglyceridemia. Fibrates are generally well tolerated, but are associated with an increase in the incidence of gallstones. Fibrates can cause myopathy, especially when combined with other lipid-lowering therapy (statins, niacin), and can raise creatinine. Fibrates should be used with caution in patients with CKD. Importantly, fibrates can potentiate the effect of warfarin and certain oral hypoglycemic agents, so the anticoagulation status and plasma glucose levels should be closely monitored in patients on these agents.

OMEGA 3 FATTY ACIDS (FISH OILS) Omega-3 fatty acids, or omega-3 polyunsaturated fatty acids (n-3 PUFAs), commonly known as fish oils, are present in high concentration in fish and in flaxseed. The most widely used n-3 PUFAs for the treatment of hyperlipidemias are the two active molecules in fish oil: eicosapentaenoic acid (EPA) and docosahexaenoic acid (DHA). n-3 PUFAs have been concentrated into tablets and in doses of 3–4 g/d are effective at lowering fasting TG levels. Fish oils are a reasonable consideration for first-line therapy in patients with severe hypertriglyceridemia (>500 mg/dL) to prevent pancreatitis. Fish oils can cause an increase in plasma LDL-C levels in some patients. In general, fish oils are well tolerated, with the major side effect being dyspepsia. They appear to be safe, at least at doses up to 3–4 g, but can be associated with a prolongation in the bleeding time.

NICOTINIC ACID Nicotinic acid, or niacin, is a B-complex vitamin that has been used as a lipid-modifying agent for more than five decades. Niacin suppresses lipolysis in the adipocyte through its effect on the niacin receptor GPR109A and has other effects on hepatic lipid metabolism that are poorly understood. Niacin reduces plasma TG and LDL-C levels and also raises the plasma concentration of HDL-C. Because it has a number of side effects and can be difficult to use, it is at best a third-line agent for the management of severe hypertriglyceridemia. Niacin therapy is generally started at lower doses and gradually titrated up to higher doses. The most frequent side effect of niacin is cutaneous flushing, which is mediated by activating GPR109A in the skin. Niacin can cause dyspepsia and can exacerbate esophageal reflux and peptic ulcer disease. Mild elevations in transaminases occur in up to 15% of patients treated with any form of niacin. Niacin can raise plasma levels of uric acid and precipitate gouty attacks in susceptible patients. Acanthosis nigricans, a dark-colored coarse skin lesion, and maculopathy are infrequent side effects of niacin.

MANAGEMENT OF CHOLESTEROL TO PREVENT CARDIOVASCULAR DISEASE

In contrast to hypertriglyceridemia and pancreatitis, there are abundant and compelling data that intervention to reduce LDL-C substantially reduces the risk of CVD, including myocardial infarction and stroke, as well as total mortality. Thus, it is imperative that patients with hypercholesterolemia be assessed for cardiovascular risk and for the need for intervention. It is also worth noting that patients at high risk for CVD who have plasma LDL-C levels in the "normal" or average range also benefit from intervention to reduce LDL-C levels.

Lifestyle The first approach to a patient with hypercholesterolemia and high cardiovascular risk is to make any necessary lifestyle changes. In obese patients, efforts should be made to reduce body weight to the ideal level. Patients should receive dietary counseling to reduce the content of saturated fats, *trans* fats, and cholesterol in the diet. Regular aerobic exercise has relatively little impact on reducing plasma LDL-C levels, although it has cardiovascular benefits independent of LDL lowering.

Pharmacologic Therapy for Hypercholesterolemia The decision to use LDL-lowering drug therapy (Table 421-5)—with a statin being first-line therapy—depends on the level of LDL-C as well as the level of cardiovascular risk. In general, patients with a Mendelian disorder of elevated LDL-C such as FH must be treated to reduce the very high lifetime risk of CVD, and treatment should be initiated as early as possible in adulthood or, in some cases, during childhood.

Otherwise, the decision to initiate LDL-lowering drug therapy is generally determined by the level of cardiovascular risk. In patients with established CVD, statin therapy is well supported by clinical trial data and should be used regardless of the LDL-C level. For patients >40 years old without clinical CVD, the AHA/ACC risk calculator *(http://my.americanheart.org/professional/StatementsGuidelines/PreventionGuidelines/Prevention-Guidelines_UCM_457698_SubHomePage.jsp)* can be used to determine the 10-year absolute risk for CVD, and current guidelines suggest that a 10-year risk >7.5% merits consideration of statin therapy regardless of plasma LDL-C level. For younger patients, the assessment of lifetime risk of CVD may help inform the decision to start a statin.

HMG-CoA REDUCTASE INHIBITORS (STATINS) Statins inhibit HMG-CoA reductase, a key enzyme in cholesterol biosynthesis. By inhibiting cholesterol biosynthesis, statins lead to increased hepatic LDL receptor activity and accelerated clearance of circulating LDL, resulting in a dose-dependent reduction in plasma levels of LDL-C. The magnitude of LDL lowering associated with statin treatment varies widely among individuals, but once a patient is on a statin, the doubling of the statin dose produces an ~6% further reduction in the level of plasma LDL-C. The statins currently available differ in their LDL-C–reducing potency (Table 421-5). Currently, there is no convincing evidence that any of the different statins confer an advantage that is independent of the effect on LDL-C. Statins also reduce plasma TGs in a dose-dependent fashion, which is roughly proportional to their LDL-C–lowering effects (if the TGs are <400 mg/dL). Statins have a modest HDL-raising effect (5–10%) that is not generally dose-dependent.

Statins are well tolerated and can be taken in tablet form once a day. Potential side effects include dyspepsia, headaches, fatigue, and muscle or joint pains. Severe myopathy and even rhabdomyolysis occur rarely with statin treatment. The risk of statin-associated myopathy is increased by the presence of older age, frailty, renal insufficiency, and coadministration of drugs that interfere with the metabolism of statins, such as erythromycin and related antibiotics, antifungal agents, immunosuppressive drugs, and fibric acid deriva-

TABLE 421-5 SUMMARY OF THE MAJOR APPROVED DRUGS USED FOR THE TREATMENT OF DYSLIPIDEMIA

Drug	Major Indications	Starting Dose	Maximal Dose	Mechanism	Common Side Effects
HMG-CoA reductase inhibitors (statins)	Elevated LDL-C; increased CV risk			↓ Cholesterol synthesis, ↑ Hepatic LDL receptors, ↓ VLDL production	Myalgias, arthralgias, elevated transaminases, dyspepsia
Lovastatin		20–40 mg daily	80 mg daily		
Pravastatin		40–80 mg daily	80 mg daily		
Simvastatin		20–40 mg daily	80 mg daily		
Fluvastatin		20–40 mg daily	80 mg daily		
Atorvastatin		20–40 mg daily	80 mg daily		
Rosuvastatin		5–20 mg daily	40 mg daily		
Pitavastatin		1–2 mg daily	4 mg daily		
Cholesterol absorption inhibitor	Elevated LDL-C			↓ Cholesterol absorption, ↑ LDL receptors	Elevated transaminases
Ezetimibe		10 mg daily	10 mg daily		
Bile acid sequestrants	Elevated LDL-C			↑ Bile acid excretion and ↑ LDL receptors	Bloating, constipation, elevated triglycerides
Cholestyramine		4 g daily	32 g daily		
Colestipol		5 g daily	40 g daily		
Colesevelam		3750 mg daily	4375 mg daily		
MTP inhibitor	HoFH			↓ VLDL production	Nausea, diarrhea, increased hepatic fat
Lomitapide		5 mg daily	60 mg daily		
ApoB inhibitor	HoFH			↓ VLDL production	Injection site reactions, flu-like symptoms, increased hepatic fat
Mipomersen		200 mg SC weekly	200 mg SC weekly		
Nicotinic acid	Elevated LDL-C, elevated TG			↓ VLDL production	Cutaneous flushing, GI upset, elevated glucose, uric acid, and elevated liver function tests
Immediate-release		100 mg tid	1 g tid		
Sustained-release		250 mg bid	1.5 g bid		
Extended-release		500 mg qhs	2 g qhs		
Fibric acid derivatives	Elevated TG			↑ LPL, ↓ VLDL synthesis	Dyspepsia, myalgia, gallstones, elevated transaminases
Gemfibrozil		600 mg bid	600 mg bid		
Fenofibrate		145 mg qd	145 mg qd		
Omega-3 fatty acids	Elevated TG			↑ TG catabolism	Dyspepsia, fishy odor to breath
Omega-3 acid ethyl esters		4 g daily	4 g daily		
Icosapent ethyl		4 g daily	4 g daily		

Abbreviations: GI, gastrointestinal; HDL-C, high-density lipoprotein cholesterol; HoFH, homozygous familial hypercholesterolemia; LDL, low-density lipoprotein; LDL-C, LDL-cholesterol; LPL, lipoprotein lipase; TG, triglyceride; VLDL, very-low-density lipoprotein.

tives (particularly gemfibrozil). Severe myopathy can usually be avoided by careful patient selection, avoidance of interacting drugs, and instructing the patient to contact the physician immediately in the event of unexplained muscle pain. In the event of muscle symptoms, the plasma creatine kinase (CK) level should be obtained to differentiate myopathy from myalgia. Serum CK levels need not be monitored on a routine basis in patients taking statins, because an elevated CK in the absence of symptoms does not predict the development of myopathy and does not necessarily suggest the need for discontinuing the drug.

Another consequence of statin therapy can be elevation in liver transaminases (alanine aminotransferase [ALT] and aspartate aminotransferase [AST]). They should be checked before starting therapy, at 2–3 months, and then annually. Substantial (greater than three times the upper limit of normal) elevation in transaminases is relatively rare, and mild-to-moderate (one to three times normal) elevation in transaminases in the absence of symptoms need not mandate discontinuing the medication. Severe clinical hepatitis associated with statins is exceedingly rare, and the trend is toward less frequent monitoring of transaminases in patients taking statins. The statin-associated elevation in liver enzymes resolves upon discontinuation of the medication.

Statins appear to be remarkably safe. Meta-analyses of large randomized controlled clinical trials with statins do not suggest an increase in any major noncardiac diseases except type 2 diabetes. A small excess percentage of those taking statins will develop diabetes but the benefits associated with the reduction in cardiovascular events outweigh the increase in incidence of diabetes. Statins are the drug class of choice for LDL-C reduction and are by far the most widely used class of lipid-lowering drugs.

CHOLESTEROL ABSORPTION INHIBITORS Cholesterol within the lumen of the small intestine is derived from the diet (about one-third) and the bile (about two-thirds) and is actively absorbed by the enterocyte through a process that involves the protein NPC1L1. Ezetimibe (Table 421-5) is a cholesterol absorption inhibitor that binds directly to and inhibits NPC1L1 and blocks the intestinal absorption of cholesterol. Ezetimibe (10 mg) inhibits cholesterol absorption by almost 60%, resulting in a reduction in delivery of dietary sterols in the liver and an increase in hepatic LDL receptor expression. The mean reduction in plasma LDL-C on ezetimibe (10 mg) is 18%, and the effect is additive when used in combination with a statin. Effects on TG and HDL-C levels are negligible. When used in combination with a statin, monitoring of liver transaminases is recommended. The only roles for ezetimibe in monotherapy are in patients who do not tolerate statins and in sitosterolemia.

BILE ACID SEQUESTRANTS (RESINS) Bile acid sequestrants bind bile acids in the intestine and promote their excretion rather than reabsorption in the ileum. To maintain the bile acid pool size, the liver diverts cholesterol to bile acid synthesis. The decreased hepatic intracellular cholesterol content results in upregulation of the LDL receptor and enhanced LDL clearance from the plasma. Bile acid sequestrants, including cholestyramine, colestipol, and colesevelam (Table 421-5), primarily reduce plasma LDL-C levels but can cause an increase in plasma TGs. Therefore, patients with hypertriglyceridemia generally should not be treated with bile acid–binding resins. Cholestyramine and colestipol are insoluble resins that must be suspended in liquids. Colesevelam is available as tablets but generally requires up to six to seven tablets per day for effective LDL-C lowering. Most side effects of resins are limited to the gastrointestinal tract and include bloating and constipation. Because bile acid sequestrants are not systemically absorbed, they are very safe and the cholesterol-lowering drug of choice in children and in women of childbearing age who are lactating, pregnant, or could become pregnant. They are effective in combination with statins and in combination with ezetimibe and are particularly useful with one or both of these drugs for patients with severe hypercholesterolemia or those with statin intolerance.

SPECIALIZED DRUGS FOR HOMOZYGOUS FH Two "orphan" drugs are approved specifically for the management of homozygous FH. They include a small-molecule inhibitor of MTP, called lomitapide, and an antisense oligonucleotide against apoB, called mipomersen. These drugs reduce VLDL production and LDL-C levels in homozygous FH patients. Due to their mechanism of action, each drug causes an increase in hepatic fat, the long-term consequences of which are unknown. In addition, lomitapide is associated with gastrointestinal-related side effects, and mipomersen is associated with skin reactions and flu-like symptoms.

LDL APHERESIS Patients who remain severely hypercholesterolemic despite optimally tolerated drug therapy are candidates for LDL apheresis. In this process, the patient's plasma is passed over a column that selectively removes the LDL, and the LDL-depleted plasma is returned to the patient. Patients on maximally tolerated combination drug therapy who have CHD and a plasma LDL-C level >200 mg/dL or no CHD and a plasma LDL-C level >300 mg/dL are candidates for every-other-week LDL apheresis and should be referred to a specialized lipid center.

422 The Metabolic Syndrome

Robert H. Eckel

The metabolic syndrome (syndrome X, insulin resistance syndrome) consists of a constellation of metabolic abnormalities that confer increased risk of cardiovascular disease (CVD) and diabetes mellitus. Evolution of the criteria for the metabolic syndrome since the original definition by the World Health Organization in 1998 reflects growing clinical evidence and analysis by a variety of consensus conferences and professional organizations. The major features of the metabolic syndrome include central obesity, hypertriglyceridemia, low levels of high-density lipoprotein (HDL) cholesterol, hyperglycemia, and hypertension (Table 422-1).

EPIDEMIOLOGY

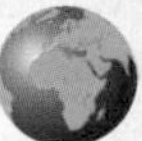

The most challenging feature of the metabolic syndrome to define is waist circumference. Intraabdominal circumference (visceral adipose tissue) is considered most strongly related to insulin resistance and risk of diabetes and CVD, and for any given waist circumference the distribution of adipose tissue between SC and visceral depots varies substantially. Thus, within and between populations, there is a lesser vs. greater risk at the same waist circumference. These differences in populations are reflected in the range of waist circumferences considered to confer risk in different geographic locations (Table 422-1).

The prevalence of the metabolic syndrome varies around the world, in part reflecting the age and ethnicity of the populations studied and the diagnostic criteria applied. In general, the prevalence of the metabolic syndrome increases with age. The highest recorded prevalence worldwide is among Native Americans, with nearly 60% of women ages 45–49 and 45% of men ages 45–49 meeting the criteria of the National Cholesterol Education Program and Adult Treatment Panel III (NCEP:ATPIII). In the United States, the metabolic syndrome is less common among African-American men and more common among Mexican-American women. Based on data from the National Health and Nutrition Examination Survey (NHANES) 2003–2006, the age-adjusted prevalence of the metabolic syndrome in U.S. adults without diabetes is 28% for men and 30% for women. In France, studies of a cohort of 30- to 60-year-olds have shown a <10% prevalence for each sex, although 17.5% of people 60–64 years of age are affected. Greater global industrialization is associated with rising rates of obesity, which are expected to increase the prevalence of the metabolic syndrome dramatically, especially as the population ages. Moreover, the rising prevalence and severity of obesity among children is reflected in features of the metabolic syndrome in a younger population.

The frequency distribution of the five components of the syndrome for the U.S. population (NHANES III) is summarized in Fig. 422-1. Increases in waist circumference predominate among women, whereas increases in fasting plasma triglyceride levels (i.e., to >150 mg/dL), reductions in HDL cholesterol levels, and hyperglycemia are more likely in men.

RISK FACTORS

Overweight/Obesity Although the metabolic syndrome was first described in the early twentieth century, the worldwide overweight/obesity epidemic has recently been the force driving its increasing recognition. Central adiposity is a key feature of the syndrome, and the syndrome's prevalence reflects the strong relationship between waist circumference and increasing adiposity. However, despite the importance of obesity, patients who are of normal weight may also be insulin resistant and may have the metabolic syndrome.

Sedentary Lifestyle Physical inactivity is a predictor of CVD events and the related risk of death. Many components of the metabolic syndrome are associated with a sedentary lifestyle, including increased adipose tissue (predominantly central), reduced HDL cholesterol, and increased triglycerides, blood pressure, and glucose in genetically susceptible persons. Compared with individuals who watch television or videos or use the computer <1 h daily, those who do so for >4 h daily have a twofold increased risk of the metabolic syndrome.

Aging The metabolic syndrome affects nearly 50% of the U.S. population older than age 50, and at >60 years of age women are more often affected than men. The age dependency of the syndrome's prevalence is seen in most populations around the world.

Diabetes Mellitus Diabetes mellitus is included in both the NCEP and the harmonizing definitions of the metabolic syndrome. It is estimated that the great majority (~75%) of patients with type 2 diabetes or impaired glucose tolerance have the metabolic syndrome. The presence of the metabolic syndrome in these populations relates to a

TABLE 422-1 NCEP:ATPIII[a] 2001 AND HARMONIZING DEFINITION CRITERIA FOR THE METABOLIC SYNDROME

NCEP:ATPIII 2001	Harmonizing Definition[b]		
Three or more of the following:	**Three of the following:**		
• Central obesity: waist circumference >102 cm (M), >88 cm (F)	• Waist circumference (cm)		
• Hypertriglyceridemia: triglyceride level ≥150 mg/dL or specific medication	**Men**	**Women**	**Ethnicity**
	≥94	≥80	Europid, sub-Saharan African, Eastern and Middle Eastern
• Low HDL[c] cholesterol: <40 mg/dL and <50 mg/dL for men and women, respectively, or specific medication	≥90	≥80	South Asian, Chinese, and ethnic South and Central American
• Hypertension: blood pressure ≥130 mmHg systolic or ≥85 mmHg diastolic or specific medication	≥85	≥90	Japanese
• Fasting plasma glucose level ≥100 mg/dL or specific medication or previously diagnosed type 2 diabetes	• Fasting triglyceride level >150 mg/dL or specific medication		
	• HDL cholesterol level <40 mg/dL and <50 mg/dL for men and women, respectively, or specific medication		
	• Blood pressure >130 mm systolic or >85 mm diastolic or previous diagnosis or specific medication		
	• Fasting plasma glucose level ≥100 mg/dL (alternative indication: drug treatment of elevated glucose levels)		

[a]National Cholesterol Education Program and Adult Treatment Panel III. [b]In this analysis, the following thresholds for waist circumference were used: white men, ≥94 cm; African-American men, ≥94 cm; Mexican-American men, ≥90 cm; white women, ≥80 cm; African-American women, ≥80 cm; Mexican-American women, ≥80 cm. For participants whose designation was "other race—including multiracial," thresholds that were once based on Europid cutoffs (≥94 cm for men and ≥80 cm for women) and on South Asian cutoffs (≥90 cm for men and ≥80 cm for women) were used. For participants who were considered "other Hispanic," the International Diabetes Federation thresholds for ethnic South and Central Americans were used. [c]High-density lipoprotein.

higher prevalence of CVD than in patients who have type 2 diabetes or impaired glucose tolerance but do not have this syndrome.

Cardiovascular Disease Individuals with the metabolic syndrome are twice as likely to die of cardiovascular disease as those who do not, and their risk of an acute myocardial infarction or stroke is threefold higher. The approximate prevalence of the metabolic syndrome among patients with coronary heart disease (CHD) is 50%, with a prevalence of ~35% among patients with premature coronary artery disease (before or at age 45) and a particularly high prevalence among women. With appropriate cardiac rehabilitation and changes in lifestyle (e.g., nutrition, physical activity, weight reduction, and—in some cases—pharmacologic therapy), the prevalence of the syndrome can be reduced.

Lipodystrophy Lipodystrophic disorders in general are associated with the metabolic syndrome. Both genetic lipodystrophy (e.g., Berardinelli-Seip congenital lipodystrophy, Dunnigan familial partial lipodystrophy) and acquired lipodystrophy (e.g., HIV-related lipodystrophy in

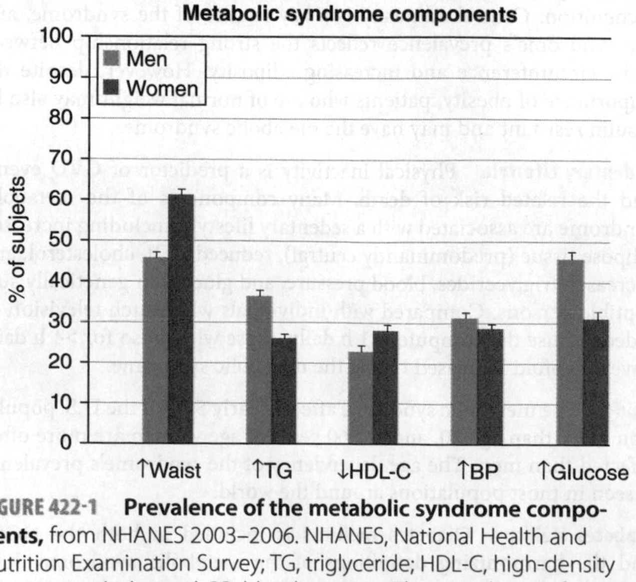

Metabolic syndrome components

Men
Women

% of subjects

↑Waist ↑TG ↓HDL-C ↑BP ↑Glucose

FIGURE 422-1 Prevalence of the metabolic syndrome components, from NHANES 2003–2006. NHANES, National Health and Nutrition Examination Survey; TG, triglyceride; HDL-C, high-density lipoprotein cholesterol; BP, blood pressure. The prevalence of elevated glucose includes individuals with known diabetes mellitus. *(Created from data in ES Ford et al: J Diabetes 2:1753, 2010.)*

patients receiving antiretroviral therapy) may give rise to severe insulin resistance and many of the components of the metabolic syndrome.

ETIOLOGY

Insulin Resistance The most accepted and unifying hypothesis to describe the pathophysiology of the metabolic syndrome is insulin resistance, which is caused by an incompletely understood defect in insulin action (Chap. 417). The onset of insulin resistance is heralded by postprandial hyperinsulinemia, which is followed by fasting hyperinsulinemia and ultimately by hyperglycemia.

An early major contributor to the development of insulin resistance is an overabundance of circulating fatty acids (Fig. 422-2). Plasma albumin-bound free fatty acids are derived predominantly from adipose-tissue triglyceride stores released by intracellular lipolytic enzymes. Fatty acids are also derived from the lipolysis of triglyceride-rich lipoproteins in tissues by lipoprotein lipase. Insulin mediates both antilipolysis and the stimulation of lipoprotein lipase in adipose tissue. Of note, the inhibition of lipolysis in adipose tissue is the most sensitive pathway of insulin action. Thus, when insulin resistance develops, increased lipolysis produces more fatty acids, which further decrease the antilipolytic effect of insulin. Excessive fatty acids enhance substrate availability and create insulin resistance by modifying downstream signaling. Fatty acids impair insulin-mediated glucose uptake and accumulate as triglycerides in both skeletal and cardiac muscle, whereas increased glucose production and triglyceride accumulation take place in the liver.

Leptin resistance has also been raised as a possible pathophysiologic mechanism to explain the metabolic syndrome. Physiologically, leptin reduces appetite, promotes energy expenditure, and enhances insulin sensitivity. In addition, leptin may regulate cardiac and vascular function through a nitric oxide–dependent mechanism. However, when obesity develops, hyperleptinemia ensues, with evidence of leptin resistance in the brain and other tissues resulting in inflammation, insulin resistance, hyperlipidemia, and a plethora of cardiovascular disorders, such as hypertension, atherosclerosis, CHD, and heart failure.

The oxidative stress hypothesis provides a unifying theory for aging and the predisposition to the metabolic syndrome. In studies of insulin-resistant individuals with obesity or type 2 diabetes, the offspring of patients with type 2 diabetes, and the elderly, a defect in mitochondrial oxidative phosphorylation that leads to the accumulation of triglycerides and related lipid molecules in muscle has been identified.

Recently, the gut microbiome has emerged as an important contributor to the development of obesity and related metabolic disorders, including the metabolic syndrome. Although the mechanism remains

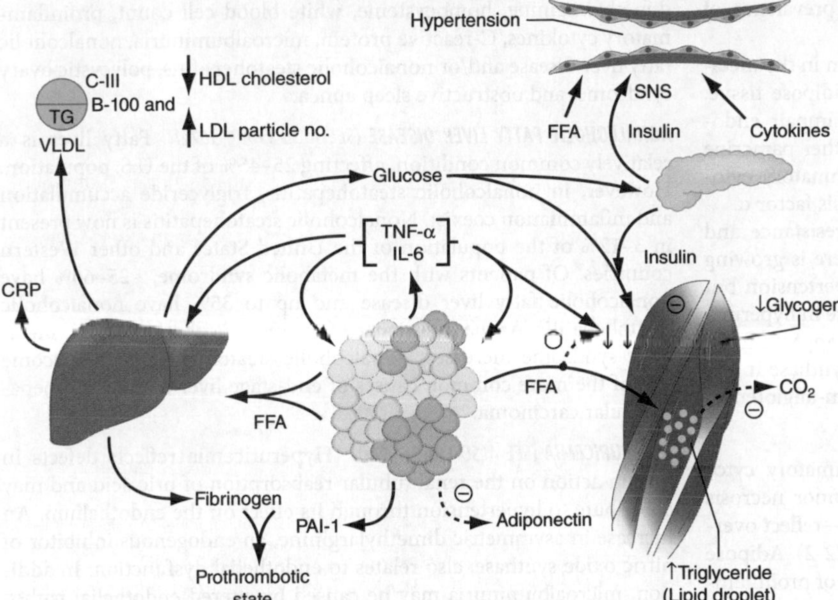

FIGURE 422-2 Pathophysiology of the metabolic syndrome. Free fatty acids (FFAs) are released in abundance from an expanded adipose tissue mass. In the liver, FFAs result in increased production of glucose and triglycerides and secretion of very low density lipoproteins (VLDLs). Associated lipid/lipoprotein abnormalities include reductions in high-density lipoprotein (HDL) cholesterol and an increased low-density lipoprotein (LDL) particle number (no.). FFAs also reduce insulin sensitivity in muscle by inhibiting insulin mediated glucose uptake. Associated defects include a reduction in glucose partitioning to glycogen and increased lipid accumulation in triglyceride (TG). The increase in circulating glucose, and to some extent FFAs, increases pancreatic insulin secretion, resulting in hyperinsulinemia. Hyperinsulinemia may result in enhanced sodium reabsorption and increased sympathetic nervous system (SNS) activity and contribute to hypertension, as might higher levels of circulating FFAs. The proinflammatory state is superimposed and contributory to the insulin resistance produced by excessive FFAs. The enhanced secretion of interleukin 6 (IL-6) and tumor necrosis factor α (TNF-α) produced by adipocytes and monocyte-derived macrophages results in more insulin resistance and lipolysis of adipose tissue triglyceride stores to circulating FFAs. IL-6 and other cytokines also enhance hepatic glucose production, VLDL production by the liver, hypertension and insulin resistance in muscle. Cytokines and FFAs also increase hepatic production of fibrinogen and adipocyte production of plasminogen activator inhibitor 1 (PAI-1), resulting in a prothrombotic state. Higher levels of circulating cytokines stimulate hepatic production of C reactive protein (CRP). Reduced production of the anti-inflammatory and insulin-sensitizing cytokine adiponectin is also associated with the metabolic syndrome. *(Modified from RH Eckel et al: Lancet 365:1415, 2005.)*

uncertain, interaction among genetic predisposition, diet, and the intestinal flora is important.

Increased Waist Circumference Waist circumference is an important component of the most recent and frequently applied diagnostic criteria for the metabolic syndrome. However, measuring waist circumference does not reliably distinguish increases in SC adipose tissue from those in visceral fat; this distinction requires CT or MRI. With increases in visceral adipose tissue, adipose tissue–derived free fatty acids are directed to the liver. In contrast, increases in abdominal SC fat release lipolysis products into the systemic circulation and avert more direct effects on hepatic metabolism. Relative increases in visceral versus SC adipose tissue with increasing waist circumference in Asians and Asian Indians may explain the greater prevalence of the syndrome in those populations than in African-American men, in whom SC fat predominates. It is also possible that visceral fat is a marker for—but not the source of—excess postprandial free fatty acids in obesity.

Dyslipidemia (See also Chap. 421) In general, free fatty acid flux to the liver is associated with increased production of ApoB-containing, triglyceride-rich, very low-density lipoproteins (VLDLs). The effect of insulin on this process is complex, but *hypertriglyceridemia* is an excellent marker of the insulin-resistant condition. Not only is hypertriglyceridemia a feature of the metabolic syndrome, but patients with the metabolic syndrome have elevated levels of ApoCIII carried on VLDLs and other lipoproteins. This increase in ApoCIII is inhibitory to lipoprotein lipase, further contributing to hypertriglyceridemia and also associated with more atherosclerotic cardiovascular disease.

The other major lipoprotein disturbance in the metabolic syndrome is a *reduction in HDL cholesterol*. This reduction is a consequence of changes in HDL composition and metabolism. In the presence of hypertriglyceridemia, a decrease in the cholesterol content of HDL is a consequence of reduced cholesteryl ester content of the lipoprotein core in combination with cholesteryl ester transfer protein–mediated alterations in triglyceride that make the particle small and dense. This change in lipoprotein composition also results in increased clearance of HDL from the circulation. These changes in HDL have a relationship to insulin resistance that is probably indirect, occurring in concert with the changes in triglyceride-rich lipoprotein metabolism.

In addition to HDLs, low-density lipoproteins (LDLs) are modified in composition in the metabolic syndrome. With fasting serum triglycerides at >2.0 mM (~180 mg/dL), there is almost always a predominance of small, dense LDLs, which are thought to be more atherogenic although their association with hypertriglyceridemia and low HDLs make their independent contribution to CVD events difficult to assess. Individuals with hypertriglyceridemia often have increases in cholesterol content of both VLDL1 and VLDL2 subfractions and in LDL particle number. Both of these lipoprotein changes may contribute to atherogenic risk in patients with the metabolic syndrome.

Glucose Intolerance (See also Chap. 417) Defects in insulin action in the metabolic syndrome lead to impaired suppression of glucose production by the liver and kidney and reduced glucose uptake and metabolism in insulin-sensitive tissues—i.e., muscle and adipose tissue. The relationship between impaired fasting glucose or impaired glucose tolerance and insulin resistance is well supported by studies of humans, nonhuman primates, and rodents. To compensate for defects in insulin action, insulin secretion and/or clearance must be modified so that euglycemia is sustained. Ultimately, this compensatory mechanism fails, usually because of defects in insulin secretion, resulting in progression from impaired fasting glucose and/or impaired glucose tolerance to diabetes mellitus.

Hypertension The relationship between insulin resistance and hypertension is well established. Paradoxically, under normal physiologic conditions, insulin is a vasodilator with secondary effects on sodium reabsorption in the kidney. However, in the setting of insulin resistance, the vasodilatory effect of insulin is lost but the renal effect on sodium reabsorption is preserved. Sodium reabsorption is increased in whites with the metabolic syndrome but not in Africans or Asians. Insulin also increases the activity of the sympathetic nervous system, an effect that may be preserved in the setting of insulin resistance. Insulin resistance is characterized by pathway-specific impairment in phosphatidylinositol-3-kinase signaling. In the endothelium, this impairment may cause an imbalance between the production of nitric oxide and the secretion of endothelin 1, with a consequent decrease in blood flow. Although these mechanisms are provocative, evaluation of insulin action by measurement of fasting insulin levels or by homeostasis model assessment shows that insulin resistance contributes only partially to the increased prevalence of hypertension in the metabolic syndrome.

Another possible mechanism underlying hypertension in the metabolic syndrome is the vasoactive role of perivascular adipose tissue. Reactive oxygen species released by NADPH oxidase impair endothelial function and result in local vasoconstriction. Other paracrine effects could be mediated by leptin or other proinflammatory cytokines released from adipose tissue, such as tumor necrosis factor α.

Hyperuricemia is another consequence of insulin resistance and is commonly observed in the metabolic syndrome. There is growing evidence not only that uric acid is associated with hypertension but also that reduction of uric acid normalizes blood pressure in hyperuricemic adolescents with hypertension. The mechanism appears to be related to an adverse effect of uric acid on nitric acid synthase in the macula densa of the kidney and stimulation of the renin-angiotensin aldosterone system.

Proinflammatory Cytokines The increases in proinflammatory cytokines—including interleukins 1, 6, and 18; resistin; tumor necrosis factor α; and the systemic biomarker C-reactive protein—reflect overproduction by the expanded adipose tissue mass (Fig. 422-2). Adipose tissue–derived macrophages may be the primary source of proinflammatory cytokines locally and in the systemic circulation. It remains unclear, however, how much of the insulin resistance is caused by the paracrine effects of these cytokines and how much by the endocrine effects.

Adiponectin Adiponectin is an anti-inflammatory cytokine produced exclusively by adipocytes. Adiponectin enhances insulin sensitivity and inhibits many steps in the inflammatory process. In the liver, adiponectin inhibits the expression of gluconeogenic enzymes and the rate of glucose production. In muscle, adiponectin increases glucose transport and enhances fatty acid oxidation, partially through the activation of AMP kinase. Adiponectin levels are reduced in the metabolic syndrome. The relative contributions of adiponectin deficiency and overabundance of the proinflammatory cytokines are unclear.

CLINICAL FEATURES

Symptoms and Signs The metabolic syndrome typically is not associated with symptoms. On physical examination, waist circumference may be expanded and blood pressure elevated. The presence of either or both of these signs should prompt the clinician to search for other biochemical abnormalities that may be associated with the metabolic syndrome. Less frequently, lipoatrophy or acanthosis nigricans is found on examination. Because these physical findings characteristically are associated with severe insulin resistance, other components of the metabolic syndrome should be expected.

Associated Diseases • *CARDIOVASCULAR DISEASE* The relative risk for new-onset CVD in patients with the metabolic syndrome who do not have diabetes averages 1.5–3 fold. However, an 8-year follow-up of middle-aged participants in the Framingham Offspring Study documented that the population-attributable CVD risk in the metabolic syndrome was 34% among men and only 16% among women. In the same study, both the metabolic syndrome and diabetes predicted ischemic stroke, with greater risk among patients with the metabolic syndrome than among those with diabetes alone (19% vs. 7%) and a particularly large difference among women (27% vs. 5%). Patients with the metabolic syndrome are also at increased risk for peripheral vascular disease.

TYPE 2 DIABETES Overall, the risk for type 2 diabetes among patients with the metabolic syndrome is increased three- to fivefold. In the Framingham Offspring Study's 8-year follow-up of middle-aged participants, the population-attributable risk for developing type 2 diabetes was 62% among men and 47% among women.

Other Associated Conditions In addition to the features specifically associated with the metabolic syndrome, other metabolic alterations accompany insulin resistance. Those alterations include increases in ApoB and ApoCIII, uric acid, prothrombotic factors (fibrinogen, plasminogen activator inhibitor 1), serum viscosity, asymmetric dimethylarginine, homocysteine, white blood cell count, proinflammatory cytokines, C-reactive protein, microalbuminuria, nonalcoholic fatty liver disease and/or nonalcoholic steatohepatitis, polycystic ovary syndrome, and obstructive sleep apnea.

***NONALCOHOLIC FATTY LIVER DISEASE** (SEE ALSO CHAP. 367e)* Fatty liver is a relatively common condition, affecting 25–45% of the U.S. population. However, in nonalcoholic steatohepatitis, triglyceride accumulation and inflammation coexist. Nonalcoholic steatohepatitis is now present in 3–12% of the population of the United States and other Western countries. Of patients with the metabolic syndrome, ~25–60% have nonalcoholic fatty liver disease and up to 35% have nonalcoholic steatohepatitis. As the prevalence of overweight/obesity and the metabolic syndrome increases, nonalcoholic steatohepatitis may become one of the more common causes of end-stage liver disease and hepatocellular carcinoma.

***HYPERURICEMIA** (SEE ALSO CHAP. 431e)* Hyperuricemia reflects defects in insulin action on the renal tubular reabsorption of uric acid and may contribute to hypertension through its effect on the endothelium. An increase in asymmetric dimethylarginine, an endogenous inhibitor of nitric oxide synthase, also relates to endothelial dysfunction. In addition, microalbuminuria may be caused by altered endothelial pathophysiology in the insulin-resistant state.

***POLYCYSTIC OVARY SYNDROME** (SEE ALSO CHAP. 412)* Polycystic ovary syndrome is highly associated with insulin resistance (50–80%) and the metabolic syndrome, with a prevalence of the syndrome between 40% and 50%. Women with polycystic ovary syndrome are two to four times more likely to have the metabolic syndrome than are women without polycystic ovary syndrome.

***OBSTRUCTIVE SLEEP APNEA** (SEE ALSO CHAP. 38)* Obstructive sleep apnea is commonly associated with obesity, hypertension, increased circulating cytokines, impaired glucose tolerance, and insulin resistance. With these associations, it is not surprising that individuals with obstructive sleep apnea frequently have the metabolic syndrome. Moreover, when biomarkers of insulin resistance are compared between patients with obstructive sleep apnea and weight-matched controls, insulin resistance is found to be more severe in those with apnea. Continuous positive airway pressure treatment improves insulin sensitivity in patients with obstructive sleep apnea.

DIAGNOSIS

The diagnosis of the metabolic syndrome relies on fulfillment of the criteria listed in Table 422-1, as assessed using tools at the bedside and in the laboratory. The medical history should include evaluation of symptoms for obstructive sleep apnea in all patients and polycystic ovary syndrome in premenopausal women. Family history will help determine risk for CVD and diabetes mellitus. Blood pressure and waist circumference measurements provide information necessary for the diagnosis.

Laboratory Tests Measurement of fasting lipids and glucose is needed in determining whether the metabolic syndrome is present. The measurement of additional biomarkers associated with insulin resistance can be individualized. Such tests might include those for ApoB, high-sensitivity C-reactive protein, fibrinogen, uric acid, urinary microalbumin, and liver function. A sleep study should be performed if symptoms of obstructive sleep apnea are present. If polycystic ovary syndrome is suspected on the basis of clinical features and anovulation, testosterone, luteinizing hormone, and follicle-stimulating hormone should be measured.

TREATMENT THE METABOLIC SYNDROME

LIFESTYLE (SEE ALSO CHAP. 416)

Obesity is the driving force behind the metabolic syndrome. Thus, weight reduction is the primary approach to the disorder. With weight reduction, improvement in insulin sensitivity is often accompanied by favorable modifications in many components of the metabolic syndrome. In general, recommendations for weight loss include a combination of caloric restriction, increased physical activity, and behavior modification. Caloric restriction is the most important component, whereas increases in physical activity are important for maintenance of weight loss. Some but not all evidence suggests that the addition of exercise to caloric restriction may promote greater weight loss from the visceral depot. The tendency for weight regain after successful weight reduction underscores the need for long-lasting behavioral changes.

Diet Before prescribing a weight-loss diet, it is important to emphasize that it has taken the patient a long time to develop an expanded fat mass; thus, the correction need not occur quickly. Given that ~3500 kcal = 1 lb of fat, ~500-kcal restriction daily equates to weight reduction of 1 lb per week. Diets restricted in carbohydrate typically provide a rapid initial weight loss. However, after 1 year, the amount of weight reduction is minimally reduced or no different from that with caloric restriction alone. Thus, adherence to the diet is more important than which diet is chosen. Moreover, there is concern about low-carbohydrate diets enriched in saturated fat, particularly for patients at risk for CVD. Therefore, a high-quality dietary pattern—i.e., a diet enriched in fruits, vegetables, whole grains, lean poultry, and fish—should be encouraged to maximize overall health benefit.

Physical Activity Before a physical activity recommendation is provided to patients with the metabolic syndrome, it is important to ensure that the increased activity does not incur risk. Some high-risk patients should undergo formal cardiovascular evaluation before initiating an exercise program. For an inactive participant, gradual increases in physical activity should be encouraged to enhance adherence and avoid injury. Although increases in physical activity can lead to modest weight reduction, 60–90 min of daily activity is required to achieve this goal. Even if an overweight or obese adult is unable to undertake this level of activity, a significant health benefit will follow from at least 30 min of moderate-intensity activity daily. The caloric value of 30 min of a variety of activities can be found at *www.heart.org/HEARTORG/GettingHealthy/WeightManagement/LosingWeight/Losing-Weight_UCM_307904_Article.jsp*. Of note, a variety of routine activities, such as gardening, walking, and housecleaning, require moderate caloric expenditure. Thus, physical activity need not be defined solely in terms of formal exercise such as jogging, swimming, or tennis.

Behavior Modification Behavioral treatment typically includes recommendations for dietary restriction and more physical activity, resulting in weight loss that benefits metabolic health. The subsequent challenge is the duration of the program because weight regain so often follows successful weight reduction. Long-term outcomes may be enhanced by a variety of methods, such as the Internet, social media, and telephone follow-up to maintain contact between providers and patients.

Obesity (See also Chap. 416) In some patients with the metabolic syndrome, treatment options need to extend beyond lifestyle intervention. Weight-loss drugs come in two major classes: appetite suppressants and absorption inhibitors. Appetite suppressants approved by the U.S. Food and Drug Administration include phentermine (for short-term use [3 months] only) as well as the more recent additions phentermine/topiramate and lorcaserin, which are approved without restrictions on the duration of therapy. In clinical trials, the phentermine/topiramate combination has resulted in ~10% weight loss in 50% of patients. Side effects include palpitations, headache, paresthesias, constipation, and insomnia. Lorcaserin results in less weight loss—typically ~5% beyond placebo—but can cause headache and nasopharyngitis. Orlistat inhibits fat absorption by ~30% and is moderately effective compared with placebo (~5% more weight loss). Orlistat has been shown to reduce the incidence of type 2 diabetes, an effect that was especially evident among patients with impaired glucose tolerance at baseline. This drug is often difficult of take because of oily leakage per rectum.

Metabolic or bariatric surgery is an option for patients with the metabolic syndrome who have a body mass index >40 kg/m^2, or >35 kg/m^2 with comorbidities. An evolving application for metabolic surgery includes patients with a body mass index as low as 30 kg/m^2 and type 2 diabetes. Gastric bypass or vertical sleeve gastrectomy results in dramatic weight reduction and improvement in the features of the metabolic syndrome. A survival benefit with gastric bypass has also been realized.

LDL CHOLESTEROL (SEE ALSO CHAP. 421)

The rationale for the NCEP:ATPIII's development of criteria for the metabolic syndrome was to go beyond LDL cholesterol in identifying and reducing the risk of CVD. The working assumption by the panel was that LDL cholesterol goals had already been achieved and that increasing evidence supports a linear reduction in CVD events as a result of progressive lowering of LDL cholesterol with statins. For patients with the metabolic syndrome and diabetes, a statin should be prescribed. For those patients with diabetes and known CVD, the current evidence supports a maximum of penultimate dose of a potent statin (e.g., atorvastatin or rosuvastatin). For those patients with the metabolic syndrome but without diabetes, a score that predicts a 10-year CVD risk exceeding 7.5% should also take a statin. With a 10-year risk of <7.5%, use of statin therapy is not evidence based.

Diets restricted in saturated fats (<7% of calories) and *trans*-fats (as few as possible) should be applied aggressively. Although less evidence exists, dietary cholesterol should also be restricted. If LDL cholesterol remains elevated, pharmacologic intervention is needed. Treatment with statins, which lower LDL cholesterol by 15–60%, is evidence based and is the first-choice medication intervention. Of note, for each doubling of the statin dose, LDL cholesterol is further lowered by only ~6%. Hepatotoxicity (more than a threefold increase in hepatic aminotransferases) is rare, and myopathy is seen in ~10% of patients. The cholesterol absorption inhibitor ezetimibe is well tolerated and should be the second-choice medication intervention. Ezetimibe typically reduces LDL cholesterol by 15–20%. The bile acid sequestrants cholestyramine, colestipol, and colesevalam may be more effective than ezetimibe but, because they can increase triglyceride levels, must be used with caution in patients with the metabolic syndrome. In general, bile sequestrants should not be administered when fasting triglyceride levels are >250 mg/dL. Side effects include gastrointestinal symptoms (palatability, bloating, belching, constipation, anal irritation). Nicotinic acid has modest LDL cholesterol–lowering capabilities (<20%). Fibrates are best employed to lower LDL cholesterol when both LDL cholesterol and triglycerides are elevated. Fenofibrate may be more effective than gemfibrozil in this setting.

TRIGLYCERIDES (SEE ALSO CHAP. 421)

The NCEP:ATPIII has focused on non-HDL cholesterol rather than on triglycerides. However, a fasting triglyceride value of <150 mg/dL is recommended. In general, the response of fasting triglycerides relates to the amount of weight reduction achieved: a weight reduction of >10% is necessary to lower fasting triglyceride levels.

A fibrate (gemfibrozil or fenofibrate) is the drug of choice to lower fasting triglyceride levels, which are typically reduced by 30–45%. Concomitant administration with drugs metabolized by the 3A4 cytochrome P450 system (including some statins) increases the risk of myopathy. In these cases, fenofibrate may be preferable to gemfibrozil. In the Veterans Affairs HDL Intervention Trial, gemfibrozil was administered to men with known CHD and levels of HDL cholesterol <40 mg/dL. A coronary disease event and mortality rate benefit was experienced predominantly among men with hyperinsulinemia and/or diabetes, many of whom were identified retrospectively as having the metabolic syndrome. Of note, the degree of triglyceride lowering in this trial did not predict benefit. Although levels of LDL cholesterol did not change, a decrease in LDL particle number correlated with benefit. Several additional clinical trials have not shown clear evidence that fibrates reduce CVD risk; however, post hoc analyses of several studies demonstrated that patients with baseline triglyceride levels >200 mg/dL and HDL cholesterol levels <35 mg/dL did benefit.

Other drugs that lower triglyceride levels include statins, nicotinic acid, and—in high doses—omega-3 fatty acids. For this purpose, an intermediate or high dose of the "more potent" statins (atorvastatin, rosuvastatin) is needed. The effect of nicotinic acid on fasting triglycerides is dose related and ~20–35%, an effect that is less pronounced than that of fibrates. In patients with the metabolic syndrome and diabetes, nicotinic acid may increase fasting glucose levels. Omega-3 fatty acid preparations that include high doses of docosahexaenoic acid plus eicosapentaenoic acid (~1.5–4.5 g/d) or eicosapentaenoic acid alone lower fasting triglyceride levels by ~30–40%. No drug interactions with fibrates or statins occur, and the main side effect of their use is eructation with a fishy taste. This taste can be partially blocked by ingestion of the nutraceutical after freezing. Clinical trials of nicotinic acid or high-dose omega-3 fatty acids in patients with the metabolic syndrome have not been reported.

HDL CHOLESTEROL (SEE ALSO CHAP. 421)

Very few lipid-modifying compounds increase HDL cholesterol levels. Statins, fibrates, and bile acid sequestrants have modest effects (5–10%), whereas ezetimibe and omega-3 fatty acids have no effect. Nicotinic acid is the only currently available drug with predictable HDL cholesterol-raising properties. The response is dose related, and nicotinic acid can increase HDL cholesterol by ~30% above baseline. After several trials of nicotinic acid versus placebo in statin-treated patients, there is still no evidence that raising HDL with nicotinic acid beneficially affects CVD events in patients with or without the metabolic syndrome.

BLOOD PRESSURE (SEE ALSO CHAP. 298)

The direct relationship between blood pressure and all-cause mortality rate has been well established in studies comparing patients with hypertension (>140/90 mmHg), patients with pre-hypertension (>120/80 mmHg but <140/90 mmHg), and individuals with normal blood pressure (<120/80 mmHg). In patients who have the metabolic syndrome without diabetes, the best choice for the initial antihypertensive medication is an angiotensin-converting enzyme (ACE) inhibitor or an angiotensin II receptor blocker, as these two classes of drugs appear to reduce the incidence of new-onset type 2 diabetes. In all patients with hypertension, a sodium-restricted dietary pattern enriched in fruits and vegetables, whole grains, and low-fat dairy products should be advocated. Home monitoring of blood pressure may assist in maintaining good blood-pressure control.

IMPAIRED FASTING GLUCOSE (SEE ALSO CHAP. 417)

In patients with the metabolic syndrome and type 2 diabetes, aggressive glycemic control may favorably modify fasting levels of triglycerides and/or HDL cholesterol. In patients with impaired fasting glucose who do not have diabetes, a lifestyle intervention that includes weight reduction, dietary fat restriction, and increased physical activity has been shown to reduce the incidence of type 2 diabetes. Metformin also reduces the incidence of diabetes, although the effect is less pronounced than that of lifestyle intervention.

INSULIN RESISTANCE (SEE ALSO CHAP. 418)

Several drug classes (biguanides, thiazolidinediones [TZDs]) increase insulin sensitivity. Because insulin resistance is the primary pathophysiologic mechanism for the metabolic syndrome, representative drugs in these classes reduce its prevalence. Both metformin and TZDs enhance insulin action in the liver and suppress endogenous glucose production. TZDs, but not metformin, also improve insulin-mediated glucose uptake in muscle and adipose tissue. Benefits of both drugs have been seen in patients with nonalcoholic fatty liver disease and polycystic ovary syndrome, and the drugs have been shown to reduce markers of inflammation.

SECTION 4 DISORDERS OF BONE AND MINERAL METABOLISM

423 Bone and Mineral Metabolism in Health and Disease

F. Richard Bringhurst, Marie B. Demay, Stephen M. Krane, Henry M. Kronenberg

BONE STRUCTURE AND METABOLISM

Bone is a dynamic tissue that is remodeled constantly throughout life. The arrangement of compact and cancellous bone provides strength and density suitable for both mobility and protection. In addition, bone provides a reservoir for calcium, magnesium, phosphorus, sodium, and other ions necessary for homeostatic functions. Bone also hosts and regulates hematopoiesis by providing niches for hematopoietic cell proliferation and differentiation. The skeleton is highly vascular and receives about 10% of the cardiac output. Remodeling of bone is accomplished by two distinct cell types: osteoblasts produce bone matrix, and osteoclasts resorb the matrix.

The extracellular components of bone consist of a solid mineral phase in close association with an organic matrix, of which 90–95% is type I collagen (Chap. 427). The noncollagenous portion of the organic matrix is heterogeneous and contains serum proteins such as albumin as well as many locally produced proteins, whose functions are incompletely understood. Those proteins include cell attachment/signaling proteins such as thrombospondin, osteopontin, and fibronectin; calcium-binding proteins such as matrix gla protein and osteocalcin; and proteoglycans such as biglycan and decorin. Some of the proteins organize collagen fibrils; others influence mineralization and binding of the mineral phase to the matrix.

The mineral phase is made up of calcium and phosphate and is best characterized as a poorly crystalline hydroxyapatite. The mineral phase of bone is deposited initially in intimate relation to the collagen fibrils and is found in specific locations in the "holes" between the collagen fibrils. This architectural arrangement of mineral and matrix results in a two-phase material well suited to withstand mechanical stresses. The organization of collagen influences the amount and type of mineral phase formed in bone. Although the primary structures of type I collagen in skin and bone tissues are similar, there are differences in posttranslational modifications and distribution of intermolecular cross-links. The holes in the packing structure of the collagen are larger in mineralized collagen of bone and dentin than in unmineralized collagens such as those in tendon. Single amino acid substitutions in the helical portion of either the α1 (*COL1A1*) or α2 (*COL1A2*) chains of type I collagen disrupt the organization of bone in osteogenesis imperfecta. The severe skeletal fragility associated with this group of disorders highlights the importance of the fibrillar matrix in the structure of bone (Chap. 427).

Osteoblasts synthesize and secrete the organic matrix and regulate its mineralization. They are derived from cells of mesenchymal origin (Fig. 423-1A). Active osteoblasts are found on the surface of newly

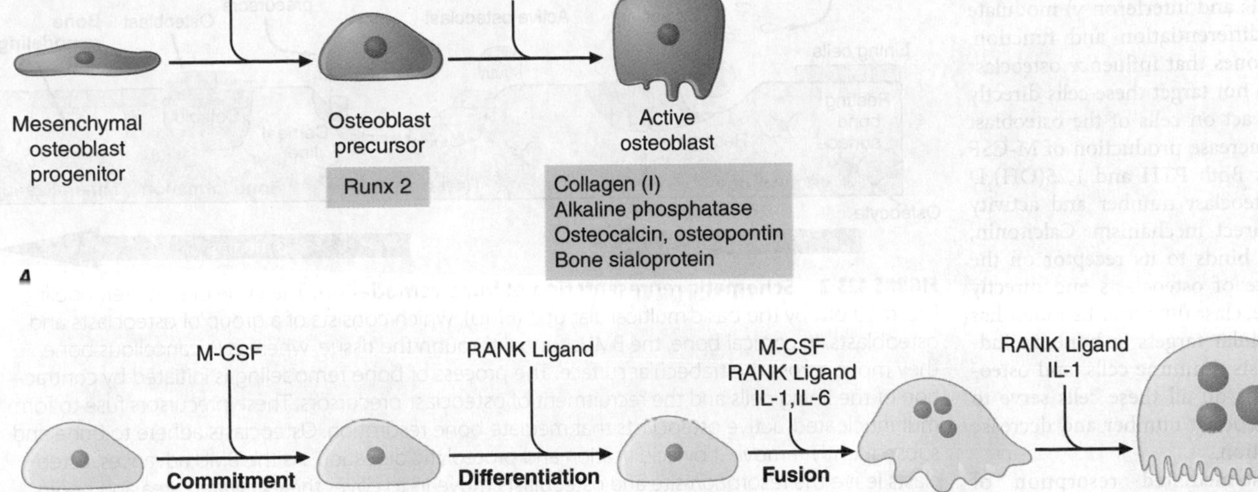

FIGURE 423-1 Pathways regulating development of (*A*) osteoblasts and (*B*) osteoclasts. Hormones, cytokines, and growth factors that control cell proliferation and differentiation are shown above the arrows. Transcription factors and other markers specific for various stages of development are depicted below the arrows. BMPs, bone morphogenic proteins; IGFs, insulin-like growth factors; IL-1, interleukin 1; IL-6, interleukin 6; M-CSF, macrophage colony-stimulating factor; NFκB, nuclear factor κB; PTH, parathyroid hormone; PU-1, a monocyte- and B lymphocyte–specific ets family transcription factor; RANK ligand, receptor activator of NFκB ligand; Runx2, Runt-related transcription factor 2; TRAF, tumor necrosis factor receptor–associated factors; Vit D, vitamin D; wnts, wingless-type mouse mammary tumor virus integration site. *(Modified from T Suda et al: Endocr Rev 20:345, 1999, with permission.)*

forming bone. As an osteoblast secretes matrix, which then is mineralized, the cell becomes an *osteocyte*, still connected with its blood supply through a series of canaliculi. Osteocytes account for the vast majority of the cells in bone. They are thought to be the mechanosensors in bone that communicate signals to surface osteoblasts and their progenitors through the canalicular network and thereby serve as master regulators of bone formation and resorption. Remarkably, osteocytes also secrete fibroblast growth factor 23 (FGF23), a major regulator of phosphate metabolism (see below). Mineralization of the matrix, both in trabecular bone and in osteones of compact cortical bone (*Haversian systems*), begins soon after the matrix is secreted (primary mineralization) but is not completed for several weeks or even longer (secondary mineralization). Although this mineralization takes advantage of the high concentrations of calcium and phosphate, already near saturation in serum, mineralization is a carefully regulated process that is dependent on the activity of osteoblast-derived alkaline phosphatase, which probably works by hydrolyzing inhibitors of mineralization.

Genetic studies in humans and mice have identified several key genes that control osteoblast development. *Runx2* is a transcription factor expressed specifically in chondrocyte (cartilage cells) and osteoblast progenitors as well as in hypertrophic chondrocytes and mature osteoblasts. *Runx2* regulates the expression of several important osteoblast proteins, including osterix (another transcription factor needed for osteoblast maturation), osteopontin, bone sialoprotein, type I collagen, osteocalcin, and receptor-activator of NFκB (RANK) ligand. *Runx2* expression is regulated in part by bone morphogenic proteins (BMPs). *Runx2*-deficient mice are devoid of osteoblasts, whereas mice with a deletion of only one allele (*Runx2* +/−) exhibit a delay in formation of the clavicles and some cranial bones. The latter abnormalities are similar to those in the human disorder *cleidocranial dysplasia*, which is also caused by heterozygous inactivating mutations in *Runx2*.

The paracrine signaling molecule, Indian hedgehog (Ihh), also plays a critical role in osteoblast development, as evidenced by Ihh-deficient mice that lack osteoblasts in the type of bone formed on a cartilage mold (endochondral ossification). Signals originating from members of the wnt (wingless-type mouse mammary tumor virus integration site) family of paracrine factors are also important for osteoblast proliferation and differentiation. Numerous other growth-regulatory factors affect osteoblast function, including the three closely related transforming growth factor βs, fibroblast growth factors (FGFs) 2 and 18, platelet-derived growth factor, and insulin-like growth factors (IGFs) I and II. Hormones such as parathyroid hormone (PTH) and 1,25-dihydroxyvitamin D (1,25[OH]$_2$D) activate receptors expressed by osteoblasts to assure mineral homeostasis and influence a variety of bone cell functions.

Resorption of bone is carried out mainly by *osteoclasts*, multinucleated cells that are formed by fusion of cells derived from the common precursor of macrophages and osteoclasts. Thus, these cells derive from the hematopoietic lineage, quite different from the mesenchymal cells that become osteoblasts. Multiple factors that regulate osteoclast development have been identified (Fig. 423-1*B*). Factors produced by osteoblasts or marrow stromal cells allow osteoblasts to control osteoclast development and activity. Macrophage colony-stimulating factor (M-CSF) plays a critical role during several steps in the pathway and ultimately leads to fusion of osteoclast progenitor cells to form multinucleated, active osteoclasts. RANK ligand, a member of the tumor necrosis factor (TNF) family, is expressed on the surface of osteoblast progenitors and stromal fibroblasts. In a process involving cell-cell interactions, RANK ligand binds to the RANK receptor on osteoclast progenitors, stimulating osteoclast differentiation and activation. Alternatively, a soluble decoy receptor, referred to as osteoprotegerin, can bind RANK ligand and inhibit osteoclast differentiation. Several growth factors and cytokines (including interleukins 1, 6, and 11; TNF; and interferon γ) modulate osteoclast differentiation and function. Most hormones that influence osteoclast function do not target these cells directly but instead act on cells of the osteoblast lineage to increase production of M-CSF and RANK. Both PTH and 1,25(OH)$_2$D increase osteoclast number and activity by this indirect mechanism. Calcitonin, in contrast, binds to its receptor on the basal surface of osteoclasts and directly inhibits osteoclast function. Estradiol has multiple cellular targets in bone, including osteoclasts, immune cells, and osteoblasts; actions on all these cells serve to decrease osteoclast number and decrease bone resorption.

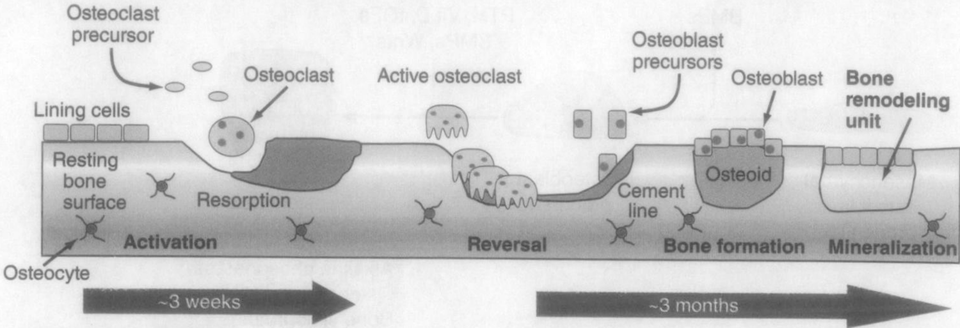

FIGURE 423-2 Schematic representation of bone remodeling. The cycle of bone remodeling is carried out by the basic multicellular unit (BMU), which consists of a group of osteoclasts and osteoblasts. In cortical bone, the BMUs tunnel through the tissue, whereas in cancellous bone, they move across the trabecular surface. The process of bone remodeling is initiated by contraction of the lining cells and the recruitment of osteoclast precursors. These precursors fuse to form multinucleated, active osteoclasts that mediate bone resorption. Osteoclasts adhere to bone and subsequently remove it by acidification and proteolytic digestion. As the BMU advances, osteoclasts leave the resorption site and osteoblasts move in to cover the excavated area and begin the process of new bone formation by secreting osteoid, which eventually is mineralized into new bone. After osteoid mineralization, osteoblasts flatten and form a layer of lining cells over new bone.

Osteoclast-mediated resorption of bone takes place in scalloped spaces (*Howship's lacunae*) where the osteoclasts are attached through a specific $\alpha_v\beta_3$ integrin to components of the bone matrix such as osteopontin. The osteoclast forms a tight seal to the underlying matrix and secretes protons, chloride, and proteinases into a confined space that has been likened to an extracellular lysosome. The active osteoclast surface forms a ruffled border that contains a specialized proton pump ATPase that secretes acid and solubilizes the mineral phase. Carbonic anhydrase (type II isoenzyme) within the osteoclast generates the needed protons. The bone matrix is resorbed in the acid environment adjacent to the ruffled border by proteases, such as cathepsin K, that act at low pH.

In the embryo and the growing child, bone develops mostly by remodeling and replacing previously calcified cartilage (endochondral bone formation) or, in a few bones, is formed without a cartilage matrix (intramembranous bone formation). During endochondral bone formation, chondrocytes proliferate, secrete and mineralize a matrix, enlarge (hypertrophy), and then die, enlarging bone and providing the matrix and factors that stimulate endochondral bone formation. This program is regulated by both local factors, such as IGF-I and -II, Ihh, PTH-related peptide (PTHrP), and FGFs, and by systemic hormones, such as growth hormone, glucocorticoids, and estrogen.

New bone, whether formed in infants or in adults during repair, has a relatively high ratio of cells to matrix and is characterized by coarse fiber bundles of collagen that are interlaced and randomly dispersed (woven bone). In adults, the more mature bone is organized with fiber bundles regularly arranged in parallel or concentric sheets (lamellar bone). In long bones, deposition of lamellar bone in a concentric arrangement around blood vessels forms the Haversian systems. Growth in length of bones is dependent on proliferation of cartilage cells and the endochondral sequence at the growth plate. Growth in width and thickness is accomplished by formation of bone at the periosteal surface and by resorption at the endosteal surface, with the rate of formation exceeding that of resorption. In adults, after the growth plates of cartilage close, growth in length and endochondral bone formation cease except for some activity in the cartilage cells beneath the articular surface. Even in adults, however, remodeling of bone (within Haversian systems as well as along the surfaces of trabecular bone) continues throughout life. In adults, ~4% of the surface of trabecular bone (such as iliac crest) is involved in active resorption, whereas 10–15% of trabecular surfaces are covered with osteoid, unmineralized new bone formed by osteoblasts. Radioisotope studies indicate that as much as 18% of the total skeletal calcium is deposited and removed each year. Thus, bone is an active metabolizing tissue that requires an intact blood supply. The cycle of bone resorption and formation is a highly orchestrated process carried out by the basic multicellular unit, which is composed of a group of osteoclasts and osteoblasts (Fig. 423-2).

The response of bone to fractures, infection, and interruption of blood supply and to expanding lesions is relatively limited. Dead bone must be resorbed, and new bone must be formed, a process carried out in association with growth of new blood vessels into the involved area. In injuries that disrupt the organization of the tissue such as a fracture in which apposition of fragments is poor or when motion exists at the fracture site, progenitor stromal cells recapitulate the endochondral bone formation of early development and form cartilage that is replaced by bone and, variably, fibrous tissue. When there is good apposition with fixation and little motion at the fracture site, repair occurs predominantly by formation of new bone without other mediating tissue.

Remodeling of bone occurs along lines of force generated by mechanical stress. The signals from these mechanical stresses are sensed by osteocytes, which transmit signals to osteoclasts and osteoblasts or their precursors. One such signal made by osteocytes is sclerostin, an inhibitor of wnt signaling. Mechanical forces suppress sclerostin production and thus increase bone formation by osteoblasts. Expanding lesions in bone such as tumors induce resorption at the surface in contact with the tumor by producing ligands such as PTHrP that stimulate osteoclast differentiation and function. Even in a disorder as architecturally disruptive as Paget's disease, remodeling is dictated by mechanical forces. Thus, bone plasticity reflects the interaction of cells with each other and with the environment.

Measurement of the products of osteoblast and osteoclast activity can assist in the diagnosis and management of bone diseases. Osteoblast activity can be assessed by measuring serum bone-specific alkaline phosphatase. Similarly, osteocalcin, a protein secreted from osteoblasts, is made virtually only by osteoblasts. Osteoclast activity can be assessed by measurement of products of collagen degradation. Collagen molecules are covalently linked to each other in the extracellular matrix through the formation of hydroxypyridinium cross-links (Chap. 427). After digestion by osteoclasts, these cross-linked peptides can be measured both in urine and in blood.

CALCIUM METABOLISM

Over 99% of the 1–2 kg of calcium present normally in the adult human body resides in the skeleton, where it provides mechanical stability and serves as a reservoir sometimes needed to maintain extracellular fluid (ECF) calcium concentration (Fig. 423-3). Skeletal calcium accretion first becomes significant during the third trimester of fetal life, accelerates throughout childhood and adolescence, reaches a peak in early adulthood, and gradually declines thereafter at rates that rarely

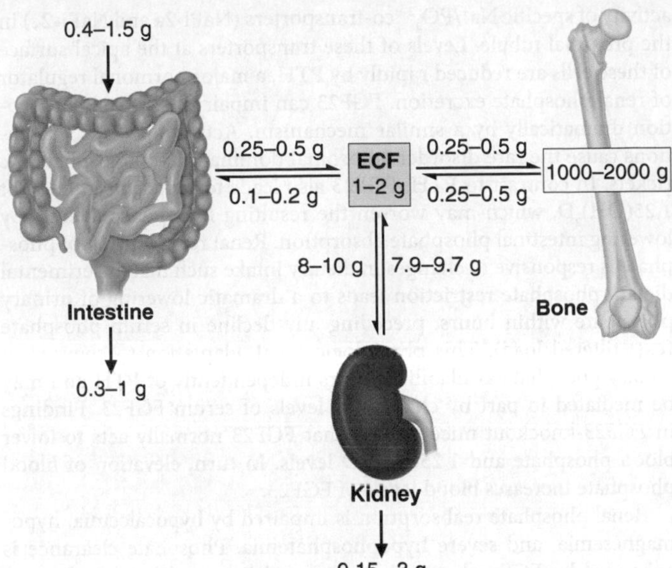

FIGURE 423-3 Calcium homeostasis. Schematic illustration of calcium content of extracellular fluid (ECF) and bone as well as of diet and feces; magnitude of calcium flux per day as calculated by various methods is shown at sites of transport in intestine, kidney, and bone. Ranges of values shown are approximate and were chosen to illustrate certain points discussed in the text. In conditions of calcium balance, rates of calcium release from and uptake into bone are equal.

exceed 1–2% per year. These slow changes in total skeletal calcium content contrast with relatively high daily rates of closely matched fluxes of calcium into and out of bone (~250–500 mg each), a process mediated by coupled osteoblastic and osteoclastic activity. Another 0.5–1% of skeletal calcium is freely exchangeable (e.g., in chemical equilibrium) with that in the ECF.

The concentration of ionized calcium in the ECF must be maintained within a narrow range because of the critical role calcium plays in a wide array of cellular functions, especially those involved in neuromuscular activity, secretion, and signal transduction. Intracellular cytosolic free calcium levels are ~100 nmol/L and are 10,000-fold lower than ionized calcium concentrations in the blood and ECF (1.1–1.3 mmol/L). Cytosolic calcium does not play the structural role played by extracellular calcium; instead, it serves a signaling function. The steep chemical gradient of calcium from outside to inside the cell promotes rapid calcium influx through various membrane calcium channels that can be activated by hormones, metabolites, or neurotransmitters, swiftly changing cellular function. In blood, total calcium concentration is normally 2.2–2.6 m*M* (8.5–10.5 mg/dL), of which ~50% is ionized. The remainder is bound ionically to negatively charged proteins (predominantly albumin and immunoglobulins) or loosely complexed with phosphate, citrate, sulfate, or other anions. Alterations in serum protein concentrations directly affect the total blood calcium concentration even if the ionized calcium concentration remains normal. An algorithm to correct for protein changes adjusts the total serum calcium (in mg/dL) upward by 0.8 times the deficit in serum albumin (g/dL) or by 0.5 times the deficit in serum immunoglobulin (in g/dL). Such corrections provide only rough approximations of actual free calcium concentrations, however, and may be misleading, particularly during acute illness. Acidosis also alters ionized calcium by reducing its association with proteins. The best practice is to measure blood ionized calcium directly by a method that employs calcium-selective electrodes in acute settings during which calcium abnormalities might occur.

Control of the ionized calcium concentration in the ECF ordinarily is accomplished by adjusting the rates of calcium movement across intestinal and renal epithelia. These adjustments are mediated mainly via changes in blood levels of the hormones, PTH and $1,25(OH)_2D$. Blood ionized calcium directly suppresses PTH secretion by activating calcium-sensing receptors (CaSRs) in parathyroid cells. Also, ionized calcium indirectly affects PTH secretion by lowering $1,25(OH)_2D$ production. This active vitamin D metabolite inhibits PTH production by an incompletely understood mechanism of negative feedback (**Chap. 424**).

Normal dietary calcium intake in the United States varies widely, ranging from 10–37 mmol/d (400–1500 mg/d). An Institute of Medicine report recommends a daily allowance of 25–30 mmol (1000–1200 mg) for most adults. Intestinal absorption of ingested calcium involves both active (transcellular) and passive (paracellular) mechanisms. Passive calcium absorption is nonsaturable and approximates 5% of daily calcium intake, whereas active absorption involves apical calcium entry via specific ion channels (TRPV5 and TRPV6), whose expression is controlled principally by $1,25(OH)_2D$, and normally ranges from 20 to 70%. Active calcium transport occurs mainly in the proximal small bowel (duodenum and proximal jejunum), although some active calcium absorption occurs in most segments of the small intestine. Optimal rates of calcium absorption require gastric acid. This is especially true for weakly dissociable calcium supplements such as calcium carbonate. In fact, large boluses of calcium carbonate are poorly absorbed because of their neutralizing effect on gastric acid. In achlorhydric subjects and for those taking drugs that inhibit gastric acid secretion, supplements should be taken with meals to optimize their absorption. Use of calcium citrate may be preferable in these circumstances. Calcium absorption may also be blunted in disease states such as pancreatic or biliary insufficiency, in which ingested calcium remains bound to unabsorbed fatty acids or other food constituents. At high levels of calcium intake, synthesis of $1,25(OH)_2D$ is reduced; this decreases the rate of active intestinal calcium absorption. The opposite occurs with dietary calcium restriction. Some calcium, ~2.5–5 mmol/d (100–200 mg/d), is excreted as an obligate component of intestinal secretions and is not regulated by calciotropic hormones.

The feedback-controlled hormonal regulation of intestinal absorptive efficiency results in a relatively constant daily net calcium absorption of ~5–7.5 mmol/d (200–400 mg/d) despite large changes in daily dietary calcium intake. This daily load of absorbed calcium is excreted by the kidneys in a manner that is also tightly regulated by the concentration of ionized calcium in the blood. Approximately 8–10 g/d of calcium is filtered by the glomeruli, of which only 2–3% appears in the urine. Most filtered calcium (65%) is reabsorbed in the proximal tubules via a passive, paracellular route that is coupled to concomitant NaCl reabsorption and not specifically regulated. The cortical thick ascending limb of Henle's loop (cTAL) reabsorbs roughly another 20% of filtered calcium, also via a paracellular mechanism. Calcium reabsorption in the cTAL requires a tight-junctional protein called paracellin-1 and is inhibited by increased blood concentrations of calcium or magnesium, acting via the CaSR, which is highly expressed on basolateral membranes in this nephron segment. Operation of the renal CaSR provides a mechanism, independent of those engaged directly by PTH or $1,25(OH)_2D$, by which serum ionized calcium can control renal calcium reabsorption. Finally, ~10% of filtered calcium is reabsorbed in the distal convoluted tubules (DCTs) by a transcellular mechanism. Calcium enters the luminal surface of the cell through specific apical calcium channels (TRPV5), whose number is regulated. It then moves across the cell in association with a specific calcium-binding protein (calbindin-D28k) that buffers cytosolic calcium concentrations from the large mass of transported calcium. Ca^{2+}-ATPases and Na^+/Ca^{2+} exchangers actively extrude calcium across the basolateral surface and thereby maintain the transcellular calcium gradient. All these processes are stimulated directly or indirectly by PTH. The DCT is also the site of action of thiazide diuretics, which lower urinary calcium excretion by inducing sodium depletion and thereby augmenting proximal calcium reabsorption. Conversely, dietary sodium loads, or increased distal sodium delivery caused by loop diuretics or saline infusion, induce calciuresis.

The homeostatic mechanisms that normally maintain a constant serum ionized calcium concentration may fail at extremes of calcium intake or when the hormonal systems or organs involved are compromised. Thus, even with maximal activity of the vitamin D–dependent intestinal active transport system, sustained calcium intakes <5 mmol/d (<200 mg/d) cannot provide enough net calcium absorption to replace obligate losses via the intestine, the kidney, sweat, and other secretions. In this case, increased blood levels of PTH and $1,25(OH)_2D$ activate osteoclastic bone resorption to obtain needed calcium from bone, which leads to progressive bone loss and negative calcium balance. Increased PTH and $1,25(OH)_2D$ also enhance renal calcium reabsorption, and $1,25(OH)_2D$ enhances calcium absorption in the gut. At very high calcium intakes (>100 mmol/d [>4 g/d]), passive intestinal absorption continues to deliver calcium into the ECF despite maximally downregulated intestinal active transport and renal tubular calcium reabsorption. This can cause severe hypercalciuria, nephrocalcinosis, progressive renal failure, and hypercalcemia (e.g., "milk-alkali syndrome"). Deficiency or excess of PTH or vitamin D, intestinal disease, and renal failure represent other commonly encountered challenges to normal calcium homeostasis (Chap. 424).

PHOSPHORUS METABOLISM

Although 85% of the ~600 g of body phosphorus is present in bone mineral, phosphorus is also a major intracellular constituent both as the free anion(s) and as a component of numerous organophosphate compounds, including structural proteins, enzymes, transcription factors, carbohydrate and lipid intermediates, high-energy stores (adenosine triphosphate [ATP], creatine phosphate), and nucleic acids. Unlike calcium, phosphorus exists intracellularly at concentrations close to those present in ECF (e.g., 1–2 mmol/L). In cells and in the ECF, phosphorus exists in several forms, predominantly as $H_2PO_4^-$ or $NaHPO_4^-$, with perhaps 10% as HPO_4^{2-}. This mixture of anions will be referred to here as "phosphate." In serum, about 12% of phosphorus is bound to proteins. Concentrations of phosphates in blood and ECF generally are expressed in terms of elemental phosphorus, with the normal range in adults being 0.75–1.45 mmol/L (2.5–4.5 mg/dL). Because the volume of the intracellular fluid compartment is twice that of the ECF, measurements of ECF phosphate may not accurately reflect phosphate availability within cells that follows even modest shifts of phosphate from one compartment to the other.

Phosphate is widely available in foods and is absorbed efficiently (65%) by the small intestine even in the absence of vitamin D. However, phosphate absorptive efficiency may be enhanced (to 85–90%) via active transport mechanisms that are stimulated by $1,25(OH)_2D$. These mechanisms involve activation of Na^+/PO_4^{2-} co-transporters that move phosphate into intestinal cells against an unfavorable electrochemical gradient. Daily net intestinal phosphate absorption varies widely with the composition of the diet but is generally in the range of 500–1000 mg/d. Phosphate absorption can be inhibited by large doses of calcium salts or by sevelamer hydrochloride (Renagel), strategies commonly used to control levels of serum phosphate in renal failure. Aluminum hydroxide antacids also reduce phosphate absorption but are used less commonly because of the potential for aluminum toxicity. Low serum phosphate stimulates renal proximal tubular synthesis of $1,25(OH)_2D$, perhaps by suppressing blood levels of FGF23 (see below).

Serum phosphate levels vary by as much as 50% on a normal day. This reflects the effect of food intake but also an underlying circadian rhythm that produces a nadir between 7:00 and 10:00 A.M. Carbohydrate administration, especially as IV dextrose solutions in fasting subjects, can decrease serum phosphate by >0.7 mmol/L (2 mg/dL) due to rapid uptake into and utilization by cells. A similar response is observed in the treatment of diabetic ketoacidosis and during metabolic or respiratory alkalosis. Because of this wide variation in serum phosphate, it is best to perform measurements in the basal, fasting state.

Control of serum phosphate is determined mainly by the rate of renal tubular reabsorption of the filtered load, which is ~4–6 g/d. Because intestinal phosphate absorption is highly efficient, urinary excretion is not constant but varies directly with dietary intake. The fractional excretion of phosphate (ratio of phosphate to creatinine clearance) is generally in the range of 10–15%. The proximal tubule is the principal site at which renal phosphate reabsorption is regulated. This is accomplished by changes in the levels of apical expression and activity of specific Na^+/PO_4^{2-} co-transporters (NaPi-2a and NaPi-2c) in the proximal tubule. Levels of these transporters at the apical surface of these cells are reduced rapidly by PTH, a major hormonal regulator of renal phosphate excretion. FGF23 can impair phosphate reabsorption dramatically by a similar mechanism. Activating *FGF23* mutations cause the rare disorder autosomal dominant hypophosphatemic rickets. In contrast to PTH, FGF23 also leads to reduced synthesis of $1,25(OH)_2D$, which may worsen the resulting hypophosphatemia by lowering intestinal phosphate absorption. Renal reabsorption of phosphate is responsive to changes in dietary intake such that experimental dietary phosphate restriction leads to a dramatic lowering of urinary phosphate within hours, preceding any decline in serum phosphate (e.g., filtered load). This physiologic renal adaptation to changes in dietary phosphate availability occurs independently of PTH and may be mediated in part by changes in levels of serum FGF23. Findings in *FGF23*-knockout mice suggest that FGF23 normally acts to lower blood phosphate and $1,25(OH)_2D$ levels. In turn, elevation of blood phosphate increases blood levels of FGF23.

Renal phosphate reabsorption is impaired by hypocalcemia, hypomagnesemia, and severe hypophosphatemia. Phosphate clearance is enhanced by ECF volume expansion and impaired by dehydration. Phosphate retention is an important pathophysiologic feature of renal insufficiency (Chap. 335).

HYPOPHOSPHATEMIA

Causes Hypophosphatemia can occur by one or more of three primary mechanisms: (1) inadequate intestinal phosphate absorption, (2) excessive renal phosphate excretion, and (3) rapid redistribution of phosphate from the ECF into bone or soft tissue (Table 423-1). Because phosphate is so abundant in foods, inadequate intestinal absorption is almost never observed now that aluminum hydroxide antacids, which bind phosphate in the gut, are no longer widely used. Fasting or starvation, however, may result in depletion of body phosphate and predispose to subsequent hypophosphatemia during refeeding, especially if this is accomplished with IV glucose alone.

Chronic hypophosphatemia usually signifies a persistent renal tubular phosphate-wasting disorder. Excessive activation of PTH/PTHrP receptors in the proximal tubule as a result of primary or secondary hyperparathyroidism or because of the PTHrP-mediated hypercalcemia syndrome in malignancy (Chap. 424) is among the more common causes of renal hypophosphatemia, especially because of the high prevalence of vitamin D deficiency in older Americans. Familial hypocalciuric hypercalcemia and Jansen's chondrodystrophy are rare examples of genetic disorders in this category (Chap. 424).

Several genetic and acquired diseases cause PTH/PTHrP-independent tubular phosphate wasting with associated rickets and osteomalacia. All these diseases manifest severe hypophosphatemia; renal phosphate wasting, sometimes accompanied by aminoaciduria; inappropriately low blood levels of $1,25(OH)_2D$; low-normal serum levels of calcium; and evidence of impaired cartilage or bone mineralization. Analysis of these diseases led to the discovery of the hormone FGF23, which is an important physiologic regulator of phosphate metabolism. FGF23 decreases phosphate reabsorption in the proximal tubule and also suppresses the 1α-hydroxylase responsible for synthesis of $1,25(OH)_2D$. FGF23 is synthesized by cells of the osteoblast lineage, primarily osteocytes. High-phosphate diets increase FGF23 levels, and low-phosphate diets decrease them. Autosomal dominant hypophosphatemic rickets (ADHR) was the first disease linked to abnormalities in FGF23. ADHR results from activating mutations in the gene that encodes FGF23. These mutations alter a cleavage site that ordinarily allows for inactivation of intact FGF23. Several other genetic disorders exhibit elevated FGF23 and hypophosphatemia. The most common of these is X-linked hypophosphatemic rickets (XLH), which results from inactivating mutations in an endopeptidase termed *PHEX* (*p*hosphate-regulating gene with *h*omologies to *e*ndopeptidases on the *X* chromosome) that is expressed most abundantly on the surface of osteocytes and mature osteoblasts. Patients with XLH usually have high FGF23 levels, and ablation of the *FGF23* gene reverses the hypophosphatemia found in the mouse version of XLH. How inactivation

TABLE 423-1 CAUSES OF HYPOPHOSPHATEMIA

I. Reduced renal tubular phosphate reabsorption
- A. PTH/PTHrP-dependent
  1. Primary hyperparathyroidism
  2. Secondary hyperparathyroidism
     - a. Vitamin D deficiency/resistance
     - b. Calcium starvation/malabsorption
     - c. Bartter's syndrome
     - d. Autosomal recessive renal hypercalciuria with hypomagnesemia
  3. PTHrP-dependent hypercalcemia of malignancy
  4. Familial hypocalciuric hypercalcemia
- B. PTH/PTHrP-independent
  1. Excess FGF23 or other "phosphatonins"
     - a. X-linked hypophosphatemic rickets (XLH)
     - b. Autosomal recessive hypophosphatemia (ARHP)
     - c. Autosomal dominant hypophosphatemic rickets (ADHR) (DMP1, ENPP1 deficiency)
     - d. Tumor-induced osteomalacia syndrome (TIO)
     - e. McCune-Albright syndrome (fibrous dysplasia)
     - f. Epidermal nevus syndrome
  2. Intrinsic renal disease
     - a. Fanconi's syndrome(s)
     - b. Cystinosis
     - c. Wilson's disease
     - d. NaPi-2a or NaPi-2c mutations
  3. Other systemic disorders
     - a. Poorly controlled diabetes mellitus
     - b. Alcoholism
     - c. Hyperaldosteronism
     - d. Hypomagnesemia
     - e. Amyloidosis
     - f. Hemolytic-uremic syndrome
     - g. Renal transplantation or partial liver resection
     - h. Rewarming or induced hyperthermia
  4. Drugs or toxins
     - a. Ethanol
     - b. Acetazolamide, other diuretics
     - c. High-dose estrogens or glucocorticoids
     - d. Heavy metals (lead, cadmium, saccharated ferric oxide)
     - e. Toluene, *N*-methyl formamide
     - f. Cisplatin, ifosfamide, foscarnet, rapamycin

II. Impaired intestinal phosphate absorption
- A. Aluminum-containing antacids
- B. Sevelamer

III. Shifts of extracellular phosphate into cells
- A. Intravenous glucose
- B. Insulin therapy for prolonged hyperglycemia or diabetic ketoacidosis
- C. Catecholamines (epinephrine, dopamine, albuterol)
- D. Acute respiratory alkalosis
- E. Gram-negative sepsis, toxic shock syndrome
- F. Recovery from starvation or acidosis
- G. Rapid cellular proliferation
  1. Leukemic blast crisis
  2. Intensive erythropoietin, other growth factor therapy

IV. Accelerated net bone formation
- A. After parathyroidectomy
- B. Treatment of vitamin D deficiency, Paget's disease
- C. Osteoblastic metastases

Abbreviations: PTH, parathyroid hormone; PTHrP, parathyroid hormone–related peptide.

of *PHEX* leads to increased levels of FGF23 has not been determined. Two rare autosomal recessive hypophosphatemic syndromes associated with elevated FGF23 are due to inactivating mutations of dentin matrix protein-1 (*DMP1*) and ectonucleotide pyrophosphatase/phosphodiesterase 1 (*ENPP1*), both of which normally are highly expressed in bone and regulate FGF23 production. An unusual hypophosphatemic disorder, tumor-induced osteomalacia (TIO), is an acquired disorder in which tumors, usually of mesenchymal origin and generally histologically benign, secrete FGF23 and/or other molecules that induce renal phosphate wasting. The hypophosphatemic syndrome resolves completely within hours to days after successful resection of the responsible tumor. Such tumors typically express large amounts of FGF23 mRNA, and patients with TIO usually exhibit elevations of FGF23 in their blood.

Dent's disease is an X-linked recessive disorder caused by inactivating mutations in *CLCN5*, a chloride transporter expressed in endosomes of the proximal tubule; features include hypercalciuria, hypophosphatemia, and recurrent kidney stones. Renal phosphate wasting is common among poorly controlled diabetic patients and alcoholics, who therefore are at risk for iatrogenic hypophosphatemia when treated with insulin or IV glucose, respectively. Diuretics and certain other drugs and toxins can cause defective renal tubular phosphate reabsorption (Table 423-1).

In hospitalized patients, hypophosphatemia is often attributable to massive redistribution of phosphate from the ECF into cells. Insulin therapy for diabetic ketoacidosis is a paradigm for this phenomenon, in which the severity of the hypophosphatemia is related to the extent of antecedent depletion of phosphate and other electrolytes (Chap. 417). The hypophosphatemia is usually greatest at a point many hours after initiation of insulin therapy and is difficult to predict from baseline measurements of serum phosphate at the time of presentation, when prerenal azotemia can obscure significant phosphate depletion. Other factors that may contribute to such acute redistributive hypophosphatemia include antecedent starvation or malnutrition, administration of IV glucose without other nutrients, elevated blood catecholamines (endogenous or exogenous), respiratory alkalosis, and recovery from metabolic acidosis.

Hypophosphatemia also can occur transiently (over weeks to months) during the phase of accelerated net bone formation that follows parathyroidectomy for severe primary hyperparathyroidism or during treatment of vitamin D deficiency or lytic Paget's disease. This is usually most prominent in patients who preoperatively have evidence of high bone turnover (e.g., high serum levels of alkaline phosphatase). Osteoblastic metastases can also lead to this syndrome.

Clinical and Laboratory Findings The clinical manifestations of severe hypophosphatemia reflect a generalized defect in cellular energy metabolism because of ATP depletion, a shift from oxidative phosphorylation toward glycolysis, and associated tissue or organ dysfunction. Acute, severe hypophosphatemia occurs mainly or exclusively in hospitalized patients with underlying serious medical or surgical illness and preexisting phosphate depletion due to excessive urinary losses, severe malabsorption, or malnutrition. Chronic hypophosphatemia tends to be less severe, with a clinical presentation dominated by musculoskeletal complaints such as bone pain, osteomalacia, pseudofractures, and proximal muscle weakness or, in children, rickets and short stature.

Neuromuscular manifestations of severe hypophosphatemia are variable but may include muscle weakness, lethargy, confusion, disorientation, hallucinations, dysarthria, dysphagia, oculomotor palsies, anisocoria, nystagmus, ataxia, cerebellar tremor, ballismus, hyporeflexia, impaired sphincter control, distal sensory deficits, paresthesia, hyperesthesia, generalized or Guillain-Barré–like ascending paralysis, seizures, coma, and even death. Serious sequelae such as paralysis, confusion, and seizures are likely only at phosphate concentrations <0.25 mmol/L (<0.8 mg/dL). Rhabdomyolysis may develop during rapidly progressive hypophosphatemia. The diagnosis of hypophosphatemia-induced rhabdomyolysis may be overlooked, as up to 30% of patients with acute hypophosphatemia (<0.7 m*M*) have creatine phosphokinase elevations that peak 1–2 days after the nadir in serum phosphate, when the release of phosphate from injured myocytes may have led to a near normalization of circulating levels of phosphate.

Respiratory failure and cardiac dysfunction, which are reversible with phosphate treatment, may occur at serum phosphate levels of 0.5–0.8 mmol/L (1.5–2.5 mg/dL). Renal tubular defects, including tubular acidosis, glycosuria, and impaired reabsorption of sodium and calcium, may occur. Hematologic abnormalities correlate with reductions in intracellular ATP and 2,3-diphosphoglycerate and may include erythrocyte microspherocytosis and hemolysis; impaired oxyhemoglobin dissociation; defective leukocyte chemotaxis, phagocytosis, and bacterial killing; and platelet dysfunction with spontaneous gastrointestinal hemorrhage.

TREATMENT HYPOPHOSPHATEMIA

Severe hypophosphatemia (<0.75 mmol/L [<2 mg/dL]), particularly in the setting of underlying phosphate depletion, constitutes a dangerous electrolyte abnormality that should be corrected promptly. Unfortunately, the cumulative deficit in body phosphate cannot be predicted easily from knowledge of the circulating level of phosphate, and therapy must be approached empirically. The threshold for IV phosphate therapy and the dose administered should reflect consideration of renal function, the likely severity and duration of the underlying phosphate depletion, and the presence and severity of symptoms consistent with those of hypophosphatemia. In adults, phosphate may be safely administered IV as neutral mixtures of sodium or potassium phosphate salts at initial doses of 0.2–0.8 mmol/kg of elemental phosphorus over 6 h (e.g., 10–50 mmol over 6 h), with doses >20 mmol/6 h reserved for those who have serum levels <0.5 mmol/L (1.5 mg/dL) and normal renal function. A suggested approach is presented in Table 423-2. Serum levels of phosphate and calcium must be monitored closely (every 6–12 h) throughout treatment. It is necessary to avoid a serum calcium-phosphorus product >50 to reduce the risk of heterotopic calcification. Hypocalcemia, if present, should be corrected before administering IV phosphate. Less severe hypophosphatemia, in the range of 0.5–0.8 mmol/L (1.5–2.5 mg/dL), usually can be treated with oral phosphate in divided doses of 750–2000 mg/d as elemental phosphorus; higher doses can cause bloating and diarrhea.

Management of chronic hypophosphatemia requires knowledge of the cause(s) of the disorder. Hypophosphatemia related to the secondary hyperparathyroidism of vitamin D deficiency usually responds to treatment with vitamin D and calcium alone. XLH, ADHR, TIO, and related renal tubular disorders usually are managed with divided oral doses of phosphate, often with calcium and $1,25(OH)_2D$ supplements to bypass the block in renal $1,25(OH)_2D$ synthesis and prevent secondary hyperparathyroidism caused by suppression of ECF calcium levels. Thiazide diuretics may be used to prevent nephrocalcinosis in patients who are managed this way. Complete normalization of hypophosphatemia is generally not possible in these conditions. Optimal therapy for TIO is extirpation of the responsible tumor, which may be localized by radiographic skeletal survey or bone scan (many are located in bone) or by radionuclide scanning using sestamibi or labeled octreotide. Successful treatment of TIO-induced hypophosphatemia with octreotide has been reported in a small number of patients.

HYPERPHOSPHATEMIA

Causes When the filtered load of phosphate and glomerular filtration rate (GFR) are normal, control of serum phosphate levels is achieved by adjusting the rate at which phosphate is reabsorbed by the proximal tubular NaPi-2 co-transporters. The principal hormonal regulators of NaPi-2 activity are PTH and FGF23. Hyperphosphatemia, defined in adults as a fasting serum phosphate concentration >1.8 mmol/L (5.5 mg/dL), usually results from impaired glomerular filtration, hypoparathyroidism, excessive delivery of phosphate into the ECF (from bone, gut, or parenteral phosphate therapy), or a combination of these factors (Table 423-3). The upper limit of normal serum phosphate concentrations is higher in children and neonates (2.4 mmol/L [7 mg/dL]). It is useful to distinguish hyperphosphatemia caused by impaired renal phosphate excretion from that which results from excessive delivery of phosphate into the ECF (Table 423-3).

In chronic renal insufficiency, reduced GFR leads to phosphate retention. Hyperphosphatemia in turn further impairs renal synthesis of $1,25(OH)_2D$, increases FGF23 levels, and stimulates PTH secretion and hypertrophy both directly and indirectly (by lowering blood ionized calcium levels). Thus, hyperphosphatemia is a major cause of the secondary hyperparathyroidism of renal failure and must be addressed early in the course of the disease (Chaps. 335 and 424).

Hypoparathyroidism leads to hyperphosphatemia via increased expression of NaPi-2 co-transporters in the proximal tubule. Hypoparathyroidism, or parathyroid suppression, has multiple potential causes, including autoimmune disease; developmental, surgical, or radiation-induced absence of functional parathyroid tissue; vitamin D intoxication or other causes of PTH-independent hypercalcemia; cellular PTH resistance (pseudohypoparathyroidism or hypomagnesemia); infiltrative disorders such as Wilson's disease and hemochromatosis; and impaired PTH secretion caused by hypermagnesemia, severe hypomagnesemia, or activating mutations in the CaSR. Hypocalcemia may also contribute directly to impaired phosphate clearance, as calcium infusion can induce phosphaturia in hypoparathyroid subjects. Increased tubular phosphate reabsorption also occurs in acromegaly, during heparin administration, and in tumoral calcinosis. Tumoral calcinosis is caused by a rare group of genetic disorders in which FGF23 is processed in a way that leads to low levels of active FGF23 in the bloodstream. This may result from mutations in the FGF23 sequence or via inactivating mutations in the *GALNT3* gene, which encodes a galactosaminyl transferase that normally adds sugar residues to FGF23 that slow its proteolysis. A similar syndrome results from FGF23 resistance due to inactivating mutations of the FGF23 co-receptor Klotho. These abnormalities cause elevated serum $1,25(OH)_2D$, parathyroid

TABLE 423-2 INTRAVENOUS THERAPY FOR HYPOPHOSPHATEMIA

Consider

Likely severity of underlying phosphate depletion

Concurrent parenteral glucose administration

Presence of neuromuscular, cardiopulmonary, or hematologic complications of hypophosphatemia

Renal function (reduce dose by 50% if serum creatinine >220 μmol/L [>2.5 mg/dL])

Serum calcium level (correct hypocalcemia first; reduce dose by 50% in hypercalcemia)

Guidelines

Serum Phosphorus, m*M* (mg/dL)	Rate of Infusion, mmol/h	Duration, h	Total Administered, mmol
<0.8 (<2.5)	2	6	12
<0.5 (<1.5)	4	6	24
<0.3 (<1)	8	6	48

Note: Rates shown are calculated for a 70-kg person; levels of serum calcium and phosphorus must be measured every 6–12 h during therapy; infusions can be repeated to achieve stable serum phosphorus levels >0.8 mmol/L (>2.5 mg/dL); most formulations available in the United States provide 3 mmol/mL of sodium or potassium phosphate.

TABLE 423-3 CAUSES OF HYPERPHOSPHATEMIA

I. Impaired renal phosphate excretion
  A. Renal insufficiency
  B. Hypoparathyroidism
    1. Developmental
    2. Autoimmune
    3. After neck surgery or radiation
    4. Activating mutations of the calcium-sensing receptor
  C. Parathyroid suppression
    1. Parathyroid-independent hypercalcemia
      a. Vitamin D or vitamin A intoxication
      b. Sarcoidosis, other granulomatous diseases
      c. Immobilization, osteolytic metastases
      d. Milk-alkali syndrome
    2. Severe hypermagnesemia or hypomagnesemia
  D. Pseudohypoparathyroidism
  E. Acromegaly
  F. Tumoral calcinosis
  G. Heparin therapy
II. Massive extracellular fluid phosphate loads
  A. Rapid administration of exogenous phosphate (intravenous, oral, rectal)
  B. Extensive cellular injury or necrosis
    1. Crush injuries
    2. Rhabdomyolysis
    3. Hyperthermia
    4. Fulminant hepatitis
    5. Cytotoxic therapy
    6. Severe hemolytic anemia
  C. Transcellular phosphate shifts
    1. Metabolic acidosis
    2. Respiratory acidosis

suppression, increased intestinal calcium absorption, and focal hyperostosis with large, lobulated periarticular heterotopic ossifications (especially at shoulders or hips) and are accompanied by hyperphosphatemia. In some forms of tumoral calcinosis, serum phosphorus levels are normal.

When large amounts of phosphate are delivered rapidly into the ECF, hyperphosphatemia can occur despite normal renal function. Examples include overzealous IV phosphate therapy, oral or rectal administration of large amounts of phosphate-containing laxatives or enemas (especially in children), extensive soft tissue injury or necrosis (crush injuries, rhabdomyolysis, hyperthermia, fulminant hepatitis, cytotoxic chemotherapy), extensive hemolytic anemia, and transcellular phosphate shifts induced by severe metabolic or respiratory acidosis.

Clinical Findings The clinical consequences of acute, severe hyperphosphatemia are due mainly to the formation of widespread calcium phosphate precipitates and resulting hypocalcemia. Thus, tetany, seizures, accelerated nephrocalcinosis (with renal failure, hyperkalemia, hyperuricemia, and metabolic acidosis), and pulmonary or cardiac calcifications (including development of acute heart block) may occur. The severity of these complications relates to the elevation of serum phosphate levels, which can reach concentrations as high as 7 mmol/L (20 mg/dL) in instances of massive soft tissue injury or tumor lysis syndrome.

TREATMENT HYPERPHOSPHATEMIA

Therapeutic options for management of severe hyperphosphatemia are limited. Volume expansion may enhance renal phosphate clearance. Aluminum hydroxide antacids or sevelamer may be helpful in chelating and limiting absorption of offending phosphate salts present in the intestine. Hemodialysis is the most effective therapeutic strategy and should be considered early in the course of severe hyperphosphatemia, especially in the setting of renal failure and symptomatic hypocalcemia.

MAGNESIUM METABOLISM

Magnesium is the major intracellular divalent cation. Normal concentrations of extracellular magnesium and calcium are crucial for normal neuromuscular activity. Intracellular magnesium forms a key complex with ATP and is an important cofactor for a wide range of enzymes, transporters, and nucleic acids required for normal cellular function, replication, and energy metabolism. The concentration of magnesium in serum is closely regulated within the range of 0.7–1 mmol/L (1.5–2 meq/L; 1.7–2.4 mg/dL), of which 30% is protein-bound and another 15% is loosely complexed to phosphate and other anions. One-half of the 25 g (1000 mmol) of total body magnesium is located in bone, only one-half of which is insoluble in the mineral phase. Almost all extraskeletal magnesium is present within cells, where the total concentration is 5 m*M*, 95% of which is bound to proteins and other macromolecules. Because only 1% of body magnesium resides in the ECF, measurements of serum magnesium levels may not accurately reflect the level of total body magnesium stores.

Dietary magnesium content normally ranges from 6 to 15 mmol/d (140–360 mg/d), of which 30–40% is absorbed, mainly in the jejunum and ileum. Intestinal magnesium absorptive efficiency is stimulated by 1,25(OH)$_2$D and can reach 70% during magnesium deprivation. Urinary magnesium excretion normally matches net intestinal absorption and is ~4 mmol/d (100 mg/d). Regulation of serum magnesium concentrations is achieved mainly by control of renal magnesium reabsorption. Only 20% of filtered magnesium is reabsorbed in the proximal tubule, whereas 60% is reclaimed in the cTAL and another 5–10% in the DCT. Magnesium reabsorption in the cTAL occurs via a paracellular route that requires both a lumen-positive potential, created by NaCl reabsorption, and tight-junction proteins encoded by members of the Claudin gene family. Magnesium reabsorption in the cTAL is increased by PTH but inhibited by hypercalcemia or hypermagnesemia, both of which activate the CaSR in this nephron segment.

HYPOMAGNESEMIA

Causes Hypomagnesemia usually signifies substantial depletion of body magnesium stores (0.5–1 mmol/kg). Hypomagnesemia can result from intestinal malabsorption; protracted vomiting, diarrhea, or intestinal drainage; defective renal tubular magnesium reabsorption; or rapid shifts of magnesium from the ECF into cells, bone, or third spaces (Table 423-4). Dietary magnesium deficiency is unlikely except possibly in the setting of alcoholism. A rare genetic disorder that causes selective intestinal magnesium malabsorption has been described (primary infantile hypomagnesemia). Another rare inherited disorder (hypomagnesemia with secondary hypocalcemia) is caused by mutations in the gene encoding TRPM6, a protein that, along with TRPM7, forms a channel important for both intestinal and distal-tubular renal transcellular magnesium transport. Malabsorptive states, often compounded by vitamin D deficiency, can critically limit magnesium absorption and produce hypomagnesemia despite the compensatory effects of secondary hyperparathyroidism and of hypocalcemia and hypomagnesemia to enhance cTAL magnesium reabsorption. Diarrhea or surgical drainage fluid may contain ≥5 mmol/L of magnesium. Proton pump inhibitors (omeprazole and others) may produce hypomagnesemia by an unknown mechanism that does not involve renal wasting of magnesium.

Several genetic magnesium-wasting syndromes have been described, including inactivating mutations of genes encoding the DCT NaCl co-transporter (Gitelman's syndrome), proteins required for cTAL Na-K-2Cl transport (Bartter's syndrome), claudin 16 or claudin 19 (autosomal recessive renal hypomagnesemia with hypercalciuria), a DCT Na^+,K^+-ATPase γ-subunit (autosomal dominant renal hypomagnesemia with hypocalciuria), DCT K^+ channels (Kv1.1, Kir4.1), and a mitochondrial gene encoding a tRNA. Activating mutations

TABLE 423-4 CAUSES OF HYPOMAGNESEMIA

I. Impaired intestinal absorption
  A. Hypomagnesemia with secondary hypocalcemia (TRPM6 mutations)
  B. Malabsorption syndromes
  C. Vitamin D deficiency
  D. Proton pump inhibitors
II. Increased intestinal losses
  A. Protracted vomiting/diarrhea
  B. Intestinal drainage, fistulas
III. Impaired renal tubular reabsorption
  A. Genetic magnesium-wasting syndromes
    1. Gitelman's syndrome
    2. Bartter's syndrome
    3. Claudin 16 or 19 mutations
    4. Potassium channel mutations (Kv1.1, Kir4.1)
    5. Na^+,K^+-ATPase γ-subunit mutations (FXYD2)
  B. Acquired renal disease
    1. Tubulointerstitial disease
    2. Postobstruction, ATN (diuretic phase)
    3. Renal transplantation
  C. Drugs and toxins
    1. Ethanol
    2. Diuretics (loop, thiazide, osmotic)
    3. Cisplatin
    4. Pentamidine, foscarnet
    5. Cyclosporine
    6. Aminoglycosides, amphotericin B
    7. Cetuximab
  D. Other
    1. Extracellular fluid volume expansion
    2. Hyperaldosteronism
    3. SIADH
    4. Diabetes mellitus
    5. Hypercalcemia
    6. Phosphate depletion
    7. Metabolic acidosis
    8. Hyperthyroidism
IV. Rapid shifts from extracellular fluid
  A. Intracellular redistribution
    1. Recovery from diabetic ketoacidosis
    2. Refeeding syndrome
    3. Correction of respiratory acidosis
    4. Catecholamines
  B. Accelerated bone formation
    1. Postparathyroidectomy
    2. Treatment of vitamin D deficiency
    3. Osteoblastic metastases
  C. Other
    1. Pancreatitis, burns, excessive sweating
    2. Pregnancy (third trimester) and lactation

Abbreviations: ATN, acute tubular necrosis; SIADH, syndrome of inappropriate antidiuretic hormone.

of the CaSR can cause hypomagnesemia as well as hypocalcemia. ECF expansion, hypercalcemia, and severe phosphate depletion may impair magnesium reabsorption, as can various forms of renal injury, including those caused by drugs such as cisplatin, cyclosporine, aminoglycosides, and pentamidine as well as the epidermal growth factor (EGF) receptor inhibitory antibody, cetuximab (EGF action is required for normal DCT apical expression of TRPM6) (Table 423-4). A rising blood concentration of ethanol directly impairs tubular magnesium reabsorption, and persistent glycosuria with osmotic diuresis leads to magnesium wasting and probably contributes to the high frequency of hypomagnesemia in poorly controlled diabetic patients. Magnesium depletion is aggravated by metabolic acidosis, which causes intracellular losses as well.

Hypomagnesemia due to rapid shifts of magnesium from ECF into the intracellular compartment can occur during recovery from diabetic ketoacidosis, starvation, or respiratory acidosis. Less acute shifts may be seen during rapid bone formation after parathyroidectomy, with treatment of vitamin D deficiency, or with osteoblastic metastases. Large amounts of magnesium may be lost with acute pancreatitis, extensive burns, or protracted and severe sweating and during pregnancy and lactation.

Clinical and Laboratory Findings Hypomagnesemia may cause generalized alterations in neuromuscular function, including tetany, tremor, seizures, muscle weakness, ataxia, nystagmus, vertigo, apathy, depression, irritability, delirium, and psychosis. Patients are usually asymptomatic when serum magnesium concentrations are >0.5 mmol/L (1 meq/L; 1.2 mg/dL), although the severity of symptoms may not correlate with serum magnesium levels. Cardiac arrhythmias may occur, including sinus tachycardia, other supraventricular tachycardias, and ventricular arrhythmias. Electrocardiographic abnormalities may include prolonged PR or QT intervals, T-wave flattening or inversion, and ST straightening. Sensitivity to digitalis toxicity may be enhanced.

Other electrolyte abnormalities often seen with hypomagnesemia, including hypocalcemia (with hypocalciuria) and hypokalemia, may not be easily corrected unless magnesium is administered as well. The hypocalcemia may be a result of concurrent vitamin D deficiency, although hypomagnesemia can cause impaired synthesis of $1,25(OH)_2D$, cellular resistance to PTH, and, at very low serum magnesium (<0.4 mmol/L [0.8 meq/L; <1 mg/dL]), a defect in PTH secretion; these abnormalities are reversible with therapy.

TREATMENT HYPOMAGNESEMIA

Mild, asymptomatic hypomagnesemia may be treated with oral magnesium salts ($MgCl_2$, MgO, $Mg[OH]_2$) in divided doses totaling 20–30 mmol/d (40–60 meq/d). Diarrhea may occur with larger doses. More severe hypomagnesemia should be treated parenterally, preferably with IV $MgCl_2$, which can be administered safely as a continuous infusion of 50 mmol/d (100 meq Mg^{2+}/d) if renal function is normal. If GFR is reduced, the infusion rate should be lowered by 50–75%. Use of IM $MgSO_4$ is discouraged; the injections are painful and provide relatively little magnesium (2 mL of 50% $MgSO_4$ supplies only 4 mmol). $MgSO_4$ may be given IV instead of $MgCl_2$, although the sulfate anions may bind calcium in serum and urine and aggravate hypocalcemia. Serum magnesium should be monitored at intervals of 12–24 h during therapy, which may continue for several days because of impaired renal conservation of magnesium (only 50–70% of the daily IV magnesium dose is retained) and delayed repletion of intracellular deficits, which may be as high as 1–1.5 mmol/kg (2–3 meq/kg).

It is important to consider the need for calcium, potassium, and phosphate supplementation in patients with hypomagnesemia. Vitamin D deficiency frequently coexists and should be treated with oral or parenteral vitamin D or 25(OH)D (but not with $1,25[OH]_2D$, which may impair tubular magnesium reabsorption, possibly via PTH suppression). In severely hypomagnesemic patients with concomitant hypocalcemia and hypophosphatemia, administration of IV magnesium alone may worsen hypophosphatemia, provoking neuromuscular symptoms or rhabdomyolysis, due to rapid stimulation of PTH secretion. This is avoided by administering both calcium and magnesium.

HYPERMAGNESEMIA

Causes Hypermagnesemia is rarely seen in the absence of renal insufficiency, as normal kidneys can excrete large amounts (250 mmol/d) of

TABLE 423-5 CAUSES OF HYPERMAGNESEMIA

I. Excessive magnesium intake
  A. Cathartics, urologic irrigants
  B. Parenteral magnesium administration
II. Rapid mobilization from soft tissues
  A. Trauma, shock, sepsis
  B. Cardiac arrest
  C. Burns
III. Impaired magnesium excretion
  A. Renal failure
  B. Familial hypocalciuric hypercalcemia
IV. Other
  A. Adrenal insufficiency
  B. Hypothyroidism
  C. Hypothermia

magnesium. Mild hypermagnesemia due to excessive reabsorption in the cTAL occurs with CaSR mutations in familial hypocalciuric hypercalcemia and has been described in some patients with adrenal insufficiency, hypothyroidism, or hypothermia. Massive exogenous magnesium exposures, usually via the gastrointestinal tract, can overwhelm renal excretory capacity and cause life-threatening hypermagnesemia (Table 423-5). A notable example of this is prolonged retention of even normal amounts of magnesium-containing cathartics in patients with intestinal ileus, obstruction, or perforation. Extensive soft tissue injury or necrosis can also deliver large amounts of magnesium into the ECF in patients who have suffered trauma, shock, sepsis, cardiac arrest, or severe burns.

Clinical and Laboratory Findings The most prominent clinical manifestations of hypermagnesemia are vasodilation and neuromuscular blockade, which may appear at serum magnesium concentrations >2 mmol/L (>4 meq/L; >4.8 mg/dL). Hypotension that is refractory to vasopressors or volume expansion may be an early sign. Nausea, lethargy, and weakness may progress to respiratory failure, paralysis, and coma, with hypoactive tendon reflexes, at serum magnesium levels >4 mmol/L. Other findings may include gastrointestinal hypomotility or ileus; facial flushing; pupillary dilation; paradoxical bradycardia; prolongation of PR, QRS, and QT intervals; heart block; and, at serum magnesium levels approaching 10 mmol/L, asystole.

Hypermagnesemia, acting via the CaSR, causes hypocalcemia and hypercalciuria due to both parathyroid suppression and impaired cTAL calcium reabsorption.

TREATMENT HYPERMAGNESEMIA

Successful treatment of hypermagnesemia generally involves identifying and interrupting the source of magnesium and employing measures to increase magnesium clearance from the ECF. Use of magnesium-free cathartics or enemas may be helpful in clearing ingested magnesium from the gastrointestinal tract. Vigorous IV hydration should be attempted, if appropriate. Hemodialysis is effective and may be required in patients with significant renal insufficiency. Calcium, administered IV in doses of 100–200 mg over 1–2 h, has been reported to provide temporary improvement in signs and symptoms of hypermagnesemia.

VITAMIN D

SYNTHESIS AND METABOLISM

1,25-Dihydroxyvitamin D (1,25[OH]$_2$D) is the major steroid hormone involved in mineral ion homeostasis regulation. Vitamin D and its metabolites are hormones and hormone precursors rather than vitamins, since in the proper biologic setting, they can be synthesized endogenously (Fig. 423-4). In response to ultraviolet radiation of the skin, a photochemical cleavage results in the formation of vitamin D from 7-dehydrocholesterol. Cutaneous production of vitamin D is decreased by melanin and high solar protection factor sunblocks, which effectively impair skin penetration by ultraviolet light. The increased use of sunblocks in North America and Western Europe and a reduction in the magnitude of solar exposure of the general population over the last several decades has led to an increased reliance on dietary sources of vitamin D. In the United States and Canada, these sources largely consist of fortified cereals and dairy products, in addition to fish oils and egg yolks. Vitamin D from plant sources is in the form of vitamin D$_2$, whereas that from animal sources is vitamin D$_3$. These two forms have equivalent biologic activity and are activated equally well by the vitamin D hydroxylases in humans. Vitamin D enters the circulation, whether absorbed from the intestine or synthesized cutaneously, bound to vitamin D–binding protein, an α-globulin synthesized in the liver. Vitamin D is subsequently 25-hydroxylated in the liver by cytochrome P450–like enzymes in the mitochondria and microsomes. The activity of this hydroxylase is not tightly regulated, and the resultant metabolite, 25-hydroxyvitamin D (25[OH]D), is the major circulating and storage form of vitamin D. Approximately 88% of 25(OH)D circulates bound to the vitamin D–binding protein, 0.03% is free, and the rest circulates bound to albumin. The half-life of 25(OH)D is approximately 2–3 weeks; however, it is shortened dramatically when vitamin D–binding protein levels are reduced, as can occur with increased urinary losses in the nephrotic syndrome.

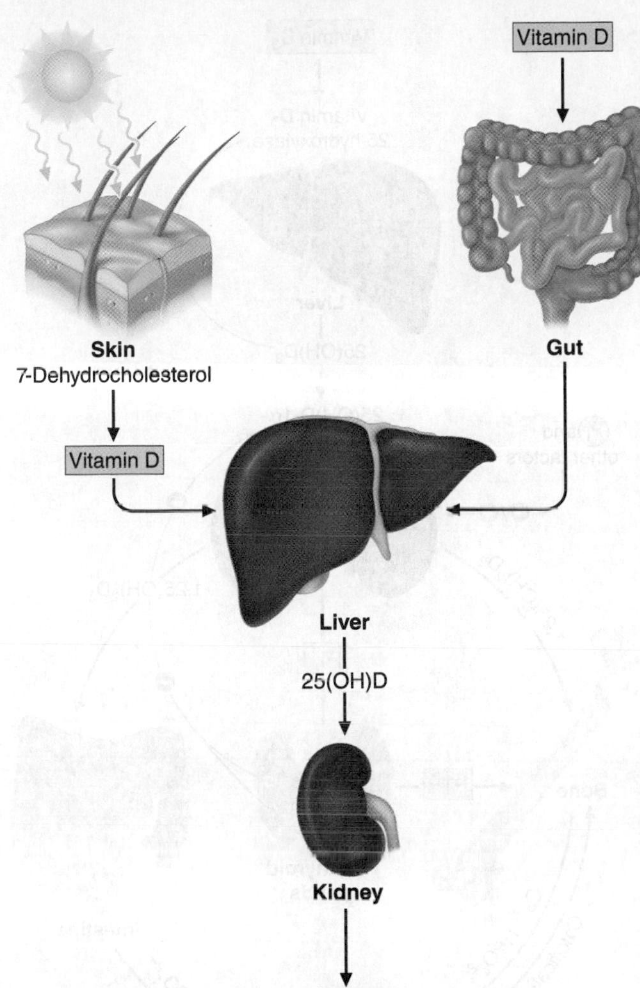

FIGURE 423-4 Vitamin D synthesis and activation. Vitamin D is synthesized in the skin in response to ultraviolet radiation and also is absorbed from the diet. It is then transported to the liver, where it undergoes 25-hydroxylation. This metabolite is the major circulating form of vitamin D. The final step in hormone activation, 1α-hydroxylation, occurs in the kidney.

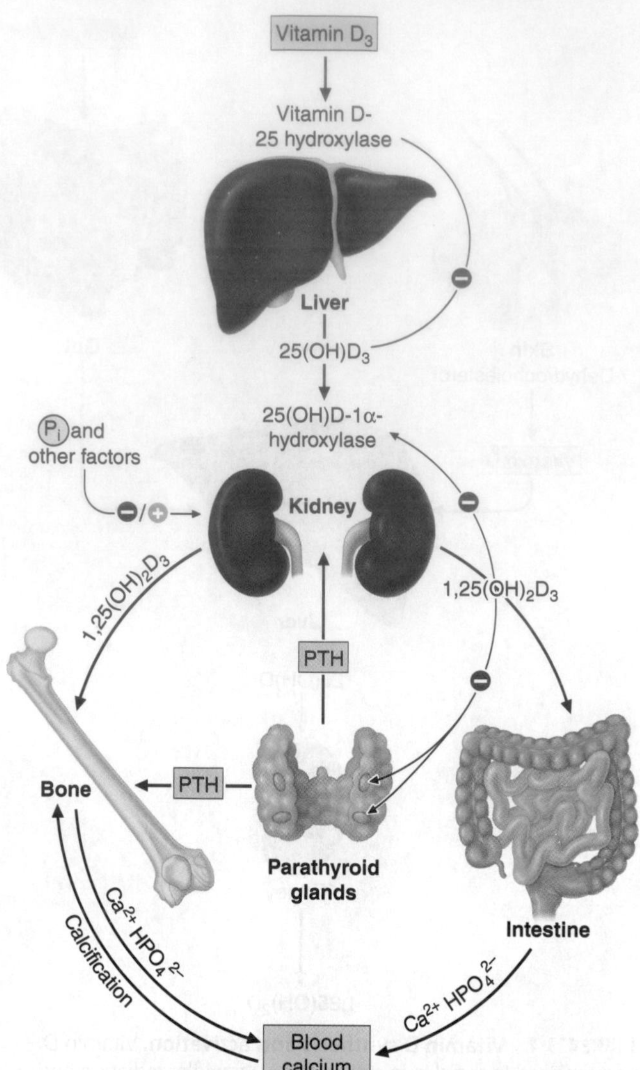

FIGURE 423-5 Schematic representation of the hormonal control loop for vitamin D metabolism and function. A reduction in the serum calcium below ~2.2 mmol/L (8.8 mg/dL) prompts a proportional increase in the secretion of parathyroid hormone (PTH) and so mobilizes additional calcium from the bone. PTH promotes the synthesis of 1,25(OH)$_2$D in the kidney, which in turn stimulates the mobilization of calcium from bone and intestine and regulates the synthesis of PTH by negative feedback.

The second hydroxylation, required for the formation of the mature hormone, occurs in the kidney (Fig. 423-5). The 25-hydroxyvitamin D-1α-hydroxylase is a tightly regulated cytochrome P450–like mixed-function oxidase expressed in the proximal convoluted tubule cells of the kidney. PTH and hypophosphatemia are the major inducers of this microsomal enzyme, whereas calcium, FGF23, and the enzyme's product, 1,25(OH)$_2$D, repress it. The 25-hydroxyvitamin D-1α-hydroxylase is also present in epidermal keratinocytes, but keratinocyte production of 1,25(OH)$_2$D is not thought to contribute to circulating levels of this hormone. In addition to being present in the trophoblastic layer of the placenta, the 1α-hydroxylase is produced by macrophages associated with granulomas and lymphomas. In these latter pathologic states, the activity of the enzyme is induced by interferon γ and TNF-α but is not regulated by calcium or 1,25(OH)$_2$D; therefore, hypercalcemia, associated with elevated levels of 1,25(OH)$_2$D, may be observed. Treatment of sarcoidosis-associated hypercalcemia with glucocorticoids, ketoconazole, or chloroquine reduces 1,25(OH)$_2$D production and effectively lowers serum calcium. In contrast, chloroquine has not been shown to lower the elevated serum 1,25(OH)$_2$D levels in patients with lymphoma.

The major pathway for inactivation of vitamin D metabolites is an additional hydroxylation step by the vitamin D 24-hydroxylase, an enzyme that is expressed in most tissues. 1,25(OH)$_2$D is the major inducer of this enzyme; therefore, this hormone promotes its own inactivation, thereby limiting its biologic effects. Mutations of the gene encoding this enzyme (CYP24A1) can lead to infantile hypercalcemia and, in those less severely affected, long-standing hypercalciuria, nephrocalcinosis, and nephrolithiasis.

Polar metabolites of 1,25(OH)$_2$D are secreted into the bile and reabsorbed via the enterohepatic circulation. Impairment of this recirculation, which is seen with diseases of the terminal ileum, leads to accelerated losses of vitamin D metabolites.

ACTIONS OF 1,25(OH)$_2$D

1,25(OH)$_2$D mediates its biologic effects by binding to a member of the nuclear receptor superfamily, the vitamin D receptor (VDR). This receptor belongs to the subfamily that includes the thyroid hormone receptors, the retinoid receptors, and the peroxisome proliferator–activated receptors; however, in contrast to the other members of this subfamily, only one VDR isoform has been isolated. The VDR binds to target DNA sequences as a heterodimer with the retinoid X receptor, recruiting a series of coactivators that modify chromatin and approximate the VDR to the basal transcriptional apparatus, resulting in the induction of target gene expression. The mechanism of transcriptional repression by the VDR varies with different target genes but has been shown to involve either interference with the action of activating transcription factors or the recruitment of novel proteins to the VDR complex, resulting in transcriptional repression.

The affinity of the VDR for 1,25(OH)$_2$D is approximately three orders of magnitude higher than that for other vitamin D metabolites. In normal physiologic circumstances, these other metabolites are not thought to stimulate receptor-dependent actions. However, in states of vitamin D toxicity, the markedly elevated levels of 25(OH)D may lead to hypercalcemia by interacting directly with the VDR and by displacing 1,25(OH)$_2$D from vitamin D–binding protein, resulting in increased bioavailability of the active hormone.

The VDR is expressed in a wide range of cells and tissues. The molecular actions of 1,25(OH)$_2$D have been studied most extensively in tissues involved in the regulation of mineral ion homeostasis. This hormone is a major inducer of calbindin 9K, a calcium-binding protein expressed in the intestine, which is thought to play an important role in the active transport of calcium across the enterocyte. The two major calcium transporters expressed by intestinal epithelia, TRPV5 and TRPV6 (transient receptor potential vanilloid), are also vitamin D responsive. By inducing the expression of these and other genes in the small intestine, 1,25(OH)$_2$D increases the efficiency of intestinal calcium absorption, and it also has been shown to have several important actions in the skeleton. The VDR is expressed in osteoblasts and regulates the expression of several genes in this cell. These genes include the bone matrix proteins osteocalcin and osteopontin, which are upregulated by 1,25(OH)$_2$D, in addition to type I collagen, which is transcriptionally repressed by 1,25(OH)$_2$D. Both 1,25(OH)$_2$D and PTH induce the expression of RANK ligand, which promotes osteoclast differentiation and increases osteoclast activity, by binding to RANK on osteoclast progenitors and mature osteoclasts. This is the mechanism by which 1,25(OH)$_2$D induces bone resorption. However, the skeletal features associated with VDR-knockout mice (rickets, osteomalacia) are largely corrected by increasing calcium and phosphorus intake, underscoring the importance of vitamin D action in the gut.

The VDR is expressed in the parathyroid gland, and 1,25(OH)$_2$D has been shown to have antiproliferative effects on parathyroid cells and to suppress the transcription of the PTH gene. These effects of 1,25(OH)$_2$D on the parathyroid gland are an important part of the rationale for current therapies directed at preventing and treating hyperparathyroidism associated with renal insufficiency.

The VDR is also expressed in tissues and organs that do not play a role in mineral ion homeostasis. Notable in this respect is the observation that 1,25(OH)$_2$D has an antiproliferative effect on several cell types, including keratinocytes, breast cancer cells, and prostate cancer cells. The effects of $1,25(OH)_2D$ and the VDR on keratinocytes are particularly intriguing. Alopecia is seen in humans and mice with mutant VDRs but is not a feature of vitamin D deficiency; thus, the effects of the VDR on the hair follicle are ligand-independent.

VITAMIN D DEFICIENCY

The mounting concern about the relationship between solar exposure and the development of skin cancer has led to increased reliance on dietary sources of vitamin D. Although the prevalence of vitamin D deficiency varies, the third National Health and Nutrition Examination Survey (NHANES III) revealed that vitamin D deficiency is prevalent throughout the United States. The clinical syndrome of vitamin D deficiency can be a result of deficient production of vitamin D in the skin, lack of dietary intake, accelerated losses of vitamin D, impaired vitamin D activation, or resistance to the biologic effects of $1,25(OH)_2D$ (Table 423-6). The elderly and nursing home residents are particularly at risk for vitamin D deficiency, since both the efficiency of vitamin D synthesis in the skin and the absorption of vitamin D from the intestine decline with age. Similarly, intestinal malabsorption of dietary fats and short bowel syndrome, including that associated with intestinal bypass surgery, can lead to vitamin D deficiency. This is further exacerbated in the presence of terminal ileal disease, which results in impaired enterohepatic circulation of vitamin D metabolites. In addition to intestinal diseases, accelerated inactivation of vitamin D metabolites can be seen with drugs that induce hepatic cytochrome P450 mixed-function oxidases such as barbiturates, phenytoin, and rifampin. Impaired 25-hydroxylation, associated with severe liver disease or isoniazid, is an uncommon cause of vitamin D deficiency. A mutation in the gene responsible for 25-hydroxylation has been identified in one kindred. Impaired 1α-hydroxylation is prevalent in the population with profound renal dysfunction due to an increase in circulating FGF23 levels and a decrease in functional renal mass. Thus, therapeutic interventions should be considered in patients whose creatinine clearance is <0.5 mL/s (30 mL/min). Mutations in the renal 1α-hydroxylase are the basis for the genetic disorder, pseudovitamin D–deficiency rickets. This autosomal recessive disorder presents with the syndrome of vitamin D deficiency in the first year of life. Patients present with growth retardation, rickets, and hypocalcemic seizures. Serum $1,25(OH)_2D$ levels are low despite normal 25(OH)D levels and elevated PTH levels. Treatment with vitamin D metabolites that do not require 1α-hydroxylation results in disease remission, although lifelong therapy is required. A second autosomal recessive disorder, hereditary vitamin D–resistant rickets, a consequence of vitamin D receptor mutations, is a greater therapeutic challenge. These patients present in a similar fashion during the first year of life, but alopecia often accompanies the disorder, demonstrating a functional role of the VDR in postnatal hair regeneration. Serum levels of $1,25(OH)_2D$ are dramatically elevated in these individuals both because of increased production due to stimulation of 1α-hydroxylase activity as a consequence of secondary hyperparathyroidism and because of impaired inactivation, since induction of the 24-hydroxylase by $1,25(OH)_2D$ requires an intact VDR. Because the receptor mutation results in hormone resistance, daily calcium and phosphorus infusions may be required to bypass the defect in intestinal mineral ion absorption.

TABLE 423-6 CAUSES OF IMPAIRED VITAMIN D ACTION

Vitamin D deficiency	Impaired 1α-hydroxylation
Impaired cutaneous production	Hypoparathyroidism
Dietary absence	Renal failure
Malabsorption	Ketoconazole
Accelerated loss of vitamin D	1α-hydroxylase mutation
Increased metabolism (barbiturates, phenytoin, rifampin)	Oncogenic osteomalacia
	X-linked hypophosphatemic rickets
Impaired enterohepatic circulation	Target organ resistance
Nephrotic syndrome	Vitamin D receptor mutation
Impaired 25-hydroxylation	Phenytoin
Liver disease, isoniazid	

Regardless of the cause, the clinical manifestations of vitamin D deficiency are largely a consequence of impaired intestinal calcium absorption. Mild to moderate vitamin D deficiency is asymptomatic, whereas long-standing vitamin D deficiency results in hypocalcemia accompanied by secondary hyperparathyroidism, impaired mineralization of the skeleton (osteopenia on x-ray or decreased bone mineral density), and proximal myopathy. Vitamin D deficiency also has been shown to be associated with an increase in overall mortality, including cardiovascular causes. In the absence of an intercurrent illness, the hypocalcemia associated with long-standing vitamin D deficiency rarely presents with acute symptoms of hypocalcemia such as numbness, tingling, and seizures. However, the concurrent development of hypomagnesemia, which impairs parathyroid function, or the administration of potent bisphosphonates, which impair bone resorption, can lead to acute symptomatic hypocalcemia in vitamin D–deficient individuals.

Rickets and Osteomalacia In children, before epiphyseal fusion, vitamin D deficiency results in growth retardation associated with an expansion of the growth plate known as *rickets*. Three layers of chondrocytes are present in the normal growth plate: the reserve zone, the proliferating zone, and the hypertrophic zone. Rickets associated with impaired vitamin D action is characterized by expansion of the hypertrophic chondrocyte layer. The proliferation and differentiation of the chondrocytes in the rachitic growth plate are normal, and the expansion of the growth plate is a consequence of impaired apoptosis of the late hypertrophic chondrocytes, an event that precedes replacement of these cells by osteoblasts during endochondral bone formation. Investigations in murine models demonstrate that hypophosphatemia, which in vitamin D deficiency is a consequence of secondary hyperparathyroidism, is a key etiologic factor in the development of the rachitic growth plate.

The hypocalcemia and hypophosphatemia that accompany vitamin D deficiency result in impaired mineralization of bone matrix proteins, a condition known as *osteomalacia*. Osteomalacia is also a feature of long-standing hypophosphatemia, which may be a consequence of renal phosphate wasting or chronic use of etidronate or phosphate-binding antacids. This hypomineralized matrix is biomechanically inferior to normal bone; as a result, patients with vitamin D deficiency are prone to bowing of weight-bearing extremities and skeletal fractures. Vitamin D and calcium supplementation have been shown to decrease the incidence of hip fracture among ambulatory nursing home residents in France, suggesting that undermineralization of bone contributes significantly to morbidity in the elderly. Proximal myopathy is a striking feature of severe vitamin D deficiency both in children and in adults. Rapid resolution of the myopathy is observed upon vitamin D treatment.

Although vitamin D deficiency is the most common cause of rickets and osteomalacia, many disorders lead to inadequate mineralization of the growth plate and bone. Calcium deficiency without vitamin D deficiency, the disorders of vitamin D metabolism previously discussed, and hypophosphatemia can all lead to inefficient mineralization. Even in the presence of normal calcium and phosphate levels, chronic acidosis and drugs such as bisphosphonates can lead to osteomalacia. The inorganic calcium/phosphate mineral phase of bone cannot form at low pH, and bisphosphonates bind to and prevent mineral crystal growth. Because alkaline phosphatase is necessary for normal mineral deposition, probably because the enzyme can hydrolyze inhibitors of mineralization such as inorganic pyrophosphate, genetic inactivation of the alkaline phosphatase gene (hereditary hypophosphatasia) also can lead to osteomalacia in the setting of normal calcium and phosphate levels.

Diagnosis of Vitamin D Deficiency, Rickets, and Osteomalacia The most specific screening test for vitamin D deficiency in otherwise healthy individuals is a serum 25(OH)D level. Although the normal ranges vary, levels of 25(OH)D <37 nmol/L (<15 ng/mL) are associated with increasing PTH levels and lower bone density. The Institute of Medicine has defined vitamin D sufficiency as a vitamin D level >50 nmol/L (>20 ng/mL), although higher levels may be required to optimize intestinal calcium absorption in the elderly and those with underlying disease states. Vitamin D deficiency leads to impaired intestinal absorption of calcium, resulting in decreased serum total and ionized calcium values. This hypocalcemia results in secondary hyperparathyroidism, a homeostatic response that initially maintains serum calcium levels at the expense of the skeleton. Due to the PTH-induced increase in bone turnover, alkaline phosphatase levels are often increased. In addition to increasing bone resorption, PTH decreases urinary calcium excretion while promoting phosphaturia. This results in hypophosphatemia, which exacerbates the mineralization defect in the skeleton. With prolonged vitamin D deficiency resulting in osteomalacia, calcium stores in the skeleton become relatively inaccessible, since osteoclasts cannot resorb unmineralized osteoid, and frank hypocalcemia ensues. Because PTH is a major stimulus for the renal 25(OH)D 1α-hydroxylase, there is increased synthesis of the active hormone, $1,25(OH)_2D$. Paradoxically, levels of this hormone are often normal in severe vitamin D deficiency. Therefore, measurements of $1,25(OH)_2D$ are not accurate reflections of vitamin D stores and should not be used to diagnose vitamin D deficiency in patients with normal renal function.

Radiologic features of vitamin D deficiency in children include a widened, expanded growth plate that is characteristic of rickets. These findings not only are apparent in the long bones but also are present at the costochondral junction, where the expansion of the growth plate leads to swellings known as the "rachitic rosary." Impairment of intramembranous bone mineralization leads to delayed fusion of the calvarial sutures and a decrease in the radiopacity of cortical bone in the long bones. If vitamin D deficiency occurs after epiphyseal fusion, the main radiologic finding is a decrease in cortical thickness and relative radiolucency of the skeleton. A specific radiologic feature of osteomalacia, whether associated with phosphate wasting or vitamin D deficiency, is pseudofractures, or Looser's zones. These are radiolucent lines that occur where large arteries are in contact with the underlying skeletal elements; it is thought that the arterial pulsations lead to the radiolucencies. As a result, these pseudofractures are usually a few millimeters wide, are several centimeters long, and are seen particularly in the scapula, the pelvis, and the femoral neck.

TREATMENT VITAMIN D DEFICIENCY

Based on the Institute of Medicine 2010 report, the recommended daily intake of vitamin D is 600 IU from 1 to 70 years of age, and 800 IU for those over 70. Based on the observation that 800 IU of vitamin D, with calcium supplementation, decreases the risk of hip fractures in elderly women, this higher dose is thought to be an appropriate daily intake for prevention of vitamin D deficiency in adults. The safety margin for vitamin D is large, and vitamin D toxicity usually is observed only in patients taking doses in the range of 40,000 IU daily. Treatment of vitamin D deficiency should be directed at the underlying disorder, if possible, and also should be tailored to the severity of the condition. Vitamin D should always be repleted in conjunction with calcium supplementation because most of the consequences of vitamin D deficiency are a result of impaired mineral ion homeostasis. In patients in whom 1α-hydroxylation is impaired, metabolites that do not require this activation step are the treatment of choice. They include $1,25(OH)_2D_3$ (calcitriol [Rocaltrol], 0.25–0.5 μg/d) and 1α-hydroxyvitamin D_2 (Hectorol, 2.5–5 μg/d). If the pathway required for activation of vitamin D is intact, severe vitamin D deficiency can be treated with pharmacologic repletion initially (50,000 IU weekly for 3–12 weeks), followed by maintenance therapy (800 IU daily). Pharmacologic doses may be required for maintenance therapy in patients who are taking medications, such as barbiturates or phenytoin, that accelerate metabolism of or cause resistance to $1,25(OH)_2D$. Calcium supplementation should include 1.5–2 g/d of elemental calcium. Normocalcemia is usually observed within 1 week of the institution of therapy, although increases in PTH and alkaline phosphatase levels may persist for 3–6 months. The most efficacious methods to monitor treatment and resolution of vitamin D deficiency are serum and urinary calcium measurements. In patients who are vitamin D replete and are taking adequate calcium supplementation, the 24-h urinary calcium excretion should be in the range of 100–250 mg/24 h. Lower levels suggest problems with adherence to the treatment regimen or with absorption of calcium or vitamin D supplements. Levels >250 mg/24 h predispose to nephrolithiasis and should lead to a reduction in vitamin D dosage and/or calcium supplementation.

424 Disorders of the Parathyroid Gland and Calcium Homeostasis

John T. Potts, Jr., Harald Jüppner

The four parathyroid glands are located posterior to the thyroid gland. They produce parathyroid hormone (PTH), which is the primary regulator of calcium physiology. PTH acts directly on bone, where it induces calcium release; on the kidney, where it enhances calcium reabsorption in the distal tubules; and in the proximal renal tubules, where it synthesizes 1,25-dihydroxyvitamin D ($1,25[OH]_2D$), a hormone that increases gastrointestinal calcium absorption. Serum PTH levels are tightly regulated by a negative feedback loop. Calcium, acting through the calcium-sensing receptor, and vitamin D, acting through its nuclear receptor, reduce PTH release and synthesis. Additional evidence indicates that fibroblast growth factor 23 (FGF23), a phosphaturic hormone, can suppress PTH secretion. Understanding the hormonal pathways that regulate calcium levels and bone metabolism is essential for effective diagnosis and management of a wide array of hyper- and hypocalcemic disorders.

Hyperparathyroidism, characterized by excess production of PTH, is a common cause of hypercalcemia and is usually the result of autonomously functioning adenomas or hyperplasia. Surgery for this disorder is highly effective and has been shown to reverse some of the deleterious effects of long-standing PTH excess on bone density. Humoral hypercalcemia of malignancy is also common and is usually due to the overproduction of parathyroid hormone–related peptide (PTHrP) by cancer cells. The similarities in the biochemical characteristics of hyperparathyroidism and humoral hypercalcemia of malignancy, first noted by Albright in 1941, are now known to reflect the actions of PTH and PTHrP through the same G protein–coupled PTH/PTHrP receptor.

The genetic basis of multiple endocrine neoplasia (MEN) types 1 and 2, familial hypocalciuric hypercalcemia (FHH), different forms of pseudohypoparathyroidism, Jansen's syndrome, disorders of vitamin D synthesis and action, and the molecular events associated with parathyroid gland neoplasia have provided new insights into the regulation of calcium homeostasis. PTH and *possibly some* of its analogues are promising therapeutic agents for the treatment of postmenopausal or senile osteoporosis, and calcimimetic agents, which activate the calcium-sensing receptor, have provided new approaches for PTH suppression.

PARATHYROID HORMONE

PHYSIOLOGY

The primary function of PTH is to maintain the extracellular fluid (ECF) calcium concentration within a narrow normal range. The hormone acts directly on bone and kidney and indirectly on the intestine through its effects on synthesis of $1,25(OH)_2D$ to increase serum calcium concentrations; in turn, PTH production is closely regulated by the concentration of serum ionized calcium. This feedback system is the critical homeostatic mechanism for maintenance of ECF calcium. Any tendency toward hypocalcemia, as might be induced by calcium- or vitamin D–deficient diets, is counteracted by an increased secretion of PTH. This in turn (1) increases the rate of dissolution of bone mineral, thereby increasing the flow of calcium from bone into blood; (2) reduces the renal clearance of calcium, returning more of the calcium and phosphate filtered at the glomerulus into ECF; and (3) increases the efficiency of calcium absorption in the intestine by stimulating the production of 1,25(OH)$_2$D. Immediate control of blood calcium is due to PTH effects on bone and, to a lesser extent, on renal calcium clearance. Maintenance of steady-state calcium balance, on the other hand, probably results from the effects of 1,25(OH)$_2$D on calcium absorption (Chap. 423). The renal actions of the hormone are exerted at multiple sites and include inhibition of phosphate transport (proximal tubule), augmentation of calcium reabsorption (distal tubule), and stimulation of the renal 25(OH)D-1α-hydroxylase. As much as 12 mmol (500 mg) of calcium is transferred between the ECF and bone each day (a large amount in relation to the total ECF calcium pool), and PTH has a major effect on this transfer. The homeostatic role of the hormone can preserve calcium concentration in blood at the cost of bone demineralization.

PTH has multiple actions on bone, some direct and some indirect. PTH-mediated changes in bone calcium release can be seen within minutes. The chronic effects of PTH are to increase the number of bone cells, both osteoblasts and osteoclasts, and to increase the remodeling of bone; these effects are apparent within hours after the hormone is given and persist for hours after PTH is withdrawn. Continuous exposure to elevated PTH (as in hyperparathyroidism or long-term infusions in animals) leads to increased osteoclast-mediated bone resorption. However, the intermittent administration of PTH, elevating hormone levels for 1–2 h each day, leads to a net stimulation of bone formation rather than bone breakdown. Striking increases, especially in trabecular bone in the spine and hip, have been reported with the use of PTH in combination with estrogen. PTH(1–34) as monotherapy caused a highly significant reduction in fracture incidence in a worldwide placebo-controlled trial.

Osteoblasts (or stromal cell precursors), which have PTH/PTHrP receptors, are crucial to this bone-forming effect of PTH; osteoclasts, which mediate bone breakdown, lack such receptors. PTH-mediated stimulation of osteoclasts is indirect, acting in part through cytokines released from osteoblasts to activate osteoclasts; in experimental studies of bone resorption in vitro, osteoblasts must be present for PTH to activate osteoclasts to resorb bone (Chap. 423).

STRUCTURE

PTH is an 84-amino-acid single-chain peptide. The amino-terminal portion, PTH(1–34), is highly conserved and is critical for the biologic actions of the molecule. Modified synthetic fragments of the amino-terminal sequence as small as PTH(1–11) are sufficient to activate the PTH/PTHrP receptor (see below). The carboxyl-terminal region of the full-length PTH(1–84) molecule also can bind to a separate binding protein/receptor (cPTH-R), but this receptor has been incompletely characterized. Fragments shortened at the amino-terminus possibly by binding to cPTH-R can reduce, directly or indirectly, some of the biologic actions of full-length PTH(1–84) and of PTH(1–34).

BIOSYNTHESIS, SECRETION, AND METABOLISM

Synthesis Parathyroid cells have multiple methods of adapting to increased needs for PTH production. Most rapid (within minutes) is secretion of preformed hormone in response to hypocalcemia. Second, within hours, PTH mRNA expression is induced by sustained hypocalcemia. Finally, protracted challenge leads within days to cellular replication to increase parathyroid gland mass.

PTH is initially synthesized as a larger molecule (preproparathyroid hormone, consisting of 115 amino acids). After a first cleavage step to remove the "pre" sequence of 25 amino acid residues, a second cleavage step removes the "pro" sequence of 6 amino acid residues before secretion of the mature peptide comprising 84 residues. Mutations in the preprotein region of the gene can cause hypoparathyroidism by interfering with hormone synthesis, transport, or secretion.

Transcriptional suppression of the PTH gene by calcium is nearly maximal at physiologic calcium concentrations. Hypocalcemia increases transcriptional activity within hours. 1,25(OH)$_2$D strongly suppresses PTH gene transcription. In patients with renal failure, IV administration of supraphysiologic levels of 1,25(OH)$_2$D or analogues of this active metabolite can dramatically suppress PTH overproduction, which is sometimes difficult to control due to severe secondary hyperparathyroidism. Regulation of proteolytic destruction of preformed hormone (posttranslational regulation of hormone production) is an important mechanism for mediating rapid (within minutes) changes in hormone availability. High calcium increases and low calcium inhibit the proteolytic destruction of stored hormone.

Regulation of PTH Secretion PTH secretion increases steeply to a maximum value of about five times the basal rate of secretion as the calcium concentration falls from normal to the range of 1.9–2.0 mmol/L (7.6–8.0 mg/dL; measured as total calcium). However, the ionized fraction of blood calcium is the important determinant of hormone secretion. Severe intracellular magnesium deficiency impairs PTH secretion (see below).

ECF calcium controls PTH secretion by interaction with a calcium-sensing receptor (CaSR), a G protein–coupled receptor (GPCR) for which Ca^{2+} ions act as the primary ligand (see below). This receptor is a member of a distinctive subgroup of the GPCR superfamily that mediates its actions through the alpha-subunits of two related signaling G proteins, namely Gq and G11, and is characterized by a large extracellular domain suitable for "clamping" the small-molecule ligand. Stimulation of the CaSR by high calcium levels suppresses PTH secretion. The CaSR is present in parathyroid glands and the calcitonin-secreting cells of the thyroid (C cells), as well as in multiple other sites, including brain and kidney. Genetic evidence has revealed a key biologic role for the CaSR in parathyroid gland responsiveness to calcium and in renal calcium clearance. Heterozygous loss-of-function mutations in CaSR cause the syndrome of FHH, in which the blood calcium abnormality resembles that observed in hyperparathyroidism but with hypocalciuria; two more recently defined variants of FHH, FHH2 and FHH3, are caused either by heterozygous mutations in G11, one of the signaling proteins downstream of the CaSR, or by heterozygous mutations in *AP2S1*. Homozygous loss-of-function mutations in the CaSR are the cause of severe neonatal hyperparathyroidism, a disorder that can be lethal if not treated within the first days of life. On the other hand, heterozygous gain-of-function mutations cause a form of hypocalcemia resembling hypoparathyroidism (see below).

Metabolism The secreted form of PTH is indistinguishable by immunologic criteria and by molecular size from the 84-amino-acid peptide (PTH[1–84]) extracted from glands. However, much of the immunoreactive material found in the circulation is smaller than the extracted or secreted hormone. The principal circulating fragments of immunoreactive hormone lack a portion of the critical amino-terminal sequence required for biologic activity and, hence, are biologically inactive fragments (so-called middle and carboxyl-terminal fragments). Much of the proteolysis of the hormone occurs in the liver and kidney. Peripheral metabolism of PTH does not appear to be regulated by physiologic states (high versus low calcium, etc.); hence, peripheral metabolism of hormone, although responsible for rapid clearance of secreted hormone, appears to be a high-capacity, metabolically invariant catabolic process.

The rate of clearance of the secreted 84-amino-acid peptide from blood is more rapid than the rate of clearance of the biologically inactive fragment(s) corresponding to the middle and carboxyl-terminal regions of PTH. Consequently, the interpretation of results obtained with earlier PTH radioimmunoassays was influenced by the nature of the peptide fragments detected by the antibodies.

Although the problems inherent in PTH measurements have been largely circumvented by use of double-antibody immunometric assays, it is now known that some of these assays detect, besides the intact molecule, large amino-terminally truncated forms of PTH, which are present in normal and uremic individuals in addition to PTH(1–84). The concentration of these fragments relative to that of intact PTH(1–84) is higher with induced hypercalcemia than in eucalcemic or hypocalcemic conditions and is higher in patients with impaired renal function. PTH(7–84) has been identified as a major component of these amino-terminally truncated fragments. Growing evidence suggests that the PTH(7–84) (and probably related amino-terminally truncated fragments) can act, through yet undefined mechanisms, as an inhibitor of PTH action and may be of clinical significance, particularly in patients with chronic kidney disease. In this group of patients, efforts to prevent secondary hyperparathyroidism by a variety of measures (vitamin D analogues, higher calcium intake, higher dialysate calcium, phosphate-lowering strategies, and calcimetic drugs) can lead to oversuppression of the parathyroid glands since some amino-terminally truncated PTH fragments, such as PTH(7–84), react in many immunometric PTH assays (now termed second-generation assays; see below under "Diagnosis"), thus overestimating the levels of biologically active, intact PTH. Such excessive parathyroid gland suppression in chronic kidney disease can lead to adynamic bone disease (see below), which has been associated with further impaired growth in children and increased bone fracture rates in adults, and can furthermore lead to significant hypercalcemia. The measurement of PTH with newer third-generation immunoassays, which use detection antibodies directed against extreme amino-terminal PTH epitopes and thus detect only full-length PTH(1–84), may provide some advantage to prevent bone disease in chronic kidney disease.

PARATHYROID HORMONE–RELATED PROTEIN (PTHrP)

PTHrP is responsible for most instances of humoral hypercalcemia of malignancy (Chap. 121), a syndrome that resembles primary hyperparathyroidism but without elevated PTH levels. Most cell types normally produce PTHrP, including brain, pancreas, heart, lung, mammary tissue, placenta, endothelial cells, and smooth muscle. In fetal animals, PTHrP directs transplacental calcium transfer, and high concentrations of PTHrP are produced in mammary tissue and secreted into milk, but the biologic significance of the very high concentrations of this hormone in breast milk is unknown. PTHrP also plays an essential role in endochondral bone formation and in branching morphogenesis of the breast, and possibly in uterine contraction and other biologic functions.

PTH and PTHrP, although products of different genes, exhibit considerable functional and structural homology (Fig. 424-1) and have evolved from a shared ancestral gene. The structure of the gene encoding human PTHrP, however, is more complex than that of PTH, containing multiple additional exons, which can undergo alternate splicing patterns during formation of the mature mRNA. Protein products of 139, 141, and 173 amino acids are produced, and other molecular forms may result from tissue-specific degradation at accessible internal cleavage sites. The biologic roles of these various molecular species and the nature of the circulating forms of PTHrP are unclear. In fact, it is uncertain whether PTHrP circulates at any significant level in adults. As a paracrine factor, PTHrP may be produced, act, and be destroyed locally within tissues. In adults, PTHrP appears to have little influence on calcium homeostasis, except in disease states, when large tumors, especially of the squamous cell type as well as renal cell carcinomas, lead to massive overproduction of the hormone and hypercalcemia.

PTH AND PTHrP HORMONE ACTION

Both PTH and PTHrP bind to and activate the PTH/PTHrP receptor. The PTH/PTHrP receptor (also known as the PTH-1 receptor, PTH1R) belongs to a subfamily of GPCRs that includes the receptors for calcitonin, glucagon, secretin, vasoactive intestinal peptide, and other peptides. Although both ligands activate the PTH1R, the two peptides induce distinct responses in the receptor, which explains how a single receptor without isoforms can serve two biologic roles. The extracellular regions of the receptor are involved in hormone binding, and the intracellular domains, after hormone activation, bind G protein subunits to transduce hormone signaling into cellular responses through the stimulation of second messenger formation. A second receptor that binds PTH, originally termed the *PTH-2 receptor* (PTH2R), is primarily expressed in brain, pancreas, and testis. Different mammalian PTH1Rs respond equivalently to PTH and PTHrP, at least when tested with traditional assays, whereas only the human PTH2R responds efficiently to PTH (but not to PTHrP). PTH2Rs from other species show little or no stimulation of second-messenger formation in response to PTH or PTHrP. The endogenous ligand of the PTH2R was shown to be a hypothalamic peptide referred to as tubular infundibular peptide of 39 residues, TIP39, that is distantly related to PTH and PTHrP. The PTH1R and the PTH2R can be traced backward in evolutionary time to fish; in fact, the zebrafish genome contains, in addition to the PTH1R and the PTH2R orthologs, a third receptor, the PTH3R, that is more closely related to the fish PTH1R than to the fish PTH2R. The evolutionary conservation of structure and function suggests important biologic roles for these receptors, even in fish, which lack discrete parathyroid glands but produce two molecules that are closely related to mammalian PTH.

Studies using the cloned PTH1R confirm that it can be coupled to more than one G protein and second-messenger pathway, apparently explaining the multiplicity of pathways stimulated by PTH. Activation of protein kinases (A and C) and calcium transport channels is associated with a variety of hormone-specific tissue responses. These responses include inhibition of phosphate and bicarbonate transport, stimulation of calcium transport, and activation of renal 1α-hydroxylase in the kidney. The responses in bone include effects on collagen synthesis, alkaline phosphatase, ornithine decarboxylase, citrate decarboxylase, and glucose-6-phosphate dehydrogenase activities; phospholipid synthesis; and calcium and phosphate transport. Ultimately, these biochemical events lead to an integrated hormonal response in bone turnover and calcium homeostasis. PTH also activates Na^+/Ca^{2+} exchangers at renal distal tubular sites and stimulates translocation of preformed calcium transport channels, moving them from the interior to the apical surface to increase tubular uptake of calcium. PTH-dependent stimulation of phosphate excretion (reducing reabsorption—the opposite effect from actions on calcium in the kidney) involves the downregulation of two sodium-dependent phosphate co-transporters, NPT2a and NPT2c, and their expression at the apical membrane, thereby reducing phosphate reabsorption in

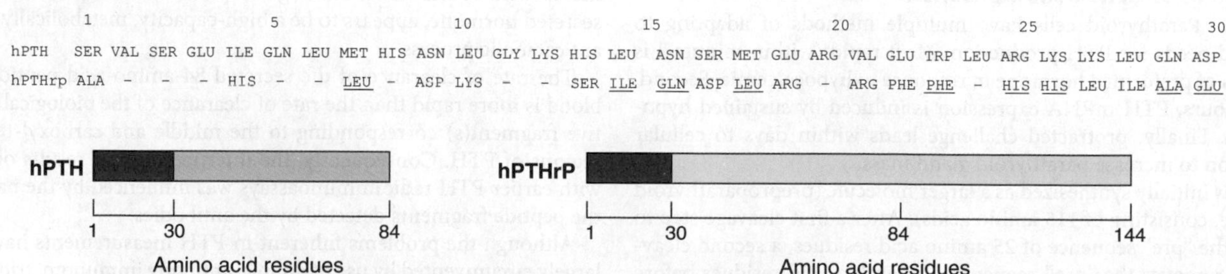

FIGURE 424-1 Schematic diagram to illustrate similarities and differences in structure of human parathyroid hormone (PTH) and human PTH-related peptide (PTHrP). Close structural (and functional) homology exists between the first 30 amino acids of hPTH and hPTHrP. The PTHrP sequence may be ≥144 amino acid residues in length. PTH is only 84 residues long; after residue 30, there is little structural homology between the two. *Dashed lines* in the PTHrP sequence indicate identity; *underlined residues*, although different from those of PTH, still represent conservative changes (charge or polarity preserved). Ten amino acids are identical, and a total of 20 of 30 are homologues.

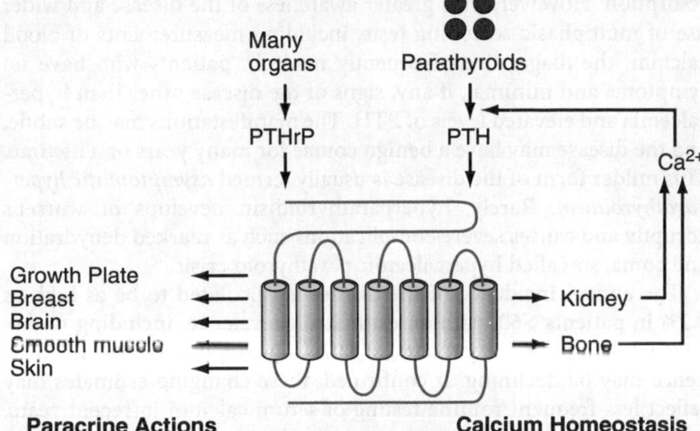

FIGURE 424-2 Dual role for the actions of the PTH/PTHrP receptor (PTH1R). Parathyroid hormone (PTH; endocrine-calcium homeostasis) and PTH-related peptide (PTHrP; paracrine–multiple tissue actions including growth plate cartilage in developing bone) use the single receptor for their disparate functions mediated by the amino-terminal 34 residues of either peptide. Other regions of both ligands interact with other receptors (not shown).

the proximal renal tubules. Similar mechanisms may be involved in other renal tubular transporters that are influenced by PTH. Recent studies reaffirm the critical linkage of blood phosphate lowering to net calcium entry into blood by PTH action and emphasize the participation of bone cells other than osteoclasts in the rapid calcium-elevating actions of PTH.

PTHrP exerts important developmental influences on fetal bone development and in adult physiology. A homozygous ablation of the gene encoding PTHrP (or disruption of the PTH1R gene) in mice causes a lethal phenotype in which animals are born with pronounced acceleration of chondrocyte maturation that resembles a lethal form of chondrodysplasia in humans that is caused by homozygous or compound heterozygous, inactivating PTH1R mutations (Fig. 424-2). Heterozygous PTH1R mutations in humans furthermore can be a cause of delayed tooth eruption, and mice that are heterozygous for ablation of the PTHrP gene display reduced mineral density consistent with osteoporosis. Experiments with these mouse models point to a hitherto unappreciated role of PTHrP as a paracrine/autocrine factor that modulates bone metabolism in adults as well as during bone development.

CALCITONIN

(See also Chap. 408) Calcitonin is a hypocalcemic peptide hormone that in several mammalian species acts as an indirect antagonist to the calcemic actions of PTH. Calcitonin seems to be of limited physiologic significance in humans, at least with regard to calcium homeostasis. It is of medical significance because of its role as a tumor marker in sporadic and hereditary cases of medullary carcinoma and its medical use as an adjunctive treatment in severe hypercalcemia and in Paget's disease of bone.

The hypocalcemic activity of calcitonin is accounted for primarily by inhibition of osteoclast-mediated bone resorption and secondarily by stimulation of renal calcium clearance. These effects are mediated by receptors on osteoclasts and renal tubular cells. Calcitonin exerts additional effects through receptors present in the brain, the gastrointestinal tract, and the immune system. The hormone, for example, exerts analgesic effects directly on cells in the hypothalamus and related structures, possibly by interacting with receptors for related peptide hormones such as calcitonin gene–related peptide (CGRP) or amylin. Both of these ligands have specific high-affinity receptors that share considerable structural similarity with the PTH1R and can also bind to and activate calcitonin receptors. The calcitonin receptor shares considerable structural similarity with the PTH1R.

The thyroid is the major source of the hormone, and the cells involved in calcitonin synthesis arise from neural crest tissue. During embryogenesis, these cells migrate into the ultimobranchial body, derived from the last branchial pouch. In submammalian vertebrates, the ultimobranchial body constitutes a discrete organ, anatomically separate from the thyroid gland; in mammals, the ultimobranchial gland fuses with and is incorporated into the thyroid gland.

The naturally occurring calcitonins consist of a peptide chain of 32 amino acids. There is considerable sequence variability among species. Calcitonin from salmon, which is used therapeutically, is 10–100 times more potent than mammalian forms in lowering serum calcium.

There are two calcitonin genes, α and β; the transcriptional control of these genes is complex. Two different mRNA molecules are transcribed from the α gene; one is translated into the precursor for calcitonin, and the other message is translated into an alternative product, CGRP. CGRP is synthesized wherever the calcitonin mRNA is expressed (e.g., in medullary carcinoma of the thyroid). The β, or CGRP-2, gene is transcribed into the mRNA for CGRP in the central nervous system (CNS); this gene does not produce calcitonin, however. CGRP has cardiovascular actions and may serve as a neurotransmitter or play a developmental role in the CNS.

The circulating level of calcitonin in humans is lower than that in many other species. In humans, even extreme variations in calcitonin production do not change calcium and phosphate metabolism; no definite effects are attributable to calcitonin deficiency (totally thyroidectomized patients receiving only replacement thyroxine) or excess (patients with medullary carcinoma of the thyroid, a calcitonin-secreting tumor) (Chap. 408). Calcitonin has been a useful pharmacologic agent to suppress bone resorption in Paget's disease (Chap. 426e) and osteoporosis (Chap. 425) and in the treatment of hypercalcemia of malignancy (see below). However, bisphosphonates are usually more effective, and the physiologic role, if any, of calcitonin in humans is uncertain. On the other hand, ablation of the calcitonin gene (combined because of the close proximity with ablation of the CGRP gene) in mice leads to reduced bone mineral density, suggesting that its biologic role in mammals is still not fully understood.

HYPERCALCEMIA

(See also Chap. 65) Hypercalcemia can be a manifestation of a serious illness such as malignancy or can be detected coincidentally by laboratory testing in a patient with no obvious illness. The number of patients recognized with asymptomatic hypercalcemia, usually hyperparathyroidism, increased in the late twentieth century.

Whenever hypercalcemia is confirmed, a definitive diagnosis must be established. Although hyperparathyroidism, a frequent cause of asymptomatic hypercalcemia, is a chronic disorder in which manifestations, if any, may be expressed only after months or years, hypercalcemia can also be the earliest manifestation of malignancy, the second most common cause of hypercalcemia in the adult. The causes of hypercalcemia are numerous (Table 424-1), but hyperparathyroidism and cancer account for 90% of all cases.

Before undertaking a diagnostic workup, it is essential to be sure that true hypercalcemia, not a false-positive laboratory test, is present. A false-positive diagnosis of hypercalcemia is usually the result of inadvertent hemoconcentration during blood collection or elevation in serum proteins such as albumin. Hypercalcemia is a chronic problem, and it is cost-effective to obtain several serum calcium measurements; these tests need not be in the fasting state.

Clinical features are helpful in differential diagnosis. Hypercalcemia in an adult who is asymptomatic is usually due to primary hyperparathyroidism. In malignancy-associated hypercalcemia, the disease is usually not occult; rather, symptoms of malignancy bring the patient to the physician, and hypercalcemia is discovered during the evaluation. In such patients, the interval between detection of hypercalcemia and death, especially without vigorous treatment, is often <6 months. Accordingly, if an asymptomatic individual has had hypercalcemia or some manifestation of hypercalcemia such as kidney stones for more than 1 or 2 years, it is unlikely that malignancy

TABLE 424-1 CLASSIFICATION OF CAUSES OF HYPERCALCEMIA

I. Parathyroid-Related
- A. Primary hyperparathyroidism
  - 1. Adenoma(s)
  - 2. Multiple endocrine neoplasia
  - 3. Carcinoma
- B. Lithium therapy
- C. Familial hypocalciuric hypercalcemia

II. Malignancy-Related
- A. Solid tumor with metastases (breast)
- B. Solid tumor with humoral mediation of hypercalcemia (lung, kidney)
- C. Hematologic malignancies (multiple myeloma, lymphoma, leukemia)

III. Vitamin D–Related
- A. Vitamin D intoxication
- B. ↑ $1,25(OH)_2D$; sarcoidosis and other granulomatous diseases
- C. ↑ $1,25(OH)_2D$; impaired $1,25(OH)_2D$ metabolism due to 24-hydroxylase deficiency

IV. Associated with High Bone Turnover
- A. Hyperthyroidism
- B. Immobilization
- C. Thiazides
- D. Vitamin A intoxication
- E. Fat necrosis

V. Associated with Renal Failure
- A. Severe secondary hyperparathyroidism
- B. Aluminum intoxication
- C. Milk-alkali syndrome

is the cause. Nevertheless, differentiating primary hyperparathyroidism from occult malignancy can occasionally be difficult, and careful evaluation is required, particularly when the duration of the hypercalcemia is unknown. Hypercalcemia not due to hyperparathyroidism or malignancy can result from excessive vitamin D action, impaired metabolism of $1,25(OH)_2D$, high bone turnover from any of several causes, or renal failure (Table 424-1). Dietary history and a history of ingestion of vitamins or drugs are often helpful in diagnosing some of the less frequent causes. Immunometric PTH assays serve as the principal laboratory test in establishing the diagnosis.

Hypercalcemia from any cause can result in fatigue, depression, mental confusion, anorexia, nausea, vomiting, constipation, reversible renal tubular defects, increased urine output, a short QT interval in the electrocardiogram, and, in some patients, cardiac arrhythmias. There is a variable relation from one patient to the next between the severity of hypercalcemia and the symptoms. Generally, symptoms are more common at calcium levels >2.9–3.0 mmol/L (11.6–12.0 mg/dL), but some patients, even at this level, are asymptomatic. When the calcium level is >3.2 mmol/L (12.8 mg/dL), calcification in kidneys, skin, vessels, lungs, heart, and stomach occurs and renal insufficiency may develop, particularly if blood phosphate levels are normal or elevated due to impaired renal excretion. Severe hypercalcemia, usually defined as ≥3.7–4.5 mmol/L (14.8–18.0 mg/dL), can be a medical emergency; coma and cardiac arrest can occur.

Acute management of the hypercalcemia is usually successful. The type of treatment is based on the severity of the hypercalcemia and the nature of associated symptoms, as outlined below.

PRIMARY HYPERPARATHYROIDISM

Natural History and Incidence Primary hyperparathyroidism is a generalized disorder of calcium, phosphate, and bone metabolism due to an increased secretion of PTH. The elevation of circulating hormone usually leads to hypercalcemia and hypophosphatemia. There is great variation in the manifestations. Patients may present with multiple signs and symptoms, including recurrent nephrolithiasis, peptic ulcers, mental changes, and, less frequently, extensive bone resorption. However, with greater awareness of the disease and wider use of multiphasic screening tests, including measurements of blood calcium, the diagnosis is frequently made in patients who have no symptoms and minimal, if any, signs of the disease other than hypercalcemia and elevated levels of PTH. The manifestations may be subtle, and the disease may have a benign course for many years or a lifetime. This milder form of the disease is usually termed *asymptomatic hyperparathyroidism*. Rarely, hyperparathyroidism develops or worsens abruptly and causes severe complications such as marked dehydration and coma, so-called hypercalcemic parathyroid crisis.

The annual incidence of the disease is calculated to be as high as 0.2% in patients >60, with an estimated prevalence, including undiscovered asymptomatic patients, of ≥1%; some reports suggest the incidence may be declining. If confirmed, these changing estimates may reflect less frequent routine testing of serum calcium in recent years, earlier overestimates in incidence, or unknown factors. The disease has a peak incidence between the third and fifth decades but occurs in young children and in the elderly.

Etiology Parathyroid tumors are most often encountered as isolated adenomas without other endocrinopathy. They may also arise in hereditary syndromes such as MEN syndromes. Parathyroid tumors may also arise as secondary to underlying disease (excessive stimulation in secondary hyperparathyroidism, especially chronic renal failure) or after other forms of excessive stimulation such as lithium therapy. These etiologies are discussed below.

SOLITARY ADENOMAS A single abnormal gland is the cause in ~80% of patients; the abnormality in the gland is usually a benign neoplasm or adenoma and rarely a parathyroid carcinoma. Some surgeons and pathologists report that the enlargement of multiple glands is common; double adenomas are reported. In ~15% of patients, all glands are hyperfunctioning; *chief cell parathyroid hyperplasia* is usually hereditary and frequently associated with other endocrine abnormalities.

HEREDITARY SYNDROMES AND MULTIPLE PARATHYROID TUMORS Hereditary hyperparathyroidism can occur without other endocrine abnormalities but is usually part of a *multiple endocrine neoplasia* (MEN) syndrome (Chap. 408). MEN 1 (Wermer's syndrome) consists of hyperparathyroidism and tumors of the pituitary and pancreas, often associated with gastric hypersecretion and peptic ulcer disease (Zollinger-Ellison syndrome). MEN 2A is characterized by pheochromocytoma and medullary carcinoma of the thyroid, as well as hyperparathyroidism; MEN 2B has additional associated features such as multiple neuromas but usually lacks hyperparathyroidism. Each of these MEN syndromes is transmitted in an apparent autosomal dominant manner, although, as noted below, the genetic basis of MEN 1 involves biallelic loss of a tumor suppressor.

The *hyperparathyroidism jaw tumor* (HPT-JT) syndrome occurs in families with parathyroid tumors (sometimes carcinomas) in association with benign jaw tumors. This disorder is caused by mutations in *CDC73* (*HRPT2*), and mutations in this gene are also observed in parathyroid cancers. Some kindreds exhibit hereditary hyperparathyroidism without other endocrinopathies. This disorder is often termed *nonsyndromic familial isolated hyperparathyroidism* (FIHP). There is speculation that these families may be examples of variable expression of the other syndromes such as MEN 1, MEN 2, or the HPT-JT syndrome, but they may also have distinctive, still unidentified genetic causes.

Pathology Adenomas are most often located in the inferior parathyroid glands, but in 6–10% of patients, parathyroid adenomas may be located in the thymus, the thyroid, the pericardium, or behind the esophagus. Adenomas are usually 0.5–5 g in size but may be as large as 10–20 g (normal glands weigh 25 mg on average). Chief cells are predominant in both hyperplasia and adenoma. With chief cell hyperplasia, the enlargement may be so asymmetric that some involved glands appear grossly normal. If generalized hyperplasia is present, however, histologic examination reveals a uniform pattern of chief cells and disappearance of fat even in the absence of an increase in gland weight. Thus, microscopic examination of biopsy specimens of several glands is essential to interpret findings at surgery.

Parathyroid carcinoma is often not aggressive. Long-term survival without recurrence is common if at initial surgery the entire gland is removed without rupture of the capsule. Recurrent parathyroid carcinoma is usually slow-growing with local spread in the neck, and surgical correction of recurrent disease may be feasible. Occasionally, however, parathyroid carcinoma is more aggressive, with distant metastases (lung, liver, and bone) found at the time of initial operation. It may be difficult to appreciate initially that a primary tumor is carcinoma; increased numbers of mitotic figures and increased fibrosis of the gland stroma may precede invasion. The diagnosis of carcinoma is often made in retrospect. Hyperparathyroidism from a parathyroid carcinoma may be indistinguishable from other forms of primary hyperparathyroidism but is usually more severe clinically. A potential clue to the diagnosis is offered by the degree of calcium elevation. Calcium values of 3.5–3.7 mmol/L (14–15 mg/dL) are frequent with carcinoma and may alert the surgeon to remove the abnormal gland with care to avoid capsular rupture. Recent findings concerning the genetic basis of parathyroid carcinoma (distinct from that of benign adenomas) indicate the need, in these kindreds, for family screening (see below).

GENETIC DEFECTS ASSOCIATED WITH HYPERPARATHYROIDISM

As in many other types of neoplasia, two fundamental types of genetic defects have been identified in parathyroid gland tumors: (1) overactivity of protooncogenes and (2) loss of function of tumor-suppressor genes. The former, by definition, can lead to uncontrolled cellular growth and function by activation (gain-of-function mutation) of a single allele of the responsible gene, whereas the latter requires loss of function of both allelic copies. Biallelic loss of function of a tumor-suppressor gene is usually characterized by a germline defect (all cells) and an additional somatic deletion/mutation in the tumor (Fig. 424-3).

Mutations in the *MEN1* gene locus, encoding the protein MENIN, on chromosome 11q13 are responsible for causing MEN 1; the normal allele of this gene fits the definition of a tumor-suppressor gene. Inheritance of one mutated allele in this hereditary syndrome, followed by loss of the other allele via somatic cell mutation, leads to monoclonal expansion and tumor development. Also, in ~15–20% of sporadic parathyroid adenomas, both alleles of the *MEN1* locus on chromosome 11 are somatically deleted, implying that the same defect responsible for MEN 1 can also cause the sporadic disease (Fig. 424-3A). Consistent with the Knudson hypothesis for two-step neoplasia in certain inherited cancer syndromes (Chap. 101e), the earlier onset of hyperparathyroidism in the hereditary syndromes reflects the need for only one mutational event to trigger the monoclonal outgrowth. In sporadic adenomas, typically occurring later in life, two different somatic events must occur before the *MEN1* gene is silenced.

Other presumptive anti-oncogenes involved in hyperparathyroidism include a still unidentified gene mapped to chromosome 1p seen in 40% of sporadic parathyroid adenomas and a gene mapped to chromosome Xp11 in patients with secondary hyperparathyroidism and renal failure, who progressed to "tertiary" hyperparathyroidism, now known to reflect monoclonal outgrowths within previously hyperplastic glands.

A more complex pattern, still incompletely resolved, arises with genetic defects and carcinoma of the parathyroids. This appears to be due to biallelic loss of a functioning copy of a gene, *HRPT2* (or CDC73), originally identified as the cause of the HPT-JT syndrome. Several inactivating mutations have been identified in *HRPT2* (located on chromosome 1q21-31), which encodes a 531-amino-acid protein called parafibromin. The responsible genetic mutations in *HRPT2* appear to be necessary, but not sufficient, for parathyroid cancer.

In general, the detection of additional genetic defects in these parathyroid tumor–related syndromes and the variations seen in

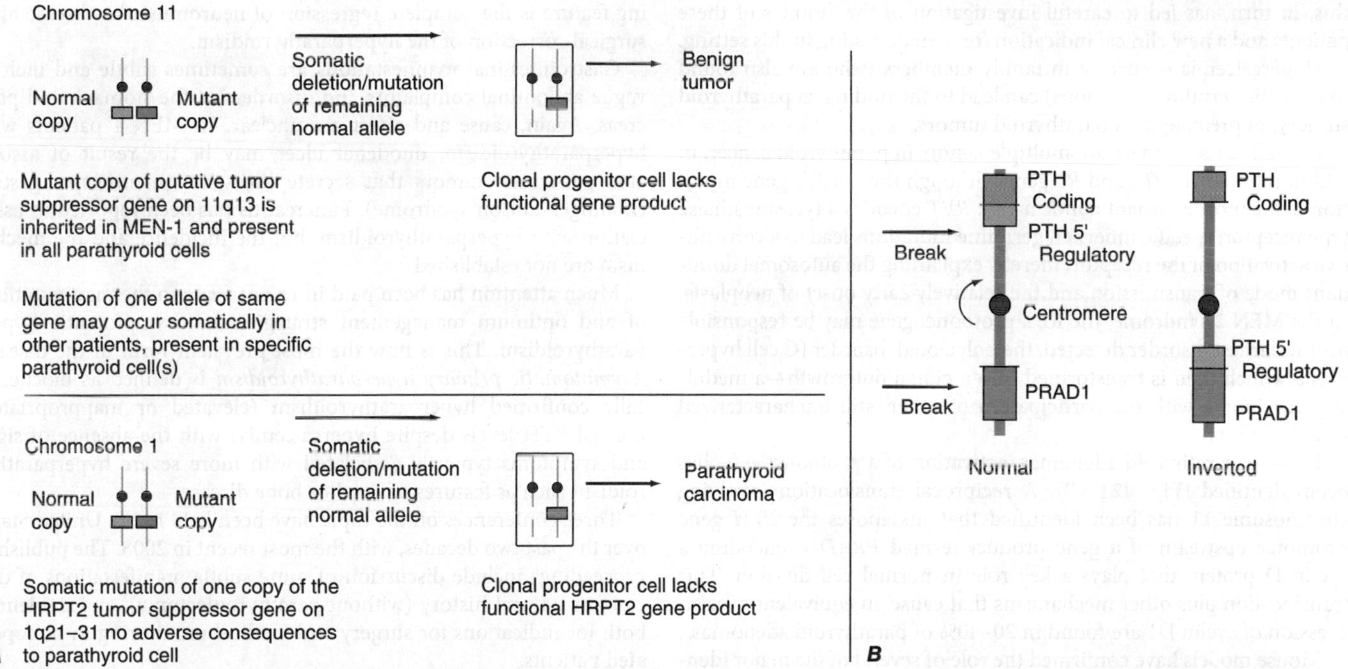

FIGURE 424-3 ***A.*** Schematic diagram indicating molecular events in tumor susceptibility. The patient with the hereditary abnormality (multiple endocrine neoplasia [MEN]) is envisioned as having one defective gene inherited from the affected parent on chromosome 11, but one copy of the normal gene is present from the other parent. In the monoclonal tumor (benign tumor), a somatic event, here partial chromosomal deletion, removes the remaining normal gene from a cell. In nonhereditary tumors, two successive somatic mutations must occur, a process that takes a longer time. By either pathway, the cell, deprived of growth-regulating influence from this gene, has unregulated growth and becomes a tumor. A different genetic locus also involving loss of a tumor-suppressor gene termed HRPT2 is involved in the pathogenesis of parathyroid carcinoma. *(From A Arnold: J Clin Endocrine Metab 77:1108, 1993. Copyright 1993, The Endocrine Society.)* ***B.*** Schematic illustration of the mechanism and consequences of gene rearrangement and overexpression of the *PRAD1* protooncogene (pericentromeric inversion of chromosome 11) in parathyroid adenomas. The excessive expression of PRAD1 (a cell cycle control protein, cyclin D_1) by the highly active parathyroid hormone (PTH) gene promoter in the parathyroid cell contributes to excess cellular proliferation. *(From J Habener et al, in L DeGroot, JL Jameson [eds]: Endocrinology, 4th ed. Philadelphia, Saunders, 2001; with permission.)*

phenotypic expression/penetrance indicate the multiplicity of the genetic factors responsible. Nonetheless, the ability to detect the presence of the major genetic contributors has greatly aided a more informed management of family members of patients identified in the hereditary syndromes such as MEN 1, MEN 2, and HPT-JT.

An important contribution from studies on the genetic origin of parathyroid carcinoma has been the realization that the mutations involve a different pathway than that involved with the benign gland enlargements. Unlike the pathogenesis of genetic alterations seen in colon cancer, where lesions evolve from benign adenomas to malignant disease by progressive genetic changes, the alterations commonly seen in most parathyroid cancers (*HRPT2* mutations) are infrequently seen in sporadic parathyroid adenomas.

Abnormalities at the *Rb* gene were the first to be noted in parathyroid cancer. The *Rb* gene, a tumor-suppressor gene located on chromosome 13q14, was initially associated with retinoblastoma but has since been implicated in other neoplasias, including parathyroid carcinoma. Early studies implicated allelic deletions of the *Rb* gene in many parathyroid carcinomas and decreased or absent expression of the Rb protein. However, because there are often large deletions in chromosome 13 that include many genes in addition to the *Rb* locus (with similar findings in some pituitary carcinomas), it remains possible that other tumor-suppressor genes on chromosome 13 may be playing a role in parathyroid carcinoma.

Study of the parathyroid cancers found in some patients with the HPT-JT syndrome has led to identification of a much larger role for mutations in the *HRPT2* gene in most parathyroid carcinomas, including those that arise sporadically, without apparent association with the HPT-JT syndrome. Mutations in the coding region have been identified in 75–80% of all parathyroid cancers analyzed, leading to the conclusion that, with addition of presumed mutations in the noncoding regions, this genetic defect may be seen in essentially all parathyroid carcinomas. Of special importance was the discovery that, in some sporadic parathyroid cancers, germline mutations have been found; this, in turn, has led to careful investigation of the families of these patients and a new clinical indication for genetic testing in this setting.

Hypercalcemia occurring in family members (who are also found to have the germline mutations) can lead to the finding, at parathyroid surgery, of premalignant parathyroid tumors.

Overall, it seems there are multiple factors in parathyroid cancer, in addition to the *HRPT2* and *Rb* gene, although the *HRPT2* gene mutation is the most invariant abnormality. *RET* encodes a tyrosine kinase type receptor; specific inherited germline mutations lead to a constitutive activation of the receptor, thereby explaining the autosomal dominant mode of transmission and the relatively early onset of neoplasia. In the MEN 2 syndrome, the *RET* protooncogene may be responsible for the earliest disorder detected, the polyclonal disorder (C cell hyperplasia, which then is transformed into a clonal outgrowth—a medullary carcinoma with the participation of other, still uncharacterized genetic defects).

In some parathyroid adenomas, activation of a protooncogene has been identified (Fig. 424-3*B*). A reciprocal translocation involving chromosome 11 has been identified that juxtaposes the *PTH* gene promoter upstream of a gene product termed *PRAD-1*, encoding a cyclin D protein that plays a key role in normal cell division. This translocation plus other mechanisms that cause an equivalent overexpression of cyclin D1 are found in 20–40% of parathyroid adenomas.

Mouse models have confirmed the role of several of the major identified genetic defects in parathyroid disease and the MEN syndromes. Loss of the *MEN1* gene locus or overexpression of the *PRAD-1* protooncogene or the mutated *RET* protooncogene have been analyzed by genetic manipulation in mice, with the expected onset of parathyroid tumors or medullary carcinoma, respectively.

Signs and Symptoms Many patients with hyperparathyroidism are asymptomatic. Manifestations of hyperparathyroidism involve primarily the kidneys and the skeletal system. Kidney involvement, due either to deposition of calcium in the renal parenchyma or to recurrent nephrolithiasis, was present in 60–70% of patients prior to 1970. With earlier detection, renal complications occur in <20% of patients in many large series. Renal stones are usually composed of either calcium oxalate or calcium phosphate. In occasional patients, repeated episodes of nephrolithiasis or the formation of large calculi may lead to urinary tract obstruction, infection, and loss of renal function. Nephrocalcinosis may also cause decreased renal function and phosphate retention.

The distinctive bone manifestation of hyperparathyroidism is *osteitis fibrosa cystica*, which occurred in 10–25% of patients in series reported 50 years ago. Histologically, the pathognomonic features are an increase in the giant multinucleated osteoclasts in scalloped areas on the surface of the bone (Howship's lacunae) and a replacement of the normal cellular and marrow elements by fibrous tissue. X-ray changes include resorption of the phalangeal tufts and replacement of the usually sharp cortical outline of the bone in the digits by an irregular outline (subperiosteal resorption). In recent years, osteitis fibrosa cystica is very rare in primary hyperparathyroidism, probably due to the earlier detection of the disease.

Dual-energy x-ray absorptiometry (DEXA) of the spine provides reproducible quantitative estimates (within a few percent) of spinal bone density. Similarly, bone density in the extremities can be quantified by densitometry of the hip or of the distal radius at a site chosen to be primarily cortical. Computed tomography (CT) is a very sensitive technique for estimating spinal bone density, but reproducibility of standard CT is no better than 5%. Newer CT techniques (spiral, "extreme" CT) are more reproducible but are currently available in a limited number of medical centers. Cortical bone density is reduced while cancellous bone density, especially in the spine, is relatively preserved. In symptomatic patients, dysfunctions of the CNS, peripheral nerve and muscle, gastrointestinal tract, and joints also occur. It has been reported that severe neuropsychiatric manifestations may be reversed by parathyroidectomy. When present in symptomatic patients, neuromuscular manifestations may include proximal muscle weakness, easy fatigability, and atrophy of muscles and may be so striking as to suggest a primary neuromuscular disorder. The distinguishing feature is the complete regression of neuromuscular disease after surgical correction of the hyperparathyroidism.

Gastrointestinal manifestations are sometimes subtle and include vague abdominal complaints and disorders of the stomach and pancreas. Again, cause and effect are unclear. In MEN 1 patients with hyperparathyroidism, duodenal ulcer may be the result of associated pancreatic tumors that secrete excessive quantities of gastrin (Zollinger-Ellison syndrome). Pancreatitis has been reported in association with hyperparathyroidism, but the incidence and the mechanism are not established.

Much attention has been paid in recent years to the manifestations of and optimum management strategies for asymptomatic hyperparathyroidism. This is now the most prevalent form of the disease. *Asymptomatic primary hyperparathyroidism* is defined as biochemically confirmed hyperparathyroidism (elevated or inappropriately normal PTH levels despite hypercalcemia) with the absence of signs and symptoms typically associated with more severe hyperparathyroidism such as features of renal or bone disease.

Three conferences on the topic have been held in the United States over the past two decades, with the most recent in 2008. The published proceedings include discussion of more subtle manifestations of disease, its natural history (without parathyroidectomy), and guidelines both for indications for surgery and medical monitoring in nonoperated patients.

Issues of concern include the potential for cardiovascular deterioration, the presence of subtle neuropsychiatric symptoms, and the longer-term status of skeletal integrity in patients not treated surgically. The current consensus is that medical monitoring rather than surgical correction of hyperparathyroidism may be justified in certain patients. The current recommendation is that patients who show mild disease, as defined by specific criteria (Table 424-2), can be safely followed under management guidelines (Table 424-3). There is, however, growing uncertainty about subtle disease manifestations and whether surgery is therefore indicated in most patients. Among the issues is the evidence of eventual (>8 years) deterioration in bone mineral density after a decade

TABLE 424-2 GUIDELINES FOR SURGERY IN ASYMPTOMATIC PRIMARY HYPERPARATHYROIDISM[a]

Parameter	Guideline
Serum calcium (above normal)	>1 mg/dL
24-h urinary calcium	No indication
Creatinine clearance (calculated)[b]	If <60 mL/min
Bone density	T score <−2.5 at any of 3 sites[c]
Age	<50

[a]JP Bilezikian et al: Guidelines for the management of asymptomatic primary hyperparathyroidism: Summary statement from the third international workshop. J Clin Endocrinol Metab 94:335, 2009. [b]Creatinine clearance calculated by Cockcroft-Gault equation or Modification of Diet in Renal Disease (MDRD) equation. [c]Spine, distal radius, hip.

of relative stability. There is concern that this late-onset deterioration in bone density in nonoperated patients could contribute significantly to the well-known age-dependent fracture risk (osteoporosis). One study reported significant and sustained improvements in bone mineral density after successful parathyroidectomy, again raising the issue regarding benefits of surgery. Other randomized studies, however, did not report major gains after surgery.

Cardiovascular disease including left ventricular hypertrophy, cardiac functional defects, and endothelial dysfunction have been reported as reversible in European patients with more severe symptomatic disease after surgery, leading to numerous studies of these cardiovascular features in those with milder disease. There are reports of endothelial dysfunction in patients with mild asymptomatic hyperparathyroidism, but the expert panels concluded that more observation is needed, especially regarding whether there is reversibility with surgery.

A topic of considerable interest and some debate is assessment of neuropsychiatric status and health-related quality of life (QOL) status in hyperparathyroid patients both before surgery and in response to parathyroidectomy. Several observational studies suggest considerable improvements in symptom score after surgery. Randomized studies of surgery versus observation, however, have yielded inconclusive results, especially regarding benefits of surgery. Most studies report that hyperparathyroidism is associated with increased neuropsychiatric symptoms, so the issue remains a significant factor in decisions regarding the impact of surgery in this disease.

DIAGNOSIS

The diagnosis is typically made by detecting an elevated immunoreactive PTH level in a patient with asymptomatic hypercalcemia (see "Differential Diagnosis: Special Tests," below). Serum phosphate is usually low but may be normal, especially if renal failure has developed.

Several modifications in PTH assays have been introduced in efforts to improve their utility in light of information about metabolism of PTH (as discussed above). First-generation assays were based on displacement of radiolabeled PTH from antibodies that reacted with PTH (often also PTH fragments). Double-antibody or immunometric assays (one antibody that is usually directed against the carboxyl-terminal portion of intact PTH to capture the hormone and a second radio- or enzyme-labeled antibody that is usually directed against the amino-terminal portion of intact PTH) greatly improved the diagnostic discrimination of the tests by eliminating interference from circulating biologically inactive fragments, detected by the original first-generation assays. Double-antibody assays are now referred to as second-generation. Such PTH assays have in some centers and testing laboratories been replaced by third-generation assays after it was discovered that large PTH fragments, devoid of only the extreme amino-terminal portion of the PTH molecule, are also present in blood and are detected, incorrectly, as intact PTH. These amino-terminally truncated PTH fragments were prevented from registering in the newer third-generation assays by use of a detection antibody directed against the extreme amino-terminal epitope. These assays may be useful for clinical research studies as in management of chronic renal disease, but the consensus is that either second- or third-generation assays are useful in the diagnosis of primary hyperparathyroidism and for the diagnosis of high-turnover bone disease in chronic kidney disease.

Many tests based on renal responses to excess PTH (renal calcium and phosphate clearance; blood phosphate, chloride, magnesium; urinary or nephrogenous cyclic AMP [cAMP]) were used in earlier decades. These tests have low specificity for hyperparathyroidism and are therefore not cost-effective; they have been replaced by PTH immunometric assays combined with simultaneous blood calcium measurements (Fig. 424-4).

TABLE 424-3 GUIDELINES FOR MONITORING IN ASYMPTOMATIC PRIMARY HYPERPARATHYROIDISM[a]

Parameter	Guideline
Serum calcium	Annually
24-h urinary calcium	Recommended
Creatinine clearance	Recommended
Serum creatinine[b]	Annually
Bone density	Annually (3 sites)[a]

[a]Updates guidelines (JP Bilezikian et al: J Clin Endocrinol Metab 2014; epub ahead of print). [b]Creatinine clearance calculated by Cockcroft-Gault equation or Modification of Diet in Renal Disease (MDRD) equation.

TREATMENT HYPERPARATHYROIDISM

Surgical excision of the abnormal parathyroid tissue is the definitive therapy for this disease. As noted above, medical surveillance without operation for patients with mild, asymptomatic disease is, however, still preferred by some physicians and patients, particularly when the patients are more elderly. Evidence favoring surgery, if medically feasible, is growing because of concerns about skeletal,

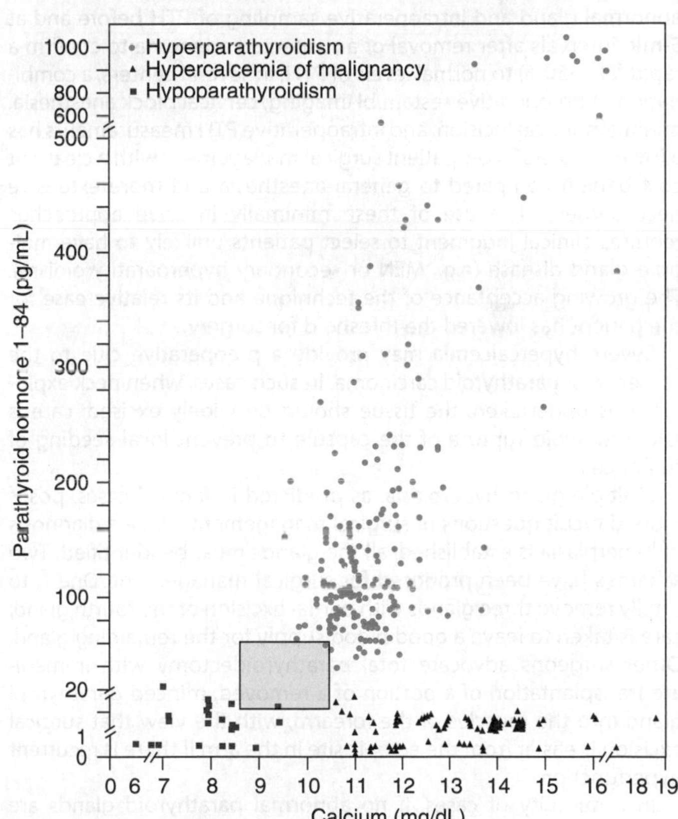

FIGURE 424-4 Levels of immunoreactive parathyroid hormone (PTH) detected in patients with primary hyperparathyroidism, hypercalcemia of malignancy, and hypoparathyroidism. *Boxed area represents the upper and normal limits of blood calcium and/or immunoreactive PTH. (From SR Nussbaum, JT Potts, Jr, in L DeGroot, JL Jameson [eds]: Endocrinology, 4th ed. Philadelphia, Saunders, 2001; with permission.)*

cardiovascular, and neuropsychiatric disease, even in mild hyperparathyroidism.

Two surgical approaches are generally practiced. The conventional parathyroidectomy procedure was neck exploration with general anesthesia; this procedure is being replaced in many centers, whenever feasible, by an outpatient procedure with local anesthesia, termed *minimally invasive parathyroidectomy*.

Parathyroid exploration is challenging and should be undertaken by an experienced surgeon. Certain features help in predicting the pathology (e.g., multiple abnormal glands in familial cases). However, some critical decisions regarding management can be made only during the operation.

With conventional surgery, one approach is still based on the view that typically only one gland (the adenoma) is abnormal. If an enlarged gland is found, a normal gland should be sought. In this view, if a biopsy of a normal-sized second gland confirms its histologic (and presumed functional) normality, no further exploration, biopsy, or excision is needed. At the other extreme is the minority viewpoint that all four glands be sought and that most of the total parathyroid tissue mass be removed. The concern with the former approach is that the recurrence rate of hyperparathyroidism may be high if a second abnormal gland is missed; the latter approach could involve unnecessary surgery and an unacceptable rate of hypoparathyroidism. When normal glands are found in association with one enlarged gland, excision of the single adenoma usually leads to cure or at least years free of symptoms. Long-term follow-up studies to establish true rates of recurrence are limited.

Recently, there has been growing experience with new surgical strategies that feature a minimally invasive approach guided by improved preoperative localization and intraoperative monitoring by PTH assays. Preoperative ^{99m}Tc sestamibi scans with single-photon emission CT (SPECT) are used to predict the location of an abnormal gland and intraoperative sampling of PTH before and at 5-min intervals after removal of a suspected adenoma to confirm a rapid fall (>50%) to normal levels of PTH. In several centers, a combination of preoperative sestamibi imaging, cervical block anesthesia, minimal surgical incision, and intraoperative PTH measurements has allowed successful outpatient surgical management with a clear-cut cost benefit compared to general anesthesia and more extensive neck surgery. The use of these minimally invasive approaches requires clinical judgment to select patients unlikely to have multiple gland disease (e.g., MEN or secondary hyperparathyroidism). The growing acceptance of the technique and its relative ease for the patient has lowered the threshold for surgery.

Severe hypercalcemia may provide a preoperative clue to the presence of parathyroid carcinoma. In such cases, when neck exploration is undertaken, the tissue should be widely excised; care is taken to avoid rupture of the capsule to prevent local seeding of tumor cells.

Multiple-gland hyperplasia, as predicted in familial cases, poses more difficult questions of surgical management. Once a diagnosis of hyperplasia is established, all the glands must be identified. Two schemes have been proposed for surgical management. One is to totally remove three glands with partial excision of the fourth gland; care is taken to leave a good blood supply for the remaining gland. Other surgeons advocate total parathyroidectomy with immediate transplantation of a portion of a removed, minced parathyroid gland into the muscles of the forearm, with the view that surgical excision is easier from the ectopic site in the arm if there is recurrent hyperfunction.

In a minority of cases, if no abnormal parathyroid glands are found in the neck, the issue of further exploration must be decided. There are documented cases of five or six parathyroid glands and of unusual locations for adenomas such as in the mediastinum.

When a second parathyroid exploration is indicated, the minimally invasive techniques for preoperative localization such as ultrasound, CT scan, and isotope scanning are combined with venous sampling and/or selective digital arteriography in one of the centers specializing in these procedures. Intraoperative monitoring of PTH levels by rapid PTH immunoassays may be useful in guiding the surgery. At one center, long-term cures have been achieved with selective embolization or injection of large amounts of contrast material into the end-arterial circulation feeding the parathyroid tumor.

A decline in serum calcium occurs within 24 h after successful surgery; usually blood calcium falls to low-normal values for 3–5 days until the remaining parathyroid tissue resumes full hormone secretion. Acute postoperative hypocalcemia is likely only if severe bone mineral deficits are present or if injury to all the normal parathyroid glands occurs during surgery. In general, there are few problems encountered in patients with uncomplicated disease such as a single adenoma (the clear majority), who do not have symptomatic bone disease or a large deficit in bone mineral, who are vitamin D and magnesium sufficient, and who have good renal and gastrointestinal function. The extent of postoperative hypocalcemia varies with the surgical approach. If all glands are biopsied, hypocalcemia may be transiently symptomatic and more prolonged. Hypocalcemia is more likely to be symptomatic after second parathyroid explorations, particularly when normal parathyroid tissue was removed at the initial operation and when the manipulation and/or biopsy of the remaining normal glands are more extensive in the search for the missing adenoma.

Patients with hyperparathyroidism have efficient intestinal calcium absorption due to the increased levels of $1,25(OH)_2D$ stimulated by PTH excess. Once hypocalcemia signifies successful surgery, patients can be put on a high-calcium intake or be given oral calcium supplements. Despite mild hypocalcemia, most patients do not require parenteral therapy. If the serum calcium falls to <2 mmol/L (8 mg/dL), *and if the phosphate level rises simultaneously*, the possibility that surgery has caused hypoparathyroidism must be considered. With unexpected hypocalcemia, coexistent hypomagnesemia should be considered, because it interferes with PTH secretion and causes functional hypoparathyroidism (Chap. 423).

Signs of hypocalcemia include symptoms such as muscle twitching, a general sense of anxiety, and positive Chvostek's and Trousseau's signs coupled with serum calcium consistently <2 mmol/L (8 mg/dL). Parenteral calcium replacement at a low level should be instituted when hypocalcemia is symptomatic. The rate and duration of IV therapy are determined by the severity of the symptoms and the response of the serum calcium to treatment. An infusion of 0.5–2 mg/kg per hour or 30–100 mL/h of a 1-mg/mL solution usually suffices to relieve symptoms. Usually, parenteral therapy is required for only a few days. If symptoms worsen or if parenteral calcium is needed for >2–3 days, therapy with a vitamin D analogue and/or oral calcium (2–4 g/d) should be started (see below). It is cost-effective to use calcitriol (doses of 0.5–1 μg/d) because of the rapidity of onset of effect and prompt cessation of action when stopped, in comparison to other forms of vitamin D. A rise in blood calcium after several months of vitamin D replacement may indicate restoration of parathyroid function to normal. It is also appropriate to monitor serum PTH serially to estimate gland function in such patients.

If magnesium deficiency was present, it can complicate the postoperative course since magnesium deficiency impairs the secretion of PTH. Hypomagnesemia should be corrected whenever detected. Magnesium replacement can be effective orally (e.g., $MgCl_2$, $MgOH_2$), but parenteral repletion is usual to ensure postoperative recovery, if magnesium deficiency is suspected due to low blood magnesium levels. Because the depressant effect of magnesium on central and peripheral nerve functions does not occur at levels <2 mmol/L (normal range 0.8–1.2 mmol/L), parenteral replacement can be given rapidly. A cumulative dose as great as 0.5–1 mmol/kg of body weight can be administered if severe hypomagnesemia is present; often, however, total doses of 20–40 mmol are sufficient.

MEDICAL MANAGEMENT

The guidelines for recommending surgical intervention, if feasible (Table 424-2), as well as for monitoring patients with asymptomatic hyperparathyroidism who elect not to undergo parathyroidectomy

(Table 424-3), reflect the changes over time since the first conference on the topic in 1990. Medical monitoring rather than corrective surgery is still acceptable, but it is clear that surgical intervention is the more frequently recommended option for the reasons noted above. Tightened guidelines favoring surgery include lowering the recommended level of serum calcium elevation, more careful attention to skeletal integrity through reference to peak skeletal mass at baseline (T scores) rather than age-adjusted bone density (*Z* scores), as well as the presence of any fragility fracture. The other changes noted in the two guidelines (Tables 424-2 and 424-3) reflect accumulated experience and practical consideration, such as a difficulty in quantity of urine collections. Despite the usefulness of the guidelines, the importance of individual patient and physician judgment and preference is clear in all recommendations.

When surgery is not selected, or not medically feasible, there is interest in the potential value of specific medical therapies. There is no long-term experience regarding specific clinical outcomes such as fracture prevention, but it has been established that bisphosphonates increase bone mineral density significantly without changing serum calcium (as does estrogen, but the latter is not favored because of reported adverse effects in other organ systems). Calcimimetics that lower PTH secretion lower calcium but do not affect bone mineral density.

OTHER PARATHYROID-RELATED CAUSES OF HYPERCALCEMIA

Lithium Therapy Lithium, used in the management of bipolar depression and other psychiatric disorders, causes hypercalcemia in ~10% of treated patients. The hypercalcemia is dependent on continued lithium treatment, remitting and recurring when lithium is stopped and restarted. The parathyroid adenomas reported in some hypercalcemic patients with lithium therapy may reflect the presence of an independently occurring parathyroid tumor; a permanent effect of lithium on parathyroid gland growth need not be implicated as most patients have complete reversal of hypercalcemia when lithium is stopped. However, long-standing stimulation of parathyroid cell replication by lithium may predispose to development of adenomas (as is documented in secondary hyperparathyroidism and renal failure).

At the levels achieved in blood in treated patients, lithium can be shown in vitro to shift the PTH secretion curve to the right in response to calcium; i.e., higher calcium levels are required to lower PTH secretion, probably acting at the calcium sensor (see below). This effect can cause elevated PTH levels and consequent hypercalcemia in otherwise normal individuals. Fortunately, there are usually alternative medications for the underlying psychiatric illness. Parathyroid surgery should not be recommended unless hypercalcemia and elevated PTH levels persist after lithium is discontinued.

GENETIC DISORDERS CAUSING HYPERPARATHYROID-LIKE SYNDROMES

Familial Hypocalciuric Hypercalcemia FHH (also called *familial benign hypercalcemia*) is inherited as an autosomal dominant trait. Affected individuals are discovered because of asymptomatic hypercalcemia. Most cases of FHH (FHH1) are caused by an inactivating mutation in a single allele of the CaSR (see below), leading to inappropriately normal or even increased secretion of PTH, whereas another hypercalcemic disorder, namely the exceedingly rare Jansen's disease, is caused by a constitutively active PTH/PTHrP receptor in target tissues. Neither FHH1 nor Jansen's disease, however, is a growth disorder of the parathyroids. Other forms of FHH are caused either by heterozygous mutations in *GNA11* (encoding G11), one of the signaling proteins downstream of the CaSR (FHH2), or by mutations in *AP2S1* (FHH3).

The pathophysiology of FHH1 is now understood. The primary defect is abnormal sensing of the blood calcium by the parathyroid gland and renal tubule, causing inappropriate secretion of PTH and excessive reabsorption of calcium in the distal renal tubules. The CaSR is a member of the third family of GPCRs (type C or type III). The receptor responds to increased ECF calcium concentration by suppressing PTH secretion through second-messenger signaling involving the G protein alpha-subunits G11 and Gq, thereby providing negative-feedback regulation of PTH secretion. Many different inactivating CaSR mutations have been identified in patients with FHH1. These mutations lower the capacity of the sensor to bind calcium, and the mutant receptors function as though blood calcium levels were low; excessive secretion of PTH occurs from an otherwise normal gland. Approximately two-thirds of patients with FHH have mutations within the protein-coding region of the CaSR gene. The remaining one-third of kindreds may have mutations in the promoter of the CaSR gene or are caused by mutations in other genes.

Even before elucidation of the pathophysiology of FHH, abundant clinical evidence served to separate the disorder from primary hyperparathyroidism; these clinical features are still useful in differential diagnosis. Patients with primary hyperparathyroidism have <99% renal calcium reabsorption, whereas most patients with FHH have >99% reabsorption. The hypercalcemia in FHH is often detectable in affected members of the kindreds in the first decade of life, whereas hypercalcemia rarely occurs in patients with primary hyperparathyroidism or the MEN syndromes who are age <10 years. PTH may be elevated in the different forms of FHH, but the values are usually normal or lower for the same degree of calcium elevation than is observed in patients with primary hyperparathyroidism. Parathyroid surgery performed in a few patients with FHH before the nature of the syndrome was understood led to permanent hypoparathyroidism; nevertheless, hypocalciuria persisted, establishing that hypocalciuria is not PTH-dependent (now known to be due to the abnormal CaSR in the kidney).

Few clinical signs or symptoms are present in patients with FHH, whereas other endocrine abnormalities are not. Most patients are detected as a result of family screening after hypercalcemia is detected in a proband. In those patients inadvertently operated upon for primary hyperparathyroidism, the parathyroids appeared normal or moderately hyperplastic. Parathyroid surgery is not appropriate, nor, in view of the lack of symptoms, does medical treatment seem needed to lower the calcium. One striking exception to the rule against parathyroid surgery in this syndrome is the occurrence, usually in consanguineous marriages (due to the rarity of the gene mutation), of a homozygous or compound heterozygote state, resulting in severe impairment of CaSR function. In this condition, neonatal severe hypercalcemia, total parathyroidectomy is mandatory, but calcimetics have been used as a temporary measure. Rare but well-documented cases of acquired hypocalciuric hypercalcemia are reported due to antibodies against the CaSR. They appear to be a complication of an underlying autoimmune disorder and respond to therapies directed against the underlying disorder.

Jansen's Disease Activating mutations in the PTH/PTHrP receptor (PTH1R) have been identified as the cause of this rare autosomal dominant syndrome. Because the mutations lead to constitutive activation of receptor function, one abnormal copy of the mutant receptor is sufficient to cause the disease, thereby accounting for its dominant mode of transmission. The disorder leads to short-limbed dwarfism due to abnormal regulation of chondrocyte maturation in the growth plates of the bone that are formed through the endochondral process. In adult life, there are numerous abnormalities in bone, including multiple cystic resorptive areas resembling those seen in severe hyperparathyroidism. Hypercalcemia and hypophosphatemia with undetectable or low PTH levels are typically observed. The pathogenesis of the growth plate abnormalities in Jansen's disease has been confirmed by transgenic experiments in which targeted expression of the mutant PTH/PTHrP receptor to the proliferating chondrocyte layer of growth plate emulated several features of the human disorder. Some of these genetic mutations in the parathyroid gland or PTH target cells that affect Ca^{2+} metabolism are illustrated in Fig. 424-5.

MALIGNANCY-RELATED HYPERCALCEMIA

Clinical Syndromes and Mechanisms of Hypercalcemia Hypercalcemia due to malignancy is common (occurring in as many as 20% of cancer patients, especially with certain types of tumor such as lung carcinoma), often severe and difficult to manage, and, on rare occasions,

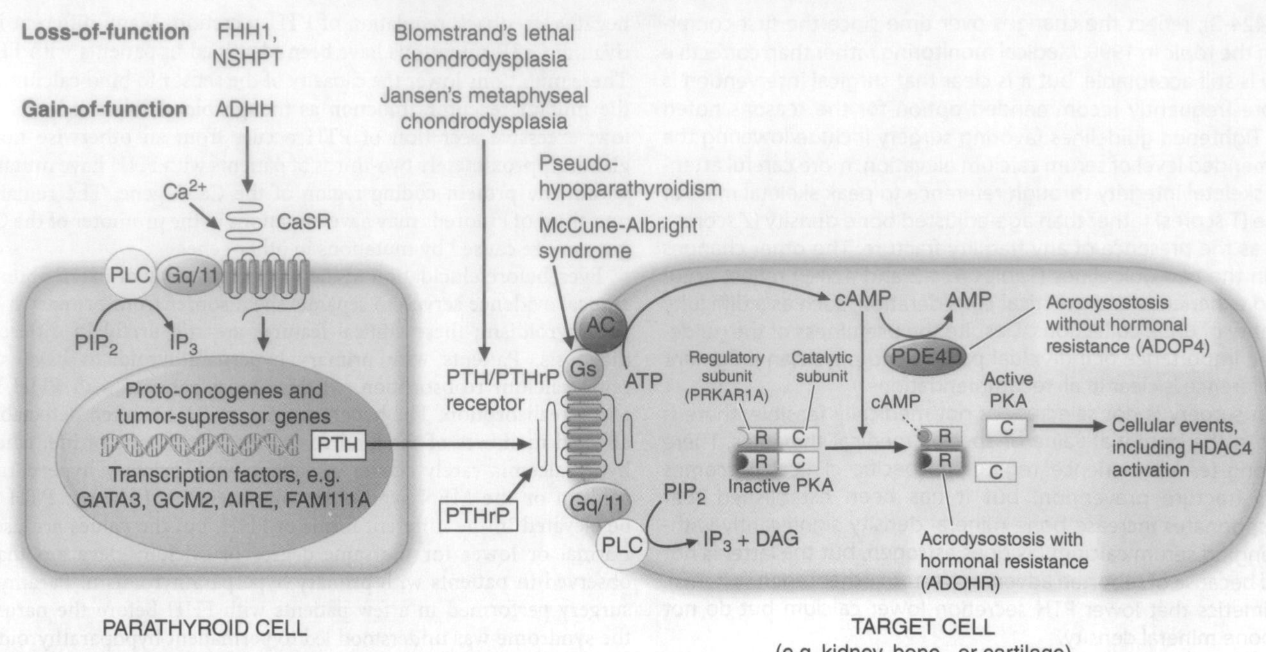

FIGURE 424-5 Illustration of some genetic mutations that alter calcium metabolism by effects on the parathyroid cell or target cells of parathyroid hormone (PTH) action. Alterations in PTH production by the parathyroid cell can be caused by changes in the response to extracellular fluid calcium (Ca^{2+}) that are detected by the calcium-sensing receptor (CaSR). Furthermore, PTH (or PTH-related peptide [PTHrP]) can show altered efficacy in target cells such as in proximal tubular cells, by altered function of its receptor (PTH/PTHrP receptor) or the signal transduction proteins, G proteins such as $G_s\alpha$, which is linked to adenylate cyclase (AC), the enzyme responsible for producing cyclic AMP (cAMP) (also illustrated are Gq/11, which activate an alternate pathway of receptor signal transmission involving the generation of inositol triphosphate [IP_3] or diacylglycerol [DAG]). Heterozygous loss-of-function mutations in the CaSR cause familial benign hypocalciuric hypercalcemia (FBHH), homozygous mutations (both alleles mutated), and severe neonatal hyperparathyroidism (NSHPT); heterozygous gain-of-function causes autosomal dominant hypercalciuric hypocalcemia (ADHH). Other defects in parathyroid cell function that occur at the level of gene regulation (oncogenes or tumor-suppressor genes) or transcription factors are discussed in the text. Blomstrand's lethal chondrodysplasia is due to homozygous or compound heterozygous loss-of-function mutations in the PTH/PTHrP receptor, a neonatally lethal disorder, while pseudohypoparathyroidism involves inactivation at the level of the G proteins, specifically mutations that eliminate or reduce $G_s\alpha$ activity in the kidney (see text for details). Acrodysostosis can occur with (acrodysostosis with hormonal resistance [ADOHR]; mutant regulatory subunit of PKA) or without hormonal resistance (ADOP4; mutant PDE4D). Jansen's metaphyseal chondrodysplasia and McCune-Albright syndrome represent gain-of-function mutations in the PTH/PTHrP receptor and $G_s\alpha$ protein, respectively.

difficult to distinguish from primary hyperparathyroidism. Although malignancy is often clinically obvious or readily detectable by medical history, hypercalcemia can occasionally be due to an occult tumor. Previously, hypercalcemia associated with malignancy was thought to be due to local invasion and destruction of bone by tumor cells; many cases are now known to result from the elaboration by the malignant cells of humoral mediators of hypercalcemia. PTHrP is the responsible humoral agent in most solid tumors that cause hypercalcemia.

The histologic character of the tumor is more important than the extent of skeletal metastases in predicting hypercalcemia. Small-cell carcinoma (oat cell) and adenocarcinoma of the lung, although the most common lung tumors associated with skeletal metastases, rarely cause hypercalcemia. By contrast, many patients with squamous cell carcinoma of the lung develop hypercalcemia. Histologic studies of bone in patients with squamous cell or epidermoid carcinoma of the lung, in sites invaded by tumor as well as areas remote from tumor invasion, reveal increased bone resorption.

Two main mechanisms of hypercalcemia are operative in cancer hypercalcemia. Many solid tumors associated with hypercalcemia, particularly squamous cell and renal tumors, produce and secrete PTHrP that causes increased bone resorption and mediate the hypercalcemia through systemic actions on the skeleton. Alternatively, direct bone marrow invasion occurs with hematologic malignancies such as leukemia, lymphoma, and multiple myeloma. Lymphokines and cytokines (including PTHrP) produced by cells involved in the marrow response to the tumors promote resorption of bone through local destruction. Several hormones, hormone analogues, cytokines, and growth factors have been implicated as the result of clinical assays, in vitro tests, or chemical isolation. The etiologic factor produced by activated normal lymphocytes and by myeloma and lymphoma cells, originally termed *osteoclast activation factor*, now appears to represent the biologic action of several different cytokines, probably interleukin 1 and lymphotoxin or tumor necrosis factor (TNF). In some lymphomas, there is a third mechanism, caused by an increased blood level of 1,25(OH)$_2$D, produced by the abnormal lymphocytes.

In the more common mechanism, usually termed *humoral hypercalcemia of malignancy*, solid tumors (cancers of the lung and kidney, in particular), in which bone metastases are absent, minimal, or not detectable clinically, secrete PTHrP measurable by immunoassay. Secretion by the tumors of the PTH-like factor, PTHrP, activates the PTH1R, resulting in a pathophysiology closely resembling hyperparathyroidism, but with normal or suppressed PTH levels. The clinical picture resembles primary hyperparathyroidism (hypophosphatemia accompanies hypercalcemia), and elimination or regression of the primary tumor leads to disappearance of the hypercalcemia.

As in hyperparathyroidism, patients with the humoral hypercalcemia of malignancy have elevated urinary nephrogenous cAMP excretion, hypophosphatemia, and increased urinary phosphate clearance. However, in humoral hypercalcemia of malignancy, immunoreactive PTH is undetectable or suppressed, making the differential diagnosis easier. Other features of the disorder differ from those of true hyperparathyroidism. Although the biologic actions of PTH and PTHrP are exerted through the same receptor, subtle differences in receptor activation by the two ligands must account for some of the discordance in pathophysiology, when an excess of one or the other peptide occurs. Other cytokines elaborated by the malignancy may contribute to the variations from hyperparathyroidism in these patients as well. Patients with humoral hypercalcemia of malignancy may have low to normal levels of 1,25(OH)$_2$D instead of elevated levels as in true hyperparathyroidism. In some patients with the humoral hypercalcemia of malignancy, osteoclastic resorption is unaccompanied by an osteoblastic or bone-forming response, implying inhibition of the normal coupling of bone formation and resorption.

Several different assays (single- or double-antibody, different epitopes) have been developed to detect PTHrP. Most data indicate that circulating PTHrP levels are undetectable (or low) in normal individuals except perhaps in pregnancy (high in human milk) and elevated in most cancer patients with the humoral syndrome. The etiologic mechanisms in cancer hypercalcemia may be multiple in the same patient. For example, in breast carcinoma (metastatic to bone) and in a distinctive type of T cell lymphoma/leukemia initiated by human T cell lymphotropic virus I, hypercalcemia is caused by direct local lysis of bone as well as by a humoral mechanism involving excess production of PTHrP. Hyperparathyroidism has been reported to coexist with the humoral cancer syndrome, and rarely, ectopic hyperparathyroidism due to tumor elaboration of true PTH is reported.

Diagnostic Issues Levels of PTH measured by the double-antibody technique are undetectable or extremely low in tumor hypercalcemia, as would be expected with the mediation of the hypercalcemia by a factor other than PTH (the hypercalcemia suppresses the normal parathyroid glands). In a patient with minimal symptoms referred for hypercalcemia, low or undetectable PTH levels would focus attention on a possible occult malignancy (except for very rare cases of ectopic hyperparathyroidism).

Ordinarily, the diagnosis of cancer hypercalcemia is not difficult because tumor symptoms are prominent when hypercalcemia is detected. Indeed, hypercalcemia may be noted incidentally during the workup of a patient with known or suspected malignancy. Clinical suspicion that malignancy is the cause of the hypercalcemia is heightened when there are other signs or symptoms of a paraneoplastic process such as weight loss, fatigue, muscle weakness, or unexplained skin rash, or when symptoms specific for a particular tumor are present. Squamous cell tumors are most frequently associated with hypercalcemia, particularly tumors of the lung, kidney, head and neck, and urogenital tract. Radiologic examinations can focus on these areas when clinical evidence is unclear. Bone scans with technetium-labeled bisphosphonate are useful for detection of osteolytic metastases; the sensitivity is high, but specificity is low; results must be confirmed by conventional x-rays to be certain that areas of increased uptake are due to osteolytic metastases per se. Bone marrow biopsies are helpful in patients with anemia or abnormal peripheral blood smears.

TREATMENT MALIGNANCY-RELATED HYPERCALCEMIA

Treatment of the hypercalcemia of malignancy is first directed to control of tumor; reduction of tumor mass usually corrects hypercalcemia. If a patient has severe hypercalcemia yet has a good chance for effective tumor therapy, treatment of the hypercalcemia should be vigorous while awaiting the results of definitive therapy. If hypercalcemia occurs in the late stages of a tumor that is resistant to antitumor therapy, the treatment of the hypercalcemia should be judicious as high calcium levels can have a mild sedating effect. Standard therapies for hypercalcemia (discussed below) are applicable to patients with malignancy.

VITAMIN D–RELATED HYPERCALCEMIA

Hypercalcemia caused by vitamin D can be due to excessive ingestion or abnormal metabolism of the vitamin. Abnormal metabolism of the vitamin is usually acquired in association with a widespread granulomatous disorder. Vitamin D metabolism is carefully regulated, particularly the activity of renal 1α-hydroxylase, the enzyme responsible for the production of 1,25(OH)$_2$D (Chap. 423). The regulation of 1α-hydroxylase and the normal feedback suppression by 1,25(OH)$_2$D seem to work less well in infants than in adults and to operate poorly, if at all, in sites other than the renal tubule; these phenomena may explain the occurrence of hypercalcemia secondary to excessive 1,25(OH)$_2$D production in infants with Williams' syndrome (see below) and in adults with sarcoidosis or lymphoma.

Vitamin D Intoxication Chronic ingestion of 40–100 times the normal physiologic requirement of vitamin D (amounts >40,000–100,000 U/d) is usually required to produce significant hypercalcemia in otherwise healthy individuals. The stated upper limit of safe dietary intake is 2000 U/d (50 μg/d) in adults because of concerns about potential toxic effects of cumulative supraphysiologic doses. These recommendations are now regarded as too restrictive, because some estimates are that in elderly individuals in northern latitudes, 2000 U/d or more may be necessary to avoid vitamin D insufficiency.

Hypercalcemia in vitamin D intoxication is due to an excessive biologic action of the vitamin, perhaps the consequence of increased levels of 25(OH)D rather than merely increased levels of the active metabolite 1,25(OH)$_2$D (the latter may not be elevated in vitamin D intoxication). 25(OH)D has definite, if low, biologic activity in the intestine and bone. The production of 25(OH)D is less tightly regulated than is the production of 1,25(OH)$_2$D. Hence concentrations of 25(OH)D are elevated several-fold in patients with excess vitamin D intake.

The diagnosis is substantiated by documenting elevated levels of 25(OH)D >100 mg/mL. Hypercalcemia is usually controlled by restriction of dietary calcium intake and appropriate attention to hydration. These measures, plus discontinuation of vitamin D, usually lead to resolution of hypercalcemia. However, vitamin D stores in fat may be substantial, and vitamin D intoxication may persist for weeks after vitamin D ingestion is terminated. Such patients are responsive to glucocorticoids, which in doses of 100 mg/d of hydrocortisone or its equivalent usually return serum calcium levels to normal over several days; severe intoxication may require intensive therapy.

Sarcoidosis and Other Granulomatous Diseases In patients with sarcoidosis and other granulomatous diseases, such as tuberculosis and fungal infections, excess 1,25(OH)$_2$D is synthesized in macrophages or other cells in the granulomas. Indeed, increased 1,25(OH)$_2$D levels have been reported in anephric patients with sarcoidosis and hypercalcemia. Macrophages obtained from granulomatous tissue convert 25(OH)D to 1,25(OH)$_2$D at an increased rate. There is a positive correlation in patients with sarcoidosis between 25(OH)D levels (reflecting vitamin D intake) and the circulating concentrations of 1,25(OH)$_2$D, whereas normally there is no increase in 1,25(OH)$_2$D with increasing 25(OH) D levels due to multiple feedback controls on renal 1α-hydroxylase (Chap. 423). The usual regulation of active metabolite production by calcium and phosphate or by PTH does not operate in these patients. Clearance of 1,25(OH)$_2$D from blood may be decreased in sarcoidosis as well. PTH levels are usually low and 1,25(OH)$_2$D levels are elevated, but primary hyperparathyroidism and sarcoidosis may coexist in some patients.

Management of the hypercalcemia can often be accomplished by avoiding excessive sunlight exposure and limiting vitamin D and calcium intake. Presumably, however, the abnormal sensitivity to vitamin D and abnormal regulation of 1,25(OH)$_2$D synthesis will persist as long as the disease is active. Alternatively, glucocorticoids in the equivalent of 100 mg/d of hydrocortisone or equivalent doses of glucocorticoids may help control hypercalcemia. Glucocorticoids appear to act by blocking excessive production of 1,25(OH)$_2$D, as well as the response to it in target organs.

Idiopathic Hypercalcemia of Infancy This rare disorder, usually referred to as *Williams' syndrome*, is an autosomal dominant disorder characterized by multiple congenital development defects, including supravalvular aortic stenosis, mental retardation, and an elfin facies, in association with hypercalcemia due to abnormal sensitivity to vitamin D. The hypercalcemia associated with the syndrome was first recognized in England after fortification of milk with vitamin D. The cardiac and developmental abnormalities were independently described, but the connection between these defects and hypercalcemia were not described until later. Levels of 1,25(OH)$_2$D can be elevated, ranging from 46 to 120 nmol/L (150–500 pg/mL). The mechanism of the abnormal sensitivity to vitamin D and of the increased circulating levels of 1,25(OH)$_2$D is still unclear. Studies suggest that genetic mutations involving microdeletions at the elastin locus and perhaps other genes on chromosome 7 may play a role in the pathogenesis. Another cause of hypercalcemia in infants and young children is a 24-hydroxylase deficiency that impairs metabolism of 1,25(OH)$_2$D.

HYPERCALCEMIA ASSOCIATED WITH HIGH BONE TURNOVER

Hyperthyroidism As many as 20% of hyperthyroid patients have high-normal or mildly elevated serum calcium concentrations; hypercalciuria is even more common. The hypercalcemia is due to increased bone turnover, with bone resorption exceeding bone formation. Severe calcium elevations are not typical, and the presence of such suggests a concomitant disease such as hyperparathyroidism. Usually, the diagnosis is obvious, but signs of hyperthyroidism may occasionally be occult, particularly in the elderly (Chap. 405). Hypercalcemia is managed by treatment of the hyperthyroidism. Reports that thyroid-stimulating hormone (TSH) itself normally has a bone-protective effect suggest that suppressed TSH levels also play a role in hypercalcemia.

Immobilization Immobilization is a rare cause of hypercalcemia in adults in the absence of an associated disease but may cause hypercalcemia in children and adolescents, particularly after spinal cord injury and paraplegia or quadriplegia. With resumption of ambulation, the hypercalcemia in children usually returns to normal.

The mechanism appears to involve a disproportion between bone formation and bone resorption; the former decreased and the latter increased. Hypercalciuria and increased mobilization of skeletal calcium can develop in normal volunteers subjected to extensive bed rest, although hypercalcemia is unusual. Immobilization of an adult with a disease associated with high bone turnover, however, such as Paget's disease, may cause hypercalcemia.

Thiazides Administration of benzothiadiazines (thiazides) can cause hypercalcemia in patients with high rates of bone turnover. Traditionally, thiazides are associated with aggravation of hypercalcemia in primary hyperparathyroidism, but this effect can be seen in other high-bone-turnover states as well. The mechanism of thiazide action is complex. Chronic thiazide administration leads to reduction in urinary calcium; the hypocalciuric effect appears to reflect the enhancement of proximal tubular resorption of sodium and calcium in response to sodium depletion. Some of this renal effect is due to augmentation of PTH action and is more pronounced in individuals with intact PTH secretion. However, thiazides cause hypocalciuria in hypoparathyroid patients on high-dose vitamin D and oral calcium replacement if sodium intake is restricted. This finding is the rationale for the use of thiazides as an adjunct to therapy in hypoparathyroid patients, as discussed below. Thiazide administration to normal individuals causes a transient increase in blood calcium (usually within the high-normal range) that reverts to preexisting levels after a week or more of continued administration. If hormonal function and calcium and bone metabolism are normal, homeostatic controls are reset to counteract the calcium-elevating effect of the thiazides. In the presence of hyperparathyroidism or increased bone turnover from another cause, homeostatic mechanisms are ineffective. The abnormal effects of the thiazide on calcium metabolism disappear within days of cessation of the drug.

Vitamin A Intoxication Vitamin A intoxication is a rare cause of hypercalcemia and is most commonly a side effect of dietary faddism (Chap. 96e). Calcium levels can be elevated into the 3–3.5-mmol/L (12–14 mg/dL) range after the ingestion of 50,000–100,000 units of vitamin A daily (10–20 times the minimum daily requirement). Typical features of severe hypercalcemia include fatigue, anorexia, and, in some, severe muscle and bone pain. Excess vitamin A intake is presumed to increase bone resorption.

The diagnosis can be established by history and by measurement of vitamin A levels in serum. Occasionally, skeletal x-rays reveal periosteal calcifications, particularly in the hands. Withdrawal of the vitamin is usually associated with prompt disappearance of the hypercalcemia and reversal of the skeletal changes. As in vitamin D intoxication, administration of 100 mg/d of hydrocortisone or its equivalent leads to a rapid return of the serum calcium to normal.

HYPERCALCEMIA ASSOCIATED WITH RENAL FAILURE

Severe Secondary Hyperparathyroidism The pathogenesis of secondary hyperparathyroidism in chronic kidney disease is incompletely understood. Resistance to the normal level of PTH is a major factor contributing to the development of hypocalcemia, which, in turn, is a stimulus to parathyroid gland enlargement. However, recent findings have indicated that an increase of FGF23 production by osteocytes (and possibly osteoblasts) in bone occurs well before an elevation in PTH is detected. FGF23 is a potent inhibitor of the renal 1-alpha hydroxylase, and the FGF23-dependent reduction in 1,25(OH)$_2$ vitamin D seems to be an important stimulus for the development of secondary hyperparathyroidism.

Secondary hyperparathyroidism occurs not only in patients with renal failure but also in those with osteomalacia due to multiple causes (Chap. 423), including deficiency of vitamin D action and pseudohypoparathyroidism (deficient response to PTH downstream of PTHR1). For both disorders, hypocalcemia seems to be the common denominator in initiating the development of secondary hyperparathyroidism. Primary (1°) and secondary (2°) hyperparathyroidism can be distinguished conceptually by the autonomous growth of the parathyroid glands in primary hyperparathyroidism (presumably irreversible) and the adaptive response of the parathyroids in secondary hyperparathyroidism (typically reversible). In fact, reversal over weeks from an abnormal pattern of secretion, presumably accompanied by involution of parathyroid gland mass to normal, occurs in patients with osteomalacia who have been treated effectively with calcium and vitamin D. However, it is now recognized that a true clonal outgrowth (irreversible) can arise in long-standing, inadequately treated chronic kidney disease (e.g., tertiary [3°] hyperparathyroidism; see below).

Patients with secondary hyperparathyroidism may develop bone pain, ectopic calcification, and pruritus. The bone disease seen in patients with secondary hyperparathyroidism and chronic kidney disease is termed *renal osteodystrophy* and affects primarily bone turnover. However, osteomalacia is frequently encountered as well and may be related to the circulating levels of FGF23.

Two other skeletal disorders have been frequently associated in the past with chronic kidney disease (CKD) patients treated by long-term dialysis, who received aluminum-containing phosphate binders. Aluminum deposition in bone (see below) leads to an osteomalacia-like picture. The other entity is a low-turnover bone disease termed "aplastic" or "adynamic" bone disease; PTH levels are lower than typically observed in CKD patients with secondary hyperparathyroidism. It is believed that the condition is caused, at least in part, by excessive PTH suppression, which may be even greater than previously appreciated in light of evidence that some of the immunoreactive PTH detected by most commercially available PTH assays is not the full-length biologically active molecule (as discussed above) but may consist of amino-terminally truncated fragments that do not activate the PTH1R.

TREATMENT SECONDARY HYPERPARATHYROIDISM

Medical therapy to reverse secondary hyperparathyroidism in CKD includes reduction of excessive blood phosphate by restriction of dietary phosphate, the use of nonabsorbable phosphate binders, and careful, selective addition of calcitriol (0.25–2 μg/d) or related analogues. Calcium carbonate became preferred over aluminum-containing antacids to prevent aluminum-induced bone disease. However, synthetic gels that also bind phosphate (such as sevelamer; Chap. 335) are now widely used, with the advantage of avoiding not only aluminum retention, but also excess calcium loading, which may contribute to cardiovascular calcifications. Intravenous calcitriol (or related analogues), administered as several pulses each week, helps control secondary hyperparathyroidism. Aggressive but carefully administered medical therapy can often, but not always, reverse hyperparathyroidism and its symptoms and manifestations.

Occasional patients develop severe manifestations of secondary hyperparathyroidism, including hypercalcemia, pruritus, extraskeletal calcifications, and painful bones, despite aggressive medical efforts to suppress the hyperparathyroidism. PTH hypersecretion no longer responsive to medical therapy, a state of severe hyperparathyroidism in patients with CKD that requires surgery, has been referred to as *tertiary hyperparathyroidism*. Parathyroid surgery is necessary to control this condition. Based on genetic evidence from examination of tumor samples in these patients, the emergence of autonomous parathyroid function is due to a monoclonal outgrowth of one or more previously hyperplastic parathyroid glands. The adaptive response has become an independent contributor to disease; this finding seems to emphasize the importance of optimal medical management to reduce the proliferative response of the parathyroid cells that enables the irreversible genetic change.

Aluminum Intoxication Aluminum intoxication (and often hypercalcemia as a complication of medical treatment) in the past occurred in patients on chronic dialysis; manifestations included acute dementia and unresponsive and severe osteomalacia. Bone pain, multiple nonhealing fractures, particularly of the ribs and pelvis, and a proximal myopathy occur. Hypercalcemia develops when these patients are treated with vitamin D or calcitriol because of impaired skeletal responsiveness. Aluminum is present at the site of osteoid mineralization, osteoblastic activity is minimal, and calcium incorporation into the skeleton is impaired. The disorder is now rare because of the avoidance of aluminum-containing antacids or aluminum excess in the dialysis regimen (Chap. 429).

Milk-Alkali Syndrome The milk-alkali syndrome is due to excessive ingestion of calcium and absorbable antacids such as milk or calcium carbonate. It is much less frequent since proton pump inhibitors and other treatments became available for peptic ulcer disease. For a time, the increased use of calcium carbonate in the management of secondary hyperparathyroidism led to reappearance of the syndrome. Several clinical presentations—acute, subacute, and chronic—have been described, all of which feature hypercalcemia, alkalosis, and renal failure. The chronic form of the disease, termed *Burnett's syndrome*, is associated with irreversible renal damage. The acute syndromes reverse if the excess calcium and absorbable alkali are stopped.

Individual susceptibility is important in the pathogenesis, because some patients are treated with calcium carbonate and alkali regimens without developing the syndrome. One variable is the fractional calcium absorption as a function of calcium intake. Some individuals absorb a high fraction of calcium, even with intakes ≥2 g of elemental calcium per day, instead of reducing calcium absorption with high intake, as occurs in most normal individuals. Resultant mild hypercalcemia after meals in such patients is postulated to contribute to the generation of alkalosis. Development of hypercalcemia causes increased sodium excretion and some depletion of total-body water. These phenomena and perhaps some suppression of endogenous PTH secretion due to mild hypercalcemia lead to increased bicarbonate resorption and to alkalosis in the face of continued calcium carbonate ingestion. Alkalosis per se selectively enhances calcium resorption in the distal nephron, thus aggravating the hypercalcemia. The cycle of mild hypercalcemia → bicarbonate retention → alkalosis → renal calcium retention → severe hypercalcemia perpetuates and aggravates hypercalcemia and alkalosis as long as calcium and absorbable alkali are ingested.

DIFFERENTIAL DIAGNOSIS: SPECIAL TESTS

Differential diagnosis of hypercalcemia is best achieved by using clinical criteria, but immunometric assays to measure PTH are especially useful in distinguishing among major causes (Fig. 424-6). The clinical features that deserve emphasis are the presence or absence of symptoms or signs of disease and evidence of chronicity. If one discounts fatigue or depression, >90% of patients with primary hyperparathyroidism have *asymptomatic hypercalcemia*; symptoms of malignancy are usually present in cancer-associated hypercalcemia. Disorders other than hyperparathyroidism and malignancy cause <10% of cases of hypercalcemia, and some of the nonparathyroid causes are associated with clear-cut manifestations such as renal failure.

Hyperparathyroidism is the likely diagnosis in patients with *chronic hypercalcemia*. If hypercalcemia has been manifest for >1 year, malignancy can usually be excluded as the cause. A striking feature of malignancy-associated hypercalcemia is the rapidity of the course,

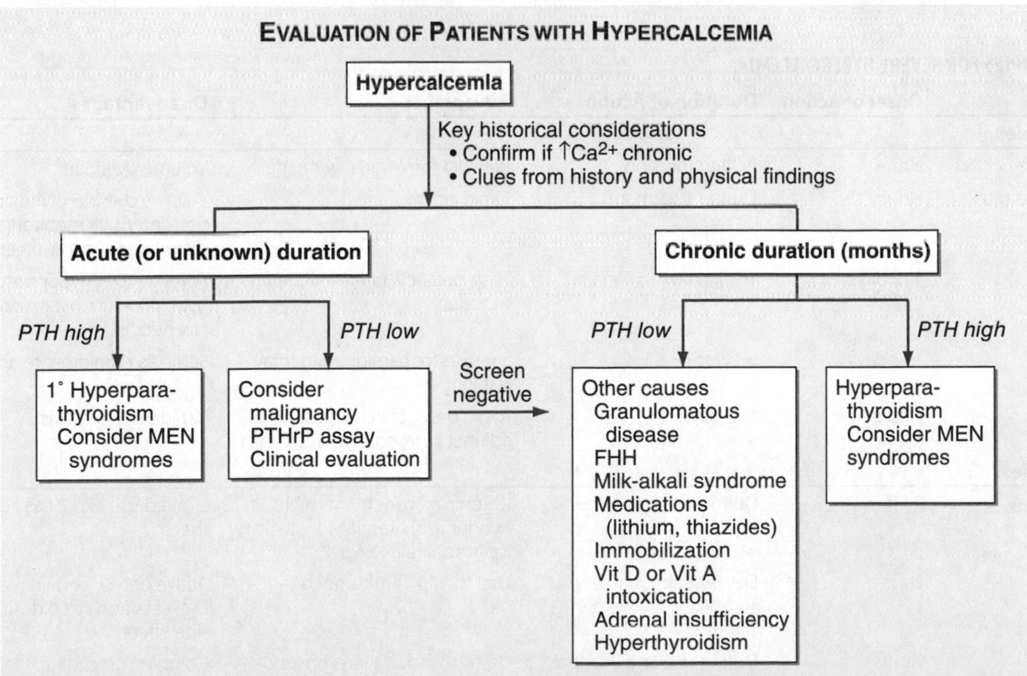

FIGURE 424-6 Algorithm for the evaluation of patients with hypercalcemia. See text for details. FHH, familial hypocalciuric hypercalcemia; MEN, multiple endocrine neoplasia; PTH, parathyroid hormone; PTHrP, parathyroid hormone–related peptide.

whereby signs and symptoms of the underlying malignancy are evident within months of the detection of hypercalcemia. Although clinical considerations are helpful in arriving at the correct diagnosis of the cause of hypercalcemia, appropriate laboratory testing is essential for definitive diagnosis. The immunoassay for PTH usually separates hyperparathyroidism from all other causes of hypercalcemia (exceptions are very rare reports of ectopic production of excess PTH by nonparathyroid tumors). Patients with hyperparathyroidism have elevated PTH levels despite hypercalcemia, whereas patients with malignancy and the other causes of hypercalcemia (except for disorders mediated by PTH such as lithium-induced hypercalcemia) have levels of hormone below normal or undetectable levels. Assays based on the double-antibody method for PTH exhibit very high sensitivity (especially if serum calcium is simultaneously evaluated) and specificity for the diagnosis of primary hyperparathyroidism (Fig. 424-4).

In summary, PTH values are elevated in >90% of parathyroid-related causes of hypercalcemia, undetectable or low in malignancy-related hypercalcemia, and undetectable or normal in vitamin D–related and high-bone-turnover causes of hypercalcemia. In view of the specificity of the PTH immunoassay and the high frequency of hyperparathyroidism in hypercalcemic patients, it is cost-effective to measure the PTH level in all hypercalcemic patients unless malignancy or a specific nonparathyroid disease is obvious. False-positive PTH assay results are rare. Immunoassays for PTHrP are helpful in diagnosing certain types of malignancy-associated hypercalcemia. Although FHH is parathyroid-related, the disease should be managed distinctively from hyperparathyroidism. Clinical features and the low urinary calcium excretion can help make the distinction. Because the incidence of malignancy and hyperparathyroidism both increase with age, they can coexist as two independent causes of hypercalcemia.

$1,25(OH)_2D$ levels are elevated in many (but not all) patients with primary hyperparathyroidism. In other disorders associated with hypercalcemia, concentrations of $1,25(OH)_2D$ are low or, at the most, normal. However, this test is of low specificity and is not cost-effective, as not all patients with hyperparathyroidism have elevated $1,25(OH)_2D$ levels and not all nonparathyroid hypercalcemic patients have suppressed $1,25(OH)_2D$. Measurement of $1,25(OH)_2D$ is, however, critically valuable in establishing the cause of hypercalcemia in sarcoidosis and certain lymphomas.

A useful general approach is outlined in Fig. 424-6. If the patient is *asymptomatic* and there is evidence of *chronicity* to the hypercalcemia, hyperparathyroidism is almost certainly the cause. If PTH levels (usually measured at least twice) are elevated, the clinical impression is confirmed and little additional evaluation is necessary. If there is only a short history or no data as to the duration of the hypercalcemia, *occult malignancy* must be considered; if the PTH levels are not elevated, then a thorough workup must be undertaken for malignancy, including chest x-ray, CT of chest and abdomen, and bone scan. Immunoassays for PTHrP may be especially useful in such situations. Attention should also be paid to clues for underlying hematologic disorders such as anemia, increased plasma globulin, and abnormal serum immunoelectrophoresis; bone scans can be negative in some patients with metastases such as in multiple myeloma. Finally, if a patient with chronic hypercalcemia is asymptomatic and malignancy therefore seems unlikely on clinical grounds, but PTH values are not elevated, it is useful to search for other chronic causes of hypercalcemia such as occult sarcoidosis. A careful history of dietary supplements and drug use may suggest intoxication with vitamin D or vitamin A or the use of thiazides.

TREATMENT HYPERCALCEMIC STATES

The approach to medical treatment of hypercalcemia varies with its severity (Table 424-4). Mild hypercalcemia, <3 mmol/L (12 mg/dL), can be managed by hydration. More severe hypercalcemia (levels of 3.2–3.7 mmol/L [13–15 mg/dL]) must be managed aggressively; above that level, hypercalcemia can be life-threatening and requires emergency measures. By using a combination of approaches in severe hypercalcemia, the serum calcium concentration can be decreased by 0.7–2.2 mmol/L (3–9 mg/dL) within 24–48 h in most patients, enough to relieve acute symptoms, prevent death from hypercalcemic crisis, and permit diagnostic evaluation. Therapy can then be directed at the underlying disorder—the second priority.

Hypercalcemia develops because of excessive skeletal calcium release, increased intestinal calcium absorption, or inadequate renal calcium excretion. Understanding the particular pathogenesis helps guide therapy. For example, hypercalcemia in patients with malignancy is primarily due to excessive skeletal calcium release and is, therefore, minimally improved by restriction of dietary calcium. On the other hand, patients with vitamin D hypersensitivity or vitamin D intoxication have excessive intestinal calcium absorption, and

TABLE 424-4 THERAPIES FOR SEVERE HYPERCALCEMIA

Treatment	Onset of Action	Duration of Action	Advantages	Disadvantages
Most Useful Therapies				
Hydration with saline	Hours	During infusion	Rehydration invariably needed	Volume overload
Forced diuresis; saline plus loop diuretic	Hours	During treatment	Rapid action	Volume overload, cardiac decompensation, intensive monitoring, electrolyte disturbance, inconvenience
Pamidronate	1–2 days	10–14 days to weeks	High potency; intermediate onset of action	Fever in 20%, hypophosphatemia, hypocalcemia, hypomagnesemia, rarely jaw necrosis
Zoledronate	1–2 days	>3 weeks	Same as for pamidronate (may last longer)	Same as pamidronate above
Calcitonin	Hours	1–2 days	Rapid onset of action; useful as adjunct in severe hypercalcemia	Rapid tachyphylaxis
Special Use Therapies				
Phosphate oral	24 h	During use	Chronic management (with hypophosphatemia); low toxicity if phosphate <4 mg/dL	Limited use except as adjuvant or chronic therapy
Glucocorticoids	Days	Days, weeks	Oral therapy, antitumor agent	Active only in certain malignancies, vitamin D excess and sarcoidosis; glucocorticoid side effects
Dialysis	Hours	During use and 24–48 h afterward	Useful in renal failure; onset of effect in hours; can immediately reverse life-threatening hypercalcemia	Complex procedure, reserved for extreme or special circumstances

restriction of dietary calcium is beneficial. Decreased renal function or ECF depletion decreases urinary calcium excretion. In such situations, rehydration may rapidly reduce or reverse the hypercalcemia, even though increased bone resorption persists. As outlined below, the more severe the hypercalcemia, the greater the number of combined therapies that should be used. Rapid-acting (hours) approaches—rehydration, forced diuresis, and calcitonin—can be used with the most effective antiresorptive agents such as bisphosphonates (since severe hypercalcemia usually involves excessive bone resorption).

HYDRATION, INCREASED SALT INTAKE, MILD AND FORCED DIURESIS

The first principle of treatment is to restore normal hydration. Many hypercalcemic patients are dehydrated because of vomiting, inanition, and/or hypercalcemia-induced defects in urinary concentrating ability. The resultant drop in glomerular filtration rate is accompanied by an additional decrease in renal tubular sodium and calcium clearance. Restoring a normal ECF volume corrects these abnormalities and increases urine calcium excretion by 2.5–7.5 mmol/d (100–300 mg/d). Increasing urinary sodium excretion to 400–500 mmol/d increases urinary calcium excretion even further than simple rehydration. After rehydration has been achieved, saline can be administered, or furosemide or ethacrynic acid can be given twice daily to depress the tubular reabsorptive mechanism for calcium (care must be taken to prevent dehydration). The combined use of these therapies can increase urinary calcium excretion to ≥12.5 mmol/d (500 mg/d) in most hypercalcemic patients. Because this is a substantial percentage of the exchangeable calcium pool, the serum calcium concentration usually falls 0.25–0.75 mmol/L (1–3 mg/dL) within 24 h. Precautions should be taken to prevent potassium and magnesium depletion; calcium-containing renal calculi are a potential complication.

Under life-threatening circumstances, the preceding approach can be pursued more aggressively, but the availability of effective agents to block bone resorption (such as bisphosphonates) has reduced the need for extreme diuresis regimens (Table 424-4). Depletion of potassium and magnesium is inevitable unless replacements are given; pulmonary edema can be precipitated. The potential complications can be reduced by careful monitoring of central venous pressure and plasma or urine electrolytes; catheterization of the bladder may be necessary. Dialysis treatment may be needed when renal function is compromised.

BISPHOSPHONATES

The bisphosphonates are analogues of pyrophosphate, with high affinity for bone, especially in areas of increased bone turnover, where they are powerful inhibitors of bone resorption. These bone-seeking compounds are stable in vivo because phosphatase enzymes cannot hydrolyze the central carbon-phosphorus-carbon bond. The bisphosphonates are concentrated in areas of high bone turnover and are taken up by and inhibit osteoclast action; the mechanism of action is complex. The bisphosphonate molecules that contain amino groups in the side chain structure (see below) interfere with prenylation of proteins and can lead to cellular apoptosis. The highly active nonamino group–containing bisphosphonates are also metabolized to cytotoxic products.

The initial bisphosphonate widely used in clinical practice, etidronate, was effective but had several disadvantages, including the capacity to inhibit bone formation as well as blocking resorption. Subsequently, a number of second- or third-generation compounds have become the mainstays of antiresorptive therapy for treatment of hypercalcemia and osteoporosis. The newer bisphosphonates have a highly favorable ratio of blocking resorption versus inhibiting bone formation; they inhibit osteoclast-mediated skeletal resorption yet do not cause mineralization defects at ordinary doses. Although the bisphosphonates have similar structures, the routes of administration, efficacy, toxicity, and side effects vary. The potency of the compounds for inhibition of bone resorption varies more than 10,000-fold, increasing in the order of etidronate, tiludronate, pamidronate, alendronate, risedronate, and zoledronate. The IV use of pamidronate and zoledronate is approved for the treatment of hypercalcemia; between 30 and 90 mg pamidronate, given as a single IV dose over a few hours, returns serum calcium to normal within 24–48 h with an effect that lasts for weeks in 80–100% of patients. Zoledronate given in doses of 4 or 8 mg/5-min infusion has a more rapid and more sustained effect than pamidronate in direct comparison.

These drugs are used extensively in cancer patients. Absolute survival improvements are noted with pamidronate and zoledronate in multiple myeloma, for example. However, although still rare, there are increasing reports of jaw necrosis, especially after dental surgery, mainly in cancer patients treated with multiple doses of the more potent bisphosphonates.

CALCITONIN

Calcitonin acts within a few hours of its administration, principally through receptors on osteoclasts, to block bone resorption. Calcitonin, after 24 h of use, is no longer effective in lowering calcium. Tachyphylaxis, a known phenomenon with this drug, seems to explain the results, since the drug is often effective in the first 24 h of use. Therefore, in life-threatening hypercalcemia, calcitonin can be used effectively within the first 24 h in combination with rehydration and saline diuresis while waiting for more sustained effects from a simultaneously administered bisphosphonate such as pamidronate. Usual doses of calcitonin are 2–8 U/kg of body weight IV, SC, or IM every 6–12 h.

OTHER THERAPIES

Denosumab, an antibody that blocks the RANK ligand (RANKL) and dramatically reduces osteoclast number and function, is approved for therapy of osteoporosis. It also appears to be an effective treatment to reverse hypercalcemia of malignancy, but is not yet approved for this indication. *Plicamycin* (formerly mithramycin), which inhibits bone resorption, and *gallium nitrate*, which exerts a hypocalcemic action also by inhibiting bone resorption, are no longer used because of superior alternatives such as bisphosphonates.

Glucocorticoids have utility, especially in hypercalcemia complicating certain malignancies. They increase urinary calcium excretion and decrease intestinal calcium absorption when given in pharmacologic doses, but they also cause negative skeletal calcium balance. In normal individuals and in patients with primary hyperparathyroidism, glucocorticoids neither increase nor decrease the serum calcium concentration. In patients with hypercalcemia due to certain osteolytic malignancies, however, glucocorticoids may be effective as a result of antitumor effects. The malignancies in which hypercalcemia responds to glucocorticoids include multiple myeloma, leukemia, Hodgkin's disease, other lymphomas, and carcinoma of the breast, at least early in the course of the disease. Glucocorticoids are also effective in treating hypercalcemia due to vitamin D intoxication and sarcoidosis. Glucocorticoids are also useful in the rare form of hypercalcemia, now recognized in certain autoimmune disorders in which inactivating antibodies against the receptor imitate FHH. Elevated PTH and calcium levels are effectively lowered by the glucocorticoids. In all the preceding situations, the hypocalcemic effect develops over several days, and the usual glucocorticoid dosage is 40–100 mg prednisone (or its equivalent) daily in four divided doses. The side effects of chronic glucocorticoid therapy may be acceptable in some circumstances.

Dialysis is often the treatment of choice for severe hypercalcemia complicated by renal failure, which is difficult to manage medically. Peritoneal dialysis with calcium-free dialysis fluid can remove 5–12.5 mmol (200–500 mg) of calcium in 24–48 h and lower the serum calcium concentration by 0.7–3 mmol/L (3–12 mg/dL). Large quantities of phosphate are lost during dialysis, and serum inorganic phosphate concentration usually falls, potentially aggravating hypercalcemia. Therefore, the serum inorganic phosphate concentration should be measured after dialysis, and phosphate supplements should be added to the diet or to dialysis fluids if necessary.

Phosphate therapy, PO or IV, has a limited role in certain circumstances (**Chap. 423**). Correcting hypophosphatemia lowers the serum calcium concentration by several mechanisms, including bone/calcium exchange. The usual oral treatment is 1–1.5 g of phosphorus per day for several days, given in divided doses. It is generally believed, but not established, that toxicity does not occur if therapy is limited to restoring serum inorganic phosphate concentrations to normal.

Raising the serum inorganic phosphate concentration above normal decreases serum calcium levels, sometimes strikingly. Intravenous phosphate is one of the most dramatically effective treatments available for severe hypercalcemia but is toxic and even dangerous (fatal hypocalcemia). For these reasons, it is used rarely and only in severely hypercalcemic patients with cardiac or renal failure where dialysis, the preferable alternative, is not feasible or is unavailable.

SUMMARY

The various therapies for hypercalcemia are listed in Table 424-4. The choice depends on the underlying disease, the severity of the hypercalcemia, the serum inorganic phosphate level, and the renal, hepatic, and bone marrow function. Mild hypercalcemia (≤3 mmol/L [12 mg/dL]) can usually be managed by hydration. Severe hypercalcemia (≥3.7 mmol/L [15 mg/dL]) requires rapid correction. Calcitonin should be given for its rapid, albeit short-lived, blockade of bone resorption, and IV pamidronate or zoledronate should be administered, although its onset of action is delayed for 1–2 days. In addition, for the first 24–48 h, aggressive sodium-calcium diuresis with IV saline should be given and, following rehydration, large doses of furosemide or ethacrynic acid, but only if appropriate monitoring is available and cardiac and renal function are adequate. Intermediate degrees of hypercalcemia between 3 and 3.7 mmol/L (12 and 15 mg/dL) should be approached with vigorous hydration and then the most appropriate selection for the patient of the combinations used with severe hypercalcemia.

HYPOCALCEMIA

(See also Chap. 65)

PATHOPHYSIOLOGY OF HYPOCALCEMIA: CLASSIFICATION BASED ON MECHANISM

Chronic hypocalcemia is less common than hypercalcemia; causes include chronic renal failure, hereditary and acquired hypoparathyroidism, vitamin D deficiency, pseudohypoparathyroidism, and hypomagnesemia (**Table 424-5**).

Acute rather than chronic hypocalcemia is seen in critically ill patients or as a consequence of certain medications and often does not require specific treatment. Transient hypocalcemia is seen with severe sepsis, burns, acute kidney injury, and extensive transfusions with citrated blood. Although as many as one-half of patients in an intensive care setting are reported to have calcium concentrations of <2.1 mmol/L (8.5 mg/dL), most do not have a reduction in ionized calcium. Patients with severe sepsis may have a decrease in ionized calcium (true hypocalcemia), but in other severely ill individuals, hypoalbuminemia is the primary cause of the reduced total calcium concentration. Alkalosis increases calcium binding to proteins, and in this setting, direct measurements of ionized calcium should be made.

Medications such as protamine, heparin, and glucagon may cause transient hypocalcemia. These forms of hypocalcemia are usually not associated with tetany and resolve with improvement in the overall medical condition. The hypocalcemia after repeated transfusions of citrated blood usually resolves quickly.

Patients with *acute pancreatitis* have hypocalcemia that persists during the acute inflammation and varies in degree with disease severity. The cause of hypocalcemia remains unclear. PTH values are

TABLE 424-5 FUNCTIONAL CLASSIFICATION OF HYPOCALCEMIA (EXCLUDING NEONATAL CONDITIONS)

PTH Absent	
Hereditary hypoparathyroidism	Hypomagnesemia
Acquired hypoparathyroidism	
PTH Ineffective	
Chronic kidney disease	Active vitamin D ineffective
Active vitamin D lacking	Intestinal malabsorption
↓ Dietary intake or sunlight	Vitamin D–dependent rickets type II
Defective metabolism:	Pseudohypoparathyroidism
Anticonvulsant therapy	
Vitamin D–dependent rickets type I	
PTH Overwhelmed	
Severe, acute hyperphosphatemia	Osteitis fibrosa after parathyroidectomy
Tumor lysis	
Acute kidney injury	
Rhabdomyolysis	

Abbreviation: PTH, parathyroid hormone.

reported to be low, normal, or elevated, and both resistance to PTH and impaired PTH secretion have been postulated. Occasionally, a chronic low total calcium and low ionized calcium concentration are detected in an elderly patient without obvious cause and with a paucity of symptoms; the pathogenesis is unclear.

Chronic hypocalcemia, however, is usually symptomatic and requires treatment. Neuromuscular and neurologic manifestations of chronic hypocalcemia include muscle spasms, carpopedal spasm, facial grimacing, and, in extreme cases, laryngeal spasm and convulsions. Respiratory arrest may occur. Increased intracranial pressure occurs in some patients with long-standing hypocalcemia, often in association with papilledema. Mental changes include irritability, depression, and psychosis. The QT interval on the electrocardiogram is prolonged, in contrast to its shortening with hypercalcemia. Arrhythmias occur, and digitalis effectiveness may be reduced. Intestinal cramps and chronic malabsorption may occur. Chvostek's or Trousseau's sign can be used to confirm latent tetany.

The classification of hypocalcemia shown in Table 424-5 is based on an organizationally useful premise that PTH is responsible for minute-to-minute regulation of plasma calcium concentration and, therefore, that the occurrence of hypocalcemia must mean a failure of the homeostatic action of PTH. Failure of the PTH response can occur if there is hereditary or acquired parathyroid gland failure, if PTH is ineffective in target organs, or if the action of the hormone is overwhelmed by the loss of calcium from the ECF at a rate faster than it can be replaced.

PTH ABSENT

Whether hereditary or acquired, hypoparathyroidism has a number of common components. Symptoms of untreated hypocalcemia are shared by both types of hypoparathyroidism, although the onset of hereditary hypoparathyroidism can be more gradual and associated with other developmental defects. Basal ganglia calcification and extrapyramidal syndromes are more common and earlier in onset in hereditary hypoparathyroidism. In previous decades, acquired hypoparathyroidism secondary to surgery in the neck was more common than hereditary hypoparathyroidism, but the frequency of surgically induced parathyroid failure has diminished as a result of improved surgical techniques that spare the parathyroid glands and increased use of nonsurgical therapy for hyperthyroidism. Pseudohypoparathyroidism, an example of ineffective PTH action rather than a failure of parathyroid gland production, may share several features with hypoparathyroidism, including extraosseous calcification and extrapyramidal manifestations such as choreoathetotic movements and dystonia.

Papilledema and raised intracranial pressure may occur in both hereditary and acquired hypoparathyroidism, as do chronic changes in fingernails and hair and lenticular cataracts, the latter usually reversible with treatment of hypocalcemia. Certain skin manifestations, including alopecia and candidiasis, are characteristic of hereditary hypoparathyroidism associated with autoimmune polyglandular failure (Chap. 408).

Hypocalcemia associated with hypomagnesemia is associated with both deficient PTH release and impaired responsiveness to the hormone. Patients with hypocalcemia secondary to hypomagnesemia have absent or low levels of circulating PTH, indicative of diminished hormone release despite a maximum physiologic stimulus by hypocalcemia. Plasma PTH levels return to normal with correction of the hypomagnesemia. Thus hypoparathyroidism with low levels of PTH in blood can be due to hereditary gland failure, acquired gland failure, or acute but reversible gland dysfunction (hypomagnesemia).

Genetic Abnormalities and Hereditary Hypoparathyroidism Hereditary hypoparathyroidism can occur as an isolated entity without other endocrine or dermatologic manifestations. More typically, it occurs in association with other abnormalities such as defective development of the thymus or failure of other endocrine organs such as the adrenal, thyroid, or ovary (Chap. 408). Hereditary hypoparathyroidism is often manifest within the first decade but may appear later.

Genetic defects associated with hypoparathyroidism serve to illuminate the complexity of organ development, hormonal biosynthesis and secretion, and tissue-specific patterns of endocrine effector function (Fig. 424-5). Often, hypoparathyroidism is isolated, signifying a highly specific functional disturbance. When hypoparathyroidism is associated with other developmental or organ defects, treatment of the hypocalcemia can still be effective.

A form of hypoparathyroidism associated with defective development of both the thymus and the parathyroid glands is termed the *DiGeorge syndrome*, or the *velocardiofacial syndrome*. Congenital cardiovascular, facial, and other developmental defects are present, and patients may die in early childhood with severe infections, hypocalcemia and seizures, or cardiovascular complications. Patients can survive into adulthood, and milder, incomplete forms occur. Most cases are sporadic, but an autosomal dominant form involving microdeletions of chromosome 22q11.2 has been described. Smaller deletions in chromosome 22 are seen in incomplete forms of the DiGeorge syndrome, appearing in childhood or adolescence, that are manifest primarily by parathyroid gland failure. The chromosome 22 defect is now termed *DSG1*; more recently, a defect in chromosome 10p is also recognized—now called *DSG2*. The phenotypes seem similar. Studies on the chromosome 22 defect have pinpointed a transcription factor, TBX1. Deletions of the orthologous mouse gene show a phenotype similar to the human syndrome.

Another autosomal dominant developmental defect, featuring hypoparathyroidism, deafness, and renal dysplasia (HDR), has been studied at the genetic level. Cytogenetic abnormalities in some, but not all kindreds, point to translocation defects on chromosome 10, as in DiGeorge syndrome. However, the lack of immunodeficiency and heart defects distinguishes the two syndromes. Mouse models, as well as deletional analysis in some HDR patients, has identified the transcription factor GATA3, which is important in embryonic development and is expressed in developing kidney, ear structures, and the parathyroids.

Another pair of linked developmental disorders involving the parathyroids is recognized. *Kenney-Caffey syndrome type I* features hypoparathyroidism, short stature, osteosclerosis, and thick cortical bones. A defect seen in Middle Eastern patients, particularly in Saudi Arabia, termed *Sanjad-Sakati syndrome*, also exhibits growth failure and other dysmorphic features. This syndrome, which is clearly autosomal recessive, involves a gene on chromosome 1q42-q43. Both syndromes apparently involve a chaperone protein, called *TBCE*, relevant to tubulin function. Recently, a defect in FAM111A was identified as the cause of *Kenney-Caffey syndrome type 2*.

Hypoparathyroidism can occur in association with a complex hereditary autoimmune syndrome involving failure of the adrenals, the ovaries, the immune system, and the parathyroids in association with recurrent mucocutaneous candidiasis, alopecia, vitiligo, and pernicious anemia (Chap. 408). The responsible gene on chromosome 21q22.3 has been identified. The protein product, which resembles a transcription factor, has been termed the *autoimmune regulator*, or AIRE. A stop codon mutation occurs in many Finnish families with the disorder, commonly referred to as *polyglandular autoimmune type 1 deficiency*, whereas another AIRE mutation (Y85C) is typically observed in Jews of Iraqi and Iranian descent.

Hypoparathyroidism is seen in two disorders associated with mitochondrial dysfunction and myopathy, one termed the *Kearns-Sayre syndrome* (KSS), with ophthalmoplegia and pigmentary retinopathy, and the other termed the *MELAS syndrome* (*m*itochondrial *e*ncephalopathy, *l*actic *a*cidosis, and *s*troke-like episodes). Mutations or deletions in mitochondrial genes have been identified.

Several forms of hypoparathyroidism, each rare in frequency, are seen as isolated defects; the genetic mechanisms are varied. The inheritance includes autosomal dominant, autosomal recessive, and X-linked modes. Three separate autosomal defects involving the parathyroid gene have been recognized: one is dominant and the other two are recessive. The dominant form has a point mutation in the signal sequence, a critical region involved in intracellular transport of the hormone precursor. An Arg for Cys mutation interferes with processing of the precursor and is believed to trigger an apoptotic cellular response, hence acting as a dominant negative. The other two forms are recessive. One point mutation also blocks cleavage of the PTH precursor but requires both alleles to cause hypoparathyroidism. The third involves a single-nucleotide base change that results in an exon splicing defect; the lost exon contains the promoter—hence, the gene is silenced. An X-linked recessive form of hypoparathyroidism has been described in males, and the defect has been localized to chromosome Xq26-q27, perhaps involving the *SOX3* gene.

Abnormalities in the CaSR are detected in three distinctive hypocalcemic disorders. All are rare, but more than 10 different gain-of-function mutations have been found in one form of hypocalcemia termed *autosomal dominant hypocalcemic hypercalciuria (ADHH)*. The receptor senses the ambient calcium level as excessive and suppresses PTH secretion, leading to hypocalcemia. The hypocalcemia is aggravated by constitutive receptor activity in the renal tubule causing excretion of inappropriate amounts of calcium. Recognition of the syndrome is important because efforts to treat the hypocalcemia with vitamin D analogues and increased oral calcium exacerbate the already excessive urinary calcium excretion (several grams or more per 24 h), leading to irreversible renal damage from stones and ectopic calcification.

Other causes of isolated hypoparathyroidism include homozygous, inactivating mutations in the parathyroid-specific transcription factor GCM2, which lead to an autosomal recessive form of the disease, or heterozygous point mutations in GCM2, which have a dominant negative effect on the wild-type protein and thus lead to an autosomal dominant form of hypoparathyroidism. Furthermore, heterozygous mutations in G11, one of the two signaling proteins downstream of the CaSR, have been identified as a cause of autosomal dominant hypoparathyroidism.

Bartter's syndrome is a group of disorders associated with disturbances in electrolyte and acid/base balance, sometimes with nephrocalcinosis and other features. Several types of ion channels or transporters are involved. Curiously, *Bartter's syndrome type V* has the electrolyte and pH disturbances seen in the other syndromes but appears to be due to a gain of function in the CaSR. The defect may be more severe than in ADHH and explains the additional features seen beyond hypocalcemia and hypercalciuria.

As with autoimmune disorders that block the CaSR (discussed above under hypercalcemic conditions), there are autoantibodies that at least transiently activate the CaSR, leading to suppressed PTH secretion and hypocalcemia. This disorder may wax and wane.

Acquired Hypoparathyroidism *Acquired chronic hypoparathyroidism* is usually the result of inadvertent surgical removal of all the parathyroid glands; in some instances, not all the tissue is removed, but the remainder undergoes vascular supply compromise secondary to fibrotic changes in the neck after surgery. In the past, the most frequent cause of acquired hypoparathyroidism was surgery for hyperthyroidism. Hypoparathyroidism now usually occurs after surgery for hyperparathyroidism when the surgeon, facing the dilemma of removing too little tissue and thus not curing the hyperparathyroidism, removes too much. Parathyroid function may not be totally absent in all patients with postoperative hypoparathyroidism.

Rare causes of acquired chronic hypoparathyroidism include radiation-induced damage subsequent to radioiodine therapy of hyperthyroidism and glandular damage in patients with hemochromatosis or hemosiderosis after repeated blood transfusions. Infection may involve one or more of the parathyroids but usually does not cause hypoparathyroidism because all four glands are rarely involved.

Transient hypoparathyroidism is frequent following surgery for hyperparathyroidism. After a variable period of hypoparathyroidism, normal parathyroid function may return due to hyperplasia or recovery of remaining tissue. Occasionally, recovery occurs months after surgery.

TREATMENT ACQUIRED AND HEREDITARY HYPOPARATHYROIDISM

Treatment involves replacement with vitamin D or $1,25(OH)_2D$ (calcitriol) combined with a high oral calcium intake. In most patients, blood calcium and phosphate levels are satisfactorily regulated, but some patients show resistance and a brittleness, with a tendency to alternate between hypocalcemia and hypercalcemia. For many patients, vitamin D in doses of 40,000–120,000 U/d (1–3 mg/d) combined with ≥1 g elemental calcium is satisfactory. The wide dosage range reflects the variation encountered from patient to patient; precise regulation of each patient is required. Compared to typical daily requirements in euparathyroid patients of 200 U/d (or in older patients as high as 800 U/d), the high dose of vitamin D (as much as 100-fold higher) reflects the reduced conversion of vitamin D to $1,25(OH)_2D$. Many physicians now use 0.5–1 μg of calcitriol in management of such patients, especially if they are difficult to control. Because of its storage in fat, when vitamin D is withdrawn, weeks are required for the disappearance of the biologic effects, compared with a few days for calcitriol, which has a rapid turnover.

Oral calcium and vitamin D restore the overall calcium-phosphate balance but do not reverse the lowered urinary calcium reabsorption typical of hypoparathyroidism. Therefore, care must be taken to avoid excessive urinary calcium excretion after vitamin D and calcium replacement therapy; otherwise, nephrocalcinosis and kidney stones can develop, and the risk of CKD is increased. Thiazide diuretics lower urine calcium by as much as 100 mg/d in hypoparathyroid patients on vitamin D, provided they are maintained on a low-sodium diet. Use of thiazides seems to be of benefit in mitigating hypercalciuria and easing the daily management of these patients.

There are now trials of parenterally administered PTH (either PTH[1–34] or PTH[1–84]) in patients with hypoparathyroidism providing greater ease of maintaining serum calcium and reducing urinary calcium excretion (desirable to protect any renal damage). However, PTH therapy for the treatment of hypoparathyroidism is not approved as of yet.

Hypomagnesemia Severe hypomagnesemia (<0.4 mmol/L; <0.8 meq/L) is associated with hypocalcemia (Chap. 423). Restoration of the total-body magnesium deficit leads to rapid reversal of hypocalcemia. There are at least two causes of the hypocalcemia—impaired PTH secretion and reduced responsiveness to PTH. **For further discussion of causes and treatment of hypomagnesemia, see Chap. 423.**

The effects of magnesium on PTH secretion are similar to those of calcium; hypermagnesemia suppresses and hypomagnesemia stimulates PTH secretion. The effects of magnesium on PTH secretion are normally of little significance, however, because the calcium effects dominate. Greater change in magnesium than in calcium is needed to influence hormone secretion. Nonetheless, hypomagnesemia might be expected to increase hormone secretion. It is therefore surprising to find that severe hypomagnesemia is associated with blunted secretion of PTH. The explanation for the paradox is that severe, chronic hypomagnesemia leads to intracellular magnesium deficiency, which interferes with secretion and peripheral responses to PTH. The mechanism of the cellular abnormalities caused by hypomagnesemia is unknown, although effects on adenylate cyclase (for which magnesium is a cofactor) have been proposed.

PTH levels are undetectable or inappropriately low in severe hypomagnesemia despite the stimulus of severe hypocalcemia, and acute repletion of magnesium leads to a rapid increase in PTH level. Serum phosphate levels are often not elevated, in contrast to the situation with acquired or idiopathic hypoparathyroidism, probably because phosphate deficiency is often seen in hypomagnesmia (Chap. 393).

Diminished peripheral responsiveness to PTH also occurs in some patients, as documented by subnormal response in urinary phosphorus and urinary cAMP excretion after administration of exogenous PTH to patients who are hypocalcemic and hypomagnesemic. Both blunted PTH secretion and lack of renal response to administered PTH can occur in the same patient. When acute magnesium repletion is undertaken, the restoration of PTH levels to normal or supranormal may precede restoration of normal serum calcium by several days.

TREATMENT HYPOMAGNESEMIA

Repletion of magnesium cures the condition. Repletion should be parenteral. Attention must be given to restoring the intracellular deficit, which may be considerable. After IV magnesium administration, serum magnesium may return transiently to the normal range, but unless replacement therapy is adequate, serum magnesium will again fall. If the cause of the hypomagnesemia is renal magnesium wasting, magnesium may have to be given long-term to prevent recurrence **(Chap. 423)**.

PTH INEFFECTIVE

PTH is not sufficiently active to fully prevent hypocalcemia (although retaining phosphaturic activity, for example). This problem occurs when the PTH1R–signaling protein complex is defective (as in the different forms of pseudohypoparathyroidism [PHP], discussed below); when PTH action to promote calcium absorption from the diet via the synthesis of $1,25(OH)_2D$ is insufficient because of vitamin D deficiency or because vitamin D is ineffective (defects in vitamin D receptor or vitamin D synthesis); or in CKD in which the calcium-elevating action of PTH is impaired.

Typically, hypophosphatemia is more severe than hypocalcemia in vitamin D deficiency states because of the increased secretion of PTH, which, although only partly effective in elevating blood calcium, is readily capable of promoting urinary phosphate excretion.

PHP, on the other hand, has a pathophysiology that is different from the other disorders of ineffective PTH action. PHP resembles hypoparathyroidism (in which PTH synthesis is deficient) and is manifested by hypocalcemia and hyperphosphatemia, yet elevated PTH levels. The cause of the disorder is defective PTH-dependent activation of the stimulatory G protein complex or the downstream effector protein kinase A, resulting in failure of PTH to increase intracellular cAMP or to respond to elevated cAMP levels (see below).

Chronic Kidney Disease Improved medical management of CKD now allows many patients to survive for decades and hence allows time enough to develop features of renal osteodystrophy, which must be controlled to avoid additional morbidity. Impaired production of $1,25(OH)_2D$ is now thought to be the principal factor that causes calcium deficiency, secondary hyperparathyroidism, and bone disease;

hyperphosphatemia typically occurs only in the later stages of the disease. Low levels of $1,25(OH)_2D$ due to increased FGF23 production in bone are critical in the development of hypocalcemia. The uremic state also causes impairment of intestinal absorption by mechanisms other than defects in vitamin D metabolism. Nonetheless, treatment with supraphysiologic amounts of vitamin D or calcitriol can correct the impaired calcium absorption. Because increased FGF23 levels are seen even in early stages of CKD and have been reported to correlate with increased mortality and left ventricular hypertrophy, there is current interest in approaches to lower intestinal phosphate absorption early during the course of kidney disease and to thereby lower FGF23 levels. However, there is concern as to whether vitamin D supplementation increases the circulating FGF23 levels in CKD patients. Although vitamin D analogs improve survival in this patient population, it is notable that there are often dramatic elevations of FGF23.

Hyperphosphatemia in CKD lowers blood calcium levels by several mechanisms, including extraosseous deposition of calcium and phosphate, impairment of the bone-resorbing action of PTH, and reduction in $1,25(OH)_2D$ production by remaining renal tissue.

TREATMENT CHRONIC KIDNEY DISEASE

Therapy of CKD (Chap. 335) involves appropriate management of patients prior to dialysis and adjustment of regimens once dialysis is initiated. Attention should be paid to restriction of phosphate in the diet; avoidance of aluminum-containing phosphate-binding antacids to prevent the problem of aluminum intoxication; provision of an adequate calcium intake by mouth, usually 1–2 g/d; and supplementation with 0.25–1 μg/d calcitriol or other activated forms of vitamin D. Each patient must be monitored closely. The aim of therapy is to restore normal calcium balance to prevent osteomalacia and severe secondary hyperparathyroidism (it is usually recommended to maintain PTH levels between 100 and 300 pg/mL) and, in light of evidence of genetic changes and monoclonal outgrowths of parathyroid glands in CKD patients, to prevent secondary hyperparathyroidism from becoming autonomous hyperparathyroidism. Reduction of hyperphosphatemia and restoration of normal intestinal calcium absorption by calcitriol can improve blood calcium levels and reduce the manifestations of secondary hyperparathyroidism. Because adynamic bone disease can occur in association with low PTH levels, it is important to avoid excessive suppression of the parathyroid glands while recognizing the beneficial effects of controlling the secondary hyperparathyroidism. These patients should probably be closely monitored with PTH assays that detect only the full-length PTH(1–84) to ensure that biologically active PTH and not inactive, inhibitory PTH fragments are measured. Use of phosphate-binding agents such as sevelamer is approved only in end-stage renal disease, but it may be necessary to initiate such treatment much earlier during the course of kidney disease to prevent the increase in FGF23 and its "off-target" effects.

Vitamin D Deficiency due to Inadequate Diet and/or Sunlight Vitamin D deficiency due to inadequate intake of dairy products enriched with vitamin D, lack of vitamin supplementation, and reduced sunlight exposure in the elderly, particularly during winter in northern latitudes, is more common in the United States than previously recognized. Biopsies of bone in elderly patients with hip fracture (documenting osteomalacia) and abnormal levels of vitamin D metabolites, PTH, calcium, and phosphate indicate that vitamin D deficiency may occur in as many as 25% of elderly patients, particularly in northern latitudes in the United States. Concentrations of 25(OH)D are low or low-normal in these patients. Quantitative histomorphometric analysis of bone biopsy specimens from such individuals reveals widened osteoid seams consistent with osteomalacia (Chap. 423). PTH hypersecretion compensates for the tendency for the blood calcium to fall but also increases renal phosphate excretion and thus causes osteomalacia.

Treatment involves adequate replacement with vitamin D and calcium until the deficiencies are corrected. Severe hypocalcemia rarely occurs in moderately severe vitamin D deficiency of the elderly, but vitamin D deficiency must be considered in the differential diagnosis of mild hypocalcemia.

Mild hypocalcemia, secondary hyperparathyroidism, severe hypophosphatemia, and a variety of nutritional deficiencies occur with gastrointestinal diseases. Hepatocellular dysfunction can lead to reduction in 25(OH)D levels, as in portal or biliary cirrhosis of the liver, and malabsorption of vitamin D and its metabolites, including $1,25(OH)_2D$, may occur in a variety of bowel diseases, hereditary or acquired. Hypocalcemia itself can lead to steatorrhea, due to deficient production of pancreatic enzymes and bile salts. Depending on the disorder, vitamin D or its metabolites can be given parenterally, guaranteeing adequate blood levels of active metabolites.

Defective Vitamin D Metabolism • ***ANTICONVULSANT THERAPY*** Anticonvulsant therapy with any of several agents induces acquired vitamin D deficiency by increasing the conversion of vitamin D to inactive compounds and/or causing resistance to its action. The more marginal the vitamin D intake in the diet, the more likely that anticonvulsant therapy will lead to abnormal mineral and bone metabolism.

VITAMIN D–DEPENDENT RICKETS TYPE I Vitamin D–dependent rickets type I, previously termed *pseudo-vitamin D–resistant rickets*, differs from true vitamin D–resistant rickets (vitamin D–dependent rickets type II, see below) in that it is typically less severe and the biochemical and radiographic abnormalities can be reversed with appropriate doses of the vitamin's active metabolite, $1,25(OH)_2D$. Physiologic amounts of calcitriol cure the disease (Chap. 423). This finding fits with the pathophysiology of the disorder, which is autosomal recessive, and is now known to be caused by mutations in the gene encoding 25(OH) D-1α-hydroxylase. Both alleles are inactivated in affected patients, and compound heterozygotes, harboring distinct mutations, are common.

Clinical features include hypocalcemia, often with tetany or convulsions, hypophosphatemia, secondary hyperparathyroidism, and osteomalacia, often associated with skeletal deformities and increased alkaline phosphatase. Treatment involves physiologic replacement doses of $1,25(OH)_2D$ (Chap. 423).

VITAMIN D–DEPENDENT RICKETS TYPE II Vitamin D–dependent rickets type II results from end-organ resistance to the active metabolite $1,25(OH)_2D$. The clinical features resemble those of the type I disorder and include hypocalcemia, hypophosphatemia, secondary hyperparathyroidism, and rickets but also partial or total alopecia. Plasma levels of $1,25(OH)_2D$ are elevated, in keeping with the refractoriness of the end organs. This disorder is caused by mutations in the gene encoding the vitamin D receptor; treatment is difficult and requires regular, usually nocturnal calcium infusions, which dramatically improve growth but do not restore hair growth (Chap. 423).

Pseudohypoparathyroidism PHP refers to a group of distinct inherited disorders. Patients affected by PHP type Ia (PHP-Ia) are characterized by symptoms and signs of hypocalcemia in association with distinctive skeletal and developmental defects. The hypocalcemia is due to a deficient response to PTH, which is probably restricted to the proximal renal tubules. Hyperplasia of the parathyroids, a response to hormone-resistant hypocalcemia, causes elevation of PTH levels. Studies, both clinical and basic, have clarified some aspects of these disorders, including the variable clinical spectrum, the pathophysiology, the genetic defects, and their mode of inheritance.

A working classification of the various forms of PHP is given in Table 424-6. The classification scheme is based on the signs of ineffective PTH action (low calcium and high phosphate), low or normal urinary cAMP response to exogenous PTH, the presence or absence of *Albright's hereditary osteodystrophy* (AHO), and assays to measure the concentration of the $G_s\alpha$ subunit of the adenylate cyclase enzyme. Using these criteria, there are four types: PHP types Ia and Ib; pseudopseudohypoparathyroidism (PPHP), and PHP-II.

TABLE 424-6 CLASSIFICATION OF PSEUDOHYPOPARATHYROIDISM (PHP) AND PSEUDOPSEUDOHYPOPARATHYROIDISM (PPHP)

Type	Hypocalcemia, Hyperphosphatemia	Response of Urinary cAMP to PTH	Serum PTH	$G_s\alpha$ Subunit Deficiency	AHO	Resistance to hormones other than PTH
PHP-Ia	Yes	↓	↑	Yes	Yes	Yes
PPHP	No	Normal	Normal	Yes	Yes	No
PHP-Ib	Yes	↓	↑	No	No	Yes (in some patients)
PHP-II	Yes	Normal	↑	No	No	No
Acrodysostosis with hormonal resistance	Yes	Normal (but ↓ phosphaturic response)	↑	No	Yes	Yes

Abbreviations: ↓, decreased; ↑, increased; AHO, Albright's hereditary osteodystrophy; PTH, parathyroid hormone.

PHP-IA AND PHP-IB Individuals with PHP-I, the most common of the disorders, show a deficient urinary cAMP response to administration of exogenous PTH. Patients with PHP-I are divided into type Ia and type Ib. Patients with PHP-Ia show evidence for AHO and reduced amounts of $G_s\alpha$ protein/activity, as determined in readily accessible tissues such as erythrocytes, lymphocytes, and fibroblasts. Patients with PHP-Ib typically lack evidence for AHO and they have normal $G_s\alpha$ activity. PHP-Ic, sometimes listed as a third form of PHP-I, is really a variant of PHP-Ia, although the mutant $G_s\alpha$ shows normal activity in certain in vitro assays.

Most patients who have PHP-Ia reveal characteristic features of AHO, which consist of short stature, round face, obesity, skeletal anomalies (brachydactyly), intellectual impairment, and/or heterotopic calcifications. Patients have low calcium and high phosphate levels, as with true hypoparathyroidism. PTH levels, however, are elevated, reflecting resistance to hormone action.

Amorphous deposits of calcium and phosphate are found in the basal ganglia in about one-half of patients. The defects in metacarpal and metatarsal bones are sometimes accompanied by short phalanges as well, possibly reflecting premature closing of the epiphyses. The typical findings are short fourth and fifth metacarpals and metatarsals. The defects are usually bilateral. Exostoses and radius curvus are frequent.

Inheritance and Genetic Defects Multiple defects at the *GNAS* locus have now been identified in PHP-Ia, PHP-Ib, and PPHP patients. This gene, which is located on chromosome 20q13.3, encodes the α-subunit of the stimulatory G protein ($G_s\alpha$), among other products (see below). Mutations include abnormalities in splice junctions associated with deficient mRNA production, point mutations, insertions, and/or deletion that all result in a protein with defective function resulting in a 50% reduction of $G_s\alpha$ activity in erythrocytes or other cells.

Detailed analyses of disease transmission in affected kindreds have clarified many features of PHP-Ia, PPHP, and PHP-Ib (Fig. 424-7). The former two entities, often traced through multiple generations, have an inheritance pattern consistent with genetic imprinting. The phenomenon of gene imprinting, involving methylation of genetic loci, independent of any mutation, impairs transcription from either the maternal or the paternal allele (Chap. 82). The $G_s\alpha$ transcript is biallelically expressed in most tissues; expression from paternal allele is silenced through as-of-yet unknown mechanisms in some tissues including the proximal renal tubules and the thyroid; consequently, inheritance of a defective paternal allele has no implications with regard to hormonal function. Thus, females affected by either PHP-Ia or PPHP will have offspring with PHP-Ia, if these children inherit the allele carrying the *GNAS* mutation; in contrast, if the mutant allele is inherited from a male affected by either disorder, the offspring will exhibit PPHP. Consistent with these data in humans, gene-ablation studies in mice have shown that inheritance of the mutant $G_s\alpha$ allele from the female causes much reduced $G_s\alpha$ protein in renal cortex, hypocalcemia, and resistance to PTH. Offspring inheriting the mutant allele from the male showed no evidence of PTH resistance or hypocalcemia.

Imprinting is tissue selective. Paternal $G_s\alpha$ expression is not silenced in most tissues. It seems likely, therefore, that the AHO phenotype recognized in PPHP as well as PHP-Ia reflects $G_s\alpha$ haploinsufficiency during embryonic or postnatal development.

The complex mechanisms that control the *GNAS* gene contribute to challenges involved in unraveling the pathogenesis of these disorders, especially that of PHP-Ib. Much intensive work with families in which multiple members are affected by PHP-Ib, as well as studies of the complex regulation of the *GNAS* gene locus, have now shown that PHP-Ib is caused by microdeletions within or upstream of the *GNAS* locus, which are associated with a loss of DNA methylation at one or several loci of the maternal allele (Table 424-6). These abnormalities in methylation silence the expression of the gene. This leads in the proximal renal tubules—where $G_s\alpha$ appears to be expressed exclusively from the maternal allele—to PTH resistance.

PHP-Ib, lacking the AHO phenotype in most instances, shares with PHP-Ia the hypocalcemia and hyperphosphatemia caused by PTH resistance, and thus the blunted urinary cAMP response to administered PTH, a standard test to assess the presence or absence of hormone resistance (Table 424-6). Furthermore, these endocrine abnormalities become apparent only if the disease-causing mutation is inherited maternally. Bone responsiveness may be excessive rather than blunted in PHP-Ib (and in PHP-Ia) patients, based on case reports that have emphasized an osteitis fibrosa–like pattern in several PHP-Ib patients.

PHP-II refers to patients with hypocalcemia and hyperphosphatemia, who have a normal urinary cAMP but an impaired urinary phosphaturic

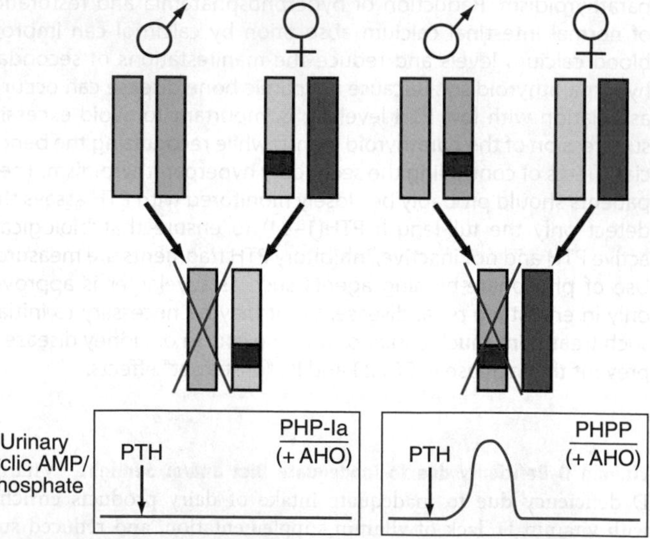

FIGURE 424-7 Paternal imprinting of renal parathyroid hormone (PTH) resistance. An impaired excretion of urinary cyclic AMP and phosphate is observed in patients with pseudohypoparathyroidism type Ia (PHP-Ia). In the renal cortex, there is selective silencing of paternal $G_s\alpha$ expression. The disease becomes manifest only in patients who inherit the defective gene from an obligate female carrier (*left*). If the genetic defect is inherited from an obligate male gene carrier, there is no biochemical abnormality; administration of PTH causes an appropriate increase in the urinary cyclic AMP and phosphate concentration (pseudo-PHP [PPHP]; *right*). Both patterns of inheritance lead to Albright's hereditary osteodystrophy (AHO), perhaps because of haplotype insufficiency—i.e., both copies of $G_s\alpha$ must be active for normal bone development.

response to PTH. In a PHP-II variant, referred to as acrodysostosis with hormonal resistance (ADOHR), patients have a defect in the regulatory subunit of PKA (PRKAR1A) that mediates the response to PTH distal to cAMP production. Acrodysostosis without hormonal resistance is caused by mutations in the cAMP-selective phosphodiesterase 4 (ADOP4). It remains unclear why the PTH-resistance in some patients, labeled as PHP-II without bony abnormalities, resolves upon treatment with vitamin D supplements.

The diagnosis of these hormone-resistant states can usually be made without difficulty when there is a positive family history for features of AHO, in association with the signs and symptoms of hypocalcemia. In both categories—PHP-Ia and PHP-Ib—serum PTH levels are elevated, particularly when patients are hypocalcemic. However, patients with PHP-Ib or PHP-II without acrodysostosis present only with hypocalcemia and high PTH levels, as evidence for hormone resistance. In PHP-Ia and PHP-Ib, the response of urinary cAMP to the administration of exogenous PTH is blunted. The diagnosis of PHP-II, in the absence of acrodysostosis, is more complex, and vitamin D deficiency must be excluded before such a diagnosis can be entertained.

TREATMENT PSEUDOHYPOPARATHYROIDISM

Treatment of PHP is similar to that of hypoparathyroidism, except that calcium and vitamin D doses are usually higher. Patients with PHP show no PTH-resistance in the distal tubules—hence, urinary calcium clearance is typically reduced, and they are not at risk of developing nephrocalcinosis as are patients with true hypoparathyroidism, unless overtreatment occurs, for example, after the completion of pubertal development and skeletal mutation, when calcium and $1,25(OH)_2D$ treatment should be reduced. Variability in response makes it necessary to establish the optimal regimen for each patient, based on maintaining appropriate blood calcium level and urinary calcium excretion and keeping the PTH level within or slightly above the normal range.

PTH OVERWHELMED

Occasionally, loss of calcium from the ECF is so severe that PTH cannot compensate. Such situations include acute pancreatitis and severe, acute hyperphosphatemia, often in association with renal failure, conditions in which there is rapid efflux of calcium from the ECF. Severe hypocalcemia can occur quickly; PTH rises in response to hypocalcemia but does not return blood calcium to normal.

Severe, Acute Hyperphosphatemia Severe hyperphosphatemia is associated with extensive tissue damage or cell destruction (Chap. 423). The combination of increased release of phosphate from muscle and impaired ability to excrete phosphorus because of renal failure causes moderate to severe hyperphosphatemia, the latter causing calcium loss from the blood and mild to moderate hypocalcemia. Hypocalcemia is usually reversed with tissue repair and restoration of renal function as phosphorus and creatinine values return to normal. There may even be a mild hypercalcemic period in the oliguric phase of renal function recovery. This sequence, severe hypocalcemia followed by mild hypercalcemia, reflects widespread deposition of calcium in muscle and subsequent redistribution of some of the calcium to the ECF after phosphate levels return to normal.

Other causes of hyperphosphatemia include hypothermia, massive hepatic failure, and hematologic malignancies, either because of high cell turnover of malignancy or because of cell destruction by chemotherapy.

TREATMENT SEVERE, ACUTE HYPERPHOSPHATEMIA

Treatment is directed toward lowering of blood phosphate by the administration of phosphate-binding antacids or dialysis, often needed for the management of CKD. Although calcium replacement may be necessary if hypocalcemia is severe and symptomatic, calcium administration during the hyperphosphatemic period tends to increase extraosseous calcium deposition and aggravate tissue damage. The levels of $1,25(OH)_2D$ may be low during the hyperphosphatemic phase and return to normal during the oliguric phase of recovery.

Osteitis Fibrosa after Parathyroidectomy Severe hypocalcemia after parathyroid surgery is rare now that osteitis fibrosa cystica is an infrequent manifestation of hyperparathyroidism. When osteitis fibrosa cystica is severe, however, bone mineral deficits can be large. After parathyroidectomy, hypocalcemia can persist for days if calcium replacement is inadequate. Treatment may require parenteral administration of calcium; addition of calcitriol and oral calcium supplementation is sometimes needed for weeks to a month or two until bone defects are filled (which, of course, is of therapeutic benefit in the skeleton), making it possible to discontinue parenteral calcium and/or reduce the amount.

DIFFERENTIAL DIAGNOSIS OF HYPOCALCEMIA

Care must be taken to ensure that true hypocalcemia is present; in addition, acute transient hypocalcemia can be a manifestation of a variety of severe, acute illnesses, as discussed above. *Chronic hypocalcemia*, however, can usually be ascribed to a few disorders associated with absent or ineffective PTH. Important clinical criteria include the duration of the illness, signs or symptoms of associated disorders, and the presence of features that suggest a hereditary abnormality. A nutritional history can be helpful in recognizing a low intake of vitamin D and calcium in the elderly, and a history of excessive alcohol intake may suggest magnesium deficiency.

Hypoparathyroidism and PHP are typically lifelong illnesses, usually (but not always) appearing by adolescence; hence, a recent onset of hypocalcemia in an adult is more likely due to nutritional deficiencies, renal failure, or intestinal disorders that result in deficient or ineffective vitamin D. Neck surgery, even long past, however, can be associated with a delayed onset of postoperative hypoparathyroidism. A history of seizure disorder raises the issue of anticonvulsive medication. Developmental defects may point to the diagnosis of PHP. Rickets and a variety of neuromuscular syndromes and deformities may indicate ineffective vitamin D action, either due to defects in vitamin D metabolism or to vitamin D deficiency.

A pattern of *low calcium with high phosphorus* in the absence of renal failure or massive tissue destruction almost invariably means hypoparathyroidism or PHP. A *low calcium and low phosphorus* pattern points to absent or ineffective vitamin D, thereby impairing the action of PTH on calcium metabolism (but not phosphate clearance). The relative ineffectiveness of PTH in calcium homeostasis in vitamin D deficiency, anticonvulsant therapy, gastrointestinal disorders, and hereditary defects in vitamin D metabolism leads to secondary hyperparathyroidism as a compensation. The excess PTH on renal tubule phosphate transport accounts for renal phosphate wasting and hypophosphatemia.

Exceptions to these patterns may occur. Most forms of hypomagnesemia are due to long-standing nutritional deficiency as seen in chronic alcoholics. Despite the fact that the hypocalcemia is principally due to an acute absence of PTH, phosphate levels are usually low, rather than elevated, as in hypoparathyroidism. Chronic renal failure is often associated with hypocalcemia and hyperphosphatemia, despite secondary hyperparathyroidism.

Diagnosis is usually established by application of the PTH immunoassay, tests for vitamin D metabolites, and measurements of the urinary cAMP response to exogenous PTH. In hereditary and acquired hypoparathyroidism and in severe hypomagnesemia, PTH is either undetectable or inappropriately in the normal range (Fig. 424-4). This finding in a hypocalcemic patient is supportive of hypoparathyroidism, as distinct from ineffective PTH action, in which even mild hypocalcemia is associated with elevated PTH levels. Hence a failure to detect elevated PTH levels establishes the diagnosis of hypoparathyroidism; elevated levels suggest the presence of secondary hyperparathyroidism, as found in many of the situations in which the hormone is ineffective due to associated abnormalities in vitamin D action. Assays for 25(OH)D can be helpful. Low or low-normal 25(OH)D indicates vitamin D deficiency due to lack of sunlight, inadequate vitamin D intake, or intestinal malabsorption. Recognition that mild hypocalcemia, rickets, and hypophosphatemia are due to anticonvulsant therapy is made by history.

TREATMENT HYPOCALCEMIC STATES

The management of hypoparathyroidism, PHP, chronic renal failure, and hereditary defects in vitamin D metabolism involves the use of vitamin D or vitamin D metabolites and calcium supplementation. Vitamin D itself is the least expensive form of vitamin D replacement and is frequently used in the management of uncomplicated hypoparathyroidism and some disorders associated with ineffective vitamin D action. When vitamin D is used prophylactically, as in the elderly or in those with chronic anticonvulsant therapy, there is a wider margin of safety than with the more potent metabolites. However, most of the conditions in which vitamin D is administered chronically for hypocalcemia require amounts 50–100 times the daily replacement dose because the formation of $1,25(OH)_2D$ is deficient. In such situations, vitamin D is no safer than the active metabolite because intoxication can occur with high-dose therapy (because of storage in fat). Calcitriol is more rapid in onset of action and also has a short biologic half-life.

Vitamin D (at least 1000 U/d [2–3 μg/d] [higher levels required in older persons]) or calcitriol (0.25–1 μg/d) is required to prevent rickets in normal individuals. In contrast, 40,000–120,000 U (1–3 mg) of vitamin D_2 or D_3 is typically required in hypoparathyroidism. The dose of calcitriol is unchanged in hypoparathyroidism, because the defect is in hydroxylation by the 25(OH)D-1α-hydroxylase. Calcitriol is also used in disorders of 25(OH)D-1α-hydroxylase; vitamin D receptor defects are much more difficult to treat.

Patients with hypoparathyroidism should be given 2–3 g of elemental calcium PO each day. The two agents, vitamin D or calcitriol and oral calcium, can be varied independently. Urinary calcium excretion needs to be monitored carefully. If hypocalcemia alternates with episodes of hypercalcemia in high-brittleness patients with hypoparathyroidism, administration of calcitriol and use of thiazides, as discussed above, may make management easier. Clinical trials with PTH(1–34) or PTH(1–84) are promising, but these alternative treatments have not yet been approved.

425 Osteoporosis

Robert Lindsay, Felicia Cosman

Osteoporosis, a condition characterized by decreased bone strength, is prevalent among postmenopausal women but also occurs in men and women with underlying conditions or major risk factors associated with bone demineralization. Its chief clinical manifestations are vertebral and hip fractures, although fractures can occur at almost any skeletal site. Osteoporosis affects almost 10 million individuals in the United States, but only a small proportion are diagnosed and treated.

DEFINITION

Osteoporosis is defined as a reduction in the strength of bone that leads to an increased risk of fractures. Loss of bone tissue is associated with deterioration in skeletal microarchitecture. The World Health Organization (WHO) operationally defines osteoporosis as a bone density that falls 2.5 standard deviations (SD) below the mean for young healthy adults of the same sex—also referred to as a *T-score* of –2.5. Postmenopausal women who fall at the lower end of the young normal range (a T-score <–1.0) are defined as having low bone density and are also at increased risk of osteoporosis. Although risk is lower in this group, more than 50% of fractures among postmenopausal women, including hip fractures, occur in this group with low bone density, because the number of individuals in this category is so much larger than that in the osteoporosis range. As a result, there are ongoing attempts to identify individuals within the low bone density range who are at high risk of fracture and might benefit from pharmacologic intervention. Furthermore, some have advocated using fracture risk as the "diagnostic" criterion for osteoporosis.

EPIDEMIOLOGY

In the United States, as many as 9 million adults have osteoporosis (T-score <–2.5 in either spine or hip), and an additional 48 million individuals have bone mass levels that put them at increased risk of developing osteoporosis (e.g., bone mass T-score <–1.0). Osteoporosis occurs more frequently with increasing age as bone tissue is lost progressively. In women, the loss of ovarian function at menopause (typically about age 50) precipitates rapid bone loss so that most women meet the diagnostic criterion for osteoporosis by age 70–80. As the population continues to age, the number of individuals with osteoporosis and fractures will also continue to increase, despite a recognized reduction in age-specific risk. It is estimated that about 2 million fractures occur each year in the United States as a consequence of osteoporosis, and that number is expected to increase as the population continues to age.

The epidemiology of fractures follows the trend for loss of bone density, with exponential increases in both hip and vertebral fractures with age. Fractures of the distal radius have a somewhat different epidemiology, increasing in frequency before age 50 and plateauing by age 60, with only a modest age-related increase thereafter. In contrast, incidence rates for hip fractures double every 5 years after age 70 (Fig. 425-1). This distinct epidemiology may be related to the way the elderly fall as they age, with fewer falls on an outstretched hand and more falls directly on the hip. About 300,000 hip fractures occur each year in the United States, most of which require hospital admission and surgical intervention. The probability that a 50-year-old white individual will have a hip fracture during his or her lifetime is 14% for women and 5% for men; the risk for African Americans is lower (about one-half those rates), and the risk for Asians is roughly equal to that for whites. Hip fractures are associated with a high incidence of deep vein thrombosis and pulmonary embolism (20–50%) and a mortality rate between 5 and 20% during the year after surgery.

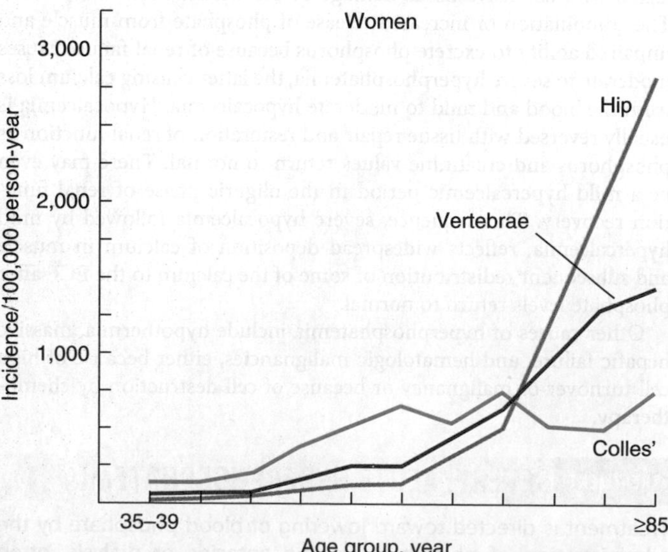

FIGURE 425-1 Epidemiology of vertebral, hip, and Colles' fractures with age. *(Adapted from C Cooper, LJ Melton III: Trends Endocrinol Metab 3:224, 1992; with permission.)*

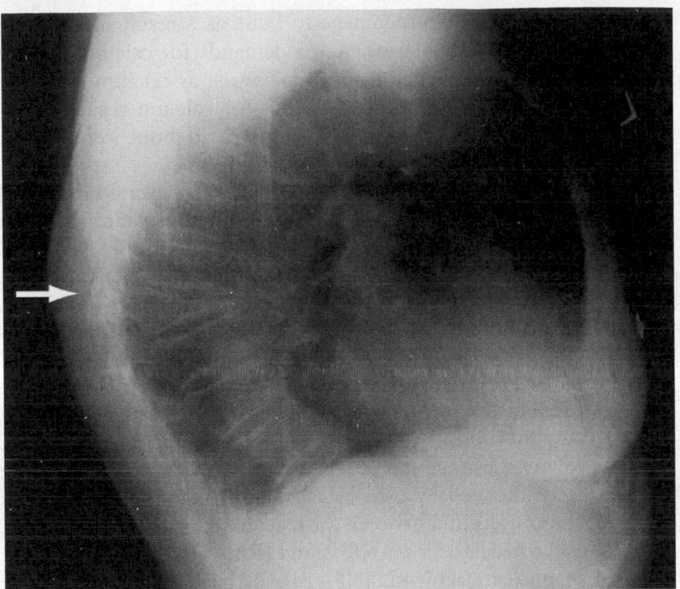

FIGURE 425-2 Lateral spine x-ray showing severe osteopenia and a severe wedge-type deformity (severe anterior compression).

There is also significant morbidity, with about 20–40% of survivors requiring long-term care, and many who are unable to function as they did before the fracture.

There are about 550,000 vertebral crush fractures per year in the United States. Only a fraction (estimated to be one-third) of them are recognized clinically, because many are relatively asymptomatic and are identified incidentally during radiography for other purposes (Fig. 425-2). Vertebral fractures rarely require hospitalization but are associated with long-term morbidity and a slight increase in mortality rates, primarily related to pulmonary disease. Multiple vertebral fractures lead to height loss (often of several inches), kyphosis, and secondary pain and discomfort related to altered biomechanics of the back. Thoracic fractures can be associated with restrictive lung disease, whereas lumbar fractures are associated with abdominal symptoms that include distention, early satiety, and constipation.

Approximately 400,000 wrist fractures and 135,000 pelvic fractures occur in the United States each year. Fractures of the humerus and other bones (estimated to be about 675,000 per year) also occur with osteoporosis; this is not surprising in light of the fact that bone loss is a systemic phenomenon. Although some fractures result from major trauma, the threshold for fracture is reduced for an osteoporotic bone (Fig. 425-3). In addition to bone density, there are a number of risk factors for fracture; the common ones are summarized in Table 425-1 Age, prior fractures (especially recent fractures), a family history of osteoporosis-related fractures, low body weight, smoking, and excessive alcohol use are all independent predictors of fracture. Chronic diseases with inflammatory components that increase skeletal remodeling such as rheumatoid arthritis, increase the risk of osteoporosis, as do

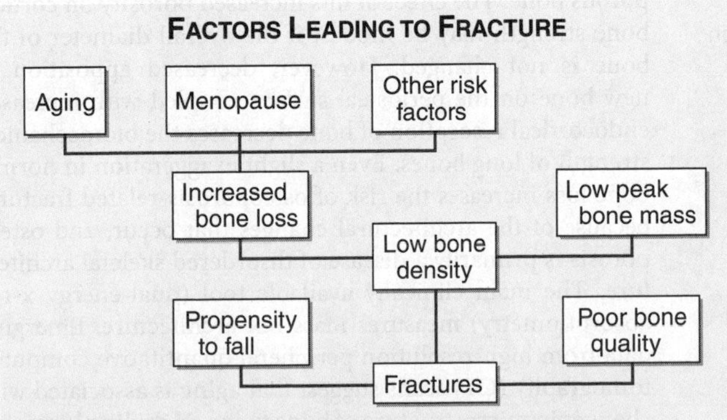

FIGURE 425-3 Factors leading to osteoporotic fractures.

diseases associated with malabsorption. Chronic diseases that increase the risk of falling or frailty, including dementia, Parkinson's disease, and multiple sclerosis, also increase fracture risk.

In the United States and Europe, osteoporosis-related fractures are more common among women than men, presumably due to a lower peak bone mass as well as postmenopausal bone loss in women. However, this sex difference in bone density and age-related increase in hip fractures is not as apparent in some other cultures, possibly due to genetics, physical activity level, or diet.

Fractures are themselves risk factors for future fractures (Table 425-1). Vertebral fractures increase the risk of other vertebral fractures as well as fractures of the peripheral skeleton such as the hip and wrist. Wrist fractures also increase the risk of vertebral and hip fractures. The risk for subsequent fractures is particularly high in the first several years after the first fracture, and the risk wanes considerably thereafter. Consequently, among individuals over age 50, any fracture should be considered as potentially related to osteoporosis regardless of the circumstances of the fracture. Osteoporotic bone is more likely to fracture than normal bone at any level of trauma, and a fracture in a person over 50 should trigger evaluation for osteoporosis. This often does not occur because postfracture care is not always well coordinated.

PATHOPHYSIOLOGY

BONE REMODELING

Osteoporosis results from bone loss due to age-related changes in bone remodeling as well as extrinsic and intrinsic factors that exaggerate this process. These changes may be superimposed on a low peak bone mass. Consequently, understanding the bone remodeling process is fundamental to understanding the pathophysiology of osteoporosis (Chap. 423). During growth, the skeleton increases in size by linear growth and by apposition of new bone tissue on the outer surfaces of the cortex (Fig. 425-4). The latter process is called *modeling*, a process that also allows the long bones to adapt in shape to the stresses placed on them. Increased sex hormone production at puberty is required for skeletal maturation, which reaches maximum mass and density in early adulthood. It is around puberty that the sexual dimorphism in skeletal size becomes obvious, although true bone density remains similar between the sexes. Nutrition and lifestyle also play an important role in growth, although genetic factors primarily determine peak skeletal mass and density. Numerous genes control skeletal growth, peak bone mass, and body size, as well as skeletal structure and density. Heritability estimates of 50–80% for bone density and size have been derived on the basis of twin studies. Although peak bone mass is often lower among individuals with a family history of osteoporosis, association studies of candidate genes (vitamin D receptor; type I collagen, the estrogen receptor [ER], and interleukin 6 [IL-6]; and insulin-like growth factor I [IGF-I]) and bone mass, bone turnover, and fracture prevalence have been inconsistent. Linkage studies suggest that a genetic locus on chromosome 11 is associated with high bone mass. Families with high bone mass and without much apparent age-related bone loss have been shown to have a point mutation in *LRP5*, a low-density lipoprotein receptor–related protein. The role of this gene in the general population is not clear, although a nonfunctional mutation results in osteoporosis-pseudoglioma syndrome, and *LRP5* signaling appears to be important in controlling bone formation. *LRP5* acts through the Wnt signaling pathway. With *LRP5* and Wnt activation, beta-catenin is translocated to the nucleus, allowing stimulation of osteoblast formation, activation, and life span as well as suppression of osteoclast activity, thereby increasing bone formation. The osteocyte product, sclerostin, is a negative inhibitor of Wnt signaling.

Genome-wide scans for low bone mass suggest multiple genes are involved, many of which are also implicated in control of body size.

In adults, bone remodeling, not modeling, is the principal metabolic skeletal process. Bone remodeling has two primary functions: (1) to repair microdamage within the skeleton to maintain skeletal strength and ensure the relative youth of the skeleton and (2) to supply calcium from the skeleton to maintain serum calcium. Remodeling may be

TABLE 425-1 CONDITIONS, DISEASES, AND MEDICATIONS THAT CONTRIBUTE TO OSTEOPOROSIS AND FRACTURES

Lifestyle factors		
Alcohol abuse	High salt intake	Falling
Low calcium intake	Inadequate physical activity	Excessive thinness
Vitamin D insufficiency	Immobilization	Prior fractures
Excess vitamin A	Smoking (active or passive)	
Genetic factors		
Cystic fibrosis	Homocystinuria	Osteogenesis imperfecta
Ehlers-Danlos syndrome	Hypophosphatasia	Parental history of hip fracture
Gaucher's disease	Idiopathic hypercalciuria	
Glycogen storage diseases	Marfan's syndrome	Porphyria
	Menkes' steely hair syndrome	Riley-Day syndrome
Hemochromatosis		
Hypogonadal states		
Androgen insensitivity	Hyperprolactinemia	Athletic amenorrhea
Anorexia nervosa and bulimia	Premature menopause	Panhypopituitarism
	Premature ovarian failure	
Turner's & Klinefelter's syndromes		
Endocrine disorders		
Adrenal insufficiency	Cushing's syndrome	Central adiposity
Diabetes mellitus (types 1 and 2)	Hyperparathyroidism	Thyrotoxicosis
Gastrointestinal disorders		
Celiac disease	Inflammatory bowel disease	Primary biliary cirrhosis
Gastric bypass	Malabsorption	
Gastrointestinal surgery	Pancreatic disease	
Hematologic disorders		
Multiple myeloma	Monoclonal gammopathies	Sickle cell disease
Hemophilia	Leukemia and lymphomas	Systemic mastocytosis
Thalassemia		
Rheumatologic and autoimmune diseases		
Ankylosing spondylitis	Lupus	Rheumatoid arthritis
Other rheumatic and autoimmune diseases		
Central nervous system disorders		
Epilepsy	Parkinson's disease	Stroke
Multiple sclerosis	Spinal cord injury	
Miscellaneous conditions and diseases		
AIDS/HIV	Congestive heart failure	Posttransplant bone disease
Alcoholism	Depression	
Amyloidosis	End-stage renal disease	Sarcoidosis
Chronic metabolic acidosis	Hypercalciuria	Weight loss
	Idiopathic scoliosis	
Chronic obstructive lung disease	Muscular dystrophy	
Medications		
Aluminum (in antacids)	Glucocorticoids (≥5 mg/d prednisone or equivalent for ≥3 months)	Tamoxifen (premenopausal use)
Anticoagulants (heparin)		
Anticonvulsants		Thiazolidinediones (such as pioglitazone and rosiglitazone)
Aromatase inhibitors	Gonadotropin-releasing hormone antagonists and agonists	
Barbiturates	Lithium	Thyroid hormones (in excess)
Cancer chemotherapeutic drugs	Methotrexate	
	Proton pump inhibitors	Parenteral nutrition
Cyclosporine A and tacrolimus	Selective serotonin reuptake inhibitors	
Depo-medroxyprogesterone (premenopausal contraception)		

Source: From the 2014 National Osteoporosis Foundation Clinician's Guide to the Prevention and Treatment of Osteoporosis. © National Osteoporosis Foundation.

activated by microdamage to bone as a result of excessive or accumulated stress. Acute demands for calcium involve osteoclast-mediated resorption as well as calcium transport by osteocytes. Chronic demands for calcium result in secondary hyperparathyroidism, increased bone remodeling, and overall loss of bone tissue.

Bone remodeling also is regulated by several circulating hormones, including estrogens, androgens, vitamin D, and parathyroid hormone (PTH), as well as locally produced growth factors such as IGF-I and immunoreactive growth hormone II (IGH-II), transforming growth factor β (TGF-β), parathyroid hormone–related peptide (PTHrP), interleukins (ILs), prostaglandins, and members of the tumor necrosis factor (TNF) superfamily. These factors primarily modulate the rate at which new remodeling sites are activated, a process that results initially in bone resorption by osteoclasts, followed by a period of repair during which new bone tissue is synthesized by osteoblasts. The cytokine responsible for communication between the osteoblasts, other marrow cells, and osteoclasts is RANK ligand (RANKL; receptor activator of nuclear factor-κB [NF-κB]). RANKL, a member of the TNF family, is secreted by osteoblasts and certain cells of the immune system (Chap. 423). The osteoclast receptor for this protein is referred to as *RANK*. Activation of RANK by RANKL is a final common path in osteoclast development, activation, and life span. A humoral decoy for RANKL, also secreted by osteoblasts, is *osteoprotegerin* (Fig. 425-5). Modulation of osteoclast recruitment and activity appears to be related to the interplay among these three factors. It appears that estrogens are pivotal in modulating secretion of osteoprotegerin (OPG) and perhaps also RANKL. Additional influences include nutrition (particularly calcium intake) and physical activity level.

In young adults, resorbed bone is replaced by an equal amount of new bone tissue. Thus, the mass of the skeleton remains constant after peak bone mass is achieved in adulthood. After age 30–45, however, the resorption and formation processes become imbalanced, and resorption exceeds formation. This imbalance may begin at different ages and varies at different skeletal sites; it becomes exaggerated in women after menopause. Excessive bone loss can be due to an increase in osteoclastic activity and/or a decrease in osteoblastic activity. In addition, an increase in remodeling activation frequency, and thus the number of remodeling sites, can magnify the small imbalance seen at each remodeling unit. Increased recruitment of bone remodeling sites produces a reversible reduction in bone tissue but also can result in permanent loss of tissue and disrupted skeletal architecture. In trabecular bone, if the osteoclasts penetrate trabeculae, they leave no template for new bone formation to occur, and, consequently, rapid bone loss ensues and cancellous connectivity becomes impaired. A higher number of remodeling sites increases the likelihood of this event. In cortical bone, increased activation of remodeling creates more porous bone. The effect of this increased porosity on cortical bone strength may be modest if the overall diameter of the bone is not changed. However, decreased apposition of new bone on the periosteal surface coupled with increased endocortical resorption of bone decreases the biomechanical strength of long bones. Even a slight exaggeration in normal bone loss increases the risk of osteoporosis-related fractures because of the architectural changes that occur, and osteoporosis is primarily a disease of disordered skeletal architecture. The main clinically available tool (dual-energy x-ray absorptiometry) measures mass not architecture. Emerging data from high-resolution peripheral quantitative computed tomography (CT) scans suggest that aging is associated with changes in microstructure of bone tissue, including increased cortical porosity and reduced cortical thickness.

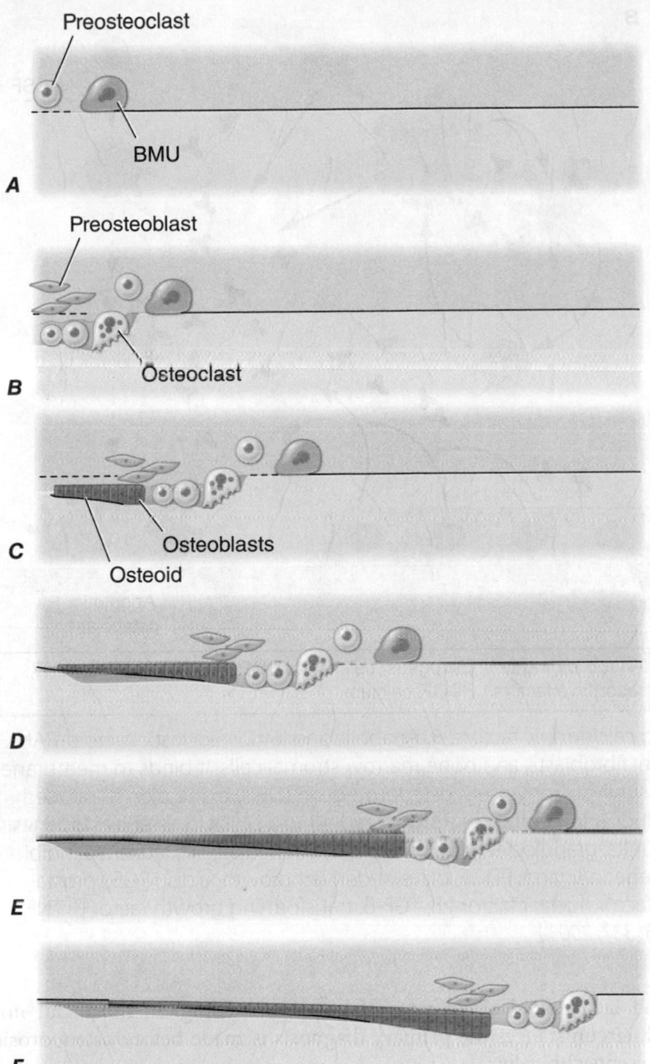

FIGURE 425-4 Mechanism of bone remodeling. The basic molecular unit (BMU) moves along the trabecular surface at a rate of about 10 μm/d. The figure depicts remodeling over ~120 days. ***A.*** Origination of BMU-lining cells contracts to expose collagen and attract preosteoclasts. ***B.*** Osteoclasts fuse into multinucleated cells that resorb a cavity. Mononuclear cells continue resorption, and preosteoblasts are stimulated to proliferate. ***C.*** Osteoblasts align at bottom of cavity and start forming osteoid (*black*). ***D.*** Osteoblasts continue formation and mineralization. Previous osteoid starts to mineralize (*horizontal lines*). ***E.*** Osteoblasts begin to flatten. ***F.*** Osteoblasts turn into lining cells; bone remodeling at initial surface (*left of drawing*) is now complete, but BMU is still advancing (*to the right*). *(Adapted from SM Ott, in JP Bilezikian et al [eds]: Principles of Bone Biology, vol. 18. San Diego, Academic Press, 1996, pp 231–241.)*

CALCIUM NUTRITION

Peak bone mass may be impaired by inadequate calcium intake during growth among other nutritional factors (calories, protein, and other minerals), leading to increased risk of osteoporosis later in life. During the adult phase of life, insufficient calcium intake contributes to relative secondary hyperparathyroidism and an increase in the rate of bone remodeling to maintain normal serum calcium levels. PTH stimulates the hydroxylation of vitamin D in the kidney, leading to increased levels of 1,25-dihydroxyvitamin D [$1,25(OH)_2D$] and enhanced gastrointestinal calcium absorption. PTH also reduces renal calcium loss. Although these are all appropriate compensatory homeostatic responses for adjusting calcium economy, the long-term effects are detrimental to the skeleton because the increased remodeling rates and the ongoing imbalance between resorption and formation at remodeling sites combine to accelerate loss of bone tissue.

Total daily calcium intakes <400 mg are detrimental to the skeleton, and intakes in the range of 600–800 mg, which is about the average intake among adults in the United States, are also probably suboptimal. The recommended daily required intake of 1000–1200 mg for adults accommodates population heterogeneity in controlling calcium balance (Chap. 95e). Such intakes should preferentially come from dietary sources, and supplements should be used only when dietary intakes fall short. The supplement should contain enough calcium to bring total intake to about 1200 mg/d.

VITAMIN D

(See also Chap. 423) Severe vitamin D deficiency causes rickets in children and osteomalacia in adults. However, there is accumulating evidence that vitamin D insufficiency may be more prevalent than previously thought, particularly among individuals at increased risk such as the elderly; those living in northern latitudes; and individuals with poor nutrition, malabsorption, or chronic liver or renal disease. Dark-skinned individuals are also at high risk of vitamin D deficiency. There is controversy regarding optimal levels of serum 25-hydroxyvitamin D [25(OH)D], with some advocating levels >20 ng/mL and others advocating optimal targets >75 nmol/L (30 ng/mL). To achieve this level for most adults requires an intake of 800–1000 units/d, particularly in individuals who avoid sunlight or routinely use ultraviolet-blocking lotions. Vitamin D insufficiency leads to compensatory secondary hyperparathyroidism and is an important risk factor for osteoporosis and fractures. Some studies have shown that >50% of inpatients on a general medical service exhibit biochemical features of vitamin D deficiency, including increased levels of PTH and alkaline phosphatase and lower levels of ionized calcium. In women living in northern latitudes, vitamin D levels decline during the winter months. This is associated with seasonal bone loss, reflecting increased bone turnover. Even among healthy ambulatory individuals, mild vitamin D deficiency is increasing in prevalence, in part due to decreased exposure to sunlight coupled with increased use of potent sunscreens. Treatment with vitamin D can return levels to normal and prevent the associated increase in bone remodeling, bone loss, and fractures. Improved muscle function and gait associated with reduced falls and fracture rates also have been documented among individuals in northern latitudes who have greater vitamin D intake and higher 25(OH)D levels (see below). Vitamin D adequacy also may affect risk and/or severity of other diseases, including cancers (colorectal, prostate, and breast), autoimmune diseases, and diabetes; however, many observational studies suggesting these potential extraskeletal benefits have not been confirmed with randomized controlled trials.

ESTROGEN STATUS

Estrogen deficiency probably causes bone loss by two distinct but interrelated mechanisms: (1) activation of new bone remodeling sites and (2) exaggeration of the imbalance between bone formation and resorption. The change in activation frequency causes a transient bone loss until a new steady state between resorption and formation is achieved. The remodeling imbalance, however, results in a permanent decrement in mass. In addition, the very presence of more remodeling sites in the skeleton increases the probability that trabeculae will be penetrated, eliminating the template on which new bone can be formed and accelerating the loss of bony tissue.

The most common estrogen-deficient state is the cessation of ovarian function at the time of menopause, which occurs on average at age 51 (Chap. 413). Thus, with current life expectancy, an average woman will spend about 30 years without an ovarian supply of estrogen. The mechanism by which estrogen deficiency causes bone loss is summarized in Fig. 425-5. Marrow cells (macrophages, monocytes, osteoclast precursors, mast cells) as well as bone cells (osteoblasts, osteocytes, osteoclasts) express ERs α and β. Loss of estrogen increases production of RANKL and may reduce production of OPG, increasing osteoclast recruitment. Estrogen also may play an important role in determining the life span of bone cells by controlling the rate of apoptosis. Thus,

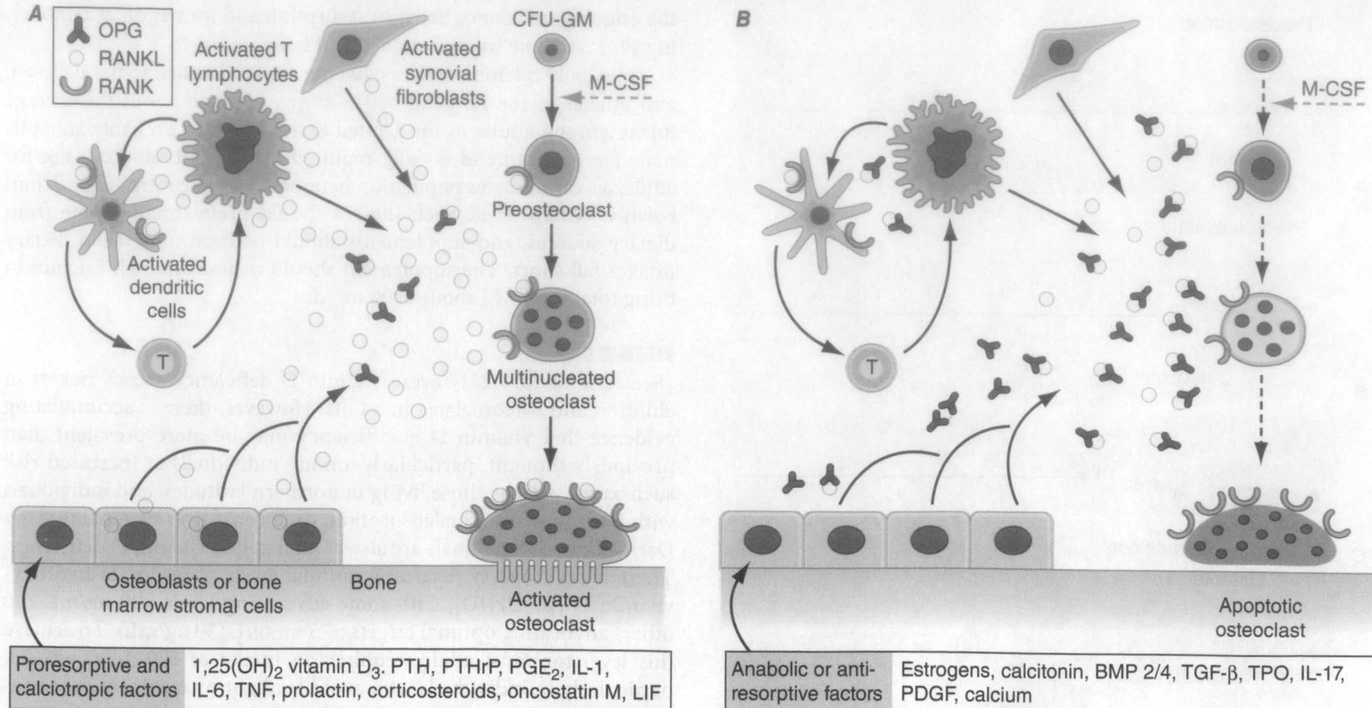

FIGURE 425-5 Hormonal control of bone resorption. ***A.*** Proresorptive and calciotropic factors. ***B.*** Anabolic and antiosteoclastic factors. RANK ligand (RANKL) expression is induced in osteoblasts, activated T cells, synovial fibroblasts, and bone marrow stromal cells. It binds to membrane-bound receptor RANK to promote osteoclast differentiation, activation, and survival. Conversely, osteoprotegerin (OPG) expression is induced by factors that block bone catabolism and promote anabolic effects. OPG binds and neutralizes RANKL, leading to a block in osteoclastogenesis and decreased survival of preexisting osteoclasts. CFU-GM, colony-forming units, granulocyte macrophage; IL, interleukin; LIF, leukemia inhibitory factor; M-CSF, macrophage colony-stimulating factor; OPG-L, osteoprotegerin-ligand; PDGF, platelet-derived growth factor; PGE_2, prostaglandin E_2; PTH, parathyroid hormone; RANKL, receptor activator of nuclear factor nuclear factor-κB; TGF-β, transforming growth factor β; TNF, tumor necrosis factor; TPO, thrombospondin. *(From WJ Boyle et al: Nature 423: 337, 2003.)*

in situations of estrogen deprivation, the life span of osteoblasts may be decreased, whereas the longevity and activity of osteoclasts are increased. The rate and duration of bone loss after menopause are heterogeneous and unpredictable. Once surfaces are lost in cancellous bone, the rate of bone loss must decline. In cortical bone, loss is slower but continues for a longer time period.

Because remodeling is initiated at the surface of bone, it follows that trabecular bone—which has a considerably larger surface area (80% of the total) than cortical bone—will be affected preferentially by estrogen deficiency. Fractures occur earliest at sites where trabecular bone contributes most to bone strength; consequently, vertebral fractures are the most common early consequence of estrogen deficiency.

PHYSICAL ACTIVITY

Inactivity, such as prolonged bed rest or paralysis, results in significant bone loss. Concordantly, athletes have higher bone mass than does the general population. These changes in skeletal mass are most marked when the stimulus begins during growth and before the age of puberty. Adults are less capable than children of increasing bone mass after restoration of physical activity. Epidemiologic data support the beneficial effects on the skeleton of chronic high levels of physical activity. Fracture risk is lower in rural communities and in countries where physical activity is maintained into old age. However, when exercise is initiated during adult life, the effects of moderate exercise on the skeleton are modest, with a bone mass increase of 1–2% in short-term studies of <2 years in duration. It is argued that more active individuals are less likely to fall and are more capable of protecting themselves upon falling, thereby reducing fracture risk.

CHRONIC DISEASE

Various genetic and acquired diseases are associated with an increase in the risk of osteoporosis (Table 425-1). Mechanisms that contribute to bone loss are unique for each disease and typically result from multiple factors, including nutrition, reduced physical activity levels, and factors that affect rates of bone remodeling. In most, but not all, circumstances the primary diagnosis is made before osteoporosis presents clinically.

MEDICATIONS

A large number of medications used in clinical practice have potentially detrimental effects on the skeleton (Table 425-1). *Glucocorticoids* are the most common cause of medication-induced osteoporosis. It is often not possible to determine the extent to which osteoporosis is related to glucocorticoids or to other factors, because treatment is superimposed on the effects of the primary disease, which in itself may be associated with bone loss (e.g., rheumatoid arthritis). Excessive doses of thyroid hormone can accelerate bone remodeling and result in bone loss.

Other medications have less detrimental effects on the skeleton than pharmacologic doses of glucocorticoids. *Anticonvulsants* are thought to increase the risk of osteoporosis, although many affected individuals have concomitant insufficiency of 1,25(OH)2D, as some anticonvulsants induce the cytochrome P450 system and vitamin D metabolism. Patients undergoing transplantation are at high risk for rapid bone loss and fracture not only from glucocorticoids but also from treatment with other *immunosuppressants* such as cyclosporine and tacrolimus (FK506). In addition, these patients often have underlying metabolic abnormalities, such as hepatic or renal failure, that predispose to bone loss.

Aromatase inhibitors, which potently block the aromatase enzyme that converts androgens and other adrenal precursors to estrogen, reduce circulating postmenopausal estrogen levels dramatically. These agents, which are used in various stages for breast cancer treatment, also have been shown to have a detrimental effect on bone density and risk of fracture. More recently a variety of agents have been implicated in increased bone loss and fractures. These include selective serotonin reuptake inhibitors, proton pump inhibitors, and thiazolidinediones. It is difficult in some cases to separate the risk accrued by the underlying disease from that attributable to the medication. For example, both depression and diabetes are risk factors for fracture by themselves.

CIGARETTE CONSUMPTION

The use of cigarettes over a long period has detrimental effects on bone mass. These effects may be mediated directly by toxic effects on osteoblasts or indirectly by modifying estrogen metabolism. On average, cigarette smokers reach menopause 1–2 years earlier than the general population. Cigarette smoking also produces secondary effects that can modulate skeletal status, including intercurrent respiratory and other illnesses, frailty, decreased exercise, poor nutrition, and the need for additional medications (e.g., glucocorticoids for lung disease).

MEASUREMENT OF BONE MASS

Several noninvasive techniques are available for estimating skeletal mass or density. They include dual-energy x-ray absorptiometry (DXA), single-energy x-ray absorptiometry (SXA), quantitative CT, and ultrasound (US). DXA is a highly accurate x-ray technique that has become the standard for measuring bone density. Although it can be used for measurement in any skeletal site, clinical determinations usually are made of the lumbar spine and hip. DXA also can be used to measure body composition. In the DXA technique, two x-ray energies are used to estimate the area of mineralized tissue, and the mineral content is divided by the area, which partially corrects for body size. However, this correction is only partial because DXA is a two-dimensional scanning technique and cannot estimate the depth or posteroanterior length of the bone. Thus, small slim people tend to have lower than average bone mineral density (BMD), a feature that is important in interpreting BMD measurements when performed in young adults, and something that must be taken into account at any age. Bone spurs, which are common in osteoarthritis, tend to falsely increase bone density of the spine and are a particular problem in measuring the spine in older individuals. Because DXA instrumentation is provided by several different manufacturers, the output varies in absolute terms. Consequently, it has become standard practice to relate the results to "normal" values by using T-scores (a T-score of 1 equals 1 SD), which compare individual results to those in a young population that is matched for race and sex. Z-scores (also measured in SD) compare individual results to those of an age-matched population that also is matched for race and sex. Thus, a 60-year-old woman with a Z-score of −1 (1 SD below mean for age) has a T-score of −2.5 (2.5 SD below mean for a young control group) (Fig. 425-6). A T-score below −2.5 in the lumbar spine, femoral neck, or total hip has been defined as a diagnosis of osteoporosis. As noted above, because more than 50% of fractures occur in individuals with low bone mass rather than BMD osteoporosis, attempts are ongoing to redefine the disease as a fracture risk rather than a specific BMD. Consistent with this concept, fractures of the spine and hip that occur in the absence of major trauma would be considered to be sufficient to diagnose osteoporosis, regardless of BMD. Fractures of other sites, such as pelvis, proximal humerus, and wrist, would be tantamount to an osteoporosis diagnosis in the presence of low BMD. CT can also be used to measure the spine and the hip, but is rarely used clinically, in part because of higher radiation exposure and cost, in addition to a lesser body of data confirming its ability to predict fracture risk, compared with BMD by DXA. High-resolution peripheral CT is used to measure bone in the forearm or tibia as a research tool to noninvasively provide some measure of skeletal architecture. Magnetic resonance imaging (MRI) can also be used in research settings to obtain some architectural information on the forearm and perhaps the hip.

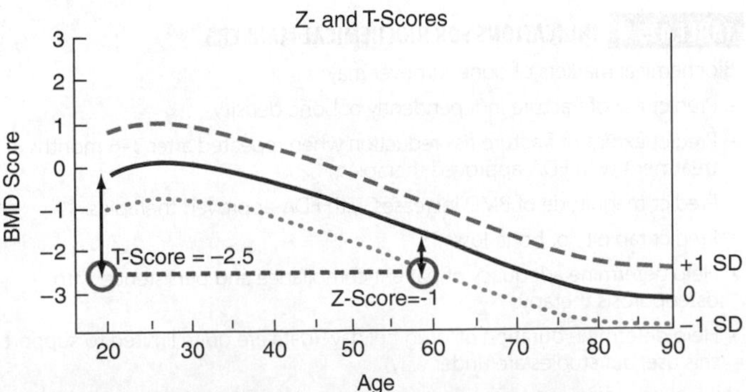

FIGURE 425-6 Relationship between Z-scores and T-scores in a 60-year-old woman. BMD, bone mineral density; SD, standard deviation.

DXA equipment can also be used to obtain lateral images of the spine, from T4 through L4, a technique called vertebral fracture assessment (VFA). Although not as definitive as radiography, it is a useful screening tool when height loss, back pain, or postural change suggests the presence of an undiagnosed vertebral fracture. Furthermore, because vertebral fractures are so prevalent with advancing age, screening vertebral imaging is recommended in women and men with low bone mass (T-score <1) by age 70 and 80, respectively.

US is used to measure bone mass by calculating the attenuation of the signal as it passes through bone or the speed with which it traverses the bone. It is unclear whether US assesses properties of bone other than mass (e.g., quality), but this is a potential advantage of the technique. Because of its relatively low cost and mobility, US is amenable for use as a screening procedure in stores or at health fairs.

All of these techniques for measuring BMD have been approved by the U.S. Food and Drug Administration (FDA) on the basis of their capacity to predict fracture risk. The hip is the preferred site of measurement in most individuals, because it predicts the risk of hip fracture, the most important consequence of osteoporosis, better than any other bone density measurement site. When hip measurements are performed by DXA, the spine can be measured at the same time. In younger individuals such as perimenopausal or early postmenopausal women, spine measurements may be the most sensitive indicator of bone loss. A risk assessment tool (FRAX) incorporates femoral neck BMD to assess 10-year fracture risk (see below).

WHEN TO MEASURE BONE MASS

Clinical guidelines have been developed for the use of bone densitometry in clinical practice. The original National Osteoporosis Foundation guidelines recommend bone mass measurements in postmenopausal women, assuming they have one or more risk factors for osteoporosis in addition to age, sex, and estrogen deficiency. The guidelines further recommend that bone mass measurement be considered in *all* women by age 65, a position ratified by the U.S. Preventive Health Services Task Force. Criteria approved for Medicare reimbursement of BMD are summarized in Table 425-2.

WHEN TO TREAT BASED ON BONE MASS RESULTS

Most guidelines suggest that patients be considered for treatment when BMD is >2.5 SD below the mean value for young adults (T-score ≤−2.5), in either spine, total hip, or femoral neck. Treatment also should also be considered in postmenopausal women with fracture risk factors even if BMD is not in the osteoporosis range. Risk factors (age, prior fracture, family history of hip fracture, low body weight, cigarette consumption, excessive alcohol use, steroid use, and rheumatoid arthritis) can be combined with BMD to assess the likelihood of a

TABLE 425-2 INDICATIONS FOR BONE DENSITY TESTING

Consider BMD testing in the following individuals:

- Women age 65 and older and men age 70 and older, regardless of clinical risk factors
- Younger postmenopausal women, women in the menopausal transition and men age 50–69 with clinical risk factors for fracture
- Adults who have a fracture after age 50
- Adults with a condition (e.g., rheumatoid arthritis) or taking a medication (e.g., glucocorticoids in a daily dose ≥5 mg prednisone or equivalent for ≥3 months) associated with low bone mass or bone loss

Source: From the 2014 National Osteoporosis Foundation Clinician's Guide to the Prevention and Treatment of Osteoporosis. © National Osteoporosis Foundation.

fracture over a 5- or 10-year period. Treatment threshold depends on cost-effectiveness analyses but probably is ~1% per year of risk in the United States.

APPROACH TO THE PATIENT: Osteoporosis

The perimenopausal transition is a good opportunity to initiate a discussion about risk factors for osteoporosis and consideration of indications for a BMD test. A careful history and physical examination should be performed to identify risk factors for osteoporosis. A low Z-score increases the suspicion of a secondary disease. Height loss >2.5–3.8 cm (>1–1.5 in.) is an indication for VFA by DXA or radiography to rule out asymptomatic vertebral fractures, as is the presence of significant kyphosis or back pain, particularly if it began after menopause. In appropriate individuals, screening BMD and screening vertebral imaging should be recommended as above, even in the absence of any specific risk factors (Table 425-3). For patients who present with fractures, it is important to ensure that the fractures are not caused by an underlying malignancy. Usually this is clear on routine radiography, but on occasion, CT, MRI, or radionuclide scans may be necessary.

ROUTINE LABORATORY EVALUATION

There is no established algorithm for the evaluation of women who present with osteoporosis. A general evaluation that includes complete blood count, serum and 24-h urine calcium, renal and hepatic function tests, and a 25(OH)D level is useful for identifying selected secondary causes of low bone mass, particularly for women with fractures or very low Z-scores. An elevated serum calcium level suggests hyperparathyroidism or malignancy, whereas a reduced serum calcium level may reflect malnutrition and osteomalacia. In the presence of hypercalcemia, a serum PTH level differentiates between hyperparathyroidism (PTH↑) and malignancy (PTH↓), and a high PTHrP level can help document the presence of humoral hypercalcemia of malignancy (Chap. 424). A low urine calcium (<50 mg/24 h) suggests osteomalacia, malnutrition, or malabsorption; a high urine calcium (>300 mg/24 h) is indicative of hypercalciuria and must be investigated further. Hypercalciuria occurs primarily in three situations: (1) a renal calcium leak, which is more common in males with osteoporosis; (2) absorptive hypercalciuria, which can be idiopathic or associated with increased $1,25(OH)_2D$ in granulomatous disease; or (3) hematologic malignancies or conditions associated with excessive bone turnover such as Paget's disease, hyperparathyroidism, and hyperthyroidism. Renal hypercalciuria is treated with thiazide diuretics, which lower urine calcium and help improve calcium economy.

Individuals who have osteoporosis-related fractures or bone density in the osteoporotic range should have a measurement of serum 25(OH)D level, because the intake of vitamin D required to achieve a target level >20–30 ng/mL is highly variable. Vitamin D levels should be optimized in all individuals being treated for osteoporosis. Hyperthyroidism should be evaluated by measuring thyroid-stimulating hormone (TSH).

When there is clinical suspicion of Cushing's syndrome, urinary free cortisol levels or a fasting serum cortisol should be measured after overnight dexamethasone. When bowel disease, malabsorption, or malnutrition is suspected, serum albumin, cholesterol, and a complete blood count should be checked. Asymptomatic malabsorption may be heralded by anemia (macrocytic—vitamin B_{12} or folate deficiency; microcytic—iron deficiency) or low serum cholesterol or urinary calcium levels. If these or other features suggest malabsorption, further evaluation is required. Asymptomatic celiac disease with selective malabsorption is being found with increasing frequency; the diagnosis can be made by testing for antigliadin, antiendomysial, or transglutaminase antibodies but may require endoscopic biopsy. A trial of a gluten-free diet can be confirmatory (Chap. 349). When osteoporosis is found associated with symptoms of rash, multiple allergies, diarrhea, or flushing, mastocytosis should be excluded by using 24-h urine histamine collection or serum tryptase.

Myeloma can masquerade as generalized osteoporosis, although it more commonly presents with bone pain and characteristic "punched-out" lesions on radiography. Serum and urine electrophoresis and or serum free light chains are required to exclude this diagnosis. More commonly, a monoclonal gammopathy of unclear significance (MGUS) is found, and the patient is subsequently monitored to ensure that this is not an incipient myeloma. Approximately 1% of patients with MGUS progress to myeloma each year. A bone marrow biopsy may be required to rule out myeloma (in patients with equivocal electrophoretic results) and also can be used to exclude mastocytosis, leukemia, and other marrow infiltrative disorders such as Gaucher's disease. MGUS syndromes, although benign, may also be associated with reduced bone mass and elevated bone turnover.

BONE BIOPSY

Tetracycline labeling of the skeleton allows determination of the rate of remodeling as well as evaluation for other metabolic bone diseases. The current use of BMD tests, in combination with hormonal evaluation and biochemical markers of bone remodeling, has largely replaced the clinical use of bone biopsy, although it remains an important tool in clinical research and assessment of mechanism of action of medication for osteoporosis.

BIOCHEMICAL MARKERS

Several biochemical tests are available that provide an index of the overall rate of bone remodeling (Table 425-4). Biochemical markers usually are characterized as those related primarily to *bone formation* or *bone resorption*. These tests measure the overall state of bone remodeling at a single point in time. Clinical use of these tests has been hampered by biologic variability (in part related to circadian rhythm) as well as analytic variability, although the latter is improving.

TABLE 425-3 INDICATIONS FOR VERTEBRAL IMAGING

Consider vertebral imaging tests in the following individuals:

- In all women age 70 and older and all men age 80 and older if bone mineral density (BMD) T-score is –1.0 or below
- In women age 65–69 and men age 75–79 if BMD T-score is –1.5 or below
- In postmenopausal women age 50–64 and men age 50–69 with specific risk factors:
  - Low-trauma fracture
  - Historical height loss of 1.5 in. or more (4 cm)
  - Prospective height loss of 0.8 in. or more (2 cm)
  - Recent or ongoing long-term glucocorticoid treatment

Source: From the 2014 National Osteoporosis Foundation Clinician's Guide to the Prevention and Treatment of Osteoporosis. © National Osteoporosis Foundation.

TABLE 425-4 INDICATIONS FOR BIOCHEMICAL MARKERS

Biochemical markers of bone turnover may:

- Predict risk of fracture independently of bone density.
- Predict extent of fracture risk reduction when repeated after 3–6 months of treatment with FDA-approved therapies.
- Predict magnitude of BMD increases with FDA-approved therapies.
- Predict rapidity of bone loss.
- Help determine adequacy of patient compliance and persistence with osteoporosis therapy.
- Help determine duration of "drug holiday" (data are quite limited to support this use, but studies are under way).

Abbreviations: BMD, bone mineral density; FDA, U.S. Food and Drug Administration.

Source: Adapted from the 2014 National Osteoporosis Foundation Clinician's Guide to the Prevention and Treatment of Osteoporosis. © National Osteoporosis Foundation.

Biochemical markers of bone resorption may help in the prediction of fracture risk, independently of bone density, particularly in older individuals. In women ≥65 years, when bone density results are greater than the usual treatment thresholds noted above, a high level of bone resorption should prompt consideration of treatment. The primary use of biochemical markers is for monitoring the response to treatment. With the introduction of antiresorptive therapeutic agents, bone remodeling declines rapidly, with the fall in resorption occurring earlier than the fall in formation. Inhibition of bone resorption is maximal within 3 months or so. Thus, measurement of bone resorption (C-telopeptide [CTX] is the preferred marker) before initiating therapy and 3–6 months after starting therapy provides an earlier estimate of patient response than does bone densitometry. A decline in resorptive markers can be ascertained after treatment with potent antiresorptive agents such as bisphosphonates, denosumab, or standard-dose estrogen; this effect is less marked after treatment with weaker agents such as raloxifene or intranasal calcitonin. A biochemical marker response to therapy is particularly useful for asymptomatic patients and may help ensure long-term adherence to treatment. Bone turnover markers are also useful in monitoring the effects of osteoanabolic agents such as 1-34hPTH, or teriparatide, which rapidly increases bone formation (P1NP is preferred, but osteocalcin is a reasonable alternative) and later bone resorption. The recent suggestion of "drug holidays" (see below) has created another use for biochemical markers, allowing evaluation of the off effect of drugs such as bisphosphonates.

TREATMENT OSTEOPOROSIS

MANAGEMENT OF PATIENTS WITH FRACTURES

Treatment of a patient with osteoporosis frequently involves management of acute fractures as well as treatment of the underlying disease. Hip fractures almost always require surgical repair if the patient is to become ambulatory again. Depending on the location and severity of the fracture, condition of the neighboring joint, and general status of the patient, procedures may include open reduction and internal fixation with pins and plates, hemiarthroplasties, and total arthroplasties. These surgical procedures are followed by intense rehabilitation in an attempt to return patients to their prefracture functional level. Long bone fractures (e.g., wrist) often require either external or internal fixation. Other fractures (e.g., vertebral, rib, and pelvic fractures) usually are managed with supportive care, requiring no specific orthopedic treatment.

Only ~25–30% of vertebral compression fractures present with sudden-onset back pain. For acutely symptomatic fractures, treatment with analgesics is required, including nonsteroidal anti-inflammatory agents and/or acetaminophen, sometimes with the addition of a narcotic agent (codeine or oxycodone). A few small, randomized clinical trials suggest that calcitonin may reduce pain related to acute vertebral compression fracture. Percutaneous injection of artificial cement (polymethylmethacrylate) into the vertebral body (vertebroplasty or kyphoplasty) may offer significant immediate pain relief in patients with severe pain from acute or subacute vertebral fractures. Safety concerns include extravasation of cement with neurologic sequelae and increased risk of fracture in neighboring vertebrae due to mechanical rigidity of the treated bone. Exactly which patients are the optimal candidates for this procedure remains unknown. Short periods of bed rest may be helpful for pain management, but in general, early mobilization is recommended because it helps prevent further bone loss associated with immobilization. Occasionally, use of a soft elastic-style brace may facilitate earlier mobilization. Muscle spasms often occur with acute compression fractures and can be treated with muscle relaxants and heat treatments.

Severe pain usually resolves within 6–10 weeks. More chronic severe pain might suggest the possibility of multiple myeloma or underlying metastatic disease. Chronic pain following vertebral fracture is probably not bony in origin; instead, it is related to abnormal strain on muscles, ligaments, and tendons and to secondary facet-joint arthritis associated with alterations in thoracic and/or abdominal shape. Chronic pain is difficult to treat effectively and may require analgesics, sometimes including narcotic analgesics. Frequent intermittent rest in a supine or semireclining position is often required to allow the soft tissues, which are under tension, to relax. Back-strengthening exercises (paraspinal) may be beneficial. Heat treatments help relax muscles and reduce the muscular component of discomfort. Various physical modalities, such as US and transcutaneous nerve stimulation, may be beneficial in some patients. Pain also occurs in the neck region, not as a result of compression fractures (which almost never occur in the cervical spine as a result of osteoporosis) but because of chronic strain associated with trying to elevate the head in a person with a significant thoracic kyphosis.

Multiple vertebral fractures often are associated with psychological symptoms; this is not always appreciated. The changes in body configuration and back pain can lead to marked loss of self-image and a secondary depression. Altered balance, precipitated by the kyphosis and the anterior movement of the body's center of gravity, leads to a fear of falling, a consequent tendency to remain indoors, and the onset of social isolation. These symptoms sometimes can be alleviated by family support and/or psychotherapy. Medication may be necessary when depressive features are present. Multiple thoracic vertebral fractures may be associated with restrictive lung disease symptoms and increased pulmonary infections. Multiple lumbar vertebral fractures are often associated with abdominal pain, constipation, protuberance, and early satiety. Multiple vertebral fractures are associated with greater age-specific mortality.

Multiple studies show that the majority of patients presenting in adulthood with fractures are not evaluated or treated for osteoporosis. Estimates suggest only about 20% of fracture patients receive follow-up care. Patients who sustain acute fractures are at dramatically elevated risk for more fractures, particularly within the first several years, and pharmacologic intervention can reduce that risk substantially. Recently, several studies have demonstrated the effectiveness of a relatively simple and inexpensive program that reduces the risk of subsequent fractures. In the Kaiser system, it is estimated that a 20% decline in hip fracture occurrence was seen with the introduction of what is called a fracture liaison service. This typically involves a health care professional (usually a nurse) whose job is to coordinate follow-up care and education of fracture patients. If the Kaiser experience can be repeated, there would be significant savings of health care dollars, as well as a dramatic drop in hip fracture incidence and a marked improvement in morbidity and mortality among the aging population.

MANAGEMENT OF THE UNDERLYING DISEASE

Patients presenting with typical osteoporosis-related fractures (certainly hip and spine) can be assumed to have osteoporosis and can be treated appropriately. Patients with osteoporosis by BMD are handled in a similar fashion. Other fracture patients and those with reduced bone mass can be classified according to their future risk of fracture and treated if that risk is sufficiently high. It must be emphasized, however, that risk assessment is an inexact science when applied to individual patients. Fractures are chance occurrences that can happen to anyone. Patients often do not understand the relative benefits of medications, compared to the perceived risks of the medications themselves.

Risk Factor Reduction Several tools exist for risk assessment. The most commonly available is the FRAX tool, developed by a working party for the WHO, and available as part of the report from many DXA machines. It is also available online *(http://www.shef.ac.uk/FRAX/tool.jsp?locationValue=9)* **(Fig. 425-7)**. In the United States, it has been estimated that it is cost-effective to treat a patient if the 10-year major fracture risk (including hip, clinical spine, proximal humerus, and tibia) from FRAX is ≥20% and/or the 10-year risk of hip fracture is ≥3%. FRAX is an imperfect tool because it does not include

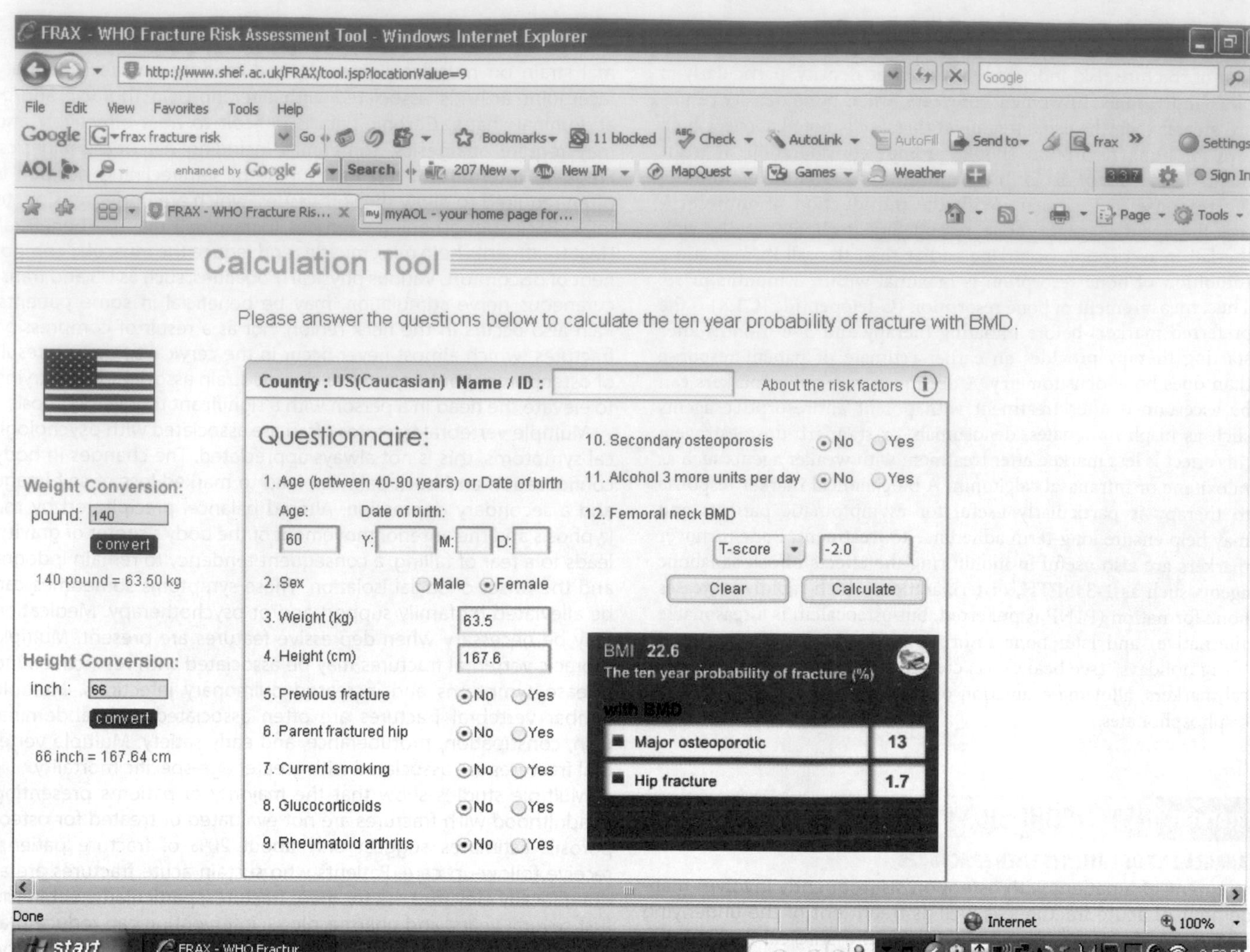

FIGURE 425-7 FRAX calculation tool. When the answers to the indicated questions are filled in, the calculator can be used to assess the 10-year probability of fracture. The calculator (available online at *http://www.shef.ac.uk/FRAX/tool.jsp?locationValue=9*) also can risk adjust for various ethnic groups.

any assessment of fall risk and secondary causes are excluded when BMD is entered. Moreover, it does not include any term for multiple fractures or recent versus remote fracture. Nonetheless, it is useful as an educational tool for patients.

After risk assessment, patients should be thoroughly educated to reduce the impact of modifiable risk factors associated with bone loss and falling. All medications that increase risk of falls, bone loss, or fractures should be reviewed to ensure that they are necessary and being used at the lowest required dose. For those on thyroid hormone replacement, TSH testing should be performed to confirm that an excessive dose is not being used, because biochemical and symptomatic thyrotoxicosis can be associated with increased bone loss. In patients who smoke, efforts should be made to facilitate smoking cessation. Reducing risk factors for falling also include alcohol abuse treatment and a review of the medical regimen for any drugs that might be associated with orthostatic hypotension and/or sedation, including hypnotics and anxiolytics. If nocturia occurs, the frequency should be reduced, if possible (e.g., by decreasing or modifying diuretic use), because arising in the middle of sleep is a common precipitant of a fall. Patients should be instructed about environmental safety with regard to eliminating exposed wires, curtain strings, slippery rugs, and mobile tables. Avoiding stocking feet on wood floors, checking carpet condition (particularly on stairs), and providing good light in paths to bathrooms and outside the home are important preventive measures. Treatment for impaired vision is recommended, particularly a problem with depth perception, which is specifically associated with increased falling risk. Elderly patients with neurologic impairment (e.g., stroke, Parkinson's disease, Alzheimer's disease) are particularly at risk of falling and require specialized supervision and care.

Nutritional Recommendations • *CALCIUM* A large body of data indicates that optimal calcium intake reduces bone loss and suppresses bone turnover. Recommended intakes from an Institute of Medicine report are shown in **Table 425-5**.

The National Health and Nutrition Examination Surveys (NHANES) have consistently documented that average calcium intakes fall considerably short of these recommendations. Food sources of calcium are dairy products (milk, yogurt, and cheese) and fortified

TABLE 425-5 ADEQUATE CALCIUM INTAKE

Life Stage Group	Estimated Adequate Daily Calcium Intake, mg/d
Young children (1–3 years)	500
Older children (4–8 years)	800
Adolescents and young adults (9–18 years)	1300
Men and women (19–50 years)	1000
Men and women (51 and older)	1200

Note: Pregnancy and lactation needs are the same as for nonpregnant women (e.g., 1300 mg/d for adolescents/young adults and 1000 mg/d for ≥19 years).

Source: Adapted from the Standing Committee on the Scientific Evaluation of Dietary Reference Intakes. Food and Nutrition Board. Institute of Medicine. Washington, DC, 1997, National Academy Press.

TABLE 425-6 SIMPLE METHOD FOR CALCULATING DIETARY CALCIUM INTAKE

STEP 1: Estimate calcium intake from calcium-rich foods

Product	# of Servings/d	Estimated calcium/ serving, in mg	Calcium in mg
Milk (8 oz.)	______	× 300	= ______
Yogurt (6 oz.)	______	× 300	= ______
Cheese (1 oz. or 1 cubic in.)	______	× 200	= ______
Fortified foods or juices	______	× 80 to 1000	= ______
	Subtotal = ______		

STEP 2: Total from above + 250 mg for nondairy sources – total dietary calcium TOTAL Calcium, in mg = ______

Source: Adapted from SM Krane, MF Holick, **Chap. 355**, in *Harrison's Principles of Internal Medicine*, 14th ed. New York, McGraw-Hill, 1998.

foods such as certain cereals, waffles, snacks, juices, and crackers. Some of these fortified foods contain as much calcium per serving as milk. Green leafy vegetables and nuts, particularly almonds, are also sources of calcium, although their bioavailability may be lower than with dairy products. Calcium intake from the diet can also be assessed **(Table 425-6)** and calculators are available at *NOF.org* or *NYSOPEP.org*.

If a calcium supplement is required, it should be taken in doses sufficient to supplement dietary intake to bring total intake to the required level (1000–1200 mg/d). Doses of supplements should be ≤600 mg at a time, because the calcium absorption fraction decreases at higher doses. Calcium supplements should be calculated on the basis of the elemental calcium content of the supplement, not the weight of the calcium salt. Calcium supplements containing carbonate are best taken with food because they require acid for solubility. Calcium citrate supplements can be taken at any time. To confirm bioavailability, calcium supplements can be placed in distilled vinegar. They should dissolve within 30 min.

Several controlled clinical trials of calcium, mostly plus vitamin D, have confirmed reductions in clinical fractures, including fractures of the hip (~20–30% risk reduction). All recent studies of pharmacologic agents have been conducted in the context of calcium replacement (± vitamin D). Thus, it is standard practice to ensure an adequate calcium and vitamin D intake in patients with osteoporosis whether they are receiving additional pharmacologic therapy or not. A systematic review confirmed a greater BMD response to antiresorptive therapy when calcium intake was adequate.

Although side effects from supplemental calcium are minimal (eructation and constipation mostly with carbonate salts), individuals with a history of kidney stones should have a 24-h urine calcium determination before starting increased calcium to avoid significant hypercalciuria. Many studies confirm a small but significant increase in the risk of renal stones with calcium supplements, but not dietary calcium. A recent analysis of published data has suggested that high intakes of calcium from supplements are associated with an increase in the risk of heart disease. This is an evolving story with additional studies that confirm or refute this finding. Because high calcium supplement intakes increase the risk of renal stones and confer no extra benefit to the skeleton, the recommendation that total intakes should be between 1000 and 1200 mg/d is reasonable.

VITAMIN D Vitamin D is synthesized in skin under the influence of heat and ultraviolet light **(Chap. 423)**. However, large segments of the population do not obtain sufficient vitamin D to maintain what is now considered an adequate supply [serum 25(OH)D consistently >75 μmol/L (30 ng/mL)]. Because vitamin D supplementation at doses that would achieve these serum levels is safe and inexpensive, the Institute of Medicine (based on obtaining a serum level of 20 ng/mL) recommends daily intakes of 200 IU for adults <50 years of age, 400 IU for those 50–70 years, and 600 IU for those >70 years. Multivitamin tablets usually contain 400 IU, and many calcium supplements also contain vitamin D. Some data suggest that higher doses (≥1000 IU) may be required in the elderly and chronically ill. The Institute of Medicine report suggests that it is safe to take up to 4000 IU/d. For those with osteoporosis or those at risk of osteoporosis, 1000–2000 IU/d can usually maintain serum 25(OH)D above 30 ng/mL.

OTHER NUTRIENTS Other nutrients such as salt, high animal protein intakes, and caffeine may have modest effects on calcium excretion or absorption. Adequate vitamin K status is required for optimal carboxylation of osteocalcin. States in which vitamin K nutrition or metabolism is impaired, such as with long-term warfarin therapy, have been associated with reduced bone mass. Research concerning cola intake is controversial but suggests a possible link to reduced bone mass through factors that are independent of caffeine. Although dark green leafy vegetables such as spinach and kale contain a fair amount of calcium, the high oxalate content reduces absorption of this calcium (but does not inhibit absorption of calcium from other food eaten simultaneously).

Magnesium is abundant in foods, and magnesium deficiency is quite rare in the absence of a serious chronic disease. Magnesium supplementation may be warranted in patients with inflammatory bowel disease, celiac disease, chemotherapy, severe diarrhea, malnutrition, or alcoholism. Dietary phytoestrogens, which are derived primarily from soy products and legumes (e.g., garbanzo beans [chickpeas] and lentils), exert some estrogenic activity but are insufficiently potent to justify their use in place of a pharmacologic agent in the treatment of osteoporosis.

Patients with hip fractures are often frail and relatively malnourished. Some data suggest an improved outcome in such patients when they are provided calorie and protein supplementation. Excessive protein intake can increase renal calcium excretion, but this can be corrected by an adequate calcium intake.

Exercise Exercise in young individuals increases the likelihood that they will attain the maximal genetically determined peak bone mass. Meta-analyses of studies performed in postmenopausal women indicate that weight-bearing exercise helps prevent bone loss but does not appear to result in substantial gain of bone mass. This beneficial effect wanes if exercise is discontinued. Most of the studies are short term, and a more substantial effect on bone mass is likely if exercise is continued over a long period. Exercise also has beneficial effects on neuromuscular function, and it improves coordination, balance, and strength, thereby reducing the risk of falling. A walking program is a practical way to start. Other activities, such as dancing, racquet sports, cross-country skiing, and use of gym equipment, are also recommended, depending on the patient's personal preference and general condition. Even women who cannot walk benefit from swimming or water exercises, not so much for the effects on bone, which are quite minimal, but because of effects on muscle. Exercise habits should be consistent, optimally at least three times a week.

PHARMACOLOGIC THERAPIES

Before the mid-1990s, estrogen treatment, either by itself or in concert with a progestin, was the primary therapeutic agent for prevention or treatment of osteoporosis. There are now a number of new medications approved for osteoporosis and more under development. Some are agents that specifically treat osteoporosis (bisphosphonates, calcitonin, denosumab, and teriparatide [1-34hPTH]); others, such as selective estrogen response modulators (SERMs) and, most recently, an estrogen/SERM combination medication, have broader effects. The availability of these drugs allows therapy to be tailored to the needs of an individual patient.

Estrogens A large body of clinical trial data indicates that various types of estrogens (conjugated equine estrogens, estradiol, estrone, esterified estrogens, ethinyl estradiol, and mestranol) reduce bone turnover, prevent bone loss, and induce small increases in bone mass of the spine, hip, and total body. The effects of estrogen are seen in women with natural or surgical menopause and in late postmenopausal women with or without established osteoporosis. Estrogens are efficacious when administered orally or transdermally. For both oral and transdermal routes of administration, combined estrogen/progestin preparations are now available in many countries, obviating the problem of taking two tablets or using a patch and oral progestin.

Dose of Estrogen For oral estrogens, the standard recommended doses have been 0.3 mg/d for esterified estrogens, 0.625 mg/d for conjugated equine estrogens, and 5 μg/d for ethinyl estradiol. For transdermal estrogen, the commonly used dose supplies 50 μg estradiol per day, but a lower dose may be appropriate for some individuals. Dose-response data for conjugated equine estrogens indicate that lower doses (0.3 and 0.45 mg/d) are effective. Doses even lower have been associated with bone mass protection.

FRACTURE DATA Epidemiologic databases indicate that women who take estrogen replacement have a 50% reduction, on average, of osteoporotic fractures, including hip fractures. The beneficial effect of estrogen is greatest among those who start replacement early and continue the treatment; the benefit declines after discontinuation to the extent that there is no residual protective effect against fracture by 10 years after discontinuation. The first clinical trial evaluating fractures as secondary outcomes, the Heart and Estrogen-Progestin Replacement Study (HERS) trial, showed no effect of hormone therapy on hip or other clinical fractures in women with established coronary artery disease. These data made the results of the Women's Health Initiative (WHI) exceedingly important (Chap. 413). The estrogen-progestin arm of the WHI in >16,000 postmenopausal healthy women indicated that hormone therapy reduces the risk of hip and clinical spine fracture by 34% and reduces the risk of all clinical fractures by 24%. There was similar antifracture efficacy seen with estrogen alone in women who had had a hysterectomy.

A few smaller clinical trials have evaluated spine fracture occurrence as an outcome with estrogen therapy. They have consistently shown that estrogen treatment reduces the incidence of vertebral compression fracture.

The WHI has provided a vast amount of data on the multisystemic effects of hormone therapy. Although earlier observational studies suggested that estrogen replacement might reduce heart disease, the WHI showed that combined estrogen-progestin treatment increased risk of fatal and nonfatal myocardial infarction by ~29%, confirming data from the HERS study. Other important relative risks included a 40% increase in stroke, a 100% increase in venous thromboembolic disease, and a 26% increase in risk of breast cancer. Subsequent analyses have confirmed the increased risk of stroke and, in a substudy, showed a twofold increase in dementia. Benefits other than the fracture reductions noted above included a 37% reduction in the risk of colon cancer. These relative risks have to be interpreted in light of absolute risk (Fig. 425-8). For example, out of 10,000 women treated with estrogen-progestin for 1 year, there will be 8 excess heart attacks, 8 excess breast cancers, 18 excess venous thromboembolic events, 5 fewer hip fractures, 44 fewer clinical fractures, and 6 fewer colorectal cancers. These numbers must be multiplied by years of hormone treatment. There was no effect of hormone treatment on the risk of uterine cancer or total mortality.

It is important to note that these WHI findings apply specifically to hormone treatment in the form of conjugated equine estrogen plus medroxyprogesterone acetate. The relative benefits and risks of unopposed estrogen in women who had hysterectomies vary somewhat. They still show benefits against fracture occurrence and increased risk of venous thrombosis and stroke, similar in magnitude to the risks for combined hormone therapy. In contrast, though, the estrogen-only arm of WHI indicated no increased risk of heart attack or breast cancer. The data suggest that at least some of the detrimental effects of combined therapy are related to the progestin component. In addition, there is the possibility, suggested by primate data, that the risk accrues mainly to women who have some years of estrogen deficiency before initiating treatment. (The average woman in the WHI was more than 10 years from the last menstrual period). Nonetheless, there is reluctance among women to use estrogen/hormone therapy, and the U.S. Preventive Services Task Force has specifically suggested that estrogen/hormone therapy not be used for disease prevention.

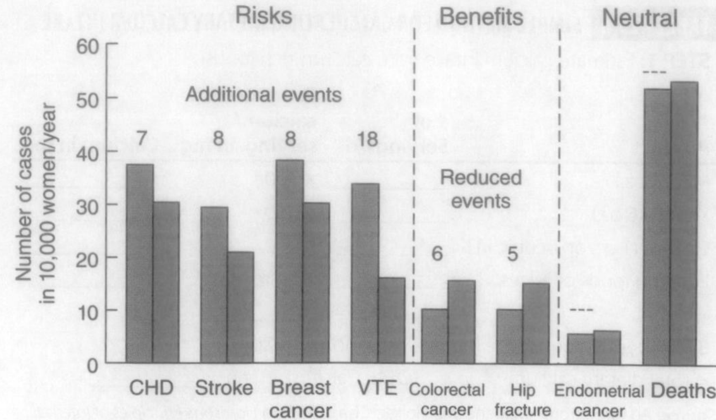

FIGURE 425-8 Effects of hormone therapy on event rates: green, placebo; purple, estrogen and progestin. CHD, coronary heart disease; VTE, venous thromboembolic events. *(Adapted from Women's Health Initiative. WHI HRT Update. Available at http://www.nhlbi.nih.gov/health/women/upd2002.htm.)*

MODE OF ACTION Two subtypes of ERs, α and β, have been identified in bone and other tissues. Cells of monocyte lineage express both ERα and ERβ, as do osteoblasts. Estrogen-mediated effects vary with the receptor type. Using ER knockout mouse models, elimination of ERα produces a modest reduction in bone mass, whereas mutation of ERβ has less of an effect on bone. A male patient with a homozygous mutation of ERα had markedly decreased bone density as well as abnormalities in epiphyseal closure, confirming the important role of ERα in bone biology. The mechanism of estrogen action in bone is an area of active investigation (Fig. 425-5). Although data are conflicting, estrogens may inhibit osteoclasts directly. However, the majority of estrogen (and androgen) effects on bone resorption are mediated through paracrine factors produced by osteoblasts and osteocytes. These actions include decreasing RANKL production and increasing OPG production by osteoblasts.

Progestins In women with a uterus, daily progestin or cyclical progestins at least 12 days per month are prescribed in combination with estrogens to reduce the risk of uterine cancer. Medroxyprogesterone acetate and norethindrone acetate blunt the high-density lipoprotein response to estrogen, but micronized progesterone does not. Neither medroxyprogesterone acetate nor micronized progesterone appears to have an independent effect on bone; at lower doses of estrogen, norethindrone acetate may have an additive benefit. On breast tissue, progestins may increase the risk of breast cancer.

SERMs

Two SERMs are used currently in postmenopausal women: raloxifene, which is approved for the prevention and treatment of osteoporosis as well as the prevention of breast cancer, and tamoxifen, which is approved for the prevention and treatment of breast cancer. A third SERM, bazedoxifene, has been complexed with conjugated estrogen, creating a tissue selective estrogen complex (TSEC). This agent has been approved for prevention of osteoporosis.

Tamoxifen reduces bone turnover and bone loss in postmenopausal women compared with placebo groups. These findings support the concept that tamoxifen acts as an estrogenic agent in bone. There are limited data on the effect of tamoxifen on fracture risk, but the Breast Cancer Prevention Study indicated a possible reduction in clinical vertebral, hip, and Colles' fractures. The major benefit of tamoxifen is on breast cancer occurrence. The breast cancer prevention trial indicated that tamoxifen administration over 4–5 years reduced the incidence of new invasive and noninvasive breast cancer by ~45% in women at increased risk of breast cancer. The incidence of ER-positive breast cancers was reduced by 65%. Tamoxifen increases the risk of uterine cancer and increases risk of venous thrombosis, cataracts, and possibly stroke in postmenopausal women, limiting its use for breast cancer prevention in women at low or moderate risk.

Raloxifene (60 mg/d) has effects on bone turnover and bone mass that are very similar to those of tamoxifen, indicating that this agent is also estrogenic on the skeleton. The effect of raloxifene on bone density (+1.4–2.8% vs placebo in the spine, hip, and total body) is somewhat less than that seen with standard doses of estrogens. Raloxifene reduces the occurrence of vertebral fracture by 30–50%, depending on the population; however, there are no data confirming that raloxifene can reduce the risk of nonvertebral fractures over 8 years of observation.

Raloxifene, like tamoxifen and estrogen, has effects in other organ systems. The most beneficial effect appears to be a reduction in invasive breast cancer (mainly decreased ER-positive) occurrence of ~65% in women who take raloxifene compared to placebo. In a head-to-head study, raloxifene was as effective as tamoxifen in preventing breast cancer in high-risk women, and raloxifene is now FDA approved for this indication. In a further study, raloxifene had no effect on heart disease in women with increased risk for this outcome. In contrast to tamoxifen, raloxifene is not associated with an increase in the risk of uterine cancer or benign uterine disease. Raloxifene increases the occurrence of hot flashes but reduces serum total and low-density lipoprotein cholesterol, lipoprotein(a), and fibrinogen. Raloxifene, with positive effects on breast cancer and vertebral fractures, has become a useful agent for the treatment of the younger asymptomatic postmenopausal woman. In some women, a recurrence of menopausal hot flashes may occur. Usually this is evanescent, but occasionally, it is sufficiently impactful on daily life and sleep that the drug must be withdrawn. Raloxifene increases the risk of deep vein thrombosis and may increase the risk of death from stroke among older women. Consequently, it is not usually recommended for women over 70 years of age.

The main advantage of the *bazedoxifene/conjugated estrogen* compound is that the bazedoxifene protects uterine tissue from the effects of estrogen and makes it possible to avoid taking a progestin, while using an estrogen primarily for control of menopausal symptoms. The TSEC prevents bone loss somewhat more potently than raloxifene alone and appears safe for the breast.

MODE OF ACTION OF SERMS All SERMs bind to the ER, but each agent produces a unique receptor-drug conformation. As a result, specific co-activator or co-repressor proteins are bound to the receptor (Chap. 400e), resulting in differential effects on gene transcription that vary depending on other transcription factors present in the cell. Another aspect of selectivity is the affinity of each SERM for the different ERα and ERβ subtypes, which are expressed differentially in various tissues. These tissue-selective effects of SERMs offer the possibility of tailoring estrogen therapy to best meet the needs and risk factor profile of an individual patient.

Bisphosphonates Alendronate, risedronate, ibandronate, and zoledronic acid are approved for the prevention and treatment of postmenopausal osteoporosis. Alendronate, risedronate, and zoledronic acid are also approved for the treatment of steroid-induced osteoporosis, and risedronate and zoledronic acid are approved for prevention of steroid-induced osteoporosis. Alendronate, risedronate, and zoledronic acid are approved for treatment of osteoporosis in men.

Alendronate has been shown to decrease bone turnover and increase bone mass in the spine by up to 8% versus placebo and by 6% versus placebo in the hip. Multiple trials have evaluated its effect on fracture occurrence. The Fracture Intervention Trial provided evidence in >2000 women with prevalent vertebral fractures that daily alendronate treatment (5 mg/d for 2 years and 10 mg/d for 9 months afterward) reduces vertebral fracture risk by about 50%, multiple vertebral fractures by up to 90%, and hip fractures by up to 50%. Several subsequent trials have confirmed these findings (Fig. 425-9). For example, in a study of >1900 women with low bone mass treated with alendronate (10 mg/d) versus placebo, the incidence of all nonvertebral fractures was reduced by ~47% after only 1 year. In the United States, the 10-mg dose is approved for treatment of osteoporosis and 5 mg/d is used for prevention.

Trials comparing once-weekly alendronate, 70 mg, with daily 10-mg dosing have shown equivalence with regard to bone mass and bone turnover responses. Consequently, once-weekly therapy generally is preferred because of the low incidence of gastrointestinal side effects and ease of administration. Alendronate should be given with a full glass of water before breakfast, because bisphosphonates are poorly absorbed. Because of the potential for esophageal irritation, alendronate is contraindicated in patients who have stricture or inadequate emptying of the esophagus. It is recommended that patients remain upright for at least 30 min after taking the medication to avoid esophageal irritation. Cases of esophagitis, esophageal ulcer, and esophageal stricture have been described, but the incidence appears to be low. In clinical trials, overall gastrointestinal symptomatology was no different with alendronate than with placebo. Alendronate is also available in a preparation that contains vitamin D.

Risedronate also reduces bone turnover and increases bone mass. Controlled clinical trials have demonstrated 40–50% reduction in vertebral fracture risk over 3 years, accompanied by a 40% reduction in clinical nonspine fractures. The only clinical trial specifically designed to evaluate hip fracture outcome (HIP) indicated that risedronate reduced hip fracture risk in women in their seventies with confirmed osteoporosis by 40%. In contrast, risedronate was not effective at reducing hip fracture occurrence in older women (80+ years) without proven osteoporosis. Studies have shown that 35 mg of risedronate administered once weekly is therapeutically equivalent to 5 mg/d and that 150 mg once monthly is therapeutically equivalent to 35 mg once weekly. Patients should take risedronate with a full glass of plain water to facilitate delivery to the stomach and should not lie down for 30 min after taking the drug. The incidence of gastrointestinal side effects in trials with risedronate was similar to that of placebo. A new preparation, which allows risedronate to be taken with food, was recently approved.

Etidronate was the first bisphosphonate to be approved, initially for use in Paget's disease and hypercalcemia. This agent has also been used in osteoporosis trials of smaller magnitude than those performed for alendronate and risedronate but is not approved by the FDA for treatment of osteoporosis. Etidronate probably has some efficacy against vertebral fracture when given as an intermittent cyclical regimen (2 weeks on, 2.5 months off). Its effectiveness against nonvertebral fractures has not been studied.

Ibandronate is the third amino-bisphosphonate approved in the United States. Ibandronate (2.5 mg/d) has been shown in clinical trials to reduce vertebral fracture risk by ~40% but with no overall effect on nonvertebral fractures. In a post hoc analysis of subjects with a femoral neck T-score of –3 or below, ibandronate reduced the risk of nonvertebral fractures by ~60%. In clinical trials, ibandronate doses of 150 mg/month PO or 3 mg every 3 months IV had greater effects on turnover and bone mass than did 2.5 mg/d. Patients should take oral ibandronate in the same way as other bisphosphonates, but with 1 h elapsing before other food or drink (other than plain water).

Zoledronic acid is a potent bisphosphonate with a unique administration regimen (5 mg by slow IV infusion annually). The data confirm that it is highly effective in fracture risk reduction. In a study of >7000 women followed for 3 years, zoledronic acid (three annual infusions) reduced the risk of vertebral fractures by 70%, nonvertebral fractures by 25%, and hip fractures by 40%. These results were associated with less height loss and disability. In the treated population, there was an increased risk of transient postdose symptoms (acute-phase reaction) manifested by fever, arthralgia, myalgias, and headache. The symptoms usually last less than 48 h. An increased risk of atrial fibrillation and transient but

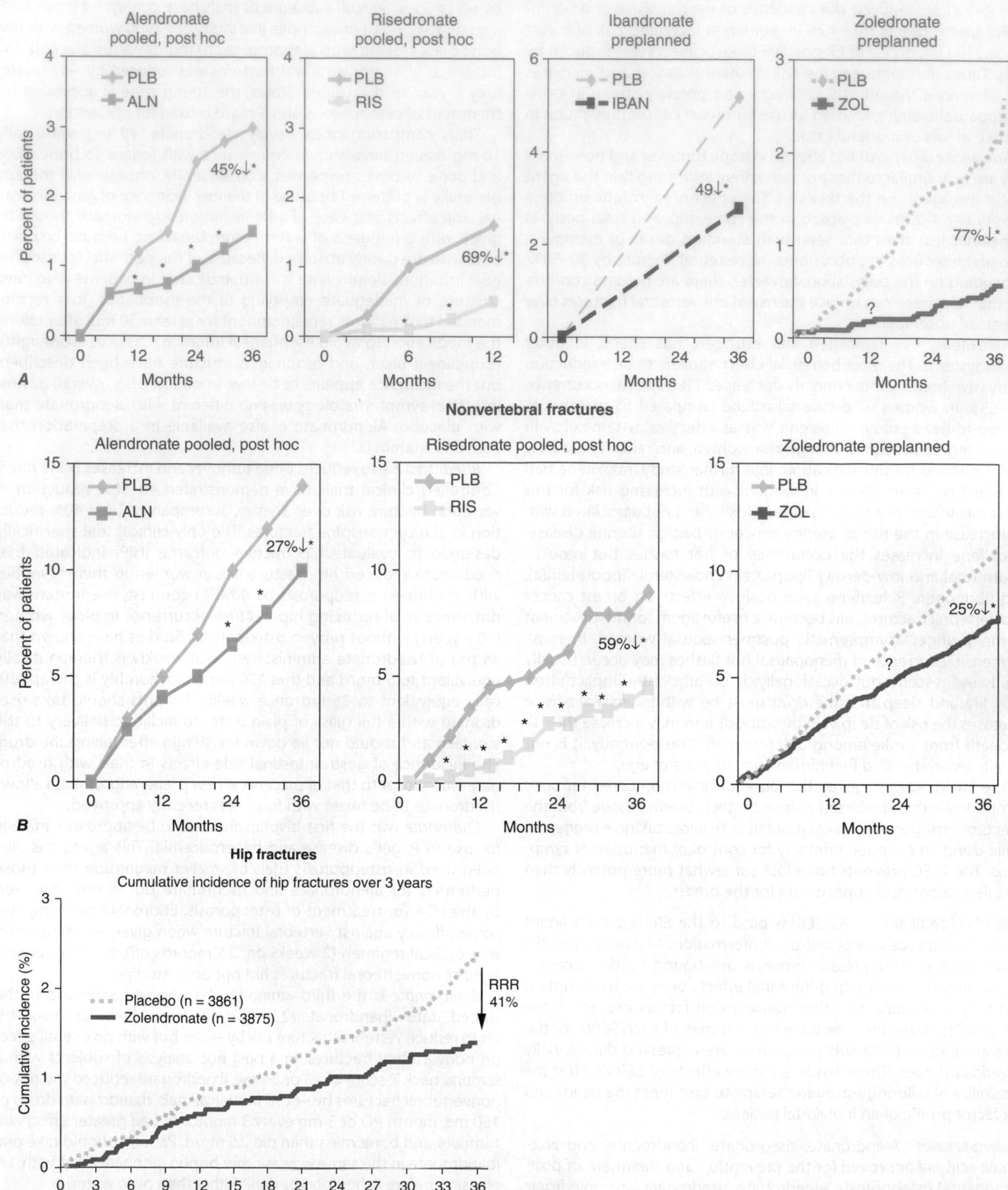

FIGURE 425-9 Effects of various bisphosphonates on clinical vertebral fractures (*A*), nonvertebral fractures (*B*), and hip fractures (*C*). PLB, placebo; RRR, relative risk reduction. *(After DM Black et al: J Clin Endocrinol Metab 85:4118, 2000; C Roux et al: Curr Med Res Opin 4:433, 2004; CH Chesnut et al: J Bone Miner Res 19:1241, 2004; DM Black et al: N Engl J Med 356:1809, 2007; JT Harrington et al: Calcif Tissue Int 74:129, 2003.)*

not permanent reduction in renal function was seen in comparison to placebo. Detailed evaluation of all bisphosphonates failed to confirm that these agents increased the risk of atrial fibrillation. Zoledronic acid is the only osteoporosis agent that has been studied in the elderly with a prior hip fracture. The risk of all clinical fractures was reduced significantly by about 35%, and there was a trend toward reduced risk of a second hip fracture (effect size similar to that seen above). There was also a reduction in mortality of about 30% that was not completely accounted for the reduced hip fracture risk.

Recently there has been concern about two potential side effects associated with bisphosphonate use. The first is osteonecrosis of the jaw (ONJ). ONJ usually follows a dental procedure in which bone is exposed (extractions or dental implants). It is presumed that the exposed bone becomes infected and dies. It is not uncommon among cancer victims with multiple myeloma or patients receiving high doses of bisphosphonates for skeletal metastases, but is rare among persons with osteoporosis on usual doses of bisphosphonates. The second side effect is called atypical femur fracture. These are unusual fractures that occur distal to the lesser trochanter and anywhere along the femoral shaft. They are often preceded by pain in the lateral thigh or groin that can be present for weeks or months before the fracture. The fractures occur with trivial trauma, sometimes completely spontaneously, and are primarily transverse, with a medial break when complete and minimally comminuted. A localized periosteal reaction, consistent with a stress fracture, is often seen in the lateral cortex (Fig. 425-10). The overall risk is low (suggested to be about one-one hundredth to one-tenth that of hip fracture) but appears to increase in incidence with long-term use of bisphosphonates. Although the fractures may be bisphosphonate related in many individuals, they clearly occur in patients with no prior bisphosphonate exposure. When complete, they require surgical fixation and may be difficult to heal. Anabolic medication may accelerate healing of these fractures in some patients, and surgery can sometimes be avoided. Patients initiating bisphosphonates need to be warned that if they develop thigh or groin pain they must notify their physician. Routine x-rays will sometimes pick up cortical thickening or even a stress fracture, but more commonly MRI or technetium bone scan is required. The presence of an abnormality requires at minimum a period of modified weight bearing and may need prophylactic rodding of the femur. It is important to realize that these fractures may be bilateral, and when an abnormality is found, the other femur should be investigated.

MODE OF ACTION Bisphosphonates are structurally related to pyrophosphates, compounds that are incorporated into bone matrix. Bisphosphonates specifically impair osteoclast function and reduce osteoclast number, in part by inducing apoptosis. Recent evidence suggests that the nitrogen-containing bisphosphonates also inhibit protein prenylation, one of the end products in the mevalonic acid pathway, by inhibiting the enzyme farnesyl pyrophosphate synthase. This effect disrupts intracellular protein trafficking and ultimately may lead to apoptosis. Some bisphosphonates have very long retention in the skeleton and may exert long-term effects. The consequences of this, if any, are unknown.

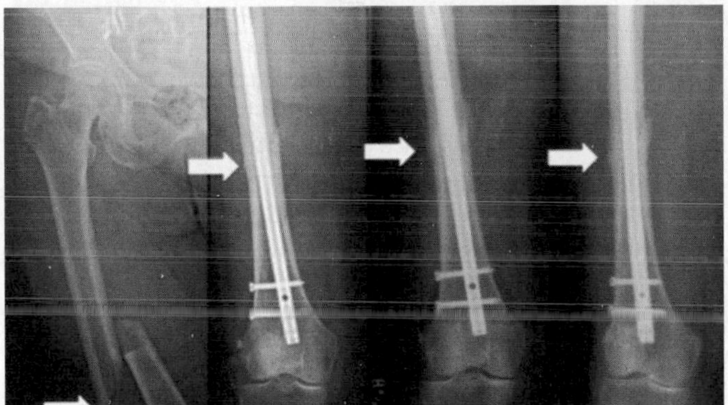

FIGURE 425-10 An atypical femur fracture (AFF) of the femoral diaphysis. ***A.*** Note the transverse fracture line in the lateral cortex that becomes oblique as it progresses medially across the femur (*white arrow*). ***B.*** On radiograph obtained immediately after intramedullary rod placement, a small area of periosteal thickening of the lateral cortex is visible (*white arrow*). ***C.*** On radiograph obtained at 6 weeks, note callus formation of the fracture site (*white arrow*). ***D.*** On radiograph obtained at 3 months, there is a mature callus that has failed to bridge the cortical gap (*white arrow*). Note the localized periosteal and/or endosteal thickening of the lateral cortex at the fracture site (*white arrow*). *(From E Shane et al: J Bone Min Res 29:1-23, 2014. Courtesy of Fergus McKiernan.)*

Calcitonin Calcitonin is a polypeptide hormone produced by the thyroid gland (Chap. 424). Its physiologic role is unclear because no skeletal disease has been described in association with calcitonin deficiency or excess. Calcitonin preparations are approved by the FDA for Paget's disease, hypercalcemia, and osteoporosis in women >5 years past menopause. Concerns have been raised about an increase in the incidence of cancer associated with calcitonin use. Initially, the cancer noted was of the prostate, but an analysis of all data suggested a more general increase in cancer risk. In Europe, the European Medicines Agency (EMA) has removed the osteoporosis indication, and an FDA Advisory Committee has voted for a similar change in the United States.

Injectable calcitonin produces small increments in bone mass of the lumbar spine. However, difficulty of administration and frequent reactions, including nausea and facial flushing, make general use limited. A nasal spray containing calcitonin (200 IU/d) is available for treatment of osteoporosis in postmenopausal women. One study suggests that nasal calcitonin produces small increments in bone mass and a small reduction in new vertebral fractures in calcitonin-treated patients versus those on calcium alone. There has been no proven effectiveness against nonvertebral fractures.

Calcitonin is not indicated for prevention of osteoporosis and is not sufficiently potent to prevent bone loss in early postmenopausal women. Calcitonin might have an analgesic effect on bone pain, both in the subcutaneous and possibly the nasal form.

MODE OF ACTION Calcitonin suppresses osteoclast activity by direct action on the osteoclast calcitonin receptor. Osteoclasts exposed to calcitonin cannot maintain their active ruffled border, which normally maintains close contact with underlying bone.

Denosumab A novel agent that was given twice yearly by SC administration in a randomized controlled trial in postmenopausal women with osteoporosis has been shown to increase BMD in the spine, hip, and forearm and reduce vertebral, hip, and nonvertebral fractures over a 3-year period by 70, 40, and 20%, respectively (Fig. 425-11). Other clinical trials indicate ability to increase bone mass in postmenopausal women with low bone mass (above osteoporosis range) and in postmenopausal women with breast cancer treated with hormonal agents. Furthermore, a study of men with prostate cancer treated with gonadotropin-releasing hormone (GnRH) agonist therapy indicated the ability of denosumab to improve bone mass and reduce vertebral fracture occurrence. Denosumab was approved by the FDA in 2010 for the treatment of postmenopausal women who have a high risk for osteoporotic fractures, including those with a history of fracture or multiple risk factors for fracture, and those who have failed or are intolerant to other osteoporosis therapy. Denosumab is also approved for the treatment of osteoporosis in men at high risk, men with prostate cancer on GnRH agonist therapy, and women with breast cancer on aromatase inhibitor therapy.

MODE OF ACTION Denosumab is a fully human monoclonal antibody to RANKL, the final common effector of osteoclast formation, activity, and survival. Denosumab binds to RANKL, inhibiting its ability to initiate formation of mature osteoclasts from osteoclast precursors and to bring mature osteoclasts to the bone surface and initiate bone resorption. Denosumab also plays a role in reducing the survival of the osteoclast. Through these actions on the osteoclast, denosumab induces potent antiresorptive action, as assessed biochemically and histomorphometrically, and may contribute to the occurrence of ONJ. Atypical femur fractures have also been noted. Serious adverse reactions include hypocalcemia, skin infections (usually cellulitis of the lower extremity), and dermatologic reactions such as dermatitis, rashes, and eczema. The effects of denosumab are rapidly reversible.

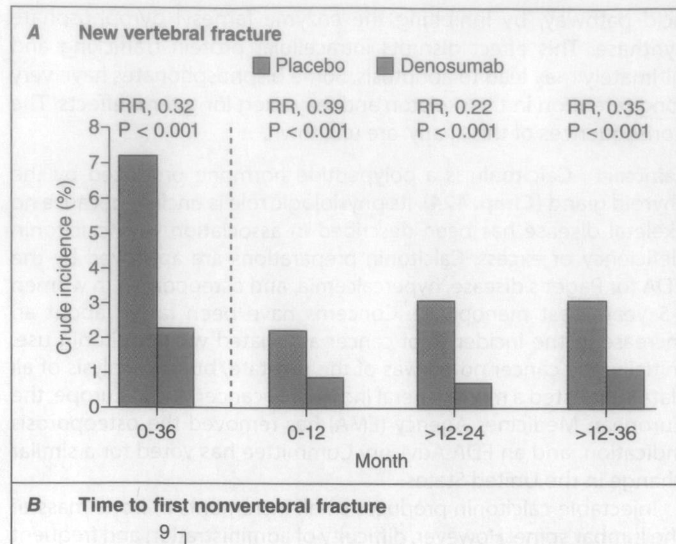

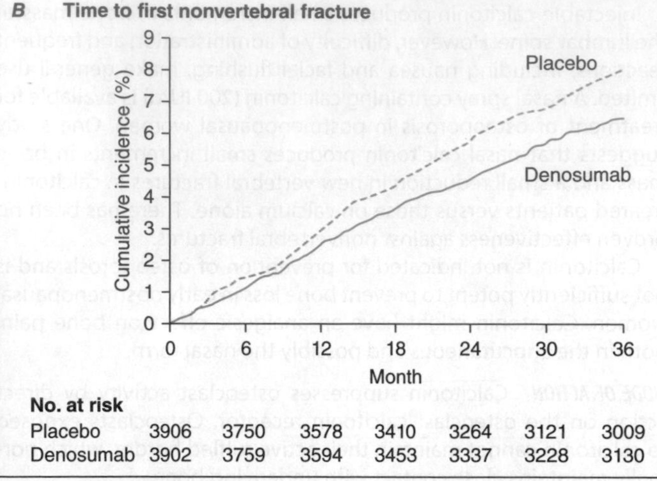

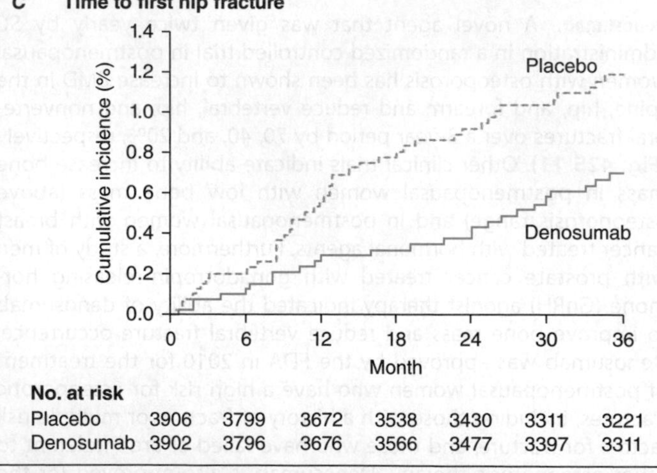

FIGURE 425-11 Effects of denosumab on new vertebral fractures (*A*) and times to nonvertebral and hip fracture (*B* and *C*). RR, relative risk. *(After SR Cummings et al: N Engl J Med 361:756, 2009.)*

If denosumab is stopped, bone will be lost rapidly if another agent is not used.

Parathyroid Hormone Endogenous PTH is an 84-amino-acid peptide that is largely responsible for calcium homeostasis **(Chap. 424)**. Although chronic elevation of PTH, as occurs in hyperparathyroidism, is associated with bone loss (particularly cortical bone), PTH when given exogenously as a daily injection exerts anabolic effects on bone. Teriparatide (1-34hPTH) is approved for the treatment of osteoporosis in both men and women at high risk for fracture. In a pivotal study (median time of treatment, 19 months' duration), 20 μg of teriparatide daily by SC injection reduced vertebral fractures by 65% and nonvertebral fractures by 45% **(Fig. 425-12)**. Treatment is administered as

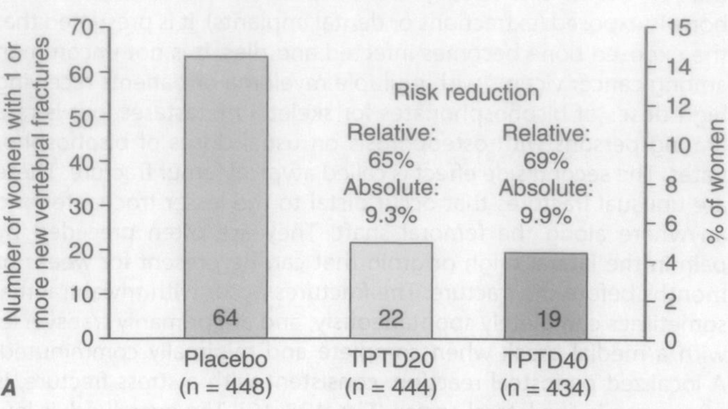

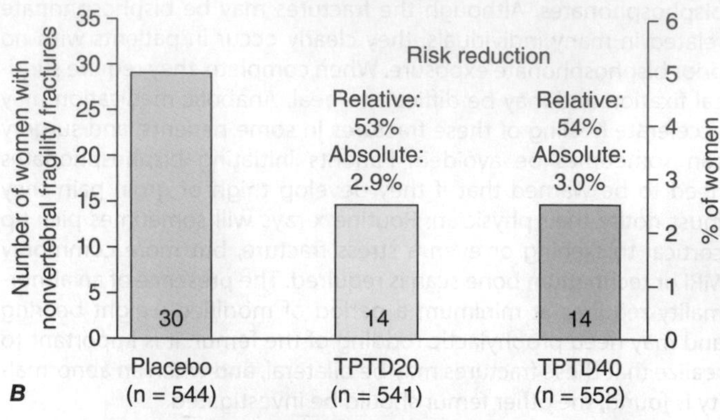

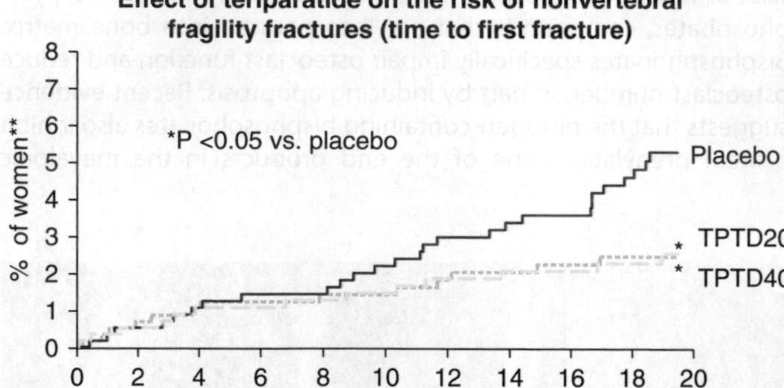

FIGURE 425-12 Effects of teriparatide (TPTD) on new vertebral fractures (*A*) and nonvertebral fragility fractures (*B* and *C*). *(After RM Neer et al: N Engl J Med 344:1434, 2001.)*

a single daily injection given for a maximum of 2 years. Teriparatide produces increases in bone mass and mediates architectural improvements in skeletal structure. These effects are lower when patients have been exposed previously to bisphosphonates, possibly in proportion to the potency of the antiresorptive effect. When teriparatide is being considered for treatment-naive patients, it is best administered as monotherapy and followed by an antiresorptive agent such as a bisphosphonate. If teriparatide treatment is not followed by an antiresorptive agent, the bone gained is rapidly lost.

Side effects of teriparatide are generally mild and can include leg cramps, muscle pain, weakness, dizziness, headache, and nausea. Rodents given prolonged treatment with PTH in relatively high doses developed osteogenic sarcomas. Long-term surveillance studies suggest no association between 2 years of teriparatide administration and osteosarcoma risk in humans.

PTH use may be limited by its mode of administration; alternative modes of delivery are being investigated. The optimal frequency of administration also remains to be established, and it is possible that

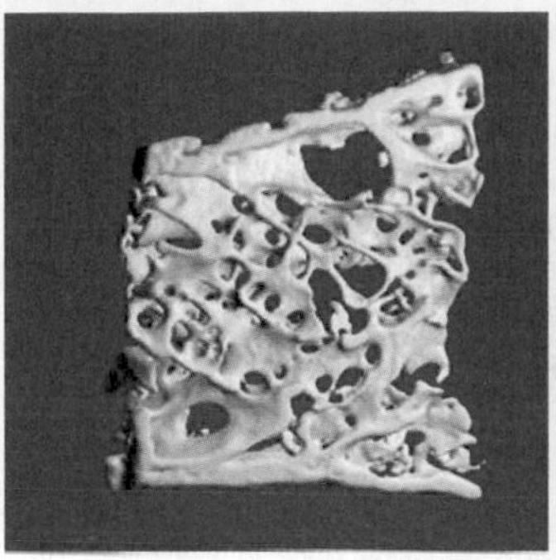

A

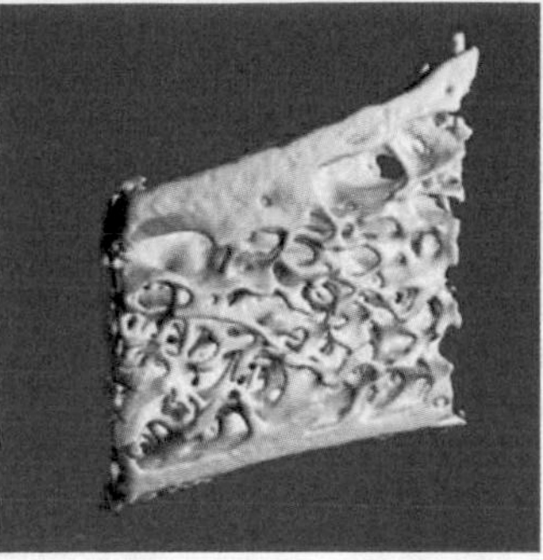

B

FIGURE 425-13 Effect of parathyroid hormone (PTH) treatment on bone microarchitecture. Paired biopsy specimens from a 64-year-old woman before (***A***) and after (***B***) treatment with PTH. *(From DW Dempster et al: J Bone Miner Res 16:1846, 2001.)*

PTH might be effective when used intermittently. Cost also may be a limiting factor. In some settings, the effect of PTH might be enhanced by combination with an antiresorptive agent. This might be particularly important in patients who have been treated previously with bisphosphonate medications.

MODE OF ACTION Exogenously administered PTH appears to have direct actions on osteoblast activity, with biochemical and histomorphometric evidence of de novo bone formation early in response to PTH, before activation of bone resorption. Subsequently, PTH activates bone remodeling but still appears to favor bone formation over bone resorption. PTH stimulates Wnt signaling, IGF-I, and collagen production and appears to increase osteoblast number by stimulating replication, enhancing osteoblast recruitment, and inhibiting apoptosis. Unlike all other treatments, PTH produces a true increase in bone tissue and an apparent restoration of bone microarchitecture **(Fig. 425-13)**.

Fluoride Fluoride has been available for many years and is a potent stimulator of osteoprogenitor cells when studied in vitro. It has been used in multiple osteoporosis studies with conflicting results, in part because of the use of varying doses and preparations. Despite increments in bone mass of up to 10%, there are no consistent effects of fluoride on vertebral or nonvertebral fracture; the latter may actually increase when high doses of fluoride are used. Fluoride remains an experimental agent despite its long history and multiple studies.

Strontium Ranelate Strontium ranelate is approved in several European countries for the treatment of osteoporosis. It increases bone mass throughout the skeleton; in clinical trials, the drug reduced the risk of vertebral fractures by 37% and that of nonvertebral fractures by 14%. It appears to be modestly antiresorptive while at the same time not causing as much of a decrease in bone formation (measured biochemically). Strontium is incorporated into hydroxyapatite, replacing calcium, a feature that might explain some of its fracture benefits. Small increased risks of venous thrombosis, sometimes severe dermatologic reactions, seizures, and abnormal cognition have been seen and require further study. An increase in risk of cardiovascular disease has also been associated with use of strontium, such that the EMA has restricted its use at present.

Other Potential Anabolic Agents Several small studies of growth hormone (GH), alone or in combination with other agents, have not shown consistent or substantial positive effects on skeletal mass. Many of these studies have been relatively short term, and the effects of GH, growth hormone–releasing hormone, and the IGFs are still under investigation. Anabolic steroids, mostly derivatives of testosterone, act primarily as antiresorptive agents to reduce bone turnover but also may stimulate osteoblastic activity. Effects on bone mass remain unclear but appear weak in general, and use is limited by masculinizing side effects. Several observational studies suggested that the statin drugs, used to treat hypercholesterolemia, may be associated with increased bone mass and reduced fractures, but conclusions from clinical trials have been largely negative. Early studies with sclerostin antibodies, which inhibit sclerostin, activate Wnt, and might be highly anabolic to bone, are under development. Odanacatib is a mixed antiresorptive, partial bone formation stimulator that is currently in the late stages of development.

NONPHARMACOLOGIC APPROACHES

In some early studies, protective pads worn around the outer thigh, which cover the trochanteric region of the hip, were able to prevent hip fractures in elderly residents in nursing homes. Randomized controlled trials of hip protectors have been unable to confirm these early findings. Therefore, the efficacy of hip protectors remains controversial at this time.

Kyphoplasty and *vertebroplasty* are also useful nonpharmacologic approaches for the treatment of painful vertebral fractures. However, no long-term data are available.

TREATMENT MONITORING

There are currently no well-accepted guidelines for monitoring treatment of osteoporosis. Because most osteoporosis treatments produce small or moderate bone mass increments on average, it is reasonable to consider BMD as a monitoring tool. Changes must exceed ~4% in the spine and 6% in the hip to be considered significant in any individual. The hip is the preferred site due to larger surface area and greater reproducibility. Medication-induced increments may require several years to produce changes of this magnitude (if they do at all). Consequently, it can be argued that BMD should be repeated at intervals >2 years. Only significant BMD reductions should prompt a change in medical regimen, because it is expected that many individuals will not show responses greater than the detection limits of the current measurement techniques.

Biochemical markers of bone turnover may prove useful for treatment monitoring, but little hard evidence currently supports this concept; it remains unclear which endpoint is most useful. If bone turnover markers are used, a determination should be made before therapy is started and repeated ≥4 months after therapy is initiated. In general, a change in bone turnover markers must be 30–40% lower than the baseline to be significant because of the biologic and technical variability in these tests. A positive change in biochemical markers and/or bone density can be useful to help patients adhere to treatment regimens.

GLUCOCORTICOID-INDUCED OSTEOPOROSIS

Osteoporotic fractures are a well-characterized consequence of the hypercortisolism associated with Cushing's syndrome. However, the therapeutic use of glucocorticoids is by far the most common form of glucocorticoid-induced osteoporosis. Glucocorticoids are used widely in the treatment of a variety of disorders, including chronic lung disorders, rheumatoid arthritis and other connective tissue diseases, inflammatory bowel disease, and after transplantation. Osteoporosis and related fractures are serious side effects of chronic glucocorticoid therapy. Because the effects of glucocorticoids on the skeleton are often superimposed on the consequences of aging and menopause, it is not surprising that women and the elderly are most frequently affected. The skeletal response to steroids is remarkably heterogeneous, however, and even young, growing individuals treated with glucocorticoids can present with fractures.

The risk of fractures depends on the dose and duration of glucocorticoid therapy, although recent data suggest that there may be no completely safe dose. Bone loss is more rapid during the early months of treatment, and trabecular bone is affected more severely than cortical bone. As a result, fractures have been shown to increase within 3 months of steroid treatment. There is an increase in fracture risk in both the axial skeleton and the appendicular skeleton, including risk of hip fracture. Bone loss can occur with any route of steroid administration, including high-dose inhaled glucocorticoids and intraarticular injections. Alternate-day delivery does not appear to ameliorate the skeletal effects of glucocorticoids.

PATHOPHYSIOLOGY

Glucocorticoids increase bone loss by multiple mechanisms, including (1) inhibition of osteoblast function and an increase in osteoblast apoptosis, resulting in impaired synthesis of new bone; (2) stimulation of bone resorption, probably as a secondary effect; (3) impairment of the absorption of calcium across the intestine, probably by a vitamin D–independent effect; (4) increase of urinary calcium loss and perhaps induction of some degree of secondary hyperparathyroidism; (5) reduction of adrenal androgens and suppression of ovarian and testicular secretion of estrogens and androgens; and (6) induction of glucocorticoid myopathy, which may exacerbate effects on skeletal and calcium homeostasis as well as increase the risk of falls.

EVALUATION OF THE PATIENT

Because of the prevalence of glucocorticoid-induced bone loss, it is important to evaluate the status of the skeleton in all patients starting or already receiving long-term glucocorticoid therapy. Modifiable risk factors should be identified, including those for falls. Examination should include testing of height and muscle strength. Laboratory evaluation should include an assessment of 24-h urinary calcium. All patients on long-term (>3 months) glucocorticoids should have measurement of bone mass at both the spine and the hip using DXA. If only one skeletal site can be measured, it is best to assess the spine in individuals <60 years and the hip in those >60 years.

PREVENTION

Bone loss caused by glucocorticoids can be prevented and the risk of fractures significantly reduced. Strategies must include using the lowest dose of glucocorticoid for disease management. Topical and inhaled routes of administration are preferred, where appropriate. Risk factor reduction is important, including smoking cessation, limitation of alcohol consumption, and participation in weight-bearing exercise, when appropriate. All patients should receive an adequate calcium and vitamin D intake from the diet or from supplements.

TREATMENT GLUCOCORTICOID-INDUCED OSTEOPOROSIS

Several bisphosphonates (alendronate, risedronate, and zoledronic acid) have been demonstrated in large clinical trials to reduce the risk of vertebral fractures in patients being treated with glucocorticoids, as well as improve bone mass in spine and hip. Teriparatide also improves bone mass and reduces fracture risk in glucocorticoid-treated osteoporosis compared to an active comparator (alendronate).

426e Paget's Disease and Other Dysplasias of Bone

Murray J. Favus, Tamara J. Vokes

This is a digital-only chapter. It is available on the DVD that accompanies this book, as well as on Access Medicine/Harrison's Online, and the eBook and "app" editions of HPIM 19e.

PAGET'S DISEASE OF BONE

Paget's disease is a localized bone-remodeling disorder that affects widespread, noncontiguous areas of the skeleton. The pathologic process is initiated by overactive osteoclastic bone resorption followed by a compensatory increase in osteoblastic new bone formation, resulting in a structurally disorganized mosaic of woven and lamellar bone. Pagetic bone is expanded, less compact, and more vascular; thus, it is more susceptible to deformities and fractures. Although most patients are asymptomatic, symptoms resulting directly from bony involvement (bone pain, secondary arthritis, fractures) or secondarily from the expansion of bone causing compression of surrounding neural tissue are not uncommon.

SECTION 5 DISORDERS OF INTERMEDIARY METABOLISM

427 Heritable Disorders of Connective Tissue

Darwin J. Prockop, John F. Bateman

CLASSIFICATION OF CONNECTIVE TISSUE DISORDERS

Some of the most common conditions that are transmitted genetically in families are disorders that produce clinically obvious changes in the skeleton, skin, or other relatively acellular tissues that have been loosely defined as connective tissues. Because of their heritability, the disorders were recognized as potentially traceable to mutated genes soon after the principles of genetics were introduced into medicine. In the last several decades, many of these disorders have been linked to mutations in several hundred different genes. However, classifying the disorders on the basis of either their clinical presentations or the mutations causing them presents a challenge for both the clinician and the geneticist.

A major development in the field was made by McKusick, who suggested that a group of disorders that included brittle bones in children (osteogenesis imperfecta), hyperextensible skin (Ehlers-Danlos syndrome), and characteristic distortions of skeleton (Marfan's syndrome) be considered as "heritable disorders of connective tissue" and that mutations causing the disorders would be found in the genes coding for proteins of the tissues.

The information on the disorders has continued to develop on two levels. The initial clinical classifications suggested by McKusick, and others, had to be refined as additional patients were examined. For example, some patients had skin changes similar to those commonly seen in Ehlers-Danlos syndrome, but this feature was overshadowed by other features such as extreme hypotonia or sudden rupture of large blood vessels. To account for the full spectrum of presentations in patients and families, many of the disorders have been reclassified several times, and each has been divided into a series of subtypes. For example, a recent effort to classify all the heritable disorders that alter the skeleton defined 456 distinctive conditions that were divided into 40 major groups.

The identification of mutations causing the diseases has developed on a parallel track. The first genes cloned for connective tissues were the two genes coding for type I collagen, the most abundant protein in bones, skin, tendons, and several other tissues. Some of the first assays in patients with osteogenesis imperfecta (OI) revealed mutations in type I collagen genes. Biochemical data developed using cultures of skin fibroblasts from affected patients demonstrated that the mutations dramatically altered the synthesis or structure of collagen fibers. The results stimulated efforts to identify additional mutations in genes coding for structural proteins. Genes for collagens provided an attractive paradigm to search for mutations, since a series of different types of collagens were found in different connective tissues and the collagen genes were readily isolated by their unique signature sequences. Also, the collagen genes are particularly vulnerable to a large number different mutations because of unusual structural requirements of the protein. The search for mutations in collagen genes proved fruitful in that mutations were found in most patients with OI, in many patients with hyperextensible skin, in some patients with dwarfism, and in patients with other disorders, including Alport's syndrome, that were not initially classified as disorders of connective tissue. Also, mutations in collagen genes were found in subset of patients with a diagnosis of osteoarthritis and a subset of patients with the diagnosis of osteoporosis. However, the search for mutations quickly expanded to hundreds of other genes that included those for other structural proteins, for the posttranslational processing of structural proteins, and for growth factors and their receptors, and other genes whose functions are still not fully understood.

In many instances, the mutations helped to define the clinical subtype of the disorder. In others, however, they did not. Some patients with the same clinical presentations were found to have mutations in different genes. Also, some patients with different manifestations were found to have mutations in the same genes. In addition, it was difficult to establish whether a change in the structure of a gene caused the phenotypic changes in patients and was not simply a neutral polymorphism. Therefore, there has been a continuing debate as to whether the disorders should be classified by their clinical presentations or by the genetic abnormalities. As an illustration of the problem, mutations in 226 genes have been found to be associated with the 456 defined disorders of the skeleton, but the latest nosology remains a "hybrid" between a list of clinically defined disorders, waiting for molecular clarification, and an annotated database documenting the phenotypic spectrum produced by mutations in a given gene. A simpler system of classification proved feasible for one rare heritable disorder of skin, epidermolysis bullosa. The disorder was first defined by the presence of friction-induced blister. It was then divided into subtypes that were defined by the ultrastructural layers of the skin that cleaved and blistered. Most patients in each subtype were subsequently shown to have mutations in genes expressed in the corresponding layer of skin. Even with these patients, however, the strength of the genotype-phenotype correlation varies, and mutations have not yet been found in every patient.

In the end, consensus reports by experts in the field and sources such as the Online Mendelian Inheritance in Man database provide valuable resources for physicians searching for diagnoses of patients with unusual clinical features. However, patients with the most common forms of the disorders have mutations in a limited number of genes. This chapter will focus primarily on these more common disorders.

COMPOSITION OF CONNECTIVE TISSUES

Connective tissues such as skin, bone, cartilage, ligaments, and tendons are the critical structural frameworks of the body important for development and function. They consist of a complex interacting extracellular matrix network of collagens, proteoglycans, and a large number of noncollagenous glycoproteins and proteins. Although these precise combinations of up to ~500 potential extracellular matrix building blocks provide tissue-specific function, there are many overarching similarities in composition, such as the role of composite collagen fibrils in providing strength and form, elastin fibrils and proteoglycans and other interacting proteins, and glycoproteins that fine-tune function (Table 427-1). The most abundant components are three similar fibrillar collagens (types I, II, and III). They have a similar tensile

TABLE 427-1 CONSTITUENTS OF CONNECTIVE TISSUES

Connective Tissue	Major Constituents	Approximate Amounts, % dry wt	Characteristics or Functions
Dermis, ligaments, tendons	Type I collagen	80	Large bundles of fibrils
	Type III collagen	5–15	Thin fibrils
	Type IV collagen, laminins, and nidogen	<5	Form basal laminae under epithelium
	Types V, VI, and VII collagens	<5	V modifies type I fibrils; VI forms beaded microfibrils, VII forms anchoring fibrils for epidermis
	Fibrillin aggregates/elastin	<5	Provide elasticity
	Fibronectin	<5	Associated with collagen fibers and cell surfaces
	Proteoglycans[a]/hyaluronan	<0.5	Provide resiliency
Bone (demineralized)	Type I collagen	90	Complex fibril network
	Type VI collagen	1–2	Beaded microfibrils
	Proteoglycans[a]hyaluronan	1	Function unclear
	Osteonectin, osteopontin, osteocalcin, α2 glycoprotein, and sialoproteins	1–5	May regulate mineralization
Aorta	Type I collagen	20–40	Fibril network
	Type III collagen	20–40	Thin fibrils
	Fibrillin aggregates/elastin	20–40	Provide elasticity
	Type IV collagen, laminins, and nidogen	<5	Form basal lamina under endothelial cells
	Types V and VI collagens	<2	V modifies type I fibrils; VI forms beaded microfibrils
	Proteoglycans[a]/hyaluronan	<3	Provide resiliency
Cartilage	Type II collagen	40–50	Arcades of thin fibrils
	Type IX collagen	5–10	Links type II fibrils and other components
	Type VI collagen	<1	Beaded microfibrils, largely pericellular
	Type X collagen	5–10	Forms pericellular network in hypertrophic growth plate cartilage
	Type XI collagen	<10	Incorporated into some type II fibrils
	Proteoglycans[a]/hyaluronan	15–50	Provide resiliency
	Small leucine-rich repeat proteins (SLRPs; >6 kinds)	<5	Multiple functions in assembly and function of the tissue

[a]Over 30 proteoglycans have been identified. They differ in the structures of their core proteins and their contents of glycosaminoglycan side chains of chondroitin-4-sulfate, chondroitin-6-sulfate, dermatan sulfate, and keratin sulfate. Basal lamina contains a proteoglycan with a side chain of heparan sulfate that resembles heparin.

strength as steel wires. The three fibrillar collagens are distributed in a tissue-specific manner: type I collagen accounts for most of the protein of dermis, ligaments, tendons, and demineralized bone; type I and type III are the most abundant proteins of large blood vessels; and type II is the most abundant protein of cartilage.

BIOSYNTHESIS AND TURNOVER OF CONNECTIVE TISSUES

Connective tissues are among the most stable components in living organisms, but they are not inert. During embryonic development, connective tissue membranes appear as early as the four-cell blastocyst to provide strength and a structural scaffold for the developing embryo. With the development of blood vessels and skeleton, there is a rapid increase in the synthesis, degradation, and resynthesis of connective tissues. The turnover continues at a slower, but still rapid pace throughout postnatal development and then spikes during the growth spurt of puberty. During adulthood, the metabolic turnover of most connective tissues is slow, but it continues at a moderate pace in bone. With age, malnutrition, physical inactivity, and low gravitational stress, the rate of degradation of most connective tissues, especially in bone and skin, begins to exceed the rate of synthesis and the tissues shrink. In starvation, a large fraction of the collagen in skin and other connective tissues is degraded and provides amino acids for gluconeogenesis (Chap. 97). In both osteoarthritis and rheumatoid arthritis, there is extensive degradation of articular cartilage collagen. Glucocorticoids weaken most tissues by decreasing collagen synthesis. In many pathologic states, however, collagen is deposited in excess. With most injuries to tissues, inflammatory and immune responses stimulate the deposition of collagen fibrils in the form of fibrotic scars. The deposition of the fibrils is largely irreversible and prevents regeneration of normal tissues in hepatic cirrhosis, pulmonary fibrosis, atherosclerosis, and nephrosclerosis.

Structure and Biosynthesis of Fibrillar Collagens The tensile strength of collagen fibers derives primarily from the self-assembly of protein monomers into large fibril structures in a process that resembles crystallization. The self-assembly requires monomers of highly uniform and relatively rigid structure. It also requires a complex series of posttranslational processing steps that maintain the solubility of the monomers until they are transported to the appropriate extracellular sites for fibril assembly. Because of the stringent requirements for correct self-assembly, it is not surprising that mutations in genes for fibrillar collagens cause many of the diseases of connective tissues.

The monomers of the three fibrillar collagens are formed from three polypeptide chains, called *α chains*, that are wrapped around each other into a rope-like triple-helical conformation. The triple helix is a unique structure among proteins, and it provides rigidity to the molecule. It also orients the side chains of amino acids in an "inside out" manner relative to most other proteins so that the charged and hydrophobic residues on the surface can direct self-assembly of the monomers into fibrils. The triple-helical conformation of the monomer is generated because each of the α chains has a repetitive amino acid sequence in which glycine (Gly) appears as every third amino acid. Each α chain contains about 1000 amino acids. Therefore, the sequence of each α chain can be designated as $(\text{-Gly-X-Y-})_n$, where X and Y represent amino acids other than glycine and n is >338. The presence of glycine, the smallest amino acid, in every third position in the sequence is critical because this residue must fit in a sterically restricted space in the middle of the helix where the three chains come together. The requirement for a glycine residue at every third position explains the severe effects of mutations that convert any of the glycine residues to an amino acid with a bulkier side chain (see below). Many of the X- and Y-position amino acids are proline and hydroxyproline, which, because of their ring structures, provide additional rigidity to the triple helix. Other X- and Y-positions are occupied by charged or hydrophobic amino acids that precisely direct lateral and longitudinal assembly of the monomers into highly ordered fibrils. Mutations that substitute amino acids in some X- and Y-positions can, in rare instances, also produce genetic diseases.

The fibers formed by the three fibrillar collagens differ in thickness and length, but they have a similar fine structure. As viewed by electron microscopy, they all have a characteristic pattern of cross-striations that are about one-quarter the length of the monomers and reflect the precise packing into fibrils. The three fibrillar collagens, however, differ in sequences found in the X- and Y-positions of the α chains and therefore in some of their physical properties. Type I collagen is composed of two identical α1(I) chains and a third α2(I) chain that differs slightly in its amino acid sequence. Type II collagen is composed of three identical α(II) chains. Type III collagen is composed of three identical α1(III) chains.

To deliver a monomer of the correct structure to the appropriate site of fibril assembly, the biosynthesis of fibrillar collagens involves a large number of unique processing steps (Fig. 427-1). The monomer, first synthesized as a soluble precursor called *procollagen*, contains an additional globular domain at each end. As the proα chains of procollagen are synthesized on ribosomes, the free N-terminal ends move into the cisternae of the rough endoplasmic reticulum. Signal peptides at the N-termini are cleaved, and additional posttranslational reactions begin. Proline residues in the Y-position of the repeating -Gly-X-Y- sequences are converted to hydroxyproline by the enzyme prolyl hydroxylase. The hydroxylation of prolyl residues is essential for the three α chains of the monomer to fold into a triple helix at body temperature. The enzyme requires ascorbic acid as one of its essential cofactors, an observation that explains why wounds fail to heal in scurvy (Chap. 96e). In scurvy, some of the underhydroxylated and unfolded protein accumulates in the cisternae of the rough endoplasmic reticulum and is degraded. Lysine residues in the Y-position are also hydroxylated to hydroxylysine by a separate lysyl hydroxylase. Many of the hydroxylysine residues are glycosylated with galactose or with galactose and glucose. A large mannose-rich oligosaccharide is assembled on the C-terminal propeptide of each chain. The proα chains are assembled by interactions among these C-terminal propeptides that control the selection of the appropriate partner chains to form hetero- or homotrimers and provide the correct chain registration required for subsequent formation of the collagen triple helix. After the C-terminal propeptides assemble the three proα chains, a nucleus of triple helix is formed near the C terminus, and the helical conformation is propagated toward the N terminus in a zipper-like manner that resembles crystallization. The folding into the triple helix is spontaneous in solution, but as discussed below, identification of rare mutations causing OI demonstrated that the folding *in cellulo* is assisted by ancillary proteins. The fully folded protein is then secreted. After secretion, procollagen is processed to collagen by cleavage of the N-propeptides and C-propeptides by two specific proteinases. The release of the propeptides decreases the solubility of the protein about 1000-fold. The entropic energy that is released drives the self-assembly of the collagen into fibrils. Self-assembled collagen fibers have considerable tensile strength, but their strength is increased further by cross-linking reactions that form covalent bonds between α chains in one molecule and α chains in adjacent molecules.

Although the assembly of collagen monomers into fibers is a spontaneous reaction, the process in tissues is modulated by the presence of less abundant collagens (type V with type I, and type XI with type II) and by other components such as a series of small leucine-rich proteins (SLRPs). Some of the less abundant components alter the rate of fibril assembly, whereas others change the morphology of the fibers or their interactions with cells and other molecules.

Collagen fibers are resistant to most proteases, but during degradation of connective tissues, they are cleaved by specific matrix metalloproteinases (collagenases) that cause partial unfolding of the triple helices into gelatin-like structures that are further degraded by less specific proteinases.

OTHER COLLAGENS AND RELATED MOLECULES

The unique properties of the triple helix are used to define a family of at least 28 collagens that contain repetitive -Gly-X-Y- sequences and form triple helices of varying length and complexity. The proteins are

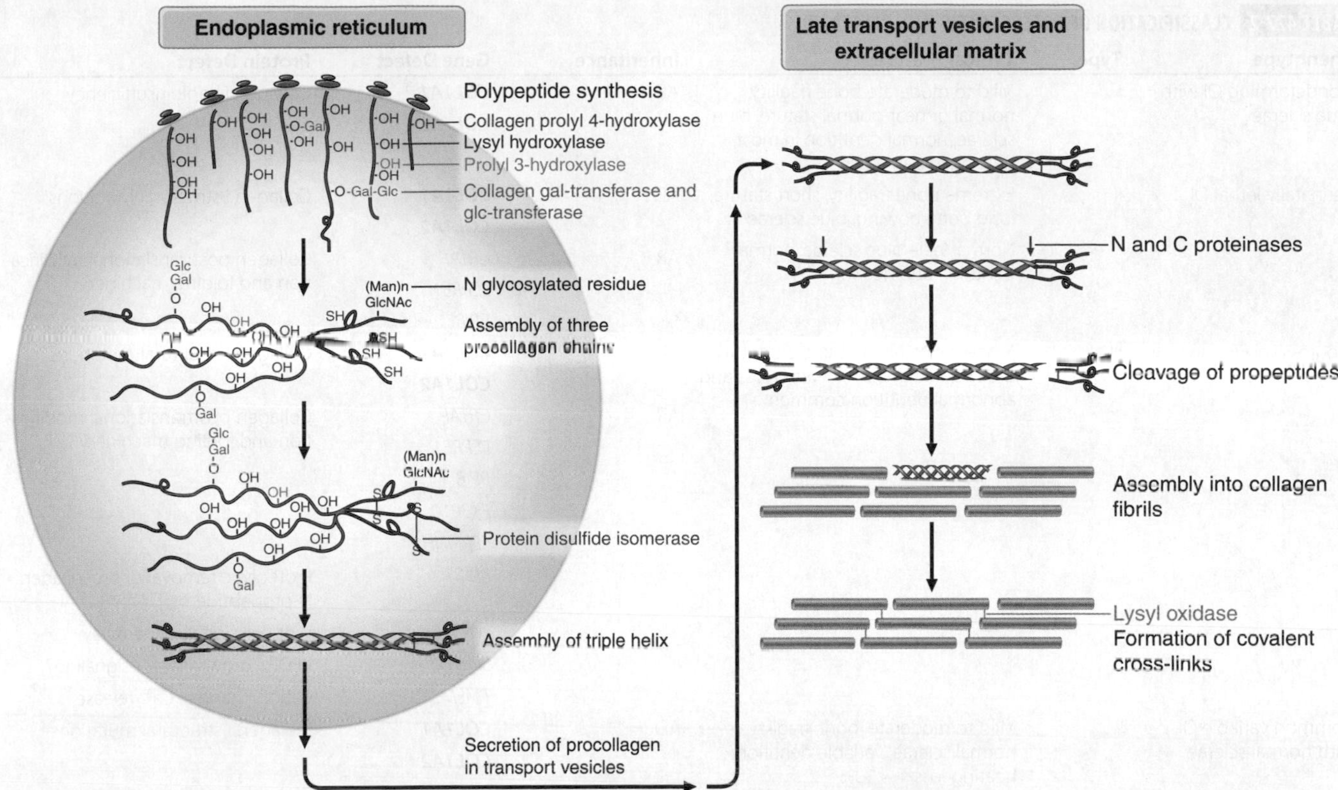

FIGURE 427-1 Schematic summary of biosynthesis of fibrillar collagens. *(Modified and reproduced with permission from J Myllyharju, KI Kivirikko: Trends in Genetics 20:33, 2004.)*

heterogeneous both in structure and function, and many are the sites of mutations causing genetic diseases. For example, the type IV collagen found in basement membranes is composed of three α chains synthesized from any of six different genes. Mutations in any of the six genes can cause Alport's syndrome.

Fibrillin Aggregates and Elastin In addition to tensile strength, many tissues such as the lung, large blood vessels, and ligaments require elasticity. The elasticity was originally ascribed to an amorphous rubber-like protein named *elastin*. Subsequent analyses, largely sparked by discoveries of mutations causing the Marfan's syndrome (MFS), demonstrated that the elasticity resided in thin fibrils composed primarily of large glycoproteins named *fibrillins*. The fibrillins contain large numbers of epidermal growth factor–like domains interspersed with characteristic cysteine-rich domains that are also found in latent transforming growth factor β (TGF-β) binding proteins. The fibrillins assemble into long beadlike strands that also contain numerous other components including small and variable amounts of elastin, bone morphogenic proteins (BMPs), and microfibril-associated glycoproteins (MAGPs). The principles whereby the fibrils provide elasticity to tissue and their biosynthetic assembly are still under investigation. As well as contributing to extracellular matrix structure, the fibrillins play a major role in TGF-β signaling.

Proteoglycans The resiliency to compression of connective tissues such as cartilage or the aorta is largely explained by the presence of proteoglycans. Proteoglycans are composed of a core protein to which are attached a large series of negatively charged polymers of disaccharides (largely chondroitin sulfates). At least 30 proteoglycans have been identified. They vary in their binding to collagens and other components of matrix, but specific functions have not been assigned to most. The major proteoglycan of cartilage, called *aggrecan*, has a core protein of 2000 amino acids that is decorated with about 100 side chains of chondroitin sulfate and keratin sulfate. The core protein, in turn, binds to long chains of the polymeric disaccharide hyaluronan to form proteoglycan aggregates, one of the largest soluble macromolecular structures in nature. Because of its highly negative charge and extended structure, the proteoglycan aggregate binds large amounts of water and small ions to distend the three-dimensional arcade of collagen fibers found in the same tissues. It thereby makes the cartilage resilient to pressure.

SPECIFIC DISORDERS

OSTEOGENESIS IMPERFECTA (OI)

The central feature of OI is a severe decrease in bone mass that makes bones brittle. The disorder is frequently associated with blue sclerae, dental abnormalities (dentinogenesis imperfecta), progressive hearing loss, and a positive family history. Most patients have mutations in one of the two genes coding for type I collagen.

Classification OI was originally classified into two subtypes of *congenita* and *tarda* depending on the age of onset of the symptoms. Sillence suggested a series of subtypes based on clinical and radiologic findings and mode of inheritance. As with the other disorders discussed here, the description of rare recessive forms of OI and discovery of mutations in new genes have opened a debate as to whether the disorders should be classified by the clinical phenotypes or by the genes at fault. For the near term, the classification based on the clinical presentations seems the most useful (Table 427-2).

Type I is the mildest subtype and can produce either mild or no apparent deformities of the skeleton. Most patients have distinctly blue sclerae. Type II produces bone so brittle that it is lethal in utero or shortly after birth; it can be subclassified into types IIA, IIB, and IIC, depending on radiologic findings. Of the nonlethal forms, type III is progressively deforming with moderate to severe bone deformity, and type IV (common variable OI with normal sclerae) has mild to moderate bone fragility.

The classifications of patients by types of OI do not consistently predict the clinical course of the disease. Some patients appear normal at birth and become progressively worse; others have multiple fractures in infancy and childhood, improve after puberty, and fracture more frequently later in life. Women are particularly prone to fracture during

TABLE 427-2 CLASSIFICATION OF OSTEOGENESIS IMPERFECTA (OI)

Phenotype	Type	Typical Features	Inheritance	Gene Defect	Protein Defect
Nondeforming OI with blue sclerae	I	Mild to moderate bone fragility, normal or near-normal stature, blue sclerae, normal dentition in most, hearing loss in ~50%	AD	***COL1A1*** ***COL1A2***	Collagen I haploinsufficiency
Perinatally lethal OI	II	Extreme bone fragility, short stature, long bone bowing, blue sclerae	AD	***COL1A1*** ***COL1A2***	Collagen I structural mutations
		Normal/pale blue sclerae, normal dentition and hearing	AR	*CRTAP* *LEPRE1* *PPIB*	Collagen posttranslational modification and folding machinery
Progressively deforming OI	III	Moderate to severe bone deformity, blue sclerae at birth, hearing loss and abnormal dentition common	AD	***COL1A1*** ***COL1A2***	Collagen I structural mutations
			AR	*CRTAP* *LEPRE1* *PPIB* *FKBP10* *SERPINH1*	Collagen posttranslational modification and folding machinery
				BMP1	Proteolytic removal of procollagen N-propeptide
				WNT1	Wnt cell signaling pathway
				SERPINF1	PEDF - growth factor signaling?
				TMEM38B	Cation channel, Ca^{2+} release
Common variable OI with normal sclerae	IV	Mild to moderate, bone fragility, normal sclerae, variable dentition, hearing loss in <10%	AD	***COL1A1*** ***COL1A2***	Collagen I structural mutations
				WNT1	Wnt cell signaling pathway
			AR	*CRTAP* *FKBP10*	Collagen posttranslational modification and folding machinery
				SP7/OSX	Transcription factor, bone formation defect
OI with calcification of the interosseous membranes	V	Calcification of the interosseous membranes in forearm and legs and/or hypertrophic callus; variable bone deformity, normal sclerae and dentition	AD	*IFITM5*	Transcription factor, bone formation defect
Bruck syndrome type 1		Contractures with pterygia, fractures in infancy or early childhood, postnatal short stature, severe limb deformity, and progressive scoliosis	AR	*FKBP10*	Collagen folding machinery
Bruck syndrome type 2		As for Bruck syndrome type 1	AR	*PLOD2*	Collagen posttranslational modification of lysine

Abbreviations: AD, autosomal dominant; AR, autosomal recessive.

Note: Predominant OI gene mutations (>90%) are in *COL1A1* and *COL1A2* (in bold typeface).

pregnancy and after menopause. A few women from families with mild variants of OI do not develop fractures until after menopause, and their disease may be difficult to distinguish from postmenopausal osteoporosis.

Incidence Type I OI has a frequency of about 1 in 15,000–20,000 births. Type II OI has a reported incidence of about 1 in 60,000. Only a limited number of patients with the severe forms of OI have been reported, and the combined incidence of the severe forms that are recognizable at birth (types II, III, and IV) may be higher than 1 in 60,000.

Skeletal Effects In type I OI, the fragility of bones may be severe enough to limit physical activity or be so mild that individuals are unaware of any disability. Radiographs of the skull in patients with mild disease may show a mottled appearance because of small islands of irregular ossification. In type II OI, ossification of many bones is frequently incomplete. Continuously beaded or broken ribs and crumpled long bones (accordina femora) may be present. For reasons that are not apparent, the long bones may be either thick or thin. In types III and IV, multiple fractures from minor physical stress can produce severe deformities. Kyphoscoliosis can impair respiration, cause cor pulmonale, and predispose to pulmonary infections. The appearance of "popcorn-like" deposits of mineral in x-rays of the ends of long bones is an ominous sign. Progressive neurologic symptoms may result from basilar compression and communicating hydrocephalus. Type V OI is recognized by the presence of dislocated radial heads and hyperplastic callus formation.

In all forms of OI, bone mineral density is decreased. However, the degree of osteopenia may be difficult to evaluate because recurrent fractures limit exercise and thereby diminish bone mass. Surprisingly, fractures appear to heal normally.

Ocular Features The sclerae can be normal, gray, slightly bluish, or bright blue. The color is probably caused by a thinness of the collagen layers of the sclerae that allows the choroid layers to be seen. Blue sclerae, however, are an inherited trait in some families who do not have increased bone fragility.

Dentinogenesis The teeth may be normal, moderately discolored, or grossly abnormal. The enamel generally appears normal, but the teeth may have a characteristic amber, yellowish brown, or translucent bluish gray color because of a deficiency of dentin that is rich in type I collagen. The deciduous teeth are usually smaller than normal, whereas permanent teeth are frequently bell-shaped and restricted at the base. In some patients, the teeth readily fracture and need to be extracted. Similar tooth defects, however, can be inherited without any evidence of OI.

Hearing Loss Hearing loss usually begins during the second decade of life and occurs in more than 50% of individuals over age 30. The loss can be conductive, sensorineural, or mixed, and it varies in severity. The middle ear usually exhibits maldevelopment, deficient ossification, persistence of cartilage in areas that are normally ossified, and abnormal calcium deposits.

Other Features Changes in other connective tissues can include thin skin that scars extensively, joint laxity with permanent dislocations indistinguishable from those of Ehlers-Danlos syndrome (EDS), and occasionally, cardiovascular manifestations such as aortic regurgitation, floppy mitral valves, mitral incompetence, and fragility of large blood vessels. For unknown reasons, some patients develop bouts of a hypermetabolic state with elevated serum thyroxine levels, hyperthermia, and excessive sweating.

Molecular Defects Of the ~1360 unique gene mutations now described in OI, more than 90% are heterozygous mutations in either *COL1A1* or *COL1A2*, the genes coding for the proα1 or proα2 chain of type I procollagen (Table 427-2).

Most patients with type I OI and blue sclerae have mutations that reduce the synthesis of proα1 chains to about one-half. Mutations that reduce the synthesis of proα2 chains produce slightly more severe phenotypes and skin defects similar to EDS.

In contrast to the null mutations found in type I OI, most of the severe variants (types II, III, and IV) are caused by mutations that produce structurally abnormal proα chains that have compromised assembly or abnormal folding of the triple helix. As with collagen mutations in other connective tissue diseases, these structural mutations generally fall into two functional categories. First, the relatively rare mutations in the C-propeptide domain can prevent or seriously impair initial assembly of the procollagen trimers. These misfolded chains are retained in the endoplasmic reticulum (ER) and targeted for degradation by the ER-associated proteasomal pathway. Because these mutations induce an ER stress response, the unfolded protein response (UPR) may have many downstream effects on cells. ER stress is a new concept in the pathophysiology of connective tissue disease and has been best characterized for chondrodysplasias (see below).

The most common type I collagen mutations, however, are single base substitutions that introduce an amino acid with a bulky side chain for one of the glycine residues that appear as every third amino acid in the triple helix. In effect, any of the 338 glycine residues in the helical domain of either the proα1 or proα2 chain of type I procollagen is a potential site for a disease-producing mutation. These mutations compromise the structural integrity of the triple helix, causing disruption to helix folding, retention of the mutant trimers in the ER, and increased posttranslational hydroxylation and glycosylation of lysines. Collagen-containing helix mutations can form insoluble aggregates in the ER that are degraded by the autophagosome-endosome system, rather than the proteasomes.

A similar sequence of events occurs with less common mutations that produce partial gene deletions, partial gene duplications, and splicing mutations. In addition to their intracellular effects, the structurally abnormal mutant-containing collagen that is secreted by the cell can also have important extracellular affects. For example, the presence of one abnormal proα chain in a procollagen molecule can interfere with cleavage of the N-propeptide from the protein. The persistence of the N-propeptide on a fraction of the molecules interferes with the self-assembly of normal collagen so that thin and irregular collagen fibrils are formed. Furthermore, if structurally abnormal collagens are incorporated into fibrils, they may have a destabilizing effect and be selectively degraded, or they may alter the interactions of collagen with other connective tissue components, disturbing architecture and stability.

Several generalizations can be made about mutations in type I collagen genes. One is that unrelated patients rarely have the same mutation in the same gene. Glycine substitutions in the N-terminal region of the triple helix tend to produce milder phenotypes, apparently because they have less effect on the zipper-like propagation of the triple-helical conformation from the C terminus. Rare substitutions of charged amino acids (Asp, Arg) or a branched amino acid (Val) in X- or Y-positions produce lethal phenotypes, apparently because they are located at sites for lateral assembly of the monomers or binding of other components of the matrix.

The search for mutations causing the less common and autosomal recessive forms of OI identified mutations in genes for a series of proteins that are essential for the timely folding of the procollagen monomer: cartilage-associated protein (*CRTAP*), prolyl-3-hydroxylase (*LEPRE1*/P3H1), cyclophilin B (*PPIB*), collagen chaperone-like protein HSP47 (*SERPINH1*), and the procollagen chaperone protein FKBP65 (*FKBP10*). Recently, mutations have been characterized in additional downstream components of the collagen fibrillogenesis pathway: *BMP1*, the gene coding for a metalloproteinase that cleaves the C-propeptide of type I procollagen, and *PLOD2* (LH2, lysyl oxidase 2), which is involved in establishing collagen cross-links. In addition to these mutations that affect the collagen assembly pathway, mutations have been characterized in genes involved in the regulation of bone formation and mineralization such as *SP7* (osterix), *IFITM5*, *WNT1*, and *TMEM38B* (Table 427-2).

Inheritance and Mosaicism in Germline Cells and in Somatic Cells Type I OI is inherited as an autosomal dominant trait. However, some patients with type I OI appear to represent sporadic new mutations or a diagnosis that was missed in earlier generations. Most lethal OI is the result of sporadic mutations that occur in the germ line in one of the parents. Because of the possibility for germline mosaicism for newly generated mutations, there is about a 7% probability that a second child could inherit a severe variant of OI.

Diagnosis OI is usually diagnosed on the basis of clinical criteria. The presence of fractures together with blue sclerae, dentinogenesis imperfecta, or family history of the disease is usually sufficient to make the diagnosis. Other causes of pathologic fractures must be excluded, including battered child syndrome, nutritional deficiencies, malignancies, and other inherited disorders such as chondrodysplasias and hypophosphatasia that can have overlapping presentations. The absence of superficial bruises can be helpful in distinguishing OI from battered child syndrome. X-rays usually reveal a decrease in bone density that can be verified by photon or x-ray absorptiometry. Bone microscopy can be helpful in the diagnosis. The diagnosis, as in other genetic disorders, is now routinely determined using targeted candidate gene sequencing and exome sequencing, but whole-genome sequencing may be used in the future.

TREATMENT OSTEOGENESIS IMPERFECTA

Many patients with OI lead productive and successful lives despite severe deformities. Those with mild forms of the disease may need little treatment when fractures decrease after puberty, but women require special attention during pregnancy and after menopause, when fractures again increase. More severely affected children require a comprehensive program of physical therapy and surgical management of fractures and skeletal deformities.

Many fractures are only slightly displaced and have little soft tissue swelling and, therefore, can be treated with minimal support or traction for a week or two followed by a light cast. If fractures are relatively painless, physical therapy can be initiated early. A judicious amount of exercise prevents loss of bone mass secondary to physical inactivity. Some physicians advocate insertion of steel rods into long bones to correct limb deformities; the risk/benefits and cost/benefits of such procedures are difficult to evaluate. Aggressive conventional intervention is usually warranted for pneumonia and cor pulmonale. For severe hearing loss, stapedectomy or replacement of the stapes with a prosthesis may be successful. Moderately to severely affected patients should be evaluated periodically to anticipate possible neurologic problems. About half of children have a substantial increase in growth when given growth hormone. Treatment with bisphosphonates to decrease bone loss has been introduced for moderate to severe forms of OI. Improvements in bone mineral density are consistently seen in patients. Some clinical trials observed improvements in bone pain and fracture incidence; however, there are still unresolved questions about the best delivery protocols and the risks associated with long-term use in OI patients. For these reasons, the current consensus is that bisphosphonate therapy should be restricted to moderate to severe OI, where the possible benefits outweigh risks. Also, a clinical trial was performed in which patients were treated by intravenous infusion of cells from bone marrow referred to as mesenchymal stem cells, or multipotential stromal cells (MSCs; see Chap. 90e). Promising results were obtained, but the trial required a prior bone marrow transplant with marrow from a normal donor who subsequently was used as a source of normal MSCs. As a result, the procedure has not been widely adopted. However, the results raise the possibility that it may be possible in the future to develop effective stem cell therapies for OI.

Counseling and emotional support are important for patients and their parents; lay organizations in some countries provide help in these areas. Prenatal ultrasonography will detect severely affected fetuses at about 16 weeks of pregnancy. Diagnosis is routinely performed on DNA from blood.

EHLERS-DANLOS SYNDROME

EDS is characterized by hyperextensible skin and hypermobile joints, but the category includes rare patients with other distinctive features. Mutations in different types of collagen are found in many patients, but other genes are at fault in rare forms. Contrary to initial expectations, no patients have been found with mutations in the gene for elastin in EDS.

Classification Several types of EDS have been defined, based on the extent to which the skin, joints, and other tissues are involved, mode of inheritance, and molecular and biochemical analysis (Table 427-3). Classical EDS includes a severe form of the disease (type I) and a milder form (type II), both characterized by joint hypermobility and skin that is velvety in texture, hyperextensible, and easily scarred. In hypermobile EDS (type III), joint hypermobility is more prominent than skin changes. In vascular-type EDS (type IV), the skin changes are more prominent than joint changes, and the patients are predisposed to sudden death from rupture of large blood vessels or other hollow organs. EDS type V is similar to EDS type II but is inherited as an X-linked trait. The ocular-scoliotic type of EDS (type VI) is characterized by scoliosis, ocular fragility, and a cone-shaped deformity of the cornea (keratoconus). The arthrochalasic type of EDS (type VIIA and VIIB) is characterized by marked joint hypermobility that is difficult to distinguish from EDS III except by the specific molecular defects in the processing of type I procollagen to collagen. The periodontotic-type EDS (type VIII) is distinguished by prominent periodontal changes. EDS types IX, X, and XI were defined on the basis of preliminary biochemical and clinical data. EDS due to tenascin X deficiency has not been assigned a type; it is an autosomal recessive form of the syndrome similar to EDS II. The cardiac valvular form of EDS has similar features to EDS II, but also involves severe changes to the aorta. The progeroid form of EDS displays features of both EDS and progeria. Because of overlapping signs and symptoms, many patients and families with some of the features of EDS cannot be assigned to any of the defined types.

Incidence The overall incidence of EDS is about 1 in 5000 births, with a higher rate for blacks. Classical and hypermobile types of EDS are the most common. Patients with milder forms frequently do not seek medical attention.

Skin Skin changes vary from thin and velvety to skin that is either dramatically hyperextensible ("rubber person" syndrome) or easily

TABLE 427-3 DIFFERENT FORMS OF EHLERS-DANLOS SYNDROME

Type	Typical Features	Inheritance	Gene Defect	Protein Defect
Classic (EDS I—severe and EDS II—mild)	Skin hyperextensibility and fragility, joint hypermobility, tissue fragility manifested by widened atrophic scarring	AD	*COL5A1* *COL5A2*	Collagen V
		AD	*COL1A1*	Proα1 (I) and proα2 (I) chains of procollagen I
		AD, AR	*COL1A2*	
Hypermobile (EDS III)	Joint hypermobility, moderate skin involvement, absence of tissue fragility	AD	*TNXB*	Tenascin X
Vascular (EDS IV)	Markedly reduced life span due to spontaneous rupture of internal organs such as arteries and intestines; skin is thin, translucent, and fragile, with extensive bruising; hypermobile minor joints; characteristic facial appearance	AD	*COL3A1*	Collagen III
X-linked EDS (EDS V)	Similar to classic type	X-linked recessive	Unknown	Unknown
Ocular-scoliotic EDS VI (EDS VIA and EDS VIB)	Features of classic EDS as well as severe muscular hypotonia after birth, progressive kyphoscoliosis, a Marfanoid habitus, osteopenia, occasionally rupture of the eye globe and great arteries	AR	*PLOD1*	Deficiency of procollagen-lysine 5-dioxygenase activity (EDS VIA)
			Unknown for EDS VIB	Unknown for EDS VIB
Arthrochalasic EDS VII (EDS VIIA and EDS VIIB)	Congenital bilateral hip dislocation, hypermobile joints, moderate skin involvement, osteopenia	AD	*COL1A1*	Mutations that prevent cleavage of the N propeptides
			COL1A2	
Dermatosparactic EDS VII C	Redundant and fragile skin, prominent hernias, joint laxity, dysmorphic features	AR	*ADAMTS2*	Deficiency of procollagen I N-terminal proteinase
Periodontotic EDS VIII	Absorptive periodontosis with premature loss of permanent teeth, fragility of the skin, skin lesions	AD	Unknown	Unknown
EDS due to tenascin X deficiency	Similar to EDS II	AR	*TNXB*	Tenascin X
EDS, progeroid form		AR?	*B4GALT7*	Deficiency of galactosyltransferase 7 (defective synthesis of dermatan sulfate proteoglycans)

Abbreviations: AD, autosomal dominant; AR, autosomal recessive.

torn or scarred. Patients with classical EDS develop characteristic "cigarette-paper" scars. In vascular-type EDS, extensive scars and hyperpigmentation develop over bony prominences, and the skin may be so thin that subcutaneous blood vessels are visible. In the periodontotic type of EDS, the skin is more fragile than hyperextensible, and it heals with atrophic, pigmented scars. Easy bruisability occurs in several types of EDS.

Ligament and Joint Changes Laxity and hypermobility of joints vary from mild to unreducible dislocations of hips and other large joints. In mild forms, patients learn to avoid dislocations by limiting physical activity. In more severe forms, surgical repair may be required. Some patients have progressive difficulty with age.

Other Features Mitral valve prolapse and hernias occur, particularly with type I. Pes planus and mild to moderate scoliosis are common. Extreme joint laxity and repeated dislocations may lead to degenerative arthritis. In the ocular-scoliotic type of EDS, the eye may rupture with minimal trauma, and kyphoscoliosis can cause respiratory impairment. Also, sclerae may be blue.

Molecular Defects Subsets of patients with different types of EDS have mutations in the structural genes for collagens (Table 427-3). These include mutations in the *COL1A1* gene in a few patients with moderately severe classical EDS (type I); mutations in *COL1A2* in rare patients with an aortic valvular form of EDS; mutations in two of the three genes (*COL5A1* and *COL5A2*) for type V collagen, a minor collagen found in association with type I collagen, in about half the patients with classical EDS (types I and II); and mutations in the *COL3A1* gene for type III collagen, which is abundant in the aorta in patients with the frequently lethal vascular EDS (type IV).

Some of the type I collagen-related mutations alter processing of the protein or genes for the processing enzymes. Arthrochalasic EDS (type VII) is caused by mutations in the amino acid sequence that make type I procollagen resistant to cleavage by procollagen N-proteinase or by mutations that decrease the activity of the enzyme. The persistence of the N propeptide causes the formation of collagen fibrils that are thin and irregular. Some of the patients have fragile bones and therefore a phenotype that overlaps with OI. The ocular-scoliotic type of EDS (type VI) is caused by homozygous or compound heterozygous mutations in the *PLOD1* gene, which encodes procollagen-lysine 5-dioxygenase (lysyl hydroxylase 1), an enzyme required for formation of stable cross-links in collagen fibers.

Some patients with the hypermobile EDS (type III) and a few with mild EDS (type II) have mutations in the *TNXB* gene, which encodes tenascin X, another minor component of connective tissue that appears to regulate the assembly of collagen fibers. Mutations in proteoglycans have been found in a few patients. The progeroid form of EDS results from autosomal recessive mutations in *B4GALT7*, the gene for β-1,4-galactosyltransferase 7, a key enzyme in the addition of glycosaminoglycan chains to proteoglycans.

Diagnosis The diagnosis is based on clinical criteria and increasingly on DNA sequencing. Correlations between genotype and phenotype can be challenging, but gene or biochemical tests are particularly useful for the diagnosis of vascular type IV EDS with its dire prognosis.

As with other heritable diseases of connective tissue, there is a large degree of variability among members of the same family carrying the same mutation. Some patients have increased fractures and are difficult to distinguish from OI. A few families with heritable aortic aneurysms have mutations in the gene for type III collagen without any evidence of EDS or OI.

TREATMENT EHLERS-DANLOS SYNDROME

Surgical repair and tightening of joint ligaments require careful evaluation of individual patients, as the ligaments frequently do not hold sutures. Patients with easy bruisability should be evaluated for bleeding disorders. Patients with type IV EDS and members of their families should be evaluated at regular intervals for early detection of aneurysms, but surgical repair may be difficult because of friable tissues. Also, women with type IV EDS should be counseled about the increased risk of uterine rupture, bleeding, and other complications of pregnancy.

CHONDRODYSPLASIAS

(See also Chap. 426e) Chondrodysplasias (CDs), also referred to as skeletal dysplasias, are heritable skeletal disorders that are characterized by dwarfism and abnormal body proportions. The category also includes some individuals with normal stature and body proportions who have features such as ocular changes or cleft palate, which are common in more severe CDs. Many patients develop degenerative joint changes, and mild CD in adults may be difficult to differentiate from primary generalized osteoarthritis. An undefined number of patients have mutations in either the most abundant collagen in cartilage (type II) or the less abundant collagens (types X or XI). Other patients have mutations in genes that code for other components of cartilage or for proteins required for the embryonic development of cartilage, including a common mutation in a gene for a fibroblast growth factor receptor.

Classification Over 200 distinct types and subtypes have been defined based on criteria such as "bringing death" (thanatophoric), causing "twisted" bones (diastrophic), affecting metaphyses (metaphyseal), affecting epiphyses (epiphyseal), affecting spine (spondylo-), and producing histologic changes such as an apparent increase in the fibrous material in the epiphyses (fibrochondrogenesis). Also, a number of eponyms are based on the first or most comprehensive case reports. Severe forms of the diseases produce dwarfism with gross distortions of most cartilaginous structures and of other structures including the eye. Mild forms are more difficult to classify. Among the features are cataracts, degeneration of the vitreous, retinal detachment, high forehead hypoplastic facies, cleft palate, short extremities, and gross distortions of the epiphyses, metaphyses, and joint surfaces. Patients with Stickler's syndrome (hereditary arthro-ophthalmopathy) have been classified into three types based on a combination of the ocular phenotype and mutated genes.

INCIDENCE

The overall incidence of all forms of CD ranges from 1 per 2500 to 1 per 4000 births. Data on the frequency of individual CDs are incomplete, but the incidence of Stickler's syndrome is 1 in 10,000. Therefore, the disease is probably among the more common heritable disorders of connective tissue.

Molecular Defects Mutations in the *COL2A1* gene for the type II collagen of cartilage are found in a fraction of patients with both mild and severe CDs. For example, a mutation in the gene substituting a cysteine residue for an arginine was found in three unrelated families with spondyloepiphyseal dysplasia (SED) and precocious generalized osteoarthritis (OA). Mutations in the gene, often glycine substitution mutations with the collagen II triple helix, were also found in some lethal CDs characterized by gross deformities of bones and cartilage, such as those found in spondyloepiphyseal dysplasia congenita, spondyloepimetaphyseal dysplasia congenita, hypochondrogenesis/achondrogenesis type II, and Kniest's syndrome. The highest incidence of *COL2A1* mutations, however, occurs in patients with the distinctive features of Stickler's syndrome, which is characterized by skeletal changes, orofacial abnormalities, and auditory abnormalities. Most of the mutations in *COL2A1* are premature stop codons that produce haploinsufficiency. In addition, some patients with Stickler's syndrome or a closely related syndrome have mutations in two genes specific for type XI collagen, which is an unusual heterotrimer formed from α chains encoded by the gene for type II collagen (*COL2A1*) and two distinctive genes for type XI collagen (*COL11A1* and *COL11A2*). Mutations in the *COL11A1* gene are also found in patients with Marshall's syndrome, which is similar to classic Stickler's syndrome, but with more severe hearing loss and dysmorphic features, such as a flat or retracted midface with a flat nasal bridge, short nose, anteverted nostrils, long philtrum, and large-appearing eyes.

CDs are also caused by mutations in the less abundant collagens found in cartilage. For example, patients with Schmid metaphyseal CD have mutations in the gene for type X collagen, a short, network-forming collagen found in the hypertrophic zone of endochondral cartilage. The syndrome is characterized by short stature, coxa vara, flaring metaphyses, and waddling gait. As with other collagen genes, the most common mutations are of two types: nonsense mutations that lead to haploinsufficiency and structural mutations that compromise collagen assembly. In type X collagen, all the structural mutations detected occur in the C-terminal NC1 domain that coordinates the formation of the trimers. This NC1 domain is functionally equivalent to the C-propeptide of the fibrillar collagens. These mutations disturb the structure of the NC1 domain, leading to misfolding and initiation of cellular ER stress via the unfolded protein response (UPR). While the UPR evolved to allow cells to adjust their ER folding capacity to differing protein folding loads, it is deployed by cells when mutant misfolded proteins accumulate in the ER. Activation of the UPR attenuates protein translation and activates mutant protein degradation pathways such as ER-associated degradation. If these strategies do not sufficiently reduce the stress response, cell death may occur. In Schmid metaphyseal CD, mutant misfolded type X collagen induces the UPR, resulting in downstream consequences that contribute to the pathophysiology. This general mechanism may also contribute to pathology in other CDs (and in other connective tissues disorders) where gene mutations lead to protein structural abnormalities.

Some patients have mutations in genes for proteins that interact with collagens. Patients with pseudoachondroplasia or autosomal dominant multiple epiphyseal dysplasia have mutations in the gene for the cartilage oligomeric matrix protein (*COMP*), a protein that interacts with both collagens and proteoglycans in cartilage. However, some families with multiple epiphyseal dysplasia have a defect in one of the three genes for type IX collagen (*COL9A1*, *COL9A2*, and *COL9A3*) or in matrilin-3, another extracellular protein found in cartilage. With misfolding mutations in *COMP* and matrilin-3, the activation of the UPR has been described, providing further evidence that the UPR is a component of pathology of these conditions.

Some CDs are caused by mutations in genes that affect early development of cartilage and related structures. The most common form of short-limbed dwarfism, achondroplasia, is caused by mutations in the gene for a receptor for a fibroblastic growth factor (*FGFR3*). The mutations in the *FGFR3* gene causing achondroplasias are unusual in several respects. The same single-base mutation in the gene that converts glycine to arginine at position 380 in the *FGFR3* gene is present in over 90% of patients. Most patients harbor sporadic new mutations, and therefore, this nucleotide change must be one of the most common recurring mutations in the human genome. The mutation causes unregulated signal transduction through the receptor and inappropriate development of cartilage. Mutations that alter other domains of *FGFR3* have been found in patients with the more severe disorders of hypochondroplasia and thanatophoric dysplasia and in a few families with a variant of craniosynostosis. However, most patients with craniosynostosis appear to have mutations in the related *FGFR2* gene. The similarities between the phenotypes produced by mutations in genes for FGF receptors and mutations in structural proteins of cartilage are probably explained by the observation that the activity of FGFs is regulated in part by binding of FGFs to proteins sequestered in the extracellular matrix. Therefore, the situation parallels the interactions between transforming growth factors (TGFs) and fibrillin in MFS (see below).

Other mutations involve the proteoglycans of cartilage, aggrecan (*AGC1*), and perlecan (*HSPG2*) and the proteoglycan posttranslational sulphation pathway (DTDST, *PAPSS2*, and *CHST3*). Mutations in more than 45 other genes have been defined in chondrodysplasias.

Diagnosis The diagnosis of CDs is made on the basis of the physical appearance, slit-lamp eye examinations, x-ray findings, histologic changes, and clinical course. Evaluation of patients by specialists in the field is usually required for a diagnosis. Targeted gene and exome sequencing or more global sequencing strategies are used for molecular diagnosis. Given the wide spectrum of CD phenotypes, these gene tests are becoming critical diagnostic tools. For Stickler's syndrome, more precise diagnostic criteria have made it possible to identify type I variants with mutations in the *COL2A1* gene with a high degree of accuracy. It has been suggested that the type II variant with mutations in the *COL11A1* gene can be identified on the basis of a "beaded" vitreous phenotype, and the type III variant with mutations in the *COL11A2* gene can be identified on the basis of the characteristic systemic features without the ocular involvement. Prenatal diagnosis based on analysis of DNA obtained from chorionic villus or amniotic fluid is possible.

TREATMENT CHONDRODYSPLASIAS

The treatment is symptomatic and is directed to secondary features such as degenerative arthritis. Many patients require joint replacement surgery and corrective surgery for cleft palate. The eyes should be monitored carefully for the development of cataracts and the need for laser therapy to prevent retinal detachment. In general, patients should be advised to avoid obesity and contact sports. Counseling for the psychological problems of short stature is critical, and support groups have formed in many countries.

MARFAN'S SYNDROME (MFS)

MFS includes features that primarily affect the skeleton, the cardiovascular system, and the eyes. Most patients have mutations in the gene for fibrillin-1.

Classification MFS was initially characterized by a triad of features: (1) skeletal changes that include long, thin extremities, frequently associated with loose joints; (2) reduced vision as the result of dislocations of the lenses (ectopia lentis); and (3) aortic aneurysms. An international panel has developed a series of revised "Ghent criteria" that are useful in classifying patients.

Incidence and Inheritance The incidence of MFS is among the highest of any heritable disorder: about 1 in 3000/5000 births in most racial and ethnic groups. The related syndromes are less common. Mutations are generally inherited as autosomal dominant traits, but about one-fourth of patients have sporadic new mutations.

Skeletal Effects Patients have long limbs and are usually tall compared to other members of the same family. The ratio of the upper segment (top of the head to the top of the pubic ramus) to the lower segment (top of the pubic ramus to the floor) is usually two standard deviations below mean for age, race, and sex. The fingers and hands are long and slender and have a spider-like appearance (arachnodactyly). Many patients have severe chest deformities, including depression (pectus excavatum), protrusion (pectus carinatum), or asymmetry. Scoliosis is frequent and usually accompanied by kyphosis. High-arched palate and high pedal arches or pes planus are common. A few patients have severe joint hypermobility similar to EDS. Computed tomography or magnetic resonance imaging examinations of the lumbar sacral region frequently reveal enlargement of the neural canal, thinning of the pedicles and laminae, widening of the foramina, or anterior meningocele (dural ectasia).

Cardiovascular Features Cardiovascular abnormalities are the major source of morbidity and mortality (Chap. 301). Mitral valve prolapse develops early in life and progresses to mitral valve regurgitation of increasing severity in about one-quarter of patients. Dilation of the root of the aorta and the sinuses of Valsalva are characteristic and ominous features of the disease that can develop at any age. The rate of dilation is unpredictable, but it can lead to aortic regurgitation, dissection of the aorta, and rupture. Dilation is probably accelerated by physical and emotional stress, as well as by pregnancy. Patients usually differ from those with familial aortic aneurysms who tend to develop aneurysms in the abdominal aorta. The location of the aneurysms, however, is somewhat variable, and the high incidence of aortic aneurysms in the general population (1 in 100) makes the differential diagnosis difficult unless other features of MFS are clearly present.

Ocular Features Upward displacement of the lens is common. It is usually not progressive but may contribute to the formation of cataracts. The ocular globe is frequently elongated, and most patients are myopic, but with adequate vision. Retinal detachment can occur.

Other Features Striae may occur over the shoulders and buttocks. A number of patients develop spontaneous pneumothorax. Inguinal and incisional hernias are common. Patients are typically thin with little subcutaneous fat, but adults may develop centripetal obesity.

Molecular Defects More than 90% of patients clinically classified as having MFS by the "Ghent criteria" have a mutation in the gene for fibrillin-1 (*FBN1*). Mutations in the same gene are found in a few patients who do not meet the Ghent criteria. Also, a few MFS patients without mutations in the *FBN1* gene have mutations in the gene for TGF-β receptor 2 (*TGFBR2*). In addition, mutations in either *TGFBR2* or *TGFBR1* are found in the related Loeys-Dietz syndrome, which is characterized by aortic aneurysms, cleft palate, and hypertelorism. Mutations in the *FBN2* gene, which is structurally similar to the *FBN1* gene, are found in patients with MFS-like syndrome of congenital contractual arachnodactyly.

FBN1 gene mutations are scattered throughout its 65 coding exons. Most are private mutations, but about 10% are recurrent new mutations that are largely located in CpG sequences known to be "hot spots." Most severe mutations are located in the central codons (24–32). About one-third of the mutations introduce premature termination codons, and about two-thirds are missense mutations that alter calcium-binding domains in the repetitive epidermal growth factor–like domains of the protein. Rarer mutations alter the processing of the protein. As in many genetic diseases, the severity of the phenotype cannot be predicted from the nature of the mutation.

The discovery that syndromes similar to MFS are caused by mutations in *TGFBR1* and *TGFBR2* refocused attention on structural similarity between fibrillin-1 and TGF-β binding proteins that sequester TGF-β in the extracellular matrix. As a result, some of the manifestations of MFS have been shown to arise from alterations in binding sites that modulate TGF-β bioavailability during development of the skeleton and other tissues. Likewise, *TGFBR1* and *TGFBR2* mutations in Loeys-Dietz syndrome alter TGF-β signaling. In both MFS and Loeys-Dietz syndrome, the pathogenic mechanisms involve increased TGF-β signaling, which contributes to aneurysm formation.

Diagnosis All patients with a suspected diagnosis of MFS should have a slit-lamp examination and an echocardiogram. Also, homocystinuria should be ruled out by amino acid analysis of plasma (Chap. 434e). The diagnosis of MFS according to the international Ghent standards places emphasis on major criteria that include presence of at least four skeletal abnormalities: ectopia lentis; dilation of the ascending aorta with or without dissection; dural ectasia; and a blood relative who meets the same criteria, with or without a DNA diagnosis. A final diagnosis is based on a balanced assessment of the major criteria together with several minor criteria. The absence of ocular changes suggests the Loeys-Dietz syndrome, and the presence of contractures with some of the signs of OI suggests congenital contractual arachnodactyly.

Diagnostic tests based on gene sequencing or detection of protein defects are available. These results are unlikely to alter the treatment or prognosis but are helpful to inform the patients and families and to rapidly exclude the diagnosis in unaffected family members.

TREATMENT MARFAN'S SYNDROME

Propranolol or other β-adrenergic blocking agents are used to lower blood pressure and thereby delay or prevent aortic dilation. Surgical correction of the aorta, aortic valve, and mitral valve has been successful in many patients, but tissues are frequently friable. Patients should be advised that the risks are increased by severe physical exertion, emotional stress, and pregnancy.

The scoliosis tends to be progressive and should be treated by mechanical bracing and physical therapy if >20° or by surgery if it progresses to >45°. Dislocated lenses rarely require surgical removal, but patients should be followed closely for retinal detachment. The finding that MFS pathophysiology involves alterations in TGF-β signaling has raised the possibility of new therapeutic strategies. Attenuation of TGF-β signaling with agents such as angiotensin II receptor blockers (e.g., losartan) was effective in animal studies and has been very promising in small observational studies on MFS patients, significantly reducing progressive aortic enlargement. Based on these results, large randomized clinical trials of angiotensin receptor blockers in MFS are under way.

ELASTIN-RELATED DISEASES

Mutations in the elastin gene (*ELN*) have been found in patients with supravalvular aortic stenosis and skin that hangs in loose and redundant folds (cutis laxa). As indicated in Table 427-3, patients with several forms of EDS have similar changes in skin that were initially thought to reflect changes in elastin.

EPIDERMOLYSIS BULLOSA (EB)

EB has been defined as the category of heritable disorders involving skin that is specifically characterized by blistering as a result of friction. Using this criterion, it was possible to define subtypes by the ultrastructural layer of skin in which the cleavage and blistering occurred. These functional and anatomical criteria made it possible to establish that most patients with a specific subtype have mutations in genes coding for a structural protein, or a cell adherence protein, expressed in the corresponding layer of skin.

Classification and Incidence The four major types of EB are: (1) EB simplex in which cleavage occurs within the epidermis, (2) junctional EB in which cleavage occurs within the lamina lucida, (3) dystrophic EB in which cleavage occurs within the sublamina densa, and (4) Kindler's syndrome with a mixed level of cleavage in different layers. Patients are then separated into major and minor subtypes based on clinical features and analysis of mutations.

The incidence of EB in the United States is about 1 in 50,000.

Molecular Defects The distinctive anatomic locations in skin have made it possible to relate the clinical subtypes of EB to mutations for specific components. In EB simplex, mutations are found primarily in the genes for the major keratins of basal epithelial cells (keratins 5 and 14) and the cell adhesion proteins plectin, α6β4 integrin, plakophilin-1, and desmoplakin. Patients with the related syndrome, epidermolytic ichthyosis, have mutations in keratin 1 and keratin 10. In junctional EB, mutations occur in type XVII collagen, a laminin (laminin-332), and α6β4 integrin. In the severe syndrome of dystrophic EB, mutations are found in the gene that codes for type VII collagen, which forms long loops anchoring the epidermis to the dermis. Patients with more complex features of what is classified as Kindler's syndrome have mutations in kindlin-1, a focal adhesion protein involved in integrin activation.

Diagnosis and Treatment The diagnosis is based on skin that readily breaks and forms blisters from minor trauma. EB simplex is generally milder than junctional EB or dystrophic EB. Dystrophic EB variants usually have large and prominent scars. Precise classification within subtypes usually requires immunofluorescent mapping. DNA diagnostic tests have been developed as research tools but are not widely available. The treatment is symptomatic. Novel therapeutic approaches such as gene therapy, protein replacement therapy, and cell therapy are being explored.

ALPORT'S SYNDROME (AS)

AS is an inherited disorder characterized by hematuria and several associated features. It was not initially considered as a disorder of connective tissue. However, the search for mutations in the genes coding for the collagen found that most patients had mutations in collagen found in basement membranes (type IV). Four forms of AS are now recognized: (1) classic AS, which is inherited as an X-linked disorder with hematuria, sensorineural deafness, and conical deformation of the anterior surface of the lens (lenticonus); (2) an X-linked form associated with diffuse leiomyomatosis; (3) an autosomal recessive form; and (4) an autosomal dominant form. Both autosomal recessive and dominant forms can cause renal disease without deafness or lenticonus.

Incidence The incidence of AS is about 1 in 10,000 births in the general population and as high as 1 in 5000 in some ethnic groups. About 80% of AS patients have the classical X-linked variant.

Molecular Defects Most patients have mutations in four of the six genes for the chains of type IV collagen (*COL4A3*, *COL4A4*, *COL4A5*, and *COL4A6*). The genes for the proteins are arranged in tandem pairs on different chromosomes in an unusual head-to-head orientation and with overlapping promoters; i.e., the *COL4A1* and *COL4A2* genes are head-to-head on chromosome 13q34, the *COL4A3* and *COL4A4* genes are on chromosome 2q35–37, and the *COL4A5* and *COL4A6* genes are on chromosome Xq22. The X-linked variants are caused by either mutations in the *COL4A5* gene or by partial deletions of both of the adjacent *COL4A4* and *COL4A5* genes. The autosomal recessive variants are caused by mutations in either the *COL4A3* or *COL4A4* gene. The mutations responsible for the autosomal dominant variants are still unknown, but they have been mapped to the same locus as the *COL4A3* and *COL4A4* genes.

Diagnosis The diagnosis of classic AS is based on X-linked inheritance of hematuria, sensorineural deafness, and lenticonus. The lenticonus together with hematuria is pathognomonic of classic AS. The sensorineural deafness is primarily in the high-tone range. It can frequently be detected only by an audiogram and is usually not progressive. Because of the X-linked transmission, women are generally underdiagnosed and are usually less severely affected than men. The hematuria usually progresses to nephritis and may cause renal failure in late adolescence in affected males and at older ages in some women. Renal transplantation is usually successful.

ACKNOWLEDGMENTS

The authors acknowledge the contributions of Helena Kuivaniemi, Gerard Tromp, Leena Ala-Kokko, and Malwina Czarny-Ratajcak to this chapter in previous editions of Harrison's. The authors also wish to thank David Sillence for his expert advice on the classifications of types of OI.

428 Hemochromatosis

Lawrie W. Powell

DEFINITION

Hemochromatosis is a common inherited disorder of iron metabolism in which dysregulation of intestinal iron absorption results in deposition of excessive amounts of iron in parenchymal cells with eventual tissue damage and impaired function in a wide range of organs. The iron-storage pigment in tissues is called *hemosiderin* because it was believed to be derived from the blood. The term *hemosiderosis* is used to describe the presence of stainable iron in tissues, but tissue iron must be quantified to assess body-iron status accurately (see below and Chap. 126). *Hemochromatosis* refers to a group of genetic diseases that predispose to iron overload, potentially leading to fibrosis and organ failure. Cirrhosis of the liver, diabetes mellitus, arthritis, cardiomyopathy, and hypogonadotropic hypogonadism are the major clinical manifestations.

Although there is debate about definitions, the following terminology is widely accepted.

1. *Hereditary hemochromatosis* is most often caused by a mutant gene, termed *HFE*, which is tightly linked to the HLA-A locus on chromosome 6p (see "Genetic Basis," below). Persons who are homozygous for the mutation are at increased risk of iron overload and account for 80–90% of clinical hereditary hemochromatosis in persons of northern European descent. In such subjects, the presence of hepatic fibrosis, cirrhosis, arthropathy, or hepatocellular carcinoma constitutes iron overload–related disease. Rarer forms of non-*HFE* hemochromatosis are caused by mutations in other genes involved in iron metabolism (Table 428-1). The disease can be recognized during its early stages when iron overload and organ damage are minimal. At this stage, the disease is best referred to as *early hemochromatosis* or *precirrhotic hemochromatosis*.
2. *Secondary iron overload* occurs as a result of an iron-loading anemia, such as thalassemia or sideroblastic anemia, in which erythropoiesis is increased but ineffective. In the acquired iron-loading disorders, massive iron deposits in parenchymal tissues can lead to the same clinical and pathologic features as in hemochromatosis.

TABLE 428-1 CLASSIFICATION OF IRON OVERLOAD STATES

Hereditary Hemochromatosis	
Hemochromatosis, *HFE*-related (type 1)	
C282Y homozygosity	
C282Y/H63D compound heterozygosity	
Hemochromatosis, non-*HFE*-related	
Juvenile hemochromatosis (type 2A) (hemojuvelin mutations)	
Juvenile hemochromatosis (type 2B) (hepcidin mutation)	
Mutated transferrin receptor 2, *TFR2* (type 3)	
Mutated ferroportin 1 gene, *SLC11A3* (type 4)	
Acquired Iron Overload	
Iron-loading anemias	Chronic liver disease
Thalassemia major	Hepatitis C
Sideroblastic anemia	Alcoholic cirrhosis, especially when advanced
Chronic hemolytic anemias	Nonalcoholic steatohepatitis
Transfusional and parenteral iron overload	Porphyria cutanea tarda
Dietary iron overload	Dysmetabolic iron overload syndrome
	Post-portacaval shunting
Miscellaneous	
Iron overload in sub-Saharan Africa	
Neonatal iron overload	
Aceruloplasminemia	
Congenital atransferrinemia	

PREVALENCE

HFE-associated hemochromatosis mutations are among the most common inherited disease alleles, although the prevalence varies in different ethnic groups. It is most common in populations of northern European extraction in whom approximately 1 in 10 persons are heterozygous carriers and 0.3–0.5% are homozygotes. However, expression of the disease is variable and modified by several factors, especially alcohol consumption and dietary iron intake, blood loss associated with menstruation and pregnancy, and blood donation. Recent population studies indicate that approximately 30% of homozygous men develop iron overload–related disease and about 6% develop hepatic cirrhosis; for women, the figure is closer to 1%. Presumably there are as yet unidentified modifying genes responsible for expression and there is some early evidence to support this. Nearly 70% of untreated patients develop the first symptoms between ages 40 and 60. The disease is rarely evident before age 20, although with family screening (see "Screening for Hemochromatosis," below) and periodic health examinations, asymptomatic subjects with iron overload can be identified, including young menstruating women.

In contrast to *HFE*-associated hemochromatosis, the non-*HFE*-associated forms of hemochromatosis (Table 428-1) are rare, but they affect all races and young people (juvenile hemochromatosis).

GENETIC BASIS

A homozygous G to A mutation in the *HFE* gene resulting in a cysteine to tyrosine substitution at position 282 (C282Y) is the most common mutation. It is identified in 85–90% of patients with hereditary hemochromatosis in populations of northern European descent but is found in only 60% of cases from Mediterranean populations (e.g., southern Italy). A second, relatively common *HFE* mutation (H63D) results in a substitution of histidine to aspartic acid at codon 63. Homozygosity for H63D is not associated with clinically significant iron overload. Some compound heterozygotes (e.g., one copy each of C282Y and H63D) have mild to moderately increased body-iron stores but develop clinical disease only in association with cofactors such as heavy alcohol intake or hepatic steatosis. Thus, *HFE*-associated hemochromatosis is inherited as an autosomal recessive trait; heterozygotes have no, or minimal, increase in iron stores. However, this slight increase in hepatic iron can act as a cofactor that may modify the expression of other diseases such as porphyria cutanea tarda (PCT) or nonalcoholic steatohepatitis.

Mutations in other genes involved in iron metabolism are responsible for non-*HFE*-associated hemochromatosis, including juvenile hemochromatosis, which affects persons in the second and third decades of life (Table 428-1). Mutations in the genes encoding hepcidin, transferrin receptor 2 (TfR2), and hemojuvelin (Fig. 428-1) result in clinicopathologic features that are indistinguishable from HFE-associated hemochromatosis. However, mutations in ferroportin, responsible for the efflux of iron from enterocytes and most other cell types, result in iron loading of reticuloendothelial cells and macrophages as well as parenchymal cells.

PATHOPHYSIOLOGY

Normally, the body-iron content of 3–4 g is maintained such that intestinal mucosal absorption of iron is equal to iron loss. This amount is approximately 1 mg/d in men and 1.5 mg/d in menstruating women. In hemochromatosis, mucosal absorption is greater than body requirements and amounts to 4 mg/d or more. The progressive accumulation of iron increases plasma iron and saturation of transferrin and results in a progressive increase of plasma ferritin (Fig. 428-2). A liver-derived peptide, hepcidin, represses basolateral iron transport in the intestine and iron release from macrophages and other cells by binding to ferroportin. Hepcidin, in turn, responds to signals in the liver mediated by HFE, TfR2, and hemojuvelin (Fig. 428-1). Thus, hepcidin is a crucial molecule in iron metabolism, linking body stores with intestinal iron absorption.

The *HFE* gene encodes a 343-amino-acid protein that is structurally related to MHC class I proteins (HFE). The basic defect in *HFE*-associated hemochromatosis is a lack of cell surface expression of HFE (due to the C282Y mutation). The normal (wild-type) HFE protein forms a complex with β_2-microglobulin and transferrin receptor 1 (TfR1). The C282Y mutation completely abrogates this interaction. As a result, the mutant HFE protein remains trapped intracellularly, reducing TfR1-mediated iron uptake by the intestinal crypt cell. This impaired TfR1-mediated iron uptake leads to upregulation of the divalent metal transporter (DMT1) on the brush border of the villus cells, causing inappropriately increased intestinal iron absorption (Fig. 428-1). In advanced disease, the body may contain 20 g or more of iron that is deposited mainly in parenchymal cells of the liver, pancreas, and heart. Iron may be increased 50- to 100-fold in the liver and pancreas

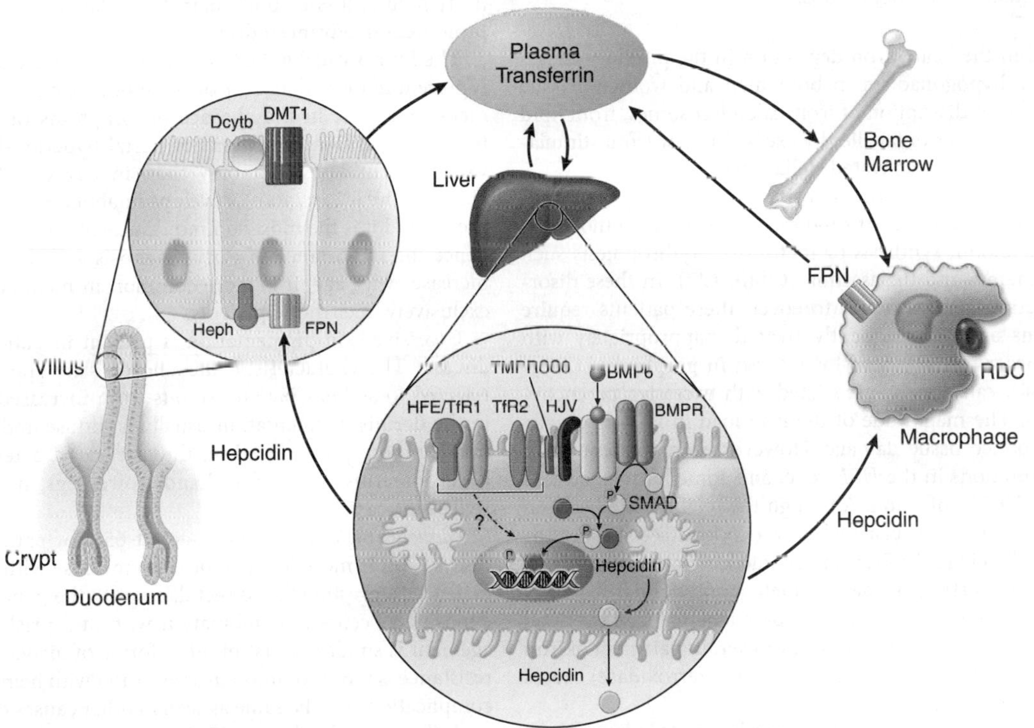

FIGURE 428-1 Pathways of normal iron homeostasis. Dietary inorganic iron traverses the brush border membrane of duodenal enterocytes via the divalent metal-ion transporter 1 (DMT1) after reduction of ferric (Fe^{3+}) iron to the ferrous (Fe^{2+}) state by duodenal cytochrome B (DcytB). Iron then moves from the enterocyte to the circulation via a process requiring the basolateral iron exporter ferroportin (FPN) and the iron oxidase hephaestin (Heph). In the circulation, iron binds to plasma transferrin and is thereby distributed to sites of iron utilization and storage. Much of the diferric transferrin supplies iron to immature erythrocyte cells in the bone marrow for hemoglobin synthesis. At the end of their life, senescent red blood cells (RBCs) are phagocytosed by macrophages, and iron is returned to the circulation after export through ferroportin. The liver-derived peptide hepcidin represses basolateral iron transport in the gut as well as iron released from macrophages and other cells and serves as a central regulator of body-iron traffic. Hepcidin responds to changes in body-iron requirements by signals mediated by diferric transferrin through two mechanisms. One involves HFE and TfR2, whereas the other involves hemojuvelin (HJV) and the bone morphogenetic protein (BMP)/SMAD pathway. TMPRSS6 is a protease that modulates HJV activity. Heme is metabolized by heme oxygenase within the enterocytes, and the released iron then follows the same pathway. Mutations in the genes encoding HFE, TfR2, hemojuvelin, and hepcidin all lead to decreased hepcidin release and increased iron absorption, resulting in hemochromatosis (Table 428-1).

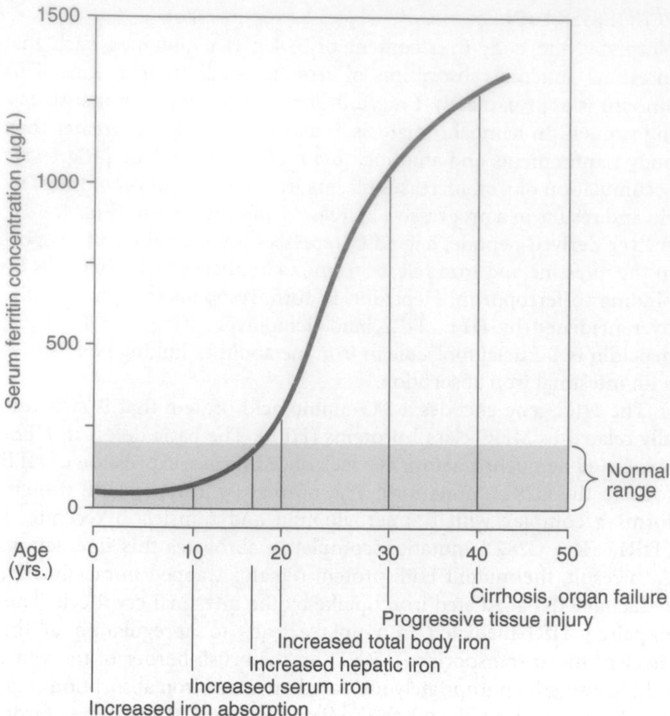

FIGURE 428-2 Sequence of events in genetic hemochromatosis and their correlation with the serum ferritin concentration. Increased iron absorption is present throughout life. Overt, symptomatic disease usually develops between ages 40 and 60, but latent disease can be detected long before this.

and 5- to 25-fold in the heart. Iron deposition in the pituitary causes hypogonadotropic hypogonadism in both men and women. Tissue injury may result from disruption of iron-laden lysosomes, from lipid peroxidation of subcellular organelles by excess iron, or from stimulation of collagen synthesis by activated stellate cells.

Secondary iron overload with deposition in parenchymal cells occurs in chronic disorders of erythropoiesis, particularly in those due to defects in hemoglobin synthesis or ineffective erythropoiesis such as sideroblastic anemia and thalassemia (Chap. 127). In these disorders, iron absorption is increased. Moreover, these patients require blood transfusions and are frequently treated inappropriately with iron. PCT, a disorder characterized by a defect in porphyrin biosynthesis (Chap. 430), can also be associated with excessive parenchymal iron deposits. The magnitude of the iron load in PCT is usually insufficient to produce tissue damage. However, some patients with PCT also have mutations in the *HFE* gene, and some have associated hepatitis C virus (HCV) infection. Although the relationship between these disorders remains to be clarified, iron overload accentuates the inherited enzyme deficiency in PCT and should be avoided along with other agents (alcohol, estrogens, haloaromatic compounds) that may exacerbate PCT. Another cause of hepatic parenchymal iron overload is hereditary aceruloplasminemia. In this disorder, impairment of iron mobilization due to deficiency of ceruloplasmin (a ferroxidase) causes iron overload in hepatocytes.

Excessive iron ingestion over many years rarely results in hemochromatosis. An important exception has been reported in South Africa among groups who brew fermented beverages in vessels made of iron. Hemochromatosis has been described in apparently normal persons who have taken medicinal iron over many years, but such individuals probably had genetic disorders.

The common denominator in all patients with hemochromatosis is *excessive amounts of iron in parenchymal tissues*. Parenteral administration of iron in the form of blood transfusions or iron preparations results predominantly in reticuloendothelial cell iron overload. This appears to lead to less tissue damage than iron loading of parenchymal cells.

In the liver, parenchymal iron is in the form of ferritin and hemosiderin. In the early stages, these deposits are seen in the periportal parenchymal cells, especially within lysosomes in the pericanalicular cytoplasm of the hepatocytes. This stage progresses to perilobular fibrosis and eventually to deposition of iron in bile-duct epithelium, Kupffer cells, and fibrous septa due to activation of stellate cells. In the advanced stage, a macronodular or mixed macro- and micronodular cirrhosis develops. Hepatic fibrosis and cirrhosis correlate significantly with hepatic iron concentration.

At autopsy, the enlarged nodular liver and pancreas are rusty in color. Histologically, iron is increased in many organs, particularly in the liver, heart, and pancreas, and, to a lesser extent, in the endocrine glands. The epidermis of the skin is thin, and melanin is increased in the cells of the basal layer and dermis. Deposits of iron are present around the synovial lining cells of the joints.

CLINICAL MANIFESTATIONS

C282Y homozygotes can be characterized by the stage of progression as follows: (1) a genetic predisposition without abnormalities; (2) iron overload without symptoms; (3) iron overload with symptoms (e.g., arthritis and fatigue); and (4) iron overload with organ damage—in particular, cirrhosis. Thus, many subjects with significant iron overload are asymptomatic. For example, in a study of 672 asymptomatic C282Y homozygous subjects—identified by either family screening or routine health examinations—there was hepatic iron overload (grades 2–4) in 56% and 34.5% of male and female subjects, respectively; hepatic fibrosis (stages 2–4) in 18.4% and 5.4%, respectively; and cirrhosis in 5.6% and 1.9%, respectively.

Initial symptoms are often nonspecific and include lethargy, arthralgia, change in skin color, loss of libido, and features of diabetes mellitus. Hepatomegaly, increased pigmentation, spider angiomas, splenomegaly, arthropathy, ascites, cardiac arrhythmias, congestive heart failure, loss of body hair, testicular atrophy, and jaundice are prominent in advanced disease.

The *liver* is usually the first organ to be affected, and hepatomegaly is present in more than 95% of symptomatic patients. Hepatic enlargement may exist in the absence of symptoms or of abnormal liver-function tests. Manifestations of portal hypertension and esophageal varices occur less commonly than in cirrhosis from other causes. Hepatocellular carcinoma develops in about 30% of patients with cirrhosis, and it is the most common cause of death in treated patients—hence the importance of early diagnosis and therapy. The incidence increases with age, it is more common in men, and it occurs almost exclusively in cirrhotic patients.

Excessive skin pigmentation is present in patients with advanced disease. The characteristic metallic or slate-gray hue is sometimes referred to as *bronzing* and results from increased melanin and iron in the dermis. Pigmentation usually is diffuse and generalized, but it may be more pronounced on the face, neck, extensor aspects of the lower forearms, dorsa of the hands, lower legs, and genital regions, as well as in scars.

Diabetes mellitus occurs in about 65% of patients with advanced disease and is more likely to develop in those with a family history of diabetes, suggesting that direct damage to the pancreatic islets by iron deposition occurs in combination with other risk factors. The management is similar to that of other forms of diabetes, although insulin resistance is more common in association with hemochromatosis. Late complications are the same as seen in other causes of diabetes mellitus.

Arthropathy develops in 25–50% of symptomatic patients. It usually occurs after age 50 but may occur as a first manifestation or long after therapy. The joints of the hands, especially the second and third metacarpophalangeal joints, are usually the first joints involved, a feature that helps to distinguish the chondrocalcinosis associated with hemochromatosis from the idiopathic form (Chap. 395). A progressive polyarthritis involving wrists, hips, ankles, and knees may also ensue. Acute brief attacks of synovitis may be associated with deposition of calcium pyrophosphate (chondrocalcinosis or pseudogout), mainly in the knees. Radiologic manifestations include cystic changes of the subchondral bones, loss of articular cartilage with narrowing of the joint space, diffuse demineralization, hypertrophic bone proliferation, and calcification of the synovium. The arthropathy tends to progress despite removal of iron by phlebotomy. Although the relation of these abnormalities to iron metabolism is not known, the fact that similar changes occur in other forms of iron overload suggests that iron is directly involved.

Cardiac involvement is the presenting manifestation in about 15% of symptomatic patients. The most common manifestation is congestive heart failure, which occurs in about 10% of young adults with the disease, especially those with juvenile hemochromatosis. Symptoms of congestive heart failure may develop suddenly, with rapid progression to death if untreated. The heart is diffusely enlarged; this may be misdiagnosed as idiopathic cardiomyopathy if other overt manifestations are absent. Cardiac arrhythmias include premature supraventricular beats, paroxysmal tachyarrhythmias, atrial flutter, atrial fibrillation, and varying degrees of atrioventricular block.

Hypogonadism occurs in both sexes and may antedate other clinical features. Manifestations include loss of libido, impotence, amenorrhea, testicular atrophy, gynecomastia, and sparse body hair. These changes are primarily the result of decreased production of gonadotropins due to impairment of hypothalamic-pituitary function by iron deposition. Adrenal insufficiency, hypothyroidism, and hypoparathyroidism are rare manifestations.

DIAGNOSIS

The association of (1) hepatomegaly, (2) skin pigmentation, (3) diabetes mellitus, (4) heart disease, (5) arthritis, and (6) hypogonadism should suggest the diagnosis. However, as stated above, significant iron overload may exist with none or only some of these manifestations. Therefore, a high index of suspicion is needed to make the diagnosis early. Treatment before permanent organ damage occurs can reverse the iron toxicity and restore life expectancy to normal.

The history should be particularly detailed in regard to disease in other family members; alcohol ingestion; iron intake; and ingestion of large doses of ascorbic acid, which promotes iron absorption (Chap. 96e). Appropriate tests should be performed to exclude iron deposition due to hematologic disease. The presence of liver, pancreatic, cardiac, and joint disease should be confirmed by physical examination, radiography, and standard function tests of these organs.

The degree of increase in total body iron stores can be assessed by (1) measurement of serum iron and the percent saturation of transferrin (or the unsaturated iron-binding capacity), (2) measurement of serum ferritin concentration, (3) liver biopsy with measurement of the iron concentration and calculation of the hepatic iron index (Table 428-2), and (4) magnetic resonance imaging (MRI) of the liver. In addition, a retrospective assessment of body-iron storage is also provided by performing weekly phlebotomy and calculating the amount of iron removed before iron stores are exhausted (1 mL blood – approximately 0.5 mg iron).

Each of these methods for assessing iron stores has advantages and limitations. The serum iron level and percent saturation of transferrin are elevated early in the course, but their specificity is reduced by significant false-positive and false-negative rates. For example, serum iron concentration may be increased in patients with alcoholic liver disease without iron overload; in this situation, however, the hepatic iron index is usually not increased as in hemochromatosis (Table 428-1). In otherwise healthy persons, a fasting serum transferrin saturation greater than 45% is abnormal and suggests homozygosity for hemochromatosis.

The serum ferritin concentration is usually a good index of body-iron stores, whether decreased or increased. In fact, an increase of 1 μg/L in serum ferritin level reflects an increase of about 5 mg in body stores. In most untreated patients with hemochromatosis, the serum ferritin level is significantly increased (Fig. 428-2 and Table 428-1), and a serum ferritin level >1000 μg/L is the strongest predictor of disease expression among individuals homozygous for the C282Y mutation. However, in patients with inflammation and hepatocellular necrosis, serum ferritin levels may be elevated out of proportion to body-iron stores due to increased release from tissues. Therefore, a repeat determination of serum ferritin should be carried out after acute hepatocellular damage has subsided (e.g., in alcoholic liver disease). Ordinarily, the combined measurements of the percent transferrin saturation and serum ferritin level provide a simple and reliable screening test for hemochromatosis, including the precirrhotic phase of the disease. If either of these tests is abnormal, genetic testing for hemochromatosis should be performed (Fig. 428-3).

The role of liver biopsy in the diagnosis and management of hemochromatosis has been reassessed as a result of the widespread availability of genetic testing for the C282Y mutation. The absence of severe fibrosis can be accurately predicted in most patients using clinical and biochemical variables. Thus, there is virtually no risk of severe fibrosis in a C282Y homozygous subject with (1) serum ferritin level less than 1000 μg/L, (2) normal serum alanine aminotransferase values, (3) no hepatomegaly, and (4) no excess alcohol intake. However, it should be emphasized that liver biopsy is the only reliable method for establishing or excluding the presence of hepatic cirrhosis, which is the critical factor determining prognosis and the risk of developing hepatocellular carcinoma. Biopsy also permits histochemical estimation of tissue iron and measurement of hepatic iron concentration. Increased density of the liver due to iron deposition can be demonstrated by computed tomography (CT) or MRI, and with improved technology, MRI has become more accurate in determining hepatic iron concentration.

SCREENING FOR HEMOCHROMATOSIS

When the diagnosis of hemochromatosis is established, it is important to counsel and screen other family members (Chap. 84). Asymptomatic and symptomatic family members with the disease usually have an increased saturation of transferrin and an increased serum ferritin concentration. These changes occur even before the iron stores are greatly increased (Fig. 428-2). All adult first-degree relatives of patients with hemochromatosis should be tested for the C282Y and H63D mutations and counseled appropriately (Fig. 428-3). In affected individuals, it is important to confirm or exclude the presence of cirrhosis and begin therapy as early as possible. For children of an identified proband, testing for *HFE* of the other parent is helpful because if

TABLE 428-2 REPRESENTATIVE IRON VALUES IN NORMAL SUBJECTS, PATIENTS WITH HEMOCHROMATOSIS, AND PATIENTS WITH ALCOHOLIC LIVER DISEASE

Determination	Normal	Symptomatic Hemochromatosis	Homozygotes with Early, Asymptomatic Hemochromatosis	Heterozygotes	Alcoholic Liver Disease
Plasma iron, μmol/L (μg/dL)	9–27 (50–150)	32–54 (180–300)	Usually elevated	Elevated or normal	Often elevated
Total iron-binding capacity, μmol/L (μg/dL)	45–66 (250–370)	36–54 (200–300)	36–54 (200–300)	Elevated or normal	45–66 (250–370)
Transferrin saturation, %	22–45	50–100	50–100	Normal or elevated	27–60
Serum ferritin, μg/L		1000–6000	200–500	Usually <500	10–500
Men	20–250				
Women	15–150				
Liver iron, μg/g dry wt	300–1400	6000–18,000	2000–4000	300–3000	300–2000
Hepatic iron index	<1.0	>2	1.5–2	<2	<2

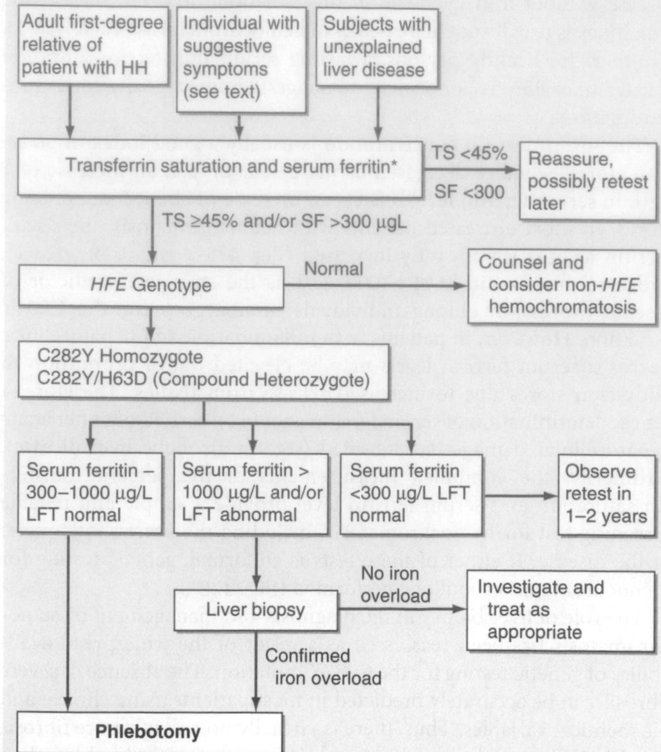

*For convenience both genotype and phenotype (iron tests) can be performed together at a single visit in first-degree relatives.

FIGURE 428-3 Algorithm for screening for *HFE*-associated hemochromatosis. HH, hereditary hemochromatosis, homozygous subject (C282Y +/+); LFT, liver function tests; SF, serum ferritin concentration; TS, transferrin saturation.

normal, the child is merely an obligate heterozygote and at no risk. Otherwise, for practical purposes, children need not be checked before they are 18 years old.

The role of population screening for hemochromatosis is controversial. Recent studies indicate that it is highly effective for primary care physicians to screen subjects using transferrin saturation and serum ferritin levels. Such screening also detects iron deficiency. Genetic screening of the normal population is feasible but is probably not cost effective.

TREATMENT HEMOCHROMATOSIS

The therapy of hemochromatosis involves removal of the excess body iron and supportive treatment of damaged organs. Iron removal is best accomplished by weekly or twice-weekly phlebotomy of 500 mL. Although there is an initial modest decline in the volume of packed red blood cells to about 35 mL/dL, the level stabilizes after several weeks. The plasma transferrin saturation remains increased until the available iron stores are depleted. In contrast, the plasma ferritin concentration falls progressively, reflecting the gradual decrease in body-iron stores. One 500-mL unit of blood contains 200–250 mg of iron, and up to 25 g of iron or more may have to be removed. Therefore, in patients with advanced disease, weekly phlebotomy may be required for 1–2 years, and it should be continued until the serum ferritin level is <50 μg/L. Thereafter, phlebotomies are performed at appropriate intervals to maintain ferritin levels between 50 and 100 μg/L. Usually one phlebotomy every 3 months will suffice.

Chelating agents such as deferoxamine, when given parenterally, remove 10–20 mg of iron per day, which is much less than that mobilized by once-weekly phlebotomy. Phlebotomy is also less expensive, more convenient, and safer for most patients. However, chelating agents are indicated when anemia or hypoproteinemia is severe enough to preclude phlebotomy. Subcutaneous infusion of deferoxamine using a portable pump is the most effective means of its administration.

An effective oral iron chelating agent, deferasirox (Exjade), has recently become available but is still in clinical trials. This agent is effective in thalassemia and secondary iron overload, but its role in primary iron overload has yet to be established.

Alcohol consumption should be severely curtailed or eliminated because it increases the risk of cirrhosis in hereditary hemochromatosis nearly tenfold. Dietary adjustments are unnecessary, although vitamin C and iron supplements should be avoided. The management of hepatic failure, cardiac failure, and diabetes mellitus is similar to conventional therapy for these conditions. Loss of libido and change in secondary sex characteristics are managed with testosterone replacement or gonadotropin therapy (**Chap. 411**).

End-stage liver disease may be an indication for liver transplantation, although results are improved if the excess iron can be removed beforehand. The available evidence indicates that the fundamental metabolic abnormality in hemochromatosis is reversed by successful liver transplantation.

PROGNOSIS

The principal causes of death are cardiac failure, hepatocellular failure or portal hypertension, and hepatocellular carcinoma.

Life expectancy is improved by removal of the excessive stores of iron and maintenance of these stores at near-normal levels. The 5-year survival rate with therapy increases from 33 to 89%. With repeated phlebotomy, the liver decreases in size, liver function improves, pigmentation of skin decreases, and cardiac failure may be reversed. Diabetes improves in about 40% of patients, but removal of excess iron has little effect on hypogonadism or arthropathy. Hepatic fibrosis may decrease, but established cirrhosis is irreversible. Hepatocellular carcinoma occurs as a late sequela in patients who are cirrhotic at presentation. The apparent increase in its incidence in treated patients is probably related to their increased life span. Hepatocellular carcinoma rarely develops if the disease is treated in the precirrhotic stage. Indeed, the life expectancy of homozygotes treated before the development of cirrhosis is normal.

The importance of family screening and early diagnosis and treatment cannot be overemphasized. Asymptomatic individuals detected by family studies should have phlebotomy therapy if iron stores are moderately to severely increased. Assessment of iron stores at appropriate intervals is also important. With this management approach, most manifestations of the disease can be prevented.

ROLE OF *HFE* MUTATIONS IN OTHER LIVER DISEASES

There is considerable interest in the role of *HFE* mutations and hepatic iron in several other liver diseases. Several studies have shown an increased prevalence of *HFE* mutations in PCT patients. Iron accentuates the inherited enzyme deficiency in PCT and clinical manifestations of PCT. The situation in nonalcoholic steatohepatitis (NASH) is less clear, but some studies have shown an increased prevalence of *HFE* mutations in NASH patients. The role of phlebotomy therapy, however, is unproven. In chronic HCV infection, *HFE* mutations are not more common, but some subjects have increased hepatic iron. Before initiating antiviral therapy in these patients, it is reasonable to perform phlebotomy therapy to remove excess iron stores, because this reduces liver enzyme levels.

HFE mutations are not increased in frequency in alcoholic liver disease. Hemochromatosis in a heavy drinker can be distinguished from alcoholic liver disease by the presence of the C282Y mutation.

End-stage liver disease may also be associated with iron overload of the degree seen in hemochromatosis. The mechanism is uncertain, although studies have shown that alcohol suppresses hepatic hepcidin secretion. Hemolysis also plays a role. *HFE* mutations are uncommon.

A recent large population study has suggested that subjects homozygous for C282Y are at increased risk of breast and colorectal cancer.

GLOBAL CONSIDERATIONS

The *HFE* mutation is of northern European origin (Celtic or Nordic) with a heterozygous carrier rate of approximately 1 in 10 (1 in 8 in Ireland). Thus, *HFE*-associated hemochromatosis is quite rare in non-European populations, e.g., Asia. However, non-*HFE*-associated hemochromatosis resulting from mutations in other genes involved in iron metabolism (Fig. 428-1) is ubiquitous and should be considered when one encounters iron overload.

429 Wilson's Disease

George J. Brewer

Wilson's disease is an autosomal recessive disorder caused by mutations in the *ATP7B* gene, which encodes a membrane-bound, copper-transporting ATPase. Clinical manifestations are caused by copper toxicity and primarily involve the liver and the brain. Because effective treatment is available, it is important to make this diagnosis early.

The frequency of Wilson's disease in most populations is about 1 in 30,000–40,000, and the frequency of carriers of *ATP7B* mutations is ~1%. Siblings of a diagnosed patient have a 1 in 4 risk of Wilson's disease, whereas children of an affected patient have about a 1 in 200 risk. Because a large number of inactivating mutations have been reported in the *ATP7B* gene, mutation screening for diagnosis is not routine, although this approach may be practical in the future. DNA haplotype analysis can be used to genotype siblings of an affected patient. A rare multisystem disorder of copper metabolism with features of both Menkes and Wilson's diseases has been reported. It is termed the MEDNIK syndrome (mental retardation, enteropathy, deafness, neuropathy, ichthyosis, keratodermia) and is caused by mutations in the *AP1S1* gene, which encodes an adaptor protein necessary for intracellular trafficking of copper pump proteins ATP7A (Menkes disease) and ATP7B (Wilson's disease).

PATHOGENESIS

ATP7B protein deficiency impairs biliary copper excretion, resulting in positive copper balance, hepatic copper accumulation, and copper toxicity from oxidant damage. Excess hepatic copper is initially bound to metallothionein; liver damage begins as this storage capacity is exceeded, sometimes by 3 years of age. Defective copper incorporation into apoceruloplasmin leads to excess catabolism and low blood levels of ceruloplasmin. Serum copper levels are usually lower than normal because of low blood levels of ceruloplasmin, which normally binds >90% of serum copper. As the disease progresses, nonceruloplasmin serum copper ("free" copper) levels increase, resulting in copper buildup in other parts of the body (e.g., in the brain, with consequent neurologic and psychiatric disease).

CLINICAL PRESENTATION

Hepatic Features Wilson's disease may present as hepatitis, cirrhosis, or hepatic decompensation. Patients typically present in the mid- to late teenage years in Western countries, although the age of presentation is quite broad and extends into the fifth decade of life. An episode of hepatitis may occur—with elevated serum aminotransferase levels, with or without jaundice—and then spontaneously regress. Hepatitis often recurs, and most of these patients eventually develop cirrhosis. Hepatic decompensation is associated with elevated serum bilirubin, reduced serum albumin and coagulation factors, ascites, peripheral edema, and hepatic encephalopathy. In severe hepatic failure, hemolytic anemia may develop because large amounts of copper derived from hepatocellular necrosis are released into the bloodstream. The association of hemolysis and liver disease makes Wilson's disease a likely diagnosis.

Neurologic Features The neurologic manifestations of Wilson's disease typically occur in patients in their early twenties, although the age of onset extends into the sixth decade of life. MRI and CT scans reveal damage in the basal ganglia and occasionally in the pons, medulla, thalamus, cerebellum, and subcortical areas. The three main movement disorders include dystonia, incoordination, and tremor. Dysarthria and dysphagia are common. In some patients, the clinical picture closely resembles that of Parkinson's disease. Dystonia can involve any part of the body and eventually leads to grotesque positions of the limbs, neck, and trunk. Autonomic disturbances may include orthostatic hypotension and sweating abnormalities as well as bowel, bladder, and sexual dysfunction. Memory loss, migraine-type headaches, and seizures may occur. Patients have difficulty focusing on tasks, but cognition usually is not grossly impaired. Sensory abnormalities and muscular weakness are not features of the disease.

Psychiatric Features Half of patients with neurologic disease have a history of behavioral disturbances with onset in the 5 years before diagnosis. The features are diverse and may include loss of emotional control (temper tantrums, crying bouts), depression, hyperactivity, or loss of sexual inhibition.

Other Manifestations Some female patients have repeated spontaneous abortions, and most become amenorrheic prior to diagnosis. Cholelithiasis and nephrolithiasis occur with increased frequency. Some patients have osteoarthritis, particularly of the knee. Microscopic hematuria is common, and levels of urinary excretion of phosphates, amino acids, glucose, or urates may increase; however, a full-blown Fanconi syndrome is rare. Sunflower cataracts and Kayser-Fleischer rings (copper deposits in the outer rim of the cornea) may be seen. Electrocardiographic and other cardiac abnormalities have been reported but are not common.

DIAGNOSIS

Diagnostic tests for Wilson's disease are listed in Table 429-1. Serum ceruloplasmin levels should not be used for definitive diagnosis, because they are normal in up to 10% of affected patients and are reduced in 20% of carriers. Kayser-Fleischer rings (Fig. 429-1) can be definitively diagnosed only by an ophthalmologist using a slit lamp. They are present in >99% of patients with neurologic/psychiatric forms of the disease and have been described very rarely in the absence of Wilson's disease. Kayser-Fleischer rings are present in only ~30–50% of patients diagnosed in the hepatic or presymptomatic state; thus, the absence of rings does not exclude the diagnosis.

Urine copper measurement is an important diagnostic tool, but urine must be collected carefully to avoid contamination. Symptomatic patients invariably have urine copper levels >1.6 μmol (>100 μg) per 24 h. Heterozygotes have values <1.3 μmol (<80 μg) per 24 h. About half of presymptomatic patients who are ultimately affected have diagnostically elevated urine copper values, but the other half have levels that are in an intermediate range between 0.9 and 1.6 μmol (60–100 μg) per 24 h. Because heterozygotes may have values up to 1.3 μmol (80 μg) per 24 h, patients in this range may require a liver biopsy for definitive diagnosis.

The gold standard for diagnosis remains liver biopsy with quantitative copper assays. Affected patients have values >3.1 μmol/g (>200 μg/g [dry weight] of liver). Copper stains are not reliable. False-positive results can occur with long-standing obstructive liver disease, which can elevate hepatic and urine copper concentrations and rarely causes Kayser-Fleischer rings.

TREATMENT WILSON'S DISEASE

Recommended anticopper treatments are listed in Table 429-2. Penicillamine was previously the primary anticopper treatment but now plays only a minor role because of its toxicity and because it often worsens existing neurologic disease if used as initial therapy. If penicillamine is given, it should always be accompanied by pyridoxine (25 mg/d). Trientine is a less toxic chelator and is supplanting penicillamine when a chelator is indicated.

TABLE 429-1 USEFUL TESTS FOR WILSON'S DISEASE

Test	Usefulness[a]	Normal Value	Heterozygous Carriers	Wilson's Disease
Serum ceruloplasmin	+	180–350 mg/L (18–35 mg/dL)	Low in 20%	Low in 90%
Kayser- Fleischer rings	++	Absent	Absent	Present in >99% if neurologic or psychiatric symptoms are present Present in 30–50% in hepatic presentation and presymptomatic state
Urine copper (24-h)	+++	0.3–0.8 μmol (20–50 μg)	Normal to 1.3 μmol (80 μg)	>1.6 μmol (>100 μg) in symptomatic patients; 0.9 to >1.6 μmol (60 to >100 μg) in presymptomatic patients
Liver copper	++++	0.3–0.8 μmol/g (20–50 μg/g of tissue)	Normal to 2.0 μmol (125 μg)	>3.1 μmol (>200 μg) (Obstructive liver disease can cause false-positive results.)
Haplotype analysis	++++ (siblings only)	0 matches	1 match	2 matches

[a]Usefulness range: + (somewhat useful) to ++++ (very useful).

For patients with hepatitis or cirrhosis but without evidence of hepatic decompensation or neurologic/psychiatric symptoms, zinc is the therapy of choice although some experts advocate therapy with trientine. Zinc has proven efficacy in Wilson's disease and is essentially nontoxic. It produces a negative copper balance by blocking intestinal absorption of copper, and it induces hepatic metallothionein synthesis, thereby sequestering additional toxic copper. All presymptomatic patients should be treated prophylactically because the disease is close to 100% penetrant.

The first step in evaluating patients presenting with hepatic decompensation is to establish disease severity, which can be estimated with the Nazer prognostic index (Table 429-3). Patients with scores <7 can usually be managed with medical therapy. Patients with scores >9 should be considered immediately for liver transplantation. For patients with scores between 7 and 9, clinical judgment is required in deciding whether to recommend transplantation or medical therapy. A combination of trientine and zinc has been used to treat patients with Nazer scores as high as 9, but such patients should be watched carefully for indications of hepatic deterioration, which mandates transplantation.

For initial medical treatment of patients with hepatic decompensation, the recommended regimen is a chelator (preferably trientine) plus zinc (Table 429-2). Zinc should not, however, be ingested simultaneously with trientine, which chelates zinc and forms therapeutically ineffective complexes. Administration of the two drugs should be separated by at least 1 h.

For initial neurologic therapy, tetrathiomolybdate is emerging as the drug of choice because of its rapid control of free copper, preservation of neurologic function, and low toxicity. Penicillamine and trientine should be avoided because both have a high risk of worsening the neurologic condition. Until tetrathiomolybdate is commercially available, zinc therapy is recommended. Although it is relatively slow-acting, zinc itself does not exacerbate neurologic abnormalities. Although hepatic transplantation may alleviate neurologic symptoms, it does so only by copper removal, which can be done more safely and inexpensively with anticopper drugs. Pregnant patients should be treated with zinc or trientine throughout pregnancy but without tight copper control because copper deficiency can be teratogenic.

Anticopper therapy must be lifelong. With treatment, liver function usually recovers after about a year although residual liver damage is usually present. Neurologic and psychiatric symptoms usually improve after 6–24 months of treatment.

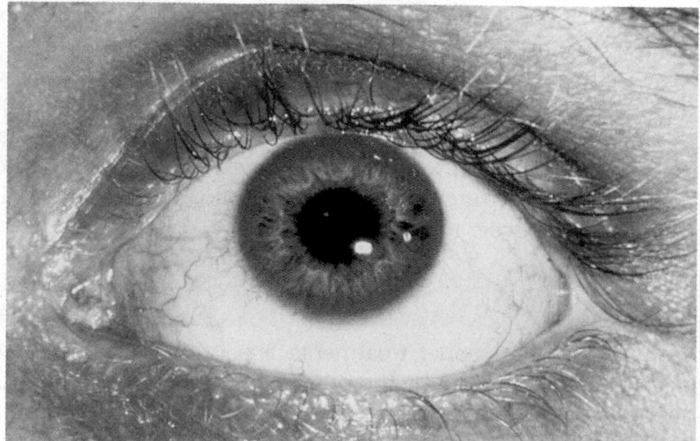

FIGURE 429-1 A Kayser-Fleischer ring. Although in this case, the brownish ring rimming the cornea is clearly visible to the naked eye, confirmation is usually made by slit-lamp examination.

MONITORING ANTICOPPER THERAPY

When trientine or penicillamine is first used, it is necessary to monitor for drug toxicity, particularly bone marrow suppression and proteinuria. Complete blood counts, standard biochemical profiles, and a urinalysis should be performed at weekly intervals for 1 month, then at twice-weekly intervals for 2 or 3 months, then at monthly intervals for 3 or 4 months, and at 4- to 6-month intervals thereafter.

The anticopper effects of trientine and penicillamine can be monitored by following 24-h "free" serum copper levels. Changes in urine copper levels are more difficult to interpret because excretion reflects the effect of the drug as well as body loading with copper. Free serum copper is calculated by subtracting the ceruloplasmin copper from

TABLE 429-2 RECOMMENDED ANTICOPPER DRUGS FOR WILSON'S DISEASE

Disease Status	First Choice	Second Choice
Initial hepatic		
Hepatitis or cirrhosis without decompensation	Zinc[a]	Trientine
Hepatic decompensation		
Mild	Trientine[b] and zinc	Penicillamine[b] and zinc
Moderate	Trientine and zinc	Hepatic transplantation
Severe	Hepatic transplantation	Trientine and zinc
Initial neurologic/ psychiatric	Tetrathiomolybdate[c] and zinc	Zinc
Maintenance	Zinc	Trientine
Presymptomatic	Zinc	Trientine
Pediatric	Zinc	Trientine
Pregnant	Zinc	Trientine

[a]Zinc acetate is supplied as Galzin, manufactured by Gate Pharmaceutical. The recommended adult dose for all the above indications is 50 mg of elemental zinc three times daily, with each dose separated by at least 1 h from consumption of food and beverages other than water as well as from trientine or penicillamine doses. [b]Trientine is supplied as Syprine and penicillamine as Cuprimine, both manufactured by Merck. The recommended adult dosage for both drugs is 500 mg twice daily, with each dose at least 0.5 h before or 2 h after meals and separated by at least 1 h from zinc administration. [c]Tetrathiomolybdate is being studied in clinical trials.

TABLE 429-3 PROGNOSTIC INDEX OF NAZER

		Score (in Points)				
Laboratory Measurement	**Normal Value**	**0**	**1**	**2**	**3**	**4**
Serum bilirubin[a]	0.2–1.2 mg/dL	<5.8	5.8–8.8	8.8–11.7	11.7–17.5	>17.5
Serum aspartate aminotransferase	10–35 IU/L	<100	100–150	151–200	201–300	>300
Prolongation of prothrombin time (sec)	—	<4	4–8	9–12	13–20	>20

[a]If hemolysis is present, serum bilirubin cannot be used as a measure of liver function until the hemolysis subsides.

Source: Modified from H Nazer et al: Gut 27:1377, 1986; with permission from BMJ Publishing Group.

the total serum copper. Each 10 mg/L (1 mg/dL) of ceruloplasmin contributes 0.5 μmol/L (3 μg/dL) of serum copper. The normal serum free copper value is 1.6–2.4 μmol/L (10–15 μg/dL); the level is often as high as 7.9 μmol/L (50 μg/dL) in untreated Wilson's disease. With treatment, the serum free copper should be <3.9 μmol/L (<25 μg/dL).

Zinc treatment does not require monitoring of blood or urine for toxicity. Its only significant side effect is gastric burning or nausea in ~10% of patients, usually with the first morning dose. This effect can be mitigated if the first dose is taken an hour after breakfast or if zinc is taken with a small amount of protein. Because zinc mainly affects stool copper, 24-h urine copper can be used to reflect body loading. The typical value in untreated symptomatic patients is >3.1 μmol (>200 μg) per 24 h. This level should decrease during the first 1–2 years of therapy to <2.0 μmol (<125 μg) per 24 h. A normal value (0.3–0.8 μmol [20–50 μg]) is rarely reached during the first decade of therapy and should raise concern about overtreatment (copper deficiency), the first sign of which is anemia and/or leukopenia.

GLOBAL CONSIDERATIONS

The age of onset of clinical disease may be considerably younger in India and the Far East; in these regions, onset often occurs in children at only 5 or 6 years of age. The incidence of the disease may be increased in certain populations as a result of founder effects. For example, in Sardinia, the incidence may be 1 in 3000. In countries where penicillamine, trientine, and zinc acetate (as Galzin) are not available or are unaffordable, zinc salts such as gluconate or sulfate provide an alternative treatment option.

430 The Porphyrias

Robert J. Desnick, Manisha Balwani

The porphyrias are metabolic disorders, each resulting from the deficiency of a specific enzyme in the heme biosynthetic pathway (Fig. 430-1 and Table 430-1).These enzyme deficiencies are inherited as autosomal dominant, autosomal recessive, or X-linked traits, with the exception of porphyria cutanea tarda (PCT), which usually is sporadic (Table 430-1). The porphyrias are classified as either *hepatic* or *erythropoietic*, depending on the primary site of overproduction and accumulation of their respective porphyrin precursors or porphyrins (Tables 430-1 and 430-2), although some have overlapping features. For example, PCT, the most common porphyria, is hepatic and presents with blistering cutaneous photosensitivity, which is typically characteristic of the erythropoietic porphyrias. The major manifestations of the acute hepatic porphyrias are neurologic, including neuropathic abdominal pain, peripheral motor neuropathy, and mental disturbances, with attacks often precipitated by dieting, certain drugs, and hormonal changes. While hepatic porphyrias are symptomatic primarily in adults, rare homozygous variants of the autosomal dominant hepatic porphyrias usually manifest clinically prior to puberty.

In contrast, the erythropoietic porphyrias usually present at birth or in early childhood with cutaneous photosensitivity, or in the case of congenital erythropoietic porphyria (CEP), even in utero as nonimmune hydrops fetalis. Cutaneous sensitivity to sunlight results from excitation of excess porphyrins in the skin by long-wave ultraviolet light, leading to cell damage, scarring, and disfigurement. Thus, the porphyrias are metabolic disorders in which environmental, physiologic, and genetic factors interact to cause disease.

Because many symptoms of the porphyrias are nonspecific, diagnosis is often delayed. Laboratory measurement of porphyrin precursors (5′-aminolevulinic acid [ALA] and porphobilinogen [PBG]) or porphyrins in urine, plasma, erythrocytes, or feces is required to confirm or exclude the various types of porphyria (see below). However, a definite diagnosis requires demonstration of the specific gene defect (Table 430-3). The genes encoding all the heme biosynthetic enzymes have been characterized, permitting identification of the mutations causing each porphyria (Table 430-2). Molecular genetic analyses now make it possible to provide precise heterozygote or homozygote identification and prenatal diagnoses in families with known mutations.

In addition to recent reviews of the porphyrias, informative and up-to-date websites are sponsored by the American Porphyria Foundation (*www.porphyriafoundation.com*) and the European Porphyria Initiative (*www.porphyria-europe.org*). An extensive list of unsafe and safe drugs for individuals with acute porphyrias is provided at the Drug Database for Acute Porphyrias (*www.drugs-porphyria.com*).

GLOBAL CONSIDERATIONS

The porphyrias are panethnic metabolic diseases that affect individuals around the globe. The acute hepatic porphyrias—acute intermittent porphyria (AIP), hereditary coproporphyria (HCP), and variegate porphyria (VP)—are autosomal dominant disorders. The frequency of AIP, the most common acute hepatic porphyria, is ~1 in 20,000 among Caucasian individuals of Western European ancestry, and it is particularly frequent in Scandinavians, with a frequency of ~1 in 10,000 in Sweden. VP is particularly frequent in South Africa, where its high prevalence (>10,000 affected patients) is in part due to a genetic "founder effect." The autosomal recessive acute hepatic porphyria, ALA dehydratase-deficient porphyria (ADP), is very rare, and less than 20 patients have been identified worldwide.

The erythropoietic protoporphyrias—CEP, erythropoietic protoporphyria (EPP), and X-linked protoporphyria (XLP)—also are panethnic. EPP is the most common porphyria in children, whereas CEP is very rare, with about 200 reported cases worldwide. The frequency of EPP varies globally because most patients have the common low expression *FECH* mutation that varies in frequency in different populations. It rarely occurs in Africans, is present in about 10% of whites, and is frequent (~30%) in the Japanese.

The autosomal recessive porphyrias—ADP, CEP, EPP, and hepatoerythropoietic porphyria (HEP)—are more frequent in regions with high rates of consanguineous unions. PCT, which is typically sporadic, occurs more frequently in countries in which its predisposing risk factors such as hepatitis C and HIV are more prevalent.

HEME BIOSYNTHESIS

Heme biosynthesis involves eight enzymatic steps in the conversion of glycine and succinyl-CoA to heme (Fig. 430-2 and Table 430-2).

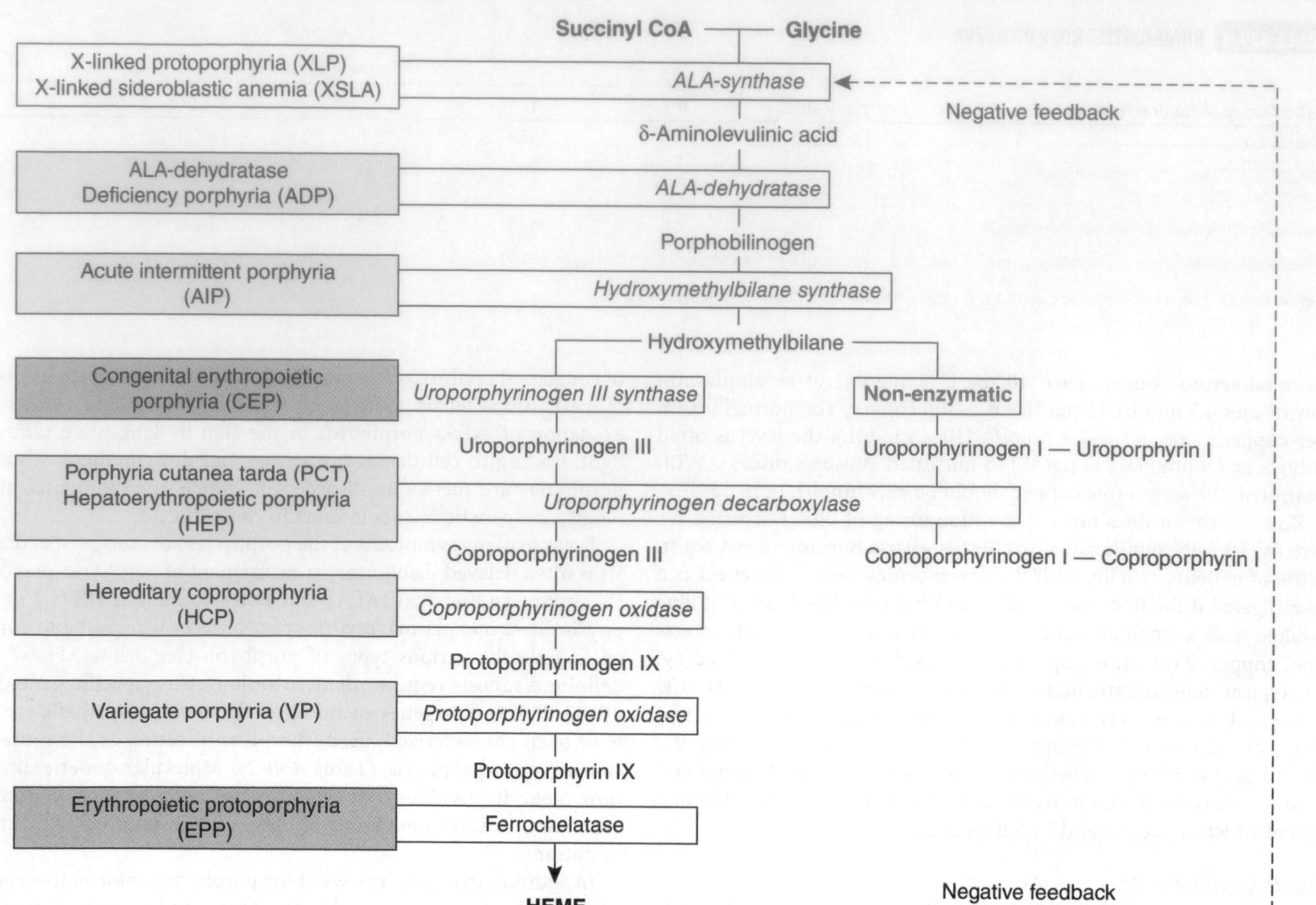

FIGURE 430-1 The human heme biosynthetic pathway indicating in *linked boxes* the enzyme that, when deficient, causes the respective porphyria. Hepatic porphyrias are shown in *yellow boxes* and erythropoietic porphyrias in *pink boxes*.

These eight enzymes are encoded by nine genes, as the first enzyme in the pathway, 5′-aminolevulinate synthase (ALA synthase), has two genes that encode unique housekeeping (*ALAS1*) and erythroid-specific (*ALAS2*) isozymes. The first and last three enzymes in the pathway are located in the mitochondrion, whereas the other four are in the cytosol. Heme is required for a variety of hemoproteins such as hemoglobin, myoglobin, respiratory cytochromes, and the cytochrome P450 enzymes (CYPs). Hemoglobin synthesis in erythroid precursor cells accounts for approximately 85% of daily heme synthesis in humans. Hepatocytes account for most of the rest, primarily for

TABLE 430-1 HUMAN PORPHYRIAS: MAJOR CLINICAL AND LABORATORY FEATURES

Porphyria	Deficient Enzyme	Inheritance	Principal Symptoms: NV or CP+	Enzyme Activity % of Normal	Increased Porphyrin Precursors and/or Porphyrins: Erythrocytes	Urine	Stool
Hepatic Porphyrias							
5-ALA dehydratase-deficient porphyria (ADP)	ALA dehydratase	AR	NV	~5	Zn-Protoporphyrin	ALA, coproporphyrin III	—
Acute intermittent porphyria (AIP)	HMB synthase	AD	NV	~50	—	ALA[a], PBG, uroporphyrin	—
Porphyria cutanea tarda (PCT)	URO decarboxylase	AD	CP	~20	—	Uroporphyrin, 7-carboxylate porphyrin	Isocoproporphyrin
Hereditary coproporphyria (HCP)	COPRO oxidase	AD	NV and CP	~50	—	ALA, PBG, coproporphyrin III	Coproporphyrin III
Variegate porphyria (VP)	PROTO oxidase	AD	NV and CP	~50	—	ALA, PBG, coproporphyrin III	Coproporphyrin III, protoporphyrin
Erythropoietic Porphyrias							
Congenital erythropoietic porphyria (CEP)	URO-synthase	AR	CP	1–5	Uroporphyrin I Coproporphyrin I	Uroporphyrin I[b] Coproporphyrin I[b]	Coproporphyrin I
Erythropoietic protoporphyria (EPP)	Ferrochelatase	AR[a]	CP	~20–30	Protoporphyrin	—	Protoporphyrin
X-linked protoporphyria (XLP)	ALA synthase 2	XL	CP	>100[c]	Protoporphyrin	—	Protoporphyrin

[a]Polymorphism in intron 3 of wild-type allele affects level of enzyme activity and clinical expression. [b]Type I isomers. [c]Increased activity due to "gain-of-function" mutations in *ALAS2* exon 11.

Abbreviations: AD, autosomal dominant; ALA, 5-aminolevulinic acid; AR, autosomal recessive; COPRO I, coproporphyrin I; COPRO III, coproporphyrin III; CP, cutaneous photosensitivity; ISOCOPRO, isocoproporphyrin; + Nv, neurovisceral; PBG, porphobilinogen; PROTO, protoporphyrin IX; URO I, uroporphyrin I; URO III, uroporphyrin III; XL, X-linked.

TABLE 430-2 HUMAN HEME BIOSYNTHETIC ENZYMES AND GENES

Enzyme	Gene Symbol	Chromosomal Location	cDNA (bp)	Gene Size (kb)	Gene Exons[a]	Protein (aa)	Subcellular Location	Known Mutations[b]	Three-Dimensional Structure[c]
ALA synthase									
Housekeeping	*ALAS1*	3p21.1	2199	17	11	640	M	—	
Erythroid-specific	*ALAS2*	Xp11.2	1937	22	11	587	M	>30	—
ALA dehydratase									
Housekeeping	*ALAD*	9q32	1149	15.9	12 (1A + 2 – 12)	330	C	12	Y
Erythroid-specific	*ALAD*	9q32	1154	15.9	12 (1B + 2 – 12)	330	C	—	
HMB synthase									
Housekeeping	*HMBS*	11q23.3	1086	11	15 (1 + 3 – 15)	361	C	>315	E
Erythroid-specific	*HMBS*	11q23.3	1035	11	15 (2 – 15)	344	C	10	
URO synthase									
Housekeeping	*UROS*	10q26.2	1296	34	10 (1 + 2B – 10)	265	C	39	H
Erythroid-specific	*UROS*	10q26.2	1216	34	10 (2A + 2B – 10)	265	C	4	
URO decarboxylase	*UROD*	1p34.1	1104	3	10	367	C	108	H
COPRO oxidase	*CPOX*	3q12.1	1062	14	7	354	M	51	H
PROTO oxidase	*PPOX*	1q23.3	1431	5.5	13	477	M	129	—
Ferrochelatase	*FECH*	18q21.31	1269	45	11	423	M	125	B

[a]Number of exons and those encoding separate housekeeping and erythroid-specific forms indicated in parentheses. [b]Number of known mutations from the Human Gene Mutation Database (*www.hgmd.org*). [c]Crystallized from human (H), murine (M), *Escherichia coli* (E), *Bacillus subtilis* (B), or yeast (Y) purified enzyme; references in Protein Data Bank (*www.rcsb.org*).

Abbreviations: C, cytoplasm; M, mitochondria.

Source: From KE Anderson et al: Disorders of heme biosynthesis. X-linked sideroblastic anemia and the porphyrias, in *The Metabolic and Molecular Bases of Inherited Diseases*, CR Scriver et al (eds). New York, McGraw-Hill, 2001, pp 2991–3062.

TABLE 430-3 DIAGNOSIS OF ACUTE AND CUTANEOUS PORPHYRIAS

Symptoms	First-Line Test: Abnormality	Possible Porphyria	Second-Line Testing if First-Line Testing Is Positive: To include: urine (U), plasma (P), and fecal (F) porphyrins; for acute porphyrias, add red blood cell (RBC) HMB synthase; for blistering skin lesions, add P and RBC porphyrins	Confirmatory Test: Enzyme Assay and/or Mutation Analysis
Neurovisceral	**Spot U:** ↑↑ALA and normal PBG	ADP	**U porphyrins:** ↑↑, mostly COPRO III **P & F porphyrins:** normal or slightly ↑ **RBC HMB synthase:** normal	Rule out other causes of elevated ALA; ↓↓RBC ALA dehydratase activity (<10%); ALA dehydratase mutation analysis
	Spot U: ↑↑PBG	AIP	**U porphyrins:** ↑↑, mostly URO and COPRO **P & F porphyrins:** normal or slightly ↑ **RBC HMB synthase:** usually ↓	HMB synthase mutation analysis
	"	HCP	**U porphyrins:** ↑↑, mostly COPRO III **P porphyrins:** normal or slightly ↑(↑ if skin lesions present) **F porphyrins:** ↑↑, mostly COPRO III	Measure RBC HMB synthase: normal activity COPRO oxidase mutation analysis
	"	VP	**U porphyrins:** ↑↑, mostly COPRO III **P porphyrins:** ↑↑(characteristic fluorescence peak at neutral pH) **F porphyrins:** ↑↑, mostly COPRO and PROTOO	Measure RBC HMB synthase: normal activity PROTO oxidase mutation analysis
Blistering skin lesions	**P:** ↑ porphyrins	PCT and HEP	**U porphyrins:** ↑↑, mostly URO and heptacarboxylate porphyrin **P porphyrins:** ↑↑ **F porphyrins:** ↑↑, including increased isocoproporphyrin **RBC porphyrins:** ↑↑ zinc PROTO in HEP[a]	RBC URO decarboxylase activity: half-normal in familial PCT (~20% of all PCT cases); substantially deficient in HEP URO decarboxylase mutation analysis: mutation(s) present in familial PCT (heterozygous) and HEP (homozygous)
	"	HCP and VP	See HCP and VP above. Also, U ALA and PBG: may be ↑	
	"	CEP	**RBC and U porphyrins:** ↑↑, mostly URO I and COPRO I **F porphyrins:** ↑↑; mostly COPRO I	↓↓ RBC URO synthase activity (<15%) URO synthase mutation analysis
Nonblistering photosensitivity	**P:** porphyrins usually ↑	EPP	**RBC porphyrins:** ↓↓, mostly free PROTO **U porphyrins:** normal **F porphyrins:** normal or ↓, mostly PROTO	*FECH* mutation analysis
	P: porphyrins usually ↑	XLP	**RBC porphyrins:** ↑↑, approximately equal free and zinc PROTO **U porphyrins:** normal **F porphyrins:** normal or ↑, mostly PROTO	*ALAS2* mutation analysis

[a]Nonspecific increases in zinc protoporphyrins are common in other porphyrias.

Abbreviations: ADP, 5-ALA dehydratase-deficient porphyria; AIP, acute intermittent porphyria; ALA, 5-aminolevulinic acid; CEP, congenital erythropoietic porphyria; COPRO I, coproporphyrin I; COPRO III, coproporphyrin III; EPP, erythropoietic protoporphyria; F, fecal; HCP, hereditary coporphyria; HEP, ; ISOCOPRO, isocoproporphyrin; P, plasma; PBG, porphobilinogen; PCT, porphyria cutanea tarda; PROTO, protoporphyrin IX; RBC, erythrocytes; U, urine; URO I, uroporphyrin I; URO III, uroporphyrin III; VP, variegate porphyria; XLP, X-linked protoporphyria.

Source: Based on KE Anderson et al: Ann Intern Med 142:439, 2005.

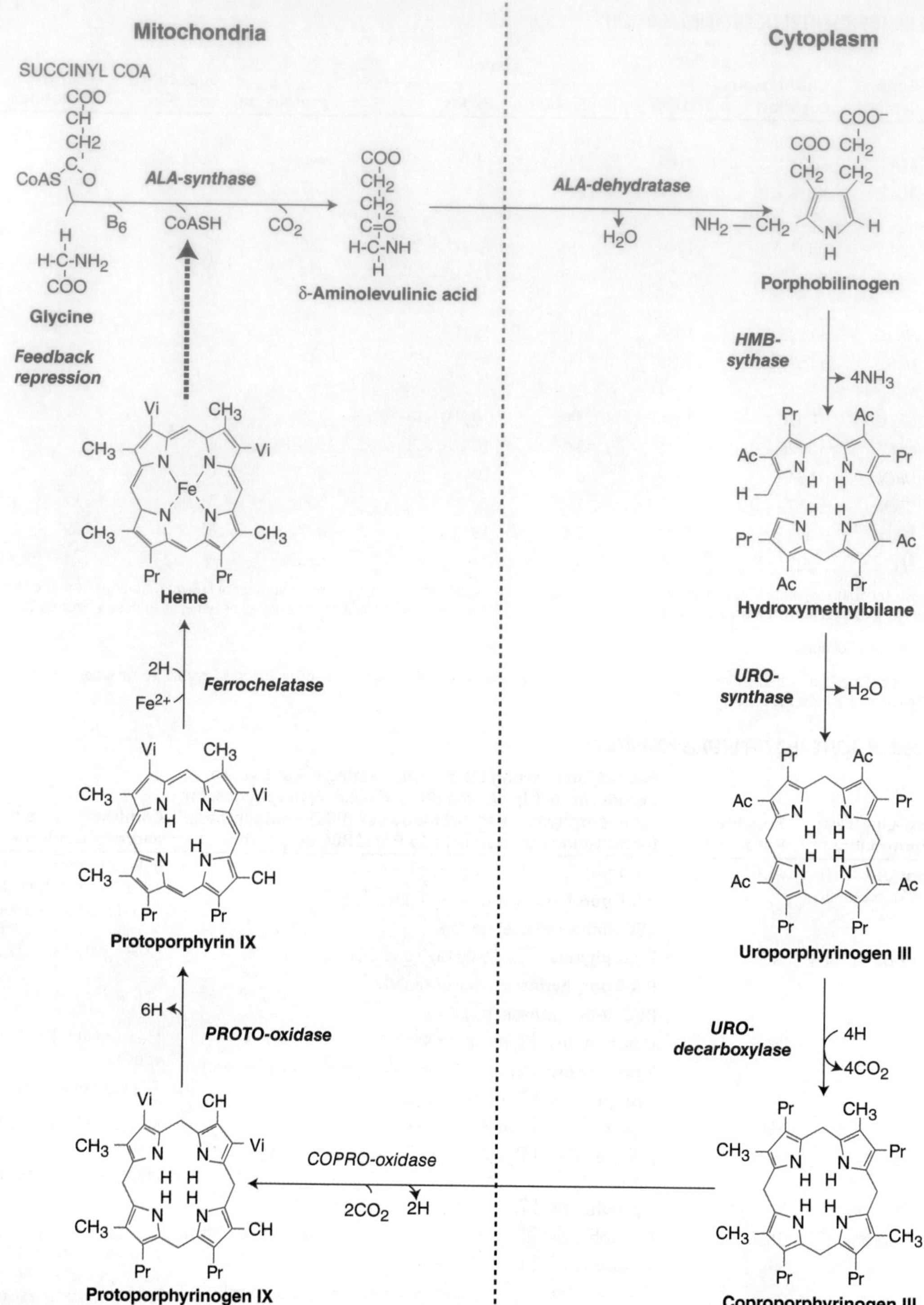

FIGURE 430-2 The heme biosynthetic pathway showing the eight enzymes and their substrates and products. Four of the enzymes are localized in the mitochondria and four in the cytosol.

the synthesis of CYPs, which are especially abundant in the liver endoplasmic reticulum, and turn over more rapidly than many other hemoproteins, such as the mitochondrial respiratory cytochromes. As shown in Fig. 430-2, pathway intermediates are the porphyrin precursors, ALA and PBG, and porphyrins (mostly in their reduced forms, known as *porphyrinogens*). At least in humans, these intermediates do not accumulate in significant amounts under normal conditions or have important physiologic functions.

The first enzyme, ALA synthase, catalyzes the condensation of glycine, activated by pyridoxal phosphate and succinyl coenzyme A, to form ALA. In the liver, this rate-limiting enzyme can be induced by a variety of drugs, steroids, and other chemicals. Distinct nonerythroid (e.g., housekeeping) and erythroid-specific forms of ALA synthase are encoded by separate genes located on chromosome 3p21.1 (*ALAS1*) and Xp11.2 (*ALAS2*), respectively. Defects in the erythroid gene *ALAS2* that decrease its activity cause X-linked sideroblastic anemia (XLSA). Recently, gain-of-function mutations in the last exon (11) of *ALAS2* that increase its activity have been shown to cause an X-linked form of EPP, known as *X-linked protoporphyria* (XLP).

The second enzyme, ALA dehydratase, catalyzes the condensation of two molecules of ALA to form PBG. Hydroxymethylbilane synthase (HMB synthase; also known as PBG deaminase) catalyzes the head-to-tail condensation of four PBG molecules by a series of deaminations to form the linear tetrapyrrole, HMB. Uroporphyrinogen III synthase

(URO synthase) catalyzes the rearrangement and rapid cyclization of HMB to form the asymmetric, physiologic, octacarboxylate porphyrinogen, uroporphyrinogen (URO'gen) III.

The fifth enzyme in the pathway, uroporphyrinogen decarboxylase (URO decarboxylase), catalyzes the sequential removal of the four carboxyl groups from the acetic acid side chains of URO'gen III to form coproporphyrinogen (COPRO'gen) III, a tetracarboxylate porphyrinogen. This compound then enters the mitochondrion via a specific transporter, ABCB6, where COPRO oxidase, the sixth enzyme, catalyzes the decarboxylation of two of the four propionic acid groups to form the two vinyl groups of protoporphyrinogen (PROTO'gen) IX, a decarboxylate porphyrinogen. Next, PROTO oxidase oxidizes PROTO gen to protoporphyrin IX by the removal of six hydrogen atoms. The product of the reaction is a porphyrin (oxidized form), in contrast to the preceding tetrapyrrole intermediates, which are porphyrinogens (reduced forms). Finally, ferrous iron is inserted into protoporphyrin to form heme, a reaction catalyzed by the eighth enzyme in the pathway, ferrochelatase (also known as heme synthetase or protoheme ferrolyase).

REGULATION OF HEME BIOSYNTHESIS

Regulation of heme synthesis differs in the two major heme-forming tissues, the liver and erythron. In the liver, the concentration of "free" heme regulates the synthesis and mitochondrial translocation of the housekeeping form of ALA synthase 1. Heme represses the synthesis of the ALA synthase 1 mRNA and interferes with the transport of the enzyme from the cytosol into mitochondria. Hepatic ALA synthase 1 is increased by many of the same chemicals that induce the cytochrome P450 enzymes in the endoplasmic reticulum of the liver. Because most of the heme in the liver is used for the synthesis of cytochrome P450 enzymes, hepatic ALA synthase 1 and the cytochrome P450s are regulated in a coordinated fashion, and many drugs that induce hepatic ALA synthase 1 also induce the CYP genes. The other hepatic heme biosynthetic enzymes are presumably expressed at constant levels, although their relative activities and kinetic properties differ. For example, normal individuals have high activities of ALA dehydratase, but low activities of HMB synthase, the latter being the second rate-limiting step in the pathway.

In the erythron, novel regulatory mechanisms allow for the production of the very large amounts of heme needed for hemoglobin synthesis. The response to stimuli for hemoglobin synthesis occurs during cell differentiation, leading to an increase in cell number. In contrast, the erythroid-specific ALA synthase 2 is expressed at higher levels than the housekeeping enzyme, and erythroid-specific control mechanisms regulate other pathway enzymes as well as iron transport into erythroid cells. Separate erythroid-specific and nonerythroid or "housekeeping" transcripts are known for the first four enzymes in the pathway. As noted above, housekeeping and erythroid-specific ALA synthases are encoded by genes on different chromosomes, but for each of the next three genes in the pathway, both erythroid and nonerythroid transcripts are transcribed by alternative promoters from their single respective genes (Table 430-2).

CLASSIFICATION OF THE PORPHYRIAS

As mentioned above, the porphyrias can be classified as either *hepatic* or *erythropoietic*, depending on whether the heme biosynthetic intermediates that accumulate arise initially from the liver or developing erythrocytes, or as *acute* or *cutaneous*, based on their clinical manifestations. Table 430-1 lists the porphyrias, their principal symptoms, and major biochemical abnormalities. Four of the five hepatic porphyrias—AIP, HCP, VP, and ADP—present during adult life with acute attacks of neurologic manifestations and elevated levels of one or both of the porphyrin precursors, ALA and PBG, and are thus classified as *acute porphyrias*. Patients with ADP have presented in infancy and adolescence. The fifth hepatic disorder, PCT, presents with blistering skin lesions. HCP and VP also may have cutaneous manifestations similar to PCT.

The erythropoietic porphyrias—CEP, EPP, and the recently described XLP—are characterized by elevations of porphyrins in bone marrow and erythrocytes and present with cutaneous photosensitivity. The skin lesions in CEP resemble PCT but are usually much more severe, whereas EPP and XLP cause a more immediate, painful, and nonblistering type of photosensitivity. EPP is the most common porphyria to cause symptoms before puberty. Around 20% of EPP patients develop minor abnormalities of liver function, with up to about 5% developing hepatic complications that can become life-threatening. XLP has a clinical presentation similar to EPP causing photosensitivity and liver disease.

DIAGNOSIS OF PORPHYRIA

A few specific and sensitive first-line laboratory tests should be used whenever symptoms or signs suggest the diagnosis of porphyria (Table 130 3). If a first-line test is significantly abnormal, more comprehensive testing should follow to establish the type of porphyria, including the specific causative gene mutation.

Acute Porphyrias An acute porphyria should be suspected in patients with neurovisceral symptoms after puberty, such as abdominal pain, and when the initial clinical evaluation does not suggest another cause. The urinary porphyrin precursors (ALA and PBG) should be measured (Fig. 430-2). Urinary PBG is virtually always increased during acute attacks of AIP, HCP, and VP and is not substantially increased in any other medical condition. Therefore, this measurement is both sensitive and specific. A method for rapid, in-house testing for urinary PBG, such as the Trace PBG kit (Thermo Scientific), can be used. Results from spot (single-void) urine specimens are highly informative because very substantial increases in PBG are expected during acute attacks of porphyria. A 24-h collection can unnecessarily delay diagnosis. The same spot urine specimen should be saved for quantitative determination of ALA, PBG, and creatinine, in order to confirm the qualitative PBG result and also to detect patients with ADP. Urinary porphyrins may remain increased longer than porphyrin precursors in HCP and VP. Therefore, it is useful to measure total urinary porphyrins in the same sample, keeping in mind that urinary porphyrin increases are often nonspecific. Measurement of urinary porphyrins alone should be avoided for screening, because these may be increased in disorders other than porphyrias, such as chronic liver disease, and misdiagnoses of porphyria can result from minimal increases in urinary porphyrins that have no diagnostic significance. Measurement of erythrocyte HMB synthase is not useful as a first-line test. Moreover, the enzyme activity is not decreased in all AIP patients, a borderline low normal value is not diagnostic, and the enzyme is not deficient in other acute porphyrias.

Cutaneous Porphyrias Blistering skin lesions due to porphyria are virtually always accompanied by increases in total plasma porphyrins. A fluorometric method is preferred, because the porphyrins in plasma in VP are mostly covalently linked to plasma proteins and may be less readily detected by high-performance liquid chromatography (HPLC). The normal range for plasma porphyrins is somewhat increased in patients with end-stage renal disease.

Although a total plasma porphyrin determination will usually detect EPP and XLP, an erythrocyte protoporphyrin determination is more sensitive. Increases in erythrocyte protoporphyrin occur in many other conditions. Therefore, the diagnosis of EPP must be confirmed by showing a predominant increase in free protoporphyrin rather than zinc protoporphyrin. In XLP, both free and zinc protoporphyrin are markedly increased in approximately equal proportions. Interpretation of laboratory reports can be difficult, because the term *free erythrocyte protoporphyrin* sometimes actually represents zinc protoporphyrin.

More extensive testing is justified when an initial test is positive. A substantial increase in PBG may be due to AIP, HCP, or VP. These acute porphyrias can be distinguished by measuring urinary porphyrins (using the same spot urine sample), fecal porphyrins, and plasma porphyrins. Assays for COPRO oxidase or PROTO oxidase are not widely available. More specifically, mutation analysis by sequencing the genes encoding HMB synthase, COPRO oxidase, and PROTO oxidase will detect almost all disease-causing mutations, and will be diagnostic even when the levels of urinary ALA and PBG have returned to normal or near normal. The various porphyrias that cause blistering skin lesions are differentiated by measuring porphyrins in urine, feces, and plasma. These porphyrias also should be confirmed at the DNA level by the demonstration of the causative gene mutation(s). It is often difficult to diagnose or "rule out" porphyria in patients who have had suggestive symptoms months or years in the past, and in relatives of patients with acute porphyrias, because porphyrin precursors and porphyrins may be normal. In those situations, detection of the specific gene mutation in the index case can make the diagnosis and facilitate the diagnosis and genetic counseling of at-risk relatives. Consultation with a specialist laboratory and physician will assist in selecting the heme biosynthetic gene or genes to be sequenced.

THE HEPATIC PORPHYRIAS

Markedly elevated plasma and urinary concentrations of the porphyrin precursors, ALA and/or PBG, which originate from the liver, are especially evident during attacks of neurologic manifestations of the four acute porphyrias—ADP, AIP, HCP, and VP. In PCT, excess porphyrins also accumulate initially in the liver and cause chronic blistering of sun-exposed areas of the skin.

ALA DEHYDRATASE-DEFICIENT PORPHYRIA (ADP)

ADP is a rare autosomal recessive acute hepatic porphyria caused by a severe deficiency of ALA dehydratase activity. To date, there are only a few documented cases, some in children or young adults, in which specific gene mutations have been identified. These affected homozygotes had <10% of normal ALA dehydratase activity in erythrocytes, but their clinically asymptomatic parents and heterozygous relatives had about half-normal levels of activity and did not excrete increased levels of ALA. The frequency of ADP is unknown, but the frequency of heterozygous individuals with <50% normal ALA dehydratase activity was ~2% in a screening study in Sweden. Because there are multiple causes for deficient ALA dehydratase activity, it is important to confirm the diagnosis of ADP by mutation analysis.

Clinical Features The clinical presentation depends on the amount of residual ALA dehydratase activity. Four of the documented patients were male adolescents with symptoms resembling those of AIP, including abdominal pain and neuropathy. One patient was an infant with more severe disease, including failure to thrive beginning at birth. The earlier age of onset and more severe manifestations in this patient reflect a more significant deficiency of ALA dehydratase activity. Another patient developed an acute motor polyneuropathy at age 63 that was associated with a myeloproliferative disorder. He was heterozygous for an *ALAD* mutation that presumably was present in erythroblasts that underwent clonal expansion due to the bone marrow malignancy.

Diagnosis All patients had significantly elevated levels of plasma and urinary ALA and urinary coproporphyrin (COPRO) III; ALAD activities in erythrocytes were <10% of normal. Hereditary tyrosinemia type 1 (fumarylacetoacetase deficiency) and lead intoxication should be considered in the differential diagnosis because either succinylacetone (which accumulates in hereditary tyrosinemia and is structurally similar to ALA) or lead can inhibit ALA dehydratase, increase urinary excretion of ALA and COPRO III, and cause manifestations that resemble those of the acute porphyrias. Heterozygotes are clinically asymptomatic and do not excrete increased levels of ALA but can be detected by demonstration of intermediate levels of erythrocyte ALA dehydratase activity or a specific mutation in the *ALAD* gene. To date, molecular studies of ADP patients have identified nine point mutations, two splice-site mutations, and a two-base deletion in the *ALAD* gene (Human Gene Mutation Database; *www.hgmd.org*). The parents in each case were not consanguineous, and the index cases had inherited a different *ALAD* mutation from each parent. Prenatal diagnosis of this disorder is possible by determination of ALA dehydratase activity and/or gene mutations in cultured chorionic villi or amniocytes.

TREATMENT ALA-DEHYDRATASE DEFICIENT PORPHYRIA

The treatment of ADP acute attacks is similar to that of AIP (see below). The severely affected infant referred to above was supported by hyperalimentation and periodic blood transfusions but did not respond to intravenous hemin and died after liver transplantation.

ACUTE INTERMITTENT PORPHYRIA (AIP)

This hepatic porphyria is an autosomal dominant condition resulting from the half-normal level of HMB synthase activity. The disease is widespread but is especially common in Scandinavia and Great Britain. Clinical expression is highly variable, and activation of the disease is often related to environmental or hormonal factors, such as drugs, diet, and steroid hormones. Attacks can be prevented by avoiding known precipitating factors. Rare homozygous dominant AIP also has been described in children (see below).

Clinical Features Induction of the rate-limiting hepatic enzyme ALA synthase in heterozygotes who have half-normal HMB synthase activity is thought to underlie the acute attacks in AIP. The disorder remains latent (or asymptomatic) in the great majority of those who are heterozygous for *HMBS* mutations, and this is almost always the case prior to puberty. In patients with no history of acute symptoms, porphyrin precursor excretion is usually normal, suggesting that half-normal hepatic HMB synthase activity is sufficient and that hepatic ALA synthase activity is not increased. However, under conditions where heme synthesis is increased in the liver, half-normal HMB synthase activity may become limiting, and ALA, PBG, and other heme pathway intermediates may accumulate and be excreted in the urine. Common precipitating factors include endogenous and exogenous steroids, porphyrinogenic drugs, alcohol ingestion, and low-calorie diets, usually instituted for weight loss.

The fact that AIP is almost always latent before puberty suggests that adult levels of steroid hormones are important for clinical expression. Symptoms are more common in women, suggesting a role for estrogens or progestins. Premenstrual attacks are probably due to endogenous progesterone. Acute porphyrias are sometimes exacerbated by exogenous steroids, including oral contraceptive preparations containing progestins. Surprisingly, pregnancy is usually well tolerated, suggesting that beneficial metabolic changes may ameliorate the effects of high levels of progesterone. Table 430-4 provides a partial list of the major drugs that are harmful in AIP (and also in HCP and VP). Extensive lists of unsafe and safe drugs are available on websites sponsored by the American Porphyria Foundation (*www.porphyriafoundation.com*) and the European Porphyria Initiative (*www.porphyria-europe.org*), and at the Drug Database for Acute Porphyrias website (*www.drugs-porphyria.com*). Reduced intake of calories and carbohydrate, as may occur with illness or attempts to lose weight, can also increase porphyrin precursor excretion and induce attacks of porphyria. Increased carbohydrate intake may ameliorate attacks. Studies in a knockout AIP mouse model indicate that the hepatic *ALAS1* gene is regulated by the peroxisome proliferator-activated receptor γ coactivator 1α (PGC-1α). Hepatic PGC-1α is induced by fasting, which in turn activates *ALAS1* transcription, resulting in increased heme biosynthesis. This finding suggests an important link between nutritional status and the attacks in acute porphyrias. Attacks also can be provoked by infections, surgery, and ethanol.

Because the neurovisceral symptoms rarely occur before puberty and are often nonspecific, a high index of suspicion is required to make the diagnosis. The disease can be disabling but is rarely fatal. Abdominal pain, the most common symptom, is usually steady and poorly localized but may be cramping. Ileus, abdominal distention, and decreased bowel sounds are common. However, increased bowel sounds and diarrhea may occur. Abdominal tenderness, fever, and leukocytosis are usually absent or mild because the symptoms are neurologic rather than inflammatory. Nausea; vomiting; constipation; tachycardia; hypertension; mental symptoms; pain in the limbs, head, neck, or chest; muscle weakness; sensory loss; dysuria; and urinary

TABLE 430-4 UNSAFE DRUGS IN PORPHYRIA

Documented Porphyrinogenic	Probably Porphyrinogenic	Possibly Porphyrinogenic	
Carbamazepine	Altretamine	Aceclofenac	Parecoxib
Carisoprodol	Aminophylline	Acitretin	Pentifylline
Chloramphenicol	Amiodarone	Acrivastine	Pentoxyverine
Clindamycin	Amitriptyline	Alfuzosin	Phenylpropanolamine + cinnarizine
Dextropropoxyphene	Amlodipine	Anastrozole	Pizotifen
Dihydralazine	Amprenavir	Auranofin	Polidocanol
Dihydroergotamine	Aprepitant	Azelastine	Polyestradiol
Drospirenone + estrogen	Atorvastatin	Benztropine	Phosphate
Dydrogesterone	Azathioprine	Benzydamine	Potassium canrenoate
Etonogestrel	Bosentan	Betaxolol	Pravastatin
Fosphenytoin sodium	Bromocriptine	Bicalutamide	Prednisolone
Hydralazine	Buspirone	Biperiden	Prilocaine
Hydroxyzine	Busulfan	Bupropion	Proguanil
Indinavir	Butylscopolamine	Carvedilol	Propafenone
Ketamine	Cabergoline	Chlorambucil	Pseudoephedrine + dexbrompheniramine
Ketoconazole	Ceftriaxone + lidocaine	Chlorcyclizine + guaifenesin	Quillaia extract
Lidocaine	Cerivastatin	Chloroquine	Quinagolide
Lynestrenol	Cetirizine	Chlorprothixene	Quinine
Lynestrenol + estrogen	Cholinetheophyllinate	Chlorzoxazone	Quinupristin + Dalfopristin
Mecillinam	Clarithromycin	Chorionic	Reboxetine
Medroxyprogesterone	Clemastine	Gonadotropin	Repaglinide
Megestrol	Clonidine	Ciclosporin	Rizatriptan
Methylergometrine	Cyclizine	Cisapride	Rofecoxib
Methyldopa	Cyproterone	Citalopram	Ropinirole
Mifepristone	Danazol	Clomethiazole	Ropivacaine
Nicotinic acid/meclozine/	Delavirdine	Clomiphene	Roxithromycin
hydroxyzine	Desogestrel + estrogen	Clomipramine	Sertraline
Nitrofurantoin	Diazepam	Clopidogrel	Sevoflurane
Norethisterone	Dienogest + estrogen	Clotrimazole	Sibutramine
Norgestimate + estrogen	Diclofenac	Cortisone	Sildenafil
Orphenadrine	Diltiazem	Cyclandelate	Sirolimus
Phenobarbital	Diphenhydramine	Cyclophosphamide	Sodium aurothiomalate
Phenytoin	Disopyramide	Cyproheptadine	Sodium oleate + chlorocymol
Pivampicillin	Disulfiram	Dacarbazine	Stavudine
Pivmecillinam	Drospirenone + estrogen	Daunorubicin	Sulindac
Primidone	Dydrogesterone	Desogestrel	Sumatriptan
Rifampicin	Ergoloid mesylate	Dichlorobenzyl alcohol	Tacrolimus
Ritonavir	Erythromycin	Dithranol	Tadalafil
Spironolactone	Estramustine	Docetaxel	Tegafur + uracil
Sulfadiazine + trimethoprim	Ethosuximide	Donepezil	Telmisartan
Tamoxifen	Etoposide	Doxycycline	Thioridazine
Testosterone, injection	Exemestane	Ebastine	Thioguanine
Thiopental	Felbamate	Econazole	Tolfenamic acid
Trimethoprim	Felodipine	Efavirenz	Tolterodine
Valproic acid	Fluconazole	Escitalopram	Torsemide
Venlafaxine	Flunitrazepam	Esomeprazole	Triamcinolone
Vinblastine	Fluvastatin	Estradiol/tablets	Trihexyphenidyl
Vincristine	Glibenclamide	Estriol/tablets	Trimipramine
Vindesine	Halothane	Estrio/vaginal crème,	Valerian
Vinorelbine	Hyoscyamine	tablet	Venlafaxine
Xylometazoline	Ifosfamide	Estrogen, conjugate	Vinblastine
Zaleplon	Imipramine	Finasteride	Vincristine
Ziprasidone	Irinotecan	Flecainide	Vindesine
Zolmitriptan	Isoniazid	Flucloxacillin	Vinorelbine
Zolpidem	Isradipine	Fluoxetine	Xylometazoline

(Continued)

TABLE 430-4 UNSAFE DRUGS IN PORPHYRIA (*CONTINUED*)

Documented Porphyrinogenic	Probably Porphyrinogenic	Possibly Porphyrinogenic	
Zuclopenthixol	Itraconazole	Flupentixol	Zaleplon
	Lamivudine + zidovudine	Flutamide	Ziprasidone
	Lansoprazole	Fluvoxamine	Zolmitriptan
	Lercanidipine	Follitropin alfa and beta	Zolpidem
	Levonorgestrel	Galantamine	Zuclopenthixol
	Lidocaine	Glimepiride	
	Lopinavir	Glipizide	
	Lutropin alfa	Gonadorelin	
	Lymecycline	Gramicidin	
	Meclozine	Guaifenesin	
	Medroxyprogesterone + estrogen	Hydrocortisone	
	Metoclopramide	Hydroxycarbamide	
	Metronidazole	Hydroxychloroquine	
	Metyrapone	Ibutilide	
	Moxonidine	Imatinib	
	Nandrolone	Indomethacin	
	Nefazodone	Ketobemidone + DDBA	
	Nelfinavir	Ketoconazole	
	Nevirapine	Ketorolac	
	Nifedipine	Lamotrigine	
	Nimodipine	Letrozole	
	Nitrazepam	Levodopa + benserazide	
	Norethisterone	Levonorgestrel intrauterine	
	Nortriptyline	Levosimendan	
	Oxcarbazepine	Lidocaine	
	Oxytetracycline	Linezolid	
	Paclitaxel	Lofepramine	
	Paroxetine	Lomustine	
	Phenazone + caffeine	Malathion	
	Pioglitazone	Maprotiline	
	Probenecid	Mebendazole	
	Progesterone, vaginal gel	Mefloquine	
	Quinidine	Melperone	
	Rabeprazole	Melphalan	
	Raloxifene	Mepenzolate	
	Rifabutin	Mepivacaine	
	Riluzole	Mercaptopurine	
	Risperidone	Methadone	
	Rosiglitazone	Methylprednisolone	
	Saquinavir	Methixene	
	Selegiline	Metolazone	
	Simvastatin	Metronidazole	
	Sulfasalazine	Mexiletine	
	Telithromycin	Mianserin	
	Terbinafine	Midazolam	
	Terfenadine	Minoxidil	
	Testosterone, transdermal patch	Mirtazapine	
	Tetracycline	Mitomycin	
	Theophylline	Mitoxantrone	
	Thiamazole	Moclobemide	
	Tibolone	Montelukast	
	Ticlopidine	Morphine + scopolamine	
	Tinidazole	Multivitamins	
	Thiotepa	Mupirocin	
	Topiramate	Nabumetone	
	Topotecan	Nafarelin	
	Toremifene		

(*Continued*)

TABLE 430-4 UNSAFE DRUGS IN PORPHYRIA (*CONTINUED*)

Documented Porphyrinogenic	Probably Porphyrinogenic	Possibly Porphyrinogenic
	Tramadol	Naltrexone
	Trimegestone + estrogen	Nateglinide
	Verapamil	Nilutamide
	Voriconazole	Noscapine
	Zidovudine/AZT	Omeprazole
		Oxybutynin
		Oxycodone
		Pantoprazole
		Papaverine

Note: Based on list in "Patient's and Doctor's Guide to Medication in Acute Porphyria," Swedish Porphyria Association and Porphyria Centre Sweden. Also see the website Drug Database for Acute Porphyrias (*www.drugs-porphyria.com*) for a searchable list of safe and unsafe drugs.

retention are characteristic. Tachycardia, hypertension, restlessness, tremors, and excess sweating are due to sympathetic overactivity.

The peripheral neuropathy is due to axonal degeneration (rather than demyelinization) and primarily affects motor neurons. Significant neuropathy does not occur with all acute attacks; abdominal symptoms are usually more prominent. Motor neuropathy affects the proximal muscles initially, more often in the shoulders and arms. The course and degree of involvement are variable and sometimes may be focal and involve cranial nerves. Deep tendon reflexes initially may be normal or hyperactive but become decreased or absent as the neuropathy advances. Sensory changes such as paresthesia and loss of sensation are less prominent. Progression to respiratory and bulbar paralysis and death occurs especially when the diagnosis and treatment are delayed. Sudden death may result from sympathetic overactivity and cardiac arrhythmia.

Mental symptoms such as anxiety, insomnia, depression, disorientation, hallucinations, and paranoia can occur in acute attacks. Seizures can be due to neurologic effects or to hyponatremia. Treatment of seizures is difficult because most antiseizure drugs can exacerbate AIP (clonazepam may be safer than phenytoin or barbiturates). Hyponatremia results from hypothalamic involvement and inappropriate vasopressin secretion or from electrolyte depletion due to vomiting, diarrhea, poor intake, or excess renal sodium loss. Persistent hypertension and impaired renal function may occur. When an attack resolves, abdominal pain may disappear within hours, and paresis begins to improve within days and may continue to improve over several years.

Homozygous dominant AIP is a rare form of AIP in which patients inherit *HMBS* mutations from each of their heterozygous parents and, therefore, have very low (<2%) enzyme activity. The disease has been described in a Dutch girl, two young British siblings, and a Spanish boy. In these homozygous affected patients, the disease presented in infancy with failure to thrive, developmental delay, bilateral cataracts, and/or hepatosplenomegaly. Urinary ALA and PBG concentrations were markedly elevated. All of these patients' *HMBS* mutations (R167W, R167Q, and R172Q) were in exon 10 within five bases of each other. Studies of the brain magnetic resonance images (MRIs) of children with homozygous AIP have suggested damage primarily in white matter that was myelinated postnatally, while tracks that myelinated prenatally were normal. Most children with homozygous AIP die at an early age.

Diagnosis ALA and PBG levels are substantially increased in plasma and urine, especially during acute attacks, and become normal only after prolonged latency. For example, urinary PBG excretion during an attack is usually 50–200 mg/24 h (220–880 μmol/24 h) (normal, 0–4 mg/24 h, [0–18 μmol/24 h]), and urinary ALA excretion is 20–100 mg/24 h (150–760 μmol/24 h) (normal, 1–7 mg/24 h [8–53 μmol/24 h]). Because levels often remain high after symptoms resolve, the diagnosis of an acute attack in a patient with biochemically proven AIP is based primarily on clinical features. Excretion of ALA and PBG decreases over a few days after intravenous hemin administration. A normal urinary PBG level before hemin effectively excludes AIP as a cause for current symptoms. Fecal porphyrins are usually normal or minimally increased in AIP, in contrast to HCP and VP. Most AIP heterozygotes with no history of symptoms have normal urinary excretion of ALA and PBG. Therefore, the detection of the family's *HMBS* mutation will diagnose asymptomatic family members.

Patients with *HMBS* mutations in the initiation of translation codon in exon 1 and in the intron 15′-splice donor site have normal enzyme levels in erythrocytes and deficient activity only in nonerythroid tissues. This occurs because the erythroid and housekeeping forms of HMB synthase are encoded by a single gene, which has two promoters. Thus, the enzyme assay may not be diagnostic, and genetic testing should be used to confirm the diagnosis.

More than 390 *HMBS* mutations have been identified in AIP, including missense, nonsense, and splicing mutations and insertions and deletions, with most mutations found in only one or a few families (Human Gene Mutation Database, *www.hgmd.org*). The prenatal diagnosis of a fetus at risk can be made with cultured amniotic cells or chorionic villi. However, this is seldom done, because the prognosis of individuals with *HMBS* mutations is generally favorable.

TREATMENT ACUTE INTERMITTENT PORPHYRIA

During acute attacks, narcotic analgesics may be required for abdominal pain, and phenothiazines are useful for nausea, vomiting, anxiety, and restlessness. Chloral hydrate can be given for insomnia, and benzodiazepines are probably safe in low doses if a minor tranquilizer is required. Carbohydrate loading, usually with intravenous glucose (at least 300 g daily), may be effective in milder acute attacks of porphyria (without paresis, hyponatremia, etc.) if hemin is not available. Intravenous hemin is more effective and should be used as first-line therapy for all acute attacks. The standard regimen is 3–4 mg/kg of heme, in the form of lyophilized hematin (Recordati Pharmaceuticals), heme albumin (hematin reconstituted with human albumin), or heme arginate (Orphan Europe), infused daily for 4 days. Heme arginate and heme albumin are chemically stable and are less likely than hematin to produce phlebitis or an anticoagulant effect. Recovery depends on the degree of neuronal damage and usually is rapid if therapy is started early. Recovery from severe motor neuropathy may require months or years. Identification and avoidance of inciting factors can hasten recovery from an attack and prevent future attacks. Inciting factors are usually multiple, and removal of one or more hastens recovery and helps prevent future attacks. Frequent attacks that occur during the luteal phase of the menstrual cycle may be prevented with a gonadotropin-releasing hormone analogue, which prevents ovulation and progesterone production, or by prophylactic hematin administration.

The long-term risk of hypertension and chronic renal disease is increased in AIP; a number of patients have undergone successful renal transplantation. Chronic, low-grade abnormalities in liver function tests are common, and the risk of hepatocellular carcinoma is increased. Hepatic imaging is recommended at least yearly for early detection of these tumors.

An allogeneic liver transplant was performed on a 19-year-old female AIP heterozygote who had 37 acute attacks in the 29 months prior to transplantation. After transplantation, her elevated urinary ALA and BPG levels returned to normal in 24 h, and she did not experience acute neurologic attacks for more than 3 years after transplant. Two AIP patients had combined liver and kidney transplants secondary to uncontrolled acute porphyria attacks, chronic peripheral neuropathy, and renal failure requiring dialysis. Both patients had a marked improvement with no attacks and normal urinary PBG levels after transplantation, as well as improvement of their neuropathic manifestations. More recently, a group from the United Kingdom reported their experience with liver transplantation in 10 AIP patients with recurrent attacks that were refractory to medical management and impaired quality of life. Patients had a complete biochemical and symptomatic resolution after transplant. The investigators reported a high rate of hepatic artery thrombosis in their series. Clearly, liver transplantation is a high-risk procedure and should be considered as a last resort in patients with severe recurrent attacks. Recently, liver-directed gene therapy has proven successful in the prevention of drug-induced biochemical attacks in a murine model of human AIP, and clinical trials of AAV-*HMBS* gene transfer have been initiated. In addition, preclinical studies of a hepatic-targeted RNA interference (RNAi) therapy directed to inhibit the markedly elevated hepatic *ALAS1* mRNA in the AIP mouse model prevented induced biochemical attacks and rapidly reduced the *ALAS1* mRNA during an ongoing attack.

PORPHYRIA CUTANEA TARDA (PCT)

PCT, the most common of the porphyrias, can be either sporadic (type 1) or familial (type 2) and can also develop after exposure to halogenated aromatic hydrocarbons. Hepatic URO decarboxylase is deficient in all types of PCT, and for clinical symptoms to manifest, this enzyme deficiency must be substantial (~20% of normal activity or less); it is currently attributed to generation of an URO decarboxylase inhibitor in the liver, which forms uroporphomethene in the presence of iron and under conditions of oxidative stress. The majority of PCT patients (~80%) have no *UROD* mutations and are said to have sporadic (type 1) disease. PCT patients heterozygous for *UROD* mutations have familial (type 2) PCT. In these patients, inheritance of a *UROD* mutation from one parent results in half-normal enzyme activity in liver and all other tissues, which is a significant predisposing factor, but is insufficient by itself to cause symptomatic PCT. As discussed below, other genetic and environmental factors contribute to susceptibility for both types of PCT. Because penetrance of the genetic trait is low, many patients with familial (type 2) PCT have no family history of the disease. HEP is an autosomal recessive form of porphyria that results from the marked systemic deficiency of URO decarboxylase activity with clinical symptoms in childhood.

Clinical Features Blistering skin lesions that appear most commonly on the backs of the hands are the major clinical feature (Fig. 430-3). These rupture and crust over, leaving areas of atrophy and scarring. Lesions may also occur on the forearms, face, legs, and feet. Skin friability and small white papules termed milia are common, especially on the backs of the hands and fingers. Hypertrichosis and hyperpigmentation, especially of the face, are especially troublesome in women. Occasionally, the skin over sun-exposed areas becomes severely thickened, with scarring and calcification that resembles systemic sclerosis. Neurologic features are absent.

A number of susceptibility factors, in addition to inherited *UROD* mutations in type 2 PCT, can be recognized clinically and can affect management. These include hepatitis C, HIV, excess alcohol, elevated iron levels, and estrogens. The importance of excess hepatic iron as a precipitating factor is underscored by the finding that the incidence of the common hemochromatosis-causing mutations, hemochromatosis gene (*HFE*) mutations C282Y and H63D, are increased in patients with types 1 and 2 PCT (Chap. 428). Excess alcohol is a long-recognized contributor, as is estrogen use in women. HIV is probably an independent but less common risk factor that, like hepatitis C, does not cause PCT in isolation. Multiple susceptibility factors that appear to act synergistically can be identified in the individual PCT patient. Patients with PCT characteristically have chronic liver disease and sometimes cirrhosis and are at risk for hepatocellular carcinoma. Various chemicals can also induce PCT; an epidemic of PCT occurred in eastern Turkey in the 1950s as a consequence of wheat contaminated with the fungicide hexachlorobenzene. PCT also occurs after exposure to other chemicals, including di- and trichlorophenols and 2,3,7,8-tetrachlorodibenzo-(*p*)-dioxin (TCDD, dioxin).

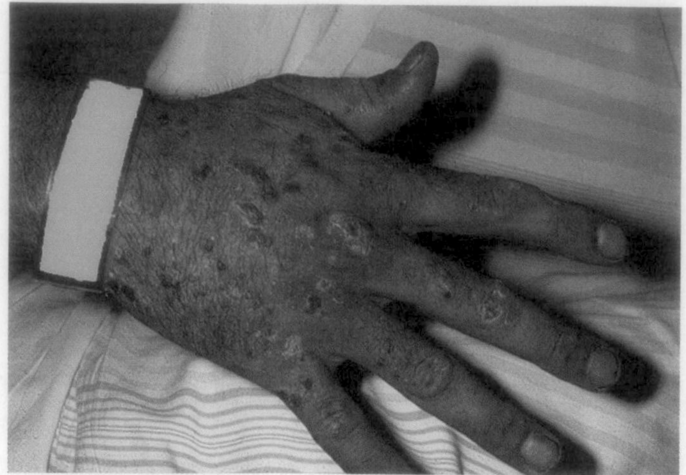

FIGURE 430-3 Typical cutaneous lesions in a patient with porphyria cutanea tarda. Chronic, crusted lesions resulting from blistering due to photosensitivity on the dorsum of the hand of a patient with porphyria cutanea tarda. *(Courtesy of Dr. Karl E. Anderson; with permission.)*

Diagnosis Porphyrins are increased in the liver, plasma, urine, and stool. The urinary ALA level may be slightly increased, but the PBG level is normal. Urinary porphyrins consist mostly of uroporphyins and heptacarboxylate porphyrin, with lesser amounts of coproporphyrin and hexa- and pentacarboxylate porphyrins. Plasma porphyrins are also increased, and fluorometric scanning of diluted plasma at neutral pH can rapidly distinguish VP and PCT (Table 430-3). Isocoproporphyrins, which are increased in feces and sometimes in plasma and urine, are diagnostic for hepatic URO decarboxylase deficiency.

Type 2 PCT and HEP can be distinguished from type 1 by finding decreased URO decarboxylase in erythrocytes. URO decarboxylase activity in liver, erythrocytes, and cultured skin fibroblasts in type 2 PCT is approximately 50% of normal in affected individuals and in family members with latent disease. In HEP, the URO decarboxylase activity is markedly deficient, with typical levels of 3–10% of normal. Over 121 mutations have been identified in the *UROD* gene (Human Gene Mutation Database; *www.hgmd.org*). Of the mutations listed in the database, ~65% are missense or nonsense and ~10% are splice-site mutations. Most *UROD* mutations have been identified in only one or two families.

TREATMENT PORPHYRIA CUTANEA TARDA

Alcohol, estrogens, iron supplements, and, if possible, any drugs that may exacerbate the disease should be discontinued, but this step does not always lead to improvement. A complete response can almost always be achieved by the standard therapy, repeated phlebotomy, to reduce hepatic iron. A unit (450 mL) of blood can be removed every 1–2 weeks. The aim is to gradually reduce excess hepatic iron until the serum ferritin level reaches the lower limits of normal. Because iron overload is not marked in most cases, remission may occur after only five or six phlebotomies; however, PCT patients with hemochromatosis may require more treatments to bring their iron levels down to the normal range. To document improvement in PCT, it is most convenient to follow the total plasma porphyrin concentration, which becomes normal some time after the target ferritin level is reached. Hemoglobin levels or hematocrits and serum ferritin should be followed closely to prevent development of iron deficiency and anemia. After remission, continued phlebotomy may not be needed. Plasma porphyrin levels are followed at 6- to 12-month intervals for early detection of recurrences, which are treated by additional phlebotomy.

An alternative when phlebotomy is contraindicated or poorly tolerated is a low-dose regimen of chloroquine or hydroxychloroquine, both of which complex with the excess porphyrins and promote their excretion. Small doses (e.g., 125 mg chloroquine phosphate twice weekly) should be given, because standard doses can induce transient, sometimes marked increases in photosensitivity and hepatocellular damage. Recent studies indicate that low-dose hydroxychloroquine is as safe and effective as phlebotomy in PCT. Hepatic imaging can diagnose or exclude complicating hepatocellular carcinoma. Treatment of PCT in patients with end-stage renal disease is facilitated by administration of erythropoietin.

HEREDITARY COPROPORPHYRIA (HCP)

HCP is an autosomal dominant hepatic porphyria that results from the half-normal activity of COPRO oxidase. The disease presents with acute attacks, as in AIP. Cutaneous photosensitivity also may occur, but much less commonly than in VP. HCP patients may have acute attacks and cutaneous photosensitivity together or separately. HCP is less common than AIP and VP. Homozygous dominant HCP and harderoporphyria, a biochemically distinguishable variant of HCP, present with clinical symptoms in children (see below).

Clinical Features HCP is influenced by the same factors that cause attacks in AIP. The disease is latent before puberty, and symptoms, which are virtually identical to those of AIP, are more common in women. HCP is generally less severe than AIP. Blistering skin lesions are identical to PCT and VP and begin in childhood in rare homozygous cases.

Diagnosis COPRO III is markedly increased in the urine and feces in symptomatic patients, and often persists, especially in feces, when there are no symptoms. Urinary ALA and PBG levels are increased (but less than in AIP) during acute attacks, but may revert to normal more quickly than in AIP when symptoms resolve. Plasma porphyrins are usually normal or only slightly increased, but they may be higher in cases with skin lesions. The diagnosis of HCP is readily confirmed by increased fecal porphyrins consisting almost entirely of COPRO III, which distinguishes it from other porphyrias.

Although the diagnosis can be confirmed by measuring COPRO oxidase activity, the assays for this mitochondrial enzyme are not widely available and require cells other than erythrocytes. To date, over 64 mutations have been identified in the *CPOX* gene, 67% of which are missense or nonsense (Human Gene Mutation Database; *www.hgmd.org*). Detection of a *CPOX* mutation in a symptomatic individual permits the identification of asymptomatic family members.

TREATMENT HEREDITARY COPROPORPHYRIA

Neurologic symptoms are treated as in AIP (see above). Phlebotomy and chloroquine are not effective for the cutaneous lesions.

VARIEGATE PORPHYRIA (VP)

VP is an autosomal dominant hepatic porphyria that results from the deficient activity of PROTO oxidase, the seventh enzyme in the heme biosynthetic pathway, and can present with neurologic symptoms, photosensitivity, or both. VP is particularly common in South Africa, where 3 of every 1000 whites have the disorder. Most are descendants of a couple who emigrated from Holland to South Africa in 1688. In other countries, VP is less common than AIP. Rare cases of homozygous dominant VP, presenting in childhood with cutaneous symptoms, also have been reported.

Clinical Features VP can present with skin photosensitivity, acute neurovisceral crises, or both. In two large studies of VP patients, 59% had only skin lesions, 20% had only acute attacks, and 22% had both. Acute attacks are identical to those in AIP and are precipitated by the same factors as AIP (see above). Blistering skin manifestations are similar to those in PCT, but are more difficult to treat and usually are of longer duration. Homozygous VP is associated with photosensitivity, neurologic symptoms, and developmental disturbances, including growth retardation, in infancy or childhood; all cases had increased erythrocyte levels of zinc protoporphyrin, a characteristic finding in all homozygous porphyrias so far described.

Diagnosis Urinary ALA and PBG levels are increased during acute attacks, but may return to normal more quickly than in AIP. Increases in fecal protoporphyrin and COPRO III and in urinary COPRO III are more persistent. Plasma porphyrin levels also are increased, particularly when there are cutaneous lesions. VP can be distinguished rapidly from all other porphyrias by examining the fluorescence emission spectrum of porphyrins in plasma since VP has a unique fluorescence peak at neutral pH.

Assays of PROTO oxidase activity in cultured fibroblasts or lymphocytes are not widely available. Over 174 mutations have been identified in the *PPOX* gene from unrelated VP patients (Human Gene Mutation Database; *www.hgmd.org*). The missense mutation R59W is the common mutation in most South Africans with VP of Dutch descent. Five missense mutations were common in English and French VP patients; however, most mutations have been found in only one or two families.

TREATMENT VARIEGATE PORPHYRIA

Acute attacks are treated as in AIP, and hemin should be started early in most cases. Other than avoiding sun exposure, there are few effective measures for treating the skin lesions. β-Carotene, phlebotomy, and chloroquine are not helpful.

THE ERYTHROPOIETIC PORPHYRIAS

In the erythropoietic porphyrias, excess porphyrins from bone marrow erythrocyte precursors are transported via the plasma to the skin and lead to cutaneous photosensitivity.

X-LINKED SIDEROBLASTIC ANEMIA (XLSA)

XLSA results from the deficient activity of the erythroid form of ALA synthase (ALA synthase 2) and is associated with ineffective erythropoiesis, weakness, and pallor.

Clinical Features Typically, males with XLSA develop refractory hemolytic anemia, pallor, and weakness during infancy. They have secondary hypersplenism, become iron overloaded, and can develop hemosiderosis. The severity depends on the level of residual erythroid ALA synthase activity and on the responsiveness of the specific mutation to pyridoxal 5′-phosphate supplementation (see below). Peripheral blood smears reveal a hypochromic, microcytic anemia with striking anisocytosis, poikilocytosis, and polychromasia; the leukocytes and platelets appear normal. Hemoglobin content is reduced, and the mean corpuscular volume and mean corpuscular hemoglobin concentration are decreased. Patients with milder, late-onset disease have been reported recently.

Diagnosis Bone marrow examination reveals hypercellularity with a left shift and megaloblastic erythropoiesis with an abnormal maturation. A variety of Prussian blue-staining sideroblasts are observed. Levels of urinary porphyrin precursors and of both urinary and fecal porphyrins are normal. The activity of erythroid ALA synthase 2 is decreased in bone marrow, but this enzyme is difficult to measure in the presence of the normal ALA synthase 1 housekeeping enzyme. Definitive diagnosis requires the demonstration of mutations in the erythroid *ALAS2* gene.

TREATMENT X-LINKED SIDEROBLASTIC ANEMIA

The severe anemia may respond to pyridoxine supplementation. This cofactor is essential for ALA synthase activity, and mutations in the pyridoxine binding site of the enzyme have been found in several responsive patients. Cofactor supplementation may make it possible to eliminate or reduce the frequency of transfusion. Unresponsive patients may be transfusion-dependent and require chelation therapy.

CONGENITAL ERYTHROPOIETIC PORPHYRIA (CEP)

CEP, also known as Günther's disease, is an autosomal recessive disorder. It is due to the markedly deficient, but not absent, activity of URO synthase and the resultant accumulation of URO I and COPRO I isomers. CEP is associated with hemolytic anemia and cutaneous lesions.

Clinical Features Severe cutaneous photosensitivity typically begins in early infancy. The skin over light-exposed areas is friable, and bullae and vesicles are prone to rupture and infection. Skin thickening, focal hypo- and hyperpigmentation, and hypertrichosis of the face and extremities are characteristic. Secondary infection of the cutaneous lesions can lead to disfigurement of the face and hands. Porphyrins are deposited in teeth and in bones. As a result, the teeth are brownish and fluoresce on exposure to long-wave ultraviolet light. Hemolysis is probably due to the marked increase in erythrocyte porphyrins and leads to splenomegaly. Adults with a milder later-onset form of the disease also have been described.

Diagnosis URO and COPRO (mostly type I isomers) accumulate in the bone marrow, erythrocytes, plasma, urine, and feces. The predominant porphyrin in feces is COPRO I. The diagnosis of CEP can be confirmed by demonstration of markedly deficient URO synthase activity and/or by the identification of specific mutations in the *UROS* gene. The disease can be detected in utero by measuring porphyrins in amniotic fluid and URO synthase activity in cultured amniotic cells or chorionic villi, or by the detection of the family's specific gene mutations. Molecular analyses of the mutant alleles from unrelated patients have revealed the presence of over 48 mutations in the *UROS* gene, including four in the erythroid-specific promoter of the *UROS* gene. Genotype/phenotype correlations can predict the severity of the disease. The CEP phenotype may be modulated by sequence variations in the erythroid specific ALA synthase 2, mutation of which typically causes XLP. One mutation (p.ArgR216WTrp) in *GATA1*, encoding the X-linked erythroid-specific transcription factor GATA binding protein 1 (*GATA1*), has been identified in an individual with CEP, thrombocytopenia, and β thalassemia.

TREATMENT CONGENITAL ERYTHROPOIETIC PORPHYRIA

Severe cases often require transfusions for anemia. Chronic transfusions of sufficient blood to suppress erythropoiesis are effective in reducing porphyrin production but result in iron overload. Splenectomy may reduce hemolysis and decrease transfusion requirements. Protection from sunlight and from minor skin trauma is important. β-Carotene may be of some value. Complicating bacterial infections should be treated promptly. Recently, bone marrow and cord blood transplantation has proven curative in several transfusion-dependent children, providing the rationale for stem cell gene therapy.

ERYTHROPOIETIC PROTOPORPHYRIA (EPP)

EPP is an inherited disorder resulting from the deficient activity of ferrochelatase (FECH), the last enzyme in the heme biosynthetic pathway. EPP is the most common erythropoietic porphyria in children and, after PCT, the second most common porphyria in adults. EPP patients have FECH activities as low as 15–25% of normal in lymphocytes and cultured fibroblasts. Protoporphyrin accumulates in bone marrow reticulocytes and then appears in plasma, is taken up in the liver, and is excreted in bile and feces. Protoporphyrin transported to the vessels in the skin causes the nonblistering photosensitivity. In most symptomatic patients (~90%) with this autosomal recessive disorder, a mutation in one *FECH* allele is inherited with a relatively common (~10% of normal whites) intronic 3 (IVS3) alteration (IVS3-48T>C) that results in the low expression of the normal enzyme. In about 10% of EPP families, two *FECH* mutations have been found. Recently, deletion mutations in exon 11 of the *ALAS2* gene have been described, causing XLP that is clinically indistinguishable from EPP. The deletion of the C-terminal amino acids of ALAS2 results in its increased activity and the accumulation of protoporphyrin. XLP accounts for approximately 2–10% of cases with the EPP phenotype in Europe and North America.

Clinical Features Skin photosensitivity, which differs from that in other porphyrias, usually begins in childhood and consists of pain, redness, and itching occurring within minutes of sunlight exposure (Fig. 430-4). Photosensitivity is associated with substantial elevations in erythrocyte protoporphyrin and occurs only in patients with genotypes that result in ferrochelatase activities below ~35% of normal. Vesicular lesions are uncommon. Redness, swelling, burning, and itching can develop shortly after sun exposure and resemble angioedema. Pain symptoms may seem out of proportion to the visible skin involvement. Sparse vesicles and bullae occur in ~10% of cases. Chronic skin changes may include lichenification, leathery pseudovesicles, labial grooving, and nail changes. Severe scarring is rare, as are pigment changes, friability, and hirsutism. Unless hepatic or other complications develop, protoporphyrin levels and symptoms of photosensitivity remain remarkably stable over many years in most patients. Factors that exacerbate the hepatic porphyrias play little or no role in EPP.

The primary source of excess protoporphyrin is the bone marrow reticulocytes. Erythrocyte protoporphyrin is free (not complexed with zinc) and is mostly bound to hemoglobin. In plasma, protoporphyrin is bound to albumin. Hemolysis and anemia are usually absent or mild.

Although EPP is an erythropoietic porphyria, up to 20% of EPP patients may have minor abnormalities of liver function, and in about 5% of these patients the accumulation of protoporphyrins causes chronic liver disease that can progress to liver failure and death. Protoporphyrin is insoluble, and excess amounts form crystalline structures in liver cells (Fig. 430-4) and can decrease hepatic bile flow. Studies in the mouse model of EPP have shown that the bile duct epithelium may be damaged by toxic bile, leading to biliary fibrosis. Thus, rapidly progressive liver disease appears to be related to the cholestatic effects of protoporphyrins and is associated with increasing hepatic protoporphyrin levels due to impaired hepatobiliary excretion and increased photosensitivity. The hepatic complications also are often characterized by increasing levels of protoporphyrins in erythrocytes and plasma as well as severe abdominal and back pains, especially in the right upper quadrant. Gallstones

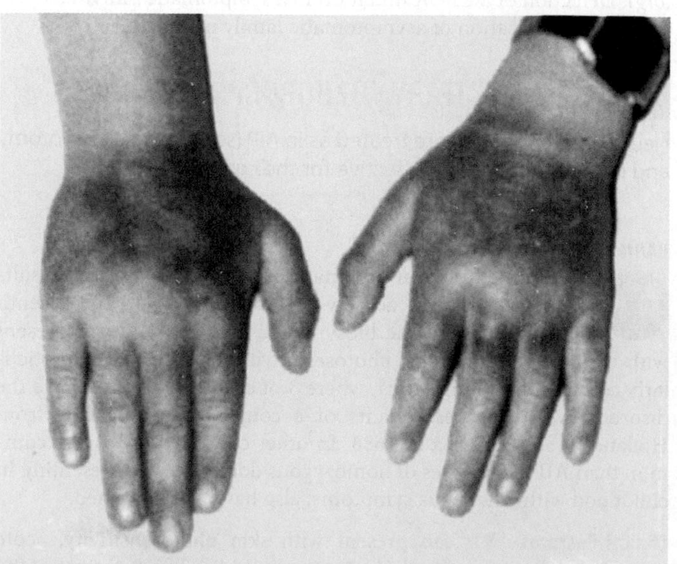

FIGURE 430-4 Erythema and edema of the hands due to acute photosensitivity in a 10-year-old boy with erythropoietic protoporphyria. *(From P Poblette-Gutierrez et al: Eur J Dermatol 16:230, 2006.)*

composed at least in part of protoporphyrin occur in some patients. Hepatic complications appear to be higher in autosomal recessive EPP due to two *FECH* mutations and in XLP.

Diagnosis A substantial increase in erythrocyte protoporphyrin, which is predominantly free and not complexed with zinc, is the hallmark of EPP. Protoporphyrin levels are also variably increased in bone marrow, plasma, bile, and feces. Erythrocyte protoporphyrin concentrations are increased in other conditions such as lead poisoning, iron deficiency, various hemolytic disorders, all homozygous forms of other porphyrias, and sometimes even in acute porphyrias. In all these conditions, however, in contrast to EPP, protoporphyrin is complexed with zinc. Therefore, after an increase in erythrocyte protoporphyrin is found in a suspected EPP patient, it is important to confirm the diagnosis by an assay that distinguishes free and zinc-complexed protoporphyrin. Erythrocytes in EPP also exhibit red fluorescence under a fluorescence microscopy at 620 nm. Urinary levels of porphyrins and porphyrin precursors are normal. Ferrochelatase activity in cultured lymphocytes or fibroblasts is decreased. DNA diagnosis by mutation analysis is recommended to detect the causative *FECH* mutation(s) and/or the presence of the IVS3-48T>C low expression allele. To date, over 190 mutations have been identified in the *FECH* gene, many of which result in an unstable or absent enzyme protein (null alleles) (Human Gene Mutation Database; *www.hgmd.org*). Studies suggest that EPP patients with a null allele (and the IVS3-48T>C low expression allele) have a greater risk for developing severe liver complications.

In XLP, the erythrocyte protoporphyrin levels appear to be higher than other forms of EPP and the proportions of free and zinc protoporphyrins may reach 50%. To date, four *ALAS2* mutations, three deletions of one to four bases, and one novel nonsense mutation have been described, which markedly increase ALA synthase 2 activity and cause XLP. XLP accounts for about 2% of patients with the EPP phenotype in Western Europe. Recent studies show that about 10% of North American patients with the EPP phenotype have XLP.

TREATMENT ERYTHROPOIETIC PROTOPORPHYRIA

Avoiding sunlight exposure and wearing clothing designed to provide protection for conditions with chronic photosensitivity are essential. Oral β-carotene (120–180 mg/dL) may improve tolerance to sunlight in some patients. The beneficial effects of β-carotene may involve quenching of singlet oxygen or free radicals. The dosage may need to be adjusted to maintain serum carotene levels in the recommended range of 10–15 mmol/L (600–800 mg/dL). Mild skin discoloration due to carotenemia is the only significant side effect. Afamelanotide, an α-melanocyte-stimulating hormone (MSH) analogue has completed phase III clinical trials in the United States for patients with EPP and XLP.

Treatment of hepatic complications, which may be accompanied by motor neuropathy, is difficult. Cholestyramine and other porphyrin absorbents such as activated charcoal may interrupt the enterohepatic circulation of protoporphyrin and promote its fecal excretion, leading to some improvement. Splenectomy may be helpful when the disease is accompanied by hemolysis and significant splenomegaly. Plasmapheresis and intravenous hemin are sometimes beneficial.

Liver transplantation has been carried out in some EPP and XLP patients with severe liver complications and is often successful in the short term. However, the disease often recurs in the transplanted liver due to continued bone marrow production of excess protoporphyrin. In a retrospective study of 17 liver-transplanted EPP patients, 11 (65%) had recurrent EPP liver disease. Posttransplantation treatment with hematin and plasmapheresis should be considered to prevent the recurrence of liver disease. However, bone marrow transplantation, which has been successful in human EPP and which prevented liver disease in a mouse model, should be considered after liver transplantation, if a suitable donor can be found.

ACKNOWLEDGMENT

The authors thank Dr. Karl E. Anderson for his review of the manuscript and helpful comments and suggestions. This work is supported in part by the Porphyrias Consortium (U54 DK083909), a part of the National Institutes of Health (NIH) Rare Disease Clinical Research Network (RDCRN), supported through collaboration between the NIH Office of Rare Diseases Research (ORDR) at the National Center for Advancing Translational Science (NCATS), and the National Institute of Diabetes and Digestive and Kidney Diseases (NIDDK). The content is solely the responsibility of the authors and does not necessarily represent the official views of the National Institutes of Health. MB is supported by a career development award K23-DK-095946

431e Disorders of Purine and Pyrimidine Metabolism

Christopher M. Burns, Robert L. Wortmann

This is a digital-only chapter. It is available on the DVD that accompanies this book, as well as on Access Medicine/Harrison's Online, and the eBook and "app" editions of HPIM 19e.

Purines (adenine and guanine) and pyrimidines (cytosine, thymine, uracil) serve fundamental roles in the replication of genetic material, gene transcription, protein synthesis, and cellular metabolism. Disorders that involve abnormalities of nucleotide metabolism range from relatively common diseases such as hyperuricemia and gout, in which there is increased production or impaired excretion of a metabolic end product of purine metabolism (uric acid), to rare enzyme deficiencies that affect purine and pyrimidine synthesis or degradation. Understanding these biochemical pathways has led, in some instances, to the development of specific forms of treatment, such as the use of allopurinol and febuxostat to reduce uric acid production.

432e Lysosomal Storage Diseases

Robert J. Hopkin, Gregory A. Grabowski

This is a digital-only chapter. It is available on the DVD that accompanies this book, as well as on Access Medicine/Harrison's Online, and the eBook and "app" editions of HPIM 19e.

Lysosomes are heterogeneous subcellular organelles containing specific hydrolyses that allow selective processing or degradation of proteins, nucleic acids, carbohydrates, and lipids. There are more than 40 different lysosomal storage diseases (LSDs), classified according to the nature of the stored material. Several of the most prevalent disorders are reviewed here: Tay-Sachs disease, Fabry disease, Gaucher disease, Niemann-Pick disease, lysosomal acid lipase deficiencies, the mucopolysaccharidoses, and Pompe disease. LSDs should be considered in the differential diagnosis of patients with neurologic, renal, or muscular degeneration and/or unexplained hepatomegaly, splenomegaly, cardiomyopathy, or skeletal dysplasias and deformations. Physical findings are disease specific, and enzyme assays or genetic testing can be used to make a definitive diagnosis. Although the nosology of LSDs segregates the variants into distinct phenotypes, these are heuristic; in the clinic, each disease exhibits—to some degree—a continuous spectrum of manifestations, from severe to attenuated variants.

433e Glycogen Storage Diseases and Other Inherited Disorders of Carbohydrate Metabolism

Priya S. Kishnani, Yuan-Tsong Chen

This is a digital-only chapter. It is available on the DVD that accompanies this book, as well as on Access Medicine/Harrison's Online, and the eBook and "app" editions of HPIM 19e.

Carbohydrate metabolism plays a vital role in cellular function by providing the energy required for most metabolic processes. Glucose is the principal substrate of energy metabolism in humans. Metabolism of glucose generates ATP through glycolysis and mitochondrial oxidative phosphorylation. The body obtains glucose through the ingestion of polysaccharides (primarily starch) and disaccharides (e.g., lactose, maltose, and sucrose). Galactose and fructose are two other monosaccharides that serve as sources of fuel for cellular metabolism; however, their role as fuel sources is much less significant than that of glucose. Galactose is derived from lactose (galactose + glucose), which is found in milk products, and is an important component of certain glycolipids, glycoproteins, and glycosaminoglycans. Fructose is found in fruits, vegetables, and honey. Sucrose (fructose + glucose) is another dietary source of fructose and is a commonly used sweetener.

434e Inherited Disorders of Amino Acid Metabolism in Adults

Nicola Longo

This is a digital-only chapter. It is available on the DVD that accompanies this book, as well as on Access Medicine/Harrison's Online, and the eBook and "app" editions of HPIM 19e.

Amino acids are not only the building blocks of proteins but also serve as neurotransmitters (glycine, glutamate, γ-aminobutyric acid) or as precursors of hormones, coenzymes, pigments, purines, or pyrimidines. Eight amino acids, referred to as *essential*, cannot be synthesized by humans and must be obtained from dietary sources. The others are formed endogenously. Each amino acid has a unique degradative pathway by which its nitrogen and carbon components are used for the synthesis of other amino acids, carbohydrates, and lipids. Disorders of amino acid metabolism and transport (Chap. 435e) are individually rare—the incidences range from 1 in 10,000 for cystinuria or phenylketonuria to 1 in 200,000 for homocystinuria or alkaptonuria—but collectively, they affect perhaps 1 in 1000 newborns. Almost all are transmitted as autosomal recessive traits.

435e Inherited Defects of Membrane Transport

Nicola Longo

This is a digital-only chapter. It is available on the DVD that accompanies this book, as well as on Access Medicine/Harrison's Online, and the eBook and "app" editions of HPIM 19e.

Specific membrane transporters mediate the passage of a wide variety of substances across cellular membranes. Classes of substrates include amino acids, sugars, cations, anions, vitamins, and water. The number of inherited disorders of membrane transport continues to increase with the identification of new transporters on the plasma membrane or intracellular organelles and the clarification of the molecular basis of diseases with previously unknown pathophysiology. The first transport disorders identified affected the gut or the kidney, but transport processes are now proving essential for the normal function of every organ. Mutations in transporter molecules cause disorders of the heart, muscle, brain, and endocrine and sensory organs. Inherited defects impairing the transport of selected amino acids that can present in adults are discussed here as examples of the abnormalities encountered; others are considered elsewhere in this text.

436e Atlas of Clinical Manifestations of Metabolic Diseases

J. Larry Jameson

This is a digital-only chapter. It is available on the DVD that accompanies this book, as well as on Access Medicine/Harrison's Online, and the eBook and "app" editions of HPIM 19e.

The term *metabolism* is derived from the Greek *metabol,* meaning "to change." This term encompasses the broad array of chemical pathways that are necessary for normal development and homeostasis. In practice, clinicians generally use the term *metabolism* in reference to energy utilization for anabolism or catabolism. Alternatively, intermediary metabolism describes the myriad cellular pathways that convert energy sources from one form to another (e.g., the citric acid cycle). The emerging field of *metabolomics* is based on the premise that the identification and measurement of metabolic products will enhance our understanding of physiology and disease.

SECTION 1 DIAGNOSIS OF NEUROLOGIC DISORDERS

437 Approach to the Patient with Neurologic Disease

Daniel H. Lowenstein, Joseph B. Martin, Stephen L. Hauser

Neurologic diseases are common and costly. According to estimates by the World Health Organization, neurologic disorders affect over 1 billion people worldwide, constitute 12% of the global burden of disease, and cause 14% of global deaths (Table 437-1). These numbers are only expected to increase as the world's population ages. Most patients with neurologic symptoms seek care from internists and other generalists rather than from neurologists. Because therapies now exist for many neurologic disorders, a skillful approach to diagnosis is essential. Errors commonly result from an overreliance on costly neuroimaging procedures and laboratory tests, which, while useful, do not substitute for an adequate history and examination. The proper approach to the patient with a neurologic illness begins with the patient and focuses the clinical problem first in anatomic and then in pathophysiologic terms; only then should a specific diagnosis be entertained. This method ensures that technology is judiciously applied, a correct diagnosis is established in an efficient manner, and treatment is promptly initiated.

THE NEUROLOGIC METHOD

DEFINE THE ANATOMY

The first priority is to identify the region of the nervous system that is likely to be responsible for the symptoms. Can the disorder be mapped to one specific location, is it multifocal, or is a diffuse process present? Are the symptoms restricted to the nervous system, or do they arise in the context of a systemic illness? Is the problem in the central nervous system (CNS), the peripheral nervous system (PNS), or both? If in the CNS, is the cerebral cortex, basal ganglia, brainstem, cerebellum, or spinal cord responsible? Are the pain-sensitive meninges involved? If in the PNS, could the disorder be located in peripheral nerves and, if so, are motor or sensory nerves primarily affected, or is a lesion in the neuromuscular junction or muscle more likely?

The first clues to defining the anatomic area of involvement appear in the history, and the examination is then directed to confirm or rule out these impressions and to clarify uncertainties. A more detailed examination of a particular region of the CNS or PNS is often indicated.

TABLE 437-1 GLOBAL DISABILITY-ADJUSTED LIFE-YEARS (DALYs) AND NUMBER OF ANNUAL DEATHS FOR SELECTED NEUROLOGIC DISORDERS IN 2010

Disorder	DALYs	Deaths
Low back and neck pain	116,704,000	—
Cerebrovascular diseases	102,232,000	5,874,000
Meningitis and encephalitis	26,540,000	541,000
Migraine	22,362,000	—
Epilepsy	17,429,000	177,000
Dementia	11,349,000	485,000
Parkinson's disease	1,918,000	111,000
% of total DALYs or deaths for all causes that are neurologic	**12.0%**	**13.6%**
% change of DALYs for neurologic disorders between 2000 and 2010	**51.6%**	**114.3%**

Source: R Lozano et al: Lancet 380: 2095, 2012.

For example, the examination of a patient who presents with a history of ascending paresthesias and weakness should be directed toward deciding, among other things, if the location of the lesion is in the spinal cord or peripheral nerves. Focal back pain, a spinal cord sensory level, and incontinence suggest a spinal cord origin, whereas a stocking-glove pattern of sensory loss suggests peripheral nerve disease; areflexia usually indicates peripheral neuropathy but may also be present with spinal shock in acute spinal cord disorders.

Deciding "where the lesion is" accomplishes the task of limiting the possible etiologies to a manageable, finite number. In addition, this strategy safeguards against making serious errors. Symptoms of recurrent vertigo, diplopia, and nystagmus should not trigger "multiple sclerosis" as an answer (etiology) but "brainstem" or "pons" (location); then a diagnosis of brainstem arteriovenous malformation will not be missed for lack of consideration. Similarly, the combination of optic neuritis and spastic ataxic paraparesis suggests optic nerve and spinal cord disease; multiple sclerosis (MS), CNS syphilis, and vitamin B_{12} deficiency are treatable disorders that can produce this syndrome. Once the question, "Where is the lesion?" is answered, then the question, "What is the lesion?" can be addressed.

IDENTIFY THE PATHOPHYSIOLOGY

Clues to the pathophysiology of the disease process may also be present in the history. Primary neuronal (gray matter) disorders may present as early cognitive disturbances, movement disorders, or seizures, whereas white matter involvement produces predominantly "long tract" disorders of motor, sensory, visual, and cerebellar pathways. Progressive and symmetric symptoms often have a metabolic or degenerative origin; in such cases lesions are usually not sharply circumscribed. Thus, a patient with paraparesis and a clear spinal cord sensory level is unlikely to have vitamin B_{12} deficiency as the explanation. A Lhermitte symptom (electric shock–like sensations evoked by neck flexion) is due to ectopic impulse generation in white matter pathways and occurs with demyelination in the cervical spinal cord; among many possible causes, this symptom may indicate MS in a young adult or compressive cervical spondylosis in an older person. Symptoms that worsen after exposure to heat or exercise may indicate conduction block in demyelinated axons, as occurs in MS. A patient with recurrent episodes of diplopia and dysarthria associated with exercise or fatigue may have a disorder of neuromuscular transmission such as myasthenia gravis. Slowly advancing visual scotoma with luminous edges, termed *fortification spectra*, indicates spreading cortical depression, typically with migraine.

THE NEUROLOGIC HISTORY

Attention to the description of the symptoms experienced by the patient and substantiated by family members and others often permits an accurate localization and determination of the probable cause of the complaints, even before the neurologic examination is performed. The history also helps to bring a focus to the neurologic examination that follows. Each complaint should be pursued as far as possible to elucidate the location of the lesion, the likely underlying pathophysiology, and potential etiologies. For example, a patient complains of weakness of the right arm. What are the associated features? Does the patient have difficulty with brushing hair or reaching upward (proximal) or buttoning buttons or opening a twist-top bottle (distal)? Negative associations may also be crucial. A patient with a right hemiparesis without a language deficit likely has a lesion (internal capsule, brainstem, or spinal cord) different from that of a patient with a right hemiparesis and aphasia (left hemisphere). Other pertinent features of the history include the following:

1. *Temporal course of the illness.* It is important to determine the precise time of appearance and rate of progression of the symptoms experienced by the patient. The rapid onset of a neurologic complaint, occurring within seconds or minutes, usually indicates a vascular event, a seizure, or migraine. The onset of sensory symptoms located in one extremity that spread over a few seconds to adjacent portions of that extremity and then to the other regions of the body suggests a seizure. A more gradual onset and less well-localized symptoms point to the possibility of a transient ischemic attack (TIA). A similar but slower temporal march of symptoms accompanied by headache, nausea, or visual disturbance suggests migraine. The presence of "positive" sensory symptoms (e.g., tingling or sensations that are difficult to describe) or involuntary motor movements suggests a seizure; in contrast, transient loss of function (negative symptoms) suggests a TIA. A stuttering onset where symptoms appear, stabilize, and then progress over hours or days also suggests cerebrovascular disease; an additional history of transient remission or regression indicates that the process is more likely due to ischemia rather than hemorrhage. A gradual evolution of symptoms over hours or days suggests a toxic, metabolic, infectious, or inflammatory process. Progressing symptoms associated with the systemic manifestations of fever, stiff neck, and altered level of consciousness imply an infectious process. Relapsing and remitting symptoms involving different levels of the nervous system suggest MS or other inflammatory processes. Slowly progressive symptoms without remissions are characteristic of neurodegenerative disorders, chronic infections, gradual intoxications, and neoplasms.
2. *Patients' descriptions of the complaint.* The same words often mean different things to different patients. "Dizziness" may imply impending syncope, a sense of disequilibrium, or true spinning vertigo. "Numbness" may mean a complete loss of feeling, a positive sensation such as tingling, or even weakness. "Blurred vision" may be used to describe unilateral visual loss, as in transient monocular blindness, or diplopia. The interpretation of the true meaning of the words used by patients to describe symptoms obviously becomes even more complex when there are differences in primary languages and cultures.
3. *Corroboration of the history by others.* It is almost always helpful to obtain additional information from family, friends, or other observers to corroborate or expand the patient's description. Memory loss, aphasia, loss of insight, intoxication, and other factors may impair the patient's capacity to communicate normally with the examiner or prevent openness about factors that have contributed to the illness. Episodes of loss of consciousness necessitate that details be sought from observers to ascertain precisely what has happened during the event.
4. *Family history.* Many neurologic disorders have an underlying genetic component. The presence of a Mendelian disorder, such as Huntington's disease or Charcot-Marie-Tooth neuropathy, is often obvious if family data are available. More detailed questions about family history are often necessary in polygenic disorders such as MS, migraine, and many types of epilepsy. It is important to elicit family history about all illnesses, in addition to neurologic and psychiatric disorders. A familial propensity to hypertension or heart disease is relevant in a patient who presents with a stroke. There are numerous inherited neurologic diseases that are associated with multisystem manifestations that may provide clues to the correct diagnosis (e.g., neurofibromatosis, Wilson's disease, mitochondrial disorders).
5. *Medical illnesses.* Many neurologic diseases occur in the context of systemic disorders. Diabetes mellitus, hypertension, and abnormalities of blood lipids predispose to cerebrovascular disease. A solitary mass lesion in the brain may be an abscess in a patient with valvular heart disease, a primary hemorrhage in a patient with a coagulopathy, a lymphoma or toxoplasmosis in a patient with AIDS, or a metastasis in a patient with underlying cancer. Patients with malignancy may also present with a neurologic paraneoplastic syndrome (Chap. 122) or complications from chemotherapy or radiotherapy. Marfan's syndrome and related collagen disorders predispose to dissection of the cranial arteries and aneurysmal subarachnoid hemorrhage; the latter may also occur with polycystic kidney disease. Various neurologic disorders occur with dysthyroid states or other endocrinopathies. It is especially important to look for the presence of systemic diseases in patients with peripheral neuropathy. Most patients with coma in a hospital setting have a metabolic, toxic, or infectious cause.
6. *Drug use and abuse and toxin exposure.* It is essential to inquire about the history of drug use, both prescribed and illicit. Sedatives, antidepressants, and other psychoactive medications are frequently associated with acute confusional states, especially in the elderly. Aminoglycoside antibiotics may exacerbate symptoms of weakness in patients with disorders of neuromuscular transmission, such as myasthenia gravis, and may cause dizziness secondary to ototoxicity. Vincristine and other antineoplastic drugs can cause peripheral neuropathy, and immunosuppressive agents such as cyclosporine can produce encephalopathy. Excessive vitamin ingestion can lead to disease; examples include vitamin A and pseudotumor cerebri or pyridoxine and peripheral neuropathy. Many patients are unaware that over-the-counter sleeping pills, cold preparations, and diet pills are actually drugs. Alcohol, the most prevalent neurotoxin, is often not recognized as such by patients, and other drugs of abuse such as cocaine and heroin can cause a wide range of neurologic abnormalities. A history of environmental or industrial exposure to neurotoxins may provide an essential clue; consultation with the patient's coworkers or employer may be required.
7. *Formulating an impression of the patient.* Use the opportunity while taking the history to form an impression of the patient. Is the information forthcoming, or does it take a circuitous course? Is there evidence of anxiety, depression, or hypochondriasis? Are there any clues to problems with language, memory, insight, comportment, or behavior? The neurologic assessment begins as soon as the patient comes into the room and the first introduction is made.

THE NEUROLOGIC EXAMINATION

The neurologic examination is challenging and complex; it has many components and includes a number of skills that can be mastered only through repeated use of the same techniques on a large number of individuals with and without neurologic disease. Mastery of the complete neurologic examination is usually important only for physicians in neurology and associated specialties. However, knowledge of the basics of the examination, especially those components that are effective in screening for neurologic dysfunction, is essential for all clinicians, especially generalists.

There is no single, universally accepted sequence of the examination that must be followed, but most clinicians begin with assessment of mental status followed by the cranial nerves, motor system, reflexes, sensory system, coordination, and gait. Whether the examination is basic or comprehensive, it is essential that it be performed in an orderly and systematic fashion to avoid errors and serious omissions. Thus, the best way to learn and gain expertise in the examination is to choose one's own approach and practice it frequently and do it in the same exact sequence each time.

The detailed description that follows describes the more commonly used parts of the neurologic examination, with a particular emphasis on the components that are considered most helpful for the assessment of common neurologic problems. Each section also includes a brief description of the minimal examination necessary to adequately screen for abnormalities in a patient who has no symptoms suggesting neurologic dysfunction. A screening examination done in this way can be completed in 3–5 min.

Several additional points about the examination are worth noting. First, in recording observations, it is important to describe what is found rather than to apply a poorly defined medical term (e.g., "patient groans to sternal rub" rather than "obtunded"). Second, subtle CNS abnormalities are best detected by carefully comparing a patient's performance on tasks that require simultaneous activation of both cerebral hemispheres (e.g., eliciting a pronator drift of an outstretched arm with the eyes closed; extinction on one side of bilaterally applied light touch, also with eyes closed; or decreased arm swing or a slight asymmetry when walking). Third, if the patient's complaint is brought on by some activity, reproduce the activity in the office. If the complaint is of dizziness when the head is turned in one direction, have the patient do this and also look for associated signs on examination (e.g., nystagmus or dysmetria). If pain occurs after walking two blocks, have the patient leave the office and walk this distance and immediately return, and repeat the relevant parts of the examination. Finally, the use of tests that are individually tailored to the patient's problem can be of value in assessing changes over time. Tests of walking a 7.5-m (25-ft) distance (normal, 5–6 s; note assistance, if any), repetitive finger or toe tapping (normal, 20–25 taps in 5 s), or handwriting are examples.

MENTAL STATUS EXAMINATION

- *The bare minimum: During the interview, look for difficulties with communication and determine whether the patient has recall and insight into recent and past events.*

The mental status examination is under way as soon as the physician begins observing and speaking with the patient. If the history raises any concern for abnormalities of higher cortical function or if cognitive problems are observed during the interview, then detailed testing of the mental status is indicated. The patient's ability to understand the language used for the examination, cultural background, educational experience, sensory or motor problems, or comorbid conditions need to be factored into the applicability of the tests and interpretation of results.

The Folstein mini-mental status examination (MMSE) is a standardized screening examination of cognitive function that is extremely easy to administer and takes <10 min to complete. Using age-adjusted values for defining normal performance, the test is ~85% sensitive and 85% specific for making the diagnosis of dementia that is moderate or severe, especially in educated patients. When there is sufficient time available, the MMSE is one of the best methods for documenting the current mental status of the patient, and this is especially useful as a baseline assessment to which future scores of the MMSE can be compared.

Individual elements of the mental status examination can be subdivided into level of consciousness, orientation, speech and language, memory, fund of information, insight and judgment, abstract thought, and calculations.

Level of consciousness is the patient's relative state of awareness of the self and the environment, and ranges from fully awake to comatose. When the patient is not fully awake, the examiner should describe the responses to the minimum stimulus necessary to elicit a reaction, ranging from verbal commands to a brief, painful stimulus such as a squeeze of the trapezius muscle. Responses that are directed toward the stimulus and signify some degree of intact cerebral function (e.g., opening the eyes and looking at the examiner or reaching to push away a painful stimulus) must be distinguished from reflex responses of a spinal origin (e.g., triple flexion response—flexion at the ankle, knee, and hip in response to a painful stimulus to the foot).

Orientation is tested by asking the person to state his or her name, location, and time (day of the week and date); time is usually the first to be affected in a variety of conditions.

Speech is assessed by observing articulation, rate, rhythm, and prosody (i.e., the changes in pitch and accentuation of syllables and words).

Language is assessed by observing the content of the patient's verbal and written output, response to spoken commands, and ability to read. A typical testing sequence is to ask the patient to name successively more detailed components of clothing, a watch, or a pen; repeat the phrase "No ifs, ands, or buts"; follow a three-step, verbal command; write a sentence; and read and respond to a written command.

Memory should be analyzed according to three main time scales: (1) immediate memory is assessed by saying a list of three items and having the patient repeat the list immediately; (2) short-term memory is tested by asking the patient to recall the same three items 5 and 15 min later; and (3) long-term memory is evaluated by determining how well the patient is able to provide a coherent chronologic history of his or her illness or personal events.

Fund of information is assessed by asking questions about major historic or current events, with special attention to educational level and life experiences.

Abnormalities of *insight and judgment* are usually detected during the patient interview; a more detailed assessment can be elicited by asking the patient to describe how he or she would respond to situations having a variety of potential outcomes (e.g., "What would you do if you found a wallet on the sidewalk?").

Abstract thought can be tested by asking the patient to describe similarities between various objects or concepts (e.g., apple and orange, desk and chair, poetry and sculpture) or to list items having the same attributes (e.g., a list of four-legged animals).

Calculation ability is assessed by having the patient carry out a computation that is appropriate to the patient's age and education (e.g., serial subtraction of 7 from 100 or 3 from 20; or word problems involving simple arithmetic).

CRANIAL NERVE EXAMINATION

- *The bare minimum: Check the fundi, visual fields, pupil size and reactivity, extraocular movements, and facial movements.*

The cranial nerves (CN) are best examined in numerical order, except for grouping together CN III, IV, and VI because of their similar function.

CN I (Olfactory) Testing is often omitted unless there is suspicion for inferior frontal lobe disease (e.g., meningioma). With eyes closed, ask the patient to sniff a mild stimulus such as toothpaste or coffee and identify the odorant.

CN II (Optic) Check visual acuity (with eyeglasses or contact lens correction) using a Snellen chart or similar tool. Test the visual fields by confrontation, i.e., by comparing the patient's visual fields to your own. As a screening test, it is usually sufficient to examine the visual fields of both eyes simultaneously; individual eye fields should be tested if there is any reason to suspect a problem of vision by the history or other elements of the examination, or if the screening test reveals an abnormality. Face the patient at a distance of approximately 0.6–1.0 m (2–3 ft) and place your hands at the periphery of your visual fields in the plane that is equidistant between you and the patient. Instruct the patient to look directly at the center of your face and to indicate when and where he or she sees one of your fingers moving. Beginning with the two inferior quadrants and then the two superior quadrants, move your index finger of the right hand, left hand, or both hands simultaneously and observe whether the patient detects the movements. A single small-amplitude movement of the finger is sufficient for a normal response. Focal perimetry and tangent screen examinations should be used to map out visual field defects fully or to search for subtle abnormalities. Optic fundi should be examined with an ophthalmoscope, and the color, size, and degree of swelling or elevation of the optic disc noted, as well as the color and texture of the retina. The retinal vessels should be checked for size, regularity, arteriovenous nicking at crossing points, hemorrhage, exudates, etc.

CN III, IV, VI (Oculomotor, Trochlear, Abducens) Describe the size and shape of pupils and reaction to light and accommodation (i.e., as the eyes converge while following your finger as it moves toward the bridge of the nose). To check extraocular movements, ask the patient to keep his or her head still while tracking the movement of the tip of your finger. Move the target slowly in the horizontal and vertical planes; observe any paresis, nystagmus, or abnormalities of smooth pursuit (saccades, oculomotor ataxia, etc.). If necessary, the relative position of the two eyes, both in primary and multidirectional gaze, can be assessed by comparing the reflections of a bright light off both pupils. However, in practice it is typically more useful to determine whether the patient describes diplopia in any direction of gaze; true diplopia should almost always resolve with one eye closed. Horizontal nystagmus is best assessed at 45° and not at extreme lateral gaze (which is uncomfortable for the patient); the target must often be held at the lateral position for at least a few seconds to detect an abnormality.

CN V (Trigeminal) Examine sensation within the three territories of the branches of the trigeminal nerve (ophthalmic, maxillary, and mandibular) on each side of the face. As with other parts of the sensory examination, testing of two sensory modalities derived from different anatomic pathways (e.g., light touch and temperature) is sufficient for a screening examination. Testing of other modalities, the corneal reflex, and the motor component of CN V (jaw clench—masseter muscle) is indicated when suggested by the history.

CN VII (Facial) Look for facial asymmetry at rest and with spontaneous movements. Test eyebrow elevation, forehead wrinkling, eye closure, smiling, and cheek puff. Look in particular for differences in the lower versus upper facial muscles; weakness of the lower two-thirds of the face with preservation of the upper third suggests an upper motor neuron lesion, whereas weakness of an entire side suggests a lower motor neuron lesion.

CN VIII (Vestibulocochlear) Check the patient's ability to hear a finger rub or whispered voice with each ear. Further testing for air versus mastoid bone conduction (Rinne) and lateralization of a 512-Hz tuning fork placed at the center of the forehead (Weber) should be done if an abnormality is detected by history or examination. Any suspected problem should be followed up with formal audiometry. For further discussion of assessing vestibular nerve function in the setting of dizziness, hearing loss, or coma, see Chaps. 28, 43, and 328, respectively.

CN IX, X (Glossopharyngeal, Vagus) Observe the position and symmetry of the palate and uvula at rest and with phonation ("aah"). The pharyngeal ("gag") reflex is evaluated by stimulating the posterior pharyngeal wall on each side with a sterile, blunt object (e.g., tongue blade), but the reflex is often absent in normal individuals.

CN XI (Spinal Accessory) Check shoulder shrug (trapezius muscle) and head rotation to each side (sternocleidomastoid) against resistance.

CN XII (Hypoglossal) Inspect the tongue for atrophy or fasciculations, position with protrusion, and strength when extended against the inner surface of the cheeks on each side.

MOTOR EXAMINATION

- *The bare minimum: Look for muscle atrophy and check extremity tone. Assess upper extremity strength by checking for pronator drift and strength of wrist or finger extensors. Assess lower extremity strength by checking strength of the toe extensors and having the patient walk normally and on heels and toes.*

The motor examination includes observations of muscle appearance, tone, and strength. Although gait is in part a test of motor function, it is usually evaluated separately at the end of the examination.

Appearance Inspect and palpate muscle groups under good light and with the patient in a comfortable and symmetric position. Check for muscle fasciculations, tenderness, and atrophy or hypertrophy. Involuntary movements may be present at rest (e.g., tics, myoclonus, choreoathetosis), during maintained posture (pill-rolling tremor of Parkinson's disease), or with voluntary movements (intention tremor of cerebellar disease or familial tremor).

Tone Muscle tone is tested by measuring the resistance to passive movement of a relaxed limb. Patients often have difficulty relaxing during this procedure, so it is useful to distract the patient to minimize active movements. In the upper limbs, tone is assessed by rapid pronation and supination of the forearm and flexion and extension at the wrist. In the lower limbs, while the patient is supine the examiner's hands are placed behind the knees and rapidly raised; with normal tone, the ankles drag along the table surface for a variable distance before rising, whereas increased tone results in an immediate lift of the heel off the surface. Decreased tone is most commonly due to lower motor neuron or peripheral nerve disorders. Increased tone may be evident as spasticity (resistance determined by the angle and velocity of motion; corticospinal tract disease), rigidity (similar resistance in all angles of motion; extrapyramidal disease), or paratonia (fluctuating changes in resistance; frontal lobe pathways or normal difficulty in relaxing). Cogwheel rigidity, in which passive motion elicits jerky interruptions in resistance, is seen in parkinsonism.

Strength Testing for pronator drift is an extremely useful method for screening upper limb weakness. The patient is asked to hold both arms fully extended and parallel to the ground with eyes closed. This position should be maintained for ~10 s; any flexion at the elbow or fingers or pronation of the forearm, especially if asymmetric, is a sign of potential weakness. Muscle strength is further assessed by having the patient exert maximal effort for the particular muscle or muscle group being tested. It is important to isolate the muscles as much as possible, i.e., hold the limb so that only the muscles of interest are active. It is also helpful to palpate accessible muscles as they contract. Grading muscle strength and evaluating the patient's effort is an art that takes time and practice. Muscle strength is traditionally graded using the following scale:

0 = no movement
1 = flicker or trace of contraction but no associated movement at a joint
2 = movement with gravity eliminated
3 = movement against gravity but not against resistance
4− = movement against a mild degree of resistance
4 = movement against moderate resistance
4+ = movement against strong resistance
5 = full power

However, in many cases, it is more practical to use the following terms:

Paralysis = no movement
Severe weakness = movement with gravity eliminated
Moderate weakness = movement against gravity but not against mild resistance
Mild weakness = movement against moderate resistance
Full strength

Noting the pattern of weakness is as important as assessing the magnitude of weakness. Unilateral or bilateral weakness of the upper limb extensors and lower limb flexors ("pyramidal weakness") suggests a lesion of the pyramidal tract, bilateral proximal weakness suggests myopathy, and bilateral distal weakness suggests peripheral neuropathy.

REFLEX EXAMINATION

- *The bare minimum: Check the biceps, patellar, and Achilles reflexes.*

Muscle Stretch Reflexes Those that are typically assessed include the biceps (C5, C6), brachioradialis (C5, C6), and triceps (C7, C8) reflexes in the upper limbs and the patellar or quadriceps (L3, L4) and Achilles (S1, S2) reflexes in the lower limbs. The patient should be relaxed and the muscle positioned midway between full contraction and extension. Reflexes may be enhanced by asking the patient to voluntarily contract other, distant muscle groups (Jendrassik maneuver). For example, upper limb reflexes may be reinforced by voluntary teeth-clenching, and the Achilles reflex by hooking the flexed fingers of the two hands together and attempting to pull them apart. For each reflex tested, the two sides should be tested sequentially, and it is important to determine the smallest stimulus required to elicit a reflex rather than the maximum response. Reflexes are graded according to the following scale:

0 = absent
1 = present but diminished
2 = normoactive
3 = exaggerated
4 = clonus

Cutaneous Reflexes The plantar reflex is elicited by stroking, with a noxious stimulus such as a tongue blade, the lateral surface of the sole of the foot beginning near the heel and moving across the ball of the foot to the great toe. The normal reflex consists of plantar flexion of the toes. With upper motor neuron lesions above the S1 level of the spinal cord, a paradoxical extension of the toe is observed, associated with fanning and extension of the other toes (termed an *extensor plantar response*, or *Babinski sign*). However, despite its popularity, the reliability and validity of the Babinski sign for identifying upper motor neuron weakness is limited—it is far more useful to rely on tests of tone, strength, stretch reflexes, and coordination. Superficial abdominal reflexes are elicited by gently stroking the abdominal surface near the umbilicus in a diagonal fashion with a sharp object (e.g., the wooden end of a cotton-tipped swab) and observing the movement of the umbilicus. Normally, the umbilicus will pull toward the stimulated quadrant. With upper motor neuron lesions, these reflexes are absent. They are most helpful when there is preservation of the upper (spinal cord level T9) but not lower (T12) abdominal reflexes, indicating a spinal lesion between T9 and T12, or when the response is asymmetric. Other useful cutaneous reflexes include the cremasteric (ipsilateral elevation of the testicle following stroking of the medial thigh; mediated by L1 and L2) and anal (contraction of the anal sphincter when the perianal skin is scratched; mediated by S2, S3, S4) reflexes. It is particularly important to test for these reflexes in any patient with suspected injury to the spinal cord or lumbosacral roots.

Primitive Reflexes With disease of the frontal lobe pathways, several primitive reflexes not normally present in the adult may appear. The suck response is elicited by lightly touching with a tongue blade the center of the lips, and the root response the corner of the lips; the patient will move the lips to suck or root in the direction of the stimulus. The grasp reflex is elicited by touching the palm between the thumb and index finger with the examiner's fingers; a positive response is a forced grasp of the examiner's hand. In many instances, stroking the back of the hand will lead to its release. The palmomental response is contraction of the mentalis muscle (chin) ipsilateral to a scratch stimulus diagonally applied to the palm.

SENSORY EXAMINATION

- *The bare minimum: Ask whether the patient can feel light touch and the temperature of a cool object in each distal extremity. Check double simultaneous stimulation using light touch on the hands. Perform the Romberg maneuver.*

Evaluating sensation is usually the most unreliable part of the examination because it is subjective and is difficult to quantify. In the compliant and discerning patient, the sensory examination can be extremely helpful for the precise localization of a lesion. With patients who are uncooperative or lack an understanding of the tests, it may be useless. The examination should be focused on the suspected lesion. For example, in spinal cord, spinal root, or peripheral nerve abnormalities, all major sensory modalities should be tested while looking for a pattern consistent with a spinal level and dermatomal or nerve distribution. In patients with lesions at or above the brainstem, screening the primary sensory modalities in the distal extremities along with tests of "cortical" sensation is usually sufficient.

The five primary sensory modalities—light touch, pain, temperature, vibration, and joint position—are tested in each limb. Light touch is assessed by stimulating the skin with single, very gentle touches of the examiner's finger or a wisp of cotton. Pain is tested using a new pin, and temperature is assessed using a metal object (e.g., tuning fork) that has been immersed in cold and warm water. Vibration is tested using a 128-Hz tuning fork applied to the distal phalanx of the great toe or index finger just below the nail bed. By placing a finger on the opposite side of the joint being tested, the examiner compares the patient's threshold of vibration perception with his or her own. For joint position testing, the examiner grasps the digit or limb laterally and distal to the joint being assessed; small 1- to 2-mm excursions can usually be sensed. The Romberg maneuver is primarily a test of proprioception. The patient is asked to stand with the feet as close together as necessary to maintain balance while the eyes are open, and the eyes are then closed. A loss of balance with the eyes closed is an abnormal response.

"Cortical" sensation is mediated by the parietal lobes and represents an integration of the primary sensory modalities; testing cortical sensation is only meaningful when primary sensation is intact. Double simultaneous stimulation is especially useful as a screening test for cortical function; with the patient's eyes closed, the examiner lightly touches one or both hands and asks the patient to identify the stimuli. With a parietal lobe lesion, the patient may be unable to identify the stimulus on the contralateral side when both hands are touched. Other modalities relying on the parietal cortex include the discrimination of two closely placed stimuli as separate (two-point discrimination), identification of an object by touch and manipulation alone (stereognosis), and the identification of numbers or letters written on the skin surface (graphesthesia).

COORDINATION EXAMINATION

- *The bare minimum: Observe the patient at rest and during spontaneous movements. Test rapid alternating movements of the hands and feet and finger to nose.*

Coordination refers to the orchestration and fluidity of movements. Even simple acts require cooperation of agonist and antagonist muscles, maintenance of posture, and complex servomechanisms to control the rate and range of movements. Part of this integration relies on normal function of the cerebellar and basal ganglia systems. However, coordination also requires intact muscle strength and kinesthetic and proprioceptive information. Thus, if the examination has disclosed abnormalities of the motor or sensory systems, the patient's coordination should be assessed with these limitations in mind.

Rapid alternating movements in the upper limbs are tested separately on each side by having the patient make a fist, partially extend the index finger, and then tap the index finger on the distal thumb as quickly as possible. In the lower limb, the patient rapidly taps the foot against the floor or the examiner's hand. Finger-to-nose testing is primarily a test of cerebellar function; the patient is asked to touch his or her index finger repetitively to the nose and then to the examiner's outstretched finger, which moves with each repetition. A similar test in the lower extremity is to have the patient raise the leg and touch the examiner's finger with the great toe. Another cerebellar test in the lower limbs is the heel-knee-shin maneuver; in the supine position the patient is asked to slide the heel of each foot from the knee down the shin of the other leg. For all these movements, the accuracy, speed, and rhythm are noted.

GAIT EXAMINATION

- *The bare minimum: Observe the patient while walking normally, on the heels and toes, and along a straight line.*

Watching the patient walk is the most important part of the neurologic examination. Normal gait requires that multiple systems—including strength, sensation, and coordination—function in a highly integrated fashion. Unexpected abnormalities may be detected that prompt the examiner to return in more detail to other aspects of the examination. The patient should be observed while walking and turning normally, walking on the heels, walking on the toes, and walking heel-to-toe along a straight line. The examination may reveal decreased arm swing on one side (corticospinal tract disease), a stooped posture and short stepped gait (parkinsonism), a broad-based unstable gait (ataxia), scissoring (spasticity), or a high-stepped, slapping gait (posterior column or peripheral nerve disease), or the patient may appear to be stuck in place (apraxia with frontal lobe disease).

NEUROLOGIC DIAGNOSIS

The clinical data obtained from the history and examination are interpreted to arrive at an anatomic localization that best explains the clinical findings (Table 437-2), to narrow the list of diagnostic possibilities, and to select the laboratory tests most likely to be informative. The laboratory assessment may include (1) serum electrolytes; complete blood count; and renal, hepatic, endocrine, and immune studies; (2) cerebrospinal fluid examination; (3) focused neuroimaging studies (Chap. 440e); or (4) electrophysiologic studies (Chap. 442e). The anatomic localization, mode of onset and course of illness, other medical data, and laboratory findings are then integrated to establish an etiologic diagnosis.

The neurologic examination may be normal even in patients with a serious neurologic disease, such as seizures, chronic meningitis, or a TIA. A comatose patient may arrive with no available history, and in such cases, the approach is as described in Chap. 328. In other patients, an inadequate history may be overcome by a succession of examinations from which the course of the illness can be inferred. In perplexing cases it is useful to remember that uncommon presentations of common diseases are more likely than rare etiologies. Thus, even in tertiary care settings, multiple strokes are usually due to emboli and not vasculitis, and dementia with myoclonus is usually Alzheimer's disease and not a prion disorder or a paraneoplastic illness. Finally, the most important task of a primary care physician

TABLE 437-2 FINDINGS HELPFUL FOR LOCALIZATIONS WITHIN THE NERVOUS SYSTEM

	Signs
Cerebrum	Abnormal mental status or cognitive impairment
	Seizures
	Unilateral weakness[a] and sensory abnormalities including head and limbs
	Visual field abnormalities
	Movement abnormalities (e.g., diffuse incoordination, tremor, chorea)
Brainstem	Isolated cranial nerve abnormalities (single or multiple)
	"Crossed" weakness[a] and sensory abnormalities of head and limbs, e.g., weakness of right face and left arm and leg
Spinal cord	Back pain or tenderness
	Weakness[a] and sensory abnormalities sparing the head
	Mixed upper and lower motor neuron findings
	Sensory level
	Sphincter dysfunction
Spinal roots	Radiating limb pain
	Weakness[b] or sensory abnormalities following root distribution **(see Figs. 31-2 and 31-3)**
	Loss of reflexes
Peripheral nerve	Mid or distal limb pain
	Weakness[b] or sensory abnormalities following nerve distribution **(see Figs. 31-2 and 31-3)**
	"Stocking or glove" distribution of sensory loss
	Loss of reflexes
Neuromuscular junction	Bilateral weakness including face (ptosis, diplopia, dysphagia) and proximal limbs
	Increasing weakness with exertion
	Sparing of sensation
Muscle	Bilateral proximal or distal weakness
	Sparing of sensation

[a]Weakness along with other abnormalities having an "upper motor neuron" pattern, i.e., spasticity, weakness of extensors > flexors in the upper extremity and flexors > extensors in the lower extremity, and hyperreflexia. [b]Weakness along with other abnormalities having a "lower motor neuron" pattern, i.e., flaccidity and hyporeflexia.

faced with a patient who has a new neurologic complaint is to assess the urgency of referral to a specialist. Here, the imperative is to rapidly identify patients likely to have nervous system infections, acute strokes, and spinal cord compression or other treatable mass lesions and arrange for immediate care.

438e The Neurologic Screening Exam

Daniel H. Lowenstein

This is a digital-only chapter. It is available on the DVD that accompanies this book, as well as on Access Medicine/Harrison's Online, and the eBook and "app" editions of HPIM 19e.

Knowledge of the basic neurologic examination is an essential clinical skill. A simple neurologic screening examination—assessment of mental status, cranial nerves, motor system, sensory system, coordination, and gait—can be reliably performed in 3–5 min. Although the components of the examination may appear daunting at first, skills usually improve rapidly with repetition and practice. In this video, the technique of performing a simple and efficient screening examination is presented.

439e Video Atlas of the Detailed Neurologic Examination

Martin A. Samuels

This is a digital-only chapter. It is available on the DVD that accompanies this book, as well as on Access Medicine/Harrison's Online, and the eBook and "app" editions of HPIM 19e.

The comprehensive neurologic examination is an irreplaceable tool for the efficient diagnosis of neurologic disorders. Mastery of its details requires knowledge of normal nervous system anatomy and physiology combined with personal experience performing orderly and systematic examinations on large numbers of patients and healthy individuals. In the hands of a great clinician, the neurologic examination also becomes a thing of beauty—the pinnacle of the art of medicine. In this video, the most commonly used components of the examination are presented in detail, with a particular emphasis on those elements that are most helpful for assessment of common neurologic problems.

440e Neuroimaging in Neurologic Disorders

William P. Dillon

This is a digital-only chapter. It is available on the DVD that accompanies this book, as well as on Access Medicine/Harrison's Online, and the eBook and "app" editions of HPIM 19e.

The clinician caring for patients with neurologic symptoms is faced with myriad imaging options, including computed tomography (CT), CT angiography (CTA), perfusion CT (pCT), magnetic resonance (MR) imaging (MRI), MR angiography (MRA), functional MRI (fMRI), MR spectroscopy (MRS), MR neurography (MRN), diffusion and diffusion tensor imaging (DTI), susceptibility-weighted MR imaging (SWI), arterial spin label MRI (ASL), and perfusion MRI (pMRI). In addition, an increasing number of interventional neuroradiologic techniques are available, including angiography catheter embolization, coiling, and stenting of vascular structures, and spine diagnostic and interventional techniques, such as diskography, transforaminal and translaminar epidural and nerve root injections, and blood patches. Multidetector CTA (MDCTA) and gadolinium-enhanced MRA have narrowed the indications for conventional angiography, which is now reserved for patients in whom small-vessel detail is essential for diagnosis or for whom concurrent interventional therapy is planned.

In general, MRI is more sensitive than CT for the detection of lesions affecting the central nervous system (CNS), particularly those of the spinal cord, cranial nerves, and posterior fossa structures. Diffusion MR, a sequence sensitive to the microscopic motion of water, is the most sensitive technique for detecting acute ischemic stroke of the brain or spinal cord, and it is also useful in the detection of encephalitis, abscesses, and prion diseases. CT, however, is quickly acquired and is widely available, making it a pragmatic choice for the initial evaluation of patients with acute changes in mental status, suspected acute stroke, hemorrhage, and intracranial or spinal trauma. CT is also more sensitive than MRI for visualizing fine osseous detail and is indicated in the initial imaging evaluation of conductive hearing loss as well as lesions affecting the skull base and calvarium. MR may, however, add important diagnostic information regarding bone marrow infiltrative processes that are difficult to detect on CT.

441e Atlas of Neuroimaging

Andre D. Furtado, William P. Dillon

This is a digital-only chapter. It is available on the DVD that accompanies this book, as well as on Access Medicine/Harrison's Online, and the eBook and "app" editions of HPIM 19e.

This atlas comprises 48 cases to assist the clinician caring for patients with neurologic symptoms. The majority of the images shown are magnetic resonance imaging (MRI) scans; other techniques illustrated include magnetic resonance (MR) and conventional angiography and computed tomography (CT) scans. Many different categories of neurologic disease are illustrated, including numerous examples of ischemic, inflammatory, inherited, vascular, and neoplastic etiologies.

442e Electrodiagnostic Studies of Nervous System Disorders: EEG, Evoked Potentials, and EMG

Michael J. Aminoff

This is a digital-only chapter. It is available on the DVD that accompanies this book, as well as on Access Medicine/Harrison's Online, and the eBook and "app" editions of HPIM 19e.

ELECTROENCEPHALOGRAPHY

The electrical activity of the brain (the electroencephalogram [EEG]) is easily recorded from electrodes placed on the scalp. The potential difference between pairs of electrodes on the scalp (bipolar derivation) or between individual scalp electrodes and a relatively inactive common reference point (referential derivation) is amplified and displayed on a computer monitor, oscilloscope, or paper. Digital systems allow the EEG to be reconstructed and displayed with any desired format and to be manipulated for more detailed analysis and also permit computerized techniques to be used to detect certain abnormalities. The characteristics of the normal EEG depend on the patient's age and level of arousal. The rhythmic activity normally recorded represents the postsynaptic potentials of vertically oriented pyramidal cells of the cerebral cortex and is characterized by its frequency. In normal awake adults lying quietly with the eyes closed, an 8- to 13-Hz alpha rhythm is seen posteriorly in the EEG, intermixed with a variable amount of generalized faster (beta) activity (>13 Hz); the alpha rhythm is attenuated when the eyes are opened. During drowsiness, the alpha rhythm is also attenuated; with light sleep, slower activity in the theta (4–7 Hz) and delta (<4 Hz) ranges becomes more conspicuous.

Activating procedures are generally undertaken while the EEG is recorded in an attempt to provoke abnormalities. Such procedures commonly include hyperventilation (for 3 or 4 min), photic stimulation, sleep, and sleep deprivation on the night prior to the recording.

Electroencephalography is relatively inexpensive and may aid clinical management in several different contexts.

443e Technique of Lumbar Puncture

Elizabeth Robbins, Stephen L. Hauser

This is a digital-only chapter. It is available on the DVD that accompanies this book, as well as on Access Medicine/Harrison's Online, and the eBook and "app" editions of HPIM 19e.

In experienced hands, lumbar puncture (LP) is usually a safe procedure. Major complications are extremely uncommon but can include cerebral herniation, injury to the spinal cord or nerve roots, hemorrhage (spinal hematoma), or infection. Minor complications occur with greater frequency and can include backache, post-LP headache, and radicular pain or numbness.

IMAGING AND LABORATORY STUDIES PRIOR TO LP

Patients with an altered level of consciousness, a focal neurologic deficit, new-onset seizure, papilledema, or an immunocompromised state are at increased risk for potentially fatal cerebellar or tentorial herniation following LP. Neuroimaging should be obtained in these patients prior to LP to exclude a focal mass lesion or diffuse swelling. Imaging studies should include the spine in patients with symptoms suggesting spinal cord compression, such as back pain, leg weakness, urinary retention, or incontinence. In patients with suspected meningitis who require neuroimaging prior to diagnostic LP, administration of antibiotics, preferably following blood culture, should precede the neuroimaging study.

LP should not be performed through infected skin, as organisms can be introduced into the subarachnoid space (SAS).

Patients with coagulation defects including thrombocytopenia are at increased risk of post-LP spinal subdural or epidural hematomas, either of which can produce permanent nerve injury and/or paralysis. If a bleeding disorder is suspected, the platelet count, international normalized ratio (INR), and partial thromboplastin time should be checked prior to LP. There are no data available to assess the safety of LP in patients with low platelet counts; a count of <20,000/μL is considered to be a contraindication to LP. Bleeding complications rarely occur in patients with platelet counts ≥50,000/μL and an INR ≤1.5. Some institutions recommend that the platelet count be > 40,000 prior to LP.

444e Biology of Neurologic Diseases

Stephen L. Hauser, Stanley B. Prusiner, M. Flint Beal

This is a digital-only chapter. It is available on the DVD that accompanies this book, as well as on Access Medicine/Harrison's Online, and the eBook and "app" editions of HPIM 19e.

The human nervous system is the organ of consciousness, cognition, ethics, and behavior; as such, it is the most intricate structure known to exist. More than one-third of the 23,000 genes encoded in the human genome are expressed in the nervous system. Each mature brain is composed of 100 billion neurons, several million miles of axons and dendrites, and $>10^{15}$ synapses. Neurons exist within a dense parenchyma of multifunctional glial cells that synthesize myelin, preserve homeostasis, and regulate immune responses. Measured against this background of complexity, the achievements of molecular neuroscience have been extraordinary. This chapter reviews selected themes in neuroscience that provide a context for understanding fundamental mechanisms underlying neurologic disorders.

445 Seizures and Epilepsy

Daniel H. Lowenstein

A *seizure* (from the Latin *sacire*, "to take possession of") is a paroxysmal event due to abnormal excessive or synchronous neuronal activity in the brain. Depending on the distribution of discharges, this abnormal brain activity can have various manifestations, ranging from dramatic convulsive activity to experiential phenomena not readily discernible by an observer. Although a variety of factors influence the incidence and prevalence of seizures, ~5–10% of the population will have at least one seizure, with the highest incidence occurring in early childhood and late adulthood.

The meaning of the term *seizure* needs to be carefully distinguished from that of epilepsy. *Epilepsy* describes a condition in which a person has *recurrent* seizures due to a chronic, underlying process. This definition implies that a person with a single seizure, or recurrent seizures due to correctable or avoidable circumstances, does not necessarily have epilepsy. Epilepsy refers to a clinical phenomenon rather than a single disease entity, because there are many forms and causes of epilepsy. However, among the many causes of epilepsy there are various *epilepsy syndromes* in which the clinical and pathologic characteristics are distinctive and suggest a specific underlying etiology.

Using the definition of epilepsy as two or more unprovoked seizures, the incidence of epilepsy is ~0.3–0.5% in different populations throughout the world, and the prevalence of epilepsy has been estimated at 5–30 persons per 1000.

CLASSIFICATION OF SEIZURES

Determining the type of seizure that has occurred is essential for focusing the diagnostic approach on particular etiologies, selecting the appropriate therapy, and providing potentially vital information regarding prognosis. The International League against Epilepsy (ILAE) Commission on Classification and Terminology, 2005–2009 has provided an updated approach to classification of seizures (Table 445-1). This system is based on the clinical features of seizures and associated electroencephalographic findings. Other potentially distinctive features such as etiology or cellular substrate are not considered in this classification system, although this will undoubtedly change in the future as more is learned about the pathophysiologic mechanisms that underlie specific seizure types.

A fundamental principle is that seizures may be either focal or generalized. *Focal seizures* originate within networks limited to one cerebral hemisphere (note that the term *partial seizures* is no longer used). *Generalized seizures* arise within and rapidly engage networks distributed across both cerebral hemispheres. Focal seizures are usually associated with structural abnormalities of the brain. In contrast, generalized seizures may result from cellular, biochemical, or structural abnormalities that have a more widespread distribution. There are clear exceptions in both cases, however.

TABLE 445-1 CLASSIFICATION OF SEIZURES

1. **Focal seizures**

   (Can be further described as having motor, sensory, autonomic, cognitive, or other features)

2. **Generalized seizures**

   a. Absence
      - Typical
      - Atypical

   b. Tonic clonic

   c. Clonic

   d. Tonic

   e. Atonic

   f. Myoclonic

3. **May be focal, generalized, or unclear**

   Epileptic spasms

FOCAL SEIZURES

Focal seizures arise from a neuronal network either discretely localized within one cerebral hemisphere or more broadly distributed but still within the hemisphere. With the new classification system, the subcategories of "simple focal seizures" and "complex focal seizures" have been eliminated. Instead, depending on the presence of cognitive impairment, they can be described as focal seizures with or without dyscognitive features. Focal seizures can also evolve into generalized seizures. In the past this was referred to as *focal seizures with secondary generalization*, but the new system relies on specific descriptions of the type of generalized seizures that evolve from the focal seizure.

The routine interictal (i.e., between seizures) electroencephalogram (EEG) in patients with focal seizures is often normal or may show brief discharges termed *epileptiform spikes*, or *sharp waves*. Because focal seizures can arise from the medial temporal lobe or inferior frontal lobe (i.e., regions distant from the scalp), the EEG recorded during the seizure may be nonlocalizing. However, the seizure focus is often detected using sphenoidal or surgically placed intracranial electrodes.

Focal Seizures Without Dyscognitive Features Focal seizures can cause motor, sensory, autonomic, or psychic symptoms without impairment of cognition. For example, a patient having a focal motor seizure arising from the right primary motor cortex near the area controlling hand movement will note the onset of involuntary movements of the contralateral, left hand. These movements are typically clonic (i.e., repetitive, flexion/extension movements) at a frequency of ~2–3 Hz; pure tonic posturing may be seen as well. Since the cortical region controlling hand movement is immediately adjacent to the region for facial expression, the seizure may also cause abnormal movements of the face synchronous with the movements of the hand. The EEG recorded with scalp electrodes during the seizure (i.e., an ictal EEG) may show abnormal discharges in a very limited region over the appropriate area of cerebral cortex if the seizure focus involves the cerebral convexity. Seizure activity occurring within deeper brain structures is sometimes not detected by the standard EEG, however, and may require intracranial electrodes for its detection.

Three additional features of focal motor seizures are worth noting. First, in some patients, the abnormal motor movements may begin in a very restricted region such as the fingers and gradually progress (over seconds to minutes) to include a larger portion of the extremity. This phenomenon, described by Hughlings Jackson and known as a "Jacksonian march," represents the spread of seizure activity over a progressively larger region of motor cortex. Second, patients may experience a localized paresis (Todd's paralysis) for minutes to many hours in the involved region following the seizure. Third, in rare instances, the seizure may continue for hours or days. This condition, termed *epilepsia partialis continua*, is often refractory to medical therapy.

Focal seizures may also manifest as changes in somatic sensation (e.g., paresthesias), vision (flashing lights or formed hallucinations), equilibrium (sensation of falling or vertigo), or autonomic function (flushing, sweating, piloerection). Focal seizures arising from the temporal or frontal cortex may also cause alterations in hearing, olfaction, or higher cortical function (psychic symptoms). This includes the sensation of unusual, intense odors (e.g., burning rubber or kerosene) or sounds (crude or highly complex sounds), or an epigastric sensation that rises from the stomach or chest to the head. Some patients describe odd, internal feelings such as fear, a sense of impending change, detachment, depersonalization, déjà vu, or illusions that objects are growing smaller (micropsia) or larger (macropsia). These subjective, "internal" events that are not directly observable by someone else are referred to as *auras*.

Focal Seizures with Dyscognitive Features Focal seizures may also be accompanied by a transient impairment of the patient's ability to maintain normal contact with the environment. The patient is unable to respond appropriately to visual or verbal commands during the seizure and has impaired recollection or awareness of the ictal phase. The seizures frequently begin with an aura (i.e., a focal seizure without cognitive disturbance) that is stereotypic for the patient. The start of the ictal phase is often a sudden behavioral arrest or motionless stare, which marks the onset of the period of impaired awareness. The behavioral arrest is usually accompanied by *automatisms*, which are involuntary, automatic behaviors that have a wide range of manifestations. Automatisms may consist of very basic behaviors such as chewing, lip smacking, swallowing, or "picking" movements of the hands, or more elaborate behaviors such as a display of emotion or running. The patient is typically confused following the seizure, and the transition to full recovery of consciousness may range from seconds up to an hour. Examination immediately following the seizure may show an anterograde amnesia or, in cases involving the dominant hemisphere, a postictal aphasia.

The range of potential clinical behaviors linked to focal seizures is so broad that extreme caution is advised before concluding that stereotypic episodes of bizarre or atypical behavior are not due to seizure activity. In such cases additional, detailed EEG studies may be helpful.

EVOLUTION OF FOCAL SEIZURES TO GENERALIZED SEIZURES

Focal seizures can spread to involve both cerebral hemispheres and produce a generalized seizure, usually of the tonic-clonic variety (discussed below). This evolution is observed frequently following focal seizures arising from a focus in the frontal lobe, but may also be associated with focal seizures occurring elsewhere in the brain. A focal seizure that evolves into a generalized seizure is often difficult to distinguish from a primary generalized-onset tonic clonic seizure, because bystanders tend to emphasize the more dramatic, generalized convulsive phase of the seizure and overlook the more subtle, focal symptoms present at onset. In some cases, the focal onset of the seizure becomes apparent only when a careful history identifies a preceding aura. Often, however, the focal onset is not clinically evident and may be established only through careful EEG analysis. Nonetheless, distinguishing between these two entities is extremely important, because there may be substantial differences in the evaluation and treatment of epilepsies associated with focal versus generalized seizures.

GENERALIZED SEIZURES

Generalized seizures are thought to arise at some point in the brain but immediately and rapidly engage neuronal networks in both cerebral hemispheres. Several types of generalized seizures have features that place them in distinctive categories and facilitate clinical diagnosis.

Typical Absence Seizures Typical absence seizures are characterized by sudden, brief lapses of consciousness without loss of postural control. The seizure typically lasts for only seconds, consciousness returns as suddenly as it was lost, and there is no postictal confusion. Although the brief loss of consciousness may be clinically inapparent or the sole manifestation of the seizure discharge, absence seizures are usually accompanied by subtle, bilateral motor signs such as rapid blinking of the eyelids, chewing movements, or small-amplitude, clonic movements of the hands.

Typical absence seizures are associated with a group of genetically determined epilepsies with onset usually in childhood (ages 4–8 years) or early adolescence and are the main seizure type in 15–20% of children with epilepsy. The seizures can occur hundreds of times per day, but the child may be unaware of or unable to convey their existence. Because the clinical signs of the seizures are subtle, especially to parents who may not have had previous experience with seizures, it is not surprising that the first clue to absence epilepsy is often unexplained "daydreaming" and a decline in school performance recognized by a teacher.

The electrophysiologic hallmark of typical absence seizures is a generalized, symmetric, 3-Hz spike-and-wave discharge that begins and ends suddenly, superimposed on a normal EEG background. Periods of spike-and-wave discharges lasting more than a few seconds usually correlate with clinical signs, but the EEG often shows many more brief bursts of abnormal cortical activity than were suspected clinically. Hyperventilation tends to provoke these electrographic discharges and even the seizures themselves and is routinely used when recording the EEG.

Atypical Absence Seizures Atypical absence seizures have features that deviate both clinically and electrophysiologically from typical absence seizures. For example, the lapse of consciousness is usually of longer duration and less abrupt in onset and cessation, and the seizure is accompanied by more obvious motor signs that may include focal or lateralizing features. The EEG shows a generalized, slow spike-and-wave pattern with a frequency of ≤2.5 per second, as well as other abnormal activity. Atypical absence seizures are usually associated with diffuse or multifocal structural abnormalities of the brain and therefore may accompany other signs of neurologic dysfunction such as mental retardation. Furthermore, the seizures are less responsive to anticonvulsants compared to typical absence seizures.

Generalized, Tonic-Clonic Seizures Generalized-onset tonic-clonic seizures are the main seizure type in ~10% of all persons with epilepsy. They are also the most common seizure type resulting from metabolic derangements and are therefore frequently encountered in many different clinical settings. The seizure usually begins abruptly without warning, although some patients describe vague premonitory symptoms in the hours leading up to the seizure. This prodrome is distinct from the stereotypic auras associated with focal seizures that generalize. The initial phase of the seizure is usually tonic contraction of muscles throughout the body, accounting for a number of the classic features of the event. Tonic contraction of the muscles of expiration and the larynx at the onset will produce a loud moan or "ictal cry." Respirations are impaired, secretions pool in the oropharynx, and cyanosis develops. Contraction of the jaw muscles may cause biting of the tongue. A marked enhancement of sympathetic tone leads to increases in heart rate, blood pressure, and pupillary size. After 10–20 s, the tonic phase of the seizure typically evolves into the clonic phase, produced by the superimposition of periods of muscle relaxation on the tonic muscle contraction. The periods of relaxation progressively increase until the end of the ictal phase, which usually lasts no more than 1 min. The postictal phase is characterized by unresponsiveness, muscular flaccidity, and excessive salivation that can cause stridorous breathing and partial airway obstruction. Bladder or bowel incontinence may occur at this point. Patients gradually regain consciousness over minutes to hours, and during this transition, there is typically a period of postictal confusion. Patients subsequently complain of headache, fatigue, and muscle ache that can last for many hours. The duration of impaired consciousness in the postictal phase can be extremely long (i.e., many hours) in patients with prolonged seizures or underlying central nervous system (CNS) diseases such as alcoholic cerebral atrophy.

The EEG during the tonic phase of the seizure shows a progressive increase in generalized low-voltage fast activity, followed by generalized high-amplitude, polyspike discharges. In the clonic phase, the high-amplitude activity is typically interrupted by slow waves to create a spike-and-wave pattern. The postictal EEG shows diffuse slowing that gradually recovers as the patient awakens.

There are a number of variants of the generalized tonic-clonic seizure, including pure tonic and pure clonic seizures. Brief tonic seizures lasting only a few seconds are especially noteworthy since they are usually associated with specific epileptic syndromes having mixed seizure phenotypes, such as the Lennox-Gastaut syndrome (discussed below).

Atonic Seizures Atonic seizures are characterized by sudden loss of postural muscle tone lasting 1–2 s. Consciousness is briefly impaired, but there is usually no postictal confusion. A very brief seizure may cause only a quick head drop or nodding movement, whereas a longer seizure will cause the patient to collapse. This can be extremely dangerous, because there is a substantial risk of direct head injury with the fall. The EEG shows brief, generalized spike-and-wave discharges followed immediately by diffuse slow waves that correlate with the loss of muscle tone. Similar to pure tonic seizures, atonic seizures are usually seen in association with known epilepsy syndromes.

Myoclonic Seizures Myoclonus is a sudden and brief muscle contraction that may involve one part of the body or the entire body. A normal, common physiologic form of myoclonus is the sudden jerking movement observed while falling asleep. Pathologic myoclonus is most commonly seen in association with metabolic disorders, degenerative CNS diseases, or anoxic brain injury (Chap. 330). Although the distinction from other forms of myoclonus is imprecise, myoclonic seizures are considered to be true epileptic events because they are caused by cortical (versus subcortical or spinal) dysfunction. The EEG may show bilaterally synchronous spike-and-wave discharges synchronized with the myoclonus, although these can be obscured by movement artifact. Myoclonic seizures usually coexist with other forms of generalized seizures but are the predominant feature of juvenile myoclonic epilepsy (discussed below).

CURRENTLY UNCLASSIFIABLE SEIZURES

Not all seizure types can be designated as focal or generalized, and they should therefore be labeled as "unclassifiable" until additional evidence allows a valid classification. *Epileptic spasms* are such an example. These are characterized by a briefly sustained flexion or extension of predominantly proximal muscles, including truncal muscles. The EEG in these patients usually shows hypsarrhythmias, which consist of diffuse, giant slow waves with a chaotic background of irregular, multifocal spikes and sharp waves. During the clinical spasm, there is a marked suppression of the EEG background (the "electrodecremental response"). The electromyogram (EMG) also reveals a characteristic rhomboid pattern that may help distinguish spasms from brief tonic and myoclonic seizures. Epileptic spasms occur predominantly in infants and likely result from differences in neuronal function and connectivity in the immature versus mature CNS.

EPILEPSY SYNDROMES

Epilepsy syndromes are disorders in which epilepsy is a predominant feature, and there is sufficient evidence (e.g., through clinical, EEG, radiologic, or genetic observations) to suggest a common underlying mechanism. Three important epilepsy syndromes are listed below; additional examples with a known genetic basis are shown in Table 445-2.

JUVENILE MYOCLONIC EPILEPSY

Juvenile myoclonic epilepsy (JME) is a generalized seizure disorder of unknown cause that appears in early adolescence and is usually characterized by bilateral myoclonic jerks that may be single or repetitive. The myoclonic seizures are most frequent in the morning after awakening and can be provoked by sleep deprivation. Consciousness is preserved unless the myoclonus is especially severe. Many patients also experience generalized tonic-clonic seizures, and up to one-third have absence seizures. Although complete remission is relatively uncommon, the seizures usually respond well to appropriate anticonvulsant medication. There is often a family history of epilepsy, and genetic linkage studies suggest a polygenic cause.

LENNOX-GASTAUT SYNDROME

Lennox-Gastaut syndrome occurs in children and is defined by the following triad: (1) multiple seizure types (usually including generalized tonic-clonic, atonic, and atypical absence seizures); (2) an EEG showing slow (<3 Hz) spike-and-wave discharges and a variety of other abnormalities; and (3) impaired cognitive function in most but not all cases. Lennox-Gastaut syndrome is associated with CNS disease or dysfunction from a variety of causes, including *de novo* mutations, developmental abnormalities, perinatal hypoxia/ischemia, trauma, infection, and other acquired lesions. The multifactorial nature of this syndrome suggests that it is a nonspecific response of the brain to diffuse neural injury. Unfortunately, many patients have a poor prognosis due to the underlying CNS disease and the physical and psychosocial consequences of severe, poorly controlled epilepsy.

MESIAL TEMPORAL LOBE EPILEPSY SYNDROME

Mesial temporal lobe epilepsy (MTLE) is the most common syndrome associated with focal seizures with dyscognitive features and is an example of an epilepsy syndrome with distinctive clinical, electroencephalographic, and pathologic features (Table 445-3). High-resolution magnetic resonance imaging (MRI) can detect the characteristic hippocampal sclerosis that appears to be essential in the pathophysiology of MTLE for many patients (Fig. 445-1). Recognition of this syndrome is especially important because it tends to be refractory to treatment with anticonvulsants but responds well to surgical intervention. Advances in the understanding of basic mechanisms of epilepsy have come through studies of experimental models of MTLE, discussed below.

THE CAUSES OF SEIZURES AND EPILEPSY

Seizures are a result of a shift in the normal balance of excitation and inhibition within the CNS. Given the numerous properties that control neuronal excitability, it is not surprising that there are many different ways to perturb this normal balance, and therefore many different causes of both seizures and epilepsy. Three clinical observations emphasize how a variety of factors determine why certain conditions may cause seizures or epilepsy in a given patient.

1. *The normal brain is capable of having a seizure under the appropriate circumstances, and there are differences between individuals in the susceptibility or threshold for seizures.* For example, seizures may be induced by high fevers in children who are otherwise normal and who never develop other neurologic problems, including epilepsy. However, febrile seizures occur only in a relatively small proportion of children. This implies there are various underlying *endogenous factors* that influence the threshold for having a seizure. Some of these factors are genetic, as a family history of epilepsy has a clear influence on the likelihood of seizures occurring in otherwise normal individuals. Normal development also plays an important role, because the brain appears to have different seizure thresholds at different maturational stages.
2. *There are a variety of conditions that have an extremely high likelihood of resulting in a chronic seizure disorder.* One of the best examples of this is severe, penetrating head trauma, which is associated with up to a 45% risk of subsequent epilepsy. The high propensity for severe traumatic brain injury to lead to epilepsy suggests that the injury results in a long-lasting pathologic change in the CNS that transforms a presumably normal neural network into one that is abnormally hyperexcitable. This process is known as *epileptogenesis*, and the specific changes that result in a lowered seizure threshold can be considered *epileptogenic factors*. Other processes associated with epileptogenesis include stroke, infections, and abnormalities of CNS development. Likewise, the genetic abnormalities associated with epilepsy likely involve processes that trigger the appearance of specific sets of epileptogenic factors.
3. *Seizures are episodic.* Patients with epilepsy have seizures intermittently and, depending on the underlying cause, many patients are completely normal for months or even years between seizures. This implies there are important provocative or *precipitating factors* that induce seizures in patients with epilepsy. Similarly, precipitating factors are responsible for causing the single seizure in someone without epilepsy. Precipitants include those due to intrinsic physiologic processes such as psychological or physical stress, sleep deprivation, or hormonal changes associated with the menstrual cycle. They also include exogenous factors such as exposure to toxic substances and certain medications.

TABLE 445-2 EXAMPLES OF GENES ASSOCIATED WITH EPILEPSY SYNDROMES[a]

Gene (Locus)	Function of Gene	Clinical Syndrome	Comments
CHRNA4 (20q13.2)	Nicotinic acetylcholine receptor subunit; mutations cause alterations in Ca^{2+} flux through the receptor; this may reduce amount of GABA release in presynaptic terminals	Autosomal dominant nocturnal frontal lobe epilepsy (ADNFLE); childhood onset; brief, nighttime seizures with prominent motor movements; often misdiagnosed as primary sleep disorder	Rare; first identified in a large Australian family; other families found to have mutations in *CHRNA2* or *CHRNB2*, and some families appear to have mutations at other loci
KCNQ2 (20q13.3)	Voltage-gated potassium channel subunits; mutation in pore regions may cause a 20–40% reduction of potassium currents, which will lead to impaired repolarization	Benign familial neonatal seizures (BFNS); autosomal dominant inheritance; onset in 1st week of life in infants who are otherwise normal; remission usually within weeks to months; long-term epilepsy in 10–15%	Rare; other families found to have mutations in *KCNQ3* or an inversion in chromosomal 5; sequence and functional homology to *KCNQ1*, mutations of which cause long QT syndrome and a cardiac-auditory syndrome
SCN1A (2q24.3)	α-Subunit of a voltage-gated sodium channel; numerous mutations affecting sodium currents that cause either gain or loss of function; network effects appear related to expression in excitatory or inhibitory cells	Generalized epilepsy with febrile seizures plus (GEFS+); autosomal dominant inheritance; presents with febrile seizures at median 1 year, which may persist >6 years, then variable seizure types not associated with fever; numerous other syndromes, including almost 80% of patients with Dravet's syndrome (severe myoclonic epilepsy of infancy) and some cases of Lennox-Gastaut syndrome	Incidence uncertain; GEFS+ identified in other families with mutations in other sodium channel subunits (*SCN2B* and *SCN2A*) and $GABA_A$ receptor subunit (*GABRG2* and *GABRA1*); significant phenotypic heterogeneity within same family, including members with febrile seizures only
LGI1 (10q24)	Leucine-rich glioma-inactivated 1 gene; previous evidence for role in glial tumor progression; recent studies suggest an influence in the postnatal development of glutamatergic circuits in the hippocampus	Autosomal dominant partial epilepsy with auditory features (ADPEAF); a form of idiopathic lateral temporal lobe epilepsy with auditory symptoms or aphasia as a major focal seizure manifestation; age of onset usually between 10 and 25 years	Mutations found in up to 50% of families containing two or more subjects with idiopathic localization-related epilepsy with ictal auditory symptoms, suggesting that at least one other gene may underlie this syndrome.
DEPDC5 (22q12.2)	Disheveled, Egl-10 and pleckstrin domain containing protein 5; exerts an inhibitory effect on mammalian target of rapamycin (mTOR)-mediated processes, such as cell growth and proliferation	Autosomal dominant familial focal epilepsy with variable foci (FFEVF); family members have seizures originating from different cortical regions; neuroimaging usually normal but may harbor subtle malformations; recent studies also suggest association with benign epilepsy with centrotemporal spikes	Study of families with limited number of affected members revealed mutations in approximately 12% of families, thus may be a relatively common cause of lesion-negative focal epilepsies with suspected genetic basis
CSTB (21q22.3)	Cystatin B, a noncaspase cysteine protease inhibitor; normal protein may block neuronal apoptosis by inhibiting caspases directly or indirectly (via cathepsins), or controlling proteolysis	Progressive myoclonus epilepsy (PME) (Unverricht-Lundborg disease); autosomal recessive inheritance; age of onset between 6 and 15 years, myoclonic seizures, ataxia, and progressive cognitive decline; brain shows neuronal degeneration	Overall rare, but relatively common in Finland and Western Mediterranean (>1 in 20,000); precise role of cystatin B in human disease unknown, although mice with null mutations of cystatin B have similar syndrome
EPM2A (6q24)	Laforin, a protein tyrosine phosphatase (PTP); involved in glycogen metabolism and may have antiapoptotic activity	Progressive myoclonus epilepsy (Lafora's disease); autosomal recessive inheritance; age of onset 6–19 years, death within 10 years; brain degeneration associated with polyglucosan intracellular inclusion bodies in numerous organs	Most common PME in Southern Europe, Middle East, Northern Africa, and Indian subcontinent; genetic heterogeneity; unknown whether seizure phenotype due to degeneration or direct effects of abnormal laforin expression
Doublecortin (Xq21-24)	*Doublecortin*, expressed primarily in frontal lobes; directly regulates microtubule polymerization and bundling	Classic lissencephaly associated with severe mental retardation and seizures in males; subcortical band heterotopia with more subtle findings in females (presumably due to random X-inactivation); X-linked dominant	Relatively rare but of uncertain incidence; recent increased ascertainment due to improved imaging techniques, relationship between migration defect and seizure phenotype unknown

[a]The first five syndromes listed in the table (ADNFLE, BFNC, GEFS+, ADPEAF, and FFEVF) are examples of idiopathic epilepsies associated with identified gene mutations. The last three syndromes are examples of the numerous Mendelian disorders in which seizures are one part of the phenotype.

Abbreviations: GABA, γ-aminobutyric acid; PME, progressive myoclonus epilepsy.

These observations emphasize the concept that the many causes of seizures and epilepsy result from a dynamic interplay between endogenous factors, epileptogenic factors, and precipitating factors. The potential role of each needs to be carefully considered when determining the appropriate management of a patient with seizures. For example, the identification of predisposing factors (e.g., family history of epilepsy) in a patient with febrile seizures may increase the necessity for closer follow-up and a more aggressive diagnostic evaluation. Finding an epileptogenic lesion may help in the estimation of seizure recurrence and duration of therapy. Finally, removal or modification of a precipitating factor may be an effective and safer method for preventing further seizures than the prophylactic use of anticonvulsant drugs.

CAUSES ACCORDING TO AGE

In practice, it is useful to consider the etiologies of seizures based on the age of the patient, because age is one of the most important factors determining both the incidence and the likely causes of seizures or epilepsy (Table 445-4). During the *neonatal period and early infancy*, potential causes include hypoxic-ischemic encephalopathy, trauma, CNS infection, congenital CNS abnormalities, and metabolic disorders. Babies born to mothers using neurotoxic drugs such as cocaine, heroin, or ethanol are susceptible to drug-withdrawal seizures in the first few days after delivery. Hypoglycemia and hypocalcemia, which can occur as secondary complications of perinatal injury, are also causes of seizures early after delivery. Seizures due to inborn errors of metabolism usually present once regular feeding begins, typically 2–3 days after birth. Pyridoxine (vitamin B_6) deficiency, an important cause of neonatal seizures, can be effectively treated with pyridoxine replacement. The idiopathic or inherited forms of benign neonatal convulsions are also seen during this time period.

The most common seizures arising in *late infancy and early childhood* are febrile seizures, which are seizures associated with fevers but without evidence of CNS infection or other defined causes. The overall prevalence

TABLE 445-3 CHARACTERISTICS OF THE MESIAL TEMPORAL LOBE EPILEPSY SYNDROME

History	
History of febrile seizures	Rare generalized seizures
Family history of epilepsy	Seizures may remit and reappear
Early onset	Seizures often intractable
Clinical Observations	
Aura common	Postictal disorientation
Behavioral arrest/stare	Memory loss
Complex automatisms	Dysphasia (with focus in dominant hemisphere)
Unilateral posturing	
Laboratory Studies	
Unilateral or bilateral anterior temporal spikes on EEG	
Hypometabolism on interictal PET	
Hypoperfusion on interictal SPECT	
Material-specific memory deficits on intracranial amobarbital (Wada) test	
MRI Findings	
Small hippocampus with increased signal on T2-weighted sequences	
Small temporal lobe	
Enlarged temporal horn	
Pathologic Findings	
Highly selective loss of specific cell populations within hippocampus in most cases	

Abbreviations: EEG, electroencephalogram; MRI, magnetic resonance imaging; PET, positron emission tomography; SPECT, single-photon emission computed tomography.

is 3–5% and even higher in some parts of the world such as Asia. Patients often have a family history of febrile seizures or epilepsy. Febrile seizures usually occur between 3 months and 5 years of age and have a peak incidence between 18 and 24 months. The typical scenario is a child who has a generalized, tonic-clonic seizure during a febrile illness in the setting of a common childhood infection such as otitis media, respiratory infection, or gastroenteritis. The seizure is likely to occur during the rising phase of the temperature curve (i.e., during the first day) rather than well into the course of the illness. A *simple* febrile seizure is a single, isolated event, brief, and symmetric in appearance. *Complex* febrile seizures are characterized by repeated seizure activity, duration >15 minutes, or by focal features. Approximately one-third of patients with febrile seizures will have a recurrence, but <10% have three or more episodes. Recurrences are much more likely when the febrile seizure occurs in the first year of life. Simple febrile seizures are not associated with an increase in the risk of developing epilepsy, while complex febrile seizures have a risk of 2–5%; other risk factors include the presence of preexisting neurologic deficits and a family history of nonfebrile seizures.

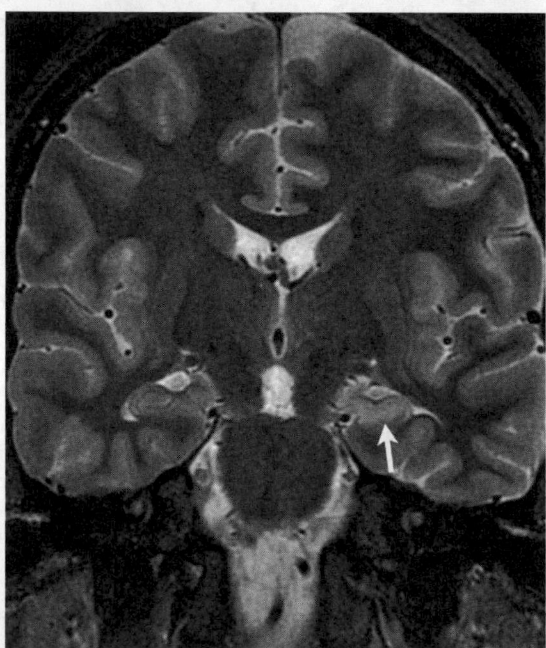

FIGURE 445-1 Mesial temporal lobe epilepsy. The electroencephalogram and seizure semiology were consistent with a left temporal lobe focus. This coronal high-resolution T2-weighted fast spin echo magnetic resonance image obtained at 3 tesla is at the level of the hippocampal bodies, and shows abnormal high signal intensity, blurring of internal laminar architecture, and reduced size of the left hippocampus (*arrow*) relative to the right. This triad of imaging findings is consistent with hippocampal sclerosis.

TABLE 445-4 CAUSES OF SEIZURES

Neonates (<1 month)	Perinatal hypoxia and ischemia
	Intracranial hemorrhage and trauma
	CNS infection
	Metabolic disturbances (hypoglycemia, hypocalcemia, hypomagnesemia, pyridoxine deficiency)
	Drug withdrawal
	Developmental disorders
	Genetic disorders
Infants and children (>1 month and <12 years)	Febrile seizures
	Genetic disorders (metabolic, degenerative, primary epilepsy syndromes)
	CNS infection
	Developmental disorders
	Trauma
Adolescents (12–18 years)	Trauma
	Genetic disorders
	Infection
	Illicit drug use
	Brain tumor
Young adults (18–35 years)	Trauma
	Alcohol withdrawal
	Illicit drug use
	Brain tumor
	Autoantibodies
Older adults (>35 years)	Cerebrovascular disease
	Brain tumor
	Alcohol withdrawal
	Metabolic disorders (uremia, hepatic failure, electrolyte abnormalities, hypoglycemia, hyperglycemia)
	Alzheimer's disease and other degenerative CNS diseases
	Autoantibodies

Abbreviation: CNS, central nervous system.

Childhood marks the age at which many of the well-defined epilepsy syndromes present. Some children who are otherwise normal develop idiopathic, generalized tonic-clonic seizures without other features that fit into specific syndromes. Temporal lobe epilepsy usually presents in childhood and may be related to mesial temporal lobe sclerosis (as part of the MTLE syndrome) or other focal abnormalities such as cortical dysgenesis. Other types of focal seizures, including those that evolve into generalized seizures, may be the relatively late manifestation of a developmental disorder, an acquired lesion such as head trauma, CNS infection (especially viral encephalitis), or very rarely a CNS tumor.

The period of *adolescence and early adulthood* is one of transition during which the idiopathic or genetically based epilepsy syndromes, including JME and juvenile absence epilepsy, become less common, while epilepsies secondary to acquired CNS lesions begin to predominate. Seizures that arise in patients in this age range may be associated with head trauma, CNS infections (including parasitic infections such as cysticercosis), brain tumors, congenital CNS abnormalities, illicit drug use, or alcohol withdrawal. Autoantibodies directed against CNS antigens such as potassium channels or glutamate receptors are a newly recognized cause of epilepsy that also begins to appear in this age group (although cases of autoimmunity are being increasingly described in the pediatric population), including patients without an identifiable cancer. This etiology should be suspected when a previously normal individual presents with a particularly aggressive seizure pattern developing over weeks to months and characterized by increasingly frequent and prolonged seizures combined with cognitive decline (Chap. 122).

Head trauma is a common cause of epilepsy in adolescents and adults. The head injury can be caused by a variety of mechanisms, and the likelihood of developing epilepsy is strongly correlated with the severity of the injury. A patient with a penetrating head wound, depressed skull fracture, intracranial hemorrhage, or prolonged post-traumatic coma or amnesia has a 30–50% risk of developing epilepsy, whereas a patient with a closed head injury and cerebral contusion has a 5–25% risk. Recurrent seizures usually develop within 1 year after head trauma, although intervals of >10 years are well known. In controlled studies, mild head injury, defined as a concussion with amnesia or loss of consciousness of <30 min, was found to be associated with only a slightly increased likelihood of epilepsy. Nonetheless, most epileptologists know of patients who have focal seizures within hours or days of a mild head injury and subsequently develop chronic seizures of the same type; such cases may represent rare examples of chronic epilepsy resulting from mild head injury.

The causes of seizures in *older adults* include cerebrovascular disease, trauma (including subdural hematoma), CNS tumors, and degenerative diseases. Cerebrovascular disease may account for ~50% of new cases of epilepsy in patients older than age 65. Acute seizures (i.e., occurring at the time of the stroke) are seen more often with embolic rather than hemorrhagic or thrombotic stroke. Chronic seizures typically appear months to years after the initial event and are associated with all forms of stroke.

Metabolic disturbances such as electrolyte imbalance, hypo- or hyperglycemia, renal failure, and hepatic failure may cause seizures at any age. Similarly, endocrine disorders, hematologic disorders, vasculitides, and many other systemic diseases may cause seizures over a broad age range. A wide variety of medications and abused substances are known to precipitate seizures as well (Table 445-5).

TABLE 445-5 DRUGS AND OTHER SUBSTANCES THAT CAN CAUSE SEIZURES

Alkylating agents (e.g., busulfan, chlorambucil)
Antimalarials (chloroquine, mefloquine)
Antimicrobials/antivirals
β-lactam and related compounds
Quinolones
Acyclovir
Isoniazid
Ganciclovir
Anesthetics and analgesics
Meperidine
Fentanyl
Tramadol
Local anesthetics
Dietary supplements
Ephedra (ma huang)
Gingko
Immunomodulatory drugs
Cyclosporine
OKT3 (monoclonal antibodies to T cells)
Tacrolimus
Interferons
Psychotropics
Antidepressants (e.g., bupropion)
Antipsychotics (e.g., clozapine)
Lithium
Radiographic contrast agents
Drug withdrawal
Alcohol
Baclofen
Barbiturates (short-acting)
Benzodiazepines (short-acting)
Zolpidem
Drugs of abuse
Amphetamine
Cocaine
Phencyclidine
Methylphenidate
Flumazenil[a]

[a]In benzodiazepine-dependent patients.

BASIC MECHANISMS

MECHANISMS OF SEIZURE INITIATION AND PROPAGATION

Focal seizure activity can begin in a very discrete region of cortex and then slowly invade the surrounding regions. The hallmark of an established seizure is typically an electrographic "spike" due to intense near-simultaneous firing of a large number of local excitatory neurons, resulting in an apparent hypersynchronization of the excitatory bursts across a relatively large cortical region. The bursting activity in individual neurons (the "paroxysmal depolarization shift") is caused by a relatively long-lasting depolarization of the neuronal membrane due to influx of extracellular calcium (Ca^{2+}), which leads to the opening of voltage-dependent sodium (Na^+) channels, influx of Na^+, and generation of repetitive action potentials. This is followed by a hyperpolarizing afterpotential mediated by γ-aminobutyric acid (GABA) receptors or potassium (K^+) channels, depending on the cell type. The synchronized bursts from a sufficient number of neurons result in a so-called spike discharge on the EEG.

The spreading seizure wavefront is slowed and ultimately halted by intact hyperpolarization and a "surround" inhibition created by feed-forward activation of inhibitory neurons. With sufficient activation, there is a recruitment of surrounding neurons via a number of synaptic and nonsynaptic mechanisms, including: (1) an increase in extracellular K^+, which blunts hyperpolarization and depolarizes neighboring neurons; (2) accumulation of Ca^{2+} in presynaptic terminals, leading to enhanced neurotransmitter release; (3) depolarization-induced activation of the *N*-methyl-D-aspartate (NMDA) subtype of the excitatory amino acid receptor, which causes additional Ca^{2+} influx and neuronal activation; and (4) ephaptic interactions related to changes in tissue osmolarity and cell swelling. The recruitment of a sufficient number of neurons leads to the propagation of excitatory currents into contiguous areas via local cortical connections and to more distant areas via long commissural pathways such as the corpus callosum.

Many factors control neuronal excitability, and thus there are many potential mechanisms for altering a neuron's propensity to have bursting activity. Mechanisms *intrinsic* to the neuron include changes in the conductance of ion channels, response characteristics of membrane receptors, cytoplasmic buffering, second-messenger systems, and protein expression as determined by gene transcription, translation, and posttranslational modification. Mechanisms *extrinsic* to the neuron include changes in the amount or type of neurotransmitters present at the synapse, modulation of receptors by extracellular ions and other molecules, and temporal and spatial properties of synaptic and nonsynaptic input. Nonneural cells, such as astrocytes and oligodendrocytes, have an important role in many of these mechanisms as well.

Certain recognized causes of seizures are explained by these mechanisms. For example, accidental ingestion of domoic acid, which is an analogue of glutamate (the principal excitatory neurotransmitter in the brain), causes profound seizures via direct activation of excitatory amino acid receptors throughout the CNS. Penicillin, which can lower the seizure threshold in humans and is a potent convulsant in experimental models, reduces inhibition by antagonizing the effects of GABA at its receptor. The basic mechanisms of other precipitating factors of seizures such as sleep deprivation, fever, alcohol withdrawal, hypoxia, and infection, are not as well understood but presumably involve analogous perturbations in neuronal excitability. Similarly, the endogenous factors that determine an individual's seizure threshold may relate to these properties as well.

Knowledge of the mechanisms responsible for initiation and propagation of most generalized seizures (including tonic-clonic, myoclonic, and atonic types) remains rudimentary and reflects the limited understanding of the connectivity of the brain at a systems level. Much more is understood about the origin of generalized spike-and-wave discharges in absence seizures. These appear to be related to oscillatory rhythms normally generated during sleep by circuits connecting the thalamus and cortex. This oscillatory behavior involves an interaction between $GABA_B$ receptors, T-type Ca^{2+} channels, and K^+ channels located within the thalamus. Pharmacologic studies indicate that modulation of these receptors and channels can induce absence seizures, and there is good evidence that the genetic forms of absence epilepsy may be associated with mutations of components of this system.

MECHANISMS OF EPILEPTOGENESIS

Epileptogenesis refers to the transformation of a normal neuronal network into one that is chronically hyperexcitable. There is often a delay of months to years between an initial CNS injury such as trauma, stroke, or infection and the first seizure. The injury appears to initiate a process that gradually lowers the seizure threshold in the affected region until a spontaneous seizure occurs. In many genetic and idiopathic forms of epilepsy, epileptogenesis is presumably determined by developmentally regulated events.

Pathologic studies of the hippocampus from patients with temporal lobe epilepsy have led to the suggestion that some forms of epileptogenesis are related to *structural changes in neuronal networks.* For example, many patients with MTLE have a highly selective loss of neurons that may contribute to inhibition of the main excitatory neurons within the dentate gyrus. There is also evidence that, in response to the loss of neurons, there is reorganization or "sprouting" of surviving neurons in a way that affects the excitability of the network. Some of these changes can be seen in experimental models of prolonged electrical seizures or traumatic brain injury. Thus, an initial injury such as head injury may lead to a very focal, confined region of structural change that causes local hyperexcitability. The local hyperexcitability leads to further structural changes that evolve over time until the focal lesion produces clinically evident seizures. Similar models have provided strong evidence for long-term alterations in *intrinsic, biochemical properties of cells* within the network such as chronic changes in glutamate or GABA receptor function. Recent work has suggested that induction of inflammatory cascades may be a critical factor in these processes as well.

GENETIC CAUSES OF EPILEPSY

The most important recent progress in epilepsy research has been the identification of genetic mutations associated with a variety of epilepsy syndromes (Table 445-2). Although most of the mutations identified to date cause rare forms of epilepsy, their discovery has led to extremely important conceptual advances. For example, it appears that many of the inherited, idiopathic epilepsies (i.e., the relatively "pure" forms of epilepsy in which seizures are the phenotypic abnormality and brain structure and function are otherwise normal) are due to mutations affecting ion channel function. These syndromes are therefore part of the larger group of channelopathies causing paroxysmal disorders such as cardiac arrhythmias, episodic ataxia, periodic weakness, and familial hemiplegic migraine. In contrast, gene mutations observed in symptomatic epilepsies (i.e., disorders in which other neurologic abnormalities such as cognitive impairment coexist with seizures) are proving to be associated with pathways influencing CNS development or neuronal homeostasis. *De novo* mutations may explain a significant proportion of these syndromes, especially those with onset in early childhood. A current challenge is to identify the multiple susceptibility genes that underlie the more common forms of idiopathic epilepsies. Recent studies suggest that ion channel mutations and copy number variants may contribute to causation in a subset of these patients.

MECHANISMS OF ACTION OF ANTIEPILEPTIC DRUGS

Antiepileptic drugs appear to act primarily by blocking the initiation or spread of seizures. This occurs through a variety of mechanisms that modify the activity of ion channels or neurotransmitters, and in most cases, the drugs have pleiotropic effects. The mechanisms include inhibition of Na^+-dependent action potentials in a frequency-dependent manner (e.g., phenytoin, carbamazepine, lamotrigine, topiramate, zonisamide, lacosamide, rufinamide), inhibition of voltage-gated Ca^{2+} channels (phenytoin, gabapentin, pregabalin), facilitating the opening of potassium channels (ezogabine), attenuation of glutamate activity (lamotrigine, topiramate, felbamate), potentiation of GABA receptor function (benzodiazepines and barbiturates), increase in the availability of GABA (valproic acid, gabapentin, tiagabine), and modulation of release of synaptic vesicles (levetiracetam). The two most effective drugs for absence seizures, ethosuximide and valproic acid, probably act by inhibiting T-type Ca^{2+} channels in thalamic neurons.

In contrast to the relatively large number of antiepileptic drugs that can attenuate seizure activity, there are currently no drugs known to prevent the formation of a seizure focus following CNS injury. The eventual development of such "antiepileptogenic" drugs will provide an important means of preventing the emergence of epilepsy following injuries such as head trauma, stroke, and CNS infection.

APPROACH TO THE PATIENT: Seizure

When a patient presents shortly after a seizure, the first priorities are attention to vital signs, respiratory and cardiovascular support, and treatment of seizures if they resume (see "Treatment: Seizures and Epilepsy"). Life-threatening conditions such as CNS infection, metabolic derangement, or drug toxicity must be recognized and managed appropriately.

When the patient is not acutely ill, the evaluation will initially focus on whether there is a history of earlier seizures (Fig. 445-2). If this is the first seizure, then the emphasis will be to: (1) establish whether the reported episode was a seizure rather than another paroxysmal event, (2) determine the cause of the seizure by identifying risk factors and precipitating events, and (3) decide whether anticonvulsant therapy is required in addition to treatment for any underlying illness.

In the patient with prior seizures or a known history of epilepsy, the evaluation is directed toward: (1) identification of the underlying cause and precipitating factors, and (2) determination of the adequacy of the patient's current therapy.

HISTORY AND EXAMINATION

The first goal is to determine whether the event was truly a seizure. An in-depth history is essential, because *in many cases the diagnosis of a seizure is based solely on clinical grounds—the examination and laboratory studies are often normal.* Questions should focus on the symptoms before, during, and after the episode in order to differentiate a seizure from other paroxysmal events (see "Differential Diagnosis of Seizures" below). Seizures frequently occur out-of-hospital, and the patient may be unaware of the ictal and immediate postictal phases; thus, witnesses to the event should be interviewed carefully.

The history should also focus on risk factors and predisposing events. Clues for a predisposition to seizures include a history of febrile seizures, earlier auras or brief seizures not recognized as such, and a family history of seizures. Epileptogenic factors such as prior head trauma, stroke, tumor, or CNS infection should be identified.

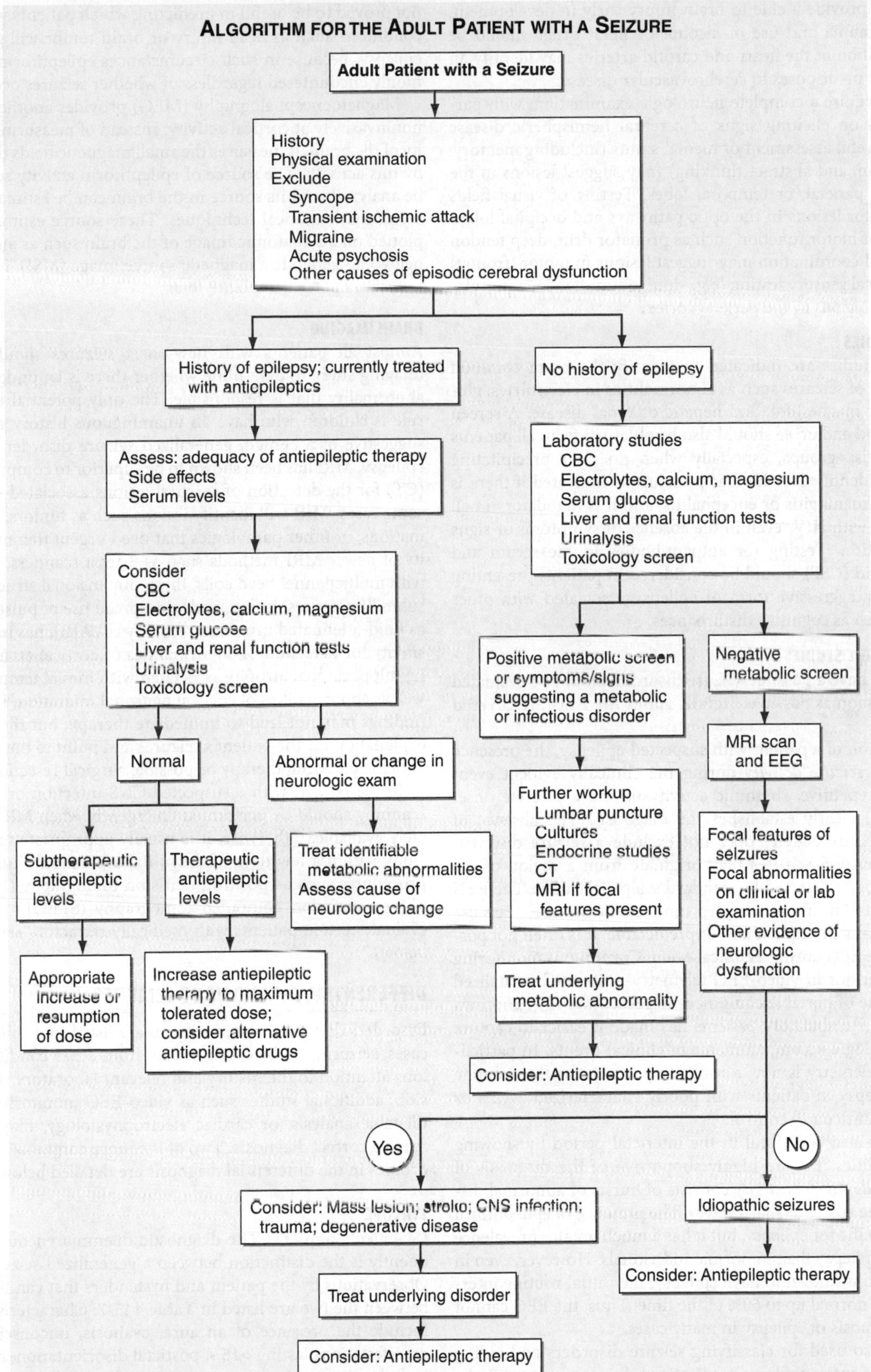

FIGURE 445-2 Evaluation of the adult patient with a seizure. CBC, complete blood count; CNS, central nervous system; CT, computed tomography; EEG, electroencephalogram; MRI, magnetic resonance imaging.

In children, a careful assessment of developmental milestones may provide evidence for underlying CNS disease. Precipitating factors such as sleep deprivation, systemic diseases, electrolyte or metabolic derangements, acute infection, drugs that lower the seizure threshold (Table 445-5), or alcohol or illicit drug use should also be identified.

The general physical examination includes a search for signs of infection or systemic illness. Careful examination of the skin may reveal signs of neurocutaneous disorders such as tuberous sclerosis or neurofibromatosis, or chronic liver or renal disease. A finding of organomegaly may indicate a metabolic storage disease, and limb asymmetry may provide a clue to brain injury early in development. Signs of head trauma and use of alcohol or illicit drugs should be sought. Auscultation of the heart and carotid arteries may identify an abnormality that predisposes to cerebrovascular disease.

All patients require a complete neurologic examination, with particular emphasis on eliciting signs of cerebral hemispheric disease (Chap. 437). Careful assessment of mental status (including memory, language function, and abstract thinking) may suggest lesions in the anterior frontal, parietal, or temporal lobes. Testing of visual fields will help screen for lesions in the optic pathways and occipital lobes. Screening tests of motor function such as pronator drift, deep tendon reflexes, gait, and coordination may suggest lesions in motor (frontal) cortex, and cortical sensory testing (e.g., double simultaneous stimulation) may detect lesions in the parietal cortex.

LABORATORY STUDIES

Routine blood studies are indicated to identify the more common metabolic causes of seizures such as abnormalities in electrolytes, glucose, calcium, or magnesium, and hepatic or renal disease. A screen for toxins in blood and urine should also be obtained from all patients in appropriate risk groups, especially when no clear precipitating factor has been identified. A lumbar puncture is indicated if there is any suspicion of meningitis or encephalitis, and it is mandatory in all patients infected with HIV, even in the absence of symptoms or signs suggesting infection. Testing for autoantibodies in the serum and cerebrospinal fluid (CSF) should be considered in patients presenting with a seemingly aggressive form of epilepsy associated with other abnormalities such as cognitive disturbances.

ELECTROPHYSIOLOGIC STUDIES

All patients who have a possible seizure disorder should be evaluated with an EEG as soon as possible. Details about the EEG are covered in Chap. 442e.

In the evaluation of a patient with suspected epilepsy, the presence of *electrographic seizure activity* during the clinically evident event (i.e., abnormal, repetitive, rhythmic activity having a discrete onset and termination) clearly establishes the diagnosis. The absence of electrographic seizure activity does not exclude a seizure disorder, however, because focal seizures may originate from a region of the cortex that cannot be detected by standard scalp electrodes. The EEG is always abnormal during generalized tonic-clonic seizures. Because seizures are typically infrequent and unpredictable, it is often not possible to obtain the EEG during a clinical event. Continuous monitoring for prolonged periods in video-EEG telemetry units for hospitalized patients or the use of portable equipment to record the EEG continuously for ≥24 h in ambulatory patients has made it easier to capture the electrophysiologic accompaniments of clinical events. In particular, video-EEG telemetry is now a routine approach for the accurate diagnosis of epilepsy in patients with poorly characterized events or seizures that are difficult to control.

The EEG may also be helpful in the interictal period by showing certain abnormalities that are highly supportive of the diagnosis of epilepsy. Such *epileptiform activity* consists of bursts of abnormal discharges containing spikes or sharp waves. The presence of epileptiform activity is not specific for epilepsy, but it has a much greater prevalence in patients with epilepsy than in normal individuals. However, even in an individual who is known to have epilepsy, the initial routine interictal EEG may be normal up to 60% of the time. Thus, the EEG cannot establish the diagnosis of epilepsy in many cases.

The EEG is also used for classifying seizure disorders and aiding in the selection of anticonvulsant medications. For example, episodic generalized spike-wave activity is usually seen in patients with typical absence epilepsy and may be seen with other generalized epilepsy syndromes. Focal interictal epileptiform discharges would support the diagnosis of a focal seizure disorder such as temporal lobe epilepsy or frontal lobe seizures, depending on the location of the discharges.

The routine scalp-recorded EEG may also be used to assess the prognosis of seizure disorders; in general, a normal EEG implies a better prognosis, whereas an abnormal background or profuse epileptiform activity suggests a poor outcome. Unfortunately, the EEG has not proved to be useful in predicting which patients with predisposing conditions such as head injury or brain tumor will go on to develop epilepsy, because in such circumstances epileptiform activity is commonly encountered regardless of whether seizures occur.

Magnetoencephalography (MEG) provides another way of looking noninvasively at cortical activity. Instead of measuring electrical activity of the brain, it measures the small magnetic fields that are generated by this activity. The source of epileptiform activity seen on MEG can be analyzed, and its source in the brain can be estimated using a variety of mathematical techniques. These source estimates can then be plotted on an anatomic image of the brain such as an MRI (discussed below), to generate a magnetic source image (MSI). MSI can be useful to localize potential seizure foci.

BRAIN IMAGING

Almost all patients with new-onset seizures should have a brain imaging study to determine whether there is an underlying structural abnormality that is responsible. The only potential exception to this rule is children who have an unambiguous history and examination suggestive of a benign, generalized seizure disorder such as absence epilepsy. MRI has been shown to be superior to computed tomography (CT) for the detection of cerebral lesions associated with epilepsy. In some cases, MRI will identify lesions such as tumors, vascular malformations, or other pathologies that need urgent therapy. The availability of newer MRI methods such as 3-tesla scanners, parallel imaging with multichannel head coils, three-dimensional structural imaging at submillimeter resolution, and widespread use of pulse sequences such as fluid-attenuated inversion recovery (FLAIR), has increased the sensitivity for detection of abnormalities of cortical architecture, including hippocampal atrophy associated with mesial temporal sclerosis, as well as abnormalities of cortical neuronal migration. In such cases, the findings may not lead to immediate therapy, but they do provide an explanation for the patient's seizures and point to the need for chronic antiepileptic drug therapy or possible surgical resection.

In the patient with a suspected CNS infection or mass lesion, CT scanning should be performed emergently when MRI is not immediately available. Otherwise, it is usually appropriate to obtain an MRI study within a few days of the initial evaluation. Functional imaging procedures such as positron emission tomography (PET) and single-photon emission computed tomography (SPECT) are also used to evaluate certain patients with medically refractory seizures (discussed below).

DIFFERENTIAL DIAGNOSIS OF SEIZURES

Disorders that may mimic seizures are listed in Table 445-6. In most cases, seizures can be distinguished from other conditions by meticulous attention to the history and relevant laboratory studies. On occasion, additional studies such as video-EEG monitoring, sleep studies, tilt-table analysis, or cardiac electrophysiology, may be required to reach a correct diagnosis. Two of the more common nonepileptic syndromes in the differential diagnosis are detailed below.

SYNCOPE

(See also Chap. 27) The diagnostic dilemma encountered most frequently is the distinction between a generalized seizure and syncope. Observations by the patient and bystanders that can help differentiate between the two are listed in Table 445-7. Characteristics of a seizure include the presence of an aura, cyanosis, unconsciousness, motor manifestations lasting >15 s, postictal disorientation, muscle soreness, and sleepiness. In contrast, a syncopal episode is more likely if the event was provoked by acute pain or anxiety or occurred immediately after arising from the lying or sitting position. Patients with syncope often describe a stereotyped transition from consciousness to unconsciousness that includes tiredness, sweating, nausea, and tunneling of vision, and they experience a relatively brief loss of consciousness. Headache or incontinence usually suggests a seizure but may on occasion also occur with syncope. A brief period (i.e., 1–10 s) of convulsive motor activity is frequently seen immediately at the onset of a syncopal episode, especially if the patient remains in an upright posture

TABLE 445-6 DIFFERENTIAL DIAGNOSIS OF SEIZURES

Syncope	**Transient ischemic attack (TIA)**
Vasovagal syncope	Basilar artery TIA
Cardiac arrhythmia	**Sleep disorders**
Valvular heart disease	Narcolepsy/cataplexy
Cardiac failure	Benign sleep myoclonus
Orthostatic hypotension	**Movement disorders**
Psychological disorders	Tics
Psychogenic seizure	Nonepileptic myoclonus
Hyperventilation	Paroxysmal choreoathetosis
Panic attack	**Special considerations in children**
Metabolic disturbances	Breath-holding spells
Alcoholic blackouts	Migraine with recurrent abdominal pain and cyclic vomiting
Delirium tremens	Benign paroxysmal vertigo
Hypoglycemia	Apnea
Hypoxia	Night terrors
Psychoactive drugs (e.g., hallucinogens)	Sleepwalking
Migraine	
Confusional migraine	
Basilar migraine	

after fainting (e.g., in a dentist's chair) and therefore has a sustained decrease in cerebral perfusion. Rarely, a syncopal episode can induce a full tonic-clonic seizure. In such cases, the evaluation must focus on both the cause of the syncopal event as well as the possibility that the patient has a propensity for recurrent seizures.

PSYCHOGENIC SEIZURES

Psychogenic seizures are nonepileptic behaviors that resemble seizures. They are often part of a conversion reaction precipitated by underlying psychological distress. Certain behaviors such as side-to-side turning of the head, asymmetric and large-amplitude shaking movements of the limbs, twitching of all four extremities without loss of consciousness, and pelvic thrusting are more commonly associated with psychogenic rather than epileptic seizures. Psychogenic seizures often last longer than epileptic seizures and may wax and wane over minutes to hours. However, the distinction is sometimes difficult on clinical grounds alone, and there are many examples of diagnostic errors made by experienced epileptologists. This is especially true for psychogenic seizures that resemble focal seizures with dyscognitive features, because the behavioral manifestations of focal seizures (especially of frontal lobe origin) can be extremely unusual, and in both cases, the routine surface EEG may be normal. Video-EEG monitoring is very useful when historic features are nondiagnostic. Generalized tonic-clonic seizures always produce marked EEG abnormalities during and after the seizure. For suspected focal seizures of temporal lobe origin, the use of additional electrodes beyond the standard scalp locations (e.g., sphenoidal electrodes) may be required to localize a seizure focus. Measurement of serum prolactin levels may also help to distinguish between organic and psychogenic seizures, because most generalized seizures and some focal seizures are accompanied by rises in serum prolactin (during the immediate 30-min postictal period), whereas psychogenic seizures are not. The diagnosis of psychogenic seizures does not exclude a concurrent diagnosis of epilepsy, because the two often coexist.

TABLE 445-7 FEATURES THAT DISTINGUISH GENERALIZED TONIC-CLONIC SEIZURE FROM SYNCOPE

Features	Seizure	Syncope
Immediate precipitating factors	Usually none	Emotional stress, Valsalva, orthostatic hypotension, cardiac etiologies
Premonitory symptoms	None or aura (e.g., odd odor)	Tiredness, nausea, diaphoresis, tunneling of vision
Posture at onset	Variable	Usually erect
Transition to unconsciousness	Often immediate	Gradual over seconds[a]
Duration of unconsciousness	Minutes	Seconds
Duration of tonic or clonic movements	30–60 s	Never more than 15 s
Facial appearance during event	Cyanosis, frothing at mouth	Pallor
Disorientation and sleepiness after event	Many minutes to hours	<5 min
Aching of muscles after event	Often	Sometimes
Biting of tongue	Sometimes	Rarely
Incontinence	Sometimes	Sometimes
Headache	Sometimes	Rarely

[a]May be sudden with certain cardiac arrhythmias.

TREATMENT SEIZURES AND EPILEPSY

Therapy for a patient with a seizure disorder is almost always multimodal and includes treatment of underlying conditions that cause or contribute to the seizures, avoidance of precipitating factors, suppression of recurrent seizures by prophylactic therapy with antiepileptic medications or surgery, and addressing a variety of psychological and social issues. Treatment plans must be individualized, given the many different types and causes of seizures as well as the differences in efficacy and toxicity of antiepileptic medications for each patient. In almost all cases, a neurologist with experience in the treatment of epilepsy should design and oversee implementation of the treatment strategy. Furthermore, patients with refractory epilepsy or those who require polypharmacy with antiepileptic drugs should remain under the regular care of a neurologist.

TREATMENT OF UNDERLYING CONDITIONS

If the sole cause of a seizure is a metabolic disturbance such as an abnormality of serum electrolytes or glucose, then treatment is aimed at reversing the metabolic problem and preventing its recurrence. Therapy with antiepileptic drugs is usually unnecessary unless the metabolic disorder cannot be corrected promptly and the patient is at risk of having further seizures. If the apparent cause of a seizure was a medication (e.g., theophylline) or illicit drug use (e.g., cocaine), then appropriate therapy is avoidance of the drug; there is usually no need for antiepileptic medications unless subsequent seizures occur in the absence of these precipitants.

Seizures caused by a structural CNS lesion such as a brain tumor, vascular malformation, or brain abscess may not recur after appropriate treatment of the underlying lesion. However, despite removal of the structural lesion, there is a risk that the seizure focus will remain in the surrounding tissue or develop *de novo* as a result of gliosis and other processes induced by surgery, radiation, or other therapies. Most patients are therefore maintained on an antiepileptic medication for at least 1 year, and an attempt is made to withdraw medications only if the patient has been completely seizure free. If seizures are refractory to medication, the patient may benefit from surgical removal of the epileptic brain region (see below).

AVOIDANCE OF PRECIPITATING FACTORS

Unfortunately, little is known about the specific factors that determine precisely when a seizure will occur in a patient with epilepsy. Some patients can identify particular situations that appear to lower their seizure threshold; these situations should be avoided. For example, a patient who has seizures in the setting of sleep deprivation should obviously be advised to maintain a normal sleep schedule. Many patients note an association between alcohol intake and seizures, and they should be encouraged to modify their drinking habits accordingly. There are also relatively rare cases of patients with seizures that are induced by highly specific stimuli such as a video game monitor, music, or an individual's voice ("reflex epilepsy"). Because there is often an association between stress and seizures, stress reduction techniques such as physical exercise, meditation, or counseling may be helpful.

ANTIEPILEPTIC DRUG THERAPY

Antiepileptic drug therapy is the mainstay of treatment for most patients with epilepsy. The overall goal is to completely prevent seizures without causing any untoward side effects, preferably with a single medication and a dosing schedule that is easy for the patient to follow. Seizure classification is an important element in designing the treatment plan, because some antiepileptic drugs have different activities against various seizure types. However, there is considerable overlap between many antiepileptic drugs such that the choice of therapy is often determined more by the patient's specific needs, especially his or her assessment of side effects.

When to Initiate Antiepileptic Drug Therapy Antiepileptic drug therapy should be started in any patient with recurrent seizures of unknown etiology or a known cause that cannot be reversed. Whether to initiate therapy in a patient with a single seizure is controversial. Patients with a single seizure due to an identified lesion such as a CNS tumor, infection, or trauma, in which there is strong evidence that the lesion is epileptogenic, should be treated. The risk of seizure recurrence in a patient with an apparently unprovoked or idiopathic seizure is uncertain, with estimates ranging from 31 to 71% in the first 12 months after the initial seizure. This uncertainty arises from differences in the underlying seizure types and etiologies in various published epidemiologic studies. Generally accepted risk factors associated with recurrent seizures include the following: (1) an abnormal neurologic examination, (2) seizures presenting as status epilepticus, (3) postictal Todd's paralysis, (4) a strong family history of seizures, or (5) an abnormal EEG. Most patients with one or more of these risk factors should be treated. Issues such as employment or driving may influence the decision whether to start medications as well. For example, a patient with a single, idiopathic seizure whose job depends on driving may prefer taking antiepileptic drugs rather than risk a seizure recurrence and the potential loss of driving privileges.

Selection of Antiepileptic Drugs Antiepileptic drugs available in the United States are shown in Table 445-8, and the main pharmacologic characteristics of commonly used drugs are listed in Table 445-9. Worldwide, older medications such as phenytoin, valproic acid, carbamazepine, phenobarbital, and ethosuximide are generally used as first-line therapy for most seizure disorders because, overall, they are as effective as recently marketed drugs and significantly less expensive overall. Most of the new drugs that have become available in the past decade are used as add-on or alternative therapy, although many are now being used as first-line monotherapy.

In addition to efficacy, factors influencing the choice of an initial medication include the convenience of dosing (e.g., once daily versus three or four times daily) and potential side effects. In this regard, a number of the newer drugs have the advantage of reduced drug-drug interactions and easier dosing. Almost all of the commonly used antiepileptic drugs can cause similar, dose-related side effects such as sedation, ataxia, and diplopia. Long-term use of some agents in adults, especially the elderly, can lead to osteoporosis. Close follow-up is required to ensure these side effects are promptly recognized and reversed. Most of the older drugs and some of the newer ones can also cause idiosyncratic toxicity such as rash, bone marrow suppression, or hepatotoxicity. Although rare, these side effects should be considered during drug selection, and patients must be instructed about symptoms or signs that should signal the need to alert their health care provider. For some drugs, laboratory tests (e.g., complete blood count and liver function tests) are recommended prior to the institution of therapy (to establish baseline values) and during initial dosing and titration of the agent. Importantly, studies have shown that Asian individuals carrying the human leukocyte antigen allele, HLA-B*1502, are at particularly high risk of developing serious skin reactions from carbamazepine and phenytoin. As a result, racial background and genotype are additional factors to consider in drug selection.

TABLE 445-8 SELECTION OF ANTIEPILEPTIC DRUGS

Generalized-Onset Tonic-Clonic	Focal	Typical Absence	Atypical Absence, Myoclonic, Atonic
First-Line			
Lamotrigine	Lamotrigine	Valproic acid	Valproic acid
Valproic acid	Carbamazepine	Ethosuximide	Lamotrigine
	Oxcarbazepine	Lamotrigine	Topiramate
	Phenytoin		
	Levetiracetam		
Alternatives			
Zonisamide[a]	Topiramate	Lamotrigine	Clonazepam
Phenytoin	Zonisamide[a]	Clonazepam	Felbamate
Carbamazepine	Valproic acid		Clobazam
Oxcarbazepine	Tiagabine[a]		Rufinamide
Topiramate	Gabapentin[a]		
Phenobarbital	Lacosamide[a]		
Primidone	Exogabine[a]		
Felbamate	Phenobarbital		
	Primidone		
	Felbamate		

[a]As adjunctive therapy.

ANTIEPILEPTIC DRUG SELECTION FOR FOCAL SEIZURES Carbamazepine (or a related drug, oxcarbazepine), lamotrigine, phenytoin, and levetiracetam are currently the drugs of choice approved for the initial treatment of focal seizures, including those that evolve into generalized seizures. Overall they have very similar efficacy, but differences in pharmacokinetics and toxicity are the main determinants for use in a given patient. For example, an advantage of carbamazepine (which is also available in an extended-release form) is that its metabolism follows first-order pharmacokinetics, which allows for a linear relationship between drug dose, serum levels, and toxicity. Carbamazepine can cause leukopenia, aplastic anemia, or hepatotoxicity and would therefore be contraindicated in patients with predispositions to these problems. Oxcarbazepine has the advantage of being metabolized in a way that avoids an intermediate metabolite associated with some of the side effects of carbamazepine. Oxcarbazepine also has fewer drug interactions than carbamazepine. Lamotrigine tends to be well tolerated in terms of side effects. However, patients need to be particularly vigilant about the possibility of a skin rash during the initiation of therapy. This can be extremely severe and lead to Stevens-Johnson syndrome if unrecognized and if the medication is not discontinued immediately. This risk can be reduced by the use of low initial doses and slow titration. Lamotrigine must be started at lower initial doses when used as add-on therapy with valproic acid, because valproic acid inhibits lamotrigine metabolism and results in a substantially prolonged half-life. Phenytoin has a relatively long half-life and offers the advantage of once or twice daily dosing compared to two or three times daily dosing for many of the other drugs. However, phenytoin shows properties of nonlinear kinetics, such that small increases in phenytoin doses above a standard maintenance dose can precipitate marked side effects. This is one of the main causes of acute phenytoin toxicity. Long-term use of phenytoin is associated with untoward cosmetic effects (e.g., hirsutism, coarsening of facial features, gingival hypertrophy) and effects on bone metabolism. Due to these side effects, phenytoin is often avoided in young patients who are likely to require the drug for many years. Levetiracetam has

TABLE 445-9 DOSAGE AND ADVERSE EFFECTS OF COMMONLY USED ANTIEPILEPTIC DRUGS

Generic Name	Trade Name	Principal Uses	Typical Dose; Dose Interval	Half-Life	Therapeutic Range	Adverse Effects: Neurologic	Adverse Effects: Systemic	Drug Interactions[a]
Carbamazepine	Tegretol[c]	Tonic-clonic Focal-onset	600–1800 mg/d (15–35 mg/kg, child); bid (capsules or tablets), tid-qid (oral suspension)	10–17 h (variable due to autoinduction: complete 3–5 wk after initiation)	4–12 μg/mL	Ataxia Dizziness Diplopia Vertigo	Aplastic anemia Leukopenia Gastrointestinal irritation Hepatotoxicity Hyponatremia	Level decreased by enzyme-inducing drugs[b] Level increased by erythromycin, propoxyphene, isoniazid, cimetidine, fluoxetine
Clobazam	Onfi	Lennox-Gastaut syndrome	10–40 mg/d (5–20 mg/d for patients <30 kg body weight); bid	36–42 h (71–82 h for less active metabolite)	Not established	Fatigue Sedation Ataxia Aggression Insomnia	Constipation Anorexia Skin rash	Level increased by CYP2C19 inhibitors
Clonazepam	Klonopin	Absence Atypical absence Myoclonic	1–12 mg/d; qd-tid	24–48 h	10–70 ng/mL	Ataxia Sedation Lethargy	Anorexia	Level decreased by enzyme-inducing drugs[b]
Ethosuximide	Zarontin	Absence	750–1250 mg/d (20-40 mg/kg); qd-bid	60 h, adult 30 h, child	40–100 μg/mL	Ataxia Lethargy Headache	Gastrointestinal irritation Skin rash Bone marrow suppression	Level decreased by enzyme-inducing drugs[b] Level increased by valproic acid
Ezogabine	Potiga	Focal-onset	800–1200 mg/d; tid	7–11 h	Not established	Dizziness Fatigue Sedation Confusion Vertigo Tremor	Retinal abnormalities Skin discoloration Cardiac conduction (QT interval prolongation) Urinary retention	Level decreased by enzyme-inducing drugs[b]
Felbamate	Felbatol	Focal-onset Lennox-Gastaut syndrome Tonic-clonic	2400–3600 mg/d, tid-qid	16–22 h	30–60 μg/mL	Insomnia Dizziness Sedation Headache	Aplastic anemia Hepatic failure Weight loss Gastrointestinal irritation	Increases phenytoin, valproic acid, active carbamazepine metabolite
Gabapentin	Neurontin	Focal-onset	900–2400 mg/d; tid-qid	5–9 h	2–20 μg/mL	Sedation Dizziness Ataxia Fatigue	Gastrointestinal irritation Weight gain Edema	No known significant interactions
Lacosamide	Vimpat	Focal-onset	200–400 mg/d; bid	13 h	Not established	Dizziness Ataxia Diplopia Vertigo	Gastrointestinal irritation Cardiac conduction (PR interval prolongation)	Level decreased by enzyme-inducing drugs[b]

(Continued)

TABLE 445-9 DOSAGE AND ADVERSE EFFECTS OF COMMONLY USED ANTIEPILEPTIC DRUGS (*CONTINUED*)

Generic Name	Trade Name	Principal Uses	Typical Dose; Dose Interval	Half-Life	Therapeutic Range	Adverse Effects		Drug Interactions[a]
						Neurologic	Systemic	
Lamotrigine	Lamictal[c]	Focal-onset Tonic-clonic Atypical absence Myoclonic Lennox-Gastaut syndrome	150–500 mg/d; bid (immediate release), daily (extended release) (lower daily dose for regimens with valproic acid; higher daily dose for regimens with an enzyme inducer)	25 h 14 h (with enzyme-inducers), 59 h (with valproic acid)	2.5–20 μg/mL	Dizziness Diplopia Sedation Ataxia Headache	Skin rash Stevens-Johnson syndrome	Level decreased by enzyme-inducing drugs[b] and oral contraceptives Level increased by valproic acid
Levetiracetam	Keppra[c]	Focal-onset	1000–3000 mg/d; bid (immediate release), daily (extended release)	6–8 h	5–45 μg/mL	Sedation Fatigue Incoordination Mood changes	Anemia Leukopenia	No known significant interactions
Oxcarbazepine[c]	Trileptal	Focal-onset Tonic-clonic	900–2400 mg/d (30–45 mg/kg, child); bid	10–17 h (for active metabolite)	10–35 μg/mL	Fatigue Ataxia Dizziness Diplopia Vertigo Headache	See carbamazepine	Level decreased by enzyme-inducing drugs[b] May increase phenytoin
Phenobarbital	Luminal	Tonic-clonic Focal-onset	60–180 mg/d; qd-tid	90 h	10–40 μg/mL	Sedation Ataxia Confusion Dizziness Decreased libido Depression	Skin rash	Level increased by valproic acid, phenytoin
Phenytoin (diphenylhydantoin)	Dilantin	Tonic-clonic Focal-onset	300–400 mg/d (3–6 mg/kg, adult; 4–8 mg/kg, child); qd-tid	24 h (wide variation, dose-dependent)	10–20 μg/mL	Dizziness Diplopia Ataxia Incoordination Confusion	Gingival hyperplasia Lymphadenopathy Hirsutism Osteomalacia Facial coarsening Skin rash	Level increased by isoniazid, sulfonamides, fluoxetine Level decreased by enzyme-inducing drugs[b] Altered folate metabolism
Primidone	Mysoline	Tonic-clonic Focal-onset	750–1000 mg/d; bid-tid	Primidone, 8–15 h Phenobarbital, 90 h	Primidone, 4–12 μg/mL Phenobarbital, 10–40 μg/mL	Same as phenobarbital		Level increased by valproic acid Level decreased by phenytoin (increased conversion to phenobarbital)

Rufinamide	Banzel	Lennox-Gastaut syndrome	3200 mg/d (45 mg/kg, child); bid	6–10 h	Not established	Sedation Fatigue Dizziness Ataxia Headache Diplopia	Gastrointestinal irritation Leukopenia Cardiac conduction (QT interval shortening)	Level decreased by enzyme-inducing drugs[b] Level increased by valproic acid May increase phenytoin
Tiagabine	Gabitril	Focal-onset	32–56 mg/d; bid-qid (as adjunct to enzyme-inducing antiepileptic drug regimen)	2–5 h (with enzyme inducer), 7–9 h (without enzyme inducer)	Not established	Confusion Sedation Depression Dizziness Speech or language problems Paresthesias Psychosis	Gastrointestinal irritation	Level decreased by enzyme-inducing drugs[b]
Topiramate	Topamax	Focal-onset Tonic-clonic Lennox-Gastaut syndrome	200–400 mg/d; bid (immediate release), daily (extended release)	20 h (immediate release), 30 h (extended release)	2–20 μg/mL	Psychomotor slowing Sedation Speech or language problems Fatigue Paresthesias	Renal stones (avoid use with other carbonic anhydrase inhibitors) Glaucoma Weight loss Hypohidrosis	Level decreased by enzyme-inducing drugs[b]
Valproic acid (valproate sodium, divalproex sodium)	Depakene Depakote[c]	Tonic-clonic Absence Atypical absence Myoclonic Focal-onset Atonic	750–2000 mg/d (20–60 mg/kg); bid-qid (immediate and delayed release), daily (extended release)	15 h	50–125 μg/mL	Ataxia Sedation Tremor	Hepatotoxicity Thrombocytopenia Gastrointestinal irritation Weight gain Transient alopecia Hyperammonemia	Level decreased by enzyme-inducing drugs[b]
Zonisamide	Zonegran	Focal-onset Tonic-clonic	200–400 mg/d; qd-bid	50–68 h	10–40 μg/mL	Sedation Dizziness Confusion Headache Psychosis	Anorexia Renal stones Hypohidrosis	Level decreased by enzyme-inducing drugs[b]

[a]Examples only; please refer to other sources for comprehensive listings of all potential drug-drug interactions. [b]Phenytoin, carbamazepine, phenobarbital. [c]Extended-release product available.

the advantage of having no known drug-drug interactions, making it especially useful in the elderly and patients on other medications. However, a significant number of patients taking levetiracetam complain of irritability, anxiety, and other psychiatric symptoms. Topiramate can be used for both focal and generalized seizures. Similar to some of the other antiepileptic drugs, topiramate can cause significant psychomotor slowing and other cognitive problems. Additionally, it should not be used in patients at risk for the development of glaucoma or renal stones.

Valproic acid is an effective alternative for some patients with focal seizures, especially when the seizures generalize. Gastrointestinal side effects are fewer when using the delayed-release formulation (Depakote). Laboratory testing is required to monitor toxicity because valproic acid can rarely cause reversible bone marrow suppression and hepatotoxicity. This drug should generally be avoided in patients with preexisting bone marrow or liver disease. Irreversible, fatal hepatic failure appearing as an idiosyncratic rather than dose-related side effect is a relatively rare complication; its risk is highest in children <2 years old, especially those taking other antiepileptic drugs or with inborn errors of metabolism.

Zonisamide, tiagabine, gabapentin, lacosamide, and ezogabine are additional drugs currently used for the treatment of focal seizures with or without evolution into generalized seizures. Phenobarbital and other barbiturate compounds were commonly used in the past as first-line therapy for many forms of epilepsy. However, the barbiturates frequently cause sedation in adults, hyperactivity in children, and other more subtle cognitive changes; thus, their use should be limited to situations in which no other suitable treatment alternatives exist.

ANTIEPILEPTIC DRUG SELECTION FOR GENERALIZED SEIZURES Lamotrigine and valproic acid are currently considered the best initial choice for the treatment of primary generalized, tonic-clonic seizures. Topiramate, zonisamide, phenytoin, carbamazepine, and oxcarbazepine are suitable alternatives. Valproic acid is also particularly effective in absence, myoclonic, and atonic seizures. It is therefore the drug of choice in patients with generalized epilepsy syndromes having mixed seizure types. Importantly, carbamazepine, oxcarbazepine, and phenytoin can worsen certain types of generalized seizures, including absence, myoclonic, tonic, and atonic seizures. Ethosuximide is a particularly effective drug for the treatment of uncomplicated absence seizures, but it is not useful for tonic-clonic or focal seizures. Periodic monitoring of blood cell counts is required since ethosuximide rarely causes bone marrow suppression. Lamotrigine appears to be particularly effective in epilepsy syndromes with mixed, generalized seizure types such as JME and Lennox-Gastaut syndrome. Topiramate, zonisamide, and felbamate may have similar broad efficacy.

INITIATION AND MONITORING OF THERAPY

Because the response to any antiepileptic drug is unpredictable, patients should be carefully educated about the approach to therapy. The goal is to prevent seizures and minimize the side effects of treatment; determination of the optimal dose is often a matter of trial and error. This process may take months or longer if the baseline seizure frequency is low. Most antiepileptic drugs need to be introduced relatively slowly to minimize side effects. Patients should expect that minor side effects such as mild sedation, slight changes in cognition, or imbalance will typically resolve within a few days. Starting doses are usually the lowest value listed under the dosage column in Table 445-9. Subsequent increases should be made only after achieving a steady state with the previous dose (i.e., after an interval of five or more half-lives).

Monitoring of serum antiepileptic drug levels can be very useful for establishing the initial dosing schedule. However, the published therapeutic ranges of serum drug concentrations are only an approximate guide for determining the proper dose for a given patient. The key determinants are the clinical measures of seizure frequency and presence of side effects, not the laboratory values. Conventional assays of serum drug levels measure the total drug (i.e., both free and protein bound). However, it is the concentration of free drug that reflects extracellular levels in the brain and correlates best with efficacy. Thus, patients with decreased levels of serum proteins (e.g., decreased serum albumin due to impaired liver or renal function) may have an increased ratio of free to bound drug, yet the concentration of free drug may be adequate for seizure control. These patients may have a "subtherapeutic" drug level, but the dose should be changed only if seizures remain uncontrolled, not just to achieve a "therapeutic" level. It is also useful to monitor free drug levels in such patients. In practice, other than during the initiation or modification of therapy, monitoring of antiepileptic drug levels is most useful for documenting adherence.

If seizures continue despite gradual increases to the maximum tolerated dose and documented compliance, then it becomes necessary to switch to another antiepileptic drug. This is usually done by maintaining the patient on the first drug while a second drug is added. The dose of the second drug should be adjusted to decrease seizure frequency without causing toxicity. Once this is achieved, the first drug can be gradually withdrawn (usually over weeks unless there is significant toxicity). The dose of the second drug is then further optimized based on seizure response and side effects. Monotherapy should be the goal whenever possible.

WHEN TO DISCONTINUE THERAPY

Overall, about 70% of children and 60% of adults who have their seizures completely controlled with antiepileptic drugs can eventually discontinue therapy. The following patient profile yields the greatest chance of remaining seizure free after drug withdrawal: (1) complete medical control of seizures for 1–5 years; (2) single seizure type, either focal or generalized; (3) normal neurologic examination, including intelligence; and (4) normal EEG. The appropriate seizure-free interval is unknown and undoubtedly varies for different forms of epilepsy. However, it seems reasonable to attempt withdrawal of therapy after 2 years in a patient who meets all of the above criteria, is motivated to discontinue the medication, and clearly understands the potential risks and benefits. In most cases, it is preferable to reduce the dose of the drug gradually over 2–3 months. Most recurrences occur in the first 3 months after discontinuing therapy, and patients should be advised to avoid potentially dangerous situations such as driving or swimming during this period.

TREATMENT OF REFRACTORY EPILEPSY

Approximately one-third of patients with epilepsy do not respond to treatment with a single antiepileptic drug, and it becomes necessary to try a combination of drugs to control seizures. Patients who have focal epilepsy related to an underlying structural lesion or those with multiple seizure types and developmental delay are particularly likely to require multiple drugs. There are currently no clear guidelines for rational polypharmacy, although in theory a combination of drugs with different mechanisms of action may be most useful. In most cases, the initial combination therapy combines first-line drugs (i.e., carbamazepine, oxcarbazepine, lamotrigine, valproic acid, levetiracetam, and phenytoin). If these drugs are unsuccessful, then the addition of other drugs such as topiramate, zonisamide, lacosamide, or tiagabine is indicated. Patients with myoclonic seizures resistant to valproic acid may benefit from the addition of clonazepam or clobazam, and those with absence seizures may respond to a combination of valproic acid and ethosuximide. The same principles concerning the monitoring of therapeutic response, toxicity, and serum levels for monotherapy apply to polypharmacy, and potential drug interactions need to be recognized. If there is no improvement, a third drug can be added while the first two are maintained. If there is a response, the less effective or less well tolerated of the first two drugs should be gradually withdrawn.

SURGICAL TREATMENT OF REFRACTORY EPILEPSY

Approximately 20–30% of patients with epilepsy continue to have seizures despite efforts to find an effective combination of antiepileptic drugs. For some, surgery can be extremely effective in substantially reducing seizure frequency and even providing complete seizure control. Understanding the potential value of surgery is especially important when a patient's seizures are not controlled with initial treatment, as such patients often do not respond to subsequent medication trials. Rather than submitting the patient to years of unsuccessful medical therapy and the psychosocial trauma and increased mortality associated with ongoing seizures, the patient should have an efficient but relatively brief attempt at medical therapy and then be referred for surgical evaluation.

The most common surgical procedure for patients with temporal lobe epilepsy involves resection of the anteromedial temporal lobe (temporal lobectomy) or a more limited removal of the underlying hippocampus and amygdala (amygdalohippocampectomy). Focal seizures arising from extratemporal regions may be abolished by a focal neocortical resection with precise removal of an identified lesion (lesionectomy). Localized neocortical resection without a clear lesion identified on MRI is also possible when other tests (e.g. MEG, PET, SPECT) implicate a focal cortical region as a seizure onset zone. When the cortical region cannot be removed, multiple subpial transection, which disrupts intracortical connections, is sometimes used to prevent seizure spread. Hemispherectomy or multilobar resection is useful for some patients with severe seizures due to hemispheric abnormalities such as hemimegalencephaly or other dysplastic abnormalities, and corpus callosotomy has been shown to be effective for disabling tonic or atonic seizures, usually when they are part of a mixed-seizure syndrome (e.g., Lennox-Gastaut syndrome).

Presurgical evaluation is designed to identify the functional and structural basis of the patient's seizure disorder. Inpatient video-EEG monitoring is used to define the anatomic location of the seizure focus and to correlate the abnormal electrophysiologic activity with behavioral manifestations of the seizure. Routine scalp or scalp-sphenoidal recordings and a high-resolution MRI scan are usually sufficient for localization of the epileptogenic focus, especially when the findings are concordant. Functional imaging studies such as SPECT, PET, and MEG are adjunctive tests that may help to reveal or verify the localization of an apparent epileptogenic region. Once the presumed location of the seizure onset is identified, additional studies, including neuropsychological testing, the intracarotid amobarbital test (Wada test), and functional MRI may be used to assess language and memory localization and to determine the possible functional consequences of surgical removal of the epileptogenic region. In some cases, standard noninvasive evaluation is not sufficient to localize the seizure onset zone, and invasive electrophysiologic monitoring, such as implanted depth or subdural electrodes, is required for more definitive localization. The exact extent of the resection to be undertaken can also be determined by performing cortical mapping at the time of the surgical procedure, allowing for a tailored resection. This involves electrocorticographic recordings made with electrodes on the surface of the brain to identify the extent of epileptiform disturbances. If the region to be resected is within or near brain regions suspected of having sensorimotor or language function, electrical cortical stimulation mapping is performed on the awake patient to determine the function of cortical regions in question in order to avoid resection of so-called eloquent cortex and thereby minimize postsurgical deficits.

Advances in presurgical evaluation and microsurgical techniques have led to a steady increase in the success of epilepsy surgery. Clinically significant complications of surgery are <5%, and the use of functional mapping procedures has markedly reduced the neurologic sequelae due to removal or sectioning of brain tissue. For example, about 70% of patients treated with temporal lobectomy will become seizure free, and another 15–25% will have at least a 90% reduction in seizure frequency. Marked improvement is also usually seen in patients treated with hemispherectomy for catastrophic seizure disorders due to large hemispheric abnormalities. Postoperatively, patients generally need to remain on antiepileptic drug therapy, but the marked reduction of seizures following resective surgery can have a very beneficial effect on quality of life.

Not all medically refractory patients are suitable candidates for resective surgery. For example, some patients have seizures arising from more than one location, making the risk of ongoing seizures or potential harm from the surgery unacceptably high. Vagus nerve stimulation (VNS) has been used in some of these cases, although the results are limited and it is difficult to predict who will benefit. A new implantable device that can detect the onset of a seizure (in some instances before the seizure becomes clinically apparent) and deliver an electrical stimulation (Responsive NeuroStimulation) has recently been approved and may be of benefit in selected patients. Studies are currently evaluating the efficacy of stereotactic radiosurgery, laser thermoablation, and deep brain stimulation (DBS) as other options for surgical treatment of refractory epilepsy.

STATUS EPILEPTICUS

Status epilepticus refers to continuous seizures or repetitive, discrete seizures with impaired consciousness in the interictal period. Status epilepticus has numerous subtypes, including generalized convulsive status epilepticus (GCSE) (e.g., persistent, generalized electrographic seizures, coma, and tonic-clonic movements) and nonconvulsive status epilepticus (e.g., persistent absence seizures or focal seizures with confusion or partially impaired consciousness, and minimal motor abnormalities). The duration of seizure activity sufficient to meet the definition of status epilepticus has traditionally been specified as 15–30 min. However, a more practical definition is to consider status epilepticus as a situation in which the duration of seizures prompts the acute use of anticonvulsant therapy. For GCSE, this is typically when seizures last beyond 5 min.

GCSE is an emergency and must be treated immediately, because cardiorespiratory dysfunction, hyperthermia, and metabolic derangements can develop as a consequence of prolonged seizures, and these can lead to irreversible neuronal injury. Furthermore, CNS injury can occur even when the patient is paralyzed with neuromuscular blockade but continues to have electrographic seizures. The most common causes of GCSE are anticonvulsant withdrawal or noncompliance, metabolic disturbances, drug toxicity, CNS infection, CNS tumors, refractory epilepsy, and head trauma.

GCSE is obvious when the patient is having overt convulsions. However, after 30–45 min of uninterrupted seizures, the signs may become increasingly subtle. Patients may have mild clonic movements of only the fingers or fine, rapid movements of the eyes. There may be paroxysmal episodes of tachycardia, hypertension, and pupillary dilation. In such cases, the EEG may be the only method of establishing the diagnosis. Thus, if the patient stops having overt seizures, yet remains comatose, an EEG should be performed to rule out ongoing status epilepticus. This is obviously also essential when a patient with GCSE has been paralyzed with neuromuscular blockade in the process of protecting the airway.

The first steps in the management of a patient in GCSE are to attend to any acute cardiorespiratory problems or hyperthermia, perform a brief medical and neurologic examination, establish venous access, and send samples for laboratory studies to identify metabolic abnormalities. Anticonvulsant therapy should then begin without delay; a treatment approach is shown in Fig. 445-3.

The treatment of nonconvulsive status epilepticus is thought to be less urgent than GCSE, because the ongoing seizures are not accompanied by the severe metabolic disturbances seen with GCSE. However, evidence suggests that nonconvulsive status epilepticus, especially that caused by ongoing, focal seizure activity, is associated with cellular injury in the region of the seizure focus; therefore this condition should be treated as promptly as possible using the general approach described for GCSE.

BEYOND SEIZURES: OTHER MANAGEMENT ISSUES

INTERICTAL BEHAVIOR

The adverse effects of epilepsy often go beyond clinical seizures, and the extent of these effects largely depends on the etiology of epilepsy, seizure frequency and severity, and side effects from antiepileptic therapy. Many epilepsy patients are completely normal between seizures

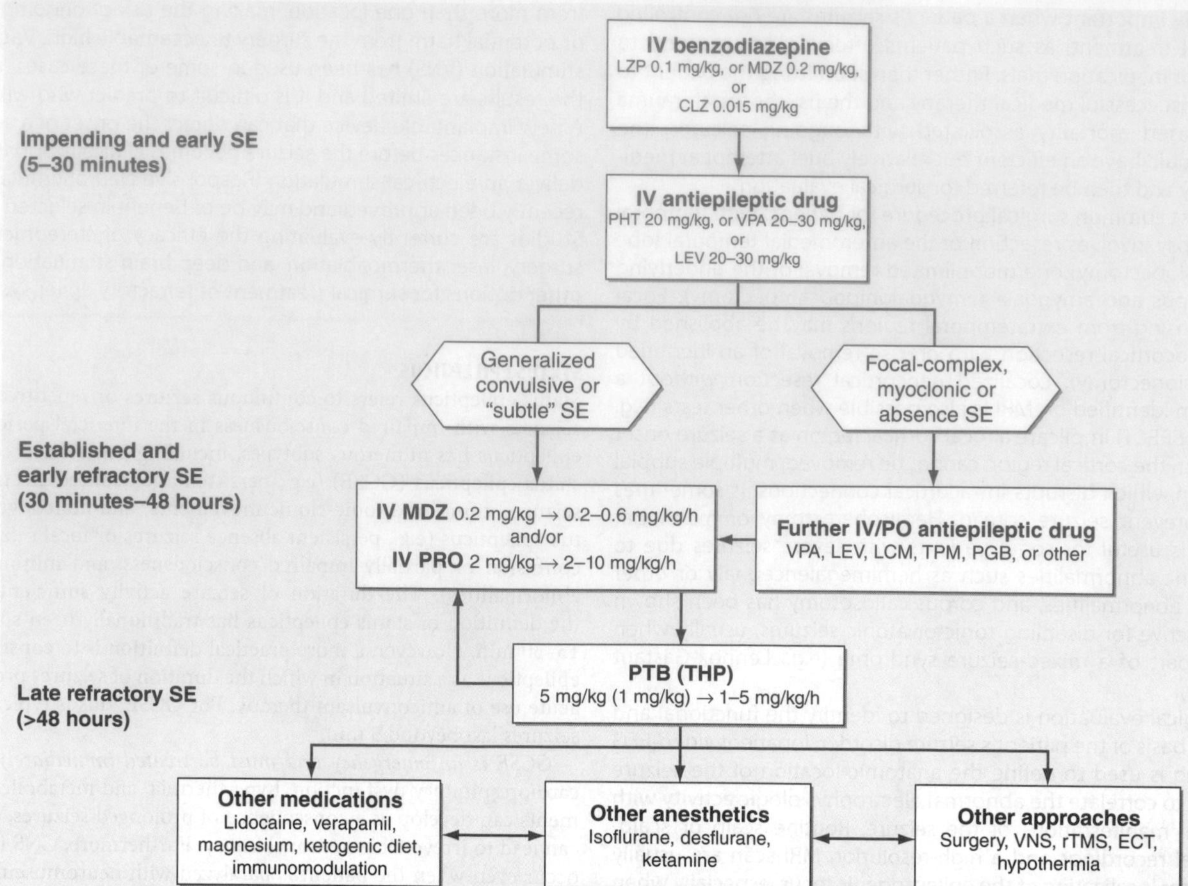

FIGURE 445-3 Pharmacologic treatment of generalized tonic-clonic status epilepticus (SE) in adults. CLZ, clonazepam; ECT, electroconvulsive therapy; LCM, lacosamide; LEV, levetiracetam; LZP, lorazepam; MDZ, midazolam; PGB, pregabalin; PHT, phenytoin or fos-phenytoin; PRO, propofol; PTB, pentobarbital; rTMS, repetitive transcranial magnetic stimulation; THP, thiopental; TPM, topiramate; VNS, vagus nerve stimulation; VPA, valproic acid. *(From AO Rossetti, DH Lowenstein: Lancet Neurol 10:922, 2011.)*

and live highly successful and productive lives. In contrast, patients with seizures secondary to developmental abnormalities or acquired brain injury may have impaired cognitive function and other neurologic deficits. Frequent interictal EEG abnormalities are associated with subtle dysfunction of memory and attention. Patients with many seizures, especially those emanating from the temporal lobe, often note an impairment of short-term memory that may progress over time.

Patients with epilepsy are at risk of developing a variety of psychiatric problems, including depression, anxiety, and psychosis. This risk varies considerably depending on many factors, including the etiology, frequency, and severity of seizures and the patient's age and previous personal or family history of psychiatric disorder. Depression occurs in ~20% of patients, and the incidence of suicide is higher in patients with epilepsy than in the general population. Depression should be treated through counseling or medication. The selective serotonin reuptake inhibitors (SSRIs) typically have minimal effect on seizures, whereas tricyclic antidepressants may lower the seizure threshold. Anxiety can be a seizure symptom, and anxious or psychotic behavior can occur during a postictal delirium. Postictal psychosis is a rare phenomenon that typically occurs after a period of increased seizure frequency. There is usually a brief lucid interval lasting up to a week, followed by days to weeks of agitated, psychotic behavior. The psychosis usually resolves spontaneously but frequently will require short-term treatment with antipsychotic or anxiolytic medications.

There is ongoing controversy as to whether some patients with epilepsy (especially temporal lobe epilepsy) have a stereotypical "interictal personality." The predominant view is that atypical personality traits occur in diverse epilepsies (e.g., generalized and frontal lobe epilepsy) and may result from an underlying structural brain lesion, antiepileptic drug effects, and psychosocial factors related to suffering from a chronic disease, as well as the epilepsy itself.

MORTALITY OF EPILEPSY

Patients with epilepsy have a risk of death that is roughly two to three times greater than expected in a matched population without epilepsy. Most of the increased mortality is due to the underlying etiology of epilepsy (e.g., tumors or strokes in older adults). However, a significant number of patients die from accidents, status epilepticus, and a syndrome known as *sudden unexpected death in epilepsy* (SUDEP), which usually affects young people with convulsive seizures and tends to occur at night. The cause of SUDEP is unknown; it may result from brainstem-mediated effects of seizures on pulmonary, cardiac, and arousal functions. Recent studies suggest that, in some cases, a genetic mutation may be the cause of both epilepsy and a cardiac conduction defect that gives rise to sudden death.

PSYCHOSOCIAL ISSUES

There continues to be a cultural stigma about epilepsy, although it is slowly declining in societies with effective health education programs. Many patients with epilepsy harbor fears such as the fear of becoming mentally retarded or dying during a seizure. These issues need to be carefully addressed by educating the patient about epilepsy and by ensuring that family members, teachers, fellow employees, and other associates are equally well informed. A useful source of educational material is the Web site *www.epilepsy.com*.

EMPLOYMENT, DRIVING, AND OTHER ACTIVITIES

Many patients with epilepsy face difficulty in obtaining or maintaining employment, even when their seizures are well controlled. Federal and state legislation is designed to prevent employers from discriminating against patients with epilepsy, and patients should be encouraged to understand and claim their legal rights. Patients in these circumstances also benefit greatly from the assistance of health providers who act as strong patient advocates.

Loss of driving privileges is one of the most disruptive social consequences of epilepsy. Physicians should be very clear about local regulations concerning driving and epilepsy, because the laws vary considerably among states and countries. In all cases, it is the physician's responsibility to warn patients of the danger imposed on themselves and others while driving if their seizures are uncontrolled (unless the seizures are not associated with impairment of consciousness or motor control). In general, most states allow patients to drive after a seizure-free interval (on or off medications) of between 3 months and 2 years.

Patients with incompletely controlled seizures must also contend with the risk of being in other situations where an impairment of consciousness or loss of motor control could lead to major injury or death. Thus, depending on the type and frequency of seizures, many patients need to be instructed to avoid working at heights or with machinery or to have someone close by for activities such as bathing and swimming.

SPECIAL ISSUES RELATED TO WOMEN AND EPILEPSY

CATAMENIAL EPILEPSY

Some women experience a marked increase in seizure frequency around the time of menses. This is believed to be mediated by either the effects of estrogen and progesterone on neuronal excitability or changes in antiepileptic drug levels due to altered protein binding or metabolism. Some patients may benefit from increases in antiepileptic drug dosages during menses. Natural progestins or intramuscular medroxyprogesterone may be of benefit to a subset of women.

PREGNANCY

Most women with epilepsy who become pregnant will have an uncomplicated gestation and deliver a normal baby. However, epilepsy poses some important risks to a pregnancy. Seizure frequency during pregnancy will remain unchanged in ~50% of women, increase in 30%, and decrease in 20%. Changes in seizure frequency are attributed to endocrine effects on the CNS, variations in antiepileptic drug pharmacokinetics (such as acceleration of hepatic drug metabolism or effects on plasma protein binding), and changes in medication compliance. It is useful to see patients at frequent intervals during pregnancy and monitor serum antiepileptic drug levels. Measurement of the unbound drug concentrations may be useful if there is an increase in seizure frequency or worsening of side effects of antiepileptic drugs.

The overall incidence of fetal abnormalities in children born to mothers with epilepsy is 5–6%, compared to 2–3% in healthy women. Part of the higher incidence is due to teratogenic effects of antiepileptic drugs, and the risk increases with the number of medications used (e.g., 10–20% risk of malformations with three drugs) and possibly with higher doses. A meta-analysis of published pregnancy registries and cohorts found that the most common malformations were defects in the cardiovascular and musculoskeletal system (1.4–1.8%). Valproic acid is strongly associated with an increased risk of adverse fetal outcomes (7–20%). Recent findings from a large pregnancy registry suggest that, other than topiramate, the newer antiepileptic drugs are far safer than valproic acid.

Because the potential harm of uncontrolled convulsive seizures on the mother and fetus is considered greater than the teratogenic effects of antiepileptic drugs, it is currently recommended that pregnant women be maintained on effective drug therapy. When possible, it seems prudent to have the patient on monotherapy at the lowest effective dose, especially during the first trimester. For some women, however, the type and frequency of their seizures may allow for them to safely wean off antiepileptic drugs prior to conception. Patients should also take folate (1–4 mg/d), because the antifolate effects of anticonvulsants are thought to play a role in the development of neural tube defects, although the benefits of this treatment remain unproved in this setting.

Enzyme-inducing drugs such as phenytoin, carbamazepine, oxcarbazepine, topiramate, phenobarbital, and primidone cause a transient and reversible deficiency of vitamin K–dependent clotting factors in ~50% of newborn infants. Although neonatal hemorrhage is uncommon, the mother should be treated with oral vitamin K (20 mg/d, phylloquinone) in the last 2 weeks of pregnancy, and the infant should receive intramuscular vitamin K (1 mg) at birth.

CONTRACEPTION

Special care should be taken when prescribing antiepileptic medications for women who are taking oral contraceptive agents. Drugs such as carbamazepine, phenytoin, phenobarbital, and topiramate can significantly decrease the efficacy of oral contraceptives via enzyme induction and other mechanisms. Patients should be advised to consider alternative forms of contraception, or their contraceptive medications should be modified to offset the effects of the antiepileptic medications.

BREAST-FEEDING

Antiepileptic medications are excreted into breast milk to a variable degree. The ratio of drug concentration in breast milk relative to serum ranges from ~5% (valproic acid) to 300% (levetiracetam). Given the overall benefits of breast-feeding and the lack of evidence for long-term harm to the infant by being exposed to antiepileptic drugs, mothers with epilepsy can be encouraged to breast-feed. This should be reconsidered, however, if there is any evidence of drug effects on the infant such as lethargy or poor feeding.

446 Cerebrovascular Diseases

Wade S. Smith, S. Claiborne Johnston, J. Claude Hemphill, III

Cerebrovascular diseases include some of the most common and devastating disorders: ischemic stroke and hemorrhagic stroke. Stroke is the second leading cause of death worldwide, causing 6.2 million deaths in 2011, and is double the rate of heart disease in China. Strokes cause ~200,000 deaths each year in the United States and are a major cause of disability. The incidence of cerebrovascular diseases increases with age, and the number of strokes is projected to increase as the elderly population grows, with a doubling in stroke deaths in the United States by 2030. A stroke, or cerebrovascular accident, is defined as an abrupt onset of a neurologic deficit that is attributable to a focal vascular cause. Thus, the definition of stroke is clinical, and laboratory studies including brain imaging are used to support the diagnosis. The clinical manifestations of stroke are highly variable because of the complex anatomy of the brain and its vasculature. *Cerebral ischemia* is caused by a reduction in blood flow that lasts longer than several seconds. Neurologic symptoms are manifest within seconds because neurons lack glycogen, so energy failure is rapid. If the cessation of flow lasts for more than a few minutes, *infarction* or death of brain tissue results. When blood flow is quickly restored, brain tissue can recover fully and the patient's symptoms are only transient: this is called a *transient ischemic attack* (TIA). The definition of TIA requires that all neurologic signs and symptoms resolve within 24 h without evidence of brain infarction on brain imaging. Stroke has occurred if the neurologic signs and symptoms last for >24 h or brain infarction is demonstrated. A generalized reduction in cerebral blood flow due to systemic hypotension (e.g., cardiac arrhythmia, myocardial infarction, or hemorrhagic shock) usually produces syncope (Chap. 27). If low cerebral blood flow persists for a longer duration, then infarction in the border zones between the major cerebral artery distributions may develop. In more severe instances, *global hypoxia-ischemia* causes widespread brain injury; the constellation of cognitive sequelae that ensues is called *hypoxic-ischemic encephalopathy* (Chap. 330). *Focal ischemia* or infarction, conversely, is usually caused by thrombosis of the cerebral vessels themselves or by emboli from a proximal arterial source or the heart. *Intracranial hemorrhage* is caused by bleeding directly into or around the brain; it produces neurologic symptoms by producing a mass effect on neural structures, from the toxic effects of blood itself, or by increasing intracranial pressure.

APPROACH TO THE PATIENT: Cerebrovascular Disease

Rapid evaluation is essential for use of time-sensitive treatments such as thrombolysis. However, patients with acute stroke often do not seek medical assistance on their own because they are rarely in pain and also may lose the appreciation that something is wrong (anosognosia); it is often a family member or a bystander who calls for help. Therefore, patients and their family members should be counseled to call emergency medical services immediately if they experience or witness the sudden onset of any of the following: loss of sensory and/or motor function on one side of the body (nearly 85% of ischemic stroke patients have hemiparesis); change in vision, gait, or ability to speak or understand; or a sudden, severe headache.

Other causes of sudden-onset neurologic symptoms that may mimic stroke include seizure, intracranial tumor, migraine, and metabolic encephalopathy. An adequate history from an observer that no convulsive activity occurred at the onset usually excludes seizure, although ongoing complex partial seizures without tonic-clonic activity can on occasion mimic stroke. Tumors may present with acute neurologic symptoms due to hemorrhage, seizure, or hydrocephalus. Surprisingly, migraine (Chap. 447) can mimic stroke, even in patients without a significant migraine history. When migraine develops without head pain (*acephalgic migraine*), the diagnosis can be especially difficult. Patients without any prior history of migraine may develop acephalgic migraine even after age 65. A sensory disturbance is often prominent, and the sensory deficit, as well as any motor deficits, tends to migrate slowly across a limb, over minutes rather than seconds as with stroke. The diagnosis of migraine becomes more secure as the cortical disturbance begins to cross vascular boundaries or if typical visual symptoms are present such as scintillating scotomata. At times it may be impossible to make the diagnosis of migraine until there have been multiple episodes with no residual symptoms or signs and no changes on brain magnetic resonance imaging (MRI). Metabolic encephalopathies typically produce fluctuating mental status changes without focal neurologic findings. However, in the setting of prior stroke or brain injury, a patient with fever or sepsis may manifest a recurrent hemiparesis, which clears rapidly when the infection is treated. The metabolic process serves to "unmask" a prior deficit.

Once the diagnosis of stroke is made, a brain imaging study is necessary to determine if the cause of stroke is ischemia or hemorrhage (Fig. 446-1). Computed tomography (CT) imaging of the brain is the standard imaging modality to detect the presence or absence of intracranial hemorrhage (see "Imaging Studies," below). If the stroke is ischemic, administration of recombinant tissue plasminogen activator (rtPA) or endovascular mechanical thrombectomy may be beneficial in restoring cerebral perfusion (see "Treatment: Acute Ischemic Stroke"). Medical management to reduce the risk of complications becomes the next priority, followed by plans for secondary prevention. For ischemic stroke, several strategies can reduce the risk of subsequent stroke in all patients, while other strategies are effective for patients with specific causes of stroke such as cardiac embolus and carotid atherosclerosis. For hemorrhagic stroke, aneurysmal subarachnoid hemorrhage (SAH) and hypertensive intracerebral hemorrhage are two important causes. The treatment and prevention of hypertensive intracerebral hemorrhage are discussed later in this chapter. SAH is discussed in Chap. 330.

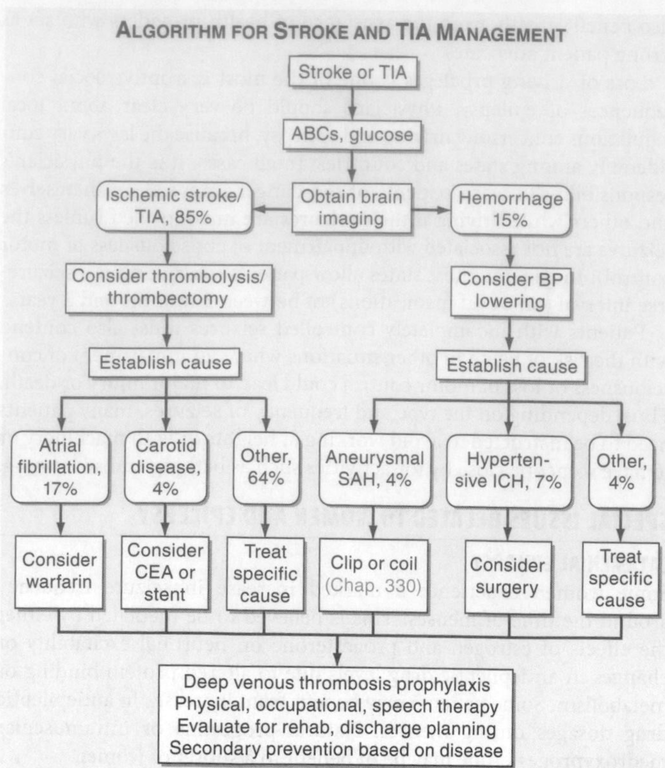

FIGURE 446-1 Medical management of stroke and TIA. *Rounded boxes* are diagnoses; *rectangles* are interventions. Numbers are percentages of stroke overall. ABCs, airway, breathing, circulation; BP, blood pressure; CEA, carotid endarterectomy; ICH, intracerebral hemorrhage; SAH, subarachnoid hemorrhage; TIA, transient ischemic attack.

ISCHEMIC STROKE

PATHOPHYSIOLOGY OF ISCHEMIC STROKE

Acute occlusion of an intracranial vessel causes reduction in blood flow to the brain region it supplies. The magnitude of flow reduction is a function of collateral blood flow, and this depends on individual vascular anatomy (which may be altered by disease), the site of occlusion, and systemic blood pressure. A decrease in cerebral blood flow to zero causes death of brain tissue within 4–10 min; values <16–18 mL/100 g tissue per minute cause infarction within an hour; and values <20 mL/100 g tissue per minute cause ischemia without infarction unless prolonged for several hours or days. If blood flow is restored to ischemic tissue before significant infarction develops, the patient may experience only transient symptoms, and the clinical syndrome is called a TIA. Another important concept is the *ischemic penumbra*, defined as the ischemic but reversibly dysfunctional tissue surrounding a core area of infarction. The penumbra can be imaged by perfusion-diffusion imaging using MRI or CT (see below and Figs. 446-15 and 446-16). The ischemic penumbra will eventually progress to infarction if no change in flow occurs, and hence saving the ischemic penumbra is the goal of revascularization therapies.

Focal cerebral infarction occurs via two distinct pathways (Fig. 446-2): (1) a necrotic pathway in which cellular cytoskeletal breakdown is rapid, due principally to energy failure of the cell; and (2) an apoptotic pathway in which cells become programmed to die. Ischemia produces necrosis by starving neurons of glucose and oxygen, which in turn results in failure of mitochondria to produce ATP. Without ATP, membrane ion pumps stop functioning and neurons depolarize, allowing intracellular calcium to rise. Cellular depolarization also causes glutamate release from synaptic terminals; excess extracellular glutamate produces neurotoxicity by activating postsynaptic glutamate receptors that increase neuronal calcium influx. Free radicals are produced by degradation of membrane lipids and mitochondrial dysfunction. Free radicals cause catalytic destruction of membranes and likely damage other vital functions of cells. Lesser degrees of ischemia, as are seen within the ischemic penumbra, favor apoptotic cellular death causing cells to die days to weeks later. Fever dramatically worsens brain injury during ischemia, as does hyperglycemia (glucose >11.1 mmol/L [200 mg/dL]), so it is reasonable to suppress fever and prevent

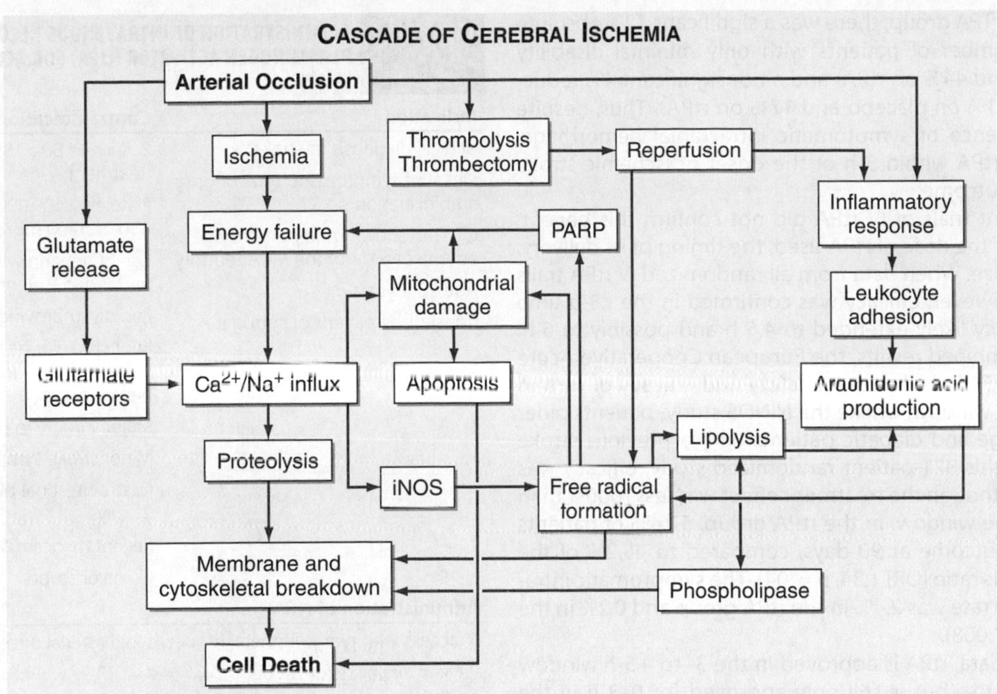

FIGURE 446-2 Major steps in the cascade of cerebral ischemia. See text for details. iNOS, inducible nitric oxide synthase; PARP, poly-A ribose polymerase.

hyperglycemia as much as possible. The value of induced mild hypothermia to improve stroke outcomes is the subject of continuing clinical research.

TREATMENT ACUTE ISCHEMIC STROKE

After the clinical diagnosis of stroke is made, an orderly process of evaluation and treatment should follow (Fig. 446-1). The first goal is to prevent or reverse brain injury. Attend to the patient's airway, breathing, and circulation (ABCs), and treat hypoglycemia or hyperglycemia if identified. Perform an emergency noncontrast head CT scan to differentiate between ischemic stroke and hemorrhagic stroke; there are no reliable clinical findings that conclusively separate ischemia from hemorrhage, although a more depressed level of consciousness, higher initial blood pressure, or worsening of symptoms after onset favor hemorrhage, and a deficit that is maximal at onset, or remits, suggests ischemia. Treatments designed to reverse or lessen the amount of tissue infarction and improve clinical outcome fall within six categories: (1) medical support, (2) IV thrombolysis, (3) endovascular revascularization, (4) antithrombotic treatment, (5) neuroprotection, and (6) stroke centers and rehabilitation.

MEDICAL SUPPORT

When ischemic stroke occurs, the immediate goal is to optimize cerebral perfusion in the surrounding ischemic penumbra. Attention is also directed toward preventing the common complications of bedridden patients—infections (pneumonia, urinary, and skin) and deep venous thrombosis (DVT) with pulmonary embolism. Subcutaneous heparin (unfractionated and low-molecular-weight) is safe and can be used concomitantly. Use of pneumatic compression stockings is of proven benefit in reducing risk of DVT and is a safe alternative to heparin.

Because collateral blood flow within the ischemic brain may be blood pressure dependent, there is controversy about whether blood pressure should be lowered acutely. Blood pressure should be lowered if there is malignant hypertension (Chap. 298) or concomitant myocardial ischemia, or if blood pressure is >185/110 mmHg and thrombolytic therapy is anticipated. When faced with the competing demands of myocardium and brain, lowering the heart rate with a β_1-adrenergic blocker (such as esmolol) can be a first step to decrease cardiac work and maintain blood pressure. Routine lowering of blood pressure has been found to worsen outcomes. Fever is detrimental and should be treated with antipyretics and surface cooling. Serum glucose should be monitored and kept at <10.0 mmol/L (180 mg/dL) using an insulin infusion if necessary.

Between 5 and 10% of patients develop enough cerebral edema to cause obtundation or brain herniation. Edema peaks on the second or third day but can cause mass effect for ~10 days. The larger the infarct, the greater the likelihood that clinically significant edema will develop. Water restriction and IV mannitol may be used to raise the serum osmolarity, but hypovolemia should be avoided because this may contribute to hypotension and worsening infarction. Combined analysis of three randomized European trials of hemicraniectomy (craniotomy and temporary removal of part of the skull) shows that hemicraniectomy markedly reduces mortality, and the clinical outcomes of survivors are acceptable. The size of the diffusion-weighted imaging volume of brain infarction during the acute stroke is a predictor of deterioration requiring hemicraniectomy.

Special vigilance is warranted for patients with cerebellar infarction. These strokes may mimic labyrinthitis because of prominent vertigo and vomiting; the presence of head or neck pain should alert the physician to consider cerebellar stroke from vertebral artery dissection. Even small amounts of cerebellar edema can acutely increase intracranial pressure (ICP) by obstructing cerebrospinal fluid (CSF) flow leading to hydrocephalus or by directly compressing the brainstem. The resulting brainstem compression can manifest as coma and respiratory arrest and require emergency surgical decompression. Prophylactic suboccipital decompression of large cerebellar infarcts before brainstem compression, although not tested rigorously in a clinical trial, is practiced at most stroke centers.

INTRAVENOUS THROMBOLYSIS

The National Institute of Neurological Disorders and Stroke (NINDS) rtPA Stroke Study showed a clear benefit for IV rtPA in selected patients with acute stroke. The NINDS study used IV rtPA (0.9 mg/kg to a 90-mg maximum; 10% as a bolus, then the remainder over 60 min) versus placebo in ischemic stroke within 3 h of onset. One-half of the patients were treated within 90 min. Symptomatic intracranial hemorrhage occurred in 6.4% of patients on rtPA and 0.6%

on placebo. In the rTPA group, there was a significant 12% absolute increase in the number of patients with only minimal disability (32% on placebo and 44% on rtPA) and a nonsignificant 4% reduction in mortality (21% on placebo and 17% on rtPA). Thus, despite an increased incidence of symptomatic intracranial hemorrhage, treatment with IV rtPA within 3 h of the onset of ischemic stroke improved clinical outcome.

Three subsequent trials of IV rtPA did not confirm this benefit, perhaps because of the dose of rtPA used, the timing of its delivery, and small sample size. When data from all randomized IV rtPA trails were combined, however, efficacy was confirmed in the <3-h time window, and efficacy likely extended to 4.5 h and possibly to 6 h. Based on these combined results, the European Cooperative Acute Stroke Study (ECASS) III explored the safety and efficacy of rtPA in the 3- to 4.5-h time window. Unlike the NINDS study, patients older than 80 years of age and diabetic patients with a previous stroke were excluded. In this 821-patient randomized study, efficacy was again confirmed, although the treatment effect was less robust than in the 0- to 3-h time window. In the rtPA group, 52.4% of patients achieved a good outcome at 90 days, compared to 45.2% of the placebo group (odds ratio [OR] 1.34, $p = .04$). The symptomatic intracranial hemorrhage rate was 2.4% in the rtPA group and 0.2% in the placebo group ($p = .008$).

Based on these data, rtPA is approved in the 3- to 4.5-h window in Europe and Canada, but is still only approved for 0–3 h in the United States and Canada. Use of IV tPA is now considered a central component of primary stroke centers (see below). It represents the first treatment proven to improve clinical outcomes in ischemic stroke and is cost-effective and cost-saving. Advanced neuroimaging techniques (see neuroimaging section below) may help to select patients beyond the 4.5-h window who will benefit from thrombolysis, but this is currently investigational. The time of stroke onset is defined as the time the patient's symptoms were witnessed to begin or the time the patient was last seen as normal. Patients who awaken with stroke have the onset defined as when they went to bed. **Table 446-1** summarizes eligibility criteria and instructions for administration of IV rtPA.

TABLE 446-1 ADMINISTRATION OF INTRAVENOUS RECOMBINANT TISSUE PLASMINOGEN ACTIVATOR (rtPA) FOR ACUTE ISCHEMIC STROKE (AIS)[a]

Indication	Contraindication
Clinical diagnosis of stroke	Sustained BP >185/110 mmHg despite treatment
Onset of symptoms to time of drug administration ≤4.5 h[b]	Platelets <100,000; HCT <25%; glucose <50 or >400 mg/dL
CT scan showing no hemorrhage or edema of >1/3 of the MCA territory	Use of heparin within 48 h and prolonged PTT, or elevated INR
Age 18 ≥ years	Rapidly improving symptoms
Consent by patient or surrogate	Prior stroke or head injury within 3 months; prior intracranial hemorrhage
	Major surgery in preceding 14 days
	Minor stroke symptoms
	Gastrointestinal bleeding in preceding 21 days
	Recent myocardial infarction
	Coma or stupor

Administration of rtPA
IV access with two peripheral IV lines (avoid arterial or central line placement)
Review eligibility for rtPA
Administer 0.9 mg/kg IV (maximum 90 mg) IV as 10% of total dose by bolus, followed by remainder of total dose over 1 h
Frequent cuff blood pressure monitoring
No other antithrombotic treatment for 24 h
For decline in neurologic status or uncontrolled blood pressure, stop infusion, give cryoprecipitate, and reimage brain emergently
Avoid urethral catheterization for ≥2 h

[a]See Activase (tissue plasminogen activator) package insert for complete list of contraindications and dosing. [b]Depending on the country, IV rtPA may be approved for up to 4.5 h with additional restrictions.

Abbreviations: BP, blood pressure; CT, computed tomography; HCT, hematocrit; INR, international normalized ratio; MCA, middle cerebral artery; PTT, partial thromboplastin time.

ENDOVASCULAR REVASCULARIZATION

Ischemic stroke from large-vessel intracranial occlusion results in high rates of mortality and morbidity. Occlusions in such large vessels (middle cerebral artery [MCA], intracranial internal carotid artery, and the basilar artery) generally involve a large clot volume and often fail to open with IV rtPA alone. Therefore, there is growing interest in using thrombolytics via an intraarterial route to increase the concentration of drug at the clot and minimize systemic bleeding complications. The Prolyse in Acute Cerebral Thromboembolism (PROACT) II trial found benefit for intraarterial prourokinase in acute MCA occlusions up to the sixth hour following onset of stroke. Intraarterial treatment of basilar artery occlusions may also be beneficial for selected patients. Intraarterial administration of a thrombolytic agent for acute ischemic stroke (AIS) is not approved by the U.S. Food and Drug Administration (FDA); however, many stroke centers offer this treatment based on these data.

Endovascular mechanical thrombectomy has been studied as an alternative or adjunctive treatment of acute stroke in patients who are ineligible for, or have contraindications to, thrombolytics or in those who failed to achieve vascular recanalization with IV thrombolytics (see Fig. 446-15). The Mechanical Embolus Removal in Cerebral Ischemia (MERCI) and multi-MERCI single-arm trials found that an endovascular thrombectomy device restored patency of occluded intracranial vessels within 8 h of ischemic stroke symptoms compared with a historical control group. Recanalization of the target vessel occurred in 48–58% of treated patients and in 60–69% of patients after use of adjuvant endovascular methods, and successful recanalization at 90 days correlated well with favorable outcomes. Based on these nonrandomized data, the FDA approved this device as the first device for revascularization of occluded vessels in AIS even if the patient has been given rtPA and that therapy has failed. The Penumbra Pivotal Stroke trial tested another mechanical device that showed even higher rates of recanalization and led to FDA clearance of the tested device as well. More recently, two Stentriever devices (nondetachable stents) were shown to significantly improve vascular recanalization compared to the first approved MERCI device, approaching recanalization rates of 90% in most large intracranial vessels.

In 2013, three randomized endovascular trials with nonendovascular controls found no benefits to endovascular therapy. The largest was the Interventional Management of Stroke III trial that randomized 656 AIS patients within 3 h of onset to IV rtPA (0.9 mg/kg) alone versus IV rtPA (0.6 mg/kg) followed by endovascular adjuvant treatment with IA rtPA, or endovascular thrombectomy as soon as possible. Outcomes between these groups were not significantly different, and there were more complications (groin bleeding chiefly) in the endovascular group. The SYNTHESIS trial based in Italy randomized 363 patients to IV rtPA versus intraarterial rtPA for patients within 3 h of stroke onset. No differences were found between the groups at 90 days. These two relatively large trials indicate that endovascular therapy using principally intraarterial rtPA is not better than IV therapy, but many questions remain. Relatively few patients received mechanical clot retraction therapies, and those who did received what we now know were inferior devices. Trials assessing more efficacious thrombectomy devices are currently ongoing.

Because use of endovascular devices in combination with rtPA appears relatively safe, some centers continue to offer endovascular therapy. This applies to patients who are not eligible for IV rtPA (recent surgery, stroke following cardiac catheterization, etc.), and some continue to use thrombectomy because of perceived better outcomes in patients with more effective devices. Comprehensive stroke centers are now obtaining credentialing to offer this therapy in distinction to primary stroke centers that offer only IV rtPA.

ANTITHROMBOTIC TREATMENT

Platelet Inhibition Aspirin is the only antiplatelet agent that has been proven effective for the acute treatment of ischemic stroke; there are several antiplatelet agents proven for the secondary prevention of stroke (see below). Two large trials, the International Stroke Trial (IST) and the Chinese Acute Stroke Trial (CAST), found that the use of aspirin within 48 h of stroke onset reduced both stroke recurrence risk and mortality minimally. Among 19,435 patients in IST, those allocated to aspirin, 300 mg/d, had slightly fewer deaths within 14 days (9.0 vs 9.4%), significantly fewer recurrent ischemic strokes (2.8 vs 3.9%), no excess of hemorrhagic strokes (0.9 vs 0.8%), and a trend toward a reduction in death or dependence at 6 months (61.2 vs 63.5%). In CAST, 21,106 patients with ischemic stroke received 160 mg/d of aspirin or a placebo for up to 4 weeks. There were very small reductions in the aspirin group in early mortality (3.3 vs 3.9%), recurrent ischemic strokes (1.6 vs 2.1%), and dependency at discharge or death (30.5 vs 31.6%). These trials demonstrate that the use of aspirin in the treatment of AIS is safe and produces a small net benefit. For every 1000 acute strokes treated with aspirin, about 9 deaths or nonfatal stroke recurrences will be prevented in the first few weeks and ~13 fewer patients will be dead or dependent at 6 months.

Clopidogrel is being tested as a way to prevent stroke following TIA and minor ischemic stroke (see below).

Anticoagulation Numerous clinical trials have failed to demonstrate any benefit of anticoagulation in the primary treatment of atherothrombotic cerebral ischemia. Several trials have investigated antiplatelet versus anticoagulant medications given within 12–24 h of the initial event. The U.S. Trial of Organon 10172 in Acute Stroke Treatment (TOAST), an investigational low-molecular-weight heparin (LMWH), failed to show any benefit over aspirin. Use of SC unfractionated heparin versus aspirin was tested in IST. Heparin given SC afforded no additional benefit over aspirin and increased bleeding rates. Several trials of LMWHs have also shown no consistent benefit in AIS. Furthermore, trials generally have shown an excess risk of brain and systemic hemorrhage with acute anticoagulation. A recent meta-analysis of all forms of heparin found no benefit for acute stroke patients at high or low risk of thrombotic events. Therefore, trials do not support the use of heparin or other anticoagulants for patients with atherothrombotic stroke.

NEUROPROTECTION

Neuroprotection is the concept of providing a treatment that prolongs the brain's tolerance to ischemia. Drugs that block the excitatory amino acid pathways have been shown to protect neurons and glia in animals, but despite multiple human trials, they have not yet been proven to be beneficial. Hypothermia is a powerful neuroprotective treatment in patients with cardiac arrest (Chap. 330) and is neuroprotective in animal models of stroke, but it has not been adequately studied in patients with ischemic stroke and is associated with an increase in pneumonia rates that could adversely impact stroke outcomes.

STROKE CENTERS AND REHABILITATION

Patient care in stroke units followed by rehabilitation services improves neurologic outcomes and reduces mortality. Use of clinical pathways and staff dedicated to the stroke patient can improve care. This includes use of standardized stroke order sets. Stroke teams that provide emergency 24-h evaluation of acute stroke patients for acute medical management and consideration of thrombolysis or endovascular treatments are essential components of primary and comprehensive stroke centers, respectively.

Proper rehabilitation of the stroke patient includes early physical, occupational, and speech therapy. It is directed toward educating the patient and family about the patient's neurologic deficit, preventing the complications of immobility (e.g., pneumonia, DVT and pulmonary embolism, pressure sores of the skin, and muscle contractures), and providing encouragement and instruction in overcoming the deficit. Use of pneumatic compression stockings is of proven benefit in reducing risk of DVT and is a safe alternative to heparin. The goal of rehabilitation is to return the patient to home and to maximize recovery by providing a safe, progressive regimen suited to the individual patient. Additionally, the use of constrained movement therapy (immobilizing the unaffected side) has been shown to improve hemiparesis following stroke, even years after the stroke, suggesting that physical therapy can recruit unused neural pathways. Newer robotic therapies appear promising as well. The human nervous system is more adaptable than previously thought, and developing physical and pharmacologic strategies to enhance long-term neural recovery is an active area of research.

ETIOLOGY OF ISCHEMIC STROKE

(Figs. 446-1 and 446-3 and Table 446-2) Although the initial management of AIS often does not depend on the etiology, establishing a cause is essential to reduce the risk of recurrence. Particular focus should be on atrial fibrillation and carotid atherosclerosis, because these etiologies have proven secondary prevention strategies. The clinical presentation and examination findings often establish the cause of stroke or narrow the possibilities to a few. Judicious use of laboratory testing and imaging studies completes the initial evaluation. Nevertheless, nearly 30% of strokes remain unexplained despite extensive evaluation.

Clinical examination should focus on the peripheral and cervical vascular system (carotid auscultation for bruits and blood pressure), the heart (dysrhythmia, murmurs), extremities (peripheral emboli), and retina (effects of hypertension and cholesterol emboli [Hollenhorst plaques]). A complete neurologic examination is performed to localize the anatomic site of stroke. An imaging study of the brain is nearly always indicated and is required for patients being considered for thrombolysis; it may be combined with CT- or MRI-based angiography to visualize the vasculature of the neck and intracranial vessels (see "Imaging Studies," below). A chest x-ray, electrocardiogram (ECG), urinalysis, complete blood count, erythrocyte sedimentation rate (ESR), serum electrolytes, blood urea nitrogen (BUN), creatinine, blood glucose, serum lipid profile, prothrombin time (PT), and partial thromboplastin time (PTT) are often useful and should be considered in all patients. An ECG may demonstrate arrhythmias or reveal evidence of recent myocardial infarction (MI). Of all these studies, only brain imaging, blood glucose, and perhaps PTT/international normalized ratio (INR) are necessary prior to IV rtPA; the results of other studies should not delay the rapid administration of IV rtPA if the patient is eligible.

Cardioembolic Stroke Cardioembolism is responsible for ~20% of all ischemic strokes. Stroke caused by heart disease is primarily due to embolism of thrombotic material forming on the atrial or ventricular wall or the left heart valves. These thrombi then detach and embolize into the arterial circulation. The thrombus may fragment or lyse quickly, producing only a TIA. Alternatively, the arterial occlusion may last longer, producing stroke. Embolic strokes tend to occur suddenly with maximum neurologic deficit present at onset. With reperfusion following more prolonged ischemia, petechial hemorrhages can occur within the ischemic territory. These are usually of no clinical significance and should be distinguished from frank intracranial hemorrhage into a region of ischemic stroke where the mass effect from the hemorrhage can cause a significant decline in neurologic function.

Emboli from the heart most often lodge in the intracranial internal carotid artery, the MCA, the posterior cerebral artery (PCA), or one of their branches; infrequently, the anterior cerebral artery (ACA) is involved. Emboli large enough to occlude the stem of the MCA (3–4 mm) lead to large infarcts that involve both deep gray and white matter and some portions of the cortical surface and its underlying white matter. A smaller embolus may occlude a small cortical or penetrating arterial branch. The location and size of an infarct within a vascular territory depend on the extent of the collateral circulation.

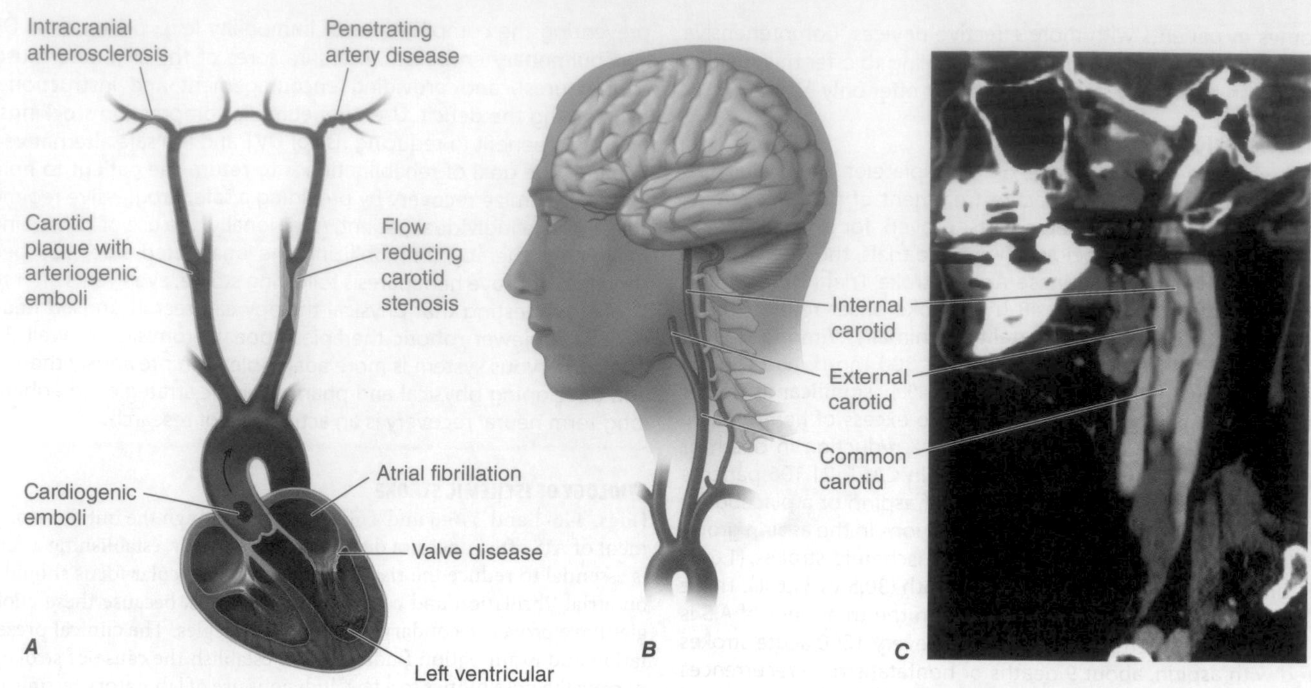

FIGURE 446-3 Pathophysiology of ischemic stroke. ***A.*** Diagram illustrating the three major mechanisms that underlie ischemic stroke: (1) occlusion of an intracranial vessel by an embolus that arises at a distant site (e.g., cardiogenic sources such as atrial fibrillation or artery-to-artery emboli from carotid atherosclerotic plaque), often affecting the large intracranial vessels; (2) in situ thrombosis of an intracranial vessel, typically affecting the small penetrating arteries that arise from the major intracranial arteries; (3) hypoperfusion caused by flow-limiting stenosis of a major extracranial (e.g., internal carotid) or intracranial vessel, often producing "watershed" ischemia. ***B.*** and ***C.*** Diagram and reformatted computed tomography angiogram of the common, internal, and external carotid arteries. High-grade stenosis of the internal carotid artery, which may be associated with either cerebral emboli or flow-limiting ischemia, was identified in this patient.

The most significant causes of cardioembolic stroke in most of the world are nonrheumatic (often called nonvalvular) atrial fibrillation, MI, prosthetic valves, rheumatic heart disease, and ischemic cardiomyopathy (Table 446-2). Cardiac disorders causing brain embolism are discussed in the chapters on heart diseases. A few pertinent aspects are highlighted here.

Nonrheumatic atrial fibrillation is the most common cause of cerebral embolism overall. The presumed stroke mechanism is thrombus formation in the fibrillating atrium or atrial appendage, with subsequent embolization. Patients with atrial fibrillation have an average annual risk of stroke of ~5%. The risk of stroke can be estimated by calculating the CHADS2 score (Table 446-3). Left atrial enlargement is an additional risk factor for formation of atrial thrombi. Rheumatic heart disease usually causes ischemic stroke when there is prominent mitral stenosis or atrial fibrillation. Recent MI may be a source of emboli, especially when transmural and involving the anteroapical ventricular wall, and prophylactic anticoagulation following MI has been shown to reduce stroke risk. Mitral valve prolapse is not usually a source of emboli unless the prolapse is severe.

Paradoxical embolization occurs when venous thrombi migrate to the arterial circulation, usually via a patent foramen ovale or atrial septal defect. Bubble-contrast echocardiography (IV injection of agitated saline coupled with either transthoracic or transesophageal echocardiography) can demonstrate a right-to-left cardiac shunt, revealing the conduit for paradoxical embolization. Alternatively, a right-to-left shunt is implied if immediately following IV injection of agitated saline, the ultrasound signature of bubbles is observed during transcranial Doppler insonation of the MCA; pulmonary arteriovenous malformations should be considered if this test is positive yet an echocardiogram fails to reveal an intracardiac shunt. Both techniques are highly sensitive for detection of right-to-left shunts. Besides venous clot, fat and tumor emboli, bacterial endocarditis, IV air, and amniotic fluid emboli at childbirth may occasionally be responsible for paradoxical embolization. The importance of a patent foramen ovale (PFO) as a cause of stroke is debated, particularly because they are present in ~15% of the general population. Some studies have suggested that the risk is only elevated in the presence of a coexisting atrial septal aneurysm. The presence of a venous source of embolus, most commonly a deep venous thrombus, may provide confirmation of the importance of a PFO with an accompanying right-to-left shunt in a particular case. Three randomized trials of PFO occlusion for secondary prevention of ischemic stroke were negative, although each lacked sufficient power to be conclusive. At present, there is no supportive evidence to offer percutaneous PFO closure for stroke prevention.

Bacterial endocarditis can be a source of valvular vegetations that give rise to septic emboli. The appearance of multifocal symptoms and signs in a patient with stroke makes bacterial endocarditis more likely. Infarcts of microscopic size occur, and large septic infarcts may evolve into brain abscesses or cause hemorrhage into the infarct, which generally precludes use of anticoagulation or thrombolytics. Mycotic aneurysms caused by septic emboli may also present as SAH or intracerebral hemorrhage.

Artery-to-Artery Embolic Stroke Thrombus formation on atherosclerotic plaques may embolize to intracranial arteries producing an artery-to-artery embolic stroke. Less commonly, a diseased vessel may acutely thrombose. Unlike the myocardial vessels, artery-to-artery embolism, rather than local thrombosis, appears to be the dominant vascular mechanism causing large-vessel brain ischemia. Any diseased vessel may be an embolic source, including the aortic arch, common carotid, internal carotid, vertebral, and basilar arteries.

CAROTID ATHEROSCLEROSIS Atherosclerosis within the carotid artery occurs most frequently within the common carotid bifurcation and proximal internal carotid artery; the carotid siphon (portion within the cavernous sinus) is also vulnerable to atherosclerosis. Male gender, older age, smoking, hypertension, diabetes, and hypercholesterolemia are risk factors for carotid disease, as they are for stroke in general (Table 446-4). Carotid atherosclerosis produces an estimated 10% of

TABLE 446-2 CAUSES OF ISCHEMIC STROKE

Common Causes	Uncommon Causes
Thrombosis	Hypercoagulable disorders
Lacunar stroke (small vessel)	Protein C deficiency[a]
Large-vessel thrombosis	Protein S deficiency[a]
Dehydration	Antithrombin III deficiency[a]
Embolic occlusion	Antiphospholipid syndrome
Artery-to-artery	Factor V Leiden mutation[a]
Carotid bifurcation	Prothrombin G20210 mutation[a]
Aortic arch	Systemic malignancy
Arterial dissection	Sickle cell anemia
Cardioembolic	β Thalassemia
Atrial fibrillation	Polycythemia vera
Mural thrombus	Systemic lupus erythematosus
Myocardial infarction	Homocysteinemia
Dilated cardiomyopathy	Thrombotic thrombocytopenic purpura
Valvular lesions	Disseminated intravascular coagulation
Mitral stenosis	Dysproteinemias[a]
Mechanical valve	Nephrotic syndrome[a]
Bacterial endocarditis	Inflammatory bowel disease[a]
Paradoxical embolus	Oral contraceptives
Atrial septal defect	Venous sinus thrombosis[b]
Patent foramen ovale	Fibromuscular dysplasia
Atrial septal aneurysm	Vasculitis
Spontaneous echo contrast	Systemic vasculitis (PAN, granulomatosis with polyangiitis [Wegener's], Takayasu's, giant cell arteritis)
Stimulant drugs: cocaine, amphetamine	Primary CNS vasculitis
	Meningitis (syphilis, tuberculosis, fungal, bacterial, zoster)
	Noninflammatory vasculopathy
	Reversible vasoconstriction syndrome
	Fabry's disease
	Angiocentric lymphoma
	Cardiogenic
	Mitral valve calcification
	Atrial myxoma
	Intracardiac tumor
	Marantic endocarditis
	Libman-Sacks endocarditis
	Subarachnoid hemorrhage vasospasm
	Moyamoya disease
	Eclampsia

[a]Chiefly cause venous sinus thrombosis. [b]May be associated with any hypercoagulable disorder.

Abbreviations: CNS, central nervous system; PAN, polyarteritis nodosa.

ischemic stroke. For further discussion of the pathogenesis of atherosclerosis, see Chap. 291e.

Carotid disease can be classified by whether the stenosis is symptomatic or asymptomatic and by the degree of stenosis (percent narrowing of the narrowest segment compared to a nondiseased segment). Symptomatic carotid disease implies that the patient has experienced a stroke or TIA within the vascular distribution of the artery, and it is associated with a greater risk of subsequent stroke than asymptomatic stenosis, in which the patient is symptom free and the stenosis is detected through screening. Greater degrees of arterial narrowing are generally associated with a higher risk of stroke, except that those with near occlusions are at lower risk of stroke.

OTHER CAUSES OF ARTERY-TO-ARTERY EMBOLIC STROKE *Intracranial atherosclerosis* produces stroke either by an embolic mechanism or by in situ thrombosis of a diseased vessel. It is more common in patients of Asian and African-American descent. Recurrent stroke risk is ~15% per year, similar to symptomatic untreated carotid atherosclerosis.

Dissection of the internal carotid or vertebral arteries or even vessels beyond the circle of Willis is a common source of embolic stroke in young (age <60 years) patients. The dissection is usually painful and precedes the stroke by several hours or days. Extracranial dissections do not cause hemorrhage, presumably because of the tough adventitia of these vessels. Intracranial dissections, conversely, may produce SAH because the adventitia of intracranial vessels is thin and pseudoaneurysms may form, requiring urgent treatment to prevent rerupture. Treating asymptomatic pseudoaneurysms following dissection is likely not necessary. The cause of dissection is usually unknown, and recurrence is rare. Ehlers-Danlos type IV, Marfan's disease, cystic medial necrosis, and fibromuscular dysplasia are associated with dissections. Trauma (usually a motor vehicle accident or a sports injury) can cause carotid and vertebral artery dissections. Spinal manipulative therapy is associated with vertebral artery dissection and stroke. Most dissections heal spontaneously, and stroke or TIA is uncommon beyond 2 weeks. Although there are no trials comparing anticoagulation to antiplatelet agents, many physicians treat acutely with anticoagulants and then convert to antiplatelet therapy after demonstration of satisfactory vascular recanalization.

SMALL-VESSEL STROKE

The term *lacunar infarction* refers to infarction following atherothrombotic or lipohyalinotic occlusion of a small artery in the brain. The term *small-vessel stroke* denotes occlusion of such a small penetrating artery and is now the preferred term. Small-vessel strokes account for ~20% of all strokes.

Pathophysiology The MCA stem, the arteries comprising the circle of Willis (A1 segment, anterior and posterior communicating arteries, and P1 segment), and the basilar and vertebral arteries all give rise to 30- to 300-μm branches that penetrate the deep gray and white matter of the cerebrum or brainstem (Fig. 446-4). Each of these small branches can occlude either by atherothrombotic disease at its origin or by the development of lipohyalinotic thickening. Thrombosis of these vessels causes small infarcts that are referred to as *lacunes* (Latin for "lake" of fluid noted at autopsy). These infarcts range in size from 3 mm to 2 cm in diameter. Hypertension and age are the principal risk factors.

Clinical Manifestations The most common small-vessel stroke syndromes are the following: (1) *Pure motor hemiparesis* from an infarct in the posterior limb of the internal capsule or the pons; the face, arm, and leg are almost always involved; (2) *pure sensory stroke* from an infarct in the ventral thalamus; (3) *ataxic hemiparesis* from an infarct in the ventral pons or internal capsule; (4) and *dysarthria and a clumsy hand* or arm due to infarction in the ventral pons or in the genu of the internal capsule.

Transient symptoms (small-vessel TIAs) may herald a small-vessel infarct; they may occur several times a day and last only a few minutes. Recovery from small-vessel strokes tends to be more rapid and complete than recovery from large-vessel strokes; in some cases, however, there is severe permanent disability.

A large-vessel source (either thrombosis or embolism) may manifest initially as a small-vessel infarction. Therefore, the search for embolic sources (carotid and heart) should not be completely abandoned in the evaluation of these patients. Secondary prevention of small-vessel stroke involves risk factor modification, specifically reduction in blood pressure (see "Treatment: Primary and Secondary Prevention of Stroke and TIA," below).

LESS COMMON CAUSES OF STROKE

(Table 446-2) *Hypercoagulable disorders* (Chap. 78) primarily increase the risk of venous, including venous sinus, thrombosis. Systemic lupus erythematosus with Libman-Sacks endocarditis can be a cause of embolic stroke. These conditions overlap with the antiphospholipid syndrome, which probably requires long-term anticoagulation to

TABLE 446-3 RECOMMENDATIONS ON CHRONIC USE OF ANTITHROMBOTICS FOR VARIOUS CARDIAC CONDITIONS

Condition	Recommendation
Nonvalvular atrial fibrillation	Calculate CHADS2[a] score
• CHADS2 score 0	Aspirin or no antithrombotic
• CHADS2 score 1	Aspirin or OAC
• CHADS2 score >1	OAC
Rheumatic mitral valve disease	
• With atrial fibrillation, previous embolization, or atrial appendage thrombus, or left atrial diameter >55 mm	OAC
• Embolization or appendage clot despite OAC	OAC plus aspirin
Mitral valve prolapse	
• Asymptomatic	No therapy
• With otherwise cryptogenic stroke or TIA	Aspirin
• Atrial fibrillation	OAC
Mitral annular calcification	
• Without atrial fibrillation but systemic embolization, or otherwise cryptogenic stroke or TIA	Aspirin
• Recurrent embolization despite aspirin	OAC
• With atrial fibrillation	OAC
Aortic valve calcification	
• Asymptomatic	No therapy
• Otherwise cryptogenic stroke or TIA	Aspirin
Aortic arch mobile atheroma	
• Otherwise cryptogenic stroke or TIA	Aspirin or OAC
Patent foramen ovale	
• Otherwise cryptogenic ischemic stroke or TIA	Aspirin
• Indication for OAC (deep venous thrombosis or hypercoagulable state)	OAC
Mechanical heart value	
• Aortic position, bileaflet or Medtronic Hall tilting disk with normal left atrial size and sinus rhythm	VKA INR 2.5, range 2–3
• Mitral position tilting disk or bileaflet valve	VKA INR 3.0, range 2.5–3.5
• Mitral or aortic position, anterior-apical myocardial infarct or left atrial enlargement	VKA INR 3.0, range 2.5–3.5
• Mitral or aortic position, with atrial fibrillation, or hypercoagulable state, or low ejection fraction, or atherosclerotic vascular disease	Aspirin plus VKA INR 3.0, range 2.5–3.5
• Systemic embolization despite target INR	Add aspirin and/or increase INR: prior target was 2.5 increase to 3.0, range 2.5–3.5; prior target was 3.0 increase to 3.5, range 3–4
Bioprosthetic valve	
• No other indication for VKA therapy	Aspirin
Infective endocarditis	Avoid antithrombotic agents
Nonbacterial thrombotic endocarditis	
• With systemic embolization	Full-dose unfractionated heparin or SC LMWH

[a]CHADS2 score calculated as follows: 1 point for age >75 years, 1 point for hypertension, 1 point for congestive heart failure, 1 point for diabetes, and 2 points for stroke or TIA; sum of points is the total CHADS2 score.

Note: Dose of aspirin is 50–325 mg/d; target INR for OAC is between 2 and 3 unless otherwise specified.

Abbreviations: INR, international normalized ratio; LMWH, low-molecular-weight heparin; OAC, oral anticoagulant (VKA, thrombin inhibitor, oral factor Xa inhibitors); TIA, transient ischemic attack; VKA, vitamin K antagonist.

Sources: Modified from DE Singer et al: Chest 133:546S, 2008; DN Salem et al: Chest 133:593S, 2008.

prevent further stroke. Homocysteinemia may cause arterial thromboses as well; this disorder is caused by various mutations in the homocysteine pathways and responds to different forms of cobalamin depending on the mutation.

Venous sinus thrombosis of the lateral or sagittal sinus or of small cortical veins (cortical vein thrombosis) occurs as a complication of oral contraceptive use, pregnancy and the postpartum period, inflammatory bowel disease, intracranial infections (meningitis), and dehydration. It is also seen in patients with laboratory-confirmed thrombophilia including polycythemia, sickle cell anemia, deficiencies of proteins C and S, factor V Leiden mutation (resistance to activated protein C), antithrombin III deficiency, homocysteinemia, and the prothrombin G20210 mutation. Women who take oral contraceptives and have the prothrombin G20210 mutation may be at particularly high risk for sinus thrombosis. Patients present with headache and may also have focal neurologic signs (especially paraparesis) and seizures. Often, CT imaging is normal unless an intracranial venous hemorrhage has occurred, but the venous sinus occlusion is readily visualized using magnetic resonance (MR) or CT venography or conventional x-ray angiography. With greater degrees of sinus thrombosis, the

TABLE 446-4 RISK FACTORS FOR STROKE

Risk Factor	Relative Risk	Relative Risk Reduction with Treatment	Number Needed to Treat[a] Primary Prevention	Secondary Prevention
Hypertension	2–5	38%	100–300	50–100
Atrial fibrillation	1.8–2.9	68% warfarin, 21% aspirin	20–83	13
Diabetes	1.8–6	No proven effect		
Smoking	1.8	50% at 1 year, baseline risk at 5 years postcessation		
Hyperlipidemia	1.8–2.6	16–30%	560	230
Asymptomatic carotid stenosis	2.0	53%	85	N/A
Symptomatic carotid stenosis (70–99%)		65% at 2 years	N/A	12
Symptomatic carotid stenosis (50–69%)		29% at 5 years	N/A	77

[a]Number needed to treat to prevent one stroke annually. Prevention of other cardiovascular outcomes is not considered here.

Abbreviation: N/A, not applicable.

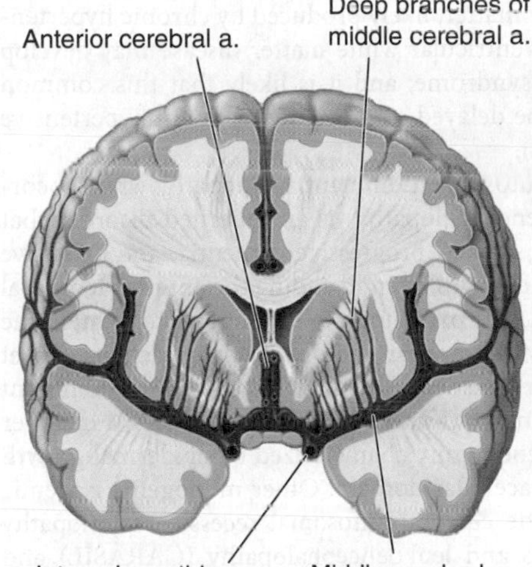

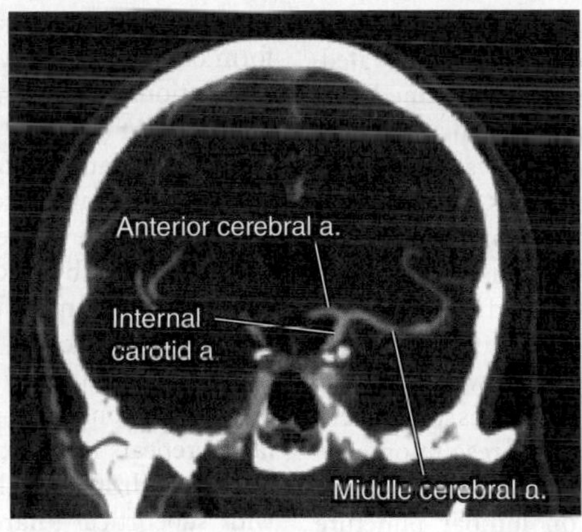

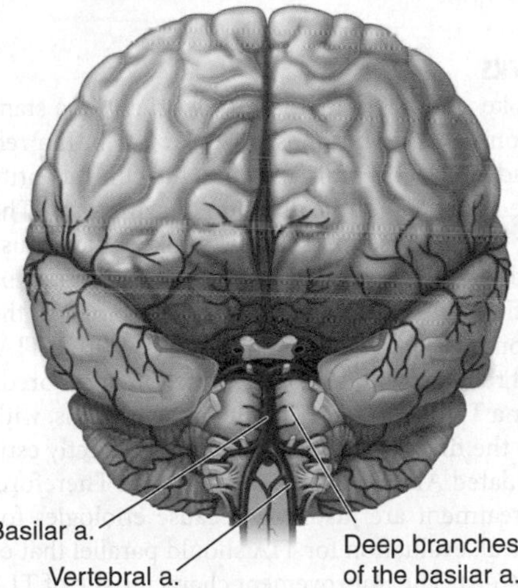

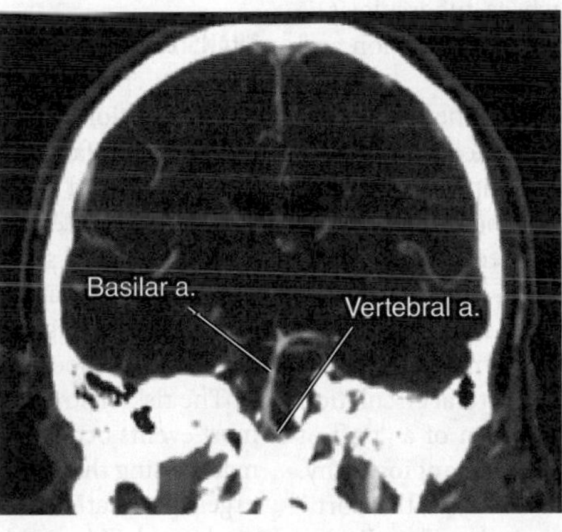

FIGURE 446-4 Diagrams and reformatted computed tomography (CT) angiograms in the coronal section illustrating the deep penetrating arteries involved in small-vessel strokes. In the anterior circulation, small penetrating arteries called *lenticulostriates* arise from the proximal portion of the anterior and middle cerebral arteries and supply deep subcortical structures (***upper panels***). In the posterior circulation, similar arteries arise directly from the vertebral and basilar arteries to supply the brainstem (***lower panels***). Occlusion of a single penetrating artery gives rise to a discrete area of infarct (pathologically termed a "lacune," or lake). Note that these vessels are too small to be visualized on CT angiography.

patient may develop signs of increased ICP and coma. Intravenous heparin, regardless of the presence of intracranial hemorrhage, reduces morbidity and mortality, and the long-term outcome is generally good. Heparin prevents further thrombosis and reduces venous hypertension and ischemia. If an underlying hypercoagulable state is not found, many physicians treat with vitamin K antagonists (VKAs) for 3–6 months and then convert to aspirin, depending on the degree of resolution of the venous sinus thrombus. Anticoagulation is often continued indefinitely if thrombophilia is diagnosed.

Sickle cell anemia (SS disease) is a common cause of stroke in children. A subset of homozygous carriers of this hemoglobin mutation develop stroke in childhood, and this may be predicted by documenting high-velocity blood flow within the MCAs using transcranial Doppler ultrasonography. In children who are identified to have high velocities, treatment with aggressive exchange transfusion dramatically reduces risk of stroke, and if exchange transfusion is ceased, their stroke rate increases again along with MCA velocities.

Fibromuscular dysplasia affects the cervical arteries and occurs mainly in women. The carotid or vertebral arteries show multiple rings of segmental narrowing alternating with dilatation. Vascular occlusion is usually incomplete. The process is often asymptomatic but occasionally is associated with an audible bruit, TIAs, or stroke. Involvement of the renal arteries is common and may cause hypertension. The cause and natural history of fibromuscular dysplasia are unknown (Chap. 302). TIA or stroke generally occurs only when the artery is severely narrowed or dissects. Anticoagulation or antiplatelet therapy may be helpful.

Temporal (giant cell) arteritis (Chap. 385) is a relatively common affliction of elderly individuals in which the external carotid system, particularly the temporal arteries, undergo subacute granulomatous inflammation with giant cells. Occlusion of posterior ciliary arteries derived from the ophthalmic artery results in blindness in one or both eyes and can be prevented with glucocorticoids. It rarely causes stroke because the internal carotid artery is usually not inflamed. Idiopathic giant cell arteritis involving the great vessels arising from the aortic arch (*Takayasu's arteritis*) may cause carotid or vertebral thrombosis; it is rare in the Western Hemisphere.

Necrotizing (or granulomatous) arteritis, occurring alone or in association with generalized polyarteritis nodosa or granulomatosis with polyangiitis (Wegener's), involves the distal small

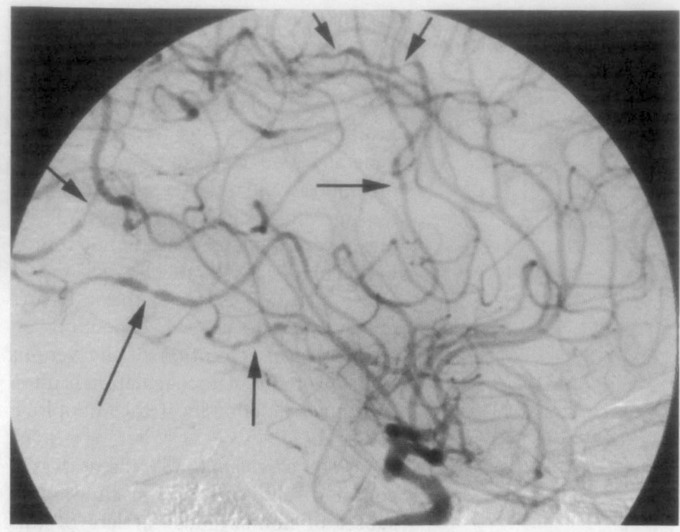

FIGURE 446-5 Cerebral angiogram from a 32-year-old male with central nervous system vasculopathy. Dramatic beading (*arrows*) typical of vasculopathy is seen.

branches (<2 mm diameter) of the main intracranial arteries and produces small ischemic infarcts in the brain, optic nerve, and spinal cord. The CSF often shows pleocytosis, and the protein level is elevated. *Primary central nervous system vasculitis* is rare; small or medium-sized vessels are usually affected, without apparent systemic vasculitis. The differential diagnosis includes other inflammatory vasculopathies including infection (tuberculous, fungal), sarcoidosis, angiocentric lymphoma, carcinomatous meningitis, and noninflammatory causes such as atherosclerosis, emboli, connective tissue disease, vasospasm, migraine-associated vasculopathy, and drug-associated causes. Some cases develop in the postpartum period and are self-limited.

Patients with any form of vasculopathy may present with insidious progression of combined white and gray matter infarctions, prominent headache, and cognitive decline. Brain biopsy or high-resolution conventional x-ray angiography is usually required to make the diagnosis (Fig. 446-5). An inflammatory profile found on lumbar puncture favors an inflammatory cause. In cases where inflammation is confirmed, aggressive immunosuppression with glucocorticoids, and often cyclophosphamide, is usually necessary to prevent progression; a diligent investigation for infectious causes such as tuberculosis is essential prior to immunosuppression. With prompt recognition and treatment, many patients can make an excellent recovery.

Drugs, in particular amphetamines and perhaps cocaine, may cause stroke on the basis of acute hypertension or drug-induced vasculopathy. No data exist on the value of any treatment. Phenylpropanolamine has been linked with intracranial hemorrhage, as has cocaine and methamphetamine, perhaps related to a drug-induced vasculopathy. *Moyamoya disease* is a poorly understood occlusive disease involving large intracranial arteries, especially the distal internal carotid artery and the stem of the MCA and ACA. Vascular inflammation is absent. The lenticulostriate arteries develop a rich collateral circulation around the occlusive lesion, which gives the impression of a "puff of smoke" (*moyamoya* in Japanese) on conventional x-ray angiography. Other collaterals include transdural anastomoses between the cortical surface branches of the meningeal and scalp arteries. The disease occurs mainly in Asian children or young adults, but the appearance may be identical in adults who have atherosclerosis, particularly in association with diabetes. Intracranial hemorrhage may result from rupture of the transdural and pial anastomotic channels; thus, anticoagulation is risky. Breakdown of dilated lenticulostriate arteries may produce intraparenchymal hemorrhage, and progressive occlusion of large surface arteries can occur, producing large-artery distribution strokes. Surgical bypass of extracranial carotid arteries to the dura or MCAs may prevent stroke and hemorrhage.

Posterior reversible encephalopathy syndrome (PRES) can occur with head injury, seizure, migraine, sympathomimetic drug use, eclampsia, and in the postpartum period (Chap. 463e). The pathophysiology is uncertain but likely involves a hyperperfusion state with widespread segmental vasoconstriction and cerebral edema. Patients complain of headache and manifest fluctuating neurologic symptoms and signs, especially visual symptoms. Sometimes cerebral infarction ensues, but typically the clinical and imaging findings suggest that ischemia reverses completely. MRI findings are characteristic with the edema present within the occipital lobes but can be generalized and do not respect any single vascular territory. A closely related *reversible cerebral vasoconstriction syndrome* (RCVS) typically presents with sudden, severe headache closely mimicking SAH. Patients may experience ischemic infarction and intracerebral hemorrhage and typically have new-onset, severe hypertension. Conventional x-ray angiography reveals changes in the vascular caliber throughout the hemispheres resembling vasculitis, but the process is noninflammatory. Oral calcium channel blockers may be effective in producing remission, and recurrence is rare.

Leukoaraiosis, or *periventricular white matter disease*, is the result of multiple small-vessel infarcts within the subcortical white matter. It is readily seen on CT or MRI scans as areas of white matter injury surrounding the ventricles and within the corona radiata. The pathophysiologic basis of the disease is lipohyalinosis of small penetrating arteries within the white matter, likely produced by chronic hypertension. Patients with periventricular white matter disease may develop a subcortical dementia syndrome, and it is likely that this common form of dementia may be delayed or prevented with antihypertensive medications (Chap. 448).

CADASIL (cerebral autosomal dominant arteriopathy with subcortical infarcts and leukoencephalopathy) is an inherited disorder that presents as small-vessel strokes, progressive dementia, and extensive symmetric white matter changes often including the anterior temporal lobes visualized by MRI. Approximately 40% of patients have migraine with aura, often manifest as transient motor or sensory deficits. Onset is usually in the fourth or fifth decade of life. This autosomal dominant condition is caused by one of several mutations in *Notch-3*, a member of a highly conserved gene family characterized by epidermal growth factor repeats in its extracellular domain. Other monogenic ischemic stroke syndromes include cerebral autosomal recessive arteriopathy with subcortical infarcts and leukoencephalopathy (CARASIL) and hereditary endotheliopathy, retinopathy, nephropathy, and stroke (HERNS). Fabry's disease also produces both a large-vessel arteriopathy and small-vessel infarctions.

TRANSIENT ISCHEMIC ATTACKS

TIAs are episodes of stroke symptoms that last only briefly; the standard definition of duration is <24 h, but most TIAs last <1 h. If a relevant brain infarction is identified on brain imaging, the clinical entity is now classified as stroke regardless of the duration of symptoms. The causes of TIA are similar to the causes of ischemic stroke, but because TIAs may herald stroke, they are an important risk factor that should be considered separately and urgently. TIAs may arise from emboli to the brain or from in situ thrombosis of an intracranial vessel. With a TIA, the occluded blood vessel reopens and neurologic function is restored.

The risk of stroke after a TIA is ~10–15% in the first 3 months, with most events occurring in the first 2 days. This risk can be directly estimated using the well-validated ABCD^2 score (Table 446-5). Therefore, urgent evaluation and treatment are justified. Because etiologies for stroke and TIA are identical, evaluation for TIA should parallel that of stroke (Figs. 446-1 and 446-3). The improvement characteristic of TIA is a contraindication to thrombolysis. However, because the risk of subsequent stroke in the first few days after a TIA is high, the opportunity to give rtPA rapidly if a stroke occurs may justify hospital admission for most patients. The combination of aspirin and clopidogrel has been recently reported to prevent stroke following TIA better than aspirin alone in a large Chinese randomized trial and is undergoing similar evaluation in an ongoing National Institutes of Health (NIH)-sponsored trial (POINT study).

TABLE 446-5 RISK OF STROKE FOLLOWING TRANSIENT ISCHEMIC ATTACK: THE ABCD² SCORE

Clinical Factor	Score
A: Age ≥60 years	1
B: SBP >140 mmHg or DBP >90 mmHg	1
C: Clinical symptoms	
Unilateral weakness	2
Speech disturbance without weakness	1
D: Duration	
>60 min	2
10–59 min	1
D: Diabetes (oral medications or insulin)	1
Total Score	**Sum Each Category**
ABCD² Score Total	3-Month Rate of Stroke (%)[a]
0	0
1	2
2	3
3	3
4	8
5	12
6	17
7	22

[a]Data ranges are from five cohorts.

Abbreviations: DBP, diastolic blood pressure; SBP, systolic blood pressure.

Source: SC Johnston et al: Validation and refinement of score to predict very early stroke risk after transient ischaemic attack. Lancet 369:283, 2007.

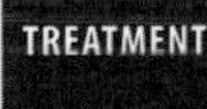

PRIMARY AND SECONDARY PREVENTION OF STROKE AND TIA

GENERAL PRINCIPLES

A number of medical and surgical interventions, as well as lifestyle modifications, are available for preventing stroke. Some of these can be widely applied because of their low cost and minimal risk; others are expensive and carry substantial risk but may be valuable for selected high-risk patients. Identification and control of modifiable risk factors, and especially hypertension, is the best strategy to reduce the burden of stroke, and the total number of strokes could be reduced substantially by these means (Table 446-4).

ATHEROSCLEROSIS RISK FACTORS

The relationship of various factors to the risk of atherosclerosis is described in **Chap. 291e**. Older age, diabetes mellitus, hypertension, tobacco smoking, abnormal blood cholesterol (particularly, low high-density lipoprotein [HDL] and/or elevated low-density lipoprotein [LDL]), and other factors are either proven or probable risk factors for ischemic stroke, largely by their link to atherosclerosis. Risk of stroke is much greater in those with prior stroke or TIA. Many cardiac conditions predispose to stroke, including atrial fibrillation and recent MI. Oral contraceptives and hormone replacement therapy increase stroke risk, and although rare, certain inherited and acquired hypercoagulable states predispose to stroke.

Hypertension is the most significant of the risk factors; in general, all hypertension should be treated to a target of less than 140–150/90 mmHg. However, many vascular neurologists recommend that guidelines for secondary prevention of stroke should aim for blood pressure reduction to 130/80 mmHg or lower. The presence of known cerebrovascular disease is not a contraindication to treatment aimed at achieving normotension. Also, the value of treating systolic hypertension in older patients has been clearly established. Lowering blood pressure to levels below those traditionally defining hypertension appears to reduce the risk of stroke even further. Data are particularly strong in support of thiazide diuretics and angiotensin-converting enzyme inhibitors.

Several trials have confirmed that statin drugs reduce the risk of stroke even in patients without elevated LDL or low HDL. The Stroke Prevention by Aggressive Reduction in Cholesterol Levels (SPARCL) trial showed benefit in secondary stroke reduction for patients with recent stroke or TIA who were prescribed atorvastatin, 80 mg/d. The primary prevention trial, Justification for the Use of Statins in Prevention: An Intervention Trial Evaluating Rosuvastatin (JUPITER), found that patients with low LDL (<130 mg/dL) caused by elevated C-reactive protein benefitted by daily use of this statin. Primary stroke occurrence was reduced by 51% (hazard ratio 0.49, $p = .004$), and there was no increase in the rates of intracranial hemorrhage. Meta-analysis has also supported a primary treatment effect for statins given acutely for ischemic stroke. Therefore, a statin should be considered in all patients with prior ischemic stroke. Tobacco smoking should be discouraged in all patients (**Chap. 470**). The use of pioglitazone (an agonist of peroxisome proliferator-activated receptor gamma) in patients with type 2 diabetes and previous stroke may lower risk of recurrent stroke, MI, or vascular death, but no trial sufficiently powered to definitively detect a significant reduction in stroke in the general diabetic population has yet been performed.

ANTIPLATELET AGENTS

Platelet antiaggregation agents can prevent atherothrombotic events, including TIA and stroke, by inhibiting the formation of intraarterial platelet aggregates. These can form on diseased arteries, induce thrombus formation, and occlude or embolize into the distal circulation. Aspirin, clopidogrel, and the combination of aspirin plus extended-release dipyridamole are the antiplatelet agents most commonly used for this purpose. Ticlopidine has been largely abandoned because of its adverse effects but may be used as an alternative to clopidogrel.

Aspirin is the most widely studied antiplatelet agent. Aspirin acetylates platelet cyclooxygenase, which irreversibly inhibits the formation in platelets of thromboxane A_2, a platelet aggregating and vasoconstricting prostaglandin. This effect is permanent and lasts for the usual 8-day life of the platelet. Paradoxically, aspirin also inhibits the formation in endothelial cells of prostacyclin, an antiaggregating and vasodilating prostaglandin. This effect is transient. As soon as aspirin is cleared from the blood, the nucleated endothelial cells again produce prostacyclin. Aspirin in low doses given once daily inhibits the production of thromboxane A_2 in platelets without substantially inhibiting prostacyclin formation. Higher doses of aspirin have not been proven to be more effective than lower doses.

Ticlopidine and clopidogrel block the adenosine diphosphate (ADP) receptor on platelets and thus prevent the cascade resulting in activation of the glycoprotein IIb/IIIa receptor that leads to fibrinogen binding to the platelet and consequent platelet aggregation. Ticlopidine is more effective than aspirin; however, it has the disadvantage of causing diarrhea, skin rash, and, in rare instances, neutropenia and thrombotic thrombocytopenic purpura (TTP). Clopidogrel rarely causes TTP but does not cause neutropenia. The Clopidogrel versus Aspirin in Patients at Risk of Ischemic Events (CAPRIE) trial, which led to FDA approval, found that it was only marginally more effective than aspirin in reducing risk of stroke. The Management of Atherothrombosis with Clopidogrel in High-Risk Patients (MATCH) trial was a large multicenter, randomized, double-blind study that compared clopidogrel in combination with aspirin to clopidogrel alone in the secondary prevention of TIA or stroke. The MATCH trial found no difference in TIA or stroke prevention with this combination, but did show a small but significant increase in major bleeding complications (3 vs 1%). In the Clopidogrel for High Atherothrombotic Risk and Ischemic Stabilization, Management, and Avoidance (CHARISMA) trial, which included a subgroup of patients with prior stroke or TIA along with other groups at high risk of cardiovascular events, there was no benefit of clopidogrel combined with aspirin compared to aspirin alone. Lastly, the SPS3 trial looked at the long-term combination of clopidogrel and aspirin versus clopidogrel alone in small-vessel stroke and found no improvement in stroke prevention and a significant increase in both hemorrhage and death. Thus, the long-term use of clopidogrel in combination with aspirin is not recommended for stroke prevention.

The short-term combination of clopidogrel with aspirin may be effective in preventing second stroke, however. A trial of 5170 Chinese patients enrolled within 24 h of TIA or minor ischemic stroke found that a clopidogrel-aspirin regimen (clopidogrel 300 mg load then 75 mg/d with aspirin 75 mg for the first 21 days) was superior to aspirin (75 mg/d) alone, with 90-day stroke risk decreased from 11.7 to 8.2% ($p < .001$) and no increase in major hemorrhage. An international NIH-sponsored trial of similar design is ongoing.

Dipyridamole is an antiplatelet agent that inhibits the uptake of adenosine by a variety of cells, including those of the vascular endothelium. The accumulated adenosine is an inhibitor of aggregation. At least in part through its effects on platelet and vessel wall phosphodiesterases, dipyridamole also potentiates the antiaggregatory effects of prostacyclin and nitric oxide produced by the endothelium and acts by inhibiting platelet phosphodiesterase, which is responsible for the breakdown of cyclic AMP. The resulting elevation in cyclic AMP inhibits aggregation of platelets. Dipyridamole is erratically absorbed depending on stomach pH, but a newer formulation combines timed-release dipyridamole, 200 mg, with aspirin, 25 mg, and has better oral bioavailability. This combination drug was studied in three trials. The European Stroke Prevention Study (ESPS) II showed efficacy of both 50 mg/d of aspirin and extended-release dipyridamole in preventing stroke, and a significantly better risk reduction when the two agents were combined. The open-label ESPRIT (European/Australasian Stroke Prevention in Reversible Ischaemia Trial) trial confirmed the ESPS-II results. After 3.5 years of follow-up, 13% of patients on aspirin and dipyridamole and 16% on aspirin alone (hazard ratio 0.80, 95% confidence index [CI] 0.66–0.98) met the primary outcome of death from all vascular causes. In the Prevention Regimen for Effectively Avoiding Second Strokes (PRoFESS) trial, the combination of extended-release dipyridamole and aspirin was compared directly with clopidogrel with and without the angiotensin receptor blocker telmisartan; there were no differences in the rates of second stroke (9% each) or degree of disability in patients with median follow-up of 2.4 years. Telmisartan also had no effect on these outcomes. This suggests that these antiplatelet regimens are similar and also raises questions about default prescription of agents to block the angiotensin pathway in all stroke patients. The principal side effect of dipyridamole is headache. The combination capsule of extended-release dipyridamole and aspirin is approved for prevention of stroke.

Many large clinical trials have demonstrated clearly that most antiplatelet agents reduce the risk of all important vascular atherothrombotic events (i.e., ischemic stroke, MI, and death due to all vascular causes) in patients at risk for these events. The overall *relative* reduction in risk of nonfatal stroke is about 25–30% and of all vascular events is about 25%. The *absolute* reduction varies considerably, depending on the particular patient's risk. Individuals at very low risk for stroke seem to experience the same relative reduction, but their risks may be so low that the "benefit" is meaningless. Conversely, individuals with a 10–15% risk of vascular events per year experience a reduction to about 7.5–11%.

Aspirin is inexpensive, can be given in low doses, and could be recommended for all adults to prevent both stroke and MI. However, it causes epigastric discomfort, gastric ulceration, and gastrointestinal hemorrhage, which may be asymptomatic or life threatening. Consequently, not every 40- or 50-year-old should be advised to take aspirin regularly because the risk of atherothrombotic stroke is extremely low and is outweighed by the risk of adverse side effects. Conversely, every patient who has experienced an atherothrombotic stroke or TIA and has no contraindication should be taking an antiplatelet agent regularly because the average annual risk of another stroke is 8–10%; another few percent will experience an MI or vascular death. Clearly, the likelihood of benefit far outweighs the risks of treatment.

The choice of antiplatelet agent and dose must balance the risk of stroke, the expected benefit, and the risk and cost of treatment. However, there are no definitive data, and opinions vary. Many authorities believe low-dose (30–75 mg/d) and high-dose (650–1300 mg/d) aspirin are about equally effective. Some advocate very low doses to avoid adverse effects, and still others advocate very high doses to be sure the benefit is maximal. Most physicians in North America recommend 81–325 mg/d, whereas most Europeans recommend 50–100 mg. Clopidogrel and extended-release dipyridamole plus aspirin are being increasingly recommended as first-line drugs for secondary prevention. Similarly, the choice of aspirin, clopidogrel, or dipyridamole plus aspirin must balance the fact that the latter are more effective than aspirin but the cost is higher, and this is likely to affect long-term patient adherence. The use of platelet aggregation studies in individual patients taking aspirin is controversial because of limited data.

ANTICOAGULATION THERAPY AND EMBOLIC STROKE

Several trials have shown that anticoagulation (INR range, 2–3) in patients with chronic nonvalvular (nonrheumatic) atrial fibrillation (NVAF) prevents cerebral embolism and stroke and is safe. For primary prevention and for patients who have experienced stroke or TIA, anticoagulation with a VKA reduces the risk by about 67%, which clearly outweighs the 1–3% risk per year of a major bleeding complication. VKAs are difficult to dose, their effects vary with dietary intake of vitamin K, and they require frequent blood monitoring of the PTT/INR. Several newer oral anticoagulants (OACs) have recently been shown to be more convenient and efficacious for stroke prevention in NVAF. A randomized trial compared the oral thrombin inhibitor dabigatran to VKAs in a noninferiority trial to prevent stroke or systemic embolization in NVAF. Two doses of dabigatran were used: 110 mg/d and 150 mg/d. Both dose tiers of dabigatran were noninferior to VKAs in preventing second stroke and systemic embolization, and the higher dose tier was superior (relative risk 0.66; 95% CI 0.53–0.82; $p < .001$) and the rate of major bleeding was lower in the lower dose tier of dabigatran compared to VKAs. Dabigatran requires no blood monitoring to titrate the dose, and its effect is independent of oral intake of vitamin K. Newer oral factor Xa inhibitors have also been found to be equivalent or safer and more effective than VKAs in NVAF stroke prevention. In the Apixaban for Reduction in Stroke and Other Thromboembolic Events in Atrial Fibrillation (ARISTOTLE) trial, patients were randomized between apixaban, 5 mg twice daily, and dose-adjusted warfarin (INR 2–3). The combined endpoint of ischemic or hemorrhagic stroke or system embolism occurred in 1.27% of patients in the apixaban group and in 1.6% in the warfarin group ($p < .001$ for noninferiority and $p < .01$ for superiority). Major bleeding was 1% less, favoring apixaban ($p < .001$). Similar results were obtained in the Rivaroxaban Once Daily Oral Direct Factor Xa Inhibition Compared with Vitamin K Antagonism for Prevention of Stroke and Embolism Trial in Atrial Fibrillation (ROCKET-AF). Here, patients with NVAF were randomized to rivaroxaban versus warfarin: 1.7% of the factor Xa group and 2.2% of the warfarin group reached the endpoint of stroke and systemic embolism ($p < .001$ for noninferiority); intracranial hemorrhage was also lower with rivaroxaban. Finally, the factor Xa inhibitor edoxaban was also found to be noninferior to warfarin. Thus, oral factor Xa inhibitors are at least a suitable alternative to VKAs, and likely are superior both in efficacy and perhaps compliance.

For patients who cannot take anticoagulant medications, clopidogrel plus aspirin was compared to aspirin alone in the Atrial Fibrillation Clopidogrel Trial with Irbesartan for Prevention of Vascular Events (ACTIVE-A). Clopidogrel combined with aspirin was more effective than aspirin alone in preventing vascular events, principally stroke, but increased the risk of major bleeding (relative risk 1.57, $p < .001$).

The decision to use anticoagulation for primary prevention is based primarily on risk factors (Table 446-3). The history of a TIA or stroke tips the balance in favor of anticoagulation regardless of other risk factors. Intermittent atrial fibrillation carries the same risk of stroke as chronic atrial fibrillation, and several ambulatory studies of seemingly "cryptogenic" stroke have found evidence of intermittent atrial fibrillation in nearly 20% of patients monitored for a few weeks. Interrogation of implanted pacemakers also confirms an association between subclinical atrial fibrillation and stroke risk. Therefore, for patients with otherwise cryptogenic embolic stroke (no evidence of any other cause for stroke), ambulatory monitoring for 3–4 weeks is a reasonable strategy to determine the best prophylactic therapy.

Because of the high annual stroke risk in untreated rheumatic heart disease with atrial fibrillation, primary prophylaxis against stroke has not been studied in a double-blind fashion. These patients generally should receive long-term anticoagulation. Dabigatran and the oral Xa inhibitors have not been studied in this population.

Anticoagulation also reduces the risk of embolism in acute MI. Most clinicians recommend a 3-month course of anticoagulation when there is anterior Q-wave infarction, substantial left ventricular dysfunction, congestive heart failure, mural thrombosis, or atrial fibrillation. OACs are recommended long-term if atrial fibrillation persists.

Stroke secondary to thromboembolism is one of the most serious complications of prosthetic heart valve implantation. The intensity of anticoagulation and/or antiplatelet therapy is dictated by the type of prosthetic valve and its location. Dabigatran may be less effective than warfarin, and the oral Xa inhibitors have not been studied in this population.

If the embolic source cannot be eliminated, anticoagulation should in most cases be continued indefinitely. Many neurologists recommend combining antiplatelet agents with anticoagulants for patients who "fail" anticoagulation (i.e., have another stroke or TIA), but the evidence basis for this is lacking.

ANTICOAGULATION THERAPY AND NONCARDIOGENIC STROKE

Data do not support the use of long-term VKAs for preventing atherothrombotic stroke for either intracranial or extracranial cerebrovascular disease. The Warfarin-Aspirin Recurrent Stroke Study (WARSS) found no benefit of warfarin sodium (INR 1.4–2.8) over aspirin, 325 mg, for secondary prevention of stroke but did find a slightly higher bleeding rate in the warfarin group; a European study confirmed this finding. The Warfarin and Aspirin for Symptomatic Intracranial Disease (WASID) study (see below) demonstrated no benefit of warfarin (INR 2–3) over aspirin in patients with symptomatic intracranial atherosclerosis and also found a higher rate of bleeding complications.

TREATMENT CAROTID ATHEROSCLEROSIS

Carotid atherosclerosis can be removed surgically (endarterectomy) or mitigated with endovascular stenting with or without balloon angioplasty. Anticoagulation has not been directly compared with antiplatelet therapy for carotid disease.

SURGICAL THERAPY

Symptomatic carotid stenosis was studied in the North American Symptomatic Carotid Endarterectomy Trial (NASCET) and the European Carotid Surgery Trial (ECST). Both showed a substantial benefit for surgery in patients with stenosis of ≥70%. In NASCET, the average cumulative ipsilateral stroke risk at 2 years was 26% for patients treated medically and 9% for those receiving the same medical treatment plus a carotid endarterectomy. This 17% *absolute* reduction in the surgical group is a 65% *relative* risk reduction favoring surgery (Table 446-4). NASCET also showed a significant, although less robust, benefit for patients with 50–70% stenosis. ECST found harm for patients with stenosis <30% treated surgically.

A patient's risk of stroke and possible benefit from surgery are related to the presence of retinal versus hemispheric symptoms, degree of arterial stenosis, extent of associated medical conditions (of note, NASCET and ECST excluded "high-risk" patients with significant cardiac, pulmonary, or renal disease), institutional surgical morbidity and mortality, timing of surgery relative to symptoms, and other factors. A recent meta-analysis of the NASCET and ECST trials demonstrated that endarterectomy is most beneficial when performed within 2 weeks of symptom onset. In addition, benefit is more pronounced in patients >75 years, and men appear to benefit more than women.

In summary, a patient with recent symptomatic hemispheric ischemia, high-grade stenosis in the appropriate internal carotid artery, and an institutional perioperative morbidity and mortality rate of ≤6% generally should undergo carotid endarterectomy. If the perioperative stroke rate is >6% for any particular surgeon, however, the benefits of carotid endarterectomy are questionable.

The indications for surgical treatment of *asymptomatic carotid disease* have been clarified by the results of the Asymptomatic Carotid Atherosclerosis Study (ACAS) and the Asymptomatic Carotid Surgery Trial (ACST). ACAS randomized asymptomatic patients with ≥60% stenosis to medical treatment with aspirin or the same medical treatment plus carotid endarterectomy. The surgical group had a risk over 5 years for ipsilateral stroke (and any perioperative stroke or death) of 5.1%, compared to a risk in the medical group of 11%. Although this demonstrates a 53% *relative* risk reduction, the *absolute* risk reduction is only 5.9% over 5 years, or 1.2% annually (Table 446-4). Nearly one-half of the strokes in the surgery group were caused by preoperative angiograms. ACST randomized asymptomatic patients with >60% carotid stenosis to endarterectomy or medical therapy. The 5-year risk of stroke in the surgical group (including perioperative stroke or death) was 6.4%, compared to 11.8% in the medically treated group (46% relative risk reduction and 5.4% absolute risk reduction).

In both ACAS and ACST, the perioperative complication rate was higher in women, perhaps negating any benefit in the reduction of stroke risk within 5 years. It is possible that with longer follow up, a clear benefit in women will emerge. At present, carotid endarterectomy in asymptomatic women remains particularly controversial.

In summary, the natural history of asymptomatic stenosis is an 2% per year stroke rate, whereas symptomatic patients experience a 13% per year risk of stroke. Whether to recommend carotid revascularization for an asymptomatic patient is somewhat controversial and depends on many factors, including patient preference, degree of stenosis, age, gender, and comorbidities. Medical therapy for reduction of atherosclerosis risk factors, including cholesterol-lowering agents and antiplatelet medications, is generally recommended for patients with asymptomatic carotid stenosis. As with atrial fibrillation, it is imperative to counsel the patient about TIAs so that therapy can be revised if symptoms develop.

ENDOVASCULAR THERAPY

Balloon angioplasty coupled with stenting is being used with increasing frequency to open stenotic carotid arteries and maintain their patency. These techniques can treat carotid stenosis not only at the bifurcation but also near the skull base and in the intracranial segments. The Stenting and Angioplasty with Protection in Patients at High Risk for Endarterectomy (SAPPHIRE) trial randomized high-risk patients (defined as patients with clinically significant coronary or pulmonary disease, contralateral carotid occlusion, restenosis after endarterectomy, contralateral laryngeal-nerve palsy, prior radical neck surgery or radiation, or age >80) with symptomatic carotid stenosis >50% or asymptomatic stenosis >80% to either stenting combined with a distal emboli-protection device or endarterectomy. The risk of death, stroke, or MI within 30 days and ipsilateral stroke or death within 1 year was 12.2% in the stenting group and 20.1% in the endarterectomy group (p = .055), suggesting that stenting is at the very least comparable to endarterectomy as a treatment option for this patient group at high risk of surgery. However, the outcomes with both interventions may not have been better than leaving the carotid stenoses untreated, particularly for the asymptomatic patients, and much of the benefit seen in the stenting group was due to a reduction in periprocedure MI. Two randomized trials comparing stents to endarterectomy in lower-risk patients have been published. The Carotid Revascularization Endarterectomy versus Stenting Trial (CREST) enrolled patients with either asymptomatic or symptomatic stenosis. The 30-day risk of stroke was 4.1% in the stent group and 2.3% in the surgical group, but the 30-day risk of MI was 1.1% in the stent group and 2.3% in the surgery group, suggesting relative equivalence of risk between the procedures. At median follow-up of 2.5 years, the combined endpoint of stroke, MI, and death was the same (7.2% stent vs 6.8% surgery). The rate of restenosis at 2 years was also similar in both groups. The International Carotid Stenting (ICSS) trial randomized symptomatic patients to stents versus endarterectomy and found a different result: At 120 days, the incidence of stroke, MI, or death was 8.5% in the stenting group versus 5.2% in the endarterectomy group ($p = .006$); longer-term follow-up is currently under way. Differences between trial designs, selection of stent, and operator experience may explain these important differences. Until more data are available, there remains controversy as to who should receive a stent or have endarterectomy; it is likely that the procedures carry similar risks if performed by experienced physicians.

BYPASS SURGERY

Extracranial-to-intracranial (EC-IC) bypass surgery has been proven ineffective for atherosclerotic stenoses that are inaccessible to conventional carotid endarterectomy. In patients with recent stroke, an associated carotid occlusion, and evidence of inadequate perfusion of the brain as measured with positron emission tomography, no benefit from EC-IC bypass was found in a trial stopped for futility.

INTRACRANIAL ATHEROSCLEROSIS

The WASID trial randomized patients with symptomatic stenosis (50–99%) of a major intracranial vessel to either high-dose aspirin (1300 mg/d) or warfarin (target INR, 2.0–3.0), with a combined primary endpoint of ischemic stroke, brain hemorrhage, or death from vascular cause other than stroke. The trial was terminated early because of an increased risk of adverse events related to warfarin anticoagulation. With a mean follow-up of 1.8 years, the primary endpoint was seen in 22.1% of patients in the aspirin group and 21.8% of the warfarin group. Death from any cause was seen in 4.3% of the aspirin group and 9.7% of the warfarin group; 3.2% of patients on aspirin experienced major hemorrhage, compared to 8.3% of patients taking warfarin.

Intracranial stenting of intracranial atherosclerosis was found to be dramatically harmful compared to aspirin in the Stenting and Aggressive Medical Management for Preventing Recurrent Stroke in Intracranial Stenosis (SAMMPRIS) trial. This trial enrolled newly symptomatic TIA or minor stroke patients with associated 70–99% intracranial stenosis to primary stenting with a self-expanding stent or to medical management. Both groups received clopidogrel, aspirin, statin, and aggressive control of blood pressure. The endpoint of stroke or death occurred in 14.7% of the stented group and 5.8% of the medically treated groups ($p = .002$). This low rate of second stroke was significantly lower than in the WASID trial and suggests that aggressive medical management had a marked influence on secondary stroke risk.

Dural Sinus Thrombosis Limited evidence exists to support short-term use of anticoagulants, regardless of the presence of intracranial hemorrhage, for venous infarction following sinus thrombosis. The long-term outcome for most patients, even those with intracerebral hemorrhage, is excellent.

STROKE SYNDROMES

A careful history and neurologic examination can often localize the region of brain dysfunction; if this region corresponds to a particular arterial distribution, the possible causes responsible for the syndrome can be narrowed. This is of particular importance when the patient presents with a TIA and a normal examination. For example, if a patient develops language loss and a right homonymous hemianopia, a search for causes of left middle cerebral emboli should be performed. A finding of an isolated stenosis of the right internal carotid artery in that patient, for example, suggests an asymptomatic carotid stenosis, and the search for other causes of stroke should continue. The following sections describe the clinical findings of cerebral ischemia associated with cerebral vascular territories depicted in **Figs. 446-4** and **446-6 through 446-14**. Stroke syndromes are divided into: (1) large-vessel stroke within the anterior circulation, (2) large-vessel stroke within the posterior circulation, and (3) small-vessel disease of either vascular bed.

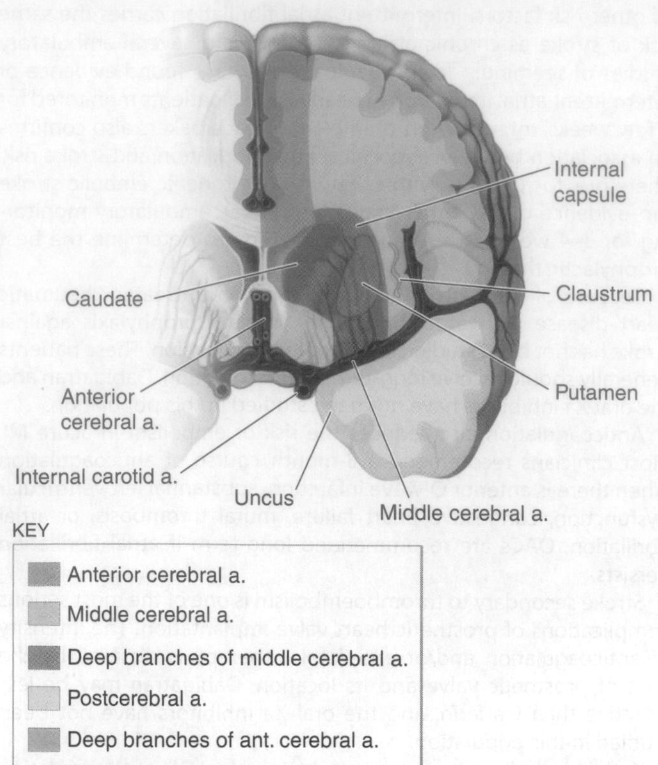

FIGURE 446-6 Diagram of a cerebral hemisphere in coronal section showing the territories of the major cerebral vessels that branch from the internal carotid arteries.

Stroke within the Anterior Circulation The internal carotid artery and its branches comprise the anterior circulation of the brain. These vessels can be occluded by intrinsic disease of the vessel (e.g., atherosclerosis or dissection) or by embolic occlusion from a proximal source as discussed above. Occlusion of each major intracranial vessel has distinct clinical manifestations.

MIDDLE CEREBRAL ARTERY Occlusion of the proximal MCA or one of its major branches is most often due to an embolus (artery-to-artery, cardiac, or of unknown source) rather than intracranial atherothrombosis. Atherosclerosis of the proximal MCA may cause distal emboli to the middle cerebral territory or, less commonly, may produce low-flow TIAs. Collateral formation via leptomeningeal vessels often prevents MCA stenosis from becoming symptomatic.

The cortical branches of the MCA supply the lateral surface of the hemisphere except for (1) the frontal pole and a strip along the superomedial border of the frontal and parietal lobes supplied by the ACA, and (2) the lower temporal and occipital pole convolutions supplied by the PCA (Figs. 446-6, 446-7, 446-8, and 446-9).

The proximal MCA (M1 segment) gives rise to penetrating branches (termed *lenticulostriate arteries*) that supply the putamen, outer globus pallidus, posterior limb of the internal capsule, adjacent corona radiata, and most of the caudate nucleus (Fig. 446-6). In the sylvian fissure, the MCA in most patients divides into *superior* and *inferior* divisions

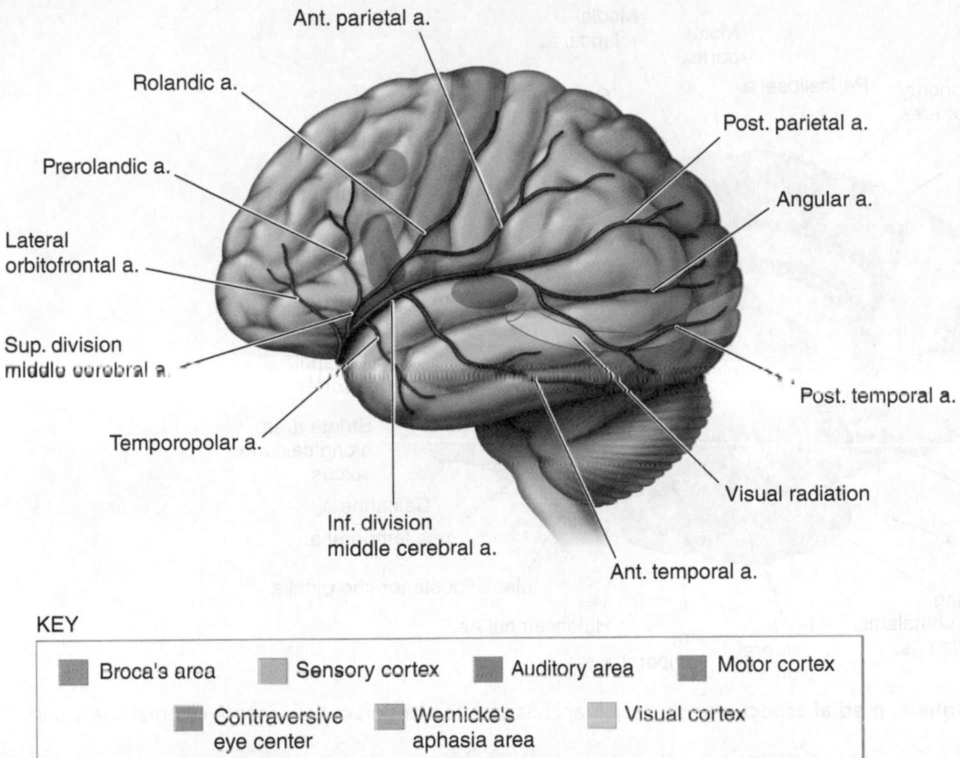

FIGURE 446-7 Diagram of a cerebral hemisphere, lateral aspect, showing the branches and distribution of the middle cerebral artery and the principal regions of cerebral localization. Note the bifurcation of the middle cerebral artery into a superior and inferior division.

Signs and symptoms: *Structures involved*

Paralysis of the contralateral face, arm, and leg; sensory impairment over the same area (pinprick, cotton touch, vibration, position, two-point discrimination, stereognosis, tactile localization, barognosis, cutaneographia): *Somatic motor area for face and arm and the fibers descending from the leg area to enter the corona radiata and corresponding somatic sensory system*

Motor aphasia: *Motor speech area of the dominant hemisphere*

Central aphasia, word deafness, anomia, jargon speech, sensory agraphia, acalculia, alexia, finger agnosia, right-left confusion (the last four comprise the Gerstmann syndrome): *Central, suprasylvian speech area and parietooccipital cortex of the dominant hemisphere*

Conduction aphasia: *Central speech area (parietal operculum)*

Apractagnosia of the nondominant hemisphere, anosognosia, hemiasomatognosia, unilateral neglect, agnosia for the left half of external space, dressing "apraxia," constructional "apraxia," distortion of visual coordinates, inaccurate localization in the half field, impaired ability to judge distance, upside-down reading, visual illusions (e.g., it may appear that another person walks through a table): *Nondominant parietal lobe (area corresponding to speech area in dominant hemisphere); loss of topographic memory is usually due to a nondominant lesion, occasionally to a dominant one*

Homonymous hemianopia (often homonymous inferior quadrantanopia): *Optic radiation deep to second temporal convolution*

Paralysis of conjugate gaze to the opposite side: *Frontal contraversive eye field or projecting fibers*

(M2 branches). Branches of the inferior division supply the inferior parietal and temporal cortex, and those from the superior division supply the frontal and superior parietal cortex (Fig. 446-7).

If the entire MCA is occluded at its origin (blocking both its penetrating and cortical branches) and the distal collaterals are limited, the clinical findings are contralateral hemiplegia, hemianesthesia, homonymous hemianopia, and a day or two of gaze preference to the ipsilateral side. Dysarthria is common because of facial weakness. When the dominant hemisphere is involved, global aphasia is present also, and when the nondominant hemisphere is affected, anosognosia, constructional apraxia, and neglect are found (Chap. 36).

Complete MCA syndromes occur most often when an embolus occludes the stem of the artery. Cortical collateral blood flow and differing arterial configurations are probably responsible for the development of many partial syndromes. Partial syndromes may also be due to emboli that enter the proximal MCA without complete occlusion, occlude distal MCA branches, or fragment and move distally.

Partial syndromes due to embolic occlusion of a single branch include hand, or arm and hand, weakness alone (brachial syndrome) or facial weakness with nonfluent (Broca) aphasia (Chap. 36), with or without arm weakness (frontal opercular syndrome). A combination of sensory disturbance, motor weakness, and nonfluent aphasia suggests that an embolus has occluded the proximal superior division and infarcted large portions of the frontal and parietal cortices (Fig. 446-7). If a fluent (Wernicke's) aphasia occurs without weakness, the inferior division of the MCA supplying the posterior part (temporal cortex) of the dominant hemisphere is probably involved. Jargon speech and an inability to comprehend written and spoken language are prominent features, often accompanied by a contralateral, homonymous superior quadrantanopia. Hemineglect or spatial agnosia without weakness indicates that the inferior division of the MCA in the nondominant hemisphere is involved.

Occlusion of a lenticulostriate vessel produces small-vessel (lacunar) stroke within the internal capsule (Fig. 446-6). This produces pure motor stroke or sensory-motor stroke contralateral to the lesion. Ischemia within the genu of the internal capsule causes primarily facial weakness followed by arm and then leg weakness as the ischemia moves posterior within the capsule. Alternatively, the contralateral hand may become ataxic, and dysarthria will be prominent (clumsy hand, dysarthria lacunar syndrome). Lacunar infarction affecting the globus pallidus and putamen often has few clinical signs, but parkinsonism and hemiballismus have been reported.

ANTERIOR CEREBRAL ARTERY The ACA is divided into two segments: the precommunal (A1) circle of Willis, or stem, which connects the internal carotid artery to the anterior communicating artery, and the postcommunal (A2) segment distal to the anterior communicating artery (Figs. 446-4, 446-6, and 446-8). The A1 segment gives rise to several deep penetrating branches that supply the anterior limb of the internal capsule, the anterior perforate substance, amygdala, anterior hypothalamus, and the inferior part of the head of the caudate nucleus (Fig. 446-6).

Occlusion of the proximal ACA is usually well tolerated because of collateral flow through the anterior communicating artery and collaterals through the MCA and PCA. Occlusion of a single A2 segment results in the contralateral symptoms noted in Fig. 446-8. If both A2 segments arise from a single anterior cerebral stem (contralateral A1 segment atresia), the occlusion may affect both hemispheres. Profound abulia (a delay in verbal and motor response) and bilateral pyramidal signs with paraparesis or quadriparesis and urinary incontinence result.

ANTERIOR CHOROIDAL ARTERY This artery arises from the internal carotid artery and supplies the posterior limb of the internal capsule and the white matter posterolateral to it, through which pass some of

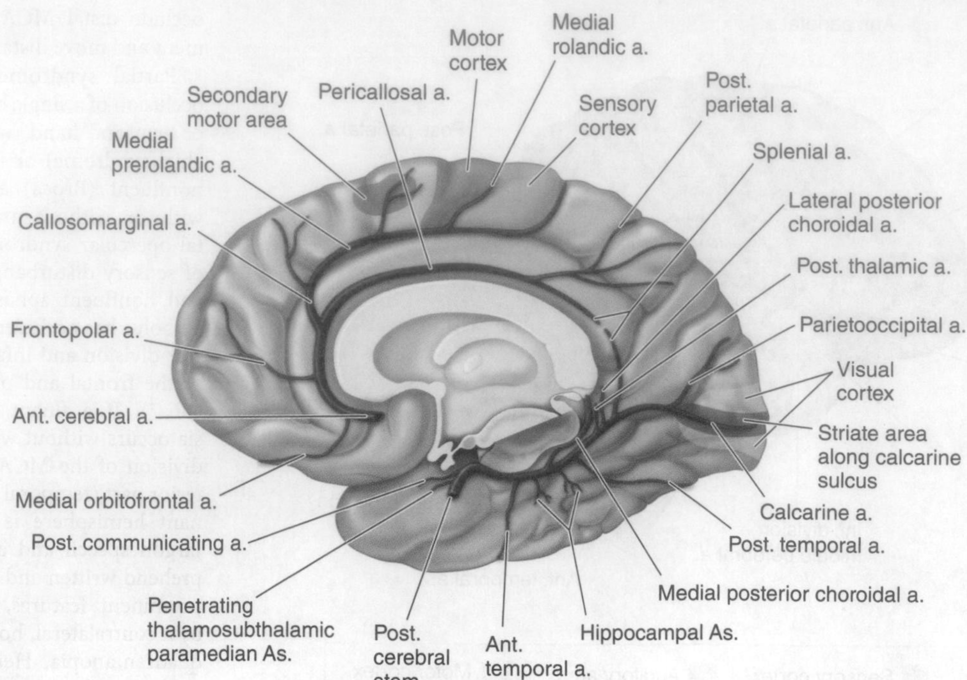

FIGURE 446-8 Diagram of a cerebral hemisphere, medial aspect, showing the branches and distribution of the anterior cerebral artery and the principal regions of cerebral localization.

Signs and symptoms: *Structures involved*

Paralysis of opposite foot and leg: *Motor leg area*

A lesser degree of paresis of opposite arm: *Arm area of cortex or fibers descending to corona radiata*

Cortical sensory loss over toes, foot, and leg: *Sensory area for foot and leg*

Urinary incontinence: *Sensorimotor area in paracentral lobule*

Contralateral grasp reflex, sucking reflex, gegenhalten (paratonic rigidity): *Medial surface of the posterior frontal lobe; likely supplemental motor area*

Abulia (akinetic mutism), slowness, delay, intermittent interruption, lack of spontaneity, whispering, reflex distraction to sights and sounds: *Uncertain localization—probably cingulate gyrus and medial inferior portion of frontal, parietal, and temporal lobes*

Impairment of gait and stance (gait apraxia): *Frontal cortex near leg motor area*

Dyspraxia of left limbs, tactile aphasia in left limbs: Corpus callosum

the geniculocalcarine fibers (Fig. 446-9). The complete syndrome of anterior choroidal artery occlusion consists of contralateral hemiplegia, hemianesthesia (hypesthesia), and homonymous hemianopia. However, because this territory is also supplied by penetrating vessels of the proximal MCA and the posterior communicating and posterior choroidal arteries, minimal deficits may occur, and patients frequently recover substantially. Anterior choroidal strokes are usually the result of in situ thrombosis of the vessel, and the vessel is particularly vulnerable to iatrogenic occlusion during surgical clipping of aneurysms arising from the internal carotid artery.

INTERNAL CAROTID ARTERY The clinical picture of internal carotid occlusion varies depending on whether the cause of ischemia is propagated thrombus, embolism, or low flow. The cortex supplied by the MCA territory is affected most often. With a competent circle of Willis, occlusion may go unnoticed. If the thrombus propagates up the internal carotid artery into the MCA or embolizes it, symptoms are identical to proximal MCA occlusion (see above). Sometimes there is massive infarction of the entire deep white matter and cortical surface. When the origins of both the ACA and MCA are occluded at the top of the carotid artery, abulia or stupor occurs with hemiplegia, hemianesthesia, and aphasia or anosognosia. When the PCA arises from the internal carotid artery (a configuration called a *fetal posterior cerebral artery*), it may also become occluded and give rise to symptoms referable to its peripheral territory (Figs. 446-8 and 446-9).

In addition to supplying the ipsilateral brain, the internal carotid artery perfuses the optic nerve and retina via the ophthalmic artery. In ~25% of symptomatic internal carotid disease, recurrent transient monocular blindness (amaurosis fugax) warns of the lesion. Patients typically describe a horizontal shade that sweeps down or up across the field of vision. They may also complain that their vision was blurred in that eye or that the upper or lower half of vision disappeared. In most cases, these symptoms last only a few minutes. Rarely, ischemia or infarction of the ophthalmic artery or central retinal arteries occurs at the time of cerebral TIA or infarction.

A high-pitched prolonged carotid bruit fading into diastole is often associated with tightly stenotic lesions. As the stenosis grows tighter and flow distal to the stenosis becomes reduced, the bruit becomes fainter and may disappear when occlusion is imminent.

COMMON CAROTID ARTERY All symptoms and signs of internal carotid occlusion may also be present with occlusion of the common carotid artery. Jaw claudication may result from low flow in the external carotid branches. Bilateral common carotid artery occlusions at their origin may occur in Takayasu's arteritis (Chap. 385).

Stroke Within the Posterior Circulation The posterior circulation is composed of the paired vertebral arteries, the basilar artery, and the paired posterior cerebral arteries. The vertebral arteries join to form the basilar artery at the pontomedullary junction. The basilar artery divides into two posterior cerebral arteries in the interpeduncular fossa (Figs. 446-4, 446-8, and 446-9). These major arteries give rise to long and short circumferential branches and to smaller deep penetrating branches that supply the cerebellum, medulla, pons, midbrain, subthalamus, thalamus, hippocampus, and medial temporal and occipital lobes. Occlusion of each vessel produces its own distinctive syndrome.

POSTERIOR CEREBRAL ARTERY In 75% of cases, both PCAs arise from the bifurcation of the basilar artery; in 20%, one has its origin from the ipsilateral internal carotid artery via the posterior communicating artery; in 5%, both originate from the respective ipsilateral internal carotid arteries (Figs. 446-8 and 446-9). The precommunal, or P1, segment of the true posterior cerebral artery is atretic in such cases.

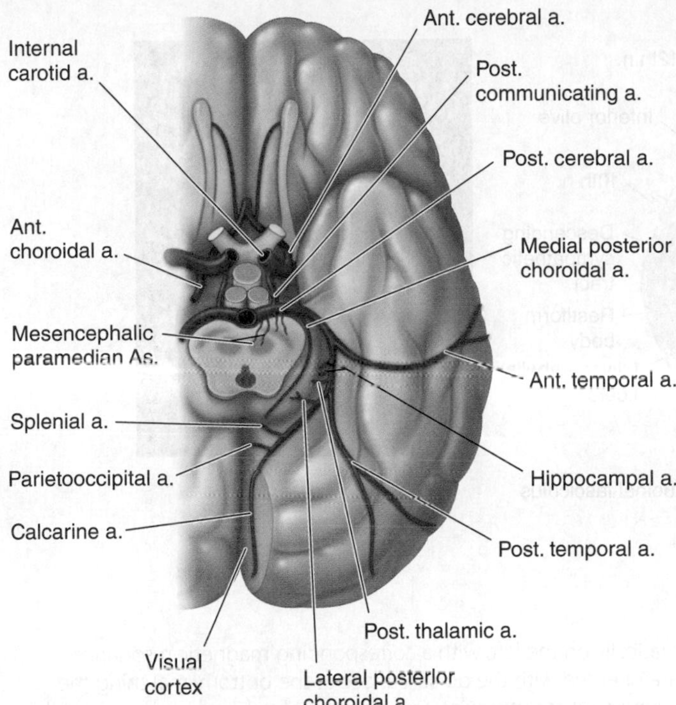

FIGURE 446-9 Inferior aspect of the brain with the branches and distribution of the posterior cerebral artery and the principal anatomic structures shown.

Signs and symptoms: *Structures involved*

Peripheral territory (see also Fig. 446-12). Homonymous hemianopia (often upper quadrantic): *Calcarine cortex or optic radiation nearby*. Bilateral homonymous hemianopia, cortical blindness, awareness or denial of blindness; tactile naming, achromatopia (color blindness), failure to see to-and-fro movements, inability to perceive objects not centrally located, apraxia of ocular movements, inability to count or enumerate objects, tendency to run into things that the patient sees and tries to avoid: *Bilateral occipital lobe with possibly the parietal lobe involved*. Verbal dyslexia without agraphia, color anomia: *Dominant calcarine lesion and posterior part of corpus callosum*. Memory defect: *Hippocampal lesion bilaterally or on the dominant side only*. Topographic disorientation and prosop agnosia: *Usually with lesions of nondominant, calcarine, and lingual gyrus*. Simultanagnosia, hemivisual neglect: *Dominant visual cortex, contralateral hemisphere*. Unformed visual hallucinations, peduncular hallucinosis, metamorphopsia, teleopsia, illusory visual spread, palinopsia, distortion of outlines, central photophobia: *Calcarine cortex*. Complex hallucinations: *Usually nondominant hemisphere*.

Central territory. Thalamic syndrome: sensory loss (all modalities), spontaneous pain and dysesthesias, choreoathetosis, intention tremor, spasms of hand, mild hemiparesis: *Posteroventral nucleus of thalamus; involvement of the adjacent subthalamus body or its afferent tracts*. Thalamoperforate syndrome: crossed cerebellar ataxia with ipsilateral third nerve palsy (Claude's syndrome): *Dentatothalamic tract and issuing third nerve*. Weber's syndrome: third nerve palsy and contralateral hemiplegia: *Third nerve and cerebral peduncle*. Contralateral hemiplegia: *Cerebral peduncle*. Paralysis or paresis of vertical eye movement, skew deviation, sluggish pupillary responses to light, slight miosis and ptosis (retraction nystagmus and "tucking" of the eyelids may be associated): *Supranuclear fibers to third nerve, interstitial nucleus of Cajal, nucleus of Darkschewitsch, and posterior commissure*. Contralateral rhythmic, ataxic action tremor; rhythmic postural or "holding" tremor (rubral tremor): *Dentatothalamic tract*.

PCA syndromes usually result from atheroma formation or emboli that lodge at the top of the basilar artery; posterior circulation disease may also be caused by dissection of either vertebral artery or fibromuscular dysplasia.

Two clinical syndromes are commonly observed with occlusion of the PCA: (1) *P1 syndrome*: midbrain, subthalamic, and thalamic signs, which are due to disease of the proximal P1 segment of the PCA or its penetrating branches (thalamogeniculate, Percheron, and posterior choroidal arteries); and (2) *P2 syndrome*: cortical temporal and occipital lobe signs, due to occlusion of the P2 segment distal to the junction of the PCA with the posterior communicating artery.

P1 SYNDROMES Infarction usually occurs in the ipsilateral subthalamus and medial thalamus and in the ipsilateral cerebral peduncle and midbrain (Figs. 446-9 and 446-14). A third nerve palsy with contralateral ataxia (Claude's syndrome) or with contralateral hemiplegia (Weber's syndrome) may result. The ataxia indicates involvement of the red nucleus or dentatorubrothalamic tract; the hemiplegia is localized to the cerebral peduncle (Fig. 446-14). If the subthalamic nucleus is involved, contralateral hemiballismus may occur. Occlusion of the artery of Percheron produces paresis of upward gaze and drowsiness and often abulia. Extensive infarction in the midbrain and subthalamus occurring with bilateral proximal PCA occlusion presents as coma, unreactive pupils, bilateral pyramidal signs, and decerebrate rigidity.

Occlusion of the penetrating branches of thalamic and thalamogeniculate arteries produces less extensive thalamic and thalamocapsular lacunar syndromes. The *thalamic Déjérine-Roussy syndrome* consists of contralateral hemisensory loss followed later by an agonizing, searing or burning pain in the affected areas. It is persistent and responds poorly to analgesics. Anticonvulsants (carbamazepine or gabapentin) or tricyclic antidepressants may be beneficial.

P2 SYNDROMES (Figs. 446-8 and 446-9) Occlusion of the distal PCA causes infarction of the medial temporal and occipital lobes. Contralateral homonymous hemianopia with macula sparing is the usual manifestation. Occasionally, only the upper quadrant of visual field is involved. If the visual association areas are spared and only the calcarine cortex is involved, the patient may be aware of visual defects. Medial temporal lobe and hippocampal involvement may cause an acute disturbance in memory, particularly if it occurs in the dominant hemisphere. The defect usually clears because memory has bilateral representation. If the dominant hemisphere is affected and the infarct extends to involve the splenium of the corpus callosum, the patient may demonstrate alexia without agraphia. Visual agnosia for faces, objects, mathematical symbols, and colors and anomia with paraphasic errors (amnestic aphasia) may also occur, even without callosal involvement. Occlusion of the posterior cerebral artery can produce *peduncular hallucinosis* (visual hallucinations of brightly colored scenes and objects).

Bilateral infarction in the distal PCAs produces cortical blindness (blindness with preserved pupillary light reaction). The patient is often unaware of the blindness or may even deny it (*Anton's syndrome*). Tiny islands of vision may persist, and the patient may report that vision fluctuates as images are captured in the preserved portions Rarely, only peripheral vision is lost and central vision is spared, resulting in "gun-barrel" vision. Bilateral visual association area lesions may result in *Balint's syndrome*, a disorder of the orderly visual scanning of the environment (Chap. 36), usually resulting from infarctions secondary to low flow in the "watershed" between the distal PCA and MCA territories, as occurs after cardiac arrest. Patients may experience persistence of a visual image for several minutes despite gazing at another scene (*palinopsia*) or an inability to synthesize the whole of an image (*asimultanagnosia*). Embolic occlusion of the top of the basilar artery can produce any or all of the central or peripheral territory symptoms. The hallmark is the sudden onset of bilateral signs, including ptosis, pupillary asymmetry or lack of reaction to light, and somnolence.

VERTEBRAL AND POSTERIOR INFERIOR CEREBELLAR ARTERIES The vertebral artery, which arises from the innominate artery on the right and the subclavian artery on the left, consists of four segments. The first (V1) extends from its origin to its entrance into the sixth or fifth transverse vertebral foramen. The second segment (V2) traverses the vertebral

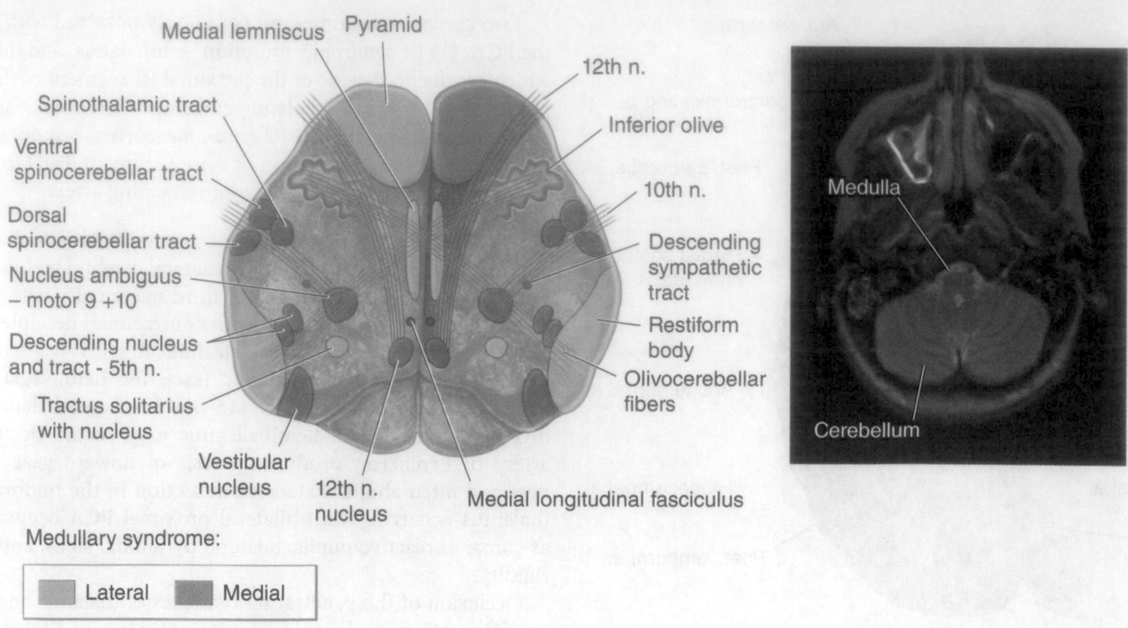

FIGURE 446-10 Axial section at the level of the medulla, depicted schematically on the left, with a corresponding magnetic resonance image on the right. Note that in Figs. 446-10 through 446-14, all drawings are oriented with the dorsal surface at the bottom, matching the orientation of the brainstem that is commonly seen in all modern neuroimaging studies. Approximate regions involved in medial and lateral medullary stroke syndromes are shown.

Signs and symptoms: *Structures involved*

1. Medial medullary syndrome (occlusion of vertebral artery or of branch of vertebral or lower basilar artery)
   On side of lesion
   Paralysis with atrophy of one-half half the tongue: *Ipsilateral twelfth nerve*
   On side opposite lesion
   Paralysis of arm and leg, sparing face; impaired tactile and proprioceptive sense over one-half the body: *Contralateral pyramidal tract and medial lemniscus*
2. Lateral medullary syndrome (occlusion of any of five vessels may be responsible—vertebral, posterior inferior cerebellar, superior, middle, or inferior lateral medullary arteries)
   On side of lesion
   Pain, numbness, impaired sensation over one-half the face: *Descending tract and nucleus fifth nerve*
   Ataxia of limbs, falling to side of lesion: *Uncertain—restiform body, cerebellar hemisphere, cerebellar fibers, spinocerebellar tract (?)*
   Nystagmus, diplopia, oscillopsia, vertigo, nausea, vomiting: *Vestibular nucleus*
   Horner's syndrome (miosis, ptosis, decreased sweating): *Descending sympathetic tract*
   Dysphagia, hoarseness, paralysis of palate, paralysis of vocal cord, diminished gag reflex: *Issuing fibers ninth and tenth nerves*
   Loss of taste: *Nucleus and tractus solitarius*
   Numbness of ipsilateral arm, trunk, or leg: *Cuneate and gracile nuclei*
   Weakness of lower face: *Genuflected upper motor neuron fibers to ipsilateral facial nucleus*
   On side opposite lesion
   Impaired pain and thermal sense over half the body, sometimes face: *Spinothalamic tract*
3. Total unilateral medullary syndrome (occlusion of vertebral artery): Combination of medial and lateral syndromes
4. Lateral pontomedullary syndrome (occlusion of vertebral artery): Combination of lateral medullary and lateral inferior pontine syndrome
5. Basilar artery syndrome (the syndrome of the lone vertebral artery is equivalent): A combination of the various brainstem syndromes plus those arising in the posterior cerebral artery distribution.
   Bilateral long tract signs (sensory and motor; cerebellar and peripheral cranial nerve abnormalities): *Bilateral long tract; cerebellar and peripheral cranial nerves*
   Paralysis or weakness of all extremities, plus all bulbar musculature: *Corticobulbar and corticospinal tracts bilaterally*

foramina from C6 to C2. The third (V3) passes through the transverse foramen and circles around the arch of the atlas to pierce the dura at the foramen magnum. The fourth (V4) segment courses upward to join the other vertebral artery to form the basilar artery; only the fourth segment gives rise to branches that supply the brainstem and cerebellum. The posterior inferior cerebellar artery (PICA) in its proximal segment supplies the lateral medulla and, in its distal branches, the inferior surface of the cerebellum.

Atherothrombotic lesions have a predilection for V1 and V4 segments of the vertebral artery. The first segment may become diseased at the origin of the vessel and may produce posterior circulation emboli; collateral flow from the contralateral vertebral artery or the ascending cervical, thyrocervical, or occipital arteries is usually sufficient to prevent low-flow TIAs or stroke. When one vertebral artery is atretic and an atherothrombotic lesion threatens the origin of the other, the collateral circulation, which may also include retrograde flow down the basilar artery, is often insufficient (Figs. 446-4 and 446-9). In this setting, low-flow TIAs may occur, consisting of syncope, vertigo, and alternating hemiplegia; this state also sets the stage for thrombosis. Disease of the distal fourth segment of the vertebral artery can promote thrombus formation manifest as embolism or with propagation as basilar artery thrombosis. Stenosis proximal to the origin of the PICA can threaten the lateral medulla and posterior inferior surface of the cerebellum.

If the subclavian artery is occluded proximal to the origin of the vertebral artery, there is a reversal in the direction of blood flow in the ipsilateral vertebral artery. Exercise of the ipsilateral arm may increase demand on vertebral flow, producing posterior circulation TIAs, or "subclavian steal."

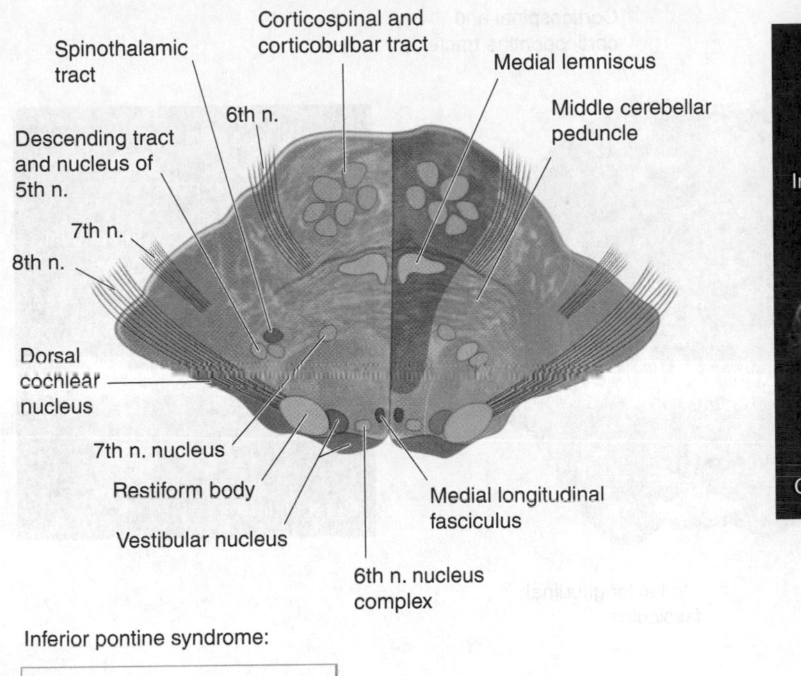

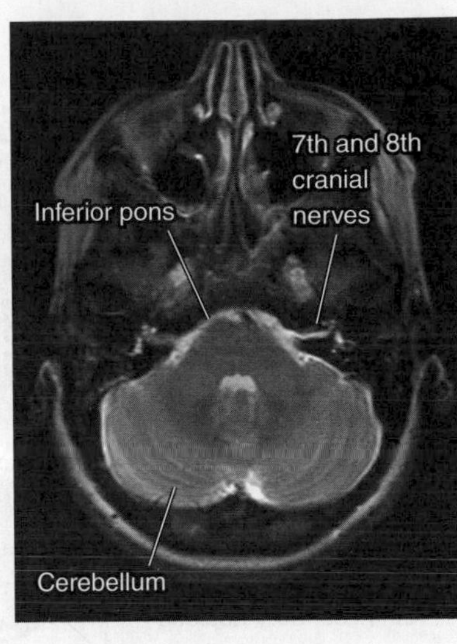

FIGURE 446-11 Axial section at the level of the inferior pons, depicted schematically on the left, with a corresponding magnetic resonance image on the right. Approximate regions involved in medial and lateral inferior pontine stroke syndromes are shown.

Signs and symptoms: *Structures involved*

1. Medial inferior pontine syndrome (occlusion of paramedian branch of basilar artery)
   On side of lesion
   Paralysis of conjugate gaze to side of lesion (preservation of convergence): *Center for conjugate lateral gaze*
   Nystagmus: *Vestibular nucleus*
   Ataxia of limbs and gait: Likely *middle cerebellar peduncle*
   Diplopia on lateral gaze: *Abducens nerve*
   On side opposite lesion
   Paralysis of face, arm, and leg: *Corticobulbar and corticospinal tract in lower pons*
   Impaired tactile and proprioceptive sense over one-half of the body: *Medial lemniscus*
2. Lateral inferior pontine syndrome (occlusion of anterior inferior cerebellar artery)
   On side of lesion
   Horizontal and vertical nystagmus, vertigo, nausea, vomiting, oscillopsia: *Vestibular nerve or nucleus*
   Facial paralysis: *Seventh nerve*
   Paralysis of conjugate gaze to side of lesion: *Center for conjugate lateral gaze*
   Deafness, tinnitus: *Auditory nerve or cochlear nucleus*
   Ataxia: *Middle cerebellar peduncle and cerebellar hemisphere*
   Impaired sensation over face: *Descending tract and nucleus fifth nerve*
   On side opposite lesion
   Impaired pain and thermal sense over one-half the body (may include face): *Spinothalamic tract*

Although atheromatous disease rarely narrows the second and third segments of the vertebral artery, this region is subject to dissection, fibromuscular dysplasia, and, rarely, encroachment by osteophytic spurs within the vertebral foramina.

Embolic occlusion or thrombosis of a V4 segment causes ischemia of the lateral medulla. The constellation of vertigo, numbness of the ipsilateral face and contralateral limbs, diplopia, hoarseness, dysarthria, dysphagia, and ipsilateral Horner's syndrome is called the *lateral medullary (or Wallenberg's) syndrome* (Fig. 446-10). Most cases result from ipsilateral vertebral artery occlusion; in the remainder, PICA occlusion is responsible. Occlusion of the medullary penetrating branches of the vertebral artery or PICA results in partial syndromes. *Hemiparesis is not a feature of vertebral artery occlusion; however, quadriparesis may result from occlusion of the anterior spinal artery.*

Rarely, a *medial medullary syndrome* occurs with infarction of the pyramid and contralateral hemiparesis of the arm and leg, sparing the face. If the medial lemniscus and emerging hypoglossal nerve fibers are involved, contralateral loss of joint position sense and ipsilateral tongue weakness occur.

Cerebellar infarction with edema can lead to *sudden respiratory arrest* due to raised ICP in the posterior fossa. Drowsiness, Babinski signs, dysarthria, and bifacial weakness may be absent, or present only briefly, before respiratory arrest ensues. Gait unsteadiness, headache, dizziness, nausea, and vomiting may be the only early symptoms and signs and should arouse suspicion of this impending complication, which may require neurosurgical decompression, often with an excellent outcome. Separating these symptoms from those of viral labyrinthitis can be a challenge, but headache, neck stiffness, and unilateral dysmetria favor stroke.

BASILAR ARTERY Branches of the basilar artery supply the base of the pons and superior cerebellum and fall into three groups: (1) paramedian, 7–10 in number, which supply a wedge of pons on either side of the midline; (2) short circumferential, 5–7 in number, that supply

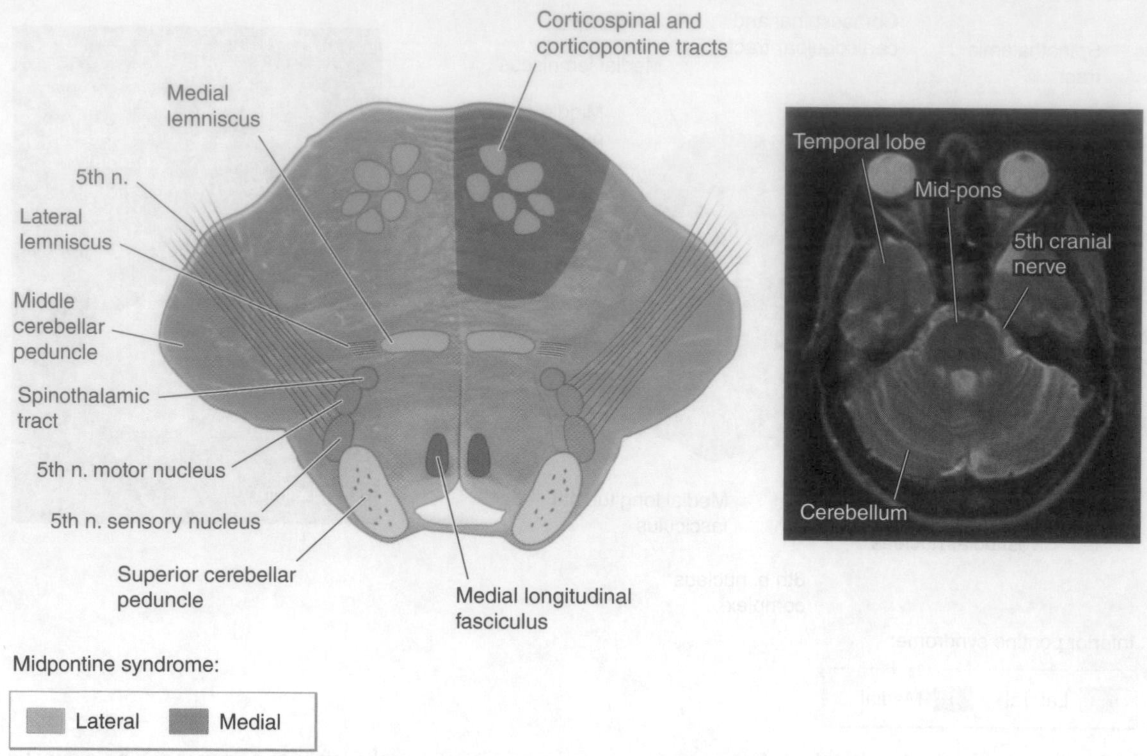

FIGURE 446-12 Axial section at the level of the midpons, depicted schematically on the left, with a corresponding magnetic resonance image on the right. Approximate regions involved in medial and lateral midpontine stroke syndromes are shown.

Signs and symptoms: *Structures involved*

1. Medial midpontine syndrome (paramedian branch of midbasilar artery)
   On side of lesion
   Ataxia of limbs and gait (more prominent in bilateral involvement): *Pontine nuclei*
   On side opposite lesion
   Paralysis of face, arm, and leg: *Corticobulbar and corticospinal tract*
   Variable impaired touch and proprioception when lesion extends posteriorly: *Medial lemniscus*
2. Lateral midpontine syndrome (short circumferential artery)
   On side of lesion
   Ataxia of limbs: *Middle cerebellar peduncle*
   Paralysis of muscles of mastication: *Motor fibers or nucleus of fifth nerve*
   Impaired sensation over side of face: *Sensory fibers or nucleus of fifth nerve*
   On side opposite lesion
   Impaired pain and thermal sense on limbs and trunk: *Spinothalamic tract*

the lateral two-thirds of the pons and middle and superior cerebellar peduncles; and (3) bilateral long circumferential (superior cerebellar and anterior inferior cerebellar arteries), which course around the pons to supply the cerebellar hemispheres.

Atheromatous lesions can occur anywhere along the basilar trunk but are most frequent in the proximal basilar and distal vertebral segments. Typically, lesions occlude either the proximal basilar and one or both vertebral arteries. The clinical picture varies depending on the availability of retrograde collateral flow from the posterior communicating arteries. Rarely, dissection of a vertebral artery may involve the basilar artery and, depending on the location of true and false lumen, may produce multiple penetrating artery strokes.

Although atherothrombosis occasionally occludes the distal portion of the basilar artery, emboli from the heart or proximal vertebral or basilar segments are more commonly responsible for "top of the basilar" syndromes.

Because the brainstem contains many structures in close apposition, a diversity of clinical syndromes may emerge with ischemia, reflecting involvement of the corticospinal and corticobulbar tracts, ascending sensory tracts, and cranial nerve nuclei (Figs. 446-11, 446-12, 446-13, and 446-14).

The symptoms of transient ischemia or infarction in the territory of the basilar artery often do not indicate whether the basilar artery itself or one of its branches is diseased, yet this distinction has important implications for therapy. *The picture of complete basilar occlusion, however, is easy to recognize as a constellation of bilateral long tract signs (sensory and motor) with signs of cranial nerve and cerebellar dysfunction.* A "locked-in" state of preserved consciousness with quadriplegia and cranial nerve signs suggests complete pontine and lower midbrain infarction. The therapeutic goal is to identify *impending* basilar occlusion before devastating infarction occurs. A series of TIAs and a slowly progressive, fluctuating stroke are extremely significant, because they often herald an atherothrombotic occlusion of the distal vertebral or proximal basilar artery.

TIAs in the proximal basilar distribution may produce vertigo (often described by patients as "swimming," "swaying," "moving," "unsteadiness," or "light-headedness"). Other symptoms that warn of basilar thrombosis include diplopia, dysarthria, facial or circumoral numbness, and hemisensory symptoms. In general, symptoms of basilar branch TIAs affect one side of the brainstem, whereas symptoms of basilar artery TIAs usually affect both sides, although a "herald" hemiparesis has been emphasized as an initial symptom of basilar occlusion. Most often, TIAs, whether due to impending occlusion of the basilar artery or a basilar branch, are short lived (5–30 min) and repetitive, occurring several times a day. The pattern suggests intermittent reduction of flow. Many neurologists treat with heparin to prevent clot propagation.

Atherothrombotic occlusion of the basilar artery with infarction usually causes *bilateral* brainstem signs. A gaze paresis or internuclear

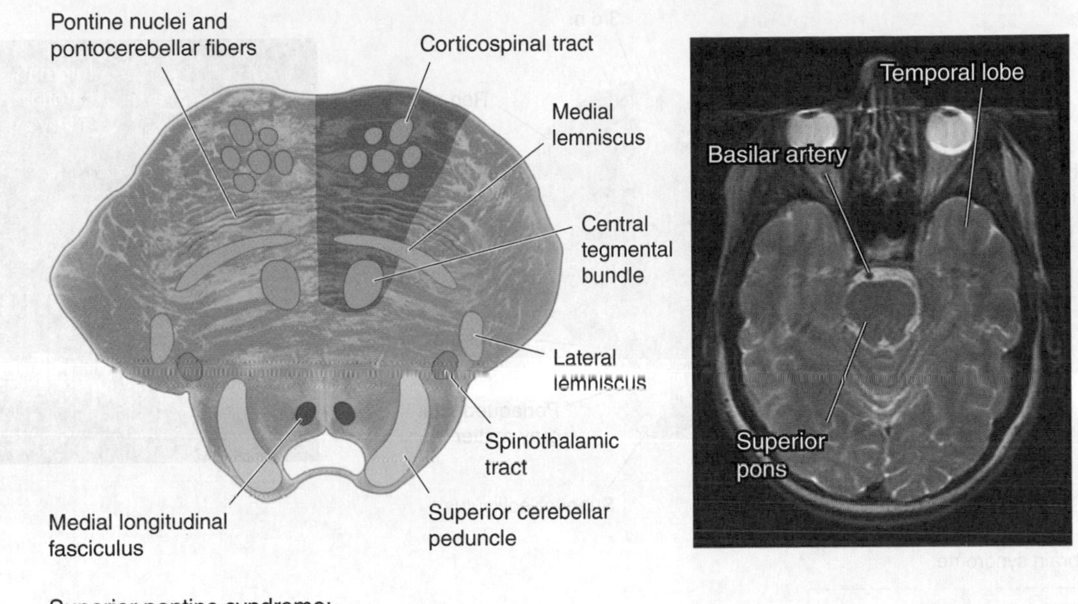

FIGURE 446-13 Axial section at the level of the superior pons, depicted schematically on the left, with a corresponding magnetic resonance image on the right. Approximate regions involved in medial and lateral superior pontine stroke syndromes are shown.

Signs and symptoms: *Structures involved*

1. Medial superior pontine syndrome (paramedian branches of upper basilar artery)
   - On side of lesion
     - Cerebellar ataxia (probably): *Superior and/or middle cerebellar peduncle*
     - Internuclear ophthalmoplegia: *Medial longitudinal fasciculus*
     - Myoclonic syndrome, palate, pharynx, vocal cords, respiratory apparatus, face, oculomotor apparatus, etc.: *Localization uncertain—central tegmental bundle, dentate projection, inferior olivary nucleus*
   - On side opposite lesion
     - Paralysis of face, arm, and leg: *Corticobulbar and corticospinal tract*
     - Rarely touch, vibration, and position are affected: *Medial lemniscus*
2. Lateral superior pontine syndrome (syndrome of superior cerebellar artery)
   - On side of lesion
     - Ataxia of limbs and gait, falling to side of lesion: *Middle and superior cerebellar peduncles, superior surface of cerebellum, dentate nucleus*
     - Dizziness, nausea, vomiting; horizontal nystagmus: *Vestibular nucleus*
     - Paresis of conjugate gaze (ipsilateral): *Pontine contralateral gaze*
     - Skew deviation: *Uncertain*
     - Miosis, ptosis, decreased sweating over face (Horner's syndrome): *Descending sympathetic fibers*
     - Tremor: *Localization unclear—Dentate nucleus, superior cerebellar peduncle*
   - On side opposite lesion
     - Impaired pain and thermal sense on face, limbs, and trunk: *Spinothalamic tract*
     - Impaired touch, vibration, and position sense, more in leg than arm (there is a tendency to incongruity of pain and touch deficits): *Medial lemniscus (lateral portion)*

ophthalmoplegia associated with ipsilateral hemiparesis may be the only manifestation of bilateral brainstem ischemia. More often, unequivocal signs of bilateral pontine disease are present. Complete basilar thrombosis carries a high mortality.

Occlusion of a branch of the basilar artery usually causes *unilateral* symptoms and signs involving motor, sensory, and cranial nerves. As long as symptoms remain unilateral, concern over pending basilar occlusion should be reduced.

Occlusion of the superior cerebellar artery results in severe ipsilateral cerebellar ataxia, nausea and vomiting, dysarthria, and contralateral loss of pain and temperature sensation over the extremities, body, and face (spino- and trigeminothalamic tract). Partial deafness, ataxic tremor of the ipsilateral upper extremity, Horner's syndrome, and palatal myoclonus may occur rarely. Partial syndromes occur frequently (Fig. 446-13). With large strokes, swelling and mass effects may compress the midbrain or produce hydrocephalus; these symptoms may evolve rapidly. Neurosurgical intervention may be lifesaving in such cases.

Occlusion of the anterior inferior cerebellar artery produces variable degrees of infarction because the size of this artery and the territory it supplies vary inversely with those of the PICA. The principal symptoms include: (1) ipsilateral deafness, facial weakness, vertigo, nausea and vomiting, nystagmus, tinnitus, cerebellar ataxia, Horner's syndrome, and paresis of conjugate lateral gaze; and (2) contralateral loss of pain and temperature sensation. An occlusion close to the origin of the artery may cause corticospinal tract signs (Fig. 446-11).

Occlusion of one of the short circumferential branches of the basilar artery affects the lateral two-thirds of the pons and middle or superior cerebellar peduncle, whereas occlusion of one of the paramedian branches affects a wedge-shaped area on either side of the medial pons (Figs. 446-11 through 446-13).

IMAGING STUDIES

See also Chap. 440e.

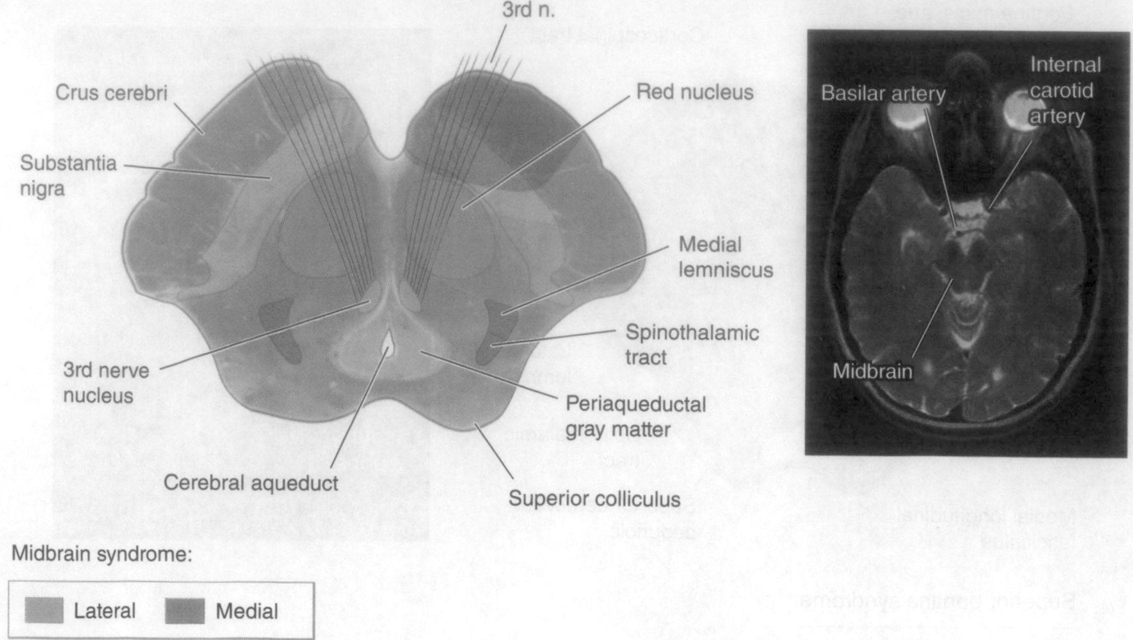

FIGURE 446-14 Axial section at the level of the midbrain, depicted schematically on the left, with a corresponding magnetic resonance image on the right. Approximate regions involved in medial and lateral midbrain stroke syndromes are shown.

Signs and symptoms: *Structures involved*

1. Medial midbrain syndrome (paramedian branches of upper basilar and proximal posterior cerebral arteries)
   On side of lesion
   Eye "down and out" secondary to unopposed action of fourth and sixth cranial nerves, with dilated and unresponsive pupil: *Third nerve fibers*
   On side opposite lesion
   Paralysis of face, arm, and leg: *Corticobulbar and corticospinal tract descending in crus cerebri*
2. Lateral midbrain syndrome (syndrome of small penetrating arteries arising from posterior cerebral artery)
   On side of lesion
   Eye "down and out" secondary to unopposed action of fourth and sixth cranial nerves, with dilated and unresponsive pupil: *Third nerve fibers and/or third nerve nucleus*
   On side opposite lesion
   Hemiataxia, hyperkinesias, tremor: *Red nucleus, dentatorubrothalamic pathway*

CT Scans CT radiographic images identify or exclude hemorrhage as the cause of stroke, and they identify extraparenchymal hemorrhages, neoplasms, abscesses, and other conditions masquerading as stroke. Brain CT scans obtained in the first several hours after an infarction generally show no abnormality, and the infarct may not be seen reliably for 24–48 h. CT may fail to show small ischemic strokes in the posterior fossa because of bone artifact; small infarcts on the cortical surface may also be missed.

Contrast-enhanced CT scans add specificity by showing contrast enhancement of subacute infarcts and allow visualization of venous structures. Coupled with multidetector scanners, CT angiography (CTA) can be performed with administration of IV iodinated contrast allowing visualization of the cervical and intracranial arteries, intracranial veins, aortic arch, and even the coronary arteries in one imaging session. Carotid disease and intracranial vascular occlusions are readily identified with this method (Fig. 446-3). After an IV bolus of contrast, deficits in brain perfusion produced by vascular occlusion can also be demonstrated (Fig. 446-15) and used to predict the region of infarcted brain and the brain at risk of further infarction (i.e., the ischemic penumbra, see "Pathophysiology of Ischemic Stroke" above). CT imaging is also sensitive for detecting SAH (although by itself does not rule it out), and CTA can readily identify intracranial aneurysms (Chap. 330). Because of its speed and wide availability, noncontrast head CT is the imaging modality of choice in patients with acute stroke (Fig. 446-1), and CTA and CT perfusion imaging may also be useful and convenient adjuncts.

MRI

MRI reliably documents the extent and location of infarction in all areas of the brain, including the posterior fossa and cortical surface. It also identifies intracranial hemorrhage and other abnormalities and, using special sequences, can be as sensitive as CT for detecting acute intracerebral hemorrhage. MRI scanners with magnets of higher field strength produce more reliable and precise images. Diffusion-weighted imaging is more sensitive for early brain infarction than standard MR sequences or CT (Fig. 446-16), as is fluid-attenuated inversion recovery (FLAIR) imaging (Chap. 440e). Using IV administration of gadolinium contrast, MR perfusion studies can be performed. Brain regions showing poor perfusion but no abnormality on diffusion provide, compared to CT, an equivalent measure of the ischemic penumbra. MR angiography is highly sensitive for stenosis of extracranial internal carotid arteries and of large intracranial vessels. With higher degrees of stenosis, MR angiography tends to overestimate the degree of stenosis when compared to conventional x-ray angiography. MRI with fat saturation is an imaging sequence used to visualize extra or intracranial arterial dissection. This sensitive technique images clotted blood within the dissected vessel wall. Iron-sensitive imaging (ISI) is helpful to detect cerebral microbleeds that may be present in cerebral amyloid angiopathy and other hemorrhagic disorders.

MRI is more expensive and time consuming than CT and less readily available. Claustrophobia and the logistics of imaging acutely critically ill patients also limit its application. Most acute stroke protocols use CT because of these limitations. However, MRI is useful outside the acute period by more clearly defining the extent of tissue injury and discriminating new from old regions of brain infarction. MRI may have particular utility in patients with TIA, because it is also more likely to identify new infarction, which is a strong predictor of subsequent stroke.

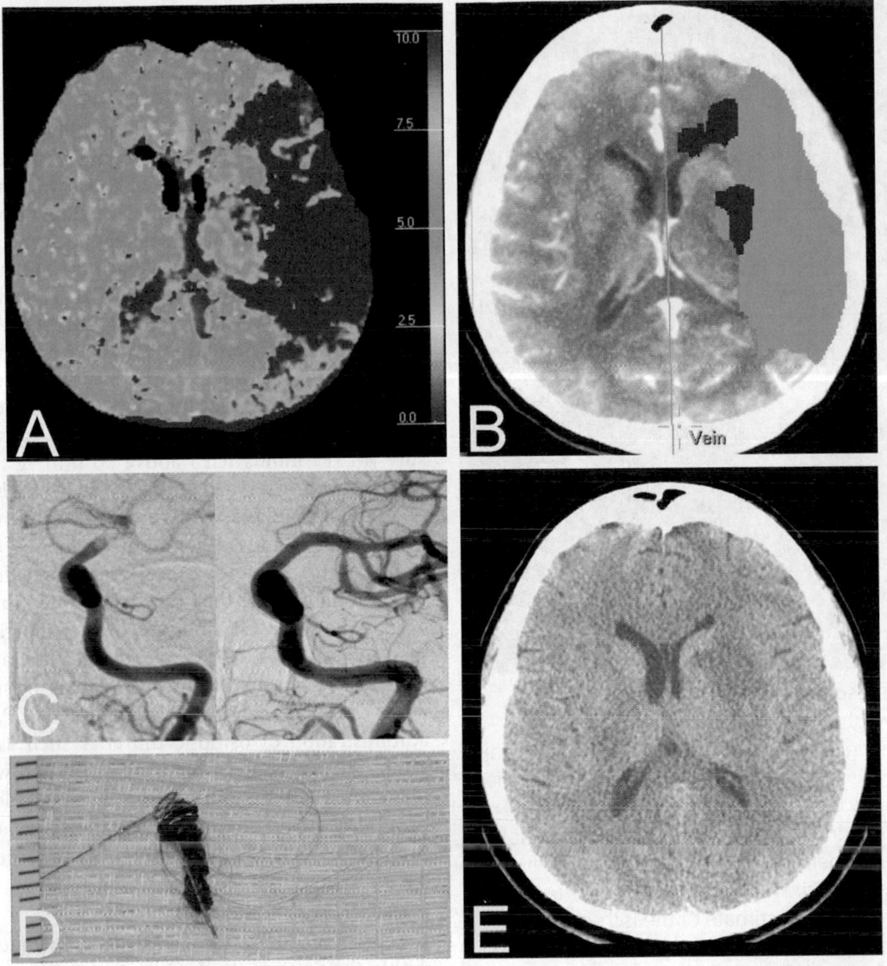

FIGURE 446-15 Acute left middle cerebral artery (MCA) stroke with right hemiplegia but preserved language. ***A.*** Computed tomography (CT) perfusion mean-transit time map showing delayed perfusion of the left MCA distribution (*blue*). ***B.*** Predicted region of infarct (*red*) and penumbra (*green*) based on CT perfusion data. ***C.*** Conventional angiogram showing occlusion of the left internal carotid–MCA bifurcation (*left panel*), and revascularization of the vessels following successful thrombectomy 8 h after stroke symptom onset (*right panel*). ***D.*** The clot removed with a thrombectomy device (L5, Concentric Medical, Inc.). ***E.*** CT scan of the brain 2 days later; note infarction in the region predicted in ***B*** but preservation of the penumbral region by successful revascularization.

Cerebral Angiography Conventional x-ray cerebral angiography is the gold standard for identifying and quantifying atherosclerotic stenoses of the cerebral arteries and for identifying and characterizing other pathologies, including aneurysms, vasospasm, intraluminal thrombi, fibromuscular dysplasia, arteriovenous fistulae, vasculitis, and collateral channels of blood flow. Conventional angiography carries risks of arterial damage, groin hemorrhage, embolic stroke, and renal failure from contrast nephropathy, so it should be reserved for situations where less invasive means are inadequate. As reviewed earlier in this chapter, endovascular stroke therapy has not been proven effective in three randomized trials, and this remains an area of ongoing investigation.

Ultrasound Techniques Stenosis at the origin of the internal carotid artery can be identified and quantified reliably by ultrasonography that combines a B-mode ultrasound image with a Doppler ultrasound assessment of flow velocity ("duplex" ultrasound). Transcranial Doppler (TCD) assessment of MCA, ACA, and PCA flow and of vertebrobasilar flow is also useful. This latter technique can detect stenotic lesions in the large intracranial arteries because such lesions increase systolic flow velocity. TCD can assist thrombolysis and improve large artery recanalization following rtPA administration; the potential clinical benefit of this treatment is the subject of ongoing study. TCD can also detect microemboli from otherwise asymptomatic carotid plaques. In many cases, MR angiography combined with carotid and transcranial ultrasound studies eliminates the need for conventional x-ray angiography in evaluating vascular stenosis. Alternatively, CT angiography of the entire head and neck can be performed during the initial imaging of acute stroke. Because this images the entire arterial system relevant to stroke, with the exception of the heart, much of the clinician's stroke workup can be completed with this single imaging study.

Perfusion Techniques Both xenon techniques (principally xenon-CT) and positron emission tomography (PET) can quantify cerebral blood flow. These tools are generally used for research (Chap. 440e) but can be useful for determining the significance of arterial stenosis and planning for revascularization surgery. Single-photon emission computed tomography (SPECT) and MR perfusion techniques report relative cerebral blood flow. As noted above, CT imaging is used as the initial imaging modality for acute stroke, and some centers combine both CT angiography and CT perfusion imaging together with the noncontrast CT scan. CT perfusion imaging increases the sensitivity for detecting ischemia and can measure the ischemic penumbra (Fig. 446-15). Alternatively, MR perfusion can be combined with MR diffusion imaging to identify the ischemic penumbra as the mismatch between these two imaging sequences (Fig. 446-16).

INTRACRANIAL HEMORRHAGE

Hemorrhages are classified by their location and the underlying vascular pathology. Bleeding into subdural and epidural spaces is

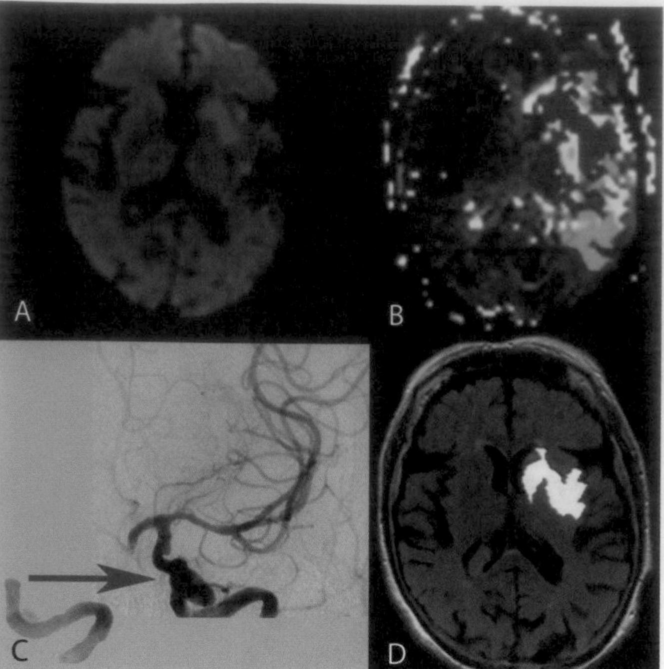

FIGURE 446-16 Magnetic resonance imaging (MRI) of acute stroke. ***A.*** MRI diffusion-weighted image (DWI) of an 82-year-old woman 2.5 h after onset of right-sided weakness and aphasia reveals restricted diffusion within the left basal ganglia and internal capsule (*colored regions*). ***B.*** Perfusion defect within the left hemisphere (*colored signal*) imaged after administration of an IV bolus of gadolinium contrast. The discrepancy between the region of poor perfusion shown in ***B*** and the diffusion deficit shown in ***A*** is called *diffusion-perfusion mismatch* and provides an estimate of the ischemic penumbra. Without specific therapy, the region of infarction will expand into much or all of the perfusion deficit. ***C.*** Cerebral angiogram of the left internal carotid artery in this patient before (*left*) and after (*right*) successful endovascular embolectomy. The occlusion is within the carotid terminus. ***D.*** Fluid-attenuated inversion recovery image obtained 3 days later showing a region of infarction (*coded as white*) that corresponds to the initial DWI image in ***A***, but not the entire area at risk shown in ***B***, suggesting that successful embolectomy saved a large region of brain tissue from infarction. *(Courtesy of Gregory Albers, MD, Stanford University; with permission.)*

principally produced by trauma. SAH results from trauma or the rupture of an intracranial aneurysm or arteriovenous malformation (AVM) (Chap. 330). Intracerebral and intraventricular hemorrhage will be considered here.

DIAGNOSIS

Intracranial hemorrhage is often discovered on noncontrast CT imaging of the brain during the acute evaluation of stroke. Because CT is more widely available and may be logistically easier, CT imaging is the preferred method for acute stroke evaluation (Fig. 446-1). The location of the hemorrhage narrows the differential diagnosis to a few entities. Table 446-6 lists the causes and anatomic spaces involved in hemorrhages.

EMERGENCY MANAGEMENT

Close attention should be paid to airway management because a reduction in the level of consciousness is common and often progressive. The initial blood pressure should be maintained until the results of the CT scan are reviewed and demonstrate an intracerebral hemorrhage (ICH). In theory, a higher blood pressure should promote hematoma expansion, but it remains unclear if lowering of blood pressure reduces hematoma growth. Recent clinical trials have shown that systolic blood pressure (SBP) can be safely lowered acutely and rapidly to <140 mmHg in patients with spontaneous ICH whose initial SBP was 150–220 mmHg. The INTERACT2 trial is the only large phase 3 clinical trial to address the effect of acute blood pressure lowering on ICH functional outcome. INTERACT2 randomized patients with spontaneous ICH within 6 h of onset and a baseline SBP of 150–220 mmHg to two different SBP targets (<140 mmHg and <180 mmHg). In those with the target SBP <140 mmHg, 52% had an outcome of death or major disability at 90 days compared with 55.6% of those with a target SBP <180 mmHg (p = .06). There was a significant shift to improved outcomes in the lower blood pressure arm, whereas both groups had a similar mortality. This study shows that it is not harmful, and may be modestly beneficial, to lower blood pressure in acute ICH. Thus, it is reasonable to target an SBP <140 mmHg initially in this group of patients. In patients who have higher SBP on presentation or who are deeply comatose with possible elevated ICP, it is unclear whether the INTERACT2 results apply. In patients who have ICP monitors in place, current recommendations are to maintain the cerebral perfusion pressure (mean arterial pressure [MAP] minus ICP) above 60 mmHg. Blood pressure should be lowered with nonvasodilating IV drugs such as nicardipine, labetalol, or esmolol. Patients with cerebellar hemorrhages or with depressed mental status and radiographic evidence of hydrocephalus should undergo urgent neurosurgical evaluation; these patients require close monitoring because they can deteriorate rapidly. Based on the clinical examination and CT findings, further imaging studies may be necessary, including MRI or conventional x-ray angiography. Stuporous or comatose patients with clinical and imaging signs of herniation are generally treated presumptively for elevated ICP, with tracheal intubation, administration of osmotic diuretics such as mannitol or hypertonic saline, and elevation of the head of the bed while surgical consultation is obtained (Chap. 330). Reversal of coagulopathy and consideration of surgical evacuation of the hematoma (detailed below) are two other principal aspects of initial emergency management.

INTRACEREBRAL HEMORRHAGE

ICH accounts for ~10% of all strokes, and about 35–45% of patients die within the first month. Incidence rates are particularly high in Asians and blacks. Hypertension, coagulopathy, sympathomimetic drugs (cocaine, methamphetamine), and cerebral amyloid angiopathy cause the majority of these hemorrhages. Advanced age and heavy alcohol consumption increase the risk, and cocaine and methamphetamine use is one of the most important causes in the young.

Hypertensive Intracerebral Hemorrhage • *PATHOPHYSIOLOGY* Hypertensive ICH usually results from spontaneous rupture of a small penetrating artery deep in the brain. The most common sites are the basal ganglia (especially the putamen), thalamus, cerebellum, and pons. The small arteries in these areas seem most prone to hypertension-induced vascular injury. When hemorrhages occur in other brain areas or in nonhypertensive patients, greater consideration should be given to other causes such as hemorrhagic disorders, neoplasms, vascular malformations, and cerebral amyloid angiopathy. The hemorrhage may be small, or a large clot may form and compress adjacent tissue, causing herniation and death. Blood may also dissect into the ventricular space, which substantially increases morbidity and may cause hydrocephalus.

Most hypertensive ICHs initially develop over 30–90 min, whereas those associated with anticoagulant therapy may evolve for as long as 24–48 h. However, it is now recognized that about a third of patients even with no coagulopathy may have significant hematoma expansion with the first day. Within 48 h, macrophages begin to phagocytize the hemorrhage at its outer surface. After 1–6 months, the hemorrhage is generally resolved to a slitlike orange cavity lined with glial scar and hemosiderin-laden macrophages.

CLINICAL MANIFESTATIONS ICH generally presents as the abrupt onset of a focal neurologic deficit. Seizures are uncommon. Although clinical symptoms may be maximal at onset, commonly the focal deficit worsens over 30–90 min and is associated with a diminishing level of consciousness and signs of increased ICP such as headache and vomiting.

The putamen is the most common site for hypertensive hemorrhage, and the adjacent internal capsule is usually damaged (Fig. 446-17). Contralateral hemiparesis is therefore the sentinel sign.

TABLE 446-6 CAUSES OF INTRACRANIAL HEMORRHAGE

Cause	Location	Comments
Head trauma	Intraparenchymal: frontal lobes, anterior temporal lobes; subarachnoid; extra-axial (subdural, epidural)	Coup and contrecoup injury during brain deceleration
Hypertensive hemorrhage	Putamen, globus pallidus, thalamus, cerebellar hemisphere, pons	Chronic hypertension produces hemorrhage from small (~30–100 μm) vessels in these regions
Transformation of prior ischemic infarction	Basal ganglion, subcortical regions, lobar	Occurs in 1–6% of ischemic strokes with predilection for large hemispheric infarctions
Metastatic brain tumor	Lobar	Lung, choriocarcinoma, melanoma, renal cell carcinoma, thyroid, atrial myxoma
Coagulopathy	Any	Risk for ongoing hematoma expansion
Drug	Any, lobar, subarachnoid	Cocaine, amphetamine
Arteriovenous malformation	Lobar, intraventricular, subarachnoid	Risk is ~2–3% per year for bleeding If previously unruptured
Aneurysm	Subarachnoid, intraparenchymal, rarely subdural	Mycotic and nonmycotic forms of aneurysms
Amyloid angiopathy	Lobar	Degenerative disease of intracranial vessels; associated with dementia, rare in patients <60 years
Cavernous angioma	Intraparenchymal	Multiple cavernous angiomas linked to mutations in *KRIT1*, *CCM2*, and *PDCD10* genes
Dural arteriovenous fistula	Lobar, subarachnoid	Produces bleeding by venous hypertension
Capillary telangiectasias	Usually brainstem	Rare cause of hemorrhage

When mild, the face sags on one side over 5–30 min, speech becomes slurred, the arm and leg gradually weaken, and the eyes deviate away from the side of the hemiparesis. The paralysis may worsen until the affected limbs become flaccid or extend rigidly. When hemorrhages are large, drowsiness gives way to stupor as signs of upper brainstem compression appear. Coma ensues, accompanied by deep, irregular, or intermittent respiration, a dilated and fixed ipsilateral pupil, and decerebrate rigidity. In milder cases, edema in adjacent brain tissue may cause progressive deterioration over 12–72 h.

Thalamic hemorrhages also produce a contralateral hemiplegia or hemiparesis from pressure on, or dissection into, the adjacent internal capsule. A prominent sensory deficit involving all modalities is usually present. Aphasia, often with preserved verbal repetition, may occur after hemorrhage into the dominant thalamus, and constructional apraxia or mutism occurs in some cases of nondominant hemorrhage. There may also be a homonymous visual field defect. Thalamic hemorrhages cause several typical ocular disturbances by virtue of extension inferiorly into the upper midbrain. These include deviation of the eyes downward and inward so that they appear to be looking at the nose, unequal pupils with absence of light reaction, skew deviation with the eye opposite the hemorrhage displaced downward and medially, ipsilateral Horner's syndrome, absence of convergence, paralysis of vertical gaze, and retraction nystagmus. Patients may later develop a chronic, contralateral pain syndrome (Déjérine-Roussy syndrome).

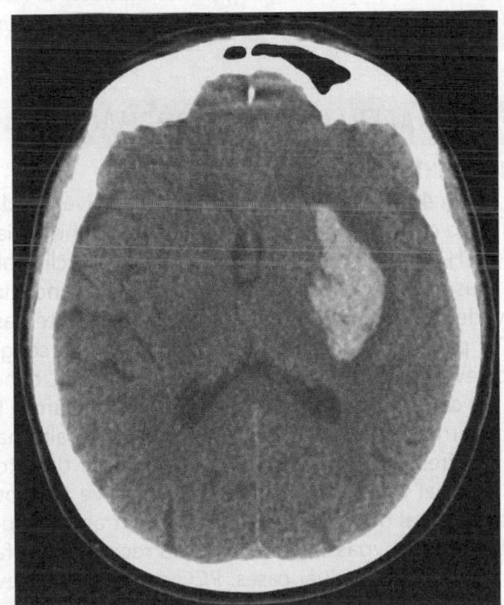

FIGURE 446-17 Hypertensive hemorrhage. Transaxial noncontrast computed tomography scan through the region of the basal ganglia reveals a hematoma involving the left putamen in a patient with rapidly progressive onset of right hemiparesis.

In pontine hemorrhages, deep coma with quadriplegia often occurs over a few minutes. Typically, there is prominent decerebrate rigidity and "pinpoint" (1 mm) pupils that react to light. There is impairment of reflex horizontal eye movements evoked by head turning (doll's-head or oculocephalic maneuver) or by irrigation of the ears with ice water (Chap. 328). Hyperpnea, severe hypertension, and hyperhidrosis are common. Most patients with deep coma from pontine hemorrhage ultimately die, but small hemorrhages are compatible with survival.

Cerebellar hemorrhages usually develop over several hours and are characterized by occipital headache, repeated vomiting, and ataxia of gait. In mild cases, there may be no other neurologic signs except for gait ataxia. Dizziness or vertigo may be prominent. There is often paresis of conjugate lateral gaze toward the side of the hemorrhage, forced deviation of the eyes to the opposite side, or an ipsilateral sixth nerve palsy. Less frequent ocular signs include blepharospasm, involuntary closure of one eye, ocular bobbing, and skew deviation. Dysarthria and dysphagia may occur. As the hours pass, the patient often becomes stuporous and then comatose from brainstem compression or obstructive hydrocephalus; immediate surgical evacuation before brainstem compression occurs may be lifesaving. Hydrocephalus from fourth ventricle compression can be relieved by external ventricular drainage, but definitive hematoma evacuation is recommended. If the deep cerebellar nuclei are spared, full recovery is common.

Lobar Hemorrhage The major neurologic deficit with an occipital hemorrhage is hemianopia; with a left temporal hemorrhage, aphasia and delirium; with a parietal hemorrhage, hemisensory loss; and with frontal hemorrhage, arm weakness. Large hemorrhages may be associated with stupor or coma if they compress the thalamus or midbrain. Most patients with lobar hemorrhages have focal headaches, and more than one-half vomit or are drowsy. Stiff neck and seizures are uncommon.

Other Causes of Intracerebral Hemorrhage *Cerebral amyloid angiopathy* is a disease of the elderly in which arteriolar degeneration occurs and amyloid is deposited in the walls of the cerebral arteries. Amyloid angiopathy causes both single and recurrent lobar hemorrhages and is probably the most common cause of lobar hemorrhage in the elderly.

It accounts for some intracranial hemorrhages associated with IV thrombolysis given for MI. This disorder can be suspected in patients who present with multiple hemorrhages (and infarcts) over several months or years or in patients with "microbleeds" seen on brain MRI sequences sensitive for hemosiderin (iron-sensitive imaging), but it is definitively diagnosed by pathologic demonstration of Congo red staining of amyloid in cerebral vessels. The ε2 and ε4 allelic variations of the apolipoprotein E gene are associated with increased risk of recurrent lobar hemorrhage and may therefore be markers of amyloid angiopathy. Currently, there is no specific therapy. OACs are typically avoided.

Cocaine and *methamphetamine* are frequent causes of stroke in young (age <45 years) patients. ICH, ischemic stroke, and SAH are all associated with stimulant use. Angiographic findings vary from completely normal arteries to large-vessel occlusion or stenosis, vasospasm, or changes consistent with vasculopathy. The mechanism of sympathomimetic-related stroke is not known, but cocaine enhances sympathetic activity causing acute, sometimes severe, hypertension, and this may lead to hemorrhage. Slightly more than one-half of stimulant-related intracranial hemorrhages are intracerebral, and the rest are subarachnoid. In cases of SAH, a saccular aneurysm is usually identified. Presumably, acute hypertension causes aneurysmal rupture.

Head injury often causes intracranial bleeding. The common sites are intraparenchymal (especially temporal and inferior frontal lobes) and into the subarachnoid, subdural, and epidural spaces. Trauma must be considered in any patient with an unexplained acute neurologic deficit (hemiparesis, stupor, or confusion), particularly if the deficit occurred in the context of a fall (Chap. 457e).

Intracranial hemorrhages associated with *anticoagulant therapy* can occur at any location; they are often lobar or subdural. Anticoagulant-related ICHs may continue to evolve over 24–48 h, especially if coagulopathy is insufficiently reversed. Coagulopathy and thrombocytopenia should be reversed rapidly, as discussed below. ICH associated with *hematologic disorders* (leukemia, aplastic anemia, thrombocytopenic purpura) can occur at any site and may present as multiple ICHs. Skin and mucous membrane bleeding may be evident and offers a diagnostic clue.

Hemorrhage into a *brain tumor* may be the first manifestation of neoplasm. Choriocarcinoma, malignant melanoma, renal cell carcinoma, and bronchogenic carcinoma are among the most common metastatic tumors associated with ICH. Glioblastoma multiforme in adults and medulloblastoma in children may also have areas of ICH.

Hypertensive encephalopathy is a complication of malignant hypertension. In this acute syndrome, severe hypertension is associated with headache, nausea, vomiting, convulsions, confusion, stupor, and coma. Focal or lateralizing neurologic signs, either transitory or permanent, may occur but are infrequent and therefore suggest some other vascular disease (hemorrhage, embolism, or atherosclerotic thrombosis). There are retinal hemorrhages, exudates, papilledema (hypertensive retinopathy), and evidence of renal and cardiac disease. In most cases, ICP and CSF protein levels are elevated. MRI brain imaging shows a pattern of typically posterior (occipital > frontal) brain edema that is reversible and termed *reversible posterior leukoencephalopathy*. The hypertension may be essential or due to chronic renal disease, acute glomerulonephritis, acute toxemia of pregnancy, pheochromocytoma, or other causes. Lowering the blood pressure reverses the process, but stroke can occur, especially if blood pressure is lowered too rapidly. Neuropathologic examination reveals multifocal to diffuse cerebral edema and hemorrhages of various sizes from petechial to massive. Microscopically, there are necrosis of arterioles, minute cerebral infarcts, and hemorrhages. The term *hypertensive encephalopathy* should be reserved for this syndrome and not for chronic recurrent headaches, dizziness, recurrent TIAs, or small strokes that often occur in association with high blood pressure.

Primary intraventricular hemorrhage is rare and should prompt investigation for an underlying vascular anomaly. Sometimes bleeding begins within the periventricular substance of the brain and dissects into the ventricular system without leaving signs of intraparenchymal hemorrhage. Alternatively, bleeding can arise from periependymal veins. Vasculitis, usually polyarteritis nodosa or lupus erythematosus, can produce hemorrhage in any region of the central nervous system; most hemorrhages are associated with hypertension, but the arteritis itself may cause bleeding by disrupting the vessel wall. Nearly one-half of patients with primary intraventricular hemorrhage have identifiable bleeding sources seen using conventional angiography.

Sepsis can cause small petechial hemorrhages throughout the cerebral white matter. *Moyamoya disease*, mainly an occlusive arterial disease that causes ischemic symptoms, may on occasion produce ICH, particularly in the young. Hemorrhages into the spinal cord are usually the result of an AVM, cavernous malformation, or metastatic tumor. *Epidural spinal hemorrhage* produces a rapidly evolving syndrome of spinal cord or nerve root compression (Chap. 456). Spinal hemorrhages usually present with sudden back pain and some manifestation of myelopathy.

Laboratory and Imaging Evaluation Patients should have routine blood chemistries and hematologic studies. Specific attention to the platelet count and PT/PTT/INR is important to identify coagulopathy. CT imaging reliably detects acute focal hemorrhages in the supratentorial space. Rarely very small pontine or medullary hemorrhages may not be well delineated because of motion and bone-induced artifact that obscure structures in the posterior fossa. After the first 2 weeks, x-ray attenuation values of clotted blood diminish until they become isodense with surrounding brain. Mass effect and edema may remain. In some cases, a surrounding rim of contrast enhancement appears after 2–4 weeks and may persist for months. MRI, although more sensitive for delineating posterior fossa lesions, is generally not necessary for primary diagnosis in most instances. Images of flowing blood on MRI scan may identify AVMs as the cause of the hemorrhage. MRI, CT angiography (CTA), and conventional x-ray angiography are used when the cause of intracranial hemorrhage is uncertain, particularly if the patient is young or not hypertensive and the hematoma is not in one of the usual sites for hypertensive hemorrhage. CTA or postcontrast CT imaging may reveal one or more small areas of enhancement within a hematoma; this "spot sign" is thought to represent ongoing bleeding. The presence of a spot sign is associated with an increased risk of hematoma expansion, increased mortality, and lower likelihood of favorable functional outcome. Some centers routinely perform CT with CTA and postcontrast CT at the time of initial imaging to rapidly identify any macrovascular etiology of the hemorrhage and provide prognostic information at the same time. Because patients typically have focal neurologic signs and obtundation and often show signs of increased ICP, a lumbar puncture is generally unnecessary and should usually be avoided because it may induce cerebral herniation.

TREATMENT INTRACEREBRAL HEMORRHAGE

ACUTE MANAGEMENT

Although about 40% of patients with a hypertensive ICH die, others have a good to complete recovery if they survive the initial hemorrhage. The ICH Score (Table 446-7) is a validated clinical grading scale that is useful for stratification of mortality risk and clinical outcome. Any identified coagulopathy should be corrected as soon as possible. For patients taking VKAs, rapid correction of coagulopathy can be achieved by infusing prothrombin complex concentrates (PCC), which can be administered quickly, with vitamin K administered concurrently. Fresh frozen plasma is an alternative but generally requires larger fluid volumes and longer time to achieve adequate reversal than PCC. There is no effective antidote to ICH associated with oral thrombin inhibitor dabigatran, although FEIBA (factor VIII inhibitor bypassing activity) and recombinant factor VIIa have been tried in individual cases. PCC may partially reverse the effects of oral factor Xa inhibitors and are reasonable to administer if available. When ICH is associated with thrombocytopenia (platelet count <50,000/μL), transfusion of fresh platelets is indicated. The role of platelet transfusions either empirically or based on urgent platelet inhibition assays remains unclear.

TABLE 446-7 THE ICH SCORE

Clinical or Imaging Factor	Point Score
Age	
<80 years	0
≥80 years	1
Hematoma Volume	
<30 cc	0
≥30 cc	1
Intraventricular Hemorrhage Present	
No	0
Yes	1
Infratentorial Origin of Hemorrhage	
No	0
Yes	1
Glasgow Coma Scale Score	
13–15	0
5–12	1
3–4	2
Total Score	Sum of each category above

ICH Score Total	% Mortality at 30 Days (95% CI)	% Walk Independently at 12 Months (95% CI)
0	0 (0–13)	70 (53–84)
1	13 (4–29)	60 (47–73)
2	26 (11–46)	33 (21–48)
3	72 (53–86)	13 (5–25)
4	97 (82–100)	3 (0–16)
5	100 (54–100)	8 (0–38)

Note: Although an ICH Score of 6 is possible with the scale, this is rarely observed and is considered highly likely to be fatal.

Abbreviations: CI, confidence interval; ICH, intracerebral hemorrhage.

Sources: JC Hemphill et al: Stroke 32:891, 2001; JC Hemphill et al: Neurology 73:1088, 2009.

Hematomas may expand for several hours following the initial hemorrhage, even in patients without coagulopathy. However, the precise mechanism is unclear. A phase 3 trial of treatment with recombinant factor VIIa reduced hematoma expansion; however, clinical outcomes were not improved, so use of this drug cannot be advocated at present. The theoretical risk of acutely elevated blood pressure on hematoma expansion forms the basis of the consideration for recently completed and ongoing clinical trials of acute blood pressure lowering.

Evacuation of supratentorial hematomas does not appear to improve outcome for most patients. The International Surgical Trial in Intracerebral Haemorrhage (STICH) randomized patients with supratentorial ICH to either early surgical evacuation or initial medical management. No benefit was found in the early surgery arm, although analysis was complicated by the fact that 26% of patients in the initial medical management group ultimately had surgery for neurologic deterioration. The follow-up study STICH-II found that surgery within 24 h of lobar, supratentorial hemorrhage did not improve overall outcome, but might have a role in select severely affected patients. Therefore, existing data do not support routine surgical evacuation of supratentorial hemorrhages in stable patients. However, many centers still consider surgery for patients deemed salvageable and who are having progressive neurologic deterioration due to herniation. Surgical techniques continue to evolve, and minimally invasive endoscopic hematoma evacuation is currently being investigated in clinical trials.

For cerebellar hemorrhages, a neurosurgeon should be consulted immediately to assist with the evaluation; most cerebellar hematomas >3 cm in diameter will require surgical evacuation. If the patient is alert without focal brainstem signs and if the hematoma is <1 cm in diameter, surgical removal is usually unnecessary. Patients with hematomas between 1 and 3 cm require careful observation for signs of impaired consciousness, progressive hydrocephalus, and precipitous respiratory failure. Hydrocephalus due to cerebellar hematoma should not be treated solely with ventricular drainage.

Tissue surrounding hematomas is displaced and compressed but not necessarily infarcted. Hence, in survivors, major improvement commonly occurs as the hematoma is reabsorbed and the adjacent tissue regains its function. Careful management of the patient during the acute phase of the hemorrhage can lead to considerable recovery.

Surprisingly, ICP is often normal even with large ICHs. However, if the hematoma causes marked midline shift of structures with consequent obtundation, coma, or hydrocephalus, osmotic agents can be instituted in preparation for placement of a ventriculostomy or parenchymal ICP monitor (**Chap. 330**). Once ICP is recorded, CSF drainage (if available), osmotic therapy, and blood pressure management can be tailored to the individual patient to keep cerebral perfusion pressure (MAP minus ICP) above 60 mmHg. For example, if ICP is found to be high, CSF can be drained from the ventricular space and osmotic therapy continued; persistent or progressive elevation in ICP may prompt surgical evacuation of the clot. Alternately, if ICP is normal or only mildly elevated, interventions such as osmotic therapy may be tapered. Because hyperventilation may actually produce ischemia by cerebral vasoconstriction, induced hyperventilation should be limited to acute resuscitation of the patient with presumptive high ICP and eliminated once other treatments (osmotic therapy or surgical treatments) have been instituted. Glucocorticoids are not helpful for the edema from intracerebral hematoma.

PREVENTION

Hypertension is the leading cause of primary ICH. Prevention is aimed at reducing chronic hypertension, eliminating excessive alcohol use, and discontinuing use of illicit drugs such as cocaine and amphetamines. Patients with amyloid angiopathy should generally avoid OACs, but antiplatelet agents may be administered if there is an indication based on atherothrombotic vascular disease.

VASCULAR ANOMALIES

Vascular anomalies can be divided into congenital vascular malformations and acquired vascular lesions.

CONGENITAL VASCULAR MALFORMATIONS

True *arteriovenous malformations* (AVMs), venous anomalies, and capillary telangiectasias are lesions that usually remain clinically silent through life. AVMs are probably congenital, but cases of acquired lesions have been reported.

True AVMs are congenital shunts between the arterial and venous systems that may present with headache, seizures, and intracranial hemorrhage. AVMs consist of a tangle of abnormal vessels across the cortical surface or deep within the brain substance. AVMs vary in size from a small blemish a few millimeters in diameter to a large mass of tortuous channels composing an arteriovenous shunt of sufficient magnitude to raise cardiac output and precipitate heart failure. Blood vessels forming the tangle interposed between arteries and veins are usually abnormally thin and histologically resemble both arteries and veins. AVMs occur in all parts of the cerebral hemispheres, brainstem, and spinal cord, but the largest ones are most frequently in the posterior half of the hemispheres, commonly forming a wedge-shaped lesion extending from the cortex to the ventricle.

Bleeding, headache, and seizures are most common between the ages of 10 and 30, occasionally as late as the fifties. AVMs are more frequent in men, and rare familial cases have been described. Familial AVM may be a part of the autosomal dominant syndrome of hereditary hemorrhagic telangiectasia (Osler-Rendu-Weber) syndrome due to mutations in either endoglin or activin receptor-like kinase 1, both involved in transforming growth factor (TGF) signaling and angiogenesis.

Headache (without bleeding) may be hemicranial and throbbing, like migraine, or diffuse. Focal seizures, with or without generalization, occur in ~30% of cases. One-half of AVMs become evident as ICHs. In most, the hemorrhage is mainly intraparenchymal with extension into the subarachnoid space in some cases. Blood is usually not deposited in the basal cisterns, and symptomatic cerebral vasospasm is rare. The risk of AVM rupture is strongly influenced by a history of prior rupture. Although unruptured AVMs have a hemorrhage rate of ~2–4% per year, previously ruptured AVMs may have a rate as high as 17% a year, at least for the first year. Hemorrhages may be massive, leading to death, or may be as small as 1 cm in diameter, leading to minor focal symptoms or no deficit. The AVM may be large enough to steal blood away from adjacent normal brain tissue or to increase venous pressure significantly to produce venous ischemia locally and in remote areas of the brain. This is seen most often with large AVMs in the territory of the MCA.

Large AVMs of the anterior circulation may be associated with a systolic and diastolic bruit (sometimes self-audible) over the eye, forehead, or neck and a bounding carotid pulse. Headache at the onset of AVM rupture is generally not as explosive as with aneurysmal rupture. MRI is better than CT for diagnosis, although noncontrast CT scanning sometimes detects calcification of the AVM and contrast may demonstrate the abnormal blood vessels. Once identified, conventional x-ray angiography is the gold standard for evaluating the precise anatomy of the AVM.

Surgical treatment of AVMs presenting with hemorrhage often done in conjunction with preoperative embolization to reduce operative bleeding is usually indicated for accessible lesions. Stereotaxic radiation, an alternative to surgery, can produce a slow sclerosis of the AVM over 2–3 years.

Several angiographic features can be used to help predict future bleeding risk. Paradoxically, smaller lesions seem to have a higher hemorrhage rate. The presence of deep venous drainage, venous outflow stenosis, and intranidal aneurysms may increase rupture risk. Because of the relatively low annual rate of hemorrhage and the risk of complications due to surgical or endovascular treatment, the indication for surgery in asymptomatic AVMs is debated. The ARUBA (A Randomized Trial of Unruptured Brain Arteriovenous Malformations) trial randomized patients to medical management versus intervention (surgery, endovascular embolization, combination embolization and surgery, or gamma-knife). The trial was stopped prematurely for harm, with the medical arm achieving the combined endpoint of death or symptomatic stroke in 10.1% of patients compared to 30.7% in the intervention group at an average follow-up time of 33 months. This highly significant finding argues against routine intervention for patients presenting without hemorrhage, although debate ensues regarding the generalizability of these results.

Venous anomalies are the result of development of anomalous cerebral, cerebellar, or brainstem venous drainage. These structures, unlike AVMs, are functional venous channels. They are of little clinical significance and should be ignored if found incidentally on brain imaging studies. Surgical resection of these anomalies may result in venous infarction and hemorrhage. Venous anomalies may be associated with cavernous malformations (see below), which do carry some bleeding risk.

Capillary telangiectasias are true capillary malformations that often form extensive vascular networks through an otherwise normal brain structure. The pons and deep cerebral white matter are typical locations, and these capillary malformations can be seen in patients with hereditary hemorrhagic telangiectasia (Osler-Rendu-Weber) syndrome. If bleeding does occur, it rarely produces mass effect or significant symptoms. No treatment options exist.

ACQUIRED VASCULAR LESIONS

Cavernous angiomas are tufts of capillary sinusoids that form within the deep hemispheric white matter and brainstem with no normal intervening neural structures. The pathogenesis is unclear. Familial cavernous angiomas have been mapped to several different genes: *KRIT1*, *CCM2*, and *PDCD10*. Both *KRIT1* and *CCM2* have roles in blood vessel formation, whereas *PDCD10* is an apoptotic gene. Cavernous angiomas are typically <1 cm in diameter and are often associated with a venous anomaly. Bleeding is usually of small volume, causing slight mass effect only. The bleeding risk for single cavernous malformations is 0.7–1.5% per year and may be higher for patients with prior clinical hemorrhage or multiple malformations. Seizures may occur if the malformation is located near the cerebral cortex. Surgical resection eliminates bleeding risk and may reduce seizure risk, but it is usually reserved for those malformations that form near the brain surface. Radiation treatment has not been shown to be of benefit.

Dural arteriovenous fistulas are acquired connections usually from a dural artery to a dural sinus. Patients may complain of a pulse-synchronous cephalic bruit ("pulsatile tinnitus") and headache. Depending on the magnitude of the shunt, venous pressures may rise high enough to cause cortical ischemia or venous hypertension and hemorrhage, particularly SAH. Surgical and endovascular techniques are usually curative. These fistulas may form because of trauma, but most are idiopathic. There is an association between fistulas and dural sinus thrombosis. Fistulas have been observed to appear months to years following venous sinus thrombosis, suggesting that angiogenesis factors elaborated from the thrombotic process may cause these anomalous connections to form. Alternatively, dural arteriovenous fistulas can produce venous sinus occlusion over time, perhaps from the high pressure and high flow through a venous structure.

447 Migraine and Other Primary Headache Disorders

Peter J. Goadsby, Neil H. Raskin

The general principles around headache as a cardinal symptom are covered elsewhere (Chap. 21); here we discuss disorders in which headache and associated features occur in the absence of any exogenous cause. The most common are migraine, tension-type headache, and the trigeminal autonomic cephalalgias, notably cluster headache; the complete list is summarized in Table 447-1.

MIGRAINE

Migraine, the second most common cause of headache, and the most common headache-related, and indeed neurologic, cause of disability in the world, afflicts approximately 15% of women and 6% of men over a 1-year period. It is usually an episodic headache associated with certain features such as sensitivity to light, sound, or movement; nausea and vomiting often accompany the headache. A useful description of migraine is a recurring syndrome of headache associated with other symptoms of neurologic dysfunction in varying admixtures (Table 447-2). Migraine can often be recognized by its activators, referred to as *triggers*.

The brain of the migraineur is particularly sensitive to environmental and sensory stimuli; migraine-prone patients do not habituate easily to sensory stimuli. This sensitivity is amplified in females during the menstrual cycle. Headache can be initiated or amplified by various triggers, including glare, bright lights, sounds, or other afferent stimulation; hunger; let-down from stress; physical exertion; stormy weather or barometric pressure changes; hormonal fluctuations during menses; lack of or excess sleep; and alcohol or other chemical stimulation, such as with nitrates. Knowledge of a patient's susceptibility to specific triggers can be useful in management strategies involving lifestyle adjustments.

Pathogenesis The sensory sensitivity that is characteristic of migraine is probably due to dysfunction of monoaminergic sensory control systems located in the brainstem and hypothalamus (Fig. 447-1).

Activation of cells in the trigeminal nucleus results in the release of vasoactive neuropeptides, particularly calcitonin gene–related peptide

TABLE 447-1 PRIMARY HEADACHE DISORDERS, MODIFIED FROM INTERNATIONAL CLASSIFICATION OF HEADACHE DISORDERS-III-BETA (HEADACHE CLASSIFICATION COMMITTEE OF THE INTERNATIONAL HEADACHE SOCIETY, 2013)

1. Migraine	1.1 Migraine without aura
	1.2 Migraine with aura
	1.2.1 Migraine with typical aura
	1.2.1.1 Typical aura with headache
	1.2.1.2 Typical aura without headache
	1.2.2 Migraine with brainstem aura
	1.2.3 Hemiplegic migraine
	1.2.3.1 Familial hemiplegic migraine (FHM)
	1.2.3.1.1 Familial hemiplegic migraine type 1
	1.2.3.1.2 Familial hemiplegic migraine type 2
	1.2.3.1.3 Familial hemiplegic migraine type 3
	1.2.3.2 Sporadic hemiplegic migraine
	1.2.4 Retinal migraine
	1.3 Chronic migraine
	1.4 Complications of migraine
	1.4.1 Status migrainosus
	1.4.2 Persistent aura without infarction
	1.4.3 Migrainous infarction
	1.4.4 Migraine aura-triggered seizure
	1.5 Probable migraine
	1.5.1 Probable migraine without aura
	1.5.2 Probable migraine with aura
	1.6 Episodic syndromes that may be associated with migraine
	1.6.1 Recurrent gastrointestinal disturbance
	1.6.1.1 Cyclical vomiting syndrome
	1.6.1.2 Abdominal migraine
	1.6.2 Benign paroxysmal vertigo
	1.6.3 Benign paroxysmal torticollis
2. Tension-type headache	2.1 Infrequent episodic tension-type headache
	2.2 Frequent episodic tension-type headache
	2.3 Chronic tension-type headache
3. Trigeminal autonomic cephalalgias	3.1 Cluster headache
	3.1.1 Episodic cluster headache
	3.1.2 Chronic cluster headache
	3.2 Paroxysmal hemicrania
	3.2.1 Episodic paroxysmal hemicrania
	3.2.2 Chronic paroxysmal hemicrania
	3.3 Short-lasting unilateral neuralgiform headache attacks
	3.3.1 Short-lasting unilateral neuralgiform headache attacks with conjunctival injection and tearing (SUNCT)
	3.3.2 Short-lasting unilateral neuralgiform headache attacks with cranial autonomic symptoms (SUNA)
	3.4 Hemicrania continua
4. Other primary headache disorders	4.1 Primary cough headache
	4.2 Primary exercise headache
	4.3 Primary headache associated with sexual activity
	4.4 Primary thunderclap headache
	4.5 Cold-stimulus headache
	4.5.1 Headache attributed to external application of a cold stimulus
	4.5.2 Headache attributed to ingestion or inhalation of a cold stimulus
	4.6 External-pressure headache
	4.6.1 External-compression headache
	4.6.2 External-traction headache
	4.7 Primary stabbing headache
	4.8 Nummular headache
	4.9 Hypnic headache
	4.10 New daily persistent headache (NDPH)

TABLE 447-2 SYMPTOMS ACCOMPANYING SEVERE MIGRAINE ATTACKS IN 500 PATIENTS

Symptom	Patients Affected, %
Nausea	87
Photophobia	82
Lightheadedness	72
Scalp tenderness	65
Vomiting	56
Visual disturbances	36
Paresthesias	33
Vertigo	33
Photopsia	26
Alteration of consciousness	18
Diarrhea	16
Fortification spectra	10
Syncope	10
Seizure	4
Confusional state	4

Source: From NH Raskin: *Headache*, 2nd ed. New York, Churchill Livingston, 1988; with permission.

(CGRP), at vascular terminations of the trigeminal nerve and within the trigeminal nucleus. CGRP receptor antagonists, *gepants*, have now been shown to be effective in the acute treatment of migraine, and monoclonal antibodies to CGRP have been shown effective in two early phase clinical trials. Centrally, the second-order trigeminal neurons cross the midline and project to ventrobasal and posterior nuclei of the thalamus for further processing. Additionally, there are projections to the periaqueductal gray and hypothalamus, from which reciprocal descending systems have established antinociceptive effects. Other brainstem regions likely to be involved in descending modulation of trigeminal pain include the nucleus locus coeruleus in the pons and the rostroventromedial medulla.

Pharmacologic and other data point to the involvement of the neurotransmitter 5-hydroxytryptamine (5-HT; also known as serotonin) in migraines. Approximately 60 years ago, methysergide was found to antagonize certain peripheral actions of 5-HT and was introduced as the first drug capable of preventing migraine attacks. The *triptans* were designed to stimulate selectively subpopulations of 5-HT receptors; at least 14 different 5-HT receptors exist in humans. The triptans are potent agonists of 5-HT_{1B} and 5-HT_{1D} receptors, and some are active at the 5-HT_{1F} receptors; the latter's exclusive agonists are called *ditans*. Triptans arrest nerve signaling in the nociceptive pathways of the trigeminovascular system, at least in the trigeminal nucleus caudalis and trigeminal sensory thalamus, in addition to cranial vasoconstriction, while *ditans*, now shown conclusively to be effective in acute migraine, act only at neural targets. An interesting range of neural targets is now being actively pursed for the acute and preventive management of migraine.

Data also support a role for dopamine in the pathophysiology of migraine. Most migraine symptoms can be induced by dopaminergic stimulation. Moreover, there is dopamine receptor hypersensitivity in migraineurs, as demonstrated by the induction of yawning, nausea, vomiting, hypotension, and other symptoms of a migraine attack by dopaminergic agonists at doses that do not affect nonmigraineurs. Dopamine receptor antagonists are effective therapeutic agents in migraine, especially when given parenterally or concurrently with other antimigraine agents. Moreover, hypothalamic activation, anterior to that seen in cluster headache, has now been shown in the

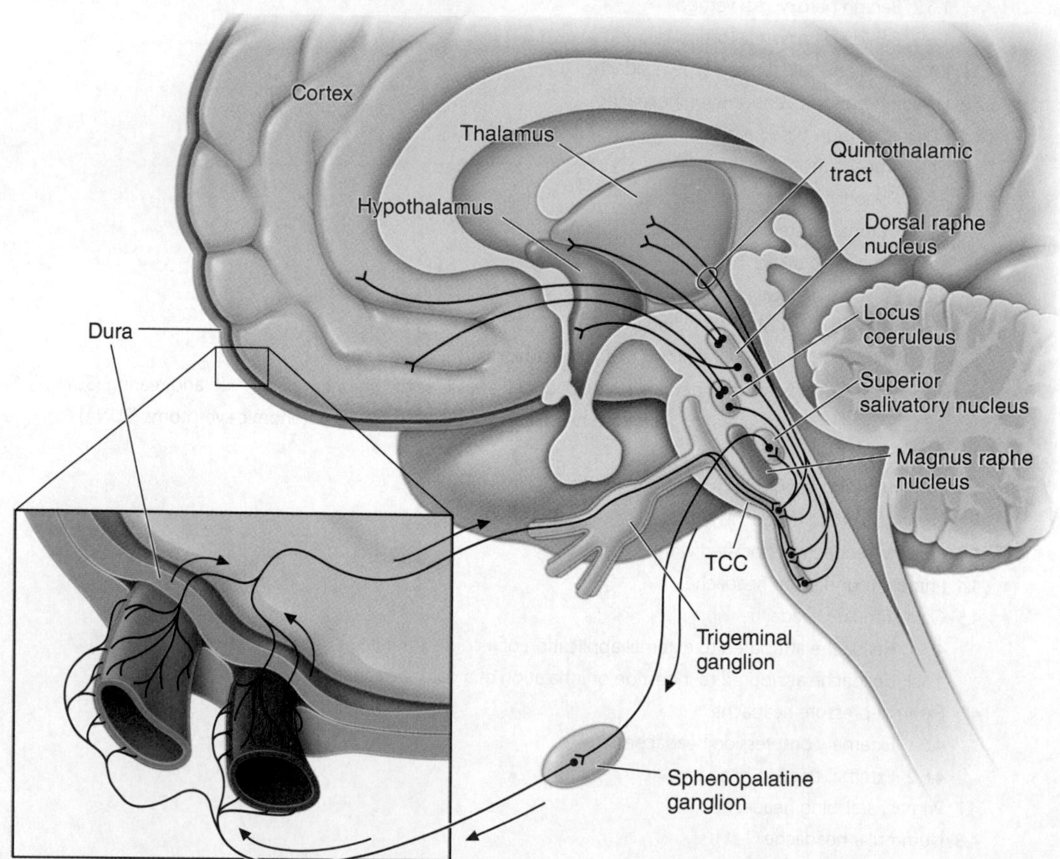

FIGURE 447-1 Brainstem pathways that modulate sensory input. The key pathway for pain in migraine is the trigeminovascular input from the meningeal vessels, which passes through the trigeminal ganglion and synapses on second-order neurons in the trigeminocervical complex (TCC). These neurons in turn project in the quintothalamic tract and, after decussating in the brainstem, synapse on neurons in the thalamus. Important modulation of the trigeminovascular nociceptive input comes from the dorsal raphe nucleus, locus coeruleus, and nucleus raphe magnus.

premonitory phase of migraine using functional imaging, and this may hold a key to understanding some part of the role of dopamine in the disorder.

Migraine genes identified by studying families with familial hemiplegic migraine (FHM) reveal involvement of ion channels, suggesting that alterations in membrane excitability can predispose to migraine. Mutations involving the $Ca_v2.1$ (P/Q)–type voltage-gated calcium channel *CACNA1A* gene are now known to cause FHM 1; this mutation is responsible for about 50% of FHMs. Mutations in the Na^+-K^+ATPase *ATP1A2* gene, designated FHM 2, are responsible for about 20% of FHMs. Mutations in the neuronal voltage-gated sodium channel *SCN1A* cause FHM 3. Functional neuroimaging has suggested that brainstem regions in migraine (Fig. 447-2) and the posterior hypothalamic gray matter region close to the human circadian pacemaker cells of the suprachiasmatic nucleus in cluster headache (Fig. 447-3) are good candidates for specific involvement in primary headache.

Diagnosis and Clinical Features Diagnostic criteria for migraine headache are listed in Table 447-3. A high index of suspicion is required to diagnose migraine: the migraine aura, consisting of visual disturbances with flashing lights or zigzag lines moving across the visual field or of other neurologic symptoms, is reported in only 20–25% of patients. A headache diary can often be helpful in making the diagnosis; this is also helpful in assessing disability and the frequency of treatment for acute attacks. Patients with episodes of migraine that occur daily or near-daily are considered to have chronic migraine (see "Chronic Daily Headache" in Chap. 21). Migraine must be differentiated from tension-type headache (discussed below), the most common primary headache syndrome seen in the population. Migraine has several forms that have been defined (Table 447-1): migraine with and without aura and chronic migraine, the latter occurring 15 days or more a month, as the most important. *Migraine at its most basic level is headache with associated features, and tension-type headache is headache that is featureless. Most patients with disabling headache probably have migraine.*

Patients with acephalgic migraine (typical aura without headache, 1.2.1.2 in Table 447-1) experience recurrent neurologic symptoms, often with nausea or vomiting, but with little or no headache. Vertigo can be prominent; it has been estimated that one-third of patients referred for vertigo or dizziness have a primary diagnosis of migraine. Migraine aura can have prominent brainstem symptoms, and the terms *basilar artery* and *basilar-type migraine* have now been replaced by *migraine with brainstem aura* (Table 447-1).

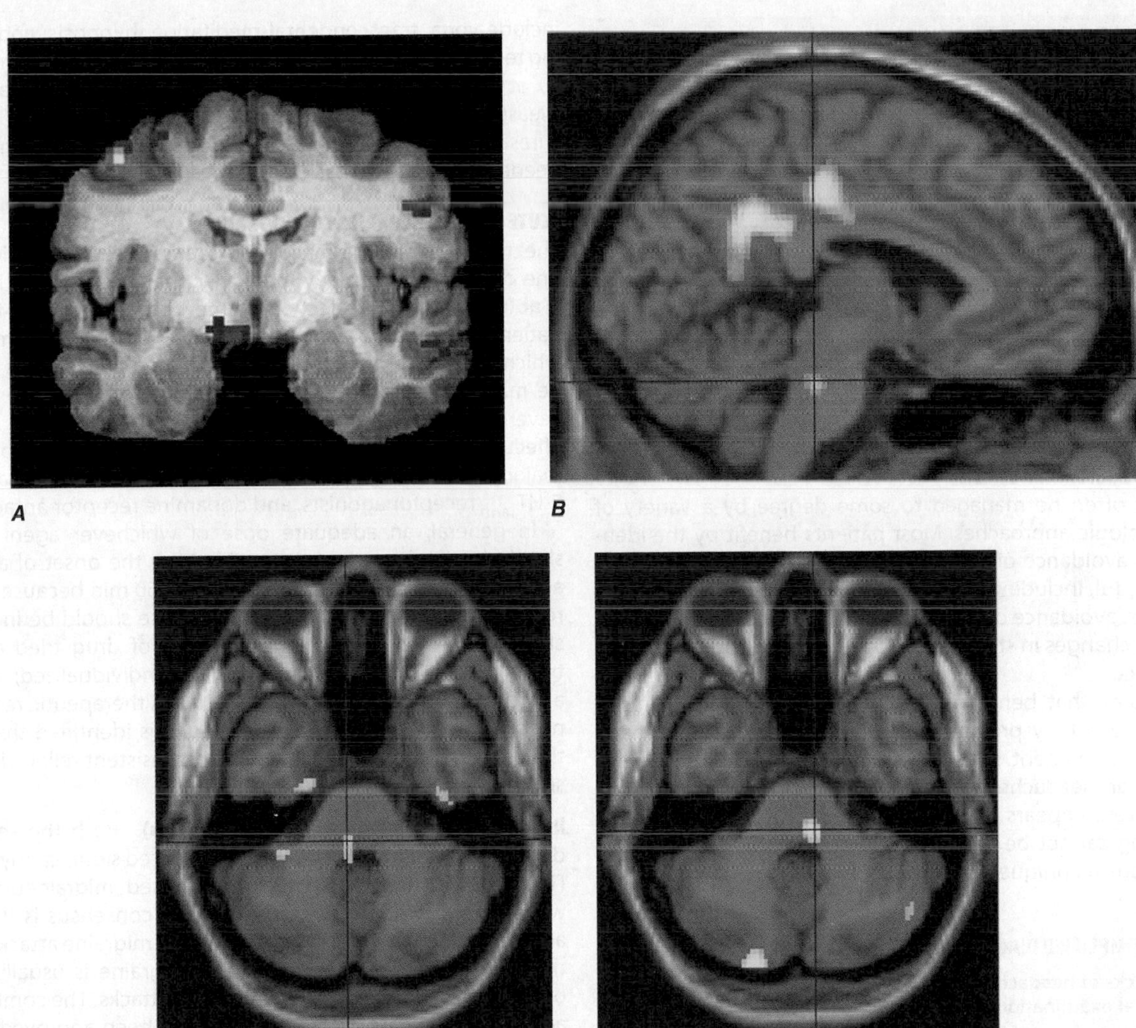

FIGURE 447-2 Positron emission tomography (PET) activation in migraine. Hypothalamic, dorsal midbrain, and dorsolateral pontine activation is seen in triggered attacks in the premonitory phase before pain, whereas in migraine attacks, dorsolateral pontine activation persists, as it does in chronic migraine (not shown). The dorsolateral pontine area, which includes the noradrenergic locus coeruleus, is fundamental to the expression of migraine. Moreover, lateralization of changes in this region of the brainstem correlates with lateralization of the head pain in hemicranial migraine; the scans shown in panels ***C*** and ***D*** are of patients with acute migraine headache on the right and left side, respectively. *(Panel A from FH Maniyar et al: Brain 137:232, 2014; panel B from SK Afridi et al: Arch Neurol 2005;62:1270; Panels C and D from SK Afridi et al: Brain 128:932, 2005.)*

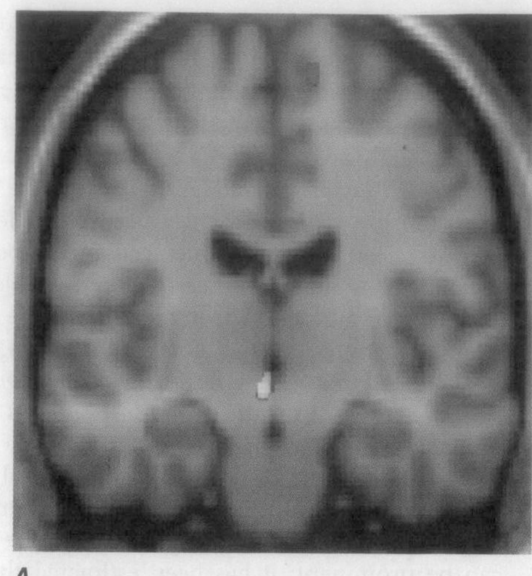

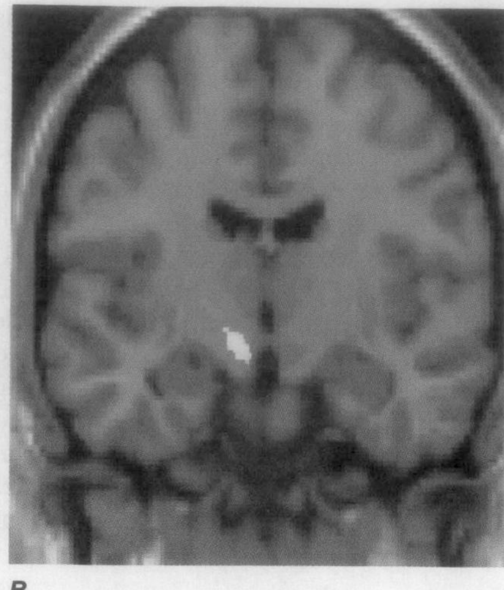

FIGURE 447-3 ***A.*** Posterior hypothalamic gray matter activation by positron emission tomography in a patient with acute cluster headache. *(From A May et al: Lancet 352:275, 1998.)* ***B.*** High-resolution T1-weighted magnetic resonance image obtained using voxel-based morphometry demonstrates increased gray matter activity, lateralized to the side of pain in a patient with cluster headache. *(From A May et al: Nat Med 5:836, 1999.)*

TREATMENT MIGRAINE HEADACHE

Once a diagnosis of migraine has been established, it is important to assess the extent of a patient's disease and disability. The Migraine Disability Assessment Score (MIDAS) is a well-validated, easy-to-use tool (Fig. 447-4).

Patient education is an important aspect of migraine management. Information for patients is available at sites such as *www.achenet.org*, the website of the American Council for Headache Education (ACHE). It is helpful for patients to understand that migraine is an inherited tendency to headache; that migraine can be modified and controlled by lifestyle adjustments and medications, but it cannot be eradicated; and that, except in some occasions in women on oral estrogens or contraceptives, migraine is not associated with serious or life-threatening illnesses.

NONPHARMACOLOGIC MANAGEMENT

Migraine can often be managed to some degree by a variety of nonpharmacologic approaches. Most patients benefit by the identification and avoidance of specific headache triggers. A regulated lifestyle is helpful, including a healthy diet, regular exercise, regular sleep patterns, avoidance of excess caffeine and alcohol, and avoidance of acute changes in stress levels, being particularly wary of the let-down effect.

The measures that benefit a given individual should be used routinely because they provide a simple, cost-effective approach to migraine management. Patients with migraine do not encounter more stress than headache-free individuals; over-responsiveness to changes in stress appears to be the issue. Because the stresses of everyday living cannot be eliminated, lessening one's response to stress by various techniques is helpful for many patients. These may include yoga, transcendental meditation, hypnosis, and conditioning techniques such as biofeedback. For most patients, this approach is, at best, an adjunct to pharmacotherapy. Nonpharmacologic measures are unlikely to prevent all migraine attacks. If these measures fail to prevent an attack, pharmacologic approaches are then needed to abort an attack.

TABLE 447-3 SIMPLIFIED DIAGNOSTIC CRITERIA FOR MIGRAINE

Repeated attacks of headache lasting 4–72 h in patients with a normal physical examination, no other reasonable cause for the headache, and:

At Least 2 of the Following Features:	Plus at Least 1 of the Following Features:
Unilateral pain	Nausea/vomiting
Throbbing pain	Photophobia and phonophobia
Aggravation by movement	
Moderate or severe intensity	

Source: Adapted from the International Headache Society Classification (Headache Classification Committee of the International Headache Society, 2013).

ACUTE ATTACK THERAPIES FOR MIGRAINE

The mainstay of pharmacologic therapy is the judicious use of one or more of the many medicines that are effective in migraine (Table 447-4). The selection of the optimal regimen for a given patient depends on a number of factors, the most important of which is the severity of the attack. Mild migraine attacks can usually be managed by oral agents; the average efficacy rate is 50–70%. Severe migraine attacks may require parenteral therapy. Most drugs effective in the treatment of migraine are members of one of three major pharmacologic classes: nonsteroidal anti-inflammatory drugs, 5-HT$_{1B/1D}$ receptor agonists, and dopamine receptor antagonists.

In general, an adequate dose of whichever agent is chosen should be used as soon as possible after the onset of an attack. If additional medication is required within 60 min because symptoms return or have not abated, the initial dose should be increased for subsequent attacks or a different class of drug tried as first-line treatment. Migraine therapy must be individualized; a standard approach for all patients is not possible. A therapeutic regimen may need to be constantly refined until one is identified that provides the patient with rapid, complete, and consistent relief with minimal side effects (Table 447-5).

Nonsteroidal Anti-Inflammatory Drugs (NSAIDs) Both the severity and duration of a migraine attack can be reduced significantly by NSAIDs (Table 447-4). Indeed, many undiagnosed migraineurs self-treat with nonprescription NSAIDs. A general consensus is that NSAIDs are most effective when taken early in the migraine attack. However, the effectiveness of these agents in migraine is usually less than optimal in moderate or severe migraine attacks. The combination of acetaminophen, aspirin, and caffeine has been approved for use by the U.S. Food and Drug Administration (FDA) for the treatment of mild to moderate migraine. The combination of aspirin and metoclopramide has been shown to be comparable to a single dose of oral sumatriptan. Important side effects of NSAIDs include dyspepsia and gastrointestinal irritation.

5-HT$_{1B/1D}$ RECEPTOR AGONISTS

Oral Stimulation of 5-HT$_{1B/1D}$ receptors can stop an acute migraine attack. Ergotamine and dihydroergotamine are nonselective receptor

***MIDAS Questionnaire**

INSTRUCTIONS: Please answer the following questions about ALL headaches you have had over the last 3 months. Write zero if you did not do the activity in the last 3 months.

1. On how many days in the last 3 months did you miss work or school because of your headaches? .... ____ days
2. How many days in the last 3 months was your productivity at work or school reduced by half or more because of your headaches *(do not include days you counted in question 1 where you missed work or school)*?........ ____ days
3. On how many days in the last 3 months did you **not** do household work because of your headaches? .... ____ days
4. How many days in the last 3 months was your productivity in household work reduced by half or more because of your headaches *(do not include days you counted in question 3 where you did not do household work)*?........ ____ days
5. On how many days in the last 3 months did you miss family, social, or leisure activities because of your headaches? .... ____ days

A. On how many days in the last 3 months did you have a headache? *(If a headache lasted more than one day, count each day.)*........ ____ days

B. On a scale of 0–10, on average how painful were these headaches? *(Where 0 = no pain at all, and 10 = pain as bad as it can be.)*........ ____

*Migraine Disability Assessment Score
(Questions 1–5 are used to calculate the MIDAS score.)
Grade I—Minimal or Infrequent Disability: 0–5
Grade II—Mild or Infrequent Disability: 6–10
Grade III—Moderate Disability: 11–20
Grade IV—Severe Disability: > 20

FIGURE 447-4 The Migraine Disability Assessment Score (MIDAS) Questionnaire.

agonists, whereas the triptans are selective 5-HT$_{1B/1D}$ receptor agonists. A variety of triptans, 5-HT$_{1B/1D}$ receptor agonists—sumatriptan, almotriptan, eletriptan, frovatriptan, naratriptan, rizatriptan, and zolmitriptan—are now available for the treatment of migraine.

Each drug in the triptan class has similar pharmacologic properties but varies slightly in terms of clinical efficacy. Rizatriptan and eletriptan are the most efficacious of the triptans currently available in the United States. Sumatriptan and zolmitriptan have similar rates of efficacy as well as time to onset, with an advantage of having multiple formulations, whereas almotriptan has a similar rate of efficacy to sumatriptan and is better tolerated, and frovatriptan and naratriptan are somewhat slower in onset and are better tolerated. Clinical efficacy appears to be related more to the t_{max} (time to peak plasma level) than to the potency, half-life, or bioavailability. This observation is consistent with a large body of data indicating that faster-acting analgesics are more effective than slower-acting agents.

Unfortunately, monotherapy with a selective oral 5-HT$_{1B/1D}$ receptor agonist does not result in rapid, consistent, and complete relief of migraine in all patients. Triptans are generally not effective in migraine with aura unless given after the aura is completed and the headache initiated. Side effects are common, although often mild and transient. Moreover, 5-HT$_{1B/1D}$ receptor agonists are contraindicated in individuals with a history of cardiovascular and cerebrovascular disease. Recurrence of headache, within usual time course of an attack, is another important limitation of triptan use and occurs at least occasionally in most patients. Evidence from randomized controlled trials show that coadministration of a longer-acting NSAID, naproxen 500 mg, with sumatriptan will augment the initial effect of sumatriptan and, importantly, reduce rates of headache recurrence.

Ergotamine preparations offer a nonselective means of stimulating 5-HT$_1$ receptors. A nonnauseating dose of ergotamine should be sought because a dose that provokes nausea is too high and may intensify head pain. Except for a sublingual formulation of ergotamine, oral formulations of ergotamine also contain 100 mg caffeine (theoretically to enhance ergotamine absorption and possibly to add additional analgesic activity). The average oral ergotamine dose for a migraine attack is 2 mg. Because the clinical studies demonstrating the efficacy of ergotamine in migraine predated the clinical trial methodologies used with the triptans, it is difficult to assess the clinical efficacy of ergotamine versus the triptans. In general, ergotamine appears to have a much higher incidence of nausea than triptans but less headache recurrence.

Nasal Nasal formulations of dihydroergotamine (Migranal), zolmitriptan (Zomig nasal), or sumatriptan can be useful in patients requiring a nonoral route of administration. The nasal sprays result in substantial blood levels within 30–60 min. Although in theory nasal sprays might provide faster and more effective relief of a migraine attack than oral formulations, their reported efficacy is only approximately 50–60%. Studies with a new inhalational formulation of dihydroergotamine indicate that its absorption problems can be overcome to produce rapid onset of action with good tolerability.

Parenteral Administration of drugs by injection, such as dihydro ergotamine and sumatriptan, is approved by the FDA for the rapid relief of a migraine attack. Peak plasma levels of dihydroergotamine are achieved 3 min after IV dosing, 30 min after IM dosing, and 45 min after SC dosing. If an attack has not already peaked, SC or IM administration of 1 mg of dihydroergotamine suffices for about 80–90% of patients. Sumatriptan, 4–6 mg SC, is effective in ~50–80% of patients, and can now be administered by a needle-free device.

DOPAMINE RECEPTOR ANTAGONISTS

Oral Oral dopamine receptor antagonists can be considered as adjunctive therapy in migraine. Drug absorption is impaired during migraine because of reduced gastrointestinal motility. Delayed absorption occurs even in the absence of nausea and is related to the severity of the attack and not its duration. Therefore, when oral NSAIDs and/or triptan agents fail, the addition of a dopamine receptor antagonist, such as metoclopramide 10 mg or domperidone 10 mg (not available in the United States), should be considered to

TABLE 447-4 TREATMENT OF ACUTE MIGRAINE

Drug	Trade Name	Dosage
Simple Analgesics		
Acetaminophen, aspirin, caffeine	Excedrin Migraine	Two tablets or caplets q6h (max 8 per day)
NSAIDs		
Naproxen	Aleve, Anaprox, generic	220–550 mg PO bid
Ibuprofen	Advil, Motrin, Nuprin, generic	400 mg PO q3–4h
Tolfenamic acid	Clotam Rapid	200 mg PO; may repeat ×1 after 1–2 h
Diclofenac K	Cambia	50 mg PO with water
5-HT$_1$ Receptor Agonists		
Oral		
Ergotamine 1 mg, caffeine 100 mg	Cafergot	One or two tablets at onset, then one tablet q½h (max 6 per day, 10 per week)
Naratriptan	Amerge	2.5-mg tablet at onset; may repeat once after 4 h
Rizatriptan	Maxalt Maxalt-MLT	5–10-mg tablet at onset; may repeat after 2 h (max 30 mg/d)
Sumatriptan	Imitrex	50–100-mg tablet at onset; may repeat after 2 h (max 200 mg/d)
Frovatriptan	Frova	2.5-mg tablet at onset, may repeat after 2 h (max 5 mg/d)
Almotriptan	Axert	12.5-mg tablet at onset, may repeat after 2 h (max 25 mg/d)
Eletriptan	Relpax	40 or 80 mg
Zolmitriptan	Zomig Zomig Rapimelt	2.5-mg tablet at onset; may repeat after 2 h (max 10 mg/d)
Nasal		
Dihydroergotamine	Migranal Nasal Spray	Prior to nasal spray, the pump must be primed 4 times; 1 spray (0.5 mg) is administered, followed in 15 min by a second spray
Sumatriptan	Imitrex Nasal Spray	5–20 mg intranasal spray as 4 sprays of 5 mg or a single 20 mg spray (may repeat once after 2 h, not to exceed a dose of 40 mg/d)
Zolmitriptan	Zomig	5 mg intranasal spray as one spray (may repeat once after 2 h, not to exceed a dose of 10 mg/d)
Parenteral		
Dihydroergotamine	DHE-45	1 mg IV, IM, or SC at onset and q1h (max 3 mg/d, 6 mg per week)
Sumatriptan	Imitrex Injection Alsuma Sumavel DosePro	6 mg SC at onset (may repeat once after 1 h for max of 2 doses in 24 h)
Dopamine Receptor Antagonists		
Oral		
Metoclopramide	Reglan,[a] generic[a]	5–10 mg/d
Prochlorperazine	Compazine,[a] generic[a]	1–25 mg/d
Parenteral		
Chlorpromazine	Generic[a]	0.1 mg/kg IV at 2 mg/min; max 35 mg/d
Metoclopramide	Reglan,[a] generic	10 mg IV
Prochlorperazine	Compazine,[a] generic[a]	10 mg IV
Other		
Oral		
Acetaminophen, 325 mg, *plus* dichloralphenazone, 100 mg, *plus* isometheptene, 65 mg	Midrin, generic	Two capsules at onset followed by 1 capsule q1h (max 5 capsules)
Nasal		
Butorphanol	Generic	1 mg (1 spray in 1 nostril), may repeat if necessary in 1–2 h
Parenteral		
Opioids	Generic[a]	Multiple preparations and dosages; **see Table 18-1**

[a]Not all drugs are specifically indicated by the FDA for migraine. Local regulations and guidelines should be consulted.

Note: Antiemetics (e.g., domperidone 10 mg or ondansetron 4 or 8 mg) or prokinetics (e.g., metoclopramide 10 mg) are sometimes useful adjuncts.

Abbreviations: 5-HT, 5-hydroxytryptamine; NSAIDs, nonsteroidal anti-inflammatory drugs.

enhance gastric absorption. In addition, dopamine receptor antagonists decrease nausea/vomiting and restore normal gastric motility.

Parenteral Dopamine receptor antagonists (e.g., chlorpromazine, prochlorperazine, metoclopramide) by injection can also provide significant acute relief of migraine; they can be used in combination with parenteral 5-HT$_{1B/1D}$ receptor agonists. A common IV protocol used for the treatment of severe migraine is the administration over 2 min of a mixture of 5 mg of prochlorperazine and 0.5 mg of dihydroergotamine.

OTHER MEDICATIONS FOR ACUTE MIGRAINE

Oral The combination of acetaminophen, dichloralphenazone, and isometheptene, one to two capsules, has been classified by the FDA

TABLE 447-5 CLINICAL STRATIFICATION OF ACUTE SPECIFIC MIGRAINE TREATMENTS

Clinical Situation	Treatment Options
Failed NSAIDs/analgesics	**First tier**
	Sumatriptan 50 mg or 100 mg PO
	Almotriptan 12.5 mg PO
	Rizatriptan 10 mg PO
	Eletriptan 40 mg PO
	Zolmitriptan 2.5 mg PO
	Slower effect/better tolerability
	Naratriptan 2.5 mg PO
	Frovatriptan 2.5 mg PO
	Infrequent headache
	Ergotamine/caffeine 1–2/100 mg PO
	Dihydroergotamine nasal spray 2 mg
Early nausea or difficulties taking tablets	Zolmitriptan 5 mg nasal spray
	Sumatriptan 20 mg nasal spray
	Rizatriptan 10 mg MLT wafer
Headache recurrence	Ergotamine 2 mg (most effective PR/usually with caffeine)
	Naratriptan 2.5 mg PO
	Almotriptan 12.5 mg PO
	Eletriptan 40 mg
Tolerating acute treatments poorly	Naratriptan 2.5 mg
	Almotriptan 12.5 mg
Early vomiting	Zolmitriptan 5 mg nasal spray
	Sumatriptan 25 mg PR
	Sumatriptan 6 mg SC
Menses-related headache	**Prevention**
	Ergotamine PO at night
	Estrogen patches
	Treatment
	Triptans
	Dihydroergotamine nasal spray
Very rapidly developing symptoms	Zolmitriptan 5 mg nasal spray
	Sumatriptan 6 mg SC
	Dihydroergotamine 1 mg IM

Abbreviation: NSAIDs, nonsteroidal anti-inflammatory drugs.

as "possibly" effective in the treatment of migraine. Because the clinical studies demonstrating the efficacy of this combination analgesic in migraine predated the clinical trial methodologies used with the triptans, it is difficult to compare the efficacy of this sympathomimetic compound to other agents.

Nasal A nasal preparation of butorphanol is available for the treatment of acute pain. As with all opioids, the use of nasal butorphanol has little role in migraine treatment.

Parenteral Opioids are modestly effective in the acute treatment of migraine. For example, IV meperidine (50–100 mg) is given frequently in the emergency room. This regimen "works" in the sense that the pain of migraine is eliminated. However, this regimen is clearly suboptimal for patients with recurrent headache. Opioids do not treat the underlying headache mechanism; rather, they act to alter the pain sensation, and there is evidence their use may decrease the likelihood of a response to triptans in the future. Moreover, in patients taking oral opioids, such as oxycodone or hydrocodone, habituation or addiction can greatly confuse the treatment of migraine. Opioid craving and/or withdrawal can aggravate and accentuate migraine. Therefore, it is recommended that opioid use in migraine be limited to patients with severe, but infrequent, headaches that are unresponsive to other pharmacologic approaches or who have contraindications to other therapies.

MEDICATION-OVERUSE HEADACHE

Acute attack medications, particularly opioid or barbiturate-containing compound analgesics, have a propensity to aggravate headache frequency and induce a state of refractory daily or near-daily headache called *medication-overuse headache*. This condition is likely not a separate headache entity but a reaction of the migraine patient to a particular medicine. Migraine patients who have two or more headache days a week should be cautioned about frequent analgesic use (see "Chronic Daily Headache" in Chap. 21).

PREVENTIVE TREATMENTS FOR MIGRAINE

Patients with an increasing frequency of migraine attacks or with attacks that are either unresponsive or poorly responsive to abortive treatments are good candidates for preventive agents. In general, a preventive medication should be considered in the subset of patients with four or more attacks a month. Significant side effects are associated with the use of many of these agents; furthermore, determination of dose can be difficult because the recommended doses have been derived for conditions other than migraine. The mechanism of action of these drugs is unclear; it seems likely that the brain sensitivity that underlies migraine is modified. Patients are usually started on a low dose of a chosen treatment; the dose is then gradually increased, up to a reasonable maximum, to achieve clinical benefit.

Drugs that have the capacity to stabilize migraine are listed in Table 447-6. Drugs must be taken daily, and there is usually a lag of between 2 to 12 weeks before an effect is seen. The drugs that have been approved by the FDA for the prophylactic treatment of migraine include propranolol, timolol, sodium valproate, topiramate, and methysergide (not available). In addition, a number of other drugs appear to display prophylactic efficacy. This group includes amitriptyline, nortriptyline, flunarizine, phenelzine, gabapentin, and cyproheptadine. Placebo-controlled trials of onabotulinum toxin type A in episodic migraine were negative, whereas, overall, placebo-controlled trials in chronic migraine were positive. Phenelzine and methysergide are usually reserved for recalcitrant cases because of their serious potential side effects. Phenelzine is a monoamine oxidase inhibitor (MAOI); therefore, tyramine-containing foods, decongestants, and meperidine are contraindicated. Methysergide may cause retroperitoneal or cardiac valvular fibrosis when it is used for >6 months, and thus monitoring is required for patients using this drug; the risk of fibrosis is about 1:1500 and is likely to reverse after the drug is stopped.

The probability of success with any one of the antimigraine drugs is 50–75%. Many patients are managed adequately with low-dose amitriptyline, propranolol, candesartan, topiramate, or valproate. If these agents fail or lead to unacceptable side effects, second-line agents such as methysergide or phenelzine can be used. Once effective stabilization is achieved, the drug is continued for ~6 months and then slowly tapered to assess the continued need. Many patients are able to discontinue medication and experience fewer and milder attacks for long periods, suggesting that these drugs may alter the natural history of migraine.

TENSION-TYPE HEADACHE

Clinical Features The term *tension-type headache* (TTH) is commonly used to describe a chronic head-pain syndrome characterized by bilateral tight, band-like discomfort. The pain typically builds slowly, fluctuates in severity, and may persist more or less continuously for many days. The headache may be episodic or chronic (present >15 days per month).

A useful clinical approach is to diagnose TTH in patients whose headaches are completely without accompanying features such as nausea, vomiting, photophobia, phonophobia, osmophobia, throbbing, and aggravation with movement. Such an approach neatly separates

TABLE 447-6 PREVENTIVE TREATMENTS IN MIGRAINE[a]

Drug	Dose	Selected Side Effects
Pizotifen[b]	0.5–2 mg qd	Weight gain Drowsiness
Beta blocker		
Propranolol	40–120 mg bid	Reduced energy
Metoprolol	25–100 mg bid	Tiredness Postural symptoms Contraindicated in asthma
Antidepressants		
Amitriptyline	10–75 mg at night	Drowsiness
Dosulepin	25–75 mg at night	
Nortriptyline	25–75 mg at night	***Note:*** Some patients may only need a total dose of 10 mg, although generally 1–1.5 mg/kg body weight is required
Venlafaxine	75–150 mg/d	
Anticonvulsants		
Topiramate	25–200 mg/d	Paresthesias Cognitive symptoms Weight loss Glaucoma Caution with nephrolithiasis
Valproate	400–600 mg bid	Drowsiness Weight gain Tremor Hair loss Fetal abnormalities Hematologic or liver abnormalities
Serotonergic drugs		
Methysergide[c]	1–4 mg qd	Drowsiness Leg cramps Hair loss Retroperitoneal fibrosis (1-month drug holiday is required every 6 months)
Other classes		
Flunarizine[b]	5–15 mg qd	Drowsiness Weight gain Depression Parkinsonism
Candesartan	16 mg daily	Dizziness
Chronic migraine		
Onabotulinum toxin type A	155 U	Loss of brow furrow
No convincing evidence from controlled trials		
Verapamil		
Controlled trials demonstrate *no effect*		
Nimodipine		
Clonidine		
Selective serotonin reuptake inhibitors: fluoxetine		

[a]Commonly used preventives are listed with typical doses and common side effects. Not all listed medicines are approved by the U.S. Food and Drug Administration; local regulations and guidelines should be consulted. [b]Not available in the United States. [c]Not currently available worldwide.

migraine, which has one or more of these features and is the main differential diagnosis, from TTH. The International Headache Society's main definition of TTH allows an admixture of nausea, photophobia, or phonophobia in various combinations, although the appendix definition does not; this illustrates the difficulty in distinguishing these two clinical entities. In clinical practice, dichotomizing patients on the basis of the presence of associated features (migraine) and the absence of associated features (TTH) is highly recommended. Indeed patients whose headaches fit the TTH phenotype and who have migraine at other times, along with a family history of migraine, migrainous illnesses of childhood, or typical migraine triggers to their migraine attacks, may be biologically different from those who have TTH headache with none of the features. TTH may be infrequent (episodic) or occur on 15 days or more a month (chronic).

Pathophysiology The pathophysiology of TTH is incompletely understood. It seems likely that TTH is due to a primary disorder of central nervous system pain modulation alone, unlike migraine, which involves a more generalized disturbance of sensory modulation. Data suggest a genetic contribution to TTH, but this may not be a valid finding: given the current diagnostic criteria, the studies undoubtedly included many migraine patients. The name *tension-type headache* implies that pain is a product of *nervous tension*, but there is no clear evidence for tension as an etiology. Muscle contraction has been considered to be a feature that distinguishes TTH from migraine, but there appear to be no differences in contraction between the two headache types.

TREATMENT TENSION-TYPE HEADACHE

The pain of TTH can generally be managed with simple analgesics such as acetaminophen, aspirin, or NSAIDs. Behavioral approaches including relaxation can also be effective. Clinical studies have demonstrated that triptans in pure TTH are not helpful, although triptans are effective in TTH when the patient also has migraine. For chronic TTH, amitriptyline is the only proven treatment (Table 447-6); other tricyclics, selective serotonin reuptake inhibitors, and the benzodiazepines have not been shown to be effective. There is no evidence for the efficacy of acupuncture. Placebo-controlled trials of onabotulinum toxin type A in chronic TTH were negative.

TRIGEMINAL AUTONOMIC CEPHALALGIAS, INCLUDING CLUSTER HEADACHE

The trigeminal autonomic cephalalgias (TACs) describe a grouping of primary headaches including cluster headache, paroxysmal hemicrania, SUNCT (*s*hort-lasting *u*nilateral *n*euralgiform headache attacks with *c*onjunctival injection and *t*earing)/SUNA (short-lasting *u*nilateral *n*euralgiform headache attacks with cranial *a*utonomic symptoms), and hemicrania continua (Table 447-1). TACs are characterized by relatively short-lasting attacks of head pain associated with cranial autonomic symptoms, such as lacrimation, conjunctival injection, or nasal congestion (Table 447-7). Pain is usually severe and may occur more than once a day. Because of the associated nasal congestion or rhinorrhea, patients are often misdiagnosed with "sinus headache" and treated with decongestants, which are ineffective.

TACs must be differentiated from short-lasting headaches that do not have prominent cranial autonomic syndromes, notably trigeminal neuralgia, primary stabbing headache, and hypnic headache. The cycling pattern and length, frequency, and timing of attacks are useful in classifying patients. Patients with TACs should undergo pituitary imaging and pituitary function tests because there is an excess of TAC presentations in patients with pituitary tumor–related headache.

Cluster Headache Cluster headache is a relatively rare form of primary headache with a population frequency of approximately 0.1%. The pain is deep, usually retroorbital, often excruciating in intensity, nonfluctuating, and explosive in quality. A core feature of cluster headache is periodicity. At least one of the daily attacks of pain recurs at about the same hour each day for the duration of a cluster bout. The typical cluster headache patient has daily bouts of one to two attacks of

TABLE 447-7 CLINICAL FEATURES OF THE TRIGEMINAL AUTONOMIC CEPHALALGIAS

	Cluster Headache	Paroxysmal Hemicrania	SUNCT/SUNA
Gender	M > F	F = M	F ~ M
Pain			
Type	Stabbing, boring	Throbbing, boring, stabbing	Burning, stabbing, sharp
Severity	Excruciating	Excruciating	Severe to excruciating
Site	Orbit, temple	Orbit, temple	Periorbital
Attack frequency	1/alternate day–8/d	1–20/d (>5/d for more than half the time)	3–200/d
Duration of attack	15–180 min	2–30 min	5–240 s
Autonomic features	Yes	Yes	Yes (prominent conjunctival injection and lacrimation)[a]
Migrainous features[b]	Yes	Yes	Yes
Alcohol trigger	Yes	No	No
Cutaneous triggers	No	No	Yes
Indomethacin effect	—	Yes[c]	—
Abortive treatment	Sumatriptan injection or nasal spray Oxygen	No effective treatment	Lidocaine (IV)
Prophylactic treatment	Verapamil Methysergide Lithium	Indomethacin	Lamotrigine Topiramate Gabapentin

[a]If conjunctival injection and tearing are not present, consider SUNA. [b]Nausea, photophobia, or phonophobia; photophobia and phonophobia are typically unilateral on the side of the pain. [c]Indicates complete response to indomethacin.

Abbreviations: SUNA, short-lasting unilateral neuralgiform headache attacks with cranial autonomic features; SUNCT, short-lasting unilateral neuralgiform headache attacks with conjunctival injection and tearing.

relatively short duration unilateral pain for 8 to 10 weeks a year; this is usually followed by a pain-free interval that averages a little less than 1 year. Cluster headache is characterized as chronic when there is less than 1 month of sustained remission without treatment. Patients are generally perfectly well between episodes. Onset is nocturnal in about 50% of patients, and men are affected three times more often than women. Patients with cluster headache tend to move about during attacks, pacing, rocking, or rubbing their head for relief; some may even become aggressive during attacks. This is in sharp contrast to patients with migraine, who prefer to remain motionless during attacks.

Cluster headache is associated with ipsilateral symptoms of cranial parasympathetic autonomic activation: conjunctival injection or lacrimation, rhinorrhea or nasal congestion, or cranial sympathetic dysfunction such as ptosis. The sympathetic deficit is peripheral and likely to be due to parasympathetic activation with injury to ascending sympathetic fibers surrounding a dilated carotid artery as it passes into the cranial cavity. When present, photophobia and phonophobia are far more likely to be unilateral and on the same side of the pain, rather than bilateral, as is seen in migraine. This phenomenon of unilateral photophobia/phonophobia is characteristic of TACs. Cluster headache is likely to be a disorder involving central pacemaker neurons in the posterior hypothalamic region (Fig. 447-3).

TREATMENT CLUSTER HEADACHE

The most satisfactory treatment is the administration of drugs to prevent cluster attacks until the bout is over. However, treatment of acute attacks is required for all cluster headache patients at some time.

ACUTE ATTACK TREATMENT

Cluster headache attacks peak rapidly, and thus a treatment with quick onset is required. Many patients with acute cluster headache respond very well to oxygen inhalation. This should be given as 100% oxygen at 10–12 L/min for 15–20 min. It appears that high flow and high oxygen content are important. Sumatriptan 6 mg SC is rapid in onset and will usually shorten an attack to 10–15 min; there is no evidence of tachyphylaxis. Sumatriptan (20 mg) and zolmitriptan (5 mg) nasal sprays are both effective in acute cluster headache, offering a useful option for patients who may not wish to self-inject daily. Oral sumatriptan is not effective for prevention or for acute treatment of cluster headache.

PREVENTIVE TREATMENTS (TABLE 447-8)

The choice of a preventive treatment in cluster headache depends in part on the length of the bout. Patients with long bouts or those with chronic cluster headache require medicines that are safe when taken for long periods. For patients with relatively short bouts, limited courses of oral glucocorticoids or methysergide (not available in the United States) can be very useful. A 10-day course of prednisone, beginning at 60 mg daily for 7 days and followed by a rapid taper, may interrupt the pain bout for many patients. Lithium (400–800 mg/d) appears to be particularly useful for the chronic form of the disorder.

Many experts favor verapamil as the first-line preventive treatment for patients with chronic cluster headache or prolonged bouts. While verapamil compares favorably with lithium in practice, some patients require verapamil doses far in excess of those administered for cardiac disorders. The initial dose range is 40–80 mg twice daily; effective doses may be as high as 960 mg/d. Side effects such as constipation and leg swelling can be problematic. Of paramount concern, however, is the cardiovascular safety of verapamil, particularly

TABLE 447-8 PREVENTIVE MANAGEMENT OF CLUSTER HEADACHE

Short-Term Prevention	Long-Term Prevention
Episodic Cluster Headache	Episodic Cluster Headache and Prolonged Chronic Cluster Headache
Prednisone 1 mg/kg up to 60 mg qd, tapering over 21 days	Verapamil 160–960 mg/d
Methysergide 3–12 mg/d	Lithium 400–800 mg/d
Verapamil 160–960 mg/d	Methysergide[a] 3–12 mg/d
Greater occipital nerve injection	Topiramate[b] 100–400 mg/d
	Gabapentin[b] 1200–3600 mg/d
	Melatonin[b] 9–12 mg/d

[a]Not available worldwide. [b]Unproven but of potential benefit.

at high doses. Verapamil can cause heart block by slowing conduction in the atrioventricular node, a condition that can be monitored by following the PR interval on a standard electrocardiogram (ECG). Approximately 20% of patients treated with verapamil develop ECG abnormalities, which can be observed with doses as low as 240 mg/d; these abnormalities can worsen over time in patients on stable doses. A baseline ECG is recommended for all patients. The ECG is repeated 10 days after a dose change in patients whose dose is being increased above 240 mg daily. Dose increases are usually made in 80-mg increments. For patients on long-term verapamil, ECG monitoring every 6 months is advised.

NEUROSTIMULATION THERAPY

When medical therapies fail in chronic cluster headache, neurostimulation strategies can be used. Deep-brain stimulation of the region of the posterior hypothalamic gray matter has proven successful in a substantial proportion of patients, although its risk-benefit ratio makes it inappropriate with so many other options now available. Favorable results have also been reported with the less-invasive approach of occipital nerve stimulation, with sphenopalatine ganglion stimulation and with a noninvasive vagal nerve stimulator.

PAROXYSMAL HEMICRANIA

Paroxysmal hemicrania (PH) is characterized by frequent unilateral, severe, short-lasting episodes of headache. Like cluster headache, the pain tends to be retroorbital but may be experienced all over the head and is associated with autonomic phenomena such as lacrimation and nasal congestion. Patients with remissions are said to have episodic PH, whereas those with the nonremitting form are said to have chronic PH. The essential features of PH are unilateral, very severe pain; short-lasting attacks (2–45 min); very frequent attacks (usually more than five a day); marked autonomic features ipsilateral to the pain; rapid course (<72 h); and excellent response to indomethacin. In contrast to cluster headache, which predominantly affects males, the male-to-female ratio in PH is close to 1:1.

Indomethacin (25–75 mg tid), which can completely suppress attacks of PH, is the treatment of choice. Although therapy may be complicated by indomethacin-induced gastrointestinal side effects, currently there are no consistently effective alternatives. Topiramate is helpful in some cases. Piroxicam has been used, although it is not as effective as indomethacin. Verapamil, an effective treatment for cluster headache, does not appear to be useful for PH. In occasional patients, PH can coexist with trigeminal neuralgia (PH-tic syndrome); similar to cluster-tic syndrome, each component may require separate treatment.

Secondary PH has been reported with lesions in the region of the sella turcica, including arteriovenous malformation, cavernous sinus meningioma, pituitary pathology and epidermoid tumors. Secondary PH is more likely if the patient requires high doses (>200 mg/d) of indomethacin. In patients with apparent bilateral PH, raised cerebrospinal fluid (CSF) pressure should be suspected. It is important to note that indomethacin reduces CSF pressure. When a diagnosis of PH is considered, magnetic resonance imaging (MRI) is indicated to exclude a pituitary lesion.

SUNCT/SUNA

SUNCT (*s*hort-lasting *u*nilateral *n*euralgiform headache attacks with *c*onjunctival injection and *t*earing) is a rare primary headache syndrome characterized by severe, unilateral orbital or temporal pain that is stabbing or throbbing in quality. Diagnosis requires at least 20 attacks, lasting for 5–240 s; ipsilateral conjunctival injection and lacrimation should be present. In some patients, conjunctival injection or lacrimation is missing, and the diagnosis of SUNA (*s*hort-lasting *u*nilateral *n*euralgiform headache attacks with cranial *a*utonomic symptoms) can be made.

DIAGNOSIS The pain of SUNCT/SUNA is unilateral and may be located anywhere in the head. Three basic patterns can be seen: single stabs, which are usually short-lived; groups of stabs; or a longer attack comprising many stabs between which the pain does not completely resolve, thus giving a "saw-tooth" phenomenon with attacks lasting many minutes. Each pattern may be seen in the context of an underlying continuous head pain. Characteristics that lead to a suspected diagnosis of SUNCT are the cutaneous (or other) triggers of attacks, a lack of refractory period to triggering between attacks, and the lack of a response to indomethacin. Apart from trigeminal sensory disturbance, the neurologic examination is normal in primary SUNCT.

The diagnosis of SUNCT/SUNA is often confused with trigeminal neuralgia (TN) particularly in first-division TN (Chap. 455). Minimal or no cranial autonomic symptoms and a clear refractory period to triggering indicate a diagnosis of TN.

SECONDARY (SYMPTOMATIC) SUNCT SUNCT can be seen with posterior fossa or pituitary lesions. All patients with SUNCT/SUNA should be evaluated with pituitary function tests and a brain MRI with pituitary views.

TREATMENT SUNCT/SUNA

ABORTIVE THERAPY

Therapy of acute attacks is not a useful concept in SUNCT/SUNA because the attacks are of such short duration. However, IV lidocaine, which arrests the symptoms, can be used in hospitalized patients.

PREVENTIVE THERAPY

Long-term prevention to minimize disability and hospitalization is the goal of treatment. The most effective treatment for prevention is lamotrigine, 200–400 mg/d. Topiramate and gabapentin may also be effective. Carbamazepine, 400–500 mg/d, has been reported by patients to offer modest benefit.

Surgical approaches such as microvascular decompression or destructive trigeminal procedures are seldom useful and often produce long-term complications. Greater occipital nerve injection has produced limited benefit in some patients. Occipital nerve stimulation is probably helpful in a subgroup of these patients. Complete control with deep-brain stimulation of the posterior hypothalamic region was reported in a single patient. For intractable cases, short-term prevention with IV lidocaine can be effective, as can occipital nerve stimulation.

Hemicrania Continua The essential features of hemicrania continua are moderate and continuous unilateral pain associated with fluctuations of severe pain; complete resolution of pain with indomethacin; and exacerbations that may be associated with autonomic features, including conjunctival injection, lacrimation, and photophobia on the affected side. The age of onset ranges from 11 to 58 years; women are affected twice as often as men. The cause is unknown.

TREATMENT HEMICRANIA CONTINUA

Treatment consists of indomethacin; other NSAIDs appear to be of little or no benefit. The IM injection of 100 mg of indomethacin has been proposed as a diagnostic tool, and administration with a placebo injection in a blinded fashion can be very useful diagnostically. Alternatively, a trial of oral indomethacin, starting with 25 mg tid, then 50 mg tid, and then 75 mg tid, can be given. Up to 2 weeks at the maximal dose may be necessary to assess whether a dose has a useful effect. Topiramate can be helpful in some patients. Occipital nerve stimulation probably has a role in patients with hemicrania continua who are unable to tolerate indomethacin.

OTHER PRIMARY HEADACHES

Primary Cough Headache Primary cough headache is a generalized headache that begins suddenly, lasts for several minutes, sometimes up to a few hours, and is precipitated by coughing; it is preventable by avoiding coughing or other precipitating events, which can include sneezing, straining, laughing, or stooping. In all patients with this syndrome, serious etiologies must be excluded before a diagnosis of "benign" primary cough headache can be established. A Chiari malformation or any lesion causing obstruction of CSF pathways or displacing cerebral structures can be the cause of the head pain. Other conditions that can present with cough or exertional headache as the initial symptom include cerebral aneurysm, carotid stenosis, and vertebrobasilar disease. Benign cough headache can resemble benign exertional headache (below), but patients with the former condition are typically older.

TREATMENT PRIMARY COUGH HEADACHE

Indomethacin 25–50 mg two to three times daily is the treatment of choice. Some patients with cough headache obtain complete cessation of their attacks with lumbar puncture; this is a simple option when compared to prolonged use of indomethacin, and it is effective in about one-third of patients. The mechanism of this response is unclear.

Primary Exercise Headache Primary exertional headache has features resembling both cough headache and migraine. It may be precipitated by any form of exercise; it often has the pulsatile quality of migraine. The pain, which can last from 5 min to 24 h, is bilateral and throbbing at onset; migrainous features may develop in patients susceptible to migraine. The duration tends to be shorter in adolescents than in older adults. Primary exertional headache can be prevented by avoiding excessive exertion, particularly in hot weather or at high altitude.

The mechanism of primary exertional headache is unclear. Acute venous distension likely explains one syndrome—the acute onset of headache with straining and breath holding, as in weightlifter's headache. Because exertion can result in headache in a number of serious underlying conditions, these must be considered in patients with exertional headache. Pain from angina may be referred to the head, probably by central connections of vagal afferents, and may present as exertional headache (cardiac cephalgia). The link to exercise is the main clinical clue that headache is of cardiac origin. Pheochromocytoma may occasionally cause exertional headache. Intracranial lesions and stenosis of the carotid arteries are other possible etiologies.

TREATMENT PRIMARY EXERTIONAL HEADACHE

Exercise regimens should begin modestly and progress gradually to higher levels of intensity. Indomethacin at daily doses from 25 to 150 mg is generally effective in benign exertional headache. Indomethacin (50 mg), ergotamine (1 mg orally), dihydroergotamine (2 mg by nasal spray), and methysergide (1–2 mg orally given 30–45 min before exercise) are useful prophylactic measures.

Primary Headache Associated with Sexual Activity Three types of sex headache are reported: a dull bilateral ache in the head and neck that intensifies as sexual excitement increases; a sudden, severe, explosive headache occurring at orgasm; and a postural headache developing after coitus that resembles the headache of low CSF pressure. The last arises from vigorous sexual activity and is a form of low CSF pressure headache (Chap. 21). Headaches developing at the time of orgasm are not always benign; 5–12% of cases of subarachnoid hemorrhage are precipitated by sexual intercourse. Sex headache is reported by men more often than women and may occur at any time during the years of sexual activity. It may develop on several occasions in succession and then not trouble the patient again, even without an obvious change in sexual activity. In patients who stop sexual activity when headache is first noticed, the pain may subside within a period of 5 min to 2 h. In about half of patients, sex headache will subside within 6 months. About half of patients with sex headache have a history of exertional headaches, but there is no excess of cough headache. Migraine is probably more common in patients with sex headache.

TREATMENT PRIMARY SEX HEADACHE

Benign sex headaches recur irregularly and infrequently. Management can often be limited to reassurance and advice about ceasing sexual activity if a mild, warning headache develops. Propranolol can be used to prevent headache that recurs regularly or frequently, but the dosage required varies from 40 to 200 mg/d. An alternative is the calcium channel–blocking agent diltiazem, 60 mg tid. Ergotamine (1 mg) or indomethacin (25–50 mg) taken 30–45 min prior to sexual activity can also be helpful.

Primary Thunderclap Headache Sudden onset of severe headache may occur in the absence of any known provocation. The differential diagnosis includes the sentinel bleed of an intracranial aneurysm, cervicocephalic arterial dissection, and cerebral venous thrombosis. Headaches of explosive onset may also be caused by the ingestion of sympathomimetic drugs or of tyramine-containing foods in a patient who is taking MAOIs, or they may be a symptom of pheochromocytoma. Whether thunderclap headache can be the presentation of an unruptured cerebral aneurysm is uncertain. When neuroimaging studies and lumbar puncture exclude subarachnoid hemorrhage, patients with thunderclap headache usually do very well over the long term. In one study of patients whose computed tomography (CT) scans and CSF findings were negative, ~15% had recurrent episodes of thunderclap headache, and nearly half subsequently developed migraine or TTH.

The first presentation of any sudden-onset severe headache should be diligently investigated with neuroimaging (CT or, when possible, MRI with MR angiography) and CSF examination. Formal cerebral angiography should be reserved for those cases in which no primary diagnosis is forthcoming and for clinical situations that are particularly suggestive of intracranial aneurysm. Reversible segmental cerebral vasoconstriction may be seen in primary thunderclap headache without an intracranial aneurysm. In the presence of posterior leukoencephalopathy, the differential diagnosis includes cerebral angiitis, drug toxicity (cyclosporine, intrathecal methotrexate/cytarabine, pseudoephedrine, or cocaine), posttransfusion effects, and postpartum angiopathy. Treatment with nimodipine may be helpful, although by definition, the vasoconstriction of primary thunderclap headache resolves spontaneously.

Cold-Stimulus Headache This refers to head pain triggered by application or ingestion/inhalation of something cold. It is bought on quickly and typically resolves within 10–30 min of the stimulus being removed. It is best recognized as "brain-freeze" headache or ice-cream headache when due to ingestion. Although cold may be uncomfortable at some level for many people, it is the reliable, severe, and somewhat prolonged nature of these pains that set them apart. The transient receptor potential cation subfamily M member 8 (TRPM8) channel, a known cold temperature sensor, may be a mediator of this syndrome.

External Pressure Headache External pressure from compression or traction on the head can produce a pain that may have some generalized component, although the pain is largely focused around the site of the pressure. It typically resolves within an hour of the stimulus being removed. Examples of stimuli include helmets, swimming goggles, or very long ponytails. Treatment is to recognize the problem and remove the stimulus.

Primary Stabbing Headache The essential features of primary stabbing headache are stabbing pain confined to the head or, rarely, the face, lasting from 1 to many seconds or minutes and occurring as a single stab or a series of stabs; absence of associated cranial autonomic features; absence of cutaneous triggering of attacks; and a pattern of recurrence at irregular intervals (hours to days). The pains have been variously described as "ice-pick pains" or "jabs and jolts." They are more common in patients with other primary headaches, such as migraine, the TACs, and hemicrania continua.

TREATMENT PRIMARY STABBING HEADACHE

The response of primary stabbing headache to indomethacin (25–50 mg two to three times daily) is usually excellent. As a general rule, the symptoms wax and wane, and after a period of control on indomethacin, it is appropriate to withdraw treatment and observe the outcome.

Nummular Headache Nummular headache is felt as a round or elliptical discomfort that is fixed in place, ranges in size from 1–6 cm, and may be continuous or intermittent. Uncommonly it may be multifocal. It may be episodic but is more often continuous during exacerbations. Accompanying the pain there may be a local sensory disturbance, such as allodynia or hypesthesia. Local dermatologic or bony lesions need to be excluded by examination and investigation. This condition can be difficult to treat; tricyclics, such as amitriptyline, or anticonvulsants, such as topiramate or valproate, are most often tried.

Hypnic Headache This headache syndrome typically begins a few hours after sleep onset. The headaches last from 15 to 30 min and are typically moderately severe and generalized, although they may be unilateral and can be throbbing. Patients may report falling back to sleep only to be awakened by a further attack a few hours later; up to three repetitions of this pattern occur through the night. Daytime naps can also precipitate head pain. Most patients are female, and the onset is usually after age 60 years. Headaches are bilateral in most, but may be unilateral. Photophobia, phonophobia, and nausea are usually absent. The major secondary consideration in this headache type is poorly controlled hypertension; 24-h blood pressure monitoring is recommended to detect this treatable condition.

TREATMENT HYPNIC HEADACHE

Patients with hypnic headache generally respond to a bedtime dose of lithium carbonate (200–600 mg). For those intolerant of lithium, verapamil (160 mg) or methysergide (1–4 mg at bedtime) may be alternative strategies. One to two cups of coffee or caffeine, 60 mg orally, at bedtime may be effective in approximately one-third of patients. Case reports also suggest that flunarizine, 5 mg nightly, can be effective.

New Daily Persistent Headache Primary new daily persistent headache (NDPH) occurs in both males and females. It can be of the migrainous type, with features of migraine, or it can be featureless, appearing as new-onset TTH. Migrainous features are common and include unilateral headache and throbbing pain; each feature is present in about one-third of patients. Nausea, photophobia, and/or phonophobia occur in about half of patients. Some patients have a previous history of migraine; however, the proportion of NDPH sufferers with preexisting migraine is no greater than the frequency of migraine in the general population. At 24 months, ~86% of patients are headache-free. Treatment of migrainous-type primary NDPH consists of using the preventive therapies effective in migraine (see above). Featureless NDPH is one of the primary headache forms most refractory to treatment. Standard preventive therapies can be offered but are often ineffective. The secondary NDPHs are discussed elsewhere (Chap. 21).

448 Alzheimer's Disease and Other Dementias

William W. Seeley, Bruce L. Miller

ALZHEIMER'S DISEASE

Approximately 10% of all persons over the age of 70 years have significant memory loss, and in more than half, the cause is Alzheimer's disease (AD). It is estimated that the median annual total cost of caring for a single patient with advanced AD is >$50,000, while the emotional toll for family members and caregivers is immeasurable. AD can manifest as young as the third decade, but it is the most common cause of dementia in the elderly. Patients most often present with an insidious loss of episodic memory followed by a slowly progressive dementia that evolves over years. In typical amnestic AD, brain imaging reveals atrophy that begins in the medial temporal lobes before spreading to lateral and medial parietal and temporal lobes and lateral frontal cortex. Microscopically, there are neuritic plaques containing amyloid beta (Aβ), neurofibrillary tangles (NFTs) composed of hyperphosphorylated tau filaments, and Aβ accumulation of in blood vessel walls in cortex and leptomeninges (see "Pathology," below). The identification of causative mutations and susceptibility genes for AD has provided a foundation for rapid progress in understanding the biological basis of the disorder. The major genetic risk for AD is apolipoprotein ε4 (Apo ε4). Carrying one E4 allele increases the risk for AD by 2- to 3-fold, whereas two alleles increase the risk 16-fold.

CLINICAL MANIFESTATIONS

The cognitive changes of AD tend to follow a characteristic pattern, beginning with memory impairment and progressing to language and visuospatial deficits. Yet, approximately 20% of patients with AD present with nonmemory complaints such as word-finding, organizational, or navigational difficulty. In other patients, upstream visual processing dysfunction (referred to as posterior cortical atrophy syndrome) or a progressive "logopenic" aphasia are the primary manifestations of AD for years before progressing to involve memory and other cognitive domains. Still other patients may present with an asymmetric akinetic-rigid-dystonic ("corticobasal") syndrome or a dysexecutive "frontal variant" of AD.

In the early stages of typical amnestic AD, the memory loss may go unrecognized or be ascribed to benign forgetfulness of aging. Once the memory loss becomes noticeable to the patient and spouse and falls 1.5 standard deviations below normal on standardized memory tests, the term mild cognitive impairment (MCI) is applied. This construct provides useful prognostic information, because approximately 50% of patients with MCI (roughly 12% per year) will progress to AD over 4 years. Increasingly, the MCI construct is being replaced by the notion of "early symptomatic AD" to signify that AD is considered the underlying disease (based on clinical or biomarker evidence) in a patient who remains functionally compensated. Even earlier in the course, "prodromal AD" refers to a person with biomarker evidence of AD (amyloid imaging positive with positron emission tomography or low cerebrospinal $A\beta_{42}$ and mildly elevated tau) in the absence of symptoms. These refinements have been developed in anticipation of early-stage treatment and prevention trials that have already begun in humans. New evidence suggests that partial and sometimes generalized seizures herald AD and can occur even prior to dementia onset.

Eventually, with AD, the cognitive problems begin to interfere with daily activities, such as keeping track of finances, following instructions on the job, driving, shopping, and housekeeping. Some patients are unaware of these difficulties (*anosognosia*), but most remain acutely attuned to their deficits. Changes in environment (travel, relocation, hospitalization) tend to destabilize the patient. Over time patients become lost on walks or while driving. Social graces, routine behavior, and superficial conversation may be surprisingly intact, even into the later stages of the illness.

In the middle stages of AD, the patient is unable to work, is easily lost and confused, and requires daily supervision. Language becomes impaired—first naming, then comprehension, and finally fluency. Word-finding difficulties and circumlocution can be evident in the early stages, even when formal testing demonstrates intact naming and fluency. *Apraxia* emerges, and patients have trouble performing learned sequential motor tasks. Visuospatial deficits begin to interfere with dressing, eating, or even walking, and patients fail to solve simple puzzles or copy geometric figures. Simple calculations and clock reading become difficult in parallel.

In the late stages, some persons remain ambulatory, wandering aimlessly. Loss of judgment and reasoning is inevitable. Delusions are common, usually simple, with common themes of theft, infidelity, or misidentification. Approximately 10% of AD patients develop *Capgras' syndrome*, believing that a caregiver has been replaced by an impostor. In contrast to dementia with Lewy bodies (DLB), where Capgras' syndrome is an early feature, in AD this syndrome emerges late. Disinhibition and uncharacteristic belligerence may occur and alternate with passivity and withdrawal. Sleep-wake patterns are disrupted, and nighttime wandering becomes disturbing to the household. Some patients develop a shuffling gait with generalized muscle rigidity associated with slowness and awkwardness of movement. Patients often look parkinsonian (Chap. 449) but rarely have a high-amplitude, low-frequency tremor at rest. There is a strong overlap between Parkinson's disease (PD) and AD, and some AD patients develop more classical PD features.

In the end stages, AD patients become rigid, mute, incontinent, and bedridden, and help is needed with eating, dressing, and toileting. Hyperactive tendon reflexes and myoclonic jerks (sudden brief contractions of various muscles or the whole body) may occur spontaneously or in response to physical or auditory stimulation. Often death results from malnutrition, secondary infections, pulmonary emboli, heart disease, or, most commonly, aspiration. The typical duration of AD is 8–10 years, but the course ranges from 1 to 25 years. For unknown reasons, some patients with AD show a steady decline in function while others have prolonged plateaus without major deterioration.

DIFFERENTIAL DIAGNOSIS

Early in the disease course, other etiologies of dementia should be excluded (see Tables 35-1, 35-3, and 35-4). Neuroimaging studies (computed tomography [CT] and magnetic resonance imaging [MRI]) do not show a single specific pattern with AD and may be normal early in the disease. As AD progresses, more distributed but usually posterior-predominant cortical atrophy becomes apparent, along with atrophy of the medial temporal memory structures (see Chap. 35, Fig. 35-1). The main purpose of imaging is to exclude other disorders, such as primary and secondary neoplasms, vascular dementia, diffuse white matter disease, and normal-pressure hydrocephalus (NPH). Imaging also helps to distinguish AD from other degenerative disorders, such as frontotemporal dementia (FTD) or Creutzfeldt-Jacob disease (CJD), which feature distinctive imaging patterns. Functional imaging studies, such as positron emission tomography (PET), reveal hypometabolism in the posterior temporal-parietal cortex in AD (see Fig. 35-1). PET can also be used to detect the presence of fibrillar amyloid in the brain (see Fig. 35-4), and amyloid PET positivity is becoming required for entry into treatment trials for AD. Barriers to interpretation continue, however, to limit the use of amyloid PET in routine clinical evaluation. Although amyloid binding with PET is typical for AD, many asymptomatic healthy older individuals show amyloid uptake, and the likelihood that these individuals will convert to clinical AD is still under study. Similarly, dementia due to a non-AD disorder can be the underlying etiology in a patient who is amyloid positive on imaging. Electroencephalogram (EEG) is normal or shows nonspecific slowing; prolonged EEG can be used to seek out intermittent nonconvulsive seizures. Routine spinal fluid examination is also normal. Cerebrospinal fluid (CSF) $A\beta_{42}$ level is reduced, whereas the tau protein is elevated, but the test characteristics of these assays still make interpretation challenging in individual patients. *Slowly progressive decline in memory and orientation, normal results on laboratory tests, and an MRI or CT scan showing only distributed or posteriorly predominant cortical and hippocampal atrophy are highly suggestive of AD.* A clinical diagnosis of AD reached after careful evaluation is confirmed at autopsy about 90% of the time, with misdiagnosed cases usually representing one of the other dementing disorders described later in this chapter, a mixture of AD with vascular pathology, or DLB.

Simple clinical clues are useful in the differential diagnosis. Early prominent gait disturbance with only mild memory loss suggests vascular dementia or, rarely, NPH (see below). Resting tremor with stooped posture, bradykinesia, and masked facies suggest PD (Chap. 449). When dementia occurs after a well-established diagnosis of PD, PD dementia (PDD) is usually the correct diagnosis, but many patients with this diagnosis will show a mixture of AD and Lewy body disease at autopsy. The early appearance of parkinsonian features in association with fluctuating alertness, visual hallucinations, or delusional misidentification suggests DLB. Chronic alcoholism should prompt the search for vitamin deficiency. Loss of joint position and vibration sensibility accompanied by Babinski signs suggests vitamin B_{12} deficiency (Chap. 456). Early onset of a focal seizure suggests a metastatic or primary brain neoplasm (Chap. 118). Previous or ongoing depression raises suspicion for depression-related cognitive impairment, although AD can feature a depressive prodrome. A history of treatment for insomnia, anxiety, psychiatric disturbance, or epilepsy suggests chronic drug intoxication. Rapid progression over a few weeks or months associated with rigidity and myoclonus suggests CJD (Chap. 453e). Prominent behavioral changes with intact navigation and focal anterior-predominant atrophy on brain imaging are typical of FTD. A positive family history of dementia suggests either one of the familial forms of AD or one of the other genetic disorders associated with dementia, such as FTD (see below), HD (see below), prion disease (Chap. 453e), or rare hereditary ataxias (Chap. 450).

EPIDEMIOLOGY

The most important risk factors for AD are old age and a positive family history. The prevalence of AD increases with each decade of adult life, reaching 20–40% of the population over the age of 85. A positive family history of dementia suggests a genetic contribution to AD, although autosomal dominant inheritance occurs in only 2% of patients. Female sex is a risk factor independent of the greater longevity of women, and women who carry an Apo ε4 allele are more susceptible than are male ε4 carriers. A history of head trauma with concussion increases the risk for AD. AD is more common in groups with low educational attainment, but education influences test-taking ability, and it is clear that AD can affect persons of all intellectual levels. One study found that the capacity to express complex written language in early adulthood correlated with a decreased risk for AD. Numerous environmental factors, including aluminum, mercury, and viruses, have been proposed as causes of AD, but rigorous studies have failed to demonstrate to a significant role for any of these exposures. Similarly, several studies suggest that the use of nonsteroidal anti-inflammatory agents is associated with a decreased risk of AD, but this risk has not been confirmed in large prospective studies. Vascular disease, and stroke in particular, seems to lower the threshold for the clinical expression of AD. Also, in many patients with AD, amyloid angiopathy can lead to microhemorrhages, large lobar hemorrhages, ischemic infarctions most often in the subcortical white matter, or in rare cases an inflammatory leukoencephalopathy. Diabetes increases the risk of AD threefold. Elevated homocysteine and cholesterol levels; hypertension; diminished serum levels of folic acid; low dietary intake of fruits, vegetables, and red wine; and low levels of exercise are all being explored as potential risk factors for AD.

PATHOLOGY

At autopsy, the earliest and most severe degeneration is usually found in the medial temporal lobe (entorhinal/perirhinal cortex and hippocampus), lateral temporal cortex, and nucleus basalis of Meynert. The characteristic microscopic findings are neuritic plaques and NFTs (Fig. 448-1). These lesions may accumulate in small numbers during

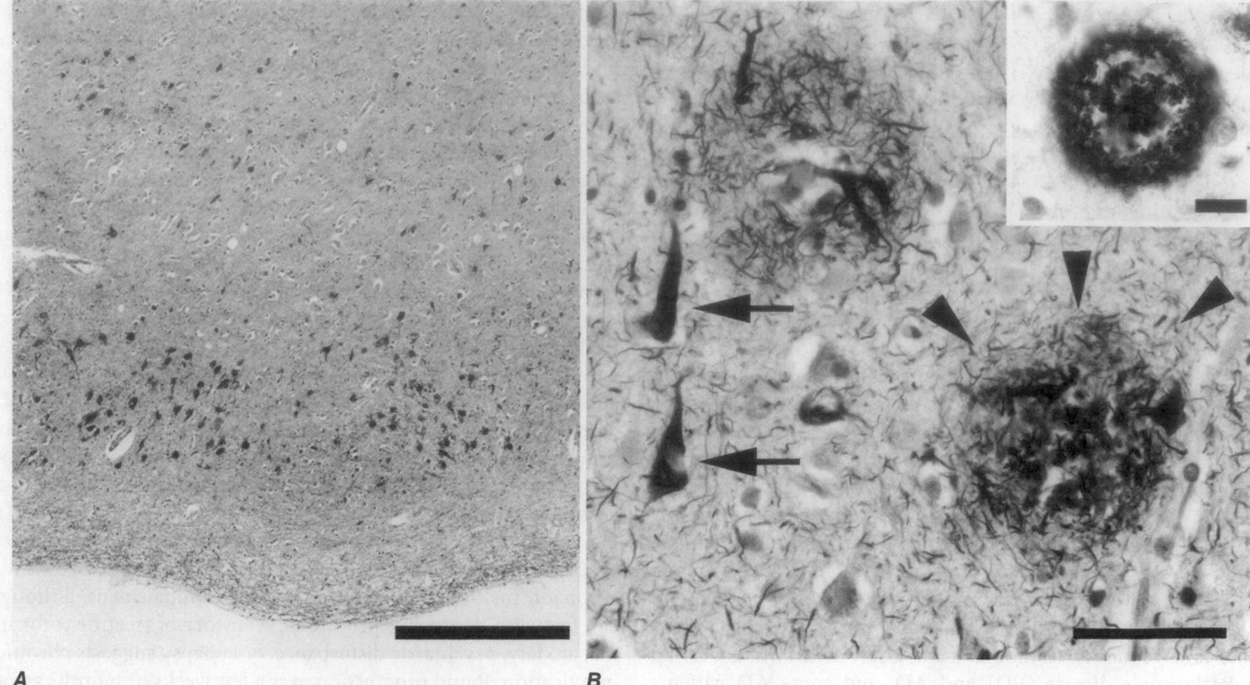

FIGURE 448-1 Neuropathology of Alzheimer's disease. ***A.*** Early neurofibrillary degeneration, consisting of neurofibrillary tangles and neuropil threads, preferentially affects the medial temporal lobes, especially the stellate pyramidal neurons that compose the layer 2 islands of entorhinal cortex, as shown. ***B.*** Higher magnification view reveals the fibrillary nature of tangles (*arrows*) and the complex structure of neuritic plaques (*arrowheads*), whose major component is Aβ (*inset* shows immunohistochemistry for Aβ). Scale bars are 500 μM in ***A***, 50 μM in ***B***, and 20 μM in ***B*** inset.

normal brain aging but dominate the picture in AD. Increasing evidence suggests that soluble amyloid species called *oligomers* may cause cellular dysfunction and represent the early toxic molecule in AD. Eventually, further amyloid polymerization and fibril formation lead to neuritic plaques, which contain a central core of amyloid, proteoglycans, Apo ε4, α-antichymotrypsin, and other proteins. Aβ is a protein of 39–42 amino acids that is derived proteolytically from a larger transmembrane protein, *amyloid precursor protein* (APP), when APP is cleaved by β and γ secretases (Fig. 448-2). The normal function of the Aβ peptides remains uncertain. APP has neurotrophic and neuroprotective properties. The plaque core is surrounded by a halo, which contains dystrophic, tau-immunoreactive neurites and activated microglia. The accumulation of Aβ in cerebral arterioles is termed *amyloid angiopathy*. NFTs are composed of silver-staining neuronal cytoplasmic fibrils composed of abnormally phosphorylated tau protein; they appear as paired helical filaments by electron microscopy. Tau binds to and stabilizes microtubules, supporting axonal transport of organelles, glycoproteins, neurotransmitters, and other important cargoes throughout the neuron. Once hyperphosphorylated, tau can no longer bind properly to microtubules and redistributes from the axon to throughout the neuronal cytoplasm and distal dendrites, compromising function. Finally, patients with AD often show comorbid DLB or vascular pathology. In animal models of AD, diminishing neuronal tau ameliorates the cognitive deficits and seizures, even though $A\beta_{42}$ continues to accumulate, raising hope for tau-lowering therapies in humans. Biochemically, AD is associated with a decrease in the cortical levels of several proteins and neurotransmitters, especially acetylcholine, its synthetic enzyme choline acetyltransferase, and nicotinic cholinergic receptors. Reduction of acetylcholine reflects degeneration of cholinergic neurons in the nucleus basalis of Meynert that project throughout the cortex. There is also noradrenergic and serotonergic depletion due to degeneration of brainstem nuclei such as the locus coeruleus and dorsal raphe, where tau-immunoreactive neuronal cytoplasmic inclusions can be identified even in individuals lacking entorhinal cortex NFTs.

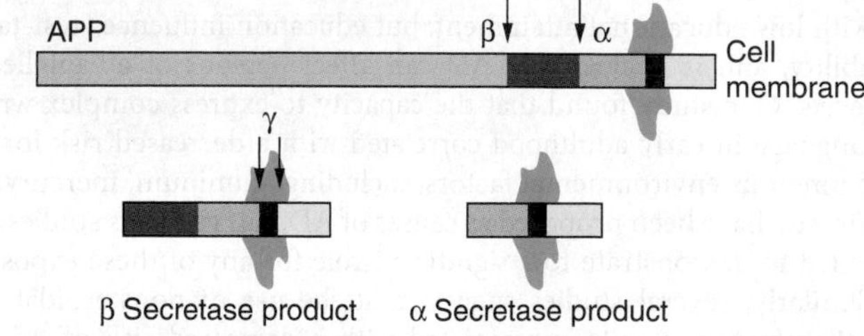

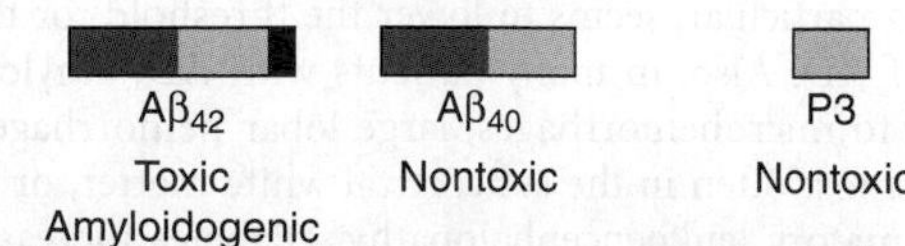

FIGURE 448-2 Amyloid precursor protein (APP) is catabolized by α, β, and γ secretases. A key initial step is the digestion by either β secretase (BASE) or α secretase (ADAM10 or ADAM17 [TACE]), producing smaller nontoxic products. Cleavage of the β secretase product by γ secretase (Step 2) results in either the toxic $A\beta_{42}$ or the nontoxic $A\beta_{40}$ peptide; cleavage of the α secretase product by γ secretase produces the nontoxic P3 peptide. Excess production of $A\beta_{42}$ is a key initiator of cellular damage in Alzheimer's disease (AD). Therapeutics for AD have focused on attempts to reduce accumulation of $A\beta_{42}$ by antagonizing β or γ secretases, promoting α secretase, or clearing $A\beta_{42}$ that has already formed by use of specific antibodies.

GENETIC CONSIDERATIONS

Several genes play an important role in the pathogenesis of AD. One is the *APP* gene on chromosome 21. Adults with trisomy 21 (Down's syndrome) consistently develop the typical neuropathologic hallmarks of AD if they survive beyond age 40 years, and many develop a progressive dementia superimposed on their baseline mental retardation. The extra dose of the *APP* gene on chromosome 21 is the initiating cause of AD in adult Down's syndrome and results in excess cerebral amyloid production. Supporting this hypothesis, some families with early age-of-onset familial AD (FAD) have point mutations in *APP*. Although very rare, these families were the first examples of single-gene autosomal dominant transmission of AD.

Investigation of large families with multigenerational FAD led to the discovery of two additional AD-causing genes, the *presenilins*. Presenilin-1 (*PS-1*) is on chromosome 14 and encodes a protein called S182. Mutations in this gene cause an early-age-of-onset AD, with onset before the age of 60 and often before age 50, transmitted in an autosomal dominant, highly penetrant fashion. More than 100 different mutations have been found in the *PS-1* gene in families from a wide range of ethnic backgrounds. Presenilin-2 (*PS-2*) is on chromosome 1 and encodes a protein called STM2. A mutation in the *PS-2* gene was first found in a group of American families with Volga German ethnic background. Mutations in *PS-1* are much more common than those in *PS-2*. The presenilins are highly homologous and encode similar proteins that at first appeared to have seven transmembrane domains (hence the designation *STM*), but subsequent studies have suggested eight such domains, with a ninth submembrane region. Both S182 and STM2 are cytoplasmic neuronal proteins that are widely expressed throughout the nervous system. They are homologous to a cell-trafficking protein, sel 12, found in the nematode *Caenorhabditis elegans*. Patients with mutations in the presenilin genes have elevated plasma levels of $A\beta_{42}$, and *PS-1* mutations produce increased $A\beta_{42}$ in the media in cell culture. There is evidence that *PS-1* is involved in the cleavage of APP at the γ secretase site and mutations in either gene (*PS-1* or *APP*) may disturb γ secretase cleavage. Mutations in *PS-1* are the most common cause of early-age-of-onset FAD, representing perhaps 40–70% of all cases. Mutations in *PS-1* tend to produce AD with an earlier age of onset (mean onset 45 years) and a shorter, more rapidly progressive course (mean duration 6–7 years) than the disease caused by mutations in *PS-2* (mean onset 53 years; duration 11 years). Although some carriers of *PS-2* mutations have had onset of dementia after the age of 70, mutations in the presenilins rarely lead to late-age-of-onset AD. Clinical genetic testing for these uncommon mutations is available but likely to be revealing only in early-age-of-onset FAD and should be performed in association with formal genetic counseling.

The *Apo* ε gene on chromosome 19 is involved in the pathogenesis of AD. The protein, apolipoprotein E, participates in cholesterol transport (Chap. 421), and the gene has three alleles: ε2, ε3, and ε4. The Apo ε4 allele confers increased risk of AD in the general population, including sporadic and late-age-of-onset familial forms. Approximately 24–30% of the nondemented white population has at least one ε4 allele (12–15% allele frequency), and about 2% are ε4/ε4 homozygotes. Among patients with AD, 40–65% have at least one ε4 allele, a highly significant elevation compared with controls. Conversely, many AD patients have no ε4 allele, and ε4 carriers may never develop AD. Therefore, ε4 is neither necessary nor sufficient to cause AD. Nevertheless, the Apo ε4 allele represents the most important genetic risk factor for sporadic AD and acts as a dose-dependent disease modifier, with the earliest age of onset associated with the ε4 homozygosity. Precise mechanisms through which Apo ε4 confers AD risk or hastens onset remain unclear, but ε4 leads to less efficient amyloid clearance and to the production of toxic fragments from cleavage of the molecule. Apo ε can be identified in neuritic plaques and may also be involved in neurofibrillary tangle formation, because it binds to tau protein. Apo ε4 decreases neurite outgrowth in dorsal root ganglion neuronal cultures, perhaps indicating a deleterious role in the brain's response to injury. Some evidence suggests that the ε2 allele may reduce AD risk. Use of Apo ε testing in AD diagnosis remains controversial. It is not indicated as a predictive test in normal persons because its precise predictive value is unclear, and many individuals with the ε4 allele never develop dementia. Many cognitively normal ε4 heterozygotes and homozygotes show decreased cerebral cortical metabolic function with PET, suggesting presymptomatic abnormalities due to AD or an inherited vulnerability of the AD-targeted network. In demented persons who meet clinical criteria for AD, finding an ε4 allele increases the reliability of diagnosis; however, the absence of an ε4 allele cannot be considered evidence against AD. Furthermore, all patients with dementia, including those with an ε4 allele, require a search for reversible causes of their cognitive impairment. Nevertheless, Apo ε4 remains the single most important biologic marker associated with AD risk, and studies of ε4's functional role and diagnostic utility are progressing rapidly. The ε4 allele is not associated with risk for FTD, DLB, or CJD, although some evidence suggests that ε4 may exacerbate the phenotype of non-AD degenerative disorders, head trauma, and other brain injuries. Additional genes are also likely to be involved in AD, especially as minor risk alleles for sporadic forms of the disease. Genome-wide association studies have implicated the clusterin (*CLU*), phosphatidylinositol-binding clathrin assembly protein (*PICALM*), and complement component (3b/4b) receptor 1 (*CR1*) genes. *CLU* may play a role in synapse turnover, *PICALM* participates in clathrin-mediated endocytosis, and *CR1* may be involved in amyloid clearance through the complement pathway. *TREM2* is a gene involved with inflammation that increases the likelihood of dementia. Homozygous mutation carriers develop a frontal dementia with bone cysts (Nasu-Hakola disease), whereas heterozygotes are predisposed to the development of AD.

TREATMENT ALZHEIMER'S DISEASE

The management of AD is challenging and gratifying despite the absence of a cure or a robust pharmacologic treatment. The primary focus is on long-term amelioration of associated behavioral and neurologic problems, as well as providing caregiver support.

Building rapport with the patient, family members, and other caregivers is essential to successful management. In the early stages of AD, memory aids such as notebooks and posted daily reminders can be helpful. Family members should emphasize activities that are pleasant while curtailing those that increase stress on the patient. Kitchens, bathrooms, stairways, and bedrooms need to be made safe, and eventually patients will need to stop driving. Loss of independence and change of environment may worsen confusion, agitation, and anger. Communication and repeated calm reassurance are necessary. Caregiver "burnout" is common, often resulting in nursing home placement of the patient or new health problems for the caregiver. Respite breaks for the caregiver help to maintain a successful long-term therapeutic milieu. Use of adult day care centers can be helpful. Local and national support groups, such as the Alzheimer's Association and the Family Caregiver Alliance, are valuable resources. Internet access to these resources has become available to clinicians and families in recent years.

Donepezil (target dose, 10 mg daily), rivastigmine (target dose, 6 mg twice daily or 9.5-mg patch daily), galantamine (target dose 24 mg daily, extended-release), and memantine (target dose, 10 mg twice daily) are approved by the Food and Drug Administration (FDA) for the treatment of AD. Due to hepatotoxicity, tacrine is no longer used. Dose escalations for each of these medications must be carried out over 4–6 weeks to minimize side effects. The pharmacologic action of donepezil, rivastigmine, and galantamine is inhibition of the cholinesterases, primarily acetylcholinesterase, with a resulting increase in cerebral acetylcholine levels. Memantine appears to act by blocking overexcited *N*-methyl-D-aspartate (NMDA) glutamate receptors. Double-blind, placebo-controlled, crossover studies with cholinesterase inhibitors and memantine in moderate to severe AD have shown them to be associated with improved caregiver ratings of patients' functioning and with an apparent decreased rate of decline in cognitive test scores over periods of up to 3 years. The average patient on an anticholinesterase inhibitor maintains his or her mini-mental state examination (MMSE) score for close to a year, whereas a placebo-treated patient declines 2–3 points over the same time period. Memantine, used in conjunction with cholinesterase inhibitors or by itself, slows cognitive deterioration and decreases caregiver burden for patients with moderate to severe AD but is not approved for mild AD. Each of these compounds has only modest efficacy for AD. Cholinesterase inhibitors are relatively easy to administer, and their major side effects are gastrointestinal symptoms (nausea, diarrhea, cramps), altered sleep with unpleasant or vivid dreams, bradycardia (usually benign), and muscle cramps.

In a prospective observational study, the use of estrogen replacement therapy appeared to protect—by about 50%—against development of AD in women. This study seemed to confirm the results of two earlier case-controlled studies. Sadly, a prospective placebo-controlled study of a combined estrogen-progesterone therapy for asymptomatic postmenopausal women increased, rather than decreased, the prevalence of dementia. This study markedly dampened enthusiasm for hormonal treatments to prevent dementia. Additionally, no benefit has been found in the treatment of AD with estrogen alone.

A controlled trial of an extract of *Ginkgo biloba* found modest improvement in cognitive function in subjects with AD and vascular dementia. Unfortunately, a comprehensive 6-year multicenter prevention study using ginkgo found no slowing of progression to dementia in the treated group.

Vaccination against $A\beta_{42}$ has proved highly efficacious in mouse models of AD, helping clear brain amyloid and preventing further amyloid accumulation. In human trials, this approach led to life-threatening complications, including meningoencephalitis, in a minority of patients. Another experimental approach to AD treatment has been the use of β and γ secretase inhibitors that diminish the production of $A\beta_{42}$, but the first two placebo-controlled trials of γ secretase inhibitors, tarenflurbil and semagacestat, were negative, and semagacestat may have accelerated cognitive decline compared to placebo. Passive immunization with monoclonal antibodies against $A\beta_{42}$ has been tried in mild to moderate AD. These studies were negative, leading some to suggest that the patients treated were too advanced to respond to amyloid-lowering therapies. Therefore, new trials have started in asymptomatic individuals with mild AD, in asymptomatic autosomal dominant forms of AD, and in cognitively normal elderly who are amyloid positive with PET. Medications that modify tau phosphorylation and aggregation, including tau antibodies, are beginning to be studied as possible treatments for both AD and non-AD tau-related disorders including FTD and progressive supranuclear palsy.

Several retrospective studies suggest that nonsteroidal anti-inflammatory agents and 3-hydroxy-3-methylglutaryl-coenzyme A (HMG-CoA) reductase inhibitors (statins) may have a protective effect on dementia if used prior to the onset of disease but do not influence clinically symptomatic AD. Finally, there is now a strong interest in the relationship between diabetes and AD, and insulin-regulating studies are being conducted.

Mild to moderate depression is common in the early stages of AD and may respond to antidepressants or cholinesterase inhibitors. Selective serotonin reuptake inhibitors (SSRIs) are commonly used due to their low anticholinergic side effects (for example, escitalopram, target dose 5–10 mg daily). Seizures can be treated with levetiracetam unless the patient had a different regimen that was effective prior to the onset of AD. Agitation, insomnia, hallucinations, and belligerence are especially troublesome characteristics of some AD patients, and these behaviors can lead to nursing home placement. The newer generation of atypical antipsychotics, such as risperidone, quetiapine, and olanzapine, are being used in low doses to treat these neuropsychiatric symptoms. The few controlled studies comparing drugs against behavioral intervention in the treatment of agitation suggest mild efficacy with significant side effects related to sleep, gait, and cardiovascular complications, including an increased risk of death. All antipsychotics carry a black box FDA warning and should be used with caution in the demented elderly; however, careful, daily, nonpharmacologic behavior management is often not available, rendering medications necessary for some patients. Finally, medications with strong anticholinergic effects should be vigilantly avoided, including prescription and over-the-counter sleep aids (e.g., diphenhydramine) or incontinence therapies (e.g., oxybutynin).

VASCULAR DEMENTIA

Dementia associated with cerebrovascular disease can be divided into two general categories: multi-infarct dementia and diffuse white matter disease (also called *leukoaraiosis, subcortical arteriosclerotic leukoencephalopathy*, or *Binswanger's disease*). Cerebrovascular disease appears to be a more common cause of dementia in Asia than in Europe and North America, perhaps due to the increased prevalence of intracranial atherosclerosis. Individuals who have had strokes may develop chronic cognitive deficits, commonly called *multi-infarct dementia*. The strokes may be large or small (sometimes lacunar) and usually involve several different brain regions. The occurrence of dementia depends partly on the total volume of damaged cortex. Patients typically report previous discrete episodes of sudden neurologic deterioration. Many patients with multi-infarct dementia have a history of hypertension, diabetes, coronary artery disease, or other manifestations of widespread atherosclerosis. Physical examination may show focal neurologic deficits such as hemiparesis, a unilateral Babinski sign, a visual field defect, or pseudobulbar palsy. Recurrent strokes result in a stepwise disease progression. Neuroimaging reveals multiple areas of infarction. Thus, the history and neuroimaging findings differentiate this condition from AD; however, both AD and multiple infarctions are common and sometimes co-occur. With normal aging, there is also an accumulation of amyloid in cerebral blood vessels, leading to a condition called *cerebral amyloid angiopathy* (without dementia), which predisposes older persons to lobar hemorrhage and brain microhemorrhages. AD patients appear to be at increased risk for amyloid angiopathy, and this association may explain some of the observed links between AD and stroke.

Some individuals with dementia are discovered on MRI to have bilateral T2 signal hyperintensities in the subcortical white matter, termed *diffuse white matter disease*, often occurring in association with lacunar infarctions (see Fig. 35-2). The dementia may be insidious in onset and progress slowly, features that distinguish it from multi-infarct dementia, but other patients show a stepwise deterioration more typical of multi-infarct dementia. Early symptoms include mild confusion, apathy, anxiety, psychosis, and memory, spatial, or executive deficits. Marked difficulties in judgment and orientation and dependence on others for daily activities develop later. Euphoria, elation, depression, or aggressive behaviors are common as the disease progresses. Pyramidal and cerebellar signs may be present, and a gait disorder is seen in at least half of these patients. With advanced disease, urinary incontinence and dysarthria with or without other pseudobulbar features (e.g., dysphagia, emotional lability) are frequent. Seizures and myoclonic jerks appear in a minority of patients. Often, this disorder results from chronic ischemia due to occlusive disease of small, penetrating cerebral arteries and arterioles (microangiopathy). Any disease-causing stenosis of small cerebral vessels may be the critical underlying factor, although hypertension is the major cause. The term *Binswanger's disease* should be used with caution, because it does not clearly identify a single entity.

Other rare causes of white matter disease also present with dementia, such as adult metachromatic leukodystrophy (arylsulfatase A deficiency) and progressive multifocal leukoencephalopathy (Chap. 164). A dominantly inherited form of white matter disease is known as *cerebral autosomal dominant arteriopathy with subcortical infarcts and leukoencephalopathy* (CADASIL), discussed later in "Other Causes of Dementia."

Mitochondrial disorders can present with stroke-like episodes and can selectively injure basal ganglia or cortex. Many such patients show other findings suggestive of a neurologic or systemic disorder such as ophthalmoplegia, retinal degeneration, deafness, myopathy, neuropathy, or diabetes. Diagnosis is difficult, but serum or (especially) CSF levels of lactate and pyruvate may be abnormal, and biopsy of affected tissue, preferably muscle, may be diagnostic.

Treatment of vascular dementia must be focused on preventing new ischemic injury by stabilizing or removing the underlying causes, such as hypertension, diabetes, smoking, or lack of exercise. Recovery of lost cognitive function is not likely, although fluctuations with periods of improvement are common.

FRONTOTEMPORAL LOBAR DEGENERATION SPECTRUM

Frontotemporal dementia (FTD) refers to a group of clinical syndromes united by underlying frontotemporal lobar degeneration (FTLD) pathology. FTD most often begins in the fifth to seventh decades and

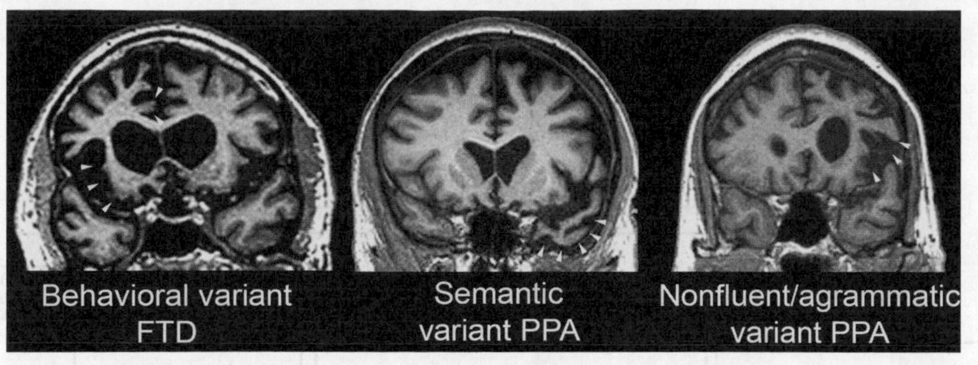

FIGURE 448-3 Three major frontotemporal dementia (FTD) clinical syndromes. Coronal magnetic resonance imaging sections from representative patients with behavioral variant FTD (*left*), semantic dementia (*center*), and progressive nonfluent aphasia (*right*). Areas of early and severe atrophy in each syndrome are highlighted (*white arrowheads*). The behavioral variant features anterior cingulate and frontoinsular atrophy, spreading to orbital and dorsolateral prefrontal cortex. Semantic variant primary progressive aphasia (PPA) shows prominent temporopolar atrophy, more often on the left. Nonfluent/agrammatic variant PPA is associated with dominant frontal opercular and dorsal insula degeneration.

is nearly as prevalent as AD in this age group. Early studies suggested that FTD may be more common in men than women, although more recent reports cast doubt on this finding. Although a family history of dementia is common, autosomal dominant inheritance is seen in only 10–20% of all FTD cases.

The clinical heterogeneity seen in familial and sporadic FTD is remarkable. Three core clinical syndromes have been described (Fig. 448-3). In the behavioral variant (bvFTD), the most common FTD syndrome, social and emotional systems dysfunction manifests as apathy, disinhibition, compulsivity, loss of empathy, and overeating, often but not always accompanied by deficits in executive control. Two forms of primary progressive aphasia (PPA), the semantic and nonfluent/agrammatic variants, are commonly due to FTLD and included under the FTD umbrella. In the semantic variant, patients slowly lose the ability to decode word, object, person-specific, and emotion meaning, whereas patients with the nonfluent/agrammatic variant develop profound inability to produce words, often with prominent motor speech impairment. Any of these three clinical syndromes, but most often bvFTD, may be accompanied by motor neuron disease (MND), in which case the term FTD-MND is applied. In addition, the corticobasal syndrome (CBS) and progressive supranuclear palsy syndrome (PSP-S) can be considered part of the FTLD clinical spectrum. Furthermore, patients may evolve from any of the major syndromes described above to have prominent features of another syndrome.

Findings at the bedside are dictated by the anatomic localization of the disorder. Right hemisphere-predominant or symmetric anterior cingulate/medial prefrontal, orbital, and anterior insular degeneration predicts bvFTD. Patients with nonfluent/agrammatic PPA show left (dominant) frontal opercular and precentral gyrus degeneration, whereas left anterior temporal atrophy presents with semantic variant PPA. Visuoconstructive ability, arithmetic calculations, and navigation may remain normal late into any FTD syndrome. Many patients with nonfluent aphasia or bvFTD later develop PSP-S, as disease spreads into diencephalic and brainstem structures, or CBS-like features, as disease moves into dorsal and lateral perirolandic cortices.

The most common autosomal dominantly inherited mutations causing FTD involve the *C9ORF72* (chromosome 9), *GRN* (chromosome 17), and *MAPT* (chromosome 17) genes. Hexanucleotide (GGGGCC) expansions in the noncoding portion of *C9ORF72* are the most recently identified and represent the most common genetic cause of familial or sporadic FTD (usually presenting as bvFTD with or without MND) and amyotrophic lateral sclerosis (ALS). The expansion is associated with reduced *C9ORF72* mRNA expression, nuclear mRNA foci containing transcribed portions of the expansion and other mRNAs, neuronal cytoplasmic inclusions containing dipeptide repeat proteins translated from the repeat mRNA, and transactive response DNA-binding protein of 43 kDa (TDP-43) neuronal cytoplasmic and glial inclusions. The pathogenic significance of these various features is a topic of vigorous investigation. *MAPT* mutations lead to a change in the alternate splicing of tau or cause loss of function in the tau molecule, thereby altering microtubule binding. With *GRN*, mutations in the coding sequence of the gene encoding progranulin protein result in mRNA degradation due to nonsense-mediated decay, providing a rare example of an autosomal dominant mutation that leads to haploinsufficiency and leads to a ~50% reduction in circulating progranulin protein levels. Intriguingly, a patient with *GRN* mutations on both chromosomes was recently reported to develop neuronal ceroid lipofuscinosis, focusing investigators on the lysosome as a site of molecular dysfunction in *GRN*-related FTD. Progranulin is a growth factor that binds to tumor necrosis factor (TNF) receptors and participates in tissue repair and tumor growth. How progranulin mutations lead to FTD remains unknown, but the most likely mechanisms include lysosomal dysfunction and enhanced neuroinflammation. Both *MAPT* and *GRN* mutations are associated with parkinsonian features, whereas ALS is rare. Infrequently, mutations in the valosin-containing protein (*VCP*, chromosome 9) and charged multivesicular body protein 2b (*CHMP2b*, chromosome 3) genes also lead to autosomal dominant familial FTD. Mutations in the *TARDBP* (encoding TDP-43) and *FUS* (encoding fused in sarcoma [FUS]) genes (see below) cause familial ALS, sometimes in association with an FTD syndrome, although a few patients presenting with FTD alone have been reported.

The gross pathologic hallmark of FTLD is a focal atrophy of frontal, insular, and/or temporal cortex, which can be visualized with neuroimaging studies (Fig. 448-3) and is often profound at autopsy. Despite the appearance of advanced disease, however, imaging studies suggest that atrophy often begins focally in one hemisphere before spreading to anatomically interconnected regions, including basal ganglia. Loss of cortical serotonergic innervation is seen in many patients. In contrast to AD, the cholinergic system is relatively spared in FTD, which accounts for the poor efficacy of acetylcholinesterase inhibitors in this group.

Although early studies suggested that 15–30% of patients with FTD showed underlying AD at autopsy, progressive refinement in clinical diagnosis has improved pathologic prediction accuracy, and most patients diagnosed with FTD at a dementia clinic with expertise in FTD will show underlying FTLD pathology. Microscopic findings seen across all patients with FTLD include gliosis, microvacuolation, and neuronal loss, but the disease is subtyped according to the protein composition of neuronal and glial inclusions, which contain either tau or TDP-43 in ~90% of patients, with the remaining ~10% showing inclusions containing FUS (Fig. 448-4).

The toxicity and spreading capacity of tau aggregates underlies the pathogenesis of many familial cases and is emerging as a key factor in sporadic tauopathies, although loss of tau microtubule stabilizing function may also play a role. TDP-43 and FUS, in contrast, are RNA/DNA binding proteins whose roles in neuronal function are still being actively investigated, but one key role may be the chaperoning of

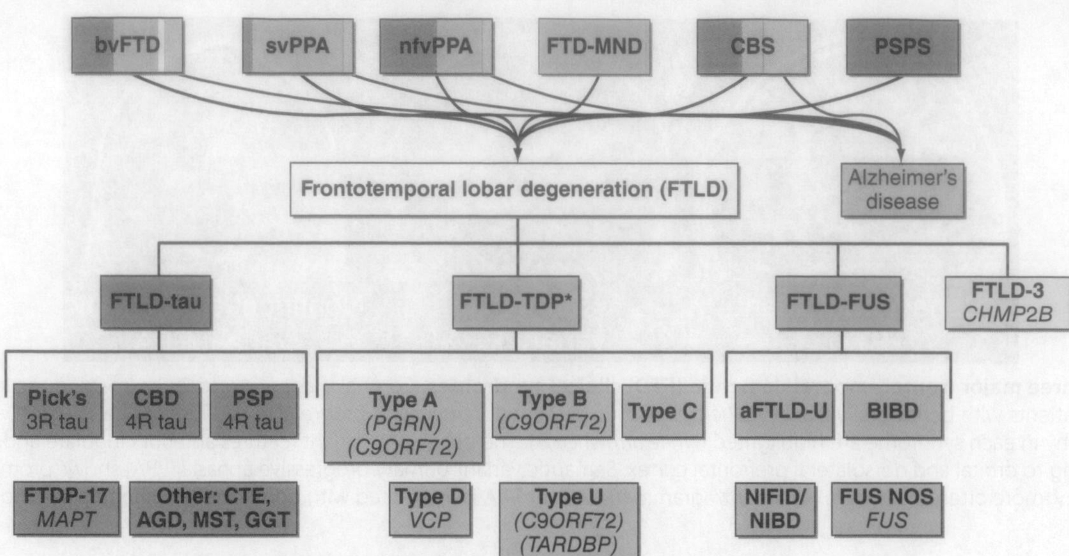

FIGURE 448-4 Frontotemporal dementia syndromes are united by underlying frontotemporal lobar degeneration pathology, which can be divided according to the presence of tau, TPD-43, or FUS-containing inclusions in neurons and glia. Correlations between clinical syndromes and major molecular classes are shown with colored shading. Despite improvements in clinical syndromic diagnosis, a small percentage of patients with some frontotemporal dementia syndromes will show Alzheimer's disease neuropathology at autopsy (*gray shading*). aFTLD-U, atypical frontotemporal lobar degeneration with ubiquitin-positive inclusions; AGD, argyrophilic grain disease; BIBD, basophilic inclusion body disease; bvFTD, behavioral variant frontotemporal dementia; CBD, corticobasal degeneration; CBS, corticobasal syndrome; CTE, chronic traumatic encephalopathy; FTD-MND, frontotemporal dementia with motor neuron disease; FTDP-17, frontotemporal dementia with parkinsonism linked to chromosome 17; FUS, fused in sarcoma; GGT, globular glial tauopathy; MST, multisystem tauopathy; nfvPPA, nonfluent/agrammatic variant primary progressive aphasia; NIBD, neurofilament inclusion body disease; NIFID, neuronal intermediate filament inclusion disease; PSP, progressive supranuclear palsy; PSPS, progressive supranuclear palsy syndrome; svPPA, semantic variant primary progressive aphasia; Type U, unclassifiable type.

mRNAs to the distal neuron for activity-dependent translation within dendritic spines. Because these proteins also form intracellular aggregates and produce similar anatomic progression, protein toxicity and spreading may also factor heavily in the pathogenesis of these FTLD-TDP and FTLD-FUS.

Increasingly, misfolded proteins in neurodegenerative disease are being recognized as having "prion-like" properties in that they can template the misfolding of their natively folded protein counterparts, a process that creates exponential amplification of protein misfolding within a cell and may promote transcellular and even transsynaptic protein propagation between cells. This hypothesis could provide a unifying explanation for the stereotypical patterns of disease spread observed in each syndrome (Chap. 444e).

Although the term *Pick's disease* was once used to describe a progressive degenerative disorder characterized by selective involvement of the anterior frontal and temporal neocortex and pathologically by intraneuronal cytoplasmic inclusions (*Pick bodies*), it is now used only in reference to a specific FTLD-tau histopathologic entity. Classical Pick bodies are argyrophilic, staining positively with the Bielschowsky silver method (but not with the Gallyas method) and also with immunostaining for hyperphosphorylated tau. Recognition of the three FTLD major molecular classes has allowed delineation of distinct FTLD subtypes within each class. These subtypes, based on the morphology and distribution of the neuronal and glial inclusions (Fig. 448-5), account for the vast majority of patients, and some subtypes show strong clinical or genetic associations (Fig. 448-4). Despite this progress, available data do not allow reliable prediction of the underlying FTLD subtype, or even the major molecular class, based on clinical features alone. Molecular PET imaging with ligands chosen to bind misfolded tau protein shows great promise and is already being applied to the study of patients with AD and FTD. Because FTLD-tau and FTLD-TDP account for 90% of FTLD patients, the ability to detect pathologic tau protein deposition in vivo will greatly improve prediction accuracy, especially when amyloid PET imaging is negative.

The burden on caregivers of patients with FTD is extremely high, especially when the illness disrupts core emotional and personality functions of the loved one. Treatment is symptomatic, and there are currently no therapies known to slow progression or improve symptoms. Many of the behaviors that may accompany FTD, such as depression, hyperorality, compulsions, and irritability, can be ameliorated with antidepressants, especially SSRIs. The co-association with motor disorders such as parkinsonism necessitates the careful use of antipsychotics, which can exacerbate this problem.

Progressive supranuclear palsy syndrome (PSP-S; also known as Steele-Richardson-Olszewski syndrome) is a degenerative disorder that involves the brainstem, basal ganglia, limbic structures, and selected areas of cortex. Clinically, PSP-S begins with falls and executive or subtle personality changes (such as mental rigidity, impulsivity, or apathy). Shortly thereafter, a progressive oculomotor syndrome ensues that begins with square wave jerks, followed by slowed saccades (vertical worse than horizontal) before resulting in progressive supranuclear ophthalmoparesis. Dysarthria, dysphagia, and symmetric axial rigidity can be prominent features that emerge at any point in the illness. A stiff, unstable posture with hyperextension of the neck and a slow, jerky, toppling gait are characteristic. Frequent unexplained and sometimes spectacular falls are common secondary to a combination of axial rigidity, inability to look down, and poor judgment. Even once patients have severely limited voluntary eye movements, they retain oculocephalic reflexes (demonstrated using a vertical doll's head maneuver); thus, the oculomotor disorder is supranuclear. The dementia overlaps with bvFTD, featuring apathy, frontal-executive dysfunction, poor judgment, slowed thought processes, impaired verbal fluency, and difficulty with sequential actions and with shifting from one task to another. These features are common at presentation and often precede the motor syndrome. Some patients with a pathologic diagnosis of PSP begin with a nonfluent aphasia or motor speech disorder and progress to classical PSP-S. Response to L-dopa is limited or absent; no other treatments exist. Death occurs within 5–10 years of onset. Like Pick's disease, increasingly the term PSP is used to refer to a specific histopathologic entity within the FTLD-tau class. In PSP, accumulation of hyperphosphorylated 4-repeat tau is seen within neurons and glia. Neuronal inclusions often take the form of NFTs, which may

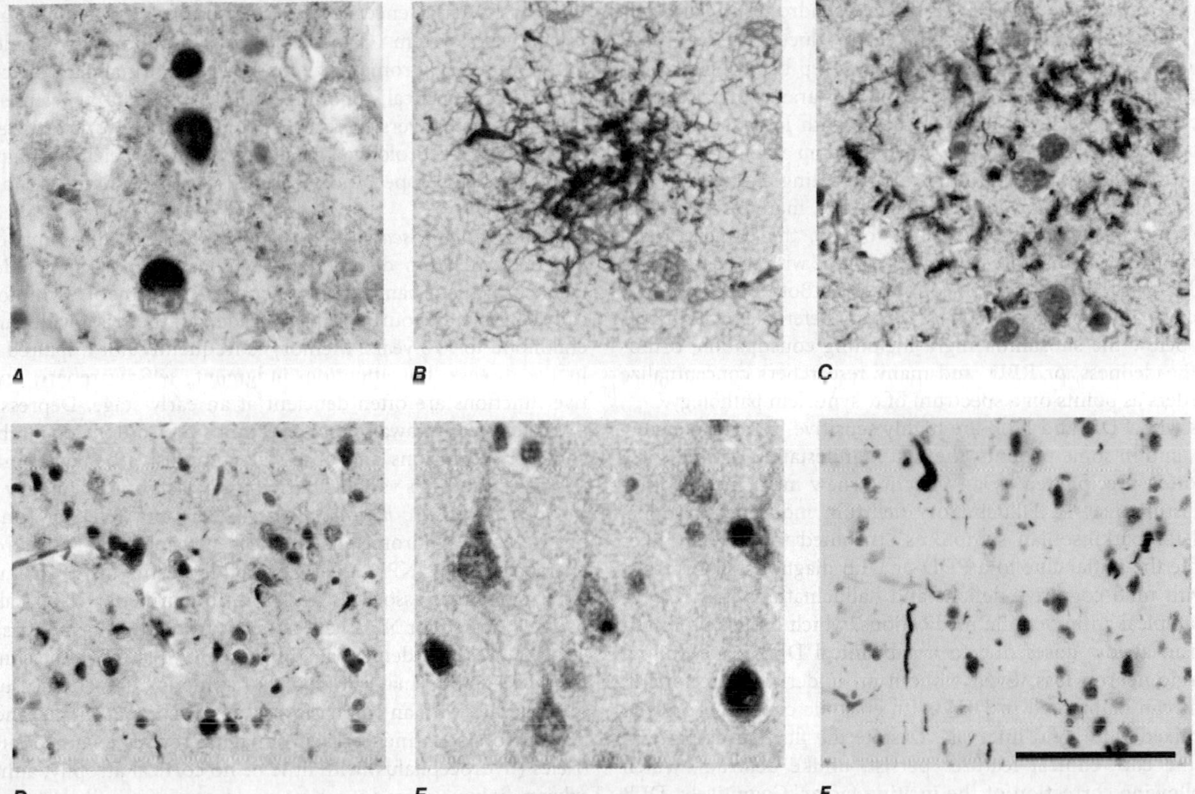

FIGURE 448-5 Neuropathology in frontotemporal lobar degeneration (FTLD). FTLD-tau (***A–C***) and FTLD-TDP (***D–F***) account for over 90% of patients with FTLD, and immunohistochemistry reveals characteristic lesions in each of the major histopathologic subtypes within each class: (***A***) Pick bodies in Pick's disease; (***B***) a tufted astrocyte in progressive supranuclear palsy; (***C***) an astrocytic plaque in corticobasal degeneration; (***D***) small compact or crescentic neuronal cytoplasmic inclusions and short, then neuropil threads in FTLD-TDP, type A; (***E***) diffuse/granular neuronal cytoplasmic inclusions (with a relative paucity of neuropil threads) in FTLD-TDP, type B; and (***F***) long, tortuous dystrophic neurites in FTLD-TDP, type C. TDP can be seen within the nucleus in neurons lacking inclusions but mislocalizes to the cytoplasm and forms inclusions in FTLD-TDP. Immunostains are 3-repeat tau (***A***), phospho-tau (***B*** and ***C***), and TDP-43 (***D–F***). Sections are counterstained with hematoxylin. Scale bar applies to all panels and represents 50 μm in ***A***, ***B***, ***C***, and ***E*** and 100 μm in ***D*** and ***F***.

be large, spherical ("globose"), and coarse in brainstem, cerebellar dentate, and diencephalic neurons. Tau deposition is most prominent in subcortical structures (including the subthalamic nucleus, globus pallidus, substantia nigra, locus coeruleus, periaqueductal gray, tectum, oculomotor nuclei, and dentate nucleus of cerebellum). Neocortical NFTs, like those in AD, often take on a more flame-shaped morphology, but on electron microscopy, PSP tangles can be shown to consist of straight tubules rather than the paired helical filaments found in AD. Furthermore, PSP is associated with prominent tau-positive glial pathologies, such as tufted astrocytes (Fig. 448-5), thorny astrocytes, and coiled oligodendroglial inclusions ("coiled bodies"). Most patients with PSP-S show PSP at autopsy, although small numbers will show another tauopathy (corticobasal degeneration [CBD] or Pick's disease; Fig. 448-4).

In addition to its overlap with FTD and CBS (see below), PSP is often confused with idiopathic *Parkinson's disease* (PD). Although elderly patients with PD may have restricted upgaze, they do not develop downgaze paresis or other abnormalities of voluntary eye movements typical of PSP. Dementia occurs in ~20% of patients with PD, often due to the emergence of a full-blown DLB-like syndrome. Furthermore, the behavioral syndromes seen with DLB differ from PSP (see below). Dementia in PD becomes more likely with increasing age, increasing severity of extrapyramidal signs, long disease duration, and the presence of depression. Patients with PD who develop dementia also show cortical atrophy on brain imaging. Neuropathologically, there may be AD-related changes in the cortex, LBD-related α-synuclein inclusions in both the limbic system and cortex, or no specific microscopic changes other than gliosis and neuronal loss. PD is discussed in detail in Chap. 449.

Corticobasal syndrome (CBS) is a slowly progressive dementia movement disorder associated with severe atrophy in perirolandic cortex and basal ganglia (substantia nigra and striatopallidum). Patients typically present with asymmetric onset of rigidity, dystonia, myoclonus, and apraxia of one limb, at times associated with *alien limb* phenomena in which the limb exhibits unintended motor actions such as grasping, groping, drifting, or undoing. Eventually CBS becomes bilateral and leads to dysarthria, slow gait, action tremor, and typically a frontal-predominant dementia. Whereas CBS refers to the clinical syndrome, CBD refers to a specific histopathologic FTLD-tau entity (Fig. 448-4). Although CBS was once thought to be pathognomonic for CBD, increasingly it has been recognize that CBS can be due to CBD, PSP, FTLD-TDP, or even AD. In CBD, the microscopic features include ballooned, achromatic, tau-positive neurons; astrocytic plaques (Fig. 448-5); and other dystrophic glial tau pathomorphologies that overlap with those seen in PSP. Most specifically, CBD features a severe tauopathy burden in the subcortical white matter, consisting of threads and oligodendroglial coiled bodies. As shown in Fig. 448-4, patients with bvFTD, nonfluent/agrammatic PPA, and PSP-S may also show CBD at autopsy, emphasizing the importance of distinguishing clinical and pathologic constructs and terminology. Treatment of CBS remains symptomatic; no disease-modifying therapies are available.

PARKINSON'S DISEASE DEMENTIA AND DEMENTIA WITH LEWY BODIES

The parkinsonian dementia syndromes are under increasing study, with many cases unified by Lewy body and Lewy neurite pathology that ascends from the low brainstem up through the substantia nigra, limbic system, and cortex. The DLB clinical syndrome is characterized by visual hallucinations, parkinsonism, fluctuating alertness, falls, and often rapid eye movement (REM) sleep behavior disorder (RBD). Dementia can precede or follow the appearance of parkinsonism. Hence, one pathway occurs in patients with long-standing PD without cognitive impairment, who slowly develop a dementia that is associated with visual hallucinations and fluctuating alertness. When this occurs after an established diagnosis of PD, many use the term *Parkinson's disease dementia* (PDD). In others, the dementia and neuropsychiatric syndrome precede or co-emerge with the parkinsonism, and this constellation is referred to as DLB. Both PDD and DLB may be accompanied or preceded by symptoms referable to brainstem pathology below the substantia nigra including constipation, orthostatic lightheadedness, or RBD, and many researchers conceptualize these disorders as points on a spectrum of α-synuclein pathology.

Patients with PDD and DLB are highly sensitive to metabolic perturbations, and in some patients, the first manifestation of illness is a delirium, often precipitated by an infection, new medicine, or other systemic disturbance. A hallucinatory delirium induced by L-dopa, prescribed for parkinsonian symptoms attributed to PD, may likewise provide the initial clue to a PDD or DLB diagnosis. Conversely, patients with mild cognitive deficits and hallucinations may receive typical or atypical antipsychotic medications, which induce profound parkinsonism at low doses due to a subclinical DLB-related nigral dopaminergic neuron loss. Even without an underlying precipitant, fluctuations can be marked in DLB, with episodic confusion or even stupor admixed with lucid intervals. Despite the fluctuating pattern, however, the core clinical features persist, unlike delirium, which resolves following correction of the inciting factor. Cognitively, DLB features relative preservation of memory but more severe visuospatial and executive deficits than seen in patients with early AD.

The key neuropathologic feature in DLB is the presence of Lewy bodies and Lewy neurites throughout specific brainstem nuclei, substantia nigra, amygdala, cingulate gyrus, and, ultimately, the neocortex. Lewy bodies are intraneuronal cytoplasmic inclusions that stain with periodic acid–Schiff (PAS) and ubiquitin but are now identified with antibodies to the presynaptic protein, α-synuclein. Lewy bodies are composed of straight neurofilaments 7–20 nm long with surrounding amorphous material and contain epitopes recognized by antibodies against phosphorylated and nonphosphorylated neurofilament proteins, ubiquitin, and α-synuclein. Lewy bodies are typically found in the substantia nigra of patients with idiopathic PD, where they can be readily seen with hematoxylin-and-eosin staining. A profound cholinergic deficit, owing to basal forebrain and pedunculopontine nucleus involvement, is present in many patients with DLB and may be a factor responsible for the fluctuations, inattention, and visual hallucinations.

Due to the frequent comorbidity with AD and the cholinergic deficit in DLB, cholinesterase inhibitors often provide significant benefit, reducing hallucinosis, stabilizing delusional symptoms, and even helping with RBD in some patients. Exercise programs maximize motor function and protect against fall-related injury. Antidepressants are often necessary. Atypical antipsychotics may be required for psychosis but can worsen extrapyramidal syndromes, even at low doses, and increase risk of death. Patients with DLB are extremely sensitive to dopaminergic medications, which must be carefully titrated; tolerability may be improved by concomitant use of a cholinesterase inhibitor.

OTHER CAUSES OF DEMENTIA

Prion diseases such as *Creutzfeldt-Jakob disease* (CJD) are rare neurodegenerative conditions (prevalence ~1 per million) that produce dementia. CJD is a rapidly progressive disorder associated with dementia, focal cortical signs, rigidity, and myoclonus, causing death <1 year after first symptoms appear. The rapidity of progression seen with CJD is uncommon in AD so that the distinction between the two disorders is usually straightforward. CBD and DLB, more rapid degenerative dementias with prominent movement abnormalities, are more likely to be mistaken for CJD. The differential diagnosis for CJD includes other rapidly progressive dementing conditions such as viral or bacterial encephalitides, Hashimoto's encephalopathy, central nervous system (CNS) vasculitis, lymphoma, or paraneoplastic/autoimmune syndromes. The markedly abnormal periodic complexes on EEG and cortical ribboning and basal ganglia hyperintensities on fluid-attenuate inversion recovery MRI are diagnostic features of CJD, although rarely, prolonged focal or generalized seizures can produce a similar imaging appearance. Prion diseases are discussed in detail in Chap. 453e.

Huntington's disease (HD) (Chap. 449) is an autosomal dominant degenerative brain disorder. HD clinical hallmarks include chorea, behavioral disturbance, and executive impairment. Symptoms typically begin in the fourth or fifth decade, but there is a wide range, from childhood to >70 years. Memory is frequently not impaired until late in the disease, but attention, judgment, self-awareness, and executive functions are often deficient at an early stage. Depression, apathy, social withdrawal, irritability, and intermittent disinhibition are common. Delusions and obsessive-compulsive behavior may occur. Disease duration is variable but typically lasts approximately 15 years.

Normal-pressure hydrocephalus (NPH) is a relatively uncommon but treatable syndrome. The clinical, physiologic, and neuroimaging characteristics of NPH must be carefully distinguished from those of other dementias associated with gait impairment. Historically, many patients treated for NPH have suffered from other dementias, particularly AD, vascular dementia, DLB, and PSP. For NPH, the clinical triad includes an abnormal gait (ataxic or apractic), dementia (usually mild to moderate, with an emphasis on executive impairment), and urinary urgency or incontinence. Neuroimaging reveals enlarged lateral ventricles (hydrocephalus) with little or no cortical atrophy, although the sylvian fissures may appear propped open (so-called "boxcarring"), which can be mistaken for perisylvian atrophy. This syndrome is a communicating hydrocephalus with a patent aqueduct of Sylvius (see Fig. 35-3), in contrast to aqueductal stenosis, in which the aqueduct is small. Lumbar puncture opening pressure falls in the high-normal range, and the CSF protein, glucose, and cell counts are normal. NPH may be caused by obstruction to normal CSF flow over the cerebral convexities and delayed resorption into the venous system. The indolent nature of the process results in enlarged lateral ventricles with relatively little increase in CSF pressure. Presumed edema, stretching, and distortion of subfrontal white matter tracts may lead to clinical symptoms, but the precise underlying pathophysiology remains unclear. Some patients provide a history of conditions that produce meningeal scarring (blocking CSF resorption) such as previous meningitis, subarachnoid hemorrhage, or head trauma. Others with long-standing but asymptomatic congenital hydrocephalus may have adult-onset deterioration in gait or memory that is confused with NPH. In contrast to AD, the patient with NPH complains of an early and prominent gait disturbance without cortical atrophy on CT or MRI.

Numerous attempts to improve NPH diagnosis with various special studies and predict the success of ventricular shunting have been undertaken. These tests include radionuclide cisternography (showing a delay in CSF absorption over the convexity) and various efforts to monitor and alter CSF flow dynamics, including a constant-pressure infusion test. None has proven to be specific or consistently useful. A transient improvement in gait or cognition may follow lumbar puncture (or serial punctures) with removal of 30–50 mL of CSF, but this finding has also not proved to be consistently predictive of postshunt improvement. Perhaps the most reliable strategy is a period of close inpatient evaluation before, during, and after lumbar CSF drainage. Occasionally, when a patient with AD presents with gait impairment (at times due to comorbid subfrontal vascular injury) and absent or only mild cortical atrophy on CT or MRI, distinguishing NPH from AD can be challenging. Hippocampal atrophy on MRI favors AD, whereas a characteristic "magnetic" gait with external hip rotation, low foot clearance, and short strides, along with prominent truncal sway or instability, favors NPH. The diagnosis of NPH should be avoided when hydrocephalus is not detected on imaging studies, even if the symptoms otherwise fit. Thirty to fifty percent of patients identified by careful diagnosis as having NPH will improve with ventricular shunting. Gait may improve more than cognition, but many reported failures to improve cognitively may have resulted from comorbid AD. Short-lasting improvement is common. Patients should be carefully selected for shunting, because subdural hematoma, infection, and shunt failure are known complications and can be a cause for early nursing home placement in an elderly patient with previously mild dementia.

Intracranial hypotension, sometimes called sagging brain syndrome, is a disorder caused by low CSF pressure, leading to downward pressure on the subcortical structures and disruption of cerebral function. It presents in a variable manner with headache, often exacerbated by coughing or a Valsalva maneuver or by moving from lying to standing. Other common symptoms include dizziness, vomiting, disruption of sleep-wake cycles, and sometimes a progressive bvFTD-like syndrome. Although sometimes idiopathic, this syndrome can be caused by CSF leaks secondary to lumbar puncture, head trauma, or spinal cord arachnoid cysts. Treatment consists of finding and patching CSF leaks.

Dementia can accompany *chronic alcoholism* (Chap. 467) and may result from associated malnutrition, especially of B vitamins, particularly thiamine. Other poorly defined aspects of chronic alcoholism may, however, also produce cerebral damage. A rare idiopathic syndrome of dementia and seizures with degeneration of the corpus callosum has been reported primarily in male Italian red wine drinkers (Marchiafava-Bignami disease).

Thiamine (vitamin B_1) deficiency causes Wernicke's encephalopathy (Chap. 330). The clinical presentation features a malnourished patient (frequently but not necessarily alcoholic) with confusion, ataxia, and diplopia resulting from inflammation and necrosis of periventricular midline structures, including dorsomedial thalamus, mammillary bodies, midline cerebellum, periaqueductal gray matter, and trochlear and abducens nuclei. Damage to the dorsomedial thalamus correlates most closely with the memory loss. Prompt administration of parenteral thiamine (100 mg intravenously for 3 days followed by daily oral dosage) may reverse the disease if given in the first days of symptom onset. Prolonged untreated thiamine deficiency can result in an irreversible and profound amnestic syndrome (Korsakoff's syndrome) or even death.

In *Korsakoff's syndrome,* the patient is unable to recall new information despite normal immediate memory, attention span, and level of consciousness. Memory for new events is seriously impaired, whereas knowledge acquired prior to the illness remains relatively intact. Patients are easily confused, disoriented, and cannot store information for more than a few minutes. Superficially, they may be conversant, engaging, and able to perform simple tasks and follow immediate commands. Confabulation is common, although not always present. There is no specific treatment because the previous thiamine deficiency has produced irreversible damage to the medial thalamic nuclei and mammillary bodies. Mammillary body atrophy may be visible on MRI in the chronic phase (see Fig. 330-6).

Vitamin B_{12} deficiency, as can occur in pernicious anemia, causes a megaloblastic anemia and may also damage the nervous system (Chaps. 128 and 456). Neurologically, it most commonly produces a spinal cord syndrome (myelopathy) affecting the posterior columns (loss of vibration and position sense) and corticospinal tracts (hyperactive tendon reflexes with Babinski signs); it also damages peripheral nerves (neuropathy), resulting in sensory loss with depressed tendon reflexes. Damage to myelinated axons may also cause dementia. The mechanism of neurologic damage is unclear but may be related to a deficiency of *S*-adenosyl methionine (required for methylation of myelin phospholipids) due to reduced methionine synthase activity or accumulation of methylmalonate, homocysteine, and propionate, providing abnormal substrates for fatty acid synthesis in myelin. Use of histamine blockers or metformin, vegan diets, autoimmunity against gastric parietal cells, and various causes of malabsorption are the typical causes for vitamin B_{12} deficiency. The neurologic sequelae of vitamin B_{12} deficiency may occur in the absence of hematologic manifestations, making it critical to avoid using the complete blood count (CBC) and blood smear as a substitute for measuring B_{12} blood levels. Treatment with parenteral vitamin B_{12} (1000 μg intramuscularly daily for a week, weekly for a month, and monthly for life for pernicious anemia) stops progression of the disease if instituted promptly, but complete reversal of advanced nervous system damage will not occur.

Deficiency of nicotinic acid (*pellagra*) is associated with skin rash over sun-exposed areas, glossitis, and angular stomatitis (Chap. 96e). Severe dietary deficiency of nicotinic acid along with other B vitamins such as pyridoxine may result in spastic paraparesis, peripheral neuropathy, fatigue, irritability, and dementia. This syndrome has been seen in prisoners of war and in concentration camps but should be considered in any malnourished individual. Low serum folate levels appear to be a rough index of malnutrition, but isolated folate deficiency has not been proved as a specific cause of dementia.

CNS infections usually cause delirium and other acute neurologic syndromes. However, some chronic CNS infections, particularly those associated with chronic meningitis (Chap. 165), may produce a dementing illness. The possibility of chronic infectious meningitis should be suspected in patients presenting with a dementia or behavioral syndrome, who also have headache, meningismus, cranial neuropathy, and/or radiculopathy. Between 20 and 30% of patients in the advanced stages of HIV infection become demented (Chap. 226). Cardinal features include psychomotor retardation, apathy, and impaired memory. This syndrome may result from secondary opportunistic infections but can also be caused by direct infection of CNS neurons with HIV. Neurosyphilis (Chap. 206) was a common cause of dementia in the preantibiotic era; it is now uncommon but can still be encountered in patients with multiple sex partners, particularly among patients with HIV. Characteristic CSF changes consist of pleocytosis, increased protein, and a positive Venereal Disease Research Laboratory (VDRL) test.

Primary and metastatic *neoplasms of the CNS* (Chap. 118) usually produce focal neurologic findings and seizures rather than dementia, but if tumor growth begins in the frontal or temporal lobes, the initial manifestations may be memory loss or behavioral changes. A paraneoplastic syndrome of dementia associated with occult carcinoma (often small-cell lung cancer) is termed *limbic encephalitis.* In this syndrome, confusion, agitation, seizures, poor memory, emotional changes, and frank dementia may occur. Paraneoplastic *encephalitis associated with NMDA receptor antibodies* presents as a progressive psychiatric disorder with memory loss and seizures; affected patients are often young women with ovarian teratoma (Chap. 122).

A *nonconvulsive seizure disorder* (Chap. 445) may underlie a syndrome of confusion, clouding of consciousness, and garbled speech. Often, psychiatric disease is suspected, but an EEG demonstrates the epileptic nature of the illness. If recurrent or persistent, the condition may be termed *complex partial status epilepticus.* The cognitive disturbance often responds to anticonvulsant therapy. The etiology may be previous small strokes or head trauma; some cases are idiopathic.

It is important to recognize *systemic diseases* that indirectly affect the brain and produce chronic confusion or dementia. Such conditions include hypothyroidism; vasculitis; and hepatic, renal, or pulmonary disease. Hepatic encephalopathy may begin with irritability and confusion and slowly progress to agitation, lethargy, and coma.

Isolated vasculitis of the CNS (CNS granulomatous angiitis) (Chaps. 385 and 446) occasionally causes a chronic encephalopathy associated with confusion, disorientation, and clouding of consciousness. Headache is common, and strokes and cranial neuropathies may occur. Brain imaging studies may be normal or nonspecifically abnormal. CSF analysis reveals a mild pleocytosis or protein elevation. Cerebral angiography can show multifocal stenoses involving medium-caliber vessels, but some patients have only small-vessel disease that is not revealed on angiography. The angiographic appearance is not specific and may be mimicked by atherosclerosis, infection, or other causes of vascular disease. Brain or meningeal biopsy demonstrates endothelial cell proliferation and mononuclear infiltrates within blood vessel walls. The prognosis is often poor, although the disorder may remit spontaneously. Some patients respond to glucocorticoids or chemotherapy.

Chronic metal exposure represents a rare cause of dementia. The key to diagnosis is to elicit a history of exposure at work or home. Chronic lead poisoning from inadequately fire-glazed pottery has been reported. Fatigue, depression, and confusion may be associated with episodic abdominal pain and peripheral neuropathy. Gray lead lines appear in the gums, usually accompanied by an anemia with basophilic stippling of red blood cells. The clinical presentation can resemble that of acute intermittent porphyria, including elevated levels of urine porphyrins as a result of the inhibition of δ-aminolevulinic acid dehydrase. The treatment is chelation therapy with agents such as ethylenediamine tetraacetic acid (EDTA). Chronic mercury poisoning produces dementia, peripheral neuropathy, ataxia, and tremulousness that may progress to a cerebellar intention tremor or choreoathetosis. The confusion and memory loss of chronic arsenic intoxication is also associated with nausea, weight loss, peripheral neuropathy, pigmentation and scaling of the skin, and transverse white lines of the fingernails (Mees' lines). Treatment is chelation therapy with dimercaprol (BAL). Aluminum poisoning is rare but was documented with the dialysis dementia syndrome, in which water used during renal dialysis was contaminated with excessive amounts of aluminum. This poisoning resulted in a progressive encephalopathy associated with confusion, nonfluent aphasia, memory loss, agitation, and, later, lethargy and stupor. Speech arrest and myoclonic jerks were common and associated with severe and generalized EEG changes. The condition has been eliminated by the use of deionized water for dialysis.

Recurrent head trauma in professional athletes may lead to a dementia previously referred to as "punch-drunk" syndrome or *dementia pugilistica* but now known as chronic traumatic encephalopathy (CTE) to signify its relevance to contact sport athletes other than boxers. The symptoms can be progressive, beginning late in an athlete's career or, more often, after retirement. Early in the course, a personality change associated with social instability and sometimes paranoia and delusions occurs. Later, memory loss progresses to full-blown dementia, often associated with parkinsonian signs and ataxia or intention tremor. At autopsy, the cerebral cortex shows changes tau-immunoreactive NFTs that are more prominent than amyloid plaques (which are usually diffuse or absent rather than neuritic). NFTs and tau-positive reactive astrocytes are often clustered in the depths of cortical sulci, and TDP-43 inclusions have also been reported, highlighting the overlap with the FTLD spectrum. Loss of neurons in the substantia nigra is a variable feature.

Chronic subdural hematoma (Chap. 457e) is also occasionally associated with dementia, often in the context of underlying cortical atrophy from conditions such as AD or HD.

Transient global amnesia (TGA) is characterized by the sudden onset of a severe episodic memory deficit, usually occurring in persons over the age of 50 years. Often the amnesia occurs in the setting of an emotional stimulus or physical exertion. During the attack, the individual is alert and communicative, general cognition seems intact, and there are no other neurologic signs or symptoms. The patient may seem confused and repeatedly ask about his or her location in place and time. The ability to form new memories returns after a period of hours, and the individual returns to normal with no recall for the period of the attack. Frequently no cause is determined, but cerebrovascular disease, epilepsy (7% in one study), migraine, or cardiac arrhythmias have all been implicated. Approximately one-quarter of patients experience recurrent attacks. Rare instances of permanent memory loss have been reported in patients with TGA-like spells, usually representing ischemic infarction of the hippocampus or dorsomedial thalamic nucleus bilaterally. Seizure activity due to AD should always be suspected in this syndrome.

The *ALS/parkinsonian/dementia complex of Guam* is a rare degenerative disease that has occurred in the Chamorro natives on the island of Guam. Individuals may have any combination of parkinsonian features, dementia, and MND. The most characteristic pathologic features are the presence of NFTs in degenerating neurons of the cortex and substantia nigra and loss of motor neurons in the spinal cord, although recent reanalysis has shown that some patients with this illness also show coexisting TDP-43 pathology. Epidemiologic evidence supports a possible environmental cause, such as exposure to a neurotoxin or an infectious agent with a long latency period. One interesting but unproven candidate neurotoxin occurs in the seed of the false palm tree, which Guamanians traditionally used to make flour. The ALS syndrome is no longer present in Guam, but a dementing illness with rigidity continues to be seen.

Rarely, adult-onset leukodystrophies, lysosomal storage diseases, and other genetic disorders can present as a dementia in middle to late life. Metachromatic leukodystrophy (MLD) causes a progressive psychiatric or dementia syndrome associated with extensive, confluent frontal white matter abnormality. MLD is diagnosed by measuring arylsulfatase A enzyme activity in white blood cells. Adult-onset presentations of adrenoleukodystrophy have been reported in female carriers, and these patients often feature spinal cord and posterior white matter involvement. Adrenoleukodystrophy is diagnosed with measurement of plasma very-long-chain fatty acids. CADASIL is another genetic syndrome associated with white matter disease, often frontally and temporally predominant. Diagnosis is made with skin biopsy, which shows osmophilic granules in arterioles, or, increasingly, through genetic testing for mutations in Notch 3. The neuronal ceroid lipofuscinoses are a genetically heterogeneous group of disorders associated with myoclonus, seizures, vision loss, and progressive dementia. Diagnosis is made by finding eosinophilic curvilinear inclusions within white blood cells or neuronal tissue.

Psychogenic amnesia for personally important memories can be seen. Whether this results from deliberate avoidance of unpleasant memories, outright malingering, or unconscious repression remains unknown and probably depends on the patient. Event-specific amnesia is more likely to occur after violent crimes such as homicide of a close relative or friend or sexual abuse. It may develop in association with severe drug or alcohol intoxication and sometimes with schizophrenia. More prolonged psychogenic amnesia occurs in fugue states that also commonly follow severe emotional stress. The patient with a fugue state suffers from a sudden loss of personal identity and may be found wandering far from home. *In contrast to neurologic amnesia, fugue states are associated with amnesia for personal identity and events closely associated with the personal past.* At the same time, memory for other recent events and the ability to learn and use new information are preserved. The episodes usually last hours or days and occasionally weeks or months while the patient takes on a new identity. On recovery, there is a residual amnesia gap for the period of the fugue. Very rarely does selective loss of autobiographic information reflect a focal injury to the brain areas involved with these functions.

Psychiatric diseases may mimic dementia. Severely depressed or anxious individuals may appear demented, a phenomenon sometimes called *pseudodementia*. Memory and language are usually intact when carefully tested, and a significant memory disturbance usually suggests an underlying dementia, even if the patient is depressed. Patients in this condition may feel confused and unable to accomplish routine tasks. Vegetative symptoms, such as insomnia, lack of energy, poor appetite, and concern with bowel function, are common. Onset is often more abrupt, and the psychosocial milieu may suggest prominent reasons for depression. Such patients respond to treatment of the underlying psychiatric illness. Schizophrenia is usually not difficult to distinguish from dementia, but occasionally the distinction can be problematic. Schizophrenia generally has a much earlier age of onset (second and third decades) than most dementing illnesses and is associated with intact memory. The delusions and hallucinations of schizophrenia are usually more complex, bizarre, and threatening than those of dementia. Some chronic schizophrenics develop an unexplained progressive dementia late in life that is not related to AD. Conversely, FTD, HD, vascular dementia, DLB, AD, or leukoencephalopathy can begin with schizophrenia-like features, leading to the misdiagnosis of a psychiatric condition. Later age of onset, significant deficits on cognitive testing, or the presence of abnormal neuroimaging suggest a degenerative condition. Memory loss may also be part of a *conversion disorder*. In this situation, patients commonly complain bitterly of memory loss, but careful cognitive testing either does not confirm the deficits or demonstrates inconsistent or unusual patterns of cognitive problems. The patient's behavior and "wrong" answers to questions often indicate that he or she understands the question and knows the correct answer.

Clouding of cognition by *chronic drug or medication use*, often prescribed by physicians, is an important cause of dementia. Sedatives, tranquilizers, and analgesics used to treat insomnia, pain, anxiety, or agitation may cause confusion, memory loss, and lethargy, especially in the elderly. Discontinuation of the offending medication often improves mentation.

449 Parkinson's Disease and Other Movement Disorders

C. Warren Olanow, Anthony H.V. Schapira, Jose A. Obeso

PARKINSON'S DISEASE AND RELATED DISORDERS

Parkinson's disease (PD) is the second commonest neurodegenerative disease, exceeded only by Alzheimer's disease (AD). Its cardinal clinical features were first described by the English physician James Parkinson in 1817. It is noteworthy that James Parkinson was a general physician who captured the essence of this condition based on a visual inspection of a mere handful of patients. It is estimated that approximately 1 million persons in the United States, 1 million in Western Europe, and 5 million worldwide suffer from this disorder. PD affects men and women of all races, all occupations, and all countries. The mean age of onset is about 60 years. The frequency of PD increases with aging, but cases can be seen in patients in their 20s and even younger. Based on the aging of the population and projected demographics, it is estimated that the prevalence of the disease will dramatically increase in the next several decades.

Clinically, PD is characterized by rest tremor, rigidity, bradykinesia (slowing), and gait impairment, known as the "cardinal features" of the disease. Additional features can include freezing of gait, postural instability, speech difficulty, autonomic disturbances, sensory alterations, mood disorders, sleep dysfunction, cognitive impairment, and dementia (Table 449-1).

Pathologically, the hallmark features of PD are degeneration of dopaminergic neurons in the substantia nigra pars compacta (SNc), reduced striatal dopamine, and intracytoplasmic proteinaceous inclusions known as Lewy bodies that primarily contain the protein alpha synuclein (Fig. 449-1). While interest has primarily focused on the dopamine system, neuronal degeneration with inclusion body formation can also affect cholinergic neurons of the nucleus basalis of Meynert (NBM), norepinephrine neurons of the locus coeruleus (LC), serotonin neurons in the raphe nuclei of the brainstem, and neurons of the olfactory system, cerebral hemispheres, spinal cord, and peripheral autonomic nervous system. This "nondopaminergic" pathology is likely responsible for the development of nondopaminergic clinical features listed in Table 449-1 characterized by their lack of satisfactory response to dopaminergic replacement therapy. There is evidence that Lewy body pathology first begins in the peripheral autonomic nervous system, olfactory system, and dorsal motor nucleus of the vagus nerve in the lower brainstem, and then spreads in a predictable and sequential manner to affect the upper brainstem and cerebral hemispheres (Braak staging). These studies suggest that degeneration of dopamine neurons develops in a mid-stage of the disease. Indeed, epidemiologic studies suggest that clinical symptoms reflecting this nondopaminergic degeneration, such as constipation, anosmia, rapid eye movement (REM) behavior sleep disorder, and cardiac denervation, can precede the onset of the classic motor features of PD.

TABLE 449-1 CLINICAL FEATURES OF PARKINSON'S DISEASE

Cardinal Motor Features	Other Motor Features	Nonmotor Features
Bradykinesia	Micrographia	Anosmia
Rest tremor	Masked facies (hypomimia)	Sensory disturbances (e.g., pain)
Rigidity	Reduced eye blinking	Mood disorders (e.g., depression)
Gait disturbance/ postural instability	Soft voice (hypophonia)	Sleep disturbances (e.g., RBD)
	Dysphagia	Autonomic disturbances
	Freezing	Orthostatic hypotension
		Gastrointestinal disturbances
		Genitourinal disturbances
		Sexual dysfunction
		Cognitive impairment (MCI/ dementia)

Abbreviations: RBD, rapid eye movement behavior disorder; MCI, mild cognitive impairment.

DIFFERENTIAL DIAGNOSIS

Parkinsonism is a generic term that is used to define a syndrome manifest as bradykinesia with rigidity and/or tremor. It has a differential diagnosis (Table 449-2) that reflects damage to different components of the basal ganglia. The basal ganglia are comprised of a group of subcortical nuclei that include the striatum (putamen and caudate nucleus), subthalamic nucleus (STN), globus pallidus pars externa (GPe), globus pallidus pars interna (GPi), and the SNc (Fig. 449-2). Among the different forms of parkinsonism, PD is the most common (approximately 75% of cases). Historically, PD was diagnosed based on the presence of two of three parkinsonian features (tremor, rigidity, bradykinesia). However, postmortem studies found a 24% error rate when diagnosis was based on these criteria. Clinicopathologic correlation studies subsequently determined that parkinsonism associated with rest tremor, asymmetry, and a good response to levodopa was more likely to predict the correct pathologic diagnosis. With these revised criteria (known as the U.K. Brain Bank Criteria), a clinical diagnosis of PD is confirmed pathologically in as many as 99% of cases. A more complete definition of PD is now needed to incorporate the fact that there is widespread pathology beyond the dopaminergic system, nondopamine and nonmotor clinical features, and a premotor stage of the disease.

Imaging of the brain dopamine system in PD with positron emission tomography (PET) or single photon emission computed tomography (SPECT) shows reduced uptake of striatal dopaminergic markers, particularly in the posterior putamen with relative sparing of the caudate nucleus (Fig. 449-3), reflecting the degeneration of nigrostriatal dopamine neurons. Imaging can be useful in patients where there is diagnostic uncertainty (e.g., dystonic tremor, essential tremor) or in research studies, but is rarely necessary in routine practice because the diagnosis can usually be established on clinical criteria alone. This may change in the future when there is a disease-modifying therapy and it is important to make the diagnosis as early as possible. Genetic testing is not routinely used at present, but can be helpful for identifying at-risk individuals in a research setting. Mutations of the *LRRK2* gene (see below) have attracted particular interest because they are the commonest cause of familial PD and are responsible for approximately 1% of typical sporadic cases of the disease. Mutations in *LRRK2* are a particularly common cause of PD in Ashkenazi Jews and North African Berber Arabs. The penetrance of the most common *LRRK2* mutation ranges from 28 to 74% and is strongly correlated to the age of the carrier, with 50% affected by age 60 years. Mutations in the *parkin* gene should be considered in patients with onset prior to 40 years of age.

Atypical and Secondary Parkinsonism Atypical parkinsonism refers to a group of neurodegenerative conditions that usually are associated with more widespread neurodegeneration than is found in PD (often involvement of striatum and/or globus pallidus as well as the SNc). As a group, they present with parkinsonism (rigidity and bradykinesia) but have a slightly different clinical picture than PD, reflecting differences in the underlying pathology. In these conditions, parkinsonism is typically characterized by early speech and gait impairment, absence of rest tremor, no motor asymmetry, poor or no response to levodopa, and an aggressive clinical course. In the early stages, they may show some modest benefit from levodopa and be difficult to distinguish from PD. Pathologically, neurodegeneration typically involves degeneration of the SNc but occurs without Lewy bodies (see below for individual conditions). Neuroimaging of the dopamine system is usually not helpful, because dopamine depletion can be seen in both PD and atypical parkinsonism. By contrast, metabolic imaging of the basal ganglia/thalamus network (using 2-F-deoxiglucose PET) may be helpful, showing a pattern of decreased activity in the GPi with increased activity in the thalamus, the reverse of what is seen in PD.

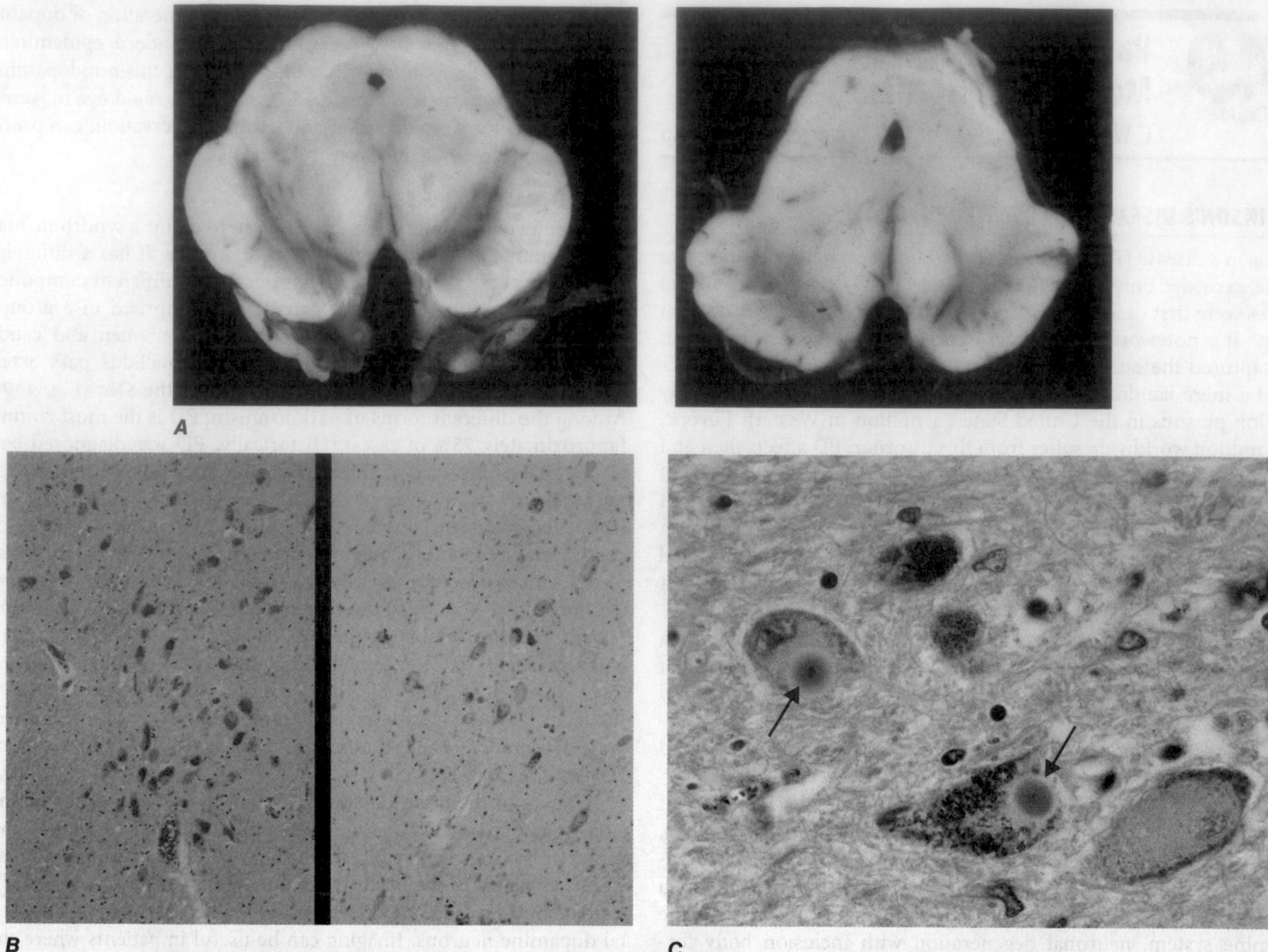

FIGURE 449-1 Pathologic specimens from a patient with Parkinson's disease (PD) compared to a normal control demonstrating (*A*) reduction of pigment in SNc in PD (*right*) versus control (*left*), (*B*) reduced numbers of cells in SNc in PD (*right*) compared to control (*left*), and (*C*) Lewy bodies (*arrows*) within melanized dopamine neurons in PD. SNc, substantia nigra pars compacta.

Multiple-system atrophy (MSA) manifests as a combination of parkinsonian, cerebellar, and autonomic features and can be divided into a predominant parkinsonian (MSA-p) or cerebellar (MSA-c) form. Clinically, MSA is suspected when a patient presents with atypical parkinsonism in conjunction with cerebellar signs and/or early and prominent autonomic dysfunction, usually orthostatic hypotension (Chap. 454). Pathologically, MSA is characterized by degeneration of the SNc, striatum, cerebellum, and inferior olivary nuclei coupled with characteristic glial cytoplasmic inclusions (GCIs) that stain for α-synuclein. Magnetic resonance imaging (MRI) can show pathologic iron accumulation in the striatum on T2-weighted scans, high signal change in the region of the external surface of the putamen (putaminal rim) in MSA-p, or cerebellar and brainstem atrophy (the pontine "hot cross buns" sign [Fig. 454-2]) in MSA-c. Mutations in the *CoQ2* gene encoding parahydroxybenzoate-polyprenyl transferase, an enzyme involved in the biosynthesis of coenzyme Q10 (CoQ10), a cofactor of the mitochondrial respiratory chain, have been identified in familial and sporadic forms of MSA.

Progressive supranuclear palsy (PSP) is a form of atypical parkinsonism that is characterized by slow ocular saccades, eyelid apraxia, and restricted eye movements with particular impairment of downward gaze. Patients frequently experience hyperextension of the neck with early gait disturbance and falls. In later stages, speech and swallowing difficulty and cognitive impairment become evident. MRI may reveal a characteristic atrophy of the midbrain with relative preservation of the pons, the "hummingbird sign" on midsagittal images. Pathologically,

TABLE 449-2 DIFFERENTIAL DIAGNOSIS OF PARKINSONISM

Parkinson's Disease	Atypical Parkinsonism	Secondary Parkinsonism	Other Neurodegenerative Disorders
Genetic	Multiple-system atrophy (MSA)	Drug-induced	Wilson's disease
Sporadic	Cerebellar type (MSA-c)	Tumor	Huntington's disease
Dementia with Lewy bodies	Parkinson type (MSA-p)	Infection	Neurodegeneration with brain iron accumulation
	Progressive supranuclear palsy	Vascular	SCA 3 (spinocerebellar ataxia)
	Corticobasal ganglionic degeneration	Normal-pressure hydrocephalus	Fragile X–associated ataxia-tremor-parkinsonism
	Frontotemporal dementia	Trauma	Prion disease
		Liver failure	Dystonia-parkinsonism (DYT3)
		Toxins (e.g., carbon monoxide, manganese, MPTP, cyanide, hexane, methanol, carbon disulfide)	Alzheimer's disease with parkinsonism

Abbreviations: MPTP, 1-methyl-4-phenyl-1,2,5,6-tetrahydropyridine.

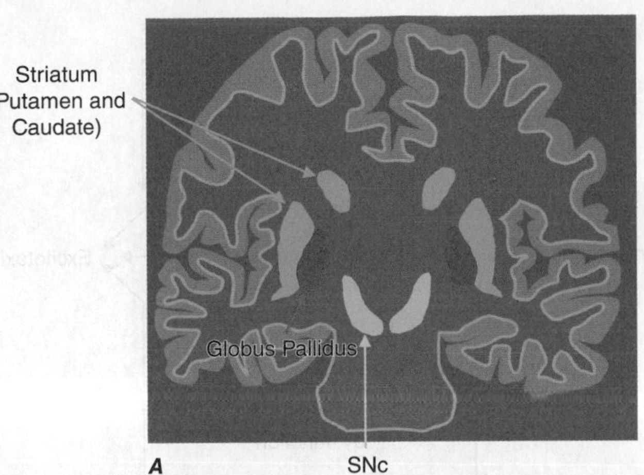

FIGURE 449-2 Basal ganglia nuclei. Schematic (*A*) and postmortem (*B*) coronal sections illustrating the various components of the basal ganglia. SNc, substantia nigra pars compacta; STN, subthalamic nucleus.

PSP is characterized by degeneration of the SNc, striatum, subthalamic nucleus, midline thalamic nuclei, and pallidum along with neurofibrillary tangles and inclusions that stain for the tau protein.

Corticobasal ganglionic degeneration is less common and is usually manifest by asymmetric dystonic contractions and clumsiness of one hand coupled with cortical sensory disturbances manifest as apraxia, agnosia, focal limb myoclonus, or alien limb phenomenon (where the limb assumes a position in space without the patient being aware of it). Dementia may occur at any stage of the disease. Both cortical and basal ganglia features are required to make this diagnosis. MRI frequently shows asymmetric cortical atrophy. Pathologic findings include achromatic neuronal degeneration with tau deposits. Because other disorders such as PSP can present with a similar clinical picture, the term corticobasal ganglia syndrome should be used until a precise diagnosis can be confirmed pathologically.

Secondary parkinsonism can occur as a result of drugs, stroke, tumor, infection, or exposure to toxins such as carbon monoxide or manganese. Dopamine-blocking agents such as the neuroleptics are the commonest cause of secondary parkinsonism. These drugs are most widely used in psychiatry, *but physicians should be aware that drugs such as metoclopramide and chlorpromazine, which are primarily used to treat gastrointestinal problems, are also neuroleptic agents* and common causes of secondary parkinsonism (as well as acute and tardive dyskinesias; see below). Other drugs that can cause secondary parkinsonism include tetrabenazine, calcium channel blockers (flunarizine, cinnarizine), amiodarone, and lithium.

Finally, parkinsonism can be seen as a feature of other degenerative disorders such as Wilson's disease, Huntington's disease (especially the juvenile form known as the Westphal variant), dopa-responsive dystonia, and neurodegenerative disorders with brain iron accumulation such as pantothenate kinase (PANK)–associated neurodegeneration (formerly known as Hallervorden-Spatz disease).

Some features that suggest parkinsonism might be due to a condition other than PD are shown in Table 449-3.

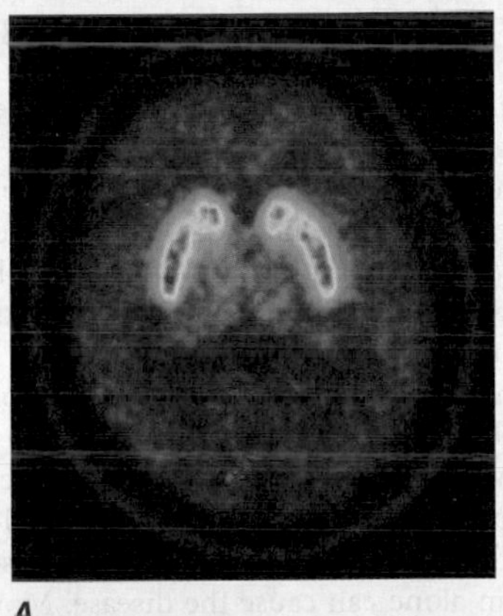

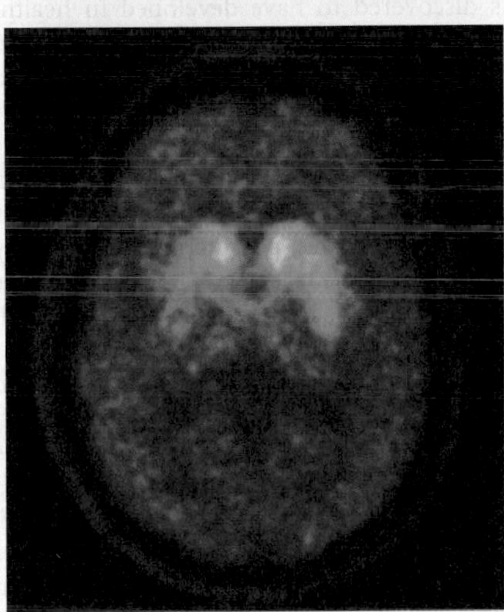

FIGURE 449-3 [^{11}C]Dihydrotetrabenazine positron emission tomography (a marker of VMAT2) in healthy control (*A*) and Parkinson's disease (*B*) patient. Note the reduced striatal uptake of tracer, which is most pronounced in the posterior putamen and tends to be asymmetric. *(Courtesy of Dr. Jon Stoessl.)*

ETIOLOGY AND PATHOGENESIS

Most PD cases occur sporadically (~85–90%) and are of unknown cause. Twin studies suggest that environmental factors likely play an important role in patients older than 50 years, with genetic factors being more important in younger patients. Epidemiologic studies also suggest increased risk with exposure to pesticides, rural living, and drinking well water and reduced risk with cigarette smoking and caffeine. However, no environmental factor has yet been proven to cause typical PD. The environmental hypothesis received support with the demonstration in the 1980s that MPTP (1-methyl-4-phenyl-1,2,5,6-tetrahydropyridine), a byproduct of the illicit manufacture of a heroin-like drug, caused a PD-like syndrome in addicts in northern California. MPTP is transported to the central nervous system, where it is oxidized to form MPP^+, a mitochondrial toxin that is selectively taken up by, and damages, dopamine neurons. However, MPTP or MPTP-like compounds have not been linked to sporadic PD.

About 10–15% of cases are familial in origin, and multiple specific mutations and gene associations have been identified (Table 449-4). Genetic factors have also been linked to sporadic cases, with several typical PD cases found to carry the *LRRK2* mutation, and genome-wide association studies (GWAS) implicating alpha synuclein, tau, and

TABLE 449-3 FEATURES SUGGESTING AN ATYPICAL OR SECONDARY CAUSE OF PARKINSONISM

Symptoms/Signs	Alternative Diagnosis to Consider
History	
Early speech and gait impairment (Lack of tremor, lack of motor asymmetry)	Atypical parkinsonism
Exposure to neuroleptics	Drug-induced parkinsonism
Onset prior to age 40	Genetic form of PD
Liver disease	Wilson's disease, non-Wilsonian hepatolenticular degeneration
Early hallucinations and dementia with later development of PD features	Dementia with Lewy bodies
Diplopia, impaired down gaze	PSP
Poor or no response to an adequate trial of levodopa	Atypical or secondary parkinsonism
Physical Exam	
Dementia as first or early feature	Dementia with Lewy bodies
Prominent orthostatic hypotension	MSA-p
Prominent cerebellar signs	MSA-c
Slow saccades with impaired down gaze	PSP
High-frequency (6–10 Hz) symmetric postural tremor with a prominent kinetic component	Essential tremor

Abbreviations: MSA-c, multiple-system atrophy–cerebellar type; MSA-p, multiple-system atrophy–Parkinson's type; PD, Parkinson's disease; PSP, progressive supranuclear palsy.

HLA as risk factors. It has been proposed that most cases of PD may be due to a "double hit" involving an interaction between a gene mutation that induces susceptibility coupled with exposure to a toxic environmental factor that may induce epigenetic or somatic DNA alterations. In this scenario, both factors are required for PD to ensue, while the presence of either one alone is not sufficient to cause the disease.

Several factors have been implicated in the pathogenesis of cell death in PD, including oxidative stress, inflammation, mitochondrial dysfunction, and proteolytic stress. Recent studies have demonstrated that with aging dopamine neurons switch from sodium to calcium pacing through calcium channels, potentially making these high-energy neurons vulnerable to calcium-mediated neurotoxicity. Whatever the pathogenic mechanism, cell death appears to occur, at least in part, by way of a signal-mediated apoptotic or "suicidal" process.

TABLE 449-4 GENETIC CAUSES OF PARKINSON'S DISEASE

Name	Chromosome	Locus	Gene	Inheritance
Park 1	Chr 4	q21-23	*α-Synuclein*	AD
Park 2	Chr 6	q25-27	*Parkin*	AR
Park 3	Chr 2	p13	Unknown	AD
Park 4	Chr 4	q21-23	*α-Synuclein*	AD
Park 5	Chr 4	p14	*UCHL-1*	AD
Park 6	Chr 1	p35-36	*PINK-1*	AR
Park 7	Chr 1	p36	*DJ-1*	AR
Park 8	Chr 12	p11-q13	*LRRK2*	AR/Sp
Park 9	Chr 1	p36	*ATP13A2*	AR
Park 10	Chr 1	p32	Unknown	Sp
Park 11	Chr 2	q36-37	*GIGYF2*	AD
Park 12	Chr X	q21-25	Unknown	Sp
Park 13	Chr 2	p13	*Omi/HtrA2*	AD
Park 14	Chr 22	q13	*PLA2G6*	AR
Park 15	Chr 22	q12-13	*FBX07*	AR
Park 16	Chr 1	q32	Unknown	Sp

Abbreviations: AD, autosomal dominant; AR, autosomal recessive; Chr, chromosome; Sp, sporadic.

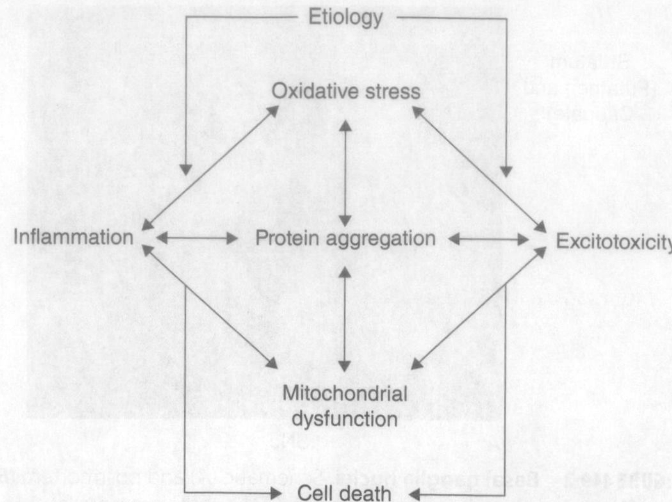

FIGURE 449-4 Schematic representation of how pathogenetic factors implicated in Parkinson's disease interact in a network manner, ultimately leading to cell death. This figure illustrates how interference with any one of these factors may not necessarily stop the cell death cascade. *(Adapted from CW Olanow: Movement Disorders 22:S-335, 2007.)*

Each of these mechanisms offers a potential target for neuroprotective drugs. However, it is not clear which of these factors is primary, if the mechanism is the same in each individual case, if they act by way of a network such that a cocktail of agents might be required to provide neuroprotection, or if the findings to date merely represent epiphenomena unrelated to the true cause of cell death that remains undiscovered (Fig. 449-4).

Gene mutations may not cause all cases of PD, but may be helpful in pointing to specific pathogenic pathways and mechanisms that are central to a neurodegenerative process that might be relevant to all forms of the disease. To date, most interest has focused on pathways implicated by mutations in *α-synuclein*, *LRRK2*, and *PINK1/Parkin*.

Most interest has focused on *α-synuclein*. Mutations in α-synuclein cause rare familial forms of PD, and α-synuclein constitutes the major component of Lewy bodies in patients with sporadic PD (Fig. 449-1). Furthermore, duplication or triplication of the wild-type *α-synuclein* can also cause a form of PD, indicating that increased production of the normal protein alone can cause the disease. More recently, Lewy pathology was discovered to have developed in healthy embryonic dopamine neurons that had been implanted into the striatum of PD patients, suggesting that the abnormal protein had transferred from affected cells to healthy unaffected dopamine neurons. Based on these findings, it has been proposed that α-synuclein is a prion and PD is a prion disorder. Here it is proposed that, like the prion protein PrP^C, α-synuclein can misfold to form β-rich sheets, generate toxic oligomers and aggregates, polymerize to form amyloid plaques (i.e., Lewy bodies), cause neurodegeneration, and spread to involve unaffected neurons. Indeed, injection of α-synuclein fibrils into the striatum promotes the development of Lewy pathology in host neurons, neurodegeneration, behavioral abnormalities, and the spread of α-synuclein pathology to anatomically connected sites. Further support for this hypothesis comes from the demonstration that inoculation of α-synuclein derived from human Lewy bodies induces widespread Lewy pathology in mice and primates. Collectively, this evidence supports the possibility that neuroprotective therapies for PD might be developed based on inhibiting accumulation or accelerating removal of α-synuclein aggregates.

Mutations in the glucocerebrosidase (*GBA*) gene associated with Gaucher's disease numerically represent the most important risk factor for the development of PD. While the responsible mechanism is not precisely known, it is noteworthy that *GBA* mutations are associated with altered autophagy and lysosomal function and could impair the clearance of α-synuclein.

Six different *LRRK2* mutations have been linked to PD, with Gly2019Ser being the most common. The mechanism responsible for cell death with this mutation is not known but is thought to involve changes in kinase activity with altered phosphorylation of target proteins (including autophosphorylation) and possibly lysosomal dysfunction. Kinase inhibitors can block toxicity associated with *LRRK2* mutations in laboratory models, and there has been much interest in developing drugs directed at this target. However, kinase inhibitors are likely to be toxic, the physiologic role of *LRRK2* is not known, and the large majority of PD patients do not carry a *LRRK2* mutation.

Mutations in *PINK1* and *parkin* have implicated mitochondrial dysfunction as a possible cause of PD. Recent studies suggest a role for parkin and PINK1 proteins in the turnover and clearance of damaged mitochondria (mitophagy), and mutations in *parkin* and *PINK1* cause mitochondrial dysfunction in transgenic animals that can be corrected with overexpression of parkin. This is a particularly attractive target because postmortem studies in PD patients show a defect in complex I of the respiratory chain in SNc neurons.

Thus, evidence is accumulating that genetics plays an important role in both familial and "sporadic" forms of PD. It is anticipated that better understanding of the pathways responsible for cell death caused by these mutations will permit the development of more relevant animal models of PD and targets for the development of neuroprotective drugs.

PATHOPHYSIOLOGY OF PD

The classic model of the organization of the basal ganglia in the normal and PD states is provided in Fig. 449-5. With respect to motor function, a series of neuronal circuits or loops link the basal ganglia nuclei with corresponding cortical motor regions in a somatotopic manner. The striatum is the major input region of the basal ganglia, while the GPi and SNr are the major output regions. The input and output regions are connected via direct and indirect pathways that have reciprocal effects on the activity of the output pathway. The output of the basal ganglia provides inhibitory (GABAergic) tone to thalamic and brainstem neurons that in turn connect to motor systems in the cerebral cortex and spinal cord that control motor function. Physiologically, decreased neuronal activity in the GPi/SNr is associated with movement facilitation and vice versa. Dopaminergic projections from SNc neurons serve to modulate neuronal firing and to stabilize the basal ganglia network. The basal ganglia and similar cortical loops are now thought to also play an important role in regulating normal behavioral, emotional, and cognitive functions.

In PD, dopamine denervation with loss of dopaminergic tone leads to increased firing of neurons in the STN and GPi, excessive inhibition of the thalamus, reduced activation of cortical motor systems, and the development of parkinsonian features (Fig. 449-5). The current role of surgery in the treatment of PD is based on this model, which predicted that lesions or high-frequency stimulation of the STN or GPi might reduce this neuronal overactivity and improve PD features.

TREATMENT PARKINSON'S DISEASE

LEVODOPA

Since its introduction in the late 1960s, levodopa has been the mainstay of therapy for PD. Experiments in the late 1950s by Carlsson demonstrated that blocking dopamine uptake with reserpine caused rabbits to become parkinsonian; this could be reversed with the dopamine precursor, levodopa. Subsequently, Hornykiewicz demonstrated a dopamine deficiency in the striatum of PD patients and suggested the potential benefit of dopaminergic replacement therapy. Dopamine does not cross the blood-brain barrier (BBB), so clinical trials were initiated with levodopa, a precursor of dopamine. Studies over the course of the next decade confirmed the value of levodopa and revolutionized the treatment of PD.

Levodopa is routinely administered in combination with a peripheral decarboxylase inhibitor to prevent its peripheral metabolism to dopamine and the development of nausea and vomiting due to activation of dopamine receptors in the area postrema that are not protected by the BBB. In the United States, levodopa is combined with the decarboxylase inhibitor carbidopa (Sinemet), whereas in

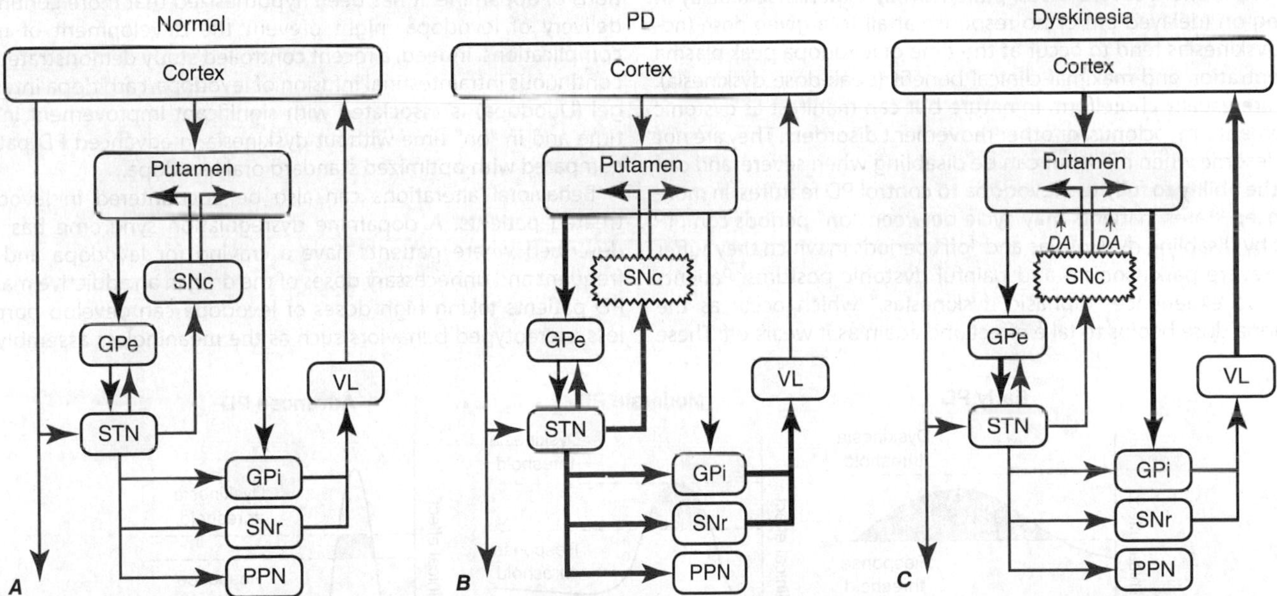

FIGURE 449-5 Basal ganglia organization. Classic model of the organization of the basal ganglia in the normal (***A***), Parkinson's disease (PD) (***B***), and levodopa-induced dyskinesia (***C***) state. Inhibitory connections are shown as *blue arrows* and excitatory connections as *red arrows*. The striatum is the major input region and receives its major input from the cortex. The GPi and SNr are the major output regions, and they project to the thalamocortical and brainstem motor regions. The striatum and GPi/SNr are connected by direct and indirect pathways. This model predicts that parkinsonism results from increased neuronal firing in the STN and GPi and that lesions or DBS of these targets might provide benefit. This concept led to the rationale for surgical therapies for PD. The model also predicts that dyskinesia results from decreased firing of the output regions, resulting in excessive cortical activation by the thalamus. This component of the model is not completely correct because lesions of the GPi ameliorate rather than increase dyskinesia in PD, suggesting that firing frequency is just one of the components that lead to the development of dyskinesia. DBS, deep brain stimulation; GPe, external segment of the globus pallidus; GPi, internal segment of the globus pallidus; PPN, pedunculopontine nucleus; SNc, substantia nigra, pars compacta; SNr, substantia nigra, pars reticulata; STN, subthalamic nucleus; VL, ventrolateral thalamus. *(Derived from JA Obeso et al: Trends Neurosci 23:S8, 2000.)*

many other countries, it is combined with benserazide (Madopar). Levodopa is also available in controlled-release formulations as well as in combination with a catechol-*O*-methyltransferase (COMT) inhibitor (see below). Levodopa remains the most effective symptomatic treatment for PD and the gold standard against which new therapies are compared. No current medical or surgical treatment provides antiparkinsonian benefits superior to what can be achieved with levodopa. Levodopa benefits the classic motor features of PD, prolongs independence and employability, improves quality of life, and increases life span. Almost all PD patients experience improvement, and failure to respond to an adequate trial should cause the diagnosis to be questioned.

There are, however, important limitations of levodopa therapy. Acute dopaminergic side effects include nausea, vomiting, and orthostatic hypotension. These are usually transient and can generally be avoided by gradual titration. If they persist, they can be treated with additional doses of a peripheral decarboxylase inhibitor (e.g., carbidopa) or a peripheral dopamine-blocking agent such as domperidone (not available in the United States). More important are motor complications (see below) that develop in the majority of patients treated long-term with levodopa. In addition, the disease continues to progress, and features such as falling, freezing, autonomic dysfunction, sleep disorders, and dementia may emerge with disease progression that are not adequately controlled by levodopa. Indeed, these nondopaminergic features (especially falling and dementia) are the primary source of disability and the main reason for nursing home placement for patients with advanced PD

Levodopa-induced motor complications consist of fluctuations in motor response ("on" episodes when the drug is working and "off" episodes when parkinsonian features return) and involuntary movements known as dyskinesias (**Fig. 449-6**). When patients initially take levodopa, benefits are long-lasting (many hours) even though the drug has a relatively short half-life (60–90 min). With continued treatment, however, the duration of benefit following an individual dose becomes progressively shorter until it approaches the half-life of the drug. This loss of benefit is known as the *wearing-off effect*. In more severe cases, patients may experience a delay in turning on (delayed-on) or no response at all to a given dose (no-on). Dyskinesias tend to occur at the time of levodopa peak plasma concentration and maximal clinical benefit (peak-dose dyskinesia). They are usually choreiform in nature but can manifest as dystonic movements, myoclonus, or other movement disorders. They are not troublesome when mild, but can be disabling when severe, and can limit the ability to fully use levodopa to control PD features. In more advanced states, patients may cycle between "on" periods complicated by disabling dyskinesias and "off" periods in which they suffer from severe parkinsonism and painful dystonic postures. Patients may also experience "diphasic dyskinesias," which occur as the levodopa dose begins to take effect and again as it wears off. These dyskinesias typically consist of transient, stereotypic, rhythmic movements that predominantly involve the lower extremities and are frequently associated with parkinsonism in other body regions. They can be relieved by increasing the dose of levodopa, although higher doses may induce more severe peak-dose dyskinesia.

The cause of levodopa-induced motor complications is not precisely known. They are more likely to occur in females, younger individuals with more severe disease, and with the use of higher doses (mg/kg) of levodopa. The classic model of the basal ganglia has been useful for understanding the origin of motor features in PD, but has proved less valuable for understanding levodopa-induced dyskinesias (Fig. 449-5). The model predicts that dopamine replacement might excessively inhibit the pallidal output system, thereby leading to increased thalamocortical activity, enhanced stimulation of cortical motor regions, and the development of dyskinesia. However, lesions of the pallidum that completely destroy its output are associated with amelioration rather than induction of dyskinesia as suggested by the classic model. It is now thought that dyskinesia results from levodopa-induced alterations in the GPi neuronal firing pattern (pauses, bursts, synchrony, etc.) and oscillatory activity, and not simply the firing frequency alone. This in turn leads to the transmission of misinformation from pallidum to thalamus/cortex, resulting in dyskinesia. Surgical lesions or high-frequency stimulation might ameliorate dyskinesia by interfering with (blocking or masking) this abnormal neuronal activity and preventing the transfer of misinformation to motor systems.

Current information suggests that altered neuronal firing patterns and motor complications relate to nonphysiologic levodopa replacement. Striatal dopamine levels are normally maintained at a relatively constant level. In PD, dopamine neurons degenerate and striatal dopamine is dependent on the peripheral availability of levodopa. Intermittent doses of short-acting levodopa result in fluctuating plasma levels because of variability in transit of the drug from the stomach to the duodenum where it is absorbed and the short half-life of the drug. This variability results in exposure of dopamine receptors to pathologically high and low concentrations of dopamine. It has been hypothesized that more continuous delivery of levodopa might prevent the development of motor complications. Indeed, a recent controlled study demonstrated that continuous intraintestinal infusion of levodopa/carbidopa intestinal gel (Duodopa) is associated with significant improvement in "off" time and in "on" time without dyskinesia in advanced PD patients compared with optimized standard oral levodopa.

Behavioral alterations can also be encountered in levodopa-treated patients. A dopamine dysregulation syndrome has been described where patients have a craving for levodopa and take frequent and unnecessary doses of the drug in an addictive manner. PD patients taking high doses of levodopa can develop purposeless, stereotyped behaviors such as the meaningless assembly and

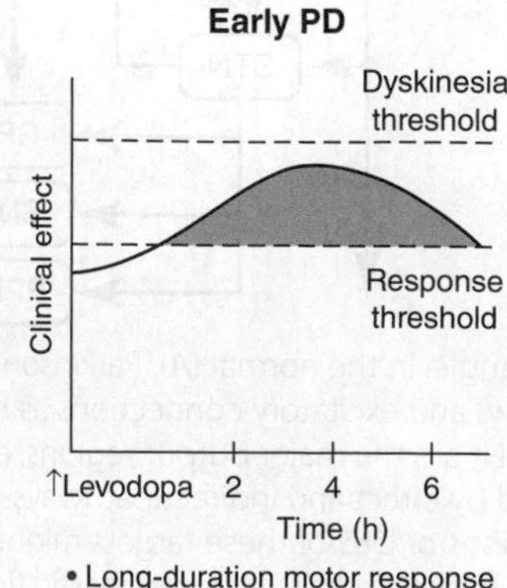

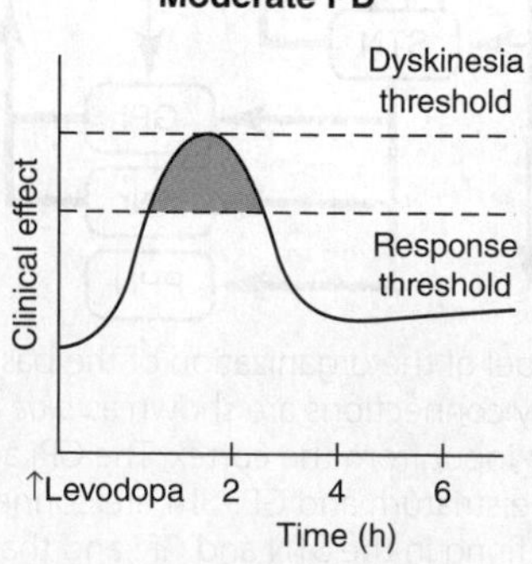

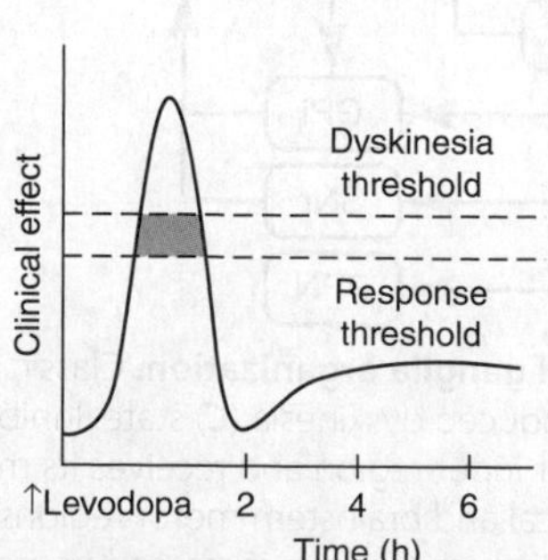

FIGURE 449-6 Changes in motor response associated with chronic levodopa treatment. Levodopa-induced motor complications. Schematic illustration of the gradual shortening of the duration of a beneficial motor response to levodopa (wearing off) and the appearance of dyskinesias complicating "on" time. PD, Parkinson's disease.

disassembly or collection and sorting of objects. This is known as punding, a term taken from the Swedish description of the meaningless behaviors seen in chronic amphetamine users. Hypersexuality and other impulse-control disorders are occasionally encountered with levodopa, although these are more commonly seen with dopamine agonists.

DOPAMINE AGONISTS

Dopamine agonists are a diverse group of drugs that act directly on dopamine receptors. Unlike levodopa, they do not require metabolism to an active product and do not undergo oxidative metabolism. Initial dopamine agonists were ergot derivatives (e.g., bromocriptine, pergolide, cabergoline) and were associated with ergot-related side effects, including cardiac valvular damage. They have largely been replaced by a second generation of nonergot dopamine agonists (e.g., pramipexole, ropinirole, rotigotine). In general, dopamine agonists do not have comparable efficacy to levodopa. They were initially introduced as adjuncts to levodopa to enhance motor function and reduce "off" time in fluctuating patients. Subsequently, it was shown that dopamine agonists, possibly because they are relatively long-acting, are less prone than levodopa to induce dyskinesia. For this reason, many physicians initiate therapy with a dopamine agonist, although supplemental levodopa is eventually required in virtually all patients. Both ropinirole and pramipexole are available as orally administered immediate (tid) and extended-release (qd) formulations. Rotigotine is administered as a once-daily transdermal patch. Apomorphine is a dopamine agonist with efficacy comparable to levodopa, but it must be administered parenterally and has a very short half-life and duration of activity (45 min). It is generally administered by injection as a rescue agent for the treatment of severe "off" episodes. Apomorphine can also be administered by continuous subcutaneous infusion and has been demonstrated to reduce both "off" time and dyskinesia in advanced patients. However, this approach has not been approved in the United States.

Dopamine agonist use is associated with a variety of side effects. Acute side effects are primarily dopaminergic and include nausea, vomiting, and orthostatic hypotension. As with levodopa, these can usually be avoided by slow titration. Side effects associated with chronic use include hallucinations and cognitive impairment. Sedation with sudden unintended episodes of falling asleep while driving a motor vehicle have been reported. Patients should be informed about this potential problem and should not drive when tired. Dopamine agonists can also be associated with impulse-control disorders, including pathologic gambling, hypersexuality, and compulsive eating and shopping. The precise cause of these problems, and why they appear to occur more frequently with dopamine agonists than levodopa, remains to be resolved, but reward systems associated with dopamine and alterations in the ventral striatum and orbitofrontal regions have been implicated. In general, chronic side effects are dose-related and can be avoided or minimized with lower doses. Injections of apomorphine and patch delivery of rotigotine can be complicated by development of skin lesions at sites of administration.

MAO-B INHIBITORS

Inhibitors of monoamine oxidase type B (MAO-B) block central dopamine metabolism and increase synaptic concentrations of the neurotransmitter. Selegiline and rasagiline are relatively selective suicide inhibitors of the MAO-B enzyme. Clinically, MAO-B inhibitors provide antiparkinsonian benefits when used as monotherapy in early disease and reduced "off" time when used as an adjunct to levodopa in patients with motor fluctuations. MAO-B inhibitors are generally safe and well tolerated. They may increase dyskinesia in levodopa-treated patients, but this can usually be controlled by down-titrating the dose of levodopa. Inhibition of the MAO-A isoform prevents metabolism of tyramine in the gut, leading to a potentially fatal hypertensive reaction known as a "cheese effect" because it can be precipitated by foods rich in tyramine such as some cheeses, aged meats, and red wine. Selegiline and rasagiline do not functionally inhibit MAO-A and are not associated with a cheese effect with doses typically used in clinical practice. There are theoretical risks of a serotonin reaction in patients receiving concomitant selective serotonin reuptake inhibitor (SSRI) antidepressants, but these are rarely encountered.

Interest in MAO-B inhibitors has also focused on their potential to have disease-modifying effects. MPTP toxicity can be prevented experimentally by coadministration of an MAO-B inhibitor that blocks its conversion to the toxic pyridinium ion MPP^+. MAO-B inhibitors also have the potential to block the oxidative metabolism of dopamine and prevent oxidative stress. In addition, both selegiline and rasagiline incorporate a propargyl ring within their molecular structure that provides antiapoptotic effects in laboratory models. The DATATOP study showed that selegiline significantly delayed the time until the emergence of disability, necessitating the introduction of levodopa, in untreated PD patients. However, it could not be determined whether this was due to a neuroprotective effect that slowed disease progression or a symptomatic effect that merely masked ongoing neurodegeneration. More recently, the ADAGIO study demonstrated that early treatment with rasagiline 1 mg/d, but not 2 mg/d, provided benefits that could not be achieved when treatment with the same drug was initiated at a later time point, consistent with a disease-modifying effect; however, the long-term significance of these findings is uncertain.

COMT INHIBITORS

When levodopa is administered with a decarboxylase inhibitor, it is primarily metabolized in the periphery by COMT. Inhibitors of COMT increase the elimination half-life of levodopa and enhance its brain availability. Combining levodopa with a COMT inhibitor reduces "off" time and prolongs "on" time in fluctuating patients while enhancing motor scores. Two COMT inhibitors have been approved, tolcapone and entacapone. There is also a combination tablet of levodopa, carbidopa, and entacapone (Stalevo).

Side effects of COMT inhibitors are primarily dopaminergic (nausea, vomiting, increased dyskinesia) and can usually be controlled by down-titrating the dose of levodopa by 20–30%. Severe diarrhea has been described with tolcapone, and to a lesser degree with entacapone, and necessitates stopping the medication in 5–10% of individuals. Cases of fatal hepatic toxicity have been reported with tolcapone, and periodic monitoring of liver function is required. This problem has not been encountered with entacapone. Discoloration of urine can be seen with both COMT inhibitors due to accumulation of a metabolite, but it is of no clinical concern.

It has been proposed that initiating levodopa in combination with a COMT inhibitor to enhance its elimination half-life could provide more continuous levodopa delivery if administered at frequent intervals and reduce the risk of motor complications. While this result has been demonstrated in a preclinical MPTP model, and continuous infusion reduces both "off" time and dyskinesia in advanced PD patients, no benefit of initiating levodopa with a COMT inhibitor compared to levodopa alone was detected in early PD patients in the STRIDE-PD study. This may have been because the combination was not administered at frequent enough intervals to provide continuous levodopa availability. For now, the main value of COMT inhibitors continues to be in patients who experience motor fluctuations.

OTHER MEDICAL THERAPIES

Centrally acting anticholinergic drugs such as trihexyphenidyl and benztropine were used historically for the treatment of PD, but they lost favor with the introduction of dopaminergic agents. Their major clinical effect is on tremor, although it is not certain that this benefit is superior to what can be obtained with agents such as levodopa and dopamine agonists. Still, they can be helpful in individual patients with severe tremor. Their use is limited particularly in the elderly, due to their propensity to induce a variety of side effects including urinary dysfunction, glaucoma, and particularly cognitive impairment.

TABLE 449-5 DRUGS COMMONLY USED FOR TREATMENT OF PARKINSON'S DISEASE[a]

Agent	Available Dosages	Typical Dosing
Levodopa[a]		
Carbidopa/levodopa	10/100, 25/100, 25/250 mg	200–1000 mg levodopa/d 2–4 times/d
Benserazide/levodopa	25/100, 50/200 mg	
Carbidopa/levodopa CR	25/100, 50/200 mg	
Benserazide/levodopa MDS	25/200, 25/250 mg	
Parcopa	10/100, 25/100, 25/250	
Carbidopa/levodopa/entacapone	12.5/50/200, 18.75/75/200, 25/100/200, 31.25/125/200, 37.5/150/200, 50/200/200 mg	
Dopamine agonists		
Pramipexole	0.125, 0.25, 0.5, 1.0, 1.5 mg	0.25–1.0 mg tid
Pramipexole ER	0.375, 0.75, 1.5. 3.0, 4.5 mg	1–3 mg/d
Ropinirole	0.25, 0.5, 1.0, 3.0 mg	6–24 mg/d
Ropinirole XL	2, 4, 6, 8 mg	6–24 mg/d
Rotigotine patch	2-, 4-, 6-, 8-mg patches	4–24 mg/d
Apomorphine SC		2–8 mg
COMT inhibitors		
Entacapone	200 mg	200 mg with each levodopa dose
Tolcapone	100, 200 mg	100–200 mg tid
MAO-B inhibitors		
Selegiline	5 mg	5 mg bid
Rasagiline	0.5, 1.0 mg	1.0 mg QAM

[a]Treatment should be individualized. Generally, drugs should be started in low doses and titrated to optimal dose.

Note: Drugs should not be withdrawn abruptly but should be gradually lowered or removed as appropriate.

Abbreviations: COMT, catechol-*O*-methyltransferase; MAO-B, monoamine oxidase type B; QAM, every morning.

Amantadine also has historical importance. Originally introduced as an antiviral agent, it was appreciated to also have antiparkinsonian effects that are now thought to be due to *N*-methyl-D-aspartate (NMDA) receptor antagonism. While some physicians use amantadine in patients with early disease for its mild symptomatic effects, it is most widely used as an antidyskinesia agent in patients with advanced PD. Indeed, it is the only oral agent that has been demonstrated in controlled studies to reduce dyskinesia without worsening parkinsonian features, although benefits may be relatively transient. Cognitive impairment is a major concern. Other side effects include livido reticularis and weight gain. Amantadine should always be discontinued gradually because patients can experience withdrawal-like symptoms.

Several new classes of drug are currently being investigated in an attempt to enhance antiparkinsonian effects, reduce off time, and treat or prevent dyskinesia. These include adenosine A_{2A} antagonists, nicotinic agonists, glutamate antagonists, and 5-HT_{1A} agonists.

A list of the major drugs and available dosage strengths is provided in **Table 449-5**.

NEUROPROTECTION

Despite the many therapeutic agents available for the treatment of PD, patients continue to experience disease progression with intolerable disability. A neuroprotective therapy that slows or stops disease progression remains the major unmet therapeutic need in PD. As noted above, trials of certain drugs (e.g., selegiline and rasagiline) have provided positive results consistent with a disease-modifying effect. However, it is not possible to determine if the positive results were due to neuroprotection with slowing of disease progression or confounding symptomatic effects that mask ongoing progression. CoQ10, a mitochondrial bioenhancer and antioxidant, attracted attention with a positive preliminary trial, but this was not replicated in larger double-blind studies.

SURGICAL TREATMENT

Surgical treatments for PD have been used for more than a century. Lesions placed in the motor cortex improved tremor but were associated with motor deficits, and this approach was abandoned. Subsequently, it was appreciated that lesions placed into the ventral intermediate (VIM) nucleus of the thalamus reduced contralateral tremor without inducing hemiparesis, but these lesions did not meaningfully help other more disabling features of PD. In the 1990s, it was shown that lesions placed in the posteroventral portion of the GPi (motor territory) improved rigidity and bradykinesia as well as tremor. Importantly, pallidotomy was also associated with marked improvement in contralateral dyskinesia. This procedure gained favor with greater understanding of the pathophysiology of PD (see above). However, this procedure is not optimal for patients with bilateral disease, because bilateral lesions are associated with side effects such as dysphagia, dysarthria, and impaired cognition, and has largely been replaced by deep brain stimulation (DBS). Unilateral lesions of the STN are associated with a larger antiparkinsonian benefit and reduced levodopa requirement, but there is a concern about the risk of hemiballismus, and this procedure is not commonly performed.

Most surgical procedures for PD performed today use DBS. Here, an electrode is placed into the target area and connected to a stimulator inserted SC over the chest wall. DBS simulates the effects of a lesion without necessitating making a brain lesion. The precise mechanism whereby DBS works is not fully resolved but may act by disrupting the abnormal signal associated with PD and motor complications. The stimulation variables can be adjusted with respect to electrode configuration, voltage, frequency, and pulse duration in order to maximize benefit and minimize adverse side effects. In cases with intolerable side effects, stimulation can be stopped and the system removed. The procedure does not require making a lesion in the brain and is thus suitable for performing bilateral procedures with relative safety.

DBS for PD primarily targets the STN or the GPi. It provides dramatic results, particularly with respect to reducing "off" time and dyskinesias, but does not improve or prevent the development of features that fail to respond to levodopa such as freezing, falling, and dementia. The procedure is thus primarily indicated for patients who suffer disability resulting from severe tremor, or levodopa-induced motor complications that cannot be satisfactorily controlled with drug manipulation. In such patients, DBS has been shown to improve quality of life in comparison to best medical therapy. Side effects can be seen with respect to the surgical procedure (hemorrhage, infarction, infection), the DBS system (infection, lead break, lead displacement, skin ulceration), or the stimulation itself (ocular and speech abnormalities, muscle twitches, paresthesias, depression, and rarely suicide). Recent studies indicate that benefits following DBS of the STN and GPi are comparable, but that GPi stimulation may be associated with a reduced frequency of depression. Although not all PD patients are candidates, the procedure is profoundly beneficial for many. Studies of DBS in early PD patients show benefits in comparison to medical therapy, but this must be weighed against the cost of the procedure and the risk of side effects. Long-term studies demonstrate continued benefits with respect to the classical motor features of PD, but DBS does not prevent the development of nondopaminergic features, which continue to be a source of disability. Studies continue to evaluate the optimal way to use DBS (low- vs high-frequency stimulation, closed systems, etc.). Comparison of DBS to other therapies aimed at improving motor function without causing dyskinesia, such as

Duodopa and apomorphine infusions, remains to be performed. Studies are examining additional DBS targets that might benefit gait dysfunction, depression, and cognitive impairment in PD patients.

EXPERIMENTAL THERAPIES FOR PD

There has been considerable scientific and public interest in a number of novel interventions that are being investigated as possible treatments for PD. These include cell-based therapies (such as transplantation of fetal nigral dopamine cells or dopamine neurons derived from stem cells), gene therapies, and trophic factors. Transplant strategies are based on the concept of implanting dopaminergic cells into the striatum to replace degenerating SNc dopamine neurons. Fetal nigral mesencephalic cells have been demonstrated to survive implantation, re-innervate the striatum in an organotypic manner, and restore motor function in PD models. However, two double-blind studies failed to show significant benefit of fetal nigral transplantation in comparison to a sham operation with respect to their primary endpoints. Additionally, grafting of fetal nigral cells is associated with a previously unrecognized form of dyskinesia that persists after lowering or even stopping levodopa. This has been postulated to be related to unregulated release of dopamine from serotonin neurons. In addition, there is evidence that after many years, transplanted healthy embryonic dopamine neurons from unrelated donors develop PD pathology and become dysfunctional, suggesting transfer of α-synuclein from affected to unaffected neurons in a prion-like manner (see discussion above). Perhaps most importantly, it is not clear how replacing dopamine cells alone will improve nondopaminergic features such as falling and dementia, which are the major sources of disability for patients with advanced disease. These same concerns apply to dopamine neurons derived from stem cells, which have not yet been properly tested in PD patients and bear the additional concern of tumors and unanticipated side effects. The short-term future for this technology as a treatment for PD, at least in its current state, is therefore not promising, and there is no scientific basis to warrant routine treatment with stem cells as is being marketed in some countries.

Trophic factors are a series of proteins that enhance neuronal growth and restore function to damaged neurons. There are several different trophic factors that have been demonstrated to have beneficial effects on dopamine neurons in laboratory studies. Glial-derived neurotrophic factor (GDNF) and neurturin have attracted particular attention as possible therapies for PD. However, double-blind trials of intraventricular and intraputaminal infusions of GDNF failed to show benefits compared to placebo in PD patients, possibly because of inadequate delivery of the trophic molecule throughout the target region.

Gene delivery offers the potential of providing widespread delivery throughout a target region and long-term expression of a therapeutic protein with a single procedure. Gene therapy involves placing the DNA of a therapeutic protein into a viral vector that can then be delivered to specific target regions. The DNA of the therapeutic protein is then incorporated into the genome of the host cells and released on a continual basis. The AAV2 virus has been most often used as the viral vector because it does not promote an inflammatory response, is not incorporated into the host genome, and is associated with long-lasting transgene expression. Clinical trials of AAV2 delivery of the trophic factor neurturin showed promising results in open label trials but failed in double-blind trials, possibly because axonal damage in PD prevented retrograde transport of the protein to dopamine neurons in the SNc where it is required to induce upregulation of repair genes required for the trophic response. However, a subsequent double-blind trial of AAV2-neurturin delivered into both the putamen and SNc also failed.

Gene delivery is also being explored as a means of delivering aromatic amino acid decarboxylase with or without tyrosine hydroxylase to the striatum to facilitate dopamine production and glutamic acid decarboxylase to the STN to inhibit overactive neuronal firing. None of these procedures has been established to be effective in PD patients. Furthermore, although gene delivery technology has great potential, this approach also carries the risk of unanticipated side effects, and current approaches directed at the nigrostriatal system do not address the nondopaminergic features of the illness.

MANAGEMENT OF THE NONMOTOR AND NONDOPAMINERGIC FEATURES OF PD

Although PD management has primarily focused on the dopaminergic features of the disease, management of the nondopaminergic features should not be ignored. Some nonmotor features, although not thought to reflect dopaminergic pathology, nonetheless benefit from dopaminergic drugs. For example, problems such as anxiety, panic attacks, depression, sweating, sensory problems, freezing, and constipation all tend to be worse during "off" periods and may improve with better dopaminergic control. Approximately 50% of PD patients suffer depression during the course of the disease, and depression is frequently underdiagnosed and undertreated. Antidepressants should not be withheld, particularly for patients with major depression. Serotonin syndromes have been a theoretical concern with the combined use of SSRIs and MAO-B inhibitors but are rarely encountered. Anxiety can be treated with short-acting benzodiazepines.

Psychosis can be a problem for some PD patients. In contrast to AD, hallucinations are typically visual, formed, and nonthreatening. Importantly, they can limit the use of dopaminergic agents to obtain satisfactory motor control. Psychosis in PD often responds to low doses of atypical neuroleptics and permits higher doses of levodopa to be tolerated. Clozapine is the most effective drug, but it can be associated with agranulocytosis, and regular monitoring is required. For this reason, many physicians start with quetiapine even though it has not been established to be effective in placebo-controlled trials. Hallucinations in PD patients are often a harbinger of a developing dementia.

Dementia in PD (PDD) is common, ultimately affecting as many as 80% of patients. Its frequency increases with aging and, in contrast to AD, primarily affects executive functions and attention, with relative sparing of language, memory, and calculations. When dementia precedes, or develops within 1 year after, the onset of motor dysfunction, it is by convention referred to as dementia with Lewy bodies (DLB; Chap. 448). These patients are particularly prone to have hallucinations and diurnal fluctuations. Pathologically, DLB is characterized by Lewy bodies distributed throughout the cerebral cortex (especially the hippocampus and amygdala) and is often also associated with AD pathology. It is likely that DLB and PDD represent a PD spectrum rather than separate disease entities. Mild cognitive impairment (MCI) frequently precedes the onset of dementia and is a more reliable index of impending dementia in PD than in the general population. Dopaminergic drugs can worsen cognitive function in demented patients and should be stopped or reduced to try and provide a compromise between antiparkinsonian benefit and preserved cognitive function. Drugs are usually discontinued in the following sequence: anticholinergics, amantadine, dopamine agonists, COMT inhibitors, and MAO-B inhibitors. Eventually, patients with cognitive impairment should be managed with the lowest dose of standard levodopa that provides meaningful antiparkinsonian effects and does not worsen mental function. Anticholinesterase agents such as rivastigmine and donepezil reduce the rate of deterioration of measures of cognitive function and can improve attention, but do not typically improve cognitive function in any meaningful way.

Autonomic disturbances are common and frequently require attention. Orthostatic hypotension can be problematic and contribute to falling. Initial treatment should include adding salt to the diet and elevating the head of the bed to prevent overnight sodium natriuresis. Low doses of fludrocortisone (Florinef) or midodrine provide control for most cases. Vasopressin, erythropoietin, and the norepinephrine precursor 3-0-methylDOPS can be used in more severe or refractory cases. If orthostatic hypotension is prominent in early disease, MSA should be considered. Sexual dysfunction can be helped with sildenafil or tadalafil. Urinary problems, especially in males, should be treated in consultation with a urologist to exclude prostate problems. Anticholinergic agents, such as oxybutynin (Ditropan), may be helpful. Constipation can be a very important problem for PD patients. Mild laxatives or enemas can be useful, but physicians should first ensure that patients are drinking adequate amounts of fluid and consuming a diet rich in bulk with green leafy vegetables and bran. Agents that promote gastrointestinal (GI) motility can also be helpful.

Sleep disturbances are common in PD patients, with many experiencing fragmented sleep with excess daytime sleepiness. Restless leg syndrome, sleep apnea, and other sleep disorders should be treated as appropriate. REM behavior disorder (RBD) is a syndrome comprised of violent movements and vocalizations during REM sleep, possibly representing acting out of dreams due to a failure of the normal inhibition of motor movements that typically accompanies REM sleep. Many PD patients have a history of antecedent RBD preceding the onset of the classic motor features of PD, and most cases of RBD go on to develop an α-synucleinopathy (PD or MSA). Low doses of clonazepam (0.5–1 mg at bedtime) are usually effective in controlling this problem. Consultation with a sleep specialist and polysomnography may be necessary to identify and optimally treat sleep problems.

NONPHARMACOLOGIC THERAPY

Gait dysfunction with falling is an important cause of disability in PD. Dopaminergic therapies can help patients whose gait is worse in "off" time, but there are currently no specific therapies available. Canes and walkers may become necessary to increase stability and reduce the risk of falling.

Freezing, where patients suddenly become stuck in place for seconds to minutes as if their feet were glued to the ground, is a major cause of falling. Freezing may occur during "on" or "off" periods. Freezing during "off" periods may respond to dopaminergic therapies, but there are no specific treatments for "on" period freezing. Some patients will respond to sensory cues such as marching in place, singing a song, or stepping over an imaginary line.

Exercise, with a full range of active and passive movements, has been shown to maintain and even improve function for PD patients, and active and passive exercises with full range of motion reduce the risk of arthritis and frozen joints. Some laboratory studies suggest the possibility that exercise might also have neuroprotective effects, but this has not been confirmed in PD. Exercise is generally recommended for all PD patients. It is less clear that physical therapy or specific exercises such as tai chi are required. It is important for patients to maintain social and intellectual activities to the extent possible. Education, assistance with financial planning, social services, and attention to home safety are important elements of the overall care plan. Information is available through numerous PD foundations and on the web, but should be reviewed with physicians to ensure accuracy. The needs of the caregiver should not be neglected. Caring for a person with PD involves a substantial work effort and there is an increased incidence of depression among caregivers. Support groups for patients and caregivers may be useful.

CURRENT MANAGEMENT OF PD

The management of PD should be tailored to the needs of the individual patient, and there is no single treatment approach that is universally accepted and applicable to all individuals. Clearly, if an agent could be demonstrated to have disease-modifying effects, it should be initiated at the time of diagnosis. Indeed, constipation, RBD, and anosmia may represent premotor features of PD and could permit the initiation of a disease-modifying therapy prior to the onset of the classical motor features of the disease. However, no therapy has yet been proved to be disease modifying. For now, physicians must use their judgment in deciding whether or not to introduce rasagiline (see above) or other drugs for their possible disease-modifying effects.

The next important issue to address is when to initiate symptomatic therapy. Several studies now suggest that it may be best to start therapy at the time of diagnosis (or soon after) in order to preserve beneficial compensatory mechanisms and possibly provide functional benefits even in the early stage of the disease. Levodopa remains the most effective symptomatic therapy for PD, and some recommend starting it immediately using low doses (≤400 mg/d), but others prefer to delay levodopa treatment, particularly in younger patients, in order to reduce the risk of inducing motor complications. An alternate approach is to begin with an MAO-B inhibitor and/or a dopamine agonist, and reserve levodopa for later stages when these drugs can no longer provide satisfactory control. In making this decision, the age, degree of disability, and side effect profile of the drug must all be considered. In patients with more severe disability, the elderly, those with cognitive impairment, or those in whom the diagnosis is uncertain, most physicians would initiate therapy with levodopa. Regardless of initial choice, it is important not to deny patients levodopa when they cannot be adequately controlled with alternative medications.

If motor complications develop, patients can initially be treated by manipulating the frequency and dose of levodopa or by combining lower doses of levodopa with a dopamine agonist, a COMT inhibitor, or an MAO-B inhibitor. Amantadine is the only drug that has been demonstrated to treat dyskinesia without worsening parkinsonism, but benefits may be short-lasting, and there are important side effects related to cognitive function. In advanced cases, it may be necessary to consider a surgical therapy such as DBS if the patient is a suitable candidate, but as described above, these procedures have their own set of complications. Continuous intraintestinal infusion of levodopa/carbidopa intestinal gel (Duodopa) appears to offer similar benefits to DBS, but also requires a surgical intervention with potentially serious complications. Continuous infusion of apomorphine is another treatment option and does not require surgery but is associated with potentially troublesome skin nodules. Comparative studies of these approaches in more advanced patients are awaited. There are ongoing efforts aimed at developing a long-acting oral or transdermal formulation of levodopa that mirrors the pharmacokinetic properties of a levodopa infusion. Such a formulation might provide all of the benefits of levodopa without motor complications and avoid the need for polypharmacy and surgical intervention.

A decision tree that considers the various treatment options and decision points for the management of PD is provided in **Fig. 449-7**.

HYPERKINETIC MOVEMENT DISORDERS

Hyperkinetic movement disorders are characterized by involuntary movements unaccompanied by weakness and occurring in isolation or in combination (Table 449-6). The major hyperkinetic movement disorders and the diseases with which they are associated are considered in this section.

TREMOR

CLINICAL FEATURES

Tremor consists of alternating contractions of agonist and antagonist muscles in an oscillating, rhythmic manner. It can be most prominent at rest (rest tremor), on assuming a posture (postural tremor), or on actively reaching for a target (kinetic tremor). Tremor is also assessed based on distribution, frequency, and related neurologic dysfunction.

PD is characterized by a resting tremor, essential tremor (ET) by a postural tremor (trying to sustain a posture), and cerebellar disease by an intention or kinetic tremor (on reaching to touch a target). Normal individuals can have a physiologic tremor that typically manifests as a mild, high-frequency (10–12 Hz), postural or action tremor that is usually of no clinical consequence and often is only appreciated with an accelerometer. An enhanced physiologic tremor (EPT) can be seen in up to 10% of the population, often in association with anxiety, fatigue, a metabolic disturbance (e.g., hyperthyroidism, electrolyte abnormalities), drugs (e.g., valproate, lithium), or toxins (e.g., alcohol). Treatment is initially directed to the control of any underlying disorder and, if necessary, can often be improved with a beta blocker.

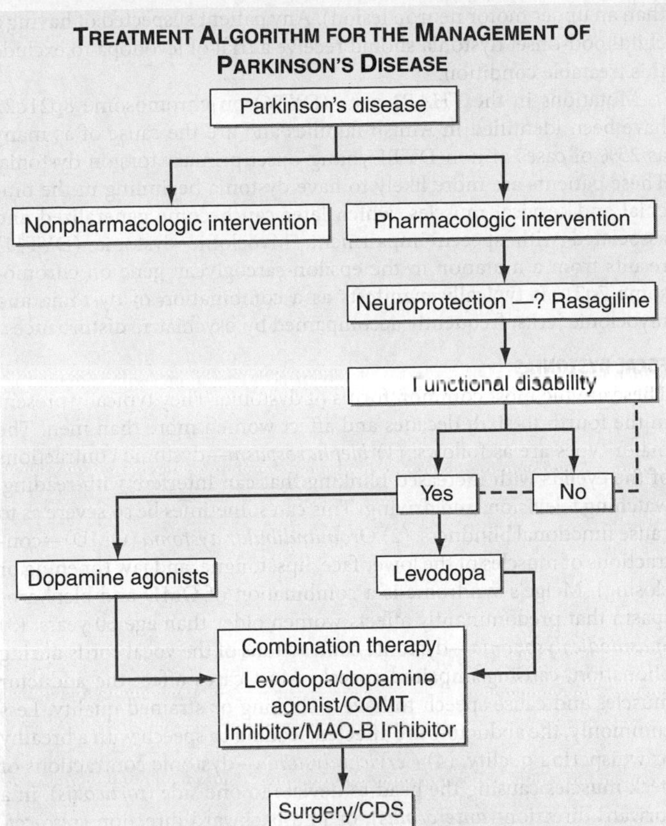

FIGURE 449-7 Treatment options for the management of Parkinson's disease (PD). Decision points include: (1) Introduction of a neuroprotective therapy: No drug has been established to have or is currently approved for neuroprotection or disease modification, but there are several agents that have this potential based on laboratory and preliminary clinical studies (e.g., rasagiline 1 mg/d, coenzyme Q10 1200 mg/d, the dopamine agonists ropinirole, and pramipexole). (2) When to initiate symptomatic therapy: There is a trend toward initiating therapy at the time of diagnosis or early in the course of the disease because patients may have some disability even at an early stage, and there is the possibility that early treatment may preserve beneficial compensatory mechanisms; however, some experts recommend waiting until there is functional disability before initiating therapy. (3) What therapy to initiate: Many experts favor starting with a monoamine oxidase type B (MAO-B) inhibitor in mildly affected patients because of the good safety profile of the drug and the potential for a disease-modifying effect; dopamine agonists for younger patients with functionally significant disability to reduce the risk of motor complications; and levodopa for patients with more advanced disease, the elderly, or those with cognitive impairment. Recent studies suggest the early employment of polypharmacy using low doses of multiple drugs to avoid side effects associated with high doses of any one agent. (4) Management of motor complications: Motor complications are typically approached with combination therapy to try and reduce dyskinesia and enhance the "on" time. When medical therapies cannot provide satisfactory control, surgical therapies such as DBS or continuous infusion of levodopa/carbidopa intestinal gel can be considered. (5) Nonpharmacologic approaches: Interventions such as exercise, education, and support should be considered throughout the course of the disease. CDS, continuous dopaminergic stimulation; COMT, catechol-*O*-methyltransferase. *(Adapted from CW Olanow et al: Neurology 72:S1, 2009.)*

ESSENTIAL TREMOR

ET is the commonest movement disorder, affecting approximately 5–10 million persons in the United States. It can present in childhood but dramatically increases in prevalence over the age of 70 years. ET is characterized by a high-frequency tremor (6–10 Hz) that predominantly affects the upper extremities. The tremor is most often manifest as a postural or action (kinetic) tremor and, in severe cases, can interfere with functions such as eating and drinking. It is typically bilateral and symmetric but may begin on one side and remain asymmetric. Patients with severe ET can have an intention tremor with overshoot and slowness of movement. Tremor involves the head in ~30% of cases, voice in ~20%, tongue in ~20%, face/jaw in ~10%, and lower limbs in ~10%. The tremor is characteristically improved by alcohol and worsened by stress. Subtle impairment of coordination or tandem walking may be present, and disturbances of hearing, cognition, personality, mood, and olfaction have also been described, but usually the neurologic examination is normal aside from tremor. The major differential is a dystonic tremor (see below) or PD. PD can usually be differentiated from ET based on the presence of bradykinesia, rigidity, micrographia, and other parkinsonian features. However, the examiner should be aware that PD patients may have a postural tremor and ET patients may develop a rest tremor. These typically begin after a latency of a few seconds (emergent tremor). The examiner must take care to differentiate the effect of tremor on measurement of tone in ET from the cogwheel rigidity found in PD.

TABLE 449-6 HYPERKINETIC MOVEMENT DISORDERS

Tremor	Rhythmic oscillation of a body part due to intermittent muscle contractions
Dystonia	Involuntary, patterned, sustained or repeated muscle contractions often associated with twisting movements and abnormal posture
Athetosis	Slow, distal, writhing, involuntary movements with a propensity to affect the arms and hands (this represents a form of dystonia with increased mobility)
Chorea	Rapid, semi-purposeful, graceful, dance-like nonpatterned involuntary movements involving distal or proximal muscle groups. When the movements are of large amplitude and predominant proximal distribution, the term *ballism* is used.
Myoclonus	Sudden, brief (<100 ms), jerk-like, arrhythmic muscle twitches
Tic	Brief, repeated, stereotyped muscle contractions that can often be suppressed for a short time. These can be simple and involve a single muscle group or complex and affect a range of motor activities.

ETIOLOGY AND PATHOPHYSIOLOGY

The etiology and pathophysiology of ET are not known. Approximately 50% of cases have a positive family history with an autosomal dominant pattern of inheritance. Linkage studies have detected loci at chromosomes 3q13 (ETM-1), 2p22-25 (ETM-2), and 6p23 (ETM-3), but no causative genes have been identified to date. GWAS demonstrated an association with the *LINGO1* gene, which is involved in oligodendrocyte differentiation and myelination, particularly in patients with young-onset ET. Recently, a nonsense mutation in the fused in sarcoma (*FUS*) gene was implicated as a cause of ET in a multigenerational family from Canada; this finding is of particular interest because different mutations in *FUS* are a known cause of familial amyotrophic lateral sclerosis (Chap. 452). It is likely that there are many other undiscovered genes for ET. The cerebellum and inferior olives have been implicated as possible sites of a "tremor pacemaker" based on the presence of cerebellar signs and increased metabolic activity and blood flow in these regions in some patients. Some pathologic studies have described cerebellar pathology with a loss of Purkinje cells and axonal torpedoes, but these findings are controversial and the precise pathologic correlate of ET remains to be defined.

TREATMENT

Many cases are mild and require no treatment other than reassurance. Occasionally, tremor can be severe and interfere with eating, writing, and activities of daily living. This is more likely to occur as the patient ages and is often associated with a reduction in tremor frequency. Beta blockers and primidone are the standard drug therapies for ET and help in about 50% of cases. Propranolol (20–120 mg daily, given in divided doses) is usually effective at relatively low doses, but higher doses may be effective in some patients. The drug is contraindicated in patients with bradycardia or asthma. Hand tremor tends to be most improved, while head tremor is often refractory. Primidone can be helpful but should be started at low doses (12.5 mg) and gradually increased (125–250 mg tid) to avoid sedation. Benefits have also been reported with gabapentin and topiramate. Botulinum toxin injections may be helpful for limb or voice tremor, but treatment can be associated with secondary muscle weakness. Surgical therapies targeting the VIM nucleus of the thalamus can be very effective for severe and drug-resistant cases.

DYSTONIA

CLINICAL FEATURES

Dystonia is a disorder characterized by sustained (>100 ms) or repetitive involuntary muscle contractions frequently associated with twisting and abnormal postures. Dystonia can range from minor contractions in an individual muscle group to severe and disabling involvement of multiple muscle groups. The frequency is estimated to be 300,000 cases in the United States but is likely to be much higher because many cases are not recognized. Dystonia is often brought out by voluntary movements (action dystonia) and can extend to involve muscle groups and body regions not required for a given action (overflow). It can be aggravated by stress and fatigue and attenuated by relaxation and sensory tricks such as touching the affected body part (geste antagoniste). Dystonia can be classified according to age of onset (childhood vs adult), distribution (focal, multifocal, segmental, or generalized), or etiology (primary or secondary).

PRIMARY DYSTONIAS

At least 16 gene mutations are associated with dystonia and classified as *DYT1–DYT16*. Idiopathic torsion dystonia (DYT1) or Oppenheim's dystonia is predominantly a childhood-onset form of dystonia with an autosomal dominant pattern of inheritance that primarily affects Ashkenazi Jewish families. The majority of patients have an age of onset younger than 26 years (mean 14 years). In young-onset patients, dystonia typically begins in the foot or the arm and in 60–70% progresses to involve other limbs as well as the head and neck. In severe cases, patients can suffer disabling postural deformities that compromise mobility. Severity can vary within family members, with some affected relatives having severe disability and others a mild dystonia that may not even be appreciated. Most childhood-onset cases are linked to a mutation in the *DYT1* gene located on chromosome 9q34, resulting in a trinucleotide GAG deletion with loss of one of a pair of glutamic acid residues in the protein torsin A. *DYT1* mutations are found in 90% of Ashkenazi Jewish patients with DYT1 dystonia and probably relate to a founder effect that occurred about 350 years ago. There is variable penetrance, with only about 30% of gene carriers expressing a clinical phenotype. Why some gene carriers express dystonia and others do not is not known. The function of torsin A is unknown, but it is a member of the AAA$^+$ (ATPase) family that resembles heat-shock proteins and may be related to protein processing and transport. The precise pathology responsible for DYT1 dystonia is not known.

Dopa-responsive dystonia (DRD) or the Segawa variant (DYT5) is a dominantly inherited form of childhood-onset dystonia caused by a mutation in the gene that encodes GTP cyclohydrolase-I, the rate-limiting enzyme for the synthesis of tetrahydrobiopterin. This mutation leads to a defect in the biochemical synthesis of tyrosine hydroxylase, the rate-limiting enzyme in the formation of dopamine. DRD typically presents in early childhood (1–12 years) and is characterized by foot dystonia that interferes with walking. Patients often experience diurnal fluctuations, with worsening of gait as the day progresses and improvement with sleep. DRD is typified by an excellent and sustained response to small doses of levodopa. Some patients may present with parkinsonian features, but can be differentiated from juvenile PD by normal striatal dopamine imaging and the absence of levodopa-induced dyskinesias. DRD may occasionally be confused with cerebral palsy because patients appear to have spasticity, increased reflexes, and Babinski responses (which likely reflect a dystonic contraction rather than an upper motor neuron lesion). Any patient suspected of having a childhood-onset dystonia should receive a trial of levodopa to exclude this treatable condition.

Mutations in the *THAP1* gene (DYT6) on chromosome 8p21q22 have been identified in Amish families and are the cause of as many as 25% of cases of non-DYT1 young-onset primary torsion dystonia. These patients are more likely to have dystonia beginning in the brachial and cervical muscles, which later can become generalized and associated with speech impairment. Myoclonic dystonia (DYT11) results from a mutation in the epsilon-sarcoglycan gene on chromosome 7q21. It typically manifests as a combination of dystonia and myoclonic jerks, frequently accompanied by psychiatric disturbances.

FOCAL DYSTONIAS

These are the most common forms of dystonia. They typically present in the fourth to sixth decades and affect women more than men. The major types are as follows: (1) *blepharospasm*—dystonic contractions of the eyelids with increased blinking that can interfere with reading, watching television, and driving. This can sometimes be so severe as to cause functional blindness. (2) *Oromandibular dystonia* (OMD)—contractions of muscles of the lower face, lips, tongue, and jaw (opening or closing). Meige's syndrome is a combination of OMD and blepharospasm that predominantly affects women older than age 60 years. (3) *Spasmodic dysphonia*—dystonic contractions of the vocal cords during phonation, causing impaired speech. Most cases affect the adductor muscles and cause speech to have a choking or strained quality. Less commonly, the abductors are affected, leading to speech with a breathy or whispering quality. (4) *Cervical dystonia*—dystonic contractions of neck muscles causing the head to deviate to one side (*torticollis*), in a forward direction (*anterocollis*), or in a backward direction (*retrocollis*). Muscle contractions can be painful and associated with a secondary cervical radiculopathy. (5) *Limb dystonias*—these can be present in either arms or legs and are often brought out by task-specific activities such as handwriting (writer's cramp), playing a musical instrument (musician's cramp), or putting (the yips). Focal dystonias can extend to involve other body regions (about 30% of cases) and are frequently misdiagnosed as psychiatric or orthopedic in origin. Their cause is not known, but genetic factors, autoimmunity, and trauma have been suggested. Focal dystonias are often associated with a high-frequency tremor that resembles ET. Dystonic tremor can usually be distinguished from ET because it tends to occur in conjunction with the dystonic contraction and disappears when the dystonia is relieved.

SECONDARY DYSTONIAS

These develop as a consequence of drugs or other neurologic disorders. Drug-induced dystonia is most commonly seen with neuroleptic drugs or after chronic levodopa treatment in PD patients and may be acute or chronic (see below). Secondary dystonia can also be observed following discrete lesions in the striatum and occasionally in the pallidum, thalamus, cortex, and brainstem due to infarction, anoxia, metabolic disorders, trauma, tumor, infection, or toxins such as manganese or carbon monoxide. In these cases, dystonia often assumes a segmental distribution, but it can be generalized when lesions are bilateral or widespread. More rarely, dystonia can develop following peripheral nerve injury and be associated with features of complex regional pain syndrome (Chap. 454). A psychogenic origin is responsible for some cases of dystonia presenting with fixed, immobile dystonic postures (see below).

DYSTONIA PLUS SYNDROMES

Dystonia may occur as a part of another neurodegenerative conditions such as Huntington's disease, PD, Wilson's disease, corticobasilar ganglionic degeneration, PSP, the Lubag form of dystonia-parkinsonism (DYT3), and mitochondrial encephalopathies. In contrast to the primary dystonias, dystonia is usually not the dominant neurologic feature in these conditions.

PATHOPHYSIOLOGY OF DYSTONIA

The pathophysiologic basis of dystonia is not completely known. The phenomenon is characterized by co-contracting synchronous bursts of agonist and antagonist muscle groups with recruitment of muscle groups that are not required for a given movement (overflow). Dystonia is characterized by derangement of the basic physiological principle of action-selection, leading to abnormal recruitment of inappropriate muscles for a given action with inadequate inhibition of this undesired motor activity. Physiologically, loss of inhibition is observed at multiple levels of the motor system (e.g., cortex, brainstem, spinal cord) accompanied by increased cortical excitability and reorganization. Attention has focused on the basal ganglia as the site of origin of at least some types of dystonia because there are alterations in blood flow and metabolism in these structures. Further, lesions of the GPi can induce dystonia, and surgical ablation or DBS of the globus pallidus can ameliorate dystonia. The dopamine system has also been implicated, because dopaminergic therapies can both induce and treat some forms of dystonia. Interestingly, no specific pathology has been consistently identified in primary dystonia.

TREATMENT DYSTONIA

Treatment of dystonia is for the most part symptomatic except in rare cases where correction of a primary underlying condition is possible. Wilson's disease should be ruled out in young patients with dystonia. Levodopa should be tried in all cases of childhood-onset dystonia to rule out DRD. High-dose anticholinergics (e.g., trihexyphenidyl 20–120 mg/d) may be beneficial in children, but adults can rarely tolerate high doses because of side effects related to cognitive impairment with hallucinations. Oral baclofen (20–120 mg) may also be helpful, but benefits, if present, are usually modest, and side effects of sedation, weakness, and memory loss can be problematic. Intrathecal infusion of baclofen is more likely to be useful, particularly for leg and trunk dystonia, but benefits are frequently not sustained, and complications can be serious and include infection, seizures, and coma. Tetrabenazine (the usual starting dose is 12.5 mg/d and the average treating dose is 25–75 mg/d) is another consideration, but use may be limited by sedation and the development of parkinsonism. Neuroleptics can improve as well as induce dystonia, but they are typically not recommended because of their potential to induce parkinsonism and other movement disorders, including tardive dystonia. Clonazepam and diazepam are rarely effective.

Botulinum toxin has become the preferred treatment for patients with focal dystonia, particularly where involvement is limited to small muscle groups such as in blepharospasm, torticollis, and spasmodic dysphonia. Botulinum toxin acts by blocking the release of acetylcholine at the neuromuscular junction, leading to reduced dystonic muscle contractions, but excessive weakness may ensue and can be troublesome particularly if it involves neck and swallowing muscles. Two serotypes of botulinum toxin are available (A and B). Both are effective, and it is not clear that there are advantages of one over the other. No systemic side effects are encountered with the doses typically used, but benefits are transient, and repeat injections are required at 2- to 5-month intervals. Some patients fail to respond after having experienced an initial benefit. This has been attributed to antibody formation, but improper muscle selection, injection technique, and inadequate dose should be excluded.

Surgical therapy is an alternative for patients with severe dystonia who are not responsive to other treatments. Peripheral procedures such as rhizotomy and myotomy were used in the past to treat cervical dystonia, but are now rarely used. DBS of the pallidum can provide dramatic benefits for patients with primary DYT1 dystonia. This represents a major therapeutic advance because previously there was no consistently effective therapy, especially for these patients who had severe disability. Benefits tend to be obtained with a lower frequency of stimulation and often occur after a relatively long latency (weeks) in comparison to PD. Better results are typically obtained in younger patients with shorter disease duration. Recent studies suggest that DBS may also be valuable for patients with focal and secondary dystonias, although results are less consistent. Supportive treatments such as physical therapy and education are important and should be a part of the treatment regimen.

Physicians should be aware of dystonic storm, a rare but potentially fatal condition that can occur in response to a stress situation such as surgery in patients with preexisting dystonia. It consists of the acute onset of generalized and persistent dystonic contractions that can involve the vocal cords or laryngeal muscles, leading to airway obstruction. Patients may experience rhabdomyolysis with renal failure and should be managed in an intensive care unit with airway protection if required. Treatment can be instituted with one or a combination of anticholinergics, diphenhydramine, baclofen, benzodiazepines, and dopaminergic agents. Spasms may be difficult to control, and anesthesia with muscle paralysis may be required. Most, if not all, cases of dystonic storm are due to a secondary cause.

CHOREAS

HUNTINGTON'S DISEASE (HD)

HD is a progressive, fatal, highly penetrant autosomal dominant disorder characterized by motor, behavioral, oculomotor, and cognitive dysfunction. The disease is named for George Huntington, a family physician who described cases on Long Island, New York, in the nineteenth century. Onset is typically between the ages of 25 and 45 years (range, 3–70 years) with a prevalence of 2–8 cases per 100,000 and an average age at death of 60 years. It is prevalent in Europe, North and South America, and Australia but is rare in African blacks and Asians. HD is characterized by rapid, nonpatterned, semipurposeful, involuntary choreiform movements, and for this reason was formerly referred to as Huntington's chorea. In the early stages, the chorea tends to be focal or segmental, but progresses over time to involve multiple body regions. Dysarthria, gait disturbance, oculomotor abnormalities, behavioral disturbance, and cognitive impairment with dementia are also common features. With advancing disease, there tends to be a reduction in chorea and the emergence of dystonia, rigidity, bradykinesia, and myoclonus. Functional decline is often predicted by progressive weight loss despite adequate calorie intake. In younger patients (~10% of cases), HD can present as an akinetic-rigid or parkinsonian syndrome (Westphal variant). HD patients eventually develop behavioral and cognitive disturbances, and the majority progress to dementia. Depression with suicidal tendencies, aggressive behavior, and psychosis can be prominent features. HD patients may also develop non-insulin-dependent diabetes mellitus and neuroendocrine abnormalities (e.g., hypothalamic dysfunction). A clinical diagnosis of HD can be strongly suspected in cases of chorea with a positive family history, but genetic testing provides the ultimate confirmation of the diagnosis. The disease predominantly affects the striatum. Progressive atrophy of the heads of the caudate nuclei, which form the lateral margins of the lateral ventricles, can be visualized by MRI (Fig. 449-8), but the putamen can be equally or even more severely affected. More diffuse cortical atrophy is seen in the middle and late stages of the disease. Supportive studies include reduced metabolic activity in the caudate nucleus and putamen. Genetic testing can be used to confirm the diagnosis and to detect at-risk individuals in the family, but must be performed with caution and in conjunction with trained counselors, because positive results can worsen depression and generate suicidal reactions. The neuropathology of HD consists of prominent neuronal loss and gliosis in the caudate nucleus and putamen; similar changes are also widespread in the cerebral cortex. Intraneuronal inclusions containing aggregates of ubiquitin and the mutant protein huntingtin are found in the nuclei of affected neurons.

In anticipation of developing neuroprotective therapies, there has been an intensive effort to define the premanifest stage of HD. Subtle motor impairment, cognitive alterations, and imaging changes can be detected in at-risk individuals who later go on to develop the manifest form of the disease. Defining the rate of progression of these features is paramount for future studies of putative disease-modifying therapies.

ETIOLOGY

HD is caused by an increase in the number of polyglutamine (CAG) repeats (>40) in the coding sequence of the huntingtin gene located on

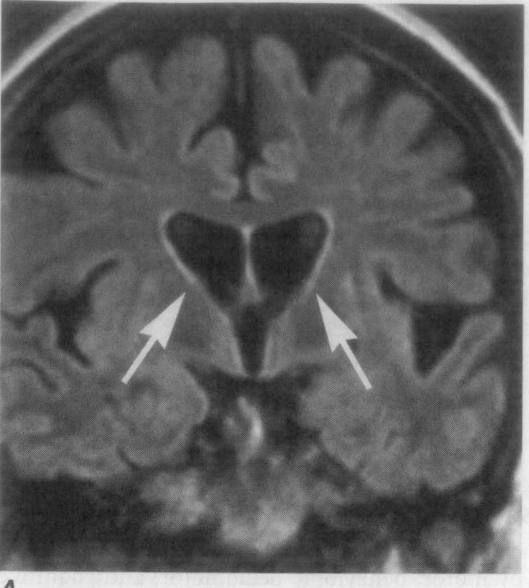

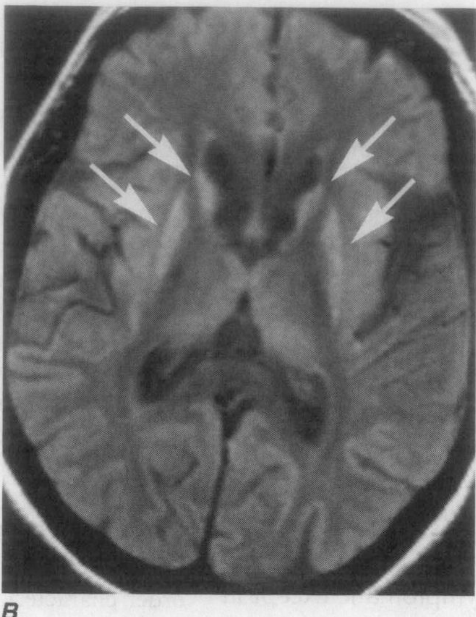

A B

FIGURE 449-8 Huntington's disease. *A.* Coronal fluid attenuated inversion recovery (FLAIR) magnetic resonance imaging shows enlargement of the lateral ventricles reflecting typical atrophy (*arrows*). ***B.*** Axial FLAIR image demonstrates abnormal high signal in the caudate and putamen (*arrows*).

the short arm of chromosome 4. The larger the number of repeats, the earlier the disease is manifest. Intermediate forms of the disease with 36–39 repeats are described in some patients, typically with less severe clinical involvement. Acceleration of the process tends to occur, particularly in males, with subsequent generations having larger numbers of repeats and earlier age of disease onset, a phenomenon referred to as anticipation. The gene encodes the highly conserved cytoplasmic protein huntingtin, which is widely distributed in neurons throughout the central nervous system (CNS) but whose function is not known. Models of HD with striatal pathology can be induced by excitotoxic agents such as kainic acid and 3-nitropoprionic acid, which promote calcium entry into the cell and cytotoxicity. Mitochondrial dysfunction has been demonstrated in the striatum and skeletal muscle of symptomatic and presymptomatic individuals. Fragments of the mutant huntingtin protein can be toxic, possibly by translocating into the nucleus and interfering with transcriptional regulation of proteins. Neuronal inclusions found in affected regions in HD may represent a protective mechanism aimed at segregating and facilitating the clearance of these toxic proteins.

TREATMENT HUNTINGTON'S DISEASE

Although the gene for HD was identified more than two decades ago, there is still no disease-modifying therapy for this disorder. Current treatment involves a multidisciplinary approach, with medical, neuropsychiatric, social, and genetic counseling for patients and their families. Dopamine-blocking agents may control the choreatic movements. Tetrabenazine (a presynaptic dopamine depleting agent) has been approved for the treatment of chorea in the United States, but can cause secondary parkinsonism. Neuroleptics are generally not recommended because of their potential to induce other more troubling movement disorders and because HD chorea tends to be self-limited and is usually not disabling. Depression and anxiety can be greater problems, and patients should be treated with appropriate antidepressant and antianxiety drugs and monitored for mania and suicidal ideations. Psychosis can be treated with atypical anti-psychotics such as clozapine (50–600 mg/d), quetiapine (50–600 mg/d), and risperidone (2–8 mg/d). There is no adequate treatment for the cognitive or motor decline. A neuroprotective therapy that slows or stops disease progression is the major unmet medical need in HD. Drugs that enhance mitochondrial function and increase the clearance of defective mitochondria are being tested as possible disease-modifying therapies. Antiglutamate agents, dopamine stabilizers, caspase inhibitors, neurotrophic factors, and transplantation of fetal striatal cells are areas of active research, but none has as yet been demonstrated to have a beneficial effect in HD. The potential to use transcriptional blockade of the mutant huntingtin gene with small interfering RNAs (siRNAs) is an exciting area currently being explored.

HUNTINGTON'S DISEASE–LIKE DISORDERS

A group of rare inherited conditions that can mimic HD, designated HD-like (HDL) disorders, have also been identified. HDL-1, -2, and -4 are autosomal dominant conditions that typically present in adulthood. HDL-1 is due to expansion of an octapeptide repeat in *PRNP*, the gene encoding the prion protein (Chap. 453e). Thus HDL-1 is properly considered a prion disease. Patients exhibit onset of personality change in the third or fourth decade, followed by chorea, rigidity, myoclonus, ataxia, and epilepsy. HDL-2 manifests in the third or fourth decade with a variety of movement disorders, including chorea, dystonia, or parkinsonism and dementia. Most patients are of African descent. Acanthocytosis can sometimes be seen in these patients, and this condition must be distinguished from neuroacanthocytosis. HDL-2 is caused by an abnormally expanded CTG/CAG trinucleotide repeat expansion in the *junctophilin-3* (*JPH3*) gene. The pathology of HDL-2 consists of intranuclear inclusions immunoreactive for ubiquitin and expanded polyglutamine repeats. HDL-4, the most common condition in this group, is caused by expansion of trinucleotide repeats in *TBP*, the gene that encodes the TATA box binding protein involved in regulating transcription; this condition is identical to spinocerebellar ataxia (SCA) 17 (Chap. 451e), and most patients present primarily with ataxia rather than chorea. Mutations of the *C9Orf* gene associated with amyotrophic lateral sclerosis have also been reported in some individuals with an HDL phenotype.

OTHER CHOREAS

Chorea can be seen in a number of additional disorders. Sydenham's chorea (originally called St. Vitus's dance) is more common in females and is typically seen in childhood (5–15 years). It often develops in association with prior exposure to group A streptococcal infection and is thought to be autoimmune in nature. It is characterized by the acute onset of choreiform movements and behavioral disturbances. With the reduction in the incidence of rheumatic fever, the incidence of Sydenham's chorea has fallen, but it can still be seen in developing countries. The chorea generally responds to dopamine-blocking agents, valproic acid, and carbamazepine, but is self-limited, and treatment is generally restricted to those with severe chorea. Chorea may recur in later life, particularly in association with pregnancy (chorea gravidarum) or treatment with sex hormones. Several reports have documented cases of chorea associated with NMDA receptor antibody–positive encephalitis following herpes simplex virus encephalitis.

Chorea-acanthocytosis (neuroacanthocytosis) is a progressive and typically fatal autosomal recessive disorder that is characterized by chorea coupled with red cell abnormalities on peripheral blood smear (acanthocytes). The chorea can be severe and associated with self-mutilating behavior, dystonia, tics, seizures, and a polyneuropathy. Mutations in the *VPS13A* gene encoding chorein have been described. A phenotypically similar X-linked form of the disorder has been described in older individuals who have reactivity with Kell blood group antigens (McLeod syndrome). A benign hereditary chorea of childhood (BHC1) due to mutations in the gene for thyroid transcription factor 1 and a late-onset benign senile chorea (BHC2) have also been described. It is important to ensure that patients with these types of choreas do not have HD.

Chorea may also occur in association with vascular diseases, hypo- and hyperglycemia, and a variety of infections and degenerative disorders. Systemic lupus erythematosus is the most common systemic disorder that causes chorea, which can last for days to years. Chorea can also be seen with hyperthyroidism, autoimmune disorders including Sjögren's syndrome, infectious disorders including HIV disease, metabolic alterations, and polycythemia rubra vera; following open-heart surgery in the pediatric population; and in association with many medications (especially anticonvulsants, cocaine, CNS stimulants, estrogens, and lithium). Chorea is commonly seen in association with chronic levodopa treatment (discussed in the section on PD above). Chorea can also be seen in paraneoplastic syndromes associated with anti-CRMP-5 or anti-Hu antibodies (Chap. 122).

HEMIBALLISMUS

Hemiballismus is a violent form of chorea comprised of wild, flinging, large-amplitude movements on one side of the body. Proximal limb muscles tend to be predominantly affected. These movements may affect just one limb (monoballism) or, more exceptionally, both upper or lower limbs (paraballism). The movements may be so severe as to cause exhaustion, dehydration, local injury, and, in extreme cases, death. Fortunately, dopamine-blocking drugs can be very helpful, and importantly, hemiballismus is usually self-limiting and tends to resolve spontaneously after weeks or months. The most common cause is a partial lesion (infarct or hemorrhage) in the STN, but cases can also be seen with lesions in the putamen, thalamus, and parietal cortex. In extreme cases, pallidotomy can be very effective. Interestingly, surgically induced lesions and DBS of the STN in PD patients are usually not associated with hemiballismus.

TICS

A *tic* is a brief, rapid, recurrent, and seemingly purposeless stereotyped motor contraction. Motor tics can be simple, with movement only affecting an individual muscle group (e.g., blinking, twitching of the nose, jerking of the neck), or complex, with coordinated involvement of multiple muscle groups (e.g., jumping, sniffing, head banging, and echopraxia [mimicking movements]). Phonic (or vocal) tics can also be simple (e.g., grunting) or complex (e.g., echolalia [repeating other people's words], palilalia [repeating one's own words], and coprolalia [expression of obscene words]). Patients may also experience sensory tics, composed of unpleasant focal sensations in the face, head, or neck. These can be mild and of little clinical consequence or severe and disabling to the patient.

TOURETTE'S SYNDROME (TS)

TS is a neurobehavioral disorder named after the French neurologist Georges Gilles de la Tourette. It predominantly affects males, and the prevalence is estimated to be 0.03–1.6%, but it is likely that many mild cases do not come to medical attention. TS is characterized by multiple motor tics often accompanied by vocalizations (phonic tics). Patients characteristically can voluntarily suppress tics for short periods of time, but then experience an irresistible urge to express them. Tics vary in intensity and may be absent for days or weeks only to recur, occasionally in a different pattern. Tics tend to present between ages 2 and 15 years (mean 7 years) and often lessen or even disappear in adulthood. Associated behavioral disturbances include anxiety, depression, attention deficit hyperactivity disorder, and obsessive-compulsive disorder. Patients may experience personality disorders, self-destructive behaviors, difficulties in school, and impaired interpersonal relationships. Tics may present in adulthood and can also be seen in association with a variety of other disorders, including PD, HD, trauma, dystonia, drugs (e.g., levodopa, neuroleptics), and toxins.

Etiology and Pathophysiology TS is thought to be a genetic disorder, but no specific gene mutation has been identified. Current evidence supports a complex inheritance pattern, with one or more major genes, multiple loci, low penetrance, and environmental influences. The risk of a family with one affected child having a second is about 25%. The pathophysiology of TS is not known, but alterations in dopamine neurotransmission, opioids, and second-messenger systems have been proposed. Some cases of TS may be the consequence of an autoimmune response to β-hemolytic streptococcal infection (pediatric autoimmune neuropsychiatric disorder associated with streptococcal infection [PANDAS]); however, this entity remains controversial.

TREATMENT TOURETTE'S SYNDROME

Patients with mild disease often only require education and counseling (for themselves and family members). Drug treatment is indicated when the tics are disabling and interfere with quality of life. Therapy is individualized, and there is no singular treatment regimen that has been properly evaluated in double-blind trials. Some physicians use the α-agonist clonidine, starting at low doses and gradually increasing the dose and frequency until satisfactory control is achieved. Guanfacine (0.5–2 mg/d) is an α-agonist that is preferred by some because it only requires once-a-day dosing. Other physicians prefer to use neuroleptics. Atypical neuroleptics are usually used initially (risperidone, olanzapine, ziprasidone) because they are thought to be associated with a reduced risk of tardive dyskinesia. If they are not effective, low doses of classical neuroleptics such as haloperidol, fluphenazine, pimozide, or tiapride can be tried because the risk of tardive dyskinesia in young people is relatively low. Botulinum toxin injections can be effective in controlling focal tics that involve small muscle groups. Behavioral features, and particularly anxiety and compulsions, can be a disabling feature of TS and should be treated. The potential value of DBS targeting the anterior portion of the internal capsule, the GPi, or the thalamus is currently being explored.

MYOCLONUS

Myoclonus is a brief, rapid (<100 ms), shock-like, jerky movement consisting of single or repetitive muscle discharges. Myoclonic jerks can be focal, multifocal, segmental, or generalized and can occur spontaneously, in association with voluntary movement (action myoclonus) or in response to an external stimulus (reflex or startle myoclonus). Negative myoclonus consists of a brief loss of muscle activity (e.g., asterixis in hepatic failure). Myoclonic jerks can be severe and interfere with normal movement or benign and of no clinical consequence as is commonly observed in normal people when waking up or falling asleep (hypnogogic jerks).

Myoclonic jerks differ from tics in that they are not typically repetitive, can interfere with normal voluntary movement, and are not suppressible. They can arise in association with abnormal neuronal discharges in cortical, subcortical, brainstem, or spinal cord regions and can be associated with lesions in each of these regions, particularly in association with hypoxemia (especially following cardiac arrest), encephalopathy, and neurodegeneration. Reversible myoclonus can be seen with metabolic disturbances (renal failure, electrolyte imbalance, hypocalcemia), toxins, and many medications. Essential myoclonus is a relatively benign familial condition characterized by multifocal, very brief, lightning-like movements that are frequently alcohol sensitive. A mutation in the epsilon-sarcoglycan gene has been associated with a variety of myoclonus seen in association with dystonia (myoclonic dystonia).

TREATMENT MYOCLONUS

Treatment primarily consists of managing the underlying condition or removing an offending agent. Pharmacologic therapy involves one or a combination of GABAergic agents such as valproic acid (800–3000 mg/d), piracetam (8–20 g/d), clonazepam (2–15 mg/d), levetiracetam (1000–3000 mg/d), or primidone (500–1000 mg/d) and may be associated with striking clinical improvement in chronic cases (e.g., postanoxic myoclonus, progressive myoclonic epilepsy). The serotonin precursor 5-hydroxitriptophan (plus carbidopa) may be useful in some cases of postanoxic myoclonus.

This important group of movement disorders is primarily associated with drugs that block dopamine receptors (neuroleptics) or central dopaminergic transmission. These drugs are widely used in psychiatry, but it is important to appreciate that drugs used in the treatment of nausea or vomiting (e.g., prochlorperazine [Compazine]) or gastroesophageal disorders (e.g., metoclopramide) are neuroleptic agents. Hyperkinetic movement disorders secondary to neuroleptic drugs can be divided into those that present acutely, subacutely, or after prolonged exposure (tardive syndromes). Dopamine-blocking drugs can also be associated with a reversible parkinsonian syndrome for which anticholinergics are often concomitantly prescribed, but there is concern that this may increase the risk of developing a tardive syndrome.

ACUTE

Dystonia is the most common acute hyperkinetic drug reaction. It is typically generalized in children and focal in adults (e.g., blepharospasm, torticollis, or oromandibular dystonia). The reaction can develop within minutes of exposure and can be successfully treated in most cases with parenteral administration of anticholinergics (benztropine or diphenhydramine), benzodiazepines (lorazepam, clonazepam, or diazepam), or dopamine agonists. The abrupt onset of severe spasms may occasionally be confused with a seizure; however, there is no loss of consciousness, automatisms, or postictal features typical of epilepsy. The acute onset of chorea, stereotypic behavior, and tics may also be seen, particularly following exposure to CNS stimulants such as methylphenidate, cocaine, or amphetamines.

SUBACUTE

Akathisia is the commonest reaction in this category. It consists of motor restlessness with a need to move that is alleviated by movement. Therapy consists of removing the offending agent. When this is not possible, symptoms may be ameliorated with benzodiazepines, anticholinergics, beta blockers, or dopamine agonists.

TARDIVE SYNDROMES

These disorders develop months to years after initiation of neuroleptic treatment. Tardive dyskinesia (TD) is most common and typically presents with choreiform movements involving the mouth, lips, and tongue. In severe cases, the trunk, limbs, and respiratory muscles may also be affected. In approximately one-third of patients, TD remits within 3 months of stopping the drug, and most patients gradually improve over the course of several years. Abnormal movements may also develop or worsen after stopping the offending agent. The movements are often mild and more upsetting to the family than to the patient, but they can be severe and disabling, particularly in the context of an underlying psychiatric disorder. Atypical antipsychotics (e.g., clozapine, risperidone, olanzapine, quetiapine, ziprasidone, and aripiprazole) are thought to be associated with a lower risk of TD in comparison to traditional antipsychotics, although this remains to be established in controlled studies. Younger patients have a lower risk of developing neuroleptic-induced TD, whereas the elderly, females, and those with underlying organic cerebral dysfunction have been reported to be at greater risk. Chronic use is associated with increased risk, and specifically, the U.S. Food and Drug Administration has warned that use of metoclopramide for more than 12 weeks increases the risk of TD. Because TD can be permanent and resistant to treatment, antipsychotics should be used judiciously, atypical neuroleptics should be the preferred agent when possible, and the need for continued use should be regularly monitored.

Treatment primarily consists of stopping the offending agent. If the patient is receiving a traditional antipsychotic and withdrawal is not possible, replacement with an atypical antipsychotic should be tried. Abrupt cessation of a neuroleptic should be avoided because acute withdrawal can induce worsening. TD can persist after withdrawal of antipsychotics and can be difficult to treat. Benefits may occasionally be achieved with valproic acid, anticholinergics, or botulinum toxin injections. In refractory cases, catecholamine depleters such as tetrabenazine may be helpful, but this drug can be associated with dose-dependent sedation and orthostatic hypotension and may induce parkinsonism as a side effect. Other approaches include baclofen (40–80 mg/d), clonazepam (1–8 mg/d), or valproic acid (750–3000 mg/d). In some cases, the abnormal movement is refractory to therapy.

Chronic neuroleptic exposure can also be associated with tardive dystonia, with preferential involvement of axial muscles and characteristic rocking movements of the trunk and pelvis. Tardive dystonia can be more troublesome than tardive dyskinesia and frequently persists despite stopping medication. Valproic acid, anticholinergics, and botulinum toxin may occasionally be beneficial, but patients are frequently refractory to medical therapy. Tardive akathisia, tardive Tourette's, and tardive tremor syndromes are rare but may also occur after chronic neuroleptic exposure.

Neuroleptic medications can also be associated with a neuroleptic malignant syndrome (NMS). NMS is characterized by the acute or subacute onset of muscle rigidity, elevated temperature, altered mental status, hyperthermia, tachycardia, labile blood pressure, renal failure, and markedly elevated creatine kinase levels. Symptoms typically evolve within days or weeks after initiating the drug. NMS can also be precipitated by the abrupt withdrawal of dopaminergic medications in PD patients. Treatment involves immediate cessation of the offending antipsychotic drug and the introduction of a dopaminergic agent (e.g., a dopamine agonist or levodopa), dantrolene, or a benzodiazepine. Treatment may need to be undertaken in an intensive care setting and include supportive measures such as control of body temperature (antipyretics and cooling blankets), hydration, electrolyte replacement, and control of renal function and blood pressure.

Drugs that have serotonin-like activity (tryptophan, MDMA or "ecstasy," meperidine) or that block serotonin reuptake can induce a rare, but potentially fatal, serotonin syndrome that is characterized by confusion, hyperthermia, tachycardia, and coma as well as rigidity, ataxia, and tremor. Myoclonus is often a prominent feature, in contrast to NMS, which it resembles. Patients can be managed with propranolol, diazepam, diphenhydramine, chlorpromazine, or cyproheptadine as well as supportive measures.

A variety of drugs can also be associated with parkinsonism (see above) and hyperkinetic movement disorders. Some examples include phenytoin (chorea, dystonia, tremor, myoclonus), carbamazepine (tics and dystonia), tricyclic antidepressants (dyskinesias, tremor, myoclonus), fluoxetine (myoclonus, chorea, dystonia), oral contraceptives (dyskinesia), β-adrenergics (tremor), buspirone (akathisia, dyskinesias, myoclonus), and digoxin, cimetidine, diazoxide, lithium, methadone, and fentanyl (dyskinesias).

PAROXYSMAL DYSKINESIAS

Paroxysmal dyskinesias are a group of rare disorders characterized by episodic, brief involuntary movements that can manifest as various types of hyperkinetic movements, including chorea, dystonia, tremor, and myoclonus. There are two main categories: (1) *paroxysmal kinesigenic dyskinesia*, where the involuntary movements are triggered by sudden movement, and (2) *paroxysmal nonkinesigenic dyskinesias*, where the attacks are not induced by movement. There are rare cases of *exercise-induced dyskinesia*, where attacks are induced by prolonged exercise.

Paroxysmal kinesigenic dyskinesia (PKD) is characterized by brief, self-limited attacks induced by movement onset such as running but also occasionally by unexpected sound or photic stimulation. Attacks may affect one side of the body, last seconds to minutes at a time, and recur several times a day. They usually manifest as dystonic posturing of a limb but may also become generalized. PKD is most commonly familial with an autosomal dominant pattern of inheritance but may also occur secondary to various brain disorders such as multiple sclerosis or hyperglycemia. PKD is more frequent in males (4:1), and the onset is typically in the first or second decade of life. About 70% report sensory symptoms such as tingling or numbness of the affected limb preceding the attack by a few milliseconds. The evolution is relatively benign, and there is a trend toward resolution of the attacks over time. The cause is not known, but a mutation in the proline-rich transmembrane protein 2 (*PRRT2*) gene that may be involved in neurotransmitter release has now been identified. Treatment with low-dose anticonvulsant therapy such as carbamazepine or phenytoin is advised when the attacks are frequent and interfere with daily life activities and is effective in about 80% of patients. Some clinical features of PKD (abrupt and short-lasting attacks preceded by an "aura") and its favorable response to anticonvulsant drugs have led to speculation that it is epileptic in origin, but this has not been established.

Paroxysmal nonkinesigenic dyskinesia (PNKD) involves attacks of generalized dyskinesias precipitated by alcohol, caffeine, stress, or fatigue. In comparison to PKD, the episodes have a relatively longer duration (minutes to hours) and are less frequent (one to three per day). PNKD is inherited as autosomal dominant with incomplete penetrance pattern in some 80% of cases. A missense mutation in the myofibrillogenesis regulator (*MR-1*) gene has been identified in several families. Recognition of the condition and elimination of the underlying precipitating factors, where possible, are the first priority. Tetrabenazine, neuroleptics, dopamine-blocking agents, propranolol, clonazepam, and baclofen may be helpful. Treatment may not be required if the condition is mild and self-limited. Most patients with PNKD do not benefit from anticonvulsant drugs, but some may respond to clonazepam or other benzodiazepines.

RESTLESS LEGS SYNDROME

Restless legs syndrome (RLS) is a neurologic disorder that affects approximately 10% of the adult population (it is rare in Asians) and can cause significant morbidity in some. It was first described in the seventeenth century by an English physician (Thomas Willis), but has only recently been recognized as being a bona fide movement disorder. The four core symptoms required for diagnosis are as follows: an urge to move the legs, usually caused or accompanied by an unpleasant sensation in the legs; symptoms that begin or worsen with rest; partial or complete relief by movement; and worsening during the evening or night.

Symptoms most commonly begin in the legs, but can spread to or even begin in the upper limbs. The unpleasant sensation is often described as a creepy-crawly feeling, paresthesia, or burning. In about 80% of patients, RLS is associated with periodic leg movements (PLMs) during sleep and occasionally while awake. These involuntary movements are usually brief, lasting no more than a few seconds, and recur every 5–90 s. The restlessness and PLMs are a major cause of sleep disturbance in patients, leading to poor-quality sleep and daytime sleepiness.

RLS is a heterogeneous condition. Primary RLS is genetic, and several loci have been found with an autosomal dominant pattern of inheritance, although penetrance may be variable. The mean age of onset in genetic forms is 27 years, although pediatric cases are recognized. The severity of symptoms is variable. Secondary RLS may be associated with pregnancy or a range of underlying disorders, including anemia, ferritin deficiency, renal failure, and peripheral neuropathy. The pathogenesis probably involves disordered dopamine function, which may be peripheral or central, in association with an abnormality of iron metabolism. Diagnosis is made on clinical grounds but can be supported by polysomnography and the demonstration of PLMs. The neurologic examination is normal. Secondary RLS should be excluded, and ferritin levels, glucose, and renal function should be measured.

Most RLS sufferers have mild symptoms that do not require specific treatment. General measures to improve sleep hygiene and quality should be attempted first. If symptoms remain intrusive, low doses of dopamine agonists, e.g., pramipexole (0.25–0.5 mg) or ropinirole (1–2 mg), are given 1–2 h before bedtime. Levodopa can be effective but is frequently associated with augmentation (spread and worsening of restlessness and its appearance earlier in the day) or rebound (reappearance sometimes with worsening of symptoms at a time compatible with the drug's short half-life). Other drugs that can be effective include anticonvulsants, analgesics, and opiates. Management of secondary RLS should be directed to correcting the underlying disorder; for example, iron replacement for anemia. Iron infusion may also be helpful for severe primary RLS but requires expert supervision.

DISORDERS THAT MAY PRESENT WITH A COMBINATION OF PARKINSONISM AND HYPERKINETIC MOVEMENTS

WILSON'S DISEASE

Wilson's disease (WD) is an autosomal recessive inherited disorder of copper metabolism that may manifest with neurologic, psychiatric, and liver disorders, alone or in combination. It is caused by mutations in the gene encoding a P-type ATPase. The disease was first comprehensively described by the English neurologist Kinnier Wilson at the beginning of the twentieth century, although at around the same time the German physicians Kayser and Fleischer separately noted the characteristic association of corneal pigmentation with hepatic and neurologic features. WD has a worldwide prevalence of approximately 1 in 30,000, with a gene carrier frequency of 1 in 90. About half of WD patients (especially younger patients) manifest with liver abnormalities. The remainder present with neurologic disease (with or without underlying liver abnormalities), and a small proportion have hematologic or psychiatric problems at disease onset.

Neurologic onset usually manifests in the second decade with tremor and rigidity. The tremor is usually in the upper limbs, bilateral, and asymmetric. Tremor can be on intention or occasionally resting and, in advanced disease, can take on a wing-beating characteristic. Other features include parkinsonism with bradykinesia, dystonia (particularly facial grimacing), dysarthria, and dysphagia. More than half of those with neurologic features have a history of psychiatric disturbances, including depression, mood swings, and overt psychosis. Kayser-Fleischer (KF) rings are seen in 80% of those with hepatic presentations and virtually all with neurologic features. KF rings represent the deposition of copper in Descemet's membrane around the cornea. They consist of a characteristic grayish rim or circle at the limbus of the cornea and are best detected by slit-lamp examination. Neuropathologic examination is characterized by neurodegeneration and astrogliosis in the basal ganglia, particularly in the striatum.

WD should always be considered in the differential diagnosis of a movement disorder in the first decades of life. Low levels of blood copper and ceruloplasmin and high levels of urinary copper may be present, but normal levels do not exclude the diagnosis. A computed tomography (CT) scan usually reveals generalized brain atrophy in established cases, and ~50% have signal hypointensity in the caudate head, putamen, globus pallidum, substantia nigra, and red nucleus on T2-weighted MRI. However, correlation of imaging changes with clinical features is not good. It is very rare for WD patients with neurologic features not to have KF rings, and therefore when the diagnosis is considered, examination by slit-lamp is essential. Liver biopsy with demonstration of high copper levels remains the gold standard for the diagnosis.

In the absence of treatment, the course is progressive and leads to severe neurologic dysfunction and early death. Treatment is directed at reducing tissue copper levels and maintenance therapy to prevent reaccumulation. There is no clear consensus on treatment, and all patients should be managed in a unit with expertise in WD. Penicillamine is frequently used to increase copper excretion, but it may lead to a worsening of symptoms in the initial stages of therapy. Side effects are common and can to some degree be attenuated by coadministration of pyridoxine. Tetrathiomolybdate blocks the absorption of copper and can be used instead of penicillamine. Trientine and zinc are useful drugs for maintenance therapy. Effective treatment can reverse the neurologic features in most patients, particularly when started early. Some patients stabilize, and a few may still progress, especially those with hepatocerebral disease. KF rings tend to decrease after 3–6 months and disappear by 2 years. Adherence to maintenance therapy is a major challenge in long-term care.

NEURODEGENERATION WITH BRAIN IRON ACCUMULATION

Neurodegeneration with brain iron accumulation (NBIA) represents a group of inherited disorders characterized by iron accumulation in the basal ganglia. Clinically, they can manifest as a progressive neurologic disorder manifesting a variety of features including parkinsonism, dystonia, neuropsychiatric abnormalities, and retinal degeneration. Cognitive disorders and cerebellar dysfunction may also be seen. Presentation is usually in childhood, but adult cases have been described. Multiple genes have been identified to date. Pantothenate kinase–associated neurodegeneration (PKAN) formerly known as Hallervorden-Spatz disease and caused by a mutation in the *PANK2* gene is the most common form of NBIA, accounting for about 50% of cases. Onset is usually in early childhood and is manifest as a combination of dystonia, parkinsonism, and spasticity. MRI shows a characteristic low signal abnormality in the center of the globus pallidus on T2-weighted scans known as the "eye of the tiger" sign caused by iron accumulation. Numerous other gene mutations have been described associated with iron accumulation including mutations in *PLA2G6, C19orf12, FA2H, ATP13A2, WDR45, FTL, CP*, and *DCAF17*. One must be cautious, however, not to assume that all cases with iron accumulation in the basal ganglia represent an NBIA, because iron accumulation in specific basal ganglia regions is normal, and excess iron accumulation may occur in the basal ganglia region as a consequence of neurodegeneration of multiple causes unrelated to a defect in iron metabolism.

OTHER DISORDERS

Acanthocytosis, some hereditary spinocerebellar atrophies and spastic parapareses, and HD can also present with parkinsonian features associated with involuntary movements. Diagnosis in these cases is best established with genetic testing.

PSYCHOGENIC DISORDERS

Virtually all movement disorders including tremor, tics, dystonia, myoclonus, chorea, ballism, and parkinsonism can be psychogenic in origin. Tremor affecting the upper limbs is the most common psychogenic movement disorder. Psychogenic movements can result from a somatoform or conversion disorder, malingering (e.g., seeking financial gain), or a factitious disorder (e.g., seeking psychological gain). Psychogenic movement disorders are common (estimated to be 2–3% of patients seen in a movement disorder clinic), more frequent in women, disabling for the patient and family, and expensive for society (estimated $20 billion annually). Clinical features suggesting a psychogenic movement disorder include an acute onset and a pattern of abnormal movement that is inconsistent with a known movement disorder. Diagnosis is based on the nonorganic quality of the movement, the absence of findings of an organic disease process, and positive features that specifically point to a psychogenic illness such as variability and distractibility. For example, the magnitude of a psychogenic tremor is increased with attention and diminishes or even disappears when the patient is distracted by being asked to perform a different task or is unaware that he or she is being observed. Other positive features suggesting a psychogenic problem include a tremor frequency that is variable or that entrains with the frequency of a designated movement in the contralateral limb, and a positive response to placebo medication. Associated features can include nonanatomic sensory findings, give-way weakness, astasia-abasia (an odd, gyrating gait; Chap. 32), and multiple somatic complaints with no underlying pathology (somatoform disorder). Comorbid psychiatric problems such as anxiety, depression, and emotional trauma may be present but are not necessary for the diagnosis of a psychogenic movement disorder to be made. Psychogenic movement disorders can occur as an isolated entity or in association with an underlying organic problem. The diagnosis can often be made based on clinical features alone, and unnecessary tests or medications can be avoided. Underlying psychiatric problems may be present and should be identified and treated, but many patients with psychogenic movement disorders have no obvious psychiatric pathology. Psychotherapy and hypnosis may be of value for patients with conversion reaction, and cognitive behavioral therapy may be helpful for patients with somatoform disorders. Patients with hypochondriasis, factitious disorders, and malingering have a poor prognosis.

450 Ataxic Disorders

Roger N. Rosenberg

APPROACH TO THE PATIENT: Ataxic Disorders

Symptoms and signs of ataxia consist of gait impairment, unclear ("scanning") speech, visual blurring due to nystagmus, hand incoordination, and tremor with movement. These result from the involvement of the cerebellum and its afferent and efferent pathways, including the spinocerebellar pathways, and the frontopontocerebellar pathway originating in the rostral frontal lobe. True cerebellar ataxia must be distinguished from ataxia associated with vestibular nerve or labyrinthine disease, as the latter results in a disorder of gait associated with a significant degree of dizziness, light-headedness, or the perception of movement (Chap. 28). True cerebellar ataxia is devoid of these vertiginous complaints and is clearly an unsteady gait due to imbalance. Sensory disturbances can also on occasion simulate the imbalance of cerebellar disease; with sensory ataxia, imbalance dramatically worsens when visual input is removed (Romberg sign). Rarely, weakness of proximal leg muscles mimics cerebellar disease. In the patient who presents with ataxia, the rate and pattern of the development of cerebellar symptoms help to narrow the diagnostic possibilities (Table 450-1). A gradual and progressive increase in symptoms with bilateral and symmetric involvement suggests a genetic, metabolic, immune, or toxic etiology. Conversely, focal, unilateral symptoms with headache and impaired level of consciousness accompanied by ipsilateral cranial nerve palsies and contralateral weakness imply a space-occupying cerebellar lesion.

SYMMETRIC ATAXIA

Progressive and symmetric ataxia can be classified with respect to onset as acute (over hours or days), subacute (weeks or months), or chronic (months to years). Acute and reversible ataxias include those caused by intoxication with alcohol, phenytoin, lithium, barbiturates, and other drugs. Intoxication caused by toluene exposure, gasoline sniffing, glue sniffing, spray painting, or exposure to methyl mercury or bismuth are additional causes of acute or subacute ataxia, as is treatment with cytotoxic chemotherapeutic drugs such as fluorouracil and paclitaxel. Patients with a postinfectious syndrome (especially after varicella) may develop gait ataxia and mild dysarthria, both of which are reversible (Chap. 458). Rare infectious causes of acquired ataxia include poliovirus, coxsackievirus, echovirus, Epstein-Barr virus, toxoplasmosis, *Legionella*, and Lyme disease.

The subacute development of ataxia of gait over weeks to months (degeneration of the cerebellar vermis) may be due to the combined effects of alcoholism and malnutrition, particularly with deficiencies of vitamins B_1 and B_{12}. Hyponatremia has also been associated with ataxia. Paraneoplastic cerebellar ataxia is associated with a number of different tumors (and autoantibodies) such as breast and ovarian cancers (anti-Yo), small-cell lung cancer (anti-PQ-type voltage-gated calcium channel), and Hodgkin's disease (anti-Tr) (Chap. 122). Another paraneoplastic syndrome associated with myoclonus and opsoclonus occurs with breast (anti-Ri) and lung cancers and neuroblastoma. Elevated serum anti-glutamic acid decarboxylase (GAD) antibodies have been associated with a progressive ataxic syndrome affecting speech and gait. For all of these paraneoplastic ataxias, the neurologic syndrome may be the presenting symptom of the cancer. Another immune-mediated progressive ataxia is associated with antigliadin (and antiendomysium) antibodies and the human leukocyte antigen (HLA) DQB1*0201 haplotype; in some affected patients, biopsy of the small intestine reveals villus atrophy consistent with gluten-sensitive enteropathy (Chap. 349). Finally, subacute progressive ataxia may be caused by a prion disorder,

TABLE 450-1 ETIOLOGY OF CEREBELLAR ATAXIA

Symmetric and Progressive Signs			Focal and Ipsilateral Cerebellar Signs		
Acute (Hours to Days)	**Subacute (Days to Weeks)**	**Chronic (Months to Years)**	**Acute (Hours to Days)**	**Subacute (Days to Weeks)**	**Chronic (Months to Years)**
Intoxication: alcohol, lithium, phenytoin, barbiturates (positive history and toxicology screen)	Intoxication: mercury, solvents, gasoline, glue; cytotoxic chemotherapeutic, hemotherapeutic drugs	Paraneoplastic syndrome	Vascular: cerebellar infarction, hemorrhage, or subdural hematoma	Neoplastic: cerebellar glioma or metastatic tumor (positive for neoplasm on MRI/CT)	Stable gliosis secondary to vascular lesion or demyelinating plaque (stable lesion on MRI/CT older than several months)
Acute viral cerebellitis (CSF supportive of acute viral infection)	Alcoholic-nutritional (vitamin B_1 and B_{12} deficiency)	Antigliadin antibody syndrome	Infectious: cerebellar abscess (mass lesion on MRI/CT, history in support of lesion)	Demyelinating: multiple sclerosis (history, CSF, and MRI are consistent)	Congenital lesion: Chiari or Dandy-Walker malformations (malformation noted on MRI/CT)
Postinfection syndrome	Lyme disease	Hypothyroidism		AIDS-related multifocal leukoencephalopathy (positive HIV test and CD4+ cell count for AIDS)	
		Inherited diseases			
		Tabes dorsalis (tertiary syphilis)			
		Phenytoin toxicity			
		Amiodarone			

Abbreviations: CSF, cerebrospinal fluid; CT, computed tomography; MRI, magnetic resonance imaging.

especially when an infectious etiology, such as transmission from contaminated human growth hormone, is responsible (Chap. 453e).

Chronic symmetric gait ataxia suggests an inherited ataxia (discussed below), a metabolic disorder, or a chronic infection. Hypothyroidism must always be considered as a readily treatable and reversible form of gait ataxia. Infectious diseases that can present with ataxia are meningovascular syphilis and tabes dorsalis due to degeneration of the posterior columns and spinocerebellar pathways in the spinal cord.

FOCAL ATAXIA

Acute focal ataxia commonly results from cerebrovascular disease, usually ischemic infarction or cerebellar hemorrhage. These lesions typically produce cerebellar symptoms ipsilateral to the injured cerebellum and may be associated with an impaired level of consciousness due to brainstem compression and increased intracranial pressure; ipsilateral pontine signs, including sixth and seventh nerve palsies, may be present. Focal and worsening signs of acute ataxia should also prompt consideration of a posterior fossa subdural hematoma, bacterial abscess, or primary or metastatic cerebellar tumor. Computed tomography (CT) or magnetic resonance imaging (MRI) studies will reveal clinically significant processes of this type. Many of these lesions represent true neurologic emergencies, as sudden herniation, either rostrally through the tentorium or caudal herniation of cerebellar tonsils through the foramen magnum, can occur and is usually devastating. Acute surgical decompression may be required (Chap. 330). Lymphoma or progressive multifocal leukoencephalopathy (PML) in a patient with AIDS may present with an acute or subacute focal cerebellar syndrome. Chronic etiologies of progressive ataxia include multiple sclerosis (Chap. 458) and congenital lesions such as a Chiari malformation (Chap. 456) or a congenital cyst of the posterior fossa (Dandy-Walker syndrome).

THE INHERITED ATAXIAS

These may show autosomal dominant, autosomal recessive, or maternal (mitochondrial) modes of inheritance. A genomic classification (Chap. 451e) has now largely superseded previous ones based on clinical expression alone.

Although the clinical manifestations and neuropathologic findings of cerebellar disease dominate the clinical picture, there may also be characteristic changes in the basal ganglia, brainstem, spinal cord, optic nerves, retina, and peripheral nerves. In large families with dominantly inherited ataxias, many gradations are observed from purely cerebellar manifestations to mixed cerebellar and brainstem disorders, cerebellar and basal ganglia syndromes, and spinal cord or peripheral nerve disease. Rarely, dementia is present as well. The clinical picture may be homogeneous within a family with dominantly inherited ataxia, but sometimes most affected family members show one characteristic syndrome, while one or several members have an entirely different phenotype.

AUTOSOMAL DOMINANT ATAXIAS

The autosomal spinocerebellar ataxias (SCAs) include SCA types 1 through 36, dentatorubropallidoluysian atrophy (DRPLA), and episodic ataxia (EA) types 1 to 7 (Chap. 451e). SCA1, SCA2, SCA3 (Machado-Joseph disease [MJD]), SCA6, SCA7, and SCA17 are caused by CAG triplet repeat expansions in different genes. SCA8 is due to an untranslated CTG repeat expansion, SCA12 is linked to an untranslated CAG repeat, and SCA10 is caused by an untranslated pentanucleotide repeat. The clinical phenotypes of these SCAs overlap. The genotype has become the gold standard for diagnosis and classification. CAG encodes glutamine, and these expanded CAG triplet repeat expansions result in expanded polyglutamine proteins, termed *ataxins*, that produce a toxic gain of function with autosomal dominant inheritance. Although the phenotype is variable for any given disease gene, a pattern of neuronal loss with gliosis is produced that is relatively unique for each ataxia. Immunohistochemical and biochemical studies have shown cytoplasmic (SCA2), neuronal (SCA1, MJD, SCA7), and nucleolar (SCA7) accumulation of the specific mutant polyglutamine-containing ataxin proteins. Expanded polyglutamine ataxins with more than ~40 glutamines are potentially toxic to neurons for a variety of reasons including: high levels of gene expression for the mutant polyglutamine ataxin in affected neurons; conformational change of the aggregated protein to a β-pleated structure; abnormal transport of the ataxin into the nucleus (SCA1, MJD, SCA7); binding to other polyglutamine proteins, including the TATA-binding transcription protein and the CREB-binding protein, impairing their functions; altering the efficiency of the ubiquitin-proteasome system of protein turnover; and inducing neuronal apoptosis. An earlier age of onset (anticipation) and more aggressive disease in subsequent generations are due to further expansion of the CAG triplet repeat and increased polyglutamine number in the mutant ataxin. The most common disorders are discussed below.

SCA1

SCA1 was previously referred to as *olivopontocerebellar atrophy*, but genomic data have shown that that entity represents several different genotypes with overlapping clinical features.

Symptoms and Signs SCA1 is characterized by the development in early or middle adult life of progressive cerebellar ataxia of the trunk and limbs, impairment of equilibrium and gait, slowness of voluntary movements, scanning speech, nystagmoid eye movements, and oscillatory tremor of the head and trunk. Dysarthria, dysphagia, and

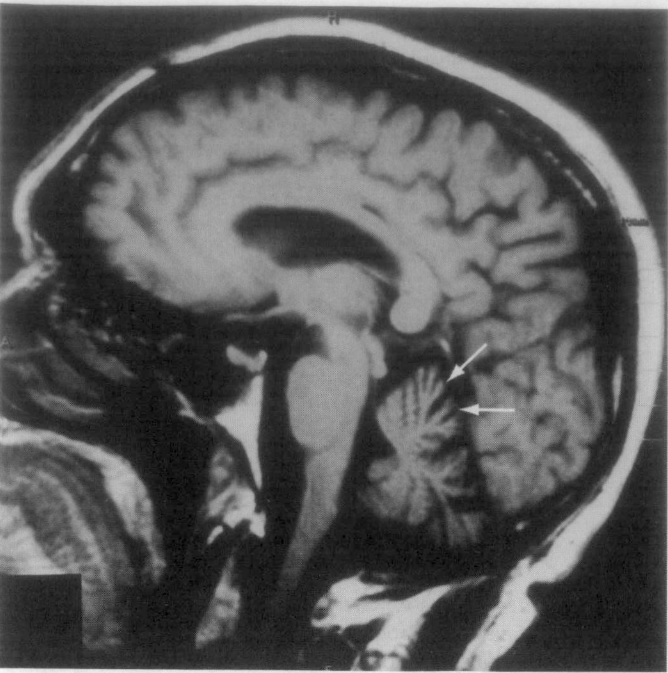
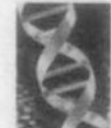

FIGURE 450-1 Sagittal magnetic resonance imaging (MRI) of the brain of a 60-year-old man with gait ataxia and dysarthria due to spinocerebellar ataxia type 1 (SCA1), illustrating cerebellar atrophy (arrows). *(Reproduced with permission from RN Rosenberg, P Khemani, in RN Rosenberg, JM Pascual [eds]: Rosenberg's Molecular and Genetic Basis of Neurological and Psychiatric Disease, 5th ed. London, Elsevier, 2015.)*

oculomotor and facial palsies may also occur. Extrapyramidal symptoms include rigidity, an immobile face, and parkinsonian tremor. The reflexes are usually normal, but knee and ankle jerks may be lost, and extensor plantar responses may occur. Dementia may be noted but is usually mild. Impairment of sphincter function is common, with urinary and sometimes fecal incontinence. Cerebellar and brainstem atrophy are evident on MRI (Fig. 450-1).

Marked shrinkage of the ventral half of the pons, disappearance of the olivary eminence on the ventral surface of the medulla, and atrophy of the cerebellum are evident on gross postmortem inspection of the brain. Variable loss of Purkinje cells, reduced numbers of cells in the molecular and granular layer, demyelination of the middle cerebellar peduncle and the cerebellar hemispheres, and severe loss of cells in the pontine nuclei and olives are found on histologic examination. Degenerative changes in the striatum, especially the putamen, and loss of the pigmented cells of the substantia nigra may be found in cases with extrapyramidal features. More widespread degeneration in the central nervous system (CNS), including involvement of the posterior columns and the spinocerebellar fibers, is often present.

GENETIC CONSIDERATIONS

SCA1 encodes a gene product, called *ataxin-1*, which is a novel protein of unknown function. The mutant allele has 40 CAG repeats located within the coding region, whereas alleles from unaffected individuals have ≤36 repeats. A few patients with 38–40 CAG repeats have been described. There is a direct correlation between a larger number of repeats and a younger age of onset for SCA1. Juvenile patients have higher numbers of repeats, and anticipation is present in subsequent generations. Transgenic mice carrying SCA1 developed ataxia and Purkinje cell pathology. Nuclear localization, but not aggregation, of ataxin-1 appears to be required for cell death initiated by the mutant protein.

SCA2

Symptoms and Signs Another clinical phenotype, SCA2, has been described in patients from Cuba and India. Cuban patients probably are descendants of a common ancestor, and the population may be the largest homogeneous group of patients with ataxia yet described. The age of onset ranges from 2–65 years, and there is considerable clinical variability within families. Although neuropathologic and clinical findings are compatible with a diagnosis of SCA1, including slow saccadic eye movements, ataxia, dysarthria, parkinsonian rigidity, optic disc pallor, mild spasticity, and retinal degeneration, SCA2 is a unique form of cerebellar degenerative disease.

GENETIC CONSIDERATIONS

The gene in SCA2 families also contains CAG repeat expansions coding for a polyglutamine-containing protein, ataxin-2. Normal alleles contain 15–32 repeats; mutant alleles have 35–77 repeats.

MACHADO-JOSEPH DISEASE/SCA3

MJD was first described among the Portuguese and their descendants in New England and California. Subsequently, MJD has been found in families from Portugal, Australia, Brazil, Canada, China, England, France, India, Israel, Italy, Japan, Spain, Taiwan, and the United States. In most populations, it is the most common autosomal dominant ataxia.

Symptoms and Signs MJD has been classified into three clinical types. In type I MJD (amyotrophic lateral sclerosis-parkinsonism-dystonia type), neurologic deficits appear in the first two decades and involve weakness and spasticity of extremities, especially the legs, often with dystonia of the face, neck, trunk, and extremities. Patellar and ankle clonus are common, as are extensor plantar responses. The gait is slow and stiff, with a slightly broadened base and lurching from side to side; this gait results from spasticity, not true ataxia. There is no truncal titubation. Pharyngeal weakness and spasticity cause difficulty with speech and swallowing. Of note is the prominence of horizontal and vertical nystagmus, loss of fast saccadic eye movements, hypermetric and hypometric saccades, and impairment of upward vertical gaze. Facial fasciculations, facial myokymia, lingual fasciculations without atrophy, ophthalmoparesis, and ocular prominence are common early manifestations.

In type II MJD (ataxic type), true cerebellar deficits of dysarthria and gait and extremity ataxia begin in the second to fourth decades along with corticospinal and extrapyramidal deficits of spasticity, rigidity, and dystonia. Type II is the most common form of MJD. Ophthalmoparesis, upward vertical gaze deficits, and facial and lingual fasciculations are also present. Type II MJD can be distinguished from the clinically similar disorders SCA1 and SCA2.

Type III MJD (ataxic-amyotrophic type) presents in the fifth to the seventh decades with a pancerebellar disorder that includes dysarthria and gait and extremity ataxia. Distal sensory loss involving pain, touch, vibration, and position senses and distal atrophy are prominent, indicating the presence of peripheral neuropathy. The deep tendon reflexes are depressed to absent, and there are no corticospinal or extrapyramidal findings.

The mean age of onset of symptoms in MJD is 25 years. Neurologic deficits invariably progress and lead to death from debilitation within 15 years of onset, especially in patients with types I and II disease. Usually, patients retain full intellectual function.

The major pathologic findings are variable loss of neurons and glial replacement in the corpus striatum and severe loss of neurons in the pars compacta of the substantia nigra. A moderate loss of neurons occurs in the dentate nucleus of the cerebellum and in the red nucleus. Purkinje cell loss and granule cell loss occur in the cerebellar cortex. Cell loss also occurs in the dentate nucleus and in the cranial nerve motor nuclei. Sparing of the inferior olives distinguishes MJD from other dominantly inherited ataxias.

GENETIC CONSIDERATIONS

The gene for MJD maps to 14q24.3-q32. Unstable CAG repeat expansions are present in the MJD gene coding for a polyglutamine-containing protein named ataxin-3, or MJD-ataxin. An earlier age of onset is associated with longer repeats. Alleles from normal individuals have between 12 and 37 CAG repeats, whereas MJD alleles have 60–84 CAG repeats. Polyglutamine-containing aggregates of ataxin-3 (MJD-ataxin) have been described in neuronal nuclei undergoing degeneration. MJD-ataxin codes for a ubiquitin protease, which is inactive due to expanded polyglutamines. Proteosome function is impaired, resulting in altered clearance of proteins and cerebellar neuronal loss.

SCA6

Genomic screening for CAG repeats in other families with autosomal dominant ataxia and vibratory and proprioceptive sensory loss have yielded another locus. Of interest is that different mutations in the same gene for the α_{1A} voltage-dependent calcium channel subunit (CACNLIA4; also referred to as the *CACNA1A* gene) at 19p13 result in different clinical disorders. CAG repeat expansions (21–27 in patients; 4–16 triplets in normal individuals) result in late-onset progressive ataxia with cerebellar degeneration. Missense mutations in this gene result in familial hemiplegic migraine. Nonsense mutations resulting in termination of protein synthesis of the gene product yield hereditary paroxysmal cerebellar ataxia or EA. Some patients with familial hemiplegic migraine develop progressive ataxia and also have cerebellar atrophy.

SCA7

This disorder is distinguished from all other SCAs by the presence of retinal pigmentary degeneration. The visual abnormalities first appear as blue-yellow color blindness and proceed to frank visual loss with macular degeneration. In almost all other respects, SCA7 resembles several other SCAs in which ataxia is accompanied by various noncerebellar findings, including ophthalmoparesis and extensor plantar responses. The genetic defect is an expanded CAG repeat in the SCA7 gene at 3p14-p21.1. The expanded repeat size in SCA7 is highly variable. Consistent with this, the severity of clinical findings varies from essentially asymptomatic to mild late-onset symptoms to severe, aggressive disease in childhood with rapid progression. Marked anticipation has been recorded, especially with paternal transmission. The disease protein, ataxin-7, forms aggregates in nuclei of affected neurons, as has also been described for SCA1 and SCA3/MJD.

SCA8

This form of ataxia is caused by a CTG repeat expansion in an untranslated region of a gene on chromosome 13q21. There is marked maternal bias in transmission, perhaps reflecting contractions of the repeat during spermatogenesis. The mutation is not fully penetrant. Symptoms include slowly progressive dysarthria and gait ataxia beginning at ~40 years of age with a range between 20 and 65 years. Other features include nystagmus, leg spasticity, and reduced vibratory sensation. Severely affected individuals are nonambulatory by the fourth to sixth decades. MRI shows cerebellar atrophy. The mechanism of disease may involve a dominant "toxic" effect occurring at the RNA level, as occurs in myotonic dystrophy.

DENTATORUBROPALLIDOLUYSIAN ATROPHY

DRPLA has a variable presentation that may include progressive ataxia, choreoathetosis, dystonia, seizures, myoclonus, and dementia. DRPLA is due to unstable CAG triplet repeats in the open reading frame of a gene named *atrophin* located on chromosome 12p12-ter. Larger expansions are found in patients with earlier onset. The number of repeats is 49 in patients with DRPLA and ≤26 in normal individuals. Anticipation occurs in successive generations, with earlier onset of disease in association with an increasing CAG repeat number in children who inherit the disease from their father. One well-characterized family in North Carolina has a phenotypic variant known as the *Haw River syndrome*, now recognized to be due to the DRPLA mutation.

EPISODIC ATAXIA

EA types 1 and 2 are two rare dominantly inherited disorders that have been mapped to chromosomes 12p (a potassium channel gene) for type 1 and 19p for type 2. Patients with EA-1 have brief episodes of ataxia with myokymia and nystagmus that last only minutes. Startle, sudden change in posture, and exercise can induce episodes. Acetazolamide or anticonvulsants may be therapeutic. Patients with EA-2 have episodes of ataxia with nystagmus that can last for hours or days. Stress, exercise, or excessive fatigue may be precipitants. Acetazolamide may be therapeutic and can reverse the relative intracellular alkalosis detected by magnetic resonance spectroscopy. Stop codon, nonsense mutations causing EA-2 have been found in the *CACNA1A* gene, encoding the α_{1A} voltage-dependent calcium channel subunit (see "SCA6," above).

AUTOSOMAL RECESSIVE ATAXIAS

Friedreich's Ataxia This is the most common form of inherited ataxia, comprising one-half of all hereditary ataxias. It can occur in a classic form or in association with a genetically determined vitamin E deficiency syndrome; the two forms are clinically indistinguishable.

SYMPTOMS AND SIGNS Friedreich's ataxia presents before 25 years of age with progressive staggering gait, frequent falling, and titubation. The lower extremities are more severely involved than the upper ones. Dysarthria occasionally is the presenting symptom; rarely, progressive scoliosis, foot deformity, nystagmus, or cardiopathy is the initial sign.

The neurologic examination reveals nystagmus, loss of fast saccadic eye movements, truncal titubation, dysarthria, dysmetria, and ataxia of trunk and limb movements. Extensor plantar responses (with normal tone in trunk and extremities), absence of deep tendon reflexes, and weakness (greater distally than proximally) are usually found. Loss of vibratory and proprioceptive sensation occurs. The median age of death is 35 years. Women have a significantly better prognosis than men.

Cardiac involvement occurs in 90% of patients. Cardiomegaly, symmetric hypertrophy, murmurs, and conduction defects are reported. Moderate mental retardation or psychiatric syndromes are present in a small percentage of patients. A high incidence of diabetes mellitus (20%) is found and is associated with insulin resistance and pancreatic β-cell dysfunction. Musculoskeletal deformities are common and include pes cavus, pes equinovarus, and scoliosis. MRI of the spinal cord shows atrophy (Fig. 450-2).

The primary sites of pathology are the spinal cord, dorsal root ganglion cells, and the peripheral nerves. Slight atrophy of the cerebellum and cerebral gyri may occur. Sclerosis and degeneration occur

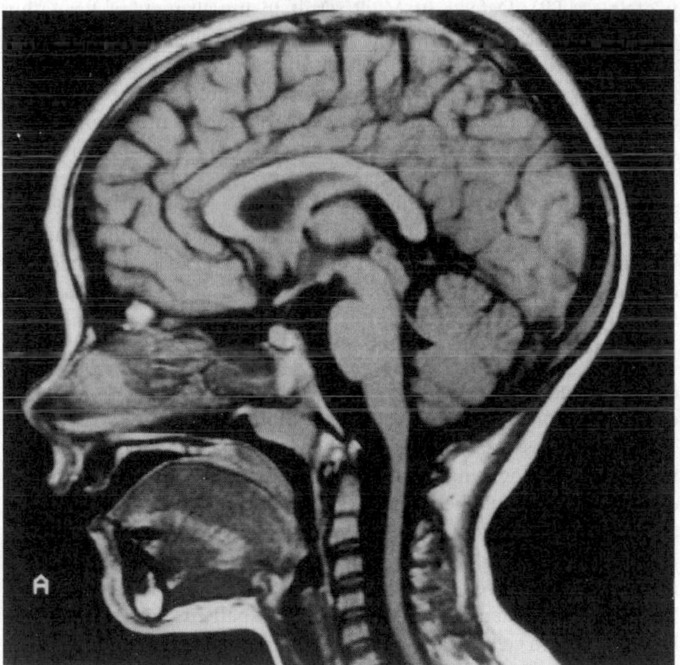

FIGURE 450-2 Sagittal magnetic resonance imaging (MRI) of the brain and spinal cord of a patient with Friedreich's ataxia, demonstrating spinal cord atrophy. *(Reproduced with permission from RN Rosenberg, P Khemani, in RN Rosenberg, JM Pascual [eds]: Rosenberg's Molecular and Genetic Basis of Neurological and Psychiatric Disease, 5th ed. London, Elsevier, 2015.)*

predominantly in the spinocerebellar tracts, lateral corticospinal tracts, and posterior columns. Degeneration of the glossopharyngeal, vagus, hypoglossal, and deep cerebellar nuclei is described. The cerebral cortex is histologically normal except for loss of Betz cells in the precentral gyri. The peripheral nerves are extensively involved, with a loss of large myelinated fibers. Cardiac pathology consists of myocytic hypertrophy and fibrosis, focal vascular fibromuscular dysplasia with subintimal or medial deposition of periodic acid-Schiff (PAS)-positive material, myocytopathy with unusual pleomorphic nuclei, and focal degeneration of nerves and cardiac ganglia.

GENETIC CONSIDERATIONS

The classic form of Friedreich's ataxia has been mapped to 9q13-q21.1, and the mutant gene, *frataxin*, contains expanded GAA triplet repeats in the first intron. There is homozygosity for expanded GAA repeats in >95% of patients. Normal persons have 7–22 GAA repeats, and patients have 200–900 GAA repeats. A more varied clinical syndrome has been described in compound heterozygotes who have one copy of the GAA expansion and the other copy a point mutation in the *frataxin* gene. When the point mutation is located in the region of the gene that encodes the amino-terminal half of frataxin, the phenotype is milder, often consisting of a spastic gait, retained or exaggerated reflexes, no dysarthria, and mild or absent ataxia.

Patients with Friedreich's ataxia have undetectable or extremely low levels of *frataxin* mRNA, as compared with carriers and unrelated individuals; thus, disease appears to be caused by a loss of expression of the frataxin protein. Frataxin is a mitochondrial protein involved in iron homeostasis. Mitochondrial iron accumulation due to loss of the iron transporter coded by the mutant *frataxin* gene results in oxidized intramitochondrial iron. Excess oxidized iron results in turn in the oxidation of cellular components and irreversible cell injury.

Two forms of hereditary ataxia associated with abnormalities in the interactions of vitamin E (α-tocopherol) with very-low-density lipoprotein (VLDL) have been delineated. These are abetalipoproteinemia (Bassen-Kornzweig syndrome) and ataxia with vitamin E deficiency (AVED). Abetalipoproteinemia is caused by mutations in the gene coding for the larger subunit of the microsomal triglyceride transfer protein (MTP). Defects in MTP result in impairment of formation and secretion of VLDL in liver. This defect results in a deficiency of delivery of vitamin E to tissues, including the central and peripheral nervous system, as VLDL is the transport molecule for vitamin E and other fat-soluble substitutes. AVED is due to mutations in the gene for α-tocopherol transfer protein (α-TTP). These patients have an impaired ability to bind vitamin E into the VLDL produced and secreted by the liver, resulting in a deficiency of vitamin E in peripheral tissues. Hence, either absence of VLDL (abetalipoproteinemia) or impaired binding of vitamin E to VLDL (AVED) causes an ataxic syndrome. Once again, a genotype classification has proved to be essential in sorting out the various forms of the Friedreich's disease syndrome, which may be clinically indistinguishable.

Ataxia Telangiectasia • *SYMPTOMS AND SIGNS* Patients with ataxia telangiectasia (AT) present in the first decade of life with progressive telangiectatic lesions associated with deficits in cerebellar function and nystagmus. The neurologic manifestations correspond to those in Friedreich's disease, which should be included in the differential diagnosis. Truncal and limb ataxia, dysarthria, extensor plantar responses, myoclonic jerks, areflexia, and distal sensory deficits may develop. There is a high incidence of recurrent pulmonary infections and neoplasms of the lymphatic and reticuloendothelial system in patients with AT. Thymic hypoplasia with cellular and humoral (IgA and IgG2) immunodeficiencies, premature aging, and endocrine disorders such as type 1 diabetes mellitus are described. There is an increased incidence of lymphomas, Hodgkin's disease, acute T cell leukemias, and breast cancer.

The most striking neuropathologic changes include loss of Purkinje, granule, and basket cells in the cerebellar cortex as well as of neurons in the deep cerebellar nuclei. The inferior olives of the medulla may also have neuronal loss. There is a loss of anterior horn neurons in the spinal cord and of dorsal root ganglion cells associated with posterior column spinal cord demyelination. A poorly developed or absent thymus gland is the most consistent defect of the lymphoid system.

GENETIC CONSIDERATIONS

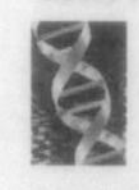

The gene for AT (the *ATM* gene) encodes a protein that is similar to several yeast and mammalian phosphatidylinositol-3′-kinases involved in mitogenic signal transduction, meiotic recombination, and cell cycle control. Defective DNA repair in AT fibroblasts exposed to ultraviolet light has been demonstrated. The discovery of *ATM* permits early diagnosis and identification of heterozygotes who are at risk for cancer (e.g., breast cancer).

MITOCHONDRIAL ATAXIAS

Spinocerebellar syndromes have been identified with mutations in mitochondrial DNA (mtDNA). Thirty pathogenic mtDNA point mutations and 60 different types of mtDNA deletions are known, several of which cause or are associated with ataxia (Chap. 462e).

TREATMENT ATAXIC DISORDERS

The most important goal in management of patients with ataxia is to identify treatable disease entities. Mass lesions must be recognized promptly and treated appropriately. Paraneoplastic disorders can often be identified by the clinical patterns of disease that they produce, measurement of specific autoantibodies, and uncovering the primary cancer; these disorders are often refractory to therapy, but some patients improve following removal of the tumor or immunotherapy (Chap. 122). Ataxia with antigliadin antibodies and gluten-sensitive enteropathy may improve with a gluten-free diet. Malabsorption syndromes leading to vitamin E deficiency may lead to ataxia. The vitamin E deficiency form of Friedreich's ataxia must be considered, and serum vitamin E levels measured. Vitamin E therapy is indicated for these rare patients. Vitamin B_1 and B_{12} levels in serum should be measured, and the vitamins administered to patients having deficient levels. Hypothyroidism is easily treated. The cerebrospinal fluid should be tested for a syphilitic infection in patients with progressive ataxia and other features of tabes dorsalis. Similarly, antibody titers for Lyme disease and *Legionella* should be measured and appropriate antibiotic therapy should be instituted in antibody-positive patients. Aminoacidopathies, leukodystrophies, urea-cycle abnormalities, and mitochondrial encephalomyopathies may produce ataxia, and some dietary or metabolic therapies are available for these disorders. The deleterious effects of phenytoin and alcohol on the cerebellum are well known, and these exposures should be avoided in patients with ataxia of any cause.

There is no proven therapy for any of the autosomal dominant ataxias (SCA1 to SCA36). There is preliminary evidence that idebenone, a free-radical scavenger, can improve myocardial hypertrophy in patients with classic Friedreich's ataxia; there is no current evidence, however, that it improves neurologic function. A small preliminary study in a mixed population of patients with different inherited ataxias raised the possibility that the glutamate antagonist riluzole may offer modest benefit. Iron chelators and antioxidant drugs are potentially harmful in Friedreich's patients because they may increase heart muscle injury. Acetazolamide can reduce the duration of symptoms of episodic ataxia. At present, identification of an at-risk person's genotype, together with appropriate family and genetic counseling, can reduce the incidence of these cerebellar syndromes in future generations (Chap. 84).

GENETIC DIAGNOSTIC LABORATORIES

1. Baylor College of Medicine; Houston, Texas, 1-713-798-6522
   http://www.bcm.edu/genetics/index.cfm?pmid=21387
2. GeneDx
   http://www.genedx.com
3. Transgenomic, 1-877-274-9432
   http://www.transgenomic.com/labs/neurology

GLOBAL FEATURES

Ataxias with autosomal dominant, autosomal recessive, X-linked, or mitochondrial forms of inheritance are present on a worldwide basis. Machado-Joseph disease (SCA3) (autosomal dominant) and Friedreich's ataxia (autosomal recessive) are the most common types in most populations. Genetic markers are now commercially available to precisely identify the genetic mutation for correct diagnosis and also for family planning. Early detection of asymptomatic preclinical disease can reduce or eliminate the inherited form of ataxia in some families on a global, worldwide basis.

451e Classification of the Spinocerebellar Ataxias

Roger N. Rosenberg

This is a digital-only chapter. It is available on the DVD that accompanies this book, as well as on Access Medicine/Harrison's Online, and the eBook and "app" editions of HPIM 19e.

Ataxias with autosomal dominant, autosomal recessive, X-linked, or mitochondrial forms of inheritance are present on a worldwide basis. Machado-Joseph disease (SCA3) (autosomal dominant) and Friedreich's ataxia (autosomal recessive) are the most common types in most populations. Mutation markers are now commercially available to identify carriers at risk in their families, which allows for precise identification of the genetic mutation for correct diagnosis and also for family planning.

452 Amyotrophic Lateral Sclerosis and Other Motor Neuron Diseases

Robert H. Brown, Jr.

AMYOTROPHIC LATERAL SCLEROSIS

Amyotrophic lateral sclerosis (ALS) is the most common form of progressive motor neuron disease. It is a prime example of a neurodegenerative disease and is arguably the most devastating of the neurodegenerative disorders.

PATHOLOGY

The pathologic hallmark of motor neuron degenerative disorders is death of lower motor neurons (consisting of anterior horn cells in the spinal cord and their brainstem homologues innervating bulbar muscles) and upper, or corticospinal, motor neurons (originating in layer five of the motor cortex and descending via the pyramidal tract to synapse with lower motor neurons, either directly or indirectly via interneurons) (Chap. 30). Although at its onset ALS may involve selective loss of function of only upper or lower motor neurons, it ultimately causes progressive loss of both categories of motor neurons. Indeed, in the absence of clear involvement of both motor neuron types, the diagnosis of ALS is questionable. In a subset of cases, ALS arises concurrently with frontotemporal dementia (Chap. 448); in these instances, there is degeneration of frontotemporal cortical neurons and corresponding cortical atrophy.

Other motor neuron diseases involve only particular subsets of motor neurons (Tables 452-1 and 452-2). Thus, in bulbar palsy and spinal muscular atrophy (SMA; also called *progressive muscular atrophy*), the lower motor neurons of brainstem and spinal cord, respectively, are most severely involved. By contrast, pseudobulbar palsy, primary lateral sclerosis (PLS), and familial spastic paraplegia (FSP) affect only upper motor neurons innervating the brainstem and spinal cord.

TABLE 452-1 ETIOLOGY OF MOTOR NEURON DISORDERS

Diagnostic Category	Investigation
Structural lesions	MRI scan of head (including foramen magnum and cervical spine)
Parasagittal or foramen magnum tumors	
Cervical spondylosis	
Chiari malformation of syrinx	
Spinal cord arteriovenous malformation	
Infections	CSF exam, culture
Bacterial—tetanus, Lyme	Lyme titer
Viral—poliomyelitis, herpes zoster	Anti-viral antibody
Retroviral—myelopathy	HTLV-1 titers
Intoxications, physical agents	24-h urine for heavy metals
Toxins—lead, aluminum, others	Serum lead level
Drugs—strychnine, phenytoin	
Electric short, x-irradiation	
Immunologic mechanisms	Complete blood count[a]
Plasma cell dyscrasias	Sedimentation rate[a]
Autoimmune polyradiculopathy	Total protein[a]
Motor neuropathy with conduction block	Anti-GM1 antibodies[a]
	Anti-Hu antibody
Paraneoplastic	MRI scan, bone marrow biopsy
Paracarcinomatous	
Metabolic	Fasting blood sugar[a]
Hypoglycemia	Routine chemistries including calcium[a]
Hyperparathyroidism	PTH
Hyperthyroidism	Thyroid function[a]
Deficiency of folate, vitamin B_{12}, vitamin E	Vitamin B_{12}, vitamin E, folate[a]
Malabsorption	Serum zinc, copper[a]
Deficiency of copper, zinc	24-h stool fat, carotene, prothrombin time
Mitochondrial dysfunction	Fasting lactate, pyruvate, ammonia
	Consider mtDNA
Hyperlipidemia	Lipid electrophoresis
Hyperglycinuria	Urine and serum amino acids
	CSF amino acids
Hereditary disorders	WBC DNA for mutational analysis
Superoxide dismutase	
TDP43	
FUS/TLS	
Androgen receptor defect (Kennedy's disease)	
Hexosaminidase deficiency	
Infantile a-glucosidase deficiency (Pompe's disease)	

[a]Should be obtained in all cases.

Abbreviations: CSF, cerebrospinal fluid; FUS/TLS, fused in sarcoma/translocated in liposarcoma; HTLV-1, human T-cell lymphotropic virus; MRI, magnetic resonance imaging; PTH, parathyroid; WBC, white blood cell.

In each of these diseases, the affected motor neurons undergo shrinkage, often with accumulation of the pigmented lipid (lipofuscin) that normally develops in these cells with advancing age. In ALS, the motor neuron cytoskeleton is typically affected early in the illness. Focal enlargements are frequent in proximal motor axons; ultrastructurally, these "spheroids" are composed of accumulations of neurofilaments and other proteins. Commonly in both sporadic and familial

TABLE 452-2 SPORADIC MOTOR NEURON DISEASES

Chronic	Entity
Upper and lower motor neuron	Amyotrophic lateral sclerosis
Predominantly upper motor neuron	Primary lateral sclerosis
Predominantly lower motor neuron	Multifocal motor neuropathy with conduction block
	Motor neuropathy with paraproteinemia or cancer
	Motor predominant peripheral neuropathies
Other	
Associated with other neurodegenerative disorders	
Secondary motor neuron disorders (see Table 452-1)	
Acute	
Poliomyelitis	
Herpes zoster	
Coxsackie virus	
West Nile virus	

ALS, the affected neurons demonstrate ubiquitin-positive aggregates, typically associated with the protein TDP43 (see below). Also seen is proliferation of astroglia and microglia, the inevitable accompaniment of all degenerative processes in the central nervous system (CNS).

The death of the peripheral motor neurons in the brainstem and spinal cord leads to denervation and consequent atrophy of the corresponding muscle fibers. Histochemical and electrophysiologic evidence indicates that in the early phases of the illness denervated muscle can be reinnervated by sprouting of nearby distal motor nerve terminals, although reinnervation in this disease is considerably less extensive than in most other disorders affecting motor neurons (e.g., poliomyelitis, peripheral neuropathy). As denervation progresses, muscle atrophy is readily recognized in muscle biopsies and on clinical examination. This is the basis for the term *amyotrophy*. The loss of cortical motor neurons results in thinning of the corticospinal tracts that travel via the internal capsule (Fig. 452-1) and brainstem to the lateral and anterior white matter columns of the spinal cord. The loss of fibers in the lateral columns and resulting fibrillary gliosis impart a particular firmness (*lateral sclerosis*). A remarkable feature of the disease is the selectivity of neuronal cell death. By light microscopy, the entire sensory apparatus, the regulatory mechanisms for the control and coordination of movement, remains intact. Except in cases of frontotemporal dementia, the components of the brain required for cognitive processing are also preserved. However, immunostaining indicates that neurons bearing ubiquitin, a marker for degeneration, are also detected in nonmotor systems. Moreover, studies of glucose metabolism in the illness also indicate that there is neuronal dysfunction outside of the motor system. Within the motor system, there is some selectivity of involvement. Thus, motor neurons required for ocular motility remain unaffected, as do the parasympathetic neurons in the sacral spinal cord (the nucleus of Onufrowicz, or Onuf) that innervate the sphincters of the bowel and bladder.

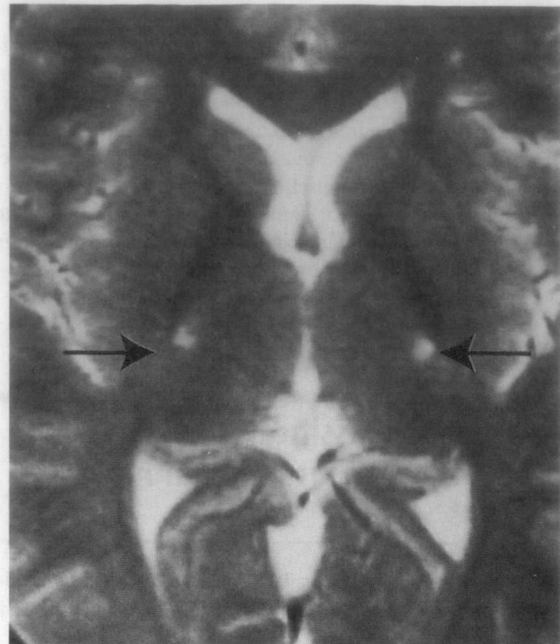

FIGURE 452-1 Amyotrophic lateral sclerosis. Axial T2-weighted magnetic resonance imaging (MRI) scan through the lateral ventricles of the brain reveals abnormal high signal intensity within the corticospinal tracts (*arrows*). This MRI feature represents an increase in water content in myelin tracts undergoing Wallerian degeneration secondary to cortical motor neuronal loss. This finding is commonly present in ALS, but can also be seen in AIDS-related encephalopathy, infarction, or other disease processes that produce corticospinal neuronal loss in a symmetric fashion.

CLINICAL MANIFESTATIONS

The manifestations of ALS are somewhat variable depending on whether corticospinal neurons or lower motor neurons in the brainstem and spinal cord are more prominently involved. With lower motor neuron dysfunction and early denervation, typically the first evidence of the disease is insidiously developing asymmetric weakness, usually first evident distally in one of the limbs. A detailed history often discloses recent development of cramping with volitional movements, typically in the early hours of the morning (e.g., while stretching in bed). Weakness caused by denervation is associated with progressive wasting and atrophy of muscles and, particularly early in the illness, spontaneous twitching of motor units, or fasciculations. In the hands, a preponderance of extensor over flexor weakness is common. When the initial denervation involves bulbar rather than limb muscles, the problem at onset is difficulty with chewing, swallowing, and movements of the face and tongue. Early involvement of the muscles of respiration may lead to death before the disease is far advanced elsewhere. With prominent corticospinal involvement, there is hyperactivity of the muscle-stretch reflexes (tendon jerks) and, often, spastic resistance to passive movements of the affected limbs. Patients with significant reflex hyperactivity complain of muscle stiffness often out of proportion to weakness. Degeneration of the corticobulbar projections innervating the brainstem results in dysarthria and exaggeration of the motor expressions of emotion. The latter leads to involuntary excess in weeping or laughing (pseudobulbar affect).

Virtually any muscle group may be the first to show signs of disease, but, as time passes, more and more muscles become involved until ultimately the disorder takes on a symmetric distribution in all regions. It is characteristic of ALS that, regardless of whether the initial disease involves upper or lower motor neurons, both will eventually be implicated. Even in the late stages of the illness, sensory, bowel and bladder, and cognitive functions are preserved. Even when there is severe brainstem disease, ocular motility is spared until the very late stages of the illness. As noted, in some cases (particularly those that are familial), ALS develops concurrently with frontotemporal dementia, characterized by early behavioral abnormalities with prominent behavioral features indicative of frontal lobe dysfunction.

A committee of the World Federation of Neurology has established diagnostic guidelines for ALS. Essential for the diagnosis is simultaneous upper and lower motor neuron involvement with progressive weakness and the exclusion of all alternative diagnoses. The disorder is ranked as "definite" ALS when three or four of the following are involved: bulbar, cervical, thoracic, and lumbosacral motor neurons. When two sites are involved, the diagnosis is "probable," and when only one site is implicated, the diagnosis is "possible." An exception is made for those who have progressive upper and lower motor neuron signs at only one site and a mutation in the gene encoding superoxide dismutase (SOD1; see below).

EPIDEMIOLOGY

The illness is relentlessly progressive, leading to death from respiratory paralysis; the median survival is from 3–5 years. There are very rare reports of stabilization or even regression of ALS. In most societies, there is an incidence of 1–3 per 100,000 and a prevalence of 3–5 per 100,000. It is striking that about 1 in 1000 adult deaths in North America and Western Europe (and probably elsewhere) are due to ALS; this finding predicts that some 300,000 individuals now alive in the United States will die of ALS. Several endemic foci of higher prevalence exist in the western Pacific (e.g., in specific regions of Guam or Papua New Guinea). In the United States and Europe, males are somewhat more frequently affected than females. Epidemiologic studies have incriminated risk factors for this disease including exposure to pesticides and insecticides, smoking, and, in one report, service in the military. Although ALS is overwhelmingly a sporadic disorder, some 5–10% of cases are inherited as an autosomal dominant trait.

FAMILIAL ALS

Several forms of selective motor neuron disease are inheritable (Table 452-3). Familial ALS (FALS) involves both corticospinal and lower motor neurons. Apart from its inheritance as an autosomal dominant trait, it is clinically indistinguishable from sporadic ALS. Genetic studies have identified mutations in multiple genes, including those encoding the protein C9orf72 (open reading frame 72 on chromosome 9), cytosolic enzyme SOD1 (superoxide dismutase), the RNA binding proteins TDP43 (encoded by the TAR DNA binding protein gene), and FUS/TLS (fused in sarcoma/translocated in liposarcoma), as the most common causes of FALS. Mutations in C9orf72 account for ~45–50% of FALS and perhaps 4–5% of sporadic ALS cases. Mutations in SOD1 explain another 20% of cases of FALS, whereas TDP43 and FUS/TLS each represent about 5% of familial cases. It has recently been reported that ~1–2% of cases are caused by mutations in genes encoding the proteins optineuron and profilin-1 as well.

Rare mutations in other genes are also clearly implicated in ALS-like diseases. Thus, a familial, dominantly inherited motor disorder that in some individuals closely mimics the ALS phenotype arises from mutations in a gene that encodes a vesicle-binding protein. A predominantly lower motor neuron disease with early hoarseness due to laryngeal dysfunction has been ascribed to mutations in the gene encoding the cellular accessory motor protein dynactin. Mutations in senataxin, a helicase, cause an early adult-onset, slowly evolving ALS variant. Kennedy's syndrome is an X-linked, adult-onset disorder that may mimic ALS, as described below.

Genetic analyses are also beginning to illuminate the pathogenesis of some childhood-onset motor neuron diseases. For example, a slowly disabling degenerative, predominantly upper motor neuron disease that starts in the first decade is caused by mutations in a gene that expresses a novel signaling molecule with properties of a guanine-exchange factor, termed *alsin*.

DIFFERENTIAL DIAGNOSIS

Because ALS is currently untreatable, it is imperative that potentially remediable causes of motor neuron dysfunction be excluded (Table 452-1). This is particularly true in cases that are atypical by virtue of (1) restriction to either upper or lower motor neurons, (2) involvement of neurons other than motor neurons, and (3) evidence of motor neuronal conduction block on electrophysiologic testing. Compression of the cervical spinal cord or cervicomedullary junction from tumors in the cervical regions or at the foramen magnum or from cervical spondylosis with osteophytes projecting into the vertebral canal can produce weakness, wasting, and fasciculations in the upper limbs and spasticity in the legs, closely resembling ALS. The absence of cranial nerve involvement may be helpful in differentiation, although some foramen magnum lesions may compress the twelfth cranial (hypoglossal) nerve, with resulting paralysis of the tongue. Absence of pain or of sensory changes, normal bowel and bladder function, normal roentgenographic studies of the spine, and normal cerebrospinal fluid (CSF) all favor ALS. Where doubt exists, magnetic resonance imaging (MRI) scans and contrast myelography should be performed to visualize the cervical spinal cord.

Another important entity in the differential diagnosis of ALS is *multifocal motor neuropathy with conduction block* (MMCB), discussed below. A diffuse, lower motor axonal neuropathy mimicking ALS sometimes evolves in association with hematopoietic disorders such as lymphoma or multiple myeloma. In this clinical setting, the presence of an M-component in serum should prompt consideration of a bone marrow biopsy. Lyme disease (Chap. 210) may also cause an axonal, lower motor neuropathy, although typically with intense proximal limb pain and a CSF pleocytosis.

Other treatable disorders that occasionally mimic ALS are chronic lead poisoning and thyrotoxicosis. These disorders may be suggested by the patient's social or occupational history or by unusual clinical features. When the family history is positive, disorders involving the genes encoding C9orf72, cytosolic SOD1, TDP43, FUS/TLS, and adult hexosaminidase A or α-glucosidase deficiency must be excluded (Chap. 432e). These are readily identified by appropriate laboratory tests. Benign fasciculations are occasionally a source of concern because on inspection they resemble the fascicular twitchings that accompany motor neuron degeneration. The absence of weakness, atrophy, or denervation phenomena on electrophysiologic examination usually excludes ALS or other serious neurologic disease. Patients who have recovered from poliomyelitis may experience a delayed deterioration of motor neurons that presents clinically with progressive weakness, atrophy, and fasciculations. Its cause is unknown, but it is thought to reflect sublethal prior injury to motor neurons by poliovirus (Chap. 228).

Rarely, ALS develops concurrently with features indicative of more widespread neurodegeneration. Thus, one infrequently encounters otherwise typical ALS patients with a parkinsonian movement disorder or frontotemporal dementia, particularly in instances of C9orf72 mutations, which strongly suggests that the simultaneous occurrence of two disorders is a direct consequence of the gene mutation. As another example, prominent amyotrophy has been described as a dominantly inherited disorder in individuals with bizarre behavior and a movement disorder suggestive of parkinsonism; many such cases have now been ascribed to mutations that alter the expression of tau protein in brain (Chap. 448). In other cases, ALS develops simultaneously with a striking frontotemporal dementia. An ALS-like disorder has also been described in some individuals with chronic traumatic encephalopathy, associated with deposition of TDP43 and neurofibrillary tangles in motor neurons.

PATHOGENESIS

The cause of sporadic ALS is not well defined. Several mechanisms that impair motor neuron viability have been elucidated in mice and rats induced to develop motor neuron disease by SOD1 transgenes with ALS-associated mutations. One may loosely group the genetic causes of ALS into three categories. In one group, the primarily problem is inherent instability of the mutant proteins, with subsequent perturbations in protein degradation (SOD1, ubiquilin-1 and -2, p62). In the second, most rapidly growing category, the causative mutant genes perturb RNA processing, transport, and metabolism (C9orf73, TDP43, FUS). In the case of C9orf72, the molecular pathology is an expansion of an intronic hexanucleotide repeat (-GGGGCC-) beyond an upper normal of 30 repeats to hundreds or more repeats. As observed in other intronic repeat disorders such as myotonic dystrophy (Chap. 462e) and spinocerebellar atrophy type 8 (Chap. 450), data suggest that the expanded intronic repeats generate expanded RNA repeats that form intranuclear foci and confer toxicity by sequestering transcription factors or by undergoing noncanonical protein translation across all possible reading frames of the expanded RNA tracts. TDP43 and FUS are multifunctional proteins that bind RNA and DNA and shuttle between the nucleus and the cytoplasm, playing multiple roles in the control of cell proliferation, DNA repair and transcription,

TABLE 452-3 GENETIC MOTOR NEURON DISEASES

Disease	Locus	Gene	Inheritance	Usual Onset	Gene Function	Unusual Features
I. Upper and Lower Motor Neurons (Familial ALS)						
ALS1	21q	Superoxide dismutase	AD	Adult	Protein antioxidant	
ALS2	2q	Alsin	AR	Juvenile	GEF signaling	Severe corticobulbar, corticospinal features
ALS4	9q	Senataxin	AD	Late juvenile	DNA helicase	Late childhood onset
ALS6	16p	FUS/TLS	AD	Adult	DNA, RNA binding	
ALS8	20q	Vesicle associated protein B	AD	Adult	Vesicular trafficking	
ALS9	14q	Angiogenin	AD	Adult	RNAse, angiogenesis	
ALS10	1q	TDP43	AD	Adult	DNA, RNA binding	
ALS12	10p	Optineurin	AD/AR	Adult	Attenuates NF-κB	
ALS13	12q	Ataxin-2	AD	Adult	Cytotoxic expanded CAG repeat	
ALS14	9p	Valosin-containing protein	AD	Adult	ATPase	
ALS18	17p	Profilin-1	AD	Adult	Involved in actin polymerization	
ALS19	2q	ErbB4	AD	Adult	Signaling molecule	
ALS20	12q	HNRNPA1	AD	Adult	Heteronuclear RNA binding protein	
ALS21	5q	MTR3	AD	Adult	Nuclear matrix protein	Early vocal/bulbar involvement
ALS	2p	Dynactin	AD	Adult	Axonal transport	
ALS	17q	Paraoxonases 1-3	AD	Adult	Detoxify intoxicants	
ALS	mtDNA	Cytochrome c oxidase	AD	Adult	ATP generation	
ALS	mtDNA	tRNA-isoleucine	AD	Adult	ATP generation	
II. Lower Motor Neurons						
Spinal muscular atrophies	5q	Survival motor neuron	AR	Infancy	RNA metabolism	
GM2-gangliosidosis						
1. Sandhoff's disease	5q	Hexosaminidase B	AR	Childhood	Ganglioside recycling	
2. AB variant	5q	GM2-activator protein	AR	Childhood	Ganglioside recycling	
3. Adult Tay-Sachs disease	15q	Hexosaminidase A	AR	Childhood	Ganglioside recycling	
X-linked spino-bulbar muscular atrophy	Xq	Androgen receptor	XR	Adult	Nuclear signaling	
III. Upper Motor Neuron (Selected FSPs)						
SPG3A	14q	Atlastin	AD	Childhood	GTPase—vesicle recycling	
SPG4	2p	Spastin	AD	Early adulthood	ATPase family—microtubule associate	Some sensory loss
SPG6	15q	NIPA1	AD	Early adulthood	Membrane transporter or receptor	Deleted in Prader-Willi, Angelman's
SPG8	8q	Strumpellin	AD	Early adulthood	Ubiquitous, spectrin-like	
SPG10	12q	Kinesin heavy chain KIF5A	AD	Second–third decade	Motor-associated protein	± Peripheral neuropathy, retardation
SPG12	19q	Reticulon 2	AD	Childhood	ER protein, interacts with spastin	
SPG13	2q	Heat shock protein 60	AD	Early adulthood	Chaperone protein	
SPG17	11q	Silver (BSCL2)	AD	Variable	Membrane protein in ER	Amyotrophy hands, feet
SPG31	2p	REEP1	AD	Early	Mitochondrial protein	Rarely, amyotrophy
SPG33	10q	ZFYVE27	AD	Adult	Interacts with spastin	Pes equinus
SPG42	3q	Acetyl-CoA-transporter	AD	Variable	Solute carrier	
SPG72	5q	REEP2	AD	Childhood	ER protein	
SPG5	8q	Cytochrome P450	AR	Variable	Degrades endogenous substances	Sensory loss
SPG7	16q	Paraplegin	AR	Variable	Mitochondrial protein	Rarely, optic atrophy, ataxia
SPG11	15q	Spatacsin	AR	Childhood	Cytosolic, ? membrane-associated	Some sensory loss, thin corpus callosum
SPG15	14q	Spastizin	AR	Childhood	Zinc finger protein	Some amyotrophy, some CNS features

(Continued)

TABLE 452-3 GENETIC MOTOR NEURON DISEASES (*CONTINUED*)

Disease	Locus	Gene	Inheritance	Usual Onset	Gene Function	Unusual Features
SPG20	13q	Spartin	AR	Childhood	Endosomal trafficking protein	
SPG21	15q	Maspardin	AR	Childhood	Endosomal trafficking protein	
SPG35	16q	Fatty acid 2 hydrolase	AR	Childhood	Membrane protein	Multiple CNS features
SPG39	19p	Neuropathy target esterase	AR	Early childhood	Esterase	
SPG44	1q	Connexin 47	AR	Childhood	Gap junction protein	Possible mild CNS features
SPG46	9p	β-Glucosidase 2	AR	Childhood	Glycoside hydrolase	Thin corpus callosum, mental retardation
SPG2	Xq	Proteolipid protein	XR	Early childhood	Myelin protein	Sometimes multiple CNS features
SPG1	Xq	L1-CAM	XR	Infancy	Cell adhesion molecule	
SPG22	Xq	SLC16A2	XR	Infancy	Monocarboxylic acid transporter	
	Xq	Adrenoleukodystrophy	XR	Early adulthood	ATP binding transporter protein	Possible adrenal insufficiency, CNS inflammation
IV. ALS-Plus Syndromes						
ALS with frontotemporal dementia, Parkinson's disease	9p	C9orf72				
Amyotrophy with behavioral disorders	17q	Tau protein				
Parkinsonism						

Abbreviations: ALS, amyotrophic lateral sclerosis; BSCL2, Bernadelli Seip congenital lipodystrophy 2B; AD, autosomal dominant; AR, autosomal recessive; CNS, central nervous system; FSP, familial spastic paraplegia; FUS/TLS, fused in sarcoma/translocated in liposarcoma; TDP43, Tar DNA binding protein 43 kd; XR, X-linked recessive.

and gene translation, both in the cytoplasm and locally in dendritic spines in response to electrical activity. How mutations in FUS/TLS provoke motor neuron cell death is not clear, although this may represent loss of function of FUS/TLS in the nucleus or an acquired, toxic function of the mutant proteins in the cytosol. In the third group of ALS genes, the primary problem is defective axonal cytoskeleton and transport (dynactin, profilin-1). It is striking that variants in other genes (e.g., EphA4) influence survival in ALS but not ALS susceptibility. Beyond the upstream, primary defects, it is also evident that the ultimate neuronal cell death process is complex involving multiple cellular processes that accelerate cell death. These include but are not limited to excitotoxicity, impairment of axonal transport, oxidative stress, activation of endoplasmic reticulum stress and the unfolded protein response, and mitochondrial dysfunction.

Multiple recent studies have convincingly demonstrated that non-neuronal cells importantly influence the disease course, at least in ALS transgenic mice. A striking additional finding in neurodegenerative disorders is that miscreant proteins arising from gene defects in familial forms of these diseases are often implicated in sporadic forms of the same disorder. For example, germline mutations in the genes encoding β-amyloid and α-synuclein cause familial forms of Alzheimer's and Parkinson's diseases, and posttranslational, noninherited abnormalities in these proteins are also central to sporadic Alzheimer's and Parkinson's diseases. Analogously, recent reports propose that nonheritable, posttranslational modifications in SOD1 are pathogenic in sporadic ALS.

TREATMENT AMYOTROPHIC LATERAL SCLEROSIS

No treatment arrests the underlying pathologic process in ALS. The drug riluzole (100 mg/d) was approved for ALS because it produces a modest lengthening of survival. In one trial, the survival rate at 18 months with riluzole was similar to placebo at 15 months. The mechanism of this effect is not known with certainty; riluzole may reduce excitotoxicity by diminishing glutamate release. Riluzole is generally well tolerated; nausea, dizziness, weight loss, and elevated liver enzymes occur occasionally. Pathophysiologic studies of mutant SOD1-related ALS in mice have disclosed diverse targets for therapy; consequently, multiple therapies are presently in clinical trials for ALS including experimental trials of small molecules, mesenchymal stem cells, and immunosuppression. Interventions such as antisense oligonucleotides (ASO) that diminish expression of mutant SOD1 protein prolong survival in transgenic ALS mice and rats and are also nearing trial now for SOD1-mediated ALS.

In the absence of a primary therapy for ALS, a variety of rehabilitative aids may substantially assist ALS patients. Foot-drop splints facilitate ambulation by obviating the need for excessive hip flexion and by preventing tripping on a floppy foot. Finger extension splints can potentiate grip. Respiratory support may be life-sustaining. For patients electing against long-term ventilation by tracheostomy, positive-pressure ventilation by mouth or nose provides transient (several weeks) relief from hypercarbia and hypoxia. Also extremely beneficial for some patients is a respiratory device (Cough Assist Device) that produces an artificial cough. This is highly effective in clearing airways and preventing aspiration pneumonia. When bulbar disease prevents normal chewing and swallowing, gastrostomy is uniformly helpful, restoring normal nutrition and hydration. Fortunately, an increasing variety of speech synthesizers are now available to augment speech when there is advanced bulbar palsy. These facilitate oral communication and may be effective for telephone use.

In contrast to ALS, several of the disorders (Tables 452-1 and 452-3) that bear some clinical resemblance to ALS are treatable. For this reason, a careful search for causes of secondary motor neuron disease is warranted.

OTHER MOTOR NEURON DISEASES

SELECTED LOWER MOTOR NEURON DISORDERS

In these motor neuron diseases, the peripheral motor neurons are affected without evidence of involvement of the corticospinal motor system (Tables 452-1, 452-2, and 452-3).

X-Linked Spinobulbar Muscular Atrophy (Kennedy's Disease) This is an X-linked lower motor neuron disorder in which progressive weakness and wasting of limb and bulbar muscles begins in males in mid-adult life and is conjoined with androgen insensitivity manifested by gynecomastia and reduced fertility (Chap. 411). In addition to gynecomastia, which may be subtle, two findings distinguishing this disorder from ALS are the absence of signs of pyramidal tract disease (spasticity) and the presence of a subtle sensory neuropathy in some patients. The underlying molecular defect is an expanded trinucleotide repeat (-CAG-) in the first exon of the androgen receptor gene on the X chromosome. DNA testing is available. An inverse correlation appears to exist between the number of -CAG- repeats and the age of onset of the disease.

Adult Tay-Sachs Disease Several reports have described adult-onset, predominantly lower motor neuropathies arising from deficiency of the enzymeβ-hexosaminidase (hex A). These tend to be distinguishable from ALS because they are very slowly progressive; dysarthria and radiographically evident cerebellar atrophy may be prominent. In rare cases, spasticity may also be present, although it is generally absent (Chap. 432e).

Spinal Muscular Atrophy The SMAs are a family of selective lower motor neuron diseases of early onset. Despite some phenotypic variability (largely in age of onset), the defect in the majority of families with SMA maps to a locus on chromosome 5 encoding a putative motor neuron survival protein (SMN, for survival motor neuron) that is important in the formation and trafficking of RNA complexes across the nuclear membrane. Neuropathologically these disorders are characterized by extensive loss of large motor neurons; muscle biopsy reveals evidence of denervation atrophy. Several clinical forms exist.

Infantile SMA (SMA I, Werdnig-Hoffmann disease) has the earliest onset and most rapidly fatal course. In some instances it is apparent even before birth, as indicated by decreased fetal movements late in the third trimester. Though alert, afflicted infants are weak and floppy (hypotonic) and lack muscle stretch reflexes. Death generally ensues within the first year of life. *Chronic childhood SMA* (SMA II) begins later in childhood and evolves with a more slowly progressive course. *Juvenile SMA* (SMA III, Kugelberg-Welander disease) manifests during late childhood and runs a slow, indolent course. Unlike most denervating diseases, in this chronic disorder, weakness is greatest in the proximal muscles; indeed, the pattern of clinical weakness can suggest a primary myopathy such as limb-girdle dystrophy. Electrophysiologic and muscle biopsy evidence of denervation distinguish SMA III from the myopathic syndromes. There is no primary therapy for SMA, although remarkable recent experimental data indicate that it may be possible to deliver the missing SMN gene to motor neurons using intravenously or intrathecally delivered adeno-associated viruses (e.g., AAV9) immediately after birth.

Multifocal Motor Neuropathy with Conduction Block In this disorder lower motor neuron function is regionally and chronically disrupted by remarkably focal blocks in conduction. Many cases have elevated serum titers of mono- and polyclonal antibodies to ganglioside GM1; it is hypothesized that the antibodies produce selective, focal, paranodal demyelination of motor neurons. MMCB is not typically associated with corticospinal signs. In contrast with ALS, MMCB may respond dramatically to therapy such as IV immunoglobulin or chemotherapy; thus, it is imperative that MMCB be excluded when considering a diagnosis of ALS.

Other Forms of Lower Motor Neuron Disease In individual families, other syndromes characterized by selective lower motor neuron dysfunction in an SMA-like pattern have been described. There are rare X-linked and autosomal dominant forms of apparent SMA. There is an ALS variant of juvenile onset, the Fazio-Londe syndrome, that involves mainly the musculature innervated by the brainstem. A component of lower motor neuron dysfunction is also found in degenerative disorders such as Machado-Joseph disease and the related olivopontocerebellar degenerations (Chap. 450).

SELECTED DISORDERS OF THE UPPER MOTOR NEURON

Primary Lateral Sclerosis This exceedingly rare disorder arises sporadically in adults in mid to late life. Clinically PLS is characterized by progressive spastic weakness of the limbs, preceded or followed by spastic dysarthria and dysphagia, indicating combined involvement of the corticospinal and corticobulbar tracts. Fasciculations, amyotrophy, and sensory changes are absent; neither electromyography nor muscle biopsy shows denervation. On neuropathologic examination, there is selective loss of the large pyramidal cells in the precentral gyrus and degeneration of the corticospinal and corticobulbar projections. The peripheral motor neurons and other neuronal systems are spared. The course of PLS is variable; although long-term survival is documented, the course may be as aggressive as in ALS, with ~3-year survival from onset to death. Early in its course, PLS raises the question of multiple sclerosis or other demyelinating diseases such as adrenoleukodystrophy as diagnostic considerations (Chap. 458). A myelopathy suggestive of PLS is infrequently seen with infection with the retrovirus human T cell lymphotropic virus 1 (HTLV-1) (Chap. 456). The clinical course and laboratory testing will distinguish these possibilities.

Familial Spastic Paraplegia In its pure form, FSP is usually transmitted as an autosomal trait; most adult-onset cases are dominantly inherited. Symptoms usually begin in the third or fourth decade, presenting as progressive spastic weakness beginning in the distal lower extremities; however, there are variants with onset so early that the differential diagnosis includes cerebral palsy. FSP typically has a long survival, presumably because respiratory function is spared. Late in the illness, there may be urinary urgency and incontinence and sometimes fecal incontinence; sexual function tends to be preserved.

In pure forms of FSP, the spastic leg weakness is often accompanied by posterior column (vibration and position) abnormalities and disturbance of bowel and bladder function. Some family members may have spasticity without clinical symptoms.

By contrast, particularly when recessively inherited, FSP may have complex or complicated forms in which altered corticospinal and dorsal column function is accompanied by significant involvement of other regions of the nervous system, including amyotrophy, mental retardation, optic atrophy, and sensory neuropathy.

Neuropathologically, in FSP, there is degeneration of the corticospinal tracts, which appear nearly normal in the brainstem but show increasing atrophy at more caudal levels in the spinal cord; in effect, the pathologic picture is of a dying-back or distal axonopathy of long neuronal fibers within the CNS.

Defects at numerous loci underlie both dominantly and recessively inherited forms of FSP (Table 452-3). More than 30 FSP genes have now been identified. The gene most commonly implicated in dominantly inherited FSP is *spastin,* which encodes a microtubule interacting protein. The most common childhood-onset dominant form arises from mutations in the *atlastin* gene. A kinesin heavy-chain protein implicated in microtubule motor function was found to be defective in a family with dominantly inherited FSP of variable-onset age.

An infantile-onset form of X-linked, recessive FSP arises from mutations in the gene for myelin proteolipid protein. This is an example of rather striking allelic variation, as most other mutations in the same gene cause not FSP but Pelizaeus-Merzbacher disease, a widespread disorder of CNS myelin. Another recessive variant is caused by defects in the *paraplegin* gene. Paraplegin has homology to metalloproteases that are important in mitochondrial function in yeast.

WEBSITES

Several websites provide valuable information on ALS including those offered by the Muscular Dystrophy Association (*www.mdausa.org*), the Amyotrophic Lateral Sclerosis Association (*www.alsa.org*), and the World Federation of Neurology and the Neuromuscular Unit at Washington University in St. Louis (*www.neuro.wustl.edu*).

453e Prion Diseases

Stanley B. Prusiner, Bruce L. Miller

This is a digital-only chapter. It is available on the DVD that accompanies this book, as well as on Access Medicine/Harrison's Online, and the eBook and "app" editions of HPIM 19e.

Prions are proteins that adopt an alternative conformation, which becomes self-propagating. Some prions cause degeneration of the central nervous system (CNS). Once relegated to causing a group of rare disorders of the CNS such as Creutzfeldt-Jakob disease (CJD), prions—as mounting evidence shows—also appear to play a key role in more common illnesses such as Alzheimer's disease (AD) and Parkinson's disease (PD). While CJD is caused by the accumulation of PrP^{Sc}, increasing data argue that Aβ prions cause AD, α-synuclein prions cause PD, and tau prions cause the frontotemporal dementias (FTDs). In this chapter, we confine our discussion to CJD, which typically presents with a rapidly progressive dementia as well as motor abnormalities. The illness is relentlessly progressive and generally causes death within 9 months of onset. Most CJD patients are between 50 and 75 years of age; however, patients as young as 17 and as old as 83 have been recorded.

454 Disorders of the Autonomic Nervous System

Phillip A. Low, John W. Engstrom

The autonomic nervous system (ANS) innervates the entire neuraxis and influences all organ systems. It regulates blood pressure (BP), heart rate, sleep, and bladder and bowel function. It operates automatically; its full importance becomes recognized only when ANS function is compromised, resulting in dysautonomia. Hypothalamic disorders that cause disturbances in homeostasis are discussed in Chaps. 23 and 401e.

ANATOMIC ORGANIZATION

The activity of the ANS is regulated by central neurons responsive to diverse afferent inputs. After central integration of afferent information, autonomic outflow is adjusted to permit the functioning of the major organ systems in accordance with the needs of the whole organism. Connections between the cerebral cortex and the autonomic centers in the brainstem coordinate autonomic outflow with higher mental functions.

The preganglionic neurons of the parasympathetic nervous system leave the central nervous system (CNS) in the third, seventh, ninth, and tenth cranial nerves as well as the second and third sacral nerves, while the preganglionic neurons of the sympathetic nervous system exit the spinal cord between the first thoracic and the second lumbar segments (Fig. 454-1). These are thinly myelinated. The postganglionic neurons, located in ganglia outside the CNS, give rise to the postganglionic unmyelinated autonomic nerves that innervate organs and tissues throughout the body. Responses to sympathetic and parasympathetic stimulation are frequently antagonistic (Table 454-1), reflecting highly coordinated interactions within the CNS; the resultant changes in parasympathetic and sympathetic activity provide more precise control of autonomic responses than could be achieved by the modulation of a single system.

Acetylcholine (ACh) is the preganglionic neurotransmitter for both divisions of the ANS as well as the postganglionic neurotransmitter of the parasympathetic neurons; the preganglionic receptors are nicotinic, and the postganglionic are muscarinic in type. Norepinephrine (NE) is the neurotransmitter of the postganglionic sympathetic neurons, except for cholinergic neurons innervating the eccrine sweat glands.

Parasympathetic | Sympathetic

III, VII, IX, X, T1–12, L1, L2, S2, 3 — Heart, Bowel, Arm, Heart, Viscera, Adrenal medulla (preganglionic supply), Leg, Terminal ganglion (coccygeal), Sympathetic chain

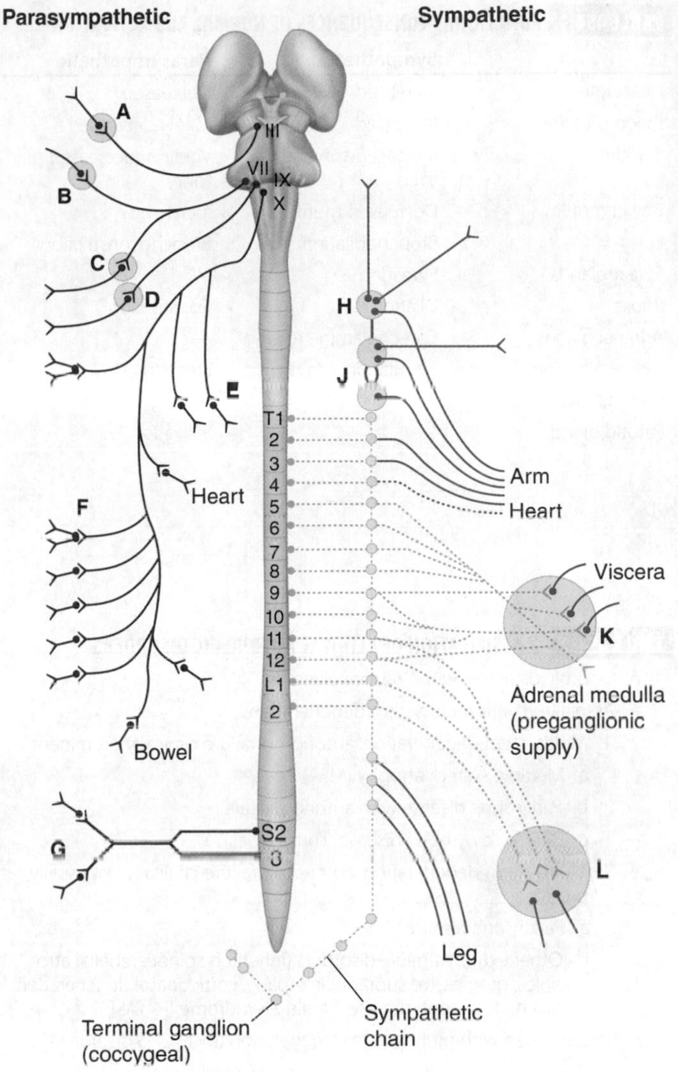

Parasympathetic system
from cranial nerves III, VII, IX, X
and from sacral nerves 2 and 3

Sympathetic system
from T1-L2
Preganglionic fibers ············
Postganglionic fibers ———

A Ciliary ganglion
B Sphenopalatine (pterygopalatine) ganglion
C Submandibular ganglion
D Otic ganglion
E Vagal ganglion cells in the heart wall
F Vagal ganglion cells in bowel wall
G Pelvic ganglia

H Superior cervical ganglion
J Middle cervical ganglion and inferior cervical (stellate) ganglion including T1 ganglion
K Coeliac and other abdominal ganglia
L Lower abdominal sympathetic ganglia

FIGURE 454-1 Schematic representation of the autonomic nervous system. *(From M Moskowitz: Clin Endocrinol Metab 6:77, 1977.)*

CLINICAL EVALUATION

CLASSIFICATION

Disorders of the ANS may result from pathology of either the CNS or the peripheral nervous system (PNS) (Table 454-2). Signs and symptoms may result from interruption of the afferent limb, CNS

TABLE 454-1 FUNCTIONAL CONSEQUENCES OF NORMAL ANS ACTIVATION

	Sympathetic	Parasympathetic
Heart rate	Increased	Decreased
Blood pressure	Increased	Mildly decreased
Bladder	Increased sphincter tone	Voiding (decreased tone)
Bowel motility	Decreased motility	Increased
Lung	Bronchodilation	Bronchoconstriction
Sweat glands	Sweating	—
Pupils	Dilation	Constriction
Adrenal glands	Catecholamine release	—
Sexual function	Ejaculation, orgasm	Erection
Lacrimal glands	—	Tearing
Parotid glands	—	Salivation

processing centers, or efferent limb of reflex arcs controlling autonomic responses. For example, a lesion of the medulla produced by a posterior fossa tumor can impair BP responses to postural changes and result in orthostatic hypotension (OH). OH can also be caused by lesions of the spinal cord or peripheral vasomotor nerve fibers (e.g., diabetic autonomic neuropathy). Lesions of the efferent limb cause the most consistent and severe OH. The site of reflex interruption is usually established by the clinical context in which the dysautonomia arises, combined with judicious use of ANS testing and neuroimaging studies. The presence or absence of CNS signs, association with sensory or motor polyneuropathy, medical illnesses, medication use, and family history are often important considerations. Some syndromes do not fit easily into any classification scheme.

SYMPTOMS OF AUTONOMIC DYSFUNCTION

Clinical manifestations can result from loss of function, overactivity, or dysregulation of autonomic circuits. Disorders of autonomic function should be considered in patients with unexplained OH, syncope, sleep dysfunction, altered sweating (hyperhidrosis or hypohidrosis), impotence, constipation or other gastrointestinal symptoms (bloating,

TABLE 454-2 CLASSIFICATION OF CLINICAL AUTONOMIC DISORDERS

I. Autonomic disorders with brain involvement
  A. Associated with multisystem degeneration
    1. Multisystem degeneration: autonomic failure clinically prominent
      a. Multiple system atrophy (MSA)
      b. Parkinson's disease with autonomic failure
      c. Diffuse Lewy body disease (some cases)
    2. Multisystem degeneration: autonomic failure clinically not usually prominent
      a. Parkinson's disease
      b. Other extrapyramidal disorders (inherited spinocerebellar atrophies, progressive supranuclear palsy, corticobasal degeneration, Machado-Joseph disease, fragile X syndrome [FXTAS])
  B. Unassociated with multisystem degeneration (focal CNS disorders)
    1. Disorders mainly due to cerebral cortex involvement
      a. Frontal cortex lesions causing urinary/bowel incontinence
      b. Focal seizures (temporal lobe or anterior cingulate)
      c. Cerebral infarction of the insula
    2. Disorders of the limbic and paralimbic circuits
      a. Shapiro's syndrome (agenesis of corpus callosum, hyperhidrosis, hypothermia)
      b. Autonomic seizures
      c. Limbic encephalitis
    3. Disorders of the hypothalamus
      a. Thiamine deficiency (Wernicke-Korsakoff syndrome)
      b. Diencephalic syndrome
      c. Neuroleptic malignant syndrome
      d. Serotonin syndrome
      e. Fatal familial insomnia
      f. Antidiuretic hormone (ADH) syndromes (diabetes insipidus, inappropriate ADH secretion)
      g. Disturbances of temperature regulation (hyperthermia, hypothermia)
      h. Disturbances of sexual function
      i. Disturbances of appetite
      j. Disturbances of BP/HR and gastric function
      k. Horner's syndrome
    4. Disorders of the brainstem and cerebellum
      a. Posterior fossa tumors
      b. Syringobulbia and Arnold-Chiari malformation
      c. Disorders of BP control (hypertension, hypotension)
      d. Cardiac arrhythmias
      e. Central sleep apnea
      f. Baroreflex failure
      g. Horner's syndrome
      h. Vertebrobasilar and lateral medullary (Wallenberg's) syndromes
      i. Brainstem encephalitis

II. Autonomic disorders with spinal cord involvement
  A. Traumatic quadriplegia
  B. Syringomyelia
  C. Subacute combined degeneration
  D. Multiple sclerosis and neuromyelitis optica
  E. Amyotrophic lateral sclerosisF. Tetanus
  G. Stiff-person syndrome
  H. Spinal cord tumors

III. Autonomic neuropathies
  A. Acute/subacute autonomic neuropathies
    1. Subacute autoimmune autonomic ganglionopathy (AAG)
      a. Subacute paraneoplastic autonomic neuropathy
      b. Guillain-Barré syndrome
      c. Botulism
      d. Porphyria
      e. Drug induced autonomic neuropathies-stimulants, drug withdrawal, vasoconstrictor, vasodilators, beta-receptor antagonists, beta-agonists
      f. Toxin-induced autonomic neuropathies
      g. Subacute cholinergic neuropathy
  B. Chronic peripheral autonomic neuropathies
    1. Distal small fiber neuropathy
    2. Combined sympathetic and parasympathetic failure
      a. Amyloid
      b. Diabetic autonomic neuropathy
      c. Autoimmune autonomic ganglionopathy (paraneoplastic and idiopathic)
      d. Sensory neuronopathy with autonomic failure
      e. Familial dysautonomia (Riley-Day syndrome)
      f. Diabetic, uremic, or nutritional deficiency
      g. Dysautonomia of old age
    3. Disorders of reduced orthostatic intolerance: reflex syncope, POTS, associated with prolonged bed rest, associated with space flight, chronic fatigue

Abbreviations: BP, blood pressure; CNS, central nervous system; HR, heart rate; POTS, postural orthostatic tachycardia syndrome.

TABLE 454-3 SYMPTOMS OF ORTHOSTATIC INTOLERANCE

Lightheadedness (dizziness)	88%
Weakness or tiredness	72%
Cognitive difficulty (thinking/concentrating)	47%
Blurred vision	47%
Tremulousness	38%
Vertigo	37%
Pallor	31%
Anxiety	29%
Palpitations	26%
Clammy feeling	19%
Nausea	18%

Source: PA Low et al: Mayo Clin Proc 70:617, 1995.

nausea, vomiting of old food, diarrhea), or bladder disorders (urinary frequency, hesitancy, or incontinence). Symptoms may be widespread or regional in distribution. An autonomic history focuses on systemic functions (BP, heart rate, sleep, fever, sweating) and involvement of individual organ systems (pupils, bowel, bladder, sexual function). The autonomic symptom profile is a self-report questionnaire that can be used for formal assessment. It is also important to recognize the modulating effects of age. For example, OH typically produces lightheadedness in the young, whereas cognitive slowing is more common in the elderly. Specific symptoms of orthostatic intolerance are diverse (Table 454-3). Autonomic symptoms may vary dramatically, reflecting the dynamic nature of autonomic control over homeostatic function. For example, OH might be manifest only in the early morning, following a meal, with exercise, or with raised ambient temperature, depending on the regional vascular bed affected by the dysautonomia.

Early symptoms may be overlooked. Impotence, although not specific for autonomic failure, often heralds autonomic failure in men and may precede other symptoms by years (Chap. 67). A decrease in the frequency of spontaneous early morning erections may occur months before loss of nocturnal penile tumescence and development of total impotence. Bladder dysfunction may appear early in men and women, particularly in those with a CNS etiology. Cold feet may indicate increased peripheral vasomotor constriction. Brain and spinal cord disease above the level of the lumbar spine results first in urinary frequency and small bladder volumes and eventually in incontinence (upper motor neuron or spastic bladder). By contrast, PNS disease of autonomic nerve fibers results in large bladder volumes, urinary frequency, and overflow incontinence (lower motor neuron flaccid bladder). Measurement of bladder volume (postvoid residual) is a useful bedside test for distinguishing between upper and lower motor neuron bladder dysfunction in the early stages of dysautonomia. Gastrointestinal autonomic dysfunction typically presents as severe constipation. Diarrhea may develop (typically in diabetes mellitus) due to rapid transit of contents or uncoordinated small-bowel motor activity, or on an osmotic basis from bacterial overgrowth associated with small-bowel stasis. Impaired glandular secretory function may cause difficulty with food intake due to decreased salivation or eye irritation due to decreased lacrimation. Occasionally, temperature elevation and vasodilation can result from anhidrosis because sweating is normally important for heat dissipation (Chap. 23). Lack of sweating after a hot bath, during exercise, or on a hot day can suggest sudomotor failure.

OH (also called *orthostatic or postural hypotension*) is perhaps the most disabling feature of autonomic dysfunction. The prevalence of OH is relatively high, especially when OH associated with aging and diabetes mellitus is included (Table 454-4). OH can cause a variety of symptoms, including dimming or loss of vision, lightheadedness, diaphoresis, diminished hearing, pallor, and weakness. Syncope results when the drop in BP impairs cerebral perfusion. Other manifestations of impaired baroreflexes are supine hypertension, a heart rate that is fixed regardless of posture, postprandial hypotension, and an excessively high nocturnal BP. Many patients with OH have a preceding

TABLE 454-4 PREVALENCE OF ORTHOSTATIC HYPOTENSION IN DIFFERENT DISORDERS

Disorder	Prevalence
Aging	14–20%
Diabetic neuropathy	10%
Other autonomic neuropathies	10–50 per 100,000
Multiple system atrophy	5–15 per 100,000
Pure autonomic failure	10–30 per 100,000

diagnosis of hypertension or have concomitant supine hypertension, reflecting the great importance of baroreflexes in maintaining postural and supine normotension. The appearance of OH in patients receiving antihypertensive treatment may indicate overtreatment or the onset of an autonomic disorder. The most common causes of OH are not neurologic in origin; these must be distinguished from the neurogenic causes (Table 454-5). Neurocardiogenic and cardiac causes of syncope are considered in Chap. 27.

APPROACH TO THE PATIENT: Orthostatic Hypotension and Other ANS Disorders

The first step in the evaluation of symptomatic OH is the exclusion of treatable causes. The history should include a review of medications that may affect the ANS (Table 454-6). The main classes of drugs that may cause OH are diuretics, antihypertensives, antidepressants, ethanol, narcotics, insulin, dopamine agonists, barbiturates, and calcium channel blocking agents. However, the precipitation of OH by medications may also be the first sign of an underlying autonomic disorder. The history may reveal an underlying cause for symptoms (e.g., diabetes, Parkinson's disease) or specific underlying mechanisms (e.g., cardiac pump failure, reduced intravascular volume). The relationship of symptoms to meals (splanchnic pooling), standing on awakening in the morning (intravascular volume depletion), ambient warming (vasodilatation), or exercise (muscle arteriolar vasodilatation)

TABLE 454-5 NONNEUROGENIC CAUSES OF ORTHOSTATIC HYPOTENSION

Cardiac pump failure	**Venous pooling**
Myocardial infarction	Alcohol
Myocarditis	Postprandial dilation of splanchnic vessel beds
Constrictive pericarditis	Vigorous exercise with dilation of skeletal vessel beds
Aortic stenosis	Heat: hot environment, hot showers and baths, fever
Tachyarrhythmias	Prolonged recumbency or standing
Bradyarrhythmias	Sepsis
Salt-losing nephropathy	**Medications**
Adrenal insufficiency	Antihypertensives
Diabetes insipidus	Diuretics
Venous obstruction	Vasodilators: nitrates, hydralazine
Reduced intravascular volume	Alpha- and beta-blocking agents
Straining or heavy lifting, urination, defecation	Central nervous system sedatives: barbiturates, opiates
Dehydration	Tricyclic antidepressants
Diarrhea, emesis	Phenothiazines
Hemorrhage	
Burns	
Metabolic	
Adrenocortical insufficiency	
Hypoaldosteronism	
Pheochromocytoma	
Severe potassium depletion	

TABLE 454-6 SOME DRUGS THAT AFFECT AUTONOMIC FUNCTION

Symptom	Drug Class	Specific Examples
Impotence	Opioids	Tylenol #3
	Anabolic steroids	—
	Some antiarrhythmics	Prazosin
	Some antihypertensives	Clonidine
	Some diuretics	Benazepril
	Some SSRIs	Venlafaxine
Urinary retention	Opioids	Fentanyl
	Decongestants	Brompheniramine
		Diphenhydramine
Diaphoresis	Some antihypertensives	Amlodipine
	Some SSRIs	Citalopram
	Opioids	Morphine
Hypotension	Tricyclics	Amitriptyline
	Beta blockers	Propranolol
	Diuretics	HCTZ
	CCBs	Verapamil

Abbreviations: CCBs, calcium channel blockers; HCTZ, hydrochlorothiazide; SSRIs, selective serotonin reuptake inhibitors.

should be sought. Standing time to first symptom and to presyncope (Chap. 27) should be followed for management.

Physical examination includes measurement of supine and standing pulse and BP. OH is defined as a sustained drop in systolic (≥20 mmHg) or diastolic (≥10 mmHg) BP after 2–3 min of standing. In nonneurogenic causes of OH (such as hypovolemia), the BP drop is accompanied by a compensatory increase in heart rate of >15 beats/min. A clue that the patient has neurogenic OH is the aggravation or precipitation of OH by autonomic stressors (a meal, hot bath, or exercise). Neurologic examination should include mental status (neurodegenerative disorders), cranial nerves (impaired downgaze with progressive supranuclear palsy; abnormal pupils with Horner's or Adie's syndrome), motor tone (Parkinson's disease and parkinsonism), and sensation (polyneuropathies). In patients without a clear diagnosis initially, follow-up evaluations every few months or whenever symptoms worsen may reveal the underlying cause.

Disorders of autonomic function should be considered in patients with symptoms of altered sweating (hyperhidrosis or hypohidrosis), gastroparesis (bloating, nausea, vomiting of old food), impotence, constipation, or bladder disturbances (urinary frequency, hesitancy, or incontinence).

AUTONOMIC TESTING

Autonomic function tests are helpful to document abnormalities when findings on history and examination are inconclusive; to detect subclinical involvement; or to follow the course of an autonomic disorder.

Heart Rate Variation with Deep Breathing This tests the parasympathetic component of cardiovascular reflexes via the vagus nerve. Results are influenced by multiple factors including the subject's position (recumbent, sitting, or standing), rate and depth of respiration (6 breaths per minute and a forced vital capacity [FVC] >1.5 L are optimal), age, medications, weight, and degree of hypocapnia. Interpretation of results requires comparison of test data with results from age-matched controls collected under identical test conditions. For example, the lower limit of normal heart rate variation with deep breathing in persons <20 years is >15–20 beats/min, but for persons over age 60 it is 5–8 beats/min. Heart rate variation with deep breathing (respiratory sinus arrhythmia) is abolished by the muscarinic ACh receptor antagonist atropine but is unaffected by sympathetic postganglionic blockade (e.g., propranolol).

Valsalva Response This response (Table 454-7) assesses the integrity of the baroreflex control of heart rate (parasympathetic) and BP (adrenergic). Under normal conditions, increases in BP at the carotid bulb trigger a reduction in heart rate (increased vagal tone), and decreases in BP trigger an increase in heart rate (reduced vagal tone). The Valsalva response is tested in the supine position. The subject exhales against a closed glottis (or into a manometer maintaining a constant expiratory pressure of 40 mmHg) for 15 s while measuring changes in heart rate and beat-to-beat BP. There are four phases of the BP and heart rate response to the Valsalva maneuver. Phases I and III are mechanical and related to changes in intrathoracic and intraabdominal pressure. In early phase II, reduced venous return results in a fall in stroke volume and BP, counteracted by a combination of reflex tachycardia and increased total peripheral resistance. Increased total peripheral resistance arrests the BP drop ~5–8 s after the onset of the maneuver. Late phase II begins with a progressive rise in BP toward or above baseline. Venous return and cardiac output return to normal in phase IV. Persistent peripheral arteriolar vasoconstriction and increased cardiac adrenergic tone result in a temporary BP overshoot and phase IV bradycardia (mediated by the baroreceptor reflex).

Autonomic function during the Valsalva maneuver can be measured using beat-to-beat BP or heart rate changes. The *Valsalva ratio* is defined as the maximum phase II tachycardia divided by the minimum phase IV bradycardia (Table 454-8). The ratio reflects the integrity of the entire baroreceptor reflex arc and of sympathetic efferents to blood vessels.

Sudomotor Function Sweating is induced by release of ACh from sympathetic postganglionic fibers. The quantitative sudomotor axon reflex test (QSART) is a measure of regional autonomic function mediated by ACh-induced sweating. A reduced or absent response indicates a lesion of the postganglionic sudomotor axon. For example, sweating may be reduced in the feet as a result of distal polyneuropathy (e.g., diabetes). The thermoregulatory sweat test (TST) is a qualitative measure of regional sweat production in response to an elevation of body temperature under controlled conditions. An indicator powder placed on the anterior surface of the body changes color with sweat production during temperature

TABLE 454-7 NORMAL BLOOD PRESSURE AND HEART RATE CHANGES DURING THE VALSALVA MANEUVER

Phase	Maneuver	Blood Pressure	Heart Rate	Comments
I	Forced expiration against a partially closed glottis	Rises; aortic compression from raised intrathoracic pressure	Decreases	Mechanical
II *early*	Continued expiration	Falls; decreased venous return to the heart	Increases (reflex tachycardia)	Reduced vagal tone
II *late*	Continued expiration	Rises; reflex increase in peripheral vascular resistance	Increases at slower rate	Requires intact efferent sympathetic response
III	End of expiration	Falls; increased capacitance of pulmonary bed	Increases further	Mechanical
IV	Recovery	Rises; persistent vasoconstriction and increased cardiac output	Compensatory bradycardia	Requires intact efferent sympathetic response

TABLE 454-8 NEURAL PATHWAYS UNDERLYING SOME STANDARDIZED AUTONOMIC TESTS

Test Evaluated	Procedure	Autonomic Function
HRDB	6 deep breaths/min	Cardiovagal function
Valsalva ratio	Expiratory pressure, 40 mmHg for 10–15 s	Cardiovagal function
QSART	Axon-reflex test 4 limb sites	Postganglionic sudomotor function
BP_{BB} to VM	BP_{BB} response to VM	Adrenergic function: baroreflex adrenergic control of vagal and vasomotor function
HUT	BP_{BB} and heart rate response to HUT	Adrenergic and cardiovagal responses to HUT

Abbreviations: BP_{BB}, beat-to-beat blood pressure; HRDB, heart rate response to deep breathing; HUT, head-up tilt; QSART, quantitative sudomotor axon reflex test; VM, Valsalva maneuver.

elevation. The pattern of color change is a measure of regional sweat secretion. A postganglionic lesion is present if both QSART and TST show absent sweating. In a preganglionic lesion, the QSART is normal but TST shows anhidrosis.

Orthostatic BP Recordings Beat-to-beat BP measurements determined in supine, 70° tilt, and tilt-back positions are useful to quantitate orthostatic failure of BP control. Allow a 20-min period of rest in the supine position before assessing changes in BP during tilting. The BP change combined with heart rate monitoring is useful for the evaluation of patients with suspected OH or unexplained syncope.

Tilt Table Testing for Syncope The great majority of patients with syncope do not have autonomic failure. Tilt table testing can be used to make the diagnosis of vasovagal syncope with sensitivity, specificity, and reproducibility. A standardized protocol is used that specifies the tilt apparatus, angle and duration of tilt, and procedure for provocation of vasodilation (e.g., sublingual or spray nitroglycerin). A positive nitroglycerin-stimulated test predicts recurrence of syncope. Recommendations for the performance of tilt studies for syncope have been incorporated in consensus guidelines.

SPECIFIC SYNDROMES OF ANS DYSFUNCTION

MULTIPLE SYSTEM ATROPHY (CHAP. 449)

Multiple system atrophy (MSA) is an entity that comprises autonomic failure (OH or a neurogenic bladder) *and* either parkinsonism (MSA-p) or a cerebellar syndrome (MSA-c). MSA-p is the more common form; the parkinsonism is atypical in that it is usually unassociated with significant tremor or a response to levodopa. Symptomatic OH within 1 year of onset of parkinsonism predicts eventual development of MSA-p in 75% of patients. There is a very high frequency of impotence in men. Although autonomic abnormalities are common in advanced Parkinson's disease (Chap. 449), the severity and distribution of autonomic failure are more severe and generalized in MSA. Brain magnetic resonance imaging (MRI) is a useful diagnostic adjunct: in MSA-p, iron deposition in the striatum may be evident as T2 hypointensity, and in MSA-c, cerebellar atrophy is present with a characteristic T2 hyperintense signal ("hot cross buns sign") in the pons (Fig. 454-2). Cardiac postganglionic adrenergic innervation, measured by uptake of fluorodopamine on positron emission tomography, is markedly impaired in the dysautonomia of Parkinson's disease (PD) but is usually normal in MSA. Neuropathologic changes include neuronal loss and gliosis in many CNS regions, including the brainstem, cerebellum, striatum, and intermediolateral cell column of the thoracolumbar spinal cord.

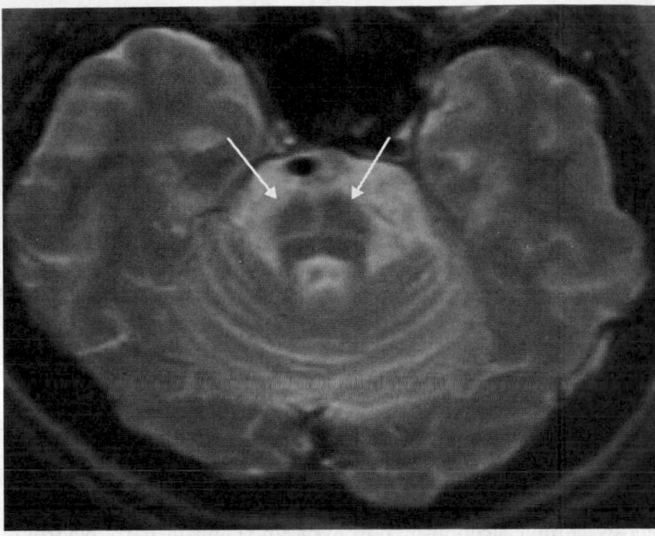

FIGURE 454-2 Multiple system atrophy, cerebellar type (MSA-c). Axial T2-weighted magnetic resonance image at the level of the pons shows a characteristic hyperintense signal, the "hot cross buns" sign. This appearance can also be seen in some spinocerebellar atrophies, as well as other neurodegenerative conditions affecting the brainstem.

MSA is uncommon, with a prevalence estimated at 2–5 per 100,000 individuals. Onset is typically in the mid-fifties, men are slightly more often affected than women, and most cases are sporadic. The diagnosis should be considered in adults over the age of 30 years who present with OH or urinary incontinence and either parkinsonism that is poorly responsive to dopamine replacement or a cerebellar syndrome. MSA generally progresses relentlessly to death 7–10 years after onset, but survival beyond 15 years has been reported. Factors that predict a worse prognosis include rapid progression of disability, bladder dysfunction, female gender, the MSA-p subtype, and an older age at onset. Attempts to slow the progression of MSA have thus far been unsuccessful, including trials of lithium, growth hormone, riluzole, rasagiline, minocycline, and a recent trail of rifampicin.

Management is symptomatic for neurogenic OH (see below), sleep disorders including laryngeal stridor, and gastrointestinal (GI) and urinary dysfunction. GI management includes frequent small meals, soft diet, stool softeners, and bulk agents. Gastroparesis is difficult to treat; metoclopramide stimulates gastric emptying but worsens parkinsonism by blocking central dopamine receptors. The peripheral dopamine (D_2 and D_3) receptor antagonist domperidone has been used patients with various GI conditions in many countries and is now available in the United States through the U.S. Food and Drug Administration's (FDA) Expanded Access to Investigational Drugs program.

Autonomic dysfunction is also a common feature in dementia with Lewy bodies (Chap. 448); the severity is usually less than that found in MSA or PD. In multiple sclerosis (MS; Chap. 458), autonomic complications reflect the CNS location of MS involvement and generally worsen with disease duration and disability.

SPINAL CORD

Spinal cord lesions from any cause may result in focal autonomic deficits or autonomic hyperreflexia (e.g., spinal cord transection or hemisection) affecting bowel, bladder, sexual, temperature-regulation, or cardiovascular functions. Quadriparetic patients exhibit both supine hypertension and OH after upward tilting. *Autonomic dysreflexia* describes a dramatic increase in BP in patients with traumatic spinal cord lesions above the T6 level, often in response to stimulation of the bladder, skin, or muscles. A distended or obstructed bladder, suprapubic palpation, catheter insertion, and urinary infection are common triggers. Associated symptoms can include facial flushing, headache, hypertension, or piloerection. Potential complications include intracranial vasospasm or hemorrhage, cardiac arrhythmia, and death. Awareness of the syndrome, identifying the trigger, and careful monitoring of BP during procedures in patients with acute or chronic spinal cord injury are essential. In patients with supine hypertension, BP can be lowered by tilting the head upward or sitting the patient up. Vasodilator drugs may be used to treat acute elevations in BP. Clonidine can be used prophylactically to reduce the hypertension resulting from bladder stimulation. Dangerous increases or decreases in body temperature may result from an inability to experience the sensory accompaniments of heat or cold exposure or control peripheral vasoconstriction or sweating below the level of the spinal cord injury.

PERIPHERAL NERVE AND NEUROMUSCULAR JUNCTION DISORDERS

Peripheral neuropathies (Chap. 459) are the most common cause of chronic autonomic insufficiency. Polyneuropathies that affect small myelinated and unmyelinated fibers of the sympathetic and parasympathetic nerves commonly occur in diabetes mellitus, amyloidosis, chronic alcoholism, porphyria, and Guillain-Barré syndrome. Neuromuscular junction disorders with autonomic involvement include botulism and Lambert-Eaton syndrome (Chap. 461).

Diabetes Mellitus Autonomic neuropathy in patients with diabetes increases the mortality rate 1.5- to 3-fold, even after adjusting for other cardiovascular risk factors. Estimates of 5-year mortality risk among these patients range from 15 to 53%. Although many deaths are due to secondary vascular disease, there are patients who specifically suffer cardiac arrest due to autonomic neuropathy. The autonomic involvement is also predictive of other complications including renal disease, stroke, and sleep apnea. Diabetes mellitus is discussed in Chaps. 417–419.

Amyloidosis Autonomic neuropathy occurs in both sporadic and familial forms of amyloidosis (Chap. 137). The AL (immunoglobulin light chain) type is associated with primary amyloidosis or amyloidosis secondary to multiple myeloma. The ATTR type, with transthyretin as the primary protein component, is responsible for the most common form of inherited amyloidosis. Although patients usually present with a distal painful polyneuropathy accompanied by sensory loss, autonomic insufficiency can precede the development of the polyneuropathy or occur in isolation. The diagnosis can be made by protein electrophoresis of blood and urine, tissue biopsy (abdominal fat pad, rectal mucosa, or sural nerve) to search for amyloid deposits, and genetic testing for transthyretin mutations in familial cases. Treatment of familial cases with liver transplantation can be successful. The response of primary amyloidosis to melphalan and stem cell transplantation has been mixed. Death is usually due to cardiac or renal involvement. Postmortem studies reveal amyloid deposition in many organs, including two sites that contribute to autonomic failure: intraneural blood vessels and autonomic ganglia. Pathologic examination reveals a loss of both unmyelinated and myelinated nerve fibers.

Alcoholic Neuropathy Abnormalities in parasympathetic vagal and efferent sympathetic function are usually mild in alcoholic polyneuropathy. OH is usually due to brainstem involvement, rather than injury to the PNS. Impotence is a major problem, but concurrent gonadal hormone abnormalities may play a role in this symptom. Clinical symptoms of autonomic failure generally appear only when the stocking-glove polyneuropathy is severe, and there is usually coexisting Wernicke's encephalopathy (Chap. 330). Autonomic involvement may contribute to the high mortality rates associated with alcoholism (Chap. 467).

Porphyria (Chap. 430) Autonomic dysfunction is most extensively documented in acute intermittent porphyria but can also occur with variegate porphyria and hereditary coproporphyria. Autonomic symptoms include tachycardia, sweating, urinary retention, abdominal pain, nausea and vomiting, insomnia, hypertension, and (less commonly) hypotension. Another prominent symptom is anxiety. Abnormal autonomic function can occur both during acute attacks and during remissions. Elevated catecholamine levels during acute attacks correlate with the degree of tachycardia and hypertension that is present.

Guillain-Barré Syndrome (Chap. 460) BP fluctuations and arrhythmias from autonomic instability can be severe. It is estimated that between 2 and 10% of patients with severe Guillain-Barré syndrome suffer fatal cardiovascular collapse. GI autonomic involvement, sphincter disturbances, abnormal sweating, and pupillary dysfunction can also occur. Demyelination has been described in the vagus and glossopharyngeal nerves, the sympathetic chain, and the white rami communicantes. Interestingly, the degree of autonomic involvement appears to be independent of the severity of motor or sensory neuropathy. Acute autonomic and sensory neuropathy is a variant that spares the motor system and presents with neurogenic OH and varying degrees of sensory loss. It is treated similarly to Guillain-Barré syndrome, but prognosis is less favorable, with persistent severe sensory deficits and variable degrees of OH in many patients.

Autoimmune Autonomic Ganglionopathy (AAG) This disorder presents with the subacute development of autonomic disturbances including OH, enteric neuropathy (gastroparesis, ileus, constipation/diarrhea), flaccid bladder, and cholinergic failure (e.g., loss of sweating, sicca complex, and a tonic pupil). A chronic form of AAG resembles pure autonomic failure (see below). Autoantibodies against the ganglionic ACh receptor (A_3 AChR), which are present in approximately half of patients, are considered diagnostic of AAG. Pathology shows preferential involvement of small unmyelinated nerve fibers, with sparing of larger myelinated ones. Onset of the neuropathy follows a viral infection in approximately half of cases. Up to one-third of untreated patients experience significant functional improvement over time. Immunotherapies that have been reported to be helpful include plasmapheresis, intravenous immune globulin, glucocorticoids, azathioprine, rituximab, and mycophenolate mofetil. OH, gastroparesis, and sicca symptoms can be managed symptomatically.

AAG can also occur on a paraneoplastic basis, with adenocarcinoma or small-cell carcinoma of the lung, lymphoma, or thymoma being the most common (Chap. 122). In the paraneoplastic cases, distinctive additional features, such as cerebellar involvement or dementia, may be present (see Tables 122-1, 122-2, and 122-3). The neoplasm may be occult and possibly suppressed by the autoantibody.

Botulism Botulinum toxin binds presynaptically to cholinergic nerve terminals and, after uptake into the cytosol, blocks ACh release. This acute cholinergic neuropathy presents as motor paralysis and autonomic disturbances that include blurred vision, dry mouth, nausea, unreactive or sluggishly reactive pupils, constipation, and urinary retention (Chap. 178).

PURE AUTONOMIC FAILURE (PAF)

This sporadic syndrome consists of postural hypotension, impotence, bladder dysfunction, and impaired sweating. The disorder begins in midlife and occurs in women more often than men. The symptoms can be disabling, but the disease does not shorten life span. The clinical and pharmacologic characteristics suggest primary involvement of postganglionic sympathetic neurons. A severe reduction in the density of neurons within sympathetic ganglia results in low supine plasma NE levels and noradrenergic supersensitivity. Some patients who are initially labeled with this diagnosis subsequently go on to develop AAG or MSA. Skin biopsies can demonstrate phosphorylated α-synuclein inclusions in postganglionic sympathetic adrenergic and cholinergic nerve fibers from some individuals with PAF, distinguishing them from AAG and suggesting that PAF is a synucleinopathy; patients with PD also have α-synuclein inclusions in sympathetic nerve biopsies.

POSTURAL ORTHOSTATIC TACHYCARDIA SYNDROME (POTS)

This syndrome is characterized by symptomatic orthostatic intolerance without OH, accompanied by either an increase in heart rate to >120 beats/min or an increase of 30 beats/min with standing that subsides on sitting or lying down. Women are affected approximately five times more often than men, and most develop the syndrome between the ages of 15 and 50. Presyncopal symptoms (lightheadedness, weakness, blurred vision) combined with symptoms of autonomic overactivity (palpitations, tremulousness, nausea) are common. Recurrent unexplained episodes of dysautonomia and fatigue also occur. The pathogenesis is unclear, but there is increasing evidence for sympathetic denervation distally in the legs with preserved cardiovascular function. Hypovolemia, venous pooling, impaired brainstem regulation, or increased sympathetic activity may play a role. Optimal treatment is uncertain, but expansion of fluid volume with water, salt, and fludrocortisone can be helpful as initial interventions. If this approach is inadequate, then midodrine, pyridostigmine, phenobarbital, beta blockers, or clonidine can be tried. Reconditioning and a sustained exercise program are important adjuncts to treatment.

INHERITED DISORDERS

There are five known hereditary sensory and autonomic neuropathies (HSAN I–V). The most important autonomic variants are HSAN I and HSAN III. HSAN I is dominantly inherited and often presents as a distal small-fiber neuropathy (burning feet syndrome) associated with sensory loss and foot ulcers. The most common responsible gene, on chromosome 9q, is *SPTLC1*. SPTLC is an important enzyme in the regulation of ceramide. Cells from HSAN I patients with the mutation produce higher-than-normal levels of glucosyl ceramide, perhaps triggering apoptosis. HSAN III (Riley-Day syndrome; familial dysautonomia) is an autosomal recessive disorder of Ashkenazi Jewish children and adults and is much less prevalent than HSAN I. Decreased tearing, hyperhidrosis, reduced sensitivity to pain, areflexia, absent fungiform papillae on the tongue, and labile BP may be present. Episodic abdominal crises and fever are common. Pathologic examination of nerves reveals a loss of sympathetic, parasympathetic, and sensory neurons. The defective gene, *IKBKAP*, may prevent normal transcription of important molecules in neural development.

PRIMARY HYPERHIDROSIS

This syndrome presents with excess sweating of the palms of the hands and soles of the feet beginning in childhood or early adulthood. The condition tends to improve with age. The disorder affects 0.6–1.0% of the population. The etiology is unclear, but there may be a genetic component because 25% of patients have a positive family history. The condition can be socially embarrassing (e.g., shaking hands) or even disabling (e.g., inability to write without soiling the paper). Topical antiperspirants are occasionally helpful. More useful are potent anticholinergic drugs such as glycopyrrolate (1–2 mg PO tid). T2 ganglionectomy or sympathectomy is successful in >90% of patients with palmar hyperhidrosis. The advent of endoscopic transaxillary T2 sympathectomy has lowered the complication rate of the procedure. The most common postoperative complication is compensatory hyperhidrosis, which improves spontaneously over months. Other potential complications include recurrent hyperhidrosis (16%), Horner's syndrome (<2%), gustatory sweating, wound infection, hemothorax, and intercostal neuralgia. Local injection of botulinum toxin has also been used to block cholinergic, postganglionic sympathetic fibers to sweat glands in patients with palmar hyperhidrosis. This approach is limited by the need for repetitive injections (the effect usually lasts 4 months before waning).

ACUTE SYMPATHETIC OVERACTIVITY SYNDROMES

The physician may be confronted occasionally with an acute state of sympathetic overactivity.

An *autonomic storm* is an acute state of sustained sympathetic surge that results in variable combinations of alterations in BP and heart rate, body temperature, respiration, and sweating. Causes of autonomic storm include brain and spinal cord injury, toxins and drugs, autonomic neuropathy, and chemodectomas (e.g., pheochromocytoma). Brain injury is the most common cause of autonomic storm and typically follows severe head trauma and postresuscitation encephalopathy anoxic-ischemic brain injury. Autonomic storm can also occur with other acute intracranial lesions such as hemorrhage, cerebral infarction, rapidly expanding tumors, subarachnoid hemorrhage, hydrocephalus, or (less commonly) an acute spinal cord lesion. The most consistent setting is that of an acute intracranial catastrophe of sufficient size and rapidity to produce a massive catecholaminergic surge. The surge can cause seizures, neurogenic pulmonary edema, and myocardial injury. Manifestations include fever, tachycardia, hypertension, tachypnea, hyperhidrosis, pupillary dilatation, and flushing. Lesions of the afferent limb of the baroreflex can result in milder recurrent autonomic storms; many of these follow neck irradiation.

Drugs and toxins may also be responsible, including sympathomimetics such as phenylpropanolamine, cocaine, amphetamines, and tricyclic antidepressants; tetanus; and, less often, botulinum toxin. Cocaine, including "crack," can cause a hypertensive state with CNS hyperstimulation. Tricyclic overdose, such as from amitriptyline, can cause flushing, hypertension, tachycardia, fever, mydriasis, anhidrosis, and a toxic psychosis. The hyperadrenergic state associated with Guillain-Barré syndrome can produce a moderate autonomic storm. Pheochromocytoma presents with a paroxysmal or sustained hyperadrenergic state, headache, hyperhidrosis, palpitations, anxiety, tremulousness, and hypertension. *Neuroleptic malignant syndrome* refers to a syndrome of muscle rigidity, hyperthermia, and hypertension in psychotic patients treated with phenothiazines (Chap. 449). Management of autonomic storm includes ruling out other causes of autonomic instability, including malignant hyperthermia, porphyria, and seizures. Sepsis and encephalitis need to be excluded with appropriate studies. An electroencephalogram (EEG) should be done to search for seizure activity; MRI of the brain and spine is often necessary. The patient should be managed in an intensive care unit. Management with morphine sulphate (10 mg every 4 h) and labetalol (100–200 mg twice daily) may be helpful. Supportive treatment may need to be maintained for several weeks. For chronic and milder autonomic storm, propranolol and/or clonidine can be effective.

MISCELLANEOUS

Other conditions associated with autonomic failure include infections, malignancy, poisoning (organophosphates), and aging. Disorders of the hypothalamus can affect autonomic function and produce abnormalities in temperature control, satiety, sexual function, and circadian rhythms (Chap. 403).

REFLEX SYMPATHETIC DYSTROPHY AND CAUSALGIA

The failure to identify a primary role of the ANS in the pathogenesis of these disorders has resulted in a change of nomenclature. The terms complex regional pain syndrome (CRPS) types I and II are now used in place of reflex sympathetic dystrophy (RSD) and causalgia.

CRPS type I is a regional pain syndrome that often develops after tissue injury and most commonly affects one limb. Examples of associated injury include minor shoulder or limb trauma, fractures, myocardial infarction, or stroke. *Allodynia* (the perception of a nonpainful stimulus as painful), *hyperpathia* (an exaggerated pain response to a painful stimulus), and spontaneous pain occur. The symptoms are unrelated to the severity of the initial trauma and are not confined to the distribution of a single peripheral nerve. CRPS type II is a regional pain syndrome that develops after injury to a specific peripheral nerve, often a major nerve trunk. Spontaneous pain initially develops within the territory of the affected nerve but eventually may spread outside the nerve distribution.

Pain (usually burning or electrical in quality) is the primary clinical feature of CRPS. Vasomotor dysfunction, sudomotor abnormalities, or focal edema may occur alone or in combination but must be present for diagnosis. Limb pain syndromes that do not meet these criteria are best classified as "limb pain—not otherwise specified." In CRPS, localized sweating (increased resting sweat output) and changes in blood flow may produce temperature differences between affected and unaffected limbs.

CRPS type I (RSD) has been classically divided into three clinical phases. Phase I consists of pain and swelling in the distal extremity occurring within weeks to 3 months after the precipitating event. The pain is diffuse, spontaneous, and either burning, throbbing, or aching in quality. The involved extremity is warm and edematous, and the joints are tender. Increased sweating and hair growth develop. In phase II (3–6 months after onset), thin, shiny, cool skin appears. After an additional 3–6 months (phase III), atrophy of the skin and subcutaneous tissue plus flexion contractures complete the clinical picture. Autonomic testing or bone scans are occasionally useful when the diagnosis is in doubt.

The natural history of typical CRPS may be more benign and more variable than previously recognized. A variety of surgical and medical treatments have been developed, with conflicting reports of efficacy. Clinical trials suggest that early mobilization with physical therapy or a brief course of glucocorticoids may be helpful for CRPS type I or II. Other medical treatments include the use of adrenergic blockers, nonsteroidal anti-inflammatory drugs, calcium channel blockers, phenytoin, opioids, and calcitonin. Stellate ganglion blockade is a commonly used invasive technique that often provides temporary pain relief, but the efficacy of repetitive blocks is uncertain.

TREATMENT AUTONOMIC FAILURE

Management of autonomic failure is aimed at specific treatment of the cause and alleviation of symptoms. Of particular importance is the removal of drugs or amelioration of underlying conditions that cause or aggravate the autonomic symptoms, especially in the elderly. For example, OH can be caused or aggravated by angiotensin-converting enzyme inhibitors, calcium channel-blocking agents, tricyclic antidepressants, levodopa, alcohol, or insulin. A summary of drugs that can cause OH by class, putative mechanism, and magnitude of the BP drop is shown in Table 454-6.

PATIENT EDUCATION

Only a minority of patients with OH require drug treatment. All patients should be taught the mechanisms of postural normotension (volume status, resistance and capacitance bed, autoregulation) and the nature of orthostatic stressors (time of day and the influence of meals, heat, standing, and exercise). Patients should learn to recognize orthostatic symptoms early (especially subtle cognitive symptoms, weakness, and fatigue) and to modify or avoid activities that provoke episodes. Other helpful measures may include keeping a BP log and dietary education (salt/fluids). Learning physical counter-maneuvers that reduce standing OH and practicing postural and resistance training are helpful measures.

SYMPTOMATIC TREATMENT

Nonpharmacologic approaches are summarized in Table 454-9. Adequate intake of salt and fluids to produce a voiding volume between 1.5 and 2.5 L of urine (containing >170 meq/L of Na^+) each 24 h is essential. Sleeping with the head of the bed elevated will minimize the effects of supine nocturnal hypertension. Prolonged recumbency should be avoided when possible. Patients are advised to sit with legs dangling over the edge of the bed for several minutes before attempting to stand in the morning; other postural stresses should be similarly approached in a gradual manner. One maneuver that can reduce OH is leg-crossing with maintained contraction of leg muscles for 30 s; this compresses leg veins and increases systemic resistance. Compressive garments, such as compression stockings or abdominal binders, are helpful on occasion but uncomfortable for many patients. For transient worsening of OH, drinking two 250-mL (8-oz) glasses of water can raise standing BP 20–30 mmHg for about 2 h, beginning ~20 min after the fluid load. The patient can increase intake of salt and fluids (bouillon treatment), increase use of physical counter-maneuvers (elevate the legs when supine), or temporarily resort to a full-body stocking (compression pressure 30–40 mmHg).

TABLE 454-9 INITIAL TREATMENT OF ORTHOSTATIC HYPOTENSION (OH)

Patient education: mechanisms and stressors of OH
High-salt diet (10–20 g/d)
High-fluid intake (2 L/d)
Elevate head of bed 10 cm (4 in.) to minimize supine hypertension
Maintain postural stimuli
Learn physical counter-maneuvers
Compression garments
Correct anemia

Anemia should be corrected with erythropoietin, administered subcutaneously at doses of 25–75 U/kg three times per week. The hematocrit increases after 2–6 weeks. A weekly maintenance dose is usually necessary. However, the increased intravascular volume that accompanies the rise in hematocrit can exacerbate supine hypertension.

If these measures are not sufficient, pharmacologic treatment may be necessary. Midodrine, a directly acting α_1-agonist that does not cross the blood-brain barrier, is effective. It has a duration of action of 2–4 h. The usual dose is 5–10 mg orally tid, but some patients respond best to a decremental dose (e.g., 15 mg on awakening, 10 mg at noon, and 5 mg in the afternoon). Midodrine should not be taken after 6:00 P.M. Side effects include pruritus, uncomfortable piloerection, and supine hypertension especially at higher doses. Droxidopa (Northera) was recently approved by the FDA for treatment of neurogenic OH associated with PAF, PD, or MSA; oral droxidopa is converted to NE and in short-term clinical trails was effective in decreasing symptoms of OH. Pyridostigmine (Mestinon) appears to improve OH without aggravating supine hypertension by enhancing ganglionic transmission (maximal when orthostatic, minimal when supine). Fludrocortisone will reduce OH but aggravates supine hypertension. At doses between 0.1 mg/d and 0.3 mg bid orally, it enhances renal sodium conservation and increases the sensitivity of arterioles to NE. Susceptible patients may develop fluid overload, congestive heart failure, supine hypertension, or hypokalemia. Potassium supplements are often necessary with chronic administration of fludrocortisone. Sustained elevations of supine BP >180/110 mmHg should be avoided. Supine hypertension (>180/110 mmHg) can be self-treated by avoiding the supine position (e.g., sleeping in a recumbent chair) and reducing fludrocortisone. A daily glass of wine, if requested by the patient, can be taken shortly before bedtime. If these simple measures are not adequate, drugs to be considered include oral hydralazine (25 mg qhs), oral nifedipine (Procardia; 10 mg qhs), or a nitroglycerin patch.

A promising drug combination (atomoxetine and yohimbine) has been studied for use in human subjects with severe OH not responsive to other agents, as can occur is some patients with diabetes and severe autonomic neuropathy not responsive to other medications. The atomoxetine blocks the NE reuptake transporter, and yohimbine blocks α_2 receptors that mediate the sympathetic feedback loop for downregulation of BP in response to atomoxetine. The result is a dramatic increase in BP and standing tolerance. This combination is not FDA approved for this purpose. It is possible that the limited drug duration of action can be used to withdraw drug treatment when the patient anticipates becoming supine (e.g., before sleep).

Postprandial OH may respond to several measures. Frequent, small, low-carbohydrate meals may diminish splanchnic shunting of blood after meals and reduce postprandial OH. Prostaglandin inhibitors (ibuprofen or indomethacin) taken with meals or midodrine (10 mg with the meal) can be helpful. The somatostatin analogue octreotide can be useful in the treatment of postprandial syncope by inhibiting the release of GI peptides that have vasodilator and hypotensive effects. The subcutaneous dose ranges from 25 μg bid to 200 μg tid.

455 Trigeminal Neuralgia, Bell's Palsy, and Other Cranial Nerve Disorders

M. Flint Beal, Stephen L. Hauser

Symptoms and signs of cranial nerve pathology are common in internal medicine. They often develop in the context of a widespread neurologic disturbance, and in such situations, cranial nerve involvement may represent the initial manifestation of the illness. In other disorders, involvement is largely restricted to one or several cranial nerves; these distinctive disorders are reviewed in this chapter. Disorders of ocular movement are discussed in Chap. 39, disorders of hearing in Chap. 43, and vertigo and disorders of vestibular function in Chap. 28.

FACIAL PAIN OR NUMBNESS

ANATOMIC CONSIDERATIONS

The trigeminal (fifth cranial) nerve supplies sensation to the skin of the face and anterior half of the head (Fig. 455-1). The motor part innervates the muscles involved in chewing (including masseters and pterygoids) as well as the tensor tympani of the middle ear (hearing especially for high-pitched tones). It is the largest of the cranial nerves. It exits in the lateral midpons and traverses the middle cranial fossa to the semilunar (gasserian, trigeminal) ganglion in Meckel's cave, where the nerve divides into three divisions (ophthalmic [V1], maxillary [V2], and mandibular [V3]). V1 and V2 traverse the cavernous sinus to exit in the superior orbital fissure and foramen rotundum, located above and below the eye socket respectively; V3 exits through the foramen ovale. The trigeminal nerve is predominantly sensory, and motor innervation is exclusively carried in V3. The cornea is primarily innervated by V1, although an inferior crescent may be V2. Upon

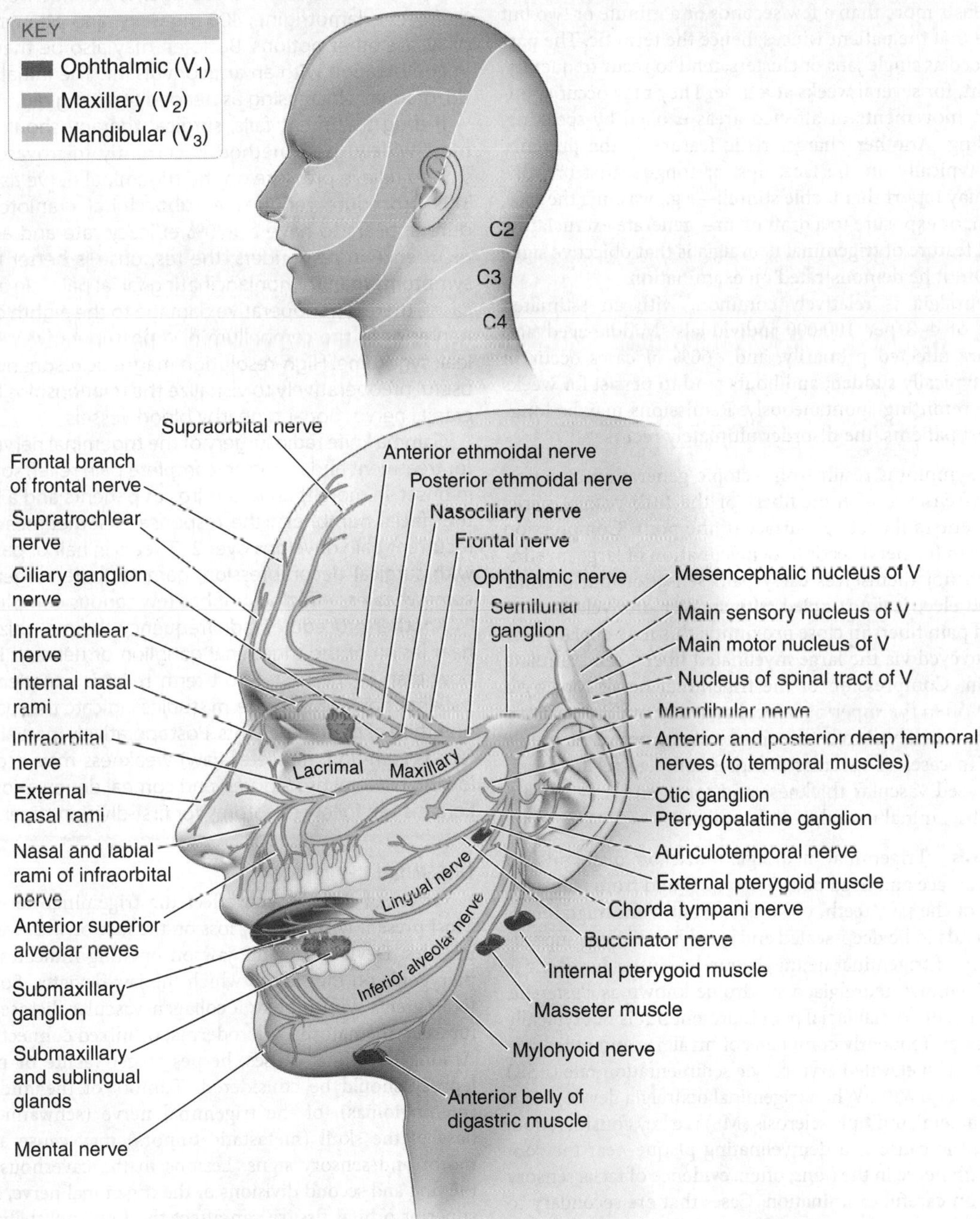

FIGURE 455-1 The trigeminal nerve and its branches and sensory distribution on the face. The three major sensory divisions of the trigeminal nerve consist of the ophthalmic, maxillary, and mandibular nerves. *(Adapted from Waxman SG: Clinical Neuroanatomy, 26th ed. http://www.accessmedicine.com. Copyright © The McGraw-Hill Companies, Inc. All rights reserved.)*

entering the pons, pain and temperature fibers descend ipsilaterally to the upper cervical spinal cord as the spinal tract of V, before synapsing with the spinal nucleus of V; this accounts for the facial numbness that can occur with spinal cord lesions above C2. In the brainstem, the spinal tract of V is also located adjacent to crossed ascending fibers of the spinothalamic tract, producing a "crossed" sensory loss for pain and temperature (ipsilateral face, contralateral arm/trunk/leg) with lesions of the lateral lower brainstem. CN V is also ensheathed by oligodendrocyte-derived, rather than Schwann cell–derived, myelin for up to 7 mm after it leaves the brainstem, unlike just a few millimeters for other cranial and spinal nerves; this may explain the high frequency of trigeminal neuralgia in multiple sclerosis (Chap. 458), a disorder of oligodendrocyte myelin.

TRIGEMINAL NEURALGIA (TIC DOULOUREUX)

Clinical Manifestations Trigeminal neuralgia is characterized by excruciating paroxysms of pain in the lips, gums, cheek, or chin and, very rarely, in the distribution of the ophthalmic division of the fifth nerve. The pain seldom lasts more than a few seconds or a minute or two but may be so intense that the patient winces, hence the term tic. The paroxysms, experienced as single jabs or clusters, tend to recur frequently, both day and night, for several weeks at a time. They may occur spontaneously or with movements of affected areas evoked by speaking, chewing, or smiling. Another characteristic feature is the presence of trigger zones, typically on the face, lips, or tongue, that provoke attacks; patients may report that tactile stimuli—e.g., washing the face, brushing the teeth, or exposure to a draft of air—generate excruciating pain. An essential feature of trigeminal neuralgia is that objective signs of sensory loss cannot be demonstrated on examination.

Trigeminal neuralgia is relatively common, with an estimated annual incidence of 4–8 per 100,000 individuals. Middle-aged and elderly persons are affected primarily, and ~60% of cases occur in women. Onset is typically sudden, and bouts tend to persist for weeks or months before remitting spontaneously. Remissions may be long-lasting, but in most patients, the disorder ultimately recurs.

Pathophysiology Symptoms result from ectopic generation of action potentials in pain-sensitive afferent fibers of the fifth cranial nerve root just before it enters the lateral surface of the pons. Compression or other pathology in the nerve leads to demyelination of large myelinated fibers that do not themselves carry pain sensation but become hyperexcitable and electrically coupled with smaller unmyelinated or poorly myelinated pain fibers in close proximity; this may explain why tactile stimuli, conveyed via the large myelinated fibers, can stimulate paroxysms of pain. Compression of the trigeminal nerve root by a blood vessel, most often the superior cerebellar artery or on occasion a tortuous vein, is now believed to be the source of trigeminal neuralgia in most patients. In cases of vascular compression, age-related brain sagging and increased vascular thickness and tortuosity may explain the prevalence of trigeminal neuralgia in later life.

Differential Diagnosis Trigeminal neuralgia must be distinguished from other causes of face and head pain (Chap. 21) and from pain arising from diseases of the jaw, teeth, or sinuses. Pain from migraine or cluster headache tends to be deep-seated and steady, unlike the superficial stabbing quality of trigeminal neuralgia; rarely, cluster headache is associated with trigeminal neuralgia, a syndrome known as *cluster-tic*. In temporal arteritis, superficial facial pain is present but is not typically shock-like, the patient frequently complains of myalgias and other systemic symptoms, and an elevated erythrocyte sedimentation rate (ESR) is usually present (Chap. 385). When trigeminal neuralgia develops in a young adult or is bilateral, multiple sclerosis (MS) is a key consideration, and in such cases, the cause is a demyelinating plaque near the root entry zone of the fifth nerve in the pons; often, evidence of facial sensory loss can be found on careful examination. Cases that are secondary to mass lesions—such as aneurysms, neurofibromas, acoustic schwannomas, or meningiomas—usually produce objective signs of sensory loss in the trigeminal nerve distribution (trigeminal neuropathy, see below).

Laboratory Evaluation An ESR is indicated if temporal arteritis is suspected. In typical cases of trigeminal neuralgia, neuroimaging studies are usually unnecessary but may be valuable if MS is a consideration or in assessing overlying vascular lesions in order to plan for decompression surgery.

TREATMENT TRIGEMINAL NEURALGIA

Drug therapy with carbamazepine is effective in ~50–75% of patients. Carbamazepine should be started as a single daily dose of 100 mg taken with food and increased gradually (by 100 mg daily in divided doses every 1–2 days) until substantial (>50%) pain relief is achieved. Most patients require a maintenance dose of 200 mg qid. Doses >1200 mg daily provide no additional benefit. Dizziness, imbalance, sedation, and rare cases of agranulocytosis are the most important side effects of carbamazepine. If treatment is effective, it is usually continued for 1 month and then tapered as tolerated. Oxcarbazepine (300–1200 mg bid) is an alternative to carbamazepine that has less bone marrow toxicity and probably is equally efficacious. If these agents are not well tolerated or are ineffective, lamotrigine, 400 mg daily, and phenytoin, 300–400 mg daily, are other options. Baclofen may also be tried, either alone or in combination with an anticonvulsant. The initial dose is 5–10 mg tid, gradually increasing as needed to 20 mg qid.

If drug treatment fails, surgical therapy should be offered. The most widely used method is currently microvascular decompression to relieve pressure on the trigeminal nerve as it exits the pons. This procedure requires a suboccipital craniotomy. This procedure appears to have a >70% efficacy rate and a low rate of pain recurrence in responders; the response is better for classic tic-like symptoms than for nonlancinating facial pains. In a small number of cases, there is perioperative damage to the eighth or seventh cranial nerves or to the cerebellum or a postoperative cerebrospinal fluid leak syndrome. High-resolution magnetic resonance angiography is useful preoperatively to visualize the relationships between the fifth cranial nerve root and nearby blood vessels.

Gamma knife radiosurgery of the trigeminal nerve root is also used for treatment and results in complete pain relief, sometimes delayed in onset, in more than two-thirds of patients and a low risk of persistent facial numbness; the response is sometimes long-lasting, but recurrent pain develops over 2–3 years in half of patients. Compared with surgical decompression, gamma knife surgery appears to be somewhat less effective but has few serious complications.

Another procedure, radiofrequency thermal rhizotomy, creates a heat lesion of the trigeminal ganglion or nerve. It is used less often now than in the past. Short-term relief is experienced by >95% of patients; however, long-term studies indicate that pain recurs in up to one-third of treated patients. Postoperatively, partial numbness of the face is common, masseter (jaw) weakness may occur especially following bilateral procedures, and corneal denervation with secondary keratitis can follow rhizotomy for first-division trigeminal neuralgia.

TRIGEMINAL NEUROPATHY

A variety of diseases can affect the trigeminal nerve (Table 455-1). Most present with sensory loss on the face or with weakness of the jaw muscles. Deviation of the jaw on opening indicates weakness of the pterygoids on the side to which the jaw deviates. Some cases are due to Sjögren's syndrome or a collagen-vascular disease such as systemic lupus erythematosus, scleroderma, or mixed connective tissue disease. Among infectious causes, herpes zoster (acute or postherpetic) and leprosy should be considered. Tumors of the middle cranial fossa (meningiomas), of the trigeminal nerve (schwannomas), or of the base of the skull (metastatic tumors) may cause a combination of motor and sensory signs. Lesions in the cavernous sinus can affect the first and second divisions of the trigeminal nerve, and lesions of the superior orbital fissure can affect the first (ophthalmic) division; the accompanying corneal anesthesia increases the risk of ulceration (neurokeratitis).

Isolated sensory loss over the chin (mental neuropathy) can be the only manifestation of systemic malignancy. Rarely, an idiopathic form of trigeminal neuropathy is observed. It is characterized by numbness

TABLE 455-1 TRIGEMINAL NERVE DISORDERS

Nuclear (brainstem) lesions	**Peripheral nerve lesions**
Multiple sclerosis	Nasopharyngeal carcinoma
Stroke	Trauma
Syringobulbia	Guillain-Barré syndrome
Glioma	Sjögren's syndrome
Lymphoma	Collagen-vascular diseases
Preganglionic lesions	Sarcoidosis
Acoustic neuroma	Leprosy
Meningioma	Drugs (stilbamidine, trichloroethylene)
Metastasis	Idiopathic trigeminal neuropathy
Chronic meningitis	
Cavernous carotid aneurysm	
Gasserian ganglion lesions	
Trigeminal neuroma	
Herpes zoster	
Infection (spread from otitis media or mastoiditis)	

and paresthesias, sometimes bilaterally, with loss of sensation in the territory of the trigeminal nerve but without weakness of the jaw. Gradual recovery is the rule. Tonic spasm of the masticatory muscles, known as trismus, is symptomatic of tetanus (Chap. 177) or may occur in patients treated with phenothiazines.

FACIAL WEAKNESS

ANATOMIC CONSIDERATIONS

(Fig. 455-2) The seventh cranial nerve supplies all the muscles concerned with facial expression. The sensory component is small (the nervus intermedius); it conveys taste sensation from the anterior two-thirds of the tongue and probably cutaneous impulses from the anterior wall of the external auditory canal. The motor nucleus of the seventh nerve lies anterior and lateral to the abducens nucleus. After leaving the pons, the seventh nerve enters the internal auditory meatus with the acoustic nerve. The nerve continues its course in its own bony channel, the facial canal, and exits from the skull via the stylomastoid foramen. It then passes through the parotid gland and subdivides to supply the facial muscles.

A complete interruption of the facial nerve at the stylomastoid foramen paralyzes all muscles of facial expression. The corner of the mouth droops, the creases and skinfolds are effaced, the forehead is unfurrowed, and the eyelids will not close. Upon attempted closure of the lids, the eye on the paralyzed side rolls upward (Bell's phenomenon). The lower lid sags and falls away from the conjunctiva, permitting tears to spill over the cheek. Food collects between the teeth and lips, and saliva may dribble from the corner of the mouth. The patient complains of a heaviness or numbness in the face, but sensory loss is rarely demonstrable and taste is intact.

If the lesion is in the middle-ear portion, taste is lost over the anterior two-thirds of the tongue on the same side. If the nerve to the stapedius is interrupted, there is hyperacusis (sensitivity to loud sounds). Lesions in the internal auditory meatus may affect the adjacent auditory and vestibular nerves, causing deafness, tinnitus, or dizziness. Intrapontine lesions that paralyze the face usually affect the abducens nucleus as well, and often the corticospinal and sensory tracts.

If the peripheral facial paralysis has existed for some time and recovery of motor function is incomplete, a continuous diffuse contraction of facial muscles may appear. The palpebral fissure becomes narrowed, and the nasolabial fold deepens. Attempts to move one group of facial muscles may result in contraction of all (associated movements, or synkinesis). Facial spasms, initiated by movements of the face, may develop (hemifacial spasm). Anomalous regeneration of seventh nerve fibers may result in other troublesome phenomena. If fibers originally connected with the orbicularis oculi come to innervate the orbicularis oris, closure of the lids may cause a retraction of the mouth, or if fibers originally connected with muscles of the face later innervate the lacrimal gland, anomalous tearing ("crocodile tears") may occur with any activity of the facial muscles, such as eating. Another facial synkinesia is triggered by jaw opening, causing closure of the eyelids on the side of the facial palsy (jaw-winking).

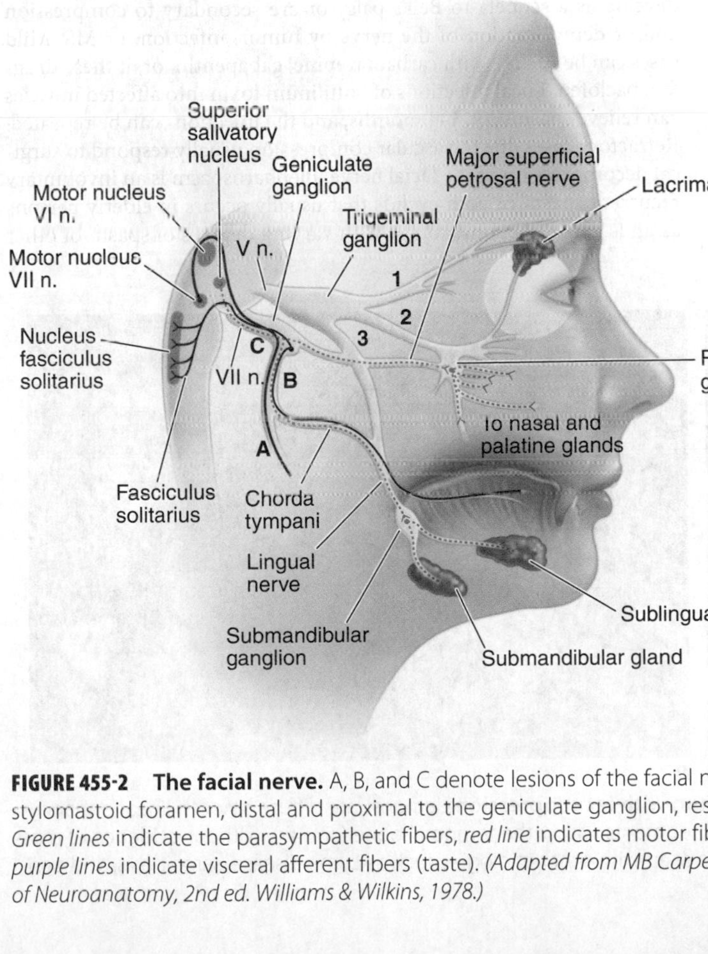

FIGURE 455-2 The facial nerve. A, B, and C denote lesions of the facial nerve at the stylomastoid foramen, distal and proximal to the geniculate ganglion, respectively. *Green lines* indicate the parasympathetic fibers, *red line* indicates motor fibers, and *purple lines* indicate visceral afferent fibers (taste). *(Adapted from MB Carpenter: Core Text of Neuroanatomy, 2nd ed. Williams & Wilkins, 1978.)*

BELL'S PALSY

The most common form of facial paralysis is Bell's palsy. The annual incidence of this idiopathic disorder is ~25 per 100,000 annually, or about 1 in 60 persons in a lifetime. Risk factors include pregnancy and diabetes mellitus.

Clinical Manifestations The onset of Bell's palsy is fairly abrupt, with maximal weakness being attained by 48 h as a general rule. Pain behind the ear may precede the paralysis for a day or two. Taste sensation may be lost unilaterally, and hyperacusis may be present. In some cases, there is mild cerebrospinal fluid lymphocytosis. Magnetic resonance imaging (MRI) may reveal swelling and uniform enhancement of the geniculate ganglion and facial nerve and, in some cases, entrapment of the swollen nerve in the temporal bone. Approximately 80% of patients recover within a few weeks or months. Electromyography may be of some prognostic value; evidence of denervation after 10 days indicates there has been axonal degeneration, that there will be a long delay (3 months as a rule) before regeneration occurs, and that it may be incomplete. The presence of incomplete paralysis in the first week is the most favorable prognostic sign. Recurrences are reported in approximately 7% of cases.

Pathophysiology In acute Bell's palsy, there is inflammation of the facial nerve with mononuclear cells, consistent with an infectious or immune cause. Herpes simplex virus (HSV) type 1 DNA was frequently detected in endoneurial fluid and posterior auricular muscle, suggesting that a reactivation of this virus in the geniculate ganglion may be responsible for most cases. Reactivation of varicella-zoster virus is associated with Bell's palsy in up to one-third of cases and may represent the second most frequent cause. A variety of other viruses have also been implicated less commonly. An increased incidence of Bell's palsy was also reported among recipients of inactivated intranasal influenza vaccine, and it was hypothesized that this could have resulted from the *Escherichia coli* enterotoxin used as adjuvant or reactivation of latent virus.

Differential Diagnosis There are many other causes of acute facial palsy that must be considered in the differential diagnosis of Bell's palsy. Lyme disease can cause unilateral or bilateral facial palsies; in endemic areas, 10% or more of cases of facial palsy are likely due to infection with *Borrelia burgdorferi* (Chap. 210). The Ramsay Hunt syndrome, caused by reactivation of herpes zoster in the geniculate ganglion, consists of a severe facial palsy associated with a vesicular eruption in the external auditory canal and sometimes in the pharynx and other parts of the cranial integument; often the eighth cranial nerve is affected as well. Facial palsy that is often bilateral occurs in sarcoidosis (Chap. 390) and in Guillain-Barré syndrome (Chap. 460). Leprosy frequently involves the facial nerve, and facial neuropathy may also occur in diabetes mellitus, connective tissue diseases including Sjögren's syndrome, and amyloidosis. The rare Melkersson-Rosenthal syndrome consists of recurrent facial paralysis; recurrent—and eventually permanent—facial (particularly labial) edema; and, less constantly, plication of the tongue. Its cause is unknown. Acoustic neuromas frequently involve the facial nerve by local compression. Infarcts, demyelinating lesions of MS, and tumors are the common pontine lesions that interrupt the facial nerve fibers; other signs of brainstem involvement are usually present. Tumors that invade the temporal bone (carotid body, cholesteatoma, dermoid) may produce a facial palsy, but the onset is insidious and the course progressive.

All these forms of nuclear or peripheral facial palsy must be distinguished from the supranuclear type. In the latter, the frontalis and orbicularis oculi muscles of the forehead are involved less than those of the lower part of the face, since the upper facial muscles are innervated by corticobulbar pathways from both motor cortices, whereas the lower facial muscles are innervated only by the opposite hemisphere. In supranuclear lesions, there may be a dissociation of emotional and voluntary facial movements, and often some degree of paralysis of the arm and leg or an aphasia (in dominant hemisphere lesions) is present.

Laboratory Evaluation The diagnosis of Bell's palsy can usually be made clinically in patients with (1) a typical presentation, (2) no risk factors or preexisting symptoms for other causes of facial paralysis, (3) absence of cutaneous lesions of herpes zoster in the external ear canal, and (4) a normal neurologic examination with the exception of the facial nerve. Particular attention to the eighth cranial nerve, which courses near to the facial nerve in the pontomedullary junction and in the temporal bone, and to other cranial nerves is essential. In atypical or uncertain cases, an ESR, testing for diabetes mellitus, a Lyme titer, angiotensin-converting enzyme and chest imaging studies for possible sarcoidosis, a lumbar puncture for possible Guillain-Barré syndrome, or MRI scanning may be indicated. MRI often shows swelling and enhancement of the facial nerve in idiopathic Bell's palsy (Fig. 455-3).

TREATMENT BELL'S PALSY

Symptomatic measures include (1) the use of paper tape to depress the upper eyelid during sleep and prevent corneal drying, and (2) massage of the weakened muscles. A course of glucocorticoids, given as prednisone 60–80 mg daily during the first 5 days and then tapered over the next 5 days, modestly shortens the recovery period and improves the functional outcome. Although large and well-controlled randomized trials found no added benefit of the antiviral agents valacyclovir (1000 mg daily for 5–7 days) or acyclovir (400 mg five times daily for 10 days) compared to glucocorticoids alone, some earlier data suggested that combination therapy with prednisone plus valacyclovir might be marginally better than prednisolone alone, especially in patients with severe clinical presentations. For patients with permanent paralysis from Bell's palsy, a number of cosmetic surgical procedures have been used to restore a relatively symmetric appearance to the face.

OTHER MOTOR DISORDERS OF THE FACE

Hemifacial spasm consists of painless irregular involuntary contractions on one side of the face. Most cases appear related to vascular compression of the exiting facial nerve in the pons. Other cases develop as a sequela to Bell's palsy or are secondary to compression and/or demyelination of the nerve by tumor, infection, or MS. Mild cases can be treated with carbamazepine, gabapentin, or, if these drugs fail, baclofen. Local injections of botulinum toxin into affected muscles can relieve spasms for 3–4 months, and the injections can be repeated. Refractory cases due to vascular compression usually respond to surgical decompression of the facial nerve. Blepharospasm is an involuntary recurrent spasm of both eyelids that usually occurs in elderly persons as an isolated phenomenon or with varying degrees of spasm of other

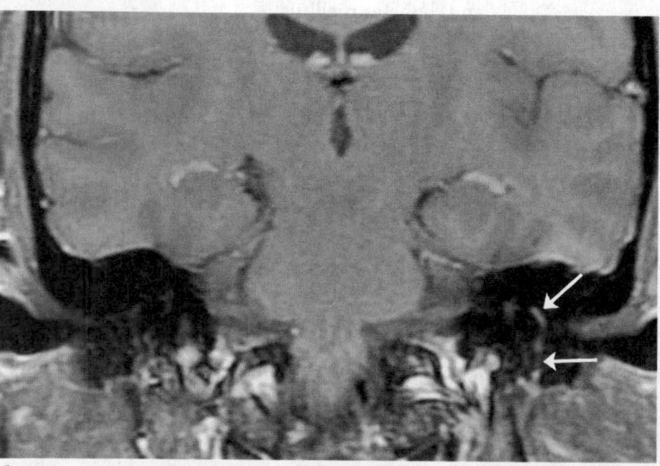

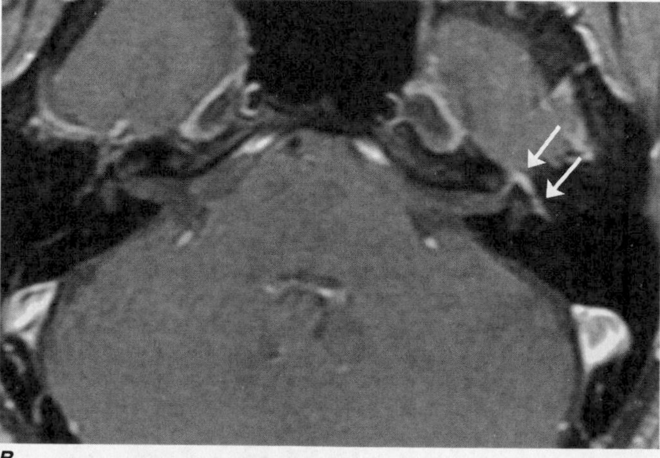

FIGURE 455-3 Axial and coronal T1-weighted images after gadolinium with fat suppression demonstrate diffuse smooth linear enhancement of the left facial nerve, involving the genu, tympanic, and mastoid segments within the temporal bone (*arrows*), without evidence of mass lesion. Although highly suggestive of Bell's palsy, similar findings may be seen with other etiologies such as Lyme disease, sarcoidosis, and perineural malignant spread.

facial muscles. Severe, persistent cases of blepharospasm can be treated by local injection of botulinum toxin into the orbicularis oculi. Facial myokymia refers to a fine rippling activity of the facial muscles; it may be caused by MS or follow Guillain-Barré syndrome (Chap. 460).

Facial hemiatrophy occurs mainly in women and is characterized by a disappearance of fat in the dermal and subcutaneous tissues on one side of the face. It usually begins in adolescence or the early adult years and is slowly progressive. In its advanced form, the affected side of the face is gaunt, and the skin is thin, wrinkled, and brown. The facial hair may turn white and fall out, and the sebaceous glands become atrophic. Bilateral involvement may occur. A limited form of systemic sclerosis (scleroderma) may be the cause of some cases. Treatment is cosmetic, consisting of transplantation of skin and subcutaneous fat.

OTHER CRANIAL NERVE DISORDERS

GLOSSOPHARYNGEAL NEURALGIA

This form of neuralgia involves the ninth (glossopharyngeal) and sometimes portions of the tenth (vagus) cranial nerves. It resembles trigeminal neuralgia in many respects but is much less common. The pain is intense and paroxysmal; it originates on one side of the throat, approximately in the tonsillar fossa. In some cases, the pain is localized in the ear or may radiate from the throat to the ear because of involvement of the tympanic branch of the glossopharyngeal nerve. Spasms of pain may be initiated by swallowing or coughing. There is no demonstrable motor or sensory deficit; the glossopharyngeal nerve supplies taste sensation to the posterior third of the tongue and, together with the vagus nerve, sensation to the posterior pharynx. Cardiac symptoms—bradycardia or asystole, hypotension, and fainting—have been reported. Glossopharyngeal neuralgia can result from vascular compression, MS, or tumors, but many cases are idiopathic. Medical therapy is similar to that for trigeminal neuralgia, and carbamazepine is generally the first choice. If drug therapy is unsuccessful, surgical procedures—including microvascular decompression if vascular compression is evident—or rhizotomy of glossopharyngeal and vagal fibers in the jugular bulb is frequently successful.

Glossopharyngeal neuropathy in conjunction with vagus and accessory nerve palsies may occur with herpes zoster infection or with a tumor or aneurysm in the posterior fossa or in the jugular foramen. Hoarseness due to vocal cord paralysis, some difficulty in swallowing, deviation of the soft palate to the intact side, anesthesia of the posterior wall of the pharynx, and weakness of the upper part of the trapezius and sternocleidomastoid muscles make up the jugular foramen syndrome (Table 455-2).

DYSPHAGIA AND DYSPHONIA

When the intracranial portion of one vagus (tenth cranial) nerve is interrupted, the soft palate droops ipsilaterally and does not rise in phonation. There is loss of the gag reflex on the affected side, as well as of the "curtain movement" of the lateral wall of the pharynx, whereby the faucial pillars move medially as the palate rises in saying "ah." The voice is hoarse and slightly nasal, and the vocal cord lies immobile midway between abduction and adduction. Loss of sensation at the external auditory meatus and the posterior pinna may also be present.

The pharyngeal branches of both vagal nerves may be affected in diphtheria; the voice has a nasal quality, and regurgitation of liquids through the nose occurs during swallowing.

Injury to the vagus nerve in the carotid sheath can also occur with carotid dissection or following endarterectomy. The vagus nerve may be involved at the meningeal level by neoplastic and infectious processes and within the medulla by tumors, vascular lesions (e.g., the lateral medullary syndrome), and motor neuron disease. This nerve may be involved by infection with varicella zoster virus. Polymyositis and dermatomyositis, which cause hoarseness and dysphagia by direct involvement of laryngeal and pharyngeal muscles, may be confused with diseases of the vagus nerves. Dysphagia is also a symptom in some patients with myotonic dystrophy. Nonneurologic causes of dysphagia are discussed in Chap. 53.

The recurrent laryngeal nerves, especially the left, are most often damaged as a result of intrathoracic disease. Aneurysm of the aortic arch, an enlarged left atrium, and tumors of the mediastinum and bronchi are much more frequent causes of an isolated vocal cord palsy than are intracranial disorders. However, a substantial number of cases of recurrent laryngeal palsy remain idiopathic.

TABLE 455-2 CRANIAL NERVE SYNDROMES

Site	Cranial Nerves	Usual Cause
Sphenoid fissure (superior orbital)	III, IV, first division V, VI	Invasive tumors of sphenoid bone; aneurysms
Lateral wall of cavernous sinus	III, IV, first division V, VI, often with proptosis	Infection, thrombosis, aneurysm, or fistula of cavernous sinus; invasive tumors from sinuses and sella turcica; benign granuloma responsive to glucocorticoids
Retrosphenoid space	II, III, IV, V, VI	Large tumors of middle cranial fossa
Apex of petrous bone	V, VI	Petrositis; tumors of petrous bone
Internal auditory meatus	VII, VIII	Tumors of petrous bone (dermoids, etc.); infectious processes; acoustic neuroma
Pontocerebellar angle	V, VII, VIII, and sometimes IX	Acoustic neuroma; meningioma
Jugular foramen	IX, X, XI	Tumors and aneurysms
Posterior laterocondylar space	IX, X, XI, XII	Tumors of parotid gland and carotid body and metastatic tumors
Posterior retroparotid space	IX, X, XI, XII, and Horner's syndrome	Tumors of parotid gland, carotid body, lymph nodes; metastatic tumor; tuberculous adenitis

When confronted with a case of laryngeal palsy, the physician must attempt to determine the site of the lesion. If it is intramedullary, there are usually other signs, such as ipsilateral cerebellar dysfunction, loss of pain and temperature sensation over the ipsilateral face and contralateral arm and leg, and an ipsilateral Horner's syndrome. If the lesion is extramedullary, the glossopharyngeal and spinal accessory nerves are frequently involved (jugular foramen syndrome). If it is extracranial in the posterior laterocondylar or retroparotid space, there may be a combination of ninth, tenth, eleventh, and twelfth cranial nerve palsies and a Horner's syndrome (Table 455-2). If there is no sensory loss over the palate and pharynx and no palatal weakness or dysphagia, the lesion is below the origin of the pharyngeal branches, which leave the vagus nerve high in the cervical region; the usual site of disease is then the mediastinum.

NECK WEAKNESS

Isolated involvement of the accessory (eleventh cranial) nerve can occur anywhere along its route, resulting in partial or complete paralysis of the sternocleidomastoid and trapezius muscles. More commonly, involvement occurs in combination with deficits of the ninth and tenth cranial nerves in the jugular foramen or after exit from the skull (Table 455-2). An idiopathic form of accessory neuropathy, akin to Bell's palsy, has been described, and it may be recurrent in some cases. Most but not all patients recover.

TONGUE PARALYSIS

The hypoglossal (twelfth cranial) nerve supplies the ipsilateral muscles of the tongue. The nucleus of the nerve or its fibers of exit may be involved by intramedullary lesions such as tumor, poliomyelitis, or most often motor neuron disease. Lesions of the basal meninges and the occipital bones (platybasia, invagination of occipital condyles, Paget's disease) may compress the nerve in its extramedullary course or in the hypoglossal canal. Isolated lesions of unknown cause can occur. Atrophy and fasciculation of the tongue develop weeks to months after interruption of the nerve.

Several cranial nerves may be affected by the same disease process. In this situation, the main clinical problem is to determine whether the lesion lies within the brainstem or outside it. Lesions that lie on the surface of the brainstem are characterized by involvement of adjacent cranial nerves (often occurring in succession) and late and rather slight involvement of the long sensory and motor pathways and segmental structures lying within the brainstem. The opposite is true of primary lesions within the brainstem. The extramedullary lesion is more likely to cause bone erosion or enlargement of the foramens of exit of cranial nerves. The intramedullary lesion involving cranial nerves often produces a crossed sensory or motor paralysis (cranial nerve signs on one side of the body and tract signs on the opposite side).

Involvement of multiple cranial nerves outside the brainstem is frequently the result of trauma, localized infections including varicella-zoster virus, infectious and noninfectious (especially carcinomatous) causes of meningitis (Chaps. 164 and 165), granulomatous diseases such as Wegener's granulomatosis, Behçet's disease, vascular disorders including those associated with diabetes, enlarging aneurysms, or locally infiltrating tumors. Among the tumors, nasopharyngeal cancers, lymphomas, neurofibromas, meningiomas, chordomas, cholesteatomas, carcinomas, and sarcomas have all been observed to involve a succession of lower cranial nerves. Owing to their anatomic relationships, the multiple cranial nerve palsies form a number of distinctive syndromes, listed in Table 455-2. Sarcoidosis is the cause of some cases of multiple cranial neuropathy; tuberculosis, the Chiari malformation, platybasia, and basilar invagination of the skull are additional causes. A purely motor disorder without atrophy always raises the question of myasthenia gravis (Chap. 461). As noted above, Guillain-Barré syndrome commonly affects the facial nerves bilaterally. In the Fisher variant of the Guillain-Barré syndrome, oculomotor paresis occurs with ataxia and areflexia in the limbs (Chap. 460). Wernicke's encephalopathy can cause a severe ophthalmoplegia combined with other brainstem signs (Chap. 330).

The cavernous sinus syndrome (Fig. 455-4) is a distinctive and frequently life-threatening disorder. It often presents as orbital or facial pain; orbital swelling and chemosis due to occlusion of the ophthalmic veins; fever; oculomotor neuropathy affecting the third, fourth, and sixth cranial nerves; and trigeminal neuropathy affecting the ophthalmic (V1) and occasionally the maxillary (V2) divisions of the trigeminal nerve. Cavernous sinus thrombosis, often secondary to infection from orbital cellulitis (frequently *Staphylococcus aureus*), a cutaneous source on the face, or sinusitis (especially with mucormycosis in diabetic patients), is the most frequent cause; other etiologies include aneurysm of the carotid artery, a carotid-cavernous fistula (orbital bruit may be present), meningioma, nasopharyngeal carcinoma, other tumors, or an idiopathic granulomatous disorder (Tolosa-Hunt syndrome). The two cavernous sinuses directly communicate via intercavernous channels; thus, involvement on one side may extend to become bilateral. Early diagnosis is essential, especially when due to infection, and treatment depends on the underlying etiology.

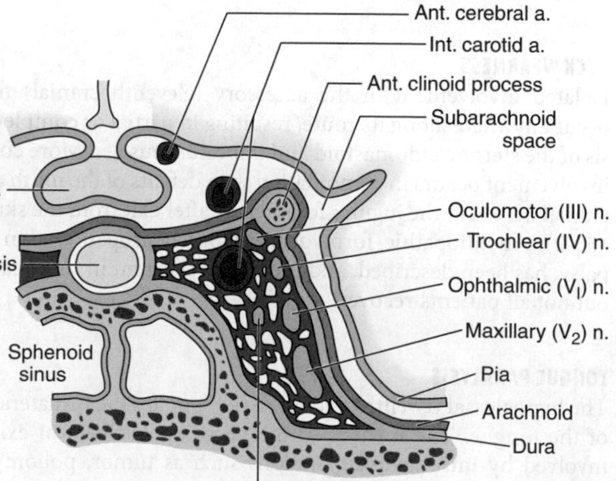

In infectious cases, prompt administration of broad-spectrum antibiotics, drainage of any abscess cavities, and identification of the offending organism are essential. Anticoagulant therapy may benefit cases of primary thrombosis. Repair or occlusion of the carotid artery may be required for treatment of fistulas or aneurysms. The Tolosa-Hunt syndrome generally responds to glucocorticoids. A dramatic improvement in pain is usually evident within a few days; oral prednisone (60 mg daily) is usually continued for 2 weeks and then gradually tapered over a month, or longer if pain recurs. Occasionally an immunosuppressive medication, such as azathioprine or methotrexate, needs to be added to maintain an initial response to glucocorticoids.

An idiopathic form of multiple cranial nerve involvement on one or both sides of the face is occasionally seen. The syndrome consists of a subacute onset of boring facial pain, followed by paralysis of motor cranial nerves. The clinical features overlap those of the Tolosa-Hunt syndrome and appear to be due to idiopathic inflammation of the dura mater, which may be visualized by MRI. The syndrome is usually responsive to glucocorticoids.

Ant. cerebral a.
Int. carotid a.
Ant. clinoid process
Subarachnoid space
Optic chiasma
Oculomotor (III) n.
Trochlear (IV) n.
Hypophysis
Ophthalmic (V_1) n.
Maxillary (V_2) n.
Sphenoid sinus
Pia
Arachnoid
Dura
Abducens (VI) n.

FIGURE 455-4 Anatomy of the cavernous sinus in coronal section, illustrating the location of the cranial nerves in relation to the vascular sinus, internal carotid artery (which loops anteriorly to the section), and surrounding structures.

456 Diseases of the Spinal Cord

Stephen L. Hauser, Allan H. Ropper

Diseases of the spinal cord are frequently devastating. They produce quadriplegia, paraplegia, and sensory deficits far beyond the damage they would inflict elsewhere in the nervous system because the spinal cord contains, in a small cross-sectional area, almost the entire motor output and sensory input of the trunk and limbs. Many spinal cord diseases are reversible if recognized and treated at an early stage (Table 456-1); thus, they are among the most critical of neurologic emergencies. The efficient use of diagnostic procedures, guided by knowledge of the anatomy and the clinical features of spinal cord diseases, is required to maximize the likelihood of a successful outcome.

APPROACH TO THE PATIENT: Spinal Cord Disease

SPINAL CORD ANATOMY RELEVANT TO CLINICAL SIGNS

The spinal cord is a thin, tubular extension of the central nervous system contained within the bony spinal canal. It originates at the medulla and continues caudally to the conus medullaris at the lumbar level; its fibrous extension, the filum terminale, terminates at the coccyx. The adult spinal cord is ~46 cm (18 in.) long, oval in shape, and enlarged in the cervical and lumbar regions, where neurons that innervate the upper and lower extremities, respectively, are located. The white matter tracts containing ascending sensory and descending motor pathways are located peripherally, whereas nerve cell bodies are clustered in an inner region of gray matter shaped like a four-leaf clover that surrounds the central canal (anatomically an extension of the fourth ventricle). The membranes that cover the spinal cord—the pia, arachnoid, and dura—are continuous with those of the brain, and the cerebrospinal fluid is contained within the subarachnoid space between the pia and arachnoid.

The spinal cord has 31 segments, each defined by an exiting ventral motor root and entering dorsal sensory root. During

TABLE 456-1 TREATABLE SPINAL CORD DISORDERS

Compressive
Epidural, intradural, or intramedullary neoplasm
Epidural abscess
Epidural hemorrhage
Cervical spondylosis
Herniated disk
Posttraumatic compression by fractured or displaced vertebra or hemorrhage
Vascular
Arteriovenous malformation and dural fistula
Antiphospholipid syndrome and other hypercoagulable states
Inflammatory
Multiple sclerosis
Neuromyelitis optica
Transverse myelitis
Sarcoidosis
Sjögren-related myelopathy
Systemic lupus erythematosus-related myelopathy
Vasculitis
Infectious
Viral: VZV, HSV-1 and -2, CMV, HIV, HTLV-1, others
Bacterial and mycobacterial: *Borrelia*, *Listeria*, syphilis, others
Mycoplasma pneumoniae
Parasitic: schistosomiasis, toxoplasmosis
Developmental
Syringomyelia
Meningomyelocele
Tethered cord syndrome
Metabolic
Vitamin B_{12} deficiency (subacute combined degeneration)
Copper deficiency

Abbreviations: CMV, cytomegalovirus; HSV, herpes simplex virus; HTLV, human T cell lymphotropic virus; VZV, varicella-zoster virus.

embryologic development, growth of the cord lags behind that of the vertebral column, and the mature spinal cord ends at approximately the first lumbar vertebral body. The lower spinal nerves take an increasingly downward course to exit via intervertebral foramina. The first seven pairs of cervical spinal nerves exit above the same-numbered vertebral bodies, whereas all the subsequent nerves exit below the same-numbered vertebral bodies because of the presence of eight cervical spinal cord segments but only seven cervical vertebrae. The relationship between spinal cord segments and the corresponding vertebral bodies is shown in Table 456-2. These relationships assume particular importance for localization of lesions that cause spinal cord compression. Sensory loss below the circumferential level of the umbilicus, for example, corresponds to the T10 cord segment but indicates involvement of the cord adjacent to the seventh or eighth thoracic vertebral body (see Figs. 31-2 and 31-3). In addition, at every level, the main ascending and descending tracts are somatotopically organized with a laminated distribution that reflects the origin or destination of nerve fibers.

TABLE 456-2 SPINAL CORD LEVELS RELATIVE TO THE VERTEBRAL BODIES

Spinal Cord Level	Corresponding Vertebral Body
Upper cervical	Same as cord level
Lower cervical	1 level higher
Upper thoracic	2 levels higher
Lower thoracic	2 to 3 levels higher
Lumbar	T10-T12
Sacral	T12-L1

Determining the Level of the Lesion The presence of a horizontally defined level below which sensory, motor, and autonomic function is impaired is a hallmark of a lesion of the spinal cord. This *sensory level* is sought by asking the patient to identify a pinprick or cold stimulus applied to the proximal legs and lower trunk and successively moved up toward the neck on each side. Sensory loss below this level is the result of damage to the spinothalamic tract on the opposite side, one to two segments higher in the case of a unilateral spinal cord lesion, and at the level of a bilateral lesion. The discrepancy in the level of a unilateral lesion is the result of the course of the second-order sensory fibers, which originate in the dorsal horn, and ascend for one or two levels as they cross anterior to the central canal to join the opposite spinothalamic tract. Lesions that transect the descending corticospinal and other motor tracts cause paraplegia or quadriplegia with heightened deep tendon reflexes, Babinski signs, and eventual spasticity (the upper motor neuron syndrome). Transverse damage to the cord also produces autonomic disturbances consisting of absent sweating below the implicated cord level and bladder, bowel, and sexual dysfunction.

The uppermost level of a spinal cord lesion can also be localized by attention to the *segmental signs* corresponding to disturbed motor or sensory innervation by an individual cord segment. A band of altered sensation (hyperalgesia or hyperpathia) at the upper end of the sensory disturbance, fasciculations or atrophy in muscles innervated by one or several segments, or a muted or absent deep tendon reflex may be noted at this level. These signs also can occur with focal root or peripheral nerve disorders; thus, they are most useful when they occur together with signs of long tract damage. With severe and acute transverse lesions, the limbs initially may be flaccid rather than spastic. This state of "spinal shock" lasts for several days, rarely for weeks, and may be mistaken for extensive damage to the anterior horn cells over many segments of the cord or for an acute polyneuropathy.

The main features of transverse damage at each level of the spinal cord are summarized below.

CERVICAL CORD Upper cervical cord lesions produce quadriplegia and weakness of the diaphragm. The uppermost level of weakness and reflex loss with lesions at C5-C6 is in the biceps; at C7, in finger and wrist extensors and triceps; and at C8, finger and wrist flexion. Horner's syndrome (miosis, ptosis, and facial hypohidrosis) may accompany a cervical cord lesion at any level.

THORACIC CORD Lesions here are localized by the sensory level on the trunk and, if present, by the site of midline back pain. Useful markers of the sensory level on the trunk are the nipples (T4) and umbilicus (T10). Leg weakness and disturbances of bladder and bowel function accompany the paralysis. Lesions at T9-T10 paralyze the lower—but not the upper—abdominal muscles, resulting in upward movement of the umbilicus when the abdominal wall contracts (*Beevor's sign*).

LUMBAR CORD Lesions at the L2-L4 spinal cord levels paralyze flexion and adduction of the thigh, weaken leg extension at the knee, and abolish the patellar reflex. Lesions at L5-S1 paralyze only movements of the foot and ankle, flexion at the knee, and extension of the thigh, and abolish the ankle jerks (S1).

SACRAL CORD/CONUS MEDULLARIS The conus medullaris is the tapered caudal termination of the spinal cord, comprising the sacral and single coccygeal segments. The distinctive conus syndrome consists of bilateral saddle anesthesia (S3-S5), prominent bladder and bowel dysfunction (urinary retention and incontinence with lax anal tone), and impotence. The bulbocavernosus (S2-S4) and anal (S4-S5) reflexes are absent (Chap. 437). Muscle strength is largely preserved. By contrast, lesions of the cauda equina, the nerve roots derived from the lower cord, are characterized by low back and radicular pain, asymmetric leg weakness and sensory loss, variable areflexia in the lower extremities, and relative sparing of bowel and bladder function. Mass lesions in the lower spinal canal often produce a mixed clinical picture with elements of both cauda equina and conus medullaris syndromes. Cauda equina syndromes are also discussed in Chap. 22.

Special Patterns of Spinal Cord Disease The location of the major ascending and descending pathways of the spinal cord are shown in Fig. 456-1. Most fiber tracts—including the posterior columns and the spinocerebellar and pyramidal tracts—are situated on the side of the body they innervate. However, afferent fibers mediating pain and temperature sensation ascend in the spinothalamic tract contralateral to the side they supply. The anatomic configurations of these tracts produce characteristic syndromes that provide clues to the underlying disease process.

BROWN-SEQUARD HEMICORD SYNDROME This consists of ipsilateral weakness (corticospinal tract) and loss of joint position and vibratory sense (posterior column), with contralateral loss of pain and temperature sense (spinothalamic tract) one or two levels below the lesion. Segmental signs, such as radicular pain, muscle atrophy, or loss of a deep tendon reflex, are unilateral. Partial forms are more common than the fully developed syndrome.

CENTRAL CORD SYNDROME This syndrome results from selective damage to the gray matter nerve cells and crossing spinothalamic tracts surrounding the central canal. In the cervical cord, the central cord syndrome produces arm weakness out of proportion to leg weakness and a "dissociated" sensory loss, meaning loss of pain and temperature sensations over the shoulders, lower neck, and upper trunk (cape distribution), in contrast to preservation of light touch, joint position, and vibration sense in these regions. Spinal trauma, syringomyelia, and intrinsic cord tumors are the main causes.

ANTERIOR SPINAL ARTERY SYNDROME Infarction of the cord is generally the result of occlusion or diminished flow in this artery. The result is bilateral tissue destruction at several contiguous levels that spares the posterior columns. All spinal cord functions—motor, sensory, and autonomic—are lost below the level of the lesion, with the striking exception of retained vibration and position sensation.

FORAMEN MAGNUM SYNDROME Lesions in this area interrupt decussating pyramidal tract fibers destined for the legs, which cross caudal to those of the arms, resulting in weakness of the legs (*crural paresis*). Compressive lesions near the foramen magnum may produce weakness of the ipsilateral shoulder and arm followed by weakness of the ipsilateral leg, then the contralateral leg, and finally the contralateral arm, an "around the clock" pattern that may begin in any of the four limbs. There is typically suboccipital pain spreading to the neck and shoulders.

INTRAMEDULLARY AND EXTRAMEDULLARY SYNDROMES It is useful to differentiate *intramedullary* processes, arising within the substance of the cord, from *extramedullary* ones that lie outside the cord and compress the spinal cord or its vascular supply. The differentiating features are only relative and serve as clinical guides. With extramedullary lesions, radicular pain is often prominent, and there is early sacral sensory loss and spastic weakness in the legs with incontinence due to the superficial location of the corresponding sensory and motor fibers in the spinothalamic and corticospinal tracts (Fig. 456-1). Intramedullary lesions tend to produce poorly localized burning pain rather than radicular pain and to spare sensation in the perineal and sacral areas ("sacral sparing"), reflecting the laminated configuration of the spinothalamic tract with sacral fibers outermost; corticospinal tract signs appear later. Regarding extramedullary lesions, a further distinction is made between extradural and intradural masses, as the former are generally malignant and the latter benign (neurofibroma being a common cause). Consequently, a long duration of symptoms favors an intradural origin.

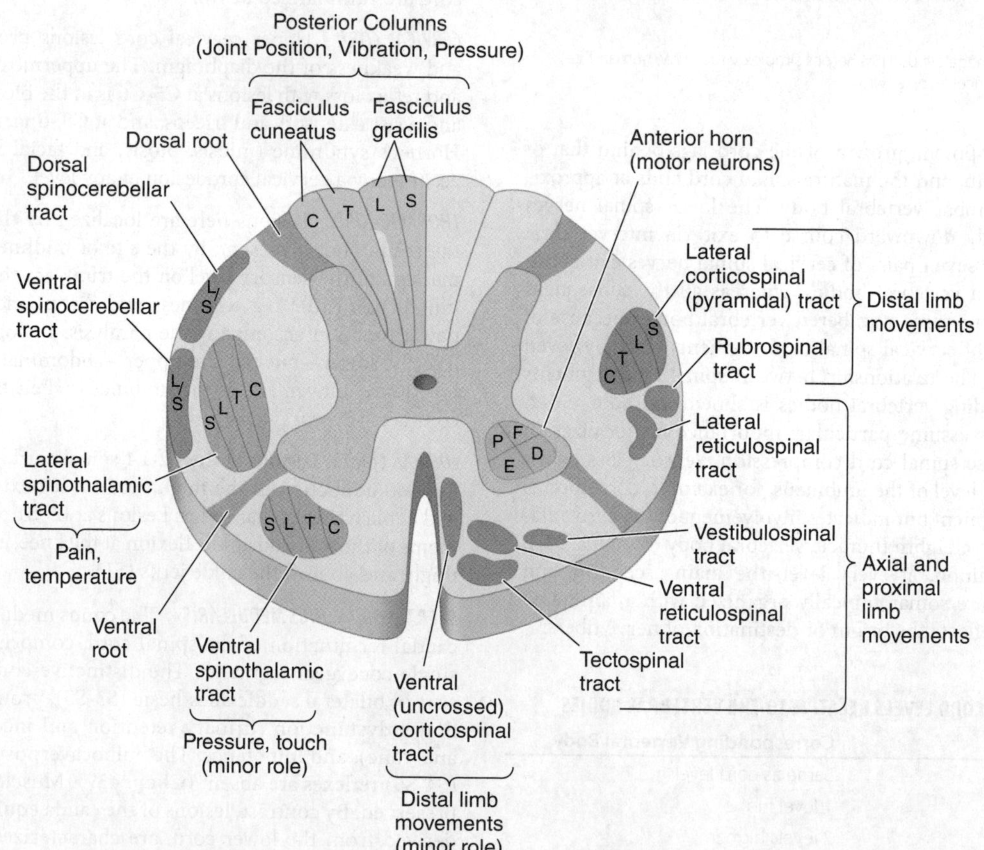

FIGURE 456-1 Transverse section through the spinal cord, composite representation, illustrating the principal ascending (*left*) and descending (*right*) pathways. The lateral and ventral spinothalamic tracts ascend contralateral to the side of the body that is innervated. C, cervical; D, distal; E, extensors; F, flexors; L, lumbar; P, proximal; S, sacral; T, thoracic.

ACUTE AND SUBACUTE SPINAL CORD DISEASES

The initial symptoms of structural diseases of the cord that evolve over days or weeks are focal neck or back pain, followed by various combinations of paresthesias, sensory loss, motor weakness, and sphincter disturbance. There may be only mild sensory symptoms or a devastating functional transection of the cord. Partial lesions selectively involve the posterior columns or anterior spinothalamic tracts or are limited to one side of the cord. Paresthesias or numbness typically begins in the feet and ascend symmetrically or asymmetrically. These symptoms simulate a polyneuropathy, but a sharply demarcated spinal cord level indicates the myelopathic nature of the process.

In severe and abrupt cases, areflexia reflecting spinal shock may be present, but hyperreflexia supervenes over days or weeks; persistent areflexic paralysis with a sensory level usually indicates necrosis over multiple segments of the spinal cord.

APPROACH TO THE PATIENT: Compressive and Noncompressive Myelopathy

DISTINGUISHING COMPRESSIVE FROM NONCOMPRESSIVE MYELOPATHY

The first priority is to exclude a treatable compression of the cord by a mass that may be amenable to treatment. The common causes are tumor, epidural abscess or hematoma, herniated disk, and vertebral pathology. Epidural compression due to malignancy or abscess often causes warning signs of neck or back pain, bladder disturbances, and sensory symptoms that precede the development of paralysis. Spinal subluxation, hemorrhage, and noncompressive etiologies such as infarction are more likely to produce myelopathy without antecedent symptoms. Magnetic resonance imaging (MRI) with gadolinium, centered on the clinically suspected level, is the initial diagnostic procedure if it is available; in some cases, it is appropriate to image the entire spine (cervical through sacral regions) to search for additional clinically inapparent lesions. Once compressive lesions have been excluded, noncompressive causes of acute myelopathy that are intrinsic to the cord are considered, primarily vascular, inflammatory, and infectious etiologies.

COMPRESSIVE MYELOPATHIES

Neoplastic Spinal Cord Compression In adults, most neoplasms are epidural in origin, resulting from metastases to the adjacent vertebral column. The propensity of solid tumors to metastasize to the vertebral column probably reflects the high proportion of bone marrow located in the axial skeleton. Almost any malignant tumor can metastasize to the spinal column, with breast, lung, prostate, kidney, lymphoma, and myeloma being particularly frequent. The thoracic spinal column is most commonly involved; exceptions are metastases from prostate and ovarian cancer, which occur disproportionately in the sacral and lumbar vertebrae, probably from spread through Batson's plexus, a network of veins along the anterior epidural space. Retroperitoneal neoplasms (especially lymphomas or sarcomas) enter the spinal canal laterally through the intervertebral foramina and produce radicular pain with signs of weakness that corresponds to the level of involved nerve roots.

Pain is usually the initial symptom of spinal metastasis; it may be aching and localized or sharp and radiating in quality and typically worsens with movement, coughing, or sneezing and characteristically awakens patients at night. A recent onset of persistent back pain, particularly if in the thoracic spine (which is uncommonly involved by spondylosis), should prompt consideration of vertebral metastasis. Rarely, pain is mild or absent. Plain radiographs of the spine and radionuclide bone scans have a limited role in diagnosis because they do not identify 15–20% of metastatic vertebral lesions and fail to detect paravertebral masses that reach the epidural space through the intervertebral foramina. MRI provides excellent anatomic resolution of the extent of spinal tumors (Fig. 456-2) and is able to distinguish between malignant lesions and other masses—epidural abscess, tuberculoma,

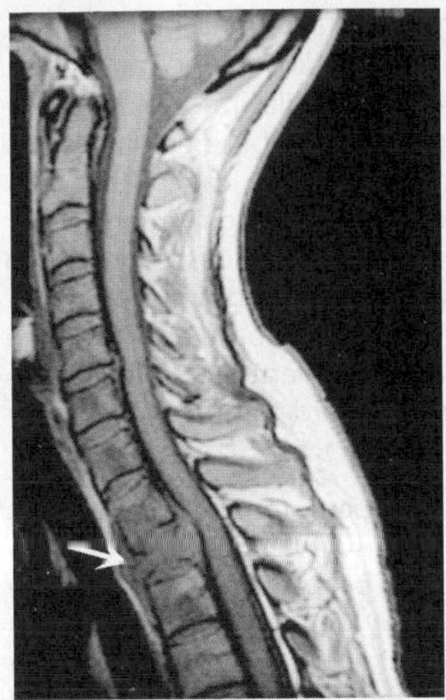

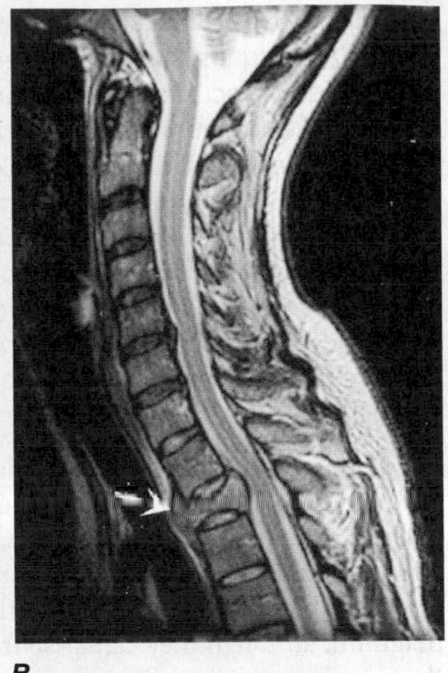

A B

FIGURE 456-2 Epidural spinal cord compression due to breast carcinoma. Sagittal T1-weighted (***A***) and T2-weighted (***B***) magnetic resonance imaging scans through the cervicothoracic junction reveal an infiltrated and collapsed second thoracic vertebral body with posterior displacement and compression of the upper thoracic spinal cord. The low-intensity bone marrow signal in ***A*** signifies replacement by tumor.

lipoma, or epidural hemorrhage, among others—that present in a similar fashion. Vertebral metastases are usually hypointense relative to a normal bone marrow signal on T1-weighted MRI; after the administration of gadolinium, contrast enhancement may deceptively "normalize" the appearance of the tumor by increasing its intensity to that of normal bone marrow. Infections of the spinal column (osteomyelitis and related disorders) are distinctive in that, unlike tumor, they often cross the disk space to involve the adjacent vertebral body.

If spinal cord compression is suspected, imaging should be obtained promptly. If there are radicular symptoms but no evidence of myelopathy, it may be safe to defer imaging for 24–48 h. Up to 40% of patients who present with cord compression at one level are found to have asymptomatic epidural metastases elsewhere; thus, the length of the spine is often imaged when epidural malignancy is in question.

TREATMENT NEOPLASTIC SPINAL CORD COMPRESSION

Management of cord compression includes glucocorticoids to reduce cord edema, local radiotherapy (initiated as early as possible) to the symptomatic lesion, and specific therapy for the underlying tumor type. Glucocorticoids (dexamethasone, up to 40 mg daily) can be administered before an imaging study if there is clinical suspicion of cord compression and the medication is continued at a lower dose until definitive treatment with radiotherapy (generally 3000 cGy administered in 15 daily fractions) and/or surgical decompression is completed. In one randomized controlled trial, initial management with surgery followed by radiotherapy was more effective than radiotherapy alone for patients with a single area of spinal cord compression by extradural tumor; however, patients with recurrent cord compression, brain metastases, radiosensitive tumors, or severe motor symptoms of >48 h in duration were excluded from this study. Radiotherapy alone may be effective even for some typically radioresistant metastases. A good response to therapy can be expected in individuals who are ambulatory at presentation. Treatment usually prevents new weakness, and some recovery of motor function occurs in up to one-third of patients. Motor deficits (paraplegia or quadriplegia), once established for >12 h, do not usually improve, and beyond 48 h the prognosis for substantial motor recovery is poor. Although most patients do not experience recurrences in the months following radiotherapy, with survival beyond 2 years, recurrence becomes increasingly likely and can be managed with additional radiotherapy. Newer techniques such as stereotactic radiosurgery can deliver high doses of focused radiation and with similar rates of response compared to traditional radiotherapy. Biopsy of the epidural mass is unnecessary in patients with known primary cancer, but it is indicated if a history of underlying cancer is lacking. Surgery, either decompression by laminectomy or vertebral body resection, is also indicated when signs of cord compression worsen despite radiotherapy, when the maximum-tolerated dose of radiotherapy has been delivered previously to the site, or when a vertebral compression fracture or spinal instability contributes to cord compression.

In contrast to tumors of the epidural space, most intradural mass lesions are slow-growing and benign. Meningiomas and neurofibromas account for most of these, with occasional cases caused by chordoma, lipoma, dermoid, or sarcoma. Meningiomas (Fig. 456-3) are often located posterior to the thoracic cord or near the foramen magnum, although they can arise from the meninges anywhere along the spinal canal. Neurofibromas are benign tumors of the nerve sheath that typically arise from the posterior root; when multiple, neurofibromatosis is the likely etiology. Symptoms usually begin with radicular sensory symptoms followed by an asymmetric, progressive spinal cord syndrome. Therapy is surgical resection.

Primary intramedullary tumors of the spinal cord are uncommon. They present as central cord or hemicord syndromes, often in the cervical region. There may be poorly localized burning pain in the extremities and sparing of sacral sensation. In adults, these lesions are ependymomas, hemangioblastomas, or low-grade astrocytomas (Fig. 456-4). Complete resection of an intramedullary ependymoma is often possible with microsurgical techniques. Debulking of an intramedullary astrocytoma can also be helpful, as these are often slowly growing lesions; the value of adjunctive radiotherapy and chemotherapy is uncertain. Secondary (metastatic) intramedullary tumors also occur, especially in patients with advanced metastatic disease (Chap. 118), although these are not nearly as frequent as brain metastases.

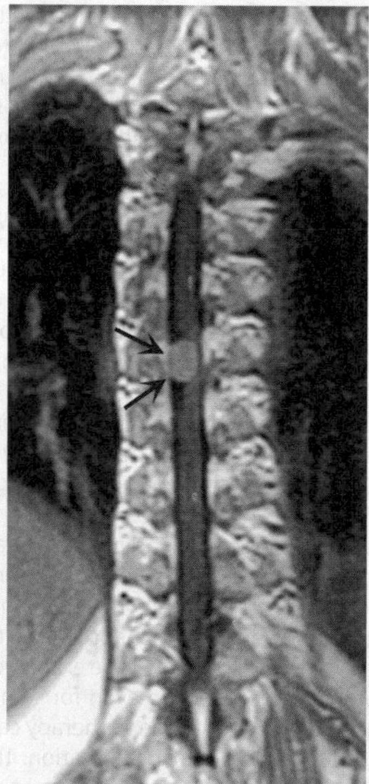

FIGURE 456-3 Magnetic resonance imaging of a thoracic meningioma. Coronal T1-weighted postcontrast image through the thoracic spinal cord demonstrates intense and uniform enhancement of a well-circumscribed extramedullary mass (*arrows*) that displaces the spinal cord to the left.

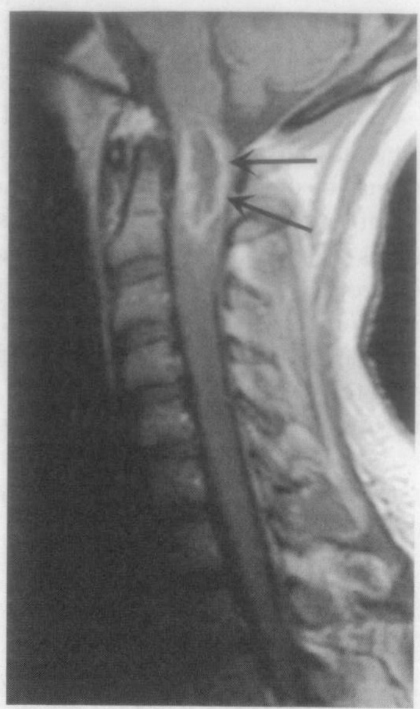

FIGURE 456-4 Magnetic resonance imaging of an intramedullary astrocytoma. Sagittal T1-weighted postcontrast image through the cervical spine demonstrates expansion of the upper cervical spine by a mass lesion emanating from within the spinal cord at the cervicomedullary junction. Irregular peripheral enhancement occurs within the mass (*arrows*).

Spinal Epidural Abscess Spinal epidural abscess presents with midline back or neck pain, fever, and progressive limb weakness. Prompt recognition of this distinctive process may prevent permanent sequelae. Aching pain is almost always present, either over the spine or in a radicular pattern. The duration of pain prior to presentation is generally ≤2 weeks but may on occasion be several months or longer. Fever is typically but not invariably present, accompanied by elevated white blood cell count, sedimentation rate, and C-reactive protein. As the abscess expands, further spinal cord damage results from venous congestion and thrombosis. Once weakness and other signs of myelopathy appear, progression may be rapid and irreversible. A more chronic sterile granulomatous form of abscess is also known, usually after treatment of an acute epidural infection.

Risk factors include an impaired immune status (HIV, diabetes mellitus, renal failure, alcoholism, malignancy), intravenous drug abuse, and infections of the skin or other tissues. Two-thirds of epidural infections result from hematogenous spread of bacteria from the skin (furunculosis), soft tissue (pharyngeal or dental abscesses; sinusitis), or deep viscera (bacterial endocarditis). The remainder arises from direct extension of a local infection to the subdural space; examples of local predisposing conditions are vertebral osteomyelitis, decubitus ulcers, lumbar puncture, epidural anesthesia, or spinal surgery. Most cases are due to *Staphylococcus aureus*; gram-negative bacilli, *Streptococcus*, anaerobes, and fungi can also cause epidural abscesses. Tuberculosis from an adjacent vertebral source (Pott's disease) remains an important cause in the developing world.

MRI (Fig. 456-5) localizes the abscess and excludes other causes of myelopathy. Blood cultures are positive in more than half of cases, but direct aspiration of the abscess at surgery is often required for a microbiologic diagnosis. Lumbar puncture is only required if encephalopathy or other clinical signs raise the question of associated meningitis, a feature that is found in <25% of cases. The level of the puncture should be planned to minimize the risk of meningitis due to passage of the needle through infected tissue. A high cervical tap is sometimes the safest approach. Cerebrospinal fluid (CSF) abnormalities in epidural and subdural abscess consist of pleocytosis with a preponderance of polymorphonuclear cells, an elevated protein level, and a reduced glucose level, but the responsible organism is not cultured unless there is associated meningitis.

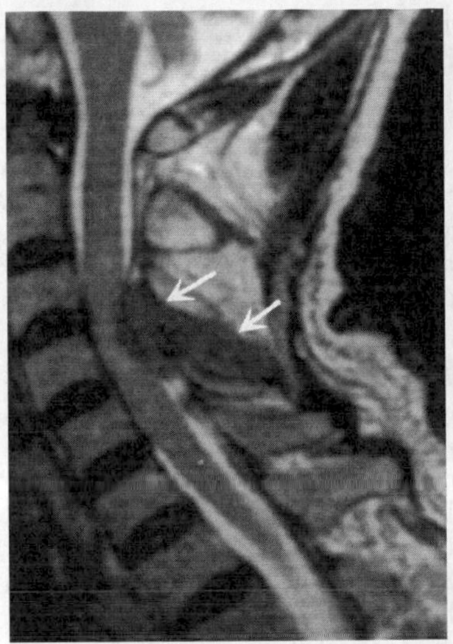

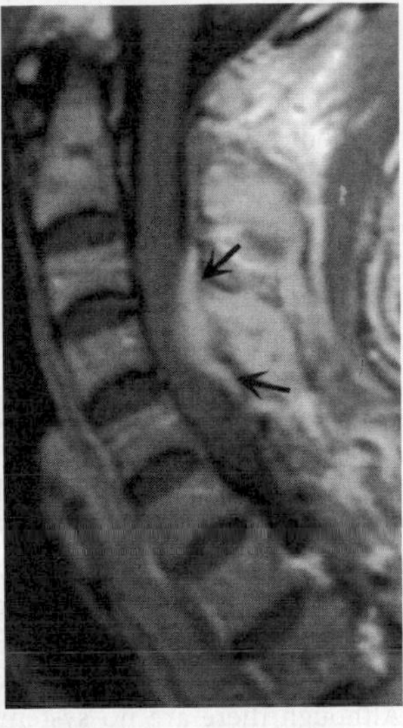

FIGURE 456-5 Magnetic resonance (MR) imaging of a spinal epidural abscess due to tuberculosis. *A.* Sagittal T2-weighted free spin-echo MR sequence. A hypointense mass replaces the posterior elements of C3 and extends epidurally to compress the spinal cord (*arrows*). ***B.*** Sagittal T1-weighted image after contrast administration reveals a diffuse enhancement of the epidural process (*arrows*) with extension into the epidural space.

TREATMENT SPINAL EPIDURAL ABSCESS

Treatment is by decompressive laminectomy with debridement combined with long-term antibiotic treatment. Surgical evacuation prevents development of paralysis and may improve or reverse paralysis in evolution, but it is unlikely to improve deficits of more than several days in duration. Broad-spectrum antibiotics should be started empirically before surgery and then modified on the basis of culture results; medication is generally continued for at least 6 weeks. If surgery is contraindicated or if there is a fixed paraplegia or quadriplegia that is unlikely to improve following surgery, long-term administration of systemic and oral antibiotics can be used; in such cases, the choice of antibiotics may be guided by results of blood cultures. Surgical management remains the treatment of choice unless the abscess is limited in size and causes few or no neurologic signs.

With prompt diagnosis and treatment of spinal epidural abscess, up to two-thirds of patients experience significant recovery.

Spinal Epidural Hematoma Hemorrhage into the epidural (or subdural) space causes acute focal or radicular pain followed by variable signs of a spinal cord or conus medullaris disorder. Therapeutic anticoagulation, trauma, tumor, or blood dyscrasias are predisposing conditions. Rare cases complicate lumbar puncture or epidural anesthesia. MRI and computed tomography (CT) confirm the clinical suspicion and can delineate the extent of the bleeding. Treatment consists of prompt reversal of any underlying clotting disorder and surgical decompression. Surgery may be followed by substantial recovery, especially in patients with some preservation of motor function preoperatively. Because of the risk of hemorrhage, lumbar puncture should be avoided whenever possible in patients with severe thrombocytopenia or other coagulopathies.

Hematomyelia Hemorrhage into the substance of the spinal cord is a rare result of trauma, intraparenchymal vascular malformation (see below), vasculitis due to polyarteritis nodosa or systemic lupus erythematosus (SLE), bleeding disorders, or a spinal cord neoplasm. Hematomyelia presents as an acute painful transverse myelopathy. With large lesions, extension into the subarachnoid space results in subarachnoid hemorrhage (Chap. 330). Diagnosis is by MRI or CT.

TABLE 456-3 EVALUATION OF ACUTE TRANSVERSE MYELOPATHY

1. MRI of spinal cord with and without contrast (exclude compressive causes).
2. CSF studies: Cell count, protein, glucose, IgG index/synthesis rate, oligoclonal bands, VDRL; Gram's stain, acid-fast bacilli, and India ink stains; PCR for VZV, HSV-2, HSV-1, EBV, CMV, HHV-6, enteroviruses, HIV; antibody for HTLV-1, *Borrelia burgdorferi*, *Mycoplasma pneumoniae*, and *Chlamydia pneumoniae*; viral, bacterial, mycobacterial, and fungal cultures.
3. Blood studies for infection: HIV; RPR; IgG and IgM enterovirus antibody; IgM mumps, measles, rubella, group B arbovirus, *Brucella melitensis*, *Chlamydia psittaci*, *Bartonella henselae*, schistosomal antibody; cultures for *B. melitensis*. Also consider nasal/pharyngeal/anal cultures for enteroviruses; stool O&P for *Schistosoma* ova.
4. Immune-mediated disorders: ESR; ANA; ENA; dsDNA; rheumatoid factor; anti-SSA; anti-SSB, complement levels; antiphospholipid and anticardiolipin antibodies; p-ANCA; antimicrosomal and antithyroglobulin antibodies; if Sjögren's syndrome suspected, Schirmer test, salivary gland scintigraphy, and salivary/lacrimal gland biopsy.
5. Sarcoidosis: Serum angiotensin-converting enzyme; serum Ca; 24-h urine Ca; chest x-ray; chest CT; total-body gallium scan; lymph node biopsy.
6. Demyelinating disease: Brain MRI scan, evoked potentials, CSF oligoclonal bands, neuromyelitis optica antibody (anti-aquaporin-4 [NMO] antibody).
7. Vascular causes: MRI, CT myelogram; spinal angiogram.

Abbreviations: ANA, antinuclear antibodies; CMV, cytomegalovirus; CSF, cerebrospinal fluid; CT, computed tomography; EBV, Epstein-Barr virus; ENA, epithelial neutrophil-activating peptide; ESR, erythrocyte sedimentation rate; HHV, human herpes virus; HSV, herpes simplex virus; HTLV, human T cell leukemia/lymphoma virus; MRI, magnetic resonance imaging; O&P, ova and parasites; p-ANCA, perinuclear antineutrophilic cytoplasmic antibodies; PCR, polymerase chain reaction; RPR, rapid plasma reagin (test); VDRL, Venereal Disease Research Laboratory; VZV, varicella-zoster virus.

Therapy is supportive, and surgical intervention is generally not useful. An exception is hematomyelia due to an underlying vascular malformation, for which spinal angiography and endovascular occlusion may be indicated, or surgery to evacuate the clot and remove the underlying vascular lesion.

NONCOMPRESSIVE MYELOPATHIES

The most frequent causes of noncompressive acute transverse myelopathy are spinal cord infarction; systemic inflammatory disorders, including SLE and sarcoidosis; demyelinating diseases, including multiple sclerosis (MS); neuromyelitis optica (NMO); postinfectious or idiopathic transverse myelitis, which is presumed to be an immune condition related to acute disseminated encephalomyelitis (Chap. 458); and infectious (primarily viral) causes. After spinal cord compression is excluded, the evaluation generally requires a lumbar puncture and a search for underlying systemic disease (Table 456-3).

Spinal Cord Infarction The cord is supplied by three arteries that course vertically over its surface: a single anterior spinal artery and paired posterior spinal arteries. The anterior spinal artery originates in paired branches of the vertebral arteries at the craniocervical junction and is fed by additional radicular vessels that arise at C6, at an upper thoracic level, and, most consistently, at T11-L2 (artery of Adamkiewicz). At each spinal cord segment, paired penetrating vessels branch from the anterior spinal artery to supply the anterior two-thirds of the cord; the posterior spinal arteries, which often become less distinct below the midthoracic level, supply the posterior columns.

Spinal cord ischemia can occur at any level; however, the presence of the artery of Adamkiewicz below, and the anterior spinal artery circulation above, creates a region of marginal blood flow in the upper thoracic segments. With hypotension or cross-clamping of the aorta, cord infarction typically occurs at the level of T3-T4, and also at boundary zones between the anterior and posterior spinal artery territories. The latter may result in a rapidly progressive syndrome over hours of weakness and spasticity with little sensory change.

Acute infarction in the territory of the *anterior spinal artery* produces paraplegia or quadriplegia, dissociated sensory loss affecting pain and temperature sense but sparing vibration and position sense, and loss of sphincter control ("anterior cord syndrome"). Onset may be sudden but more typically is progressive over minutes or a few hours, quite unlike stroke in the cerebral hemispheres. Sharp midline or radiating back pain localized to the area of ischemia is frequent. Areflexia due to spinal shock is often present initially; with time, hyperreflexia and spasticity appear. Less common is infarction in the territory of the *posterior spinal arteries*, resulting in loss of posterior column function either on one side or bilaterally.

Causes of spinal cord infarction include aortic atherosclerosis, dissecting aortic aneurysm, vertebral artery occlusion or dissection in the neck, aortic surgery, or profound hypotension from any cause. A "surfer's myelopathy" in the cervical region is probably vascular in origin. Cardiogenic emboli, vasculitis (Chap. 385), and collagen vascular disease (particularly SLE [Chap. 378], Sjögren's syndrome [Chap. 383], and the antiphospholipid antibody syndrome [Chap. 379]) are other etiologies. Occasional cases develop from *embolism of nucleus pulposus* material into spinal vessels, usually from local spine trauma. In a substantial number of cases, no cause can be found, and thromboembolism in arterial feeders is suspected. MRI may fail to demonstrate infarctions of the cord, especially in the first day, but often the imaging becomes abnormal at the affected level.

In cord infarction due to presumed thromboembolism, acute anticoagulation is not indicated, with the possible exception of the unusual transient ischemic attack or incomplete infarction with a stuttering or progressive course. The antiphospholipid antibody syndrome is treated with anticoagulation (Chap. 379). Lumbar drainage of spinal fluid has reportedly been successful in some cases of cord infarction and has been used prophylactically during aortic surgery, but it has not been studied systematically.

Inflammatory and Immune Myelopathies (Myelitis) This broad category includes the demyelinating conditions MS, NMO, and postinfectious myelitis, as well as sarcoidosis and systemic autoimmune disease. In approximately one-quarter of cases of myelitis, no underlying cause can be identified. Some will later manifest additional symptoms of an immune-mediated disease. *Recurrent episodes of myelitis* are usually due to one of the immune-mediated diseases or to infection with herpes simplex virus (HSV) type 2 (below).

MULTIPLE SCLEROSIS MS may present with acute myelitis, particularly in individuals of Asian or African ancestry. In Caucasians, MS attacks rarely cause a transverse myelopathy (i.e., attacks of bilateral sensory disturbances, unilateral or bilateral weakness, and bladder or bowel symptoms), but it is among the most common causes of a partial cord syndrome. MRI findings in MS-associated myelitis typically consist of mild swelling of the cord and diffuse or multifocal "shoddy" areas of abnormal signal on T2-weighted sequences. Contrast enhancement, indicating disruption in the blood-brain barrier associated with inflammation, is present in many acute cases. A brain MRI is most helpful in gauging the likelihood that a case of myelitis represents an initial attack of MS. A normal scan indicates that the risk of evolution to MS is low, ~10–15% over 5 years; in contrast, the finding of multiple periventricular T2-bright lesions indicates a much higher risk, >50% over 5 years and >90% by 14 years. The CSF may be normal, but more often there is a mild mononuclear cell pleocytosis, with normal or mildly elevated CSF protein levels; the presence of oligoclonal bands is variable, but when they are found, a diagnosis of MS is more likely.

There are no adequate trials of therapy for MS-associated transverse myelitis. Intravenous methylprednisolone (500 mg qd for 3 days) followed by oral prednisone (1 mg/kg per day for several weeks, then gradual taper) has been used as initial treatment. A course of plasma exchange may be indicated for severe cases if glucocorticoids are ineffective. MS is discussed in Chap. 458.

NEUROMYELITIS OPTICA NMO is an immune-mediated demyelinating disorder consisting of a severe myelopathy that is typically longitudinally extensive, meaning that the lesion spans three or more vertebral segments. NMO is associated with optic neuritis that is often bilateral and may precede or follow myelitis by weeks or months, and also by brainstem and, in some cases, hypothalamic involvement. Recurrent myelitis without optic nerve involvemement can also occur in NMO; affected individuals are usually female and often of Asian ancestry. CSF studies reveal a variable mononuclear pleocytosis of up to several hundred cells per microliter; unlike MS, oligoclonal bands are generally absent. Diagnostic serum autoantibodies against the water channel protein aquaporin-4 are present in 60–70% of patients with NMO. NMO has also been associated with SLE and antiphospholipid antibodies (see below) as well as with other systemic autoimmune diseases; rare cases are paraneoplastic in origin. Treatment is with glucocorticoids and, for refractory cases, plasma exchange (as for MS, above). Preliminary studies suggest that treatment with azathioprine, mycophenylate, or anti-CD20 (anti–B cell) monoclonal antibody may protect against subsequent relapses; treatment for 5 years or longer is generally recommended. NMO is discussed in Chap. 458.

SYSTEMIC IMMUNE-MEDIATED DISORDERS Myelitis occurs in a small number of patients with SLE, many cases of which are associated with antibodies to antiphospholipids and/or to aquaporin-4. Patients with aquaporin-4 antibodies are likely to have longitudinally extensive myelitis by MRI, are considered to have an NMO-spectrum disorder, and are at high risk of developing future episodes of myelitis and/or optic neuritis. The CSF in SLE myelitis is usually normal or shows a mild lymphocytic pleocytosis; oligoclonal bands are a variable finding. Although there are no systematic trials of therapy for SLE myelitis, based on limited data, high-dose glucocorticoids followed by cyclophosphamide have been recommended. Acute severe episodes of transverse myelitis that do not initially respond to glucocorticoids are often treated with a course of plasma exchange. Sjögren's syndrome (Chap. 383) can also be associated with NMO spectrum disorder and also with cases of acute transverse or chronic progressive myelopathy. Other immune-mediated myelitides include antiphospholipid antibody syndrome (Chap. 379), mixed connective tissue disease (Chap. 382), Behçet's syndrome (Chap. 387), and vasculitis related to polyarteritis nodosa, perinuclear antineutrophilic cytoplasmic (p-ANCA) antibodies, or primary central nervous system vasculitis (Chap. 385).

Another important consideration in this group is sarcoid myelopathy that may present as a slowly progressive or relapsing disorder. MRI reveals an edematous swelling of the spinal cord that may mimic tumor; there is almost always gadolinium enhancement of active lesions and in some cases nodular enhancement of the adjacent surface of the cord; lesions may be single or multiple, and on axial images, enhancement of the central cord is usually present. The typical CSF profile consists of a mild lymphocytic pleocytosis and mildly elevated protein level; in a minority of cases, reduced glucose and oligoclonal bands are found. The diagnosis is particularly difficult when systemic manifestations of sarcoid are minor or absent (nearly 50% of cases) or when other typical neurologic manifestations of the disease—such as cranial neuropathy, hypothalamic involvement, or meningeal enhancement visualized by MRI—are lacking. A slit-lamp examination of the eye to search for uveitis, chest x-ray and CT to assess pulmonary involvement and mediastinal lymphadenopathy, serum or CSF angiotensin-converting enzyme (ACE; CSF values elevated in only a minority of cases), serum calcium, and a gallium scan may assist in the diagnosis. The usefulness of spinal fluid ACE is uncertain. Initial treatment is with oral glucocorticoids; immunosuppressant drugs, including the tumor necrosis factor α inhibitor infliximab, have been used for resistant cases. Sarcoidosis is discussed in Chap. 390.

POSTINFECTIOUS MYELITIS Many cases of myelitis, termed *postinfectious* or *postvaccinal*, follow an infection or vaccination. Numerous organisms have been implicated, including Epstein-Barr virus (EBV), cytomegalovirus (CMV), mycoplasma, influenza, measles, varicella, rubeola, and mumps. As in the related disorder acute disseminated encephalomyelitis (Chap. 458), postinfectious myelitis often begins as the patient appears to be recovering from an acute febrile infection, or in the subsequent days or weeks, but an infectious agent cannot be isolated from the nervous system or CSF. The presumption is that the myelitis represents an autoimmune disorder triggered by infection and is not due to direct infection of the spinal cord. No randomized controlled trials of therapy exist; treatment is usually with glucocorticoids or, in fulminant cases, plasma exchange.

ACUTE INFECTIOUS MYELITIS Many viruses have been associated with an acute myelitis that is infectious in nature rather than postinfectious. Nonetheless, the two processes are often difficult to distinguish. Herpes zoster is the best characterized viral myelitis, but HSV types 1 and 2, EBV, CMV, and rabies virus are other well-described causes. HSV-2 (and less commonly HSV-1) produces a distinctive syndrome of recurrent sacral cauda equina neuritis in association with outbreaks of genital herpes (Elsberg's syndrome). Poliomyelitis is the prototypic viral myelitis, but it is more or less restricted to the anterior gray matter of the cord containing the spinal motoneurons. A polio-like syndrome can also be caused by a large number of enteroviruses (including enterovirus 71 and coxsackie), and with West Nile virus and other flaviviruses. Recently, cases of paralysis in children and adolescents were associated with enterovirus D-68 infection but a causal role for this virus has not been established. Chronic viral myelitic infections, such as those due to HIV or human T cell lymphotropic virus type 1 (HTLV-1), are discussed below.

Bacterial and mycobacterial myelitis (most are essentially abscesses) are less common than viral causes and much less frequent than cerebral bacterial abscess. Almost any pathogenic species may be responsible, including *Borrelia burgdorferi* (Lyme disease), *Listeria monocytogenes*, *Mycobacterium tuberculosis*, and *Treponema pallidum* (syphilis). *Mycoplasma pneumoniae* may be a cause of myelitis, but its status is uncertain because many cases are more properly classified as postinfectious.

Schistosomiasis (Chap. 259) is an important cause of parasitic myelitis in endemic areas. The process is intensely inflammatory and granulomatous, caused by a local response to tissue digesting enzymes from the ova of the parasite, typically *Schistosoma mansoni*. Toxoplasmosis (Chap. 253) can occasionally cause a focal myelopathy, and this diagnosis should especially be considered in patients with AIDS (Chap. 226).

In cases of suspected viral myelitis, it may be appropriate to begin specific therapy pending laboratory confirmation. Herpes zoster, HSV, and EBV myelitis are treated with intravenous acyclovir (10 mg/kg q8h) or oral valacyclovir (2 g tid) for 10–14 days; CMV is treated with ganciclovir (5 mg/kg IV bid) plus foscarnet (60 mg/kg IV tid) or cidofovir (5 mg/kg per week for 2 weeks).

High-Voltage Electrical Injury Spinal cord injuries are prominent following electrocution from lightning strikes or other accidental electrical exposures. The syndrome consists of transient weakness acutely (often with an altered sensorium and focal cerebral disturbances), followed several days or even weeks later by a myelopathy that can be severe and permanent. This is a rare injury type, and limited data incriminate a vascular pathology involving the anterior spinal artery and its branches in some cases. Therapy is supportive.

CHRONIC MYELOPATHIES

SPONDYLOTIC MYELOPATHY

Spondylotic myelopathy is one of the most common causes of chronic cord compression and of gait difficulty in the elderly. Neck and shoulder pain with stiffness are early symptoms; impingement of bone and soft tissue overgrowth on nerve roots results in radicular arm pain, most often in a C5 or C6 distribution. Compression of the cervical cord, which occurs in fewer than one-third of cases, produces a slowly progressive spastic paraparesis, at times asymmetric and often accompanied by paresthesias in the feet and hands. Vibratory sense is diminished in the legs, there is a Romberg sign, and occasionally there is a sensory level for vibration or pinprick on the upper thorax. In some cases, coughing or straining produces leg weakness or radiating arm or shoulder pain. Dermatomal sensory loss in the arms, atrophy of intrinsic hand muscles, increased deep-tendon reflexes in the legs, and extensor plantar responses are common. Urinary urgency or incontinence occurs in advanced cases, but there are many alternative causes of these problems in older individuals. A tendon reflex in the arms is often diminished at some level; most often at the biceps (C5-C6). In individual cases, radicular, myelopathic, or combined signs may predominate. The diagnosis should be considered in appropriate cases of progressive cervical myelopathy, paresthesias of the feet and hands, or wasting of the hands.

Diagnosis is usually made by MRI and may be suspected from CT images; plain x-rays are less helpful. Extrinsic cord compression and deformation are appreciated on axial MRI views, and T2-weighted sequences may reveal areas of high signal intensity within the cord adjacent to the site of compression. A cervical collar may be helpful in milder cases, but definitive therapy consists of surgical decompression. Posterior laminectomy or an anterior approach with resection of the protruded disk and bony material may be required. Cervical spondylosis and related degenerative diseases of the spine are discussed in Chap. 22.

VASCULAR MALFORMATIONS OF THE CORD AND DURA

Vascular malformations of the cord and overlying dura are treatable causes of progressive myelopathy. Most common are fistulas located within the dura or posteriorly along the surface of the cord. Most dural arteriovenous (AV) fistulas are located at or below the midthoracic level, usually consisting of a direct connection between a radicular feeding artery in the nerve root sleeve with dural veins. The typical presentation is a middle-aged man with a progressive myelopathy that worsens slowly or intermittently and may have periods of remission, sometimes mimicking MS. Acute deterioration due to hemorrhage into the spinal cord (hematomyelia) or subarachnoid space may also occur but is rare. A saltatory progression is most common and appears to be the result of local ischemia and edema from venous congestion. Most patients have incomplete sensory, motor, and bladder disturbances. The motor disorder may predominate and produce a mixture of upper and restricted lower motor neuron signs, simulating amyotrophic lateral sclerosis (ALS). Pain over the dorsal spine, dysesthesias, or radicular pain may be present. Other symptoms suggestive of AV malformation (AVM) or dural fistula include intermittent claudication; symptoms that change with posture, exertion, Valsalva maneuver, or menses; and fever.

Less commonly, AVM disorders are intramedullary rather than dural. One unusual disorder is a progressive thoracic myelopathy with paraparesis developing over weeks or months, characterized pathologically by abnormally thick, hyalinized vessels within the cord (subacute necrotic myelopathy, or Foix-Alajouanine syndrome).

Spinal bruits are infrequent but may be sought at rest and after exercise in suspected cases. A vascular nevus on the overlying skin may indicate an underlying vascular malformation as occurs with Klippel-Trenaunay-Weber syndrome. High-resolution MRI with contrast administration detects the draining vessels of many but not all AVMs (Fig. 456-6). An uncertain proportion may be visualized by CT myelography as enlarged vessels along the surface of the cord. Definitive diagnosis requires selective spinal angiography, which defines the feeding vessels and the extent of the malformation. Endovascular embolization of the major feeding vessels may stabilize a progressive neurologic deficit or allow for gradual recovery. Some lesions, especially small dural fistulas, can be resected surgically.

RETROVIRUS-ASSOCIATED MYELOPATHIES

The myelopathy associated with HTLV-1, formerly called tropical spastic paraparesis, is a slowly progressive spastic syndrome with variable sensory and bladder disturbance. Approximately half of patients have mild back or leg pain. The neurologic signs may be asymmetric, often lacking a well-defined sensory level; the only sign in the arms may be hyperreflexia after several years of illness. The onset is insidious, and the illness is slowly progressive at a variable rate; most patients are unable to walk within 10 years of onset. This presentation may resemble primary progressive MS or a thoracic AVM. Diagnosis is made by demonstration of HTLV-1-specific antibody in serum by enzyme-linked immunosorbent assay (ELISA), confirmed by radioimmunoprecipitation or Western blot analysis. Especially in endemic areas, a finding of HTLV-1 seropositivity in a patient with myelopathy does not necessarily prove that HTLV-1 is causative. The CSF/serum antibody index may provide support by establishing intrathecal synthesis of antibodies favoring HTVL-1 myelopathy over asymptomatic carriage. Measuring proviral DNA by polymerase chain reaction (PCR) in serum and CSF cells can be useful as an ancillary part of diagnosis, because proviral DNA levels may be higher in patients with myelopathy. The myelopathy appears to result from an

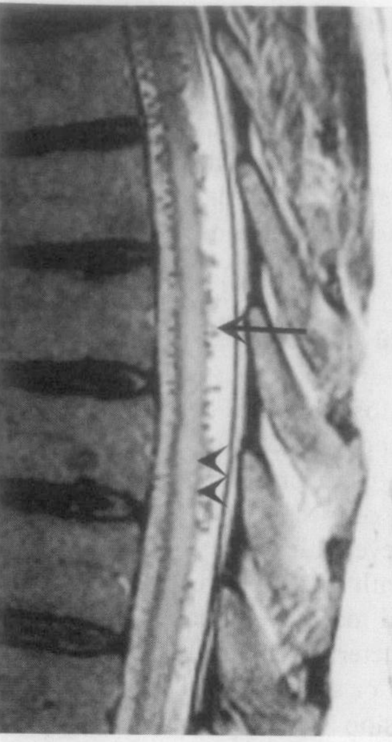

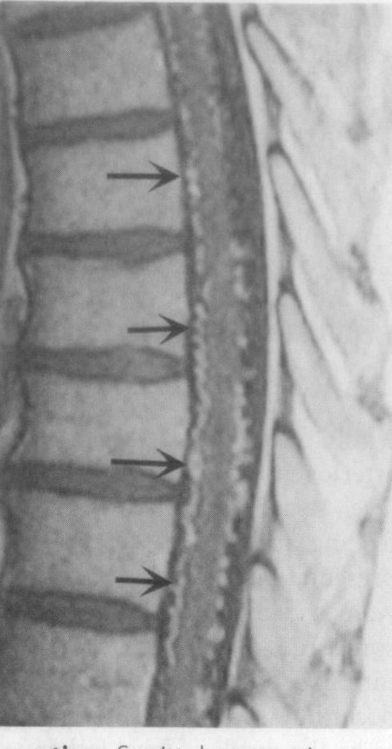

FIGURE 456-6 Arteriovenous malformation. Sagittal magnetic resonance scans of the thoracic spinal cord: T2 fast spin-echo technique (*left*) and T1 postcontrast image (*right*). On the T2-weighted image (*left*), abnormally high signal intensity is noted in the central aspect of the spinal cord (*arrowheads*). Numerous punctate flow voids indent the dorsal and ventral spinal cord (*arrow*). These represent the abnormally dilated venous plexus supplied by a dural arteriovenous fistula. After contrast administration (*right*), multiple, serpentine, enhancing veins (*arrows*) on the ventral and dorsal aspect of the thoracic spinal cord are visualized, diagnostic of arteriovenous malformation. This patient was a 54-year-old man with a 4-year history of progressive paraparesis.

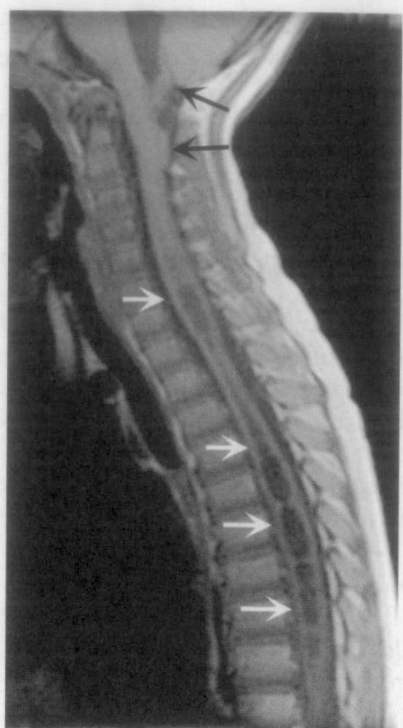

FIGURE 456-7 Magnetic resonance imaging of syringomyelia associated with a Chiari malformation. Sagittal T1-weighted image through the cervical and upper thoracic spine demonstrates descent of the cerebellar tonsils below the level of the foramen magnum (*black arrows*). Within the substance of the cervical and thoracic spinal cord, a cerebrospinal fluid collection dilates the central canal (*white arrows*).

immune-mediated attack on the spinal cord rather than the result of direct viral infection. There is no effective treatment, but symptomatic therapy for spasticity and bladder symptoms may be helpful.

A progressive myelopathy may also result from HIV infection (Chap. 226). It is characterized by vacuolar degeneration of the posterior and lateral tracts, resembling subacute combined degeneration (see below).

SYRINGOMYELIA

Syringomyelia is a developmental cavity of the cervical cord that may enlarge and produce progressive myelopathy or may remain asymptomatic. Symptoms begin insidiously in adolescence or early adulthood, progress irregularly, and may undergo spontaneous arrest for several years. Many young patients acquire a cervical-thoracic scoliosis. More than half of all cases are associated with Chiari type 1 malformations in which the cerebellar tonsils protrude through the foramen magnum and into the cervical spinal canal. The pathophysiology of syrinx expansion is controversial, but some interference with the normal flow of CSF seems likely, perhaps by the Chiari malformation. Acquired cavitations of the cord in areas of necrosis are also termed *syrinx cavities*; these follow trauma, myelitis, necrotic spinal cord tumors, and chronic arachnoiditis due to tuberculosis and other etiologies.

The presentation is a central cord syndrome consisting of a regional dissociated sensory loss (loss of pain and temperature sensation with sparing of touch and vibration) and areflexic weakness in the upper limbs. The sensory deficit has a distribution that is "suspended" over the nape of the neck, shoulders, and upper arms (cape distribution) or in the hands. Most cases begin asymmetrically with unilateral sensory loss in the hands that leads to injuries and burns that are not appreciated by the patient. Muscle wasting in the lower neck, shoulders, arms, and hands with asymmetric or absent reflexes in the arms reflects expansion of the cavity in the gray matter of the cord. As the cavity enlarges and compresses the long tracts, spasticity and weakness of the legs, bladder and bowel dysfunction, and a Horner's syndrome appear. Some patients develop facial numbness and sensory loss from damage to the descending tract of the trigeminal nerve (C2 level or above). In cases with Chiari malformations, cough-induced headache and neck, arm, or facial pain may be reported. Extension of the syrinx into the medulla, syringobulbia, causes palatal or vocal cord paralysis, dysarthria, horizontal or vertical nystagmus, episodic dizziness or vertigo, and tongue weakness with atrophy.

MRI accurately identifies developmental and acquired syrinx cavities and their associated spinal cord enlargement (Fig. 456-7). Images of the brain and the entire spinal cord should be obtained to delineate the full longitudinal extent of the syrinx, assess posterior fossa structures for the Chiari malformation, and determine whether hydrocephalus is present.

TREATMENT SYRINGOMYELIA

Treatment of syringomyelia is generally unsatisfactory. The Chiari tonsillar herniation may be decompressed, generally by suboccipital craniectomy, upper cervical laminectomy, and placement of a dural graft. Fourth ventricular outflow is reestablished by this procedure. If the syrinx cavity is large, some surgeons recommend direct decompression or drainage by one of a number of methods, but the added benefit of this procedure is uncertain, and complications are common. With Chiari malformations, shunting of hydrocephalus generally precedes any attempt to correct the syrinx. Surgery may stabilize the neurologic deficit, and some patients improve. Patients with few symptoms and signs from the syrinx do not require surgery and are followed by serial clinical and imaging examinations.

Syrinx cavities secondary to trauma or infection, if symptomatic, are treated with a decompression and drainage procedure in which a small shunt is inserted between the cavity and subarachnoid space; alternatively, the cavity can be fenestrated. Cases due to intramedullary spinal cord tumor are generally managed by resection of the tumor.

CHRONIC MYELOPATHY OF MULTIPLE SCLEROSIS

A chronic progressive myelopathy is the most frequent cause of disability in both primary progressive and secondary progressive forms of MS. Involvement is typically bilateral but asymmetric and produces motor, sensory, and bladder/bowel disturbances. Fixed motor disability appears to result from extensive loss of axons in the corticospinal tracts. Diagnosis is facilitated by identification of earlier attacks such as optic neuritis. MRI, CSF, and evoked response testing are confirmatory. Disease-modifying therapy is indicated for patients with progressive myelopathy who also have coexisting MS relapses. Therapy is sometimes offered to patients who have a progressive course without relapses but with "active" MRI scans (e.g., the presence of new focal demyelinating lesions) despite the lack of evidence supporting the value of treatment in this setting. MS is discussed in Chap. 458.

SUBACUTE COMBINED DEGENERATION (VITAMIN B_{12} DEFICIENCY)

This treatable myelopathy presents with subacute paresthesias in the hands and feet, loss of vibration and position sensation, and a progressive spastic and ataxic weakness. Loss of reflexes due to an associated peripheral neuropathy in a patient who also has Babinski signs is an important diagnostic clue. Optic atrophy and irritability or other cognitive changes may be prominent in advanced cases and are occasionally the presenting symptoms. The myelopathy of subacute combined degeneration tends to be diffuse rather than focal; signs are generally symmetric and reflect predominant involvement of the posterior and lateral tracts, including Romberg's sign. The diagnosis is confirmed by the finding of macrocytic red blood cells, a low serum B_{12} concentration, elevated serum levels of homocysteine and methylmalonic acid, and in uncertain cases, testing for anti–parietal cell antibodies and a Schilling test. Treatment is by replacement therapy, beginning with 1000 μg of intramuscular vitamin B_{12} repeated at regular intervals or by subsequent oral treatment (Chap. 128).

HYPOCUPRIC MYELOPATHY

This myelopathy is similar to subacute combined degeneration (described above), except there is no neuropathy, and explains cases with normal serum levels of B_{12}. Low levels of serum copper are found, and often there is also a low level of serum ceruloplasmin. Some cases follow gastrointestinal procedures, particularly bariatric surgery, that result in impaired copper absorption; others have been associated with excess zinc from health food supplements or, until recently, zinc-containing denture creams, all of which impair copper absorption via induction of metallothionein, a copper-binding protein. Many cases are idiopathic. Improvement or at least stabilization may be expected with reconstitution of copper stores by oral supplementation. There is microcytic or macrocytic anemia. The pathophysiology and pathology of the idiopathic form are not known.

TABES DORSALIS

The classic syphilitic syndromes of tabes dorsalis and meningovascular inflammation of the spinal cord are now less frequent than in the past but must be considered in the differential diagnosis of spinal cord disorders. The characteristic symptoms of tabes are fleeting and repetitive lancinating pains, primarily in the legs or less often in the back, thorax, abdomen, arms, and face. Ataxia of the legs and gait due to loss of position sense occurs in half of patients. Paresthesias, bladder disturbances, and acute abdominal pain with vomiting (visceral crisis) occur in 15–30% of patients. The cardinal signs of tabes are loss of reflexes in the legs; impaired position and vibratory sense; Romberg's sign; and, in almost all cases, bilateral Argyll Robertson pupils, which fail to constrict to light but accommodate. Diabetic polyradiculopathy may simulate tabes.

FAMILIAL SPASTIC PARAPLEGIA

Many cases of slowly progressive myelopathy are genetic in origin (Chap. 452). More than 30 different causative loci have been identified, including autosomal dominant, autosomal recessive, and X-linked forms. Especially for the recessive and X-linked forms, a family history of myelopathy may be lacking. Most patients present with almost imperceptibly progressive spasticity and weakness in the legs, usually but not always symmetrical. Sensory symptoms and signs are absent or mild, but sphincter disturbances may be present. In some families, additional neurologic signs are prominent, including nystagmus, ataxia, or optic atrophy. The onset may be as early as the first year of life or as late as middle adulthood. Only symptomatic therapies are available.

ADRENOMYELONEUROPATHY

This X-linked disorder is a variant of adrenoleukodystrophy. Most affected males have a history of adrenal insufficiency and then develop a progressive spastic (or ataxic) paraparesis beginning in early or sometimes middle adulthood; some patients also have a mild peripheral neuropathy. Female heterozygotes may develop a slower, insidiously progressive spastic myelopathy beginning later in adulthood and without adrenal insufficiency. Diagnosis is usually made by demonstration of elevated levels of very-long-chain fatty acids in plasma and in cultured fibroblasts. The responsible gene encodes the adrenoleukodystrophy protein (ADLP), a peroxisomal membrane transporter involved in carrying long-chain fatty acids to peroxisomes for degradation. Corticosteroid replacement is indicated if hypoadrenalism is present, and bone marrow transplantation and nutritional supplements have been attempted for this condition without clear evidence of efficacy.

OTHER CHRONIC MYELOPATHIES

Primary lateral sclerosis (Chap. 452) is a degenerative disorder characterized by progressive spasticity with weakness, eventually accompanied by dysarthria and dysphonia; bladder symptoms occur in approximately half of patients. Sensory function is spared. The disorder resembles ALS and is considered a variant of the motor neuron degenerations, but without the characteristic lower motor neuron disturbance. Some cases may represent familial spastic paraplegia, particularly autosomal recessive or X-linked varieties in which a family history may be absent.

Tethered cord syndrome is a developmental disorder of the lower spinal cord and nerve roots that rarely presents in adulthood as low back pain accompanied by a progressive lower spinal cord and/or nerve root syndrome. Some patients have a small leg or foot deformity indicating a long-standing process, and in others, a dimple, patch of hair, or sinus tract on the skin overlying the lower back is the clue to a congenital lesion. Diagnosis is made by MRI, which demonstrates a low-lying conus medullaris and thickened filum terminale. The MRI may also reveal diastematomyelia (division of the lower spinal cord into two halves), lipomas, cysts, or other congenital abnormalities of the lower spine coexisting with the tethered cord. Treatment is with surgical release.

There are a number of rare toxic causes of spastic myelopathy, including lathyrism due to ingestion of chickpeas containing the excitotoxin β-*N*-oxalylamino-L-alanine (BOAA), seen primarily in the developing world, and nitrous oxide inhalation producing a myelopathy identical to subacute combined degeneration. SLE, Sjögren's syndrome, and sarcoidosis may each cause a myelopathy without overt evidence of systemic disease. Cancer-related causes of chronic myelopathy, besides the common neoplastic compressive myelopathy discussed earlier, include radiation injury (Chap. 118) and rare paraneoplastic myelopathies. The last of these are most often associated with lung or breast cancer and anti-Hu antibodies (Chap. 122) or with lymphoma that causes a syndrome of destruction of anterior horn cells; NMO (Chap. 458) can also rarely be paraneoplastic in origin. Metastases to the cord are probably more common than either of these in patients with cancer. Often, a cause of intrinsic myelopathy can be identified only through periodic reassessment.

REHABILITATION OF SPINAL CORD DISORDERS

The prospects for recovery from an acute destructive spinal cord lesion fade after ~6 months. There are currently no effective means to

TABLE 456-4 EXPECTED NEUROLOGIC FUNCTION FOLLOWING COMPLETE CORD LESIONS

Level	Self-Care	Transfers	Maximum Mobility
High quadriplegia (C1-C4)	Dependent on others; requires respiratory support	Dependent on others	Motorized wheelchair
Low quadriplegia (C5-C8)	Partially independent with adaptive equipment	May be dependent or independent	May use manual wheelchair, drive an automobile with adaptive equipment
Paraplegia (below T1)	Independent	Independent	Ambulates short distances with aids

Source: Adapted from JF Ditunno, CS Formal: Chronic spinal cord injury. N Engl J Med 330:550, 1994; with permission.

promote repair of injured spinal cord tissue; promising but entirely experimental approaches include the use of factors that influence reinnervation by axons of the corticospinal tract, nerve and neural sheath graft bridges, forms of electrical stimulation at the site of injury, and the local introduction of stem cells. The disability associated with irreversible spinal cord damage is determined primarily by the level of the lesion and by whether the disturbance in function is complete or incomplete (Table 456-4). Even a complete high cervical cord lesion may be compatible with a productive life. The primary goals are development of a rehabilitation plan framed by realistic expectations and attention to the neurologic, medical, and psychological complications that commonly arise.

Many of the usual symptoms associated with medical illnesses, especially somatic and visceral pain, may be lacking because of the destruction of afferent pain pathways. Unexplained fever, worsening of spasticity, or deterioration in neurologic function should prompt a search for infection, thrombophlebitis, or an intraabdominal pathology. The loss of normal thermoregulation and inability to maintain normal body temperature can produce recurrent fever (*quadriplegic fever*), although most episodes of fever are due to infection of the urinary tract, lung, skin, or bone.

Bladder dysfunction generally results from loss of supraspinal innervation of the detrusor muscle of the bladder wall and the sphincter musculature. Detrusor spasticity is treated with anticholinergic drugs (oxybutynin, 2.5–5 mg qid) or tricyclic antidepressants with anticholinergic properties (imipramine, 25–200 mg/d). Failure of the sphincter muscle to relax during bladder emptying (urinary dyssynergia) may be managed with the α-adrenergic blocking agent terazosin hydrochloride (1–2 mg tid or qid), with intermittent catheterization, or, if that is not feasible, by use of a condom catheter in men or a permanent indwelling catheter. Surgical options include the creation of an artificial bladder by isolating a segment of intestine that can be catheterized intermittently (enterocystoplasty) or can drain continuously to an external appliance (urinary conduit). Bladder areflexia due to acute spinal shock or conus lesions is best treated by catheterization. Bowel regimens and disimpaction are necessary in most patients to ensure at least biweekly evacuation and avoid colonic distention or obstruction.

Patients with acute cord injury are at risk for venous thrombosis and pulmonary embolism. Use of calf-compression devices and anticoagulation with low-molecular-weight heparin is recommended. In cases of persistent paralysis, anticoagulation should probably be continued for 3 months.

Prophylaxis against decubitus ulcers should involve frequent changes in position in a chair or bed, the use of special mattresses, and cushioning of areas where pressure sores often develop, such as the sacral prominence and heels. Early treatment of ulcers with careful cleansing, surgical or enzyme debridement of necrotic tissue, and appropriate dressing and drainage may prevent infection of adjacent soft tissue or bone.

Spasticity is aided by stretching exercises to maintain mobility of joints. Drug treatment is effective but may result in reduced function, as some patients depend on spasticity as an aid to stand, transfer, or walk. Baclofen (up to 240 mg/d in divided doses) is effective; it acts by facilitating γ-aminobutyric acid–mediated inhibition of motor reflex arcs. Diazepam acts by a similar mechanism and is useful for leg spasms that interrupt sleep (2–4 mg at bedtime). Tizanidine (2–8 mg tid), an α_2 adrenergic agonist that increases presynaptic inhibition of motor neurons, is another option. For nonambulatory patients, the direct muscle inhibitor dantrolene (25–100 mg qid) may be used, but it is potentially hepatotoxic. In refractory cases, intrathecal baclofen administered via an implanted pump, botulinum toxin injections, or dorsal rhizotomy may be required to control spasticity.

Despite the loss of sensory function, many patients with spinal cord injury experience chronic pain sufficient to diminish their quality of life. Randomized controlled studies indicate that gabapentin or pregabalin is useful in this setting. Epidural electrical stimulation and intrathecal infusion of pain medications have been tried with some success. Management of chronic pain is discussed in Chap. 18.

A paroxysmal autonomic hyperreflexia may occur following lesions above the major splanchnic sympathetic outflow at T6. Headache, flushing, and diaphoresis above the level of the lesion, as well as hypertension with bradycardia or tachycardia, are the major symptoms. The trigger is typically a noxious stimulus—for example, bladder or bowel distention, a urinary tract infection, or a decubitus ulcer—below the level of the cord lesion. Treatment consists of removal of offending stimuli; ganglionic blocking agents (mecamylamine, 2.5–5 mg) or other short-acting antihypertensive drugs are useful in some patients.

Attention to these details allows longevity and a productive life for patients with complete transverse myelopathies.

457e Concussion and Other Traumatic Brain Injuries

Allan H. Ropper

This is a digital-only chapter. It is available on the DVD that accompanies this book, as well as on Access Medicine/Harrison's Online, and the eBook and "app" editions of HPIM 19e.

Almost 10 million head injuries occur annually in the United States, about 20% of which are serious enough to cause brain damage. Among men <35 years, accidents, usually motor vehicle collisions, are the chief cause of death and >70% of these involve head injury. Furthermore, minor head injuries are so common that almost all physicians will be called upon to provide immediate care or to see patients who are suffering from various sequelae.

Medical personnel caring for head injury patients should be aware that (1) spinal injury often accompanies head injury, and care must be taken in handling the patient to prevent compression of the spinal cord due to instability of the spinal column; (2) intoxication is frequently associated with traumatic brain injury, and thus testing for drugs and alcohol should be carried out when appropriate; and (3) additional injuries, including rupture of abdominal organs, may produce vascular collapse, shock, or respiratory distress that requires immediate attention.

458 Multiple Sclerosis and Other Demyelinating Diseases

Stephen L. Hauser, Douglas S. Goodin

Demyelinating disorders are immune-mediated conditions characterized by preferential destruction of central nervous system (CNS) myelin. The peripheral nervous system (PNS) is spared, and most patients have no evidence of an associated systemic illness. Multiple sclerosis, the most common disease in this category, is second only to trauma as a cause of neurologic disability beginning in early to middle adulthood.

MULTIPLE SCLEROSIS

Multiple sclerosis (MS) is an autoimmune disease of the CNS characterized by chronic inflammation, demyelination, gliosis (scarring), and neuronal loss; the course can be relapsing-remitting or progressive. Lesions of MS typically develop at different times and in different CNS locations (i.e., MS is said to be disseminated in time and space). Approximately 350,000 individuals in the United States and 2.5 million individuals worldwide are affected. The clinical course can be extremely variable, ranging from a benign condition to a rapidly evolving and incapacitating disease requiring profound lifestyle adjustments.

PATHOGENESIS

Pathology New MS lesions begin with perivenular cuffing by inflammatory mononuclear cells, predominantly T cells and macrophages, which also infiltrate the surrounding white matter. At sites of inflammation, the blood-brain barrier (BBB) is disrupted, but unlike vasculitis, the vessel wall is preserved. Involvement of the humoral immune system is also evident; small numbers of B lymphocytes also infiltrate the nervous system, myelin-specific autoantibodies are present on degenerating myelin sheaths, and complement is activated. Demyelination is the hallmark of the pathology, and evidence of myelin degeneration is found at the earliest time points of tissue injury. A remarkable feature of MS plaques is that oligodendrocyte precursor cells survive—and in many lesions are present in even greater numbers than in normal tissue—but these cells fail to differentiate into mature myelin-producing cells. In some lesions, surviving oligodendrocytes or those that differentiate from precursor cells partially remyelinate the surviving naked axons, producing so-called *shadow plaques*. As lesions evolve, there is prominent astrocytic proliferation (gliosis). Over time, ectopic lymphocyte follicle-like structures, consisting of aggregates of T and B cells resembling secondary lymphoid tissue, appear in the meninges and especially overlying deep cortical sulci and also in perivascular spaces. Although relative sparing of axons is typical of MS, partial or total axonal destruction can also occur, especially within highly inflammatory lesions. Thus MS is not solely a disease of myelin, and neuronal pathology is increasingly recognized as a major contributor to irreversible neurologic disability. Inflammation, demyelination, and plaque formation are also present in the cerebral cortex, and significant axon loss indicating death of neurons is widespread, especially in advanced cases (see "Neurodegeneration," below).

Physiology Nerve conduction in myelinated axons occurs in a saltatory manner, with the nerve impulse jumping from one node of Ranvier to the next without depolarization of the axonal membrane underlying the myelin sheath between nodes (Fig. 458-1). This produces considerably faster conduction velocities (~70 m/s) than the slow velocities (~1 m/s) produced by continuous propagation in unmyelinated nerves. Conduction block occurs when the nerve impulse is unable to traverse the demyelinated segment. This can happen when the resting axon membrane becomes hyperpolarized due to the exposure of voltage-dependent potassium channels that are normally buried underneath the myelin sheath. A temporary conduction block often follows a demyelinating event before sodium channels (originally concentrated at the nodes) redistribute along the naked axon (Fig. 458-1). This redistribution ultimately allows continuous propagation of nerve action potentials through the demyelinated segment. Conduction block may be incomplete, affecting high- but not low-frequency volleys of impulses. Variable conduction block can occur with raised body temperature or metabolic alterations and may explain clinical fluctuations that vary from hour to hour or appear with fever or exercise. Conduction slowing occurs when the demyelinated segments of the axonal membrane are reorganized to support continuous (slow) nerve impulse propagation.

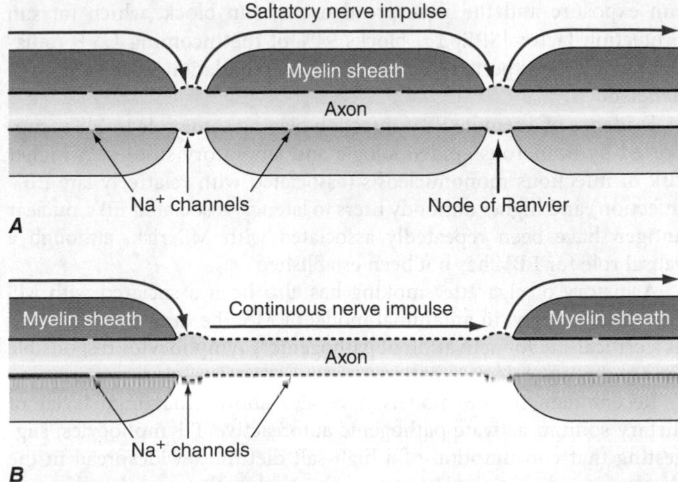

FIGURE 458-1 Nerve conduction in myelinated and demyelinated axons. ***A.*** Saltatory nerve conduction in myelinated axons occurs with the nerve impulse jumping from one node of Ranvier to the next. Sodium channels (shown as breaks in the solid black line) are concentrated at the nodes where axonal depolarization occurs. ***B.*** Following demyelination, additional sodium channels are redistributed along the axon itself, thereby allowing continuous propagation of the nerve action potential despite the absence of myelin.

Epidemiology MS is approximately threefold more common in women than men. The age of onset is typically between 20 and 40 years (slightly later in men than in women), but the disease can present across the lifespan. Approximately 10% of cases begin before age 18 years of age, and a small percentage of cases begin before the age of 10 years.

Geographical gradients have been repeatedly observed in MS, with the highest known prevalence for MS (250 per 100,000) in the Orkney Islands, located north of Scotland. In other temperate zone areas (e.g., northern North America, northern Europe, southern Australia, and southern New Zealand), the prevalence of MS is 0.1–0.2%. By contrast, in the tropics (e.g., Asia, equatorial Africa, and the Middle East), the prevalence is often 10- to 20-fold less.

The prevalence of MS has increased steadily (and dramatically) in several regions around the world over the past half-century, presumably reflecting the impact of some environmental shift. Moreover, the fact that this increase has occurred primarily (or exclusively) in women indicates that women are more responsive to this environmental change.

Well-established risk factors for MS include vitamin D deficiency, exposure to Epstein-Barr virus (EBV) after early childhood, and cigarette smoking.

Vitamin D deficiency is associated with an increase in MS risk, and data suggest that ongoing deficiency may also increase disease activity after MS begins. Immunoregulatory effects of vitamin D could explain these apparent relationships. Exposure of the skin to ultraviolet-B (UVB) radiation from the sun is essential for the biosynthesis of vitamin D, and this endogenous production is the most important source of vitamin D in most individuals; a diet rich in fatty fish represents another source of vitamin D. At high latitudes, the amount of UVB radiation reaching the earth's surface is often insufficient, particularly during winter months, and consequently, low serum levels of vitamin D are common in temperate zones. The common practice to avoid direct sun exposure and the widespread use of sun block, which (at sun protection factor [SPF] 15) blocks 94% of the incoming UVB radiation, would be expected to exacerbate any population-wide vitamin D deficiency.

Evidence of a remote EBV infection playing some role in MS is supported by numerous epidemiologic and laboratory studies. A higher risk of infectious mononucleosis (associated with relatively late EBV infection) and higher antibody titers to latency-associated EBV nuclear antigen have been repeatedly associated with MS risk, although a causal role for EBV has not been established.

A history of cigarette smoking has also been associated with MS risk. Interestingly, in an animal model of MS, the lung was identified as a critical site for activation of pathogenic T lymphocytes responsible for autoimmune demyelination.

Recent data in MS models have also shown that high levels of dietary sodium activate pathogenic autoreactive T lymphocytes, suggesting that consumption of a high-salt diet, now widespread in the Western world, might be part of the explanation for the observed increase in the prevalence of MS in recent years.

GENETIC CONSIDERATIONS

Whites are inherently at higher risk for MS than Africans or Asians, even when residing in a similar environment. MS also aggregates within some families, and adoption, half-sibling, twin, and spousal studies indicate that familial aggregation is due to genetic, and not environmental, factors (Table 458-1).

Susceptibility to MS is polygenic, with each gene contributing a relatively small amount to the overall risk. The strongest susceptibility signal in genome-wide studies maps to the HLA-DRB1 gene in the class II region of the major histocompatibility complex (MHC), and this association accounts for approximately 10% of the disease risk. This HLA association, which was first described several decades ago, suggests that MS, at its core, is an antigen-specific autoimmune disease. Whole-genome association studies have now identified approximately 110 other MS susceptibility variants, each of which individually has only a modest effect on MS risk. Most of these MS-associated genes have known roles in the adaptive immune system, for example the genes for the interleukin (IL) 7 receptor (CD127), IL-2 receptor (CD25), and T cell costimulatory molecule LFA-3 (CD58); some variants also influence susceptibility to other autoimmune diseases in addition to MS. The variants identified so far all lack specificity and sensitivity for MS; thus, at present, they are not useful for diagnosis or to predict the future course of the disease.

IMMUNOLOGY A proinflammatory autoimmune response directed against a component of CNS myelin, and perhaps other neural elements as well, remains the cornerstone of current concepts of MS pathogenesis.

AUTOREACTIVE T LYMPHOCYTES Myelin basic protein (MBP), an intracellular protein involved in myelin compaction, is an important T cell antigen in experimental allergic encephalomyelitis (EAE), a laboratory model, and probably also in human MS. Activated MBP-reactive T cells have been identified in the blood, in cerebrospinal fluid (CSF), and within MS lesions. Moreover, *DRB1*15:01* may influence the autoimmune response because it binds with high affinity to a fragment of MBP (spanning amino acids 89–96), stimulating T cell responses to this self-protein. Two different populations of proinflammatory T cells are likely to mediate autoimmunity in MS. T-helper type 1 (T_H1) cells producing interferon γ (IFN-γ) are one key effector population, and more recently, a role for highly proinflammatory T_H17 T cells has been established. T_H17 cells are induced by transforming growth factor β (TGF-β) and IL-6 and are amplified by IL-21 and IL-23. T_H17 cells, and levels of their corresponding cytokine IL-17, are increased in MS lesions and also in the circulation of people with active MS. High circulating levels of IL-17 may also be a marker of a more severe course of MS. T_H1 cytokines, including IL-2, tumor necrosis factor (TNF)-α, and IFN-γ, also play key roles in activating and maintaining autoimmune responses, and TNF-α and IFN-γ may directly injure oligodendrocytes or the myelin membrane.

TABLE 458-1 RISK OF DEVELOPING MULTIPLE SCLEROSIS (MS)

1 in 3	If an identical twin has MS
1 in 15	If a fraternal twin has MS
1 in 25	If a sibling has MS
1 in 50	If a parent or half-sibling has MS
1 in 100	If a first cousin has MS
1 in 1000	If a spouse has MS
1 in 1000	If no one in the family has MS

HUMORAL AUTOIMMUNITY B cell activation and antibody responses also appear to be necessary for the full development of demyelinating lesions to occur, both in experimental models and in human MS. Clonally restricted populations of activated, antigen-experienced, memory B cells and plasma cells are present in MS lesions, in lymphoid follicle-like structures in the meninges overlying the cerebral cortex, and in the CSF. Similar or identical clonal populations are found in each compartment, indicating that a highly focused B cell response is occurring locally within the CNS in MS. Myelin-specific autoantibodies, some directed against an extracellular myelin protein, myelin oligodendrocyte glycoprotein (MOG), have been detected bound to vesiculated myelin debris in MS plaques. In the CSF, elevated levels of locally synthesized immunoglobulins and oligoclonal antibodies, derived from clonally restricted CNS B cells and plasma cells, are also characteristic of MS. The pattern of oligoclonal banding is unique to each individual, and attempts to identify the targets of these antibodies have been largely unsuccessful.

TRIGGERS Serial magnetic resonance imaging (MRI) studies in early relapsing-remitting MS reveal that bursts of focal inflammatory disease activity occur far more frequently than would have been predicted by the frequency of relapses. Thus, early in MS, most disease activity is clinically silent. Although the triggers causing these bursts are unknown, molecular mimicry between environmental agents, presumably pathogens, and myelin antigens activating pathogenic T cells may be responsible (Chap. 377e).

Neurodegeneration Axonal damage occurs in every newly formed MS lesion, and cumulative axonal loss is considered to be one important cause of irreversible neurologic disability in MS. As many as 70% of axons are lost from the lateral corticospinal (e.g., motor) tracts in patients with advanced paraparesis from MS, and longitudinal MRI studies suggest there is progressive axonal loss over time within established, inactive lesions. Demyelination can result in reduced trophic support for axons, redistribution of ion channels, and destabilization of action potential membrane potentials. Axons can adapt initially to these injuries, but over time, distal and retrograde degeneration often occurs. Therefore, promoting remyelination remains an important therapeutic goal.

In progressive MS, a key unresolved question is whether the primary neurodegenerative process occurs primarily in the cerebral cortex, the white matter, or in some combination of the two sites. As noted above, meningeal infiltrates of B and T cells are particularly prominent in progressive MS cases, and these "lymphoid follicles" are associated with underlying microglial activation, gray matter plaques, and loss of cortical neurons. White matter lesions may also contribute to late progressive MS; inactive plaques are often noninflammatory at the center, but at the edges, microglia and macrophages and evidence of ongoing axonal injury can be found. This suggests that a simmering, and possibly concentrically expanding, axonopathy may be present, even in the most chronic cases. In addition, a diffuse low-grade inflammation across large areas of white matter may be present, associated with reduced myelin staining and axonal injury ("dirty white matter"). Another characteristic of progressive MS is that inflammation is often present without a concomitant disruption of the BBB; possibly, this feature might explain the failure of immunotherapies not capable of crossing the BBB to benefit patients with progressive MS.

Evidence supports a role of one, or more likely several, of the following mechanisms in progressive MS. Axonal and neuronal death may result from glutamate-mediated excitotoxicity, oxidative injury, iron accumulation, and/or mitochondrial failure either occurring as a consequence of free-radical damage or due to accumulation of deletions in mitochondrial DNA.

CLINICAL MANIFESTATIONS

The onset of MS may be abrupt or insidious. Symptoms may be severe or seem so trivial that a patient may not seek medical attention for months or years. Indeed, at autopsy, approximately 0.1% of individuals who were asymptomatic during life will be found, unexpectedly, to have pathologic evidence of MS. Similarly, in the modern era, an MRI scan obtained for an unrelated reason may show evidence of asymptomatic MS. Symptoms of MS are extremely varied and depend on the location and severity of lesions within the CNS (Table 458-2). Examination often reveals evidence of neurologic dysfunction, often in asymptomatic locations. For example, a patient may present with symptoms in one leg but signs in both.

Weakness of the limbs may manifest as loss of strength, speed, or dexterity, as fatigue, or as a disturbance of gait. Exercise-induced weakness is a characteristic symptom of MS. The weakness is of the upper motor neuron type (Chap. 30) and is usually accompanied by other pyramidal signs such as spasticity, hyperreflexia, and Babinski signs. Occasionally a tendon reflex may be lost (simulating a lower motor neuron lesion) if an MS lesion disrupts the afferent reflex fibers in the spinal cord (see Fig. 30-2).

Spasticity (Chap. 30) is commonly associated with spontaneous and movement-induced muscle spasms. More than 30% of MS patients have moderate to severe spasticity, especially in the legs. This is often accompanied by painful spasms interfering with ambulation, work, or self-care. Occasionally spasticity provides support for the body weight during ambulation, and in these cases, treatment of spasticity may actually do more harm than good.

Optic neuritis (ON) presents as diminished visual acuity, dimness, or decreased color perception (desaturation) in the central field of vision. These symptoms can be mild or may progress to severe visual loss. Rarely, there is complete loss of light perception. Visual symptoms are generally monocular but may be bilateral. Periorbital pain (aggravated by eye movement) often precedes or accompanies the visual loss. An afferent pupillary defect (Chap. 39) is usually present. Funduscopic examination may be normal or reveal optic disc swelling (papillitis). Pallor of the optic disc (optic atrophy) commonly follows ON. Uveitis is uncommon and should raise the possibility of alternative diagnoses such as sarcoid or lymphoma.

Visual blurring in MS may result from ON or diplopia (double vision); if the symptom resolves when either eye is covered, the cause is diplopia.

Diplopia may result from internuclear ophthalmoplegia (INO) or from palsy of the sixth cranial nerve (rarely the third or fourth). An INO consists of impaired adduction of one eye due to a lesion in the ipsilateral medial longitudinal fasciculus (Chaps. 41e and 42).

TABLE 458-2 INITIAL SYMPTOMS OF MS

Symptom	Percentage of Cases	Symptom	Percentage of Cases
Sensory loss	37	Lhermitte	3
Optic neuritis	36	Pain	3
Weakness	35	Dementia	2
Paresthesias	24	Visual loss	2
Diplopia	15	Facial palsy	1
Ataxia	11	Impotence	1
Vertigo	6	Myokymia	1
Paroxysmal attacks	4	Epilepsy	1
Bladder	4	Falling	1

Source: After WB Matthews et al: *McAlpine's Multiple Sclerosis*. New York, Churchill Livingstone, 1991.

Prominent nystagmus is often observed in the abducting eye, along with a small skew deviation. A bilateral INO is particularly suggestive of MS. Other common gaze disturbances in MS include (1) a horizontal gaze palsy, (2) a "one and a half" syndrome (horizontal gaze palsy plus an INO), and (3) acquired pendular nystagmus.

Sensory symptoms are varied and include both paresthesias (e.g., tingling, prickling sensations, formications, "pins and needles," or painful burning) and hypesthesia (e.g., reduced sensation, numbness, or a "dead" feeling). Unpleasant sensations (e.g., feelings that body parts are swollen, wet, raw, or tightly wrapped) are also common. Sensory impairment of the trunk and legs below a horizontal line on the torso (a sensory level) indicates that the spinal cord is the origin of the sensory disturbance. It is often accompanied by a bandlike sensation of tightness around the torso. Pain is a common symptom of MS, experienced by >50% of patients. Pain can occur anywhere on the body and can change locations over time.

Ataxia usually manifests as cerebellar tremors (Chap. 450). Ataxia may also involve the head and trunk or the voice, producing a characteristic cerebellar dysarthria (scanning speech).

Bladder dysfunction is present in >90% of MS patients, and in a third of patients, dysfunction results in weekly or more frequent episodes of incontinence. During normal reflex voiding, relaxation of the bladder sphincter (α-adrenergic innervation) is coordinated with contraction of the detrusor muscle in the bladder wall (muscarinic cholinergic innervation). *Detrusor hyperreflexia*, due to impairment of suprasegmental inhibition, causes urinary frequency, urgency, nocturia, and uncontrolled bladder emptying. *Detrusor sphincter dyssynergia*, due to loss of synchronization between detrusor and sphincter muscles, causes difficulty in initiating and/or stopping the urinary stream, producing hesitancy, urinary retention, overflow incontinence, and recurrent infection.

Constipation occurs in >30% of patients. Fecal urgency or *bowel incontinence* is less common (<15%) but can be socially debilitating.

Cognitive dysfunction can include memory loss; impaired attention; difficulties in executive functioning, memory, and problem solving; slowed information processing; and problems shifting between cognitive tasks. Euphoria (elevated mood) was once thought to be characteristic of MS but is actually uncommon, occurring in <20% of patients. Cognitive dysfunction sufficient to impair activities of daily living is rare.

Depression, experienced by approximately half of patients, can be reactive, endogenous, or part of the illness itself and can contribute to fatigue.

Fatigue (Chap. 29) is experienced by 90% of patients; this symptom is the most common reason for work-related disability in MS. Fatigue can be exacerbated by elevated temperatures, depression, expending exceptional effort to accomplish basic activities of daily living, or sleep disturbances (e.g., from frequent nocturnal awakenings to urinate).

Sexual dysfunction may manifest as decreased libido, impaired genital sensation, impotence in men, and diminished vaginal lubrication or adductor spasms in women.

Facial weakness due to a lesion in the pons may resemble idiopathic Bell's palsy (Chap. 455). Unlike Bell's palsy, facial weakness in MS is usually not associated with ipsilateral loss of taste sensation or retroauricular pain.

Vertigo may appear suddenly from a brainstem lesion, superficially resembling acute labyrinthitis (Chap. 28). *Hearing loss* (Chap. 43) may also occur in MS but is uncommon.

Ancillary Symptoms *Heat sensitivity* refers to neurologic symptoms produced by an elevation of the body's core temperature. For example, unilateral visual blurring may occur during a hot shower or with physical exercise (*Uhthoff's symptom*). It is also common for MS symptoms to worsen transiently, sometimes dramatically, during febrile illnesses (see "Acute Attacks or Initial Demyelinating Episodes," below). Such heat-related symptoms probably result from transient conduction block (see above).

Lhermitte's symptom is an electric shock–like sensation (typically induced by flexion or other movements of the neck) that radiates down the back into the legs. Rarely, it radiates into the arms. It is generally self-limited but may persist for years. Lhermitte's symptom can also occur with other disorders of the cervical spinal cord (e.g., cervical spondylosis).

Paroxysmal symptoms are distinguished by their brief duration (10 s to 2 min), high frequency (5–40 episodes per day), lack of any alteration of consciousness or change in background electroencephalogram during episodes, and a self-limited course (generally lasting weeks to months). They may be precipitated by hyperventilation or movement. These syndromes may include Lhermitte's symptom; tonic contractions of a limb, face, or trunk (tonic seizures); paroxysmal dysarthria and ataxia; paroxysmal sensory disturbances; and several other less well-characterized syndromes. Paroxysmal symptoms probably result from spontaneous discharges, arising at the edges of demyelinated plaques and spreading to adjacent white matter tracts.

Trigeminal neuralgia, hemifacial spasm, and *glossopharyngeal neuralgia* (Chap. 455) can occur when the demyelinating lesion involves the root entry (or exit) zone of the fifth, seventh, and ninth cranial nerve, respectively. Trigeminal neuralgia (tic douloureux) is a very brief lancinating facial pain often triggered by an afferent input from the face or teeth. Most cases of trigeminal neuralgia are not MS related; however, atypical features such as onset before age 50 years, bilateral symptoms, objective sensory loss, or nonparoxysmal pain should raise the possibility that MS could be responsible.

Facial myokymia consists of either persistent rapid flickering contractions of the facial musculature (especially the lower portion of the orbicularis oculus) or a contraction that slowly spreads across the face. It results from lesions of the corticobulbar tracts or brainstem course of the facial nerve.

DISEASE COURSE

Four clinical types of MS exist (Fig. 458-2):

1. *Relapsing/remitting MS* (RRMS) accounts for 85% of MS cases at onset and is characterized by discrete attacks that generally evolve over days to weeks (rarely over hours). With initial attacks, there is often substantial or complete recovery over the ensuing weeks to months, but as attacks continue over time recovery may be less evident (Fig. 458-2*A*). Between attacks, patients are neurologically stable.
2. *Secondary progressive MS* (SPMS) always begins as RRMS (Fig. 458-2*B*). At some point, however, the clinical course changes so that the patient experiences a steady deterioration in function unassociated with acute attacks (which may continue or cease during the progressive phase). SPMS produces a greater amount of fixed neurologic disability than RRMS. For a patient with RRMS, the risk of developing SPMS is ~2% each year, meaning that the great majority of RRMS ultimately evolves into SPMS. SPMS appears to represent a late stage of the same underlying illness as RRMS.
3. *Primary progressive MS* (PPMS) accounts for ~15% of cases. These patients do not experience attacks but only a steady functional decline from disease onset (Fig. 458-2*C*). Compared to RRMS, the sex distribution is more even, the disease begins later in life (mean age ~40 years), and disability develops faster (at least relative to the onset of the first clinical symptom). Despite these differences, PPMS appears to represent the same underlying illness as RRMS.
4. *Progressive/relapsing MS* (PRMS) overlaps PPMS and SPMS and accounts for ~5% of MS patients. Like patients with PPMS, these patients experience a steady deterioration in their condition from disease onset. However, like SPMS patients, they experience occasional attacks superimposed upon their progressive course (Fig. 458-2*D*).

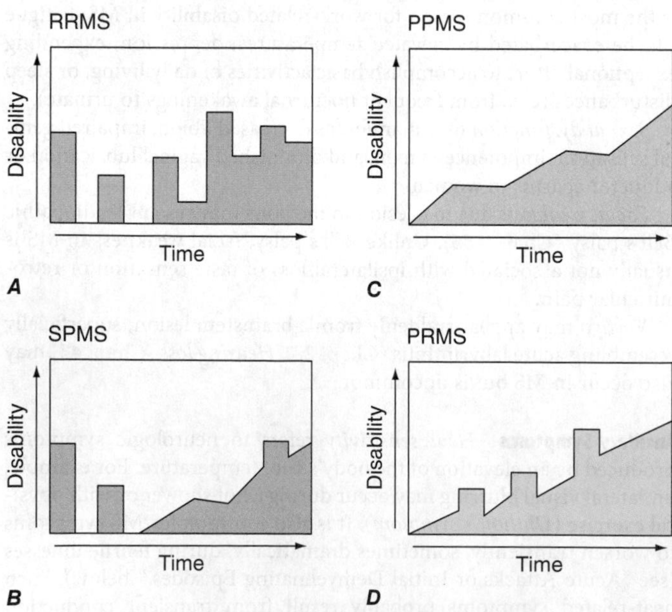

FIGURE 458-2 Clinical course of multiple sclerosis (MS). ***A.*** Relapsing/remitting MS (RRMS). ***B.*** Secondary progressive MS (SPMS). ***C.*** Primary progressive MS (PPMS). ***D.*** Progressive/relapsing MS (PRMS).

DIAGNOSIS

There is no definitive diagnostic test for MS. Diagnostic criteria for clinically definite MS require documentation of two or more episodes of symptoms and two or more signs that reflect pathology in anatomically noncontiguous white matter tracts of the CNS (Table 458-3). Symptoms must last for >24 h and occur as distinct episodes that are separated by a month or more. In patients who have only one of the two required signs on neurologic examination, the second may be documented by abnormal tests such as MRI or evoked potentials (EPs). Similarly, in the most recent diagnostic scheme, the second clinical event (in time) may be supported solely by MRI findings, consisting of either the development of new focal white matter lesions on MRI or the simultaneous presence of both an enhancing lesion and a nonenhancing lesion in an asymptomatic location. In patients whose course is progressive from onset for ≥6 months without superimposed relapses, documentation of intrathecal IgG synthesis may be used to support a diagnosis of PPMS.

DIAGNOSTIC TESTS

Magnetic Resonance Imaging MRI has revolutionized the diagnosis and management of MS (Fig. 458-3); characteristic abnormalities are found in >95% of patients, although more than 90% of the lesions visualized by MRI are asymptomatic. An increase in vascular permeability from a breakdown of the BBB is detected by leakage of intravenous gadolinium (Gd) into the parenchyma. Such leakage occurs early in the development of an MS lesion and serves as a useful marker of inflammation. Gd enhancement typically persists for approximately 1 month, and the residual MS plaque remains visible indefinitely as a focal area of hyperintensity (a lesion) on spin-echo (T2-weighted) and proton-density images. Lesions are frequently oriented perpendicular to the ventricular surface, corresponding to the pathologic pattern of perivenous demyelination (Dawson's fingers). Lesions are multifocal within the brain, brainstem, and spinal cord. Lesions larger than 6 mm located in the corpus callosum, periventricular white matter, brainstem, cerebellum, or spinal cord are particularly helpful diagnostically. Current criteria for the use of MRI in the diagnosis of MS are shown in Table 458-3.

The total volume of T2-weighted signal abnormality (the "burden of disease") shows a significant (albeit weak) correlation with clinical disability, as do measures of brain atrophy. Approximately one-third of T2-weighted lesions appear as hypointense lesions (black holes) on T1-weighted imaging. Black holes may be a marker of irreversible demyelination and axonal loss, although even this measure depends on the timing of the image acquisition (e.g., most acute Gd-enhancing T2 lesions are T1 dark).

Newer MRI methods such as magnetization transfer ratio (MTR) imaging and proton magnetic resonance spectroscopic imaging (MRSI) may ultimately serve as surrogate markers of clinical disability. MRSI can quantitate molecules such as *N*-acetyl aspartate, which

TABLE 458-3 DIAGNOSTIC CRITERIA FOR MULTIPLE SCLEROSIS (MS)

Clinical Presentation	Additional Data Needed for MS Diagnosis
2 or more attacks; objective clinical evidence of 2 or more lesions or objective clinical evidence of 1 lesion with reasonable historical evidence of a prior attack	None
2 or more attacks; objective clinical evidence of 1 lesion	Dissemination in space, demonstrated by • ≥1 T2 lesion on MRI in at least 2 out of 4 MS-typical regions of the CNS (periventricular, juxtacortical, infratentorial, or spinal cord) OR • Await a further clinical attack implicating a different CNS site
1 attack; objective clinical evidence of 2 or more lesions	Dissemination in time, demonstrated by • Simultaneous presence of asymptomatic gadolinium-enhancing and nonenhancing lesions at any time OR • A new T2 and/or gadolinium-enhancing lesion(s) on follow-up MRI, irrespective of its timing with reference to a baseline scan OR • Await a second clinical attack
1 attack; objective clinical evidence of 1 lesion (clinically isolated syndrome)	Dissemination in space and time, demonstrated by: For dissemination in space • ≥1 T2 lesion in at least 2 out of 4 MS-typical regions of the CNS (periventricular, juxtacortical, infratentorial, or spinal cord) OR • Await a second clinical attack implicating a different CNS site AND For dissemination in time • Simultaneous presence of asymptomatic gadolinium-enhancing and nonenhancing lesions at any time OR • A new T2 and/or gadolinium-enhancing lesion(s) on follow-up MRI, irrespective of its timing with reference to a baseline scan OR • Await a second clinical attack
Insidious neurologic progression suggestive of MS (PPMS)	1 year of disease progression (retrospectively or prospectively determined) PLUS 2 out of the 3 following criteria Evidence for dissemination in space in the brain based on ≥1 T2+ lesions in the MS-characteristic periventricular, juxtacortical, or infratentorial regions Evidence for dissemination in space in the spinal cord based on ≥2 T2+ lesions in the cord Positive CSF (isoelectric focusing evidence of oligoclonal bands and/or elevated IgG index)

Abbreviations: CNS, central nervous system; CSF, cerebrospinal fluid; MRI, magnetic resonance imaging; PPMS, primary progressive multiple sclerosis.

Source: From CH Polman et al: Diagnostic Criteria for Multiple Sclerosis: 2010 Revisions to the "McDonald Criteria." Ann Neurol 69:292, 2011.

is a marker of axonal integrity, and MTR may be able to distinguish demyelination from edema.

Evoked Potentials EP testing assesses function in afferent (visual, auditory, and somatosensory) or efferent (motor) CNS pathways. EPs use computer averaging to measure CNS electric potentials evoked by repetitive stimulation of selected peripheral nerves or of the brain. These tests provide the most information when the pathways studied are clinically uninvolved. For example, in a patient with a remitting and relapsing spinal cord syndrome with sensory deficits in the legs, an abnormal somatosensory EP following posterior tibial nerve stimulation provides little new information. By contrast, an abnormal visual EP in this circumstance would permit a diagnosis of clinically definite MS (Table 458-3). Abnormalities on one or more EP modalities occur in 80–90% of MS patients. EP abnormalities are not specific to MS, although a marked delay in the latency of a specific EP component (as opposed to a reduced amplitude or distorted wave-shape) is suggestive of demyelination.

Cerebrospinal Fluid CSF abnormalities found in MS include a mononuclear cell pleocytosis and an increased level of intrathecally synthesized IgG. The total CSF protein is usually normal. Various formulas distinguish intrathecally synthesized IgG from IgG that may have entered the CNS passively from the serum. One formula, the CSF IgG index, expresses the ratio of IgG to albumin in the CSF divided by the same ratio in the serum. The IgG synthesis rate uses serum and CSF IgG and albumin measurements to calculate the rate of CNS IgG synthesis. The measurement of oligoclonal bands (OCBs) by agarose gel electrophoresis in the CSF also assesses intrathecal production of IgG. Two or more discrete OCBs, not present in a paired serum sample, are found in >75% of patients with MS. OCBs may be absent at the onset of MS, and in individual patients, the number of bands may increase with time.

A mild CSF pleocytosis (>5 cells/μL) is present in ~25% of cases, usually in young patients with RRMS. A pleocytosis of >75 cells/μL, the presence of polymorphonuclear leukocytes, or a protein concentration >1 g/L (>100 mg/dL) in CSF should raise concern that the patient may not have MS.

DIFFERENTIAL DIAGNOSIS

No single clinical sign or test is diagnostic of MS. The diagnosis is readily made in a young adult with relapsing and remitting symptoms involving different areas of CNS white matter. The possibility of an alternative diagnosis should always be considered (Table 458-4), particularly when (1) symptoms are localized exclusively to the posterior fossa, craniocervical junction, or spinal cord; (2) the patient is <15 or >60 years of age; (3) the clinical course is progressive from onset; (4) the patient has never experienced visual, sensory, or bladder symptoms; or (5) laboratory findings (e.g., MRI, CSF, or EPs) are atypical. Similarly, uncommon or rare symptoms in MS (e.g., aphasia, parkinsonism, chorea, isolated dementia, severe muscular atrophy, peripheral neuropathy, episodic loss of consciousness, fever, headache, seizures, or coma) should increase concern about an alternative diagnosis. Diagnosis is also difficult in patients with a rapid or explosive (stroke-like) onset or with mild symptoms and a normal neurologic examination. Rarely, intense inflammation and swelling may produce a mass lesion that mimics a primary or metastatic tumor. In the current era, the disorders most likely to be mistaken for MS are neuromyelitis optica (see below), sarcoid, vascular disorders (including antiphospholipid syndrome and vasculitis), and rarely CNS lymphoma. The specific tests required to exclude alternative diagnoses will vary with each clinical situation; however, an erythrocyte sedimentation rate, serum B_{12} level, ANA, and treponemal antibody should probably be obtained in all patients with suspected MS.

PROGNOSIS

Most patients with clinically evident MS ultimately experience progressive neurologic disability. In older studies conducted mostly before disease-modifying therapies for MS were widely available, 15 years after onset, only 20% of patients had no functional limitation, and between one-third and one-half progressed to SPMS and required assistance with ambulation; furthermore, 25 years after onset, ~80% of MS patients reached this level of disability. The long-term prognosis for untreated MS appears to have improved in recent years, at least in part because of the development of therapies for the early relapsing form of the disease. Although the prognosis in an individual is

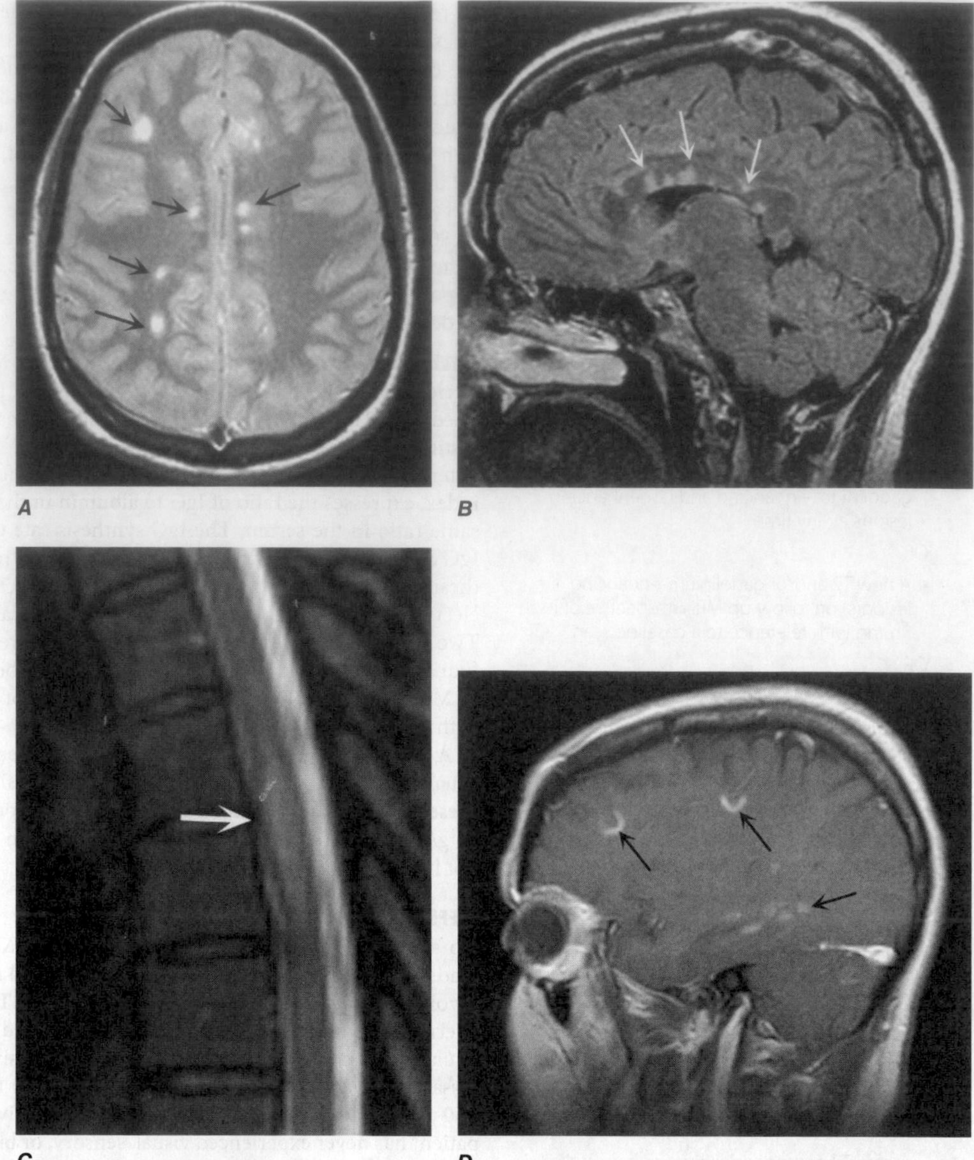

FIGURE 458-3 Magnetic resonance imaging findings in multiple sclerosis (MS). ***A.*** Axial first-echo image from T2-weighted sequence demonstrates multiple bright signal abnormalities in white matter, typical for MS. ***B.*** Sagittal T2-weighted fluid-attenuated inversion recovery (FLAIR) image in which the high signal of cerebrospinal fluid (CSF) has been suppressed. CSF appears dark, whereas areas of brain edema or demyelination appear high in signal as shown here in the corpus callosum (*arrows*). Lesions in the anterior corpus callosum are frequent in MS and rare in vascular disease. ***C.*** Sagittal T2-weighted fast spin echo image of the thoracic spine demonstrates a fusiform high-signal-intensity lesion in the midthoracic spinal cord. ***D.*** Sagittal T1-weighted image obtained after the intravenous administration of gadolinium DTPA reveals focal areas of blood-brain barrier disruption, identified as high-signal-intensity regions (*arrows*).

difficult to establish, certain clinical features suggest a more favorable prognosis. These include ON or sensory symptoms at onset; fewer than two relapses in the first year of illness; and minimal impairment after 5 years. By contrast, patients with truncal ataxia, action tremor, pyramidal symptoms, or a progressive disease course are more likely to become disabled. Patients with a long-term favorable course are likely to have developed fewer MRI lesions during the early years of disease, and vice versa. Importantly, some MS patients have a benign variant of MS and never develop neurologic disability. The likelihood of having benign MS is thought to be <20%. Patients with benign MS 15 years after onset who have entirely normal neurologic examinations are likely to maintain their benign course

In patients with their first demyelinating event (i.e., a clinically isolated syndrome), the brain MRI provides prognostic information. With three or more typical T2-weighted lesions, the risk of developing MS after 20 years is ~80%. Conversely, with a normal brain MRI, the likelihood of developing MS is <20%. Similarly, the presence of two or more Gd-enhancing lesions at baseline is highly predictive of future MS, as is the appearance of either new T2-weighted lesions or new Gd enhancement ≥3 months after the initial episode.

Mortality as a direct consequence of MS is uncommon, although it has been estimated that the 25-year survival is only 85% of expected. Death can occur during an acute MS attack, although this is distinctly rare. More commonly, death occurs as a complication of MS (e.g., pneumonia in a debilitated individual). Death can also result from suicide. Early disease-modifying therapy seems to reduce this excess mortality.

Effect of Pregnancy Pregnant MS patients experience fewer attacks than expected during gestation (especially in the last trimester), but more attacks than expected in the first 3 months postpartum. When considering the pregnancy year as a whole (i.e., 9 months of pregnancy plus 3 months postpartum), the overall disease course is unaffected. Decisions about childbearing should thus be made based on (1) the mother's physical state, (2) her ability to care for the child, and (3) the availability of social support. Disease-modifying therapy is

TABLE 458-4 DISORDERS THAT CAN MIMIC MULTIPLE SCLEROSIS (MS)

Acute disseminated encephalomyelitis (ADEM)
Antiphospholipid antibody syndrome
Behçet's disease
Cerebral autosomal dominant arteriopathy, subcortical infarcts, and leukoencephalopathy (CADASIL)
Congenital leukodystrophies (e.g., adrenoleukodystrophy, metachromatic leukodystrophy)
Human immunodeficiency virus (HIV) infection
Ischemic optic neuropathy (arteritic and nonarteritic)
Lyme disease
Mitochondrial encephalopathy with lactic acidosis and stroke (MELAS)
Neoplasms (e.g., lymphoma, glioma, meningioma)
Sarcoid
Sjögren's syndrome
Stroke and ischemic cerebrovascular disease
Syphilis
Systemic lupus erythematosus and related collagen vascular disorders
Tropical spastic paraparesis (HTLV-1/2 infection)
Vascular malformations (especially spinal dural AV fistulas)
Vasculitis (primary CNS or other)
Vitamin B_{12} deficiency

Abbreviations: AV, arteriovenous; CNS, central nervous system; HTLV, human T cell lymphotropic virus.

generally discontinued during pregnancy, although the actual risk from the interferons and glatiramer acetate (see below) appears to be low.

TREATMENT MULTIPLE SCLEROSIS

Therapy for MS can be divided into several categories: (1) treatment of acute attacks, (2) treatment with disease-modifying agents that reduce the biologic activity of MS, and (3) symptomatic therapy. Treatments that promote remyelination or neural repair do not currently exist, but several promising approaches are being actively investigated.

The Expanded Disability Status Score (EDSS) is a widely used measure of neurologic impairment in MS (Table 458-5). Most patients with EDSS scores <3.5 have RRMS, walk normally, and are generally not disabled; by contrast, patients with EDSS scores >5.5 have progressive MS (SPMS or PPMS), are gait-impaired, and, typically, are occupationally disabled.

ACUTE ATTACKS OR INITIAL DEMYELINATING EPISODES

When patients experience acute deterioration, it is important to consider whether this change reflects new disease activity or a "pseudoexacerbation" resulting from an increase in ambient temperature, fever, or an infection. When the clinical change is thought to reflect a pseudoexacerbation, glucocorticoid treatment is inappropriate. Glucocorticoids are used to manage either first attacks or acute exacerbations. They provide short-term clinical benefit by reducing the severity and shortening the duration of attacks. Whether treatment provides any long-term benefit on the course of the illness is less clear. Therefore, mild attacks are often not treated. Physical and occupational therapy can help with mobility and manual dexterity.

Glucocorticoid treatment is usually administered as intravenous methylprednisolone, 500–1000 mg/d for 3–5 days, either without a taper or followed by a course of oral prednisone beginning at a dose of 60–80 mg/d and gradually tapered over 2 weeks. Orally administered methylprednisolone or dexamethasone (in equivalent dosages) can be substituted for the intravenous portion of the therapy, although gastrointestinal complications are more common by this route. Outpatient treatment is almost always possible.

Side effects of short-term glucocorticoid therapy include fluid retention, potassium loss, weight gain, gastric disturbances, acne, and emotional lability. Concurrent use of a low-salt, potassium-rich diet and avoidance of potassium-wasting diuretics are advisable. Lithium carbonate (300 mg orally bid) may help to manage emotional lability and insomnia associated with glucocorticoid therapy. Patients with a history of peptic ulcer disease may require cimetidine (400 mg bid) or ranitidine (150 mg bid). Proton pump inhibitors such as pantoprazole (40 mg orally bid) may reduce the likelihood of gastritis, especially when large doses are administered orally. Plasma exchange (five to seven exchanges: 40–60 mL/kg per exchange, every other day for 14 days) may benefit patients with fulminant attacks of demyelination that are unresponsive to glucocorticoids. However, the cost is high, and conclusive evidence of efficacy is lacking.

DISEASE-MODIFYING THERAPIES FOR RELAPSING FORMS OF MS (RRMS, SPMS WITH EXACERBATIONS)

Ten such agents are approved by the U.S. Food and Drug Administration (FDA): (1) IFN-β-1a (Avonex), (2) IFN-β-1a (Rebif), (3) IFN-β-1b (Betaseron or Extavia), (4) glatiramer acetate (Copaxone), (5) natalizumab (Tysabri), (6) fingolimod (Gilenya), (7) dimethyl fumarate (Tecfidera), (8) teriflunomide (Aubagio), (9) mitoxantrone (Novantrone), and (10) alemtuzumab (Lemtrada). Several other promising agents are in varying stages of product development. Each of these treatments can also be used in SPMS patients who continue to experience attacks, both because SPMS can be difficult to distinguish from RRMS and because the available clinical trials, although not definitive, suggest that such patients may sometimes derive therapeutic benefit. Thus, in several phase 3 clinical trials, recipients of each of these agents experienced fewer clinical exacerbations and fewer new MRI lesions compared to placebo recipients (Table 458-6). Because of its potential toxicity as an immunosuppressant, mitoxantrone is generally reserved for patients with progressive disability who have failed other treatments. When considering the data in Table 458-6, however, it is important to note that the relative efficacy of the different agents cannot be determined by cross-trial comparisons. Relative efficacy can only be assessed from nonbiased head-to-head clinical trials.

Interferon-β IFN-β is a class I interferon originally identified by its antiviral properties. Efficacy in MS probably results from immunomodulatory properties including (1) downregulating expression of MHC molecules on antigen-presenting cells, (2) reducing proinflammatory and increasing regulatory cytokine levels, (3) inhibiting T cell proliferation, and (4) limiting the trafficking of inflammatory cells in the CNS. IFN-β reduces the attack rate and improves disease severity measures such as EDSS progression and MRI-documented disease burden. IFN-β should be considered in patients with either RRMS or SPMS with superimposed relapses. In patients with SPMS but without relapses, efficacy has not been established. Head-to-head trials suggest that dosing IFN-β more frequently and at higher doses has better efficacy but is also more likely to induce neutralizing antibodies (see below). IFN-β-1a (Avonex), 30 μg, is administered by intramuscular injection once every week. IFN-β-1a (Rebif), 44 μg, is administered by subcutaneous injection three times per week. IFN-β-1b (Betaseron or Extavia), 250 μg, is administered by subcutaneous injection every other day.

Common side effects of IFN-β therapy include flulike symptoms (e.g., fevers, chills, and myalgias) and mild abnormalities on routine laboratory evaluation (e.g., elevated liver function tests or lymphopenia). Rarely, more severe hepatotoxicity may occur. Subcutaneous IFN-β also causes reactions at the injection site (e.g., pain, redness, induration, or, rarely, skin necrosis). Side effects can usually be managed with concomitant nonsteroidal anti-inflammatory medications. Depression, increased spasticity, and cognitive changes have been reported, although these symptoms can also be due to the underlying disease. In any event, side effects due to IFN-β therapy usually subside over time.

TABLE 458-5 SCORING SYSTEMS FOR MULTIPLE SCLEROSIS (MS)

Kurtzke Expanded Disability Status Score (EDSS)

- 0.0 = Normal neurologic exam (all grade 0 in functional status [FS])
- 1.0 = No disability, minimal signs in one FS (i.e., grade 1)
- 1.5 = No disability, minimal signs in more than one FS (more than one grade 1)
- 2.0 = Minimal disability in one FS (one FS grade 2, others 0 or 1)
- 2.5 = Minimal disability in two FS (two FS grade 2, others 0 or 1)
- 3.0 = Moderate disability in one FS (one FS grade 3, others 0 or 1) or mild disability in three or four FS (three/four FS grade 2, others 0 or 1) although fully ambulatory
- 3.5 = Fully ambulatory but with moderate disability in one FS (one grade 3) and one or two FS grade 2; or two FS grade 3; or five FS grade 2 (others 0 or 1)
- 4.0 = Ambulatory without aid or rest for ~500 m
- 4.5 = Ambulatory without aid or rest for ~300 m
- 5.0 = Ambulatory without aid or rest for ~200 m
- 5.5 = Ambulatory without aid or rest for ~100 m
- 6.0 = Unilateral assistance required to walk about 100 m with or without resting
- 6.5 = Constant bilateral assistance required to walk about 20 m without resting
- 7.0 = Unable to walk beyond about 5 m even with aid; essentially restricted to wheelchair; wheels self and transfers alone
- 7.5 = Unable to take more than a few steps; restricted to wheelchair; may need aid to transfer
- 8.0 = Essentially restricted to bed or chair or perambulated in wheelchair, but out of bed most of day; retains many self-care functions; generally has effective use of arms
- 8.5 = Essentially restricted to bed much of the day; has some effective use of arm(s); retains some self-care functions
- 9.0 = Helpless bed patient; can communicate and eat
- 9.5 = Totally helpless bed patient; unable to communicate or eat
- 10.0 = Death due to MS

Functional Status (FS) Score

A. Pyramidal functions

- 0 = Normal
- 1 = Abnormal signs without disability
- 2 = Minimal disability
- 3 = Mild or moderate paraparesis or hemiparesis, or severe monoparesis
- 4 = Marked paraparesis or hemiparesis, moderate quadriparesis, or monoplegia
- 5 = Paraplegia, hemiplegia, or marked quadriparesis
- 6 = Quadriplegia

B. Cerebellar functions

- 0 = Normal
- 1 = Abnormal signs without disability
- 2 = Mild ataxia
- 3 = Moderate truncal or limb ataxia
- 4 = Severe ataxia all limbs
- 5 = Unable to perform coordinated movements due to ataxia

C. Brainstem functions

- 0 = Normal
- 1 = Signs only
- 2 = Moderate nystagmus or other mild disability
- 3 = Severe nystagmus, marked extraocular weakness, or moderate disability of other cranial nerves
- 4 = Marked dysarthria or other marked disability
- 5 = Inability to swallow or speak

D. Sensory functions

- 0 = Normal
- 1 = Vibration or figure-writing decrease only, in 1 or 2 limbs
- 2 = Mild decrease in touch or pain or position sense, and/or moderate decrease in vibration in 1 or 2 limbs, or vibratory decrease alone in 3 or 4 limbs
- 3 = Moderate decrease in touch or pain or position sense, and/or essentially lost vibration in 1 or 2 limbs, or mild decrease in touch or pain, and/or moderate decrease in all proprioceptive tests in 3 or 4 limbs
- 4 = Marked decrease in touch or pain or loss of proprioception, alone or combined, in 1 or 2 limbs or moderate decrease in touch or pain and/or severe proprioceptive decrease in more than 2 limbs
- 5 = Loss (essentially) of sensation in 1 or 2 limbs or moderate decrease in touch or pain and/or loss of proprioception for most of the body below the head
- 6 = Sensation essentially lost below the head

E. Bowel and bladder functions

- 0 = Normal
- 1 = Mild urinary hesitancy, urgency, or retention
- 2 = Moderate hesitancy, urgency, retention of bowel or bladder, or rare urinary incontinence
- 3 = Frequent urinary incontinence
- 4 = In need of almost constant catheterization
- 5 = Loss of bladder function
- 6 = Loss of bowel and bladder function

F. Visual (or optic) functions

- 0 = Normal
- 1 = Scotoma with visual acuity (corrected) better than 20/30
- 2 = Worse eye with scotoma with maximal visual acuity (corrected) of 20/30 to 20/59
- 3 = Worse eye with large scotoma, or moderate decrease in fields, but with maximal visual acuity (corrected) of 20/60 to 20/99
- 4 = Worse eye with marked decrease of fields and maximal acuity (corrected) of 20/100 to 20/200; grade 3 plus maximal acuity of better eye of 20/60 or less
- 5 = Worse eye with maximal visual acuity (corrected) less than 20/200; grade 4 plus maximal acuity of better eye of 20/60 or less
- 6 = Grade 5 plus maximal visual acuity of better eye of 20/60 or less

G. Cerebral (or mental) functions

- 0 = Normal
- 1 = Mood alteration only (does not affect EDSS score)
- 2 = Mild decrease in mentation
- 3 = Moderate decrease in mentation
- 4 = Marked decrease in mentation
- 5 = Chronic brain syndrome—severe or incompetent

Source: Adapted from JF Kurtzke: Rating neurologic impairment in multiple sclerosis: An expanded disability status scale (EDSS). Neurology 33:1444, 1983.

Approximately 2–10% of IFN-β-1a (Avonex) recipients, 15–25% of IFN-β-1a (Rebif) recipients, and 30–40% of IFN-β-1b (Betaseron/Extavia) recipients develop neutralizing antibodies to IFN-β, which may disappear over time. Two very large randomized trials (one with >2000 patients) provide unequivocal evidence that neutralizing antibodies reduce efficacy as determined by several MRI outcomes. Paradoxically, however, these same trials, despite abundant statistical power, failed to demonstrate any concomitant impact on the clinical outcomes of disability and relapse rate. The reason for this clinical-radiologic dissociation is unresolved. For a patient doing well on therapy, the presence of antibodies should not affect treatment. Conversely, for a patient doing poorly on therapy, alternative treatment should be considered, even if there are no detectable antibodies.

Glatiramer Acetate Glatiramer acetate is a synthetic, random polypeptide composed of four amino acids (L-glutamic acid, L-lysine, L-alanine, and L-tyrosine). Its mechanism of action may include (1) induction of antigen-specific suppressor T cells; (2) binding to MHC molecules, thereby displacing bound MBP; or (3) altering

TABLE 458-6 TWO-YEAR OUTCOMES FOR FDA-APPROVED THERAPIES FOR MULTIPLE SCLEROSIS[a]

	Clinical Outcomes[b]		MRI Outcomes[c]	
Dose, Route, and Schedule	Attack Rate, Mean	Change in Disease Severity	New T2 Lesions[d]	Total Burden of Disease
IFN-β-1b, 250 μg SC qod	−34%[e]	−29% (NS)	−83%[f]	−17%[e]
IFN-β-1a, 30 μg IM qw	−18%[g]	−37%[g]	−36%[f]	−4% (NS)
IFN-β-1a, 44 μg SC tiw	−32%[e]	−30%[g]	−78%[e]	−15%[e]
GA, 20 mg SC qd	−29%[f]	−12% (NS)	−38%[f]	−8%[f]
MTX, 12 mg/m² IV q3mo	−66%[e]	−75%[g]	−79%[g]	NR
NTZ, 300 mg IV qmo	−68%[e]	−42%[e]	−83%[e]	−18%[e]
FGM, 0.5 mg PO qd	−55%[e]	−34%[f]	−74%[e]	−23%[e]
DMF, 240 mg PO bid	−52%[e]	−40%[f]	−71%[e]	NR
TF, 14 mg PO qd	−31%[e]	−26%[g]	−70%[e]	−20%[g]

[a]Percentage reductions (or increases) have been calculated by dividing the reported rates in the treated group by the comparable rates in the placebo group, except for magnetic resonance imaging (MRI) disease burden, which was calculated as the difference in the median percent change between the treated and placebo groups. [b]Severity = 1 point Expanded Disability Status Score progression, sustained for 3 months (in the IFN-β-1a 30 μg qw trial, this change was sustained for 6 months; in the IFN-β-1b trial, this was over 3 years). [c]Different studies measured these MRI measures differently, making comparisons difficult (numbers for new T2 represent the best case scenario for each trial). [d]New lesions seen on T2-weighted MRI. [e]$p = .001$. [f]$p = .01$. [g]$p = .05$.

Abbreviations: DMF, dimethyl fumarate; FDA, U.S. Food and Drug Administration; FGM, fingolimod; GA, glatiramer acetate; IFN-β, interferon β; IM, intramuscular; IV, intravenous; MTX, mitoxantrone; NR, not reported; NS, not significant; NTZ, natalizumab; PO, oral; q3mo, once every 3 months; qd, daily; qmo, once per month; qod, every other day; qw, once per week; qyr, once per year; SC, subcutaneous; TF, teriflunomide; tiw, three times per week.

the balance between proinflammatory and regulatory cytokines. Glatiramer acetate reduces the attack rate (whether measured clinically or by MRI) in RRMS. Glatiramer acetate also benefits disease severity measures, although, for clinical disability, this is less well established than for IFN-β. Nevertheless, two very large head-to-head trials demonstrated that the impact of glatiramer acetate on clinical relapse rates and disability was comparable to high-dose, high-frequency IFN-β. Therefore, glatiramer acetate should be considered as an equally effective alternative to IFN-β in RRMS patients. Its usefulness in progressive disease is unknown. Glatiramer acetate is administered by subcutaneous injection of either 20 mg every day or 40 mg thrice weekly. Injection-site reactions also occur with glatiramer acetate. Initially, these were thought to be less severe than with IFN-β, although two recent head-to-head comparisons of high-dose, high-frequency IFN-β to daily glatiramer acetate did not bear out this impression. In addition, approximately 15% of patients experience one or more episodes of flushing, chest tightness, dyspnea, palpitations, and anxiety after injection. This systemic reaction is unpredictable, brief (duration <1 h), and tends not to recur. Finally, some patients experience lipoatrophy, which, on occasion, can be disfiguring and require cessation of treatment.

Natalizumab Natalizumab is a humanized monoclonal antibody directed against the α_4 subunit of $\alpha_4\beta_1$ integrin, a cellular adhesion molecule expressed on the surface of lymphocytes. It prevents lymphocytes from binding to endothelial cells, thereby preventing lymphocytes from penetrating the BBB and entering the CNS. Natalizumab is highly effective in reducing the attack rate and significantly improves all measures of disease severity in MS (both clinical and MRI). Moreover, it is well-tolerated, and the dosing schedule of monthly intravenous infusions makes it very convenient for patients. However, progressive multifocal leukoencephalopathy (PML), a life-threatening condition resulting from infection by the John Cunningham (JC) virus, has occurred in approximately 0.3% of patients treated with natalizumab. The incidence of PML is very low in the first year of treatment but then rises by the second year to reach a level of about 2 cases per 1000 patients per year. Nevertheless, the measurement of antibodies against the JC virus in the serum can be used to stratify this risk. Thus, in patients who do not have these antibodies, the risk of PML is either minimal or nonexistent (as long as they remain JC antibody free). Conversely, in patients who have these antibodies (especially those who have them in high titer), the risk may be as high as 0.6% or greater. The risk is also high in patients who have previously received immunosuppressive therapy. Natalizumab is currently recommended only for JC antibody–negative patients, unless they have failed alternative therapies or if they have a particularly aggressive disease course. Head-to-head data show that natalizumab is superior to low-dose (weekly) IFN-β-1a in RRMS. However, its relative efficacy compared to other agents has not been established conclusively.

Natalizumab, 300 mg, is administered by IV infusion each month. Treatment with natalizumab is, in general, well tolerated. A small percentage (<10%) of patients experience hypersensitivity reactions (including anaphylaxis), and 6% develop neutralizing antibodies to the molecule (only half of which persist).

The major concern with long-term treatment is the risk of PML. Approximately half of the adult population is JC antibody positive, indicating that they experienced an asymptomatic infection with the JC virus at some time in the past. Nevertheless, because the risk is extremely low during the first year of treatment with natalizumab (regardless of antibody status), natalizumab can still be used safely in JC antibody–positive patients for a period of 12 months. After this time, in antibody-positive patients, a change to another disease-modifying therapy should be strongly considered. By contrast, persistently antibody-negative patients can be continued on treatment indefinitely. Up to 2% of seronegative MS patients undergoing treatment with natalizumab seroconvert annually; thus it is recommended that JC antibody status be assessed at 6-month intervals in all patients receiving treatment with this agent.

Fingolimod Fingolimod is a sphingosine-1-phosphate (S1P) inhibitor that prevents the egress of lymphocytes from the secondary lymphoid organs such as the lymph nodes and spleen. Its mechanism of action is probably due, in part, to the trapping of lymphocytes in the periphery and inhibiting their trafficking to the CNS. Fingolimod reduces the attack rate and significantly improves all measures of disease severity in MS. It is well tolerated, and the daily oral dosing schedule makes it very convenient for patients. A large head-to-head phase 3 randomized study demonstrated the superiority of fingolimod over low-dose (weekly) IFN-β-1a. However, its relative efficacy compared to other agents has not been established conclusively.

Fingolimod, 0.5 mg, is administered orally each day. Treatment with fingolimod is also, in general, well tolerated. Mild abnormalities on routine laboratory evaluation (e.g., elevated liver function tests or lymphopenia) are more common than in controls, sometimes requiring discontinuation of the medication. First- and second-degree heart block and bradycardia can also occur when fingolimod therapy is initiated. A 6-h period of observation (including electrocardiogram monitoring) is recommended for all patients receiving their first dose, and individuals with preexisting cardiac disease should probably not be treated with this agent. Other side effects include macular edema and, rarely, disseminated varicella-zoster virus (VZV) infection; prior to initiating therapy with fingolimod, an ophthalmic exam and VZV vaccination for seronegative individuals are indicated.

Dimethyl Fumarate (DMF) Although the precise mechanisms of action of DMF are not fully understood, it seems to have anti-inflammatory effects through its modulation of the expression of proinflammatory and anti-inflammatory cytokines. Also, DMF inhibits the ubiquitylation and degradation of nuclear factor E2-related factor 2 (Nrf2)—a transcription factor that binds to the antioxidant response elements (AREs) located on the DNA and thereby induces the transcription of several antioxidant proteins. DMF reduces the attack rate and significantly improves all measures of disease severity in MS patients. However, its twice-daily oral dosing schedule makes it somewhat less convenient for patients than daily oral therapies. In addition, compliance is likely to be less with a twice-daily dosing regimen—a factor that could be of concern given the observation (in a small clinical trial) that once-daily DMF lacks efficacy. A head-to-head trial provided evidence that DMF was superior to glatiramer acetate on some outcome measures.

DMF, 240 mg, is administered orally twice each day. Gastrointestinal side effects (abdominal discomfort, nausea, vomiting, flushing, and diarrhea) are common at the start of therapy but generally subside with continued administration. Other adverse events included mild decreases in neutrophil and lymphocyte counts and mild elevations in liver enzymes. Nevertheless, in general, treatment with DMF is well tolerated after an initial period of adjustment. Following the release of DMF, four cases of PML were reported in patients receiving other products (not Tecfidera) that contained DMF. Each of these patients was lymphocytopenic, and most had received previous immunosuppressant therapy so that the relationship of DMF to the PML (if any) in these cases is uncertain. Nevertheless, these reports underscore the fact, stated previously, that long-term safety can never be guaranteed by the results of short-term trials. In the case of DMF for MS, only time and experience will tell us whether or not there is any cause for concern.

Teriflunomide Teriflunomide inhibits the mitochondrial enzyme dihydro-orotate dehydrogenase, which is a key part of the pathway for de novo pyrimidine biosynthesis from carbamoyl phosphate and aspartate. It is the active metabolite of the drug leflunomide (FDA-approved for rheumatoid arthritis), and it exerts its anti-inflammatory effects by limiting the proliferation of rapidly dividing T and B cells. This enzyme is not involved in the so-called "salvage pathway," by which existing pyrimidine pools are recycled for DNA and RNA synthesis in resting and homeostatically proliferating cells. Consequently, teriflunomide is considered to be cytostatic rather than cytotoxic. Teriflunomide reduces the attack rate and significantly improves all measures of disease severity in MS patients. It is well tolerated, and its daily oral dosing schedule makes it very convenient for patients. A head-to-head trial suggested the equivalence, but not superiority, of teriflunomide and high-dose (thrice-weekly) IFN-β-1a. Teriflunomide, either 7 or 14 mg, is administered orally each day. In the pivotal clinical trials, mild hair thinning and gastrointestinal symptoms (nausea and diarrhea) were more common than in controls, but in general, treatment with teriflunomide was well tolerated. As with any new agent, the long-term safety is not guaranteed by the results of short-term trials. A major limitation, especially in women of childbearing age, is its possible teratogenicity (pregnancy category X); teriflunomide can remain in the bloodstream for 2 years, and it is recommended that exposed men and women who wish to conceive receive cholestyramine or activated charcoal to eliminate residual drug.

Mitoxantrone Hydrochloride Mitoxantrone, an anthracenedione, exerts its antineoplastic action by (1) intercalating into DNA and producing both strand breaks and interstrand cross-links, (2) interfering with RNA synthesis, and (3) inhibiting topoisomerase II (involved in DNA repair). The FDA approved mitoxantrone on the basis of a single (relatively small) phase 3 clinical trial in Europe, in addition to an even smaller phase 2 study completed earlier. Mitoxantrone received (from the FDA) the broadest indication of any current treatment for MS. Thus, mitoxantrone is indicated for use in SPMS, in PRMS, and in patients with worsening RRMS (defined as patients whose neurologic status remains significantly abnormal between MS attacks). Despite this broad indication, however, the data supporting its efficacy are weaker than for other approved therapies.

Mitoxantrone can be cardiotoxic (e.g., cardiomyopathy, reduced left ventricular ejection fraction, and irreversible congestive heart failure). As a result, a cumulative dose <140 mg/m^2 is not recommended. At currently approved doses (12 mg/m^2 every 3 months), the maximum duration of therapy can be only 2–3 years. Furthermore, >40% of women will experience amenorrhea, which may be permanent. Finally, there is risk of acute leukemia from mitoxantrone, estimated as at least a 1% lifetime risk, and this complication has been reported in several mitoxantrone-treated MS patients.

Because of these risks, and a growing list of alternative therapies, mitoxantrone is now only rarely used for MS. It should not be used as a first-line agent in either RRMS or relapsing SPMS, but might be considered in selected patients with a progressive course who have failed other therapies.

Alemtuzumab Alemtuzumab is a humanized monoclonal antibody directed against the CD52 antigen, which is expressed on both monocytes and lymphocytes. It causes lymphocyte depletion (of both B and T cells) and a change in the composition of lymphocyte subsets. Both of these changes, particularly the impact on lymphocyte subsets, are long lasting. In preliminary trials, alemtuzumab markedly reduced the attack rate and significantly improved all measures of disease severity in MS patients. In two phase 3 trials, however, its impact on clinical disability was less convincing. Notably, both trials used the active comparator of thrice-weekly, high-dose IFN-β-1a. The European and Canadian drug agencies were the first to approve this agent for use in RRMS; the FDA has also approved alemtuzumab, but only after an appeal following initial disapproval. The reasons for the initial disapproval were based on a perceived lack of a convincing disability effect and concerns over potential toxicity. The toxicities of concern were the occurrence (during the trial or thereafter) of (1) autoimmune diseases including thyroiditis, Graves' disease, thrombocytopenia, hemolytic anemia, pancytopenia, antiglomerular basement membrane disease, and membranous glomerulonephritis; (2) malignancies including thyroid cancer, melanoma, breast cancer, and human papillomavirus (HPV)–related cancers; (3) serious infections; and (4) infusion reactions.

Initiating and Changing Treatment Previously, most patients with relapsing forms of MS received injectable agents (IFN-β or glatiramer acetate) as first-line therapy. However, with the introduction of effective and probably safe oral agents, including DMF, fingolimod, and teriflunomide, this has begun to change. In addition, the monthly infusion therapy natalizumab, which is highly effective, well tolerated, and apparently safe in JC antibody–negative patients, provides an attractive option in many cases. As noted above, with the exception of the first-generation injectable agents, long-term safety data are not available, and for the most part, comparative data are lacking. The value of combination therapy is also largely unknown, although a recent clinical trial demonstrated no added benefit to the combination of glatiramer acetate with low-dose, once-weekly IFN-β-1a.

Despite these unknowns, clinicians need to make decisions based on the best available evidence, coupled with practical considerations. One reasonable approach stratifies initial decision-making based on two levels of disease aggressiveness (Fig. 458-4).

MILD INITIAL COURSE In the case of recent onset, normal exam or minimal impairment (EDSS ≤2.5 or less), or low disease activity, either an injectable (IFN-β or glatiramer acetate) or an oral (DMF,

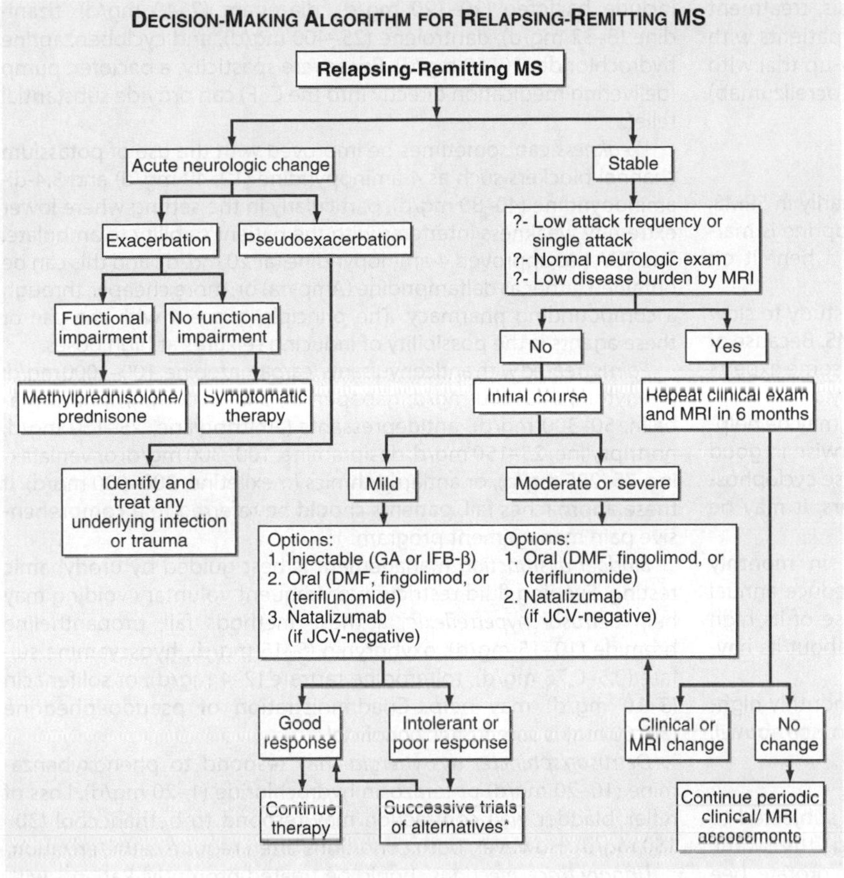

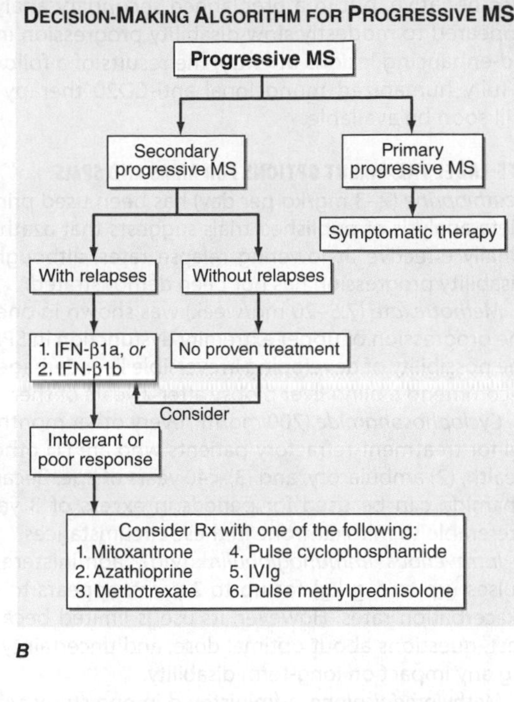

FIGURE 458-4 Therapeutic decision-making for multiple sclerosis (MS). *Can include trials of different preparations of interferon β (IFN-β, particularly advancing from once-weekly (Avonex) to a more frequent (e.g., Rebif, Betaseron/Extavia) dosing regimen. Options also include use of natalizumab in JC virus–positive patients. MRI, magnetic resonance imaging.

fingolimod, or teriflunomide) agent is reasonable. Although head-to-head comparisons are not available, natalizumab is thought to be more effective than these other agents, and therefore, this therapy can be considered even in minimally affected, JCV antibody–seronegative patients. The injectable agents (IFN-β and glatiramer acetate) have a superb track record for safety but have a high nuisance factor due to the need for frequent injections, as well as bothersome side effects that contribute to noncompliance. Some of the oral agents (DMF and fingolimod) are probably more effective than the injectables, but long-term risks are mostly unknown; DMF produces bothersome gastrointestinal symptoms in many patients at least initially (can be mitigated by beginning at one-quarter strength and gradually advancing to full dose), and fingolimod can lead to bradycardia and other cardiac disturbances of unclear clinical significance. Teriflunomide may be less effective than the other oral agents, and there are concerns about its possible long-lasting pregnancy risks. Nevertheless, its long-term safety has likely been established because of its extensive human exposure as the active metabolite of leflunomide—a drug long approved by the FDA.

MODERATE OR SEVERE INITIAL COURSE In highly active disease or moderate impairment (EDSS >2.5), either a highly effective oral agent (DMF or fingolimod) or, if the patient is JC virus antibody seronegative, infusion therapy with natalizumab is recommended.

Regardless of which agent is chosen first, treatment should probably be changed in patients who continue to have relapses, progressive neurologic impairment or, arguably, ongoing evidence of subclinical MRI activity (Fig. 458-4).

The long-term impact of these treatments on the disease course remains controversial, although several recent studies have shown that these agents improve the long-term outcome of MS including a prolongation of the time to reach certain disability outcomes (e.g., SPMS and requiring assistance to ambulate) and reduction in MS-related mortality. These benefits seem most conspicuous when treatment begins early in the RRMS stage of the illness. Unfortunately, however, already established progressive symptoms do not respond well to treatment with these disease-modifying therapies. Because progressive symptoms are likely to result from accumulated axonal and neuronal loss, many experts now believe that very early treatment with a disease-modifying drug is appropriate for most MS patients. It may also be reasonable to delay initiating treatment in patients with (1) normal neurologic exams, (2) a single attack or a low attack frequency, and (3) a low burden of disease as assessed by brain MRI. Untreated patients, however, should be followed closely with periodic brain MRI scans; the need for therapy is reassessed if scans reveal evidence of ongoing, subclinical disease. Finally, vitamin D deficiency should be corrected in all patients with MS, and generally this requires oral supplementation with vitamin D_3, 4000 to 5000 IU daily.

DISEASE-MODIFYING THERAPIES FOR PROGRESSIVE MS

SPMS High-dose IFN-β probably has a beneficial effect in patients with SPMS who are still experiencing acute relapses. IFN-β is probably ineffective in patients with SPMS who are not having acute attacks. All of the other agents have not yet been studied in this patient population. Although mitoxantrone has been approved for patients with progressive MS, this is not the population studied in the pivotal trial. Therefore no evidence-based recommendation can be made with regard to its use in this setting.

PPMS No therapies have been convincingly shown to modify the course of PPMS. A phase 3 clinical trial of glatiramer acetate in PPMS was stopped because of lack of efficacy. A phase 2/3 trial of the monoclonal antibody rituximab (anti-CD20) in PPMS was also negative, but in a preplanned secondary analysis, treatment appeared to modestly slow disability progression in patients with Gd-enhancing lesions at entry; the results of a follow-up trial with a fully humanized monoclonal anti-CD20 therapy (ocrelizumab) will soon be available.

OFF-LABEL TREATMENT OPTIONS FOR RRMS AND SPMS

Azathioprine (2–3 mg/kg per day) has been used primarily in SPMS. Meta-analysis of published trials suggests that azathioprine is marginally effective at lowering relapse rates, although a benefit on disability progression has not been demonstrated.

Methotrexate (7.5–20 mg/week) was shown in one study to slow the progression of upper extremity dysfunction in SPMS. Because of the possibility of developing irreversible liver damage, some experts recommend a blind liver biopsy after 2 years of therapy.

Cyclophosphamide (700 mg/m^2, every other month) may be helpful for treatment-refractory patients who are (1) otherwise in good health, (2) ambulatory, and (3) <40 years of age. Because cyclophosphamide can be used for periods in excess of 3 years, it may be preferable to mitoxantrone in these circumstances.

Intravenous immunoglobulin (IVIg), administered in monthly pulses (up to 1 g/kg) for up to 2 years, appears to reduce annual exacerbation rates. However, its use is limited because of its high cost, questions about optimal dose, and uncertainty about its having any impact on long-term disability.

Methylprednisolone, administered in one study as monthly high-dose intravenous pulses, reduced disability progression (see above).

OTHER THERAPEUTIC CLAIMS

Many purported treatments for MS have never been subjected to scientific scrutiny. These include dietary therapies (e.g., the Swank diet, in addition to others), megadose vitamins, calcium orotate, bee stings, cow colostrum, hyperbaric oxygen, procarin (a combination of histamine and caffeine), chelation, acupuncture, acupressure, various Chinese herbal remedies, and removal of mercury-amalgam tooth fillings, among many others. Patients should avoid costly or potentially hazardous unproven treatments. Many such treatments lack biologic plausibility. For example, no reliable case of mercury poisoning resembling typical MS has ever been described.

Although potential roles for EBV, human herpesvirus (HHV) 6, or chlamydia have been suggested for MS, these reports are unconfirmed, and treatment with antiviral agents or antibiotics is not recommended.

Most recently, chronic cerebrospinal insufficiency (CCSVI) has been proposed as a cause of MS, and vascular-surgical intervention is recommended. However, the failure of independent investigators to even approximate the initial claims of 100% sensitivity and 100% specificity for the diagnostic procedure have raised considerable doubt that CCSVI is a real entity. Certainly, any potentially dangerous surgery should be avoided until more rigorous science is available.

SYMPTOMATIC THERAPY

For all patients, it is useful to encourage attention to a healthy lifestyle, including maintaining an optimistic outlook, a healthy diet, and regular exercise as tolerated (swimming is often well-tolerated because of the cooling effect of cold water). It is reasonable also to correct vitamin D deficiency with oral vitamin D and to recommend dietary supplementation with long-chain (omega-3) unsaturated fatty acids (present in oily fish such as salmon), because of their biologic plausibility for MS pathogenesis, safety, and general health benefits.

Ataxia/tremor is often intractable. Clonazepam, 1.5–20 mg/d; primidone, 50–250 mg/d; propranolol, 40–200 mg/d; or ondansetron, 8–16 mg/d, may help. Wrist weights occasionally reduce tremor in the arm or hand. Thalamotomy or deep-brain stimulation has been tried with mixed success.

Spasticity and *spasms* may improve with physical therapy, regular exercise, and stretching. Avoidance of triggers (e.g., infections, fecal impactions, bed sores) is extremely important. Effective medications include baclofen (20–120 mg/d), diazepam (2–40 mg/d), tizanidine (8–32 mg/d), dantrolene (25–400 mg/d), and cyclobenzaprine hydrochloride (10–60 mg/d). For severe spasticity, a baclofen pump (delivering medication directly into the CSF) can provide substantial relief.

Weakness can sometimes be improved with the use of potassium channel blockers such as 4-aminopyridine (10–40 mg/d) and 3,4-diaminopyridine (40–80 mg/d), particularly in the setting where lower extremity weakness interferes with the patient's ability to ambulate. The FDA has approved 4-aminopyridine (at 20 mg/d), and this can be obtained either as dalfampridine (Ampyra) or, more cheaply, through a compounding pharmacy. The principle concern with the use of these agents is the possibility of inducing seizures at high doses.

Pain is treated with anticonvulsants (carbamazepine, 100–1000 mg/d; phenytoin, 300–600 mg/d; gabapentin, 300–3600 mg/d; or pregabalin, 50–300 mg/d), antidepressants (amitriptyline, 25–150 mg/d; nortriptyline, 25–150 mg/d; desipramine, 100–300 mg/d; or venlafaxine, 75–225 mg/d), or antiarrhythmics (mexiletine, 300–900 mg/d). If these approaches fail, patients should be referred to a comprehensive pain management program.

Bladder dysfunction management is best guided by urodynamic testing. Evening fluid restriction or frequent voluntary voiding may help *detrusor hyperreflexia*. If these methods fail, propantheline bromide (10–15 mg/d), oxybutynin (5–15 mg/d), hyoscyamine sulfate (0.5–0.75 mg/d), tolterodine tartrate (2–4 mg/d), or solifenacin (5–10 mg/d) may help. Coadministration of pseudoephedrine (30–60 mg) is sometimes beneficial.

Detrusor/sphincter dyssynergia may respond to phenoxybenzamine (10–20 mg/d) or terazosin hydrochloride (1–20 mg/d). Loss of reflex bladder wall contraction may respond to bethanechol (30–150 mg/d). However, both conditions often require catheterization.

Urinary tract infections should be treated promptly. Patients with large postvoid residual urine volumes are predisposed to infections. Prevention by urine acidification (with cranberry juice or vitamin C) inhibits some bacteria. Prophylactic administration of antibiotics is sometimes necessary but may lead to colonization by resistant organisms. Intermittent catheterization may help to prevent recurrent infections.

Treatment of *constipation* includes high-fiber diets and fluids. Natural or other laxatives may help. *Fecal incontinence* may respond to a reduction in dietary fiber.

Depression should be treated. Useful drugs include the selective serotonin reuptake inhibitors (fluoxetine, 20–80 mg/d, or sertraline, 50–200 mg/d), the tricyclic antidepressants (amitriptyline, 25–150 mg/d; nortriptyline, 25–150 mg/d; or desipramine, 100–300 mg/d), and the nontricyclic antidepressants (venlafaxine, 75–225 mg/d).

Fatigue may improve with assistive devices, help in the home, or successful management of spasticity. Patients with frequent nocturia may benefit from anticholinergic medication at bedtime. Primary MS fatigue may respond to amantadine (200 mg/d), methylphenidate (5–25 mg/d), or modafinil (100–400 mg/d).

Cognitive problems may respond to the cholinesterase inhibitor donepezil hydrochloride (10 mg/d).

Paroxysmal symptoms respond dramatically to low-dose anticonvulsants (acetazolamide, 200–600 mg/d; carbamazepine, 50–400 mg/d; phenytoin, 50–300 mg/d; or gabapentin, 600–1800 mg/d).

Heat sensitivity may respond to heat avoidance, air-conditioning, or cooling garments.

Sexual dysfunction may be helped by lubricants to aid in genital stimulation and sexual arousal. Management of pain, spasticity, fatigue, and bladder/bowel dysfunction may also help. Sildenafil (50–100 mg), tadalafil (5–20 mg), or vardenafil (5–20 mg), taken 1–2 h before sex, is now the standard treatment for maintaining erections.

PROMISING EXPERIMENTAL THERAPIES

Numerous clinical trials are currently under way. These include studies on (1) monoclonal antibodies against CD20 to deplete B cells and against the IL-2 receptor; (2) selective oral sphingosine-1-phosphate receptor antagonists to sequester lymphocytes in secondary lymphoid organs; (3) estriol to induce a pregnancy-like state; (4) molecules to promote remyelination; and (4) bone marrow transplantation.

CLINICAL VARIANTS OF MS

Acute MS (*Marburg's variant*) is a fulminant demyelinating process that in some cases progresses inexorably to death within 1–2 years. Typically, there are no remissions. When acute MS presents as a solitary, usually cavitary, lesion, a brain tumor is often suspected. In such cases, a brain biopsy is usually required to establish the diagnosis. An antibody-mediated process appears to be responsible for most cases. Marburg's variant does not seem to follow infection or vaccination, and it is unclear whether this syndrome represents an extreme form of MS or another disease altogether. No controlled trials of therapy exist; high-dose glucocorticoids, plasma exchange, and cyclophosphamide have been tried, with uncertain benefit.

NEUROMYELITIS OPTICA

Neuromyelitis optica (NMO; Devic's disease) is an aggressive inflammatory disorder characterized by recurrent attacks of ON and myelitis (Table 458-7). NMO is more frequent in women than men (>3:1), typically begins in childhood or early adulthood but can arise at any age, and is uncommon in whites compared with individuals of Asian and African ancestry. Attacks of ON can be bilateral (rare in MS) or unilateral; myelitis can be severe and transverse (rare in MS) and is typically longitudinally extensive, involving three or more contiguous vertebral segments. Also in contrast to MS, progressive symptoms do not occur in NMO. The brain MRI was earlier thought to be normal in NMO, but it is now recognized that in approximately half of cases, there are lesions involving the hypothalamus causing an endocrinopathy; the lower brainstem presenting as intractable hiccoughs or vomiting from involvement of the area postrema in the lower medulla; or the cerebral hemispheres producing focal symptoms, encephalopathy, or seizures. Large MRI lesions in the cerebral hemispheres can be asymptomatic, sometimes have a "cloud-like" appearance and, unlike MS lesions, are often not destructive, and can resolve completely. Spinal cord MRI lesions typically consist of focal enhancing areas of swelling and tissue destruction, extending over three or more spinal cord segments, and on axial sequences, these are centered on the gray matter of the cord. CSF findings include pleocytosis greater than that observed in MS, with neutrophils and eosinophils present in some cases; OCBs are uncommon, occurring in fewer than 30% of NMO patients. The pathology of NMO is a distinctive astrocytopathy with inflammation, a loss of astrocytes, and an absence of staining of the water channel protein aquaporin-4 by immunohistochemistry, plus thickened blood vessel walls, demyelination, and deposition of antibody and complement.

NMO is best understood as a syndrome with diverse causes. Up to 40% of patients have a systemic autoimmune disorder, often systemic lupus erythematosus, Sjögren's syndrome, perinuclear antineutrophil cytoplasmic antibody (p-ANCA)–associated vasculitis, myasthenia gravis, Hashimoto's thyroiditis, or mixed connective tissue disease. In others, onset may be associated with acute infection with VZV, EBV, HIV, or tuberculosis. Rare cases appear to be paraneoplastic and associated with breast, lung, or other cancers. NMO is often idiopathic, however. NMO is usually disabling over time; in one series, respiratory failure from cervical myelitis was present in one-third of patients, and 8 years after onset, 60% of patients were blind and more than half had permanent paralysis of one or more limbs.

TABLE 458-7 DIAGNOSTIC CRITERIA FOR NEUROMYELITIS OPTICA

Required:

1. Optic neuritis
2. Acute transverse myelitis

Supportive (2 of 3 criteria required):

1. Longitudinally extensive cord lesion extending over 3 or more vertebral segments
2. Brain magnetic resonance imaging normal or not meeting criteria for multiple sclerosis
3. Aquaporin-4 seropositivity

Source: Adapted from DM Wingerchuk et al: Neurology 66:1485, 2006.

A highly specific autoantibody directed against aquaporin-4 is present in the sera of approximately two-thirds of patients with a clinical diagnosis of NMO. Seropositive patients have a very high risk for future relapses; more than half will relapse within 1 year if untreated. Aquaporin-4 is localized to the foot processes of astrocytes in close apposition to endothelial surfaces, as well as at paranodal regions near nodes of Ranvier. It is likely that aquaporin-4 antibodies are pathogenic, as passive transfer of antibodies from NMO patients into laboratory animals reproduce histologic features of the disease.

When MS affects individuals of African or Asian ancestry, there is a propensity for demyelinating lesions to involve predominantly the optic nerve and spinal cord, an MS subtype termed *opticospinal MS*. Interestingly, some individuals with opticospinal MS are seropositive for aquaporin-4 antibodies, suggesting that such cases represent an NMO spectrum disorder.

TREATMENT NEUROMYELITIS OPTICA

Disease-modifying therapies have not been rigorously studied in NMO. Acute attacks of NMO are usually treated with high-dose glucocorticoids (solumedrol 1–2 g/d for 5–10 days followed by a prednisone taper). Plasma exchange (typically 7 qod exchanges of 1.5 plasma volumes) has also been used empirically for acute episodes that fail to respond to glucocorticoids. Given the unfavorable natural history of untreated NMO, prophylaxis against relapses is recommended for most patients using one of the following regimens: mycophenylate mofetil (250 mg bid gradually increasing to 1000 mg bid); B cell depletion with anti-CD20 monoclonal antibody (rituximab); or a combination of glucocorticoids (500 mg IV methylprednisolone daily for 5 days; then oral prednisone 1 mg/kg per day for 2 months, followed by slow taper) plus azathioprine (2 mg/kg per day started on week 3). Available evidence suggests that use of IFN-β is ineffective and paradoxically may increase the risk of NMO relapses.

ACUTE DISSEMINATED ENCEPHALOMYELITIS

Acute disseminated encephalomyelitis (ADEM) has a monophasic course and is most frequently associated with an antecedent infection (postinfectious encephalomyelitis); approximately 5% of ADEM cases follow immunization (postvaccinal encephalomyelitis). ADEM is far more common in children than adults, and many adult cases initially thought to represent ADEM subsequently experience late relapses qualifying as either MS or another chronic inflammatory disorder such as vasculitis, sarcoid, or lymphoma. The hallmark of ADEM is the presence of widely scattered small foci of perivenular inflammation and demyelination, in contrast to larger confluent demyelinating lesions typical of MS. In the most explosive form of ADEM, acute hemorrhagic leukoencephalitis, the lesions are vasculitic and hemorrhagic, and the clinical course is devastating.

Postinfectious encephalomyelitis is most frequently associated with the viral exanthems of childhood. Infection with measles virus is the most common antecedent (1 in 1000 cases). Worldwide, measles encephalomyelitis is still common, although use of the live measles vaccine has dramatically reduced its incidence in developed countries. An ADEM-like illness rarely follows vaccination with live measles vaccine (1–2 in 10^6 immunizations). ADEM is now most frequently associated with varicella (chickenpox) infections (1 in 4000–10,000 cases). It may also follow infection with rubella, mumps, influenza, parainfluenza, EBV, HHV-6, HIV, other viruses, and *Mycoplasma pneumoniae*. Some patients may have a nonspecific upper respiratory infection or no known antecedent illness. In addition to measles, postvaccinal encephalomyelitis may also follow the administration of vaccines for smallpox (5 cases per million), the Semple rabies, and Japanese encephalitis. Modern vaccines that do not require viral culture in CNS tissue have reduced the ADEM risk.

All forms of ADEM presumably result from a cross-reactive immune response to the infectious agent or vaccine that then triggers an inflammatory demyelinating response. Autoantibodies to MBP and to other myelin antigens have been detected in the CSF from some patients with ADEM. Attempts to demonstrate direct viral invasion of the CNS have been unsuccessful.

CLINICAL MANIFESTATIONS

In severe cases, onset is abrupt and progression rapid (hours to days). In postinfectious ADEM, the neurologic syndrome generally begins late in the course of the viral illness as the exanthem is fading. Fever reappears, and headache, meningismus, and lethargy progressing to coma may develop. Seizures are common. Signs of disseminated neurologic disease are consistently present (e.g., hemiparesis or quadriparesis, extensor plantar responses, lost or hyperactive tendon reflexes, sensory loss, and brainstem involvement). In ADEM due to chickenpox, cerebellar involvement is often conspicuous. CSF protein is modestly elevated (0.5–1.5 g/L [50–150 mg/dL]). Lymphocytic pleocytosis, generally 200 cells/μL or greater, occurs in 80% of patients. Occasional patients have higher counts or a mixed polymorphonuclear-lymphocytic pattern during the initial days of the illness. Transient CSF oligoclonal banding has been reported. MRI usually reveals extensive changes in the brain and spinal cord, consisting of white matter hyperintensities on T2 and fluid-attenuated inversion recovery sequences with Gd enhancement on T1-weighted sequences.

DIAGNOSIS

The diagnosis is most reliably established when there is a history of recent vaccination or viral exanthematous illness. In severe cases with predominantly cerebral involvement, acute encephalitis due to infection with herpes simplex or other viruses including HIV may be difficult to exclude (Chap. 164); other considerations include hypercoagulable states including the antiphospholipid antibody syndrome, vasculitis, neurosarcoid, primary CNS lymphoma, or metastatic cancer. An explosive presentation of MS can mimic ADEM, and especially in adults, it may not be possible to distinguish these conditions at onset. The simultaneous onset of disseminated symptoms and signs is common in ADEM and rare in MS. Similarly, meningismus, drowsiness, coma, and seizures suggest ADEM rather than MS. Unlike MS, in ADEM, optic nerve involvement is generally bilateral and transverse myelopathy complete. MRI findings that favor ADEM include extensive and relatively symmetric white matter abnormalities, basal ganglia or cortical gray matter lesions, and Gd enhancement of all abnormal areas. By contrast, OCBs in the CSF are more common in MS. In one study of adult patients initially thought to have ADEM, 30% experienced additional relapses over a follow-up period of 3 years, and they were reclassified as having MS. Occasional patients with "recurrent ADEM" have also been reported, especially children; however, it is not possible to distinguish this entity from atypical MS.

TREATMENT ACUTE DISSEMINATED ENCEPHALOMYELITIS

Initial treatment is with high-dose glucocorticoids as for exacerbations of NMO (see above); depending on the response, treatment may need to be continued for 8 weeks. Patients who fail to respond within a few days may benefit from a course of plasma exchange or intravenous immunoglobulin. The prognosis reflects the severity of the underlying acute illness. In recent case series of presumptive ADEM in adults, mortality rates of 5–20% are reported, and many survivors have permanent neurologic sequelae.

SECTION 3 NERVE AND MUSCLE DISORDERS

459 Peripheral Neuropathy

Anthony A. Amato, Richard J. Barohn

Peripheral nerves are composed of sensory, motor, and autonomic elements. Diseases can affect the cell body of a neuron or its peripheral processes, namely the axons or the encasing myelin sheaths. Most peripheral nerves are mixed and contain sensory and motor as well as autonomic fibers. Nerves can be subdivided into three major classes: large myelinated, small myelinated, and small unmyelinated. Motor axons are usually large myelinated fibers that conduct rapidly (approximately 50 m/s). Sensory fibers may be any of the three types. Large-diameter sensory fibers conduct proprioception and vibratory sensation to the brain, while the smaller-diameter myelinated and unmyelinated fibers transmit pain and temperature sensation. Autonomic nerves are also small in diameter. Thus, peripheral neuropathies can impair sensory, motor, or autonomic function, either singly or in combination. Peripheral neuropathies are further classified into those that primarily affect the cell body (e.g., neuronopathy or ganglionopathy), myelin (myelinopathy), and the axon (axonopathy). These different classes of peripheral neuropathies have distinct clinical and electrophysiologic features. This chapter discusses the clinical approach to a patient suspected of having a peripheral neuropathy, as well as specific neuropathies, including hereditary and acquired neuropathies. The inflammatory neuropathies are discussed in Chap. 460.

GENERAL APPROACH

In approaching a patient with a neuropathy, the clinician has three main goals: (1) identify where the lesion is, (2) identify the cause, and (3) determine the proper treatment. The first goal is accomplished by obtaining a thorough history, neurologic examination, and electrodiagnostic and other laboratory studies (Fig. 459-1). While gathering this information, seven key questions are asked (Table 459-1), the answers to which can usually identify the category of pathology that is present (Table 459-2). Despite an extensive evaluation, in approximately half of patients, no etiology is ever found; these patients typically have a predominately sensory polyneuropathy and have been labeled as having idiopathic or cryptogenic sensory polyneuropathy (CSPN).

INFORMATION FROM THE HISTORY AND PHYSICAL EXAMINATION: SEVEN KEY QUESTIONS (TABLE 459-1)

1. What Systems are Involved? It is important to determine if the patient's symptoms and signs are motor, sensory, autonomic, or a combination of these. If the patient has only weakness without any evidence of sensory or autonomic dysfunction, a motor neuropathy, neuromuscular junction abnormality, or myopathy should be considered. Some peripheral neuropathies are associated with significant autonomic nervous system dysfunction. Symptoms of autonomic involvement include fainting spells or orthostatic lightheadedness; heat intolerance; or any bowel, bladder, or sexual dysfunction (Chap. 454). There will typically be an orthostatic fall in blood pressure without an appropriate increase in heart rate. Autonomic dysfunction in the absence of diabetes should

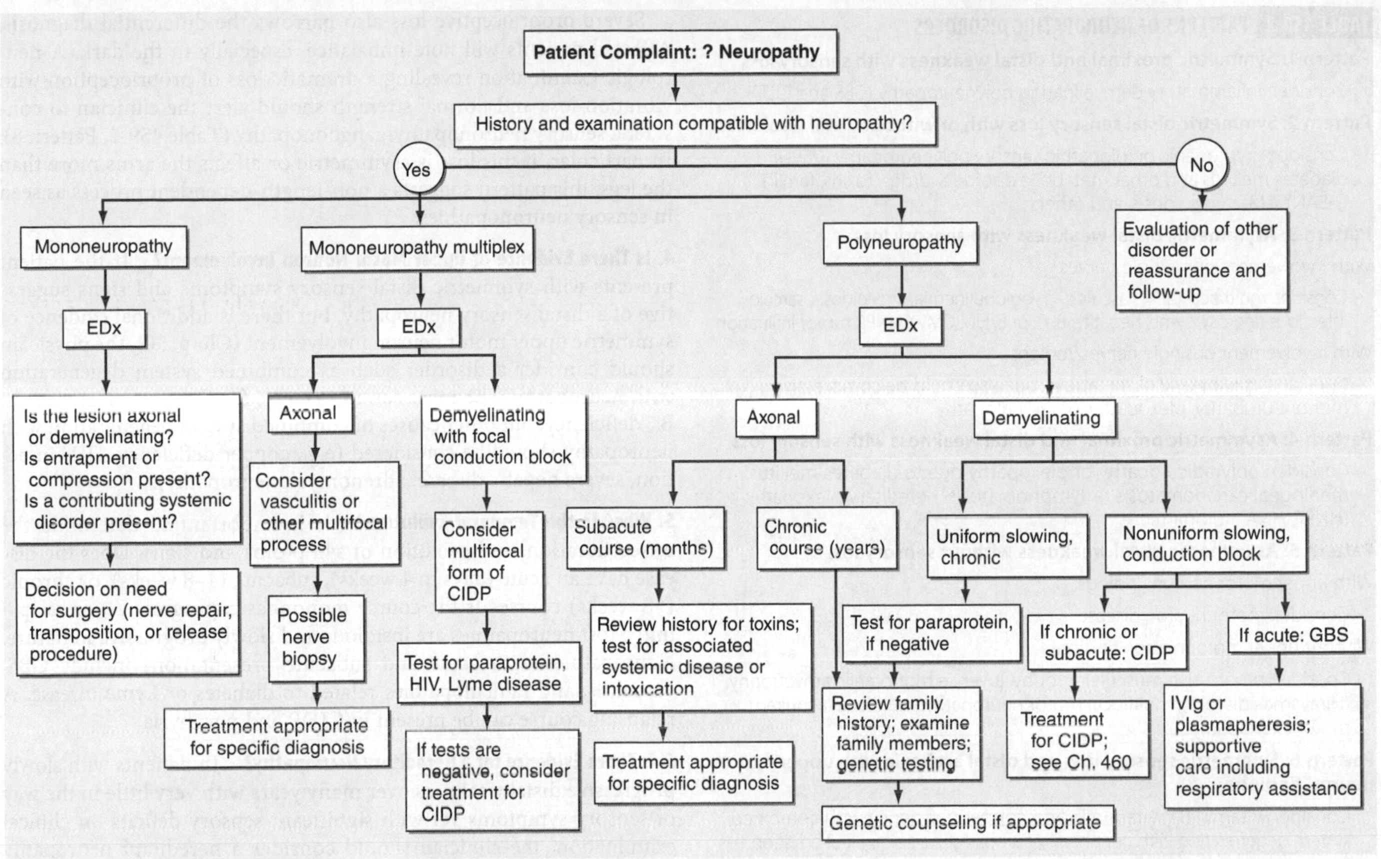

FIGURE 459-1 Approach to the evaluation of peripheral neuropathies. CIDP, chronic inflammatory demyelinating polyradiculoneuropathy; EDx, electrodiagnostic; GBS, Guillain-Barré syndrome; IVIg, intravenous immunoglobulin.

alert the clinician to the possibility of amyloid polyneuropathy. Rarely, a pandysautonomic syndrome can be the only manifestation of a peripheral neuropathy without other motor or sensory findings. The majority of neuropathies are predominantly sensory in nature.

TABLE 459-1 APPROACH TO NEUROPATHIC DISORDERS: SEVEN KEY QUESTIONS

1. What systems are involved?
- Motor, sensory, autonomic, or combinations

2. What is the distribution of weakness?
- Only distal versus proximal and distal
- Focal/asymmetric versus symmetric

3. What is the nature of the sensory involvement?
- Temperature loss or burning or stabbing pain (e.g., small fiber)
- Vibratory or proprioceptive loss (e.g., large fiber)

4. Is there evidence of upper motor neuron involvement?
- Without sensory loss
- With sensory loss

5. What is the temporal evolution?
- Acute (days to 4 weeks)
- Subacute (4–8 weeks)
- Chronic (>8 weeks)
- Monophasic, progressive, or relapsing-remitting

6. Is there evidence for a hereditary neuropathy?
- Family history of neuropathy
- Lack of sensory symptoms despite sensory signs

7. Are there any associated medical conditions?
- Cancer, diabetes mellitus, connective tissue disease or other autoimmune diseases, infection (e.g., HIV, Lyme disease, leprosy)
- Medications including over-the-counter drugs that may cause a toxic neuropathy
- Preceding events, drugs, toxins

2. What is the Distribution of Weakness? Delineating the pattern of weakness, if present, is essential for diagnosis, and in this regard two additional questions should be answered: (1) Does the weakness only involve the distal extremity, or is it both proximal and distal? and (2) Is the weakness focal and asymmetric, or is it symmetric? Symmetric proximal and distal weakness is the hallmark of acquired immune demyelinating polyneuropathies, both the acute form (acute inflammatory demyelinating polyneuropathy [AIDP], also known as Guillain-Barré syndrome [GBS]) and the chronic form (chronic inflammatory demyelinating polyneuropathy [CIDP]). The importance of finding symmetric proximal and distal weakness in a patient who presents with both motor and sensory symptoms cannot be overemphasized because this identifies the important subset of patients who may have a treatable acquired demyelinating neuropathic disorder (i.e., AIDP or CIDP).

Findings of an asymmetric or multifocal pattern of weakness narrow the differential diagnosis. Some neuropathic disorders may present with unilateral extremity weakness. In the absence of sensory symptoms and signs, such weakness evolving over weeks or months would be worrisome for motor neuron disease (e.g., amyotrophic lateral sclerosis [ALS]), but it would be important to exclude multifocal motor neuropathy that may be treatable (Chap. 452). In a patient presenting with asymmetric subacute or acute sensory and motor symptoms and signs, radiculopathies, plexopathies, compressive mononeuropathies, or multiple mononeuropathies (e.g., mononeuropathy multiplex) must be considered.

3. What is the Nature of the Sensory Involvement? The patient may have loss of sensation (numbness), altered sensation to touch (hyperpathia or allodynia), or uncomfortable spontaneous sensations (tingling, burning, or aching) (Chap. 31). Neuropathic pain can be burning, dull, and poorly localized (protopathic pain), presumably transmitted by polymodal C nociceptor fibers, or sharp and lancinating (epicritic pain), relayed by A-delta fibers. If pain and temperature perception are lost, while vibratory and position sense are preserved along with

TABLE 459-2 PATTERNS OF NEUROPATHIC DISORDERS

Pattern 1: Symmetric proximal and distal weakness with sensory loss

Consider: inflammatory demyelinating polyneuropathy (GBS and CIDP)

Pattern 2: Symmetric distal sensory loss with or without distal weakness

Consider: cryptogenic or idiopathic sensory polyneuropathy (CSPN), diabetes mellitus and other metabolic disorders, drugs, toxins, familial (HSAN), CMT, amyloidosis, and others

Pattern 3: Asymmetric distal weakness with sensory loss

With involvement of multiple nerves

Consider: multifocal CIDP, vasculitis, cryoglobulinemia, amyloidosis, sarcoid, infectious (leprosy, Lyme, hepatitis B, C, or E, HIV, CMV), HNPP, tumor infiltration

With involvement of single nerves/regions

Consider: may be any of the above but also could be compressive mononeuropathy, plexopathy, or radiculopathy

Pattern 4: Asymmetric proximal and distal weakness with sensory loss

Consider: polyradiculopathy or plexopathy due to diabetes mellitus, meningeal carcinomatosis or lymphomatosis, hereditary plexopathy (HNPP, HNA), idiopathic

Pattern 5: Asymmetric distal weakness without sensory loss

With upper motor neuron findings

Consider: motor neuron disease

Without upper motor neuron findings

Consider: progressive muscular atrophy, juvenile monomelic amyotrophy (Hirayama's disease), multifocal motor neuropathy, multifocal acquired motor axonopathy

Pattern 6: Symmetric sensory loss and distal areflexia with upper motor neuron findings

Consider: Vitamin B_{12}, vitamin E, and copper deficiency with combined system degeneration with peripheral neuropathy, hereditary leukodystrophies (e.g., adrenomyeloneuropathy)

Pattern 7: Symmetric weakness without sensory loss

With proximal and distal weakness

Consider: SMA

With distal weakness

Consider: hereditary motor neuropathy ("distal" SMA) or atypical CMT

Pattern 8: Asymmetric proprioceptive sensory loss without weakness

Consider causes of a sensory neuronopathy (ganglionopathy):

Cancer (paraneoplastic)

Sjögren's syndrome

Idiopathic sensory neuronopathy (possible GBS variant)

Cisplatin and other chemotherapeutic agents

Vitamin B_6 toxicity

HIV-related sensory neuronopathy

Pattern 9: Autonomic symptoms and signs

Consider neuropathies associated with prominent autonomic dysfunction:

Hereditary sensory and autonomic neuropathy

Amyloidosis (familial and acquired)

Diabetes mellitus

Idiopathic pandysautonomia (may be a variant of Guillain-Barré syndrome)

Porphyria

HIV-related autonomic neuropathy

Vincristine and other chemotherapeutic agents

Abbreviations: CIDP, chronic inflammatory demyelinating polyneuropathy; CMT, Charcot-Marie-Tooth disease; CMV, cytomegalovirus; GBS, Guillain-Barré syndrome; HIV, human immunodeficiency virus; HNA, hereditary neuralgic amyotrophy; HNPP, hereditary neuropathy with liability to pressure palsies; HSAN, hereditary sensory and autonomic neuropathy; SMA, spinal muscular atrophy.

muscle strength, deep tendon reflexes, and normal nerve conduction studies, a small-fiber neuropathy is likely. This is important, because the most likely cause of small-fiber neuropathies, when one is identified, is diabetes mellitus or glucose intolerance. Amyloid neuropathy should be considered as well in such cases, but most of these small-fiber neuropathies remain idiopathic in nature despite extensive evaluation.

Severe proprioceptive loss also narrows the differential diagnosis. Affected patients will note imbalance, especially in the dark. A neurologic examination revealing a dramatic loss of proprioception with vibration loss and normal strength should alert the clinician to consider a sensory neuronopathy/ganglionopathy (Table 459-2, Pattern 8). In particular, if this loss is asymmetric or affects the arms more than the legs, this pattern suggests a non-length-dependent process as seen in sensory neuronopathies.

4. Is There Evidence of Upper Motor Neuron Involvement? If the patient presents with symmetric distal sensory symptoms and signs suggestive of a distal sensory neuropathy, but there is additional evidence of symmetric upper motor neuron involvement (Chap. 30), the physician should consider a disorder such as combined system degeneration with neuropathy. The most common cause for this pattern is vitamin B_{12} deficiency, but other causes of combined system degeneration with neuropathy should be considered (e.g., copper deficiency, HIV infection, severe hepatic disease, adrenomyeloneuropathy).

5. What is the Temporal Evolution? It is important to determine the onset, duration, and evolution of symptoms and signs. Does the disease have an acute (days to 4 weeks), subacute (4–8 weeks), or chronic (>8 weeks) course? Is the course monophasic, progressive, or relapsing? Most neuropathies are insidious and slowly progressive in nature. Neuropathies with acute and subacute presentations include GBS, vasculitis, and radiculopathies related to diabetes or Lyme disease. A relapsing course can be present in CIDP and porphyria.

6. Is There Evidence for a Hereditary Neuropathy? In patients with slowly progressive distal weakness over many years with very little in the way of sensory symptoms yet with significant sensory deficits on clinical examination, the clinician should consider a hereditary neuropathy (e.g., Charcot-Marie-Tooth disease [CMT]). On examination, the feet may show arch and toe abnormalities (high or flat arches, hammertoes); scoliosis may be present. In suspected cases, it may be necessary to perform both neurologic and electrophysiologic studies on family members in addition to the patient.

7. Does the Patient Have Any Other Medical Conditions? It is important to inquire about associated medical conditions (e.g., diabetes mellitus, systemic lupus erythematosus); preceding or concurrent infections (e.g. diarrheal illness preceding GBS); surgeries (e.g., gastric bypass and nutritional neuropathies); medications (toxic neuropathy), including over-the-counter vitamin preparations (B_6); alcohol; dietary habits; and use of dentures (e.g., fixatives contain zinc that can lead to copper deficiency).

PATTERN RECOGNITION APPROACH TO NEUROPATHIC DISORDERS

Based on the answers to the seven key questions, neuropathic disorders can be classified into several patterns based on the distribution or pattern of sensory, motor, and autonomic involvement (Table 459-2). Each pattern has a limited differential diagnosis. A final diagnosis is established by using other clues such as the temporal course, presence of other disease states, family history, and information from laboratory studies.

ELECTRODIAGNOSTIC STUDIES

The electrodiagnostic (EDx) evaluation of patients with a suspected peripheral neuropathy consists of nerve conduction studies (NCS) and needle electromyography (EMG). In addition, studies of autonomic function can be valuable. The electrophysiologic data provide additional information about the distribution of the neuropathy that will support or refute the findings from the history and physical examination; they can confirm whether the neuropathic disorder is a mononeuropathy, multiple mononeuropathy (mononeuropathy multiplex), radiculopathy, plexopathy, or generalized polyneuropathy. Similarly, EDx evaluation can ascertain whether the process involves only sensory fibers, motor fibers, autonomic fibers, or a combination of these. Finally, the electrophysiologic data can help distinguish axonopathies from myelinopathies as well as axonal degeneration secondary to ganglionopathies from the more common length-dependent axonopathies.

TABLE 459-3 ELECTROPHYSIOLOGIC FEATURES: AXONAL DEGENERATION VERSUS SEGMENTAL DEMYELINATION

	Axonal Degeneration	Segmental Demyelination
Motor Nerve Conduction Studies		
CMAP amplitude	Decreased	Normal (except with CB or distal dispersion)
Distal latency	Normal	Prolonged
Conduction velocity	Normal	Slow
Conduction block	Absent	Present
Temporal dispersion	Absent	Present
F wave	Normal or absent	Prolonged or absent
H reflex	Normal or absent	Prolonged or absent
Sensory Nerve Conduction Studies		
SNAP amplitude	Decreased	Normal or decreased
Distal latency	Normal	Prolonged
Conduction velocity	Normal	Slow
Needle EMG		
Spontaneous activity		
Fibrillations	Present	Absent
Fasciculations	Present	Absent
Motor unit potentials		
Recruitment	Decreased	Decreased
Morphology	Long duration/polyphasic	Normal

Abbreviations: CB, conduction block; CMAP, compound motor action potential; EMG, electromyography; SNAP, sensory nerve action potential.

NCS are most helpful in classifying a neuropathy as being due to axonal degeneration or segmental demyelination (Table 459-3). In general, low-amplitude potentials with relatively preserved distal latencies, conduction velocities, and late potentials, along with fibrillations on needle EMG, suggest an axonal neuropathy. On the other hand, slow conduction velocities, prolonged distal latencies and late potentials, relatively preserved amplitudes, and the absence of fibrillations on needle EMG imply a primary demyelinating neuropathy. The presence of nonuniform slowing of conduction velocity, conduction block, or temporal dispersion further suggests an acquired demyelinating neuropathy (e.g., GBS or CIDP) as opposed to a hereditary demyelinating neuropathy (e.g., CMT type 1).

Autonomic studies are used to assess small myelinated (A-delta) or unmyelinated (C) nerve fiber involvement. Such testing includes heart rate response to deep breathing, heart rate, and blood pressure response to both the Valsalva maneuver and tilt-table testing and quantitative sudomotor axon reflex testing (Chap. 454). These studies are particularly useful in patients who have pure small-fiber neuropathy or autonomic neuropathy in which routine NCS are normal.

OTHER IMPORTANT LABORATORY INFORMATION

In patients with generalized symmetric peripheral neuropathy, a standard laboratory evaluation should include a complete blood count, basic chemistries including serum electrolytes and tests of renal and hepatic function, fasting blood glucose (FBS), HbA_{1c}, urinalysis, thyroid function tests, B_{12}, folate, erythrocyte sedimentation rate (ESR), rheumatoid factor, antinuclear antibodies (ANA), serum protein electrophoresis (SPEP) and immunoelectrophoresis or immunofixation, and urine for Bence Jones protein. Quantification of the concentration of serum free light chains and the kappa/lambda ratio is more sensitive than SPEP, immunoelectrophoresis, or immunofixation in looking for a monoclonal gammopathy and therefore should be done if one suspects amyloidosis. A skeletal survey should be performed in patients with acquired demyelinating neuropathies and M-spikes to look for osteosclerotic or lytic lesions. Patients with monoclonal gammopathy should also be referred to a hematologist for consideration of a bone marrow biopsy. An oral glucose tolerance test is indicated in patients with painful sensory neuropathies even if FBS and HbA_{1c} are normal, as the test is abnormal in about one-third of such patients. In addition to the above tests, patients with a mononeuropathy multiplex pattern of involvement should have a vasculitis workup, including antineutrophil cytoplasmic antibodies (ANCA), cryoglobulins, hepatitis serology, Western blot for Lyme disease, HIV, and occasionally a cytomegalovirus (CMV) titer.

There are many autoantibody panels (various antiganglioside antibodies) marketed for screening routine neuropathy patients for a treatable condition. These autoantibodies have no proven clinical utility or added benefit beyond the information obtained from a complete clinical examination and detailed EDx. A heavy metal screen is also not necessary as a screening procedure, unless there is a history of possible exposure or suggestive features on examination (e.g., severe painful sensorimotor and autonomic neuropathy and alopecia—thallium; severe painful sensorimotor neuropathy with or without gastrointestinal [GI] disturbance and Mee's lines—arsenic; wrist or finger extensor weakness and anemia with basophilic stippling of red blood cells—lead).

In patients with suspected GBS or CIDP, a lumbar puncture is indicated to look for an elevated cerebral spinal fluid (CSF) protein. In idiopathic cases of GBS and CIDP, there should not be pleocytosis in the CSF. If cells are present, one should consider HIV infection, Lyme disease, sarcoidosis, or lymphomatous or leukemic infiltration of nerve roots. Some patients with GBS and CIDP have abnormal liver function tests. In these cases, it is important to also check for hepatitis B and C, HIV, CMV, and Epstein-Barr virus (EBV) infection. In patients with an axonal GBS (by EMG/NCS) or those with a suspicious coinciding history (e.g., unexplained abdominal pain, psychiatric illness, significant autonomic dysfunction), it is reasonable to screen for porphyria.

In patients with a severe sensory ataxia, a sensory ganglionopathy or neuronopathy should be considered. The most common causes of sensory ganglionopathies are Sjögren's syndrome and a paraneoplastic neuropathy. Neuropathy can be the initial manifestation of Sjögren's syndrome. Thus, one should always inquire about dry eyes and mouth in patients with sensory signs and symptoms. Further, some patients can manifest sicca complex without full-blown Sjögren's syndrome. Thus, patients with sensory ataxia should have a senile systemic amyloidosis (SSA) and single strand binding (SSB) in addition to the routine ANA. To work up a possible paraneoplastic sensory ganglionopathy, antineuronal nuclear antibodies (e.g., anti-Hu antibodies) should be obtained (Chap. 122). These antibodies are most commonly seen in patients with small-cell carcinoma of the lung but are seen also in breast, ovarian, lymphoma, and other cancers. Importantly, the paraneoplastic neuropathy can precede the detection of the cancer, and detection of these autoantibodies should lead to a search for malignancy.

NERVE BIOPSIES

Nerve biopsies are now rarely indicated for evaluation of neuropathies. The primary indication for nerve biopsy is suspicion for amyloid neuropathy or vasculitis. In most instances, the abnormalities present on biopsies do not help distinguish one form of peripheral neuropathy from another (beyond what is already apparent by clinical examination and the NCS). Nerve biopsies should only be done if the NCS are abnormal. The sural nerve is most commonly biopsied because it is a pure sensory nerve and biopsy will not result in loss of motor function. In suspected vasculitis, a combination biopsy of a superficial peroneal nerve (pure sensory) and the underlying peroneus brevis muscle obtained from a single small incision increases the diagnostic yield. Tissue can be analyzed by frozen section and paraffin section to assess the supporting structures for evidence of inflammation, vasculitis, or amyloid deposition. Semithin plastic sections, teased fiber preparations, and electron microscopy are used to assess the morphology of the nerve fibers and to distinguish axonopathies from myelinopathies.

SKIN BIOPSIES

Skin biopsies are sometimes used to diagnose a small-fiber neuropathy. Following a punch biopsy of the skin in the distal lower extremity, immunologic staining can be used to measure the density of small unmyelinated fibers. The density of these nerve fibers is reduced in patients with small-fiber neuropathies in whom NCS and routine nerve biopsies are often normal. This technique may allow for an objective measurement in patients with mainly subjective symptoms. However, it adds little to what one already knows from the clinical examination and EDx.

SPECIFIC DISORDERS

HEREDITARY NEUROPATHIES

Charcot-Marie-Tooth (CMT) disease is the most common type of hereditary neuropathy. Rather than one disease, CMT is a syndrome of several genetically distinct disorders (Table 459-4). The various subtypes of CMT are classified according to the nerve conduction velocities and predominant pathology (e.g., demyelination or axonal degeneration), inheritance pattern (autosomal dominant, recessive, or X-linked), and the specific mutated genes. Type 1 CMT (or CMT1) refers to inherited demyelinating sensorimotor neuropathies, whereas the axonal sensory neuropathies are classified as CMT2. By definition, motor conduction velocities in the arms are slowed to less than 38 m/s in CMT1 and are greater than 38 m/s in CMT2. However, most cases of CMT1 actually have motor nerve conduction velocities (NCVs) between 20 and 25 m/s. CMT1 and CMT2 usually begin in childhood or early adult life; however, onset later in life can occur, particularly in CMT2. Both are associated with autosomal dominant inheritance, with a few exceptions. CMT3 is an autosomal dominant neuropathy that appears in infancy and is associated with severe demyelination or hypomyelination. CMT4 is an autosomal recessive neuropathy that typically begins in childhood or early adult life. There are no medical therapies for any of the CMTs, but physical and occupational therapy can be beneficial, as can bracing (e.g., ankle-foot orthotics for footdrop) and other orthotic devices.

CMT1 CMT1 is the most common form of hereditary neuropathy, with the ratio of CMT1:CMT2 being approximately 2:1. Affected individuals usually present in the first to third decade of life with distal leg weakness (e.g., footdrop), although patients may remain asymptomatic even late in life. People with CMT generally do not complain of numbness or tingling, which can be helpful in distinguishing CMT from acquired forms of neuropathy in which sensory symptoms usually predominate. Although usually asymptomatic in this regard, reduced sensation to all modalities is apparent on examination. Muscle stretch reflexes are unobtainable or reduced throughout. There is often atrophy of the muscles below the knee (particularly the anterior compartment), leading to so-called inverted champagne bottle legs.

Motor NCVs are usually in the 20–25 m/s range. Nerve biopsies usually are not performed on patients suspected of having CMT1, because the diagnosis usually can be made by less invasive testing (e.g., NCS and genetic studies). However, when done, the biopsies reveal reduction of myelinated nerve fibers with a predilection for the loss of the large-diameter fibers and Schwann cell proliferation around thinly or demyelinated fibers, forming so-called onion bulbs.

CMT1A is the most common subtype of CMT1, representing 70% of cases, and is caused by a 1.5-megabase (Mb) duplication within chromosome 17p11.2-12 wherein the gene for peripheral myelin protein-22 (PMP-22) lies. This results in patients having three copies of the PMP-22 gene rather than two. This protein accounts for 2–5% of myelin protein and is expressed in compact portions of the peripheral myelin sheath. Approximately 20% of patients with CMT1 have CMT1B, which is caused by mutations in the myelin protein zero (MPZ). CMT1B is for the most part clinically, electrophysiologically, and histologically indistinguishable from CMT1A. MPZ is an integral myelin protein and accounts for more than half of the myelin protein in peripheral nerves. Other forms of CMT1 are much less common and again indistinguishable from one another clinically and electrophysiologically.

CMT2 CMT2 tends to present later in life compared to CMT1. Affected individuals usually become symptomatic in the second decade of life; some cases present earlier in childhood, whereas others remain asymptomatic into late adult life. Clinically, CMT2 is for the most part indistinguishable from CMT1. NCS are helpful in this regard; in contrast to CMT1, the velocities are normal or only slightly slowed. The most common cause of CMT2 is a mutation in the gene for mitofusin 2 (MFN2), which accounts for one-third of CMT2 cases overall. MFN2 localizes to the outer mitochondrial membrane, where it regulates the mitochondrial network architecture by fusion of mitochondria. The other genes associated with CMT2 are much less common.

CMTDI In dominant-intermediate CMTs (CMTDIs), the NCVs are faster than usually seen in CMT1 (e.g., >38 m/s) but slower than in CMT2.

CMT3 CMT3 was originally described by Dejerine and Sottas as a hereditary demyelinating sensorimotor polyneuropathy presenting in infancy or early childhood. Affected children are severely weak. Motor NCVs are markedly slowed, typically 5–10 m/s or less. Most cases of CMT3 are caused by point mutations in the genes for PMP-22, MPZ, or ERG-2, which are also the genes responsible for CMT1.

CMT4 CMT4 is extremely rare and is characterized by a severe, childhood-onset sensorimotor polyneuropathy that is usually inherited in an autosomal recessive fashion. Electrophysiologic and histologic evaluations can show demyelinating or axonal features. CMT4 is genetically heterogenic (Table 459-4).

CMT1X CMT1X is an X-linked dominant disorder with clinical features similar to CMT1 and CMT2, except that the neuropathy is much more severe in men than in women. CMT1X accounts for approximately 10–15% of CMT overall. Men usually present in the first two decades of life with atrophy and weakness of the distal arms and legs, areflexia, pes cavus, and hammertoes. Obligate women carriers are frequently asymptomatic, but can develop signs and symptoms. Onset in women is usually after the second decade of life, and the neuropathy is milder in severity.

NCS reveal features of both demyelination and axonal degeneration that are more severe in men compared to women. In men, motor NCVs in the arms and legs are moderately slowed (in the low to mid 30-m/s range). About 50% of men with CMT1X have motor NCVs between 15 and 35 m/s with about 80% of these falling between 25 and 35 m/s (intermediate slowing). In contrast, about 80% of women with CMT1X have NCVs in the normal range and 20% have NCVs in the intermediate range. CMT1X is caused by mutations in the connexin 32 gene. Connexins are gap junction structural proteins that are important in cell-to-cell communication.

Hereditary Neuropathy with Liability to Pressure Palsies (HNPP) HNPP is an autosomal dominant disorder related to CMT1A. Although CMT1A is usually associated with a 1.5-Mb duplication in chromosome 17p11.2 that results in an extra copy of PMP-22 gene, HNPP is caused by inheritance of the chromosome with the corresponding 1.5-Mb deletion of this segment, and thus affected individuals have only one copy of the PMP-22 gene. Patients usually manifest in the second or third decade of life with painless numbness and weakness in the distribution of single peripheral nerves, although multiple mononeuropathies can occur. Symptomatic mononeuropathy or multiple mononeuropathies are often precipitated by trivial compression of nerve(s) as can occur with wearing a backpack, leaning on the elbows, or crossing one's legs for even a short period of time. These pressure-related mononeuropathies may take weeks or months to resolve. In addition, some affected individuals manifest with a progressive or relapsing, generalized and symmetric, sensorimotor peripheral neuropathy that resembles CMT.

Hereditary Neuralgic Amyotrophy (HNA) HNA is an autosomal dominant disorder characterized by recurrent attacks of pain, weakness, and sensory loss in the distribution of the brachial plexus often beginning in childhood. These attacks are similar to those seen with idiopathic brachial plexitis (see below). Attacks may occur in the postpartum period, following surgery, or at other times of stress. Most patients recover over several weeks or months. Slightly dysmorphic features, including hypotelorism, epicanthal folds, cleft palate, syndactyly, micrognathia, and facial asymmetry, are evident in some individuals. EDx demonstrate an axonal process. HNA is caused by mutations in septin 9 (*SEPT9*). Septins may be important in formation of the

TABLE 459-4 CLASSIFICATION OF CHARCOT-MARIE-TOOTH DISEASE AND RELATED NEUROPATHIES

Name	Inheritance	Gene Location	Gene Product
CMT1			
CMT1A	AD	17p11.2	PMP-22 (usually duplication of gene)
CMT1B	AD	1q21-23	MPZ
CMT1C	AD	16p13.1-p12.3	LITAF
CMT1D	AD	10q21.1-22.1	ERG2
CMT1E (with deafness)	AD	17p11.2	Point mutations in PMP 22 gene
CMT1F	AD	8p13-21	Neurofilament light chain
CMT1G	AD	14q32.33	INF2
CMT1X	X-linked dominant	Xq13	Connexin-32
HNPP	AD	17p11.2 1q21-23	PMP-22 MPZ
CMT dominant-intermediate (CMTD1)			
CMTD1A	AD	10q24.1-25.1	?
CMTD1B	AD	19.p12-13.2	Dynamin 2
CMTD1C	AD	1p35	YARS
CMTD1D	AD	1q22	MPZ
CMT2			
CMT2A2 (allelic to HMSN VI with optic atrophy)	AD	1p36.2	MFN2
CMT2B	AD	3q13-q22	RAB7
CMT2B1 (allelic to LGMD 1B)	AR	1q21.2	Lamin A/C
CMT2B2	AR and AD	19q13	MED25 for AR Unknown for AD
CMT2C (with vocal cord and diaphragm paralysis)	AD	12q23-24	TRPV4
CMT2D (allelic to distal SMA5)	AD	7p14	Glycine tRNA synthetase
CMT2E (allelic to CMT 1F)	AD	8p21	Neurofilament light chain
CMT2F	AD	7q11-q21	Heat-shock 27-kDa protein-1
CMT2G	AD	12q23	Unknown
CMT2I (allelic to CMT1B)	AD	1q22	MPZ
CMT2J	AD	1q22	MPZ
CMT2H, CMT2K (allelic to CMT4A)	AD	8q13-q21	GDAP1
CMT2L (allelic to distal hereditary motor neuropathy type 2)	AD	12q24	Heat-shock protein 8
CMT2M	AD	16q22	Dynamin-2
CMT2N	AD	16q22.1	AARS
CMT2O	AD	14q32.31	DYNC1H1
CMT2P	AD	9q34.13	LRSAM1
CMT2P-Okinawa (HSMN2P)	AD	3q13-q14	TFG
CMT2X	X-linked	Xq22-24	PRPS1
CMT3 (Dejerine-Sottas disease, congenital hypomyelinating neuropathy)	AD AD AR AR	17p11.2 1q21-23 10q21.1-22.1 19q13	PMP-22 MPZ ERG2 Periaxon
CMT4			
CMT4A	AR	8q13-21.1	GDAP1
CMT4B1	AR	11q23	MTMR2
CMT4B2	AR	11p15	MTMR13
CMT4C	AR	5q23-33	SH3TC2
CMT4D (HMSN-Lom)	AR	8q24	NDRG1
CMT4E (congenital hypomyelinating neuropathy)	AR	Multiple	Includes PMP22, MPZ, and ERG-2
CMT4F	AR	19q13.1-13.3	Periaxin
CMT4G	AR	10q23.2	HKI
CMT4H	AR	12q12-q13	Frabin
CMT4J	AR	6q21	FIG4
HNA	AD	17q24	SEPT9
HSAN1A	AD	9q22	SPTLC1
HSAN1B	AD	3q21	RAB7
HSAN1C	AD	14q24.3	SPTLC2
HSAN1D	AD	14q21.3	ATL1
HSAN1E	AD	19p13.2	DNMT1

(Continued)

TABLE 459-4 CLASSIFICATION OF CHARCOT-MARIE-TOOTH DISEASE AND RELATED NEUROPATHIES (CONTINUED)

Name	Inheritance	Gene Location	Gene Product
HSAN2A	AR	12p13.33	PRKWNK1
HSAN2B	AR	5p15.1	FAM134B
HSAN2C	AR	12q13.13	KIF1A
HSAN3	AR	9q21	IKAP
HSAN4	AR	3q	trkA/NGF receptor
HSAN5	AD or AR	1p11.2-p13.2	NGFb
HSAN6	AR	6p12.1	Dystonin

Abbreviations: AARS, alanyl-tRNA synthetase; AD, autosomal dominant; AR, autosomal recessive; ATL, atlastin; CMT, Charcot-Marie-Tooth; DNMT1, DNA methyltransferase 1; DYNC1HI, cytoplasmic dynein 1 heavy chain 1; ERG2, early growth response-2 protein; FAM134B, family with sequence similarity 134, member B; FIG4, FDG1-related F actin-binding protein; GDAP1, ganglioside-induced differentiation-associated protein-1; HK1, hexokinase 1; HMSN-P, hereditary motor and sensory neuropathyproximal; HNA, hereditary neuralgic amyotrophy; HNPP, hereditary neuropathy with liability to pressure palsies; HSAN; hereditary sensory and autonomic neuropathy; IFN2, inverted formin-2; IKAP, $_k$B kinase complex-associated protein; LGMD, limb girdle muscular dystrophy; LITAF, lipopolysaccharide-induced tumor necrosis factor α factor; LRSAM1, E3 ubiquitin-protein ligase; MED25, mediator 25; MFN2, mitochondrial fusion protein mitofusin 2 gene; MPZ, myelin protein zero protein; MTMR2, myotubularin-related protein-2; NDRG1, N-myc downstream regulated 1; PMP-22, peripheral myelin protein-22; PRKWNK1, protein kinase, lysine deficient 1; PRPS1, phosphoribosylpyrophosphate synthetase 1; RAB7, Ras-related protein 7; SEPT9, Septin 9; SH3TC2, SH3 domain and tetratricopeptide repeats 2; SMA, spinal muscular atrophy; SPTLC, serine palmitoyltransferase long-chain base; TFG, TRK-fused gene; TrkA/NGF, tyrosine kinase A/nerve growth factor; tRNA, transfer ribonucleic acid; TRPV4, transient receptor potential cation channel, subfamily V, member 4; WNK1, WNK lysine deficient; YARS, tyrosyl-tRNA synthetase.

Source: Modified from AA Amato, J Russell: *Neuromuscular Disease*. New York, McGraw-Hill, 2008.

neuronal cytoskeleton and have a role in cell division, but the mechanism of causing HNA is unclear.

Hereditary Sensory and Autonomic Neuropathy (HSAN) The HSANs are a very rare group of hereditary neuropathies in which sensory and autonomic dysfunction predominates over muscle weakness, unlike CMT, in which motor findings are most prominent (Table 459-4). Nevertheless, affected individuals can develop motor weakness and there can be overlap with CMT. There are no medical therapies available to treat these neuropathies, other than prevention and treatment of mutilating skin and bone lesions.

Of the HSANs, only HSAN1 typically presents in adults. HSAN1 is the most common of the HSANs and is inherited in an autosomal dominant fashion. Affected individuals with HSAN1 usually manifest in the second through fourth decades of life. HSAN1 is associated with the degeneration of small myelinated and unmyelinated nerve fibers leading to severe loss of pain and temperature sensation, deep dermal ulcerations, recurrent osteomyelitis, Charcot joints, bone loss, gross foot and hand deformities, and amputated digits. Although most people with HSAN1 do not complain of numbness, they often describe burning, aching, or lancinating pains. Autonomic neuropathy is not a prominent feature, but bladder dysfunction and reduced sweating in the feet may occur. HSAN1A, which is most common, is caused by mutations in the serine palmitoyltransferase long-chain base 1 (*SPTLC1*) gene.

OTHER HEREDITARY NEUROPATHIES (TABLE 459-5)

FABRY'S DISEASE

Fabry's disease (angiokeratoma corporis diffusum) is an X-linked dominant disorder. Although men are more commonly and severely affected, women can also show severe signs of the disease. Angiokeratomas are reddish-purple maculopapular lesions that are usually found around the umbilicus, scrotum, inguinal region, and perineum. Burning or lancinating pain in the hands and feet often develops in males in late childhood or early adult life. However, the neuropathy is usually overshadowed by complications arising from the associated premature atherosclerosis (e.g., hypertension, renal failure, cardiac disease, and stroke) that often lead to death by the fifth decade of life. Some patients also manifest primarily with a dilated cardiomyopathy.

Fabry's disease is caused by mutations in the a-galactosidase gene that leads to the accumulation of ceramide trihexoside in nerves and blood vessels. A decrease in a-galactosidase activity is evident in leukocytes and cultured fibroblasts. Glycolipid granules may be appreciated in ganglion cells of the peripheral and sympathetic nervous systems and in perineurial cells. Enzyme replacement therapy with a-galactosidase B can improve the neuropathy if patients are treated early, before irreversible nerve fiber loss.

ADRENOLEUKODYSTROPHY/ADRENOMYELONEUROPATHY

Adrenoleukodystrophy (ALD) and adrenomyeloneuropathy (AMN) are allelic X-linked dominant disorders caused by mutations in the peroxisomal transmembrane adenosine triphosphate-binding cassette (ABC) transporter gene. Patients with ALD manifest with central nervous system (CNS) abnormalities. However, 30% with mutations in this gene present with the AMN phenotype that typically manifests in the third to fifth decade of life with mild to moderate peripheral neuropathy combined with progressive spastic paraplegia (Chap. 456). Rare patients present with an adult-onset spinocerebellar ataxia or only with adrenal insufficiency.

EDx is suggestive of a primary axonopathy with secondary demyelination. Nerve biopsies demonstrate a loss of myelinated and unmyelinated nerve fibers with lamellar inclusions in the cytoplasm of Schwann cells. Very long chain fatty acid (VLCFA) levels (C24, C25, and C26) are increased in the urine. Laboratory evidence of adrenal insufficiency is evident in approximately two-thirds of patients. The diagnosis can be confirmed by genetic testing.

Adrenal insufficiency is managed by replacement therapy; however, there is no proven effective therapy for the neurologic manifestations

TABLE 459-5 RARE HEREDITARY NEUROPATHIES

Hereditary Disorders of Lipid Metabolism
Metachromatic leukodystrophy
Krabbe's disease (globoid cell leukodystrophy)
Fabry's disease
Adrenoleukodystrophy/adrenomyeloneuropathy
Refsum's disease
Tangier disease
Cerebrotendinous xanthomatosis
Hereditary Ataxias with Neuropathy
Friedreich's ataxia
Vitamin E deficiency
Spinocerebellar ataxia
Abetalipoproteinemia (Bassen-Kornzweig disease)
Disorders of Defective DNA Repair
Ataxia-telangiectasia
Cockayne's syndrome
Giant Axonal Neuropathy
Porphyria
Acute intermittent porphyria (AIP)
Hereditary coproporphyria (HCP)
Variegate porphyria (VP)
Familial Amyloid Polyneuropathy (FAP)
Transthyretin-related
Gelsolin-related
Apolipoprotein A1-related

of ALD/AMN. Diets low in VLCFAs and supplemented with Lorenzo's oil (erucic and oleic acids) reduce the levels of VLCFAs and increase the levels of C22 in serum, fibroblasts, and liver; however, several large, open-label trials of Lorenzo's oil failed to demonstrate efficacy.

REFSUM'S DISEASE

Refsum's disease can manifest in infancy to early adulthood with the classic tetrad of (1) peripheral neuropathy, (2) retinitis pigmentosa, (3) cerebellar ataxia, and (4) elevated CSF protein concentration. Most affected individuals develop progressive distal sensory loss and weakness in the legs leading to footdrop by their 20s. Subsequently, the proximal leg and arm muscles may become weak. Patients may also develop sensorineural hearing loss, cardiac conduction abnormalities, ichthyosis, and anosmia.

Serum phytanic acid levels are elevated. Sensory and motor NCS reveal reduced amplitudes, prolonged latencies, and slowed conduction velocities. Nerve biopsy demonstrates a loss of myelinated nerve fibers, with remaining axons often thinly myelinated and associated with onion bulb formation.

Refsum disease is genetically heterogeneous but autosomal recessive in nature. Classical Refsum disease with childhood or early adult onset is caused by mutations in the gene that encodes for phytanoyl-CoA α-hydroxylase (*PAHX*). Less commonly, mutations in the gene encoding peroxin 7 receptor protein (PRX7) are responsible. These mutations lead to the accumulation of phytanic acid in the central and peripheral nervous systems. Refsum's disease is treated by removing phytanic precursors (phytols: fish oils, dairy products, and ruminant fats) from the diet.

TANGIER DISEASE

Tangier disease is a rare autosomal recessive disorder that can present as (1) asymmetric multiple mononeuropathies, (2) a slowly progressive symmetric polyneuropathy predominantly in the legs, or (3) a pseudo-syringomyelia pattern with dissociated sensory loss (i.e., abnormal pain/temperature perception but preserved position/vibration in the arms [Chap. 456]). The tonsils may appear swollen and yellowish-orange in color, and there may also be splenomegaly and lymphadenopathy.

Tangier disease is caused by mutations in the ATP-binding cassette transporter 1 (ABC1) gene, which leads to markedly reduced levels of high-density lipoprotein (HDL) cholesterol levels, whereas triacylglycerol levels are increased. Nerve biopsies reveal axonal degeneration with demyelination and remyelination. Electron microscopy demonstrates abnormal accumulation of lipid in Schwann cells, particularly those encompassing umyelinated and small myelinated nerves. There is no specific treatment.

PORPHYRIA

Porphyria is a group of inherited disorders caused by defects in heme biosynthesis (Chap. 430). Three forms of porphyria are associated with peripheral neuropathy: acute intermittent porphyria (AIP), hereditary coproporphyria (HCP), and variegate porphyria (VP). The acute neurologic manifestations are similar in each, with the exception that a photosensitive rash is seen with HCP and VP but not in AIP. Attacks of porphyria can be precipitated by certain drugs (usually those metabolized by the P450 system), hormonal changes (e.g., pregnancy, menstrual cycle), and dietary restrictions.

An acute attack of porphyria may begin with sharp abdominal pain. Subsequently, patients may develop agitation, hallucinations, or seizures. Several days later, back and extremity pain followed by weakness ensues, mimicking GBS. Weakness can involve the arms or the legs and can be asymmetric, proximal, or distal in distribution, as well as affecting the face and bulbar musculature. Dysautonomia and signs of sympathetic overactivity are common (e.g., pupillary dilation, tachycardia, and hypertension). Constipation, urinary retention, and incontinence can also be seen.

The CSF protein is typically normal or mildly elevated. Liver function tests and hematologic parameters are usually normal. Some patients are hyponatremic due to inappropriate secretion of antidiuretic hormone (Chap. 401e). The urine may appear brownish in color secondary to the high concentration of porphyrin metabolites. Accumulation of intermediary precursors of heme (i.e., d-aminolevulinic acid, porphobilinogen, uroporphobilinogen, coproporphyrinogen, and protoporphyrinogen) is found in urine. Specific enzyme activities can also be measured in erythrocytes and leukocytes. The primary abnormalities on EDx are marked reductions in compound motor action potential (CMAP) amplitudes and signs of active axonal degeneration on needle EMG.

The porphyrias are inherited in an autosomal dominant fashion. AIP is associated with porphobilinogen deaminase deficiency, HCP is caused by defects in coproporphyrin oxidase, and VP is associated with protoporphyrinogen oxidase deficiency. The pathogenesis of the neuropathy is not completely understood. Treatment with glucose and hematin may reduce the accumulation of heme precursors. Intravenous glucose is started at a rate of 10–20 g/h. If there is no improvement within 24 h, intravenous hematin 2–5 mg/kg per day for 3–14 days should be given.

FAMILIAL AMYLOID POLYNEUROPATHY

Familial amyloid polyneuropathy (FAP) is phenotypically and genetically heterogeneous and is caused by mutations in the genes for transthyretin (TTR), apolipoprotein A1, or gelsolin (Chap. 137). The majority of patients with FAP have mutations in the TTR gene. Amyloid deposition may be evident in abdominal fat pad, rectal, or nerve biopsies. The clinical features, histopathology, and EDx reveal abnormalities consistent with a generalized or multifocal, predominantly axonal but occasionally demyelinating, sensorimotor polyneuropathy.

Patients with TTR-related FAP usually develop insidious onset of numbness and painful paresthesias in the distal lower limbs in the third to fourth decade of life, although some patients develop the disorder later in life. Carpal tunnel syndrome (CTS) is common. Autonomic involvement can be severe, leading to postural hypotension, constipation or persistent diarrhea, erectile dysfunction, and impaired sweating. Amyloid deposition also occurs in the heart, kidneys, liver, and corneas. Patients usually die 10–15 years after the onset of symptoms from cardiac failure or complications from malnutrition. Because the liver produces much of the body's TTR, liver transplantation has been used to treat FAP related to TTR mutations. Serum TTR levels decrease after transplantation, and improvement in clinical and EDx features has been reported.

Patients with apolipoprotein A1-related FAP (Van Allen type) usually present in the fourth decade with numbness and painful dysesthesias in the distal limbs. Gradually, the symptoms progress, leading to proximal and distal weakness and atrophy. Although autonomic neuropathy is not severe, some patients develop diarrhea, constipation, or gastroparesis. Most patients die from systemic complications of amyloidosis (e.g., renal failure) 12–15 years after the onset of the neuropathy.

Gelsolin-related amyloidosis (Finnish type) is characterized by the combination of lattice corneal dystrophy and multiple cranial neuropathies that usually begin in the third decade of life. Over time, a mild generalized sensorimotor polyneuropathy develops. Autonomic dysfunction does not occur.

ACQUIRED NEUROPATHIES

PRIMARY OR AL AMYLOIDOSIS (SEE CHAP. 137)

Besides FAP, amyloidosis can also be acquired. In primary or AL amyloidosis, the abnormal protein deposition is composed of immunoglobulin light chains. AL amyloidosis occurs in the setting of multiple myeloma, Waldenström's macroglobulinemia, lymphoma, other plasmacytomas, or lymphoproliferative disorders, or without any other identifiable disease.

Approximately 30% of patients with AL primary amyloidosis present with a polyneuropathy, most typically painful dysesthesias and burning sensations in the feet. However, the trunk can be involved, and some patients manifest with a mononeuropathy multiplex pattern. CTS occurs in 25% of patients and may be the initial manifestation. The neuropathy is slowly progressive, and eventually weakness develops along with large-fiber sensory loss. Most patients develop autonomic involvement with postural hypertension, syncope, bowel and bladder incontinence, constipation, impotence, and impaired sweating. Patients generally die from their systemic illness (renal failure, cardiac disease).

The monoclonal protein may be composed of IgG, IgA, IgM, or only free light chain. Lambda (λ) is more common than κ light chain (>2:1) in AL amyloidosis. The CSF protein is often increased (with normal cell count), and thus the neuropathy may be mistaken for CIDP (Chap. 460). Nerve biopsies reveal axonal degeneration and amyloid deposition in either a globular or diffuse pattern infiltrating the perineurial, epineurial, and endoneurial connected tissue and in blood vessel walls.

The median survival of patients with primary amyloidosis is less than 2 years, with death usually from progressive congestive heart failure or renal failure. Chemotherapy with melphalan, prednisone, and colchicine, to reduce the concentration of monoclonal proteins, and autologous stem cell transplantation may prolong survival, but whether the neuropathy improves is controversial.

DIABETIC NEUROPATHY

Diabetes mellitus (DM) is the most common cause of peripheral neuropathy in developed countries. DM is associated with several types of polyneuropathy: distal symmetric sensory or sensorimotor polyneuropathy, autonomic neuropathy, diabetic neuropathic cachexia, polyradiculoneuropathies, cranial neuropathies, and other mononeuropathies. Risk factors for the development of neuropathy include long-standing, poorly controlled DM and the presence of retinopathy and nephropathy.

Diabetic Distal Symmetric Sensory and Sensorimotor Polyneuropathy (DSPN)

DSPN is the most common form of diabetic neuropathy and manifests as sensory loss beginning in the toes that gradually progresses over time up the legs and into the fingers and arms. When severe, a patient may develop sensory loss in the trunk (chest and abdomen), initially in the midline anteriorly and later extending laterally. Tingling, burning, deep aching pains may also be apparent. NCS usually show reduced amplitudes and mild to moderate slowing of conduction velocities (CVs). Nerve biopsy reveals axonal degeneration, endothelial hyperplasia, and, occasionally, perivascular inflammation. Tight control of glucose can reduce the risk of developing neuropathy or improve the underlying neuropathy. A variety of medications have been used with variable success to treat painful symptoms associated with DSPN, including antiepileptic medications, antidepressants, sodium channel blockers, and other analgesics (Table 459-6).

Diabetic Autonomic Neuropathy Autonomic neuropathy is typically seen in combination with DSPN. The autonomic neuropathy can manifest as abnormal sweating, dysfunctional thermoregulation, dry eyes and mouth, pupillary abnormalities, cardiac arrhythmias, postural hypotension, GI abnormalities (e.g., gastroparesis, postprandial bloating, chronic diarrhea or constipation), and genitourinary dysfunction (e.g., impotence, retrograde ejaculation, incontinence). Tests of autonomic function are generally abnormal, including sympathetic skin responses and quantitative sudomotor axon reflex testing. Sensory and motor NCS generally demonstrate features described above with DSPN.

Diabetic Radiculoplexus Neuropathy (Diabetic Amyotrophy or Bruns-Garland Syndrome) Diabetic radiculoplexus neuropathy is the presenting manifestation of DM in approximately one-third of patients. Typically, patients present with severe pain in the low back, hip, and thigh in one leg. Rarely, the diabetic polyradiculoneuropathy begins in both legs at the same time. Atrophy and weakness of proximal and distal muscles in the affected leg become apparent within a few days or weeks. The neuropathy is often accompanied or heralded by severe weight loss. Weakness usually progresses over several weeks or months, but can continue to progress for 18 months or more. Subsequently, there is slow recovery but many are left with residual weakness, sensory loss, and pain. In contrast to the more typical lumbosacral radiculoplexus neuropathy, some patients develop thoracic radiculopathy or, even less commonly, a cervical polyradiculoneuropathy. CSF protein is usually elevated, while the cell count is normal. ESR is often increased. EDx reveals evidence of active denervation in affected proximal and distal muscles in the affected limbs and in paraspinal muscles. Nerve biopsies may demonstrate axonal degeneration along with perivascular inflammation. Patients with severe pain are sometimes treated in the acute period with glucocorticoids, although a randomized controlled trial

TABLE 459-6 TREATMENT OF PAINFUL SENSORY NEUROPATHIES

Therapy	Route	Dose	Side Effects
First-Line			
Lidoderm 5% patch	Apply to painful area	Up to 3 patches qd	Skin irritation
Tricyclic antidepressants (e.g., amitriptyline, nortriptyline)	PO	10–100 mg qhs	Cognitive changes, sedation, dry eyes and mouth, urinary retention, constipation
Gabapentin	PO	300–1200 mg tid	Cognitive changes, sedation, peripheral edema
Pregabalin	PO	50–100 mg tid	Cognitive changes, sedation, peripheral edema
Duloxetine	PO	30–60 mg qd	Cognitive changes, sedation, dry eyes, diaphoresis, nausea, diarrhea, constipation
Second-Line			
Carbamazepine	PO	200–400 mg q 6–8 h	Cognitive changes, dizziness, leukopenia, liver dysfunction
Phenytoin	PO	200–400 mg qhs	Cognitive changes, dizziness, liver dysfunction
Venlafaxine	PO	37.5–150 mg/d	Asthenia, sweating, nausea, constipation, anorexia, vomiting, somnolence, dry mouth, dizziness, nervousness, anxiety, tremor, and blurred vision as well as abnormal ejaculation/orgasm and impotence
Tramadol	PO	50 mg qid	Cognitive changes, gastrointestinal upset
Third-Line			
Mexiletine	PO	200–300 mg tid	Arrhythmias
Other Agents			
EMLA cream 2.5% lidocaine 2.5% prilocaine	Apply cutaneously	qid	Local erythema
Capsaicin 0.025–0.075% cream	Apply cutaneously	qid	Painful burning skin

Source: Modified from AA Amato, J Russell: *Neuromuscular Disease*. New York, McGraw-Hill, 2008.

has yet to be performed, and the natural history of this neuropathy is gradual improvement.

Diabetic Mononeuropathies or Multiple Mononeuropathies The most common mononeuropathies are median neuropathy at the wrist and ulnar neuropathy at the elbow, but peroneal neuropathy at the fibular head, and sciatic, lateral femoral, cutaneous, or cranial neuropathies also occur. In regard to cranial mononeuropathies, seventh nerve palsies are relatively common but may have other, nondiabetic etiologies. In diabetics, a third nerve palsy is most common, followed by sixth nerve, and, less frequently, fourth nerve palsies. Diabetic third nerve palsies are characteristically pupil-sparing (Chap. 39).

HYPOTHYROIDISM

Hypothyroidism is more commonly associated with a proximal myopathy, but some patients develop a neuropathy, most typically CTS. Rarely, a generalized sensory polyneuropathy characterized by painful paresthesias and numbness in both the legs and hands can occur. Treatment is correction of the hypothyroidism.

SJÖGREN'S SYNDROME

Sjögren's syndrome, characterized by the sicca complex of xerophthalmia, xerostomia, and dryness of other mucous membranes, can be complicated by neuropathy (Chap. 383). Most common is a length-dependent axonal sensorimotor neuropathy characterized mainly by sensory loss in the distal extremities. A pure small-fiber neuropathy or a cranial neuropathy, particularly involving the trigeminal nerve, can also be seen. Sjögren's syndrome is also associated with sensory neuronopathy/ganglionopathy. Patients with sensory ganglionopathies develop progressive numbness and tingling of the limbs, trunk, and face in a non-length dependent manner such that symptoms can involve the face or arms more than the legs. The onset can be acute or insidious. Sensory examination demonstrates severe vibratory and proprioceptive loss leading to sensory ataxia.

Patients with neuropathy due to Sjögren's syndrome may have ANAs, SS-A/Ro, and SS-B/La antibodies in the serum, but most do not. NCS demonstrate reduced amplitudes of sensory studies in the affected limbs. Nerve biopsy demonstrates axonal degeneration. Nonspecific perivascular inflammation may be present, but only rarely is there necrotizing vasculitis. There is no specific treatment for neuropathies related to Sjögren's syndrome. When vasculitis is suspected, immunosuppressive agents may be beneficial. Occasionally, the sensory neuronopathy/ganglionopathy stabilizes or improves with immunotherapy, such as IVIg.

RHEUMATOID ARTHRITIS

Peripheral neuropathy occurs in at least 50% of patients with rheumatoid arthritis (RA) and may be vasculitic in nature (Chap. 380). Vasculitic neuropathy can present with a mononeuropathy multiplex, a generalized symmetric pattern of involvement, or a combination of these patterns (Chap. 385). Neuropathies may also be due to drugs used to treat the RA (e.g., tumor necrosis blockers, leflunomide). Nerve biopsy often reveals thickening of the epineurial and endoneurial blood vessels as well as perivascular inflammation or vasculitis, with transmural inflammatory cell infiltration and fibrinoid necrosis of vessel walls. The neuropathy often is responsive to immunomodulating therapies.

SYSTEMIC LUPUS ERYTHEMATOSUS (SLE)

Between 2 and 27% of individuals with SLE develop a peripheral neuropathy (Chap. 378). Affected patients typically present with a slowly progressive sensory loss beginning in the feet. Some patients develop burning pain and paresthesias with normal reflexes, and NCS suggest a pure small-fiber neuropathy. Less common are multiple mononeuropathies presumably secondary to necrotizing vasculitis. Rarely, a generalized sensorimotor polyneuropathy meeting clinical, laboratory, electrophysiologic, and histologic criteria for either GBS or CIDP may occur. Immunosuppressive therapy is beneficial in SLE patients with neuropathy due to vasculitis. Immunosuppressive agents are less likely to be effective in patients with a generalized sensory or sensorimotor polyneuropathy without evidence of vasculitis. Patients with a GBS or CIDP-like neuropathy should be treated accordingly (Chap. 385).

SYSTEMIC SCLEROSIS (SCLERODERMA)

A distal symmetric, mainly sensory, polyneuropathy complicates 5–67% of scleroderma cases (Chap. 382). Cranial mononeuropathies can also develop, most commonly of the trigeminal nerve, producing numbness and dysesthesias in the face. Multiple mononeuropathies also occur. The EDx and histologic features of nerve biopsy are those of an axonal sensory greater than motor polyneuropathy.

MIXED CONNECTIVE TISSUE DISEASE (MCTD)

A mild distal axonal sensorimotor polyneuropathy occurs in approximately 10% of patients with MCTD.

SARCOIDOSIS

The peripheral or central nervous system is involved in about 5% of patients with sarcoidosis (Chap. 390). The most common cranial nerve involved is the seventh nerve, which can be affected bilaterally. Some patients develop radiculopathy or polyradiculopathy. With a generalized root involvement, the clinical presentation can mimic GBS or CIDP. Patients can also present with multiple mononeuropathies or a generalized, slowly progressive, sensory greater than motor polyneuropathy. Some have features of a pure small-fiber neuropathy. EDx reveals an axonal neuropathy. Nerve biopsy can reveal noncaseating granulomas infiltrating the endoneurium, perineurium, and epineurium along with lymphocytic necrotizing angiitis. Neurosarcoidosis may respond to treatment with glucocorticoids or other immunosuppressive agents.

HYPEREOSINOPHILIC SYNDROME

Hypereosinophilic syndrome is characterized by eosinophilia associated with various skin, cardiac, hematologic, and neurologic abnormalities. A generalized peripheral neuropathy or a mononeuropathy multiplex occurs in 6–14% of patients.

CELIAC DISEASE (GLUTEN-INDUCED ENTEROPATHY OR NONTROPICAL SPRUE)

Neurologic complications, particularly ataxia and peripheral neuropathy, are estimated to occur in 10% of patients with celiac disease (Chap. 349). A generalized sensorimotor polyneuropathy, pure motor neuropathy, multiple mononeuropathies, autonomic neuropathy, small-fiber neuropathy, and neuromyotonia have all been reported in association with celiac disease or antigliadin/antiendomysial antibodies. Nerve biopsy may reveal a loss of large myelinated fibers. The neuropathy may be secondary to malabsorption of vitamins B_{12} and E. However, some patients have no appreciable vitamin deficiencies. The pathogenic basis for the neuropathy in these patients is unclear but may be autoimmune in etiology. The neuropathy does not appear to respond to a gluten-free diet. In patients with vitamin B_{12} or vitamin E deficiency, replacement therapy may improve or stabilize the neuropathy.

INFLAMMATORY BOWEL DISEASE

Ulcerative colitis and Crohn's disease may be complicated by GBS, CIDP, generalized axonal sensory or sensorimotor polyneuropathy, small-fiber neuropathy, or mononeuropathy (Chap. 351). These neuropathies may be autoimmune, nutritional (e.g., vitamin B_{12} deficiency), treatment related (e.g., metronidazole), or idiopathic in nature. An acute neuropathy with demyelination resembling GBS, CIDP, or multifocal motor neuropathy may occur in patients treated with tumor necrosis factor α blockers.

UREMIC NEUROPATHY

Approximately 60% of patients with renal failure develop a polyneuropathy characterized by length-dependent numbness, tingling, allodynia, and mild distal weakness. Rarely, a rapidly progressive weakness and sensory loss very similar to GBS can occur that improves with an increase in the intensity of renal dialysis or with transplantation. Mononeuropathies can also occur, the most common of which is CTS.

Ischemic monomelic neuropathy (see below) can complicate arteriovenous shunts created in the arm for dialysis. EDx in uremic patients reveals features of a length-dependent, primarily axonal, sensorimotor polyneuropathy. Sural nerve biopsies demonstrate a loss of nerve fibers (particularly large myelinated nerve fibers), active axonal degeneration, and segmental and paranodal demyelination. The sensorimotor polyneuropathy can be stabilized by hemodialysis and improved with successful renal transplantation.

CHRONIC LIVER DISEASE

A generalized sensorimotor neuropathy characterized by numbness, tingling, and minor weakness in the distal aspects of primarily the lower limbs commonly occurs in patients with chronic liver failure. EDx studies are consistent with a sensory greater than motor axonopathy. Sural nerve biopsy reveals both segmental demyelination and axonal loss. It is not known if hepatic failure in isolation can cause peripheral neuropathy, as the majority of patients have liver disease secondary to other disorders, such as alcoholism or viral hepatitis, which can also cause neuropathy.

CRITICAL ILLNESS POLYNEUROPATHY

The most common causes of acute generalized weakness leading to admission to a medical intensive care unit (ICU) are GBS and myasthenia gravis (Chap. 461). However, weakness developing in critically ill patients while in the ICU is usually caused by critical illness polyneuropathy (CIP) or critical illness myopathy (CIM) or, much less commonly, by prolonged neuromuscular blockade. From a clinical and EDx standpoint, it can be quite difficult to distinguish these disorders. Most specialists suggest that CIM is more common. Both CIM and CIP develop as a complication of sepsis and multiple organ failure. They usually present as an inability to wean a patient from a ventilator. A coexisting encephalopathy may limit the neurologic exam, in particular the sensory examination. Muscle stretch reflexes are absent or reduced.

Serum creatine kinase (CK) is usually normal; an elevated serum CK would point to CIM as opposed to CIP. NCS reveal absent or markedly reduced amplitudes of motor and sensory studies in CIP, whereas sensory studies are relatively preserved in CIM. Needle EMG usually reveals profuse positive sharp waves and fibrillation potentials, and it is not unusual in patients with severe weakness to be unable to recruit motor unit action potentials. The pathogenic basis of CIP is not known. Perhaps circulating toxins and metabolic abnormalities associated with sepsis and multiorgan failure impair axonal transport or mitochondrial function, leading to axonal degeneration.

LEPROSY (HANSEN'S DISEASE)

Leprosy, caused by the acid-fast bacteria *Mycobacterium leprae*, is the most common cause of peripheral neuropathy in Southeast Asia, Africa, and South America (Chap. 203). Clinical manifestations range from tuberculoid leprosy at one end to lepromatous leprosy at the other end of the spectrum, with borderline leprosy in between. Neuropathies are most common in patients with borderline leprosy. Superficial cutaneous nerves of the ears and distal limbs are commonly affected. Mononeuropathies, multiple mononeuropathies, or a slowly progressive symmetric sensorimotor polyneuropathy may develop. Sensory NCS are usually absent in the lower limb and are reduced in amplitude in the arms. Motor NCS may demonstrate reduced amplitudes in affected nerves but occasionally can reveal demyelinating features. Leprosy is usually diagnosed by skin lesion biopsy. Nerve biopsy can also be diagnostic, particularly when there are no apparent skin lesions. The tuberculoid form is characterized by granulomas, and bacilli are not seen. In contrast, with lepromatous leprosy, large numbers of infiltrating bacilli, T_H2 lymphocytes, and organism-laden, foamy macrophages with minimal granulomatous infiltration are evident. The bacilli are best appreciated using the Fite stain, where they can be seen as red-staining rods often in clusters free in the endoneurium, within macrophages, or within Schwann cells.

Patients are generally treated with multiple drugs: dapsone, rifampin, and clofazimine. Other medications that are used include thalidomide, pefloxacin, ofloxacin, sparfloxacin, minocycline, and clarithromycin. Patients are generally treated for 2 years. Treatment is sometimes complicated by the so-called reversal reaction, particularly in borderline leprosy. The reversal reaction can occur at any time during treatment and develops because of a shift to the tuberculoid end of the spectrum, with an increase in cellular immunity during treatment. The cellular response is upregulated as evidenced by an increased release of tumor necrosis factor α, interferon γ, and interleukin 2, with new granuloma formation. This can result in an exacerbation of the rash and the neuropathy as well as in appearance of new lesions. High-dose glucocorticoids blunt this adverse reaction and may be used prophylactically at treatment onset in high-risk patients. Erythema nodosum leprosum (ENL) is also treated with glucocorticoids or thalidomide.

LYME DISEASE

Lyme disease is caused by infection with *Borrelia burgdorferi*, a spirochete usually transmitted by the deer tick *Ixodes dammini* (Chap. 210). Neurologic complications may develop during the second and third stages of infection. Facial neuropathy is most common and is bilateral in about half of cases, which is rare for idiopathic Bell's palsy. Involvement of nerves is frequently asymmetric. Some patients present with a polyradiculoneuropathy or multiple mononeuropathies. EDx is suggestive of a primary axonopathy. Nerve biopsies can reveal axonal degeneration with perivascular inflammation. Treatment is with antibiotics (Chap. 210).

DIPHTHERITIC NEUROPATHY

Diphtheria is caused by the bacteria *Corynebacterium diphtheriae* (Chap. 175). Infected individuals present with flulike symptoms of generalized myalgias, headache, fatigue, low-grade fever, and irritability within a week to 10 days of the exposure. About 20–70% of patients develop a peripheral neuropathy caused by a toxin released by the bacteria. Three to 4 weeks after infection, patients may note decreased sensation in their throat and begin to develop dysphagia, dysarthria, hoarseness, and blurred vision due to impaired accommodation. A generalized polyneuropathy may manifest 2 or 3 months following the initial infection, characterized by numbness, paresthesias, and weakness of the arms and legs and occasionally ventilatory failure. CSF protein can be elevated with or without lymphocytic pleocytosis. EDx suggests a diffuse axonal sensorimotor polyneuropathy. Antitoxin and antibiotics should be given within 48 h of symptom onset. Although early treatment reduces the incidence and severity of some complications (i.e., cardiomyopathy), it does not appear to alter the natural history of the associated peripheral neuropathy. The neuropathy usually resolves after several months.

HUMAN IMMUNODEFICIENCY VIRUS (HIV)

HIV infection can result in a variety of neurologic complications, including peripheral neuropathies (Chap. 226). Approximately 20% of HIV-infected individuals develop a neuropathy either as a direct result of the virus itself, other associated viral infections (e.g., CMV), or neurotoxicity secondary to antiviral medications (see below). The major presentations of peripheral neuropathy associated with HIV infection include (1) distal symmetric polyneuropathy, (2) inflammatory demyelinating polyneuropathy (including both GBS and CIDP), (3) multiple mononeuropathies (e.g., vasculitis, CMV-related), (4) polyradiculopathy (usually CMV-related), (5) autonomic neuropathy, and (6) sensory ganglionitis.

HIV-Related Distal Symmetric Polyneuropathy (DSP) DSP is the most common form of peripheral neuropathy associated with HIV infection and usually is seen in patients with AIDS. It is characterized by numbness and painful paresthesias involving the distal extremities. The pathogenic basis for DSP is unknown but is not due to actual infection of the peripheral nerves. The neuropathy may be immune mediated, perhaps caused by the release of cytokines from surrounding inflammatory cells. Vitamin B_{12} deficiency may contribute in some instances but is not a major cause of most cases of DSP. Some antiretroviral agents (e.g., dideoxycytidine, dideoxyinosine, stavudine) are also neurotoxic and can cause a painful sensory neuropathy.

HIV-Related Inflammatory Demyelinating Polyradiculoneuropathy Both AIDP and CIDP can occur as a complication of HIV infection. AIDP usually develops at the time of seroconversion, whereas CIDP can occur any time in the course of the infection. Clinical and EDx features are indistinguishable from idiopathic AIDP or CIDP (discussed in Chap. 460). In addition to elevated protein levels, lymphocytic pleocytosis is evident in the CSF, a finding that helps distinguish this HIV-associated polyradiculoneuropathy from idiopathic AIDP/CIDP.

HIV-Related Progressive Polyradiculopathy An acute, progressive lumbosacral polyradiculoneuropathy usually secondary to CMV infection can develop in patients with AIDS. Patients present with severe radicular pain, numbness, and weakness in the legs, which is usually asymmetric. CSF is abnormal, demonstrating an increased protein along with reduced glucose concentration and notably a neutrophilic pleocytosis. EDx studies reveal features of active axonal degeneration. The polyradiculoneuropathy may improve with antiviral therapy.

HIV-Related Multiple Mononeuropathies Multiple mononeuropathies can also develop in patients with HIV infection, usually in the context of AIDS. Weakness, numbness, paresthesias, and pain occur in the distribution of affected nerves. Nerve biopsies can reveal axonal degeneration with necrotizing vasculitis or perivascular inflammation. Glucocorticoid treatment is indicated for vasculitis directly due to HIV infection.

HIV-Related Sensory Neuronopathy/Ganglionopathy Dorsal root ganglionitis is a very rare complication of HIV infection, and neuronopathy can be the presenting manifestation. Patients develop sensory ataxia similar to idiopathic sensory neuronopathy/ganglionopathy. NCS reveal reduced amplitudes or absence of sensory nerve action potentials (SNAPs).

HERPES VARICELLA-ZOSTER VIRUS

Peripheral neuropathy from herpes varicella-zoster (HVZ) infection results from reactivation of latent virus or from a primary infection (Chap. 217). Two-thirds of infections in adults are characterized by dermal zoster in which severe pain and paresthesias develop in a dermatomal region followed within a week or two by a vesicular rash in the same distribution. Weakness in muscles innervated by roots corresponding to the dermatomal distribution of skin lesions occurs in 5–30% of patients. Approximately 25% of affected patients have continued pain (postherpetic neuralgia [PHN]). A large clinical trial demonstrated that vaccination against zoster reduces the incidence of HVZ among vaccine recipients by 51% and reduces the incidence of PHN by 67%. Treatment of PHN is symptomatic (Table 459-6).

CYTOMEGALOVIRUS

CMV can cause an acute lumbosacral polyradiculopathy and multiple mononeuropathies in patients with HIV infection and in other immune deficiency conditions (Chap. 219).

EPSTEIN-BARR VIRUS

EBV infection has been associated with GBS, cranial neuropathies, mononeuropathy multiplex, brachial plexopathy, lumbosacral radiculoplexopathy, and sensory neuronopathies (Chap. 218).

HEPATITIS VIRUSES

Hepatitis B and C can cause multiple mononeuropathies related to vasculitis, AIDP, or CIDP (Chap. 362).

NEUROPATHIES ASSOCIATED WITH MALIGNANCY

Patients with malignancy can develop neuropathies due to (1) a direct effect of the cancer by invasion or compression of the nerves, (2) remote or paraneoplastic effect, (3) a toxic effect of treatment, or (4) as a consequence of immune compromise caused by immunosuppressive medications. The most common associated malignancy is lung cancer, but neuropathies also complicate carcinoma of the breast, ovaries, stomach, colon, rectum, and other organs, including the lymphoproliferative system.

PARANEOPLASTIC SENSORY NEURONOPATHY/GANGLIONOPATHY

Paraneoplastic encephalomyelitis/sensory neuronopathy (PEM/SN) usually complicates small-cell lung carcinoma (Chap. 122). Patients usually present with numbness and paresthesias in the distal extremities that are often asymmetric. The onset can be acute or insidiously progressive. Prominent loss of proprioception leads to sensory ataxia. Weakness can be present, usually secondary to an associated myelitis, motor neuronopathy, or concurrent Lambert-Eaton myasthenic syndrome (LEMS). Many patients also develop confusion, memory loss, depression, hallucinations or seizures, or cerebellar ataxia. Polyclonal antineuronal antibodies (IgG) directed against a 35- to 40-kDa protein or complex of proteins, the so-called Hu antigen, are found in the sera or CSF in the majority of patients with paraneoplastic PEM/SN. CSF may be normal or may demonstrate mild lymphocytic pleocytosis and elevated protein. PEM/SN is probably the result of antigenic similarity between proteins expressed in the tumor cells and neuronal cells, leading to an immune response directed against both cell types. Treatment of the underlying cancer generally does not affect the course of PEM/SN. However, occasional patients may improve following treatment of the tumor. Unfortunately, plasmapheresis, intravenous immunoglobulin, and immunosuppressive agents have not shown benefit.

NEUROPATHY SECONDARY TO TUMOR INFILTRATION

Malignant cells, in particular leukemia and lymphoma, can infiltrate cranial and peripheral nerves, leading to mononeuropathy, mononeuropathy multiplex, polyradiculopathy, plexopathy, or even a generalized symmetric distal or proximal and distal polyneuropathy. Neuropathy related to tumor infiltration is often painful; it can be the presenting manifestation of the cancer or the heralding symptom of a relapse. The neuropathy may improve with treatment of the underlying leukemia or lymphoma or with glucocorticoids.

NEUROPATHY AS A COMPLICATION OF BONE MARROW TRANSPLANTATION

Neuropathies may develop in patients who undergo bone marrow transplantation (BMT) because of the toxic effects of chemotherapy, radiation, infection, or an autoimmune response directed against the peripheral nerves. Peripheral neuropathy in BMT is often associated with graft-versus-host disease (GVHD). Chronic GVHD shares many features with a variety of autoimmune disorders, and it is possible that an immune-mediated response directed against peripheral nerves is responsible. Patients with chronic GVHD may develop cranial neuropathies, sensorimotor polyneuropathies, multiple mononeuropathies, and severe generalized peripheral neuropathies resembling AIDP or CIDP. The neuropathy may improve by increasing the intensity of immunosuppressive or immunomodulating therapy and resolution of the GVHD.

LYMPHOMA

Lymphomas may cause neuropathy by infiltration or direct compression of nerves or by a paraneoplastic process. The neuropathy can be purely sensory or motor, but most commonly is sensorimotor. The pattern of involvement may be symmetric, asymmetric, or multifocal, and the course may be acute, gradually progressive, or relapsing and remitting. EDx can be compatible with either an axonal or demyelinating process. CSF may reveal lymphocytic pleocytosis and an elevated protein. Nerve biopsy may demonstrate endoneurial inflammatory cells in both the infiltrative and the paraneoplastic etiologies. A monoclonal population of cells favors lymphomatous invasion. The neuropathy may respond to treatment of the underlying lymphoma or immunomodulating therapies.

MULTIPLE MYELOMA

Multiple myeloma (MM) usually presents in the fifth to seventh decade of life with fatigue, bone pain, anemia, and hypercalcemia (Chap. 136). Clinical and EDx features of neuropathy occur in as many as 40% of patients. The most common pattern is that of a distal, axonal, sensory, or sensorimotor polyneuropathy. Less frequently, a chronic demyelinating polyradiculoneuropathy may develop (see POEMS, Chap. 460). MM can be complicated by amyloid polyneuropathy and should be considered in patients with painful paresthesias, loss of pinprick and temperature discrimination, and autonomic dysfunction (suggestive of a small-fiber neuropathy) and CTS. Expanding plasmacytomas can compress cranial nerves and spinal roots as well. A monoclonal protein, usually composed of γ or μ heavy chains or κ light chains, may be identified in the serum or urine. EDx usually shows reduced amplitudes with normal or only mildly abnormal distal latencies and conduction velocities. A superimposed median neuropathy at the wrist is common. Abdominal fat pad, rectal, or sural nerve biopsy can be performed to look for amyloid deposition. Unfortunately, the treatment of the underlying MM does not usually affect the course of the neuropathy.

NEUROPATHIES ASSOCIATED WITH MONOCLONAL GAMMOPATHY OF UNCERTAIN SIGNIFICANCE (SEE CHAP. 460)

Toxic Neuropathies Secondary to Chemotherapy Many of the commonly used chemotherapy agents can cause a toxic neuropathy (Table 459-7). The mechanisms by which these agents cause toxic neuropathies vary, as does the specific type of neuropathy produced. The risk of developing a toxic neuropathy or more severe neuropathy appears to be greater in patients with a preexisting neuropathy (e.g., Charcot-Marie-Tooth disease, diabetic neuropathy) and those who also take other potentially neurotoxic drugs (e.g., nitrofurantoin, isoniazid, disulfiram, pyridoxine). Chemotherapeutic agents usually cause a sensory greater than motor length-dependent axonal neuropathy or neuronopathy/ganglionopathy.

OTHER TOXIC NEUROPATHIES

Neuropathies can develop as complications of toxic effects of various drugs and other environmental exposures (Table 459-8). The more common neuropathies associated with these agents are discussed here.

CHLOROQUINE AND HYDROXYCHLOROQUINE

Chloroquine and hydroxychloroquine can cause a toxic myopathy characterized by slowly progressive, painless, proximal weakness and atrophy, which is worse in the legs than the arms. In addition, neuropathy can also develop with or without the myopathy leading to sensory loss and distal weakness. The "neuromyopathy" usually appears in patients taking 500 mg daily for a year or more but has been reported with doses as low as 200 mg/d. Serum CK levels are usually elevated due to the superimposed myopathy. NCS reveal mild slowing of motor and sensory NCVs with a mild to moderate reduction in the amplitudes, although NCS may be normal in patients with only the myopathy. EMG demonstrates myopathic muscle action potentials (MUAPs), increased insertional activity in the form of positive sharp waves, fibrillation potentials, and occasionally myotonic potentials, particularly in the proximal muscles. Neurogenic MUAPs and reduced recruitment are found in more distal muscles. Nerve biopsy demonstrates autophagic vacuoles within Schwann cells. Vacuoles may also be evident in muscle biopsies. The pathogenic basis of the neuropathy is not known but may be related to the amphiphilic properties of the drug. These agents contain both hydrophobic and hydrophilic regions

TABLE 459-7 TOXIC NEUROPATHIES SECONDARY TO CHEMOTHERAPY

Drug	Mechanism of Neurotoxicity	Clinical Features	Nerve Histopathology	EMG/NCS
Vinca alkaloids (vincristine, vinblastine, vindesine, vinorelbine)	Interfere with axonal microtubule assembly; impairs axonal transport	Symmetric, S-M, large-/small-fiber PN; autonomic symptoms common; infrequent cranial neuropathies	Axonal degeneration of myelinated and unmyelinated fibers; regenerating clusters, minimal segmental demyelination	Axonal sensorimotor PN; distal denervation on EMG; abnormal QST, particularly vibratory perception
Cisplatin	Preferential damage to dorsal root ganglia: ? binds to and cross-links DNA ? inhibits protein synthesis ? impairs axonal transport	Predominant large-fiber sensory neuronopathy; sensory ataxia	Loss of large > small myelinated and unmyelinated fibers; axonal degeneration with small clusters of regenerating fibers; secondary segmental demyelination	Low-amplitude or unobtainable SNAPs with normal CMAPs and EMG; abnormal QST, particularly vibratory perception
Taxanes (paclitaxel, docetaxel)	Promotes axonal microtubule assembly; interferes with axonal transport	Symmetric, predominantly sensory PN; large-fiber modalities affected more than small-fiber	Loss of large > small myelinated and unmyelinated fibers; axonal degeneration with small clusters of regenerating fibers; secondary segmental demyelination	Axonal sensorimotor PN; distal denervation on EMG; abnormal QST, particularly vibratory perception
Suramin				
Axonal PN	Unknown; ? inhibition of neurotrophic growth factor binding; ? neuronal lysosomal storage	Symmetric, length-dependent, sensory-predominant PN	None described	Abnormalities consistent with an axonal S-M PN
Demyelinating PN	Unknown; ? immunomodulating effects	Subacute, S-M PN with diffuse proximal and distal weakness; areflexia; increased CSF protein	Loss of large and small myelinated fibers with primary demyelination and secondary axonal degeneration; occasional epi- and endoneurial inflammatory cell infiltrates	Features suggestive of an acquired demyelinating sensorimotor PN (e.g., slow CVs, prolonged distal latencies and F-wave latencies, conduction block, temporal dispersion)
Cytarabine (ARA-C)	Unknown; ? selective Schwann cell toxicity; ? immunomodulating effects	GBS-like syndrome; pure sensory neuropathy; brachial plexopathy	Loss of myelinated nerve fibers; axonal degeneration; segmental demyelination; no inflammation	Axonal, demyelinating, or mixed S-M PN; denervation on EMG
Etoposide (VP-16)	Unknown; ? selective dorsal root ganglia toxicity	Length-dependent, sensory-predominant PN; autonomic neuropathy	None described	Abnormalities consistent with an axonal S-M PN
Bortezomib (Velcade)	Unknown	Length-dependent, sensory, predominantly small-fiber PN	Not reported	Abnormalities consistent with an axonal sensory neuropathy with early small-fiber involvement (abnormal autonomic studies)

Abbreviations: CMAP, compound motor action potential; CSF, cerebrospinal fluid; CVs, conduction velocities; EMG, electromyography; GBS, Guillain-Barré syndrome; NCS, nerve conduction studies; PN, polyneuropathy; QST, quantitative sensory testing; S-M, sensorimotor; SNAP, sensory nerve action potential.

Source: From AA Amato, J Russell: *Neuromuscular Disease*. New York, McGraw-Hill, 2008.

TABLE 459-8 TOXIC NEUROPATHIES

Drug	Mechanism of Neurotoxicity	Clinical Features	Nerve Histopathology	EMG/NCS
Misonidazole	Unknown	Painful paresthesias and loss of large- and small-fiber sensory modalities and sometimes distal weakness in length-dependent pattern	Axonal degeneration of large myelinated fibers; axonal swellings; segmental demyelination	Low-amplitude or unobtainable SNAPs with normal or only slightly reduced CMAPs amplitudes
Metronidazole	Unknown	Painful paresthesias and loss of large- and small-fiber sensory modalities and sometimes distal weakness in length-dependent pattern	Axonal degeneration	Low-amplitude or unobtainable SNAPs with normal CMAPs
Chloroquine and hydroxychloroquine	Amphiphilic properties may lead to drug-lipid complexes that are indigestible and result in accumulation of autophagic vacuoles	Loss of large- and small-fiber sensory modalities and distal weakness in length-dependent pattern; superimposed myopathy may lead to proximal weakness	Axonal degeneration with autophagic vacuoles in nerves as well as muscle fibers	Low-amplitude or unobtainable SNAPs with normal or reduced CMAP amplitudes; distal denervation on EMG; irritability and myopathic-appearing MUAPs proximally in patients with superimposed toxic myopathy
Amiodarone	Amphiphilic properties may lead to drug-lipid complexes that are indigestible and result in accumulation of autophagic vacuoles	Paresthesias and pain with loss of large- and small-fiber sensory modalities and distal weakness in length-dependent pattern; superimposed myopathy may lead to proximal weakness	Axonal degeneration and segmental demyelination with myeloid inclusions in nerves and muscle fibers	Low-amplitude or unobtainable SNAPs with normal or reduced CMAP amplitudes; can also have prominent slowing of CVs; distal denervation on EMG; irritability and myopathic-appearing MUAPs proximally in patients with superimposed toxic myopathy
Colchicine	Inhibits polymerization of tubulin in microtubules and impairs axoplasmic flow	Numbness and paresthesias with loss of large-fiber modalities in a length-dependent fashion; superimposed myopathy may lead to proximal in addition to distal weakness	Nerve biopsy demonstrates axonal degeneration; muscle biopsy reveals fibers with vacuoles	Low-amplitude or unobtainable SNAPs with normal or reduced CMAP amplitudes; irritability and myopathic-appearing MUAPs proximally in patients with superimposed toxic myopathy
Podophyllin	Binds to microtubules and impairs axoplasmic flow	Sensory loss, tingling, muscle weakness, and diminished muscle stretch reflexes in length-dependent pattern; autonomic neuropathy	Axonal degeneration	Low-amplitude or unobtainable SNAPs with normal or reduced CMAP amplitudes
Thalidomide	Unknown	Numbness, tingling, and burning pain and weakness in a length-dependent pattern	Axonal degeneration; autopsy studies reveal degeneration of dorsal root ganglia	Low-amplitude or unobtainable SNAPs with normal or reduced CMAP amplitudes
Disulfiram	Accumulation of neurofilaments and impaired axoplasmic flow	Numbness, tingling, and burning pain in a length-dependent pattern	Axonal degeneration with accumulation of neurofilaments in the axons	Low-amplitude or unobtainable SNAPs with normal or reduced CMAP amplitudes
Dapsone	Unknown	Distal weakness that may progress to proximal muscles; sensory loss	Axonal degeneration and segmental demyelination	Low-amplitude or unobtainable CMAPs with normal or reduced SNAP amplitudes
Leflunomide	Unknown	Paresthesias and numbness in a length-dependent pattern	Unknown	Low-amplitude or unobtainable SNAPs with normal or reduced CMAP amplitudes
Nitrofurantoin	Unknown	Numbness, painful paresthesias, and severe weakness that may resemble GBS	Axonal degeneration; autopsy studies reveal degeneration of dorsal root ganglia and anterior horn cells	Low-amplitude or unobtainable SNAPs with normal or reduced CMAP amplitudes
Pyridoxine (vitamin B_6)	Unknown	Dysesthesias and sensory ataxia; impaired large-fiber sensory modalities on examination	Marked loss of sensory axons and cell bodies in dorsal root ganglia	Reduced amplitudes or absent SNAPs
Isoniazid	Inhibits pyridoxal phosphokinase leading to pyridoxine deficiency	Dysesthesias and sensory ataxia; impaired large fiber sensory modalities on examination	Marked loss of sensory axons and cell bodies in dorsal root ganglia and degeneration of the dorsal columns	Reduced amplitudes or absent SNAPs and, to a lesser extent, CMAPs
Ethambutol	Unknown	Numbness with loss of large-fiber modalities on examination	Axonal degeneration	Reduced amplitudes or absent SNAPs
Antinucleosides	Unknown	Dysesthesia and sensory ataxia; impaired large-fiber sensory modalities on examination	Axonal degeneration	Reduced amplitudes or absent SNAPs
Phenytoin	Unknown	Numbness with loss of large-fiber modalities on examination	Axonal degeneration and segmental demyelination	Low-amplitude or unobtainable SNAPs with normal or reduced CMAP amplitudes
Lithium	Unknown	Numbness with loss of large-fiber modalities on examination	Axonal degeneration	Low-amplitude or unobtainable SNAPs with normal or reduced CMAP amplitudes

(Continued)

TABLE 459-8 TOXIC NEUROPATHIES (*CONTINUED*)

Drug	Mechanism of Neurotoxicity	Clinical Features	Nerve Histopathology	EMG/NCS
Acrylamide	Unknown; may be caused by impaired axonal transport	Numbness with loss of large-fiber modalities on examination; sensory ataxia; mild distal weakness	Degeneration of sensory axons in peripheral nerves and posterior columns, spinocerebellar tracts, mammillary bodies, optic tracts, and corticospinal tracts in the CNS	Low-amplitude or unobtainable SNAPs with normal or reduced CMAP amplitudes
Carbon disulfide	Unknown	Length-dependent numbness and tingling with mild distal weakness	Axonal swellings with accumulation of neurofilaments	Low-amplitude or unobtainable SNAPs with normal or reduced CMAP amplitudes
Ethylene oxide	Unknown; may act as alkylating agent and bind DNA	Length-dependent numbness and tingling; may have mild distal weakness	Axonal degeneration	Low-amplitude or unobtainable SNAPs with normal or reduced CMAP amplitudes
Organophosphates	Bind and inhibit neuropathy target esterase	Early features are those of neuromuscular blockade with generalized weakness; later axonal sensorimotor PN ensues	Axonal degeneration along with degeneration of gracile fasciculus and corticospinal tracts	Early: repetitive firing of CMAPs and decrement with repetitive nerve stimulation; late: axonal sensorimotor PN
Hexacarbons	Unknown; may lead to covalent cross-linking between neurofilaments	Acute, severe sensorimotor PN that may resemble GBS	Axonal degeneration and giant axons swollen with neurofilaments	Features of a mixed axonal and/or demyelinating sensorimotor axonal PN—reduced amplitudes, prolonged distal latencies, conduction block, and slowing of CVs
Lead	Unknown; may interfere with mitochondria	Encephalopathy; motor neuropathy (often resembles radial neuropathy with wrist and finger drop); autonomic neuropathy; bluish-black discoloration of gums	Axonal degeneration of motor axons	Reduction of CMAP amplitudes with active denervation on EMG
Mercury	Unknown; may combine with sulfhydryl groups	Abdominal pain and nephrotic syndrome; encephalopathy; ataxia; paresthesias	Axonal degeneration; degeneration of dorsal root ganglia, calcarine, and cerebellar cortex	Low-amplitude or unobtainable SNAPs with normal or reduced CMAP amplitudes
Thallium	Unknown	Encephalopathy; painful sensory symptoms; mild loss of vibration; distal or generalized weakness may also develop; autonomic neuropathy; alopecia	Axonal degeneration	Low-amplitude or unobtainable SNAPs with normal or reduced CMAP amplitudes
Arsenic	Unknown; may combine with sulfhydryl groups	Abdominal discomfort, burning pain, and paresthesias; generalized weakness; autonomic insufficiency; can resemble GBS	Axonal degeneration	Low-amplitude or unobtainable SNAPs with normal or reduced CMAP amplitudes; may have demyelinating features: prolonged distal latencies and slowing of CVs
Gold	Unknown	Distal paresthesias and reduction of all sensory modalities	Axonal degeneration	Low-amplitude or unobtainable SNAPs

Abbreviations: CMAP, compound motor action potential; CVs, conduction velocities; EMG, electromyography; GBS, Guillain-Barré syndrome; MUAP, muscle action potential; NCS, nerve conduction studies; PN, polyneuropathy; S-M, sensorimotor; SNAP, sensory nerve action potential

Source: From AA Amato, J Russell: *Neuromuscular Disease*. New York, McGraw-Hill, 2008.

that allow them to interact with the anionic phospholipids of cell membranes and organelles. The drug-lipid complexes may be resistant to digestion by lysosomal enzymes, leading to the formation of autophagic vacuoles filled with myeloid debris that may in turn cause degeneration of nerves and muscle fibers. The signs and symptoms of the neuropathy and myopathy are usually reversible following discontinuation of medication.

AMIODARONE

Amiodarone can cause a neuromyopathy similar to chloroquine and hydroxychloroquine. The neuromyopathy typically appears after patients have taken the medication for 2–3 years. Nerve biopsy demonstrates a combination of segmental demyelination and axonal loss. Electron microscopy reveals lamellar or dense inclusions in Schwann cells, pericytes, and endothelial cells. The inclusions in muscle and nerve biopsies have persisted as long as 2 years following discontinuation of the medication.

COLCHICINE

Colchicine can also cause a neuromyopathy. Patients usually present with proximal weakness and numbness and tingling in the distal extremities. EDx reveals features of an axonal polyneuropathy. Muscle biopsy reveals a vacuolar myopathy, whereas sensory nerves demonstrate axonal degeneration. Colchicine inhibits the polymerization of tubulin into microtubules. The disruption of the microtubules probably leads to defective intracellular movement of important proteins, nutrients, and waste products in muscle and nerves.

THALIDOMIDE

Thalidomide is an immunomodulating agent used to treat multiple myeloma, GVHD, leprosy, and other autoimmune disorders. Thalidomide is associated with severe teratogenic effects as well as peripheral neuropathy that can be dose-limiting. Patients develop numbness, painful tingling, and burning discomfort in the feet and hands and less commonly muscle weakness and atrophy. Even after stopping the drug for 4–6 years, as many as 50% patients continue to have significant symptoms. NCS demonstrate reduced amplitudes or complete absence of SNAPs, with preserved conduction velocities when obtainable. Motor NCS are usually normal. Nerve biopsy reveals a loss of large-diameter myelinated fibers and axonal degeneration. Degeneration of dorsal root ganglion cells has been reported at autopsy.

PYRIDOXINE (VITAMIN B_6) TOXICITY

Pyridoxine is an essential vitamin that serves as a coenzyme for transamination and decarboxylation. However, at high doses (116 mg/d), patients can develop a severe sensory neuropathy with dysesthesias and sensory ataxia. NCS reveal absent or markedly reduced SNAP amplitudes with relatively preserved CMAPs. Nerve biopsy reveals axonal loss of fiber at all diameters. Loss of dorsal root ganglion cells with subsequent degeneration of both the peripheral and central sensory tracts have been reported in animal models.

ISONIAZID

One of the most common side effects of isoniazid (INH) is peripheral neuropathy. Standard doses of INH (3–5 mg/kg per day) are associated with a 2% incidence of neuropathy, whereas neuropathy develops in at least 17% of patients taking in excess of 6 mg/kg per day. The elderly, malnourished, and "slow acetylators" are at increased risk for developing the neuropathy. INH inhibits pyridoxal phosphokinase, resulting in pyridoxine deficiency and the neuropathy. Prophylactic administration of pyridoxine 100 mg/d can prevent the neuropathy from developing.

ANTIRETROVIRAL AGENTS

The nucleoside analogues zalcitabine (dideoxycytidine or ddC), didanosine (dideoxyinosine or ddI), stavudine (d4T), lamivudine (3TC), and antiretroviral nucleoside reverse transcriptase inhibitor (NRTI) are used to treat HIV infection. One of the major dose-limiting side effects of these medications is a predominantly sensory, length-dependent, symmetrically painful neuropathy. Zalcitabine (ddC) is the most extensively studied of the nucleoside analogues, and at doses greater than 0.18 mg/kg per day, it is associated with a subacute onset of severe burning and lancinating pains in the feet and hands. NCS reveal decreased amplitudes of the SNAPs with normal motor studies. The nucleoside analogues inhibit mitochondrial DNA polymerase, which is the suspected pathogenic basis for the neuropathy. Because of a "coasting effect," patients can continue to worsen even 2–3 weeks after stopping the medication. Following dose reduction, improvement in the neuropathy is seen in most patients after several months (mean time about 10 weeks).

HEXACARBONS (*n*-HEXANE, METHYL *n*-BUTYL KETONE)/GLUE SNIFFER'S NEUROPATHY

n-Hexane and methyl *n*-butyl ketone are water-insoluble industrial organic solvents that are also present in some glues. Exposure through inhalation, accidentally or intentionally (glue sniffing), or through skin absorption can lead to a profound subacute sensory and motor polyneuropathy. NCS demonstrate decreased amplitudes of the SNAPs and CMAPs with slightly slow CVs. Nerve biopsy reveals a loss of myelinated fibers and giant axons that are filled with 10-nm neurofilaments. Hexacarbon exposure leads to covalent cross-linking between axonal neurofilaments that result in their aggregation, impaired axonal transport, swelling of the axons, and eventual axonal degeneration.

LEAD

Lead neuropathy is uncommon, but it can be seen in children who accidentally ingest lead-based paints in older buildings and in industrial workers exposed to lead-containing products. The most common presentation of lead poisoning is an encephalopathy; however, symptoms and signs of a primarily motor neuropathy can also occur. The neuropathy is characterized by an insidious and progressive onset of weakness usually beginning in the arms, in particular involving the wrist and finger extensors, resembling a radial neuropathy. Sensation is generally preserved; however, the autonomic nervous system can be affected. Laboratory investigation can reveal a microcytic hypochromic anemia with basophilic stippling of erythrocytes, an elevated serum lead level, and an elevated serum coproporphyrin level. A 24-h urine collection demonstrates elevated levels of lead excretion. The NCS may reveal reduced CMAP amplitudes, while the SNAPs are typically normal. The pathogenic basis may be related to abnormal porphyrin metabolism. The most important principle of management is to remove the source of the exposure. Chelation therapy with calcium disodium ethylene-diaminetetraacetic acid (EDTA), British anti-Lewisite (BAL), and penicillamine also demonstrates variable efficacy.

MERCURY

Mercury toxicity may occur as a result of exposure to either organic or inorganic mercurials. Mercury poisoning presents with paresthesias in hands and feet that progress proximally and may involve the face and tongue. Motor weakness can also develop. CNS symptoms often overshadow the neuropathy. EDx shows features of a primarily axonal sensorimotor polyneuropathy. The primary site of neuromuscular pathology appears to be the dorsal root ganglia. The mainstay of treatment is removing the source of exposure.

THALLIUM

Thallium can exist in a monovalent or trivalent form and is primarily used as a rodenticide. The toxic neuropathy usually manifests as burning paresthesias of the feet, abdominal pain, and vomiting. Increased thirst, sleep disturbances, and psychotic behavior may be noted. Within the first week, patients develop pigmentation of the hair, an acne-like rash in the malar area of the face, and hyperreflexia. By the second and third week, autonomic instability with labile heart rate and blood pressure may be seen. Hyporeflexia and alopecia also occur but may not be evident until the third or fourth week following exposure. With severe intoxication, proximal weakness and involvement of the cranial nerves can occur. Some patients require mechanical ventilation due to respiratory muscle involvement. The lethal dose of thallium is variable, ranging from 8 to 15 mg/kg body weight. Death can result in less than 48 h following a particularly large dose. NCS demonstrate features of a primarily axonal sensorimotor polyneuropathy. With acute intoxication, potassium ferric ferrocyanide II may be effective in preventing absorption of thallium from the gut. However, there may be no benefit once thallium has been absorbed. Unfortunately, chelating agents are not very efficacious. Adequate diuresis is essential to help eliminate thallium from the body without increasing tissue availability from the serum.

ARSENIC

Arsenic is another heavy metal that can cause a toxic sensorimotor polyneuropathy. The neuropathy manifests 5–10 days after ingestion of arsenic and progresses for several weeks, sometimes mimicking GBS. The presenting symptoms are typically an abrupt onset of abdominal discomfort, nausea, vomiting, pain, and diarrhea followed within several days by burning pain in the feet and hands. Examination of the skin can be helpful in the diagnosis as the loss of the superficial epidermal layer results in patchy regions of increased or decreased pigmentation on the skin several weeks after an acute exposure or with chronic low levels of ingestion. Mee's lines, which are transverse lines at the base of the fingernails and toenails, do not become evident until 1 or 2 months after the exposure. Multiple Mee's lines may be seen in patients with long fingernails who have had chronic exposure to arsenic. Mee's lines are not specific for arsenic toxicity as they can also be seen following thallium poisoning. Because arsenic is cleared from blood rapidly, the serum concentration of arsenic is not diagnostically helpful. However, arsenic levels are increased in the urine, hair, and fingernails of patients exposed to arsenic. Anemia with stippling of erythrocytes is common, and occasionally pancytopenia and aplastic anemia can develop. Increased CSF protein levels without pleocytosis can be seen; this can lead to misdiagnosis as GBS. NCS are usually suggestive of an axonal sensorimotor polyneuropathy; however, demyelinating features can be present. Chelation therapy with BAL has yielded inconsistent results; therefore, it is not generally recommended.

NUTRITIONAL NEUROPATHIES

COBALAMIN (VITAMIN B_{12})

Pernicious anemia is the most common cause of cobalamin deficiency. Other causes include dietary avoidance (vegetarians), gastrectomy, gastric bypass surgery, inflammatory bowel disease, pancreatic insufficiency, bacterial overgrowth, and possibly histamine-2 blockers and proton pump inhibitors. An underappreciated cause of cobalamin deficiency is food-cobalamin malabsorption. This typically occurs in older individuals and results from an inability to adequately absorb cobalamin in food protein. No apparent cause of deficiency is identified in a significant number of patients with cobalamin deficiency. The use of nitrous oxide as an anesthetic agent or as a recreational drug can produce acute cobalamin deficiency neuropathy and subacute combined degeneration.

Complaints of numb hands typically appear before lower extremity paresthesias are noted. A preferential large-fiber sensory loss affecting proprioception and vibration with sparing of small-fiber modalities is present; an unsteady gait reflects sensory ataxia. These features, coupled with diffuse hyperreflexia and absent Achilles reflexes, should always focus attention on the possibility of cobalamin deficiency. Optic atrophy and, in severe cases, behavioral changes ranging from mild irritability and forgetfulness to severe dementia and frank psychosis may appear. The full clinical picture of subacute combined degeneration is uncommon. CNS manifestations, especially pyramidal tract signs, may be missing, and in fact some patients may only exhibit symptoms of peripheral neuropathy.

EDx shows an axonal sensorimotor neuropathy. CNS involvement produces abnormal somatosensory and visual evoked potential latencies. The diagnosis is confirmed by finding reduced serum cobalamin levels. In up to 40% of patients, anemia and macrocytosis are lacking. Serum methylmalonic acid and homocysteine, the metabolites that accumulate when cobalamin-dependent reactions are blocked, are elevated. Antibodies to intrinsic factor are present in approximately 60%, and antiparietal cell antibodies in about 90%, of individuals with pernicious anemia.

Cobalamin deficiency can be treated with various regimens of cobalamin. One typical regimen consists of 1000 μg cyanocobalamin IM weekly for 1 month and monthly thereafter. Patients with food cobalamin malabsorption can absorb free cobalamin and therefore can be treated with oral cobalamin supplementation. An oral cobalamin dose of 1000 μg per day should be sufficient. Treatment for cobalamin deficiency usually does not completely reverse the clinical manifestations, and at least 50% of patients exhibit some permanent neurologic deficit.

THIAMINE DEFICIENCY

Thiamine (vitamin B_1) deficiency is an uncommon cause of peripheral neuropathy in developed countries. It is now most often seen as a consequence of chronic alcohol abuse, recurrent vomiting, total parenteral nutrition, and bariatric surgery. Thiamine deficiency polyneuropathy can occur in normal, healthy young adults who do not abuse alcohol but who engage in inappropriately restrictive diets. Thiamine is water-soluble. It is present in most animal and plant tissues, but the greatest sources are unrefined cereal grains, wheat germ, yeast, soybean flour, and pork. Beriberi means "I can't, I can't" in Singhalese, the language of natives of what was once part of the Dutch East Indies (now Sri Lanka). *Dry beriberi* refers to neuropathic symptoms. The term *wet beriberi* is used when cardiac manifestations predominate (in reference to edema). Beriberi was relatively uncommon until the late 1800s when it became widespread among people for whom rice was a dietary mainstay. This epidemic was due to a new technique of processing rice that removed the germ from the rice shaft, rendering the so-called polished rice deficient in thiamine and other essential nutrients.

Symptoms of neuropathy follow prolonged deficiency. These begin with mild sensory loss and/or burning dysesthesias in the toes and feet and aching and cramping in the lower legs. Pain may be the predominant symptom. With progression, patients develop features of a nonspecific generalized polyneuropathy, with distal sensory loss in the feet and hands.

Blood and urine assays for thiamine are not reliable for diagnosis of deficiency. Erythrocyte transketolase activity and the percentage increase in activity (in vitro) following the addition of thiamine pyrophosphate (TPP) may be more accurate and reliable. EDx shows nonspecific findings of an axonal sensorimotor polyneuropathy. When a diagnosis of thiamine deficiency is made or suspected, thiamine replacement should be provided until proper nutrition is restored. Thiamine is usually given intravenously or intramuscularly at a dose of 100 mg/d. Although cardiac manifestations show a striking response to thiamine replacement, neurologic improvement is usually more variable and less dramatic.

VITAMIN E DEFICIENCY

The term *vitamin E* is usually used for a-tocopherol, the most active of the four main types of vitamin E. Because vitamin E is present in animal fat, vegetable oils, and various grains, deficiency is usually due to factors other than insufficient intake. Vitamin E deficiency usually occurs secondary to lipid malabsorption or in uncommon disorders of vitamin E transport. One hereditary disorder is abetalipoproteinemia, a rare autosomal dominant disorder characterized by steatorrhea, pigmentary retinopathy, acanthocytosis, and progressive ataxia. Patients with cystic fibrosis may also have vitamin E deficiency secondary to steatorrhea. There are genetic forms of isolated vitamin E deficiency not associated with lipid malabsorption. Vitamin E deficiency may also occur as a consequence of various cholestatic and hepatobiliary disorders as well as short-bowel syndromes resulting from the surgical treatment of intestinal disorders.

Clinical features may not appear until many years after the onset of deficiency. The onset of symptoms tends to be insidious, and progression is slow. The main clinical features are spinocerebellar ataxia and polyneuropathy, thus resembling Friedreich's ataxia or other spinocerebellar ataxias. Patients manifest progressive ataxia and signs of posterior column dysfunction, such as impaired joint position and vibratory sensation. Because of the polyneuropathy, there is hyporeflexia, but plantar responses may be extensor as a result of the spinal cord involvement. Other neurologic manifestations may include ophthalmoplegia, pigmented retinopathy, night blindness, dysarthria, pseudoathetosis, dystonia, and tremor. Vitamin E deficiency may present as an isolated polyneuropathy, but this is very rare. The yield of checking serum vitamin E levels in patients with isolated polyneuropathy is extremely low, and this test should not be part of routine practice.

Diagnosis is made by measuring a-tocopherol levels in the serum. EDx shows features of an axonal neuropathy. Treatment is replacement with oral vitamin E, but high doses are not needed. For patients with isolated vitamin E deficiency, treatment consists of 1500–6000 IU/d in divided doses.

VITAMIN B_6 DEFICIENCY

Vitamin B_6, or pyridoxine, can produce neuropathic manifestations from both deficiency and toxicity. Vitamin B_6 toxicity was discussed above. Vitamin B_6 deficiency is most commonly seen in patients treated with isoniazid or hydralazine. The polyneuropathy of vitamin B_6 is nonspecific, manifesting as a generalized axonal sensorimotor polyneuropathy. Vitamin B_6 deficiency can be detected by direct assay. Vitamin B_6 supplementation with 50–100 mg/d is suggested for patients being treated with isoniazid or hydralazine. This same dose is appropriate for replacement in cases of nutritional deficiency.

PELLAGRA (NIACIN DEFICIENCY)

Pellagra is produced by deficiency of niacin. Although pellagra may be seen in alcoholics, this disorder has essentially been eradicated in most Western countries by means of enriching bread with niacin. Nevertheless, pellagra continues to be a problem in a number of underdeveloped regions, particularly in Asia and Africa, where corn is the main source of carbohydrate. Neurologic manifestations are variable; abnormalities can develop in the brain and spinal cord as well as peripheral nerves. When peripheral nerves are involved, the neuropathy is usually mild and resembles beriberi. Treatment is with niacin 40–250 mg/d.

COPPER DEFICIENCY

A syndrome that has only recently been described is myeloneuropathy secondary to copper deficiency. Most patients present with lower limb paresthesias, weakness, spasticity, and gait difficulties. Large-fiber sensory function is impaired, reflexes are brisk, and plantar responses are extensor. In some cases, light touch and pinprick sensation are affected, and NCS indicate sensorimotor axonal polyneuropathy in addition to myelopathy.

Hematologic abnormalities are a known complication of copper deficiency; these can include microcytic anemia, neutropenia, and occasionally pancytopenia. Because copper is absorbed in the stomach and proximal jejunum, many cases of copper deficiency are in the setting of prior gastric surgery. Excess zinc is an established cause of copper deficiency. Zinc upregulates enterocyte production of metallothionine, which results in decreased absorption of copper. Excessive dietary zinc supplements or denture cream containing zinc can produce this clinical picture. Other potential causes of copper deficiency include malnutrition, prematurity, total parenteral nutrition, and ingestion of copper-chelating agents.

Following oral or IV copper replacement, some patients show neurologic improvement, but this may take many months or not occur at all. Replacement consists of oral copper sulfate or gluconate 2 mg one to three times a day. If oral copper replacement is not effective, elemental copper in the copper sulfate or copper chloride forms can be given as 2 mg IV daily for 3–5 days, then weekly for 1–2 months until copper levels normalize. Thereafter, oral daily copper therapy can be resumed. In contrast to the neurologic manifestations, most of the hematologic indices completely normalize in response to copper replacement therapy.

NEUROPATHY ASSOCIATED WITH GASTRIC SURGERY

Polyneuropathy may occur following gastric surgery for ulcer, cancer, or weight reduction. This usually occurs in the context of rapid, significant weight loss and recurrent, protracted vomiting. The clinical picture is one of acute or subacute sensory loss and weakness. Neuropathy following weight loss surgery usually occurs in the first several months after surgery. Weight reduction surgical procedures include gastrojejunostomy, gastric stapling, vertical banded gastroplasty, and gastrectomy with Roux-en-Y anastomosis. The initial manifestations are usually numbness and paresthesias in the feet. In many cases, no specific nutritional deficiency factor is identified.

Management consists of parenteral vitamin supplementation, especially including thiamine. Improvement has been observed following supplementation, parenteral nutritional support, and reversal of the surgical bypass. The duration and severity of deficits before identification and treatment of neuropathy are important predictors of final outcome.

CRYPTOGENIC (IDIOPATHIC) SENSORY AND SENSORIMOTOR POLYNEUROPATHY

CSPN is a diagnosis of exclusion, established after a careful medical, family, and social history; neurologic examination; and directed laboratory testing. Despite extensive evaluation, the cause of polyneuropathy in as many as 50% of all patients is idiopathic. CSPN should be considered a distinct diagnostic subset of peripheral neuropathy. The onset of CSPN is predominantly in the sixth and seventh decades. Patients complain of distal numbness, tingling, and often burning pain that invariably begins in the feet and may eventually involve the fingers and hands. Patients exhibit a distal sensory loss to pinprick, touch, and vibration in the toes and feet, and occasionally in the fingers. It is uncommon to see significant proprioception deficits, even though patients may complain of gait unsteadiness. However, tandem gait may be abnormal in a minority of cases. Neither subjective nor objective evidence of weakness is a prominent feature. Most patients have evidence of both large- and small-fiber loss on neurologic exam and EDx. Approximately 10% of patients have only evidence of small-fiber involvement. The ankle muscle stretch reflex is frequently absent, but in cases with predominantly small-fiber loss, this may be preserved. The EDx findings range from isolated sensory nerve action potential abnormalities (usually with loss of amplitude), to evidence for an axonal sensorimotor neuropathy, to a completely normal study (if primarily small fibers are involved). Therapy primarily involves the control of neuropathic pain (Table 459-6) if present. These drugs should not be used if the patient has only numbness and tingling but no pain.

Although no treatment is available that can reverse an idiopathic distal peripheral neuropathy, the prognosis is good. Progression often does not occur or is minimal, with sensory symptoms and signs progressing proximally up to the knees and elbows. The disorder does not lead to significant motor disability over time. The relatively benign course of this disorder should be explained to patients.

MONONEUROPATHIES/PLEXOPATHIES/RADICULOPATHIES

MEDIAN NEUROPATHY

CTS is a compression of the median nerve in the carpal tunnel at the wrist. The median nerve enters the hand through the carpal tunnel by coursing under the transverse carpal ligament. The symptoms of CTS consist of numbness and paresthesias variably in the thumb, index, middle, and half of the ring finger. At times, the paresthesias can include the entire hand and extend into the forearm or upper arm or can be isolated to one or two fingers. Pain is another common symptom and can be located in the hand and forearm and, at times, in the proximal arm. CTS is common and often misdiagnosed as thoracic outlet syndrome. The signs of CTS are decreased sensation in the median nerve distribution; reproduction of the sensation of tingling when a percussion hammer is tapped over the wrist (Tinel's sign) or the wrist is flexed for 30–60 s (Phalen's sign); and weakness of thumb opposition and abduction. EDx is extremely sensitive and shows slowing of sensory and, to a lesser extent, motor median potentials across the wrist. Treatment options consist of avoidance of precipitating activities; control of underlying systemic-associated conditions if present; nonsteroidal anti-inflammatory medications; neutral (volar) position wrist splints, especially for night use; glucocorticoid/anesthetic injection into the carpal tunnel; and surgical decompression by dividing the transverse carpal ligament. The surgical option should be considered if there is a poor response to nonsurgical treatments; if there is thenar muscle atrophy and/or weakness; and if there are significant denervation potentials on EMG.

Other proximal median neuropathies are very uncommon and include the pronator teres syndrome and anterior interosseous neuropathy. These often occur as a partial form of brachial plexitis.

ULNAR NEUROPATHY AT THE ELBOW—"CUBITAL TUNNEL SYNDROME"

The ulnar nerve passes through the condylar groove between the medial epicondyle and the olecranon. Symptoms consist of paresthesias, tingling, and numbness in the medial hand and half of the fourth and the entire fifth fingers, pain at the elbow or forearm, and weakness. Signs consist of decreased sensation in an ulnar distribution, Tinel's sign at the elbow, and weakness and atrophy of ulnar-innervated hand muscles. The Froment sign indicates thumb adductor weakness and consists of flexion of the thumb at the interphalangeal joint when attempting to oppose the thumb against the lateral border of the second digit. EDx may show slowing of ulnar motor NCV across the elbow with prolonged ulnar sensory latencies. Treatment consists of avoiding aggravating factors, using elbow pads, and surgery to decompress the nerve in the cubital tunnel. Ulnar neuropathies can also rarely occur at the wrist in the ulnar (Guyon) canal or in the hand, usually after trauma.

RADIAL NEUROPATHY

The radial nerve winds around the proximal humerus in the spiral groove and proceeds down the lateral arm and enters the forearm, dividing into the posterior interosseous nerve and superficial nerve. The symptoms and signs consist of wristdrop; finger extension weakness; thumb abduction weakness; and sensory loss in the dorsal web between the thumb and index finger. Triceps and brachioradialis strength is often normal, and triceps reflex is often intact. Most cases of radial neuropathy are transient compressive (neuropraxic) injuries that recover spontaneously in 6–8 weeks. If there has been prolonged compression and severe axonal damage, it may take several months to recover. Treatment consists of cock-up wrist and finger splints, avoiding further compression, and physical therapy to avoid flexion contracture. If there is no improvement in 2–3 weeks, an EDx study is recommended to confirm the clinical diagnosis and determine the degree of severity.

LATERAL FEMORAL CUTANEOUS NEUROPATHY (MERALGIA PARESTHETICA)

The lateral femoral cutaneous nerve arises from the upper lumbar plexus (spinal levels L2/3), crosses through the inguinal ligament near its attachment to the iliac bone, and supplies sensation to the anterior lateral thigh. The neuropathy affecting this nerve is also known as meralgia paresthetica. Symptoms and signs consist of paresthesias, numbness, and occasionally pain in the lateral thigh. Symptoms are increased by standing or walking and are relieved by sitting. There is normal strength, and knee reflexes are intact. The diagnosis is clinical, and further tests usually are not performed. EDx is only needed to rule out lumbar plexopathy, radiculopathy, or femoral neuropathy. If the symptoms and signs are classic, EMG is not necessary. Symptoms often resolve spontaneously over weeks or months, but the patient may be left with permanent numbness. Treatment consists of weight loss and avoiding tight belts. Analgesics in the form of a lidocaine patch, nonsteroidal agents, and occasionally medications for neuropathic pain can be used (Table 459-6). Rarely, locally injecting the nerve with an anesthetic can be tried. There is no role for surgery.

FEMORAL NEUROPATHY

Femoral neuropathies can arise as complications of retroperitoneal hematoma, lithotomy positioning, hip arthroplasty or dislocation, iliac artery occlusion, femoral arterial procedures, infiltration by hematogenous malignancy, penetrating groin trauma, pelvic surgery including hysterectomy and renal transplantation, and diabetes (a partial form of lumbosacral diabetic plexopathy); some cases are idiopathic. Patients with femoral neuropathy have difficulty extending their knee and flexing the hip. Sensory symptoms occurring either on the anterior thigh and/or medial leg occur in only half of reported cases. A prominent painful component is the exception rather than the rule, may be delayed, and is often self-limited in nature. The quadriceps (patellar) reflex is diminished.

SCIATIC NEUROPATHY

Sciatic neuropathies commonly complicate hip arthroplasty, pelvic procedures in which patients are placed in a prolonged lithotomy position, trauma, hematomas, tumor infiltration, and vasculitis. In addition, many sciatic neuropathies are idiopathic. Weakness may involve all motions of the ankles and toes as well as flexion of the leg at the knee; abduction and extension of the thigh at the hip are spared. Sensory loss occurs in the entire foot and the distal lateral leg. The ankle jerk and on occasion the internal hamstring reflex are diminished or more typically absent on the affected side. The peroneal subdivision of the sciatic nerve is typically involved disproportionately to the tibial counterpart. Thus, patients may have only ankle dorsiflexion and eversion weakness with sparing of knee flexion, ankle inversion, and plantar flexion; these features can lead to misdiagnosis of a common peroneal neuropathy.

PERONEAL NEUROPATHY

The sciatic nerve divides at the distal femur into the tibial and peroneal nerve. The common peroneal nerve passes posterior and laterally around the fibular head, under the fibular tunnel. It then divides into the superficial peroneal nerve, which supplies the ankle evertor muscles and sensation over the anterolateral distal leg and dorsum of the foot, and the deep peroneal nerve, which supplies ankle dorsiflexors and toe extensor muscles and a small area of sensation dorsally in the area of the first and second toes.

Symptoms and signs consist of footdrop (ankle dorsiflexion, toe extension, and ankle eversion weakness) and variable sensory loss, which may involve the superficial and deep peroneal pattern. There is usually no pain. Onset may be on awakening in the morning. Peroneal neuropathy needs to be distinguished from L5 radiculopathy. In L5 radiculopathy, ankle invertors and evertors are weak and needle EMG reveals denervation. EDx can help localize the lesion. Peroneal motor conduction velocity shows slowing and amplitude drop across the fibular head. Management consists of rapid weight loss and avoiding leg crossing. Footdrop is treated with an ankle brace. A knee pad can be worn over the lateral knee to avoid further compression. Most cases spontaneously resolve over weeks or months.

RADICULOPATHIES

Radiculopathies are most often due to compression from degenerative joint disease and herniated disks, but there are a number of unusual etiologies (Table 459-9). Degenerative spine disease affects a number of different structures, which narrow the diameter of the neural foramen or canal of the spinal column and compromise nerve root integrity; these are discussed in detail in Chap. 22.

PLEXOPATHIES

BRACHIAL PLEXUS

The brachial plexus is composed of three trunks (upper, middle, and lower), with two divisions (anterior and posterior) per trunk (Fig. 459-2). Subsequently, the trunks divide into three cords (medial, lateral, and posterior), and from these arise the multiple terminal nerves innervating the arm. The anterior primary rami of C5 and C6 fuse to form the upper trunk; the anterior primary ramus of C7 continues as the middle trunk, while the anterior rami of C8 and T1 join to form the lower trunk. There are several disorders commonly associated with brachial plexopathy.

Immune-Mediated Brachial Plexus Neuropathy Immune-mediated brachial plexus neuropathy (IBPN) goes by various terms, including *acute brachial plexitis*, *neuralgic amyotrophy*, and *Parsonage-Turner syndrome*. IBPN usually presents with an acute onset of severe pain in the shoulder region. The intense pain usually lasts several days to a few weeks, but a dull ache can persist. Individuals who are affected may not appreciate weakness of the arm early in the course because the pain limits movement. However, as the pain dissipates, weakness and often sensory loss are appreciated. Attacks can occasionally recur.

Clinical findings are dependent on the distribution of involvement (e.g., specific trunk, divisions, cords, or terminal nerves). The most common pattern of IBPN involves the upper trunk or a single or multiple mononeuropathies primarily involving the suprascapular, long thoracic, or axillary nerves. Additionally, the phrenic and anterior interosseous nerves may be concomitantly affected. Any of these nerves may also be affected in isolation. EDx is useful to confirm and localize the site(s) of involvement. Empirical treatment of severe pain with glucocorticoids is often used in the acute period.

Brachial Plexopathies Associated with Neoplasms Neoplasms involving the brachial plexus may be primary nerve tumors, local cancers expanding into the plexus (e.g., Pancoast lung tumor or lymphoma),

TABLE 459-9 CAUSES OF RADICULOPATHY

- Herniated nucleus pulposus
- Degenerative joint disease
- Rheumatoid arthritis
- Trauma
- Vertebral body compression fracture
- Pott's disease
- Compression by extradural mass (e.g., meningioma, metastatic tumor, hematoma, abscess)
- Primary nerve tumor (e.g., neurofibroma, schwannoma, neurinoma)
- Carcinomatous meningitis
- Perineurial spread of tumor (e.g., prostate cancer)
- Acute inflammatory demyelinating polyradiculopathy
- Chronic inflammatory demyelinating polyradiculopathy
- Sarcoidosis
- Amyloidoma
- Diabetic radiculopathy
- Infection (Lyme disease, herpes zoster, cytomegalovirus, syphilis, schistosomiasis, strongyloides)

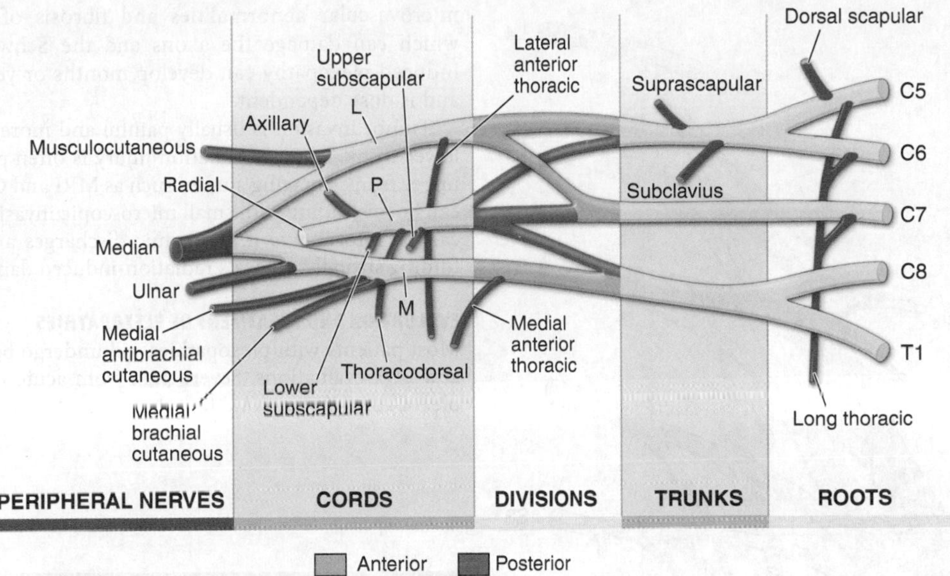

FIGURE 459-2 Brachial plexus anatomy. L, lateral; M, medial; P, posterior. *(From J Goodgold: Anatomical Correlates of Clinical Electromyography. Baltimore, Williams and Wilkins, 1974, p. 126, with permission.)*

and metastatic tumors. Primary brachial plexus tumors are less common than the secondary tumors and include schwannomas, neurinomas, and neurofibromas. Secondary tumors affecting the brachial plexus are more common and are always malignant. These may arise from local tumors, expanding into the plexus. For example, a Pancoast tumor of the upper lobe of the lung may invade or compress the lower trunk, whereas a primary lymphoma arising from the cervical or axillary lymph nodes may also infiltrate the plexus. Pancoast tumors typically present as an insidious onset of pain in the upper arm, sensory disturbance in the medial aspect of the forearm and hand, and weakness and atrophy of the intrinsic hand muscles along with an ipsilateral Horner's syndrome. Chest computed tomography (CT) scans or magnetic resonance imaging (MRI) can demonstrate extension of the tumor into the plexus. Metastatic involvement of the brachial plexus may occur with spread of breast cancer into the axillary lymph nodes with local spread into the nearby nerves.

Perioperative Plexopathies (Median Sternotomy) The most common surgical procedures associated with brachial plexopathy as a complication are those that involve median sternotomies (e.g., open-heart surgeries and thoracotomies). Brachial plexopathies occur in as many as 5% of patients following a median sternotomy and typically affect the lower trunk. Thus, individuals manifest with sensory disturbance affecting the medial aspect of forearm and hand along with weakness of the intrinsic hand muscles. The mechanism is related to the stretch of the lower trunk, so most individuals who are affected recover within a few months.

Lumbosacral Plexus The lumbar plexus arises from the ventral primary rami of the first to the fourth lumbar spinal nerves (Fig. 459-3). These nerves pass downward and laterally from the vertebral column within the psoas major muscle. The femoral nerve derives from the dorsal branches of the second to the fourth lumbar ventral rami. The obturator nerve arises from the ventral branches of the same lumbar rami. The lumbar plexus communicates with the sacral plexus by the lumbosacral trunk, which contains some fibers from the fourth and all of the fibers from the fifth lumbar ventral rami (Fig. 459-4).

The sacral plexus is the part of the lumbosacral plexus that is formed by the union of the lumbosacral trunk with the ventral rami of the first to fourth sacral nerves. The plexus lies on the posterior and posterolateral wall of the pelvis with its components converging toward the sciatic notch. The lateral trunk of the sciatic nerve (which forms the common peroneal nerve) arises from the union of the dorsal branches of the lumbosacral trunk (L4, L5) and the dorsal branches of the S1 and S2 spinal nerve ventral rami. The medial trunk of the sciatic nerve (which forms the tibial nerve) derives from the ventral branches of the same ventral rami (L4-S2).

LUMBOSACRAL PLEXOPATHIES

Plexopathies are typically recognized when motor, sensory, and if applicable, reflex deficits occur in multiple nerve and segmental distributions confined to one extremity. If localization within the lumbosacral plexus can be accomplished, designation as a lumbar plexopathy, a sacral plexopathy, a lumbosacral trunk lesion, or a panplexopathy is the best localization that can be expected. Although lumbar plexopathies may be bilateral, usually occurring in a stepwise and chronologically dissociated manner, sacral plexopathies are more likely to behave in this manner due to their closer anatomic proximity. The differential diagnosis of plexopathy includes disorders of the conus medullaris and cauda equina (polyradiculopathy). If there is a paucity of pain and sensory involvement, motor neuron disease should be considered as well.

The causes of lumbosacral plexopathies are listed in Table 459-10. Diabetic radiculopathy (discussed above) is a fairly common cause of painful leg weakness. Lumbosacral plexopathies are a well-recognized

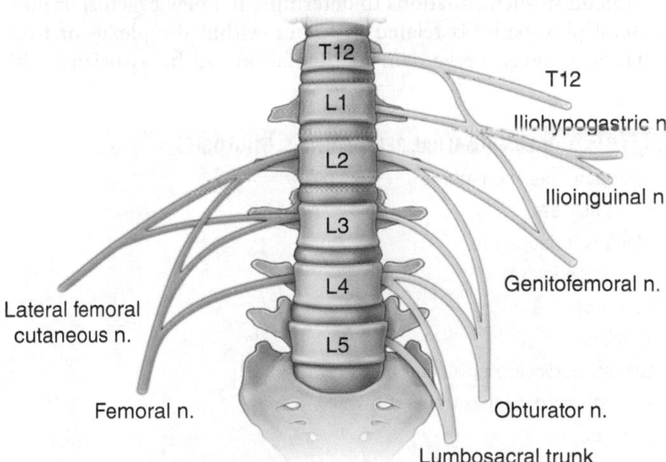

FIGURE 459-3 Lumbar plexus. Posterior divisions are in orange, and anterior divisions are in yellow. *(From J Goodgold: Anatomical Correlates of Clinical Electromyography.Baltimore, Williams and Wilkins, 1974, p. 126, with permission.)*

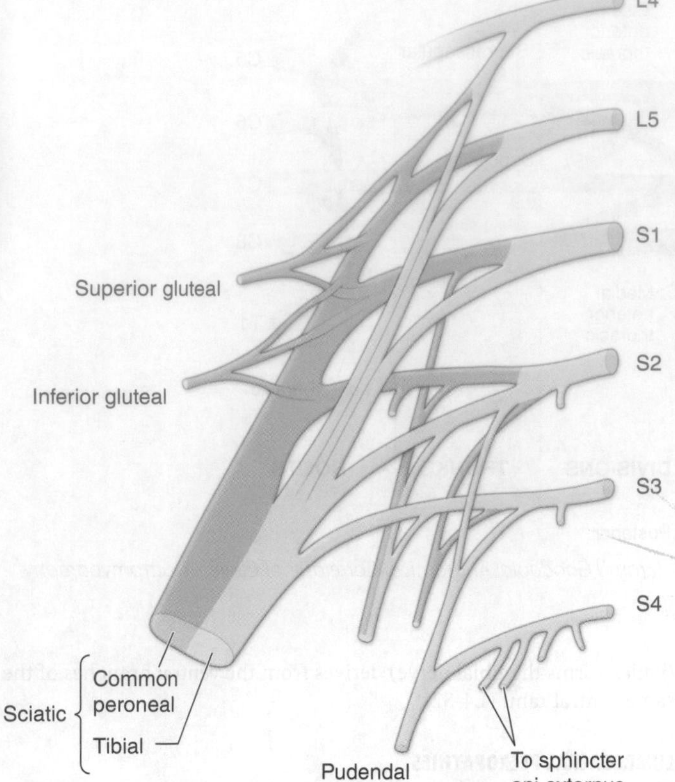

FIGURE 459-4 Lumbosacral plexus. Posterior divisions are in orange, and anterior divisions are in yellow. *(From J Goodgold: Anatomical Correlates of Clinical Electromyography. Baltimore, Williams and Wilkins, 1974, p. 126, with permission.)*

complication of retroperitoneal hemorrhage. Various primary and metastatic malignancies can affect the lumbosacral plexus as well; these include carcinoma of the cervix, endometrium, and ovary; osteosarcoma; testicular cancer; multiple myeloma; lymphoma; acute myelogenous leukemia; colon cancer; squamous cell carcinoma of the rectum; adenocarcinoma of unknown origin; and intraneural spread of prostate cancer.

RECURRENT NEOPLASTIC DISEASE OR RADIATION-INDUCED PLEXOPATHY

The treatment for various malignancies is often radiation therapy, the field of which may include parts of the brachial plexus. It can be difficult in such situations to determine if a new brachial or lumbosacral plexopathy is related to tumor within the plexus or from radiation-induced nerve damage. Radiation can be associated with microvascular abnormalities and fibrosis of surrounding tissues, which can damage the axons and the Schwann cells. Radiation-induced plexopathy can develop months or years following therapy and is dose dependent.

Tumor invasion is usually painful and more commonly affects the lower trunk, whereas radiation injury is often painless and affects the upper trunk. Imaging studies such as MRI and CT scans are useful but can be misleading with small microscopic invasion of the plexus. EMG can be informative if myokymic discharges are appreciated, as this finding strongly suggests radiation-induced damage.

TABLE 459-10 LUMBOSACRAL PLEXOPATHIES: ETIOLOGIES

- Retroperitoneal hematoma
- Psoas abscess
- Malignant neoplasm
- Benign neoplasm
- Radiation
- Amyloid
- Diabetic radiculoplexus neuropathy
- Idiopathic radiculoplexus neuropathy
- Sarcoidosis
- Aortic occlusion/surgery
- Lithotomy positioning
- Hip arthroplasty
- Pelvic fracture
- Obstetric injury

EVALUATION AND TREATMENT OF PLEXOPATHIES

Most patients with plexopathies will undergo both imaging with MRI and EDx evaluations. Severe pain from acute idiopathic lumbosacral plexopathy may respond to a short course of glucocorticoids.

460 Guillain-Barré Syndrome and Other Immune-Mediated Neuropathies

Stephen L. Hauser, Anthony A. Amato

GUILLAIN-BARRÉ SYNDROME

Guillain-Barré syndrome (GBS) is an acute, frequently severe, and fulminant polyradiculoneuropathy that is autoimmune in nature. It occurs year-round at a rate of between 1 and 4 cases per 100,000 annually; in the United States, ~5000–6000 cases occur per year. Males are at slightly higher risk for GBS than females, and in Western countries, adults are more frequently affected than children.

Clinical Manifestations GBS manifests as a rapidly evolving areflexic motor paralysis with or without sensory disturbance. The usual pattern is an ascending paralysis that may be first noticed as rubbery legs. Weakness typically evolves over hours to a few days and is frequently accompanied by tingling dysesthesias in the extremities. The legs are usually more affected than the arms, and facial diparesis is present in 50% of affected individuals. The lower cranial nerves are also frequently involved, causing bulbar weakness with difficulty handling secretions and maintaining an airway; the diagnosis in these patients may initially be mistaken for brainstem ischemia. Pain in the neck, shoulder, back, or diffusely over the spine is also common in the early stages of GBS, occurring in ~50% of patients. Most patients require hospitalization, and in different series, up to 30% require ventilatory assistance at some time during the illness. The need for mechanical ventilation is associated with more severe weakness on admission, a rapid tempo of progression, and the presence of facial and/or bulbar weakness during the first week of symptoms. Fever and constitutional symptoms are absent at the onset and, if present, cast doubt on the diagnosis. Deep tendon reflexes attenuate or disappear within the first few days of onset. Cutaneous sensory deficits (e.g., loss of pain and temperature sensation) are usually relatively mild, but functions subserved by large sensory fibers, such as deep tendon reflexes and proprioception, are more severely affected. Bladder dysfunction may occur in severe cases but is usually transient. If bladder dysfunction is a prominent feature and comes early in the course, diagnostic possibilities other than GBS should be considered, particularly spinal cord disease. Once clinical worsening stops and the patient reaches a plateau (almost always within 4 weeks of onset), further progression is unlikely.

Autonomic involvement is common and may occur even in patients whose GBS is otherwise mild. The usual manifestations are loss of vasomotor control with wide fluctuation in blood pressure, postural

TABLE 460-1 SUBTYPES OF GUILLAIN-BARRÉ SYNDROME (GBS)

Subtype	Features	Electrodiagnosis	Pathology
Acute inflammatory demyelinating polyneuropathy (AIDP)	Adults affected more than children; 90% of cases in Western world; recovery rapid; anti-GM1 antibodies (<50%)	Demyelinating	First attack on Schwann cell surface; widespread myelin damage, macrophage activation, and lymphocytic infiltration; variable secondary axonal damage
Acute motor axonal neuropathy (AMAN)	Children and young adults; prevalent in China and Mexico; may be seasonal; recovery rapid; anti-GD1a antibodies	Axonal	First attack at motor nodes of Ranvier; macrophage activation, few lymphocytes, frequent periaxonal macrophages; extent of axonal damage highly variable
Acute motor sensory axonal neuropathy (AMSAN)	Mostly adults; uncommon; recovery slow, often incomplete; closely related to AMAN	Axonal	Same as AMAN, but also affects sensory nerves and roots; axonal damage usually severe
Miller Fisher syndrome (MFS)	Adults and children; ophthalmoplegia, ataxia, and areflexia; anti-GQ1b antibodies (90%)	Axonal or demyelinating	Few cases examined; resembles AIDP

hypotension, and cardiac dysrhythmias. These features require close monitoring and management and can be fatal. Pain is another common feature of GBS; in addition to the acute pain described above, a deep aching pain may be present in weakened muscles that patients liken to having overexercised the previous day. Other pains in GBS include dysesthetic pain in the extremities as a manifestation of sensory nerve fiber involvement. These pains are self-limited and often respond to standard analgesics (Chap. 18).

Several subtypes of GBS are recognized, as determined primarily by electrodiagnostic (Edx) and pathologic distinctions (Table 460-1). The most common variant is acute inflammatory demyelinating polyneuropathy (AIDP). Additionally, there are two axonal variants, which are often clinically severe the acute motor axonal neuropathy (AMAN) and acute motor sensory axonal neuropathy (AMSAN) subtypes. In addition, a range of limited or regional GBS syndromes are also encountered. Notable among these is the Miller Fisher syndrome (MFS), which presents as rapidly evolving ataxia and areflexia of limbs without weakness, and ophthalmoplegia, often with pupillary paralysis. The MFS variant accounts for ~5% of all cases and is strongly associated with antibodies to the ganglioside GQ1b (see "Immunopathogenesis," below). Other regional variants of GBS include (1) pure sensory forms; (2) ophthalmoplegia with anti-GQ1b antibodies as part of severe motor-sensory GBS; (3) GBS with severe bulbar and facial paralysis, sometimes associated with antecedent cytomegalovirus (CMV) infection and anti-GM2 antibodies; and (4) acute pandysautonomia (Chap. 454).

Antecedent Events Approximately 70% of cases of GBS occur 1–3 weeks after an acute infectious process, usually respiratory or gastrointestinal. Culture and seroepidemiologic techniques show that 20–30% of all cases occurring in North America, Europe, and Australia are preceded by infection or reinfection with *Campylobacter jejuni*. A similar proportion is preceded by a human herpes virus infection, often CMV or Epstein-Barr virus. Other viruses (e.g., HIV, hepatitis E) and also *Mycoplasma pneumoniae* have been identified as agents involved in antecedent infections, as have recent immunizations. The swine influenza vaccine, administered widely in the United States in 1976, is the most notable example. Influenza vaccines in use from 1992 to 1994, however, resulted in only one additional case of GBS per million persons vaccinated, and the more recent seasonal influenza vaccines appear to confer a GBS risk of <1 per million. Epidemiologic studies looking at H1N1 vaccination demonstrated at most only a slight increased risk of GBS. Meningococcal vaccinations (Menactra) does not appear to carry an increased risk. Older-type rabies vaccine, prepared in nervous system tissue, is implicated as a trigger of GBS in developing countries where it is still used; the mechanism is presumably immunization against neural antigens. GBS also occurs more frequently than can be attributed to chance alone in patients with lymphoma (including Hodgkin's disease), in HIV-seropositive individuals, and in patients with systemic lupus erythematosus (SLE). *C. jejuni* has also been implicated in summer outbreaks of AMAN among children and young adults exposed to chickens in rural China.

Immunopathogenesis Several lines of evidence support an autoimmune basis for acute inflammatory demyelinating polyneuropathy (AIDP), the most common and best-studied type of GBS; the concept extends to all of the subtypes of GBS (Table 460-1).

It is likely that both cellular and humoral immune mechanisms contribute to tissue damage in AIDP. T cell activation is suggested by the finding that elevated levels of cytokines and cytokine receptors are present in serum (interleukin [IL] 2, soluble IL-2 receptor) and in cerebrospinal fluid (CSF) (IL-6, tumor necrosis factor α, interferon γ). AIDP is also closely analogous to an experimental T cell–mediated immunopathy designated *experimental allergic neuritis* (EAN). EAN is induced in laboratory animals by immune sensitization against protein fragments derived from peripheral nerve proteins, and in particular against the P2 protein. Based on analogy to EAN, it was initially thought that AIDP was likely to be primarily a T cell–mediated disorder; however, abundant data now suggest that autoantibodies directed against nonprotein determinants may be central to many cases.

Circumstantial evidence suggests that all GBS results from immune responses to nonself antigens (infectious agents, vaccines) that misdirect to host nerve tissue through a resemblance-of-epitope (molecular mimicry) mechanism (Fig. 460-1). The neural targets are likely to be glycoconjugates, specifically gangliosides (Table 460-2; Fig. 460-2). Gangliosides are complex glycosphingolipids that contain one or more sialic acid residues; various gangliosides participate in cell-cell interactions (including those between axons and glia), modulation of receptors, and regulation of growth. They are typically exposed on the plasma membrane of cells, rendering them susceptible to an antibody-mediated attack. Gangliosides and other glycoconjugates are present in large quantity in human nervous tissues and in key sites, such as nodes of Ranvier. Antiganglioside antibodies, most frequently to GM1, are common in GBS (20–50% of cases), particularly in AMAN and AMSAN and in those cases preceded by *C. jejuni* infection. Furthermore, isolates of *C. jejuni* from stool cultures of patients with GBS have surface glycolipid structures that antigenically cross react with gangliosides, including GM1, concentrated in human nerves. Sialic acid residues from pathogenic *C. jejuni* strains can also trigger activation of dendritic cells via signaling through a toll-like receptor (TLR4), promoting B cell differentiation and further amplifying humoral autoimmunity. Another line of evidence is derived from experience in Europe with parenteral use of purified bovine brain gangliosides for treatment of various neuropathic disorders. Between 5 and 15 days after injection, some recipients developed acute motor axonal GBS with high titers of anti-GM1 antibodies that recognized epitopes at nodes of Ranvier and motor endplates. Experimentally, anti-GM1 antibodies can trigger complement-mediated injury at paranodal axon-glial junctions, disrupting the clustering of sodium channels and likely contributing to conduction block (see "Pathophysiology," below).

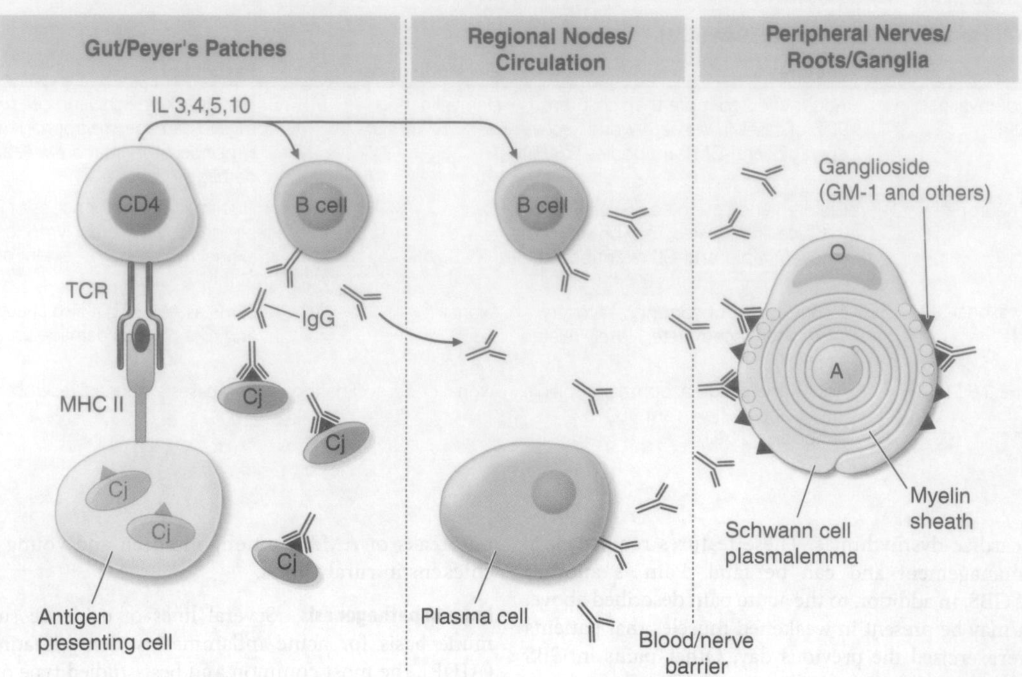

FIGURE 460-1 Postulated immunopathogenesis of Guillain-Barré syndrome (GBS) associated with *Campylobacter jejuni* infection. B cells recognize glycoconjugates on *C. jejuni* (Cj) (*triangles*) that cross-react with ganglioside present on Schwann cell surface and subjacent peripheral nerve myelin. Some B cells, activated via a T cell–independent mechanism, secrete primarily IgM (not shown). Other B cells (*upper left side*) are activated via a partially T cell–dependent route and secrete primarily IgG; T cell help is provided by CD4 cells activated locally by fragments of Cj proteins that are presented on the surface of antigen-presenting cells (APCs). A critical event in the development of GBS is the escape of activated B cells from Peyer's patches into regional lymph nodes. Activated T cells probably also function to assist in opening of the blood-nerve barrier, facilitating penetration of pathogenic autoantibodies. The earliest changes in myelin (*right*) consist of edema between myelin lamellae and vesicular disruption (*shown as circular blebs*) of the outermost myelin layers. These effects are associated with activation of the C5b-C9 membrane attack complex and probably mediated by calcium entry; it is possible that the macrophage cytokine tumor necrosis factor (TNF) also participates in myelin damage. A, axon; B, B cell; MHC II, class II major histocompatibility complex molecule; O, oligodendrocyte; TCR, T cell receptor.

TABLE 460-2 PRINCIPAL ANTIGLYCOLIPID ANTIBODIES IMPLICATED IN IMMUNE NEUROPATHIES

Clinical Presentation	Antibody Target	Usual Isotype
Acute Immune Neuropathies (Guillain-Barré Syndrome)		
Acute inflammatory demyelinating polyneuropathy (AIDP)	No clear patterns	IgG (polyclonal)
	GM1 most common	
Acute motor axonal neuropathy (AMAN)	GD1a, GM1, GM1b, GalNAc–GD1a (<50% for any)	IgG (polyclonal)
Miller Fisher syndrome (MFS)	GQ1b (>90%)	IgG (polyclonal)
Acute pharyngeal cervicobrachial neuropathy (APCBN)	GT1a (? most)	IgG (polyclonal)
Chronic Immune Neuropathies		
Chronic inflammatory demyelinating polyneuropathy (CIDP) (75%)	P0, myelin P2 protein, PMP22, neurofascin	No clear pattern
CIDP-M (MGUS associated) (25%)	Neural binding sites	IgG, IgA (monoclonal)
Chronic sensory > motor neuropathy	SPGP, SGLPG (on MAG) (50%)	IgM (monoclonal)
	Uncertain (50%)	IgM (monoclonal)
Multifocal motor neuropathy (MMN)	GM1, GalNAc–GD1a, others (25–50%)	IgM (polyclonal, monoclonal)
Chronic sensory ataxic neuropathy	GD1b, GQ1b, and other b-series gangliosides	IgM (monoclonal)

Abbreviations: CIDP-M, CIDP with a monoclonal gammopathy; MAG, myelin-associated glycoprotein; MGUS, monoclonal gammopathy of undetermined significance.

Source: Modified from HJ Willison, N Yuki: Brain 125:2591, 2002.

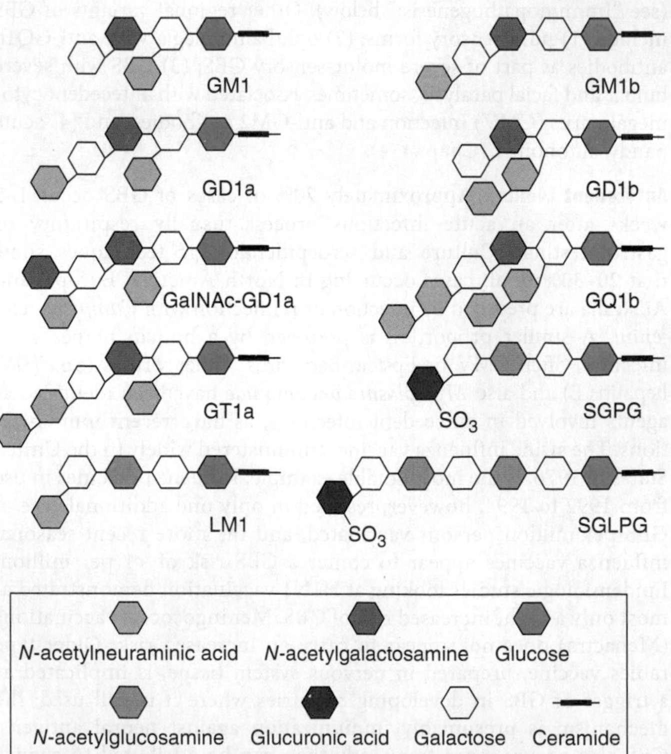

FIGURE 460-2 Glycolipids implicated as antigens in immune-mediated neuropathies. (*Modified from HJ Willison, N Yuki: Brain 125: 2591, 2002.*)

Anti-GQ1b IgG antibodies are found in >90% of patients with MFS (Table 460-2; Fig. 460-2), and titers of IgG are highest early in the course. Anti-GQ1b antibodies are not found in other forms of GBS unless there is extraocular motor nerve involvement. A possible explanation for this association is that extraocular motor nerves are enriched in GQ1b gangliosides in comparison to limb nerves. In addition, a monoclonal anti-GQ1b antibody raised against *C. jejuni* isolated from a patient with MFS blocked neuromuscular transmission experimentally.

Taken together, these observations provide strong but still inconclusive evidence that autoantibodies play an important pathogenic role in GBS. Although antiganglioside antibodies have been studied most intensively, other antigenic targets may also be important. One report identified IgG antibodies against Schwann cells and neurons (nerve growth cone region) in some GBS cases. Proof that these antibodies are pathogenic requires that they be capable of mediating disease following direct passive transfer to naïve hosts; this has not yet been demonstrated, although one case of possible maternal-fetal transplacental transfer of GBS has been described.

In AIDP, an early step in the induction of tissue damage appears to be complement deposition along the outer surface of the Schwann cell. Activation of complement initiates a characteristic vesicular disintegration of the myelin sheath and also leads to recruitment of activated macrophages, which participate in damage to myelin and axons. In AMAN, the pattern is different in that complement is deposited along with IgG at the nodes of Ranvier along large motor axons. Interestingly, in cases of AMAN, antibodies against GD1a appear to have a fine specificity that favors binding to motor rather than sensory nerve roots, even though this ganglioside is expressed on both fiber types.

Pathophysiology In the demyelinating forms of GBS, the basis for flaccid paralysis and sensory disturbance is conduction block. This finding, demonstrable electrophysiologically, implies that the axonal connections remain intact. Hence, recovery can take place rapidly as remyelination occurs. In severe cases of demyelinating GBS, secondary axonal degeneration usually occurs; its extent can be estimated electrophysiologically. More secondary axonal degeneration correlates with a slower rate of recovery and a greater degree of residual disability. When a severe primary axonal pattern is encountered electrophysiologically, the implication is that axons have degenerated and become disconnected from their targets, specifically the neuromuscular junctions, and must therefore regenerate for recovery to take place. In motor axonal cases in which recovery is rapid, the lesion is thought to be localized to preterminal motor branches, allowing regeneration and reinnervation to take place quickly. Alternatively, in mild cases, collateral sprouting and reinnervation from surviving motor axons near the neuromuscular junction may begin to reestablish physiologic continuity with muscle cells over a period of several months.

Laboratory Features CSF findings are distinctive, consisting of an elevated CSF protein level (1–10 g/L [100–1000 mg/dL]) without accompanying pleocytosis. The CSF is often normal when symptoms have been present for ≤48 h; by the end of the first week, the level of protein is usually elevated. A transient increase in the CSF white cell count (10–100/μL) occurs on occasion in otherwise typical GBS; however, a sustained CSF pleocytosis suggests an alternative diagnosis (viral myelitis) or a concurrent diagnosis such as unrecognized HIV infection, leukemia or lymphoma with infiltration of nerves, or neurosarcoidosis. Edx features are mild or absent in the early stages of GBS and lag behind the clinical evolution. In AIDP, the earliest features are prolonged F-wave latencies, prolonged distal latencies, and reduced amplitudes of compound muscle action potentials (CMAPs), probably owing to the predilection for involvement of nerve roots and distal motor nerve terminals early in the course. Later, slowing of conduction velocity, conduction block, and temporal dispersion may be appreciated (Table 460-1). Occasionally, sensory nerve action potentials (SNAPs) may be normal in the feet (e.g., sural nerve) when abnormal in the arms. This is also a sign that the patient does not have one of the more typical "length-dependent" polyneuropathies. In cases with primary axonal pathology, the principal Edx finding is reduced amplitude of CMAPs (and also SNAPS with AMSAN) without conduction slowing or prolongation of distal latencies.

Diagnosis GBS is a descriptive entity. The diagnosis of AIDP is made by recognizing the pattern of rapidly evolving paralysis with areflexia, absence of fever or other systemic symptoms, and characteristic antecedent events. In 2011, the Brighton Collaboration developed a new set of case definitions for GBS in response to needs of epidemiologic studies of vaccination and assessing risks of GBS (Table 460-3). These criteria have subsequently been validated. Other disorders that may enter into the differential diagnosis include acute myelopathies (especially with prolonged back pain and sphincter disturbances); diphtheria (early oropharyngeal disturbances); Lyme polyradiculitis and other tick-borne paralyses; porphyria (abdominal pain, seizures, psychosis); vasculitic neuropathy (check erythrocyte sedimentation rate, described below); poliomyelitis (fever and meningismus common); West Nile virus; CMV polyradiculitis (in immunocompromised patients); critical illness neuropathy or myopathy; neuromuscular junction disorders such as myasthenia gravis and botulism (pupillary reactivity lost early); poisonings with organophosphates, thallium, or arsenic; paralytic shellfish poisoning; or severe hypophosphatemia (rare). Laboratory tests are helpful primarily to exclude mimics of GBS. Edx features may be minimal, and the CSF protein level may not rise until the end of the first week. If the diagnosis is strongly suspected, treatment should be initiated without waiting for evolution of the characteristic Edx and CSF findings to occur. GBS patients with risk factors for HIV or with CSF pleocytosis should have a serologic test for HIV.

TREATMENT GUILLAIN-BARRÉ SYNDROME

In the vast majority of patients with GBS, treatment should be initiated as soon after diagnosis as possible. Each day counts; ~2 weeks after the first motor symptoms, it is not known whether immunotherapy is still effective. If the patient has already reached the plateau stage, then treatment probably is no longer indicated, unless the patient has severe motor weakness and one cannot exclude the possibility that an immunologic attack is still ongoing. Either high-dose intravenous immune globulin (IVIg) or plasmapheresis can be initiated, as they are equally effective for typical GBS. A combination of the two therapies is not significantly better than either alone. IVIg is often the initial therapy chosen because of its ease of administration and good safety record. Anecdotal data have also suggested that IVIg may be preferable to plasma exchange (PE) for the AMAN and MFS variants of GBS. IVIg is administered as five daily infusions for a total dose of 2 g/kg body weight. There is some evidence that GBS autoantibodies are neutralized by anti-idiotypic antibodies present in IVIg preparations, perhaps accounting for the therapeutic effect. A course of plasmapheresis usually consists of ~40–50 mL/kg PE four to five times over a week. Meta-analysis of randomized clinical trials indicates that treatment reduces the need for mechanical ventilation by nearly half (from 27% to 14% with PE) and increases the likelihood of full recovery at 1 year (from 55% to 68%). Functionally significant improvement may occur toward the end of the first week of treatment or may be delayed for several weeks. The lack of noticeable improvement following a course of IVIg or PE is not an indication to treat with the alternate treatment. However, there are occasional patients who are treated early in the course of GBS and improve, who then relapse within a month. Brief retreatment with the original therapy is usually effective in such cases. Glucocorticoids have not been found to be effective in GBS. Occasional patients with very mild forms of GBS, especially those who appear to have already reached a plateau when initially seen, may be managed conservatively without IVIg or PE.

In the worsening phase of GBS, most patients require monitoring in a critical care setting, with particular attention to vital capacity, heart rhythm, blood pressure, nutrition, deep vein thrombosis prophylaxis, cardiovascular status, early consideration (after 2 weeks

TABLE 460-3 BRIGHTON CRITERIA FOR DIAGNOSIS OF GUILLAIN-BARRÉ SYNDROME (GBS) AND MILLER FISHER SYNDROME

Clinical case definitions for diagnosis of GBS

Level 1 of diagnostic certainty

Bilateral AND flaccid weakness of the limbs

AND

Decreased or absent deep tendon reflexes in weak limbs

AND

Monophasic illness pattern and interval between onset and nadir of weakness between 12 h and 28 days and subsequent clinical plateau

AND

Electrophysiologic findings consistent with GBS

AND

Cytoalbuminologic dissociation (i.e., elevation of CSF protein level above laboratory normal value AND CSF total white cell count <50 cells/μL)

AND

Absence of an identified alternative diagnosis for weakness

Level 2 of diagnostic certainty

Bilateral AND flaccid weakness of the limbs

AND

Decreased or absent deep tendon reflexes in weak limbs

AND

Monophasic illness pattern and interval between onset and nadir of weakness between 12 h and 28 days and subsequent clinical plateau

AND

CSF total white cell count <50 cells/μL (with or without CSF protein elevation above laboratory normal value)

OR

If CSF not collected or results not available, electrophysiologic studies consistent with GBS

AND

Absence of identified alternative diagnosis for weakness

Level 3 of diagnostic certainty

Bilateral and flaccid weakness of the limbs

AND

Decreased or absent deep tendon reflexes in weak limbs

AND

Monophasic illness pattern and interval between onset and nadir of weakness between 12 h and 28 days and subsequent clinical plateau

AND

Absence of identified alternative diagnosis for weakness

Clinical case definitions for diagnosis of Miller Fisher syndrome

Level 1 of diagnostic certainty

Bilateral ophthalmoparesis and bilateral reduced or absent tendon reflexes, and ataxia

AND

Absence of limb weakness

AND

Monophasic illness pattern and interval between onset and nadir of weakness between 12 h and 28 days and subsequent clinical plateau

AND

Cytoalbuminologic dissociation (i.e., elevation of cerebrospinal protein above the laboratory normal and total CSF white cell count <50 cells/μL)

AND

Nerve conduction studies are normal, OR indicate involvement of sensory nerves only

AND

No alterations in consciousness or corticospinal tract signs

AND

Absence of identified alternative diagnosis

Level 2 of diagnostic certainty

Bilateral ophthalmoparesis and bilateral reduced or absent tendon reflexes and ataxia

AND

Absence of limb weakness

AND

Monophasic illness pattern and interval between onset and nadir of weakness between 12 h and 28 days and subsequent clinical plateau

AND

CSF with a total white cell count <50 cells/μL) (with or without CSF protein elevation above laboratory normal value)

OR

Nerve conduction studies are normal, OR indicate involvement of sensory nerves only

AND

No alterations in consciousness or corticospinal tract signs

AND

Absence of identified alternative diagnosis

Level 3 of diagnostic certainty

Bilateral ophthalmoparesis and bilateral reduced or absent tendon reflexes and ataxia

AND

Absence of limb weakness

AND

Monophasic illness pattern and interval between onset and nadir of weakness between 12 h and 28 days and subsequent clinical plateau

AND

No alterations in consciousness or corticospinal tract signs

AND

Absence of identified alternative diagnosis

Abbreviation: CSF, cerebrospinal fluid.

Source: From JJ Sejvar et al: Guillain-Barré syndrome and Fisher syndrome: case definitions and guidelines for collection, analysis, and presentation of immunization safety data. Vaccine 29:599, 2011. Validation study published by C Fokke et al: Diagnosis of Guillain-Barré syndrome and validation of Brighton criteria. Brain 137:33, 2014.

of intubation) of tracheotomy, and chest physiotherapy. As noted, ~30% of patients with GBS require ventilatory assistance, sometimes for prolonged periods of time (several weeks or longer). Frequent turning and assiduous skin care are important, as are daily range-of-motion exercises to avoid joint contractures and daily reassurance as to the generally good outlook for recovery.

Prognosis and Recovery Approximately 85% of patients with GBS achieve a full functional recovery within several months to a year, although minor findings on examination (such as areflexia) may persist and patients often complain of continued symptoms, including fatigue. The mortality rate is <5% in optimal settings; death usually results from secondary pulmonary complications. The outlook is worst in patients with severe proximal motor and sensory axonal damage. Such axonal damage may be either primary or secondary in nature (see "Pathophysiology," above), but in either case successful regeneration cannot occur. Other factors that worsen the outlook for recovery are advanced age, a fulminant or severe attack, and a delay in the onset of treatment. Between 5 and 10% of patients with typical GBS have one or more late relapses; such cases are then classified as chronic inflammatory demyelinating polyneuropathy (CIDP).

CHRONIC INFLAMMATORY DEMYELINATING POLYNEUROPATHY

CIDP is distinguished from GBS by its chronic course. In other respects, this neuropathy shares many features with the common demyelinating form of GBS, including elevated CSF protein levels and the Edx findings of acquired demyelination. Most cases occur in adults, and males are affected slightly more often than females. The incidence of CIDP is lower than that of GBS, but due to the protracted course, the prevalence is greater.

Clinical Manifestations Onset is usually gradual over a few months or longer, but in a few cases, the initial attack is indistinguishable from that of GBS. An acute-onset form of CIDP should be considered when GBS deteriorates >9 weeks after onset or relapses at least three times. Symptoms are both motor and sensory in most cases. Weakness of the limbs is usually symmetric but can be strikingly asymmetric in multifocal acquired demyelinating sensory and motor (MADSAM) neuropathy variant (Lewis-Sumner syndrome) in which discrete peripheral nerves are involved. There is considerable variability from case to case. Some patients experience a chronic progressive course, whereas others, usually younger patients, have a relapsing and remitting course. Some have only motor findings, and a small proportion present with a relatively pure syndrome of sensory ataxia. Tremor occurs in ~10% and may become more prominent during periods of subacute worsening or improvement. A small proportion have cranial nerve findings, including external ophthalmoplegia. CIDP tends to ameliorate over time with treatment; the result is that many years after onset, nearly 75% of patients have reasonable functional status. Death from CIDP is uncommon.

Diagnosis The diagnosis rests on characteristic clinical, CSF, and electrophysiologic findings. The CSF is usually acellular with an elevated protein level, sometimes several times normal. As with GBS, a CSF pleocytosis should lead to the consideration of HIV infection, leukemia or lymphoma, and neurosarcoidosis. Edx findings reveal variable degrees of conduction slowing, prolonged distal latencies, distal and temporal dispersion of CMAPs, and conduction block as the principal features. In particular, the presence of conduction block is a certain sign of an acquired demyelinating process. Evidence of axonal loss, presumably secondary to demyelination, is present in >50% of patients. Serum protein electrophoresis with immunofixation is indicated to search for monoclonal gammopathy and associated conditions (see "Monoclonal Gammopathy of Undetermined Significance," below). In all patients with presumptive CIDP, it is also reasonable to exclude vasculitis, collagen vascular disease (especially SLE), chronic hepatitis, HIV infection, amyloidosis, and diabetes mellitus. Other associated conditions include inflammatory bowel disease and lymphoma.

Pathogenesis Although there is evidence of immune activation in CIDP, the precise mechanisms of pathogenesis are unknown. Biopsy typically reveals little inflammation and onion-bulb changes (imbricated layers of attenuated Schwann cell processes surrounding an axon) that result from recurrent demyelination and remyelination (Fig. 460-1). The response to therapy suggests that CIDP is immune-mediated; CIDP responds to glucocorticoids, whereas GBS does not. Passive transfer of demyelination into experimental animals has been accomplished using IgG purified from the serum of some patients with CIDP, lending support for a humoral autoimmune pathogenesis. A minority of patients have serum antibodies against P0, myelin P2 protein, PMP22, or neurofascin. It is also of interest that a CIDP-like illness developed spontaneously in the nonobese diabetic (NOD) mouse when the immune co-stimulatory molecule B7-2 (CD86) was genetically deleted; this suggests that CIDP can result from altered triggering of T cells by antigen-presenting cells.

Approximately 25% of patients with clinical features of CIDP also have a monoclonal gammopathy of undetermined significance (MGUS). Cases associated with monoclonal IgA or IgG kappa usually respond to treatment as favorably as cases without a monoclonal gammopathy. Patients with IgM monoclonal gammopathy and antibodies directed against myelin-associated glycoprotein (MAG) have a distinct polyneuropathy, tend to have more sensory findings and a more protracted course, and usually have a less satisfactory response to treatment.

TREATMENT CHRONIC INFLAMMATORY DEMYELINATING POLYNEUROPATHY

Most authorities initiate treatment for CIDP when progression is rapid or walking is compromised. If the disorder is mild, management can be expectant, awaiting spontaneous remission. Controlled studies have shown that high-dose IVIg, PE, and glucocorticoids are all more effective than placebo. Initial therapy is usually with IVIg, administered as 2.0 g/kg body weight given in divided doses over 2–5 days; three monthly courses are generally recommended before concluding a patient is a treatment failure. If the patient responds, the infusion intervals can be gradually increased or the dosage decreased (e.g., 1 g/kg per month). PE, which appears to be as effective as IVIg, is initiated at two to three treatments per week for 6 weeks; periodic re-treatment may also be required. Treatment with glucocorticoids is another option (60–80 mg prednisone PO daily for 1–2 months, followed by a gradual dose reduction of 10 mg per month as tolerated), but long-term adverse effects including bone demineralization, gastrointestinal bleeding, and cushingoid changes are problematic. As many as one-third of patients with CIDP fail to respond adequately to the initial therapy chosen; a different treatment should then be tried. Patients who fail therapy with IVIg, PE, and glucocorticoids may benefit from treatment with immunosuppressive agents such as azathioprine, methotrexate, cyclosporine, and cyclophosphamide, either alone or as adjunctive therapy. Early experience with anti-CD20 (rituximab) has also shown promise. Use of these therapies requires periodic reassessment of their risks and benefits. In patients with a CIDP-like neuropathy who fail to respond to treatment, it is important to evaluate for POEMS syndrome (*p*olyneuropathy, *o*rganomegaly, *e*ndocrinopathy, *m*onoclonal gammopathy, *s*kin changes; see below).

MULTIFOCAL MOTOR NEUROPATHY

Multifocal motor neuropathy (MMN) is a distinctive but uncommon neuropathy that presents as slowly progressive motor weakness and atrophy evolving over years in the distribution of selected nerve trunks, associated with sites of persistent focal motor conduction block in the same nerve trunks. Sensory fibers are relatively spared. The arms are affected more frequently than the legs, and >75% of all patients are male. Some cases have been confused with lower motor neuron forms of amyotrophic lateral sclerosis (Chap. 452). Less than 50% of patients present with high titers of polyclonal IgM antibody to the ganglioside GM1. It is uncertain how this finding relates to the discrete foci of persistent motor conduction block, but high concentrations of GM1 gangliosides are normal constituents of nodes of Ranvier in peripheral nerve fibers. Pathology reveals demyelination and mild inflammatory changes at the sites of conduction block.

Most patients with MMN respond to high-dose IVIg (dosages as for CIDP, above); periodic re-treatment is required (usually at least monthly) to maintain the benefit. Some refractory patients have responded to rituximab or cyclophosphamide. Glucocorticoids and PE are not effective.

NEUROPATHIES WITH MONOCLONAL GAMMOPATHY

MULTIPLE MYELOMA

Clinically overt polyneuropathy occurs in ~5% of patients with the commonly encountered type of multiple myeloma, which exhibits either lytic or diffuse osteoporotic bone lesions. These neuropathies are sensorimotor, are usually mild and slowly progressive but may be severe, and generally do not reverse with successful suppression of the myeloma. In most cases, Edx and pathologic features are consistent with a process of axonal degeneration.

In contrast, myeloma with osteosclerotic features, although representing only 3% of all myelomas, is associated with polyneuropathy in one-half of cases. These neuropathies, which may also occur with solitary plasmacytoma, are distinct because they (1) are usually demyelinating in nature and resemble CIDP; (2) often respond to radiation therapy or removal of the primary lesion; (3) are associated with different monoclonal proteins and light chains (almost always lambda as opposed to primarily kappa in the lytic type of multiple myeloma); (4) are typically refractory to standard treatments of CIDP; and (5) may occur in association with other systemic findings including thickening of the skin, hyperpigmentation, hypertrichosis, organomegaly, endocrinopathy, anasarca, and clubbing of fingers. These are features of the POEMS syndrome (*p*olyneuropathy, *o*rganomegaly, *e*ndocrinopathy, *m*onoclonal gammopathy, and *s*kin changes). Levels of vascular endothelial growth factor (VEGF) are increased in the serum, and this factor is felt to somehow play a pathogenic role in this syndrome. Treatment of the neuropathy is best directed at the osteosclerotic myeloma using surgery, radiotherapy, chemotherapy, or autologous peripheral blood stem cell transplantation.

Neuropathies are also encountered in other systemic conditions with gammopathy, including Waldenström's macroglobulinemia, primary systemic amyloidosis, and cryoglobulinemic states (mixed essential cryoglobulinemia, some cases of hepatitis C).

MONOCLONAL GAMMOPATHY OF UNDETERMINED SIGNIFICANCE

Chronic polyneuropathies occurring in association with MGUS are usually associated with the immunoglobulin isotypes IgG, IgA, and IgM. Most patients present with isolated sensory symptoms in their distal extremities and have Edx features of an axonal sensory or sensorimotor polyneuropathy. These patients otherwise resemble idiopathic sensory polyneuropathy, and the MGUS might just be coincidental. They usually do not respond to immunotherapies designed to reduce the concentration of the monoclonal protein. Some patients, however, present with generalized weakness and sensory loss and Edx studies indistinguishable from CIDP without monoclonal gammopathy (see "Chronic Inflammatory Demyelinating Polyneuropathy," above), and their response to immunosuppressive agents is also similar. An exception is the syndrome of IgM kappa monoclonal gammopathy associated with an indolent, longstanding, sometimes static sensory neuropathy, frequently with tremor and sensory ataxia. Most patients are male and older than age 50 years. In the majority, the monoclonal IgM immunoglobulin binds to a normal peripheral nerve constituent, MAG, found in the paranodal regions of Schwann cells. Binding appears to be specific for a polysaccharide epitope that is also found in other normal peripheral nerve myelin glycoproteins, P0 and PMP22, and also in other normal nerve-related glycosphingolipids (Fig. 460-1). In the MAG-positive cases, IgM paraprotein is incorporated into the myelin sheaths of affected patients and widens the spacing of the myelin lamellae, thus producing a distinctive ultrastructural pattern. Demyelination and remyelination are the hallmarks of the lesions, but axonal loss develops over time. These anti-MAG polyneuropathies are typical refractory to immunotherapy. In a small proportion of patients (30% at 10 years), MGUS will in time evolve into frankly malignant conditions such as multiple myeloma or lymphoma.

VASCULITIC NEUROPATHY

Peripheral nerve involvement is common in polyarteritis nodosa (PAN), appearing in half of all cases clinically and in 100% of cases at postmortem studies (Chap. 385). The most common pattern is multifocal (asymmetric) motor-sensory neuropathy (mononeuropathy multiplex) due to ischemic lesions of nerve trunks and roots; however, some cases of vasculitic neuropathy present as a distal, symmetric sensorimotor polyneuropathy. Symptoms of neuropathy are a common presenting complaint in patients with PAN. The Edx findings are those of an axonal process. Small- to medium-sized arteries of the vasa nervorum, particularly the epineural vessels, are affected in PAN, resulting in a widespread ischemic neuropathy. A high frequency of neuropathy occurs in allergic angiitis and granulomatosis (Churg-Strauss syndrome [CSS]).

Systemic vasculitis should always be considered when a subacute or chronically evolving mononeuropathy multiplex occurs in conjunction with constitutional symptoms (fever, anorexia, weight loss, loss of energy, malaise, and nonspecific pains). Diagnosis of suspected vasculitic neuropathy is made by a combined nerve and muscle biopsy, with serial section or skip-serial techniques.

Approximately one-third of biopsy-proven cases of vasculitic neuropathy are "nonsystemic" in that the vasculitis appears to affect only peripheral nerves. Constitutional symptoms are absent, and the course is more indolent than that of PAN. The erythrocyte sedimentation rate may be elevated, but other tests for systemic disease are negative. Nevertheless, clinically silent involvement of other organs is likely, and vasculitis is frequently found in muscle biopsied at the same time as nerve.

Vasculitic neuropathy may also be seen as part of the vasculitis syndrome occurring in the course of other connective tissue disorders (Chap. 385). The most frequent is rheumatoid arthritis, but ischemic neuropathy due to involvement of vasa nervorum may also occur in mixed cryoglobulinemia, Sjögren's syndrome, granulomatosis with polyangiitis (Wegener's), hypersensitivity angiitis, systemic lupus erythematosus, and progressive systemic sclerosis.

Some vasculitides are associated with antineutrophil cytoplasmic antibodies (ANCAs), which in turn, are subclassified as cytoplasmic (cANCA) or perinuclear (pANCA). cANCAs are directed against proteinase 3 (PR3), whereas pANCAs target myeloperoxidase (MPO). PR3/cANCAs are associated with granulomatosis with polyangiitis (Wegener's), whereas MPO/pANCAs are typically associated with microscopic polyangiitis, CSS, and less commonly PAN. Of note, MPO/pANCA has also been seen in minocycline-induced vasculitis.

Management of these neuropathies, including the "nonsystemic" vasculitic neuropathy, consists of treatment of the underlying condition as well as the aggressive use of glucocorticoids and cyclophosphamide. Use of these immunosuppressive agents has resulted in dramatic improvements in outcome, with 5-year survival rates now greater than 80%. Recent clinical trials found that the combination of rituximab and glucocorticoids is not inferior to cyclophosphamide and glucocorticoids. Thus, combination therapy with glucocorticoids and rituximab is increasingly recommended as the standard initial treatment, particularly for ANCA-associated vasculitis.

ANTI-Hu PARANEOPLASTIC NEUROPATHY (CHAP. 122)

This uncommon immune-mediated disorder manifests as a sensory neuronopathy (i.e., selective damage to sensory nerve bodies in dorsal root ganglia). The onset is often asymmetric with dysesthesias and sensory loss in the limbs that soon progress to affect all limbs, the torso, and the face. Marked sensory ataxia, pseudoathetosis, and inability to walk, stand, or even sit unsupported are frequent features and are secondary to the extensive deafferentation. Subacute sensory neuronopathy may be idiopathic, but more than half of cases are paraneoplastic, primarily related to lung cancer, and most of those are small-cell lung cancer (SCLC). Diagnosis of the underlying SCLC requires awareness of the association, testing for the paraneoplastic antibody, and often positron emission tomography (PET) scanning for the tumor. The target antigens are a family of RNA-binding proteins (HuD, HuC, and Hel-N1) that in normal tissues are only expressed by neurons. The same proteins are usually expressed by SCLC, triggering in some patients an immune response characterized by antibodies and cytotoxic T cells that cross-react with the Hu proteins of the dorsal root ganglion neurons, resulting in immune-mediated neuronal destruction. An encephalomyelitis may accompany the sensory neuronopathy and presumably has the same pathogenesis. Neurologic symptoms usually precede, by ≤6 months, the identification of SCLC. The sensory neuronopathy runs its course in a few weeks or months and stabilizes, leaving the patient disabled. Most cases are unresponsive to treatment with glucocorticoids, IVIg, PE, or immunosuppressant drugs.

461 Myasthenia Gravis and Other Diseases of the Neuromuscular Junction

Daniel B. Drachman, Anthony A. Amato

Myasthenia gravis (MG) is a neuromuscular disorder characterized by weakness and fatigability of skeletal muscles. The underlying defect is a decrease in the number of available acetylcholine receptors (AChRs) at neuromuscular junctions due to an antibody-mediated autoimmune attack. Treatment now available for MG is highly effective, although a specific cure has remained elusive.

PATHOPHYSIOLOGY

At the neuromuscular junction (**Fig. 461-1, Video 461-1**), acetylcholine (ACh) is synthesized in the motor nerve terminal and stored in vesicles (quanta). When an action potential travels down a motor nerve and reaches the nerve terminal, ACh from 150 to 200 vesicles is released and combines with AChRs that are densely packed at the peaks of postsynaptic folds. The AChR consists of five subunits (2α, 1β, 1δ, and 1γ or ε) arranged around a central pore. When ACh combines with the binding sites on the α subunits of the AChR, the channel in the AChR opens, permitting the rapid entry of cations, chiefly sodium, which produces depolarization at the end-plate region of the muscle fiber. If the depolarization is sufficiently large, it initiates an action potential that is propagated along the muscle fiber, triggering muscle contraction. This process is rapidly terminated by hydrolysis of ACh by acetylcholinesterase (AChE), which is present within the synaptic folds, and by diffusion of ACh away from the receptor.

In MG, the fundamental defect is a decrease in the number of available AChRs at the postsynaptic muscle membrane. In addition, the postsynaptic folds are flattened, or "simplified." These changes result in decreased efficiency of neuromuscular transmission. Therefore, although ACh is released normally, it produces small end-plate potentials that may fail to trigger muscle action potentials. Failure of transmission at many neuromuscular junctions results in weakness of muscle contraction.

The amount of ACh released per impulse normally declines on repeated activity (termed *presynaptic rundown*). In the myasthenic patient, the decreased efficiency of neuromuscular transmission combined with the normal rundown results in the activation of fewer and fewer muscle fibers by successive nerve impulses and hence increasing weakness, or *myasthenic fatigue*. This mechanism also accounts for the decremental response to repetitive nerve stimulation seen on electrodiagnostic testing.

The neuromuscular abnormalities in MG are caused by an autoimmune response mediated by specific anti-AChR antibodies. The anti-AChR antibodies reduce the number of available AChRs at neuromuscular junctions by three distinct mechanisms: (1) accelerated turnover of AChRs by a mechanism involving cross-linking and rapid endocytosis of the receptors; (2) damage to the postsynaptic muscle membrane by the antibody in collaboration with complement; and (3) blockade of the active site of the AChR, i.e., the site that normally binds ACh. An immune response to muscle-specific kinase (MuSK), a protein involved in AChR clustering at neuromuscular junctions, can also result in MG, with reduction of AChRs demonstrated experimentally. Anti-MuSK antibody occurs in about 40% of patients without AChR antibody. A small proportion of patients whose sera are negative for both AChR and MuSK antibodies have antibodies to another protein at the neuromuscular junction—low-density lipoprotein receptor-related protein 4 (lrp4)—that is important for clustering of AChRs. The pathogenic antibodies are IgG and are T cell dependent. Thus, immunotherapeutic strategies directed against either the antibody-producing B cells or helper T cells are effective in this antibody-mediated disease.

How the autoimmune response is initiated and maintained in MG is not completely understood, but the thymus appears to play a role in this process. The thymus is abnormal in ~75% of patients with AChR antibody–positive MG; in ~65% the thymus is "hyperplastic," with the presence of active germinal centers detected histologically, although the hyperplastic thymus is not necessarily enlarged. An additional 10% of patients have thymic tumors (thymomas). Muscle-like cells within the thymus (myoid cells), which express AChRs on their surface, may serve as a source of autoantigen and trigger the autoimmune reaction within the thymus gland.

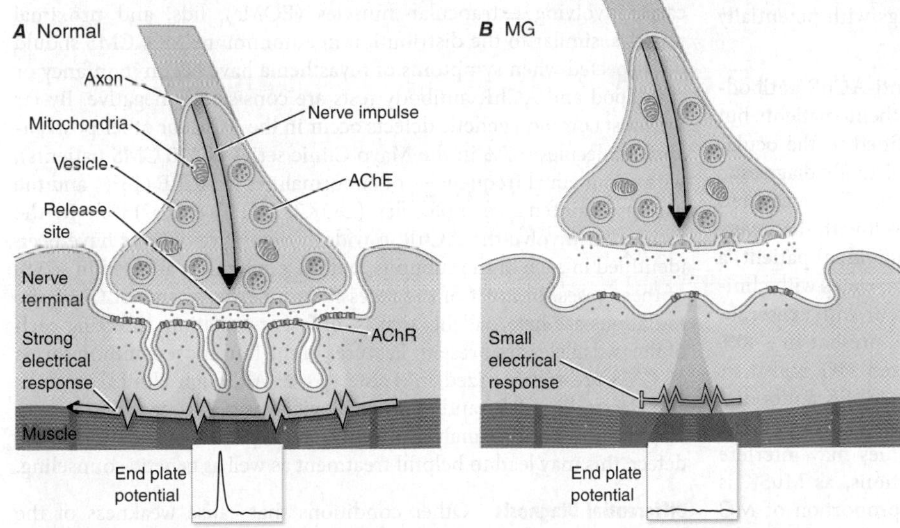

FIGURE 461-1 Diagrams of (*A*) normal and (*B*) myasthenic neuromuscular junctions. AChE, acetylcholinesterase. See text for description of normal neuromuscular transmission. The myasthenia gravis (MG) junction demonstrates a normal nerve terminal; a reduced number of acetylcholine receptors (AChRs) (stippling); flattened, simplified postsynaptic folds; and a widened synaptic space. **See Video 461-1 also.** *(Modified from DB Drachman: N Engl J Med 330:1797, 1994; with permission.)*

CLINICAL FEATURES

MG is not rare, having a prevalence as high as 2–7 in 10,000. It affects individuals in all age groups, but peaks of incidence occur in women in their twenties and thirties and in men in their fifties and sixties. Overall, women are affected more frequently than men, in a ratio of ~3:2. The cardinal features are *weakness* and *fatigability* of muscles. The weakness increases during repeated use (fatigue) or late in the day and may improve following rest or sleep. The course of MG is often variable. Exacerbations and remissions may occur, particularly during the first few years after the onset of the disease. Remissions are rarely complete or permanent. Unrelated infections or systemic disorders can lead to increased myasthenic weakness and may precipitate "crisis" (see below).

The distribution of muscle weakness often has a characteristic pattern. The cranial muscles, particularly the lids and extraocular muscles, are typically involved early in the course of MG; diplopia and ptosis are common initial complaints. Facial weakness produces a "snarling" expression when the patient attempts to smile. Weakness in chewing is most noticeable after prolonged effort, as in chewing meat. Speech may have a nasal timbre caused by weakness of the palate or a dysarthric "mushy" quality due to tongue weakness. Difficulty in swallowing may occur as a result of weakness of the palate, tongue, or pharynx, giving rise to nasal regurgitation or aspiration of liquids or food. Bulbar weakness is especially prominent in MuSK antibody–positive MG. In ~85% of

TABLE 461-1 DIAGNOSIS OF MYASTHENIA GRAVIS (MG)

History
- Diplopia, ptosis, dysarthria, dysphagia, dyspnea
- Weakness in characteristic distribution: proximal limbs, neck extensors, generalized
- Fluctuation and fatigue: worse with repeated activity, improved by rest
- Effects of previous treatments

Physical examination
- Ptosis, diplopia
- Motor power survey: quantitative testing of muscle strength
- Forward arm abduction time (5 min)
- Vital capacity measurement
- Absence of other neurologic signs

Laboratory testing
- Anti-AChR radioimmunoassay: ~85% positive in generalized MG; 50% in ocular MG; definite diagnosis if positive; negative result does not exclude MG; ~40% of AChR antibody–negative patients with generalized MG have anti-MuSK antibodies
- Repetitive nerve stimulation: decrement of >15% at 3 Hz: highly probable
- Single-fiber electromyography: blocking and jitter, with normal fiber density; confirmatory, but not specific
- Edrophonium chloride (Enlon®) 2 mg + 8 mg IV; highly probable diagnosis if unequivocally positive
- For ocular or cranial MG: exclude intracranial lesions by CT or MRI

Abbreviations: AChR, acetylcholine receptor; CT, computed tomography; MRI, magnetic resonance imaging; MuSK, muscle-specific tyrosine kinase.

patients, the weakness becomes generalized, affecting the limb muscles as well. If weakness remains restricted to the extraocular muscles for 3 years, it is likely that it will not become generalized, and these patients are said to have *ocular MG*. The limb weakness in MG is often proximal and may be asymmetric. Despite the muscle weakness, deep tendon reflexes are preserved. If weakness of respiration becomes so severe as to require respiratory assistance, the patient is said to be in *crisis*.

DIAGNOSIS AND EVALUATION

(Table 461-1) The diagnosis is suspected on the basis of weakness and fatigability in the typical distribution described above, without loss of reflexes or impairment of sensation or other neurologic function. The suspected diagnosis should always be confirmed definitively before treatment is undertaken; this is essential because (1) other treatable conditions may closely resemble MG and (2) the treatment of MG may involve surgery and the prolonged use of drugs with potentially adverse side effects.

Antibodies to AChR, MuSK, or lrp4 As noted above, anti-AChR antibodies are detectable in the serum of ~85% of all myasthenic patients but in only about 50% of patients with weakness confined to the ocular muscles. The presence of anti-AChR antibodies is virtually diagnostic of MG, but a negative test does not exclude the disease. The measured level of anti-AChR antibody does not correspond well with the severity of MG in different patients. However, in an individual patient, a treatment-induced fall in the antibody level often correlates with clinical improvement, whereas a rise in the level may occur with exacerbations. Antibodies to MuSK have been found to be present in ~40% of AChR antibody–negative patients with generalized MG, and their presence is a useful diagnostic test in these patients. MuSK antibodies are rarely present in AChR antibody–positive patients or in patients with MG limited to ocular muscles. These antibodies may interfere with clustering of AChRs at neuromuscular junctions, as MuSK is known to do during early development. A small proportion of MG patients without antibodies to AChR or MuSK may have antibodies to lrp4, although a test for lrp4 antibodies is not yet commercially available. Finally, antibodies against agrin have recently been found in some patients with MG. Agrin is a protein derived from motor nerves that normally binds to lrp4 and thus may also interfere with clustering of AChRs at neuromuscular junctions. There may well be other—as yet undefined—antibodies that impair neuromuscular transmission.

Electrodiagnostic Testing Repetitive nerve stimulation may provide helpful diagnostic evidence of MG. Anti-AChE medication is stopped 6–24 h before testing. It is best to test weak muscles or proximal muscle groups. Electric shocks are delivered at a rate of two or three per second to the appropriate nerves, and action potentials are recorded from the muscles. In normal individuals, the amplitude of the evoked muscle action potentials does not change at these rates of stimulation. However, in myasthenic patients, there is a rapid reduction of >10–15% in the amplitude of the evoked responses.

Anticholinesterase Test Drugs that inhibit the enzyme AChE allow ACh to interact repeatedly with the limited number of AChRs in MG, producing improvement in muscle strength. Edrophonium is used most commonly for diagnostic testing because of the rapid onset (30 s) and short duration (~5 min) of its effect. An objective end point must be selected to evaluate the effect of edrophonium, such as weakness of extraocular muscles, impairment of speech, or the length of time that the patient can maintain the arms in forward abduction. An initial IV dose of 2 mg of edrophonium is given. If definite improvement occurs, the test is considered positive and is terminated. If there is no change, the patient is given an additional 8 mg IV. The dose is administered in two parts because some patients react to edrophonium with side effects such as nausea, diarrhea, salivation, fasciculations, and rarely with severe symptoms of syncope or bradycardia. Atropine (0.6 mg) should be drawn up in a syringe and ready for IV administration if these symptoms become troublesome. The edrophonium test is now reserved for patients with clinical findings that are suggestive of MG but who have negative antibody and electrodiagnostic test results. False-positive tests occur in occasional patients with other neurologic disorders, such as amyotrophic lateral sclerosis, and in placebo-reactors. False-negative or equivocal tests may also occur. In some cases, it is helpful to use a longer-acting drug such as neostigmine (15 mg PO), because this permits more time for detailed evaluation of strength.

Inherited Myasthenic Syndromes The congenital myasthenic syndromes (CMS) comprise a heterogeneous group of disorders of the neuromuscular junction that are not autoimmune but rather are due to genetic mutations in which virtually any component of the neuromuscular junction may be affected. Alterations in function of the presynaptic nerve terminal, in the various subunits of the AChR, AChE, or the other molecules involved in end-plate development or maintenance, have been identified in the different forms of CMS. These disorders share many of the clinical features of autoimmune MG, including weakness and fatigability of skeletal muscles, in some cases involving extraocular muscles (EOMs), lids, and proximal muscles, similar to the distribution in autoimmune MG. CMS should be suspected when symptoms of myasthenia have begun in infancy or childhood and AChR antibody tests are consistently negative. By far the most common genetic defects occur in the AChR or other postsynaptic molecules (67% in the Mayo Clinic series of 350 CMS patients), with about equal frequencies of abnormalities in AChE (13%) and the various maintenance molecules (DOK7, GFPT, etc.; ~14%). In the forms that involve the AChR, a wide variety of mutations have been identified in each of the subunits, but the ε subunit is affected in ~75% of these cases. In most of the recessively inherited forms of CMS, the mutations are heteroallelic; that is, different mutations affecting each of the two alleles are present. Features of the four most common forms of CMS are summarized in Table 461-2. Although clinical features and electrodiagnostic and pharmacologic tests may suggest the correct diagnosis, molecular analysis is required for precise elucidation of the defect; this may lead to helpful treatment as well as genetic counseling.

Differential Diagnosis Other conditions that cause weakness of the cranial and/or somatic musculature include the nonautoimmune CMS discussed above, drug-induced myasthenia, Lambert-Eaton myasthenic syndrome (LEMS), neurasthenia, hyperthyroidism (Graves' disease), botulism, intracranial mass lesions, oculopharyngeal dystrophy, and mitochondrial myopathy (Kearns-Sayre syndrome, progressive external ophthalmoplegia). Treatment with penicillamine (used for scleroderma or rheumatoid arthritis) may result in true autoimmune

TABLE 461-2 THE CONGENITAL MYASTHENIC SYNDROMES

Type	Clinical Features	Electrophysiology	Genetics	End-Plate Effects	Treatment
Slow channel	Most common; weak forearm extensors; onset second to third decade; variable severity	Repetitive muscle response on nerve stimulation; prolonged channel opening and MEPP duration	Autosomal dominant; α, β, ε; AChR mutations	Excitotoxic end-plate myopathy; decreased AChRs; postsynaptic damage	Quinidine, fluoxetine: decrease end-plate damage; made worse by anti-AChE
Low-affinity fast channel	Onset early; moderately severe; ptosis, EOM involvement; weakness and fatigue	Brief and infrequent channel openings; opposite of slow channel syndrome	Autosomal recessive; may be heteroallelic	Normal end-plate structure	3,4-DAP; anti-AChE
Severe AChR deficiencies	Early onset; variable severity; fatigue; typical MG features	Decremental response to repetitive nerve stimulation; decreased MEPP amplitudes	Autosomal recessive; ε mutations most common; many different mutations	Increased length of end plates; variable synaptic folds	Anti-AChE; 3,4-DAP
AChE deficiency	Early onset; variable severity; scoliosis; may have normal EOM, absent pupillary responses	Decremental response to repetitive nerve stimulation	Mutant gene for AChE's collagen anchor (COLQ)	Small nerve terminals; degenerated junctional folds	Worse with anti-AChE drugs; use albuterol, ephedrine, 3,4-DAP

Abbreviations: AChE, acetylcholinesterase; AChR, acetylcholine receptor; EOM, extraocular muscles; MEPP, miniature end plate potentials; MG, myasthenia gravis; 3,4-DAP, 3,4-diaminopyridine.

MG, but the weakness is usually mild, and recovery occurs within weeks or months after discontinuing its use. Aminoglycoside antibiotics or procainamide can cause exacerbation of weakness in myasthenic patients; very large doses can cause neuromuscular weakness in normal individuals.

LEMS is a presynaptic disorder of the neuromuscular junction that can cause weakness similar to that of MG. The proximal muscles of the lower limbs are most commonly affected, but other muscles may be involved as well. Cranial nerve findings, including ptosis of the eyelids and diplopia, occur in up to 70% of patients and resemble features of MG. However, the two conditions are usually readily distinguished, because patients with LEMS have depressed or absent reflexes and experience autonomic changes such as dry mouth and impotence. Nerve stimulation produces an initial low-amplitude response and, at low rates of repetitive stimulation (2–3 Hz), decremental responses like those of MG; however, at high rates (50 Hz), or following exercise, incremental responses occur. LEMS is caused by autoantibodies directed against P/Q-type calcium channels at the motor nerve terminals, which can be detected in ~85% of LEMS patients by radioimmunoassay. These autoantibodies result in impaired release of ACh from nerve terminals. Many patients with LEMS have an associated malignancy, most commonly small-cell carcinoma of the lung, which may express calcium channels that stimulate the autoimmune response. The diagnosis of LEMS may signal the presence of a tumor long before it would otherwise be detected, permitting early removal. Treatment of LEMS involves plasmapheresis and immunosuppression, as for MG. 3,4-Diaminopyridine (3,4-DAP) and pyridostigmine may also be symptomatically helpful. 3,4-DAP acts by blocking potassium channels, which results in prolonged depolarization of the motor nerve terminals and thus enhances ACh release. Pyridostigmine prolongs the action of ACh, allowing repeated interactions with AChRs.

Botulism (Chap. 178) is due to potent bacterial toxins produced by any of eight different strains of *Clostridium botulinum*. The toxins enzymatically cleave specific proteins essential for the release of ACh from the motor nerve terminal, thereby interfering with neuromuscular transmission. Most commonly, botulism is caused by ingestion of improperly prepared food containing toxin. Rarely, the nearly ubiquitous spores of *C. botulinum* may germinate in wounds. In infants, the spores may germinate in the gastrointestinal (GI) tract and release toxin, causing muscle weakness. Patients present with myasthenia-like bulbar weakness (e.g., diplopia, dysarthria, dysphagia) and lack sensory symptoms and signs. Weakness may generalize to the limbs and may result in respiratory failure. Reflexes are present early, but they may be diminished as the disease progresses. Mentation is normal. Autonomic findings include paralytic ileus, constipation, urinary retention, dilated or poorly reactive pupils, and dry mouth. The demonstration of toxin in serum by bioassay is definitive, but the results usually take a relatively long time to be completed and may be negative. Nerve stimulation studies reveal findings of presynaptic neuromuscular blockade with reduced compound muscle action potentials (CMAPs) that increase in amplitude following high-frequency repetitive stimulation. Treatment includes ventilatory support and aggressive inpatient supportive care (e.g., nutrition, deep vein thrombosis prophylaxis) as needed. Antitoxin should be given as early as possible to be effective and can be obtained through the Centers for Disease Control and Prevention. A preventive vaccine is available for laboratory workers or other highly exposed individuals.

Neurasthenia is the historic term for a myasthenia-like fatigue syndrome without an organic basis. These patients may present with subjective symptoms of weakness and fatigue, but muscle testing usually reveals the "give-away weakness" characteristic of nonorganic disorders; the complaint of fatigue in these patients means tiredness or apathy rather than decreasing muscle power on repeated effort. Hyperthyroidism is readily diagnosed or excluded by tests of thyroid function, which should be carried out routinely in patients with suspected MG. Abnormalities of thyroid function (hyper- or hypothyroidism) may increase myasthenic weakness. Diplopia resembling that in MG may occasionally be due to an intracranial mass lesion that compresses nerves to the EOMs (e.g., sphenoid ridge meningioma), but magnetic resonance imaging (MRI) of the head and orbits usually reveals the lesion.

Progressive external ophthalmoplegia is a rare condition resulting in weakness of the EOMs, which may be accompanied by weakness of the proximal muscles of the limbs and other systemic features. Most patients with this condition have mitochondrial disorders that can be detected on muscle biopsy (Chap. 462e).

Search for Associated Conditions (Table 461-3) Myasthenic patients have an increased incidence of several associated disorders. Thymic abnormalities occur in ~75% of AChR antibody–positive patients, as noted above. Neoplastic change (thymoma) may produce enlargement of the thymus, which is detected by computed tomography (CT) scanning of the anterior mediastinum. A thymic shadow on CT scan may normally be present through young adulthood, but enlargement of the thymus in a patient age >40 years is highly suspicious of thymoma. Hyperthyroidism occurs in 3–8% of patients and may aggravate the myasthenic weakness. Thyroid function tests should be obtained in all patients with suspected MG. Because of the association of MG with other autoimmune disorders, blood tests for rheumatoid factor and antinuclear antibodies should also be carried out. Chronic infection of any kind can exacerbate MG and should be sought carefully. Finally, measurements of ventilatory function are valuable because of the frequency and seriousness of respiratory impairment in myasthenic patients.

Because of the side effects of glucocorticoids and other immunosuppressive agents used in the treatment of MG, a thorough medical

TABLE 461-3 DISORDERS ASSOCIATED WITH MYASTHENIA GRAVIS AND RECOMMENDED LABORATORY TESTS

Associated disorders

Disorders of the thymus: thymoma, hyperplasia

Other autoimmune disorders: Hashimoto's thyroiditis, Graves' disease, rheumatoid arthritis, lupus erythematosus, skin disorders, family history of autoimmune disorder

Disorders or circumstances that may exacerbate myasthenia gravis: hyperthyroidism or hypothyroidism, occult infection, medical treatment for other conditions (see Table 461-4)

Disorders that may interfere with therapy: tuberculosis, diabetes, peptic ulcer, gastrointestinal bleeding, renal disease, hypertension, asthma, osteoporosis, obesity

Recommended laboratory tests or procedures

CT or MRI of chest

Tests for lupus erythematosus, antinuclear antibody, rheumatoid factor, antithyroid antibodies

Thyroid function tests

PPD skin test

Fasting blood glucose, hemoglobin A1c

Pulmonary function tests

Bone densitometry

Abbreviations: CT, computed tomography; MRI, magnetic resonance imaging; PPD, purified protein derivative.

investigation should be undertaken, searching specifically for evidence of chronic or latent infection (such as tuberculosis or hepatitis), hypertension, diabetes, renal disease, and glaucoma.

TREATMENT MYASTHENIA GRAVIS

The prognosis has improved strikingly as a result of advances in treatment. Nearly all myasthenic patients can be returned to full productive lives with proper therapy. The most useful treatments for MG include anticholinesterase medications, immunosuppressive agents, thymectomy, and plasmapheresis or intravenous immunoglobulin (IVIg) **(Fig. 461-2)**.

ANTICHOLINESTERASE MEDICATIONS

Anticholinesterase medication produces at least partial improvement in most myasthenic patients, although improvement is complete in only a few. Patients with anti-MuSK MG generally obtain less benefit from anticholinesterase agents than those with AChR antibodies. Pyridostigmine is the most widely used anticholinesterase drug. The beneficial action of oral pyridostigmine begins within 15–30 min and lasts for 3–4 h, but individual responses vary. Treatment is begun with a moderate dose, e.g., 30–60 mg three to four times daily. The frequency and amount of the dose should be tailored to the patient's individual requirements throughout the day. For example, patients with weakness in chewing and swallowing may benefit by taking the medication before meals so that peak strength coincides with mealtimes. Long-acting pyridostigmine may occasionally be useful to get the patient through the night but should not be used for daytime medication because of variable absorption. The maximum useful dose of pyridostigmine rarely exceeds 120 mg every 4–6 h during daytime. Overdosage with anticholinesterase medication may cause increased weakness and other side effects. In some patients, muscarinic side effects of the anticholinesterase medication (diarrhea, abdominal cramps, salivation, nausea) may limit the dose tolerated. Atropine/diphenoxylate or loperamide is useful for the treatment of GI symptoms.

THYMECTOMY

Two separate issues should be distinguished: (1) surgical removal of thymoma, and (2) thymectomy as a treatment for MG. Surgical removal of a thymoma is necessary because of the possibility of local tumor spread, although most thymomas are histologically benign.

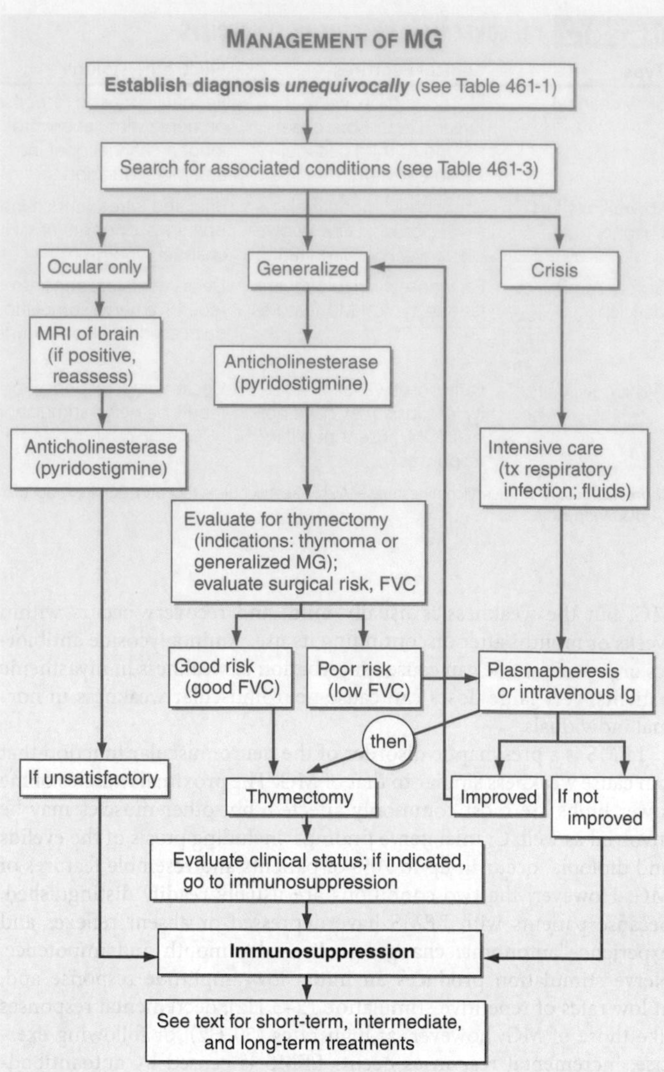

FIGURE 461-2 Algorithm for the management of myasthenia gravis. FVC, forced vital capacity; MRI, magnetic resonance imaging.

In the absence of a tumor, the available evidence suggests that up to 85% of patients experience improvement after thymectomy; of these, ~35% achieve drug-free remission. However, the improvement is typically delayed for months to years. The advantage of thymectomy is that it offers the possibility of long-term benefit, in some cases diminishing or eliminating the need for continuing medical treatment. Review of the published studies showed that following thymectomy, MG patients were 1.7 times as likely to improve and twice as likely to attain remission as those who did not have surgical thymectomy. In view of these potential benefits and of the negligible risk in skilled hands, thymectomy has gained widespread acceptance in the treatment of MG. It is the consensus that thymectomy should be carried out in all patients with generalized MG who are between the ages of puberty and at least 55 years. Whether thymectomy should be recommended in children, in adults >55 years of age, and in patients with weakness limited to the ocular muscles is still a matter of debate. There is also evidence that patients with MuSK antibody–positive MG respond less well to thymectomy than those with AChR antibody. Thymectomy must be carried out in a hospital where it is performed regularly and where the staff is experienced in the pre- and postoperative management, anesthesia, and surgical techniques of total thymectomy. Thymectomy should never be carried out as an emergency procedure, but only when the patient is adequately prepared. If necessary, treatment with IVIg or plasmapheresis may be used before surgery, but it is helpful to try to avoid immunosuppressive agents because of the risk of infection.

IMMUNOSUPPRESSION

Immunosuppression using one or more of the available agents is effective in nearly all patients with MG. The choice of drugs or other immunomodulatory treatments should be guided by the relative benefits and risks for the individual patient and the urgency of treatment. It is helpful to develop a treatment plan based on short-term, intermediate-term, and long-term objectives. For example, if immediate improvement is essential either because of the severity of weakness or because of the patient's need to return to activity as soon as possible, IVIg should be administered or plasmapheresis should be undertaken. For the intermediate term, glucocorticoids and cyclosporine or tacrolimus generally produce clinical improvement within a period of 1–3 months. The beneficial effects of azathioprine and mycophenolate mofetil usually begin after many months (as long as a year), but these drugs have advantages for the long-term treatment of patients with MG. There is a growing body of evidence that rituximab is effective in many MG patients, especially those with MuSK antibody.

Glucocorticoid Therapy Glucocorticoids, when used properly, produce improvement in myasthenic weakness in the great majority of patients. To minimize adverse side effects, prednisone should be given in a single dose rather than in divided doses throughout the day. The initial dose should be relatively low (15–25 mg/d) to avoid the early weakening that occurs in up to one-third of patients treated initially with a high-dose regimen. The dose is increased stepwise, as tolerated by the patient (usually by 5 mg/d at 2- to 3-day intervals), until there is marked clinical improvement or a dose of 50–60 mg/d is reached. This dose is maintained for 1–3 months and then is gradually modified to an alternate-day regimen over the course of an additional 1–3 months; the goal is to reduce the dose on the "off day" to zero or to a minimal level. Generally, patients begin to improve within a few weeks after reaching the maximum dose, and improvement continues to progress for months or years. The prednisone dosage may gradually be reduced, but usually months or years may be needed to determine the minimum effective dose, and close monitoring is required. Few patients are able to do without immunosuppressive agents entirely. Patients on long-term glucocorticoid therapy must be followed carefully to prevent or treat adverse side effects. The most common errors in glucocorticoid treatment of myasthenic patients include (1) insufficient persistence—improvement may be delayed and gradual; (2) tapering the dosage too early, too rapidly, or excessively; and (3) lack of attention to prevention and treatment of side effects.

The management of patients treated with glucocorticoids is discussed in Chap. 406.

Other Immunosuppressive Drugs Mycophenolate mofetil, azathioprine, cyclosporine, tacrolimus, rituximab, and occasionally cyclophosphamide are effective in many patients, either alone or in various combinations.

Mycophenolate mofetil has become one of the most widely used drugs in the treatment of MG because of its effectiveness and relative lack of side effects. A dose of 1–1.5 g bid is recommended. Its mechanism of action involves inhibition of purine synthesis by the de novo pathway. Since lymphocytes have only the de novo pathway, but lack the alternative salvage pathway that is present in all other cells, mycophenolate inhibits proliferation of lymphocytes but not proliferation of other cells. It does not kill or eliminate preexisting autoreactive lymphocytes, and therefore clinical improvement may be delayed for many months to a year, until the preexisting autoreactive lymphocytes die spontaneously. The advantage of mycophenolate lies in its relative lack of adverse side effects, with only occasional production of GI symptoms, rare development of leukopenia, and very small risks of malignancy or progressive multifocal leukoencephalopathy inherent in nearly all immunosuppressive treatments. Although two published studies did not show positive outcomes, most experts attribute the negative results to flaws in the trial designs, and mycophenolate is widely used for long-term treatment of myasthenic patients.

Until recently, azathioprine has been the most commonly used immunosuppressive agent for MG because of its relative safety in most patients and long track record. Its therapeutic effect may add to that of glucocorticoids and/or allow the glucocorticoid dose to be reduced. However, up to 10% of patients are unable to tolerate azathioprine because of idiosyncratic reactions consisting of flu-like symptoms of fever and malaise, bone marrow suppression, or abnormalities of liver function. An initial dose of 50 mg/d should be used for several days to test for these side effects. If this dose is tolerated, it is increased gradually to about 2–3 mg/kg of total body weight, or until the white blood count falls to 3000–4000/μL. The beneficial effect of azathioprine takes 3–6 months to begin and even longer to peak. In patients taking azathioprine, allopurinol should never be used to treat hyperuricemia. Because the two drugs share a common degradation pathway, the result may be severe bone marrow suppression due to increased effects of the azathioprine.

The calcineurin inhibitors cyclosporine and tacrolimus (FK506) are approximately as effective as azathioprine and are being used increasingly in the management of MG. Their beneficial effect appears more rapidly than that of azathioprine. Either drug may be used alone, but they are usually used as an adjunct to glucocorticoids to permit reduction of the glucocorticoid dose. The usual dose of cyclosporine is 4–5 mg/kg per day, and the average dose of tacrolimus is 0.07–0.1 mg/kg per day, given in two equally divided doses (to minimize side effects). Side effects of these drugs include hypertension and nephrotoxicity, which must be closely monitored. "Trough" blood levels are measured 12 h after the evening dose. The therapeutic range for the trough level of cyclosporine is 150–200 ng/L, and for tacrolimus, it is 5–15 ng/L.

Rituximab (Rituxan) is a monoclonal antibody that binds to the CD20 molecule on B lymphocytes. It has been widely used for the treatment of B cell lymphomas and has also proven successful in the treatment of several autoimmune diseases including rheumatoid arthritis, pemphigus, and some IgM-related neuropathies. There is now an extensive literature on the benefit of rituximab in MG. It is particularly effective in MuSK antibody–positive MG, although some patients with AChR antibody MG respond to it as well. The usual dose is 375 mg/m^2, given IV in 4 weekly infusions, or 1 g, given IV on two occasions 2 weeks apart.

For the occasional patient with MG that is genuinely refractory to optimal treatment with conventional immunosuppressive agents, a course of high-dose cyclophosphamide may induce long-lasting benefit by "rebooting" the immune system. At high doses, cyclophosphamide eliminates mature lymphocytes but spares hematopoietic precursors (stem cells), because they express the enzyme aldehyde dehydrogenase, which hydrolyzes cyclophosphamide. At present, this procedure is reserved for refractory patients and should be administered only in a facility fully familiar with this approach. Maintenance immunotherapy after rebooting is usually required to sustain the beneficial effect.

PLASMAPHERESIS AND INTRAVENOUS IMMUNOGLOBULIN

Plasmapheresis has been used therapeutically in MG. Plasma, which contains the pathogenic antibodies, is mechanically separated from the blood cells, which are returned to the patient. A course of five exchanges (3–4 L per exchange) is generally administered over a 10- to 14-day period. Plasmapheresis produces a short-term reduction in anti-AChR antibodies, with clinical improvement in many patients. It is useful as a temporary expedient in seriously affected patients or to improve the patient's condition prior to surgery (e.g., thymectomy).

The indications for the use of IVIg are the same as those for plasma exchange: to produce rapid improvement to help the patient through a difficult period of myasthenic weakness or prior to surgery. This treatment has the advantages of not requiring special equipment or large-bore venous access. The usual dose is 2 g/kg, which is typically administered over 5 days (400 mg/kg per day). If tolerated, the total dose of IVIg can be given over a 3- to 4-day period. Improvement occurs in ~70% of patients, beginning during treatment, or within a week, and continuing for weeks to months. The mechanism of action of IVIg is not known; the treatment has no consistent effect on the measurable amount of circulating AChR antibody. Adverse reactions are generally not serious but may include headache, fluid overload, and rarely aseptic meningitis or renal failure. IVIg should rarely be used as a long-term treatment in place of rationally managed immunosuppressive therapy. Unfortunately, there is a tendency for physicians unfamiliar with immunosuppressive treatments to rely on repeated IVIg infusions, which usually produce only intermittent benefit, do not reduce the underlying autoimmune response, and are very costly. The intermediate and long-term treatment of myasthenic patients requires other methods of therapy outlined earlier in this chapter.

MANAGEMENT OF MYASTHENIC CRISIS

Myasthenic crisis is defined as an exacerbation of weakness sufficient to endanger life; it usually consists of respiratory failure caused by diaphragmatic and intercostal muscle weakness. Crisis rarely occurs in properly managed patients. Treatment should be carried out in intensive care units staffed with teams experienced in the management of MG, respiratory insufficiency, infectious disease, and fluid and electrolyte therapy. The possibility that deterioration could be due to excessive anticholinesterase medication ("cholinergic crisis") is best excluded by temporarily stopping anticholinesterase drugs. The most common cause of crisis is intercurrent infection. This should be treated immediately, because the mechanical and immunologic defenses of the patient can be assumed to be compromised. The myasthenic patient with fever and early infection should be treated like other immunocompromised patients. Early and effective antibiotic therapy, respiratory assistance (preferably noninvasive, using bilevel positive airway pressure), and pulmonary physiotherapy are essentials of the treatment program. As discussed above, plasmapheresis or IVIg is frequently helpful in hastening recovery.

DRUGS TO AVOID IN MYASTHENIC PATIENTS

Many drugs have been reported to exacerbate weakness in patients with MG (Table 461-4), but not all patients react adversely to all of these. Conversely, not all "safe" drugs can be used with impunity in patients with MG. As a rule, the listed drugs should be avoided *whenever possible*, and myasthenic patients should be followed closely when *any new drug* is introduced.

TABLE 461-4 DRUGS WITH INTERACTIONS IN MYASTHENIA GRAVIS (MG)

Drugs That May Exacerbate MG
Antibiotics
Aminoglycosides: e.g., streptomycin, tobramycin, kanamycin
Quinolones: e.g., ciprofloxacin, levofloxacin, ofloxacin, gatifloxacin
Macrolides: e.g., erythromycin, azithromycin
Nondepolarizing muscle relaxants for surgery
D-Tubocurarine (curare), pancuronium, vecuronium, atracurium
Beta-blocking agents
Propranolol, atenolol, metoprolol
Local anesthetics and related agents
Procaine, Xylocaine in large amounts
Procainamide (for arrhythmias)
Botulinum toxin
Botox exacerbates weakness
Quinine derivatives
Quinine, quinidine, chloroquine, mefloquine (Lariam)
Magnesium
Decreases acetylcholine release
Penicillamine
May cause MG
Drugs with Important Interactions in MG
Cyclosporine
Broad range of drug interactions, which may raise or lower cyclosporine levels.
Azathioprine
Avoid allopurinol—combination may result in myelosuppression.

Myasthenia Gravis Worksheet

History				
General	Normal	Good	Fair	Poor
Diplopia	None	Rare	Occasional	Constant
Ptosis	None	Rare	Occasional	Constant
Arms	Normal	Slightly limited	Some ADL impairment	Definitely limited
Legs	Normal	Walks/runs fatigues	Can walk limited distances	Minimal walking
Speech	Normal	Dysarthric	Severely dysarthric	Unintelligible
Voice	Normal	Fades	Impaired	Severely impaired
Chew	Normal	Fatigue on normal foods	Fatigue on soft foods	Feeding tube
Swallow	Normal	Normal foods	Soft foods only	Feeding tube
Respiration	Normal	Dyspnea on unusual effort	Dyspnea on any effort	Dyspnea at rest

Examination

BP ____ Pulse ____ Wt ____	Arm abduction time R ____ L ____
Edema ____	Deltoids R ____ L ____
Vital capacity ____	Biceps R ____ L ____
Cataracts? R ____ L ____	Triceps R ____ L ____
EOMS ____	Grip R ____ L ____
Ptosis time ____	Iliopsoas R ____ L ____
Face ____	Quadriceps R ____ L ____
	Hamstrings R ____ L ____
	Other R ____ L ____

FIGURE 461-3 Abbreviated interval assessment form for use in evaluating treatment for myasthenia gravis.

PATIENT ASSESSMENT

To evaluate the effectiveness of treatment as well as drug-induced side effects, it is important to assess the patient's clinical status systematically at baseline and on repeated interval examinations. Because of the variability of symptoms of MG, the interval history and physical findings on examination must be taken into account. The most useful clinical tests include forward arm abduction time (up to a full 5 min), spirometry with determination of forced vital capacity, range of eye movements, and time to development of ptosis on upward gaze. Manual muscle testing or, preferably, quantitative dynamometry of limb muscles, especially proximal muscles, is also important. An interval form can provide a succinct summary of the patient's status and a guide to treatment results; an abbreviated form is shown in Fig. 461-3. A progressive reduction in the patient's AChR antibody level also provides clinically valuable confirmation of the effectiveness of treatment; conversely, a rise in AChR antibody levels during tapering of immunosuppressive medication may predict clinical exacerbation. For reliable quantitative measurement of AChR antibody levels, it is best to compare antibody levels from prior frozen serum aliquots with current serum samples in simultaneously run assays.

462e Muscular Dystrophies and Other Muscle Diseases

Anthony A. Amato, Robert H. Brown, Jr.

This is a digital-only chapter. It is available on the DVD that accompanies this book, as well as on Access Medicine/Harrison's Online, and the eBook and "app" editions of HPIM 19e.

Skeletal muscle diseases, or myopathies, are disorders with structural changes or functional impairment of muscle. These conditions can be differentiated from other diseases of the motor unit (e.g., lower motor neuron or neuromuscular junction pathologies) by characteristic clinical and laboratory findings.

Myasthenia gravis and related disorders are discussed in Chap. 461; dermatomyositis, polymyositis, and inclusion body myositis are discussed in Chap. 388.

CLINICAL FEATURES

Most myopathies present with proximal, symmetric limb weakness (arms or legs) with preserved reflexes and sensation. However, asymmetric and predominantly distal weakness can be seen in some myopathies. An associated sensory loss suggests injury to a peripheral nerve or the central nervous system (CNS) rather than myopathy. On occasion, disorders affecting the motor nerve cell bodies in the spinal cord (anterior horn cell disease), the neuromuscular junction, or peripheral nerves can mimic findings of myopathy.

463e Special Issues in Inpatient Neurologic Consultation

S. Andrew Josephson, Martin A. Samuels

This is a digital-only chapter. It is available on the DVD that accompanies this book, as well as on Access Medicine/Harrison's Online, and the eBook and "app" editions of HPIM 19e.

Inpatient neurologic consultations usually involve questions regarding specific disease processes or prognostication after various cerebral injuries. Common reasons for neurologic consultation include stroke (Chap. 446), seizures (Chap. 445), altered mental status (Chap. 34), headache (Chap. 21), and management of coma and other neurocritical care conditions (Chaps. 328 and 330). This chapter focuses on additional common reasons for consultation that are not addressed elsewhere in the text.

CONSULTATIONS REGARDING CENTRAL NERVOUS SYSTEM DYSFUNCTION

HYPERPERFUSION STATES LEADING TO POSTERIOR REVERSIBLE ENCEPHALOPATHY SYNDROME

A group of neurologic disorders shares the common feature of hyperperfusion, probably related to endothelial dysfunction, playing a key role in pathogenesis. These seemingly diverse syndromes include hypertensive encephalopathy, eclampsia, postcarotid endarterectomy syndrome, and toxicity from calcineurin-inhibitor and other medications. Modern imaging techniques and experimental models suggest that vasogenic edema is typically the primary process leading to neurologic dysfunction; therefore, prompt recognition and management of this condition should allow for clinical recovery as long as superimposed hemorrhage or infarction has not occurred.

SECTION 4 CHRONIC FATIGUE SYNDROME

464e Chronic Fatigue Syndrome

Gijs Bleijenberg, Jos W. M. van der Meer

This is a digital-only chapter. It is available on the DVD that accompanies this book, as well as on Access Medicine/Harrison's Online, and the eBook and "app" editions of HPIM 19e.

DEFINITION

Chronic fatigue syndrome (CFS) is a disorder characterized by persistent and unexplained fatigue resulting in severe impairment in daily functioning. Besides intense fatigue, most patients with CFS report concomitant symptoms such as pain, cognitive dysfunction, and unrefreshing sleep. Additional symptoms can include headache, sore throat, tender lymph nodes, muscle aches, joint aches, feverishness, difficulty sleeping, psychiatric problems, allergies, and abdominal cramps. Criteria for the diagnosis of CFS have been developed by the U.S. Centers for Disease Control and Prevention.

465e Biology of Psychiatric Disorders

Robert O. Messing, Eric J. Nestler

This is a digital-only chapter. It is available on the DVD that accompanies this book, as well as on Access Medicine/Harrison's Online, and the eBook and "app" editions of HPIM 19e.

Psychiatric disorders are central nervous system diseases characterized by disturbances in emotion, cognition, motivation, and socialization. They are highly heritable, with genetic risk comprising 20–90% of disease vulnerability. As a result of their prevalence, early onset, and persistence, they contribute substantially to the burden of illness worldwide. All psychiatric disorders are broad heterogeneous syndromes that currently lack well-defined neuropathology and *bona fide* biologic markers. Therefore, diagnoses continue to be made solely from clinical observations using criteria in the *Diagnostic and Statistical Manual of Mental Disorders* (DSM) of the American Psychiatric Association, which is in its fifth edition as of 2013.

466 Mental Disorders

Victor I. Reus

Mental disorders are common in medical practice and may present either as a primary disorder or as a comorbid condition. The prevalence of mental or substance use disorders in the United States is approximately 30%, but only one-third of affected individuals are currently receiving treatment. Global burden of disease statistics indicate that 4 of the 10 most important causes of morbidity and attendant health care costs worldwide are psychiatric in origin.

Changes in health care delivery underscore the need for primary care physicians to assume responsibility for the initial diagnosis and treatment of the most common mental disorders. Prompt diagnosis is essential to ensure that patients have access to appropriate medical services and to maximize the clinical outcome. Validated patient-based questionnaires have been developed that systematically probe for signs and symptoms associated with the most prevalent psychiatric diagnoses and guide the clinician into targeted assessment. The Primary Care Evaluation of Mental Disorders (PRIME-MD; and a self-report form, the Patient Health Questionnaire) and the Symptom-Driven Diagnostic System for Primary Care (SDDS-PC) are inventories that require only 10 min to complete and link patient responses to the formal diagnostic criteria of anxiety, mood, somatoform, and eating disorders and to alcohol abuse or dependence.

A physician who refers patients to a psychiatrist should know not only when doing so is appropriate but also how to refer, because societal misconceptions and the stigma of mental illness impede the process. Primary care physicians should base referrals to a psychiatrist on the presence of signs and symptoms of a mental disorder and not simply on the absence of a physical explanation for a patient's complaint. The physician should discuss with the patient the reasons for requesting the referral or consultation and provide reassurance that he or she will continue to provide medical care and work collaboratively with the mental health professional. Consultation with a psychiatrist or transfer of care is appropriate when physicians encounter evidence of psychotic symptoms, mania, severe depression, or anxiety; symptoms of posttraumatic stress disorder (PTSD); suicidal or homicidal preoccupation; or a failure to respond to first-order treatment. This chapter reviews the clinical assessment and treatment of some of the most common mental disorders presenting in primary care and is based on the *Diagnostic and Statistical Manual of Mental Disorders*, Fifth Edition (DSM-5), the framework for categorizing psychiatric illness used in the United States. Eating disorders are discussed later in this chapter, and the biology of psychiatric and addictive disorders is discussed in Chap. 465e.

GLOBAL CONSIDERATIONS

The DSM-5 and the tenth revision of the International Classification of Diseases (ICD-10), which is used more commonly worldwide, have taken somewhat differing approaches to the diagnosis of mental illness, but considerable effort has been expended to provide an operational translation between the two nosologies. Both systems are in essence purely descriptive and emphasize clinical pragmatism, in distinction to the Research Domain Criteria (RDOC) proposed by National Institute of Mental Health, which aspires to provide a causal framework for classification of behavioral disturbance. None of these diagnostic systems has as yet achieved adequate validation. The Global Burden of Disease Study 2010, using available epidemiologic data, nevertheless has reinforced the conclusion that, regardless of nosologic differences, mental and substance abuse disorders are the major cause of life-years lost to disability among all medical illnesses. There is general agreement that high-income countries will need to build capacity in professional training in low- and middle-income countries in order to provide an adequate balanced care model for the delivery of evidence-based therapies for mental disorders. Recent surveys that indicate a dramatic increase in mental disorder prevalence in rapidly developing countries, such as China, may reflect both an increased recognition of the issue, but also the consequence of social turmoil, stigma, and historically inadequate resources. The need for improved prevention strategies and for more definitive and effective interventional treatments remains a global concern.

ANXIETY DISORDERS

Anxiety disorders, the most prevalent psychiatric illnesses in the general community, are present in 15–20% of medical clinic patients. Anxiety, defined as a subjective sense of unease, dread, or foreboding, can indicate a primary psychiatric condition or can be a component of, or reaction to, a primary medical disease. The primary anxiety disorders are classified according to their duration and course and the existence and nature of precipitants.

When evaluating the anxious patient, the clinician must first determine whether the anxiety antedates or postdates a medical illness or is due to a medication side effect. Approximately one-third of patients presenting with anxiety have a medical etiology for their psychiatric symptoms, but an anxiety disorder can also present with somatic symptoms in the absence of a diagnosable medical condition.

PANIC DISORDER

Clinical Manifestations Panic disorder is defined by the presence of recurrent and unpredictable panic attacks, which are distinct episodes of intense fear and discomfort associated with a variety of physical symptoms, including palpitations, sweating, trembling, shortness of breath, chest pain, dizziness, and a fear of impending doom or death. Paresthesias, gastrointestinal distress, and feelings of unreality are also common. Diagnostic criteria require at least 1 month of concern or worry about the attacks or a change in behavior related to them. The lifetime prevalence of panic disorder is 2–3%. Panic attacks have a sudden onset, developing within 10 min and usually resolving over the course of an hour, and they occur in an unexpected fashion. Some may occur when waking from sleep. The frequency and severity of panic attacks vary, ranging from once a week to clusters of attacks separated by months of well-being. The first attack is usually outside the home, and onset is typically in late adolescence to early adulthood. In some individuals, anticipatory anxiety develops over time and results in a generalized fear and a progressive avoidance of places or situations in which a panic attack might recur. *Agoraphobia*, which occurs commonly in patients with panic disorder, is an acquired irrational fear of being in places where one might feel trapped or unable to escape. It may, however, be diagnosed even if panic disorder is not present. Typically, it leads the patient into a progressive restriction in lifestyle and, in a literal sense, in geography. Frequently, patients are embarrassed that they are housebound and dependent on the company of others to go out into the world and do not volunteer this information; thus, physicians will fail to recognize the syndrome if direct questioning is not pursued.

Differential Diagnosis A diagnosis of panic disorder is made after a medical etiology for the panic attacks has been ruled out. A variety of cardiovascular, respiratory, endocrine, and neurologic conditions can present with anxiety as the chief complaint. Patients with true panic disorder will often focus on one specific feature to the exclusion of others. For example, 20% of patients who present with syncope as a primary medical complaint have a primary diagnosis of a mood, anxiety, or substance abuse disorder, the most common being panic disorder. The differential diagnosis of panic disorder is complicated by a high rate of comorbidity with other psychiatric conditions, especially alcohol and benzodiazepine abuse, which patients initially use in an attempt at self-medication. Some 75% of panic disorder patients will also satisfy criteria for major depression at some point in their illness.

When the history is nonspecific, physical examination and focused laboratory testing must be used to rule out anxiety states resulting from medical disorders such as pheochromocytoma, thyrotoxicosis, or hypoglycemia. Electrocardiogram (ECG) and echocardiogram may detect some cardiovascular conditions associated with panic such as paroxysmal atrial tachycardia and mitral valve prolapse. In two studies, panic disorder was the primary diagnosis in 43% of patients with chest pain who had normal coronary angiograms and was present in 9% of all outpatients referred for cardiac evaluation. Panic disorder has also been diagnosed in many patients referred for pulmonary function testing or with symptoms of irritable bowel syndrome.

Etiology and Pathophysiology The etiology of panic disorder is unknown but appears to involve a genetic predisposition, altered autonomic responsivity, and social learning. Panic disorder shows familial aggregation; the disorder is concordant in 30–45% of monozygotic twins, and genome-wide screens have identified suggestive risk loci. Acute panic attacks appear to be associated with increased noradrenergic discharges in the locus coeruleus. Intravenous infusion of sodium lactate evokes an attack in two-thirds of panic disorder patients, as do the α_2-adrenergic antagonist yohimbine, cholecystokinin tetrapeptide (CCK-4), and carbon dioxide inhalation. It is hypothesized that each of these stimuli activates a pathway involving noradrenergic neurons in the locus coeruleus and serotonergic neurons in the dorsal raphe. Agents that block serotonin reuptake can prevent attacks. Patients with panic disorder have a heightened sensitivity to somatic symptoms, which triggers increasing arousal, setting off the panic attack; accordingly, therapeutic intervention involves altering the patient's cognitive interpretation of anxiety-producing experiences as well as preventing the attack itself.

TREATMENT PANIC DISORDER

Achievable goals of treatment are to decrease the frequency of panic attacks and to reduce their intensity. The cornerstone of drug therapy is antidepressant medication (Tables 466-1 through 466-3). Selective serotonin reuptake inhibitors (SSRIs) benefit the majority of panic disorder patients and do not have the adverse effects of tricyclic antidepressants (TCAs). Fluoxetine, paroxetine, sertraline, and the selective serotonin-norepinephrine reuptake inhibitor (SNRI) venlafaxine have received approval from the U.S. Food and Drug Administration (FDA) for this indication. These drugs should be started at one-third to one-half of their usual antidepressant dose (e.g., 5–10 mg fluoxetine, 25–50 mg sertraline, 10 mg paroxetine, venlafaxine 37.5 mg). Monoamine oxidase inhibitors (MAOIs) are also effective and may specifically benefit patients who have comorbid features of atypical depression (i.e., hypersomnia and weight gain). Insomnia, orthostatic hypotension, and the need to maintain a low-tyramine diet (avoidance of cheese and wine) have limited their use, however. Antidepressants typically take 2–6 weeks to become effective, and doses may need to be adjusted based on the clinical response.

Because of anticipatory anxiety and the need for immediate relief of panic symptoms, benzodiazepines are useful early in the course of treatment and sporadically thereafter (Table 466-4). For example, alprazolam, starting at 0.5 mg qid and increasing to 4 mg/d in divided doses, is effective, but patients must be monitored closely, as some develop dependence and begin to escalate the dose of this medication. Clonazepam, at a final maintenance dose of 2–4 mg/d, is also helpful; its longer half-life permits twice-daily dosing, and patients appear less likely to develop dependence on this agent.

Early psychotherapeutic intervention and education aimed at symptom control enhance the effectiveness of drug treatment. Patients can be taught breathing techniques, be educated about physiologic changes that occur with panic, and learn to expose themselves voluntarily to precipitating events in a treatment program spanning 12–15 sessions. Homework assignments and monitored compliance are important components of successful treatment. Once patients have achieved a satisfactory response, drug treatment should be maintained for 1–2 years to prevent relapse. Controlled trials indicate a success rate of 75–85%, although the likelihood of complete remission is somewhat lower.

GENERALIZED ANXIETY DISORDER

Clinical Manifestations Patients with generalized anxiety disorder (GAD) have persistent, excessive, and/or unrealistic worry associated with muscle tension, impaired concentration, autonomic arousal, feeling "on edge" or restless, and insomnia (Table 466-5). Onset is usually before age 20 years, and a history of childhood fears and social inhibition may be present. The lifetime prevalence of GAD is 5–6%; the risk is higher in first degree relatives of patients with the diagnosis. Interestingly, family studies indicate that GAD and panic disorder segregate independently. More than 80% of patients with GAD also suffer from major depression, dysthymia, or social phobia. Comorbid substance abuse is common in these patients, particularly alcohol and/or sedative/hypnotic abuse. Patients with GAD worry excessively over minor matters, with life-disrupting effects; unlike in panic disorder, complaints of shortness of breath, palpitations, and tachycardia are relatively rare.

Etiology and Pathophysiology All anxiogenic agents act on the γ-aminobutyric acid $(GABA)_A$ receptor/chloride ion channel complex, implicating this neurotransmitter system in the pathogenesis of anxiety and panic attacks. Benzodiazepines are thought to bind two separate $GABA_A$ receptor sites: type I, which has a broad neuroanatomic distribution, and type II, which is concentrated in the hippocampus, striatum, and neocortex. The antianxiety effects of the various benzodiazepines are influenced by their relative binding to alpha 2 and 3 subunits of the $GABA_A$ receptor, and sedation and memory impairment to the alpha 1 subunit, Serotonin (5-hydroxytryptamine [5-HT]) and 3α-reduced neuroactive steroids (allosteric modulators of $GABA_A$) also appear to have a role in anxiety, and buspirone, a partial 5-HT_{1A} receptor agonist, and certain 5-HT_{2A} and 5-HT_{2C} receptor antagonists (e.g., nefazodone) may have beneficial effects.

TREATMENT GENERALIZED ANXIETY DISORDER

A combination of pharmacologic and psychotherapeutic interventions is most effective in GAD, but complete symptomatic relief is rare. A short course of a benzodiazepine is usually indicated, preferably lorazepam, oxazepam, or alprazolam. (The first two of these agents are metabolized via conjugation rather than oxidation and thus do not accumulate if hepatic function is impaired; the latter

TABLE 466-1 ANTIDEPRESSANTS

Name	Usual Daily Dose, mg	Side Effects	Comments
SSRIs			
Fluoxetine (Prozac)	10–80	Headache; nausea and other GI effects; jitteriness; insomnia; sexual dysfunction; can affect plasma levels of other medicines (except sertraline); akathisia rare	Once-daily dosing, usually in the morning; fluoxetine has very long half-life; must not be combined with MAOIs
Sertraline (Zoloft)	50–200		
Paroxetine (Paxil)	20–60		
Fluvoxamine (Luvox)	100–300		
Citalopram (Celexa)	20–60		
Escitalopram (Lexapro)	10–30		
TCAs			
Amitriptyline (Elavil)	150–300	Anticholinergic (dry mouth, tachycardia, constipation, urinary retention, blurred vision); sweating; tremor; postural hypotension; cardiac conduction delay; sedation; weight gain	Once-daily dosing, usually qhs; blood levels of most TCAs available; can be lethal in overdose (lethal dose = 2 g); nortriptyline best tolerated, especially by elderly
Nortriptyline (Pamelor)	50–200		
Imipramine (Tofranil)	150–300		
Desipramine (Norpramin)	150–300		
Doxepin (Sinequan)	150–300		
Clomipramine (Anafranil)	150–300		FDA approved for OCD
Mixed Norepinephrine/Serotonin Reuptake Inhibitors (SNRI) and Receptor Blockers			
Venlafaxine (Effexor)	75–375	Nausea; dizziness; dry mouth; headaches; increased blood pressure; anxiety and insomnia	Bid-tid dosing (extended release available); lower potential for drug interactions than SSRIs; contraindicated with MAOIs
Desvenlafaxine (Pristiq)	50–400	Nausea, dizziness, insomnia	Primary metabolite of venlafaxine; no increased efficacy with higher dosing
Duloxetine (Cymbalta)	40–60	Nausea, dizziness, headache, insomnia, constipation	May have utility in treatment of neuropathic pain and stress incontinence
Mirtazapine (Remeron)	15–45	Somnolence, weight gain; neutropenia rare	Once a day dosing
Vilazodone (Viibryd)	40	Nausea, diarrhea, headache; dosage adjustment if given with CYP3A4 inhibitor/stimulator	Also 5-HT_{1a} receptor partial agonist
Vortioxetine (Brintellix)	5–20	Nausea, diarrhea, sweating, headache; low incidence of sedation or weight gain	No specific p450 effects; 5-HT_{3a} and 5-HT_7 receptor antagonist, 5-HT_{1b} partial agonist, and 5-HT_{1a} agonist
Levomilnacipran (Fetzima)	40–120	Nausea, constipation, sweating; rare increase in blood pressure/pulse	Most noradrenergic of SNRIs
Mixed-Action Drugs			
Bupropion (Wellbutrin)	250–450	Jitteriness; flushing; seizures in at-risk patients; anorexia; tachycardia; psychosis	Tid dosing, but sustained release also available; fewer sexual side effects than SSRIs or TCAs; may be useful for adult ADD
Trazodone (Desyrel)	200–600	Sedation; dry mouth; ventricular irritability; postural hypotension; priapism rare	Useful in low doses for sleep because of sedating effects with no anticholinergic side effects
Trazodone extended release (Oleptro)	150–375	Daytime somnolence, dizziness, nausea	
Amoxapine (Asendin)	200–600	Sexual dysfunction	Lethality in overdose; EPS possible
MAOIs			
Phenelzine (Nardil)	45–90	Insomnia; hypotension; edema; anorgasmia; weight gain; neuropathy; hypertensive crisis; toxic reactions with SSRIs; narcotics	May be more effective in patients with atypical features or treatment-refractory depression
Tranylcypromine (Parnate)	20–50		
Isocarboxazid (Marplan)	20–60		Less weight gain and hypotension than phenelzine
Transdermal selegiline (Emsam)	6–12	Local skin reaction hypertension	No dietary restrictions with 6 mg dose

Abbreviations: ADD, attention deficit disorder; EPS, extrapyramidal symptoms; FDA, U.S. Food and Drug Administration; GI, gastrointestinal; MAOIs, monoamine oxidase inhibitors; OCD, obsessive-compulsive disorder; SSRIs, selective serotonin reuptake inhibitors; TCAs, tricyclic antidepressants.

also has limited active metabolites.) Treatment should be initiated at the lowest dose possible and prescribed on an as-needed basis as symptoms warrant. Benzodiazepines differ in their milligram per kilogram potency, half-life, lipid solubility, metabolic pathways, and presence of active metabolites. Agents that are absorbed rapidly and are lipid soluble, such as diazepam, have a rapid onset of action and a higher abuse potential. Benzodiazepines should generally not be prescribed for >4–6 weeks because of the development of tolerance and the risk of abuse and dependence. Withdrawal must be closely monitored as relapses can occur. It is important to warn patients that concomitant use of alcohol or other sedating drugs may exacerbate side effects and impair their ability to function. An optimistic approach that encourages the patient to clarify environmental precipitants, anticipate his or her reactions, and plan effective response strategies is an essential element of therapy.

Adverse effects of benzodiazepines generally parallel their relative half-lives. Longer-acting agents, such as diazepam, chlordiazepoxide, flurazepam, and clonazepam, tend to accumulate active metabolites, with resultant sedation, impairment of cognition, and poor psychomotor performance. Shorter-acting compounds, such as alprazolam, lorazepam, and oxazepam, can produce daytime anxiety, early morning insomnia, and, with discontinuation, rebound anxiety and insomnia. Although patients develop tolerance to the sedative effects of benzodiazepines, they are less likely to habituate to the adverse psychomotor effects. Withdrawal from the longer half-life benzodiazepines can be accomplished through gradual, stepwise dose reduction (by 10% every 1–2 weeks) over 6–12 weeks. It is usually more difficult to taper patients off shorter-acting benzodiazepines. Physicians may need to switch the patient to a benzodiazepine with a longer half-life or use an

TABLE 466-2 MANAGEMENT OF ANTIDEPRESSANT SIDE EFFECTS

Symptoms	Comments and Management Strategies
Gastrointestinal	
Nausea, loss of appetite	Usually short-lived and dose-related; consider temporary dose reduction or administration with food and antacids
Diarrhea	Famotidine, 20–40 mg/d
Constipation	Wait for tolerance; try diet change, stool softener, exercise; avoid laxatives
Sexual dysfunction	Consider dose reduction; drug holiday
Anorgasmia/ impotence; impaired ejaculation	Bethanechol, 10–20 mg, 2 h before activity, or cyproheptadine, 4–8 mg 2 h before activity, or bupropion, 100 mg bid, or amantadine, 100 mg bid/tid
Orthostasis	Tolerance unlikely; increase fluid intake, use calf exercises/support hose; fludrocortisone, 0.025 mg/d
Anticholinergic	Wait for tolerance
Dry mouth, eyes	Maintain good oral hygiene; use artificial tears, sugar-free gum
Tremor/jitteriness	Antiparkinsonian drugs not effective; use dose reduction/slow increase; lorazepam, 0.5 mg bid, or propranolol, 10–20 mg bid
Insomnia	Schedule all doses for the morning; trazodone, 50–100 mg qhs
Sedation	Caffeine; schedule all dosing for bedtime; bupropion, 75–100 mg in afternoon
Headache	Evaluate diet, stress, other drugs; try dose reduction; amitriptyline, 50 mg/d
Weight gain	Decrease carbohydrates; exercise; consider fluoxetine
Loss of therapeutic benefit over time	Related to tolerance? Increase dose or drug holiday; add amantadine, 100 mg bid, buspirone, 10 mg tid, or pindolol, 2.5 mg bid

adjunctive medication such as a beta blocker or carbamazepine, before attempting to discontinue the benzodiazepine. Withdrawal reactions vary in severity and duration; they can include depression, anxiety, lethargy, diaphoresis, autonomic arousal, and, rarely, seizures.

TABLE 466-3 POSSIBLE DRUG INTERACTIONS WITH SELECTIVE SEROTONIN REUPTAKE INHIBITORS

Agent	Effect
Monoamine oxidase inhibitors	Serotonin syndrome—absolute contraindication
Serotonergic agonists, e.g., tryptophan, fenfluramine, tryptans	Potential serotonin syndrome
Drugs that are metabolized by P450 isoenzymes: tricyclics, other SSRIs, antipsychotics, beta blockers, codeine, triazolobenzodiazepines, calcium channel blockers	Delayed metabolism resulting in increased blood levels and potential toxicity
Drugs that are bound tightly to plasma proteins, e.g., warfarin	Increased bleeding secondary to displacement
Drugs that inhibit the metabolism of SSRIs by P450 isoenzymes, e.g., quinidine	Increased SSRI side effects

Abbreviation: SSRIs, selective serotonin reuptake inhibitors.

Buspirone is a nonbenzodiazepine anxiolytic agent. It is nonsedating, does not produce tolerance or dependence, does not interact with benzodiazepine receptors or alcohol, and has no abuse or disinhibition potential. However, it requires several weeks to take effect and requires thrice-daily dosing. Patients who were previously responsive to a benzodiazepine are unlikely to rate buspirone as equally effective, but patients with head injury or dementia who have symptoms of anxiety and/or agitation may do well with this agent. Escitalopram, paroxetine, and venlafaxine are FDA approved for the treatment of GAD, usually at doses that are comparable to their efficacy in major depression, and may be preferable to usage of benzodiazepines in the treatment of chronic anxiety. Benzodiazepines are contraindicated during pregnancy and breast-feeding.

Anticonvulsants with GABAergic properties may also be effective against anxiety. Gabapentin, oxcarbazepine, tiagabine, pregabalin, and divalproex have all shown some degree of benefit in a variety of anxiety-related syndromes in off-label usage. Agents that selectively target $GABA_A$ receptor subtypes are currently under development, and it is hoped that these will lack the sedating, memory-impairing, and addicting properties of benzodiazepines.

TABLE 466-4 ANXIOLYTICS

Name	Equivalent PO Dose, mg	Onset of Action	Half-Life, h	Comments
Benzodiazepines				
Diazepam (Valium)	5	Fast	20–70	Active metabolites; quite sedating
Flurazepam (Dalmane)	15	Fast	30–100	Flurazepam is a prodrug; metabolites are active; quite sedating
Triazolam (Halcion)	0.25	Intermediate	1.5–5	No active metabolites; can induce confusion and delirium, especially in elderly
Lorazepam (Ativan)	1	Intermediate	10–20	No active metabolites; direct hepatic glucuronide conjugation; quite sedating; FDA approved for anxiety with depression
Alprazolam (Xanax)	0.5	Intermediate	12–15	Active metabolites; not too sedating; FDA approved for panic disorder and anxiety with depression; tolerance and dependence develop easily; difficult to withdraw
Chlordiazepoxide (Librium)	10	Intermediate	5–30	Active metabolites; moderately sedating
Oxazepam (Serax)	15	Slow	5–15	No active metabolites; direct glucuronide conjugation; not too sedating
Temazepam (Restoril)	15	Slow	9–12	No active metabolites; moderately sedating
Clonazepam (Klonopin)	0.5	Slow	18–50	No active metabolites; moderately sedating; FDA approved for panic disorder
Clorazepate (Tranxene)	15	Fast	40–200	Low sedation; unreliable absorption
Nonbenzodiazepines				
Buspirone (BuSpar)	7.5	2 weeks	2–3	Active metabolites; tid dosing—usual daily dose 10–20 mg tid; nonsedating; no additive effects with alcohol; useful for controlling agitation in demented or brain-injured patients

Abbreviation: FDA, U.S. Food and Drug Administration.

TABLE 466-5 DIAGNOSTIC CRITERIA FOR GENERALIZED ANXIETY DISORDER

A. Excessive anxiety and worry (apprehensive expectation), occurring more days than not for at least 6 months, about a number of events or activities (such as work or school performance).

B. The individual finds it difficult to control the worry.

C. The anxiety and worry are associated with three (or more) of the following six symptoms (with at least some symptoms present for more days than not for the past 6 months): (1) restlessness or feeling keyed up or on edge; (2) being easily fatigued; (3) difficulty concentrating or mind going blank; (4) irritability; (5) muscle tension; (6) sleep disturbance (difficulty falling or staying asleep, or restless, unsatisfying sleep).

D. The anxiety, worry, or physical symptoms cause clinically significant distress or impairment in social, occupational, or other important areas of functioning.

E. The disturbance is not attributable to the physiologic effects of a substance (e.g., a drug of abuse, a medication) or another medical condition (e.g., hyperthyroidism).

F. The disturbance is not better explained by another mental disorder (e.g., anxiety or worry about having panic attacks in panic disorder, negative evaluation in social anxiety disorder [social phobia], contamination or other obsessions in obsessive-compulsive disorder, separation from attachment figures in separation anxiety disorder, reminders of traumatic events in posttraumatic stress disorder, gaining weight in anorexia nervosa, physical complaints in somatic symptom disorder, perceived appearance flaws in body dysmorphic disorder, having a serious illness in illness anxiety disorder, or the content of delusional beliefs in schizophrenia or delusional disorder).

Source: *Diagnostic and Statistical Manual of Mental Disorders*, 5th ed. Washington, DC, American Psychiatric Association, 2013.

PHOBIC DISORDERS

Clinical Manifestations The cardinal feature of phobic disorders is a marked and persistent fear of objects or situations, exposure to which results in an immediate anxiety reaction. The patient avoids the phobic stimulus, and this avoidance usually impairs occupational or social functioning. Panic attacks may be triggered by the phobic stimulus or may occur spontaneously. Unlike patients with other anxiety disorders, individuals with phobias usually experience anxiety only in specific situations. Common phobias include fear of closed spaces (claustrophobia), fear of blood, and fear of flying. Social phobia is distinguished by a specific fear of social or performance situations in which the individual is exposed to unfamiliar individuals or to possible examination and evaluation by others. Examples include having to converse at a party, use public restrooms, and meet strangers. In each case, the affected individual is aware that the experienced fear is excessive and unreasonable given the circumstance. The specific content of a phobia may vary across gender, ethnic, and cultural boundaries.

Phobic disorders are common, affecting ~7–9% of the population. Twice as many females are affected than males. Full criteria for diagnosis are usually satisfied first in early adulthood, but behavioral avoidance of unfamiliar people, situations, or objects dating from early childhood is common.

In one study of female twins, concordance rates for agoraphobia, social phobia, and animal phobia were found to be 23% for monozygotic twins and 15% for dizygotic twins. A twin study of fear conditioning, a model for the acquisition of phobias, demonstrated a heritability of 35–45%. Animal studies of fear conditioning have indicated that processing of the fear stimulus occurs through the lateral nucleus of the amygdala, extending through the central nucleus and projecting to the periaqueductal gray region, lateral hypothalamus, and paraventricular hypothalamus.

TREATMENT PHOBIC DISORDERS

Beta blockers (e.g., propranolol, 20–40 mg orally 2 h before the event) are particularly effective in the treatment of "performance anxiety" (but not general social phobia) and appear to work by blocking the peripheral manifestations of anxiety such as perspiration, tachycardia, palpitations, and tremor. MAOIs alleviate social phobia independently of their antidepressant activity, and paroxetine, sertraline, and venlafaxine have received FDA approval for treatment of social anxiety. Benzodiazepines can be helpful in reducing fearful avoidance, but the chronic nature of phobic disorders limits their usefulness.

Behaviorally focused psychotherapy is an important component of treatment because relapse rates are high when medication is used as the sole treatment. Cognitive-behavioral strategies are based on the finding that distorted perceptions and interpretations of fear-producing stimuli play a major role in perpetuation of phobias. Individual and group therapy sessions teach the patient to identify specific negative thoughts associated with the anxiety-producing situation and help to reduce the patient's fear of loss of control. In desensitization therapy, hierarchies of feared situations are constructed, and the patient is encouraged to pursue and master gradual exposure to the anxiety-producing stimuli.

Patients with social phobia, in particular, have a high rate of comorbid alcohol abuse, as well as of other psychiatric conditions (e.g., eating disorders), necessitating the need for parallel management of each disorder if anxiety reduction is to be achieved.

STRESS DISORDERS

Clinical Manifestations Patients may develop anxiety after exposure to extreme traumatic events such as the threat of personal death or injury or the death of a loved one. The reaction may occur shortly after the trauma (*acute stress disorder*) or be delayed and subject to recurrence (PTSD) (**Table 466-6**). In both syndromes, individuals experience associated symptoms of detachment and loss of emotional responsivity. The patient may feel depersonalized and unable to recall specific aspects of the trauma, although typically it is reexperienced through intrusions in thought, dreams, or flashbacks, particularly when cues of the original event are present. Patients often actively avoid stimuli that precipitate recollections of the trauma and demonstrate a resulting increase in vigilance, arousal, and startle response. Patients with stress disorders are at risk for the development of other disorders related to anxiety, mood, and substance abuse (especially alcohol). Between 5 and 10% of Americans will at some time in their life satisfy criteria for PTSD, with women more likely to be affected than men.

Risk factors for the development of PTSD include a past psychiatric history and personality characteristics of high neuroticism and extroversion. Twin studies show a substantial genetic influence on all symptoms associated with PTSD, with less evidence for an environmental effect.

Etiology and Pathophysiology It is hypothesized that in PTSD there is excessive release of norepinephrine from the locus coeruleus in response to stress and increased noradrenergic activity at projection sites in the hippocampus and amygdala. These changes theoretically facilitate the encoding of fear-based memories. Greater sympathetic responses to cues associated with the traumatic event occur in PTSD, although pituitary adrenal responses are blunted.

TREATMENT STRESS DISORDERS

Acute stress reactions are usually self-limited, and treatment typically involves the short-term use of benzodiazepines and supportive/expressive psychotherapy. The chronic and recurrent nature of PTSD, however, requires a more complex approach using drug and behavioral treatments. PTSD is highly correlated with peritraumatic dissociative symptoms and the development of an acute stress disorder at the time of the trauma. The SSRIs (paroxetine and sertraline are FDA approved for PTSD), venlafaxine, and topiramate can all reduce anxiety, symptoms of intrusion, and avoidance behaviors, as can prazosin, an α_1 antagonist. Propranolol and opiates such as morphine, given during the acute stress period, may have beneficial effects in preventing the development of PTSD, and adjunctive naltrexone can be effective when comorbid alcoholism is present. Trazodone, a sedating antidepressant, is frequently used at night

TABLE 466-6 DIAGNOSTIC CRITERIA FOR POSTTRAUMATIC STRESS DISORDER

A. Exposure to actual or threatened death, serious injury, or sexual violence in one (or more) of the following ways:
  1. Directly experiencing the traumatic event(s).
  2. Witnessing, in person, the event(s) as it occurred to others.
  3. Learning that the traumatic event(s) occurred to a close family member or close friend. In cases of actual or threatened death of a family member or friend, the event(s) must have been violent or accidental.
  4. Experiencing repeated or extreme exposure to aversive details of the traumatic event(s) (e.g., first responders collecting human remains; police officers repeatedly exposed to details of child abuse).

B. Presence of one (or more) of the following intrusion symptoms associated with the traumatic event(s), beginning after the traumatic event(s) occurred:
  1. Recurrent, involuntary, and intrusive distressing memories of the traumatic event(s).
  2. Recurrent distressing dreams in which the content and/or affect of the dream are related to the traumatic event(s).
  3. Dissociative reactions (e.g., flashbacks) in which the individual feels or acts as if the traumatic event(s) were recurring. (Such reactions may occur on a continuum, with the most extreme expression being a complete loss of awareness of present surroundings.)
  4. Intense or prolonged psychological distress at exposure to internal or external cues that symbolize or resemble an aspect of the traumatic event(s).
  5. Marked physiologic reactions to internal or external cues that symbolize or resemble an aspect of the traumatic event(s).

C. Persistent avoidance of stimuli associated with the traumatic event(s), beginning after the traumatic event(s) occurred, as evidenced by one or both of the following:
  1. Avoidance of or efforts to avoid distressing memories, thoughts, or feelings about or closely associated with the traumatic event(s).
  2. Avoidance of or efforts to avoid external reminders (people, places, conversations, activities, objects, situations) that arouse distressing memories, thoughts, or feelings about or closely associated with the traumatic event(s).

D. Negative alterations in cognitions and mood associated with the traumatic event(s), beginning or worsening after the traumatic event(s) occurred as evidenced by two (or more) of the following:
  1. Inability to remember an important aspect of the traumatic event(s) (typically due to dissociative amnesia and not to other factors such as head injury, alcohol, or drugs).
  2. Persistent and exaggerated negative beliefs or expectations about oneself, others, or the world (e.g., "I am bad," "No one can be trusted," "The world is completely dangerous," "My whole nervous system is permanently ruined").
  3. Persistent, distorted cognitions about the cause or consequences of the traumatic event(s) that lead the individual to blame himself/herself or others.
  4. Persistent negative emotional state (e.g., fear, horror, anger, guilt, or shame).
  5. Markedly diminished interest or participation in significant activities.
  6. Feelings of detachment or estrangement from others.
  7. Persistent inability to experience positive emotions (e.g., inability to experience happiness, satisfaction, or loving feelings).

E. Marked alterations in arousal and reactivity associated with the traumatic event(s), beginning or worsening after the traumatic event(s) occurred, as evidenced by two (or more) of the following:
  1. Irritable behavior and angry outbursts (with little or no provocation) typically expressed as verbal or physical aggression toward people or objects.
  2. Reckless or self-destructive behavior.
  3. Hypervigilance.
  4. Exaggerated startle response.
  5. Problems with concentration.
  6. Sleep disturbance (e.g., difficulty falling or staying asleep or restless sleep).

F. Duration of the disturbance (criteria B, C, D, and E) is more than 1 month.

G. The disturbance causes clinically significant distress or impairment in social, occupational, or other important areas of functioning.

H. The disturbance is not attributable to the physiologic effects of a substance (e.g., medication, alcohol) or another medical condition.

Source: *Diagnostic and Statistical Manual of Mental Disorders*, 5th ed. Washington, DC, American Psychiatric Association, 2013.

to help with insomnia (50–150 mg qhs). Carbamazepine, valproic acid, and alprazolam have also independently produced improvement in uncontrolled trials. Psychotherapeutic strategies for PTSD help the patient overcome avoidance behaviors and demoralization and master fear of recurrence of the trauma; therapies that encourage the patient to dismantle avoidance behaviors through stepwise focusing on the experience of the traumatic event, such as trauma-focused cognitive-behavioral therapy, exposure therapy, and eye movement desensitization and reprocessing, are the most effective.

OBSESSIVE-COMPULSIVE DISORDER

Clinical Manifestations Obsessive-compulsive disorder (OCD) is characterized by obsessive thoughts and compulsive behaviors that impair everyday functioning. Fears of contamination and germs are common, as are handwashing, counting behaviors, and having to check and recheck such actions as whether a door is locked. The degree to which the disorder is disruptive for the individual varies, but in all cases, obsessive-compulsive activities take up >1 h per day and are undertaken to relieve the anxiety triggered by the core fear. Patients often conceal their symptoms, usually because they are embarrassed by the content of their thoughts or the nature of their actions. Physicians must ask specific questions regarding recurrent thoughts and behaviors, particularly if physical clues such as chafed and reddened hands or patchy hair loss (from repetitive hair pulling, or trichotillomania) are present. Comorbid conditions are common, the most frequent being depression, other anxiety disorders, eating disorders, and tics. OCD has a lifetime prevalence of 2–3% worldwide. Onset is usually gradual, beginning in early adulthood, but childhood onset is not rare. The disorder usually has a waxing and waning course, but some cases may show a steady deterioration in psychosocial functioning.

Etiology and Pathophysiology A genetic contribution to OCD is suggested by twin studies, but no susceptibility gene for OCD has been identified to date. Family studies show an aggregation of OCD with Tourette's disorder, and both are more common in males and in first-born children.

The anatomy of obsessive-compulsive behavior is thought to include the orbital frontal cortex, caudate nucleus, and globus pallidus. The caudate nucleus appears to be involved in the acquisition and maintenance of habit and skill learning, and interventions that are successful in reducing obsessive-compulsive behaviors also decrease metabolic activity measured in the caudate.

TREATMENT OBSESSIVE-COMPULSIVE DISORDER

Clomipramine, fluoxetine, fluvoxamine, and sertraline are approved for the treatment of OCD in adults (fluvoxamine is also approved for children). Clomipramine is a TCA that is often tolerated poorly owing to anticholinergic and sedative side effects at the doses required to treat the illness (25–250 mg/d); its efficacy in OCD is unrelated to its antidepressant activity. Fluoxetine (5–60 mg/d), fluvoxamine (25–300 mg/d), and sertraline (50–150 mg/d) are as effective as clomipramine and have a more benign side effect profile. Only 50–60% of patients with OCD show adequate improvement with pharmacotherapy alone. In treatment-resistant cases, augmentation with other serotonergic agents such as buspirone, or with a neuroleptic or benzodiazepine, may be beneficial, and in severe cases, deep brain stimulation has been found to be effective. When a therapeutic response is achieved, long-duration maintenance therapy is usually indicated.

For many individuals, particularly those with time-consuming compulsions, behavior therapy will result in as much improvement as that afforded by medication. Effective techniques include the gradual increase in exposure to stressful situations, maintenance of a diary to clarify stressors, and homework assignments that substitute new activities for compulsive behaviors.

MOOD DISORDERS

Mood disorders are characterized by a disturbance in the regulation of mood, behavior, and affect. Mood disorders are subdivided into (1) depressive disorders, (2) bipolar disorders, and (3) depression in association with medical illness or alcohol and substance abuse (Chaps. 467 through 471e). Major depressive disorder (MDD) is differentiated from bipolar disorder by the absence of a manic or hypomanic episode. The relationship between pure depressive syndromes and bipolar disorders is not well understood; MDD is more frequent in families of bipolar individuals, but the reverse is not true. In the Global Burden of Disease Study conducted by the World Health Organization, unipolar major depression ranked fourth among all diseases in terms of disability-adjusted life-years and was projected to rank second by the year 2020. In the United States, lost productivity directly related to mood disorders has been estimated at $55.1 billion per year.

DEPRESSION IN ASSOCIATION WITH MEDICAL ILLNESS

Depression occurring in the context of medical illness is difficult to evaluate. Depressive symptomatology may reflect the psychological stress of coping with the disease, may be caused by the disease process itself or by the medications used to treat it, or may simply coexist in time with the medical diagnosis.

Virtually every class of *medication* includes some agent that can induce depression. Antihypertensive drugs, anticholesterolemic agents, and antiarrhythmic agents are common triggers of depressive symptoms. Iatrogenic depression should also be considered in patients receiving glucocorticoids, antimicrobials, systemic analgesics, antiparkinsonian medications, and anticonvulsants. To decide whether a causal relationship exists between pharmacologic therapy and a patient's change in mood, it may sometimes be necessary to undertake an empirical trial of an alternative medication.

Between 20 and 30% of *cardiac* patients manifest a depressive disorder; an even higher percentage experience depressive symptomatology when self-reporting scales are used. Depressive symptoms following unstable angina, myocardial infarction, cardiac bypass surgery, or heart transplant impair rehabilitation and are associated with higher rates of mortality and medical morbidity. Depressed patients often show decreased variability in heart rate (an index of reduced parasympathetic nervous system activity), which may predispose individuals to ventricular arrhythmia and increased morbidity. Depression also appears to increase the risk of developing coronary heart disease, possibly through increased platelet aggregation. TCAs are contraindicated in patients with bundle branch block, and TCA-induced tachycardia is an additional concern in patients with congestive heart failure. SSRIs appear not to induce ECG changes or adverse cardiac events and thus are reasonable first-line drugs for patients at risk for TCA-related complications. SSRIs may interfere with hepatic metabolism of anticoagulants, however, causing increased anticoagulation.

In patients with *cancer*, the mean prevalence of depression is 25%, but depression occurs in 40–50% of patients with cancers of the pancreas or oropharynx. This association is not due to the effect of cachexia alone, as the higher prevalence of depression in patients with pancreatic cancer persists when compared to those with advanced gastric cancer. Initiation of antidepressant medication in cancer patients has been shown to improve quality of life as well as mood. Psychotherapeutic approaches, particularly group therapy, may have some effect on short-term depression, anxiety, and pain symptoms.

Depression occurs frequently in patients with *neurologic disorders*, particularly cerebrovascular disorders, Parkinson's disease, dementia, multiple sclerosis, and traumatic brain injury. One in five patients with left-hemisphere stroke involving the dorsolateral frontal cortex experiences major depression. Late-onset depression in otherwise cognitively normal individuals increases the risk of a subsequent diagnosis of Alzheimer's disease. All classes of antidepressant agents are effective against these depressions, as are, in some cases, stimulant compounds.

The reported prevalence of depression in patients with *diabetes mellitus* varies from 8 to 27%, with the severity of the mood state correlating with the level of hyperglycemia and the presence of diabetic complications. Treatment of depression may be complicated by effects of antidepressive agents on glycemic control. MAOIs can induce hypoglycemia and weight gain, whereas TCAs can produce hyperglycemia and carbohydrate craving. SSRIs and SNRIs, like MAOIs, may reduce fasting plasma glucose, but they are easier to use and may also improve dietary and medication compliance.

Hypothyroidism is frequently associated with features of depression, most commonly depressed mood and memory impairment. Hyperthyroid states may also present in a similar fashion, usually in geriatric populations. Improvement in mood usually follows normalization of thyroid function, but adjunctive antidepressant medication is sometimes required. Patients with subclinical hypothyroidism can also experience symptoms of depression and cognitive difficulty that respond to thyroid replacement.

The lifetime prevalence of depression in *HIV-positive* individuals has been estimated at 22–45%. The relationship between depression and disease progression is multifactorial and likely to involve psychological and social factors, alterations in immune function, and central nervous system (CNS) disease. Chronic hepatitis C infection is also associated with depression, which may worsen with interferon-α treatment.

Some chronic disorders of uncertain etiology, such as chronic fatigue syndrome (Chap. 464e) and fibromyalgia (Chap. 396), are strongly associated with depression and anxiety; patients may benefit from antidepressant treatment or anticonvulsant agents such as pregabalin.

DEPRESSIVE DISORDERS

Clinical Manifestations Major depression is defined as depressed mood on a daily basis for a minimum duration of 2 weeks (Table 466-7). An episode may be characterized by sadness, indifference, apathy, or irritability and is usually associated with changes in sleep patterns, appetite, and weight; motor agitation or retardation; fatigue; impaired concentration and decision making; feelings of shame or guilt; and thoughts of death or dying. Patients with depression have a profound loss of pleasure in all enjoyable activities, exhibit early morning awakening, feel that the dysphoric mood state is qualitatively different from sadness, and often notice a diurnal variation in mood (worse in morning hours). Patients experiencing bereavement or grief may exhibit many of the same signs and symptoms of major depression, although the emphasis is usually on feelings of emptiness and loss, rather than

TABLE 466-7 CRITERIA FOR A MAJOR DEPRESSIVE EPISODE

A. Five (or more) of the following symptoms have been present during the same 2-week period and represent a change from previous functioning; at least one of the symptoms is either (1) depressed mood or (2) loss of interest or pleasure. ***Note:*** Do not include symptoms that are clearly attributable to another medical condition.

1. Depressed mood most of the day, nearly every day, as indicated by either subjective report (e.g., feels sad, empty, hopeless) or observation made by others (e.g., appears tearful).
2. Markedly diminished interest or pleasure in all, or almost all, activities most of the day, nearly every day (as indicated by either subjective account or observation).
3. Significant weight loss when not dieting or weight gain (e.g., a change of >5% of body weight in a month), or decrease or increase in appetite nearly every day.
4. Insomnia or hypersomnia nearly every day.
5. Psychomotor agitation or retardation nearly every day (observable by others, not merely subjective feelings of restlessness or being slowed down).
6. Fatigue or loss of energy nearly every day.
7. Feelings of worthlessness or excessive or inappropriate guilt (which may be delusional) nearly every day (not merely self-reproach or guilt about being sick).
8. Diminished ability to think or concentrate, or indecisiveness, nearly every day (either by subjective account or as observed by others).
9. Recurrent thoughts of death (not just fear of dying), recurrent suicidal ideation without a specific plan, or a suicide attempt or a specific plan for committing suicide

B. The symptoms cause clinically significant distress or impairment in social, occupational, or other important areas of functioning

C. The episode is not attributable to the physiologic effects of a substance or to another medical condition.

D. The occurrence of the major depressive episode is not better explained by seasonal affective disorder, schizophrenia, schizophreniform disorder, delusional disorder, or other specified and unspecified schizophrenia spectrum and other psychotic disorders.

E. There has never been a manic episode or a hypomanic episode.

Source: *Diagnostic and Statistical Manual of Mental Disorders*, 5th ed. Washington, DC, American Psychiatric Association, 2013.

anhedonia and loss of self-esteem, and the duration is usually limited. In certain cases, however, the diagnosis of major depression may be warranted even in the context of a significant loss.

Approximately 15% of the population experiences a major depressive episode at some point in life, and 6–8% of all outpatients in primary care settings satisfy diagnostic criteria for the disorder. Depression is often undiagnosed, and even more frequently, it is treated inadequately. If a physician suspects the presence of a major depressive episode, the initial task is to determine whether it represents unipolar or bipolar depression or is one of the 10–15% of cases that are secondary to general medical illness or substance abuse. Physicians should also assess the risk of suicide by direct questioning, as patients are often reluctant to verbalize such thoughts without prompting. If specific plans are uncovered or if significant risk factors exist (e.g., a past history of suicide attempts, profound hopelessness, concurrent medical illness, substance abuse, or social isolation), the patient must be referred to a mental health specialist for immediate care. The physician should specifically probe each of these areas in an empathic and hopeful manner, being sensitive to denial and possible minimization of distress. The presence of anxiety, panic, or agitation significantly increases near-term suicidal risk. Approximately 4–5% of all depressed patients will commit suicide; most will have sought help from physicians within 1 month of their deaths.

In some depressed patients, the mood disorder does not appear to be episodic and is not clearly associated with either psychosocial dysfunction or change from the individual's usual experience in life. Persistent depressive disorder (*dysthymic disorder*) consists of a pattern of chronic (at least 2 years), ongoing depressive symptoms that are usually less severe and/or less numerous than those found in major depression, but the functional consequences may be equivalent to or even greater; the two conditions are sometimes difficult to separate and can occur together ("double depression"). Many patients who exhibit a profile of pessimism, disinterest, and low self-esteem respond to antidepressant treatment. Persistent and chronic depressive disorders occur in approximately 2% of the general population.

Depression is approximately twice as common in women as in men, and the incidence increases with age in both sexes. Twin studies indicate that the liability to major depression of early onset (before age 25) is largely genetic in origin. Negative life events can precipitate and contribute to depression, but genetic factors influence the sensitivity of individuals to these stressful events. In most cases, both biologic and psychosocial factors are involved in the precipitation and unfolding of depressive episodes. The most potent stressors appear to involve death of a relative, assault, or severe marital or relationship problems.

Unipolar depressive disorders usually begin in early adulthood and recur episodically over the course of a lifetime. The best predictor of future risk is the number of past episodes; 50–60% of patients who have a first episode have at least one or two recurrences. Some patients experience multiple episodes that become more severe and frequent over time. The duration of an untreated episode varies greatly, ranging from a few months to ≥1 year. The pattern of recurrence and clinical progression in a developing episode are also variable. Within an individual, the nature of episodes (e.g., specific presenting symptoms, frequency and duration) may be similar over time. In a minority of patients, a severe depressive episode may progress to a psychotic state; in elderly patients, depressive symptoms may be associated with cognitive deficits mimicking dementia ("pseudodementia"). A seasonal pattern of depression, called *seasonal affective disorder*, may manifest with onset and remission of episodes at predictable times of the year. This disorder is more common in women, whose symptoms are anergy, fatigue, weight gain, hypersomnia, and episodic carbohydrate craving. The prevalence increases with distance from the equator, and improvement may occur by altering light exposure.

Etiology and Pathophysiology Although evidence for genetic transmission of unipolar depression is not as strong as in bipolar disorder, monozygotic twins have a higher concordance rate (46%) than dizygotic siblings (20%), with little support for any effect of a shared family environment.

Neuroendocrine abnormalities that reflect the neurovegetative signs and symptoms of depression include: (1) increased cortisol and corticotropin-releasing hormone (CRH) secretion, (2) an increase in adrenal size, (3) a decreased inhibitory response of glucocorticoids to dexamethasone, and (4) a blunted response of thyroid-stimulating hormone (TSH) level to infusion of thyroid-releasing hormone (TRH). Antidepressant treatment leads to normalization of these abnormalities. Major depression is also associated with changes in levels of pro-inflammatory cytokines and neurotrophins.

Diurnal variations in symptom severity and alterations in circadian rhythmicity of a number of neurochemical and neurohumoral factors suggest that biologic differences may be secondary to a primary defect in regulation of biologic rhythms. Patients with major depression show consistent findings of a decrease in rapid eye movement (REM) sleep onset (REM latency), an increase in REM density, and, in some subjects, a decrease in stage IV delta slow-wave sleep.

Although antidepressant drugs inhibit neurotransmitter uptake within hours, their therapeutic effects typically emerge over several weeks, implicating adaptive changes in second messenger systems and transcription factors as possible mechanisms of action.

The pathogenesis of depression is discussed in detail in Chap. 465e.

TREATMENT DEPRESSIVE DISORDERS

Treatment planning requires coordination of short-term strategies to induce remission combined with longer term maintenance designed to prevent recurrence. The most effective intervention

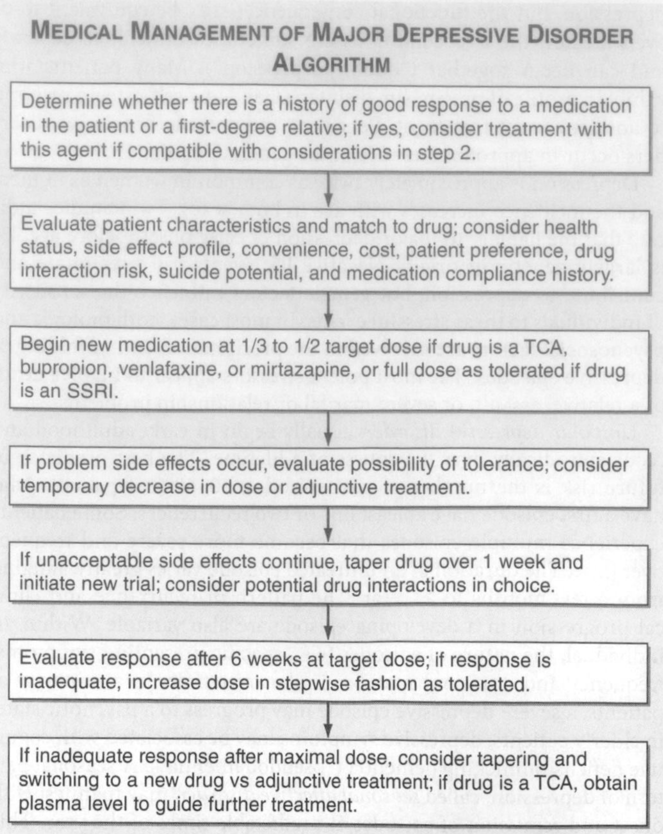

Medical Management of Major Depressive Disorder Algorithm

Determine whether there is a history of good response to a medication in the patient or a first-degree relative; if yes, consider treatment with this agent if compatible with considerations in step 2.

↓

Evaluate patient characteristics and match to drug; consider health status, side effect profile, convenience, cost, patient preference, drug interaction risk, suicide potential, and medication compliance history.

↓

Begin new medication at 1/3 to 1/2 target dose if drug is a TCA, bupropion, venlafaxine, or mirtazapine, or full dose as tolerated if drug is an SSRI.

↓

If problem side effects occur, evaluate possibility of tolerance; consider temporary decrease in dose or adjunctive treatment.

↓

If unacceptable side effects continue, taper drug over 1 week and initiate new trial; consider potential drug interactions in choice.

↓

Evaluate response after 6 weeks at target dose; if response is inadequate, increase dose in stepwise fashion as tolerated.

↓

If inadequate response after maximal dose, consider tapering and switching to a new drug vs adjunctive treatment; if drug is a TCA, obtain plasma level to guide further treatment.

FIGURE 466-1 A guideline for the medical management of major depressive disorder. SSRI, selective serotonin reuptake inhibitor; TCA, tricyclic antidepressant.

for achieving remission and preventing relapse is medication, but combined treatment, incorporating psychotherapy to help the patient cope with decreased self-esteem and demoralization, improves outcome (Fig. 466-1). Approximately 40% of primary care patients with depression drop out of treatment and discontinue medication if symptomatic improvement is not noted within a month, unless additional support is provided. Outcome improves with (1) increased intensity and frequency of visits during the first 4–6 weeks of treatment, (2) supplemental educational materials, and (3) psychiatric consultation as indicated. Despite the widespread use of SSRIs and other second-generation antidepressant drugs, there is no convincing evidence that these classes of antidepressants are more efficacious than TCAs. Between 60 and 70% of all depressed patients respond to any drug chosen, if it is given in a sufficient dose for 6–8 weeks.

A rational approach to selecting which antidepressant to use involves matching the patient's preference and medical history with the metabolic and side effect profile of the drug (Tables 466-4 and 466-5). A previous response, or a family history of a positive response, to a specific antidepressant often suggests that that drug be tried first. Before initiating antidepressant therapy, the physician should evaluate the possible contribution of comorbid illnesses and consider their specific treatment. In individuals with suicidal ideation, particular attention should be paid to choosing a drug with low toxicity if taken in overdose. Newer antidepressant drugs are distinctly safer in this regard; nevertheless, the advantages of TCAs have not been completely superseded. The existence of generic equivalents makes TCAs relatively cheap, and for secondary tricyclics, particularly nortriptyline and desipramine, well-defined relationships among dose, plasma level, and therapeutic response exist. The steady-state plasma level achieved for a given drug dose can vary more than 10-fold between individuals, and plasma levels may help in interpreting apparent resistance to treatment and/or unexpected drug toxicity. The principal side effects of TCAs are antihistamine (sedation) and anticholinergic (constipation, dry mouth, urinary hesitancy, blurred vision). TCAs are contraindicated in patients with serious cardiovascular risk factors, and overdoses of tricyclic agents can be lethal, with desipramine carrying the greatest risk. It is judicious to prescribe only a 10-day supply when suicide is a risk. Most patients require a daily dose of 150–200 mg of imipramine or amitriptyline or its equivalent to achieve a therapeutic blood level of 150–300 ng/mL and a satisfactory remission; some patients show a partial effect at lower doses. Geriatric patients may require a low starting dose and slow escalation. Ethnic differences in drug metabolism are significant, with Hispanic, Asian, and black patients generally requiring lower doses than whites to achieve a comparable blood level. P450 profiling using genetic chip technology may be clinically useful in predicting individual sensitivity.

Second-generation antidepressants are similar to tricyclics in their effect on neurotransmitter reuptake, although some also have specific actions on catecholamine and indolamine receptors as well. Amoxapine is a dibenzoxazepine derivative that blocks norepinephrine and serotonin reuptake and has a metabolite that shows a degree of dopamine blockade. Long-term use of this drug carries a risk of tardive dyskinesia. Maprotiline is a potent noradrenergic reuptake blocker that has little anticholinergic effect but may produce seizures. Bupropion is a novel antidepressant whose mechanism of action is thought to involve enhancement of noradrenergic function. It has no anticholinergic, sedating, or orthostatic side effects and has a low incidence of sexual side effects. It may, however, be associated with stimulant-like side effects, may lower seizure threshold, and has an exceptionally short half-life, requiring frequent dosing. An extended-release preparation is available.

SSRIs such as fluoxetine, sertraline, paroxetine, citalopram, and escitalopram cause a lower frequency of anticholinergic, sedating, and cardiovascular side effects but a possibly greater incidence of gastrointestinal complaints, sleep impairment, and sexual dysfunction than do TCAs. Akathisia, involving an inner sense of restlessness and anxiety in addition to increased motor activity, may also be more common, particularly during the first week of treatment. One concern is the risk of "serotonin syndrome," which is thought to result from hyperstimulation of brainstem 5-HT_{1A} receptors and characterized by myoclonus, agitation, abdominal cramping, hyperpyrexia, hypertension, and potentially death. Serotonergic agonists taken in combination should be monitored closely for this reason. Considerations such as half-life, compliance, toxicity, and drug-drug interactions may guide the choice of a particular SSRI. Fluoxetine and its principal active metabolite, norfluoxetine, for example, have a combined half-life of almost 7 days, resulting in a delay of 5 weeks before steady-state levels are achieved and a similar delay for complete drug excretion once its use is discontinued. All the SSRIs may impair sexual function, resulting in diminished libido, impotence, or difficulty in achieving orgasm. Sexual dysfunction frequently results in noncompliance and should be asked about specifically. Sexual dysfunction can sometimes be ameliorated by lowering the dose, by instituting weekend drug holidays (two or three times a month), or by treatment with amantadine (100 mg tid), bethanechol (25 mg tid), buspirone (10 mg tid), or bupropion (100–150 mg/d). Paroxetine appears to be more anticholinergic than either fluoxetine or sertraline, and sertraline carries a lower risk of producing an adverse drug interaction than the other two. Rare side effects of SSRIs include angina due to vasospasm and prolongation of the prothrombin time. Escitalopram is the most specific of currently available SSRIs and appears to have no specific inhibitory effects on the P450 system.

Venlafaxine, desvenlafaxine, duloxetine, vilazodone, vortioxetine, and levomilnacipran block the reuptake of both norepinephrine and serotonin but produce relatively little in the way of traditional tricyclic side effects. Unlike the SSRIs, venlafaxine and vortioxetine have relatively linear dose-response curves. Patients on immediate release venlafaxine should be monitored for a possible increase in diastolic blood pressure, and multiple daily dosing is required because of the drug's short half-life. An extended-release form is available and has a somewhat lower incidence of gastrointestinal side effects. Mirtazapine is a TCA that has a unique spectrum of activity. It increases noradrenergic and serotonergic neurotransmission through a blockade of central α_2-adrenergic receptors and postsynaptic 5-HT_2 and 5-HT_3 receptors. It is also strongly antihistaminic and, as such, may produce sedation. Levomilnacipran is the most noradrenergic of the SNRIs and theoretically may be appropriate for patients with more severe fatigue and anergia.

With the exception of citalopram and escitalopram, each of the SSRIs may inhibit one or more cytochrome P450 enzymes. Depending on the specific isoenzyme involved, the metabolism of a number of concomitantly administered medications can be dramatically affected. Fluoxetine and paroxetine, for example, by inhibiting 2D6, can cause dramatic increases in the blood level of type 1C antiarrhythmics, whereas sertraline, by acting on 3A4, may alter blood levels of carbamazepine or digoxin. Depending on drug specificity for a particular CYP enzyme for its own metabolism, concomitant medications or dietary factors, such as grapefruit juice, may in turn affect the efficacy or toxicity of the SSRI.

The MAOIs are highly effective, particularly in atypical depression, but the risk of hypertensive crisis following intake of tyramine-containing food or sympathomimetic drugs makes them inappropriate as first-line agents. Transdermal selegiline may avert this risk at low dose. Common side effects include orthostatic hypotension, weight gain, insomnia, and sexual dysfunction. MAOIs should not be used concomitantly with SSRIs, because of the risk of serotonin syndrome, or with TCAs, because of possible hyperadrenergic effects.

Electroconvulsive therapy is at least as effective as medication, but its use is reserved for treatment-resistant cases and delusional depressions. Transcranial magnetic stimulation (TMS) is approved for treatment-resistant depression and has been shown to have efficacy in several controlled trials. Vagus nerve stimulation (VNS) has also recently been approved for treatment-resistant depression, but its degree of efficacy is controversial. Deep brain stimulation and ketamine, a glutamatergic antagonist, are experimental approaches for treatment-resistant cases.

Regardless of the treatment undertaken, the response should be evaluated after ~2 months. Three-quarters of patients show improvement by this time, but if remission is inadequate, the patient should be questioned about compliance, and an increase in medication dose should be considered if side effects are not troublesome. If this approach is unsuccessful, referral to a mental health specialist is advised. Strategies for treatment then include selection of an alternative drug, combinations of antidepressants, and/or adjunctive treatment with other classes of drugs, including lithium, thyroid hormone, atypical antipsychotic agents, and dopamine agonists. A large randomized trial (STAR-D) was unable to show preferential efficacy, but the addition of certain atypical antipsychotic drugs (quetiapine extended-release; aripiprazole) has received FDA approval, as has usage of a combined medication, olanzapine and fluoxetine (Symbyax). Patients whose response to an SSRI wanes over time may benefit from the addition of buspirone (10 mg tid) or pindolol (2–5 mg tid) or small amounts of a TCA such as desipramine (25 mg bid or tid). Most patients will show some degree of response, but aggressive treatment should be pursued until remission is achieved, and drug treatment should be continued for at least 6–9 more months to prevent relapse. In patients who have had two or more episodes of depression, indefinite maintenance treatment should be considered.

It is essential to educate patients both about depression and the benefits and side effects of medications they are receiving. Advice about stress reduction and cautions that alcohol may exacerbate depressive symptoms and impair drug response are helpful. Patients should be given time to describe their experience, their outlook, and the impact of the depression on them and their families. Occasional empathic silence may be as helpful for the treatment alliance as verbal reassurance. Controlled trials have shown that cognitive-behavioral and interpersonal therapies are effective in improving psychological and social adjustment and that a combined treatment approach is more successful than medication alone for many patients.

BIPOLAR DISORDER

Clinical Manifestations Bipolar disorder is characterized by unpredictable swings in mood from mania (or hypomania) to depression. Some patients suffer only from recurrent attacks of *mania*, which in its pure form is associated with increased psychomotor activity; excessive social extroversion; decreased need for sleep; impulsivity and impairment in judgment; and expansive, grandiose, and sometimes irritable mood (Table 466-8). In severe mania, patients may experience delusions and paranoid thinking indistinguishable from schizophrenia. One-half of patients with bipolar disorder present with a mixture of psychomotor agitation and activation with dysphoria, anxiety, and irritability. It may be difficult to distinguish *mixed mania* from *agitated depression*. In some bipolar patients (*bipolar II disorder*), the full criteria for mania are lacking, and the requisite recurrent depressions are separated by periods of mild activation and increased energy (hypomania). In *cyclothymic disorder*, there are numerous hypomanic periods, usually of relatively short duration, alternating with clusters of depressive symptoms that fail, either in severity or duration, to meet the criteria of major depression. The mood fluctuations are chronic and should be present for at least 2 years before the diagnosis is made.

Manic episodes typically emerge over a period of days to weeks, but onset within hours is possible, usually in the early morning hours. An untreated episode of either depression or mania can be as short as several weeks or last as long as 8–12 months, and rare patients have an unremitting chronic course. The term *rapid cycling* is used for patients who have four or more episodes of either depression or mania in a given year. This pattern occurs in 15% of all patients, almost all of whom are women. In some cases, rapid cycling is linked to an underlying thyroid dysfunction, and in others, it is iatrogenically triggered by prolonged antidepressant treatment. Approximately one-half of patients have sustained difficulties in work performance and psychosocial functioning, with depressive phases being more responsible for impairment than mania.

TABLE 466-8 CRITERIA FOR A MANIC EPISODE

A. A distinct period of abnormally and persistently elevated, expansive, or irritable mood and abnormally and persistently increased goal directed activity or energy, lasting at least 1 week and present most of the day, nearly every day (or any duration if hospitalization is necessary).

B. During the period of the mood disturbance and increased energy or activity, three (or more) of the following symptoms (four if the mood is only irritable) are present to a significant degree and represent a noticeable change from usual behavior:

1. Inflated self-esteem or grandiosity.
2. Decreased need for sleep (e.g., feels rested after only 3 h of sleep).
3. More talkative than usual or pressure to keep talking.
4. Flight of ideas or subjective experience that thoughts are racing.
5. Distractibility (i.e., attention too easily drawn to unimportant or irrelevant external stimuli), as reported or observed.
6. Increase in goal-directed activity (either socially, at work or school, or sexually) or psychomotor agitation (i.e., purposeless non-goal-directed activity).
7. Excessive involvement in activities that have a high potential for painful consequences (e.g., engaging in unrestrained buying sprees, sexual indiscretions, or foolish business investments).

C. The mood disturbance is sufficiently severe to cause marked impairment in social or occupational functioning or to necessitate hospitalization to prevent harm to self or others, or there are psychotic features.

D. The episode is not attributable to the physiologic effects of a substance (e.g., a drug of abuse, a medication, or other treatment) or another medical condition.

Source: *Diagnostic and Statistical Manual of Mental Disorders*, 5th ed. Washington, DC, American Psychiatric Association, 2013.

Bipolar disorder is common, affecting ~1.5% of the population in the United States. Onset is typically between 20 and 30 years of age, but many individuals report premorbid symptoms in late childhood or early adolescence. The prevalence is similar for men and women; women are likely to have more depressive and men more manic episodes over a lifetime.

Differential Diagnosis The differential diagnosis of mania includes secondary mania induced by stimulant or sympathomimetic drugs, hyperthyroidism, AIDS, and neurologic disorders such as Huntington's or Wilson's disease and cerebrovascular accidents. Comorbidity with alcohol and substance abuse is common, either because of poor judgment and increased impulsivity or because of an attempt to self-treat the underlying mood symptoms and sleep disturbances.

Etiology and Pathophysiology Genetic predisposition to bipolar disorder is evident from family studies; the concordance rate for monozygotic twins approaches 80%. Patients with bipolar disorder also appear to have altered circadian rhythmicity, and lithium may exert its therapeutic benefit through a resynchronization of intrinsic rhythms keyed to the light/dark cycle.

TREATMENT BIPOLAR DISORDER

(Table 466-9) Lithium carbonate is the mainstay of treatment in bipolar disorder, although sodium valproate and carbamazepine, as well as a number of second-generation antipsychotic agents (aripiprazole, asenapine, olanzapine, quetiapine, risperidone, ziprasidone), also have FDA approval for the treatment of acute mania. Oxcarbazepine is not FDA approved, but appears to enjoy carbamazepine's spectrum of efficacy. The response rate to lithium carbonate is 70–80% in acute mania, with beneficial effects appearing in 1–2 weeks. Lithium also has a prophylactic effect in prevention of recurrent mania and, to a lesser extent, in the prevention of recurrent depression. A simple cation, lithium is rapidly absorbed from the gastrointestinal tract and remains unbound to plasma or tissue proteins. Some 95% of a given dose is excreted unchanged through the kidneys within 24 h.

Serious side effects from lithium are rare, but minor complaints such as gastrointestinal discomfort, nausea, diarrhea, polyuria, weight gain, skin eruptions, alopecia, and edema are common. Over time, urine-concentrating ability may be decreased, but significant nephrotoxicity does not usually occur. Lithium exerts an antithyroid effect by interfering with the synthesis and release of thyroid hormones. More serious side effects include tremor, poor concentration and memory, ataxia, dysarthria, and incoordination. There is suggestive, but not conclusive, evidence that lithium is teratogenic, inducing cardiac malformations in the first trimester.

In the treatment of acute mania, lithium is initiated at 300 mg bid or tid, and the dose is then increased by 300 mg every 2–3 days to achieve blood levels of 0.8–1.2 meq/L. Because the therapeutic effect of lithium may not appear until after 7–10 days of treatment, adjunctive usage of lorazepam (1–2 mg every 4 h) or clonazepam (0.5–1 mg every 4 h) may be beneficial to control agitation. Antipsychotics are indicated in patients with severe agitation who respond only partially to benzodiazepines. Patients using lithium should be monitored closely, since the blood levels required to achieve a therapeutic benefit are close to those associated with toxicity.

Valproic acid may be better than lithium for patients who experience rapid cycling (i.e., more than four episodes a year) or who present with a mixed or dysphoric mania. Tremor and weight gain are the most common side effects; hepatotoxicity and pancreatitis are rare toxicities.

The recurrent nature of bipolar mood disorder necessitates maintenance treatment. A sustained blood lithium level of at least 0.8 meq/L is important for optimal prophylaxis and has been shown to reduce the risk of suicide, a finding not yet apparent for other mood stabilizers. Combinations of mood stabilizers together or with atypical antipsychotic drugs are sometimes required to maintain mood stability. Quetiapine extended release, olanzapine, risperidone, and lamotrigine have been approved for maintenance treatment as sole agents, in combination with lithium and with aripiprazole and ziprasidone as adjunctive drugs. Lurasidone, olanzapine/fluoxetine, and quetiapine are also approved to treat acute depressive episodes in bipolar disorder. Compliance is frequently an issue and often requires enlistment and education of concerned family members. Efforts to identify and modify psychosocial factors that may trigger episodes are important, as is an emphasis on lifestyle regularity. Antidepressant medications are sometimes required for the treatment of severe breakthrough depressions, but their use should generally be avoided during maintenance treatment because of the risk of precipitating mania or accelerating the cycle frequency. Loss of efficacy over time may be observed with any of the mood-stabilizing agents. In such situations, an alternative agent or combination therapy is usually helpful.

TABLE 466-9 CLINICAL PHARMACOLOGY OF MOOD STABILIZERS

Agent and Dosing	Side Effects and Other Effects
Lithium	**Common Side Effects**
Starting dose: 300 mg bid or tid	Nausea/anorexia/diarrhea, fine tremor, thirst, polyuria, fatigue, weight gain, acne, folliculitis, neutrophilia, hypothyroidism
Therapeutic blood level: 0.8–1.2 meq/L	Blood level is increased by thiazides, tetracyclines, and NSAIDs
	Blood level is decreased by bronchodilators, verapamil, and carbonic anhydrase inhibitors
	Rare side effects: Neurotoxicity, renal toxicity, hypercalcemia, ECG changes
Valproic Acid	**Common Side Effects**
Starting dose: 250 mg tid	Nausea/anorexia, weight gain, sedation, tremor, rash, alopecia
Therapeutic blood level: 50–125 μg/mL	Inhibits hepatic metabolism of other medications
	Rare side effects: Pancreatitis, hepatotoxicity, Stevens-Johnson syndrome
Carbamazepine/ Oxcarbazepine	**Common Side Effects**
Starting dose: 200 mg bid for carbamazepine, 150 mg bid for oxcarbazepine	Nausea/anorexia, sedation, rash, dizziness/ ataxia
Therapeutic blood level: 4–12 μg/mL for carbamazepine	Carbamazepine, but not oxcarbazepine, induces hepatic metabolism of other medications
	Rare side effects: Hyponatremia, agranulocytosis, Stevens-Johnson syndrome
Lamotrigine	**Common Side Effects**
Starting dose: 25 mg/d	Rash, dizziness, headache, tremor, sedation, nausea
	Rare side effect: Stevens-Johnson syndrome

Abbreviations: ECG, electrocardiogram; NSAIDs, nonsteroidal anti-inflammatory drugs.

SOMATIC SYMPTOM DISORDER

Many patients presenting in general medical practice, perhaps as many as 5–7%, will experience a somatic symptom(s) as particularly distressing and preoccupying, to the point that it comes to dominate their thoughts, feelings, and beliefs and interferes to a varying degree with everyday functioning. Although the absence of a medical explanation for these complaints was historically emphasized as a diagnostic element, it has been recognized that the patient's interpretation and elaboration of the experience is the critical defining factor and that patients with well-established medical causation may qualify for the diagnosis. Multiple complaints are typical, but severe single symptoms can occur as well. Comorbidity with depressive and anxiety disorders is common and may affect the severity of the experience and its functional consequences. Personality factors may be a significant risk factor, as may a low level of educational or socioeconomic status or a history of recent stressful life events. Cultural factors are relevant as well and should be incorporated into the evaluation. Individuals who have persistent preoccupations about having or acquiring a serious illness, but who do not have a specific somatic complaint, may qualify for a related diagnosis—illness anxiety disorder. The diagnosis of conversion disorder (functional neurologic symptom disorder) is used to specifically identify those individuals whose somatic complaints involve one or more symptoms of altered voluntary motor or sensory function that cannot be medically explained and that causes significant distress or impairment or requires medical evaluation.

In *factitious illnesses*, the patient consciously and voluntarily produces physical symptoms of illness. The term *Munchausen's syndrome* is reserved for individuals with particularly dramatic, chronic, or severe factitious illness. In true factitious illness, the sick role itself is gratifying. A variety of signs, symptoms, and diseases have been either simulated or caused by factitious behavior, the most common including chronic diarrhea, fever of unknown origin, intestinal bleeding or hematuria, seizures, and hypoglycemia. Factitious disorder is usually not diagnosed until 5–10 years after its onset, and it can produce significant social and medical costs. In *malingering*, the fabrication derives from a desire for some external reward such as a narcotic medication or disability reimbursement.

TREATMENT SOMATIC SYMPTOM DISORDER AND RELATED DISORDERS

Patients with somatic symptom disorder are frequently subjected to many diagnostic tests and exploratory surgeries in an attempt to find their "real" illness. Such an approach is doomed to failure and does not address the core issue. Successful treatment is best achieved through behavior modification, in which access to the physician is tightly regulated and adjusted to provide a sustained and predictable level of support that is less clearly contingent on the patient's level of presenting distress. Visits can be brief and should not be associated with a need for a diagnostic or treatment action. Although the literature is limited, some patients may benefit from antidepressant treatment.

Any attempt to confront the patient usually creates a sense of humiliation and causes the patient to abandon treatment from that caregiver. A better strategy is to introduce psychological causation as one of a number of possible explanations in the differential diagnoses that are discussed. Without directly linking psychotherapeutic intervention to the diagnosis, the patient can be offered a face-saving means by which the pathologic relationship with the health care system can be examined and alternative approaches to life stressors developed. Specific medical treatments also may be indicated and effective in treating some of the functional consequences of conversion disorder.

FEEDING AND EATING DISORDERS

CLINICAL MANIFESTATIONS

Feeding and eating disorders constitute a group of conditions in which there is a persistent disturbance of eating or associated behaviors that significantly impair an individual's physical health or psychosocial functioning. In DSM-5 the described categories (with the exception of pica) are defined to be mutually exclusive in a given episode, based on the understanding that although they are phenotypically similar in some ways, they differ in course, prognosis, and effective treatment interventions. Compared with DSM-IV-TR, three disorders (i.e., avoidant/restrictive food intake disorder, rumination disorder, pica) that were previously classified as disorders of infancy or childhood have been grouped together with the disorders of anorexia and bulimia nervosa. Binge-eating disorder is also now included as a formal diagnosis; the intent of each of these modifications is to encourage clinicians to be more specific in their codification of eating and feeding pathology.

PICA

Pica is diagnosed when the individual, over age 2, eats one or more nonnutritive, nonfood substances for a month or more and requires medical attention as a result. There is usually no specific aversion to food in general but a preferential choice to ingest substances such as clay, starch, soap, paper, or ash. The diagnosis requires the exclusion of specific culturally approved practices and has not been commonly found to be caused by a specific nutritional deficiency. Onset is most common in childhood but the disorder can occur in association with other major psychiatric conditions in adults. An association with pregnancy has been observed, but the condition is only diagnosed when medical risks are increased by the behavior.

RUMINATION DISORDER

In this condition, individuals who have no demonstrable associated gastrointestinal or other medical condition repeatedly regurgitate their food after eating and then either rechew or swallow it or spit it out. The behavior typically occurs on a daily basis and must persist for at least 1 month. Weight loss and malnutrition are common sequelae, and individuals may attempt to conceal their behavior, either by covering their mouth or through social avoidance while eating. In infancy, the onset is typically between 3 to 12 months, and the behavior may remit spontaneously, although in some it appears to be recurrent.

AVOIDANT/RESTRICTIVE FOOD INTAKE DISORDER

The cardinal feature of this disorder is avoidance or restriction of food intake, usually stemming from a lack of interest in or distaste of food and associated with weight loss, nutritional deficiency, dependency on nutritional supplementation, or marked impairment in psychosocial functioning, either alone or in combination. Culturally approved practices, such as fasting, or a lack of available food must be excluded as possible causes. The disorder is distinguished from anorexia nervosa by the presence of emotional factors, such as a fear of gaining weight and distortion of body image in the latter condition. Onset is usually in infancy or early childhood, but avoidant behaviors may persist into adulthood. The disorder is equally prevalent in males and females and is frequently comorbid with anxiety and cognitive and attention-deficit disorders and situations of familial stress. Developmental delay and functional deficits may be significant if the disorder is long-standing and unrecognized.

ANOREXIA NERVOSA

Individuals are diagnosed with anorexia nervosa if they restrict their caloric intake to a degree that their body weight deviates significantly from age, gender, health, and developmental norms and if they also exhibit a fear of gaining weight and an associated disturbance in body image. The condition is further characterized by differentiating those who achieve their weight loss predominantly through restricting intake or by excessive exercise (restricting type) from those who engage in recurrent binge eating and/or subsequent purging, self-induced vomiting, and usage of enemas, laxatives, or diuretics (binge-eating/purging type). Such subtyping is more state than trait specific, as individuals may transition from one profile to the other over time. Determination of whether an individual satisfies the primary criterion of significant low weight is complex and must be individualized, using all available historical information and comparison of body habitus to international body mass norms and guidelines.

Individuals with anorexia nervosa frequently lack insight into their condition and are in denial about possible medical consequences; they often are not comforted by their achieved weight loss and persist in their behaviors despite having met previously self-designated weight goals. Recent research has identified alterations in the circuitry of reward sensitivity and executive function in anorexia and implicated disturbances in frontal cortex and anterior insula regulation of interoceptive awareness of satiety and hunger. Neurochemical findings, including the role of ghrelin, remain controversial.

Onset is most common in adolescence, although onset in later life can occur. Many more females than males are affected, with a lifetime prevalence in women of up to 4%. The disorder appears most prevalent in postindustrialized and urbanized countries and is frequently comorbid with preexisting anxiety disorders. The medical consequences of prolonged anorexia nervosa are multisystemic and can be life-threatening in severe presentations. Changes in blood chemistry include leukopenia with lymphocytosis, elevations in blood urea nitrogen, and metabolic alkalosis and hypokalemia when purging is present. History and physical examination may reveal amenorrhea in females, skin abnormalities (petechiae, lanugo hair, dryness), and signs of hypometabolic function, including hypotension, hypothermia, and sinus bradycardia. Endocrine effects include hypogonadism, growth hormone resistance, and hypercortisolemia. Osteoporosis is a longer-term concern.

The course of the disorder is variable, with some individuals recovering after a single episode, while others exhibit recurrent episodes or a chronic course. Untreated anorexia has a mortality of 5.1/1000, the highest among psychiatric conditions. Maudsley family-based therapy has proven to be an effective therapy in younger individuals, with strict behavioral contingencies used when weight loss becomes critical. No pharmacologic intervention has proven to be specifically beneficial, but comorbid depression and anxiety should be treated. Weight gain should be undertaken gradually with a goal of 0.5 to 1 pound per week to prevent refeeding syndrome. Most individuals are able to achieve remission within 5 years of the original diagnosis.

BULIMIA NERVOSA

Bulimia nervosa describes individuals who engage in recurrent and frequent (at least once a week for 3 months) periods of binge eating and who then resort to compensatory behaviors, such as self-induced purging, enemas, use of laxatives, or excessive exercise to avoid weight gain. Binge eating itself is defined as excessive food intake in a prescribed period of time, usually <2 h. As in anorexia nervosa, disturbances in body image occur and promote the behavior, but unlike in anorexia, individuals are of normal weight or even somewhat overweight. Subjects typically describe a loss of control and express shame about their actions, and often relate that their episodes are triggered by feelings of negative self-esteem or social stresses. The lifetime prevalence in women is approximately 2%, with a 10:1 female-to-male ratio. The disorder typically begins in adolescence and may be persistent over a number of years. Transition to anorexia occurs in only 10–15% of cases. Many of the medical risks associated with bulimia nervosa parallel those of anorexia nervosa and are a direct consequence of purging, including fluid and electrolyte disturbances and conduction abnormalities. Physical examination often results in no specific findings, but dental erosion and parotid gland enlargement may be present. Effective treatment approaches include SSRI antidepressants, usually in combination with cognitive-behavioral, emotion regulation, or interpersonal-based psychotherapies.

BINGE-EATING DISORDER

Binge-eating disorder is distinguished from bulimia nervosa by the absence of compensatory behaviors to prevent weight gain after an episode and by a lack of effort to restrict weight gain between episodes. Other features are similar, including distress over the behavior and the experience of loss of control, resulting in eating more rapidly or in greater amounts than intended or eating when not hungry. The 12-month prevalence in females is 1.6%, with a much lower female-to-male ratio than bulimia nervosa. Little is known about the course of the disorder, given its recent categorization, but its prognosis is markedly better than for other eating disorders, both in terms of its natural course and response to treatment. Transition to other eating disorder conditions is thought to be rare.

PERSONALITY DISORDERS

CLINICAL MANIFESTATIONS

Personality disorders are characteristic patterns of thinking, feeling, and interpersonal behavior that are relatively inflexible and cause significant functional impairment or subjective distress for the individual. The observed behaviors are not secondary to another mental disorder, nor are they precipitated by substance abuse or a general medical condition. This distinction is often difficult to make in clinical practice, because personality change may be the first sign of serious neurologic, endocrine, or other medical illness. Patients with frontal lobe tumors, for example, can present with changes in motivation and personality while the results of the neurologic examination remain within normal limits. Individuals with personality disorders are often regarded as "difficult patients" in clinical medical practice because they are seen as excessively demanding and/or unwilling to follow recommended treatment plans. Although DSM-5 portrays personality disorders as qualitatively distinct categories, there is an alternative perspective that personality characteristics vary as a continuum between normal functioning and formal mental disorder.

Personality disorders have been grouped into three overlapping clusters. *Cluster A* includes paranoid, schizoid, and schizotypal personality disorders. It includes individuals who are odd and eccentric and who maintain an emotional distance from others. Individuals have a restricted emotional range and remain socially isolated. Patients with schizotypal personality disorder frequently have unusual perceptual experiences and express magical beliefs about the external world. The essential feature of paranoid personality disorder is a pervasive mistrust and suspiciousness of others to an extent that is unjustified by available evidence. *Cluster B* disorders include antisocial, borderline, histrionic, and narcissistic types and describe individuals whose behavior is impulsive, excessively emotional, and erratic. *Cluster C* incorporates avoidant, dependent, and obsessive-compulsive personality types; enduring traits are anxiety and fear. The boundaries between cluster types are to some extent artificial, and many patients who meet criteria for one personality disorder also meet criteria for aspects of another. The risk of a comorbid major mental disorder is increased in patients who qualify for a diagnosis of personality disorder.

TREATMENT PERSONALITY DISORDERS

Dialectical behavior therapy (DBT) is a cognitive-behavioral approach that focuses on behavioral change while providing acceptance, compassion, and validation of the patient. Several randomized trials have demonstrated the efficacy of DBT in the treatment of personality disorders. Antidepressant medications and low-dose antipsychotic drugs have some efficacy in cluster A personality disorders, whereas anticonvulsant mood-stabilizing agents and MAOIs may be considered for patients with cluster B diagnoses who show marked mood reactivity, behavioral dyscontrol, and/or rejection hypersensitivity. Anxious or fearful cluster C patients often respond to medications used for axis I anxiety disorders (see above). It is important that the physician and the patient have reasonable expectations vis-à-vis the possible benefit of any medication used and its side effects. Improvement may be subtle and observable only over time.

SCHIZOPHRENIA

CLINICAL MANIFESTATIONS

Schizophrenia is a heterogeneous syndrome characterized by perturbations of language, perception, thinking, social activity, affect, and volition. There are no pathognomonic features. The syndrome commonly begins in late adolescence, has an insidious (and less commonly acute) onset, and, often, a poor outcome, progressing from social withdrawal and perceptual distortions to recurrent delusions and hallucinations. Patients may present with positive symptoms (such as conceptual disorganization, delusions, or hallucinations) or negative symptoms (loss of function, anhedonia, decreased emotional expression, impaired concentration, and diminished social engagement) and must have at least two of these for a 1-month period and continuous signs for at least 6 months to meet formal diagnostic criteria. Disorganized thinking or speech and grossly disorganized motor behavior, including catatonia, may also be present. As individuals age, positive psychotic symptoms tend to attenuate, and some measure of social and occupational function may be regained. "Negative" symptoms predominate in one-third of the schizophrenic population and are associated with a poor long-term outcome and a poor response to drug treatment. However, marked variability in the course and individual character of symptoms is typical.

The term *schizophreniform disorder* describes patients who meet the symptom requirements but not the duration requirements for schizophrenia, and *schizoaffective disorder* is used for those who manifest symptoms of schizophrenia and independent periods of mood disturbance. The terms "schizotypal" and "schizoid" refer to specific personality disorders and are discussed in that section. The diagnosis of delusional disorder is used for individuals who have delusions of various content for at least 1 month but who otherwise do not meet criteria for schizophrenia. Patients who experience a sudden onset of a brief (<1 month) alteration in thought processing, characterized by delusions, hallucinations, disorganized speech, or gross motor behavior, are most appropriately designated as having a brief psychotic disorder. Catatonia is recognized as a nonspecific syndrome that can occur as a consequence of other severe psychiatric/medical disorders and is diagnosed by the documentation of three or more of a cluster of motor and behavioral symptoms, including stupor, cataplexy, mutism, waxy flexibility, and stereotypy, among others. Prognosis depends not on symptom severity but on the response to antipsychotic medication. A permanent remission without recurrence does occasionally occur. About 10% of schizophrenic patients commit suicide.

Schizophrenia is present in 0.85% of individuals worldwide, with a lifetime prevalence of ~1–1.5%. An estimated 300,000 episodes of acute schizophrenia occur annually in the United States, resulting in direct and indirect costs of $62.7 billion.

DIFFERENTIAL DIAGNOSIS

The diagnosis is principally one of exclusion, requiring the absence of significant associated mood symptoms, any relevant medical condition, and substance abuse. Drug reactions that cause hallucinations, paranoia, confusion, or bizarre behavior may be dose-related or idiosyncratic; parkinsonian medications, clonidine, quinacrine, and procaine derivatives are the most common prescription medications associated with these symptoms. Drug causes should be ruled out in any case of newly emergent psychosis. The general neurologic examination in patients with schizophrenia is usually normal, but motor rigidity, tremor, and dyskinesias are noted in one-quarter of untreated patients.

EPIDEMIOLOGY AND PATHOPHYSIOLOGY

Epidemiologic surveys identify several risk factors for schizophrenia, including genetic susceptibility, early developmental insults, winter birth, and increasing parental age. Genetic factors are involved in at least a subset of individuals who develop schizophrenia. Schizophrenia is observed in ~6.6% of all first-degree relatives of an affected proband. If both parents are affected, the risk for offspring is 40%. The concordance rate for monozygotic twins is 50%, compared to 10% for dizygotic twins. Schizophrenia-prone families are also at risk for other psychiatric disorders, including schizoaffective disorder and *schizotypal* and *schizoid personality disorders*, the latter terms designating individuals who show a lifetime pattern of social and interpersonal deficits characterized by an inability to form close interpersonal relationships, eccentric behavior, and mild perceptual distortions.

TREATMENT SCHIZOPHRENIA

Antipsychotic agents (Table 466-10) are the cornerstone of acute and maintenance treatment of schizophrenia and are effective in the treatment of hallucinations, delusions, and thought disorders, regardless of etiology. The mechanism of action involves, at least in part, binding to dopamine D_2/D_3 receptors in the ventral striatum; the clinical potencies of traditional antipsychotic drugs parallel their affinities for the D_2 receptor, and even the newer "atypical" agents exert some degree of D_2 receptor blockade. All neuroleptics induce expression of the immediate-early gene *c-fos* in the nucleus accumbens, a dopaminergic site connecting prefrontal and limbic cortices. The clinical efficacy of newer atypical neuroleptics, however, may involve *N*-methyl-D-aspartate (NMDA) receptor blockade, α_1- and α_2-noradrenergic activity, altering the relationship between 5-HT_2 and D_2 receptor activity, and faster dissociation of D_2 binding and effects on neuroplasticity.

Conventional neuroleptics differ in their potency and side effect profile. Older agents, such as chlorpromazine and thioridazine, are more sedating and anticholinergic and more likely to cause orthostatic hypotension, whereas higher potency antipsychotics, such as haloperidol, perphenazine, and thiothixene, are more likely to induce extrapyramidal side effects. The model "atypical" antipsychotic agent is *clozapine*, a dibenzodiazepine that has a greater potency in blocking the 5-HT_2 than the D_2 receptor and a much higher affinity for the D_4 than the D_2 receptor. Its principal disadvantage is a risk of blood dyscrasias. Paliperidone is a recently approved agent that is a metabolite of risperidone and shares many of its properties. Unlike other antipsychotics, clozapine does not cause a rise in prolactin level. Approximately 30% of patients who do not benefit from conventional antipsychotic agents will have a better response to this drug, which also has a demonstrated superiority to other antipsychotic agents in preventing suicide; however, its side effect profile makes it most appropriate for treatment-resistant cases. *Risperidone*, a benzisoxazole derivative, is more potent at 5-HT_2 than D_2 receptor sites, like clozapine, but it also exerts significant α_2 antagonism, a property that may contribute to its perceived ability to improve mood and increase motor activity. Risperidone is not as effective as clozapine in treatment-resistant cases but does not carry a risk of blood dyscrasias. *Olanzapine* is similar neurochemically to clozapine but has a significant risk of inducing weight gain. *Quetiapine* is distinct in having a weak D_2 effect but potent α_1 and histamine blockade. *Ziprasidone* causes minimal weight gain and is unlikely to increase prolactin but may increase QT prolongation. *Aripiprazole* also has little risk of weight gain or prolactin increase but may increase anxiety, nausea, and insomnia as a result of its partial agonist properties. Asenapine is associated with minimal weight gain and anticholinergic effect but may have a higher than expected risk of extrapyramidal symptoms.

Antipsychotic agents are effective in 70% of patients presenting with a first episode. Improvement may be observed within hours or days, but full remission usually requires 6–8 weeks. The choice of agent depends principally on the side effect profile and cost of treatment or on a past personal or family history of a favorable response to the drug in question. Atypical agents appear to be more effective in treating negative symptoms and improving cognitive function. An equivalent treatment response can usually be achieved with relatively low doses of any drug selected (i.e., 4–6 mg/d of haloperidol, 10–15 mg of olanzapine, or 4–6 mg/d of risperidone). Doses in this range result in >80% D_2 receptor blockade, and there is little evidence that higher doses increase either the rapidity or degree of response. Maintenance treatment requires careful attention to the possibility of relapse and monitoring for the development of a movement disorder. Intermittent drug treatment is less effective than regular dosing, but gradual dose reduction is likely to improve social functioning in many schizophrenic patients who have been maintained at high doses. If medications are completely discontinued, however, the relapse rate is 60% within 6 months. Long-acting injectable preparations (risperidone, paliperidone, olanzapine, aripiprazole) are considered when noncompliance with oral therapy leads to relapses but should not be considered interchangeable, because the agents differ in their indications, injection intervals and sites/volumes, and possible adverse reactions, among other factors. In treatment-resistant patients, a transition to clozapine usually results in rapid improvement, but a prolonged delay in response in some cases necessitates a 6- to 9-month trial for maximal benefit to occur.

Antipsychotic medications can cause a broad range of side effects, including lethargy, weight gain, postural hypotension, constipation, and dry mouth. Extrapyramidal symptoms such as dystonia, akathisia, and akinesia are also frequent with first-generation agents and may contribute to poor adherence if not specifically

TABLE 466-10 ANTIPSYCHOTIC AGENTS

Name	Usual PO Daily Dose, mg	Side Effects	Sedation	Comments
First-Generation Antipsychotics				
Low potency				
Chlorpromazine (Thorazine)	100–1000	Anticholinergic effects; orthostasis; photosensitivity; cholestasis; QT prolongation	+++	EPSEs usually not prominent; can cause anticholinergic delirium in elderly patients
Thioridazine (Mellaril)	100–600			
Midpotency				
Trifluoperazine (Stelazine)	2–50	Fewer anticholinergic side effects	++	Well tolerated by most patients
Perphenazine (Trilafon)	4–64	Fewer EPSEs than with higher potency agents	++	
Loxapine (Loxitane)	30–100	Frequent EPSEs	++	
Molindone (Moban)	30–100	Frequent EPSEs	0	Little weight gain
High potency				
Haloperidol (Haldol)	5–20	No anticholinergic side effects; EPSEs often prominent	0/+	Often prescribed in doses that are too high; long-acting injectable forms of haloperidol and fluphenazine available
Fluphenazine (Prolixin)	1–20	Frequent EPSEs	0/+	
Thiothixene (Navane)	2–50	Frequent EPSEs	0/+	
Second-Generation Antipsychotics				
Clozapine (Clozaril)	150–600	Agranulocytosis (1%); weight gain; seizures; drooling; hyperthermia	++	Requires weekly WBC count for first 6 months, then biweekly if stable
Risperidone (Risperdal)	2–8	Orthostasis	+	Requires slow titration; EPSEs observed with doses >6 mg qd
Olanzapine (Zyprexa)	10–30	Weight gain	++	Mild prolactin elevation
Quetiapine (Seroquel)	350–800	Sedation; weight gain; anxiety	+++	Bid dosing
Ziprasidone (Geodon)	120–200	Orthostatic hypotension	+/++	Minimal weight gain; increases QT interval
Aripiprazole (Abilify)	10–30	Nausea, anxiety, insomnia	0/+	Mixed agonist/antagonist
Paliperidone (Invega)	3–12	Restlessness, EPSEs, increased prolactin, headache	+	Active metabolite of risperidone
Iloperidone (Fanapt)	12–24	Dizziness, hypotension	0/+	Requires dose titration; long acting injectable available
Asenapine (Saphris)	10–20	Dizziness, anxiety, EPSEs, minimal weight gain	++	Sublingual tablets; bid dosing
Lurasidone (Latuda)	40–80	Nausea, EPSEs	++	Uses CYP3A4

Abbreviations: EPSEs, extrapyramidal side effects; WBC, white blood cell.

addressed. Anticholinergic and parkinsonian symptoms respond well to trihexyphenidyl, 2 mg bid, or benztropine mesylate, 1–2 mg bid. Akathisia may respond to beta blockers. In rare cases, more serious and occasionally life-threatening side effects may emerge, including hyperprolactinemia, ventricular arrhythmias, gastrointestinal obstruction, retinal pigmentation, obstructive jaundice, and neuroleptic malignant syndrome (characterized by hyperthermia, autonomic dysfunction, muscular rigidity, and elevated creatine phosphokinase levels). The most serious adverse effects of clozapine are agranulocytosis, which has an incidence of 1%, and induction of seizures, which has an incidence of 10%. Weekly white blood cell counts are required, particularly during the first 3 months of treatment.

The risk of type 2 diabetes mellitus appears to be increased in schizophrenia, and second-generation agents as a group produce greater adverse effects on glucose regulation, independent of effects on obesity, than traditional agents. Clozapine, olanzapine, and quetiapine seem more likely to cause hyperglycemia, weight gain, and hypertriglyceridemia than other atypical antipsychotic drugs. Close monitoring of plasma glucose and lipid levels are indicated with the use of these agents.

A serious side effect of long-term use of first-generation antipsychotic agents is *tardive dyskinesia*, characterized by repetitive, involuntary, and potentially irreversible movements of the tongue and lips (bucco-linguo-masticatory triad) and, in approximately half of cases, choreoathetosis. Tardive dyskinesia has an incidence of 2–4% per year of exposure and a prevalence of 20% in chronically treated patients. The prevalence increases with age, total dose, and duration of drug administration. The risk associated with second-generation agents appears to be much lower. The cause may involve formation of free radicals and perhaps mitochondrial energy failure. Vitamin E may reduce abnormal involuntary movements if given early in the syndrome.

The CATIE study, a large-scale investigation of the effectiveness of antipsychotic agents in "real-world" patients, revealed a high rate of discontinuation of treatment over 18 months. Olanzapine showed greater effectiveness than quetiapine, risperidone, perphenazine, or ziprasidone but also a higher discontinuation rate due to weight gain and metabolic effects. Surprisingly, perphenazine, a first-generation agent, showed little evidence of inferiority to newer drugs.

Drug treatment of schizophrenia is by itself insufficient. Educational efforts directed toward families and relevant community resources have proved to be necessary to maintain stability and optimize outcome. A treatment model involving a multidisciplinary case-management team that seeks out and closely follows the patient in the community has proved particularly effective.

ASSESSMENT AND EVALUATION OF VIOLENCE

Primary care physicians may encounter situations in which family, domestic, or societal violence is discovered or suspected. Such an awareness can carry legal and moral obligations; many state laws mandate reporting of child, spousal, and elder abuse. Physicians are frequently the first point of contact for both victim and abuser. Approximately 2 million older Americans and 1.5 million U.S. children are thought to experience some form of physical maltreatment each year. Spousal abuse is thought to be even more prevalent. An interview study of 24,000 women in 10 countries found a lifetime prevalence of physical or sexual violence that ranged from 15 to 71%; these individuals are more likely to suffer from depression, anxiety, and substance abuse and to have attempted suicide. In addition, abused individuals frequently express low self-esteem, vague somatic symptomatology, social isolation, and a passive feeling of loss of control. Although it is essential to treat these elements in the victim, the first obligation is to ensure that the perpetrator has taken responsibility for preventing any further violence. Substance abuse and/or dependence and serious mental illness in the abuser may contribute to the risk of harm and require direct intervention. Depending on the situation, law enforcement agencies, community resources such as support groups and shelters, and individual and family counseling can be appropriate components of a treatment plan. A safety plan should be formulated with the victim, in addition to providing information about abuse, its likelihood of recurrence, and its tendency to increase in severity and frequency. Antianxiety and antidepressant medications may sometimes be useful in treating the acute symptoms, but only if independent evidence for an appropriate psychiatric diagnosis exists.

MENTAL HEALTH PROBLEMS IN THE HOMELESS

There is a high prevalence of mental disorders and substance abuse among homeless and impoverished individuals. Depending on the definition used, estimates of the total number of homeless individuals in the United States range from 800,000 to 2 million, one-third of whom qualify as having a serious mental disorder. Poor hygiene and nutrition, substance abuse, psychiatric illness, physical trauma, and exposure to the elements combine to make the provision of medical care challenging. Only a minority of these individuals receives formal mental health care; the main points of contact are outpatient medical clinics and emergency departments. Primary care settings represent a critical site in which housing needs, treatment of substance dependence, and evaluation and treatment of psychiatric illness can most efficiently take place. Successful intervention is dependent on breaking down traditional administrative barriers to health care and recognizing the physical constraints and emotional costs imposed by homelessness. Simplifying health care instructions and follow-up, allowing frequent visits, and dispensing medications in limited amounts that require ongoing contact are possible techniques for establishing a successful therapeutic relationship.

467 Alcohol and Alcoholism

Marc A. Schuckit

Alcohol (beverage ethanol) distributes throughout the body, affecting almost all systems and altering nearly every neurochemical process in the brain. This drug is likely to exacerbate most medical problems, affect medications metabolized in the liver, and temporarily mimic many medical (e.g., diabetes) and psychiatric (e.g., depression) conditions. The lifetime risk for repetitive alcohol problems is almost 20% for men and 10% for women, regardless of a person's education or income. Although low doses of alcohol might have healthful benefits, greater than three standard drinks per day enhances the risk for cancer and vascular disease, and alcohol use disorders decrease the life span by about 10 years. Unfortunately, most clinicians have had only limited training regarding alcohol-related disorders. This chapter presents a brief overview of clinically useful information about alcohol use and problems.

PHARMACOLOGY AND NUTRITIONAL IMPACT OF ETHANOL

Ethanol blood levels are expressed as milligrams or grams of ethanol per deciliter (e.g., 100 mg/dL = 0.10 g/dL), with values of ~0.02 g/dL resulting from the ingestion of one typical drink. In round figures, a standard drink is 10–12 g, as seen in 340 mL (12 oz) of beer, 115 mL (4 oz) of nonfortified wine, and 43 mL (1.5 oz) (a shot) of 80-proof beverage (e.g., whisky); 0.5 L (1 pint) of 80-proof beverage contains ~160 g of ethanol (about 16 standard drinks), and 750 mL of wine contains ~60 g of ethanol. These beverages also have additional components (*congeners*) that affect the drink's taste and might contribute to adverse effects on the body. Congeners include methanol, butanol, acetaldehyde, histamine, tannins, iron, and lead. Alcohol acutely decreases neuronal activity and has similar behavioral effects and cross-tolerance with other depressants, including benzodiazepines and barbiturates.

Alcohol is absorbed from mucous membranes of the mouth and esophagus (in small amounts), from the stomach and large bowel (in modest amounts), and from the proximal portion of the small intestine (the major site). The rate of absorption is increased by rapid gastric emptying (as seen with carbonation); by the absence of proteins, fats, or carbohydrates (which interfere with absorption); and by dilution to a modest percentage of ethanol (maximum at ~20% by volume).

Between 2% (at low blood alcohol concentrations) and 10% (at high blood alcohol concentrations) of ethanol is excreted directly through the lungs, urine, or sweat, but most is metabolized to acetaldehyde, primarily in the liver. The most important pathway occurs in the cell cytosol where alcohol dehydrogenase (ADH) produces acetaldehyde, which is then rapidly destroyed by aldehyde dehydrogenase (ALDH) in the cytosol and mitochondria (Fig. 467-1). A second pathway occurs in the microsomes of the smooth endoplasmic reticulum (the microsomal ethanol-oxidizing system, or MEOS) that is responsible for ≥10% of ethanol oxidation at high blood alcohol concentrations.

Although a drink contains ~300 kJ, or 70–100 kcal, these are devoid of minerals, proteins, and vitamins. In addition, alcohol interferes with absorption of vitamins in the small intestine and decreases their storage in the liver with modest effects on folate (folacin or folic acid), pyridoxine (B_6), thiamine (B_1), nicotinic acid (niacin, B_3), and vitamin A.

Heavy drinking in a fasting, healthy individual can produce transient hypoglycemia within 6–36 h, secondary to the acute actions of ethanol on gluconeogenesis. This can result in temporary abnormal glucose tolerance tests (with a resulting erroneous diagnosis of diabetes mellitus) until the alcoholic has abstained for 2–4 weeks. Alcohol ketoacidosis, probably reflecting a decrease in fatty acid oxidation coupled with poor diet or recurrent vomiting, can be misdiagnosed as diabetic ketosis. With the former, patients show an increase in serum ketones along with a mild increase in glucose but a large anion gap, a mild to moderate increase in serum lactate, and a β-hydroxybutyrate/lactate ratio of between 2:1 and 9:1 (with normal being 1:1).

In the brain, alcohol affects almost all neurotransmitter systems, with acute effects that are often the opposite of those seen following desistance after a period of heavy drinking. The most prominent actions relate to boosting γ-aminobutyric acid (GABA) activity,

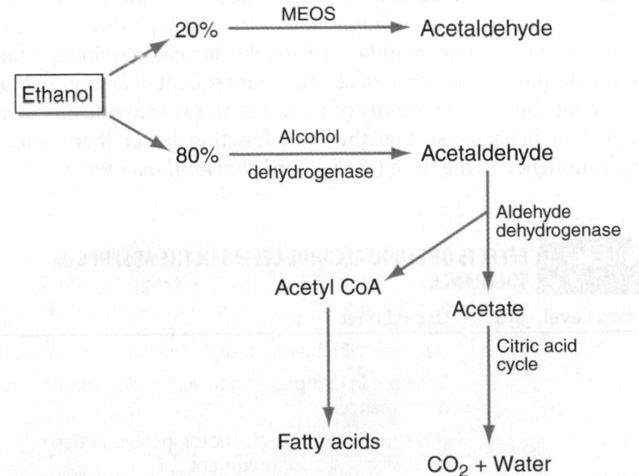

FIGURE 467-1 The metabolism of alcohol. CoA, coenzyme A; MEOS, microsomal ethanoloxidizing system.

especially at $GABA_A$ receptors. Enhancement of this complex chloride channel system contributes to anticonvulsant, sleep-inducing, antianxiety, and muscle relaxation effects of all GABA-boosting drugs. Acutely administered alcohol produces a release of GABA, and continued use increases density of $GABA_A$ receptors, whereas alcohol withdrawal states are characterized by decreases in GABA-related activity. Equally important is the ability of acute alcohol to inhibit postsynaptic *N*-methyl-D-aspartate (NMDA) excitatory glutamate receptors, whereas chronic drinking and desistance are associated with an upregulation of these excitatory receptor subunits. The relationships between greater GABA and diminished NMDA receptor activity during acute intoxication and diminished GABA with enhanced NMDA actions during alcohol withdrawal explain much of intoxication and withdrawal phenomena.

As with all pleasurable activities, alcohol acutely increases dopamine levels in the ventral tegmentum and related brain regions, and this effect plays an important role in continued alcohol use, craving, and relapse. The changes in dopamine pathways are also linked to increases in "stress hormones," including cortisol and adrenocorticotropic hormone (ACTH) during intoxication and withdrawal. Such alterations are likely to contribute to both feelings of reward during intoxication and depression during falling blood alcohol concentrations. Also closely linked to alterations in dopamine (especially in the nucleus accumbens) are alcohol-induced changes in opioid receptors, with acute alcohol causing release of beta endorphins.

Additional neurochemical changes include increases in synaptic levels of serotonin during acute intoxication and subsequent upregulation of serotonin receptors. Acute increases in nicotinic acetylcholine systems contribute to the impact of alcohol in the ventral tegmental region, which occurs in concert with enhanced dopamine activity. In the same regions, alcohol impacts on cannabinol receptors, with resulting release of dopamine, GABA, and glutamate as well as subsequent effects on brain reward circuits.

BEHAVIORAL EFFECTS, TOLERANCE, AND WITHDRAWAL

The acute effects of a drug depend on the dose, the rate of increase in plasma, the concomitant presence of other drugs, and past experience with the agent. "Legal intoxication" with alcohol in most states requires a blood alcohol concentration of 0.08 g/dL, but levels of 0.04 are cited in some other countries. However, behavioral, psychomotor, and cognitive changes are seen at 0.02–0.04 g/dL (i.e., after one to two drinks) (Table 467-1). Deep but disturbed sleep can be seen at twice the legal intoxication level, and death can occur with levels between 0.30 and 0.40 g/dL. Beverage alcohol is probably responsible for more overdose deaths than any other drug.

Repeated use of alcohol contributes to acquired tolerance, a phenomenon involving at least three compensatory mechanisms. (1) After 1–2 weeks of daily drinking, *metabolic or pharmacokinetic tolerance* can be seen, with up to 30% increases in the rate of hepatic ethanol metabolism. This alteration disappears almost as rapidly as it develops. (2) *Cellular or pharmacodynamic tolerance* develops through neurochemical changes that maintain relatively normal physiologic functioning despite the presence of alcohol. Subsequent decreases in blood levels contribute to symptoms of withdrawal. (3) Individuals learn to adapt their behavior so that they can function better than expected under influence of the drug (*learned or behavioral tolerance*).

TABLE 467-1 EFFECTS OF BLOOD ALCOHOL LEVELS IN THE ABSENCE OF TOLERANCE

Blood Level, g/dL	Usual Effect
0.02	Decreased inhibitions, a slight feeling of intoxication
0.08	Decrease in complex cognitive functions and motor performance
0.20	Obvious slurred speech, motor incoordination, irritability, and poor judgment
0.30	Light coma and depressed vital signs
0.40	Death

The cellular changes caused by chronic ethanol exposure may not resolve for several weeks or longer following cessation of drinking. Rapid decreases in blood alcohol levels before that time can produce a withdrawal syndrome, which is most intense during the first 5 days, but some symptoms (e.g., disturbed sleep and anxiety) can take up to 4–6 months to resolve.

THE EFFECTS OF ETHANOL ON ORGAN SYSTEMS

Relatively low doses of alcohol (one or two drinks per day) have potential beneficial effects of increasing high-density lipoprotein cholesterol and decreasing aggregation of platelets, with a resulting decrease in risk for occlusive coronary disease and embolic strokes. Red wine has additional potential health-promoting qualities at relatively low doses due to flavinols and related substances. Modest drinking might also decrease the risk for vascular dementia and, possibly, Alzheimer's disease. However, any potential healthful effects disappear with the regular consumption of three or more drinks per day, and knowledge about the deleterious effects of alcohol can both help the physician to identify patients with an alcohol use disorder and to supply them with information that might help motivate a change in behavior.

NERVOUS SYSTEM

Approximately 35% of drinkers (and a much higher proportion of alcoholics) experience a *blackout*, an episode of temporary anterograde amnesia, in which the person forgets all or part of what occurred during a drinking evening. Another common problem, one seen after as few as one or two drinks shortly before bedtime, is disturbed sleep. Although alcohol might initially help a person fall asleep, it disrupts sleep throughout the rest of the night. The stages of sleep are altered, and time spent in rapid eye movement (REM) and deep sleep is reduced. Alcohol relaxes muscles in the pharynx, which can cause snoring and exacerbate sleep apnea; symptoms of the latter occur in 75% of alcoholic men older than age 60 years. Patients may also experience prominent and sometimes disturbing dreams later in the night. All of these sleep problems are more pronounced in alcoholics, and their persistence may contribute to relapse.

Another common consequence of alcohol use is impaired judgment and coordination, increasing the risk of injury. In the United States, ~40% of drinkers have at some time driven while intoxicated. Heavy drinking can also be associated with headache, thirst, nausea, vomiting, and fatigue the following day, a hangover syndrome that is responsible for much missed time and temporary cognitive deficits at work and school.

Chronic high doses cause *peripheral neuropathy* in ~10% of alcoholics: similar to diabetes, patients experience bilateral limb numbness, tingling, and paresthesias, all of which are more pronounced distally. Approximately 1% of alcoholics develop *cerebellar degeneration or atrophy*, producing a syndrome of progressive unsteady stance and gait often accompanied by mild nystagmus; neuroimaging studies reveal atrophy of the cerebellar vermis. Fortunately, very few alcoholics (perhaps as few as 1 in 500 for the full syndrome) develop *Wernicke's* (ophthalmoparesis, ataxia, and encephalopathy) and *Korsakoff's* (retrograde and anterograde amnesia) *syndromes*, although a higher proportion have one or more neuropathologic findings related to these conditions. These result from low levels of thiamine, especially in predisposed individuals with transketolase deficiencies. Alcoholics can manifest *cognitive problems* and temporary memory impairment lasting for weeks to months after drinking heavily for days or weeks. Brain atrophy, evident as ventricular enlargement and widened cortical sulci on magnetic resonance imaging (MRI) and computed tomography (CT) scans, occurs in ~50% of chronic alcoholics; these changes are usually reversible if abstinence is maintained. There is no single alcoholic dementia syndrome; rather, this label describes patients who have irreversible cognitive changes (possibly from diverse causes) in the context of chronic alcoholism.

Psychiatric Comorbidity As many as two-thirds of individuals with alcohol use disorders meet the criteria for another psychiatric syndrome in the fifth edition of the *Diagnostic and Statistical Manual of Mental Disorders* (DSM-5) of the American Psychiatric Association

(Chap. 466). Half of these relate to a preexisting antisocial personality manifesting as impulsivity and disinhibition that contribute to both alcohol and drug use disorders. The lifetime risk is 3% in males, and ≥80% of such individuals demonstrate alcohol- and/or drug-related conditions. Another common comorbidity occurs with problems regarding illicit substances. The remainder of alcoholics with psychiatric syndromes have preexisting conditions such as schizophrenia or manic-depressive disease and anxiety syndromes such as panic disorder. The comorbidities of alcoholism with independent psychiatric disorders might represent an overlap in genetic vulnerabilities, impaired judgment in the use of alcohol from the independent psychiatric condition, or an attempt to use alcohol to alleviate symptoms of the disorder or side effects of medications.

Many psychiatric syndromes can be seen *temporarily* during heavy drinking and subsequent withdrawal. These alcohol-induced conditions include an intense *sadness* lasting for days to weeks in the midst of heavy drinking seen in 40% of alcoholics, which tends to disappear over several weeks of abstinence (alcohol-induced mood disorder); temporary severe *anxiety* in 10–30% of alcoholics, often beginning during alcohol withdrawal, which can persist for a month or more after cessation of drinking (alcohol-induced anxiety disorder); and auditory *hallucinations* and/or paranoid delusions in a person who is alert and oriented, seen in 3–5% of alcoholics (*alcohol-induced psychotic disorder*).

Treatment of all forms of alcohol-induced psychopathology includes helping patients achieve abstinence and offering supportive care, as well as reassurance and "talk therapy" such as cognitive-behavioral approaches. However, with the exception of short-term antipsychotics or similar drugs for substance-induced psychoses, substance-induced psychiatric conditions only rarely require medications. Recovery is likely within several days to 4 weeks of abstinence. Conversely, because alcohol-induced conditions are temporary and do not indicate a need for long-term pharmacotherapy, a history of alcohol intake is an important part of the workup for any patient with one of these psychiatric symptoms.

THE GASTROINTESTINAL SYSTEM

Esophagus and Stomach Alcohol can cause inflammation of the esophagus and stomach causing epigastric distress and gastrointestinal bleeding, making alcohol one of the most common causes of hemorrhagic gastritis. Violent vomiting can produce severe bleeding through a Mallory-Weiss lesion, a longitudinal tear in the mucosa at the gastroesophageal junction.

Pancreas and Liver The incidence of acute pancreatitis (~25 per 1000 per year) is almost threefold higher in alcoholics than in the general population, accounting for an estimated 10% or more of the total cases. Alcohol impairs gluconeogenesis in the liver, resulting in a fall in the amount of glucose produced from glycogen, increased lactate production, and decreased oxidation of fatty acids. This contributes to an increase in fat accumulation in liver cells. In healthy individuals these changes are reversible, but with repeated exposure to ethanol, especially daily heavy drinking, more severe changes in the liver occur, including alcohol-induced hepatitis, perivenular sclerosis, and cirrhosis, with the latter observed in an estimated 15% of alcoholics (Chap. 363). Perhaps through an enhanced vulnerability to infections, alcoholics have an elevated rate of hepatitis C, and drinking in the context of that disease is associated with more severe liver deterioration.

CANCER

As few as 1.5 drinks per day increases a woman's risk of breast cancer 1.4-fold. For both genders, four drinks per day increases the risk for oral and esophageal cancers approximately threefold and rectal cancers by a factor of 1.5; seven to eight or more drinks per day produces an approximately fivefold increased risk for many cancers. These consequences may result directly from cancer-promoting effects of alcohol and acetaldehyde or indirectly by interfering with immune homeostasis.

HEMATOPOIETIC SYSTEM

Ethanol causes an increase in red blood cell size (mean corpuscular volume [MCV]), which reflects its effects on stem cells. If heavy drinking is accompanied by folic acid deficiency, there can also be hypersegmented neutrophils, reticulocytopenia, and a hyperplastic bone marrow; if malnutrition is present, sideroblastic changes can be observed. Chronic heavy drinking can decrease production of white blood cells, decrease granulocyte mobility and adherence, and impair delayed-hypersensitivity responses to novel antigens (with a possible false-negative tuberculin skin test). Associated immune deficiencies can contribute to vulnerability toward infections, including hepatitis and HIV, and interfere with their treatment. Finally, many alcoholics have mild thrombocytopenia, which usually resolves within a week of abstinence unless there is hepatic cirrhosis or congestive splenomegaly.

CARDIOVASCULAR SYSTEM

Acutely, ethanol decreases myocardial contractility and causes peripheral vasodilation, with a resulting mild decrease in blood pressure and a compensatory increase in cardiac output. Exercise-induced increases in cardiac oxygen consumption are higher after alcohol intake. These acute effects have little clinical significance for the average healthy drinker but can be problematic when persisting cardiac disease is present.

The consumption of three or more drinks per day results in a dose-dependent increase in blood pressure, which returns to normal within weeks of abstinence. Thus, heavy drinking is an important factor in mild to moderate hypertension. Chronic heavy drinkers also have a sixfold increased risk for coronary artery disease, related, in part, to increased low-density lipoprotein cholesterol, and carry an increased risk for cardiomyopathy through direct effects of alcohol on heart muscle. Symptoms of the latter include unexplained arrhythmias in the presence of left ventricular impairment, heart failure, hypocontractility of heart muscle, and dilation of all four heart chambers with associated mural thrombi and mitral valve regurgitation. Atrial or ventricular arrhythmias, especially paroxysmal tachycardia, can also occur temporarily after heavy drinking in individuals showing no other evidence of heart disease—a syndrome known as the "holiday heart."

GENITOURINARY SYSTEM CHANGES, SEXUAL FUNCTIONING, AND FETAL DEVELOPMENT

Drinking in adolescence can affect normal sexual development and reproductive onset. At any age, modest ethanol doses (e.g., blood alcohol concentrations of 0.06 g/dL) can increase sexual drive but also decrease erectile capacity in men. Even in the absence of liver impairment, a significant minority of chronic alcoholic men show irreversible testicular atrophy with shrinkage of the seminiferous tubules, decreases in ejaculate volume, and a lower sperm count (Chap. 411).

The repeated ingestion of high doses of ethanol by women can result in amenorrhea, a decrease in ovarian size, absence of corpora lutea with associated infertility, and an increased risk of spontaneous abortion. Heavy drinking during pregnancy results in the rapid placental transfer of both ethanol and acetaldehyde, which may contribute to a range of consequences known as fetal alcohol spectrum disorder (FASD). One severe result is the *fetal alcohol syndrome* (FAS), seen in ~5% of children born to heavy-drinking mothers, which can include any of the following: facial changes with epicanthal eye folds; poorly formed ear concha; small teeth with faulty enamel; cardiac atrial or ventricular septal defects; an aberrant palmar crease and limitation in joint movement; and microcephaly with mental retardation. Less pervasive FASD conditions include combinations of low birth weight, a lower intelligence quotient (IQ), hyperactive behavior, and some modest cognitive deficits. The amount of ethanol required and the time of vulnerability during pregnancy have not been defined, making it advisable for pregnant women to abstain completely.

OTHER EFFECTS

Between one-half and two-thirds of alcoholics have skeletal muscle weakness caused by acute *alcoholic myopathy*, a condition that improves but which might not fully remit with abstinence. Effects of repeated heavy drinking on the *skeletal system* include changes in calcium metabolism, lower bone density, and decreased growth in the epiphyses, leading to an increased risk for fractures and osteonecrosis of the femoral head. *Hormonal changes* include an increase in cortisol levels, which can remain elevated during heavy drinking; inhibition of vasopressin secretion at rising blood alcohol concentrations and enhanced secretion at falling blood alcohol concentrations (with the final result that most alcoholics are likely to be slightly overhydrated); a modest and reversible decrease in serum thyroxine (T_4); and a more marked decrease in serum triiodothyronine (T_3). Hormone irregularities should be reevaluated because they may disappear after a month of abstinence.

ALCOHOLISM (ALCOHOL USE DISORDER)

Because many drinkers occasionally imbibe to excess, temporary alcohol-related problems are common in nonalcoholics, especially in the late teens to the late twenties. However, repeated problems in multiple life areas can indicate an alcohol use disorder as defined in DSM-5.

DEFINITIONS AND EPIDEMIOLOGY

An *alcohol use disorder* is defined as repeated alcohol-related difficulties in at least 2 of 11 life areas that cluster together in the same 12-month period (Table 467-2). Ten of the 11 items were taken directly from the 7 dependence and 4 abuse criteria in DSM-IV, after deleting legal problems and adding craving. Severity of an alcohol use disorder is based on the number of items endorsed: mild is two or three items; moderate is four or five; and severe is six or more of the criterion items. The new diagnostic approach is similar enough to DSM-IV that the following descriptions of associated phenomena are still accurate.

The lifetime risk for an alcohol use disorder in most Western countries is about 10–15% for men and 5–8% for women. Rates are similar in the United States, Canada, Germany, Australia, and the United Kingdom, tend to be lower in most Mediterranean countries, such as Italy, Greece, and Israel, and may be higher in Ireland, France, and Scandinavia. An even higher lifetime prevalence has been reported for most native cultures, including American Indians, Eskimos, Maori groups, and aboriginal tribes of Australia. These differences reflect both cultural and genetic influences, as described below. In Western countries, the typical alcoholic is more often a blue- or white-collar worker or homemaker. The lifetime risk for alcoholism among physicians is similar to that of the general population.

GENETICS

Approximately 60% of the risk for alcohol use disorders is attributed to genes, as indicated by the fourfold higher risk in children of alcoholics (even if adopted early in life and raised by nonalcoholics) and a higher risk in identical twins compared to fraternal twins of alcoholics. The genetic variations operate primarily through intermediate characteristics that subsequently combine with environmental influences to alter the risk for heavy drinking and alcohol problems. These include genes relating to a high risk for all substance use disorders that operate through impulsivity, schizophrenia, and bipolar disorder. Another characteristic, an intense flushing response when drinking, decreases the risk for only alcohol use disorders through gene variations for several alcohol-metabolizing enzymes, especially aldehyde dehydrogenase (a mutation only seen in Asians), and to a lesser extent, variations in ADH.

An additional genetically influenced characteristic, a low sensitivity to alcohol, affects the risk for heavy drinking and may operate, in part, through variations in genes relating to calcium and potassium channels, GABA, nicotinic, and serotonin systems. A low response per drink is observed early in the drinking career and before alcohol use disorders develop. All follow-up studies have demonstrated that this need for higher doses of alcohol to achieve effects predicts future heavy drinking, alcohol problems, and alcohol use disorders. The impact of a low response to alcohol on adverse drinking outcomes is partially mediated by a range of environmental influences, including the selection of heavier-drinking friends, more positive expectations of the effects of high doses of alcohol, and suboptimal ways of coping with stress.

TABLE 467-2 *DIAGNOSTIC AND STATISTICAL MANUAL OF MENTAL DISORDERS*, FIFTH EDITION, CLASSIFICATION OF ALCOHOL USE DISORDER (AUD)

Criteria
Two or more of the following items occurring in the same 12-month period must be endorsed for the diagnosis of an alcohol use disorder[a]:
Drinking resulting in recurrent failure to fulfill role obligations
Recurrent drinking in hazardous situations
Continued drinking despite alcohol-related social or interpersonal problems
Tolerance
Withdrawal, or substance use for relief/avoidance of withdrawal
Drinking in larger amounts or for longer than intended
Persistent desire/unsuccessful attempts to stop or reduce drinking
Great deal of time spent obtaining, using, or recovering from alcohol
Important activities given up/reduced because of drinking
Continued drinking despite knowledge of physical or psychological problems caused by alcohol
Alcohol craving

[a]*Mild AUD*: 2–3 criteria required; *Moderate AUD*: 4–5 items endorsed; *severe AUD*: 6 or more items endorsed.

NATURAL HISTORY

Although the age of the first drink (~15 years) is similar in most alcoholics and nonalcoholics, a slightly earlier onset of regular drinking and drunkenness, especially in the context of conduct problems, is associated with a higher risk for later alcohol use disorders. By the mid-twenties, most nonalcoholic men and women moderate their drinking (perhaps learning from problems), whereas alcoholics are likely to escalate their patterns of drinking despite difficulties. The first major life problem from alcohol often appears in the late teens to early twenties, and a pattern of multiple alcohol difficulties by the midtwenties. Once established, the course of alcoholism is likely to include exacerbations and remissions, with little difficulty in temporarily stopping or controlling alcohol use when problems develop, but without help, desistance usually gives way to escalations in alcohol intake and subsequent problems. Following treatment, between half and two-thirds of alcoholics maintain abstinence for years, and often permanently. Even without formal treatment or self-help groups, there is at least a 20% chance of spontaneous remission with long-term abstinence. However, should the alcoholic continue to drink heavily, the life span is shortened by ~10 years on average, with the leading causes of death being heart disease, cancer, accidents, and suicide.

TREATMENT

The approach to treating alcohol-related conditions is relatively straightforward: (1) recognize that at least 20% of all patients have an alcohol use disorder; (2) learn how to identify and treat acute alcohol-related conditions; (3) know how to help patients begin to address their alcohol problems; and (4) know enough about treating alcoholism to appropriately refer patients for additional help.

IDENTIFICATION OF THE ALCOHOLIC

Even in affluent locales, ~20% of patients have an alcohol use disorder. These men and women can be identified by asking questions about *alcohol problems* and noting laboratory test results that can reflect regular consumption of six to eight or more drinks per day. The two blood tests with ≥60% sensitivity and specificity for heavy alcohol consumption are γ-glutamyl transferase (GGT) (>35 U) and carbohydrate-deficient transferrin (CDT) (>20 U/L or >2.6%); the combination of the two is likely to be more accurate than either alone. The values for these serologic markers are likely to return toward normal within several weeks of abstinence. Other useful blood tests include high-normal MCVs (≥91 μm³) and serum uric acid (>416 mol/L, or 7 mg/dL).

The diagnosis of an alcohol use disorder ultimately rests on the documentation of a pattern of repeated difficulties associated with alcohol (Table 467-2). Thus, in screening, it is important to probe for marital or job problems, legal difficulties, histories of accidents, medical problems, evidence of tolerance, and so on, and then attempt to tie in use

TABLE 467-3 THE ALCOHOL USE DISORDERS IDENTIFICATION TEST (AUDIT)[a]

Item	5-Point Scale (Least to Most)
1. How often do you have a drink containing alcohol?	Never (0) to 4+ per week (4)
2. How many drinks containing alcohol do you have on a typical day?	1 or 2 (0) to 10+ (4)
3. How often do you have six or more drinks on one occasion?	Never (0) to daily or almost daily (4)
4. How often during the last year have you found that you were not able to stop drinking once you had started?	Never (0) to daily or almost daily (4)
5. How often during the last year have you failed to do what was normally expected from you because of drinking?	Never (0) to daily or almost daily (4)
6. How often during the last year have you needed a first drink in the morning to get yourself going after a heavy drinking session?	Never (0) to daily or almost daily (4)
7. How often during the last year have you had a feeling of guilt or remorse after drinking?	Never (0) to daily or almost daily (4)
8. How often during the last year have you been unable to remember what happened the night before because you had been drinking?	Never (0) to daily or almost daily (4)
9. Have you or someone else been injured as a result of your drinking?	No (0) to yes, during the last year (4)
10. Has a relative, friend, doctor or other health worker been concerned about your drinking or suggested that you should cut down?	No (0) to yes, during the last year (4)

[a]The AUDIT is scored by simply summing the values associated with the endorsed response. A score ≥8 may indicate harmful alcohol use.

of alcohol or another substance. Some standardized questionnaires can be helpful, including the 10-item Alcohol Use Disorders Identification Test (AUDIT) (Table 467-3), but these are only screening tools, and a face-to-face interview is still required for a meaningful diagnosis.

TREATMENT ALCOHOL-RELATED CONDITIONS

ACUTE INTOXICATION

The first priority in treating severe intoxication is to assess vital signs and manage respiratory depression, cardiac arrhythmias, or blood pressure instability, if present. The possibility of intoxication with other drugs should be considered by obtaining toxicology screens for other central nervous system (CNS) depressants such as benzodiazepines and for opioids. Aggressive behavior should be handled by offering reassurance but also by considering a possible show of force with an intervention team. If the aggressive behavior continues, relatively low doses of a short-acting benzodiazepine such as lorazepam (e.g., 1–2 mg PO or IV) may be used and can be repeated as needed, but care must be taken not to destabilize vital signs or worsen confusion. An alternative approach is to use an antipsychotic medication (e.g., 0.5–5 mg of haloperidol PO or IM every 4–8 h as needed, or olanzapine 2.5–10 mg IM repeated at 2 and 6 h, if needed).

INTERVENTION

There are two main elements to intervention in a person with alcoholism: motivational interviewing and brief interventions. During motivational interviewing, the clinician helps the patient to think through the assets (e.g., comfort in social situations) and liabilities (e.g., health- and interpersonal-related problems) of the current pattern of drinking. The patient's responses are key, and the clinician should listen empathetically, helping to weigh options and encouraging the patient to take responsibility for needed changes. Patients should be reminded that only they can decide to avoid the consequences that will occur without changes in drinking. The process of brief intervention has been summarized by the acronym FRAMES: *F*eedback to the patient; *R*esponsibility to be taken by the patient; *A*dvice, rather than orders, on what needs to be done; *M*enus of options that might be considered; *E*mpathy for understanding the patient's thoughts and feelings; and *S*elf-efficacy, i.e., offering support for the capacity of the patient to make changes.

Once the patient begins to consider change, the emphasis shifts to brief interventions designed to help them understand more about potential actions. Discussions focus on consequences of high alcohol consumption, suggested approaches to stopping drinking, and help in recognizing and avoiding situations likely to lead to heavy drinking. Both motivational interviewing and brief interventions can be carried out in 15 min sessions, but because patients do not always change behavior immediately, multiple meetings are often required to explain the problem, discuss optimal treatments, and explain the benefits of abstinence.

ALCOHOL WITHDRAWAL

If the patient agrees to stop drinking, sudden decreases in alcohol intake can produce withdrawal symptoms, many of which are the opposite of those produced by intoxication. Features include tremor of the hands (shakes); agitation and anxiety; autonomic nervous system overactivity including an increase in pulse, respiratory rate, sweating, and body temperature; and insomnia. These symptoms usually begin within 5–10 h of decreasing ethanol intake, peak on day 2 or 3, and improve by day 4 or 5, although mild levels of these problems may persist for 4–6 months as a protracted abstinence syndrome.

About 2% of alcoholics experience a withdrawal seizure, with the risk increasing in the context of concomitant medical problems, misuse of additional drugs, and higher alcohol quantities. The same risk factors also contribute to a similar rate of *delirium tremens* (DTs), where the withdrawal includes delirium (mental confusion, agitation, and fluctuating levels of consciousness) associated with a tremor and autonomic overactivity (e.g., marked increases in pulse, blood pressure, and respirations). The risks for seizures and DTs can be diminished by identifying and treating any underlying medical conditions early in the course of withdrawal.

Thus, the first step is a thorough physical examination in all alcoholics considering abstinence, including a search for evidence of liver failure, gastrointestinal bleeding, cardiac arrhythmia, infection, and glucose or electrolyte imbalances. It is also important to offer adequate nutrition and oral multiple B vitamins, including 50–100 mg of thiamine daily for a week or more. Because most alcoholics who enter withdrawal are either normally hydrated or mildly overhydrated, IV fluids should be avoided unless there is a relevant medical problem or significant recent bleeding, vomiting, or diarrhea.

The next step is to recognize that because withdrawal symptoms reflect the rapid removal of a CNS depressant, alcohol, the symptoms can be controlled by administering any depressant in doses that decrease symptoms (e.g., a rapid pulse and tremor) and then tapering the dose over 3–5 days. Although most depressants are effective, benzodiazepines (Chap. 466) have the highest margin of safety and lowest cost and are, therefore, the preferred class of drugs. Short-half-life benzodiazepines can be considered for patients with serious liver impairment or evidence of significant brain damage, but they must be given every 4 h to avoid abrupt blood-level fluctuations that may increase the risk for seizures. Therefore, most clinicians use drugs with longer half-lives (e.g., chlordiazepoxide), adjusting the dose if signs of withdrawal escalate, and withholding the drug if the patient is sleeping or has orthostatic hypotension. The average patient requires 25–50 mg of chlordiazepoxide or 10 mg of diazepam given PO every 4–6 h on the first day, with doses then decreased to zero over the next 5 days. Although alcohol withdrawal can be treated in a hospital, patients in good physical condition who demonstrate mild signs of withdrawal despite low blood alcohol concentrations and who have no prior history of DTs or withdrawal seizures can be considered for outpatient detoxification. For the next

4 or 5 days, these patients should return daily for evaluation of vital signs and can be hospitalized if signs and symptoms of withdrawal escalate.

Treatment of patient with DTs can be challenging, and the condition is likely to run a course of 3–5 days regardless of the therapy used. The focus of care is to identify and correct medical problems and to control behavior and prevent injuries. Many clinicians recommend the use of high doses of a benzodiazepine (as much as 800 mg/d of chlordiazepoxide has been reported), a treatment that will decrease agitation and raise the seizure threshold but probably does little to improve the confusion. Other clinicians recommend the use of antipsychotic medications, such as haloperidol or olanzapine as discussed above, although these drugs have not been directly evaluated for DTs. Antipsychotics are less likely to exacerbate confusion but may increase the risk of seizures; they have no place in the treatment of mild withdrawal symptoms.

Generalized withdrawal seizures rarely require more than giving an adequate dose of benzodiazepines. There is little evidence that anticonvulsants such as phenytoin or gabapentin are more effective in drug-withdrawal seizures, and the risk of seizures has usually passed by the time effective drug levels are reached. The rare patient with status epilepticus must be treated aggressively (**Chap. 445**).

REHABILITATION OF ALCOHOLICS

An Overview After completing alcoholic rehabilitation, ≥60% of alcoholics, especially middle-class patients, maintain abstinence for at least a year, and many achieve lifetime sobriety. The core of treatment uses cognitive-behavioral approaches to help patients recognize the need to change, while working with them to alter their behaviors to enhance compliance. A key step is to optimize motivation toward abstinence through education about alcoholism and instructions to family members to stop protecting the patient from problems caused by alcohol. After years of heavy drinking, many patients also need counseling, some require vocational or avocational help to structure their days, and all should try self-help groups such as Alcoholics Anonymous (AA) to help them develop a sober peer group and learn how to deal with life's stresses while sober. A third component, *relapse prevention*, helps the patient identify situations in which a return to drinking is likely, formulate ways of managing these risks, and develop coping strategies that increase the chances of a return to abstinence if a slip occurs.

Although many can be treated as outpatients, more intense interventions are more effective, and some alcoholics do not respond to AA or outpatient groups. Whatever the setting, subsequent contact with outpatient treatment staff should be maintained for at least 6 months and preferably a year after abstinence. Counseling focuses on areas of improved functioning in the absence of alcohol (i.e., why it is a good idea to continue abstinence) and helping the patient to manage free time without alcohol, develop a nondrinking peer group, and handle stresses.

The physician serves an important role in identifying the alcoholic, diagnosing and treating associated medical and psychiatric syndromes, overseeing detoxification, referring the patient to rehabilitation programs, providing counseling, and, if appropriate, selecting which (if any) medication might be needed. For insomnia, patients should be reassured that troubled sleep is normal after alcohol withdrawal and will improve over subsequent weeks. They should be taught the elements of "sleep hygiene" including maintaining consistent schedules for bedtime and awakening. Sleep medications have the danger of being misused and of rebound insomnia when stopped. Sedating antidepressants (e.g., trazodone) should not be used because they interfere with cognitive functioning the next morning and disturb the normal sleep architecture, but occasional use of over-the-counter sleeping medications (sedating antihistamines) can be considered. Anxiety can be addressed by increasing the patient's insight into the temporary nature of the symptoms and helping the patient to develop strategies to achieve relaxation by using forms of cognitive therapy.

Medications for Rehabilitation Several medications have modest benefits when used for the first 6 months of recovery. The opioid antagonist, naltrexone, 50–150 mg/d orally, may shorten subsequent relapses, whether used in the oral form or as a once-per-month 380-mg injection, especially in individuals with the G allele of the AII8G polymorphism of the μ opioid receptor. By blocking opioid receptors, naltrexone decreases activity in the dopamine-rich ventral tegmental reward system and decreases the feeling of pleasure if alcohol is imbibed. A second medication, acamprosate (Campral) at ~2 g/d divided into three oral doses, has similar modest effects; acamprosate inhibits NMDA receptors, decreasing mild symptoms of protracted withdrawal. Several trials of combined naltrexone and acamprosate have reported that the combination may be superior to either drug alone, although not all studies agree.

It is more difficult to establish the asset-to-liability ratio of a third drug, disulfiram, an ALDH inhibitor, used at doses of 250 mg/d. This drug produces vomiting and autonomic nervous system instability in the presence of alcohol as a result of rapidly rising blood levels of acetaldehyde. This reaction can be dangerous, especially for patients with heart disease, stroke, diabetes mellitus, or hypertension. The drug itself carries potential risks of depression, psychotic symptoms, peripheral neuropathy, and liver damage. Disulfiram is best given under supervision by someone (such as a spouse), especially during high-risk drinking situations (such as the Christmas holiday). Other drugs under investigation include another opioid antagonist nalmefene, the nicotinic receptor agonist varenicline, the serotonin antagonist ondansetron, the α-adrenergic agonist prazosin, the $GABA_B$ receptor agonist baclofen, the anticonvulsant topiramate, and cannabinol receptor antagonists. At present, there are insufficient data to determine the asset-to-liability ratio for these medications in treating alcoholism and, therefore, no data to offer solid support for their use in routine clinical settings.

GLOBAL CONSIDERATIONS

As described above, rates of alcohol use disorders differ across sex, age, ethnicity, and country. There are also differences across countries regarding the definition of a standard drink (e.g., 10–12 g of ethanol in the United States and 8 g in the United Kingdom) and the definition of being legally drunk. The preferred alcoholic beverage also varies across groups, even within countries. That said, regardless of sex, ethnicity, or country, the actual drug in the drink is still ethanol, and the risks for problems, course of alcohol use disorders, and approaches to treatment are similar across the world.

468e Opioid-Related Disorders

Thomas R. Kosten, Colin N. Haile

This is a digital-only chapter. It is available on the DVD that accompanies this book, as well as on Access Medicine/Harrison's Online, and the eBook and "app" editions of HPIM 19e.

Opiate analgesics have been abused since at least 300 B.C. Nepenthe (Greek "free from sorrow") helped the hero of the *Odyssey*, but widespread opium smoking in China and the Near East has caused harm for centuries. Since the first chemical isolation of opium and codeine 200 years ago, a wide range of synthetic opioids have been developed, and opioid receptors were cloned in the 1990s. Two of the most important adverse effects of all these agents are the development of opioid use disorder and overdose. The 0.1% annual prevalence of heroin dependence in the United States is only about one-third the rate of prescription opiate use and is substantially lower than the 2% rate of morphine users in Southeast and Southwest Asia.

Prescription opiates are primarily used for pain management, but due to ease of availability, adolescents procure and use these drugs with dire consequences. In 2011, for example, 11 million individuals in the United States used nonmedically prescribed pain killers that were linked to over 420,000 emergency department visits and nearly 17,000 overdose deaths. Although these rates are low relative to other abused substances, their disease burden is substantial, with high rates of morbidity and mortality; disease transmission; increased health care, crime, and law enforcement costs; and less tangible costs of family distress and lost productivity.

469e Cocaine and Other Commonly Abused Drugs

Nancy K. Mello[1], Jack H. Mendelson[1]

This is a digital-only chapter. It is available on the DVD that accompanies this book, as well as on Access Medicine/Harrison's Online, and the eBook and "app" editions of HPIM 19e.

The abuse of cocaine and other psychostimulants reflects a complex interaction between the pharmacology of the drug, the personality and expectations of the user, and the environmental context in which the drug is used. Polydrug abuse involving the concurrent use of several drugs with different pharmacologic effects is increasingly common. Sometimes one drug is used to enhance the effects of another, as with the combined use of cocaine and nicotine, benzodiazepines and methadone, or cocaine and heroin in methadone-maintained patients. Some forms of polydrug abuse, such as the combined use of IV heroin and cocaine, are especially dangerous and account for many hospital emergency room visits.

470 Nicotine Addiction

David M. Burns

The use of tobacco leaf to create and satisfy nicotine addiction was introduced to Columbus by Native Americans and spread rapidly to Europe. Use of tobacco as cigarettes, however, only became popular in the twentieth century and so is a modern phenomenon, as is the epidemic of disease caused by this form of tobacco use.

Nicotine is the principal constituent of tobacco responsible for its addictive character, but other smoke constituents and behavioral associations contribute to the strength of the addiction. Addicted smokers regulate their nicotine intake by adjusting the frequency and intensity of their tobacco use both to obtain the desired psychoactive effects and avoid withdrawal.

Unburned cured tobacco used orally contains nicotine, carcinogens, and other toxicants capable of causing gum disease, oral and pancreatic cancers, and an increase in the risk of heart disease. When tobacco is burned, the resultant smoke contains, in addition to nicotine, more than 7000 other compounds that result from volatilization, pyrolysis, and pyrosynthesis of tobacco and various chemical additives used in making different tobacco products. The smoke is composed of a fine aerosol and a vapor phase; aerosolized particles are of a size range that results in deposition in the airways and alveolar surfaces of the lungs.

[1]Deceased

The aggregate of particulate matter, after subtracting nicotine and moisture, is referred to as tar.

The alkaline pH of smoke from blends of tobacco used for pipes and cigars allows sufficient absorption of nicotine across the oral mucosa to satisfy the smoker's need for this drug. Therefore, smokers of pipes and cigars tend not to inhale the smoke into the lung, confining the toxic and carcinogenic exposure (and the increased rates of disease) largely to the upper airway for most users of these products. The acidic pH of smoke generated by the tobacco used in cigarettes dramatically reduces absorption of nicotine in the mouth, necessitating inhalation of the smoke into the larger surface of the lungs in order to absorb quantities of nicotine sufficient to satisfy the smoker's addiction. The shift to using tobacco as cigarettes, with resultant increased deposition of smoke in the lung, has created the epidemic of heart disease, lung disease, and lung cancer that dominates the current disease manifestations of tobacco use.

Several genes have been associated with nicotine addiction. Some reduce the clearance of nicotine, and others have been associated with an increased likelihood of becoming dependent on tobacco and other drugs as well as a higher incidence of depression. Rates of smoking cessation have increased, and rates of nicotine addiction have decreased dramatically, since the mid-1950s, suggesting that factors other than genetics are important. It is likely that genetic susceptibility can influence the probability that adolescent experimentation with tobacco will lead to addiction as an adult.

Adult cigarette smoking prevalence has declined to about 19% in the United States, with 20–40% of those smokers not smoking every day. Male smoking prevalence is falling but remains high in most Asian countries, with increasing smoking prevalence among women in those countries. The highest rates of smoking and least cessation are observed in eastern European countries. Of particular concern is the rapidly rising smoking rate observed in the developing world. The World Health Organization Framework Convention on Tobacco Control is encouraging effective tobacco control approaches in these countries with the hope of preventing a future epidemic of tobacco-related illness.

DISEASE MANIFESTATIONS OF CIGARETTE SMOKING

More than 400,000 individuals die prematurely each year in the United States from cigarette use; this represents almost one of every five deaths in the United States. Approximately 40% of cigarette smokers will die prematurely due to cigarette smoking unless they are able to quit.

The major diseases caused by cigarette smoking are listed in Table 470-1. The ratio of smoking-related disease rates in smokers compared to never smokers (relative risk) is greater at younger ages, particularly for coronary artery disease and stroke. At older ages, the background rate of disease in nonsmokers increases, diminishing the fractional contribution of smoking and the relative risk; however, absolute excess rates of disease mortality found in smokers compared to nonsmokers increase with increasing age. The organ damage caused by smoking and the number of smokers who die from smoking are both greater among the elderly, as one would expect from a process of cumulative injury.

CARDIOVASCULAR DISEASES

Cigarette smokers are more likely than nonsmokers to develop both large-vessel atherosclerosis and small-vessel disease. Approximately 90% of peripheral vascular disease in the nondiabetic population can be attributed to cigarette smoking, as can ~50% of aortic aneurysms. In contrast, 20–30% of coronary artery disease and ~10% of ischemic and hemorrhagic strokes are caused by cigarette smoking. There is a multiplicative interaction between cigarette smoking and other cardiac risk factors such that the increment in risk produced by smoking among individuals with hypertension or elevated serum lipids is substantially greater than the increment in risk produced by smoking for individuals without these risk factors.

In addition to its role in promoting atherosclerosis, cigarette smoking also increases the likelihood of myocardial infarction and sudden cardiac death by promoting platelet aggregation and vascular occlusion. Reversal of these effects on coagulation may explain the rapid

TABLE 470-1 RELATIVE RISKS FOR CURRENT SMOKERS OF CIGARETTES

	Current Smokers	
Disease or Condition	Males	Females
Coronary heart disease		
Age 35–64	2.8	3.1
Age ≥65	1.5	1.6
Cerebrovascular disease		
Age 35–64	3.3	4
Age ≥65	1.6	1.5
Aortic aneurysm	6.2	7.1
Chronic airway obstruction	10.6	13.1
Cancer		
Lung	23.3	12.7
Larynx	14.6	13
Lip, oral cavity, pharynx	10.9	5.1
Esophagus	6.8	7.8
Bladder, other urinary organs	3.3	2.2
Kidney	2.7	1.3
Pancreas	2.3	2.3
Stomach	2	1.4
Liver	1.7	1.7
Colorectal	1.2	1.2
Cervix		1.6
Acute myeloid leukemia	1.4	1.4
Sudden infant death syndrome		2.3
Infant respiratory distress syndrome		1.3
Low birth weight at delivery		1.8

benefit of smoking cessation for a new coronary event demonstrable among those who have survived a first myocardial infarction. This effect may also explain the substantially higher rates of graft occlusion among continuing smokers following vascular bypass surgery for cardiac or peripheral vascular disease.

Cessation of cigarette smoking reduces the risk of a second coronary event within 6–12 months; rates of first myocardial infarction and death from coronary heart disease also decline within the first few years following cessation among those with no prior cardiovascular history. After 15 years of abstinence, the risk of a new myocardial infarction or death from coronary heart disease in former smokers is similar to that for those who have never smoked.

CANCER

Tobacco smoking causes cancer of the lung; oral cavity; naso-, oro-, and hypopharynx; nasal cavity and paranasal sinuses; larynx; esophagus; stomach; pancreas; liver (hepatocellular); colon and rectum; kidney (body and pelvis); ureter; urinary bladder; and uterine cervix, and also causes myeloid leukemia. There is evidence suggesting that cigarette smoking may play a role in increasing the risk of breast cancer. There does not appear to be a causal link between cigarette smoking and cancer of the endometrium, and there is a lower risk of uterine cancer among postmenopausal women who smoke. The risks of cancer increase with the increasing number of cigarettes smoked per day and with increasing duration of smoking. Additionally, there are synergistic interactions between cigarette smoking and alcohol use for cancer of the oral cavity and esophagus. Several occupational exposures synergistically increase lung cancer risk among cigarette smokers, most notably occupational asbestos and radon exposure.

Cessation of cigarette smoking reduces the risk of developing cancer relative to continuing smoking, but even 20 years after cessation, there is a modest persistent increased risk of developing lung cancer.

RESPIRATORY DISEASE

Cigarette smoking is responsible for 90% of chronic obstructive pulmonary disease. Within 1–2 years of beginning to smoke regularly, many young smokers will develop inflammatory changes in their small airways, although lung function measures of these changes do not predict development of chronic airflow obstruction. After 20 years of smoking, pathophysiologic changes in the lungs develop and progress proportional to smoking intensity and duration. Chronic mucous hyperplasia of the larger airways results in a chronic productive cough in as many as 80% of smokers >60 years of age. Chronic inflammation and narrowing of the small airways and/or enzymatic digestion of alveolar walls resulting in pulmonary emphysema can result in reduced expiratory airflow sufficient to produce clinical symptoms of respiratory limitation in ~15–25% of smokers.

Changes in the small airways of young smokers will reverse after 1–2 years of cessation. There may also be a small increase in measures of expiratory airflow following cessation among individuals who have developed chronic airflow obstruction, but the major change following cessation is a slowing of the rate of decline in lung function with advancing age rather than a return of lung function toward normal.

PREGNANCY

Cigarette smoking is associated with several maternal complications of pregnancy: premature rupture of membranes, abruptio placentae, and placenta previa; there is also a small increase in the risk of spontaneous abortion among smokers. Infants of smoking mothers are more likely to experience preterm delivery, have a higher perinatal mortality rate, be small for their gestational age, and have higher rates of infant respiratory distress syndrome; they are more likely to die of sudden infant death syndrome and appear to have a developmental lag for at least the first several years of life.

OTHER CONDITIONS

Smoking delays healing of peptic ulcers; increases the risk of developing diabetes, active tuberculosis, rheumatoid arthritis, osteoporosis, senile cataracts, and neovascular and atrophic forms of macular degeneration; and results in premature menopause, wrinkling of the skin, gallstones and cholecystitis in women, and male impotence.

ENVIRONMENTAL TOBACCO SMOKE

Long-term exposure to environmental tobacco smoke increases the risk of lung cancer and coronary artery disease among nonsmokers. It also increases the incidence of respiratory infections, chronic otitis media, and asthma in children and causes exacerbation of asthma in children. Some evidence suggests that environmental tobacco smoke exposure may increase the risk of premenopausal breast cancer. Patients who continue to smoke during treatment for cancer with chemotherapy or radiation have poorer outcomes and reduced survival.

PHARMACOLOGIC INTERACTIONS

Cigarette smoking may interact with a variety of other drugs (Table 470-2). Cigarette smoking induces the cytochrome P450 system, which may alter the metabolic clearance of drugs such as theophylline. This may result in inadequate serum levels in smokers as outpatients when the dosage is established in the hospital under nonsmoking conditions. Correspondingly, serum levels may rise when smokers are hospitalized and not allowed to smoke. Smokers may also have higher first-pass clearance for drugs such as lidocaine, and the stimulant effects of nicotine may reduce the effect of benzodiazepines or beta blockers.

OTHER FORMS OF TOBACCO USE

Other major forms of tobacco use are moist snuff deposited between the cheek and gum, chewing tobacco, pipes and cigars, and recently bidi (tobacco wrapped in tendu or temburni leaf; commonly used in India), clove cigarettes, and water pipes. Oral tobacco use leads to gum disease and can result in oral and pancreatic cancer as well as heart disease, with dramatic differences in the risks evident for products used in Africa and Asia as compared to those in the United States and Europe.

TABLE 470-2 INTERACTIONS OF SMOKING AND PRESCRIPTION DRUGS

Drug	Interaction
Amitriptyline	Increased clearance
Benzodiazepines	Less sedation
Beta blockers	Reduced lowering of heart rate and blood pressure
Caffeine	Faster metabolic clearance
Chlorpromazine	Decreased serum concentrations[a]
Clomipramine	Decreased serum concentrations[a]
Clozapine	Decreased serum concentrations[a]
Dextropropoxyphene	Less analgesia
Estrogens (oral)	Increased hepatic clearance
Flecainide	Increased first-pass clearance
Fluphenazine	Decreased serum concentrations[a]
Fluvoxamine	Decreased serum concentrations[a]
Haloperidol	Decreased serum concentrations[a]
Heparin	Faster clearance
Imipramine	Decreased serum concentrations[a]
Insulin	Delayed absorption due to skin vasoconstriction
Lidocaine	Increased first-pass clearance
Mexiletine	Increased first-pass clearance
Naratriptan	Increased clearance
Olanzapine	Faster clearance
Pentazocine	Less analgesia, possible increased clearance
Propranolol	Increased first-pass clearance
Propoxyphene	Increased hepatic metabolism
Rivastigmine	Increased clearance
Tacrine	Increased clearance
Tacrine	Faster metabolic clearance
Theophylline	Faster metabolic clearance
Thiothixene	Faster metabolic clearance
Trazodone	Decreased serum concentrations[a]
Verapamil	Increased clearance

[a]Clinical implications uncertain.

All forms of burned tobacco generate toxic and carcinogenic smoke similar to that of cigarette smoke. The differences in disease consequences of use relate to frequency of use and depth of inhalation. The risk of upper airway cancers is similar among cigarette, pipe, and cigar smokers, whereas those who have smoked only pipes and cigars have a much lower risk of lung cancer, heart disease, and chronic obstructive pulmonary disease. However, cigarette smokers who switch to pipes or cigars do tend to inhale the smoke, increasing their risk; and it is likely that comparable inhalation and frequency of exposure to tobacco smoke from any of these forms of tobacco use will lead to comparable disease outcomes.

A resurgence of cigar, bidi, and water pipe use among adolescents of both genders has raised concerns that these older forms of tobacco use are once again causing a public health problem. A variety of devices are currently sold that deliver nicotine by electronically heating materials containing nicotine, the so-called electronic cigarettes. Although these devices are marketed as substitutes for cigarettes and as cessation tools, the composition of the vapor and nicotine delivery varies widely from product to product, raising questions of both safety and efficacy in the absence of regulatory oversight.

LOWER TAR AND NICOTINE CIGARETTES

Filtered cigarettes with lower machine-measured yields of tar and nicotine commonly use ventilation holes in the filters and other engineering designs to artificially lower the machine measurements. Smokers compensate for the lowered nicotine delivery by changing the manner in which they puff on the cigarette or the number of cigarettes smoked per day, and tar and nicotine deliveries are not reduced with use of these products. Cigarette design changes that reduce machine-measured tar and nicotine lead to deeper inhalation of the smoke and an increase in the carcinogenicity of the smoke inhaled by smokers. The presentation of more carcinogenic smoke to the alveolar portions of the lung has resulted in an increase in the risk of lung cancer, and possibly chronic obstructive pulmonary disease, among smokers over the past six decades. This change in cigarette product is also one cause of the dramatic rise in rates of adenocarcinoma of the lung observed over the past half century. There has been no increase in risk of lung cancer or adenocarcinoma of the lung in never smokers over time.

CESSATION

The process of stopping smoking is commonly a cyclical one, with the smoker sometimes making multiple attempts to quit and failing before finally being successful. Approximately 70–80% of smokers would like to quit smoking. More than one-half of current smokers attempted to quit in the last year, but only 6% quit for 6 months, and only 3% remain abstinent for 2 years. Clinician-based smoking interventions should repeatedly encourage smokers to try to quit and to use different forms of cessation assistance with each new cessation attempt rather than focusing exclusively on immediate cessation at the time of the first visit.

Advice from a physician to quit smoking, particularly at the time of an acute illness, is a powerful trigger for cessation attempts, with up to half of patients who are advised to quit making a cessation effort. Other triggers include the cost of cigarettes, media campaigns, and changes in rules to restrict smoking in the workplace.

PHYSICIAN INTERVENTION (TABLE 470-3)

All patients should be asked whether they smoke, how much they smoke, how long they have smoked, their past experience with quitting, and whether they are currently interested in quitting. Intensity of smoking and smoking within 30 min of waking are useful measures of the intensity of nicotine addiction. Even those who are not interested in quitting should be encouraged and motivated to quit; provided a clear, strong, and personalized message by the clinician that smoking

TABLE 470-3 CLINICAL PRACTICE GUIDELINES

Physician Actions
Ask: Systematically identify all tobacco users at every visit
Advise: Strongly urge all smokers to quit
Identify smokers willing to quit
Assist the patient in quitting
Arrange follow-up contact
Effective Pharmacologic Interventions[a]
First-line therapies
Nicotine gum (1.5)
Nicotine patch (1.9)
Nicotine nasal inhaler (2.7)
Nicotine oral inhaler (2.5)
Nicotine lozenge (2.0)
Bupropion (2.1)
Varenicline (2.7)
Second-line therapies
Clonidine (2.1)
Nortriptyline (3.2)
Other Effective Interventions[a]
Physician or other medical personnel counseling (10 min) (1.3)
Intensive smoking cessation programs (at least 4–7 sessions of 20- to 30-min duration lasting at least 2 and preferably 8 weeks) (2.3)
Clinic-based smoking status identification system (3.1)
Counseling by nonclinicians and social support by family and friends
Telephone counseling (1.2)

[a]Numerical value following the intervention is the multiple for cessation success compared to no intervention.

is an important health concern; and offered assistance if they become interested in quitting in the future. Many of those not currently expressing an interest in quitting may nevertheless make an attempt to quit in the subsequent year. For those interested in quitting, a quit date should be negotiated, usually not the day of the visit but within the next few weeks, and a follow-up contact by office staff around the time of the quit date should be provided. There is a relationship between the amount of assistance a patient is willing to accept and the success of the cessation attempt.

There are a variety of nicotine-replacement products, including over-the-counter nicotine patches, gum, and lozenges, as well as nicotine nasal and oral inhalers available by prescription. These products can be used for up to 3–6 months, and some products are formulated to allow a gradual step-down in dosage with increasing duration of abstinence. Antidepressants such as bupropion (300 mg in divided doses for up to 6 months) have also been shown to be effective, as has varenicline, a partial agonist for the nicotinic acetylcholine receptor (initial dose 0.5 mg daily increasing to 1 mg twice daily at day 8; treatment duration up to 6 months). Severe psychiatric symptoms, including suicidal ideation, have been reported with varenicline, resulting in a U.S. Food and Drug Administration–mandated warning and a recommendation for closer therapeutic supervision, but evidence to establish the frequency of these responses and the specificity of their association with varenicline remains unclear. Some evidence supports the combined use of nicotine-replacement therapy (NRT) and antidepressants as well as the use of gum or lozenges for acute cravings in patients using patches. Pretreatment with antidepressants or varenicline is recommended for 1–2 weeks prior to the quit date, and pretreatment with nicotine-replacement products is also being explored, as is longer duration of nicotine replacement as a maintenance therapy for those who are unsuccessful in quitting with a shorter duration of use. NRT is provided in different dosages, with higher doses being recommended for more intense smokers. Clonidine or nortriptyline may be useful for patients who have failed on first-line pharmacologic treatment or who are unable to use other therapies. Antidepressants are more effective in those with a history of depression symptoms.

Current recommendations are to offer pharmacologic treatment, usually with NRT or varenicline, to all who will accept it and to provide counseling and other support as a part of the cessation attempt. There are some data to suggest that longer term use of NRT may enable cessation in some smokers who are unable to quit with shorter duration use and that some individuals are able to achieve abstinence from tobacco through use of NRT chronically. Cessation advice alone by a physician or his or her staff is likely to increase success compared with no intervention; a more comprehensive approach with advice, pharmacologic assistance, and counseling can increase cessation success nearly threefold.

Incorporation of cessation assistance into a practice requires a change of the care delivery infrastructure. Simple changes include (1) adding questions about smoking and interest in cessation on patient-intake questionnaires, (2) asking patients whether they smoke as part of the initial vital sign measurements made by office staff, (3) listing smoking as a problem in the medical record, and (4) automating follow-up contact with the patient on the quit date. These changes are essential to institutionalizing smoking intervention within the practice setting; without this institutionalization, the best intentions of physicians to intervene with their patients who smoke are often lost in the time crush of a busy practice.

PREVENTION

Approximately 85% of individuals who become cigarette smokers initiate the behavior during adolescence. Factors that promote adolescent initiation are parental or older-sibling cigarette smoking, tobacco advertising and promotional activities, the availability of cigarettes, and the social acceptability of smoking. The need for an enhanced self-image and to imitate adult behavior is greatest for those adolescents who have the least external validation of their self-worth, which may explain in part the enormous differences in adolescent smoking prevalence by socioeconomic and school performance strata.

Prevention of smoking initiation must begin early, preferably in the elementary school years. Physicians who treat adolescents should be sensitive to the prevalence of this problem even in the pre-teen population. Physicians should ask all adolescents whether they have experimented with tobacco or currently use tobacco, reinforce the fact that most adolescents and adults do not smoke, and explain that all forms of tobacco are both addictive and harmful.

471e Neuropsychiatric Illnesses in War Veterans

Charles W. Hoge

This is a digital-only chapter. It is available on the DVD that accompanies this book, as well as on Access Medicine/Harrison's Online, and the eBook and "app" editions of HPIM 19e.

Neuropsychiatric sequelae are common in combat veterans. Advances in personal protective body armor, armored vehicles, battlefield resuscitation, and the speed of evacuation to tertiary care have considerably improved the survivability of battlefield injuries, resulting in a greater awareness of the "silent wounds" associated with service in a combat zone. Although psychiatric and neurologic problems have been well documented in veterans of prior wars, the conflicts in Iraq and Afghanistan that began after September 11, 2001, were unique in terms of the level of commitment by the U.S. Department of Defense (DoD) and Department of Veterans Affairs (VA), Veterans Health Administration (VHA) to support research as the wars unfolded and to use that knowledge to guide population-level screening, evaluation, and treatment initiatives.

The Iraq and Afghanistan conflicts produced over 2.5 million combat veterans, many of whom have received or will need care in government and civilian medical facilities in the future. Studies clearly showed that service in the Iraq and Afghanistan theaters was associated with significantly elevated rates of mental disorders. Two conditions in particular have been labeled the signature injuries related to these wars: posttraumatic stress disorder (PTSD) and mild traumatic brain injury (mTBI)—also known as concussion. Although particular emphasis will be given in this chapter to PTSD and concussion/mTBI, it is important to understand that the neuropsychiatric sequelae of war are much broader than these two conditions. Wartime service is associated with a number of health concerns that coexist and overlap, and a multidisciplinary patient-centered approach to care is necessary.

472e Heavy Metal Poisoning

Howard Hu

This is a digital-only chapter. It is available on the DVD that accompanies this book, as well as on Access Medicine/Harrison's Online, and the eBook and "app" editions of HPIM 19e.

Metals pose a significant threat to health through low-level environmental as well as occupational exposures. One indication of their importance relative to other potential hazards is their ranking by the U.S. Agency for Toxic Substances and Disease Registry, which maintains an updated list of all hazards present in toxic waste sites according to their prevalence and the severity of their toxicity. The first, second, third, and seventh hazards on the list are heavy metals: lead, mercury, arsenic, and cadmium, respectively (*http://www.atsdr.cdc.gov/spl/*).

Metals are inhaled primarily as dusts and fumes (the latter defined as tiny particles generated by combustion). Metal poisoning can also result from exposure to vapors (e.g., mercury vapor in creating dental amalgams). When metals are ingested in contaminated food or drink or by hand-to-mouth activity (implicated especially in children), their gastrointestinal absorption varies greatly with the specific chemical form of the metal and the nutritional status of the host. Once a metal is absorbed, blood is the main medium for its transport, with the precise kinetics dependent on diffusibility, protein binding, rates of biotransformation, availability of intracellular ligands, and other factors. Some organs (e.g., bone, liver, and kidney) sequester metals in relatively high concentrations for years. Most metals are excreted through renal clearance and gastrointestinal excretion; some proportion is also excreted through salivation, perspiration, exhalation, lactation, skin exfoliation, and loss of hair and nails. The intrinsic stability of metals facilitates tracing and measurement in biologic material, although the clinical significance of the levels measured is not always clear.

473e Poisoning and Drug Overdose

Mark B. Mycyk

This is a digital-only chapter. It is available on the DVD that accompanies this book, as well as on Access Medicine/Harrison's Online, and the eBook and "app" editions of HPIM 19e.

Poisoning refers to the development of dose-related adverse effects following exposure to chemicals, drugs, or other xenobiotics. To paraphrase Paracelsus, the dose makes the poison. In excessive amounts, substances that are usually innocuous, such as oxygen and water, can cause toxicity. Conversely, in small doses, substances commonly regarded as poisons, such as arsenic and cyanide, can be consumed without ill effect. Although most poisons have predictable dose-related effects, individual responses to a given dose may vary because of genetic polymorphism, enzymatic induction or inhibition in the presence of other xenobiotics, or acquired tolerance. Poisoning may be local (e.g., skin, eyes, or lungs) or systemic depending on the route of exposure, the chemical and physical properties of the poison, and its mechanism of action. The severity and reversibility of poisoning also depend on the functional reserve of the individual or target organ, which is influenced by age and preexisting disease.

474 Disorders Caused by Venomous Snakebites and Marine Animal Exposures

Charles Lei, Natalie J. Badowski, Paul S. Auerbach, Robert L. Norris

This chapter outlines general principles for the evaluation and management of victims of envenomation and poisoning by venomous snakes and marine animals. Because the incidence of serious bites and stings is relatively low in developed nations, there is a paucity of relevant clinical research; as a result, therapeutic decision making often is based on anecdotal information.

VENOMOUS SNAKEBITE

EPIDEMIOLOGY

The venomous snakes of the world belong to the families Viperidae (subfamily Viperinae: Old World vipers; subfamily Crotalinae: New World and Asian pit vipers), Elapidae (including cobras, coral snakes, sea snakes, kraits, and all Australian venomous snakes), Lamprophiidae (subfamily Atractaspidinae: burrowing asps), and Colubridae (a large family in which most species are nonvenomous and only a few are dangerously toxic to humans). Most snakebites occur in developing countries with temperate and tropical climates in which populations subsist on agriculture and fishing. Recent estimates indicate that somewhere between 1.2 million and 5.5 million snakebites occur worldwide each year, with 421,000–1,841,000 envenomations and 20,000–94,000 deaths. Such wide-ranging estimates reflect the challenges of collecting accurate data in the regions most affected by venomous snakes; many victims do not seek hospital treatment, and reporting and record keeping are generally poor.

SNAKE ANATOMY/IDENTIFICATION

The typical snake venom delivery apparatus consists of bilateral venom glands situated below and behind the eyes and connected by ducts to hollow anterior maxillary fangs. In viperids (vipers and pit vipers), these fangs are long and highly mobile; they are retracted against the roof of the mouth when the snake is at rest and brought to an upright position for a strike. In elapids, the fangs are smaller and are relatively fixed in an erect position. Approximately 20% of pit viper bites and higher percentages of other snakebites (up to 75% for sea snakes) are "dry" bites, meaning no venom is released. Significant envenomation probably occurs in ~50% of all venomous snakebites.

Differentiation of venomous from nonvenomous snake species can be difficult. Viperids are characterized by somewhat triangular heads (a feature shared with many harmless snakes), elliptical pupils (also seen in some nonvenomous snakes, such as boas and pythons), enlarged maxillary fangs, and, in pit vipers, heat-sensing pits (foveal organs) on each side of the head that assist with locating prey and aiming strikes. The New World rattlesnakes possess a series of interlocking keratin plates (the rattle) on the tip of the tail that emits a buzzing sound when the snake rapidly vibrates its tail; this sound serves as a warning signal to perceived threats. Identifying venomous snakes by color pattern is notoriously misleading, as many harmless snakes have color patterns that closely mimic those of venomous snakes found in the same region.

VENOMS AND CLINICAL MANIFESTATIONS

Snake venoms are highly variable and complex mixtures of enzymes, low-molecular-weight polypeptides, glycoproteins, and other constituents. Among the deleterious components are hemorrhagins that promote vascular leakage and cause both local and systemic bleeding.

Proteolytic enzymes cause local tissue necrosis, affect the coagulation pathway at various steps, and impair organ function. Hyaluronidases promote the spread of venom through connective tissue. Myocardial depressant factors reduce cardiac output, and bradykinins cause vasodilation and hypotension. Neurotoxins act either pre- or postsynaptically to block transmission at the neuromuscular junction, causing muscle paralysis. Most snake venoms have multisystem effects on their victims.

After a venomous snakebite, the time to symptom onset and clinical presentation can be quite variable and depend on the species involved, the anatomic location of the bite, and the amount of venom injected. Envenomations by most viperids and some elapids with necrotizing venoms cause progressive local pain, swelling, ecchymosis (Fig. 474-1), and (over a period of hours to days) hemorrhagic or serum-filled vesicles and bullae. In serious bites, tissue loss can be significant (Figs. 474-2 and 474-3). Systemic findings are extremely variable and can include tachycardia or bradycardia, hypotension, generalized weakness, changes in taste, mouth numbness, muscle fasciculations, pulmonary edema, renal dysfunction, and spontaneous hemorrhage (from essentially any anatomic site). Envenomations by neurotoxic elapids such as kraits (*Bungarus* species), many Australian elapids (e.g., death adders [*Acanthophis* species] and tiger snakes [*Notechis* species]), some cobras (*Naja* species), and some viperids (e.g., the South American rattlesnake [*Crotalus durissus*] and some Indian Russell's vipers [*Daboia russelii*]) cause neurologic dysfunction. Early findings may consist of nausea and vomiting, headache, paresthesias or numbness, and altered mental status. Victims may develop cranial nerve abnormalities (e.g., ptosis, difficulty swallowing) followed by peripheral motor weakness. Severe envenomation may result in muscle paralysis, including the muscles of respiration, and lead to death from respiratory failure and aspiration. Sea snake envenomation results in local pain (variable), generalized myalgias, trismus, rhabdomyolysis, and progressive flaccid paralysis; these manifestations can be delayed for several hours.

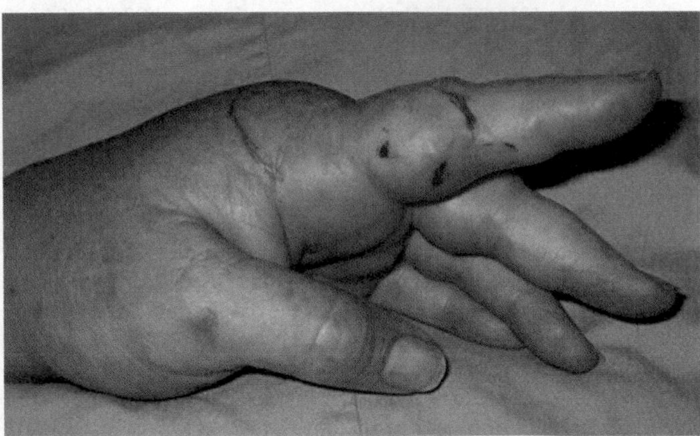

A

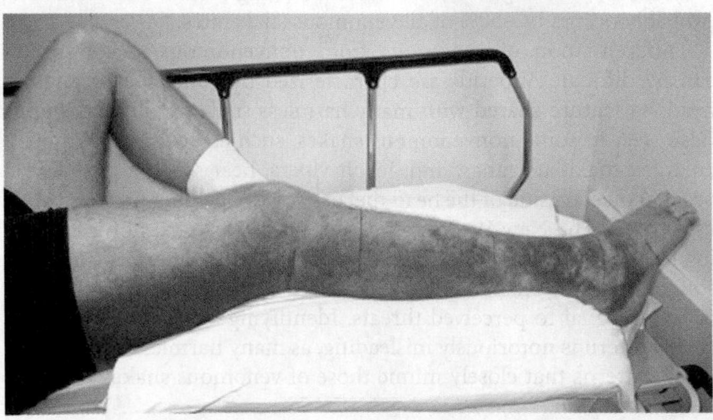

B

FIGURE 474-1 Northern Pacific rattlesnake (*Crotalus oreganus oreganus*) envenomations. *A.* Moderately severe envenomation. Note edema and early ecchymosis 2 h after a bite to the finger. ***B.*** Severe envenomation. Note extensive ecchymosis 5 days after a bite to the ankle.

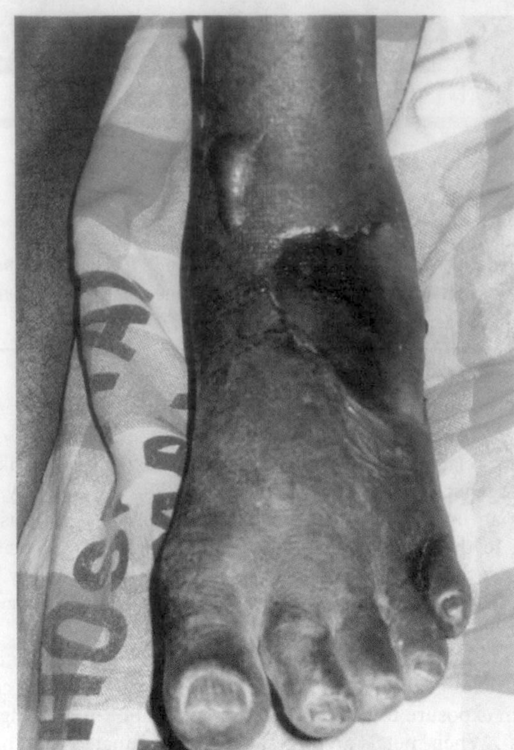

FIGURE 474-2 Early stages of severe, full-thickness necrosis 5 days after a Russell's viper (*Daboia russelii*) bite in southwestern India.

TREATMENT VENOMOUS SNAKEBITE

FIELD MANAGEMENT

The most important aspect of prehospital care of a person bitten by a venomous snake is rapid transport to a medical facility equipped to provide supportive care (airway, breathing, and circulation) and antivenom therapy. Most of the first-aid measures recommended in the past are of little benefit, and some actually worsen outcome. It is reasonable to apply a splint to the bitten extremity to lessen bleeding and discomfort and, if possible, to keep the extremity at approximately heart level. In developing countries, indigenous people should be encouraged to seek immediate care at a health care

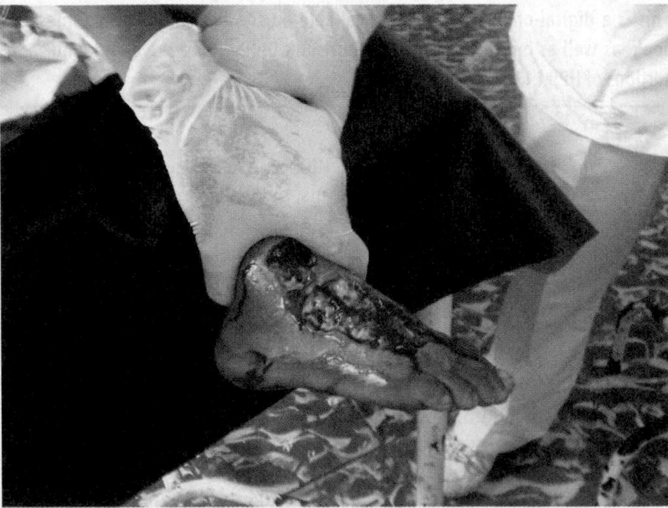

FIGURE 474-3 Severe necrosis 10 days after a pit viper bite in a young child in Colombia. *(Courtesy of Jay R. Stanka; with permission.)*

facility equipped with antivenom instead of consulting traditional healers and thus incurring significant delays in reaching appropriate care. Attempting to capture and transport the offending snake, alive or dead, is not advised; instead, digital photographs of the snake taken from a safe distance may assist with snake identification and treatment decisions.

Incising and/or applying suction to the bite site should be avoided, as these measures are ineffective and exacerbate local tissue damage. Similarly ineffective and potentially harmful are the application of poultices, ice, and electric shock. Techniques or devices used in an effort to limit venom spread (e.g., lymphoocclusive bandages or tourniquets) are ineffective and may result in greater local tissue damage by restricting the spread of potentially necrotizing venom. Tourniquet use can result in loss of function and amputation even in the absence of envenomation.

Elapid venoms that are primarily neurotoxic and have no significant effects on local tissue may be localized by pressure-immobilization, a technique in which the entire limb is wrapped immediately with a bandage (e.g., crepe or elastic) and then immobilized. For this technique to be effective, the wrap pressure must be precise (40–70 mmHg in upper-extremity application and 55–70 mmHg in lower-extremity application) and the victim must be carried out of the field because walking generates muscle-pumping activity that—regardless of the anatomic site of the bite—will disperse venom into the systemic circulation. Pressure-immobilization should be used only in cases in which the offending snake is reliably identified and known to be primarily neurotoxic, the rescuer is skilled in pressure-wrap application, the necessary supplies are readily available, and the victim can be fully immobilized and carried to medical care—an uncommon combination of conditions, particularly in the regions of the world where such bites are most common.

HOSPITAL MANAGEMENT

In the hospital, the victim should be closely monitored (vital signs, cardiac rhythm, oxygen saturation, urine output) while a history is quickly obtained and a rapid, thorough physical examination is performed. To objectively evaluate the progression of local envenomation, the level of swelling in the bitten extremity should be marked and limb circumference should be measured every 15 min until the swelling has stabilized. During this period of observation, the extremity should be positioned at approximately heart level. Measures applied in the field (such as bandages or wraps) should be removed once IV access has been obtained, with cognizance that the release of such ligatures may result in hypotension or dysrhythmias when stagnant acidotic blood containing venom is released into the systemic circulation. Two large-bore IV lines should be established in unaffected extremities. Because of the potential for coagulopathy, venipuncture attempts should be minimized, and noncompressible sites (e.g., a subclavian vein) should be avoided. Early hypotension is due to pooling of blood in the pulmonary and splanchnic vascular beds. Later, systemic bleeding, hemolysis, and loss of intravascular volume into the soft tissues may play important roles. Fluid resuscitation with isotonic saline (20–40 mL/kg IV) should be initiated if there is any evidence of hemodynamic instability, and a trial of 5% albumin (10–20 mL/kg IV) may be given if the response to saline infusion is inadequate. Only after aggressive volume resuscitation and antivenom administration (see below) are accomplished should vasopressors (e.g., dopamine) be added. Invasive hemodynamic monitoring (central venous and/or continuous arterial pressures) can be helpful in such cases, although obtaining central vascular access is risky if coagulopathy has developed. Victims of neurotoxic envenomation should be watched carefully for evidence of cranial nerve dysfunction (e.g., ptosis) that may precede the onset of difficulty swallowing or respiratory insufficiency that necessitates definitive airway protection by endotracheal intubation.

Blood should be drawn for typing and cross-matching and for laboratory evaluation as soon as possible. Important studies include a complete blood count to determine the degree of hemorrhage or hemolysis and to identify thrombocytopenia; studies of renal and hepatic function; coagulation studies to diagnose consumptive coagulopathy; creatine kinase for suspected rhabdomyolysis; and testing of urine for blood or myoglobin. In developing regions, the 20-min whole-blood clotting test can be used to reliably diagnose coagulopathy. A few milliliters of fresh blood are placed in a new, clean, plain glass receptacle (e.g., a test tube) and left undisturbed for 20 min. The tube is then tipped once to 45° to determine whether a clot has formed. If it has not, coagulopathy is diagnosed. Arterial blood gas studies, electrocardiography, and chest radiography may be helpful in severe envenomations or when there is significant comorbidity. Any arterial puncture in the setting of coagulopathy requires great caution and must be performed at an anatomic site amenable to direct-pressure tamponade. After antivenom therapy (see below), laboratory values should be rechecked every 6 h until clinical stability is achieved. If initial laboratory values are normal, the complete blood count and coagulation studies should be repeated every hour until it is clear that no systemic envenomation has occurred.

The mainstay of treatment of a venomous snakebite resulting in significant envenomation is prompt administration of specific antivenom. Antivenoms are produced by injecting animals (generally horses or sheep) with venoms from medically important snakes. Once the stock animals develop antibodies to the venoms, their serum is harvested and the antibodies are isolated for antivenom preparation, which may involve varying degrees of digestion and purification of the IgG molecules. The goal of antivenom administration is to allow antibodies (or antibody fragments) to bind and deactivate circulating venom components before they can attach to target tissues and cause deleterious effects. Antivenoms may be monospecific (directed against a particular snake species) or polyspecific (covering several medically important species in the region) but rarely offer cross-protection against snake species other than those used in their production unless the species are known to have homologous venoms. Thus, antivenom selection must be specific for the offending snake; if the antivenom chosen does not contain antibodies to that snake's venom components, it will provide no benefit and may lead to unnecessary complications (see below). In the United States, assistance in finding appropriate antivenom can be obtained from regional poison control centers.

For victims of bites by viperids or cytotoxic elapids, indications for antivenom administration include significant progressive local findings (e.g., soft tissue swelling crossing a joint or involving more than half the bitten limb) and any evidence of systemic envenomation (systemic symptoms or signs, laboratory abnormalities). Caution must be used in determining the significance of isolated soft tissue swelling after the bite of an unidentified snake because the saliva of some relatively harmless species can cause mild edema at the bite site; in such bites, antivenoms are useless and potentially harmful. Antivenoms have limited efficacy in preventing tissue damage caused by necrotizing venoms, as venom components bind to local tissues very quickly, before antivenom administration can be initiated. Nevertheless, antivenom should be administered as soon as the need for it is identified to limit further tissue damage and systemic effects. Antivenom administration after bites by neurotoxic elapids is indicated at the first sign of any evidence of neurotoxicity (e.g., cranial nerve dysfunction, peripheral neuropathy). In general, antivenom is effective only in reversing active venom toxicity; it is of no benefit in reversing effects that already have been established (e.g., renal failure, established paralysis) and that will improve only with time and other supportive therapies.

Specific comments related to the management of venomous snakebites in the United States and Canada appear in Table 474-1. The package insert for the selected antivenom can be consulted regarding species covered, method of administration, starting dose, and need (if any) for re-dosing. The information in antivenom package inserts, however, is not always accurate and reliable. Whenever possible, it is advisable for treating physicians to seek advice from experts in snakebite management regarding indications for and dosing of antivenom.

TABLE 474-1 MANAGEMENT OF VENOMOUS SNAKEBITE IN THE UNITED STATES AND CANADA[a]

Pit viper bites (rattlesnakes [*Crotalus* and *Sistrurus* spp.], cottonmouth water moccasins [*Agkistrodon piscivorus*], and copperheads [*Agkistrodon contortrix*])

- Stabilize airway, breathing, and circulation.
- Institute monitoring (vital signs, cardiac rhythm, and oxygen saturation).
- Establish two large-bore IV lines.
  - If the patient is hypotensive, administer a normal saline bolus (20–40 mL/kg IV).
  - If hypotension persists, consider 5% albumin (10–20 mL/kg IV).
- Take rapid history and perform thorough physical examination.
- Identify offending snake if possible.
- Measure and record circumference of bitten extremity every 15 min until swelling has stabilized.
- Send laboratory studies (CBC, metabolic panel, PT/INR/PTT, fibrinogen level, FDP, blood type and cross-matching, urinalysis).
  - If normal, repeat CBC and coagulation studies every hour until it is clear that no systemic envenomation has occurred.
  - If abnormal, repeat 6 h after antivenom administration (see below).
- Determine severity of envenomation.
  - None: fang marks only ("dry" bite)
  - Mild: local findings only (e.g., pain, ecchymosis, nonprogressive swelling)
  - Moderate: swelling that is clearly progressing, systemic symptoms or signs, and/or laboratory abnormalities
  - Severe: neurologic dysfunction, respiratory distress, and/or cardiovascular instability/shock
- Contact regional poison control center.
- Locate and administer antivenom as indicated: Crotalidae Polyvalent Immune Fab (CroFab) (Ovine) (BTG International Inc., West Conshohocken, PA).
  - Starting dose
    - Based on severity of envenomation
      - None or mild: none
      - Moderate: 4–6 vials
      - Severe: 6 vials
    - Dilute reconstituted vials in 250 mL of normal saline.
    - No pretesting for potential hypersensitivity; no pretreatment
    - Infuse IV over 1 h (with physician in close attendance).
  - If acute reaction to antivenom:
    - Stop infusion.
    - Treat with standard doses of epinephrine (IM or IV; latter route only in setting of severe hypotension), antihistamines (IV), and glucocorticoids (IV).
    - When reaction is controlled, restart antivenom as soon as possible (may further dilute in larger volume of normal saline).
  - Monitor clinical status over 1 h.
    - Stabilized or improved: Admit to hospital.
    - Progressing or unimproved: Repeat starting dose (and continue this pattern until patient's condition is stable or improved).
- Blood products are rarely needed; if required, they should be given only after antivenom administration.
- Update tetanus immunization as needed.
- Prophylactic antibiotics are unnecessary unless prehospital care included incision or mouth suction.
- Pain management: acetaminophen and/or narcotics as needed; avoidance of salicylates and nonsteroidal anti-inflammatory agents
- Admit to hospital. (If no evidence of envenomation, monitor for 8 h before discharge.)
  - Give additional CroFab (2 vials every 6 h for 3 additional doses, with close monitoring).
  - Monitor for evidence of rising intracompartmental pressures (see text).
  - Provide wound care (see text).
  - Start physical therapy (see text).
- At discharge, warn patient of possible recurrent coagulopathy and symptoms/signs of delayed serum sickness.

Coral snakebites (*Micrurus* spp. and *Micruroides euryxanthus*)

- Stabilize airway, breathing, and circulation.
- Institute monitoring (vital signs, cardiac rhythm, and oxygen saturation).
- Establish one large-bore IV line and initiate normal saline infusion.
- Take rapid history and perform thorough physical examination.
- Identify offending snake if possible.
- Laboratory studies are unlikely to be helpful.
- Contact regional poison control center.
- Locate and administer antivenom as indicated: Antivenin (*Micrurus fulvius*) (equine) (commonly referred to as North American Coral Snake Antivenin; Wyeth Pharmaceuticals, New York, NY).[b]
  - Refer to antivenom package insert.
  - Dilute 3–5 reconstituted vials of antivenom in 250 mL of normal saline.
  - Infuse IV over 1 h (with physician in close attendance).
  - If signs of envenomation progress despite initial antivenom, repeat the starting dose (up to 10 vials total may be required).

(Continued)

TABLE 474-1 MANAGEMENT OF VENOMOUS SNAKEBITE IN THE UNITED STATES AND CANADA[a] (CONTINUED)

- If acute adverse reaction to antivenom:
  - Stop infusion.
  - Treat with standard doses of epinephrine (IM or IV; latter route only in setting of severe hypotension), antihistamines (IV), and glucocorticoids (IV).
  - When reaction is controlled, restart antivenom as soon as possible (may further dilute in larger volume of normal saline).
- If any evidence of neurologic dysfunction (e.g., any cranial nerve abnormalities such as ptosis):
  - Trial of acetylcholinesterase inhibitors (see Table 474-2)
  - With any evidence of difficulty swallowing or breathing, proceed with endotracheal intubation and ventilatory support (may be required for days or weeks).
- Update tetanus immunization as needed.
- Prophylactic antibiotics are unnecessary unless prehospital care included incision or mouth suction.
- Admit to hospital (intensive care unit) even if there is no evidence of envenomation; monitor for at least 24 h.

[a]These recommendations are specific to the care of victims of venomous snakebites in the United States and Canada and should not be applied to bites in other regions of the world. [b]At the time of publication, a single lot of antivenom remains, with an extended expiration date of April 30, 2015.

Abbreviations: CBC, complete blood count; FDP, fibrin degradation products; PT/INR/PTT, prothrombin time/international normalized ratio/partial thromboplastin time.

Antivenom should be administered only by the IV route, and the infusion should be started slowly, with the physician at the bedside ready to intervene immediately at the first signs of an acute adverse reaction. In the absence of an adverse reaction, the rate of infusion can be increased gradually until the full starting dose has been administered (over a total period of ~1 h). Further antivenom may be necessary if the patient's acute clinical condition worsens or fails to stabilize or if venom effects that were initially controlled recur. The decision to administer further antivenom to a stabilized patient should be based on clinical evidence of persistent circulation of unbound venom components. For viperid bites, antivenom administration generally should be continued until the victim shows definite improvement (e.g., stabilized vital signs, reduced pain, restored coagulation). Neurotoxicity from elapid bites may be more difficult to reverse with antivenom. Once neurotoxicity is established and endotracheal intubation is required, further doses of antivenom are unlikely to be beneficial. In such cases, the victim must be maintained on mechanical ventilation until recovery, which may take days or weeks.

Adverse reactions to antivenom administration include immediate (nonallergic and, less commonly, allergic anaphylaxis) and delayed-type hypersensitivity reactions (serum sickness). Clinical manifestations of immediate hypersensitivity include urticaria, laryngeal edema, bronchospasm, and hypotension. Skin testing for potential hypersensitivity, although recommended by some antivenom manufacturers, is insensitive and nonspecific and should be omitted. Worldwide, the quality of antivenoms is highly variable. Rates of acute nonallergic anaphylactic reactions to some of these products exceed 50%. For this reason, some authorities have recommended pretreatment with IV antihistamines (e.g., diphenhydramine, 1 mg/kg to a maximum of 100 mg; and cimetidine, 5–10 mg/kg to a maximum of 300 mg) or even a prophylactic SC or IM dose of epinephrine (0.01 mg/kg, up to 0.3 mg). Further research is necessary, however, to determine whether any pretreatment measures are truly beneficial. Modest expansion of the patient's intravascular volume with crystalloids may blunt acute adverse blood pressure decline. Epinephrine and airway equipment should always be immediately available during antivenom infusion. An acute anaphylactic reaction may be heralded by a single hive or mild itching or may present as bronchospasm or acute cardiovascular collapse. If the patient develops an acute reaction to antivenom, the infusion should be temporarily stopped and the reaction immediately treated with IM epinephrine and IV antihistamines and glucocorticoids. Once the reaction has been controlled, if the severity of the envenomation warrants additional antivenom, the dose should be diluted further in isotonic saline and restarted as soon as possible. Rarely, in cases of recalcitrant hypotension, a concomitant IV infusion of epinephrine may be initiated and titrated to clinical effect while antivenom is administered. The patient must be monitored very closely during such therapy, preferably in an intensive care setting. Serum sickness typically develops 1–2 weeks after antivenom administration and may present as fever, chills, urticaria, myalgias, arthralgias, lymphadenopathy, and renal or neurologic dysfunction. Treatment of serum sickness consists of systemic glucocorticoids (e.g., oral prednisone, 1–2 mg/kg daily) until all symptoms have resolved, followed by a taper over 1–2 weeks. Oral antihistamines and analgesics may provide additional relief of symptoms.

Blood products are rarely necessary in the management of an envenomed patient. The venoms of many snake species can deplete coagulation factors and cause a decrease in platelet count or hematocrit. Nevertheless, these components usually rebound within hours after administration of adequate antivenom. If the need for blood products is thought to be great (e.g., a dangerously low platelet count in a hemorrhaging patient), these products should be given only after adequate antivenom administration to avoid fueling ongoing consumptive coagulopathy.

Rhabdomyolysis and hemolysis should be managed in standard fashion. Victims who develop acute renal failure should be evaluated by a nephrologist and referred for hemodialysis or peritoneal dialysis as needed. Such renal failure, which usually is due to acute tubular necrosis, is frequently reversible. If bilateral cortical necrosis occurs, however, the prognosis for renal recovery is less favorable, and long-term dialysis with possible renal transplantation may be necessary.

Acetylcholinesterase inhibitors (e.g., edrophonium and neostigmine) may promote neurologic improvement in patients bitten by snakes with postsynaptic neurotoxins. Snakebite victims with objective evidence of neurologic dysfunction should receive a test dose of acetylcholinesterase inhibitors, as outlined in **Table 474-2**. If they exhibit improvement, additional doses of long-acting neostigmine can be administered as needed. Close monitoring is required to prevent aspiration if repetitive dosing of neostigmine is used in an

TABLE 474-2 USE OF ACETYLCHOLINESTERASE INHIBITORS IN NEUROTOXIC SNAKE ENVENOMATION

1. Patients with clear, objective evidence of neurotoxicity (e.g., ptosis or inability to maintain upward gaze) should receive a test dose of edrophonium (if available) or neostigmine.
   a. Pretreat with atropine: 0.6 mg IV (children, 0.02 mg/kg with a minimum of 0.1 mg)
   b. Treat with:
      Edrophonium: 10 mg IV (children, 0.25 mg/kg)
      or
      Neostigmine: 1.5–2.0 mg IM (children, 0.025–0.08 mg/kg)
2. If objective improvement is evident after 5 min, treat with:
   a. Neostigmine: 0.5 mg IV or SC (children, 0.01 mg/kg) every 30 min as needed
   b. Atropine: 0.6 mg IV continuous infusion over 8 h (children, 0.02 mg/kg over 8 h)
3. Closely monitor the airway and perform endotracheal intubation as needed.

attempt to obviate endotracheal intubation. Acetylcholinesterase inhibitors are not a substitute for administration of an appropriate antivenom when available.

Care of the bite wound includes simple cleansing with soap and water; application of a dry, sterile dressing; and splinting of the affected extremity with padding between the digits. Once antivenom therapy has been initiated, the extremity should be elevated above heart level to reduce swelling. Tetanus immunization should be updated as appropriate. Prophylactic antibiotics are generally unnecessary after bites by North American snakes, as the incidence of secondary infection is low. In some regions, secondary bacterial infection is more common and the consequences are dire; in these regions, prophylactic antibiotics (e.g., cephalosporins) are used commonly. Antibiotics may also be considered if misguided first aid efforts have included incision or mouth suction of the bite site. Pain control should be achieved with acetaminophen or narcotic analgesics. Salicylates and nonsteroidal anti-inflammatory agents should be avoided because of their effects on blood clotting.

Most snake envenomations involve SC deposition of venom. On occasion, however, venom can be injected more deeply into muscle compartments, particularly if the offending snake was large and the bite occurred on the lower leg, forearm, or hand. Intramuscular swelling of the affected extremity may be accompanied by severe pain, decreased strength, altered sensation, cyanosis, and apparent pulselessness—signs suggesting a muscle compartment syndrome. If there is clinical concern that subfascial muscle edema may be impeding tissue perfusion, intracompartmental pressures should be measured by a minimally invasive technique (e.g., wick catheter or digital readout device). If the intracompartmental pressure is high (>30–40 mmHg), the extremity should be kept elevated while antivenom is administered. A dose of IV mannitol (1 g/kg) can be given in an effort to reduce muscle edema if the patient is hemodynamically stable. If the intracompartmental pressure remains elevated after 1 h of such therapy, a surgical consultation should be obtained for possible fasciotomy. Although evidence from animal studies suggests that fasciotomy may actually worsen myonecrosis, compartmental decompression is still necessary to preserve nerve function. Fortunately, the incidence of compartment syndrome is very low after a snakebite, with fasciotomies required in <1% of cases. Nevertheless, vigilance is essential. If a fasciotomy is deemed necessary, it should be undertaken with the patient's informed consent whenever possible.

Wound care in the days after the bite should include careful aseptic debridement of clearly necrotic tissue once coagulation has been restored. Intact serum-filled vesicles or hemorrhagic blebs should be left undisturbed. If ruptured, they should be debrided with sterile technique. Any debridement of damaged muscle should be conservative because there is evidence that such muscle may recover to a significant degree after antivenom therapy.

Physical therapy should be started as soon as possible so that the victim can return to a functional state. The incidence of long-term loss of function (e.g., reduced range of motion, impaired sensory function) is unclear but is probably quite high (>30%), particularly after viperid bites.

Any patient with signs of envenomation should be observed in the hospital for at least 24 h. In North America, a patient with an apparently "dry" viperid bite should be watched for at least 8 h before discharge, as significant toxicity occasionally develops after a delay of several hours. The onset of systemic symptoms commonly is delayed for a number of hours after bites by several of the elapids (including coral snakes, *Micrurus* species), some non–North American viperids (e.g., the hump-nosed pit viper [*Hypnale hypnale*]), and sea snakes. Patients bitten by these snakes should be observed in the hospital for at least 24 h. Patients whose condition is not stable should be admitted to an intensive care setting.

At hospital discharge, victims of venomous snakebites should be warned about symptoms and signs of wound infection, antivenom-related serum sickness, and potential long-term sequelae, such as pituitary insufficiency from Russell's viper (*D. russelii*) bites. If coagulopathy developed in the acute stages of envenomation, it can recur during the first 2–3 weeks after the bite. In such cases, victims should be warned to avoid elective surgery or activities posing a high risk of trauma during this period. Outpatient analgesic treatment, wound management, and physical therapy should be provided.

MORBIDITY AND MORTALITY

The overall mortality rates for victims of venomous snakebites are low in regions with rapid access to medical care and appropriate antivenoms. In the United States, for example, the mortality rate is <1% for victims who receive antivenom. Eastern and western diamondback rattlesnakes (*Crotalus adamanteus* and *Crotalus atrox*, respectively) are responsible for the majority of snakebite deaths in the United States. Snakes responsible for large numbers of deaths in other countries include cobras (*Naja* spp.), carpet and saw-scaled vipers (*Echis* spp.), Russell's vipers (*D. russelii*), large African vipers (*Bitis* spp.), lancehead pit vipers (*Bothrops* spp.), and tropical rattlesnakes (*C. durissus*).

The incidence of morbidity—defined as permanent functional loss in a bitten extremity—is difficult to estimate but is substantial. Morbidity may be due to muscle, nerve, or vascular injury or to scar contracture. Such morbidity can have devastating consequences for victims in the developing world when they lose the ability to work and provide for their families. In the United States, functional loss tends to be more common and severe after rattlesnake bites than after bites by copperheads (*Agkistrodon contortrix*) or water moccasins (*Agkistrodon piscivorus*).

GLOBAL CONSIDERATIONS

In many developing countries where snakebites are common, scarce access to medical care and antivenom resources contributes to high rates of morbidity and mortality. In many countries, the available antivenoms are inappropriate and ineffective against the venoms of medically important indigenous snakes. In those regions, further research is necessary to determine the actual impact of venomous snakebites and the specific antivenom needs in terms of both quantity and spectrum of coverage. Without accurate statistics, it is difficult to persuade antivenom manufacturers to begin and sustain production of appropriate antisera in developing nations. There is evidence that antivenoms can be produced in much more cost-effective ways than those currently being used. Just as important as getting the correct antivenoms into underserved regions is the need to educate populations about snakebite prevention and to train medical care providers in proper management approaches. Local protocols written with significant input from experienced providers in the region of concern should be developed and distributed. Appropriate antivenoms must be available at the likely first point of medical contact for patients (e.g., primary health centers) in order to minimize the common practice of referring victims to more distant, higher levels of care for the initiation of antivenom therapy. Those who care for snakebite victims in these often-remote clinics must have the skills and confidence required to begin antivenom treatment (and to treat possible reactions) as soon as possible when needed.

MARINE ENVENOMATIONS

Much of the management of envenomation by marine creatures is supportive in nature. A specific marine antivenom can be used when appropriate.

INVERTEBRATES

Cnidarians The Golgi apparatus of the cnidoblast cells within cnidarians, such as hydroids, fire coral, jellyfish, Portuguese men-of-war, and sea anemones, secretes specialized living stinging organelles called *cnidae* (also referred to as *cnidocysts*, a term that encompasses nematocysts, ptychocysts, and spirocysts). Within each organelle resides a stinging mechanism ("thread tube") and venom. In the stinging process, cnidocysts are released and discharged upon mechanosensory stimulation. The venoms from these organisms contain bioactive substances such as tetramine, 5-hydroxytryptamine, histamine, serotonin, and high-molecular-weight toxins, all of which can, among other effects, change the permeability of cells to ions. Victims usually report immediate prickling or burning, pruritus, paresthesias, and painful throbbing with radiation. The skin becomes reddened, darkened, edematous, and blistered and may show signs of superficial necrosis. A legion of neurologic, cardiovascular, respiratory, rheumatologic, gastrointestinal, renal, and ocular symptoms has been described, especially following stings from anemones, *Physalia* species, and scyphozoans. Anaphylaxis is possible. Hundreds of deaths have been reported, many of them caused by *Chironex fleckeri, Stomolophus nomurai, Physalia physalis,* and *Chiropsalmus quadrumanus*. Irukandji syndrome, associated with the Australian jellyfish *Carukia barnesi* and other species, is a potentially fatal condition that most commonly is characterized by hypertension; severe back, chest, and abdominal pain; nausea and vomiting; headache; sweating; and, in the most serious cases, myocardial troponin leak, pulmonary edema, and ultimately hypotension. This syndrome is thought to be mediated, at least in part, by the release of endogenous catecholamines followed by cytokines and nitric oxide.

Rescuers should note that envenomations by different cnidarians (typified by jellyfish) may respond differently to similar topical therapies; thus, the recommendations in this chapter must be tailored to local species and clinical practices. During stabilization, the skin should be decontaminated immediately with a generous application of lidocaine (up to 4%), an all-purpose agent that appears to be useful for relieving pain caused by a large number of species. Vinegar (5% acetic acid), rubbing alcohol (40–70% isopropyl alcohol), baking soda (sodium bicarbonate, especially for sea nettle stings), papain (unseasoned meat tenderizer), fresh lemon or lime juice, olive oil, or sugar may be effective, depending on the species of stinging creature. Household ammonia may in and of itself cause skin irritation.

The pressure-immobilization technique is no longer recommended for venom containment in the setting of any jellyfish sting. For the sting of the venomous box jellyfish (*C. fleckeri*), vinegar should be used. Local application of heat (up to 45°C/113°F), commonly by immersion in hot water, may be as effective. A baking soda slurry (50% baking soda, 50% water) has been recommended for *Cyanea* and *Chrysaora* species. Commercial (chemical) cold packs or real ice packs applied over a thin dry cloth or a plastic membrane have been shown to be effective in alleviating mild or moderate *Physalia utriculus* (bluebottle jellyfish) stings but may be less effective than application of heat. Perfume, aftershave lotion, and high-proof ethanol are not efficacious and may be detrimental; formalin, ether, gasoline, and other organic solvents should not be used. Shaving the skin helps remove remaining nematocysts. Freshwater irrigation and rubbing lead to further stinging by adherent nematocysts and should be avoided.

After decontamination, topical application of an anesthetic ointment (lidocaine, benzocaine), an antihistamine (diphenhydramine), or a glucocorticoid (hydrocortisone) may be helpful. Persistent severe pain after decontamination may be treated with morphine, meperidine, fentanyl, or another narcotic analgesic. Muscle spasms may respond to diazepam (2–5 mg, titrated upward as necessary) or 10% calcium gluconate (5–10 mL) given IV. An ovine-derived IgG antivenom is available from Commonwealth Serum Laboratories (see "Sources of Antivenoms and Other Assistance," below) for stings from the box jellyfish found in Australian and Indo-Pacific waters. However, despite its reported clinical efficacy, one school of thought holds that perhaps the antivenom is unable to bind the venom rapidly enough to account for its effects. Until further notice, current recommendations for its use apply. Treatment for Irukandji syndrome may require administration of opioid analgesics and $MgSO_4$ as well as aggressive treatment (phentolamine, 5 mg IV) of hypertension. All victims with systemic reactions should be observed for at least 6–8 h for rebound from any therapy, and all elderly adults should be checked for cardiac arrhythmias. Patients may suffer postinflammatory hyperpigmentation and persistent cutaneous hypersensitivity in areas of skin contact.

Safe Sea, a "jellyfish-safe" sunblock (*www.nidaria.com*) applied to the skin before an individual enters the water, inactivates the recognition and discharge mechanisms of nematocysts, has been tested successfully against a number of marine stingers, and may prevent or diminish the effects of coelenterate stings. Whenever possible, a dive skin or wet suit should be worn when entering ocean waters.

Sea Sponges Many sponges produce crinotoxins that are present on their surface or in their internal secretions. As a result, touching a sea sponge may result in dermatitis or "sponge diver's disease," a necrotic skin reaction. Irritant dermatitis may result if small spicules of silica or calcium carbonate penetrate the skin. It is impossible to distinguish between the allergic and spicule reactions, so the treatment is the same for both. Afflicted skin should be gently dried and adhesive tape used to remove embedded spicules. Vinegar should be applied immediately and then for 10–30 min three or four times a day. Rubbing alcohol may be used if vinegar is unavailable. After spicule removal and skin decontamination, glucocorticoid or antihistamine cream may be applied to the skin. Severe vesiculation should be treated with a 2-week tapering course of systemic glucocorticoids. Mild reactions subside in 3–7 days, while involvement of large areas of the skin may result in systemic symptoms of fever, dizziness, nausea, muscle cramps, and formication.

Annelid Worms Annelid worms (bristleworms) possess rows of soft, cactus-like spines capable of inflicting painful stings. Contact results in symptoms similar to those of nematocyst envenomation. Without treatment, pain usually subsides over several hours, but inflammation may persist for up to a week (Fig. 474-4). Victims should resist the urge to scratch because scratching may fracture retrievable spines. Visible bristles should be removed with forceps and adhesive tape or a commercial facial peel; alternatively, a thin layer of rubber cement can be used to entrap and then peel away the spines. Use of vinegar or rubbing alcohol or a brief application of lidocaine or unseasoned meat tenderizer (papain) may provide additional relief. Local inflammation should be treated with topical or systemic glucocorticoids.

Sea Urchins Venomous sea urchins possess either hollow, venom-filled calcified spines or triple-jawed, globiferous pedicellariae with venom glands. Venom may also be found within the integumentary sheath on the external spine surface of certain species. The venom contains toxic components, including steroid glycosides, hemolysins, proteases, serotonin, and cholinergic substances. Contact with either venom apparatus produces immediate and intensely painful stings. One or more spines entering a joint can cause synovitis that may, over time, progress to arthritis if the spine(s) remain in or near the joint. If multiple spines penetrate the skin, the patient may develop systemic symptoms, including nausea, vomiting, numbness, muscular paralysis, and respiratory distress. A delayed hypersensitivity reaction 7–10 days after resolution of primary symptoms has been described.

The affected part should be immersed immediately in hot water to tolerance (up to 45°C/113°F). Pedicellariae should be removed by shaving so that envenomation cannot continue. Accessible embedded spines should be removed but may break off and remain lodged in

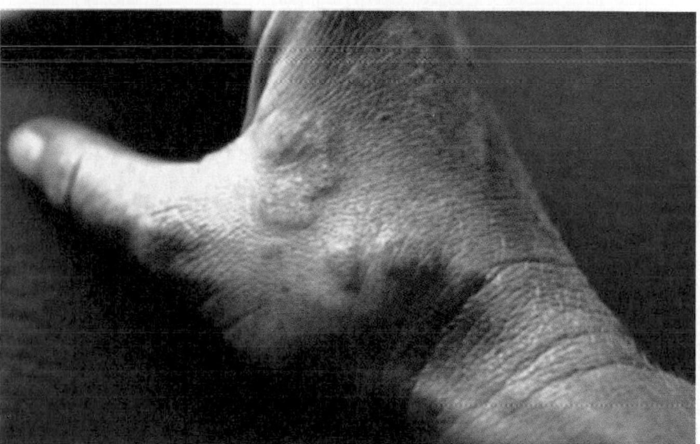

FIGURE 474-4 Rash on the hand of a diver from the spines of a bristleworm. *(Courtesy of Paul Auerbach, with permission.)*

the victim. Residual dye from the surface of a spine remaining after the spine's removal may mimic a retained spine but is otherwise of no consequence. Soft tissue radiography or MRI can confirm the presence of retained spines, which may warrant referral for attempted surgical removal if the spines are near vital structures (e.g., joints, neurovascular bundles). Retained spines may cause the formation of granulomas that are amenable to excision or to intralesional injection with triamcinolone hexacetonide (5 mg/mL). Chronic granulomatous arthritis of the proximal interphalangeal joints has been treated with synovectomy and removal of granulation tissue. Erbium-YAG laser ablation has been deployed to destroy multiple sea urchin spines embedded in the foot and identified visually at the surface level without causing thermal necrosis of the adjacent tissues. Eosinophilic pneumonia and local and diffuse neuropathies have been observed separately after penetration by multiple spines of the black sea urchin (presumed *Diadema* species). The pathophysiologies of these phenomena have not been determined.

Starfish The crown-of-thorns *Acanthaster planci* produces venom in glandular tissue underneath the epidermis, which is released via its spiny surfaces (Fig. 474-5). Skin puncture causes pain, bleeding, and local edema, usually with remission over 30–180 min. Multiple punctures may result in reactions such as local muscle paralysis; retained fragments may cause granulomatous lesions and synovitis. There has also been a case report of elevated liver enzymes after *A. planci* envenomation. Envenomed persons benefit from acute immersion therapy in hot water, local anesthesia, wound cleansing, and possible exploration to remove foreign material.

Sea Cucumbers Sea cucumbers produce holothurin (a cantharin-like liquid toxin) in their body walls. This toxin is concentrated in the tentacular organs that are projected when the animal is threatened. Underwater, holothurin induces minimal contact dermatitis in the skin but can cause significant corneal and conjunctival irritation. A severe reaction can lead to blindness. Skin should be detoxified with 5% acetic acid (vinegar), papain, or isopropyl alcohol. The eye should be anesthetized with one or two drops of 0.5% proparacaine and irrigated with 100–250 mL of normal saline, with subsequent slit-lamp examination to identify corneal defects.

Cone Snails Cone snails use a detachable dartlike tooth to inject conotoxins into prey, inducing tetanus followed by paralysis. In an unknowing handler, stings result in small, burning punctate wounds followed by local ischemia, cyanosis, and numbness. Dysphagia, syncope, dysarthria, ptosis, blurred vision, and pruritus have also been documented. Some envenomations induce paralysis leading to respiratory failure, coma, and death. There is no antivenom. Pressure-immobilization (see "Octopuses," below), hot-water soaks, and local anesthetics have been used empirically with success. The wound should be inspected for a foreign body. Edrophonium has been recommended as therapy for paralysis if a Tensilon test is positive.

Octopuses Serious envenomations and deaths have followed bites of Australian blue-ringed octopuses (*Octopus maculosus* and *Octopus lunulata*). Although these animals rarely exceed 20 cm in length, their salivary venom contains a potent neurotoxin (maculotoxin) that inhibits peripheral nerve transmission by blocking sodium conductance. Oral numbness and facial numbness develop within several minutes of a serious envenomation and rapidly progress to total flaccid paralysis, including failure of respiratory muscles. Immediately after envenomation, a circumferential pressure-immobilization dressing 15 cm wide should be applied over a gauze pad (~7 × 7 × 2 cm) that has been placed directly over the sting. The dressing should be applied at venous-lymphatic pressure, with the preservation of distal arterial pulses. The limb should then be splinted. Once the victim has been transported to the nearest medical facility, the bandage can be released. Because there is no antidote and passive immunotherapy (rabbit IgG antibody) has been proven effective only against tetrodotoxin in mice, treatment is supportive. Patients with respiratory failure may need to be mechanically ventilated. If respirations are assisted, the victim may remain awake although completely paralyzed. Even with serious envenomations, significant recovery often takes place within 4–10 h, although complete recovery may require 2–4 days. Sequelae are uncommon unless related to hypoxia.

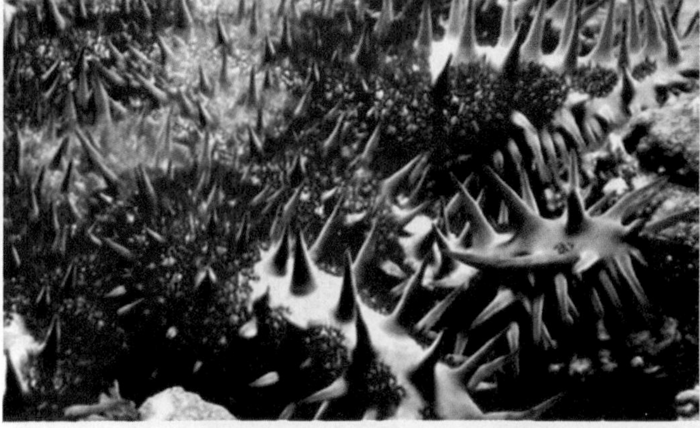

FIGURE 474-5 Spines on the crown-of-thorns sea star (*Acanthaster planci*). *(Courtesy of Paul Auerbach, with permission.)*

VERTEBRATES

As for all penetrating injuries, first-aid care should be undertaken. In addition, consideration must be given to local wound infection by marine *Vibrio* species and freshwater *Aeromonas hydrophila* as well as other "aquatic bacteria," particularly if spines and needles remain embedded.

Stingrays A stingray injury is both an envenomation and a traumatic wound. Thoracic and cardiac penetration, major vessel laceration, and compartment syndrome have all been observed. The venom, which contains serotonin, 5′-nucleotidase, and phosphodiesterase, causes immediate, intense pain that may last up to 48 h. The wound is very painful (with the pain peaking at 30–60 min and lasting up to 48 h), often becomes ischemic in appearance, and heals poorly, with adjacent soft tissue swelling and prolonged disability. Systemic effects include weakness, diaphoresis, nausea, vomiting, diarrhea, dysrhythmias, syncope, hypotension, muscle cramps, fasciculations, paralysis, and (in rare cases) death. Because of differences in the toxins present on the tissues covering the stingers, freshwater stingrays may cause more severe injuries than marine stingrays.

Scorpionfish The designation *scorpionfish* encompasses members of the family Scorpaenidae and includes not only scorpionfish but also lionfish and stonefish. A complex venom with neuromuscular toxicity is delivered through 12 or 13 dorsal, 2 pelvic, and 3 anal spines. In general, the sting of a stonefish is regarded as the most serious (severe to life-threatening); that of the scorpionfish is of intermediate seriousness; and that of the lionfish is the least serious. Like that of a stingray, the sting of a scorpionfish is immediately and intensely painful. Pain from a stonefish envenomation may last for days. Systemic manifestations of scorpionfish stings are similar to those of stingray envenomations but may be more pronounced, particularly in the case of a stonefish sting, which may cause severe local tissue necrosis in addition to vital organ failure. The rare deaths that follow stonefish envenomation usually occur within 6–8 h. There is a commercially available stonefish antivenom.

Other Fish Three species of marine catfish—*Plotosus lineatus* (oriental catfish), *Bagre marinus* (sail catfish), and *Galeichthys felis* (common sea catfish)—as well as several species of freshwater catfish are capable of stinging humans. Venom is delivered through a single dorsal spine and two pectoral spines. Clinically, a catfish sting is comparable to that of a stingray, although marine catfish envenomations are generally more severe than those of their freshwater counterparts. Surgeonfish (doctorfish, tang), weeverfish, ratfish, and horned venomous sharks have also envenomed humans.

Platypus The platypus is a venomous mammal. The male has a keratinous spur on each hind limb; the spur is connected to a venom gland within the upper thigh. Skin puncture causes soft tissue edema and pain that may last for days or weeks. Care is supportive, and hot-water therapy does not appear to benefit the victim.

TREATMENT MARINE VERTEBRATE STINGS

The stings of all marine vertebrates are treated in a similar fashion. Except for stonefish and serious scorpionfish envenomations (see below), no antivenom is available. The affected part should be immersed immediately in nonscalding hot water (45°C/113°F) for 30–90 min or until there is significant relief from pain. Recurrent pain may respond to repeated hot-water treatment. Cryotherapy is contraindicated, and no data support the use of antihistamines or steroids. Opiates will help alleviate the pain, as will local wound infiltration or regional nerve block with 1% lidocaine, 0.5% bupivacaine, and sodium bicarbonate mixed in a 5:5:1 ratio. After soaking and anesthetic administration, the wound must be explored and debrided. Radiography (in particular, MRI) may be helpful in identification of foreign bodies. After exploration and debridement, the wound should be irrigated vigorously with warm sterile water, saline, or 1% povidone-iodine in solution. Bleeding usually can be controlled by sustained local pressure for 10–15 min. In general, wounds should be left open to heal by secondary intention or treated by delayed primary closure. Tetanus immunization should be updated. Antibiotic treatment should be considered for serious wounds and for envenomation in immunocompromised hosts. The initial antibiotics should cover *Staphylococcus* and *Streptococcus* species. If the victim is immunocompromised, if a wound is primarily repaired and is more than minor, or if an infection develops, antibiotic coverage should be broadened to include *Vibrio* species. Infection with *Aeromonas* species is of similar concern for wounds associated with natural freshwater.

APPROACH TO THE PATIENT: Marine Envenomations

It is useful to be familiar with the local marine fauna and to recognize patterns of injury.

A large puncture wound or jagged laceration (particularly on the lower extremity) that is more painful than one would expect from the size and configuration of the wound is likely to be a stingray envenomation. Smaller punctures, as described above, represent the activity of a sea urchin (Fig. 474-6) or starfish. Stony corals cause rough abrasions and, in rare instances, lacerations or puncture wounds.

Coelenterate (marine invertebrate) stings sometimes create diagnostic skin patterns. A diffuse urticarial rash on exposed skin is often indicative of exposure to fragmented hydroids or larval anemones. A linear, whiplike print pattern appears where a jellyfish tentacle has contacted the skin. In the case of the dreaded box jellyfish, a cross-hatched appearance, followed by development of dark purple coloration within a few hours of the sting, heralds skin necrosis. A frosted appearance may be created by aluminum salt–based remedies applied to the wound. An encounter with fire coral causes immediate pain and swollen red skin irritation in the pattern of contact, similar to but more severe than the imprint left by exposure to an intact feather hydroid. Seabather's eruption, caused by thimble jellyfishes and larval anemones, may produce a diffuse rash that consists of clusters of erythematous macules or raised papules and is accompanied by intense itching (Fig. 474-7). Toxic sponges create a burning and painful red rash on exposed skin, which may blister and later desquamate. Because virtually all marine stingers invoke the sequelae of inflammation, local erythema, swelling, and adenopathy are fairly nonspecific.

SOURCES OF ANTIVENOMS AND OTHER ASSISTANCE

The best way to locate a specific antivenom in the United States is to call a regional poison control center and ask for assistance.

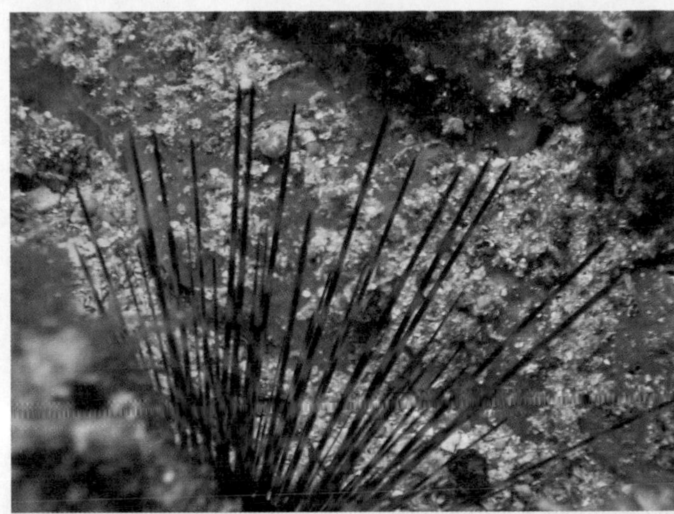

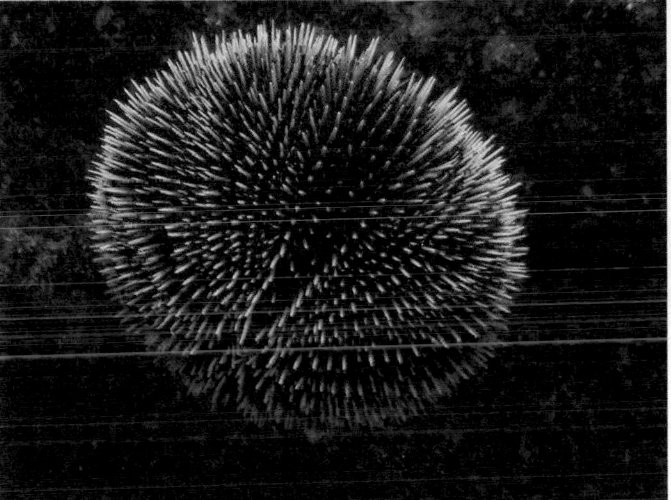

FIGURE 474-6 Spiny sea urchins. *(Courtesy of Dr. Paul Auerbach, with permission.)*

Divers Alert Network, a nonprofit organization designed to assist in the care of injured divers, also may help with the treatment of marine injuries. The network can be reached on the Internet at *www.diversalertnetwork.org* or by telephone 24 h a day at (919) 684-9111. An antivenom for the box jellyfish (*C. fleckeri*) and another for stonefish

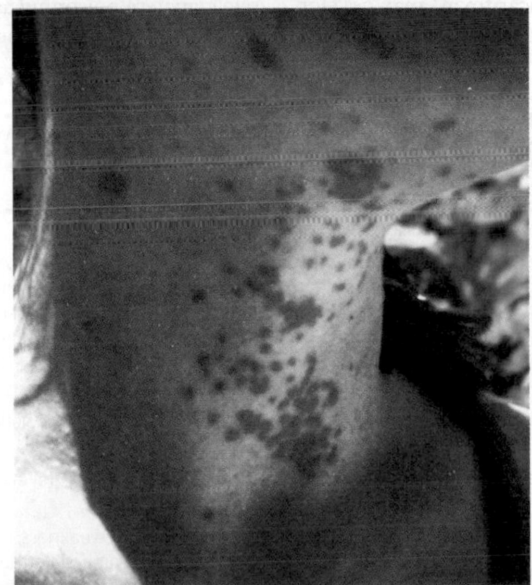

FIGURE 474-7 Erythematous, papular rash typical of seabather's eruption caused by thimble jellyfish and larval anemones.

(and severe scorpionfish) envenomation are made in Australia by the Commonwealth Serum Laboratories (CSL; 45 Poplar Road, Parkville, Victoria, Australia 3052; *www.csl.com.au*; 61-3-9389-1911). When administering the box jellyfish antivenom, time is of the essence. For cardiac or respiratory decompensation, give a minimum of one ampoule and up to six ampoules consecutively IV, preferably in a 1:10 dilution with normal saline. For stonefish (or severe scorpionfish) envenomation, give one ampoule of specific antivenom IM for every one or two punctures, to a maximum of three ampoules.

MARINE POISONINGS

CIGUATERA

Epidemiology and Pathogenesis Ciguatera poisoning is the most common nonbacterial food poisoning associated with fish in the United States; most U.S. cases occur in Florida and Hawaii, although, with transportation of imported fish nationwide, all clinicians need to be aware of ciguatera. The poisoning almost exclusively involves tropical and semitropical marine coral reef fish common in the Indian Ocean, the South Pacific, and the Caribbean Sea. Global estimates predict that 20,000–50,000 people may be affected by this poisoning each year. More than 400 different fish have been associated with ciguatera toxicity, but 75% of poisonings involve the reef-dwelling barracuda, snapper, jack, or grouper. Ciguatera toxin is created by warm-water ocean reef microalgae of the genus *Gambierdiscus toxicus*, whose consumption by grazing fish allows the toxin to bioaccumulate in the food chain. Three major ciguatoxins are found in the flesh and viscera of ciguateric fish: CTX-1, -2, and -3. Recent research suggests that CTX-1 activates astrocytes and astroglia. In addition, TRPV1, a nonselective cation channel expressed in nociceptive neurons, may play a role in the neurologic disturbances unique to ciguatera poisoning. Most, if not all, ciguatoxins are unaffected by freeze-drying, heat, cold, and gastric acid. None of the toxins affects the odor, color, or taste of fish. Cooking methods may alter the relative concentrations of the various toxins.

Clinical Manifestations The onset of symptoms may come within 15–30 min of ingestion and typically takes place within 2–6 h. Symptoms increase in severity over the ensuing 4–6 h. Most victims develop symptoms within 12 h of ingestion, and virtually all are afflicted within 24 h. The more than 150 signs and symptoms reported include those shown in Table 474-3. Diarrhea, vomiting, and abdominal pain usually develop 3–6 h after ingestion of a ciguatoxic fish. Symptoms may persist for 48 h and then generally resolve (even without treatment). A pathognomonic symptom is the reversal of hot and cold tactile perception, which develops in some persons after 3–5 days and may last for months. More severe reactions tend to occur in persons previously stricken with the disease. Persons who have ingested parrotfish (scaritoxin) may develop classic ciguatera poisoning as well as a "second-phase" syndrome (after 5–10 days' delay) of disequilibrium with locomotor ataxia, dysmetria, and resting or kinetic tremor. This syndrome may persist for 2–6 weeks.

TABLE 474-3 REPRESENTATIVE SIGNS AND SYMPTOMS OF CIGUATERA POISONING

System	Signs/Symptoms
Gastrointestinal	Abdominal pain, nausea, vomiting, diarrhea
Neurologic	Paresthesias, pruritus, tongue and throat numbness or burning, sensation of "carbonation" during swallowing, odontalgia or dental dysesthesias, dysphagia, tremor, fasciculations, athetosis, meningismus, aphonia, ataxia, vertigo, pain and weakness in the lower extremities, visual blurring, transient blindness, hyporeflexia, seizures, coma
Dermatologic	Conjunctivitis, maculopapular rash, skin vesiculations, dermatographism
Cardiovascular	Bradycardia, heart block, hypotension, central respiratory failure[a]
Other	Chills, dysuria, dyspnea, dyspareunia, weakness, fatigue, nasal congestion and dryness, insomnia, sialorrhea, diaphoresis, headache, arthralgias, myalgias

[a]Tachycardia and hypertension may occur after potentially severe transient bradycardia and hypotension. Death is rare.

Diagnosis The differential diagnosis of ciguatera includes paralytic shellfish poisoning, eosinophilic meningitis, type E botulism, organophosphate insecticide poisoning, tetrodotoxin poisoning, and psychogenic hyperventilation. At present, the diagnosis of ciguatera poisoning is made on clinical grounds because no routinely used laboratory test detects ciguatoxin in human blood. Liquid chromatography–mass spectrometry is available for ciguatoxins but is of limited clinical value because most health care institutions do not have the equipment needed to perform the test. A ciguatoxin enzyme immunoassay or radioimmunoassay may be used to test small portions of the suspected fish, but even these tests may not detect the very small amount of toxin (0.1 ppb) necessary to render fish flesh toxic. A newer neuroblastoma assay may be sufficiently sensitive to detect small amounts of toxin but is not readily available for clinical use.

TREATMENT CIGUATERA POISONING

Therapy is supportive and based on symptoms. Nausea and vomiting may be controlled with an antiemetic such as ondansetron (4–8 mg IV). Syrup of ipecac and activated charcoal are not recommended for ciguatera poisoning. Hypotension may require the administration of IV crystalloid and, in rare cases, a pressor drug. Bradyarrhythmias that lead to cardiac insufficiency and hypotension generally respond well to atropine (0.5 mg IV, up to 2 mg). Goal-directed combination cardiovascular fluid and pressor therapy may be required. Cool showers or the administration of hydroxyzine (25 mg PO every 6–8 h) may relieve pruritus. Amitriptyline (25 mg PO twice a day) reportedly alleviates pruritus and dysesthesias. In three cases unresponsive to amitriptyline, tocainide has appeared to be efficacious. Nifedipine has been used to treat headache and poor circulation in order to prevent hypotension, but only after the initial acute phase of the poisoning has passed. IV infusion of mannitol may be beneficial in moderate or severe cases in fluid-repleted patients, particularly for the relief of distressing neurologic or cardiovascular symptoms, although the efficacy of this therapy has been challenged and has not been definitively proved. The infusion is rendered initially as 1 g/kg per day over 45–60 min during the acute phase (days 1–5). If symptoms improve, a second dose may be given within 3–4 h and a third dose may be administered the next day. Care must be taken to avoid dehydration in a treated patient. The mechanism of the benefit against ciguatera intoxication is perhaps hyperosmotic water-drawing action, which reverses ciguatoxin-induced Schwann cell edema. Mannitol may also act in some fashion as a "hydroxyl scavenger" or may competitively inhibit ciguatoxin at the cell membrane.

During recovery from ciguatera poisoning, the victim should exclude the following from the diet for 6 months: fish (fresh or preserved), fish sauces, shellfish, shellfish sauces, alcoholic beverages, nuts, and nut oils. Consumption of fish in ciguatera-endemic regions should be avoided. All oversized fish of any predacious reef species should be suspected of harboring ciguatoxin. Neither moray eels nor the viscera of tropical marine fish should ever be eaten.

DIARRHETIC SHELLFISH POISONING

Diarrhetic shellfish poisoning occurs with consumption of shellfish producing diarrheal illness. The first suspected incident, which occurred in the Netherlands in 1961, was followed by outbreaks in Japan, the United Kingdom, and (most recently) China. The causative agents are the lipophilic compound okadaic acid and the dinophysistoxins, which inhibit serine and threonine protein phosphatases, with consequent protein accumulation and continued secretion of fluid in intestinal cells leading to diarrhea. Shellfish acquire these toxins by feeding on dinoflagellates, particularly of the genera *Dinophysis* and *Prorocentrum*.

Symptoms include diarrhea, nausea, vomiting, abdominal pain, and chills. Onset occurs within 30 min to 12 h. The illness is usually self-limited; most patients recover in 3 or 4 days, and only a few require hospitalization. Treatment is supportive and focused on hydration. Toxins can be detected in food samples by a mouse bioassay, an immunoassay, and high-performance liquid chromatography with fluorometric detection (HPLC-FLD).

PARALYTIC SHELLFISH POISONING

Paralytic shellfish poisoning is induced by ingestion of any of a variety of feral or aquacultured filter-feeding organisms, including clams, oysters, scallops, mussels, chitons, limpets, starfish, and sand crabs. The origin of their toxicity is the chemical toxin they accumulate and concentrate by feeding on various planktonic dinoflagellates (e.g., *Protogonyaulax, Ptychodiscus,* and *Gymnodinium*) and protozoan organisms. The unicellular phytoplanktonic organisms form the foundation of the food chain, and in warm summer months these organisms "bloom" in nutrient-rich coastal temperate and semitropical waters. In the United States, paralytic shellfish poisoning is acquired primarily from seafood harvested in the Northeast, the Pacific Northwest, and Alaska. These planktonic species can release massive amounts of toxic metabolites into the water and cause mortality in bird and marine populations. The paralytic shellfish toxins are water soluble as well as heat and acid stable; they cannot be destroyed by ordinary cooking or freezing. Contaminated seafood looks, smells, and tastes normal. The best-characterized, most potent, and most frequently identified paralytic shellfish toxin is saxitoxin, which takes its name from the Alaska butter clam *Saxidomus giganteus.* Saxitoxin appears to block sodium conductance, inhibiting neuromuscular transmission at the axonal and muscle membrane levels. A toxin concentration of >75 μg/100 g of foodstuff is considered hazardous to humans. In the 1972 New England "red tide," the concentration of saxitoxin in blue mussels exceeded 9000 μg/100 g of foodstuff.

The onset of intraoral and perioral paresthesias (notably of the lips, tongue, and gums) comes within minutes to a few hours after ingestion of contaminated shellfish, and these paresthesias progress rapidly to involve the neck and distal extremities. The tingling or burning sensation later changes to numbness. Other symptoms rapidly develop and include light-headedness, disequilibrium, incoordination, weakness, hyperreflexia, incoherence, dysarthria, sialorrhea, dysphagia, thirst, diarrhea, abdominal pain, nausea, vomiting, nystagmus, dysmetria, headache, diaphoresis, loss of vision, chest pain, and tachycardia. Flaccid paralysis and respiratory insufficiency may follow 2–12 h after ingestion. In the absence of hypoxia, the victim often remains alert but paralyzed. Up to 12% of patients die.

TREATMENT PARALYTIC SHELLFISH POISONING

Treatment is supportive and based on symptoms. If the victim comes to medical attention within the first few hours after poison ingestion, the stomach should be emptied by gastric lavage and then irrigated with 2 L (in 200-mL aliquots) of a solution of 2% sodium bicarbonate; this intervention has not been proved to be of benefit but is based on the notion that gastric acidity may enhance the potency of saxitoxin. Because breathing difficulty can be rapid in onset, induction of emesis is not advised. The administration of activated charcoal (50–100 g) and a cathartic (sorbitol, 20–50 g) makes empirical sense because these shellfish toxins are believed to bind well to charcoal. Some authors advise against administration of magnesium-based solutions (e.g., certain cathartics), cautioning that hypermagnesemia may contribute to suppression of nerve conduction.

The most serious problem is respiratory paralysis. The victim should be closely observed for respiratory distress for at least 24 h in a hospital. With prompt recognition of ventilatory failure, endotracheal intubation, and assisted ventilation, anoxic myocardial and brain injury may be prevented. If the patient survives for 18 h, the prognosis is good for a complete recovery.

A direct human serum assay to identify the toxin responsible for paralytic shellfish poisoning is not yet clinically available; the mouse bioassay in widespread use may be replaced by an automated tissue-culture bioassay. A polyclonal enzyme-linked immunosorbent assay (ELISA) to measure specific toxins is under development, as is HPLC-FLD. In addition, an inhibition immunoassay that may be able to simultaneously detect paralytic shellfish, diarrhetic shellfish, and amnesic shellfish toxins is being investigated.

DOMOIC ACID INTOXICATION (AMNESTIC SHELLFISH POISONING)

In late 1987 in eastern Canada, an outbreak of gastrointestinal and neurologic symptoms (amnestic shellfish poisoning) was documented in persons who had consumed mussels found to be contaminated with domoic acid. In this outbreak, the source of the toxin was *Nitzschia pungens,* a diatom ingested by the mussels. Since the Canadian outbreak, the toxin has been found in shellfish from the United States, the United Kingdom, and Spain. In 1991, an epidemic of domoic acid poisoning in the state of Washington was attributed to the consumption of razor clams. A water-soluble, heat-stable neuroexcitatory amino acid with biochemical analogues of kainic acid and glutamic acid, domoic acid binds to the kainate type of glutamate receptor with three times the affinity of kainic acid and is 20 times as powerful a toxin. Shellfish can be tested for domoic acid by mouse bioassay and HPLC. The regulatory limit for domoic acid in shellfish is 20 parts per million.

The abnormalities noted within 24 h of ingesting contaminated mussels (*Mytilus edulis*) include arousal, confusion, disorientation, and memory loss. The median time of onset is 5.5 h. Other prominent signs and symptoms include severe headache, nausea, vomiting, diarrhea, abdominal cramps, hiccups, arrhythmias, hypotension, seizures, ophthalmoplegia, pupillary dilation, piloerection, hemiparesis, mutism, grimacing, agitation, emotional lability, coma, copious bronchial secretions, and pulmonary edema. Histologic study of brain tissue taken at autopsy has shown neuronal necrosis or cell loss and astrocytosis, most prominently in the hippocampus and the amygdaloid nucleus—findings similar to those in animals poisoned with kainic acid. Several months after the primary intoxication, victims still display chronic residual memory deficits and motor neuronopathy or axonopathy. Nonneurologic illness does not persist.

TREATMENT DOMOIC ACID INTOXICATION

Therapy is supportive and based on symptoms. Because kainic acid neuropathology seems to be nearly entirely seizure mediated, the emphasis should be on anticonvulsive therapy, for which diazepam appears to be as effective as any other drug.

SCOMBROID POISONING

Scombroid fish poisoning may be the most common type of seafood poisoning worldwide. It follows consumption of scombroid (mackerel-like) fish, which include albacore, bluefin, and yellowfin tuna; mackerel; saury; needlefish; wahoo; skipjack; and bonito, as well as nonscombroid fish, such as dolphinfish (Hawaiian mahimahi, *Coryphaena hippurus*), kahawai, sardine, black marlin, pilchard, anchovy, herring, amberjack, and Australian ocean salmon. In the northeastern and mid-Atlantic United States, bluefish (*Pomatomus saltatrix*) has been linked to scombroid poisoning. Because greater numbers of nonscombroid fish are being recognized as scombrotoxic, the syndrome may more appropriately be called *pseudoallergic fish poisoning.*

Under conditions of inadequate preservation or refrigeration, the musculature of these dark- or red-fleshed fish undergoes decomposition by *Proteus morganii* and *Klebsiella pneumoniae* bacteria, with consequent decarboxylation of the amino acid L-histidine to histamine, histamine phosphate, and histamine hydrochloride. Histamine levels of 20–50 mg/100 g are noted in toxic fish, with levels >400 mg/100 g on occasion. However, it is possible that some other compound may be responsible for this intoxication, because large doses of oral histamine do not reproduce the affliction. It is proposed that this unknown agent works by inhibiting the metabolism of histamine, promoting degranulation of mast cells to release endogenous histamine, or acting as a histamine receptor agonist. Whatever toxin or toxins are involved are heat stable and are not destroyed by domestic or commercial cooking. Affected fish typically have a sharply metallic or peppery taste; however, they may be normal in appearance, color, and flavor. Not all persons who eat a contaminated fish necessarily become ill, perhaps because of uneven distribution of decay within the fish.

Symptoms develop within 15–90 min of ingestion. Most cases are mild, with tingling of lips and mouth, mild abdominal discomfort, and nausea. The more severe and commonly described presentation includes flushing (sharply demarcated; exacerbated by ultraviolet exposure; particularly pronounced on the face, neck, and upper trunk), a sensation of warmth without elevated core temperature, conjunctival hyperemia, pruritus, urticaria, and angioneurotic edema. This syndrome may progress to bronchospasm, nausea, vomiting, diarrhea, epigastric pain, abdominal cramps, dysphagia, headache, thirst, pharyngitis, gingival burning, palpitations, tachycardia, dizziness, and hypotension. Without treatment, the symptoms generally resolve within 8–12 h. Because of blockade of gastrointestinal tract histaminase, the reaction may be more severe in a person who is concurrently ingesting isoniazid.

TREATMENT SCOMBROID POISONING

Therapy is directed at reversing the histamine effect with antihistamines, either H-1 or H-2. If bronchospasm is severe, an inhaled bronchodilator—or in rare, extremely severe circumstances, injected epinephrine—may be used. Glucocorticoids are of no proven benefit. Protracted nausea and vomiting, which may empty the stomach of toxin, may be controlled with a specific antiemetic, such as ondansetron or prochlorperazine. The persistent headache of scombroid poisoning may respond to cimetidine or a similar antihistamine if standard analgesics are not effective.

475 Ectoparasite Infestations and Arthropod Injuries

Richard J. Pollack, Scott A. Norton

Ectoparasites include arthropods and creatures from other phyla that infest the skin or hair of animals; the host animals provide them with sustenance and shelter. The ectoparasites may penetrate within or beneath the surface of the host or may attach by mouthparts and specialized claws. These organisms may inflict direct mechanical injury, consume blood or nutrients, induce hypersensitivity reactions, inoculate toxins, transmit pathogens, and incite fear or disgust. Humans are the sole or obligate hosts for many kinds of ectoparasites and serve as facultative or paratenic (accidental) hosts for many others.

Arthropods that are ectoparasitic or otherwise cause injury include insects (such as lice, fleas, bedbugs, wasps, ants, bees, and flies), arachnids (spiders, scorpions, mites, and ticks), millipedes, and centipedes. Certain nematodes (helminths), such as the hookworms (Chap. 256), are ectoparasitic in that they penetrate and migrate through the skin. Infrequently encountered ectoparasites in other phyla include the pentastomes (tongue worms) and leeches.

Arthropods may also cause injury when they attempt to take a blood meal or as they defend themselves by biting, stinging, or exuding venoms. Various arachnids (spiders and scorpions), insects (bees, hornets, wasps, ants, flies, true bugs, caterpillars, and beetles), millipedes, and centipedes produce ill effects during these behaviors. Similarly, certain ectoparasites (e.g., ticks, biting mites, and fleas) that typically infest nonhuman animals can be medically significant. In the United States, lesions caused by arthropod bites and stings are so diverse and variable that it is rarely possible to identify the precise causative organism without a bona fide specimen and taxonomic expertise.

SCABIES

The human itch mite, *Sarcoptes scabiei* var. *hominis,* is a common cause of itching dermatosis, infesting ~300 million persons worldwide at any one time. Gravid female mites (~0.3 mm in length) burrow superficially within the stratum corneum, depositing three or fewer eggs per day. Six-legged larvae mature to eight-legged nymphs and then to adults. Gravid adult females emerge to the surface of the skin about 8 days later and then (re)invade the skin of the same or another host. Newly fertilized female mites are transferred from person to person mainly by direct skin-to-skin contact; transfer is facilitated by crowding, poor hygiene, and sex with multiple partners. Generally, these mites die within a day or so in the absence of host contact. Transmission via sharing of contaminated bedding or clothing occurs far less frequently than is often thought. In the United States, scabies may account for up to 5% of visits to dermatologists. Outbreaks occur in preschools, hospitals, nursing homes, and other residential institutions.

The itching and rash associated with scabies derive from a sensitization reaction to the mites and their secretions/excretions. A person's initial infestation remains asymptomatic for up to 6 weeks before the onset of intense pruritus, but a reinfestation produces a hypersensitivity reaction without delay. Burrows become surrounded by inflammatory infiltrates composed of eosinophils, lymphocytes, and histiocytes, and a generalized hypersensitivity rash later develops in remote sites. Immunity and associated scratching limit most infestations to <15 mites per person. Hyperinfestation with thousands of mites, a condition known as *crusted scabies* (formerly termed *Norwegian scabies*), may result from glucocorticoid use, immunodeficiency, and neurologic or psychiatric illnesses that limit the itch and/or the scratch response.

Pruritus typically intensifies at night and after hot showers. Classic burrows are often difficult to find because they are few in number and may be obscured by excoriations. Burrows appear as dark wavy lines in the upper epidermis and are 3–15 mm long. Scabetic lesions are most common on the volar wrists and along the digital web spaces. In males, the penis and scrotum become involved. Small papules and vesicles, often accompanied by eczematous plaques, pustules, or nodules, appear symmetrically at those sites; within intertriginous areas; around the navel and belt line; in the axillae; and on the buttocks and upper thighs. Except in infants, the face, scalp, neck, palms, and soles are usually spared. Crusted scabies often resembles psoriasis: both are characterized by widespread thick keratotic crusts, scaly plaques, and dystrophic nails. Characteristic burrows are not seen in crusted scabies, and patients usually do not itch, although their infestations are highly contagious and have been responsible for outbreaks of classic scabies in hospitals.

Scabies should be considered in patients with pruritus and symmetric superficial, excoriated, papulovesicular skin lesions in characteristic locations, particularly if there is a history of household contact with an infested person. Burrows should be sought and unroofed with a sterile needle or scalpel blade, and the scrapings should be examined microscopically for mites, eggs, and fecal pellets. Examination of skin biopsies (including superficial cyanoacrylate biopsy) or scrapings, dermatoscopic imaging of papulovesicular lesions, and microscopic inspection of clear cellophane tape lifted from lesions also may be diagnostic. In the absence of identifiable mites or eggs, the diagnosis is based on a history of pruritus, a clinical examination, and an epidemiologic link. Diverse kinds of dermatitis from other causes frequently are misdiagnosed as scabies, particularly in presumed "outbreak" situations. Scabies mites of other animals may cause transient irritation, but they do not reside or reproduce in human hosts.

TREATMENT SCABIES

Permethrin cream (5%) is less toxic than 1% lindane preparations and is effective against lindane-tolerant infestations. Scabicides are applied thinly but thoroughly behind the ears and from the neck down after bathing—with careful application to interdigital spaces and the umbilicus and under the fingernails—and are removed

8–14 h later with soap and water. Successful treatment of crusted scabies requires preapplication of a keratolytic agent such as 6% salicylic acid and then of scabicides to the scalp, face, and ears. Repeated treatments or the sequential use of several agents may be necessary. Ivermectin has not been approved by the U.S. Food and Drug Administration (FDA) for treatment of any form of scabies, but a single oral dose (200 μg/kg) is effective in otherwise healthy persons; patients with crusted scabies may require two doses separated by an interval of 1–2 weeks. All FDA-approved scabicides are available solely by prescription.

Within 1 day of effective treatment, scabies infestations become noncommunicable, but the pruritic hypersensitivity dermatitis induced by the now-dead mites and their remnant products frequently persists for weeks. Unnecessary re-treatment with topical agents may provoke contact dermatitis. Antihistamines, salicylates, and calamine lotion relieve itching during treatment, and topical glucocorticoids are useful for pruritus that lingers after effective treatment. To prevent reinfestations, bedding and clothing should be washed and dried on high heat or heat-pressed. Close contacts of confirmed cases, even if asymptomatic, should be treated simultaneously.

CHIGGERS AND OTHER BITING MITES

Chiggers are the larvae of trombiculid (harvest) mites that normally feed on mice in grassy or brush-covered sites in tropical, subtropical, and (less frequently) temperate areas during warm months. They reside on low vegetation and attach themselves to passing mammalian hosts. While feeding, larvae secrete saliva with proteolytic enzymes to create a tube-like invagination in the host's skin; this *stylostome* allows the mite to imbibe tissue fluids. The stylostomal saliva is highly antigenic and causes exceptionally pruritic papular, papulovesicular, or papulourticarial lesions (≤2 cm in diameter). In people previously sensitized to salivary antigens, the papules develop within hours of attachment. While attached, mites appear as tiny red vesicles on the skin. Generally, lesions vesicate and develop a hemorrhagic base. Scratching, however, invariably destroys the body of a mite. Itching and burning often persist for weeks. The rash is common on the ankles and areas where clothing obstructs the further wanderings of the mites. Repellents are useful for preventing chigger bites.

Many kinds of mites that are associated with peridomestic birds and rodents are particularly bothersome when they invade homes and bite people. In North America, the northern fowl mite, chicken mite, tropical rat mite, and house mouse mite normally feed on poultry, various songbirds, and small mammals and are abundant in and around their hosts' nests. After their natural hosts die or leave the nest, these mites frequently invade human habitations. Although the mites are rarely seen because of their small size, their bites can be painful and pruritic. Once confirmed as the cause of irritation, rodent- and bird-associated mites are best eliminated by excluding their hosts, removing the nests, and cleaning and treating the nesting area with appropriate acaricides. *Pyemotes* and other mites that infest grain, straw, cheese, hay, or other products occasionally produce similar episodes of rash and discomfort and may produce a unique dermatologic "comet sign" lesion—a paisley-shaped urticarial plaque.

Diagnosis of mite-induced dermatitides (including those caused by chiggers) relies on confirmation of the mite's identity or elicitation of a history of exposure to the mite's source. Oral antihistamines or topical steroids may suppress mite-induced pruritus temporarily but do not eliminate the mites.

TICK BITES AND TICK PARALYSIS

Ticks attach superficially to skin and feed painlessly; blood is their only food. Their salivary secretions are biologically active and can produce local reactions, induce fevers, and cause paralysis in addition to transmitting diverse pathogens. The two main families of ticks are the hard (*ixodid*) and soft (*argasid*) ticks. Generally, soft ticks attach for <1 h, leaving red macules after they drop off. Some species in Africa, the western United States, and Mexico produce painful hemorrhagic lesions. Hard ticks are much more common and transmit most of the tick-borne infections that are familiar to physicians and patients. Hard ticks attach to the host and feed for several days or sometimes for >1 week. At the site of hard-tick bites, small areas of induration, often purpuric, develop and may be surrounded by an erythematous rim. A necrotic eschar, called a *tâche noire*, occasionally develops. Chronic nodules (persistent tick-bite granulomas) can be several centimeters in diameter and may linger for months after the feeding tick has been removed. These granulomas can be treated with injected intralesional glucocorticoids or by surgical excision. Tick-induced fever, unassociated with transmission of any pathogen, is often accompanied by headache, nausea, and malaise but usually resolves ≤36 h after the tick is removed.

Tick paralysis, an acute ascending flaccid paralysis that resembles Guillain-Barré syndrome, is believed to be caused by one or more toxins in tick saliva that block neuromuscular transmission and decrease nerve conduction. This rare complication has followed the bites of more than 60 kinds of ticks, although in the United States dog and wood ticks (*Dermacentor* species) are most commonly involved. Weakness begins symmetrically in the lower extremities ≤6 days after the tick's attachment, ascends symmetrically during several days, and may culminate in complete paralysis of the extremities and cranial nerves. Deep tendon reflexes are diminished or absent, but sensory examination and findings on lumbar puncture are typically normal. Removal of the tick generally leads to rapid improvement within a few hours and complete recovery after several days, although the patient's condition may continue to deteriorate for a full day. Failure to remove the tick may lead to dysarthria, dysphagia, and ultimately death from aspiration or respiratory paralysis. Diagnosis depends on finding the tick, which is often hidden beneath scalp hair. An antiserum to the saliva of *Ixodes holocyclus*, the usual cause of tick paralysis in Australia, effectively reverses paralysis caused by these ticks.

Removal of hard ticks during the first 36 h of attachment nearly always prevents transmission of the agents of Lyme disease, babesiosis, anaplasmosis, and ehrlichiosis, although several tick-borne viruses may be transmitted more quickly. Ticks should be removed by traction with fine-tipped forceps placed firmly around the tick's mouthparts. Careful handling (to avoid rupture of ticks) and use of gloves may avert accidental contamination with pathogens contained in tick fluids. Use of occlusive dressings, heat, or other substances (in an attempt to induce the tick to detach) merely delay tick removal. Afterward, the site of attachment should be disinfected. Tick mouthparts sometimes remain in the skin but generally are shed spontaneously within days without excision. Although somewhat controversial, current guidelines from the Centers for Disease Control and Prevention suggest that, rather than awaiting the onset of erythema migrans, the results of tick testing, or seroconversion to antigens diagnostic for Lyme disease, administering prophylaxis with a single oral dose of doxycycline (200 mg) within 72 h of tick removal is appropriate in adult patients with bites thought to be associated with deer ticks (Fig. 475-1) in Lyme disease–endemic areas from Maryland to Maine and in Wisconsin and Minnesota.

LOUSE INFESTATION (PEDICULIASIS AND PTHIRIASIS)

Nymphs and adults of all three kinds of human lice feed at least once a day, ingesting human blood exclusively. Head lice (*Pediculus capitis*) infest mainly the hair of the scalp, body lice (*Pediculus humanus*) the clothing, and crab or pubic lice (*Pthirus pubis*) mainly the hair of the pubis. The saliva of lice produces a pruritic morbilliform or urticarial rash in some sensitized persons. Female head and pubic lice cement their eggs (nits) firmly to hair, whereas female body lice cement their eggs to clothing, particularly to threads along clothing seams. After ~10 days of development within the egg, a nymph hatches. Empty eggs may remain affixed for months thereafter.

In North America, head lice infest ~1% of elementary school-age children. Head lice are transmitted mainly by direct head-to-head contact rather than by fomites such as shared headgear, bed linens, hairbrushes, and other grooming implements. Chronic infestations by head lice tend to be asymptomatic. Pruritus, due mainly to hypersensitivity to the louse's saliva, generally is transient and mild. Head lice

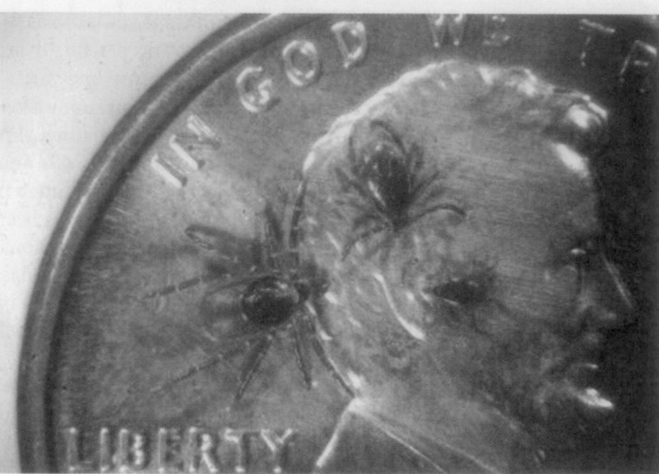

FIGURE 475-1 Deer ticks (*Ixodes scapularis*, black-legged ticks) on a U.S. penny: larva (*below ear*), nymph (*right*), adult male (*above*), and adult female (*left*).

removed from a person succumb to desiccation and starvation within ~1 day. Head lice are not known to serve as a natural vector for any pathogens.

Body lice remain on clothing except when feeding and generally succumb in ≤2 days if separated from their host. In most Western countries, body lice are generally found on a small proportion of indigent persons but may become increasingly prevalent after upheaval associated with natural or human-caused disasters, when homeless victims are in close contact with infested individuals with whom they share accommodations. Body lice are acquired by direct contact or by sharing of infested clothing and bedding. These lice are vectors for the agents of louse-borne (epidemic) typhus (Chap. 211), louse-borne relapsing fever (Chap. 209), and trench fever (Chap. 197). Pruritic lesions from their bites are particularly common around the neckline. Chronic infestations result in a postinflammatory hyperpigmentation and thickening of skin known as *vagabond's disease*.

The crab or pubic louse is transmitted mainly by sexual contact. These lice occur predominantly on pubic hair and less frequently on axillary or facial hair, including the eyelashes. Children and adults may acquire pubic lice by sexual or close nonsexual contact. Intensely pruritic, bluish macules ~3 mm in diameter (*maculae ceruleae*) develop at the site of bites. Blepharitis commonly accompanies infestations of the eyelashes.

Pediculiasis is often suspected upon the detection of nits firmly cemented to hairs or in clothing. Many bona fide nits, however, are dead or hatched relics of prior infestation, and pseudo-nits are frequently misconstrued to be signs of a louse infestation. Confirmation of a louse infestation, therefore, best relies on the discovery of a live louse.

TREATMENT LOUSE INFESTATION

Generally, treatment is warranted only if live lice are discovered. The presence of nits alone is evidence of a former—not necessarily current—infestation. Mechanical removal of lice and their eggs with a fine-toothed louse or nit comb (Fig. 475-2) often fails to eliminate infestations. Treatment of newly identified active infestations generally relies on a 10-min topical application of ~1% permethrin or pyrethrins, with a second application ~10 days later. Lice persisting after this treatment may be resistant to pyrethroids. Chronic infestations may be treated for ≤12 h with 0.5% malathion. Lindane is applied for just 4 min but seems less effective and may pose a greater risk of adverse reactions, particularly when misused. Resistance of head lice to permethrin, malathion, and lindane has been reported. Newer FDA-approved topical pediculicides contain benzyl alcohol, dimethicone, spinosad, and ivermectin. Although children infested by head lice—or those who simply have remnant nits from a prior infestation—are frequently isolated or excluded

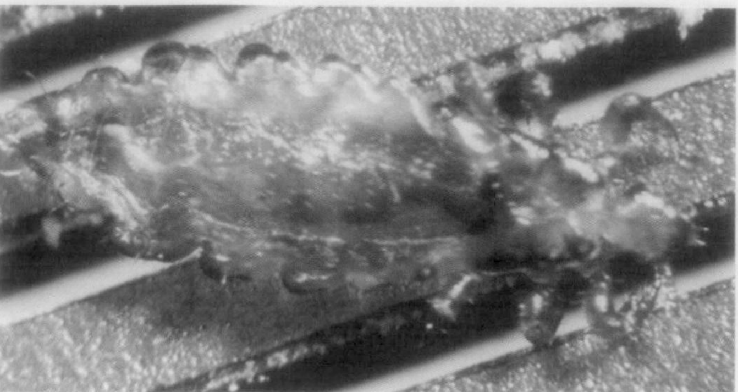

FIGURE 475-2 Adult female human head louse (*Pediculus capitis*) on a nit (louse-egg) comb.

from school, this practice increasingly is seen as unjustified and ineffective.

Body lice usually are eliminated by bathing and by changing to laundered clothes. Application of topical pediculicides from head to foot may be necessary for hirsute patients. Clothes and bedding are effectively deloused by heating in a clothes dryer at ≥55°C (≥131°F) for 30 min or by heat-pressing. Emergency mass delousing of persons and clothing may be warranted during periods of civil strife and after natural disasters to reduce the risk of pathogen transmission by body lice.

Pubic louse infestations are treated with topical pediculicides, except for eyelid infestations (*pthiriasis palpebrum*), which generally respond to a coating of petrolatum applied for 3–4 days.

MYIASIS (FLY INFESTATION)

Myiasis refers to infestations by several kinds of fly larvae (maggots) that invade living or necrotic tissues or body cavities and produce different clinical syndromes, depending on the species of fly.

In forested parts of Central and South America, larvae of the human botfly (*Dermatobia hominis*) produce furuncular (boil-like) papules or subcutaneous nodules ≤3 cm in diameter. A gravid adult female botfly captures a mosquito or another bloodsucking insect and deposits her eggs on its abdomen. When the carrier insect attacks a human or bovine host several days later, the warmth and moisture of the host's skin stimulate the eggs to hatch. The emerging larvae promptly penetrate intact skin. After 6–12 weeks of development, mature larvae emerge from the skin and drop to the ground to pupate and then become adults.

The African tumbu fly (*Cordylobia anthropophaga*) deposits its eggs on damp sand or leaf litter or on drying laundry, particularly that contaminated by urine or sweat. Larvae hatch from eggs upon contact with a host's body and penetrate the skin, producing boil-like lesions from which mature larvae emerge ~9 days later. Furuncular myiasis is suggested by uncomfortable lesions with a central breathing pore that emits bubbles when submerged in water. A sensation of movement under the patient's skin may cause severe emotional distress.

Larvae that cause furuncular myiasis may be induced to emerge if the air pore is coated with petrolatum or another occlusive substance. Removal may be facilitated by injection of a local anesthetic into the surrounding tissue, but surgical excision is sometimes necessary because upward-pointing spines of some species hold the larvae firmly in place.

Other fly larvae cause nonfuruncular myiasis. For example, larvae of the horse botfly (*Gasterophilus intestinalis*) emerge from eggs deposited on the horse's flanks and may come into contact with and infest human beings. After penetrating human skin, these larvae rarely mature but instead may migrate for weeks in the dermis. The resulting pruritic and serpiginous eruption resembles cutaneous larva migrans caused by canine or feline hookworms (Chap. 256). Larvae of rabbit and rodent botflies (*Cuterebra* species) occasionally cause dermal or tracheopulmonary myiasis.

Certain flies are attracted to blood and pus, laying their eggs on open or draining sores. Newly hatched larvae enter wounds or diseased skin. Larvae of several types of green bottle flies (*Lucilia/Phaenicia* species) usually remain superficial and confined to necrotic tissue. Specially raised, sterile "surgical maggots" are sometimes used intentionally for wound debridement. Larvae of screwworm flies, *Cochliomyia*, and the flesh fly invade viable tissues more deeply and produce large suppurating lesions. Larvae that infest wounds also may enter body cavities such as the mouth, nose, ears, sinuses, anus, vagina, and lower urinary tract, particularly in unconscious or otherwise debilitated patients. The consequences range from harmless colonization to destruction of the nose, meningitis, and deafness. Treatment involves removal of maggots and debridement of tissue.

The maggots responsible for furuncular and wound myiasis also may cause ophthalmomyiasis. Sequelae include nodules in the eyelid, retinal detachment, and destruction of the globe. Most instances in which maggots are found in human feces result from deposition of eggs or larvae by flies on recently passed stools, not from an intestinal maggot infestation.

PENTASTOMIASIS

Pentastomids (tongue worms) inhabit the respiratory passages of reptiles and carnivorous mammals. Human infestation by *Linguatula serrata* is common in the Middle East and results from the consumption of encysted larval stages in raw liver or lymph nodes of sheep and goats, which are true intermediate hosts for the tongue worms. Larvae migrate to the nasopharynx and produce an acute self-limiting syndrome—known as *halzoun* or *marrara*—characterized by pain and itching of the throat and ears, coughing, hoarseness, dysphagia, and dyspnea. Severe edema may cause obstruction that requires tracheostomy. In addition, ocular invasion has been described. Diagnostic larvae measuring ≤10 mm in length appear in copious nasal discharge or vomitus. Individuals become infected with another type of tongue worm, *Armillifer armillatus*, by consuming its eggs in contaminated food or drink or after handling the definitive host, the African python. Larvae encyst in various organs but rarely cause symptoms. Cysts may require surgical removal as they enlarge during molting, but they usually are encountered as an incidental finding at autopsy. Parasite-induced lesions may be misinterpreted as a malignancy, with the correct diagnosis confirmed histopathologically. Cutaneous larva migrans–type syndromes of other pentastomes have been reported from Southeast Asia and Central America.

LEECH INFESTATIONS

Medically important leeches are annelid worms that attach to their hosts with chitinous cutting jaws and draw blood through muscular suckers. The medicinal leech (*Hirudo medicinalis*) is still used occasionally for medical purposes to reduce venous congestion in surgical flaps or replanted body parts. This practice has been complicated by intractable bleeding, wound infections, myonecrosis, and sepsis due to *Aeromonas hydrophila*, which colonizes the gullets of commercially available leeches.

Ubiquitous aquatic leeches that parasitize fish, frogs, and turtles readily attach to the skin of human beings and avidly suck blood. More notorious are arboreal land leeches that live among moist vegetation of tropical rain forests. Attachment is usually painless, and the leeches will detach themselves when satiated with a blood meal. Hirudin, a powerful anticoagulant secreted by the leech, causes continued bleeding after the leech has detached. Healing of a leech-bite wound is slow, and bacterial infections are not uncommon. Several kinds of aquatic leeches in Africa, Asia, and southern Europe can enter the mouth, nose, and genitourinary tract and attach to mucosal surfaces at sites as deep as the esophagus and trachea. Externally attached leeches generally drop off after they have engorged, but removal is hastened by gentle scraping aside of the anterior and posterior suckers the leech uses for attachment and feeding. Some authorities dispute the wisdom of removing leeches with alcohol, salt, vinegar, insect repellent, a flame or heated instrument, or applications of other noxious substances. Internally attached leeches may detach on exposure to gargled saline or may be removed by forceps.

SPIDER BITES

Of the more than 30,000 recognized species of spiders, only ~100 defend themselves aggressively and have fangs sufficiently long to penetrate human skin. The venom that some spiders use to immobilize and digest their prey can cause necrosis of skin and systemic toxicity. Whereas the bites of most spiders are painful but not harmful, envenomations by recluse or fiddleback spiders (*Loxosceles* species) and widow spiders (*Latrodectus* species) may be life-threatening. Identification of the offending spider is important because specific treatments exist for bites of widow spiders and because injuries attributed to spiders are frequently due to other causes. Except in cases where the patient actually observes a spider immediately associated with the bite or fleeing from the site, lesions reported as spider-bite reactions are most often due to other injuries or to infections with bacteria such as methicillin-resistant *Staphylococcus aureus* (MRSA).

Recluse Spider Bites and Necrotic Arachnidism Brown recluse spiders live mainly in the south-central United States and have close relatives in Central and South America, Africa, and the Middle East. Bites by brown recluse spiders usually cause only minor injuries, with edema and erythema. Envenomation, however, occasionally causes severe necrosis of skin and subcutaneous tissue and more rarely causes systemic hemolysis. These spiders are not aggressive toward humans and will bite only if threatened or pressed against the skin. They hide under rocks and logs or in caves and animal burrows. They invade homes and seek dark and undisturbed hiding spots in closets, in folds of clothing, or under furniture and rubbish in storage rooms, garages, and attics. Despite their impressive abundance in some homes, these spiders rarely bite humans. Bites tend to occur while the victim is dressing and are sustained primarily on the hands, arms, neck, and lower abdomen.

Initially, the bite is painless or may produce a stinging sensation. Within the next few hours, the site becomes painful and pruritic, with central induration surrounded by a pale ischemic zone that itself is encircled by a zone of erythema. In most cases, the lesion resolves without treatment in just a few days. In severe cases, the erythema spreads, and the center of the lesion becomes hemorrhagic or necrotic with an overlying bulla. A black eschar forms and sloughs several weeks later, leaving an ulcer that eventually may create a depressed scar. Healing usually takes place in ≤6 months but may take as long as 3 years if adipose tissue is involved. Local complications include injury to nerves and secondary bacterial infection. Fever, chills, weakness, headache, nausea, vomiting, myalgia, arthralgia, maculopapular rash, and leukocytosis may develop ≤72 h after the bite. Reports of deaths attributed to bites of North American brown recluse spiders have not been verified.

TREATMENT RECLUSE SPIDER BITES

Initial management includes RICE (rest, ice, compression, elevation). Analgesics, antihistamines, antibiotics, and tetanus prophylaxis should be administered if indicated. Early debridement or surgical excision of the wound without closure delays healing. Routine use of antibiotics or dapsone is unnecessary. Patients should be monitored closely for signs of hemolysis, renal failure, and other systemic complications.

Widow Spider Bites The black widow spider, common in the southeastern United States, measures ≤1 cm in body length and 5 cm in leg span and is shiny black with a red hourglass marking on the ventral abdomen. Other dangerous *Latrodectus* species occur elsewhere in temperate and subtropical parts of the world. The bites of the female widow spiders are notorious for their potent neurotoxins.

Widow spiders spin their webs under stones, logs, plants, or rock piles and in dark spaces in barns, garages, and outhouses. Bites are most common in the summer and early autumn and occur when a web is disturbed or a spider is trapped or provoked. The initial bite is perceived as a sharp pinprick or may go unnoticed. Fang-puncture marks are uncommon. The venom that is injected does not produce local necrosis, and some persons experience no other symptoms. α-Latrotoxin, the most active component of the venom, binds irreversibly to presynaptic nerve terminals and causes release and eventual depletion of acetylcholine, norepinephrine, and other neurotransmitters from those terminals. Painful cramps may spread within 60 min from the bite site to large muscles of the extremities and trunk. Extreme rigidity of the abdominal muscles and excruciating pain may suggest peritonitis, but the abdomen is not tender on palpation and surgery is not warranted. The pain begins to subside during the first 12 h but may recur during several days or weeks before resolving spontaneously. A wide range of other neurologic sequelae may include salivation, diaphoresis, vomiting, hypertension, tachycardia, labored breathing, anxiety, headache, weakness, fasciculations, paresthesia, hyperreflexia, urinary retention, uterine contractions, and premature labor. Rhabdomyolysis and renal failure have been reported, and respiratory arrest, cerebral hemorrhage, or cardiac failure may end fatally, especially in very young, elderly, or debilitated persons.

TREATMENT WIDOW SPIDER BITES

Treatment consists of RICE and tetanus prophylaxis. Hypertension that does not respond to analgesics and antispasmodics (e.g., benzodiazepines or methocarbamol) requires specific antihypertensive medication. The efficacy and safety of antivenoms for black widow and redback spiders are controversial because of concerns about potential anaphylaxis or serum sickness.

Tarantulas and Other Spiders Tarantulas are hairy spiders of which 30 species are found in the United States, mainly in the Southwest. The tarantulas that have become popular household pets are usually imported from Central or South America. Tarantulas bite only when threatened and usually cause no more harm than a bee sting, but on occasion the venom causes deep pain and swelling. Several species of tarantulas are covered with urticating hairs that are brushed off in the thousands when a threatened spider rubs its hind legs across its dorsal abdomen. These hairs can penetrate human skin and produce pruritic papules that may persist for weeks. Failure to wear gloves or to wash the hands after handling the Chilean Rose tarantula, a popular pet spider, has resulted in transfer of hairs to the eye with subsequent devastating ocular inflammation. Treatment of bites includes local washing and elevation of the bitten area, tetanus prophylaxis, and analgesic administration. Antihistamines and topical or systemic glucocorticoids are given for exposure to urticating hairs.

Atrax robustus, a funnel-web spider of Australia, and *Phoneutria* species, the South American banana spiders, are among the most dangerous spiders in the world because of their aggressive behavior and potent neurotoxins. Envenomation by *A. robustus* causes a rapidly progressive neuromotor syndrome that can be fatal within 2 h. The bite of a banana spider causes severe local pain followed by profound systemic symptoms and respiratory paralysis that can lead to death within 2–6 h. Specific antivenoms for use after bites by each of these spiders are available. Yellow sac spiders (*Cheiracanthium* species) are common in homes worldwide. Their bites, though painful, generally lead to only minor erythema, edema, and pruritus.

SCORPION STINGS

Scorpions are arachnids that feed on ground-dwelling arthropods and small lizards. They paralyze their prey and defend themselves by injecting venom from a stinger on the tip of the tail. Painful but relatively harmless scorpion stings need to be distinguished from the potentially lethal envenomations that are produced by ~30 of the ~1000 known species and that cause more than 5000 deaths worldwide each year. Scorpions are nocturnal and remain hidden during the day in crevices or burrows or under wood, loose bark, or rocks. They occasionally enter houses and tents and may hide in shoes, clothing, or bedding. Scorpions sting humans only when threatened.

Of the 40 or so scorpion species in the United States, only bark scorpions—e.g., *Centruroides sculpturatus* (*C. exilicauda*) in the Southwest—produce venom that is potentially lethal to humans. This venom contains neurotoxins that cause sodium channels to remain open. Such envenomations usually are associated with little swelling, but prominent pain, paresthesia, and hyperesthesia can be accentuated by tapping on the affected area (the *tap test*). These symptoms soon spread to other locations; dysfunction of cranial nerves and hyperexcitability of skeletal muscles develop within hours. Patients present with restlessness, blurred vision, abnormal eye movements, profuse salivation, lacrimation, rhinorrhea, slurred speech, difficulty in handling secretions, diaphoresis, nausea, and vomiting. Muscle twitching, jerking, and shaking may be mistaken for a seizure. Complications include tachycardia, arrhythmias, hypertension, hyperthermia, rhabdomyolysis, and acidosis. Symptoms progress to maximal severity in ~5 h and subside within a day or two, although pain and paresthesia can last for weeks. Fatal respiratory arrest is most common among young children and the elderly.

Envenomations by *Leiurus quinquestriatus* in the Middle East and North Africa, by *Mesobuthus tamulus* in India, by *Androctonus* species along the Mediterranean littoral and in North Africa and the Middle East, and by *Tityus serrulatus* in Brazil cause massive release of endogenous catecholamines with hypertensive crises, arrhythmias, pulmonary edema, and myocardial damage. Acute pancreatitis occurs with stings of *Tityus trinitatis* in Trinidad, and central nervous toxicity complicates stings of *Parabuthus* and *Buthotus* scorpions of South Africa. Tissue necrosis and hemolysis may follow stings of the Iranian *Hemiscorpius lepturus*.

Stings of most other species cause immediate sharp local pain followed by edema, ecchymosis, and a burning sensation. Symptoms typically resolve within a few hours, and skin does not slough. Allergic reactions to the venom sometimes develop.

TREATMENT SCORPION STINGS

Identification of the offending scorpion helps to determine the course of treatment. Stings of nonlethal species require at most ice packs, analgesics, or antihistamines. Because most victims experience only local discomfort, they can be managed at home with instructions to return to the emergency department if signs of cranial-nerve or neuromuscular dysfunction develop. Aggressive supportive care and judicious use of antivenom can reduce or eliminate deaths from more severe envenomations. Keeping the patient calm and applying pressure dressings and cold packs to the sting site are measures that decrease the absorption of venom. A continuous IV infusion of midazolam controls the agitation, flailing, and involuntary muscle movements produced by scorpion stings. Close monitoring during treatment with this drug and other sedatives or narcotics is necessary for persons with neuromuscular symptoms because of the risk of respiratory arrest. Hypertension and pulmonary edema respond to nifedipine, nitroprusside, hydralazine, or prazosin. Dangerous bradyarrhythmias can be controlled with atropine.

Commercially prepared antivenoms are available in several countries for some of the most dangerous species. An FDA-approved *C. sculpturatus* antivenom in horse serum is now available. IV administration of antivenom rapidly reverses cranial-nerve dysfunction and muscular symptoms. Although effective, cost analyses suggest that antivenoms should be reserved for only the most severe envenomations.

HYMENOPTERA STINGS

Insects that sting in defense or to subdue their prey belong to the order Hymenoptera, which includes bees, wasps, hornets, yellow jackets, and ants. Their venoms contain a wide array of amines, peptides, and enzymes that cause local and systemic reactions. Although the toxic effect of multiple stings can be fatal to a human, nearly all of the ≥100 deaths due to hymenopteran stings in the United States each year result from allergic reactions.

Bee and Wasp Stings The stinger of the honeybee (*Apis mellifera*) is unique in being barbed. When a bee stings a foe, its stinging apparatus and attached venom sac tear loose from its body. Muscular contraction of the venom sac continues to inject venom into the skin. Other kinds of bees, ants, and wasps have smooth stinging mechanisms and can sting numerous times in succession. Honeybees, bumblebees, and social wasps generally attack only when a colony is disturbed. Africanized honeybees (now present in South and Central America and the southern and western United States) respond to minimal intrusions more aggressively. Whereas the sting of an Africanized bee contains less venom than that of its non-Africanized relatives, victims tend to sustain far more stings and therefore to receive a far greater overall volume of venom. Most patients who report having sustained a "bee sting," however, are more likely to have encountered stinging wasps instead.

The venoms of different species of hymenopterans are biochemically and immunologically distinct. Direct toxic effects are mediated by mixtures of low-molecular-weight compounds such as serotonin, histamine, acetylcholine, and several kinins. Polypeptide toxins in honeybee venom include mellitin that damages cell membranes, mast cell–degranulating protein that causes histamine release, the neurotoxin apamin, and the anti-inflammatory compound adolapin. Enzymes in venom include hyaluronidase and phospholipases. There appears to be little cross-sensitization between the venoms of honeybees and wasps.

Uncomplicated hymenopteran stings cause immediate pain, a wheal-and-flare reaction, and local edema, all of which usually subside in a few hours. Multiple stings can lead to vomiting, diarrhea, generalized edema, dyspnea, hypotension, and non-anaphylactic circulatory collapse. Rhabdomyolysis and intravascular hemolysis may cause renal failure. Death from the direct (nonallergic) effects of venom has followed stings of several hundred honeybees. Stings to the tongue or mouth may induce life-threatening edema of the upper airways.

Large local reactions accompanied by erythema, edema, warmth, and tenderness that spread ≥10 cm around the sting site over 1–2 days are not uncommon. These reactions may resemble bacterial cellulitis but are caused by hypersensitivity rather than by secondary infection. Such reactions tend to recur on subsequent exposure but are seldom accompanied by anaphylaxis and are not prevented by venom immunotherapy.

An estimated 0.4–4.0% of the U.S. population exhibits clinical immediate-type hypersensitivity to hymenopteran stings, and 15% may have asymptomatic sensitization manifested by positive skin tests. Persons who experience severe allergic reactions are likely to have similar reactions after subsequent stings by the same or closely related species. Occasionally, persons who have had mild reactions earlier in life will experience more serious reactions to subsequent stings. Mild anaphylactic reactions from insect stings, as from other causes, consist of nausea, abdominal cramping, generalized urticaria, flushing, and angioedema. Serious reactions, including upper airway edema, bronchospasm, hypotension, and shock, may be rapidly fatal. Severe reactions usually begin within 10 min of the sting and only rarely develop after 5 h.

TREATMENT BEE AND WASP STINGS

Honeybee stingers embedded in the skin should be removed as soon as possible to limit the quantity of venom delivered. The stinger and venom sac may be scraped off with a blade, the edge of a credit card, or a fingernail or may be removed with forceps. The site should be cleansed and disinfected and ice packs applied to slow the spread of venom. Elevation of the affected site and administration of analgesics, oral antihistamines, and topical calamine lotion help relieve symptoms. Large local reactions may require a short course of oral therapy with glucocorticoids. Patients with numerous stings should be monitored for 24 h for evidence of renal failure or coagulopathy.

Anaphylaxis is treated with SC injection of 0.3–0.5 mL of epinephrine hydrochloride in a 1:1000 dilution; treatment is repeated every 20–30 min as necessary. IV epinephrine (2–5 mL of a 1:10,000 solution administered by slow push) is indicated for profound shock. A tourniquet may slow the spread of venom. Parenteral antihistamines, fluid resuscitation, bronchodilators, supplemental oxygen, intubation, and vasopressors may be required. Patients should be observed for 24 h for recurrent anaphylaxis.

Persons with a history of allergy to insect stings should carry an anaphylaxis kit with a preloaded syringe containing epinephrine for self-administration. These patients should seek medical attention immediately after using the kit.

Repeated injections of purified venom produce a blocking IgG antibody response to venom and reduce the incidence of recurrent anaphylaxis. Honeybee, wasp, and yellow jacket venoms are commercially available for desensitization and for skin testing. Results of skin tests and venom-specific radioallergosorbent tests (RASTs) aid in the selection of patients for immunotherapy and guide the design of such treatment.

STINGING ANTS

Stinging fire ants are an important medical problem in the United States. Imported fire ants (*Solenopsis* species) infest southern states from Texas to North Carolina, with colonies now established in California, New Mexico, Arizona, and Virginia. Slight disturbances of their mound nests have provoked massive outpourings of ants and as many as 10,000 stings on a single person. Elderly and immobile persons are at high risk for attacks when fire ants invade dwellings.

Fire ants attach to skin with powerful mandibles and rotate their bodies while repeatedly injecting venom with posteriorly situated stingers. The alkaloid venom consists of cytotoxic and hemolytic piperidines and several proteins with enzymatic activity. The initial wheal-and-flare reaction, burning, and itching resolve in ~30 min, and a sterile pustule develops within 24 h. The pustule ulcerates over the next 48 h and then heals in ≥1 week. Large areas of erythema and edema lasting several days are not uncommon and in extreme cases may compress nerves and blood vessels. Anaphylaxis occurs in fewer than 2% of victims; seizures and mononeuritis have been reported. Stings are treated with ice packs, topical glucocorticoids, and oral antihistamines. Pustules should be cleansed and then covered with bandages and antibiotic ointment to prevent bacterial infection. Epinephrine administration and supportive measures are indicated for anaphylactic reactions. Fire ant whole-body extracts are available for skin testing and immunotherapy, which appears to lower the rate of anaphylactic reactions.

European fire (red) ants (*Myrmica rubra*) have recently become public health pests in the northeastern United States and southern Canada. The western United States is home to harvester ants (*Pogonomyrmex* species). The painful local reaction that follows harvester ant stings often extends to lymph nodes and may be accompanied by anaphylaxis. The bullet or conga ant (*Paraponera clavata*) of South America is known locally as *hormiga veinticuatro* ("24-hour ant"), a designation that refers to the 24 h of throbbing, excruciating pain following a sting that delivers the potent paralyzing neurotoxin poneratoxin.

DIPTERAN (FLY AND MOSQUITO) BITES

In the process of feeding on vertebrate blood and tissue fluids, adults of certain flies inflict painful bites, produce local allergic reactions, and may transmit pathogenic agents. Bites of mosquitoes, tiny "no-see-um" (ceratopogonid) midges, and phlebotomine sand flies typically produce a wheal and a pruritic papule. Small humpbacked black flies (simuliids) lacerate skin, resulting in a lesion with serosanguineous discharge that is often painful and pruritic. Regional lymphadenopathy, fever, or anaphylaxis occasionally ensues. The widely distributed deerflies and horseflies as well as the tsetse flies of Africa are stout flies measuring ≤25 mm in length that attack during the day and produce large and painful bleeding punctures. Houseflies (*Musca domestica*) do not consume blood but use rasping mouthparts to scarify skin and feed upon tissue fluids and salt. Beyond direct injury from bites of any kind of fly, risks include transmission of diverse pathogens and secondary infection of the lesion.

TREATMENT FLY AND MOSQUITO BITES

Treatment of fly bites is symptom based. Topical application of antipruritic agents, glucocorticoids, or antiseptic lotions may relieve itching and pain. Allergic reactions may require oral antihistamines. Antibiotics may be necessary for the treatment of large bite wounds that become secondarily infected.

FLEA BITES

Common human-biting fleas include the dog and cat fleas (*Ctenocephalides* species) and the rat flea (*Xenopsylla cheopis*), which infest their respective hosts and the hosts' nests and resting sites. Sensitized persons develop erythematous pruritic papules (*papular urticaria*) and occasionally vesicles and bacterial superinfection at the site of the bite. Symptom-based treatment consists of antihistamines, topical glucocorticoids, and topical antipruritic agents.

Flea infestations are eliminated by removal and treatment of animal nests, frequent cleaning of pet bedding, and application of contact and systemic insecticides to pets and the dwelling. Flea infestations in the home may be abated or prevented if pets are regularly treated with veterinary antiparasitic agents and insect growth regulators.

Tunga penetrans, like other fleas, is a wingless, laterally flattened insect that feeds on blood. Also known as the chigoe flea, sand flea, or jigger (not to be confused with the chigger), it occurs in tropical regions of Africa and the Americas. Adult female chigoes live in sandy soil and burrow under the skin, usually between toes, under nails, or on the soles of bare feet. Gravid chigoes engorge on the host's blood and grow from pinpoint to pea size during a 2-week interval. They produce lesions that resemble a white pustule with a central black depression and that may be pruritic or painful. Occasional complications include tetanus, bacterial infections, and autoamputation of toes (*ainhum*). Tungiasis is treated by removal of the intact flea with a sterile needle or scalpel, tetanus vaccination, and topical application of antibiotics.

HEMIPTERAN (TRUE BUG) BITES

Several true bugs of the family Reduviidae inflict bites that produce allergic reactions and are sometimes painful. The cone-nose bugs, so called because of their elongated heads, include the assassin and wheel bugs, which feed on other insects and bite vertebrates only in self-defense, and the kissing bugs, which routinely feed on vertebrate blood. The bites of the night-feeding kissing bugs are painless. Reactions to such bites depend on prior sensitization and include tender and pruritic papules, vesicular or bullous lesions, extensive urticaria, fever, lymphadenopathy, and (rarely) anaphylaxis. Bug bites are treated with topical antipruritics or oral antihistamines. Persons with anaphylactic reactions to reduviid bites should keep an epinephrine kit available. Some reduviids transmit *Trypanosoma cruzi*, the agent of New World trypanosomiasis (also called *Chagas disease*) (Chap. 252).

The cosmopolitan bedbugs (*Cimex* species) hide in crevices of mattresses, bed frames and other furniture, walls, and picture frames and under loose wallpaper. Bedbug populations have resurged, recently attaining levels and spreading to an extent not encountered since the mid-twentieth century. These bugs are now a common pest in homes, dormitories, and hotels; on cruise ships; and even in medical facilities. Generally, the bugs hide during the day and take blood meals at night. Their bite is painless, but minutes to days later, sensitized persons develop erythema, itching, and wheals around a central hemorrhagic punctum. Bedbugs are not known to transmit pathogens.

CENTIPEDE BITES AND MILLIPEDE DERMATITIS

The fangs of centipedes of the genus *Scolopendra* can penetrate human skin and deliver a venom that produces intense burning pain, swelling, erythema, and sterile lymphangitis. Dizziness, nausea, and anxiety are described occasionally, and rhabdomyolysis and renal failure have been reported. Treatment includes washing of the site, application of cold dressings, oral analgesic administration or local lidocaine infiltration, and tetanus prophylaxis.

Millipedes are docile and do not bite, but some secrete defensive fluids that may burn and discolor human skin. Affected skin turns brown overnight and may blister and exfoliate. Secretions in the eye cause intense pain and inflammation that can result in corneal ulcers and even blindness. Management includes irrigation with copious amounts of water or saline, use of analgesics, and local care of denuded skin.

CATERPILLAR STINGS AND DERMATITIS

Caterpillars of several moth species are covered with hairs or spines that produce mechanical irritation and may contain or be coated with venom. Contact with these caterpillars or their hairs may lead to lepidopterism or caterpillar envenomation. The response typically consists of an immediate burning sensation followed by local swelling and erythema and occasionally by regional lymphadenopathy, nausea, vomiting, and headache. A rare reaction to a South American caterpillar, *Lonomia obliqua*, can cause disseminated coagulopathy and fatal hemorrhagic shock. In the United States, dermatitis is most often associated with caterpillars of the io, puss, saddleback, and brown-tail moths. Even contact with detached hairs of other caterpillars, such as gypsy moth larvae, can later produce a pruritic urticarial or papular rash called *erucism*. Spines may be deposited on tree trunks or drying laundry or may be airborne and cause irritation of the eyes and upper airways. Treatment of caterpillar stings consists of repeated application of adhesive or cellophane tape to remove the hairs, which can then be identified microscopically. Local ice packs, topical glucocorticoids, and oral antihistamines relieve symptoms.

BEETLE VESICATION AND DERMITITIS

Several families of beetles have independently developed the ability to produce chemically unrelated vesicating toxins. When disturbed, blister beetles (family Meloidae) extrude cantharidin, a low-molecular-weight toxin that produces thin-walled blisters (≤5 cm in diameter) 2–5 h after contact. The blisters are not painful or pruritic unless broken and resolve without treatment in ≤10 days. Nephritis may follow unusually heavy cantharidin exposure. Contact occurs when individuals sit on the ground, work in the garden, or deliberately handle the beetles. The hemolymph of certain rove beetles (Staphylinidae) contains pederin, a potent vesicant. When these beetles are crushed or brushed against the skin, the released fluid causes painful, red, flaccid bullae. These beetles occur worldwide but are most numerous and problematic in parts of Africa (where they are called "Nairobi fly") and southwestern Asia. Ocular lesions may develop after impact with flying beetles at night or unintentional transfer of the vesicant on the fingers. Treatment is rarely necessary, although ruptured blisters should be kept clean and bandaged.

Larvae of common carpet beetles are adorned with dense arrays of ornate hairs called *hastisetae*. Contact with these larvae or their setae results in delayed dermal reactions in sensitized individuals. The lesions are commonly mistaken as bites of bedbugs.

DELUSIONAL INFESTATIONS

The groundless conviction that one is infested with arthropods or other parasites (Ekbom's syndrome, delusory parasitosis, delusions of parasitosis, and perhaps Morgellons syndrome) is extremely difficult to treat and, unfortunately, is not uncommon. Patients describe uncomfortable sensations of something moving in or on their skin. Excoriations and self-induced ulcerations typically accompany the pruritus, dysesthesias, and imaginary insect bites. Patients often believe that some invisible or as yet undescribed creatures are infesting their skin, clothing, homes, or environment in general. Frequently, patients submit as evidence of infestation specimens that consist of plant-feeding and nonbiting peridomestic arthropods, pieces of skin, vegetable matter, lint, and other inanimate detritus. When evaluating a patient with possible delusional parasitosis, it is imperative to rule out true infestations and bites by arthropods, endocrinopathies, sensory disorders due to neuropathies, opiate and other drug use, environmental irritants (e.g., fiberglass threads), and other causes of tingling or prickling sensations. Frequently, such patients repeatedly seek medical consultations, resist alternative explanations for their symptoms, and exacerbate their discomfort by self-treatment. Long-term pharmacotherapy with pimozide or other psychotropic agents has been more helpful than psychotherapy in treating this disorder. Patients with delusional parasitosis often develop the unshakeable conviction that they are infested by a previously unknown pathogen, while their personal lives, family support, and employment collapse around them.

Acknowledgment

The substantial contributions of Andrew Spielman and James H. Maguire to this chapter in previous editions are gratefully acknowledged.

476e Altitude Illness

Buddha Basnyat, Geoffrey Tabin

This is a digital-only chapter. It is available on the DVD that accompanies this book, as well as on Access Medicine/Harrison's Online, and the eBook and "app" editions of HPIM 19e.

EPIDEMIOLOGY

Mountains cover one-fifth of the earth's surface; 38 million people live permanently at altitudes ≥2400 m, and 100 million people travel to high-altitude locations each year. Skiers in the Alps or Aspen; religious pilgrims to Lhasa or Kailash; trekkers and climbers to Kilimanjaro, Aconcagua, or Everest; and military personnel deployed to high-altitude locations are all at risk of developing acute mountain sickness (AMS), high-altitude cerebral edema (HACE), high-altitude pulmonary edema (HAPE), and other altitude-related problems. AMS is the benign form of altitude illness, whereas HACE and HAPE are life-threatening. Altitude illness is likely to occur above 2500 m but has been documented even at 1500–2500 m. In the Mount Everest region of Nepal, ~50% of trekkers who walk to altitudes >4000 m over ≥5 days develop AMS, as do 84% of people who fly directly to 3860 m. The incidences of HACE and HAPE are much lower than that of AMS, with estimates in the range of 0.1–4%.

477e Hyperbaric and Diving Medicine

Michael H. Bennett, Simon J. Mitchell

This is a digital-only chapter. It is available on the DVD that accompanies this book, as well as on Access Medicine/Harrison's Online, and the eBook and "app" editions of HPIM 19e.

WHAT IS HYPERBARIC AND DIVING MEDICINE?

Hyperbaric medicine is the treatment of health disorders using whole-body exposure to pressures greater than 101.3 kPa (1 atmosphere or 760 mmHg). In practice, this almost always means the administration of *hyperbaric oxygen therapy* (HBO_2T). The Undersea and Hyperbaric Medical Society (UHMS) defines HBO_2T as: "a treatment in which a patient breathes 100% oxygen … while inside a treatment chamber at a pressure higher than sea level pressure (i.e., >1 atmosphere absolute or ATA)." The treatment chamber is an airtight vessel variously called a hyperbaric chamber, recompression chamber, or decompression chamber, depending on the clinical and historical context. Such chambers may be capable of compressing a single patient (a monoplace chamber) or multiple patients and attendants as required (a multiplace chamber). Historically, these compression chambers were first used for the treatment of divers and compressed air workers suffering decompression sickness (DCS; "the bends"). Although the prevention and treatment of disorders arising after decompression in diving, aviation, and space flight has developed into a specialized field of its own, it remains closely linked to the broader practice of hyperbaric medicine.

Despite an increased understanding of mechanisms and an improving evidence basis, hyperbaric medicine has struggled to achieve widespread recognition as a "legitimate" therapeutic measure. There are several contributing factors, but high among them are a poor grounding in general oxygen physiology and oxygen therapy at medical schools and a continuing tradition of charlatans advocating hyperbaric therapy (often using air) as a panacea. Funding for both basic and clinical research has been difficult in an environment where the pharmacologic agent under study is abundant, cheap, and unpatentable. Recently, however, there are signs of an improved appreciation of the potential importance of HBO_2T with significant National Institutes of Health (NIH) funding for mechanisms research and from the U.S. military for clinical investigation.

478e Hypothermia and Frostbite

Daniel F. Danzl

This is a digital-only chapter. It is available on the DVD that accompanies this book, as well as on Access Medicine/Harrison's Online, and the eBook and "app" editions of HPIM 19e.

HYPOTHERMIA

Accidental hypothermia occurs when there is an unintentional drop in the body's core temperature below 35°C (95°F). At this temperature, many of the compensatory physiologic mechanisms that conserve heat begin to fail. *Primary accidental hypothermia* is a result of the direct exposure of a previously healthy individual to the cold. The mortality rate is much higher for patients who develop *secondary hypothermia* as a complication of a serious systemic disorder.

479e Heat-Related Illnesses

Daniel F. Danzl

This is a digital-only chapter. It is available on the DVD that accompanies this book, as well as on Access Medicine/Harrison's Online, and the eBook and "app" editions of HPIM 19e.

Heat-related illnesses include a spectrum of disorders ranging from heat syncope, muscle cramps, and heat exhaustion to medical emergencies such as heatstroke. The core body temperature is normally maintained within a very narrow range. Although significant levels of hypothermia are tolerated (Chap. 478e), multiorgan dysfunction occurs rapidly at temperatures >41°–43°C. In contrast to severe hyperthermia, the far more common sign of fever reflects intact thermoregulation.

APPENDIX: Laboratory Values of Clinical Importance

Alexander Kratz, Michael A. Pesce, Robert C. Basner, Andrew J. Einstein

This Appendix contains tables of reference values for common laboratory tests. A variety of factors can influence reference values. Such variables include the population studied, the duration and means of specimen transport, laboratory methods and instrumentation, and even the type of container used for the collection of the specimen. The reference or "normal" ranges given in this appendix may therefore not be appropriate for all laboratories, and these values should only be used as general guidelines. Whenever possible, reference values provided by the laboratory performing the testing should be used in the interpretation of laboratory data. Values supplied in this Appendix reflect typical reference ranges in nonpregnant adults. Pediatric reference ranges and values in pregnant patients may vary significantly from the data presented in the Appendix.

In preparing the Appendix, the authors have taken into account the fact that the system of international units (SI, système international d'unités) is used in most countries and in some medical journals. However, clinical laboratories may continue to report values in "traditional" or conventional units. Therefore, both systems are provided in the Appendix. The dual system is also used in the text except for those instances in which the numbers remain the same and only the terminology is changed (mmol/L for meq/L or IU/L for mIU/mL), when only the SI units are given.

TABLE 1 HEMATOLOGY AND COAGULATION

Analyte	Specimen	SI Units	Conventional Units
Activated clotting time	WB	70–180 s	70–180 s
Activated protein C resistance (factor V Leiden)	P	Not applicable	Ratio >2.1
ADAMTS13 activity	P	≥0.67	≥67%
ADAMTS13 inhibitor activity	P	Not applicable	≤0.4 U
ADAMTS13 antibody	P	Not applicable	≤18 U
Alpha$_2$ antiplasmin	P	0.87–1.55	87–155%
Antiphospholipid antibody panel			
PTT-LA (lupus anticoagulant screen)	P	Negative	Negative
Platelet neutralization procedure	P	Negative	Negative
Dilute viper venom screen	P	Negative	Negative
Anticardiolipin antibody	S		
IgG		0–15 arbitrary units	0–15 GPL
IgM		0–15 arbitrary units	0–15 MPL
Beta-2 glycoprotein 1 antibodies	S		
IgG		0–20 arbitrary units	0–20 SGU
IgM		0–20 arbitrary units	0–20 SMU
Antithrombin III	P		
Antigenic		220–390 mg/L	22–39 mg/dL
Functional		0.7–1.30 U/L	70–130 %
Anti-Xa assay (heparin assay)	P		
Unfractionated heparin		0.3–0.7 kIU/L	0.3–0.7 IU/mL
Low-molecular-weight heparin		0.5–1.0 kIU/L	0.5–1.0 IU/mL
Danaparoid (Orgaran)		0.5–0.8 kIU/L	0.5–0.8 IU/mL
Autohemolysis test	WB	0.004–0.045	0.4–4.50%
Autohemolysis test with glucose	WB	0.003–0.007	0.3–0.7%
Bleeding time (adult)		<7.1 min	<7.1 min
C4 binding protein	P	305–695 mg/L	30.5–69.5 mg/dL
	S	275–604 mg/L	27.5–60.4 mg/dL
Clot retraction	WB	0.50–1.00/2 h	50–100%/2 h
Cryofibrinogen	P	Negative	Negative
D-dimer	P	220–740 ng/mL FEU	220–740 ng/mL FEU
Differential blood count	WB		
Relative counts:			
Neutrophils		0.40–0.70	40–70%
Bands		0.0–0.05	0–5%
Lymphocytes		0.20–0.50	20–50%
Monocytes		0.04–0.08	4–8%
Eosinophils		0.0–0.6	0–6%
Basophils		0.0–0.02	0–2%

(Continued)

TABLE 1 HEMATOLOGY AND COAGULATION (*CONTINUED*)

Analyte	Specimen	SI Units	Conventional Units
Absolute counts:			
Neutrophils		1.42–6.34 × 10^9/L	1420–6340/mm^3
Bands		0–0.45 × 10^9/L	0–450/mm^3
Lymphocytes		0.71–4.53 × 10^9/L	710–4530/mm^3
Monocytes		0.14–0.72 × 10^9/L	140–720/mm^3
Eosinophils		0–0.54 × 10^9/L	0–540/mm^3
Basophils		0–0.18 × 10^9/L	0–180/mm^3
Erythrocyte count	WB		
Adult males		4.30–5.60 × 10^{12}/L	4.30–5.60 × 10^6/mm^3
Adult females		4.00–5.20 × 10^{12}/L	4.00–5.20 × 10^6/mm^3
Erythrocyte life span	WB		
Normal survival		120 days	120 days
Chromium labeled, half-life ($t_{1/2}$)		25–35 days	25–35 days
Erythrocyte sedimentation rate	WB		
Females		0–20 mm/h	0–20 mm/h
Males		0–15 mm/h	0–15 mm/h
Euglobulin lysis time	P	7200–14400 s	120–240 min
Factor II, prothrombin	P	0.50–1.50	50–150%
Factor V	P	0.50–1.50	50–150%
Factor VII	P	0.50–1.50	50–150%
Factor VIII	P	0.50–1.50	50–150%
Factor IX	P	0.50–1.50	50–150%
Factor X	P	0.50–1.50	50–150%
Factor XI	P	0.50–1.50	50–150%
Factor XII	P	0.50–1.50	50–150%
Factor XIII screen	P	Not applicable	Present
Factor Inhibitor assay	P	<0.5 Bethesda Units	<0.5 Bethesda Units
Fibrin(ogen) degradation products	P	0–1 mg/L	0–1 μg/mL
Fibrinogen	P	2.33–4.96 g/L	233–496 mg/dL
Glucose-6-phosphate dehydrogenase (erythrocyte)	WB	<2400 s	<40 min
Ham's test (acid serum)	WB	Negative	Negative
Hematocrit	WB		
Adult males		0.388–0.464	38.8–46.4
Adult females		0.354–0.444	35.4–44.4
Hemoglobin			
Plasma	P	6–50 mg/L	0.6–5.0 mg/dL
Whole blood:	WB		
Adult males		133–162 g/L	13.3–16.2 g/dL
Adult females		120–158 g/L	12.0–15.8 g/dL
Hemoglobin electrophoresis	WB		
Hemoglobin A		0.95–0.98	95–98%
Hemoglobin A_2		0.015–0.031	1.5–3.1%
Hemoglobin F		0–0.02	0–2.0%
Hemoglobins other than A, A_2, or F		Absent	Absent
Heparin-induced thrombocytopenia antibody	P	Negative	Negative
Immature platelet fraction (IPF)	WB	0.011–0.061	1.1–6.1%
Joint fluid crystal	JF	Not applicable	No crystals seen
Joint fluid mucin	JF	Not applicable	Only type I mucin present
Leukocytes			
Alkaline phosphatase (LAP)	WB	0.2–1.6 μkat/L	13–100 μ/L
Count (WBC)	WB	3.54–9.06 × 10^9/L	3.54–9.06 × 10^3/mm^3
Mean corpuscular hemoglobin (MCH)	WB	26.7–31.9 pg/cell	26.7–31.9 pg/cell
Mean corpuscular hemoglobin concentration (MCHC)	WB	323–359 g/L	32.3–35.9 g/dL
Mean corpuscular hemoglobin of reticulocytes (CH)	WB	24–36 pg	24–36 pg
Mean corpuscular volume (MCV)	WB	79–93.3 fL	79–93.3 $μm^3$
Mean platelet volume (MPV)	WB	9.00–12.95 fL	9.00–12.95

(*Continued*)

TABLE 1 HEMATOLOGY AND COAGULATION (*CONTINUED*)

Analyte	Specimen	SI Units	Conventional Units
Osmotic fragility of erythrocytes	WB		
Direct		0.0035–0.0045	0.35–0.45%
Indirect		0.0030–0.0065	0.30–0.65%
Partial thromboplastin time, activated	P	26.3–39.4 s	26.3–39.4 s
Plasminogen	P		
Antigen		84–140 mg/L	8.4–14.0 mg/dL
Functional		0.70–1.30	70–130%
Plasminogen activator inhibitor 1	P	4–43 μg/L	4–43 ng/mL
Platelet aggregation	PRP	Not applicable	>65% aggregation in response to adenosine diphosphate, epinephrine, collagen, ristocetin, and arachidonic acid
Platelet count	WB	165–415 × 10^9/L	165–415 × 10^3/mm^3
Platelet, mean volume	WB	6.4–11 fL	6.4–11.0 μm^3
Prekallikrein assay	P	0.50–1.5	50–150%
Prekallikrein screen	P		No deficiency detected
Protein C	P		
Total antigen		0.70–1.40	70–140%
Functional		0.70–1.30	70–130%
Protein S	P		
Total antigen		0.70–1.40	70–140%
Functional		0.65–1.40	65–140%
Free antigen		0.70–1.40	70–140%
Prothrombin gene mutation G20210A	WB	Not applicable	Not present
Prothrombin time	P	12.7–15.4 s	12.7–15.4 s
Protoporphyrin, free erythrocyte	WB	0.28–0.64 μmol/L of red blood cells	16–36 μg/dL of red blood cells
Red cell distribution width	WB	<0.145	<14.5%
Reptilase time	P	16–23.6 s	16–23.6 s
Reticulocyte count	WB		
Adult males		0.008–0.023 red cells	0.8–2.3% red cells
Adult females		0.008–0.020 red cells	0.8–2.0% red cells
Reticulocyte hemoglobin content	WB	>26 pg/cell	>26 pg/cell
Ristocetin cofactor (functional von Willebrand factor)	P		
Blood group O		0.75 mean of normal	75% mean of normal
Blood group A		1.05 mean of normal	105% mean of normal
Blood group B		1.15 mean of normal	115% mean of normal
Blood group AB		1.25 mean of normal	125% mean of normal
Serotonin release assay	S	<0.2 release	<20% release
Sickle cell test	WB	Negative	Negative
Sucrose hemolysis	WB	<0.1	<10% hemolysis
Thrombin time	P	15.3–18.5 s	15.3–18.5 s
Thrombin-antithrombin (TAT) complex	P	<4 μg/L	<4 ng/mL
Total eosinophils	WB	150–300 × 10^6/L	150–300/mm^3
Transferrin receptor	S, P	9.6–29.6 nmol/L	9.6–29.6 nmol/L
Viscosity			
Plasma	P	1.7–2.1	1.7–2.1
Serum	S	1.4–1.8	1.4–1.8
von Willebrand factor (VWF) antigen (factor VIII:R antigen)	P		
Blood group O		0.75 mean of normal	75% mean of normal
Blood group A		1.05 mean of normal	105% mean of normal
Blood group B		1.15 mean of normal	115% mean of normal
Blood group AB		1.25 mean of normal	125% mean of normal
von Willebrand factor collagen binding	P	590–2490 units/L	59–249 units/dL
von Willebrand factor multimers	P	Normal distribution	Normal distribution
White blood cells: see "Leukocytes"			

Abbreviations: JF, joint fluid; P, plasma; PRP, platelet-rich plasma; S, serum; WB, whole blood.

TABLE 2 CLINICAL CHEMISTRY AND IMMUNOLOGY

Analyte	Specimen	SI Units	Conventional Units
Acetoacetate	P	49–294 μmol/L	0.5–3.0 mg/dL
Adrenocorticotropin (ACTH)	P	1.3–16.7 pmol/L	6.0–76.0 pg/mL
Alanine aminotransferase (ALT, SGPT)	S	0.12–0.70 μkat/L	7–41 U/L
Albumin	S	40–50 g/L	4.0–5.0 mg/dL
Aldolase	S	26–138 nkat/L	1.5–8.1 U/L
Aldosterone (adult)			
Supine, normal sodium diet	S, P	<443 pmol/L	<16 ng/dL
Upright, normal.	S, P	111–858 pmol/L	4–31 ng/dL
Alpha fetoprotein (adult)	S	0–8.5 μg/L	0–8.5 ng/mL
Alpha-1-acid glycoprotein	S	0.50–1.2 g/L	50–120 mg/dL
Alpha$_1$ antitrypsin	S	1.0–2.0 g/L	100–200 mg/dL
Ammonia, as NH_3	P	11–35 μmol/L	19–60 μg/dL
Amylase (method dependent)	S	0.34–1.6 μkat/L	20–96 U/L
Androstenedione (adult)	S		
Males		0.81–3.1 nmol/L	23–89 ng/dL
Females			
Premenopausal		0.91–7.5 nmol/L	26–214 ng/dL
Postmenopausal		0.46–2.9 nmol/L	13–82 ng/dL
Angiotensin-converting enzyme (ACE)	S	0.15–1.1 μkat/L	9–67 U/L
Anion gap	S	7–16 mmol/L	7–16 mmol/L
Apolipoprotein A-1	S		
Male		0.94–1.78 g/L	94–178 mg/dL
Female		1.01–1.99 g/L	101–199 mg/dL
Apolipoprotein B	S		
Male		0.55–1.40 g/L	55–140 mg/dL
Female		0.55–1.25 g/L	55–125 mg/dL
Arterial blood gases	WB		
(HCO_3^-)		22–30 mmol/L	22–30 meq/L
Pco_2 (Sea Level, Fio_2 0.21)		4.7–6.0 kPa	35–45 mmHg
pH		7.35–7.45	7.35–7.45
Po_2 (Sea Level, Fio_2 0.21, age related)		8.9–13.8 kPa	67–104 mmHg
Carboxyhemoglobin and methemoglobin at pH 7.40 and 37°C		≤0.01	≤1%
Aspartate aminotransferase (AST, SGOT)	S	0.20–0.65 μkat/L	12–38 U/L
Autoantibodies	S		
Anti-centromere antibody IgG		≤29 AU/mL	≤29 AU/mL
Anti-double-strand (native) DNA		<25 IU/L	<25 IU/L
Anti-glomerular basement membrane antibodies			
Qualitative IgG, IgA		Negative	Negative
Quantitative IgG antibody		≤19 AU/mL	≤19 AU/mL
Anti-histone antibodies		<1.0 U	<1.0 U
Anti-Jo-1 antibody		≤29 AU/mL	≤29 AU/mL
Anti-mitochondrial antibody		Not applicable	<20 Units
Anti neutrophil cytoplasmic autoantibodies		Not applicable	<1:20
Serine proteinase 3 antibodies		≤19 AU/mL	≤19 AU/mL
Myeloperoxidase antibodies		≤19 AU/mL	≤19 AU/mL
Antinuclear antibody		Not applicable	Negative at 1:40
Anti-parietal cell antibody		Not applicable	None detected
Anti-RNP antibody		Not applicable	<1.0 U
Anti-Scl 70 antibody		Not applicable	<1.0 U
Anti-Smith antibody		Not applicable	<1.0 U
Anti-smooth muscle antibody		Not applicable	<1.0 U
Anti-SSA antibody		Not applicable	<1.0 U
Anti-SSB antibody		Not applicable	Negative
Anti-thyroglobulin antibody		<40 KIU/mL	<40 IU/mL
Anti-thyroid peroxidase antibody		<35 KIU/L	<35 IU/L

(Continued)

TABLE 2 CLINICAL CHEMISTRY AND IMMUNOLOGY (*CONTINUED*)

Analyte	Specimen	SI Units	Conventional Units
B-type natriuretic peptide (BNP)	P	Age and gender specific: <100 ng/L	Age and gender specific: <100 pg/mL
Bence Jones protein, serum qualitative	S	Not applicable	None detected
Bence Jones protein, serum quantitative	S		
Free kappa		3.3–19.4 mg/L	0.33–1.94 mg/dL
Free lambda		5.7–26.3 mg/L	0.57–2.63 mg/dL
K/L ratio		0.26–1.65	0.26–1.65
Beta-2-microglobulin	S	1.1–2.4 mg/L	1.1–2.4 mg/L
Bile acids	S		
Cholic acid		0–1.9 μmol/L	0–1.9 μmol/L
Chenodeoxycholic acid		0–3.4 μmol/L	0–3.4 μmol/L
Deoxycholic acid		0–2.5 μmol/L	0–2.5 μmol/L
Ursodeoxycholic acid		0–1.0 μmol/L	0–1.0 μmol/L
Total		0–7.0 μmol/L	0–7.0 μmol/L
Bilirubin	S		
Total		5.1–22 μmol/L	0.3–1.3 mg/dL
Direct		1.7–6.8 μmol/L	0.1–0.4 mg/dL
Indirect		3.4–15.2 μmol/L	0.2–0.9 mg/dL
C peptide	S	0.27–1.19 nmol/L	0.8–3.5 ng/mL
C1-esterase-inhibitor protein	S	210–390 mg/L	21–39 mg/dL
CA 125	S	<35 kU/L	<35 U/mL
CA 19-9	S	<37 kU/L	<37 U/mL
CA 15-3	S	<33 kU/L	<33 U/mL
CA 27-29	S	0–40 kU/L	0–40 U/mL
Calcitonin	S		
Male		0–7.5 ng/L	0–7.5 pg/mL
Female		0–5.1 ng/L	0–5.1 pg/mL
Calcium	S	2.2–2.6 mmol/L	8.7–10.2 mg/dL
Calcium, ionized	WB	1.12–1.32 mmol/L	4.5–5.3 mg/dL
Carbon dioxide content (TCO_2)	P (sea level)	22–30 mmol/L	22–30 meq/L
Carboxyhemoglobin (carbon monoxide content)	WB		
Nonsmokers (in a nonsmoking environment)		0.0–0.025	0–2.5% of total hemoglobin (Hgb) value
Smokers		0.04–0.09	4–9% of total Hgb value
Loss of consciousness and death		>0.50	>50% of total Hgb value
Carcinoembryonic antigen (CEA)	S		
Nonsmokers		0.0–3.0 μg/L	0.0–3.0 ng/mL
Smokers		0.0–5.0 μg/L	0.0–5.0 ng/mL
Ceruloplasmin	S	250–630 mg/L	25–63 mg/dL
Chloride	S	102–109 mmol/L	102–109 meq/L
Cholesterol (LCL, Total, HDL): Ranges depend on individual patient factors; see 2013 ACC/AHA Guideline on the Treatment of Blood Cholesterol			
Cholinesterase	S	5–12 kU/L	5–12 U/mL
Chromogranin A	S	0–95 μg/L	0–95 ng/mL
Complement	S		
C3		0.83–1.77 g/L	83–177 mg/dL
C4		0.16–0.47 g/L	16–47 mg/dL
Complement total		60–144 CAE units	60–144 CAE units
Cortisol			
Fasting, 8 A.M.–12 noon	S	138–690 nmol/L	5–25 μg/dL
12 noon–8 P.M.		138–414 nmol/L	5–15 μg/dL
8 P.M.–8 A.M.		0–276 nmol/L	0–10 μg/dL
C-reactive protein	S	<10 mg/L	<10 mg/L
C-reactive protein, high sensitivity	S	Cardiac risk Low: <1.0 mg/L Average: 1.0–3.0 mg/L High: >3.0 mg/L	Cardiac risk Low: <1.0 mg/L Average: 1.0–3.0 mg/L High: >3.0 mg/L

(*Continued*)

TABLE 2 CLINICAL CHEMISTRY AND IMMUNOLOGY (*CONTINUED*)

Analyte	Specimen	SI Units	Conventional Units
Creatine kinase (total)	S		
Females		0.66–4.0 µkat/L	39–238 U/L
Males		0.87–5.0 µkat/L	51–294 U/L
Creatine kinase-MB	S		
Mass		0.0–5.5 µg/L	0.0–5.5 ng/mL
Fraction of total activity (by electrophoresis)		0–0.04	0–4.0%
Creatinine	S		
Female		44–80 µmol/L	0.5–0.9 mg/dL
Male		53–106 µmol/L	0.6–1.2 mg/dL
Cryoglobulins	S	Not applicable	None detected
Cyclic citrullinated peptide (CCP) antibody (IgG)	S	Negative: <20 Units Weak positive: 20–39 Units Moderate positive: 40–59 Units Strong positive: ≥60 Units	Negative: <20 Units Weak positive: 20–39 Units Moderate positive: 40–59 Units Strong positive: ≥60 Units
Cystatin C	S	0.5–1.0 mg/L	0.5–1.0 mg/L
Deamidated gliadin peptide (DGP) antibody, IgA	S		
Negative		≤19 Units	≤19 Units
Weak positive		20–30 Units	20–30 Units
Positive		≥31 Units	≥31 Units
Deamidated gliadin peptide (DGP) antibody, IgG	S		
Negative		≤19 Units	≤19 Units
Weak positive		20–30 Units	20–30 Units
Positive		≥31 Units	≥31 Units
Dehydroepiandrosterone (DHEA) (adult)			
Male	S	6.2–43.4 nmol/L	180–1250 ng/dL
Female		4.5–34.0 nmol/L	130–980 ng/dL
Dehydroepiandrosterone (DHEA) sulfate	S		
Male (adult)		100–6190 µg/L	10–619 µg/dL
Female (adult, premenopausal)		120–5350 µg/L	12–535 µg/dL
Female (adult, postmenopausal)		300–2600 µg/L	30–260 µg/dL
11-Deoxycortisol (adult) (compound S)	S	0.34–4.56 nmol/L	12–158 ng/dL
Dihydrotestosterone			
Male	S, P	1.03–2.92 nmol/L	30–85 ng/dL
Female		0.14–0.76 nmol/L	4–22 ng/dL
Dopamine	P	0–130 pmol/L	0–20 pg/mL
Endomysial antibody, IgA	S	<1:10	<1:10
Endomysial antibody, IgG	S	<1:10	<1:10
Epinephrine	P		
Supine (30 min)		<273 pmol/L	<50 pg/mL
Sitting		<328 pmol/L	<60 pg/mL
Standing (30 min)		<491pmol/L	<90 pg/mL
Erythropoietin	S	4–27 U/L	4–27 U/L
Estradiol	S, P		
Female			
Menstruating:			
Follicular phase		74–532 pmol/L	<20–145 pg/mL
Midcycle peak		411–1626 pmol/L	112–443 pg/mL
Luteal phase		74–885 pmol/L	<20–241 pg/mL
Postmenopausal		217 pmol/L	<59 pg/mL
Male		74 pmol/L	<20 pg/mL
Estrone	S, P		
Female			
Menstruating:			
Follicular phase		<555 pmol/L	<150 pg/mL
Luteal phase		<740 pmol/L	<200 pg/mL
Postmenopausal		11–118 pmol/L	3–32 pg/mL
Male		33–133 pmol/L	9–36 pg/mL

(*Continued*)

Analyte	Specimen	SI Units	Conventional Units
Fatty acids, free (nonesterified)	P	0.1–0.6 mmol/L	2.8–16.8 mg/dL
Ferritin	S		
Female		10–150 μg/L	10–150 ng/mL
Male		29–248 μg/L	29–248 ng/mL
Follicle-stimulating hormone (FSH)	S, P		
Female			
Menstruating			
Follicular phase		3.0–20.0 IU/L	3.0–20.0 mIU/mL
Ovulatory phase		9.0–26.0 IU/L	9.0–26.0 mIU/mL
Luteal phase		1.0–12.0 IU/L	1.0–12.0 mIU/mL
Postmenopausal		18.0–153.0 IU/L	18.0–153.0 mIU/mL
Male		1.0–12.0 IU/L	1.0–12.0 mIU/mL
Fructosamine	S	<285 μmol/L	<285 μmol/L
Galectin-3	S		
Low risk		≤17.8 μg/L	≤17.8 ng/mL
Intermediate risk		17.9–25.9 μg/L	17.9–25.9 ng/mL
Higher risk		>25.9 μg/L	>25.9 ng/mL
Gamma glutamyltransferase	S	0.15–0.99 μkat/L	9–58 U/L
Gastrin	S	<100 ng/L	<100 pg/mL
Glucagon	P	40–130 ng/L	40–130 pg/mL
Glucose	WB	3.6–5.3 mmol/L	65–95 mg/dL
Glucose (fasting)	P		
Normal		4.2–5.6 mmol/L	75–100 mg/dL
Increased risk for diabetes		5.6–6.9 mmol/L	100–125 mg/dL
Diabetes mellitus		Fasting ≥7.0 mmol/L A 2-h level of ≥11.1 mmol/L during an oral glucose tolerance test A random glucose level of ≥11.1 mmol/L in patients with symptoms of hyperglycemia	Fasting ≥126 mg/dL A 2-h level of ≥200 mg/dL during an oral glucose tolerance test A random glucose level of ≥200 mg/dL in patients with symptoms of hyperglycemia
Growth hormone	S	0–5 μg/L	0–5 ng/mL
Hemoglobin A_{1c}	WB	0.04–0.06 Hgb fraction	4.0–5.6%
Prediabetes		0.057–0.064 Hgb fraction	5.7–6.4%
Diabetes mellitus		A hemoglobin A_{1c} level of ≥0.065 Hgb fraction as suggested by the American Diabetes Association	A hemoglobin A_{1c} level of ≥6.5% as suggested by the American Diabetes Association
Hemoglobin A_{1c} with estimated average glucose (eAG)	WB	eAg mmoL/L = 1.59 × HbA_{1c} – 2.59	eAg (mg/dL) = 28.7 × HbA_{1c} – 46.7
Homocysteine	P	4.4–10.8 μmol/L	4.4–10.8 μmol/L
Human chorionic gonadotropin (HCG)	S		
Nonpregnant female		<5 IU/L	<5 mIU/mL
1–2 weeks postconception		9–130 IU/L	9–130 mIU/mL
2–3 weeks postconception		75–2600 IU/L	75–2600 mIU/mL
3–4 weeks postconception		850–20,800 IU/L	850–20,800 mIU/mL
4–5 weeks postconception		4000–100,200 IU/L	4000–100,200 mIU/mL
5–10 weeks postconception		11,500–289,000 IU/L	11,500–289,000 mIU/mL
10–14 weeks postconception		18,300–137,000 IU/L	18,300–137,000 mIU/mL
Second trimester		1400–53,000 IU/L	1400–53,000 mIU/mL
Third trimester		940–60,000 IU/L	940–60,000 mIU/mL
Human epididymis protein 4 (HE-4)	S	0–150 pmol/L	0–150 pmol/L
β-Hydroxybutyrate	P	60–170 μmol/L	0.6–1.8 mg/dL
17-Hydroxyprogesterone (adult)	S		
Male		<4.17 nmol/L	<139 ng/dL
Female			
Follicular phase		0.45–2.1 nmol/L	15–70 ng/dL
Luteal phase		1.05–8.7 nmol/L	35–290 ng/dL
Immunofixation	S	Not applicable	No bands detected

(Continued)

TABLE 2 CLINICAL CHEMISTRY AND IMMUNOLOGY (*CONTINUED*)

Analyte	Specimen	SI Units	Conventional Units
Immunoglobulin, quantitation (adult)			
IgA	S	0.70–3.50 g/L	70–350 mg/dL
IgD	S	0–140 mg/L	0–14 mg/dL
IgE	S	1–87 KIU/L	1–87 IU/mL
IgG	S	7.0–17.0 g/L	700–1700 mg/dL
IgG_1	S	2.7–17.4 g/L	270–1740 mg/dL
IgG_2	S	0.3–6.3 g/L	30–630 mg/dL
IgG_3	S	0.13–3.2 g/L	13–320 mg/dL
IgG_4	S	0.11–6.2 g/L	11–620 mg/dL
IgM	S	0.50–3.0 g/L	50–300 mg/dL
Inhibin A	S		
Males		≤2.0 ng/L	≤2.0 pg/mL
Females			
Early follicular phase		1.8–17.3 ng/L	1.8–17.3 pg/mL
Mid follicular phase		3.5–31.7 ng/L	3.5–17.3 pg/mL
Late follicular phase		9.8–90.3 ng/L	9.8–90.3 pg/mL
Midcycle		16.9–91.8 ng/L	16.9–91.8 pg/mL
Early luteal phase		16.1–97.5 ng/L	16.1–97.5 pg/mL
Mid luteal phase		3.9–87.7 ng/L	3.9–87.7 pg/mL
Late luteal phase		2.7–47.1 ng/L	2.7–47.1 pg/mL
Postmenopausal		<1.0–2.1 ng/L	<1.0–2.1 pg/mL
Insulin	S, P	14.35–143.5 pmol/L	2–20 μU/mL
Iron	S	7–25 μmol/L	41–141 μg/dL
Iron-binding capacity	S	45–73 μmol/L	251–406 μg/dL
Iron-binding capacity saturation	S	0.16–0.35	16–35%
Ischemia modified albumin	S	<85 KU/L	<85 U/mL
Joint fluid crystal	JF	Not applicable	No crystals seen
Joint fluid mucin	JF	Not applicable	Only type I mucin present
Ketone (acetone)	S	Negative	Negative
Lactate	P, arterial	0.5–1.6 mmol/L	4.5–14.4 mg/dL
	P, venous	0.5–2.2 mmol/L	4.5–19.8 mg/dL
Lactate dehydrogenase	S	2.0–3.8 μkat/L	115–221 U/L
Lamellar body count	AMF		
Immature		<15,000/μL	<15,000/μL
Indeterminate		15,000–50,000/μL	15,000-50,000/μL
Mature		>50,000/μL	>50,000/μL
Lecithin/sphingomyelin (L/S) ratio	AMF		
Immature		≤1.5	≤1.5
Transitional		1.5–1.9	1.5–1.9
Mature		2.0–2.5 or greater	2.0–2.5 or greater
Lipase	S	0.51–0.73 μkat/L	3–43 U/L
Lipoprotein (a)	S	0–300 mg/L	0–30 mg/dL
Lipoprotein associated phospholipase A2	S, P	0–234 μg/L	0-234 ng/mL
Luteinizing hormone (LH)	S, P		
Female			
Menstruating			
Follicular phase		2.0–15.0 U/L	2.0–15.0 mIU/mL
Ovulatory phase		22.0–105.0 U/L	22.0–105.0 mIU/mL
Luteal phase		0.6–19.0 U/L	0.6–19.0 mIU/mL
Postmenopausal		16.0–64.0 U/L	16.0–64.0 mIU/mL
Male		2.0–12.0 U/L	2.0–12.0 mIU/mL
Magnesium	S	0.62–0.95 mmol/L	1.5–2.3 mg/dL
Metanephrine	P	<0.5 nmol/L	<100 pg/mL
Methemoglobin	WB	0.0–0.01	0–1% of total Hgb value

(Continued)

TABLE 2 CLINICAL CHEMISTRY AND IMMUNOLOGY (*CONTINUED*)

Analyte	Specimen	SI Units	Conventional Units
Myoglobin	S		
Male		20–71 μg/L	20–71 μg/L
Female		25–58 μg/L	25–58 μg/L
Norepinephrine	P		
Supine (30 min)		650–2423 pmol/L	110–410 pg/mL
Sitting		709–4019 pmol/L	120–680 pg/mL
Standing (30 min)		739–4137 pmol/L	125–700 pg/mL
N-telopeptide (cross-linked), NTx	S		
Female, premenopausal		6.2–19.0 nmol BCE	6.2–19.0 nmol BCE
Male		5.4–24.2 nmol BCE	5.4–24.2 nmol BCE
BCE = bone collagen equivalent			
NT-proBNP	S, P	<125 ng/L up to 75 years	<125 pg/mL up to 75 years
		<450 ng/L >75 years	<450 pg/mL >75 years
5′ Nucleotidase	S	0.00–0.19 μkat/L	0–11 U/L
Osmolality	P	275–295 mOsmol/kg serum water	275–295 mOsmol/kg serum water
Osteocalcin	S	11–50 μg/L	11–50 ng/mL
Oxygen content (age and gender related)	WB		
Arterial (sea level)		17–21 mL/dL	17–21 vol%
Venous (sea level)		10–16 mL/dL	10–16 vol%
Oxygen saturation (sea level)	WB	Fraction:	Percent:
Arterial		0.91–1.0	91–100%
Venous, arm		0.60–0.85	60–85%
Parathyroid hormone (intact)	S	8–51 ng/L	8–51 pg/mL
Phosphatase, alkaline	S	0.56–1.63 μkat/L	33–96 U/L
Phosphatase, alkaline bone	S		
Male		≤20 μg/L	≤20 ng/mL
Female			
Premenopausal		≤14 μg/L	≤14 ng/mL
Postmenopausal		≤22 μg/L	≤22 ng/mL
Phosphorus, inorganic	S	0.81–1.4 mmol/L	2.5–4.3 mg/dL
Potassium	S	3.5–5.0 mmol/L	3.5–5.0 meq/L
Prealbumin (transthyretin)	S	170–340 mg/L	17–34 mg/dL
Procalcitonin	S	<0.1 μg/L	<0.1 ng/mL
Progesterone	S, P		
Female: Follicular		<3.18 nmol/L	<1.0 ng/mL
Midluteal		9.54–63.6 nmol/L	3–20 ng/mL
Male		<3.18 nmol/L	<1.0 ng/mL
Prolactin	S		
Male		53–360 mg/L	2.5–17 ng/mL
Female		40–530 mg/L	1.9–25 ng/mL
Prostate-specific antigen (PSA)	S	0.0–4.0 μg/L	0.0–4.0 ng/mL
Prostate-specific antigen, free	S	With total PSA between 4 and 10 μg/L and when the free PSA is:	With total PSA between 4 and 10 ng/mL and when the free PSA is:
		>0.25 decreased risk of prostate cancer	>25% decreased risk of prostate cancer
		<0.10 increased risk of prostate cancer	<10% increased risk of prostate cancer
Protein fractions:	S		
Albumin		35–55 g/L	3.5–5.5 g/dL (50–60%)
Globulin		20–35 g/L	2.0–3.5 g/dL (40–50%)
$Alpha_1$		2–4 g/L	0.2–0.4 g/dL (4.2–7.2%)
$Alpha_2$		5–9 g/L	0.5–0.9 g/dL (6.8–12%)
Beta		6–11 g/L	0.6–1.1 g/dL (9.3–15%)
Gamma		7–17 g/L	0.7–1.7 g/dL (13–23%)
Protein, total	S	67–86 g/L	6.7–8.6 g/dL
Pyruvate	P	40–130 μmol/L	0.35–1.14 mg/dL
Retinol-binding protein	S	0.71–2.9 μmol /L	1.5–6.0 mg/dL
Rheumatoid factor	S	<15 kIU/L	<15 IU/mL
Serotonin	WB	0.28–1.14 μmol/L	50–200 ng/mL

(Continued)

TABLE 2 CLINICAL CHEMISTRY AND IMMUNOLOGY (*CONTINUED*)

Analyte	Specimen	SI Units	Conventional Units
Serum protein electrophoresis	S	Not applicable	Normal pattern
Sex hormone–binding globulin (adult)	S		
Male		11–80 nmol/L	11–80 nmol/L
Female		30–135 nmol/L	30–135 nmol/L
Sodium	S	136–146 mmol/L	136–146 meq/L
Somatomedin-C (IGF-1) (adult)	S		
16 years		226–903 μg/L	226–903 ng/mL
17 years		193–731 μg/L	193–731 ng/mL
18 years		163–584 μg/L	163–584 ng/mL
19 years		141–483 μg/L	141–483 ng/mL
20 years		127–424 μg/L	127–424 ng/mL
21–25 years		116–358 μg/L	116–358 ng/mL
26–30 years		117–329 μg/L	117–329 ng/mL
31–35 years		115–307 μg/L	115–307 ng/mL
36–40 years		119–204 μg/L	119–204 ng/mL
41–45 years		101–267 μg/L	101–267 ng/mL
46–50 years		94–252 μg/L	94–252 ng/mL
51–55 years		87–238 μg/L	87–238 ng/mL
56–60 years		81–225 μg/L	81–225 ng/mL
61–65 years		75–212 μg/L	75–212 ng/mL
66–70 years		69–200 μg/L	69–200 ng/mL
71–75 years		64–188 μg/L	64–188 ng/mL
76–80 years		59–177 μg/L	59–177 ng/mL
81–85 years		55–166 μg/L	55–166 ng/mL
Somatostatin	P	<25 ng/L	<25 pg/mL
Testosterone, free			
Female, adult	S	10.4–65.9 pmol/L	3–19 pg/mL
Male, adult		312–1041 pmol/L	90–300 pg/mL
Testosterone, total,	S		
Female		0.21–2.98 nmol/L	6–86 ng/dL
Male		9.36–37.10 nmol/L	270–1070 ng/dL
Thyroglobulin	S	13–318 μg/L	1.3–31.8 ng/mL
Thyroid-binding globulin	S	13–30 mg/L	1.3–3.0 mg/dL
Thyroid-stimulating hormone (thyrotropin)	S	0.34–4.25 mIU/L	0.34–4.25 μIU/mL
Thyrotropin receptor antibody	S	≤1.75 IU/L	≤1.75 mIU/mL
Thyroxine, free (fT_4)	S	9.0–16 pmol/L	0.7–1.24 ng/dL
Thyroxine, total (T_4)	S	70–151 nmol/L	5.4–11.7 μg/dL
Thyroxine index (free)	S	6.7–10.9	6.7–10.9
Tissue transglutaminase (tTG) Antibody, IgA	S		
Negative		<4.0 Units/mL	<4.0 Units/mL
Weak positive		4.0–10.0 Units/mL	4.0–10.0 Units/mL
Positive		>10.0 Units/mL	>10.0 Units/mL
Tissue transglutaminase (tTG) antibody, IgG	S		
Negative		<6.0 Units/mL	<6.0 Units/mL
Weak positive		6.0–9.0 Units/mL	6.0–9.0 Units/mL
Positive		>9.0 Units/mL	>9.0 Units/mL
Transferrin	S	2.0–4.0 g/L	200–400 mg/dL
Transferrin, carbohydrate deficient, for alcohol use	S	0.017	1.7%
Triglycerides	S	0.34–2.26 mmol/L	30–200 mg/dL
Triiodothyronine, free (fT_3)	S	3.7–6.5 pmol/L	2.4–4.2 pg/mL
Triiodothyronine, total (T_3)	S	1.2–2.1 nmol/L	77–135 ng/dL
Troponin I	S, P		
99th percentile of a healthy population		Method-dependent	Method-dependent
Troponin T	S, P		
99th percentile of a healthy population		0–14 ng/L	0–14 ng/L
Urea nitrogen	S	2.5–7.1 mmol/L	7–20 mg/dL

(*Continued*)

TABLE 2 CLINICAL CHEMISTRY AND IMMUNOLOGY (*CONTINUED*)

Analyte	Specimen	SI Units	Conventional Units
Uric acid	S		
Females		0.15–0.33 mmol/L	2.5–5.6 mg/dL
Males		0.18–0.41 mmol/L	3.1–7.0 mg/dL
Vasoactive intestinal polypeptide	P	0–60 ng/L	0–60 pg/mL
Zinc protoporphyrin	WB	0–400 μg/L	0–40 μg/dL
Zinc protoporphyrin (ZPP)-to-heme ratio	WB	0–69 μmol ZPP/mol heme	0–69 μmol ZPP/mol heme

Abbreviations: AMF, amniotic fluid; P, plasma; S, serum; WB, whole blood.

Source: NJ Stone et al: J Am Coll Cardiol 63:2889-2934, 2014.

TABLE 3 TOXICOLOGY AND THERAPEUTIC DRUG MONITORING

	Therapeutic Range		Toxic Level	
Drug	SI Units	Conventional Units	SI Units	Conventional Units
Acetaminophen	66–199 μmol/L	10–30 μg/mL	>1320 μmol/L	>200 μg/mL
Amikacin				
Peak	34–51 μmol/L	20–30 μg/mL	>60 μmol/L	>35 μg/mL
Trough	0–17 μmol/L	0–10 μg/mL	>17 μmol/L	>10 μg/mL
Amitriptyline/nortriptyline (total drug)	430–900 nmol/L	120–250 ng/mL	>1800 nmol/L	>500 ng/mL
Amphetamine	150–220 nmol/L	20–30 ng/mL	>1500 nmol/L	>200 ng/mL
Bromide	9.4–18.7 mmol/L	75–150 mg/dL	>18.8 mmol/L	>150 mg/dL
Mild toxicity			6.4–18.8 mmol/L	51–150 mg/dL
Severe toxicity			>18.8 mmol/L	>150 mg/dL
Lethal			>37.5 mmol/L	>300 mg/dL
Caffeine	25.8–103 μmol/L	5–20 μg/ml	>206 μmol/L	>40 μg/mL
Carbamazepine	17–42 μmol/L	4–10 μg/mL	> 85 μmol/L	>20 μg/mL
Chloramphenicol				
Peak	31–62 μmol/L	10–20 μg/mL	>77 μmol/L	>25 μg/mL
Trough	15–31 μmol/L	5–10 μg/mL	>46 μmol/L	>15 μg/mL
Chlordiazepoxide	1.7–10 μmol/L	0.5–3.0 μg/mL	>17 μmol/L	>5.0 μg/mL
Clonazepam	32–240 nmol/L	10–75 ng/mL	>320 nmol/L	>100 ng/mL
Clozapine	0.6–2.1 μmol/L	200–700 ng/mL	>3.7 μmol/L	>1200 ng/mL
Cocaine			>3.3 μmol/L	>1.0 μg/mL
Codeine	43–110 nmol/mL	13–33 ng/mL	>3700 nmol/mL	>1100 ng/mL (lethal)
Cyclosporine				
Renal transplant				
0–6 months	208–312 nmol/L	250–375 ng/mL	>312 nmol/L	>375 ng/mL
6–12 months after transplant	166–250 nmol/L	200–300 ng/mL	>250 nmol/L	>300 ng/mL
>12 months	83–125 nmol/L	100–150 ng/mL	>125 nmol/L	>150 ng/mL
Cardiac transplant				
0–6 months	208–291 nmol/L	250–350 ng/mL	>291 nmol/L	>350 ng/mL
6–12 months after transplant	125–208 nmol/L	150–250 ng/mL	>208 nmol/L	>250 ng/mL
>12 months	83–125 nmol/L	100–150 ng/mL	>125 nmol/L	150 ng/mL
Lung transplant				
0–6 months	250–374 nmol/L	300–450 ng/mL	>374 nmol/L	>450 ng/mL
Liver transplant				
Initiation	208–291 nmol/L	250–350 ng/mL	>291 nmol/L	>350 ng/mL
Maintenance	83–166 nmol/L	100–200 ng/mL	>166 nmol/L	>200 ng/mL
Desipramine	375–1130 nmol/L	100–300 ng/mL	>1880 nmol/L	>500 ng/mL
Diazepam (and metabolite)				
Diazepam	0.7 –3.5 μmol/L	0.2–1.0 μg/mL	>7.0 μmol/L	>2.0 μg/mL
Nordiazepam	0.4– 6.6 μmol/L	0.1–1.8 μg/mL	>9.2 μmol/L	>2.5 μg/mL
Digoxin	0.64–1.6 nmol/L	0.5–1.2 ng/mL	>3.1 nmol/L	>2.4 ng/mL
Disopyramide	5.3–14.7 μmol/L	2–5 μg/mL	>20.6 μmol/L	>7 μg/mL
Doxepin and nordoxepin				
Doxepin	0.36–0.98 μmol/L	101–274 ng/mL	>1.8 μmol/L	>503 ng/mL
Nordoxepin	0.38–1.04 μmol/L	106–291 ng/mL	>1.9 μmol/L	>531 ng/mL

(*Continued*)

TABLE 3 TOXICOLOGY AND THERAPEUTIC DRUG MONITORING (*CONTINUED*)

Drug	Therapeutic Range		Toxic Level	
	SI Units	Conventional Units	SI Units	Conventional Units
Ethanol				
Behavioral changes			>4.3 mmol/L	>20 mg/dL
Legal limit			≥17 mmol/L	≥80 mg/dL
Critical with acute exposure			>54 mmol/L	>250 mg/dL
Ethylene glycol				
Toxic			>2 mmol/L	>12 mg/dL
Lethal			>20 mmol/L	>120 mg/dL
Ethosuximide	280–700 μmol/L	40–100 μg/mL	>700 μmol/L	>100 μg/mL
Everolimus (trough)				
Kidney transplant	3.1–8.34 nmol/L	3–8 ng/mL	>12.5 nmol/L	>12 ng/mL
Oncology	5.2–10.4 nmol/L	5.0–10.0 ng/mL	>12.5 nmol/L	>12 ng/mL
Felbamate (trough)	126–252 μmol/L	30–60 μg/mL	Toxic range not well established	
Flecainide	0.5–2.4 μmol/L	0.2–1.0 μg/mL	>3.6 μmol/L	>1.5 μg/mL
Gabapentin (trough)	11.7–116.8 μmol/L	2–20 μg/mL	Toxic range not well established	
Gentamicin				
Peak	10–21 μmol/mL	5–10 μg/mL	>25 μmol/mL	>12 μg/mL
Trough	0–4.2 μmol/mL	0–2 μg/mL	>4.2 μmol/mL	>2 μg/mL
Heroin (diacetyl morphine)			>700 μmol/L	>200 ng/mL (as morphine)
Ibuprofen	49–243 μmol/L	10–50 μg/mL	>970 μmol/L	>200 μg/mL
Imipramine (and metabolites)				
Desimipramine	375–1130 nmol/L	100–300 ng/mL	>1880 nmol/L	>500 ng/mL
Total imipramine + desimipramine	563–1130 nmol/L	150–300 ng/mL	>1880 nmol/L	>500 ng/mL
Isopropanol			>8.3 mmol/L	>50 mg/dL
Lamotrigine	11.7–54.7 μmol/L	3–14 μg/mL	>58.7 μmol/L	>15 μg/mL
Levetiracetam (Keppra)	29–176 μmol/L	5–30 μg/mL	Toxic range not well established	
Lidocaine	5.1–21.3 μmol/L	1.2–5.0 μg/mL	>38.4 μmol/L	>9.0 μg/mL
Lithium	0.5–1.3 mmol/L	0.5–1.3 meq/L	>2 mmol/L	>2 meq/L
Methadone	1.0–3.2 μmol/L	0.3–1.0 μg/mL	>6.5 μmol/L	>2 μg/mL
Methamphetamine	0.07–0.34 μmol/L	0.01–0.05 μg/mL	>3.35 μmol/L	>0.5 μg/mL
Methanol			>6 mmol/L	>20 mg/dL
Methotrexate				
Low-dose	0.01–0.1 μmol/L	0.01–0.1 μmol/L	>0.1 μmol/L	>0.1 μmol/L
High-dose (24h)	<5.0 μmol/L	<5.0 μmol/L	>5.0 μmol/L	>5.0 μmol/L
High-dose (48h)	<0.50 μmol/L	<0.50 μmol/L	>0.5 μmol/L	>0.5 μmol/L
High-dose (72h)	<0.10 μmol/L	<0.10 μmol/L	>0.1 μmol/L	>0.1 μmol/L
Morphine	232–286 μmol/L	65–80 ng/mL	>720 μmol/L	>200 ng/mL
Mycophenolic acid	3.1–10.9 μmol/L	1.0–3.5 ng/mL	>37 μmol/L	>12 ng/mL
Nitroprusside (as thiocyanate)	103–499 μmol/L	6–29 μg/mL	860 μmol/L	>50 μg/mL
Nortriptyline	190–569 nmol/L	50–150 ng/mL	>1900 nmol/L	>500 ng/mL
Phenobarbital	65–172 μmol/L	15–40 μg/mL	>258 μmol/L	>60 μg/mL
Phenytoin	40–79 μmol/L	10–20 μg/mL	>158 μmol/L	>40 μg/mL
Phenytoin, free	4.0–7.9 μg/mL	1–2 μg/mL	>13.9 μg/mL	>3.5 μg/mL
% Free	0.08–0.14	8–14%		
Primidone and metabolite				
Primidone	23–55 μmol/L	5–12 μg/mL	>69 μmol/L	>15 μg/mL
Phenobarbital	65–172 μmol/L	15–40 μg/mL	>215 μmol/L	>50 μg/mL
Procainamide				
Procainamide	17–42 μmol/L	4–10 μg/mL	>43 μmol/L	>10 μg/mL
NAPA (*N*-acetylprocainamide)	22–72 μmol/L	6–20 μg/mL	>126 μmol/L	>35 μg/mL
Quinidine	6.2–15.4 μmol/L	2.0–5.0 μg/mL	>19 μmol/L	>6 μg/mL
Salicylates	145–2100 μmol/L	2–29 mg/dL	>2900 μmol/L	>40 mg/dL
Sirolimus (trough level)				
Kidney transplant	4.4–15.4 nmol/L	4–14 ng/mL	>16 nmol/L	>15 ng/mL

(*Continued*)

TABLE 3 TOXICOLOGY AND THERAPEUTIC DRUG MONITORING (*CONTINUED*)

	Therapeutic Range		Toxic Level	
Drug	**SI Units**	**Conventional Units**	**SI Units**	**Conventional Units**
Tacrolimus (FK506) (trough)				
Kidney and liver transplant				
Initiation	12–19 nmol/L	10–15 ng/mL	>25 nmol/L	>20 ng/mL
Maintenance	6–12 nmol/L	5–10 ng/mL	>25 nmol/L	>20 ng/mL
Heart transplant				
Initiation	19–25 nmol/L	15–20 ng/mL		
Maintenance	6–12 nmol/L	5–10 ng/mL		
Theophylline	56–111 μg/mL	10–20 μg/mL	>168 μg/mL	>30 μg/mL
Thiocyanate				
After nitroprusside infusion	103–499 μmol/L	6–29 μg/mL	860 μmol/L	>50 μg/mL
Nonsmoker	17–69 μmol/L	1–4 μg/mL		
Smoker	52–206 μmol/L	3–12 μg/mL		
Tobramycin				
Peak	11–22 μg/L	5–10 μg/mL	>26 μg/L	>12 μg/mL
Trough	0–4.3 μg/L	0–2 μg/mL	>4.3 μg/L	>2 μg/mL
Topiramate (trough)	5.9–58.9 μmol/L	2.0–20.0 μg/mL	Toxic range not well established	
Valproic acid	346–693 μmol/L	50–100 μg/mL	>693 μmol/L	>100 μg/mL
Vancomycin				
Peak	14–28 μmol/L	20–40 μg/mL	>55 μmol/L	>80 μg/mL
Trough	3.5–10.4 μmol/L	5–15 μg/mL	>14 μmol/L	>20 μg/mL
Zonisamide (trough)	47–188 μmol/L	10–40 μg/ mL	Toxic range not well established	

TABLE 4 VITAMINS AND SELECTED TRACE MINERALS

		Reference Range	
Specimen	**Analyte**	**SI Units**	**Conventional Units**
Aluminum	S	<0.2 μmol/L	<5.41 μg/L
Arsenic	WB	0.0–0.17 μmol/L	0–13 μg/L
Cadmium	WB	<44.5 nmol/L	<5.0 μg/L
Coenzyme Q10 (ubiquinone)	P	433–1532 μg/L	433–1532 μg/L
β-Carotene	S	0.07–1.43 μmol/L	4–77 μg/dL
Copper	S	11–22 μmol/L	70–140 μg/dL
Folic acid	RC	340–1020 nmol/L cells	150–450 ng/mL cells
Folic acid	S	12.2–40.8 nmol/L	5.4–18.0 ng/mL
Lead	S		
Adult		<0.5 μmol/L	<10 μg/dL
Children		<0.25 μmol/L	<5 μg/dL
Mercury	WB	0–50 μmol/L	0–10 μg/L
Selenium	S	0.8–2.0 μmol/L	63–160 μg/L
Vitamin A	S	0.7–3.5 μmol/L	20–100 μg/dL
Vitamin B_1 (thiamine)	S	0–75 nmol/L	0–2 μg/dL
Vitamin B_2 (riboflavin)	S	106–638 nmol/L	4–24 μg/dL
Vitamin B_6	P	20–121 nmol/L	5–30 ng/mL
Vitamin B_{12}	S	206–735 pmol/L	279–996 pg/mL
Vitamin C (ascorbic acid)	S	23–57 μmol/L	0.4–1.0 mg/dL
Vitamin D 1,25-dihydroxy, total	S, P	36–180 pmol/L	15–75 pg/mL
Vitamin D 25-hydroxy, total	P	75–250 nmol/L	30–100 ng/mL
Vitamin E	S	12–42 μmol/L	5–18 μg/mL
Vitamin K	S	0.29–2.64 nmol/L	0.13–1.19 ng/mL
Zinc	S	11.5–18.4 μmol/L	75–120 μg/dL

Abbreviations: P, plasma; RC, red cells; S, serum; WB, whole blood.

TABLE 5 CEREBROSPINAL FLUID[a]

Constituent	Reference Range	
	SI Units	**Conventional Units**
Osmolarity	292–297 mmol/kg water	292–297 mOsm/L
Electrolytes		
Sodium	137–145 mmol/L	137–145 meq/L
Potassium	2.7–3.9 mmol/L	2.7–3.9 meq/L
Calcium	1.0–1.5 mmol/L	2.1–3.0 meq/L
Magnesium	1.0–1.2 mmol/L	2.0–2.5 meq/L
Chloride	116–122 mmol/L	116–122 meq/L
CO_2 content	20–24 mmol/L	20–24 meq/L
Pco_2	6–7 kPa	45–49 mmHg
pH	7.31–7.34	
Glucose	2.22–3.89 mmol/L	40–70 mg/dL
Lactate	1–2 mmol/L	10–20 mg/dL
Total protein:		
Lumbar	0.15–0.5 g/L	15–50 mg/dL
Cisternal	0.15–0.25 g/L	15–25 mg/dL
Ventricular	0.06–0.15 g/L	6–15 mg/dL
Albumin	0.066–0.442 g/L	6.6–44.2 mg/dL
IgG	0.009–0.057 g/L	0.9–5.7 mg/dL
IgG index[b]	0.29–0.59	
Oligoclonal bands (OGB)	<2 bands not present in matched serum sample	
Ammonia	15–47 μmol/L	25–80 μg/dL
Creatinine	44–168 μmol/L	0.5–1.9 mg/dL
Myelin basic protein	<4 μg/L	
Cerebrospinal fluid pressure		50–180 mmH_2O
Cerebrospinal fluid volume (adult)	~150 mL	
Red blood cells	0	0
Leukocytes		
Total	0–5 mononuclear cells per μL	
Differential		
Lymphocytes	60–70%	
Monocytes	30–50%	
Neutrophils	None	

[a]Since cerebrospinal fluid (CSF) concentrations are equilibrium values, measurements of the same parameters in blood plasma obtained at the same time are recommended. However, there is a time lag in attainment of equilibrium, and cerebrospinal levels of plasma constituents that can fluctuate rapidly (such as plasma glucose) may not achieve stable values until after a significant lag phase. [b]IgG index = CSF IgG (mg/dL) × serum albumin (g/dL)/serum IgG (g/dL) × CSF albumin (mg/dL).

TABLE 6 URINE ANALYSIS AND RENAL FUNCTION TESTS

	Reference Range	
	SI Units	**Conventional Units**
Acidity, titratable	20–40 mmol/d	20–40 meq/d
Aldosterone	Normal diet: 6–25 μg/d	Normal diet: 6–25 μg/d
	Low-salt diet: 17–44 μg/d	Low-salt diet: 17–44 μg/d
	High-salt diet: 0–6 μg/d	High-salt diet: 0–6 μg/d
Aluminum	0.19–1.11 μmol/L	5–30 μg/L
Ammonia	30–50 mmol/d	30–50 meq/d
Amylase		4–400 U/L
Amylase/creatinine clearance ratio ($[Cl_{am}/Cl_{cr}] \times 100$)	1–5	1–5
Arsenic	0.07–0.67 μmol/d	5–50 μg/d
Bence Jones protein, urine, qualitative	Not applicable	None detected
Bence Jones protein, urine, quantitative		
Free kappa	1.4–24.2 mg/L	0.14–2.42 mg/dL
Free lambda	0.2–6.7 mg/L	0.02–0.67 mg/dL
K/L ratio	2.04–10.37	2.04–10.37
Calcium (10 meq/d or 200 mg/d dietary calcium)	<7.5 mmol/d	<300 mg/d
Chloride	140–250 mmol/d	140–250 mmol/d
Citrate	320–1240 mg/d	320–1240 mg/d
Copper	<0.95 μmol/d	<60 μg/d
Coproporphyrins (types I and III)	0–20 μmol/mol creatinine	0–20 μmol/mol creatinine
Cortisol, free	55–193 nmol/d	20–70 μg/d
Creatine, as creatinine		
Female	<760 μmol/d	<100 mg/d
Male	<380 μmol/d	<50 mg/d
Creatinine	8.8–14 mmol/d	1.0–1.6 g/d
Dopamine	392–2876 nmol/d	60–440 μg/d
Eosinophils	<100 eosinophils/mL	<100 eosinophils/mL
Epinephrine	0–109 nmol/d	0–20 μg/d
Glomerular filtration rate	>60 mL/min/1.73 m^2	>60 mL/min/1.73 m^2
	For African Americans, multiply the result by 1.21	For African Americans, multiply the result by 1.21
Glucose (glucose oxidase method)	0.3–1.7 mmol/d	50–300 mg/d
5-Hydroindoleacetic acid (5-HIAA)	0–78.8 μmol/d	0–15 mg/d
Hydroxyproline	53–328 μmol/d	53–328 μmol/d
Iodine, spot urine		
WHO classification of iodine deficiency:		
Not iodine deficient	>100 μg/L	>100 μg/L
Mild iodine deficiency	50–100 μg/L	50–100 μg/L
Moderate iodine deficiency	20–49 μg/L	20–49 μg/L
Severe iodine deficiency	<20 μg/L	<20 μg/L
Ketone (acetone)	Negative	Negative
17 Ketosteroids	3–12 mg/d	3–12 mg/d
Metanephrines		
Metanephrine	30–350 μg/d	30–350 μg/d
Normetanephrine	50–650 μg/d	50–650 μg/d
Microalbumin		
Normal	0.0–0.03 g/d	0–30 mg/d
Microalbuminuria	0.03–0.30 g/d	30–300 mg/d
Clinical albuminuria	>0.3 g/d	>300 mg/d
Microalbumin/creatinine ratio		
Normal	0–3.4 g/mol creatinine	0–30 μg/mg creatinine
Microalbuminuria	3.4–34 g/mol creatinine	30–300 μg/mg creatinine
Clinical albuminuria	>34 g/mol creatinine	>300 μg/mg creatinine
β_2-Microglobulin	0–160 μg/L	0–160 μg/L
Norepinephrine	89–473 nmol/d	15–80 μg/d

(Continued)

TABLE 6 URINE ANALYSIS AND RENAL FUNCTION TESTS (*CONTINUED*)

	Reference Range	
	SI Units	**Conventional Units**
N-telopeptide (cross-linked), NTx		
Female, premenopausal	17–94 nmol BCE/mmol creatinine	17–94 nmol BCE/mmol creatinine
Female, postmenopausal	26–124 nmol BCE/mmol creatinine	26–124 nmol BCE/mmol creatinine
Male	21–83 nmol BCE/mmol creatinine	21–83 nmol BCE/mmol creatinine
Osmolality	100–800 mosm/kg	100–800 mosm/kg
Oxalate		
Male	80–500 μmol/d	7–44 mg/d
Female	45–350 μmol/d	4–31 mg/d
pH	5.0–9.0	5.0–9.0
Phosphate (phosphorus) (varies with intake)	12.9–42.0 mmol/d	400–1300 mg/d
Porphobilinogen	None	None
Potassium (varies with intake)	25–100 mmol/d	25–100 meq/d
Protein	<0.15 g/d	<150 mg/d
Protein/creatinine ratio	Male: 15–68 mg/g Female: 10–107 mg/g	Male: 15–68 mg/g Female: 10–107 mg/g
Sediment		
Red blood cells	0–2/high-power field	
White blood cells	0–2/high-power field	
Bacteria	None	
Crystals	None	
Bladder cells	None	
Squamous cells	None	
Tubular cells	None	
Broad casts	None	
Epithelial cell casts	None	
Granular casts	None	
Hyaline casts	0–5/low-power field	
Red blood cell casts	None	
Waxy casts	None	
White cell casts	None	
Sodium (varies with intake)	100–260 mmol/d	100–260 meq/d
Specific gravity:		
After 12-h fluid restriction	>1.025	>1.025
After 12-h deliberate water intake	≤1.003	≤1.003
Tubular reabsorption, phosphorus	0.79–0.94 of filtered load	79–94% of filtered load
Urea nitrogen	214–607 mmol/d	6–17 g/d
Uric acid (normal diet)	1.49–4.76 mmol/d	250–800 mg/d
Vanillylmandelic acid (VMA)	<30 μmol/d	<6 mg/d

Abbreviation: BCE = bone collagen equivalent.

Acknowledgment

The contributions of Drs. Daniel J. Fink, Patrick M. Sluss, James L. Januzzi, Kent B. Lewandrowski, Amudha Palanisamy, and Scott Fink to this chapter in previous editions are gratefully acknowledged. We also express our gratitude to Drs. Alex Rai and Jeffrey Jhang for helpful suggestions.

480e The Clinical Laboratory in Modern Health Care

Anthony A. Killeen

This is a digital-only chapter. It is available on the DVD that accompanies this book, as well as on Access Medicine/Harrison's Online, and the eBook and "app" editions of HPIM 19e.

Modern medicine relies extensively on the clinical laboratory as a key component of health care. It is estimated that, in current practice, at least 60–70% of all clinical decisions rely to some extent on a laboratory result. For many diseases, the clinical laboratory provides essential diagnostic information. As an example, histopathologic analysis provides basic information about histologic type and classification of tumors and their degree of invasion into adjacent tissues. Microbiologic testing is required to identify infectious organisms and determine antibiotic susceptibility. For many common diseases, expert groups have produced standard guidelines for diagnosis that rely on defined clinical laboratory values, e.g., blood glucose or hemoglobin A_{1C} levels form the basis for diagnosis of diabetes mellitus; the presence of specific serum antibodies is required for diagnosis of many rheumatologic diseases; and serum levels of cardiac markers are a mainstay in diagnosis of acute coronary syndromes.

With their ever-increasing number and scope, clinical laboratory tests provide the clinician with a powerful set of tools but pose challenges in terms of appropriate selection and judicious, cost-effective use to deliver effective patient care.

481e Clinical Procedure Tutorial: Central Venous Catheter Placement

Maria A. Yialamas, William E. Corcoran, Gyorgy Frendl, Kurt Fink

482e Clinical Procedure Tutorial: Thoracentesis

Charles A. Morris, Andrea S. Wolf

483e Clinical Procedure Tutorial: Abdominal Paracentesis

Maria A. Yialamas, Anna E. Rutherford, Lindsay King

484e Clinical Procedure Tutorial: Endotracheal Intubation

Charles A. Morris, Emily Page Nelson

485e Clinical Procedures Tutorial: Percutaneous Arterial Blood Gas Sampling

Christian D. Becker
Medical Editors: Sean Sadikot, Jeremy Matloff

486e Clinical Procedures Tutorial: Lumbar Puncture

Beth Rapaport, Stephen Krieger, Corey McGraw
Medical Editors: Sean Sadikot, Jeremy Matloff

These are digital-only chapters. These chapters are available on the DVD that accompanies this book, as well as on Access Medicine/Harrison's Online, and the eBook and "app" editions of HPIM 19e.

Clinical procedures are an important component of medical student and resident training, and some are required for board and hospital certification. In these *Harrison's* Chaps. 481e–486e, video tutorials are presented for performing abdominal paracentesis, thoracentesis, endotracheal intubation, central venous catheter placement, percutaneous arterial blood gas sampling, and lumbar puncture. These videos have been created specifically for *Harrison's*. Each includes the indications, contraindications, equipment, potential complications, and related patient safety considerations. Additional video tutorials covering clinical procedures such as breast biopsy, IV line insertion, phlebotomy, arterial line insertion, arthrocentesis, bone marrow biopsy, pelvic examination, thyroid aspiration, basic suturing, and urethral catheterization are available to subscribers of *Harrison's Online* and AccessMedicine (available at *www.accessmedicine.com*).

Page numbers in **bold** indicate the start of the main discussion of the topic. Page numbers followed by "f" or "t" refer to the page location of figures and tables, respectively, and a "v" indicates a video on the DVD. Numbers containing "e-" followed by a number (e.g., 91e-3) refer to pages in the e-chapters on the DVD.

INDEX

INDEX

INDEX

INDEX

INDEX

INDEX

INDEX

INDEX

INDEX

INDEX

INDEX

INDEX

F

INDEX

INDEX

INDEX

INDEX

INDEX

INDEX

INDEX

INDEX

INDEX

INDEX

INDEX

INDEX

INDEX

INDEX

INDEX

INDEX

INDEX

INDEX

INDEX

INDEX

INDEX

INDEX

INDEX

INDEX

INDEX

INDEX

INDEX

INDEX

INDEX

INDEX

ENDOCRINOLOGY AND METABOLISM

GASTROENTEROLOGY AND HEPATOLOGY

HEMATOLOGY AND ONCOLOGY

INFECTIOUS DISEASES

NEPHROLOGY

NEUROLOGY AND PSYCHIATRY

PULMONOLOGY

SYSTEMIC CONDITIONS